CANCER

Principles & Practice of Oncology

7th Edition

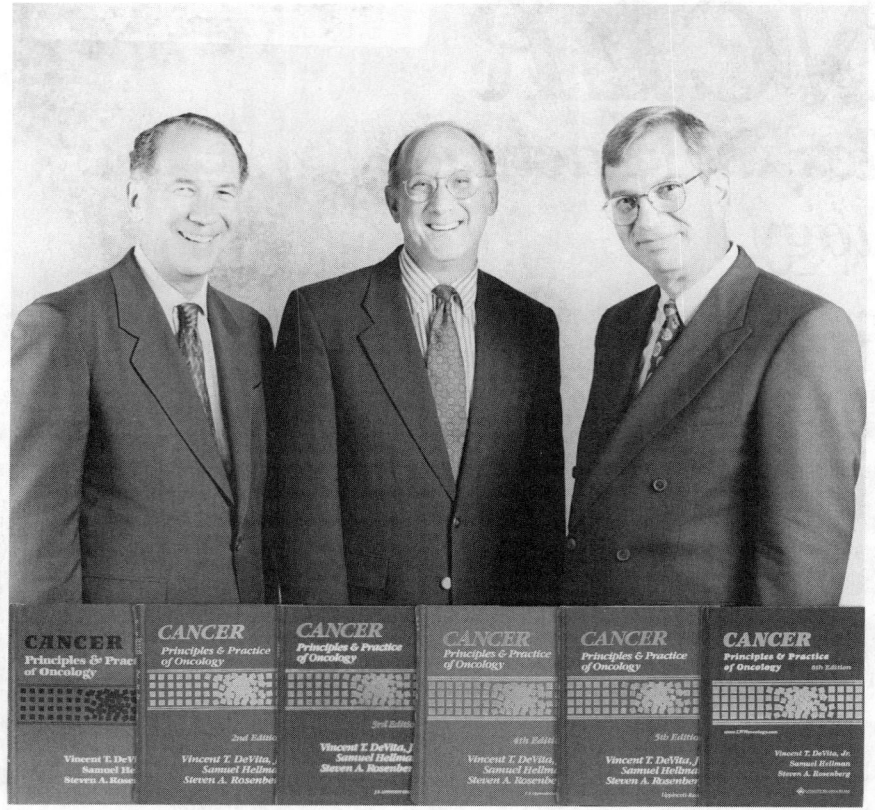

EDITED BY

Vincent T. DeVita, Jr., MD

Amy and Joseph Perella Professor of Medicine, Yale Cancer Center, Yale University School of Medicine; Professor of Epidemiology and Public Health, Yale University School of Public Health, New Haven, Connecticut

Samuel Hellman, MD

A. N. Pritzker Distinguished Service Professor, Department of Radiation and Cellular Oncology, University of Chicago, Chicago, Illinois

Steven A. Rosenberg, MD, PhD

Chief of Surgery, National Cancer Institute, National Institutes of Health; Professor of Surgery, Uniformed Services University of the Health Sciences School of Medicine, Bethesda, Maryland; Professor of Surgery, George Washington University School of Medicine, Washington, DC

With 355 Contributing Authors

CANCER
Principles & Practice of Oncology

7th Edition

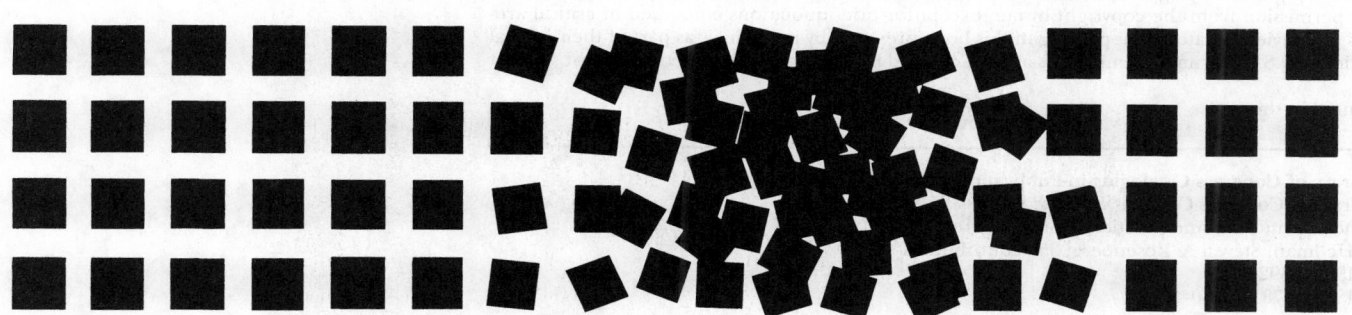

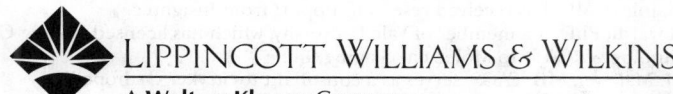

LIPPINCOTT WILLIAMS & WILKINS
A **Wolters Kluwer** Company

Philadelphia • Baltimore • New York • London
Buenos Aires • Hong Kong • Sydney • Tokyo

Executive Editor: Jonathan Pine
Developmental Editors: Joyce Murphy and Stacey Sebring
Project Manager: Nicole Walz
Production Editors: Brooke Begin and Amanda Yanovitch, Silverchair Science + Communications
Senior Manufacturing Manager: Ben Rivera
Senior Marketing Manager: Adam Glazer
Compositor: Silverchair Science + Communications
Printer: Quebecor World-Versailles

© 2005 by LIPPINCOTT WILLIAMS & WILKINS
530 Walnut Street
Philadelphia, PA 19106 USA
LWW.com

Library of Congress Cataloging-in-Publication Data
Library of Congress Control Number: 89-649-721
Cancer: principles and practice of oncology [edited by] Vincent T. DeVita, Jr., Samuel
    Hellman, Steven A. Rosenberg; 355 contributors.—7th
    ISSN 0892-0567
    ISBN 0-781-74450-4

Care has been taken to confirm the accuracy of the information presented and to describe generally accepted practices. However, the authors, editors, and publisher are not responsible for errors or omissions or for any consequences from application of the information in this book and make no warranty, expressed or implied, with respect to the currency, completeness, or accuracy of the contents of the publication. Application of this information in a particular situation remains the professional responsibility of the practitioner.

The authors, editors, and publisher have exerted every effort to ensure that drug selection and dosage set forth in this text are in accordance with current recommendations and practice at the time of publication. However, in view of ongoing research, changes in government regulations, and the constant flow of information relating to drug therapy and drug reactions, the reader is urged to check the package insert for each drug for any change in indications and dosage and for added warnings and precautions. This is particularly important when the recommended agent is a new or infrequently employed drug.

Some drugs and medical devices presented in this publication have Food and Drug Administration (FDA) clearance for limited use in restricted research settings. It is the responsibility of health care providers to ascertain the FDA status of each drug or device planned for use in their clinical practice.

10 9 8 7 6 5 4 3 2

Author Disclosure

All authors of *Cancer: Principles & Practice of Oncology*, Seventh Edition, are expected to disclose any significant financial interest or other relationship with the manufacturer(s) of any commercial product(s) and/or provider(s) of commercial services discussed in the book.
Janet L. Abrahm, MD, has served as a consultant to Medtronic and Endo and has been on the speaker's bureau for Purdue Pharma, Orthobiotech, and Merck.
George D. Demetri, MD, has received research support from Novartis and Pfizer Oncology.
Vincent T. DeVita, Jr., MD, serves on the Boards of Directors of ImClone Systems, CuraGen Corporation, and Oncotech.
Lee M. Ellis, MD, FACS, has served as a consultant to Genentech BioOncology, Novartis, and ImClone Systems.
Samuel Hellman, MD, serves on the Boards of Directors of Varian Medical Systems and of Insightec. He is a scientific adviser to GenVec.
Ferenc A. Jolesz, MD, has received research support from Insightec.
Paul M. Lizardi, PhD, is a member of Yale University, which has licensed Rolling Circle Amplification Technology (RCAT) to Molecular Staging, Inc.
Martin M. Malawer, MD, FACS, serves as a consultant to Stryker Orthopedics.
Paul A. Marks, MD, was founder of Aton Pharma Inc., a biotechnology company that has been acquired by Merck. Dr. Marks is a scientific consultant to Merck.
Steven A. Rosenberg, MD, PhD, is a consultant to RITA Corporation.
Vernon K. Sondak, MD, serves on the Speakers Bureau of Schering Oncology Biotech.
Ronald M. Summers, MD, PhD, has patents in the subject area of his chapter.

To
Mary Kay
Rusty
Alice

CONTRIBUTING AUTHORS

Sumaira Z. Aasi, MD
Assistant Professor
Department of Dermatology
Yale University School of Medicine
New Haven, Connecticut

Janet L. Abrahm, MD
Associate Professor of Medicine and Anesthesia
Co-Director, Pain and Palliative Care Program
Department of Medical Oncology
Harvard Medical School
Dana-Farber Cancer Institute
Brigham and Women's Hospital
Boston, Massachusetts

Ross A. Abrams, MD
Professor and Chairman
Department of Radiation Oncology
Rush Medical College of Rush University
Chicago, Illinois

Gregory Paul Adams, PhD
Associate Member
Department of Medical Oncology, Division of Medical Sciences
Fox Chase Cancer Center
Philadelphia, Pennsylvania

Jaffer A. Ajani, MD
Professor of Medicine
Department of Gastrointestinal Medical Oncology
The University of Texas M. D. Anderson Cancer Center
Houston, Texas

Oguz Akin, MD
Assistant Professor of Radiology
Memorial Sloan-Kettering Cancer Center
New York, New York

Daniel M. Albert, MD, MS
F. A. Davis Professor and Lorenz E. Zimmerman Professor
of Ophthalmology
Emeritus Chair of Ophthalmology
Department of Ophthalmology and Visual Sciences
University of Wisconsin Medical School
University of Wisconsin Hospital and Clinics
Madison, Wisconsin

H. Richard Alexander, Jr., MD
Head, Surgical Metabolism Section
Deputy Director
Center for Cancer Research
Surgery Branch
National Cancer Institute
National Institutes of Health
Bethesda, Maryland

Nasser K. Altorki, MD
Professor of Cardiothoracic Surgery
Cornell University Joan and Sanford I. Weill Medical College
New York-Presbyterian Hospital
New York, New York

Kenneth C. Anderson, MD
Kraft Family Professor of Medicine
Harvard Medical School
Chief, Division of Hematologic Neoplasia
Director, Jerome Lipper Multiple Myeloma Center
Department of Medical Oncology
Dana-Farber Cancer Institute
Boston, Massachusetts

Susanne M. Arnold, MD
Assistant Professor of Medicine
Department of Internal Medicine and Radiation Medicine
University of Kentucky College of Medicine
Markey Cancer Center
Lexington, Kentucky

Michael B. Atkins, MD
Professor of Medicine
Division of Hematology-Oncology
Harvard Medical School
Beth Israel Deaconess Medical Center
Boston, Massachusetts

Richard M. Auchter, MD
Associate Professor of Human Oncology
Section of Radiotherapy
University of Wisconsin Medical School
Madison, Wisconsin

Robert B. Avery, MD, PhD
Assistant Professor
Department of Surgery
Division of Ophthalmology
University of New Mexico School of Medicine
Albuquerque, New Mexico

Joachim M. Baehring, MD
Assistant Professor of Neurology and Neurosurgery
Yale University School of Medicine
New Haven, Connecticut

Dean F. Bajorin, MD, FACP
Professor of Medicine
Cornell University Joan and Sanford I. Weill Medical College
Attending Physician
Department of Medicine
Genitourinary Oncology Service
Division of Solid Tumor Oncology
Memorial Hospital for Cancer and Allied Diseases
Member, Memorial Sloan-Kettering Cancer Center
New York, New York

Charles M. Balch, MD
Professor of Surgery and Oncology
Johns Hopkins Medical Institutions
Baltimore, Maryland
Executive Vice President and Chief Executive Officer
American Society of Clinical Oncology
Alexandria, Virginia

Fred G. Barker II, MD
Assistant Professor of Surgery (Neurosurgery)
Harvard Medical School
Boston, Massachusetts

David L. Bartlett, MD
Associate Professor of Surgery
University of Pittsburgh School of Medicine
Chief, Division of Surgical Oncology
University of Pittsburgh Medical Centers
Pittsburgh, Pennsylvania

Ethan M. Basch, MD, MPhil
President
Natural Standard Research Collaboration
Cambridge, Massachusetts

Susan E. Bates, MD
Senior Investigator
Cancer Therapeutics Branch
Center for Cancer Research
National Cancer Institute
National Institutes of Health
Bethesda, Maryland

Luba Benimetskaya, PhD
Assistant Professor
Department of Oncology
Albert Einstein-Montefiore Cancer Center
New York, New York

Jonathan S. Berek, MD, MMSc
Professor and Chair, College of Applied Anatomy
Executive Vice-Chair, Department of Obstetrics and Gynecology
Chief, Division of Gynecologic Oncology and Gynecology Service
Director, UCLA Women's Reproductive Cancer Program
University of California, Los Angeles, David Geffen School of
    Medicine at UCLA
Los Angeles, California

Ann M. Berger, MSN, MD
Bethesda, Maryland

George J. Bosl, MD
Professor of Medicine
Cornell University Joan and Sanford I. Weill Medical College
Member, Memorial Sloan-Kettering Cancer Center
New York, New York

Michelle S. Bradbury, MD, PhD
Instructor in Radiology
Department of Diagnostic Radiology
Memorial Sloan-Kettering Cancer Center
New York, New York

Murray F. Brennan, MD
Chairman, Department of Surgery
Memorial Sloan-Kettering Cancer Center
New York, New York

Karen T. Brown, MD
Associate Professor of Radiology
Memorial Sloan-Kettering Cancer Center
New York, New York

Kevin M. Brown, PhD
Post-Doctoral Fellow
Department of Molecular Diagnostics and Target Validation
Translational Genomics Research Institute (TGen)
Phoenix, Arizona

Gary L. Buchschacher, Jr., MD, PhD
Assistant Clinical Professor
Department of Medicine
University of California, Los Angeles, David Geffen School of
    Medicine at UCLA
Associate Physician
Department of Hematology/Oncology
Los Angeles Medical Center, SCPMG
Los Angeles, California

Kenneth H. Buetow, PhD
Director, National Cancer Institute Center for Bioinformatics
Chief, Laboratory of Population Genetics
Department of Health and Human Services
National Cancer Institute
National Institutes of Health
Bethesda, Maryland

Thomas W. Burke, MD
Professor of Gynecologic Oncology
The University of Texas M. D. Anderson Cancer Center
Houston, Texas

Katherine R. Calvo, MD, PhD
Clinical Fellow in Pathology
Laboratory of Pathology
National Institutes of Health, Clinical Center
Bethesda, Maryland

Robert B. Cameron, MD
Associate Professor of Clinical Surgery
Divisions of Thoracic Surgery and Surgical Oncology
Chief, Division of Thoracic Surgery
University of California, Los Angeles, David Geffen School
    of Medicine at UCLA
Department of Surgery
West Los Angeles VA Medical Center
Los Angeles, California

Lewis C. Cantley, PhD
Professor of Systems Biology
Harvard Medical School
Chief, Division of Signal Transduction
Department of Medicine
Beth Israel Deaconess Medical Center
Boston, Massachusetts

Marcia I. Canto, MD, MHS
Assistant Professor of Medicine and Oncology
Director of Therapeutic Endoscopy and Endoscopic Ultrasonography
Johns Hopkins University School of Medicine
Johns Hopkins Hospital
Baltimore, Maryland

Michele Carbone, MD, PhD
Associate Professor of Pathology
Loyola University Medical Center
Cardinal Bernardin Cancer Center
Maywood, Illinois

Tobias Carling, MD, PhD
Surgical Resident
Yale University School of Medicine
New Haven, Connecticut
Associate Professor of Experimental Surgical Research
Uppsala University
Uppsala, Sweden

Giselle D. Carnaby (Mann), BAppSci, MPH, PhD
Research Scientist
Department of Communicative Disorders
College of Public Health and Health Professions
University of Florida
Gainesville, Florida

Christopher L. Carpenter, MD, PhD
Assistant Professor of Medicine
Harvard Medical School
Beth Israel Deaconess Medical Center
Boston, Massachusetts

Brian I. Carr, MD, PhD, FRCP
Professor and Co-Director
Liver Cancer Center
Department of Surgery
Starzl Transplant Institute
University of Pittsburgh School of Medicine
Pittsburgh, Pennsylvania

Darryl Carter, MD
Professor Emeritus
Department of Pathology
Yale University School of Medicine
New Haven, Connecticut

Nicholas J. Cassisi, MD, DDS
Kenneth W. Grader Professor
Department of Otolaryngology
Senior Associate Dean for Clinical Affairs
Dean's Office
University of Florida College of Medicine
Shands HealthCare at University of Florida
Gainesville, Florida

Webster K. Cavenee, PhD
Professor and Director
Ludwig Institute for Cancer Research
University of California, San Diego, School of Medicine
La Jolla, California

R. S. K. Chaganti, PhD
Member, William E. Snee Chair
Professor of Genetics in Pathology
Professor of Cell Biology and Genetics
Department of Medicine
Cornell University Joan and Sanford I. Weill Medical College
Memorial Sloan-Kettering Cancer Center
New York, New York

Jonathan D. Cheng, MD
Associate Member
Department of Medical Oncology
Fox Chase Cancer Center
Philadelphia, Pennsylvania

Richard W. Childs, MD
Senior Investigator, Stem Cell Transplantation
Hematology Branch
National Heart, Lung, and Blood Institute
National Institutes of Health
Bethesda, Maryland

Edward Chu, MD
Professor of Medicine and Pharmacology
Yale University School of Medicine
Chief, Section of Medical Oncology
Director, VACT Cancer Center
Yale Cancer Center
New Haven, Connecticut

Rebecca A. Clark-Snow, RN, BSN, OCN
Coordinator, Clinical Oncology Research Program
University of Kansas Cancer Center
Kansas City, Kansas

Graham A. Colditz, MD, DrPH
Professor of Medicine
Channing Laboratory
Harvard Medical School
Brigham and Women's Hospital
Boston, Massachusetts

Jonathan A. Coleman, MD
Senior Clinical Investigator
Urology Oncology Branch
National Cancer Institute
National Institutes of Health
Bethesda, Maryland

O. Michael Colvin, MD
William Shingleton Professor of Cancer Research
Professor of Pharmacology and Cancer Biology
Department of Medicine
Director Emeritus, Duke Comprehensive Cancer Center
Duke University Medical Center
Durham, North Carolina

Philip P. Connell, MD
Assistant Professor
Department of Radiation and Cellular Oncology
University of Chicago Pritzker School of Medicine
Chicago, Illinois

Dennis L. Cooper, MD
Professor of Medicine
Department of Internal Medicine
Yale University School of Medicine
New Haven, Connecticut

Mehmet Sitki Copur, MD, FACP
Assistant Professor of Medicine
University of Nebraska College of Medicine
Medical Director of Oncology
Department of Medical Oncology
Saint Francis Cancer Center

Saint Francis Medical Center
University of Nebraska Medical Center
Grand Island, Nebraska

Carlos Cordon-Cardo, MD, PhD
Director, Division of Molecular Pathology
Department of Pathology
Memorial Sloan-Kettering Cancer Center
New York, New York

José C. Costa, MD
Professor of Pathology
Director of Anatomic Pathology
Vice-Chair, Department of Pathology
Deputy Director, Yale Cancer Center
Yale University School of Medicine
New Haven, Connecticut

Anne M. Covey, MD
Assistant Professor
Department of Diagnostic Radiology
Memorial Sloan-Kettering Cancer Center
New York, New York

Michael A. Crary, PhD, MMS
Professor of Speech Pathology
Department of Communicative Disorders
University of Florida Health Science Center
Gainesville, Florida

Bernard J. Cummings, MBChB, FRCPC, FRCR, FRANZCR
Professor of Radiation of Oncology
University of Toronto Faculty of Medicine
Princess Margaret Hospital
University Health Network
Toronto, Ontario, Canada

Douglas M. Dahl, MD
Assistant Professor of Surgery
Department of Urology
Harvard Medical School
Massachusetts General Hospital
Boston, Massachusetts

Christopher K. Daugherty, MD
Associate Professor of Medicine
Section of Hematology/Oncology
Vice-Chair, Institutional Review Board
University of Chicago Pritzker School of Medicine
McLean Center for Clinical Medical Ethics
Chicago, Illinois

Lisa M. DeAngelis, MD
Chair, Department of Neurology
Memorial Sloan-Kettering Cancer Center
New York, New York

George D. Demetri, MD
Associate Professor of Medicine
Harvard Medical School
Director, Center for Sarcoma and Bone Oncology
Dana-Farber Cancer Institute
Boston, Massachusetts

Marc de Perrot, MD, MSc
Assistant Professor of Surgery
Division of Thoracic Surgery
University of Toronto Faculty of Medicine
Toronto General Hospital
Toronto, Ontario, Canada

Ronald A. DePinho, MD
Professor of Medicine (Genetics)

Department of Medical Oncology
Harvard Medical School
American Cancer Society Research Professor
Dana-Farber Cancer Institute
Boston, Massachusetts

Melvin Deutsch, MD
Raul Mercado Professor of Radiation Oncology
University of Pittsburgh Medical Center
University of Pittsburgh Medical Center Presbyterian Shadyside
Pittsburgh, Pennsylvania

Vincent T. DeVita, Jr., MD
Amy and Joseph Perella Professor of Medicine
Yale Cancer Center
Yale University School of Medicine
Professor of Epidemiology and Public Health
Yale University School of Public Health
New Haven, Connecticut

Robert B. Dickson, PhD
Professor and Vice-Chair of Oncology
Lombardi Comprehensive Cancer Center
Georgetown University Medical Center
Washington, DC

Volker Diehl, MD
Professor of Medicine and Oncology
German Hodgkin Study Lymphoma Group, Haus Lebens Wert
Universität zu Köln
Köln, Germany

Beth L. Dinoff, PhD
Clinical Psychologist
Department of Medicine and Rehabilitation
Birmingham VA Medical Center
Birmingham, Alabama

Joseph J. Disa, MD, FACS
Associate Professor of Surgery
Cornell University Joan and Sanford I. Weill Medical College
Associate Attending Surgeon
Plastic and Reconstructive Surgery Service
Memorial Hospital for Cancer and Allied Diseases
New York, New York

Gerard M. Doherty, MD
N. W. Thompson Professor of Surgery
University of Michigan Medical School
Ann Arbor, Michigan

Marisa Dolled-Filhart, MPhil
Department of Genetics and Pathology
Yale University School of Medicine
New Haven, Connecticut

Brian J. Druker, MD
Investigator, Howard Hughes Medical Institute
JELD-WEN Chair of Leukemia Research
Oregon Health Sciences University Cancer Institute
Portland, Oregon

Mark E. Dudley, PhD
Director, Cell Production Facility
Surgery Branch
Center for Cancer Research
National Cancer Institute
National Institutes of Health
Bethesda, Maryland

David H. Ebb, MD
Assistant Professor of Pediatric Hematology-Oncology
Harvard Medical School

Massachusetts General Hospital
Boston, Massachusetts

Richard L. Edelson, MD
Professor of Dermatology
Chair, Department of Dermatology
Yale University School of Medicine
Director, Yale Cancer Center
New Haven, Connecticut

Patricia J. Eifel, MD, FACR
Professor of Radiation Oncology
The University of Texas M. D. Anderson Cancer Center
Houston, Texas

Albert B. Einstein, Jr., MD, FACP
Executive Director, Swedish Cancer Institute
Swedish Medical Center
Seattle, Washington

Lee M. Ellis, MD
Professor of Surgery and Cancer Biology
The University of Texas M. D. Anderson Cancer Center
Houston, Texas

Charles Erlichman, MD, FACP, FRCPC
Professor of Oncology
Chair, Department of Oncology
Mayo Medical School
Associate Director, Mayo Clinic Comprehensive Cancer Center
Rochester, Minnesota

Stefan Faderl, MD
Assistant Professor
Department of Leukemia
The University of Texas M. D. Anderson Cancer Center
Houston, Texas

Jane M. Fall-Dickson, RN, MSN, PhD
Investigator, National Institute of Nursing Research
Laboratory of Symptom Management
Formerly Clinical Research Fellow
Pain and Neurosurgery Mechanisms Branch
National Institute of Dental and Craniofacial Research
National Institutes of Health
Bethesda, Maryland

Isaiah J. Fidler, DVM, PhD
R. E. "Bob" Smith Distinguished Chair in Cell Biology
Professor and Chairman
Professor of Urology
Director, Cancer Metastasis Research Center
Department of Cancer Biology
The University of Texas M. D. Anderson Cancer Center
Houston, Texas

Howard A. Fine, MD
Senior Investigator
Neuro-Oncology Branch
National Cancer Institute
National Institute for Neurologic Disorders and Stroke
National Institutes of Health
Bethesda, Maryland

Steven E. Finkelstein, MD
Fellow in Surgery
Surgery Branch, Center for Cancer Research
National Cancer Institute
National Institutes of Health
Bethesda, Maryland

Laurie B. Fisher, SM
Research Associate

Department of Medicine
Harvard Medical School
Brigham and Women's Hospital
Boston, Massachusetts

Richard I. Fisher, MD
Samuel E. Durand Professor of Medicine
Chief, Hematology-Oncology Unit
University of Rochester School of Medicine and Dentistry
Director of Cancer Services
Strong Health
Director, James P. Wilmot Cancer Center
Rochester, New York

Antonio Tito Fojo, MD, PhD
Senior Investigator
Cancer Therapeutics Branch
Center for Cancer Research
National Cancer Institute
National Institutes of Health
Bethesda, Maryland

Kathleen M. Foley, MD
Professor of Neurology, Neuroscience, and Clinical Pharmacology
Cornell University Joan and Sanford I. Weill Medical College
Department of Neurology, Pain and Palliative Care Service
Memorial Sloan-Kettering Cancer Center
New York, New York

Judah Folkman, MD
Andrus Professor of Pediatric Surgery
Professor of Cell Biology
Department of Surgery
Harvard Medical School
Director, Vascular Biology Program
Children's Hospital Boston
Boston, Massachusetts

Kwun M. Fong, PhD, MBBS
Associate Professor
Department of Thoracic Medicine
University of Queensland School of Medicine
Thoracic Physician
The Prince Charles Hospital
Brisbane, Australia

Kenneth A. Foon, MD
Professor of Medicine
University of Pittsburgh School of Medicine
Internal Medicine
Division of Hematology and Oncology
University of Pittsburgh Medical Center Cancer Pavilion
Pittsburgh, Pennsylvania

Arlene A. Forastiere, MD
Professor of Oncology
Sidney Kimmel Comprehensive Cancer Center at Johns Hopkins
Johns Hopkins University School of Medicine
Baltimore, Maryland

Douglas L. Fraker, MD
Jonathan E. Rhoads Professor of Surgery
University of Pennsylvania School of Medicine
Philadelphia, Pennsylvania

David Frankenfield, MS, RD, CNSD
Chief Clinical Dietitian
Nutrition Support Specialist
Department of Clinical Nutrition
Milton S. Hershey Medical Center
Hershey, Pennsylvania

Jonathan W. Friedberg, MD, MMSc
Assistant Professor of Medicine and Oncology
University of Rochester School of Medicine and Dentistry
Associate Director of Lymphoma Clinical Research
James P. Wilmot Cancer Center
Rochester, New York

Henry S. Friedman, MD
James B. Powell, Jr., Professor of Neurooncology
Department of Surgery
Duke University Medical Center
Durham, North Carolina

Zvi Fuks, MD
Professor of Radiation Oncology
Cornell University Joan and Sanford I. Weill Medical
    College
Memorial Sloan-Kettering Cancer Center
New York, New York

Don Ganem, MD
Professor of Microbiology and Medicine
University of California, San Francisco, School of Medicine
San Francisco, California

Patricia A. Ganz, MD
Professor
Department of Medicine
Division of Hematology/Oncology and Health Services
University of California, Los Angeles, David Geffen School
    of Medicine at UCLA
UCLA School of Public Health
Director, Cancer Prevention and Control
Jonsson Comprehensive Cancer Center
UCLA Medical Center
Los Angeles, California

Juan C. Gea-Banacloche, MD
Head, Infectious Diseases Section
Experimental Transplantation and Immunology Branch
National Cancer Institute
National Institutes of Health
Bethesda, Maryland

Alan C. Geller, MPH, RN
Research Associate Professor
Departments of Dermatology and Epidemiology
Boston University School of Medicine
Boston University School of Public Health
Boston, Massachusetts

Lynn H. Gerber, MD
Chief, Rehabilitation Medicine
Warren G. Magnuson Clinical Center
National Institutes of Health
Bethesda, Maryland

D. Gary Gilliland, MD, PhD
Professor of Medicine
Department of Hematology
Harvard Medical School
Director, Leukemia Program
Dana-Farber Cancer Institute
Investigator, Howard Hughes Medical Institute
Boston, Massachusetts

Michael Girardi, MD
Associate Professor of Dermatology
Yale University School of Medicine
New Haven, Connecticut

Matthew P. Goetz, MD
Assistant Professor of Oncology

Mayo Clinic
Rochester, Minnesota

Michael Goggins, MD
Associate Professor of Pathology, Medicine, and
    Oncology
Department of Pathology
Johns Hopkins Medical Institutions
Baltimore, Maryland

Boon-Cher Goh, MBBS, MRCP(UK)
Consultant, Medical Oncology
Department of Hematology-Oncology
National University Hospital
Singapore

Leonard G. Gomella, MD
Bernard W. Godwin Professor of Urology
Jefferson Medical College of Thomas Jefferson University
Director of Urologic Oncology
Kimmel Cancer Center
Philadelphia, Pennsylvania

F. Anthony Greco, MD
Director, Sarah Cannon Cancer Center
Nashville, Tennessee

Daniel M. Green, MD, BS
Professor of Pediatrics
University at Buffalo State University School of Medicine and
    Biomedical Sciences
Physician
Department of Pediatrics
Roswell Park Cancer Institute
Buffalo, New York

Peter Greenwald, MD, DrPH
Director, Division of Cancer Prevention
National Cancer Institute
National Institutes of Health
Bethesda, Maryland

Martin E. Gutierrez, MD
Head, Office of Navy Oncology
Head, Lung Cancer Research Section
Medical Oncology Clinical Research Unit
National Cancer Institute
National Institutes of Health
Bethesda, Maryland

Stephen M. Hahn, MD
Associate Professor
Department of Radiation Oncology
Division of Hematology-Oncology
Department of Medicine
University of Pennsylvania School of Medicine
Philadelphia, Pennsylvania

John D. Hainsworth, MD
Director, Clinical Research
Sarah Cannon Cancer Center
Nashville, Tennessee

Peter Harper, MD, FRCP
Consultant Medical Oncologist
Guy's Hospital
London, England, United Kingdom

Nancy Lee Harris, MD
Austin L. Vickery Professor of Pathology
Harvard Medical School
Massachusetts General Hospital
Boston, Massachusetts

Peter W. Heald, MD
Professor of Dermatology
Yale University School of Medicine
New Haven, Connecticut

John H. Healey, MD
Professor of Orthopedic Surgery
Cornell University Joan and Sanford I. Weill Medical College
Chief of Orthopedic Surgery
Memorial Sloan-Kettering Cancer Center
New York, New York

Ingrid A. Hedenfalk, PhD
Fellow, Department of Laboratory Medicine
Division of Pathology
Lund University
Malmö University Hospital
Malmö, Sweden

Samuel Hellman, MD
A. N. Pritzker Distinguished Service Professor
Department of Radiation and Cellular Oncology
University of Chicago
Chicago, Illinois

Lee J. Helman, MD
Chief, Pediatric Oncology Branch
National Cancer Institute
National Institutes of Health
Bethesda, Maryland

S. Jane Henley, MSPH
Epidemiologist
Epidemiology and Surveillance Research
American Cancer Society
Atlanta, Georgia

Claudia L. Henschke, MD, PhD
Professor of Radiology
Chest Imaging Division
Cornell University Joan and Sanford I. Weill Medical College
New York Presbyterian Hospital
New York, New York

Meenhard Herlyn, DVM, DSc
Professor and Chairman
Program of Molecular and Cellular Oncogenesis
The Wistar Institute
Philadelphia, Pennsylvania

Robert A. Hiatt, MD, PhD
Professor of Epidemiology and Biostatistics
Director of Population Sciences
Deputy Director, UCSF Comprehensive Cancer Center
Comprehensive Cancer Center
University of California, San Francisco, School of Medicine
San Francisco, California

Manuel Hidalgo, MD, PhD
Associate Professor of Oncology
Co-Director, Drug Development Program
Johns Hopkins University School of Medicine
Baltimore, Maryland

Steven M. Holland, MD
Chief, Laboratory of Clinical Infectious Diseases
National Institute of Allergy and Infectious Disease
National Institutes of Health
Bethesda, Maryland

Jennifer L. Holter, MD
Chief Fellow, Hematology/Oncology
University of Oklahoma Medical Center
University of Oklahoma Cancer Center
Oklahoma City, Oklahoma

Richard B. Hostetter, MD, FACS
Associate Medical Director
Surgical Oncology
Center for Cancer Care at Goshen Health System
Goshen, Indiana

Peter M. Howley, MD
Shattuck Professor of Anatomical Pathology
Department of Pathology
Harvard Medical School
Boston, Massachusetts

Hedvig Hricak, MD, PhD
Professor of Radiology
Cornell University Joan and Sanford I. Weill Medical College
Chairman, Department of Radiology
Memorial Sloan-Kettering Cancer Center
New York, New York

Ralph H. Hruban, MD
Professor of Pathology and Oncology
Department of Pathology
Johns Hopkins University School of Medicine
Baltimore, Maryland

Patrick Hwu, MD
Professor and Chair
Department of Melanoma Medical Oncology
The University of Texas M. D. Anderson Cancer Center
Houston, Texas

Kullervo H. Hynynen, PhD
Professor of Radiology
Harvard Medical School
Director, Focused Ultrasound Laboratory
Brigham and Women's Hospital
Boston, Massachusetts

Christine A. Iacobuzio-Donohue, MD, PhD
Assistant Professor of Oncology and Pathology
Department of Gastrointestinal/Liver Pathology
Johns Hopkins Hospital
Baltimore, Maryland

Bonnie A. Indeck, MSW, LCSW
Clinical Instructor
Department of Internal Medicine
Yale New Haven Hospital
Yale Cancer Center
New Haven, Connecticut

Elizabeth M. Jaffee, MD
Professor of Oncology
Sidney Kimmel Comprehensive Cancer Center at Johns Hopkins
Baltimore, Maryland

Ahmedin Jemal, DVM, PhD
Program Director, Cancer Surveillance
Department of Epidemiology and Surveillance Research
American Cancer Society
Atlanta, Georgia

Robert T. Jensen
Chief, Digestive Diseases Branch
Digestive and Kidney Diseases
National Institute of Diabetes
National Institutes of Health
Bethesda, Maryland

Steven W. Johnson, PhD
Research Assistant Professor
Department of Pharmacology
University of Pennsylvania School of Medicine
Philadelphia, Pennsylvania

Michael R. Johnston, MD, FRCSC
Associate Professor of Surgery
University of Toronto Faculty of Medicine
Division of Thoracic Surgery
Toronto General Hospital
Department of Surgical Oncology
Princess Margaret Hospital
Toronto, Ontario, Canada

Ferenc A. Jolesz, MD
B. Leonard Holman Professor of Radiology
Harvard Medical School
Brigham and Women's Hospital
Boston, Massachusetts

Glenn W. Jones, MD, FRCP(C), MSc
Associate Professor
Department of Medicine
McMaster University School of Medicine
Hamilton, Ontario, Canada
Credit Valley Hospital
Mississauga, Ontario, Canada

Robert J. Kaner, MD
Associate Professor of Clinical Medicine
Department of Medicine
Division of Pulmonary and Critical Care Medicine
Cornell University Joan and Sanford I. Weill Medical College
New York, New York

Hagop M. Kantarjian, MD
Professor and Chair
Department of Leukemia
The University of Texas M. D. Anderson Cancer Center
Houston, Texas

Joyson Karakunnel, MD
Fellow in Pain and Palliative Care
National Institutes of Health
Bethesda, Maryland

Beth Y. Karlan, MD
Professor of Obstetrics and Oncology
University of California, Los Angeles, David Geffen School
   of Medicine at UCLA
Cedars-Sinai Medical Center
Los Angeles, California

Donald S. Kaufman, MD
Clinical Professor of Medicine
Harvard Medical School
Director, The Claire and John Bertucci Center for Genitourinary
   Cancers
Department of Hematology/Oncology
Massachusetts General Hospital
Boston, Massachusetts

Michael J. Keating, MD
Professor of Medicine
Department of Leukemia
The University of Texas M. D. Anderson Cancer Center
Houston, Texas

Patricia Keegan, MD
Division Director
Division of Therapeutic Biological Oncology Products
Center for Drug Evaluation and Review

U.S. Food and Drug Administration
Rockville, Maryland

Wm. Kevin Kelly, DO
Assistant Attending Physician
Department of Medicine
Genitourinary Oncology Service
Division of Solid Tumor Oncology
Memorial Sloan-Kettering Cancer Center
New York, New York

David P. Kelsen, MD
Professor of Medicine
Cornell University Joan and Sanford I. Weill Medical College
Edward S. Gordon Chair in Medical Oncology
Chief, Gastrointestinal Oncology Service
Memorial Sloan-Kettering Cancer Center
New York, New York

Nancy E. Kemeny, MD
Professor of Medicine
Division of Gastrointestinal Oncology
Cornell University Joan and Sanford I. Weill Medical College
Attending Physician
Memorial Sloan-Kettering Cancer Center
New York, New York

Robert S. Kerbel, PhD
Professor
Department of Medical Biophysics
University of Toronto Faculty of Medicine
Senior Scientist
Molecular and Cellular Biology Research
Sunnybrook and Women's College Health Sciences Centre
Canada Research Chair in Molecular Medicine
Toronto, Ontario, Canada

Scott E. Kern, MD
Professor of Oncology and Pathology
Department of Oncology
Sidney Kimmel Comprehensive Cancer Center at
   Johns Hopkins
Baltimore, Maryland

David Khayat, MD, PhD
Professor of Oncology
Department of Medical Oncology
Pierre et Marie Curie University
President of the National Cancer Institute (France)
Salpetrièrè Hospital
Paris, France

Elliot Kieff, MD, PhD
Albee Professor of Medicine and Microbiology and Molecular
   Genetics
Harvard Medical School
Director of Infectious Disease
Brigham and Women's Hospital
Boston, Massachusetts

Albert S. Ko, MD
Surgical Oncology Fellow
Department of Surgery
Division of Surgical Oncology
Cedars-Sinai Medical Center
Los Angeles, California

Howard K. Koh, MD, MPH
Professor of Health Policy and Management
Director, Division of Public Health Practice
Associate Dean for Public Health Practice
Harvard School of Public Health
Boston, Massachusetts

Stanley J. Korsmeyer, MD
Sidney Farber Professor of Pathology and Professor of Medicine
Investigator, Howard Hughes Medical Institute
Harvard Medical School
Director, Program in Molecular Oncology
Department of Cancer Immunology and AIDS
Dana-Farber Cancer Institute
Boston, Massachusetts

Shivaani Kummar, MBBS
Senior Staff Clinician
Medical Oncology Clinical Research Unit (MOCRU)
National Cancer Institute
National Institutes of Health
Bethesda, Maryland

Daniel A. Laheru, MD
Assistant Professor of Oncology
Department of Medical Oncology
Johns Hopkins University School of Medicine
Sidney Kimmel Comprehensive Cancer Center at
    Johns Hopkins
Baltimore, Maryland

Terry C. Lairmore, MD
Associate Professor of Surgery
Department of Endocrine and Oncologic Surgery
Washington University School of Medicine
Barnes-Jewish Hospital
St. Louis, Missouri

Robert R. Langley, PhD
Instructor
Department of Cancer Biology
The University of Texas M. D. Anderson Cancer Center
Houston, Texas

David A. Larson, MD, PhD
Professor of Radiation Oncology
University of California, San Francisco, School of Medicine
San Francisco, California

Steven M. Larson, MD
Professor of Radiology
Cornell University Joan and Sanford I. Weill Medical College
Attending, Department of Radiology
Chief, Nuclear Medicine Service
Head, Nuclear Medicine Research Laboratory
Co-Leader, Imaging and Radiation Sciences Bridge Program
Director, Radiology Research
Member, Memorial Sloan-Kettering Cancer Center
New York, New York

Theodore S. Lawrence, MD, PhD
Isadore Lampe Professor and Chair
Department of Radiation Oncology
University of Michigan Medical School
Ann Arbor, Michigan

Stephanie J. Lee, MD, MPH
Assistant Professor of Medicine
Department of Medical Oncology
Dana-Farber Cancer Institute
Boston, Massachusetts

David J. Leffell, MD
Professor of Dermatology and Surgery
Yale University School of Medicine
New Haven, Connecticut

Alan T. Lefor, MD, MPH
Professor of Clinical Surgery
Department of Surgery

University of California, Los Angeles, David Geffen School
    of Medicine at UCLA
Director, Division of Surgical Oncology
Department of Surgery
Cedars-Sinai Medical Center
Los Angeles, California

Steven A. Leibel, MD
Professor of Radiation Oncology
Medical Director, Stanford Cancer Center
Stanford Hospital and Clinics
Stanford, California

Jonathan J. Lewis, MD, PhD
CEO and Executive Chair
ZIOPHARM, Inc.
New Haven, Connecticut

Laura Liberman, MD, FACR
Professor of Radiology
Cornell University Joan and Sanford I. Weill Medical College
Director of Breast Imaging Research Programs
Department of Radiology
Memorial Sloan-Kettering Cancer Center
New York, New York

Steven K. Libutti, MD
Senior Investigator
Surgery Branch
National Cancer Institute
National Institutes of Health
Bethesda, Maryland

Frank S. Lieberman, MD
Associate Professor of Neurology and Medical Oncology
Chief, Adult Neurooncology Service
Department of Neurology
University of Pittsburgh Cancer Institute
Pittsburgh, Pennsylvania

W. Marston Linehan, MD
Chief, Urologic Surgery
Urologic Oncology Branch
Center for Cancer Research
National Cancer Institute
National Institutes of Health
Warren Grant Magnusson Clinical Center
Bethesda, Maryland

Jonathan D. Linkous, MPA
Executive Director
American Telemedicine Association
Washington, DC

Lance A. Liotta, MD, PhD
Laboratory Chief
Laboratory of Pathology
Center for Cancer Research
National Cancer Institute
National Institutes of Health
Bethesda, Maryland

Marc E. Lippman, MD
John G. Searle Professor and Chair
Department of Internal Medicine
University of Michigan Medical School
Ann Arbor, Michigan

Scott M. Lippman, MD
Anderson Clinical Faculty Chair for Cancer Treatment and Research
Professor of Medicine and Cancer Prevention
Chair, Department of Clinical Cancer Prevention
Department of Thoracic/Head and Neck Medical Oncology

The University of Texas M. D. Anderson Cancer Center
Houston, Texas

Larry I. Lipshultz, MD
Professor of Urology
Lester and Sue Smith Chair in Reproductive Medicine
Chief, Division of Male Reproductive Medicine and Surgery
Scott Department of Urology
Baylor College of Medicine
Houston, Texas

Richard F. Little, MD, MPH
Senior Clinical Investigator
HIV and AIDS Malignancy Branch
Center for Cancer Research
National Cancer Institute
National Institutes of Health
Bethesda, Maryland

Mark S. Litwin, MD, MPH
Professor of Urology and Health Services
University of California, Los Angeles, David Geffen School of Medicine
    at UCLA and School of Public Health
Los Angeles, California

Zhao-Jun Liu, MD, PhD
Senior Scientist
Program of Molecular and Cellular Oncogenesis
The Wistar Institute
Philadelphia, Pennsylvania

Paul M. Lizardi, PhD
Professor of Pathology
Yale University School of Medicine
New Haven, Connecticut

Jay S. Loeffler, MD
Herman and Joan Suit Professor of Radiation Oncology
Harvard Medical School
Chief, Department of Radiation Oncology
Massachusetts General Hospital
Boston, Massachusetts

Patrick J. Loehrer, Sr., MD
Bruce Kenneth Wiseman Professor of Medicine
Chair, Section of Hematology-Oncology
Indiana University School of Medicine
Indiana University Hospital
Indianapolis, Indiana

Charles L. Loprinzi, MD
Professor of Oncology
Mayo Medical School
Mayo Clinic
Rochester, Minnesota

David N. Louis, MD
Professor and Associate Chief
Department of Pathology
Harvard Medical School
Massachusetts General Hospital
Boston, Massachusetts

Douglas R. Lowy, MD
Deputy Director
Chief, Laboratory of Cellular Oncology
Center for Cancer Research
National Cancer Institute
National Institutes of Health
Bethesda, Maryland

Xiaomei Ma, PhD
Assistant Professor of Epidemiology

Department of Epidemiology and Public Health
Yale University School of Medicine
New Haven, Connecticut

Anirban Maitra, MBBS
Assistant Professor of Pathology, Oncology, and Genetic Medicine
Department of Pathology
Johns Hopkins University School of Medicine
Baltimore, Maryland

Robert G. Maki, MD, PhD
Assistant Member
Department of Medicine
Memorial Sloan-Kettering Cancer Center
New York, New York

Martin M. Malawer, MD, FACS
Professor (Clinical Scholar)
Department of Orthopedics
Professor of Orthopedic Surgery
Director, Orthopedic Oncology
Georgetown University School of Medicine
Director, Orthopedic Oncology
Washington Cancer Institute
Washington Hospital Center
Washington, DC
Consultant, Pediatric and Surgery Branch
National Cancer Institute
National Institutes of Health
Baltimore, Maryland

David Malkin, MD, FRCP(C)
Professor of Pediatrics and Medical Biophysics
University of Toronto Faculty of Medicine
Director, Cancer Genetics Program
Division of Hematology/Oncology
Hospital for Sick Children
Toronto, Ontario, Canada

Sridhar Mani, MD
Associate Professor of Medicine, Oncology, and Molecular Genetics
Director, Phase I Program
Albert Einstein College of Medicine of Yeshiva University
Bronx, New York

Mark W. Manoso, MD
Fellow, Orthopedic Oncology
Department of Surgery
Orthopedic Service
Memorial Sloan-Kettering Cancer Center
New York, New York

Francesco M. Marincola, MD
Senior Investigator
Department of Transfusion Medicine
National Institutes of Health
Bethesda, Maryland

James M. Markert, MD
Associate Professor of Surgery
Neurosurgery, Physiology and Biophysics, and Pediatrics
University of Alabama School of Medicine
Birmingham, Alabama

Maurie A. Markman, MD
Professor of Medicine
Vice President for Clinical Research
The University of Texas M. D. Anderson Cancer Center
Houston, Texas

Paul A. Marks, MD
Member and President Emeritus
Department of Developmental Cell Biology

Memorial Sloan-Kettering Cancer Center
New York, New York

J. Wallis Marsh, MD, MBA
Professor of Surgery
Thomas E. Starzl Transplantation Institute
University of Pittsburgh School of Medicine
Pittsburgh, Pennsylvania

Mary K. Martel, PhD
Associate Professor of Radiation and Cellular Oncology
University of Chicago Pritzker School of Medicine
Chicago, Illinois

Peter G. Maslak, MD
Associate Member
Clinical Laboratories and Department of Medicine
Memorial Sloan-Kettering Cancer Center
New York, New York

Daniel R. Masys, MD
Professor of Medicine
Director, Biomedical Informatics
University of California, San Diego, School of Medicine
La Jolla, California

Ellen T. Matloff, MS
Associate Research Scientist
Director, Cancer Genetic Counseling
Department of Genetics
Yale University School of Medicine
Yale Cancer Center
New Haven, Connecticut

Peter M. Mauch, MD
Professor
Department of Radiation Oncology
Harvard Medical School
Senior Physician
Department of Radiation Oncology
Brigham and Women's Hospital
Boston, Massachusetts

Susan T. Mayne, PhD, FACE
Associate Professor of Epidemiology and Public Health
Yale University School of Medicine
Associate Director for Cancer Prevention and Control
    Research
Yale Cancer Center
New Haven, Connecticut

Mark McClellan, MD, PhD
Administrator
Centers for Medicare and Medicaid Services
Baltimore, Maryland

Michael W. McDermott, MD, FRCSC
Associate Professor
Vice-Chair and Robert and Ruth Halperin Chair
Department of Neurosurgery
University of California, San Francisco, School of Medicine
San Francisco, California

W. Scott McDougal, MD, AM(Hon)
Walter S. Kerr, Jr., Professor of Urology
Harvard Medical School
Chief of Urology
Massachusetts General Hospital
Boston, Massachusetts

Howard L. McLeod, PharmD
Associate Professor
Department of Medicine, Genetics, and Pharmacology

Washington University School of Medicine
St. Louis, Missouri

Minesh P. Mehta, MD
Professor
Department of Human Oncology
University of Wisconsin Medical School
Madison, Wisconsin

Marvin L. Meistrich, PhD
Professor of Experimental Radiation Oncology
The University of Texas M. D. Anderson Cancer
    Center
Houston, Texas

William M. Mendenhall, MD
Professor of Radiation Oncology
University of Florida College of Medicine
Shands HealthCare at University of Florida
Gainesville, Florida

Wells Messersmith, MD
Assistant Professor of Oncology
Department of Medical Oncology
Johns Hopkins University School of Medicine
Baltimore, Maryland

Beth E. Meyerowitz, PhD
Professor of Psychology
University of Southern California
Los Angeles, California

M. Dror Michaelson, MD, PhD
Instructor in Medicine
Harvard Medical School
Clinical Associate in Medicine
Department of Hematology and Oncology
Massachusetts General Hospital
Boston, Massachusetts

Karin B. Michels, ScD, MSc, MPH
Associate Professor
Obstetrics and Gynecology Epidemiology Center
Harvard Medical School
Brigham and Women's Hospital
Department of Epidemiology
Harvard School of Public Health
Boston, Massachusetts

James W. Mier, MD
Associate Professor
Department of Medicine
Beth Israel Deaconess Medical Center
Boston, Massachusetts

Thomas A. Miller, PhD
Director, Chemistry
Aton Pharma
New York, New York

John D. Minna, MD
Professor of Internal Medicine and Pharmacology
Director, Hamon Center for Therapeutic Oncology
    Research
University of Texas Southwestern Medical Center
Dallas, Texas

Bruce D. Minsky, MD
Professor of Radiation Oncology
Cornell University Joan and Sanford I. Weill Medical
    College
Vice-Chair
Department of Radiation Oncology

Memorial Sloan-Kettering Cancer Center
New York, New York

Jeffrey F. Moley, MD
Professor of Surgery
Washington University School of Medicine
Associate Director
Siteman Cancer Center
St. Louis, Missouri

Richard A. Morgan, PhD
Staff Scientist, Surgery Branch
National Cancer Institute
National Institutes of Health
Bethesda, Maryland

Robert J. Motzer, MD
Attending Physician
Department of Medicine
Genitourinary Oncology Section
Memorial Sloan-Kettering Cancer Center
New York, New York

Franco M. Muggia, MD
David H. Cogan and Anné Murnick Professor of
    Oncology
Department of Medicine
New York University School of Medicine
New York, New York

Arno J. Mundt, MD
Associate Professor
Department of Radiation and Cellular Oncology
University of Chicago Pritzker School of Medicine
University of Illinois College of Medicine
Chicago, Illinois

Nikhil C. Munshi, MD
Associate Director
Jerome Lipper Myeloma Center
Harvard Medical School
Dana-Farber Cancer Institute
Boston, Massachusetts

John R. Murren, MD
Associate Professor
Department of Medicine
Yale University School of Medicine
New Haven, Connecticut

Hyman B. Muss, MD
Professor of Medicine
University of Vermont College of Medicine
Director, Hematology/Oncology
Fletcher Allen Health Care
Burlington, Vermont

Dao M. Nguyen, MD
Tenure-Track Principle Investigator
Section of Thoracic Oncology
Surgery Branch
Center for Cancer Research
National Cancer Institute
National Institutes of Health
Bethesda, Maryland

Vanita Noronha, MD
Postdoctoral Fellow in Medical Oncology
Internal Medicine
Yale University School of Medicine
Yale Cancer Center
New Haven, Connecticut

Jeffrey A. Norton, MD
Professor of Surgery
Chief, Surgical Oncology
Department of General Surgery
Stanford University Medical Center
Stanford, California

Susan O'Brien, MD
Professor of Medicine
Department of Leukemia
The University of Texas M. D. Anderson Cancer
    Center
Houston, Texas

Peter J. O'Dwyer, MD
Professor of Medicine
University of Pennsylvania School of Medicine
Program Director, Developmental Therapeutics
Abramson Cancer Center
Vice-Chair, Eastern Cooperative Oncology Group
Philadelphia, Pennsylvania

Neil R. P. Ogden, MS
Chief, General Surgery Device Branch
Division of General, Restorative, and Neurological
    Devices
Office of Device Evaluation
Center for Devices and Radiological Health
U.S. Food and Drug Administration
Department of Health and Human Services
Rockville, Maryland

Olufunmilayo I. Olopade, MBBS, FACP
Professor of Medicine
Department of Medicine and Human Genetics
University of Chicago Pritzker School of Medicine
Chicago, Illinois

Brian O'Sullivan, MD, FRCPC
Professor of Radiation Oncology
Head, Sarcoma Section
University of Toronto Faculty of Medicine
Princess Margaret Hospital
Toronto, Ontario, Canada

Howard Ozer, MD, PhD
Professor of Medicine
Easton Chair and Chief
Director, Fellowship Program
Section of Hematology/Oncology
Director, University of Oklahoma Cancer Center
University of Oklahoma Medical Center
Oklahoma City, Oklahoma

Harvey I. Pass, MD
Professor of Surgery and Medicine
Wayne State University School of Medicine
Barbara Ann Karmanos Cancer Institute
Harper University Hospital
Detroit, Michigan

Richard Pazdur, MD
Director, Oncology Drug Products
Center for Drug Evaluation and Research
U.S. Food and Drug Administration
Rockville, Maryland

Peter L. Perrotta, MD
Assistant Professor of Pathology
Stony Brook University School of Medicine
University Hospital
Stony Brook, New York

Richard G. Pestell, MD, PhD, MBB
Director, Lombardi Cancer Comprehensive Center
Chairman, Department of Oncology
Georgetown University Medical Center
Washington, DC

Jeanne A. Petrek, MD
Professor of Surgery
Cornell University Joan and Sanford I. Weill Medical
    College
Memorial Sloan-Kettering Cancer Center
New York, New York

Emanuel F. Petricoin III, PhD
Co-Director, U.S. Food and Drug Administration–National
    Cancer Institute Clinical Proteomics Program
Center for Biologics Evaluation and Research
U.S. Food and Drug Administration
Bethesda, Maryland

James F. Pingpank, Jr., MD
Senior Investigator
Surgery Branch
National Cancer Institute
National Institutes of Health
Bethesda, Maryland

Peter W. T. Pisters, MD
Professor of Surgery
Department of Surgical Oncology
The University of Texas M. D. Anderson Cancer Center
Houston, Texas

Carol S. Portlock, MD
Professor of Clinical Medicine
Cornell University Joan and Sanford I. Weill Medical
    College
Attending Physician, Lymphoma Service
Memorial Sloan-Kettering Cancer Center
New York, New York

Mitchell C. Posner, MD
Professor of Surgery
Chief, Surgical Oncology
University of Chicago Pritzker School of
    Medicine
Chicago, Illinois

Steven M. Powell, MD
Associate Professor of Medicine
Division of Gastroenterology
University of Virginia School of Medicine
Charlottesville, Virginia

Mazin B. Qumsiyeh, PhD
Associate Professor
Department of Genetics
Yale University School of Medicine
New Haven, Connecticut

Glen David Raffel, MD, PhD
Instructor in Medicine
Division of Hematology/Oncology
Beth Israel Deaconess Medical Center
Boston, Massachusetts

Ramesh K. Ramanathan, MD
Associate Professor of Medicine
Division of Hematology/Oncology
University of Pittsburgh School of Medicine
University of Pittsburgh Medical Center
Pittsburgh, Pennsylvania

Sanjay Razdan, MD, MCh
Director of Endourology and Minimally Invasive
    Oncology
Department of Urology
Carrion Urological Center
Miami, Florida

Bruce G. Redman, DO
Professor of Medicine
Department of Internal Medicine
Division of Hematology/Oncology
University of Michigan Medical School
Ann Arbor, Michigan

Steven I. Reed, PhD
Professor of Molecular Biology
The Scripps Research Institute
La Jolla, California

Nicholas P. Restifo, MD
Principal Investigator
National Cancer Institute
National Institutes of Health
Bethesda, Maryland

Victoria M. Richon, PhD
Executive Director
Department of Biology
Aton Pharma
Tarrytown, New York

Stanley R. Riddell, MD
Member, Program in Immunology
Clinical Research Division
Fred Hutchinson Cancer Research Center
Seattle, Washington

Charles E. Riggs, Jr., MD
Associate Professor of Medicine
Shands HealthCare at University of Florida
Gainesville, Florida

Barbara K. Rimer, MPH, DrPH
Alumni Distinguished Professor
Health Behavior and Health Education
University of North Carolina School of Public
    Health
Chapel Hill, North Carolina

David L. Rimm, MD, PhD
Associate Professor
Program Director, Cytopathology Fellowship
Facility Director, Yale Cancer Center Tissue
    Microarray
Department of Pathology
Yale University School of Medicine
New Haven, Connecticut

Olivier Rixe, MD, PhD
Professor of Medical Oncology
Pierre et Marie Curie University
Salpêtrière Hospital
Paris, France

Matthew K. Robinson, PhD
Staff Scientist
Department of Medical Oncology
Fox Chase Cancer Center
Philadelphia, Pennsylvania

Michal G. Rose, MD
Assistant Professor of Medicine

Section of Medical Oncology
Yale University School of Medicine
Cancer Center
VA Connecticut Healthcare System
West Haven, Connecticut

Steven A. Rosenberg, MD, PhD
Chief of Surgery
National Cancer Institute
National Institutes of Health
Professor of Surgery
Uniformed Services University of the Health Sciences
    School of Medicine
Bethesda, Maryland
Professor of Surgery
George Washington University School of Medicine
Washington, DC

Eric K. Rowinsky, MD
Clinical Professor of Medicine
University of Texas Medical School at San Antonio
Director, Institute for Drug Development
Cancer Therapy and Research Center
San Antonio, Texas

James L. Rubenstein, MD, PhD
Assistant Professor
Department of Medicine
Hematology/Oncology
University of California, San Francisco, School of
    Medicine
San Francisco, California

Anil K. Rustgi, MD
T. Grier Miller Professor of Medicine and
    Genetics
Chief, Gastroenterology
Department of Medicine
University of Pennsylvania School of Medicine
Philadelphia, Pennsylvania

Leonard B. Saltz, MD
Attending Physician and Member
Department of Medicine
Gastrointestinal Oncology Service
Division of Solid Tumor Oncology
Memorial Sloan-Kettering Cancer Center
New York, New York

Jay H. Sanders, MD
Adjunct Professor of Medicine
Johns Hopkins University School of Medicine
Baltimore, Maryland

Richard M. Satava, MD, MS(Surg), FACS
Professor of Surgery
University of Washington Medical Center
Seattle, Washington
Program Manager
Advanced Biomedical Technologies
Defense Advanced Research Projects Agency
Arlington, Virginia

Peter T. Scardino, MD
Chair, Department of Urology
Memorial Sloan-Kettering Cancer Center
New York, New York

David A. Scheinberg, MD, PhD
Chair, Molecular Pharmacology and
    Chemistry
Department of Medicine

Memorial Sloan-Kettering Cancer Center
New York, New York

Howard I. Scher, MD
Professor of Medicine
D. Wayne Calloway Chair in Urologic Oncology
Cornell University Joan and Sanford I. Weill Medical
    College
Chief, Genitourinary Oncology Service
Department of Medicine
Memorial Sloan-Kettering Cancer Center
New York, New York

Joellen M. Schildkraut, MPH, PhD
Associate Professor
Department of Community and Family Medicine
Duke University Medical Center
Durham, North Carolina

John T. Schiller, PhD
Principal Investigator
Laboratory of Cellular Oncology
Center for Cancer Research
National Cancer Institute
National Institutes of Health
Bethesda, Maryland

David S. Schrump, MD
Senior Investigator
Surgery Branch
Thoracic Oncology Section
National Cancer Institute
National Institutes of Health
Bethesda, Maryland

Lawrence H. Schwartz, MD
Associate Professor of Radiology
Cornell University Joan and Sanford I. Weill Medical
    College
Memorial Sloan-Kettering Cancer Center
New York, New York

Douglas J. Schwartzentruber, MD
Medical Director, Center for Cancer Care
Goshen Health System
Goshen, Indiana

Brahm H. Segal, MD
Chief, Infectious Diseases
Department of Medicine
Roswell Park Cancer Institute
Buffalo, New York

Yoshitaka Sekido, MD, PhD
Assistant Professor
Department of Clinical Preventative
    Medicine
Nagoya University School of Medicine
Nagoya, Japan

Stuart Seropian, MD
Assistant Professor
Department of Internal Medicine
Yale University School of Medicine
New Haven, Connecticut

Robert C. Shamberger, MD
Robert E. Gross Professor of Surgery
Harvard Medical School
Chief of Surgery
Children's Hospital, Boston
Boston, Massachusetts

Joel Sheinfeld, MD
Vice-Chair
Department of Urology
Memorial Sloan-Kettering Cancer Center
New York, New York

Richard M. Sherry, MD
Senior Investigator
Surgery Branch
National Cancer Institute
National Institutes of Health
Bethesda, Maryland

Peter G. Shields, MD
Professor of Oncology and Medicine
Department of Oncology
Lombardi Comprehensive Cancer Center
Georgetown University School of Medicine
Washington, DC

William U. Shipley, MD
Andres Soriano Professor of Radiation Oncology
Harvard Medical School
The Claire and John Bertucci Center for Genitourinary Cancers
Head, Genitourinary Oncology Unit
Department of Radiation Oncology
Massachusetts General Hospital
Boston, Massachusetts

John L. Shuster, MD
Clinical Professor of Psychiatry
University of Alabama
Birmingham, Alabama
Research Physician
Tuscaloosa VA Medical Center
Tuscaloosa, Alabama

David Sidransky, MD
Director, Head and Neck Cancer Research Division
Department of Otolaryngology
Johns Hopkins University School of Medicine
Baltimore, Maryland

Richard M. Simon, DSc
Chief, Biometric Research Branch
Head, Computational Biology Group
Division of Cancer Treatment and Diagnosis
National Cancer Institute
National Institutes of Health
Bethesda, Maryland

Samuel Singer, MD
Associate Professor of Surgery
Cornell University Joan and Sanford I. Weill Medical College
Associate Attending
Department of Surgery
Sarcoma Disease Management Program
Memorial Sloan-Kettering Cancer Center
New York, New York

William Small, Jr., MD
Associate Professor of Clinical Radiology
Department of Radiation Oncology
Robert H. Lurie Comprehensive Cancer Center of Northwestern University
Chicago, Illinois

J. Stanley Smith, MD
Professor of Surgery
Pennsylvania State University College of Medicine
Milton S. Hershey Medical Center
Hershey, Pennsylvania

Rebecca G. Smith, MD, MS
Clinical Director, Musculoskeletal and Pain Rehabilitation Programs
MossRehab
Albert Einstein Healthcare at Elkins Park
Elkins Park, Pennsylvania

Edward L. Snyder, MD
Professor of Laboratory Medicine
Yale University School of Medicine
Director, Blood Bank/Apheresis/Stem Cell Processing Laboratory
Yale-New Haven Hospital
New Haven, Connecticut

Arthur J. Sober, MD
Professor of Dermatology
Harvard Medical School
Massachusetts General Hospital
Boston, Massachusetts

Lawrence J. Solin, MD, FACR
Professor
Department of Radiation Oncology
University of Pennsylvania School of Medicine
Philadelphia, Pennsylvania

Vernon K. Sondak, MD
Professor
Program Leader, Cutaneous Oncology
Department of Interdisciplinary Oncology
University of South Florida College of Medicine
H. Lee Moffitt Cancer Center and Research Institute
Tampa, Florida

Wiley W. Souba, MD, ScD
John A. and Marian T. Waldhausen Professor and Chair
Department of Surgery
Pennsylvania State University College of Medicine
Surgeon-in-Chief
Milton S. Hershey Medical Center
Hershey, Pennsylvania

C. A. Stein, MD, PhD
Professor of Medicine, Urology, and Molecular Pharmacology
Department of Oncology
Albert Einstein College of Medicine of Yeshiva University
Montefiore Medical Center
Bronx, New York

William G. Stetler-Stevenson, MD, PhD
Senior Investigator
Cell and Cancer Biology Branch
Center for Cancer Research
National Cancer Institute
National Institutes of Health
Bethesda, Maryland

Diane E. Stover, MD
Professor of Clinical Medicine
Cornell University Joan and Sanford I. Weill Medical College
Head, Division of General Medicine
Chief, Pulmonary Service
Memorial Sloan-Kettering Cancer Center
New York, New York

Ronald M. Summers, MD, PhD
Senior Investigator and Staff Radiologist
Chief, Clinical Image Processing Service

Chief, Virtual Endoscopy and Computer-Aided Diagnosis
Laboratory
Department of Radiology
National Institutes of Health
Bethesda, Maryland

Carol J. Swallow, MD, PhD
Associate Professor
Department of Surgery
University of Toronto Faculty of Medicine
Attending Surgeon
Department of Surgical Oncology
Princess Margaret Hospital
Toronto, Ontario, Canada

Chris H. Takimoto, MD, PhD
Associate Professor
Department of Medicine
Division of Medical Oncology
University of Texas Medical School at San Antonio
San Antonio, Texas

Nancy J. Tarbell, MD
Professor of Radiation Oncology
Department of Pediatric Radiation Oncology
Massachusetts General Hospital
Boston, Massachusetts

Robert Temple, MD
Director, Office of Drug Evaluation
Food and Drug Administration
Rockville, Maryland

Joel E. Tepper, MD
Professor and Chair
Department of Radiation Oncology
University of North Carolina at Chapel Hill School of Medicine
Chapel Hill, North Carolina

Charles R. Thomas, Jr., MD
Professor and Vice-Chair
Department of Radiation Oncology
University of Texas Health Science Center at San Antonio
San Antonio, Texas

Michael J. Thun, MD, MS
Vice President
Epidemiology and Surveillance Research
American Cancer Society
Atlanta, Georgia

Anthony W. Tolcher, MD, FRCP(C)
Clinical Professor of Medicine
Department of Medical Oncology
Institute for Drug Development
Cancer Therapy and Research Center
University of Texas Health Science Center San Antonio
San Antonio, Texas

Lois B. Travis, MD, ScD
Adjunct Professor of Oncology
Lombardi Cancer Center
Georgetown University Medical Center
Washington, DC
Senior Investigator
Division of Cancer Epidemiology and Genetics
National Cancer Institute
National Institutes of Health
Bethesda, Maryland

Jeffrey M. Trent, PhD
President and Scientific Director

Translational Genomics Research Institute
Phoenix, Arizona

Margaret A. Tucker, MD
Chief, Genetic Epidemiology Branch
Division of Cancer Epidemiology and Genetics
National Cancer Institute
National Institutes of Health
Bethesda, Maryland

Andrew T. Turrisi, MD
Professor and Chair
Department of Radiation Oncology
Wayne State University School of Medicine
Karmanos Comprehensive Cancer Center
Detroit Medical Center
Detroit, Michigan

Robert Udelsman, MD, MBA
Lampman Professor of Surgery and Oncology
Chairman, Department of Surgery
Yale University School of Medicine
Surgeon-in-Chief
Yale-New Haven Hospital
New Haven, Connecticut

Catherine E. Ulbricht, PharmD, RPh, MBA(c)
Assistant Professor
Northeastern University
Boston, Massachusetts
Massachusetts College of Pharmacy
Boston, Massachusetts
University of Rhode Island
Kinston, Rhode Island
Chief Editor
Natural Standard Research Collaboration
(http://www.naturalstandard.com)
Journal of Herbal Pharmacotherapy
(http://www.haworthpress.com)
Cambridge, Massachusetts
Senior Attending Pharmacist
Massachusetts General Hospital
Boston, Massachusetts

Robert L. Ullrich, PhD
Barbara Cox Anthony University Chair in Oncology
Departments of Environmental and Radiological Health
Sciences and Clinical Sciences
Colorado State University
Fort Collins, Colorado

Flora E. van Leeuwen, PhD
Professor of Cancer Epidemiology
Netherlands Cancer Institute
Amsterdam, The Netherlands

Mary M. Vargo, MD
Assistant Professor
Department of Physical Medicine and Rehabilitation
Case Western Reserve University at Metro Health Medical
Center
Cleveland, Ohio

Rena Vassilopoulou-Sellin, MD
Professor
Endocrine Neoplasia and Hormonal Disorders
The University of Texas M. D. Anderson Cancer Center
Houston, Texas

Nicholas J. Vogelzang, MD
Director, Nevada Cancer Institute
Las Vegas, Nevada

Andrew C. von Eschenbach, MD
Director, National Cancer Institute
National Institutes of Health
Bethesda, Maryland

Thomas J. Walsh, MD
Head, Immunocompromised Host Section
Pediatric Oncology Branch
National Cancer Institute
National Institutes of Health
Bethesda, Maryland

McClellan M. Walther, MD
Staff Physician
Urologic Oncology Branch
National Cancer Institute
National Institutes of Health
Bethesda, Maryland

Elizabeth M. Ward, PhD
Director, Surveillance Research
Department of Epidemiology and Surveillance
    Research
American Cancer Society
Atlanta, Georgia

Irving Waxman, MD
Professor of Medicine
Director of Endoscopy
Department of Medicine
University of Chicago Pritzker School of
    Medicine
Chicago, Illinois

Louis M. Weiner, MD
Vice President
Translational Research
Chairman, Department of Medical Oncology
G. Morris Dorrance, Jr., Endowed Chair in Medical
    Science
Fox Chase Cancer Center
Philadelphia, Pennsylvania

Howard J. Weinstein, MD
Professor of Pediatrics
Harvard Medical School
Chief, Pediatric Hematology-Oncology
Massachusetts General Hospital for Children
Boston, Massachusetts

Mark A. Weiss, MD
Associate Attending Physician
Department of Medicine
Memorial Sloan-Kettering Cancer Center
New York, New York

Raymond B. Weiss, MD, FACP
Clinical Professor of Medicine
Lombardi Cancer Center
Georgetown University Medical Center
Washington, DC

Walter C. Willett, MD, DrPH
Professor of Epidemiology and Nutrition
Chair, Department of Nutrition
Harvard School of Public Health
Boston, Massachusetts

Grant A. Williams, MD
Deputy Director
Division of Oncology Drug Products
Center for Drug Evaluation and Research

U.S. Food and Drug Administration
Rockville, Maryland

Lynn D. Wilson, MD, MPH
Associate Professor
Department of Therapeutic Radiology
Yale University School of Medicine
Yale Comprehensive Cancer Center
New Haven, Connecticut

Kathleen Yaus Wolin, BA
Department of Epidemiology
Harvard School of Public Health
Channing Laboratory
Brigham and Women's Hospital
Boston, Massachusetts

Kwok-Kin Wong, MD, PhD
Instructor of Medical Oncology
Dana-Farber Cancer Institute
Brigham and Women's Hospital
Boston, Massachusetts

Flossie Wong-Staal, PhD
Professor of Medicine
University of California, San Diego, School of
    Medicine
La Jolla, California

William C. Wood, MD
Professor and Chairman
Department of Surgery
Emory University School of Medicine
Atlanta, Georgia

YanYun Wu, MD, PhD
Assistant Professor
Department of Laboratory Medicine
Yale University School of Medicine
Assistant Director
Blood Bank/Apheresis/Stem Cell Processing
    Laboratory
Yale-New Haven Hospital
New Haven, Connecticut

John R. Wunderlich, MD
Surgery Branch
National Cancer Institute
National Institutes of Health
Bethesda, Maryland

Joachim Yahalom, MD
Professor of Radiation Oncology
Cornell University Joan and Sanford I. Weill Medical
    College
Member and Attending
Memorial Sloan-Kettering Cancer Center
New York, New York

James C. Yang, MD
Senior Investigator
Surgery Branch
National Cancer Institute
National Institutes of Health
Bethesda, Maryland

Robert Yarchoan, MD
Chief, HIV and AIDS Malignancy Branch
Center for Cancer Research
National Cancer Institute
National Institutes of Health
Bethesda, Maryland

Charles J. Yeo, MD
Professor of Surgery and Oncology
Chief, Division of General and Gastrointestinal Surgery
Johns Hopkins Medical Institutions
Baltimore, Maryland

Theresa Pluth Yeo, MPH, MSN
Assistant Professor
Johns Hopkins University School of Nursing
Acute Care Nurse Practitioner
Sidney Kimmel Cancer Center at Johns Hopkins
Baltimore, Maryland

Yesim Yilmaz, MD
Postdoctoral Associate in Clinical Cytogenetics
Department of Genetics
Yale University School of Medicine
New Haven, Connecticut

Stuart H. Yuspa, MD
Chief, Laboratory of Cellular Carcinogenesis and
    Tumor Promotion
Deputy Director, Center for Cancer
    Research
National Cancer Institute
National Institutes of Health
Bethesda, Maryland

Herbert J. Zeh III, MD
Assistant Professor of Surgery
Division of Surgical Oncology
University of Pittsburgh School of Medicine
Pittsburgh, Pennsylvania

Anthony L. Zietman, MD
Professor of Radiation Oncology
Harvard Medical School
Massachusetts General Hospital
Boston, Massachusetts

Sandra S. Zinkel, MD, PhD
Instructor in Medicine
Dana-Farber Cancer Institute
Boston, Massachusetts

PREFACE

The practice of oncology is being transformed by the increasing application of scientific advances to the management of cancer patients and by increased emphasis on well-designed clinical trials as a guide to evidence-based clinical practice. As in each of the prior editions of this text, this seventh edition of *Cancer: Principles and Practice of Oncology* has been carefully constructed to help oncologists in all fields keep abreast of the latest scientific advances in oncology as they apply to clinical practice, as well as to provide a critical and practical guide to the optimal management of cancer patients.

To meet these goals, the text has been divided into four main parts.

PART 1: **Molecular Biology of Cancer** describes molecular assays used in oncologic studies, such as complementary DNA arrays, tissue arrays, and DNA amplification techniques, and has an extensive discussion of the emerging fields of genomics and proteomics as they apply to research and clinical application in oncology. Approaches to the development of new treatments are based on an understanding of specific molecular targets. PART 1 also deals with the basic mechanisms of signal transduction, the cell cycle, apoptosis, angiogenesis, cancer immunology, and other areas that form the foundations of current and emerging treatments for cancer patients.

PART 2: **Principles of Oncology** deals with the principles that provide the basis for efforts in cancer prevention, diagnosis, and treatment. The viral, chemical, and physical factors involved in cancer etiology and the pharmacology of chemical, biologic, and endocrine agents involved in cancer treatment are described. The principles underlying the practice of surgical, medical, and radiation oncology are discussed, as well as information on the design and analysis of clinical trials.

PART 3: **Practice of Oncology** is designed to provide the practical information needed to provide state-of-the-art care to cancer patients. Chapters on cancer prevention deal with practical approaches to the prevention of tobacco-related cancers, as well as the role of dietary factors and chemopreventive agents. Diagnostic issues deal with cancer screening, advanced molecular diagnostic approaches, and advanced imaging modalities. A hallmark of this and all previous editions of this text is the careful integration of all treatment modalities in the management of cancer patients. Thus, chapters dealing with the major cancer organ sites have been coauthored by surgeons, medical oncologists, and radiation therapists to provide the practicing oncologist with an integrated multimodality approach to cancer care by stage of disease to optimize outcomes. The optimal management of the symptoms caused by cancer or its treatment is dealt with in detail. Increased emphasis has been placed on supportive treatments that are increasingly effective in improving the quality of life of cancer patients.

PART 4: **Newer Approaches in Cancer Treatment** describes emerging areas that will have an increasing impact on the practice of oncology in the future. Thus, chapters on gene therapy, immunotherapy, and antiangiogenesis, as well as emerging molecular treatments for cancer, provide the oncologist with a glimpse into treatments under development.

The incidence and mortality of cancer are decreasing, due not only to scientific and clinical improvements in care, but also as a result of the dissemination of information concerning the prevention, the diagnosis, and the coordinated multimodality approach to cancer treatment that is required to optimize patient outcome. We believe that the prior six editions of *Cancer: Principles and Practice of Oncology* since 1982 have played a role in these improvements by educating oncologists in the scientific basis of oncology and by always presenting the leading edge of the state-of-the-art care of cancer patients. We thank the many hundreds of scientists and clinicians—all experts in their fields—who have contributed to this effort. The editors are proud to present this seventh edition of *Cancer: Principles and Practice of Oncology*, aimed at providing the best possible care for each individual cancer patient.

Vincent T. DeVita, Jr., MD
Samuel Hellman, MD
Steven A. Rosenberg, MD, PhD

ACKNOWLEDGMENTS

The editors would like to acknowledge the extraordinary contributions of Zia Raven, who played a vital role in the preparation of this edition. Ms. Raven assumed responsibility for the organization and compilation of all of the chapters in this text. We are grateful for her dedication and hard work. We also thank Jonathan W. Pine, Jr., Senior Executive Editor at Lippincott Williams & Wilkins, for his excellent help in the production of this text.

VTD
SH
SAR

CONTENTS

PART 1

MOLECULAR BIOLOGY OF CANCER

1

14

Principles of Medical Oncology **295**

EDWARD CHU
VINCENT T. DEVITA, JR.

Historical Perspective *295*
Clinical Application of Chemotherapy *296*
Clinical End Points in Evaluating Response to Chemotherapy *297*
Cancer Cell Kinetics and Response to Chemotherapy *298*
Principles Governing the Use of Chemotherapy *298*
Concept of Dose Intensity *300*
Apoptosis, Cell-Cycle Control, and Resistance to Chemotherapy *301*

15

Pharmacology of Cancer Chemotherapy **307**

SECTION **1** **Drug Development** *307*
EDWARD CHU

Drug Discovery *307*
Combinatorial Chemistry *309*
Drug Screening *311*
Molecularly Targeted Screening *312*
Preclinical Pharmacology *313*
Formulation Studies *314*
Preclinical Toxicology *315*
Clinical Development *315*
Conclusion *316*

SECTION **2** **Pharmacokinetics** *317*
CHRIS H. TAKIMOTO

Introduction *317*
Pharmacokinetic Concepts *319*
Pharmacodynamic Concepts *323*
Special Topics in Pharmacokinetics and Pharmacodynamics *324*
Pharmacokinetics and Pharmacodynamics in Oncology Drug Development *325*
Conclusion *326*

SECTION **3** **Pharmacogenomics** *327*
HOWARD L. MCLEOD
BOON-CHER GOH

Pharmacogenomics of Chemotherapy Drug Toxicity *327*
Pharmacogenomics of Tumor Response *330*
Conclusion *331*

SECTION **4** **Alkylating Agents** *332*
O. MICHAEL COLVIN
HENRY S. FRIEDMAN

History of the Alkylating Agents *332*

PART *3*

PRACTICE OF ONCOLOGY

20

Cancer Prevention: Diet and Chemopreventive Agents **507**

29

Cancers of the Gastrointestinal Tract **861**

30
Cancers of the Genitourinary System **1139**

36
Benign and Malignant Mesothelioma **1687**

HARVEY I. PASS
NICHOLAS J. VOGELZANG
STEPHEN M. HAHN
MICHELE CARBONE

37
Cancer of the Skin **1717**

SUMAIRA Z. AASI
DAVID J. LEFFELL

38
Melanoma **1745**

ZHAO-JUN LIU
MEENHARD HERLYN

CHARLES M. BALCH
MICHAEL B. ATKINS
ARTHUR J. SOBER

SECTION **3**   *Intraocular Melanoma*   *1809*

ROBERT B. AVERY
MINESH P. MEHTA
RICHARD M. AUCHTER
DANIEL M. ALBERT

39
Neoplasms of the Central Nervous System **1827**

SECTION **1**   *Molecular Biology of Central Nervous System Neoplasms*   *1827*

DAVID N. LOUIS
WEBSTER K. CAVENEE

47

48

49

51
Treatment of Metastatic Cancer **2323**

PART **4**

NEWER APPROACHES IN CANCER TREATMENT

CANCER
Principles & Practice of Oncology

7th Edition

MOLECULAR BIOLOGY OF CANCER

Molecular Methods in Oncology

SECTION **1**   PAUL M. LIZARDI

Amplification Techniques

Advances in molecular biology together with new information about gene organization and sequence, derived from the Human Genome Project, are dramatically expanding the repertoire of analytical approaches that are available to study genetic alterations in cancer. As new analytical strategies undergo testing and validation in clinical research settings, they increasingly acquire the potential to drive significant advances in oncology. DNA-based assays are rapidly evolving as a result of an expansion in the repertoire of nucleic acid amplification methods and the availability of accurate gene annotation and sequences. The development of low-cost instruments and probes for real-time fluorescence monitoring of DNA amplification reactions is facilitating the application of these new methods. Improved methodology for whole genome amplification has removed former technical hurdles for the analysis of very small tissue samples. Additionally, the introduction of microarray formats for the analysis of DNA as well as proteins has stimulated the adoption of *comprehensive molecular analysis* as a valid research paradigm in oncology. The cancer investigator need no longer limit analysis to a few genes of interest but is readily able to gather information about thousands of molecular targets in parallel. In this chapter, some of the salient developments in the use of amplification technologies, alone or in combination with microarray readouts, are visited. The impact of these developments in the expansion of cancer diagnosis and treatment options is considered.

IMPROVED ANALYSIS OF MUTATIONS IN ONCOGENES AND TUMOR SUPPRESSOR GENES

Malignant tumors are caused by a multiplicity of genetic disturbances in somatic cells. The analysis of somatic mutations is greatly facilitated by amplification techniques, and the preferred method in many instances continues to be the polymerase chain reaction (PCR). Specific primer pairs can be targeted to any gene locus of interest, and primer design can be optimized *in silico* using appropriate software. Over the last few years, some of the most significant advances in DNA amplification technology have been in two key areas: (1) the ability to perform assays that interrogate a large number of cancer-related DNA alterations in parallel and (2) the ability to detect somatic mutations and other genetic alterations in the presence of a large excess of normal DNA.

Significant advances have been made in software and instrumentation for performing multiplex real-time PCR. The investigator can choose to use so-called TaqMan probes, which generate fluorescent signals in proportion to the amount of PCR product and are readily available from commercial sources to quantify a variety of target genes. Another option is to use custom-designed molecular beacons, which undergo a conformational change on hybridization with PCR amplicons and generate a fluorescent signal that is highly sequence specific. Molecular beacons with as many as four different fluorophores can be designed to detect different point mutations in cancer genes. It has been reported that, using molecular beacon assays, the measured signal ratios are proportional to the amount of the minor allele over a wider range than with the TaqMan assay.[1]

If the research objective is to detect a large number of mutations, and high throughput is a requirement, an attractive option is the use of ligation-dependent assays with readout based on zip-code arrays.[2] Zip-code arrays are more economical than standard microarrays because they contain universal probe sequences that do not change as different genes need to be targeted. Exons of interest are first amplified by PCR, and pools containing a mixture of different amplicons are interrogated using a mutation-specific ligation assay. Mutation detection is based on oligonucleotide probe pairs that contain gene-complementary sequences, which are ligated only if there is perfect base pairing. In addition, one of the two oligonucleotides comprising each ligation probe pair is tethered to a sequence that is complementary to a zip-code array element. After ligation, the joined probes are detected by hybridization to the complementary zip-code elements in the universal array. Ligation-dependent point mutation detection has been combined with rolling circle amplification (RCA) signal enhancement and universal zip-code arrays to enable detection of up to 17 different mutated alleles in parallel. The improved limit of detection and dynamic range available with RCA signal enhancement permits the detection of mutant alleles in the presence of a 100-fold excess of wild-type DNA.[3]

An endonuclease/ligase mutation scanning method[4] is particularly well suited for the analysis of neoplastic tissues. DNA loci of interest are amplified by PCR, using two primers with different fluorescent labels. The amplified DNA is denatured and reannealed to form heteroduplexes, and these are digested with endonuclease V to generate nicks that, in mismatched DNA, are preferentially located one base toward the 3' side of the mismatch. Thermostable ligase is then added to reseal background nicking artifacts that are present at otherwise perfectly matched regions. Finally, the digested and resealed PCR amplicons are separated in a sequencing gel to reveal the sites of mismatch-induced nicking. The method enables scanning for detection of mutations in fragments as long as 1.7 kb and does not require preexisting knowledge of the mutated sequence. Thus, it could be used for the detection of virtually any mutation in an oncogene or tumor suppressor gene. A particularly attractive application of this method is mutational scanning using complementary DNA derived from messenger RNA (mRNA), as this would permit detection of mutations in the majority of exons of any gene of moderate size, in a single assay.

The detection of mutant alleles in the presence of a very large excess (greater than 100-fold) of normal DNA is a challenging goal. An elegant solution to this problem has been devised, based on the ability of the PCR to amplify single DNA molecules. In so-called digital PCR,[5,6] DNA is diluted to the point that amplification by PCR reports the presence of single molecules, present in highly dilute DNA samples. In this situation, a rare mutant DNA molecule, sampled (and thus purified) by terminal dilution, generates amplicons that are 100% mutant. Although this method is extremely powerful, it is also expensive and technically demanding because hundreds (or even thousands) of PCR reactions must be performed to generate data for a single sample. In other words, if mutant DNA is present at a level of 1%, it is necessary to perform more than 300 individual PCR reactions to have a reasonable chance of detecting the mutant molecule. An alternative to digital PCR is the use of novel methods that enable isolation of mutant DNA before amplification. A powerful approach has been described[7] that begins with the generation of heteroduplexes with A/G mismatches in renatured DNA obtained from cancer tissue. *Escherichia coli* M*utY* is used to generate aldehydes at mismatched adenines, and subsequent treatment with a biotinylated hydroxylamine results in highly specific biotinylation at the site of every

mismatch. Biotinylated DNA, which represents the mutated DNA subset, is isolated and then amplified by PCR, using synthetic linkers. This method allows large-scale, whole genome detection of genetic alterations without any preexisting assumptions as to the affected gene locus.

HIGHLY PARALLELIZED SINGLE-NUCLEOTIDE POLYMORPHISM ASSAYS CAN ALSO BE USED FOR SOMATIC GENOTYPING

Hardenbol et al.[8] have described a novel method for single-nucleotide polymorphism (SNP) detection that can be highly parallelized. The method, which the authors call *sequence-tagged molecular inversion probes*, is unique because of its potential for high throughput. It is based on the use of a multiplicity of circularizable, or "padlock," probes that carry unique identifier tags and are designed to hybridize specifically to individual SNP sequences. As shown in Figure 1.1-1, a mixture of padlock probes is hybridized with total human DNA, ligated to form circles, relinearized by cleavage at a site distal from the ligation site, and finally amplified by PCR. The mixture of PCR amplicons is interrogated for specific SNP readout by hybridization on microarrays that decode each probe's identifier sequence codes. This elegant parallel amplification/decoding method is capable of rapidly interrogating several thousand SNPs using four separate gap-fill reactions (see Fig. 1.1-1) and a single microarray. The method can readily be applied to the problem of somatic mutation analysis in cancer.

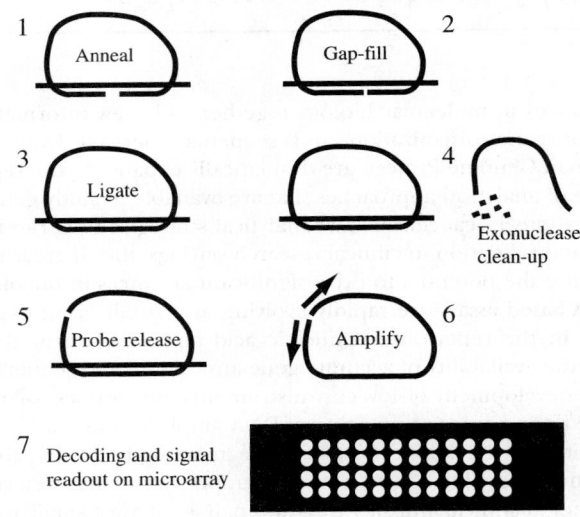

FIGURE 1.1-1. Scheme for assays based on sequence-tagged molecular inversion probes. **1:** A unique "padlock" probe, present in a mixture of probes, anneals specifically at its intended target. **2:** The gap is filled by extension with DNA polymerase. *Four different allele-discriminating gap-fill reactions are performed, each in a different tube, with a single deoxyribonucleoside triphosphate.* **3:** The probes with correctly extended gaps are circularized by ligation. **4:** Noncircularized excess probes are destroyed by digestion with exonuclease. **5:** The probe is released by cleavage with uracyl glycosylase. **6:** The probe is amplified by polymerase chain reaction. **7:** Because different probes carry different sequence codes, they can be sorted by hybridization on a microarray of complementary decoding probes. Finally, the array is scanned to measure fluorescent signal intensities.

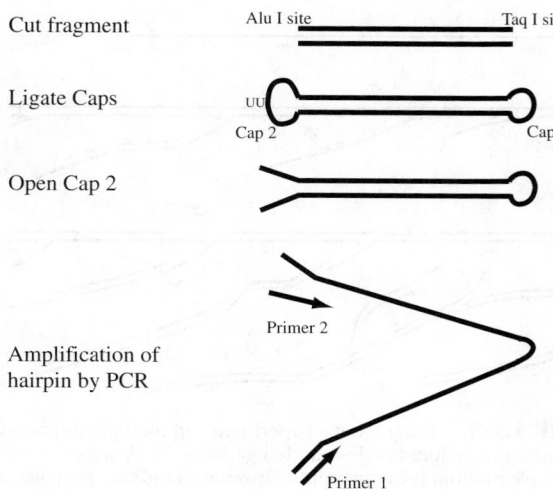

Cut fragment   Alu I site   Taq I site

Ligate Caps

Cap 2   Cap 1

Open Cap 2

Primer 2

Amplification of
hairpin by PCR

Primer 1

FIGURE 1.1-2. Diagram outlining the hairpin–polymerase chain reaction (PCR) method. DNA is fragmented with two different restriction endonucleases. The termini of those fragments that are flanked by two different cleavage sites (Taq I, Alu I) are capped by hairpin oligonucleotides, using DNA ligase. The enzyme uracyl glycosidase is then used to depurinate one of the caps, which contains two uracyl residues. On heating, the abasic site is cleaved by beta-elimination. The open DNA structure can now be amplified by PCR. After amplification, the hairpin structure renatures, and the small fraction of amplicons where the polymerase introduced copying errors has one mismatched base.

INCREASING THE ACCURACY OF SEQUENCE INFORMATION DERIVED FROM POLYMERASE CHAIN REACTION AMPLIFICATION

Errors introduced during PCR amplification set an artificial limit for the analysis of genetic alterations, because polymerase misincorporation invariably gets confused with genuine mutations. A new form of PCR, termed *hairpin-PCR*,[9] completely separates genuine mutations from errors generated by misincorporation. The method (Fig. 1.1-2) is based on ligation of an artificial DNA hairpin to the DNA target of interest before the PCR. During the DNA elongation step, the polymerase copies both DNA strands of the hairpin in a single pass. When a misincorporation occurs, it forms a mismatch after amplification, and these mismatched molecules can be distinguished from genuine mutations, which remain perfectly matched to the opposite strand of the hairpin-amplicon. Error-free DNA is subsequently isolated using a separation procedure capable of separating mismatched duplexes from perfectly matched duplexes, such as denaturing high-performance liquid chromatography.

MULTIPLEX REAL-TIME POLYMERASE CHAIN REACTION AMPLIFICATION FOR DETECTION OF MINIMAL RESIDUAL DISEASE OR VIRAL LOAD

The *in vitro* amplification of tumor-specific DNA or RNA sequences by PCR allows identification of a few neoplastic cells in as many as a million normal cells. Depending on the under-

lying malignant disease and therapeutic treatment, the presence of residual tumor cells in the blood of an individual patient may indicate a possibility of relapse. Monitoring of residual leukemia and lymphoma cells can provide important information about the effectiveness of treatment and the risk of recurrent disease, as shown by minimal residual disease (MRD) analysis in patients with various malignant diseases (reviewed in ref. 10). Such diseases include childhood acute lymphoblastic leukemia, after induction therapy; acute promyelocytic leukemia, during and after chemotherapy; and chronic myelogenous leukemia, during treatment with interferon-α and after allogeneic bone marrow transplantation. Improvements in multiplex real-time PCR now make it fairly simple to target as many as four markers of MRD in a single amplification reaction, expanding the power of MRD detection after treatment for patients whose cancers display molecular heterogeneity and cannot be monitored by single-gene targeting.

Multiplex PCR has greatly improved the ability to perform viral load determinations and viral genotyping for oncogenic viruses. DNA amplification assays have enabled screening for a broad spectrum of human papillomavirus types in clinical specimens using a single PCR reaction. After amplification using consensus primers, individual human papillomavirus genotypes are identified via a variety of methods. Using consensus primers in real-time quantitative PCR, it is possible to generate viral load (concentration) data from reaction curves generated by monitoring PCR reaction kinetics in real time. For example, the simultaneous detection of three different human papillomavirus genotypes (16, 18, 45) using molecular beacons has been reported.[11]

MUTATION DETECTION USING *IN SITU* HYBRIDIZATION METHODS COUPLED WITH DNA AMPLIFICATION

Unique gene loci are very difficult to detect using standard fluorescent probes. Two methods are available that enable the detection of such loci *in situ* by amplifying the probe signal. The tyramide signal amplification method, which is based on chemical amplification, can be extended to a two-color system to enable the simultaneous detection of two genes. An alternative system, which is capable of fourfold signal multiplexing, consists of surface-anchored DNA amplification. Hybridized DNA probes can be coupled to RCA *in situ* to generate fluorescent signal enhancement of approximately 300-fold. In this system, signals are generated by specific fluorescent oligonucleotides that bind to the *in situ* amplified DNA. One of the implementations of the *in situ* RCA detection system uses bipartite probes that are only capable of signal generation after ligation.[12] This system is capable of discriminating point mutations in cells fixed with methanol/acetic acid, but its efficiency is diminished when formalin-fixed tissue is used. An alternative implementation of surface-anchored RCA[13] uses circularizable (padlock) probes. It is claimed that this modified version of the RCA method can detect gene copy number changes and point mutations with efficiencies that approach 90% using methanol/acetic acid–fixed cells. The potential utility of the multicolor *in situ* RCA systems for detection of gene copy number changes and point mutations in formalin-fixed tissues remains to be determined.

HIGH-THROUGHPUT METHODS FOR MEASURING GENE DOSAGE ALTERATIONS

Gene dosage measurements are often performed using microsatellite assays or comparative genomic hybridization. The former provides high resolution, whereas the latter enables genome-wide coverage of allele losses and gains. A drawback of microsatellite-based assays for detection of loss of heterozygosity has been the requirement for patient DNA to be heterozygous at each microsatellite locus of interest, as homozygous loci are not informative. Dumur et al.[14] have demonstrated the use of the Affymetrix (Santa Clara, CA) SNP chip as a tool for loss of heterozygosity analysis. Multiple SNP loci were amplified by PCR, and the copy number status of each SNP was measured by hybridization of PCR amplicons on the SNP probe microarrays. As is the case for microsatellite-based loss of heterozygosity analysis, those loci that were homozygous for an SNP were not informative. However, as the content of SNP microarrays increases to many thousands of probes, the number of informative loci will become larger and larger, and the main limitation will be the number of PCR reactions required to amplify individual loci.

WHOLE GENOME AMPLIFICATION OF MICRODISSECTED TISSUE

The analysis of regions of dysplasia or small neoplasms surrounded by normal tissue is best performed using advanced microdissection methods, ideally laser-capture microdissection. Here the challenge is to perform comprehensive genetic analysis using a sample that may consist of just a few hundred cells. In this situation it is advantageous to perform whole genome amplification before genetic analysis. Methods have been introduced that enable the amplification of the whole human genome, with relatively unbiased representation of gene loci. In a method called *balanced PCR*,[15] two distinct genomic DNA samples are tagged with oligonucleotides that contain a common and a unique DNA sequence. The genomic DNA samples are pooled and amplified in a single PCR tube using the common DNA tag. Because both samples are amplified in the same PCR reaction, representational distortion is reduced. The PCR-amplified pooled samples are then separated using the DNA tag unique to each individual genomic DNA sample.

A remarkably simple method for whole genome amplification uses a reaction that relies on random primers to drive DNA replication by a strand-displacing DNA polymerase. Because newly replicated DNA strands are driven apart by DNA polymerase itself (Fig. 1.1-3), there is no need for temperature cycling, and the reaction proceeds *isothermally*. This reaction, called *multiple displacement amplification*, has been shown to generate DNA with relatively little representation bias. This has been demonstrated for 47 gene loci using real-time PCR[16] and for thousands of gene loci using microarray-based comparative genomic hybridization.[17] The latter studies demonstrated that it is possible to detect gene amplification in cell lines derived from breast tumors using as few as 500 cells as starting material. Regions of chromosome 17 and chromosome 20 that showed increased gene dosage in breast cancer cell lines were detected reliably in DNA generated by the isothermal multiple displacement amplification method.

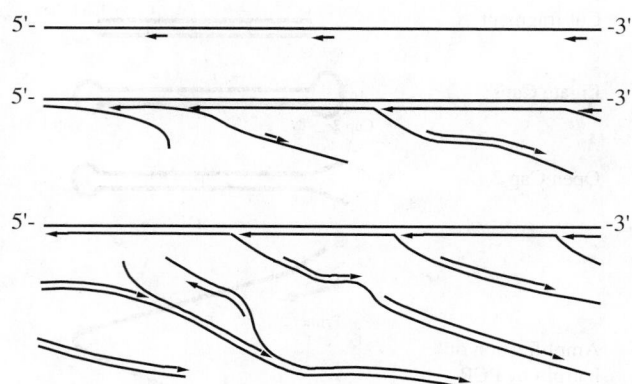

FIGURE 1.1-3. Diagram of a hyperbranched multiple displacement amplification reaction. Single-stranded genomic DNA serves as a target for multiple random priming events. Growing strands are propagated by a DNA polymerase with strand displacement activity. The 5'-end of each strand is displaced by another upstream strand, growing in the same direction. Displaced strands are now targeted by new random priming events, and these new strands are elongated in the opposite direction. As the reaction proceeds, the hyperbranched network expands dramatically, generating thousands of copies of the original DNA.

AMPLIFICATION OF GENOMIC REPRESENTATIONS FOR ANALYSIS OF GENE GAIN/LOSS

An alternative method for studying gene gain or gene loss at the level of the entire human genome is the analysis of genomic representations. Total human DNA is digested with a six-cutter (or four-cutter) restriction endonuclease, and oligonucleotide adaptors are ligated at the multiple DNA termini generated by digestion. Using primers specific for the adaptor sequences, PCR amplification is performed, generating predominantly a subset of unique amplicons that harbor genomic DNA sequence "representations." The genomic DNA loci captured in each representation tend to be highly reproducible across different amplification experiments, and this property implies that representations derived from different experiments can be compared to each other. The preferred method for comparing genomic representations generated from different tumor samples is a microarray that contains thousands of DNA probes, each specific for those gene loci that are present in a representation. Suitable probes are 60-base synthetic oligonucleotides. Using the genomic representation approach, Lucito et al.[18] have demonstrated the detection of gene gains and losses in tumor DNA. An advantage of this approach is that the complexity of the DNA present in a pool of genomic representations is significantly lower than that of total genomic DNA, and this leads to improved quantitative performance at the level of DNA microarray analysis. Hence, this method enables robust detection of hemizygous gene losses, which are often difficult to measure accurately with other methods.

TUMOR CLASSIFICATION USING REAL-TIME POLYMERASE CHAIN REACTION TO MEASURE MESSENGER RNA LEVELS

Microarray methods are wonderful tools for obtaining a global view of mRNA expression in tissue. RNA amplification methods (see Chapter 1.3) make possible microarray expression analysis starting from very small RNA samples. However, there are two main drawbacks of microarray methods: (1) the relatively high expense, which will remain a problem until microarrays are commoditized, and (2) the relatively poor precision, because typical microarray coefficients of variation for genes expressed at low levels are on the order of 15% to 25%. As a result of these drawbacks, investigators often use microarrays as the tools for initial global surveying of tumor gene expression and then shift to real-time PCR as the method of choice for obtaining very accurate measurements of gene expression for a limited set of genes of interest. It has been shown that the accurate classification of tumor types can be performed using a limited subset of genes, numbering in the range of 5 to 50. For repeated analysis of such small sets, real-time PCR is often the tool of choice. For example, quantitative PCR has been used as a validation tool to identify five genes with expression patterns that could be used to distinguish four types of adenocarcinomas.[19] Quantitative real-time PCR expression data obtained from the validation set clustered tumor samples in an unsupervised manner, generating a self-organized map with distinctive tumor site-specific domains. Quantitative PCR is not necessarily limited to the analysis of a small number of genes. Notably, Muro et al.[20] have analyzed the expression levels of 1536 genes in 100 colorectal cancer and 11 normal tissues using adaptor-tagged competitive PCR, a high-throughput reverse transcription–PCR technique. Different RNA samples are processed to generate separate complementary DNA libraries, using different adaptors, and the libraries are then pooled. Five tester samples and two controls that serve as calibration inputs are processed in a single PCR amplification reaction. PCR amplicons from each of the seven different samples are generated, and the predesigned complementary DNA adaptor length differences enable post-PCR separation of the different amplicons in an ABI 3700 analyzer (Foster City, CA).

A report demonstrates how an analytical capability to measure the expression levels of RNA transcripts that differ in only a single base can be exploited to find novel prognostic markers for breast cancer. The β subunit of human chorionic gonadotropin (HCG) is encoded by four genes, of which the β–HCG-3, -5, and -8 gene variants differ by a single nucleotide. Applying a molecular beacon reverse transcription real-time PCR assay,[21] it has been possible to measure the expression levels of β–HCG-3, -5, and -8 gene transcripts in 129 sporadic unilateral breast cancer samples. Multivariate survival analysis, including the analysis of follow-up samples from the same patients, showed that expression of β–HCG-3, -5, and -8 may help identify node-negative patients with poor prognosis.

BIOMARKER DETECTION USING DNA-AMPLIFIED IMMUNOASSAYS

It is possible to achieve dramatic increases in the sensitivity in microarray-based assays by using RCA.[22] This application of RCA is based on surface-anchored amplification of DNA and permits the detection of individual molecular recognition events on solid surfaces. The utility of RCA for dramatic improvements in the sensitivity of immunoassays (immuno-RCA) has been demonstrated.[23] Antibodies with covalently bound DNA primers were used to generate fluorescent signals on a protein microarray sandwich immunoassay format and attained antigen detection sensitivities in the range of 0.001 ng/mL. This application of immuno-RCA technology involved the detection of a panel of 75 different cytokines that were present at levels in the range of 0.1 to 20.0 pg/mL.[23] In the future, antibody microarray signal amplification based on immuno-RCA technology may find interesting applications in the detection of cancer biomarkers present at extremely low concentrations in human serum.

AMPLIFICATION-BASED APPROACHES FOR DNA METHYLATION ANALYSIS IN CANCER

Epigenetic alterations are frequently found in tumors. DNA methylation at 5-methylcytosine is a faithfully propagated epigenetic modification of certain DNA elements, particularly heterochromatic repeats. In cancer cells there is often an abnormally low level of methylation in highly and moderately repeated DNA sequences, including heterochromatic DNA repeats, dispersed retrotransposons, and endogenous retroviral elements. However, the functional significance of this remarkable hypomethylated epigenetic state with regard to neoplasia is not well understood.

A second type of epigenetic alteration concerns sequences rich in CG dinucleotides (CpG islands), which are commonly found in the immediate vicinity of gene promoters. The normal status of most CpG islands is a lack of methylation. However, in many tumors there is evidence for increased methylation of a multiplicity of CpG islands. Hypermethylation of CpG islands is known to be involved in promoter inactivation and is a frequent event implicated in the silencing of tumor suppressor genes. Because promoters number in the tens of thousands, it is quite challenging to devise assays that are capable of interrogating methylation status at all CpG islands, to find the specific subset of CpG islands that undergoes cancer-related changes in any given tumor type. Several approaches are available for studying the CpG island methylation. A widely used approach is based on the use of restriction endonucleases whose ability to cleave DNA is altered by methylation of 5-methylcytosine. The absence of cleavage at a CpG island can be coupled to PCR amplification, yielding amplicons enriched in methylated DNA. An alternative approach is based on the use of a bisulfite modification reaction to convert 5-methylcytosine to uracyl. This reaction generates DNA with different sequences (after uracyl is replaced by thymidine during PCR amplification) depending on the presence or absence of methylated bases. Both approaches can be readily enhanced by the use of microarray-based signal readouts, to increase assay throughput.

A report[24] describes a microarray-based technique for the simultaneous detection of multiple CpG islands, using colorectal cancer as a model. Amplicons from tumor and control samples were pooled and differentially methylated CpG island fragments hybridized to a panel of approximately 8000 CpG island probes. Data analysis identified 694 CpG island loci hypermethylated in a group of 14 colorectal tumors. A hierarchical clustering algorithm segregated the tumors into two subgroups, one of which exhibited a high level of concurrent hypermethylation and the other of which had little or no methylation. This is in agreement with previous observations of a CpG island methylation phenotype present in a subset of colorectal tumors.

A similar approach combining PCR amplification of CpG islands followed by microarray readout has been used[25] to profile methylation alterations of CpG islands in ovarian tumors. Analysis was performed on 19 patients with stage III and IV ovarian carcinomas. Hierarchical clustering of the microarray data identified two groups of patients with distinct methylation profiles. Tumors from group 1 contained high levels of concurrent methylation, whereas group 2 tumors had lower tumor methylation levels. The data suggest that a higher degree of CpG island methylation is associated with early disease recurrence after chemotherapy.

REFERENCES

1. Tapp I, Malmberg L, Rennel E, et al. Homogeneous scoring of single-nucleotide polymorphisms: comparison of the 5'-nuclease TaqMan assay and Molecular Beacon probes. *Biotechniques* 2000;28:732.
2. Gerry NP, Witowski NE, Day J, et al. Universal DNA microarray method for multiplex detection of low abundance point mutations. *J Mol Biol* 1999;292:251.
3. Ladner DP, Leamon JH, Hamann S, et al. Multiplex detection of hotspot mutations by rolling circle-enabled universal microarrays. *Lab Invest* 2001;81:1079.
4. Huang J, Kirk B, Favis R, et al. An endonuclease/ligase based mutation scanning method especially suited for analysis of neoplastic tissue. *Oncogene* 2002;21:1909.
5. Vogelstein B, Kinzler KW. Digital PCR. *Proc Natl Acad Sci U S A* 1999;96:9236.
6. Zhou W, Galizia G, Lieto E, et al. Counting alleles reveals a connection between chromosome 18q loss and vascular invasion. *Nat Biotechnol* 2001;19:78.
7. Chakrabarti S, Price BD, Tetradis S, et al. Highly selective isolation of unknown mutations in diverse DNA fragments: toward new multiplex screening in cancer. *Cancer Res* 2000;60:3732.
8. Hardenbol P, Baner J, Jain M, et al. Multiplexed genotyping with sequence-tagged molecular inversion probes. *Nat Biotechnol* 2003;21:673.
9. Kaur M, Makrigiorgos GM. Novel amplification of DNA in a hairpin structure: towards a radical elimination of PCR errors from amplified DNA. *Nucleic Acids Res* 2003;31:e26.
10. Dolken G. Detection of minimal residual disease. *Adv Cancer Res* 2001;82:133.
11. Szuhai K, Sandhaus E, Kolkman-Uljee SM, et al. A novel strategy for human papillomavirus detection and genotyping with SybrGreen and molecular beacon polymerase chain reaction. *Am J Pathol* 2001;159:1651.
12. Zhong XB, Lizardi PM, Huang XH, et al. Visualization of oligonucleotide probes and point mutations in interphase nuclei and DNA fibers using rolling circle DNA amplification. *Proc Natl Acad Sci U S A* 2001;98:3940.
13. Christian AT, Pattee MS, Attix CM, et al. Detection of DNA point mutations and mRNA expression levels by rolling circle amplification in individual cells. *Proc Natl Acad Sci U S A* 2001;98:14238.
14. Dumur CI, Dechsukhum C, Ware JL, et al. Genome-wide detection of LOH in prostate cancer using human SNP microarray technology. *Genomics* 2003;81:260.
15. Makrigiorgos GM, Chakrabarti S, Zhang Y, et al. A PCR-based amplification method retaining the quantitative difference between two complex genomes. *Nat Biotechnol* 2002;20:936.
16. Hosono S, Faruqi AF, Dean FB, et al. Unbiased whole-genome amplification directly from clinical samples. *Genome Res* 2003;13:954.
17. Lage JM, Leamon JH, Pejovic T, et al. Whole genome analysis of genetic alterations in small DNA samples using hyperbranched strand displacement amplification and array-CGH. *Genome Res* 2003;13:294.
18. Lucito R, Healy J, Alexander J, et al. Representational oligonucleotide microarray analysis: a high-resolution method to detect genome copy number variation. *Genome Res* 2003;13:2291.
19. Buckhaults P, Zhang Z, Chen YC, et al. Identifying tumor origin using a gene expression-based classification map. *Cancer Res* 2003;63:4144.
20. Muro S, Takemasa I, Oba S, et al. Identification of expressed genes linked to malignancy of human colorectal carcinoma by parametric clustering of quantitative expression data. *Genome Biol* 2003;4:R21.
21. Span PN, Manders P, Heuvel JJ, et al. Molecular beacon reverse transcription-PCR of human chorionic gonadotropin-beta-3, -5, and -8 mRNAs has prognostic value in breast cancer. *Clin Chem* 2003;49:1074.
22. Lizardi PM, Huang X, Zhu Z, et al. Mutation detection and single-molecule counting using isothermal rolling-circle amplification. *Nat Genet* 1998;19:225.
23. Schweitzer B, Roberts S, Grimwade B, et al. Multiplexed protein profiling on microarrays by rolling-circle amplification. *Nat Biotechnol* 2002;20:359.
24. Yan PS, Efferth T, Chen HL, et al. Use of CpG island microarrays to identify colorectal tumors with a high degree of concurrent methylation. *Methods* 2002;27:162.
25. Wei SH, Chen CM, Strathdee G, et al. Methylation microarray analysis of late-stage ovarian carcinomas distinguishes progression-free survival in patients and identifies candidate epigenetic markers. *Clin Cancer Res* 2002;8:2246.

SECTION **2**

RICHARD A. MORGAN

RNA Interference

The explosion of interest in RNA interference (RNAi) in the past few years has taken many researchers by surprise. A field once relegated to the backwaters of plant and invertebrate genetics has now been hailed as a potential revolution in molecular medicine and genomics.[1-3] This chapter describes why this change has occurred and attempts to put into perspective the potential applications of this new technology without overstating the promise of RNAi.

The underlying mechanisms involved in RNAi are conserved in vertebrates, invertebrates, fungi, and plants, suggesting that RNAi may be an intrinsic part of eukaryotic cell biochemistry. The first real detailed understanding of RNAi came from work that resulted from a discovery made by Andrew Fire while attempting to silence gene expression in *Caenorhabditis elegans*.[4] In these experiments, it was discovered that double-stranded RNAs (dsRNAs) inhibited gene expression 100-fold better than standard antisense RNAs. Only a few copies of RNA could be injected into the worms to result in global inhibition of gene expression, and, most remarkably, this inhibition was passed on to progeny animals. In addition to these findings, researchers involved in plant genetic engineering described a phenomenon called *cosuppression* in which

transgenes could repress the expression of endogenous genes[5] and further demonstrated that plant viruses were kept in check by mechanisms involving RNA destruction. These seemingly unrelated observations were then combined with data from studies in the fungi *Neurospora* and fruit fly *Drosophila*, leading to a proposal for an underlying mechanism to account for these diverse observations.[1-3]

BIOCHEMISTRY AND FUNCTION

When dsRNA is present in cells, it can associate with an adenosine triphosphate (ATP)-dependent RNase III–like nuclease called *Dicer*. Dicer processes the dsRNA to short interfering RNAs (siRNAs) that are 22 to 25 nucleotides (nt) in length with 2-nt 3' overhangs (Fig. 1.2-1). These siRNAs then incorporate into a larger multicomponent RNA-inducing silencing complex (RISC). The precise nature of RISC is still to be elucidated, but it contains at least four components (in addition to the siRNA): a protein of the Argonaute-2 gene family with potential helicase activity, a putative RNA-binding protein related to the *Drosophila VIG* gene, a micrococcal nuclease-homologue protein termed *Tudor-SN*, and a protein related to the human fragile X mental retardation protein.[6] The association of the fragile X mental retardation protein–related proteins in the RISC is intriguing, as the fragile X protein has been implicated in the posttranscription gene regulation, suggesting a possible link between RNAi-like biochemistry and this human

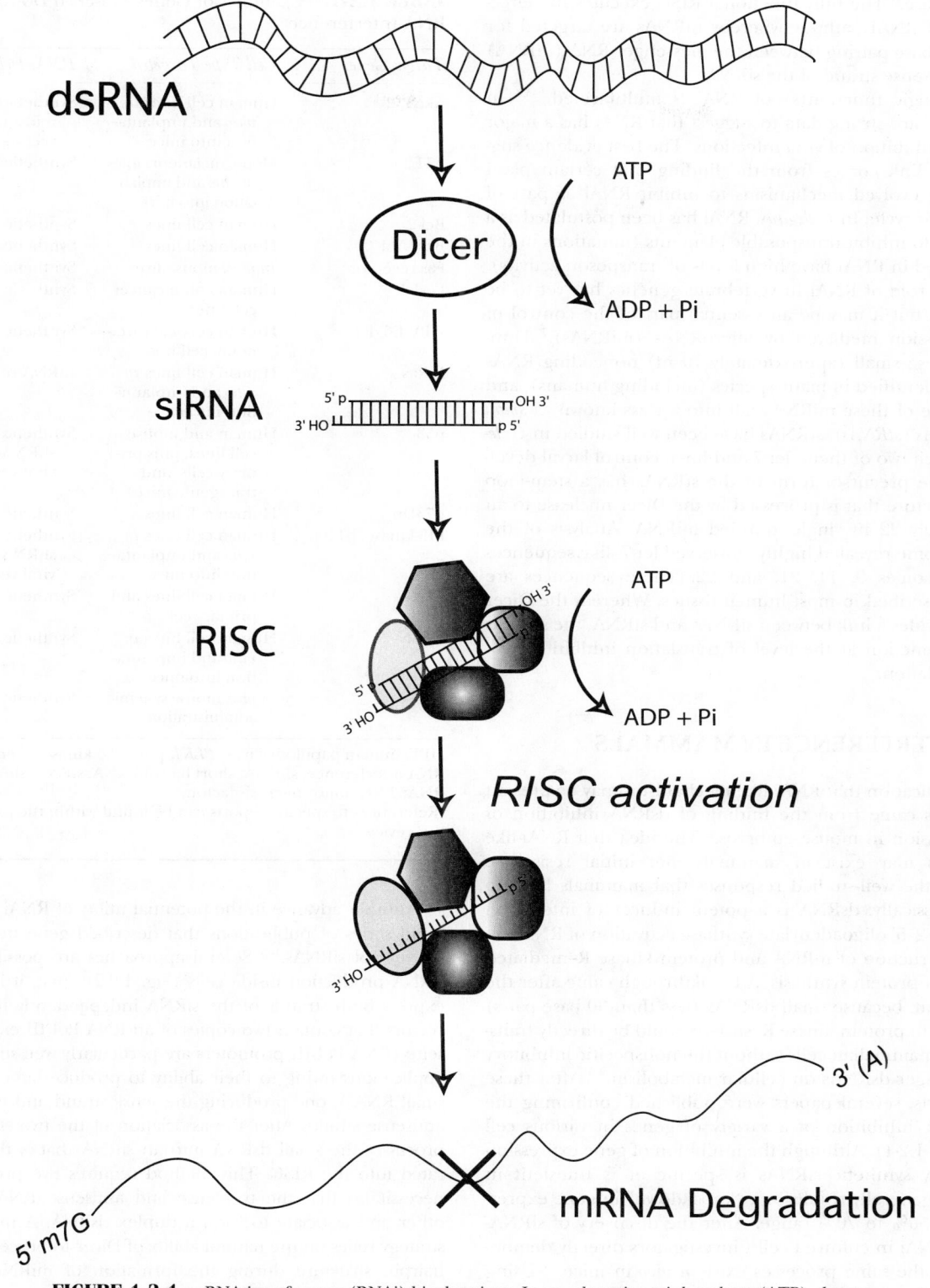

FIGURE 1.2-1. RNA interference (RNAi) biochemistry. In an adenosine triphosphate (ATP)–dependent process, double-stranded RNA (dsRNA) is brought into association with the Dicer nuclease. Dicer processes the long dsRNA into short (22 to 25 nt) dsRNAs with characteristic two nucleotide 3' overhangs [short interfering RNA (siRNA)]. The siRNA then associates with the multicomponent RNA-inducing silencing complex (RISC), which requires ATP to form an active effector complex. The activated RISC uses the antisense strand of the siRNA to target specific messenger RNAs (mRNAs) for cleavage and subsequent degradation. ADP, adenosine diphosphate; Pi, inorganic phosphate.

genetic disease.[6] The fully functional RISC executes the effector phase of RNAi pathway whereby mRNAs are targeted for cleavage by base pairing between the messenger RNA (mRNA) and the antisense strand of the siRNA.

The biologic function(s) of RNAi is multifaceted.[1–3,6] In plants, there are strong data to suggest that RNAi has a major role in the inhibition of viral infections. The best evidence suggesting this link comes from the finding that certain plant viruses have evolved mechanisms to inhibit RNAi as part of their viral life cycle. In *C elegans*, RNAi has been postulated as a mechanism to inhibit transposable elements (mutations in the gene involved in RNAi have high levels of transposon activity). A definitive role of RNAi in vertebrate genetics has yet to be understood, but it may be an essential part of the control of gene expression mediated by microRNAs (miRNAs).[7] Hundreds of these small (approximately 70 nt) noncoding RNAs have been identified in many species (including humans), and at least some of these miRNAs fall into a class known as *small temporal RNAs* (*stRNAs*). stRNAs have been well studied in *C elegans*, in which two of them, let-7 and lin-4, control larval development. The precursor form of the stRNAs has a stem-loop hairpin structure that is processed by the Dicer nuclease to an approximately 22 nt single-stranded miRNA. Analysis of the human genome revealed highly conserved let-7–like sequences on chromosomes 9, 11, 21, and 22. These sequences are actively transcribed in most human tissues. Whereas the Dicer protein provides a link between siRNAs and stRNA, the stRNAs appear to function at the level of translation inhibition, not RNA degradation.

RNA INTERFERENCE IN MAMMALS

The first indication that RNAi-like mechanisms may be present in mammals came from the finding of dsRNA inhibition of gene expression in mouse embryos.[2] The idea that RNAi-like mechanisms may exist in mammals met initial resistance because of the well-studied responses that mammals have to dsRNA. Classically, dsRNA is a potent inducer of interferon and leads to 2'-5' oligoadenylate synthase activation of RNase L, causing destruction of mRNA and protein kinase R–mediated inhibition of protein synthesis. A breakthrough came after the discovery that, because small dsRNAs (less than 30 base pairs) do not bind to protein kinase R, siRNAs could be directly transfected into mammalian cells without the nonspecific inhibitory effects of larger dsRNAs on cellular metabolism.[8,9] After these initial reports, several papers were published confirming the gene-specific inhibition of a variety of genes in various cell types (Table 1.2-1). Although the inhibition of gene expression mediated by synthetic siRNAs is specific, it is transient in nature and generally results in a "knockdown" in gene expression in the 50% to 70% range. After the discovery of siRNA-mediated RNAi in cultured cells, investigators directly demonstrated that the same processes exist *in vivo* in mice.[10] Using hydrodynamic-mediated gene delivery to the liver, two groups reported that siRNAs could be injected into mouse livers with resultant knockdown in gene expression. Further reports went on to demonstrate *in vivo* protection against autoimmune hepatitis via injection of siRNA against *Fas* and reduction in hepatitis B virus production by codelivery of cloned hepatitis B virus DNA along with siRNA against hepatitis B virus.[11]

TABLE 1.2-1.   Examples of Genes Knocked Down by RNA Interference[a]

Target Gene	Cell Type Targeted	RNAi Delivery Method
Akt 1, 2	Human cell lines *in vitro* and implantation into mice	Synthetic siRNA, plasmid and viral shRNA vectors
ATF2	Mouse melanoma lines *in vitro* and implantation into mice	Synthetic siRNA
Bcl-2	Human cell lines	Synthetic siRNA
Bcr/Abl	Human cell lines	Synthetic siRNA
Fas receptor	*In vivo*, mouse liver	Synthetic siRNA
FosL1	Human colon cancer cell lines	Synthetic siRNA
HPV E6, E7	Human cervical carcinoma cell lines	Synthetic siRNA
K-Ras	Human cell lines *in vitro* and implantation into mice	shRNA retroviral vector
p53	Human and mouse cell lines, plus primary cells, and transgenic mice	Synthetic siRNA, shRNA plasmid and viral vectors
p73Dn	Human cell lines	Synthetic siRNA
PI3-kinase, p110β	Human cell lines *in vitro* and implantation into mice	Synthetic siRNA, shRNA plasmid and viral vectors
PLK1	Human cell lines and primary cells	Synthetic siRNA
PTEN	Human cell lines *in vitro* and implantation into mice	Synthetic siRNA
TNF-α	*In vivo*, mouse systemic administration	Synthetic siRNA

HPV, human papillomavirus; *PLK1*, polo-like kinase-1 gene; RNAi, RNA interference; shRNA, short hairpin RNA; siRNA, short interfering RNA; TNF, tumor necrosis factor.
[a]References to specific reports can be found within the papers cited in this review.

Another advance in the potential utility of RNAi came with a rapid series of publications that described gene transfer vector delivery of siRNAs.[1–3] Several approaches are possible to direct siRNA production inside cells (Fig. 1.2-2). First, it is possible to express both strands of the siRNA independently in cells using vectors that contain two copies of an RNA Pol III expression cassette (RNA Pol III promoters are particularly well suited to these applications owing to their ability to produce large amounts of small RNAs), one producing the sense strand and the other the antisense strand. After the association of the two strands, Dicer processes the small dsRNA into an siRNA that is then incorporated into the RISC. This method requires two promoters and necessitates that the two-sense and antisense RNAs find each other and associate to form a duplex dsRNA. A more effective strategy relies on the natural ability of Dicer to process the stRNA hairpin structure during the formation of miRNAs. In these approaches, a single RNA Pol III or Pol II promoter is used to drive the synthesis of the sense and the antisense target sequences, which are separated by a spacer sequence, allowing them to form a hairpin stem-loop structure. After Dicer processing of these short hairpin RNAs (shRNAs) to siRNA, effective knockdown target gene expression can be achieved. A variety of viral and nonviral vectors have been used to deliver these hairpin expression

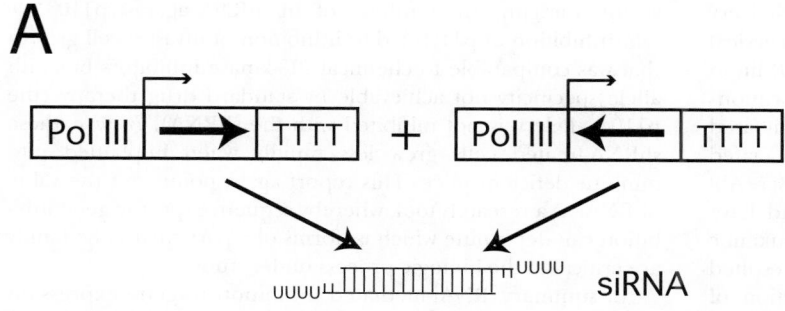

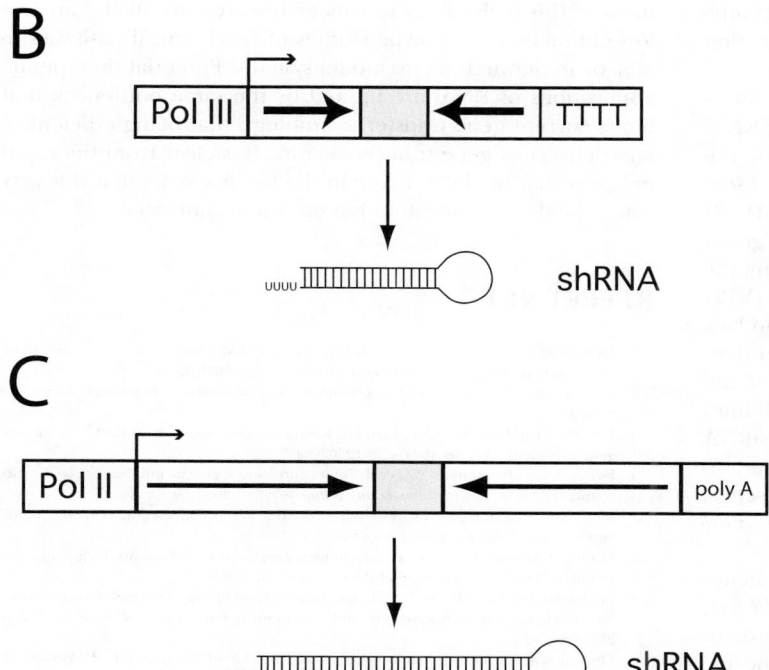

FIGURE 1.2-2. RNA interference expression systems. **A:** In this system, two RNA Pol III expression cassettes are designed to produce sense and antisense RNAs (as indicated by the *arrows*). RNA Pol III transcription is terminated by a run of consecutive Ts in the expression cassette design. The independent RNAs then need to associate, at which time they can be processed by Dicer to a short interfering RNA (siRNA). **B:** Using a single RNA Pol III promoter construct, it is possible to physically join the sense and antisense RNAs (shown by *arrows*) separated by a nonhomologous spacer sequence. These short hairpin transcripts (shRNAs) fold to form a stable stem loop, which is processed by Dicer to the siRNA. **C:** Similar in design to the RNA Pol III expression cassettes, an RNA Pol II promoter can produce a transcript with sense and antisense sequences separated by a spacer region. These transcripts use the poly A termination signal of messenger RNAs. After folding, an shRNA can be processed to siRNA by Dicer. RNA Pol II expression cassettes are generally greater in length than RNA Pol III–expressed transcripts.

cassettes, including adenoviral vectors, oncoretroviral vectors, and lentiviral vectors. In these reports, knockdown of gene expression was durable (measured in months), and in some cases the amount of inhibition was greater than 90%.

CANCER APPLICATIONS

Given that RNAi-like mechanisms may be involved in gene regulation, it has been speculated that defects in RNAi-related enzymes may be involved in transformation and in the development of cancer.[12] At present, there is little direct evidence to suggest this potential, but a region of chromosome 1 that is frequently deleted in Wilms' tumor (1p34-35) contains three Argonaute family genes, which may be involved in formation of RISC. The potential therapeutic applications of RNAi in human cancer come from its use as a research tool and its potential use as a direct cancer therapeutic. RNAi knockdown of gene expression is extremely specific, and this specificity permits allele-specific targeting of nearly any gene. With the completed sequence of the human genome, it is now theoretically possible to use RNAi as a reverse genetic

approach to functionally knock down virtually any gene and observe the resultant phenotype. The power of this large-scale functional genomics approach to gene knockdown is currently in the process of evaluation in *C elegans*, in which all of the approximately 19,000 genes are being targeted using RNAi. Similar strategies could be applied to the human genome using the appropriate high-throughput methods that are currently used for other small-molecule drug screening.

The potential for siRNA to knock down gene expression can be applied at a variety of levels in cancer research. The types of intervention for which this technology might logically be pursued include viral-induced oncogenesis, transformation associated with specific oncogene or tumor suppressor point mutations, and cancers associated with chromosomal translocations. Of the viral-associated malignancies, human papillomavirus–induced cervical cancer is a logical target for the application of RNAi technology. In work by Jiang and Milner,[13] siRNAs were designed to target the E6 and E7 genes of human papillomavirus-16. In cervical carcinoma cell lines, the silencing of E6 by siRNAs resulted in accumulation of p53 protein, activation of p21, and reduction in cell growth, whereas E7 knockdown induced apoptotic cell death. If appropriate delivery methods can be developed, localized cancers such as cervical cancer may be likely targets of siRNA therapeutics. In addition to viral-induced malignancies, cancer-associated translocations and common point mutations are obvious targets to RNAi-based interventions. Chronic myeloid leukemia is often associated with the t(9;22) translocation of the *Bcr* and *Abl* genes. Bcr/Abl fusion transcripts are unique to the leukemic cells and have been targets of siRNA knockdown.[14] Treatment of leukemic cells with siRNA specific for the translocation junction resulted in reduction of Bcr/Abl mRNA, proteins, and induction of apoptosis. In comparison to the tyrosine kinase inhibitor STI 571 (imatinib), siRNA was less effective, but transfection efficiencies in this report were only 80%. Interestingly, the combination of STI 572 and siRNA did not show enhanced induction of apoptosis.

Mutations of protooncogenes and tumor suppressors associated with cell transformation have been an active area of RNAi research. Brummelkamp et al.[15] used an shRNA-expressing retroviral vector to specifically target a mutated form of the *K-Ras* oncogene. An shRNA designed to knock down the *K-Ras* (V12) allele (which differs by one base pair from the wild-type gene) was shown to specifically inhibit the mutated *K-Ras*, leaving the wild-type allele unaffected. Stable inhibition of the *K-Ras* (V12) leads to loss of anchorage-independent growth *in vitro* and lack of tumorigenicity in nude mice *in vivo*. At least six independent groups have reported on RNAi-mediated knockdown of the p53. siRNA knockdown of p53 expression in multiple cell lines was demonstrated by Bergamaschi et al.,[16] and, further, siRNA potentiated the induction of apoptosis in cells exposed to doxorubicin or cisplatin. Using shRNA expression cassettes, stable inhibition of p53 expression has been reported *in vitro* and *in vivo* using retroviral and lentiviral vectors.[2,3]

Other examples using RNAi to target cancer-related genes include silencing Fra1, ATF2, polo-like kinase-1 gene (*PLK1*), and the PI3-kinase pathway. The Fra1 protein (a Fos protein family member) was targeted by Vial et al.[17] using siRNA specific to its gene (*FosL1*). In colon cancer cell lines BE and Hct-116, Fra1 protein was knocked down 90% to 95% 2 days after transfection with siRNAs; this resulted in a significant reduction (less than 80%) in the ability of these cells to migrate in a Matrigel matrix assay, and cell motility decreased tenfold (from 18 μm/h to 1.8 μm/h). *ATF2* is a transcription factor implicated in the progression of melanoma. Bhoumik et al.[18] report that *ATF2* inhibition by siRNA in SW melanoma cells resulted in up-regulation of *c-Jun* expression and the sensitization of these cells to apoptosis induction in response to anisomycin treatment. In several unrelated cancer cell lines, Spankuch-Schmitt et al.[19] demonstrated that the *PLK1* gene was inhibited as much as 95% with siRNA. The siRNA acted as an antiproliferative agent in these cells, as knockdown of *PLK1* resulted in aberrant microtubule function, negatively affecting cell division and inducing apoptosis. As a final example of RNAi applications, Czauderna et al.[20] demonstrated that the phosphatidylinositol PI3-kinase pathway member p110β could be stably knocked down using RNA Pol III

vectors directing the synthesis of an shRNA against p110β. *In vitro* inhibition of p110β led to inhibition of invasive cell growth that was comparable to chemical PI3-kinase inhibitors but with allele specificity not achievable by standard drug therapy (the p110α allele was not inhibited with the shRNA). *In vivo*, these shRNA-treated cells grew less rapidly when implanted into immune-deficient mice. This report again points out the value of RNAi as a research tool, whereby sequence-specific gene inhibition can determine which isoforms of a particular gene family are critical to the biologic process under study.

In summary, RNAi-mediated inhibition of gene expression is a sequence-specific method to knock down the expression of a given gene at the RNA level. At present, the main applications of this technology in cancer research are in the area of loss-of-function phenotype studies of biochemical pathways *in vitro* or in defined *in vivo* model systems. Potential therapeutic applications of RNAi are limited by the same bottleneck that limits current gene transfer technology, that being efficient *in vivo* delivery of gene transfer vectors. It is clear from the rapid progress that has been made in the last few years that this very young field of investigation has enormous potential.

REFERENCES

1. Lieberman J, Song E, Lee SK, et al. Interfering with disease: opportunities and roadblocks to harnessing RNA interference. *Trends Mol Med* 2003;9:397.
2. Paddison PJ, Hannon GJ. RNA interference: the new somatic cell genetics? *Cancer Cell* 2002;2:17.
3. Dykxhoorn DM, Novina CD, Sharp PA. Killing the messenger: short RNAs that silence gene expression. *Nat Rev Mol Cell Biol* 2003;4:457.
4. Fire A, Xu S, Montgomery MK, et al. Potent and specific genetic interference by double-stranded RNA in *Caenorhabditis elegans*. *Nature* 1998;391:806.
5. Jorgensen R. Altered gene expression in plants due to trans interactions between homologous genes. *Trends Biotechnol* 1990;8:340.
6. Denli AM, Hannon GJ. RNAi: an ever-growing puzzle. *Trends Biochem Sci* 2003;28:196.
7. Dennis C. The brave new world of RNA. *Nature* 2002;418:122.
8. Caplen NJ, Parrish S, Imani F, et al. Specific inhibition of gene expression by small double-stranded RNAs in invertebrate and vertebrate systems. *Proc Natl Acad Sci U S A* 2001;98:9742.
9. Elbashir SM, Harborth J, Lendeckel W, et al. Duplexes of 21-nucleotide RNAs mediate RNA interference in cultured mammalian cells. *Nature* 2001;411:494.
10. Lewis DL, Hagstrom JE, Loomis AG, et al. Efficient delivery of siRNA for inhibition of gene expression in postnatal mice. *Nat Genet* 2002;32:107.
11. Song E, Lee SK, Wang J, et al. RNA interference targeting Fas protects mice from fulminant hepatitis. *Nat Med* 2003;9:347.
12. Carmell MA, Xuan Z, Zhang MQ, et al. The Argonaute family: tentacles that reach into RNAi, developmental control, stem cell maintenance, and tumorigenesis. *Genes Dev* 2002;16:2733.
13. Jiang M, Milner J. Selective silencing of viral gene expression in HPV-positive human cervical carcinoma cells treated with siRNA, a primer of RNA interference. *Oncogene* 2002;21:6041.
14. Wilda M, Fuchs U, Wossmann W, et al. Killing of leukemic cells with a BCR/ABL fusion gene by RNA interference (RNAi). *Oncogene* 2002;21:5716.
15. Brummelkamp TR, Bernards R, Agami R. Stable suppression of tumorigenicity by virus-mediated RNA interference. *Cancer Cell* 2002;2:243.
16. Bergamaschi D, Gasco M, Hiller L, et al. p53 polymorphism influences response in cancer chemotherapy via modulation of p73-dependent apoptosis. *Cancer Cell* 2003;3:387.
17. Vial E, Sahai E, Marshall CJ. ERK-MAPK signaling coordinately regulates activity of Rac1 and RhoA for tumor cell motility. *Cancer Cell* 2003;4:67.
18. Bhoumik A, Huang TG, Ivanov V, et al. An ATF2-derived peptide sensitizes melanomas to apoptosis and inhibits their growth and metastasis. *J Clin Invest* 2002;110:643.
19. Spankuch-Schmitt B, Bereiter-Hahn J, Kaufmann M, et al. Effect of RNA silencing of polo-like kinase-1 (PLK1) on apoptosis and spindle formation in human cancer cells. *J Natl Cancer Inst* 2002;94:1863.
20. Czauderna F, Fechtner M, Aygun H, et al. Functional studies of the PI(3)-kinase signaling pathway employing synthetic and expressed siRNA. *Nucleic Acids Res* 2003;31:670.

KEVIN M. BROWN
INGRID A. HEDENFALK
JEFFREY M. TRENT

SECTION **3**

cDNA Arrays

DNA MICROARRAYS AND THE MOLECULAR PROFILING OF HUMAN CANCERS

The seminal publication of a series of papers in the journals *Nature* and *Science* has heralded a new era in medicine.[1,2] The sequence of more than 98% of the three billion nucleotides of the human genome[3] has illustrated that an estimated 34,000 genes are present, and, counting splice variants, the number of functionally distinct proteins is likely to exceed 100,000.[2] We now have access to the "kit of parts" of human biology; however, this is only the first stage in understanding how humans develop and function and what happens to our bodies when disease strikes. The sequence of human genes provides first-order understanding of their corresponding protein products. The genome sequence does not, however, allow an immediate understanding of the physiologic circumstances under which these proteins are produced and function in the cell.

Genes are regulated at multiple levels (transcriptional, posttranscriptional, translational, and posttranslational) to produce the delicate balance of a fully functional organism. Nevertheless, gene-specific transcription is one of the major gene regulatory steps in the cell and is influenced by cell type and differentiation stage, as well as external stimuli. Although it may not be currently understood how all of the circuits regulating gene expression function, defects in these circuits that characterize biologically distinct disease states can be identified by ascertaining the amount of each transcript that is being produced.

Using DNA microarrays to simultaneously evaluate the level of transcription of thousands of genes ("expression profiling") is one means to visualize cellular transcriptional circuitry and has tremendous potential for advancing the understanding of human cancers. The vast majority of human cancers display marked aneuploidy, multiple genetic alterations, and/or genetic instability; this complexity most likely attributes to the diversity in clinical outcome of histopathologically similar cancers. The downstream effects of these complex changes, however, have proven difficult to investigate with traditional gene-by-gene methods. Because many of these genetic changes alter the transcription of specific groups of genes, expression microarrays are an attractive platform for characterizing the changes associated with specific cancers as well as facilitating a global, comprehensive view of the biologic changes attributable to these alterations.

A major focus in cancer research today, now greatly aided by the use of microarrays, lies in identifying genetic markers that can be used for precise diagnosis and as targets for novel therapies and in translating these findings into the clinic. Microarrays can be used to subclassify tumors into homogeneous entities based on gene expression profiles; such subgroups of specific cancers may represent distinct disease states that respond differently to currently used therapies. In addition, genome-wide expression data can help in further characterizing the biology of these "new" subgroups. Finally, microarray experiments can aid in the search for new therapeutic targets and in the identification of novel diagnostic markers. Significant strides have been made toward these goals for several types of malignancies for which large numbers of frozen samples suitable for RNA analysis had been previously assembled. As a result, the use of DNA microarrays is now nearing implementation into clinical practice for several such malignancies, as are promising new therapies whose target was identified through expression profiling.

MICROARRAY TECHNOLOGY

MICROARRAY EXPERIMENT OVERVIEW

Figure 1.3-1 details the general strategy of a microarray experiment. Although various microarray platforms [complementary DNA (cDNA) and oligonucleotide] may use diverse manufacturing, labeling, and analysis methods, the general principle of a microarray experiment remains the same. For each sample to be analyzed, RNA is first extracted. The messenger RNA (mRNA) is subsequently copied in an enzymatic reaction using a reverse transcriptase and labeled nucleotides (usually fluorescent), thereby generating labeled cDNA. This labeled cDNA is subsequently applied to the surface of a microarray, which contains thousands of cDNA or oligonucleotide probes, each derived from the coding sequence of individual human genes and located at a unique location on the array surface. As the cDNA is incubated on the microarray, labeled cDNA molecules hybridize to the microarray spot representing their respective genes. After hybridization, the array is washed and scanned using a fluorescence microscope, and the degree of fluorescence at each microarray spot is quantitated. Thus, a disparity in the abundance of any specific gene transcript between two samples is reflected by differences in the fluorescent intensity at the spot representing that gene on the microarray.

DATA ANALYSIS: CLASSIFICATION OF HUMAN TUMORS

Although new array analysis methods to classify tumors are continuously being developed and are becoming increasingly sophisticated and computationally intensive,[4] two approaches, in general, are commonly used to classify cancers using gene expression profiling data. Unsupervised analyses typically use pattern-recognition algorithms to define groups of samples that have similar global patterns of gene expression. Likewise, such analysis also identifies genes whose expression pattern is similar across a set of samples. Unsupervised analyses minimize *a priori* assumptions about the data and thus identify structure in array data without regard to known clinical parameters. Thus, such analysis is useful for distinguishing subgroups of cancer that differ from each other in the expression of large numbers of genes, presumably unique biologic entities. Indeed, unsupervised analysis of microarray data has successfully separated subgroups of cancer that are known to differ significantly in terms of biology as well as clinical outcome, for example, estrogen receptor–positive (ER+) and –negative (ER–) breast cancers (Fig. 1.3-2A).[5] Despite the fact that the genes selected for this analysis were not chosen in advance on the basis of correlation with any clinical parameter, tumors with a similar phenotypic characteristic (ER status) were largely grouped

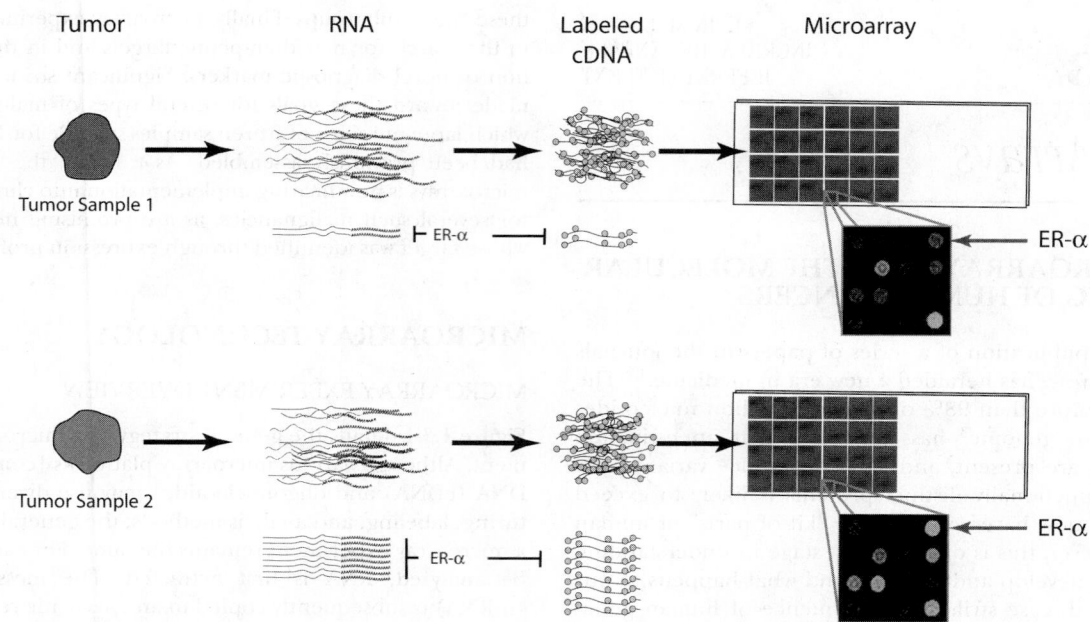

FIGURE 1.3-1. Schematic of a microarray experiment. From each tumor sample to be analyzed, RNA is first extracted. The messenger RNA (mRNA) is enzymatically copied into complementary DNA (cDNA) using labeled nucleotides, and the cDNA is subsequently hybridized to a microarray. During hybridization, cDNA molecules hybridize to the microarray spot representing their respective genes. Thus, differences in the abundance of any given mRNA transcript between two tumors, for example, the estrogen receptor-α (ER-α), are reflected by a disparity in the fluorescent intensities at the spot representing that gene on the microarrays. (See Color Fig. 1.3-1 in the CD-ROM.)

together on the basis of global patterns of gene expression, suggesting that these samples are biologically similar. Likewise, genes with similar patterns of expression, including those that distinguish ER+ and ER– tumors, are grouped, suggesting that these genes may be commonly regulated in an ER-dependent manner.

Although unsupervised analyses are effective at classifying tumors that have similar expression patterns for a large number of genes, such analyses are far less effective at identifying differences in the expression of small numbers of genes that nonetheless correlate with clinical parameters, including response to therapy. Such genes may be useful as markers for the development of differentiating tests that refine our ability to classify tumors and predict response to therapy beyond that achievable using current clinical data or array-based unsupervised classification methods, or both. Identifying these relationships often requires supervised analysis, in which statistical algorithms are used to identify genes whose expression is significantly correlated with a specific clinical parameter such as outcome. The power of these genes may be subsequently validated on an independent set of tumors by clinically classifying these samples based only on the expression levels of these preselected genes alone. For example, Golub et al.[6] used a supervised analysis in their study that provided the proof-in-principle that morphologically indistinct human cancers [acute lymphoblastic leukemia (ALL) and acute myeloid leukemia (AML)] could be distinguished by their gene expression alone. A statistical measure of correlation was first used to identify genes whose expression was most indicative of the ALL versus AML distinction (Fig. 1.3-3). Based on the expression levels of this set of genes, an independent set of ALL and AML samples could be blindly assigned to ALL or AML categories with high accuracy. Of these genes, many are clearly relevant to the ALL versus AML distinc-

tion, with myeloid-specific genes such as *CD33* and *NAZC* expressed at high levels in AML and lymphocyte-specific genes such as *MB1* strongly expressed in ALL. Still, the differential expression of other discriminating genes cannot be readily explained in terms of hematopoietic lineage. Many of these genes, however, have known roles in human cancer and may speak to the biologic differences between these two types of cancer. Because supervised analyses use only those genes that best correlate with specific clinical parameters, they frequently classify tumors according to those parameters better than do unsupervised methods. In the case of breast cancers, for example, ER+ and ER– tumors are better classified when only the genes that best distinguish these two subgroups are considered (see Fig. 1.3-2B).[7]

TOWARD TRANSLATION OF MICROARRAY RESEARCH TO THE CLINIC

Retrospective expression profiling of human cancers has in recent years led to a greater understanding of the heterogeneity underlying numerous types of malignancies, particularly those that are readily resectable and for which frozen biopsies were frequently archived in the past (e.g., leukemias). Several malignancies, in particular, have been quite well studied, leading to improvements in the ability to subclassify clinically heterogeneous cancers and predict patient outcome and, in some cases, to the identification of novel therapies. Presented here is a synopsis of the progress made through microarray expression profiling for three well-studied cancers: ALL; diffuse large B-cell lymphoma (DLBCL); and breast cancer. The advancements made for these cancers are slowly being translated into clinical practice, and for breast cancer in particular, microarray-based diagnostics

A

Clustering of ~5000 significant genes

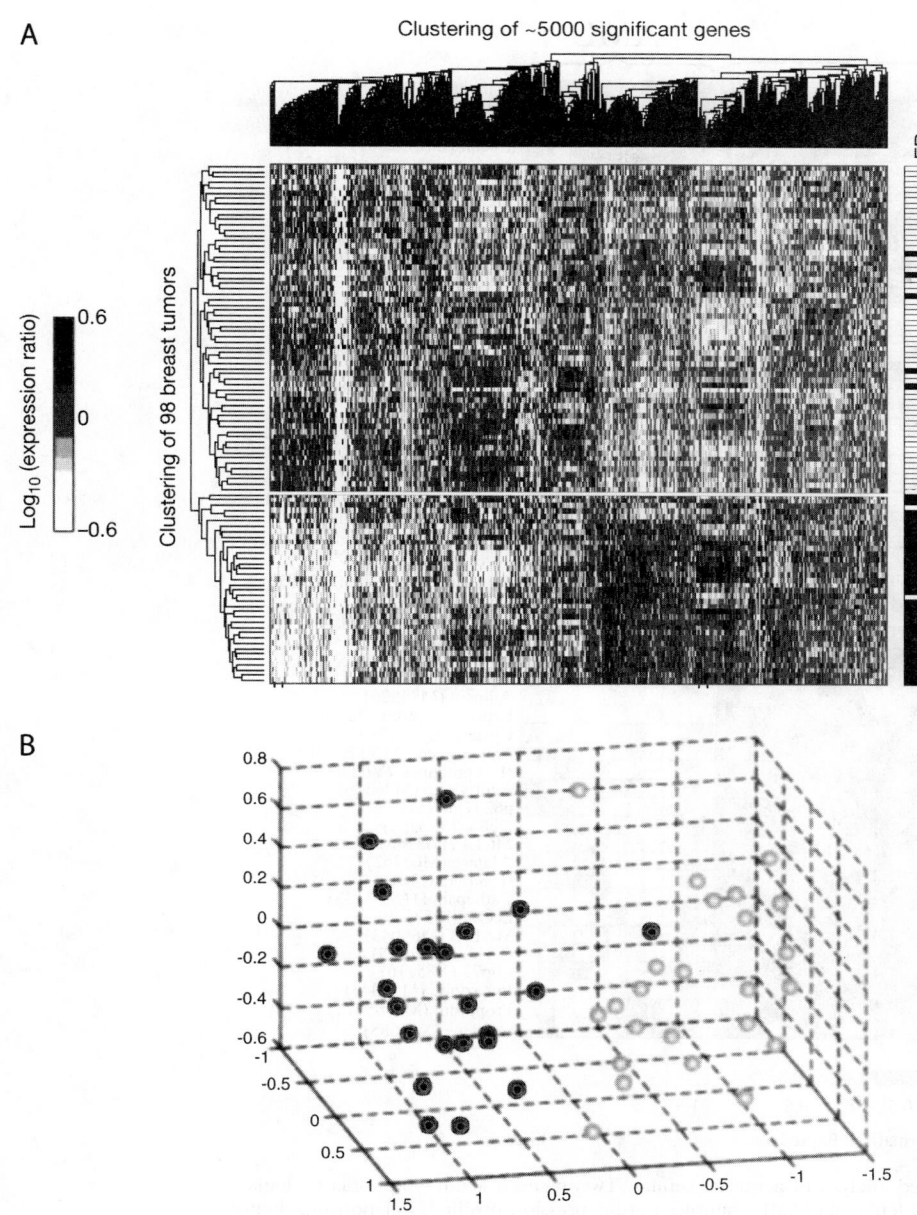

FIGURE 1.3-2. Classification of human breast tumors. **A:** Ninety-eight breast tumors were expression profiled, and the data representing the expression levels of approximately 5000 genes for these samples were organized using an *unsupervised* algorithm (hierarchical clustering). Each column represents one gene in the genome, and each row represents an individual tumor. Each colored block represents the expression of a single gene within the respective tumor; red represents high-level expression of a gene (black on grayscale version), and green represents low-level expression (white on grayscale version). The dendrogram on the horizontal axis reveals the relationship between tumor samples in terms of overall gene expression. Thus, unsupervised clustering reveals large differences in gene expression between most of the estrogen receptor–positive (ER+) and –negative (ER–) tumors. The actual ER status of tumors is listed to the right: ER+ tumors in white and ER– tumors in black. (From van't Veer LJ, Dai H, van de Vijver MJ, et al. Gene expression profiling predicts clinical outcome of breast cancer. *Nature* 2002;415:530, with permission. Copyright 2002 Nature Publishing Group.) **B:** Fifty-eight node-negative breast tumors were expression profiled and classified using a *supervised* methodology. One hundred thirteen genes that best distinguished ER+ and ER– tumors were preselected. The relationship between each tumor in terms of the expression of the 113 discriminator genes is represented via multidimensional scaling. ER+ (blue/dark) and ER– (yellow/light) tumors are represented in three-dimensional euclidean space, in which the distance between any two tumors reflects the degree of correlation in gene expression between the two samples. With the exception of a single ER+ sample, ER+ and ER– tumors are well separated from each other. (From Gruvberger S, Ringner M, Chen Y, et al. Estrogen receptor status in breast cancer is associated with remarkably distinct gene expression patterns. *Cancer Res* 2001;61:5979, with permission. Copyright 2001 AACR.) (See Color Fig. 1.3-2 in the CD-ROM.)

are now being used to identify good-prognosis patients who do not need to receive adjuvant therapy after surgery.[8] Finally, insights into the process of metastasis, revealed by comparative analyses of large microarray-based studies in numerous malignancies, including lung, breast, prostate, and brain cancer, are discussed. Such analyses are beginning to lead to a better understanding of common mechanisms that influence the progression of multiple types of tumors. The work presented here demonstrates the potential of genomic expression analysis to revolutionize the diagnosis and treatment of human cancers.

PEDIATRIC ACUTE LYMPHOBLASTIC LEUKEMIA

ALL is the most common childhood malignancy and the second leading cause of death from childhood cancer in the

United States.[9] It is a heterogeneous disease; numerous clinical parameters have been shown to be associated with risk of relapse, including age of onset, spread of leukemia to the cerebrospinal fluid, and initial response to induction therapy. Additionally, several molecular characteristics of these cancer cells are correlated with disease relapse. Specifically, patients with T-lineage ALL (T-ALL), as defined by immunophenotyping, have a higher risk of relapse than those with B-lineage ALL (B-ALL). For B-ALL, specific recurrent chromosomal abnormalities are frequently observed [t(9;22) (*BCR-ABL*) and the mixed-lineage leukemia gene (*MLL*) rearrangements] and appear to confer poor prognosis, whereas others [t(12;21) (*TEL-AML1*) and hyperdiploid karyotypes] are associated with a favorable outcome.[10] Based on these factors, therapy for ALL patients is already tailored to the individual; intensified therapy for high-risk patients has been shown to result in better survival than standard protocols.[11]

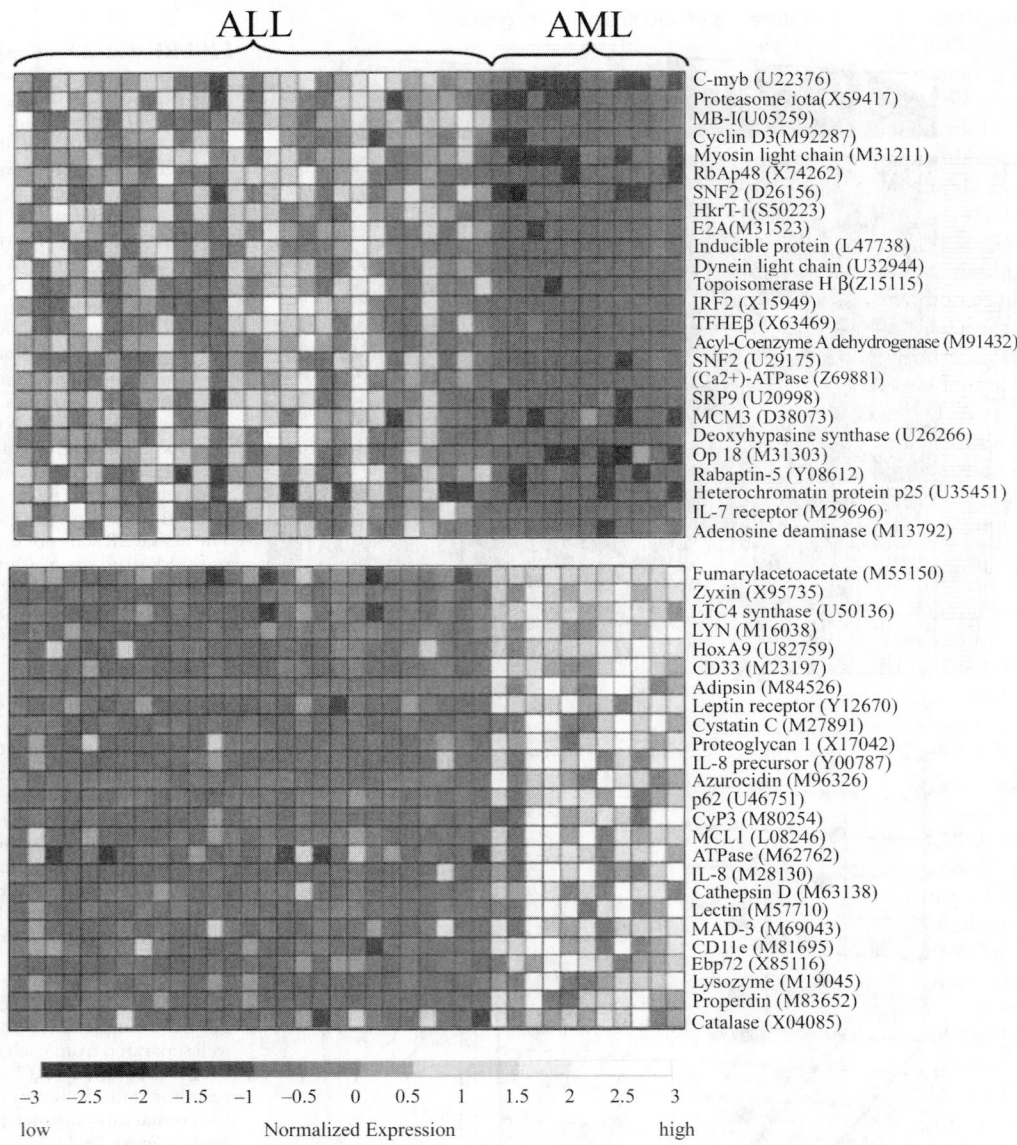

FIGURE 1.3-3. Supervised analysis of acute leukemias. Twenty-seven acute lymphoblastic leukemia (ALL) and 11 acute myeloid leukemia (AML) samples were expression profiled. Relationships between gene expression and the ALL versus AML distinction were revealed by supervised analysis. A statistical analysis revealed the 25 genes whose overexpression, represented by red and pink coloring (light colors on grayscale version), was most significantly associated with ALL specimens (*top*) as well as the 25 genes whose overexpression was most associated with AML (*bottom*). By examining the expression levels of these 50 genes, an independent set of ALL and AML samples could be blindly assigned to ALL and AML categories with high accuracy. (From Golub TR, Slonim DK, Tamayo P, et al. Molecular classification of cancer: class discovery and class prediction by gene expression monitoring. *Science* 1999;286:531, with permission. Copyright 1999 AAAS.) (See Color Fig. 1.3-3 in the CD-ROM.)

Treatment of patients who relapse is significantly more difficult than initial treatment of ALL. For children who experience a relapse involving the bone marrow less than 24 months after their initial diagnosis, prognosis remains poor, with fewer than 10% achieving disease-free survival despite intensive treatment including bone marrow transplantation. Patients who relapse more than 24 months after initial diagnosis have a better prognosis. Still, salvage therapy only results in disease-free survival for about 40% of these children.[12] The propensity of relapsed ALL to be drug resistant, poor efficacy of salvage therapy for relapsed patients, and lack of effective treatment alternatives for relapsed individuals have led many to suggest that the best chance for successful treatment is the identification of patients at high risk for relapse and administration of intensified therapy at the time of initial diagnosis.

Despite current success in classifying ALL patients, 20% of standard-risk patients eventually relapse. This suggests that the heterogeneity of ALL is not adequately explained by the immunophenotypic and cytogenetic subgroups discovered to date and that the current classification system could be further improved. Specifically, some genetic events not detectable by routine cytogenetic analysis may nonetheless act in a functionally similar manner to commonly observed chromosomal abnormalities, thereby influencing survival. Alternatively, uncharacterized genetic events may influence clinical outcome independently of common chromosomal aberrations.

Because bone marrow biopsies from pediatric leukemia patients have routinely been frozen and banked for decades by clinical centers, large numbers of samples suitable for microarray analysis have been available to the research community. To date, numerous studies have been published using global expression profiling with the aim of improving on our ability to diagnose and tailor treatment for ALL patients. Significant strides have been made in terms of improving classification accuracy, and this work is beginning to lead to the identification of novel molecular targets for the treatment of specific ALL subgroups.

DISCOVERY OF DISEASE SUBCLASSES

Gene expression profiling was first shown to be capable of classifying ALL patients by disease immunophenotype by Golub et al.,[6] who first reported that T-ALL could be distinguished from B-ALL on the basis of gene expression patterns. Subsequently, other microarray studies have similarly demonstrated this capability with varying degrees of accuracy.[13–15] Not surprisingly, many of the genes that best distinguish T-ALL from B-ALL are known to be specifically expressed in the respective hematopoietic lineage.

Of importance, B-ALL samples can also be further subclassified accurately according to their cytogenetic subtypes via global gene expression patterns. Intriguingly, although accurate classification of patient samples was best achieved via supervised analysis, most of these subgroups could largely be distinguished from each other by unsupervised analysis, with each group characterized by a distinct molecular signature consisting of a large number of genes. These data support the hypothesis that these leukemia subtypes are biologically distinct entities. Armstrong et al.[16] first demonstrated that B-ALL samples harboring rearrangements of the *MLL* gene could be accurately distinguished from those that did not harbor such changes. In a subsequent large study of 327 diagnostic bone marrow samples from ALL patients, Yeoh et al.[13] significantly expanded on this concept, demonstrating the ability to predict immunophenotype and cytogenetic subgroups [t(9;22)(*BCR-ABL*); t(1;19)(*E2A-PBX*); t(12;21)(*TEL-AML1*); *MLL* gene rearrangements; and hyperdiploidy] with 96% to 100% accuracy. This same research group later reprofiled 132 of these samples on microarrays with a much higher density of oligonucleotide probes representing the majority of genes in the genome and were able to catalog an even larger number of genes that distinguish these groups.[14] Importantly, a small proportion of the B-ALL specimens demonstrated unique molecular signatures quite different from those that distinguish the common cytogenetically defined subgroups; thus, there is likely at least one additional biologically distinct but previously undefined subgroup of ALL that occurs at a relatively low frequency.[13,14]

A microarray-based classification method for diagnosis of ALL is particularly attractive, as a sizable proportion of ALL biopsies do not grow in culture sufficiently well for cytogenetic analysis. Notably, two of these studies identified samples demon-

strating an expression profile indicative of common cytogenetic translocations that were not originally detected at the time of diagnosis; the presence of the translocations in these samples was subsequently confirmed, highlighting the usefulness of an expression-based diagnostic.[13,16] Intriguingly, several samples that did not harbor the t(12;21)(*TEL-AML1*) translocation were nonetheless found to be grouped together with *TEL-AML1*–positive samples. Subsequent analysis revealed unique genetic alterations of *TEL*, suggesting that such changes may be functionally similar to those of t(12;21).[13]

PREDICTING CLINICAL OUTCOME

Ferrando et al.[17] adopted a hypothesis-driven approach to identify novel biologic subgroups of T-ALL via microarray analysis within a cohort of 59 T-ALL patients. Recurrent chromosomal translocations in T-ALL frequently join promoters that are responsible for high expression levels of T-cell–specific genes with transcription factors involved in development (including *HOX11*, *TAL1*, and *LYL1*), resulting in inappropriate expression of these genes. Array analysis revealed that a significant proportion of samples that lacked any such rearrangements nonetheless overexpressed one of these three genes. Strikingly, samples that individually overexpressed one of these three genes coexpressed molecular markers specific for three respective stages of normal thymocyte development. Samples overexpressing *LYL1* coexpressed markers characteristic of normal immature T-cell precursors, and *HOX11* and *TAL1* overexpression coincided with expression of markers of normal early- and late-cortical thymocytes, respectively. In contrast to *HOX11* overexpressing T-ALL cases, those with overexpression of *LYL1* and *TAL1* had a poor outcome. Such correlations have been observed for other cancers, in which distinct molecular subgroups correlating with specific stages of cell development were found to have markedly different outcomes.[18]

In contrast to T-ALL, expression signatures reflecting specific immunophenotypically defined stages of B-cell differentiation have not been observed to date in B-ALL. Instead, Yeoh et al.[13] adopted a supervised approach to predicting relapse in their cohort of B-ALL and T-ALL specimens. Expression profiling did indeed appear to provide sufficient information to predict which patients would relapse and which would go into complete remission. Despite a large sample size, no single-expression patterns were found that predicted relapse for both immunophenotypes of ALL or for all cytogenetically defined subtypes of B-ALL. Instead, unique subsets of genes predicted outcome for T-ALL and each individual cytogenetic subclass of ALL with 97% to 100% accuracy. These data reinforce the hypothesis that cytogenetically defined subgroups of ALL represent biologically and clinically distinct entities. Although the number of relapsed patients represented in this data set is small, these data are nonetheless promising and suggest that larger studies will validate and possibly further refine this microarray-based risk stratification model.

IDENTIFICATION OF NOVEL THERAPIES

Despite an improved ability to predict response to therapy and modulate treatment intensity accordingly, some ALL patients will nonetheless relapse. The ability to predict disease outcome is of little use to these patients unless effective alternative therapies are available to treat their poor-prognosis cancer. Microarray analysis is beginning to lead to protocols for testing these new therapeutic approaches. The expression profiling of a cohort of ALL patients harboring *MLL* gene rearrangements, a subgroup with poor prognosis, identified overexpression of the tyrosine kinase receptor *FLT3* as a key feature of *MLL*-rearranged disease.[16] This finding led to the discovery that approximately 15% of *MLL*-rearranged leukemias harbored activating mutations in *FLT3*. Inhibition of FLT3 signal transduction with the FLT3 inhibitor PKC412 is cytotoxic *in vitro* to B-ALL cells with rearranged *MLL* and high *FLT3*, but not those without *MLL* rearrangements. Likewise, PKC412 was an effective treatment *in vivo* against a murine xenograft model of *MLL*-rearranged ALL.[19] Based on these data, FLT3 inhibitors are now moving into clinical trials for the treatment of relapsed patients with *MLL* rearrangements. Similar approaches targeting tyrosine kinases found to be overexpressed in other cancers are being pursued[20] and may prove to be a useful strategy for other subgroups of ALL as well.

DIFFUSE LARGE B-CELL LYMPHOMA

DLBCL is the most common diagnostic category of non-Hodgkin's lymphoma. It is a clinically heterogeneous disease, and, like ALL, numerous factors have been shown to be associated with outcome, including the age at diagnosis, the presence or absence of systemic symptoms, performance status, serum lactate dehydrogenase concentration, the number of nodal and extranodal sites of disease, tumor size, and the distinction between localized disease and advanced disease.[21] Nonetheless, the currently used International Prognostic Index (IPI) risk stratification model that incorporates these factors is far from perfect.[22] Currently, standard chemotherapy cures only 40% of DLBCL patients. The marked heterogeneity in terms of DLBCL treatment response has suggested to many that DLBCL may be, in fact, a classification comprised of multiple molecularly distinct lymphomas.

DISCOVERY OF DISEASE SUBTYPES

In an attempt to identify novel subgroups of DLBCL and perhaps to relate such subgroups to various stages of normal B-cell development, Alizadeh et al.[18] expression profiled a cohort of 42 DLBCL samples that had been biopsied before chemotherapy, as well as additional human lymphocyte cell samples representing distinct stages of normal lymphocyte development, on custom cDNA microarrays enriched for genes expressed by hematopoietic cells (i.e., the "lymphochip"). Based on the hypothesis that DLBCLs are derived from normal B cells located within germinal centers (GC), the authors examined the expression levels of genes that distinguish normal GC B cells from other stages of B-cell development. Only a subset of DLBCLs expressed these genes (GC B-like DLBCL; GCB), whereas the remaining samples tended to be distinguished instead by expression of genes characteristic of *in vitro*–activated peripheral B cells from blood (activated B-like DLBCL; ABC). More recently, this same research group profiled a much larger cohort of 240 DLBCL biopsies.[23] Classification of these samples using the genes that characterize the GCB and ABC subgroups revealed that not all DLBCLs fit into these two categories (Fig. 1.3-4A). A small but significant proportion of

DLBCL samples (classified as "type 3") do not significantly express any of the genes that define GCB and ABC, suggesting the presence of at least one additional biologically distinct DLBCL subclass.

PREDICTING CLINICAL OUTCOME

The discovery of DLBCL subgroups that express genes specific for different stages of B-cell development is in itself intriguing. More importantly, however, this distinction revealed subgroups with markedly different survival after standard multiagent chemotherapy in both studies (see Fig. 1.3-4B); GCB DLBCL patients have better 5-year survival rates than those with activated B-like or type 3 DLBCL (60% vs. 35% vs. 39%).[23] Incorporation of the GCB and ABC signatures improves risk stratification for patients classified as low risk by the IPI, suggesting that the gene expression data contain additional information associated with outcome not reflected by the IPI alone.[18,23]

Because this biologically based distinction does not completely explain survival in DLBCL patients, Rosenwald et al.[23] sought to further improve accuracy of risk stratification by performing a supervised analysis, identifying additional gene expression markers that are associated with survival after standard multiagent chemotherapy, but whose expression is statistically independent of those genes that define the GCB/ABC/type 3 distinction. This analysis revealed four unique expression patterns, each consisting of coordinately expressed genes whose expression correlated with patient response to chemotherapy. These four expression patterns were significantly different from each other and from those that define the GCB/ABC/type 3 distinction, suggesting that each may contain additional independent survival information that can be used to refine predictors of response to therapy. Notably, each pattern was comprised of genes that share a similar biologic function. Firstly, the expression of a cluster of coordinately regulated genes commonly associated with cell proliferation correlated with poor outcome in DLBCL patients. These data are consistent with previous work indicating that a high cell proliferation rate is associated with poor survival in DLBCL.[24] Secondly, expression of several coordinately expressed genes involved in antigen presentation to T-helper cells by major histocompatibility complex (MHC) class II was observed to be associated with a favorable outcome. Past data have shown that loss of MHC class II antigen expression on the cell surface results in poor treatment outcome, suggesting that antigen presentation by tumors to the immune system may mediate therapeutic response.[25] Also supporting a role for the immune system in response to therapy, a "lymph node" signature, consisting of genes previously observed to characterize cells isolated from normal human lymph nodes,[18] was correlated with good prognosis. This cluster of genes includes markers of macrophages and natural killer cells, suggesting that an innate immune response to lymphoma may work in concert with cytotoxic drugs. Finally, expression of a single additional gene, *BMP6*, also predicted poor outcome. Based on these observations, the GCB/ABC/type 3 signature was combined with *BMP6*, proliferation, MHC class II, and lymph node signatures into an accurate, multivariate risk stratification model to predict outcome. Importantly, when the gene expression and IPI models were considered together, risk stratification was considerably improved.[23]

In contrast to hypothesis-driven class-discovery methods used for DLBCL,[18] another microarray study of 58 diagnostic DLBCL

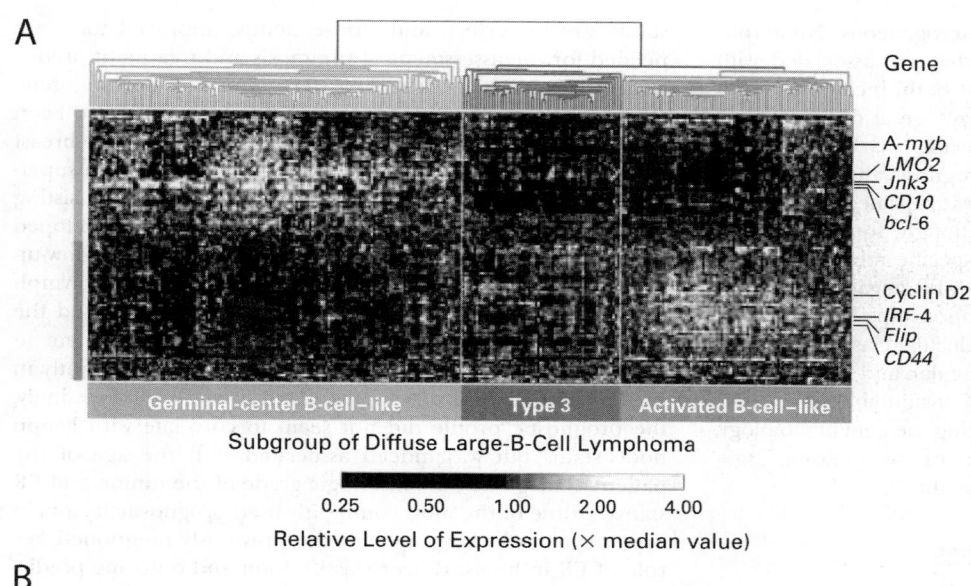

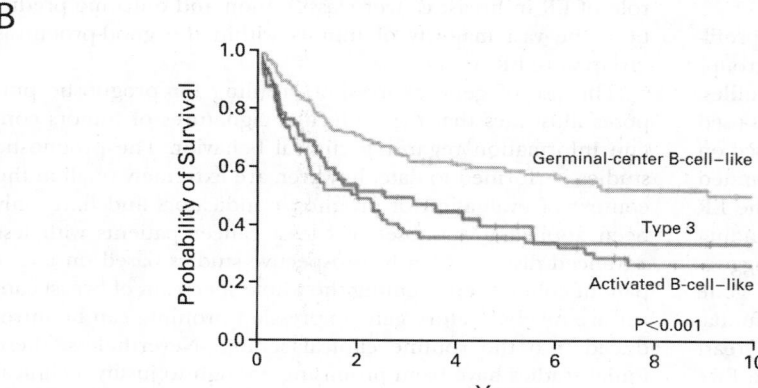

FIGURE 1.3-4. Supervised analysis of diffuse large B-cell lymphomas (DLBCLs) reveals disease subclasses with differences in survival. **A:** Two hundred forty DLBCL biopsies were expression profiled and classified based on the expression of 70 genes previously determined to correlate with activated B-cell–like (ABC) and germinal center B-cell–like (GCB) subclasses of DLBCL.[18] Individual lymphoma samples (columns) were organized into GCB, ABC subclasses, as well as into a novel molecular subclass of lymphomas that do not preferentially express the 70 discriminating genes (type 3). **B:** Kaplan-Meier survival analysis of patients comprising the ABC, GCB, and type 3 subgroups. Patients with GCB DLBCL had a significantly better survival after chemotherapy than those assigned to ABC and type 3 subclasses. (From Rosenwald A, Wright G, Chan WC, et al. The use of molecular profiling to predict survival after chemotherapy for diffuse large-B-cell lymphoma. *N Engl J Med* 2002;346:1937, with permission. Copyright 2002 Massachusetts Medical Society.) (See Color Fig. 1.3-4 in the CD-ROM.)

biopsies adopted a strictly supervised approach to predicting disease outcome.[26] This study identified a relatively small number of genes (n = 13) that could be used to predict patient survival after chemotherapy. Much like the GCB/ABC/type 3 distinction, this 13-gene predictor also improved on the accuracy of the IPI stratification model, particularly for patients in the low, low-intermediate, and high-intermediate IPI groups. The authors subsequently attempted to validate their predictor using the independent data set generated by Alizadeh et al.[18] Although only 3 of the 13 genes were present in this validation data set, all 3 were significantly correlated with outcome. Interestingly, this same data set of 58 DLBCL samples has subsequently been used to successfully validate the cell-of-origin (GCB/ABC/type 3) expression patterns as predictors of clinical outcome.[27] The results from all these studies, although they use different statistical methodology, suggest that gene expression profiling at the time of diagnosis can be successfully used to identify subgroups of patients with a high risk of treatment failure.

IDENTIFICATION OF NOVEL THERAPIES

Analysis of microarray data has uncovered a potential novel therapeutic target for the treatment of activated B-cell–like DLBCL, a welcome advance given the dismal prognosis of this DLBCL subgroup. Activated B-cell–like DLBCLs are characterized by expression of a large group of genes typically expressed by acti-

vated peripheral B cells signaling through the B-cell receptor. B-cell receptor signaling is known to activate the NFκB pathway, a pathway that results in the expression of genes that desensitize cells to stimuli that trigger apoptotic cell death. Given that constitutive activation of antiapoptotic pathways by a cancer could greatly influence the effectiveness of chemotherapeutic agents that trigger cancer cell apoptosis, Davis et al.[28] specifically looked at the expression of NFκB target genes in DLBCL samples. Indeed, a number of genes that are known to be induced by NFκB were preferentially expressed in ABC DLBCL. Subsequent *in vitro* work revealed that in ABC-DLBCLs, but not GCB-DLBCLs, NFκB is constitutively activated, and inhibition of the NFκB pathway is cytotoxic. Based on these data, protocols combining NFκB inhibitors with chemotherapy are now moving into clinical trials for relapsed or refractory DLBCL; expression profiling of pretreatment biopsies from patients entering these trials will be used subsequently to develop a predictor of patient response to this new therapeutic option.

BREAST CANCER

Breast cancer is one of the most common malignancies affecting women in the Western world today, with one million cases diagnosed annually worldwide and the lifetime risk for an individual woman being approximately 10%. Breast cancer is clinically, genetically, and histopathologically heterogeneous. Numerous clinical factors have been identified that are associated with patient survival, response to therapy, or both, including lymph node status, tumor size, tumor histology, age at diagnosis, and cellular proliferation rate. Several molecular markers have also been found to correlate with patient prognosis, the most important of which is expression of the ER, with ER negativity associated with poor patient survival. Although some histologic subgroups are clearly associated with specific molecular markers, for example, comedocarcinoma with ER negativity and with *ERBB2* overexpression, other such relationships are less clear; most commonly used histologic and molecular classifications fail to account for the wide histologic, molecular, and clinical heterogeneity observed in breast cancers. Considerable effort over the last few years has gone into elucidating the genetics, biology, pathology, and clinical outcome of breast cancer using high-throughput gene expression profiling methods.

DISCOVERY OF DISEASE SUBCLASSES

Some of the earliest studies using global gene expression profiling dealt with the classification of breast cancer into subgroups representing breast tumors with similar transcriptional profiles. In a study of invasive ductal breast carcinomas, investigators used unsupervised analyses, identifying five distinct subtypes based on gene expression profiling.[29,30] These analyses largely separated breast tumors into two main groups: those positive for the ER expression (ER+) and those negative for ER (ER–). This finding has since been recapitulated in several other studies,[7,31] suggesting that ER status makes the strongest impact on the gene expression patterns of breast cancers and reinforcing the fundamental role of ER in the development and progression of breast cancer. The unsupervised analyses further subdivided the ER+ and ER– groups into unique subgroups with differences in patient survival.[29,30] ER+ tumors, which are characterized by expression of several molecular markers of normal luminal epithelial cells, can be further divided into two or three smaller "luminal" subgroups. Patients who comprise the luminal subgroup defined by the highest expression levels of luminal/ER-associated genes have a poorer 5-year survival after adjuvant therapy than those with low to moderate expression of these genes.[30] The ER– group was likewise divided into three subgroups, characterized by expression of markers of adipose-enriched normal breast tissues, markers of normal breast basal epithelial cells, or high-level expression of the oncogene *ERBB2*, respectively.[29,30] The suggestion that ductal breast carcinomas can be derived from two distinct cell types (basal or luminal) is intriguing, especially in the light of suggestions of the presence of a breast stem cell, and warrants further investigation.[32,33] The clinical significance of these proposed novel subgroups remains an open question; however, the prognostic heterogeneity suggested in these studies illustrates the need for more targeted treatment regimens for subsets of patients with breast cancer and also demonstrates the potential for gene expression profiling in identifying these subgroups.

PREDICTING CLINICAL OUTCOME

Currently available criteria used to predict disease progression and clinical outcome in breast cancer, including tumor size, age at diagnosis, lymph node status, histologic grade, and ER status, are imperfect, and, consequently, improved tools are needed for the assessment of prognosis and treatment prediction in breast cancer. The first steps toward associating gene expression patterns with survival in breast cancer have been reported. In a study comprised of lymph node–negative breast cancer patients who did not receive adjuvant therapy, a supervised analysis was used to identify a genetic signature consisting of 70 genes that distinguished between patients who developed metastases within 5 years from those who did not.[5] A follow-up study performed by the same investigators, including lymph node–positive and –negative breast cancer patients, used the expression levels of these same 70 genes to assign them to good- and poor-prognosis groups that differed significantly in the rate of metastasis development and survival.[34] Interestingly, the prognostic profile did not seem to correlate with lymph node status but was indeed associated with the age of the patient at diagnosis, the histologic grade of the tumor, and ER status—three of the most commonly used prognostic factors in breast cancer. In keeping with the previously mentioned key role of ER in breast cancer classification and outcome prediction, the vast majority of tumors within the good-prognosis group were ER positive.

The use of gene expression profiling for prognostic purposes illustrates that the molecular signatures of tumors contain information regarding clinical behavior. The prognostic studies performed to date, however, are extremely small in the context of evaluation of prognostic indicators and have only been applied to a subset of breast cancer patients with less advanced disease. Clearly, prospective studies based on larger patient cohorts representing the whole spectrum of breast cancer are needed before gene expression profiling can be introduced into the routine clinical setting. Nevertheless, these initial studies have been promising enough to justify a clinical trial in which this array-based diagnostic will be used to guide decisions as to whether patients will receive adjuvant therapy after surgery.[8] Further studies aimed at elucidating the effect of different treatment regimens on disease outcome, combined with efforts to develop targeted therapies, are needed to identify those patients who are most likely to benefit from available and novel adjuvant treatments.

USE OF MICROARRAYS TO DETECT FAMILIAL PREDISPOSITION GENES

Approximately 5% to 10% of breast cancers are of hereditary origin, and two major breast cancer susceptibility genes have been identified to date, *BRCA1* and *BRCA2*.[35,36] Mutation screening in these two genes for hereditary breast cancer families has become commonplace at oncology clinics across the world, allowing gene carriers to make informed decisions regarding intensive surveillance programs, prophylactic treatments, or both. The techniques used for screening are, however, time consuming, laborious, and expensive, especially because both genes are large and mutations are spread across the entire coding region. Although *BRCA1*-derived breast cancers display certain histopathologic characteristics that may aid in the characterization of *BRCA1* tumors, these tumors do not constitute an entirely uniform group. Moreover, *BRCA2* breast cancers make up a considerably more heterogeneous group. An alternative means of identifying *BRCA1*- or *BRCA2*-associated tumors would greatly facilitate the identification of patients who carry mutations in these genes, particularly those with an unknown family history. Finally, extended knowledge of the defect(s) causing the development of breast cancer may greatly improve treatment schemes and intervention strategies for the affected individuals.

Investigations of gene expression profiles in hereditary breast cancers have illustrated that tumors derived from individuals with *BRCA1* mutations can be distinguished from those with *BRCA2* mutations based on gene expression profiles.[37] This finding could have clinical implications in that it may become possible to perform gene expression profiling analyses based on a set of highly informative genes (a *BRCA1/2* diagnostic gene chip) to determine if a potential mutation carrier belongs to the *BRCA1* or *BRCA2* group. The most intriguing finding in this study was the discovery of a *BRCA1*-like gene expression profile in a tumor from a patient without a germline mutation in the gene. Instead, the promoter of the *BRCA1* gene showed aberrant methylation resulting in silencing of gene expression, and this was found to be the underlying cause of the *BRCA1*-like gene expression profile of the tumor. Because epigenetic events such as promoter methylation can be important in tumorigenesis, this finding points to the use of expression profiling for identifying such events in the absence of germline alterations. It also illustrates the high degree of sensitivity of transcriptional profiling and demonstrates that defects in individual genes give rise to unique and characteristic genetic changes that may, on further investigation, shed light on the functional relationship between specific genetic or epigenetic defects and disease.

Although *BRCA1* and *BRCA2* were initially proposed to be responsible for the majority of inherited breast cancer,[35,36] more recent population-based studies suggest that they account for a far smaller portion of familial breast cancer, with considerable variation between different populations.[38] Presumably, non-*BRCA1/2* (*BRCAx*) hereditary breast tumors may arise as a result of mutations in other high-penetrance genes,[39] or perhaps as a result of low-penetrance alleles (e.g., *CHEK2*).[40] The non-*BRCA1/2* subgroup of breast cancer appears to comprise a histologically heterogeneous group, indicating the presence of multiple underlying alterations. The heterogeneity of cancer-predisposing mutations in *BRCAx* families has severely limited the power of traditional linkage analysis. With no current means to identify subgroups of *BRCAx* families with cancer-predisposing mutations in a common gene, the search for new breast cancer predisposition genes has been confounded. Although in many cases frozen tumor material is unavailable, studies have demonstrated the power of expression profiling for this purpose. Familial *BRCAx* tumors can indeed be subclassified into homogeneous subsets, separate from *BRCA1* and *BRCA2* tumors, based on gene expression patterns.[41] Furthermore, copy-number analysis of genomic DNA from these same tumors using microarray-based comparative genomic hybridization (CGH) revealed that these subgroups were each associated with specific somatic genetic alterations, further supporting the hypothesis that there are multiple distinct subclasses of *BRCAx* tumors.[41] These findings illustrate that gene expression–based profiling can be used to identify distinct and homogeneous subclasses within the non-*BRCA1/2* (*BRCAx*) familial breast cancers, and microarray-based CGH can be used to identify distinct chromosomal aberrations within these subgroups, thereby potentially increasing the power of conventional genetic analysis by enabling the search for novel breast cancer genes within homogeneous subsets of families.[41]

MICROARRAYS, TUMOR AGGRESSIVENESS, AND METASTASIS

In addition to leading to a better understanding of the molecular events involved in tumorigenesis of specific cancers, microarray studies are beginning to reveal clues to genetic influences that affect tumor progression across a broad spectrum of cancers. To date, several microarray studies have attempted to correlate gene expression with aggressive tumor phenotypes. Expression profiling studies have thus identified gene expression signatures associated with tumor cell aggressiveness in melanoma.[42] Among the genes most preferentially expressed by highly invasive melanoma cells, *WNT5A* expression and signaling through the *WNT5A* receptor (*FZD5*) have been shown to have a functional role in mediating the invasive phenotype.[43]

Likewise, expression profiling studies have identified expression signatures associated with the eventual development of metastases in primary breast tumors,[5] as well as signatures correlating with the presence of metastases at the time of diagnosis in childhood medulloblastoma.[20] Most recently, Ramaswamy et al.[44] expression profiled a collection of primary lung adenocarcinomas as well as lung adenocarcinoma metastases and identified a 17-gene molecular signature preferentially expressed by metastases. Strikingly, a small proportion of primary tumors expressed this metastasis signature, leading the authors to hypothesize that these specific primary tumors may have an inherent "metastatic program." In support of this hypothesis, individuals with primary tumors that expressed this metastasis signature had a much poorer outcome than those with a nonmetastatic signature. To determine whether this 17-gene signature held any relevance for other types of cancer, the authors subsequently applied this metastasis predictor to previously published microarray data sets from breast cancer, prostate cancer, medulloblastoma, and lymphoma. Intriguingly, for the three solid tumor types, stratification of patients based on the expression of these genes resulted in groups that differed significantly in clinical outcome, with the metastasis signature associated with poor survival.

The observation of "metastasis signatures" in primary tumors has led many to suggest that the prevailing model of metastasis, in which only rare cells in a tumor acquire the metastatic phenotype, may need to be reconsidered.[44,45] Because of limitations in the sensitivity of DNA microarrays, the presence of a metastasis signature in a primary tumor suggests that the proportion of cells in the tumor that have acquired metastatic characteristics must be large; metastasis-specific changes in expression that occur in only a very rare population of cells would not likely be detectable. That a large proportion of cells in a tumor express metastasis marker genes, then, suggests that at least some of the changes that potentiate metastasis may be early changes that also promote noninvasive growth.

This hypothesis is supported by the results of a genetic screen for metastatic potential in *Drosophila*, in which the oncogenic background of a tumor was shown to contribute toward metastasis formation. Although inactivation of specific cell polarity genes promotes the formation of metastases in eye disc tumors initiated by mutations to the *Ras* oncogene, inactivation of these same cell polarity genes did not influence metastasis development in the context of tumor-initiating mutations to the *lats* tumor suppressor gene.[46] It has alternatively been suggested that a patient's inherited genetic background, reflected within the gene expression of their tumor, may contribute to metastatic potential; the genetic background of mice appears to influence the frequency of metastasis in a transgene-induced mouse tumor model.[47] Still, it is a point of contention whether any of these data are truly inconsistent with the prevalent model of metastasis; it has been suggested that although many of the cells may acquire *some* of the characteristics that allow for successful metastasis early during progression, it is still the rare cell that acquires *all* of these characteristics.[48] Nonetheless, these data highlight the fact that early genetic events critical for early tumor progression may also influence the later potential of a tumor to metastasize.

ARE DNA MICROARRAYS READY FOR ROUTINE CLINICAL MANAGEMENT OF PATIENTS WITH CANCER?

The accuracy of some standard diagnostic assays currently used for tumor classification is subject to variability between institutions. For example, cytogenetic analyses rely heavily on the individual skill level of the technician. Widespread interobserver variation also exists for immunohistochemistry, where discordance rates in the scoring of tumors for single antigens are as high as 25% between pathologists,[49] and similar variability has been reported in the morphologic classification of tumors.[50] Clinicians frequently rely on several such assays to make informed decisions regarding therapy for some cancers. A single, standardized assay capable not only of replacing all of these tests, but providing more accurate prognostic information, would clearly be an attractive option in the clinic. Given the promising results for gene expression–based prediction of breast cancer outcome, microarray diagnostics are indeed moving into the clinic to guide decisions as to whether or not patients need to receive adjuvant therapy after surgery.[8] As such gene expression–based tests are translated to the clinical setting, several issues relating to the accuracy of such predictors need to be considered.

INTRABIOPSY HETEROGENEITY

The issues of sample heterogeneity and the impact of "contaminating" normal cell types are frequently raised in the context of global gene expression profiling of tumors and represent an important issue for the translation of expression-based risk stratification methods to the clinic. In considering the use of array-based diagnostics for clinical implementation, the consequences of such heterogeneity to prediction accuracy need to be defined. For example, biopsies frequently vary in the content of genetically normal, noncancerous cells including lymphocytes and stromal cells. Because heterogeneity may confound the biologic interpretation of expression profiling experiments, many have recommended the use of techniques that are capable of enriching tumor cells, including microdissection or flow-sorting, before expression profiling to ensure that only malignant cells are being profiled. The need for such techniques in the clinic

would clearly complicate array-based diagnostics and in some cases reintroduce variability attributable to the individual skill of the practitioner. In fact, cell enrichment may not be warranted in many cancers. Tumor samples from the same tumor or patient, as well as microdissected and grossly dissected samples from the same tumor, have been found to be more highly related to each other on a global gene expression level than to tumors from other individuals, despite treatment or tumor evolution between samplings.[29,41,51,52] Moreover, the contribution to the gene expression profile from specific cell types other than the cancer cells can be used for the *in silico* identification of each cellular component of a tumor. Because genetically normal cells such as lymphocytes, stromal cells, macrophages, and fibroblasts may significantly influence tumor behavior, information regarding the contribution of additional cell types toward global gene expression of a tumor may, in fact, provide useful prognostic information. Indeed, such expression signatures, for example, the lymph node signature in DLBCL, have been shown to be associated with disease outcome.[23] Thus, this approach has the potential to reveal the complex network of cellular and molecular interactions that drive tumor growth or to reveal tumor-host interactions that mediate response to cancer therapies.

The inherent genetic heterogeneity of tumors may also potentially confound array-based diagnostics. Such heterogeneity is clearly observed, for instance, in the expression of molecular markers of metastasis in medulloblastoma, which are often not expressed by the entire tumor.[20] Theoretically, expression profiles from different regions of a tumor may vary, and thus the expression profiles derived from small biopsies of a tumor may not always completely reflect the biologic characteristics of the tumor as a whole. Nonetheless, a tissue microarray analysis has suggested that heterogeneity may not negatively impact predictive power for many markers, as analysis of single breast tumor tissue cores for ER, progesterone-receptor, and p53 protein expression yielded nearly as much prognostic information as multiple tumor samplings.[53] Similar analyses for newly identified molecular markers will be critical for evaluating the effect of tumor heterogeneity on classification accuracy.

LARGE-SCALE CLINICAL TRIALS TO VALIDATE PREDICTORS

Larger clinical trials validating the accuracy of expression profiling as a prognostic tool are clearly warranted. Even in studies of large patient cohorts, some biologically distinct groups of patients may be represented in only small numbers. Robust classifiers that work well for predicting outcome in well-represented patient populations may not, in fact, work well in underrepresented groups. For example, in the breast cancer classifier developed by van't Veer et al.,[5] the prognostic profile developed was associated with, among other parameters, ER status. Consistent with the key role of ER in breast cancer outcome, the vast majority of tumors examined within the good-prognosis group were ER+. Thus, it is not altogether clear how well this predictor will work with a larger cohort of ER– samples. Because the etiology of cancer is complex and in many cases influenced by environmental exposures and genetic background, future studies aimed at validating outcome predictors for various cancers will also need to address accuracy across diverse ethnic or geographic populations, or both. Clearly, prospective microarray studies based on larger patient cohorts representing the whole spectrum of any given cancer are needed to refine prognostic models that are truly ready for routine clinical use.

NEW THERAPIES FOR HIGH-RISK PATIENTS

For many cancers, the ability to better predict outcome may immediately improve patient survival; high-risk patients may receive intensified therapy at the time of diagnosis, whereas groups of low-risk patients who do not require such therapy to be cured may be spared treatment-related risks. However, for many diseases that lack effective alternative therapies for high-risk subgroups, such prognostics are of little immediate value to the patient. Identification of therapeutic targets for the treatment of these subgroups is of critical importance. In the short term, many of the genes that define high-risk subgroups may prove to be viable targets for drugs that are currently in development or already in clinical trials for other types of cancer. Overexpressed kinases that already have pharmacologically characterized inhibitors are currently particularly attractive targets, for example, *FLT3* in ALL.[19]

Still, the development of new therapies based on microarray data has been a slow process, on the whole, for several reasons. Effective therapies against many potentially attractive therapeutic targets identified via microarray experiments, for example, DNA-binding transcription factors, are lacking. The development of agents that effectively target these molecular markers is required for the potential of these therapeutic targets to be realized. Still other genes whose expression defines a high-risk cancer subgroup may not themselves be attractive therapeutic targets at all, as altering the expression or function of these genes alone may not dramatically impact the tumorigenic process. The altered expression of such genes may instead be a downstream readout of more important upstream oncogenic events critical to tumorigenesis, for example, the preferential expression of NFκB target genes reflecting constitutive NFκB activation in activated B cell–like DLBCL.[28] Numerous bioinformatic tools that may recognize gene expression patterns attributable to such "hidden" oncogenic events are currently in development. These tools, however, will be much improved in the future with the continued generation of basic research data characterizing cellular transcriptional responses to various oncogenic stimuli, particularly in controlled *in vitro* systems. Finally, when a new druggable therapeutic target is identified, a tremendous amount of validation work may be required, in *in vitro* and in animal models, before any such novel therapies are moved into human clinical trials. Thus, the larger impact of microarray technology on clinical practice may be felt more in the long term.

LOW-DENSITY VERSUS HIGH-DENSITY MICROARRAYS

Many have proposed that, as gene expression–based diagnostics move into the clinic, the process of expression profiling can and should be simplified for routine clinical practice. Because many cancer subclasses are predictable using even a small handful of genes, the arrays needed for clinical diagnosis can be greatly reduced in complexity. Still, high-density microarrays will be indispensable tools to characterize expression correlates of patient response to new therapies. For example, cytokine therapy with high-dose interleukin-2 (IL-2) has been shown to be an effective therapy for a minority of patients with metastatic melanoma for whom standard therapy failed.[54] High-density microarrays have identified an expression signature that correlated with lasting clinical remission in patients with metastatic melanoma who were treated using various immunotherapy protocols (most including systemic IL-2), suggesting that expression profiling may eventually be used to identify patients likely to respond to high-dose IL-2.[55] These data highlight the potential benefit of incorporating genome-scale expression analysis into clinical trials; high-density arrays will be needed more than ever in the "discovery" mode to constantly evaluate the genes whose expression defines patient response to a diverse array of treatment protocols.

In the long term, as extremely robust, validated expression-based predictors of response to a wide variety of therapies are developed, simplified microarrays will undoubtedly be used in the clinic. Importantly, work is under way to create integrated diagnostic systems that automate the entire process of expression profiling and data analysis into a simple and inexpensive device, assaying a limited number of genes (Fig. 1.3-5). Similar automated devices integrating amplification, hybridization, and washing steps have already been created for polymerase chain reaction–based hybridization assays for the detection of bacterial DNA.[56] Such devices are clearly attractive for clinical use, as their accuracy will not rely on the skill level of its operator.

INTEGRATION OF DATA FROM OTHER GENOMIC TECHNOLOGIES

A number of other relatively new genomic technologies are emerging that stand poised to contribute significantly to the goal of improving cancer diagnosis and survival. Importantly, these methods may provide unique prognostic and biologic insight into the pathogenesis of human cancers that cannot be derived from expression microarray data. Specifically, somatic changes associated with specific cancers may dramatically influence tumor phenotype. As mentioned earlier in Use of Microarrays to Detect Familial Predisposition Genes, array-based CGH for identifying DNA copy number changes in individual genes may provide a useful tool for cancer classification and prediction of response to therapy. Array CGH can be used in conjunction with expression arrays to quantitate the impact of genomic changes on gene expression.[41] Likewise, mutation detection methods have already proved to be useful, revealing common mechanisms of tumor progression. In some cases, such as activating *KIT* mutations in gastrointestinal stromal tumors,[57] the discovery of such mutations has led to the implementation of new therapies.

Inherited differences in an individual's genetic background may also dramatically influence tumor growth and metastasis, as well as response to therapy (drug metabolism by the body). Such differences may not be substantially reflected in tumor gene expression levels but could nonetheless have a dramatic effect on treatment outcome. Thus, large-scale efforts to identify single-nucleotide polymorphisms that are responsible for, or associated with, such differences will doubtless be important; such information would greatly complement gene expression–based diagnostics.

Lastly, proteomic methods have tremendous potential to detect differences between tumors in regard to the complement of proteins expressed by a cell, as well as their respective

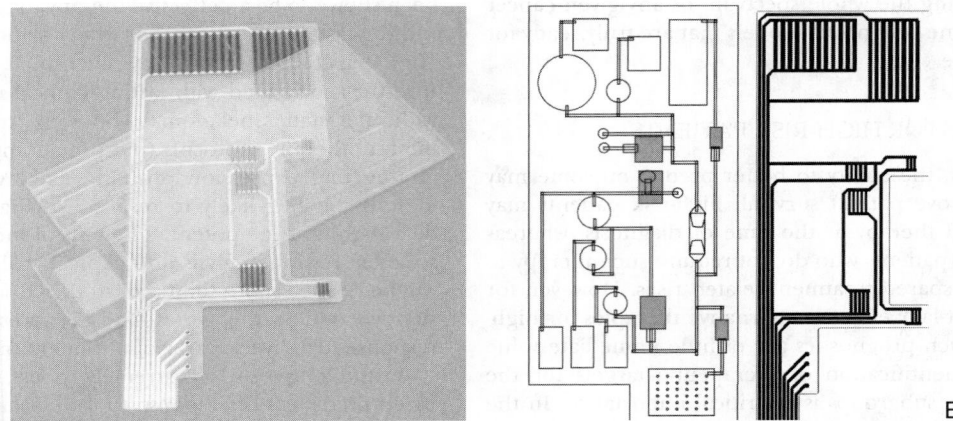

FIGURE 1.3-5. An integrated, automated expression-based diagnostic system: "Lab-on-a-Chip." **A:** Photograph of a prototype Lab-on-a-Chip for gene expression–based classification of human cancers. The device integrates enzymatic labeling of RNA, hybridization, and washing steps into a single automated device made of inexpensive polycarbonate plastic (opaque). Reagent and sample pumping, as well as incubations, are controlled using a reusable circuit board (yellow) with integrated Peltier devices. **B:** Schematic of prototype Lab-on-a-Chip polycarbonate microarray (*left*) and circuit board with Peltier devices (*right*). (Figure courtesy of Dr. Frederic Zenhausern, Center for Applied NanoBioscience, Arizona State University, Tempe, AZ.) (See Color Fig. 1.3-5 in the CD-ROM.)

states of posttranslational modification. Protein spectra of individual tumors can be used in a similar manner to microarrays for the classification of tumors and identification of molecular therapeutic targets. Furthermore, the tremendous sensitivity associated with some proteomic methods also makes them ideal for the identification of serum markers for the detection of residual disease, circulating metastases, or the early detection of cancers.[58]

CONCLUDING REMARKS

As a result of the power of DNA microarray analysis, the future will likely continue to bring substantial changes to the molecular and pathologic classification of tumors. Although progress has certainly been made in the study of many cancers, gene expression in numerous malignancies remains minimally studied on a genome-wide level. Tissue access remains perhaps the largest hurdle for the study of most of these cancers. For many cancers, tumor tissue is not easily resected or biopsied, precluding the assembly of large sample sets for expression profiling. For other tumors, biopsies are small, and many institutions or researchers are understandably reluctant to part with such precious tissue, some or all of which may be consumed by a single microarray experiment. Ongoing advances in RNA amplification and microarray labeling methods promise to greatly reduce the amount of tissue needed for reliable genome-scale expression analysis down to perhaps 100 cells. Last, although many individual clinicians and clinical institutions have begun to archive frozen specimens regularly with the goal of amassing sample sets large enough for genomic analysis, a single institution may not amass a cohort of specimens large enough to sample a genetically heterogeneous tumor type adequately, even after years of prospective collection. Efforts are under way to address this concern, including a National Biospecimen Network. Although no consensus on a specimen acquisition platform has yet been reached, the National Biospecimen Network

would serve to collect well-annotated tissue specimens and distribute these resources to the research community.

The pooling of resources from multiple clinical institutions is clearly required to accelerate the discovery process for cancer research. The pace of tissue accrual would be quickened by the regular archiving of frozen tissues by all clinical institutions, not just those with genomic research programs. Clinicians at these institutions could be benefited by entering into collaborations with genomics research groups that are actively amassing large, multi-institutional sample sets for microarray study; indeed, many of the large sample sets published to date represent such multi-institutional collaborations. Alternatively, such institutions could also benefit the research community as a whole by submission of well-annotated, frozen specimens to cooperative tissue banks that distribute these samples to the research community (e.g., the Cooperative Human Tissue Network at the National Cancer Institute). Finally, such samples could also be submitted to large molecular profiling organizations that expression profile cancers and publicly disseminate expression profiling data free of charge (e.g., International Genomics Consortium: http://www.intgen.org).

Continuing efforts to study the gene expression of cancers on a genome-wide scale will ultimately result in advances in patient treatment. Past microarray studies have demonstrated that gene expression profiles are capable of confirming the major histopathologic distinctions described in cancer, as well as further defining phenotypically indistinguishable tumor subsets as biologically distinguishable entities. These novel subsets sometimes harbor subtle molecular changes that appear to have a significant impact on prognosis and response to therapy. Indeed, the variability in clinical behavior reflects the heterogeneity of tumors, and it appears likely that the introduction of transcriptional profiling technologies into the clinical setting will make possible the individualization of treatments and greatly improve the efficacy of anticancer therapy. Moreover, large-scale expression analysis will likely become increasingly useful in the search for novel therapeutic targets, as well as in the establishment of new prognostic markers for disease. The initial studies in this exciting field of genetic cancer research await confirmation in independent analyses, but it appears likely that molecular profiling using disease-specific microarrays will regularly be incorporated into clinical practice within the not-too-distant future.

REFERENCES

1. Venter JC, Adams MD, Myers EW, et al. The sequence of the human genome. *Science* 2001;291:1304.
2. Lander ES, Linton LM, Birren B, et al. Initial sequencing and analysis of the human genome. *Nature* 2001;409:860.
3. International Consortium Completes Human Genome Project. National Human Genome Research Institute, National Institutes of Health, 2003.
4. Kim S, Dougherty ER, Shmulevich L, et al. Identification of combination gene sets for glioma classification. *Mol Cancer Ther* 2002;1:1229.
5. van't Veer LJ, Dai H, van de Vijver MJ, et al. Gene expression profiling predicts clinical outcome of breast cancer. *Nature* 2002;415:530.
6. Golub TR, Slonim DK, Tamayo P, et al. Molecular classification of cancer: class discovery and class prediction by gene expression monitoring. *Science* 1999;286:531.
7. Gruvberger S, Ringner M, Chen Y, et al. Estrogen receptor status in breast cancer is associated with remarkably distinct gene expression patterns. *Cancer Res* 2001;61:5979.
8. Schubert CM. Microarray to be used as routine clinical screen. *Nat Med* 2003;9:9.
9. Ries LAG, Smith MA, Gurney JG, et al. Cancer Incidence and Survival among Children and Adolescents: United States SEER Program 1975–1995. Bethesda: National Cancer Institute, SEER Program, NIH, 1999.
10. Ferrando AA, Look AT. Clinical implications of recurring chromosomal and associated molecular abnormalities in acute lymphoblastic leukemia. *Semin Hematol* 2000;37:381.
11. Nachman JB, Sather HN, Sensel MG, et al. Augmented post-induction therapy for children with high-risk acute lymphoblastic leukemia and a slow response to initial therapy. *N Engl J Med* 1998;338:663.
12. Gaynon, PS, Qu RP, Chappell RJ, et al. Survival after relapse in childhood acute lymphoblastic leukemia: impact of site and time to first relapse—the Children's Cancer Group Experience. *Cancer* 1998;82:1387.
13. Yeoh EJ, Ross ME, Shurtleff SA, et al. Classification, subtype discovery, and prediction of outcome in pediatric acute lymphoblastic leukemia by gene expression profiling. *Cancer Cell* 2002;1:133.
14. Ross ME, Zhou X, Song G, et al. Classification of pediatric acute lymphoblastic leukemia by gene expression profiling. *Blood* 2003;102(8):2951.
15. Moos PJ, Raetz EA, Carlson MA, et al. Identification of gene expression profiles that segregate patients with childhood leukemia. *Clin Cancer Res* 2002;8(10):3118.
16. Armstrong SA, Staunton JE, Silverman LB, et al. MLL translocations specify a distinct gene expression profile that distinguishes a unique leukemia. *Nat Genet* 2002;30(1):41.
17. Ferrando AA, Neuberg DS, Staunton J, et al. Gene expression signatures define novel oncogenic pathways in T cell acute lymphoblastic leukemia. *Cancer Cell* 2002;1:75.
18. Alizadeh AA, Eisen MB, Davis RE, et al. Distinct types of diffuse large B-cell lymphoma identified by gene expression profiling. *Nature* 2000;403:503.
19. Armstrong SA, Kung AL, Mabon ME, et al. Inhibition of FLT3 in MLL. Validation of a therapeutic target identified by gene expression based classification. *Cancer Cell* 2003;3:173.
20. MacDonald TJ, Brown KM, LaFleur B, et al. Expression profiling of medulloblastoma: PDGFRA and the RAS/MAPK pathway as therapeutic targets for metastatic disease. *Nat Genet* 2001;29:143.
21. The International Non-Hodgkin's Lymphoma Prognostic Factors Project. A predictive model for aggressive non-Hodgkin's lymphoma. *N Engl J Med* 1993;329:987.
22. Shipp MA, Abeloff MD, Antman KH, et al. International Consensus Conference on High-Dose Therapy with Hematopoietic Stem Cell Transplantation in Aggressive Non-Hodgkin's Lymphomas: report of the jury. *J Clin Oncol* 1999;17:423.
23. Rosenwald A, Wright G, Chan WC, et al. The use of molecular profiling to predict survival after chemotherapy for diffuse large-B-cell lymphoma. *N Engl J Med* 2002;346:1937.
24. Silvestrini R, Costa A, Boracchi P, et al. Cell proliferation as a long-term prognostic factor in diffuse large-cell lymphomas. *Int J Cancer* 1993;54:231.
25. Miller TP, Lippman SM, Spier CM, et al. HLA-DR (Ia) immune phenotype predicts outcome for patients with diffuse large cell lymphoma. *J Clin Invest* 1988;82:370.
26. Shipp MA, Ross KN, Tamayo P, et al. Diffuse large B-cell lymphoma outcome prediction by gene-expression profiling and supervised machine learning. *Nat Med* 2002;8:68.
27. Wright G, Tan B, Rosenwald A, et al. A gene expression-based method to diagnose clinically distinct subgroups of diffuse large B cell lymphoma. *Proc Natl Acad Sci U S A* 2003;100:9991.
28. Davis RE, Brown KD, Siebenlist U, et al. Constitutive nuclear factor kappaB activity is required for survival of activated B cell-like diffuse large B cell lymphoma cells. *J Exp Med* 2001;194:1861.
29. Perou CM, Sorlie T, Eisen MB, et al. Molecular portraits of human breast tumours. *Nature* 2000;406:747.
30. Sorlie T, Perou CM, Tibshirani R, et al. Gene expression patterns of breast carcinomas distinguish tumor subclasses with clinical implications. *Proc Natl Acad Sci U S A* 2001;98:10869.
31. West M, Blanchette C, Dressman H, et al. Predicting the clinical status of human breast cancer by using gene expression profiles. *Proc Natl Acad Sci U S A* 2001;98:11462.
32. Kordon EC, Smith GH. An entire functional mammary gland may comprise the progeny from a single cell. *Development* 1998;125:1921.
33. Gudjonsson T, Villadsen R, Nielsen HL, et al. Isolation, immortalization, and characterization of a human breast epithelial cell line with stem cell properties. *Genes Dev* 2002;16:693.
34. van de Vijver MJ, He YD, van't Veer LJ, et al. A gene-expression signature as a predictor of survival in breast cancer. *N Engl J Med* 2002;347:1999.
35. Wooster R, Bignell G, Lancaster J, et al. Identification of the breast cancer susceptibility gene BRCA2. *Nature* 1995;378:789.
36. Miki Y, Swensen J, Shattuck-Eidens D, et al. A strong candidate for the breast and ovarian cancer susceptibility gene BRCA1. *Science* 1994;266:66.
37. Hedenfalk I, Duggan D, Chen Y, et al. Gene-expression profiles in hereditary breast cancer. *N Engl J Med* 2001;344:539.
38. Szabo CI, King MC. Population genetics of BRCA1 and BRCA2. *Am J Hum Genet* 1997;60:1013.
39. Kainu T, Juo SH, Desper R, et al. Somatic deletions in hereditary breast cancers implicate 13q21 as a putative novel breast cancer susceptibility locus. *Proc Natl Acad Sci U S A* 2000;97:9603.
40. Meijers-Heijboer H, Van Den Ouweland A, Klijn J, et al. Low-penetrance susceptibility to breast cancer due to CHEK2(*)1100delC in noncarriers of BRCA1 or BRCA2 mutations. *Nat Genet* 2002;31:55.
41. Hedenfalk I, Ringner M, Ben-Dor A, et al. Molecular classification of familial non-BRCA1/BRCA2 breast cancer. *Proc Natl Acad Sci U S A* 2003;100:2532.
42. Bittner M, Meltzer P, Chen Y, et al. Molecular classification of cutaneous malignant melanoma by gene expression profiling. *Nature* 2000;406:536.
43. Weeraratna AT, Jiang Y, Hostetter G, et al. Wnt5a signaling directly affects cell motility and invasion of metastatic melanoma. *Cancer Cell* 2002;1:279.
44. Ramaswamy S, Ross KN, Lander ES, et al. A molecular signature of metastasis in primary solid tumors. *Nat Genet* 2003;33:49.
45. Bernards R, Weinberg RA. A progression puzzle. *Nature* 2002;418:823.
46. Pagliarini RA, Xu T. A genetic screen in Drosophila for metastatic behavior. *Science* 2003;302:1227.
47. Hunter K, Welch DR, Liu ET. Genetic background is an important determinant of metastatic potential. *Nat Genet* 2003;34:23.
48. Fidler IJ, Kripke ML. Genomic analysis of primary tumors does not address the prevalence of metastatic cells in the population. *Nat Genet* 2003;34:23.
49. Chebil G, Bendahl PO, Ferno M. Estrogen and progesterone receptor assay in paraffin-embedded breast cancer—reproducibility of assessment. *Acta Oncol* 2003;42:43.
50. Terry MB, Neugut AI, Bostick RM, et al. Reliability in the classification of advanced colorectal adenomas. *Cancer Epidemiol Biomarkers Prev* 2002;11:660.
51. Sgroi DC, Teng S, Robinson G, et al. In vivo gene expression profile analysis of human breast cancer progression. *Cancer Res* 1999;59:5656.
52. Sotiriou C, Khanna C, Jazaeri AA, et al. Core biopsies can be used to distinguish differences in expression profiling by cDNA microarrays. *J Mol Diagn* 2002;4:30.
53. Torhorst J, Bucher C, Kononen J, et al. Tissue microarrays for rapid linking of molecular changes to clinical endpoints. *Am J Pathol* 2001;159:2249.
54. Rosenberg SA, Lotze MT, Muul LM, et al. A progress report on the treatment of 157 patients with advanced cancer using lymphokine-activated killer cells and interleukin-2 or high-dose interleukin-2 alone. *N Engl J Med* 1987;316:889.
55. Wang E, Miller LD, Ohnmacht GA, et al. Prospective molecular profiling of melanoma metastases suggests classifiers of immune responsiveness. *Cancer Res* 2002;62:3581.
56. Liu Y, Rauch CB, Stevens RL, et al. DNA amplification and hybridization assays in integrated plastic monolithic devices. *Anal Chem* 2002;74:3063.
57. Hirota S, Isozaki K, Moriyama Y, et al. Gain-of-function mutations of c-kit in human gastrointestinal stromal tumors. *Science* 1998;279:577.
58. Petricoin EF, Ardekani AM, Hitt BA, et al. Use of proteomic patterns in serum to identify ovarian cancer. *Lancet* 2002;359:572.

SECTION **4**

MARISA DOLLED-FILHART
DAVID L. RIMM

Tissue Arrays

A long-standing problem in the analysis of tissue samples is the time-consuming and tedious process of histologic preparation and pathologist-based review of sections. These two critical factors, inherent nonuniformity in preparation and subjectivity of analysis, have historically limited the scientific and statistical rigor of studies involving tissue. Tissue microarrays provide a potential solution to each of these problems. This chapter discusses the mechanism of the solution, including the methods used to create tissue microarrays, the advantages and disadvantages of the technology, analysis methods, and future applications.

The idea of piecing different tissue specimens together into one block was first published by Battifora in 1986.[1] One hundred or more different samples were cut into small pieces with a razor blade and then arranged for paraffin embedding into a multitumor "sausage" block. This was followed by modifications for precise localization of tissue samples by Wan et al.[2] They placed skin biopsy–type cores in spatially fixed positions, resulting in the first true tissue microarray pictures in the literature. Early applications of tissue arrays in breast cancer included the study of Her2-neu expression and amplification in breast cancer by Press et al.[3,4]

In the shadow of the development of massively parallel high-throughput analyses by microarrays, Kononen et al.[5] published an updated version with the description of a new mechanical device dedicated to precise tissue microarray construction. This manual micrometer-driven arraying device can core histologic blocks and place the cores into a recipient array block. These tissue microarrays can contain up to approximately 800 individual 0.6-mm cylindrical tissue cores in a single paraffin "recipient" block that can then be sectioned and analyzed. The resulting sectioned slide allows simultaneous processing and high-throughput analysis of DNA, RNA, and protein expression on hundreds of samples, representing hundreds of patients. In contrast to complementary DNA (cDNA) microarrays, in which hundreds or thousands of genes are evaluated from a single tissue sample or cell line, tissue microarrays allow the examination of a single gene (or gene product) on hundreds or thousands of patients.

TISSUE MICROARRAY CONSTRUCTION

ARRAY CONSTRUCTION

Tissue microarray construction generally begins with the collection of cases with tissue samples that have been fixed and paraffin embedded. For each tissue block, a section is cut and stained with a standard hematoxylin and eosin (H&E) stain. A pathologist reviews the H&E slide to mark the region of the tissue to be included in the array (e.g., by circling the region of interest). The specimen blocks ("donor" tissue) are then organized and arranged in the order in which they will be arrayed into the "recipient" paraffin block according to row and column assignment within the array. Arrays can be designed in many ways, usu-

ally including control spots (either tissue or cell line cell blocks) and redundancy (multiple cores from the same patient).

Once tissue selection and grid organization have been completed, the tissue samples can be arrayed onto a recipient block by using a Beecher Instruments (Sun Prairie, WI) or Chemicon (Temecula, CA) manual arraying device. The overall process is illustrated in Figure 1.4-1. The H&E slide from each selected tissue is used to guide the location of the needle biopsy that will be removed from each sample. The tissue block is placed on the stage of the arraying device, with the H&E slide aligned with the tissue so that an appropriate region can be selected for coring. Before a core biopsy is taken from the tissue block, the H&E slide is removed. The arraying device results in reproducible circular cores of 0.6 mm in diameter and 3 to 5 mm in height (depending on donor tissue thickness) to be removed from the donor tissue and embedded into the recipient block. The 0.6-mm circular spots have an area of 0.282 mm², which is the equivalent of two to three high-power fields, although larger and smaller needles have been used, ranging from 0.2 mm to 2.0 mm. The manual arraying device allows the user to control the location of the punches with an X-Y micrometer coordinate system on the device. Typical spacing of these cores in an array is 0.8 to 1.0 mm between the centers of the spots (0.2 to 0.4 mm from the edge of one spot to the edge of the next spot). As the space between cores is decreased, more cores can be placed into a single block. However, when spaced too closely together, some cores can be damaged in sectioning, which contributes to the loss of tissue cores. A maximum of approximately 800 cores can be placed in a standard-sized single-recipient block. Beecher Instruments also manufactures an automated arraying device. This device allows for the construction of tissue microarrays with up to seven hundred seventy-five 0.6-mm cores in each recipient block. The current device requires imaging the tissue on the block (a few more steps) and has a maximum batch size of only 26 donor blocks. The automated device does not significantly increase either the speed or accuracy of production of a single-tissue microarray master block. However, if two or more master

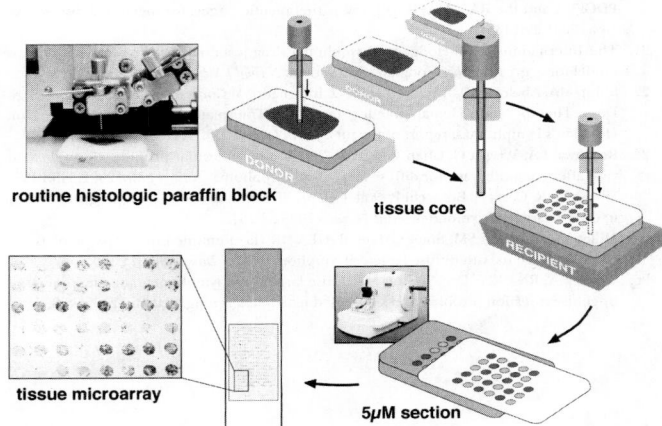

routine histologic paraffin block

tissue core

tissue microarray

5μM section

FIGURE 1.4-1. Overview of tissue microarray construction. Cores are removed from a set of paraffin-embedded tissue "donor" blocks and placed into a "recipient" block. The recipient block is then sliced at a thickness of 5 μm on a microtome and transferred onto a slide, often using a tape-assisted transfer method. A sample of a stained tissue microarray is shown in the inset. (See Color Fig. 1.4-1 in the CD-ROM.)

blocks are desired for each case, the automated device can significantly improve speed and possibly accuracy.

Accurate recording of the tumor specimen and its grid location is critical for future data analysis that is linked to the clinical information from each specimen. It is helpful to use a defined layout that makes the tissue microarrays easier to read by eye. Some methods that have been used include dividing up the tissue into groups,[6] using a red crayon core as a place marker at a standard incremental number of rows or columns or for orientation,[7] or using different normal tissues to identify each row based on morphology.[8] A final consideration in layout is redundancy. It is generally unwise to place samples from the same case in pairs or triplets, because artifacts or mishaps that affect one region of the slide then affect all representations of a single case rather than decrease the redundancy of a few cases. On the other hand, redundancy is common, because it has been shown to increase the likelihood of the core specimens being representative of the entire tumor, as discussed in Tissue Microarray Validation, later in this chapter.

SECTIONING OF TISSUE MICROARRAYS

After the master (recipient) block has been constructed, the tissue microarray needs to be sectioned. A piece of adhesive-coated tape from Instrumedics (Hackensack, NJ) is placed onto the tissue microarray such that the microtome knife can cut a 3- to 5-μm section that is thereby adhered to the tape. The adhesive-coated tape with the tissue microarray section is then transferred by use of a small roller onto a positively charged glass slide that is coated with an ultraviolet cross-linkable adhesive. The slides are then cross-linked under ultraviolet light to adhere the tissue cores strongly onto the slide, and the tape is removed in a degreasing solvent. Many investigators have experimented with other coatings, variable section thickness, and floating sections rather than using tape, but the method above is the most widely used. Slide storage after sectioning is also an issue, because it has been shown that tissue loses antigenicity on sectioning (presumably as a result of oxidation).[9] To minimize this problem, in some laboratories the slide is placed in xylene, coated with paraffin, and stored in an air-tight nitrogen container to prevent tissue oxidation before use of the tissue microarray slides,[7] whereas other laboratories store slides wrapped in parafilm in freezers. Typically, an H&E stain is done on the first section and on later sections (e.g., every tenth section) to assess the morphology through later sections and to assess for the exhaustion of the tissue within the core. Generally, tissue microarray blocks can be sectioned approximately 100 to 150 times before the block becomes exhausted. The high sections (from 150 to 250 or more), although not useful for general analysis, can still be used for titering or other testing, because 30% to 50% of the cases often still have evaluable tissue present.

The use of archived specimens leads to the question of antigen preservation of tissues over many decades of storage, although this issue is not unique to tissue microarrays but rather to retrospective analysis of pathology samples. Using archived tissue allows the generation of large cohorts of patients with long-term follow-up information. Late recurrence information is important to consider in outcome studies using tissue microarrays, which is not possible with short-term follow-up of more recent cases. In addition to the benefit of long-term follow-up and recurrence information, archived tissue allows researchers the ability to study a larger number of rare tumors that may be unlikely to collect

within a short amount of time for a study. Camp et al.[10] found no significant changes in the levels of antigen expression of HER2, Ki-67, PR, and cytokeratin in breast cancer tissue that was archived at different decades from 1932 to the present. Overall, it was found that the antigenicity of breast cancer tissue for protein expression studies was retained by formalin fixation and paraffin-embedded preservation for more than 60 years.

To overcome some of the limitations of RNA preservation in archived tissue, Hoos and Cordon-Cardo[8] developed a cryoarray consisting of frozen tissues embedded in an optimal cutting temperature compound (Sakura Finetek, Torrance, CA). This method uses a specially designed set of 48 pins of 3-mm diameter that is placed in a cryomold, creating a grid of holes framed by the optimal cutting temperature, limiting each array to 48 specimens. The use of an optimal cutting temperature compound for making tissue microarrays from frozen tissue (described with 1-mm cores) has also been described by Schoenberg Fejzo and Slamon[11] for the improved detection of DNA, RNA, and protein.

ADVANTAGES OF TISSUE MICROARRAYS

Tissue microarrays have several significant advantages over conventional tumor tissue block sectioning and staining. The most compelling advantage is tissue amplification. A standard tissue block is generally exhausted after 60 to 80 cuts (depending on the skill of the histotechnologist), resulting in a maximum of 80 assays per tissue block. Taking core biopsies allows for a high number of samples to be taken from a tumor block (approximately 300 to 400 punches for a 1-cm × 1-cm tissue sample) while still maintaining the histologic integrity of the tumor tissue. This exponentially amplifies the amount of experimental work that can be done with each tumor, as each tissue microarray block can be sectioned productively up to 200 times. Thus, instead of 60 to 80 assays, one can obtain 60,000 to 80,000 assays, or 1000-fold amplification. To date, more than 250 papers have reported using tissue microarrays for examination of DNA, RNA, or protein expression in large numbers of tissue specimens.

The second most compelling advantage is reproducibility. Processing specimens in an array results in equal and simultaneous conditions for antigen retrieval and staining reagents. This reduces the inherent slide-to-slide variability that occurs with large cohorts of conventional tissue section processing. In addition, because only one slide contains all of the tumor samples, only small amounts of reagent are necessary for analysis of large cohorts. Other advantages include greater access to automated analysis as described in Tissue Microarray Analysis, later in this chapter; internal controls; and the subtle advantage of limited tissue size. When pathologists judge expression on whole tissue sections, they can be biased by selection of strong- or weak-staining areas. Although some argue that evaluation of a larger tissue specimen is critical, the current standard of care for evaluation of a 1-cm tumor in surgical pathology practice is a single 5-μm section. This represents less than 0.03% of the tissue in a 1-cm^3 tumor. Thus, across a population of tumors, the defined section area of a single tissue spot tends to standardize, rather than misrepresent, expression levels.

TISSUE MICROARRAY VALIDATION

Tissue microarray technology has given rise to numerous criticisms, including, most significantly, the issue of representation.

This issue includes the problem of tumor heterogeneity with respect to protein expression as well as the problem of validity, or the number of cores required to represent a tumor with respect to assessment of outcome.

Multiple groups have examined each of these issues. The first study to address this issue was a high-redundancy array of 38 invasive breast cancer blocks that was constructed with up to ten cores from each of the breast cancer cases.[10] Antibodies to HER2, Ki-67, ER, PR, and cytokeratin were used to test this array by immunohistochemistry and showed that the staining of two microarray cores was comparable to analysis of the whole tissue section in greater than 95% of cases. A similar study by Torhorst et al.[12] of the number of cores needed for tissue representatively in tissue microarrays looked at ER, PR, and p53 staining in breast cancer tissue microarrays. They found that a single core sample from each tumor was sufficient to identify ER staining in 95% of the cases, PR in 75% to 81% of the cases, and p53 in 70% to 74% of the cases compared to whole tissue section analysis. In addition, a single sample of each tumor was also enough to be representative of the association between molecular changes (staining level) and clinical end points (patient survival). The number of interpretable tumors for all three markers of interest increased from 86% using one tissue microarray block to up to 97% using information from each of four replicate arrays, with most tumors showing identical results from all four replicate arrayed samples.

In a study by Nocito et al.,[13] Ki-67 labeling index and histologic grade in bladder cancer tumors were studied by using a set of 2137 bladder cancer tumors and comparing large sections to the tissue microarrays. They found that the information of the whole sections were reproduced on the tissue microarrays for every association between grade, Ki-67 labeling index, tumor stage, prognosis, and clinical information, thereby showing that intratumor heterogeneity did not affect the ability to detect correlations of a clinical or pathologic nature.

More than 20 other studies of this nature have been done in many different tumor tissue types. Several studies have described the construction, validation, and use of tissue microarrays using larger core sizes of 1 to 2 mm in diameter; however, there is no published evidence that these larger cores are more representative. All of these studies together suggest that tissue microarrays, when constructed with care and attention to detail along with appropriate controls, can be an accurate method for a high-throughput analysis of markers with negligible damage to tissue resources.

CONTROLS

The inclusion of control tissue in each array is considered essential, but the type of control and the number are widely variable. Paraffin-embedded specimens of normal tissue can be arrayed as controls in tumor array experiments or analyzed on their own to determine the tissue distribution of normal tissue expression levels.[14] Cell lines,[8] blood,[7] xenografts,[15] synthetic messenger RNA (mRNA) control blocks,[16] and fluid that are prepared as cell blocks can also be embedded in paraffin to serve as controls. Whole arrays of control tissues can be used as well, to test antibody reactivity[2] so that future antibodies can be rated based on comparison of their expression with control arrays. Although there are many ways of adding control cores, tissue microarrays themselves can be used as controls when analyzing clinical specimens. An example of this application is by Packeisen et al.[17] with the construction of a tissue microarray of 12 different tissues with a wide antigen expression profile. This tissue microarray was mounted at the end of slides near the tumor sample, thereby creating an internal positive control for immunohistochemical staining in each assay and serving as a diagnostic quality control method for each individual patient specimen to be analyzed.

TISSUE MICROARRAY VISUALIZATION

Traditional histochemical, immunohistochemical, DNA, and RNA methods can be used on tissue microarrays by chromogen-based methods, radioisotope-based methods, and fluorescence-based methods. Many techniques have been applied and adapted for *in situ* use on tissue microarrays just as they have been used on conventional tissue sections. In addition, precise coupling of DNA, mRNA, and protein extraction (for methods such as Western blotting, etc.) from tissues along with the construction of tissue microarrays from the same exact samples can allow direct sample comparison through different detection methods.[18]

DNA VISUALIZATION

An inherent difficulty exists in using fluorescence *in situ* hybridization (FISH) on formalin-fixed paraffin-embedded tissues. Variations in sample age, fixation time, section thickness, and differences between types of tissue use in the same tissue microarray construction all contribute to the range of uninterpretable spots after FISH hybridizations.[6] FISH has been used in more than 35 tissue microarray studies for successful determination of chromosomal amplification or loss in those samples. An example of FISH for HER2 amplification on tissue microarrays is shown in Figure 1.4-2A. Chromogenic *in situ* hybridization (CISH) was described by Tanner et al.[19] as an alternate method of DNA detection. Their studies show that CISH results are highly concordant with FISH on a 177-case tissue microarray.

RNA VISUALIZATION

Although reliable analysis of mRNA on archival tissue has been questioned[6] due to cross-linking and degradation of mRNA by formalin fixation,[20] several studies have successfully analyzed mRNA expression in formalin-fixed paraffin-embedded tissue despite the limitations using radioactive and chromogenic methods. Kononen et al.[5] used a probe against HER2 mRNA on their breast cancer tissue microarray and found that all HER2-amplified tumors (based on FISH results) overexpressed HER2 mRNA as well as overexpressed the protein (as detected by immunohistochemistry). ISH for mRNA has been done using radioactive and chromogenic methods, but neither method allows visualization of tissue morphology. An example of a chromogen-based method of RNA detection is shown in Figure 1.4-2B. It should be noted that the morphology is substantially degraded by the proteases and other reagents required for the ISH reactions but that general tissue architecture is preserved. It is important to select control genes to screen for mRNA integrity as well as to use positive controls to ensure probe specificity. Finally, another method of assessment

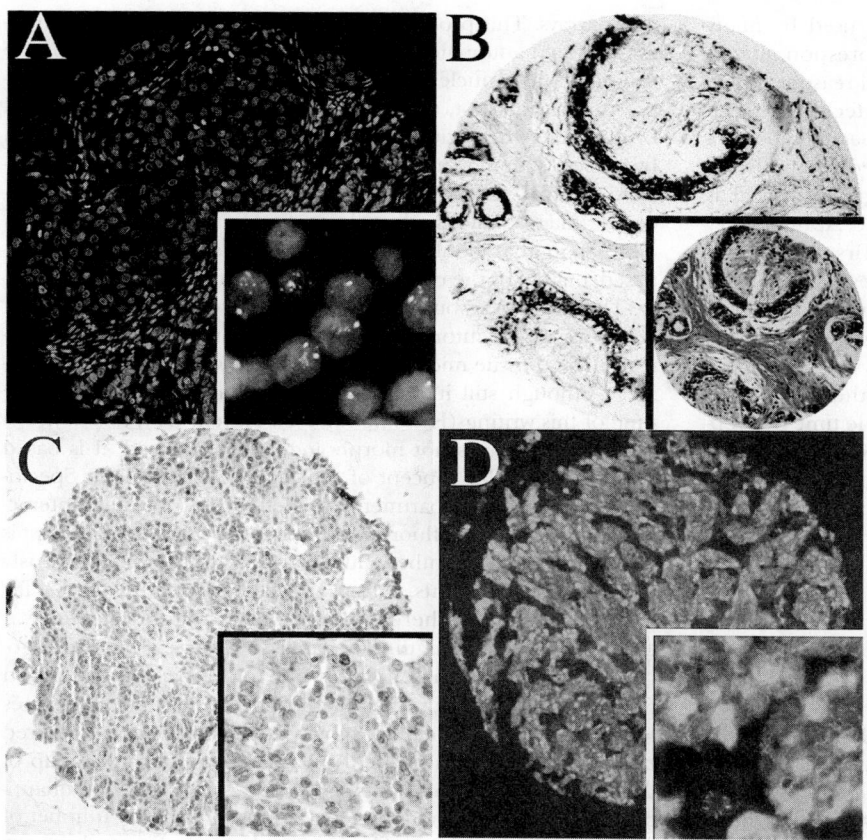

FIGURE 1.4-2. Visualization of tissue microarrays. Tissue microarrays can be used for DNA (**A**), RNA (**B**), and protein analyses (**C** and **D**). **A:** A low-power view of an archival breast cancer tissue microarray spot that was hybridized for HER2 and chromosome 17 by fluorescence *in situ* hybridization (FISH) and counterstained with 4',6'-diamidino-2-phenylindole (DAPI). Inset is a high-power view of nuclei showing HER2 amplification (red), chromosome 17 centromere (green), and DAPI (blue). Note that there are two copies of chromosome 17 in most cells but many copies of HER2, indicating amplification. Some signals appear slightly out of focus because of the thickness of the section. **B:** U6 RNA ISH detection (dark staining) by chromogenic ISH is shown on an archival breast cancer tissue microarray. Inset is a hematoxylin and eosin stain of the spot. The messenger RNA ISH procedure results in some degradation of the histology, but general architectural features are preserved. **C:** A low-power (10× objective) light microscopic image of Mart-1 using the immunoperoxidase (brown stain) method for visualization on a melanoma tissue microarray shows cytoplasmic expression. The inset is 40× original magnification. **D:** A low-power (10× objective) epifluorescent microscope image of a melanoma tissue microarray stained with β-catenin by immunofluorescence. The inset is 40× original magnification. (See Color Fig. 1.4-2 in the CD-ROM.)

of RNA levels in tissue microarrays is by quantitative *in situ* reverse transcriptase polymerase chain reaction, as described by Stamps et al.[21] They successfully analyzed spondin-2 RNA levels on commercially available multitissue microarrays using *in situ* reverse transcriptase polymerase chain reaction by eliminating extensive DNAse treatment to better preserve tissue structure morphology and by using lower numbers of polymerase chain reaction cycles.

PROTEIN VISUALIZATION

Although any technique that can be done on a formalin-fixed, paraffin-embedded section can also be used on a tissue microarray, immunohistochemistry is the most common application. Either visualization with a chromogen/brown stain by light microscopy (see Fig. 1.4-2*C*) or with fluorescent molecules by epifluorescent microscopy (see Fig. 1.4-2*D*) allows the detection of the protein(s) of interest. Initially, the standard was use of the conventional diaminobenzidine-based methods of visualization. However, a broad array of new technologies for visualization by light microscopy has emerged, including the DAKO EnVision[22] (Carpinteria, CA) and NEN (NEN Life Science Products, Boston, MA) tyramide-based amplification techniques.[23] Immunofluorescence techniques have also been applied to tissue microarrays. Although there is some endogenous autofluorescence, careful selection of fluorophores, inclusion of internal controls, and careful antibody titering make this method comparable or better than bright-field technologies. Potential advantages of fluorescence include ease of signal quantification and the potential to use multiple markers on a single slide. As many as 5 markers

can be used with simple technologies, and with special optics, more than 20 markers can be visualized on a single slide.

TISSUE MICROARRAY ANALYSIS

TRADITIONAL, PATHOLOGIST-BASED ANALYSIS

Traditional semiquantitative scoring of immunohistochemical staining on whole tissue sections involves multiplying the percentage of positive cells by the intensity of the stain (usually ranging from 0 to 3).[24,25] This traditional method for scoring pathology sections, or similar methods based on a three- or four-point scale, are subject to considerable intra- and interobserver variability. However, they still largely represent the standard of care for routine pathology and thus have been used extensively for tissue microarray analysis. As the sections of tissue on tissue microarrays are smaller than whole sections and are often homogeneous, no area variable is taken into account in scoring of tissue microarray samples.

QUANTITATIVE CHROMOGENIC ANALYSIS OF PROTEIN EXPRESSION

Quantitative analysis of chromogen-based antigen detection systems has a long and somewhat checkered past. Quantitative biochemical methods for measurement of proteins (i.e., estrogen receptor) gave way to immunologic mechanisms as average tumor size decreased, often leaving insufficient material for biochemical analysis. The CAS system, originally designed by

James Bacus, was validated[26] and then widely used by many laboratories to determine estrogen receptor expression quantitatively. Probably largely for political or financial reasons, usage of this test has decreased, but some of the same technology can be found in the BLISS system [produced by Bacus Laboratories, Inc. (Lombard, IL)], which has generated methods for automated analysis of tissue microarrays. This group, as well as ChromaVision (San Juan Capistrano, CA), and Apreio [now part of DAKO Cytomation (Carpinteria, CA)] first focused on imaging and cataloging tissue microarray images, which would be presented on a computer monitor for scoring. However, each has now incorporated feature extraction technologies, combined with density-based quantitative analysis. Although a fair number of abstracts have appeared using these technologies, the first papers were not yet published at the time of preparation of this chapter. Other tissue microarray analysis instrument makers include Tripath (Burlington, NC), TissueInformatics (Pittsburgh, PA), and BioGenex (San Ramon, CA); however, these companies focus mainly on services for the pharmaceutical industry.

QUANTITATIVE FLUORESCENT ANALYSIS OF PROTEIN EXPRESSION

The use of fluorophores conjugated to antibodies has long been a popular method for protein visualization in cell biology, largely due to its quantitative nature. Numerous software packages are available for quantitative analysis of fluorescence. However, the application of this technology to tissue microarrays has been somewhat slower than the use of chromogens. Although this mirrors general use in pathology practice, fluorescence offers some significant advantages for quantification of protein expression.

Rao et al.[27] have used a device built by Applied Imaging (Santa Clara, CA) with a method called *quantitative fluorescence image analysis* to quantitatively assess protein expression on tissue microarrays. This process uses manual selection of cells of interest and then automated image analysis. Rao et al. used it for the examination of nuclear *BRCA1* protein expression. For each tissue microarray spot, the epithelial cells were manually selected by outline of the region of interest, definition of nuclear region by nuclear staining, and background subtraction based on a negative control. These authors found that quantitative fluorescence image analysis was able to detect subtle differences in expression that would not be seen with standard pathologist-based analysis of the chromogen-based immunohistochemistry.

The authors' group has developed a set of algorithms that allows for rapid, automated quantitative analysis of immunofluorescence on tissue microarrays called *automated quantitative analysis*.[28] Although still in the process of commercialization at the time of this writing (Histometrix, New Haven, CT), this device is unique in that it is not morphology based. Instead, it is based completely on the concept of molecular colocalization. Specifically, subcellular compartments are defined by molecular interactions using one set of fluorophores; then the protein of interest is quantified using another fluorophore within the previously defined compartments. Often Cy5, a fluorophore in the far red, is used because there is minimal tissue autofluorescence at this emission wavelength. The analysis is based on two algorithms, one for colocalization and one to compensate for section thickness. The colocalization algorithm defines and normalizes for area. The exponential subtraction algorithm is required because the thickness of the tissue sections results in overlap of the subcellular compartments. The result is an automated quantitative analysis score that is directly proportional to the number of molecules per unit area. The images shown in Figure 1.4-3 are of a breast cancer tissue microarray core immunofluorescently stained with a rabbit pancytokeratin antibody (Fig. 1.4-3A), 4'-6'-diamidino-2-phenylindole (DAPI) (Fig. 1.4-3B), and an estrogen receptor antibody (Fig. 1.4-3C), allowing for differential fluorescent tagging of each. In this example, keratin defines a tumor

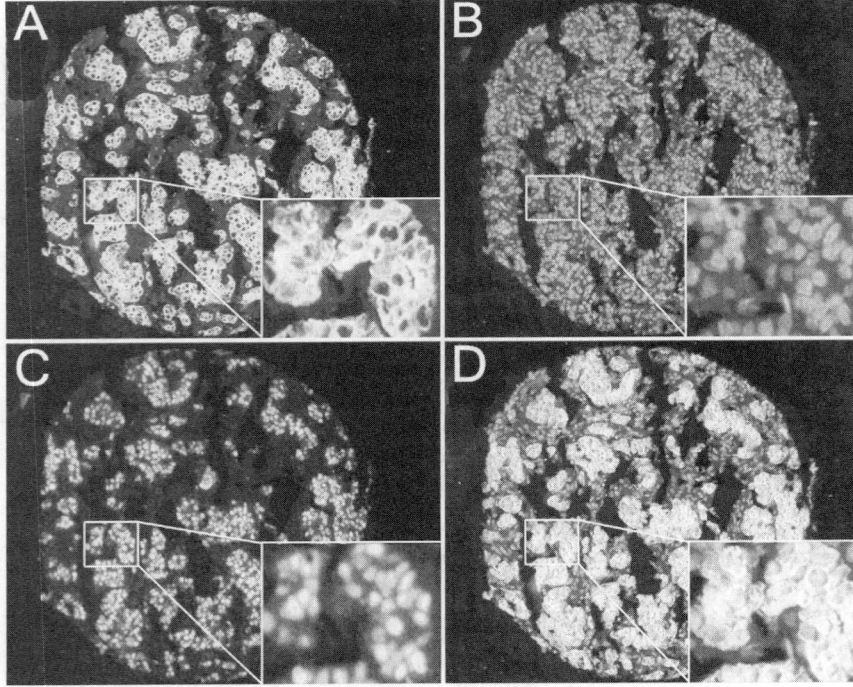

FIGURE 1.4-3.   Immunofluorescent images used in automated quantitative analysis of tissue microarrays. The antibodies used for immunofluorescence were rabbit pancytokeratin antibody from DAKO (Glostrup, Denmark), estrogen receptor (ER) antibody (mAb clone 1D5, DAKO), and 4',6'-diamidino-2-phenylindole (DAPI), allowing for differential fluorescent tagging of each. **A:** Cytokeratin staining (Cy2, green) of the breast cancer tissue microarray core shows strong staining of epithelial tissue, which is used to define a binary mask for the tumor region to separate it from the surrounding stroma. **B:** DAPI (blue) stains all nuclei in the specimen within tumor and stromal regions. This is used to define the subcellular compartment of "nuclei." **C:** Estrogen receptor staining (Cy5, red) shows nuclear staining. Cy5 is used as for the staining of the target of interest because it is outside the autofluorescence spectrum of tissue. **D:** This three-color overlay image illustrates the separation of epithelial tumor (green regions) from the stroma, which stained only with DAPI. The overlay of the ER staining onto the cytokeratin and DAPI images shows that ER stains nuclei only within the breast tumor region and not the stromal nuclei, resulting in a magenta color. (See Color Fig. 1.4-3 in the CD-ROM.)

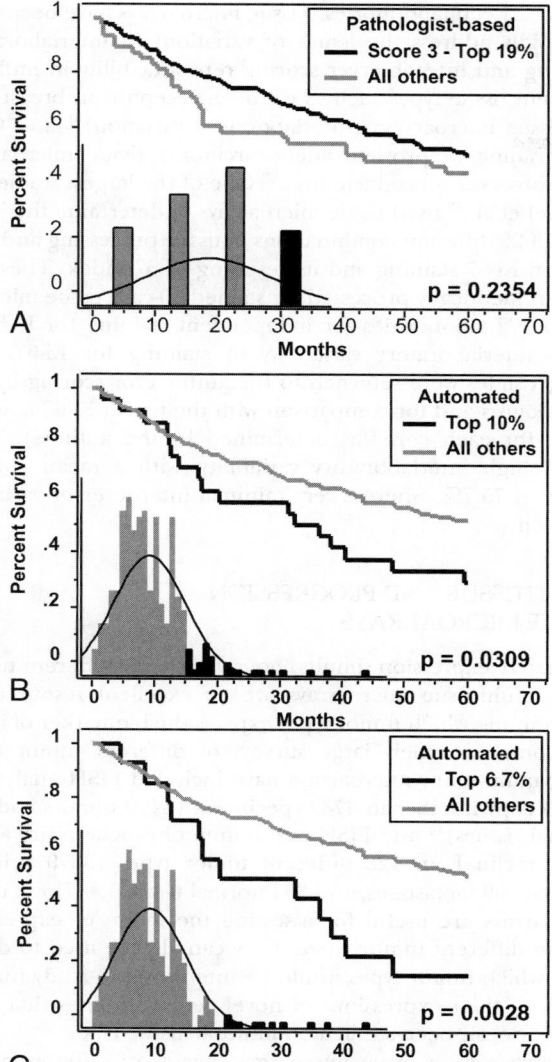

FIGURE 1.4-4. Automated quantitative analysis (AQUA) with subcellular localization of β-catenin identifies prognostic classes in colon carcinoma that were not discernible by pathologist-based analysis. A cohort of 310 colon carcinomas was analyzed for the relative amount of nuclear-localized β-catenin. **A:** Analysis of nuclear β-catenin levels in a pathologist-based analysis using a four-point scale (0 to 3+) fails to find a significant survival difference when comparing tumors with the highest levels of nuclear localized β-catenin (3+, 19% of cases) versus the remaining cases (P = .2354). **B,C:** In contrast, automated analysis of tumor subsets with progressively higher levels of β-catenin show increasingly poorer survival, with increasing significance: **B,** top 10%, P = .0309; **C,** top 6.7%, P = .0028. Insets show the frequency distribution of intensity scores for each analysis, with the selected subset in black (the x-axes for the insets are not shown but represent the AQUA score and extend linearly from 1 to 1000).

mask, DAPI defines a nuclear compartment, and estrogen receptor is measured quantitatively within the pixels in the keratin mask within the DAPI compartment. This objective and continuous scoring technology has revealed numerous associations with outcome that were not previously discernible to pathologists using nominal "bye-eye" scoring methods,[28,29] as illustrated in Figure 1.4-4.

PROTEIN ANALYSIS BY LASER IMAGING

The application of laser imaging systems has been used for automated evaluation of protein expression in tissue microarrays. Laser scanning cytometry has been applied by LaSalle et al.[30] to determine the level and distribution in human and mouse tissue microarray samples with immunofluorescence staining of MeCP2. Haedicke et al.[31] describe the use of a two-color DNA microarray laser scanner for quantitative immunofluorescence. They use cytokeratin to normalize for the amount of epithelial tissue per tissue microarray core and quantify the levels of their marker of interest within each core. Although this allows the application of devices and software that are available in many DNA microarray facilities for the analysis of tissue microarrays, it does not provide high-resolution images, information about subcellular localization of markers, or the ability to analyze more than two different markers/fluorophores.

Use of a high-resolution (5 μm² × 5 μm² pixel resolution) flat bed scanner for the automated acquisition of tissue microarrays was described by Vrolijk et al.[32] This method also uses low-resolution image analysis to define the location of tissue cores, followed by high-resolution quantification for individual cores. The high resolution was not suitable for individual cell analysis and is therefore limited to feature extraction and total levels of markers rather than subcellular specific analysis. Lack of cytokeratin positivity was used to eliminate nonepithelial containing cores in their analysis of colorectal cancer tissue microarrays. Similar methods used by the Genentech group[16] showed high correlation with pathologist scoring for p53 and CD31 but was lower for Ki-67 and was complicated by stromal expression fluorescence for hMLH1, because there was no epithelial and stromal separation in the analysis. The limiting factor for this technology is the lower resolution of laser scanning as compared to microscopy.

DNA AND RNA IMAGING METHODS

Although FISH-based detection of gene amplification has also been traditionally scored by eye, automated FISH scoring has been described as well.[33] Grigoryan et al.[33] use a confocal fluorescence microscope and an image analysis algorithm and show a high correlation between traditional and automated scoring results of HER2 FISH on breast cancer tissue microarrays. Methods are also available to quantify mRNA ISH results. Frantz et al.[34] demonstrated the success of mRNA in *in situ* hybridization by radioactive detection in human formalin-fixed paraffin-embedded tissues using phosphate-33–labeled prostate-specific antigen mRNA riboprobes, which were quantified by radioactivity detection measurements by phosphorimage analysis. This method has also been used by the Genentech group for the analysis of vascular endothelial cell growth factor-A, hepatocyte growth factor, and c-Met mRNA expression.[16]

INFORMATION MANAGEMENT

Digital storage of tissue microarray images in databases that allow Web viewing and include complete clinical, pathologic, and demographic parameters was the first approach to the streamlining of tissue microarray analysis. Tissue microarray cataloging and digital microscopy programs are available from many different companies, including Bacus Laboratories, Inc.; ChromaVision; and others. Also, numerous custom software packages have been developed at academic centers. An example is the relational database structure by Manley et al.[35] Nineteen tissue microarray blocks and their associated spot location information were linked to patient, tissue, clinical, diagnostic, and pathology information in Microsoft Access databases by a unique identifier and then analyzed for immunohistochemical staining intensity on the Web for several biomarkers. Several other approaches have been used to manage tissue microarray data and images, such as a Web-based prototype for automated imaging and archiving of tissue microarray samples that allows for access by multiple users on a network[36] and a relational database for integrated image viewing, scoring, and analysis.[37] To more easily facilitate the use of tissue microarray data for clustering or other analyses, Liu et al.[38] developed the TMA-Deconvoluter program, which reformats tissue microarray staining results for use in other programs. In addition, their Stainfinder software links their digital tissue microarray image database with scoring information with the clustered data, which currently has archived more than 3000 cases and 65,000 different staining results. Cowan and Tuck at Yale University (*personal communication*) have developed a similar MySQL-based, Java-interfaced program for tissue microarray data management that is optimized for future data mining–type applications. A similar effort has been led by Angelo DeMarzo at Johns Hopkins Medical Institutions (*personal communication*). Berman et al.[39] have proposed the standardization of tissue microarray data for uniform reporting and submission to journals. They describe a community-based open source tool for tissue microarray data sharing and exchange that evolved from a series of workshops (sponsored by the Association of Pathology Informatics and the National Cancer Institute).

TISSUE MICROARRAY APPLICATIONS

TISSUE MICROARRAYS AS VALIDATION TOOLS FOR PROGNOSTIC/PREDICTIVE MARKERS

In this era in which there are multiple methods for target discovery, technologies for high-throughput validation of these targets are required. Tissue microarrays have been used by many groups to validate a range of targets generated by cDNA microarray or similar technologies. The Rubin/Chinnaiyan group has illustrated this concept in a number of cases in which a prostate-specific marker that was discovered by cDNA array-based analysis was validated using a large cohort prostate tissue microarray.[40] These large, highly clinically annotated tissue microarrays have also been used for validation of numerous conventional biomarkers. The main advantage of using tissue microarrays in this context is the number of assays obtainable from each tissue sample. Because extensive effort is required to collect complete demographic, pathologic, and outcome information, it is highly desirable to minimize tissue used for each assay. Use of tissue microarrays instead of conventional slides in this context results in approximately 1000-fold amplification of the number of assays per tissue sample (as discussed in Advantages of Tissue Microarrays, earlier in this chapter).

INTEROBSERVER REPRODUCIBILITY, TISSUE PROCESSING, AND STAINING VARIATION ANALYSIS

Many factors, including different antigen retrieval methods, reagents, and detection methods, can result in staining differ-ences between laboratories. Tissue microarrays have been used to rapidly address the issues of variations in interlaboratory staining and interobserver scoring reproducibility in multiple different tissue types such as estrogen receptor on breast cancer tissue microarrays (interlaboratory variation)[41] and Gleason grading of prostate adenocarcinoma tissue microarrays (interobserver reproducibility).[42] One of the largest studies, by Mengel et al.,[43] used tissue microarrays to determine the influence of 22 different combinations of tissue processing and fixation on Ki-67 staining and its resulting Ki-67 index. They also sent an identically processed, unstained 30-case tissue microarray to 172 laboratories for independent staining for Ki-67 to assess interlaboratory variability in staining for Ki-67. The stained slides were returned to the authors for scoring by two pathologists and for comparison with the preset Ki-67 labeling index for each core (as determined by the authors). They found high interlaboratory variability, with a mean concordance of 75.7%, whereas very minimal interobserver variation was seen.

MULTITISSUE AND PROGRESSION TISSUE MICROARRAYS

To analyze expression simultaneously on many different tumor types, multitissue microarrays are an excellent resource for determining which tumor types express the biomarker of interest. Some extremely large surveys of different tumor types using multitumor microarrays have included FISH analysis of 17q23 copy number in 4788 specimens (4429 tumors and 359 normal tissues)[44] and FISH and immunohistochemistry analysis of cyclin E in 128 different tumor types (3670 primary tumors, 709 metastases, and 354 normal tissues).[45] These tissue microarrays are useful for assessing the range of expression among different tumor types. They can also be used to determine which tumor types would be interesting to study further based on their expressions of novel genes or genes that have not previously been studied on multiple tissue types.

A progression tissue microarray consists of different stages and states of tumors all on one slide. This type of tissue microarray has been used in numerous prostate cancer studies[46,47] such that combinations of samples from normal prostate, benign prostatic hyperplasia, primary tumors, recurrences, metastases, hormone refractory samples, different Gleason grades, and different stages have been examined simultaneously for particular alterations or expression patterns. Progression studies using tissue microarrays have also been done in colon cancer, melanoma, breast cancer, renal cell carcinoma, hepatocellular carcinoma, and other tumor types.

CLUSTERING AND PATHWAY ANALYSIS

One of the advantages of tissue microarrays is the ease with which multiple pathway components or multiple markers can be analyzed on large cohorts of tumors. Generation of data on tissue microarrays with many markers allows for clustering of the results, similar to analyses done with cDNA microarray data, to generate biomarker expression-specific clusters, pathway "fingerprints," or disease classifications. A set of 166 breast cancer cases that had previously been analyzed by comparative genomic hybridization were evaluated by Korsching et al.[48] on tissue microarrays. They analyzed HER2 amplification by CISH and 15 antibodies using traditional immunohistochemistry to look at the relationship between protein expression and patterns of cytogenetic alterations. The markers included antibodies to standard breast cancer clinical biomarkers, cyclins, cytokeratins, and others. The semiquantitative scores of staining on the tissue microarrays were clustered, resulting in three main clusters of tumors (an HER2 amplification and overexpression cluster, a cytokeratin 8/18 cluster, and a "basal" cytokeratin 5/6–positive cluster), with the different clusters showing higher frequency of expression for different markers. With 21 antibodies, Alkushi et al.[49] found cytokeratins, along with estrogen receptor, vimentin, and carcinoembryonic antigen, to be important cluster components in immunoprofile analysis of immunohistochemical staining of cervical and endometrial adenocarcinoma tissue microarrays. A panel of 22 antibodies used in a multitumor tissue microarray study by Hsu et al.[50] allowed the analysis of interlaboratory variability for S-100 staining in five different laboratories as well as for hierarchical clustering, which was able to group many tumors based on their site of origin. They used software designed for clustering of microarray analysis by Eisen et al.[51] by adapting tissue microarray data for clustering analysis.[38] Clustering analysis to date has been limited by semiquantitative, discontinuous, and subjective nominal data from pathologist-based scoring of tissue microarrays. Future studies with data from automated quantitative analysis of tissue microarrays should allow for more robust data sets for complex multivariable analysis.

Pathway analysis has also been done to examine many members from the same biologic pathway on a single patient cohort. Examples include analysis of the hepatocyte growth factor/Met pathway components in node-negative breast cancer tissue microarrays[52] and the PI3K pathway in glioblastoma tissue microarrays.[53] This approach allows investigators to find correlations between individual nodes of a pathway as well as multivariate analyses with multiple components to identify pathway keystones or signatures.

FUTURE APPLICATIONS

Tissue microarrays are quite versatile and have many other potential future applications. One striking potential use is the analysis of expression of many genes or proteins toward the goal of target discovery, in a manner analogous to that used for cDNA arrays. The potential targets might include known genes (particular pathways, functional groups, or other genes already known to be related to carcinoma) as well as large numbers of unknown genes (expressed sequence tags) for gene discovery on tissue microarrays. By compiling together results of many markers, with the added benefit of large cohort size, it may be possible to discover relationships or targets not easily found using nucleic acid–based arrays.

Other applications are also under way or anticipated. Tissue from transgenic animals is being analyzed using microarrays to allow for rapid assessment of the status of expression of the gene(s) of interest in many different tissue types simultaneously. Tissue microarrays can be constructed to study cardiovascular, neurologic, adipose, or inflammatory tissue. Cell line and blood as tissue microarrays provide a valuable way to simultaneously assess for biomarkers of interest as controls, as well as a basis for studies of their own, and some companies are already marketing

cell line arrays. Additionally, tissue microarray spots can be individually microdissected and sequenced for assessment of mutation status of genes of interest.[54] In spite of the many uses of tissue microarrays that have been proposed, it seems unlikely that they will ever be used for routine clinical testing. However, tissue microarrays have already been incorporated into routine clinical tests as calibration standards and controls. In summary, it seems highly likely that tissue microarray technology will change the criterion standard for protein expression studies, especially those that rely on formalin-fixed, paraffin-embedded tissue.

REFERENCES

1. Battifora H. The multitumor (sausage) tissue block: novel method for immunohistochemical antibody testing. *Lab Invest* 1986;55:244.
2. Wan WH, Fortuna MB, Furmanski P. A rapid and efficient method for testing immunohistochemical reactivity of monoclonal antibodies against multiple tissue samples simultaneously. *J Immunol Methods* 1987;103:121.
3. Press MF, Hung G, Godolphin W, et al. Sensitivity of HER-2/neu antibodies in archival tissue samples: potential source of error in immunohistochemical studies of oncogene expression. *Cancer Res* 1994;54:2771.
4. Press MF, Bernstein L, Thomas PA, et al. HER-2/neu gene amplification characterized by fluorescence in situ hybridization: poor prognosis in node-negative breast carcinomas. *J Clin Oncol* 1997;15:2894.
5. Kononen J, Bubendorf L, Kallioniemi A, et al. Tissue microarrays for high-throughput molecular profiling of tumor specimens. *Nat Med* 1998;4:844.
6. Bubendorf L, Nocito A, Moch H, et al. Tissue microarray (TMA) technology: miniaturized pathology archives for high-throughput in situ studies. *J Pathol* 2001;195:72.
7. Rimm DL, Camp RL, Charette LA, et al. Amplification of tissue by construction of tissue microarrays. *Exp Mol Pathol* 2001;70:255.
8. Hoos A, Cordon-Cardo C. Tissue microarray profiling of cancer specimens and cell lines: opportunities and limitations. *Lab Invest* 2001;81:1331.
9. Jacobs TW, Prioleau JE, Stillman IE, et al. Loss of tumor marker-immunostaining intensity on stored paraffin slides of breast cancer. *J Natl Cancer Inst* 1996;88:1054.
10. Camp RL, Charette LA, Rimm DL. Validation of tissue microarray technology in breast carcinoma. *Lab Invest* 2000;80:1943.
11. Schoenberg Fejzo M, Slamon DJ. Frozen tumor tissue microarray technology for analysis of tumor RNA, DNA, and proteins. *Am J Pathol* 2001;159:1645.
12. Torhorst J, Bucher C, Kononen J, et al. Tissue microarrays for rapid linking of molecular changes to clinical endpoints. *Am J Pathol* 2001;159:2249.
13. Nocito A, Bubendorf L, Maria Tinner E, et al. Microarrays of bladder cancer tissue are highly representative of proliferation index and histological grade. *J Pathol* 2001;194:349.
14. Oberst MD, Singh B, Ozdemirli M, et al. Characterization of matriptase expression in normal human tissues. *J Histochem Cytochem* 2003;51:1017.
15. Mousses S, Bubendorf L, Wagner U, et al. Clinical validation of candidate genes associated with prostate cancer progression in the CWR22 model system using tissue microarrays. *Cancer Res* 2002;62:1256.
16. Jubb AM, Landon TH, Burwick J, et al. Quantitative analysis of colorectal tissue microarrays by immunofluorescence and in situ hybridization. *J Pathol* 2003;200:577.
17. Packeisen J, Buerger H, Krech R, et al. Tissue microarrays: a new approach for quality control in immunohistochemistry. *J Clin Pathol* 2002;55:613.
18. Li H, Sun Y, Kong QY, et al. Combination of nucleic acid and protein isolation with tissue array construction: using defined histologic regions in single frozen tissue blocks for multiple research purposes. *Int J Mol Med* 2003;12:299.
19. Tanner M, Gancberg D, Di Leo A, et al. Chromogenic in situ hybridization: a practical alternative for fluorescence in situ hybridization to detect HER-2/neu oncogene amplification in archival breast cancer samples. *Am J Pathol* 2000;157:1467.
20. Kallioniemi OP, Wagner U, Kononen J, et al. Tissue microarray technology for high-throughput molecular profiling of cancer. *Hum Mol Genet* 2001;10:657.
21. Stamps AC, Terrett JA, Adam PJ. Application of in situ reverse transcriptase-polymerase chain reaction (RT-PCR) to tissue microarrays. *J Nanobiotechnology* 2003;1:3.
22. Sabattini E, Bisgaard K, Ascani S, et al. The EnVision++ system: a new immunohistochemical method for diagnostics and research. Critical comparison with the APAAP, ChemMate, CSA, LABC, and SABC techniques. *J Clin Pathol* 1998;51:506.
23. Toda Y, Kono K, Abiru H, et al. Application of tyramide signal amplification system to immunohistochemistry: a potent method to localize antigens that are not detectable by ordinary method. *Pathol Int* 1999;49:479.
24. McCarty KS Jr, Szabo E, Flowers JL, et al. Use of a monoclonal anti-estrogen receptor antibody in the immunohistochemical evaluation of human tumors. *Cancer Res* 1986;46:4244s.
25. Allred DC, Harvey JM, Berardo M, et al. Prognostic and predictive factors in breast cancer by immunohistochemical analysis. *Mod Pathol* 1998;11:155.
26. Esteban JM, Battifora H, Warsi Z, et al. Quantification of estrogen receptors on paraffin-embedded tumors by image analysis. *Mod Pathol* 1991;4:53.
27. Rao J, Seligson D, Hemstreet GP. Protein expression analysis using quantitative fluorescence image analysis on tissue microarray slides. *Biotechniques* 2002;32:924.
28. Camp RL, Chung GG, Rimm DL. Automated subcellular localization and quantification of protein expression in tissue microarrays. *Nat Med* 2002;8:1323.

29. Camp RL, Dolled-Filhart M, King BL, et al. Quantitative analysis of breast cancer tissue microarrays shows that both high and normal levels of HER2 expression are associated with poor outcome. *Cancer Res* 2003;63:1445.

30. LaSalle JM, Goldstine J, Balmer D, et al. Quantitative localization of heterogeneous methyl-CpG-binding protein 2 (MeCP2) expression phenotypes in normal and Rett syndrome brain by laser scanning cytometry. *Hum Mol Genet* 2001;10:1729.

31. Haedicke W, Popper HH, Buck CR, et al. Automated evaluation and normalization of immunohistochemistry on tissue microarrays with a DNA microarray scanner. *Biotechniques* 2003;35:164.

32. Vrolijk H, Sloos W, Mesker W, et al. Automated acquisition of stained tissue microarrays for high-throughput evaluation of molecular targets. *J Mol Diagn* 2003;5:160.

33. Grigoryan AM, Dougherty ER, Kononen J, et al. Morphological spot counting from stacked images for automated analysis of gene copy numbers by fluorescence in situ hybridization. *J Biomed Opt* 2002;7:109.

34. Frantz GD, Pham TQ, Peale FV Jr, et al. Detection of novel gene expression in paraffin-embedded tissues by isotopic in situ hybridization in tissue microarrays. *J Pathol* 2001;195:87.

35. Manley S, Mucci NR, De Marzo AM, et al. Relational database structure to manage high-density tissue microarray data and images for pathology studies focusing on clinical outcome: the prostate specialized program of research excellence model. *Am J Pathol* 2001;159:837.

36. Chen W, Foran DJ, Reiss M. Unsupervised imaging, registration and archiving of tissue microarrays. *Proc AMIA Symp* 2002:136.

37. Shaknovich R, Celestine A, Yang L, et al. Novel relational database for tissue microarray analysis. *Arch Pathol Lab Med* 2003;127:492.

38. Liu CL, Prapong W, Natkunam Y, et al. Software tools for high-throughput analysis and archiving of immunohistochemistry staining data obtained with tissue microarrays. *Am J Pathol* 2002;161:1557.

39. Berman JJ, Edgerton ME, Friedman BA. The tissue microarray data exchange specification: a community-based, open source tool for sharing tissue microarray data. *BMC Med Inform Decis Mak* 2003;3:5.

40. Rubin MA, Zhou M, Dhanasekaran SM, et al. Alpha-methylacyl coenzyme A racemase as a tissue biomarker for prostate cancer. *JAMA* 2002;287:1662.

41. Parker RL, Huntsman DG, Lesack DW, et al. Assessment of interlaboratory variation in the immunohistochemical determination of estrogen receptor status using a breast cancer tissue microarray. *Am J Clin Pathol* 2002;117:723.

42. De La Taille A, Viellefond A, Berger N, et al. Evaluation of the interobserver reproducibility of Gleason grading of prostatic adenocarcinoma using tissue microarrays. *Hum Pathol* 2003;34:444.

43. Mengel M, von Wasielewski R, Wiese B, et al. Inter-laboratory and inter-observer reproducibility of immunohistochemical assessment of the Ki-67 labeling index in a large multi-centre trial. *J Pathol* 2002;198:292.

44. Andersen CL, Monni O, Wagner U, et al. High-throughput copy number analysis of 17q23 in 3520 tissue specimens by fluorescence in situ hybridization to tissue microarrays. *Am J Pathol* 2002;161:73.

45. Schraml P, Bucher C, Bissig H, et al. Cyclin E overexpression and amplification in human tumours. *J Pathol* 2003;200:375.

46. Bubendorf L, Kononen J, Koivisto P, et al. Survey of gene amplifications during prostate cancer progression by high-throughout fluorescence in situ hybridization on tissue microarrays. *Cancer Res* 1999;59:803.

47. Rubin MA, Mucci NR, Figurski J, et al. E-cadherin expression in prostate cancer: a broad survey using high-density tissue microarray technology. *Hum Pathol* 2001;32:690.

48. Korsching E, Packeisen J, Agelopoulos K, et al. Cytogenetic alterations and cytokeratin expression patterns in breast cancer: integrating a new model of breast differentiation into cytogenetic pathways of breast carcinogenesis. *Lab Invest* 2002;82:1525.

49. Alkushi A, Irving J, Hsu F, et al. Immunoprofile of cervical and endometrial adenocarcinomas using a tissue microarray. *Virchows Arch* 2003;442:271.

50. Hsu FD, Nielsen TO, Alkushi A, et al. Tissue microarrays are an effective quality assurance tool for diagnostic immunohistochemistry. *Mod Pathol* 2002;15:1374.

51. Eisen MB, Spellman PT, Brown PO, et al. Cluster analysis and display of genome-wide expression patterns. *Proc Natl Acad Sci U S A* 1998;95:14863.

52. Kang JY, Dolled-Filhart M, Ocal IT, et al. Tissue microarray analysis of hepatocyte growth factor/Met pathway components reveals a role for Met, matriptase, and hepatocyte growth factor activator inhibitor 1 in the progression of node-negative breast cancer. *Cancer Res* 2003;63:1101.

53. Choe G, Horvath S, Cloughesy TF, et al. Analysis of the phosphatidylinositol 3'-kinase signaling pathway in glioblastoma patients in vivo. *Cancer Res* 2003;63:2742.

54. Rimm DL, Camp RL, Charette LA, et al. Tissue microarray: a new technology for amplification of tissue resources. *Cancer J* 2001;7:24.

MAZIN B. QUMSIYEH

YESIM YILMAZ

SECTION 5

Cytogenetics

Boveri proposed the paradigm that mutations in somatic cells cause uncontrolled cell proliferation. This ushered in an era of a more rational approach to oncology.[1] This theoretic underpinning was validated after technical improvements allowed chromosomes to be examined in detail in cancer cells. Between 1956 and 1960, researchers identified specific chromosome abnormalities associated with congenital abnormalities (e.g., Down, Turner's, and Klinefelter's syndromes) and with cancer. The opening salvo in cancer clinical cytogenetics was finding a characteristic marker for chronic myelogenous leukemia (CML): the Philadelphia chromosome. Developments in banding techniques in 1969 and 1970 allowed characterization of this aberration as caused by a balanced translocation involving chromosomes 9 and 22. Developments in molecular techniques allowed cloning of the affected genes by positional cloning. In the last three decades, the knowledge of human cancer cytogenetics has expanded significantly with the addition of new molecular methodologies such as *in situ* hybridization and with the revolution made possible by the Human Genome Project. The field is now most aptly described as *molecular cytogenetics.*

Classifications of tumors by the World Health Organization emphasize the importance of cytogenetic and genetic data.[2,3] It is thus not surprising that cytogenetic testing is one of the fastest-growing areas in laboratory medicine. The authors estimate that the total number of cytogenetic tests in the United States is close to 400,000 per year. In this chapter, we do not review the molecular cytogenetic knowledge in particular diseases or discuss the biologic effect of cancer chromosome abnormalities (e.g., oncogene activation or tumor suppressor genes) because these are covered in detail in the chapters that deal with specific diseases. The aim is to provide a concise overview of basic tools and application of cancer cytogenetics. Included are terminology, chromosome structure, mechanisms of formation of chromosome abnormalities, new technical developments in the field, and some genetic topics that are not covered in other chapters. The continuous advances in techniques of molecular cytogenetics are emphasized.

CHROMOSOME STRUCTURE AND FUNCTION

CHROMOSOME ARCHITECTURE

The human genome consists of approximately 6.8×10^9 base pairs (bp) of nuclear DNA in each cell. If stretched end to end, this length of DNA would span 2 m. In a normal human somatic cell, this DNA is packaged into 44 autosomes and the two sex chromosomes in a compact nucleus. The first level of packaging involves a wrapping of 146 bp in 1.75 turns around a histone core, resulting in the complexes called *nucleosomes*, with a diameter of 10 nm. This basic DNA fiber is then further condensed in a spiral of 30-nm diameter called a *solenoid fiber.* The solenoid in turn forms larger fibers that are visible with the light microscope as chromatin fibers. Chromatin loops of 60 to 90 kilobases are anchored at scaffold attachment regions. These loops also appear to represent functional replication domains called *replicons.*

Human nuclear DNA is organized into 46 chromosomes. This diploid chromosome number is reduced to 23 (haploid) during meiosis, a specialized cell division during gametogenesis in the ovaries and testes. At conception, haploid cells from each parent combine to form a new diploid cell (zygote), which then divides via mitosis (somatic nuclear division) to produce the cells of the developing embryo. During metaphase, the characteristic chromosome structures can be observed: Each chromosome represents two chromatids joined in an area of constriction known as the *centromere.*

The development of various banding techniques between 1969 and 1971 revealed that chromosomal segments respond differently to biochemical and physical treatments. Banding can be produced by various treatments such as denaturation or enzymatic digestion, or both, followed by staining with DNA-binding dyes, suggesting that there is a higher-order structure for human chromosomes. One of the first recognized divisions of chromatin is into the categories of euchromatin and heterochromatin. Heterochromatin was the material that stained dark (heteropycnotic) with various staining techniques, giving rise to chromocenters in interphase. We now know that this dark staining results from the more condensed DNA structure in these regions picking up more DNA dyes. Two types of heterochromatin exist. Constitutive heterochromatin is chromatin that is constitutionally condensed in all cells and cell types. Facultative heterochromatin can switch from condensed to decondensed and vice versa. An example of the latter type is the inactivation of the X chromosome in female cells for gene dosage compensation. Banding is produced along the chromosomal length because of structural and functional differences in light and dark euchromatic G bands.

CENTROMERES

The centromeric DNA is vital to the attachment of specialized proteins to form a functioning structure called the *kinetochore.* Kinetochores are responsible for the segregation of the chromatids to the opposite poles of the dividing nucleus during anaphase of mitosis and the segregation of the homologous chromosomes during anaphase of the first meiotic division. The centromere provides a useful landmark along the chromosome axis, dividing each chromosome into two segments or arms: a short arm (known as the *p arm* from the French "petit") and a long arm (the *q arm*, named after the next letter in the alphabet). By convention, chromosomes are identified by their centromeres even when they contain noncentromeric material from other chromosomes. Although human chromosomes are normally monocentric, patients with robertsonian translocations may have dicentric chromosomes, and cancer cells occasionally have dicentric and even polycentric chromosomes. Chromosomes are classified by their centromere positions and size (Fig. 1.5-1). Metacentric chromosomes have equal or almost equal arms (centromere at or almost at the middle of the chromosome). Acrocentrics (chromosomes 13, 14, 15, 20, 21) have a very tiny short arm carrying a satellite of repeat sequences and the nucleolar organizer region and the DNA coding for ribosomal RNA. A submetacentric is a chromosome with a short arm that is less than half the length of the long arm.

TELOMERES AND TELOMERASE

In humans, telomeres contain 15 to 20 kilobase pairs (at birth) of a repeat of six nucleotides (TTAGGG). Telomeres cap the

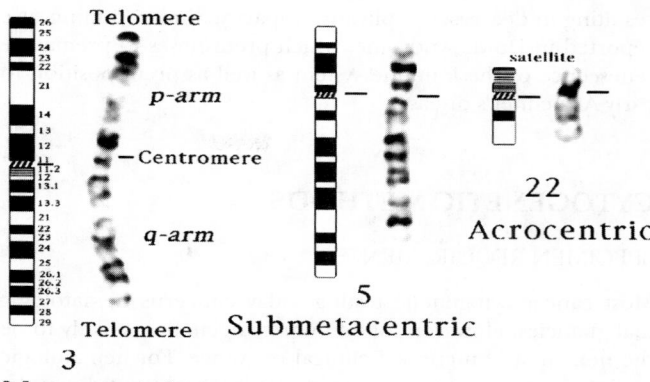

FIGURE 1.5-1. Chromosomes are numbered according to size and centromere position, and the bands are numbered from centromere toward telomere. Examples of a metacentric, submetacentric, and acrocentric chromosome are shown.

ends of chromosomes and protect the integrity of chromosomal DNA. The telomere sequence is synthesized by a specialized DNA polymerase called *telomerase* (reviewed in reference 4). The telomerase function includes an enzymatic protein component as well as an RNA component. Telomerase is responsible for programmed end healing *in vivo* after breaks and in maintaining telomere length. The telomeres contain other specific proteins that function in protecting the ends of the chromosomes from recombination, nuclease attack, activation of cell-cycle checkpoints, and end-to-end fusions.

Hayflick and Moorhead[5] recognized that fibroblast cells grown in culture have limited replicative potential (50 to 100 cell divisions). This "Hayflick phenomenon" is now understood as being due to age-related deterioration of telomeres. In the absence of telomerase, the ends of the chromosomes would shorten gradually (by 25 to 200 bp in each replication) because of the end-replication problem. It is thought that in normal cells, this deterioration of telomeres can eventually lead to cell-cycle arrest and thus cellular senescence. The reverse is also true; it was shown that telomerase reactivation is important in immortalization of cell lines and in cancer development and metastasis.[6] A technique developed by Kim et al.[7] called *telomeric repeat amplification protocol* is used to detect telomerase activity in cell extracts.

It is now recognized that telomerase activity is found in the majority of primary human tumors and may provide a target for cancer therapy.[6] Data are available that strongly suggest prognostic and therapeutic value in examining telomerase activity in certain cancers.[8] One complicating factor is that there are other pathways for developing "immortality" besides telomere maintenance or for maintaining telomeres without detectable telomerase activity (e.g., involving recombination). In fact, some human cancer cells even at metastasis have decreased telomeres and are susceptible to end-to-end attachments in metaphase. This phenomenon was recognized very early in human cytogenetics as "sticky" chromosomal ends. Furthermore, genetically engineered mice that lack telomerase RNA lose their telomeres but are still capable of developing tumors.[9]

Some human premature aging syndromes result from decreased replicative capacity of the cells. In the example of Hutchinson-Gilford progeria, telomeres are markedly reduced, resulting in decreased replicative capacity. Similar findings are reported in Down syndrome, which predisposes to premature senescence of the immune system as well as predisposition to early Alzheimer's disease.

CYTOGENETIC METHODS

SPECIMEN REQUIREMENTS

Most cancer cytogenetic testing today concerns hematologic malignancies. However, solid-tumor cytogenetics is likely to be the next area of increased clinical relevance. For hematologic malignancies, a bone marrow aspirate is the preferred sample. Success can also be achieved in some difficult cases using core biopsies. Peripheral blood samples can be useful if there are circulating blast cells. A lymph node biopsy can also be used in cases with lymph node involvement. Other types of specimens can be studied, including infiltrates, pleural effusion, spinal fluid, and basically any tissue that may have cancer cells. Technologies have developed such that even fine-needle aspirates can be tested for cytogenetic abnormalities.

It is important to provide clinical information on specimens submitted for testing. This helps select appropriate culture and analysis procedures and in some cases suggests additional tests. Examples include (1) the need to stimulate cultures with B-cell mitogens (e.g., Epstein-Barr virus, lipopolysaccharide, or 12-O-tetradecanoyl-phorbol-13-acetate) in B-cell malignancies, (2) the importance of longer culture time in some myeloid disorders [e.g., for detection of t(15;17) in acute myeloid leukemia (AML)], and (3) offering fluorescence *in situ* hybridization (FISH) tests in cases of certain translocations should the routine cytogenetics be negative [e.g., inv(16) or t(9;22)]. It is recommended that cytogenetic studies be performed at diagnosis and for follow-up of cancer progression. Occasionally, failure to obtain results can be due to the fact that a patient is under treatment and cell proliferation has thus been suppressed. Because the study requires viable cells, specimen handling is important in cytogenetics. Drawing of a bone marrow or a blood sample should be done in sterile collection tools and containers with sodium heparin as an anticoagulant. For bone marrow aspirates volumes can be from 0.25 to 1.0 mL; for blood, 3 to 5 mL is adequate. However, smaller specimens can be processed in some cases. Referring physicians should check with the laboratory for detailed information.

BANDING TECHNIQUES (CLASSIC CYTOGENETICS)

Banding requires fixed cells in the process of mitosis in which the chromosome structure is most clearly defined (most commonly in late prophase or early metaphase). Spontaneously dividing tissues such as in hematopoiesis or in cancer would be expected to provide mitotic cells for analysis even in a direct harvest of the material submitted. In practice, the quality of such preparations is suboptimal, and cell culture may be required in some cases. The time required for culture and analysis varies depending on the tissue sampled and specific testing requested. Average turnaround time for studies can be as low as 2 to 3 days for bone marrows, 4 to 7 days for blood, and up to 3 weeks for some solid-tissue biopsies. Chromosomes are prepared on glass slides and are treated by digestion or high temperature and then stained with Wright's or Giemsa's stain. The most commonly used staining techniques are G banding and R banding, which produce characteristic banding patterns for each human chromosome. These techniques, in combination with the physical chromosomal structure, allow for the identification of individual chromosomes.

FLUORESCENCE *IN SITU* HYBRIDIZATION

Under appropriate conditions, the double-stranded DNA can be resolved to single strands and the complementary single-stranded DNA can be reannealed or annealed to other complementary single-stranded sequences. This property is used in various molecular methods involving DNA hybridization. By merging the nucleic acid hybridization onto metaphase chromosome spreads, FISH has established a solid technical foundation for the field of molecular cancer cytogenetics.[10] FISH involves hybridization of a DNA probe with an incorporated reporter molecule (hapten) to a chromosomal locus containing the complementary sequence. This is followed by detection of the reporter molecule. The reporter molecule can be a protein such as biotin or digoxigenin or a fluorescent molecule such as rhodamine or fluoroisothiocyanate. Incorporation of the reporter molecule as labeled nucleotides in the probe is performed using nick translation or primer extension.

FISH analysis extends routine cytogenetic banding methods by resolving ambiguous diagnosis and providing a new tool to diagnose submicroscopic abnormalities. FISH is a relatively simple, fast, and reliable procedure. Depending on the sequence complexity of labeled DNA probe and the content of tested specimen, FISH has variable signal sensitivity and spatial resolution. Hybridization probes range from very small DNA fragments (500 bp) to large yeast artificial chromosomes or bacterial artificial chromosomes. The spatial resolution measured by the closest separable signals could range from 5 megabase pairs on metaphase chromosomes to 100 kilobase pairs on interphase chromatin. Specimens that can be used for FISH include peripheral blood cells, cultured cell lines, bone marrow cells, paraffin-embedded tissue sections, and frozen tissues. Specific applications of FISH include

1. Delineation of chromosomal numerical abnormalities. For example, interphase FISH has been used for detection of trisomy 8 in myeloid disorders, trisomy 7 in prostate cancer, and trisomy 12 in CLL.
2. Detection of specific translocations (Fig. 1.5-2*A*).
3. Determining degree of engraftment after sex-mismatched bone marrow and cord blood transplants (Fig. 1.5-2*B*).
4. Determining the origin of specific translocations and marker chromosomes using paint probes in cases in which G banding cannot identify the origin (Fig. 1.5-2*C*).
5. Revealing cases with gene amplification (e.g., Fig. 1.5-2*D*).

MULTICOLOR FLUORESCENCE *IN SITU* HYBRIDIZATION AND SPECTRAL KARYOTYPING

In the past few years, new development of FISH allowed for detection of different chromosomes using probes that were combinatorially labeled with several fluorescent dyes. One method of analysis of this technique is to image each fluorophore separately and then allow a computer to translate the different ratio of color combination to a pseudocolor. This

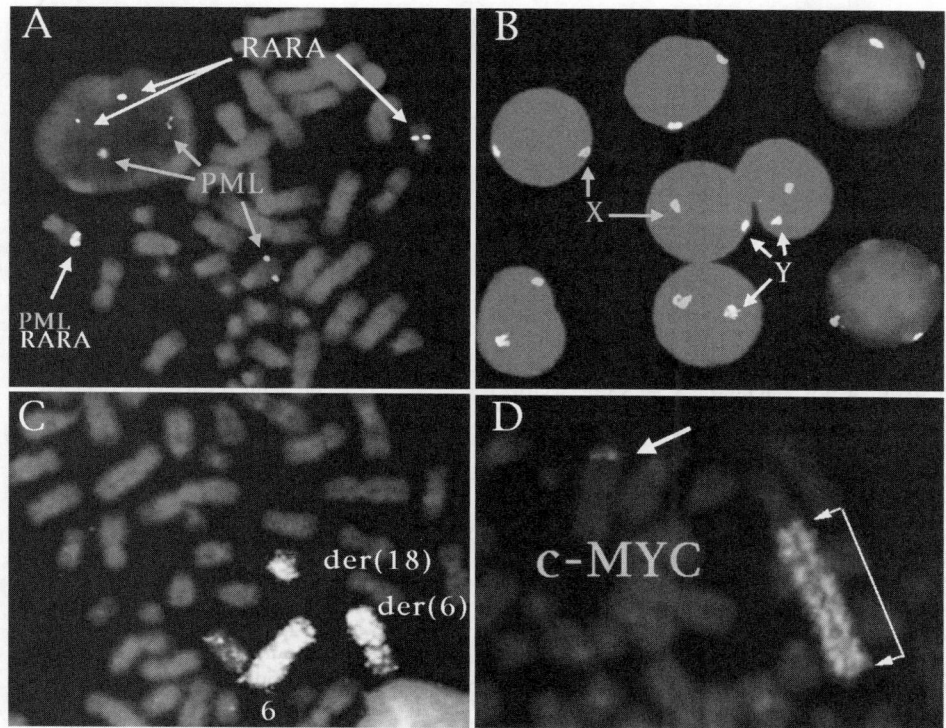

FIGURE 1.5-2. Examples of application of molecular cytogenetics. **A:** Fluorescence *in situ* hybridization (FISH) using probes for PML gene at 15q22 (red) and RARA gene at 17q21 (green). Shown are a negative interphase nucleus (two reds, two greens) and a positive metaphase with one red, one green, and one fused red/green (yellowish) signal. **B:** Use of probes for repeat sequences on the X (red) and Y (green) in sex-mismatched bone marrow transplant. In this case, all cells were donor male cells. **C:** A painting probe (green) for chromosome 6 used to identify translocations (in this case to chromosome 18). **D:** Illustration of FISH use in gene amplification using a probe for c-myc on 8q24. The probe labels the distal 8q in this case (*thick arrow*) plus an amplified area on the homologous 8q (*between thin arrows*). (See Color Fig. 1.5-2 in the CD-ROM.)

multicolor FISH (M-FISH) technique can be used to identify derivative and marker chromosomes.

A similar technique named *spectral karyotyping* (SKY) was also introduced by using a combination of epifluorescence microscopy, the charge-coupled device imaging, and Fourier spectroscopic measurement.[11] The only difference between M-FISH and SKY is the imaging system used to discriminate the fluorophore combination. M-FISH and SKY cannot detect some intrachromosomal anomalies such as inversions. These techniques still require metaphases of good quality and have a limited resolution. A combined binary ratio approach, combinatorial and ratio labeling, achieves good separation using only four fluorophores.[12]

PRIMED *IN SITU* LABELING

Primed *in situ* labeling is a method that combines complementary DNA hybridization and *in situ* primer extension. The method consists of annealing DNA primers to complementary sequences on fixed chromosomes, followed by a primer extension reaction catalyzed by DNA polymerase to incorporate labeled nucleotides and then visualization of synthesized DNA by image analysis. Primed *in situ* labeling has been used in interphase analysis of aneuploidy in cancer cell lines[13] and in the detection and sizing of telomeric repeat DNA *in situ*.[14]

COMPARATIVE GENOMIC HYBRIDIZATION

Comparative genomic hybridization (CGH) is a molecular cytogenetic approach with the potential of detecting chromosomal imbalance without the need for dividing cells in the test sample. The method entails isolating DNA from a test sample (can be a few cells from any source, including fixed material and even paraffin sections), labeling this test DNA with one color, and cohybridizing this DNA with a control DNA labeled with another color to

normal metaphases. The ratio of the colors on each chromosomal segment reflects the ratio of test DNA to control DNA on that segment. The differences in fluorescence intensities along the chromosomes on the reference metaphase are measured through a digital image analysis and shown as a ratio of the two distinct fluorophores. The decreased and increased ratios of fluorescent intensities for the test DNA probes represent the deletion (losses) and amplification (gains) of the chromosomal regions in the cancer genome, respectively.[15] Thus, using CGH, the entire genome can be scanned to identify chromosomal imbalance. This technique is more involved than FISH and requires the use of specific software to allow the calculation of color ratios along each chromosome.

CGH technique provides a genomic fingerprint at a megabase level of resolution for detecting gains and losses of DNA sequences. Therefore, it is particularly appropriate for cancer studies to identify recurrent chromosomal gains and losses, which serve as starting points for the characterization and isolation of pathogenetically relevant genes such as oncogene amplifications or the deletion of segments containing tumor suppressor gene. CGH could also be used to detect imbalances correlated with tumor progression, to analyze markers of genomic instability, and to identify clonal differences within a specimen. A review by Knuutila et al.[16] showed rapid adoption of these techniques in diverse neoplasms, including detecting abnormalities of 1p32-p36, 1q and 12q13-q21 in sarcomas; 2p13-p16 and 18q in non-Hodgkin's lymphoma; 2p23-p25 in neuroblastomas and small cell lung cancer; and 3q, 5p, 8q, 12p, 17p11.2-p12, 17q12-q21, 17q22-qter, 20q, and Xp11-q13 in prostate cancer. CGH analysis also reveals unique genomic response toward clinical treatment. Using CGH, Visakorpi et al.[17] demonstrated that an Xp11-q13 amplicon containing the androgen receptor is present in relapsed but not in primary prostate cancer. When prostate cancer is treated with androgen depletion therapy, amplification of the androgen receptor gene enables the cell to recover from the depletion therapy. This finding has evident therapeutic implications.

MICROARRAYS

Conventional CGH has a limited resolution of approximately 10 megabytes simply because DNA is hybridized to human metaphases. In array CGH, equal amounts of normal and test DNA (e.g., tumor DNA) that are differentially fluorophore labeled are hybridized simultaneously to arrayed cloned DNAs immobilized on a solid surface. For each spot, one would expect a ratio of 1:1 green-red unless that locus is over- or underrepresented in the test DNA as compared to the control DNA.[18] The number of arrayed sequences can range from a few selected ones to thousands covering the genome. Higher resolution can also be obtained by using complementary DNA arrays. Analysis of messenger RNA expression patterns of thousands of genes is also possible with the high-density oligonucleotide microarray technique. One study has used gene expression profiling technology in multiple myeloma and identified four distinct subgroups on the basis of their gene expression pattern.[19]

CHROMOSOME ABNORMALITIES IN CANCER

As indicated earlier in the section Centromeres, chromosomes are classified by size and centromere position. The bands along each chromosome are numbered consecutively, by region, starting at the centromere, and each individual band is given a region and a band number from the centromere toward the telomere (see Fig. 1.5-1). Bands can also be divided into subbands. Thus, in this international nomenclature, a description 3q22.3 indicates the long arm of chromosome 3, region 2, band 2, subband 3. Occasionally, more sophisticated techniques such as high-resolution banding of late-prophase chromosomes or *in situ* hybridization with DNA probes are called for to identify chromosome abnormalities beyond the resolution limits of the routine banding methods. An International System of Cytogenetic Nomenclature[20] ensures uniformity of the terminology used to describe cytogenetic results. Table 1.5-1 lists examples of the karyotype designations based on the International System of Cytogenetic Nomenclature. It should be noted that the order of listing of abnormalities is sex chromosomes first followed by numerical order (regardless of abnormality). The order of clone presentation is to list the main clonal abnormalities followed by any sidelines (derived clones) and finally by the normal cells.

Not all variations in chromosome structure are pathologic. Some morphologic variations in chromosomes are considered normal and carry no clinical significance. Increased amounts of repetitive DNA in the heterochromatic regions on chromosomes 1, 9, 16, and the Y are seen frequently and are not associated with any clinical manifestations. A large Y chromosome is common in Asian populations and some Bedouin tribes and is entirely due to a large heterochromatic region on the distal long arm. Another common nonpathogenic variant is a pericentric (around the centromere) inversion of the heterochromatic region of chromosome 9. These normal or acceptable variations in chromosome structure are called *polymorphisms*. Other changes may be seen that have little or no pathologic

TABLE 1.5-1. Examples of the International System of Cytogenetic Nomenclature

47,XY,+21	Male with trisomy 21
45,X,-X[15]/46,XX[5]	Loss of X chromosome seen in 15 cells (not a constitutional event)
45,Xc[15]/46,XX[5]	A mosaic monosomy X (constitutional), as may be seen in a patient with Turner's syndrome (no somatic mutations)
46,XY,t(9;22)(q34;q11.2)	Male with the Philadelphia translocation
46,XX,-7,t(9;22)(q34;q11.2), Philadelphia +der(22)t(9;22)	Monosomy 7, the Philadelphia translocation, and an extra chromosome (the small deleted 22 occurs in two copies)
46,XX,del(11)(q23)	Deletion of the distal end of the long arm of chromosome 11 with breakpoint at 11q23 [most are likely interstitial deletions (see text)]
46,XY,dup(1)(q22q25)	Duplication of the segment of 1q extending from q22 to q25
46,X,ins(5;X)(p14;q21q25)	Insertion of material from chromosome X (from Xq21 to Xq25) into chromosome 5 at 5p14
46,XY,+21c,-7	A male patient with a constitutional trisomy 21 (Down syndrome) and a malignancy-related monosomy 7
ISH 9q34(ABLx2),22q11.2 (BCRx2)(ABL con BCRx1)	*In situ* hybridization showing evidence for juxtaposition of the ABL gene on 9q34 and the BCR gene on 22q11-2

significance. In normal individuals of advanced age, the loss of one of the two X chromosomes in lymphocytes of women and the Y chromosome in men is a common observation.

Beyond the polymorphic and normal variations, structural or numerical abnormalities can be causative of congenital anomalies (if constitutional) or malignancy (if somatic or acquired) (Fig. 1.5-3). Somatic or acquired chromosomal abnormalities occur after conception and are commonly present only in specific tissues. Constitutional abnormalities are determined at conception and may be present in all somatic tissues of an individual (rarely as tissue-limited mosaicism).

NUMERICAL ABNORMALITIES

During anaphase of meiosis I in germ cells, the homologous chromosomes separate (disjoin) after accomplishing recombination (crossover). During anaphase of mitosis and the second meiotic division, chromatids separate (disjoin) and migrate to the opposite poles of the cell. A failure of separation in either of these situations is termed *nondisjunction*. Rather than both daughter cells receiving the expected number of chromosomes, there will be gain of material in one daughter nucleus and loss of genetic material in the other daughter nucleus. For human autosomes, the normal situation is disomy (two copies of each chromosome). Thus, trisomy refers to having an extra chromosome and monosomy to having a missing chromosome. Another mechanism for producing a chromosome abnormality is anaphase lag, in which a chromosome lags at anaphase and fails to be included in daughter nuclei and is thus lost. This can result only in monosomy. Trisomies and monosomies are common in human cancers. Polyploidy occurs when cells have more than the normal two sets of chromosomes (diploidy). Thus, a triploid cell has three sets of chromosomes (modal

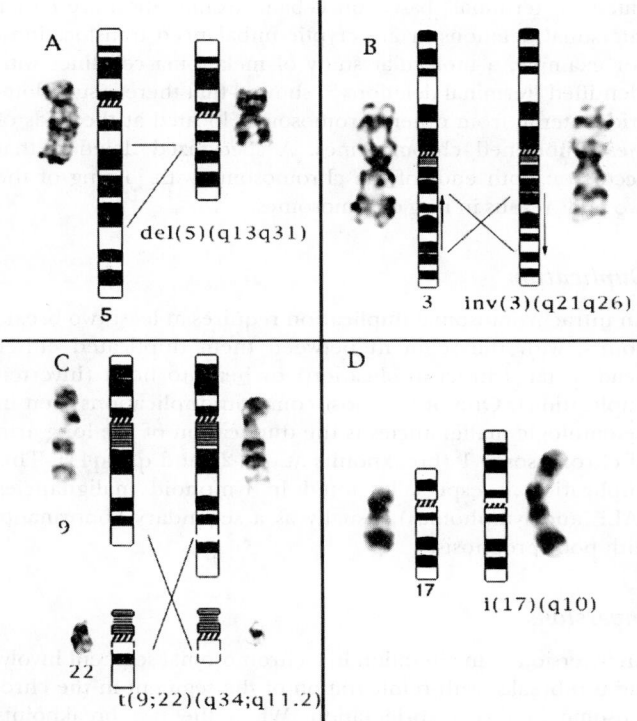

FIGURE 1.5-3. Structural chromosome abnormalities seen in cancer cytogenetics. **A:** Interstitial deletion of chromosome 5 seen in myeloid disorders, including the 5q- syndrome. **B:** Paracentric inversion of chromosome 3 seen in acute myeloid leukemia (AML). **C:** Balanced translocation t(9;22), resulting in a small chromosome 22 dubbed the *Philadelphia chromosome* seen primarily in chronic myelogenous leukemia (but also in AML and acute lymphocytic leukemia). **D:** Isochromosome for the long arm of 17 seen in AML.

number of chromosomes 69) and a tetraploid cell four sets (modal chromosome number 92). Polyploidy is noted in hematologic malignancies and in solid tumors and is usually seen duplicating a set of chromosomes that already have abnormal chromosomes (structural or numerical).

Our understanding of the impact of numerical abnormalities on development and progression of cancer has lagged behind that of structural abnormalities. For monosomy, speculation about loss of tumor suppressor genes on these chromosomes abound, but for the most common monosomies (e.g., monosomy 7 in myeloid disorders), no confirmed tumor suppressor genes cloned have yet been proven to be directly related to these monosomies. Trisomies are even more problematic because it is difficult to show that specific genes on the extra chromosome are responsible for cell proliferation as a result of a dosage effect (three vs. two copies of the gene). It has been demonstrated that the extra chromosome 7 in papillary renal carcinomas with trisomy 7 includes the mutant MET allele.[21] This indicates that one mechanism for the effect of a trisomy is duplication of mutant oncogenes. Other involved mechanisms include gene interactions, imprinting, and/or position effects.[22,23]

STRUCTURAL ABNORMALITIES

Numerical chromosome abnormalities entail having loss or gain of whole chromosomes. By contrast, structural abnor-malities involve changes in part of one or more chromosomes. By definition, structural chromosome aberrations require one or more breaks in the DNA sequence. Chromosome rearrangements are expected to be deleterious. Thus, it is not surprising that strong selective forces in evolution resulted in numerous mechanisms to reduce the rate of chromosome aberrations. Pathways of cell-cycle arrest after DNA breaks and DNA repair are exemplified by p53-mediated response to double-strand DNA breaks. Other evolutionary mechanisms for protection of genome integrity include a nuclear architecture with chromosome domains, increased nuclear size in the gametocytes, and asynchrony of DNA replication. Despite all these mechanisms, many abnormalities escape negative selection, resulting in disease. Constitutional chromosome abnormalities are found in an estimated 1% of newborns, and somatic chromosome abnormalities are key factors in development of many cancers.

Although DNA breaks can occur in any sequence, there are clear preferential sites for DNA rearrangements. Several studies on recurrent cancer translocations are particularly illustrative of possible mechanisms for the origin of these abnormalities. In lymphoid neoplasms, it is now well established that many translocations in the immunoglobulin family of genes occur during genomic DNA rearrangements normally seen in those cells. These translocations occur because of errors during the process of recombination that is responsible for creating immunoglobulin diversity. In other structural abnormalities, there is evidence of the role of interchromosomal recombination between repeat sequences after double-strand break repair.[24,25] The observation of proximity of these genes during certain stages of the cell cycle and differentiation of hematopoietic cells suggests a possible mechanism for their formation by illegitimate pairing and exchange.[26]

The mechanisms by which structural chromosome rearrangements exert an effect on the phenotype are varied. Clearly, and as detailed in other chapters, balanced translocations in cancer lead to fusion products or gene regulation changes that have a direct impact on cellular proliferation, escape from cell-cycle arrest, and/or apoptosis. In the case of deletions, duplications, trisomies, and monosomies, a gene dosage effect can also be involved. However, gene regulation at the translocation breakpoint and gene dosage effects probably do not explain all cancers. Accumulated data suggest that structural chromosome abnormalities can impact gene expression not only of the affected chromosomes but also of nearby chromosomal regions. In cancer, the acquisition of "suites" of particular chromosome rearrangements in cancers after the presumed initial cancer genetic change may be explained by nuclear position effects.[23] Another example is cited for the repeated establishment of isochromosome 17q in certain cancers.[27] However, gene alterations at or near the breakpoints clearly explain the effects of the majority of translocations in cancer cytogenetics. This still provides a veritable gold mine for positional cloning of new cancer-related genes.

Common target gene groups for oncogenic activity that results from chromosomal translocations are transcription factors. Leukemias are frequently caused by mutations or chromosomal translocations, or both, that alter the expression or function of the hematopoietic transcription factors.[28] In addition to transcriptional activation, translocations might cause fusions that usually result in production of a chimeric protein.[29]

Reciprocal Translocations

A common type of structural chromosome change is the reciprocal translocation. This translocation involves breakage of two chromosomes, a reciprocal exchange, and resealing of the broken ends (see Fig. 1.5-3C). Considering the size of the genome and the small percentage of DNA that is coding, most random breaks resulting in balanced translocations would not produce a phenotypic effect because no genetic material is lost or gained in the process and no genes are disrupted or affected. Most carriers of constitutional reciprocal translocations are phenotypically normal but may have an increased risk of producing chromosomally unbalanced offspring. A clinically significant abnormality may result when a translocation causes disruption or activation of genes or has a long-range effect. Somatic (acquired) translocations in cancer usually result in fusion gene products or in activation of an oncogene, or both. These are discussed in the appropriate chapters. Three examples here illustrate the effects of such balanced translocations. The t(14;18)(q32;q21) is found in a majority of lymphomas with follicular center cell morphology and in one-third of diffuse large cell lymphomas. The translocation is associated with overexpression of the BCL2 gene at 18q21. The BCL-2 protein is localized in mitochondria, the endoplasmic reticulum, and the nuclear envelope and is involved in cell-cycle regulation. Various rearrangements involving 11q23 occur in acute lymphocytic leukemia (ALL) and a subset of cases with AML. The disrupted MLL gene at 11q23 has more than 30 different partner genes involved (hence, MLL is called a *promiscuous oncogene*). The t(11;22)(q24;q12) is found in greater than 90% of cases of Ewing's sarcoma and can be very diagnostic. FISH can be used to detect all these translocations using dual-color probes (see example in Fig. 1.5-2A).

Robertsonian Translocations

Robertsonian translocations (initially described by Robertson) specifically involve breakage at or near the centromeres of two acrocentric chromosomes, with the long arms joining to form a novel metacentric or submetacentric chromosome. Because the short arms of these acrocentric chromosomes carry only ribosomal genes, these translocations can reduce the chromosome number without causing a phenotypic abnormality. Although these are the most common constitutional translocations, they are very rare as somatic mutations in cancer. When noted in cancer, they seem to exert an effect by being unbalanced translocations resulting in trisomies for the long arms of the acrocentric chromosomes.

Deletions

Deletions are common in cancer cells. At the G-band level they may appear as terminal deletions (i.e., one breakpoint with loss of material distal to the breakpoint, e.g., see Fig. 1.5-3A). However, most, if not all, are likely not true terminal deletions, and no proof has been found that terminal deletions exist in cancer, probably because of cell-cycle arrest due to failure to correct breaks. Very rare examples of telomere regeneration have been seen. The single confirmed recapping by telomeres of a terminally deleted chromosome is that reported for chromosome 16 deletion noted in rare cases of patients with mental retardation and hemoglobin abnormalities. Deletions designated as "terminal" based on G-band examination are either interstitial deletions or are cryptic unbalanced translocations. For example, a molecular study of melanoma cell lines with identified "terminal deletions"[30] showed that there is subtelomeric material from other chromosomes located at the ends of these shortened chromosomes. A specialized deletion that occurs on both ends of the chromosome with joining of the two ends results in ring chromosomes.

Duplication

An intrachromosomal duplication requires at least two breakpoints, with the segment between them duplicated either head to tail (direct duplication) or head to head (inverted duplication). One of the most common duplications seen in hematologic malignancies is the duplication of the long arm of chromosome 1 (breakpoints at q12-21 and q31-q44). This duplication is especially noted in lymphoid malignancies (ALL and lymphomas), usually as a secondary abnormality with poor prognosis.

Inversions

An inversion is an alteration in a chromosomal segment involving two breaks, with reintegration of the segment in the chromosome in reverse orientation. When the two breakpoints occur on one side of the centromere, this is termed *paracentric inversion*. A good example is the paracentric inversion of the long arm of chromosome 3 seen in AML with the concomitant dysregulation of the EVI1 gene at 3q26 (see Fig. 1.5-3B). If the two breaks surround the centromere (pericentric inversion), a change in arm ratio of the chromosome may occur. The pericentric inversion of chromosome 16 seen in acute myelomonocytic leukemia with abnormal eosinophils (M4eo) is a good example. The result of the inversion is a fusion between the myosin heavy-chain gene (MYH11) on 16p13 and the core binding factor b, a transcription factor at 16q22. In a subset of patients with inv(16), the breakpoints also appear to cause loss of a gene for a multidrug resistance protein.[31] Because this inversion is rather difficult to see in suboptimal chromosome preparations, FISH is an ideal tool for detection of this inversion. Although a number of FAB classes have been noted, most cases of inv(16) are classified as M4eo and carry a favorable prognosis. In these patients, trisomy 8, trisomy 22, and deletion of 7 may also occur.

Isochromosomes and Dicentrics

An isochromosome is derived by breaks in one arm of a chromosome followed by rearrangement of the chromatids to produce duplications of the other arm of the chromosome. These are usually dicentric chromosomes, with the net effect being a loss of material from one arm and duplication of the other arm. A classic example is the common observation of isochromosome 17q seen in myeloid and lymphoid malignancies as well as in adenocarcinomas (different organs) and neuroectodermal tumors. In all these cases, the presence of i(17)(q10) carries a poor prognosis. An i(1)(q10) is noted in adenocarcinomas (breast, kidney, intestine, uterus) and less so in hematologic malignancies. A variation is the break involving two nonhomologous chromosomes forming a dicentric chromosome (see Fig. 1.5-3D).

Gene Amplification

Molecular genetic methods allowed for rigorous study of variations in gene copy number in mammalian cells. This led to the understanding of the earlier cytogenetic observation of "double minutes" (DMs) and of homogenously staining regions in cancer cells and drug-resistant cell lines. Homogenously staining regions and other forms of chromosomal DNA amplification are notable as unusually banded regions on the chromosomes. DMs are extrachromosomal, acentric (lacking centromeres), circular DNA molecules (lacking telomeres) and can be variable in size. Generally, DMs are less stable than homogenously staining regions in culture, which is expected because DMs lack centromeres and would not segregate properly to daughter nuclei in mitosis. Gene amplification is noted in many biologic phenomena, including amplification of insecticide detoxification genes in insects, induced amplification of certain genes in cultured cells (used to produce certain proteins industrially), amplification of developmental genes in *Xenopus* and other organisms, and amplification of drug resistance genes and certain oncogenes in cancer. It is the latter topic that is of interest here. Duplication of a chromosome or a chromosome region is not considered here under amplification (e.g., CML patients can have two or three Philadelphia chromosomes harboring the fusion abl-bcr gene). An example of gene amplification in cancer drug resistance is dihydrofolate reductase amplification in methotrexate resistance. Another interesting example is the amplification of the p-glycoprotein gene (chromosome 7) in multidrug resistance causing failure of cancer chemotherapy.[32] Researchers have identified many genes that are amplified in cancer. Following are a few examples of gene amplification in specific cancers:

c-myc (8q24): small cell lung carcinoma
N-myc (2p23-24): neuroblastoma (advanced stages), small cell lung carcinoma
Cholinesterases (3q26): ovarian carcinoma
HER-2/neu (C-erbB-2, 17q11.2): breast cancer
CAS (cellular apoptosis susceptibility at 20q13): breast cancer
Epidermal growth factor receptor (7p12.1-12.3): glioma and non–small cell lung cancer
PRAD1/cyclin D1, bcl-1, HST-1, INT-2 (11q13): breast cancer, non–small cell lung cancer, head and neck cancer, and other cancers
MDM2 (12q13-14): neuroblastoma, sarcoma, glioma
Primase 1 (12q13): osteosarcoma

CAUTIONS TO EXERCISE IN INTERPRETING CHROMOSOME ABNORMALITIES SEEN IN CANCER STUDIES

In examining a sample from a presumed malignant tissue, one must always remember that normal cells are found mixed with the malignant cells and thus can significantly complicate the analysis. A report of 20 normal metaphases should be read with caution because these metaphases could be those of normal surrounding cells. In some malignancies, normal cells in the submitted sample can give much better chromosome morphology than abnormal cells. This is especially true in acute lymphoblastic leukemia. Experienced cytogenetic technologists learn to analyze fuzzy, poor metaphases and quickly identify these abnormalities even in poor cells. Further variations are expected between laboratories due to different referral bases.

Physicians differ in their referral pattern, and individual referral may vary depending on such factors as patient-specific situation, stage of the disease, and even financial considerations. As more data have accumulated, there are now clearer indications for cytogenetic studies, which should decrease (but not eliminate) variation in the rate of detection of chromosome abnormalities by different laboratories.

Failure to note the aberration in routine analysis may also occur because the abnormality involves a small amount of chromosomal material or produces little change in perceived banding patterns. The t(15;17)(q22;q22) in AML M3 and inv(16)(p13q22) seen in AML M4eo are not easily noted in short or poorly banded chromosomes. A more interesting example is the complete failure of detection of t(12;21) by banding methods because the exchange is between segments of these chromosomes that stain similar (light) by G-banding. The translocation resulting in a fusion of ETV6 (TEL) gene at 12p13 and CBFA2 (AML1) gene at 21q22 is variably reported in 16% to 36% of cases of childhood ALL. This t(12;21)(p13;q22) is reported to be associated with B-cell precursor ALL with favorable prognosis. FISH using probes for ETV6 and CBFA2 is the method of choice for identifying this translocation.

Some chromosome abnormalities are present at birth and are not related to neoplasia. These include balanced translocations, robertsonian translocations, inversions, and insertions that are found at some level in normal-appearing individuals (but in most cases affecting their reproductive success or resulting in the birth of children with congenital abnormalities, or both). Other constitutional abnormalities can be associated with an abnormal phenotype, and some predispose to cancer development (e.g., Down, Klinefelter's, and chromosome breakage syndromes). These abnormalities are usually found in all cells in a person and are not limited to a particular tissue type. Thus, when we find such abnormalities in all examined cells, we are suspicious of a potential constitutional translocation. Obvious exceptions to this assumption are translocations that are classically noted in certain cancers such as t(9;22) in CML, in which all examined cells may have the translocation but it is not a constitutional translocation. To distinguish between a constitutional translocation and a novel translocation found in all sampled cells, a cytogeneticist may request a constitutional chromosome study. The simplest is to get a peripheral blood sample cultured for 48 to 96 hours using B- or T-cell stimulants (mitogens) to ensure adequate numbers of actively dividing cells for analysis. Chromosome studies can also be performed using other cells such as skin fibroblasts.

CLONAL EVOLUTION AND CHROMOSOME EVOLUTION

Early studies using X inactivation as a marker for clonality in female cells suggested that most if not all cancers originate clonally. Later chromosome studies confirmed the clonal origin of cancer cells with specific chromosome abnormalities. However, there are published cases of apparently independent clones with distinct chromosome abnormalities (occurring in approximately 1% of cases of leukemias and lymphomas). The generally accepted explanation for most of these cases is that a unifying submicroscopic event occurred, with further genetic alterations appearing as unique events (i.e., they are an evolution of the original clone). True multiclonal cancers are indeed rare. In testing, the authors usually examine a minimum of 20 metaphases in an attempt to locate a clone with a chromosome abnormality. According to the International System for Human Cytogenetic Nomenclature,[20] a clone is recognized if three or more cells have the same missing chromosome or two or more cells with the same additional chromosome or structural abnormality. The reason for the difference in number of cells needed to define a clone with a missing chromosome (monosomy) versus one with trisomy relates to the possibility in cytogenetic preparation of overspreading of chromosomes and hence artifactual "missing" chromosomes. If one of the first 20 cells showed a particular aberration likely related to the cancer, a count of additional cells can be initiated or molecular cytogenetic methods used to confirm the presence of a clone. In any case, once a clone is identified this can provide a baseline for diagnosis and prognosis and also for follow-up study of relapse.

Many cancers are seen with only simple aberrations, such as the t(9;22) in CML. However, these early events can progress to more complex karyotypes. The stepwise progression of cancer by acquiring additional abnormalities is now well established for a number of cancers. A good example of this is colorectal carcinoma, which involves a successive series of genetic alterations. One must caution, however, that simplistic multistage scenarios usually are not the common pattern seen. For many solid tumors, chromosome instability results in massive karyotypic changes that appear totally unrelated to selective advantage. One possible explanation is that a genetic event resulting in cancer or predisposition to cancer removes a cell-cycle checkpoint involved in preventing damaged cells from dividing. An example is that cells missing p53 can accumulate chromosome abnormalities because of the absence of p53-mediated cell-cycle arrest after double-strand DNA breaks.

CONSTITUTIONAL CHROMOSOME ABNORMALITIES PREDISPOSING TO CANCER DEVELOPMENT

Hereditary cancer syndromes due to gene mutation (e.g., hereditary breast cancer and Li-Fraumeni syndrome) are reviewed elsewhere in this book (e.g., Chapter 33). A partial listing of syndromes with microscopically visible chromosome abnormalities that predispose to cancer is shown in Table 1.5-2. Knowledge of many of these syndromes and their underlying biology continues to expand, and updates can be found in the Online Mendelian Inheritance in Man database (Table 1.5-3).

DATA MINING IN CANCER CYTOGENETICS

The proliferation of information in this rapidly growing field of cytogenetics has been a great asset to clinicians and researchers. Fortunately, the development of information technology has made it easier to keep abreast of the rapid changes in this field. Commercial or semicommercial databases for cancer cytogenetics are available. An example is the software called *Cancer Cytogenetics Lookup*, published by Gilbert B. Coté. Further, the large text by Mitelman titled *Catalogue of Chromosome Aberration in Cancer* is also available in a CD (John Wiley & Sons). However, the proliferation of free Internet resources with on-line direct access to continuously updated data has mushroomed. Table 1.5-3 lists some specialized Web pages of interest. Many other resources are also

TABLE 1.5-2. Syndromes Associated with Cytogenetic Defects That Predispose to Cancer Development

Syndrome	Associated Cancers
13q14 deletion	Retinoblastoma
45,X/46,XY or 45,X/ 46,X,der(Y)	Gonadoblastoma
Ataxia telangiectasia	Leukemia (especially T cell), lymphoma, breast
Bloom	Leukemia, lymphoma, colon, breast, stomach, Wilms' tumor
Cockayne	Skin, aging-related cancers
Denys-Drash	Wilms' tumor
Diamond-Blackfan anemia	AML primarily, many others
Down (trisomy 21)	Leukemia
Fanconi's anemia	Leukemia, myelodysplastic syndromes, hepatocellular carcinoma
Flamm (dysplastic nevus syndrome)	Melanoma
Frasier	Gonadoblastoma, Wilms' tumor
Gardner (familial adenomatous polyposis)	Colorectal, hepatoblastoma, medulloblastoma, thyroid
Gorlin (nevoid basal cell carcinoma)	Multiple basal cell carcinoma, medulloblastoma, ovarian
Hemihyperplasia, isolated	Wilms' tumor, hepatoblastoma, neuroblastoma, adrenocorticocarcinoma
ICF	T-cell leukemia
Klinefelter (47,XXY)	Germ cell tumors, breast cancer
Multiple endocrine neoplasia type 2B	Thyroid cancer, pheochromocytoma
N syndrome	T-cell leukemia
Neurofibromatosis type 1	Malignant peripheral nerve sheath tumors, leukemia, neural tumors
Neurofibromatosis type 2	Schwannomas, meningiomas
Nijmegen	Lymphoma (especially B cell)
Peutz-Jeghers	Gastrointestinal and other malignancies (including breast, pancreatic, reproductive tract)
Reifenstein	Male breast
Renal cell carcinoma, hereditary papillary	Papillary renal cell carcinoma
Rothmund-Thomson	Osteosarcoma, skin (squamous and basal cell carcinomas)
Rubinstein-Taybi	Medulloblastoma
Simpson-Golabi-Behmel	Wilms' tumor
Tuberous sclerosis	Renal, cardia rhabdomyomata, brain, retina
von Hippel-Lindau	CNS hemangioblastomas, renal, pancreas
WAGR (Wilms' tumor, aniridia, genital anomalies, mental retardation)	Wilms' tumor
Werner	Osteosarcoma, meningioma
Wiedemann-Beckwith	Wilms' tumor, hepatoblastoma, neuroblastoma, adrenocorticocarcinoma
Xeroderma pigmentosum	Skin and corneal cancers
XYY (extra Y syndrome)	Myelomonocytic leukemia, RAEB
XY gonadal dysgenesis	Gonadoblastoma, dysgerminoma

AML, acute myeloid leukemia; CNS, central nervous system; ICF, immunodeficiency, centromeric instability, facial anomalies; RAEB, refractory anemia with excess blasts.

available to the student of cancer cytogenetics, including subscriptions to bibliographic updates (e.g., Current Contents, now available on the Web), running search engines for Web pages (e.g., Google, Yahoo, Infoseek, Excite, etc.), and local and national library search engines (e.g., Medline).

TABLE 1.5-3. Web Sites of Interest in Molecular Cytogenetics

American Cancer Society, informative site for basic cancer material: http://www.cancer.org

Atlas of Genetics and Cytogenetics in Oncology and Hematology (excellent resource): http://www.infobiogen.fr/services/chromcancer/

Breakpoint map of recurrent chromosome aberrations in cancer at National Center for Biotechnology Information: http://cgap.nci.nih.gov/Chromosomes/Mitelman

Cancer Web information from the United Kingdom and National Cancer Institute: http://cancerweb.ncl.ac.uk

Common cytogenetic findings in hematologic disorders from Michigan State University: http://www.phd.msu.edu/cyto/hemat.htm

European Molecular Biology Laboratory (includes sequence information): http://www2.ebi.ac.uk/

Genomics lexicon (terms and definitions): http://www.phrma.org/genomics/lexicon/

Genome link; a site to allow access to genome databases, genome project sites, and approximately two dozen genetic sites of interest: http://www-ls.lanl.gov/HGhotlist.html

Human Chromosome Launchpad (information on each human chromosome): http://www.ornl.gov/hgmis/launchpad/

Human chromosome maps; linkage mapping information, tools, etc.: http://www.genlink.wustl.edu/chrmaps/

Human Genome Chromosome Databases at Medical Research Council: http://www.hgmp.mrc.ac.uk/GenomeWeb/human-gen-db-chromosomes.html#0

Human genome links to other sites; very concise if you know what you want: http://www.ornl.gov/TechResources/Human_Genome/links.html

National Cancer Institute informative sites on various cancers and links to databases for loci: http://www.ncbi.nlm.nih.gov/disease/Cancer.html

Online Mendelian Inheritance in Man; detailed with references and histories: http://www.ncbi.nlm.nih.gov/entrez/query.fcgi?db=OMIM

U.S. Department of Energy, Oak Ridge National Laboratory: http://www.ornl.gov/hgmis/

Specialized list servers are also available that help facilitate communications between researchers and clinicians. For example, one could get onto the Molecular Genetics list serve at http://www.hum-molgen.de and be able to ask and answer questions for various areas of molecular genetics. More on this topic will be found in Chapter 1.6.

REFERENCES

1. Boveri T. *Zur frage der entstehung maligner tumoren.* Jena: Gustav Fischer, 1914.
2. Jaffe ES, Harris NL, Stein H, et al, eds. *Pathology and genetics of tumours of haematopoetic and lymphoid tissues. WHO classification of tumours.* Lyon: IARC Press, 2001.
3. Fletcher DM, et al, eds. *Pathology and genetics of tumours of soft tissue and bone. WHO classification of tumours.* Lyon: IARC Press, 2002.
4. Kipling D. *The telomere.* Oxford: Oxford University Press, 1995:208.
5. Hayflick L, Moorhead PS. The serial cultivation of human diploid strains. *Exp Cell Res* 1961;25:585.
6. Shay WJ, Wright WE. Telomerase: a target for cancer therapeutics. *Cancer Cell* 2002;2:257.
7. Kim NW, Piatyszek MA, Prowse KR, et al. Specific association of human telomerase activity with immortal cells and cancer. *Science* 1994;266:2011.
8. Lavelle F, Riou JF, Laoui A, et al. Telomerase: a therapeutic target for the third millennium? *Crit Rev Oncol Hematol* 2000;34:111.
9. Blasco MA, Lee HW, Hande MP, et al. Telomere shortening and tumor formation by mouse cells lacking telomerase RNA. *Cell* 1997;91:25.
10. Weier HU, Greulich-Bode KM, Ito Y, et al. FISH in cancer diagnosis and prognostication: from cause to course of disease. *Expert Rev Mol Diagn* 2002;2:109.
11. Ried T, Liyanage M, duManoir S, et al. Tumor cytogenetics revisited: comparative genomic hybridization and spectral karyotyping. *J Molecular Med Imm* 1997;75:801.
12. Tanke HJ, Wiegant J, van Gijlswijk RPM, et al. New strategy for multi-colour fluorescence in situ hybridization: COBRA: combined binary ratio labeling. *Eur J Hum Genet* 1999;7:2.
13. Pellestor F, Andreo B, Coullin P. Interphasic analysis of aneuploidy in cancer cell lines using primer in situ labeling. *Cancer Genet Cytogenet* 1999;111:111.
14. Serakinci N, Koch J. Detection and sizing of telomeric repeat DNA in situ. *Nat Biotech* 1999;17:200.
15. Kallioniemi A, Kallioniemi O, Sudar D, et al. Comparative genomic hybridization for molecular cytogenetic analysis of solid tumors. *Science* 1992;258:18.
16. Knuutila S, Bjorkqvist AM, Autio K, et al. DNA copy number amplifications in human neoplasms: review of comparative genomic hybridization studies. *Am J Pathol* 1998;152:1107.
17. Visakorpi T, Kallioniemi AH, Syvanen AC, et al. Genetic changes in primary and recurrent prostate cancer by comparative genomic hybridization. *Cancer Res* 1995;55:342.
18. Pollack JR, Perou CM, Alizadeh AA, et al. Genome-wide analysis of DNA copy-number changes using cDNA microarrays. *Nat Genet* 1999;23:41.
19. Zhan F, Hardin J, Kordsmeier B, et al. Global gene expression profiling of multiple myeloma, monoclonal gammopathy of undetermined significance, and normal bone marrow plasma cells. *Blood* 2002;99:1745.
20. Harnden DG, Klinger HP. ISCN. An international system for human cytogenetic nomenclature. *Cytogenet Cell Genet* 1995;21:117.
21. Zhuang ZP, Park WS, Pack S, et al. Trisomy 7-harbouring non-random duplication of the mutant MET allele in hereditary papillary renal carcinomas. *Nat Genet* 1998;20:66.
22. Qumsiyeh MB. Impact of rearrangements on function and position of chromosomes in the interphase nucleus and on human genetic disorders. *Chromosome Res* 1995;3:455.
23. Qumsiyeh MB. Structure and function of the nucleus: anatomy and physiology of chromatin. *Cell Mol Life Sci* 1999;55:1129.
24. Kolomietz E, Meyn SM, Pandita A, et al. The role of Alu repeat clusters as mediators of recurrent chromosomal aberrations in tumors. *Genes Chromosomes Cancer* 2002;35:97.
25. Deininger PL, Batzer MA. Alu repeats and human disease. *Mol Genet Metab* 1999;67:183.
26. Neves H, Ramos C, da Silva M, et al. The nuclear topography of ABL, BCR, PML, and RAR alpha genes: evidence for gene proximity in specific phases of the cell cycle and stages of hematopoietic differentiation. *Blood* 1999;93:1197.
27. Matioli GT. On a mechanism for isochromatid 17q in a subset of Ph+ chronic myeloid leukemia patients. *Med Hypotheses* 1998;50(5):375.
28. Crans HN, Sakamoto KM. Transcription factors and translocations in lymphoid and myeloid leukemia. *Leukemia* 2001;15:313.
29. Rowley JD. The role of chromosomal translocations in leukemogenesis. *Semin Hematol* 1999;36[Suppl 7]:59.
30. Meltzer PS, Guan XY, Trent JM. Telomere capture stabilizes chromosome breakage. *Nat Genet* 1993;4(3):252.
31. Kuss BJ, Deeley RG, Cole SPC, et al. The biological significance of the multidrug resistance gene MRP in inversion 16 leukemias. *Leuk Lymphoma* 1996;20:357.
32. Trambas CM, Muller HK, Woods GM. P-glycoprotein mediated multidrug resistance and its implications for pathology. *Pathology* 1997;29:122.

SECTION **6**   KENNETH H. BUETOW

Bioinformatics

Information technology has become ubiquitous in the field of biomedicine. It is difficult to envision a research investigation that does not require the use of some form of computer application. It is increasingly impractical to practice medicine without the use of computer-related technology.

The volume of information of potential use to the oncologist has become overwhelming. Not only has the magnitude of information grown, but it has also grown in complexity. More and more, oncologists must digest not only the literature of their chosen specialty but must also consume of information from fields such as genomics and proteomics.

These new areas of molecular medicine generate rapidly changing perspectives as well as mountains of data. Information technology provides a valuable tool for the capture, processing, and integration of the rapidly expanding universe of biomedical data.

The application of information technology to address problems in biomedicine is called *bioinformatics*. Bioinformatics facilitates the electronic representation, redistribution, and integration of biomedical data. It makes information accessible within and between the allied fields associated with oncology. It integrates disparate pieces of information into knowledge. Bioinformatics is at the core of a new direction in biomedicine, *in silico* biology. Within *in silico* biology, virtual experiments are conducted using the large collection of data that are available to the cancer community. The linear nature of science is transformed into a spiral, with bioinformatics joining the loose ends and facilitating progressive cycles of hypothesis generation and knowledge creation.

Bioinformatics provides solutions to many of the challenges faced by the oncology community. The large bodies of data that are required by the field are amenable to computer storage and manipulation. Information science can be used to bridge the different languages and concepts that are present among the oncology disciplines. The knowledge of experts can be captured in computer models. Information technology can be used to generate tools that integrate information and display it in a manner that informs experts and novices alike. Most provocatively, there is the potential for the computational creation of new models that distill the novel insights present in these large and diverse collections of data. The computer, with its access to these models and rich data, is becoming a full partner with the oncologist in searching for new clues to the etiology of cancer and new approaches to its prevention and treatment.

"FLAVORS" OF BIOINFORMATICS

Bioinformatics is becoming an independent discipline within biomedicine. However, the ubiquity of information technology in biomedicine makes it difficult to have bounded discussions of what constitutes this discipline. For the purpose of this chapter, several boundaries are set. For example, although unquestionably one cannot do bioinformatics without the use of physical computing infrastructure, the discipline of bioinformatics is not formally about hardware platforms and network components. It is increasingly the case that an Internet-connected computer is as standard to an office as is a desktop phone. The continued explosion of the World Wide Web (WWW) and its related technologies renders many of the differences a matter of personal choice for an individual user.

An incredible universe of computer-based applications and activities of potential use to the oncologist is available. For the sake of discussion, these can be classified into three broad categories: (1) productivity applications, (2) biostatistics, and (3) biomedical informatics.

Productivity applications (word processing, spreadsheets, and databases, as well as electronic mail, calendars, and WWW browsers) represent tools used within multiple disciplines. Although these applications have had a remarkable impact on the practice of oncology, the provision and support of these generic productivity tools do not require specialized knowledge of biomedicine.

Biostatistics and bioinformatics are commonly combined in the thinking of most communities. Biostatisticians are heavy con-

sumers of information technology and commonly have significant experience in its use. Biostatistical applications represent some of the most sophisticated use of computer technology. These applications range from clinical trials design and analysis (http://www.cytel.com/East) to the interpretation of microarray gene expression experiments (http://linus.nci.nih.gov/BRB-ArrayTools.html). Biostatistics is a discipline in its own right, one that is separate from bioinformatics. By analogy, a biostatistician may work closely with an oncologist in conducting a clinical trial, but that does not make the biostatistician an oncologist. The discipline of bioinformatics represents a special collection of skills and tools.

BIOMEDICAL INFORMATICS

Biomedical informatics represents the unique core of the discipline of bioinformatics. It has two broad subclasses that are intimately intertwined. The first is electronic information provisioning. More and more information required by oncologists is accessible in an electronic form. In its most basic form, Gutenberg's printing press has been transformed into electronic publications. These publications are commonly generated by and are accessible through the productivity applications mentioned in the previous section, "Flavors" of Bioinformatics. Electronic publication, however, represents only the tip of the iceberg of electronic information. WWW sites and Internet-accessible databases dwarf the volume of information captured in the published literature.

The second component of biomedical informatics is *in silico* biomedical applications. This component transforms raw data through infrastructure and applications into insight. It is the challenge, as well as the promise, of the field of bioinformatics. Most commonly, *in silico* biomedical applications take the form of individual or institution-based databases and applications. In this form, they facilitate practice or research by permitting individuals to extract new information from data electronically captured through normal operations. This additional information can range from value-added annotations, which could influence patterns of care, all the way to hypothesis generation, fueling the creation of the next clinical trial or research investigation. As these individual resources are joined via the Internet, they raise the possibility of new paradigms of practice and research.

As with the discussion above, the edges of these subcategories are fuzzy. As *in silico* biomedical applications become more sophisticated, raw data of various sources will be accessible to the practicing oncologist in real time to inform care decisions. Complex information will be integrated and presented in digestible form to facilitate the use of the vast array of new technologies driving the development of next-generation understanding, treatment, and prevention paradigms.

ELECTRONIC INFORMATION PROVISIONING

The real-time electronic sharing of information had its genesis with the establishment of ARPAnet in 1969. The forerunner of today's Internet, it enabled the creation of the WWW in 1991.[1] It is surprisingly difficult to estimate the current size of the Web.[2] In the summer of 2003, more than 3 billion Web pages were indexed by Google (http://www.google.com). More than 26 million of these pages contained the word *cancer*, and 2.5 million used the word *oncology*. It is worth noting that these numbers dramatically underestimate available information, as they only reach that which is publicly accessible. Information requiring registration or subscription, such as electronic journals, or information generated in response to completing forms is not represented in such totals.

As the above indicates, there is no shortage of electronic oncology information available. In fact, the sheer volume of cancer-related resources almost renders them unusable. A strategy for dealing with this complexity is to recover information through a single, comprehensive authoritative source. At least two such WWW sources exist for cancer information: the government-supported National Cancer Institute (NCI) site (http://www.cancer.gov) and the privately supported American Cancer Society (ACS) site (http://www.cancer.org). The NCI's WWW resources are arguably the most comprehensive.

From the NCI's homepage, one can access information on cancer research programs; research funding; detailed and authoritative information on cancer etiology, treatment, and prevention; clinical trials resources; and cancer statistics. It is difficult to overstate the volume and diversity of oncology-related resources available through the NCI site. The site provides detailed descriptions of different types of cancer, current NCI recommendations for treatment, summaries of cancer screening guidelines, information on prevention, summaries of current knowledge of cancer causes, and information on coping with cancer. One of the more valuable resources is the NCI's Physician Data Query (PDQ), a carefully curated section that summarizes the opinions of expert panels on various cancer subjects. The NCI site provides access to supported clinical trials and cancer incidence/mortality statistics, with maps showing geographic distributions of different cancer types throughout the United States. Finally, through a sidebar resources section, one can search the cancer literature, obtain information on cancer concepts though the NCI's terminology thesaurus, and traverse to other cancer-related WWW resources not maintained by the NCI.

The NCI is certainly not the only authoritative source of cancer information. The ACS (http://www.cancer.org) has a rich collection of information, including the annual *Cancer Facts and Figures* publication. Other sources include Oncolink (http://www.oncolink.org), the CancerSource (http://cancersourcemd.com)—which includes the American Joint Committee on Cancer's staging tools, and The National Coalition for Cancer Survivorship (http://www.canceradvocacy.org). Different segments of the cancer community also post information on the WWW. These include the American Society of Clinical Oncology (http://www.asco.org); the various cooperative groups—including their umbrella organization, the Coalition of National Cancer Cooperative groups (http://www.cancertrialshelp.org); and various cancer centers.

The majority of the sites described above have a decided clinical focus, with target audiences of practicing physicians or cancer patients seeking information about their disease and treatment options. This represents only a small fraction of WWW sites containing cancer-related information. A large collection of sites contain information relevant to cancer researchers. The diversity and complexity of these sites is daunting.

The majority of these sites represent microrepositories of data generated by an investigator or institution that were cre-

ated for the purpose of sharing with the oncology research community (e.g., http://www.microarray.org—Stanford's gene expression microarray database and tools). Several notable exceptions exist.

Perhaps the largest and most diverse research site is the NCI's Cancer Genome Anatomy Project (CGAP) site (http://cgap.nci.nih.gov). This site provides data on cancer genes, gene expression differences in cancer, cancer-related gene pathways, catalogs of gene variation, and Mitelman's database on cytogenetic alterations associated with cancer. It provides access to a vast array of genomic analysis reagents.

The NCI has constructed a repository for the experimental models being generated by the cancer research community. The repository is called the Cancer Models Database (CMD) (http://cancermodels.nci.nih.gov). It contains models that can be used to further explore cancer's origins and to test new therapies. The CMD allows researchers to share the insights that they have gained in their investigations. It also permits additional investigators to extend the work of the model generators, building directly on the base that they have constructed. Models submitted to the CMD are curated by the NCI's Mouse Models of Human Cancer Consortium. The CMD is one part of a larger Internet portal (http://emice.nci.nih.gov) where the community can electronically interact, exchange, and share resources. This portal has the unique feature of providing e-papers generated by the Mouse Models of Human Cancer Consortium that integrate and synthesize information on different cancer types. Within a specific cancer area, each e-report captures the current knowledge of human cancer of that type, the mouse models that exist for this cancer, and how the models relate to human cancer genetically and histopathologically. The reports are annotated with images of human and mouse cancer histology that can be examined by researchers.

The NCI has also created a WWW resource to assist in the redefinition of how cancer is classified (http://caArray.nci.nih.gov). These efforts are using the genes within the tumor itself to define molecular systems of taxonomy. The site contains a repository for experimental data called the Gene Expression Database Portal (http://gedp.nci.nih.gov). This site is available for use by the entire cancer research community. The caArray WWW site also provides access to a rich collection of data management and analytic tools. These tools can be used to analyze data generated by an individual investigator and to explore data present in the repository. They include gene expression analysis tools and tools that evaluate gene copy number through comparative genomic hybridization (CGH) experiments.

A WWW site supported by the Institute of Pathology, University Hospital Charité Humboldt–University of Berlin (http://amba.charite.de/cgh) complements this resource and specializes exclusively in supporting CGH data. It collects and distributes cytogenetically based CGH data for a variety of cancer types.

More clinically oriented research data are available through the NCI's Developmental Therapeutics Program WWW site (http://dtp.nci.nih.gov). Through this site, one can access information on molecular targets, structures of cancer treatment compounds, and the results of screening compounds on the NCI's drug-screening panel of cell lines. The site contains a tool that permits the search of targets or compounds whose patterns correlate with a therapeutic target of interest and links to various databases with information (function, sequences, disease associations) about the target.

The difficulty with using the collection of authoritative WWW resources above is that one must consume of the information along the retrieval paths built into the WWW sites. This strategy provides structure but may make access to information nonintuitive. It is not always obvious what content is present on a site or what path one must traverse to obtain it.

An alternative strategy is the use of a WWW search engine. These engines index key words contained on WWW pages and rapidly return the page when those words are provided to the engine. One can search for any type of information that can be represented electronically (documents, images, slide presentations, tutorials). A large number of search engines index the content of the Internet (e.g., http://www.yahoo.com, http://www.msn.com, http://www.altavista.com). The current leader in coverage of the public WWW is http://www.google.com. At the Google site, one can perform simple searches simply by typing a word into the search box and pressing "Enter." A more sophisticated search technique allows one to search for phrases (by placing the phrase in quotes). One can also require that the page contain a given word (or collection of words) by placing the "+" character in front of the word or words. Similarly, pages that contain given words can be excluded by placing a "–" in front of the word. This latter technique can be quite useful when attempting to eliminate sites that overlap with the information one is interested in obtaining. The Google site itself has instructions for performing sophisticated searches. It also has the desirable feature of presenting tabs at the top of its page that let one distinguish text searches of the WWW (Web) from image searches (Images).

The WWW has an almost incomprehensible volume of resources, but it is also littered with highly unreliable information. As such, when obtaining information through an *ad hoc* search it is important to ask a number of questions of the site returning the information. These include

- Who is responsible for the site and its information?
- What is the original source of the information?
- What are the credentials of the people who prepare or review the material on the site?
- What will the site do and not do with personal information collected?

A complete set of guidelines for using information from the WWW is available at the NCI WWW site.

The ACS site offers an application that overcomes many of the above difficulties and joins the electronic information provisioning and *in silico* biomedical application worlds. A section of the ACS site's homepage, "Interactive Help—Make Treatment Decisions," allows one to enter patient characteristics, in high or low degree of detail (http://www.cancer.org/docroot/ETO/eto_1_1a.asp). It then uses computer models to match these characteristics to a database of clinical trials treatment outcomes of individuals with similar characteristics that have been extracted from the literature by NEXcura (http://www.NEXcura.com). These outcomes are then presented as graphics showing likely outcomes for the various treatment options. It also provides the opportunity for this patient to be matched to ongoing clinical trials.

IN SILICO BIOMEDICAL APPLICATIONS

In silico biomedical applications do more than simply present a user with precompiled data. They integrate, interpret, and meaningfully present information back to a user. To generate *in silico* biomedical applications, bioinformatics requires the use of principles of information engineering. These include

- Introduction of formal business processes
- Use of information models
- Development of knowledge models

Interestingly, although these software engineering approaches are new to biomedicine, these strategies are well developed in support of business and e-commerce.

FORMAL BUSINESS PROCESSES

To integrate information electronically, it is necessary to have knowledge not only of the outcome of an experiment or trial, but also the design and protocols used in the experiment/trial. The use of electronic laboratory and trials management systems [LIMS/CTMS (laboratory information management systems/clinical trials management systems)] facilitates the routine collection of this metadata. LIMS/CTMS faithfully and efficiently communicate protocols, as well as observations. Differences in outcome can then be electronically mined for differences in experiment/trial structure.

Electronic capture of data and metadata represents only a part of the solution. To integrate data, it is necessary for them to be accessible in common forms. It is impractical to assume that rapidly developing fields such as biomedicine are able to anticipate all required data formats or to standardize all data collection. As such, it is necessary to develop software adapters that facilitate the translation and transformation of data. Multitiered computer systems architecture, in which data are separated from user interfaces by software layers, permit control of access and allow researchers to map new data collections to existing data concepts.

Barriers to communication and sharing of data can be reduced further through the adoption of Internet service models. Given ubiquitous academic access to high-speed Internet connections, researchers could share their data through standard service interfaces. These could include WWW services or other peer-to-peer technologies. The electronic data would be available to the larger research community with standard technology and interfaces with minimum individual effort required to package and redistribute.

INFORMATION MODELING

To create connections ("semantic interfaces") between data generated by different cancer research communities, it is necessary to develop tools and infrastructure that enable the information modeling of data. Information modeling itself is a multilayered process. Ideally, data would be collected using controlled, standard vocabularies. However, given the extent of scientific dialects that already exist, it is impractical to assume that standardization is achievable in the near term. As such, it is necessary to cross-map terminologies that exist among the different disciplines. This cross-mapping can serve as a "Rosetta stone" to translate between the different disciplines. This Rosetta stone, however, needs to be tied to a unifying common ontology, whose concepts are represented in a computable form.

To capture data systematically, it is advantageous to obtain it in common, structured form. Therefore, infrastructure to facilitate the creation and use of common data elements is desirable. These elements would be named using controlled vocabulary and populated with defined values from these vocabularies. Much of scientific data is not represented by terminology but by numeric values. The data elements would then define the units in which the data were captured and the format in which the data are represented.

Structured data elements represent a primitive component of the required connections (semantic interfaces). The actual interface is composed of aggregations of these elements in the form of information objects. These objects expose data and methods for processing data. The objects have relationships with other objects so that expert information about data structure and relationships can be captured and shared in computer software. The joining of these objects in novel ways demonstrates emergent properties not necessarily considered by the generator of the original object.

KNOWLEDGE MODELING

A key goal of the application of information technology is to facilitate the generation of knowledge. The most straightforward application in this context is visualization. Graphic display of information can dramatically increase its interpretation. These graphic displays can take the form of plots, histograms, or other presentations of the interrelationships of concepts. They can also capture the visual metaphors used to communicate complex concepts. Concepts as diverse as biologic pathway diagrams or geographic maps can be linked to underlying information objects. Information can then be displayed and constrained in familiar contexts.

In addition to visualization, information technology can assist in the capture and mining of knowledge from complex information stores. Through statistical or mathematical modeling, or both, complex relationships can be identified and captured in the form of equations. The equations objectively capture hypotheses, which can then be tested with future observations. Information technology can be used to generate the equations and to act as an electronic repository that can be used for future testing of the model.

Computers can also help to create objective, software-based models of the metaphors used to communicate complex concepts. If created as simple, modular units, these software models can be joined to make computer models of arbitrary complexity. Such models can be used to rigorously test assumptions by "computing" on input data and observing output outcomes. Missing components and errors in models can then be identified. These models can also be used to test how perturbations of the system may influence outcome. Using techniques such as genetic algorithms, they can be systematically altered to search for emergent system properties.

CONSTRUCTING A CANCER KNOWLEDGE RESOURCE

To tackle the disparate nature of the large oncologic data collections, the NCI has developed a knowledge "stack." By processing data through the stack, they are transformed into information components, which can be combined to generate knowledge. This stack is called the cancer Common Ontologic Reference Environment (caCORE) (http://ncicb.nci.nih.gov/core).[3]

The caCORE is composed of three interacting layers. At its foundation is the NCI's Enterprise Vocabulary Services (EVS) (http://ncicb.nci.nih.gov/core/EVS). The EVS organizes and translates the cancer research communities' distinct, but overlapping, terminology. It is composed of two related components. The first, the NCI Metathesaurus, helps in translating among vocabularies used in different scientific specialties. More specifically, the Metathesaurus cross-maps medical vocabularies such as MEDRA, SNOMED, and ICD with other scientific vocabularies/ontologies such as the Gene Ontology and the histopathology nomenclature used by the National Library of Medicine's National Center for Biotechnology Information (NCBI). The second, the NCI Thesaurus, builds a common, enterprise-wide vocabulary. The EVS is currently implementing the use of a description logic framework that facilitates computer-based processing and reasoning using the concepts modeled in the vocabularies.

The middle tier of caCORE is composed of common data elements, standard ways of collecting scientific data. The common data elements are composed using the EVS and provide a standard means for the cancer research community to exchange information. The cancer Data Standards Repository (http://ncicb.nci.nih.gov/core/caDSR) has been created to store and redistribute the elements. The repository has been built in adherence with international standards (ISO 11179). These efforts ensure that data from NCI Center for Bioinformatics–supported programs can be easily shared, whether from clinical trials, animal model programs, basic research, or any other discipline.

The top layer of caCORE is composed of models of information—the cancer Bioinformatics Infrastructure Objects (caBIO) (http://ncicb.nci.nih.gov/core/caBIO). This tier is being constructed mimicking the strategy nature uses to build complex systems. Biomedical concepts are captured as simple software components. Complexity is generated through the joining of combinations of these components. The objects capture the expertise of the different disciplines that constitute cancer research, allowing the knowledge to be shared through computer tools. The current collection of objects captures knowledge in the areas of genomics, genetics, animal models, and clinical trials. caBIO is built with open source software and is available without restriction.

IN SILICO BIOMEDICAL APPLICATIONS: GENOMICS

Genomics research arguably required the development of bioinformatics as a sister discipline. Genomics, by definition, creates large volumes of diverse data. It has seen the development of large public and private databases of genomic information ranging from the human genetic sequence to catalogs of genes found in cancer cells. These databases supplement the standard publication forums as repositories of raw genomic data. The genomic repositories are complemented by analytic tools and WWW portals that process and present these data to the community. Given its genomics legacy, much of the current thinking within the bioinformatics field is colored by the experiences of genomics.

BASIC LOCAL ALIGNMENT SEARCH TOOL: A CASE STUDY IN IN SILICO BIOMEDICAL APPLICATIONS

Perhaps the most widely used application in genomic research is the basic local alignment search tool (BLAST) (http://www.ncbi.nlm.nih.gov/BLAST).[4] The characteristics that underlie the success of the BLAST application usefully demonstrate many of the components required to build oncology-related *in silico* biomedical applications.

First, BLAST is based on an implicit conceptual model. Given its genomic origins, this model assumes that the DNA sequence of organisms is stable over evolutionary time periods and that it changes in a predictable manner. As such, one can "search" for DNA sequences looking for lexical matches to its alphabet and draw conclusions about the identity of sequences and the evolutionary relationship of genes and organisms. The conceptual model of BLAST is captured in a mathematical/statistical model, allowing it to be instantiated as a computer application. As such, the technical knowledge necessary to perform sequence searches objectively is made available to nonexperts, empowering them to perform complex operations without acquiring detailed knowledge of the domain used to create BLAST.

Use of the BLAST application requires adherence to a common semantic representation of DNA data (A, C, T, G) and standard data structure (text of a specific format). It is available as a service via the WWW. The application returns its information in tabular form but also in an intuitive, graphic presentation. The graphic presentation is linked to other genetic and genomic information. One of the key factors influencing the success of the BLAST application is that it can access and analyze the world's collection of genome sequence data. It achieves access to this data set through a single, centralized repository maintained by the National Library of Medicine. The agreement of the research community to share data in a common format has empowered the whole field of biomedical research to consume of genomic information. Before the availability of these collections of large data sets, BLAST was merely one of many interesting analytic tools available to the isolated scientific community of gene sequencers.

Of interest, most of the properties associated with the success of this application did not result from conscious information engineering. The semantic and conceptual models of DNA are inherent in the genome. The genomics community was initially quite small and grew up assuming a common set of information exchange standards. Unfortunately, the complexity of the information that must be processed in oncology is much greater, the diversity of data types much larger, and the community much bigger and more established. Nevertheless, BLAST helps illustrate the components required to build *in silico* biomedical applications in oncology.

GENERAL GENOMICS RESOURCES

Genomics research is supported by a vast number of electronic applications. An excellent collection of reviews of the current tools and resources available to human genomic researchers has been compiled as "The User's Guide to the Human Genome" (http://www.nature.com/cgi-taf/DynaPage.taf?file=/ng/journal/v32/n1s/index.html).[5] Although these resources are unquestionably invaluable to the larger biomedical research community, their immediate use in oncology is often indirect. Nevertheless, any discussion of bioinformatics would be incomplete without their description.

National Center for Biotechnology Information

NCBI (http://www.ncbi.nlm.nih.gov) is the primary holder and curator of public genomic information in the United States. It hosts GenBank—the repository of sequence data for organisms ranging from humans to bacteria, dbSNP—a repository of sequence variation, the OMIM (McKusick's Online Mendelian Inheritance in Man) catalog of genetic diseases, and protein and protein structure databases. These data repositories are accessed through the ENTREZ retrieval system (http://www.ncbi.nlm.nih.gov/Entrez), which allows text-based queries from all of the databases supported by NCBI, including the PubMed literature database. NCBI also supports various data-mining tools, including the BLAST tool (described in Basic Local Alignment Search Tool: A Case Study in *In Silico* Biomedical Applications, earlier in this chapter), a Map Viewer for displaying genome maps for different organisms, and LocusLink, which combines descriptive and sequence information on genetic loci.

European Bioinformatics Institute

The European Bioinformatics Institute (EBI) (http://www.ebi.ac.uk) represents the major bioinformatics group in Europe. Like NCBI, EBI maintains genome data repositories and tools that support its analysis and interpretation. These tools include sequence analysis, protein function analysis, and protein structure analysis. EBI's Ensembl (http://www.ensembl.org) is an integration engine that maintains automatic annotation of the genomes it maintains. It permits text- and sequence-based searching of these resources.

University of California Santa Cruz Golden Path Database

Arguably the best example of an *in silico* biomedical application in the area of genomics, University of California Santa Cruz Genome Browser (http://genome.ucsc.edu) and associated tools provide an integrated view of genomes and their annotations. The site serves the genome data deposited at the repositories described above. Its key feature is a browser that integrates various types of information through projection against the human genome, based on their sequence coordinates. Types of information include genes, polymorphisms, various genetic and genomic markers, and gene expression patterns for selected tissues.

Cancer Genome Analysis through the Cancer Genome Anatomy Project

The CGAP resource (http://cgap.nci.nih.gov) represents a cancer-specific view of genomic data. In addition to provisioning data, it contains tools that permit an investigator to perform *in silico* experiments in cancer genomics. Using the rich collections of diverse data provisioned, it permits an investigator to examine gene expression patterns in different tissues, normal as well as cancer. It can be used to identify genes whose expression patterns differ in cancer. Display of these data takes multiple forms. The data can be visualized in an anatomic viewer that indicates by color the relative expression of a gene in different organs. One can also display the information in a virtual Northern blot in a manner analogous to what the data would look like if an actual experiment has been conducted. Finally, the data can output as tables or spreadsheets for further analysis. Once a gene is identified, one can electronically determine where the gene is located, the pathways and biologic processes in which it participates, similar genes in other organisms, and whether DNA-based variation is associated with it.

ONCOLOGY-BASED ELECTRONIC PROVISIONING/ *IN SILICO* APPLICATION: BIOGOPHER

The NCI has constructed a tool that bridges the information provisioning and *in silico* biomedical application spaces. The BIOgopher (http://biogopher.nci.nih.gov) "goes for" various types of information stored in the NCI's knowledge management framework caBIO (described earlier in Constructing a Cancer Knowledge Resource). The application allows one to browse the information model, returning user-specified information ranging from gene sequence to clinical trials. It returns the information in the form of an Excel spreadsheet so that further analysis can be performed using standard biostatistical tools. One can also start with user-generated data captured in Excel spreadsheet and add annotations to the data from information present in the knowledge environment. For example, a gene list that represents a molecular pathology signature could be provided to the application. The BIOgopher could then return information ranging from pathways of which the genes are members to agents that have been described to therapeutically target these genes.

PROTOTYPIC *IN SILICO* APPLICATION FOR ONCOLOGIC RESEARCH: CANCER MOLECULAR ANALYSIS PROJECT

The genome presents an important but incomplete framework for organizing oncology information. Oncology spans many additional disciplines whose insights are critical for understanding cancer. The true promise of the application of information technology lies in its ability to integrate information between the different research disciplines. To explore this opportunity, the NCI has undertaken the Cancer Molecular Analysis Project (CMAP) (http://cmap.nci.nih.gov).[6] CMAP's primary goal is to facilitate the identification and evaluation of molecular targets in cancer. To achieve this goal, CMAP integrates comprehensive molecular characterizations of cancer. CMAP is built using the NCI's caCORE infrastructure.

CMAP currently draws data from multiple resources. Genomic information is obtained from the NCBI, University of California Santa Cruz, and the CGAP. Information on molecular pathways is obtained from BioCarta (http://www.biocarta.com). Functional classification of genes is obtained from the Gene Ontology Consortium (http://www.geneontology.org). Information on gene expression comes from CGAP's serial analysis of gene expression data and from the NCI's Developmental Therapeutics Program's cDNA microarray evaluation of the NCI 60 cell lines (NCI60) used for drug screening. Molecularly targeted therapeutic agent information is obtained from the NCI's Cancer Therapy Evaluation Program (http://ctep.info.nih.gov). Preclinical efficacy of agents on the NCI60 is obtained from the Developmental Therapeutics Program. Information on clinical trials is obtained from the Cancer Therapy Evaluation Program and the NCI's Office of Cancer Communications. The CMAP data and infrastructure are publicly accessible.

The information is accessed through different high-level organizational views that help researchers approach the fully integrated data set within a contextually familiar environment.

Currently, there are four entry points to CMAP information: molecular profiles, molecular targets, targeted agents, and trials of targeted agents. These entry points roughly approximate the steps associated with selection, development, and validation of a targeted therapy. The molecular profiles section presents the molecular description of tumors. The molecular targets section organizes and presents molecular information by functional ontologies and molecular pathways. The agents section provides access to information on molecularly targeted therapeutics. Finally, the trials section catalogs and describes NCI-supported clinical trials using molecularly targeted agents.

Orthogonal to these entry points is the ability to determine the cancer context through which information is obtained and integrated. Information retrieval spans the continuum from all cancers of all types to specific histologic subtypes of cancer of a given tissue type. This variability enables two different lines of inquiry. When queried from a histologically specific perspective, it is possible to discover molecular heterogeneity within a cancer type. Alternatively, a query that aggregates over multiple cancer types facilitates the identification of commonalities among their molecular architectures.

Each of the individual sections provides opportunities to discover patterns, view information in biologic contexts, and/ or integrate across the various cancer research disciplines. Within the molecular profiles section, one can examine molecular signatures of cancer and normal tissue. It is possible to identify collections of genes that show high or low patterns of relative expression in different tissues for cancer or normal histology. For a given gene, one can identify other genes that have statistically similar expression patterns. It is possible to search for similar expression patterns for a given collection of genes across tissue or histology. By browsing this section one can identify genes that may be candidate targets by virtue of their expression patterns, collections of genes with similar expression patterns, and tissues that share profiles.

Within the molecular targets section, a researcher can examine data through alternative means of classification. One can view gene information through functional classifications or through biologic pathways. Through these views, one can see relative expression patterns in a biologically relevant context. One can ask whether expression is related to cellular role. In the context of pathways, it is possible to see whether over- or underexpression patterns cluster within pathway components. Overlaid on this is information on anomalies (when available) for genes within the pathway. Combining this information helps elucidate potential molecular targets. Within this section, one sees agents that have been suggested to act on a given gene target, suggesting possible interventions for these targets.

The molecular targeted agents section allows one to search the collection of agents. By selecting an agent one can find the results of its screening against the NCI's Human Tumor Cell Line Screening Panel, conducted through the NCI's Developmental Therapeutics Program. The expression information for this panel represents one of the data sources used to identify signatures. As such, it is possible to identify genes that show expression patterns correlated with the target gene on which the agent is speculated to act. Detailed information about the molecular target is available through this section, permitting the identification of other agents that may act against this target or agents that would act against genes with related expression patterns. Finally, a listing of clinical trials associated with the agent is presented.

The final section provides a clinical trials–oriented view of information. In this section, one can identify trials of molecularly targeted agents constrained by tissue, histology, agent, and/or key word. By drilling down in this space, it is possible to recover information on the agents on which the trial is based or molecular targets at which the trial is aimed.

THE FUTURE

It is very clear that the promise of bioinformatics requires the involvement of the entire cancer research community. To this end, the NCI is developing the cancer Biomedical Informatics Grid (http://caBIG.nci.nih.gov). Through these partnerships it will broaden the base of components, interoperable tools, data, and infrastructure. It also will foster research in informat-

ics built on this foundation, using these tools and data sources. With success, it is hoped that a network of plug-and-play applications, data sources, and services will be available. Such a network would increase the efficiency of cancer research as well as integration of information, which is so critical for the generation of knowledge.

REFERENCES

1. Berners-Lee TJ, et al. World-Wide Web: Information Universe. Electronic Publishing: Research, Applications and Policy, April 1992.
2. Lawrence S, Giles CL. Searching the World Wide Web. *Science* 1998;280:98.
3. Covitz, PA, Hartel F, Schaefer C, et al. caCORE: a common infrastructure for cancer informatics. *Bioinformatics* 2003;19:2404.
4. Altschul SF, Gish W, Miller W, et al. Basic local alignment search tool. *J Mol Biol* 1990;215:403.
5. Wolfsberg TG, Wetterstrand KA, Guyer MS, et al. A user's guide to the human genome. *Nat Genet* 2003;35[Suppl 1]:4.
6. Buetow KH, Klausner RD, Fine H, et al. Cancer molecular analysis project: weaving a rich cancer research tapestry. *Cancer Cell* 2002;1:315.

Katherine R. Calvo
Emanuel F. Petricoin III
Lance A. Liotta

CHAPTER **2**

Genomics and Proteomics

UNDERSTANDING CANCER AT THE MOLECULAR LEVEL: AN EVOLVING FRONTIER

Functional genomic and proteomic research will launch the next era of cancer molecular medicine. The ongoing revolution in molecular medicine can be divided into three phases. The first phase is gene discovery, in which the tools of molecular biology have been used to identify and sequence previously unknown genes. The major achievement of this phase culminated in the completion of the Human Genome Project in 2003,[1-3] 50 years after the discovery of the DNA double helix. The second phase is molecular fingerprinting, which correlates the genomic state, the complementary DNA (cDNA) expression pattern, and the protein repertoire with the functional status of the cells or tissue. The promise of this phase is that expression profiles can uncover clues to functionally important molecules in the development of human disease and generate information to subclassify human tumors and tailor a treatment to the individual patient. The third phase is the synthesis of proteomic information into functional pathways and circuits in cells and tissues. This must take into account the dynamic state of protein posttranslational modifications and protein–protein or protein–DNA interactions that allow molecular dissection of tumors to identify the specific dysregulated pathways driving tumorigenesis. Through an integrated genomic/proteomic analysis, the ultimate outcome will be an actual functional understanding of the molecular events underlying normal development and disease pathophysiology. This higher level of functional understanding will be the basis for true rational therapeutic design that specifically targets the molecular lesions underlying human disease.

Progress in these three phases of molecular medicine is largely driven by new technologies. The development of polymerase chain reaction (PCR), high-throughput sequencing, and bioinformatics has been a driving force in the first phase. In the second phase, microhybridization arrays applied to genetic analysis and gene expression[4-6] represent a powerful tool that has entered the commercial sector, and it is widely available to researchers. As genes are identified and their functions elucidated, specialized gene and protein arrays will be offered that are specific for a tissue type (e.g., mammary gland chip), physiologic process (e.g., apoptosis chip, angiogenesis chip, invasion chip), or class of genes (e.g., suppressor gene chip, oncogene chip). This chapter begins with a review of the current understanding of the molecular pathogenesis of cancer. It then proceeds to describe new technologies in genomics and proteomics and the implications for early cancer diagnostics from the drop of a patient's blood, to the molecular dissection of a patient's individual tumor cells, to the development of individualized molecularly targeted therapies.

GENETIC MECHANISMS OF CANCER PROGRESSION

Cancer is a genetic disease in its origins. Progression from normal tissue to invasive cancer is thought to take place over 5 to 20 years and is influenced by hereditary genetic factors as well as somatic genetic changes (Table 2-1). Cancer progression is a multistep process driven by a series of accumulating genetic or epigenetic changes. The hallmark of cancer is uncontrolled growth. Genetic oncogenic changes induce persistent activation of growth stimulatory signal transduction pathways, suppression of death (apopto-

TABLE 2-1.   Genes Involved in Cancer Susceptibility

Disorder	Gene
Familial retinoblastoma	Rb
Li-Fraumeni syndrome	p53
Familial breast and ovarian cancer	BRCA1
Familial breast cancer	BRCA2
Cowden's disease	PTEN
Familial adenomatous polyposis	APC
Hereditary nonpolyposis colorectal cancer	MSH2, MLH1, PMS1, PMS2
von Hippel-Lindau syndrome	VHL
Familial papillary renal cell carcinoma	MET
Nevoid basal cell carcinoma	PTCH
Familial melanoma	p16
MEN1	MEN1
MEN2	RET
Neurofibromatosis	NF1 and NF2
Ataxia-telangiectasia	ATM
Wilms' tumor	WT-1

MEN, multiple endocrine neoplasia.

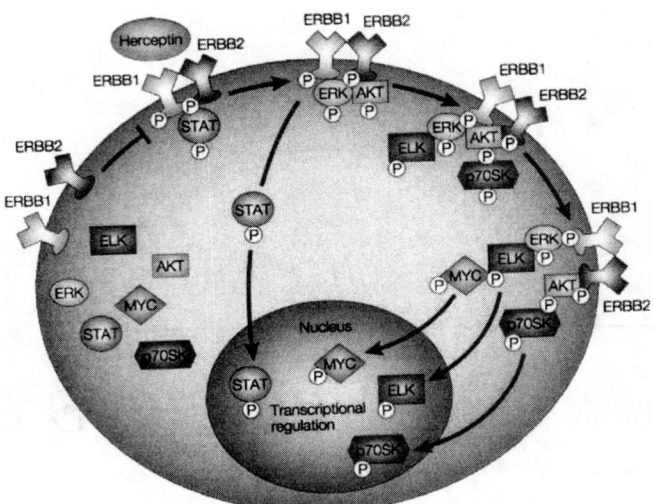

FIGURE 2-1.   Example of a protein-signaling pathway. Protein-signaling pathways and networks consist of protein complexes that assemble in response to a stimulus. Information transfer occurs through posttranslational modification (e.g., phosphorylation) of protein-binding partners. Example components of the ERBB1 and -2 pathways are shown. This pathway is a target for treatment with Herceptin, an antibody that recognizes ERBB2. AKT, v-akt murine thymoma viral oncogene homologue; ELK, member of the ETS family of transcription factors; ERBB, avian erythroblastic leukemia viral oncogene homologue; ERK, extracellular signal–regulated kinase; MYC, avian v-myc myelocytomatosis viral oncogene homologue; p70SK, 70-kD ribosomal protein S6 kinase; STAT, signal transducer and activator of transcription. (See Color Fig. 2-1 in the CD-ROM.)

sis) or senescence, alteration of critical nodes in the cell cycle, and/or downstream deregulation at the level of DNA transcription factors. Oncogenic factors can also dysregulate other cellular processes, contributing to the malignant phenotype. Some oncogenes cause a block or alteration in cell differentiation, promoting an immature phenotype that possesses self-renewal capacity. Other oncogenes block apoptosis or programmed cell death, conferring long-term survival or immortality. Epigenetic changes, such as DNA methylation, histone acetylation, or gene imprinting, can alter gene expression patterns, contributing to uncontrolled growth. Single oncogenic changes may result in a precancerous atypical or dysplastic phenotype. However, multiple accumulated oncogenic changes cooperate to induce a fully transformed malignant phenotype. Once a malignant phenotype is reached, separate genetic changes (beyond those causing uncontrolled growth) are required for tumor invasion and metastasis. Invasion and metastasis are a multistep cascade involving positive and negative regulatory pathways. Cancer invasion and angiogenesis are an uncontrolled version of physiologic invasion performed by non-malignant cells, such as surveillance cells of the immune system and stem cells.

Genetic instability may predispose the premalignant cell to generate malignant offspring. Instability can take place at the macro (chromosome karyotype) level, resulting in changes such as translocations, inversions, and chromosome loss or gain. Chromosomal rearrangement can activate silent oncogenes through creation of chimeric oncogenes (portions of two different genes fused together as one) or by altering expression patterns of the normal protooncogene through regulation by an inappropriate translocated promoter. Chromosomal rearrangements can also disrupt regions containing suppressor genes. Loss of heterozygosity is a hallmark of suppressor gene inactivation in cancer progression. Instability can also occur on the micro level, as with altered function of DNA sequence copy fidelity repair. Defects in DNA repair mechanisms contribute to the accumulation of genetic defects, fueling cancer progression through activation of oncogenes or inactivation of tumor suppressor genes. Defects in telomerase may affect growth control as well as genetic instability.

Cooperating genetic defects disrupting multiple pathways regulating proliferation, differentiation, and cell death are significant mechanisms in tumorigenesis.

PERTURBATIONS IN SIGNALING

Viral oncogenes provided the first evidence that host genes can directly cause cancer. Normal cellular genes (protooncogenes, identified by the c prefix) are "picked up" or transduced by the retrovirus and mutated through the error-prone process of the retroviral replication. This results in a functional viral oncogene (v-onc) that is arrested in a biochemically activated form. Early studies revealed that the oncogene precursors, the protooncogenes, act as biochemical switches in the command and control processes of a cell, specifically, transmitting signals from the outside of the cell to the nucleus. The normal and controlled transfer of extracellular signals is bypassed when one of the relay members is mutated and is made constitutively activated, resulting in the characteristic of a cancer cell–dysregulated growth.

In cancer, many oncogenic mutations are members of signaling pathways[7] (Fig. 2-1). For example, the receptor tyrosine kinase epidermal growth factor receptor (mutated or overexpressed in brain and epithelial cancers; related retroviral oncogene, v-erbB), when stimulated with one of its ligands, transforming growth factor-α (TGF-α) (overexpressed in some human cancers), interacts with ras (retroviral homologue, v-H-ras or v-K-ras; mutated in 10 to 20% of human cancers) through bridging proteins. Ras is controlled by guanosine triphosphatase–activating proteins (oncogenic homologue is NF1, the gene involved in neurofibromatosis) and transmits signals by activating raf (retroviral homologue, v-raf). Stimulation of the ras/raf pathway results in increased expression of the nuclear proteins jun, fos, and myc (retroviral homologues, v-jun, v-fos, v-myc; myc is mutated and rearranged in lymphoid malignancies and amplified in breast cancers), which are transcription factors that can induce the expression of other genes, thereby altering cellular physiology. Thus, every relay node in this signal transduction pathway is a potential site for oncogenic conversion. The complexity of the transformation process is reflected in the multiple parallel signaling pathways that are promiscuous in their selection of biochemical partners.

For example, the receptor tyrosine kinase HER-2 physically associates with itself or with related receptor tyrosine kinases, such as epidermal growth factor receptor, HER-3, and HER-4. Ras can be regulated by either ras–guanosine triphosphatase–activating proteins or NF1. Stimulation of the ras pathway activates a number of mitogen-activated protein kinases, inducing proliferation.

Oncogenesis can be initiated by a molecular lesion that disrupts critical regulatory signaling cascades at any level, from the ligand or receptor at the cell surface to the nuclear transcription factor directly targeting gene expression (Table 2-2).

TABLE 2-2. Selected Oncogenes and Their Proteins

| Type/Name | Oncogene Found in | | Subcellular Location of Protein | Nature of Encoded Protein |
	Animal Retrovirus	Nonviral Tumor		
CLASS I: GROWTH FACTORS				
sis	Simian sarcoma	—	Secreted	A form of platelet-derived growth factor
CLASS II: RECEPTORS				
Cell surface receptors with tyrosine kinase activity				
fms	McDonough feline sarcoma	—	Plasma membrane	CSF-1 receptor
erbB	Avian erythroblastosis	—	Plasma membrane	EGFR
neu (*erb-2*)	—	Neuroblastoma	Plasma membrane	Related to EGFR
ros	URII avian sarcoma	—	Plasma membrane	Related to insulin receptor
Intracellular receptors				
erbA	Avian erythroblastosis	—	Nuclear	Thyroid hormone receptor
CLASS III: INTRACELLULAR TRANSDUCERS				
Protein tyrosine kinases				
src	Rous avian sarcoma	—	Cytoplasm	Protein kinases that phosphorylate tyrosine residues
abl	Abelson murine leukemia	Chronic myelogenous leukemia	Cytoplasm and nucleus	Protein kinases that phosphorylate tyrosine residues
fps (*fes*)	Fujinami avian sarcoma and feline leukemia	—	Cytoplasm	Protein kinases that phosphorylate tyrosine residues
met	—	Murine osteosarcoma	Cytoplasm	Protein kinases that phosphorylate tyrosine residues
Protein serine-threonine kinases				
mos	Moloney murine sarcoma	—	Cytoplasm	Protein kinases that phosphorylate serine or threonine
raf (*mil*)	3611 murine sarcoma	—	Cytoplasm	Protein kinases that phosphorylate serine or threonine
***Ras* proteins**				
Ha-*ras*	Harvey murine sarcoma	Bladder, mammary, and skin carcinomas	Plasma membrane inner face	Guanine nucleotide-binding protein with GTPase activity
Ki-*ras*	Kirsten murine sarcoma	Lung and colon carcinomas	Plasma membrane inner face	Guanine nucleotide-binding protein with GTPase activity
N-*ras*	—	Neuroblastomas and leukemias	Plasma membrane inner face	Guanine nucleotide-binding protein with GTPase activity
Phospholipase C related				
crk	Avian sarcoma virus	—	Cytoplasm	Homologous to phospholipase C with src-related regions
CLASS IV: NUCLEAR TRANSCRIPTION FACTORS				
jun	Avian sarcoma virus 17	—	Nucleus	Transcription factor AP-1
fos	Osteosarcoma	—	Nucleus	Transcription factor AP-1
myc	Avian MC29 myelocytomatosis	—	Nuclear matrix	Regulation of transcription
N-myc	—	Neuroblastoma	Nuclear matrix	Regulation of transcription
myb	Avian myeloblastosis	Leukemia	Nuclear matrix	Regulation of transcription
rel	—	Avian reticuloendotheliosis	Nucleus and cytoplasm	Regulation of transcription
hox genes	—	Leukemia	Nucleus	Regulation of transcription
Rb	—	Retinoblastoma	Nucleus	Tumor suppressor
p53	—	—	Nucleus	Tumor suppressor

AP-1, transcription factor; CSF, colony-stimulating factor; EGFR, epidermal growth factor receptor; GTP, guanosine triphosphate.

Ample evidence has been shown of direct mutational activation of transcription factors in the genesis and maintenance of the cancerous state. Myc, AML1, MLL (mixed-lineage leukemia gene), and the homeobox proteins are all examples of altered transcriptional machinery in the induction of human cancers.

In human cancers, although mutations in protooncogenes result in altered function, inappropriate expression of structurally normal proteins (that may have no role in the biology of a specific tissue) can also lead to cancer. Several transcription factors are in this category: myc, tal-1/SCL, lyl-1, Tig-1, and Tig-2. These oncoproteins are structurally identical to their normal forms but are either inappropriately expressed in the cell cycle or in inappropriate tissues. Myc is expressed in all cells and plays a role in cell division and differentiation. Activation of myc due to the t(8;14) (q24;q32) seen in Burkitt's lymphomas and B-cell acute lymphocytic leukemias deregulates myc expression, and exquisite control of myc transcription is lost. In lymphoid tissues, this leads to the expansion of pre-B cells in transgenic mice inappropriately expressing myc, which ultimately results in the emergence of a lymphoid malignancy. Other members on this list (tal-1/lyl-1 and Tig-2) are linked to T-cell acute lymphocytic leukemia. In this group, oncogenic activation is through expression in an inappropriate cell type: tal-1 is normally expressed in erythroid and myeloid precursors and not in T cells; lyl-1 is expressed in myeloid and B-lymphoid cells; and Tig-2 transcripts are found in liver, spleen, and kidney but not in activated T cells. In these examples, the inappropriate expression of a transcription factor serves as a molecular switch to induce a malignancy.

LOSS OF SUPPRESSION AND GENETIC INSTABILITY

Whereas protooncogenes are identified by a gain of function after mutational damage, another class of cancer genes, tumor suppressor genes, contributes to cancer induction by a loss of function. To this end, tumor suppressor genes, such as the retinoblastoma gene (Rb-1) and p53, block cellular proliferation, and each appears to function through distinct pathways. Rb-1 negatively regulates the important transcription factor E2F, and the deletion of the Rb gene (seen in congenital retinoblastoma) releases the suppression of E2F. p53 enhances the expression of p21/CIP1, which is a suppressor of cell-cycle regulatory kinases [cyclin-dependent kinases (CDKs)]. Activation of these CDKs is necessary for progression through the cell cycle, and CDK inhibitors, such as p21/CI1, block the process. Thus, the loss of p53 and the attenuation of p21/CIP1 expression result in unmanaged progression through the cell cycle.

That Rb and p53 both are involved in the genesis of cancer is evidenced by the identification of germline mutations of these genes in individuals with cancer predisposition syndromes, such as congenital retinoblastoma ([a]Rb) and the Li-Fraumeni multicancer syndrome (p53). As with oncogenes, the presence of a single abnormal tumor suppressor allele alone is insufficient for cancer to develop; lesions at other genetic loci are necessary. For example, Rb and p53 may both need to be inactivated for some normal cells to be rendered immortal. The DNA tumor virus, the human papillomavirus (HPV) that is the causative agent in many cervical, anal, and penile carcinomas, inhibits both these critical proteins through binding with and inactivation by the HPV viral proteins E6 and E7. In this manner, HPV biochemically achieves the same outcome that carcinogens accomplish through inactivating genetic mutations. In colon cancers, mutations in p53 are frequently associated with other genetic lesions, including those involved in cytoskeletal organization (APC), signal transduction (ras), and cell motility (DCC) as a polyp progresses over time toward an invasive cancer.

A tumor suppression gene can be defined as any gene whose loss of function contributes to cancer progression. One category of genes is the inhibitors of the CDKs, which are enzymes that control the progression through the cell cycle. They, in turn, are controlled by protein activators (called *cyclins*) and inhibitors (called *CDK inhibitors*). The attenuation of expression of CDK inhibitors, such as p16, p27, and p57, has been associated with a diverse range of cancers, from lung to head and neck, breast, and pancreas cancers, as well as melanoma. In malignant melanoma, the loss of both p16 alleles is found in most primary tumors, and inactivating germline mutations in p16 segregate with familial melanoma syndromes. Therefore, CDK inhibitors, such as p16, maintain the normal cellular state by regulating cell proliferation, and disruption of its inhibitor function leads to cancer.

The subsequent discovery and analysis of other tumor suppressor genes have uncovered other mechanisms to inhibit cancer formation. In fact, it now seems that the inhibition of growth may not be the only important function of these genetic suppressors. In the case of p53, one role is in DNA repair.[8] As nature devised it, the regulation of growth is coupled with the regulation of DNA repair. When cells suffer DNA damage, cellular "hibernation," manifested by an arrest at the G_1 or G_2 checkpoints, permits repair to take place and prevents the accumulation of mutant sequences.[9] Cells bearing mutant p53 genes lose the ability to arrest in G_1 after exposure to γ-irradiation or other genotoxins.[10] Mice with p53 gene disruptions are completely viable but exhibit an accelerated rate of tumor formation and a loss of the G_1 checkpoint after treatment with DNA damaging agents.[11] Arrest at the G_1 and G_2 checkpoints by p53 may partially be achieved via direct inhibition of key transcriptional activators, such as p300.[12] p53 also appears to be involved in two other critical functions: genomic stability and apoptosis. Cells without a functional p53 show a dramatically increased ability to amplify DNA, which is a measure of the genetic plasticity characteristic of cancer.[13] Moreover, a mutant p53 renders cells less likely to undergo apoptosis after cellular stress, including chemotherapeutic agents and γ-irradiation. A high level of DNA damage in normal cells that overwhelms its repair capabilities triggers cell death. This self-destruct mechanism is another way to prevent the accumulation of cells harboring mutant genes. p53-mediated apoptosis can be achieved via positive transcriptional regulation of the phosphatase PTEN[14] or negative transcriptional regulation of phosphoinositide 3 kinase.[15] Taken together, these data suggest that the primary role of p53 is not only to regulate growth but to maintain the genetic integrity of a cell as the "guardian of the genome."[16]

Other important tumor suppressors have similar policing functions. BRCA1 and BRCA2 are genetically distinct and structurally unrelated genes with a convergent effect: Disabling mutations in either gene render an individual more susceptible to breast and ovarian cancers. In gene transfection experiments, the ability of BRCA1 to inhibit cellular growth is limited to certain cell lines[17] and, possibly, only to those with an intact

Rb gene.[18] In other experiments, however, BRCA1 and BRCA2 appear to be associated with signs of growth promotion. Both proteins are increased at S phase, and knockout mouse embryos that die *in utero* exhibit an increase in p21, a decrease in cyclin E, and a reduction in proliferating cells.[19] These data suggest that BRCA1 and BRCA2 serve to support rather than to suppress proliferation. More important, however, are the observations that BRCA1 and BRCA2 are both associated with each other and with the same components of DNA repair, RAD51 and PCNA, especially after DNA damage.[20] The functional consequences of this association are also clear. Cells from a BRCA1 null mouse are defective in transcription-coupled DNA repair.[21] BRCA2 null cells are exquisitely sensitive to γ-irradiation[22] and to chemotherapeutic agents.[23] It is remarkable that two structurally dissimilar genes interact with the same biochemical entities and lead to similar disease phenotypes. The fundamental lessons learned from investigating the BRCA1 and BRCA2, however, are that the primary causes of breast cancer may be related to DNA damage and repair and not to excessive growth.

A characteristic of a cancer cell is the ability to accumulate and survive genetic mutations. Normal cells not only have the ability to identify and repair DNA damage but also to prevent the expansion of mutation-laden daughter cells by suicide mechanisms, such as apoptosis. Defects in DNA repair found in rare disorders such as xeroderma pigmentosum and ataxia-telangiectasia are associated with cancer risk. More recently, however, common human cancers have been linked to abnormalities in repair processes. One example is the hereditary nonpolyposis colorectal cancer (HNPCC) syndrome. HNPCC is an inherited syndrome characterized by increased risk for colon cancer without the associated polyposis seen in carriers of another hereditable cancer syndrome, adenomatous polyposis coli. Affected individuals with HNPCC show signs of a defect in the repair of DNA mismatches. Additions of reductions in the number of two nucleotide repeats found in human DNA (called *microsatellite instability*) are clonally detected in their tumors. This type of DNA abnormality is a signature for a form of repair defect previously studied in bacteria and yeast. When incorrectly paired nucleotides occur in a DNA duplex, either through misincorporations or nucleotide damage, cells use a mismatch repair system to identify and remove the mismatch. This recognition and cleavage is mediated by the protein products of the MSH2, MSH3, MSH6, MLH1, PMS1, and PMS2 genes. HNPCC patients have mutations primarily in MSH2 and MLH1, although mutations in the other mismatch repair genes also are found. The clinical consequence of this molecular defect in humans is the emergence of colon cancers that differ from the sporadic variety and that are characterized by fewer ras and p53 mutations as well as allelic losses. Moreover, colon cancer in HNPCC patients appears to have a better prognosis than their sporadic counterparts.

Advances in molecular biology and their application to cancer research have yielded a wealth of new knowledge uncovering molecular mechanisms that can trigger and sustain uncontrolled growth. From the clinical perspective, it is astonishing that the molecular pathways that lead to cancer can be different in different types of neoplasms, in different tissues, and even in the same type of pathology. Thus, a molecular understanding of cancer clarifies why curing this disease is so difficult, whereas, at the same time, this knowledge provides single targets as well as entire networks of targets for treatments in the future.

INHIBITION OF APOPTOSIS

Earlier on, the study of molecular oncogenesis concentrated on processes that stimulated growth. However, the accumulation of cancer cells can also be accomplished by a decrease in cell loss as well as by an increase in cell proliferation. Current evidence suggests that the abrogation of programmed cell death (apoptosis) is an important mechanism for neoplastic transformation. Normal cells have self-policing mechanisms that activate suicide programs under various conditions. Such conditions are thought to include points where the mutational load of the cell exceeds a critical point. Other processes, such as cytokine signaling (e.g., tumor necrosis factor, interleukin-3 withdrawal) or DNA damage, can trigger a cascade of events culminating in activation of intracellular proteases. These activated proteases lead to the regulated cleavage and destruction of cellular components, including proteins and DNA, and, ultimately, to cell death. The cell exerts exquisite control of this process, using redundant systems to induce or block apoptosis. Some of these control switches are involved in cancer progression and are promising targets for cancer treatment.

The clearest example of an oncogene modulating the apoptotic process is Bcl-2. Bcl-2 is the oncogene involved in the t(14q;18q) translocation frequently found in follicular lymphomas. Bcl-2 blocks apoptosis when overexpressed or inappropriately expressed. In lymphomas, inappropriate expression of bcl-2 may be among the earliest oncogene abnormalities that act to prolong the life span of cells that are prone to accumulate genetic mutations. In experimental lymphomas, bcl-2 does not cause cancer directly but is followed by rearrangements of other oncogenes, such as c-myc, which results in accelerated progression of the tumor. This bcl-2/myc cooperativity highlights another principle of oncogene action—that is, more than one cancer gene must be perturbed for a malignancy to arise. Other bcl-2–related proteins have been identified, all of which are capable of physically interacting with each other as homo- or heterodimers. Bcl-X and bcl-2 are antiapoptotic, whereas overexpression of bax, bak, bcl-X, and BAD induces apoptosis. Thus, the ratio of antiapoptotic to proapoptotic factors determines the cell's "set point" triggering apoptosis. This set point can modulate a cell's responsiveness to injury from radiation and chemotherapy.

More recently, growth factor receptors and other surface signaling molecules have been shown to affect the apoptotic process directly. Many receptor kinases, such as platelet-derived growth factor receptor and Met, recruit and activate phosphatidylinositol 3 kinase. p13-kinase activates the Akt protein kinase, which supports cell survival through its phosphorylation and inactivation of BAD, one of the bcl-2–related proteins that promotes cell death. Therefore, augmented Akt function induced by ligand receptor interactions is predicted to have an antiapoptotic effect. It is not clear why certain tumors genetically alter bcl-2 to alter apoptotic potential, whereas others use alternative biochemical pathways to accomplish the same ends. Nevertheless, cancer may result when genetically abnormal cells are not cleared via apoptosis but are allowed to proliferate, thus accumulating mutations that favor malignant progression and resistance to apoptosis-inducing chemotherapy.

The cancer susceptibility gene, PTEN/MMAC localized to 10q23, is an example of another genetic "guardian" that functions to regulate aspects of cell death and survival. PTEN was identified through position cloning as the gene responsible for Cowden's syndrome. Cowden's syndrome is characterized by gastrointestinal hamartomas, cutaneous trichilemmomas, and increased rates of breast (25% to 50%) and thyroid (3% to 10%) cancers, as well as uterine leiomyomas. Although germline PTEN mutations are operative in a relatively rare disorder, somatic mutations leading to the loss of PTEN function are found in a large number of sporadic cancers, including high-grade gliomas, thyroid cancers, and endometrial cancers, and are circumstantially associated in gastrointestinal, breast, and prostate cancers as well.[24] Transfection of the wild-type PTEN cDNA reduces growth and cell spreading in established cell lines, and mice that have one disrupted PTEN allele have a high rate of tumor formation in the form of lymphomas, teratocarcinomas, and liver and prostatic cancer.[25] Thus, PTEN satisfies the classic definition of a tumor suppressor. The function of PTEN is as a multifunctional phosphatase that removes phosphorylates from tyrosine and serine residues, as well as from phosphatidylinositols, especially phosphatidylinositol(3,4,5)triphosphate. The most important biochemical consequence of PTEN action is to disarm the PI3'-kinase/AKT pathway.[26,27] Specifically, mutations in PTEN are associated with an increase in AKT activity, which is a pivotal member of a pathway that induces cell survival and motility. It is thought that AKT phosphorylates the BCL2 proapoptotic homologue, BAD, resulting in a block to apoptosis.[28] Evidence also suggests that activated AKT mediates cell-cycle progression by phosphorylation of the CDK inhibitor p27, resulting in its inactivation via cytosolic sequestration.[29] Thus, PTEN mutations render cells more resistant to cell death signals. This mode of cancer induction is akin to the antiapoptotic effects of the bcl2 oncogene up-regulated by the t(14;18) in follicular lymphoma.

COOPERATIVITY OF ONCOGENES AND TUMOR SUPRESSOR GENES

The current state of knowledge of tumor suppressors/genetic guardians paints a complex picture of how multiple suppressor genes interact with each other and with oncogenes to generate the cancer state. For example, BRCA1 and BRCA2 bind with each other and with RAD51 and PCNA, and PTEN intersects with AKT, which was originally found as a retroviral oncogene, v-akt, that causes lymphomas in infected mice. The AKT protooncogene has also been noted to be amplified in human ovarian cancers. Thus, activation of the PI3'-kinase/AKT pathway, either through crippling the tumor-suppressing phosphatase PTEN or augmenting the activity of the AKT kinase, can lead to cancer.

A more dramatic example of the confluence of oncogenic processes has been uncovered in the analysis of the TGF-β pathway in gastrointestinal carcinogenesis. It has long been known that the peptide factor, TGF-β, can inhibit tumor formation and that tumor progression is associated with loss of response to TGF-β. This loss of response now appears to be due to the disruption of the type II TGF-β receptor. TGF-β acts by heterodimerizing the cognate type I and II receptors (TGF-βRI and TGF-βRII), leading to the phosphorylation of the type I receptor and engagement of the downstream pathway. Many tumors, especially colorectal cancers, have frameshift mutations in a short polyadenine tract within the gene that generates a truncated TGF-β protein that lacks kinase activity.[30] Interestingly, this frameshift mutation occurs most commonly in cancers that bear aberrations in mismatch repair, including those from patients with HNPCC, and occurs at the switch from colonic adenoma to malignant carcinoma.[30] The TGF-β signaling pathway requires engagement and phosphorylation by the activated receptors with cytoplasmic SMAD proteins. Activated SMADs form heterodimers between SMAD1 or SMAD2 with SMAD4, enter the nucleus, and interact with DNA-binding proteins to induce transcription of TGF-β–responsive genes.[31,32] The importance of this sequence is that SMAD4, which is an essential component in the signaling pathway, is a major tumor suppressor gene found to be disrupted in 50% of human pancreatic cancers and, to a lesser extent, in gastric, breast, ovarian, and prostatic cancers. Thus, the TGF-β pathway alone involves three functional nodes that have significant roles in human cancers: mismatch repair, TGF-βRII, and SMAD4.

EPIGENETICS AND CANCER

Epigenetics refers to heritable modifications in gene function that do not involve a change in DNA sequence. One very important epigenetic mechanism involves DNA methylation at the carbon-5 position of cytosine, where the cytosine is followed on the same strand by guanine. Between 2% and 7% of cytosines in human DNA are modified by methylation. The pattern of DNA methylation is passed on to progeny when DNA replicates and a cell divides. DNA methylation is typically associated with genes that are silent, whereas DNA that is actively transcribed is relatively undermethylated. Genome-wide hypomethylation of DNA has long been associated with tumor cells.[33] Interestingly, specific regions of hypermethylation in tumor cells have been proposed to function in the silencing of tumor suppressor genes.[34] Gaudet et al.[35,36] created knockout mice with levels of DNA methyltransferase 1 (Dnmt1, the enzyme that maintains DNA methylation patterns in somatic cells) that were reduced by 90%. This resulted in mice that developed aggressive T-cell lymphomas at 4 to 8 months accompanied by a high frequency of trisomy 15. Hence, DNA hypomethylation may play a role in tumorigenesis and chromosomal instability.

Gene imprinting is another epigenetic phenomenon. Each human cell contains two copies (or alleles) of each gene, a maternal copy and a paternal copy. Imprinting is an epigenetic process occurring in some genes during embryonic development whereby one of the parental alleles is silenced while the other parental allele remains active. Errors in gene imprinting have been attributed to congenital diseases, such as Beckwith-Wiedemann syndrome, and to human cancer.[37] The IGF-2 gene is normally maternally imprinted, with expression occurring from the paternal allele. Development of the pediatric Wilms' tumor is associated with biallelic IGF-2 expression.[38] Epigenetic imprinting can become altered over time, resulting in disease. Loss of IGF-2 imprinting is found in up to 40% of colon cancers and is believed to produce higher expression levels of growth factor, resulting in dysregulated proliferation.[39]

Chromatin remodeling is an epigenetic process involved in the regulation of gene transcription, which may play a role in oncogenesis or tumor progression. Histones can be modified by acetylation, methylation, ADP-ribosylation, phosphorylation, and ubiquitinylation. Such modifications appear be important in regulating gene function. For a gene to be transcribed, it must become physically accessible to transcriptional machinery. Hence, genes that are tightly wrapped around histones are functionally repressed. Histone acetyl-transferases (HATs), such as core-binding protein (CBP/p300), are important in acetylating histones and acting as coactivators in promoting gene transcription.[40,41] HATs putatively function to unwind DNA and allow access of transcription factors to their DNA sequence-specific regulatory elements. Conversely, histone acetylases (HDACs), such as N-COR and SMRT, remodel chromatin by deacetylating histones, functioning as corepressors in silencing gene expression.[42,43] Altered function of HATs and HDACs is associated with several human cancers. CBP is targeted in chromosomal translocations in human leukemias [t(11;16) and t(8;16)], whereas several oncoproteins (Aml1-Eto, PML-RAR) have been shown to interact with N-COR to repress gene expression, resulting in a loss of cell-cycle control or block in cell differentiation.[44] HDAC inhibitors have shown some promise in the treatment of certain cancers as promoters of differentiation.

STEM CELLS AND DIFFERENTIATION ARREST

Tumor cells possess unique properties that distinguish them from the surrounding normal tissue cells. Interestingly, many of these properties (self-renewal, immortality, lack of differentiation, invasion potential) are also attributed to stem cells and some committed progenitor cells. Given the similarity in properties, it has been hypothesized that cancer may begin as alterations in stem cells[45] or committed progenitors and may constitute an aberration in organogenesis involving differentiation arrest. This concept has been most explored in the hematopoietic system, in which different forms of acute leukemias are manifested by tumor cells arrested at specific stages in well-characterized maturation lineages. For example, acute lymphoblastic pre-B-cell leukemia is comprised of tumor cells arrested at the pre-B-cell stage of maturation. Acute promyelocytic leukemia is made up of tumor cells that are blocked in differentiation at the promyelocyte stage of myeloid maturation. Acute promyelocytic leukemia is a consequence of the t(15;17) translocation, which creates the chimeric oncoprotein PML-RAR, believed to repress normal retinoid acid–responsive gene transcription required for maturation.[46] Interestingly, treatment with supraphysiologic levels of all-*trans*-retinoic acid is able to overcome the repression and permit differentiation of tumor cells corresponding with decreased tumor load. Unfortunately, over time, tumor cells generally become resistant to treatment with all-*trans*-retinoic acid.

Homeobox genes encode transcription factors that are master regulators of differentiation in development and are targets of chromosomal translocations in some leukemias. HoxA9 and Meis1 are constitutively expressed in the majority of acute myeloid leukemias. *In vitro* myeloid assays suggest that HoxA9 and Meis1 cooperate to block myeloid differentiation along the signaling pathways initiated by the cytokines granulocyte colony-stimulating factor and macrophage colony-stimulating factor, in addition to promoting self-renewal in response to stem cell factor.[47,48] MLL is a common target for translocations in acute leukemias and forms chimeric oncoproteins with up to 30 distinct partners. MLL fusions in early hematopoietic stem cells or progenitors appear to drive aberrant Hox gene expression,[49] leading to differentiation arrest in acute leukemia.

Hematopoietic stem cells have been isolated and used in transplants for the treatment of hematopoietic cancers for many years. It is likely that epithelial stem cell counterparts and committed progenitors (that have yet to be isolated) exist in each organ system. Epithelial and mesenchymal stem cells and their downstream progenitors may play a role in the tumorigenesis of carcinomas and sarcomas. Such cells are likely to possess proliferative, self-renewal, immortal, and invasion properties attributed to the respective cancers of their lineages. The more that is understood about stem cells, committed progenitors, normal differentiation, and organogenesis, the better insight might be gained into the etiology of cancer and opportunities for novel stem cell–based therapies.

POSTGENOME CHALLENGE FOR MOLECULAR MEDICINE

Sequencing the human genome has provided new tools and insights that will continue to enhance the understanding of the genetic mechanisms underlying cancer. Before the completion of the human genome, a leading method for rapid gene discovery used single-pass partial sequencing of cDNA clones from one or both ends to generate expressed sequence tags. This strategy was widely successful when applied to humans and other species.[50] Before 1991 and the development of the expressed sequence tag method, sequence data existed for fewer than 3000 human genes (GenBank release 68, June 1991). In less than 13 years (2003), the entire human genome sequence, containing on the order of six billion DNA base pairs, had been elucidated. Analysis of the human genome reveals an estimate of 30,000 to 40,000 genes, fewer than the 100,000 previously predicted.[1,3] The combination of data on gene expression and putative gene functions inferred from sequence similarities and motif analysis will provide a powerful means of assessing the transcriptional activity of the genome in the cells and tissue before, during, and after disease. For the next generation of scientists and clinicians, identification of a new gene will be as rare as finding a new species of mammal. Future challenges include understanding the function of proteins encoded by genes, the multiplicity of regulated protein pathways controlling cellular physiology, the specific lesions in these pathways that result in human disease, and development of molecularly targeted therapeutics to restore appropriate regulation.

Completion of the human genome sequence[1,3] is just the beginning of what promises to be a new era in medicine.[2] The current challenge is to generate a comprehensive understanding of the "software and the hardware" of the cell and the organism. Less than 2% of the noninfectious human disease burden is monogenic in nature. The rest (98%) is polygenic—caused by multiple genes at once, or is epigenetic—caused by nongenetic or postgenetic alterations in cellular molecules. Consequently, elucidating disease mechanisms, and full penetration of the causal mechanisms driving carcinogenesis and cancer progression, requires analysis tools ranging from direct DNA sequencing, to messenger RNA (mRNA) expression monitoring, to protein sequencing, to protein localization studies, and, finally, metabolic or physiologic profiling and the development of molecular network maps.

A further essential phase will be a description of the normal range of human polymorphisms (base variations in the genome), which may provide a starting point for correlating genetic variance with disease states or predisposition to disease. The final physiologic state is further complicated because biologic diversity causally associated with disease may be due to posttranslational processes regulated by the cellular environment. These changes cannot be inferred from known DNA variance. Hence, elucidation of the human proteome will involve identification of all human proteins, with corresponding repertoire of potential modifications and functional correlation. Thus, a complete understanding of the molecular basis of cancer depends on a multidisciplinary approach combining genetics, pathology, protein structure and function, cell biology, bioinformatics, computer science, and clinical medicine.

Finding all the expressed human genes is a different task from sequencing the genome itself. This is because only a small proportion of the genome comprises the actual expressed genes and their regulatory elements in any given cell type. The actual number of human genes expressed during a lifetime may be 30,000 to 40,000. However, at any time, for any individual cell in any given tissue, the number of genes "in use" may be as few as 4000. Of this 4000, only a small proportion may be susceptible to the influence of carcinogenic events. These may be genes whose protein products are critical regulators of pathways controlling proliferation, differentiation, or apoptosis. Thus, an important goal for molecular profiling of cancer is to identify a subset of expressed genes that are correlated with, or causally related to, the development and progression of cancer. Setting aside hereditary susceptibility, it is likely that the majority of cancers may originate in tissue that starts with a completely normal genome. Carcinogenic events produce heritable genetic alterations that expand in microscopic premalignant states, such as hyperplasia and dysplasia, before frank malignant cancer ensues. Identification of the important genetic derangements and the causally important genes and proteins depends on direct analysis of actual human cancer tissues, combined with insights gained using animal and cell culture methods. The massive profiling of genes associated with cancer progression is now possible using new technology for microdissection and array hybridization.

TISSUE MICRODISSECTION TECHNOLOGY BRINGS MOLECULAR ANALYSIS TO THE TISSUE LEVEL

Molecular analysis of pure cell populations in their native tissue environment will be an important component of the next generation of medical genetics. Accomplishing this goal is much more difficult than just grinding up a piece of tissue and applying the extracted molecules to a panel of assays. This is because tissues are complicated three-dimensional structures composed of large numbers of different types of interacting cell populations. The cell subpopulation of interest may constitute a tiny fraction of the total tissue volume. For example, a biopsy of breast tissue harboring a malignant tumor usually contains the following types of cell populations: (1) fat cells in the abundant adipose tissue surrounding the ducts, (2) normal

epithelium and myoepithelium in the branching ducts, (3) fibroblasts and endothelial cells in the stroma and blood vessels, (4) premalignant carcinoma cells in the *in situ* lesions, and (5) clusters of invasive carcinoma. If the goal is to analyze the genetic changes in the premalignant cells or the malignant cells, these subpopulations are frequently located in microscopic regions occupying less than 5% of the tissue volume. After the computer adage "garbage in, garbage out," if the extract of a complex tissue is analyzed using a sophisticated technology, the output will be severely compromised if the input material is contaminated by the wrong cells. Culturing cell populations from fresh tissue is one approach to reducing contamination. However, cultured cells may not accurately represent the molecular events taking place in the actual tissue from which they were derived. Assuming methods are successful to isolate and grow the tissue cells of interest, the gene expression pattern of the cultured cells is influenced by the culture environment and can be quite different from the genes expressed in the native tissue state. This is because the cultured cells are separated from the tissue elements that regulate gene expression, such as soluble factors, extracellular matrix molecules, and cell-cell communication. Thus, the problem of cellular heterogeneity has been a significant barrier to the molecular analysis of normal and diseased tissue. This problem can now be overcome by new developments in the field of tissue microdissection.

Analysis of critical gene expression and protein patterns in normal developing and diseased tissue progression requires the microdissection and extraction of a microscopic homogeneous cellular subpopulation from its complex tissue milieu.[51,52] This subpopulation can then be compared to adjacent, interacting, but distinct, subpopulations of cells in the same tissue. The method of procurement of pure cell populations from heterogeneous tissue should fully preserve the state of the cell molecules if it is to allow quantitative analysis, particularly in sensitive amplification methods based on PCR, reverse transcriptase-PCR, or enzymatic function. Laser capture microdissection (LCM) has been developed to provide scientists with a fast and dependable method of capturing and preserving specific cells from tissue, under direct microscopic visualization. With the ease of procuring a homogeneous population of cells from a complex tissue using the LCM, the approaches to molecular analysis of pathologic processes are significantly enhanced.[51–54] The mRNA from microdissected cancer lesions has been used as the starting material to produce cDNA libraries, microchip microarrays, differential display, and other techniques to find new genes or mutations.

The development of LCM allows investigators to determine specific gene expression patterns from tissues of individual patients. Pure populations of cells can be obtained and RNA extracted, copied to cDNA, and hybridized to thousands of genes on a cDNA microchip microarray. In this manner, an individualized molecular profile can be obtained for each histologically identified pathology (Fig. 2-2). Using such multiplex analysis, investigators will be able to correlate the pattern of expressed genes with the etiology and response to treatment. A patient's risk for disease and appropriate choice of treatment could, in the future, be personalized based on the profile. A growing clinical database of such results could be used to develop a minimal subset of key markers that will lead to a revolutionary approach for early detection and accurate diagnosis of disease.

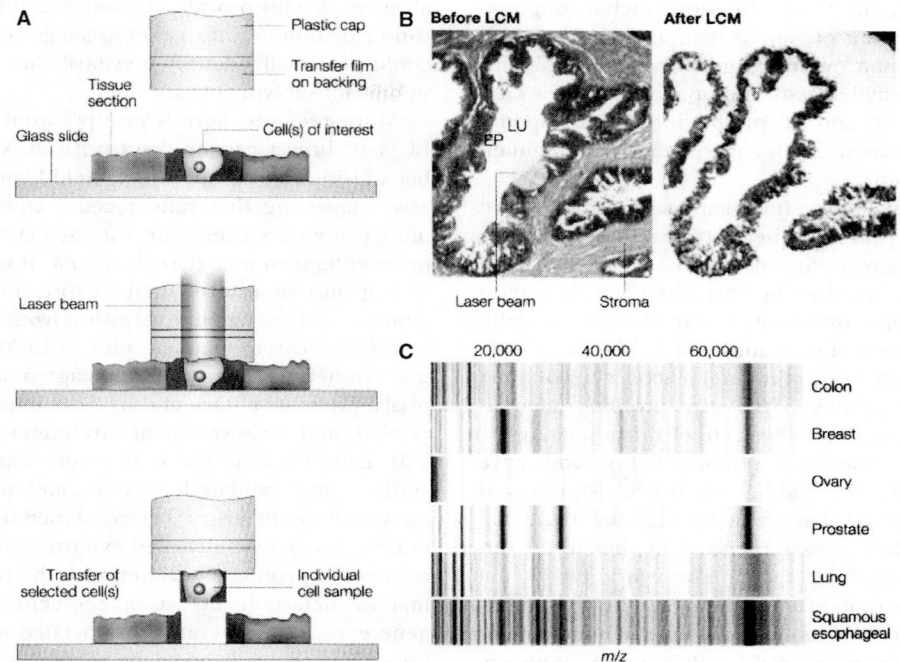

FIGURE 2-2. Laser capture microdissection (LCM). LCM is a technology for procuring pure cell populations from a stained tissue section under direct microscopic visualization. Tissues contain heterogeneous cellular populations (e.g., epithelium, cancer cells, fibroblasts, endothelium, and immune cells). The diseased cellular population of interest usually comprises only a small percentage of the tissue volume. LCM directly procures the subpopulation of cells selected for study, while leaving behind all of the contaminating cells. A stained section of the heterogeneous tissue is mounted on a glass microscope slide and viewed under high magnification (**A**). The experimenter selects the individual cell(s) to be studied using a joystick. The chosen cells are lifted out of the tissue by the action of a laser pulse. The infrared laser, mounted in the optical axis of the microscope, locally expands a thermoplastic polymer to reach down and capture the cell beneath the laser pulse. When the film is lifted from the tissue section, only the pure cells for study are excised from the heterogeneous cellular population (**B**). The DNA, RNA, and proteins of the captured cells remain intact and unperturbed. Using LCM, one to several thousand tissue cells can be captured in less than 5 minutes. Using appropriate buffers, the cellular constituents are solubilized and subjected to microanalysis methods. Proteins from all compartments of the cell can be readily procured. Protein conformation and enzymatic activity are retained if the tissues are frozen or fixed in ethanol before sectioning. The extracted proteins can be analyzed by any method that has sufficient sensitivity. An example is shown for surface-enhanced laser-desorption ionization fingerprinting of microdissected cancer cells (**C**). Each histologic type of cancer has a characteristic ion spectrum. The character of the spectra might reflect cancer-specific differences in proteomic composition. EP, epithelium; LU, lumen. (See Color Fig. 2-2 in the CD-ROM.)

Efficient coupling of LCM of serial tissue sections with multiplex molecular analysis techniques should lead to sensitive and quantitative methods to visualize three-dimensional interactions between morphologic elements of the tissue. For example, it will be possible to trace the gene expression pattern along the length of a prostate gland or breast duct to examine the progression of neoplastic development. The end result will be a new era in the integration of molecular biology with tissue morphogenesis and pathology.

COMPLEMENTARY DNA MICROARRAYS AS A TOOL TO ANALYZE GENE EXPRESSION PATTERNS IN HUMAN CANCER

Every oncologist is faced daily with the biologic heterogeneity of cancer emergence, aggressiveness, and treatment response in individual patients. Every pathologist is faced daily with the enormous histologic diversity of human neoplasms. In the last

century, diagnostic determination of malignancy by pathologists has been largely achieved via microscopic morphologic characterization of paraffin sections of tumor samples. The advent of immunohistochemistry in the last century and use of antibody stains to histologically subclassify tumors further has added a significant dimension to clinical diagnostics. However, tumor diagnostics are largely still made by morphologic patterns recognized by the well-trained human eye. It is assumed that the morphologic microscopic appearance (e.g., staining pattern, nuclear shape and contour, cellular configuration, and pleomorphism) of a particular neoplastic lesion that "spells" cancer is the outward manifestation of molecular changes that are occurring inside the interacting tissue cell populations. It is further assumed that scores of molecules and genes can be involved in the behavior of an individual patient's tumor. When examining cancer at the genetic level, one also sees heterogeneity. This is evident in the variable presence of chromosomal translocations, deletions of suppressor genes, and numbers of chromosomes. Consequently, it is critical for molecular oncology of the future to adopt high-throughput technology to survey panels of genes,[5] ranging from hundreds to even the whole human expressed gene set, and apply this technology to (1) accurately classify tumor and pathologic entities in individual patients and (2) predict individual response to current varying treatment regimens to choose the regimen best suited for the patient.

In response to this challenge, investigators in the public and the private sector have sought to perfect gene-chip arrays that can be used to survey great patterns of gene expression. The change in the pattern can then be correlated with histomorphology, clinical behavior, or response to treatment. Typically, the analysis takes the form of rows and rows of oligonucleotide strands lined up in dots on a miniature silicon chip or glass slide or sheet of nitrocellulose. Transcript profiling microarrays work as follows: First, the RNA is extracted from the tumor tissue, amplified, and labeled with a fluorescent or radioactive probe. This assumes that the highly labeled RNA is preserved when the tissue is extracted. The labeled tissue total RNA, containing the mRNA of the expressed genes, is applied to the surface of the chip or sheet. After appropriate hybridization, the relative intensity of the signal for each spot on the chip corresponds to the abundance of its matching mRNA species and, hence, reflects the expression level for its gene. With appropriate pattern recognition software, it is then possible to assemble a global score for the gene study set represented on the substratum.[4,5,55,56]

Tremendous progress has been made in the use of DNA/RNA arrays to analyze gene expression patterns in human cancer cell lines and human cancer tissue. In early studies, Brown's group used cDNA microarrays to study 60 cancer cell lines used by the National Cancer Institute to screen anticancer drugs.[56] When they classified the cell lines based on the gene expression subclasses, they obtained a correspondence to the ostensible cell-type origin of the cancer cell line (i.e., epithelial or fibroblast or hematopoietic). Specific features of the cell line expression pattern appeared to correlate with the growth rate in culture or drug metabolism. These investigators then went on to use the cultured cell gene expression pattern as a template for comparison to RNA extracted from actual pieces of cancer tissue. They found that the gene pattern of the cancer tissue varied greatly from one cancer type to the next. Moreover, the pattern of a carcinoma gene expression appeared to correspond with the cell lines that had an epithelial origin. This study provided direct evidence that tissue pathology was heterogeneous at the level of gene expression patterns and offered hope that this information could potentially be applied to predict patient outcome.

The first major clinical correlation of gene expression patterns with disease outcome was provided by Staudt's group.[55] Diffuse, large B-cell lymphoma (DLBCL), the most common subtype of non-Hodgkin's lymphoma, is clinically heterogeneous. Sixty percent of the patients die from the disease, and the remainder respond well to the current therapy and have prolonged survival. This variability in natural history correlated with a distinct pattern of gene expression revealed by DNA arrays. The group identified two molecularly distinct forms of DLBCL, one that had a gene expression pattern indicative of a B-cell differentiation pattern. The second type expressed genes induced during *in vitro* activation of peripheral B cells. Patients with the germinal B-like DLBCL had a significantly better over-

all survival. This provided evidence that the molecular classification of tumors into general categories of gene expression could potentially identify previously undetected and clinically significant subtypes of cancer.

More recently, Sgroi's group[57] went further to combine LCM of breast cancer tissue with cDNA arrays. This study began with a test of the widely held hypothesis of tumorigenesis, suggesting that cancer cells acquire inherently malignant properties over time with selection of mutations that favor enhanced malignancy, such as invasion and metastasis. The group monitored gene expression to observe which genes would change in expression from precancerous lesions to invasive carcinoma. Samples of LCM-procured pure normal epithelium, premalignant stage of atypical ductal hyperplasia, preinvasive stage of ductal carcinoma (ductal carcinoma *in situ*), and invasive ductal carcinoma were compared (Fig. 2-3). Differences in the *in vivo* gene expression profile were verified and validated by real-time quantitative PCR and immunohistochemistry. The combined use of LCM and cDNA microarray analysis revealed extensive similarities in the gene expression profiles associated with the progression from normal to metastatic breast cancer cells. This suggested that gene expression alterations associated with the potential for invasive growth observed in invasive ductal carcinoma are already present in preinvasive stages (atypical ductal hyperplasia and ductal carcinoma *in situ*)! This study demonstrated that *in vivo* gene expression profiling can be done on specific tissue cell populations and that the results of the cDNA arrays correlated well with the RTQ-PCR analysis and immunohistochemistry. Consequently, cDNA arrays can be used to (1) uncover patterns that correlate with the biology and may generate new hypotheses explaining cancer progression and (2) find lead candidate genes that may serve as future markers or drug targets.

Cancer researchers have made significant progress in the identification of molecular signatures of cancer through the use of genomic technologies. The use of DNA microarrays has created molecular phenotypes for many tumors, including brain, breast, colon, gastric, kidney, leukemia, lymphoma, lung, melanoma, ovary, prostate, and small, round blue-cell tumors of childhood. In a subset of these studies, the gene expression profiles strongly suggest that this information would improve diagnosis and predict clinical outcome when compared with the standardized prognostic criteria, such as tumor grade, tumor size, patient age, and patient performance status. However, these breakthroughs have been qualified successes. The lack of a standardized method for data collection, data analysis, and validation has made it difficult to rigorously compare studies from different laboratories and has thus hampered the introduction of this type of data into clinical medicine. Ntzani and Ioannidis[58] conducted a study evaluating the predictive performances of DNA microarray molecular profiling studies in oncology published between 1995 and April 2003. They found variable prognostic performances with the median number of samples being only 25, with only 26% of studies attempting independent validation or cross-validation of their proposed findings and only 23% adjusting for other known predictors. Conclusions of their study include the need for larger studies with appropriate clinical designs, adjustment for known predictors, and proper validation.

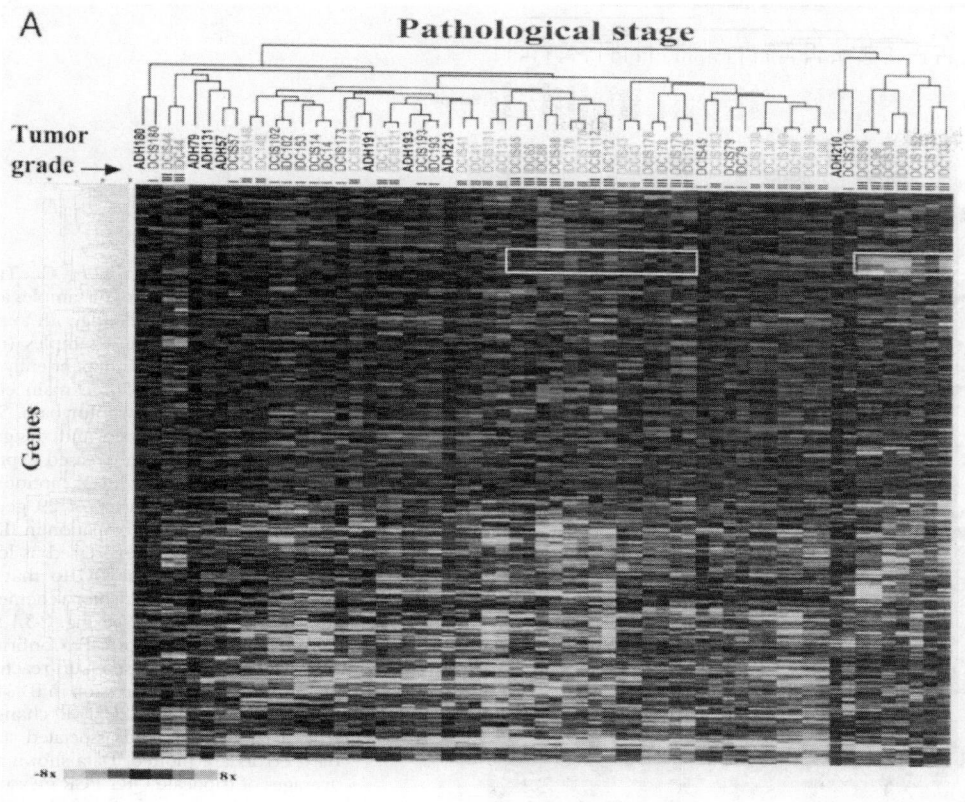

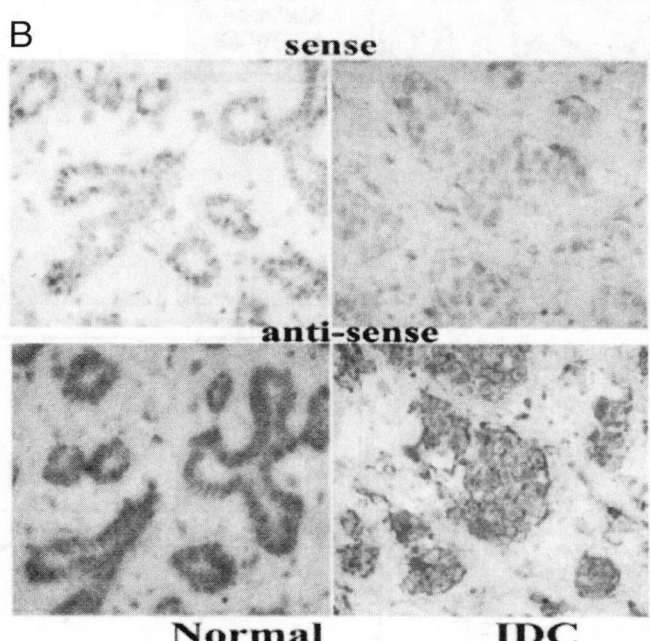

FIGURE 2-3. **A,B:** Gene expression profiles of breast cancer progression. **A:** Two-dimensional hierarchic clustering of the data matrix consisting of 1940 genes by 61 samples of different pathologic stages. Rows represent genes, and columns represent samples, which are color-coded by tumor grade (blue, green, and red correspond to grades I, II, and III, respectively). Color scale is shown at bottom left. **B:** *In situ* hybridization of CRIP1 messenger RNA. DIG-labeled RNA probes from the antisense and the sense (negative control) strands of CRIP1 transcript were hybridized to sections of normal and invasive ductal carcinoma (IDC) components of case 179. Hybridization signals were visualized by alkaline phosphatase–conjugated anti-DIG antibody using fast red as substrate. (*Figure continues*)

Despite the need for universal standardization guidelines for the clinical use of DNA microarray technology, several validated studies have demonstrated great utility for clinical applications. Based on the published work of van't Veer et al.[59,60] and van de Vijver et al.,[61] which predicted potential for metastasis in stage I to II breast cancer patients based on the expression profiles of key 70 genes, the Netherlands Cancer Institute in Amsterdam announced in 2003 that it would become the first institution in the world to use DNA microarray analysis to make treatment decisions regarding women with breast cancer.[62] In 2003, four major university hospitals in the United States were incorporating gene expression patterns into clinical trials of breast cancer. However, the integration of clinical genomics with developing clinical proteomic technologies[63] holds the most promise for the ultimate goal of developing personalized cancer diagnostics and individualized therapies.

C

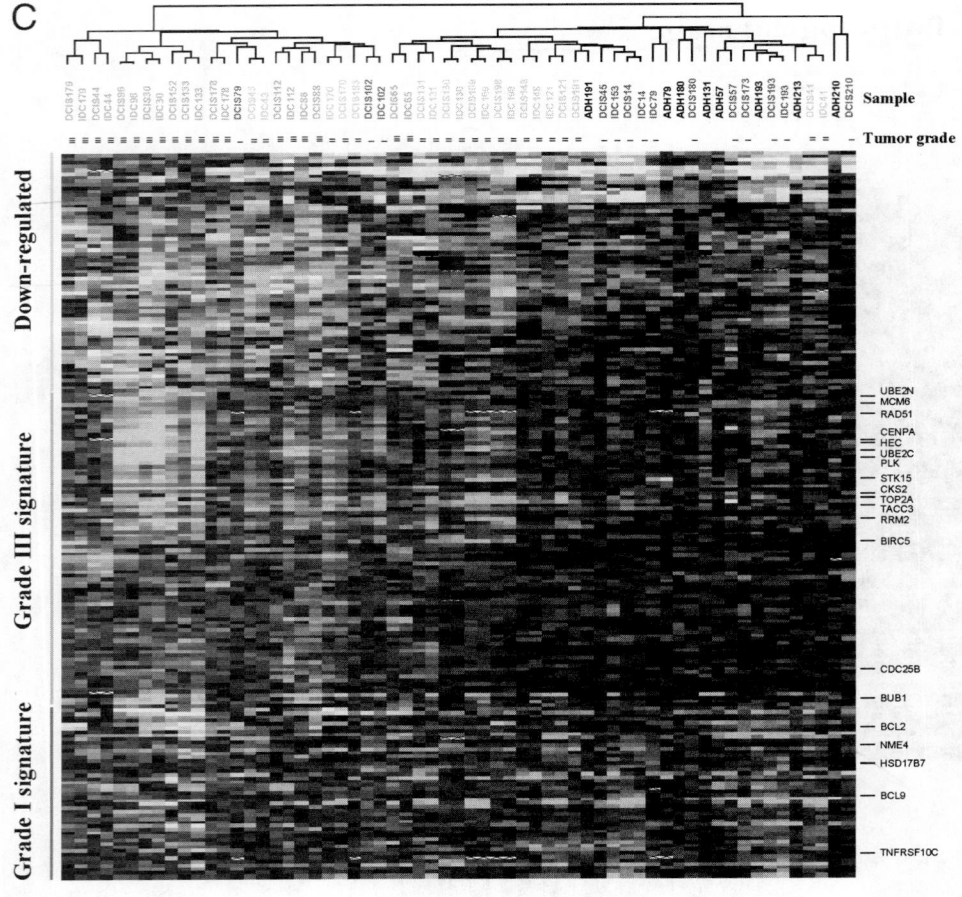

FIGURE 2-3. (*Continued*) **C:** Two-dimensional clustering of 61 samples and the top 200 genes correlating with tumor grade. Genes (rows) and samples (columns) were clustered independently by hierarchic clustering. Three main clusters are highlighted by color bars. See Fig. 2-3*A* for color scale and designations. **D,E:** Genes with increased expression in IDC relative to ductal carcinoma *in situ* (DCIS). **D:** Cluster of 29 genes showing consistent up-regulation in IDC. Expression values are expressed as log2 ratios of expression in IDC to that in patient-matched DCIS. Color scheme is shown at bottom left; see Fig. 2-3*A* for sample color designations. **E:** Confirmation by QRT–polymerase chain reaction (PCR) of increased expression in IDC for CKS2, RRM2, and UBE2C. Fold changes from DCIS to IDC and associated standard errors are plotted. Data shown are averages of triplicate QRT-PCR measurements. *Values outside the scale in the y-axis. (From ref. 57, with permission.) (See Color Fig. 2-3*A–D* in the CD-ROM.)

D   E

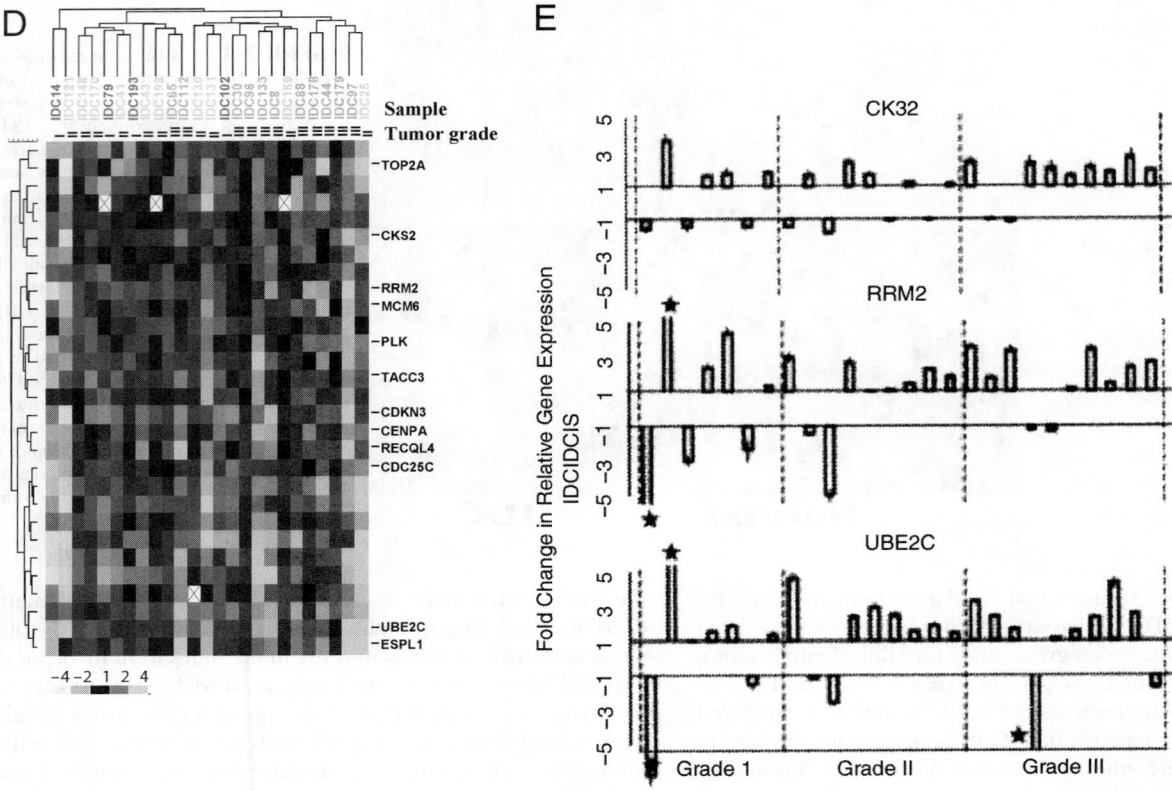

BEYOND FUNCTIONAL GENOMICS TO CANCER PROTEOMICS

Whereas DNA is an information archive, proteins do all the work of the cell. The existence of a given DNA sequence does not guarantee the synthesis of a corresponding protein. The DNA sequence is also not sufficient to describe protein structure, function, and cellular location.[64] This is because protein complexity and versatility stem from context-dependent posttranslational processes, such as phosphorylation, sulfation, or glycosylation. Moreover, the DNA code does not provide information about how proteins link together into networks and functional machines in the cell. In fact, the activation of a protein signal pathway, causing a cell to migrate, die, or initiate division, can immediately take place before any changes occur in DNA/RNA gene expression. Consequently, the technology to drive the Molecular Medicine Revolution into the third phase is emerging from protein analytic methods.

The term *proteome*, which denotes all the proteins expressed by a genome, was first coined in late 1994 at the Siena two-dimensional (2D) gel electrophoresis meeting. *Proteomics* is proclaimed as the next step after genomics. A goal of investigators in this exciting field is to assemble a complete library of all the proteins. Only a small percentage of the proteome has been cataloged. Because "PCR for proteins" does not exist, sequencing the order of 20 possible amino acids in a given protein remains relatively slow and labor intensive compared to nucleotide sequencing. Although a number of new technologies are being introduced for high-throughput protein characterization and discovery,[54,65,66] the mainstay of protein identification continues to be 2D gel electrophoresis. 2D electrophoresis can separate proteins by molecular weight in one dimension and charge in a second dimension. When a mixture of proteins is applied to the 2D gel, individual proteins in the mixture are separated out into signature locations on the display, depending on their individual size and charge. Each signature is a "spot" on the gel that can constitute a unique single-protein species. The protein spot can be procured from the gel, and a partial amino acid sequence can be read. In this manner, known proteins can be monitored for changes in abundance under treatment or new proteins can be identified. An experimental 2D gel image can be captured and overlayed digitally with known archived 2D gels. In this way it is possible to immediately highlight proteins that are differentially abundant in one state versus another (e.g., tumor vs. normal or before and after hormone treatment).

2D gels have traditionally required large amounts of protein-starting material equivalent to millions of cells. Thus, their application has been limited to cultured cells or ground-up heterogeneous tissue. Not unexpectedly, this approach does not provide an accurate picture of the proteins that are in use by cells in real tissue. Tissues are complicated structures composed of hundreds of interacting cell populations in specialized spatial configurations. The fluctuating proteins expressed by cells in tissues may bear little resemblance to the proteins made by cultured cells that are torn from their tissue context and reacting to a new culture environment. Proteins extracted from ground-up tissue represent an averaging-out of proteins from all the heterogeneous tissue subpopulations. For example, in the case of breast tissue, the glandular epithelium constitutes a small proportion of the tissue: The vast majority is stroma and adipose. Thus, it has previously been impossible to obtain a clear snapshot of gene or protein expression within normal or diseased tissue cell subpopulations.

To address the tissue-context problem, new technology is again coming to the rescue; creating *tissue proteomics* is an exciting expanding discipline. Two major technologic approaches have been successfully used to sample macromolecules directly from subpopulations of human tissue cells. The first technology is LCM, used to procure specific tissue cell subpopulations under direct microscopic visualization of a standard stained frozen or fixed tissue section on a glass microscope slide. Tissue cells procured by LCM have been used for highly sensitive and reproducible proteomic analysis using 2D gels and other analytic methods.[66,67]

A second major approach to isolate tissue cell subpopulations is affinity cell sorting of disaggregated cells from pieces of fresh tissue. A highly notable application of this technology in the field of breast physiology is the result of a collaboration between Oxford Glycosciences and the Ludwig Institute.[54] In this study the investigators separated and purified normal human breast luminal and myoepithelial cells from reduction mammoplasty specimens using double-antibody magnetic affinity cell sorting and Dynabead magnetic sedimentation. After using enzymatic treatments and various incubation, separation, and washing steps, the investigators obtained purified luminal and myoepithelial cells in yields of 5×10^6 to 2×10^7. Proteins from these cell populations were then analyzed by using 2D gels. A master image for each cell type comprising a total of 1738 distinct proteins was derived. The investigators found 170 protein spots that were elevated twofold or more between the two populations; 51 of these were further characterized by tandem mass spectroscopy. The proteins preferential to the myoepithelial cells contained muscle-specific enzymes and structural proteins consistent with the contractile muscle–related derivation of these cell types.

A pathologic hallmark of early cancer progression from carcinoma *in situ* to invasive cancer is the loss or redistribution of myoepithelial cells. The conspicuous absence of myoepithelial cells in breast cancer progression could mean that these cells produce suppressor proteins that normally keep the malignant cells in check. Thus, one or more of the proteins identified in tissue myoepithelial cells could be candidate cancer prevention molecules.

The complicated changing pattern of protein expression should contain important information about the pathologic process taking place in the cells of the actual tissue. This pattern of protein information could provide correlates with pathologic state or response to therapy. Using a protein biochip that classified protein populations into molecular weight classes, Paweletz et al.[68] showed distinct protein patterns of normal, premalignant, and malignant cancer cells microdissected from human tissue. Furthermore, they reported that different histologic types of cancer and tissue (ovarian, esophageal, prostate, breast, and hepatic) exhibited distinct protein profiles. Such a means to rapidly display a pattern of expressed proteins from microscopic tissue cellular populations will potentially be an important enabling technology for pharmacoproteomics, molecular pathology, and drug intervention monitoring.

MOLECULAR DIAGNOSTICS AND INDIVIDUALIZED CANCER THERAPY

The evolution of human disease, on a functional level, involves alterations on genomic and corresponding proteomic levels. Genetic or epigenetic defects are selected during cancer progression because they cooperate to orchestrate alterations in protein networks generating a survival advantage for the target cell. Altered signal transduction pathways may lead to increased growth of tumor cells, blockage of apoptosis, differentiation aberrations, or invasion and metastasis. A goal of functional proteomics is to develop "circuit maps" of protein pathways regulating proliferation, apoptosis, and differentiation in normal cells and diseased cells. The advantage of the emerging technology of protein microarrays is the possibility of profiling cellular signaling pathways in a manner not possible by gene arrays. In the future, it may be possible to map the functional state of key pathways within a patient's tumor cells, allowing the identification of molecular lesions within cooperating dysregulated pathways. The advancement of this technology may serve as a foundation for the development of personalized cancer therapies. It is theoretically feasible to administer combination therapy targeting multiple interdependent points along a pathogenic pathway or targeting multiple distinct yet cooperating dysregulated pathways. The success of the Bcr-Abl tyrosine kinase inhibitor Gleevec (STI 571) in targeting the proliferative signaling pathway altered in chronic myelogenous leukemia[69–71] is a groundbreaking model for the development of additional molecular inhibitors to target key pathways that are altered in oncogenesis.

PROTEIN MICROARRAYS: DIAGNOSING ABERRANT PROTEIN SIGNALING CIRCUITS IN CANCER

Proteins assemble themselves into networks through a variety of protein–protein interactions and posttranslational modifications. The amino acid sequence of a protein determines its three-dimensional shape. It is this shape, and the surface presentation of nested amino acid motifs [e.g., SH2 (src homology) and SH3 domains and zinc fingers], that enables the highly selective recognition between protein partners in a communication circuit. These domains provide specific coupling points for defined regulated protein–protein interactions, resulting in changes in protein conformation or states of activity. Disruption of these dysregulated interactions in cancer cells may serve as important targets of drug therapy.[72]

Normal tissue cells exist within a microecology of intercommunicating cell subpopulations. Cells communicate with each other through a variety of protein-mediated channels, such as cell–cell contacts, soluble hormone and enzyme exchange, and remodeling of the extracellular matrix. Cell lines cultured in the laboratory may not accurately reflect the physiologic state of the tissue microenvironment because they are missing the appropriate communication inputs. Until recently, it was impossible to reliably analyze the individual cellular subpopulations within actual human clinical tissue specimens. With the advent of high-throughput microdissection technology (e.g., LCM), individual tissue cells can be studied directly.

Protein microarrays offer the advantage of allowing the evaluation of native proteins in normal and diseased cells and the posttranslational modifications associated with protein–protein interactions in the context of communication networks regulating cellular processes such as growth, differentiation, apoptosis, and invasion and metastasis.[73,74] Assuming that information flow through a specific node in the proteomic network requires the phosphorylation of a known protein at a specific amino acid sequence, by measuring the proportion of those protein molecules that are phosphorylated, the level of activity of that signal node can be inferred. If one compares this measurement over time, at stages of disease progression, or before and after treatment, a correlation can be made between the activity of the node and the biologic or disease state. The development of highly sensitive protein microarrays now makes it possible to profile the states of protein signal pathways in tissue biopsies, aspirates, or body fluid samples.

The application of this technology to clinical molecular diagnostics will be greatly enhanced by increasing numbers of high-quality antibodies that are specific for the modification or activation state of target proteins within key pathways. Antibody specificity is particularly critical, given the complex array of biologic proteins at vastly different concentrations contained in cell lysates. Because there are no PCR-like direct amplification methods for proteins, the sensitivity of antibodies must be achieved in near femtomolar range. Moreover, the labeling and amplification method must be linear and reproducible. A cubic centimeter of biopsy tissue may contain approximately 10^9 cells, whereas a needle biopsy or cell aspirate may contain less than 100,000 cells. If the cell population of the specimen is heterogeneous, the final number of actual tumor cells microdissected or procured for analysis may be as low as a few thousand. Assuming that the proteins of interest,

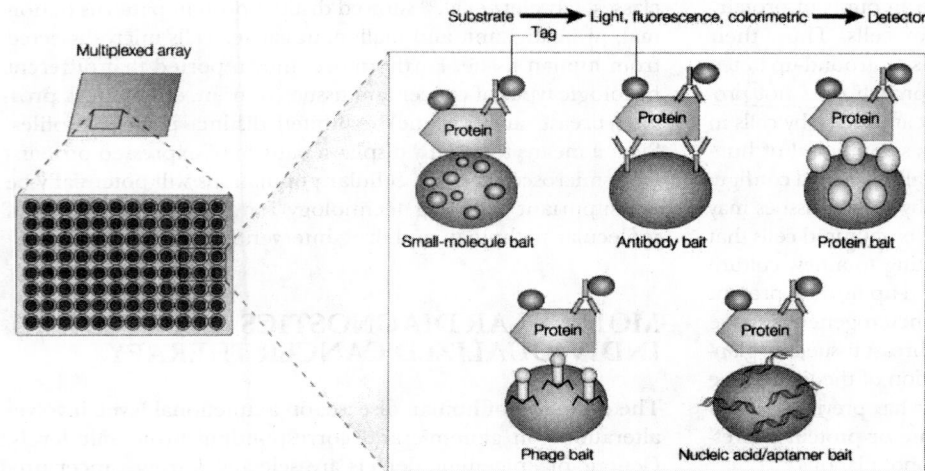

FIGURE 2-4. Protein microarray. Protein microarrays consist of an array of protein samples, or protein baits, immobilized on a solid phase. The array is queried with a mixture of labeled proteins containing analytes of interest. The analyte proteins are captured and can be detected using fluorescence or chemiluminescence means. (See Color Fig. 2-4 in the CD-ROM.)

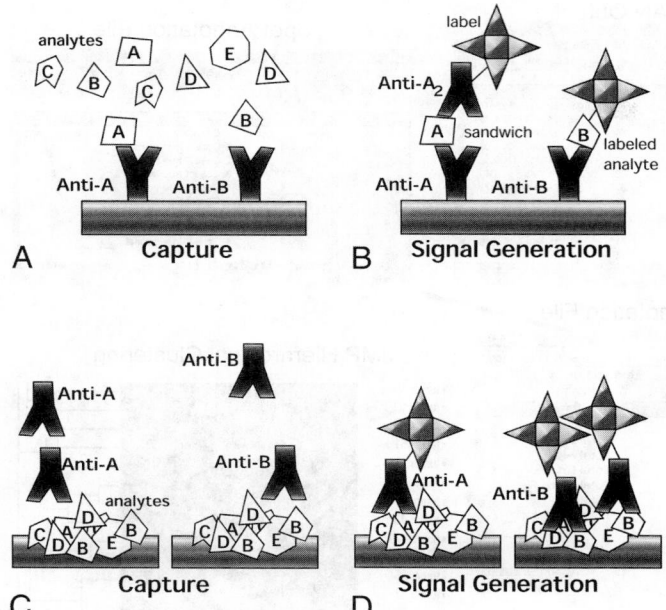

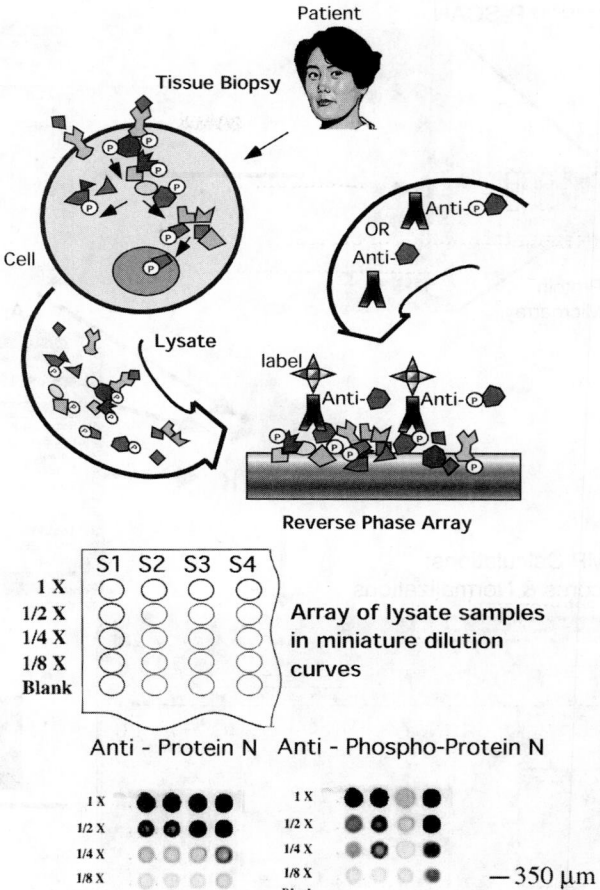

FIGURE 2-5. Classes of protein microarray platforms. Forward phase arrays (**A,B**) immobilize a bait molecule such as an antibody designed to capture specific analytes with a mixture of test sample proteins. The bound analytes are detected by a second sandwich antibody or by labeling the analyte directly (**B**). Reverse phase arrays immobilize the test sample analytes on the solid phase. An analyte-specific ligand (e.g., antibody; **C**) is applied in solution phase. Bound antibodies are detected by secondary tagging and signal amplification (**D**). (See Color Fig. 2-5 in the CD-ROM.)

FIGURE 2-6. Reverse phase array design applied to analyze phosphorylation states of signal pathway proteins. After tissue procurement and microdissection, the cancer cells are lysed, and the entire cellular proteomic repertoire is immobilized onto a solid phase. The immobilized analyte proteins containing those phosphorylated during signal transduction are probed with two classes of antibodies that specifically recognize (1) the phosphorylated (modified) form of the protein or (2) the total protein regardless of its modified state. Each test sample S1–S4 is arrayed and immobilized in a miniature dilution curve. On signal development and imaging, the relative proportion of the analyte protein molecules, which are phosphorylated, can be compared between test samples on the same array. For example, S3 has a low ratio of phosphorylated to total protein, whereas sample S4 has a high ratio. (See Color Fig. 2-6 in the CD-ROM.)

and their phosphorylated counterparts, exist in low abundance, the total concentration of analyte proteins in the sample will be very low. If the sensitivity of an analytic system is s (moles per volume), and the number of analyte molecules per cell is x (molecules per cell), then the threshold for cell procurement per volume will be

$$T = \frac{(A*s)}{x}$$

where T = threshold for cell procurement per volume (cells per volume) and A = Avogadro's number (6.02 * 1023 molecules per mole). Newer generations of protein microarrays with highly sensitive and specific antibodies are now able to achieve adequate levels of sensitivity for analysis of clinical specimens.

PROTEIN MICROARRAY FORMATS

Protein microarrays currently fall into two major classes, forward phase arrays (FPA) and reverse phase arrays (RPA). In FPAs, the capture molecules, usually antibodies, are immobilized onto the substratum (e.g., nitrocellulose-coated glass slides) and act as bait (Fig. 2-4). Each spot on an array contains one type of immobilized antibody or bait. In the FPA format, each array is incubated with one test sample (e.g., patient's cellular lysate), and multiple analytes spotted on the array are measured at once. Similar to sandwich assays, the analyte is captured between an immobilized antibody recognizing one epitope and a second labeled antibody recognizing a different

epitope on the same analyte. The linear detection range can only be achieved if the concentration of the analyte and the antibody/ligand is properly matched to the affinity. Because there are two sets of affinity constants for each analyte, the use of this format doubles the stringency placed on detection linearity for each spot across the array. A common experimental strategy for antibody arrays requires direct conjugation of the analyte proteins with a fluorescent, nucleic acid, or biotin tag, which becomes the basis for subsequent detection or signal amplification. Unfortunately, the conjugation method may denature, damage, or mask the epitope.

In contrast, with the RPA format (Fig. 2-5), each spot on an array immobilizes an individual test sample so that many patient samples are contained on one array. Each array is incubated with one detection protein (e.g., antibody), and a single analyte end

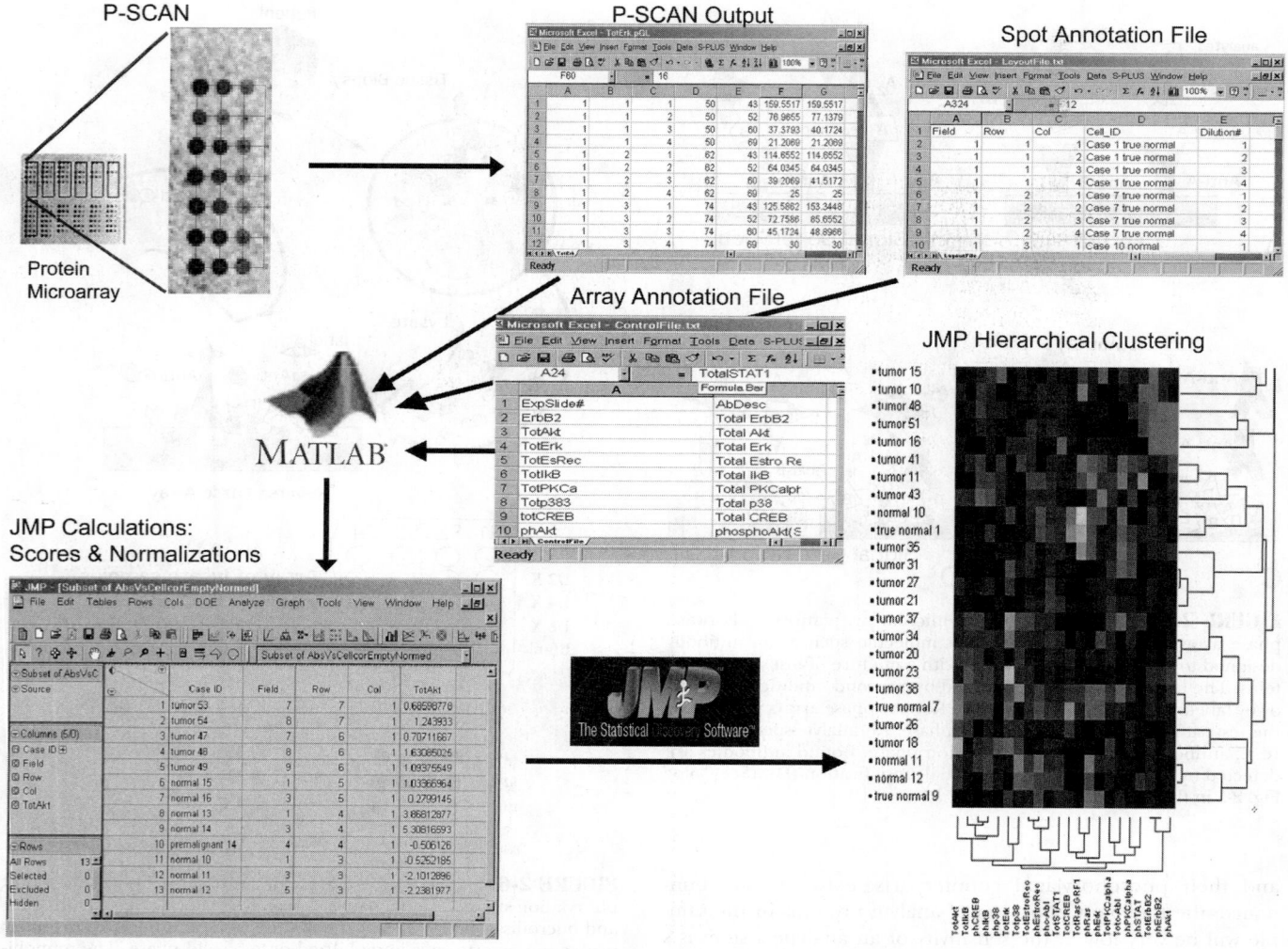

FIGURE 2-7. Scanning and bioinformatic analysis of reverse phase tissue protein arrays. The example shown displays a cluster analysis of microdissected human breast cancer and normal breast epithelium (vertical axis) compared across the phosphorylation states of a series of proteins within the epidermal growth factor receptor family signal pathway (horizontal axis, *lower right*). The data collection steps depicted are described in the text. (See Color Fig. 2-7 in the CD-ROM.)

point is measured and directly compared across many samples. RPAs do not require direct labeling of the sample analyte and do not use a two-site antibody sandwich. Therefore, no experimental variability is introduced due to labeling yield, efficiency, or epitope masking. As each array is comprised of dozens or hundreds of experimental samples, subtle differences in an analyte can be measured because each sample is exposed for the same amount of time to the same concentration of primary and secondary antibody and amplification reagents.

A critical factor in determining the linearity of a protein array, common to all immunoassays, is the match between the antibody probe concentration (affinity constant) and the unknown concentration of an analyte. In the RPA format, each sample can be applied in a miniature dilution curve on the array. This provides an improved means of matching the antibody concentration with the analyte concentration so that the linear range of each analyte measurement is ensured (Fig. 2-6). The high sensitivity of RPAs is in part because the detection probe can be tagged and the signal amplified independent from the immobilized analyte. For exam-

ple, coupling the detection antibody with highly sensitive tyramide-based avidin/biotin signal amplification systems can yield detection sensitivities down to fewer than 1000 to 5000 molecules per spot. A biopsy of 10,000 cells can yield 100 RPA arrays, with each array being probed with a different antibody. RPAs have been successfully applied to analyze the state of apoptosis and mitogenesis pathways within microdissected premalignant lesions, compared to adjacent normal epithelium, invasive carcinoma, and host stroma.[53,75,76]

BIOINFORMATIC ANALYSIS OF PROTEIN ARRAY DATA

A variety of bioanalytic methods have been successfully used for protein microarrays,[77–81] mainly by adopting methods used in gene microarray analysis. Analyzing RPAs presents a new set of challenges compared with conventional spotted arrays. Using the flexible, open source program P-SCAN,[78] an analysis strategy tailored specifically to these arrays has been developed (Fig. 2-7). Multiple RPAs, each analyzing a different phosphorylated protein, are scanned, spot intensities are calculated and normalized, and the dilution curve is collapsed to a single intensity value. This value is then assigned a relative normalized intensity value referenced to the other patient samples on the array. The data output is in the form suitable for traditional unsupervised and supervised computer software learning systems. In this way, protein array data are displayed as traditional "heat maps" and can use powerful bayesian clustering analysis for signal pathway profiling.

SERUM PROTEOMICS

The recognition that cancer is a product of the proteomic tissue microenvironment and involves communication networks has important implications. First, it shifts the emphasis away from therapeutic targets being directed solely against individual molecules within pathways and focuses the effort on targeting "nodes" in multiple pathways inside and outside the cancer cell that cooperate to orchestrate the malignant phenotype. Second, the tumor-host communication system may involve unique enzymatic events and sharing of growth factors. Consequently, the microenvironment of the tumor-host interaction could be a source for biomarkers that could ultimately be shed into the serum proteome (Fig. 2-8).

APPLICATION OF SERUM PROTEOMICS TO EARLY DIAGNOSIS

Unfortunately, in many cases, cancer is diagnosed and treated too late, when the tumor cells have already invaded and metastasized throughout the body. More than 60% of patients with breast, lung, colon, and ovarian cancer already have hidden or overt metastatic colonies. At this stage, therapeutic modalities are limited in their success. Detecting cancers at their earliest stages, even in the premalignant state, means that current or future treatment modalities might have a higher likelihood of a true cure. Ovarian cancer is a prime example of this clinical dilemma. More than two-thirds of cases of ovarian cancer are detected at an advanced stage, when the ovarian cancer cells have spread away from the ovary surface and have disseminated throughout the peritoneal cavity. Although the disease at this stage is advanced, it rarely produces specific or diagnostic symptoms. Consequently, ovarian cancer is usually treated when it is at an advanced stage. The resulting 5-year survival rate is 35% to 40% for patients with late-stage disease who receive the best possible surgical and chemotherapeutic intervention. By contrast, if ovarian cancer is detected when it is still confined to the ovary (stage I), conventional therapy produces a high rate (95%) of 5-year survival. Thus, early detection of ovarian cancer, by itself, could have a profound effect on the successful treatment of this disease. Unfortunately, early-stage ovarian cancer lacks a specific symptom or a specific biomarker and accurate and reliable diagnostic, noninvasive modalities. Because of such profound clinical need, a principal focus of protein marker discovery has been ovarian cancer.[82]

An effective, clinically useful biomarker should be measurable in a readily accessible body fluid, such as serum, urine, or saliva. The field of clinical proteomics is especially well suited to discovering such biomarkers, as serum is a protein-rich information reservoir that contains the traces of what has been encountered by the blood during its constant perfusion and percolation throughout the body. However, until now, the search for cancer-related biomarkers for early disease detection has been a "one-at-a-time" approach, which has looked for overexpressed proteins in blood that are shed into the circulation as a consequence of the disease process. Unfortunately, this method is laborious and time consuming, as there are potentially thousands of intact and cleaved proteins in the human serum proteome. Finding a single disease-related pro-

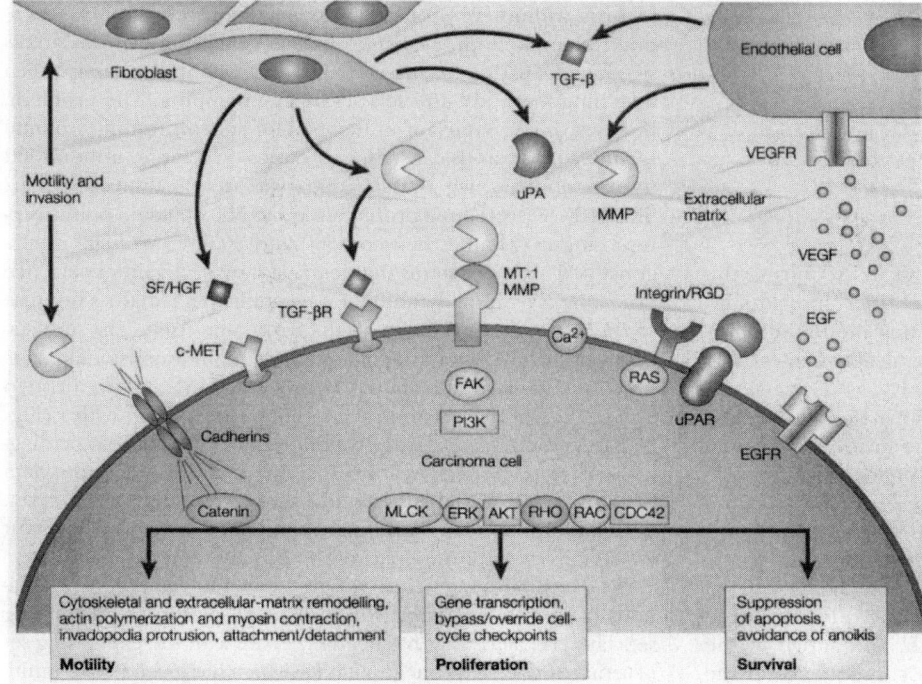

FIGURE 2-8. Tumor-host interaction. Cancer is a disease of the tissue microenvironment. Interactions between the cancer cell and the host (cellular and extracellular matrix) promote tumor cell growth, invasion, and angiogenesis and survival. Examples include the exchange of growth factors, degradative enzymes, and motility-stimulating molecules. AKT, v-akt murine thymoma viral oncogene homologue; CDC42, cell division cycle 42; c-MET, MET protooncogene; EGF, epidermal growth factor; EGFR, EGF receptor; ERK, extracellular-signal–regulated kinase; FAK, focal adhesion kinase; MLCK, myosin light-chain kinase; MMP, matrix metalloproteinase; MT-1, metallothionein 1; PI3K, phosphatidylinositol 3 kinase; RAC, a member of the RAS superfamily of small G proteins; RGD, Arg-Gly-Asp motif; RHO, a member of the RAS superfamily of small G proteins; SF/HGF, scatter factor/hepatocyte growth factor; TGF-β, transforming growth factor-β; TGF-βR, TGF-β receptor; uPA, urokinase plasminogen activator; uPAR, uPA receptor; VEGF, vascular endothelial growth factor; VEGFR, VEGF receptor. (See Color Fig. 2-8 in the CD-ROM.)

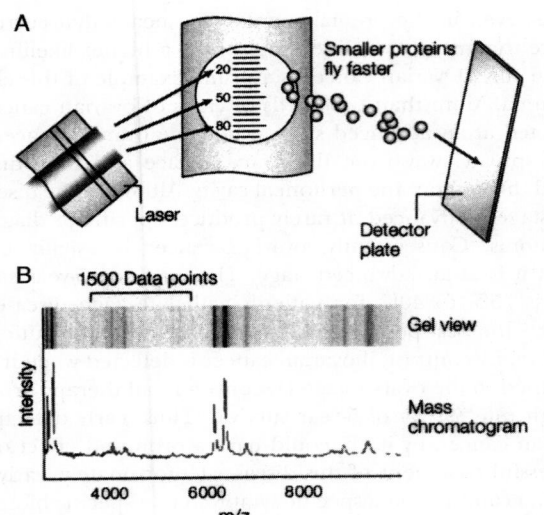

FIGURE 2-9. Surface enhanced laser-desorption ionization time-of-flight (SELDI-TOF) mass spectrometry. Using a robotic sample dispenser/processor to increase reproducibility, accuracy, and speed for sample handling and delivery, 1 μL raw, unfractionated serum is applied to the surface of a protein-binding chip. Depending on the type of chromatographic matrix used (weak cation, strong anion, or immobilized metal affinity), a subset of the proteins in the sample binds to the surface of the chip (**A**). This interaction is specific, as the chromatographic binding is based on the inherent amino acid sequence of any given protein, as well as on the pH, detergent, and salt concentration in the binding reaction buffer. Decreasing the amount of time allowed for incubation also allows the researcher to minimize nonspecific binding, as the high-affinity interactions occur more quickly than low-affinity binding. The chip is rinsed to remove unbound proteins, and the bound proteins are treated with a matrix compound, washed, and dried (**A**). The chip, containing many patient samples, is inserted into a vacuum chamber, where it is irradiated with a laser. The laser desorbs the adherent proteins, which causes them to be launched as protonated and charged ions. The TOF of the ion, before it is detected by an electrode, is a measure of the mass to charge (m/z) value of the ion. The ion spectra can be analyzed by computer-assisted tools to classify a subset of the spectra by their characteristic patterns of relative intensity. Using this method, 1 μL raw, unfractionated serum from a patient is analyzed by SELDI-TOF to create a proteomic signature of the serum (**B**). This serum proteomic bar code is comprised of potentially tens of thousands of protein ion signatures, which then require high-order data-mining operations for analysis. A typical low-resolution SELDI-TOF proteomic profile has up to 15,500 data points that comprise the recordings of data between 500 and 20,000 m/z, with higher-resolution mass-spectrometry instruments generating as many as 400,000 data points for 500 to 12,000 m/z. (See Color Fig. 2-9 in the CD-ROM.)

tein is like searching for a needle in a haystack, requiring the separation and identification of these entities individually. Serum-based proteomic pattern analysis, a new method in diagnostics and disease detection, offers several advantages over previous technologies.[83]

The diagnostic end point for the detection of ovarian cancer using serum proteomics was a pattern that comprised many individual proteins, none of which could independently differentiate diseased from healthy individuals. These patterns reflect the blood proteome without specific knowledge of what the proteins are. The blood proteome is changing constantly as a consequence of perfusion of the diseased organ. These disease-related differences in protein levels could be the result of proteins being overexpressed or abnormally shed, or both, and added to the serum proteome, clipped or modified as a consequence of the

disease process, or subtracted from the proteome owing to abnormal activation of the proteolytic degradation pathway. Quaternary effects due to disease-related protein–protein interactions and protein complex formation can also modify and subtly change the serum proteome.

One microliter of raw, unfractionated serum from patients can be analyzed by surface enhanced laser-desorption ionization time-of-flight (SELDI-TOF) spectrometry to give a proteomic signature of the serum (Fig. 2-9). The experimenter applies unfractionated serum directly to the surface of a treated metal bar. A subset of the proteins in the serum binds to the surface of the bar, and the unbound proteins are washed away. The adherent proteins are treated with acid (so that they become ionized by the laser energy) and are then dried down onto the bar surface. The bar containing the individual, captured serum protein samples as a row of spots is then inserted into a vacuum chamber, and a laser beam is fired at each spot. The laser energy desorbs the ionized proteins, and the launched proteins fly down the vacuum tube toward an oppositely charged electrode. Each ion that strikes the electrode registers as a component of the data spectrum that emerges from the analysis. The mass-charge ratio (m/z) of each ion can be estimated by the time it takes for the launched ion to reach the electrode—small ions travel faster. The MS spectrum provides a TOF "bar code" of ions ordered by size. This serum proteomic bar code consists of thousands of protein ion signatures, which require highly ordered data-mining operations for analysis.

Many bioinformatics data-mining systems are being developed, but most fall into two main types of approach. The first approach involves supervised systems that require a corpus of knowledge or data to train on, for which the outcome or classification is known ahead of time. Training is a process in which a computer-driven system is provided data from a training set in which the outcome is known and is unblinded. Examples of such approaches are linear regression models, nonlinear feed-forward neural networks, and genetic algorithms. The second type of approach involves unsupervised systems that cluster or group records without previous knowledge of outcome or classification. Example approaches are k-means nearest-neighbor analysis, euclidean distance-based nonlinear methods, fuzzy-pattern matching methods, and self-organizing mapping. The problem, however, is the same for either type of system: finding optimal feature sets or, in this instance, proteins, in a large, unbounded information archive that is unknown at this time. A typical SELDI-TOF proteomic profile has up to 350,000 data points representing m/z values between 500 and 20,000. Artificial intelligence (AI)-based systems that learn, adapt, and gain experience over time are uniquely suited to proteomic data analysis because of the huge dimensionality of the proteome itself. The application of these AI systems to analyzing high-dimensional mass-spectral data derived from the serum proteome has given rise to a new analytic paradigm: proteomic pattern diagnostics (Fig. 2-10). As each new patient is validated through pathologic diagnosis using retrospective or prospective study sets, the input data from the patient can be added to an ever-expanding training set. An AI tool that adapts and gains experience through constant learning is an important part of the process.

It is possible to generate not just one, but multiple combinations of proteomic patterns from a single mass-spectral training set. This is exactly what has been observed with the expanding set of sera from ovarian cancer patients, which has given rise to multi-

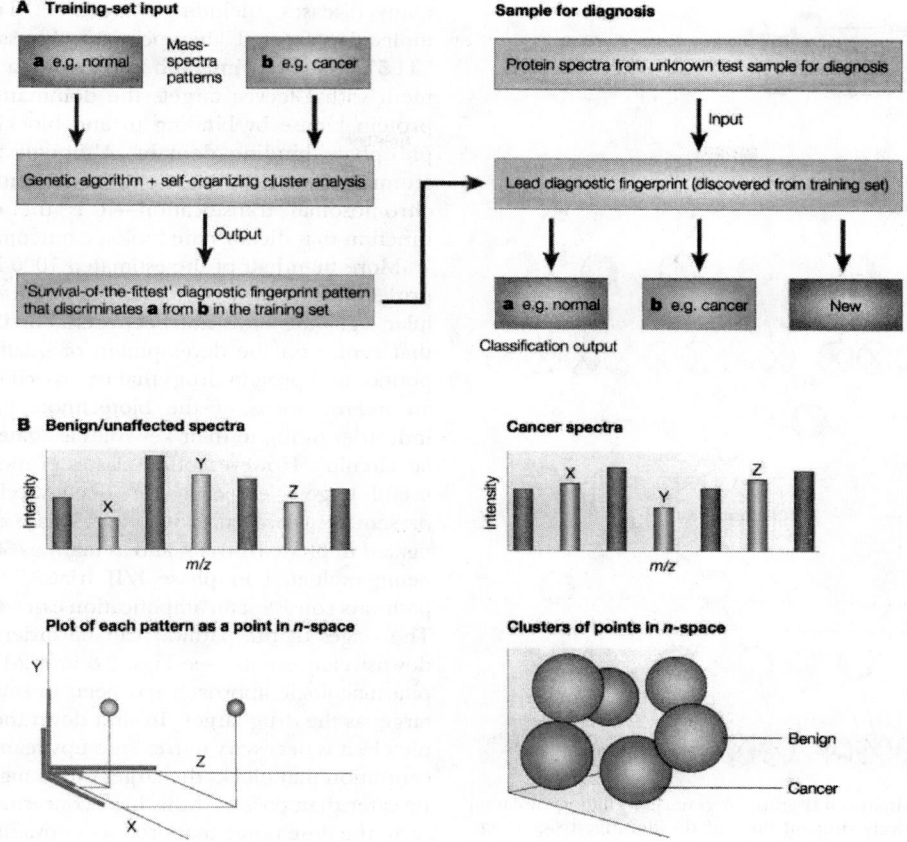

FIGURE 2-10. Proteomic pattern diagnostics. Proteomic pattern analysis begins with artificial intelligence (AI)–based computer searching of mass-spectrometry data to find the "most fit" combination of proteins through the use of a training set and a blinded test set **(A)**. The training sets comprise serum from individuals who are healthy or have active disease at the time of serum collection. The AI engine first uses a genetic algorithm to search through the 15,500 data points by parsing the data into "data packets" that contain 5 to 20 m/z (protein ion mass–charge ratio) values. The engine then searches through combinations of protein signatures within the training set until it finds the best combination of 5 to 20 proteins with combined relative abundance that are different in the disease cohort relative to the healthy population. Because much of the mass spectrum is background noise, identifying true protein ion signatures requires a system that can rapidly and iteratively search through the decision space. The parsing of data into packages of 5 to 20 values creates $15,500 \times 10^5$ to $15,500 \times 10^{20}$ combinations, or about 1.5×10^9 to 1.5×10^{24} patterns. If each of these combinations was explored one at a time, it would take a computer performing 1×10^9 operations per second more than 47 million years to find the optimal discriminatory pattern. Genetic algorithms can find near-optimal solutions to these massive sets in only a few days through iterative searching, remating, and recombination of the data packets and applying "selective pressure." The systems use a fitness test, such as an unsupervised self-organizing mapping–based adaptive clustering program. Clusters are formed in fifth- to twentieth-dimensional space by the vector plots of the euclidean distance values obtained by the combined relative peak intensities that are selected at the m/z values chosen by the genetic algorithm **(B)**. Once an optimal combination pattern has been found, incoming (blinded) data are analyzed rapidly by the software, simply by plotting in the fifth- to twentieth-dimensional vector space the combined relative amplitudes of the subset of the key discriminatory proteins and finding whether they fall into the clusters formed by the training set. If the blinded spectral plot falls within an existing cluster that contains only cancer patients, the sample is classified as cancerous; if it falls into an existing cluster that contains only healthy patients, it is classified as normal. If the n-dimensional vector plot falls outside any cluster, it forms its own new cluster, and the model adapts on the basis of the unblinded classification. (See Color Fig. 2-10 in the CD-ROM.)

ple combinations of proteomic patterns that are more than 98% sensitive and specific. The initial and reported discriminatory pattern had a sensitivity of 100% and a specificity of 95% for ovarian cancer at all stages. One of the newer discriminatory patterns, which has key discriminatory values at m/z ratios of 554, 601, 834, 5134, and 16,292, was shown to be 100% sensitive and specific in a blinded set of 52 healthy individuals and 92 cancer patients (with stage I, II, or III ovarian cancer), including 15 patients with stage I

ovarian cancer. These new spectra are posted on the Web site of the Clinical Proteomics Program Databank (http://clinicalproteomics.steem.com).

PERSONALIZED MEDICINE

Evidence is emerging to support the concept that each patient's cancer might have a unique complement of pathogenic molecu-

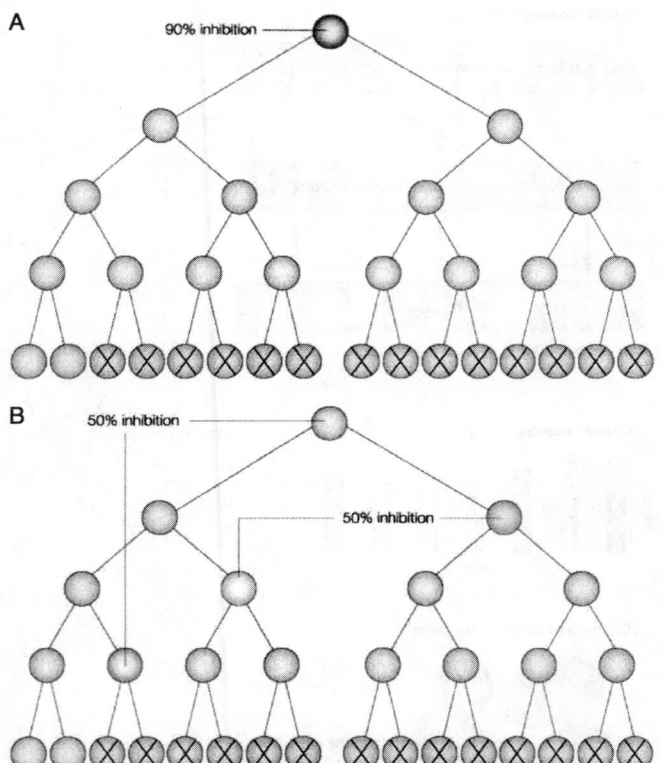

FIGURE 2-11. Combinatorial therapy. A generic signaling cascade is depicted. **A:** To effectively shut off 90% of the deranged signaling emanating from the activated node, a high dose of a single drug (*filled green circle*) is required to shut down that one node and the pathway. **B:** By contrast, targeting with a combination of drugs, each shutting off unique but interconnected nodes (*colored circles*) within the pathway that flows from the single derangement, can achieve the same efficacy with a lower dose of each drug. (See Color Fig. 2-11 in the CD-ROM.)

lar derangements. Consequently, a given class of therapy might be effective for only a subset of patients who harbor tumors with susceptible molecular derangements. With this insight, there is a strong justification to develop a strategy that could select from a menu of treatment choices, or treatment combinations, those that best match the individual molecular profile of a tumor. Molecular profiling using gene arrays has shown considerable potential for the classification of patient populations according to disease stage or survival outcome. Nevertheless, transcript profiling, by itself, might provide an incomplete picture. This is because gene-transcript level might bear no relationship to the phosphorylated or otherwise functional state of the encoded protein. Moreover, gene transcripts provide little information about protein–protein interactions and the state of the cellular signaling circuitry. Thus, the application of molecular profiling to select the appropriate treatment strategy must include direct proteomic pathway analysis of the biopsy material.

At present, cancer therapy has been directed at a single molecular target. In the future, the authors can imagine targeting an entire set of nodes all along the pathogenic signaling pathway (Fig. 2-11). Such an approach could, theoretically, achieve a higher efficacy with a lower toxicity. Protein kinases are the key molecules that make up these nodes in the cellular circuitry, and their aberrant function is often at the center of

many diseases, including cancer.[84–87] The narrowly focused molecular-targeted therapeutics addresses this concept.[88–91] STI 571 (Gleevec, imatinib mesylate) is a key example.[71] Treatment with Gleevec targets the dominant activity of the ABL protein kinase by binding to and blocking its adenosine triphosphate–binding domain. Although this pathogenic proteomic circuit has a genetic underpinning—in this case, a chromosomal translocation—it is the deranged proteomic function that dictates the biologic outcome.

More than half of the estimated 1000 kinases in the human proteome have yet to be identified, and their central roles in cellular signaling have not been defined. Drug discovery efforts that center on the development of small-molecular-mass compounds and protein drugs that can specifically block kinases are an intense focus of the biotechnology and pharmaceutical industries owing to their key roles as "gatekeepers" of the cellular circuitry. However, other classes of molecules might also be useful targets, especially for T-cell vaccine-based therapy. At present, four molecules that block kinase activity are being investigated in phase III trials, and as many as 30 kinase inhibitors are being evaluated in phase I/II trials.[92,93] Proteomic signaling pathways consist of an amplification cascade of enzymatic events. The stages of the pathway can be ordered from upstream to downstream events (see Figs. 2-8 and 2-11). The conventional pharmacologic approach has been to select a single upstream target as the drug target. To shut down the entire pathway completely, it is necessary to treat the upstream target at a drug concentration that blocks the target with a high degree of efficiency (greater than 85%). At this high concentration, the drug might be in the dose range that produces unwanted toxic side effects.

Combinatorial therapy, an alternative approach to single-agent therapy, offers the promise of higher specificity at lower treatment doses.[94–96] A correctly chosen series of inhibitors that act at several points along the signaling pathway can be used at low concentrations, yet the result can be a complete shutdown of the pathway. The advantage is realized because the inhibitors work in series at different points along the pathway. This means that output of one node in the pathway is inhibited before it reaches the next node. Consequently, a lower concentration of inhibitor is required at each successive level. With this concept in mind, a redefined goal of molecular profiling is to map the cellular circuit so as to define the optimal set of interconnected drug targets. The use of combinatorial therapy for increased efficacy could also yield a decrease in unwanted toxic side effects, as each drug can now be given at a lower treatment dose. However, this needs to be proved and requires a higher degree of vigilance during implementation of the regime to monitor the combined toxic effects of the drugs on normal cell populations.

FRONTIERS OF NANOTECHNOLOGY AND MEDICINE

The advent of nanotechnology has heralded a new frontier for medical diagnostics and therapeutics. The development of inorganic nanoparticles that bind specific tumor markers that exist at very low concentrations in serum may be able to be used as serum "harvesting" agents. In the future, patients may be injected with such nanoparticles that seek out and bind tumor or disease markers of interest. Once the nanoparticles have bound their targets, they can be "harvested" from the serum to enable diagnosis or to monitor disease progression.[97]

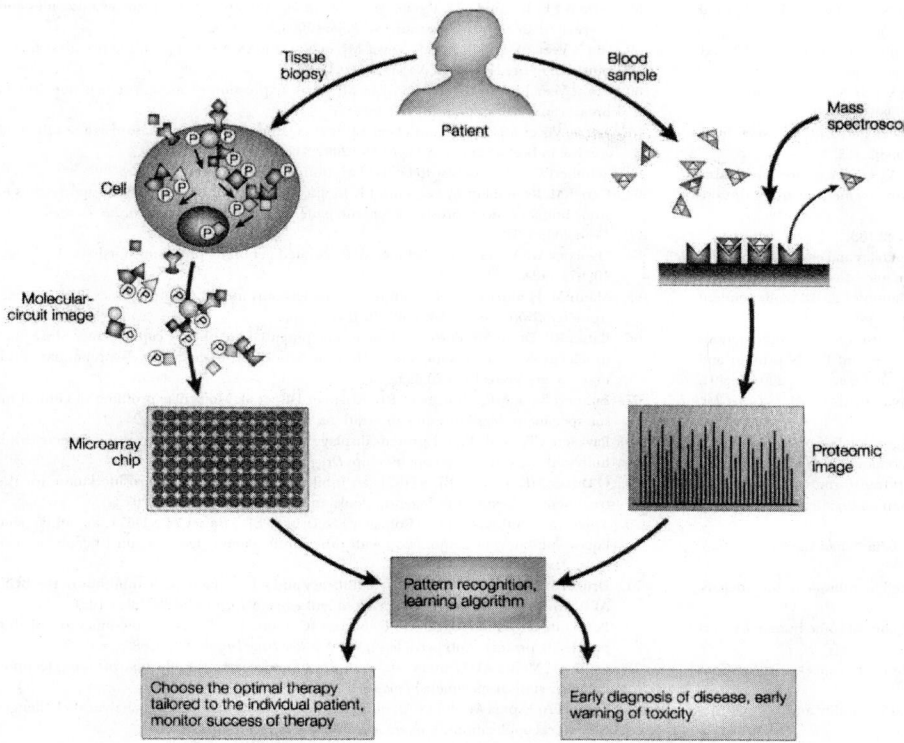

FIGURE 2-12. Proteomic technology applied to management of the cancer patient. Proteomic pattern analysis of serum has the potential to detect early-stage disease, toxicity, or recurrence. Once the disease has been diagnosed and biopsied, protein microarrays coupled with laser capture microdissection offer a means to profile the individual signal pathways that are deranged in the tumor cells of the patient. In this manner, the combinatorial therapy can be tailored to, and monitored in, the individual patient. (See Color Fig. 2-12 in the CD-ROM.)

Evidence suggests that each organ and tumor has its unique "molecular address" encoded within the vasculature.[98] Peptides that recognize organ-specific vascular beds have been identified via the screening of phage libraries *in vivo*.[99,100] With the synthesis of peptide carriers designed to transport drug therapies to specific vascular beds, treatments can be designed to treat specific tissues or tumor sites leaving nonmalignant tissues unaffected. The use of homing nanoparticles, or semiconductor quantum dots,[101] may be an important part of imaging diagnostics, in addition to drug delivery, in the health care of the future.

FUTURE OF CLINICAL PROTEOMICS

Clinical proteomics can have important direct "bedside" applications. There may well be a future in which the pathologist and the patient's clinical team, together, will use these different proteomic analyses at many points of disease management. The pathologist of the future will detect early manifestations of disease using proteomic patterns of body-fluid samples and will provide the primary physician a diagnosis based on proteomic signatures as a complement to histopathology. He or she will be able to dissect a patient's individual tumor molecularly, identifying the specific regulatory pathways that are deranged in the cell cycle, differentiation, apoptosis, and invasion and metastasis. Based on this knowledge, recommendations will be made for an individualized selection of therapeutic combinations of molecularly targeted agents that best strike the entire disease-specific protein network of the tumor. The pathologist and the diagnostic imaging physician will assist the clinical team to perform real-time assessment of therapeutic efficacy and toxicity. Proteomic and genomic analysis of recurrent tumor lesions could be the basis for rational redirection of therapy because it could reveal

changes in the diseased protein network that are associated with drug resistance. The paradigm shift will directly affect clinical practice, as it has an impact on all of the crucial elements of patient care and management (Fig. 2-12).

REFERENCES

1. Lander ES, Linton LM, Birren B, et al. Initial sequencing and analysis of the human genome. *Nature* 2001;409:860.
2. Collins FS, Green ED, Guttmacher AE, Guyer MS. A vision for the future of genomics research. *Nature* 2003;422:835.
3. Venter JC, Adams MD, Myers EW, et al. The sequence of the human genome. *Science* 2001;291:1304.
4. DeRisi J, Penland L, Brown PO, et al. Use of a cDNA microarray to analyse gene expression patterns in human cancer. *Nat Genet* 1996;14:457.
5. Golub TR, Slonim DK, Tamayo P, et al. Molecular classification of cancer: class discovery and class prediction by gene expression monitoring. *Science* 1999;286:531.
6. Holloway AJ, van Laar RK, Tothill RW, Bowtell DD. Options available–from start to finish–for obtaining data from DNA microarrays II. *Nat Genet* 2002;32[Suppl]:481.
7. Hunter T. Signaling–2000 and beyond. *Cell* 2000;100:113.
8. Vogelstein B, Lane D, Levine AJ. Surfing the p53 network. *Nature* 2000;408:307.
9. O'Connor PM. Mammalian G1 and G2 phase checkpoints. *Cancer Surv* 1997;29:151.
10. O'Connor PM, Jackman J, Bae I, et al. Characterization of the p53 tumor suppressor pathway in cell lines of the National Cancer Institute anticancer drug screen and correlations with the growth-inhibitory potency of 123 anticancer agents. *Cancer Res* 1997;57:4285.
11. Donehower LA, Godley LA, Aldaz CM, et al. The role of p53 loss in genomic instability and tumor progression in a murine mammary cancer model. *Prog Clin Biol Res* 1996;395:1.
12. Avantaggiati ML, Ogryzko V, Gardner K, et al. Recruitment of p300/CBP in p53-dependent signal pathways. *Cell* 1997;89:1175.
13. Livingstone LR, White A, Sprouse J, et al. Altered cell cycle arrest and gene amplification potential accompany loss of wild-type p53. *Cell* 1992;70:923.
14. Stambolic V, MacPherson D, Sas D, et al. Regulation of PTEN transcription by p53. *Mol Cell* 2001;8:317.
15. Singh B, Reddy PG, Goberdhan A, et al. p53 regulates cell survival by inhibiting PIK3CA in squamous cell carcinomas. *Genes Dev* 2002;16:984.
16. Levine AJ. p53, the cellular gatekeeper for growth and division. *Cell* 1997;88:323.
17. Holt JT, Thompson ME, Szabo C, et al. Growth retardation and tumour inhibition by BRCA1. *Nat Genet* 1996;12:298.
18. Aprelikova ON, Fang BS, Meissner EG, et al. BRCA1-associated growth arrest is RB-dependent. *Proc Natl Acad Sci U S A* 1999;96:11866.

19. Hakem R, de la Pompa JL, Sirard C, et al. The tumor suppressor gene Brca1 is required for embryonic cellular proliferation in the mouse. *Cell* 1996;85:1009.

20. Chen J, Silver DP, Walpita D, et al. Stable interaction between the products of the BRCA1 and BRCA2 tumor suppressor genes in mitotic and meiotic cells. *Mol Cell* 1998;2:317.

21. Gowen LC, Avrutskaya AV, Latour AM, Koller BH, Leadon SA. BRCA1 required for transcription-coupled repair of oxidative DNA damage. *Science* 1998;281:1009.

22. Sharan SK, Bradley A. Functional characterization of BRCA1 and BRCA2: clues from their interacting proteins. *J Mammary Gland Biol Neoplasia* 1998;3:413.

23. Abbott DW, Thompson ME, Robinson-Benion C, et al. BRCA1 expression restores radiation resistance in BRCA1-defective cancer cells through enhancement of transcription-coupled DNA repair. *J Biol Chem* 1999;274:18808.

24. Eng C. PTEN: one gene, many syndromes. *Hum Mutat* 2003;22:183.

25. Suzuki A, de la Pompa JL, Stambolic V, et al. High cancer susceptibility and embryonic lethality associated with mutation of the PTEN tumor suppressor gene in mice. *Curr Biol* 1998;8:1169.

26. Stambolic V, Suzuki A, de la Pompa JL, et al. Negative regulation of PKB/Akt-dependent cell survival by the tumor suppressor PTEN. *Cell* 1998;95:29.

27. Zhou XP, Waite KA, Pilarski R, et al. Germline PTEN promoter mutations and deletions in Cowden/Bannayan-Riley-Ruvalcaba syndrome result in aberrant PTEN protein and dysregulation of the phosphoinositol-3-kinase/Akt pathway. *Am J Hum Genet* 2003;73:404.

28. Datta SR, Brunet A, Greenberg ME. Cellular survival: a play in three Akts. *Genes Dev* 1999;13:2905.

29. Shin I, Yakes FM, Rojo F, et al. PKB/Akt mediates cell-cycle progression by phosphorylation of p27(Kip1) at threonine 157 and modulation of its cellular localization. *Nat Med* 2002;8:1145.

30. Grady WM, Rajput A, Myeroff L, et al. Mutation of the type II transforming growth factor-beta receptor is coincident with the transformation of human colon adenomas to malignant carcinomas. *Cancer Res* 1998;58:3101.

31. Massague J, Wotton D. Transcriptional control by the TGF-beta/Smad signaling system. *EMBO J* 2000;19:1745.

32. Shi Y, Massague J. Mechanisms of TGF-beta signaling from cell membrane to the nucleus. *Cell* 2003;113:685.

33. Feinberg AP, Vogelstein B. Hypomethylation distinguishes genes of some human cancers from their normal counterparts. *Nature* 1983;301:89.

34. Jones PA, Baylin SB. The fundamental role of epigenetic events in cancer. *Nat Rev Genet* 2002;3:415.

35. Eden A, Gaudet F, Waghmare A, Jaenisch R. Chromosomal instability and tumors promoted by DNA hypomethylation. *Science* 2003;300:455.

36. Gaudet F, Hodgson JG, Eden A, et al. Induction of tumors in mice by genomic hypomethylation. *Science* 2003;300:489.

37. Walter J, Paulsen M. Imprinting and disease. *Semin Cell Dev Biol* 2003;14:101.

38. Weksberg R, Smith AC, Squire J, Sadowski P. Beckwith-Wiedemann syndrome demonstrates a role for epigenetic control of normal development. *Hum Mol Genet* 2003;12:R61.

39. Issa JP, Vertino PM, Boehm CD, Newsham IF, Baylin SB. Switch from monoallelic to biallelic human IGF2 promoter methylation during aging and carcinogenesis. *Proc Natl Acad Sci U S A* 1996;93:11757.

40. Mayr B, Montminy M. Transcriptional regulation by the phosphorylation-dependent factor CREB. *Nat Rev Mol Cell Biol* 2001;2:599.

41. Korzus E, Torchia J, Rose DW, et al. Transcription factor-specific requirements for coactivators and their acetyltransferase functions. *Science* 1998;279:703.

42. Lunyak VV, Burgess R, Prefontaine GG, et al. Corepressor-dependent silencing of chromosomal regions encoding neuronal genes. *Science* 2002;298:1747.

43. Nagy L, Kao HY, Chakravarti D, et al. Nuclear receptor repression mediated by a complex containing SMRT, mSin3A, and histone deacetylase. *Cell* 1997;89:373.

44. Lin RJ, Nagy L, Inoue S, et al. Role of the histone deacetylase complex in acute promyelocytic leukaemia. *Nature* 1998;391:811.

45. Reya T, Morrison SJ, Clarke MF, Weissman IL. Stem cells, cancer, and cancer stem cells. *Nature* 2001;414:105.

46. Lin RJ, Evans RM. Acquisition of oncogenic potential by RAR chimeras in acute promyelocytic leukemia through formation of homodimers. *Mol Cell* 2000;5:821.

47. Calvo KR, Sykes DB, Pasillas M, Kamps MP. Hoxa9 immortalizes a granulocyte-macrophage colony-stimulating factor-dependent promyelocyte capable of biphenotypic differentiation to neutrophils or macrophages, independent of enforced meis expression. *Mol Cell Biol* 2000;20:3274.

48. Calvo KR, Knoepfler PS, Sykes DB, Pasillas MP, Kamps MP. Meis1a suppresses differentiation by G-CSF and promotes proliferation by SCF: potential mechanisms of cooperativity with Hoxa9 in myeloid leukemia. *Proc Natl Acad Sci U S A* 2001;98:13120.

49. Ayton PM, Cleary ML. Transformation of myeloid progenitors by MLL oncoproteins is dependent on Hoxa7 and Hoxa9. *Genes Dev* 2003;17:2298.

50. Adams MD, Kerlavage AR, Fleischmann RD, et al. Initial assessment of human gene diversity and expression patterns based upon 83 million nucleotides of cDNA sequence. *Nature* 1995;377[Suppl 6547]:3.

51. Sgroi D, Teng S, Robinson G, et al. In vivo gene expression profile analysis of human breast cancer progression. *Cancer Res* 1999;59:5656.

52. Emmert-Buck MR, Bonner RF, Smith PD, et al. Laser capture microdissection. *Science* 1996;274:998.

53. Paweletz CP, Liotta LA, Petricoin EF 3rd. New technologies for biomarker analysis of prostate cancer progression: Laser capture microdissection and tissue proteomics. *Urology* 2001;57[Suppl 1]:160.

54. Page MJ, Amess B, Townsend RR, et al. Proteomic definition of normal human luminal and myoepithelial breast cells purified from reduction mammoplasties. *Proc Natl Acad Sci U S A* 1999;96:12589.

55. Alizadeh AA, Eisen MB, Davis RE, et al. Distinct types of diffuse large B-cell lymphoma identified by gene expression profiling. *Nature* 2000;403:503.

56. Perou CM, Jeffrey SS, van de Rijn M, et al. Distinctive gene expression patterns in human mammary epithelial cells and breast cancers. *Proc Natl Acad Sci U S A* 1999;96:9212.

57. Ma XJ, Salunga R, Tuggle JT, et al. Gene expression profiles of human breast cancer progression. *Proc Natl Acad Sci U S A* 2003;100:5974.

58. Ntzani EE, Ioannidis JP. Predictive ability of DNA microarrays for cancer outcomes and correlates: an empirical assessment. *Lancet* 2003;362:1439.

59. van 't Veer LJ, Dai H, van de Vijver MJ, et al. Gene expression profiling predicts clinical outcome of breast cancer. *Nature* 2002;415:530.

60. van 't Veer LJ, Dai H, van de Vijver MJ, et al. Expression profiling predicts outcome in breast cancer. *Breast Cancer Res* 2003;5:57.

61. van de Vijver MJ, He YD, van't Veer LJ, et al. A gene-expression signature as a predictor of survival in breast cancer. *N Engl J Med* 2002;347:1999.

62. Schubert CM. Microarray to be used as routine clinical screen. *Nat Med* 2003;9:9.

63. Carr KM, Rosenblatt K, Petricoin EF, Liotta LA. Genomic and proteomic approaches to study human cancer: prospects for true patient-tailored therapy. *Annu Rev Genomics Hum Genet* 2003;1:32.

64. Hancock W, Apffel A, Chakel J, et al. Integrated genomic/proteomic analysis. *Anal Chem* 1999;71:742A.

65. Mann M, Hendrickson RC, Pandey A. Analysis of proteins and proteomes by mass spectrometry. *Annu Rev Biochem* 2001;70:437.

66. Banks RE, Dunn MJ, Forbes MA, et al. The potential use of laser capture microdissection to selectively obtain distinct populations of cells for proteomic analysis—preliminary findings. *Electrophoresis* 1999;20:689.

67. Emmert-Buck MR, Strausberg RL, Krizman DB, et al. Molecular profiling of clinical tissue specimens: feasibility and applications. *Am J Pathol* 2000;156:1109.

68. Paweletz CP, et al. Rapid protein display profiling of cancer progression directly from human tissue using a protein biochip. *Drug Dev Res* 2000;49:34.

69. O'Dwyer ME, Druker BJ. STI571: an inhibitor of the BCR-ABL tyrosine kinase for the treatment of chronic myelogenous leukaemia. *Lancet Oncol* 2000;1:207.

70. Thiesing JT, Ohno-Jones S, Kolibaba KS, Druker BJ. Efficacy of STI571, an abl tyrosine kinase inhibitor, in conjunction with other antileukemic agents against bcr-abl-positive cells. *Blood* 2000;96:3195.

71. Druker BJ, Talpaz M, Resta DJ, et al. Efficacy and safety of a specific inhibitor of the BCR-ABL tyrosine kinase in chronic myeloid leukemia. *N Engl J Med* 2001;344:1031.

72. Petricoin EF, Zoon KC, Kohn EC, Barrett JC, Liotta LA. Clinical proteomics: translating benchside promise into bedside reality. *Nat Rev Drug Discov* 2002;1:683.

73. Espina V, Mehta AI, Winters ME, et al. Protein microarrays: molecular profiling technologies for clinical specimens. *Proteomics* 2003;3:2091.

74. Liotta LA, Espina V, Mehta AI, et al. Protein microarrays: meeting analytical challenges for clinical applications. *Cancer Cell* 2003;3:317.

75. Wulfkuhle JD, Aquino JA, Calvert VS, et al. Signal pathway profiling of ovarian cancer from human tissue specimens using reverse-phase protein microarrays. *Proteomics* 2003;3:2085.

76. Grubb RL, Calvert VS, Wulkuhle JD, et al. Signal pathway profiling of prostate cancer using reverse phase protein arrays. *Proteomics* 2003;3:2142.

77. Brazma A, Hingamp P, Quackenbush J, et al. Minimum information about a microarray experiment (MIAME)-toward standards for microarray data. *Nat Genet* 2001;29:365.

78. Carlisle AJ, Prabhu VV, Elkahloun A, et al. Development of a prostate cDNA microarray and statistical gene expression analysis package. *Mol Carcinog* 2000;28:12.

79. Cutler P. Protein arrays: the current state-of-the-art. *Proteomics* 2003;3:3.

80. Sreekumar A, Nyati MK, Varambally S, et al. Profiling of cancer cells using protein microarrays: discovery of novel radiation-regulated proteins. *Cancer Res* 2001;61:7585.

81. Miller JC, Zhou H, Kwekel J, et al. Antibody microarray profiling of human prostate cancer sera: antibody screening and identification of potential biomarkers. *Proteomics* 2003;3:56.

82. Rapkiewicz AV, Petricoin EF, Liotta LA. Biomarkers in ovarian cancer. *Eur J Cancer* 2004 (in press).

83. Wulfkuhle JD, Liotta LA, Petricoin EF. Proteomic applications for the early detection of cancer. *Nat Rev Cancer* 2003;3:267.

84. Blume-Jensen P, Hunter T. Oncogenic kinase signaling. *Nature* 2001;411:355.

85. Ponder BA. Cancer genetics. *Nature* 2001;411:336.

86. Cavenee WK, Ponder B, Solomon E. Genetics and cancer. *Eur J Cancer* 1991;27:1706.

87. Evan GI, Vousden KH. Proliferation, cell cycle and apoptosis in cancer. *Nature* 2001;411:342.

88. Kaptain S, Tan LK, Chen B. Her-2/neu and breast cancer. *Diagn Mol Pathol* 2001;10:139.

89. Leyland-Jones B. Trastuzumab: hopes and realities. *Lancet Oncol* 2002;3:137.

90. Sebolt-Leopold JS. Development of anticancer drugs targeting the MAP kinase pathway. *Oncogene* 2000;19:6594.

91. Santen RJ, Song RX, McPherson R, et al. The role of mitogen-activated protein (MAP) kinase in breast cancer. *J Steroid Biochem Mol Biol* 2002;80:239.

92. Traxler P, Bold G, Buchdunger E, et al. Tyrosine kinase inhibitors: from rational design to clinical trials. *Med Res Rev* 2001;21:499.

93. Zwick E, Bange J, Ullrich A. Receptor tyrosine kinases as targets for anticancer drugs. *Trends Mol Med* 2002;8:17.

94. Normanno N, Campiglio M, De LA, et al. Cooperative inhibitory effect of ZD1839 (Iressa) in combination with trastuzumab (Herceptin) on human breast cancer cell growth. *Ann Oncol* 2002;13:65.

95. Moasser MM, Basso A, Averbuch SD, Rosen N. The tyrosine kinase inhibitor ZD1839 ("Iressa") inhibits HER2-driven signaling and suppresses the growth of HER2-overexpressing tumor cells. *Cancer Res* 2001;61:7184.

96. Cuello M, Ettenberg SA, Clark AS, et al. Down-regulation of the erbB-2 receptor by trastuzumab (Herceptin) enhances tumor necrosis factor-related apoptosis-inducing ligand-mediated apoptosis in breast and ovarian cancer cell lines that overexpress erbB-2. *Cancer Res* 2001;61:4892.

97. Liotta LA, Ferrari M, Petricoin E. Clinical proteomics: written in blood. *Nature* 2003;425:905.

98. Ruoslahti E. Specialization of tumour vasculature. *Nat Rev Cancer* 2002;2:83.

99. Akerman ME, Chan WC, Laakkonen P, Bhatia SN, Ruoslahti E. Nanocrystal targeting in vivo. *Proc Natl Acad Sci U S A* 2002;99:12617.

100. Ruoslahti E. Targeting tumor vasculature with homing peptides from phage display. *Semin Cancer Biol* 2000;10:435.

101. Alivisatos A. Less is more in medicine. *Sci Am* 2001;285:67.

CHAPTER 3

Molecular Targets in Oncology

SECTION **1**

CHRISTOPHER L. CARPENTER
LEWIS C. CANTLEY

Signal Transduction Systems

Signal transduction is the chemistry that allows communication at the cellular level. Cells sense signals from the extracellular and intracellular environments, as well as directly from other cells. In response, they regulate protein expression and function. Protein levels are controlled by rates of transcription, translation, and proteolysis, whereas protein activities are affected by location, covalent modifications, and noncovalent interactions. Signal transduction pathways regulate differentiation, division, and death in the mature and in the developing organism. They are involved in pathways common to all cells, as well as particular functions of specialized cells (e.g., synthesis and secretion of insulin by the pancreas, migration and phagocytosis by neutrophils) and the abnormal behavior of diseased cells (e.g., invasion and growth of cancer cells).

To emphasize the essentials of signal transduction, the focus in this chapter is on the variety of solutions to the two common problems faced by cells and organisms in signal transduction:

1. How is a signal sensed?
2. How are the levels and activities of proteins modified in response to the signal?

Most signals are transmitted by ligands and are sensed by the receptors to which they bind. Binding of a ligand to a receptor stimulates the activities of proteins necessary to continue the transmission of the signal, through the formation of multiprotein complexes and the generation of small-molecule second messengers. Integration of signals from multiple pathways determines the cell's responses to competing and complementary signals.

SENSORY MACHINERY: LIGANDS AND RECEPTORS

SIGNALS

Signal transduction pathways have evolved to respond to an enormous variety of stimuli. Molecules that initiate signaling cascades include proteins, amino acids, lipids, nucleotides, gases, and light (Table 3.1-1). Most extracellular signals, such as growth factors, bind to receptors on the plasma membrane, but others, such as cortisol, diffuse into the cell and bind to receptors in the cytoplasm and nucleus. Some signals are continuous, such as those sent by the extracellular matrix, whereas others are episodic, such as the secretion of insulin by pancreatic β cells in response to increases in blood glucose. Signaling molecules originate from a variety of sources. Some, such as neurotransmitters, are stored in the cell and are released to provide communication with other cells under specific conditions. Other ligands are stored outside the cell (e.g., in the extracellular matrix) and become accessible in response to tissue damage or remodeling. Traditionally, signals have been divided into those that affect distant cells (endocrine), nearby cells (paracrine), or the same cell that sends a signal (autocrine). Cells also respond to signals that arise from within. Important examples include the checkpoint pathways that ensure the orderly progression of the cell cycle and the pathways that sense and repair damaged DNA.[1]

73

TABLE 3.1-1.   Ligands That Stimulate Signal Transduction Pathways

Types of Ligands	Examples
PROTEINS	
Soluble	Insulin
Matrix	Fibronectin
Bound to other cells	Ephrins
AMINO ACIDS	Glutamate
NUCLEOTIDES	
Soluble	Adenosine triphosphate
DNA	Double-strand breaks
LIPIDS	Prostaglandins
GASES	Nitric oxide
LIGHT	Rhodopsin, visual system

RECEPTORS

The plasma membrane of eukaryotic cells serves to insulate the cell from the outside environment, but this barrier must be breached to signal to the cell. Signals transverse the plasma membrane either by activating by transmembrane receptors or by using ligands that are membrane permeable (Table 3.1-2). Cells are exquisitely sensitive to most ligands. The affinity of receptors for ligands generally is in the picomolar to nanomolar range, and very few receptors have to be occupied to transmit a signal. It has been estimated that activation of ten T-cell receptors is sufficient to send a maximal signal. Cytokine-responsive cells may express only a few hundred receptors on the cell surface. Given the small number of receptors that are activated, amplification of most signals is necessary for the cell to respond. A requirement for signal amplification also allows opposing signals to affect signal strength more efficiently. As a result of ligand binding, receptors undergo conformational changes or oligomerization, or both, and the intrinsic activity of the receptor or of associated proteins is stimulated. Receptors may bind and respond to more than one ligand [e.g., the epidermal growth factor (EGF) receptor binds to transforming growth factor (TGF)-α, EGF, heparin-binding EGF (HB-EGF), betacellulin, epiregulin, epigen, and amphiregulin]. The stimulation of most receptors leads to the activation of several downstream pathways that either function cooperatively to activate a common target or stimulate distinct targets.

Generally, some of the pathways activated are counterregulatory and serve to attenuate the signal. Receptors may also activate other receptors. A well-studied example is the activation of the EGF receptor by G protein–coupled receptors (GPCR), which occurs as a result of protease cleavage and activation of HB-EGF.

Receptor Tyrosine Kinases

Receptor tyrosine kinases are transmembrane proteins that have an extracellular ligand-binding domain, a transmembrane domain, and a cytoplasmic tyrosine kinase domain.[2,3] The ligands for these receptors are proteins or peptides. Most receptor tyrosine kinases are monomeric, but the insulin receptor family are heterotetramers in which the subunits are linked by disulfide bonds. Receptor tyrosine kinases have been divided into six classes, primarily on the basis of the sequence of extracytoplasmic domain. Examples of tyrosine kinase receptors include the insulin receptor, the platelet-derived growth factor (PDGF) receptor, the EGF receptor family, and the fibroblast growth factor (FGF) receptor family.

Activation of receptor tyrosine kinases generally requires tyrosine phosphorylation of the receptor. In the case of the insulin receptor, an insulin-stimulated conformational change activates the kinase. Most other tyrosine kinases are activated by oligomerization, which brings the kinase domains into close proximity so that they cross-phosphorylate. Auto- or transphosphorylation of a tyrosine in the activation loop of the kinase domain locks the kinase into a high-activity conformation, stimulating phosphorylation of other sites on the receptor, as well as other substrates.

Ligands stimulate receptor oligomerization in a variety of ways (Fig. 3.1-1). Some ligands, such as PDGF, are dimeric, so that the ligand is able to bind two receptors simultaneously.[4] Other ligands, such as growth hormone, are monomeric but have two receptor-binding sites that allow them to induce receptor dimerization.[5] FGFs are also monomeric but have only a single receptor-binding site. FGF molecules bind to heparin sulfate proteoglycans, which concentrates FGF and facilitates dimerization of the FGF receptor.[6] EGF is also monomeric, but binding of EGF to the receptor changes the receptor conformation and promotes interaction with a second ligand/receptor dimer leading to activation.[7] Ligands not only stimulate receptor-depen-

TABLE 3.1-2.   Receptors in Signal Transduction

Types of Receptors	Examples	Types of Ligands
Tyrosine kinase	PDGF, EGF, FGF, insulin	Peptide growth factors
Serine kinase	TGF-β	Activin
Heterotrimeric G protein–coupled receptors	Thrombin, smell receptors	Thrombin
Receptors bound to tyrosine kinases	IL-2, interferon	IL-2
TNF family	Fas receptor	Fas
Notch	Notch	Delta-Serrate-LAG-2
Guanylate cyclase	—	Atrial natriuretic factor, NO
Tyrosine phosphatase	CD45, LAR	Contactin
Nuclear receptors	Estrogen, prostaglandins	Estrogen
Adhesion receptors	Integrins, CD44	Fibronectin, hyaluronic acid

EGF, epidermal growth factor; FGF, fibroblast growth factor; IL-2, interleukin-2; PDGF, platelet-derived growth factor; TGF-β, transforming growth factor-β; TNF, tumor necrosis factor.

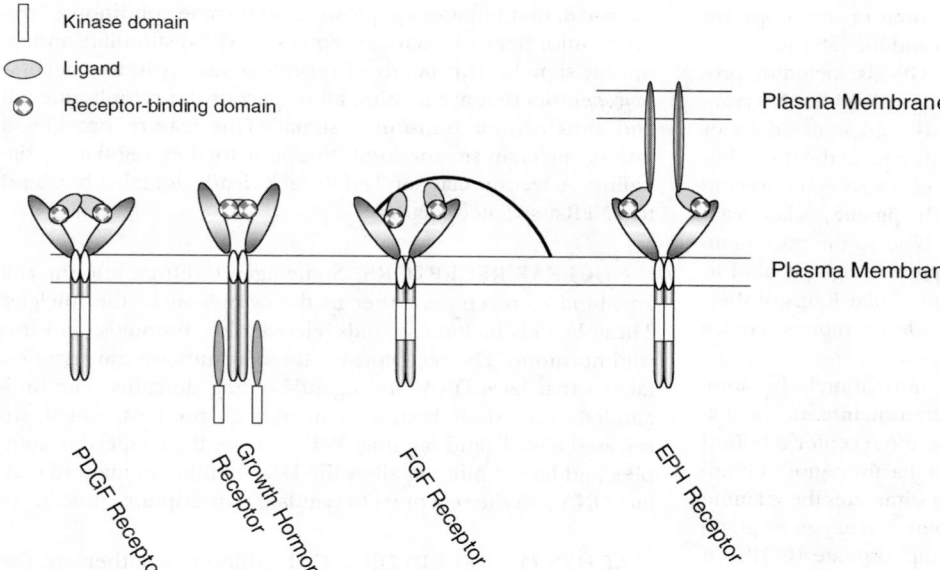

Kinase domain

Ligand

Receptor-binding domain

Plasma Membrane

Plasma Membrane

PDGF Receptor

Growth Hormone Receptor

FGF Receptor

EPH Receptor

FIGURE 3.1-1. Dimerization of tyrosine kinase receptors. Most tyrosine kinase receptors are activated by ligand-induced dimerization. Some ligands, such as platelet-derived growth factor (PDGF), are dimeric and induce dimerization using the two receptor-binding domains. Other ligands, such as growth hormone, contain two receptor-binding domains in the same molecule. The fibroblast growth factors (FGFs) rely on proteoglycans to aid the formation of ligand dimers. Some ligands, such as the ephrins (EPHs), are present on nearby cells and, when the cells come into contact, bind to the receptors and promote clustering.

dent signaling, but also some ligand-receptor interactions result in signaling by the ligand. Ephrins are ligands for the protein tyrosine kinase EPH receptors. Ephrins are expressed on the surface of adjacent cells, and interaction of EPH receptors and ephrins activates the tyrosine kinase activity of the receptor and leads to stimulation of signaling by the ligand in the adjacent cell.[8]

Studies of the EGF receptor family illustrate some important concepts in signal transduction. The EGF-signaling pathways involve four known receptors (EGF receptor, erbB2, erbB3, and erbB4) and many ligands.[9] EGF stimulates homodimerization of the EGF receptor, but, under certain conditions, heterodimerization with other family members also occurs. The same ligand activates different signaling pathways, depending on the subgroups of EGF receptor family members expressed in a cell. For example, HB-EGF–like growth factor stimulates mitogenesis but not chemotaxis when it activates the EGF receptor but is a mitogen and chemotactic factor when it activates Erb4.[10] One study also suggests that different ligands binding to the same receptors activate distinct downstream-signaling pathways.[11] These findings suggest that different ligands may cause distinct conformational changes that lead to the phosphorylation of different sets of tyrosine residues on the receptor and could lead also to phosphorylation of distinct sets of substrates.

RECEPTORS THAT ACTIVATE TYROSINE KINASES. A number of receptors do not have intrinsic enzymatic activity but stimulate associated tyrosine kinases. Important examples of this type of receptor include the cytokine and interferon receptors that associate constitutively with members of the Jak family of tyrosine kinases[12] and the multichain immune recognition receptors that activate SFK and Syk family tyrosine kinases.[13,14] The kinases appear to be inactive in the absence of ligand, but, as happens in receptors with intrinsic tyrosine kinase activity, signaling is initiated by ligand-stimulated heterodimerization and conformational changes of the receptors.

SERINE-THREONINE KINASE RECEPTORS. The TGF-β family of receptors are transmembrane proteins with intrinsic serine-threonine kinase activity.[15] TGF-β ligands are dimers that lead to oligomerization of type I and type II receptors. The type I and type II receptors are homologous but distinctly regulated. The type II receptors seem to be constitutively active but do not normally phosphorylate substrates, whereas the type I receptors are normally inactive. On ligand-mediated dimerization of the type I and type II receptors, the active type II receptor phosphorylates the type I receptor and converts it to an active kinase. Subsequent signal propagation is dependent on the kinase activity of the type I receptor and the phosphorylation of downstream substrates.

Receptor Phosphotyrosine Phosphatases

Receptor protein tyrosine phosphatases (RPTPs) have an extracellular domain, a single transmembrane-spanning domain, and cytoplasmic catalytic domains.[16] The extracellular domains of some receptor tyrosine phosphatases contain fibronectin and immunoglobulin repeats, suggesting that some of these receptors may recognize adhesion molecules as ligands. Several RPTPs are capable of homotypic interaction, but no true ligands are yet known for RPTPs. Most receptor tyrosine phosphatases have two catalytic domains, and both are active in at least some receptors. Functional and structural evidence suggests that the phosphatase activity of some of these receptors is inhibited by dimerization. These receptors may be constitutively active as tyrosine phosphatases but lose that activity after ligand binding. Inhibition of tyrosine phosphatase activity would enhance signals emanating from tyrosine kinases. RPTPs do not always function in strict opposition to tyrosine kinases, however. For example, CD45 is necessary for signaling by the B-cell receptor, which also requires tyrosine kinase activity.[17]

G PROTEIN–COUPLED RECEPTORS. GPCRs[18] are by far the most numerous receptors. Almost 700 GPCRs are present in the human genome.[19] The number of GPCRs is so high because they encode the light, smell, and taste receptors, all of which require great diversity. These receptors have seven membrane-spanning domains: The N-terminus and three of the loops are extracellular, whereas the other three loops and the C-terminus are cytoplasmic. A wide variety of ligands bind GPCRs, including proteins and peptides, lipids, amino acids, and nucleotides. No common binding domain exists for all ligands, and interactions of ligands with GPCRs are fairly distinct.[20] In the case of the thrombin receptor, thrombin cleaves the N-terminus of the receptor, freeing a new N-terminus that self-associates with the ligand pocket, leading to activation. Amines and eicosanoids bind to the transmembrane domains of their GPCRs, whereas peptide ligands bind to the transmembrane domains and the extracellular loops of their GPCRs. Neurotransmitters and some peptide hormones require the N-terminus for binding and activation.

GPCRs basally are kept in an inactive conformation by intramolecular bonds involving residues in the transmembrane or juxtamembrane regions.[21] In the inactive state, the receptor is bound to a heterotrimeric G protein, which is also inactive. Agonist binding results in a conformational change that stimulates the guanine nucleotide exchange activity of the receptor. Exchange of guanosine triphosphate (GTP) for guanosine diphosphate (GDP) on the α subunit of the heterotrimeric G proteins initiates signaling. Ultimately, GPCRs stimulate the same downstream pathways as other receptor types, including protein tyrosine and serine kinases, phospholipases (PLs A, C, and D), and ion channels.[18] Certain GPCRs also activate receptor tyrosine kinases. As mentioned earlier in the section Signals, GPCR-dependent cleavage of HB-EGF stimulates the EGF receptor, which is necessary for the GPCR to activate the mitogen-activated kinase (MAP kinase) pathway.

NOTCH FAMILY OF RECEPTORS. The Notch receptor has a large extracellular domain, a single transmembrane domain, and a cytoplasmic domain.[22] Ligands for the Notch receptor are proteins expressed on the surface of adjacent cells, and activation results in two separate proteolytic cleavages of Notch. Initial cleavage by ADAM family proteases removes the extracellular domain and causes endocytosis. Subsequent proteolysis by the preselinin protease family releases the cytoplasmic region of Notch as a soluble signal. This fragment moves to the nucleus, where it complexes with the transcriptional repressor CBF1, relieving its inhibitory effects and stimulating transcription.

GUANYLATE CYCLASES. Cyclic nucleotides are important second messengers and allosteric regulators of enzyme activities.[23] The synthesis of cyclic adenosine monophosphate (cAMP) by adenylate cyclase is regulated principally by heterotrimeric G proteins, but the synthesis of cyclic guanosine monophosphate is regulated directly by ligands. Plasma membrane guanylate cyclases are receptors for atrial natriuretic hormone. Nitrous oxide binds to soluble guanylate cyclases. Both stimuli increase cyclic guanosine monophosphate levels.

TUMOR NECROSIS FACTOR RECEPTOR FAMILY. The tumor necrosis factor family of receptors has a conserved cysteine-rich region in the extracellular domain, a transmembrane domain, and a domain called the *death domain* in the cytoplasmic tail.[24] The receptors undergo oligomerization after ligand binding, which is necessary for signaling. These receptors are distinct in several respects. Stimulation of the receptor leads to recruitment of cytoplasmic proteins that bind to each other and the receptor through death domains, activating a protease,

caspase 8, that initiates apoptosis. Under some conditions, however, tumor necrosis factor receptors (TNFRs) stimulate antiapoptotic signals. This family of receptors also includes "decoys" or receptors that are missing all or part of the cytoplasmic tail and thus cannot transmit a signal. This feature provides a unique mechanism for inhibiting and further regulating signaling. A second class of TNFRs lack death domains but bind to TNFR-associated factors.

NUCLEAR RECEPTORS. Some ligands diffuse into the cell and bind to receptors either in the cytoplasm or the nucleus. These ligands include steroids, eicosanoids, retinoids, and thyroid hormone. The receptors for these ligands are transcription factors that have DNA- and ligand-binding domains. The unliganded receptor is bound to heat-shock proteins, which are released after ligand binding. Release from the chaperone complex and ligand binding allow the DNA-binding domain to contact DNA and the receptors to regulate transcription directly.

ADHESION RECEPTORS. Cell adherence either to the extracellular matrix or to other cells is mediated by receptors that function mechanically and stimulate intracellular signaling pathways, primarily through tyrosine kinases.[25] Integrins, which mediate adherence to extracellular matrix, are composed of heterodimers of α and β subunits and bind to an arginine, glycine, aspartate, or leucine aspartate valine motif found in matrix molecules. Activation of integrin signaling involves binding to ligand and clustering of integrins. Structural studies have shown that inactive integrins adopt a conformation that inhibits ligand binding, and the intracellular regions are also hindered from binding to effector molecules.[26] Binding of ligand opens the intracellular regions so that they bind to the molecules required to transmit integrin-dependent signals. Similarly, modification of the intracellular region, such as phosphorylation, affects the conformation of the extracellular region to favor ligand binding. Integrin signaling is necessary for cell movement, but, in contrast to other pathways, adherence in nonmotile cells provides a continuous signal. This signal appears to be necessary for survival of most cells. The ability to circumvent the requirement for adherence-dependent survival plays a major role in the development of human cancers by allowing tumor survival in inappropriate locations.

PROPAGATION OF SIGNALS TO THE CELL INTERIOR

Eukaryotic cells use a varied collection of receptors and ligands to initiate cell signaling, but most receptors activate a common set of downstream molecules to transmit their signals. These molecules include protein and lipid kinases, GTPases, phospholipases, proteases, adaptors, and adenylate cyclases (Table 3.1-3). These pathways lead to a broad array of responses, including changes in transcription and translation, enzymatic activities, and cell motility.

REGULATION OF PROTEIN KINASES

Proteins undergo several covalent modifications, but phosphorylation is the most common covalent modification involved in the

TABLE 3.1-3. Enzyme Classes Stimulated by Activated Receptors

Enzyme Classes	Examples
PROTEIN KINASES	
Tyrosine	Jak
Serine, threonine	ERKs
PROTEIN PHOSPHATASES	
Tyrosine	SHP-2
Serine, threonine	Calcineurin
LIPID KINASES	
Phosphatidylinositol	PI3-kinase
LIPID PHOSPHATASES	
Phosphatidylinositol	SHIP, PTEN
PHOSPHOLIPASES	
A	CPLA2
C	PLC γ
D	
G PROTEINS	
Heterotrimeric	Gs, Gi
Ras-like	Ras, Rac
NUCLEOTIDE CYCLASES	
Adenylate	
Guanylate	

ERKs, extracellular signaling–regulated kinases; PI3-kinase, phosphoinositide 3 kinase; PLC, phospholipase C.

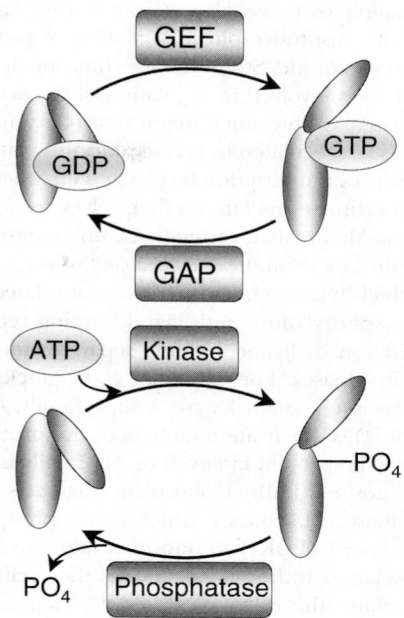

FIGURE 3.1-2. Regulation of protein activity by phosphate. The exchange of guanosine triphosphate (GTP) for guanosine diphosphate (GDP) bound to G proteins induces an activating conformational change dependent on the additional γ phosphate of GTP. Guanine nucleotide exchange factors catalyze GDP/GTP exchange. GTPase-activating proteins (GAPs) accelerate the hydrolysis of GTP to GDP to remove the γ phosphate and attenuate G-protein signaling. Protein kinases add phosphate to proteins, resulting in conformational changes and changes in enzymatic activity. Protein phosphatases remove the phosphate to inhibit the signal. G proteins and protein kinase substrates undergo a similar cycle of phosphate addition and removal to regulate their activity. ATP, adenosine triphosphate; GEF, guanine nucleotide exchange factor.

regulation of protein function. Phosphorylation by kinases and the addition of a phosphate moiety in the form of GTP exchange for GDP result in conformational changes that regulate protein activity (Fig. 3.1-2). The balance between kinase and phosphatase activity controls protein phosphorylation.[27] Protein kinases themselves, transcription factors, and cytoskeletal components are a few examples of proteins regulated by phosphorylation. Protein kinases in eukaryotic cells are divided into three classes on the basis of residues they phosphorylate: protein tyrosine kinases, protein serine-threonine kinases, and dual-specificity kinases that phosphorylate serine, threonine, and tyrosine residues. Important issues in understanding the role and regulation of protein phosphorylation are how specificities of kinases and phosphatases are determined and how phosphorylation alters the function of proteins. Work at the structural and functional levels has provided preliminary answers to these questions.

Most signal transduction pathways activate tyrosine kinases. Receptors that are not themselves tyrosine kinase use several cytoplasmic tyrosine kinases, including the Src, Syk, and Jak families. Phosphorylation of proteins on tyrosine can result in either the stimulation or inhibition of enzymatic activity and also provides sites for protein–protein interaction. An example of how tyrosine phosphorylation regulates enzymatic activity is the Src family of protein tyrosine kinases, which are regulated positively and negatively by tyrosine phosphorylation.[28] Phosphorylation of a tyrosine residue in the C-terminus leads to an intramolecular bond involving this phosphotyrosine and the Src homology 2 (SH2) domain that blocks access of substrate to the catalytic domain. In contrast, phosphorylation of a tyrosine in the telomere loop (T loop) of the catalytic domain stimulates the kinase activity by stabilizing the catalytic pocket in an active conformation.

A common theme in the regulation of the activity of tyrosine and serine-threonine protein kinases is phosphorylation of the activation, or T, loop as a mechanism of activation. The T loop forms a lip of the catalytic pocket and may occlude the active site, preventing access of the substrate. In the case of the insulin receptor, the unphosphorylated T loop also appears to interfere with adenosine triphosphate (ATP) binding.[29] Crystallographic studies indicate that the T loop is mobile and thus is probably not always in an inhibitory confirmation, providing kinases with some constitutive activity. This low level of activity is sufficient to phosphorylate a nearby kinase (e.g., autophosphorylation of a partner in a dimeric receptor). After phosphorylation, the T loop undergoes a conformational change that allows much more efficient substrate access to the catalytic site.

Once a protein kinase is active, only specific substrates are phosphorylated. This specificity rests on two properties: colocalization of the kinase with the substrate (discussed in Efficiency and Specificity: Formation of Multiprotein Signaling Complexes, later in this chapter) and the presence of sequences in a potential substrate that can be phosphorylated by the kinase. Particular motifs have been identified in substrates that in some cases govern whether a protein will be a substrate. A proline following the phosphorylated serine or threonine is absolutely required for substrates of MAP kinases. In other cases, particular motifs are favored as phosphorylation sites.[30] These motifs probably fit best into the catalytic cleft of the kinase. In some cases, sequences distant from the site of phosphorylation mediate low-affinity association of a kinase with its substrate and thereby enhance phosphorylation.

Most signaling pathways also activate serine kinases, but a higher level of constitutive phosphorylation of proteins occurs on serine and threonine. Still unclear is how much of this basal phosphorylation is involved in regulation of the activity or location of proteins and how much might be irrelevant. Myriad cellular functions are regulated by serine phosphorylation, ranging from the activity of transcription factors and enzymes to the polymerization of actin. Serine kinases themselves are regulated in a variety of ways. Mammalian serine-threonine kinases have been subdivided into 11 subfamilies on the basis of primary sequence homology, which has also been predictive of related function.[31] Location, phosphorylation, and ligand binding regulate serine kinases. Activation by ligand binding separates some classes of serine protein kinases. For example, cyclic nucleotides (e.g., cAMP) activate the protein kinase A superfamily. Calcium and diacylglycerol (DAG) activate members of the protein kinase C (PKC) family. The protein kinase B or Akt family is activated by phosphatidylinositol (PtdIns) phosphate products of phosphoinositide 3 kinase (PI3-kinase), which allows phosphoinositide-dependent kinase 1 (PDK1) to phosphorylate the activation, or T, loop. Association with cyclins activates the cyclin-dependent kinase family, and the calcium-calmodulin–dependent kinases are activated by calcium. Kinase cascades also are important in allowing multiple levels of regulation and amplification of serine kinase activity. For example, MAP kinases are activated by phosphorylation of the T loop after activation of upstream kinases: Activation of Raf leads to phosphorylation and activation of MEK1, which phosphorylates and activates the extracellular signaling–regulated kinases (ERKs) (Fig. 3.1-3).

Protein kinase signals are generally attenuated by phosphatases, metabolism of activating second messengers, or both. Dephosphorylation of the T-loop site markedly reduces the activity of most kinases, and dephosphorylation of motifs required for protein–protein binding prevents kinases from interacting with their substrates. Phosphatases also counteract the phosphorylation of substrate molecules, reversing the effects of the kinases.

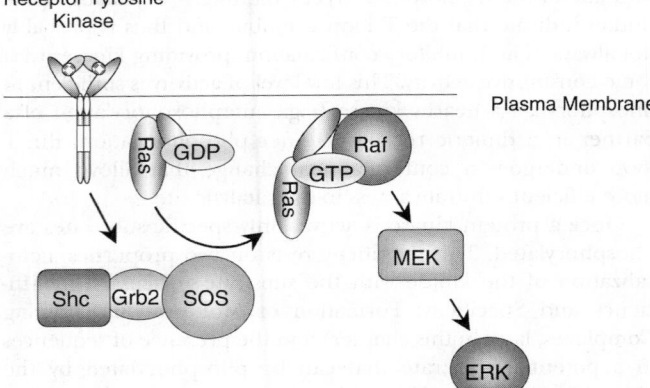

Receptor Tyrosine Kinase

Plasma Membrane

FIGURE 3.1-3.   Activation of the extracellular signaling–regulated kinase (ERK) pathway. Many receptors activate the ERKs. Most receptor tyrosine kinases stimulate the activity of the Ras guanine nucleotide exchange factor son of sevenless (SOS), which associates with the linker proteins Shc and Grb2. The activation of Ras by SOS stimulates a protein serine kinase cascade initiated by Raf, which stimulates MEK. MEK then activates the ERKs. ERKs phosphorylate transcription factors to regulate gene expression. GDP, guanosine diphosphate; GTP, guanosine triphosphate.

REGULATION OF PROTEIN PHOSPHATASES

Protein phosphatases remove the phosphate residues from proteins and activate and inhibit signaling pathways, depending on the sites that are dephosphorylated. Protein phosphatases are divided into the same three groups as the kinases, on the basis of their substrates: tyrosine phosphatases, serine-threonine phosphatases, and dual-specificity phosphatases. Tyrosine phosphatases and dual-specificity phosphatases use a cysteinylphosphate intermediate, whereas the serine-threonine phosphatases are metal-requiring enzymes that dephosphorylate in a single step.[32]

Structural work has revealed how the activity of some nonreceptor tyrosine phosphatases is regulated.[33] The SHP-2 phosphatase has, in addition to the catalytic domain, two SH2 domains. These domains (discussed in more detail in Domains That Mediate Protein–Protein Binding, later in this chapter) mediate binding to other proteins by direct association with phosphorylated tyrosine residues. In the inactive state, the catalytic cleft of SHP-2 is blocked by the N-terminal SH2 domain. Binding of the N-terminal SH2 domain to a phosphotyrosine residue of a target protein induces a conformational change that allows substrate access to the catalytic domain. Tyrosine phosphatases act to attenuate signals that require tyrosine phosphorylation and to activate pathways inhibited by tyrosine phosphorylation. An example of the negative regulatory function of tyrosine phosphatases is the role of SHP-1 (a homologue of SHP-2) in inhibiting cytokine and B-cell receptor signaling. In contrast, SHP-2 is necessary for cytokine stimulation of cells. On the basis of the ability of phosphatase inhibitors (e.g., vanadate) to activate tyrosine kinase–dependent signaling in the absence of ligands, acute inactivation of specific tyrosine phosphatases may play a more important role than previously appreciated in regulating the balance of tyrosine phosphorylation and dephosphorylation that controls signaling pathways.

Protein phosphatase 1 (PP1), PP2A, PP2B, and PP2C are the major serine-threonine phosphatase activities *in vivo*.[33] PP1 and PP2A are composed of catalytic and regulatory subunits. PP1 affects many pathways, from glycogen metabolism to the cell cycle. PP2B binds to calmodulin and is regulated by calcium. Phosphorylation of either the regulatory or catalytic subunit regulates the activity of serine phosphatases. More than 100 PP1 regulatory subunits function to target the catalytic domain to different cellular locations and mediate activation or inhibition. This action provides an example of how a single catalytic activity can perform multiple specific functions as a result of targeting by a regulatory subunit.

GUANOSINE TRIPHOSPHATE–BINDING PROTEINS

Just as covalent modification as a mechanism of protein activity regulation is important, so is noncovalent binding to proteins. A number of small molecules regulate protein function, as does protein–protein interaction. G proteins are the best-studied protein mediators that regulate other proteins.

GTP-binding proteins function as digital switches. They are inactive when bound to GDP, but GTP binding results in a conformational change that allows binding to effector molecules and transmission of a signal (see Fig. 3.1-2). GTP hydrolysis to GDP ultimately returns the protein to its basal state. GTP-binding proteins regulate the same molecules activated by receptors: protein and lipid kinases, phosphatases, and phospholipases. GTP-binding proteins are categorized into two large classes: the heterotrimeric GTP-binding proteins and the Ras-like GTP-binding proteins. Activation of GTP-binding proteins is regulated by guanine nucleotide exchange factors that catalyze the release of GDP and allow GTP to bind to and activate the protein. GTPase-activating proteins (GAPs) accelerate GTP hydrolysis and regulate inactivation of GTP-binding proteins. All GTP-binding proteins have lipid modifications that promote membrane association.

Heterotrimeric GTP-binding proteins have three subunits and are activated by GPCR.[34] In the inactive state, the α, β, and γ subunits are associated as a heterotrimer. In mammalian cells, 20 α subunits, 6 β subunits, and 12 γ subunits are known. The heterotrimeric forms are divided into four classes on the basis of function. Gαs stimulates adenylate cyclase, Gαi inhibits adenylate cyclase, and Gαq activates PLC β. G12 and G13 form a related group whose function is not yet known, although Gα_{13} does couple to the lysophosphatidic acid receptor. Activation of GPCRs allows them to catalyze GDP/GTP exchange on the α subunit of heterotrimeric G proteins. In response to GTP loading, the α and β/γ subunits dissociate. The β and γ subunits do not dissociate *in vivo*. The α subunit and the β/γ complex send signals. The α subunit undergoes a conformational change in response to GTP that allows it to bind to effectors. The β/γ dimer does not undergo a conformational change, but release from the α subunit exposes surfaces that allow it to bind to effectors. The α and β/γ subunits affect the activity of a wide range of downstream effectors, including ion channels, protein kinases, and phospholipases. Domains termed *regulators of G-protein signaling* act as GAPs toward the α subunit and attenuate the signal by catalyzing hydrolysis of GTP to GDP.[35]

Ras-like GTP-binding proteins are monomeric and usually of lower molecular weight than are the heterotrimeric GTP-binding proteins. Ras-like GTP-binding proteins are classified into five families: the Ras,[36] Rho,[37] Rab,[38] Arf,[39] and Ran families.[40] The Ras and Rho families regulate cell growth, transcription, and the actin cytoskeleton; the Arf family regulates PLD and vesicle trafficking; the Rab family regulates vesicle trafficking; and the Ran family regulates nuclear import. Ras-like GTP-binding proteins are activated in a manner similar to that of the α subunit of heterotrimeric G proteins. Exchange of GTP for GDP results in a conformational change that promotes binding to effector molecules. In contrast to heterotrimeric G proteins, nucleotide exchange for Ras-like GTP-binding proteins is not catalyzed directly by receptors. Specific exchange factors are activated downstream of receptors or in response to specific cellular events. Signals are attenuated by the action of GAPs, analogous to regulators of the G protein–signaling domain–containing proteins that catalyze GTP hydrolysis.

GTP-binding proteins affect the activity of their targets by causing conformational changes and perhaps by serving to localize the target. Crystal structures of the catalytic domain of adenylate cyclase bound to G proteins illustrate the conformational change.[41] Gαs binds to the C2a domain of adenylate cyclase, causing rotation of the C1a domain, which positions the catalytic residues more favorably for conversion of ATP to cAMP. Although crystal structures of small G proteins bound to portions of their targets also have been solved, the effect on the activity of target molecules as a result of binding has not yet been explained. Studies of the role of Ras in the interaction of Raf suggest that an important role of Ras is localization of Raf to the membrane, but Ras also may help to activate Raf directly.[42]

SMALL-MOLECULE SECOND MESSENGERS

Small molecules transmit signals by binding noncovalently to protein targets and affecting their function. These molecules are called *second messengers* because they are generated within the cell in response to a first messenger, such as a growth factor, binding to a cell surface receptor.

cAMP was the first second messenger discovered. Adenylate cyclase, activated by heterotrimeric G proteins, catalyzes the synthesis of cAMP from ATP.[65] The primary target of cAMP is protein kinase A, and the activation of protein kinase A by cAMP demonstrates how second messengers function.[40] The inactive form of protein kinase A is a tetramer of two catalytic and two regulatory subunits; the regulatory subunit inhibits the activity of the catalytic subunit. The regulatory subunit contains two cAMP-binding sites. Binding of cAMP to the first site causes a conformational change that exposes the second site. Binding of cAMP to the second site results in dissociation of the regulatory and catalytic subunits. The free catalytic subunits are then active.

PLCs are common downstream effectors, which cleave PtdIns-4,5-P_2 to generate inositol-1,4,5-trisphosphate (IP$_3$) and DAG.[43] All three families of PLC—β, γ, and δ—are activated by calcium. PLC β is activated by the α and the β/γ subunits of heterotrimeric G proteins, and PLC γ is activated by tyrosine phosphorylation. DAG interacts with the C1 domain of PKC to mediate their membrane localization and activation. IP$_3$ binds to a calcium channel in the endoplasmic reticulum (ER) and stimulates the release of calcium from intracellular stores.[44] The initial increase in cytoplasmic calcium is followed by an influx of extracellular calcium via capacitive calcium channels at the plasma membrane. In unstimulated cells, cytosolic calcium is much lower than in the extracellular space or ER (100 nM vs. 1 mM), and therefore opening channels in the ER or plasma membrane allows calcium to flood into the cytoplasm, temporarily raising the cytoplasmic calcium to micromolar concentrations. Ultimately, calcium returns to basal levels as a result of closing of the channels and removal of cytosolic calcium by extracellular transport and pumping calcium into intracellular compartments. Calcium has a multitude of cellular effects, including directly regulating enzymatic activities, ion channels, and transcription. Several calcium-binding domains are known, including the C2 domain and EF hands. Calcium binds directly to enzymes and regulates their activity or to regulatory subunits, such as calmodulin.

Eicosanoids are ubiquitous signaling molecules that bind to GPCR and to transcription factors.[45] Eicosanoid synthesis occurs in response to a number of stimuli and is an example of rapid cell-to-cell signaling. Unlike most second messengers, eicosanoids produced in one cell escape that cell and diffuse to nearby cells and either bind to receptors or are metabolized further. Eicosanoid synthesis is regulated by the production of arachidonic acid, which is produced from DAG via diglyceride lipases or from phospholipids by PLA. PLA2 cleave the sn-2 acyl group of phospholipids to produce a free fatty acid and a lysophospholipid. The calcium-regulated form of PLA2 shows a preference for substrates containing arachidonic acid. The further metabolism of arachidonic acid results in the synthesis of prostaglandins and leukotrienes.

EFFICIENCY AND SPECIFICITY: FORMATION OF MULTIPROTEIN SIGNALING COMPLEXES

COMPARTMENTATION

The ability of a signal transduction pathway to transmit a signal is dependent on the probability that a protein finds its target. The likelihood of any two proteins coming into contact is proportional to their concentrations. Recruiting a protein to a specific compartment in a cell markedly increases the local concentration of that protein, thereby enhancing the probability that it will interact with other proteins or small molecules that are recruited to or generated in the same compartment. Colocalization of proteins in a signaling pathway is achieved by recruitment to the same membrane surface or organelle (e.g., plasma membrane vs. ER) and by protein–protein interactions. Conversely, separating proteins or second messengers (or both) into distinct compartments turns off signaling pathways.

Transport of signaling proteins into the nucleus is important in a number of signal transduction pathways and illustrates the concept of colocalization in the same organelle.[46] Nuclear transport proceeds through nuclear pores. Proteins of less than 40 kD cross by simple diffusion, but transport of larger molecules requires a nuclear localization signal to which the importin proteins bind. The importins target the protein to the nuclear pore, and the complex is transported into the nucleus. The Ran G protein dissociates the importins from their cargo once they are in the nucleus. Regulated export of proteins from the nucleus is similar to import. A nuclear export signal is recognized by the protein exportin, which then transports the cargo out of the nucleus. A specific example is nuclear localization of the transcription factor nuclear factor of activated T cells (NFAT), which is required for its transcriptional activity.[47] In response to T-cell activation and a rise in intracellular calcium, NFAT is dephosphorylated by the calcium-responsive phosphatase calcineurin. Dephosphorylation allows the nuclear localization signal in NFAT to bind to the importins, and NFAT, along with calcineurin, is imported into the nucleus. NFAT also contains a nuclear export signal, and phosphorylation appears to allow the nuclear export signal to bind to exportin, resulting in transport to the cytoplasm.

Protein compartmentation also occurs on a smaller scale in the form of protein–protein complexes, which serve either to target proteins to particular parts of the cell or to promote efficient signal transmission. Well-studied examples of the use of protein–protein interaction to determine the localization of enzymes include the A kinase anchoring proteins that bind to protein kinase A, a family of proteins that bind to PKC[48] and the subunits of PP2A.[49]

Lipid rafts are regions where sphingolipids and cholesterol are concentrated in the outer leaflet of the plasma membrane and are important sites for signaling.[50,51] The lipid composition provides structural cohesiveness. Rafts concentrate and exclude proteins, promoting the formation of signaling complexes. Glycosylphosphatidylinositol-linked proteins on the extracellular surface of the plasma membrane concentrate in lipid rafts, as do acylated proteins on the intracellular surface.

Transmembrane receptors can be recruited into rafts following their activation, along with their targets, leading to efficient signal generation.

DOMAINS THAT MEDIATE PROTEIN–PROTEIN BINDING

The regulated assembly of protein–protein complexes has several functions in signal transduction, including the formation of complexes involving proteins that signal to each other, forming a "solid state" module that does not require diffusion to transmit a signal. Protein–protein interactions also localize an enzyme near its substrate: The binding of PLC γ1 to the PDGF receptor brings the enzyme to the plasma membrane where its substrate, PtdIns-4,5-P_2, is concentrated. These interactions are often mediated by conserved domains that recognize phosphorylated tyrosine or serine residues or proline-rich sequences (Table 3.1-4).

SH2 domains and phosphotyrosine-binding domains bind to motifs containing phosphorylated tyrosine residues.[52] The crystal structures of several SH2 domains have been determined and reveal a pocket that binds the phosphotyrosine and a groove that determines binding specificity based on the fit of the residue's C-terminal (or, in a few cases, N-terminal) to the phosphotyrosine.[53,54] Tyrosine kinases and phosphatases regulate the formation of complexes involving these domains. Tyrosine kinases themselves serve as docking sites for other proteins, which is most evident with tyrosine kinase receptors that recruit PI3-kinase, p120 Ras GAP, PLC γ, and SHP-2 through SH2 domain–dependent interactions. Tyrosine kinases phosphorylate adaptors such as the IRS[55] and Gab families of proteins[56] that also recruit other signaling molecules through phosphotyrosine-based interactions. In addition to mediating protein–protein interactions, binding of SH2 domains to phosphotyrosine residues stimulates the enzymatic activities of such proteins as PI3-kinase and Src kinases. SH2 domains also bind to intramolecular phosphotyrosines, as in the case of Src, to inhibit catalytic activity.

Phosphotyrosine-binding domains are functionally analogous to SH2 domains in that they bind phosphotyrosine residues to assemble multiprotein complexes, but they have no sequence or structural similarity to SH2 domains. Thus, they represent an independent evolutionary solution to phosphotyrosine-dependent assembly of protein complexes. A few phos-

TABLE 3.1-4. Protein–Protein Interaction Domains and Motifs

Motifs	Domains That Bind Motif	Examples of Proteins That Contain the Domain
Phosphotyrosine	SH2	Src, PI3-kinase, SHP-2
	PTB	IRS family, SHC
Phosphoserine	WD40 14-3-3	Telomerase, APAF-1, coatamer
	WW	Pin1
	FHA	Rad53
Proline-rich	SH3	Src, PI3-kinase
	WW	YAP, dystrophin
	EVH1	VASP, ENA, WASp
C-terminal sequences	PDZ	ZO-1, lim kinase

PI3-kinase, phosphoinositide 3 kinase; SH2, src homology 2; SH3, src homology 3.

photyrosine-binding and SH2 domains bind to a tyrosine-containing motif in the absence of phosphorylation.

Recognition of phosphoserine motifs is also an important means of protein–protein interaction. Forkhead-associated domains, 14-3-3 proteins, and some WD40 and WW domains bind to regions of proteins containing phosphoserine.[57] WD40 domains in proteins that are members of the F-box and WD40 repeat family are important in regulating ubiquitination and subsequent proteolysis of proteins, such as the inhibitor of κB (IκB), which regulates the activity of the transcription factor nuclear factor κB (NFκB). 14-3-3 proteins are a family of small proteins whose primary function appears to be binding to phosphoserine motifs. An example of the importance of this interaction is the role of 14-3-3 in regulating the nuclear location of the phosphatase Cdc25 that regulates the cell cycle. Binding of 14-3-3 to phosphorylated Cdc25 leads to its export from the nucleus and a block in the cell cycle.

Src homology 3 (SH3), WW, and ena-vasp homology domains are structurally distinct, but all bind to proline-rich sequences.[58] Many proteins that contain SH3 domains also have proline-rich regions that could be involved in intramolecular binding, suggesting that a conformational change in the protein could disrupt intramolecular binding and allow the SH3 domain to interact with other proteins. Similarly, the accessibility of proline-rich regions to SH3 domains may be regulated by conformational changes that expose the proline-rich region or disrupt an intramolecular interaction.

PDZ domains recognize motifs in the C-termini of proteins, as well as each other and lipids.[59] These motifs are found in cytoplasmic proteins, and many also contain multiple PDZ domains. PDZ domain–containing proteins function to aggregate transmembrane proteins, such as the glutamate receptor. Group I PDZ domains bind to a consensus sequence, T/S-X-V/I, where V/I is the C-terminus of the protein. Phosphorylation of the S or T in this motif disrupts PDZ binding in some cases. For example, phosphorylation of this serine in the β_2-adrenergic receptor was shown to lead to a loss of PDZ domain–mediated binding to EBP50, which regulates endocytic sorting of the receptor.

DOMAINS THAT MEDIATE PROTEIN BINDING TO MEMBRANE LIPIDS

Localization of proteins to membranes greatly limits the space in which proteins diffuse and increases the probability that enzymes and substrates will contact each other. A variety of domains have evolved to bind phospholipids (Table 3.1-5). C1 domains present in PKC and some other signaling molecules bind to DAG, thereby recruiting PKC to the membrane.[60] Membrane recruitment of PKC is aided also by the C2 domain, which binds to anionic phospholipids in the presence of calcium. This pathway is controlled by DAG production, and the primary source is DAG produced by PLC hydrolysis of PtdIns-4,5-P_2.

Several different domains bind to phosphoinositides and serve to localize the proteins that contain them to membranes.[61] These domains include pleckstrin homology (PH), Phox, FYVE, FERM, and ENTH domains. Particular PH domains bind specific phosphoinositides, including PtdIns-3-P, PtdIns-4,5-P_2, PtdIns-3,4-P_2, and PtdIns-3,4,5-P_3. Phox and FYVE domains bind to PtdIns-3-P. FERM and ENTH domains bind PtdIns-4,5-P_2. The accessibility of the domain and the availability of PtdIns phosphates regulate

TABLE 3.1-5. Domains That Bind Phospholipids

Phospholipid	Domains That Bind
Diacylglycerol	C1
Phosphatidic acid	PX
PtdIns-4-P	PH
PtdIns-3-P	PX, PH, FYVE
PtdIns-3,4-P_2	PH
PtdIns-3,5-P_2	PH
PtdIns-4,5-P_2	PH, Tubby, FERM, Sprouty, ENTH, ANTH
PtdIns-3,4,5-P_3	PH

PH, pleckstrin homology.

these interactions. Phosphoinositide kinases synthesize phosphoinositides. PtdIns 4-kinases synthesize PtdIns-4-P from PtdIns. Type I PtdIns phosphate kinases phosphorylate PtdIns-4-P at the 5 position to make PtdIns-4,5-P_2. Phosphoinositide 3 kinases phosphorylate PtdIns, PtdIns-4-P, and PtdIns-4,5-P_2 at the 3 position of the inositol ring to make PtdIns-3-P, PtdIns-3,4-P_2, and PtdIns-3,4,5-P_3, respectively. Phosphoinositide levels also are regulated by phosphatases. PTEN and related phosphatases remove the phosphate from the 3 position of PtdIns-3,4-5-P_3, PtdIns-3,4-P_2, and PtdIns-3-P.[62] PTEN thus counteracts PI3-kinase signals, and cells from which PTEN is absent have increased signaling through PI3-kinase–dependent pathways. A family of phosphatases that removes the phosphate from the 5 position of PtdIns-3,4-5-P_3, the SH2 inositol phosphatases (SHIP1 and SHIP2), also regulates phosphoinositide signaling pathways.[63]

Acute production of specific phosphoinositides in a membrane compartment results in the recruitment of proteins containing a PH domain that recognizes the phosphoinositide. Colocalization of a subset of proteins allows them to interact more efficiently. An example of the role of PH domains in such a pathway is the activation of akt by PDK1.[64] PDK1 and akt are protein serine-threonine kinases that contain PH domains that bind PtdIns-3,4-P_2 or PtdIns-3,4,5-P_3. Activation of PI3-kinase leads to local synthesis of PtdIns-3,4-P_2 and PtdIns-3,4,5-P_3 that causes recruitment of akt and PDK1 to the same membrane location. This localization facilitates phosphorylation and activation of akt by PDK1.

REGULATION OF PROTEIN LEVELS: TRANSCRIPTION, TRANSLATION, AND PROTEOLYSIS

In addition to influencing the activity of proteins in the cell, signal transduction pathways also regulate the type and levels of proteins expressed in cells. This sort of regulation is necessary for development, differentiation, and the specific function of distinct cell types. Whether a protein is expressed at all in a cell is regulated at the transcriptional level, whereas transcription, translation, and proteolysis have a role in determining the amount of an expressed protein present in a cell.

Ultimately, most signal transduction pathways regulate gene transcription and, thus, the level and type of proteins expressed in the cell. The magnitude of the effect of a signaling pathway on the transcriptional output of a cell is illustrated by the effects of stimuli on gene expression profiles using microarray analysis.

A single stimulus affects the transcription of hundreds of genes. The ability to transcribe a gene is regulated at multiple levels, including the structure of chromatin in the region of the gene, modifications of the promoter regions, and the activity of transcription factors and coactivators. Signal transduction pathways regulate histone acetylases and deacetylases that determine the accessibility of chromatin to the transcriptional apparatus. Recent work has shown that a number of signals lead to histone hyperacetylation that disrupts the nucleosome to allow transcription. These pathways cooperate with the activation of transcription factor to induce transcription.

Signal transduction pathways activate transcription factors in numerous ways. The binding of ligands to the nuclear receptor family of transcription factors causes dissociation of the receptor from a complex with heat-shock proteins and allows the receptor to bind to DNA. Tyrosine phosphorylation of the STAT family of transcription factors by Jak kinases in response to stimulation of cytokine receptors allows them to dimerize through their SH2 domains and enter the nucleus to bind DNA.[65] TGF-β receptors activate transcription by phosphorylating SMAD proteins on serine residues.[15] Phosphorylation of SMAD proteins promotes heterodimerization with SMAD4 and exposes the DNA-binding domain. Activated SMADs translocate to the nucleus complex with a protein called *Fast1* and bind to DNA to regulate transcription.

Activation of transcription factors also occurs much farther downstream from the receptor. Stimulation of the transcriptional activity of Elk-1 by EGF requires activation of a Ras exchange factor, which leads to activation of Ras. Active Ras promotes the stimulation of Raf activity. Raf in turn phosphorylates and activates MEK1, which phosphorylates and activates ERK. Active ERK translocates to the nucleus and phosphorylates and stimulates the activity of the transcription factor elk-1.

Translation is also controlled at several levels.[66] The sequences of some RNAs result in stable tertiary structures that bind proteins to regulate location or translation. The ability of these types of RNAs to be translated is regulated by protein kinase cascades. A common target of signal transduction pathways is phosphorylation of initiation factor eIF-4E and availability of eIF-4E. p70^{S6} kinase regulates the translation of specific RNAs containing a 5' terminal oligopyrimidine tract by phosphorylation of the ribosomal S6 protein. This increases the ability of the ribosome to process such messages.

The levels of particular proteins in the cell are also regulated by proteolysis, which occurs either via the proteosome or the lysosome. Ubiquitination targets proteins to the proteosome but can also regulate other aspects of protein function.[67] An example of the role of ubiquitination is the regulation of IκB levels. Phosphorylation of IκB is stimulated by a number of receptor-mediated signaling pathways. This action leads to its dissociation from NFκB and allows NFκB to enter the nucleus and bind DNA. After phosphorylation, the β transducin repeat–containing protein binds to IκB, recruiting ubiquitin ligase that catalyzes the ubiquitination of IκB and leads to its recognition and degradation by the proteosome.

The second major pathway of protein degradation is the lysosomal pathway, which is also important in signal transduction. An early response to the stimulation of receptors is their internalization into endosomes; some evidence suggests that signaling persists at this location after endocytosis.[68] In the case of receptor tyrosine kinases, ligand-dependent kinase activity is necessary for endocytosis, mediated by clathrin-coated pits. After endocytosis, either receptors may recycle to the plasma membrane or the endosomes may fuse with lysosomes, leading to degradation of the receptor.

REFERENCES

1. Nyberg KA, Michelson RJ, Putnam CW, et al. Toward maintaining the genome: DNA damage and replication checkpoints. *Annu Rev Genet* 2002;36:617.
2. van der Geer P, Hunter T, Lindberg RA. Receptor protein-tyrosine kinases and their signal transduction pathways. *Annu Rev Cell Biol* 1994;10:251.
3. Schlessinger J. Cell signaling by receptor tyrosine kinases. *Cell* 2000;103:211.
4. Fretto LJ, Snape AJ, Tomlinson JE, et al. Mechanism of platelet-derived growth factor (PDGF) AA, AB, and BB binding to alpha and beta PDGF receptor. *J Biol Chem* 1993;268:3625.
5. de Vos AM, Ultsch M, Kossiakoff AA. Human growth hormone and extracellular domain of its receptor: crystal structure of the complex. *Science* 1992;255:306.
6. Spivak-Kroizman T, Lemmon MA, Dikic I, et al. Heparin-induced oligomerization of FGF molecules is responsible for FGF receptor dimerization, activation, and cell proliferation. *Cell* 1994;79:1015.
7. Schlessinger J. Ligand-induced, receptor-mediated dimerization and activation of EGF receptor. *Cell* 2002;110:669.
8. Kullander K, Klein R. Mechanisms and functions of Eph and ephrin signaling. *Nat Rev Mol Cell Biol* 2002;3:475.
9. Harris RC, Chung E, Coffey RJ. EGF receptor ligands. *Exp Cell Res* 2003;284:2.
10. Elenius K, Paul S, Allison G, et al. Activation of HER4 by heparin-binding EGF-like growth factor stimulates chemotaxis but not proliferation. *EMBO J* 1997;16:1268.
11. Crovello CS, Lai C, Cantley LC, et al. Differential signaling by the epidermal growth factor-like growth factors neuregulin-1 and neuregulin-2. *J Biol Chem* 1998;273:26954.
12. Kerr IM, Costa-Pereira AP, Lillemeier BF, et al. Of JAKs, STATs, blind watchmakers, jeeps and trains. *FEBS Lett* 2003;546:1.
13. Mustelin T, Abraham RT, Rudd CE, et al. Protein tyrosine phosphorylation in T cell signaling. *Front Biosci* 2002;7:d918.
14. Gauld SB, Dal Porto JM, Cambier JC. B cell antigen receptor signaling: roles in cell development and disease. *Science* 2002;296:1641.
15. Shi Y, Massague J. Mechanisms of TGF-beta signaling from cell membrane to the nucleus. *Cell* 2003;113:685.
16. Fischer EH. Cell signaling by protein tyrosine phosphorylation. *Adv Enzyme Regul* 1999;39:359.
17. Hermiston ML, Xu Z, Weiss A. CD45: a critical regulator of signaling thresholds in immune cells. *Annu Rev Immunol* 2003;21:107.
18. Pierce KL, Premont RT, Lefkowitz RJ. Seven-transmembrane receptors. *Nat Rev Mol Cell Biol* 2002;3:639.
19. Foord SM. Receptor classification: post genome. *Curr Opin Pharmacol* 2002;2:561.
20. Ji TH, Grossmann M, Ji I. G protein-coupled receptors. I. Diversity of receptor-ligand interactions. *J Biol Chem* 1998;273:17299.
21. Hamm HE. The many faces of G protein signaling. *J Biol Chem* 1998;273:669.
22. Baron M. An overview of the Notch signaling pathway. *Semin Cell Dev Biol* 2003;14:113.
23. Wedel B, Garbers D. The guanylyl cyclase family at Y2K. *Annu Rev Physiol* 2001;63:215.
24. Aggarwal BB. Signaling pathways of the TNF superfamily: a double-edged sword. *Nat Rev Immunol* 2003;3:745.
25. Damsky CH, Ilic D. Integrin signaling: it's where the action is. *Curr Opin Cell Biol* 2002;14:594.
26. Humphries MJ, McEwan PA, Barton SJ, et al. Integrin structure: heady advances in ligand binding, but activation still makes the knees wobble. *Trends Biochem Sci* 2003;28:313.
27. Hunter T. Protein kinases and phosphatases: the yin and yang of protein phosphorylation and signaling. *Cell* 1995;80:225.
28. Bjorge JD, Jakymiw A, Fujita DJ. Selected glimpses into the activation and function of Src kinase. *Oncogene* 2000;19:5620.
29. Hubbard SR. Protein tyrosine kinases: autoregulation and small-molecule inhibition. *Curr Opin Struct Biol* 2002;12:735.
30. Manning BD, Cantley LC. Hitting the target: emerging technologies in the search for kinase substrates. *Sci STKE* 2002;2002:PE49.
31. Manning G, Whyte DB, Martinez R, et al. The protein kinase complement of the human genome. *Science* 2002;298:1912.
32. Barford D. Protein phosphatases. *Curr Opin Struct Biol* 1995;5:728.
33. Barford D, Neel BG. Revealing mechanisms for SH2 domain mediated regulation of the protein tyrosine phosphatase SHP-2. *Structure* 1998;6:249.
34. Neves SR, Ram PT, Iyengar R. G protein pathways. *Science* 2002;296:1636.
35. Druey KM. Bridging with GAPs: receptor communication through RGS proteins. *Sci STKE* 2001;2001:RE14.
36. Wolfman A. Ras isoform-specific signaling: location, location, location. *Sci STKE* 2001;2001:PE2.
37. Etienne-Manneville S, Hall A. Rho GTPases in cell biology. *Nature* 2002;420:629.
38. Pfeffer SR. Rab GTPases: specifying and deciphering organelle identity and function. *Trends Cell Biol* 2001;11:487.
39. Randazzo PA, Nie Z, Miura K, et al. Molecular aspects of the cellular activities of ADP-ribosylation factors. *Sci STKE* 2000;2000:RE1.
40. Dasso M. The Ran GTPase: theme and variations. *Curr Biol* 2002;12:R502.
41. Simonds WF. G protein regulation of adenylate cyclase. *Trends Pharmacol Sci* 1999;20:66.

42. Chong H, Vikis HG, Guan KL. Mechanisms of regulating the Raf kinase family. *Cell Signal* 2003;15:463.

43. Rhee SG. Regulation of phosphoinositide-specific phospholipase C. *Annu Rev Biochem* 2001;70:281.

44. Taylor CW. Controlling calcium entry. *Cell* 2002;111:767.

45. Soberman RJ, Christmas P. The organization and consequences of eicosanoid signaling. *J Clin Invest* 2003;111:1107.

46. Lei EP, Silver PA. Protein and RNA export from the nucleus. *Dev Cell* 2002;2:261.

47. Crabtree GR, Olson EN. NFAT signaling: choreographing the social lives of cells. *Cell* 2002;109[Suppl]:S67.

48. Bauman AL, Scott JD. Kinase- and phosphatase-anchoring proteins: harnessing the dynamic duo. *Nat Cell Biol* 2002;4:E203.

49. Virshup DM. Protein phosphatase 2A: a panoply of enzymes. *Curr Opin Cell Biol* 2000;12:180.

50. Lai EC. Lipid rafts make for slippery platforms. *J Cell Biol* 2003;162:365.

51. Dykstra M, Cherukuri A, Sohn HW, et al. Location is everything: lipid rafts and immune cell signaling. *Annu Rev Immunol* 2003;21:457.

52. Schlessinger J, Lemmon MA. SH2 and PTB domains in tyrosine kinase signaling. *Sci STKE* 2003;2003:RE12.

53. Waksman G, Shoelson SE, Pant N, et al. Binding of a high affinity phosphotyrosyl peptide to the Src SH2 domain: crystal structures of the complexed and peptide-free forms. *Cell* 1993;72:779.

54. Eck MJ, Shoelson SE, Harrison SC. Recognition of a high-affinity phosphotyrosyl peptide by the Src homology-2 domain of p56lck. *Nature* 1993;362:87.

55. White MF, Yenush L. The IRS-signaling system: a network of docking proteins that mediate insulin and cytokine action. *Curr Top Microbiol Immunol* 1998;228:179.

56. Gu H, Neel BG. The Gab in signal transduction. *Trends Cell Biol* 2003;13:122.

57. Yaffe MB, Elia AE. Phosphoserine/threonine-binding domains. *Curr Opin Cell Biol* 2001;13:131.

58. Zarrinpar A, Bhattacharyya RP, Lim WA. The structure and function of proline recognition domains. *Sci STKE* 2003;2003:RE8.

59. Nourry C, Grant SG, Borg JP. PDZ domain proteins: plug and play! *Sci STKE* 2003;2003:RE7.

60. Kazanietz MG. Novel nonkinase phorbol ester receptors: the C1 domain connection. *Mol Pharmacol* 2002;61:759.

61. Lemmon MA. Phosphoinositide recognition domains. *Traffic* 2003;4:201.

62. Maehama T, Taylor GS, Dixon JE. PTEN and myotubularin: novel phosphoinositide phosphatases. *Annu Rev Biochem* 2001;70:247.

63. Rohrschneider LR, Fuller JF, Wolf I, et al. Structure, function, and biology of SHIP proteins. *Genes Dev* 2000;14:505.

64. Vanhaesebroeck B, Alessi DR. The PI3K-PDK1 connection: more than just a road to PKB. *Biochem J* 2000;346:561.

65. Levy DE, Darnell JE Jr. Stats: transcriptional control and biological impact. *Nat Rev Mol Cell Biol* 2002;3:651.

66. Dever TE. Gene-specific regulation by general translation factors. *Cell* 2002;108:545.

67. Schwartz DC, Hochstrasser M. A superfamily of protein tags: ubiquitin, SUMO and related modifiers. *Trends Biochem Sci* 2003;28:321.

68. Di Fiore PP, De Camilli P. Endocytosis and signaling: an inseparable partnership. *Cell* 2001;106:1.

SECTION 2

STEVEN I. REED

Cell Cycle

Cell division is a process that must be carried out with absolute fidelity. The program of generating an adult organism from a single zygote involves countless cell duplications, each requiring the precise partitioning of genetic material and most other cellular components to daughter cells. The division process then continues during adult life to replenish essential cells restricted to a limited life span. As a result, organisms have evolved cell duplication strategies that include redundant safeguards to prevent errors or, if errors occur, to correct them. Nevertheless, errors do occur at a measurable frequency, and mutations accumulated over time can weaken protective mechanisms, rendering the genome increasingly vulnerable to challenges. The resulting loss of genetic and genomic stability has serious implications for survival in that it is a major contributing factor to the development of malignancy. Indeed, cancer is one of the leading causes of mortality in humans.

In this chapter, the basic principles of mammalian cell division and the mechanisms that have evolved to safeguard the integrity of the process are reviewed. Then, there is a discussion on how the normal control mechanisms of cell division and protective safeguards become subverted in cancer cells. It is hoped that, ultimately, detailed knowledge of cell division in normal and cancer cells will lead to rational effective therapeutic approaches.

CELL-CYCLE ENGINE

Although the details of cell division vary considerably across phylogenetic lines and even in different cell types within the same organism, the underlying infrastructure that mediates and controls the cell division process is remarkably conserved. If one compares yeast cells and mammalian cells in culture, perhaps the two most aggressively studied model cell division systems, are not only the respective cell division cycles organized along a similar scheme, but many of the proteins used in the cell division pathway are easily recognizable as being evolutionarily related. Indeed, some of these proteins are so highly conserved that they are functional in the heterologous organism despite a billion years of divergent evolution.

PHASES OF THE CELL CYCLE

As alluded to above, the basic organization of the cell cycle is highly conserved in eukaryotic evolution. In 1951, Howard and Pelc,[1] studying the division of plant root cells, separated the process into four phases eventually referred to as *GAP1, synthetic phase, GAP2,* and *mitosis.* The shorthand that emerged from this descriptive work (G_1, S phase, G_2, and M phase or mitosis) has been the lens through which all subsequent dividing cells have been observed, and the four successive phases are referred to collectively as the *cell cycle.* The key observation made by these investigators was that the events that together make up the cell division process do not all occur continuously. Specifically, although growth and protein synthesis occur constantly for the most part, synthesis of DNA occurs only during a discrete interval. The preceding phase was designated *GAP1* or G_1, and the subsequent phase before cell division was referred to as *GAP2* or G_2. Although at the time little could be said concerning what a cell did during these silent "gap" phases, it is now known that these are not idle periods in a cell's life but the intervals in which most regulation of the cell cycle is specifically exerted. A large amount of information, originating from the external environment and the cell's internal milieu, is integrated during the G_1 and G_2 intervals and used to determine whether and when to proceed into S phase and M phase, respectively.

Mitosis, the most visibly dynamic interval of the cell cycle, has itself been traditionally subdivided into five phases: prophase, prometaphase, metaphase, anaphase, and telophase. In metazoans and plants (as opposed to fungi) mitosis entails a particularly dramatic change of state for the cell. During prophase most of the internal membranous compartments of the cell, including the nucleus, are disassembled and dispersed. Replicated chromosomes (chromatids) are condensed into paired compact rods, and a bipolar microtubule spindle is assembled. Biosynthesis of proteins (transcription and translation) ceases. During prometaphase, chromosomes form bivalent attachments to the spindle, driving them to the cellular equator. Proper alignment of paired chromatids on the spindle is indicative of metaphase. During anaphase, the paired sister chromatids lose cohesion and microtubule forces separate the chromatids and pull them to opposite poles of the cell. During telophase, the events of prophase are reversed: The nuclei and other membrane structures reassemble, the chromosomes decondense, and protein synthesis resumes. After mitosis, the two daughter cells pull apart and separate in a process known as *cytokinesis.*

Current knowledge of the cell cycle has accrued historically from a number of different experimental approaches and systems. In the early 1970s, experiments carried out by fusing mammalian cells in different cell-cycle phases revealed the existence of dominant inductive activities for the S phase and the M phase.[2,3] Shortly thereafter, similar inductive activities were isolated from mature frog eggs arrested at meiotic metaphase II and shown to be capable of inducing G_2 oocytes to enter into meiotic divisions,[4] equivalent in many respects to mitosis. At the same time, genetic analysis of cell division in yeast revealed that the products of individual genes controlled specific events in the cell cycle and that these events could be organized in pathways, much like metabolic pathways.[5] Eventually, all of these lines of investigation converged in the 1980s, leading to the discovery of cyclin-dependent kinases (cdks).

CYCLIN-DEPENDENT KINASES

Arguably the most significant advance in understanding cell-cycle regulation was the discovery of cdks.[6] These are binary proline-directed serine-threonine–specific protein kinases that consist of a catalytic subunit (the cdk) that has little if any intrinsic enzymatic activity and a requisite positive regulatory subunit known as a *cyclin.* In yeast, one cdk and numerous cyclins carry out cell-cycle regulatory functions, whereas in mammals, these same functions are carried out by a number of different cdks and cyclins. In yeast, in which multiple cyclins activate the same cdk (cdk1) for distinct cell-cycle tasks, it is clear that most if not all substrate specificity beyond a rather degenerate primary structure target consensus lies in the cyclin subunit. In mammals, it is likely that substrate specificity is shared by cdk and cyclin subunits. Although not all pairwise combinations are permitted, there are enough combinatorial possibilities to create a significant level of substrate specificity.

Cdks have a structure similar to that of other protein kinases, consisting of two globular domains (the N-lobe and C-lobe) held together by a semiflexible hinge region. Protein substrates bound by the active enzyme are thought to fit into a cleft between the two domains. The N-lobe contains the adenosine triphosphate (ATP)–binding site. Studies comparing cdks and cdk-cyclin complexes based on x-ray diffraction crystallography indicate that the primary role of the cyclin, in addition to substrate docking functions, is to realign critical active site residues into an active configuration and to open the catalytic

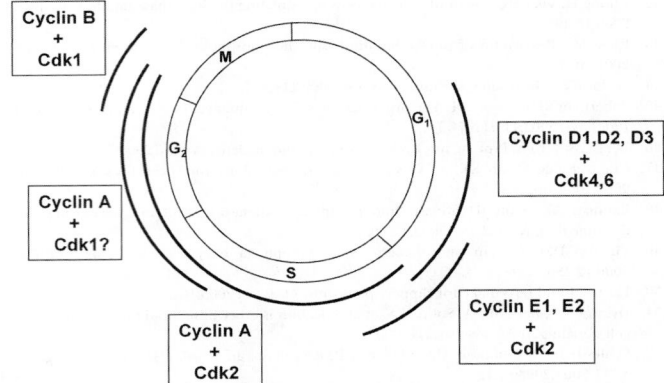

FIGURE 3.2-1. Windows of cyclin-dependent kinase (cdk) function in the cell cycle. D-type cyclins (cyclins D1, D2, and D3) activate cdk4 and cdk6 for functions extending from mid G_1 to the G_1/S-phase transition. E-type cyclins (cyclins E1 and E2) activate cdk2 for functions at the G_1/S-phase boundary, probably extending into early S phase. Cyclin A activates cdk2 for functions extending from the G_1/S-phase boundary and extending into G_2. Cyclin A is known to interact with cdk1 as well; however, no specific function for this complex has been identified. Finally, cyclin B activates cdk1 at the G_2/M-phase boundary with activity that lasts until cyclin B is degraded during anaphase.

cleft to accommodate substrates.[7] Once bound to a cyclin, the cdk active site is configured similarly to other protein kinases that do not require cyclin binding.

The known cdks and cyclins and their presumptive intervals of function in the mammalian cell cycle are summarized in Figure 3.2-1. For the most part, the functional intervals of cdks are determined by the accumulation and disappearance of cyclins. Whereas cdks tend to be expressed at a constant level through the cell cycle, cyclin accumulation is usually dynamic, regulated at the level of biosynthesis and degradation (discussed in greater detail in Cell-Cycle Machinery, later in this chapter). To summarize, three partially redundant D-type cyclins (D1, D2, and D3) activate two partially redundant cdks (cdk4 and cdk6). Although, unlike most other cyclins, D-type cyclins do not appear to be expressed with high periodicity in cycling cells, the interval at which their primary activating function is thought to occur is from mid to late G_1 to direct phosphorylation of the cell-cycle inhibitor pRb and related proteins p107 and p130. Phosphorylation of these proteins by cyclin D–cdk4/6 inactivates their negative regulatory functions, allowing progression into S phase.[8,9]

Unlike D-type cyclins, E-type cyclins (E1 and E2) are expressed with high cell-cycle periodicity, accumulating in late G_1 and declining during S phase. E-type cyclins activate cdk2, and the fact that premature expression of cyclin E1 leads to accelerated entry into S phase[10,11] has suggested that the target(s) must be proteins responsible for initiation of DNA replication. However, the essentiality of cyclin E–cdk2 in this context has been put into question by the demonstration that cells from cyclin E1/E2 nullizygous mouse embryos can cycle with reasonably normal kinetics and can certainly initiate DNA replication.[12] The most likely explanation for the dispensability of E-type cyclins for S-phase functions is redundancy with cyclin A, which also activates cdk2.

Cyclin A accumulates initially at the G_1/S-phase boundary and persists until prometaphase of mitosis. It has been best characterized as an activator of cdk2; however, it has also been reported to form complexes with cdk1. It is presumed that cdk2, activated by E-type cyclins and cyclin A, promotes cell-cycle progression from the G_1-S boundary through the G_2 interval.

At this time, B-type cyclins, in conjunction with cdk1, are responsible for getting cells into and through mitosis. Although mammalian cells express a number of B-type cyclins, only cyclin B1 appears to be essential. Cyclin B1 accumulates through S phase and G_2 and then is degraded at the metaphase-anaphase transition. It should be pointed out that the cdk family is extensive and that eukaryotes possess many additional cdks that ostensibly have nothing to do with cell-cycle regulation.

MODES OF CYCLIN-DEPENDENT KINASE REGULATION

Because the activity of cdks is central to cell survival, these enzymes are of necessity highly regulated.[6] As a result, a number of diverse regulatory mechanisms have evolved to allow for integration of environmental and internal signals (Fig. 3.2-2). A primary mode of cdk regulation is the availability of activating cyclins, as alluded to above. For most cell-cycle regulatory cdks, the relevant cyclins exhibit a distinct temporal program of accumulation and degradation, determining a precise window of cdk activation. Although D-type cyclins tend not to be highly regulated in cycling cells, they are strongly down-regulated as cells exit the cell cycle into a nonproliferative state and then resynthesized in response to mitogen stimulation and cell-cycle reentry. The genes encoding cyclin E1 and E2 are transcribed periodically late in G_1 and up to the G_1/S-phase transition. This, coupled with ubiquitin-mediated proteolysis of cyclin E in active cyclin E–cdk2 complexes, creates the observed window of cyclin E accumulation from late G_1 to mid S phase. Like cyclin E, the accumulation of cyclin A is determined by periodic transcription. However, unlike cyclin E, cyclin A remains stable in active cdk2 complexes. The timing of ubiquitin-mediated proteolysis of cyclin A is determined by activation of a protein-ubiquitin ligase known as the *anaphase-promoting complex/cyclosome* (APC/C) in prometaphase. Thus, the window of cyclin A accumulation is from the G_1-S transition until early in mitosis. Finally, B-type cyclin accumulation is also linked to periodic transcription. In this case, transcription

begins in late S phase and persists through G_2. Similarly to cyclin A, B-type cyclins are targeted for ubiquitin-mediated proteolysis by the APC/C during mitosis, although their disappearance occurs slightly later in mitosis than that of cyclin A.

A second important mode of cdk regulation is by phosphorylation. cdks require an activating phosphorylation on a structural feature designated the *T loop*. Phosphorylation induces a movement of the T loop that has global effects on cdk2 structure, including an increase in cdk-cyclin contacts and changes in the substrate-binding site.[13] In most if not all instances, T-loop phosphorylation appears to constitute a housekeeping function that occurs concomitant with cyclin binding. However, negative regulatory phosphorylation of cdks is a highly dynamic process. Proper cell-cycle regulation of cdk1, in particular, requires phosphorylation on two residues within the N-lobe, adjacent to the ATP-binding site: threonine 14 and tyrosine 15. During the normal course of the cell cycle, as cyclin B–cdk1 complexes accumulate, they are immediately phosphorylated at these sites and thereby kept inactive. This allows stockpiling of the large numbers of cyclin B–cdk1 complexes required for efficient entry into mitosis and maintaining them in an inactive state during late S phase and G_2. At the G_2/M-phase boundary, there is concerted dephosphorylation of these residues, causing cells to advance rapidly into mitosis. Although cdk2 and cdk4 have also been reported to undergo negative regulatory phosphorylation at the homologous residues, the function(s) of this regulation are not as clear-cut (but see DNA Damage Checkpoints, later in this chapter).

A third mode of cdk regulation is through the action of inhibitory proteins that can form either binary complexes with cdks or ternary complexes with cyclin-cdk dimers. These exist in three major families. The INK4 family consists of four members (p15, p16, p18, and p19). All are composed of a series of conserved structural motifs known as *ankyrin repeats* and specifically target cdk4 and cdk6. The mechanism of action of these inhibitors is to bind the cdk subunit and, by causing a rotation of the N-lobe relative to the C-lobe, constraining the kinase in an inactive conformation and, in addition, precluding cyclin binding.[14] The Cip/Kip family consists of three members in mammals,

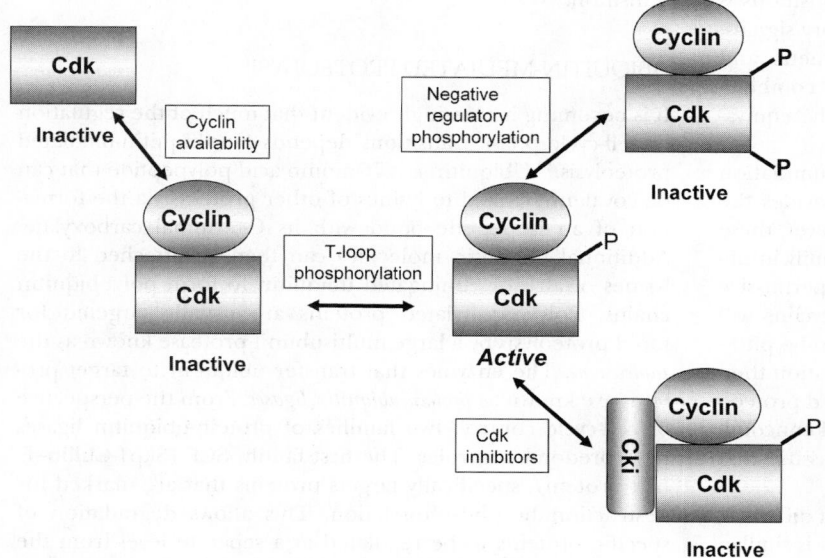

FIGURE 3.2-2. Principles of cyclin-dependent kinase (cdk) regulation. Because cdk catalytic subunits are inactive when unbound to cyclins, the first level of regulation is through the expression and availability of cyclins. The second level of regulation appears to constitute a housekeeping function in that cyclin binding stimulates an essential phosphorylation of a threonine within a structural feature known as the *T loop*. Binary complexes with phosphorylated T loops are active. Such active kinase complexes can be subjected to negative regulation in two ways. Additional phosphorylation events on threonine 14 and tyrosine 15 (or the equivalent residues) renders the kinase inactive. In addition, the formation of ternary complexes with cdk inhibitory proteins (Ckis) promotes an inactive state. One class of Cki, INK4, specific for cdk4 and cdk6, can inhibit by forming binary complexes directly with the cdk.

p21^{Cip1}, p27^{Kip1}, and p57^{Kip2}. All contain a conserved amino-terminal cyclin-cdk–binding inhibitory domain and a divergent C-terminal domain possessing other less well-characterized functions. Although these are potent inhibitors of cdk2, the case for inhibition of cdk4 and cdk6 is less certain. Whereas Cip/Kip inhibitors are clearly capable of inhibiting cdk4 and cdk6 at high concentration, it is not clear that these conditions are met *in vivo*, and the situation is further complicated by the finding that Cip/Kip inhibitor binding is actually required as a chaperonin or assembly factor for the efficient formation of active cyclin D–cdk4 complexes.[15,16] In the case of cyclin A–cdk2, where structural studies have been carried out, it appears that the Cip/Kip inhibitors first anchor via a high-affinity interaction with the cyclin.[16] This then allows the inhibitor polypeptide to invade and deform the N-lobe, thus interfering with ATP binding and catalysis.[16] The final class of inhibitors consists of two members of the pRb protein family, p107 and p130. Although these proteins have well-characterized functions as transcriptional inhibitors, they also are potent cyclin E/A–cdk2 inhibitors. p107 and p130 each contain cyclin-binding and cdk-binding sites that collaborate to confer inhibitory activity.

A final mode of cdk regulation is via control of nuclear import/export. This level of regulation is most obvious for cyclin B–cdk1 complexes, which are kept out of the nucleus via active nuclear export until late G_2, when phosphorylation inactivates cis-acting nuclear export signals allowing nuclear accumulation.[17] Sequestration of cyclin B–cdk1 in the cytoplasm is a redundant mechanism, along with negative regulatory phosphorylation of cdk1, for preventing premature phosphorylation of mitotic targets.

INDUCTION OF CELL-CYCLE PHASE TRANSITIONS

The cell cycle is composed of two action phases, S phase and M phase, in which the genetic material is duplicated and the components of a mother cell are divided into two daughter cells, respectively. The intervening phases, G_1 and G_2, are thought to exist primarily to allow time for cell growth and for regulatory inputs. Therefore, from the point of view of regulatory theory, cell proliferation is controlled operationally at two key transitions: that between G_1 and S phase and that between G_2 and M phase. The important characteristic of these two transitions is that, once initiated based on integration of regulatory signals, they must be executed decisively to maintain genetic and genomic integrity. This is accomplished by using a combination of positive and negative modulators to set up the equivalent of a molecular capacitor.

In cycling mammalian cells, the programmed accumulation of cyclins E and A via transcriptional induction provides the positive impetus for the G_1/S-phase transition. However, these kinases are kept in check by the action of Cip/Kip family inhibitors. If the internal and external environments are permissive for proliferation, the continued accumulation of cyclins will eventually titrate the inhibitors, allowing the latter to be phosphorylated by free cyclin-cdk complexes. Phosphorylation then marks these inhibitors as targets of ubiquitin-mediated proteolysis. The concerted destruction of cdk inhibitors and concomitant activation of the entire pool of cdk complexes assure that the transition into S phase is rapid and irreversible.

Although the details of its regulation are somewhat different, the strategy underlying control of the G_2-M transition is similar.

Cyclin B–cdk1 complexes accumulate starting near the end of S phase but are held in check not by cdk inhibitors but by negative regulatory phosphorylation of cdk1. This phosphorylation on threonine 14 and tyrosine 15 is carried out by kinases Wee1 and Myt1. Entry into M phase is signaled by the rapid dephosphorylation of T14 and Y15, resulting in activation of cdk1. This dephosphorylation is carried out by specialized protein phosphatases cdc25B and cdc25C. The concerted dephosphorylation of cdk1 depends on activation of cdc25 isoforms by phosphorylation, as well as ubiquitin-mediated proteolysis of Wee1, also in response to phosphorylation. Although the initial activation of CDC25 isoforms is thought to be carried out by other protein kinases, such as Plk1, CDC25B and C are also activated by cyclin B–cdk1, establishing a positive feedback loop. These positive feedback dynamics leading to the simultaneous activation of a large accumulated pool of cyclin B–cdk1 assures that entry into mitosis is decisive. The turnover of Wee1 enforces irreversibility. Because entry into mitosis involves dismantling many of the cell's components and organelles, as well as construction and use of a complex apparatus for segregating the cell's genetic material, mitosis is a period of particular vulnerability, and therefore it is important that this transition and subsequent events be carried out rapidly and efficiently.

An important secondary transition that occurs within M phase is that between metaphase and anaphase (Fig. 3.2-3).[18] To preserve genomic integrity, all duplicated chromosomes must be aligned along the cell's equator and properly attached to microtubules of the mitotic spindle. The trigger for separation of sister chromatids and their movement to opposite poles of the cell is the activation of the protein-ubiquitin ligase APC/C. This is achieved via cdk1 activation, but more importantly by the binding of a key cofactor, cdc20, whose availability is linked to the proper attachment of chromosomes and the integrity of the spindle. The target of the APC/C is a protein known as *securin*, which binds to and inhibits a specialized protease, separase. The key target of separase is a complex that binds sister chromatids together: cohesin. Cleavage of the Scc1 subunit of cohesin leads to a rapid execution of anaphase. It is the ability to stockpile a large pool of inactive securin-separase complexes that can be rapidly mobilized by irreversible proteolysis of securin that allows for a rapid irreversible metaphase-anaphase transition.

UBIQUITIN-MEDIATED PROTEOLYSIS

It is becoming increasingly evident that much of the regulation of cell-cycle phase transitions depends on ubiquitin-mediated proteolysis.[19] Ubiquitin is a 76 amino acid polypeptide that can be covalently linked to lysines of other proteins via the formation of an isopeptide bond with its C-terminal carboxylate. Additional ubiquitin molecules can then be attached to the lysines of already conjugated ubiquitin to form polyubiquitin chains. Polyubiquitylated proteins are usually targeted for rapid proteolysis by a large multisubunit protease known as the *proteasome*. The enzymes that transfer ubiquitin to target proteins are known as *protein-ubiquitin ligases*. From the perspective of cell-cycle control, two families of protein-ubiquitin ligases have predominant roles. The first family, SCF (Skp1-Cullin–F-box protein), specifically targets proteins that are marked for destruction by phosphorylation. This allows degradation of specific proteins to be regulated at a separate level from the

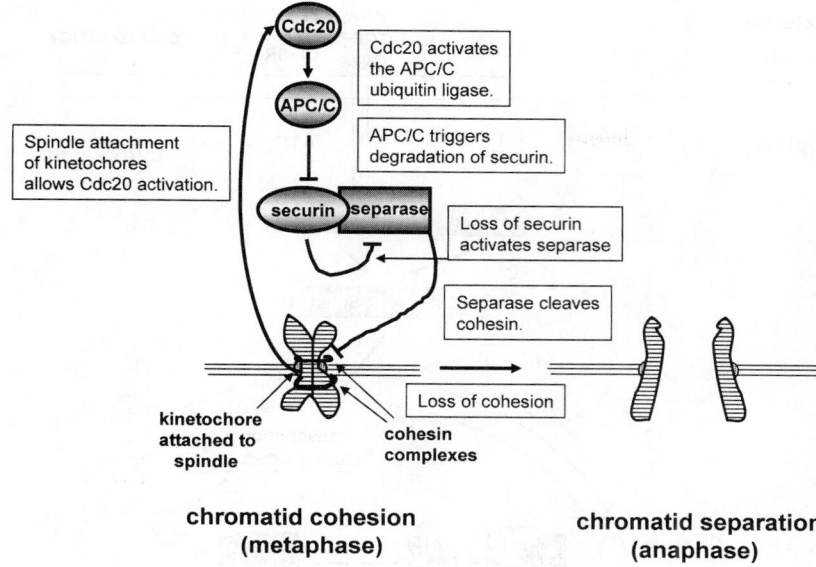

**chromatid cohesion
(metaphase)**   **chromatid separation
(anaphase)**

FIGURE 3.2-3. Regulation of the metaphase-anaphase transition. After replication, paired sister chromatids are held together by a complex of proteins, known collectively as *cohesin*, thus preventing anaphase. However, once paired chromatids have formed bivalent attachments to a functional mitotic spindle, inhibition of cdc20 mediated by the chromosome kinetochores is relieved. cdc20 is an essential cofactor of the protein-ubiquitin ligase anaphase-promoting complex/cyclosome (APC/C), which now becomes active. The primary initial target of the APC/C is securin, an inhibitor of the protease separase. Ubiquitin-mediated proteolysis of securin releases separase to cleave the cohesin subunit Scc1. This event releases paired chromatids from cohesion, thereby allowing anaphase to proceed.

protein-ubiquitin ligase itself, which can be expressed constitutively and used to target a large number of substrates independently. SCF ligases consist of three invariant core components and one of a number of specificity factors (F-box proteins) that recognize phosphorylated substrates. A few notable examples of SCF protein-ubiquitin ligases are SCF[Skp2] (containing the F-box protein Skp2), which targets p27[20] and p130,[21] and SCF[cdc4] (containing the F-box protein cdc4), which targets cyclin E.[22–24] The second family of protein-ubiquitin ligases that is critical for cell-cycle control is known collectively as the *APC/C*. The APC/C is a large complex consisting of 12 core subunits and one of two specificity factors, cdc20 and Cdh1. Unlike SCF ubiquitin ligases, targeting of substrates by the APC/C is determined by ligase activation rather than substrate activation. APC[cdc20] is active from metaphase until the end of mitosis, whereas APC[Cdh1] is active during the subsequent G_1 interval. In this manner, important mitotic targets, such as cyclin A, cyclin B, and securin (as well as many others), are degraded during mitosis and prevented from reaccumulating during the subsequent G_1 interval.

REGULATION OF THE CELL CYCLE

To preserve organismic function and integrity, the cell cycle must be regulated at a number of levels. These include entry into and exit from proliferation mode, coordination of cell-cycle events, and specialized responses that increase the probability of surviving a variety of environmental and internally generated insults.

QUIESCENCE AND DIFFERENTIATION

The most fundamental aspect of cell-cycle control is the regulation of entry and exit. For mammalian cells, the decision to enter or exit the proliferative mode is based on environmental signals such as mitogens, growth factors, hormones, and cell-cell contact, as well as on internal differentiation programs. If the state of cell-cycle exit is reversible, it is referred to as *quiescence*. If it is in the

context of terminal differentiation, cell-cycle exit may merely be one component of a differentiation program. Although cells entering quiescence and postmitotic differentiation differ from each other in many respects, from the perspective of cell-cycle control, they have much in common. First, cell-cycle exit is usually associated, at least initially, with an accumulation of G_1/S cdk inhibitors. Members of the INK4 family, targeting cdk4 and cdk6 and members of the Cip/Kip family, as well as the Rb-related protein p130, all targeting cdk2, are up-regulated. This causes accumulation of cells in G_1, from where cell-cycle exit can occur. Next, or simultaneously, the positive cell-cycle machinery is dismantled by down-regulation of cdks and cyclins, primarily at the transcriptional level. In the case of quiescence, cell-cycle exit is paralleled by a reduced rate of protein synthesis, indicative that cells have entered the resting state. Entry into and exit from quiescence are mediated largely by growth factors and mitogens that interact with cell surface receptors. These in turn are linked to intracellular signaling cascades that up-regulate the rate of protein synthesis as well as the transcription of genes that promote proliferation, such as cdks and cyclins. The two best-characterized signaling pathways in this context are the mitogen-activated protein kinase/extracellular signaling–regulated kinase pathway[25] and the phosphoinositide 3 (PI3) kinase/AKT pathway,[26] shown in Figure 3.2-4. Whereas the mitogen-activated protein kinase/extracellular signaling–regulated kinase pathway tends to stimulate expression of genes required for proliferation, the PI3-kinase/AKT pathway primarily stimulates protein synthesis and growth but also affects key cell-cycle regulatory proteins. Just as the presence of growth factors and mitogens stimulates these pathways, promoting cell-cycle entry, their removal shuts down these pathways, promoting quiescence. This is the basis for the reversibility of the quiescent state.

ANTIMITOGENIC SIGNALS

An important aspect of control of cell division in mammals is antimitogenic signaling. Just as mitogens and growth factors bind to transmembrane receptors and use signal transduction pathways and downstream transcriptional programs to stimulate proliferation, parallel systems antagonize proliferation.

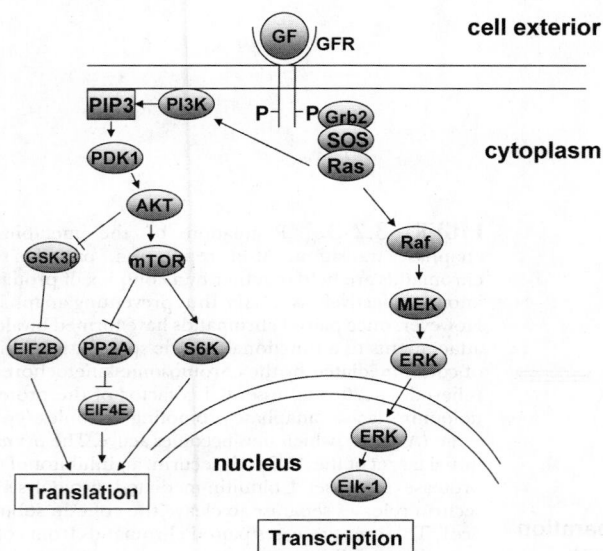

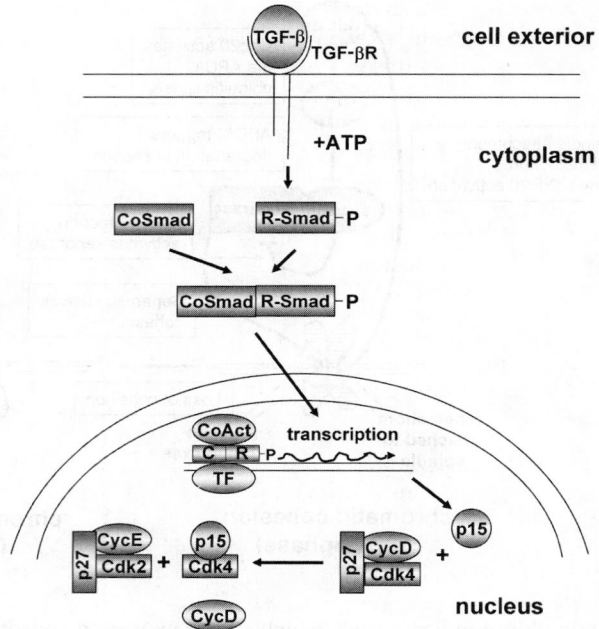

FIGURE 3.2-4. Growth factor (GF)/mitogen stimulation via Ras. Occupancy of many GF receptors (GFR) by ligand depends on the small guanosine triphosphatase transducer Ras. Receptor activation leads to phosphorylation of the receptor cytoplasmic domain. The phosphorylated receptor assembles a complex that includes Ras and its activated nucleotide exchange factor, son of sevenless (SOS), leading to activation of Ras. Activated Ras can then stimulate two important signal transduction pathways: the extracellular signaling–regulated kinase (ERK) pathway and the phosphoinositide 3 kinase (PI3K) pathway. Activated Ras stimulates the protein kinase activity of Raf, activating a protein kinase cascade consisting of Raf, MEK, and ERK. Activated ERK then translocates into the nucleus, where it phosphorylates and activates transcription factors, notably Elk-1. Genes important for growth and division are then transcribed. Activated Ras also stimulates PI3K activity, leading to the accumulation of phosphatidylinositol 3,4,5-triphosphate. This in turn stimulates the protein kinase activity of phosphoinositide-dependent kinase 1 (PDK1), activating a protein kinase cascade consisting of PDK1, AKT, and mTOR. Activation of this signal transduction pathway has the effect of stimulating translation and growth. AKT phosphorylates and inhibits the protein kinase glycogen synthase kinase-3β (GSK3β), thereby activating EIF2B required for translational initiation. mTOR phosphorylates and inhibits the protein phosphatase PP2A, thereby activating EIF4E, also required for translational initiation. Finally, mTOR phosphorylates and activates pp70S6 kinase, which in turn phosphorylates and activates ribosomal subunit S6.

FIGURE 3.2-5. Transforming growth factor-β (TGF-β) antimitogenic pathway. Occupancy of the heterodimeric TGF-β receptor by ligand leads to phosphorylation of a class of transcription factor known collectively as *R-SMADs*. Phosphorylated R-SMADs then dimerize with nontargeted cofactors known as *CoSMADs* and translocate to the nucleus. There the R-SMAD/CoSMAD dimers complex with DNA-binding transcription factors and transcriptional coactivators to stimulate transcription of specific genes. One of the key targets of TGF-β signaling is the gene encoding p15/INK4b, a cdk4/6 inhibitor. p15, by binding to cdk4 and cdk6, inhibits these kinases and displaces a large pool of cdk4/6-bound p27, which is then free to inhibit cdk2 complexes. The result is G_1 arrest. ATP, adenosine triphosphate.

The classic example of an antimitogenic signal is the effect of transforming growth factor-β (TGF-β) on epithelial cells (Fig. 3.2-5).[27] TGF-β, a cytokine, binds to a specific heterodimeric transmembrane receptor that, when occupied by ligand, phosphorylates a class of transcription factors, known as *SMADs*. These phosphorylated SMADs heterodimerize with nonreceptor-interactive SMADs and translocate to the nucleus, where they complex with DNA-binding transcription factors and coactivators to transactivate specific genes. Relevant to cell-cycle regulation, stimulation of the TGF-β signaling pathway promotes transcription of the gene encoding p15. p15 is an INK4 class cdk inhibitor that specifically inactivates cdk4 and cdk6. However, the effects of p15 accumulation on cell-cycle regulators are more global than inhibition of cdk4/6.[28] INK4 inhibitors such as p15 have a secondary effect of displacing a pool of the Cip/Kip inhibitor p27 from cyclin D–cdk4/6 complexes, allowing it to then target and inactivate cyclin E–cdk2 and cyclin A–cdk2 (see Fig. 3.2-5). Thus, exposure of epithelial cells to

TGF-β has the effect of inhibiting G_1 and S-phase cdk activities, thereby causing G_1 arrest. Interestingly, in many cancers of epithelial origin, the response to TGF-β has been abrogated, suggesting that this and similar response pathways have an important role in maintaining control of proliferation. Interferons comprise another class of cytokines that have antiproliferative effects on many cell types. Although the receptors used and signaling pathways are distinct from those used by TGF-β, the ultimate effects on the cell-cycle machinery are similar: up-regulation of cdk inhibitors and down-regulation of cyclins.

CHECKPOINTS

Cells are constantly faced with insults resulting in damage that can threaten their survival. These insults can be generated internally as by-products of metabolism or can originate in the external environment—for example, chemical agents or radiation. As a result, mechanisms have evolved to remove damaged molecules and make necessary repairs. In instances in which cell-cycle progression would be harmful or catastrophic before repair of damage, further mechanisms have evolved to delay progression pending repair. These are called *cell-cycle checkpoints*.[29] The necessity of checkpoints can be easily envisioned for genotoxic agents. Cells are particularly susceptible to the harmful effects of DNA damage at two points in the cell cycle: S phase and M phase. Unrepaired DNA damage poses a number of problems for cells undergoing DNA replication. Chromosomal lesions present physical barriers to replication forks. Replication that does traverse regions of DNA damage is likely to be error prone, resulting in accumulation of mutations. Likewise, segregation of severely damaged chromosomes at mitosis might lead to loss of genetic information, seriously threatening the survival of daughter cells. Therefore, cells possess mechanisms for preventing DNA replication and mitosis in response to genotoxic stress. Although the scope of this review does not permit a detailed description of all known checkpoints, those thought to be most basic to cell survival are characterized later.

DNA Damage Checkpoints

Although DNA damage exists in many forms, ranging from chemical adducts to double-strand breaks, they all pose similar problems for proliferating cells. As stated above, impeded and error-prone DNA replication and loss of genetic material during mitosis are some of the likely consequences in the absence of DNA damage checkpoints. Therefore, cell-cycle progression is blocked at three points: before S-phase entry (the G_1 DNA damage checkpoint), during S phase (the intra–S phase DNA damage checkpoint), and before M-phase entry (the G_2 DNA damage checkpoint). Although the responses to different types of DNA damage are not identical, they are similar enough to generalize. DNA damage of various forms is first detected by DNA-bound protein complexes that serve as sensors. In mammalian cells, two related atypical protein kinases that share homology with lipid kinases, ATM and ATR,[30] are primary signal transducers that are activated by DNA damage at all points in the cell cycle. A key effector of the G_1 and G_2 checkpoint responses is a transcription factor known as *p53*.[31] In response to DNA damage, p53 is activated and stabilized leading to increased levels. The principal transcriptional target of p53 in the context of the G_1 checkpoint is the Cip/Kip inhibitor p21[Cip1]. The resulting high levels of p21 block cdk2 activity and possibly cdk4 and cdk6 activity, leading to G_1 arrest. Another transcriptional target of p53, GADD45, inhibits cdk1, thereby contributing to the G_2 DNA damage checkpoint. However, the primary mechanism underlying the G_2 DNA damage checkpoint is p53 independent. It involves one of two effector protein kinases known as *chk1* and *chk2* that have the effect of inhibiting CDC25C,[32] which carries out the activating dephosphorylation of cdk1. Therefore, in response to DNA damage, G_2 cells accumulate inhibited cyclin B–cdk1 complexes and are incapable of entering into mitosis. The intra–S-phase DNA damage checkpoint response appears to be p53 independent but requires the chk1 or chk2 kinases, or both. A key target is CDC25A, responsible for activating dephosphorylation of cdk2. In response to DNA damage, phosphorylation of CDC25A by chk1 or chk2 leads to its destabilization and the accumulation of inactive cdk2 complexes[33] phosphorylated on threonine 14 and tyrosine 15. Because ongoing DNA replication requires the activity of cdk2, DNA synthesis ceases until damage is repaired.

Replication Checkpoint

Under normal circumstances, DNA replication is complete well before the time when the accumulation and activation of cyclin B–cdk1 would drive cells into mitosis. However, through the action of toxins or the rare but finite probability that the duration of S phase will be excessively long, situations can be encountered in which completion of replication extends beyond the normal time of mitotic induction or replication is blocked entirely. Under such circumstances, it is necessary to delay or block entrance into M phase accordingly, as segregation of incompletely replicated chromosomes would be catastrophic. Although the signaling pathways are somewhat different, the replication checkpoint ultimately functions like the G_2 DNA damage checkpoint in that mitotic entry is blocked by inhibiting CDC25C via the action of chk1, thus preventing activation of cdk1.

Spindle Integrity Checkpoint

The actual act of division is a dangerous time for a cell. It requires aligning duplicated chromosomes by attaching them via bipolar attachments to the spindle and then separating the chromatids so that each daughter cell gets a full complement. Errors result in aneuploidy, an extremely undesirable outcome. As a result, assembling a mitotic spindle and attaching chromosomes to it are extensively monitored processes. The mechanism of delay at prometaphase or metaphase in response to spindle defects or improper chromosome attachment is referred to as the *spindle integrity checkpoint*.[34] The sensor for this checkpoint consists of a number of proteins that reside at the chromosome kinetochores, sites of spindle microtubule attachment. The target is the essential APC/C cofactor, cdc20. Unattached or improperly attached kinetochores not experiencing an appropriate level of tension indicative of biopolar attachment inhibit cdc20 function. This in turn prevents the ubiquitylation and degradation of the anaphase inhibitor, securin. As a result, cells are prevented from initiating anaphase until all kinetochores are properly attached to a bipolar spindle (see Fig. 3.2-3).

Restriction Point

Cells deprived of an essential nutrient or growth factor are blocked from cell-cycle progression at a point in mid G_1.[35] Cells that have already passed this point, termed the *restriction point* or *R*, enter into S phase and complete the current cell cycle before arresting in the subsequent G_1 interval. In contrast, G_1 cells that have not reached the restriction point arrest immediately. The molecular basis for the restriction point has remained elusive. Initially, it was thought that passage through the restriction point was a manifestation of G_1 cdk activation. However, more recent work has indicated that cdk activation occurs after passage through the restriction point.[36] Significantly, most malignant cells do not have a functional restriction point, which presumably helps them evade normal growth control signals.

SENESCENCE

All normal mammalian cells have a finite proliferative life span. As cells approach the end of their proliferative capacity, they enter a state referred to as *replicative senescence*.[37,38] Although the reasons for programmed senescence are not known, it has been speculated that restricting cells to a finite number of divisions may be a protective mechanism against malignant growth. Although the rationale for senescence is not known, the mechanism has been largely elucidated, particularly for human cells. It is based on the requirement for a specialized replicase, telomerase, in the replication of the ends of chromosomes known as *telomeres*. Whereas germline cells express telomerase, most if not all somatic cells do not. As a result, because of the topology of telomeres and the requirements of conventional DNA replication, progressive telomere shortening or attrition occurs with each cell cycle. Although linear chromosome ends create a discontinuity, which topologically is indistinguishable from a chromosome break, telomere-specific DNA sequences are shielded from the DNA damage checkpoints. However, when sufficient telomere attrition has removed these protected sequences, cells enter into a chronic checkpoint response, which is the molecular basis for senescence. Senescence is characterized by the accumulation of high levels of cdk inhibitors and ultimately permanent G_1 arrest. It should be noted that one of the requirements of malignant transformation of cells is to overcome the senescence barrier so as to provide tumor cells with unlimited proliferative capacity.

REGULATION OF DNA REPLICATION

Entry into S phase is one of the key regulatory points of the cell cycle. The actual triggering of replication is attributed to the activation of cdk2 by cyclins E and A. However, the transcription of a large number of genes whose products are required for DNA replication requires the activity of cdk4 or cdk6, or both, driven by D-type cyclins. Mechanistically, this is based on the function of pRb and related proteins p130 and p107 serving as transcriptional repressors when bound to E2F family transcription factors (Fig. 3.2-6).[8] Phosphorylation by cyclin D–cdk4/6

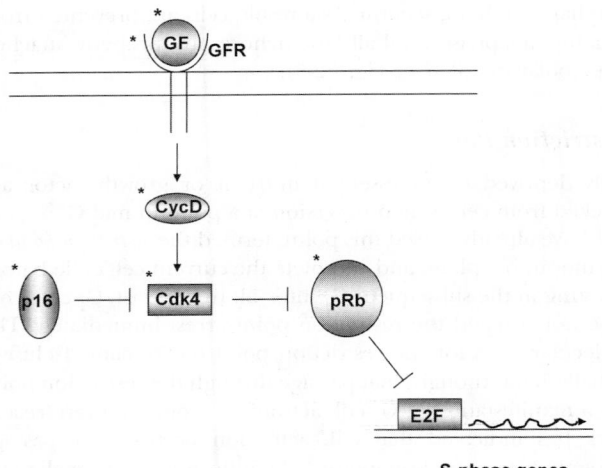

S-phase genes

FIGURE 3.2-6. pRb pathway. pRb is a critical negative cell-cycle regulator that links growth factor signaling pathways to cell-cycle progression. One of the principal functions of pRb is to interact with E2F family transcription factors and, by recruitment of corepressors, to maintain many genes encoding proteins that are important for cell-cycle progression in a tightly repressed state. Growth factor (GF) and mitogen-signaling pathways relieve this repression by stimulating accumulation of D-type cyclins on receptor occupancy. The resulting activation of cdk4 and cdk6 leads to phosphorylation of pRb and concomitant inactivation of its repressive functions. p16 is a cdk inhibitor of the INK4 family that down-regulates this pathway by inhibiting cdk4. It should be noted that all elements marked by an asterisk are found mutated or deregulated, or both, in human cancer. GFs, GF receptors (GFRs), and D-type cyclins are frequently overexpressed or deregulated. p16 is often not expressed or is underexpressed. Mutant versions of cdk4 that cannot bind p16 have been identified in human cancers. Finally, the gene encoding pRb is frequently mutated in cancer.

relieves this repression. Once cells have synthesized all the necessary enzymes and initiated DNA replication, another serious regulatory problem is encountered. To maintain genomic integrity, cells must replicate all genomic sequences only once per cell cycle, necessitating that origins of replication, sites where DNA synthesis begins, are used once during each S phase. This is accomplished by requiring that replication origin preparation and firing are mediated, respectively, by distinct cdk environments.[39] Prereplication complex assembly is triggered by low or absent cdk activity and therefore normally occurs as cells exit mitosis. This process requires the successive loading of proteins, cdc6, ctd1, and six MCM proteins (MCM2–7) to another complex of proteins, known as the *origin recognition complex* (ORC), which marks the origin site. Because of the requirement for low cdk activity, the permissive window for this process extends from the end of mitosis (telophase) until the point in G_1 when cdk activity begins to rise. The activation of cdk2 in late G_1 has the dual effect of blocking further prereplication complex assembly and causing DNA replication to initiate at primed origins. The maintenance of high levels of cdk activity (cdk2 followed by cdk1) for the remainder of the cell cycle assures that no new prereplication complex assembly can occur until the end of mitosis, when cdk levels once again decline, and in doing so restricts origin function to once per cell cycle.

CELL CYCLE AND CANCER

Cancer is in part a disease of uncontrolled proliferation. Because the proliferation of cells within an organism is normally tightly controlled by redundant regulatory pathways, it is not surprising that cell-cycle and checkpoint genes are often found misregulated or mutated in cancer. Genes in which mutations give rise to a gain of function or an enhanced level of function, leading to malignancy, are referred to as *protooncogenes*. Protooncogenes usually encode growth- or division-promoting proteins. Genes that give rise to loss of function mutations that lead to malignancy are referred to as *tumor suppressor genes*. Tumor suppressor genes usually encode negative regulators of growth and proliferation that protect cells from malignancy. Some cell-cycle genes commonly mutated or misregulated in cancer are listed in Table 3.2-1. Whereas mutations that create oncogenes tend to be dominant, mutations in tumor suppressor genes are usually recessive. This has led to the two-hit model of carcinogenesis (Fig. 3.2-7).[40] Briefly, recessive mutations occur in tumor suppressor genes but are latent due to the persistence of a wild-type allele. The tumor suppressor phenotype, therefore, requires mutation or loss of the second allele, a process known as *loss of heterozygosity*. A number of genes encoding negative regulators of the cell cycle conform to this two-hit paradigm.

In theory, to achieve uncontrolled cell division, two basic requirements must be met. First, cells need a strong constitutive proliferation signal capable of overriding the environmental and internal restraints on division that normal cells experience. Second, the barrier of senescence needs to be dismantled to render tumor cells immortal. Mutations in a large variety of cell-cycle control and related genes are associated with malignancy, and most of these can be accommodated within this framework. This model of tumorigenesis has been confirmed in rodent tissue culture–based *in vitro* models. Transfection of primary rodent fibroblasts with individual plasmids programmed to express proteins

TABLE 3.2-1. Cell-Cycle Genes Commonly Mutated or Altered in Expression in Human Cancer

Gene	Protein	Function	Alteration in Cancer
CCND1,2,3	D cyclins	Positive regulator of cdk4/6	Overexpressed
CCNE1	Cyclin E1	Positive regulator of cdk2	Overexpressed, deregulated
CDKN2A	p16, INK4a[a]	cdk4/6 inhibitor	Mutated, deleted, methylated
CDKN1B	p27[Kip1]	cdk2 inhibitor	Underexpressed
CDKN1C	p57[Kip2]	cdk2 inhibitor	Underexpressed, methylated
SKP2	Skp2	Turnover of p27	Overexpressed
CDK4	cdk4	Inactivates pRb	p16-resistant mutations
hCDC4	hCdc4	Turnover of cyclin E	Mutated, deleted
RB1	pRb	Represses E2F transcription	Mutated, deleted
RB2	p130	Inhibits cdks, represses E2F	Mutated, deleted
CKS1,2	cks1, cks2	cdk-binding proteins	Overexpressed
AURKA	Aurora A	Mitotic kinase	Overexpressed
PLK	Plk1	Mitotic kinase	Overexpressed
PTTG1	Securin	Anaphase inhibitor	Overexpressed
TP53	p53	Checkpoints, apoptosis	Mutated, deleted
MTBP	MDM-2	Inhibitor of p53	Overexpressed
CDKN2A	p14[Arf, a]	Activator of p53	Mutated, deleted
ATM	ATM	Checkpoints, repair	Mutated, deleted
CHK2	chk2	Checkpoints	Mutated
NBS1	Nbs1	Checkpoints, repair	Mutated

[a]Interestingly, the p16[INK4A] and p14[Arf] are encoded by the same gene via alternative reading frames and different promoters.

that promote either growth or immortalization does not result in malignant transformation. However, cotransfection of two plasmids, one in each category, does promote transformation (Fig. 3.2-8). However, these results need to be interpreted cautiously in the context of human cancer because immortalization of rodent cells in culture most likely does not involve telomeres.[41] One idea that has emerged is that strong growth signals

and other environmental pressures exerted on premalignant cells produce potent stress responses, leading to cell-cycle blockade or cell death.[41] Therefore, genetic alterations are likely required to neutralize these stress responses to immortalize rodent cells. Transformation of human cells requires these same genetic alterations, but also telomere attrition must be reckoned with, requiring additional mutations.

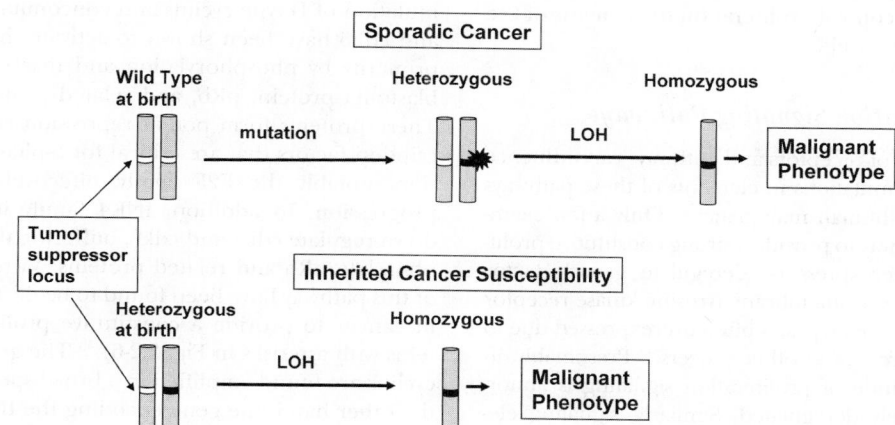

FIGURE 3.2-7. The two-hit model of tumor suppression. Tumor suppressors are proteins that are thought to provide protection from malignancy. Depicted is a chromosome carrying a tumor suppressor–encoding locus shown in white. At birth, normal individuals carry two wild-type alleles (*white bands*) at tumor suppressor loci. Over time, however, spontaneous mutations occur at these loci (*black flash*) that render one allele nonfunctional (*black band*). However, because such mutations are expected to be recessive to the wild-type allele that is still present, there is no phenotypic consequence. Over time, additional events can lead to loss of the wild-type allele, a phenomenon referred to as *loss of heterozygosity* (LOH). LOH then provides a tangible contribution to the malignant phenotype. However, because spontaneous mutations at specific loci and specific secondary allelic losses are rare events, malignancy usually only develops after a very long latency period. On the other hand, some individuals are born with inherited tumor suppressor mutations. Because only LOH is then required for expression of the tumor suppressor–null phenotype, cancer with decreased latency and higher penetrance develops in such individuals.

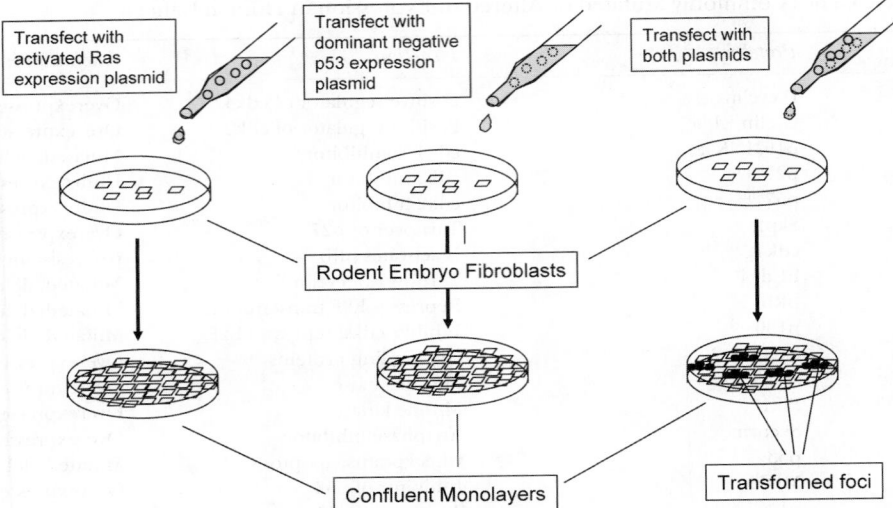

FIGURE 3.2-8. Malignant transformation requires multiple genetic alterations. Depicted is an *in vitro* experiment using primary rodent embryonic fibroblasts. Cells transfected with a plasmid programmed to express an activated Ras allele eventually grow to form a confluent monolayer, at which time proliferation ceases because of inhibition mediated by cell-cell contact. Similarly, cells transfected with a plasmid are programmed to express a dominant-negative allele of p53 (encoding a protein that can complex with and inactivate endogenous wild-type p53) from a confluent monolayer. However, cells transfected simultaneously with both plasmids form a confluent monolayer out of which grow transformed foci. These piles of cells are no longer subject to the controls that restrict fibroblast proliferation and, as such, resemble cancer cells. The requirement for two perturbations in this system supports a mechanism whereby activated Ras stimulates growth and proliferation and dominant negative p53 inactivates stress pathways that would cause these cells to have a limited proliferative life span.

ALTERATIONS IN PATHWAYS AFFECTING GROWTH AND PROLIFERATION

Mutations that regulate cell growth and proliferation can occur at many levels, ranging from cell surface receptor–mediated signaling pathways that control proliferation to elements of the core cell-cycle machinery itself.

Growth and Proliferation Signaling Pathways

Because a large number of receptors and pathways can influence cell proliferation, many mutations in elements of these pathways have been recovered in human malignancies. Only a few examples are cited here. One way to provide a strong constitutive proliferation signal is to overexpress or deregulate growth factor receptors. HER2/neu, a transmembrane tyrosine kinase receptor found on many epithelial cell types, is often overexpressed due to gene amplification in breast and other cancers.[42] Presumably, in such tumors the amplitude of proliferation signaling is abnormally high or completely deregulated. Similarly, signaling elements downstream of mitogen receptors can be mutated to produce constitutive signaling. Perhaps the best-known example is the case of the Ras guanosine triphosphatases, which serve as signal transducers for a number of key proliferation pathways. Dominant mutations in Ras isoforms that stabilize the activated state confer strong constitutive proliferation signaling. One of the pathways stimulated by Ras is the PI3-kinase pathway. A PI3 phosphatase, PTEN, normally reverses this phosphorylation, keeping the signal in check. However, mutational loss of PTEN similarly to oncogenic mutations in Ras can lead to constitutive signaling contributing to carcinogenesis.

Cell-Cycle Machinery

Signaling pathways that stimulate proliferation impinge on the cell-cycle machinery by stimulating the biosynthesis of D-type cyclins and promoting the degradation of cdk inhibitors. Accumulation of D-type cyclins and concomitant activation of cdk4 and cdk6 have been shown to activate the cell-cycle program primarily by phosphorylation and inactivation of the retinoblastoma protein, pRb, and related proteins p107 and p130. These proteins form potent repression complexes with transcription factors that are critical for S-phase entry and progression, notably the E2F family, effectively blocking cell-cycle progression. In addition, INK4 family inhibitors specifically down-regulate cdk4 and cdk6, buffering their capacity to phosphorylate pRb and related proteins. Virtually all components of this pathway have been found to be misregulated or mutated in cancer to provide a constitutive proliferation signal (proteins with asterisks in Fig. 3.2-6).[43] The genes encoding D-type cyclins are found amplified in a broad spectrum of tumors. On the other hand, the gene encoding the INK4 inhibitor, p16, is mutated and lost in some types of cancer, whereas cdk4 has been found to be mutated so as not to bind p16. In many instances p16, although not genetically altered, is down-regulated at the epigenetic level. The p16 promoter contains a CpG island that is subject to repression via methylation. Finally, pRb is the tumor suppressor on which the so-called two-hit hypothesis was originally formulated. Inherited mutations in the *RB* gene and subsequent loss of heterozygosity invariably lead to childhood retinoblastoma and eventually other malignancies. However, somatic mutation of *RB1* and loss of heterozygosity are found in many sporadic noninherited cancers.

Like D-type cyclins, cyclin E is frequently found up-regulated in cancer. The fact that deregulated expression of cyclin E can drive cells prematurely into S phase suggests that cyclin E provides a growth/division stimulus during carcinogenesis. Furthermore, cells from cyclin E nullizygous mice are resistant to malignant transformation in tissue culture models.[12] However, other evidence suggests that deregulation of cyclin E may promote carcinogenesis principally by inducing genomic instability rather than by promoting growth (see Mutations Causing Genetic and Genomic Instability, later in this chapter). Likewise, the cdk2 inhibitor p27[Kip1] is often found down-regulated in cancer, although never behaving as a classic tumor suppressor inactivated through mutation and allelic loss. However, as with cyclin E deregulation, it is not clear whether low p27 levels have an impact on carcinogenesis by promoting growth or genomic instability.

ALTERATIONS IN PATHWAYS AFFECTING SENESCENCE

In addition to a constitutive growth stimulus that overrides natural restraints, tumors need to have the capacity for unlimited proliferation. Normally, the limited life span of somatic cells imposed by the process of clonal senescence constitutes a natural barrier to tumorigenesis. Therefore, genes that mediate senescence are commonly mutated in cancer. However, the issue of senescence is complicated by functional overlap between senescence pathway genes and stress pathway genes that also require inactivation. Because senescence is a result of checkpoint responses to acute telomere attrition, genes that encode DNA checkpoint signaling elements and transducers are targeted. One of the most commonly mutated genes in human cancer encodes the checkpoint effector p53.[31] Inherited mutations in *TP53*, the gene encoding p53, confer a syndrome known as *Li-Fraumeni* characterized by early-onset cancer.[44] However, the majority of sporadic cancers are also mutated at the p53 locus. The role of p53 mutation in cancer as a promoter of immortalization is supported by the finding that cells from p53 nullizygous mice are immortal.[45] However, this conclusion is complicated by the fact that p53 is central to cellular stress responses that also require inactivation during malignant transformation. Nevertheless, an observation supporting the idea that checkpoint genes likely to be triggered by telomere attrition are targeted to immortalize premalignant cells is that chk2, a signaling element of the DNA damage checkpoint response, is mutated in a subset of Li-Fraumeni patients[44] rather than p53. Mutation of the gene encoding Nbs1, required for activation of chk1 and chk2 kinases, is also associated with a hereditary cancer syndrome,[46] Nijmegen disease, as well as sporadic cancers, although the interpretation of this result is complicated by the fact that Nbs1 is also involved in DNA damage repair (see Mutations Causing Genetic and Genomic Instability, later in this chapter). However, the most direct strategy to bypass senescence is to induce directly the expression of telomerase in somatic cells. c-Myc, a transcription factor linked to stimulation of proliferation, has also been shown to be a positive regulator of the gene encoding telomerase reverse transcriptase (hTERT), the catalytic subunit of telomerase.[47] This readily explains the high frequency of human tumors exhibiting c-Myc amplification or overexpression, or both. However, there appear to be a number of different mutational targets that can lead to derepression of the *hTERT* gene.[48]

MUTATIONS NEUTRALIZING STRESS RESPONSES

As stated in Alterations in Pathways Affecting Senescence, cellular stress responses are intimately related to checkpoint responses. Therefore, it is difficult to clearly categorize mutations that affect both. An example is p53, which is required for DNA damage checkpoint responses but also is a key effector of cellular stress responses.[31] Murine double-minute gene-2, which is frequently amplified and overexpressed in human cancer, promotes turnover of p53, consistent with a role in neutralizing stress responses.[49] Conversely, p14[Arf], a protein that stabilizes p53 by antagonizing murine double-minute gene-2, is frequently found mutated or underexpressed in cancer.[49] Indeed, the p53 pathway is so frequently inactivated in human cancer most likely because loss of p53 function simultaneously antagonizes stress pathways and helps override cellular responses to telomere attrition.

MUTATIONS CAUSING GENETIC AND GENOMIC INSTABILITY

The pathway to malignancy minimally requires several mutations. In the case of tumor suppressor mutations, secondary genetic events mediating allelic loss are necessary. Therefore, any mutation that itself can confer genetic or genomic instability, or both, is likely to promote carcinogenesis.[50,51] Mutations in genes required for DNA repair result in a mutator phenotype linked to hyperaccumulation of secondary mutations. In this context, strong association between mutation of the gene encoding Nbs1, which is required for efficient DNA repair as well as checkpoint signaling, and carcinogenesis is easily understood.[46] Similarly, the association between mutation of components of the spindle integrity checkpoint, such as Bub1, and carcinogenesis can be rationalized.[52] Cells defective in this checkpoint experience deregulated mitosis, leading to chromosome instability and ultimately aneuploidy. In principle, aneuploidy potentiates amplification at oncogenic loci and allelic losses at tumor suppressor loci. An interesting link between the core cell-cycle machinery and genomic instability is the case of cyclin E. Cyclin E is found overexpressed and deregulated in a broad spectrum of malignancies.[53] Although this correlation might be interpreted in the context of simply promoting proliferation, experiments on cells in culture have revealed that deregulation of cyclin E expression causes chromosome instability and aneuploidy.[54] Interestingly, an essential component of the ubiquitin ligase responsible for cell cycle–dependent targeting of cyclin E for proteolysis, hcdc4, is often found mutated in cancer.[22,24,55] Thus, genetic alterations that interfere with proper regulation of cell-cycle machinery have the potential of affecting not only the cell cycle itself, but also the genetic and genomic integrity of the cell.

CELL CYCLE AS A TARGET FOR THERAPY

Because cancer cells must proliferate, essential cell-cycle proteins have been suggested as targets for therapeutic exploitation. Notably, cdks have been extensively screened for small-molecule inhibitors, some of which are in clinical trials. It is too early, however, to judge the efficacy of this approach beyond its success using *in vitro* models. An alternative approach being explored is to develop agents that undermine checkpoint responses. The presumption is that cancer cells, due to their highly proliferative state, might be more susceptible to loss of essential controls. This idea remains to be confirmed. However, it is noteworthy that many therapeutic approaches currently use compounds that normally trigger checkpoint responses, such as genotoxic agents or spindle poisons. It is assumed that these treatments are effective because tumor cells are actually impaired in their defensive checkpoint responses.

CONCLUSION

Cell division is a process that is essential for all living organisms. Yet, in the intrinsic ability of cells to divide lies a risk that the process will become deregulated, leading to excessive accumulation of cells that have lost their functional and positional context. In animals, this phenomenon is referred to as *cancer*. Because cancer always has deleterious, usually fatal, consequences for an animal, layers of safeguards have been superimposed on the pathways that execute and control cell division. As a result, cancer is a complex genetic disease that invariably requires multiple genetic lesions to breach these safeguards. Even in individuals with inherited mutations in critical protective tumor suppressor genes, cancer usually does not develop for many or even tens of years. Yet, the inexorable accumulation of mutations during a lifetime ensures that some form of malignant disease will eventually develop in many if not most humans. Even though the workings of the cell-cycle machinery and the checkpoints that protect genetic and genomic integrity during division have been largely elucidated, there has been little progress as of yet in translating this knowledge into dramatic advances in cancer protection or treatment. Because tumors are usually highly genetically unstable and therefore inherently difficult to treat, it seems that the best hope for having a significant impact will be to use increasing knowledge concerning growth and cell-cycle control, checkpoints, and immortalization to develop protective strategies that bolster our extensive intrinsic defenses against cancer.

REFERENCES

1. Howard A, Pelc SR. Nuclear incorporation of p32 as demonstrated by autoradiographs. *Exp Cell Res* 1951;2:178.
2. Johnson RT, Rao PN. Mammalian cell fusion: induction of premature chromosome condensation in interphase nuclei. *Nature* 1970;226:717.
3. Rao PN, Johnson RT. Mammalian cell fusion: studies on the regulation of DNA synthesis and mitosis. *Nature* 1970;225:159.
4. Masui Y, Markert CL. Cytoplasmic control of nuclear behavior during meiotic maturation of frog oocytes. *J Exp Zool* 1971;177:129.
5. Hartwell LH, Culotti J, Pringle JR, et al. Genetic control of the cell division cycle in yeast. *Science* 1974;183:46.
6. Harper JW, Adams PD. Cyclin-dependent kinases. *Chem Rev* 2001;101:2511.
7. Jeffrey PD, Russo AA, Polyak K, et al. Mechanism of CDK activation revealed by the structure of a cyclinA-CDK2 complex. *Nature* 1995;376:313.
8. Stevens C, La Thangue NB. E2F and cell cycle control: a double-edged sword. *Arch Biochem Biophys* 2003;412:157.
9. Stiegler P, Giordano A. The family of retinoblastoma proteins. *Crit Rev Eukaryot Gene Expr* 2001;11:59.
10. Ohtsubo M, Roberts JM. Cyclin-dependent regulation of G1 in mammalian fibroblasts. *Science* 1993;259:1908.
11. Resnitzky D, Gossen M, Bujard H, et al. Acceleration of the G1/S phase transition by expression of cyclins D1 and E with an inducible system. *Mol Cell Biol* 1994;14:1669.
12. Geng Y, Yu Q, Sicinska E, et al. Cyclin E ablation in the mouse. *Cell* 2003;114:431.
13. Russo AA, Jeffrey PD, Pavletich NP. Structural basis of cyclin-dependent kinase activation by phosphorylation. *Nat Struct Biol* 1996;3:696.
14. Russo AA, Tong L, Lee JO, et al. Structural basis for inhibition of the cyclin-dependent kinase Cdk6 by the tumour suppressor p16INK4a. *Nature* 1998;395:237.
15. Cheng M, Olivier P, Diehl JA, et al. The p21(Cip1) and p27(Kip1) CDK inhibitors are essential activators of cyclin D-dependent kinases in murine fibroblasts. *EMBO J* 1999;18:1571.
16. Russo AA, Jeffrey PD, Patten AK, et al. Crystal structure of the p27Kip1 cyclin-dependent-kinase inhibitor bound to the cyclin A-Cdk2 complex. *Nature* 1996;382:325.
17. Yang J, Bardes ES, Moore JD, et al. Control of cyclin B1 localization through regulated binding of the nuclear export factor CRM1. *Genes Dev* 1998;12:2131.
18. Nasmyth K. Disseminating the genome: joining, resolving, and separating sister chromatids during mitosis and meiosis. *Annu Rev Genet* 2001;35:673.
19. Reed SI. Ratchets and clocks: the cell cycle, ubiquitylation and protein turnover. *Nat Rev Mol Cell Biol* 2003;4:855.
20. Carrano AC, Eytan E, Hershko A, et al. SKP2 is required for ubiquitin-mediated degradation of the CDK inhibitor p27. *Nat Cell Biol* 1999;1:193.
21. Tedesco D, Lukas J, Reed SI. The pRb-related protein p130 is regulated by phosphorylation-dependent proteolysis via the protein-ubiquitin ligase SCF(Skp2). *Genes Dev* 2002;16:2946.
22. Strohmaier H, Spruck CH, Kaiser P, et al. Human F-box protein hCdc4 targets cyclin E for proteolysis and is mutated in a breast cancer cell line. *Nature* 2001;413:316.
23. Koepp DM, Schaefer LK, Ye X, et al. Phosphorylation-dependent ubiquitination of cyclin E by the SCFFbw7 ubiquitin ligase. *Science* 2001;294:173.
24. Moberg KH, Bell DW, Wahrer DC, et al. Archipelago regulates cyclin E levels in Drosophila and is mutated in human cancer cell lines. *Nature* 2001;413:311.
25. Davis RJ. Transcriptional regulation by MAP kinases. *Mol Reprod Dev* 1995;42:459.
26. Chang F, Lee JT, Navolanic PM, et al. Involvement of PI3K/Akt pathway in cell cycle progression, apoptosis, and neoplastic transformation: a target for cancer chemotherapy. *Leukemia* 2003;17:590.
27. Shi Y, Massague J. Mechanisms of TGF-beta signaling from cell membrane to the nucleus. *Cell* 2003;113:685.
28. Reynisdottir I, Polyak K, Iavarone A, et al. Kip/Cip and Ink4 Cdk inhibitors cooperate to induce cell cycle arrest in response to TGF-beta. *Genes Dev* 1995;9:1831.
29. Elledge SJ. Cell cycle checkpoints: preventing an identity crisis. *Science* 1996;274:1664.
30. Yang J, Yu Y, Hamrick HE. ATM, ATR, and DNA-PK: initiators of the cellular genotoxic stress responses. *Carcinogenesis* 2003;24:1571.
31. Vousden KH. Activation of the p53 tumor suppressor protein. *Biochim Biophys Acta* 2002;1602:47.
32. Bartek J, Lukas J. Chk1 and Chk2 kinases in checkpoint control and cancer. *Cancer Cell* 2003;3:421.
33. Sorensen CS, Syljuasen RG, Falck J, et al. Chk1 regulates the S phase checkpoint by coupling the physiological turnover and ionizing radiation-induced accelerated proteolysis of Cdc25A. *Cancer Cell* 2003;3:247.
34. Allshire RC. Centromeres, checkpoints and chromatid cohesion. *Curr Opin Genet Dev* 1997;7:264.
35. Blagosklonny MV, Pardee AB. The restriction point of the cell cycle. *Cell Cycle* 2002;1:103.
36. Ekholm SV, Zickert P, Reed SI, et al. Accumulation of cyclin E is not a prerequisite for passage through the restriction point. *Mol Cell Biol* 2001;21:3256.
37. Smith JR, Pereira-Smith OM. Replicative senescence: implications for in vivo aging and tumor suppression. *Science* 1996;273:63.
38. Harley CB, Sherwood SW. Telomerase, checkpoints and cancer. *Cancer Surv* 1997;29:263.
39. Woo RA, Poon RY. Cyclin-dependent kinases and S phase control in mammalian cells. *Cell Cycle* 2003;2:316.
40. Knudson AG Jr. Hereditary cancer. *JAMA* 1979;241:279.
41. Sherr CJ, DePinho RA. Cellular senescence: mitotic clock or culture shock? *Cell* 2000;102:407.
42. Yarden Y. Biology of HER2 and its importance in breast cancer. *Oncology* 2001;61[Suppl 2]:1.
43. Ortega S, Malumbres M, Barbacid M. Cyclin D-dependent kinases, INK4 inhibitors and cancer. *Biochim Biophys Acta* 2002;1602:73.
44. Varley JT. TP53, hChk2, and the Li-Fraumeni syndrome. *Methods Mol Biol* 2003;222:117.
45. Tsukada T, Tomooka Y, Takai S, et al. Enhanced proliferative potential in culture of cells from p53-deficient mice. *Oncogene* 1993;8:3313.
46. D'Amours D, Jackson SP. The Mre11 complex: at the crossroads of DNA repair and checkpoint signaling. *Nat Rev Mol Cell Biol* 2002;3:317.
47. Kyo S, Takakura M, Taira T, et al. Sp1 cooperates with c-Myc to activate transcription of the human telomerase reverse transcriptase gene (hTERT). *Nucleic Acids Res* 2000;28:669.
48. Lin SY, Elledge SJ. Multiple tumor suppressor pathways negatively regulate telomerase. *Cell* 2003;113:881.
49. Zhang Y, Xiong Y. Control of p53 ubiquitination and nuclear export by MDM2 and ARF. *Cell Growth Differ* 2001;12:175.
50. Loeb KR, Loeb LA. Significance of multiple mutations in cancer. *Carcinogenesis* 2000;21:379.
51. Vessey CJ, Norbury CJ, Hickson ID. Genetic disorders associated with cancer predisposition and genomic instability. *Prog Nucleic Acid Res Mol Biol* 1999;63:189.
52. Jallepalli PV, Lengauer C. Chromosome segregation and cancer: cutting through the mystery. *Nat Rev Cancer* 2001;1:109.
53. Donnellan R, Chetty R. Cyclin E in human cancers. *FASEB J* 1999;13:773.
54. Spruck CH, Won KA, Reed SI. Deregulated cyclin E induces chromosome instability. *Nature* 1999;401:297.
55. Spruck CH, Strohmaier H, Sangfelt O, et al. hCDC4 gene mutations in endometrial cancer. *Cancer Res* 2002;62:4535.

SANDRA S. ZINKEL
STANLEY J. KORSMEYER

SECTION **3**

Apoptosis

Multicellular organisms have developed a highly organized and carefully regulated mechanism of cell suicide to craft the development of multiple lineages and to maintain cellular homeostasis. Normal development and morphogenesis proceed by the production of excess cells, which are then removed by a genetically programmed, evolutionarily conserved process. This same program of cell death is used by the organism to remove pathologically damaged cells, including virally infected cells.

Programmed cell death may have first been recognized in the developing neuronal system of the toad by Carl Vogt.[1] Kerr, Wyllie, and Currie described cell deaths with distinct ultrastructural features involving plasma membrane blebbing, volume contraction, nuclear condensation, and endonucleolytic cleavage of DNA. They noted that these features were consistent with an active, regulated process and coined the term *apoptosis* from the Greek word used to describe "dropping off" or "falling off" of petals from flowers or leaves from trees.[1-3]

Studies of chromosomal translocations in human lymphoid malignancies yielded the *BCL-2* gene, the first component of the cell death pathway to be cloned and identified. The most common chromosomal translocation found in these malignancies is the t(14;18): (q32;q21), harbored by 85% of follicular and 20% of diffuse B-cell lymphomas.[4,5] The breakpoint proved to be the result of aberrant immunoglobulin (Ig) heavy-chain rearrangements[6-8] in which *BCL-2* was introduced from chromosome 18. The consequence of this rearrangement is to place *BCL-2* under the transcriptional control of the Ig heavy-chain locus. B cells that harbor this translocation express inappropriately elevated levels of BCL-2 protein.[9]

Clues to the biologic consequence of BCL-2 overexpression reside in the natural history of follicular lymphoma.[10] The disease usually follows an indolent course, with symptoms that wax and wane over years. Transformation to a high-grade lymphoma with diffuse mixed or diffuse large cell morphology often occurs within the first decade. When a *BCL-2–Ig* minigene that recapitulated the t(14;18) breakpoint was inserted into the germline of a mouse, follicular hyperplasia resulted (Fig. 3.3-1). This polyclonal expansion of small resting B cells was principally in G_0, G_1 of the cell cycle.[11,12] Over time, these mice progress to diffuse, large cell immunoblastic lymphoma. Long latency followed by progression to high-grade malignancy is essentially diagnostic of the acquisition of second genetic abnormalities. Indeed, approximately half of the high-grade tumors have acquired an additional translocation, placing *c-myc* under the control of the Ig heavy-chain locus, thus combining an inherent survival advantage (*Bcl-2*) with a gene that promotes proliferation (*c-myc*).[13] Further evidence for the potent synergy of such a combination emerged when *Bcl-2* transgenic mice were mated to myc transgenic mice, resulting in the rapid appearance of an undifferentiated hematolymphoid leukemia.[14] BCL-2 extends cell survival by specifically blocking apoptosis.[15,16] The oncogenic potential of BCL-2 is not restricted to the B-cell lineage; overexpression in T cells results in peripheral T-cell lymphomas.[17]

Tumorigenesis reflects the accumulation of excess cells that formally results from increased cell proliferation or decreased cell death, or both.[18] The first oncogenes to be discovered were genes involved in signal transduction or regulation of transcription. Gain of function mutations in these genes results in oncogenesis by increased proliferation. A second class of oncogenes was subsequently identified whose normal function is to inhibit growth and proliferation. It is often loss-of-function mutations in this class of genes that result in tumors. *BCL-2* represents the cardinal member of a third class of oncogenes, which regulate cell death, resulting in resistance to apoptosis that enables the accumulation of additional genetic aberrations.[19]

GENETICS OF CELL DEATH

A genetic program for developmental cell deaths emerged from the study of the nematode *Caenorhabditis elegans*. These worms are particularly well suited to the study of cell fates, as they are transparent, allowing visualization of individual cells in living organisms. During the development of the *C elegans* hermaphrodite, 1090 cells are generated, and 131 of these cells undergo programmed cell death.[20] Genes have been identified that reside in a common, core pathway responsible for the regulation of all 131 cell deaths. Moreover, lineage-specific genes that reside in private pathways more upstream are responsible for initiating the cell deaths. Furthermore, two complementary sets of genes have been identified that control the phagocytosis of cell corpses.

Functional mammalian counterparts to many of these genes have been identified (Fig. 3.3-2), indicating that the basic tenets of apoptosis are conserved from nematodes to humans. The *ced-9* (for cell death abnormal) gene confers resistance to cell death. Loss of function mutations of *ced-9* result in massive cell death, leading to death of the worm. Conversely, overexpression of *ced-9* inhibits cell death. Thus, ced-9 is a structural and a functional homologue of *Bcl-2*.[21]

Three additional genes required for apoptosis have been identified: *egl-1* (egg-laying abnormal), *ced-3*, and *ced-4*. Loss-of-function mutations in either *ced-3* or *ced-4* can rescue cells from death.[22] *Egl-1* functions as an upstream, negative regulator of the *BCL-2* homologue *ced-9*.[23] Whereas the killing activity of *ced-4* requires functional *ced-3*, the killing activity of *ced-3* is independent of active *ced-4*. *ced-4* thus appears to function upstream of *ced-3* in this genetic pathway. An overall genetic pathway consistent with all the observations would be *Egl-1→ced-9→ced-4→ced-3*.

ced-3 encodes a cysteine protease homologous to the mammalian ICE or caspase 1, required for the proteolytic activation of prointerleukin-1β.[24-26] Transient expression of either CED-3 or ICE induces apoptosis in mammalian cells, suggesting that this family of proteases plays a critical role in programmed cell death.[27]

BCL-2 FAMILY

The Bcl-2 family of proteins is situated upstream of irreversible cellular damage in the apoptotic pathway[28] (Fig. 3.3-3), providing a pivotal decisional checkpoint in the fate of a cell after a death stimulus. Pro- and antiapoptotic family members have

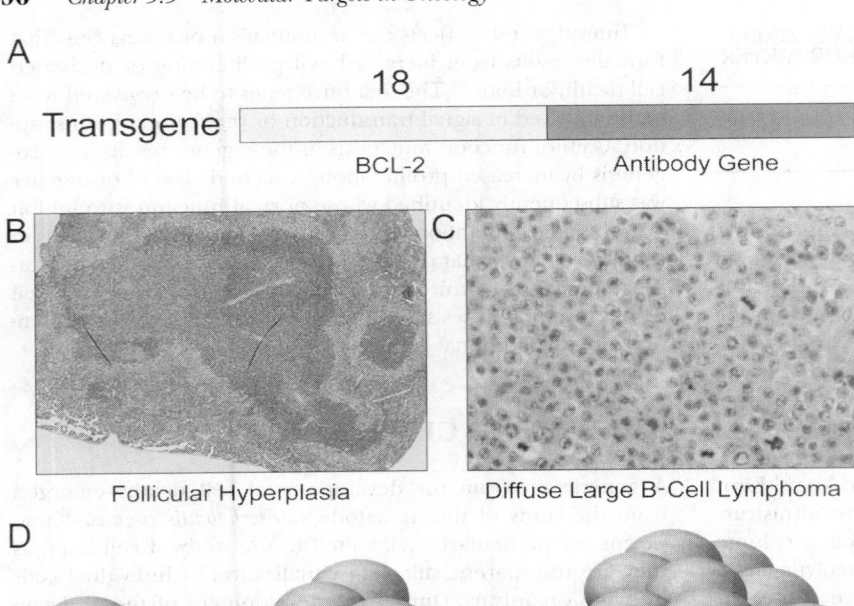

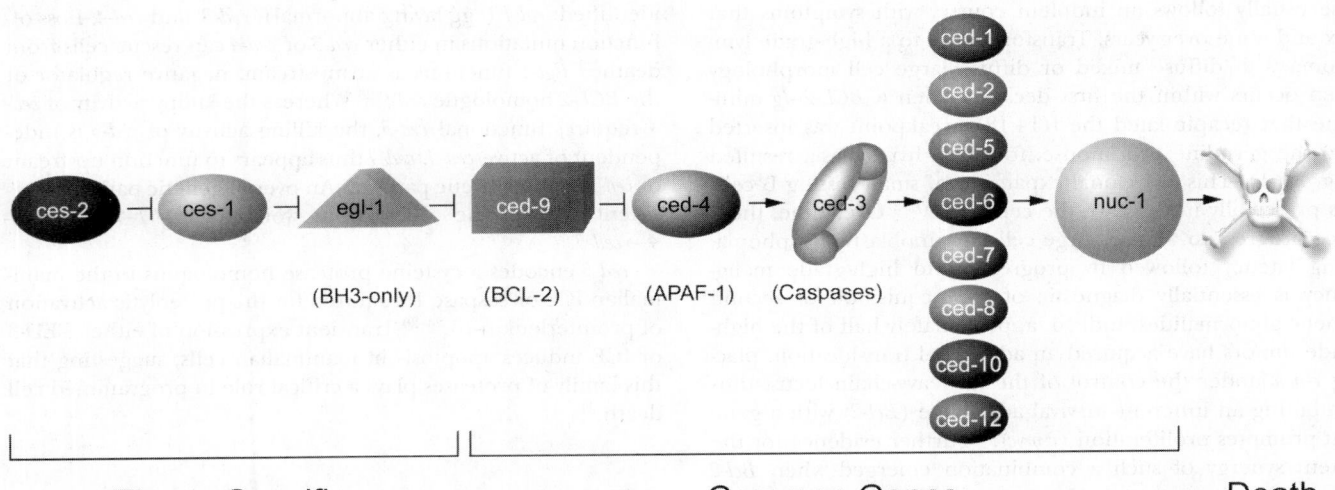

FIGURE 3.3-1. *Bcl-2–Ig* transgenic mice. **A:** The *Bcl-2–Ig* minigene recapitulates the t(14;18) chromosomal translocation of follicular B-cell lymphoma. Gain of function *Bcl-2* leads to B-cell expansion and an enlarged white pulp in follicular hyperplasia (**B**) that progress to diffuse large B-cell lymphoma (**C**). **D:** B cells accumulate as a result of extended cell survival, and their resistance to dying is complemented by a translocation of the myc gene that promotes cell division. (See Color Fig. 3.3-1 in the CD-ROM.)

been identified. Members of the family possess up to four conserved α-helical domains, designated *BH1*, *BH2*, *BH3*, and *BH4*.[29–31] Mutagenesis studies of BCL-2 indicate that the conserved domains are necessary for the interaction with proapoptotic members for the inhibition of cell death.[32] BAX and BAK are more highly conserved prodeath members of the BCL-2 family bearing BH1, BH2, and BH3 domains. A subset of proapoptotic BCL-2 family members possess sequence homol-

ogy only within the BH3 domain, further emphasizing the concept that this region forms a critical death domain.

The "multidomain" proapoptotic proteins BAX and BAK serve as a critical gateway in the intrinsic pathway of apoptosis operating at the mitochondria and endoplasmic reticulum (ER).[33,34] Cells doubly deficient for BAX and BAK are resistant to multiple intrinsic death stimuli. On activation by "BH3-only" proteins, proapoptotic BAX translocates from the cytosol to the

FIGURE 3.3-2. Genetic pathway regulating developmental cell death in the nematode *Caenorhabditis elegans* begins with upstream tissue-specific genes followed by a common, core gene pathway. Cell death in the nematode transpires by a single protease (ced-3), whose activity is regulated by a single activator (ced-4) and an inhibitor (ced-9). Mammalian counterparts of the genes in *C elegans* are indicated in parentheses. ced-1 through ced-12 regulate the phagocytosis of dead cells. (See Color Fig. 3.3-2 in the CD-ROM.)

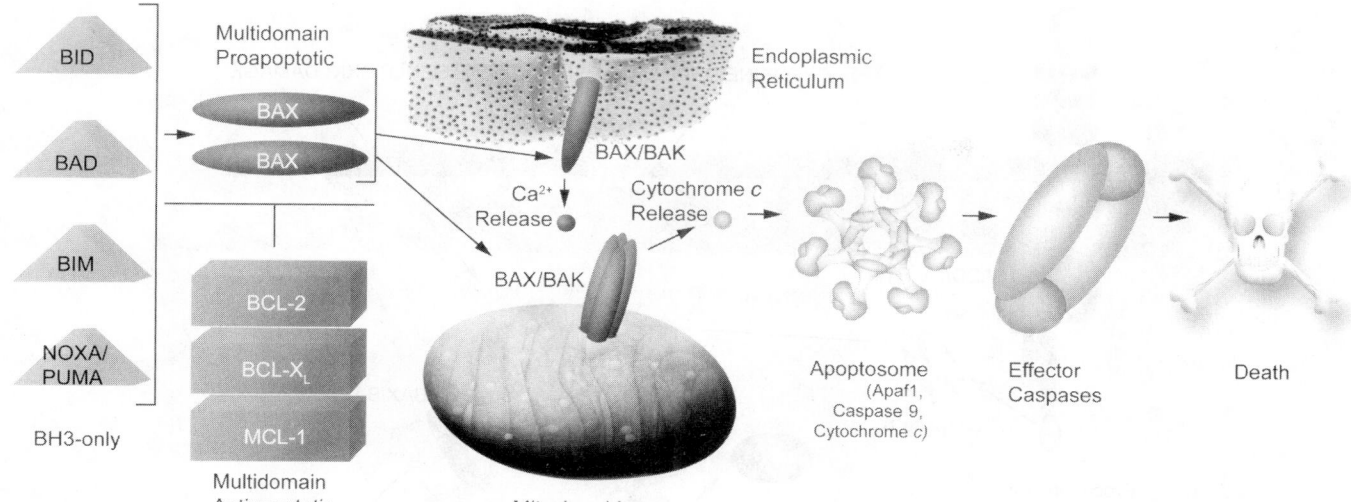

FIGURE 3.3-3.   Mammalian apoptotic pathway. Activated BH3-only proteins either directly or indirectly trigger the activation of the "multidomain" proapoptotic members BAX/BAK. In contrast, BH3-only members can be bound and sequestered by the multidomain antiapoptotic members BCL-2, BCL-X$_L$, or MCL-1. If proapoptotic activation is in excess of antiapoptotic protection, BAX/BAK homo-oligomerize in the mitochondrial outer membrane, resulting in its permeabilization and the release of intermembrane space proteins, especially cytochrome *c*. This prompts the assemblage of the heptameric apoptosome complex with the amplifier/adapter Apaf-1 and initiator caspase 9 that catalyzes activation of effector caspases and cell death. A second gateway exists for BAX/BAK, where 10% to 15% localizes to and functions at the endoplasmic reticulum (ER), the currency there being the regulation of steady-state intraluminal ER Ca^{2+} levels and consequently the amount of Ca^{2+} released on a death stimulus. (See Color Fig. 3.3-3 in the CD-ROM.)

mitochondrion and inserts into the mitochondrial outer membrane, where its oligomerization and permeabilization of the mitochondrial outer membrane culminate in release of proteins such as cytochrome *c* and second mitochondrial activator of caspases (SMAC)/ direct inhibitor of apoptosis binding protein with low pI (DIABLO) from the intermembrane space (IMS). BAK is already resident at the mitochondrial membrane in viable cells but is activated after death stimuli, either directly or indirectly, by BH3-only molecules, resulting in BAK oligomerization and release of IMS proteins including cytochrome *c*.

The three-dimensional structures for an antiapoptotic and the proapoptotic molecules have been determined.[35–37] In their closed, monomeric forms, the α helices comprising domains BH1-3 of the multidomain antiapoptotic members are juxtaposed to form a binding pocket or groove. This pocket binds the hydrophobic face of a BH3 amphipathic α helix from a proapoptotic family member.[38,39]

Many of the proapoptotic molecules, especially the BH3-only subset, are localized to the cytosol or cytoskeleton and undergo posttranslational modification, after a death signal, which allows them to target and integrate into the mitochondrial membrane.[40–43] BH3-only molecules link upstream death signals to the checkpoint of BCL-2 multidomain members (Fig. 3.3-4).

In support of this thesis, the BH3-only protein BAD is modified by phosphorylation on two serine residues in the presence of survival factors.[44] In its phosphorylated form, BAD is inactive and can be bound and sequestered by 14-3-3. On exposure to a death stimulus such as the deprivation of survival factors, BAD is dephosphorylated, resulting in the interaction of its BH3 domain with the pocket of antiapoptotic BCL-2/BCL-XL at the mitochondrial membrane.[39] Distinct kinases appear to be responsible for the

phosphorylation of the two serine sites in BAD. The phosphoinositol 3 kinase pathway regulates the phosphorylation of serine 136 in BAD. AKT, a serine-threonine survival signaling kinase in that pathway, can phosphorylate BAD serine 136.[45–48] AKT can also phosphorylate and inactivate the proapoptotic transcription factor FKHRL1 and caspase 9.[48,49] The phosphorylation and inactivation of serine 112 are mediated at the mitochondrial membrane by cyclic adenosine monophosphate–dependent protein kinase that is tethered to this locale by mitochondrial-based A kinase anchoring proteins.[50] Thus, a single proapoptotic molecule BAD has multiple signal transduction pathways that converge to inactivate it. This example indicates how complex the regulation of this pathway will be and offers additional sites for therapeutic intervention.

Another BH3-only protein, BID, connects the death signal through the tumor necrosis factor-α (TNF-α) receptor or Fas to downstream death effectors. BID exists in the cytoplasm as an inactive 22-kD protein. After exposure to TNF-α or FasL, BID is cleaved in an unstructured loop by caspase 8 to expose a new myristoylation site. Myristoylation facilitates BID's translocation to the mitochondrial membrane.[51] Once targeted, the activated p15tBID fragment's exposed BH3 domain serves as a ligand for binding multidomain members. Activated BH3-only proteins such as tBID either directly or indirectly result in the activation of multidomain BAX and BAK, which are required for the release of cytochrome *c* and the downstream apoptotic program. Protection of cells by antiapoptotics such as BCL-2/BCL-X$_L$ serves a principal, although perhaps not an exclusive, role of binding and sequestering BH3-only molecules, thus preventing activation of BAX, BAK.[52]

Additional studies using α-helical BH3 peptides to release cytochrome *c* from purified mitochondria suggest that BH3-only

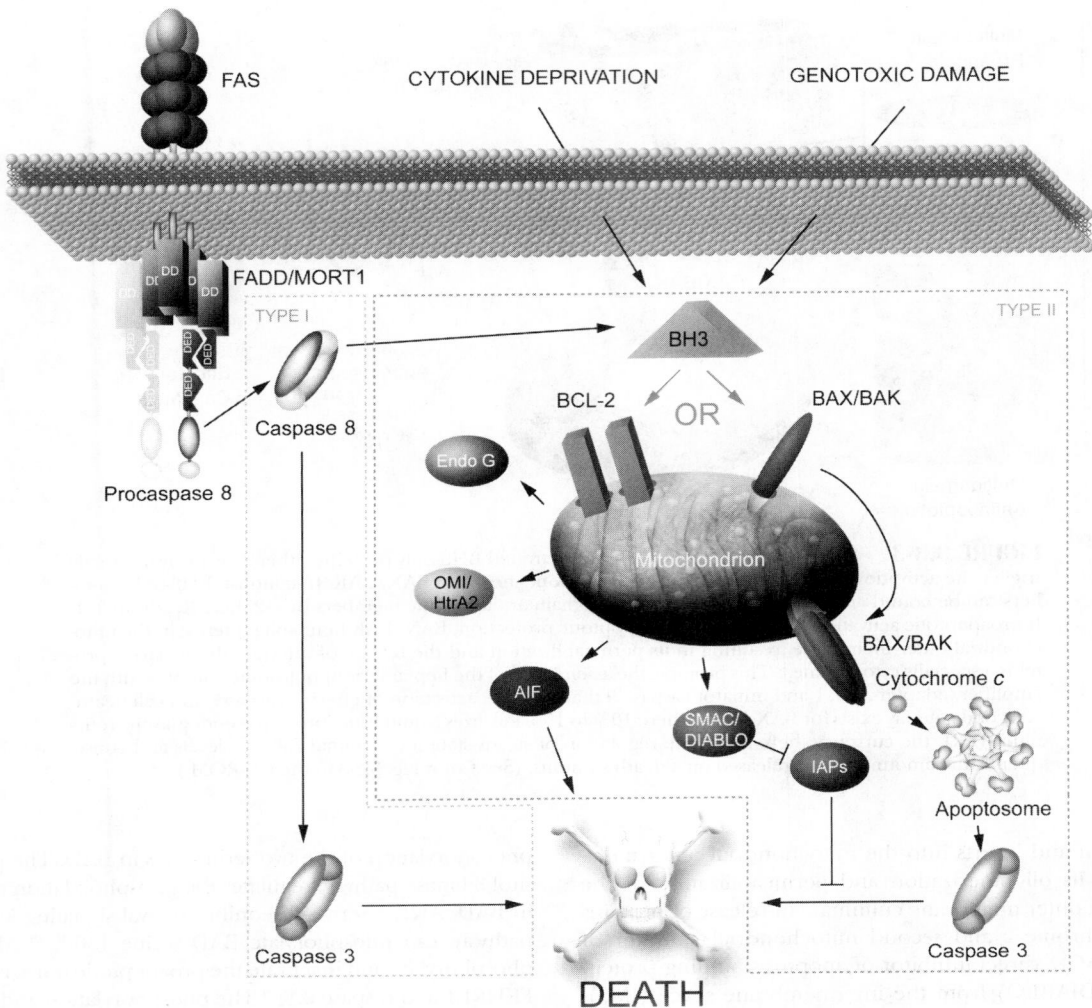

FIGURE 3.3-4. Caspase pathway and mitochondrial dysfunction. Two principal apoptotic execution programs follow death receptor signals. Whether a cell will live or die is determined by a balance of positive versus negative regulators from the proximal death signals to the core apoptotic pathway. (See Color Fig. 3.3-4 in the CD-ROM.)

molecules can be further subdivided into "activators" of BAX and BAK, such as BID, or "sensitizers," such as BAD. Sensitizers exert their effect by binding to the pocket of antiapoptotic molecules, thereby displacing "activator" proteins to activate BAX and BAK.[53] BH3 mimetics, whether engineered peptidomimetics or chemical small molecules that occupy BCL-2 member binding pockets, represent prototype therapeutics.

CRITICAL ROLE OF APOPTOSIS IN TISSUE HOMEOSTASIS

The most stringent test of the role of a gene in normal development and homeostasis is an animal in which the gene of interest has been disrupted. Newborn *Bcl-2* knockout mice are viable, but the majority die within a few weeks of birth.[54–56] Renal failure develops in the surviving mice as a result of severe polycystic kidney disease. BCL-2 functions in the normal fetal kidney to maintain cell survival during inductive epithelial-

mesenchymal interactions. At 5 to 6 weeks, the animals turn gray as a result of apoptosis of melanocytes. The hematopoietic system is initially normal, but thymus and spleen subsequently undergo massive involution resulting from apoptosis, reflecting a failure to maintain homeostasis in B and T cells. Mice that lack $Bcl-X_L$ are unable to complete normal development, with embryos dying of erythroid and neuronal apoptosis.[57,58] It thus appears that different antiapoptotic family members predominate in a tissue- and developmental-specific manner.

Loss of the proapoptotic gene *Bax* resulted in hyperplasia of thymocytes and B cells and accumulation of atrophic granulosa cells and excess primordial follicles that failed to undergo apoptosis.[59] The male mice were infertile due to failure of normal postnatal death of spermatogonia. This led to a markedly disorganized seminiferous tubule and to the failure to complete meiosis successfully. Increased numbers of neurons are also present in Bax-deficient animals, indicating that cells that normally would have died during embryonic development due to inadequate innervation are saved in the absence of *Bax*.[60]

When challenged with lethal doses of agonistic anti-Fas antibody, mice without the BH3-only BID are resistant to the ensuing Fas-induced hepatocellular apoptosis, indicating a critical role for a BID-dependent mitochondrial amplification loop in this Fas-signaled death.[61] Despite this dramatic phenotype on anti-Fas challenge, *Bid*-deficient mice successfully complete embryonic development and appear grossly normal. However, as these *Bid*-deficient mice age, a myeloproliferative disorder develops that progresses to a fatal disease resembling chronic myelomonocytic leukemia, indicating an essential role for BID in maintaining myeloid homeostasis and suppressing oncogenesis.[62]

Loss of proapoptotic *Bim* as well as *Bad* manifest predominantly in the lymphoid lineage. *Bim*-deficient mice display abnormal thymocyte development and deletion of autoreactive thymocytes and B cells.[63–67] Loss of proapoptotic *Bad* displays a more subtle phenotype, with normal lymphocyte development and death. However, the mice develop diffuse large B-cell lymphomas with age[68] as well as defects in glycolysis.[69]

Biochemical and genetic studies reveal tiering of antiapoptotic members, where MCL-1 is an apical checkpoint working upstream to BCL-2/BCL-XL and BAX/BAK.[70,71] MCL-1 is the singularly required antiapoptotic needed for survival factors to save cells in early development. MCL-1, which selectively counters the activator BH3-only BIM, must undergo degradation to enable cell death.

CASPASES

Caspases are a large family of proteases whose members function in inflammation or apoptosis.[72] Caspases are expressed as inactive proenzymes and activated by proteolytic cleavage after a death stimulus. Members of the caspase family possess a common structural design consisting of three domains: an amino-terminal domain, a large subunit, and a small subunit, separated by caspase cleavage consensus sites. After cleavage of the proenzyme, the large and small subunits associate to form a heterodimer. Crystallographic analyses of caspase 1 and caspase 3 show association of two heterodimers to form a tetramer. The large and small subunits contribute residues that are important for substrate binding and specificity. The two catalytic sites of the tetramer appear to function independently.[73–75]

The caspase catalytic site contains a conserved pentapeptide, QACXG, surrounding the active site cysteine residue. Caspases all strongly prefer an aspartic acid residue at the P_1 position of their cleavage site. Specificity of individual caspase substrate binding pockets varies, which dictates the preferred amino acids at the P_2-P_4 sites amino terminal to the substrate cleavage site.[76,77] In the case of caspase 1, a relatively large pocket is consistent with the substrate preference for bulky hydrophobic residues, whereas the smaller pocket of caspase 3 is consistent with its preference for an Asp residue at the P_4 site.

Caspases function in initiation of apoptosis in response to proapoptotic signals and in the subsequent effector pathway to disassemble the cell (see Fig. 3.3-4). On this basis they can be separated into initiator caspases, which link death signals to the cellular death program, and effector caspases that carry out a coordinated program of proteolysis, resulting in the destruction of critical cell structures involved in homeostasis and repair. Caspase prodomains play a key role in specifically transducing death signals to result in caspase activation. Two distinct structural domains have been identified within these prodomains that mediate specific protein–protein interactions. Death effector domains (DED), found on the initiator caspases 8 and 10, mediate recruitment of these initiator caspases to death receptors. The multiprotein complex thus formed induces proximity of monomers of caspase 8. Cellular and biophysical studies have suggested that oligomerization is the driving force behind activation.[78–80] Caspase activation and recruitment domains (CARD) are found on caspases 9 and 2. In the case of caspase 9, the CARD domain facilitates recruitment to a multiprotein complex composed of cytochrome *c*, Apaf-1, and caspase 9 termed the *apoptosome*. This suggests a unified model for the activation of apical caspases.[80–82] After activation, these upstream caspases initiate a proteolytic cascade, rapidly transmitting and exponentially amplifying the death signal through effector caspases 3 and 7. The culmination of these events leads to destruction of the cell by apoptosis.

DEATH RECEPTORS

In mammals, one mechanism by which initiation of cell death can occur is through interaction of death ligands, such as TNF-α, FasL, or TNF-related apoptosis-inducing ligand (TRAIL).[83] After interaction with their respective ligands, death receptors recruit adaptor proteins such as Fas-associated death domain protein (FADD) and TNF receptor–associated death domain protein (TRADD) to a plasma membrane complex called the *death-inducing signaling complex*. Death receptor and adaptor proteins interact via their death domain, present on the receptor and the adaptor proteins.[84–87] For example, in the case of CD95 Fas/FasL, this activated receptor through its adaptor FADD recruits caspase 8 by way of interaction via its DED to activate it, resulting in cleavage of downstream substrates, including effector caspases (Fig. 3.3-5). In type I cells, such as lymphocytes, Fas-induced apoptosis is mediated via caspase 8 activation of caspase 3, 7. In contrast, type II cells, such as hepatocytes, require a mitochondrial amplification loop in which cleavage and activation of BID are needed.[88] The outcome of death versus survival appears to be decided in part by the formation of different complexes by various death domain or DEDs containing proteins. A temporal time course of TNFR1 complexes has been noted.[89] Complex 1 containing TRADD, TRAF2, C-IAP1, and the kinase RIP1 assembles quickly, leading to nuclear factor κB (NFκB) activation and survival. Later, complex II forms with FADD-recruited caspase 8. In this model the balance between complex I (survival) and complex II (death) is influenced by the level of c-FLIP, an inhibitor of caspase 8 regulated by NFκB. A further pair of death receptors (DR4/5) shares a unique death ligand entitled *APO2L/TRAIL*.[90] Reports suggest that cancer cells display differential sensitivity to TRAIL-mediated apoptosis. Death-inducing signaling complex formation is similar for DR4/5 that appears to emphasize the mitochondrial and post-mitochondrial amplification steps.

APOPTOSOME

A number of death stimuli, including those we regard as being intrinsic to the cell, trigger the release of cytochrome *c* from the mitochondrial IMS, resulting in the formation of a caspase 3 activating complex, termed the *apoptosome*. The requisite members of

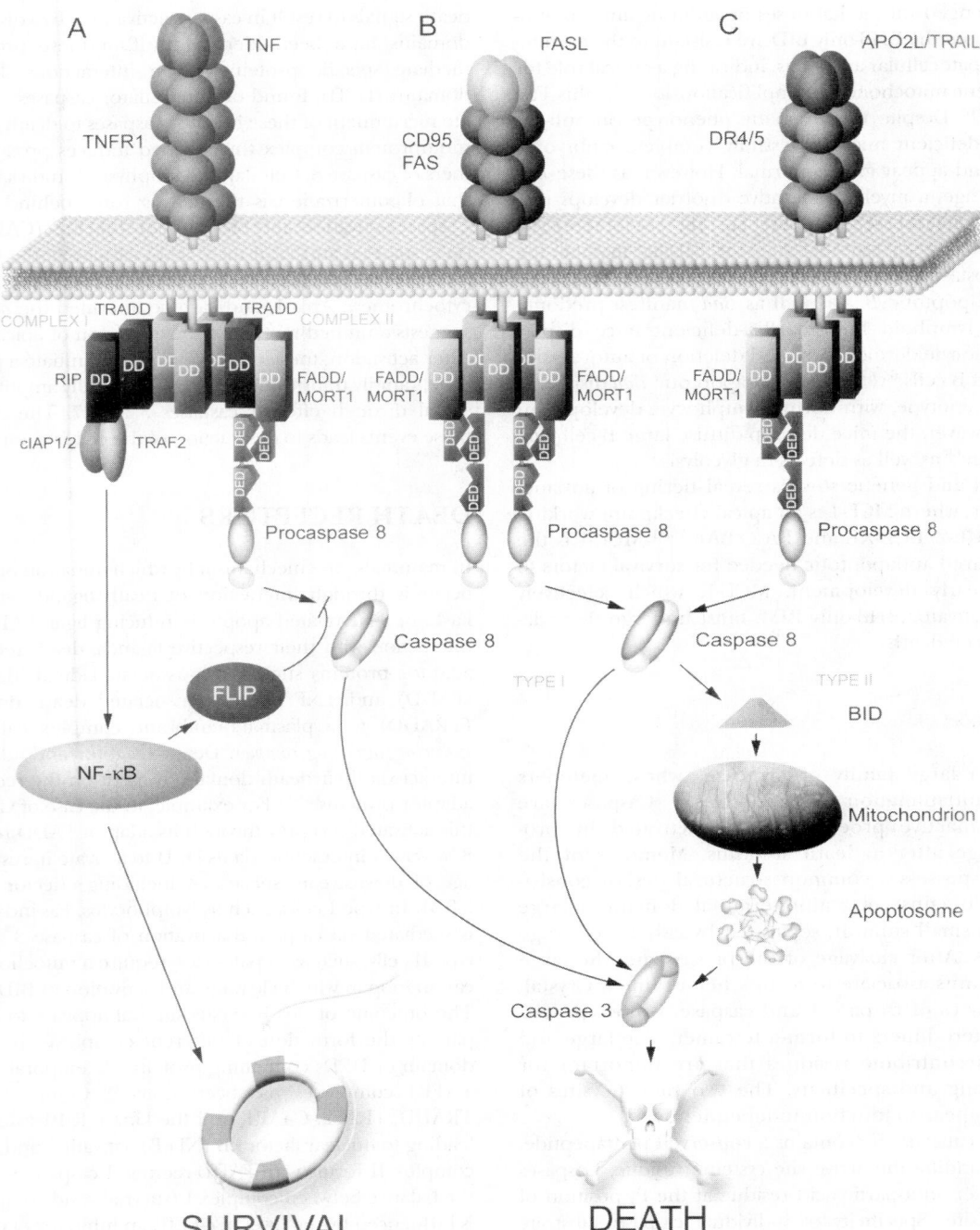

FIGURE 3.3-5. Signaling apoptosis through death receptors. The compositions of death-inducing-signaling complex (DISC) downstream of different death receptor family members are distinct. **A:** A temporal time course of TNFR1 complexes has been noted in which complex I [TNF receptor–associated death domain protein (TRADD), TRAF2, C-IAP1, and the kinase RIP1] leads to nuclear factor κB (NFκB) activation and survival, whereas complex II forms with Fas-associated death domain protein (FADD)–recruited caspase 8 by way of interaction via its death effector domain. The balance between complex I and complex II activity is influenced by the level of c-FLIP. **B:** In the case of CD95 Fas/FasL, the adaptor FADD recruits caspase 8. Type I cells mediate apoptosis via caspase 8 activation of caspase 3, 7, whereas type II cells require a mitochondrial amplification loop. **C:** A pair of death receptors (DR4/5) share a unique death ligand entitled *APO2L/TRAIL* (tumor necrosis factor–related apoptosis-inducing ligand). DISC complex formation is similar for DR4/5 and appears to emphasize the mitochondrial and postmitochondrial amplification steps. (See Color Fig. 3.3-5 in the CD-ROM.)

the apoptosome include cytochrome *c*, dATP, APAF-1 (a mammalian homologue of CED-4), and the initiator, caspase 9.[91–93] In the presence of cytochrome *c* and dATP, APAF-1 forms a multiprotein complex with procaspase 9 via CARD domains.[94] Procaspase 9 is subsequently activated and in turn activates caspase 3. Activated effector caspases carry out their role in cell death through the proteolytic cleavage of antiapoptotic proteins and repair proteins, as well as the degradation of cell structures such as the nuclear lamina.

INHIBITORS OF APOPTOSIS

Given the potentially devastating effects of inappropriate caspase activation, cells devised an additional level of caspase control. Inhibitors of apoptosis (IAPs) are a family of proteins characterized by a zinc-binding region rich in cystidine and histidine residues termed the baculoviral IAP repeat (BIR). Members of the family include proteins such as XIAP, c-IAP1, and c-IAP2 that bind and inhibit caspases as well as proteins such as survivin, which function primarily in the control of cytokinesis. The prototype IAP p35 was identified in baculovirus as a protein that inhibits caspases. Orthologues have been identified in organisms from flies to humans, indicating that this regulatory mechanism is highly conserved.

XIAP is a representative mammalian IAP whose BIR domain binds directly to caspases 3, 7, and 9, which is required for its antiapoptotic function. Structural studies indicate that the region immediately adjacent to the BIR3 domain of XIAP mediates binding to caspase 9.[95–97] Proteolytic processing exposes a region of caspase 9 used to associate with XIAP.[96] A linker region between BIR domains of XIAP inhibits caspases 3 and 7 through high-affinity binding and steric occlusion. In the case of caspase 7, the binding directly occludes the catalytic groove of the enzyme.[98,99] Thus, XIAP inhibits the various caspases by distinct mechanisms.

IAP activity is itself tightly regulated at transcriptional and posttranscriptional levels in certain situations. IAPs such as survivin that exert effects during cytokinesis are subject to cell cycle–dependent transcriptional regulation. NFκB induces the expression of c-IAP2 and XIAP, providing a transcriptional regulatory mechanism.[100] Posttranscriptional regulation of IAPs occurs at the level of translation, protein degradation, and regulatory protein–protein interactions. The ubiquitin-proteasome system of protein degradation regulates levels of XIAP, c-IAP1, and survivin. Cells undergoing apoptosis degrade XIAP and c-IAP1 by autoubiquitination followed by proteosomal degradation. A number of regulatory proteins have been identified that bind to IAPs. Two classes of IAP regulatory proteins are released from the mitochondria on receipt of an apoptotic signal. SMAC/DIABLO[101,102] binds to the same pocket of XIAP as caspase 9.[103] A second protein that is released from mitochondria, Omi/HtrA2, is a proapoptotic serine protease, which requires IAP binding and serine protease functions for activity.[104]

ROLE OF INTRACELLULAR ORGANELLES: MITOCHONDRIA AND ENDOPLASMIC RETICULUM

Many of the critical control steps in the intrinsic apoptotic pathway are localized to the surface of intracellular organelles. The mitochondrial dysfunction that occurs in cell death is manifest as altered transmembrane potential ($\Delta\psi m$), the release of proteins from the IMS and the production of reactive oxygen species. Prior studies of necrotic death and at least late stages of apoptotic cell death have noted mitochondrial swelling attributed to the opening of a mitochondrial permeability transition pore that allows the passage of solutes and dissipation of the transmembrane gradient. The localization of antiapoptotic molecules such as BCL-2 as well as the translocation of proapoptotic proteins to the mitochondrial membrane emphasizes the importance of mitochondrial dysfunction in the action of these molecules. Cellular energy metabolism and the core apoptotic pathway are two major determinants of cellular survival. Growth/survival factors such as insulin-like growth factor-1 or interleukin-3 also stimulate glucose transport and the translocation of hexokinases to mitochondria, stimulating glycolysis as well as inhibiting apoptosis.[105,106] Antiapoptotic BCL-2/BCL-X_L blocks apoptosis in a glucose-independent fashion but does not prevent metabolic decline when growth/survival factors are withdrawn. Proteomics studies indicate a more intimate integration of glucose metabolism and apoptosis. At liver mitochondria, BAD nucleates a macromolecular complex containing hexokinase IV, a resident kinase (cyclic adenosine monophosphate–dependent protein kinase)/phosphatase (PP1α) pair, and an A-kinase anchoring protein (WAVE-1).[69] BAD plays an unexpected role in regulating glucose homeostasis, suggesting that BH3-only proteins serve as specific sentinels for death signals, by being embedded as integral participants in the pathways they monitor. Another link between the core apoptotic pathway and mitochondrial physiology has been established by VDAC2 (voltage-dependent anion channel) binding and inhibiting the potentially lethal BAK molecule at the mitochondria of viable cells.[107]

The ER also serves as a critical control point in the intrinsic apoptotic pathway. Antiapoptotic BCL-2 and proapoptotic BAX/BAK localize to the ER. Ca^{2+} appears to be the currency regulated at the ER by the BCL-2 family that controls cell death.[34,108,109] Certain death signals rely on an ER Ca^{2+} gateway rather than the mitochondrial gateway, including Ca^{2+}-dependent lipid second messengers as well as pathologic oxidative stress. Many death stimuli, including some physiologic cues, engage the ER and the mitochondrial gateways to apoptosis (see Fig. 3.3-3).

CELL PROLIFERATION AND APOPTOSIS

Apoptosis represents a brake on cellular expansion, which counters cell proliferation. Substantial evidence exists for crosstalk between proliferation and apoptosis pathways.[110] The oncoproteins c-Myc and adenovirus E1A, both potent inducers of proliferation, have also been shown to possess proapoptotic properties.[111–114] The mitogenic and apoptotic properties of c-Myc and adenovirus E1A are genetically inseparable.[111,115,116] E1A induces proliferation and apoptosis by interacting with the retinoblastoma protein (Rb), a regulator of cell-cycle progression, or the transcriptional corepressor p300.[117–121] c-Myc appears to promote apoptosis by multiple pathways.[111]

Rb itself also provides a link between cell proliferation and apoptosis. Rb functions as a cell-cycle checkpoint between G_1 and S phase and mediates its effect through interaction with a family of transcription factors that control the expression of genes required for cell-cycle progression, the E2F proteins.[122–124] Complexes containing E2Fs and Rb have been shown to bind to target DNA sequences in a number of promoters and actively repress transcription.[125–128] Entry into S phase induced by ectopic expression of E2F, or mutagenesis, which abolishes interaction with Rb, results in increased apoptosis.[128–130] Mice in which the Rb gene has been knocked out by homologous recombination die at embryonic days 12 to 13 and exhibit proliferation and apoptosis of the liver, central nervous system, lens, and skeletal muscle cells.[131,132] E2F-1 knockout mice develop a broad spectrum of tumors, including lymphomas, and display decreased apoptosis in double-positive thymocytes, further establishing the link between cell proliferation, apoptosis, and tumorigenesis.[133,134] Oncogenes have been shown to sensitize cells to a wide variety of stimuli, including DNA damage, hypoxia, TNF-α and FasL, and growth factor withdrawal.[111,135–139] It appears that the cellular machinery directing cell proliferation and apoptosis are coupled, suggesting that the decision of a cell to undergo apoptosis or proliferation is tightly coupled.

One link between these two processes is the p53 tumor suppressor. Loss of p53 has been observed in numerous tumor types, and p53 function is abrogated in a large percentage of tumors.[140] p53 expression is induced in response to a variety of cellular stresses, including DNA damage, hypoxia, and oncogene activation, resulting in cell-cycle arrest or apoptosis. Mice deficient for p53 are developmentally normal, but spontaneous tumors develop in 75% by 6 months of age.[141] Germline mutation of p53 in humans results in Li-Fraumeni syndrome, and tumors develop in greater than 50% of these individuals by age 30.[142]

The majority of p53 mutations in human tumors cluster within the DNA-binding domain, suggesting that p53 exerts its effects at least in part through transcriptional regulation of target genes.[142,143] The mechanism by which p53 exerts its apoptotic effect appears to be multifactorial. It is able to induce the expression of *NOXA*, *PUMA*, *BAX*, and *FAS*, and another member of the TNF family of death receptors, DR5.[144] p53 also appears to induce apoptosis by posttranslational mechanisms.[52,144]

POSSIBILITIES FOR THERAPEUTIC INTERVENTION

Death receptors in theory constitute attractive targets for therapeutic intervention in cancer. Unfortunately, infusion of TNF-α causes a lethal inflammatory response resembling septic shock, resulting in proinflammatory activation of macrophages and endothelial cells,[145,146] and infusion of agonistic anti-Fas antibody causes lethal hepatic apoptosis. The related death ligand TRAIL (APO2L) appears to possess the ability to induce apoptosis in a wide variety of tumor cell lines. *In vivo* administration of a leucine zipper modified form of TRAIL in which the molecule is stabilized as a trimer suppresses the growth of a mammary adenocarcinoma cell line in SCID mice.[147] Similarly, recombinant TRAIL administered shortly after tumor xenograft injection markedly reduced tumor incidence. A synergistic effect was noted with TRAIL and 5-fluorouracil or CPT-11.[146,148]

BCL-2 and other family members provide promising targets for therapeutic intervention.[149] The strategy of antisense oligonucleotide therapy has been used to "silence" *BCL-2* expression. Antisense oligonucleotides are short stretches of DNA, approximately 16 to 20 bases in length. The oligonucleotides are internalized by cells through a saturable endocytosis pathway. On injection into a host, expression of a specific gene can be blocked by hybridization with the target messenger RNA through Watson-Crick base pairing. The result is either degradation of the RNA-DNA complex by RNAse H or block in translation of the RNA.

An 18-base-pair antisense oligonucleotide G3139 (Genta, San Diego, CA) was designed against *BCL-2* for the treatment of follicular lymphoma.[150] Initial studies in a t(14;18) murine xenograft lymphoma model were encouraging, and clinical trials of G3139 that will reveal its ultimate utility are under way.

Another strategy to promote apoptosis of cancer cells is to inhibit the antiapoptotic BCL-2 members. Mimics of BH3 domains that compete for the binding pockets of antiapoptotic members such as BCL-2 or BCL-X$_L$ would displace proapoptotic members triggering cell death. Cancer cells, which often display a reset antiapoptotic/proapoptotic rheostat, might prove differentially susceptible to such an approach. Peptidomimetics derived from the BH3 domains of proapoptotic members as well as chemical small molecules selected for their capacity to bind the pockets of antiapoptotic BCL-2 members are under development.

CONCLUSION

Apoptosis is a highly regulated pathway that is critical for maintaining homeostasis in multicellular organisms. Numerous signals are capable of modulating cell death. Apoptosis can be initiated through extrinsic pathway engaging death receptors, which often trigger a caspase cascade that is capable of killing the cell. Intracellular damage proceeds through an intrinsic pathway of apoptosis that relies on amplification loops, especially the release of cytochrome *c* from the mitochondrion to further activate caspases. The BCL-2 family of proteins is situated upstream to the irreversible damage of cellular constituents, providing a pivotal checkpoint in the fate of a cell. The proapoptotic BH3-only members such as BID, BAD, and BIM serve as upstream sentinels that recognize specific death signals and are proximal to the multidomain BCL-2 members of the common, core apoptotic pathway. Activated BH3-only molecules either directly or indirectly activate multidomain BAX/BAK that constitute the requisite gateway to the intrinsic pathway operative at the surface of the mitochondrion and ER. In contrast, antiapoptotics such as BCL-2, BCL-X$_L$, and MCL-1 bind and sequester BH3-only molecules, protecting BAX/BAK from activation. Downstream of the mitochondrion, amplification is achieved via the apoptosome to generate further caspase activity. Layers of postmitochondrial regulation include the IAPs as well as their inhibitors SMAC/OMI. Cancer cells frequently and possibly invariably possess apoptotic defects. It is conceivable that defects are always required in proliferation and cell death pathways, as single defects tend to be self-correcting in their net effect on cell number. If genetic events inherent to the transformation process always violate physiologic checkpoints that would trigger apoptosis, it is conceivable that cancer cells will prove to be addicted to their apoptotic defects for their own maintenance. In this context, apoptotic pathways provide exciting molecular targets for the rational design of new therapeutic agents to specifically promote apoptosis of cancer cells.

REFERENCES

1. Vogt C. *Untersuchungen uber die Entwicklungsgeschichte der Geburtshelferkroete.* Solothurn, Switzerland: Jent und Gassman, 1842.
2. Kerr JF, Wyllie AH, Currie AR. Apoptosis: a basic biological phenomenon with wide-ranging implications in tissue kinetics. *Br J Cancer* 1972;26:239.
3. Wyllie AH. Apoptosis: cell death in tissue regulation. *J Pathol* 1987;153:313.
4. Fukuhara S, Rowley JD, Variakojis D, et al. Chromosome abnormalities in poorly differentiated lymphocytic lymphoma. *Cancer Res* 1979;39:3119.
5. Yunis JJ, Frizzera G, Oken MM, et al. Multiple recurrent genomic defects in follicular lymphoma. A possible model for cancer. *N Engl J Med* 1987;316:79.
6. Tsujimoto Y, Gorham J, Cossman J, et al. The t(14;18) chromosome translocations involved in B-cell neoplasms result from mistakes in VDJ joining. *Science* 1985;229:1390.
7. Bakhshi A, Jensen JP, Goldman P, et al. Cloning the chromosomal breakpoint of t(14;18) human lymphomas: clustering around JH on chromosome 14 and near a transcriptional unit on 18. *Cell* 1985;41:899.
8. Cleary ML, Sklar J. Nucleotide sequence of a t(14;18) chromosomal breakpoint in follicular lymphoma and demonstration of a breakpoint-cluster region near a transcriptionally active locus on chromosome 18. *Proc Natl Acad Sci U S A* 1985;82:7439.
9. Korsmeyer SJ. BCL-2 gene family and the regulation of programmed cell death. *Cancer Res* 1999;59:1693s.
10. Horning SJ. Natural history of and therapy for the indolent non-Hodgkin's lymphomas. *Semin Oncol* 1993;20:75.
11. McDonnell TJ, Nunez G, Platt FM, et al. Deregulated Bcl-2-immunoglobulin transgene expands a resting but responsive immunoglobulin M and D-expressing B-cell population. *Mol Cell Biol* 1990;10:1901.
12. McDonnell TJ, Deane N, Platt FM, et al. bcl-2-immunoglobulin transgenic mice demonstrate extended B cell survival and follicular lymphoproliferation. *Cell* 1989;57:79.
13. McDonnell TJ, Korsmeyer SJ. Progression from lymphoid hyperplasia to high-grade malignant lymphoma in mice transgenic for the t(14;18). *Nature* 1991;349:254.
14. Strasser A, Harris AW, Bath ML, et al. Novel primitive lymphoid tumours induced in transgenic mice by cooperation between myc and bcl-2. *Nature* 1990;348:331.
15. Vaux DL, Cory S, Adams JM. Bcl-2 gene promotes haemopoietic cell survival and cooperates with c-myc to immortalize pre-B cells. *Nature* 1988;335:440.
16. Hockenbery D, Nunez G, Milliman C, et al. Bcl-2 is an inner mitochondrial membrane protein that blocks programmed cell death. *Nature* 1990;348:334.
17. Linette GP, Hess JL, Sentman CL, et al. Peripheral T-cell lymphoma in lckpr-bcl-2 transgenic mice. *Blood* 1995;86:1255.
18. Bishop JM. The molecular genetics of cancer. *Science* 1987;235:305.
19. Korsmeyer SJ. Bcl-2 initiates a new category of oncogenes: regulators of cell death. *Blood* 1992;80:879.
20. Sulston JE, Horvitz HR. Post-embryonic cell lineages of the nematode, *Caenorhabditis elegans. Dev Biol* 1977;56:110.
21. Hengartner MO, Horvitz HR. *C. elegans* cell survival gene ced-9 encodes a functional homolog of the mammalian proto-oncogene bcl-2. *Cell* 1994;76:665.
22. Cryns V, Yuan J. Proteases to die for. *Genes Dev* 1998;12:1551.
23. Conradt B, Horvitz HR. The *C. elegans* protein EGL-1 is required for programmed cell death and interacts with the Bcl-2-like protein CED-9. *Cell* 1998;93:519.
24. Cerretti DP, Kozlosky CJ, Mosley B, et al. Molecular cloning of the interleukin-1 beta converting enzyme. *Science* 1992;256:97.
25. Thornberry NA, Bull HG, Calaycay JR, et al. A novel heterodimeric cysteine protease is required for interleukin-1 beta processing in monocytes. *Nature* 1992;356:768.
26. Yuan J, Shaham S, Ledoux S, et al. The *C. elegans* cell death gene ced-3 encodes a protein similar to mammalian interleukin-1 beta-converting enzyme. *Cell* 1993;75:641.
27. Miura M, Zhu H, Rotello R, et al. Induction of apoptosis in fibroblasts by IL-1 beta-converting enzyme, a mammalian homolog of the *C. elegans* cell death gene ced-3. *Cell* 1993;75:653.
28. Gross A, McDonnell JM, Korsmeyer SJ. BCL-2 family members and the mitochondria in apoptosis. *Genes Dev* 1999;13:1899.
29. Adams JM, Cory S. The Bcl-2 protein family: arbiters of cell survival. *Science* 1998;281:1322.
30. Kelekar A, Thompson CB. Bcl-2-family proteins: the role of the BH3 domain in apoptosis. *Trends Cell Biol* 1998;8:324.
31. Reed JC. Bcl-2 family proteins. *Oncogene* 1998;17:3225.
32. Yin XM, Oltvai ZN, Korsmeyer SJ. BH1 and BH2 domains of Bcl-2 are required for inhibition of apoptosis and heterodimerization with Bax. *Nature* 1994;369:321.
33. Wei MC, Zong WX, Cheng EH, et al. Proapoptotic BAX and BAK: a requisite gateway to mitochondrial dysfunction and death. *Science* 2001;292:727.
34. Scorrano L, Oakes SA, Opferman JT, et al. BAX and BAK regulation of endoplasmic reticulum Ca2+: a control point for apoptosis. *Science* 2003;300:135.
35. Muchmore SW, Sattler M, Liang H, et al. X-ray and NMR structure of human Bcl-xL, an inhibitor of programmed cell death. *Nature* 1996;381:335.
36. Chou JJ, Li H, Salvesen GS, et al. Solution structure of BID, an intracellular amplifier of apoptotic signaling. *Cell* 1999;96:615.
37. McDonnell JM, Fushman D, Milliman CL, et al. Solution structure of the proapoptotic molecule BID: a structural basis for apoptotic agonists and antagonists. *Cell* 1999;96:625.
38. Sattler M, Liang H, Nettesheim D, et al. Structure of Bcl-xL-Bak peptide complex: recognition between regulators of apoptosis. *Science* 1997;275:983.
39. Zha J, Harada H, Osipov K, et al. BH3 domain of BAD is required for heterodimerization with BCL-XL and pro-apoptotic activity. *J Biol Chem* 1997;272:24101.
40. Zhu W, Cowie A, Wasfy GW, et al. Bcl-2 mutants with restricted subcellular location reveal spatially distinct pathways for apoptosis in different cell types. *EMBO J* 1996;15:4130.
41. Hsu YT, Wolter KG, Youle RJ. Cytosol-to-membrane redistribution of Bax and Bcl-X(L) during apoptosis. *Proc Natl Acad Sci U S A* 1997;94:3668.
42. Gross A, Jockel J, Wei MC, et al. Enforced dimerization of BAX results in its translocation, mitochondrial dysfunction and apoptosis. *EMBO J* 1998;17:3878.
43. Puthalakath H, Huang DC, O'Reilly LA, et al. The proapoptotic activity of the Bcl-2 family member Bim is regulated by interaction with the dynein motor complex. *Mol Cell* 1999;3:287.
44. Zha J, Harada H, Yang E, et al. Serine phosphorylation of death agonist BAD in response to survival factor results in binding to 14-3-3 not BCL-X(L). *Cell* 1996;87:619.
45. Datta SR, Dudek H, Tao X, et al. Akt phosphorylation of BAD couples survival signals to the cell-intrinsic death machinery. *Cell* 1997;91:231.
46. del Peso L, Gonzalez-Garcia M, Page C, et al. Interleukin-3-induced phosphorylation of BAD through the protein kinase Akt. *Science* 1997;278:687.
47. Blume-Jensen P, Janknecht R, Hunter T. The kit receptor promotes cell survival via activation of PI 3-kinase and subsequent Akt-mediated phosphorylation of Bad on Ser136. *Curr Biol* 1998;8:779.
48. Brunet A, Bonni A, Zigmond MJ, et al. Akt promotes cell survival by phosphorylating and inhibiting a Forkhead transcription factor. *Cell* 1999;96:857.
49. Cardone MH, Roy N, Stennicke HR, et al. Regulation of cell death protease caspase-9 by phosphorylation. *Science* 1998;282:1318.
50. Harada H, Becknell B, Wilm M, et al. Phosphorylation and inactivation of BAD by mitochondria-anchored protein kinase A. *Mol Cell* 1999;3:413.
51. Zha J, Weiler S, Oh KJ, et al. Posttranslational N-myristoylation of BID as a molecular switch for targeting mitochondria and apoptosis. *Science* 2000;290:1761.
52. Cheng EH, Wei MC, Weiler S, et al. BCL-2, BCL-X(L) sequester BH3 domain-only molecules preventing BAX- and BAK-mediated mitochondrial apoptosis. *Mol Cell* 2001;8:705.
53. Letai A, Bassik MC, Walensky LD, et al. Distinct BH3 domains either sensitize or activate mitochondrial apoptosis, serving as prototype cancer therapeutics. *Cancer Cell* 2002;2:183.
54. Veis DJ, Sorenson CM, Shutter JR, et al. Bcl-2-deficient mice demonstrate fulminant lymphoid apoptosis, polycystic kidneys, and hypopigmented hair. *Cell* 1993;75:229.
55. Nakayama K, Negishi I, Kuida K, et al. Targeted disruption of Bcl-2 alpha beta in mice: occurrence of gray hair, polycystic kidney disease, and lymphocytopenia. *Proc Natl Acad Sci U S A* 1994;91:3700.
56. Kamada S, Shimono A, Shinto Y, et al. bcl-2 deficiency in mice leads to pleiotropic abnormalities: accelerated lymphoid cell death in thymus and spleen, polycystic kidney, hair hypopigmentation, and distorted small intestine. *Cancer Res* 1995;55:354.
57. Motoyama N, Wang F, Roth KA, et al. Massive cell death of immature hematopoietic cells and neurons in Bcl-x-deficient mice. *Science* 1995;267:1506.
58. Ma A, Pena JC, Chang B, et al. Bclx regulates the survival of double-positive thymocytes. *Proc Natl Acad Sci U S A* 1995;92:4763.
59. Knudson CM, Tung KS, Tourtellotte WG, et al. Bax-deficient mice with lymphoid hyperplasia and male germ cell death. *Science* 1995;270:96.
60. Deckwerth TL, Elliott JL, Knudson CM, et al. BAX is required for neuronal death after trophic factor deprivation and during development. *Neuron* 1996;17:401.
61. Yin XM, Wang K, Gross A, et al. Bid-deficient mice are resistant to Fas-induced hepatocellular apoptosis. *Nature* 1999;400:886.
62. Zinkel SS, Ong CC, Ferguson DO, et al. Proapoptotic BID is required for myeloid homeostasis and tumor suppression. *Genes Dev* 2003;17:229.
63. Hildeman DA, Zhu Y, Mitchell TC, et al. Activated T cell death in vivo mediated by proapoptotic bcl-2 family member bim. *Immunity* 2002;16:759.
64. Enders A, Bouillet P, Puthalakath H, et al. Loss of the pro-apoptotic BH3-only Bcl-2 family member Bim inhibits BCR stimulation-induced apoptosis and deletion of autoreactive B cells. *J Exp Med* 2003;198:1119.
65. Bouillet P, Purton JF, Godfrey DI, et al. BH3-only Bcl-2 family member Bim is required for apoptosis of autoreactive thymocytes. *Nature* 2002;415:922.
66. Bouillet P, Huang DC, O'Reilly LA, et al. The role of the pro-apoptotic Bcl-2 family member bim in physiological cell death. *Ann N Y Acad Sci* 2000;926:83.
67. Strasser A, Puthalakath H, Bouillet P, et al. The role of bim, a proapoptotic BH3-only member of the Bcl-2 family in cell-death control. *Ann N Y Acad Sci* 2000;917:541.
68. Ranger AM, Zha J, Harada H, et al. Bad-deficient mice develop diffuse large B cell lymphoma. *Proc Natl Acad Sci U S A* 2003;100:9324.
69. Danial NN, Gramm CF, Scorrano L, et al. BAD and glucokinase reside in a mitochondrial complex that integrates glycolysis and apoptosis. *Nature* 2003;424:952.
70. Nijhawan D, Fang M, Traer E, et al. Elimination of Mcl-1 is required for the initiation of apoptosis following ultraviolet irradiation. *Genes Dev* 2003;17:1475.
71. Opferman JT, Letai A, Beard C, et al. Development and maintenance of B and T lymphocytes requires antiapoptotic MCL-1. *Nature* 2003;426:671.
72. Thornberry NA, Lazebnik Y. Caspases: enemies within. *Science* 1998;281:1312.
73. Walker NP, Talanian RV, Brady KD, et al. Crystal structure of the cysteine protease interleukin-1 beta-converting enzyme: a (p20/p10)2 homodimer. *Cell* 1994;78:343.
74. Wilson KP, Black JA, Thomson JA, et al. Structure and mechanism of interleukin-1 beta converting enzyme. *Nature* 1994;370:270.
75. Rotonda J, Nicholson DW, Fazil KM, et al. The three-dimensional structure of apopain/CPP32, a key mediator of apoptosis. *Nat Struct Biol* 1996;3:619.
76. Talanian RV, Quinlan C, Trautz S, et al. Substrate specificities of caspase family proteases. *J Biol Chem* 1997;272:9677.
77. Thornberry NA, Rano TA, Peterson EP, et al. A combinatorial approach defines specificities of members of the caspase family and granzyme B. Functional relationships established for key mediators of apoptosis. *J Biol Chem* 1997;272:17907.
78. Chen M, Orozco A, Spencer DM, et al. Activation of initiator caspases through a stable dimeric intermediate. *J Biol Chem* 2002;277:50761.
79. Donepudi M, Mac Sweeney A, Briand C, et al. Insights into the regulatory mechanism for caspase-8 activation. *Mol Cell* 2003;11:543.
80. Boatright KM, Renatus M, Scott FL, et al. A unified model for apical caspase activation. *Mol Cell* 2003;11:529.

81. Renatus M, Stennicke HR, Scott FL, et al. Dimer formation drives the activation of the cell death protease caspase 9. *Proc Natl Acad Sci U S A* 2001;98:14250.
82. Shi Y. Mechanisms of caspase activation and inhibition during apoptosis. *Mol Cell* 2002;9:459.
83. Nagata S. Apoptosis by death factor. *Cell* 1997;88:355.
84. Chinnaiyan AM, O'Rourke K, Tewari M, et al. FADD, a novel death domain-containing protein, interacts with the death domain of Fas and initiates apoptosis. *Cell* 1995;81:505.
85. Chinnaiyan AM, Tepper CG, Seldin MF, et al. FADD/MORT1 is a common mediator of CD95 (Fas/APO-1) and tumor necrosis factor receptor-induced apoptosis. *J Biol Chem* 1996;271:4961.
86. Hsu H, Xiong J, Goeddel DV. The TNF receptor 1-associated protein TRADD signals cell death and NF-kappa B activation. *Cell* 1995;81:495.
87. Stanger BZ, Leder P, Lee TH, et al. RIP: a novel protein containing a death domain that interacts with Fas/APO-1 (CD95) in yeast and causes cell death. *Cell* 1995;81:513.
88. Scaffidi C, Fulda S, Srinivasan A, et al. Two CD95 (APO-1/Fas) signaling pathways. *EMBO J* 1998;17:1675.
89. Micheau O, Tschopp J. Induction of TNF receptor I-mediated apoptosis via two sequential signaling complexes. *Cell* 2003;114:181.
90. Ashkenazi A, Dixit VM. Death receptors: signaling and modulation. *Science* 1998;281:1305.
91. Liu X, Kim CN, Yang J, et al. Induction of apoptotic program in cell-free extracts: requirement for dATP and cytochrome c. *Cell* 1996;86:147.
92. Li F, Srinivasan A, Wang Y, et al. Cell-specific induction of apoptosis by microinjection of cytochrome c. Bcl-xL has activity independent of cytochrome c release. *J Biol Chem* 1997;272:30299.
93. Zou H, Henzel WJ, Liu X, et al. Apaf-1, a human protein homologous to C. elegans CED-4, participates in cytochrome c-dependent activation of caspase-3. *Cell* 1997;90:405.
94. Zou H, Li Y, Liu X, et al. An APAF-1.cytochrome c multimeric complex is a functional apoptosome that activates procaspase-9. *J Biol Chem* 1999;274:11549.
95. Shiozaki EN, Chai J, Rigotti DJ, et al. Mechanism of XIAP-mediated inhibition of caspase-9. *Mol Cell* 2003;11:519.
96. Srinivasula SM, Hegde R, Saleh A, et al. A conserved XIAP-interaction motif in caspase-9 and Smac/DIABLO regulates caspase activity and apoptosis. *Nature* 2001;410:112.
97. Sun C, Cai M, Meadows RP, et al. NMR structure and mutagenesis of the third Bir domain of the inhibitor of apoptosis protein XIAP. *J Biol Chem* 2000;275:33777.
98. Sun C, Cai M, Gunasekera AH, et al. NMR structure and mutagenesis of the inhibitor-of-apoptosis protein XIAP. *Nature* 1999;401:818.
99. Chai J, Shiozaki E, Srinivasula SM, et al. Structural basis of caspase-7 inhibition by XIAP. *Cell* 2001;104:769.
100. Wang CY, Mayo MW, Korneluk RG, et al. NF-kappaB antiapoptosis: induction of TRAF1 and TRAF2 and c-IAP1 and c-IAP2 to suppress caspase-8 activation. *Science* 1998;281:1680.
101. Du C, Fang M, Li Y, et al. Smac, a mitochondrial protein that promotes cytochrome c-dependent caspase activation by eliminating IAP inhibition. *Cell* 2000;102:33.
102. Verhagen AM, Ekert PG, Pakusch M, et al. Identification of DIABLO, a mammalian protein that promotes apoptosis by binding to and antagonizing IAP proteins. *Cell* 2000;102:43.
103. Liston P, Fong WG, Korneluk RG. The inhibitors of apoptosis: there is more to life than Bcl2. *Oncogene* 2003;22:8568.
104. Ravagnan L, Roumier T, Kroemer G. Mitochondria, the killer organelles and their weapons. *J Cell Physiol* 2002;192:131.
105. Gottlieb E, Armour SM, Thompson CB. Mitochondrial respiratory control is lost during growth factor deprivation. *Proc Natl Acad Sci U S A* 2002;99:12801.
106. Vander Heiden MG, Plas DR, Rathmell JC, et al. Growth factors can influence cell growth and survival through effects on glucose metabolism. *Mol Cell Biol* 2001;21:5899.
107. Cheng EH, Sheiko TV, Fisher JK, et al. VDAC2 inhibits BAK activation and mitochondrial apoptosis. *Science* 2003;301:513.
108. Lam M, Dubyak G, Chen L, et al. Evidence that BCL-2 represses apoptosis by regulating endoplasmic reticulum-associated Ca2+ fluxes. *Proc Natl Acad Sci U S A* 1994;91:6569.
109. Pinton P, Ferrari D, Rapizzi E, et al. The Ca2+ concentration of the endoplasmic reticulum is a key determinant of ceramide-induced apoptosis: significance for the molecular mechanism of Bcl-2 action. *EMBO J* 2001;20:2690.
110. Evan G, Littlewood T. A matter of life and cell death. *Science* 1998;281:1317.
111. Evan GI, Wyllie AH, Gilbert CS, et al. Induction of apoptosis in fibroblasts by c-myc protein. *Cell* 1992;69:119.
112. Sakamuro D, Eviner V, Elliott KJ, et al. c-Myc induces apoptosis in epithelial cells by both p53-dependent and p53-independent mechanisms. *Oncogene* 1995;11:2411.
113. Shi Y, Glynn JM, Guilbert LJ, et al. Role for c-myc in activation-induced apoptotic cell death in T cell hybridomas. *Science* 1992;257:212.
114. White E, Cipriani R, Sabbatini P, et al. Adenovirus E1B 19-kilodalton protein overcomes the cytotoxicity of E1A proteins. *J Virol* 1991;65:2968.
115. Amati B, Littlewood TD, Evan GI, et al. The c-Myc protein induces cell cycle progression and apoptosis through dimerization with Max. *EMBO J* 1993;12:5083.
116. Raychaudhuri P, Bagchi S, Devoto SH, et al. Domains of the adenovirus E1A protein required for oncogenic activity are also required for dissociation of E2F transcription factor complexes. *Genes Dev* 1991;5:1200.
117. Flint J, Shenk T. Viral transactivating proteins. *Annu Rev Genet* 1997;31:177.
118. Samuelson AV, Lowe SW. Selective induction of p53 and chemosensitivity in RB-deficient cells by E1A mutants unable to bind the RB-related proteins. *Proc Natl Acad Sci U S A* 1997;94:12094.
119. Shisler J, Duerksen-Hughes P, Hermiston TM, et al. Induction of susceptibility to tumor necrosis factor by E1A is dependent on binding to either p300 or p105-Rb and induction of DNA synthesis. *J Virol* 1996;70:68.
120. Querido E, Teodoro JG, Branton PE. Accumulation of p53 induced by the adenovirus E1A protein requires regions involved in the stimulation of DNA synthesis. *J Virol* 1997;71:3526.
121. Johnson DG, Schneider-Broussard R. Role of E2F in cell cycle control and cancer. *Front Biosci* 1998;3:d447.
122. Weinberg RA. The retinoblastoma protein and cell cycle control. *Cell* 1995;81:323.
123. Nevins JR. E2F: a link between the Rb tumor suppressor protein and viral oncoproteins. *Science* 1992;258:424.
124. La Thangue NB. DRTF1/E2F: an expanding family of heterodimeric transcription factors implicated in cell-cycle control. *Trends Biochem Sci* 1994;19:108.
125. Weintraub SJ, Prater CA, Dean DC. Retinoblastoma protein switches the E2F site from positive to negative element. *Nature* 1992;358:259.
126. Lam EW, Watson RJ. An E2F-binding site mediates cell-cycle regulated repression of mouse B-myb transcription. *EMBO J* 1993;12:2705.
127. Dynlacht BD, Flores O, Lees JA, et al. Differential regulation of E2F transactivation by cyclin/cdk2 complexes. *Genes Dev* 1994;8:1772.
128. Qin XQ, Livingston DM, Kaelin WG Jr, et al. Deregulated transcription factor E2F-1 expression leads to S-phase entry and p53-mediated apoptosis. *Proc Natl Acad Sci U S A* 1994;91:10918.
129. Adams PD, Kaelin WG Jr. The cellular effects of E2F overexpression. *Curr Top Microbiol Immunol* 1996;208:79.
130. Shan B, Lee WH. Deregulated expression of E2F-1 induces S-phase entry and leads to apoptosis. *Mol Cell Biol* 1994;14:8166.
131. Jacks T, Fazeli A, Schmitt EM, et al. Effects of an Rb mutation in the mouse. *Nature* 1992;359:295.
132. Clarke AR, Maandag ER, van Roon M, et al. Requirement for a functional Rb-1 gene in murine development. *Nature* 1992;359:328.
133. Yamasaki L, Jacks T, Bronson R, et al. Tumor induction and tissue atrophy in mice lacking E2F-1. *Cell* 1996;85:537.
134. Field SJ, Tsai FY, Kuo F, et al. E2F-1 functions in mice to promote apoptosis and suppress proliferation. *Cell* 1996;85:549.
135. Nip J, Strom DK, Fee BE, et al. E2F-1 cooperates with topoisomerase II inhibition and DNA damage to selectively augment p53-independent apoptosis. *Mol Cell Biol* 1997;17:1049.
136. Lowe SW, Ruley HE, Jacks T, et al. p53-dependent apoptosis modulates the cytotoxicity of anticancer agents. *Cell* 1993;74:957.
137. Klefstrom J, Vastrik I, Saksela E, et al. c-Myc induces cellular susceptibility to the cytotoxic action of TNF-alpha. *EMBO J* 1994;13:5442.
138. Hueber AO, Zornig M, Lyon D, et al. Requirement for the CD95 receptor-ligand pathway in c-Myc-induced apoptosis. *Science* 1997;278:1305.
139. Harrington EA, Fanidi A, Evan GI. Oncogenes and cell death. *Curr Opin Genet Dev* 1994;4:120.
140. Hollstein M, Sidransky D, Vogelstein B, et al. p53 mutations in human cancers. *Science* 1991;253:49.
141. Donehower LA, Harvey M, Slagle BL, et al. Mice deficient for p53 are developmentally normal but susceptible to spontaneous tumours. *Nature* 1992;356:215.
142. Malkin D, Li FP, Strong LC, et al. Germ line p53 mutations in a familial syndrome of breast cancer, sarcomas, and other neoplasms. *Science* 1990;250:1233.
143. Cho Y, Gorina S, Jeffrey PD, et al. Crystal structure of a p53 tumor suppressor-DNA complex: understanding tumorigenic mutations. *Science* 1994;265:346.
144. Fridman JS, Lowe SW. Control of apoptosis by p53. *Oncogene* 2003;22:9030.
145. Tartaglia LA, Goeddel DV. Two TNF receptors. *Immunol Today* 1992;13:151.
146. Ashkenazi A, Pai RC, Fong S, et al. Safety and antitumor activity of recombinant soluble Apo2 ligand. *J Clin Invest* 1999;104:155.
147. Walczak H, Miller RE, Ariail K, et al. Tumoricidal activity of tumor necrosis factor-related apoptosis-inducing ligand in vivo. *Nat Med* 1999;5:157.
148. Smyth MJ, Takeda K, Hayakawa Y, et al. Nature's TRAIL—on a path to cancer immunotherapy. *Immunity* 2003;18:1.
149. Cotter FE. Antisense therapy of hematologic malignancies. *Semin Hematol* 1999;36:9.
150. Webb A, Cunningham D, Cotter F, et al. BCL-2 antisense therapy in patients with non-Hodgkin lymphoma. *Lancet* 1997;349:1137.

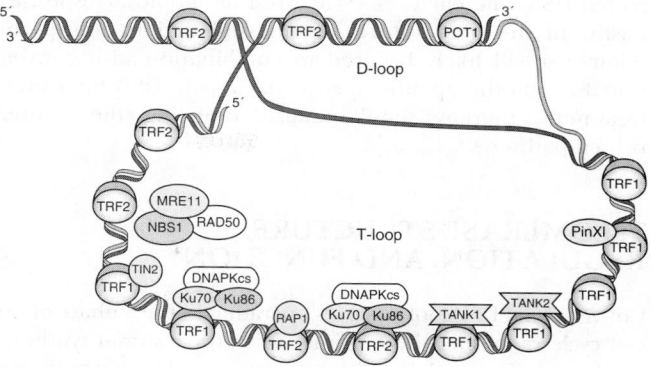

SECTION 4

KWOK-KIN WONG
RONALD A. DEPINHO

Telomerase

Our knowledge of the basic biology of telomeres is now beginning to yield fundamental insights into the pathophysiology of complex diseases, as studies in humans and model organisms have demonstrated that telomere maintenance and the cellular response to telomere dysfunction play crucial roles in processes of genomic instability, organ homeostasis, chronic diseases, aging, and tumorigenesis. With respect to the latter, the study of telomeres has begun to provide mechanistic insights into how advancing age fuels the development of epithelial cancers as well as how chronic inflammation and degeneration may engender increased cancer risk in affected organs. These advances in the basic understanding of telomere maintenance are now being translated into clinically relevant applications that may have an impact on the diagnosis and management of a broad spectrum of cancers.

TELOMERES

Telomeres are specialized nucleoprotein complexes at the ends of linear chromosomes consisting of long arrays of double-stranded TTAGGG repeats, a G-rich 3' single-strand overhang, and associated telomeric repeat binding proteins.[1,2] The work of Muller and McClintock in the 1930s led to the concept that telomeres function to "cap" chromosomal termini and prevent end-to-end recombination, thereby maintaining chromosomal integrity. Subsequent work has substantiated this model across the animal and plant kingdom, underscoring the critical roles served by the telomere complex.

Telomere structure and function have been studied extensively in mammals. Although the overall structural features of telomeres are preserved among different mammalian organisms, lengths can vary considerably from species to species: for example, 5 to 15 kilobases (kb) for humans and 20 to 80 kb for the laboratory mouse. On the structural level, electron microscopy and other studies show that telomeres form complex secondary and tertiary structures via DNA-DNA interactions between the telomeric repeats, DNA-protein interactions between the telomeric DNA and the telomeric repeat binding proteins, and protein–protein interactions between the telomeric repeat binding proteins themselves and other associated proteins (Fig. 3.4-1). The formation of this well-documented higher-order DNA-protein complex has provided a working model of how the telomere functions as a capping structure, preventing the ends of linear chromosomal DNA from being recognized and repaired as a double-strand DNA break (DSB), thereby avoiding the formation of chromosomal end-to-end fusions.

Paradoxically, many DSB repair proteins, involved in nonhomologous end joining and homologous recombination processes, have been found to be physically associated with the telomeres.[3,4] These findings have fueled speculation that DSB repair proteins are somehow reprogrammed to assume

FIGURE 3.4-1. Human telomere structure. Human telomeres form telomere loop (T loop) and displacement loop (D loop) secondary structures. Long stretches of telomeric repeats create a loopback structure (T loop), completed by the invasion of the single GT-rich 3' overhang into the double-stranded DNA molecule (D loop), thus protecting the chromosome terminus. In human cells, double-stranded telomeric repeats are bound directly by two proteins, TRF1 (TTAGG repeat binding factor 1) and TRF2. Cell culture studies have suggested that TRF1's main function is to regulate telomere length, whereas TRF2 functions to protect telomeres from activating nonhomologous end joining (NHEJ) and other DNA repair or DNA damage response pathways. Biochemical studies also suggest that the formation of the T loop is dependent on TRF2. Another protein, Pot1 (protection of telomere 1), has been shown to bind to the single-stranded human telomeric 3' overhang. Pot1 has been proposed to interact with TRF1 complexes to regulate telomere length. Thus, there is significant interplay between telomeric binding proteins and the formation of the secondary/tertiary structures that protect the ends of chromosomes. Several other proteins have been shown to localize to the telomeres via protein–protein interactions with TRF1 and TRF2. Three TRF1-interacting proteins have been identified: PinX1, tankyrase1/2, and TRF1-interacting nuclear protein 2 (TIN2). TRF2 also interacts with the human Rap1 protein (hRap), the DNA-damage response Mre11 complex composed of Mre11, Rad50, and the Nbs1 protein. Chromatin precipitation experiments have shown that Ku70, Ku86, and DNA-PKcs proteins, involved in NHEJ repair of double-stranded DNA break, are also localized to the telomeres.

a protective role at the telomere, for example, by sequestering the telomere end from the DNA damage surveillance/repair machinery. Experimental support for this hypothesis has emerged from the mouse, in which germline inactivation of various repair proteins (e.g., Ku and DNA-PK) results in reduced telomere length or loss of capping function, or both, leading to increased end-to-end fusions.[5] Correspondingly, in cultured human cells, experimental disruption of telomere-binding proteins results in the unraveling of higher-order nucleoprotein structure and telomere localization of DNA DSB surveillance/repair proteins (e.g., 53BP1, gamma-H2AX, Rad17, ATM, and Mre11), establishing that dysfunctional telomeres can indeed serve as substrates for the classic DNA repair machinery.[6] A further understanding of the molecular mechanisms governing the repression versus activation of the DNA DSB surveillance/repair apparatus at the telomere could lead to the development of novel cancer therapeutic options. For example, the design of agents that can uncap telomeres while preserving the DNA damage checkpoint response yet neutralize the actual DNA damage repair process would be ideal, as they would produce unrepaired DSBs and elicit cell-cycle arrest or apoptosis responses. Lastly, in the near future, agents designed to uncap the telomeres will likely be used in combination with conventional chemotherapeutic agents that create DSB for cancer treatment, thereby simultaneously targeting these intertwined pathways.

TELOMERASE STRUCTURE, REGULATION, AND FUNCTION

Conventional DNA polymerases operating in the S phase of the cell cycle require an RNA primer for reverse strand synthesis, resulting in incomplete DNA replication of telomeres during each cell division. The solution to this "end-replication problem" is the telomere-synthesizing telomerase enzyme, a specialized ribonucleoprotein complex with reverse transcriptase activity. The functional telomerase holoenzyme is a large multisubunit complex that includes an essential telomerase RNA (hTERC) component serving as a template for the addition of telomere repeats and a telomerase reverse transcriptase (hTERT) catalytic subunit.[7] In normal human cells, telomerase levels are insufficient to maintain telomere length, resulting in progressive attrition with each cell division. This forms the basis for the theory that the metered loss of telomeres can serve as a cellular mitotic clock that ultimately limits the number of cell divisions and cellular life span.

Many normal somatic human cells and differentiated tissues express readily detectable levels of the hTERC component. In contrast, hTERT expression and activity are more restricted due to stringent regulation on the levels of transcriptional initiation, alternative RNA processing, posttranslational modification, and subcellular localization. With the identification of an increasing number of TERT-associated proteins, it is likely that additional regulatory mechanisms will surface, such as those governing the accessibility of the telomerase holoenzyme onto the telomere end.[8] Here again, a more complete elucidation of these regulatory mechanisms may provide additional therapeutic strategies that can preferentially target telomerase activity in cancer cells. Indeed, the development of such selective strategies may become paramount because studies have revealed low telomerase levels in cycling somatic human cells that were previously thought to have no telomerase activity.[9] Eradication of residual telomerase function in these primary cells alters the maintenance of the 3' single-strand telomeric overhang without changing the rate of overall telomere shortening, resulting in diminished proliferation rates and overall reduction in proliferative capacity. These studies support an additional protective function of telomerase at the telomeres[10] and raise concerns that generalized antitelomerase therapy could lead to the immediate uncapping of telomeres in normal cells, thus limiting the use of antitelomerase therapy in cancer patients.

CRISIS, TELOMERASE REACTIVATION, AND ALTERNATIVE LENGTHENING OF TELOMERES

In human cell culture, the first cell division barrier triggered by critically shortened telomeres manifests as a cellular senescence response, termed the *Hayflick limit* (or mortality stage 1, M1). Because the loss of RB or p53 pathway function, or both, in primary human cells permits additional cell divisions beyond the Hayflick limit, these pathways appear to be involved in the activation of this senescence program brought about by the "shortened telomere" signal. Under circumstances of extended cell divisions, progressive telomere erosion ultimately leads to loss of capping function, resulting in increasing chromosomal instability. This leads to progressive loss of cell viability and proliferative capacity across the cell population, ultimately resulting in "cellular crisis" (or mortality stage 2, M2). The cellular phenotypes of massive cell death and growth arrest are a likely by-product of rampant chromosomal instability and associated loss of essential genetic material. Emergence from crisis is a rare event in human cell culture and requires restoration of telomere function to a level compatible with cell viability, achieved either by up-regulation of telomerase activity or activation of the alternative lengthening of telomeres (ALT) mechanism.[11] Finally, the extent to which normal tissues experience Hayflick and crisis transitions is a subject of ongoing study. Although clear evidence of the presence of telomere-activated Hayflick limit is still lacking, support is mounting for telomere-based crisis, particularly during early stages of neoplastic development.

Transcriptional up-regulation of the TERT gene seems to be a key rate-limiting step in telomerase reactivation, whereas the telomerase-independent ALT pathway appears to be executed via a homologous recombination pathway. The analysis of pathways regulating TERT gene transcription has forged links to well-known oncoproteins and tumor suppressors including Myc, Mad, and Menin, among others, demonstrating the capacity of these proteins to engage the TERT gene promoter directly.[12–14] The regulation of ALT remains a mystery. It appears to be most often activated in the setting of p53 deficiency and in tumors of mesenchymal origin.[15] Studies in yeast have also shown that ALT is enhanced in mismatch repair-deficient cells, owing to increased homologous recombination between chromosomes.[16] The rare use of ALT by epithelial-derived tumors, coupled with functional comparisons of telomerase- versus ALT-mediated telomere maintenance, has shown that ALT may not be as biologically robust in advancing malignancy, a finding that diminishes the theoretic concern that ALT may provide a robust resistance mechanism to antitelomerase therapy in advanced malignancy. The idea that ALT may be a less effective telomere maintenance mechanism derives additional support from studies in human cell culture and the mouse revealing that telomerase per se is needed for full malignant transformation, including metastatic potential. The fundamental mechanistic differences between ALT and telomerase reactivation in telomere maintenance may provide an explanation for the report of more favorable clinical outcomes for ALT-positive compared to telomerase-positive glioblastomas,[17] although analysis of 71 human osteosarcoma cases failed to show a more favorable clinical outcome for the ALT-positive subset.[18] However, it should be noted that in the latter, the absence of any telomere maintenance mechanism was more associated with improved survival than stage or response to chemotherapy, further emphasizing the general importance of telomere maintenance in cancer.

TELOMERE MAINTENANCE AND CANCER

Robust telomerase activity is observed in greater than 80% of all human cancers,[19] a profile consistent with its role in promoting malignant progression. However, another side to the telomerase-cancer connection has emerged from mouse models and correlative data in staged human tumors. These data have indicated that a lack of telomerase and associated telomere attrition during the early stages of neoplastic growth may provide a mutator mechanism that enables would-be cancer cells to achieve a threshold of cancer-promoting changes required to traverse the benign to malignant transition. Indeed, telomeres of human cancer cells are often significantly shorter than their normal tissue counterparts, suggesting that telomere attrition has occurred at some time during the life history of these cancers, presumably during early phases when telomerase activity is low. The subsequent reactivation of telomerase appears to restore telomere function, albeit at a shorter set length. Thus, although reactivation of telomerase is critical to the emergence of immortal human cells, a preceding and transient period of telomere shortening and dysfunction appears to contribute to carcinogenesis by leading to the formation of chromosomal rearrangements through breakage-fusion-bridge (BFB) cycles. Serial BFB in turn begets rapid and wholesale genetic changes in the population, with rare cells incurring a threshold number of relevant procarcinogenic changes needed to initiate the transformation process. Although, at first glance, the cancer-promoting effects of telomere-based

crisis seem contradictory to the hackneyed role of telomerase activation in cancer progression, this mechanism is less paradoxic if one considers that many early-stage cancers deactivate pathways essential for telomere checkpoint responses, thus increasing the survival and proliferation of cells with increasing genomic instability[20,21] (Fig. 3.4-2). This hypothesis of "episodic instability"–derived support from genetic studies in the mouse shows that telomere-based crisis coupled with loss of the p53-dependent DNA damage response can act cooperatively to effect malignant transformation. In humans, the accumulation of oncogenic lesions during normal aging or accelerated accumulation of DNA damage (e.g., environmental carcinogen exposure or oxidative damage) may deactivate the telomere checkpoint response, accelerate telomere attrition, and drive the affected premalignant cells into crisis. It is the rare transformed cell that may emerge from this process with reactivated telomerase. Thus, telomeric shortening can be viewed as a barrier to cancer development in the presence of intact checkpoint response and as a facilitator for numerous genetic changes necessary for the emergence of nascent cancer cells in the absence of the checkpoint response pathways.

AGING AND CANCER

The study of telomeres has also provided some insights into the link between advancing age and increased cancer risk. In humans, there is a dramatic escalation in cancer risk between the ages of 40 and 80, resulting primarily from a marked increase in epithelial malignancies such as carcinomas of the breast, lung, colon, and prostate. A conventional view is that the cancer-prone phenotype of older humans reflects the combined effects of cumulative mutational load, decreased DNA repair capabilities, increased epigenetic gene silencing, and altered hormonal and stromal milieus. Although these factors are almost certain to contribute to increasing cancer incidence in aged humans, it is less evident why such processes would spur the preferential development of epithelial cancers. Moreover, these mechanisms do not readily explain one of the cardinal features of adult epithelial carcinomas—namely, a radically altered genome typified by marked aneuploidy and complex nonreciprocal chromosomal translocations.

The study of telomere dynamics in normal and neoplastic cells of the mouse has provided a potential explanation for the observed tumor spectrum and associated cytogenetic profiles in aged humans. In *Terc p53* compound mutant mice, the presence of telomere dysfunction results in a dramatic shift in the tumor spectrum toward epithelial cancers, including those of the lung, colon, and skin. Moreover, in contrast to the somewhat normal cytogenetic profiles of cancers arising in mice with intact telomeres, the cancers generated in the *Terc p53* compound mutant mice had cytogenetic profiles with a striking resemblance to human epithelial cancer genomes.[22]

In attempting to assign relevance of these murine studies to humans, it is worth considering that the typical adult cancer, an epithelial carcinoma, derives from a compartment that has undergone continued renewal throughout the

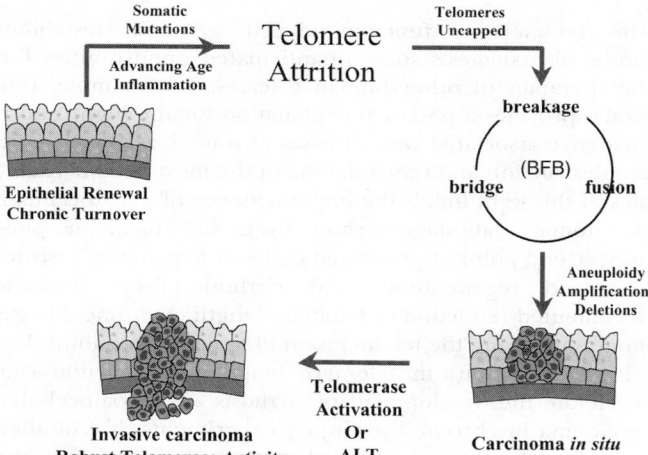

FIGURE 3.4-2. Dysfunctional telomere-induced genomic instability model of epithelial carcinogenesis. Continuous epithelial turnover during aging coupled with somatic mutations inactivating checkpoint responses is thought to lead to critical telomere erosion, resulting in telomere uncapping and the initiation of breakage-fusion-bridge (BFB) cycles. The double-strand breaks created by the BFB cycles are nidi for amplifications and deletions for the resulting daughter cells. The broken chromosome may become fused to another chromosome, generating a second dicentric chromosome and perpetuating the BFB cycle. This facilitation of the accumulation of genetic changes (via aneuploidy, nonreciprocal translocations, amplifications, and deletions) by the BFB cycles coupled with the reactivation of telomerase enables cells to emerge from crisis and proceed to malignancy. ALT, alternative lengthening of telomeres. (See Color Fig. 3.4-2 in the CD-ROM.)

human life span. Against this backdrop of physiologic cell turnover, combined with the occasional proproliferative oncogenic mutation, telomere lengths would shorten in self-renewing progenitor cells of these epithelial tissues. If somatic mutations also neutralize RB/INK4a/p53-dependent senescence checkpoints, continued growth beyond the Hayflick limit further drives telomere erosion and loss of the capping function, culminating in cellular crisis with attendant genomic instability. In this manner, telomere-based crisis provides the means to generate many additional mutations required to reach the early stages of malignant transformation. The subsequent reactivation of telomerase in transformed clones would serve to stabilize the genome to a level compatible with cell viability, allowing these initiated neoplasms to mature further.[23] It is unclear whether additional somatic mutations, beyond telomerase activation, would be needed to produce a fully malignant phenotype that includes invasive and metastatic potential. Thus, a transient period of explosive chromosomal instability before telomerase reactivation appears to be required for the stochastic acquisition of the relatively high number of mutations thought to be required for adult epithelial carcinogenesis.

The episodic instability model of epithelial carcinogenesis fits well with current knowledge regarding the timing of telomerase activation and evolving genomic changes during various stages of human carcinoma development, particularly those of the breast, esophagus, and colon. Comparative genome hybridization has demonstrated that dysplastic human breast, esophageal, and colon lesions sustain widespread gains and losses of regions of chromosomes early in their development, often well before these tissues exhibit carcinoma *in situ* or invasive growth.[24–26] The ploidy changes detected by comparative genome hybridization appear to correlate tightly with the presence of complex chromosomal rearrangements, and these markers of genomic instability are evident in the stages of advanced dysplasia of these tissues (e.g., ductal carcinoma *in situ*, Barrett's esophagus, etc.). As these cancers progress through invasive and metastatic stages, genomic instability continues, apparently at a moderate rate, but further mutations would be predicted to derive from nontelomere-based mechanisms. Correspondingly, the measurement of telomerase activity in adenomatous polyps and colorectal cancers has established that telomerase activity is low or undetectable in small- and intermediate-sized polyps, reflecting less intact telomere function. In contrast, telomerase increases markedly in large adenomas and colorectal carcinomas, reflecting stabilization of telomere function.[27] Therefore, it appears that widespread and severe chromosomal instability is present early on during human tumorigenesis at a time when telomerase activity is low.

Additional support for this episodic instability model derives from the documentation of anaphase bridging (a reasonable correlate of telomere-based crisis) in evolving human colorectal cancers and in genomically unstable pancreatic cancers.[28,29] This suggests that the DSB-induced conditions (including but not limited to telomere dysfunction), coupled with mutations that allow survival in the face of a DSB, could provide amplification/deletion mechanisms across the genome. Biologic forces would in turn lead to the selection of clones with the amplifications and deletions that

target cancer-relevant loci. Studies in the telomerase mutant mouse have begun to provide mechanistic insight into how BFB leads to cancer-relevant changes. In particular, telomerase p53 compound mutant mice with telomere dysfunction have increased end-to-end fusions, and the ensuing BFB process is associated with chromosomal regional gains and losses that appear linked to nonreciprocal translocations.[30,31]

In future human studies, it will be important to document telomere attrition in renewing epithelial stem cells and to perform a simultaneous comparison of telomere status, telomerase activity, and chromosomal instability in the same tumor samples, particularly during the earliest stages of human epithelial cell transformation. Defining the temporal point at which telomerase is reactivated in the genesis and progression of the different cancers may also lead to the development of biomarkers for diagnosis, prognosis, and outcomes prediction. Such studies are needed to more firmly establish a causal link between telomere dysfunction and early chromosomal instability in human neoplasms.

The importance of telomere dysfunction in human epithelial carcinogenesis is also gaining experimental support from research of other human diseases. The discovery that germline mutations of the telomerase complex cause dyskeratosis congenita, a progeroid syndrome characterized by increased susceptibility to a variety of malignancies, lends additional support to the hypothesis that telomere dynamics are intricately linked to aging and cancer.[32]

TELOMERE DYNAMICS, INFLAMMATORY DISEASES, AND CANCER

The telomere dysfunction-induced genomic instability model also suggests some unanticipated opportunities for the therapies of other human diseases. For example, this model provides a potential explanation for the high cancer incidence associated with diseases characterized by chronic cell destruction and renewal. One of the most notable examples of this tight link is the high incidence of hepatocellular carcinoma in late-stage cirrhotic livers. Cirrhosis is the phenotypic end point of prolonged cycles of hepatocyte destruction and regeneration, and cirrhotic livers show a documented reduction in telomere length over time. Mouse models involving the telomerase null mouse have shown that critical reductions in telomere length and function can accelerate the development of cirrhosis and hepatocellular carcinoma in chronic liver injury experiments.[33,34] Another example of a telomere-based pathogenetic relationship between chronic tissue turnover, telomere-based crisis, and increased cancer risk is ulcerative colitis, a condition characterized by rapid cell turnover and oxidative injury to the intestines, and a high incidence of intestinal dysplasia or cancer.[28] In addition to the progressive telomere attrition resulting from the cell turnover, accelerated telomere attrition might occur via increased oxidative stress and from the altered inflammatory microenvironment milieu. Together, such observations suggest the intriguing possibility that early somatic reconstitution of telomerase could attenuate telomere attrition and paradoxically reduce the occurrence of cancers in these high-turnover disease states, a theory that requires additional preclinical studies. In addition, serial

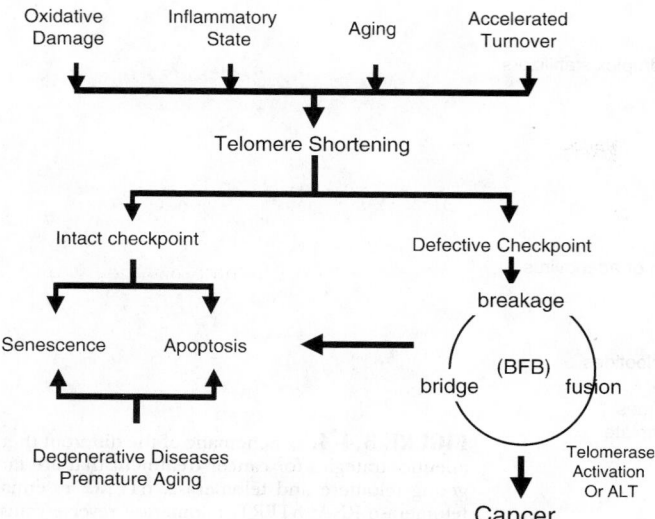

FIGURE 3.4-3. Schematic of the roles of telomere maintenance in cancer, chronic diseases, and aging. ALT, alternative lengthening of telomeres; BFB, breakage-fusion-bridge.

analyses of telomere length from these tissues may provide prognostic information regarding the rising risk of cancer development. Thus, progress in our understanding of telomere biology has mechanistically connected diverse fields in medicine involving chronic inflammatory diseases, degenerative diseases, geriatrics, and oncology (Fig. 3.4-3).

TELOMERE STATUS AS A BIOMARKER FOR CANCER

Given the important roles of telomerase and telomere maintenance in the development of various cancers, intense efforts have been made to develop assays based on telomerase activity or telomere length to ascertain malignant progression, to detect malignant cells, and to predict clinical outcome. Using the polymerase chain reaction–based telomerase assay, telomeric repeat amplification protocol, telomerase activity is detected in approximately 80% to 90% of the most common cancers, such as breast, prostate, lung, liver, pancreatic, and colon.[35] Therefore, it is a near universal marker of human cancer, with low or absent expression in normal somatic cells. Accordingly, the telomeric repeat amplification protocol assay for hTERT expression is being used for the diagnosis of various cancers from cells obtained from biopsy specimens or from cytologic specimens obtained from secretion samples, washing or brushing samples, and fine-needle aspirates. In a group of cancers, such as non–small cell lung cancer, gastric cancers, and neuroblastoma, in which telomerase activity is up-regulated during cancer progression, telomerase expression is not only useful to evaluate malignant grade of the tumors but also correlates with the prognosis of the patients.[36] However, these advances must be tempered with the fact that some normal differentiated cell types as well as stem cells in various organ compartments also express telomerase. Thus, the specificity of these tests must be evaluated

closely before they are widely applied in the clinical diagnostic field.

Efforts have also been directed toward assessing whether telomere length itself in the tissue of interest could serve as a biomarker for the risk of developing cancer and other diseases or serve as a prognostic marker in the setting of established disease, or both. In addition, several studies have begun to explore the use of telomere length determination in accessible peripheral blood lymphocytes (PBL) rather than the diseased tissue per se. Such studies in nonneoplastic diseases have suggested that PBL telomere lengths can provide predictive information on the risk of developing atherosclerosis, premature myocardial infarctions, coronary artery disease, Alzheimer's disease status, and overall mortality. It has also been shown that the presence of short telomeres in PBL is associated with increased risk for the development of carcinomas of the head and neck, kidney, bladder, and lung.[37] Further substantiation of the use of PBL telomere length determination is necessary before it can serve as a reliable and noninvasive surrogate marker that predicts the malignant propensity of epithelial lineages.

In the years ahead, basic telomere science discoveries will continue to yield mechanistic insights into cancer pathogenesis that can then translate into new tools for the screening and diagnosis of cancer. Parallel advances in technology may make possible the determination of telomere length *in vivo* at the level of a single cell, improving its sensitivity and specificity for diagnosis. Such advances in telomere-based biomarkers may greatly enhance general screening for cancer. For example, periodic screening for the rate of telomere attrition in specific organs may eventually be used to assign risk of cancer development in those organs. This approach would be particularly appealing for the assessment of cancer risk for patients with chronic hepatitis or ulcerative colitis, as an accelerated rate of telomere attrition has been documented for these conditions. It seems likely that serial telomere length measurements in such premalignant conditions will be useful as a biomarker to stratify more accurately where these patients lie on the risk curve.

TELOMERASE AND TELOMERE MAINTENANCE AS THERAPEUTIC TARGETS

A significant body of evidence supports the view that telomerase-mediated telomere maintenance represents an ideal and near universal therapeutic target for cancer. Indeed, cell culture–based studies of human cancer cells have established that inhibition of telomerase culminates in cell death after extended cell divisions. The past few years have witnessed intense efforts to design therapeutic strategies capable of targeting telomere structure and the telomerase holoenzyme[38,39] (Fig. 3.4-4).

Many natural compounds and small molecules that have inhibitory activity against the reverse transcriptase enzymatic function of telomerase have been identified. However, all these compounds have a significant lag time (measured in months) between the inhibition of telomerase and the time telomeres in the cancer cell are shortened sufficiently to produce an effect on tumor growth. Such a lag time is not necessarily a hurdle to telomerase therapy, as the median survival of many

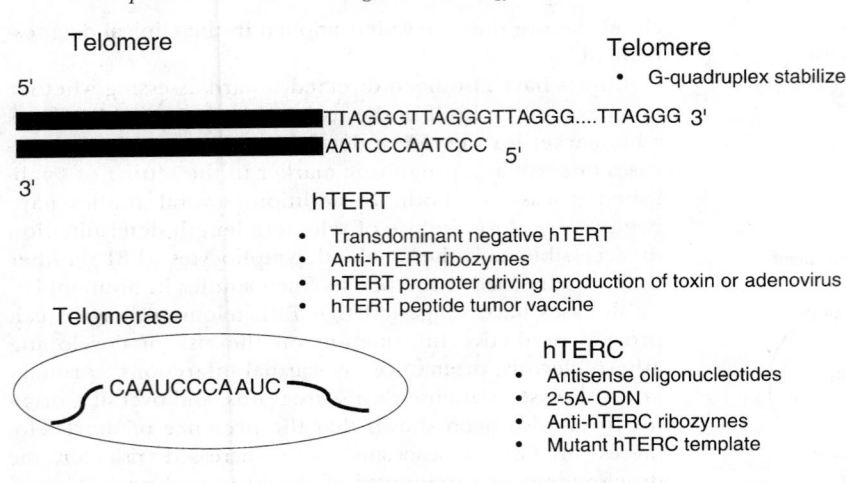

FIGURE 3.4-4. Schematic of the different therapeutic strategies for cancer treatment that are targeting telomere and telomerase. hTERC, essential telomerase RNA; hTERT, telomerase reverse transcriptase.

metastatic epithelial cancers such as breast and colon now significantly exceeds 1 year. However, this lag time could pose significant economic and logistic challenges for the clinical development of these compounds.

Several different classes of agents have been developed to target the two components of the core telomerase enzyme, namely the RNA (hTERC) or the catalytic subunit (hTERT). Antisense oligonucleotides or hammerhead ribozymes that target hTERC RNA have had limited success in preclinical studies because of pharmacokinetic and long lag time issues. Second-generation antisense oligonucleotides against hTERC, chemically modified (bonded to 5'-phosphorylated 2'-5'–linked oligoadenylate) to activate the cellular RNase L system to cleave single-stranded RNA, have been shown to induce apoptosis in telomerase-positive cancer cells within 3 to 6 days after the treatment. This effect was not seen in cells that lack telomerase and occurred before telomere length shortening. One explanation for this rapid response independent of telomere shortening is that this treatment may cause degradation of the core telomerase enzyme, which, as described above, appears to have other cellular activities independent of its enzymatic activity (including capping of the telomeres). The safety profile in humans of this agent, particularly the impact on tissue stem cell reserves, will only become evident with completion of human phase I studies.

Similar approaches have been used to target the hTERT component of telomerase. One strategy uses a ribozyme against the hTERT RNA that, on application of cultured cancer cells, results in the immediate induction of apoptosis independent of initial telomere length in these cancer cells. Interestingly, several studies have also shown that expression of mutant hTERT in human cancer cells exerts a strong transdominant negative effect that rapidly causes increased apoptosis and decreased cell viability independent of telomere shortening. The presumed mechanism for this effect is altered telomere structure stemming from altered DNA-protein or DNA-DNA interactions that uncap the telomeres. Again, the effects of these approaches on normal human cells that possess telomerase activity await entry into clinical trials.

The physical structure of the telomere itself has provided another potential therapeutic target. The G-rich 3' overhang at the ends of telomeres can form a core stack of guanines arranged in an almost planar hydrogen-bonded tetrad, called a G-quadruplex structure. This structure may hinder telomerase from elongating the 3' overhang of the telomere. Chemical compounds such as telomestatin, TMPyP4, and specific oligonucleotides that can facilitate and stabilize the formation of the G-quadruplex structure have been shown to be effective telomerase inhibitors. One potential advantage of some members of this class of compounds, such as TMPyP4, is that they appear to suppress ALT-positive cells in addition to telomerase-positive cells. However, many studies have demonstrated that these compounds also have a significant lag time in achieving antiproliferation effects. The effects of these compounds on normal human cells and organs are also not known.

Other approaches to devise tumor-specific gene delivery have exploited the restricted expression pattern of hTERT in normal cells and its nearly universal expression in most advanced cancers. Studies using adenoviral vectors or plasmids to deliver toxic genes such as FADD, Bax, and caspases driven by the hTERT promoter have shown that expression of these toxic gene products is limited to telomerase-expressing cells. The clinical application of this delivery system is limited, as only a small subset of cancer cells can feasibly be infected with adenoviral vectors or transfected with plasmids using current delivery technologies. A more promising alternative strategy is the construction of adenoviral vectors under the control of the hTERT promoter that could infect normal and cancer cells, but the virus would only replicate in those cells that are expressing telomerase activity. The hTERT-driven adenovirus would replicate and eventually lyse the infected cells and release additional viral particles to continue the next round of infection of the neighboring cells. However, given the discoveries that most cycling human somatic cells express a low level of hTERT, it is not clear whether this strategy will have detrimental effects *in vivo*. Furthermore, this is one area in telomere biology in which clinical research is ahead of the basic science, as little is known about the regulation of hTERT in different tissues.

Lastly, another telomerase-related cancer treatment strategy is immunotherapy, targeting immune recognition and the destruction of cells that express telomerase. Immune responses, specifically cytotoxic T-cell responses, have been generated against peptide sequences of the hTERT protein, and it has been demonstrated that these cytotoxic T cells are capable of selectively lysing target cells that express TERT peptides presented on the cell surface in the context of major histocompatibility complex class I molecules. Preclinical studies suggest that telomerase is a poor autoantigen either due to the low level of hTERT protein or, alternatively, the inefficient processing of the hTERT peptide in these normal cells. Several phase I trials using peptides from telomerase as a vaccine are ongoing. Although there are no reports of severe toxicity including autoimmunity, the clinical efficacy of this approach is not yet known.

Overall, in contrast to the diagnostic areas, the cancer therapeutic applications are not firmly anchored on the basics of telomere biology. Many unresolved questions still exist regarding the exact targets and mechanisms of action for all these approaches. An important caveat is that analyses of the telomerase-deficient (*mTerc−/−*) mouse with ample telomere reserve showed that the cells from the various organ compartments are phenotypically normal and viable in the absence of telomerase activity. (It remains to be seen whether the deletion of the mTert catalytic protein subunit will yield a similarly benign phenotypic outcome.) The proposed alternative capping or other functions of telomerase that are independent of its enzymatic function have not been fully elucidated. (This would also suggest that there might be use in the disruption of the telomerase protein even in ALT cancer cells.) It is also not totally clear whether the induction of telomere dysfunction in the absence of intact p53 checkpoint response would cause reentry into a phase of rampant genomic instability from which more aggressive and resistant tumors would emerge. Last, inhibition of telomerase activity might cause the cancer cells to activate the ALT.

RATIONAL CLINICAL TRIAL DESIGNS OF TELOMERE- AND TELOMERASE-BASED THERAPEUTICS

The large body of knowledge accumulated in telomere biology should provide a foundation for the improved design and assessment of future clinical trials of telomere- and telomerase-based agents. The class of agents that inhibits telomerase activity is expected to exhibit a long lag time but may be effective in the setting of minimal residual disease after the administration of standard chemotherapeutic agents and surgery. In addition, clinical assays capable of assessing inhibition of telomerase activity in individual patients are needed.

Presently, the most promising classes of agents are those that uncap the telomeres and those that disrupt the formation of the telomerase holoenzyme, as these two strategies cause immediate apoptosis and decreased cell viability. The safety profile of these agents remains unclear, however, as they may be too nonspecific and toxic to be used safely in the clinical setting.

Experience with the telomerase mutant mouse model and human cell culture systems should serve as a guide for the design of human clinical trials. Evidence of germ cell defects, proliferation, and organ homeostasis defects, as well as an increased rate of spontaneous malignancy, in telomerase null mice with telomere dysfunction suggests that clinical trials should actively monitor patients for these sequelae. The issue of secondary malignancy in other organs should be monitored carefully, as critical telomere shortening in the absence of appropriate checkpoint responses may lead to crisis where wholesale genomic changes can occur, and transformed cells may emerge even in the absence of telomerase reactivation (via the ALT pathway). Furthermore, the tumors of candidates for clinical trials may need to be characterized to determine the status of p53 before enrollment into these clinical trials; mouse modeling studies with telomerase- and p53-deficient compound mutant mice suggest that the combination of p53 deficiency with telomere dysfunction generates greater genomic instability. When the p53 pathway is intact, critical telomere shortening should induce p53-dependent apoptosis. The final answers to these safety questions reside in the analyses of current and future clinical trials with humans.

Conversely, data from the telomerase null mice model have demonstrated that telomerase-deficient cells and animals with telomere dysfunction are more sensitive to ionizing radiation and DNA double-stranded break chemotherapeutic agents; thus, telomerase activity inhibitors should be paired with radiation or certain classes of chemotherapy that produce DSBs, as they might produce synergistic effects. Again, however, particular care is warranted here, as the combination of increased DNA damage with reduced capacity for normal repair may produce marked increases in the toxicity of chemoradiotherapy.[40]

Thus, based on the knowledge obtained from mouse modeling and human cell culture, the ideal initial clinical trial design can be structured as follows: (1) lymphoid malignancies, as this organ compartment has shown the greatest sensitivity to telomere dysfunction in telomerase-deficient mouse models; (2) tumors that retain a competent p53 response to DNA damage (e.g., p14/p19 ARF-deficient tumors) wherein a robust p53-dependent telomere checkpoint response is retained; and (3) tumors with uniform robust telomerase activity yet short telomeres. It remains to be seen whether such trials should couple the telomerase inhibitor with a DSB-inducing chemotherapeutic agent such as doxorubicin to achieve maximal synergistic therapeutic effect. Additionally, clinical assays with appropriate biomarkers for monitoring the effectiveness of the tested agents need to be developed to help guide and facilitate these clinical trials.

Recent years have witnessed significant progress in the telomere field that is now maturing into new opportunities for improved diagnostics and novel therapeutic applications in oncology. Discoveries in telomere biology have also provided new mechanistic insights into the pathogenesis of human cancer. However, many fundamental questions regarding telomere dynamics still need to be addressed. Further advances in this rapidly evolving arena will fuel new opportunities for clinical applications in cancer and other human diseases. An integration of laboratory and clinical approaches, combined with rational clinical trial design incorporating scientifically based biologic end points, will allow these new agents and applications to be tested quickly and efficiently.

REFERENCES

1. Greider CW. Telomere length regulation. *Annu Rev Biochem* 1996;65:337.
2. Rhodes D, Fairall L, Simonsson T, et al. Telomere architecture. *EMBO Rep* 2002;3:1139.
3. de Lange T. Protection of mammalian telomeres. *Oncogene* 2002;21:532.
4. Zhu XD, Kuster B, Mann M, et al. Cell-cycle-regulated association of RAD50/MRE11/NBS1 with TRF2 and human telomeres. *Nat Genet* 2000;25:347.
5. Goytisolo FA, Blasco MA. Many ways to telomere dysfunction: in vivo studies using mouse models. *Oncogene* 2002;21:584.
6. Takai H, Smogorzewska A, de Lange T. DNA damage foci at dysfunctional telomeres. *Curr Biol* 2003;13:1549.
7. Cong YS, Wright WE, Shay JW. Human telomerase and its regulation. *Microbiol Mol Biol Rev* 2002;66:407.
8. Pennock E, Buckley K, Lundblad V. Cdc13 delivers separate complexes to the telomere for end protection and replication. *Cell* 2001;104:387.
9. Masutomi K, Yu EY, Khurts S, et al. Telomerase maintains telomere structure in normal human cells. *Cell* 2003;114:241.
10. Blackburn EH. Telomere states and cell fates. *Nature* 2000;408:53.
11. Stewart SA, Weinberg RA. Telomerase and human tumorigenesis. *Semin Cancer Biol* 2000;10:399.
12. Lin SY, Elledge SJ. Multiple tumor suppressor pathways negatively regulate telomerase. *Cell* 2003;113:881.
13. Blasco MA. Telomerase beyond telomeres. *Nat Rev Cancer* 2002;2:627.
14. O'Hagan RC, Schreiber-Agus N, Chen K, et al. Gene-target recognition among members of the myc superfamily and implications for oncogenesis. *Nat Genet* 2000;24:113.
15. Henson JD, Neumann AA, Yeager TR, et al. Alternative lengthening of telomeres in mammalian cells. *Oncogene* 2002;21:598.
16. Rizki A, Lundblad V. Defects in mismatch repair promote telomerase-independent proliferation. *Nature* 2001;411:713.
17. Hakin-Smith V, Jellinek DA, Levy D, et al. Alternative lengthening of telomeres and survival in patients with glioblastoma multiforme. *Lancet* 2003;361:836.
18. Ulaner GA, Huang HY, Otero J, et al. Absence of a telomere maintenance mechanism as a favorable prognostic factor in patients with osteosarcoma. *Cancer Res* 2003;63:1759.
19. Shay JW, Bacchetti S. A survey of telomerase activity in human cancer. *Eur J Cancer* 1997;33:787.
20. Feldser DM, Hackett JA, Greider CW. Telomere dysfunction and the initiation of genome instability. *Nat Rev Cancer* 2003;3:623.
21. Maser RS, DePinho RA. Connecting chromosomes, crisis, and cancer. *Science* 2002;297:565.
22. Artandi SE, Chang S, Lee SL, et al. Telomere dysfunction promotes non-reciprocal translocations and epithelial cancers in mice. *Nature* 2000;406:641.
23. Campisi J, Kim SH, Lim CS, et al. Cellular senescence, cancer and aging: the telomere connection. *Exp Gerontol* 2001;36:1619.
24. Yen CC, Chen YJ, Chen JT, et al. Comparative genomic hybridization of esophageal squamous cell carcinoma: correlations between chromosomal aberrations and disease progression/prognosis. *Cancer* 2001;92:2769.
25. Buerger H, Otterbach F, Simon R, et al. Comparative genomic hybridization of ductal carcinoma in situ of the breast—evidence of multiple genetic pathways. *J Pathol* 1999;187:396.
26. Al-Mulla F, Keith WN, Pickford IR, et al. Comparative genomic hybridization analysis of primary colorectal carcinomas and their synchronous metastases. *Genes Chromosomes Cancer* 1999;24:306.
27. Tang R, Cheng A-J, Wang J-Y, et al. Close correlation between telomerase expression and adenomatous polyp progression in multistep colorectal carcinogenesis. *Cancer Res* 1998;58:4052.
28. O'Sullivan JN, Bronner MP, Brentnall TA, et al. Chromosomal instability in ulcerative colitis is related to telomere shortening. *Nat Genet* 2002;32:280.
29. Gisselsson D, Jonson T, Petersen A, et al. Telomere dysfunction triggers extensive DNA fragmentation and evolution of complex chromosome abnormalities in human malignant tumors. *Proc Natl Acad Sci U S A* 2001;98:12683.
30. Chin L, Artandi SE, Shen Q, et al. p53 deficiency rescues the adverse effects of telomere loss and cooperates with telomere dysfunction to accelerate carcinogenesis. *Cell* 1999;97:527.
31. O'Hagan RC, Chang S, Maser RS, et al. Telomere dysfunction provokes regional amplification and deletion in cancer genomes. *Cancer Cell* 2002;2:149.
32. Wong JM, Collins K. Telomere maintenance and disease. *Lancet* 2003;362:983.
33. Rudolph KL, Millard M, Bosenberg MW, et al. Telomere dysfunction and evolution of intestinal carcinoma in mice and humans. *Nat Genet* 2001;28:155.
34. Farazi PA, Glickman J, Jiang S, et al. Differential impact of telomere dysfunction on initiation and progression of hepatocellular carcinoma. *Cancer Res* 2003;63:5021.
35. Nicol Keith W, Jeffry Evans TR, Glasspool RM. Telomerase and cancer: time to move from a promising target to a clinical reality. *J Pathol* 2001;195:404.
36. Hiyama E, Hiyama K. Telomerase as tumor marker. *Cancer Lett* 2003;194:221.
37. Wong KK, DePinho RA. Walking the telomere plank into cancer. *J Natl Cancer Inst* 2003;95:1184.
38. Shay JW, Wright WE. Telomerase: a target for cancer therapeutics. *Cancer Cell* 2002;2:257.
39. Saretzki G. Telomerase inhibition as cancer therapy. *Cancer Lett* 2003;194:209.
40. McCaul JA, Gordon KE, Clark LJ, et al. Telomerase inhibition and the future management of head-and-neck cancer. *Lancet Oncol* 2002;3:280.

William G. Stetler-Stevenson

CHAPTER **4**

Invasion and Metastases

Metastasis formation is the spread of cancer cells from a primary tumor to vital organs and distant sites in the cancer patient's body. This process is the end result of a complex series of genetic alterations, epigenetic events, and host responses. The tendency of a primary tumor to form a metastasis is the hallmark of malignant cancer. Metastasis formation associated with malignant transformation has significant diagnostic, prognostic, and therapeutic implications. After a diagnosis of cancer, the primary tumor is resected and histologic examination of this tissue is performed for evidence of metastatic potential (local invasion). The patient also undergoes clinical staging for evidence of metastatic involvement of other organs. Major factors dictating the course of cancer treatment are the malignant potential of the primary tumor (i.e., presence of local invasion and regional lymph node involvement) and the presence of distant metastases. One of the major obstacles to effective cancer diagnosis is the detection of clinically occult metastatic disease. Once the primary tumor is resected, cancer therapy is directed at the elimination of metastases. The variation in size, age, dispersed anatomic location, and heterogeneous composition of metastases makes complete eradication of metastatic disease by currently available therapeutic strategies extremely difficult. Patients with metastases succumb to organ failure secondary to anatomic compromise of organ function by nonfunctional tumor tissue or to complications associated with systemic therapy directed against the metastatic disease.

The principal objectives of current research in cancer invasion and metastasis are improvement of diagnostic markers for detection of malignant potential and clinically silent (occult) metastasis formation, as well as the design of more effective therapies to treat metastatic disease. These goals require a better understanding of the molecular events, cellular processes, and host responses involved in metastasis formation. The focus of current research efforts is directed at understanding the origins of cancer metastasis, definition of malignant potential (i.e., delineating the metastatic propensity of a primary tumor from any given patient), and identification of genes specifically associated with metastasis formation as potential therapeutic targets.

TUMOR PROGRESSION AND GENETIC INSTABILITY

It is widely accepted that tumor formation, or tumorigenesis, requires several genetic alterations, either somatic or inherited, that confer a selective growth advantage to the neoplastic cell population.[1] This concept is supported by studies on the molecular changes in oncogenes and tumor suppressor genes that are associated with distinct pathologic lesions, for example, epithelial dysplasia, adenoma, or carcinoma *in situ*, before the development of invasive carcinoma.[2,3] During tumor development, initial random genetic alterations result in a tumor cell population with a proliferative advantage. These tumor cells become the progenitors of a clonal population that eventually dominates the tumor mass. Subsequently, a second random genetic event occurs that is again clonally selected on the basis of improved fitness. In this view, tumor progression is analogous to Darwinian selection, with repeated mutations and subsequent dominance of the daughter cell population via expression of a phenotypic advantage—that is, growth autonomy, resistance to apoptosis, and so forth.[1,4] As these random, advantageous mutations are selected, they become fixed in future generations of the tumor cell population, as it is the daughter cell that eventually overtakes the remaining nonmutant tumor cells. However, this clonal selection is an ongoing process, and the domi-

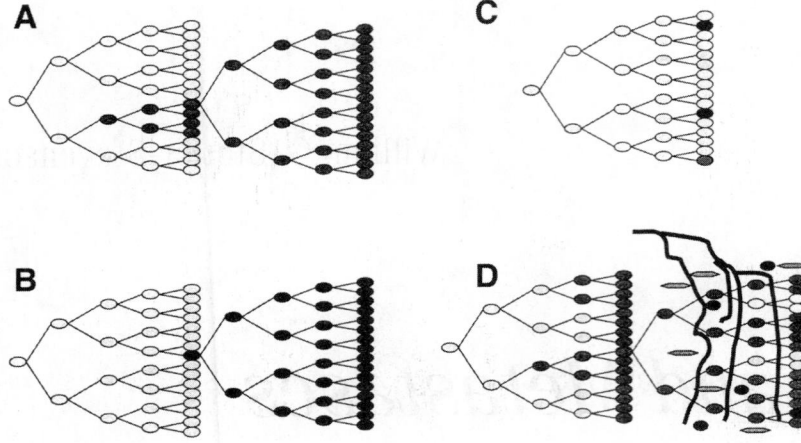

FIGURE 4-1. Current models of tumor progression and metastatic origins. **A:** Clonal progression model of tumorigenesis. **B:** Clonal dominance theory of tumor progression. **C:** Metastatic variant model of tumor progression. **D:** Current working hypothesis of tumor progression.

nant tumor cell population in the primary tumor changes through continuous accrual of new genetic events (Fig. 4-1).

Analysis of the age-dependent incidence of most types of cancer suggests that at least four to seven rate-limiting, stochastic events are requisite for tumor formation.[5] The mutation of specific genes is a highly inefficient process, and acquisition of the genetic changes required for tumorigenesis may require 20 to 40 years. This is in contrast to the large number of genetic alterations that have been documented in human tumors, many more than are likely to occur within a human life span. The limited series of mutations required for tumor formation compared with the relatively large number of genetic changes observed in many cancers suggests that most tumors acquire an inherent genetic instability, sometimes referred to as the *mutator phenotype*.[6] The acquisition of genetic instability combined with an enhanced proliferative capacity would provide a mechanism that accounts for the large number of accrued genetic changes seen in many tumors. It has been suggested that acquisition of this genetic instability, evidenced by subtle sequence changes, alterations in chromosome number, chromosomal translocations, or gene amplification, is the engine of tumor progression and of tumor heterogeneity.[6] Initial stochastic mutations conferring enhanced proliferative capacity are complemented by defects in DNA repair mechanisms (loss of p53 function), resulting in acceleration of the Darwinian selection process that leads to clonal expansion. This role for genetic instability also accounts for the observation that humans and animals with inherent genetic instability (e.g., those with xeroderma pigmentosa, adenomatous polyposis coli), secondary to defects in DNA repair or chromosomal segregation, or both, are prone to development of cancers. The relative contributions of genetic instability and somatic mutation mechanisms to the process of tumor progression and metastasis remain controversial.[7]

ORIGINS OF METASTATIC TUMOR CELLS

The central question with regard to metastasis formation, and with significant clinical implications for the diagnosis and treatment of cancer metastasis, is how metastases arise from the primary tumor. Two dominant hypotheses have been formulated regarding the evolution of cancer metastases. The following section briefly reviews the origins of these hypotheses.

Metastasis formation is the final step in tumor progression. This suggests that, like tumorigenesis, neoplastic cells with metastatic capacity arise through a process analogous to Darwinian natural selection aided by genetic instability. Initial genetic changes, mutations in specific oncogenes, and inactivation of tumor suppressor genes result in acquisition of a selective growth advantage that produces a dominant descendent population within the primary tumor mass. Subsequent genetic changes confer additional advantageous phenotypes that include self-sufficiency in growth signals (growth autonomy), insensitivity to antigrowth signals, evasion of apoptosis, sustained angiogenesis, limitless replicative potential, and the capacity for tissue invasion and metastasis.[8] These changes and subsequent genetic or epigenetic alterations would dominate the primary tumor cell population through clonal expansion (see Fig. 4-1). This clonal progression model is consistent with numerous studies demonstrating similar patterns of gene expression in the primary tumor and metastases derived from the same patient. This model of metastatic progression suggests that evolution of metastatic competence is a generic predisposition that can be expressed at any time during the process of tumor development and that this phenotype will predominate in the primary tumor through clonal expansion.

In contrast, a second model suggests that metastases arise from rare, highly metastatic variants within the primary tumor. In this model, metastatic competence does not confer a selective growth advantage within the primary so that these rare tumor cells with metastatic capacity remain a minor cell population in the primary tumor (see Fig. 4-1). This model is principally based on classic animal model experiments of Fidler et al.[9,10] showing that multiple variants of metastatic potential can be isolated from the primary tumor population by subcloning *in vitro* or by *in vivo* selection. This is an important concept in that it suggests that metastatic variants "preexist" in the primary tumor, that not all cells of the primary tumor population share the same propensity for metastasis formation, and that metastasis results from selection of an aggressive, rare subpopulation of tumor cells from the primary tumor population. Furthermore, this model of tumor progression suggests that the metastatic potential of the primary tumor would be determined by the size or behavior, or both, of this highly aggressive subpopulation. Therefore, detection of such rare variant cells within the primary tumor population would be of significant prognostic value. This would suggest that determination of the average metastatic potential of the entire primary tumor cell population, by assessment of molecular markers associated with metastatic potential, may not reflect the presence of these highly metastatic variants.

Are the clonal expansion and rare variant models for the origin of metastatic tumor cells mutually exclusive, or are they two conceptual frameworks in a continuous spectrum of mechanisms for metastasis formation? To study this experimentally, Kerbel[11] exploited the random integration of foreign DNA into the tumor cell genome to tag metastatic cells isolated from a primary tumor population. Tumor cell clones tagged with different integration sites were mixed with a single tagged metastatic clone and inoculated subcutaneously into syngeneic experimental animals. The clonal evolution of primary tumors and metastatic foci were then followed over time by restriction fragment length polymorphism analysis of the foreign DNA integration sites. The results of these experiments indicate that a single clone, initially present in the mixture in as low as 1% to 2% of the tumor cell inoculum, grows to dominate the primary tumor and that this clone is metastatically competent. This suggested that if a rare metastatic variant preexists within the tumor cell population, it can, over time, overgrow the primary tumor mass. This mechanism is referred to as the *clonal dominance theory of cancer progression.*[11]

The underlying implication of these studies is that metastatic competence and growth dominance in the primary tumor are somehow linked. If, instead of a single metastatic clone mixed with tagged primary tumor cells, the experiment was conducted by pooling a large number (10^4 or 10^5) of metastatically competent tumor cell clones, the results were similar, in that the tumor cell populations in primary and metastatic tumors were dominated by a few (less than 10) clones. These findings suggest that cells within the primary tumor that obtain metastatic potential also have a selective growth advantage. It must be noted, however, that the seemingly "genetically" convergent dominant clones, although homogeneous with respect to the tag used to identify them, are still heterogeneous in other characteristics due to the ongoing process of genetic instability. These other characteristics may be secondary, unrelated to growth or metastatic potential (referred to as *carrier mutations*), or primary in that they enhance the metastatic phenotype. Finally, the clonal dominance model of Kerbel suggests that the clonal progression and metastatic variant models for the evolution of metastatic tumor cells may contribute to the development of metastatic tumor cells and that these models are not mutually exclusive.

The consideration of these models of tumor progression and origin of metastatic tumor cells is increasingly important for the design of experiments to isolate and identify genes involved in tumor metastasis. With the advent of complementary DNA (cDNA) microarray technologies, researchers can simultaneously screen for the differential expression of thousands of genes in a single experiment. However, to obtain useful information from these experiments, we must understand the potential relationships between primary tumors and metastasis. For example, cDNA microarray experiments comparing the differential gene expression between a primary tumor and metastatic lesion from the same patient yield different information than an experiment that compares a series of nonmetastatic and metastatic tumors from different patients.

MICROARRAY ANALYSIS OF TUMOR PROGRESSION AND METASTASIS

The introduction of cDNA microarray technology affords investigators the opportunity to examine changes in expression of thousands of genes in a single experiment. Such experiments have been used to explore the process of tumor progression and identify genes that may be involved in metastasis formation. Patterns of gene expression have been analyzed for a variety of primary tumors and their metastases. These studies include microarray profiling of primary tumor cells and metastatic lesions in animal models of tumor progression, as well as analysis of human tumor samples. The results of these experiments clearly indicate that specific patterns of gene expression can be associated with specific tumor subsets and clinical outcomes. However, these experiments also present new insights into the origins of metastatic tumor cells and the relationship between primary tumors and their metastases.

cDNA microarray (transcriptome) analysis of primary breast tumors and comparison of the gene expression profiles of nonmetastatic and metastatic primary tumors result in identification of a gene expression signature that predicts the probability of metastases.[12] In these experiments the gene expression profiles across approximately 25,000 genes were conducted using primary breast cancer tissue from two groups of patients: those in whom distant metastasis developed within 5 years and those who remained disease free after a period of at least 5 years. All of these patients with sporadic breast cancer were lymph node negative and under age 55 at the time of diagnosis. The authors found that some 5000 genes were significantly regulated across this group of patient samples and that simple hierarchic cluster analysis revealed two distinct groups of patients. In one group, only 34% of patients had metastasis within 5 years, in comparison with the second group, in which 70% of patients had metastatic progression. From this study the authors identified a set of 70 genes to establish a prognosis profile that would predict clinical outcome in node-negative primary breast cancer. Application of this gene expression profile demonstrated that it was a more powerful predictor of disease outcome than standard prognostic systems based on clinical and histologic criteria.[13]

Researchers have also compared the gene expression profiles of adenocarcinomas of multiple tumor types to unmatched primary adenocarcinomas.[14] In this study, the investigators examined the expression profiles of metastatic nodules and compared these with primary adenocarcinomas of similar tissue origin. These authors found a gene expression signature that distinguished primary from metastatic adenocarcinomas and that was associated with metastasis and poor clinical outcome. Further refinement of the initial gene set identified 17 unique genes that recapitulated the distinction of primary tumors and metastasis across the entire set of tumor types. Application of this subset of 17 genes to specific tumor types, for example, breast cancer, lung cancer, prostate adenocarcinoma, and medulloblastomas (brain tumors), revealed the general utility of this subset in identifying primary tumors that were more likely to develop distant metastases, demonstrating the prognostic value of this approach.[14] This study also found a subset of primary tumors in which the gene expression signatures were identical to the metastatic tumors, an observation consistent with the clonal evolution model of cancer metastasis.

Primary breast carcinomas and metastases from the same patient may also show very similar gene expression profiles.[15]

Examination of premalignant, preinvasive, and malignant mammary lesions, obtained by laser capture microdissection, revealed extensive similarities in the gene expression patterns (transcriptome) between these distinct stages of breast cancer progression.[16] Collectively, these findings suggest that the molecular program of a primary tumor may generally be retained in its metastasis, which is again consistent with the clonal evolution model for the origin of metastatic tumor cells. However, these methods cannot detect rare, highly metastatic variants within the primary tumor population and so do not exclude the presence of these variants or their contribution to metastasis formation.

Transcriptome analysis (cDNA microarrays) has also been used to examine the changes in gene expression that are associated with *in vivo* selection of highly metastatic tumor cell variants.[17] These experiments used techniques for the isolation of highly metastatic variants, for example, *in vivo* selection, identical to those originally used by Fidler et al.[9,10] Poorly metastatic melanoma cell lines, either the murine B16F0 or human A375P, were injected intravenously into the tail vein of host mice. Pulmonary metastases were isolated and reinjected via tail vein either two (A375) or three (B16) times for selection of highly metastatic tumor cell lines. The gene expression profiles of pulmonary metastasis were compared with the parental A375P or B16F0 cell lines grown as subcutaneous tumors. The results define a pattern of gene expression that involved 15 genes, independent of tumor site, that correlate with progression to a metastatic phenotype, independent of the tumor microenvironment. However, many of the differentially expressed genes that were identified in this study encode extracellular matrix (ECM) proteins, suggesting that enhanced expression of specific ECM proteins may promote tumor cell survival or angiogenesis, or both.[17] The pattern of transcriptome alterations observed in this animal model of progression are distinct and more restricted than those observed in studies of human clinical material. Although this is due in part to the use of tumor cell lines as a starting point, it also suggests that many of the cells within the heterogeneous tumorigenic populations of the parental tumor cell lines (A375P or B15F0) are genetically primed for acquisition of metastatic ability. This was demonstrated by additional experiments in which introduction of a single gene (RhoC), identified in the original screen, back into the parental cell population was sufficient to confer a high level of metastatic capacity.

These findings are supported by a study on the formation of osteolytic bone metastases in breast cancer. Kang et al.[18] intravenously injected the human breast cancer cell line MDA-MB-231 into athymic nude mice, which resulted in formation of metastasis in bone and the adrenal medulla. The authors isolated the cells from osteolytic bone metastasis and reinjected them to obtain cells with a stable elevated capacity to form bone metastasis. Transcriptome analysis (cDNA microarray) revealed that the parental MDA-MB-231 cell line, derived from a patient with metastatic breast cancer, demonstrated the poor prognosis gene expression signature previously defined using human clinical samples.[12] No enhanced expression of this poor prognosis pattern occurred in the osteolytic metastasis, but this comparison did yield a bone metastasis signature composed of a set of four genes. These four genes included the chemokine receptor CXCR4, interleukin-11, connective tissue growth factor, and matrix metalloproteinase 1 (MMP-1). Tumor cell populations expressing only one of these four genes were not more aggressive than the parental MDA-MB-231 cells, but expression

of any three of the four genes resulted in metastatic activity that was intermediate between the parental cell and fully metastatic population (expressing all four genes). These findings suggest that the parental MDA-MB-231 cell population contains evidence of clonal evolution for the entire primary tumor cell population to a "poor prognosis" pattern of gene expression. However, superimposed on this poor prognosis signature are variant cells of high metastatic potential with gene expression profiles for metastasis at a specific tissue or organ site. These findings are consistent with our hypothesis that the "clonal evolution" and "metastatic variant" models of metastatic progression represent nonexclusive mechanisms for the development of site-specific metastatic tumor cells and that these models should not be considered mutually exclusive but rather opposite ends in the spectrum for the origin of tumor metastases.

Collectively, cDNA microarray data support the concept that clonal evolution and metastatic variants occur within the same tumor (see Fig. 4-1). The clonal evolution of this primary tumor results in a poor prognosis profile in tumors with enhanced metastatic potential. Superimposition of additional genetic changes (metastatic variants) on the poor prognosis profile of gene expression increases the potential for metastasis to a specific site or organ. These findings suggest that tumor formation and metastasis may be under independent genetic control.

TUMORIGENESIS AND METASTASIS ARE UNDER SEPARATE GENETIC CONTROL: TUMOR SUPPRESSOR GENES

It has been demonstrated that transfection of oncogenic sequences into the correct recipient cell can result in acquisition of an invasive phenotype and metastatic competence. This was first demonstrated by transfection of Ras sequences into fetal mouse fibroblasts and has been confirmed for fibroblast and epithelial cells. Similar findings have been observed with transfection of Mos, Raf, Src, Fes, and Fms. At first, these results might suggest that the metastatic phenotype might arise from genetic alterations associated with tumor development and progression (tumorigenicity). However, not all tumor cells acquire metastatic competence after oncogene transfection. Furthermore, metastatic competence could be dissociated from tumorigenicity in ras-transfected rat embryo fibroblasts by adenovirus 2E1A gene expression. These findings can be explained by the fact that metastasis requires activation of additional "metastasis effector genes" or inactivation of "metastasis suppressor genes" over and above genetic alterations required for tumorigenesis. This concept is also consistent with the findings of Kang et al.,[18] which suggest that primary tumors may present a poor prognosis profile of gene expression, but formation of site-specific metastasis requires additional changes in gene expression.

Inherent in this concept is the idea that, just as there are tumor suppressor genes, for example, retinoblastoma gene or von Hippel-Lindau gene, there may also be a metastasis suppressor gene. Several metastasis suppressor genes have been identified through their reduced expression in highly metastatic tumor cells compared with tumorigenic but poorly or nonmetastatic tumor cells.[19] By definition, reexpression of the metastasis suppressor gene in a tumor cell line results in loss of metastatic competence *in vivo*, without a significant reduction in tumorigenicity. At least eight tumor suppressor genes have been identified to date through a variety of methods, including subtractive hybridization, differential display, serial analysis of gene expression, and mircroarray analysis.[19] These tumor suppressor genes affect many aspects of signal transduction, including growth factor receptor signaling, cell-cell communication, mitogen-activated protein kinase (MAPK) pathway, and transcription. The identity and functions of tumor suppressor genes have been reviewed in detail elsewhere.[19]

METASTATIC CASCADE

Investigators refer to the process of metastasis formation as the *metastatic cascade* (Fig. 4-2). This conceptual framework divides the process into a series of discrete steps that can then be investigated for identification of cellular and molecular events requisite for metastasis to occur. It is well established, from clinical observations and from mechanistic studies, that metastasis formation is an inefficient process. What is the source of this inefficiency?

Large numbers of tumor cells and tumor cell clumps are shed into the vascular drainage of a primary tumor.[20] It has been demonstrated experimentally that, after intravenous injection of highly metastatic tumor cells, only approximately 0.01% of these cells will form tumor foci. The number of circulating tumor cells and tumor emboli correlates with the size and age of the primary tumor; that is, larger tumors shed more tumor cells and emboli. However, the number of circulating tumor cells does not correlate with the clinical outcome of metastases.

The inefficiency of tumor cells in completing the metastatic cascade is, in part, the result of the fact that successful forma-tion of metastatic foci consists of several highly complex and interdependent steps. Each step is rate limiting in that failure to complete any of these events completely disrupts metastasis formation. Thus, the steps involved in metastasis formation also represent a Darwinian selection process. Only those tumor cells that have acquired sufficient genetic changes and accompanying alterations in gene expression can successfully complete the requisite events to allow metastasis formation.

Another source of inefficiency in the metastatic cascade is revealed by studies on tumor cells shedding into the circulation.[21] In these experiments, highly metastatic tumor cells were grown subcutaneously in athymic nude mice and perfused *in vivo* to collect shed tumor cells. The shed tumor cells were collected and analyzed for clonogenicity in soft agar, resistance to apoptosis, and ability to form tumors *in vivo* after *in vitro* expansion and reinjection subcutaneously. These properties of the tumor cells shed into the circulation were compared with those of tumor cells isolated directly from the primary tumors by excision and dissociation into single-cell suspensions. Somewhat surprisingly, the authors found that shed tumor cells have a low metastatic potential compared to cells isolated directly from the primary tumor. Specifically, cells in shed tumor cell populations showed an increase in apoptosis (48%), compared with an average apoptotic fraction of 20% in the native tumors. This suggests that an additional source of inefficiency in the metastatic cascade is due to the fact that most of the tumor cells shed into the circulation are in the process of dying as they exit the tumor.[21] Thus, not all circulating tumor cells represent metastatically competent tumor cells capable of colonizing distant tissue sites.

As might be expected from the highly complex nature of metastasis formation, no single gene product is exclusively

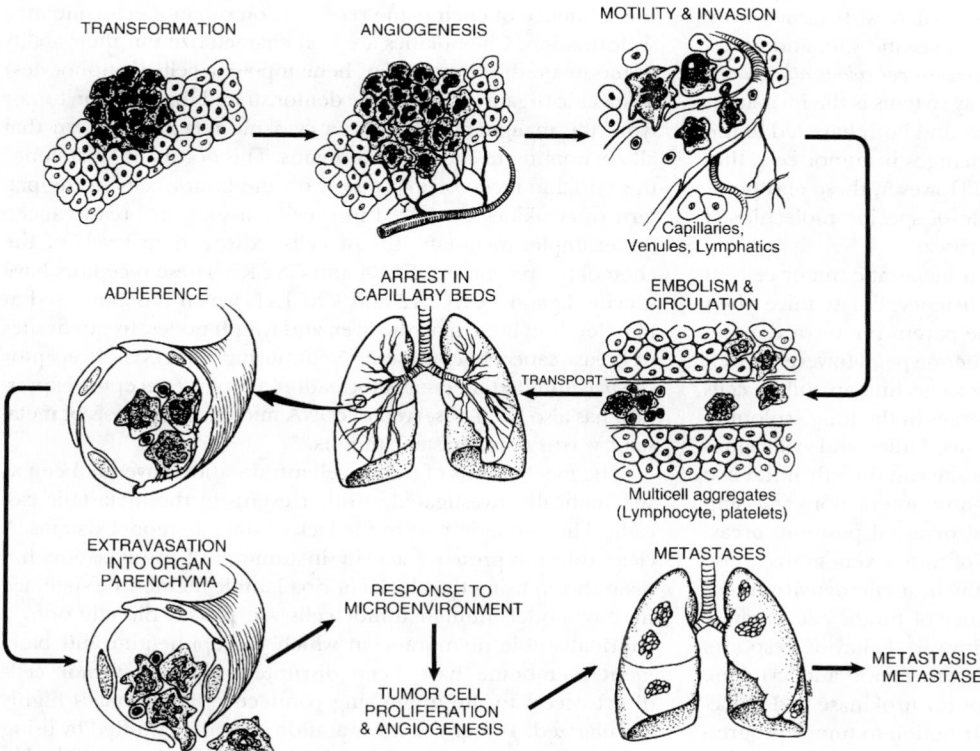

FIGURE 4-2. The pathogenesis of cancer metastasis. To produce metastases, tumor cells must detach from the primary tumor, invade the extracellular basement membrane and enter the circulation, survive in the circulation to arrest in the capillary bed, adhere to subendothelial basement membrane, gain entrance into the organ parenchyma, respond to paracrine growth factors, proliferate and induce angiogenesis, and evade host defenses. The pathogenesis of metastasis is therefore complex and consists of multiple sequential, selective, and interdependent steps whose outcome depends on the interaction of tumor cells with homeostatic factors.

responsible for metastasis formation. Successful completion of many of the steps of the metastatic cascade is the result of acquisition of both positive effectors, as well as the loss of negative regulators. Unrestrained growth is not sufficient to result in tumor metastasis. Tumor metastasis is not a passive process secondary to tumor growth and requires additional genetic changes other than those associated with the tumorigenicity. Tumorigenicity and metastatic competence have some overlapping features but are clearly under separate genetic control. Ongoing research into the steps of the metastatic cascade has identified gene products that can facilitate completion of each of the steps outlined above. These are the molecular effectors of tumor metastasis. In many cases, research has also identified gene products that function to block successful completion of each of the steps in the metastatic cascade—that is, metastasis suppressor genes. The idea that there is loss of negative effectors, as well as positive phenotypic changes associated with malignant progression and metastasis formation, is now well established.

TUMOR MICROENVIRONMENT: DETERMINANT OF METASTATIC POTENTIAL AND SITE OF METASTASIS

During investigation of the molecular events associated with specific steps in the metastatic cascade, investigators frequently use animal models of metastasis. In these assays, tumor cells are either injected into experimental animals to form a primary tumor site that subsequently metastasizes or directly into the circulation to model the later phases of metastasis formation. Animal models in which there is formation of a primary tumor and subsequent metastasis formation are known as *spontaneous metastasis* models. Intravenous injection of tumor cells, bypassing the molecular and cellular events associated with tumor invasion, focuses on colonization of the metastatic site, and assays that use this technique are referred to as *tumor colonization* models. The end point in both types of assay systems is the formation of visible metastases at a secondary site, and both have led to the identification of specific molecular changes in tumor cells that contribute to metastatic competence. However, these end point assays are unable to examine the role of specific molecules at each individual step in the metastatic cascade.

Subcutaneous xenografts of human metastatic tumor cells in nude or severe combined immunodeficiency disease mice often fail to recapitulate the behavior of the parent tumor or demonstrate a spontaneously metastatic phenotype. However, when injected intravenously, many of these same human tumor cells are capable of forming metastatic colonies in the lung (colonization assays). In pioneering experiments, Fidler and colleagues demonstrated that the primary tumor site can directly influence metastatic potential through tumor-host interactions.[22] Using orthotopic (defined as in the normal or usual position, breast tumors in breast tissue) implantation of tumor xenografts, these investigators have demonstrated that the host microenvironment has a profound influence on a number of tumor cell parameters.[22] These include tumor growth, invasive behavior, response to chemotherapeutic agents, and growth factor and cytokine production, as well as protease profiles for urokinase and metalloproteinases. An important host contribution to tumor progression is the frequent association of MMP production by stimulated stromal fibroblasts adjacent to invading tumor cells.[23] In more recent studies, Fidler[24] has extended these findings to demonstrate that tumor-host interactions also influence gene expression patterns in metastatic foci and may contribute to tumor progression at these sites. These findings are supported by transcriptome analysis of metastatic human tumors in murine models, which show that successful formation of metastatic foci is associated with alterations in gene expression of host tissues.[18]

These findings suggest that favorable tumor-host interactions may facilitate the outgrowth of metastatic tumor cells, whereas unfavorable interactions would suppress metastasis formation. This concept is embodied in the "seed-soil" hypothesis of metastasis originally put forth by Paget.[25] Paget noted the propensity for some types of cancer to produce metastasis in specific organs and that the metastatic site was not simply a matter of chance. This idea was later challenged by the proposal of James Ewing,[26] who suggested that the pattern of blood circulation leaving the site of the primary tumor was a principal determinant for the site of metastases.

However, these theories are not mutually exclusive, and evidence from more recent studies supports contributions from both mechanisms. For example, the direct drainage of the portal circulation through the liver can account for this organ as a principal site of metastatic involvement in patients with advanced colorectal carcinomas. However, in a study in which colorectal cancer cells of differing metastatic ability were implanted into the liver, it was found that growth regulation in the liver microenvironment influenced tumor cell growth, although the molecular basis for these differences remains to be elucidated. As described above, the organ microenvironment can influence gene expression and response to chemotherapy. Investigators have identified soluble cytokines and cell-adhesion molecules in the tissue microenvironment that modulate tumor cell responses to chemotherapy and therapy-induced cell death. Another example is the influence of chemokine receptors on organ-specific metastasis formation. Chemokines are well characterized in their ability to modulate the "homing" of hematopoietic cells (lymphocytes) to specific organs. Studies have demonstrated that in some tumor types the malignant cells have a cytokine receptor pattern that allows homing to specific end organs. This occurs by "matching" the cytokine receptor expression on the tumor cells to the pattern of cytokines expressed in specific tissues. In breast cancer, for example, metastatic tumor cells express high levels of the chemokine receptors CXCR4 and CXCR7. These receptors have specific ligands, CXCL12 and CXCL21, which are expressed at high levels in bone marrow, liver, and lymph nodes, frequent sites of breast cancer metastases.[27] Neutralizing the CXCR4 receptor *in vivo* inhibited metastasis formation. Cytokine receptor expression has also been observed in cDNA microarray analysis of metastatic versus nonmetastatic tumors.[18]

The mechanisms of tumor cell intravasation have not been as systematically investigated as other events in the metastatic cascade. This is due in part to the lack of suitable model systems. A clear role for protease activity in tumor cell intravasation has been shown using the chick chorioallantoic membrane system.[28] In this model, human tumor cells are placed directly onto a chorioallantoic membrane in which the epithelium and basement membrane have been disrupted, allowing tumor cells direct access to the underlying connective tissue that is highly vascularized. Tumor cell intravasation is then quantified by using polymerase chain reaction amplification of human-specific Alu genomic DNA sequences of tumor cells present in the chorioallantoic membrane on the other side of the chick embryo from the initial tumor cell inoculation. These experiments demonstrate that MMPs, as well as urokinase-type plasminogen activator and the urokinase-type plasminogen activator-receptor, are involved in the escape of cells from the primary tumor.

Chambers et al.[29] have used intravital videomicroscopy to study the events and mechanisms involved in tumor cell exit from the circulation (extravasation). The results of these studies have profoundly changed current thinking about the metastatic process. It appears that circulating tumor cells may remain viable in the circulation and extravasate up to 3 days after their introduction into the circulation. Surprisingly, metastatic and nonmetastatic cells extravasate, and this process is not protease dependent. However, only a small subset (1 in 40) of cells grow and expand to form micrometastases, and even fewer (1 in 100) continue to grow, forming macroscopic tumors. Almost 40% of injected tumor cells remained as dormant solitary cancer cells. These findings suggest that the control of postextravasation growth of individual cancer cells is a dominant effect in metastatic inefficiency. Collectively, these data, as well as the studies on orthotropic effects, demonstrate that the local environment of the target organ and primary tumor may profoundly influence the growth potential and metastatic competence of both the primary tumor and its metastases.

For the remainder of this chapter, the molecular events associated with tumor cell invasion and migration are examined, with the aim of identifying the molecular mechanisms, as well as effector and suppressor genes, that may become targets for new and effective cancer therapies. Immune modulation of cancer is discussed elsewhere, as is the process of tumor-associated angiogenesis.

TUMOR CELL MOTILITY

Cell motility is a critical component of the invasive phenotype. Understanding the molecular mechanisms that confer tumor cell motility should allow identification of novel targets for disrupting this process and preventing tumor dissemination. Tumor cell motility can be correlated with metastatic behavior. When parameters such as pseudopod extension, membrane ruffling, or vectorial translation are measured, there is a quantitative increase in metastatic tumor cells when compared with their nonmetastatic counterparts. A variety of stimuli have been shown to stimulate tumor cell motility *in vitro*, including host-derived factors, growth factors, and tumor-secreted factors that function in an autocrine fashion to stimulate tumor cell motility. Autocrine motility factor (AMF) is a 60-kD glycoprotein produced by human melanoma cells that stimulates tumor cell migration. AMF has been identified as neuroleukin/phosphohexose isomerase. Autotaxin (ATX), another autocrine motility agent, is a 125-kD glycoprotein that elicits chemotactic and chemokinetic responses at picomolar to nanomolar concentrations in human melanoma cells. ATX possesses 5'-nucleotide PDE (EC 3.1.4.1) activity,[30] binds adenosine triphosphate (ATP), and is phosphorylated only on threonine (Thr210), which is required for motility-stimulating activities. ATX possesses no detectable protein kinase activity toward histone, myelin basic protein, or casein. These results have led to the proposal that ATX is capable of at least two alternative reaction mechanisms, threonine (T-type) ATPase and 5'-nucleotide PDE/ATP pyrophosphatase, with a common site (Thr210) for the formation of covalently bound reaction intermediates, threonine phosphate and threonine adenylate, respectively.[30] The identification of AMF and ATX suggests that stimulation of tumor cell movement occurs in response to autocrine mechanisms that are unique to metastatic tumor cells.

TUMOR INVASION OF THE BASEMENT MEMBRANE

During the transition from benign to invasive carcinoma, extensive changes occur in the quantity, organization, and distribution of the subepithelial basement membrane. A primary histopathologic feature of malignant tumors is the disruption of the epithelial basement membrane and the presence of cancer cells in the stromal compartment.[31] Benign proliferative disorders such as fibrocystic disease, sclerosing adenosis, intraductal hyperplasia, intraductal papilloma, and fibroadenoma are all characterized by disorganization of the normal epithelial architecture. No matter how extensive this disorganization may become, however, these benign lesions are always characterized by a continuous basement membrane that separates the neoplastic epithelium from the stroma.[31] In contrast, malignant tumors are characterized by a loss of basement membrane around the invasive tumor cells in the stromal compartment. Once the basement membrane barrier is compromised, it is impossible to determine the quantity or location of tumor cells that may have escaped from the primary tumor. Thus, local invasion is paramount to metastatic competence, which is the hallmark of malignant conversion.

The ability to invade across basement membrane barriers is not unique to malignant tumor cells, however. During an inflammatory response, nonneoplastic immune cells regularly cross the subendothelial basement membranes, as do endothelial cells during the angiogenic response. Trophoblasts invade the endometrial stroma and blood vessels to establish contact with the maternal circulation during development of the hemochorial placenta. Nonneoplastic invasive cells, such as trophoblasts, endothelial cells, and inflammatory cells, all use mechanisms for invasion that are functionally similar to those of tumor cells. The difference between these normal invasive processes and the pathologic nature of tumor metastasis is therefore one of regulation. An understanding of the factors that control cellular processes essential to cell invasion should allow identification of novel targets for therapeutic intervention to prevent and treat angiogenesis and inflammatory diseases, as well as tumor metastases.

INITIATION OF CELL MIGRATION

The initial events in cellular migration are changes in cell adhesion. These changes consist of alterations in cell-cell adhesion as well as interactions of cells with the ECM. A variety of cell surface receptors that mediate these interactions have been characterized. These include the cadherins, integrins, immunoglobulin (Ig) superfamily members, and CD44. Tumor cells must decrease cell- and matrix-adhesive interactions to escape from the primary tumor. However, at later stages in the metastatic cascade, tumor cells may need to increase adhesive interactions with cells or ECM, or both, such as during arrest and extravasation at a distant site. The apparent contribution of each class of cell-adhesion molecule to invasive behavior will, in some way, be dependent on the tumor cell population and model system used to study these interactions. This chapter reviews the contribution of changes in cell-cell adhesion to tumor progression before considering alterations in tumor cell adhesion to the ECM.

CELL–CELL ADHESION: METASTASIS SUPPRESSOR

The majority of human cancers arise in epithelial cells. Several types of junctional structures, such as desmosomes, tight junctions, and adherens-type junctions, tightly interconnect normal epithelial cells. The formation and maintenance of these contacts require Ca^{2+}-dependent homophilic interactions mediated by the cell-adhesion molecules known as *cadherins* (Fig. 4-3). Cadherins are a superfamily of single-pass transmembrane glycoproteins that mediate Ca^{2+}-dependent cell–cell adhesion. The cadherin superfamily now consists of five subfamilies. These are the classic type I and type II cadherins, desmosomal cadherins,

protocadherins, and cadherin-related proteins.[32] The classic cadherin, epithelial cadherin (E-cadherin) mediates homotypic cell adhesion in epithelial cells. E-cadherin is a transmembrane glycoprotein that has five extracellular homologous domains (ectodomains), a single membrane-spanning region, and a cytosolic domain. E-cadherin is physically anchored to the actin cytoskeleton by cytoplasmic proteins termed *catenins*. β-Catenin is also a major component of the wnt signaling pathway.

Any disruption of the intracellular E-cadherin–catenin complex results in loss of cell adhesion. This includes changes in E-cadherin expression or function, as well as genes other than E-cadherin required for junctional complex formation and function. Abundant evidence has been shown that E-cadherin function is frequently lost during progression of many human cancers, including those arising in the breast, prostate, esophagus, stomach, colon, skin, kidney, lung, and liver.[33] This loss of E-cadherin function arises via several different mechanisms. In familial gastric carcinomas, germline mutations in the E-cadherin gene predispose an individual to the development of malignant cancer. Mutations in β-catenin are found in many primary tumors, including prostatic cancer and melanoma, as well as gastric and colon cancer. Another mechanism disrupting E-

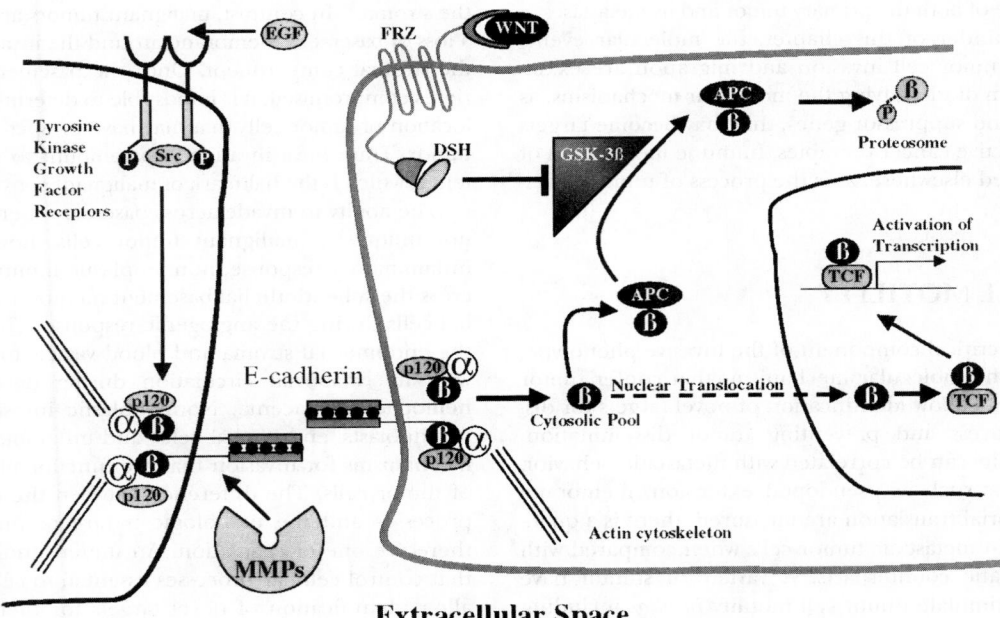

FIGURE 4-3.   Disruption of cell-cell adhesion concomitant with tumor progression. Epithelial cadherin (E-cadherin) is a homotypic cell-adhesion molecule containing five homologous, extracellular domains (ectodomains) that bind divalent calcium ions. Calcium binding promotes homophilic cell–cell E-cadherin complexes found in such structures as desmosomes, tight junctions, and adherens-type junctions. The cytoplasmic tail of E-cadherin involved in cell–cell adhesion interacts with β-catenin, α-catenin, and p120[CAS] (p120). Loss of E-cadherin function, by germline mutation, promoter hypermethylation, or destruction of the ectodomains by matrix metalloproteinase (MMP) activity, results in an increase in free cytosolic β-catenin levels. Increased cytoplasmic β-catenin can be directed to the proteosome complex by glycogen synthase kinase-3β (GSK3β) phosphorylation and subsequent interaction with the adenomatous polyposis coli (APC) gene product. The frizzled (FRZ)-disheveled (DSH) pathway for WNT signaling can down-regulate the activity of GSK3β. Activation of the WNT signaling pathway or loss of APC function facilitates the increase in cytosolic β-catenin levels that are associated with loss of E-cadherin function or mutations of the β-catenin gene that result in reduced association with E-cadherin cytoplasmic domain. Translocation of β-catenin to the nucleus results in association with members of the TCF/LEF-1 transcription factor family. This is associated with gene expression associated with cell transformation and tumor growth (i.e., c-Myc, cyclin D1). It is noteworthy that this cascade of cellular transformation can be initiated by expression of an extracellular protease that culminates in enhanced chromosomal instability. EGF, epidermal growth factor; P, phosphorylated amino acid residues; TCF, tissue coding factor. (From ref. 36, with permission.)

cadherin function during tumor progression is hypermethylation of the E-cadherin promoter, resulting in decreased gene expression. This has been found to be a major mechanism in papillary thyroid cancer in that 83% of cases demonstrated hypermethylation of the E-cadherin promoter.[34] Yet another mechanism to alter E-cadherin function is proteolytic modification. Lochter et al.[35] reported that E-cadherin function can be disrupted by degradation of E-cadherin extracellular domains by stromelysin-1, a member of the MMP family that has been closely linked with tumor progression. Constitutive expression of active stromelysin in mammary epithelial cells results in cleavage of E-cadherin and progressive phenotypic changes *in vitro*, including loss of catenins from cell-cell contacts, down-regulation of cytokeratins, up-regulation of vimentin, and MMP-9. These changes result in a stable epithelial-to-mesenchymal transition of cellular phenotype. *In vivo* stromelysin expression promotes mammary carcinogenesis that includes genomic changes that are distinct from those seen in other mouse breast cancer models.[36] It has been reported that loss of H-cadherin expression occurs during the progression of breast cancer, but little is known about the function of other cadherin family members during tumor progression. In summary, a decrease in cell–cell adhesion is associated with malignant conversion. Forced expression of E-cadherin in tumor cell lines results in reversion from an invasive to a benign tumor cell phenotype,[33] implicating E-cadherin as a metastasis suppressor.

In normal cells, β-catenin is sequestered in the intracellular adhesion complex with the cytoplasmic domain of E-cadherin, α-catenin, γ-catenin, and p120[CAS]. Loss of cell–cell adhesion results in disruption of the adhesion complex and an increase in free cytosolic β-catenin. This free β-catenin is bound by the adenomatous polyposis coli (APC) gene product and is rapidly phosphorylated by glycogen synthase kinase-3β. Phosphorylated β-catenin is subsequently degraded in the ubiquitin-proteosome pathway. In many colon cancer cells, the tumor suppressor gene APC is nonfunctional. This can lead to accumulation of high levels of cytoplasmic β-catenin that are subsequently translocated to the nucleus. The wnt-1 protooncogene-initiated signaling pathway, which includes the frizzled and disheveled gene products, blocks the activity of the glycogen synthase kinase-β and results in accumulation of β-catenin. In the nucleus, free nonphosphorylated β-catenin can bind to members of the TCF/LEF-1 family of transcription factors. It has been demonstrated that, after inactivation of APC function, the increase in available cytosolic β-catenin results in translocation to the nucleus, where it complexes with transcription factor Tcf-4 and up-regulates c-Myc expression.[37] It has also been shown that β-catenin activates transcription from the cyclin D1 promoter and contributes to neoplastic transformation by causing accumulation of cyclin D1.[38] These findings link changes in cell–cell adhesion with intracellular signaling, oncogene expression, and tumor cell growth. Thus, loss of cadherin-mediated cell–cell adhesion is an important event that has many far-reaching consequences for acquisition of the invasive phenotype and tumor progression.

Other types of cell–cell adhesive interactions can actually facilitate metastasis formation. They may be particularly important during tumor cell arrest and extravasation. These molecules include members of the Ig superfamily such as NCAM and VCAM-1. This superfamily has a wide variety of members involved in cellular immunity and signal transduction, as well as cell adhesion. Members of the Ig superfamily share the Ig homology unit that consists of 70- to 110-amino acid residues organized into seven to nine β-sheet structures. The diversity of superfamily members precludes generalization about their role in tumor cell invasion and metastasis. However, the role of one family member seems straightforward. VCAM-1 is an endothelial cell, cytokine-inducible, counter-receptor for VLA-4 integrin, also known as $\alpha_4\beta_1$-*integrin receptor*. The role of integrin receptors is discussed separately in Role of Integrins in Tumor Progression, later in this chapter. Normally, VLA-4 is expressed on leukocytes and functions in mediating leukocyte attachment to endothelial cells. VLA-4 is also found on tumor cells in malignant melanoma and metastatic sarcoma, but not in adenocarcinomas. It is thought that expression of VLA-4 may facilitate interaction of circulating tumor cells with endothelium before tumor cell extravasation. This was demonstrated by intravenous injection of human melanoma cells into nude mice pretreated with VLA-4–inducing cytokines, which results in an enhanced number of lung metastases compared with no cytokine pretreatment of the mice.[39] Cell-cell adhesive interactions can either suppress or facilitate metastasis formation. Either role is dependent on the specific context and molecular mechanisms of cell–cell interaction.

CELL MATRIX INTERACTIONS AND TUMOR CELL MIGRATION

As stated previously in Initiation of Cell Migration, the interaction of the tumor cell with the ECM, in particular the basement membrane, defines the invasive phenotype, and tumor invasion is paramount to metastasis. It is now recognized that the ECM exerts a profound influence on the behavior of nonneoplastic cells and that cells can direct the assembly/disassembly of the matrix. This concept is known as *dynamic reciprocity* and also applies to the interaction of malignant tumor cells with the ECM. During the process of metastasis formation, malignant tumor cells must interact with a variety of different types of ECM. These include the subepithelial basement membrane of the tissue of origin, stromal elements of the tissue of origin, subendothelial basement membranes during extravasation, and the stromal matrix and basement membranes of the organ(s) at the site of metastasis growth. Attachment of nonneoplastic cells to the ECM is prerequisite for cell survival. A fundamental difference for neoplastic cells is the loss of anchorage requirement for cell survival and growth. The anchorage-independent growth of tumor cells may result from an uncoupling of cell survival signals transduced from the ECM via ECM receptors together with autonomous growth mechanisms associated with neoplastic transformation. Tumor cell interactions with the ECM have profound implications for cell-cycle regulation and for migration.

ROLE OF CD44 IN TUMOR INVASION AND METASTASIS

CD44 is a transmembrane glycoprotein with a large ectodomain and single cytoplasmic domain. CD44 is involved in cell adhesion to hyaluronan (HA). The gene encoding CD44 is on the short arm of human chromosome 11 and contains constant and variable exons.[40] As a result of this gene structure, a number of differentially spliced isoforms of CD44 can be generated. The isoform containing no variant exon sequences is referred to as *standard CD44* (CD44s). A total of nine variant regions can encode protein sequences v2 to v10. Alternatively, spliced messenger RNA variants of CD44 (CD44v) can contain one or more variant coding regions. More than 30 different splice variants have been detected by polymerase chain reaction analysis. In addition to these variants, there are also cell type–specific differences in glycosylation of the core protein. The pattern of glycosylation and presence of variant exons influence the ability of CD44 to function in HA binding.

Several lines of evidence suggest that CD44 expression plays a role in metastasis formation. Clinical studies demonstrate that a variety of different types of cancer express high cell surface levels of CD44, which correlate with a poorer clinical outcome compared with tumors that have low CD44 surface expression.[41,42] Forced expression of CD44 v4 to v7 confers metastatic ability to a nonmetastasizing rat pancreatic carcinoma cell line, and metastasis formation could be blocked using anti-CD44 variant–specific antibodies. However, the exact role of CD44v in metastasis formation remains elusive.

In some tumors, CD44-associated increases in tumor growth and metastatic potential correlate with CD44-mediated cell attachment to HA.[43] CD44 also functions in HA uptake and degradation correlated with invasive tumor cell behavior.[44] These studies demonstrate that CD44 aggregation on the cell surface creates a binding site for the active MMP-9. It is postulated that bound MMP-9 may liberate ECM-bound HA and facilitates tumor cell HA uptake and degradation. These findings link cell adhesion and ECM turnover. In addition, they suggest that CD44 may function at different stages of tumor cell invasion and metastasis and that the specific CD44 role may depend on the specific stage of metastasis formation that is examined.

ROLE OF INTEGRINS IN TUMOR PROGRESSION

Integrins are heterodimeric transmembrane proteins that are formed by the noncovalent association of α and β subunits.[45,46] Considerable redundancy within cell-ECM interaction mediated by integrins exists, as most integrins bind to several individual matrix proteins, and ECM components, such as laminin, fibronectin, vitronectin, and collagens, can bind to several different integrin receptors. This suggests that integrins are capable of providing the cell with detailed information about the surrounding ECM environment, which is then integrated at the cellular level to generate a cellular response (Fig. 4-4). It is now well established that integrins can signal across the cell membrane in both directions.[47] Binding of ECM ligands to integrins is known to initiate signal transduction pathways that can result in cell proliferation, differentiation, migration, or cell death (apoptosis, anoikis). This is referred to as *outside-in signaling*. It is also known that intracellular events can modulate the binding activity of integrins for their ligands in the ECM; this is referred to as *inside-out signaling*. Integrin clustering and ligand occupancy are crucial for the initiation of intracellular integrin-mediated signal pathways.

The roles of specific integrins in tumor progression and metastasis formation are dichotomous. The decreased expression of some integrins is associated with cellular transformation and tumorigenesis. These include $\alpha_5\beta_1$ and $\alpha_2\beta_1$ integrins. HT-29 colon carcinoma cells lacking $\alpha_5\beta_1$ expression were either significantly less tumorigenic or completely nontumorigenic when forced to express α_5.[48] Loss of $\alpha_2\beta_1$ expression in breast epithelial cells correlates with the transformed phenotype, and reexpression of this integrin abrogates the malignant phenotype.[49] On the other hand, expression of some integrins directly correlates with tumorigenicity and tumor progression. For example, the $\alpha_v\beta_3$ integrin is expressed in metastatic melanoma but not in benign melanocytic lesions.[50] Antibodies against α_v integrins blocked the growth of human melanoma xenografts in nude mice.[51] Integrin α_6 expression is increased in oropharyngeal and bladder cancers as well as lung tumors.[39] Tumor progression is associated with expression of $\alpha_3\beta_1$ in 82% of tumors. The molecular events associated with enhanced expression of this integrin and tumor progression are not well defined. The role of integrins in tumor invasion and metastasis may only be secondarily related to growth control. Integrins are also directly involved in cell migration.

Integrin-mediated signal transduction involves direct activation of signaling pathways and collaborative signaling (also referred to as *cooperative signaling*), in which integrins modulate signaling events initiated through receptor tyrosine kinases.[52] The *cis* association of integrins with other receptors on the same cell surface results in formation of multireceptor complexes. Little evidence has been shown that these complexes signal exclusively through integrin-specific pathways; instead they cooperate with the other receptors to influence a variety of signaling pathways. Direct integrin signaling starts after the engagement of these receptors with their cognate ECM ligands, which results in lateral clustering of the integrin receptors. Lateral aggregation leads to interaction of the integrin cytoplasmic domains to form complexes that link to the cytoskeleton. This results in organization of cell structures known as *focal adhesions*.

Autophosphorylation of the focal adhesion kinase (FAK) was among the first integrin-mediated signaling events to be identified. This autophosphorylation event on tyrosine 397 results in recruitment of Src family protein kinases that in turn leads to phosphorylation of additional tyrosine residues on FAK. Phosphorylation of FAK can result in activation of the extracellular signal–regulated kinase/MAPK pathway. Activation of the MAPK pathway has been linked to induction of cell migration. The activation of MAPK can be mediated by Grb-2 recruitment to FAK, which then binds Sos, a guanine nucleotide exchange factor, for Ras.[53] Alternatively, activation of the MAPK pathway can result from FAK phosphorylation of paxillin and the Crk-associated substrate (p130Cas) that leads to binding of link proteins, such as Nck. In addition, phosphorylation of FAK at tyrosine 397 creates a binding site for the regulatory subunit of phosphoinositol 3 kinase and triggers activation of this signaling pathway.

The knowledge that FAK is tyrosine phosphorylated on integrin activation suggests that focal adhesion-associated protein tyrosine phosphatases (PTP) could modulate Fak function. Several PTPs that interact with components of the focal adhesion complex have been identified. These are PTP α and PTP-PEST (PTP rich in proline, glutamic acid, serine, and threonine), which negatively regulate Src and paxillin, respectively.[54] It has been shown that PTP-PEST–deficient cells have a defect in cell motility that correlates with an increase in the size

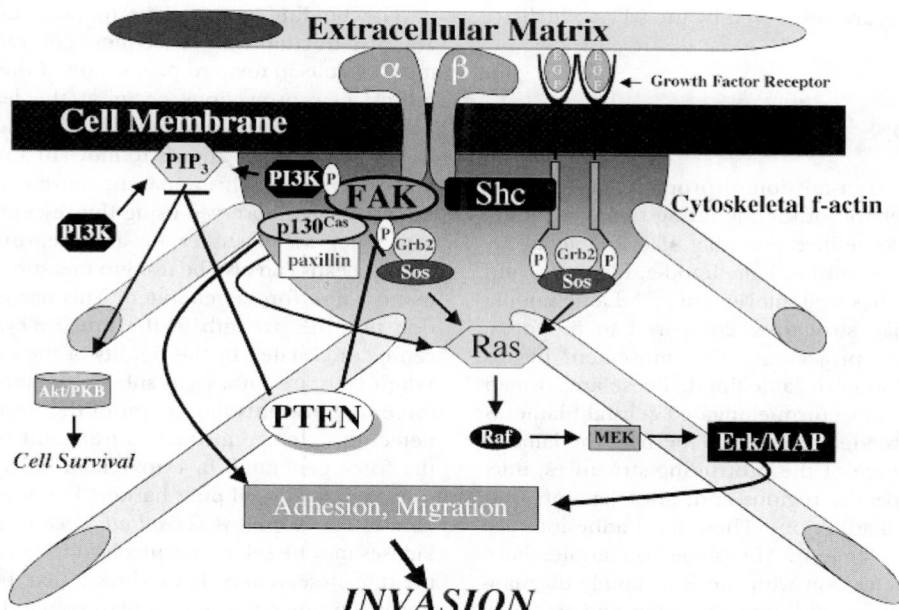

FIGURE 4-4. Role of integrins in tumor cell invasion and metastasis: integration of kinase and phosphatase activities. Binding of extracellular matrix (ECM) components to integrin receptors initiates an intracellular signaling cascade that results in formation of a focal adhesion complex that consists of cytoskeletal and signal transduction molecules. Ligand binding to the integrin receptor results in integrin clustering and association of signal transduction molecules. Integrin receptor clustering induces autophosphorylation of focal adhesion kinase (FAK) on tyrosine 397. Subsequently, an Src homology 2 (SH2)-containing (Shc) adapter protein of the Src kinase family that binds to specific phosphotyrosine residues (Y397) on FAK is recruited to the integrin-FAK complex. Recruitment of additional proteins, such as α-actinin, talin, and paxillin, to this complex connects the focal adhesion complex to the filamentous actin cytoskeleton. Interaction of Shc with FAK results in additional sites of phosphorylation on the FAK molecule and subsequent recruitment of additional SH2 adapter proteins, such as Grb2 and the nucleotide exchange factor Sos. These interactions lead to activation of the mitogen-activated protein (MAP) pathway that stimulates tumor cell growth, adhesion, and migration. Similarly, receptors for growth factors can transiently associate with the focal adhesion complex to synergistically activate the MAP kinase pathway.

FAK activation also acts upstream of the Akt/protein kinase B (PKB) signaling pathway that promotes cell survival. Association of the p85 subunit of phosphatidylinositol 3 kinase (PI3K) with tyrosine 397 in FAK mediates this effect. The rapid elevation of phosphatidylinositol(3,4,5)triphosphate (PIP$_3$) lipid product of PI3K activity stimulates the Akt/PKB pathway, leading to enhanced cell survival.

Crk-associated substrate (p130[CAS]) is another SH2- and SH3-containing signal transduction that associates with FAK on integrin binding to the ECM. Interaction of p130[CAS] with FAK is mediated by a proline-rich region on FAK (residues 712-178) that interacts with the SH3 domain of p130[CAS]. Activation of p130[CAS] promotes cell migration and invasion, which are associated with enhanced metastatic behavior.

The tumor suppressor gene PTEN inhibits cell adhesion, migration, and invasion. This inhibition is mediated by direct PTEN dephosphorylation of FAK and Shc. This leads to negative regulation of the p130[CAS] pathway that affects cell attachment, migration, and invasion. Down-regulation of the MAPK pathway by PTEN dephosphorylation of FAK and Shc negatively affects cell growth in addition to attachment and migration. PTEN is also known to directly dephosphorylate PIP$_3$ and negatively regulate the downstream Akt/PKB cell survival pathway. PTEN may also disrupt this pathway indirectly by dephosphorylation of FAK, which alters PI3K activation. Thus, integrin-mediated regulation of cell growth, adhesion, migration, and invasion is a complex network of signal transduction cascades that have positive (kinase) and negative (phosphatase) regulatory elements. EGF, epidermal growth factor; Erk, extracellular signal–regulated kinase; MEK, MAP kinase or ERK kinase.

and number of focal adhesions.[55] This defect appears to be due to in part to the constitutive increase in tyrosine phosphorylation of paxillin, as well as p130CAS and FAK.

A PTP that interacts directly with FAK is PTEN. PTEN was identified as a tumor suppressor gene on human chromosome 10q23, which is frequently mutated or deleted in a wide variety of human cancers, including gliomas, prostate, breast, lung, bladder, endometrial, kidney, and oropharyngeal cancers.[53,56] This gene encodes a phosphatase domain and also has extensive sequence homology to the cytoskeletal protein, tensin. PTEN functions as a dual-specificity phosphatase in that not only is it a PTP but it also dephosphorylates the lipid phosphatidylinositol(3,4,5)triphosphate (PIP3). The current view is that phosphatase activities function as tumor suppressor activities. The lipid phosphatase activity regulates levels of PIP3 that in turn regulate activation of the protein kinase B (PKB/Akt) pathway, which is protective against programmed cell death (apoptosis, anoikis). As a PTP, PTEN can also regulate the phosphorylation status of FAK and Shc, which, in turn, regulate cell adhesion, migration, cytoskeletal organization, and MAPK activation.

To summarize, loss of PTEN function results in alterations in integrin-mediated signaling via the FAK and PIP3 pathways, which results in a migratory and invasive phenotype.[53,56] The protein kinase activities function to promote cell invasion. The activities of these kinases are countered by the PTPs, which act as tumor suppressors.

CELL MIGRATION

Cell migration requires transmission of propulsive force from the ECM to the cytoskeleton of the migrating tumor or endothelial cell (Fig. 4-5). Repetitive assembly of cytoskeletal elements to form membrane ruffles, lamellipodia, filopodia, and pseudopodia accomplishes cell movement.[57,58] Lamellipodia are broad, flat sheet-like structures, compared to filopodia, which are thin cylindric projections. Cell movement begins with protrusion of a filopod or lamellipod. These are formed by polymerization of actin to form elongated central filaments in the filopod and a broader cross-weave mesh in the lamellipod.[59] At the leading edge of the protruding structures, integrins concentrate in specific regions and, after ligation with ECM ligands, form focal adhesions. These focal adhesions are anchored to the actin filaments. Microinjection studies have shown that integrin association with the Rho family of guanosine triphosphatases is critical for organization and assembly of the actin cytoskeleton. It has been demonstrated that there is a hierarchic cascade among these guanosine triphosphatases that controls formation of specific cytoskeletal structures. Cdc42 and Rac control formation of filopodia and lamellipodia, respectively, whereas Rho controls stress fiber formation and focal adhesions.[60]

The binding of integrins to their ECM ligands provides adhesive traction. The subsequent contraction of the actin filaments results in forward propulsion of the cell body. As the cell moves, new projections occur at the leading edge and are anchored with new focal adhesion. As the cell moves forward, the focal adhesions appear to move in a retrograde fashion on the cell surface. This apparent movement of the focal adhesions has been observed using fluorescent-tagged beads coated with integrin substrates or antiintegrin antibodies.[61] These coated beads can also be used to measure the integrin-cytoskeletal traction forces generated. This has led to the demonstration that the strength of the integrin-cytoskeletal interaction can be modulated by the rigidity of the extracellular substrate. When cells are on a rigid substrate, there is more restraining force that prevents movement of the focal adhesion. Cells can detect this change in the substrate and respond by increasing the force generated by cytoskeletal linkage to the focal adhesion so that the cell pulls harder. This is referred to as *reinforcement of the integrin-cytoskeletal attachments.* Data suggest that Src kinases may be selectively involved in regulating this reinforcement.[61] Researchers have shown that beads binding to the fibronectin receptor in fibroblast containing either wild-type or Src-deficient cells show similar reinforcement of the fibronectin-receptor–actin cytoskeletal linkage. In contrast, when they use vitronectin, there is little reinforcement of the vitronectin receptor in wild-type Src-expressing cells, but a strong reinforcement in the Src-deficient fibroblasts. These authors also show that kinase-defective Src selectively associates with the α_v

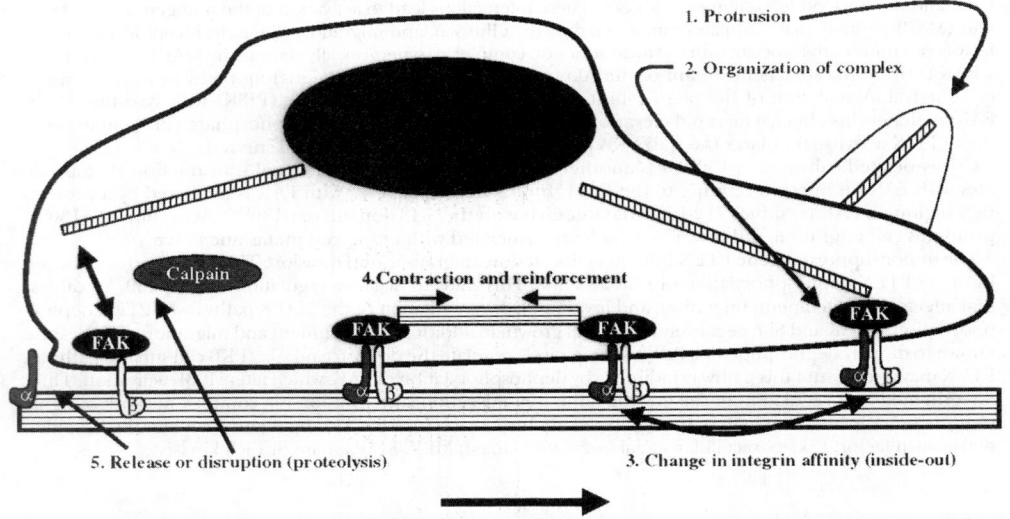

Net force and direction of movement

FIGURE 4-5. Cell migration requires transmission of force from the extracellular matrix (ECM) to the cytoskeleton. This is accomplished in distinct steps, several of which are illustrated. First, there is protrusion of a cellular projection (filopodia or lamellipodia) that is mediated by actin polymerization. The second step involves organization of the focal adhesion complex and connection with the actin cytoskeleton. This is accomplished via mechanisms described in Figure 4-4. Evidence suggests that if the integrin component of these complexes is not activated, they continually recycle across the cell surface without cell movement. Step 3 entails engagement of the integrin with the ECM that is mediated by a change in integrin affinity. Traction force is generated and transmitted by the contraction and reinforcement of the actin cytoskeleton. The final step in cell locomotion is the release or disruption of the focal adhesion complex at the trailing edge of the migrating cell. Step 5 is accomplished by release of components of the integrin complex or via proteolytic disruption of focal adhesion kinase (FAK) connections with the filamentous action cytoskeleton.

integrin subunit of the vitronectin receptor, but not with the fibronectin receptor. This observation suggests that either Src is normally a selective inhibitor of reinforcement during force generation through the vitronectin receptor or that Src promotes the turnover of links between cytoskeletal and integrin components of the focal adhesion complex.

Investigators have used a β_1 integrin–GFP chimera to follow focal adhesion cycling over the cell surface.[62] These experiments demonstrate that in stationary cells focal adhesions were highly motile and moved in a linear fashion to the cell center. In motile cells, the focal adhesions remained stationary and only moved at the trailing edge of the cell. These authors postulate a cellular "clutch-like mechanism" in which there is alteration in integrin affinity in response to migratory stimulus. Regulation of integrin-ligand interactions by inside-out signaling helps determine the nature of cellular responses to the ECM, that is, whether a cell becomes migratory or remains stationary.

The last step in integrin-mediated cell migration is the release of the ECM-integrin-cytoskeletal attachments at the trailing edge of the cell.[57] Two mechanisms have been identified in this detachment. The first involves the release of the integrins from the cell surface. Integrin release from the cell membrane has been observed in fibroblast migration and by tumor cell lines *in vitro*.[63] A second mechanism that mediates release of the trailing edge of the cell is destabilization of cytoskeletal linkages intracellularly by either proteolytic activity or phosphatase activity. Calpain is a Ca^{2+}-dependent protease that localizes to focal adhesions and regulates retraction in CHO cells migrating on fibronectin by destabilizing cytoskeletal linkages.[64]

PROTEASES IN TUMOR CELL INVASION

Proteolytic remodeling of the ECM has been recognized as essential for tumor cell invasion. Tumor cells must be able to move through connective tissue barriers such as the basement membrane and interstitial matrix to spread from their site of origin. Although a variety of proteases have been implicated in this process, the family of proteases that has received the most attention has been the MMPs. MMPs and their specific inhibitors, the tissue inhibitors of metalloproteinases (TIMPs), play important roles in physiologic remodeling of the ECM. Approximately 26 MMPs and four TIMPs have been characterized in humans and other animals.[23,65] The MMPs share a common domain structure (Fig. 4-6), although not all domains are represented in all family members. All of the enzymes have a signal peptide sequence; a propeptide domain (prodomain); a catalytic domain, which includes a highly conserved binding site for the catalytic zinc ion; and a hemopexin-like domain. Two family members, MMP-2 and MMP-9, have a gelatin-binding domain containing three fibronectin type II repeats inserted into the catalytic domain just on the amino side of the active site sequence. Five family members have a carboxy-terminal transmembrane domain after the hemopexin domain. This subgroup is also known as the *membrane-type MMPs*, or *MT-*

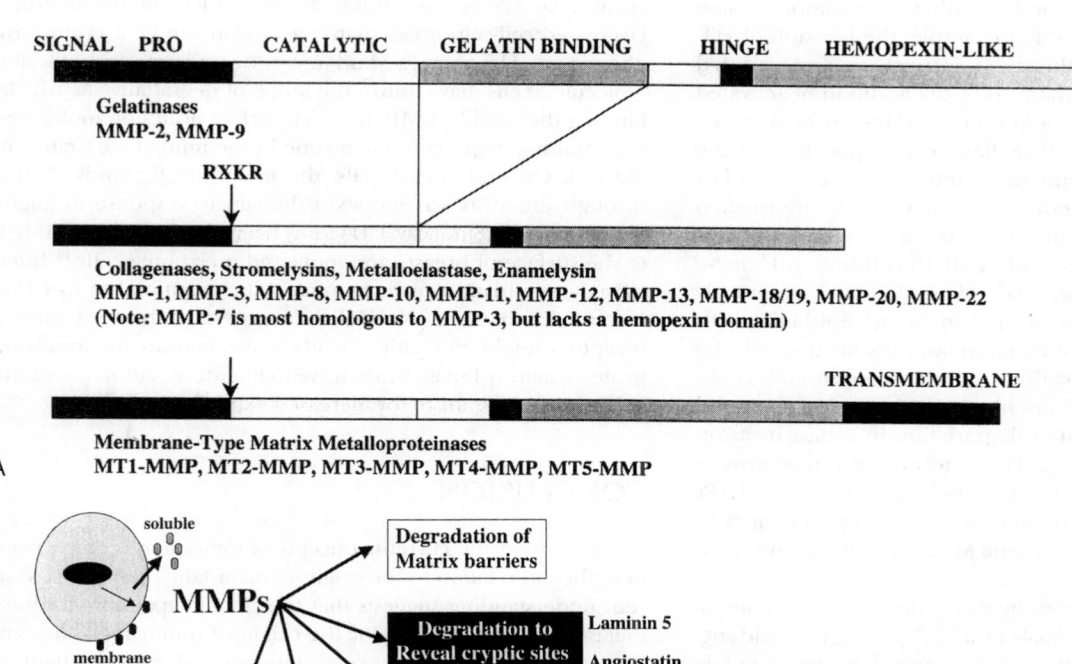

FIGURE 4-6. Matrix metalloproteinase (MMP) family members. **A:** Domain structure of MMPs. Simplified schematic domain structure of the MMPs. Most MMPs have the same basic domain structure, consisting of signal, pro, catalytic, hinge, and hemopexin-like domains. MMP-7 lacks the hemopexin-like domain, and the gelatinases and membrane-type MMPs have additional domains. The arrow indicates the location of the furin RXKR cleavage site of MMP-11 and the membrane-type MMPs. The length of each segment is roughly proportional to the number of amino acids that comprise the domain. **B:** Emerging roles of MMPs in tumor progression.

MMPs. These MT-MMPs reside on the cell surface, in contrast to the other family members, which are all secreted as proenzymes into the extracellular milieu.

The TIMPs also share a high level of homology, including 12 conserved cysteine residues that are all involved in intramolecular disulfide bonds. TIMPs are divided into two domains by the disulfide-bonding pattern. An amino-terminal domain contains the inhibitory site and a carboxy-terminal domain has other binding interactions. Because most of these enzymes are secreted in their proenzyme forms, activation is a key regulatory step. Many of the MMPs are activated by an initial protease cleavage with the prodomain by another MMP or by a serine protease such as plasmin or urokinase-type plasminogen activator. This destabilizes the bond between a conserved prodomain cysteine sulfhydryl group and the catalytic zinc in the active site. The bond breaks and the prodomains are released, which frees the active site for catalysis. Unlike the other family members, which are typically activated outside the cell, MMP-13 and the MT-MMP subgroup are activated intracellularly by a furin-dependent cleavage of a conserved RXKR sequence that lies between the prodomain and the catalytic domain. The activation mechanisms have been the subject of a review.[66]

An early indication of the importance of MMPs in tumor biology was the characterization in 1980 of an MMP secreted from a melanoma cell line that was able to degrade basement membrane collagen type IV and was initially referred to as *type IV collagenase* (now MMP-2).[67] This was followed by numerous studies showing that secretion of MMPs enhanced tumor cell invasion in experimental model systems and that inhibition of protease activity by TIMPs or by synthetic metalloproteinase inhibitors impeded invasion. For example, the invasion of HT-1080 fibrosarcoma cells through Matrigel (a reconstituted basement membrane) is enhanced by the addition of activated MMP-2 and inhibited by the addition of TIMP-2 or by zinc chelators.[68] Such *in vitro* evidence has been supported by the results of *in vivo* experiments using transfected cell lines. For example, when MYU3L bladder carcinoma cells are transfected with *mmp-2*, they have enhanced metastatic potential, whereas transfecting the highly metastatic LMC19 cell line with *timp-2* reduces its metastatic potential. Mice that are genetically engineered to overexpress MMP-3 in breast epithelial cells develop spontaneous breast carcinomas, possibly through the effects of MMP-3 on the E-cadherin/β-catenin system.[36] These experiments and many others like them have demonstrated the key role of MMP-initiated degradation in tumor invasion and metastasis. The ability of TIMPs to inhibit tumor growth and metastasis suggests that targeted inhibition of MMPs could be an effective therapeutic strategy for cancer therapy. However, clinical trials of synthetic MMP inhibitors have been disappointing.[23]

The role of these enzymes in this process is more complicated than a "degradation equals invasion" paradigm would suggest. Uninhibited matrix degradation may lead to complete dissolution of matrix proteins and would prevent tumor cells from being able to form attachments to each other or to matrix proteins, which is a necessary part of the tumor invasion mechanism. Thus, there is an implied balance between active proteases and inhibitors that would result in an optimal invasive phenotype. As a demonstration of this principle, when A2058 melanoma cells are transfected with either sense or antisense *timp-2*, the invasive potential is decreased. Increasing TIMP-2 expression in this cell line enhances cell attachment and decreases motility, whereas decreasing expression decreases cell attachment and motility. Thus, although protease activity in tumor cell invasion is abnormal, it cannot be totally unregulated.

Another possible explanation for the ineffectiveness of synthetic metalloproteinase inhibitors in clinical trials is that MMPs have been shown to have effects other than removal of structural barriers to invasion.[65] For example, some MMPs act on other proteins to reveal hidden biologic activities. MMPs, such as MMP-2 and MT-1-MMP, specifically degrade the γ2 chain of laminin-5, a structural protein in the basement membrane, to reveal a site on the α3 chain that has chemotactic properties.[69] Although the physiologic role of this fragment may be to act as a wound-related chemoattractant, in tumors this peptide may attract tumor cells to breaks in the basement membrane. In contrast, MMPs have also been shown to process monocyte chemoattractant protein-3 (MCP-3).[70] However, in this case the MMP processing of MCP-3, which results in removal of five amino acids from the N-terminus, results in loss of chemoattractant function and conversion of MCP-3 into an agonist that blocks inflammatory cell recruitment. Further complicating their role in tumor progression, MMPs have been shown to degrade plasminogen into angiostatin, the angiogenesis inhibitor.[71] Studies have focused on the interaction between cell surface adhesion molecules and the MMP family. One obvious interaction is the simple degradation of cell surface adhesion molecules. For example, MMP-3 degrades E-cadherin on mammary epithelial cells, inducing an increased expression of vimentin and decreased expression of keratin.[35] The cell matrix adhesion molecule CD44 is also cleaved by MMPs, permitting detachment from the matrix.[72] Decreased cell-cell or cell matrix adhesion can be a proinvasive phenotype. However, beyond mere degradation of adhesion molecules, cells may control the scope of degradative activity by binding the soluble MMPs with cell surface adhesion molecules, thus limiting degradation to a zone in the immediate vicinity of the cell. On endothelial cells, the integrin $\alpha_v\beta_3$ binds MMP-2 through the MMP's hemopexin domain in response to angiogenic stimuli.[73] Similarly, CD44 has been shown to bind MMP-9 to the surface of breast carcinoma and melanoma cells.[44] Interestingly, stimulation of melanoma cells by antibodies to CD44 increased expression of MMP-2,[74] suggesting that cell surface receptors might not only provide a mechanism for localizing protease activity but also may serve to initiate an autocrine-stimulating loop mechanism for increased expression of MMPs.

CONCLUSION

In this chapter the current concepts of tumorigenesis have been described in relation to the origin of metastatic tumor cells. Current understanding suggests that the clonal expansion and rare metastatic variant models for the origin of tumor metastasis are not mutually exclusive but represent two ends of a mechanistic spectrum. Primary cancers evolve through a process that contains elements of both theories, as well as a profound influence from tumor cell-host cell interactions (microenvironment). Studies using cDNA microarray analysis demonstrate that specific patterns of overall gene expression can reveal the prognosis and eventual outcome in some tumor types. Additional studies show that metastatic propensity for a specific site (osteolytic metastasis) can also be identified by a small subset of gene expression superimposed on the poor prognosis profile. Interestingly, the molecular mechanisms that mediate invasive growth and metastasis are also found in embryonic development and tissue repair processes. This suggests that tumor progression and metastasis formation represent an exaggeration of the normal developmental processes that has become dysregulated. Finally, it is increasingly apparent that the stromal microenvironment profoundly influences the process of tumor progression including metastasis formation. However, the understanding of how the many cellular events are integrated and coordinated between tumor cells and host stromal components remains incomplete.

REFERENCES

1. Nowell PC. The clonal evolution of tumor cell populations. *Science* 1976;194:23.
2. Fearon ER, Vogelstein B. A genetic model for colorectal tumorigenesis. *Cell* 1990;61:759.
3. Kinzler KW, Vogelstein B. Lessons from hereditary colorectal cancer. *Cell* 1996;87:159.
4. Bernards R, Weinberg RA. A progression puzzle. *Nature* 2002;418:823.
5. Renan MJ. How many mutations are required for tumorigenesis? Implications from human cancer data. *Mol Carcinog* 1993;7:139.
6. Loeb LA. Mutator phenotype may be required for multistep carcinogenesis. *Cancer Res* 1991;51:3073.
7. Rajagopalan H, Nowak MA, Vogelstein B, et al. The significance of unstable chromosomes in colorectal cancer. *Nat Rev Cancer* 2003;3:695.
8. Hanahan D, Weinberg RA. The hallmarks of cancer. *Cell* 2000;100:57.
9. Fidler IJ, Kripke ML. Metastasis results from pre-existing cells within a malignant tumor. *Science* 1977;197:893.
10. Fidler IJ, Hart IR. Biological diversity in metastatic neoplasms: origins and implications. *Science* 1982;217:998.
11. Kerbel RS. Growth dominance of the metastatic cancer cell: cellular and molecular aspects. *Adv Cancer Res* 1990;55:87.
12. van't Veer LJ, Dai H, van de Vijver MJ, et al. Gene expression profiling predicts clinical outcome of breast cancer. *Nature* 2002;415:530.
13. van de Vijver MJ, He YD, van't Veer LJ, et al. A gene-expression signature as a predictor of survival in breast cancer. *N Engl J Med* 1992;347:1999.
14. Ramaswamy S, Ross KN, Lander ES, et al. A molecular signature of metastasis in primary solid tumors. *Nat Genet* 2003;33:49.
15. Perou CM, Sorlie T, Eisen MB, et al. Molecular portraits of human breast tumours. *Nature* 2000;406:747.
16. Ma X-J, Salunga R, Tuggle JT, et al. Gene expression profiles of human breast cancer progression. *Proc Natl Acad Sci U S A* 2003;100:5974.
17. Clark EA, Golub TR, Lander ES, et al. Genomic analysis of metastasis reveals an essential role for RhoC. *Nature* 2000;406:532.
18. Kang Y, Siegel PM, Shu W, et al. A multigenic program mediating breast cancer metastasis to bone. *Cancer Cell* 2003;3:537.
19. Steeg PS. Metastasis suppressors alter the signal transduction of cancer cells. *Nat Rev Cancer* 2003;3:55.
20. Liotta LA, Kleinerman J, Saidel G. Quantitative relationships of intravascular tumor cells, tumor vessels and pulmonary metastasis. *Cancer Res* 1974;34:977.
21. Swartz MA, Kristensen CA, Melder RJ, et al. Cells shed from tumours show reduced clonogenicity, resistance to apoptosis, and in vivo tumorigenicity. *Br J Cancer* 1999;81:756.
22. Stephenson RA, Dinney CP, Gohji K, et al. Metastatic model for human prostate cancer using orthotopic implantation in nude mice. *J Natl Cancer Inst* 1992;84:951.
23. Coussens LM, Fingleton B, Matrisian LM. Matrix metalloproteinase inhibitors and cancer: trials and tribulations. *Science* 2002;295:2387.
24. Fidler IJ. The organ microenvironment and cancer metastasis. *Differentiation* 2002;70:498.
25. Paget S. The distribution of secondary growths in cancer of the breast. *Lancet* 1889;1:99.
26. Ewing J. Neoplastic diseases. *A treatise on tumors*. London: W.B. Saunders, 1928.
27. Müller A, Homey B, Soto H, et al. Involvement of chemokine receptor in breast cancer metastasis. *Nature* 2001;410:50.
28. Kim J, Yu W, Kovalski K, et al. Requirement for specific proteases in cancer cell intravasation as revealed by a novel semiquantitative PCR-based assay. *Cell* 1998;94:353.
29. Chambers AF, MacDonald IC, Schmidt EE, et al. Steps in tumor metastasis: new concepts from intravital videomicroscopy. *Cancer Metastasis Rev* 1995;14:279.
30. Clair T, Lee HY, Liotta LA, et al. Autotaxin is an exoenzyme possessing 5'-nucleotide phosphodiesterase/ATP pyrophosphatase and ATPase activities. *J Biol Chem* 1997; 272:996.
31. Liotta LA, Steeg PS, Stetler-Stevenson WG. Cancer metastasis and angiogenesis: an imbalance of positive and negative regulation. *Cell* 1991;64:327.
32. Suzuki ST. Protocadherins and diversity of the cadherin superfamily. *J Cell Sci* 1996;109:2609.
33. Bracke MC, van Roy FM, Mareel MM. The E-cadherin/catenin complex in invasion and metastasis. *Curr Top Microbiol Immunol* 1996;213:123.
34. Graff JR. Distinct patterns of E-cadherin CpG island methylation in papillary, follicular, Hurthle's cell, and poorly differentiated human thyroid carcinoma. *Cancer Res* 1998;58:2063.
35. Lochter A, Galosy S, Muschler J, et al. Matrix metalloproteinase stromelysin-1 triggers a
cascade of molecular alterations that lead to stable-epithelial-to-mesenchymal conversion and a premalignant phenotype in mammary epithelial cells. *J Cell Biol* 1997;139:1861.
36. Sternlicht MD, Lochter A, Sympson CJ, et al. The stromal proteinase mmp3/stromelysin-1 promotes mammary carcinogenesis. *Cell* 1999;98:137.
37. He T-C, Sparks AB, Rago C, et al. Identification of c-myc as a target of the APC pathway. *Science* 1998;281:1509.
38. Tetsu O, McCormick F. β-catenin regulated expression of cyclin d1 in colon carcinoma cells. *Nature* 1999;398:422.
39. Garofolo A, Chirivi RGS, Fogelieni C, et al. Involvement of the very late antigen 4-integrin on melanoma in interleukin-1-augmented experimental metastasis. *Cancer Res* 1995;55:414.
40. Screaton GR, Bell MV, Jackson DG, et al. Genomic structure of DNA encoding the lymphocyte homing receptor cd44 reveals at least 12 alternatively spliced exons. *Proc Natl Acad Sci U S A* 1992;89:12160.
41. Jalkanen S, Joensuu H, Soderstrom KO, et al. Lymphocyte homing and clinical behavior of non-Hodgkin's lymphoma. *J Clin Invest* 1991;87:1835.
42. Pals ST, Horst E, Ossekoppele GJ, et al. Expression of lymphocyte homing receptor as a mechanism of dissemination in non-Hodgkin's lymphoma. *Blood* 1989;73:885.
43. Sy MS, Guo YJ, Stamenkovic I. Distinct effects of two cd44 isoforms on tumor growth in vivo. *J Exp Med* 1991;174:859.
44. Yu Q, Toole BP, Stamenkovic I. Induction of apoptosis of metastatic mammary carcinoma cells in vivo by disruption of tumor cell surface cd44 function. *J Exp Med* 1997;186:1985.
45. Yamada KM. Integrin signaling. *Matrix Biol* 1997;16:137.
46. Giancotti FG, Ruoslahti E. Integrin signaling. *Science* 1999;285:1028.
47. Hughes PE, Renshaw MW, Pfaff M, et al. Suppression of integrin activation: a novel function of a Ras/Raf-initiated MAP kinase pathway. *Cell* 1997;88:521.
48. Varner JA, Emerson DA, Juliano RL. Integrin alpha 5 beta 1 expression negatively regulates cell growth: reversal by attachment to fibronectin. *Mol Biol Cell* 1995;6:725.
49. Zutter MM, Santoro SA, Staatz WD, et al. Re-expression of the alpha 2 beta 1 integrin abrogates the malignant phenotype of breast carcinoma cells. *Proc Natl Acad Sci U S A* 1995;92:7411.
50. Albelda SM, Mette SA, Elder DE, et al. Integrin distribution in malignant melanoma: association of the beta 3 subunit with tumor progression. *Cancer Res* 1990;50:6757.
51. Mitjans F, Sander D, Adan J, et al. An anti-alpha v-integrin antibody that blocks integrin function inhibits the development of a human melanoma in nude mice. *J Cell Sci* 1995;108:2825.
52. Porter JC, Hogg N. Integrins take partners: cross-talk between integrins and other membrane receptors. *Trends Cell Biol* 1998;8:390.
53. Tamura M, Gu J, Tran H, et al. PTEN gene and integrin signaling in cancer. *J Natl Cancer Inst* 1999;91:1820.
54. Shen Y, Schneider G, Cloutier JF, et al. Direct association of protein-tyrosine phosphatase PTP-PEST with paxillin. *J Biol Chem* 1998;273:6474.
55. Angers-Loustau A, Cote JF, Charest A, et al. Protein tyrosine phosphatase-pest regulates focal adhesion disassembly, migration, and cytokinesis in fibroblasts. *J Cell Biol* 1999;144:1019.
56. Tamura M, Gu J, Matsumoto K, et al. Inhibition of cell migration, spreading, and focal adhesions by tumor suppressor PTEN. *Science* 1998;280:1614.
57. Lauffenburger DA, Horowitz AF. Cell migration: a physically integrated molecular process. *Cell* 1996;84:359.
58. Gumbiner BM. Cell adhesion: the molecular basis of tissue architecture and morphogenesis. *Cell* 1996;84:345.
59. Mitchison TJ, Cramer LP. Actin-base cell motility and cell locomotion. *Cell* 1996;84:371.
60. Tapon N, Hall A. Rho, Rac and Cdc42 GTPases regulate the organization of the actin cytoskeleton. *Curr Opin Cell Biol* 1997;9:86.
61. Felsenfeld DP, Schwartzberg PL, Venegas A, et al. Selective regulation of integrin–cytoskeleton interactions by the tyrosine kinase Src. *Nat Cell Biol* 1999;1:200.
62. Smilenov LB, Mikhailov A, Pelham RJ, et al. Focal adhesion motility revealed in stationary fibroblasts. *Science* 1999;286:1172.
63. Palecek SP, Schmidt CE, Lauffenburger DA, et al. Integrin dynamics on the tail region of migrating fibroblasts. *J Cell Sci* 1996;109:941.
64. Huttenlocher A, Palecek SP, Lu Q, et al. Regulation of cell migration by the calcium-dependent protease calpain. *J Biol Chem* 1997;272:32719.
65. Egeblad M, Werb Z. New functions for the matrix metalloproteinases in cancer progression. *Nat Rev Cancer* 2002;2:161.
66. Murphy G, Stanton H, Cowell S, et al. Mechanisms for pro matrix metalloproteinase activation. *AMPIS* 1999;107:38.
67. Liotta LA, Tryggvason K, Garbisa S, et al. Metastatic potential correlates with enzymatic degradation of basement membrane collagen. *Nature* 1980;284:67.
68. Albini A, Melchiori A, Santi L, et al. Tumor cell invasion inhibited by timp-2. *J Natl Cancer Inst* 1991;83:775.
69. Giannelli G, Falk-Marzillier J, Schiraldi O, et al. Induction of cell migration by matrix metalloprotease-2 cleavage of laminin-5. *Science* 1997;277:225.
70. McQuibban GA, Gong JH, Tam EM, et al. Inflammation dampened by gelatinase a cleavage of monocyte chemoattractant protein-3. *Science* 2000;289:1202.
71. O'Reilly MS, Wiederschain D, Stetler-Stevenson WG, et al. Regulation of angiostatin production by matrix metalloproteinase-2 in a model of concomitant resistance. *J Biol Chem* 1999;274:29568.
72. Okamoto I, Kawano Y, Tsuiki H, et al. Cd44 cleavage induced by a membrane-associated metalloprotease plays a critical role in tumor cell migration. *Oncogene* 1999;18:1435.
73. Brooks PC, Stromblad S, Sanders LC, et al. Localization of matrix metalloproteinase mmp-2 to the surface of invasive cells by interaction with integrin alpha v beta 3. *Cell* 1996;85:683.
74. Takahashi K, Eto H, Tanabe KK. Involvement of cd44 in matrix metalloproteinase-2 regulation in human melanoma cells. *Int J Cancer* 1999;80:387.

Isaiah J. Fidler
Robert R. Langley
Robert S. Kerbel
Lee M. Ellis

CHAPTER **5**

Angiogenesis

The progressive growth of neoplasms and the production of metastasis depend on the establishment of adequate blood supply—that is, angiogenesis.[1,2] The process of angiogenesis consists of multiple, sequential, and interdependent steps. It begins with local degradation of the basement membrane surrounding capillaries, which is followed by invasion of the surrounding stroma by the underlying endothelial cells in the direction of the angiogenic stimulus. Endothelial cell migration is accompanied by the proliferation of endothelial cells and their organization into three-dimensional structures that join with other similar structures to form a network of new blood vessels (Fig. 5-1). This is sometimes referred to as *sprouting angiogenesis*, which is a local process. In addition, endothelial cells can be generated not only by the division of preexisting differentiated endothelial cells but also by the influx of bone marrow–derived circulating endothelial progenitor cells, a process sometimes referred to as *systemic vasculogenesis*.[2]

The diffusion coefficient of oxygen within tissues is 150 to 200 μm.[3] Double labeling of tissue sections for bromodeoxyuridine uptake (cell division) and CD31 reactivity (endothelium) and end-labeling assay (terminal uridine nick end labeling, or TUNEL) to detect apoptotic cells revealed that all dividing tumor cells within autochthonous human lung cancer brain metastases were located within 75 μm of the nearest vessel (Fig. 5-2A), whereas apoptotic tumor cells in autochthonous human lung cancer brain metastases were located 150 to 170 μm from the nearest blood vessel (Fig. 5-2B).[4] These data clearly demonstrate that the location of both dividing and apoptotic tumor cells within autochthonous brain metastases is related to the diffusion coefficient of oxygen within tissues. Hence, a tumor mass that is less than 0.5 mm in diameter can receive oxygen and nutrients by diffusion, but any increase in tumor mass beyond 0.5 mm requires the proliferation and morphogenesis of vascular endothelial cells.[4]

NEOPLASTIC ANGIOGENESIS

The onset of angiogenesis involves an alteration in the balance between proangiogenic and antiangiogenic molecules in the local tissue microenvironment.[1,2,5] These molecules mediate multiple steps in the process of angiogenesis by selectively altering the characteristics of endothelial cells and associated perivascular structures (i.e., pericytes, vascular smooth muscle cells). Angiogenesis can occur by either sprouting or nonsprouting processes.[5] Sprouting angiogenesis involves the branching of new capillaries from preexisting vessels. Nonsprouting angiogenesis results from the enlargement, splitting, and fusion of preexisting vessels produced by the proliferation of endothelial cells within the wall of a vessel. Transvascular bridges are sometimes observed in enlarged vessels produced by nonsprouting angiogenesis.[5] This type of angiogenesis can occur concurrently with sprouting angiogenesis in the vascularization of organs or tissues such as the lung and heart. The mechanism of nonsprouting angiogenesis was found in brain metastases, and vascular endothelial growth factor (VEGF), also called *vascular permeability factor* (VPF),[6–8] has a pivotal role in developmental, physiologic, and pathologic neovascularization.

VEGF/VPF was initially detected as a factor secreted by tumor cells into tissue culture medium or ascites fluid *in vivo*.[7] The factor was identified as a heparin-binding protein with a molecular weight of 34 to 42 kD and was termed VPF. It was later demonstrated that VPF also stimulated endothelial cell division. Independently, several groups isolated a secreted

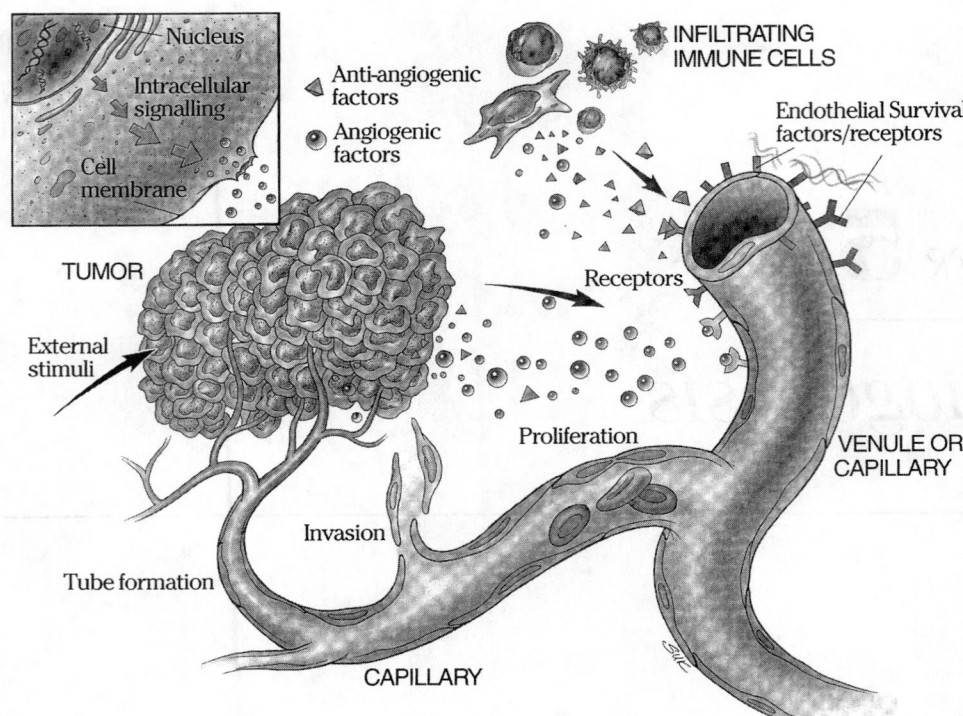

FIGURE 5-1. The angiogenic process. The process of angiogenesis is a series of linked and sequential steps that ultimately leads to the development of a neovascular blood supply to the tumor mass. Different steps in the angiogenic process may be occurring in different parts of the tumor at the same time. Tumor cells or host cells (infiltrating immune cells or adjacent normal tissue) secrete angiogenic growth factors, which then bind to specific receptors on endothelial cells. This ligand-receptor interaction leads to endothelial cell proliferation, migration, invasion, and eventually capillary tube formation. Factors also affect endothelial cell survival under adverse conditions that occur in tumors. The proangiogenic process is balanced by the activity of antiangiogenic molecules that are necessary for homeostatic processes. When the activity of the proangiogenic molecules exceeds the activity of the antiangiogenic molecules, new blood vessel formation occurs. Proangiogenic factors may be constitutively expressed, but their expression may be increased by certain stimuli such as hypoxia, low pH, cytokines, growth factors, tumor size, activated oncogenes, signal transduction pathways, or loss of tumor suppressor gene function.

protein that had selective mitogenic activity for cultured endothelial cells, which they called VEGF.[8] On the basis of amino acid and complementary DNA sequence analysis, it is now known that VEGF and VPF are the same protein, and VEGF is now the term more commonly used to describe this angiogenic factor.

VEGF is a homodimeric heparin-binding glycoprotein that exists in at least four isoforms due to alternative splicing of the primary messenger RNA transcript. The isoforms are designated $VEGF_{121}$, $VEGF_{165}$, $VEGF_{189}$, and $VEGF_{205}$ according to the number of amino acids each protein contains. The vascular permeability induced by VEGF/VPF is 50,000 times that induced by histamine, the standard for induction of permeability. Induction of permeability by VEGF allows for the diffusion of proteins into the interstitium on which endothelial cells migrate.

There are at least four other members of the VEGF family. The aforementioned VEGF is referred to as VEGF-A. VEGF-B most likely plays an important role in vasculogenesis but may have other functions such as activation of invasive enzymes on endothelial cells.[8,9] VEGF-C is most commonly associated with lymphangiogenesis, but more recently, its expression has been associated with tumor angiogenesis in several systems. The role of VEGF-D is less well defined, but this protein may bind to VEGF receptor-2 (VEGFR-2) and VEGFR-3 and may induce *in vivo* angiogenesis. Little is known about VEGF-E, except that it binds to VEGFR-2 and can induce endothelial cell mitosis and angiogenesis.[9]

The receptors for VEGF are expressed on endothelial cells and some tumor cells.[8] Three VEGF/VPF receptors have been identified. The fms-like tyrosine kinase (Flt-1) and fetal liver kinase 1 (Flk-1)/kinase insert domain–containing receptor (KDR) are high-affinity VEGF/VPF receptors with an extracellular domain containing seven immunoglobulin-like domains and a split tyrosine kinase intracellular domain.[8] Flk-1 has 85% homology with the human homologue, KDR. Both Flt-1 and Flk-1/KDR have been shown to be important regulatory systems for vasculogenesis and physiologic angiogenesis.[8,9] However, the interaction of VEGF/VPF with Flk-1/KDR is thought to be the more important interaction for tumor angiogenesis because it is essential for induction of the full spectrum of VEGF/VPF functions.[8] Blockade of VEGF/VPF activities mediated by Flk-1/KDR has been shown to have antiangiogenic activity,[10] and VEGFR-3 (Flt-4) has been shown to be the receptor for VEGF-C.[9]

Another family of endothelial cell-specific molecules is the angiopoietin (Ang) family. The best characterized are Ang-1 and Ang-2, which bind to the specific tyrosine kinase receptor Tie-2 on endothelial cells. Ang-1 acts as an agonist and is involved in endothelial cell differentiation and stabilization, whereas Ang-2 binds to Tie-2 and blocks the binding of Ang-1 to this receptor, which leads to endothelial cell destabilization and vascular regression.[10]

The development of knockout mice has provided a useful method to study the role of various factors in angiogenesis. Homozygous knockout mice for VEGF or any of the VEGFRs leads to embryonic death due to defective vascular development.[10,11] Knockout for Ang-1, Ang-2, Tie-1, and Tie-2 also lead to defective vascular development and embryonic lethality. Numerous nonspecific angiogenic molecules affect not only the growth of endothelial cells but the growth of other cell types as well. These factors include the fibroblast growth factors (FGFs) (acidic and basic); transforming growth factor-α; epidermal growth factor (EGF); platelet-derived growth factor (PDGF); platelet-derived endothelial cell growth factor; angiogenin; and the CXC chemokines interleukin-8, macrophage inflammatory

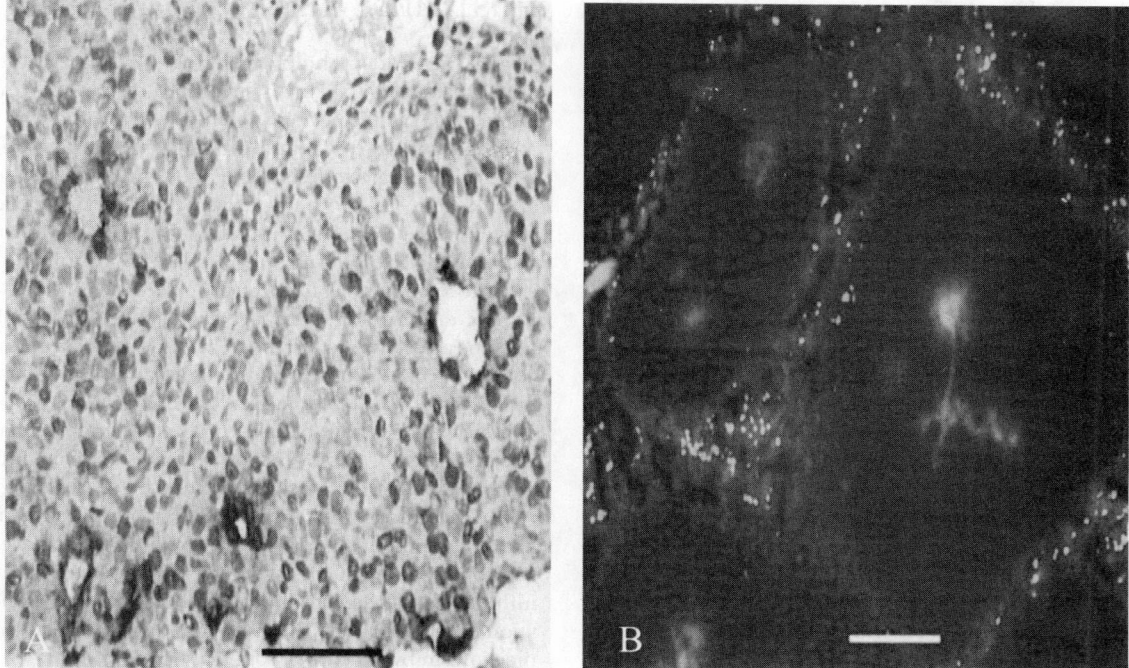

FIGURE 5-2. Dividing and apoptotic tumor cells in brain metastasis. Location of dividing and apoptotic lung cancer cells in relation to blood vessels in autochthonous brain metastases. **A:** Cells staining positive for bromodeoxyuridine uptake are red. Mean distance from nearest blood vessel is 74 μm. **B:** Apoptotic cells staining positive with terminal uridine nick end labeling (TUNEL) are bright green. Mean distance from nearest blood vessel is 167 μm. Bars = 100 μm. (From ref. 4, with permission.) (See Color Fig. 5-2 in the CD-ROM.)

protein, platelet factor-4, and growth-related oncogene-α. These multiple factors regulate different aspects of angiogenesis.[12] For example, basic FGF (bFGF) is the most potent mitogen for endothelial cells, followed by VEGF and platelet-derived endothelial cell growth factor. VEGF, bFGF, and PDGF are also potent survival factors for endothelial cells.[1] However, bFGF is the angiogenic factor most associated with increasing activity of degradative enzymes. Hepatocyte growth factor enhances endothelial cell motility more than any other angiogenic factor studied. The more recent recognition of Ang-1 and Ang-2 and their role in endothelial cell stabilization suggests that these molecules are also important in endothelial cell survival.[10]

PHENOTYPIC DIVERSITY OF ORGAN-SPECIFIC ENDOTHELIAL CELLS

Hematopoietic stem cells and endothelial progenitor cells that originate from either the bone marrow or other tissues may also participate in the neovascularization process of wound healing, limb ischemia, arteriosclerosis, postmyocardial infarction, and cancer. At present, considerable effort is directed toward determining the factors that mobilize and direct these cells to sites of neovascularization. Regardless of their origin, endothelial cells in the vasculature of different organs express different receptors.[13] Phage-display technology has enabled *in vivo* identification of organ-specific tumor vessels' "zip codes."[13] Because the initial establishment of

metastasis involves recognition of endothelial cell receptors by circulating metastatic tumor cells,[14] understanding these interactions is a major goal of research. Until recently, efforts to isolate and propagate organ-specific endothelial cells have not been successful because the cells fail to proliferate multiple times under *in vitro* conditions.

Commercially available endothelial cell lines may alleviate some of the purification concerns, but at present, cells from only a very few tissues are available. For these reasons, many of the examinations between tumor and endothelial cells have been performed on human umbilical vein endothelial cell lines. Because these cells are from a tissue that is not associated with metastasis, it remains unclear whether these cells provide a relevant model system. To overcome these limitations, the authors used two-color flow cytometry to identify and select microvascular endothelial cells from primary cultures obtained from different organs of mice whose tissues harbor a temperature-sensitive SV40 large T antigen (*H-2K^b-ts*A58 mice; ImmortoMice). The selection strategy targeted cell populations expressing the inducible endothelial cell adhesion molecules E-selectin and vascular cell adhesion molecule-1, and proved successful in generating microvascular endothelial cell lines from a number of different organs. When cultured under a permissive temperature (33°C), the cells rapidly proliferated. At a nonpermissive temperature (37°C), the cells differentiated and entered a quiescent state. The cell lines exhibited many inherent endothelial properties and formed loop structures on Matrigel surfaces.[15] The endothelial cell lines of different organs possess distinct growth factor profiles. For example, the most potent mitogen for endothelial cells of the bone is bFGF, whereas for those of the uterus, it is EGF. PDGF is a potent survival factor for endothelial cells of the bone but not those of the lung. The availability of endothelial cells from different organs may be useful for identifying factors that regulate proliferation and tumor cell adhesion in different vascular beds.

TUMOR VASCULATURE

The vasculature in progressively growing neoplasms is often associated with inefficient blood supply.[4] Because tumor cell proliferation can often exceed development of new blood vessels, the vascular space can decrease as tumors enlarge.[1,4] Consequently, most tumors are hypoxic and rely on physiologic hypoxia-sensing mechanisms such as hypoxia-inducible factor-1 (HIF-1).[16] HIF-1 is comprised of an $\alpha\beta$ heterodimer in which the α subunits are inducible by hypoxia, whereas the β subunits are constitutively expressed nuclear proteins. Declining oxygen tension stabilizes HIF-1α and promotes its accumulation in the nucleus, where it heterodimerizes with HIF-1β to initiate the transcription of a number of genes implicated in angiogenesis, invasion, and metastasis.

Hypoxia also induces that expression of PDGF.[17] To date, four PDGF polypeptide chains have been identified that combine to form five PDGF isoforms: PDGF-AA, -AB, -BB, -CC, and -DD. The isoforms bind to and activate their tyrosine kinase receptors, α and β. The specific role of the PDGF isoforms in neoplastic angiogenesis depends on the specific organ microenvironment. For example, in pancreatic carcinomas, PDGF signaling provides integrity to developing vascular networks by recruiting mural cells to support the immature vessel wall.[18] In gliomas, PDGF promotes the neovascularization of cerebral lesions by stimulating the release of VEGF from tumor-associated endothelium. Tumors growing in the subcutaneous space, however, rely on PDGF-BB to regulate the level of interstitial fluid pressure within the tumor. In the bone microenvironment, activation of PDGF receptor (PDGFR) on tumor-associated vessels has been shown to be essential for progression of androgen-independent prostate tumors.[19] In normal tissues, endothelial cells rarely proliferate, whereas in neoplasms, endothelial cell turnover is common.[20] The rate of endothelial cell proliferation varies among different human neoplasms. Data from a detailed study using a double-labeling immunohistochemical approach to measure proliferating endothelial cells in a broad panel of autochthonous human tumors documented that glioblastomas and renal cell carcinomas possess the highest density of capillary beds with endothelial cell proliferation of 9.6% and 9.4%, respectively. The rate of endothelial cell proliferation in lung and prostate tumors is the lowest (2.6% and 2.0%, respectively). The magnitude of tumor angiogenesis was 4 to 20 times less intense than the physiologic angiogenesis associated with the growing ovarian rubrum.[20] Collectively, this study emphasizes the need for caution when attempting to compare the results generated from murine tumors that grow exponentially over a period of a few weeks (usually in the subcutis) to human neoplasms that progressively grow over months or even years.

HOST-MEDIATED ANGIOGENESIS

Physiologic and pathologic angiogenesis can be regulated by positive and negative factors released by parenchymal cells and circulating lymphoid cells such as T lymphocytes, mast cells, and macrophages.[21] Immunologic mechanisms involved in physiologic angiogenesis occur subsequent to wound healing,[21] and systemic chemotherapy has been shown to retard the process of wound healing, possibly by decreasing angiogenesis mediated by circulating lymphoid cells. Tumor vascularization is retarded in mice myelosuppressed by systemic administration of doxorubicin compared with that in control mice.[22] In mice treated with doxorubicin and injected with normal spleen cells 1 day before tumor challenge, tumor growth was comparable to that in control mice.[22]

Macrophages have been recognized as important angiogenesis effector cells for a number of years.[21] They may influence new capillary growth by several different mechanisms. First, macrophages produce factors that act directly to influence angiogenesis-linked endothelial cell functions. *In vitro* studies have shown that macrophages produce in excess of 20 molecules that reportedly influence endothelial cell proliferation, migration, and differentiation *in vitro* and that are potentially angiogenic *in vivo*. A second mechanism by which macrophages might modulate angiogenesis is by modifying the extracellular matrix (ECM). The composition of the ECM has been shown to influence endothelial cell shape and morphology dramatically and may profoundly influence new capillary growth.[23] Macrophages can influence the composition of the ECM either through the direct production of ECM components or through the production of proteases, which effectively alter the structure and composition of the ECM. A third mechanism is by producing substances that suppress angiogenesis.

Activated macrophages influence the angiogenic process by secreting enzymes that can break down the ECM and by secreting angiogenic molecules and growth factors such as bFGF, transforming growth factor-α and -β, insulin-like growth factor-1, PDGF, and VEGF/VPF.[24] These factors induce endothelial cells to migrate and proliferate. The number of macrophages infiltrating human ovarian cancers has been shown to directly correlate with the microvessel density, and macrophages isolated from ascitic fluid aspirated from women with advanced ovarian cancer have been shown to produce angiogenic effects *in vitro* and *in vivo*.[25] Moreover, the expression of matrix metalloprotease-9 (MMP-9) in clinical samples of ovarian tumors is associated with epithelial and stromal cells.[25]

High levels of MMP-2 and MMP-9 (also called *type IV collagenases* or *gelatinases*) in tissues have been associated with active neovascularization.[26] Indeed, inhibitors of MMPs, such as tissue inhibitor of MMP-2 (TIMP-2), have been shown to inhibit *in vitro* proliferation and tube formation by endothelial cells. TIMP-2 as well as tissue inhibitor of MMP-1 (TIMP-1) have been shown to suppress *in vivo* angiogenesis.

To determine the source of MMP-2 and MMP-9 in neoplastic angiogenesis, human ovarian cancer cells SKOV3.ip1 and HEY-A8, which express low and high levels of MMP-9, respectively, were implanted into the peritoneal cavities of nude mice that lacked the gene for MMP-9 (MMP-9$^{-/-}$) or had wild-type MMP-9 (MMP-9$^{+/+}$). Regardless of the expression level of MMP-2 and MMP-9 by ovarian tumor cells, progressive tumor growth and carcinomatosis were statistically significantly lower in MMP-9$^{-/-}$ mice than in MMP-9$^{+/+}$ mice.[27] Reconstitution of

MMP-9$^{-/-}$ mice with spleen cells collected from postnatal MMP-9$^{+/+}$ mice led to increased angiogenesis and tumorigenicity of human ovarian cancer. Double immunofluorescence staining demonstrated that the growing tumors contained MMP-9$^{+/+}$ macrophages.[27] These data suggest that deficiency of MMP-9 in host cells (but not in tumor cells) inhibited neoplastic angiogenesis and, hence, the carcinomatosis of human ovarian cancers. Targeting MMP-9 in tumor cells, and more so in host cells, may therefore be an effective approach to controlling angiogenesis and carcinomatosis of human ovarian tumors.

OVERVIEW OF ANTIANGIOGENIC AND ANTIVASCULAR THERAPIES

ANTI–VASCULAR ENDOTHELIAL GROWTH FACTOR APPROACHES

Most of the novel antiangiogenic agents currently being evaluated in the clinic target the VEGF/VPF ligand-receptor system. VEGF is an attractive target because its receptors are expressed almost exclusively on endothelial cells and are up-regulated on tumor endothelium compared to the surrounding normal endothelium.[8] Agents that target the VEGF ligand-receptor system are currently being studied in clinical trials (summarized in Table 5-1). Many of these agents, specifically the tyrosine kinase inhibitors, also demonstrate some (albeit less) activity against other tyrosine kinase receptors, such as the EGF receptor or PDGFR. Thus far, agents that target the VEGF ligand-receptor system have shown relatively little toxicity in clinical trials compared to the toxicity of standard chemotherapy; however, adverse effects such as hypertension, headaches, nausea, proteinuria, and thrombotic events have been reported. The long-term effects of antiangiogenic therapy are as yet unknown.

ENDOGENOUS ANTIANGIOGENIC AGENTS

One class of antiangiogenic agents, currently in various phases of preclinical and clinical trials, are proteins or cleavage products of proteins known to be produced *in vivo*. Many of these agents, such as angiostatin and endostatin, were discovered as products of primary tumors that could inhibit the growth and angiogenesis of distant metastases.[1] Numerous potential explanations for the mechanism of action of endogenous antiangiogenic agents have been proposed, including inhibition of activation of MMPs, dephosphorylation of endothelial nitric oxide synthase, and changes in endothelial cell proliferation and adhesion via binding to adenosine triphosphate synthase. However, the exact mechanism of action for many of these agents remains unknown.

Thrombospondin (TSP) is a high-molecular-weight multifunctional glycoprotein that was first described as a product of platelets in response to activation of thrombin.[28] TSP is present in the ECM of a wide variety of tissues and contains binding sites for several ECM- and cell-associated molecules. TSP is synthesized and secreted by fibroblasts, vascular smooth muscle cells, monocytes, and macrophages as well as neoplastic cells. Of the five subtypes of TSP (TSP-1, -2, -3, -4, and -5), TSP-1 and TSP-2 have been implicated in the inhibition of angiogenesis. The expression of TSP-1 and TSP-2 has been inversely related to vessel counts in numerous tumor systems.[28]

A large, growing, and structurally diverse family of endogenous protein inhibitors of angiogenesis has been discovered, for example, TSP-1[29]; interferon-α, interferon-β, and interferon-γ[30]; and angiostatin, endostatin, and vasostatin.[30] Some of these are internal fragments of various proteins that normally lack any antiangiogenic activity; for example, the active component of angiostatin comprises one or more fragments of plasminogen, and endostatin is a fragment of type XVIII collagen.[31]

The generation of angiostatin by subcutaneous Lewis lung carcinoma requires the presence of macrophages and is directly correlated with their metalloelastase activity.[32] For example, the addition of plasminogen to Lewis lung carcinoma cells cultured *in vitro* did not result in generation of angiostatin, whereas the addition of plasminogen to co-cultures of macrophages and 3LL cells did. Elastase activity in macrophages was up-regulated by the cytokine granulocyte-macrophage colony-stimulating factor. Granulocyte-macrophage colony-stimulating factor secreted by Lewis lung carcinoma cells significantly enhanced the produc-

TABLE 5-1. Partial List of Antiangiogenic Agents Directly Targeting the VEGFR, EGFR, and PDGFR Pathways

Agent	Company	Phase of Trial	Mechanism of Action
IMC1121	ImClone Systems	I	Antibody against VEGFR-2
Bevacizumab (Avastin)	Genentech	II/III[a]	Antibody against VEGF
CEP-7055	Cephalon	I	RTK against VEGFR
PTK787/ZK222584	Novartis/Schering	III	RTK against VEGFR
SU11248	Pfizer	I	RTK against VEGFR, PDGFR
VEGF Trap	Regeneron/Aventis	I/II	Soluble receptor hybrid of VEGF
ZD6474	Astra Zeneca	II	RTK against VEGFR, EGFR
AG013736	Pfizer	I	RTK against VEGFR, PDGFR
AEE788	Novartis	I	RTK against VEGFR, EGFR
CP-547,632	Pfizer	I	RTK against VEGFR, bFGFR
STI 571 [imatinib (Gleevec)]	Novartis	I/II	RTK against PDGFR

bFGFR, basic fibroblast growth factor receptor; EGFR, epidermal growth factor receptor; PDGFR, platelet-derived growth factor receptor; RTK, receptor tyrosine kinase; VEGF, vascular endothelial growth factor; VEGFR, vascular endothelial growth factor receptor.
Note: The authors' intent is to provide a general overview of the many agents in clinical trials at this time. The status of these agents may change by the time of publication. For an update, please visit http://www.cancertrials.gov.
Receptor tyrosine kinase inhibitors are not specific but preferentially target receptors at concentrations far below that of other tyrosine kinases.
[a]Under U.S. Food and Drug Administration review for colorectal cancer.

tion of elastase by macrophages and hence the generation of angiostatin from plasminogen.[32] These data suggest that elastase released from tumor-infiltrating macrophages is responsible for the angiostatin production in this tumor model and the angiogenesis-inhibiting role of macrophages.

As stated in Neoplastic Angiogenesis, earlier in this chapter, neoplastic angiogenesis is triggered as a result of a shift in the balance of stimulators to inhibitors. When the ratio is low, tumor angiogenesis is blocked or modest in magnitude; in contrast, when the ratio is high, the angiogenic switch is turned to the On position. For example, the loss of wild-type p53 gene function can result in a loss of TSP expression.[29] Furthermore, it is now increasingly recognized that oncogenes such as mutant ras or src may also contribute to tumor angiogenesis by influencing (i.e., enhancing) the production of proangiogenic molecules such as VEGF/VPF, bFGF, and PDGF.

Paracrine EGF signaling from tumor cells to microvascular endothelial cells has also been shown to be an important component of the growth of pancreatic metastases in the liver. Use of either a monoclonal antibody blocking strategy (C225) or protein tyrosine kinase that specifically inhibit EGF-R signaling in combination with gemcitabine has been shown to dramatically reduce both primary pancreatic cancer (L3.6pl) growth and liver metastatic burden. These combination therapies were associated with down-regulation of VEGF in the tumor region and apoptosis of tumor-associated endothelial cells.[33]

VASCULAR TARGETING AGENTS

Antiangiogenic agents act to specifically inhibit endothelial cell function, which leads to a decrease in the formation of new vessels. In contrast, vascular targeting agents attack the *existing* neovasculature and are intended to induce tumor endothelial cell apoptosis and subsequent microvessel thrombosis. Examples of vascular targeting agents include antibodies that specifically target antigens expressed on tumor endothelium, derivatives of flavone acetic acid, and agents that bind the colchicine site of tubulin.[34,35]

Other vascular targeting agents, such as the tubulin-binding agents, act to selectively destroy the tumor vasculature via polymerization of the endothelial cell microtubules. This polymerization causes a disruption of the endothelial cell cytoskeleton, which results in microvessel thrombosis and secondary tumor cell death.[36]

ANTIVASCULAR THERAPY FOR BONE METASTASIS

PDGF and the PDGFR are coexpressed in many human carcinomas, including those of the stomach, pancreas, lung, and prostate. The binding of PDGF to PDGFR can stimulate cell division, cell migration, and angiogenesis.[37] PDGF binding causes PDGFR activation, which involves dimerization and autophosphorylation (i.e., activation) of specific tyrosines in the cytoplasmic domain of PDGFR. The phosphotyrosines serve as targets for cytoplasmic effector proteins involved in signal transduction. Activation of PDGFR has also been shown to inhibit some apoptotic pathways in normal cells and in tumor cells.[38] Hence, inhibition of PDGFR activation may decrease cell proliferation and increase the rate of cell death. PDGF and PDGFR may play criti-

cal roles in the osteotropism of human prostate cancer cells and the development of bone metastases.

STI 571, a derivative of 2-phenylaminopyrimidine, was originally developed as a competitor for an adenosine triphosphate–binding site of the Abl protein tyrosine kinase.[39] STI 571 is also a potent inhibitor of the tyrosine kinase activities of c-KIT and PDGFR, and it inhibits cell proliferation and induces apoptosis.[40]

The authors examined whether oral administration of STI 571, with or without intraperitoneal injections of paclitaxel, could inhibit the growth of androgen-independent human prostate cancer cells in the bone of nude mice. The data show that these cells growing in the tibia of nude mice express high levels of PDGF and the PDGFR, and that the PDGFR was autophosphorylated. After the bone lysed, tumor cells grew in the surrounding musculature. The tumor cells that grew in the musculature of the leg (distant from bony tissue) expressed low levels of PDGF and PDGFR. The endothelial cells within the bone lesions expressed activated PDGFR, whereas the endothelial cells in uninvolved bone or in the human prostate cancer–derived lesions in the muscles did not. Oral administration of STI 571 in combination with paclitaxel (Taxol) (administered by intraperitoneal injection) was associated with a reduction in the phosphorylation of PDGFR and an increase in apoptosis in endothelial cells and tumor cells that expressed PDGFR; treatment with STI 571 plus paclitaxel was associated with a statistically significant inhibition of the growth of bone lesions (tumors) and preservation of bone structure as determined by digital radiography and histologic examinations.[19] The finding that the prostate cancer cells growing adjacent to the bone expressed PDGF and PDGFR, whereas cells growing in the muscle or in long-term culture did not, provides an example of the "seed and soil" hypothesis, which states that the organ microenvironment can influence the phenotype of tumor cells.[14]

Treatment of mice with STI 571 plus paclitaxel was associated with a decrease in the incidence and size of tumors in the bone and musculature compared with treatment of mice with water or paclitaxel alone. Mice treated with STI 571 plus paclitaxel had statistically significantly fewer dividing tumor cells in bone lesions than mice treated with paclitaxel alone or with water. PDGF directly depolymerizes microtubules during the initiation of DNA synthesis and cell division.[41] STI 571 inhibits PDGF-mediated receptor phosphorylation and hence stabilizes microtubules in the target cells, a process similar to the mechanism of action of paclitaxel—that is, lowering the critical concentration of tubulin monomers for polymerization and promotion of tubulin assembly into distinct microtubule bundles with stability against depolymerization. Thus, combining the two drugs produces additive therapeutic effects.

Endothelial cell function, proliferation, and survival depend on the expression of specific receptors to these and other factors, and inhibition of the interactions of these factors with their receptors can lead to endothelial cell apoptosis.[42] Destruction of vasculature within neoplasms is known to produce necrosis of actively growing tumors. Hence, the induction of apoptosis in tumor-associated endothelial cells (within the bone lesions) produces regression of the tumors.

Blockade of the EGF receptor or PDGFR can alter phosphatidylinositol 3' kinase activity and lead to a change in interstitial fluid homeostasis, which results in a reduction of interstitial hypertension with an increase in transcapillary transport.[43] The role of EGF and PDGF in angiogenesis has been reported for several human tumors, and destruction of the vasculature within neoplasms can produce necrosis of actively growing tumors.[44] The induction of apoptosis in tumor-associated endothelial cells suggests that this regimen of therapy is directed against tumor vasculature. Activation of the PDGFR has been shown to increase expression of Bcl-2 and PI3K/Akt and to decrease the level of caspase in cells, that is, increase resistance to apoptosis. Because treatment of cells with STI 571 increases their sensitivity to an anticycling drug (e.g., paclitaxel), the results support the hypothesis that PDGF could be a survival factor for tumor cells.

CLINICAL STUDIES OF IMATINIB

To translate the preclinical observations of PDGFR inhibition with imatinib [STI 571 (Gleevec)] in combination with cytotoxic therapy, a modular phase I trial including men with androgen-independent prostate cancer was carried out.[45] Twenty-eight men, who were largely pretreated with chemotherapy, were recruited to this study. A lead-in period of 30 days with imatinib alone at 600 mg daily was followed by weekly docetaxel for 4 weeks in 6-week cycles. During the lead-in period with imatinib alone, 7% of patients showed a decline in prostate-specific antigen (PSA) levels of less than 50% whereas 89% showed a progression in PSA levels. Twenty-one patients were subsequently treated with the imatinib plus docetaxel combination therapy, and of these 38% had a greater than 50% decline in PSA levels, 29% had a less than 50% decline in PSA levels, and 33% had progression in PSA level. These results indicate that treatment with imatinib and docetaxel lowers PSA levels with greater efficacy than imatinib alone (67% vs. 7%, respectively). Toxicity appeared manageable at docetaxel levels of 30 mg/m² and lower. Long-term responders with combination therapy were observed in this heavily pretreated group. A decline in PDGFR-expressing tumor was seen in serial bone biopsies after combination therapy but not after imatinib alone.[45] These results support the rationale that a heterogeneous disease such as cancer should be treated by combination therapy targeting both tumor cells and the host microenvironmental factors, such as the tumor vasculature.

DISCREPANCY BETWEEN RESULTS OF PRECLINICAL AND CLINICAL TRIALS

Preclinical studies have shown great promise for antiangiogenic therapy, even in single-agent studies. Clinical trials of antiangiogenic agents have yielded mixed results.[33] For example, disappointing results from a phase III clinical trial with SU5416, a VEGFR-2 tyrosine kinase inhibitor, plus chemotherapy led to the decision that this agent would be dropped from further clinical development. The poor results with SU5416 were surprising, because preclinical studies demonstrated that this agent had promise in treating experimental metastasis.[46] These findings raise the question of why an agent that produces significant therapy in preclinical studies fails to produce significant effects in cancer patients.

There are several potential reasons why success in preclinical studies has not translated to success in the clinical setting. First, in preclinical models, tumors are not always grown in the ortho-

topic site. The site of tumor growth is an important determinant of efficacy in preclinical studies and may also be important in evaluating the efficacy of antiangiogenic therapy in clinical trials. Endothelium from different organs clearly is phenotypically distinct,[13–15] and therefore therapy that is effective at one site may be ineffective at another. Hence, the most relevant models for evaluating antiangiogenic therapy in preclinical studies are orthotopic or transgenic models in which the tumor is growing in the appropriate host microenvironment.

Second, the age and maturity of the vasculature in preclinical studies may not be equivalent to that found in clinical cancer. Tumor xenografts contain newly formed blood vessels, usually only days to weeks old, whereas in patients, tumors become clinically apparent (i.e., 1 to 2 cm) when the vasculature has been present for years—that is, the vasculature in human tumors is more mature and differentiated than that found in experimental animal models. One indicator of a more mature vasculature bed is the formation of a layer of smooth muscle cells surrounding the endothelium.[47] Data suggest that these pericytes may protect endothelial cells from apoptosis. Indeed, in preclinical studies in which expression of VEGF in transgenic mice was under the control of an inducible vector, withdrawal of VEGF led to apoptosis of endothelial cells, many of which were not associated with pericytes.[47]

Third, in preclinical studies evaluating antiangiogenic agents in mice, the agent is usually delivered when tumors are so small that they would be undetectable by current imaging methods (less than 1 to 2 mm in diameter). In contrast, patients enrolled in clinical trials of antiangiogenic agents have widespread, bulky disease. Because antiangiogenic agents are expected to have cytostatic effects, it might be more beneficial to determine the clinical benefit of these agents in the adjuvant setting.[47] In addition, patients enrolled in phase I and II clinical trials often have been heavily pretreated with either standard-of-care or new therapies and have relapsed with drug-resistant, refractory disease, which may be less responsive to new therapeutic agents. It is very rare, in preclinical studies, to mimic this type of situation.[48]

BASIC PRINCIPLES FOR DESIGN OF CLINICAL TRIALS OF ANTIANGIOGENIC AGENTS

The vast majority of preclinical studies demonstrate that antiangiogenic therapy leads to inhibition of tumor growth rather than regression of established tumors.[1] The ability to interpret experimental studies appropriately is critical to ensure that extrapolations to the clinical setting are not fraught with unrealistic expectations. Single-agent therapy with antiangiogenic agents may not show efficacy as determined by current standards of tumor regression yet may still induce antitumor effects as determined by increased time to progression and increased overall survival. A potential method for maximizing the impact of antiangiogenic therapy is to use antiangiogenic agents in combination with agents that induce tumor regression, such as cytotoxic chemotherapy or vascular targeting agents.[49]

Preclinical and ongoing clinical trials have suggested that the combination of antiangiogenic agents and standard chemotherapy has enhanced effects.[50,51] The combination of these two types of agents has enabled the dosages of both to be lowered, which leads to fewer adverse side effects and improved quality of life. However, care must be taken in selecting the agents to combine. For example, the combination of SU5416 with gemcitabine and cisplatin in cancer patients has been associated with an increase in adverse cardiovascular events that was not seen with any of these drugs administered as single agents.[52]

In current clinical trials investigating the efficacy of cytotoxic agents, patient response rates are used as a surrogate marker of patient survival. Given that the goal of cancer therapy is also to transform an acute disease into a chronic disease, measurement of other intermediate parameters may be more appropriate. By definition, antiangiogenic agents are intended to prevent the formation of new blood vessels and hence limit tumor growth. Thus, time to progression and quality of life may be reasonable secondary end points in clinical trials of antiangiogenic agents. However, the gold standard as the primary end point for these trials remains overall survival. With respect to development of surrogate markers that may be useful for monitoring antiangiogenic activity of drugs and helping to guide proper, optimal dosing, several promising avenues are currently being explored, including functional imaging, which measures changes in tumor blood flow[53] and changes in the levels or viability of circulating endothelial cells, or both, or of bone marrow–derived circulating endothelial progenitor cells, as illustrated by the "metronomic" antiangiogenic chemotherapy study by Bertolini et al.[54]

Overall, antiangiogenic therapy remains a promising modality for antineoplastic therapy. A better understanding of the biology of angiogenesis will help determine appropriate antiangiogenic therapy for different tumors growing in different sites. At this stage, it appears that antiangiogenic therapy will be most beneficial when combined with another antineoplastic modality or radiation therapy, or both. The best approach to antiangiogenic therapy remains to be determined, but continued study of these agents in phase III clinical trials will not only help optimize antineoplastic regimens but will also help elucidate the biologic principles that underlie tumor angiogenesis in progression. Chapter 63 is devoted to current studies of antiangiogenic agents.

CONCLUSION

The process of angiogenesis is a dynamic process essential for the growth of primary and metastatic malignancies as well as hematopoietic cancers. Understanding the basic principles of the biology of angiogenesis has led to the development of new prognostic factors, tumor markers, imaging techniques, and therapeutic modalities. The challenge lies in integrating this knowledge into the care of patients with malignant diseases of all types and stages. Understanding the basic biology of angiogenesis and tumor biology will ultimately lead to the rational implementation of new paradigms for the treatment of patients with cancer.

REFERENCES

1. Folkman J. Angiogenesis in cancer, vascular, rheumatoid and other diseases. *Nat Med* 1995;1:27.
2. Kerbel RS, Folkman J. Clinical translation of angiogenesis inhibitors. *Nat Rev Cancer* 2002;2:727.
3. Brown JM, Giaccia AJ. The unique physiology of solid tumours: opportunities (and problems) for cancer therapy. *Cancer Res* 1998;58:1408.
4. Fidler IJ, Yano S, Zhang R, et al. The seed and soil hypothesis: vascularization and brain metastasis. *Lancet Oncol* 2002;3:53.
5. Risau W. Mechanisms of angiogenesis. *Nature* 1997;386:671.
6. Thomas KA. Vascular endothelial growth factor, a potent and selective angiogenic agent. *J Biol Chem* 1996;271:603.
7. Senger DR, Galli SJ, Dvorak AM, et al. Tumor cells secrete a vascular permeability factor that promotes accumulation of ascites fluid. *Science* 1983;219:983.
8. Ferrara N, Gerber HP, LeCouter J. The biology of VEGF and its receptors. *Nat Med* 2003;9:669.
9. Veikkola T, Karkkainen M, Claesson-Welsh L, et al. Regulation of angiogenesis via vascular endothelial growth factor receptors. *Cancer Res* 2000;60:203.
10. Davis S, Yancopoulos GD. The angiopoietins: Yin and Yang in angiogenesis. *Curr Top Microbiol Immunol* 1999;237:173.
11. Yoon YS, Murayama T, Gravereaux E, et al. VEGF-C gene therapy augments postnatal lymphangiogenesis and ameliorates secondary lymphedema. *J Clin Invest* 2003;111:717.
12. Kumar R, Yoneda J, Bucana CD, et al. Regulation of distinct steps of angiogenesis by different angiogenic molecules. *Int J Oncol* 1998;12:7498.
13. Ruoslahti E. Specialization of tumor vasculature. *Nat Rev Cancer* 2002;2:83.
14. Fidler IJ. The pathogenesis of cancer metastasis: the 'seed and soil' hypothesis revisited (Timeline). *Nat Rev Cancer* 2003;3:453.
15. Langley RR, Ramirez KM, Tsan RZ, et al. Tissue specific microvascular endothelial cell lines from H-2Kᵇ-tsA58 mice for studies of angiogenesis and metastasis. *Cancer Res* 2003;63:2971.
16. Pugh CW, Ratcliffe PJ. Regulation of angiogenesis by hypoxia: role of the HIF system. *Nat Med* 2003;9:677.
17. Harris AL. Hypoxia—a key regulatory factor in tumor growth. *Nat Rev Cancer* 2002;2:38.
18. Bergers G, Song S, Meyer-Morse N, et al. Benefits of targeting both pericytes and endothelial cells in the tumor vasculature with kinase inhibitors. *J Clin Invest* 2003;111:1287.
19. Uehara H, Kim SJ, Karashima T, et al. Effects of blocking platelet-derived growth factor-receptor signaling in a mouse model of experimental prostate cancer bone metastases. *J Natl Cancer Inst* 2003;95:458.
20. Eberhard A, Kahlert S, Goede V, et al. Heterogeneity of angiogenesis and blood vessel maturation in human tumors: implications for antiangiogenic tumor therapies. *Cancer Res* 2000;60:1388.
21. Sunderkotter C, Steinbrink K, Goebeler M, et al. Macrophages and angiogenesis. *J Leukoc Biol* 1994;55:410.
22. Gutman M, Singh RK, Yoon S, et al. Leukocyte-induced angiogenesis and subcutaneous growth of B16 melanoma. *Cancer Biother* 1994;56:423.
23. Polverini PJ. How the extracellular matrix and macrophages contribute to angiogenesis-dependent diseases. *Eur J Cancer* 1996;32A:2430.
24. Mantovani A, Bottazzi B, Colotta F, et al. The origin and function of tumor-associated macrophages. *Immunol Today* 1992;13:265.
25. Naylor MS, Stamp GW, Davies BD, et al. Expression and activity of MMPs and their regulators in ovarian cancer. *Int J Cancer* 1994;58:50.
26. Liotta LA, Kohn EC. The microenvironment of the tumor-host invasion field. *Nature* 2001;411:375.
27. Huang S, Van Arsdall M, Tedjarati S, et al. Contributions of stromal metalloproteinase-9 to angiogenesis and growth of human ovarian carcinoma in mice. *J Natl Cancer Inst* 2002;94:1134.
28. Qian X, Tuszynski GP. Expression of thrombospondin-1 in cancer: a role in tumor progression. *Proc Soc Exp Biol Med* 1996;212:199.
29. Dameron KM, Volpert OV, Tainsky MA, et al. Control of angiogenesis in fibroblasts by p53 regulation of thrombospondin-1. *Science* 1994;265:1502.
30. Ezekowitz RAB, Mulliken JB, Folkman J. Interferon alfa-2a therapy for life-threatening hemangiomas of infancy. *N Engl J Med* 1992;326:1456.
31. Folkman J. Angiogenesis inhibitors generated by tumors. *Mol Med* 1995;1:120.
32. Dong Z, Kumar R, Yang X, et al. Macrophage-derived metalloelastase is responsible for the generation of angiostatin in Lewis lung carcinoma. *Cell* 1997;88:801.
33. Rosen LS. Clinical experience with angiogenesis signaling inhibitors: focus on vascular endothelial growth factor (VEGF) blockers. *Cancer Control* 2002;9:36.
34. Herbst RS, O'Reilly MS. The rationale and potential of combining novel biologic therapies with radiotherapy: focus on non-small cell lung cancer. *Semin Oncol* 2003;30:113.
35. Bloemendal HJ, Logtenbert T, Voest EE. New strategies in antivascular cancer therapy. *Eur J Clin Invest* 1999;29:802.
36. Blakey DC, Westwood FR, Walker M, et al. Antitumor activity of the novel vascular targeting agent ZD6126 in a panel of tumor models. *Clin Cancer Res* 2002;8:1974.
37. Plate KH, Breier G, Farrell CL, et al. Platelet-derived growth factor receptor-beta is induced during tumor development and upregulated during tumor progression in endothelial cells in human gliomas. *Lab Invest* 1992;67:529.
38. Zha J, Harada H, Yang E, et al. Serine phosphorylation of death agonist BAD in response to survival factor results in binding to 14-3-3 not BCL-X(L). *Cell* 1996;87:619.
39. Druker BJ, Tamura S, Buchdunger E, et al. Effects of a selective inhibitor of the Abl tyrosine kinase on the growth of Bcr-Abl positive cells. *Nat Med* 1996;2:561.
40. Buchdunger E, Cioffi CL, Law N, et al. Abl protein-tyrosine kinase inhibitor STI571 inhibits *in vitro* signal transduction mediated by c-kit and platelet-derived growth factor receptors. *J Pharmacol Exp Ther* 2000;295:139.
41. Yoon SY, Tefferi A, Li CY. Cellular distribution of platelet-derived growth factor, transforming growth factor-beta, basic fibroblast growth factor, and their receptors in normal bone marrow. *Acta Haematol* 2000;104:151.
42. Watanabe Y, Dvorak HV. Vascular permeability factor/vascular endothelial growth factor inhibits anchorage-disruption-induced apoptosis in microvessel endothelial cells by inducing scaffold formation. *Exp Cell Res* 1997;233:340.
43. Traxler P, Bold G, Buchdunger E, et al. Tyrosine kinase inhibitors: from rational design to clinical trials. *Med Res Rev* 2001;21:499.
44. Morioka H, Weissbach L, Vogel T, et al. Anti-angiogenesis treatment combined with chemotherapy produces chondrosarcoma necrosis. *Clin Cancer Res* 2003;9:1211.

45. Mathew P, Thall P, Jones D, et al. Targeting the platelet-derived growth factor receptor (PDGFf) in androgen-independent prostate cancer (AIPCa) bone metastasis: results of a phase I trial. *Proc Am Soc Clin Oncol* 2003;22:410(abst).

46. Shaheen RM, Davis DW, Liu W, et al. Antiangiogenic therapy targeting the tyrosine kinase receptor for vascular endothelial growth factor receptor inhibits the growth of colon cancer liver metastasis and induces tumor and endothelial cell apoptosis. *Cancer Res* 1999;59:5412.

47. Benjamin LE, Golijanin D, Itin A, et al. Selective ablation of immature blood vessels in established human tumors follows vascular endothelial growth factor withdrawal. *J Clin Invest* 1999;103:159.

48. Kerbel RS. Human tumor xenografts as predictive preclinical models for anticancer drug activity in humans. *Cancer Biol Ther* 2003;2:S134.

49. Ellis LM, Liu W, Fan F, et al. Role of angiogenesis inhibitors in cancer treatment. *Oncology* 2001;15:39.

50. Browder T, Butterfield CE, Kraling BM, et al. Antiangiogenic scheduling of chemotherapy improves efficacy against experimental drug-resistant cancer. *Cancer Res* 2000;60:1878.

51. Eskens FA, Verweij J. Clinical studies in the development of new anticancer agents exhibiting growth inhibition in models: facing the challenge of a proper study design. *Crit Rev Oncol Hematol* 2000;34:83.

52. Kuenen BC, Levi M, Meijers JC, et al. Potential role of platelets in endothelial damage observed during treatment with cisplatin, gemcitabine, and the angiogenesis inhibitor, SU5416. *J Clin Oncol* 2003;21:2192.

53. Ellis LM. Antiangiogenic therapy: more promise and, yet again, more questions (*editorial*). *J Clin Oncol* 2003;21:1.

54. Bertolini F, Paul S, Mancuso P, et al. Maximum tolerable dose and low-dose metronomic chemotherapy have opposite effects on the mobilization and viability of circulating endothelial progenitor cells. *Cancer Res* 2003;63:4342.

Nicholas P. Restifo
John R. Wunderlich

CHAPTER **6**

Cancer Immunology

Potentially harmful challenges to the body include viruses, bacteria, unicellular and multicellular pathogens, and cancer cells. In response to these challenges, the body has evolved active defenses that compose the immune system. Although the immune system is composed of a wide range of distinct cell types, lymphocytes play a central role by providing the specificity of immune recognition. Through its various appendages, the immune system is capable of interacting, directly or indirectly, with nearly every cell in the body.

The focus of this chapter is on how the immune system, particularly adaptive immune responses, can potentially recognize and destroy tumor cells. Adaptive immunity provides the host defenses with the means to recognize specific pathogens, including a growing number of tumor cell sources. The time course of adaptive immune responses involves a delay during which they develop. Once initiated, however, these responses are specific for particular pathogens, closely regulated, and long lasting through the development of memory for the pathogen, and they generally do not react against normal autologous cells. In contrast, innate immune responses provide immediate reactions against pathogens. Although they lack memory and are not as closely regulated as adaptive responses, the innate responses are commonly critical to the process of starting adaptive immune responses.[1-3]

If naturally occurring immune responses protect humans against cancer, the incidence of cancer in immunosuppressed transplant patients may rise, providing support for the cancer immunosurveillance hypothesis.[4] Indeed, the incidence is significantly higher for cancers associated with virus infections. Evidence is also accumulating for a higher incidence of cancers not associated with viral infections; however, at this stage, the data are preliminary. Thus, this chapter also considers tumor immunology from the perspective of what the immune system may accomplish if it is perturbed by vaccinations or adoptive immunotherapy and not just what may be accomplished if the immune system is left to its own devices in a natural environment.

A central division is found in the immune system between the humoral branch, which is largely composed of B lymphocytes and their products, and the cellular branch, many functions of which are performed by T lymphocytes. The humoral (from the Latin word *umor*, meaning *fluid*) branch of the immune system is involved with the production of antibodies that are capable of neutralizing or destroying harmful challenges to the body.

A great deal of work has established that the cellular branch of the immune system is particularly relevant to human tumor immunology, thus expanding the decades-old recognition of the association in animal models of cellular immunity with delayed-type hypersensitivity[5] and with the rejection of foreign grafts[6] and tumors.[7] As techniques for isolating and identifying cells associated with immune responses developed, it became clear that T cells, or thymus-derived lymphocytes, are essential for cellular immune responses. Thus, understanding the principles of cellular immunity has largely come to mean understanding the development, function, and regulation of T cells.

Fundamental differences are seen in the ways that the cellular and the humoral immune systems recognize antigens* (Table 6-1). B cells can recognize antigens not presented in the

---

*We use *antigen* in this chapter for a substance if it or one of its components binds specifically to the combining site of an antibody or a T-cell receptor. Some of these structures elicit immune responses (*immunogens*), whereas others do not. Exceptions to this terminology, such as superantigens, are found. T cells recognize peptide–major histocompatibility complexes (MHC) and not the peptide apart from an MHC partner. Nevertheless, the peptide and its parent protein often are called *antigens* in the literature. The antigenic peptide is also called an *epitope*. We use *self-antigens* to refer to antigens that are products of the host's normal cells, and we use foreign antigens to refer to antigens that are alien to the normal host but gain access from the outside environment (e.g., products of infectious microbes) or arise internally (e.g., various products of cancer cells that are not produced by normal host cells).

TABLE 6-1. Toward a Molecular Understanding of Immune Recognition of Antigen

	Humoral	*Cellular[a]*
Recognizing cell	B lymphocyte	T lymphocyte
Recognizing molecule	Immunoglobulin	T-cell receptor
Self-molecules required?	No	Yes
Chemical identity of antigen	Protein, nucleic acid, polysaccharide, other	Protein
Phase of antigen	Fluid or solid	Solid
State of antigen	Native or denatured	"Processed"

[a]Various exceptions are presented in the text.

context of other molecules. T cells, on the other hand, generally recognize antigens in the context of cell surface glycoproteins encoded in a group of genes referred to as the *major histocompatibility complex* (*MHC*). T cells use structures on their surfaces called *T-cell receptors* (*TCRs*) to recognize antigen/MHC molecule complexes; B cells use immunoglobulin (Ig) molecules to react specifically with antigens. Whereas Ig is secreted, sometimes in extremely large quantities, few, if any, TCRs are shed by T cells. Underlying the difference in the molecules used for recognition is an important difference in the types of antigens recognized: Whereas B cells can recognize antigen in its native conformation, T cells generally recognize antigen that has been "processed" by another cell and then presented on the surface of the cell by MHC molecules. More specifically, antigen is denatured, cleaved within the cell, and transported into specific subcellular compartments, where it is bound by MHC molecules. After a complex of antigen and MHC completes its journey to the cell surface, it is potentially recognizable by a T cell. The source of antigens is critical to T-cell responses against tumors: Unlike antigens recognized by antibodies, antigens recognized by T cells can arise from the multitude of intracellular proteins that are not expressed on the cell surface as intact proteins.

ANTITUMOR T CELLS

T lymphocytes were first identified as a functional subset of lymphocytes, the development of which depends on the existence of a thymus.[8] In conditions of congenital absence of the thymus or after neonatal thymectomy in animal models, a number of immune responses were found to be impaired, including cell-mediated killing and transplantation reactions such as graft-versus-host disease and allograft rejection. Subsequent to this functional definition of T lymphocytes, differentiation antigens were identified on T cells using antibodies. The ability to identify T cells and thus isolate T cells and their subsets, and the ability to selectively grow these cells in culture, has resulted in a body of experimental evidence that reveals many mechanisms of activation and effector functions of this population.

Early experiments showed that the growth of a syngeneic tumor in a mouse could be prevented by prior immunization with that same tumor.[9–12] Since then, the mechanisms involved in antitumor immune responses have been partially elucidated, and T cells have been shown to play a critical role.[13–15] Guided by results from animal model studies, human T cells have been shown to be capable of specifically lysing autologous tumor cells *in vitro*.[16,17] T cells can also specifically secrete cytokines, such as interleukin-2 (IL-2), interferon-γ (IFN-γ), granulocyte-macrophage colony-stimulating factor, and tumor necrosis factor-α (TNF-α), and proliferate in response to stimulation with autologous tumor cells.[18,19] Antitumor T cells can be grown to large numbers *in vitro* and adoptively transferred to treat even substantial tumor burdens in humans and mice.[20,21] Finally, tumor antigens recognized by autologous human T cells have been identified by a variety of independent techniques.[13,14,22] Taken together, these findings provide nearly incontrovertible evidence that a T-cell immune response can occur against an autologous tumor.

BIOLOGIC SOURCES OF TUMOR-ASSOCIATED ANTIGENS

Antigens of special interest have the potential to trigger tumor-selective clinical responses as a result of humoral or cellular immune reactions. Most of these antigens are tumor associated and are expressed in total or in part (e.g., as peptides) on the tumor cell surface.

TUMOR-ASSOCIATED ANTIGENS TARGETED WITH MONOCLONAL ANTIBODIES

Lineage-selective markers can serve as therapeutic targets for humanized, mouse monoclonal antibodies (MAbs), generated in part in the laboratory, as long as the cell lineage is not a vital one or can be replaced in a timely fashion from stem cells. These therapeutic targets are normal proteins that generally are not immunogenic in the autologous human host, and consequently the MAbs are commonly induced in mice. Structural genes for the MAbs are modified in the laboratory to make them as human-like as possible, without changing their antigen specificity. Whole or essential parts of MAbs have been used alone or fused to a toxin to treat selected B-cell malignancies (e.g., anti-CD20–rituximab and anti-CD25).[23,24] Other tumor antigens are overexpressed by particular malignancies, such as the protooncogene product and growth factor receptor HER-2/neu, which is overexpressed by selected breast cancers and can mediate clinically evident responses to MAbs (trastuzumab).[23]

Still other antigens are targeted not because they are on the surface of tumor cells but because blocking their biologic activity interferes with tumor growth. Thus, treating selected cancer patients with MAbs that block the activity of cell-free, diffusible vascular endothelial growth factor[25,26] or the activity of CTLA-4 (cytotoxic T lymphocyte–associated antigen),[27,28] a cell surface receptor with inhibitory functions on activated T cells, has resulted in clinically evident responses. In addition, antigens are being targeted to prevent cancer rather than treat it. Early vaccination against hepatitis B appears to be successful in reducing the incidence of hepatocellular carcinoma,[29] and vaccination programs have started against papillomavirus, which is associated with cervical cancer.[30]

TUMOR-ASSOCIATED ANTIGENS
TARGETED WITH T CELLS

Reports of successful clinical trials based on T-cell antitumor activity[31] and rigorous criteria for identifying clinical responses[32] are at an early stage. Thus, the following summary includes tumor antigens recognized by T cells that have not been tested in clinical trials. Antigens recognized by T cells and described below may be expressed on the cell surface only by tumor cells (*tumor-specific antigens*), or they may be shared by multiple tumors and a limited group of normal cells.[13,14,22,33–36]

One study of human colorectal carcinoma indicated genomic damage at a mean of approximately 11,000 events per cell.[37] Thus, many tumor-associated antigens derived from abnormal proteins result from the inherent genetic instability of tumor cells reflected by, for example, somatic single-base mutations within the coding region, mutations in stop codons that extend the normal open reading frame, deletion mutations resulting in frameshifts, use of alternative open reading frames, gene rearrangements leading to fusion proteins, antisense transcription of normal genes, and aberrant splicing of the messenger RNA (mRNA) such that introns are included in the coding sequence. Some tumor-specific antigens that are caused by a particular point mutation and are recognized by T cells have been found in multiple independent tumors. In these cases the mutated protein is commonly one that promotes the development or growth of malignant cells.[33,38] Posttranslational modifications also contribute to the generation of tumor antigens, including a melanoma antigen caused by posttranslational conversion of an amino acid[39] and a renal cancer antigen caused by posttranslational protein splicing.[40] In the latter case, the antigen was derived from fibroblast growth factor-5 and was expressed by multiple sources of renal cell cancer cell lines, as well as by some prostate and breast carcinoma cell lines.[41]

As an additional source of tumor antigens, abnormal proteins may arise from extrinsic sources, such as found in virus-associated malignancies. Epstein-Barr virus–lymphoproliferative disease, for example, can be treated successfully by adoptive immunotherapy with T cells specific for selected viral antigens.[42]

The advancing strategies for identifying tumor antigens and the studies of cancer genomics and proteomics are greatly improving our understanding of the nature of alterations at the DNA, mRNA, and protein-peptide levels; the potential antigens resulting from these changes; and the distribution of the antigens between tumor and normal tissues.[43,44]

Two major sources of normal proteins provide tumor-shared antigens recognized by T cells.[14,36,46] First, *cancer/testis antigens* are expressed by many types of tumors, and they are products of genes that are inactive in normal tissues, except in male germline cells and occasionally in the placenta. T cells do not recognize the antigens on male germline cells, because these cells do not express MHC class I or II molecules.[47] The impetus for expression of cancer/testis antigens appears to be demethylation of the promoter genes. This event is part of the widespread, deregulated methylation of genes that is frequently observed in cancer cells.[14,48] Tumors that more commonly express cancer/testes antigens include melanomas, lung carcinomas, and cancers of the head and neck, esopha-

gus, and bladder. Second, tumor antigens can be expressed by multiple sources of tumor in a tissue-specific fashion (*differentiation antigens* or, alternatively, *tissue-specific antigens*). In melanomas, in which these and other human tumor antigens recognized by T cells have been studied most, antigen expression by normal tissues is limited to melanocytes and pigment-producing cells in the retina. Where function has been established, the antigens are associated with melanin production. Of note, the most common T-cell antitumor reactivity found in melanoma patients has been against one of these antigens, MART-1/Melan-A.[46]

Antigens other than peptides, particularly lipids or glycolipids and relatively low-molecular-weight phosphorylated metabolites, can be recognized by appropriate TCRs on T cells and may contribute to antitumor responses.[49–51] Investigation of the roles of these antigens in mediating antitumor responses is at a relatively early stage.

Considering the highly varied sources of tumor antigens recognized by T cells, several aspects of the antigens are of particular interest with respect to potential tumor responses to immunotherapy. For example, is the antigen unique or is it shared by multiple sources of tumor, thus being relevant to many patients? As another example, is the antigen expressed only by tumor cells or also by normal cells? This question relates to the challenges of addressing responses to self-antigens. In addition, what proportion of malignant cells in a tumor stably express the antigen at a level that triggers antitumor effector T cells? This issue relates to the survival and growth of immunoresistant tumor cells. Moreover, can T cells recognize the antigen as expressed by native tumor cells? T-cell recognition of native tumor cells is required for clinical responses, in contrast, for example, to recognition of a surrogate target cell pulsed with the antigenic peptide. As a further example, does the parent antigenic molecule yield different antigenic epitopes, some stimulating CD8+ T cells and others CD4+ T cells? This issue raises not only the possibility of immune responses against many different antigens expressed by a tumor cell and a reduced likelihood of emerging immunoresistant tumor cells but also the possibility of needing CD8+ as well as CD4+ T-cell responses to generate T cells that will destroy the tumor.

PRESENTATION OF TUMOR ANTIGENS TO T CELLS

MAJOR HISTOCOMPATIBILITY COMPLEX MOLECULES AS ANTIGEN RECEPTORS

In this section we describe the presentation of antigens to T cells. The presentation of tumor antigens appears to follow the same general mechanisms used for other antigens, such as viral proteins. Tumor-associated antigens recognized by T cells are fragments of proteins produced by malignant cells that are presented by MHC molecules. Understanding the molecular structure of MHC molecules has made clear their function with respect to antigen recognition by T cells: MHC molecules are receptors for peptide antigens.[52–54] X-ray crystallographic data have shown that MHC molecules have peptide-binding domains consisting of a deep groove that runs between two long α helices found on the outward-facing surface of the

MHC molecule.[52,53,55] Structural data have since been refined and extended to include x-ray images of particular peptides lying in the clefts of MHC molecules in an extended conformation.[56-63] Supporting the structural data, peptides of the appropriate size for MHC binding have been eluted from MHC preparations purified from a variety of human cancer cell lines, including melanoma,[64] ovarian adenocarcinoma,[65] and breast[66] and colon carcinomas.[67] Investigators identified the peptides physically and in several of the studies showed that the eluted peptides, or synthetic copies of the peptides, served as T-cell epitopes.

Sequence studies indicate that MHC class I and class II molecules are among the most highly polymorphic molecules in the genome. The polymorphism of MHC molecules is concentrated in the peptide-binding grooves.[68,69] MHC diversity is what makes the job of the transplant surgeon so difficult and must be taken into account by the cancer immunotherapist. For example, tyrosinase, which is a tumor antigen associated with normal melanocytes and with melanoma cells, has an epitope that is presented to lytic CD8+ T lymphocytes in the context of the HLA-A24.[70] Use of this peptide in a patient not expressing this class I molecule is likely to be ineffective, because the appropriate MHC molecule for presenting the peptide would not be available and because that particular peptide would be unlikely to bind efficiently to other class I alleles.

DIFFERENCES BETWEEN MAJOR HISTOCOMPATIBILITY COMPLEX CLASS I AND CLASS II MOLECULES

Although class I and class II molecules are united by their function as receptors for antigenic peptides, their differences are critical to the nature of T-cell immune responses. Class I and class II molecules have different tissue distributions, and they present bound peptides to different T-cell subsets, thus eliciting different types of immune responses. They arise from different gene clusters, and they differ structurally. Class I and class II molecules also differ in their requirements for binding peptide antigens, and these peptides originate from different sources. Finally, the two types of MHC molecules follow different intracellular routes on their way to the cell surface and noncovalently associate with peptides in different subcellular compartments.

These issues bear on how tumor cell antigens initiate immune responses and how they mediate tumor cell destruction. They relate to whether tumor antigens activate immune effector cells that mediate tumor cell destruction or cells that primarily regulate immune responses.

Whereas class I molecules are found on most tumor cells and somatic cells, class II molecules are found in high concentrations on only a subset of tumor cells and on B cells, bone marrow–derived phagocytic cells (e.g., macrophages), dendritic cells (DCs), and, in lesser quantities, other cells, including subpopulations of thymocytes, activated peripheral T cells, and certain epithelial cells.

Class I molecules present antigenic peptides to CD8+ T lymphocytes; class II molecules perform the same function for CD4+ T lymphocytes. CD8+ T lymphocytes are sometimes termed *cytotoxic T lymphocytes* (CTLs), in reference to a major subpopulation of these cells that can lyse target cells directly through the release of lytic granules as well as through triggering "death"

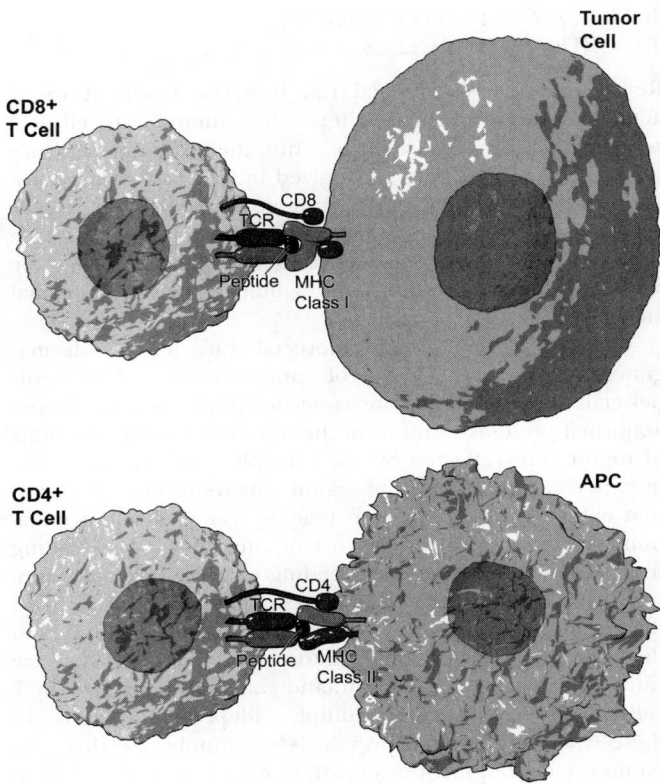

FIGURE 6-1. Model for stimulation of CD4+ and CD8+ T-cell antitumor immunity, based on CD8+ T cells interacting with tumor cells and CD4+ T cells interacting with host antigen-presenting cells (APCs). MHC, major histocompatibility complex; TCR, T-cell receptor. (Illustration by Emily Green Shaw.)

receptors, such as Fas, on target cells. CD4+ T cells, although also capable of cytotoxic activity in some cases, are called *helper T cells* because they commonly enhance immune responses by promoting the activation of B cells, other T cells, and other important cells in the immune system, such as DCs and macrophages.

A model of how the two major types of T lymphocytes may interact with target cells is depicted in Figure 6-1. A CD8+ T cell is shown interacting directly with a tumor cell, and a CD4+ T cell is shown interacting with an antigen-presenting cell (APC) expressing class II molecules.

GENE CLUSTERS AND PROTEIN STRUCTURE. The major locations, or loci, for class I genes are named *A*, *B*, and *C* in the human and *K*, *D*, and *L* in the mouse (Fig. 6-2). Class II molecules originate from three major subregions in the human, designated *DP*, *DQ*, and *DR*, and two in the mouse, designated *I-A* and *I-E*. MHC molecules from these major subregions are codominantly expressed. The extent of MHC polymorphism present in the human gene pool usually results in heterozygosity for most individuals at nearly every major class I and class II locus. Because there are three different major class I loci and three different major class II loci in the human, individuals may express six different class I alleles and six different class II alleles. Codominant expression in a single individual of MHC molecules originating from multiple loci enhances that individual's ability to present a variety

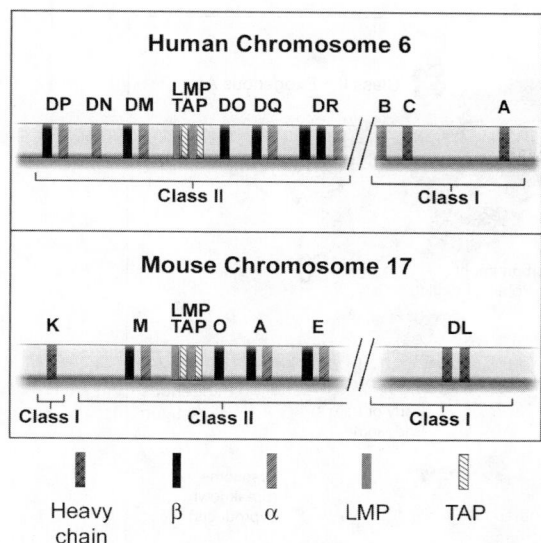

FIGURE 6-2.   Highly schematic map of the genomic arrangement of the major histocompatibility complex in humans and mice. Heavy chain, class I α chain; β, class II β chain; α, class II α chain; LMP, low-molecular-weight protein; TAP, transporter associated with antigen processing. LMP and TAP are genes whose products are involved with antigen processing for MHC class I presentation. For simplicity, class Ib genes and the class III regions are not shown. (Illustration by Emily Green Shaw.)

of antigens. For tumor cells, another consequence of heterozygosity and codominance is that loss of expression of a single allele for an MHC locus can result in loss of presentation of a particular tumor antigen, as the pairing of antigenic peptides with MHC molecules is selective.

Class I molecules are heterodimers composed of an extremely polymorphic, approximately 45-kD α chain and a 12-kD β₂-microglobulin. Class I molecules are considered by some to be true heterotrimers, as a peptide eight to ten amino acids long having a molecular weight of approximately 1 kD is required for stability and proper expression.

The α chains of class I molecules (also called *heavy chains*) have three large extracellular domains. The α_1 and α_2 domains are directly involved in the binding of peptides. The α_3 domain contains the nonpolymorphic region that is the ligand for the CD8 molecule. A 25-amino acid transmembrane region, connected to the α_3 domain, forms a hydrophobic α helix that anchors class I into the cell membrane. A short intracytoplasmic segment, 30 amino acids long, is involved in the intracellular trafficking of class I molecules and contains regions that interact with the cytoskeleton as well as residues that can be phosphorylated.

β₂-microglobulin is a structural component of the MHC class I molecule, which is noncovalently associated with the α chain. It plays an indispensable role in the proper folding of the α chain. The β₂-microglobulin gene is not encoded within the MHC and has minimal polymorphism, even among mammalian species.

The class II molecule is very similar to the class I molecule in its general shape, but it is composed of a 34-kD α chain and a 28-kD β chain, both of which are integral membrane glycoproteins. The α and β chains have transmembrane regions as well as short intracytoplasmic regions. The α_1 and β_1 domains of the class II molecule correspond with the α_1 and α_2 domains of the class I molecule and thus are directly involved in the binding of the presented peptide. The α_2 domain of class II corresponds with the β₂-microglobulin light chain of class I. Finally, the β_2 domain of class II corresponds with the α_3 domain of class I and is involved in the binding of CD4.

Although the general architecture of the peptide-binding grooves of MHC class I and class II are almost identical, critical differences fundamentally change the way peptides are bound. Class I molecules bind shorter peptides of defined lengths (generally 8 to 10 residues), whereas class II molecules bind peptides that are more variable in length (often 12 to 20 amino acids but occasionally longer).[71] In fact, class II molecules often bind a core motif of an antigen that can vary in content in either direction from the core (also referred to as *nested sets* of peptides). The binding cleft of class I molecules is closed at both ends, enabling the molecule to make hydrogen bonds with the bound peptides at the N-terminal and the C-terminal. Class II molecules, on the other hand, have a peptide-binding cleft that is open on both ends. In the class I and the class II molecules, peptides are bound by pockets in the binding site. These peptides bind to MHC molecules with affinities that can range from the picomolar to micromolar range.

It is now possible to forecast which epitopes within a protein will bind to particular MHC molecules. Allele-specific epitope forecasting has been done with a large number of MHC molecules,[72,73] which are characterized by strong preferences for particular amino acid side chains at some positions in the bound peptides and a wide tolerance for amino acid side chains at other positions. Although the anchor positions are critically important in predicting which peptides will bind to particular MHC molecules, the amino acid side chains at other positions can play a role and cannot be disregarded.[74] Nevertheless, in clinical trials investigators have increased the capacity of a melanoma peptide to activate antitumor T cells that react with the native peptide, by modifying an anchor residue to enhance the binding of the peptide to its HLA-restriction molecule, the HLA molecule that normally presents the peptide at the cell surface.[46]

ANTIGEN PROCESSING FOR PRESENTATION BY MAJOR HISTOCOMPATIBILITY COMPLEX CLASS I AND II MOLECULES

Understanding how tumor cell proteins, like other proteins, are processed into peptides that are complexed with MHC molecules and expressed on cell surfaces as T-cell antigens has had a central role in advancing the understanding of tumor immunology. Antigenic peptides complexed with MHC class I and class II molecules originate from two different sources (Fig. 6-3). Class I molecules generally present antigens derived from intracellular cytosolic proteins, such as self-proteins and products of intracellular viruses and other microorganisms in the cytosol. By contrast, class II peptides are derived primarily from membrane glycoproteins or extracellular proteins that enter the acidic vacuolar compartment by endocytosis.[71] Clear examples exist, however, that contradict this distinction, as noted below in this section. A more precise understanding of the difference between the sources

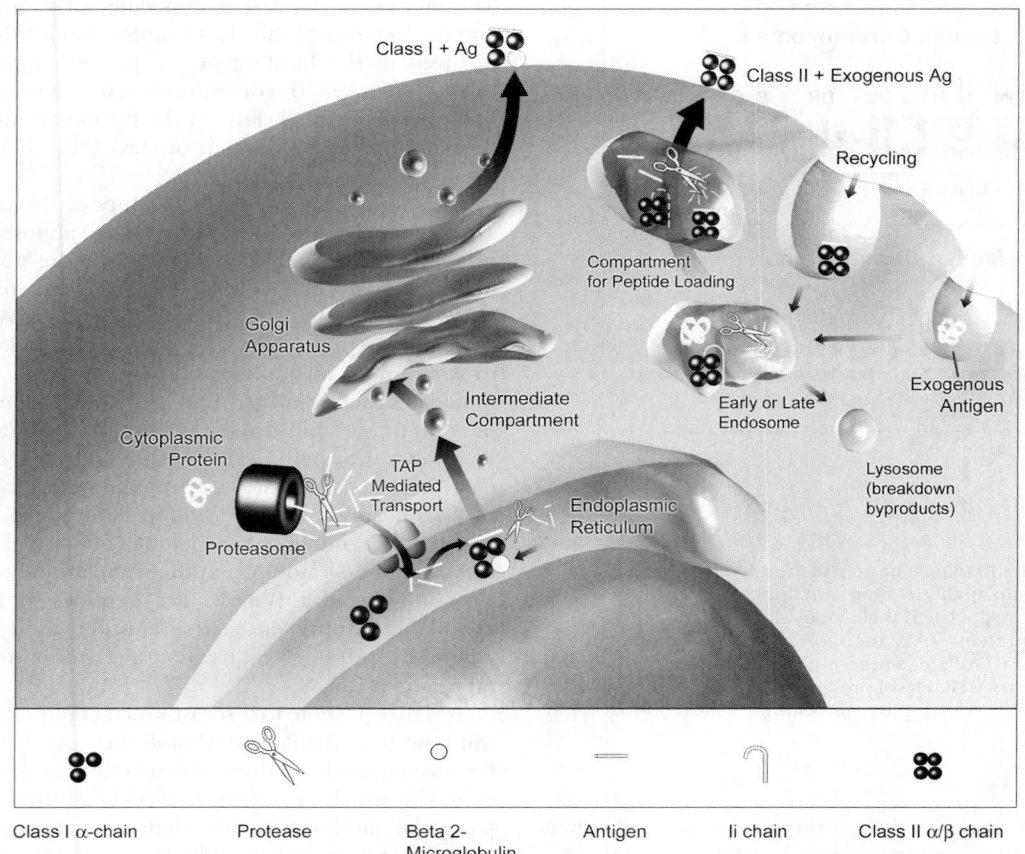

At the bottom of the figure, icons labeled:

Class I α-chain   Protease   Beta 2-Microglobulin   Antigen   Ii chain   Class II α/β chain

FIGURE 6-3.   Intracellular trafficking pathways in the presentation of endogenous and exogenous antigen. Cytoplasmic proteins are digested by proteases in the proteasome molecular complex, trimmed, and transported into the endoplasmic reticulum by TAP (transporter associated with antigen-processing) molecules. Accessory proteins facilitate assembly of the peptide–major histocompatibility complex (MHC) class I complex. The complexes pass through the Golgi apparatus to the cell surface for presentation of antigen to CD8+ T cells. Exogenous antigen (Ag) uptake occurs by endocytosis in immature dendritic cells, macrophages, and B lymphocytes. Acid-dependent proteases digest antigens in acidified lysosomes, where peptides form complexes with MHC class II molecules. The assembled complexes move to the cell surface for presentation of antigen to CD4+ T cells. CPL, compartment for peptide loading; SRP, signal recognition particle. (Illustration by Emily Green Shaw.)

of antigens results from an understanding of patterns of intracellular trafficking of these two sets of molecules: Class II molecules intersect endocytosed antigen, whereas class I molecules efficiently bind to intracellular antigens in the endoplasmic reticulum (ER).[75,76] Thus, antigens or antigenic fragments intersecting the ER can be presented by class I molecules; those that intersect the endosomal subcellular compartment can be presented by class II molecules.

Peptide fragments from intracellular proteins are prepared for MHC class I binding by a series of processing events.[77,78] Proteins from the cytosol are digested in the cytosol by proteases in a molecular complex known as the *proteasome* (see Fig. 6-3), enzymatically trimmed, and then transported into the ER by TAP (transporter associated with antigen processing) molecules. Peptides with the proper affinity may bind to class I molecules, the α chains, and β₂-microglobulin to form peptide-MHC complex. Among the many factors that determine which antigenic peptides from a protein will be immunodominant for T-cell responses are the peptide-MHC–binding affinities, availability of the reactants, and level of competition among different peptides

for the same MHC-binding site. Of note, the forecasted immunodominant peptides may not be the ones of choice for finding antitumor activity, as the maturing T cells with specificity for these peptides may have been deleted during their maturation in the thymus.[79] Additional specialized mechanisms, involving chaperone proteins, commonly facilitate MHC binding to peptide in the ER. The complexes pass from the ER through the Golgi complex to the cell surface, where they are expressed and present peptides to CD8+ T lymphocytes.

Although the class I pathway generally presents peptides of cytoplasmic origin, selected APCs, namely DCs, can also express MHC class I–peptide complexes generated from extracellular proteins. This mechanism is particularly important for activating naive CD8+ T cells and is often referred to as *cross-priming or cross-presentation*.[80–82] *Naive T cells* are those that have left the thymus but as mature cells have not encountered their specific antigen. Mechanisms have been proposed to account for cross-presentation, including proteins in endocytic vacuoles gaining access to the cytosol and peptides from digested proteins in endocytic vacuoles gaining access to recycling MHC class I molecules without entering the cytosol. Alternatively, peptides may bind to heat-shock proteins (HSPs) in the cells of origin, leave the cells as peptide-HSP complexes, enter APCs through HSP receptors, and finally enter the cytosol and processing mechanisms in the standard class I pathway.[83] HSPs derived from tumor cells may be useful in this fashion for stimulating antitumor CTLs.

Antigen processing is generally necessary for the expression of class I molecules at the cell surface, because class I α chains do not efficiently exit the ER in large quantities unless they are fully assembled with peptide and β_2-microglobulin. The ability of a cell to process antigens via the class II pathway (see Fig. 6-3) is more specialized than the almost ubiquitous ability of nucleated cells to process antigen via the class I pathway. Class II–bearing cells include DCs, macrophages, and B lymphocytes.

Proteins whose peptides are destined for presentation by MHC class II molecules generally are acquired from outside the cell by immature DCs, macrophages, and B lymphocytes.[71,84,85] Antigen uptake occurs by means of endocytosis, which commonly is mediated by cell surface receptors and ranges from the engulfment of fluid with soluble materials (pinocytosis) to the uptake of particulate materials, including whole dying cells (phagocytosis). As the early endosome containing extracellular material moves away from the periphery of the cell toward the nucleus, it becomes more acidic and the activity of acid-dependent proteolytic enzymes rises in the organelle, likely brought about by endosome fusion with enzyme-containing lysosomes. Agents that block acidification, such as chloroquine, inhibit antigen processing. Proteins acquired from outside the cell are progressively denatured and enzymatically fragmented; some of them fit into open, antigen-binding grooves of class II αβ heterodimers present in the same organelle. The peptides or denatured proteins may be modified by enzymatic trimming after binding to the class II molecules.

Class II molecules arrive in the acidified endosome/lysosome organelles from the ER as a complex containing the α and β class II chains and a third chain (*invariant chain or Ii*), a nonpolymorphic, non-MHC–encoded glycoprotein. The invariant chain combines with the class II molecules soon after their synthesis in the ER and supports antigen processing by (1) facilitating the folding and assembly of class II molecules in the ER, (2) shielding the peptide-binding site from premature peptide binding, and (3) promoting movement of the complex from the ER through the Golgi complex to the acidified endosome/lysosome organelles rather than to the secretory pathway. In the acidified endosome/lysosome organelles, the invariant chain is degraded and released, the last stage of which is promoted by a class II–like molecule, HLA-DM in humans, allowing the class II molecules to bind the exogenous peptides. The assembled MHC class II–peptide complexes move to the surface of the cell, where they are expressed and are available for interacting with CD4+ T cells. The multiple stages and mechanisms required for antigen processing offer numerous opportunities for virus infections and tumor cell abnormalities to interfere with the expression of peptide-MHC complexes.[86–88]

Nonclassic Major Histocompatibility Complex Class I Molecules

Humans and mice express β_2-microglobulin–associated, MHC class I–like molecules with an unusual set of features that dis-

tinguish these "nonclassic" MHC–class Ib products from the "classic" MHC–class Ia products, such as HLA-A, -B, and -C molecules.[89–93] As a group, nonclassic MHC molecules generally are expressed at low levels, and their role in the antitumor immune response is at an early stage of investigation. They are characterized by limited polymorphism, in stark contrast to MHC class I or class II molecules, which are the most polymorphic genes to be described.

Role of Interferon-γ

Genetic evidence supports the point that many of the various molecules described in the class I pathway have related functions. TAP and proteasome component molecules appear to be very closely associated with the MHC region encoding class I α chains and class II α and β chains on chromosome 17 in the mouse or chromosome 6 in the human. Many of these groups of molecules appear to be regulated in concert with IFN-γ as the conductor. IFN-γ changes the proteolytic activity of proteasomes, perhaps to favor the production of peptides capable of binding to MHC class I. Molecules known to be up-regulated by IFN-γ include at least two, probably three, proteasome component and regulatory molecules, the peptide transporters, class I heavy chain, and β_2-microglobulin.[77,94] In addition, some HSPs are inducible with IFN-γ.[95] Class Ib genes also can respond to IFN-γ.[96] Finally, IFN-γ also induces the expression of MHC class II molecules in many cell types and tissues.[97] Thus, these groups of molecules appear to share the ability to be regulated together.

DISRUPTIONS OF ANTIGEN PRESENTATION IN MALIGNANCY

As noted in preceding sections, most cells in the body express MHC class I–peptide complexes, which are ligands for the TCRs on CD8+ T cells. Some tumor cells clearly present antigenic peptides in the context of class I, because specific recognition of tumor cells by cytolytic CD8+ T cells results in their destruction *in vitro* and *in vivo*. Tumor cells that fail to process or present antigen recognized by cytotoxic T cells may enjoy a selective advantage, because they are not susceptible to antigen-specific T cells.[98]

Tumor cells can escape antigen-specific, T-cell recognition by different mechanisms, which often are abnormalities reflecting genetic instability.[98–101] Genetic changes in tumor cells can reduce their ability to present antigens by any of a variety of ways without impairing cell viability or growth. Antigen presentation by class I molecules in humans requires the class I α chain encoded by genes on chromosome 6, the β_2-microglobulin chain encoded by genes on chromosome 15, and peptide from the processed antigen. Failure to generate, assemble, and transport the complete complex to the cell surface results in loss of antigen presentation. A prominent example is loss of the expression of relevant MHC genes. Loss of class I expression by tumor cells in a specimen ranges from partial to total loss, from specific class I alleles to all class I expression, and from a portion of the tumor cells to all of the tumor cells. Many studies focus on freshly explanted tumors, as cultured lines can accumulate additional genetic alterations *in vitro*. Tumor lines are also used, however, for detailed analysis of the numerous genetic changes that can alter MHC expression. For example, some tumor cells derived from epithelium have greatly reduced or undetectable levels of class I molecules on their surfaces. These histologies include embryonal carcinomas, choriocarcinomas, cervical carcinomas, mammary carcinomas, small cell carcinomas of the lung, neuroblastomas, colorectal carcinomas, and some melanomas. Other tumors, including melanoma and renal cell carcinoma, express virtually no class I on their cell surfaces as a result of absent or mutated β$_2$-microglobulin.[98,102,103] Thus, in these cell lines, the class I α chain molecules do not fold properly, never leave the ER, and are degraded rapidly. β$_2$-microglobulin–deficient mice have been found to express little, if any, functional class I antigen and have no mature CD8+ T cells.[104] The frequencies of HLA class I antigen alterations in human cervical carcinomas, breast carcinomas, and colorectal carcinomas have been reported to be 87% or higher of tumor samples examined.[99] Other tumors can down-regulate the expression of particular class I loci[105] or lose the genes for particular class I α chains.[106] Still other tumors, including small cell carcinoma of the lung, can down-regulate the proteasome component molecules or other specialized mechanisms that serve important roles in generating and expressing peptide-MHC complexes.[107] Moreover, tumors may escape T-cell recognition because of mutations in the portion of the gene coding for a critical antigenic peptide (antigenic drift), resulting in failure of the peptide to bind to the MHC molecule or in failure of T cells to recognize the peptide-MHC complex.[108]

ROLE OF ANTIGEN-PRESENTING CELLS IN ACTIVATING ANTITUMOR T CELLS

Which cells initiate T-cell immune responses to tumor antigens? Although most tumor cells express MHC class I molecules and some tumor cells also express MHC class II molecules, they generally do not express an important set of products called *costimulatory molecules*, such as B7-1 (CD80) and B7-2 (CD86), which are believed to be critical for the activation of many T cells resting from prior stimulation and for the activation of naive T cells. In addition, tumor cells, as a rule, do not release immunostimulatory cytokines (e.g., IL-12) that may be essential for initiating T-cell responses leading to antitumor cytotoxic T cells.

Specialized APCs, designated as *accessory cells*, can help T lymphocytes respond to tumor antigens. The most effective of these cells is a group often referred to as *professional antigen-presenting cells*,[109] which are represented principally by mature DCs. These APCs are distinguished functionally from the vast majority of somatic cells, which can present antigens in the context of MHC only for recognition as target cells by effector T cells. Professional APCs are also distinguished from APCs that are unable to stimulate naive T cells. For example, immature DCs and resting B cells express low or undetectable levels of the costimulatory molecules B7-1 and B7-2 on their cell surfaces, are poor sources of APCs, and have been associated with the induction of T-cell tolerance. Effective antigen presentation by APCs is closely regulated, as APCs continuously process normal cell products and present self-antigens that could promote autoimmunity.

DENDRITIC CELLS

Mature or maturing DCs are the most effective APCs for initiating naive T-cell responses. DCs were so named because of the

stellate or branch-like appearance of a particular subpopulation of murine adherent cells from peripheral lymphoid organs,[110] reminiscent of dendrites in neural tissue. These processes presumably increase the DC's surface area and its ability to sample surrounding tissues. Understanding the differentiation pathways and detailed function of DCs *in situ* has been challenging because of the existence of the different progenitors, the different DC migration patterns, and particularly the web of interacting DC regulatory factors, such as pathogens, cells, cytokines, and cytokine feedback loops.

DCs are of hematopoietic origin, arising in humans from at least two distinct circulating precursors: myeloid (including monocytes) and plasmacytoid cells, which can be identified by cell surface markers. As immature cells, myeloid-derived DCs are widely distributed among the body's tissues, where they steadily endocytose and process potential antigens. After activation, these DCs mature and migrate into T cell–rich areas of draining lymph nodes, where they contact and activate T cells expressing appropriate TCRs. Activated DCs that have migrated into lymph nodes appear to die after a few days. Some immature DCs, without the enhanced expression of peptide-MHC complexes and costimulatory molecules needed for the activation of naive T cells, are able to migrate to lymph nodes, indicating that DC migration and maturation can be regulated independently. Plasmacytoid-derived DCs are found in T cell–rich areas of peripheral lymphoid organs, but they do not appear to serve as sentinels in the general tissues of the body.

In the course of presenting MHC-associated, antigenic peptides to T cells, DCs appear to mediate two opposing functions that are of vital importance to the immune system.[111–114] As potent stimulators of naive T cells, they initiate primary immune responses. They also provide strong stimulation for previously stimulated T cells that are resting. By contrast, they also support tolerance to self-antigens. These two conflicting activities, activation and tolerance, appear to relate to different stages of DC maturation. Endocytosis, including phagocytosis, is a prominent feature of immature DCs, and they express MHC class I molecules bearing peptides likely processed by cross-presenting mechanisms (see earlier in Antigen Processing for Presentation by Major Histocompatibility Class I and II Molecules). Indeed, studies with mice show that cross-presentation *in vivo* is mainly by DCs.[85] By receptor-mediated phagocytosis, immature DCs can engulf live cells (e.g., opsonized cells), dying cells (e.g., apoptotic cells), and necrotic cells, including tumor cells and infected cells.[115] The expression of MHC class II and costimulatory molecules by immature DCs, however, is relatively low.

Immature DCs can be activated by a variety of stimuli to transform into mature DCs. The responding DCs greatly enhance their cell surface expression of MHC class I and class II molecules, costimulatory molecules such as B7-1 and B7-2, and chemokine receptors that promote migration toward T-cell–rich regions of the draining lymphoid organs. For example, *Langerhans cells*, which are immature DCs particularly evident in the epidermis of the skin and in the epithelium of mucosal surfaces, mature and migrate becoming activated to the regional lymph nodes. Many of the DC-activating microbial products act through toll-like receptors that induce primordial defenses against various pathogens, including the release of proinflammatory cytokines.[1,116–119] Some cytokines [e.g., IL-10 and transforming growth factor-β (TGF-β)] inhibit the maturation of DCs. Antigen uptake falls in mature DCs. However, antigens processed by immature DCs accumulate in the endosomes, and with DC maturation the stores of antigens are expressed on the cell surface as increased levels of MHC class I and II complexed with antigenic peptides.

Maturing and mature DCs, which appear to have a life span of just a few days, can activate naive T cells in the lymph nodes in an antigen-specific fashion, including T cells destined to develop very different functions. They can activate naive CD4+ T cells and selectively influence, or perhaps determine, which broad function the cells will develop. Thus, activated naive CD4+ T cells may become *Th1 CD4+ helper T cells* that support cellular immune responses, *Th2 CD4+ helper T cells* that support humoral immune responses, or regulatory T cells that cause unresponsiveness to antigens.[111,120–122] During their brief life span, mature DCs appear to maintain a particular polarizing effect on the development of helper T cells, and various designations have been used to refer to the DCs displaying these activities, such as *Th-1 promoting, Th-1 cell inducing, Th-1 polarizing,* and *DC1.*

Numerous factors appear to influence whether maturing DCs become professional APCs with DC1 or DC2 cell functions or whether the T cell–stimulating ability of DCs is inhibited and tolerogenic activity dominates. A decisive factor is the level of IL-12 produced by the DCs early in the course of maturation. High levels of IL-12 are associated with DC1 activity and low levels with DC2 activity, if antigen presentation by peptide-MHC complexes and costimulatory activity (e.g., by B7-1 and B7-2) remain high. If microbial products are contributing to DC maturation, the nature of the organism is important. Cytokines in the microenvironment of the maturing DCs are important; for example, DC production of IL-12 is promoted by IFN-γ and inhibited by TGF-β, prostaglandin E_2 (PGE_2), and IL-10. The time course of DC maturation is important: The production of IL-12 is highest early after the initiation of maturation.

Activated DCs are also the most effective APCs for stimulating naive CD8+ T cells, including human peripheral blood T cells with TCRs specific for a melanoma differentiation antigen.[123] In at least one model, optimal stimulation of naive CD8+ T cells by mature DCs that results in not just proliferation but also cytolytic effector activity depends particularly on the presence of IL-12.[124] This association may relate to IL-12 released by DCs that also promote Th-1 CD4+ T cells, which help cellular immune responses. Like DCs promoting naive CD4+ Th-1 cell responses, those promoting naive CD8+ T-cell responses express high levels of costimulatory molecules and produce high levels of IL-12; however, the CD8+ T cells specifically recognize MHC class I–peptide complexes rather than MHC class II–peptide complexes on DCs. As reported for DC stimulation of naive CD4+ T cells, persistent presentation of antigen to naive CD8+ T cells in a reported mouse model had an important role, and in this study an essential role, in promoting tolerance.[125]

With growing evidence that immature DCs and a subset of mature DCs help establish and maintain T-cell tolerance to self-antigens, several mechanisms have been proposed for DC-mediated deletion or inactivation of T cells, including (1) antigen presentation with insufficient costimulation, (2) DC tryptophan metabolism resulting in either a product toxic for bound T cells or else insufficient tryptophan levels essential for proliferation of the T cells, and (3) the induction of several different populations of regulatory T cells—including CD4+CD25+ cells—that suppress the activities of other T cells.[112,114,125,126] The presence of IL-10 during DC maturation and chronic antigenic stimulation of T cells by immature DCs appear to have roles in the development of suppressor T cells.

B CELLS AND MACROPHAGES AS ANTIGEN-PRESENTING CELLS

B cells are particularly adept at taking in soluble antigens, present at low concentrations, after specific antigen binding to their cell surface Ig receptors and subsequent receptor-mediated endocytosis.[71] Moreover, B cells constitutively express high levels of MHC class II molecules, and after activation they can also express large quantities of the costimulatory molecules B7-1 and B7-2. Thus, B cells can present exogenous antigens to CD4+ T cells via their class II molecules and stimulate antigen-specific T-cell help. They are not known for cross-presentation of antigen, however, and before activation they may tolerize naive T cells because of insufficient expression of costimulatory molecules.

As they enter various tissues, circulating monocytes differentiate into macrophages.[85,127,128] Macrophages are represented in all tissues, especially in areas surrounding blood vessels and near epithelial cells. Under normal circumstances they do not divide or recirculate. Resident macrophages in some tissues have specific identifications, such as Kupffer cells in the liver sinusoids and microglia in the central nervous system. Tissue macrophages and myeloid DCs are closely related, as sources of both include a common myeloid progenitor and examples of both can be generated from monocytes.

Immunologically, macrophages participate as APCs. Resting, unstimulated macrophages, as represented by microglia from healthy central nervous system tissue, express low levels of MHC class II and costimulatory molecules. Without activation they are relatively poor APCs for T-cell stimulation and may induce tolerance.[129] The APC function of macrophages is regulated. Exposing macrophages to inflammatory cytokines (e.g., IFN-γ or TNF-α) enhances cell surface expression of MHC class I and II molecules, costimulatory molecules, and APC activity. Exposing macrophages to a variety of pathogens, bacterial products, and necrotic cell debris has the same effect. Macrophages, like DCs, can engulf cells by phagocytosis through a wide variety of cell surface receptors and present antigenic peptides that complex with MHC class II. In contrast to DCs, however, macrophages do not appear to cross-present antigens on MHC class I molecules. Phagocytosis of apoptotic (but not infected) cells before their lysis commonly is associated with macrophage release of antiinflammatory cytokines (e.g., TGF-β, PGE_2, and platelet-activating factor) that would tend to suppress APC activity.[130]

ANTIGEN-PRESENTING CELLS IN THE TUMOR MICROENVIRONMENT

Tissue injury has long been associated with inflammation and infiltration of host leukocytes. Cancer is no exception.[98,128,131,132] Leukocytes are drawn to the tumor site by particular chemokines, which are chemoattractant proteins for cells with appropriate receptors. Macrophages in particular, derived from circulating monocytes, and immature DCs are among the infiltrating leukocytes. Early findings indicate that tumor-associated macrophages commonly release cytokines, including IL-10, that inhibit antigen presentation; they have relatively poor antigen-presenting ability; and they may promote tumor growth. The tumor cytokine environment, including IL-10, PGE_2, and TGF-β, may inhibit the activation of DCs and consequently their migration to the draining lymph nodes and maturation of their APC activity. In this environment, APCs would tend to be Th-1 promoting. However, the naturally occurring inflammatory infiltrate, including the APCs, may contribute to rather than inhibit cancer growth and spread.

T-CELL RECOGNITION OF TUMOR ANTIGENS

Antitumor T cells are stimulated after they interact with tumor cells or with APCs that initiate antitumor responses. A variety of receptor-ligand interactions occur between the two cell surfaces that initiate T-cell activation. The most important of these is between TCRs and MHC-antigen complexes on the opposing cell surface.

TUMOR ANTIGEN–SPECIFIC T-CELL RECEPTOR

Antitumor T cells express receptors (TCRs) that react with tumor-associated antigens. The antigens and their recognition by TCRs are often called *cognate antigens* and *cognate recognition* (from the Latin word *cognatus* meaning "born together"), respectively, which refer to the interaction of a native ligand (antigen) with its receptor (TCR), that is, molecules that typically interact. The TCR consists of two paired proteins that form a transmembrane, nonsecreted heterodimer. The heterodimer is unique for each clone of T cells and determines the antigen specificity of the TCR.[133] Two types of TCRs and their crystal structures have been identified, the αβ heterodimer and the γδ heterodimer.[50,133,134] The crystal structures, determined for multiple TCRs complexed with peptide-MHC class I and class II ligands, demonstrate the structural basis for a TCR recognizing (contacting) the bound peptide and the adjacent MHC molecule (MHC-restricted antigen recognition).[135–137] In this chapter, we emphasize T cells expressing TCR αβ, because they are the main T cell reported among tumor-infiltrating lymphocytes[138] and their development and function have been widely reported.

The affinity of the TCR for the peptide-MHC complex is far weaker than that of most antibody-antigen interactions, a property consistent with an important role for other antigen-independent, T-cell surface receptors acting as accessory molecules in promoting the triggering process.[139,140] TCR-peptide-MHC complex interactions have low affinities and rapid off-rates, thus allowing for a rapid scanning-type interaction.[140,141] Soluble, fluorescent peptide-MHC tetramers can identify individual T cells with a particular antigen reactivity, including human tumor antigens.[142–144]

Antitumor TCRs recognize the three-dimensional structure of the contact surface provided by a peptide-MHC complex. A TCR can show great specificity for a peptide-MHC complex. For example, a very minor change in the structure of the complex can alter the contact surface sufficiently to convert a reactive complex to one that will not react with the TCR. Alternatively, different peptides presented by the same or different MHC molecules can activate the same TCR, showing marked degeneracy in antigen recognition. Studies of crystal structures of TCR-peptide-MHC complexes appear to explain the seemingly inconsistent properties of TCR specificity, where a TCR can recognize a variety of different peptide-MHC complexes. Cross-reactivity may occur if the altered peptide-MHC complex presents a structural TCR recognition surface similar to the native peptide-MHC[145] or if the TCR is physically flexible, allowing adaptable binding.[146] Activation of the same TCR by different peptide-MHC complexes is sometimes referred to as *antigenic cross-reactivity* or *antigenic mimicry*. The well-established observation that at least some TCRs can show considerable degeneracy or plasticity in antigen recognition changes the rule in these cases from "one cell–one specificity" used for B cells and humoral immunity to "one cell–many specificities" for T cells.[147] Several factors may promote degeneracy in tumor-antigen recognition by a T cell: if only a few TCR molecules on a T cell's surface need to be bound by antigen to activate the T cell; if the density of antigen on the APC is high; if the TCR-peptide-MHC complexes can activate the T cell when the "fit" between the TCR and peptide-MHC complex is relatively poor, reflecting a low binding affinity; and if the TCR-binding sites can change conformation to adapt to the antigen-binding site.[147] An intriguing aspect of TCR degeneracy may apply to antitumor immunity: A peptide antigen modified at a residue associated with TCR binding, instead of one that is critical for MHC binding, may activate naive antitumor T cells that are not activated by the native tumor antigen, but nevertheless as differentiated effector cells will react with the native tumor antigen.[148,149]

STRUCTURE OF TUMOR-SPECIFIC T-CELL RECEPTORS

Through a process of differentiation in the thymus, a mature receptor-bearing T cell, with the potential capability of recognizing a tumor-associated antigen, generally expresses an αβ heterodimeric TCR.[133] On the cell surface, α and β chains, each approximately 40 to 45 kD molecular weight, are disulfide linked. Each mature T cell expresses only one β chain, because productive rearrangement of a TCR β gene prevents subsequent full rearrangements of other β genes (allelic exclusion), with rare exceptions.[150,151] The TCR α gene is not subject to allelic exclusion, and T cells have the potential to express two different α-chain genes, one from each allele.[152] Most individual T cells, however, appear to be limited to the functional expression of antigen receptors with the same α chains.[153]

A high frequency of T-cell clones react not only with the foreign antigens against which they were intentionally immunized but also with allo-MHC determinants.[154] This dual reactivity may represent cross-reactivity of a single TCR with different antigens, which would maintain the rule of one cell–one receptor. Nevertheless, the possibility of significant numbers of T cells expressing two TCR αβ receptors has not been excluded.[155,156]

Each of the TCR α and β chains expressed on the surface of a T cell consists of a C-terminal constant region and an extracellular N-terminal variable region. The constant region anchors each chain to the cell surface membrane and promotes signal transduction. Unlike antibodies, the constant region of TCR chains does not have different regions that

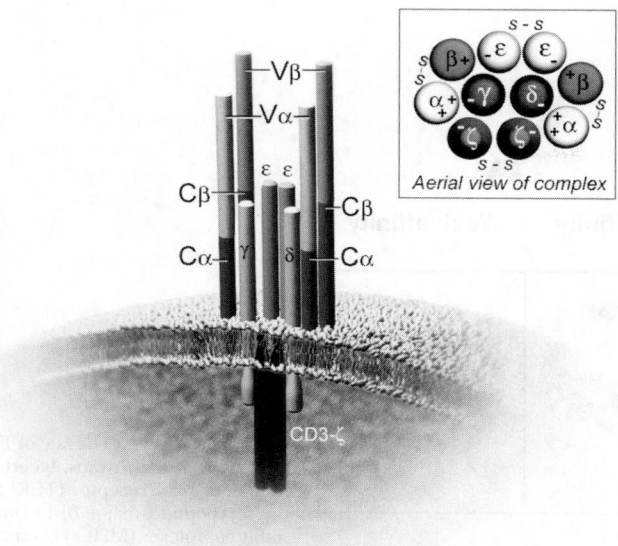

Aerial view of complex

FIGURE 6-4. T-cell receptor (TCR) complex. α, α chain of the TCR; β, β chain of the TCR; V, polypeptide variable region; C, polypeptide constant region; ε, γ, δ, and ξ, chains that constitute the CD3 complex. (An alternative nomenclature includes only ε, γ, and δ chains in the CD3 complex.) (Illustration by Emily Green Shaw.)

relate to differences in function, such as binding complement or binding to receptors on the surfaces of other cells. The paired variable regions from the two TCR chains provide binding specificity for MHC-restricted antigens. The generation process for the variable region is based on sequential somatic recombination of gene segments from three basic families of variable region germline genes, each of which contributes a gene segment to the variable region of a TCR chain. The ability of the immune system's T cells to recognize a vast range of MHC-restricted antigens appears to result from the generation and selection of a large number of different TCRs during T-cell maturation in the thymus, combined with TCR degeneracy in antigen recognition.

T-CELL RECEPTOR–CD3 COMPLEX

Expression of TCRs at the cell surface and also triggering of T cells after the cross-linking of TCRs through binding with antigen depend on the close but noncovalent association of TCRs with the CD3 complex, which consists of several invariant proteins (Fig. 6-4).[157] Cytoplasmic portions of this complex are critical to TCR-initiated signal transduction, and particular extracellular portions provide serologic markers commonly used to define mature T cells with anti-CD3 antisera.

MATURATION OF ANTITUMOR T CELLS

Precursors of T cells with the potential to participate in the antitumor response generally migrate from the bone marrow to the thymus, where they mature.[158,159] A series of important events, which define specific functions of mature T cells, occur in the thymus. Here, among a considerable amount of cell pro-

liferation and cell death, T cells first express antigen reactivity, develop MHC restriction for antigen recognition, and express the cell surface CD4 or CD8 molecules that relate closely to whether the T cell will recognize MHC class I– or class II–restricted antigens. It is here that individual T cells are limited to the expression of one TCR reactivity, or perhaps two in a few cases. It is also here that the first round of selection occurs against maturing T cells that react against the body's normal tissue antigens.

Much of the current understanding of T-cell maturation is based on models that involve genetic changes related specifically to T-cell function, such as transgenic or "knockout" mice with added or deleted germline genes, respectively, and natural mutants that affect the immune system.[160–162]

MARKERS AND PHENOTYPES OF TUMOR ANTIGEN-SPECIFIC T CELLS

Cell surface markers based on antibody reactivity have been identified that permit detecting individual T cells with a particular stage of maturation.[163,164] The markers are cell surface molecules, which present a characteristic identifying phenotype of the cell when expressed individually or in a certain combination. For example, the TCR/CD3 complex is now commonly used as a marker for T cells. Thy-1 (mouse) and CD2 are expressed rather ubiquitously, but not exclusively on T cells. Co-receptors CD4 and CD8 are expressed differently by distinct T-cell subpopulations, and mature T cells generally express one but not both.

THYMIC DEVELOPMENT OF ANTITUMOR T CELLS

The TCRs that mediate MHC-restricted recognition of tumor-associated antigens are encoded by germline genes that, with the few exceptions of extrathymic maturation, are first expressed in the thymus. The functional TCR repertoire that is expressed by mature T cells as a whole in an individual, however, is molded during at least two points in T-cell development. The first point occurs in the thymus. The second occurs with mature T cells that have left the thymus, and it is discussed later in How Peripheral T-Cell Tolerance Reduces the Antitumor T-Cell Repertoire.

The CD4+CD8+ double-positive T cells in the thymus undergo selection that results in their deletion or continued maturation. Positive selection favors the survival of T cells that, outside the thymus (commonly called the *periphery*), will react with foreign antigens presented by the same MHC determinants that are expressed in the thymic environment. MHC-bound peptides that promote positive selection are derived primarily from the endogenous pool of normal proteins within the thymus rather than from foreign proteins. Positive selection may depend on an appropriate level of signaling triggered by TCRs and determined by relatively low affinity (or avidity*) TCRs for MHC/self-peptide ligands. The nature of the peptide-MHC ligands driving positive selection in the thymus and their relationship to the peptide-MHC

---

*Avidity may be more relevant here than affinity, because *affinity* relates to the binding strength of an isolated monovalent ligand-receptor interaction, whereas *avidity* addresses a multimolecular binding surface and allows for the summation of numerous independent affinities with ongoing binding, disassociation, and rebinding.

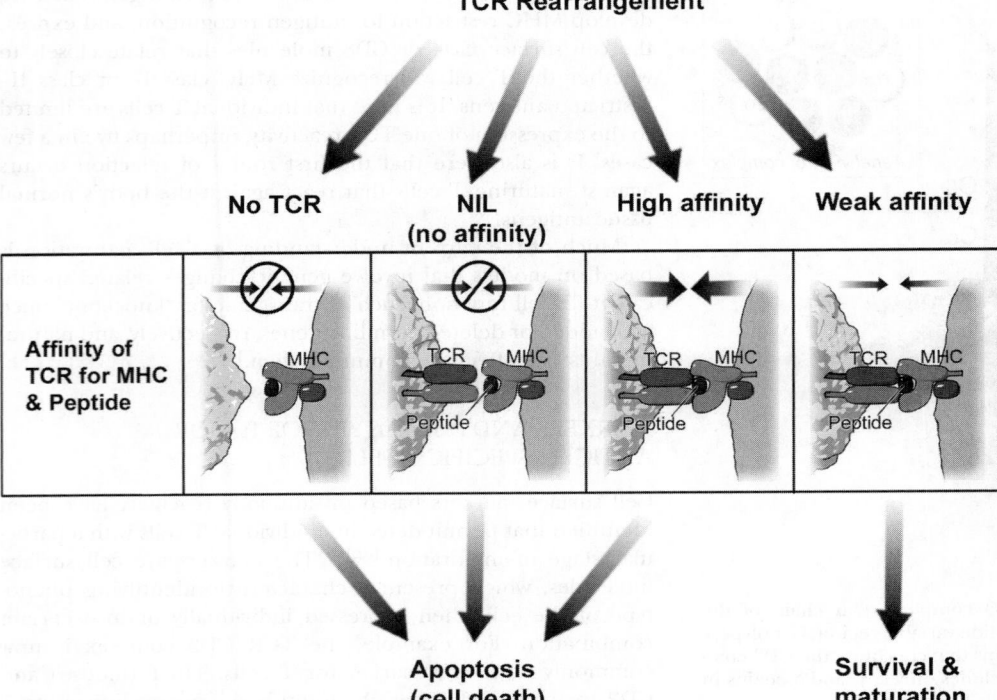

FIGURE 6-5. The fate of T cells maturing in the thymus, based on a model of T-cell receptor (TCR) affinity for peptide–major histocompatibility complexes (MHCs) on antigen-presenting cells. The figure illustrates TCR engagement of MHC class I–peptide complexes. The same basic model applies to TCR engagement of MHC class II–peptide complexes. Possible sources of co-signals for selection are not included. (Illustration by Emily Green Shaw.)

ligands activating T cells in the periphery have not been established. The relationship may include a TCR cross-reactivity between MHC/self-peptide complexes in the thymus and an MHC/foreign peptide complex in the periphery.

ELIMINATION OF POTENTIALLY TUMOR-REACTIVE T CELLS IN THE THYMUS

It appears that three paths end in the disappearance of T cells in the thymus (Fig. 6-5). First, immature T cells die if they fail to express a functional TCR. Second, they die if the TCR fails to react with MHC-antigen complexes. Third, negative selection, brought about by relatively high-affinity (or avidity) TCRs for self-MHC/self-peptide ligands, deletes many of the T cells in the thymus that would otherwise be reactive against normal tissues. Several explanations have been offered for negative selection of T cells whose TCRs react with high affinity against tissue-specific antigens,[165] such as gp100 and MART-1/Melan-A shared between melanoma cells and normal melanocytes. Tissue-specific antigens may be carried into the thymus through the circulation and then processed and presented to T cells. In addition, they may be ectopically expressed by cells within the thymus, resulting in the deletion of T cells with high avidity for "self"-antigens. Also, TCRs with high affinity against tissue-specific antigens may cross-react with other self-antigens expressed in the thymus, resulting in negative selection. Coupling negative selection to cross-reactive TCR binding, however, would also shrink the T-cell repertoire for foreign antigens.[166]

CD4 and CD8 co-receptors appear to contribute to the triggering of negative selection, as does the lymphocyte function-associated antigen 1/intracellular adhesion molecule (LFA-1/ICAM) interaction. Evidence suggests that clonal T-cell deletion in the thymus has a lower activation threshold than that required for the activation of mature peripheral T cells. This balance would reduce the likelihood of mature peripheral T cells that can react against normal tissues.

T cells in the thymus that are not selected for further maturation die by apoptosis, a process resulting in programmed cell death.[167–171] The vast majority of thymocytes die. Potentially tumor-reactive T cells with high affinities for self-antigens die after engagement of the TCR. Immature T cells whose TCRs fail to bind to other cells in the thymus appear to be preprogrammed for death by apoptosis. The differences in events between positive and negative selection that result in T-cell survival or apoptosis are not clear, but apoptosis may be initiated simply by a strong signal or set of signals delivered to the immature thymic T cells by a combination of the TCRs and other receptors.

ACTIVATION OF MATURE ANTITUMOR T CELLS

SIGNAL REQUIREMENTS FOR T-CELL ACTIVATION

The responses of mature antitumor T cells to activation commonly include combinations of cell proliferation, up-regulation of selected surface molecules, cytokine production and release, cytotoxic activity, and cell anergy or death. The initiation of antigen-specific T-cell activation requires cross-linking and clustering of the TCR/CD3 complex with an antigenic ligand, which generally consists of an antigenic peptide in association with a self-MHC product on the surface of another cell—the APC. The minimum number of MHC molecules that must be occupied by a particular peptide to activate a responsive T cell appears to be extremely low—on the order of 10, but it may be as low as 1 for some cells.[172] A single peptide-MHC complex can serially trigger many low-affinity TCRs, which are then internalized, degraded, and replaced by new cell surface TCRs. Full T-cell activation, resulting in cell proliferation and differentiation into effector functions, depends on many factors. Important variables include the concentration of antigenic peptide-MHC complexes on the APC and also the duration of interaction between the T cell and the APC.[173] Full activation requires a relatively long period of TCR triggering, which may be a day or more for naive T cells.[174] A shorter period of TCR triggering may result in a partial response (e.g., cytokine production but no proliferation) or no response.

CD8 and CD4 Molecules as Co-Receptors for Antitumor T Cells

CD8 and CD4 are cell surface glycoproteins that provide markers for the two major lineages of mature T cells. Functionally, they serve as co-receptors for delivering the TCR signals.[175–180] Although no clear structural or sequence differences have been discovered between TCRs detecting antigens associated with MHC class I versus class II molecules, a clear difference has been found in the ligands for the CD8 and CD4 molecules. CD8 and CD4 bind to invariable regions of MHC molecules that are away from the TCR-binding site and do not relate to antigen specificity. They are designated *co-receptors*, because a single peptide-MHC complex on the target cell is able to bind, simultaneously, a TCR and either a CD8 or CD4 molecule. They stabilize the TCR-peptide-MHC complex and enhance the level, the duration, or both, of TCR-mediated intracellular signaling. Their role as co-receptors is required for most immune responses by naive T cells and by some activated effector T cells. In several studies, high-affinity TCR binding does not appear to require CD8 for effective T-cell activation. In contrast, TCRs that recognize tumor-associated antigens shared with normal cells generally bind the peptide-MHC complexes with a relatively low affinity. The low-affinity TCR-peptide-MHC complex interactions commonly require co-receptor participation for T-cell activation.

Adhesion Molecules in the T-Cell Recognition of Tumor Antigens

The relatively weak interactions between TCRs and self-antigens expressed by tumors are strengthened by the binding of neighboring molecules to ligands on APCs, such as LFA-1 to ICAMs, CD2 to LFA-3, and CD5 to CD72. These interactions enhance the conjugation of T cells and APCs, thereby raising the likelihood of interactions between the TCR and the peptide-MHC complexes (Fig. 6-6).[181,182]

Molecules that facilitate the binding of a lymphocyte to its target cell have been referred to as *adhesion molecules*. However, an increasing number of these molecules also appear to provide signaling activity after engagement with their ligands, either by enhancing the signal generated by the TCR or by contributing independent stimulatory signals.[164,183–186] CD28, CD2, CD5, LFA-1, CD44, CD69, CD4, and CD8 are examples of cell surface receptors that contribute to the signaling events. Optimal activation of T cells expressing TCRs with low affinities for antigen is thus dependent on receptor-ligand interactions that promote the binding of T cells to APCs and that contribute to the T-cell activating signals.

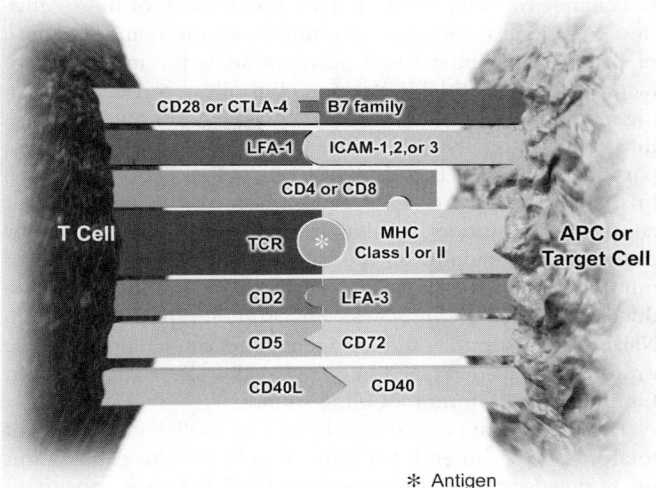

* Antigen

FIGURE 6-6. Selection of cell surface molecules associated with the mature T-cell immunologic synapse and receptor-ligand pairing during T-cell recognition of antigens on antigen-presenting cells (APCs). The physical ordering of receptor-ligand pairs in the figure is not intended to reflect that in the natural synapse. CTLA, cytotoxic T lymphocyte–associated antigen; ICAM, intracellular adhesion molecule; LFA, lymphocyte function-associated antigen; MHC, major histocompatibility complex; TCR, T-cell receptor. (Illustration by Emily Green Shaw.)

The transmembrane receptor-ligand pairs that contribute to antigen-mediated activation of T cells are highly enriched in the area of contact between T cells and APCs.[187–191] Within minutes of initial TCR triggering by peptide-MHC ligand, a mature micron-scale "immunologic synapse" forms in the area of contact between the T cell and the APC. The synapse consists of a central area of redistributed, relatively small molecules—TCR-peptide-MHC, CD4/CD8:MHC, CD28:B7, and CD2:LFA-3 (in humans)—surrounded by a ring of larger molecules such as LFA-1:ICAM-3 (in humans). Cytoplasmic participants in signaling also move toward the synapse. The existence of the synapse and some of its properties has become apparent from studies using new cell-imaging techniques and a variety of labeling probes. The role of the synapse in T-cell activation is controversial, because the synapse is not required for TCR signaling. Nevertheless, the clustering and enrichment of receptor-ligand pairs and cytoplasmic signal transduction proteins has raised several possibilities, such as increasing the antigen sensitivity of T cells expressing low-affinity receptors or reacting against APCs with low antigen densities. The synapse appears to increase the avidity of ligand-receptor interactions critical to T-cell activation. The synapse also provides the contact structure through the center of which cytotoxic T cells deliver cytotoxic secretory granules to target cells, thus limiting the innocent bystander effects of the otherwise nonspecifically toxic product.

HOW CYTOKINES AND COSTIMULATORY MOLECULES ACTIVATE ANTITUMOR T CELLS

Triggering TCRs on naive CD4+ T cells commonly induces expression of the high-affinity IL-2 receptor and rouses cells to move from the G_0 resting stage of the cell cycle into the G_1 stage. Triggering TCRs can activate effector functions of CTL, but changes in gene expression are not needed for these activities. TCR signals alone do not stimulate synthesis and secretion of IL-2. IL-2, a single 15-kD polypeptide, is the major growth factor for T cells.[192–194] IL-2 is now clinically approved for treating metastatic melanoma and kidney cancer. Although not produced by resting T cells, IL-2 is generated after cell activation, particularly by the Th1 subset of CD4+ helper T cells. Extracellular levels of IL-2 are tightly regulated by the requirement for continuous activation signaling for transcription of its gene, by the controlled half-life of its mRNA, by its serum half-life of minutes, and by the short life span of the activated T cells producing IL-2. IL-2 stimulates cell proliferation and survival. Naive T cells, stimulated by antigen alone, can become anergic without IL-2, as described later in Possible Role of Anergy in Limiting the Antitumor T-Cell Response.

Loss of IL-2 function results in immunodeficiencies, but not total loss of peripheral T-cell function.[195,196] The explanation for reduced but not absent mature T-cell function appears to be the partially redundant functions of cytokines belonging to the IL-2 family, particularly the overlap in function between IL-2 and IL-15. IL-2 and IL-15 stimulate proliferation of activated T cells and promote the development of cytolytic effector T cells. IL-15 worked as well as IL-2 in supporting rejection of large tumor growths by adoptive transfer of CD8+ T antitumor cells in a mouse model using a syngeneic tumor expressing differentiation antigens.[197] Critical differences in function exist, however, that probably result from differences between one of the three subunits that make up the IL-2 and IL-15 cell surface receptors.[193] The receptors have in common two of the three subunits. Thus, in mouse models IL-2 contributes to activation-induced cell death (AICD) of T cells, whereas IL-15 inhibits it (discussed later in Deletion of Mature, Tumor-Specific T Cells). IL-15 promotes the homeostasis (maintenance) of CD8+ memory T cells, whereas IL-2 inhibits it (discussed later in Naive, Effector, and Memory T Cells).

Triggering the TCR is often referred to as the *first signal* for T-cell activation. With naive CD4+ and CD8+ T cells and many memory cells as well, the first signal alone is commonly not sufficient for stimulating a full T-cell response. CD28 molecules on the T-cell surface can provide a critical second or costimulatory signal by engaging the B7 family of ligands on the APCs, particularly at sites where the APCs are optimally activated, such as inflamed sites or the draining lymph nodes.[198,199] B7 ligands are expressed by mature DCs, monocyte-macrophages, and activated B cells, as described earlier in Role of Antigen-Presenting Cells in Activating Antitumor T Cells.

For naive and many memory T cells, the signaling pathway associated with triggering CD28 completes the pathway for T-cell activation that was initiated by TCR triggering.[200–202] Triggering CD28 appears to reduce the threshold of TCR signaling needed for T-cell activation. In addition, the second signal appears to stimulate prolonged IL-2 production by increasing the half-life of its mRNA and by increasing the rate of gene transcription. Also, the second signal activates genes whose products, particularly Bcl-xl, promote cell survival.[170,203,204] Finally, triggering CD28 appears to control the development of CD25+CD4+ regulatory T cells in the thymus and has a prominent role in maintaining the cells in the periphery.[202] Normal cells that express a TCR-reactive antigen but lack a second signal ligand will generally not activate naive T cells; indeed, these cells may induce anergy, as described later in Possible Role of Anergy in Limiting the Antitumor T-Cell Response. Thus, TCR engagement initiates the response in an antigen-specific fashion, whereas the requirement for a second signal tends to restrict the response of naive T cells to APCs that provide antigen and second signals.[109]

In the absence of the CD28-B7 interaction, costimulatory molecules on APCs can provide second signals for previously stimulated, but generally not naive, T cells.[205,206] ICOS, which is structurally related to CD28, serves this purpose. Receptors in the TNF family, such as 4-1BB, OX40, and CD27, can also act in this fashion. Other costimulatory ligands have been reported, such as ICAM-1 (the ligand for LFA-1) and heat-stable antigen.[207] They apparently are not, however, the usual primary source of second signals, and the T-cell response is commonly partial and suboptimal. Alternative sources of costimulation are most effective when combined with a strong primary signal from the TCR.

Activation of T cells stimulates the expression of CTLA-4, a structural homologue of CD28, but one with opposite effects. CTLA-4 has a lower level of surface expression than CD28 but a far higher avidity for ligands in the B7 family.[208–210] Cross-linking CTLA-4 by B7 ligand can inhibit T-cell activation, IL-2 production, and subsequent cell proliferation. Mice lacking CTLA-4 experience severe, generalized T-cell lymphoproliferation and die within several weeks after birth. Consequently, CTLA-4 can provide a mechanism for down-regulating a T-cell response.

The stimulation requirements of one T-cell population can differ substantially from those of another. For example, naive CD8+ and CD4+ T cells generally need TCR triggering as well as second signals to proliferate and generate activated effector cells. Activated effector cells, however, do not require second signals to engage and kill target cells or release cytokines.[211–214] These functions do not require IL-2 production or cell proliferation.

FACTORS THAT CAN END THE RESPONSE OF ACTIVATED ANTITUMOR T CELLS

Eliminating most of the activating antigen generally results in death by apoptosis for the responding T cells, except for the relatively few cells remaining as memory cells.[170,215–217] After antigen clearance, the priorities of the antigen repertoire of a body's T cells return toward their baseline levels, with emphasis represented by memory cells. Many factors appear to contribute to the death of T cells activated in an immune response.

Perhaps the foremost factor is that in the absence of antigen, the stimulation for producing supportive cytokines—particularly IL-2—disappears, resulting in death of the activated T cells.[217] Also, antiapoptosis factors in the Bcl-2 family, which raise the threshold for death from IL-2 withdrawal, diminish without the T-cell activation signals. In addition, activated T cells express CTLA-4 at the cell surface, and triggered CTLA-4 can interfere with CD28-induced activation signals, as described earlier in How Cytokines and Costimulatory Molecules Activate Antitumor T Cells. Activated T cells also express higher levels of members of the TNF receptor family with death domains—"death receptors," such as Fas, which can trigger apoptosis when cross-linked. Activated T cells also express higher levels of ligands for the death receptors. Thus, activated T cells are more at risk for apoptotic death than are resting cells. Other factors are at work, too, which act by inhibiting the response even as it is developing. Regulatory T cells may interfere with activated T cells or their generation, as described later in CD4+CD25+ Regulatory T Cells. T-cell responses may also be inhibited by mechanisms associated with peripheral T-cell tolerance.

HOW PERIPHERAL T-CELL TOLERANCE REDUCES THE ANTITUMOR T-CELL REPERTOIRE

The concepts and observations underlying tolerance are central to T-cell responses to human cancer, because many human cancer antigens associated with clinical responses to T-cell immunity are from normal autologous proteins (see Tumor-Associated Antigens Targeted with T Cells, earlier in this chapter).[31] Consequently, T cells specific for these tumor antigens are confined by many of the mechanisms of tolerance that resist the development of autoimmunity. Activating these T cells may require breaking restrictions of tolerance in a selective fashion that does not unleash autoimmunity.

Tolerance is the failure of the immune system to respond to an antigen, particularly an antigen from normal autologous tissues. Failure can be measured anywhere between the response of a single T cell and the response of the entire immune system. Investigators specify their criteria with each study. In this section we comment on failure of T-cell responses to reject tumors because of mechanisms associated with tolerance.

The potential for mature T-cell responses to self-antigens is reduced in the thymus in an antigen-specific fashion by negative selection, resulting in central tolerance (see Elimination of Potentially Tumor-Reactive T Cells in the Thymus, earlier in this chapter). However, some T cells leaving the thymus have the potential to react against self-antigens in the periphery. Escape of self-reactive T cells from the thymus is particularly likely for cells that can react in the periphery with tissue-specific antigens that are not presented adequately or imitated in the thymus in a fashion sufficient to induce clonal deletion. The escaped T cells may encounter more potent immunizing conditions in the periphery, which are sufficient to stimulate T-cell activity against MHC/self-peptide complexes on normal host cells that otherwise would be ignored. For example, an inflamed environment occurring naturally or as part of intentional immunization might activate APCs. The associated enhancement of antigen presentation to T cells by the activated APCs might reach the threshold necessary for triggering otherwise unresponsive T cells. Without the nonspecific immunostimulation associated with inflammation, the T cells and normal cells expressing the appropriate self-antigens might simply coexist without evidence of an immune response. This state is often referred to as *immunologic ignorance*, which could represent simply a lack of contact between the immune system and the antigen or could represent self-antigen at too low a concentration or too low an avidity for the TCR to trigger a T-cell response. Tolerance among mature T cells can also be induced in the periphery in an antigen-specific fashion by causing cellular anergy or by deleting the T cells. These possibilities are addressed in the following sections.

POSSIBLE ROLE OF ANERGY IN LIMITING THE ANTITUMOR T-CELL RESPONSE

In a variety of models, primary T-cell responses to antigen by either CD4+ or CD8+ T cells may result in antigen-specific anergy, in which the T cells are functionally inactivated but continue to exist in a hyporesponsive state for an extended period of time.[218] Anergic cells do not produce IL-2 or proliferate, even under optimal conditions for normal activation. Otherwise, anergic cells may differ in a variety of important ways. Addition of IL-2 or removal of antigen may or may not end the anergy, depending on how the anergy was induced. Suboptimal TCR triggering by peptide-MHC complexes, for example by low TCR affinity or low concentrations, may induce anergy. T cells may become anergic after TCR triggering without costimulatory signals, or they may become anergic after TCR triggering followed by negative signals from cell surface T-cell receptors in the CD28 (T-cell)-B7 (APC) superfamily. For example, CTLA-4 signaling, triggered by a B7 ligand, blocks cell-cycle progression. Like the receptor-ligand pairs other than CD28-B7 that may provide costimulation signals for T-cell activation, there are receptor-ligand pairs other than CTLA-4–B7 that may inhibit T-cell activation.[219] The balance between positive versus negative co-signaling may be particularly relevant to T-cell tolerance to cancer *in vivo*. Indeed, treatment of melanoma patients by blockade of CTLA-4 combined with a concurrent or previous melanoma vaccine has resulted in objective cancer regression and also signs of autoimmunity.[27,28]

DELETION OF MATURE, TUMOR-SPECIFIC T CELLS

After activation, mature peripheral T cells can be deleted by apoptosis as a result of repetitive restimulation with high concentrations of antigen.[220–224] Tumor antigens, T-cell mitogens, and antibodies against the TCR/CD3 complex have all been associated with the outcome. The process, often referred to as *activation-induced cell death* (AICD), can affect CD4+ and CD8+ T cells.[166,217,225,226] In most cases, T-cell deletion is preceded several days by strong antigenic restimulation of already activated T cells, by IL-2 release from the activated cells, and by rapid proliferation possibly driven by the IL-2. When activated, proliferating T cells pass into the late G_1 or S phase of the cell cycle, where they appear to be far more susceptible to apoptosis than in the resting stage.

The roles of factors contributing to death of the T cells in this situation are unsettled, such as the strength of the TCR stimulation, the role of other cytokines in the IL-2 family, and co-signals delivered by accessory cells. The T-cell deletion appears to be caused by apoptosis triggered primarily by Fas ligand, but also by other TNF-like ligands whose receptors are up-regulated on activated T cells. Because a T cell can express Fas ligand as well as Fas, T cells can kill themselves (suicide) and each other (fratricide). Fas-mediated apoptosis in this situation affects primarily the activated T cells with TCRs bound to antigen at the time that Fas is triggered. Activated T cells from mice with a defect in the Fas gene are less susceptible to AICD than activated T cells from normal mice.[227] AICD may serve a normal physiologic function by limiting the height and duration of a T-cell response. In selected situations AICD may also contribute to tolerance; for example, it may abort a response to persistently high levels of antigen, such as might occur in a host with widely spread cancer. IL-2 is likely the primary natural stimulus for the T-cell proliferation that is required for AICD. This possibility could contribute to the unanticipated observations that loss of IL-2 function resulted in lymphoproliferative disorders and autoimmunity in mice and in one patient.[195,196] An alternative interpretation is based on the possible role of IL-2 in promoting regulatory T-cell activity and that loss of

IL-2 function and regulatory cell activity results in the immune disorders (discussed later in CD4+CD25+ Regulatory T Cells).

ACTIVATION STATES OF ANTITUMOR T CELLS

NAIVE, EFFECTOR, AND MEMORY T CELLS

Three populations of T cells—naive T cells, effector T cells, and memory T cells—constitute the antigen repertoire of the pool of mature T cells.[228] They differ by their state of activation and by prior exposure to antigen. The T cells commonly referred to as *naive* or *virgin* are immunocompetent T cells that have not been activated by antigen in the periphery, such as those that have just emerged from the thymus—the primary (central) lymphoid organ for generating mature T cells from nonfunctional precursors. After activation, these cells may develop specific functions associated with cytotoxic activity or the release of particular cytokines. In this activated state they are referred to as *effector* cells. After a short period in the activated state, most of the cells die, but some appear to become *memory* cells. The extent of T-cell death depends, in part, on the dose of antigen, with lower doses resulting in less death.

Naive T cells are long lived and circulate through the blood stream and lymphatics between the secondary (peripheral) lymphoid organs (such as lymph nodes, the spleen, and lymphoid tissue associated with the mucosa of the small intestine), where they may encounter APCs presenting their specific antigens and be activated. The long life span of naive T cells appears to depend on their TCRs interacting with normal cells expressing complexes of MHC/self-peptide; otherwise, the naive cells die by apoptosis.[229,230] The interaction does not trigger cell activation and the generation of effector functions, perhaps because TCR triggering is relatively weak, as with positive selection in the thymus. Naive T cells are uncommon in nonlymphoid tissues. They are primarily resting cells that do not proliferate rapidly without antigen stimulation, which would change them to the activated or effector category. Consequently, little of the antigen repertoire represented by naive T cells is against a particular pathogen. In response to general T-cell depletion, the body's naive T-cell population approximately expands back to its baseline numbers.[216]

Effector T cells are activated, can proliferate rapidly, act immediately after target cell contact (e.g., cytolysis or cytokine release), and are short lived. Exhibiting different homing properties than naive T cells, they are commonly found in nonlymphoid, extravascular tissues.

Memory T cells are characterized by their ability to generate an immune response that is earlier, more intense, and longer lasting than that of naive cells, after reexposure of the host to the same antigen or a cross-reacting antigen.[231,232] The nature of the progenitors has not been settled, such as naive cells, effector cells, and intermediate cells. Memory cells have been divided in the literature into two major groupings called *central memory* and *effector memory*. These distinctions are based on their homing to different tissues and their expression of different cell surface molecules. Central and effector memory cells home to secondary lymphoid and nonlymphoid tissues (including sites of inflammation), respectively.

The generation of functional CD8+ T-cell memory may require CD4+ T-cell help. T-cell memory appears to involve intermittent proliferation of T cells responding to cytokines, particularly IL-7 and IL-15. As discussed earlier in the sections Possible Role of Anergy in Limiting the Antitumor T-Cell Response and Deletion of Mature Tumor-Specific T Cells, T cells specifically reactive with the antigen can be deleted or functionally inactivated. In response to general T-cell depletion, the body's memory T cells expand back to their baseline numbers, independent of that for naive T cells and that for B lymphocytes.[216]

PHENOTYPES OF ANTIGEN-STIMULATED ANTITUMOR T CELLS

Characteristic cell surface markers have greatly facilitated tracking antigen-activated, effector T cells and distinguishing them from naive T cells. The activated mature peripheral T cells express CD45RO, a low-molecular-weight isoform of CD45, and relatively little of the higher-molecular-weight form (CD45RA) associated with naive cells. They may also express a variety of cell surface molecules at higher levels than are found on naive T cells, including CD2, LFA-1, LFA-3, CD27, CD29, CD44, CD69, adhesion molecules in the very late activation antigen (VLA) series that react with extracellular matrix proteins, the IL-2R α chain associated with high-affinity IL-2 receptor activity, and MHC class II molecules. CD44 is commonly used as a marker for memory cells because of persistent expression by the cells. As the activated cells revert to a resting stage, many of the activation markers are lost. An unsettled issue is how well cell surface markers can distinguish between activated cells and memory cells; consequently, the two types of cells are grouped together here.

MIGRATION OF ANTITUMOR T CELLS

The antigen repertoire of peripheral T cells can be partitioned, to an extent, in the body through the selected migration of T cells out of the circulation. Naive T cells exit the circulation directly into lymphoid tissues through a specialized type of venule designated *high endothelial venules*.[233–235] The movement of the T cells through the endothelium occurs in several sequential steps that involve progressively tighter binding of the lymphocytes to the endothelial wall and, finally, migration through the endothelium into the extravascular space. Specialized adhesion molecules on circulating T cells (e.g., L-selectin), binding to particular mucin-like molecules on the high endothelial venules, provide specificity for the exit site. This process is also called *homing*.

Effector and most memory cells do not bear receptors (e.g., L-selectin) associated with migration directly into normal secondary lymphoid tissues. Instead, they migrate to other selected sites, such as the gastrointestinal wall, the skin, and sites of inflammation. Other receptors, not expressed by naive cells, have been identified (e.g., VLA-4 for inflamed sites and cutaneous lymphocyte antigen for skin) that contribute to the selective exit sites for memory and effector T cells.

Chemotactic cytokines, or *chemokines*, contribute to the exit sites for cells by binding to specific determinants on the endothelial wall, such as macrophage inflammatory protein-1β, which binds to selected proteoglycans on the endothelium and promotes T-cell adhesion, particularly of CD8+ T cells.[236] Inflammation and associated cytokines also up-regulate lymphocyte-binding ligands expressed by the endothelial cells.

The tissue migration of lymphocytes, and leukocytes in general, is largely influenced by chemokines.[237–241] These small proteins belong to a family of at least 40 members in humans. On the basis of a cysteine motif, most of the chemokines and their receptors are classified as in the CXC (α) or CC (β) subfamilies. At least 15 cell surface, G protein–coupled receptors for chemokines have been identified. Chemokines in the CXC subfamily act primarily on neutrophils and other selected leukocytes, whereas those in the CC subfamily generally act on a different spectrum of leukocytes and not on neutrophils. Within a subfamily there is redundancy in receptor-ligand pairing in that most receptors bind more than one chemokine, and several chemokines can bind to more than one receptor. A single cell can express different chemokine receptors; thus, cell migration may respond to combinatorial patterns and gradients of chemokines. Cells activated by chemokines may change in other ways too, such as modulating the expression of cell surface adhesion molecules. Although the conditions have not been resolved under which several types of cells do or do not express particular chemokine receptors, a general pattern is emerging in which chemokine receptor expression, and thus responsiveness to chemokines, may vary with the subtype of cell, such as Th1 versus Th2 T cells, with resting or immature versus activated or mature cells, and with the source of activation. For example, immature DCs express receptors for chemokines commonly produced at sites of inflammation by resident cells and infiltrating leukocytes and, hence, may home to these sites, where they gather antigens, are activated by cytokines associated with inflammation, and appear to alter their expression of receptors to ones associated with chemokines produced constitutively in normal lymphoid tissues, with subsequent homing to these sites. Consequently, the recruitment of particular combinations of cells to selected sites, such as naive CD8+ T cells, CD4+ Th1 helper cells, and APCs, is strongly influenced by an integrated combination of cytokines and chemokines. By regulating lymphocyte migration to particular anatomic sites, chemokines affect not only the activation of lymphocytes by antigens but also the development and maturation of normal lymphoid tissues.

FUNCTIONS OF MATURE ANTITUMOR T CELLS

CD4+ T-CELL SUBSETS

Helper T Cells

The generation of CTL *in situ* generally benefits from help from other T cells.[242,243] The helper T cells, activated by APCs, may provide IL-2, other cytokines, or cell surface ligands for nearby CTL precursor cells attached to the same APCs. The predominant activity of helper T cells, however, may be to promote progressive self-activation and APC activation through TCR-peptide-MHC coupling and CD40/CD40L coupling, respectively, between conjugated helper T cells and APCs, followed by the activated APCs instigating the critical first (TCR triggering) and second (e.g., CD28 triggering) signals for activating attached naive CTL precursors.[244–246] In addition, the activated APCs may provide important cytokines, such as IL-12, for CTL activation. DCs, the key APCs for inducing CD8+ T-cell responses against tumor antigens, can be activated by factors other than helper T cells (see Dendritic Cells, earlier in this chapter). Indeed, CD4+ T cells are not necessary in a variety of studies of primary responses by CD8+ T cells; however, support from CD4+ T helper cells reduces the need for CD28 costimulatory signals in the responding T cell.[247–250] Helper T cells may be required in these systems for the generation of CD8+ memory T cells. The life span of memory CD8+ T cells, and their ability to proliferate and function in response to antigen, may be impaired seriously by the absence of help from CD4+ T cells during the primary response, irrespective of the maturity of the DCs.

CD4+ helper T cells have been further subdivided into two groups of cells, Th1 and Th2, on the basis of the patterns of cytokines that they secrete after being stimulated.[251–258] CD4+CD25+ regulatory T cells are described in the following section. In contrast to the TCR, which determines the specificity of the T cell, the secreted cytokines affect the function of the targeted T cells. One group promotes primarily cellular immune responses (Th1) and the other group humoral immune responses (Th2). In human models, IFN-γ is secreted by Th1 cells, whereas IL-4, IL-5, and IL-9 are secreted by Th2 cells. Many helper T cells secrete Th1 and Th2 cytokines and are referred to as *Th0 cells*, which may represent an earlier stage of differentiation. Naive T cells generate primarily IL-2 after stimulation, and the pattern of cytokines surrounding these stimulated T cells strongly influences whether a Th1 or Th2 type of response develops.

The responses of the two classes of helper T cells are influenced differently by many factors, including the nature of the antigen and its dose, the type of APC and its membrane-bound costimulatory signals, and various pharmacologic agents. As with humoral and cellular immunity, the responses of the two classes of helper T cells often are regulated in a reciprocal fashion, and here the influence of cytokines is critical. For example, in mouse models, the presence of IFN-γ and IL-12 and the absence of IL-4 tend to promote the activation of Th1 cells, whereas IL-4 and IL-10 tend to promote the activation of Th2 cells. Reciprocal roles for individual cytokines have been observed, in that IFN-γ can directly inhibit the proliferation of Th2 cells, and IL-10 can inhibit cytokine production by Th1 cells indirectly by inhibiting macrophage activation of the Th1 cells.

CD4+CD25+ Regulatory T Cells

Regulatory T cells are capable of inhibiting the activities of other cells, including CD4+ and CD8+ T cells. It remains unclear whether early observations on "suppressor" T cells account for the phenomenon that can be induced by "regulatory" T cells; however, recent work has brought clarity on the cellular and molecular levels to these earlier studies. The most studied of the regulatory T-cell subpopulations have a CD4+CD25+ phenotype and express a transactivator gene called *FOXP3* (*Foxp3* in mice).[259–261] These regulatory T cells suppress the functions of other T cells largely through a mechanism that requires cell-to-cell contact.

It has been reported that regulatory T cells can have specificity for tumor-associated antigens.[262] Depletion of regulatory T cells in rodents can be accomplished through a variety of genetic means, and the absence of regulatory T cells triggers autoimmunity. Regulatory T cells may inhibit antitumor responses, and depletion of regulatory T cells is a promising approach to the immunotherapy of cancer. It is possible and even likely that in addition to the CD4+CD25+ population of regulatory T cells, other types of inhibitory or suppressor T-cell subsets exist.[263]

CYTOTOXIC T LYMPHOCYTES

Different host mechanisms for destroying target cells have evolved, resulting in a diverse collection of cytotoxic cells capable of reacting against a wide variety of foreign cells and organisms. A common feature among them, however, is that cytotoxicity is a regulated process. They are generally activated as a result of cell surface ligands on the target cells binding and triggering selected cell surface receptor molecules on the effector cells. The primary sources of antitumor cytotoxic effector cells are CTLs and natural killer (NK) lymphocytes.

Most reported human antitumor CTLs are activated CD8+ effector T cells, and most of the reported human tumor antigens are MHC class I restricted.[33,34] The class of MHC molecule with which the tumor antigen is associated correlates with whether the CTL is CD8+ or CD4+; the antigen-specific receptors (TCRs) of CD8+ CTLs recognize primarily MHC class I–associated antigens, and the antigen-specific receptors of CD4+ CTLs recognize primarily MHC class II–associated antigens. Most tumors express MHC class I but not class II molecules. Nevertheless, several reports provide evidence that CD4+ T cells can act as antitumor effector cells,[264–266] in addition to serving as helper cells, by promoting the generation of CTL and activating APCs.[267,268]

CTL-mediated antitumor reactions generally are triggered by cross-linking of the TCRs on CTLs after contact with tumor cell antigens expressed on the tumor cell surface. A variety of adhesion and accessory molecules may not only facilitate the binding of CTLs to target cells but may contribute to T-cell triggering by the TCRs. Consequently, the activation of only a few TCRs or TCRs with low affinity for MHC-antigen complexes may be capable of triggering T cells with the support of other receptor-ligand pairs. Death of the tumor cells usually includes apoptosis, with distinguishing characteristics such as membrane blebbing, chromatin condensation, and DNA fragmentation, followed by lysis. In addition, CTLs are not destroyed during the cytolytic reaction. They commonly deliver a "lethal hit" to target cells within minutes and then recycle to kill more target cells. Their life span, however, is relatively short.

CTLs appear to use two significantly different ways of destroying target cells during cytolytic reactions that occur within a few hours. These include (1) granule exocytosis and (2) the triggering of target cell receptors by particular TNF-related ligands expressed by the CTLs, such as Fas ligand and the *TNF-related apoptosis-inducing ligand* (TRAIL).[269,270]

With respect to granule exocytosis, the contents of specialized granules are secreted into areas of close contact with target cells after triggering of the TCRs. The granules contain two types of proteins that contribute in a cooperative fashion to the destruction of target cells: perforin, which is related to the terminal component of complement and forms pores in the outer membrane of the target cells, and granzymes, a subfamily of serine proteases in lymphocytes that appear to be necessary for apoptosis of the target cells. The cytotoxicity is generally antigen specific, because of TCR-mediated triggering and focused delivery of the cytotoxic granule contents at the point of contact between the CTL and the target cell. Additional factors contribute to the specificity of apoptosis: the short burst, local concentration gradients, and short half-lives of perforin and the granzymes.

Other rapid cytolytic reactions of CTLs with target cells, however, lack features of the granule secretion mechanism and appear to depend on the triggering of receptors for TNF-like molecules on the target cells. A well-characterized example of these receptors is Fas, which is expressed on the surface of a wide variety of cell types.[171,271–276] Cross-linking Fas commonly triggers apoptosis in cells expressing these molecules. A Fas ligand that is a transmembrane protein belonging to the TNF family has been identified on the surface of activated CTLs, particularly among CD8+ T cells and CD4+ Th1 T cells. The antigen specificity of Fas-mediated cytolysis by CTLs may depend on TCR-mediated stimulation of the CTL for brief expression of the Fas ligand in a functional form at the site of contact with the TCR-triggering target cell.[277,278]

Exceptions to the antigen specificity of CTL-mediated lysis of target cells have been described.[232,269,270,279–282] For example, Fas ligands may be expressed at cell surface sites other than the point of contact with the TCR-triggering target cell. Also, Fas ligand expression may continue after TCR contact with antigen is lost and TCR stimulation ends. Consequently, CTL could continue to destroy innocent bystander cells that express Fas and are in contact with the CTL. This mechanism may be particularly relevant to tumor destruction (1) by CD4+ Th1 CTL, which recognize tumor antigens in the context of MHC class II molecules, and (2) by CD8+ that recognize tumor antigens expressed only by a portion of the neighboring tumor cells. In addition, nonspecificity may result from lymphotoxin/TNF-α–like molecules whose release from CTL is triggered by MHC-restricted antigens but, given an opportunity to accumulate in the intercellular space, are nonspecifically toxic. The TNF-related, apoptosis-inducing ligand, TRAIL, may be an exception, as the soluble form appears to be more toxic for cancer cells than for normal cells.[283]

Tests of gene-knockout and gene-reconstitution mouse models have clearly established the importance of granule exocytosis and the Fas-mediated pathways.[277,278,284–286] Perforin-deficient mice are impaired in their resistance to tumors.[287,288] Whereas the granule exocytosis pathway may be used more against pathogens, the Fas-mediated pathway may be more involved with down-regulating immune responses.[168,171,215,224,270,289,290] Of note, Fas is markedly up-regulated on activated T cells. However, not all Fas-expressing lymphocytes are susceptible to apoptosis through this pathway; prolonged stimulation for at least a period of days may be needed.

Studies indicate that antigen-stimulated T cells can express cell surface receptors, originally found on NK cells, that augment or suppress TCR-mediated cell activation.[291] Investigations are at an early stage to determine if receptor ligands expressed by tumor cells will affect antigen-specific antitumor T-cell activity.

NATURAL KILLER CELLS

NK cells are a relatively small population of lymphocytes distinct from T and B lymphocytes.[2,3,292–294] They generally are large granular lymphocytes that originate in the bone marrow. NK cells share a common progenitor with T cells, and NK cell precursors have been identified in the thymus. They do not, however, require the thymus for maturation, and they do not express the TCR/CD3 complex. They probably diverge from the T-cell lineage at an early stage of differentiation.[294a]

NK cells are the host's major source of cell-mediated antitumor cytotoxic activity that is not triggered by antigen-specific recognition. They are part of the host's innate or front-line defense mechanisms, because to function they require no antigen-specific adaptation of the host or immunization. NK cells have no memory response. In addition to their potential for direct antitumor cytotoxicity, their production of cytokines and chemokines as part of the early, innate host defense response can strongly promote subsequent adaptive immune responses.

Although the picture is far from complete, the basic cytotoxic mechanisms of NK cells and CTLs appear to be similar.[272,295–299] Granule exocytosis, perforin, and granzymes have well-established roles in cytotoxicity mediated by NK cells. NK cells also kill tumor cells by TNF-related ligands, such as Fas ligand.[300–302] As with T cells, activation of NK cells increases the cytotoxic activity.

An NK cell expresses a variety of receptors that either stimulate or inhibit cytotoxic acitivity *in vitro* against different sources of tumor. Many of the receptors and ligands have been identified. An important feature of NK cells is that some of the receptors react with MHC class I molecules on target cells, resulting in inhibition of cytotoxic activity. This feature has raised the possibility of combined T-cell and NK cell attacks against tumor cells expressing or lacking MHC class I molecules, respectively. Efforts are in progress to establish a therapeutic effectiveness of NK cells against established tumors.

CONCLUSION

The immune system has evolved as a highly complex, regulated, and adaptive mechanism for distinguishing between foreign cells and autologous normal cells and for reacting against the foreign cells. Tumor cells that are sensitive to the adaptive immune system are recognized and destroyed primarily by cellular immune responses. These responses depend on the clonally distributed TCR for specific recognition of cell surface tumor antigens and for triggering T-cell activities that kill the tumor cells either directly or through recruitment of other host cells.

T cells that directly kill tumor cells are commonly CD8+ and generally recognize tumor antigens as cell surface complexes of MHC class I molecules and antigenic peptides derived primarily from intracellular proteins processed in the tumor cells. T cells that help immune responses against tumors are commonly CD4+ and generally recognize cell surface complexes of MHC class II molecules and tumor-derived antigenic peptides. Like the mature T-cell precursors to CD8+ killer T cells, mature T-cell precursors to CD4+ helper T cells are activated primarily by host APCs, particularly activated DCs, activated B lymphocytes, and activated macrophages. These three sources of host APCs or their precursors can process tumor proteins acquired by endocytosis. Activated DCs, however, appear to be unique in being able to activate T cells for the first time against tumor antigens after leaving the thymus as mature, but freshly minted, naive T cells.

Stimulating T lymphocytes, particularly naive T cells, in an antigen-specific fashion commonly requires two different cell surface signals. The first signal is from the tumor antigen, which selects the T cell to respond and provides specificity as a result of triggering the antigen-specific receptor (TCR) on the T-cell surface. The second signal is an essential (but by itself insufficient) costimulatory signal from APCs, such as DCs, which adds stringency and reduces the likelihood of careless T-cell responses. The immune response is promoted or limited by regulatory cells through their secreted cytokines and cell surface ligands, which, as a group, form a network of overlapping activities that reduce the likelihood of general failure of an immune response or of an immune response getting out of hand.

Antitumor T cells can recognize non–self-antigens or self-antigens. Non–self-tumor antigens are mainly derived from (1) proteins that have an abnormal structure resulting from the genetic instability of tumors, (2) proteins that are products of viral genes within the tumor, and (3) proteins that are not produced in normal cells at an immunogenic threshold level. The TCRs of mature T cells that react with these antigens commonly do so with a high affinity.

In contrast, many tumor proteins are self-proteins shared with normal cells, and T cells with high affinities for these antigenic peptides appear to be largely deleted during their maturation in the thymus. Stimulating an immune response against these antigens is difficult and generally requires breaking tolerance, which is the failure of the immune system to respond to an antigen. In addition to deletion of T cells in the thymus, a variety of mechanisms outside the thymus prevent cellular immune responses against self-antigens. Antigen-specific activation of naive T cells is limited primarily to antigenic peptides presented by activated DCs, and these cells generally function in locations where inflammation and a source of antigen are present. Deletion or anergy is a fate common to naive T cells that respond to antigen in the absence of costimulatory signals. Regulatory T cells may block the proliferation and function of antitumor T cells.

REFERENCES

1. Janeway CA, Jr, Medzhitov R. Innate immune recognition. *Annu Rev Immunol* 2002; 20:197.
2. Diefenbach A, Raulet DH. The innate immune response to tumors and its role in the induction of T-cell immunity. *Immunol Rev* 2002;188:9.
3. Wu J, Lanier LL. Natural killer cells and cancer. *Adv Cancer Res* 2003;90:127.
4. Dunn GP, Bruce AT, Ikeda H, et al. Cancer immunoediting: from immunosurveillance to tumor escape. *Nat Immunol* 2002;3:991.
5. Landsteiner K, Chase MW. Experiments on transfer of cutaneous sensitivity to simple compounds. *Proc Soc Exp Biol Med* 1942;49:688.
6. Billingham RE, Brent L, Medawar PB. Quantitative studies on tissue transplantation immunity. II. The origin, strength, and duration of actively and adoptively acquired immunity. *Proc Roy Soc London* 1954;B143:58.
7. Mitchison NA. Passive transfer of transplantation immunity. *Proc Roy Soc London* 1954; B142:72.
8. Miller JF. The thymus and its role in immunity. *Chem Immunol* 1990;49:51.
9. Gross L. Intradermal immunization of C3H mice against a sarcoma that originated in an animal of the same line. *Cancer Res* 1943;3:326.
10. Foley EJ. Antigenic properties of methylcholanthrene-induced tumors in mice of the strain of origin. *Cancer Res* 1953;13:835.
11. Prehn RT, Main JM. Immunity to methylcholanthrene-induced sarcomas. *J Natl Cancer Inst* 1957;18:769.
12. Klein G, Sjögren HO, Klein E, et al. Demonstration of resistance against methylcholanthrene-induced sarcomas in the primary autochthonous host. *Cancer Res* 1960;20:1561.
13. Rosenberg SA. Progress in human tumour immunology and immunotherapy. *Nature* 2001;411:380.
14. Van Der BP, Zhang Y, Chaux P, et al. Tumor-specific shared antigenic peptides recognized by human T cells. *Immunol Rev* 2002;188:51.

15. Pardoll D. Does the immune system see tumors as foreign or self? *Annu Rev Immunol* 2003;21:807.
16. Itoh K, Platsoucas DC, Balch CM. Autologous tumor-specific cytotoxic T lymphocytes in the infiltrate of human metastatic melanomas: activation by interleukin 2 and autologous tumor cells and involvement of the T cell receptor. *J Exp Med* 1988;168:1419.
17. Topalian SL, Solomon D, Rosenberg SA. Tumor-specific cytolysis by lymphocytes infiltrating human melanomas. *J Immunol* 1989;142:3714.
18. Barth RJ Jr, Mule JJ, Spiess PJ, et al. Interferon gamma and tumor necrosis factor have a role in tumor regressions mediated by murine CD8+ tumor-infiltrating lymphocytes. *J Exp Med* 1991;173:647.
19. Toes RE, Ossendorp F, Offringa R, et al. CD4 T cells and their role in antitumor immune responses. *J Exp Med* 1999;189:753.
20. Dudley ME, Wunderlich JR, Robbins PF, et al. Cancer regression and autoimmunity in patients after clonal repopulation with antitumor lymphocytes. *Science* 2002;298:850.
21. Overwijk WW, Theoret MR, Finkelstein SE, et al. Tumor regression and autoimmunity after reversal of a functionally tolerant state of self-reactive CD8+ T cells. *J Exp Med* 2003;198:569.
22. Rammensee HG, Weinschenk T, Gouttefangeas C, et al. Towards patient-specific tumor antigen selection for vaccination. *Immunol Rev* 2002;188:164.
23. Waldmann TA, Levy R, Coller BS. Emerging therapies: spectrum of applications of monoclonal antibody therapy. *Hematology (Am Soc Hematol Educ Program)* 2000;394.
24. Press OW, Leonard JP, Coiffier B, et al. Immunotherapy of Non-Hodgkin's lymphomas. *Hematology (Am Soc Hematol Educ Program)* 2001;221.
25. Yang JC, Haworth L, Sherry RM, et al. A randomized trial of bevacizumab, an anti-vascular endothelial growth factor antibody, for metastatic renal cancer. *N Engl J Med* 2003;349:427.
26. Fernando NH, Hurwitz HI. Inhibition of vascular endothelial growth factor in the treatment of colorectal cancer. *Semin Oncol* 2003;30:39.
27. Phan GQ, Yang JC, Sherry RM, et al. Cancer regression and autoimmunity induced by cytotoxic T lymphocyte-associated antigen 4 blockade in patients with metastatic melanoma. *Proc Natl Acad Sci U S A* 2003;100:8372.
28. Hodi FS, Mihm MC, Soiffer RJ, et al. Biologic activity of cytotoxic T lymphocyte-associated antigen 4 antibody blockade in previously vaccinated metastatic melanoma and ovarian carcinoma patients. *Proc Natl Acad Sci U S A* 2003;100:4712.
29. Chang MH, Chen CJ, Lai MS, et al. Universal hepatitis B vaccination in Taiwan and the incidence of hepatocellular carcinoma in children. Taiwan Childhood Hepatoma Study Group. *N Engl J Med* 1997;336:1855.
30. Koutsky LA, Ault KA, Wheeler CM, et al. A controlled trial of a human papillomavirus type 16 vaccine. *N Engl J Med* 2002;347:1645.
31. Dudley ME, Rosenberg SA. Adoptive-cell-transfer therapy for the treatment of patients with cancer. *Nat Rev Cancer* 2003;3:666.
32. Therasse P, Arbuck SG, Eisenhauer EA, et al. New guidelines to evaluate the response to treatment in solid tumors. European Organization for Research and Treatment of Cancer, National Cancer Institute of the United States, National Cancer Institute of Canada. *J Natl Cancer Inst* 2000;92:205.
33. Robbins PF, Wang RF. Tumor antigens recognized by cytotoxic lymphocytes. In: Sitkovsky MV, Henkart PA, eds. *Cytotoxic cells: basic mechanisms and medical applications.* Philadelphia: Lippincott Williams & Wilkins, 2000:363.
34. Renkvist N, Castelli C, Robbins PF, et al. A listing of human tumor antigens recognized by T cells. *Cancer Immunol Immunother* 2001;50:3.
35. Wang RF, Zeng G, Johnston SF, et al. T cell-mediated immune responses in melanoma: implications for immunotherapy. *Crit Rev Oncol Hematol* 2002;43:1.
36. Scanlan MJ, Gure AO, Jungbluth AA, et al. Cancer/testis antigens: an expanding family of targets for cancer immunotherapy. *Immunol Rev* 2002;188:22.
37. Stoler DL, Chen N, Basik M, et al. The onset and extent of genomic instability in sporadic colorectal tumor progression. *Proc Natl Acad Sci U S A* 1999;96:15121.
38. Sharkey MS, Lizée G, Gonzales MI, et al. CD4+ T-cell recognition of mutated B-RAF in melanoma patients harboring the V599E mutation. *Cancer Res* 2004;64:1595.
39. Skipper JC, Hendrickson RC, Gulden PH, et al. An HLA-A2-restricted tyrosinase antigen on melanoma cells results from posttranslational modification and suggests a novel pathway for processing of membrane proteins. *J Exp Med* 1996;183:527.
40. Hanada K, Yewdell JW, Yang JC. Immune recognition of a human renal cancer antigen through post-translational protein splicing. *Nature* 2004;427:252.
41. Hanada K, Perry-Lalley DM, Ohnmacht GA, et al. Identification of fibroblast growth factor-5 as an overexpressed antigen in multiple human adenocarcinomas. *Cancer Res* 2001;61:5511.
42. Gottschalk S, Heslop HE, Roon CM. Treatment of Epstein-Barr virus-associated malignancies with specific T cells. *Adv Cancer Res* 2002;84:175.
43. Strausberg RL, Simpson AJ, Wooster R. Sequence-based cancer genomics: progress, lessons and opportunities. *Nat Rev Genet* 2003;4:409.
44. Hanash S. Disease proteomics. *Nature* 2003;422:226.
45. Sprent J, Tough DF. T cell death and memory. *Science* 2001;293:245.
46. Rosenberg SA. A new era for cancer immunotherapy based on the genes that encode cancer antigens. *Immunity* 1999;10:281.
47. Jassim A, Ollier W, Payne A, et al. Analysis of HLA antigens on germ cells in human semen. *Eur J Immunol* 1989;19:1215.
48. Maio M, Coral S, Fratta E, et al. Epigenetic targets for immune intervention in human malignancies. *Oncogene* 2003;22:6484.
49. Vincent MS, Gumperz JE, Brenner MB. Understanding the function of CD1-restricted T cells. *Nat Immunol* 2003;4:517.
50. Allison TJ, Garboczi DN. Structure of gammadelta T cell receptors and their recognition of non-peptide antigens. *Mol Immunol* 2002;38:1051.
51. Ferrarini M, Ferrero E, Dagna L, et al. Human gammadelta T cells: a nonredundant system in the immune-surveillance against cancer. *Trends Immunol* 2002;23:14.
52. Bjorkman PJ, Saper MA, Samraoui B, et al. Structure of the human class I histocompatibility antigen, HLA-A2. *Nature* 1987;329:506.
53. Bjorkman PJ, Saper MA, Samraoui B, et al. The foreign antigen binding site and T cell recognition regions of class I histocompatibility antigens. *Nature* 1987;329:512.
54. Rammensee HG, Falk K, Rotzschke O. MHC molecules as peptide receptors. *Curr Opin Immunol* 1993;5:35.
55. Brown JH, Jardetzky TS, Gorga JC, et al. Three-dimensional structure of the human class II histocompatibility antigen HLA-DR1. *Nature* 1993;364:33.
56. Fremont DH, Stura EA, Matsumura M, et al. Crystal structure of an H-2Kb-ovalbumin peptide complex reveals the interplay of primary and secondary anchor positions in the major histocompatibility complex binding groove. *Proc Natl Acad Sci U S A* 1995;92:2479.
57. Wilson IA, Fremont DH. Structural analysis of MHC class I molecules with bound peptide antigens. *Semin Immunol* 1993;5:75.
58. Stura EA, Matsumura M, Fremont DH, et al. Crystallization of murine major histocompatibility complex class I H-2Kb with single peptides. *J Mol Biol* 1992;228:975.
59. Matsumura M, Fremont DH, Peterson PA, et al. Emerging principles for the recognition of peptide antigens by MHC class I molecules. *Science* 1992;257:927.
60. Fremont DH, Matsumura M, Stura EA, et al. Crystal structures of two viral peptides in complex with murine MHC class I H-2Kᵇ. *Science* 1992;257:919.
61. Stern LJ, Brown JH, Jardetzky TS, et al. Crystal structure of the human class II MHC protein HLA-DR1 complexed with an influenza virus peptide. *Nature* 1994;368:215.
62. Collins EJ, Garboczi DN, Wiley DC. Three-dimensional structure of a peptide extending from one end of a class I MHC binding site. *Nature* 1994;371:626.
63. Smith KJ, Pyrdol J, Gauthier L, et al. Crystal structure of HLA-DR2 (DRA*0101, DRB1*1501) complexed with a peptide from human myelin basic protein. *J Exp Med* 1998;188:1511.
64. Cox AL, Skipper J, Chen Y, et al. Identification of a peptide recognized by five melanoma-specific human cytotoxic T cell lines. *Science* 1994;264:716.
65. Ramakrishna V, Ross MM, Petersson M, et al. Naturally occurring peptides associated with HLA-A2 in ovarian cancer cell lines identified by mass spectrometry are targets of HLA-A2-restricted cytotoxic T cells. *Int Immunol* 2003;15:751.
66. Pascolo S, Schirle M, Guckel B, et al. A MAGE-A1 HLA-A A*0201 epitope identified by mass spectrometry. *Cancer Res* 2001;61:4072.
67. Schirle M, Keilholz W, Weber B, et al. Identification of tumor-associated MHC class I ligands by a novel T cell-independent approach. *Eur J Immunol* 2000;30:2216.
68. Barber LD, Parham P. Peptide binding to major histocompatibility complex molecules. *Annu Rev Cell Biol* 1993;9:163.
69. Parham P. HLA, anthropology, and transplantation. *Transplant Proc* 1993;25:159.
70. Kang X, Kawakami Y, El-Gamil M, et al. Identification of a tyrosinase epitope recognized by HLA-A24-restricted, tumor-infiltrating lymphocytes. *J Immunol* 1995;155:1343.
71. Pieters J. MHC class II-restricted antigen processing and presentation. *Adv Immunol* 2000;75:159.
72. Parker KC, Bednarek MA, Coligan JE. Scheme for ranking potential HLA-A2 binding peptides based on independent binding of individual peptide side-chains. *J Immunol* 1994;152:163.
73. Rammensee H, Bachmann J, Emmerich NP, et al. SYFPEITHI: database for MHC ligands and peptide motifs. *Immunogenetics* 1999;50:213.
74. Ruppert J, Sidney J, Celis E, et al. Prominent role of secondary anchor residues in peptide binding to HLA-A2.1 molecules. *Cell* 1993;74:929.
75. Yewdell JW, Bennink JR. Cell biology of antigen processing and presentation to major histocompatibility complex class I molecule-restricted T lymphocytes. *Adv Immunol* 1992;52:1.
76. Germain RN. MHC-dependent antigen processing and peptide presentation: providing ligands for T lymphocyte activation. *Cell* 1994;76:287.
77. Rock KL, York IA, Saric T, et al. Protein degradation and the generation of MHC class I-presented peptides. *Adv Immunol* 2002;80:1.
78. Berzofsky JA, Berkower IJ. Immunogenicity and antigen structure. In: Paul WE, ed. *Fundamental immunology,* 5th ed. Philadelphia: Lippincott Williams & Wilkins, 2003:631.
79. Restifo NP. Hierarchy, tolerance, and dominance in the antitumor T-cell response. *J Immunother* 2001;24:193.
80. Guermonprez P, Valladeau J, Zitvogel L, et al. Antigen presentation and T cell stimulation by dendritic cells. *Annu Rev Immunol* 2002;20:621.
81. den Haan JM, Bevan MJ. Antigen presentation to CD8+ T cells: cross-priming in infectious diseases. *Curr Opin Immunol* 2001;13:437.
82. Belz GT, Carbone FR, Heath WR. Cross-presentation of antigens by dendritic cells. *Crit Rev Immunol* 2002;22:439.
83. Castelli C, Rivoltini L, Rini F, et al. Heat shock proteins: biological functions and clinical application as personalized vaccines for human cancer. *Cancer Immunol Immunother* 2003;53:227.
84. Bryant PW, Lennon-Dumenil AM, Fiebiger E, et al. Proteolysis and antigen presentation by MHC class II molecules. *Adv Immunol* 2002;80:71.
85. Watts C, Amigorena S. Phagocytosis and antigen presentation. *Semin Immunol* 2001;13:373.
86. Seliger B, Cabrera T, Garrido F, et al. HLA class I antigen abnormalities and immune escape by malignant cells. *Semin Cancer Biol* 2002;12:3.
87. Hewitt EW. The MHC class I antigen presentation pathway: strategies for viral immune evasion. *Immunology* 2003;110:163.
88. Yewdell JW, Hill AB. Viral interference with antigen presentation. *Nat Immunol* 2002;3:1019.
89. Braud VM, Allan DS, McMichael AJ. Functions of nonclassical MHC and non-MHC-encoded class I molecules. *Curr Opin Immunol* 1999;11:100.
90. O'Callaghan CA, Bell JI. Structure and function of the human MHC class Ib molecules HLA-E, HLA-F and HLA-G. *Immunol Rev* 1998;163:129.

91. Menier C, Saez B, Horejsi V, et al. Characterization of monoclonal antibodies recognizing HLA-G or HLA-E: new tools to analyze the expression of nonclassical HLA class I molecules. *Hum Immunol* 2003;64:315.

92. Allan DS, Lepin EJ, Braud VM, et al. Tetrameric complexes of HLA-E, HLA-F, and HLA-G. *J Immunol Methods* 2002;268:43.

93. Carosella ED, Moreau P, Le Maoult J, et al. HLA-G molecules: from maternal-fetal tolerance to tissue acceptance. *Adv Immunol* 2003;81:199.

94. Kessler BM, Glas R, Ploegh HL. MHC class I antigen processing regulated by cytosolic proteolysis—short cuts that alter peptide generation. *Mol Immunol* 2002;39:171.

95. Anderson SL, Shen T, Lou J, et al. The endoplasmic reticular heat shock protein gp96 is transcriptionally upregulated in interferon-treated cells. *J Exp Med* 1994;180:1565.

96. Howcroft TK, Singer DS. Expression of nonclassical MHC class Ib genes: comparison of regulatory elements. *Immunol Res* 2003;27:1.

97. Ting JP, Trowsdale J. Genetic control of MHC class II expression. *Cell* 2002;109 [Suppl]:S21.

98. Marincola FM, Jaffee EM, Hicklin DJ, et al. Escape of human solid tumors from T-cell recognition: molecular mechanisms and functional significance. *Adv Immunol* 2000;74:181.

99. Garcia-Lora A, Algarra I, Garrido F. MHC class I antigens, immune surveillance, and tumor immune escape. *J Cell Physiol* 2003;195:346.

100. Campoli M, Chang CC, Ferrone S. HLA class I antigen loss, tumor immune escape and immune selection. *Vaccine* 2002;20[Suppl 4]:A40.

101. Khong HT, Restifo NP. Natural selection of tumor variants in the generation of "tumor escape" phenotypes. *Nat Immunol* 2002;3:999.

102. Restifo NP, Marincola FM, Kawakami Y, et al. Loss of functional beta 2-microglobulin in metastatic melanomas from five patients receiving immunotherapy. *J Natl Cancer Inst* 1996;88:100.

103. Jakobsen MK, Restifo NP, Cohen PA, et al. Defective major histocompatibility complex class I expression in a sarcomatoid renal cell carcinoma cell line. *J Immunother Emphasis Tumor Immunol* 1995;17:222.

104. Zijlstra M, Bix M, Simister NE, et al. B2-microglobulin deficient mice lack CD4⁻ CD8⁺ cytolytic T cells. *Nature* 1990;344:742.

105. Marincola FM, Shamamian P, Simonis TB, et al. Locus-specific analysis of human leukocyte antigen class I expression in melanoma cell lines. *J Immunother Emphasis Tumor Immunol* 1994;16:13.

106. Marincola FM, Shamamian P, Alexander RB, et al. Loss of HLA haplotype and B locus down-regulation in melanoma cell lines. *J Immunol* 1994;153:1225.

107. Restifo NP, Esquivel F, Kawakami Y, et al. Identification of human cancers deficient in antigen processing. *J Exp Med* 1993;177:265.

108. Bai XF, Liu J, Li O, et al. Antigenic drift as a mechanism for tumor evasion of destruction by cytolytic T lymphocytes. *J Clin Invest* 2003;111:1487.

109. Matzinger P. Tolerance, danger, and the extended family. *Annu Rev Immunol* 1994;12:991.

110. Steinman RM, Cohn ZA. Identification of a novel cell type in peripheral lymphoid organs of mice. I. Morphology, quantitation, tissue distribution. *J Exp Med* 1973;137:1142.

111. Lanzavecchia A, Sallusto F. Regulation of T cell immunity by dendritic cells. *Cell* 2001;106:263.

112. Moser M. Dendritic cells in immunity and tolerance—do they display opposite functions? *Immunity* 2003;19:5.

113. Mellman I, Steinman RM. Dendritic cells: specialized and regulated antigen processing machines. *Cell* 2001;106:255.

114. Steinman RM, Hawiger D, Nussenzweig MC. Tolerogenic dendritic cells. *Annu Rev Immunol* 2003;21:685.

115. Fonteneau JF, Larsson M, Bhardwaj N. Interactions between dead cells and dendritic cells in the induction of antiviral CTL responses. *Curr Opin Immunol* 2002;14:471.

116. Aderem A, Ulevitch RJ. Toll-like receptors in the induction of the innate immune response. *Nature* 2000;406:782.

117. Bell JK, Mullen GE, Leifer CA, et al. Leucine-rich repeats and pathogen recognition in Toll-like receptors. *Trends Immunol* 2003;24:528.

118. Sabroe I, Read RC, Whyte MK, et al. Toll-like receptors in health and disease: complex questions remain. *J Immunol* 2003;171:1630.

119. Takeda K, Kaisho T, Akira S. Toll-like receptors. *Annu Rev Immunol* 2003;21:335.

120. Moser M, Murphy KM. Dendritic cell regulation of TH1-TH2 development. *Nat Immunol* 2000;1:199.

121. Kapsenberg ML. Dendritic-cell control of pathogen-driven T-cell polarization. *Nat Rev Immunol* 2003;3:984.

122. Liu YJ, Kanzler H, Soumelis V, et al. Dendritic cell lineage, plasticity and cross-regulation. *Nat Immunol* 2001;2:585.

123. Salio M, Shepherd D, Dunbar PR, et al. Mature dendritic cells prime functionally superior melan-A-specific CD8+ lymphocytes as compared with nonprofessional APC. *J Immunol* 2001;167:1188.

124. Curtsinger JM, Lins DC, Mescher MF. Signal 3 determines tolerance versus full activation of naive CD8 T cells: dissociating proliferation and development of effector function. *J Exp Med* 2003;197:1141.

125. Redmond WL, Hernandez J, Sherman LA. Deletion of naive CD8 T cells requires persistent antigen and is not programmed by an initial signal from the tolerogenic APC. *J Immunol* 2003;171:6349.

126. Jonuleit H, Schmitt E, Steinbrink K, et al. Dendritic cells as a tool to induce anergic and regulatory T cells. *Trends Immunol* 2001;22:394.

127. Gordon S. Alternative activation of macrophages. *Nat Rev Immunol* 2003;3:23.

128. Mantovani A, Sozzani S, Locati M, et al. Macrophage polarization: tumor-associated macrophages as a paradigm for polarized M2 mononuclear phagocytes. *Trends Immunol* 2002;23:549.

129. Aloisi F, Ria F, Adorini L. Regulation of T-cell responses by CNS antigen-presenting cells: different roles for microglia and astrocytes. *Immunol Today* 2000;21:141.

130. Fadok VA, Bratton DL, Guthrie L, et al. Differential effects of apoptotic versus lysed cells on macrophage production of cytokines: role of proteases. *J Immunol* 2001;166:6847.

131. Balkwill F, Mantovani A. Inflammation and cancer: back to Virchow? *Lancet* 2001;357:539.

132. Coussens LM, Werb Z. Inflammation and cancer. *Nature* 2002;420:860.

133. Davis MM, Chien YH. T-cell antigen receptors. In: Paul WE, ed. *Fundamental immunology*, 5th ed. Philadelphia: Lippincott Williams and Wilkins Publishers, 2003:227.

134. Bentley GA, Mariuzza RA. The structure of the T cell antigen receptor. *Annu Rev Immunol* 1996;14:563.

135. Reinherz EL, Tan K, Tang L, et al. The crystal structure of a T cell receptor in complex with peptide and MHC class II. *Science* 1999;286:1913.

136. Garcia KC, Teyton L, Wilson IA. Structural basis of T cell recognition. *Annu Rev Immunol* 1999;17:369.

137. Hennecke J, Wiley DC. T cell receptor-MHC interactions up close. *Cell* 2001;104:1.

138. Whiteside TL, Parmiani G. Tumor-infiltrating lymphocytes: their phenotype, functions and clinical use. *Cancer Immunol Immunother* 1994;39:15.

139. Khilko SN, Jelonek MT, Corr M, et al. Measuring interactions of MHC class I molecules using surface plasmon resonance. *J Immunol Methods* 1995;183:77.

140. Corr M, Slanetz AE, Boyd LF, et al. T cell receptor-MHC class I peptide interactions: affinity, kinetics, and specificity. *Science* 1994;265:946.

141. Boniface JJ, Reich Z, Lyons DS, et al. Thermodynamics of T cell receptor binding to peptide-MHC: evidence for a general mechanism of molecular scanning. *Proc Natl Acad Sci U S A* 1999;96:11446.

142. Yee C, Savage PA, Lee PP, et al. Isolation of high avidity melanoma-reactive CTL from heterogeneous populations using peptide-MHC tetramers. *J Immunol* 1999;162:2227.

143. Altman JD, Moss PH, Goulder PR, et al. Phenotypic analysis of antigen-specific T lymphocytes. *Science* 1996;274:94.

144. Morgan RA, Dudley ME, Yu YY, et al. High efficiency TCR gene transfer into primary human lymphocytes affords avid recognition of melanoma tumor antigen glycoprotein 100 and does not alter the recognition of autologous melanoma antigens. *J Immunol* 2003;171:3287.

145. Lang HL, Jacobsen H, Ikemizu S, et al. A functional and structural basis for TCR cross-reactivity in multiple sclerosis. *Nat Immunol* 2002;3:940.

146. Reiser JB, Darnault C, Gregoire C, et al. CDR3 loop flexibility contributes to the degeneracy of TCR recognition. *Nat Immunol* 2003;4:241.

147. Eisen HN. Specificity and degeneracy in antigen recognition: yin and yang in the immune system. *Annu Rev Immunol* 2001;19:1.

148. Tangri S, Ishioka GY, Huang X, et al. Structural features of peptide analogs of human histocompatibility leukocyte antigen class I epitopes that are more potent and immunogenic than wild-type peptide. *J Exp Med* 2001;194:833.

149. Slansky JE, Rattis FM, Boyd LF, et al. Enhanced antigen-specific antitumor immunity with altered peptide ligands that stabilize the MHC-peptide-TCR complex. *Immunity* 2000;13:529.

150. Padovan E, Giachino C, Cella M, et al. Normal T lymphocytes can express two different T cell receptor beta chains: implications for the mechanism of allelic exclusion. *J Exp Med* 1995;181:1587.

151. Davodeau F, Peyrat MA, Romagne F, et al. Dual T cell receptor beta chain expression on human T lymphocytes. *J Exp Med* 1995;181:1391.

152. Padovan E, Casorati G, Dellabona P, et al. Expression of two T cell receptor alpha chains: dual receptor T cells. *Science* 1993;262:422.

153. Malissen M, Trucy J, Jouvin-Marche E, et al. Regulation of TCR alpha and beta gene allelic exclusion during T-cell development. *Immunol Today* 1992;13:315.

154. Ashwell JD, Chen C, Schwartz RH. High frequency and nonrandom distribution of alloreactivity in T cell clones selected for recognition of foreign antigen in association with self class II molecules. *J Immunol* 1986;136:389.

155. Heath WR, Carbone FR, Bertolino P, et al. Expression of two T cell receptor alpha chains on the surface of normal murine T cells. *Eur J Immunol* 1995;25:1617.

156. Padovan E, Casorati G, Dellabona P, et al. Dual receptor T-cells. Implications for alloreactivity and autoimmunity. *Ann N Y Acad Sci* 1995;756:66.

157. Malissen B, Ardouin L, Lin SY, et al. Function of the CD3 subunits of the pre-TCR and TCR complexes during T cell development. *Adv Immunol* 1999;72:103.

158. Rothenberg EV, Yui MA, Telfer JC. T-cell developmental biology. In: Paul WE, ed. *Fundamental immunology*, 5th ed. Philadelphia: Lippincott Williams & Wilkins, 2003:259.

159. von Boehmer H, Aifantis I, Gounari F, et al. Thymic selection revisited: how essential is it? *Immunol Rev* 2003;191:62.

160. Buckley RH. Primary cellular immunodeficiencies. *J Allergy Clin Immunol* 2002;109:747.

161. Mak TW, Penninger JM, Ohashi PS. Knockout mice: a paradigm shift in modern immunology. *Nat Rev Immunol* 2001;1:11.

162. Fischer A. Human primary immunodeficiency diseases: a perspective. *Nat Immunol* 2004;5:23.

163. Barclay AN, Brown MH, Law SK, et al. *The leucocyte antigen factsbook*, 2nd ed. London: Academic Press, 1997.

164. Protein reviews on the Web. Zola H, Swart B, Katz KS, Shaw S, eds. World Wide Web URL: http://www.ncbi.nlm.nih.gov/prow/, 2002.

165. Kyewski B, Derbinski J, Gotter J, et al. Promiscuous gene expression and central T-cell tolerance: more than meets the eye. *Trends Immunol* 2002;23:364.

166. Walker LS, Abbas AK. The enemy within: keeping self-reactive T cells at bay in the periphery. *Nat Rev Immunol* 2002;2:11.

167. King LB, Ashwell JD. Thymocyte and T cell apoptosis: is all death created equal? *Thymus* 1994;23:209.

168. Penninger JM, Kroemer G. Molecular and cellular mechanisms of T lymphocyte apoptosis. *Adv Immunol* 1998;68:51.

169. Moulian N, Berrih-Aknin S. Fas/APO-1/CD95 in health and autoimmune disease: thymic and peripheral aspects. *Semin Immunol* 1998;10:449.

170. Rathmell JC, Thompson CB. The central effectors of cell death in the immune system. *Annu Rev Immunol* 1999;17:781.

171. Nagata S. Apoptosis by death factor. *Cell* 1997;88:355.

172. Davis MM, Krogsgaard M, Huppa JB, et al. Dynamics of cell surface molecules during T cell recognition. *Annu Rev Biochem* 2003;72:717.

173. Lanzavecchia A, Sallusto F. Progressive differentiation and selection of the fittest in the immune response. *Nat Rev Immunol* 2002;2:982.

174. Lanzavecchia A, Sallusto F. Antigen decoding by T lymphocytes: from synapses to fate determination. *Nat Immunol* 2001;2:487.

175. Konig R. Interactions between MHC molecules and co-receptors of the TCR. *Curr Opin Immunol* 2002;14:75.

176. Gao GF, Jakobsen BK. Molecular interactions of coreceptor CD8 and MHC class I: the molecular basis for functional coordination with the T-cell receptor. *Immunol Today* 2000;21:630.

177. Kerry SE, Buslepp J, Cramer LA, et al. Interplay between TCR affinity and necessity of coreceptor ligation: high-affinity peptide-MHC/TCR interaction overcomes lack of CD8 engagement. *J Immunol* 2003;171:4493.

178. Hutchinson SL, Wooldridge L, Tafuro S, et al. The CD8 T cell coreceptor exhibits disproportionate biological activity at extremely low binding affinities. *J Biol Chem* 2003;278: 24285.

179. Cho BK, Lian KC, Lee P, et al. Differences in antigen recognition and cytolytic activity of CD8(+) and CD8(-) T cells that express the same antigen-specific receptor. *Proc Natl Acad Sci U S A* 2001;98:1723.

180. Germain RN. T-cell activation: the power of one. *Curr Biol* 2003;13:R137.

181. Shimizu Y, Shaw S. T lymphocyte adhesion molecules. *Year Immunol* 1990;6:69.

182. Dustin ML, Springer TA. Role of lymphocyte adhesion receptors in transient interactions and cell locomotion. *Annu Rev Immunol* 1991;9:27.

183. Fraser JD, Straus D, Weiss A. Signal transduction events leading to T-cell lymphokine gene expression. *Immunol Today* 1993;14:357.

184. Linsley PS, Ledbetter JA. The role of the CD28 receptor during T cell responses to antigen. *Annu Rev Immunol* 1993;11:191.

185. Schwartz RH. Costimulation of T lymphocytes: the role of CD28, CTLA-4, and B7/BB1 in interleukin-2 production and immunotherapy. *Cell* 1992;71:1065.

186. Watts TH, DeBenedette MA. T cell co-stimulatory molecules other than CD28. *Curr Opin Immunol* 1999;11:286.

187. Delon J, Germain RN. Information transfer at the immunological synapse. *Curr Biol* 2000;10:R923.

188. Shaw AS. FERMing up the synapse. *Immunity* 2001;15:683.

189. van der Merwe PA. Formation and function of the immunological synapse. *Curr Opin Immunol* 2002;14:293.

190. Dustin ML, Colman DR. Neural and immunological synaptic relations. *Science* 2002; 298:785.

191. Huppa JB, Davis MM. T-cell-antigen recognition and the immunological synapse. *Nat Rev Immunol* 2003;3:973.

192. Nelson BH, Willerford DM. Biology of the interleukin-2 receptor. *Adv Immunol* 1998;70:1.

193. Waldmann TA, Dubois S, Tagaya Y. Contrasting roles of IL-2 and IL-15 in the life and death of lymphocytes: implications for immunotherapy. *Immunity* 2001;14:105.

194. Leonard WJ. Type I cytokines and interferons and their receptors. In: Paul WE, ed. *Fundamental immunology*, 5th ed. Philadelphia: Lippincott Williams & Wilkins, 2003:701.

195. Nelson BH. IL-2, regulatory T cells, and tolerance. *J Immunol* 2004;172:3983.

196. Grunebaum E, Roifman CM. Signal-transduction defects in T cells. *Clin Rev Allergy Immunol* 2001;20:27.

197. Klebanoff CA, Finkelstein SE, Surman DR, et al. IL-15 enhances the in vivo antitumor activity of tumor-reactive CD8+ T cells. *Proc Natl Acad Sci U S A* 2004;101:1969.

198. Powell JD, Ragheb JA, Kitagawa-Sakakida S, et al. Molecular regulation of interleukin-2 expression by CD28 co-stimulation and anergy. *Immunol Rev* 1998;165:287.

199. Chambers CA, Allison JP. Co-stimulation in T cell responses. *Curr Opin Immunol* 1997;9:396.

200. Acuto O, Michel F. CD28-mediated co-stimulation: a quantitative support for TCR signaling. *Nat Rev Immunol* 2003;3:939.

201. Kane LP, Lin J, Weiss A. It's all Rel-ative: NF-kappaB and CD28 costimulation of T-cell activation. *Trends Immunol* 2002;23:413.

202. Bour-Jordan H, Blueston JA. CD28 function: a balance of costimulatory and regulatory signals. *J Clin Immunol* 2002;22:1.

203. Cory S. Regulation of lymphocyte survival by the bcl-2 gene family. *Annu Rev Immunol* 1995;13:513.

204. Broome HE, Dargan CM, Krajewski S, et al. Expression of Bcl-2, Bcl-x, and Bax after T cell activation and IL-2 withdrawal. *J Immunol* 1965;155:2311.

205. Sharpe AH, Freeman GJ. The B7-CD28 superfamily. *Nat Rev Immunol* 2002;2:116.

206. Croft M. Co-stimulatory members of the TNFR family: keys to effective T-cell immunity? *Nat Rev Immunol* 2003;3:609.

207. Watts TH, DeBenedette MA. T cell co-stimulatory molecules other than CD28. *Curr Opin Immunol* 1999;11:286.

208. Oosterwegel MA, Greenwald RJ, Mandelbrot DA, et al. CTLA-4 and T cell activation. *Curr Opin Immunol* 1999;11:294.

209. Thompson CB, Allison JP. The emerging role of CTLA-4 as an immune attenuator. *Immunity* 1997;7:445.

210. Bluestone JA. Is CTLA-4 a master switch for peripheral T cell tolerance? *J Immunol* 1997;158:1989.

211. Chen L, McGowan P, Ashe S, et al. Tumor immunogenicity determines the effect of B7 costimulation on T cell-mediated tumor immunity. *J Exp Med* 1994;179:523.

212. Chen L, Ashe S, Brady WA, et al. Costimulation of antitumor immunity by the B7 counterreceptor for the T lymphocyte molecules CD28 and CTLA-4. *Cell* 1992;71:1093.

213. Townsend SE, Allison JP. Tumor rejection after direct costimulation of CD8+ T cells by B7-transfected melanoma cells. *Science* 1993;259:368.

214. Baskar S, Ostrand-Rosenberg S, Nabavi N, et al. Constitutive expression of B7 restores immunogenicity of tumor cells expressing truncated major histocompatibility complex class II molecules. *Proc Natl Acad Sci U S A* 1993;90:5687.

215. Van Parijs L, Abbas AK. Homeostasis and self-tolerance in the immune system: turning lymphocytes off. *Science* 1998;280:243.

216. Goldrath AW, Bevan MJ. Selecting and maintaining a diverse T-cell repertoire. *Nature* 1999;402:255.

217. Rathmell JC, Thompson CB. Pathways of apoptosis in lymphocyte development, homeostasis, and disease. *Cell* 2002;109[Suppl]:S97.

218. Schwartz RH. T cell anergy. *Annu Rev Immunol* 2003;21:305.

219. Greenwald RJ, Latchman YE, Sharpe AH. Negative co-receptors on lymphocytes. *Curr Opin Immunol* 2002;14:391.

220. Kabelitz D, Pohl T, Pechhold K. Activation-induced cell death (apoptosis) of mature peripheral T lymphocytes. *Immunol Today* 1993;14:338.

221. Green DR, Scott DW. Activation-induced apoptosis in lymphocytes. *Curr Opin Immunol* 1994;6:476.

222. Vacchio MS, Ashwell JD. T cell tolerance. *Chem Immunol* 1994;58:1.

223. Webb DR, Kraig E, Devens BH. Suppressor cells and immunity. *Chem Immunol* 1994;58: 146.

224. Lenardo M, Chan KM, Hornung F, et al. Mature T lymphocyte apoptosis—immune regulation in a dynamic and unpredictable antigenic environment. *Annu Rev Immunol* 1999;17:221.

225. Green DR, Droin N, Pinkoski M. Activation-induced cell death in T cells. *Immunol Rev* 2003;193:70.

226. Hildeman DA, Zhu Y, Mitchell TC, et al. Molecular mechanisms of activated T cell death in vivo. *Curr Opin Immunol* 2002;14:354.

227. Russell JH, Rush B, Weaver C, et al. Mature T cells of autoimmune lpr/lpr mice have a defect in antigen-stimulated suicide. *Proc Natl Acad Sci U S A* 1993;90:4409.

228. Ahmed R, Gray D. Immunological memory and protective immunity: understanding their relation. *Science* 1996;272:54.

229. Freitas AA, Rocha B. Peripheral T cell survival. *Curr Opin Immunol* 1999;11:152.

230. Ernst B, Lee DS, Chang JM, et al. The peptide ligands mediating positive selection in the thymus control T cell survival and homeostatic proliferation in the periphery. *Immunity* 1999;11:173.

231. Sprent J, Surh CD. T cell memory. *Annu Rev Immunol* 2002;20:551.

232. Sallusto F, Geginat J, Lanzavecchia A. Central memory and effector memory T cell subsets: function, generation, and maintenance. *Annu Rev Immunol* 2004;22:745.

233. Picker LJ, Butcher EC. Physiological and molecular mechanisms of lymphocyte homing. *Annu Rev Immunol* 1992;10:561.

234. Shimizu Y, Newman W, Tanaka Y, et al. Lymphocyte interactions with endothelial cells. *Immunol Today* 1992;13:106.

235. Springer TA. Traffic signals on endothelium for lymphocyte recirculation and leukocyte emigration. *Annu Rev Physiol* 1995;57:827.

236. Tanaka Y, Adams DH, Shaw S. Proteoglycans on endothelial cells present adhesion-inducing cytokines to leukocytes. *Immunol Today* 1993;14:111.

237. Baggiolini M. Chemokines and leukocyte traffic. *Nature* 1998;392:565.

238. Muller G, Lipp M. Concerted action of the chemokine and lymphokine system in secondary lymphoid-organ development. *Curr Opin Immunol* 2003;15:217.

239. Sallusto F, Lanzavecchia A, Mackay CR. Chemokines and chemokine receptors in T-cell priming and Th1/Th2-mediated responses. *Immunol Today* 1998;19:568.

240. Zlotnik A, Morales J, Hedrick JA. Recent advances in chemokines and chemokine receptors. *Crit Rev Immunol* 1999;19:1.

241. Rot A, Von Andrian UH. Chemokines in innate and adaptive host defense: basic chemokinese grammar for immune cells. *Annu Rev Immunol* 2004;22:891.

242. Hodes RJ. T-cell-mediated regulation: help and suppression. In: Paul WE, ed. *Fundamental immunology*, 2nd ed. New York: Raven Press, 1989:587.

243. Oxenius A, Zinkernagel RM, Hengartner H. CD4+ T-cell induction and effector functions: a comparison of immunity against soluble antigens and viral infections. *Adv Immunol* 1998;70:313.

244. Lanzavecchia A. Immunology. Licence to kill. *Nature* 1998;393:413.

245. Heath WR, Carbone FR. Cytotoxic T lymphocyte activation by cross-priming. *Curr Opin Immunol* 1999;11:314.

246. Guerder S, Matzinger P. A fail-safe mechanism for maintaining self-tolerance. *J Exp Med* 1992;176:553.

247. Sun JC, Bevan MJ. Defective CD8 T cell memory following acute infection without CD4 T cell help. *Science* 2003;300:339.

248. Shedlock DJ, Shen H. Requirement for CD4 T cell help in generating functional CD8 T cell memory. *Science* 2003;300:337.

249. Janssen EM, Lemmens EE, Wolfe T, et al. CD4+ T cells are required for secondary expansion and memory in CD8+ T lymphocytes. *Nature* 2003;421:852.

250. Bourgeois C, Tanchot C. Mini-review CD4 T cells are required for CD8 T cell memory generation. *Eur J Immunol* 2003;33:3225.

251. Fitch FW, McKisic MD, Lancki DW, et al. Differential regulation of murine T lymphocyte subsets. *Annu Rev Immunol* 1993;11:29.

252. Seder RA, Mosmann TM. Differentiation of effector phenotypes of CD4+ and CD8+ T cells. In: Paul WE, ed. *Fundamental immunology*, 4th ed. Philadelphia: Lippincott–Raven Publishers, 1999:879.

253. Romagnani S. The Th1/Th2 paradigm. *Immunol Today* 1997;18:263.

254. Seder RA, Paul WE. Acquisition of lymphokine-producing phenotype by CD4+ T cells. *Annu Rev Immunol* 1994;12:635.

255. Carter LL, Swain SL. Single cell analyses of cytokine production. *Curr Opin Immunol* 1997;9:177.

256. Constant SL, Bottomly K. Induction of Th1 and Th2 CD4+ T cell responses: the alternative approaches. *Annu Rev Immunol* 1997;15:297.

257. O'Garra A. Cytokines induce the development of functionally heterogeneous T helper cell subsets. *Immunity* 1998;8:275.

258. Abbas AK, Murphy KM, Sher A. Functional diversity of helper T lymphocytes. *Nature* 1996;383:787.

259. Shevach EM. CD4+ CD25+ suppressor T cells: more questions than answers. *Nat Rev Immunol* 2002;2:389.

260. Sakaguchi S. Naturally arising CD4+ regulatory T cells for immunologic self-tolerance and negative control of immune responses. *Annu Rev Immunol* 2004;22:531.

261. Ramsdell F. Foxp3 and natural regulatory T cells: key to a cell lineage? *Immunity* 2003;19:165.

262. Wang HY, Lee DA, Peng G, et al. Tumor-specific human CD4+ regulatory T cells and their ligands: implications for immunotherapy. *Immunity* 2004;20:107.

263. Schwartz RH, Mueller DL. Immunological tolerance. In: Paul WE, ed. *Fundamental immunology*, 5th ed. Philadelphia: Lippincott Williams and Wilkins Publishers, 2003:901.

264. Greenberg PD. Adoptive T cell therapy of tumors: mechanisms operative in the recognition and elimination of tumor cells. *Adv Immunol* 1991;49:281.

265. Cohen PA, Peng L, Plautz GE, et al. CD4+ T cells in adoptive immunotherapy and the indirect mechanism of tumor rejection. *Crit Rev Immunol* 2000;20:17.

266. Thomas WD, Hersey P. TNF-related apoptosis-inducing ligand (TRAIL) induces apoptosis in Fas ligand-resistant melanoma cells and mediates CD4 T cell killing of target cells. *J Immunol* 1998;161:2195.

267. Hung K, Hayashi R, Lafond-Walker A, et al. The central role of CD4(+) T cells in the antitumor immune response. *J Exp Med* 1998;188:2357.

268. Pardoll DM, Topalian SL. The role of CD4+ T cell responses in antitumor immunity. *Curr Opin Immunol* 1998;10:588.

269. Henkart PA, Sitkovsky MV. Cytotoxic T-lymphocytes. In: Paul WE, ed. *Fundamental immunology*, 5th ed. Philadelphia: Lippincott Williams & Wilkins, 2003:1127.

270. Russell JH, Ley TJ. Lymphocyte-mediated cytotoxicity. *Annu Rev Immunol* 2002;20:323.

271. Rouvier E, Luciani MF, Golstein P. Fas involvement in Ca(2+)-independent T cell-mediated cytotoxicity. *J Exp Med* 1993;177:195.

272. Griffiths GM, Schopp J. *Pathways for cytolysis*. Berlin: Springer-Verlag, 1995.

273. Berke G. The CTL's kiss of death. *Cell* 1995;81:9.

274. Henkart PA. Lymphocyte-mediated cytotoxicity: two pathways and multiple effector molecules. *Immunity* 1994;1:343.

275. Crispe IN. Fatal interactions: Fas-induced apoptosis of mature T cells. *Immunity* 1994;1:347.

276. Nagata S, Golstein P. The Fas death factor. *Science* 1995;267:1449.

277. Kojima H, Shinohara N, Hanaoka S, et al. Two distinct pathways of specific killing revealed by perforin mutant cytotoxic T lymphocytes. *Immunity* 1994;1:357.

278. Walsh CM, Matloubian M, Liu CC, et al. Immune function in mice lacking the perforin gene. *Proc Natl Acad Sci U S A* 1994;91:10854.

279. Paul NL, Ruddle NH. Lymphotoxin. *Annu Rev Immunol* 1988;6:407.

280. Aggarwal BB, Vilcek J. *Tumor necrosis factors: structure, function, and mechanism of action.* New York: Dekker, 1992.

281. Beutler B. *Tumor necrosis factors: the molecules and their emerging role in medicine.* New York: Raven Press, 1992.

282. Ratner A, Clark WR. Role of TNF-alpha in CD8+ cytotoxic T lymphocyte-mediated lysis. *J Immunol* 1993;150:4303.

282a. Spiotto MT, Rowley DA, Schreiber H. Bystander elimination of antigen loss variants in established tumors. *Nat Med* 2004;10:294.

283. Ashkenazi A. Targeting death and decoy receptors of the tumour-necrosis factor superfamily. *Nat Rev Cancer* 2002;2:420.

284. Lowin B, Hahne M, Mattmann C, et al. Cytolytic T-cell cytotoxicity is mediated through perforin and Fas lytic pathways. *Nature* 1994;370:650.

285. Kagi D, Vignaux F, Ledermann B, et al. Fas and perforin pathways as major mechanisms of T cell-mediated cytotoxicity. *Science* 1994;265:528.

286. Henkart PA, Williams MS, Nakajima H. Degranulating cytotoxic lymphocytes inflict multiple damage pathways on target cells. *Curr Top Microbiol Immunol* 1995;198:75.

287. Kagi D, Ledermann B, Burki K, et al. Molecular mechanisms of lymphocyte-mediated cytotoxicity and their role in immunological protection and pathogenesis in vivo. *Annu Rev Immunol* 1996;14:207.

288. van den Broek ME, Kagi D, Ossendorp F, et al. Decreased tumor surveillance in perforin-deficient mice. *J Exp Med* 1996;184:1781.

289. Crispe IN. Death and destruction of activated T lymphocytes. *Immunol Res* 1999;19:143.

290. Alderson MR, Lynch DH. Receptors and ligands that mediate activation-induced death of T cells. *Springer Semin Immunopathol* 1998;19:289.

291. McMahon CW, Raulet DH. Expression and function of NK cell receptors in CD8+ T cells. *Curr Opin Immunol* 2001;13:465.

292. McQueen KL, Parham P. Variable receptors controlling activation and inhibition of NK cells. *Curr Opin Immunol* 2002;14:615.

293. Basse PH, Whiteside TL, Chambers W, et al. Therapeutic activity of NK cells against tumors. *Int Rev Immunol* 2001;20:439.

294. Moretta L, Biassoni R, Bottino C, et al. Human NK cells and their receptors. *Microbes Infect* 2002;4:1539.

294a. Spits H, Lanier LL, Phillips JH. Development of human T and natural killer cells. *Blood* 1995;85:2654.

295. Berke G. The functions and mechanisms of action of cytolytic lymphocytes. In: Paul WE, ed. *Fundamental immunology*, 3rd ed. New York: Raven Press Publishers, 1993:965.

296. Henkart PA, Hayes MP, Shiver JW. The granule exocytosis model for lymphocyte cytotoxicity and its relevance to target cell DNA breakdown. In: Sitkovsky MV, Henkart P, eds. *Cytotoxic cells: recognition, effector function, generation, and methods*. Boston: Birkhauser Publishers, 1993:153.

297. Yagita H, Nakata M, Kawasaki A, et al. Role of perforin in lymphocyte-mediated cytolysis. *Adv Immunol* 1992;51:215.

298. Lanier LL, Phillips JH. Natural killer cells. *Curr Opin Immunol* 1992;4:38.

299. Shi L, Kraut RP, Aebersold R, et al. A natural killer cell granule protein that induces DNA fragmentation and apoptosis. *J Exp Med* 1992;175:553.

300. Arase H, Arase N, Saito T. Fas-mediated cytotoxicity by freshly isolated natural killer cells. *J Exp Med* 1995;181:1235.

301. Kashii Y, Giorda R, Herberman RB, et al. Constitutive expression and role of the TNF family ligands in apoptotic killing of tumor cells by human NK cells. *J Immunol* 1999;163:5358.

302. Zamai L, Ahmad M, Bennett IM, et al. Natural killer (NK) cell-mediated cytotoxicity: differential use of TRAIL and Fas ligand by immature and mature primary human NK cells. *J Exp Med* 1998;188:2375.

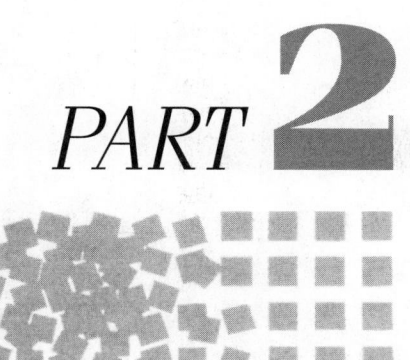

PART 2

PRINCIPLES OF ONCOLOGY

CHAPTER 7

Etiology of Cancer: Viruses

SECTION **1**

GARY L. BUCHSCHACHER, JR.
FLOSSIE WONG-STAAL

RNA Viruses

Viruses have long been hypothesized to cause some cancers. Although several DNA viruses are associated with the development of malignancy, members of only two RNA virus families—*Retroviridae* and *Flaviviridae*—have thus far been associated with development of neoplastic disease.[1–3] In humans, these viruses include the retroviruses human T-lymphotropic virus (HTLV) and human immunodeficiency virus (HIV) and the flavivirus hepatitis C virus (HCV). HTLV type 1 (HTLV-1) appears to contribute directly to the development of adult T-cell leukemia (ATL); HIV and HCV are associated with human malignancy but likely contribute to its development in an indirect manner.

However, a number of animal retroviruses cause cancer in their natural hosts and have been important tools for understanding oncogenesis in humans and animals.[4] The discovery and characterization of oncogenes and the subsequent elucidation of protooncogene functions have been closely intertwined and made possible by the study of retroviruses. In this section, the discussion focuses on the molecular genetics and the characteristics of retroviruses relevant to oncogenesis and explores the roles of the retroviruses HTLV-1, HTLV-2, and HIV and the flavivirus HCV in human cancers. In many examples, although these viruses may play key initiating or contributing roles to carcinogenesis, additional events are needed for infection to yield the full malignant phenotype.

RETROVIRUSES: BACKGROUND, REPLICATION CYCLE, AND MOLECULAR GENETICS

In the past, retroviruses had been classified on the basis of pathogenesis into the oncoretrovirus (the retroviruses associated with tumor formation), lentivirus, and spumavirus groups or on the basis of virus particle morphology (virus types A through D). Now, however, the retroviruses are organized into seven genera based on molecular genetic analysis: *Alpha-, Beta-, Gamma-, Delta-,* and *Epsilon-retroviruses; Lentiviruses;* and *Spumaviruses.* This taxonomic system divides the oncoretroviruses into five genera. Few human retroviruses are known: the *Deltaretroviruses* HTLV-1 and HTLV-2 and the *Lentiviruses* HIV-1 and HIV-2. The spumavirus formerly termed *human foamy virus* is, in fact, a simian retrovirus isolated from contaminated human cell cultures (it is now termed *chimpanzee foamy virus human isolate*). Human endogenous retroviruses (HERVs) are endogenous retroviral elements contained within the human genome but are not classified as retroviruses per se.

Retroviruses are unique among animal viruses in having an RNA genome that replicates through a DNA intermediate.[5,6] Retroviral virions contain two identical plus-sense RNA molecules. The RNA genome (Fig. 7.1-1) contains a 5' untranslated region; the three genes common to all retroviruses—*gag, pol,* and *env;* and a 3' untranslated region and polyadenylated tail. In general, the *gag* gene encodes viral structural proteins, *pol* encodes viral enzymatic proteins, and *env* encodes viral envelope glycoproteins.

After entry into a cell, the single-stranded viral genome is converted to a double-stranded DNA copy by reverse transcriptase,[7] an RNA-dependent DNA polymerase (see Fig. 7.1-1). Then, the retro-

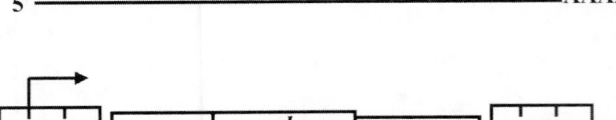

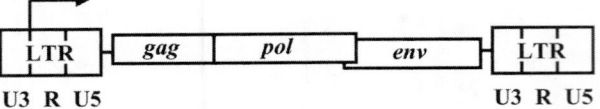

FIGURE 7.1-1. Retrovirus genetic organization. General genome structure of a typical replication-competent oncoretrovirus. The structure of the double-stranded DNA copy (provirus) is shown below that of the genomic RNA. In the provirus, *gag* (encoding viral structural proteins), *pol* (viral replication enzymes), and *env* (viral envelope glycoproteins) genes are flanked on each end by the long terminal repeats (LTRs). The viral promoter/enhancer is located in the 5' U3, with transcription termination and polyadenylation signals located in the 3' LTR. The arrow indicates point and direction of transcription initiation. R, repeat; U3, unique 3' region; U5, unique 5' region.

viral integrase protein inserts the double-stranded DNA viral genome into a host cell chromosome, where it permanently resides as a provirus.[8] An integrated retroviral provirus resembles cellular genes in that it is duplicated along with the cell's genome, passed on to daughter cells during mitosis, and subsequently transcribed and processed into messenger RNA (mRNA).

Reverse transcription is a complicated process that can use both viral RNA molecules as templates for DNA synthesis and involves RNA and DNA template strand-switching events during nucleotide polymerization. This process results in duplication of the 5' and 3' ends of the genome, thus forming the long terminal repeats (LTRs), which are composed of the unique 3'(U3), repeat (R), and unique 5' (U5) regions. The viral promoter and enhancer functions reside within the LTR. Transcription initiates in the 5' LTR and proceeds to the polyadenylation signal, usually located in the 3' LTR.

In summary, a number of features unique to the retroviral replication cycle demonstrate how retroviruses may be involved in the development of or be used for the study of the molecular basis of cell transformation.[9,10] Integration of the provirus into the cellular genome can permanently introduce genes into a cell or can result in mutation or altered regulation of genes. In addition, the molecular mechanism by which reverse transcription occurs is a fertile environment in which alterations of genes or the creation of cancer-causing genes might take place.[11,12]

MECHANISMS OF RETROVIRAL ONCOGENESIS

Infection by members of the *Alpha-, Beta-, Gamma-, Delta-,* and *Epsilon-retrovirus* genera may lead to the development of neoplastic disease in different ways (the genera are classified based on variations in genetic structure, not by shared mechanisms of pathogenesis), but, in general, individual members of each genus can be thought of as either acutely or slowly transforming viruses. In the case of the acutely transforming retroviruses, virtually all infected cells are swiftly transformed, whereas for other retroviruses, transformation is an unusual and much delayed outcome that often depends on the cell's accrual of additional alteration of its

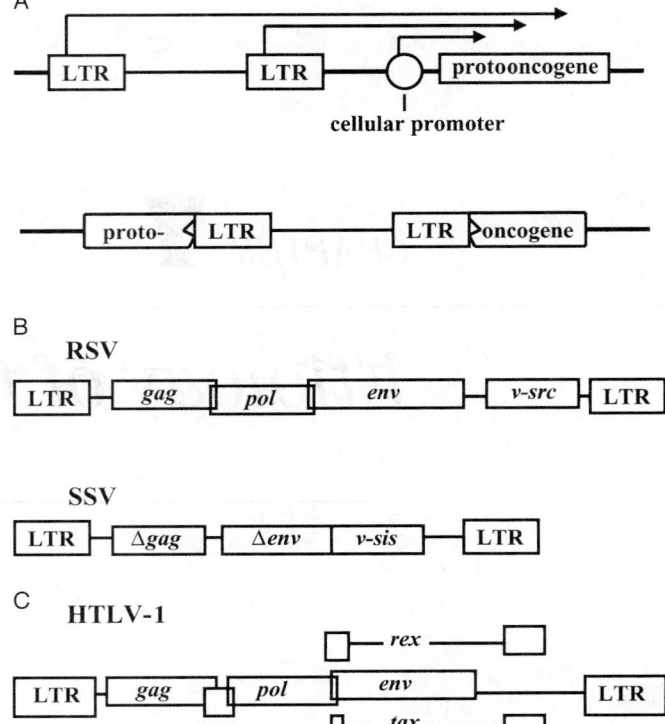

FIGURE 7.1-2. Three types of oncogenic retroviruses. **A:** Slowly transforming retroviruses. In the upper example, a provirus has integrated upstream of a cellular protooncogene. The viral promoters may alter protooncogene expression directly [via read-through transcription originating from the 5' long terminal repeat (LTR) or from transcripts aberrantly originating in the 3' LTR] or indirectly via the effect of viral enhancers increasing transcription from cellular promoters (the viral enhancer can also affect expression of cellular genes 5' to and in the opposite orientation of the site of provirus integration). In the second example, insertional mutagenesis and consequent gene disruption are illustrated. This process may lead to inactivation of a tumor suppressor or to production of a mutant cellular protein that could lead to oncogenesis. In both cases, aberrant splicing could result in production of chimeric viral-cellular proteins. Arrows indicate points of initiation and direction of transcription. **B:** Acutely transforming retroviruses. Rous sarcoma virus (RSV) and simian sarcoma virus (SSV), retroviruses that contain oncogenes, are shown. RSV is unique in that the oncogene, *v-src*, has been added to the viral genome without concomitant loss of replicative genes. SSV, an example of the more common oncogene-containing retroviruses, is not replication competent; the recombination that led to *v-sis* insertion resulted in deletion of some viral sequences. **C:** *Trans*-acting retroviruses. In addition to *gag, pol,* and *env,* the human T-lymphotropic virus type 1 (HTLV-1) genome encodes the proteins Tax, Rev, p12[I], p13[I], and p30[II], derived from open reading frames I to IV located in the pX region. Tax (and possibly p12[I]) is implicated in the genesis of adult T-cell leukemia through interactions with cellular transcription factors, resulting in alteration of expression of many T-cell growth regulation genes, including cytokines and cell-cycle control elements.

DNA. This latter group includes the classic slowly transforming retroviruses and the *trans*-acting retroviruses. Reverse transcription and integration of the viral genome into the cell favor the three major mechanisms by which oncogenic retroviruses may participate in the malignant transformation process (Fig. 7.1-2):

1. Slowly transforming viruses [e.g., avian leukosis virus (ALV), an *Alpharetrovirus*] alter cellular gene expres-

sion by random integration of a provirus within or adjacent to cellular protooncogenes (insertional mutagenesis). Direct physical disruption of a gene or effects of viral promoters and enhancers on cellular gene expression can lead to a malignant phenotype in infected cells.

2. Acutely transforming retroviruses [e.g., Rous sarcoma virus (RSV), an *Alpharetrovirus*] have incorporated into their genomes viral oncogenes derived from cellular protooncogenes (protooncogene capture) and subsequently transfer these altered or deregulated oncogenes into newly infected cells, thus leading to development of a malignant phenotype.

3. *Trans*-acting retroviruses (e.g., HTLV-1, a *Deltaretrovirus*) alter cellular gene expression and function and, consequently, the control of cell growth via viral protein(s) that act in *trans*.

SLOWLY TRANSFORMING RETROVIRUSES: INSERTIONAL MUTAGENESIS

Simple integration of a provirus into the genome of a cell can, rarely, be tumorigenic by leading to aberrant activity of cellular genes. Retroviruses that act in this manner have been termed *chronic, or slow-acting, tumor viruses.* They do not transform cells in tissue culture and, *in vivo*, a long latency period between infection and tumorigenesis is typical. In general, in addition to the mutagenesis caused by provirus integration, tumors produced by slowly transforming retroviruses require additional mutagenic events to take place for their transforming properties to become apparent.

Most proviral integrations have no effect on the phenotype of the infected cell but rarely can lead to phenotypically evident insertional mutagenesis in one of a number of ways.[13,14] Proviral integration might disrupt a gene (typically a tumor suppressor gene) by integrating within the gene (in an exon or intron) or by disrupting the promoter of the gene, thereby preventing production of a functional protein. Alternatively, insertion upstream or within a gene can also result in aberrant production of a cellular protein if the retroviral promoters in either the 5' or 3' LTRs are active and, because of read-through transcription, result in production of chimeric viral/cellular mRNAs. The protein derived from this mRNA may be wild type but produced in increased amounts, or may be a truncated or viral/cellular chimeric protein due to read-through transcription and aberrant RNA splicing. The enhancers present in the retroviral LTRs also can affect expression of cellular genes either upstream or downstream of the provirus integration site and genes in either the sense or antisense orientation relative to the provirus.

With the exception of rare cases of T-cell malignancy that appear to involve a monoclonal expansion of an HIV-1–infected cell, naturally occurring retroviruses have not been shown to cause malignancy by insertional mutagenesis in humans. However, humans are clearly susceptible to malignancy associated with retroviral-mediated insertional mutagenesis. In a gene transfer clinical trial using a murine leukemia virus (MLV) (a *Gammaretrovirus*) vector, two of the treated pediatric patients developed T-cell acute lymphoblastic leukemia (T-ALL) that appears to have been caused, at least in part, by insertion of the MLV vector provirus within or near the *LMO-2* gene.[15,16]

ACUTELY TRANSFORMING RETROVIRUSES: ONCOGENE TRANSDUCTION

Acutely transforming retroviruses have taken the oncogenic potential of slow-acting retroviruses one step further and are capable of rapidly transforming infected cells, which is followed by subsequent tumor formation. Although there are no known acutely transforming human retroviruses, the animal viruses are important because of the roles they played in the discovery of oncogenes and in the continued study of the molecular mechanisms of tumor formation.

Acutely transforming retroviruses are mutant retroviruses that encode oncogenes that, when integrated into the genome of an infected cell and subsequently expressed, result in cell transformation. These viral oncogenes are derivatives of cellular protooncogenes that were "captured" from the genome of a previously infected cell and incorporated into the retroviral genome, thereby creating a recombinant retrovirus containing a cancer-causing gene.

Many acutely transforming retroviruses contain different oncogenes. RSV is the prototype of such viruses. In fact, it was the study of RSV (and then other transforming retroviruses) that eventually led to the discovery of cellular protooncogenes and their potential roles in cancer development.[17,18]

RSV arose when a retrovirus incorporated an oncogene into its genome; it is unique among acutely transforming retroviruses in that it encodes an oncogene (*v-src*) and functional retroviral *gag*, *pol*, and *env* genes. Typically, the recombination events that incorporate the oncogene into the retroviral genome also result in deletion of some or all of the retroviral genes. Therefore, the recombinant viruses are only capable of being propagated and infecting new cells when cells are coinfected with the parental, wild-type virus, which can produce all necessary retroviral proteins.

Acutely transforming retroviruses are believed to be formed after a number of complex events due to recombination during reverse transcription. The first such event is the integration of a wild-type retroviral provirus within or near a cellular protooncogene, as has been described for slowly transforming retroviruses. The next step involves formation of chimeric retroviral/cellular protooncogene mRNA, resulting from transcription from the 5' LTR, with subsequent read-through transcription into the cellular protooncogene. This chimeric viral/cellular mRNA can then be copackaged into a virion (which normally contains two identical copies of the viral genome) capable of infecting a new cell. Then, because reverse transcription of the retroviral genome involves template strand-switching events and also may lead to recombination events, nonhomologous recombination between wild-type and chimeric molecules can occur, thereby resulting in a novel provirus with an oncogene incorporated into its genome.

A protooncogene generally is not transduced intact from the cell to the retroviral genome: Deletion, frameshift, and point mutations are likely to occur during the process. In addition, the chimeric molecule can result in production of a viral/cellular fusion protein. Any or all of these alterations to the cellular protooncogene might contribute to altering the activity, level of expression, stability, function, or localization of the resulting protein, therefore resulting in the conversion of a cellular protooncogene with the potential to cause cancer into a viral oncogene fully capable of doing so.

TRANS-ACTIVATING RETROVIRUSES

A third manner of transformation involves *trans*-acting viral proteins that affect the expression or function of cellular growth and differentiation genes. This mechanism of oncogenesis is illustrated by HTLV-1, the only human retrovirus known to directly cause cancer.

HUMAN T-LYMPHOTROPIC VIRUS TYPE 1

HISTORY AND EPIDEMIOLOGY

ATL, an aggressive malignancy of CD4+ T cells, originally was believed confined to southern Japan. The geographic clustering of ATL suggested an infectious etiology. Serologic testing of Japanese ATL patients with antigens prepared from a newly discovered retrovirus (now called *HTLV-1*) revealed nearly 100% seropositivity, and subsequent isolations of the virus from ATL patients soon were reported.[19] Other epidemiologic clusters consistent with an etiologic role for endemic HTLV-1 infection have since been documented, most notably in the Caribbean basin, the southeastern United States, northeastern South America, Central Africa, and Papua New Guinea. It is estimated that 10 to 20 million people are infected with HTLV-1. Transmission of HTLV-1 by blood transfusion (but, unlike HIV, not cell-free blood products), needle sharing, and breast feeding, and from male to female (rarely the reverse) by sexual intercourse, has been documented.

In addition to seroepidemiologic studies of patients and their close contacts, several lines of evidence support a causal role for HTLV-1 in ATL: The virus can be isolated reproducibly from ATL patients; leukemic cells contain an HTLV-1 provirus, whereas other cells from these patients do not; and infected individuals born in an endemic region carry their risk of developing ATL with them if they move elsewhere. In addition, infection clearly precedes transformation, because the tumor cells carry monoclonal or oligoclonal insertions of HTLV-1 DNA and have a single T-cell antigen receptor-β gene rearrangement. This monoclonality also provides additional evidence that transformation is a rare sequel to infection.

VIRAL REPLICATION CYCLE AND ITS IMPLICATIONS FOR VIRUS SPREAD

Although HTLV-1 shares many features with other oncoretroviruses, it is considerably more complex genetically and biologically. In addition to *gag*, *pol*, and *env*, the virus genome contains additional open reading frames (ORF I to IV) located in the pX region of the genome.[20] The two best characterized are the *trans*-regulating proteins Tax and Rex. Both proteins are expressed early in the viral replication cycle and are important for expression of viral genes; as such, they are analogous to the HIV proteins Tat and Rev. Rex promotes the cytoplasmic accumulation of singly spliced (*env*) and unspliced (genomic) mRNAs. Tax activates transcription from the HTLV-1 LTR by associating with a number of cellular transcription factors.

Additional HTLV-1 proteins (p12[I], p13[II], p30[II]) derived from translation of alternatively spliced RNA of the pX region also exist; their precise roles in the viral replication cycle are not clear, but they appear to be required for *in vivo* infectivity of the virus.

Although HTLV-1 shares a number of features with HIV—a complex genetic structure, tropism for CD4+ T lymphocytes, induction of syncytia in cultured T cells, and similar routes of transmission between individuals—HTLV-1 infection is not associated with marked cellular immunodeficiency unless ATL develops. In addition, although there are points during the course of HIV infection at which cell-to-cell transmission of the virus is important, infection by free virions occurs, with high levels of viremia detected in HIV-1–infected individuals. By contrast, in individuals infected with HTLV-1, significant viremia is not detected; it appears that, in culture and *in vivo*, virus spreads to uninfected cells by cell-to-cell transmission of the virus. This cell-to-cell spread of HTLV-1 appears to involve polarization of the cytoskeleton of infected cells to a cell-cell junction, promoting spread of virus to new cells.[21] In addition to cell-to-cell virus transmission, the number of HTLV-1–infected cells within an individual increases by simple mitosis of provirus-containing T cells, thereby amplifying the number of infected T cells.

The *in vivo* latency and low levels of viremia in HTLV-1 patients have implications for virus spread and for evolution and represent one factor in the less efficient, endemic transmission of HTLV-1 compared to the epidemic spread of HIV-1, even though the same routes of infection appear to be operative. Unlike HIV-1, there is remarkably little genetic variability among HTLV-1 isolates.

MODELS FOR HUMAN T-LYMPHOTROPIC VIRUS TYPE 1 LEUKEMOGENESIS

The most common outcome of HTLV-1 infection is an asymptomatic carrier state; HTLV-1 carriers have an estimated lifetime risk of developing ATL of approximately 3% to 5%, with a latency period from time of infection to development of malignancy of 30 to 50 years. Given these facts, it is apparent that factors other than simple viral infection must be necessary for leukemogenesis. The sites of proviral insertion are random from patient to patient, indicating that *cis*-acting insertional mutagenesis does not play a role in tumorigenesis. Furthermore, the virus does not appear to encode a host-derived oncogene: No homologies between human cellular genes and nonstructural HTLV-1 genes have been observed. A third genetic mechanism for tumorigenesis, which appears to be a multistep process, is thus implicated, with the Tax protein being central to transformation.[22–25]

Tax promotes viral gene expression by indirectly activating the viral promoter in the LTR via interaction with cellular transcription proteins. However, the interaction of Tax with various transcription factors also transactivates numerous cellular gene promoters.[26] The cellular transcription pathways activated by Tax include activating transcription factor/cyclic adenosine monophosphate–responsive element-binding protein (ATF/CREB), nuclear factor κB/c-Rel, and serum response factor. Tax is able to bind directly to the TATA-binding protein, a component of the transcriptional complex, and to p300 and CREB-binding protein, both of which are transcriptional coactivators.

Among the cellular genes transactivated by Tax, the most relevant are the interleukin (IL)-2 and IL-2 receptor genes.

Unlike normal resting T cells, ATL cells and T cells transformed *in vitro* by HTLV-1 constitutively express the α chain of the IL-2 receptor at high levels, which can stimulate proliferation of infected cells. In addition, possible interactions between another HTLV-1 protein (p12^I) and the gamma subunit of the IL-2 receptor may contribute to ligand-independent activation of this receptor, potentially resulting in stimulation and expansion of the pool of infected cells.

Tax has also been shown to down-regulate expression of a cellular DNA repair enzyme, β-DNA polymerase, a potentially straightforward link to accelerated accumulation of mutations. In addition, expression of a large number of genes involved in cell proliferation is transactivated by Tax, including granulocyte-macrophage colony-stimulating factor, the protooncogenes *c-fos* and *c-sis*, HLA class I, vimentin, and tumor necrosis factor.

The IL-2 independence of HTLV-1–infected T-cell proliferation involves a cell signaling pathway in which receptor-associated protein kinases in the Janus kinase (Jak) family phosphorylate cytoplasmic transcription factors called *STATs* (signal transducers and activators of transcription).[27] After phosphorylation, STATs translocate to the cell nucleus and bind to specific DNA elements to modulate transcription. The Jak-STAT pathway is triggered by IL-2 in normal T cells; however, transition to IL-2 independence after HTLV-1 infection was associated with constitutive activation of the pathway.

Tax also has been shown to interact with and presumably inactivate a number of cell cycle–related proteins,[28] including the cyclin-dependent kinase (CDK) inhibitor p16^{INK4a} and the cell-cycle checkpoint protein MAD1. Tax activates the promoter of p21$^{waf1/cip1}$, also a CDK inhibitor, and, through the activation of the ATF/CREB pathway, suppresses the activity of p53, which can prevent p53-induced apoptosis. It also has been suggested that constitutive action of the IL-2 receptor pathway allows cells, through an unknown mechanism, to avoid apoptosis.

In summary, although the exact steps in HTLV-1–induced leukemogenesis are unclear, Tax (and probably p12^I) seems to play a critical role by direct interaction with cellular proteins involved in transcription, cell-cycle regulation, cell proliferation, and apoptosis. It appears that additional mutational events are necessary for the transition from cell immortalization to monoclonality and acute ATL. Immortalization and propagation of clones of infected cells probably allow alterations in the cell-cycle and apoptosis pathways to accumulate, permitting a dominant transformed clone to emerge. Further work to determine the key events in the complex network of cell-cycle/apoptosis pathways will help elucidate the fundamental cell biology leading to HTLV-1 leukemogenesis.

CLINICAL FEATURES OF HUMAN T-LYMPHOTROPIC VIRUS TYPE 1 DISEASE

In acute ATL, tumor cells aggressively infiltrate multiple organs, commonly involving lymph nodes, liver, spleen, skin, and lung. Median survival is measured in months. The age of onset averages 58 years (range, 24 to 85), with a male-female ratio of 1.4:1.0. Either a leukemic or a non-Hodgkin's T-cell lymphoma presentation may predominate. Leukemic cells are morphologically distinct, with lobulated ("flower") nuclei. Leukemic cells typically are CD2+, CD3+, CD4+, CD8–, CD25+, and HLA-DR+. However, there is evidence that in addition to CD4+ T cells (the phenotype of the majority of ATLs) HTLV-1 can also infect and transform CD8+ T cells, as well as immature CD4– CD8– T-cell precursors in bone marrow.

ATL has been classified into four stages: acute, chronic, smoldering, and lymphomatous. Characteristics of the malignancy may include hypercalcemia, elevated lactate dehydrogenase levels, cutaneous leukemic infiltrates, lytic bone lesions, lymphadenopathy, and liver or spleen lesions. Death is often the result of opportunistic infection.

The differential diagnosis includes mycosis fungoides, Sézary syndrome, Hodgkin's disease, and T-cell chronic lymphocytic leukemia. HTLV-1 seropositivity, negative TdT staining, and CD4 positivity are characteristic of ATL. Detection of a mono- or oligoclonally integrated HTLV-1 provirus makes the diagnosis definitive.

In addition to ATL, HTLV-1 is also associated with tropical spastic paraparesis/HTLV-associated myelopathy (TSP/HAM), a chronic progressive neurologic disorder.[29] HTLV-1 carriers are estimated to have a lifetime risk of developing TSP/HAM of less than 2%. Features of the disorder include leg weakness, sensory deficits, hyperreflexia, incontinence, and impotence. Although it is not clear how HTLV-1 infection leads to TSP/HAM, the most likely scenarios involve immune mechanisms, either cell-mediated destruction of infected cells within the central nervous system (CNS) or the autoimmune destruction of cells expressing cross-reactive antigens, with subsequent cytokine release in both cases. Early on, disease progression may be slowed with corticosteroid treatment, but no curative therapy is known to exist.

HUMAN T-LYMPHOTROPIC VIRUS TYPE 2

HTLV-2 is closely related to HTLV-1, sharing the same overall genetic organization and 70% homology at the amino acid level. Although it also infects and transforms T cells *in vitro*, HTLV-2 is preferentially tropic *in vitro* for the CD8+ subset. The virus was isolated from a patient with atypical T-cell variant hairy cell leukemia and subsequently from two other individuals. Other disease associations have been reported; however, convincing epidemiologic data for an etiologic role for HTLV-2 in human disease are lacking. Most patients with either T- or B-cell hairy cell leukemia are not infected with HTLV-2, and so far no disease has a demonstrated increased incidence in HTLV-2–infected populations. In contrast to HTLV-1, HTLV-2 is able to transform T cells in a manner not dependent on activation of the Jak/STAT pathway,[30] although the exact mechanism of cell transformation by HTLV-2 remains unknown.

HTLV-2 is transmitted by the same routes as HTLV-1: contaminated blood, breast feeding, and sexual intercourse (nearly always male to female). In the general U.S. population, HTLV-2 is present in fewer than 0.01% of blood donors and in a larger proportion of intravenous drug users. HTLV-2 is recognized to be endemic in African pygmies and in many indigenous New World populations, including the Navajo, Pueblo, and Seminole Indians in North America; the Guyami Indians in Panama; and various quite widely separated and remote tribes in South America.[31]

HUMAN IMMUNODEFICIENCY VIRUS

HIV-1 and HIV-2 are members of the *Lentivirus* genus of retroviruses. Both viruses became human pathogens after zoonotic

HIV-1

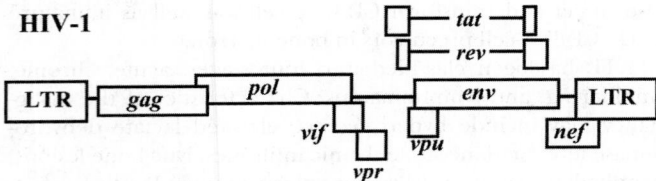

FIGURE 7.1-3. Human immunodeficiency virus type 1 (HIV-1) genome. Overall genomic organization of HIV is the same as for the simpler retroviruses, with *gag*, *pol*, and *env* genes flanked on each end by long terminal repeats (LTRs). HIV also encodes other proteins involved in the viral replication cycle.

transmission to humans from primate reservoirs. Although HIV-2 can also cause AIDS in humans and monkeys, the majority of AIDS cases worldwide are the result of HIV-1 infection. Therefore, this discussion focuses on HIV-1 disease.

As with HTLV-1, the HIV genome (Fig. 7.1-3) and replication cycle are complex.[32,33] In sharp contrast to HTLV-1, however, HIV replicates actively after initial infection, which results in high levels of viremia. The high rate of viral replication, combined with a high mutation rate due to lack of proofreading ability of reverse transcriptase during reverse transcription, results in the extreme genetic variability that has been documented for HIV-1. This genetic variability occurs within individual patients (resulting in formation of quasispecies from which drug-resistant mutants are easily selected) and among patients. In addition, HIV, unlike HTLV-1, is highly cytopathic for CD4-positive T cells.

HIV encodes two *trans*-acting proteins, Tat and Rev, analogous in function to the HTLV-1 proteins Tax and Rex. Like HTLV-1 Tax, HIV Tat is necessary for efficient expression from the viral promoter in the 5' LTR. At a molecular level, however, Tat and Tax act through different mechanisms. Instead of interacting indirectly with a region of the proviral LTR via interactions with cellular transcription factors, Tat interacts directly with a 5' LTR region of HIV RNA known as the *trans*-activating region (TAR) and promotes processive transcription through further interactions with cellular factors that modify RNA polymerase II function.

HTLV Rex and HIV Rev use similar mechanisms to promote expression of viral structural and enzymatic proteins, binding to their respective RNA response elements, *rxre* and *rre*, to mediate the export of full-length and singly spliced viral transcripts from the nucleus to the cytoplasm. In addition to Tat and Rev, HIV-1 encodes a number of accessory proteins not found in other retroviruses. These include Vif, Vpu, and Nef, the functions of which are not yet fully elucidated. The protein Vpr contributes to the ability of HIV to infect nondividing cells, a property unique to lentiviruses. Although none of the accessory genes are absolutely necessary for generating infectious virions *in vitro*, they may contribute to transmissibility, viral burden, and pathogenicity *in vivo*.

The immunodeficiency resulting from HIV infection can contribute to the development of malignancies.[34,35] However, there has been little evidence to suggest that HIV is directly oncogenic. Although HIV infection may contribute to the pathogenesis or complicate the treatment of neoplastic diseases, no viral protein has been shown to be directly transforming. Transduction of cellular oncogenes has not been observed. Despite rare reports of insertional mutagenesis resulting in T-cell lymphoma, this disease does not occur disproportionately in HIV-infected individuals. Given the high level of sustained viral replication, one might expect that insertional activation of oncogenes or disruption of tumor suppressor genes and resultant oncogenesis might be observed more frequently; however, it is possible that the limited cell tropism of HIV and the cytopathic effects of the virus may limit or mask the frequency at which insertional mutagenesis occurs.

In HIV-infected persons, non-Hodgkin's lymphoma (NHL; Burkitt's, immunoblastic, and primary CNS types), Kaposi's sarcoma (KS), and cervical cancer are all AIDS-defining illnesses. In addition, anal squamous cell carcinoma is commonly seen in AIDS patients. Many of the neoplasms common to AIDS patients are associated with infection by DNA viruses. These viruses include KS-associated herpesvirus/human herpesvirus-8 (KSHV/HHV-8), Epstein-Barr virus (EBV), and human papillomavirus. These viruses and their associations with oncogenesis are discussed in detail in section 7.2 (DNA Viruses) and elsewhere in this book and are mentioned only briefly here.

Four epidemiologic patterns of KS appear to exist. The classic form occurs in elderly men of Mediterranean background. A second form exists in sections of equatorial Africa. KS associated with these epidemiologic groups is not associated with apparent immune deficiency. A third group at risk for development of KS consists of immunosuppressed organ transplant recipients. AIDS patients make up the last group in which KS has been identified. In fact, a high incidence of KS in young men was one of the first epidemiologic clues signaling the onset of the AIDS epidemic. Although evidence supports KSHV/HHV-8 as an etiologic agent of KS, HIV is clearly an important cofactor in the development of AIDS-associated KS.

The tumor biology of KS is complex and not completely understood. Unlike most tumors that have readily identifiable neoplastic cells, KS tumors are histologically complex. The predominant cell and the most likely candidate tumor cell of KS is the spindle cell, but other cells, including infiltrating leukocytes, are present in the tumor. It is unclear how much of the tumor is made up of true neoplastic versus hyperplastic, secondary inflammatory, or angiogenic cells. A polyclonal, multicentric proliferative process seems to occur, which is reflected in the frequently observed waxing and waning clinical course of KS. For example, lesions may disappear in one region only to be supplanted by new lesions elsewhere.

In addition to the immunodeficiency caused by HIV infection, Tat and dysregulation of cytokines appear to be involved in the pathogenesis of KS.[36] Tat is secreted from HIV-infected cells and can promote growth of endothelial spindle cells, at least in part by affecting extracellular matrix proteins and matrix metalloproteinases. Tat can directly or indirectly increase the levels of a variety of cytokines and angiogenic substances, including interferon-γ, tumor necrosis factor-α, IL-1, IL-6, basic fibroblast growth factor (bFGF), vascular endothelial growth factor (VEGF), and platelet-derived growth factor (PDGF). These factors may promote growth of endothelial cells and further production of angiogenic substances by acting in either an autocrine or paracrine manner. In addition to its activity within HIV-infected cells, Tat protein that is released from HIV-infected cells can be taken up by other cells, thereby widening its potential effects. It appears that a complex interplay between HIV, the cytokines induced by HIV infection, and KSHV/HHV-8 (which encodes the viral protein vIL-6, an IL-6 homologue) provides the microenvironment and stimulus for KS development.[37,38]

AIDS patients are also at increased risk for the development of NHLs, including Burkitt's or Burkitt's-like, immunoblastic, and primary CNS types. The majority of these lymphomas are of B-cell origin, and many, but not all, are associated with EBV infection. In general, these malignancies carry a poor prognosis. Primary CNS lymphoma is rare in the general population. Unlike the systemic lymphomas, primary CNS NHL is nearly universally associated with EBV infection. In this respect it is similar to the posttransplant lymphoproliferative disorder seen in immunosuppressed organ transplant recipients. Another form of systemic NHL, primary effusion lymphoma, has been associated with infection by HHV-8; coinfection of cells with EBV also has been observed. Multicentric Castleman's disease also is associated with HHV-8 infection. The role that HIV itself might play in the genesis of the AIDS-associated lymphoproliferative disorders is not clear. In addition to the immunosuppression caused by T-cell depletion, it has been theorized that HIV may contribute to lymphomagenesis via dysregulation of cytokine production and subsequent alteration of B-cell growth regulation.[39]

Cervical carcinoma and anal squamous cell carcinoma are two other malignancies seen in AIDS patients; both are associated with human papillomavirus infection. These malignancies may present in a more advanced or invasive form than in non-HIV–infected patients. Immune suppression may support development of and can complicate treatment of these tumors, but at this time there is no evidence that HIV plays a more direct role in their genesis.

HEPATITIS C VIRUS

HCV infection is a well-established risk factor for the development of hepatocellular carcinoma (HCC).[40,41] However, its major role in oncogenesis is likely to be indirect. HCV belongs to the *Hepacivirus* genus of the *Flaviviridae* family of viruses. Virions consist of a single-stranded plus-sense RNA molecule surrounded by a nucleocapsid and envelope. The viral genome (Fig. 7.1-4) has a single, large ORF encoding viral proteins.[42] The 5' leader sequence of the viral genome is highly conserved among HCV isolates and contains stem-loop structures, one of

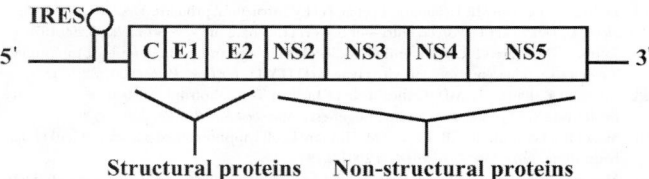

FIGURE 7.1-4. Hepatitis C virus (HCV) genome. The HCV genome consists of 5' and 3' untranslated regions and a single open reading frame encoding a protein precursor that is proteolytically processed into individual viral structural and enzymatic proteins. Structural proteins include the nucleocapsid (C) and envelope proteins (E1, E2). The metalloprotease (NS2) and serine protease (NS3) perform most of the proteolytic processing of the polyprotein precursor. NS5 encodes the RNA-dependent RNA polymerase. Major protein domains are shown; further proteolytic processing also takes place. The 5' untranslated region contains an internal ribosome binding site (IRES) that allows translation of the uncapped viral RNA.

which acts as an internal ribosome entry site. HCV encodes a polyprotein precursor that is proteolytically processed into viral structural and enzymatic proteins: the capsid (C) protein, envelope (E1, E2) glycoproteins, a metalloprotease (NS2), a serine protease and helicase (both encoded by NS3), and the RNA-dependent RNA polymerase (NS5B) responsible for viral nucleic acid replication. Additional proteins and peptides, some of whose functions are not known, also are encoded by the ORF. The extreme 3' end of the RNA genome contains a short untranslated region (composed of the VR, polyU/UC, and 3'X segments) important for viral nucleic acid replication.[43]

After entry into cells, the viral genome is replicated by the viral-encoded RNA-dependent RNA polymerase via a minus-strand RNA intermediate; unlike the case with retroviruses, there is no DNA intermediate in the replication cycle.[44,45] Plus-strand viral RNA molecules lack the usual CAP modification at the 5' end of mRNAs and are translated into a single polyprotein, using the internal ribosome entry site to initiate translation. The polyprotein produced is processed to yield all HCV enzymatic and structural proteins. Genomic RNA and structural proteins associate to form progeny virus particles, which are released from cells, most likely through the endoplasmic reticulum and host cell secretory pathways.

HCV is transmitted percutaneously in the majority of cases.[46] Before 1989, when screening for HCV began, use of contaminated blood products accounted for a significant fraction of new infections; spread via contaminated needles used by intravenous drug users continues to be a major problem. The virus also can be transmitted perinatally and via sexual routes; in approximately 10% of cases, known risk factors for transmission are not identified. It is estimated that about three million people in the United States are chronically infected with HCV.

HCV infection is strongly associated with the development of hepatic cirrhosis and HCC, although the regional prevalence of HCV infection in HCC varies. In Italy, Spain, and Japan, approximately 50% to 70% of HCC cases are associated with HCV infection, compared to only about 30% in the United States. Not all individuals infected with HCV go on to develop HCC (or, for that matter, cirrhosis). After initial infection by HCV, approximately 25% of people develop acute clinical hepatitis, whereas others are asymptomatic. HCV infection is chronic in 50% to 80% of cases. Of these patients, 60% to 70% will develop chronic hepatitis, with approximately 20% of this group progressing to cirrhosis. The estimated proportion of individuals chronically infected with HCV in whom HCC develops is estimated to be 1% to 5%. The rate of HCC development in those with cirrhosis is estimated to be 1% to 4% per year. Given the number of people infected with HCV (estimated to be approximately 170 million worldwide), such a percentage accounts for a large number of HCC cases per year. However, an individual patient's risk for progression to HCC development is difficult to assess, because additional factors may affect the likelihood of HCC development. For example, alcohol consumption or coinfection with hepatitis B virus greatly increases the relative risk for development of HCC. Diabetes and obesity also have been suggested to increase the risk of HCC development, although this effect has not yet been confirmed.

The role of HCV in HCC pathogenesis is not entirely clear.[47] It is unlikely that HCV itself is directly oncogenic, that is, capable of fully transforming normal hepatocytes into neoplastic clones on its own. After initial HCV infection, there is an approximately 10- to 20-year period before development of cirrhosis and a 20- to 30-year period before development of HCC. It appears likely that HCC largely develops indirectly as a result of the cellular turnover occurring during the inflammatory responses that lead to hepatocyte destruction, regeneration, and fibrosis characteristic of cirrhosis.

It has been postulated, however, that the virus may play a more direct role in neoplastic transformation of hepatocytes. For example, results have suggested that the HCV core protein may contribute to tumor development: Mice transgenic for the core gene developed tumors histologically similar to those of early HCV-associated HCC. The core protein also has been suggested to affect expression of genes that are ultimately involved in regulation of the cell cycle via the CDK pathway and to inhibit apoptosis. Further studies are required to determine the clinical significance of these observations. In addition, infection by different strains of HCV may also pose different levels of risk for HCC development. Many groups have reported that HCV genotype 1b confers an elevated risk for development of HCC.[48] However, the observed effects were variable and not seen in all studies.

Because of the morbidity and mortality of associated cirrhosis and HCC, HCV is a major public health problem. Even though new infection rates have declined due to screening of blood donors, a large number of currently infected people are expected to progress to HCC. An effective vaccine to prevent new HCV infections is being pursued. For those infected with HCV, combined therapy with interferon-α and ribavirin, a synthetic guanosine analogue, can be effective in stably reducing viral load and improving histologic hepatic changes, with sustained response rates varying from approximately 50% to 80% (sustained response rates for genotype 1 are lower than for genotypes 2 and 3). In this subgroup of patients, the risk of HCC development may be decreased but not eliminated; it is still not clear if this treatment can decrease permanently the risk of developing HCV-associated HCC.

Even so, given that many patients do not have sustained responses to current therapy but may experience significant side effects, improved therapies for HCV infection are needed. Lack of an *in vitro* culture system has hindered study of HCV replication, but the development of a replicon system for HCV will enable more detailed investigation of viral replication and potential antiviral agents. Areas of investigation include inhibitors of the viral protease, helicase or polymerase. In addition, the possible utility of ribozymes and antisense RNA molecules targeting viral RNA is being investigated. Finally, functional genomics approaches are being used to identify essential HCV cellular cofactors that may serve as therapeutic targets.[49]

Surgical resection of tumors and liver transplantation are the only two curative therapies for HCC; therefore, early detection of HCC is important. Unfortunately, attempts at early detection of HCV-associated HCC by screening hepatic ultrasound or computed tomographic scans or by measurement of serum α-fetoprotein levels have not proved effective in reducing HCC-related mortality.[50]

In addition to infecting hepatocytes, HCV can infect hematopoietic cells, including lymphocytes and CD34-positive precursor cells. Patients infected with HCV are suggested to be at increased risk for the development of B-cell NHL. This association, however, has not been observed in all studies. The disparity could be due to variations of geographic locales and ethnicity of subjects in different studies. Furthermore, different HCV genotypes potentially could pose a greater or lesser risk for development of lymphoma, and different histologic subtypes of B-cell malignancies might have greater or lesser association with HCV infection. For example, HCV infection is associated with mixed cryoglobulinemia, a condition that has been postulated to result from chronic HCV antigen stimulation of B cells. This stimulation may contribute to a clonal B-cell expansion, predisposing patients to development of low-grade B-cell malignancies. Further studies are needed to resolve fully the potential contribution of HCV infection to the development of some subtypes of B-cell lymphoproliferative disorders.

REFERENCES

1. Blattner WA. Human retroviruses: their role in cancer. *Proc Assoc Am Physicians* 1999;111:563.
2. Klein G. Perspectives in studies of human tumor viruses. *Front Biosci* 2002;7:d268.
3. Burmeister T. Oncogenic retroviruses in animals and humans. *Rev Med Virol* 2001;11:369.
4. Kim R, Trbetskoy A, Suzuki T, et al. Genome-based identification of cancer genes by proviral tagging in mouse retrovirus-induced T-cell lymphomas. *J Virol* 2003;77:2056.
5. Buchschacher GL Jr. Introduction to retroviruses and retroviral vectors. *Somat Cell Mol Genet* 2001;26:1.
6. Goff SP. Retroviridae: the retroviruses and their replication. In: Knipe DM, Howley PM, eds. *Fundamental virology*, 4th ed. Philadelphia: Lippincott Williams & Wilkins, 2001:843.
7. Temin, HM, Mizutani S. RNA-dependent DNA polymerase in virions of RNA tumour viruses. *Nature* 1970;226:1211.
8. Trono D. Picking the right spot. *Science* 2003;300:1670.
9. Dudley JP, Mertz JA, Rajan L, et al. What retroviruses teach us about the involvement of c-Myc in leukemias and lymphomas. *Leukemia* 2002;16:1086.
10. Neil JC, Cameron ER. Retroviral insertion sites and cancer: fountain of all knowledge? *Cancer Cell* 2002;2:253.
11. Zhang J, Temin HM. Rate and mechanism of nonhomologous recombination during a single cycle of retroviral replication. *Science* 1993;259:234.
12. Hu W-S, Rhodes T, Dang Q, et al. Retroviral recombination: review of genetic analysis. *Front Biosci* 2003;8:143.
13. Hayward WS, Neel BG, Astrin SM. Activation of a cellular onc gene by promoter insertion in ALV-induced lymphoid leukosis. *Nature* 1981;290:475.
14. Nilsen TW, Maroney PA, Goodwin RG, et al. c-erbB activation in ALV-induced erythroblastosis: novel RNA processing and promoter insertion result in expression of an amino-truncated EGF receptor. *Cell* 1985;41:719.
15. Buchschacher GL Jr. Safety considerations associated with development and clinical application of lentiviral vector systems for gene transfer. *Curr Genomics* 2004;5:19.
16. *Letter from NIH Office of Biotechnology Activities to principal investigators for human gene transfer trials employing retroviral vectors.* World Wide Web URL: http://www4.od.nih.gov/oba/rac/documents1.htm, 2004.
17. Parker RC, Varmus HE, Bishop JM. Expression of v-src and chicken c-src in rat cells demonstrates qualitative differences between pp60vsrc and pp60c-src. *Cell* 1984;37:131.
18. Irby RB, Yeatman TJ. Role of Src expression and activation in human cancer. *Oncogene* 2000;19:5636.
19. Poiesz BJ, Ruscetti FW, Reitz MS, et al. Isolation of a new type C retrovirus (HTLV) in primary uncultured cells of a patient with Sézary T-cell leukemia. *Nature* 1981;294:268.
20. Le Blanc I, Grange MP, Delamarre L, et al. HTLV-1 structural proteins. *Virus Res* 2001;78:5.
21. Derse D, Heidecker G. Forced entry—or does HTLV-I have the key? *Science* 2003;299:1670.
22. Johnson JM, Harrod R, Franchini G. Molecular biology and pathogenesis of the human T-cell-leukaemia/lymphotropic virus type-1 (HTLV-1). *Int J Exp Pathol* 2001;82:135.
23. Albrecht B, Lairmore MD. Critical role of human T-lymphotropic virus type 1 accessory proteins in viral replication and pathogenesis. *Microbiol Mol Biol Rev* 2002;66:396.
24. Siegel RS, Gartenhaus RB, Kuzel TM. Human T-cell lymphotropic-I-associated leukemia/lymphoma. *Curr Treat Options Oncol* 2001;2:291.
25. Mortreux F, Gabet A-S, Wattel E. Molecular and cellular aspects of HTLV-1 associated leukemogenesis in vivo. *Leukemia* 2003;17:26.
26. Gatza ML, Watt JC, Marriott SJ. Cellular transformation by the HTLV-I tax protein, a jack-of-all-trades. *Oncogene* 2003;22:5141.
27. Takemoto S, Mulloy JC, Cereseto A, et al. Proliferation of adult T cell leukemia/lymphoma cells is associated with the constitutive activation of JAK/STAT proteins. *Proc Natl Acad Sci U S A* 1997;94:13897.
28. Neuveut C, Jeang KT. Cell cycle dysregulation by HTLV-I: role of the tax oncoprotein. *Front Biosci* 2002;7:157.
29. Jacobson S. Immunopathogenesis of human T cell lymphotropic virus type I-associated neurologic disease. *J Infect Dis* 2002;186:S187.
30. Mulloy JC, Migone T-S, Ross TM, et al. Human and simian T-cell leukemia viruses type 2 (HTLV-2 and STLV-2(pan-p)) transform T cells independently of Jak/STAT activation. *J Virol* 1998;72:4408.

31. Lewis GW, Sheremata WA, Minagar A. Epidemiologic features of HTLV-II: serologic and molecular evidence. *Ann Epidemiol* 2002;12:46.
32. Freed EO. HIV-1 replication. *Somat Cell Mol Genet* 2001;26:13.
33. Gummuluru S, Emerman M. Advances in HIV molecular biology. *AIDS* 2002;16:S17.
34. Scadden DT. AIDS-related malignancies. *Annu Rev Med* 2003;54:285.
35. Dal Maso L, Franceschi S. Epidemiology of non-Hodgkin lymphomas and haemolymphopoietic neoplasms in people with AIDS. *Lancet North Am Ed* 2003;4:110.
36. Barillari G, Ensoli B. Angiogenic effects of extracellular human immunodeficiency virus type 1 Tat protein and its role in the pathogenesis of AIDS-associated Kaposi's sarcoma. *Clin Microbiol Rev* 2002;15:310.
37. Dezube BJ. The role of human immunodeficiency virus-1 in the pathogenesis of acquired immunodeficiency syndrome-related Kaposi's sarcoma: the importance of an inflammatory and angiogenic milieu. *Semin Oncol* 2000;27:420.
38. Yen-Moore A, Hudnall SD, Rady PL, et al. Differential expression of the HHV-8 vGCR cellular homolog gene in AIDS-associated and classic Kaposi's sarcoma: potential role of HIV-1 Tat. *Virology* 2000;267:247.
39. Martinez-Maza O, Breen EC. B-cell activation and lymphoma in patients with HIV. *Curr Opin Oncol* 2002;14:528.
40. El-Serag HB. Hepatocellular carcinoma and hepatitis C in the United States. *Hepatology* 2002;36:S74.
41. Flamm SL. Chronic hepatitis C virus infection. *JAMA* 2003;289:2413.
42. Rosenberg S. Recent advances in the molecular biology of hepatitis C virus. *J Mol Biol* 2001;313:451.
43. Yi M, Lemon SM. 3' Untranslated RNA signals required for replication of hepatitis C virus RNA. *J Virol* 2003;77:3557.
44. Bartenschlager R, Lohmann V. Replication of hepatitis C virus. *J Gen Virol* 2000;81:1631.
45. Moradpour D, Brass V, Gosert R, et al. Hepatitis C: molecular virology and antiviral targets. *Trends Mol Med* 2002;8:476.
46. Centers for Disease Control and Prevention. Recommendations for prevention and control of hepatitis C (HCV) infection and HCV-related chronic disease. *MMWR Morb Mortal Wkly Rep* 1998;47:1.
47. Koike K, Tsutsumi T, Fujie H, et al. Molecular mechanism of viral hepatocarcinogenesis. *Oncology* 2002;62:S29.
48. Reid AE, Koziel MJ, Aiza I, et al. Hepatitis C virus genotypes and viremia and hepatocellular carcinoma in the United States. *Am J Gastroenterol* 1999;94:1619.
49. Tang H, Peng T, Wong-Staal, F. Novel technologies for studying virus-host interaction and discovering new drug targets for HCV and HIV. *Curr Opin Pharmacol* 2002;2:541.
50. Gebo KA, Chandler G, Jenckes MW, et al. Screening tests for hepatocellular carcinoma in patients with chronic hepatitis C: a systematic review. *Hepatology* 2002;36:S84.

SECTION **2**

PETER M. HOWLEY
DON GANEM
ELLIOT KIEFF

DNA Viruses

Viral oncology has its foundations in scientific observations made at the turn of the last century defining the transmissibility of avian leukemia in Denmark in 1908 and of an avian sarcoma in chickens in 1911. These important discoveries were not appreciated at the time and their impact on virology and medicine was not recognized for decades. The importance of the work of Peyton Rous[1] showing that cell-free extracts from sarcoma in chickens could, within a few weeks, induce tumors in chickens injected with the extracts even when passed through filters that retained bacteria was recognized by a Nobel prize in 1968. Rous's original work pointed out that this infectious agent was not only capable of inducing tumors but also imprinted the phenotypic characteristics of the original tumor on the recipient cell. This early work, however, was at the time relegated to the rank of avian curiosities, and its importance was not recognized for several decades.

In the 1930s Richard Shope published a series of papers demonstrating cell-free transmission of tumors in rabbits. The first studies involved fibromatous tumors found in the footpads of wild cottontail rabbits that could be transmitted by injecting cell-free extracts into either wild or domestic rabbits. Subsequent studies have shown that this virus, now referred to as the Shope fibroma virus, is a poxvirus. Additional studies carried out by Shope demonstrated that cutaneous papillomatosis in wild cottontail rabbits could also be transmitted by cell-free extracts. In a number of cases, these benign papillomas progressed spontaneously into squamous cell carcinomas in infected domestic rabbits or in the infected cottontail rabbits.[2,3]

In general, however, the field of viral oncology lay dormant until the early 1950s with the discovery of the murine leukemia viruses by Ludwig Gross and of the mouse polyomavirus by Gross, Sarah Stewart, and Bernice Eddy. These findings of tumor viruses in mice led many cancer researchers and virolo-

gists to the field of viral oncology. These researchers had the hope that these initial observations in mammals could be extended to humans and that a fair proportion of human tumors might also be found to have a viral etiology. The Special Viral Cancer Program at the National Cancer Institute grew from this intense interest in viral oncology and the hope that human tumor viruses would be identified.

The year 1964, when Tony Epstein and colleagues demonstrated herpesvirus-like particles in human lymphoblasts derived from Burkitt's lymphoma (BL), marks the starting point of active research in human cancer viruses. During the 1970s evidence accumulated for a role for hepatitis B virus (HBV) in primary hepatocellular carcinoma (HCC) in humans. Molecular biologic analyses, however, revealed that only a portion of HCCs contained HBV nucleic acids, and subsequent studies have shown a role for hepatitis C virus in many of these HCCs. In the 1970s specific human papillomaviruses (HPVs) were linked by Orth and Jablonska to skin cancers in patients with a rare skin disease called *epidermodysplasia verruciformis* (EV). In 1980, human T-cell leukemia virus type 1 was isolated by the Gallo group and subsequently linked to adult T-cell leukemia. In the mid-1980s specific HPVs were identified in human cervical cancers by zur Hausen and his colleagues. In the 1990s, a new herpesvirus was linked to Kaposi's sarcoma [KS; KS-associated herpesvirus (KSHV), also known as *human herpesvirus-8* (HHV-8)]. The details surrounding these discoveries are discussed in this chapter.

Because of the important role of retroviruses in murine tumors, much of the initial focus of the Special Viral Cancer Program at the National Cancer Institute was on the identification of human retroviruses in human cancers. However, with the exception of human T-cell leukemia virus type 1, no other retroviruses have been directly linked as causative agents for human cancers. The human immunodeficiency virus (HIV), however, is an important cofactor in many human cancers, in part by causing immunosuppression. General characteristics that have emerged for many human cancer viruses are the following: (1) the viruses that have been implicated in human carcinogenesis are frequently ubiquitous [e.g., Epstein-Barr virus (EBV), HPV, hepatitis viruses]; (2) cancer is a rare outcome of virus infection, and only a small percentage of infected individ-

TABLE 7.2-1. Human Viruses with Oncogenic Properties

Virus Family	Type	Human Tumor	Cofactors
Adenoviruses	Types 2, 5, 12	None	—
Flaviviruses	HCV	Hepatocellular carcinoma	—
Hepadnavirus	HBV	Hepatocellular carcinoma	Aflatoxin, alcohol, smoking
Herpesviruses	EBV	Burkitt's lymphoma	Malaria
		Immunoblastic lymphoma	Immunodeficiency
		Nasopharyngeal carcinoma	Nitrosamines, HLA genotype
		Hodgkin's disease	—
		Leiomyosarcomas	—
		Gastric cancers	—
	HHV-8	Kaposi's sarcoma	HIV infection
		Body cavity–based lymphoma	HIV infection
		Castleman's disease	HIV infection
Papillomaviruses	HPV-16, -18, -33, -39	Anogenital cancers and some upper airway cancers	Smoking, ? other factors
	HPV-5, -8, -17	Skin cancer	EV, sunlight, immune suppression
Polyomaviruses	SV40, JC, BK	? Brain tumors	—
		? Insulinomas	—
		? Mesotheliomas	—
Retroviruses	HTLV-I	Adult T-cell leukemia/lymphoma	Uncertain
	HTLV-II	Hairy cell leukemia	Unknown

EBV, Epstein-Barr virus; EV, epidermodysplasia verruciformis; HBV, hepatitis B virus; HCV, hepatitis C virus; HHV, human herpesvirus; HIV, human immunodeficiency virus; HPV, human papillomavirus; HTLV, human T-cell leukemia virus; SV40, simian vacuolating virus 40.

uals develop cancer; (3) the time interval between the initial infection and cancer development is long (usually decades); (4) the cancers are usually clonal; and (5) chemical or physical agents have been implicated as playing cofactor roles.

Furthermore, many of the most important developments in modern molecular biology derive from studies in viral oncology done in the 1960s and 1970s. The discovery of reverse transcriptase, the development of recombinant DNA technology, the discovery of messenger RNA splicing, and the discovery of oncogenes and later tumor suppressor genes were all developments that derive directly from studies in viral oncology. Oncogenes were first recognized as cellular genes that had been acquired by retroviruses through recombinational processes to convert them into acute transforming RNA tumor viruses. It is now recognized that oncogenes participate in many different types of tumor and can be involved at different stages of tumorigenesis and viral oncology. This has contributed significantly to the concepts of nonviral carcinogenesis. It is likely that the direct transforming, oncogene-transducing retroviruses do not play a major causative role in naturally occurring cancers in animals or in humans, but rather represent laboratory-generated recombinants. A list of human viruses with oncogenic properties is presented in Table 7.2-1. This list includes viruses such as the transforming adenoviruses that are capable of transforming normal cells into malignant cells in the laboratory but that have not been associated with any known human tumors. The list also includes viruses such as the papillomaviruses that have been etiologically associated with specific human cancers and that have been shown to encode transforming viral oncogenes. Finally, it includes viruses such as HBV and hepatitis C virus that have been closely linked with a specific human tumor, HCC, for which the evidence of a bona fide viral oncogene is still unclear. This chapter focuses primarily on the DNA viruses that have been associated with specific human cancers and discusses the biology and pertinent molec-

ular biology of these viruses. Chapter 7.1 deals with the RNA viruses and in particular the human retroviruses. The evidence pertaining to the association of each of these viruses with specific types of human neoplasia is presented, and the mechanisms by which these viruses may contribute to malignant transformation are discussed.

HEPADNAVIRUSES AND HEPATOCELLULAR CARCINOMA

HCC is one of the world's most common malignancies. Although rare in the West, the disease is highly prevalent in Southeast Asia and sub-Saharan Africa. In the 1970s, this distribution was recognized to mirror the distribution of chronic HBV infection. This fact, and the long-recognized histopathologic association between HCC and chronic hepatitis in the surrounding nontumorous liver, led to the strong presumption that chronic HBV infection predisposes to hepatic cancer. This presumption has been strikingly validated in large prospective epidemiologic studies in Taiwan, in which chronically infected individuals were followed for deaths due to this tumor.[4] These studies showed that chronic HBV infection is associated with a 100-fold increase in HCC risk over that of controls who are not chronically infected.

HBV is a small DNA virus classified as a member of the hepadnavirus family (for *hepatotropic DNA viruses*). HBV is the only human virus in this family, which also includes related viruses of woodchucks (woodchuck hepatitis virus, or WHV), ground squirrels (ground squirrel hepatitis virus), and ducks (duck HBV). Primary HBV infection produces either a subclinical infection or acute liver injury, but irrespective of their clinical manifestations 95% of such infections resolve, with clearance of virus from liver and blood and the induction of lasting immunity to re-infection.[5] However, 5% of patients go on to have persistent (usually lifelong) hepatic infection and viremia, and most of the demonstrated HCC risk falls within this subgroup of infected individuals. In fact, patients with the highest levels of HBV viremia display the highest HCC risk.[6]

Another factor that adds to risk is the severity of chronic liver injury: Asymptomatic carriers have lower HCC risk than those with chronic active hepatitis or cirrhosis. In chronic hepatitis B, hepatocyte injury is due to host immune responses triggered by recognition of viral antigens presented on the surface of infected cells.[5,7] The induction of hepatocellular injury is thought to be important in HCC pathogenesis because it triggers in the liver a stereotyped proliferative response. Such proliferation increases opportunities for replicative errors (mutations) that over time can contribute to the loss of normal cellular growth control; cells harboring such mutations have a selective advantage that further perpetuates this cycle. In this conceptualization, HBV serves indirectly as an agent of oncogenesis, chiefly by provoking cellular proliferation in response to immune-mediated injury; no direct genetic contribution is made by viral sequences acting in *cis* or viral gene products acting in *trans*. This view accords well with the fact that HCC risk is increased in every condition that provokes chronic liver injury and regeneration—including diseases as diverse as alcoholism, α_1-antitrypsin deficiency, Wilson's disease, and HCV infection.

Despite strong experimental support for the pathogenetic scheme described, there is reason to believe that hepadnaviruses may also make a more direct genetic contribution to HCC. Phylogenetic analyses of hepadnaviral genome organization reveal that the structure of the oncogenic mammalian viruses differs from that of the nononcogenic avian viruses in an important way: The mammalian viruses all harbor an additional coding region, termed *ORF X* (for *open reading frame X*; Fig. 7.2-1). This gene encodes a small regulatory protein (HBx) implicated in signal transduction and transcriptional activation. This open reading frame is absent in the avian viruses, which fail to induce HCC in their native hosts despite the regular induction of persistent infection. Interestingly, in several lines of transgenic mice displaying constitutive hepatic expression of HBx, HCC arises with increased frequency.[8] Tumors in such mice do not begin until midlife, which suggests that additional genetic changes are necessary for loss of normal growth control. In addition, in many HBV-related HCCs, the HBx coding region is deleted or inactivated in the retained HBV DNA. Thus, if HBx expression is important in carcinogenesis *in vivo*, it must be involved at early stages and become dispensable during later tumor progression.

Another class of more direct genetic contributions that HBV might make to HCC derives from the existence of integrated copies of viral DNA in the tumor cells. Unlike retroviruses, hepadnaviruses do not specify genetic functions directing genomic integration, and such integration is not essential for HBV replication. In fact, because every nucleotide of the viral genome is in a coding region, integration of HBV DNA generally disrupts essential genes and is incompatible with replication. Yet, most hepatoma cells arising in HBV-infected patients harbor multiple integrated HBV genomes, and in general active viral replication has been extinguished. The tumors are clonal with respect to these viral insertions: All cells of the tumor bear the same pattern of integrants, which indicates that integration preceded or accompanied the final transforming event. But close inspection of these integrants indicates that they are usually highly rearranged, with multiple deletions, inversions, reduplications, or

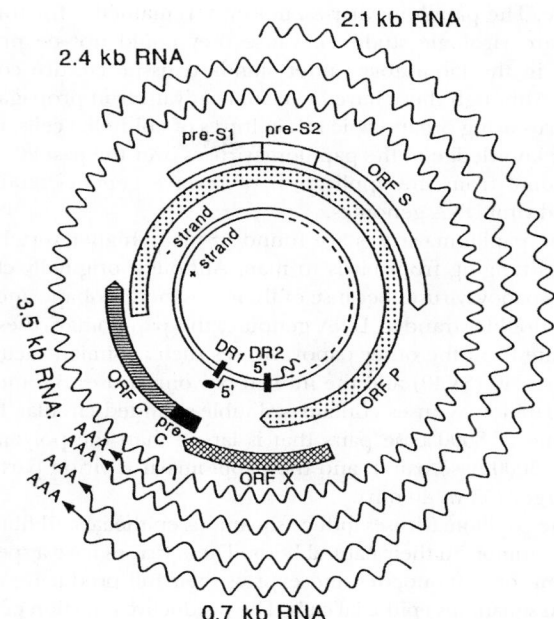

FIGURE 7.2-1. Genomic and transcriptional organization of the human hepatitis B virus. The inner circle represents the partially double-stranded virion DNA, with dashes specifying the single-stranded genomic region. The locations of the direct repeat (DR1 and DR2) regions are indicated. The boxed arcs specify the viral coding regions, and the arrows indicate the direction of translation. The outermost wavy lines depict the viral RNAs identified in infected cells with the arrows indicating the direction of transcription and the AAAs indicating the polyadenylated 3' tails. ORF, open reading frame.

other mutations typically present.[9] Although individual integrants may retain certain coding functions, no one viral coding region is invariably preserved, as are E6 and E7 of the HPVs.

These facts have led to interest in the model that the viral sequences might be contributing *cis*-acting regulatory signals rather than *trans*-acting proteins to the host cell. Strong evidence that hepadnaviruses can mediate such activation events in *cis* has been proffered for WHV. WHV is strikingly oncogenic in its native host: Virtually 100% of woodchucks chronically infected from birth develop HCC.[10] As in HBV-induced cancer, the tumors display multiple viral insertions, often highly rearranged, and in a clonal pattern. But here, remarkably, the vast majority of tumors can be shown to harbor at least one viral insertion in *cis* to the protooncogene N-myc2.[11] This gene, normally silent in adult liver, is strongly up-regulated by this insertion, and this activation can be seen early in the oncogenic sequence, even in premalignant lesions. Clearly, insertional activation of N-myc plays a major role in WHV oncogenesis. However, similar efforts to identify common integration sites for integrated HBV genomes in human HCC have not met with comparable success. It is well to remember that, despite its many similarities to HBV, WHV differs strikingly in its oncogenic potency; it is possible that insertional activation of N-myc loci is responsible for this difference.

PAPILLOMAVIRUSES AND HUMAN CANCER

The viral nature of human warts was first demonstrated at the turn of the last century by transmission studies using a cell-free filtrate. The papillomaviruses, however, remained refractory to standard virologic studies because they could not be propagated in the laboratory under standard tissue culture conditions. Although there have been some advances in propagating the virus using organotypic raft cultures of epithelial cells, most of the knowledge of the papillomaviruses over the past 20 years has come from the application of reverse genetics studying cloned viral DNA genomes.

The papillomaviruses are found in many higher vertebrate species ranging from birds to man. Although originally classified as papovaviruses because of their icosahedral shape and circular, double-stranded DNA genome, the papillomaviruses are separate from the other papovaviruses such as simian vacuolating virus 40 (SV40) and the human polyomaviruses BK and JC. The papillomaviruses contain a double-stranded circular DNA genome of 8000 base pairs that is larger than the polyomaviruses (5000 base pairs), and the papillomavirus virion particles are larger (55 vs. 40 nm).

The papillomaviruses induce squamous epithelial and fibroepithelial tumors in their natural hosts. These viruses have a specific tropism for keratinocytes and express their full productive cycle only in squamous epithelial cells. The productive infection of cells by papillomaviruses is divided into stages, and these stages are linked to the differentiation state of the epithelial cell. In the squamous epithelium, the basal cell is the only cell normally capable of supporting cellular DNA synthesis and undergoing cellular division. The virus must therefore infect the basal cell to induce a lesion that can persist. *In situ* hybridization experiments have demonstrated that the papillomavirus DNA is indeed present within the basal cells of a papilloma. As the cells of an HPV-infected lesion migrate upward through the epithelium into the granular layer, they undergo a program of differentiation. The control of papillomavirus late gene expression is tightly linked to the differentiation state of the squamous epithelial cells. Vegetative viral DNA synthesis and expression of the capsid proteins occur only in the most terminally differentiated epithelial cells.[12]

Over 140 different HPV types have now been recognized, and each of them is associated with specific clinical lesions.[13] All HPV types have a similar genomic organization. The DNA genomes of each of the HPVs sequenced as well as the other animal papillomaviruses are approximately 8000 base pairs in size. All of the open reading frames that could serve to encode proteins for these viruses are located on only one of the two viral DNA strands. RNA studies have indicated that only one strand is transcribed. A more detailed description of the molecular biology of the papillomaviruses can be found in the fourth edition of *Fields' Virology*.[12]

The HPV genome can be divided into two distinct regions: an "early" region, which encodes the viral proteins involved in viral DNA replication, transcriptional regulation, and cellular transformation, and a "late" region, which encodes the viral capsid proteins. The genomic map of HPV-16 is shown in Figure 7.2-2. The genes located in the early region are designated as E1, E2, and so on, and the two genes located in the late region encoding the capsid proteins are designated L1 and L2. From studies of the HPVs, it is likely that E4 encodes a late gene that is expressed only in productively infected keratinocytes. Thus, although this gene is located within the early region, its function may be important only in the vegetative replication of the virus. A listing of the functions assigned to the HPV-16 open reading frames is provided in Table 7.2-2.

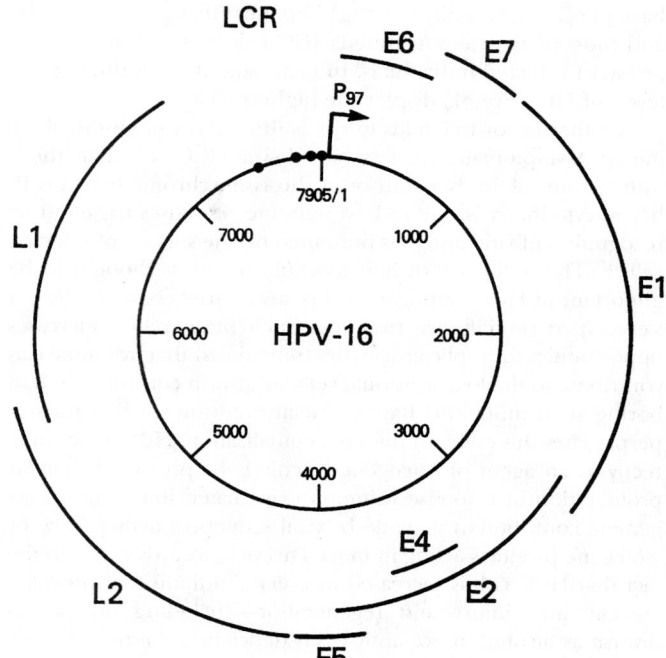

FIGURE 7.2-2. The genomic map of human papillomavirus-16 (HPV-16) deduced from the DNA sequence. The nucleotide numbers are noted within the circular maps, transcription proceeds clockwise, and the major open reading frames (E1 to E7, L1, and L2) are indicated. The only transcriptional promoter mapped to data for HPV-16 is designated P_{97}. The viral long control region (LCR) containing the putative viral transcriptional and replication regulatory elements is noted. The closed circles on the genome represent the four E2 binding sites that have been noted in the LCR.

Much of the understanding of the molecular biology of papillomaviruses derives from studies with bovine papillomavirus-1 (BPV-1), which is capable of transforming a variety of rodent fibroblast cell lines in tissue culture. In these transformed cells, the DNA remains as a stable extrachromosomal plasmid, and this system has served as an excellent model for studying latent infection by papillomavirus. BPV-1 has served as the prototype

TABLE 7.2-2.   Human Papillomavirus-16 Gene Functions

Open Reading Frame	Function
L1	L1 protein, major capsid protein
L2	L2 protein, minor capsid protein
E1	Initiation of viral DNA replication, helicase, adenosine triphosphatase
E2	Transcriptional regulatory protein, auxiliary role in viral DNA replication, genome maintenance
E4	Late protein; disrupts cytokeratins
E5	Membrane transforming protein; interacts with growth factor receptors
E6	Transforming protein of human papillomaviruses (HPVs); targets degradation of p53; activates telomerase
E7	Transforming protein of HPVs; binds to the retinoblastoma protein, affects centrosome duplication

for unraveling important aspects of the biology of the papillomaviruses over the past 20 years. Two independent transforming activities have been mapped in BPV-1: one to the E5 gene and the other to the E6 and E7 genes. Transformation by the BPV-1 E5 oncoprotein appears to be mediated through the activation by binding of the platelet-derived growth factor-β receptor.[14] The mechanisms by which the E6 and E7 genes of BPV-1 transform cells have not yet been as well elucidated. It is noteworthy, however, that unlike their HPV-16 counterparts, the BPV-1 E6 and E7 proteins do not directly bind the p53 and retinoblastoma (RB) tumor suppressor gene proteins (as discussed later).

The functions of the papillomavirus E1 and E2 genes appear to be highly conserved among different papillomaviruses, and much of what is known about these genes derives from BPV-1.[12] The papillomavirus E2 gene has roles in the regulation of viral transcription, enhancing the activity of E1 in viral DNA replication and in ensuring the maintenance of the viral genome in persistently infected cells. E2 is a DNA-binding protein and can function as a transcriptional activator or a transcriptional repressor depending on the context of its cognate sites in the promoter. In addition, E2 has a direct role in viral DNA replication. E2 forms a complex with the viral E1 protein to direct replication origin binding by E1 and to enhance E1-dependent replication. The E1 gene encodes a protein necessary for initiating viral DNA replication. E1 has DNA-binding, DNA helicase, and adenosine triphosphatase activities and binds components of the host cell replication machinery for recruitment to the viral DNA. Papillomaviruses do not encode a viral DNA polymerase and are dependent on the host cell replication machinery to replicate the viral genomes. L1 encodes the major caption protein and L2 encodes a minor caption protein. The L1 and L2 genes are expressed only in the terminally differentiated keratinocytes of a productively infected lesion.

Because of their association with human cervical cancer, studies on the mechanisms of transformation have extensively focused on HPV-16 and HPV-18. Although the genomic organization of the HPVs is quite similar to that of BPV-1, there appear to be important differences in the mechanisms by which they transform cells. The principal transforming genes for the cancer-associated HPVs have been mapped to E6 and E7.[15] E7 is by itself sufficient for the transformation of primary rodent cells. E7 is also capable of cooperating with an activated ras oncogene to transform primary rodent cells. Expression of E6 and E7 together is sufficient for the efficient immortalization of primary human cells, most notably primary human keratinocytes, which are the normal host cell for the HPVs. Cellular targets for the HPV E6 and E7 proteins have been identified, as discussed later (see Fig. 7.2-3). HPV E5 may also have transforming activities, but it has not been as well studied as BPV E5 and does not appear to function through interaction with the platelet-derived growth factor-β receptor.

Only a subset of the papillomaviruses associated with lesions may progress to cancer. This is true for the HPVs as well as papillomaviruses in other animal species. The Shope papillomavirus (CRPV) that infects cottontail rabbits in nature was the first papillomavirus to be identified and is the etiologic agent of cutaneous papillomatosis in rabbits. CRPV has also been extensively studied as a model for papillomavirus-induced carcinogenesis. One of the features of carcinogenic progression with the papillomaviruses is the synergy between the virus and car-

cinogenic external factors. For instance, in the case of CRPV, carcinomas develop at an increased frequency in virus-induced papillomas that are painted with cool tar or methylcholanthrene.[16,17] CRPV-associated carcinomas contain viral DNA that is transcriptionally active, an observation which supports the hypothesis that these viruses play an active role in the cancers that develop.

Other animal papillomaviruses have also been associated with naturally occurring cancers. Of note is BPV-4, which has been associated with esophageal papillomatosis in cattle and is also associated with squamous cell carcinomas of the upper alimentary tract. Interestingly, however, only those cattle from the highlands of Scotland that are infected with BPV-4 and that also feed on bracken fern (which is known to contain a radiomimetic substance) have a high incidence of squamous cell carcinomas of the esophagus and of the foregut. In contrast to the CRPV-associated carcinomas, in which the viral DNA can invariably be found, extensive analysis of the squamous cell carcinomas of the upper alimentary tract in cattle infected with BPV-4 have failed to reveal a consistent pattern of viral DNA sequences within the malignant tumors. In the case of these alimentary tract tumors, it is possible that the continued presence of BPV-4 DNA sequences is not required for the maintenance of the cancer.[18]

The first evidence that HPVs were associated with human cancer came from studies of skin cancers in patients with EV, a rare lifelong disease in humans that usually begins in infancy or childhood (reviewed in ref. 19). The disease is characterized by disseminated polymorphic cutaneous lesions that resemble flat warts and also appear as reddish macules sometimes referred to as *pityriasis-like lesions*. Approximately half of the patients with EV develop multiple skin cancers, usually during the third of fourth decades of their lives. Papillomavirus particles have been detected within the benign lesions and not in the carcinomas. More than 20 different HPV types have now been demonstrated in individual lesions in patients with this rare disease. EV is linked to a rare, recessive, abnormal allele of an X-linked gene. Patients with EV often have impaired cell-mediated immunity, which is believed to play a role in the lifelong infection by papillomaviruses. The carcinomas that develop in these patients arise in sun-exposed areas, and it is suspected that ultraviolet radiation plays a co-carcinogenic role with the papillomaviruses in the etiology of these cancers. Two genes, EVER1 and EVER2, have now been associated with the disease.[20] The gene products EVER1 and EVER2 have features of integral membrane proteins and are localized in the endoplasmic reticulum, but the mechanisms by which mutations in these genes contribute to EV have not yet been elucidated. EV is a very rare disease, yet it has been under intense study by dermatologists and virologists.

The role of HPVs in cutaneous cancers in humans may extend beyond EV patients to other patients, both immunosuppressed and immunocompetent. New HPV types have been found in squamous and basal cell carcinomas of immunosuppressed patients and in some of the same tumors in immunocompetent patients. The same HPV types that have been seen in skin cancers of patients with EV are also found in skin cancers seen in some immunosuppressed patients, such as renal transplant patients.

The major interest in HPV and cancer, however, comes from its association with cervical cancer. This cancer is one of the most common cancers among women worldwide, with approximately 500,000 newly diagnosed cases each year, which account for approximately a quarter of a million cancer deaths per year. Despite its worldwide distribution, the frequency of cervical cancer varies considerably. Cervical cancer is the most common cancer of women in most developing countries. It occurs less frequently in developed countries because of effective screening programs. In the United States, there are approximately 13,000 newly diagnosed cases annually, and approximately one-third of these women die of their malignant disease.

Epidemiologic studies long implicated an infectious agent in the etiology of human cervical carcinoma.[21] Venereal transmission of a carcinogenic factor with a long latency had been suggested by epidemiologic studies. Sexual promiscuity, an early age of onset of sexual activity, and poor sexual hygienic conditions are known risk factors for cervical carcinoma. There was also a correlation between the incidence rates of cervical cancer and penile carcinoma in different geographic areas, although the incidence rates for penile carcinoma are 20-fold lower than those of cervical carcinoma. A similar ratio of incidence between cervical carcinoma and penile carcinoma is maintained, however, in areas of high, medium, and low prevalence, which suggests that the etiologic factors for penile and cervical carcinoma may be the same. In addition, the "male factor" implicated a venereally transmitted agent: Women who are monogamous are at a higher risk for cervical carcinoma if their spouses have multiple sexual partners.

In the late 1960s and early 1970s genital infection by herpes simplex virus (HSV) type 2 was considered as a possible etiologic candidate. Support for the notion that HSV might be a cancer-associated virus came from studies demonstrating the ability of HSV to transform certain rodent cells in the laboratory *in vitro* and from serologic studies suggesting a higher frequency of antibodies to HSV-2 in patients with cervical carcinoma. However, subsequent carefully done molecular studies attempting to demonstrate HSV RNA or HSV DNA in cervical cancer tissues could not provide convincing evidence for a role for HSV in cervical cancer.[22] Subsequent prospective epidemiologic studies have also failed to support the involvement of HSV infections as the major etiologic agent in human cervical cancer.

In the mid-1970s, zur Hausen suggested an association between papillomaviruses and genital cancers.[23] The initial evidence that linked an HPV infection with cervical carcinoma came from the recognition that the morphologic changes previously interpreted on Papanicolaou smears and tissue sections of the cervix as cervical dysplasia were due to a papillomavirus infection.[24] The association of an HPV with cervical dysplasia (also referred to as *cervical intraepithelial neoplasia* or *squamous epithelial lesions*) sparked an examination of cervical cancers for HPV sequences. The natural history linking cervical intraepithelial neoplasia to carcinoma *in situ* and to invasive squamous cell carcinoma of the cervix had already been well established. Initial experiments from a number of laboratories revealed HPV sequences in occasional cases of cervical carcinoma and of anogenital carcinoma, but no consistent pattern of positivity emerged. Some initial studies focused on HPV-6 and HPV-11, which are related HPV types found in venereal warts (also known as *condyloma acuminata*). The majority of cervical carcinomas and other genital tract carcinomas, however, are negative for HPV-6 and HPV-11. Nonetheless, there are rare genital tract tumors that are positive for HPV-6 or HPV-11 in which

there is malignant conversion of condyloma acuminata into squamous cell carcinoma. These lesions are referred to as *Buschke-Löwenstein tumors* and sometimes designated as *giant condylomas.* These tumors have characteristics similar to those of a locally invasive squamous cell carcinoma.

Using radioactively labeled HPV-11 DNA under conditions of hybridization of low stringency, zur Hausen and his colleagues identified two new papillomavirus DNAs, for HPV-16 and HPV-18, in cellular DNA from human cervical cancers.[25,26] Using these HPV DNAs as probes, HPV types 16 and 18 could be demonstrated in approximately 70% of cervical carcinomas[27] and are the two HPV types associated with the majority of human cervical cancers. The use of low-stringency hybridization and polymerase chain reaction (PCR) with degenerate primers has led to the identification of approximately 25 different HPVs now associated with genital tract lesions. These additional HPV types, including HPV-31, HPV-33, HPV-39, and HPV-42, among others, are each associated with a small percentage of cervical carcinomas. A causal role for HPV infections in cervical cancer has been documented beyond reasonable doubt, and the association is present in virtually all cervical cancer cases worldwide.[28] Specific HPVs can also be found in a lower percentage of other human genital carcinomas, including penile carcinomas, vulvar carcinomas, and perianal carcinomas.

Molecular studies of cervical cancers and derived cell lines have indicated that the HPV DNA is usually integrated, although there are some cases in which DNA is apparently also extrachromosomal. In those cases in which the DNA is integrated, the pattern of integration is clonal, which indicates that the association of the HPV preceded the clonal outgrowth of the tumor. Integration of the viral DNA is not at specific sites in the host chromosome, although in some cell lines the integration event has occurred in the vicinity of known oncogenes. For instance, in the HeLa cell line (which is an HPV-18–positive cervical carcinoma cell line), the integration of the viral genome has occurred within approximately 50 kilobases of the c-myc locus on human chromosome 8. It is not known whether such an integration event provides a selective advantage to the regression of a preneoplastic lesion to a cancer; however, it seems quite plausible that in some individual cancers, the integration of the viral DNA could result in genetic changes that could contribute to carcinogenic progression.

In HPV-positive cancers there appears to be a selection for the integrity of the E6 and E7 coding region and the upstream regulatory region. Furthermore, the E6 and E7 genes are regularly expressed in HPV-positive cervical cancers. Furthermore, integration of the HPV DNA into the host chromosome in the cancers is often associated with disruption of the viral E1 or E2 genes. HPV E2 is an important viral regulatory factor that can negatively regulate the transcriptional promoter directing the E6 and E7 genes.[12] Disruption of the E2 gene by the integration event releases the viral promoter of the E6 and E7 genes from the inhibitory activity of E2, which results in the dysregulated and increased expression of E6 and E7.

The E6 and E7 proteins encoded by the high-risk HPVs are oncoproteins and contribute, at least in part, to cellular transformation by binding to the cell-regulatory proteins p53 and RB, respectively (Fig. 7.2-3). The E7 proteins encoded by the high-risk HPVs share sequence similarity to adenovirus E1A and to SV40 large T-antigen transforming proteins. In all three proteins, these regions of similarity are critical for their trans-

Polyomaviruses

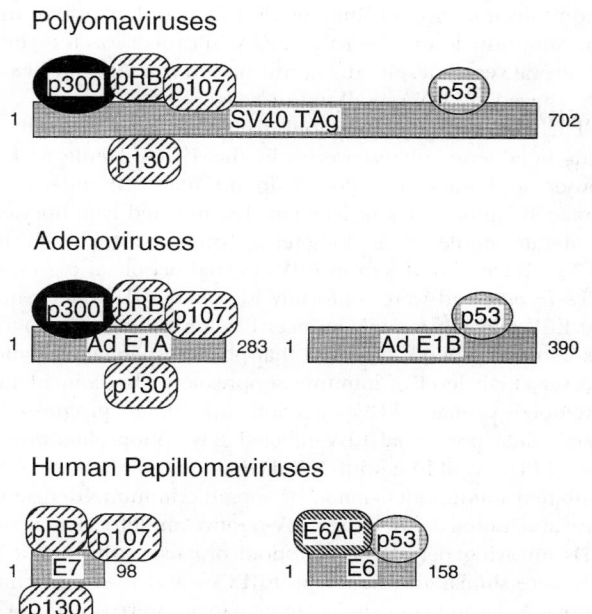

Adenoviruses

Human Papillomaviruses

FIGURE 7.2-3. The transforming proteins encoded by three distinct groups of DNA tumor viruses target similar cellular proteins. The binding of human papillomavirus E6 oncoproteins to p53 is mediated by a cellular protein called *E6-AP*. SV40, simian virus 40.

formational properties. The regions of amino acid sequence similarity between E7 and adenovirus E1A that are shared with SV40 large T antigen are regions that participate in the binding to the product of the RB tumor suppressor gene (pRB) and the related "pocket" proteins, p107 and p130.[15] One consequence of the interaction of E7 with pRB is the disruption of a complex between pRB and E2F transcription factors. The E7-mediated release of E2F from these complexes activates the expression of genes required for cell-cycle progression from G_1 into S. However, mutational analyses with E7 indicate that there must be other cellular targets of E7 and that complex formation between E7 and the pocket proteins, including pRB, is not sufficient to account for the immortalization and transforming functions of this viral oncoprotein. A number of additional cellular targets have been proposed for HPV-16 E7.[15]

HPV-16 E7 has been shown to induce abnormal centrosome duplication resulting in multipolar, abnormal mitoses and aneuploidy.[29] The mechanism by which E7 affects centrosome homeostasis is not yet known, but it is a property that is not shared by the E7 proteins of the non–cancer-associated HPV types. Abnormal centrosome duplication induced by HPV E7 rapidly results in genomic instability and aneuploidy, two of the hallmarks of a cancer cell.[30] This activity may be functionally relevant to the contribution of high-risk HPVs to malignant progression.

The transforming properties of the E6 protein were first revealed by studies using primary human cells, most importantly, the normal host cell for the HPVs, the keratinocyte. Efficient immortalization of primary human cells requires both the E6 and E7 genes of the high-risk HPVs. The ability of the E6 and E7 proteins together to extend the life span of primary human keratinocytes is a characteristic of the high-risk HPVs, but not of the low-risk HPVs.[12] Like SV40 large T antigen and

the 55-kD protein encoded by adenovirus E1B, the E6 proteins of the high-risk HPVs can enter into a complex with the tumor suppressor protein p53, and it can promote the degradation of p53 *in vitro*. The interaction of E6 with p53 is mediated by a cellular protein, called the E6-associated protein (E6AP), which promotes the ubiquitination of p53, leading to its proteolysis. E6 has other activities. It has immortalization and transformation properties that cannot be fully explained through its interaction with p53.

Cells expressing E6 do not exhibit a functional p53 response. The p53 tumor suppressor is not required for normal cellular proliferation but rather functions as "guardian of the human genome" by integrating various signal transduction pathways that can sense cellular stress, including genotoxic and cytotoxic insults. The interaction of E6 with p53 appears to contribute to the chromosomal instability observed in cells infected by a high-risk HPV.[31] E6, however, has functions other than targeting the proteolysis of p53 that are important in cellular transformation and carcinogenesis. One important function that is p53 independent is that E6 causes the activation of the cellular telomerase in infected cells.[32] In addition, a number of laboratories have identified additional E6-interacting proteins, some of which may prove relevant to its transforming activities.[15]

It is clear that infection by a specific HPV is itself not sufficient for the development of cervical cancer. Only a small fraction of those individuals who are infected by a specific HPV eventually develop cancer, and the time interval between infection and invasive cancer can be several decades. Thus, the genetic information carried by the virus per se does not result in cancer; rather, it initiates a process that can ultimately result in cancer. Other factors must be involved in the progression of virus-associated lesions to these genital tract cancers, and there is a clear requirement for additional genetic mutations in the infected cell for a cancer to arise. Epidemiologic studies have suggested that smoking is a risk factor for development of cervical carcinoma.[33] The recognition that other factors are involved in the progression to cervical carcinomas suggests that papillomavirus infections may work synergistically with these other factors.

Consistent with the multistep nature of tumorigenesis, cervical cancers have been shown to harbor cytogenetic alterations.[34] Certain cytogenetic changes have been found in a relatively high proportion of tumors.[35] Between one-fourth and one-half of cervical cancers show loss of heterozygosity in chromosome regions 3p14, 4p16, 4q21-35, 6p21-22, 11p15, 11q23, 17p13.3, and 18q12-22. Loss of heterozygosity in 3p has also been implicated in cervical dysplasias adjacent to cancers. This observation implies that inactivation of a putative tumor suppressor gene in this region may occur as an early event that could predispose to further progression, although the specific gene has not yet been identified.

The availability of specific HPV DNA probes has provided investigators the opportunity to carry out extensive screenings of a variety of human cancers for HPV sequences.[13] Based on the animal models, it seems likely that any carcinomas of any squamous epithelium or an epithelium that can undergo squamous metaplasia would be a potential candidate for an association with an HPV. Studies examining oral, upper airway, and tonsillar carcinomas have revealed some HPV-positive carcinomas. HPV DNA has been found in benign oral papillomas, and oral focal epithelial hyperplasia has been firmly established as having a papillomavirus etiology. In addition, papillomavirus DNA sequences have been found associated with some cases of oral leukoplasia. Esophageal carcinomas in humans have not yet been convincingly shown to be associated with an HPV. The esophagus is lined by a squamous epithelium, and squamous cell papillomas of the esophagus have been described in humans. Additional studies would seem warranted to investigate a possible role of HPV in human esophageal cancers. There are also sporadic reports in the literature associating occasional human tumors, including colon cancer, ovarian cancer, prostate cancer, and even melanomas, with the presence of HPV DNA. In general, it seems prudent to be skeptical of such reports until systematic and well-performed studies provide confirmation in multiple laboratories.

Significant advances have been made in the development of vaccines against papillomavirus infections. The expression in yeast and in insect cells of the major capsid protein L1, either alone or together with L2, leads to the assembly of virus-like particles (VLPs) that are morphologically identical to native virion particles.[36,37] Furthermore, these VLPs present the conformational epitopes that are necessary for the development of a high-titer neutralizing antisera. Such VLPs are now being used in clinical trials in humans and have been shown to prevent infection with HPV. In a randomized placebo-controlled HPV-16 VLP vaccine study involving young sexually active women, protection against HPV-16 persistent infection has been demonstrated over a 12- to 18-month period.[38] This study demonstrates proof of principle for a VLP-based HPV vaccine. An eventual vaccine will need to be multivalent against multiple HPV types, however, because there is no evidence of protection across HPV types. Additional studies are also needed to determine the length of protection. In addition, there is interest in the development of therapeutic vaccines directed against the E6 and E7 proteins expressed in cancers and preneoplastic lesions. A variety of approaches have now been described in the literature, including the use of vaccinia virus vectors, DNA vaccines, and chimeric virus-like particles containing additional epitopes fused to L1 for therapeutic vaccines.[39]

EPSTEIN-BARR VIRUS

In 1964, Epstein and Barr discovered a new herpesvirus (EBV) in BL cells that they had succeeded in growing in culture (for reviews, see refs. 40, 41). This lent support to Burkitt's hypothesis that this endemic lymphoma of children in equatorial Africa is caused by an infectious agent. EBV became the first candidate human cancer virus. In culture, a small fraction of the latently infected BL cells undergo lytic infection. This enabled the Henle, Klein, and Epstein groups[41] to use viral antigens in the lytically infected cells (EBV viral capsid antigen) for seroepidemiologic surveys of EBV-specific antibody levels in normal populations and in people with malignancies. Surprisingly, most people have EBV-specific antibody, but Africans with BL, Chinese with anaplastic nasopharyngeal carcinoma (NPC), and people from the United States, Europe, or South America with Hodgkin's disease (HD) frequently have higher EBV antibody titers. Using the same assay, Henle[41] discovered that primary EBV infection is the cause of infectious mononucleosis, a disease that he had been studying for decades. Given the nearly

ubiquitous infection of humans with EBV and its role in infectious mononucleosis, the role of EBV in cancer was less certain for several years, despite the confirmation that African BLs and NPCs have EBV DNA in all tumor cells.

The role of EBV in lymphoid malignancies was brought into focus by a series of discoveries in the 1970s. Henle and zur-Hausen and Moss and Pope[41] found that EBV infection of human B lymphocytes *in vitro* enabled infected lymphocytes to proliferate endlessly as long-term lymphoblastoid cell lines (LCLs). B lymphocytes from EBV-infected people also grew into LCLs *in vitro* and were uniformly EBV infected. Miller[41] noted that EBV injection rapidly induces B-cell lymphomas in marmosets. Ho and others[41] observed that posttransplantation patients at a very high level of immune suppression who coincidentally developed primary EBV infection sometimes progressed to acutely fatal polyclonal EBV-infected B-lymphoproliferative disease (LPD). Children with X-linked immunodeficiency, severe combined immunodeficiency, or sporadic immune deficiencies were also noted to develop EBV-positive multifocal malignant LPDs involving peripheral lymphoid organs or the brain. The cells were similar in phenotype to LCLs and to the marmoset tumors. A decade later similar malignancies were noted in CD4-depleted HIV-infected people or patients with acquired immunodeficiency syndrome (AIDS). EBV latent gene expression in LCLs and in LPD was found to include six nuclear proteins, termed *Epstein-Barr nuclear antigens* (EBNAs); two integral membrane proteins, termed *latent infection–associated membrane proteins* (LMPs); two small RNAs, termed *EBV-encoded small RNAs* (EBERs); and RNAs of uncertain function, termed *BARF0*. This type of latent EBV infection is now called *latency III*. Later-onset posttransplantation lymphomas, many of the peripheral lymphomas in HIV-infected people, and African BLs have c-myc translocations. Although these cells are also usually EBV infected, EBV gene expression in BLs is usually restricted to latency I, characterized by expression of EBNA1, EBV-encoded small RNAs, and sometimes BARF0 RNAs. The Moss, Rickinson, Klein, and McMichael groups[41] discovered that normal humans have an unusually robust T-cell response to EBV latency III infection. The T-cell response persists lifelong at a high level. Rooney and O'Reilley[41] used normal or *in vitro* augmented EBV-specific donor T cells to prevent or treat LPD after T-cell–depleted bone marrow transplantation.

EBV is a remarkably unusual virus that induces potentially malignant infected B-lymphocyte proliferation in normal primary human infection.[40,41] In acute infection, latency III infected B lymphocytes may be up to 10% of peripheral blood B lymphocytes. These cells then seed into lymphatic organs. Infected B-cell proliferation is dependent on EBNAs and LMP1 expression. The EBNAs concomitantly induce high level CD4+ and CD8+ T-lymphocyte responses. EBV-immune T cells kill most of the latency III proliferating cells. Some latency III infected cells exit from cell cycle, revert to latency I, and express only EBNA1 or EBNA1 and LMP2. EBNA1 is poorly processed into the class I pathway, and infected cells that express only EBNA1 can survive in the face of high-level CD4+ and CD8+ T-cell immunity directed primarily against the other EBNAs. EBV-infected B cells are the source of reactivated lytic virus infection.[42] Lytic reactivations enable EBV to frequently replicate in the oropharynx of infected people. The saliva of EBV-seropositive people is frequently positive for EBV DNA. In the context of the key role of CD4+ and CD8+ T lymphocytes in normally effective immune responses to EBV-infected cells,[43] EBV-associated LPD, EBV-associated BL, EBV-associated HD, and even NPC are probably partial failures of the normally protective EBV-specific T-lymphocyte response (for reviews see refs. 43, 44).

Recombinant EBV–based analyses of the role of EBV genes in the conversion of primary B lymphocytes to LCLs indicate that EBNA2, EBNALP, EBNA3A, EBNA3C, EBNA1, and LMP1 are critical, but other EBV genes are not.[40] When EBV infects a human B lymphocyte, the genome enters the nucleus and circularizes by joining the terminal direct repeats. EBNA2 and EBNALP are the first EBV genes expressed in B lymphocytes. EBNA2 and EBNALP act together to up-regulate virus and cell gene transcription. EBNA2 gets to specific promoters by direct interaction with cell-encoded DNA sequence–specific transcription factors RBPJκ/CBF1, PU.1, and AUF1. EBNA2 then activates transcription through its acidic activation domain, which binds basal and activation-related transcription factors. EBNALP binds to a different component of the EBNA2 acidic activation domain and coregulates transcription with EBNA2. EBNA2, EBNA3A, EBNA3B, and EBNA3C stably associate with RBPJκ/CBF1 at high levels and therefore likely coregulate overlapping sets of promoters. The Notch receptor signaling domain also activates transcription through RBPJκ/CBF1. Overexpressed Notch1 signaling domain is a cause of acute leukemia consistent with the importance of this pathway in cell growth. EBNA2, EBNALP, EBNA3A, and EBNA3C jointly constitutively regulate the viral LMP1 promoter and the cellular c-myc promoter, through RBPJκ/CBF1.[45,46] EBNA1 is also essential for efficient conversion of lymphocytes to LCLs, because of its role in enabling EBV episomes to replicate and persist in dividing cells.[47,48]

LMP1 is the other key transforming component in EBV's constitutive proliferative effects. LMP1 has six hydrophobic transmembrane domains that enable constitutive self-aggregation in cytoplasmic membranes, including the plasma membrane. LMP1 has two important C-terminal cytoplasmic signaling domains: One domain engages tumor necrosis factor receptor–associated cytoplasmic factors TRAF3, TRAF1, TRAF2, and TRAF5, and the other domain engages death domain proteins, including TRADD and RIP, without propagating a death signal. Both domains activate IKKα and IKKβ, JNK, and p38, although the TRAF interacting domain appears to be the principal IKKα activator. The TRAF domain is also particularly important for LCL outgrowth as well as for up-regulation of TRAF1 and EGF receptor expression.[49] NFκB activation is critical for LCL survival but may not have a significant role in cell proliferation. Although not important for LCL growth or survival, LMP2 mimics a constitutively active immunoglobulin receptor and desensitizes cells to immunoglobulin receptor signaling. LMP2 can also enhance cell survival as a result of low-level forward signaling through phosphatidylinositol 3 kinase, particularly in differentiating B lymphocytes or epithelial cells.[44]

After primary infection, EBV is also associated with LPD in heart, lung, liver, pancreas, or T-cell–depleted bone marrow transplant recipients, CD4-depleted HIV-infected people, almost all Africans with BL, approximately 20% of non-Africans with BL, and approximately 50% of those with classical HD tumors, particularly individuals with Reed-Sternberg cell–positive HD or young or Hispanic people with HD.[41] EBV is also associated with almost all NPCs worldwide, approximately 5% of gastric cancers, unusual T-cell lymphomas, and leiomyomas. Latency III EBV infection is confined to LPD, unusual BLs, and rare T-cell lymphomas, whereas latency II infection, characterized by expres-

sion of EBNA1, LMP1, and LMP2, is evident in many NPCs and almost all EBV-associated HD. Latency I infection is characteristic of most EBV-associated BL. EBV appears to be present at the onset of EBV-associated BL, HD, NPC, and gastric cancer, because all tumor cells in the same patient have EBV genomes with the same number of terminal repeats, whereas variability in terminal repeat number is a characteristic of independent EBV infection events. EBV is also the cause of oral hairy leukoplakia (OHL), a wart-like lesion on the tongue of HIV-infected people and transplant recipients. Surprisingly, OHL is a site for lytic, but not latent, EBV infection. OHL lesions have wild-type and defective EBV genomes.[50] The lesions disappear in response to suppression of EBV replication with acyclovir.

EBV is an important factor in the evolution of EBV-associated BLs, HD, and gastric cancer, and an almost universal factor in NPC.[41] Cellular changes that accompany the presumed transformation from an EBV-infected cell or normal B cell to BL have been partially characterized and include changes in cell DNA that result in up-regulation of expression of c-myc, Bcl-6, or Rel.[51–53] EBV-infected HD tumor cells are similar to non–EBV-infected HD cells in having nonproductive immunoglobulin mutations and up-regulated NFκB and AP-1 transcription.[54,55] Serologic testing has been useful in population-based surveys for early detection of primary NPC and for detecting recurrences.[56] Unfortunately, the serologic tests vary among institutions and over time; the utility of serologic testing is dependent on recent clinical validation. EBV LMP1 and LMP2 are likely to have important roles in early survival of NPC cells. Loss of heterozygosity, chromosomal amplification, and hypermethylation have been described in NPC cell lines and tumors.[57] Among people from southern China, NPC is a very common malignancy. Families have been described with multiple affected members, which has permitted a familial genetic analysis and localization of a risk factor to 4p15.1-q12.[58] Because of the frequent expression of LMP1 and LMP2 in NPC and EBV-associated HD and the potential recognition of LMP1 or LMP2 epitopes on NPC or HD cells, attempts are being made at T-cell immune prevention and therapy.[59,60]

KAPOSI'S SARCOMA–ASSOCIATED HERPESVIRUS

KS has long been known as an uncommon and indolent tumor of elderly Mediterranean and African men. More recently, it has been recognized to occur at higher frequency in immunosuppressed organ transplant recipients and AIDS patients. In all cases, the histologic picture of the disease is similar—and highly distinctive. KS is a composite of three processes: a proliferative component (made up of spindle-shaped endothelial cells), an inflammatory component (T and B cells and monocytes), and an angiogenic component (comprising highly aberrant, slit-like neovascular spaces). In advanced KS, the spindle cell proliferation dominates, resulting in nodule formation, but even in such cases, the disease is often oligoclonal or polyclonal.[61] This is one of many ways in which KS differs from classical neoplasms. For example, cultured KS spindle cells are not fully tumorigenic: Most do not produce stable transplantable tumors in nude mice or grow in soft agar. In fact, unlike most transformed cells, they continue to display a strong dependence on exogenous growth factors. (In turn, they themselves produce a large array of growth and angiogenic factors.) When transplanted into nude mice, they survive only transiently, but during their period of viability they recruit host inflammatory cells and neovascular structures very reminiscent of KS.[62] When the human spindle cells involute, the entire lesion disappears. This suggests a model for KS in which the entire process consists of paracrine signaling loops between its several components, no one of which is completely autonomous.[63,64]

KS has long been suspected to have a viral etiology. Early models attempted to relate spindle cell growth to HIV infection. Certainly, HIV infection is an enormous risk factor for KS development. However, spindle cells themselves are not targets of HIV infection, and KS epidemiology indicates that the lesion cannot depend solely on HIV infection. First, of course, KS often arises in HIV-negative hosts, especially in the Mediterranean basin and Africa. More importantly, even within HIV-infected populations there are large differences in KS risk that must be attributed to factors other than HIV infection.[65] KS risk is highest in homosexual men with untreated AIDS: 20% to 30% of such individuals will develop KS in the course of their HIV disease if no anti-HIV treatment is instituted. By contrast, fewer than 1% to 2% of individuals with AIDS related to blood product administration are similarly afflicted, and KS is rarer still in pediatric AIDS cases in which HIV infection is acquired vertically from infected mothers. These and other data suggested the possibility of a sexually transmitted cofactor in KS etiology or pathogenesis. Inspired by these clues,[66] Chang et al. used a PCR-based method to search for the putative causal virus by looking for DNA sequences that were present in DNA extracted from an AIDS-related KS specimen but absent in normal genomic DNA from the same patient. This search led to the discovery of the genome of the virus now known as *KSHV* or *HHV-8*.

Strong epidemiologic and molecular evidence indicates a pivotal role for this virus in KS development.[67] First, KSHV sequences are present in virtually all KS tumors, irrespective of the individual's HIV status. Moreover, unlike HIV, in KS lesions KSHV DNA is found primarily in the spindle cells—the key cell type in KS pathogenesis. Most such cells display latent infection, although a small subpopulation is in the lytic cycle. In HIV-positive populations studied prospectively, KSHV infection precedes the development of KS, and prior infection with KSHV is strongly predictive of increased KS risk. Worldwide, there is a strong correlation between KSHV prevalence and KS risk: Countries with high rates of classical KS display high rates of seropositivity for KSHV, and areas at low risk for KS typically have low prevalences of KSHV seropositivity. These data clearly indicate that KSHV is the agent predicted by KS epidemiology and strongly implicate KSHV in KS pathogenesis. KS is virtually never observed in the absence of documented KSHV infection, which leads most experts in the field to conclude that KSHV is necessary for KS development. However, there is also strong consensus that it is not sufficient for this process. For example, 5% to 7% of the general population in the United States is infected by KSHV, yet this population has no significant KS risk. Clearly, therefore, one or more cofactors in addition to KSHV are required to promote tumorigenesis. In the case of AIDS-related KS, of course, that cofactor is HIV infection, although exactly what HIV contributes to pathogenesis is much debated. The nature of the cofactor(s) in the HIV-negative forms of KS remains unknown.

Studies of KSHV seroepidemiology conducted in the developing world have yielded additional insights. First, the prevalence of KSHV in the general population is remarkably elevated in countries in which classical KS is common. For example, in Southern Italy, Sicily, and Sardinia, KSHV antibodies are found in over 20% of the general population; in many populations in sub-Saharan Africa, where classical KS was common even in the pre-AIDS era, 60% to 80% of the population is seropositive. These numbers also reflect major epidemiologic differences between KSHV infection in Africa and the Mediterranean versus that in Western Europe and America. In the latter areas, gay men represent a major reservoir of infection, with much lower rates in women and very little infection in prepubertal children. By contrast, in Africa and the Mediterranean, seroconversions begin in childhood, and the seroprevalence rises nearly continuously throughout the first four to five decades of life. Moreover, seroprevalences are equal in males and females, in sharp contrast to the developed world. The basis for this strikingly different epidemiology is not yet understood. The frequent occurrence of infection in young children in the Mediterranean and Africa suggest the existence of nonsexual routes of spread, and the equal infection rates in adult males and females also suggests different routes of spread from those observed in the West. Exactly what these routes are remains conjectural, but the presence of virus in high titer in the saliva of infected subjects suggests that a salivary route—as has been postulated for EBV transmission—is likely.

How does KSHV infection predispose to KS? The understanding of this association at the molecular level is still fragmentary and has been reviewed elsewhere.[68-70] Because most KS tumor cells are latently infected, efforts to identify and characterize KSHV latency genes have been made on the presumption that, as in EBV, these genes play strong roles in spindle cell growth deregulation. Several interesting genes have been identified in this fashion. One latency cluster expresses a set of three genes from a common promoter. Their products include (1) LANA, an antigen that appears to function in KSHV genomic maintenance in latency but also can impair p53 and RB function as well as up-regulate the β-catenin pathway; expression of LANA in primary endothelial cells extends their survival, although it does not immortalize or transform them; (2) V-cyclin, a viral homologue of cellular cyclin D1 that can bind and activate cdk6, which indicates that it is a functional cyclin; its activity displays reduced sensitivity to the inhibitory effects of certain cdk inhibitors, which suggests that it might be refractory to normal regulatory controls imposed on its host counterparts; (3) V-FLIP, a homologue of cellular inhibitors of caspase activation (Flice-inhibitory protein, or FLIP), which can also bind the IκB kinase complex and result in constitutive NFκB activation. The latter activity has been shown to be important in promoting cell survival. Other latent viral proteins include the kaposin family. These are transmembrane and soluble proteins that appear to be active in signal transduction. One of them, kaposin A, activates cytohesin-1, a protein involved in cell signaling cascades regulating cell shape. Kaposins B and C appear to be involved in the regulation of signaling pathways that govern cytokine production.

As already noted, KS tumors also harbor smaller numbers of lytically infected cells. The significance of lytic infection in KS tumorigenesis is unknown, but there are reasons to believe that the lytic cycle may play a more profound role in KS than in other herpesvirus-induced malignancies. First, a clinical trial has shown that even in patients with advanced AIDS, treatment with ganciclovir, which is active only against lytic herpesviral infection, profoundly reduces the subsequent development of KS over the ensuing 6 to 12 months.[71] Although this result might mean simply that lytic reactivation from the lymphoid reservoir is necessary for spread to the endothelium to initiate latent infection there, it is also compatible with a requirement for ongoing KSHV replication in KS pathogenesis. The latter is an attractive notion, because the virus contains numerous genes that are potent signaling molecules expressed principally during lytic growth.[72,73] Some of these are secreted factors (e.g., homologues of interleukin-6, CC chemokines, and other factors), whereas others (e.g., the K1 protein and a virus-specific G protein–coupled receptor) are transmembrane proteins that trigger deregulated signal transduction in the host, which often leads to secretory products that can influence surrounding cells. For example, virus-specific G protein–coupled receptor expression induces the release of vascular endothelial growth factor, a protein long speculated to play a role in the angiogenic phenotype of KS. Some of the viral chemokines can trigger angiogenesis as well; moreover, these molecules would be expected to contribute to the influx of inflammatory cells in the lesion—another hallmark of KS. Defining the relative contributions of latency and lytic growth to KS pathogenesis will be a major focus of KSHV research in the coming decade.

The homologies to EBV and HVS place KSHV/HHV-8 within the lymphotropic herpesvirus subfamily, an assignment supported by the finding of viral DNA in the B-cell compartment of the peripheral blood mononuclear cell population. This raises the possibility that the virus might participate in lymphoid neoplasia as well, and in recent years viral infection has in fact been associated with at least two lymphoproliferative conditions. The first is a rare B-cell lymphoma, termed *primary effusion lymphoma*, that has thus far been limited to HIV-positive hosts.[74] These lesions present as ascites tumors in the pleural and peritoneal cavities, often without clinically evident lymphadenopathy or bone marrow involvement. Primary effusion lymphoma cells are uniformly latently infected with KSHV; many (but not all) also bear latent EBV genomes as well. The other lymphoid lesion associated with KSHV is multicentric Castleman's disease, a complex and poorly understood lymphoproliferative syndrome that can occur in both HIV-positive and HIV-negative individuals. The HIV-positive form appears to be uniformly associated with KSHV, whereas only approximately one-half of the HIV-negative forms can be shown to harbor the virus.[75] It is interesting that an association of Castleman's disease with KS has long been recognized, although little discussed.

Study of viral gene expression in multicentric Castleman's disease has revealed some provocative surprises. Within the involved tissue, viral DNA is confined to B cells in the mantle zones surrounding the lymphoid follicles. There, both latently and lytically infected cells can be found, with a rather larger proportion of the infected cell population being in the lytic cycle compared with KS.[76,77] Lytically infected cells produce large quantities of viral interleukin-6, as well as host interleukin-6, and it is thought that these factors drive the polyclonal expansion of B cells that is the hallmark of this disorder. This is not to say that other viral gene products pay no role in multicentric Castleman's disease—it seems likely that latency products are also involved, but the relative contributions of different viral gene products to pathogenesis are still being explored.

SIMIAN VACUOLATING VIRUS 40 AND THE HUMAN POLYOMAVIRUSES

There have been occasional reports for the past three decades suggesting the presence of SV40 or human polyomavirus DNA or antigens in a variety of different human cancers, including renal carcinomas, osteosarcomas, mesotheliomas, pancreatic tumors, and brain tumors. The possibility that these polyomaviruses might play an etiologic role in specific human cancers has received some interest from the National Cancer Institute and from the Institute of Medicine.[78] All of these studies are not summarized here; instead, the reader is referred to a number of reviews and articles on this subject.[79–81]

SV40 is a nonhuman primate virus that naturally infects Asian macaques. The major source of human exposure to SV40 was through contaminated poliovirus vaccines that were given between 1955 and 1963.[82] It is a highly oncogenic virus in rodent cells and has served as an extremely valuable model for determining the various mechanisms by which DNA tumor viruses transform cells and contribute to tumor formation. There is no epidemiologic evidence indicating a higher risk of cancers among the populations of individuals who received the SV40-contaminated vaccine, however.

There are no compelling data that the virus is circulating among human communities. Much of the data claiming an association of SV40 DNA with human tumors has been gathered by the use of the PCR assays, which are error prone, and has been difficult to confirm. In fact, the only double-blind study conducted thus far, involving nine different laboratories, was unable to confirm a correlation.[83] The possibility that SV40 (or any virus, for that matter) is involved in the etiology of human cancer is strengthened when multiple lines of evidence (including epidemiology, as well as pathogenic and molecular mechanisms) converge. Thus, it is premature to consider SV40 a human cancer virus. Additional blinded studies are necessary.

REFERENCES

1. Rous PA. Sarcoma of the fowl transmissible by an agent separable from the tumor cells. *J Exp Med* 1911;13:397.
2. Shope RE, Hurst EW. Infectious papillomatosis of rabbits; with a note on the histopathology. *J Exp Med* 1933;58:607.
3. Rous P, Beard JW. Carcinomatous changes in virus-induced papillomas of rabbits. *Proc Soc Exp Biol Med* 1935;32:578.
4. Beasley RP. Hepatitis B virus—the major etiology of the hepatocellular carcinoma. *Cancer* 1988;61:1942.
5. Ganem D, Prince AM. Hepatitis B virus infection—natural history and clinical consequences. *N Engl J Med* 2004;350:1118.
6. Yang HI, Lu SN, Liaw YF, et al. Hepatitis B e antigen and the risk of hepatocellular carcinoma. *N Engl J Med* 2002;347:168.
7. Chisari FV, Ferrari C. Hepatitis B virus immunopathogenesis. *Ann Rev Immunol* 1995;13:29.
8. Kim C-Y, Koike K, Saito I, Miyamura T, Jay G. HBx gene of hepatitis B virus induces liver cancer in transgenic mice. *Nature* 1991;351:317.
9. Nagaya T, Nakamura T, Tokino T, et al. The mode of hepatitis B virus DNA integration in chromosomes of human hepatocellular carcinoma. *Genes Dev* 1987;1:773.
10. Popper H, Roth L, Purcell RH, Tennant BC, Gerin JL. Hepatocarcinogenicity of the woodchuck hepatitis virus. *Proc Natl Acad Sci U S A* 1987;84:866.
11. Fourel G, Trepo C, Bougueleret L, et al. Frequent activation of N-myc genes by hepadnavirus insertion in woodchuck liver tumours. *Nature* 1990;347:294.
12. Howley PM, Lowy DR. Papillomaviruses and their replication. In: Knipe DM, Howley PM, eds. *Fields' virology.* Philadelphia: Lippincott Williams & Wilkins, 2001:2197.
13. Lowy DR, Howley PM. Papillomaviruses. In: Knipe DM, Howley PM, eds. *Fields' virology.* Philadelphia: Lippincott Williams & Wilkins, 2001:2231.
14. DiMaio D, Lai C-C, Mattoon D. The platelet-derived growth factor b receptor as a target of the bovine papillomavirus E5 protein. *Cytokine Growth Factor Rev* 2000;11:283.
15. Munger K, Howley PM. Human papillomavirus immortalization and transformation functions. *Virus Res* 2002;89:213.
16. Rous P, Kidd JG. The carcinogenic effect of a virus upon tarred skin. *Science* 1936;83:468.

17. Rous P, Beard JW. The progression to carcinoma of virus-induced rabbit papillomas (Shope). *J Exp Med* 1935;62:523.
18. Campo MS. Animal models of papillomavirus pathogenesis. *Virus Res* 2002;89:249.
19. Jablonska S, Majewski S. Epidermoplasia verruciformis: immunological and clinical aspects. *Curr Topics Microbiol Immunol* 1994;186:157.
20. Ramoz N, Rueda LA, Bouadjar B, et al. Mutations in two adjacent novel genes are associated with epidermodysplasia verruciformis. *Nat Genet* 2002;32:579.
21. Kessler IL. Human cervical cancer as a venereal disease. *Cancer Res* 1976;36:783.
22. zur Hausen H. Herpes simplex virus in human genital cancer. *Int Rev Exp Pathol* 1983;25:307.
23. zur Hausen H. Condylomata acuminata and human genital cancer. *Cancer Res* 1976; 36:530.
24. Meisels A, Fortin R. Condylomatous lesions of the cervix and vagina. I. Cytologic patterns. *Acta Cytol* 1976;20:505.
25. Durst M, Gissmann L, Idenburg H, zur Hausen H. A papillomavirus DNA from a cervical carcinoma and its prevalence in cancer biopsy samples from different geographic regions. *Proc Natl Acad Sci U S A* 1983;80:3812.
26. Boshart M, Gissman L, Ikenberg H, et al. A new type of papillomavirus DNA, its presence in genital cancer biopsies and in cell lines derived from cervical cancer. *EMBO J* 1984;3:1151.
27. Gissmann L, Schwarz E. Persistence and expression of human papillomavirus DNA in genital cancer. In: Evered D, Clark S, eds. *Papillomaviruses.* Chichester: John Wiley & Sons, 1986:190.
28. Bosch FX, Lorincz A, Munoz N, Meijer CJ, Shah KV. The causal relation between human papillomavirus and cervical cancer. *J Clin Pathol* 2002;55:244.
29. Duensing S, Lee LY, Duensing A, et al. The human papillomavirus type 16 E6 and E7 oncoproteins cooperate to induce mitotic defects and genomic instability by uncoupling centrosome duplication from the cell division cycle. *Proc Natl Acad Sci U S A* 2000;97:10002.
30. Duensing A, Crum CP, Munger K, Duensing S. Centrosome abnormalities, genomic instability and carcinogenic progression. *Cancer Res* 2001;61:2356.
31. White A, Livanos EM, Tlsty TD. Differential disruption of genomic integrity and cell cycle regulation in normal human fibroblasts by the HPV oncoproteins. *Genes Dev* 1994;8:666.
32. Klingelhutz AJ, Foster SA, McDougall JK. Telomerase activation by the E6 gene product of human papillomavirus type 16. *Nature* 1996;380:79.
33. Clarke EA, Morgan RW, Newman AM. Smoking as a risk factor in cancer of the cervix: additional evidence from a case control study. *Am J Epidemiol* 1982;115:59.
34. Kersemaekers AM, van de Vijver MJ, Kenter GG, Fleuren GJ. Genetic alterations during the progression of squamous cell carcinomas of the uterine cervix. *Genes Chromosomes Cancer* 1999;26:346.
35. Lazo PA. The molecular genetics of cervical carcinoma. *Br J Cancer* 1999;80:2008.
36. Zhou J, Stenzel DJ, Sun XY, Frazer IH. Synthesis and assembly of infectious bovine papillomavirus particles in vitro. *J Gen Virol* 1993;74:763.
37. Kirnbauer R, Booy F, Cheng N, Lowy DR, Schiller JT. Papillomavirus L1 major capsid protein self-assembles into virus-like particles that are highly immunogenic. *Proc Natl Acad Sci U S A* 1992;89:12180.
38. Koutsky LA, Ault KA, Wheeler CM, et al. A controlled trial of a human papillomavirus type 16 vaccine. *N Engl J Med* 2002;347:1645.
39. Frazer IH. Prevention of cervical cancer through papillomavirus vaccination. *Nat Rev Immunol* 2004;4:46.
40. Kieff E, Rickinson AB. Epstein-Barr virus and its replication. In: Knipe D, Howley PM, eds. *Fields virology.* Philadelphia: Lippincott Williams & Wilkins, 2001:2511.
41. Rickinson AB, Kieff E. Epstein-Barr virus. In: Knipe D, Howley PM, eds. *Fields' virology.* Philadelphia: Lippincott Williams & Wilkins, 2001:2575.
42. Faulkner GC, Burrows SR, Khanna R. X-Linked agammaglobulinemia patients are not infected with Epstein-Barr virus: implications for the biology of the virus. *J Virol* 1999;73:1555.
43. Amyes E, Hatton C, Montamat-Sicotte D. Characterization of the CD4+ T cell response to Epstein-Barr virus during primary and persistent infection. *J Exp Med* 2003;198:903.
44. Caldwell RG, Brown RC, Longnecker R. Epstein-Barr virus LMP2A-induced B-cell survival in two unique classes of EmuLMP2A transgenic mice. *J Virol* 2000;74:1101.
45. Cooper A, Johannsen E, Maruo S, et al. EBNA3A association with RBP-Jkappa down-regulates c-myc and Epstein-Barr virus-transformed lymphoblast growth. *J Virol* 2003;77:999.
46. Gordadze AV, Peng R, Tan J, et al. Notch1IC partially replaces EBNA2 function in B cells immortalized by Epstein-Barr virus. *J Virol* 2001;75:5899.
47. Humme S, Reisbach G, Feederle R, et al. The EBV nuclear antigen 1 (EBNA1) enhances B cell immortalization several thousandfold. *Proc Natl Acad Sci U S A* 2003;100:10989.
48. Kang MS, Hung SC, Kieff E. Epstein-Barr virus nuclear antigen 1 activates transcription from episomal but not integrated DNA and does not alter lymphocyte growth. *Proc Natl Acad Sci U S A* 2001;98:15233.
49. Luftig M, Yasui T, Soni V, et al. Epstein-Barr virus latent infection membrane protein 1 TRAF-binding site induces NIK/IKK alpha-dependent noncanonical NF-kappaB activation EBNA3A association with RBP-Jkappa down-regulates c-myc and Epstein-Barr virus-transformed lymphoblast growth. *Proc Natl Acad Sci U S A* 2004;101:141.
50. Walling DM, Flaitz CM, Nichols CM. Epstein-Barr virus replication in oral hairy leukoplakia: response, persistence, and resistance to treatment with valacyclovir. *J Infect Dis* 2003;188:883.
51. Houldsworth J, Olshen AB, Cattoretti G, et al. Relationship between REL amplification, REL function, and clinical and biologic features in diffuse large B-cell lymphomas. *Blood* 2004;103:1862.
52. Kuppers R, Dalla-Favera R. Mechanisms of chromosomal translocations in B cell lymphomas. *Oncogene* 2001;20:5580.
53. Kuppers R, Klein U, Schwering I, et al. Identification of Hodgkin and Reed-Sternberg cell-specific genes by gene expression profiling. *J Clin Invest* 2003;111:529.
54. Hinz M, Lemke P, Anagnostopoulos I, et al. Nuclear factor kappaB-dependent gene expression profiling of Hodgkin's disease tumor cells, pathogenetic significance, and link to constitutive signal transducer and activator of transcription 5a activity. *J Exp Med* 2002;196:605.
55. Mathas S, Hinz M, Anagnostopoulos I, et al. Aberrantly expressed c-Jun and JunB are a hallmark of Hodgkin lymphoma cells, stimulate proliferation and synergize with NF-kappa B. *EMBO J* 2002;21:4104.
56. Chan KH, Gu YL, Ng F, et al. EBV specific antibody-based and DNA-based assays in serologic diagnosis of nasopharyngeal carcinoma. *Int J Cancer* 2003;105:706.
57. Wong N, Hui AB, Fan B, et al. Molecular cytogenetic characterization of nasopharyngeal carcinoma cell lines and xenografts by comparative genomic hybridization and spectral karyotyping. *Cancer Genet Cytogenet* 2003;140:124.
58. Feng BJ, Huang W, Shugart YY, et al. Genome-wide scan for familial nasopharyngeal carcinoma reveals evidence of linkage to chromosome 4. *Nat Genet* 2002;31:395.
59. Chua D, Huang J, Zheng B, et al. Adoptive transfer of autologous Epstein-Barr virus-specific cytotoxic T cells for nasopharyngeal carcinoma. *Int J Cancer* 2001;94:73.
60. Timms JM, Bell A, Flavell JR, et al. Target cells of Epstein-Barr-virus (EBV)-positive post-transplant lymphoproliferative disease: similarities to EBV-positive Hodgkin's lymphoma. *Lancet* 2003;361:217.
61. Gill PS, Tsai YC, Rao AP, et al. Evidence for multiclonality in multicentric Kaposi's sarcoma. *Proc Natl Acad Sci U S A* 1998;95:8257.
62. Salahuddin SZ, Nakamura S, Biberfeld P, et al. Angiogenic properties of Kaposi's sarcoma-derived cells after longterm culture in vitro. *Science* 1988;242:430.
63. Ensoli B, Sirianni MC. Kaposi's sarcoma pathogenesis: a link between immunology and tumor biology. *Crit Rev Oncog* 1998;9:107.
64. Cesarman E, Mesri EA, Gershengorn MC. Viral G protein-coupled receptor and Kaposi's sarcoma: a model of paracrine neoplasia? *J Exp Med* 2000;191:417.
65. Beral V, Peterman T, Berkelman R, Jaffe HW. Kaposi's sarcoma among persons with AIDS: a sexually transmitted infection? *Lancet* 1990;335:123.
66. Chang Y, Cesarman E, Pessin MS, et al. Identification of herpesvirus-like DNA sequences in AIDS-associated Kaposi's sarcoma. *Science* 1994;266:1865.
67. Schulz TF. Kaposi's sarcoma-associated herpesvirus (human herpesvirus-8). *J Gen Virol* 1998;79:1573.
68. Jenner RG, Boshoff C. The molecular pathology of Kaposi's sarcoma-associated herpesvirus. *Biochim Biophys Acta* 2002;1602:1.
69. Schulz TF, Sheldon J, Greensill J. Kaposi's sarcoma associated herpesvirus (KSHV) or human herpesvirus 8 (HHV8). *Virus Res* 2002;82:115.
70. Moore PS, Chang Y. Kaposi's sarcoma-associated herpesvirus immunoevasion and tumorigenesis: two sides of the same coin? *Annu Rev Microbiol* 2003;57:609.
71. Martin DF, Kuppermann BD, Wolitz RA, et al. Roche Ganciclovir Study Group. Oral ganciclovir for patients with cytomegalovirus retinitis treated with a ganciclovir implant. *N Engl J Med* 1999;340:1063.
72. Moore PS, Boshoff C, Weiss RA, Chang Y. Molecular mimicry of human cytokine and cytokine response pathway genes by KSHV. *Science* 1996;274:1739.
73. Nicholas J. Human herpesvirus-8-encoded signaling ligands and receptors. *J Biomed Sci* 2003;10:475.
74. Cesarman E. The role of Kaposi's sarcoma-associated herpesvirus (KSHV/HHV-8) in lymphoproliferative diseases. *Recent Results Cancer Res* 2002;159:27.
75. Soulier J, Grollet L, Oksenhendler E, et al. Kaposi's sarcoma-associated herpesvirus-like DNA sequences in multicentric Castleman's disease. *Blood* 1995;86:1276.
76. Dupin N, Fisher C, Kellam P, et al. Distribution of human herpesvirus-8 latently infected cells in Kaposi's sarcoma, multicentric Castleman's disease, and primary effusion lymphoma. *Proc Natl Acad Sci U S A* 1999;96:4546.
77. Parravicini C, Chandran B, Corbellino M, et al. Differential viral protein expression in Kaposi's sarcoma herpesvirus-associated diseases: Kaposi's sarcoma, primary effusion lymphoma, and multicentric Castleman's disease. *Am J Pathol* 2000;156:743.
78. Stratton K, Alamario DA, McCormick MC. *Immunization safety review—SV40 contamination of polio vaccine and cancer.* Washington, D.C.: National Academies Press, 2003:101.
79. Garcea RL, Imperiale MJ. Simian virus 40 infection of humans. *J Virol* 2003;77:5039.
80. Carbone M, Pass HI, Miele L, Bocchetta M. New developments about the association of SV40 with human mesothelioma. *Oncogene* 2003;22:5173.
81. Vilchez RA, Kozinetz CA, Arrington AS, Madden CR, Butel JS. Simian virus 40 in human cancers. *Am J Med* 2003;114:675.
82. Shah KV, Nathanson N. Human exposure to SV40: review and comment. *Am J Epidemiol* 1976;103:1.
83. Strickler HD. A multicenter evaluation of assays for detection of SV40 DNA and results in masked mesothelioma specimens. *Cancer Epidemiol Biomarkers Prev* 2001;10:523.

Stuart H. Yuspa
Peter G. Shields

CHAPTER **8**

Etiology of Cancer: Chemical Factors

The chemical origin of human malignancies was recognized by observations of unusual cancer incidences in certain occupational groups. The capacity for chemicals to cause cancer was subsequently confirmed in numerous experimental animal studies. The extent to which chemical exposures contribute to cancer incidence was not fully appreciated until population-based studies documented differing organ-specific cancer rates among geographically distinct populations. Changes in cancer frequency among migrating ethnic groups, high cancer rates associated with specific occupations, and the high risk of smoking-associated cancers confirmed that environmental and lifestyle exposures were major determinants of human cancer risk. Current data indicate that changing lifestyles and exposures can modify cancer risk.[1] Although genetic factors dictate a very high cancer risk for a small group of individuals with hereditary cancer syndromes, the general population carries hereditary susceptibility genes that increase cancer risk for particular exposures. Thus, most human cancer is not simply a genetically determined sequela of aging but rather the manifestation of personal and cultural behavior, superimposed on individually determined hereditary susceptibility.

The experimental induction of tumors in animals and neoplastic transformation of cultured cells by chemicals and the analysis of environmentally induced human tumors have revealed important concepts regarding the pathogenesis of cancer and the consistency of pathways impacted for cancer development in rodent and human species (see refs. 2–5 for more extensive reviews). Chemical carcinogens are often organ specific, target epithelial cells, and cause genetic damage (genotoxic). Chemically related DNA damage and consequent somatic mutations relevant to human cancer can occur either directly from environmental exposures or indirectly by activation of endogenous mutagenic pathways (e.g., nitric

oxide and oxyradicals).[3] The risk of developing a chemically induced tumor may be modified by nongenotoxic exogenous and endogenous exposures and factors and by accumulated exposure to the same or different genotoxic carcinogens.[2]

Analysis of the chemical induction of cancer in animal models and human populations has had a major impact on human health. Experimental studies have been instrumental in validating hypotheses generated from human studies. Animal experiments confirmed the carcinogenic and tumor-promoting properties of cigarette smoke and identified the active chemical and gaseous components.[6] The transplacental carcinogenicity of diethylstilbestrol and the hazards of specific occupational carcinogens, such as vinyl chloride, benzene, aromatic amines, and bis(chloromethyl)ether, led to the removal of the suspected human carcinogens from the environment and reduction of cancer rate. Dietary factors that enhance or inhibit cancer development and the contribution of obesity to specific organ sites have been identified in models of chemical carcinogenesis, resulting in a reduction of cancer incidence through nutritional alterations. The application of cancer chemoprevention strategies, particularly retinoids, antiestrogens, and inhibitors of the arachidonic acid cascade, is the direct result of studies conducted in models of chemical carcinogenesis[7] and is reducing the tumor incidence in high-risk populations.

NATURE OF CHEMICAL CARCINOGENS: CHEMISTRY AND METABOLISM

Although a wide variety of chemicals and chemical classes can cause cancer in animals and humans[8] (Table 8-1), the process is very specific. Most chemicals are not known to be carcinogenic.

TABLE 8-1. Known or Suspected Chemical Carcinogens in Humans

Target Organ	Agents	Industries	Tumor Type
Lung	Tobacco smoke, arsenic, asbestos, crystalline silica, benzo[a]pyrene, beryllium, *bis*(chloro)methyl ether, 1,3-butadiene, chromium VI compounds, coal tar and pitch, nickel compounds, soots, mustard gas	Aluminum production, coal gasification, coke production, hematite mining, painters	Squamous, large cell and small cell cancer, and adenocarcinoma
Pleura	Asbestos, erionite		Mesothelioma
Oral cavity	Tobacco smoke, alcoholic beverages, nickel compounds	Boot and shoe production, furniture manufacturer, isopropyl alcohol production	Squamous cell cancer
Esophagus	Tobacco smoke, alcoholic beverages		Squamous cell cancer
Gastric system	Smoked, salted, and pickled foods	Rubber industry	Adenocarcinoma
Colon	Heterocyclic amines, asbestos	Pattern makers	Adenocarcinoma
Liver	Aflatoxin, vinyl chloride, tobacco smoke, alcoholic beverages, thorium dioxide		Hepatocellular carcinoma, hemangiosarcoma
Kidney	Tobacco smoke, phenacetin		Renal cell cancer
Bladder	Tobacco smoke, 4-aminobiphenyl, benzidine, 2-naphthylamine, phenacetin	Magenta manufacture, auramine manufacture	Transitional cell cancer
Prostate	Cadmium	—	Adenocarcinoma
Skin	Arsenic, benzo[a]pyrene, coal tar and pitch, mineral oils, soots, cyclosporin A, PUVA	Coal gasification, coke production	Squamous cell cancer, basal cell cancer
Bone marrow	Benzene, tobacco smoke, ethylene oxide, antineoplastic agents, cyclosporin A	Rubber workers	Leukemia, lymphoma

PUVA, psoralen and ultraviolet A light.
Note: These carcinogen designations are determined by regulatory or review agencies based on public health needs. They do not imply proof of carcinogenicity in individuals. This table is not all-inclusive. For additional information, the reader is referred to agency documents and publications.[8]

Within chemical classes, stereoisomers may vary widely in carcinogenicity. Genotoxic carcinogens have high chemical reactivity (such as alkylating agents) or can be metabolized to reactive intermediates by the host. They form covalent adducts with macromolecules and target DNA in the nucleus and mitochondria.[9] Because there is a good correlation between the ability to form DNA adducts and the potency to induce tumors in laboratory animals, DNA is considered the ultimate target for most carcinogens. Genotoxic carcinogens may transfer simple alkyl or complexed (aryl) alkyl groups to specific sites on DNA bases.[3] These alkylating and arylalkylating agents include, but are not limited to, N-nitrosocompounds, aliphatic epoxides, aflatoxins, mustards, polycyclic aromatic hydrocarbons (PAHs), and other combustion products of fossil fuels and vegetable matter. Others transfer arylamine residues to DNA as exemplified by aryl aromatic amines, aminoazodyes, and heterocyclic aromatic amines; the latter is produced by overcooking meat, poultry, or fish at high temperatures. For genotoxic carcinogens, the interaction with DNA is not random, and each class of agents reacts selectively with purine and pyrimidine targets.[9] Furthermore, targeting of carcinogens to particular sites in DNA is determined by nucleotide sequence, by host cell, and by selective DNA repair processes (see DNA Repair Protects the Most from Chemical Carcinogens, later in this chapter), making some genetic material at risk over others. As expected from this chemistry, genotoxic carcinogens are potent mutagens, particularly adept at causing base mispairing or small deletions, leading to missense or nonsense mutations. Others may cause macrogenetic damage such as chromosome breaks and large deletions.[10] In all cases, mutations detected in tumors represent a combination of the effect of the mutagenic change on the function of the protein product and the effect of the functional alteration on the behavior of the specific host cell type.

A number of chemicals that cause cancers in laboratory rodents are not demonstrably genotoxic. Synthetic pesticides and herbicides fall within this group, as do a number of natural products that are ingested. In general, these agents are carcinogenic in laboratory animals at high doses and require prolonged exposure. The mechanism of action by nongenotoxic carcinogens is controversial and may be related in some cases to toxic cell death and regenerative hyperplasia. Induction of endogenous mutagenic mechanisms such as DNA oxyradical damage,[3] depurination, and deamination of 5-methylcytosine by exposure to nongenotoxic carcinogens may contribute to carcinogenicity of these agents. In other cases, nongenotoxic carcinogens may have hormonal effects, influencing hormone-dependent tissues directly. Although the contribution of nongenotoxic carcinogens to human cancer causation is not certain, they may also serve as modifiers in concert with genotoxic agents, altering tissue homeostasis to provide an environment conducive to the selective expansion of a neoplastic clone. A number of endogenous metabolic enzymes activate or detoxify carcinogens and procarcinogens (chemicals that can be transformed into active carcinogens).[11] These pathways are complex and interactive, and genetic polymorphisms in animal models and humans are thought to be major determinants of cancer susceptibility and indications of risk for particular exposures.[11] Furthermore, a number of metabolic pathways are inducible and modified by diet, hormones, and additional exposures, adding further complexity to the process of environmental carcinogenesis.

ANIMAL MODEL SYSTEMS AND CHEMICAL CARCINOGENESIS

Virtually every major form of human cancer can be reproduced in experimental animals by exposure to specific chemical carcinogens. In many cases, the cell of origin, morphogenesis, phenotypic markers, and genetic alterations are qualitatively identical to those of corresponding human cancers.[2] Furthermore, animal models have revealed the constancy of carcinogen-host interaction among mammalian species by reproducing organ-specific cancers in animals with chemicals identified as human carcinogens, such as coal tar and squamous cell carcinomas, vinyl chloride and hepatic angiosarcomas, aflatoxin and hepatocarcinoma, and aromatic amines and bladder cancer. The introduction of genetically modified mice designed to reproduce specific human cancer syndromes has accelerated the understanding of the contributions of chemicals to cancer causation and the identification of potential exogenous carcinogens.[12] Together, these studies have indicated that carcinogenic agents can directly activate oncogenes, inactivate tumor suppressor genes, and cause the genomic changes that are associated with autonomous growth, enhanced survival, and modified gene expression profiles that are required for the malignant phenotype.[5]

DNA REPAIR PROTECTS THE HOST FROM CHEMICAL CARCINOGENS

DNA repair defects have been identified in a number of cancer-prone individuals, and repair-deficient mammalian cells are susceptible to transformation by chemical and physical carcinogens.[13] Nucleotide excision repair commonly removes carcinogen-DNA adducts or ultraviolet photoproducts by a complex process involving at least ten gene products, each potentially associated with mutations that lead to human DNA repair defect syndromes and increased cancer rates. Nucleotide excision repair commonly favors adduct removal on the transcribed strand to protect protein synthesis. Genetically engineered mice deficient in genes involved in nucleotide excision repair are particularly sensitive to chemical and ultraviolet carcinogenesis at particular organ sites. The highly mutagenic O^6-methylguanine, a consequence of exposure to certain methylating agents, is repaired by O^6-alkyl-deoxyguanine-DNA-alkyltransferase, an enzyme that protects the host from thymic lymphomas, colonic preneoplastic lesions, and colonic K-*ras* mutations after exposure of mice to methylating agents. Mutations in genes involved in nucleotide mismatch repair increase risk for colon cancer in humans, and engineered mice that are null for a gene in this pathway are predisposed to development of tumors.[14] The human cancer susceptibility genes BRCA1 and -2 and ATM participate in repair of carcinogen-induced DNA double-strand breaks in pathways linked to homologous recombination.[13]

GENETIC SUSCEPTIBILITY TO CHEMICAL CARCINOGENESIS

The identification and characterization of genes that modify risks for cancer development have been facilitated by substantial variation in susceptibility to chemically induced carcinogenesis at specific tissue sites among inbred strains of rodents and spontaneous or genetically modified mutant strains.[15,16] For a variety of tissue sites, including lung, liver, breast, and skin, pairs of inbred mice that differ by 100-fold in risk for tumor development after carcinogen exposure have been characterized. Genetically determined difference in the affinity for the aryl hydrocarbon hydroxylase (Ah) receptor or other differences in metabolic processing of car-

cinogens is one modifier that has a major impact on experimental cancer risk.[11] Other loci regulate the growth of premalignant foci, the response to tumor promoters, the immune response to metastatic cells, and the basal proliferation rate of target cells.[15] In mice susceptible to colon cancer due to a carcinogen-induced constitutive mutation in the *apc* gene, a locus on mouse chromosome 4 confers resistance to colon cancer.[16] The identification of the phospholipase A_2 gene at this locus and subsequent functional testing in transgenic mice revealed an interesting paracrine protective influence on tumor development.[16] This gene and several other genes mapped for susceptibility to chemically induced mouse tumors (*ptprj*—a receptor-type tyrosine phosphatase and *STK6/ STK15*—an aurora kinase) have now been shown to influence susceptibility to organ-specific cancer induction in humans.[15,16]

DETERMINATION OF CHEMICAL CARCINOGENS FOR HUMANS AND POPULATION-BASED RISK ASSESSMENT

Our current understanding of carcinogenesis and risk to human health comes from a variety of models and methods, including mutagenesis assays, mammalian cell culture experiments, animal studies, classic epidemiology, and molecular epidemiology. The goal of these studies is to elucidate cancer etiologies, define cancer risks in humans (population and individual), and identify more rational cancer prevention methods. Physicians are challenged when they attempt to determine what causes a cancer in a particular individual. This process requires an accurate history and physical examination and interpretation of research data. Several types of research models are used to identify potential human carcinogens. Extrapolating cell culture and animal data to human cancer risk has limitations, however, and epidemiology remains the best evidence toward conclusions of causation. Using available studies of any type, guidelines for assessing causality have been proposed.[17] Physicians can look to various regulatory, governmental, or review organizations for extensive evaluation of the scientific literature, but this can be problematic, as their charge is to assess risk across the general population and not for individual risk assessment. These agencies perform formal quantitative risk assessments to estimate the risk to a population that is exposed to a particular carcinogen at a specific dose. Risk assessments usually include four general steps: (1) hazard assessment, which qualitatively reviews scientific literature to decide whether a hazard might exist; (2) dose-response assessment, which evaluates the doses used in scientific studies and relates them to human exposures through modeling; (3) exposure assessment, which examines a population thought to be at risk regarding the quantity, duration, and routes of exposure; and (4) risk characterization, which incorporates the above information and evaluates the assumptions used and the uncertainties to estimate risk. These processes, however, cannot account for individual characteristics and genetic susceptibilities. Some known and potential human carcinogens, as reported by various regulatory and research organizations, are listed in Table 8-1.

CHEMICAL CARCINOGENESIS AND CANCER RISK

In recent years, new technologies have allowed epidemiologic studies to improve testing of biologically based hypotheses. An important goal has been to identify cancer risk based on individual exposures and genetically determined susceptibilities to cancer, namely gene-environment interactions. Still, the authors remain challenged because cancer is a complex disease of diverse etiologies, which is actually caused by multiple exposures causing damage in different genes, for example, gene^n-environment^n interactions, for which how many "n" is not known. Two fundamental principles underlie current studies of molecular epidemiology. First, carcinogenesis is a multistage process in which behind each stage are steps of numerous genetic events. Thus, characterizing a specific risk factor against a background of many risk factors is difficult and limits statistical power. Second, wide interindividual variation in response to carcinogen exposure and other carcinogenic processes indicate that the human response is not homogeneous, so that experimental models and epidemiology (e.g., the use of a single cell clone to study a gene's effect experimentally or the assumption that the population responds similarly to the mean in epidemiology studies) might not be representative of susceptible and resistant groups within a population.

BIOMARKERS OF CANCER RISK

The evaluation of cancer risk can include four components: external exposure measurements, internal exposure measurements, biomarkers estimating the biologically effective dose,[18] and biomarkers of harm. The latter three measurements improve on the first by quantifying exposure at the cellular level to characterize low-dose exposures in low-risk populations, providing a relative contribution of individual chemical carcinogens from complex mixtures and estimating total burden of a particular exposure where there are many sources.[19]

Chemicals cause genetic damage in different ways, namely, the formation of carcinogen-DNA adducts, leading to base mutations, or gross chromosomal changes. Adducts are formed when a mutagen, or part of it, irreversibly binds to DNA so that it can cause a base substitution, insertion, or deletion during DNA replication. Gross chromosomal mutations are chromosome breaks, gaps, or translocations. The level of DNA damage is the biologically effective dose in a target organ and reflects the net result of carcinogen exposure, activation, lack of detoxification, lack of DNA repair, and lack of programmed cell death. A variety of assays are available to identify carcinogen-macromolecular adducts in human tissues—for example, for assessing risk from tobacco smoking.[20] Important considerations for the assessment of biomarkers include sensitivity, specificity, reproducibility, accessibility for human use, and whether it represents a risk measured in a target organ or surrogate tissue. No single biomarker has been considered to be sufficiently validated for use as a cancer risk marker in an individual as it relates to chemical carcinogenesis. However, there has been some consistency in the literature.[21]

People are commonly exposed to N-nitrosamine and other N-nitrosocompounds from dietary and tobacco exposures, which are associated with DNA adduct formation and cancer.[6,22,23] Exposure can occur through endogenous formation of N-nitrosamines from nitrates in food or directly from dietary sources, cosmetics, drugs, household commodities, and tobacco smoke. The greatest source of exposure in the United States is from processed meats and, until recently, beer. Endogenous formation occurs in the stomach from the reaction of nitrosatable amines and nitrate, used as a preservative, which is converted to nitrites by bacteria. N-

nitrosamines undergo metabolic activation by cytochrome P-450s (*CYP2E1*, *CYP2A6*, and *CYP2D6*) and form DNA adducts that have been identified in target tissues.

Other examples of mutagens from the food, in addition to N-nitrosamines, occur as contaminants or from cooking practices. Heterocyclic amines are formed from the overheating of food with creatine, such as meat, chicken, and fish.[23-25] Heterocyclic amines, estimated as consumption of well-done meat, have been associated with breast and colon cancer. Aflatoxins are suspected human liver carcinogens and are considered to be a major contributor to liver cancer in China and parts of Africa.[26] Urinary aflatoxin adduct levels vary among regions of the world, depending on dietary exposures, which are predictors of liver cancer risk, especially as an interaction with hepatitis B infection.

SMOKING AND OCCUPATIONAL EXPOSURES THAT CAN LEAD TO CANCER

PAHs are associated with an increased risk of lung and skin cancer.[6,27] Wide interindividual variation is seen in individuals for metabolizing PAHs such that some are more susceptible than others. Several methods are available for detecting PAH DNA adducts as well as measuring PAH metabolites in the urine. Aromatic amines are another class of human carcinogens.[28] Aryl aromatic amines have been implicated in bladder carcinogenesis, especially in occupationally exposed cohorts (e.g., dye workers) and tobacco smokers. The quantitative assessment using biomarkers has been more difficult, but some persons have studied DNA adducts as well.

Genetic Susceptibility

The determination of genetic susceptibility can be by phenotyping or genotyping. Phenotypes generally represent complex genotypes. The cancer risk from chemical carcinogen exposure related to heritability can range from small to large, depending on its penetrance, and the study of gene-environment interactions is complicated.[29,30] Highly penetrant cancer susceptibility genes cause familial cancers and account for fewer than 1% of all cancers. Low-penetrant genes cause common sporadic cancers, which have large public health consequences. A *genetic polymorphism* [e.g., single-nucleotide polymorphisms (SNPs)] is defined as a genetic variant present in at least 1% of the population. Table 8-2 lists several investigated genetic polymorphisms and their association with cancer risk. The focus of current research for genetic susceptibilities tends to focus on pathways leading to cancer. These include carcinogen metabolism, DNA repair, oxidative damage, and cell-cycle control.

Lung cancer has been the most extensively studied for gene-environment interactions.[31] Examples of frequently studied genetic polymorphisms in tobacco-related cancers that have been shown in some studies to modify smoking-related disease risk include the glutathione S-transferase M1 (*GSTM1*), cytochrome P-450 1A1 (*CYP1A1*) genes, glutathione S-transferase Pi, and those involved in DNA repair. These genetic polymorphisms, and others, are believed to affect biomarker levels, such as DNA adducts.

Breast cancer is clearly related to endogenous and exogenous estrogens, but these factors explain less than half of the excess risk, and genetic susceptibilities have been implicated.[32,33] For hormonal etiologies, it can be hypothesized that variation in

TABLE 8-2. Inherited Susceptibility Determinants for Human Cancer: Selected Examples

Gene	Examples of Substrate	Associated Cancer	Comments
METABOLIC ACTIVATION			
CYP1A1	Polycyclic aromatic hydrocarbons	Lung, breast, oral cavity	Different polymorphisms exist in different racial populations; several studies relate a functionally active polymorphism to lung cancer.
CYP2E1	N-nitrosamines, benzene, urethane, 1,3-butadiene	Lung	Different polymorphisms exist in different racial groups; functional polymorphisms exist.
CYP2A6	N-nitrosamines	Lung	Genotyping method available but technically difficult and may not be accurate. New polymorphisms associated with nicotine metabolism that controls smoking.
CYP3A4	Polycyclic aromatic hydrocarbons, aflatoxin	Breast	Phenotyping methods available; racial variation exists.
N-acetyltransferase-1	Aryl and heterocyclic aromatic amines	Bladder, oral cavity, colon	Phenotyping methods available; genotype may not correlate with phenotype; multiple variants exist with different and complex pathways for different substrates.
N-acetyltransferase-2	Aryl and heterocyclic aromatic amines	Bladder, colon, breast	Phenotyping methods available; multiple polymorphisms known; wide racial variation; polymorphisms can alter activity in both directions.
Epoxide hydrolase	Polycyclic aromatic hydrocarbons, aflatoxin	Liver, oral cavity, lung	Two variants known, each can affect activity; also considered a detoxification enzyme (aflatoxin).
CYP17	Estrogens	Breast	Related to age at menarche; might increase transcription.
CYP19	Estrogens	Breast	—
Catechol-methyl-transferase	Estrogens	Breast	Opposite results reported in literature.
Nitroquinone oxoreductase	Benzene	Leukemia	Functional polymorphism.
DETOXICATION ENZYMES			
Glutathione S-transferase M1	Polycyclic aromatic hydrocarbons, aromatic amines, others	Lung, breast	The polymorphism results in the deletion of the entire gene; other glutathione S-transferases also are important but are not polymorphic.
Glutathione S-transferase Pi	Polycyclic aromatic hydrocarbons	Lung, oral cavity	Phenotype questionable associated with genotype.
Alcohol dehydrogenase	Ethanol	Oral cavity, breast, liver	Two polymorphisms are known that determine detoxication of alcoholic beverages.
Aldehyde dehydrogenase	Acetaldehyde	Liver	Two separate polymorphisms are known that determine detoxication of alcoholic beverages.
Uradine diphosphate-glucuronosyl transferases	Aromatic amines, polycyclic aromatic hydrocarbons, phenols, steroids	Unknown	Interindividual variation known but appears to be unimodal.
REPLICATION/REPAIR			
O^6-alkyl-deoxyguanine-DNA-alkyl-transferase	N-nitrosamine–related damage	Lung	Wide interindividual variation exists.
HOGG1	Free radical damage	Lung	—
XRCC3	Recombination repair	Lung, breast	—
XPD	Excision repair	Lung, breast	—

estrogen metabolism by cytochrome P-450s (*CYP1A1*, *CYP1B1*, *CYP1A2*, and *CYP17*) and other genes can affect hormonal levels, resulting in altered cell proliferation or DNA damage and subsequent cancer risk.

The role for genetic determinants of carcinogen metabolism in cancer risk is established for other cancers. Some consistency is seen in the literature for bladder cancer, and other data exist for oropharyngeal and prostate cancer.[34,35]

Interest has been shown in determining if haplotypes that combine multiple SNP data are more predictive for cancer than studying individual SNPs. Haplotypes might be more representative for protein structure, for example. Using two to three SNPs might characterize the haplotype, and high-throughput genotyping makes this possible to do in epidemiologic studies.

TUMOR SUPPRESSOR GENES IN HUMAN CANCER

The study of mutations in human tumors and experimental models is elucidating important carcinogenic mechanisms. *In vitro* studies using prokaryotic and simple eukaryotic assays, including human cells (e.g., site-specific mutagenesis assays), indicate that human exposure to mutagens might result in a narrow spectrum of mutations that are nonrandom. Some carcinogenic agents produce a "fingerprint" of mutations, although, given that different chemicals may contribute to cancer as a gene[n]-environment[n] interaction, the mutational spectrum in cancers is typically broad. A fingerprint tends to be the exception rather than the rule. The study of mutations in the p53 tumor suppressor gene is uniquely suited for the study of cancer etiology, exposure, and susceptibility, because p53 is involved in many cellular processes, including maintenance of genomic stability, programmed cell death, DNA repair, and others. The p53 mutation frequency varies by organ site and histologic subtype,[36] indicating that cancers occur through different pathways and different exposures at the cellular level. Several examples of particular carcinogenic exposures are linked to cancers via a p53 mutational mechanism, especially the demonstration that ultraviolet light exposure and skin cancer are associated with cytosine-cytosine to thymine-thymine tandem transitions. Another example is dietary aflatoxin B_1 exposure and a consistent finding of mutations in the third nucleotide pair of codon 249 of liver cancers in regions with endemic exposure to aflatoxin B_1. An interactive effect of alcohol drinking and cigarette use in oral cavity cancers yields different types of p53 mutations.

Among the most exciting areas in molecular epidemiology is the potential ability to identify mutations and preneoplastic lesions before the development of cancer or as a diagnostic test for early cancer. Analyses of stool from patients with cancer have found cells with the same K-*ras* mutations present in the cancer.[37] Similar findings have been reported in sputum samples from head and neck cancers.[38] Analysis of codon 12 mutations in the K-*ras* gene of bronchoalveolar cells has shown a 33% rate of detection in cancer patients, with an acceptable specificity, and many of the positive samples were cytologically negative for cancer.[39] Archived sputum samples also have revealed mutations in K-*ras* that were later matched to a confirmed diagnosis of lung cancer.[40]

DNA methylation in gene promoter regions is an important regulator of gene expression. Hypermethylation is a common finding in breast, colon, lung, and other cancers. Overall, methylation is thought to be one of the most common molecular alterations in cancer. The p16 gene is a tumor suppressor gene whose protein is a cyclin-dependent kinase inhibitor that blocks the transcription of cell-cycle regulatory proteins. The p16 gene is more commonly methylated in normal lung cells of smokers and predicts the subsequent development of lung cancer.[41] A quantitative relation with smoking and hypermethylation has been variably reported, and the larger studies show a positive correlation (i.e., with pack-years, $P = .007$ in 185 subjects).[42]

TOBACCO SMOKING AND CANCER RISK

Tobacco smoking is the major cause of cancer and accounts for almost 96% of all male lung cancers in whites. Although the risk of lung cancer decreases after smoking cessation, it never returns to that for nonsmokers. Tobacco smoke contains more than 3500 chemicals, of which more than 20 are carcinogens. Specific chemicals in tobacco smoke include PAHs and N-nitrosamines, aromatic amines, ethylene oxide, 1,3-butadiene, and agents that cause oxyradical damage. PAHs and tobacco-specific nitrosamines are considered to be the most potent carcinogens in tobacco smoke. During the last 40 years, although the tar (which contains PAHs) and nicotine content has decreased approximately threefold, there also has been an increase of other carcinogens including tobacco-specific nitrosamines.[43] Today, light cigarettes dominate the market, and, until recently, it was believed that they were less harmful than regular cigarettes. However, because smokers must maintain their nicotine addiction, the smoking of lower-nicotine cigarettes results in having to smoke more (numbers of cigarettes per day and inhalation). Also, the chemical composition of the smoke is different for light and regular cigarettes, yielding more mutagenic tar and different mixtures of carcinogens. As a result, light cigarettes are not less harmful and are considered to be the reason why lung cancer histology has changed from squamous cell cancers to mostly peripheral adenocarcinomas.

Convincing laboratory animal and human studies have demonstrated a relationship between tobacco smoke constituents, carcinogen-DNA adduct formation, and cancer.[44] Several determinants of tobacco carcinogen exposure and cancer risk are known, including the number of cigarettes smoked per day, years smoked, cigarette type [e.g., tar content (the total dry particulate component of smoke)], and smoking topography (e.g., how much smoke enters the lung, measured by puff volume, number of puffs per cigarette, puff duration, and interpuff interval). However, wide interindividual variation for carcinogen metabolism and DNA adduct formation affects lung cancer risk. The evaluation of cancer risk has more recently focused on biomarkers that can be used to assess different levels of carcinogen exposure, but no single biomarker is sufficient for this.[20] Importantly, not all smokers have the same carcinogenic risks; lung cancer develops in only one in ten heavy smokers, and some heavy smokers live to their 90s. This is thought to be due to genetic polymorphisms relating to DNA carcinogen metabolism, DNA repair, and cell-cycle control.

REFERENCES

1. Wingo PA, Ries LA, Giovino GA, et al. Annual report to the nation on the status of cancer, 1973–1996, with a special section on lung cancer and tobacco smoking. *J Natl Cancer Inst* 1999;91:675.
2. Yuspa SH, Poirier MC. Chemical carcinogenesis: from animal models to molecular models in one decade. *Adv Cancer Res* 1988;50:25.
3. Weston A, Harris CC. Chemical carcinogenesis. In: Holland JF, Frei E, Bast R, et al., eds. *Cancer medicine*, 6th ed. Ontario: BC Decker, Inc., 2003:267.
4. Stanley LA. Molecular aspects of chemical carcinogenesis: the roles of oncogenes and tumour suppressor genes. *Toxicology* 1995;96:173.
5. Hanahan D, Weinberg RA. The hallmarks of cancer. *Cell* 2000;100:57.
6. Hecht SS. Tobacco smoke carcinogens and lung cancer. *J Natl Cancer Inst* 1999;91:1194.
7. Sporn MB, Suh N. Chemoprevention: an essential approach to controlling cancer. *Nat Rev Cancer* 2002;2:537.
8. U.S. Department of Health and Human Services, Public Health Service, National Toxicology Program. *Report on carcinogens*, 10th ed. World Wide Web URL: http://ehp.niehs.nih.gov/roc/toc10.html, 2004.
9. Dipple A. DNA adducts of chemical carcinogens. *Carcinogenesis* 1995;16:437.
10. Loeb LA, Loeb KR, Anderson JP. Multiple mutations and cancer. *Proc Natl Acad Sci U S A* 2003;100:776.
11. Lash LH, Hines RN, Gonzalez FJ, et al. Genetics and susceptibility to toxic chemicals: do you (or should you) know your genetic profile? *J Pharmacol Exp Ther* 2003;305:403.
12. Gulezian D, Jacobson-Kram D, McCullough CB, et al. Use of transgenic animals for carcinogenicity testing: considerations and implications for risk assessment. *Toxicol Pathol* 2000;28:482.
13. Yu Z, Chen J, Ford BN, et al. Human DNA repair systems: an overview. *Environ Mol Mutagen* 1999;33:3.
14. Edelmann W, Yang K, Umar A, et al. Mutation in the mismatch repair gene Msh6 causes cancer susceptibility. *Cell* 1997;91:467.
15. Demant P. Cancer susceptibility in the mouse: genetics, biology and implications for human cancer. *Nat Rev Genet* 2003;4:721.
16. Klatt P, Serrano M. Engineering cancer resistance in mice. *Carcinogenesis* 2003;24:817.
17. Hill AB. The environment and disease: association or causation. *Proc R Soc Med* 1965;58:295.
18. Perera FP. Molecular cancer epidemiology: a new tool in cancer prevention. *J Natl Cancer Inst* 1987;78:887.
19. Vineis P, Porta M. Causal thinking, biomarkers, and mechanisms of carcinogenesis. *J Clin Epidemiol* 1996;49:951.
20. Shields PG. Tobacco smoking, harm reduction, and biomarkers. *J Natl Cancer Inst* 2002;94:1435.
21. Veglia F, Matullo G, Vineis P. Bulky DNA adducts and risk of cancer: a meta-analysis. *Cancer Epidemiol Biomarkers Prev* 2003;12:157.
22. Goldman R, Shields PG. Food mutagens. *J Nutr* 2003;133[Suppl 3]:965S.
23. Ferguson LR. Natural and human-made mutagens and carcinogens in the human diet. *Toxicology* 2002;181–182:79.

24. Sugimura T. Food and cancer. *Toxicology* 2002;181:17.

25. Sinha R, Norat T. Meat cooking and cancer risk. *IARC Sci Publ* 2002;156:181.

26. Wild CP, Turner PC. The toxicology of aflatoxins as a basis for public health decisions. *Mutagenesis* 2002;17:471.

27. Phillips DH. Polycyclic aromatic hydrocarbons in the diet. *Mutat Res* 1999;443:139.

28. Vineis P, Pirastu R. Aromatic amines and cancer. *Cancer Causes Control* 1997;8:346.

29. Vineis P. The relationship between polymorphisms of xenobiotic metabolizing enzymes and susceptibility to cancer. *Toxicology* 2002;181:457.

30. Brennan P. Gene-environment interaction and a etiology of cancer: what does it mean and how can we measure it? *Carcinogenesis* 2002;23:381.

31. Shields PG. Molecular epidemiology of smoking and lung cancer. *Oncogene* 2002;21:6870.

32. Rebbeck TR. The contribution of inherited genotype to breast cancer. *Breast Cancer Res* 2002;4:85.

33. Mitrunen K, Hirvonen A. Molecular epidemiology of sporadic breast cancer. The role of polymorphic genes involved in oestrogen biosynthesis and metabolism. *Mutat Res* 2003;544:9.

34. Coughlin SS, Hall IJ. A review of genetic polymorphisms and prostate cancer risk. *Ann Epidemiol* 2002;12:182.

35. Sturgis EM, Wei Q. Genetic susceptibility—molecular epidemiology of head and neck cancer. *Curr Opin Oncol* 2002;14:310.

36. Greenblatt MS, Bennett WP, Hollstein M, et al. Mutations in the p53 tumor suppressor gene: clues to cancer etiology and molecular pathogenesis. *Cancer Res* 1994;54:4855.

37. Sidransky D, Tokino T, Hamilton SR, et al. Identification of ras oncogene mutations in the stool of patients with curable colorectal tumors. *Science* 1992;256:102.

38. Boyle JO, Mao L, Brennan JA, et al. Gene mutations in saliva as molecular markers for head and neck squamous cell carcinomas. *Am J Surg* 1994;168:429.

39. Mills NE, Fishman CL, Scholes J, et al. Detection of K-ras oncogene mutations in bronchoalveolar lavage fluid for lung cancer diagnosis. *J Natl Cancer Inst* 1995;87:1056.

40. Mao L, Hruban RH, Boyle JO, et al. Detection of oncogene mutations in sputum precedes diagnosis of lung cancer. *Cancer Res* 1994;54:1634.

41. Palmisano WA, Divine KK, Saccomanno G, et al. Predicting lung cancer by detecting aberrant promoter methylation in sputum. *Cancer Res* 2000;60:5954.

42. Kim DH, Nelson HH, Wiencke JK, et al. p16(INK4a) and histology-specific methylation of CpG islands by exposure to tobacco smoke in non-small cell lung cancer. *Cancer Res* 2001;61:3419.

43. Hoffmann D, Hoffmann I. The changing cigarette, 1950–1995. *J Toxicol Environ Health* 1997;50:307.

44. Shields PG, Harris CC. Cancer risk and low-penetrance susceptibility genes in gene-environment interactions. *J Clin Oncol* 2000;18:2309.

Graham A. Colditz
Laurie B. Fisher

CHAPTER **9**

Etiology of Cancer: Tobacco Use

Tobacco use is the leading preventable cause of death worldwide. In the United States alone, the use of tobacco, primarily in the form of cigarette smoking, causes over 440,000 deaths each year and is responsible for approximately 30% of all cancer-related deaths (Fig. 9-1).[1,2] Worldwide, the numbers are even more staggering. The World Health Organization estimates that in 1998 there were 4 million deaths worldwide linked to tobacco use.[3] By 2020, this number is expected to more than double.[4]

Smoking takes a toll on the health of not only individual smokers, but also those around them. Every year, approximately 40,000 deaths in the United States are caused by secondhand smoke, 1000 infant deaths are related to smoking during pregnancy, and a further 1000 deaths are caused by residential fires attributable to smoking. The devastation in loss of lives due to tobacco use is compounded by economic losses to society. In the United States, annual health-related costs attributed to smoking amount to $157 billion.[4]

This chapter discusses the health effects of smoking and the benefits of cessation as related to more than 20 types of cancer. Trends in smoking as well as disparities in smoking among special populations are described. Current issues of interest, including the effects of secondhand smoke and harm reduction, are explored. Finally, effective strategies to curb tobacco use are highlighted. The clinician plays a critical role in these strategies, not only in the patient setting but also as a member of his or her local community.

EFFECTS OF TOBACCO USE AND CESSATION ON CANCER RISK

The causal link between smoking and cancer was established as early as 1964, when the first Surgeon General's report on smoking and health was released.[5] At that time, data were available to sup-

port a causal link with only two cancers: lung cancer and laryngeal cancer. Since then, however, enough evidence has accrued that smoking is now known to cause eight cancers: bladder, esophageal, kidney, laryngeal, lung, oropharyngeal, pancreatic, and stomach cancers. In addition, the most recent literature on the topic provides sufficient evidence to implicate tobacco use as a probable cause of additional cancers, including acute leukemia, cervical cancer, colorectal cancer, and liver cancer. Smoking has also been identified as a probable cause of prostate cancer mortality, by increasing the risk of developing aggressive, deadly forms of the disease. Although few studies are currently available, smoking may also increase the risk of cancers of the adrenal gland, gallbladder, genitals, nasal cavity, and sinuses. Active smoking is not causally related to brain cancer, breast cancer, Hodgkin's lymphoma, ovarian cancer, skin cancers, soft tissue sarcomas, testicular cancer, or childhood cancers. Smoking has a small protective effect with regard to endometrial cancer. Using the criteria outlined by the World Cancer Research Fund and the American Institute of Cancer Research, Table 9-1 categorizes the epidemiologic associations between smoking and each type of cancer as either convincing, probable, possible, or unlikely.

Although never starting to smoke is the best approach to avoiding tobacco-related diseases, there are substantial health benefits for smokers who quit. The risk of most smoking-related cancers decreases within a few years of cessation.

BLADDER CANCER

Smoking is a well-known risk factor for bladder cancer, causing 30% of cases in women and 50% in men.[6] Overall, a strong dose-response relationship is seen, with risk increasing as duration and amount of smoking increase.[6] Moderate to heavy smokers tend to have two to five times the risk of nonsmokers.

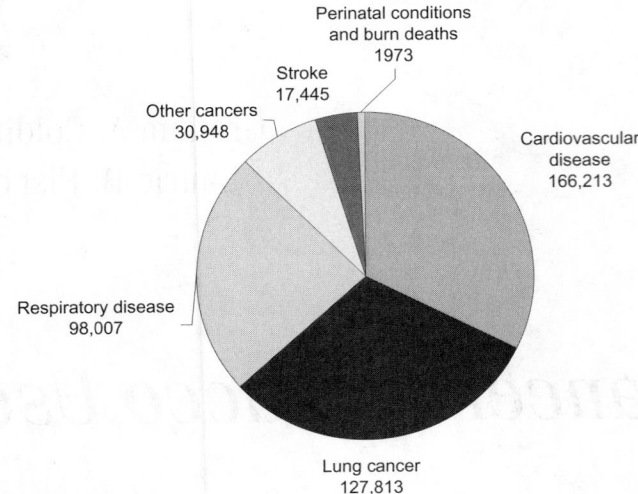

FIGURE 9-1. Tobacco-related mortality in the United States, 1995 to 1999. (Adapted from ref. 2.) (See Color Fig. 9-1 in the CD-ROM.)

The most likely causal pathway between tobacco use and bladder cancer is the exposure of bladder tissue to the carcinogenic by-products of tobacco metabolism found in urine.

Smoking cessation has been shown to lower the risk of bladder cancer in former smokers. In a pooled analysis of 11 case-control studies, the International Agency for Research on Cancer found that the risk of bladder cancer in former smokers compared with current smokers began to decrease almost immediately after cessation and continued to decline over time.[7] Although the risk never reached that of nonsmokers, it dropped 35% in the first 4 years after quitting—and 60% over the next 25 years.[7]

BREAST CANCER

Overall, the evidence does not support a link between active smoking and breast cancer risk.[8] Although a few studies have suggested that smoking at a young age or smoking for a long duration may increase the risk of breast cancer, these results have not been confirmed.[8]

CERVICAL CANCER

Studies have consistently found that smoking increases the risk of cervical cancer. Compared with nonsmokers, smokers appear to have approximately a fivefold increase in risk. However, a major challenge in studying smoking and cervical cancer is potential confounding by other risk factors, particularly infection with human papilloma virus, which is more common among smokers than nonsmokers. The extent to which smoking is a risk factor, independent of human papilloma virus infection, remains uncertain.[9]

Evidence points to a probable inverse association between smoking cessation and cervical cancer.[10] Taken collectively, the data suggest that former smokers experience a lower risk of cervical cancer than do current smokers.[11] The effect of the time since quitting on risk is unclear at present.

CHILDHOOD CANCERS

The weight of evidence does not support a link between parental smoking and childhood cancers in offspring. Neither parental smoking before conception nor smoking during pregnancy appear to increase risk for childhood leukemia, lymphoma, or brain tumors.[12]

COLORECTAL CANCER

Based on available epidemiologic evidence, it is likely that a positive association exists between long-term smoking and an increased risk of colorectal cancer incidence and mortality. Compared with never smoking, being a current smoker appears to increase the risk of death from colorectal cancer by 20% to 50% in men and 10% to 40% in women.[9] Risk of both incidence and mortality increases with number of years of smoking and younger age at initiation.[9] In addition, smoking is associated with an increased risk for adenomatous colorectal polyps in both men and women, with odds ratio estimates ranging between 1.5 and 3.8.[13]

Evidence suggests that smoking cessation can lower the risk of colorectal cancer mortality. Data from the Cancer Prevention Study II suggest that the risk of dying from the disease decreases with additional years since cessation and younger age at cessation.[14] Quitting smoking for 20 years or more appears to lower the risk of mortality to that of an individual who never smoked.[9]

ENDOMETRIAL CANCER

Endometrial cancer is the only type of cancer for which smoking reduces risk.[8] This is primarily because smokers tend to be

TABLE 9-1. Level of Evidence for a Causal Association between Smoking and Cancer

Convincing	*Probable*	*Possible*	*Unlikely*
Bladder cancer	Acute myeloid leukemia	Adrenal gland cancer	Acute lymphocytic leukemia
Esophageal cancer	Cervical cancer	Gallbladder cancer	Breast cancer
Kidney (renal) cancer	Colorectal cancer	Genital cancers	Childhood cancers
Laryngeal cancer	Liver cancer	Sinonasal cancers	Ovarian cancer
Lung cancer	Prostate cancer mortality	Thyroid cancer	Skin cancer
Oropharyngeal cancer			Testicular cancer
Pancreatic cancer			
Stomach cancer			

leaner and to have lower serum estrogen levels, both of which are associated with a lower risk of endometrial cancer.[8]

ESOPHAGEAL CANCER

Tobacco use is an established cause of esophageal cancer.[1] The rate of disease is seven times higher among current smokers than among nonsmokers. At particularly high risk are heavy smokers, whose rates of esophageal cancer are 15 times that of nonsmokers.[15] For those who quit smoking, the excess risk of esophageal cancer starts to drop significantly within 3 to 4 years of cessation.[16] The most likely causal pathway between tobacco use and cancer of the esophagus is direct contact with the carcinogens in tobacco and its smoke.

KIDNEY (RENAL) CANCER

Convincing evidence exists that smoking is causally associated with the development of renal cancer, including cancer of the renal pelvis. As reviewed in the 1989 report of the Surgeon General, the relative risk of kidney cancer for smokers compared with nonsmokers ranged from 1 to 5 and rose with the number of cigarettes smoked.[1] As with bladder cancer, the likely causal pathway is through exposure of renal tissue to the carcinogenic by-products of tobacco metabolism in urine.

There is good evidence that former smokers have a lower risk of renal cancer (including cancer of the renal pelvis) than do current smokers. The International Renal-Cell Cancer Study found that, after 15 years of cessation, former smokers had a 15% to 25% lower risk than did current smokers.[17] Moreover, evidence suggests that after more than 20 years of cessation, the risk of renal cell cancer in former smokers may be lowered to the level of those who never smoked.[18]

LARYNGEAL CANCER

Smoking is causally associated with laryngeal cancer incidence and mortality in both men and women.[1] The risk of death due to laryngeal cancer is 10 to 13 times higher among smokers than among nonsmokers and is exacerbated by heavy alcohol consumption.[1,8] In addition, a strong dose-response relationship exists, such that risk rises with increasing number of cigarettes smoked and increasing number of years of smoking.[1,8] Cancer of the larynx is most likely caused by direct contact between tissues of the larynx and the carcinogens contained in tobacco smoke. Numerous studies have demonstrated significant drops in risk for former smokers compared with current smokers. This decline in risk begins 3 to 4 years after cessation and risk decreases steadily thereafter.[16]

LEUKEMIA

Evidence suggests that smoking probably raises the risk of certain types of leukemia.[12] Smoking is most strongly associated with acute myeloid leukemia but has no effect on the incidence of acute lymphocytic leukemia or multiple myeloma.[8,9] Overall, smoking likely increases the risk of acute myeloid leukemia by 30% to 50%.[9] Several studies have found that heavier smokers are at greater risk of disease and that longer durations of use may further increase risk.[8] The chemical benzene, which is found in cigarette smoke, is one of the most likely causal links

between smoking and leukemia. In both human and animal studies, benzene has been shown to promote cancerous changes in white blood cells.[9]

There is limited evidence that smoking cessation decreases the risk of leukemia.[8] Inconsistencies in study results may be due to the varying effects of smoking on different types of leukemia.

LIVER CANCER

Although the current body of evidence is suggestive of a positive relationship between cigarette smoking and liver cancer, further study is needed to clarify this association.[8] Estimates vary from no increase in risk to a threefold increase in risk among smokers, compared with nonsmokers. The major challenge in inferring causation is that many studies on smoking and liver cancer have not adequately controlled for alcohol intake and hepatitis status, two key factors that can potentially confound the relationship. However, several studies that have examined risk among individuals with hepatitis B have found increases in the risk of liver cancer mortality. This suggests that smoking may indeed be an independent risk factor for liver cancer.[9] Many carcinogens found in tobacco smoke are metabolized in the liver, and this direct exposure to toxins may lead to the development of cancer.[9] In terms of cessation, there is growing but not convincing evidence that the risk of liver cancer is lower in former smokers than in current smokers.[8,11]

LUNG CANCER

Convincing epidemiologic evidence links smoking to an increased risk of lung cancer. Smoking is responsible for over 90% of lung cancer cases and is the strongest risk factor for the disease. Compared with nonsmokers, smokers have a 10- to 20-fold increase in risk, depending on smoking habits and duration of smoking. A positive dose-response relationship has been consistently observed with number of cigarettes smoked, deepness of inhalation, and duration of cigarette use.[1,8] Carcinogens in tobacco smoke interact with DNA and promote genetic mutations in the cells of the lung, leading to the development of cancer.[9]

Although smoking dramatically increases the risk of lung cancer, there is convincing evidence that cessation lessens much of the harmful effect.[11] Former smokers have a lower risk of lung cancer than do current smokers. Risk begins to decrease within 2 to 3 years after quitting and steadily declines for the next 10 years. Although risk will never return to that of a person who never smoked—and may remain elevated for up to 30 years after cessation—the risk is still dramatically lower than that of a current smoker.[19] Cessation is beneficial for nearly all smokers, regardless of gender, age, and level of habit. Those who quit smoking before middle age benefit the most, avoiding 90% of the excess risk of lung cancer linked to tobacco use. However, those who stop between ages 50 and 60 also benefit substantially.[20]

OROPHARYNGEAL CANCER

A strong causal link exists between smoking and cancers of the oral cavity and pharynx. The relative risk of oropharyngeal cancer associated with smoking ranges from 3 to 13, depending on amount and duration of cigarette use.[1] In addition, consumption of alcohol can greatly enhance this risk. Although smoking is an independent risk factor for oropharyngeal cancer, alcohol and tobacco use together are thought to account for approximately 75% of oral cancers in the United States.[21] The most likely causal pathway between tobacco use and these cancers is the direct contact of carcinogens with tissues of the oral cavity and pharynx.

There is convincing evidence that cessation reduces the smoking-related risk of oropharyngeal cancer. Former smokers have a lower risk of disease than do current smokers, and this risk decreases steadily with the number of years since cessation (after the first few years). Some studies have suggested that within 10 years of quitting, this risk might even return to that of a person who never smoked.[8] As with lung cancer, the younger the smoker at the time of cessation, the more the individual avoids the excess risk of oropharyngeal cancer associated with smoking.[22]

OVARIAN CANCER

The majority of studies have found no association between active smoking and ovarian cancer. Although there is some evidence that smoking may affect risk for certain histologic subtypes of ovarian cancer, data remain inconclusive.[9]

PANCREATIC CANCER

Epidemiologic evidence supports a causal association between smoking and pancreatic cancer. Overall, smokers are two to three times more likely to develop this disease than nonsmokers. The risk increases with increasing number of cigarettes smoked but declines with cessation.[23] A large prospective study in men found that risk dropped nearly 50% within 2 years of cessation. After fewer than 10 years, risk declined to approximately that of men who never smoked.[24]

PROSTATE CANCER

Studies on smoking and prostate cancer incidence have yielded inconsistent results such that a causal association does not appear likely.[12] However, a number of large, prospective cohort studies have documented a link between smoking and prostate cancer mortality, with some demonstrating a dose-response relationship with number of cigarettes smoked.[12] Cessation appears to reduce the excess risk of mortality associated with smoking. Studies suggest that within 10 years of cessation, a former smoker's risk of prostate cancer mortality returns to that of a nonsmoker.[25]

STOMACH CANCER

Since 1982, reports of the Surgeon General on smoking and health have documented a positive association between smoking and stomach cancer.[26] It is estimated that 11% of stomach cancers worldwide can be attributed to tobacco smoking.[27] Compared with nonsmokers, male smokers have an almost 60% increase in risk, and female smokers have an 11% increase in risk. A number of possible causal pathways exist between smoking and stomach cancer, including a link between smoking and *Helicobacter pylori* infection, a major risk factor for stomach cancer worldwide, as well as decreased serum levels of certain micronutrients that may help protect against the disease.[27]

A growing body of evidence supports a lower risk of stomach cancer in former versus current smokers.[27,28] As time since cessation increases, the risk of stomach cancer decreases. After approximately 20 years of cessation, risk approaches the level of a person who never smoked.[28]

THYROID CANCER

Smokers appear to have a slight reduction in risk of thyroid cancer compared with nonsmokers. Although the biologic mechanism of the effect of smoking and thyroid cancer remains unclear, the relationship may be due to lower levels of thyroid-stimulating hormone among smokers. Because thyroid cancer is more common among women and high estrogen levels may promote the disease, the association may be due to the antiestrogenic effect of smoking. It has further been hypothesized that nonsmoking women are more likely to be health conscious and are therefore more likely to be diagnosed with the disease.[8]

OTHER CANCERS

Current evidence suggests a possible link between smoking and cancers of the adrenal gland, gallbladder, and sinonasal cavity. Because these cancers are rare, however, there are few data on these associations. Plausible biologic mechanisms exist for gallbladder cancer and sinonasal cancer.[12] Smoking also appears to be related to genital cancers, including cancer of the penis and vulva. Both of these relationships may be confounded by human papilloma virus infection, and, therefore, further study is needed to clarify the strength and independence of these associations.[8] To date, research has shown no relationship between smoking and melanoma or smoking and testicular cancer.[12]

EFFECT OF TOBACCO USE ON CARDIOVASCULAR DISEASE

Smoking is a primary cause of cardiovascular disease (CVD), including coronary heart disease and stroke. Approximately one-third of all smoking-related deaths in the United States are due to CVD.[2] Smokers are 70% more likely than nonsmokers to develop CVD, and those who smoke two or more packs per day have a two- to threefold greater risk.[29] Fortunately, quitting smoking can greatly decrease many CVD risks. After only 1 year of cessation, the risk of coronary heart disease decreases by 25% to 50%. After 15 years, the relative risk of dying from a coronary event is approximately that of a person who never smoked.[16]

CIGARS, PIPES, AND SMOKELESS TOBACCO

Cigarette smoking is by far the preferred use of tobacco in the United States. However, a substantial number of people also use tobacco in pipes and in the form of cigars and smokeless tobacco. Like cigarette use, cigar use is more prevalent among younger adults aged 18 to 25 than among older adults. In 2002, 11% of young adults reported use of cigars during the previous month, compared with fewer than 5% of older adults.[30] Pipe use is not highly prevalent, with approximately 1% of adults

TABLE 9-2. Cigar Smoking and Risk of Cancer

Cancer	Relative Risk (95% Confidence Interval)
Lung	5.1 (4.0–6.6)
Oral cavity/pharynx	4.0 (1.5–10.3)
Larynx	10.3 (2.6–41.0)
Pancreas	2.7 (1.5–4.8)[a]
Bladder	3.6 (1.3–9.9)[a]

[a]Subset of cigar smokers who inhale.
(From ref. 31, with permission.)

and fewer than 1% of adolescents reporting use during the previous month in 2002.[30] Both pipe use and cigar use are more common among men than among women.[30]

Although cigar use is seemingly less dangerous and less addictive than cigarette use, an analysis of data from the American Cancer Society's Cancer Prevention Study II cohort found that current cigar smoking in men substantially increased the risk of lung, oral, and laryngeal cancers.[31] As detailed in Table 9-2, risks of pancreatic and bladder cancer were also significantly increased in current cigar smokers who inhaled. An analysis of the U.S. veterans cohort found that cigar and pipe use increased the risk of liver cancer approximately threefold.[32] Pipe smoking also increases the risk of oral cancer and lung cancer, although generally to a lesser degree than cigarette smoking.[1,5]

Although use of smokeless tobacco is fairly low nationwide (prevalence of less than 5%), it is quite common in certain subpopulations, especially among low-income, young adult men living in rural areas.[30,33] Past month chewing tobacco use among teens has remained fairly steady in the past decade, with 2001 rates at 8.2%.[34]

As reviewed in detail in the 1986 Surgeon General's report *The Health Consequences of Using Smokeless Tobacco*, there is convincing evidence that smokeless tobacco use causes cancer of the oral cavity.[35] Although data are less substantial, some evidence exists for a link with other cancers as well as with cardiovascular disease.[36]

SECONDHAND TOBACCO SMOKE

Categorized in 1992 as a known human carcinogen by the Environment Protection Agency, secondhand tobacco smoke poses significant threats to health. Numerous studies have found that secondhand smoke significantly increases the risk of lung cancer and is responsible for 3000 lung cancer deaths among nonsmokers each year. Secondhand smoke is also linked to other diseases, such as heart disease and respiratory illness in children. Children exposed to secondhand smoke are at increased risk of asthma, ear infections, hospitalizations for pneumonia, and other childhood illnesses.[37] Overall, secondhand smoke is responsible for 40,000 deaths annually in the United States.

NATIONAL TRENDS IN SMOKING PREVALENCE

Current smoking among U.S. adults has remained steady over the past decade. Once quite pronounced, the gender disparity in smoking rates is now relatively small and has been stable since 1990. In 2002, 25.7% of men were current smokers compared with 20.8% of women.[38] Although smoking rates among adults appear to be stable, smoking among certain populations is on the rise.

During the 1990s, an escalation in smoking behaviors among the young adult and college-aged populations prompted concern in the medical and public health communities.[39,40] Among smokers aged 35 years and older, smoking declined somewhat over this period, but among younger adults (aged 18 to 25 years), smoking rates rose to an alarming level.[38] After the tobacco industry was specifically prohibited from marketing to youth under provisions in the Master Settlement Agreement, the use of strategies targeting the college-aged population increased. Tobacco industry tactics such as promotions in bars and on college campuses appear to be contributing to the rise in smoking among this age group. Traditionally, almost 90% of adult smokers began smoking by age 18. However, young adults now appear to be at risk for initiating smoking after age 18.[38]

Smoking among adolescents is showing signs of declining. In 2001, 28.5% of U.S. high school students were defined as current smokers—that is, having smoked a cigarette in the previous 30 days.[34] This marked the first time in 10 years that adolescent smoking rates dipped below 30%.

Rates of smoking also vary with race and ethnicity. In 2001, the National Health Interview Survey found that Alaskan Natives and American Indians had the highest rates of smoking (36%), whereas Asians and Hispanics had the lowest (14% and 19%, respectively).[41] In that same year, approximately 24% of whites and approximately 23% of African Americans were current smokers.[41]

DISPARITIES IN ACTIVE TOBACCO USE AND CESSATION

Smoking rates are closely tied to measures of socioeconomic status, including income and education level. Across both gender and race, people of lower income are more likely to smoke than are people of higher income.[8,41] When education level is examined, women with only 9 to 11 years of education are found to be approximately three times more likely to smoke than are women with a college education.[8] The influence of low socioeconomic status on smoking is particularly apparent in vulnerable populations, such as pregnant women. The effect of socioeconomic status on smoking habits is not limited to adults. Adolescents who grow up in low-income households or who have parents with low levels of educational attainment are more likely to begin smoking.[8,42]

Occupation is strongly linked to rates of smoking as well, even after controlling for age, income, gender, and race or ethnicity.[43] The 1997 National Health Interview Survey found that the prevalence of cigarette smoking was 36.4% for blue-collar workers, 32.3% for service industry workers, 27.4% for farm workers, and 20.8% for white-collar workers.[43] Although such disparities have persisted for many years, data suggest that the gap in smoking rates between blue-collar workers and white-collar workers may be widening.[43]

As with active tobacco use, there are gender and racial disparities in smoking cessation. Women are less likely than men to quit smoking successfully. Women's concerns about weight gain associated with cessation and stress related to family care may contribute to this gender disparity.

CIGARETTE PRODUCT MODIFICATION— HARM REDUCTION

One of the most controversial topics in the realm of tobacco control is the concept of harm reduction. The development of less carcinogenic cigarettes is seen by some as an opportunity to offer a less toxic alternative to smokers who are not interested in quitting or are not able to quit with available cessation methods. For these smokers, a safer alternative might offer some health benefit. However, many believe that smokers who do want to quit will instead choose to smoke these products. Because no cigarette is safe or free of health consequences, smokers who use these products instead of quitting lose the health benefits of cessation.

TOBACCO AND NICOTINE ADDICTION

The 1988 Surgeon General's report concluded that nicotine was an addictive drug, similar to heroin and cocaine.[44] The cigarette is a highly effective drug delivery device, ingenuously engineered to deliver nicotine efficiently into the lungs, where it is absorbed into the blood stream and quickly reaches the brain. Once in the brain, it interacts with nicotine receptors and causes a variety of biochemical and electrocortical effects that affect the body's neuroendocrine systems.[44]

Physical addiction occurs quickly in most people and has proven extremely challenging to overcome. Although 70% of smokers wish to quit smoking, fewer than 10% are able to do so on their own.[45] Even with the aid of cessation treatment, the average smoker makes multiple attempts to quit before he or she is successful. Withdrawal can be severe and includes both physical and psychological symptoms such as cravings, depression, irritability, fatigue, sleeping difficulties, headache, and increased appetite.[16]

ROLE OF THE CLINICIAN

Physicians play a vital role in curbing tobacco use on an individual patient level as well as on the community level. Studies in primary care settings have found that providing even brief cessation counseling (3 minutes or less) can increase smoking cessation rates by 30%, and longer periods of counseling can increase these rates further.[46] Moreover, physicians have the opportunity to offer cessation advice to patients who smoke, because the majority of smokers visit a physician every year.[45] Being familiar with effective cessation methods is therefore important for clinicians. The U.S. Public Health Service issues clinical practice guidelines for the treatment of nicotine dependence. These guidelines include the 5 As: Ask (about smoking habits to identify smokers), Advise (smokers to quit), Assess (whether or not the patient is willing to make an attempt to quit), Assist (with designing and implementing a cessation plan), and Arrange (follow-up contact).[46] Implementation of an office-based chart system is a useful way to ensure that physicians are reminded to ask patients about smoking.[45]

TABLE 9-3. Effective Strategies for Tobacco Control

To reduce youth initiation of smoking and promote smoking cessation:
- Increase the price of tobacco products, particularly through increases in state and federal excise taxes.
- Develop mass media campaigns, especially when part of a comprehensive program.
- Reduce the cost of effective cessation treatment.
- Include telephone counseling as a component of community-wide cessation interventions.

To decrease the effects of secondhand smoke:
- Enact legislation restricting smoking in workplaces and general areas used by the public.

To assist with smoking cessation from a clinical perspective:
- Increase the screening of patients for tobacco use by promoting provider education and implementation of reminder systems.
- Deliver counseling for cessation.
- Recommend pharmacologic treatments (nicotine replacement and/or bupropion) as first-line therapies.

(Adapted from ref. 48.)

The Public Health Service recommends two primary forms of treatment for cessation: counseling and pharmaceutical therapy. Counseling sessions are offered in a variety of settings (one-on-one counseling, group sessions, telephone quit lines), all of which are effective in increasing cessation rates. Pharmaceutical treatments help alleviate the withdrawal symptoms associated with quitting. The most common form is nicotine replacement therapy (NRT). The U.S. Food and Drug Administration has approved NRT in five forms: gum, patch, inhalant, lozenge, and nasal spray.[47] The use of the antidepressant bupropion has also been shown to be an effective cessation aid. It can be used alone or in conjunction with NRT.[46] Although many forms of NRT are available over the counter, bupropion is available only by prescription at this time. When combined with counseling, both NRT and bupropion have been shown to double cessation rates among smokers.[45] Using these tools, physicians can influence healthy behavior change in smokers.

STRATEGIES FOR TOBACCO CONTROL

Although individual-level strategies are crucial to the well-being of smokers, community-level programs and policies are necessary to promote and protect the health of smokers and nonsmokers alike. A number of tobacco control strategies have been shown to be effective in promoting smoking prevention and cessation, as well as in reducing exposure to secondhand smoke. Summarized in Table 9-3, these include increased taxation of tobacco products, mass media antitobacco campaigns, reductions in costs of cessation treatments, and workplace smoking restrictions. As active supporters of programs and policies at the state and local levels, physicians can play an integral role in advancing tobacco control.

CONCLUSION

Tobacco use is the leading preventable cause of mortality worldwide. Although all forms of tobacco use are deleterious to health, cigarette smoking is the most widespread and causes the most harm. Cigarette smoking is causally related to many types of cancer, as well as cardiovascular disease, and many of these diseases exhibit a dose-response relationship. Cessation leads to significant reductions in both risk of incidence of disease and mortality for most types of cancer within a few years after cessation. Similar benefits are seen for cardiovascular disease.

Increasing evidence regarding the health hazards of secondhand smoke has emerged in the past several decades. Now causally linked to lung cancer, as well as other respiratory diseases in nonsmokers, secondhand smoke exposure has become a major health concern.

Smoking is of special concern among populations that appear to be particularly susceptible to initiation and continued use of cigarettes. Although smoking rates among older adults and adolescents in the United States appear to be decreasing or holding steady, smoking rates among young adults appear to be on the rise. Smoking rates remain high among those of low socioeconomic status and those employed in blue-collar professions and the service industry. Those at higher risk for smoking are often those who have difficulties accessing cessation treatments. Physicians are in a key position to offer counseling and pharmaceutical treatment to smokers of all ages, ethnicities, and socioeconomic status.

On a broader level, state and local tobacco control strategies are crucial to reducing both smoking and exposure to tobacco smoke. Cigarette taxation is the most effective way to reduce smoking in both adults and adolescents. Restricting smoking in workplaces and public areas not only can greatly reduce exposure to secondhand smoke but also can help mold social norms. A comprehensive tobacco control strategy at the state or community level can enhance individual-level strategies that prevent smoking initiation and promote cessation.

REFERENCES

1. US Department of Health and Human Services, Public Health Service, Centers for Disease Control and Prevention, Center for Chronic Disease Prevention and Health Promotion, Office on Smoking and Health. Reducing the health consequences of smoking: 25 years of progress. A report of the Surgeon General. Atlanta, GA,1989.
2. Centers for Disease Control and Prevention. Annual smoking attributable mortality, years of potential life lost and economic costs—United States, 1995–1999. *JAMA* 2002;287:2355.
3. World Health Organization. World health report 1999. Geneva, Switzerland: World Health Organization, 1999.
4. Murray C, Lopez A. Alternative projections of mortality and disability by cause 1990–2020: Global Burden of Disease Study. *Lancet* 1997;349:1498.
5. US Department of Health, Education, and Welfare, Public Health Service. Smoking and health: report of the Advisory Committee to the Surgeon General of the Public Health Service. Washington, DC, 1964.
6. Silverman, DT, Hartge P, Morrison AS, et al. Epidemiology of bladder cancer. *Hematol Oncol Clin North Am* 1992;6:1.
7. Brennan P, Bogillot O, Greiser E, et al. The contribution of cigarette smoking to bladder cancer in women (pooled European data). *Cancer Causes Control* 2001;12:411.
8. US Department of Health and Human Services, Public Health Service, Office of the Surgeon General, Centers for Disease Control and Prevention, National Center for Chronic Disease Prevention and Health Promotion, Office on Smoking and Health. Women and smoking: a report of the Surgeon General. Washington, DC, 2001.
9. US Department of Health and Human Services, Public Health Service, Office of the Surgeon General. The health consequences of tobacco use. A report of the Surgeon General *(in press)*.
10. Haverkos HW, Soon G, Steckley SL, et al. Cigarette smoking and cervical cancer: part I: a meta-analysis. *Biomed Pharmacother* 2003;57:67.
11. US Department of Health and Human Services, Center for Chronic Disease Prevention and Health Promotion, Office on Smoking and Health, United States Public Health Service, Office of the Surgeon General. Smoking and health: a national status report. A report to congress. Atlanta, GA: Centers for Disease Control and Prevention, 1990.
12. Kuper H, Boffetta P, Adami HO. Tobacco use and cancer causation: association by tumour type. *J Intern Med* 2002;252:206.
13. Giovannucci E, Martinez ME. Tobacco, colorectal cancer, and adenomas: a review of the evidence. *J Natl Cancer Inst* 1996;88:1717.
14. Chao A, Thun MJ, Jacobs EJ, et al. Cigarette smoking and colorectal cancer mortality in the cancer prevention study II. *J Natl Cancer Inst* 2000;92:1888.
15. Doll R, Peto R, Wheatley K, et al. Mortality in relation to smoking: 40 years' observations on male British doctors. *BMJ* 1994;309:901.
16. US Department of Health and Human Services, Public Health Service, Centers for Disease Control and Prevention, Center for Chronic Disease Prevention and Health Promotion, Office on Smoking and Health. The health benefits of smoking cessation: a report of the Surgeon General. Rockville, MD, 1990.
17. McLaughlin JK, Lindblad P, Mellemgaard A, et al. International Renal-Cell Cancer Study. I. Tobacco use. *Int J Cancer* 1995;60:194.
18. Parker AS, Cerhan JR, Janney CA, et al. Smoking cessation and renal cell carcinoma. *Ann Epidemiol* 2003;13:245.
19. Ebbert JO, Yang P, Vachon CM, et al. Lung cancer risk reduction after smoking cessation: observations from a prospective cohort of women. *J Clin Oncol* 2003;21:921.
20. Peto R, Darby S, Deo H, et al. Smoking, smoking cessation, and lung cancer in the UK since 1950: combination of national statistics with two case-control studies. *BMJ* 2000;321:323.
21. Blot WJ, McLaughlin JK, Winn DM, et al. Smoking and drinking in relation to oral and pharyngeal cancer. *Cancer Res* 1988;48:3282.
22. Blanchaert RH Jr. Oral and oral pharyngeal cancer: an update on incidence and epidemiology, identification, advances in treatment, and outcomes. *Compend Contin Educ Dent* 2002;23[Suppl 12]:25.
23. Andersson SO, Baron J, Bergstrom R, et al. Lifestyle factors and prostate cancer risk: a case-control study in Sweden. *Cancer Epidemiol Biomarkers Prev* 1996;5:509.
24. Fuchs CS, Colditz GA, Stampfer MJ, et al. A prospective study of cigarette smoking and the risk of pancreatic cancer. *Arch Intern Med* 1996;156;2255.
25. Giovannucci E, Rimm EB, Ascherio A, et al. Smoking and risk of total and fatal prostate cancer in United States health professionals. *Cancer Epidemiol Biomarkers Prev* 1999;8:277.
26. US Department of Health and Human Services, US Public Health Service, Office on Smoking and Health, Office of the Surgeon General, Office on Smoking and Health. The health consequences of smoking. Cancer: a report of the Surgeon General. Washington, DC, 1982.
27. Tredaniel J, Boffetta P, Buiatti E, et al. Tobacco smoking and gastric cancer: review and meta-analysis. *Int J Cancer* 1997;72:565.
28. Chao A, Thun MJ, Henley SJ, et al. Cigarette smoking, use of other tobacco products and stomach cancer mortality in US adults: The Cancer Prevention Study II. *Int J Cancer* 2002;101:380.
29. Hahn RA, Heath GW, Chang MH. Cardiovascular disease risk factors and preventive practices among adults—United States, 1994: a behavioral risk factor atlas. Behavioral Risk Factor Surveillance System State Coordinators. *MMWR CDC Surveill Summ* 1998;47:35.
30. Substance Abuse and Mental Health Services Administration. Results from the 2002 National Survey on Drug Use and Health: National Findings. Rockville, MD: Office of Applied Studies NHSDA, 2003.
31. Shapiro JA, Jacobs EJ, Thun MJ. Cigar smoking in men and risk of death from tobacco-related cancers. *J Natl Cancer Inst* 2000;92:333.
32. Hsing AW, McLaughlin JK, Hrubec Z, et al. Cigarette smoking and liver cancer among US veterans. *Cancer Causes Control* 1990;1:217.
33. Bell RA, Spangler JG, Quandt SA. Smokeless tobacco use among adults in the Southeast. *South Med J* 2000;93:456.
34. Centers for Disease Control and Prevention. Youth risk behavior surveillance system. World Wide Web URL: http://apps.nccd.cdc.gov/yrbss, 2003.
35. US Department of Health and Human Services, US Bureau of Maternal and Child Health and Resources Development, Office of Maternal and Child Health. The health consequences of using smokeless tobacco: a report of the Advisory Committee to the Surgeon General—1986. Bethesda, MD: United States Public Health Service, 1986.
36. Winn DM. Epidemiology of cancer and other systemic effects associated with the use of smokeless tobacco. *Adv Dent Res* 1997;11:313.
37. US Department of Health and Human Services, Public Health Service, Centers for Disease Control and Prevention, Center for Health Promotion and Education, Office on Smoking and Health. The health consequences of involuntary smoking: a report of the Surgeon General. Rockville, MD, 1986.
38. Centers for Disease Control and Prevention. Behavioral risk factor surveillance system. World Wide Web URL: http://apps.nccd.cdc.gov/brfss/, 2004.
39. Rigotti, NA, Lee JE, Wechsler H. US college students' use of tobacco products: results of a national survey. *JAMA* 2000;284:699.
40. Wechsler H, Rigotti NA, Gledhill-Hoyt J, et al. Increased levels of cigarette use among college students: a cause for national concern. *JAMA* 1998;280:1673.
41. Centers for Disease Control and Prevention. Cigarette smoking among adults—United States, 2000. *MMWR Morb Mortal Wkly Rep* 2002;51:642.
42. US Department of Health and Human Services, Public Health Service, Centers for Disease Control and Prevention, National Center for Chronic Disease Prevention and Health Promotion, Office on Smoking and Health. Preventing tobacco use among young people: a report of the Surgeon General. Atlanta, GA, 1994.
43. Centers for Disease Control and Prevention. Cigarette smoking among adults—United States, 1998. *MMWR Morb Mortal Wkly Rep* 2000;49:881.
44. US Department of Health and Human Services. Public Health Service, Centers for Disease Control and Prevention, Center for Health Promotion and Education, Office on Smoking and Health. The health consequences of smoking: nicotine addiction. A report of the Surgeon General. Rockville, MD, 1988.
45. Rigotti NA. Clinical practice. Treatment of tobacco use and dependence. *N Engl J Med* 2002;346:506.
46. US Public Health Service. Treating tobacco use and dependence. World Wide Web URL: http://www.surgeongeneral.gov/tobacco, 1994.
47. US Food and Drug Administration. CDER new and generic drug approvals: 1998–2003. World Wide Web URL: http://www.fda.gov, 2004.
48. Curry S, Byers T, Hewitt M, eds. *Institute of Medicine and National Research Council fulfilling the potential of cancer prevention and early detection.* Washington, DC: The National Academy Press, 2003.

Robert L. Ullrich

CHAPTER **10**

Etiology of Cancer: Physical Factors

Among the best-known and well-characterized carcinogens that are known from direct evidence to increase the risk of cancer in humans are physical agents, including ionizing radiation, ultraviolet (UV) light, and asbestos. For all these agents the evidence that exposure will increase the risk for cancer development is clear and unequivocal. Because their carcinogenic potential is well known, questions about these agents tend to focus on the degree of risk to humans as a function of exposure level or dose and on underlying mechanisms. The issue of risk as a function of exposure level or dose is not an academic exercise; rather it is an extremely important consideration in medicine for which the techniques using ionizing radiation are powerful tools in the diagnosis and treatment of a wide range of diseases. Risks from radiation exposures that result from the application of these medical procedures must be weighed against the potential or real benefits of the procedure. Although the doses to individuals are generally low, without knowledge of the relationship between radiation dose and subsequent cancer risk such decisions cannot be made with confidence. This risk-versus-benefit issue is exacerbated when procedures result in relatively large numbers of individuals being exposed. In this instance, although the risk to any particular individual might be low, because the numbers of individuals exposed is very large, the potential for significantly increasing the cancer risk in the population as a whole may be substantial. Mechanistic studies provide insight into potential risks at low levels of exposure, for which effects cannot be directly measured by epidemiologic studies and provide information on approaches to reducing or preventing the carcinogenic effects of these agents. Such studies are also helpful in identifying potential sensitive subpopulations. As will be seen, focusing on sensitive subpopulations is

helpful for reducing risks but has also been important in dissecting underlying mechanisms.

Exposures to ionizing radiation can come from natural and from human-made sources. We are continuously exposed to naturally occurring radioisotopes contained in soil, rocks, and plants and, as a result, in building materials. One of the greatest sources of naturally occurring radiation is radon. In addition, we are exposed to cosmic rays. The amount of exposure is related to where we live. At higher altitudes the amount of exposure from cosmic rays is higher than at sea level. The levels of this naturally occurring radiation, often referred to as *background radiation*, varies with altitude, geology, and the predominant type of materials used to construct homes and other materials. It is often not appreciated that the most significant human-made source of radiation exposure comes from medical procedures, including diagnostic imaging, nuclear medicine, and therapeutic procedures. On average, the dose to the general population from medical procedures is similar to that received from background radiation. However, the medical contribution to radiation exposure is rapidly increasing. This is a result of the wider application of more powerful imaging tools, such as helical computed tomography (CT) scans and the movement to the use of digital images rather than film and from the application of techniques such as intensity-modulated radiation therapy (IMRT).

UV light from the sun is responsible for an increasing number of skin cancers throughout the world. Risks for skin cancer vary with altitude, latitude, and pigmentation, all of which modify the dose of UV light delivered to target cells in the skin. The understanding of the underlying mechanisms of UV-induced skin cancer has benefited greatly from the identification and study of

201

individuals who are extremely sensitive to the effects of ionizing radiation. More recently, the development of genetically engineered mice with specific gene defects has also proved to be invaluable in the dissection of underlying mechanisms.

Although asbestos fibers have a chemical composition, they have generally been classified as a physical carcinogen because it is believed that their physical interactions with cells rather than specific chemical interactions are responsible for their carcinogenic effects. Asbestos is a naturally occurring mineral silicone that results from fibrous crystallization. Health effects, including lung cancer, are well documented from high occupational exposures from its commercial uses. More controversial and uncertain are the health effects at low levels to which the general public might be exposed.

INTERACTIONS OF RADIATION WITH CELLS AND TISSUES

Gamma rays, x-rays, and UV light are all part of the electromagnetic spectrum shown in Figure 10-1.[1] Their interactions with biologic material depend on the frequency or wavelength of the radiation. UV light and electromagnetic forms of ionizing radiation have the highest frequencies and energies. At the short wavelengths of x-rays and gamma rays, electromagnetic radiation has sufficient energy to produce ionizations as a result of removal of electrons from atoms. At the longer wavelengths including low-level electric and magnetic fields up to and including UV light, the energy deposition is insufficient to produce ionizations, and these forms of energy are generally referred to as *nonionizing radiations*.

IONIZING RADIATION

In addition to the electromagnetic forms of ionizing radiation (such as gamma rays and x-rays), there are particulate forms of ionizing radiation, including electrons, protons, α-particles, and neutrons. A full discussion of how these different radiations interact with matter is beyond the scope of this chapter, and the reader is referred to other books on this subject.[1,2] The spatial distribution of the ionizations produced by these different forms

of ionizing radiation provides an additional means of classification based on their interactions in matter including biologic material. This classification is of particular relevance to the biologic effects of the different forms of ionizing radiation. This spatial distribution of ionizations is measured as the energy transferred per unit track length [linear energy transfer (LET)] in units of kiloelectronvolt per millimeter. On this basis, x-rays, gamma rays, and electrons are classified as sparsely ionizing radiation, whereas α-particles (such as those associated with radon) and neutrons are densely ionizing. The density of the ionizing radiation can have a substantial impact on the biologic effects of the radiation exposure. These differences can be qualitative as well as quantitative. The quantitative differences are measured by comparing the dose of a test radiation (e.g., α-particles) to produce the same level of effect as a specific dose of x-rays (or sometimes gamma rays). The ratio of these doses is called the *relative biologic effectiveness* (RBE).[3] For cell-killing effects, RBE values for α-particles and neutrons have been found to be in the range of 3 to 5. An RBE for cell killing after irradiation with α-particles on the order of 5 would mean that an alpha dose of 1 Gy would result in the same level of cell killing as that produced by an x-ray dose of 5 Gy. For cancer induction, estimates for RBE values from experimental studies can be 20 or higher for α-particles and neutrons. RBE tends to increase as a function of LET to a maximum of approximately 100 keV/mm. At this LET, the average separation of ionizing events is approximately the diameter of the double helix, which would tend to maximize the probability that a single track of radiation can produce a double-strand break (DSB). Qualitative differences between high and low LET radiations are suggested by the observation that, for all effects examined (including cell killing, chromosome aberrations, mutation induction, and cancer induction), the radiation damage responsible for these effects appears to be less easily repaired by the cell or organism after exposure to high LET radiation.[3]

Energy deposited in biologic material can produce ionizations in target molecules, such as DNA, directly through production of ionizations in those molecules or indirectly through interactions with water molecules that result in the formation of free radicals. These free radicals then produce the damage to the DNA. Because ionizing events from low LET radiations are

Wavelength

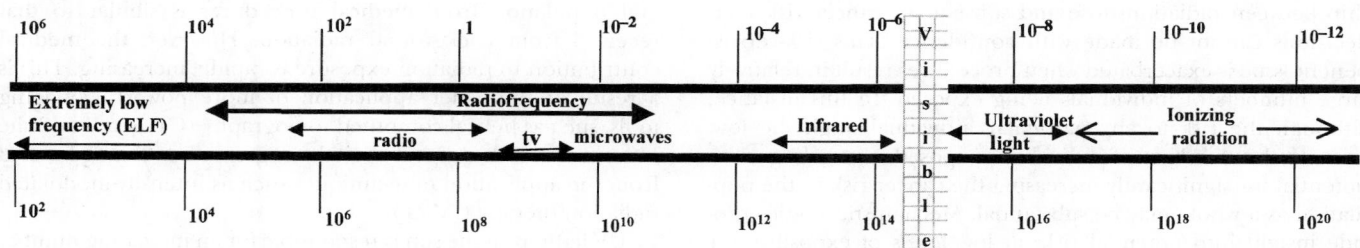

Frequency

FIGURE 10-1. Electromagnetic spectrum.

more sparsely distributed, damage to DNA and other targets is less likely to be a result of direct ionizations but rather is principally a result of indirect mechanisms mediated by free radicals. Because of the density of the ionizations, high LET effects are more generally mediated via direct effects on target molecules.

Whether these effects are directly or indirectly produced, ionizing radiation results in base damage and single-strand breaks and DSBs in DNA. As discussed earlier, for low LET radiation, these effects are mediated via reactive oxygen species much like those produced by normal cellular processes. The reason that ionizing radiations are able to cause the degree of damage that they do is because of the differences in spatial distribution of energy that result in a markedly different distribution of these reactive oxygen species than occurs during normal cellular processes. Exposure to ionizing radiation results in highly clustered ionization events. As such the damage produced by ionizing radiation either directly or indirectly is more complex, with localized areas of DNA molecules with multiple and complex lesions consisting of a combination of base damage and single-strand breaks and DSBs.[4–7] These complex lesions are less easily repaired with fidelity than are more simple forms of DNA damage.[8] For high LET radiations, because of the density of the ionizations, the molecular damage can be particularly complex and difficult to repair.

ULTRAVIOLET LIGHT

UV radiation does not have sufficient energy to produce ionizations. Rather, its effects are the result of molecular excitation after absorption of energy by the target molecule. UV light can be categorized into three types, based on wavelength: UVC with wavelengths ranging from 240 to 290 nm, UVB ranging from 290 to 320 nm, and UVA ranging from 320 to 400 nm. UVC is not in sunlight that reaches the earth because it is readily absorbed by the earth's atmosphere. It has proven to be useful, however, for a number of applications. It is produced by low-pressure mercury lamps commonly used for sterilization. Because the peak wavelength for these lamps (254 nm) is very close to the peak for absorption in DNA molecules (260 nm), it has been an important experimental tool in photobiology for studies of the effects of UV light on DNA. UVB, as is discussed later in Sunlight and Skin Cancer, appears to be primarily responsible for skin cancer induction after sunlight exposure. This appears to be a result of direct damage to DNA mediated by UVB.

The amount of UV light to which an individual or a population is exposed depends on many factors, including the ozone layer. Effects of UVB and UVC appear to be mediated via effects on DNA interactions that result in a number of molecular changes, the most prevalent of which are dimers between adjacent pyrimidines.[9] The most biologically important of these are the cyclobutane dimer and the 6-4 photoproduct. Although other products are produced, these two, especially the cyclobutane dimer, appear to play the major role in the mutagenic and carcinogenic effects of UVB.[10] UVA is not absorbed by the atmosphere and penetrates deeper into the skin than UVB. Because of its wavelength, DNA and proteins only weakly absorb UVA, but, interestingly, it has been shown to be carcinogenic. It is speculated that this carcinogenic effect is due to the production of reactive oxygen species through its interactions with target chromophores. These reactive oxygen species are then able to produce DNA damage indirectly.[11]

For UVC and UVB, the distribution of specific changes in genomic DNA depends on base sequence and secondary and tertiary genomic structure. For example, cytosine absorbs higher wavelengths of UV radiation than thymine. As a result, dimers containing cytosine are more readily formed after UVB radiation. Data have shown that methylation at specific sequences in the p53 molecule enhance formation of dimers in specific regions as well.[12] This results in mutations in p53 that are relatively specific for UV damage and that have been found to be relatively early events in certain forms of skin cancer.[10,13]

IONIZING RADIATION AND CANCER

Studies of Cancer in Exposed Human Populations

The benefits of ionizing radiation in the diagnosis and treatment of disease were recognized by the medical community very soon after the discovery of x-rays and radioactivity. Almost as quickly, the risks of exposure began to be recognized as well. The first cancers that were related to radiation exposure were skin cancers detected only a few years after the discovery of x-rays.[14,15] These cancers were the result of high skin doses received by early workers, who often used their hands to test the output of x-ray tubes. These cases were followed by cases of radiation-induced leukemias among radiologists and radioisotope workers. These early studies provided clear evidence that radiation exposure could result in the development of cancer in humans, but the extent of the risk as a function of dose was not known. Because these early cancers were a result of relatively high levels of exposures, it was thought that tissue injury was probably required to increase cancer risk. Potential risks at low doses were not appreciated. This began to change with the study of the Japanese survivors of the atomic bombs, the study of patient populations exposed to radiation for therapeutic and diagnostic procedures, and occupationally exposed populations such as radiologists, uranium miners, and nuclear industry workers.[16] A partial list of principal sources of information on cancer risks in humans after radiation exposure is shown in Table 10-1. Studies of such populations began in the

TABLE 10-1. Studies of Radiation-Exposed Populations

ATOMIC BOMB
Japanese survivors
OCCUPATIONAL EXPOSURES
Radiologists
Underground miners
Radium dial painters
Nuclear workers
Radiation technologists
MEDICAL EXPOSURES
Ankylosing spondylitis patients
Tinea capitis
Thymic enlargement
Benign breast disease
Benign gynecologic disease
Fluoroscopy during treatment for tuberculosis
Cervical cancer
Hodgkin's disease
Breast cancer
Childhood cancer

1950s and 1960s and continue today. Such studies have provided and continue to provide information on risks as a function of dose, organ and tissue sensitivity, and risk-modifying factors, such as age and genetic background.

The largest population studied and the one that continues to serve as the primary source for understanding risks for cancer development in humans after exposure to radiation are the populations in Hiroshima and Nagasaki, Japan, who survived the atomic bombings of these two cities.[16–18] The doses received were single acute exposures of a mixture of gamma rays and a small amount of neutrons to the entire body. Although the doses received to those very close to the bomb were quite large and often acutely lethal, the survivors of the bombings received a range of doses that has provided substantial information on the relationship between cancer risk and radiation dose. What is generally not appreciated is that the majority of the survivors were not exposed to very large radiation doses. The average dose received by survivors was less than 0.3 Sv. As a result, this population represents the major source of information for determining potential risks at low doses. It is also not appreciated that approximately half of the individuals, those who were children, adolescents, and young adults at the time of the bombing, are still alive today. As is discussed later in Tissue Sensitivity and Latent Period, because the latent period for the development of solid tumors is quite long, important information on solid cancer risks at low doses is just beginning to emerge from these studies. Although the study is not complete, ongoing analyses of this population have provided the majority of the information available on the risk of cancer in humans as a function of dose as well as insight into variations in tissue and organ sensitivity. Because the age distribution of the population was wide, including the old and very young (as well as children exposed *in utero*), this study is also an important source of information about the effects of age on risks and on the tumor latent period, that is, the time between exposure and the appearance of radiation-induced tumors.

Information about radiation cancer risks in humans has also come from the study of patient populations exposed to ionizing radiation as a result of therapeutic or diagnostic procedures.[16,19] The numbers of patients in each individual study are smaller, but the number of such studies is relatively large. Nevertheless, only a few have been useful for the quantification of risks as a function of dose. Because such populations generally receive localized exposures, these groups generally can provide information on risks in specific organs and tissues. Such populations have also provided insight into modifying factors such as age and genetic background. In the past, radiation was used to treat a variety of diseases and medical disorders, including enlarged thymus glands and tonsils, tinea capitis, ankylosing spondylitis, and peptic ulcers. Epidemiologic studies of these populations have provided information on radiation-induced leukemia, as well as thyroid, breast, and stomach cancers. In general, diagnostic procedures result in very low radiation doses; however, a few studies have provided evidence for increased cancer risks. In one of the most extensive studies, tuberculosis patients were subjected to multiple diagnostic fluoroscopies during the course of being treated for their tuberculosis. Although the individual doses were low, the large numbers of procedures resulted in the accumulation of relatively large total doses. In these studies, females have been shown to be at a significantly increased risk for breast cancer.

No increase in lung cancer risk was observed, although from the doses received it might have been expected. An increased risk of childhood cancer has also been attributed to diagnostic radiation exposures *in utero*.

As is the case for other carcinogenic agents, occupational exposures are a valuable source of information.[20,21] Studies of uranium miners and other underground miners have been a particularly important source of information on cancer risks associated with exposure to radon. The analysis of nuclear workers has also provided and will continue to provide an important source of information of risks after chronic prolonged exposure to ionizing radiation. Likewise, because a major source of exposure is from medical procedures, medical workers, including radiologists, technicians, and nurses, are being studied intensively.[22]

Tissue Sensitivity and Latent Period

Although ionizing radiation can, in theory, induce virtually any type of cancer, certain organs, tissues, and cell types are more sensitive than others.[16] Acute and chronic myelogenous leukemia are very sensitive to induction, as is acute lymphocytic leukemia, whereas no evidence indicates that chronic lymphocytic leukemia or Hodgkin's disease is induced after radiation exposure. Among solid cancers, cancers of the thyroid gland, female breast, and lung cancer are among the most sensitive. Evidence also suggests an increased risk for salivary gland tumors, colon cancer, stomach cancer, and cancers of the liver, ovary, bladder, esophagus, skin, and central nervous system. However, these sites do not appear to be as sensitive. Most skin cancers are basal cell carcinomas with less evidence for a dose-related increase in squamous cell carcinoma or malignant melanoma. Some evidence has been shown for an increased risk of malignant melanoma as a second cancer after high doses of radiation therapy, although it is not clear that this increase is directly attributable to the radiation exposure.[15] In general, bone sarcoma and other sarcomas require relatively high doses before a significant increase can be detected. No clear evidence exists for the induction of cancers of the pancreas, prostate, uterine cervix, and small intestine.

The period of time between radiation exposure and the appearance of a radiation-induced tumor is referred to as the *latent period*. The latent period for radiation-induced leukemias is generally shorter than that for the appearance of solid tumors.[16] Depending on dose, leukemias can begin to appear as early as 2 years after exposure, with a peak incidence occurring between 4 and 8 years after exposure. After this peak, the risk begins to decline toward baseline levels. This pattern would suggest that the increased risk for leukemia is mainly limited to a specific period of time after exposure and does not remain high over the entire lifetime of an individual exposed to ionizing radiation. Studies indicate a minimum latent period of 5 to 10 years for solid tumors. At low doses, solid cancers do not appear until 10 or more years after radiation exposure, and it is not unusual for the latent period to exceed 20 years. This latent period can be affected by age at time of irradiation, the dose, and a variety of host factors. For example, the appearance of radiation-induced breast cancer is relatively short for a woman exposed in her late twenties or early thirties, whereas it can be quite long for a prepubertal or adolescent girl. A close look at the relationship between age at exposure and time of appearance of solid cancers suggests that these radiation-induced cancers appear at a time when the natural incidence of these tumors is also rising. This suggests that host factors play a strong role in influencing the ultimate expression of radiation-initiated cells. These data have important implications for potential mechanisms of radiation-induced cancer and for risks at very low doses. On a more practical level, these very long latent periods, particularly for younger exposed individuals, should be remembered when assessing risks associated with specific treatment protocols. Because of the long latent period for solid tumors, the relationship between risk and time after irradiation is less certain than for radiation-induced leukemia. At present, it is considered prudent to assume that an increased risk for solid tumors remains elevated over the lifetime of the individual. As studies are able to examine risk in large populations over their entire lifetime, for example, when the population of the atomic bomb survivors has lived out their lives and the study is completed, this important question will be able to be answered with more confidence.

Dose-Response Relationships and Low-Dose Risks

LOW LINEAR ENERGY TRANSFER RADIATION. Understanding the relationship between cancer frequency or risk and radiation dose is fundamental for estimating risks at the low doses normally encountered by the general population and for which effects may not be able to be directly determined from experimental or epidemiologic studies. Accurate risk estimates at low doses are essential for regulating environmental and occupational exposures. Table 10-2 provides a list of dose levels for selected exposures to ionizing radiation. It is also required in decisions about medical uses of radiation when weighing the benefits of a procedure versus its risks. Three examples are worth noting in this regard. The first is the debate over the use of mammography as a general screen for breast cancer and the age at which screening should be initiated and practiced routinely. The question of whether the benefits of this screening approach to detect early breast cancers outweigh the risks for inducing new breast cancers depends on many complex issues, but central to this debate is the risk of breast cancer from the doses received. It is virtually impossible to measure directly the risks for induction of breast cancer at the low doses received as a result of a single mammographic procedure. Even the lifetime accumulated dose from this procedure is quite low and still below a dose at which risks for radiation-induced breast cancer can be directly determined with any level of confidence.

TABLE 10-2.   Approximate Mean Doses for Selected Exposures to Ionizing Radiation

Exposure	Mean Individual Dose (mSv)
Round-trip flight, New York to London	0.1
Single screening mammogram (breast dose)	3
Background dose due to natural radiation exposure	3/y
Pediatric computed tomography scan (stomach dose from abdominal scan)	25
Radiation worker exposure limit	20/y
Exposure on international space station	170/y

As a result estimates of risk and risk-benefit decisions must be based on models of dose-response relationships that allow estimates to be derived. The second, more recent example is for risks associated with pediatric CT scans. For this procedure, doses to individual children have been estimated to be 10 to 15 times those of a mammographic procedure, which put the doses in the range for which there is direct evidence of an increased risk of cancer.[16,23] Because of the rapidly increasing use of CT scans in pediatric medicine and the known higher sensitivity to radiation-induced cancer in children (see Modifiers of Risk, later in this chapter), studies were conducted to assess the potential risks involved. These studies have suggested a significant number of new cancers attributable to this procedure. Although these studies have been controversial, they have stimulated a more careful examination of pediatric doses resulting from CT scans and have motivated radiologists to consider approaches to reducing numbers of procedures and individual doses received by pediatric patients. Although the mammography issue is focused on individual risk-versus-benefit concerns, the impetus for the pediatric CT debate was not motivated by concerns over individual risk-versus-benefit considerations but rather by a public health perspective when considering long-term population-based risks. In this regard it is worth noting that an epidemiologic study has suggested a small but significant increase in risk for leukemia associated with two or more pediatric CT scans. A third example is not related to low-dose risks from diagnostic procedures but applies to potential risks of second cancers after radiation therapy. The key question here is related to the shape of the dose response after high total doses of radiation, where there is as much uncertainty as there is in the low-dose range with respect to what the risks might be. This is discussed in more detail in Second Cancers after Radiation Therapy, later in this chapter.[24]

From theoretic models of radiation interactions at the cellular and molecular levels, and from experimental and epidemiologic studies, two dose-response models are most prominent: the linear model and the linear-quadratic model.[2,16,18,24] As suggested by its name, the linear model cancer risk is directly proportional to radiation dose (incidence = αD). With the linear-quadratic model, risk at low dose is proportional to dose, whereas at higher dose, the risk increases more rapidly as a function of the square of the dose (incidence = $\alpha D + \beta D^2$). The linear-quadratic model is based on biophysical theories of radiation action and is compatible with results from laboratory studies examining the dose response for a variety of end points relevant to the etiology of cancer, including induction of chromosome aberrations and induction of cancer in laboratory animals.[2,16,24,25] For this model the βD^2 component represents effects produced by multiple ionization tracks, whereas the αD component represents effects produced by single ionization tracks. For sparsely ionizing low LET radiation at low doses, the probability is that only a few ionization tracks will traverse a cell (at very low doses, perhaps only one). Therefore, any effects observed, such as a DSB or a chromosome aberration, must be a result of such single tracks. At higher doses effects would be a result of the interaction of multiple events occurring in close proximity. Because the probability of inducing complex damage such as a chromosome aberration is more likely with multiple events in close proximity, the dose response would be predicted to rise more rapidly than at low doses.

Irrespective of the model, the prediction at low doses is that the dose response is linear. This prediction implies that any dose of radiation has a probability of inducing molecular damage that may be of significance for transforming a normal cell into a cell with the capability of progressing into a cancer cell. On this basis, any dose would be expected to result in an increase in cancer risk. Some argument about this assumption has been raised at very low doses because of the repair and damage response capabilities of cells and the potential for eliminating radiation-altered cells through apoptotic mechanisms.[26] However, current understanding of mechanisms of cancer induction by ionizing radiation, discussed later in Mechanisms of Radiation-Induced Cancer, would tend to support the view that any dose of radiation confers some degree of risk.

Both models also suggest that at low total doses, for example, in the range of 200 mGy or less, multiple low-dose exposures should be additive and risks would be equivalent whether the dose was received all at once or accumulated over a long period of time. At doses of 2 to 3 Gy, the linear quadratic model would predict differences in risks depending on the time over which the total dose was received.[2,27] Single acute exposures would result in the highest risk, because such doses would be in the region of the dose response where the βD^2 component predominates. Fractionating the exposure or delivering the dose over a long period of time at low-dose rates would result in a reduction of the βD^2 component (because the likelihood of the interaction of 2 track events would be low when the dose is delivered over a long period of time) and a more linear dose response over a wider range of doses. As a result, the cancer-inducing effects of a radiation dose of 2 to 3 Gy or higher delivered as a fractionated or low-dose rate exposure would be less than that observed if the dose were delivered all at once.[25,27,28] Linear models would predict no such reduction in risks in this dose range irrespective of the time over which the dose was received. Experimental studies indicate that the prediction of the linear-quadratic model of reduced effects after fractionation in the moderate- to high-dose range is generally true. Carcinogenic risks after low-dose rate or fractionated exposures after total doses in the range of 2 to 3 Gy or higher are lower than after single acute exposures by a factor of 2 to 3. This difference in effects depending on time over which the dose is received is called the *dose rate reduction factor* (DREF).[16,25] Limited epidemiologic studies also provide evidence for a reduced effect when doses are accumulated over a long period of time rather than delivered as a single acute exposure. A report of cancer risk in radiologists, exposed for 40 or more years, indicated a cancer risk at least two times lower than that for A-bomb survivors.[22] Experimental and epidemiologic studies indicate that the DREF is dependent on type of cancer. Studies suggest a clear reduction in risk for leukemia after fractionated or protracted exposures. However, studies comparing cancer risks in the tuberculosis fluoroscopy patients who received multiple low-dose fractions to A-bomb survivors suggest a reduced risk for lung cancer but no reduction in risk for breast cancer.[29] Although this issue has been an area of considerable debate over many years, it is fast becoming less important with respect to low-dose risks. Arguments in the past have focused on the need to take this reduction factor of 2 to 3 into account when extrapolating epidemiologic data down to low doses for risk estimation for two closely linked reasons: First, data in the 2- to 3-Gy dose range or even higher predominated in epidemiologic data. Second, most estimates relied heavily on data derived from the A-bomb survivor studies, for which exposures were all instantaneous. Because of these two factors, it has been argued that the predicted reduced effects in the 2- to 3-Gy dose range when doses were protracted over a period of time should be

taken into account when extrapolating to low-dose risks. However, epidemiologic data are now sufficiently precise in the 0.10- to 1.0-Gy dose range to make direct estimates of risk.[18] Irrespective of the overall shape of the dose response, it is generally agreed that over this dose range a linear dose response should predominate and effects should be relatively dose rate independent. As a result, many of the arguments regarding extrapolation from high doses now appear moot. These dose rate and fractionation effects are quite real; however, at moderate to high total doses they are clearly important when considering risks from second cancers after radiation therapy. Based on linear extrapolations current estimates of risk in the general population are 10% per Sv for acute exposures. Application of a DREF of 2 has generally been applied for exposures that are received over a long period of time, resulting in estimate of risk of 5% per Sv under these circumstances. This means that the risk of developing cancer is increased by 10% over the normal risk after receiving a single acute exposure of 1 Sv. If the risk of developing cancer were 10% over an individual's lifetime, that risk would be increased to 11% after exposure to a single dose of 1 Gy.

Until recently, most of the emphasis on studies of dose-response relationships has focused on risks at low to moderate doses of ionizing radiation. At high doses (greater than approximately 4 Gy), it has been assumed that the risk would decline because of killing of target cells. A close look at this assumption suggests that this is not the case, at least with regard to solid cancers. Rather, the dose response appears to peak and then plateau over a wide dose range. In other words, at high total doses the risk appears to be constant over a wide range of total doses. The shape of the dose response at these high total doses becomes an issue when considering risks of second cancers after radiation therapy. If the dose response tends to bend over and decrease as a function of dose at high total doses, the risk of second cancers might be expected to be relatively low. On the other hand, if the risk remains constant, risk would be predicted to be higher than presently predicted and be highly dependent on volume of tissue irradiated.[24]

HIGH LINEAR ENERGY TRANSFER RADIATION. For densely ionizing radiation, ionization tracks through an individual cell are few but the density of the ionization is sufficient to produce complex effects with a high probability with single tracks. As a result the dose response is predicted to be linear (because of the single-track nature of the events) with a steeper slope (because of the higher effectiveness of the radiation for inducing such effects).[2] A further prediction is that there would be no difference in effects when the dose is fractionated or protracted. Experimental evidence tends to support these predictions. Studies of fission spectrum neutrons with an average LET in the range of approximately 100 keV/mm have found linear dose responses for the induction of leukemia and a variety of solid tumors over the range of 0.02 to 0.50 Gy. At higher doses, the response tends to plateau (again, not decline). Fractionating the exposure or reducing the dose rate in general has little effect on cancer risks over the 0.02- to 0.50-Gy dose range. However, at higher total doses the risks tend to remain linear over a wider dose range and do not plateau. This results in a greater risk after fractionation at doses greater than approximately 0.5 Gy. This has been termed an *inverse dose rate effect.* Comparing the low-dose linear portions of the dose-response relationships for cancer induction after exposure to neutrons or gamma rays, one can obtain estimates of the RBE of these neutrons with respect to cancer induction. Such analyses suggest RBE values in the range of 20 to 40, although higher values have been reported.[25,31]

The major source of exposure to high LET radiation for the general population is from exposure to radon.[20] Radon is a gas that comes from naturally occurring rocks and soil. As a gas, it is able to flow from these rocks and soil into the air, and because of this, underground mines, especially uranium mines, often contain high levels of radon. Homes in many areas of the world also contain measurable levels of radon because of the makeup of the rocks and soil in the area. Radon, although radioactive, is chemically inert and uncharged. The spontaneous decay of radon results in radon progeny that are also radioactive but electrically charged. These charged particles attach to dust particles and, when inhaled, can deposit in the lung, where decay of the progeny results in irradiation of the lung with α-particles.

Studies of underground miners exposed to high levels of radon have clearly demonstrated an increased risk for lung cancer. The risk is specific for lung cancer, and no increase has been observed for leukemia or other solid cancers. These studies suggest a linear dose-response relationship between lung cancer risk and radon exposure, but there is a clear indication of an inverse dose rate effect in these miners if the relatively high doses they receive are protracted. Risks at the lower doses received from radon in homes has been more controversial, but analyses have provided clear evidence for such risks and appear to confirm that the exposure response relationship derived for underground miner studies adequately predicts risks at low radon levels as well. All of these risks are complicated by the overwhelming risk associated with smoking that must be taken into account in many study groups. On the basis of estimates from miners and studies of risks in homes, it is estimated that 10% to 15% of lung cancer cases in the U.S. population may be attributable to radon.

Of interest with respect to radon risks have been studies of so-called bystander effects in cells after low-dose exposures of high LET radiation.[18] In the bystander effect, cells directly hit by radiation, such as an α-particle, send out signals to neighboring cells not directly hit by the radiation. These signals have been shown to result in cryptogenic, mutagenic, and oncogenic damage to these nonirradiated cells. This only applies at very low doses at which all cells are not directly hit by an α-particle. At higher doses the effect is not applicable because all cells are irradiated. Because the target for effects is increased to include not just irradiated cells but also a portion of the adjacent cells, the dose response for effects such as cytogenetic, mutagenic, and oncogenic effects is steeper at low doses than at higher total doses. These effects have been extensively demonstrated experimentally for α-particles and have important implications for low-dose risks for radon and other high LET radiations. The relevance of the bystander effects with respect to low-dose risks for low LET radiations is not clear.

Modifiers of Risk

AGE. The age at the time of exposure has a significant impact on susceptibility to radiation-induced cancer.[16] Increased risks for thyroid cancer are primarily found after exposure of children to radiation, whereas the risk in adults is small if not negligible. For breast cancer, young children and adolescents are at

the highest risk. Although still increased, risks are lower for young adult women in their twenties and thirties compared with younger individuals. For women over the age of 45 to 50 years of age, radiation appears to have little influence on risk. Although not as dramatic, risks for induction of acute leukemia, colon cancer, cancer of the central nervous system, and skin cancer are all greater if the exposure occurs earlier in life. Estimates of overall cancer risks would suggest that young children may be 10 to 15 times as sensitive as middle-aged adults.[24]

Reports in the mid-1950s suggested for the first time an increased risk of childhood leukemia and all childhood cancers as a result of *in utero* exposures from diagnostic procedures. Initial concerns of a selection bias that might have resulted in more *in utero* exposures for children at risk of childhood leukemia because of an underlying medical problem that was the actual risk factor were essentially dispelled by confirmation of these results in a study of twins in which such a selection bias could be minimized. It is now generally accepted that an increased risk exists for childhood cancers of approximately 6% per Sv from *in utero* exposures.[32,33] Whether the cancer risk for exposed individuals remains elevated throughout life and results in increased risks for solid tumors in adults remains to be determined. The reason this has yet to be determined is because of the long latent periods for solid tumors discussed earlier in Tissue Sensitivity and Latent Period. Individuals exposed in the late 1940s and 1950s are only now at the age when solid cancers are beginning to develop and potential increased risks can be determined.

GENETIC SUSCEPTIBILITY AND RADIATION-INDUCED CANCER. It has been recognized for many years that there are individuals within the population who have a higher risk for spontaneous cancer. Studies of these individuals and their families have led to the discovery of a number of genes involved in heritable susceptibility to specific cancers and also provided substantial insight into the pathogenesis of cancer in general. In individuals with such susceptibilities, the probability of developing a specific tumor during their lifetime can exceed 50%, and in some instances the probability is higher.[34,35] Fortunately, mutations so markedly affecting cancer susceptibility are relatively rare. Currently, known high-penetrance genes appear to account for approximately 5% of the total cancers in the population. A major area of uncertainty and increasing interest is the potential impact of low-penetrance mutations or polymorphisms that are likely to be much more common in the general population. The existence of such functional polymorphisms and their impact are difficult to detect using conventional epidemiologic approaches. However, experimental studies in animal models and human cells have provided evidence for their existence and implicated a potential role in radiation-induced cancer. On the basis of known mechanisms of radiation-induced damage and cancer development, it would be predicted that alterations in genes associated with repair of DSBs and those associated with increased sensitivity to chromosome aberrations would be high on the list of potential candidates.

Most information from human exposures to radiation on susceptibility genes and radiation risks has come from studies of second cancers after radiation therapy. Studies have demonstrated increased risks for radiation-induced osteosarcoma and soft tissue sarcoma in patients with the hereditary form of retinoblastoma.[36] Studies of patients with basal cell nevus carcinoma syndrome have been found to be at an increased risk for basal cell carcinoma and ovarian tumors in the irradiated field.[37] In addition, patients with Li-Fraumeni syndrome appear to be at an increased risk for radiation-induced cancer.[38,39] In each instance these patients have defects in genes known to be tumor suppressor genes, the retinoblastoma gene, the human homologue of the patched gene (PTCH), and the p53 gene, respectively. Similarly, studies in murine models heterozygous for deficiencies in Tp53, *ptch*, and apc also are at an increased risk for radiation-induced cancer.[40–42] The human and mouse data support the view that germline mutations in tumor suppressor genes not only increase the risk for spontaneous cancers but also increase the risks for radiation-induced cancers. This increased radiation sensitivity appears to be generally a result of large deletions in the normal wild-type allele of the tumor suppressor gene.

It has been proposed that defects in the gene involved in the disease ataxia-telangiectasia may also confer sensitivity for radiation-induced cancer, particularly breast cancer.[43,44] Ataxia-telangiectasia is a recessively inherited syndrome that results in hypersensitivity to acute radiation effects, such as cell killing, because of mutations or deletions in the ATM gene. This gene is a critical component of the DNA damage signaling and response pathway. Patients homozygous for defects in this gene are at a much higher risk for the development of cancer and are also at an increased risk for cancer after radiation exposure. What are more uncertain are the risks in individuals who are heterozygous for mutated forms of ATM. The sensitivity of these individuals for acute effects is generally considered to be in the normal range. Numerous epidemiologic studies have been performed with no definitive overall conclusions. Some studies have found an association between ATM heterozygotes and increased cancer risk, whereas others have not. Animal studies, using mice containing specific mutated forms of ATM that have been observed at a higher frequency in breast cancer patients, suggest a reason for the disparity of results.[44] Data from this study would suggest that particular subsets of mutations are likely to increase the risk of breast cancer, whereas other mutations, particularly truncation mutations, are not. It appears that critical mutations involve the activation of protein product of the ATM gene into a dominant negative form that specifically acts on critical kinase activities of the protein product of the ATM gene, whereas truncation mutations have no such effect on normal activity. Critical tests of this hypothesis are currently under way.

Second Cancers after Radiation Therapy

As the treatment of cancer has improved, long-term survivors have begun to develop second cancers as a result of treatment. Given the long latent period for the development of solid tumors after radiation exposure (often 10 years or more), it is only recently that there are sufficient numbers of individuals living long enough to develop a second cancer. The study of such populations can provide information on the nature of potential risks and suggest new approaches to treatment that may reduce such risks. A number of studies have now been reported on risks of second cancers arising after treatment for childhood cancer, cervical cancer, Hodgkin's disease, and breast cancer. Data are also available regarding risks of second cancers after whole body irradiation for bone marrow transplants. After radiation therapy two types of second cancer risks must be considered: first, the development of sarcomas in, or adjacent to, the heavily irradiated treatment field; second, the development of carcinomas in tissues and organs at a distance from the treatment site. Sarcomas are rarely seen in studies at low doses. It is not likely that this is because the target cells are particularly resistant to the oncogenic effects of ionizing radiation. Rather, it has been speculated that large doses are required for the induction of sarcomas because tissue injury is necessary to stimulate proliferation of radiation-initiated cells.

Obtaining reliable estimates of risks for cancer induction, particularly carcinomas, is difficult because of statistical problems of sample size that normally hamper studies limited to experience at a single institution and because of potential complicating factors of lifestyle or genetic predisposition that could have been associated with their first tumor. Two large studies of second cancers after radiation therapy are both statistically adequate to examine second cancer risks and appear to control for potential confounding factors. In both cases, adequate surgical control groups were available to facilitate analyses.

The first study examined the development of second cancers in patients with cervical cancer treated with high doses of ionizing radiation.[45] Although small, increased risks were detected for leukemia and for a few solid cancers compared to nonirradiated surgically treated controls. It was speculated that the small increased risk for leukemia was related to the fact that the dose to the majority of potential target cells in bone marrow away from the high-dose area was relatively small and the dose to any target cells within the treatment field was likely sufficiently high to result in cell killing. The authors were, in fact, able to construct a dose response for leukemia induction that rose linearly up to approximately 4 Gy and then began to decline. A minimum latent period for leukemia of approximately 2 years was seen, and the risk remained elevated for up to 15 years. At very high doses, in addition to an increased risk for sarcomas, increased risks for the development of cancer of the bladder, rectum, bone, and vagina were observed. Away from the treatment area, an increased risk for cancers of the stomach was observed as a result of scatter of approximately 1 Gy.

The second large study examined second cancers after radiotherapy of the prostate.[46] In this study, using the National Cancer Institute's Surveillance, Epidemiology, and End Results program, the investigators reported that the risk of a second solid cancer developing was significantly elevated in patients receiving radiation therapy compared to matched controls treated with surgery alone. This risk increases with time after treatment up through at least 10 years after treatment. The most dramatic increases in risk were for sarcomas and cancers of the bladder and rectum.

Several studies have reported increased risk for breast cancer in the contralateral breast after radiation treatment for breast cancer.[47,48] These studies are made difficult because of the clear increased risk for the development of breast cancer in the contralateral breast in women with breast cancer in general. Despite this potential confounding factor, in women under age 45 at the time of treatment, the risk was elevated to a similar extent as that predicted from A-bomb survivor studies. Significantly, for women older than 45 at the time of treatment, no increased risk was observed. In addition to breast cancer, an increased risk for lung cancer in all age groups was reported.[49]

In long-term survivors of Hodgkin's disease, the risk of leukemia appears mainly to be associated with the use of alkylating agents.[19] Radiation in combination with chemotherapy does not appear to increase the risk for development of leukemia over that associated with chemotherapy alone. Studies of solid cancers, however, indicate increased risks for a number of solid cancers, including cancers of the breast, thyroid, stomach, bone, and skin. As would be expected, the risk of developing second cancers of the breast is particularly pronounced in women treated at young ages. The relative risk for women treated when they were younger than 15 years is 136. For those treated between the ages of 15 and 24, the relative risk is 19; for ages 25 to 29, a relative risk of 7.3 has been reported. Women treated at older ages did not appear to be at an increased risk.[19,50–52] It is also important to note that the time between treatment and disease onset was long. The risk was higher at times beyond 15 years after treatment than before 15 years. An excess risk for lung cancer has also been reported. Unlike breast, lung cancers have been reported as early as 5 years after treatment. As might be expected, a strong interaction between smoking and radiation with respect to lung cancer risk has been seen.[53,54] An increased risk for thyroid cancer has been reported in patients treated at young ages, but not in adults. An increased risk for bone cancers has been reported mainly in patients treated as adolescents.

Studies have been reported for patients receiving whole body irradiation for bone marrow transplantations in the dose range of 10 to 15 Gy.[55] Those surviving 10 or more years had an increased risk for developing a second cancer that was eight times greater than expected. Risks were higher in those treated at younger ages than in those treated at older ages. Included among cancers for which an increased risk was observed were cancers of the buccal cavity, liver, brain and central nervous system, thyroid, bone, connective tissue, and malignant melanoma.

Relatively little information is available on risks for second cancers among long-term survivors of childhood cancer.[19] Interpretation of studies is complicated by the fact that many of these cancers are associated with germinal mutations that can influence susceptibility to the development of additional cancers independent of radiation exposure or perhaps enhance susceptibility to radiation exposure. Another complicating factor is that many patients with childhood cancers receive chemotherapeutic agents as well. Furthermore, in many instances insufficient time has passed for the development of second cancers. The most common cancers to date after treatment of childhood cancers are bone and soft tissue sarcomas. The largest source of information on induction of these sarcomas comes from studies of patients with retinoblastoma, many of whom have an elevated risk of such cancers independent of radiation exposure because of heritable mutations in the retinoblastoma gene. In these children, risk of sarcomas after radiation therapy can be as high as 50%. Although genetic susceptibility of these children can complicate interpretation when they have the familial form of retinoblastoma, studies of patients with the spontaneous form of retinoblastoma and other forms of childhood cancer also show increased risk for the development of sarcomas. Increased risk of other cancers has also been reported, including thyroid, breast, and skin cancer as well as tumors of the central nervous system.

Concern has been raised about potential increases in the risk of second cancers as a result of the shift from three-dimensional conformal radiation therapy to IMRT.[24] This change in approaches results in a decrease in the volume of normal tissue receiving a high dose. As a result it is likely that an overall reduction in sarcomas appearing as second tumors would result. At the same time, the use of IMRT is likely to result in a larger volume of normal tissues receiving lower doses. This is for two reasons: (1) The increased number of fields will result

in an increased volume of normal tissue receiving low-dose irradiation, and (2) the increased time required for the linear accelerator to be energized to deliver each treatment will result in an increased whole body patient dose by a factor of 2 to 3 because of leakage radiation. This increase in normal tissue volume receiving low-dose radiation exposure is likely to result in an increase in overall risks for the development of cancers in tissues outside of the treatment field. One study has suggested an increase in the incidence of second cancers from the current estimate of 1.0% to 1.75% of all patients surviving 10 years. These numbers would be expected to be higher for young patients and for those who survive longer than 10 years.

Mechanisms of Radiation-Induced Cancer

Although radiation-induced tumorigenesis in experimental animals and in humans has been the subject of intense study for many years, until recently direct evidence with respect to underlying mechanisms of radiation carcinogenesis has been lacking and models have relied heavily on indirect inferential data. For example, it has been suggested for many years that low LET ionizing radiation acts principally on early events; that is, radiation's primary effect is as a tumor-initiating agent. This is based on several observations. First, the generally increased sensitivity of animals and humans to the tumorigenic effects of ionizing radiation at young ages is more consistent with effects on tumor initiation than with promotional effects that accelerate the development of preexisting neoplasms.[16,56–59] Second, experimental animal data on skin cancer development specifically designed to examine the influence of radiation on different stages of tumorigenesis show radiation to only weakly promote the development and progression of chemically initiated tumors while having significant initiating activity.[60] Finally, the observation in humans and animals that single acute doses of low LET radiation are sufficient to produce a dose-dependent increase in cancer risk and that in quantitative animal studies dose protraction decreases that risk also supports the view that the major effect of radiation is on early events in the carcinogenic process.[16,31] Although this inference appears to be logically based, until recently there has been no direct evidence.

Advances in cell biology, cytogenetics, molecular biology, and mouse genetics over the past several years have made it possible to more directly investigate events in the tumorigenic process after radiation exposure. Such studies are providing valuable insights into mechanisms as well as a better understanding of potential risks by linking cell and molecular effects directly to the tumorigenic process. Of particular importance in this regard have been animal studies using newly developed models in inbred mice and rats and in genetically engineered rodents. Quantitative studies using mouse and rat models for radiation-induced mammary cancer and for thyroid cancer in rats have provided direct evidence to indicate that the principal effects of ionizing radiation are on early events.[60–69] Cellular, cytogenetic, and molecular data for acute myeloid leukemia, intestinal tumors, and mammary tumors also provide evidence for early monoclonal development of radiation-induced preneoplasms, implying an initial, single cell target.[65,70,71] Cytogenetic and molecular studies on the induction of acute myeloid leukemia and mammary tumors in inbred mouse strains and a variety of tumors in transgenic mouse models have provided more specific information on the potential nature of these early events.[40,41,71–74] These studies provide direct support for the view that the critical radiation-associated events in the tumorigenic process are predominantly early events involving DNA losses targeting specific genomic regions harboring critical genes. Because many of the radiation-associated DNA loss events in these tumorigenesis models involve large chromosomal regions within the genome, it can be concluded that mechanisms for radiation-induced chromosome aberration induction involving DNA DSB induction and postirradiation error-prone nonhomologous end-joining repair appear to play a critical role in the pathogenesis of cancer. More recently, experimental studies have questioned whether the initiating events produced by radiation are direct chromosomal or mutational effects or whether the mutations and chromosomal rearrangements result indirectly as a consequence of genomic instability induced by the radiation exposure.[75–79]

It is well known that the development of tumors is frequently accompanied by the acquisition of genomic instability phenotypes that serve to promote the mutational evolution involved in neoplastic progression. This form of genomic instability is increasingly well understood, and many of the responsible tumor gene mutations have been identified.[80] This instability, however, differs from radiation-induced genomic instability described during the last decade.[78] Over this time, evidence has accumulated that, under certain experimental conditions, the progeny of cells surviving radiation appear to express new chromosomal and gene mutations over many postirradiation cell generations. The observation of genomic instability induced by radiation is relatively recent. It has been generally believed that all mutagenic and cytogenetic effects of ionizing radiation occurred in the first few cell divisions. It has now been shown that increased mutation rates and new cytogenetic damage can occur in a large proportion of the progeny of irradiated cells many generations later (Fig. 10-2). What

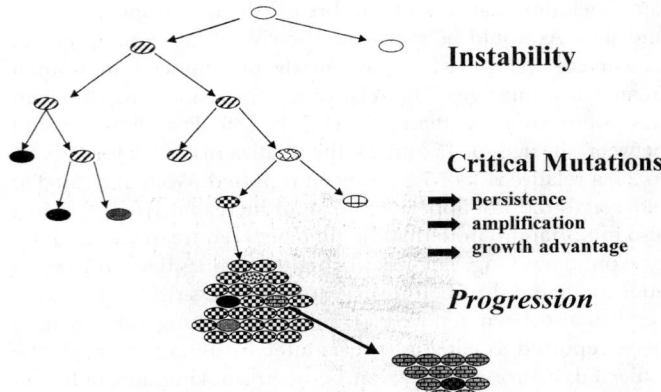

FIGURE 10-3. Proposed role of radiation-induced cytogenetic instability in radiation-induced cancer. Radiation exposure induces instability in a high percentage of the progeny of the irradiated cells (*striped* cells represent unstable progeny). As a result of this instability, the rate of chromosome aberrations and mutations is increased. Some mutations result in cell death (black) or slow-growing cells (gray), whereas some occur in critical genes involved in the regulation of cell growth and differentiation or in the maintenance of the stability of the genome. These mutations result in the persistence and amplification of genomic instability or in cells with a growth advantage. As these cells continue to develop into a clonal outgrowth, further mutations result in additional cellular changes, which lead to death or progression toward neoplasia. Cells with other patterns represent cells with specific mutations or sets of mutations that arise subsequent to radiation exposure.

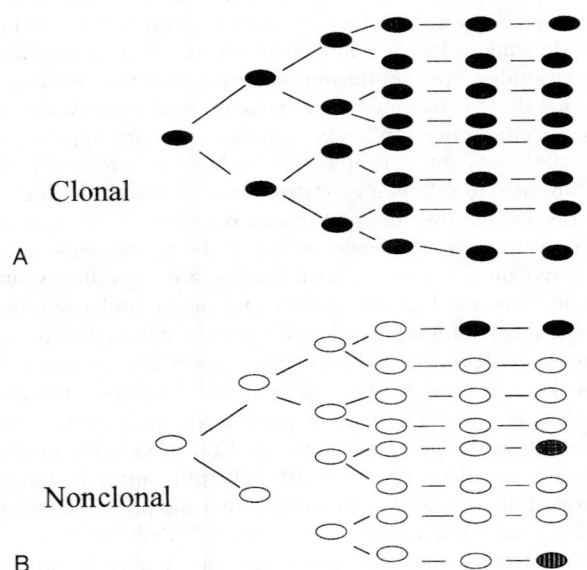

FIGURE 10-2. Comparison of mutations and cytogenetic damage as a result of direct radiation damage or radiation-induced genomic instability. **A:** Directly induced mutations or chromosome aberrations are passed to all progeny (i.e., the alterations are clonal). **B:** In contrast, mutations or aberrations arising as a result of radiation-induced instability arise in the progeny of irradiated cells that have not been directly irradiated. This leads to a nonclonal, or mosaic, pattern. Because the alterations arise in the progeny of the cells, another characteristic of instability is that the mutational or clastogenic effects are delayed with respect to the radiation exposure.

may be unique about radiation-induced instability with respect to its potential role in tumorigenesis is that, because of the high frequencies of instability observed after radiation exposure (10% to 50% of irradiated cells), such instability would not appear to be a result of radiation-induced mutations in a specific gene or family of genes.[78,81,82] On the basis of data discussed earlier in Mechanisms of Radiation-Induced Cancer on radiation-induced genomic instability and the previously reported high frequency of neoplastic cell transformation,[78,83] it has been suggested that such can serve to destabilize the genomes of a substantial fraction of the progeny of irradiated cells and that it is the elevated postirradiation mutation rates in cell progeny rather than gene-specific initial mutations that act to drive radiation tumorigenesis[78] (Fig. 10-3).

One form of instability that appears to be of particular relevance to tumorigenesis is that associated with telomere dysfunction.[77,84–90] Such dysfunction can be manifest in several forms. Telomeric repeat sequences $(TTAGGG)_n$ cap the ends of mammalian chromosomes and serve to protect against replicative erosion and chromosomal fusion; in normal human cells in culture, telomere shortening and instability are natural features of replicative cell senescence. In often degenerate forms, telomeric repeats are also found in subtelomeric and interstitial chromosomal locations, and there is some evidence that these loci may act as sites at which radiation-induced and other forms of genomic damage are preferentially resolved. Good evidence has also been shown that telomeric instability is a recurrent feature of tumorigenic development. Of particular relevance to the question of unstable translocation junctions are the so-called segmental jumping translocations, which have been well characterized in spontaneously arising human leukemias. With respect to radiation-induced leukemia, detailed cytogenetic analyses suggest an excess of complex aberrations and segmental jumping translocations in leukemias arising at old ages in high-dose–exposed A-bomb survivors.[91] Telomeric instability at radiation-associated deletion/translocation breakpoints in mouse myeloid leukemia has also been reported, but this is not a general characteristic of these tumor-associated events. Interestingly, excess spontaneous telomeric instability is often found to be associated with DNA repair or damage response deficiency.[84]

Evidence for the involvement of telomeric sequences in the pathogenesis of at least some forms of radiation-induced instability comes from several laboratories. Early studies on the postirradiation development of chromosomal instability in *in vitro* passaged human diploid fibroblasts were among the first to suggest a link between telomeres and instability. Initial studies using this *in vitro* model were suggestive of instability effects in a high proportion of irradiated cells.[92,93] Subsequent studies by the same research group have served to address issues related to the pathogenesis of instability as well as to its frequency.[86,87,89,94] Detailed cytogenetic analyses suggested that passage-dependent instability in cultured human fibroblasts primarily represented telomeric events expressed in cell clones naturally selected by growth rate during passage. Overall, the data obtained can be interpreted as initial radiation exposure bringing forward in time the natural process of clonal telomeric instability associated with cell senescence and telomere shortening. Equally important is the suggestion that selection processes lead to an overestimate with respect to the frequency of induction of instability by radiation. Whether selection processes impact estimates of the frequency of instability in other systems remains to be addressed.

A different form of postirradiation telomere-associated instability is expressed in a hamster-human hybrid cell system in which, in some clones, chromosomal instability is persistently expressed at translocations that have telomeric sequences at their junction.[77] Similar unstable structures have been observed in nonirradiated hamster cells undergoing gene amplification. Such data suggest that radiation is inducing genomic structures that enhance the natural expression of instability. A number of other reports have also suggested that radiation-associated chromosomal exchange can lead to the formation of unstable junctions that undergo secondary change leading to the formation of complex chromosomal aberrations.[77,85–88]

Although the role of radiation-induced genomic instability in radiation-induced cancer is still a matter of investigation, several observations provide a framework for its potential role in cancer development after radiation exposure. In the case of radiation-associated persistent telomeric rearrangement and unstable chromosome translocation junctions, a strong case can be made that a certain fraction of misrepaired genomic damage after radiation may be prone to ongoing secondary change in clonal progeny. Because there is evidence that such secondary genomic rearrangement can be a normal component of tumor development, it is reasonable to assume that instability of this type would be involved in the pathogenesis of some radiation-associated tumors. The question of whether it plays a major role and for which tumor types is unclear. The genetic evidence from mouse mammary studies that postirradiation instability can associate with mammary tumor development supports a role for genomic instability in this system. Thus, in certain genetic settings, such as individuals harboring specific types of DNA repair deficiencies, a role for postirradiation instability in tumorigenesis appears reasonable.

Of interest, recent data in the SCID and in the BALB/c mouse, both of which have defects in DNA-PKcs (catalytic subunit of DNA-dependent protein kinase), suggest that telomeric instability may be the underlying mechanism for the induction of instability, with the resulting cytogenetic instability playing an important role in early carcinogenic events in the mouse mammary carcinogenesis model discussed above. In particular, it appears that dysfunctional telomeres have a propensity to interact with sites of radiation-induced DSBs, increasing the probability of the misrepair.[84,95,96] It would be predicted that mechanisms involving DNA DSB and telomeric sequence interactions would be particularly important at low doses at which DNA DSBs are in relatively low abundance. This appears to be consistent with observations that instability is induced in a dose-dependent manner at radiation below 50 cGy but no dose dependence is observed at higher doses, at which the response appears to plateau. Importantly, the emerging evidence suggests a role for radiation-induced DSBs in the induction of instability and provides a mechanistic link between DSBs, chromosome aberrations, and cancer not unlike that for more directly induced effects.

It is well known that the probability that individual initiated cells will progress to become tumors can be modulated by interactions with surrounding cell and tissue components as well as systemic host factors.[97] Studies have also provided evidence that radiation can influence these cell–cell, cell–tissue, and host factor interactions.[97–101] Renewed interest has been shown in these effects as a result of studies that have begun to identify potential underlying mechanisms involved in modulation of tumorigenic progression and expression.[97,100,102,103] Research in this area will be extremely important in understanding the overall processes involved in neoplastic development, but a clear understanding of their potential impact on radiation-induced cancer remains to be determined.

ULTRAVIOLET LIGHT

Skin cancer is one of the most common forms of cancer, and its incidence is rising.[104–106] Although it is difficult to estimate overall incidence rates for nonmelanoma skin cancer, it is estimated that the annual incidence is in excess of one million new cases per year. Approximately 80% of all nonmelanoma skin cancers are basal cell carcinomas, with squamous cell carcinoma comprising the other 20%. Mortality for these cancers is low. However, this is not the case for cutaneous malignant melanoma, the incidence of which has been rising increasingly rapidly over the last few decades. Current estimates suggest that more than 54,000 individuals will be diagnosed with malignant melanoma in the last year, with more than 7000 of these resulting in death. A major cause of all forms of skin cancer is UV light from the sun.

SUNLIGHT AND SKIN CANCER

The evidence that UV light is responsible for a large proportion of skin cancer is considerable. Skin cancer is more frequent in populations in regions with high ambient solar radiation and in individuals exposed to sunlight as a result of their occupations (e.g., farmers). Nonmelanoma skin cancer is most frequent in sites that are the most exposed to sunlight, such as the head, neck, and arms. Pigmented skin is less susceptible to nonmelanoma skin cancer, and lack of pigment increases risk. In the United States, the incidence of basal cell carcinoma and squamous cell carcinoma increase by 2% to 3% for every 1% increase in ambient UV light, and malignant melanoma increases by 0.5% to 1.0%.[107] On a worldwide level, the incidence of skin cancer is extremely dependent on latitude, which directly equates with level of UV light. Specifically, it is seen that the closer to the equator one lives, the greater is the risk. This is exacerbated in countries, such as Australia, in which a large proportion of the population is lightly pigmented.[108] In addition to family history, the known risk factors for skin cancer are all related to increased propensity for damage from UV light from the sun: light pigmentation, inability to tan, propensity to burn, history of sunburns, and/or cumulative exposure to UV radiation.

Malignant melanoma appears less dependent on total exposure, and the site of development is not related to chronically exposed anatomic sites. Rather, risk for malignant melanoma appears to be more related to a history of acute sunburn rather than accumulated dose.[109,110] Interestingly, it has been observed that children who move to countries with high ambient sunlight are at an increased risk for melanoma, whereas this does not appear to be true when individuals move at older ages.[108] This observation suggests that exposure factors and age influence risk. Similarly, a greater risk for nonmelanoma skin cancer is seen in children and adolescents compared with adults.

GENETICS AND RISK

A high incidence of skin cancer associated with sunlight exposure is seen in young individuals who have xeroderma pigmentosum. Besides extraordinary sensitivity to sunlight exposure and skin cancer, individuals with this disease have premature aging of the skin and buccal cavity and progressive neurologic symptoms. One of the critical discoveries that mechanistically linked UV light, DNA damage, and skin cancer was that patients with xeroderma pigmentosum are defective in nucleotide excision repair.[10,111,112] XP is now categorized into at least eight complementation groups according to the capacity of the individuals to repair DNA damage. Nucleotide excision repair is the repair pathway that removes cyclobutane pyrimidine dimers produced in DNA by exposure to UV light and repairs the damaged site. This pathway is complex and involves a number of sequential steps. These steps include lesion recognition; assembly of the enzymes that make up the excision complex, which then excises a 27-29 nucleotide region containing the photoproduct; removal of the oligonucleotide sequence containing the damaged site; and finally replacement and filling of the gap by polymerization and ligation. Another pathway, termed *base excision repair*, removes less complex base damage. Both pathways are influenced by many factors, including transcriptional activity of the genomic region, the nucleotide sequence surrounding the damaged site, and DNA conformation.

In addition to xeroderma pigmentosum, a number of other disorders have been identified that result in acute sensitivity to UVC or UVB.[10] These include Cockayne's syndrome, and trichothiodystrophy. Both are related to disorders in genes involved in DNA damage repair, but individuals with these diseases are not at an increased risk for skin cancer after exposure to UV light. Studies of these disorders and the various complementation groups of xeroderma pigmentosum are providing important addi-

tional insights into details of the underlying mechanisms of UV-induced skin cancer. For example, it has been found that cells from patients with Cockayne's syndrome are able to repair only transcriptionally inactive genes.[113] This would suggest that repair of transcriptionally active genes is more important for prevention of UV-induced mutagenesis and carcinogenesis.

MECHANISMS

Squamous Cell and Basal Cell Carcinoma

The development of squamous cell and basal cell carcinomas is strongly associated with chronic exposure to UV light. In other words, multiple exposures are necessary for the development of these forms of skin cancer. This observation is consistent with the observation that UV radiation (UVB and UVC) acts as an initiator and a promoter for squamous cell tumors.[60] Essentially, UV light creates UV-specific dipyrimidine photoproducts in the DNA of the target cells. When these are not sufficiently repaired, errors in replication can result in characteristic mutations in critical genes. These mutations are likely the initiating events in skin cancer development. Squamous cell and basal cell carcinomas undergo specific and characteristic molecular changes in specific genes and gene pathways that are pathognomonic for each tumor type. Prolonged exposure of the skin to UV light creates damage that facilitates clonal expansion of these initiated cells, which subsequently undergo additional genomic changes that ultimately lead to cancer development. For squamous cell carcinoma, UV-induced mutations in p53 appear to be early events in this process. Further exposures may lead to additional mutations as well as clonal expansion of initiated cells through killing effects on normal but not p53 mutant cells.[10,114,115] Exposure to UV light also has been shown to suppress the ability of the immune system to suppress tumor growth. High doses of UV radiation apparently affect the ability of Langerhans' cells to efficiently transfer antigenic signals to T cells in local lymph nodes.[116]

Studies of patients with basal cell nevus syndrome have provided insight into early events in the development of basal cell carcinoma.[117] These patients are highly susceptible to the development of basal cell carcinoma after exposure to either ionizing or UV radiations, but keratinocytes from these patients show no difference in sensitivity to cell killing. It has been shown that the gene associated with this syndrome is PTCH, the human homologue of the *Drosophila* patched gene.[118] In *Drosophila*, this gene plays a role in cell–cell communication and transforming growth factor-β signaling. The most common genetic alteration in nonfamilial basal cell carcinoma is loss of heterozygosity at chromosome 9q22, which contains the PTCH locus. Mutations in PTCH and loss of heterozygosity in the 9q22 region are observed even in the smallest tumors, suggesting that alterations in PTCH are an early event in the pathogenesis of basal cell carcinoma.

Melanoma

Epidemiologic evidence has established a causal relationship between sunlight exposure and malignant melanoma that appears to be primarily a function of acute sunburn rather than chronic exposures.[119] A history of five or more sunburns as an adolescent has been found to double the risk for malignant melanoma. Experimental studies suggest that the majority of malignant melanomas are induced by UVA rather than UVB or UVC.[120] If this is the case, damage to DNA would be predicted to be a result of the production of reactive oxygen species rather than dipyrimidine photoproducts. In the familial form of malignant melanoma, susceptibility is associated with alterations in chromosome 9p21, which contains CDKN2A, the gene encoding the tumor suppressor genes, p16 and p19.[121] In sporadic and familial forms, additional alterations have been identified in several chromosomes in addition to 9p, including 6, 8, and 10.[122] As yet, there is no evidence that these changes are a direct result of damage produced by UV light.

INTERACTIONS BETWEEN IONIZING ULTRAVIOLET RADIATIONS AND SKIN CANCER RISKS

A biologically interesting and potentially clinically relevant question is whether UV radiation and ionizing radiation have potentially carcinogenic interaction.[15,123] Experimental studies suggest that ionizing radiation is able to initiate skin cancers that can be subsequently promoted by chronic exposure to UV light; the reverse did not obtain. Skin cancers did not develop after initiation of skin cells with a single dose of UV followed by chronic exposure of the skin to ionizing radiation. At present, epidemiologic studies are equivocal. At least one study has suggested a greater risk in individuals whose scalps were irradiated for tinea capitis in areas of skin that were subsequently exposed to UV light than in UV-shielded skin. In addition, a comparison of risks for the development of basal cell carcinoma in a population of white and African American individuals exposed to ionizing radiation for tinea capitis demonstrated that the whites were at a ten times higher risk than were the African Americans. Studies of A-bomb survivors, on the other hand, suggest greater risks in areas not exposed to UV light than on the face and hands.

ASBESTOS

Asbestos use has spanned many centuries. Major industrial use began in the late 1800s and became widespread during World War II. Use peaked in the 1970s, and recognition of its deleterious health effects has led to major reductions in mining and use of asbestos. It has also led to large programs aimed at removing asbestos from existing structures. The carcinogenic effects of asbestos have been clearly demonstrated in studies of individuals exposed in the mining and industrial uses of asbestos.[124]

FIBER TYPE AND DISEASE

Asbestos is actually a group of fiber types, with each type having a unique structure and chemical composition (Table 10-3). Each type also appears to differ in its chemical reactivity. Not unexpectedly, each type also appears to have differing biologic properties and effects. The two main subgroups are chrysolite fibers, which are long, curly, snake-like fibers, and amphibole fibers, which are shorter and rod-like in structure. The most common amphibole types include crocidolite, amosite, and tremolite. Few malignant mesotheliomas are associated with exposure to chrysolite fibers, probably because they do not tend to persist in the lung. The persistence of amphibole fibers, more commonly linked with mesothelioma, is significantly greater.[125]

TABLE 10-3. Characteristics of Asbestos Fibers

Name	Type	Chemical Composition
Chrysotile	Serpentine (curly)	$Mg_6Si_4O_{10}(OH)_8$
Crocidolite	Amphibole (rod-like)	$Na_2(Fe^{3+})_2(Fe^{2+})_3Si_8O_{22}(OH)_2$
Amosite	Amphibole (rod-like)	$(Fe,Mg)_7Si_8O_{22}(OH)_2$
Tremolite	Amphibole (rod-like)	$Ca_2Mg_5Si_8O_{22}(OH)_2$
Anthophyllite	Amphibole (rod-like)	$(Mg,Fe)_7Si_8O_{22}(OH)_2$
Actinolite	Amphibole (rod-like)	$Ca_2Mg_5Si_8O_{22}(OH)_2$

CANCER RISK AND ASBESTOS EXPOSURE

The most common form of cancer associated with asbestos exposure is malignant mesothelioma, but the risk of bronchogenic cancer is also significantly elevated. Although it is lung cancer that is generally associated with asbestos exposure, other cancers that have been reported to occur at an increased frequency include cancers of the larynx, oropharynx, kidney, esophagus, and gallbladder/bile duct.

Because it is very rare, it has been relatively easy to link the risk of mesothelioma with asbestos exposure. Occupational exposure can be linked to 50% to 80% of all patients with malignant mesotheliomas.[125] In a study of tile workers exposed to asbestos over a 50-year period, it was found that the incidence of mesothelioma was as high as 2%.[126] A study of a large group of asbestos insulation workers found that mesothelioma was responsible for approximately 8% of all deaths. The latent period between exposure and development of malignant mesothelioma is usually quite long, typically 30 to 40 years.[125] Approximately half of all malignant mesotheliomas are epithelioid, and the other half are sarcomatoid, mesenchymal, or mixed.

A link between asbestos and bronchogenic carcinomas was first reported in the 1930s and has been subsequently confirmed in several investigations.[125,127] Although the vast majority of bronchogenic carcinomas are related to smoking, it has been estimated that from 3% to 17% of such cancers are from occupational exposure, including asbestos. Asbestos and smoking appear to interact in a multiplicative manner, and the risk is decreased when exposure to either agent is stopped. Whereas the majority of smoking-related tumors are squamous cell carcinomas originating in the upper lobes of the lung, those associated with asbestos are more often adenocarcinomas located in the lower lobes. The asbestos-related tumors are also often associated with areas of fibrosis.

MECHANISMS

Asbestos fibers are cytotoxic and genotoxic.[128] They have been shown to induce DNA damage, including DSBs, mutations, and chromosomal damage. Evidence also indicates that asbestos fibers can impair mitosis and chromosomal segregation, which can result in aneuploidy. The majority of these effects are believed to be due to oxidoreductive processes that result in the formation of reactive oxygen species.[129,130] Support for this view comes from studies showing that the amount of damage induced is increased if iron is present in the chemical structure of the fibers. Besides the direct induction of reactive oxygen species, these effects may also be indirectly induced as a result of phagocytosis of the asbestos fibers. Fibers also tend to induce inflammatory response, resulting in the release of cytokines. Such inflammatory responses may facilitate the growth, clonal selection, and expansion of initiated cells.

Loss of one copy of chromosome 22 is one of the most common chromosomal alterations in malignant melanoma.[131] A wide range of other changes have also been reported, including deletions in chromosomes 1p, 3p, 6q, 9q, 13q, 15, and 22q. Analyses of tumors have found some common features. First, deletions of CDKN2A, located on chromosome 9p, have been observed. Second, mutations in NF2 (the neurofibromatosis type 2 gene, located on chromosome 22q) have been found; such mutations are often coupled with the loss of the normal NF2 allele as a result of one copy of chromosome 22.

REFERENCES

1. Johns H, Cunningham J. *The physics of radiology.* 4th ed. Springfield, IL: Charles C. Thomas, 1983.
2. Hall E. *Radiobiology for the radiologist,* 5th ed. New York: JB Lippincott, 2000.
3. National Committee on Radiation Protection and Measurements. *NCRP 104. Relative biological effectiveness of radiations of different quality.* Washington, DC: National Committee on Radiation Protection and Measurements, 2004.
4. Ward JF. DNA damage produced by ionizing radiation in mammalian cells: identities, mechanisms of formation, and reparability. *Prog Nucleic Acid Res Mol Biol* 1988;35:95.
5. Ward JF. DNA damage in mammalian cells. *Free Radic Res Commun* 1989;6:179.
6. Ward JF. Radiation mutagenesis: the initial DNA lesions responsible. *Radiat Res* 1995;142:362.
7. Nickjoo, H, O'Neil P, Wilson W, Goodhead DT. Computational approach for determining the spectrum of DNA damage induced by ionizing radiation. *Radiat Res* 2001;156:577.
8. Jeggo PA. DNA breakage and repair. *Adv Genet* 1998;38:185.
9. Niggli HJ, Cerutti P. Cyclobutane pyrimidine photodimer production in human skin fibroblasts after irradiation with 313 nm ultraviolet light. *Biochemistry* 1983;22:1390.
10. Cleaver JE, Crowley E. UV damage, DNA repair and skin carcinogenesis. *Front Biosci* 2002;7:1024.
11. Tyrrell RM, Pidoux M. Action spectra for human skin cell: estimates of the relative cytotoxicity of the middle ultraviolet, near ultraviolet, and violet regions of sunlight on epidermal keratinocytes. *Cancer Res* 1987;47:1825.
12. Tommasi S, Denissenko MF, Pfeifer GP. Sunlight induces pyrimidine dimers preferentially at 5-methylcytosine bases. *Cancer Res* 1997;57:4727.
13. Ziegler A, Jonason AS, Leffell DJ, et al. Sunburn and p53 in the onset of skin cancer. *Nature* 1994;372:773.
14. Miller RW. Delayed effects of external radiation exposure: a brief history. *Radiat Res* 1995;144:160.
15. Shore RE. Radiation-induced skin cancer in humans. *Med Pediatr Oncol* 2001;36:549.
16. *UNSCEAR: sources and effects of ionizing radiation.* New York: United Nations, 2000.
17. Preston DL, Shimizu Y, Pierce DA, Suyama A, Mabuchi K. Studies of mortality of atomic bomb survivors. Report 13: Solid cancer and noncancer disease mortality: 1950–1997. *Radiat Res* 2003;160:381.
18. Brenner D, Doll R, Goodhead DT, et al. Cancer risks attributable to low doses of ionizing radiation: assessing what we really know. *Proc Natl Acad Sci U S A* 2003;100:13761.
19. Inskip PD. *Second cancers following radiation therapy 91.* Philadelphia: Lippincott Williams & Wilkins, 1999.
20. National Council Committee on Health Risks of Exposure to Radon (BEIR IV). *Health effects of exposure to radon: time for reassessment.* Washington, DC: National Academy of Sciences, USA, 1994.
21. Gilbert ES. Invited commentary: studies of workers exposed to low doses of radiation. *Am J Epidemiol* 2001;153:319.
22. Berrington A, Darby SC, Weiss HA, Doll R. 100 years of observation on British radiologists: mortality from cancer and other causes 1897–1997. *Br J Radiol* 2001;74:507.
23. Brenner D, Elliston CD, Hall EJ, Berdon WE. Estimated risks of radiation-induced fatal cancer from pediatric CT. *Am J Radiol* 2001;176:289.
24. Hall EJ, Wuu C. Radiation-induced second cancers: the impact of 3D-CRT and IMRT. *Int J Radiat Oncol Biol Phys* 2003;56:83.
25. National Council on Radiation Protection and Measurements. NCRP Report No. 64. Influence of dose and its distribution in time on dose-response relationships for low LET radiations. Washington, DC: National Council on Radiation Protection and Measurements, 1980.
26. Ferguson DO, Sekiguchi JM, Chang S, et al. The nonhomologous end-joining pathway of DNA repair is required for genomic stability and the suppression of translocations. *Proc Natl Acad Sci U S A* 2000;97:6630.
27. Ullrich RL, Jernigan MC, Satterfield LC, Bowles ND. Radiation carcinogenesis: time-dose relationships. *Radiat Res* 1987;111:179.
28. Ullrich RL, Storer JB. Influence of gamma irradiation on the development of neoplastic disease in mice. III. Dose-rate effects. *Radiat Res* 1979;80:325.
29. Boice JD. Ionizing radiation. In: Harras A. *Cancer: rate and risks,* 4th ed. Washington, DC: U.S. Department of Health and Human Services, Public Health Service, National Institutes of Health, 1996:90.
30. Reference deleted.
31. IARC Monographs on the evaluation of carcinogenic risks to humans. Vol. 75, ionizing radiation. Part 1: x- and gamma radiation and neutrons. Lyon, France: IARC, 2000.
32. Doll R, Wakeford R. Risk of childhood cancer from fetal irradiation. *Br J Radiol* 1997;70:771.
33. Doll R, Wakeford R. Risk of childhood cancer from fetal irradiation. *Br J Radiol* 1997;70:130.
34. Sankaranarayanan K, Chakraborty R. Cancer predisposition, radiosensitivity and the risk of radiation-induced cancers. I. Background. *Radiat Res* 1995;143:121.
35. Sharp C, Cox R. Genetic susceptibility to radiation effects: possible implication for medical ionizing radiation exposures. *Euro J Nucl Med* 1999;26:425.
36. Wong F, Boice JD Jr, Abramson DH, et al. Cancer incidence after retinoblastoma: radiation dose and sarcoma risk. *JAMA* 1997;278:1262.
37. Strong LC. Theories of pathogenesis: mutation and cancer. *Genetics of human cancer 401.* New York: Raven Press, 1977.
38. Li FP, Fraumeni JF Jr, Mulvihill JJ, et al. A cancer family syndrome in twenty-four kindreds. *Cancer Res* 1988;48:5358.
39. Srivastava S, Zou ZQ, Pirollo K, Blattner W, Chang EH. Germ-line transmission of a mutated P53 gene in a cancer-prone family with Li-Fraumeni syndrome. *Nature* 1990;348:747.
40. Kemp CJ, Wheldon T, Balmain A. P53-deficient mice are extremely susceptible to radiation-induced tumorigenesis. *Nature Genet* 1994;8:66.
41. Pazzaglia S, Mancuso M, Atkinson MJ, et al. High incidence of medulloblastoma following X-ray-irradiation of newborn Ptc1 heterozygous mice. *Oncogene* 2002;21:7580.
42. Haines J, Dunford R, Moody J, et al. Loss of heterozygosity in spontaneous and X-ray-induced intestinal tumors arising in FI hybrid min mice: evidence for sequential loss of Apc(+) and Dpc4 in tumor development. *Genes Chromosomes Cancer* 2000;28:387.
43. Swift M, Morrell D, Massey RB, Chase CL. Incidence of cancer in 161 families affected by ataxia-telangiectasia. *N Engl J Med* 1991;325:1831.
44. Spring K, Ahangari F, Scott SP, et al. Mice heterozygous for mutation in Atm, the gene involved in ataxia-telangiectasia, have heightened susceptibility to cancer. *Nature Genet* 2002;32:185.
45. Boice JD, et al. Second cancers following radiation treatment for cervical-cancer—an international collaboration among cancer registries. *J Natl Cancer Inst* 1985;74:955.
46. Brenner DJ, Curtis RE, Hall EJ, Ron E. Second malignancies in prostate carcinoma patients after radiotherapy compared with surgery. *Cancer* 2000;88:398.
47. Boice JD, Stovall M, Blettner M. Cancer in the contralateral breast after radiotherapy for breast-cancer. *N Engl J Med* 1992;327:431.
48. Boice JD, Harvey EB, Blettner M, Stovall M, Flannery JT. Cancer in the contralateral breast after radiotherapy for breast-cancer. *N Engl J Med* 1992;326:781.
49. Inskip PD, Stovall M, Flannery JT. Lung-cancer risk and radiation-dose among women treated for breast-cancer. *J Natl Cancer Inst* 1994;86:983.
50. Hancock SL, Tucker MA, Hoppe RT. Breast-cancer after treatment of Hodgkin's disease. *J Natl Cancer Inst* 1993;85:25.
51. Bhatia S, Robison LL, Meadows AT. Late effects of treatment for childhood Hodgkin's disease. *N Engl J Med* 1996;335:353.
52. Bhatia S, Robison LL, Oberlin O, et al. Breast cancer and other second neoplasms after childhood Hodgkin's disease. *N Engl J Med* 1996;334:745.
53. Vanleeuwen FE, et al. Roles of radiotherapy and smoking in lung-cancer following Hodgkin's disease. *J Natl Cancer Inst* 1995;87:1530.
54. Boivin JF, Hutchison GB, Zauber AG, et al. Incidence of second cancers in patients treated for Hodgkin's disease. *J Natl Cancer Inst* 1995;87:732.
55. Curtis RE, Rowlings PA, Deeg HJ, et al. Solid cancers after bone marrow transplantation. *N Engl J Med* 1997;336:897.
56. Clifton KH, Tanner MA, Gould MN. Assessment of radiogenic cancer initiation frequency per clonogenic rat mammary cell in vivo. *Cancer Res* 1986;46:2390.
57. Fry RJM, et al. Age-dependency of radiation-induced late effects. *Radiat Res* 1977;70:609.
58. Fry RJM, Storer JB. External radiation carcinogenesis. *Advan Radiat Biol* 1987;13:31.
59. Fry RJM. The role of animal experiments in estimates of radiation risk. In: Lett JT, Sinclair WK, eds. *Advances in radiation research.* New York, 1992:181.
60. Jaffe D, Bowden GT. Ionizing-radiation as an initiator—effects of proliferation and promotion time on tumor-incidence in mice. *Cancer Res* 1987;47:6692.
61. Adams LM, Ethier SP, Ullrich RL. Enhanced in vitro proliferation and in vivo tumorigenic potential of mammary epithelium from BALB/c mice exposed in vivo to gamma-radiation and/or 7,12-dimethylbenz[a]anthracene. *Cancer Res* 1987;47:4425.
62. Bouffler SD, Meijne EIM, Huiskamp R, Cox R. Chromosomal abnormalities in neutron-induced acute myeloid leukemias in CBA/H mice. *Radiat Res* 1996;146:349.
63. Bouffler SD, Meijne EIM, Morris DJ, Papworth D. Chromosome 2 hypersensitivity and clonal development in murine radiation acute myeloid leukaemia. *Int J Radiat Biol* 1997;72:181.
64. Ethier SP, Ullrich RL. Factors influencing expression of mammary ductal dysplasia in cell dissociation-derived murine mammary outgrowths. *Cancer Res* 1984;44:4523.
65. Ullrich RL, Bowles ND, Satterfield LC, Davis CM. Strain-dependent susceptibility to radiation-induced mammary cancer is a result of differences in epithelial cell sensitivity to transformation. *Radiat Res* 1996;146:353.
66. Domann FE, Freitas MA, Gould MN, Clifton KH. Quantifying the frequency of radiogenic thyroid-cancer per clonogenic cell in-vivo. *Radiat Res* 1994;137:330.
67. Gould MN, Watanabe H, Kamiya K, Clifton KH. Modification of expression of the malignant phenotype in radiation-initiated cells. *Int J Radiat Biol* 1987;51:1081.
68. Watanabe H, Tanner MA, Gould MN, Clifton KH. Suppression of cancer progression in radiation initiated rat-thyroid cells by normal thyroid-cells. *Proc AACR* 1986;27:97.
69. Mulcahy RT, Gould MN, Clifton KH. Radiogenic initiation of thyroid-cancer—a common cellular event. *Int J Radiat Biol* 1984;45:419.

70. Bouffler SD, Meijne EIM, Morris DJ, Papworth D. Chromosome 2 hypersensitivity and clonal development in murine radiation acute myeloid leukaemia. *Int J Radiat Biol* 1997;72:181.

71. Haines J, Dunford R, Moody J, et al. Loss of heterozygosity in spontaneous and X-ray-induced intestinal tumors arising in FI hybrid min mice: evidence for sequential loss of Apc(+) and Dpc4 in tumor development. *Genes Chromosomes Cancer* 2000;28:387.

72. Bouffler SD, Breckon G, Cox R. Chromosomal mechanisms in murine radiation acute myeloid leukaemogenesis. *Carcinogenesis* 1996;17:655.

73. Selvanayagam CS, Davis CM, Cornforth MN, Ullrich RL. Latent expression of p53 mutations and radiation-induced mammary cancer. *Cancer Res* 1995;55:3310.

74. Silver A, Moody J, Dunford R, et al. Molecular mapping of chromosome 2 deletions in murine radiation-induced AML localizes a putative tumor suppressor gene to a 1.0 cM region homologous to human chromosome segment 11p11-12. *Genes Chromosomes Cancer* 1999;24:95.

75. Little JB, Nagasawa H, Pfenning T, Vetrovs H. Radiation-induced genomic instability: delayed mutagenic and cytogenetic effects of X rays and alpha particles. *Radiat Res* 1997;148:299.

76. Little JB, Gorgojo L, Vetrovs H. Delayed appearance of lethal and specific gene mutations in irradiated mammalian cells. *Int J Radiat Oncol Biol Phys* 1990;19:1425.

77. Morgan WF, Day JP, Kaplan MI, McGhee EM, Limoli CL. Genomic instability induced by ionizing radiation. *Radiat Res* 1996;146:247.

78. Selvanayagam CS, Davis CM, Cornforth MN, Ullrich RL. Latent expression of P53 mutations and radiation-induced mammary-cancer. *Cancer Res* 1995;55:3310.

79. Yu Y, Okayasu R, Weil MM, et al. Elevated breast cancer risk in irradiated BALB/c mice associates with unique functional polymorphism of the Prkdc (DNA-dependent protein kinase catalytic subunit) gene. *Cancer Res* 2001;61:1820.

80. Loeb LA. A mutator phenotype in cancer. *Cancer Res* 2001;61:3230.

81. Kadim MA, et al. Transmission of chromosomal instability after plutonium α-particle irradiation. *Nature* 1991;355:738.

82. Wright EG. Radiation-induced genetic instability in stem cells. Tenth International Congress of Radiation Research. 1995;37(abst).

83. Kennedy AR, Fox M, Murphy G, Little JB. Relationship between x-ray exposure and malignant transformation of C3H 10T1/2 cells. *Proc Natl Acad Sci U S A* 1980;77:7262.

84. Mills KD, Ferguson DO, Alt FW. The role of DNA breaks in genomic instability and tumorigenesis. *Immunol Rev* 2003;194:77.

85. Desmaze C, Soria JC, Freulet-Marriere MA, Mathieu N, Sabatier L. Telomere-driven genomic instability in cancer cells. *Cancer Lett* 2003;194:173.

86. Lo AWI, et al. DNA amplification by breakage/fusion/bridge cycles initiated by spontaneous telomere loss in a human cancer cell line. *Neoplasia* 2002;4:531.

87. Lo AWI, et al. Chromosome instability as a result of double-strand breaks near telomeres in mouse embryonic stem cells. *Molec Cell Biol* 2002;22:4836.

88. Desmaze C, Alberti C, Martins L, et al. The influence of interstitial telomeric sequences on chromosome instability in human cells. *Cytogenet Cell Genet* 1999;86:288.

89. Ducray C, Pommier JP, Martins L, Boussin FD, Sabatier L. Telomere dynamics, end-to-end fusions and telomerase activation during the human fibroblast immortalization process. *Oncogene* 1999;18:4211.

90. Bouffler SD, Blasco MA, Cox R, Smith PJ. Telomeric sequences, radiation sensitivity and genomic instability. *Int J Radiat Biol* 2001;77:995.

91. Nakanishi M, Tanaka K, Shintani T, Takahashi T, Kamada N. Chromosomal instability in acute myelocytic leukemia and myelodysplastic syndrome patients among atomic bomb survivors. *J Radiat Res* 1999;40:159.

92. Sabatier L, et al. Specific sites of chromosomal radiation-induced rearrangements. *New trends in genetic risk assessment.* New York: Academic Press, 1989:213.

93. Sabatier L, Durtillaux B, Martin MB. Chromosomal instability. *Nature* 1992;357:548.

94. Desmaze C, Alberti C, Martins L, et al. The influence of interstitial telomeric sequences on chromosome instability in human cells. *Cytogenet Cell Genet* 1999;86:288.

95. Bailey SM, Meyne J, Chen DJ, et al. DNA double-strand break repair proteins are required to cap the ends of mammalian chromosomes. *Proc Natl Acad Sci U S A* 1999;96:14899.

96. Bailey SM, Cornforth MN, Kurimasa A, Chen DJ, Goodwin EH. Strand-specific postreplicative processing of mammalian telomeres. *Science* 2001;293:2462.

97. Bissell MJ, Radisky D. Putting tumors in context. *Nat Rev Cancer* 2001;1:46.

98. Barcellos-Hoff MH. How do tissues respond to damage at the cellular level? The role of cytokines in irradiated tissues. *Radiat Res* 1998;150[suppl]:S109.

99. Barcellos-Hoff MH. It takes a tissue to make a tumor: epigenetics, cancer and the microenvironment. *J Mammary Gland Biol Neoplasia* 2001;6:213.

100. Barcellos-Hoff MH, Brooks AL. Extracellular signaling through the microenvironment: a hypothesis relating carcinogenesis, bystander effects, and genomic instability. *Radiat Res* 2001;156:618.

101. Park CC, et al. Ionizing radiation induces heritable disruption of epithelial cell interactions. *Proc Natl Acad Sci U S A* 2003;100:10728.

102. Barcellos-Hoff MH. Latency and activation in the control of TGF-beta. *J Mammary Gland Biol Neoplasia* 1996;1:353.

103. Barcellos-Hoff MH, Ewan KB. Transforming growth factor-beta and breast cancer: mammary gland development. *Breast Cancer Res* 2000;2:92.

104. American Cancer Society. *Cancer facts and figures, 2002.* American Cancer Society, 2002.

105. Jemal A, Devesa SS, Fears TR, Hartge P. Cancer surveillance series: changing patterns of cutaneous malignant melanoma mortality rates among whites in the United States. *J Natl Cancer Inst* 2000;92:811.

106. Jemal A, Devesa SS, Hartge P, Tucker MA. Recent trends in cutaneous melanoma incidence among whites in the United States. *J Natl Cancer Inst* 2001;93:678.

107. Landis SH, Murray T, Bolden S, Wingo PA. Cancer statistics, 1998. *CA Cancer J Clin* 1998;48:6.

108. Armstrong BK, Kricker A. Epidemiology of sun exposure and skin cancer. *Cancer Surv* 1996;26:133.

109. Urbach F. Ultraviolet radiation and skin cancer of humans. *J Photochem Photobiol B* 1997;40:3.

110. Urbach F. Phototoxic skin reaction to UVR—is "sunburn" a "burn"? *Photodermatol Photoimmunol Photomed* 1996;12:219.

111. Cleaver JE. Defective repair replications of DNA in xeroderma pigmentosum. *Nature* 1968;218:642.

112. Cleaver JE. Common pathways for ultraviolet skin carcinogenesis in the repair and replication defective groups of xeroderma pigmentosum. *J Dermatol Sci* 2000;23:1.

113. Venema J, Mullenders LHF, Natarajan AT, van Zeeland AA, Mayne LV. The genetic defect in Cockayne syndrome is associated with a defect in repair of UV-induced DNA damage in transcriptionally active DNA. *Proc Natl Acad Sci U S A* 1990;87:4707.

114. Berg RJW, et al. Early p53 alterations in mouse skin carcinogenesis by UVB radiation: immunohistochemical detection of mutant p53 protein in clusters of preneoplastic epidermal cells. *Proc Natl Acad Sci U S A* 1996;93:274.

115. Brash DE. Sunlight and the onset of skin cancer. *TIG* 1997;13:410.

116. Daynes RA, Bernhard EJ, Gurish MF, Lynch DH. Experimental photo-immunology—immunological ramifications of UV-induced carcinogenesis. *J Invest Dermatol* 1981;77:77.

117. Stacey M, Thacker S, Taylor AMR. Cultured skin keratinocytes from both normal individuals and basal-cell nevus syndrome patients are more resistant to gamma-rays and UV-light compared with cultured skin fibroblasts. *Int J Radiat Biol* 1989;56:45.

118. Gailani MR, Bale AE. Developmental genes and cancer: role of patched in basal cell carcinoma of the skin. *J Natl Cancer Inst* 1997;89:1103.

119. Weinstock MA. Controversies in the role of sunlight in the pathogenesis of cutaneous melanoma. *Photochem Photobiol* 1996;63:406.

120. Jhappan C, Noonan FP, Merlino G. Ultraviolet radiation and cutaneous malignant melanoma. *Oncogene* 2003;22:3099.

121. Monzon J, Liu L, Brill H, et al. CDKN2A mutations in multiple primary melanomas. *N Engl J Med* 1998;338:879.

122. Bastian BC, LeBoit PE, Hamm H, Brocker EB, Pinkel D. Chromosomal gains and losses in primary cutaneous melanomas detected by comparative genomic hybridization. *Cancer Res* 1998;58:2170.

123. Shore RE, Albert RE, Reed M, Harley N, Pasternack BS. Skin-cancer incidence among children irradiated for ringworm of the scalp. *Radiat Res* 1984;100:192.

124. Albin M, Magnani C, Krstev S, Rapiti E, Shefer I. Asbestos and cancer: an overview of current trends in Europe. *Environ Health Perspect* 1999;107:289.

125. Mossman BT, Kemp DW, Weitzman SA. Mechanisms of carcinogenesis and clinical features of asbestos associated cancers. *Cancer Invest* 1996;14:466.

126. Peto J, et al. Relationship of mortality to measures of environmental asbestos pollution in an asbestos textile factory. *Ann Occup Hyg* 1985;29:305.

127. Enterline PE. Changing attitudes and opinions regarding asbestos and cancer. *Am J Ind Med* 1997;20:685.

128. Okayasu R, Takahashi S, Yamada S, Hei TK, Ullrich RL. Asbestos and DNA double strand breaks. *Cancer Res* 1999;59:298.

129. Kamp DW, Preusen SE, Weitzman SA. Asbestos causes DNA strand breaks in cultured human pulmonary epithelial-like cells. *Clin Res* 1992;40:A721.

130. Kamp DW, Graceffa P, Pryor WA, Weitzman SA. The role of free-radicals in asbestos-induced diseases. *Free Radic Biol Med* 1992;12:293.

131. Murthy SS, Testa JR. Asbestos, chromosomal deletions, and tumor suppressor gene alterations in human malignant mesothelioma. *J Cell Physiol* 1999;180:150.

CHAPTER 11

Epidemiology of Cancer

SECTION **1**

XIAOMEI MA
MARGARET A. TUCKER

Epidemiologic Methods

Epidemiology is the study of the distribution and determinants of health-related states or events in specified populations and the application of this study to control health problems.[1] Epidemiologic principles and methods have long been applied to cancer research, with the assumptions that cancer does not occur at random and that the nonrandomness of carcinogenesis can be elucidated through systematic research. An example of such applications is the lung cancer study conducted by Doll and Hill[2] in the early 1950s, which linked tobacco smoking to an increased mortality from lung cancer in more than 40,000 medical professionals in the United Kingdom. The observation from this study and many similar observations from other studies, in conjunction with basic laboratory findings regarding the underlying biologic mechanisms for the effect of tobacco smoking, helped establish the role of tobacco smoking in the etiology of lung cancer and formed the rationale for preventive strategies. Epidemiologic methods are also widely used in clinical settings, where trials are conducted to evaluate the efficacy of new treatment protocols or preventive measures and observational studies of prognostic factors are done.

Epidemiologic studies can take different forms, but generally they can be classified into two broad categories, observational studies and experimental studies (Fig. 11.1-1). In experimental studies, an investigator allocates different study regimens to the subjects, usually with randomization (experimental studies without randomization are sometimes referred to as *quasi-experiments*[3]).

Experimental studies can be individual-based or community-based. An experimental study most closely resembles laboratory experiments in that the investigator has control over the study condition. In a well-designed randomized trial with a large enough sample size, other factors that may affect the relationship between the study factor (e.g., a new drug) and the outcome (e.g., cured or not) are balanced between the group with the study factor (e.g., the treatment group) and the group without the study factor (e.g., the placebo group). Therefore, the difference observed in the treatment outcome between the two groups can be attributed to the study factor. In practice, experimental studies can be used to evaluate the efficacy of various treatment protocols (e.g., low-dose compared with standard-dose chemotherapy for non-Hodgkin's lymphoma[4]) or preventive measures (e.g., tamoxifen for women at an increased risk of breast cancer[5]; supplementary β-carotene for patients at risk for second head and neck cancer[6]). Although experimental studies are often considered the "gold standard" because of well-controlled study situations, they are only suitable for the evaluation of effects that are beneficial or at least not harmful due to ethical concerns. Experimental studies are discussed in detail in other chapters of this book. This chapter focuses on observational studies.

Observational studies, as the name indicates, do not involve artificial manipulation of study regimens. In an observational study, an investigator stands by to observe what happens or happened to the subjects in terms of exposure and outcome. Observational studies can be further divided into two subcategories, descriptive studies and analytic studies (see Fig. 11.1-1). Descriptive studies focus on the distribution of diseases with respect to person, place, and time, that is, who, where, and when, whereas analytic studies focus on the determinants of diseases. Descriptive studies are often used to generate hypotheses, whereas analytic studies are frequently used to test hypotheses. However, the

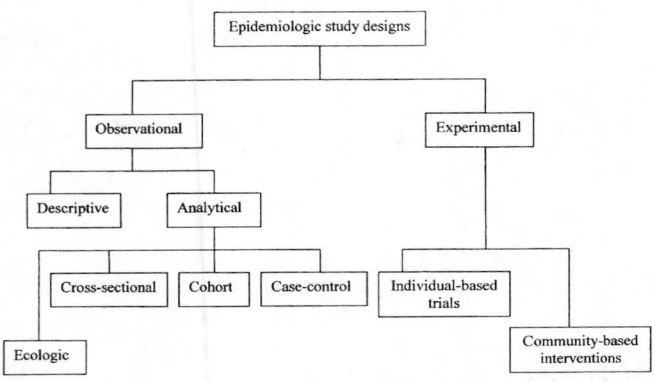

FIGURE 11.1-1. Classification of epidemiologic study designs.

two types of studies should not be considered mutually exclusive entities; rather, they are the opposite ends of a continuum. Investigators seldom describe something just for the purpose of description—there is usually an implicit or explicit indication for analysis. On the other hand, no matter how complicated an analysis is, it usually begins with simple descriptions.

DESCRIPTIVE STUDIES

Monitoring trends in disease frequency is essential in descriptive studies. The different measures of disease frequency mainly include prevalence, incidence, and mortality. Prevalence is the proportion of individuals in a population who have the disease at a given point (point prevalence) or during a specified period of time (period prevalence). Prevalence is calculated by dividing the number of existing cases by the total population. Incidence can be measured in two ways, cumulative incidence and incidence density (also known as *incidence rate*). Cumulative incidence is the proportion of people in whom the disease develops during a specified period of time and is calculated by dividing the number of new cases that occurred during a period by the total population *at risk*. Incidence density is the instantaneous rate of developing the disease in a population, which can only be calculated when there are data on the exact individual person-time under observation. Mortality is analogous to incidence where the outcome of interest is death instead of the occurrence of new disease. Because mortality data are usually easier to obtain than incidence data, sometimes disease-specific mortality is used as a proxy measure of incidence. Under certain circumstances (e.g., when there is better reporting of causes of death than of new cases of cancer), mortality may be a more reliable measure than incidence. Nevertheless, it is important to note that the mortality approximates incidence only when the disease is highly fatal and the interval between disease occurrence and death is short.[7] Prevalence reflects the public health burden of a disease (i.e., how many patients must be treated or followed up by the medical care system), whereas incidence is considered a more relevant measure of disease frequency for etiologic evaluation. A change in incidence over time or a difference in incidence between different populations or different geographic regions usually leads to hypotheses involving changes or differences in possible risk factors of the disease.

The quality of descriptive studies depends on the quality of data collected. The quality of incidence data varies substantially, depending on the medical care systems, the thoroughness with which a diagnosis of a specific type of cancer is pursued, the completeness of reporting a new diagnosis of cancer to whatever institution is collecting the data, and the accuracy of the population numbers. The percentage of histologic confirmation of new cancer diagnoses also varies widely among health care systems and among tumor registries. The ideal population for evaluating cancer rates would be a large, diverse one in which there is little in or out migration, one health care system provides high-quality care from birth to death, and each individual has a unique identifier for life.

The Surveillance, Epidemiology, and End Results (SEER) program of the National Cancer Institute (NCI) is an authoritative source of information on new cancer cases and cancer survival in the United States. Case ascertainment for SEER began on January 1, 1973, and with several subsequent expansions, it now covers approximately 26% of the U.S. population (http://seer.cancer.gov). Geographic areas were selected for inclusion in the SEER program based on their ability to operate and maintain a high-quality population-based cancer reporting system and for their epidemiologically significant population subgroups. According to information from the Web site, the population covered by SEER is comparable to the general U.S. population with regard to measures of poverty and education. SEER data provide population-based incidence rates, survival, and mortality. Furthermore, SEER data include information on the demographic characteristics of cancer cases and characteristics of the cancer (site, morphology, and stage). A large amount of information can be accessed through the SEER Web site, and many important reports can be downloaded, such as the Joint NCI/Centers for Disease Control and Prevention report: U.S. Cancer Statistics, 2000 Incidence. The Cancer Mortality Maps & Graphs Web site of the NCI (http://www3.cancer.gov/atlasplus/) provides interactive maps, graphs, text, tables, and figures showing geographic patterns and time trends of cancer death rates for the time period 1950 to 1994 for more than 40 cancers. The American Cancer Society also publishes an annual report called *Cancer Facts and Figures*, which can be accessed from the Web site http://www.cancer.org/statistics. Outside the United States, the World Health Organization's International Agency for Research on Cancer and the International Association of Cancer Registries publishes *Cancer Incidence in Five Continents*, which is extremely useful in evaluating the variation in cancer incidence worldwide. The observed variation, if any, may help provide insight into the etiology of different types of cancer.[8]

When comparing incidence or mortality measures across different populations or over time, it may be misleading to use the crude measure directly. This is because different populations may have different structures with respect to age and other factors. For example, if population A has a much larger percentage of older people than population B and the age-specific incidences are exactly the same in population A and population B, the crude incidence from population A will be higher than the crude incidence from population B (given that the incidence of most types of cancer increases with age). In this situation, one can choose a standard population and use the age distribution of the standard population and the age-specific rates of the population under study to calculate an adjusted rate. The adjusted rate is a fictional one, representing what the crude rate would have been if the study population had the same age distribution as the standard population. For comparisons involving two populations, two adjusted rates must be calculated using the same standard population and then compared with each other. The comparison of the adjusted rates, rather than the actual value of each adjusted rate, is the focus. Choice of standard population may affect the result of the comparison. Age is probably the most commonly adjusted factor, but sometimes standardizations are also made for other factors, such as gender and race.

Age, period, and cohort effects can be evaluated when analyzing time trends in disease. An age effect is present when the disease rate varies by age, regardless of when the individuals were born. A period effect is present when the disease rate varies by period (i.e., calendar time), regardless of age or when the individuals were born. A cohort effect is present when the disease rate varies by year of birth, regardless of age.[3] Assessing these effects is important in understanding the trends we observe. For example, there may appear to be an increased incidence of a specific type of cancer (e.g., prostate cancer) after the introduction of a new screening technique (e.g., prostate-specific antigen) at a given point in time (i.e., a period effect), but this apparent increase may very well be an artifact; that is, the observed increase could be due to an increase in its diagnosis instead of a real increase in incidence. Similarly, if a period effect coincides with a change of the disease definition or a change in the cancer reporting system (e.g., from voluntary to mandatory), the coincidence must be taken into account when the observed trend is interpreted. Under many circumstances, the age, period, and cohort effects are difficult to disentangle because the three effects are related. In practice, these effects can be assessed by graphically displaying age-specific rates by period or cohort, or both, as well as fitting regression models.

Robertson et al.[9] used graphic and regression analyses to evaluate the trends in breast cancer incidence in Slovenia, and the results suggested that the increase in incidence (1971 to 1993) was mostly due to cohort effects. The researchers predicted a decrease in future incidence because more recent birth cohorts have a more favorable reproductive pattern (e.g., a lower percentage of women who are nulliparous).[9] In another study, age-period-cohort Poisson regression analyses were used to gain etiologic clues regarding the increased incidence in salivary gland cancers, and the rising trend was largely attributed to period effects and artifactual changes, such as a shift in the designation of cancer sites (from floor of mouth and lower gum to salivary gland), an increased use of needle aspirate biopsies, and a greater access to medical care for the elderly.[10]

ANALYTIC STUDIES

ECOLOGIC STUDIES

As in experimental studies, the unit of analysis can be individuals or groups of people in observational studies. Studies that use groups of people as the unit of analysis are called *ecologic studies*. Ecologic studies are relatively easy to carry out when group level measures of exposure or outcome, or both, are available. However, a relationship observed between variables on a group level does not necessarily reflect the relationship that exists at an indi-

vidual level. For example, the fraction of energy supply from animal products was found to be positively correlated with breast cancer mortality in an ecologic study, which used preexisting data on dietary supply and breast cancer mortality from 35 countries.[11] Because the data were country based, no reliable inference can be made at an individual level. Within each country, it could be that the people who had a low fraction of energy supply from animal products were actually dying from breast cancer. Results from ecologic studies are useful for inference at an individual level only when the within-group variability of the exposure is low so a group-level measure can reasonably reflect exposure at an individual level. On the other hand, if the implications for prevention or intervention are at a group level (e.g., regulations regarding advertisements or taxation of cigarettes to prevent or reduce smoking), results from ecologic studies are very useful.

CROSS-SECTIONAL STUDIES

In three main types of analytic studies, the unit of analysis is individuals: cross-sectional studies, cohort studies, and case-control studies. In a cross-sectional study, the information on various factors is collected from the study population at a given point in time. In other words, a cross-sectional study is a snapshot of what is happening at the moment of the study. From a public health perspective, data collected in cross-sectional studies can be of great value in assessing the general health status of a population and allocating resources. For example, the third National Health and Nutrition Examination Survey conducted by the National Center for Health Statistics between 1988 and 1994 has provided valuable national estimates of health and nutritional status of the U.S. civilian, noninstitutionalized population.[12] Findings from cross-sectional studies can also help generate hypotheses that can be tested later in other types of studies. However, it should be noted that cross-sectional studies have serious methodologic limitations if the research purpose is etiologic inference. Because exposures and disease status are evaluated simultaneously, it is usually not possible to know the temporality of events, unless the exposure cannot change over time (e.g., blood type, skin color, race, country of birth, etc.). If one observes that more patients with brain cancer are depressed than people without brain cancer in a cross-sectional study, the correlation does not necessarily mean that depression causes brain cancer. Depression may simply have resulted from the pathogenesis and diagnosis of brain cancer, or depression may have caused brain cancer in some patients and resulted from brain cancer in other patients. Without obtaining additional information on the timing of events, no conclusions can be made. Another methodologic concern in cross-sectional studies is the enrollment of prevalent cases—that is, cases of patients who survived different lengths of time after the incidence of disease. Factors that affect survival may also influence incidence. Prevalent cases may not be representative of incident cases, which makes etiologic inferences based on cross-sectional studies suspect at best. These limitations are probably the reasons that cross-sectional studies, together with ecologic studies, are sometimes categorized as descriptive studies. As discussed in the introductory section, the line dividing descriptive studies and analytic studies is rather blurry.

COHORT STUDIES

In a cohort study, a study population free of a specific disease (or any other health-related condition) is grouped based on their exposure status and followed up for a certain period of time, and then the exposed and unexposed subjects are compared with respect to disease status at the end of the follow-up. The objective of a cohort study is usually to evaluate whether the incidence of a disease is associated with an exposure. The cohort design is fundamental in observational epidemiology and is considered "ideal" in that, if unbiased, cohort data reflect the real-life cause-effect sequence of disease.[13] Subjects in cohort studies may be a sample of the general population in a geographic area, a group of workers who are exposed to certain occupational hazards in a specific industry, or people who are considered at high risk for a specific disease. A cohort study is considered prospective or concurrent if the investigator starts following up the cohort from the present time into the future and retrospective or historic if the cohort is established in the past based on existing records (e.g., an occupational cohort based on employment records) and the follow-up ends before or at the time of the study. Alternatively, a cohort study can be ambidirectional in that data collection goes in both directions.[14] Whether a cohort study is prospective, retrospective, or ambidirectional, the key feature is that all the subjects were free of the disease at the beginning of the follow-up and the study tracks the subjects from exposure to disease. Time is an essential element in cohort studies. Follow-up time in cohort studies can range from days to decades.

In a cohort study, the incidence of disease in the exposed group and the unexposed group is compared. The incidence measure can be cumulative incidence or incidence density, depending on the availability of data. When comparing the incidence in the two groups, relative differences and absolute differences can be assessed. In cohort studies, the relative risk of developing the disease is expressed as the ratio of the cumulative incidence in the exposed group to that in the unexposed group, which is also called *cumulative incidence ratio* or *risk ratio.* If we have data on the exact person-time of follow-up for every subject, we can also calculate an incidence density ratio (also called *rate ratio*) in a similar way. A risk or rate ratio above 1 indicates that the exposed group has a higher risk of developing the disease than the unexposed group, and therefore, the exposure is a risk factor. A risk or rate ratio equal to 1 suggests that the two groups have the same risk of developing the disease. A risk or rate ratio below 1 indicates that the exposed group has a lower risk of developing the disease than the unexposed group, and therefore, the exposure is a protective factor. The numeric value of the risk or rate ratio reflects the magnitude of the association between an exposure and a disease. For example, a risk ratio of 2 would be interpreted as exposed individuals having doubled risk of developing a disease over unexposed individuals, whereas a risk ratio of 5 indicates that exposed individuals have five times greater risk of developing a disease than do unexposed individuals. Put in another way, a factor with a risk ratio of 5 has a stronger effect than another factor with a risk ratio of 2. In addition to risk ratio and rate ratio, another relative measure called *probability odds ratio* can be calculated in cohort studies. The probability odds of disease is the number of subjects who developed a disease divided by the number of subjects who did not develop the disease, and the probability odds ratio is the probability odds in the exposed group divided by the probability odds in the unexposed group. The probability odds ratio tends to exaggerate the association between an exposure and a disease in that the numeric value of a probability odds

ratio will be further away from 1 than the risk ratio, but the difference between probability odds ratio and risk ratio is often negligible if the disease is rare. Many investigators prefer risk ratio or rate ratio to probability odds ratio in cohort studies, because the ability to directly measure the risk of developing a disease is one of the most significant advantages in cohort studies. In practice, however, probability odds ratio is often used as an approximation for risk or rate ratio, especially when multivariate logistic regression models are used to adjust for the effect of other factors that may influence the relationship between an exposure and a disease.

As for absolute differences, a commonly used measure is called *attributable risk* in the exposed, which is the incidence in the exposed group minus the incidence in the unexposed group. Attributable risk reflects the disease incidence that could be attributed to the exposure in exposed individuals and the reduction in incidence that we would expect if the exposure can be removed from the exposed individuals, provided that there is a causal relationship between the exposure and the disease. Another absolute measure called *population attributable risk* extends this concept to the general population: It estimates the disease incidence that could be attributed to an exposure in the general population. Population attributable risk is lower than attributable risk in the exposed, but it becomes close to attributable risk in the exposed when an exposure is common in the general population.

Because relative differences and absolute differences can be assessed in cohort studies, a natural question to ask is what measures to choose. In general, the relative differences are used more often if the main research objective is etiologic inference, and they can be used for the judgment of causality. Once causality is established or at least assumed, measures of absolute differences are more important from the perspective of public health administration and policy. This point can be illustrated using the following hypothetical example: Assuming toxin X in the environment triples the risk of bladder cancer and toxin Y doubles the risk of bladder cancer, the effects of X and Y are entirely independent of each other, the prevalence of exposure to toxin Y in the general population is 20 times higher than the prevalence of exposure to toxin X, and there are only resources available to reduce the exposure to one toxin, it would be more effective to use the resources to reduce the exposure to toxin Y instead of toxin X. This is because the population attributable risk due to Y is higher than that due to X, although the risk ratio associated with toxin Y is smaller than that associated with toxin X.

Cohort studies have many advantages. A cohort design is the best way to ascertain the incidence and the natural history of a disease.[14] A clear temporal relationship is usually seen between an exposure and a disease, because all the subjects are free of the disease at the beginning of the follow-up (a problem may arise if a subject has a subclinical disease such as undetected prostate cancer). Furthermore, multiple diseases can be studied with respect to the same exposure. On the other hand, cohort studies, especially prospective cohort studies, are usually costly in terms of time and money. A cohort design requires the follow-up of a large number of study participants over a sometimes extremely lengthy period of time and usually extensive data collection through questionnaires, physical measurements, and/or biologic specimens at regular intervals. Participants may be "lost" during the follow-up because they become tired of the study, move away from the study area, or die from some causes other than the disease under study. If the subjects who are lost during the follow-up are different from those who remain under observation with respect to exposure, disease, or other factors that may influence the relationship between the exposure and the disease, results from the study will be biased. To date, cohort studies have been used to study the etiology of a wide spectrum of diseases, including different types of cancer. However, if the disease of interest is rare or takes a long time to develop, a cohort design is not efficient. Most types of cancer are uncommon and involve a long induction time. If a cohort study is conducted to evaluate the etiology of cancer, the study sample size would usually need to be very large and the follow-up time would need to be long, unless the cohort selected is a high-risk population.

For simplicity, we have discussed cohort studies in which the outcome of interest is the incidence of a specific disease and there are only two exposure groups. In practice, any health-related event can be the outcome of interest, and multiple exposure groups can be compared.

CASE-CONTROL STUDIES

Case-control design is an alternative to cohort design for the evaluation of the relationship between an exposure and a disease (or any other health condition). A case-control approach compares the odds of past exposure between cases and non-cases (controls) and uses the exposure odds ratio as an estimate for relative risk. A primary goal in a case-control study is to reach the same conclusions as would have been obtained from a cohort study if one had been done.[15] If appropriately designed and conducted, a case-control study can optimize speed and efficiency, as the need for follow-up is avoided.[13] The starting point of a case-control study is a source population from which the cases arise. The source population represents a hypothetical population in which a cohort study might have been conducted. Instead of obtaining the denominators for the calculation of risks or rates in a cohort study, a control group is sampled from the entire source population. After selecting control subjects, who ideally would have become cases had they developed the disease, an investigator collects data on past exposures from the cases and the controls and then calculates an exposure odds ratio, which is the odds of exposure in the cases divided by the odds of exposure in the controls. In case-control studies, exposure odds ratio equals disease odds ratio (odds of disease in the exposed divided by the odds of disease in the unexposed), and, therefore, it can be used to estimate relative risk. It is important to note that for the exposure odds ratio to be a valid estimate of relative risk, controls must be selected independent of their exposure status.

The two main types of case-control studies are case-based case-control studies and case-control studies within defined cohorts.[13] Some variations of the case-control design also exist. For instance, if the effect of an exposure is transient, a case can sometimes be used as his or her own control (case-crossover design). In case-based case-control studies, cases and controls are selected at a given point in time from a hypothetical cohort (i.e., at the end of follow-up). A cross-sectional ascertainment of cases results in a case group that mostly contains prevalent cases, who may have survived for different lengths of time after disease incidence. Cases who died before an investigator began

subject ascertainment would not be eligible to be included in the study. As a result, the cases finally included in the study may not be representative of all the cases from the entire hypothetical cohort, with respect to the exposure or other factors that may influence the relationship between the exposure and the disease. Another disadvantage of enrolling prevalent cases is that cases who were diagnosed a long time ago will likely have difficulties recalling exposures that occurred before disease incidence (exposures that occurred after disease incidence are irrelevant for etiologic inference). In case-control studies it is preferable to ascertain incident cases as soon as they are diagnosed and to select controls as soon as cases are identified. Case-control studies that enroll only incident cases are sometimes called *prospective case-control studies* in that the investigators must wait for the incident cases to develop and get diagnosed. For cancer studies, the cases can be ascertained from population-based cancer registries or hospitals. A major advantage of using a cancer registry is the completeness of case ascertainment, but the reporting of cancer cases to registries is usually not instantaneous. A lag time of several months or even over a year could occur, and some cases could have died during the lag time. If the cancer under study has a poor survival or clinical specimens must be obtained in a timely manner, or both, it may be preferable to identify cases directly from hospitals using a rapid ascertainment protocol. If all or most hospitals within a given geographic area are included in a rapid ascertainment system, cases identified from the system will be approximately population based.

As for the selection of controls, the key issue is that controls should be representative of the source population from which the cases arise, and theoretically the controls would have been ascertained as cases had they developed the disease. The most common types of controls include population-based controls (often selected through random digit dialing in case-control studies of cancer etiology), hospital controls, and friend controls. The advantages and disadvantages of different types of controls have been nicely summarized by Wacholder et al.[16] No matter what type of control is chosen, it is challenging to ensure a truly representative sample because the source population from which the cases arise is sometimes difficult to define and the participation rate of potential controls is usually lower than that of the cases. Because no follow-up is involved in case-based case-control studies, incidence risk or rate cannot be calculated directly for case and control groups. The odds ratio is usually the effect measure. In case-based case-control studies, the odds ratio will be a good estimate of relative risk if the disease is uncommon.

In addition to case-based case-control studies, there are also case-control studies within defined cohorts (also known as *hybrid or ambidirectional designs*), including case-cohort studies and nested case-control studies. In case-cohort studies, cases are identified from a well-defined cohort after some follow-up time, and controls are selected from the baseline cohort. In nested case-control studies, cases are also identified from a cohort, but controls are selected from the individuals at risk at the time each case occurs (i.e., incidence density sampling).[13] In these types of designs, controls are a sample of the cohort and the controls selected can theoretically become cases at some point. The possibility of selection bias in case-control studies within defined cohorts is lower than that in case-based case-control studies because the cases and the controls are selected from the same source population. Because of an increased awareness of the methodologic issues inherent in the design of case-based case-control studies and the availability of a growing number of large cohorts, case-control studies within defined cohorts have become more common in recent years. Such designs have been applied to the evaluation of cancer etiology.[17] The advantage of case-control studies within cohorts over traditional cohort studies is mainly the efficiency in additional data collection. For instance, a nested case-control study evaluated the relationship between endogenous sex hormones and prostate cancer risk.[17] Instead of measuring the serum hormone levels of the entire cohort (more than 12,000 subjects), investigators chose to measure only 300 cases and 300 controls selected from the cohort. Doing so not only significantly reduced the cost of measurements and the time it took to address the research question but also helped preserve valuable serum samples for possible analyses in the future. As in case-based case-control studies, the odds ratio is also the effect measure in case-control studies within cohorts. In a case-cohort design, an odds ratio estimates risk ratio; in a nested case-control design, an odds ratio estimates rate ratio. In both designs, the disease under study does not have to be rare for the odds ratio to be a good estimate of the risk ratio or rate ratio.[13,18] This is different from case-based case-control studies.

The biggest advantage of a case-control design is the speed and efficiency in obtaining data. It is claimed that investigators implement case-control studies more frequently than any other analytic epidemiologic study.[19] Because most types of cancer are not common and take a long time to develop, to date most epidemiologic studies of cancer have been case-control instead of cohort in design. A case-control study can be conducted to evaluate the relationship between many different exposures and a specific disease, but the study will have limited statistical power if the exposure is rare. In general, a case-control design tends to be more susceptible to biases than a cohort design. Such biases include but are not limited to selection bias when choosing and enrolling subjects (especially controls) and recall bias when obtaining data from the subjects. The status of the subjects, that is, case or control, may affect how they recall and report previous exposures, some of which occurred years or even decades ago. In a way, case-control studies are easier to do, but they are also easier to do wrong.[19] It is important for investigators to explicitly define the diagnostic and eligibility criteria for cases; to select controls from the same population as the cases independent of the exposures of interest; to blind data collection staff to the case or control status of subjects or, if impossible, at least to blind them to the main hypotheses of the study; to ascertain exposure in a similar manner from cases and controls; and to take into account other factors that may influence the relationship between an exposure and a disease.[19]

INTERPRETATION OF EPIDEMIOLOGIC FINDINGS

Measures of effects in various study designs have been discussed. However, a risk ratio of 3 from a cohort study or an odds ratio of 2.5 from a case-control study does not necessarily mean that there is an association between an exposure and a disease. Several alternative explanations must be assessed, including chance (random error), bias (systematic error), and confounding. Potential interaction also must be evaluated.

Statistical methods are required to evaluate the role of chance. A usual way is to calculate the upper and lower limits of a 95% confidence interval around a point estimate for relative risk (risk ratio, rate ratio, or odds ratio). If the confidence interval does not include 1, one would say that the observed association is statistically significant; if the confidence interval includes 1, one would say that the observed relationship is not statistically significant. The width of a confidence interval is directly related to the number of participants in a study, which is called *sample size*. A larger sample size leads to less variability in the data, a tighter confidence interval, and a higher possibility in finding a statistically significant relationship, if one truly exists. A 95% confidence interval means that if the data collection and analysis could be replicated many times, the confidence interval should include the correct value of the measure 95% of the time.[20] The choice of 95% is almost a default in the literature, but the upper and lower limits of an interval with a different level of confidence (e.g., 90%, 99%) can certainly be calculated and interpreted accordingly. The calculation of confidence interval involves two assumptions: (1) The only thing that would differ in hypothetical replications of the study would be the statistical, or chance, element in the data; and (2) the variability in the data can be described adequately by statistical methods, and biases are nonexistent.[20] Because these assumptions are fairly unrealistic in epidemiologic studies, it is more useful to consider a confidence interval to be a general guide to the amount of random error in the data but not necessarily a literal measure of statistical variability.[20]

Bias can be defined as any systematic error in an epidemiologic study that results in an incorrect estimate of the association between exposure and disease, and it can occur in every type of epidemiologic study design. The two main types of bias are selection bias and information bias. Selection bias is present when individuals included in a study are systematically different from the target population, for example, if a study aimed to generate a sample representing all women in the United States, of the women contacted more with a family history of breast cancer agreed to participate. This sample would be at a higher risk for breast cancer than the target population. Refusal to participate poses a constant challenge in epidemiologic studies. As individuals have become more concerned about privacy issues and as studies have become more demanding of time, biologic specimens, and other impositions, participation rates have dropped substantially in recent years. If nonparticipants are different from the participants with respect to study-related characteristics, the validity of the study is threatened. In cohort studies, selection bias often manifests through differential losses to follow up with respect to disease in the exposed and unexposed groups. In case-control studies, selection bias can occur if the selection of cases and controls is influenced by exposure status, prevalent cases are included, or the controls are selected from a population with different characteristics than the population to which the cases belong.

Information bias occurs when the data collected from the study subjects are erroneous. Information bias is also known as *misclassification* if the variable is measured on a categoric scale and the error causes a subject to be placed in a wrong category. Misclassification can happen to exposure and to disease. For example, in a case-control study of previous reproductive history and ovarian cancer, a woman who had an extremely early pregnancy loss may not even realize that she was ever pregnant and would mistakenly report no pregnancy, and another woman who has only subclinical presentations of ovarian cancer may be mistakenly selected as a control. Misclassification can be differential or nondifferential. An exposure misclassification is considered differential if it is related to disease status and nondifferential if not related to disease status. Similarly, a disease misclassification is considered differential if it is related to exposure status and nondifferential if not related to exposure status. If a binary exposure variable and a binary disease variable are analyzed, nondifferential misclassification will result in an underestimate of the true association. Differential misclassification can either exaggerate or underestimate a true effect. In a cohort study, differential misclassification can occur if the ascertainment of disease by the observer is influenced by the exposure status (e.g., a physician may examine a subject more thoroughly if he or she knows that the subject is exposed and likely has a higher risk, and exposed subjects may visit doctors more often if they think that they are at a higher risk). In case-control studies, differential misclassification can occur if cases and controls recall and report their past exposure in a systematically different way (e.g., cases overreport exposure and controls report the truth).

Usually not much can be done to control or correct selection and information bias at the data analysis stage; therefore, it is important for investigators to establish research protocols that are not prone to bias. The evaluation of potential bias is critical to the interpretation of study results. An invalid estimate is worse than no estimate.

Confounding refers to a situation in which the association between an exposure and a disease (or any health-related condition) is influenced by a third variable. This third variable is considered a confounding variable or confounder. A confounder must fulfill three criteria: (1) be associated with the exposure, (2) be associated with the disease independent of the exposure, and (3) not be an intermediate step between the exposure and the disease (i.e., not on the causal pathway). Unlike bias, which is primarily introduced by the investigator or study participants, confounding is a function of the complex interrelationship between various exposures and disease.[7] In a hypothetical case-control study of the effect of alcohol drinking on lung cancer, we may observe an odds ratio of 2.5 (usually called a *crude* odds ratio in the sense that no other variables were taken into account), which indicates that alcohol drinking increases the risk of lung cancer by 1.5-fold. However, if we classify all study subjects into two strata based on history of cigarette smoking and then calculate the odds ratio in the two strata (smokers and nonsmokers) separately, we may have two stratum-specific odds ratios both equal to 1, indicating that alcohol drinking is not associated with lung cancer risk. In this example, the crude odds ratio calculated to estimate the association between alcohol drinking and lung cancer without considering smoking is simply misleading. Being associated with the exposure (i.e., alcohol drinking) and the disease (i.e., lung cancer), smoking acted as a confounder in this example.

A stratified analysis is needed to evaluate the potential confounding effect of a third variable, whether it is done with pencil and paper or statistical modeling. Usually, data are stratified based on the level of a third variable. If the stratum-specific effect measures are similar to each other but different from the crude effect measure, confounding is said to be present. In this chapter, we have illustrated basic epidemiologic principles using an overly simplified scenario and only considered a single exposure. In practice, most, if not all, diseases, cancer included, have a multifactorial etiology. Consequently, it is usually necessary to

assess the potential confounding effect of a group of variables simultaneously using multivariate statistical models. However, the essence of multivariate modeling is still a stratified analysis. The effect measure derived from a multivariate model is then called an *adjusted* one in the sense that the effect of other factors was also adjusted for. Without controlling for the potential effect of other variables, an investigator cannot really judge whether an observed association between a given exposure and a specific disease is spurious.

If the effect of an exposure on the risk of a disease is not homogeneous in strata formed by a third variable, the third variable is considered an effect modifier, and the situation is called *interaction* or *effect modification*. Put in other words, interaction exists when the stratum-specific effect measures are different from each other. In the lung cancer example above, if the odds ratio for alcohol drinking is 1 in smokers but 3 in nonsmokers, interaction has occurred and smoking is an effect modifier. The evaluation of interaction is essentially a stratified analysis, which is similar to the evaluation of confounding. Confounding and interaction can both be present in a given study. However, when interaction occurs, the stratum-specific effect measures should be reported. It is no longer appropriate to report an adjusted summary effect measure in the presence of interaction. Interaction can be evaluated on an additive scale and a multiplicative scale. Unlike confounding, a nuisance that an investigator hopes to remove, interaction is a more detailed description of the true relationship between an exposure and a disease. The evaluation of gene-environment interaction has captured considerable attention in recent years. Gene-environment interaction can obscure environmental effects (which may be evident only in genetically susceptible persons) and genetic effects (which may be evident only in those with certain histories of environmental exposure). Therefore, study of gene-environment interaction is important for improving accuracy and precision in the assessment of genetic and environmental influences.[21]

A primary goal of epidemiology is to identify the causes of disease, that is, to make causal inferences based on observations and experiments. No simple procedure is available to follow to determine whether an observed relationship is causal. A commonly cited list of nine criteria (strength, consistency, specificity, temporality, biologic gradient, plausibility, coherence, experimental evidence, and analogy) is attributed to Dr. Branford Hill, although he did not propose these criteria as a checklist for evaluating whether a reported association might be interpreted as causal.[20] These criteria provide a starting point from which to examine claims of causal associations, but with the exception of temporality, no other criterion can bring indisputable evidence for or against a cause-and-effect hypothesis. The sufficient and component cause model proposed by Rothman[20] offers an alternative way of thinking. Relatively new tools have been suggested for causal inferences, including causal diagrams[22] and marginal structural models.[23]

SPECIAL TOPIC: MOLECULAR AND GENETIC EPIDEMIOLOGY

The incorporation of molecular, cellular, and other biologic measurements into epidemiologic research has given rise to a relatively new field, molecular epidemiology. Molecular epidemiologic studies generally include (1) studies that directly assay exposure to specific substances, (2) those that evaluate phenotype or genotype information about metabolic pathways that may alter the effective dose of an exposure or other host susceptibility factors, and (3) those that use markers of a specific effect (for instance gene expression) to refine disease categories for analyses (of heterogeneity, prognosis, etiology, etc.). The type of specimen collected is determined by the exposure of interest and the methods available to quantify that exposure. Some investigations focus on directly measuring exposure, such as blood levels of substances (e.g., toxins, carcinogens, nutrients, micronutrients, viral titers), DNA adducts, levels of metabolites in urine, and the like. These data are then correlated with measures of exposure from occupational records, questionnaire responses, medical records, and other sources of data. If metabolic pathways of the exposure of interest are known, often genes with variations (polymorphisms) are evaluated and correlated with either biologic measurements of dose or historic measures, or both. Newer technologies such as gene expression to define subtypes of tumors[24] or protein patterns specific for cancers[25] have been used in clinical studies and are being considered for large-scale epidemiologic studies. Other host susceptibility factors (for instance immune function) may be related to time to progression, disease severity, or other parameters.

Molecular epidemiologic studies have all of the logistic and methodologic characteristics of conventional epidemiologic studies. They also have the added constraints of laboratory components.[26,27] Molecular epidemiologic studies are, by definition, interdisciplinary and require investigators from highly divergent fields to collaborate closely from study design to completion. The complexity of these investigations manifests in the epidemiologic and the laboratory components.

Many of the early molecular epidemiologic investigations were relatively small, exploratory studies to determine the feasibility of this approach, to validate biologic markers, and to estimate level of risk.[26] Even when assessing polymorphisms present in one-half of the population, these relatively small studies do not have statistical power to evaluate modest risks, especially in subgroup analyses.[28,29] With the advances in laboratory techniques and the identification of many genetic variations that alter effective dose of exposure, much larger studies now are necessary to test adequately hypotheses involving complex exposures.[30,31] Careful estimates of sample size to detect the level of risk expected, given the frequency of exposure expected and the variation in biologic measures, must be accomplished as part of the early planning. The epidemiologic study design is directly affected by the sample size necessary for molecular studies. These investigations typically must include hundreds or thousands of study subjects to detect a significant difference in, for instance, the effect of a genetic polymorphism that occurs in one-third of the population or a difference in adduct levels when one-half of the population is exposed. Even larger numbers are necessary to try to evaluate gene exposure or gene-gene interactions. The appropriate controls for these molecular epidemiologic studies have also been under extensive discussion. Although some have argued strongly for the use of cases' relatives as controls to avoid population stratification,[32] others have demonstrated that population stratification is unlikely to cause problems in a carefully conducted study and analysis.[33] The type and quantity of biologic specimens to be collected has to be decided together with the laboratory investigators. The specimens requested will have an effect not only on the study design and cost but on the response rate of the potential participants.[34] Adequate consent procedures are complex and essential. Because many of the exact laboratory assays may not have been selected (or developed) at the time the participant is enrolled in the study, specifying exactly what will be done with the specimen may be somewhat problematic. Many investigators now use a consent that allows for different levels of use of the specimen (e.g., for only the specified assays or for other assays related to the disease of interest) or for any future use. Analytic methods to incorporate complex laboratory information such as haplotype data or expression arrays as well as traditional epidemiologic data must be developed and refined.

The additional complexity of the laboratory components begins with establishing methods for appropriate collection, processing, and transportation of biologic specimens with necessary quality control measures. Because many of the specimens must be stored for various lengths of time before being assayed, some type of repository system is needed to locate and track specimens. As laboratory assays are completed for the samples, each sample becomes more valuable because of the laboratory information in combination with the epidemiologic information connected to each sample. Repository functions, including proper identification and tracking of each sample, remain essential. All the routine difficulties of validity and reproducibility of the laboratory techniques being used on the specimens must be resolved before analysis of the samples. Many of the assays of particular interest may be technically challenging, quite complex, or very expensive. The laboratory collaborators often have to develop the methods to conduct the assays or genotyping on large numbers of samples (hundreds or thousands). When costs may be prohibitive in very large studies, carefully designed subgroup analyses may be useful. Despite the challenges of these complex studies, they hold the promise of more closely integrating biologic measures of exposure to the more traditional questionnaire and record abstraction of exposure information.

Many investigators conducting cohort studies try to collect biologic specimens for future use. One major advantage of these collections is that specimen collection occurs before disease onset. Because, in large cohorts, a majority of individuals will not develop the diseases of interest, many specimens will not be informative about the diseases the study was designed to investigate. With the sequential information gathered over time, new hypotheses and different outcomes can be evaluated in these cohorts, however. Collection and storage of large numbers of specimens for decades is costly, especially because relatively few of the samples will actually be assayed (in nested case-control or case-cohort analyses). Storage costs are proportional to volume of material and number of specimens collected. For cohort studies with large numbers and continuing contact with the study participants, the type of specimen collected is a trade-off between imposition costs for the participants, the storage needs and costs of the specimen, and the potential uses of those specimens. For low-cost blood storage for DNA, limited quantities of blood (100 to 150 µL) can be stored on collection cards.[35] For noninvasive collection of genetic materials, buccal cell collection is a reasonable option with limitations.[36] For most cohort studies, specimen collections will be relatively limited with finite quantities; extremely careful selective use of samples for assays is therefore essential. As new laboratory techniques develop that consume less of the total sample, these invaluable resources can be increasingly informative. For DNA-based analyses, new whole genome amplification techniques may extend the sample.

Case-control studies may offer more efficient collection and storage of specimens, but these samples may be altered by the presence of disease in the cases or by hospital-related exposures. A relative advantage is that the specimens will be quickly informative. In contrast to cohort studies, there is not a long latency before cases occur and samples are potentially useful for proposed laboratory tests. Greater volumes of specimens (e.g., blood) can possibly be collected and stored, because the participants are not being sequentially contacted and long-term storage (for decades) before use is not anticipated. Storage issues for thousands of samples accrued over a several-year period are not trivial, however. Consent issues may still be problematic, as with cohort studies, because new hypotheses or laboratory tests may be developed that were not originally anticipated when participants were accrued. Case-control studies may be a more efficient design to investigate interactions between host susceptibility factors and exposures (gene exposure and gene-gene interactions), especially when the type of cancer being studied is relatively rare.[26]

Genetic epidemiologic studies overlap substantially with molecular epidemiologic studies, particularly when the "molecular" component is evaluating variations in genes, expression of genes, or gene products. The field of genetic epidemiology has rapidly increased with the advent of gene identification and large-scale genotyping. Genetic epidemiology in its broad context, however, includes family studies, molecular epidemiologic studies with genetic components, and more traditional cohort and case-control studies with family history components. Similar to the molecular epidemiologic studies, genetic epidemiologic studies are multidisciplinary from the outset and involve clinicians, geneticists, epidemiologists, and laboratory investigators. These studies include all the complications of molecular epidemiologic studies, often with the additional complexity of having to deal with family dynamics.[37]

Family studies have been essential for mapping and identifying the many major cancer susceptibility genes found in the past decade. Once the contribution of genetic variation to disease within the families has been established, however, these variations should be evaluated in relation to known exposure factors for the specific cancers of interest (parity, reproductive factors for breast cancer; sun for melanoma, etc.). Complex analytic techniques that incorporate genotype information and environmental risk factors into a regressive model have been developed.[38] Again, large numbers of families are necessary for these gene-environment and, potentially, gene-gene interactions. To facilitate these studies, international consortia have been formed.[39,40] Care must be taken in these analyses to account for familial relationships, as the observations within families are not necessarily independent. Families share not only genes but environmental exposures and lifestyles. Within high-risk families, selected because there are many living members, penetrance (risk of developing disease associated with carrying an altered gene) estimates will be high but useful for determining an upper limit on the risk associated with alteration of a specific gene.

Larger population studies are important for estimating the effect of an altered gene outside of high-risk families selected for linkage analyses. Because most cancers are adult-onset, complex diseases, even when a major susceptibility gene is mutated, other factors may be important. Large epidemiologic studies are needed to identify these additional risk factors so that the complex chain of events that results in cancer development can be interrupted. One approach is to conduct a large case-control study in which usual risk factors are obtained and large genes, such as *BRCA1* or *BRCA2* (each having hundreds of mutations throughout the gene), are analyzed.[41] This is logistically challenging, laboratory time intensive, and costly. Even though mutations in such genes as *BRCA1* and *BRCA2* account for a percentage of familial breast cancer and are important for understanding the biology of breast cancer development, they represent only a small fraction of breast cancer in the general population.[41] Sample sizes for these studies must, therefore, be large, and, even then, the limitation is the number of mutation carriers in the referent (control) population.

Another approach to understanding the role of mutations in the development of cancers is to take advantage of the opportunity afforded by relatively isolated populations with so-called founder mutations, recurrent mutations prevalent in a specific group. Unlike other populations in which an entire gene must be sequenced, these founder mutations can be more easily genotyped because the laboratory searches for one or a limited number of specific mutations.[35] It is thus feasible to screen thousands of samples for the specific mutation. Founder mutations have been identified in a number of populations worldwide. For example, breast, ovarian, and prostate cancer risk associated with prevalent mutations in *BRCA1* and *BRCA2* was estimated in volunteers from the Jewish community of Washington, DC, and found to be much lower than estimates from high-risk families.[35] Populations with founder mutations in which participants in a study are not selected because of family history can also be informative about gene-exposure relationships. In a population-based study of ovarian cancer in Israel, almost one-third of the cases had one of the founder mutations. Among individuals carrying one of these mutations, parity was protective against ovarian cancer, but oral contraceptives were not. Among noncarriers, parity and oral contraceptive use were both protective.[42]

Family history data from case-control or cohort studies can be used to evaluate clustering of cancers in families. Information on first-degree relatives is usually accurate among well-educated Americans,[43,44] but this type of information is culture specific. In cultures in which notification of cancer diagnoses is not routine, information on cancer diagnoses in relatives will not be accurate. One approach to identifying families with known ascertainment for clustering studies or linkage analyses is to identify individuals from case-control or cohort studies with a family history of interest, contact the individual to ask for permission to contact other family members, and then evaluate the family members who are willing to participate. Another approach to systematic identification of families at increased risk of specific cancers is through population registries,[37] where genetic findings can be extrapolated to the population from which the cases are derived.[37,45] Individuals with a disease of interest are identified at the time of registration, and family history is obtained. If the family meets the criteria, family members are invited to participate in a family registry study.

This approach is being developed to provide resources for the research community.

Genetic epidemiologic studies that investigate other genes not considered among the major susceptibility genes are similar to those described in molecular epidemiology. Genetic epidemiologic studies have special issues, however.[35] Informed consent is complex. A growing concern among potential participants in any type of genetic epidemiologic study is the implementation of confidentiality practices to protect the privacy of genetic information. Another concern is notifying participants of results and the approach of this notification. If all identifiers are removed, individual notification becomes impossible. In most large studies, it is not feasible to counsel participants individually about their genotype status, even if it were possible to interpret the meaning of such variation. One approach is to notify participants about aggregate results so that they can then pursue clinical, rather than research, genetic testing with their physicians.

REFERENCES

1. Last J. *A dictionary of epidemiology.* New York: Oxford University Press, 1995.
2. Doll R, Hill AB. Lung cancer and other causes of death in relation to smoking; a second report on the mortality of British doctors. *BMJ* 1956;12:1071.
3. Kleinbaum D, Kupper L, Morgenstern H. *Epidemiologic research.* New York: Van Nostrand Reinhold, 1982.
4. Kaplan LD, et al. Low-dose compared with standard-dose m-BACOD chemotherapy for non-Hodgkin's lymphoma associated with human immunodeficiency virus infection. National Institute of Allergy and Infectious Diseases AIDS Clinical Trials Group. *N Engl J Med* 1997;336:1641.
5. Dunn BK, Kramer BS, Ford LG. Phase III, large-scale chemoprevention trials. Approach to chemoprevention clinical trials and phase III clinical trial of tamoxifen as a chemopreventive for breast cancer—the US National Cancer Institute experience. *Hematol Oncol Clin North Am* 1998;12:1019.
6. Mayne ST, et al. Randomized trial of supplemental beta-carotene to prevent second head and neck cancer. *Cancer Res* 2001;61:1457.
7. Hennekens C, Buring J. *Epidemiology in medicine.* In: Mayrent S, et al. Boston: Little, Brown and Company, 1987.
8. Corley DA, Buffler PA. Oesophageal and gastric cardia adenocarcinomas: analysis of regional variation using the Cancer Incidence in Five Continents database. *Int J Epidemiol* 2001;30:1415.
9. Robertson C, Perone C, Primic-Zakelj M, Kirn VP, Boyle P. Breast cancer incidence rates in Slovenia 1971–1993. *Int J Epidemiol* 2000;29:969.
10. Zheng T, et al. Are cancers of the salivary gland increasing? Experience from Connecticut, USA. *Int J Epidemiol* 1997;26:264.
11. Grant WB. An ecologic study of dietary and solar ultraviolet-B links to breast carcinoma mortality rates. *Cancer* 2002;94:272.
12. US Department of Health and Human Services (DHHS). National Center for Health Statistics. *Third National Health and Nutrition Examination Survey, 1988–1994.* Hyattsville, MD: Centers for Disease Control and Prevention, 1996.
13. Szklo M, Nieto F. *Epidemiology: beyond the basics.* Gaithersburg, MD: Aspen Publishers, 2000.
14. Grimes DA, Schulz KF. Cohort studies: marching towards outcomes. *Lancet* 2002;359:341.
15. Mantel N, Haenszel W. Statistical aspects of the analysis of data from retrospective studies of disease. *J Natl Cancer Inst* 1959;22:719.
16. Wacholder S, Silverman DT, McLaughlin JK, Mandel JS. Selection of controls in case-control studies. II. Types of controls. *Am J Epidemiol* 1992;135:1029.
17. Chen C, et al. Endogenous sex hormones and prostate cancer risk: a case-control study nested within the Carotene and Retinol Efficacy Trial. *Cancer Epidemiol Biomarkers Prev* 2003;12:1410.
18. Pearce N. What does the odds ratio estimate in a case-control study? *Int J Epidemiol* 1993;22:1189.
19. Schulz KF, Grimes DA. Case-control studies: research in reverse. *Lancet* 2002;359:431.
20. Rothman K. *Epidemiology: an introduction.* New York: Oxford University Press, 2002.
21. Ottman R. Gene-environment interaction: definitions and study designs. *Prev Med* 1996; 25:764.
22. Greenland S, Pearl J, Robins JM. Causal diagrams for epidemiologic research. *Epidemiology* 1999;10:37.
23. Robins JM, Hernan MA, Brumback B. Marginal structural models and causal inference in epidemiology. *Epidemiology* 2000;11:550.
24. Wright G, et al. A gene expression-based method to diagnose clinically distinct subgroups of diffuse large B cell lymphoma. *Proc Natl Acad Sci U S A* 2003;100:9991.
25. Petricoin EF, et al. Use of proteomic patterns in serum to identify ovarian cancer. *Lancet* 2002;359:572.
26. Caporaso N, Rothman N, Wacholder S. Case-control studies of common alleles and environmental factors. *J Natl Cancer Inst Monogr* 1999;25.
27. Schaid DJ, et al. Discovery of cancer susceptibility genes: study designs, analytic approaches, and trends in technology. *J Natl Cancer Inst Monogr* 1999;1.
28. Le Marchand L, et al. Associations of CYP1A1, GSTM1, and CYP2E1 polymorphisms with lung cancer suggest cell type specificities to tobacco carcinogens. *Cancer Res* 1998;58:4858.
29. London SJ, et al. Lung cancer risk in African-Americans in relation to a race-specific CYP1A1 polymorphism. *Cancer Res* 1995;55:6035.
30. Garcia-Closas M, Rothman N, Lubin J. Misclassification in case-control studies of gene-environment interactions: assessment of bias and sample size. *Cancer Epidemiol Biomarkers Prev* 1999;8:1043.
31. Garcia-Closas M, Lubin JH. Power and sample size calculations in case-control studies of gene-environment interactions: comments on different approaches. *Am J Epidemiol* 1999; 149:689.
32. Thomas DC, Witte JS. Point: population stratification: a problem for case-control studies of candidate-gene associations? *Cancer Epidemiol Biomarkers Prev* 2002;11:505.
33. Wacholder S, Rothman N, Caporaso N. Counterpoint: bias from population stratification is not a major threat to the validity of conclusions from epidemiological studies of common polymorphisms and cancer. *Cancer Epidemiol Biomarkers Prev* 2002;11:513.
34. Hunter D. *Methodological issues in the use of biological markers in cancer epidemiology: cohort studies.* Lyon, France: IARC, 1997.
35. Struewing JP, et al. The risk of cancer associated with specific mutations of BRCA1 and BRCA2 among Ashkenazi Jews. *N Engl J Med* 1997;336:1401.
36. Lum A, Le Marchand L. A simple mouthwash method for obtaining genomic DNA in molecular epidemiological studies. *Cancer Epidemiol Biomarkers Prev* 1998;7:719.
37. Whittemore AS, Nelson LM. Study design in genetic epidemiology: theoretical and practical considerations. *J Natl Cancer Inst Monogr* 1999:61.
38. Demenais F, Lathrop M. Use of the regressive models in linkage analysis of quantitative traits. *Genet Epidemiol* 1993;10:587.
39. Easton DF, Ford D, Bishop DT. Breast and ovarian cancer incidence in BRCA1-mutation carriers. Breast Cancer Linkage Consortium. *Am J Hum Genet* 1995;56:265.
40. Bishop DT, et al. Geographical variation in the penetrance of CDKN2A mutations for melanoma. *J Natl Cancer Inst* 2002;94:894.
41. Newman B, et al. Frequency of breast cancer attributable to BRCA1 in a population-based series of American women. *JAMA* 1998;279:915.
42. Modan B, et al. Parity, oral contraceptives, and the risk of ovarian cancer among carriers and noncarriers of a BRCA1 or BRCA2 mutation. *N Engl J Med* 2001;345:235.
43. Bondy ML, Strom SS, Colopy MW, Brown BW, Strong LC. Accuracy of family history of cancer obtained through interviews with relatives of patients with childhood sarcoma. *J Clin Epidemiol* 1994;47:89.
44. Novakovic B, Goldstein AM, Tucker MA. Validation of family history of cancer in deceased family members. *J Natl Cancer Inst* 1996;88:1492.
45. Hopper JL, et al. Design and analysis issues in a population-based, case-control-family study of the genetic epidemiology of breast cancer and the Co-operative Family Registry for Breast Cancer Studies (CFRBCS). *J Natl Cancer Inst Monogr* 1999:95.

AHMEDIN JEMAL
ELIZABETH M. WARD
MICHAEL J. THUN

SECTION 2

Cancer Statistics

Descriptive epidemiology of cancer, or cancer surveillance, characterizes cancer incidence and mortality by person, place, and time. By monitoring cancer patterns according to demographic characteristics (age, sex, race, socioeconomic status), geographic location, and trends over time, descriptive epidemiology provides clues about the causes of cancer and helps to set priorities and monitor the effectiveness of cancer control efforts.

MEASURES OF THE CANCER BURDEN

INCIDENCE AND MORTALITY

Incidence and mortality are two frequently used measures of cancer occurrence. These indices quantify the number of new

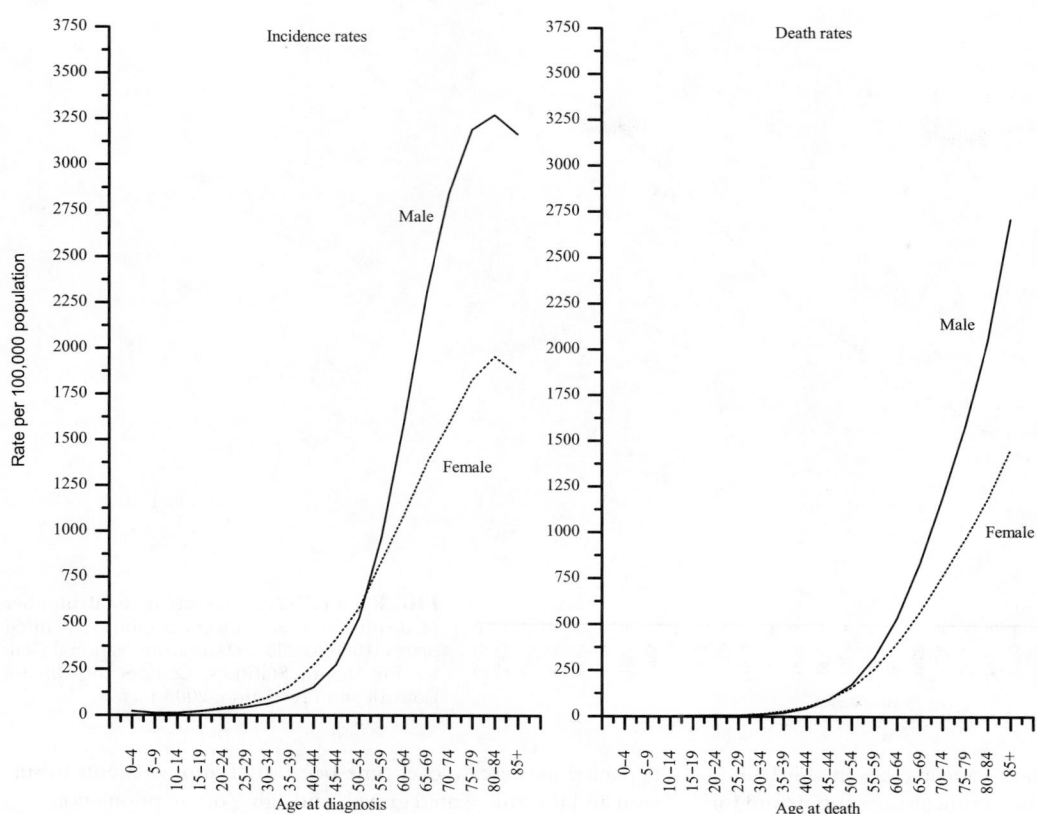

FIGURE 11.2-1. Age- and sex-specific incidence and death rates from all cancers combined, United States, 2000. [Incidence rates from Surveillance, Epidemiology, and End Results (SEER) program (http://www.seer.cancer.gov) SEER*Stat Database, 1973–2000. National Cancer Institute, 2003. Death rates from National Center for Health Statistics, Centers for Disease Control and Prevention, 2003.]

cancer cases or deaths, respectively, in a specified population over a defined time period. Incidence and mortality are commonly expressed as counts per 100,000 people per year to allow comparisons across populations of varying size and length of observation.

The incidence and death rates from all cancers combined increases exponentially with age from approximately 10 to 84 years (Fig. 11.2-1). Because age is such an important determinant of risk, vital statistics data usually present either age-specific data or rates that have been adjusted or standardized for age. Age standardization (described later in Data Sources and Age Standardization) serves two purposes: It summarizes the age-specific rates into a single number, and it allows valid comparisons to be made across populations with different age distributions.

NUMBER OF NEW CANCER CASES AND DEATHS

Another measure of the cancer burden in a population is the total number of new cases and deaths that occur in a given year in a specified community, irrespective of its size or age distribution. This measure reflects the absolute number of new cases that must be cared for by medical providers and social services. In the United States, as in most developed countries, the number of people who develop or die from cancer has increased substantially over time (Fig. 11.2-2) because of the growth and aging of the population. The increase in the total number of cancer deaths has occurred despite the decrease in the age-adjusted death rate from all cancers combined during the 1990s. Similarly, the projected number of new cancer cases

diagnosed in each year will double in 50 years if current age-adjusted incidence rates remain unchanged, from 1.3 million in 2000 to 2.6 million in 2050.[1]

Each year the American Cancer Society estimates the total number of new cancer cases and deaths that will occur in the nation and in each state in the current year (Fig. 11.2-3). These estimates are of interest because actual mortality statistics do not become available for approximately 3 years and incidence data are not collected nationwide in the United States. The American Cancer Society projections are more readily understood by the public than are projections of cancer rates and are frequently cited by cancer control planners and researchers.[2] The estimates are produced by modeling historic information on the observed number of cancer cases and deaths in past years and modeling trends over time.[3,4]

PREVALENCE

In contrast to incidence rates, which measure the rate at which new cancer cases are diagnosed in a specified population and time interval, prevalence measures the proportion of people who live with cancer at a certain point in time. In principle, the number of prevalent cases includes newly diagnosed cases, those who are under treatment, and people who are in remission. It is a function of the incidence rate and of survival or cure of the particular cancer. In practice, estimates of the number of prevalent cases cannot distinguish precisely between people who have been cured and those with active disease. Nevertheless, prevalence is a useful measure of the health care burden for planning future medical care needs.

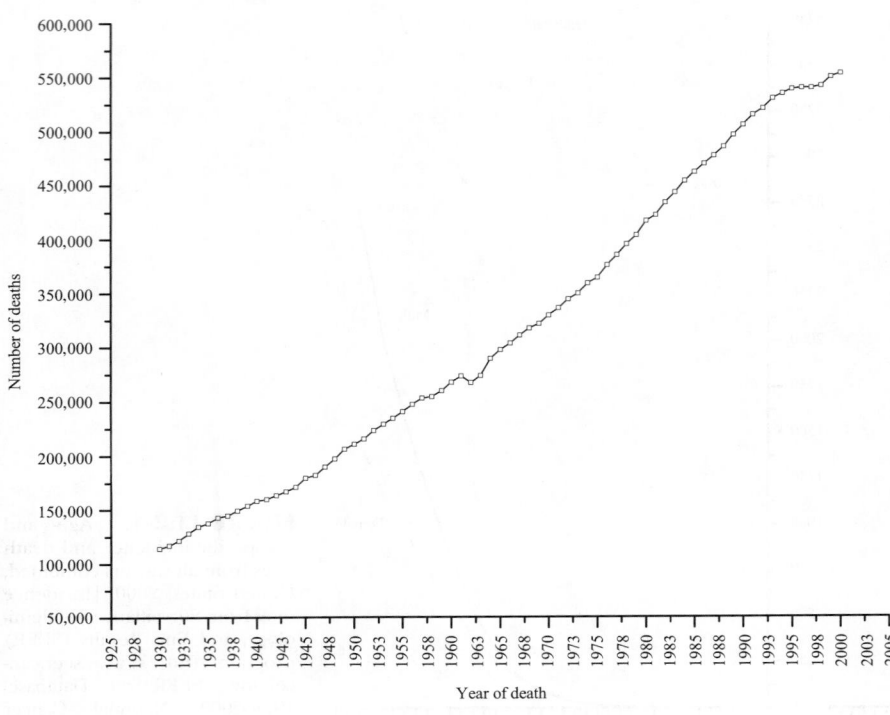

FIGURE 11.2-2. Trends in total number of deaths from all cancers combined, United States, 1930 to 2000. (Data from National Center for Health Statistics, Centers for Disease Control and Prevention, 2003.)

The exact number of prevalent cancer cases in the United States is unknown for lack of national cancer registration and follow-up for cure. However, based on extrapolated data from the nine oldest Surveillance, Epidemiology, and End Results (SEER) cancer registries of the National Cancer Institute, approximately 9.6 million people were alive in the United States who were diagnosed with cancer before January 1, 2000.[5] This number is

expected to increase over time because of improvements in survival and the anticipated growth and aging of the population.

According to the National Cancer Institute estimates, there were more prevalent cancer cases in women (5.3 million) than in men (4.2 million) in the year 2000. This largely reflects high survival rates of women with early-stage breast cancers and the greater longevity of women than men. Approximately 20.6 million U.S.

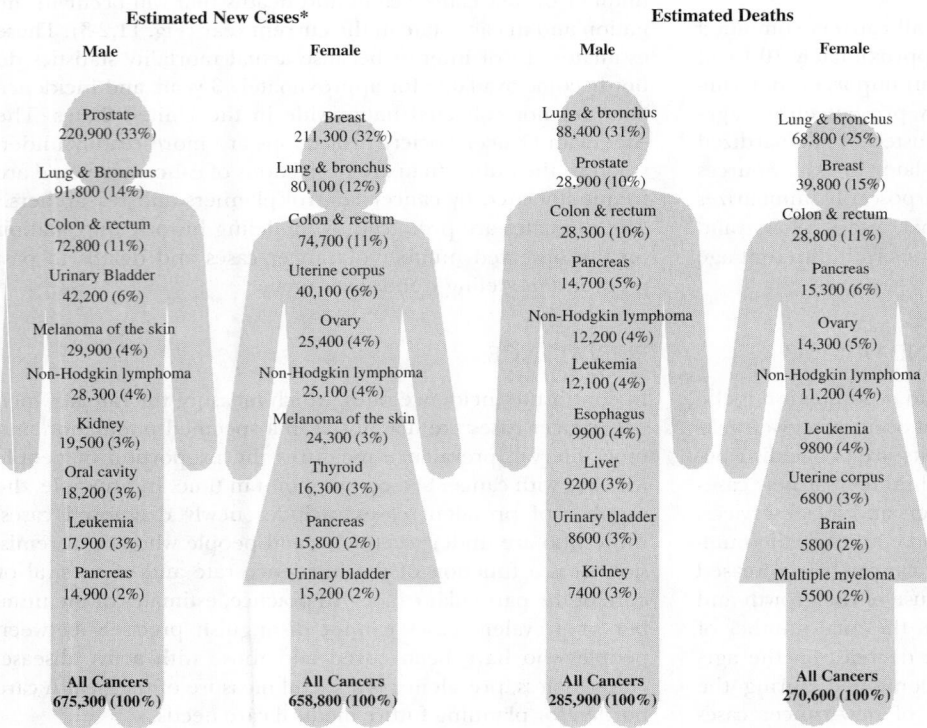

FIGURE 11.2-3. Leading sites of new cancer cases and deaths—2003 estimates. *Excludes basal and squamous cell skin cancer and *in situ* carcinomas except urinary bladder. Percentage may not total 100%. (Data from Cancer Facts and Figures, 2003. American Cancer Society.)

TABLE 11.2-1. Estimated Number of Prevalent Cases for Selected Cancer Types, by Sex, United States, 2000

Cancer Type	Male No.	Male %	Female No.	Female %	Total No.	Total %
All sites	4,241,699	100	5,313,613	100	9,555,312	100
Breast			2,197,504	41.4	2,197,504	23.0
Cervix			231,064	4.3	231,064	2.4
Colon and rectum	499,018	11.8	542,481	10.2	1,041,499	10.9
Esophagus	16,038	0.4	5,490	0.1	21,528	0.2
Leukemia	99,956	2.4	78,450	1.5	178,406	1.9
Lung and bronchus	174,547	4.1	167,910	3.2	342,457	3.6
Melanoma	267,432	6.3	283,428	5.3	550,860	5.8
Pancreas	11,364	0.3	12,170	0.2	23,534	0.2
Prostate	1,637,208	38.6			1,637,208	17.1
Thyroid	65,022	1.5	227,533	4.3	292,555	3.1

[Data from Surveillance, Epidemiology, and End Results (SEER) program, 1973–2000, Division of Cancer Control and Population Sciences, National Cancer Institute, 2003.]

women were 65 and older in the year 2000, compared to 14.4 million men. The number of prevalent cases of specific cancer sites varies according to incidence and survival rates for that cancer. Prostate and breast cancers are the most prevalent cancers in men and women, respectively (Table 11.2-1). The number of prevalent cases of thyroid cancer, which is uncommon but highly curable, was greater than the number of prevalent cases of pancreatic cancer, which is much more common but the most fatal of all cancers.

PROBABILITY OF DEVELOPING CANCER

The probability that an individual will develop or die from cancer by a certain age is another measure used to describe average risk in the general population (Table 11.2-2). The probability, usually expressed as percentage, can also be expressed as one person in X persons. For example, the lifetime risk of developing lung cancer in U.S. men, 7.7%, can be expressed as 1 in 13 men developing lung cancer in his lifetime. These estimates are based on the average experience of the general population and may over- or underestimate individual risk because of family history or individual risk factors. For example, the estimate that lung cancer will develop in 1 man in 13 in a lifetime overestimates the risk for nonsmokers and underestimates the risk for smokers. Software to estimate probability of developing or dying from cancer within specified age ranges is available at http://srab.cancer.gov/devcan.

TABLE 11.2-2. Probability of Developing Invasive Cancers over Selected Age Intervals, by Sex, 1998 to 2000[a]

Cancer Type	Sex	Birth to 39 Y (%)	40–59 Y (%)	60–79 Y (%)	Birth to Death (%)
All sites[b]	Male	1.36 (1 in 73)	8.03 (1 in 12)	33.92 (1 in 3)	44.77 (1 in 2)
	Female	1.92 (1 in 52)	9.01 (1 in 11)	22.61 (1 in 4)	38.03 (1 in 3)
Bladder[c]	Male	0.02 (1 in 4603)	0.40 (1 in 250)	2.36 (1 in 42)	3.46 (1 in 29)
	Female	0.01 (1 in 9557)	0.12 (1 in 831)	0.64 (1 in 157)	1.10 (1 in 91)
Breast	Female	0.44 (1 in 229)	4.14 (1 in 24)	7.53 (1 in 13)	13.36 (1 in 7)
Colon and rectum	Male	0.06 (1 in 1678)	0.86 (1 in 116)	3.94 (1 in 25)	5.88 (1 in 17)
	Female	0.06 (1 in 1651)	0.67 (1 in 150)	3.05 (1 in 33)	5.49 (1 in 18)
Leukemia	Male	0.15 (1 in 649)	0.20 (1 in 495)	0.82 (1 in 122)	1.45 (1 in 70)
	Female	0.13 (1 in 789)	0.14 (1 in 706)	0.46 (1 in 219)	1.00 (1 in 100)
Lung and bronchus	Male	0.03 (1 in 3439)	1.02 (1 in 98)	5.80 (1 in 17)	7.69 (1 in 13)
	Female	0.03 (1 in 3046)	0.79 (1 in 126)	3.93 (1 in 25)	5.73 (1 in 17)
Melanoma of the skin	Male	0.12 (1 in 809)	0.49 (1 in 205)	0.97 (1 in 103)	1.81 (1 in 55)
	Female	0.19 (1 in 532)	0.39 (1 in 255)	0.51 (1 in 197)	1.22 (1 in 82)
Non-Hodgkin's lymphoma	Male	0.14 (1 in 739)	0.45 (1 in 224)	1.27 (1 in 79)	2.10 (1 in 48)
	Female	0.08 (1 in 1258)	0.30 (1 in 332)	0.98 (1 in 102)	1.76 (1 in 57)
Prostate	Male	0.01 (1 in 12,833)	2.28 (1 in 44)	14.20 (1 in 7)	17.15 (1 in 6)
Uterine cervix	Female	0.16 (1 in 632)	0.31 (1 in 322)	0.27 (1 in 368)	0.78 (1 in 128)
Uterine corpus	Female	0.05 (1 in 1832)	0.69 (1 in 144)	1.57 (1 in 64)	2.60 (1 in 38)

[a]For persons free of cancer at beginning of age interval. Based on cancer cases diagnosed during 1998 to 2000. The "1 in" statistics and the inverse of the percentage may not be equivalent due to rounding.
[b]All sites exclude basal and squamous cell skin cancer and *in situ* cancers except urinary bladder.
[c]Includes invasive and *in situ* cancer cases.
(From DEVCAN Software, Probability of Developing or Dying of Cancer software, Version 5.1. Statistical Research and Application Branch, National Cancer Institute, 2003. http://srab.cancer.gov/devcan.)

SURVIVAL RATES

The survival rate reflects the proportion of people alive at a specified period after diagnosis, usually 5 years. The two basic measures of survival are observed and relative. The observed survival rate quantifies the proportion of cancer patients alive after 5 years of follow-up since diagnosis, irrespective of deaths from conditions other than cancer. In contrast, relative survival rates compare the proportion of cancer patients alive 5 years after diagnosis to the corresponding proportions in persons of the same age and sex without cancer. Thus, the relative survival rate reflects the specific effects of cancer on shortened survival. For instance, the 87% 5-year relative survival rate for breast cancer translates to 13% fewer breast cancer patients surviving for 5 years compared to their peers in the general population. Whereas the observed survival rate is commonly used in evaluating the effectiveness of new cancer treatments in age-matched randomized clinical trials, relative survival rates are used to measure progress in early detection and cancer treatment in the general population.

DATA SOURCES AND AGE STANDARDIZATION

DATA SOURCES

Incidence data are collected by regional and national population-based cancer registries. Population-based cancer registries collect data from all medical facilities, including hospitals, doctors' offices, radiation facilities, and diagnostic laboratories. The type of cancer is coded according to the International Classification of Diseases for Oncology, which assigns an anatomic site and a histologic code.[6] In the United States, the SEER program has been collecting information in nine population-based cancer registries since 1973 on demographic characteristics of new cancer patients, anatomic site of the tumor, histologic type, extent of disease at the time of diagnosis, first course of treatment, and follow-up for vital status. These registries, which provide the information on temporal trends, cover approximately 10% of the U.S. population. Subsequent expansions of the SEER program provide coverage of approximately 26% of the U.S. population (http://www.seer.cancer.gov).

The Centers for Disease Control and Prevention's National Program of Cancer Registries (NPCR) was established in 1994 to improve existing non-SEER population-based cancer registries and to establish new statewide cancer registries (http://www.cdc.gov/cancer/npcr). Currently, NPCR funds central cancer registries in 45 states, the District of Columbia, and the territories of Puerto Rico, the Republic of Palau, and the Virgin Islands. Through the NPCR and SEER programs, cancer data are collected in almost all parts of the United States, although data quality varies across registries. The National Association of Central Cancer Registries (NAACCR) develops and promotes standardized methods of cancer registration and evaluates the quality of data collected by population-based registries. Forty states and the District of Columbia (more than 70% of the U.S. population) met the NAACCR criteria for highest quality for data collected in the year 2000.

Hospital-based cancer registries provide data to state and national surveillance systems and information on care delivered by individual hospitals. However, it is generally not possible to calculate accurate incidence rates from hospital data because the populations from which cases are drawn are not well defined. The compositions of cancer cases seen at a particular hospital are influenced by referral patterns. The National Cancer Data Base is the largest compilation of hospital-based cancer registration in the United States (http://www.facs.org/dept/cancer/ncdb). It collects incidence and outcome data from more than 1500 hospitals in 50 states, covering approximately 50% (600,000) of estimated new cancer cases diagnosed annually in the United States. These data can be used to compare treatment patterns in participating hospitals. However, comparisons of survival across hospitals require great care to adjust for stage at diagnosis and other prognostic variables, comorbidities, age, and other demographic characteristics of the populations being served.

Mortality data have been collected for most of the United States since 1930, based on information from death certificates. The underlying cause of death is classified according to the most current International Statistical Classification of Diseases (ICD).[7] Deaths that occurred since 1999 in the United States are classified according to ICD-10, replacing ICD-9, used from 1979 to 1998. The classification of deaths due to cancer is highly accurate in the United States, with approximately 90% agreement between death certificates and pathology reports.[8] Mortality data are available from the National Center for Health Statistics (http://www.cdc.gov/nchs/nvss.html).

The International Agency for Research on Cancer (IARC; http://www.iarc.fr) compiles worldwide data on cancer incidence, mortality, and prevalence. This information can be accessed through the GLOBOCAN database.[9] Incidence data in most countries are collected at regional levels only. Few countries have a nationwide cancer registry. For countries with no cancer registry (the case in most developing countries), incidence data are obtained by converting mortality data or by borrowing information from neighboring countries.[10] A limitation of this method is that it assumes equal survival across neighboring countries.

AGE STANDARDIZATION

Age standardization is widely used to summarize age-specific rates for comparisons of incidence and death rates between two or more populations with differing age composition. This is achieved by applying the age-specific rates in the populations of interest to a standard set of weights based on a common age distribution. Standardization removes the effect of the differences in age in the populations being compared. The standardized rate is a hypothetical rate that would be observed in each population were the age composition the same as in the standard population.

Beginning with cancer cases and deaths that occurred in 1999, incidence and mortality rates in the United States have been standardized to the 2000 U.S. standard population.[11] Previously, rates were standardized to the 1970 standard population. The purpose of shifting from the 1970 standard to the 2000 standard was to approximate the current age distribution of the U.S. population so that the age-standardized rates would more closely resemble contemporary incidence and death rates. The new standard reflects the aging of the population between 1970 and 2000 and gives more weight to older age groups. Consequently, the introduction of the new standard increased overall incidence rates by approximately 20% (Table 11.2-3). The effect of the new standard on the rate of a particular cancer type, how-

TABLE 11.2-3. Effect of Change in Standard Population on Age-Adjusted Incidence Rates, United States, 2000

| | Incidence Rates | | |
| | Standard Population | | |
Cancer Type	1970	2000	% Change
All sites	397.8	472.9	18.9
Colon and rectum	42.4	53.1	25.1
Lung and bronchus	52.6	62.3	18.6
Female breast	115.2	135.1	17.2
Prostate	151.2	176.9	16.9
Acute lymphocytic leukemia	1.5	1.4	−7.0

ever, depends on whether the cancer predominantly affects younger or older individuals. Rates increased by as much as 25% for cancer sites that increase with age such as lung and colon cancers, whereas they decreased by as much as 7% for childhood cancers such as acute lymphocytic leukemia (see Table 11.2-3). Age-adjusted rates from published reports using the 1970 standard should not be compared with rates based on the 2000 standard. The new standard does not affect either the age-specific rates or the total number of cases or deaths, but only the age-standardized rate.

TEMPORAL TRENDS

INCIDENCE AND MORTALITY

The incidence and mortality for all cancers combined have changed substantially over time (Fig. 11.2-4). The increase in the incidence rate among men from 1975 through 1988 (see Fig. 11.2-4) reflects the rise in lung cancer from smoking and in the diagnosis of prostate cancer from transurethral resection (Fig. 11.2-5).[12] In contrast, the sharp increase and subsequent decrease in incidence from 1988 through 1992 (see Fig. 11.2-4) reflect the introduction of prostate-specific antigen (PSA) testing and rapid increase and subsequent decrease in the diagnosis of prostate cancer (see Fig. 11.2-5).[13] The increase in overall incidence rate among women (see Fig. 11.2-4) reflects lung and breast cancer trends (see Fig. 11.2-5). Lung cancer incidence rates have continued to increase among women, although the rate of increase has slowed in the most recent time period.[14] The long-term increase in breast cancer incidence rates reflects changes in reproductive factors (delayed childbearing)[15] and increases in mammography use.[16] Recent patterns may also reflect increased prevalence of underlying risk factors, such as hormone replacement therapy and obesity.[17]

After increasing since 1930, the overall cancer death rate declined in the 1990s among men (see Fig. 11.2-4), predominantly reflecting declines in smoking-related cancer mortality (Fig. 11.2-6) caused by long-term reductions in cigarette consumption.[18] Cancers caused by smoking include oro- and nasopharynx, larynx, lung, esophagus, stomach, liver, pancreas, urinary bladder, kidney, cervix, and myeloid leukemia,[19] accounting for approximately 30% to 40% of the total cancer deaths in the United States.[20,21] Colorectal cancer death rates have continued to decline since the 1980s because of detection and removal of precancerous polyps,[22,23] earlier diagnosis, and improved treatment and supportive care. Reasons for the decline in prostate cancer death rates since the early 1990s are not fully understood[24] but are thought to include earlier detection due to PSA testing[25] and advances in treatment. The dramatic decrease in stomach cancer mortality, which has occurred in most industrialized countries, is

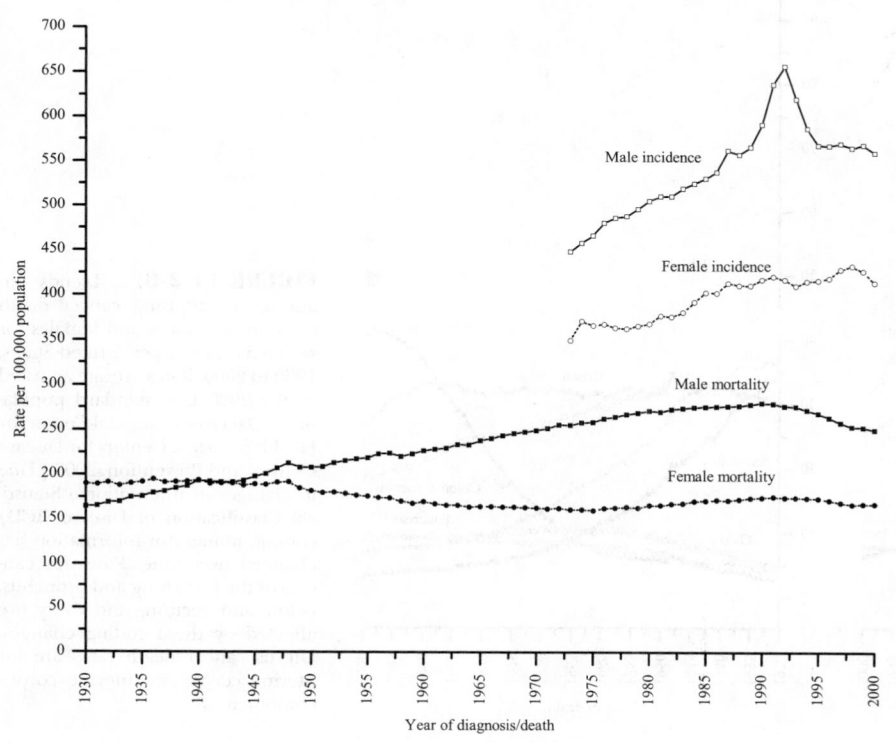

FIGURE 11.2-4. Trends in all cancers, combined incidence and mortality, United States. Rates are age adjusted to the 2000 U.S. standard population. [Incidence rates from Surveillance, Epidemiology, and End Results (SEER) program (http://www.seer.cancer.gov) SEER*Stat Database, 1973–2000. National Cancer Institute, 2003. Death rates from National Center for Health Statistics, Centers for Disease Control and Prevention, 2003.]

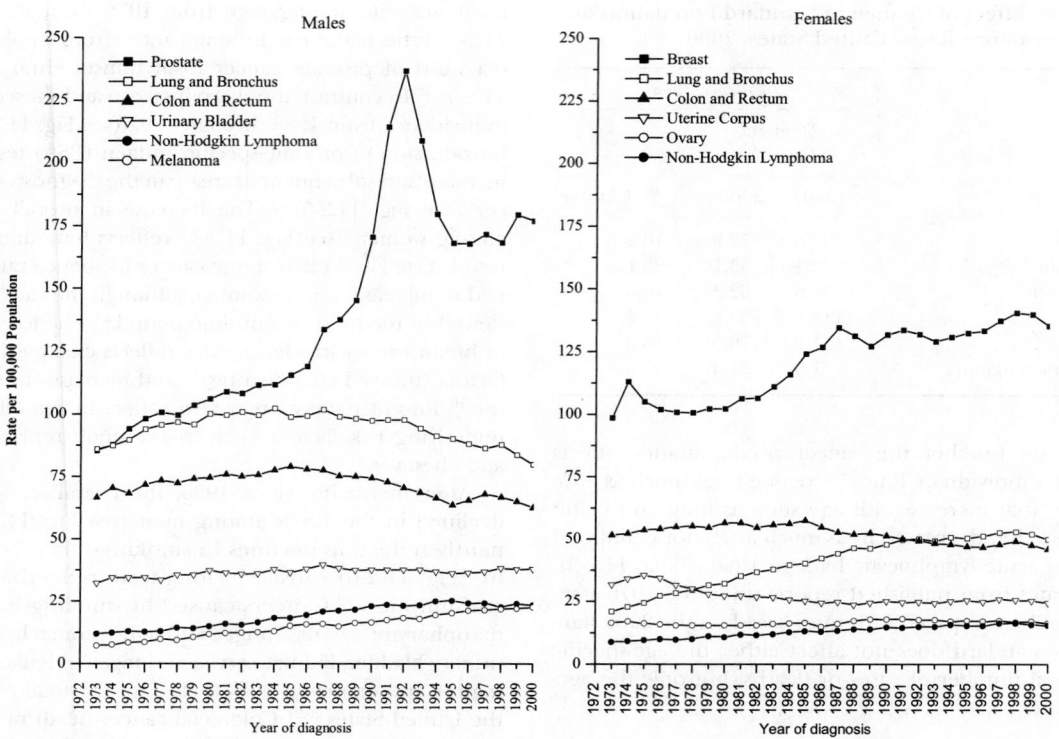

FIGURE 11.2-5. Annual age-adjusted cancer incidence rates among males and females for selected cancer sites, United States, 1973 to 2000. Rates are age adjusted to the 2000 U.S. standard population. [Incidence rates from Surveillance, Epidemiology, and End Results (SEER) program (http://www.seer.cancer.gov) SEER*Stat Database, 1973–2000. National Cancer Institute, 2003.]

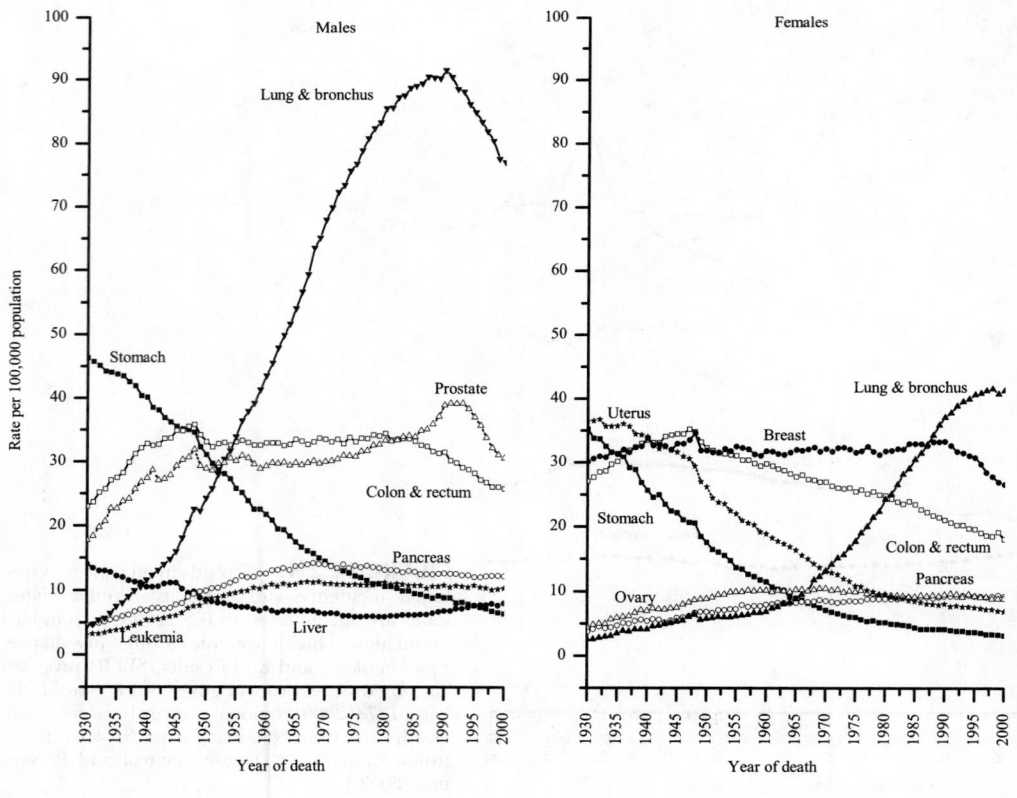

FIGURE 11.2-6. Trends in annual age-adjusted cancer death rates among males and females for selected cancer types, United States, 1930 to 2000. Rates are age adjusted to the 2000 U.S. standard population. (Data from National Center for Health Statistics, Centers for Disease Control and Prevention, 2003.) Due to changes in International Statistical Classification of Disease (ICD) coding, numerator information has changed over time. Rates for cancers of the liver, lung and bronchus, colon and rectum, and ovary are affected by these coding changes. Uterus cancer death rates are for uterine cervix and uterine corpus combined.

thought to be a result of better food preservation procedures and reduced prevalence of *Helicobacter pylori* infection.[26]

Among women, the overall cancer death rate decreased from the 1930s through early 1970s, increased until the early 1990s, and stabilized thereafter (see Fig. 11.2-4). The long-term decline before the 1970s reflects decreases in deaths from cancer of the stomach, cervix-uterus, and colon and rectum (see Fig. 11.2-6). The historic decreases in mortality from stomach and cervix-uterus cancers were offset by the increases in lung cancer mortality after 1960.[27] A substantial decrease in female breast cancer mortality has occurred since the early 1990s, which is thought to reflect early detection[28] and improvements in treatment.[29] The rapid decline in colorectal cancer death rates since the mid 1980s may reflect screening (with removal of precancerous polyps)[22,23] and improvements in treatment. It is interesting to note that cancer death rates were higher in women than in men during the turn of the twentieth century, presumably because of higher death rates from female reproductive cancers.

SURVIVAL RATES

Relative survival rates measure the proportion of cancer patients who are alive a specified duration since diagnosis after adjusting for other causes of death. Relative survival rate is frequently used to measure the effectiveness and dissemination of improved treat-ments and early detection. Table 11.2-4 shows the changes in 5-year relative survival rates for selected cancer sites in patients diagnosed during two time intervals, 1974 to 1976 and 1992 to 1999. For all races combined, the 5-year survival rate for cancer patients diagnosed during 1992 to 1999 varied from 4% for pancreatic cancer to 98% for prostate cancer. Survival rates increased over the two periods for all cancer types except for corpus uterine and larynx, with prostate cancer showing the highest increase (31%).

The observed increases in 5-year survival reflect a complex mixture of actual improvements in prognosis and artifactual effects of screening. Ideally, early detection will lead to a more favorable prognosis and improved survival because treatment given before onset of clinical symptoms is more effective than after, when the disease is at a more advanced stage. At the population level, this translates to reductions in mortality. However, early detection can increase survival in the absence of effective treatments by merely advancing the time of diagnosis. This is often referred as *lead-time bias*, with "lead time" referring to the interval between when the cancer is diagnosed because of screening and when it would have been diagnosed clinically. Screening may also increase survival by changing the case mix, that is, by detecting tumors that would not otherwise have been detected during the person's lifetime. For example, the increase in 5-year relative survival rate from 67% for prostate cancer patients diagnosed in 1974 to 1976 to 98% for those diagnosed in 1992 to 1999 in part reflects the detection of tumors that

TABLE 11.2-4. Changes in 5-Year Relative Survival Rates[a] (%) by Race and Year of Diagnosis, United States, 1974 to 1999

Site	All Races			White			African American		
	1974–1976	1992–1999	Diff.	1974–1976	1992–1999	Diff.	1974–1976	1992–1999	Diff.
All cancers	50	63	13[b]	51	64	13[b]	39	53	14[b]
Brain	22	33	11[b]	22	32	10[b]	27	39	12[b]
Breast (female)	75	87	12[b]	75	88	13[b]	63	74	11[b]
Cervix uteri	69	71	2[b]	70	73	3[b]	64	61	−3
Colon	50	62	12[b]	51	63	12	46	53	7[b]
Corpus uterine	88	84	−4[b]	89	86	−3[b]	62	60	−2
Esophagus	5	14	9[b]	5	15	10[b]	4	9	5[b]
Hodgkin's disease	71	84	13[b]	72	85	13[b]	69	78	9[b]
Kidney	52	63	11[b]	52	63	11[b]	49	61	12[b]
Larynx	66	65	−1	66	67	1	60	53	−7
Leukemia	34	46	12[b]	35	48	13[b]	31	39	8
Liver	4	7	3[b]	4	7	3[b]	1	5	4
Lung and bronchus	13	15	2[b]	13	15	2[b]	11	12	1[b]
Melanoma of the skin	80	90	10[b]	81	90	9[b]	67	64	−3
Multiple myeloma	24	32	8[b]	24	31	7[b]	28	33	5
Non-Hodgkin's lymphoma	47	56	9[b]	48	57	9[b]	49	47	−2
Oral cavity	54	57	3[b]	55	60	5[b]	36	36	0
Ovary	37	53	16[b]	37	52	15[b]	41	52	11[b]
Pancreas	3	4	1[b]	3	4	1[b]	3	4	1
Prostate	67	98	31[b]	68	98	30[b]	58	93	35[b]
Rectum	49	62	13[b]	49	62	13[b]	42	53	11[b]
Stomach	15	23	8[b]	15	21	6[b]	17	21	4
Testis	79	96	17[b]	79	96	17[b]	76	87	11
Thyroid	92	96	4[b]	92	96	4[b]	88	94	6
Urinary bladder	73	82	9[b]	74	83	9[b]	48	64	16[b]

Diff., difference.

[a]Survival rates are adjusted for normal life expectancy and are based on cases diagnosed from 1974 to 1976 and 1992 to 1999 and followed through 2000.
[b]The difference in rates between 1974 to 1976 and 1992 to 1999 is statistically significant (*P* <.05).
[Data from Surveillance, Epidemiology, and End Results (SEER) program, 1973 to 2000, Division of Cancer Control and Population Sciences, National Cancer Institute, 2003.]

might otherwise have remained clinically inapparent but were discovered because of PSA testing.

The overall 5-year relative survival rate increased approximately equally in whites and blacks (see Table 11.4-4). However, survival rates in the most recent time period are still substantially lower among blacks than whites, reflecting later stage at diagnosis and poorer stage-specific survival among blacks compared to whites. These differences are thought to largely reflect economic, structural, and cultural barriers to high-quality medical care for the black population. Poorer survival has also been observed for members of other racial and ethnic minority groups. Relative survival rates cannot be calculated for other groups because reliable life tables do not exist to predict survival in the general population. However, an analysis of cause-specific survival rate for patients in the SEER registry diagnosed between 1988 and 1997 found that, in general, all minority populations (Hispanic whites, blacks, American Indians/Alaskan Natives, and Hawaiian natives) have an increased probability of dying from cancer within 5 years of diagnosis compared to non-Hispanic whites diagnosed at the same age and stage.[30]

DEMOGRAPHIC AND GEOGRAPHIC PATTERNS

Cancer occurrence is heavily influenced by demographic characteristics, such as age, race/ethnicity, socioeconomic status, and place of residence.

AGE AND SEX

Cancer incidence rates generally increase with age, although the incidence rate for age 0 to 4 is twice that for ages 5 to 9 and

10 to 14, and the rates of cancer diagnosis (if not true incidence) decrease after age 84 (see Fig. 11.2-1). Specific cancers that contribute to higher incidence rates at ages 0 to 4, compared to 5 to 9 and 10 to 14 years, include acute lymphocytic leukemia, neuroblastoma, and retinoblastoma. The decrease in age 85 and older largely reflects underdiagnosis. The age-specific incidence pattern is slightly different for males and females. Rates are higher and rise faster in women than in men from ages 20 to 54, but after age 54, rates are higher and rise more steeply in men. Breast and thyroid cancers, in addition to gynecologic cancers, contribute to higher incidence rates in females than in males before age 55.

The age-specific mortality pattern is generally similar to the incidence pattern (see Fig. 11.2-1). Cancer death rates are higher in women than in men between ages 30 and 49, although the differences are smaller than those for incidence rates. In contrast to incidence rates, the death rate at age 0 to 4 is not higher than rates at ages 5 to 9 and 10 to 14, and rates continue to increase through age 85 and older.

Although cancer occurs less frequently in the young and is generally assumed to be a disease of old people, it ranks as an important cause of death at younger ages in the United States. Cancer is one of the five leading causes of death in every age group, categorized in 20-year age intervals, among males and females.[31] Further, it is the leading cause of death before age 65, followed by heart disease (Fig. 11.2-7). A total of 160,714 people under age 65 died from cancer in the United States in 2000, compared to 116,994 people from heart disease.

For all ages combined, the three most commonly diagnosed cancers in the United States in 2003 will be prostate, lung, and colon and rectum in men and breast, lung and bronchus, and colon and rectum in females (see Fig. 11.2-3). These cancers account for more than 55% of the new cases in males and in

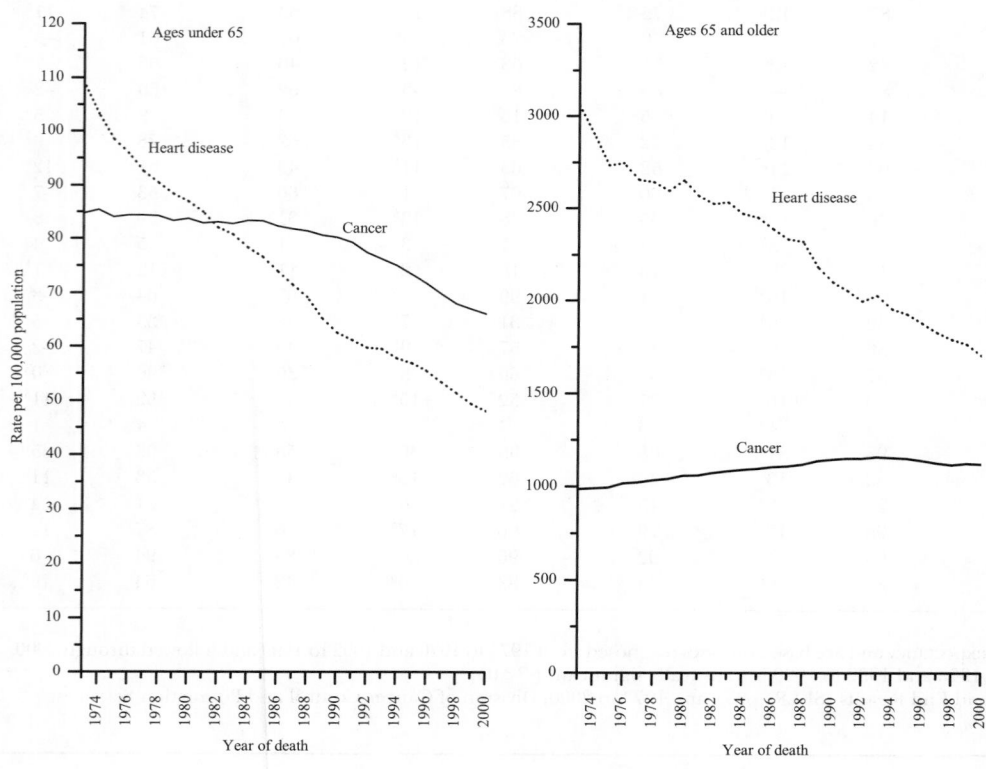

FIGURE 11.2-7. Death rates from cancer and heart disease for ages under 65 and 65 and older, United States, 1973 to 2000. Rates are age adjusted to the 2000 U.S. standard population. (Data from National Center for Health Statistics, Centers for Disease Control and Prevention, 2003.)

TABLE 11.2-5.   Age-Standardized Incidence and Death Rates[a] for Selected Cancer Sites by Race and Ethnicity, United States, 1996 to 2000

	White	*Black*	*Asian/Pacific Islander*	*American Indian/Alaskan Native*	*Hispanic Latino[b]*
INCIDENCE					
All sites					
Males	555.9	696.8	392.0	259.0	419.3
Females	431.8	406.3	306.9	229.2	312.2
Breast (female)	140.8	121.7	97.2	58.0	89.8
Colon and rectum					
Males	64.1	72.4	57.2	37.5	49.8
Females	46.2	56.2	38.8	32.6	32.9
Lung and bronchus					
Males	79.4	120.4	62.1	45.6	46.1
Females	51.9	54.8	28.4	23.4	24.4
Prostate	164.3	272.1	100.0	53.6	137.2
Stomach					
Males	11.2	19.9	23.0	14.4	18.1
Females	5.1	9.9	12.8	8.3	10.0
Liver					
Males	7.3	11.0	21.1	6.1	13.8
Females	2.8	3.9	7.7	5.5	5.6
Cervix	9.2	12.4	10.2	6.9	16.8
MORTALITY					
All sites					
Males	249.5	356.2	154.8	172.3	176.7
Females	166.9	198.6	102.0	115.8	112.4
Breast (female)	27.2	35.9	12.5	14.9	17.9
Colon and rectum					
Males	25.3	34.6	15.8	18.5	18.4
Females	17.5	24.6	11.0	12.1	11.4
Lung and bronchus					
Males	78.1	107.0	40.9	52.9	40.7
Females	41.5	40.0	19.1	26.2	15.1
Prostate	30.2	73.0	13.9	21.9	24.1
Stomach					
Males	6.1	14.0	12.5	7.0	9.9
Females	2.9	6.5	7.4	4.2	5.3
Liver					
Males	6.0	9.3	16.1	7.6	10.5
Females	2.7	3.7	6.7	4.3	5.0
Cervix	2.7	5.9	2.9	2.9	3.7

[a]Per 100,000, age adjusted to 2000 U.S. standard population.
[b]Hispanic Latinos are not mutually exclusive from whites, blacks, Asian/Pacific Islanders, and American Indian/Alaska Natives.
[Data from Surveillance, Epidemiology, and End Results (SEER) program, 1973 to 2000, Division of Cancer Control and Population Sciences, National Cancer Institute, 2003.]

females. Lung and bronchus cancer is the leading cause of cancer death in men and in women, followed by prostate cancer in men, breast cancer in women, and colorectal cancer in men and in women. For both sexes combined, colorectal cancer is the second leading cause of cancer death.

RACE AND ETHNICITY

Cancer rates vary widely across racial and ethnic groups (Table 11.2-5). Cancer incidence and death rates are 25% and 43% higher, respectively, in black men than in white men. Similarly, cancer death rates are nearly 20% higher in black women than white women, despite lower incidence. Most notable is the striking divergence in mortality from certain cancers between blacks and whites over time (Fig. 11.2-8). Death rates for female breast and colorectal cancers were approximately equal between whites and blacks around 1980. Subsequently, the gap in mortality widened over time, so that in 2000 the female breast and colorectal cancers were 32% and 30% higher in blacks than in whites, respectively. These trends occurred during a period of substantial improvement in early detection and treatment for breast and colorectal cancers. Historically, the use of mammography, which has contributed to reduction in deaths from breast cancer, has been lower in black women than in white women, although the rate has become comparable more recently.[32] There is also some evidence that black women are less likely than white women to receive radiation therapy after breast-conserving surgery,[33,34] a regimen that is known to

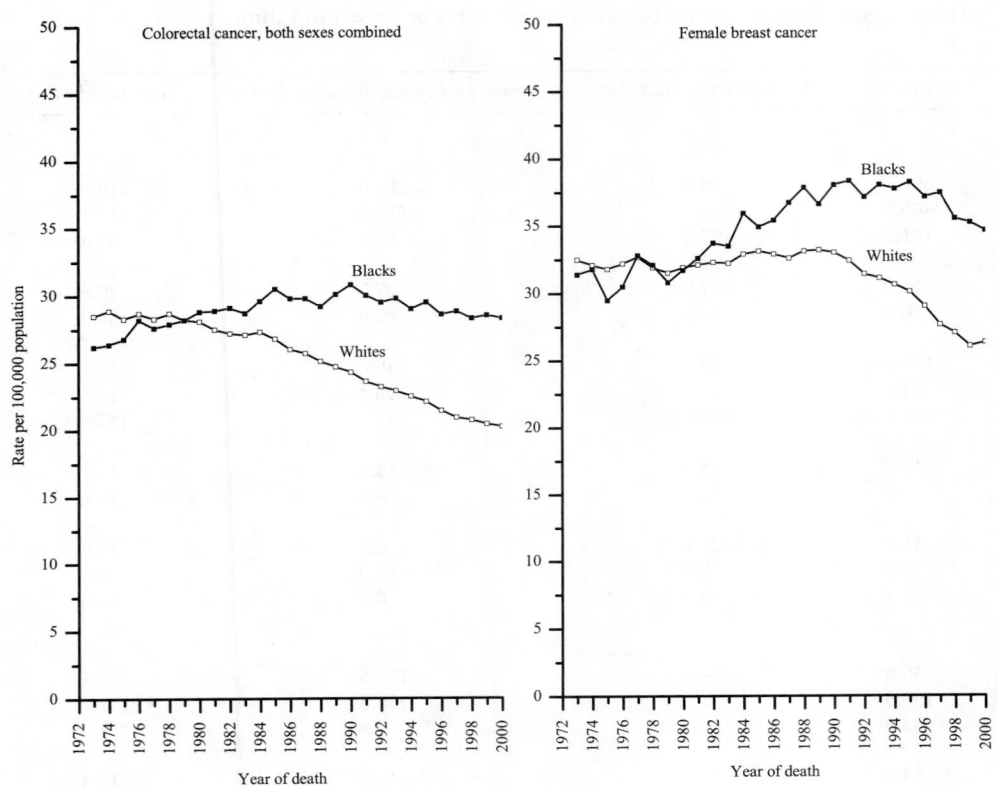

FIGURE 11.2-8. Trends in colorectal and female breast cancers: death rates by race, United States, 1973 to 2000. Rates are age adjusted to the 2000 U.S. standard population. (Data from National Center for Health Statistics, Centers for Disease Control and Prevention, 2003.)

improve survival.[35] The diverging trends in mortality suggest that not all segments of the population have benefited equally from medical advances.

Other racial ethnic groups have lower incidence and mortality for all sites combined and for the four most common cancer sites (lung and bronchus, colon and rectum, prostate, and female breast) compared to whites and blacks. The rates of certain cancers (stomach, liver and intrahepatic bile duct, cervix) are generally higher in minority populations than in whites. This is thought to reflect greater exposure to specific infectious agents (in the case of stomach and liver cancers), lower use of screening (for cervical cancer), and higher consumption of preserved rather than fresh foods (for stomach cancer).

Biologic or inherited characteristics are thought to be less important than socioeconomic factors in explaining differences in cancer incidence and mortality among the major racial and ethnic populations in the United States.[36] Differences in cancer occurrence by race and ethnicity generally reflect a complex interplay of socioeconomic factors, social injustice, and culture, where poverty and lack of access to medical care play a key role.

POVERTY

In the United States and internationally, socioeconomic status is known to influence cancer occurrence. Individual-level data on socioeconomic variables, such as educational attainment and income, are not available in cancer surveillance data in the United States. However, indirect measures of socioeconomic status have been derived by linking the cancer patient's address at the time of diagnosis with socioeconomic variables defined at the census tract or county level. A study of SEER data analyzed cancer mortality, incidence, stage at diagnosis, and survival by area poverty rate [the percentage of the population below the poverty level, categorized as low (less than 10%), medium (10% to 20%), and high (greater than 20%)].[37] For most cancers, residents of higher poverty areas were at increased risk of developing or dying from cancer, or both. For example, incidence and mortality rates for lung cancer among men were substantially higher for residents of high-poverty compared to low-poverty areas. Although much of the excess incidence and mortality can be explained by higher smoking rates among the less affluent, differences in stage at diagnosis for lung cancer and 5-year survival rates by area socioeconomic status were also noted. In contrast, incidence rates for melanoma of the skin were more than twice as high among residents of counties where poverty was uncommon, probably reflecting increased opportunity for recreational sun exposure, the major risk factor for melanoma. Detection may also play a role, as residents of more affluent counties were substantially more likely to be screened for melanoma.

The combination of later detection and lower-quality treatment results in lower 5-year survival for cancer of all sites combined for residents of poorer compared to more affluent counties. For example, for men diagnosed in 1988 to 1994, 5-year cause-specific survival rates were 49% for residents of high poverty census tracts, 55% for residents of medium poverty census tracts, and 61.0% for residents of low poverty census tracts.[37] For all cancer sites combined, differential survival by area socioeconomic status was consistently seen within racial and ethnic groups. Differences in survival for major cancers by area poverty rate were also apparent when stage-specific survival rates are analyzed.

TABLE 11.2-6. International Variations in Cancer Death Rates for Selected Cancer Sites

Country	Lung		Colon/Rectum		Stomach		Breast	Cervix Uteri	Prostate
	Male	Female	Male	Female	Male	Female	Female		
United States	53.2	27.2	15.9	12.0	4.5	2.3	21.2	3.3	17.9
Chile	20.3	7.0	7.0	7.1	30.1	12.7	12.7	10.6	19.9
China	33.2	13.5	7.2	5.3	27.0	13.0	4.5	3.1	1.0
Czech Republic	65.3	11.5	34.2	18.5	13.5	7.5	21.0	6.2	15.7
Denmark	50.0	26.7	23.8	18.5	7.5	3.6	29.2	4.1	23.1
France	48.5	6.7	18.3	12.1	8.0	3.6	21.4	3.5	19.2
Germany	46.2	9.6	21.7	17.0	12.9	7.8	23.7	4.2	18.4
Hungary	86.2	20.0	33.5	20.9	21.0	10.1	25.3	7.7	17.9
Israel	27.5	9.3	19.7	15.3	9.3	5.6	26.2	3.1	14.2
Japan	33.1	9.6	17.6	11.0	31.2	13.8	7.7	3.0	5.5
Mexico	22.1	8.2	4.7	4.6	13.2	9.8	12.2	17.1	16.6
Norway	31.7	12.8	22.0	18.0	9.6	5.5	20.7	3.3	26.8
Russian Federation	68.2	6.8	17.5	12.7	35.6	15.2	16.7	5.2	6.8
Spain	49.4	4.2	17.3	11.1	12.6	6.2	18.1	2.7	15.0
United Kingdom	48.6	21.1	18.7	13.8	10.1	4.8	26.8	3.9	18.5
Venezuela	19.4	9.2	5.8	6.1	17.5	10.0	11.6	15.2	18.2

(From Ferlay J, et al. GLOBOCAN 2000: Cancer Incidence, Mortality and Prevalence Worldwide, Version 1.0. IARC CancerBase No. 5. Lyons: IARC Press, 2001, with permission.)

GEOGRAPHIC PATTERNS

Analyzing cancer occurrence patterns by geographic location has provided information on the preventability of cancers and clues about the etiology of many cancers.[38,39] Geographic comparisons are also important in identifying places where cancer prevention and early detection efforts should be strengthened.

Table 11.2-6 shows death rates from certain cancers in the United States and selected other countries. The age-adjusted rates were calculated using the world standard population for 1960 rather than the U.S. standard population. Cancer rates vary across countries because of differences in exposures (tobacco use, nutrition, infectious agents) and diagnosis. The especially high lung cancer rates in eastern European countries, such as Hungary and the Czech Republic, reflect very high prevalence of long-term cigarette smoking. Cervical cancer death rate is highest in Mexico and Central and South America because of lack of screening and early treatment for cervical cancer. In contrast, female breast cancer death rates are higher in Scandinavian countries and western Europe, in part due to increased underlying risk factors, such as late age at childbearing. The highest female breast cancer death rates in Israel suggest greater genetic susceptibility.

Migrant studies are a powerful technique for assessing whether variations in cancer rates across countries are due to environmental factors or genetic factors. For example, Table 11.2-7 shows cancer mortality risks for colon, stomach, and liver among Japanese in Japan, first (Issei)- and second (Nisei)-generation Japanese in California, and native California whites.[40] Compared to whites in California, cancers of the stomach and liver were more common and cancer of the colon was less common in Japan between 1950 and 1960. However, the risk of dying from stomach and liver cancer among the first-generation Japanese men in California was substantially lower than among Japanese living in Japan, although higher than that among California white men. The risk among Japanese migrants and whites became more similar by the second generation. The risk

of colon cancer was twofold higher in the first-generation Japanese in California than in Japanese in Japan, with risk in the second generation approaching that of California white men. Of interest is the higher rate of male colorectal cancer death rates in Japan in 2000 compared to the United States (see Table 11.2-6), presumably reflecting changing dietary patterns.

Cancer rates also vary within smaller geographic areas, such as country and state. Regional variations in cancer rates have been reported widely in the United States.[41] Besides providing clues to etiologic hypotheses,[42] geographic comparisons can be used to identify where cancer-screening and control efforts should be enhanced. For example, the high cervical cancer mortality in Appalachia[41] motivated the U.S. Congress to create the Centers for Disease Control's National Breast and Cervical Cancer Early Detection Program, which improves access to breast and cervical cancer screening and diagnostic services for low-income women.[43] In an attempt to measure the effectiveness of state tobacco control efforts using lung cancer rate in young adults, a study found that lung cancer rates in young adults were higher in states with low tobacco control efforts than in states with high tobacco control efforts.[44]

TABLE 11.2-7. Stomach, Colon, and Liver Cancer Risks in Japanese in Japan and in California and in California Whites Aged 45 to 64 Years, between 1956 and 1962

Cancer Site	California Whites	Japanese		
		2nd Generation in California	1st Generation in California	In Japan
Stomach	1.0	2.8	3.8	8.4
Colon	1.0	0.9	0.4	0.2
Liver	1.0	2.2	2.7	4.1

(Adapted from ref. 40.)

Geographic information system (GIS) is a new tool for describing cancer patterns by place of residence through coding address at diagnosis or death. It is a powerful automated system for the capture, storage, retrieval, analysis, and display of spatial data. Examples of GIS application in cancer epidemiology include identification of geographic areas with a high proportion of distant stage breast cancer in New Jersey[45] and an inverse relationship between travel distance to radiation therapy and receipt of radiotherapy after breast-conserving surgery in New Mexico.[46]

ISSUES IN THE INTERPRETATION AND UNDERSTANDING OF TEMPORAL TRENDS

National organizations involved in cancer surveillance in the United States use a common method to evaluate long-term trends in cancer incidence and mortality. The method, known as the *joinpoint model*,[47] was developed by investigators at the National Cancer Institute. Each year, when the *Annual Report to the Nation on the Status of Cancer* reports on incidence and mortality trends,[14] the slope and the statistical significance of the last segment determine whether incidence and mortality are described as increasing, decreasing, or stable.

FACTORS THAT AFFECT TRENDS

Decreases in incidence rates not only reflect the impact of primary preventive strategies, such as reduction in cigarette smoking, but may also result from increased screening for cancers with known precursors (polyps for colorectal cancer and superficial cellular abnormalities for cervical cancer). Increases in incidence rates may signal increased exposure to risk factors or increased detection due to introduction of screening. Reductions in mortality are easier to interpret and less susceptible to artifact than are trends in incidence and survival. Such decreases generally reflect the effectiveness of cancer prevention, early detection, and treatment improvements over past decades. Trends in incidence rates can also be influenced by methodologic factors, including delay in reporting of cancer cases to registries, revision of population estimates, and changes in diagnosis and disease classification; of these, the latter two factors may also affect mortality trends.

Incidence rates and trends are known to be affected by delays in reporting.[48] Population-based registries usually calculate and report rates 3 years after the year of diagnosis, to allow time for data collection and coding. However, cancer types that are commonly diagnosed in outpatient settings, such as prostate cancer and melanoma, may be reported to registries even later. A method has been developed to adjust for delayed reporting in analyzing cancer incidence trends from the SEER registry database.[48] Delayed reporting may cause the incidence rates for melanoma and prostate cancer to be underestimated by as much as 14% in the most recent 1 to 2 years.[48] Consideration of delay adjustment in the 2003 *Annual Report to the Nation on the Status of Cancer* caused the overall incidence trend for all cancers combined for the period 1995 to 2000 to change from stable to slightly increasing.[14] It should be noted that the impact of delays in reporting in SEER registry data is probably less than the impact for other population-based registries, because they are long-standing registries of very high quality.

The introduction of new diagnostic or screening techniques can also influence trends in cancer incidence rates. Typically, the introduction of a new screening technique leads to a rise in incidence rate for a brief period, with subsequent decline and return to the baseline; this is because existing cases are diagnosed earlier than would have been the case in the absence of screening. For example, the rapid increase and subsequent decrease in prostate cancer incidence rates between 1998 and 1992 (see Fig. 11.2-5) largely reflects the broad dissemination and use of PSA testing[13] rather than a real increase in disease occurrence. The corresponding rise in prostate cancer mortality, which was unexpected, is thought to result from attribution bias by physicians in recording cause of death.[49]

Change in disease classification may also influence interpretation of incidence and mortality. The World Health Organization updates international statistical classification of diseases approximately every 10 years to stay abreast of medical advances. The introduction of ICD-10 beginning with deaths occurring in 1999 increased the proportion of deaths attributed to cancer by 0.7% relative to ICD-9.[50] This change disrupted the downward trend in mortality that began in 1992, with the decline appearing to end in 1998.[14] When the change in ICD-10 was accounted for, however, the decrease in rate continued from 1992 to 2000.[51]

Cancer rates are also influenced by the accuracy of population estimates. During the years that follow the most recent decennial census, the population at risk is unknown and must be projected by the U.S. Census Bureau based on the last census. Projections based on the last census become increasingly inaccurate as the time from the census increases, particularly in smaller geographic areas. For example, in the late 1990s, cancer rates were thought to be as much as 17% higher among blacks in Atlanta than among blacks in other parts of the United States (Fig. 11.2-9), based on population estimates projected from the 1990 census. However, when the population estimates for the 1990s were revised using interpolated data from the 1990 and 2000 censuses, cancer rates among blacks in Atlanta were found to be lower than rates among blacks residing in other parts of the United States. The erroneous impression from the 1990 projections resulted from underestimation of the black population in the Atlanta area by the census projections, which were unable to take into account a large migration of blacks into the Atlanta metropolitan area during the 1990s.

UNDERSTANDING TEMPORAL TRENDS

As discussed above, long-term temporal trends in cancer incidence rates can be influenced by several factors, the most prominent of which are changes in underlying risk factors and introduction of new screening techniques. Mortality is influenced by these factors as well as by the introduction of more effective treatments.

In describing temporal trends, epidemiologists often refer to time period and cohort effects. A period effect results from medical advances (the introduction of a new screening technique or improved treatment) or changes in disease classification that increase or decrease the incidence rate across all age groups in the same calendar period. A striking contemporary example of a period effect is the sharp increase and subsequent decrease in prostate cancer incidence rates in almost all age groups between the late 1980s and early 1990s in the United States (Fig. 11.2-10),

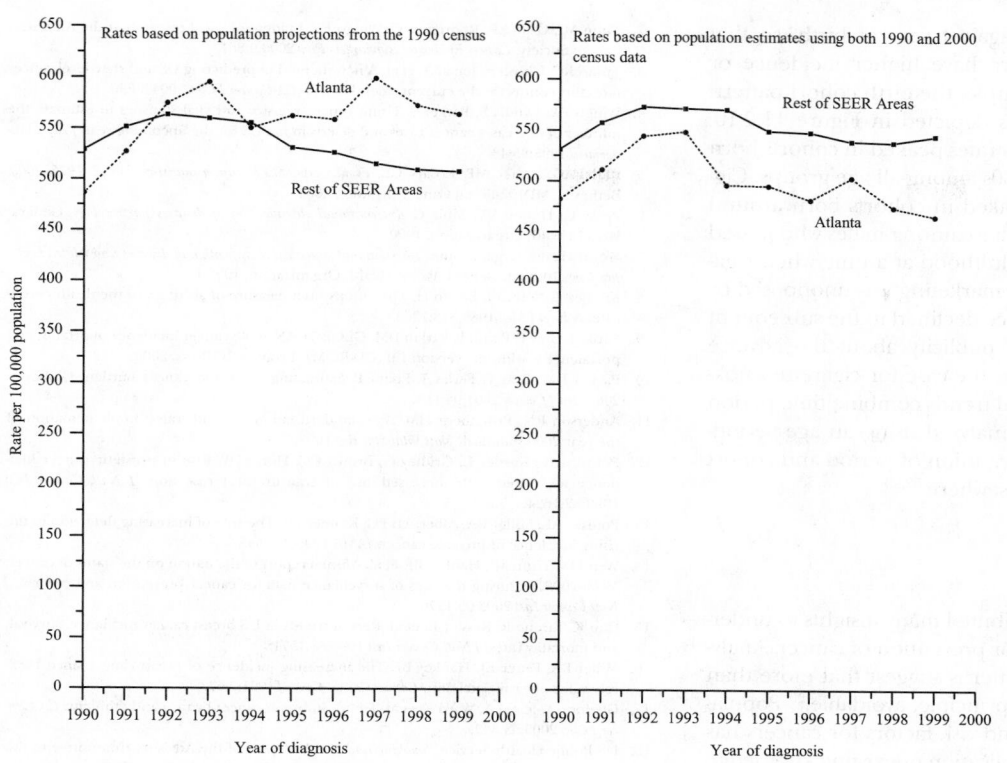

FIGURE 11.2-9. The influence of population estimates on cancer incidence rates among blacks in Atlanta, 1990 to 2000. Rates are age adjusted to the 2000 U.S. standard population. [Data from Surveillance, Epidemiology, and End Results (SEER) program (http://www.seer.cancer.gov) SEER*Stat Database, 1973–2000. National Cancer Institute, 2003.]

reflecting the introduction and broad use of PSA testing in the late 1980s.[13]

In contrast, a birth cohort effect typically results from the introduction (or increased prevalence) of a risk factor that becomes established at a young age in people born during the same time period. In birth cohort patterns, the disease consequences from these exposures become manifest later in life as each birth cohort ages. Birth cohort effects are often identified

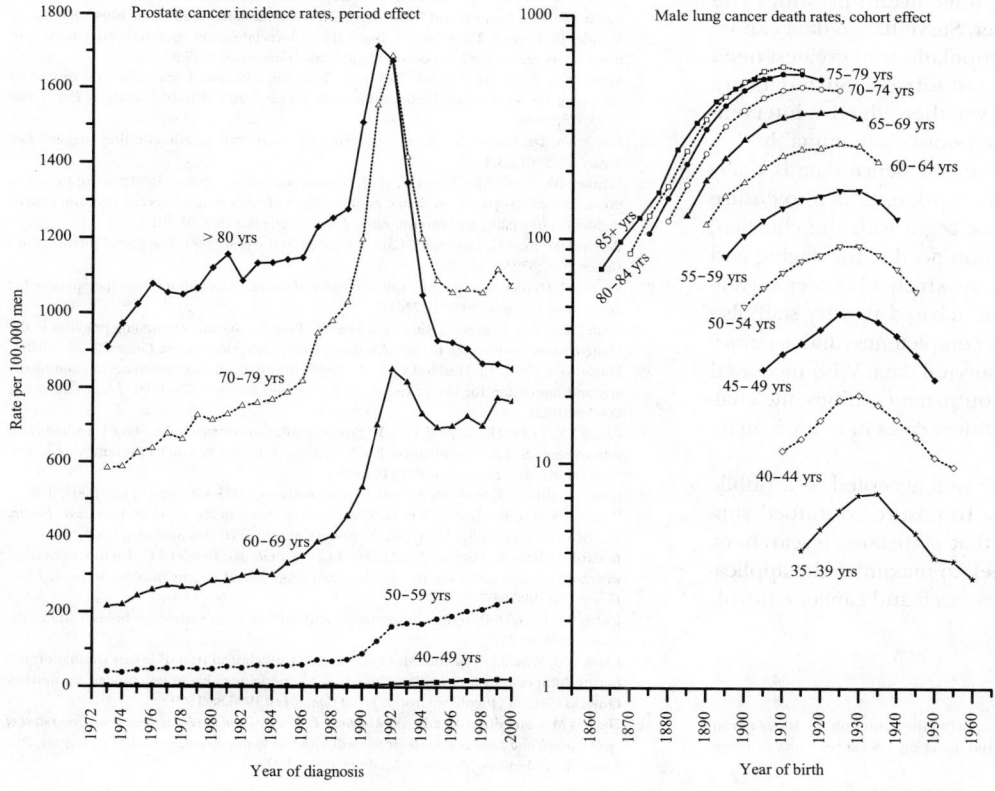

FIGURE 11.2-10. Trends in age-specific rates showing period and birth cohort effects. [Incidence rates from Surveillance, Epidemiology, and End Results (SEER) program (http://www.seer.cancer.gov) SEER*Stat Database, 1973–2000. National Cancer Institute, 2003. Death rates from National Center for Health Statistics, Centers for Disease Control and Prevention, 2003.]

by plotting the age-specific rates against year of birth, so that birth cohorts with higher exposure have higher incidence or death rates at a given age. For example, the birth cohort pattern in lung cancer mortality in men is depicted in Figure 11.2-10. Age-specific male lung cancer death rates peaked in cohorts born around the late 1920s and early 1930s among all age groups. Cigarette smoking prevalence also peaked in cohorts born around this period. Smoking rates were highest among males who passed through adolescence and young adulthood at a time when cigarettes were plentiful and aggressive marketing was unopposed by health concerns. Smoking prevalence declined in the subsequent birth cohorts because of growing publicity about the adverse effects of smoking on health.[18] As is the case for cigarette smoking and lung cancer, many temporal trends combine time period and cohort effects. These can be analyzed using an age-period-cohort model to partition the contribution of period and cohort effects. This method is described elsewhere.[52,53]

CONCLUSION

Descriptive epidemiology has contributed many insights to understanding the causes and potential for prevention of cancer. Analyses of temporal and geographic patterns suggest that more than two-thirds of cancer deaths are, in principle, avoidable.[20] Population-based surveillance of cancer and risk factors for cancers has great potential to accelerate the application of existing knowledge about cancer prevention, screening, and treatment. Cancer surveillance data can be used to convince legislators of the impact of cancer and potential benefit of allocating resources to cancer control programs.

The advent of nearly national coverage of the U.S. population by cancer registries in the 1990s has expanded the use of descriptive epidemiology in setting public health priorities and in monitoring progress against cancer. Surveillance data can be used to target existing resources to populations in greatest need of prevention, screening, and treatment services. Such data are also critically important in assessing whether effective interventions are reaching all segments of the population equitably.

The collection of high-quality cancer incidence data is vitally important in characterizing the cancer burden. Efforts to ensure the quality of cancer surveillance data begin with the clinician, whose accurate recording of information needed for staging and histologic diagnosis is the foundation on which all cancer surveillance depends. Hospital and population-based registry staff also play a critical function in assuring the completeness and accuracy of cancer incidence, treatment, and survival data. With increased diagnosis and treatment of cancer in outpatient settings, the challenge of collecting data on incident cancer cases in a timely manner is even greater.

Cancer registration appears to be well accepted as a public health priority in the United States. To ensure continued support of this activity, it is important that clinicians, researchers, and the public health community seek to maximize the application of cancer surveillance data for research and cancer control.

REFERENCES

1. Edwards BK, Howe HL, Ries LA, et al. Annual report to the nation on the status of cancer, 1973–1999, featuring implications of age and aging on US cancer burden. *Cancer* 2002;94:2766.
2. Thun MJ, Calle EE, Rodriguez C, Wingo PA. Epidemiological research at the American Cancer Society. *Cancer Epidemiol Biomarkers Prev* 2000;9:861.
3. Tiwari RC, Ghosh K, Jemal A, et al. A new method of predicting US and state-level cancer mortality counts for the current calendar year. *CA Cancer J Clin* 2004;54:30.
4. Wingo PA, Landis S, Parker S. Using cancer registry and vital statistics to estimate the number of new cases cancer cases and deaths in the US for the upcoming year. *J Reg Management* 1998;25:43.
5. Ries LAG, Eisner MP, Kosary CL, et al., eds. *SEER cancer statistics review, 1975–2000.* Bethesda, MD: National Cancer Institute, 2003.
6. Percy C, Holten VV, Muir C. *International classification of diseases for oncology.* Geneva: World Health Organization, 1990.
7. World Health Organization. *International statistical classification of diseases and related health problems*, 10th ed. Geneva: World Health Organization, 1992:1.
8. Kircher T, Nelson J, Burdo H. The autopsy as a measure of accuracy of the death certificate. *N Engl J Med* 1985;313:1263.
9. Ferlay J, Bray F, Pisani P, Parkin DM. GLOBOCAN 2000: cancer incidence, mortality, and prevalence worldwide, version 1.0 (CD-ROM). Lyon: IARC Press, 2000.
10. Parkin DM, Bray F, Ferlay J, Pisani P. Estimating the world cancer burden: Globocan 2000. *Int J Cancer* 2001;94:153.
11. Anderson RN, Rosenberg HM. Age standardization of death rates: implementation of the year 2000 standard. *Natl Vital Stat Rep* 1998;47:1.
12. Potosky AL, Kessler L, Gridley G, Brown CC, Horm JW. Rise in prostatic cancer incidence associated with increased use of transurethral resection. *J Natl Cancer Inst* 1990;82:1624.
13. Potosky AL, Miller BA, Albertsen PC, Kramer BS. The role of increasing detection in the rising incidence of prostate cancer. *JAMA* 1995;273:548.
14. Weir HK, Thun MJ, Hankey BF, et al. Annual report to the nation on the status of cancer, 1975–2000, featuring the uses of surveillance data for cancer prevention and control. *J Natl Cancer Inst* 2003;95:1276.
15. Chu K, Tarone R, Kessler L, et al. Recent trends in US breast cancer incidence, survival, and mortality rates. *J Natl Cancer Inst* 1996;88:1571.
16. Miller BA, Feuer EJ, Hankey BF. The increasing incidence of breast cancer since 1982: relevance of early detection. *Cancer Causes Control* 1991;2:67.
17. Ghafoor A, Jemal A, Ward E, et al. Trends in breast cancer by race and ethnicity. *CA Cancer J Clin* 2003;53:342.
18. US Public Health Service. *Smoking and health.* Report of the Advisory Committee to the Surgeon General of the Public Health Service. Washington, DC: US Department of Health, Education, and Welfare, Public Health Service, Centers for Disease Control and Prevention, 1964.
19. *International Agency for Research on Cancer (IARC).* Tobacco smoke and involuntary smoking. Lyons: IARC Press, 2002:83. World Wide Web URL: http://monographs.iarc.fr/htdocs/monographs/vol83/02-involuntary.html, 2004.
20. Doll R, Peto R. The causes of cancer: quantitative estimates of avoidable risks of cancer in the United States today. *J Natl Cancer Inst* 1981;66:1191.
21. US Department of Health and Human Services. *A Surgeon General's report on the Health Consequences of smoking.* Atlanta, GA: US Department of Health and Human Services, Centers for Disease Control and Prevention, Office of Smoking and Health 2004 (in press).
22. Mandel JS, Church TR, Ederer F, Bond JH. Colorectal cancer mortality: effectiveness of biennial screening for fecal occult blood. *J Natl Cancer Inst* 1999;91:434.
23. Mandel JS, Bond JH, Church TR, et al. Reducing mortality from colorectal cancer by screening for fecal occult blood. Minnesota Colon Cancer Control Study. *N Engl J Med* 1993;328:1365.
24. Hsing AW, Devesa SS. Trends and patterns of prostate cancer: what do they suggest? *Epidemiol Rev* 2001;23:3.
25. Hankey BF, Feuer EJ, Clegg LX, et al. Cancer surveillance series: interpreting trends in prostate cancer—part I: evidence of the effects of screening in recent prostate cancer incidence, mortality, and survival rates. *J Natl Cancer Inst* 1999;91:1017.
26. Parkin DM, Bray FI, Devesa SS. Cancer burden in the year 2000. The global picture. *Eur J Cancer* 2001;37:[Suppl 8]S4.
27. Thun MJ, Henley SJ, Calle EE. Tobacco use and cancer: an epidemiologic perspective for geneticists. *Oncogene* 2002;21:7307.
28. Swan J, Breen N, Coates RJ, Rimer BK, Lee NC. Progress in cancer screening practices in the United States: results from the 2000 National Health Interview Survey. *Cancer* 2003;97:1528.
29. Mariotto A, Feuer EJ, Harlan LC, et al. Trends in use of adjuvant multi-agent chemotherapy and tamoxifen for breast cancer in the United States: 1975–1999. *J Natl Cancer Inst* 2002;94:1626.
30. Clegg LX, Li FP, Hankey BF, Chu K, Edwards BK. Cancer survival among US whites and minorities: a SEER (Surveillance, Epidemiology, and End Results) Program population-based study. *Arch Intern Med* 2002;162:1985.
31. Jemal A, Murray T, Samuels A, et al. Cancer statistics, 2003. *CA Cancer J Clin* 2003;53:5.
32. Pastor PN MD, Reuben C, Xia H. *Chart book on trends in the health of Americans. Health, United States.* Hyattsville, Maryland: National Center for Health Statistics, 2002.
33. Ballard-Barbash R, Potosky AL, Harlan LC, Nayfield SG, Kessler LG. Factors associated with surgical and radiation therapy for early stage breast cancer in older women. *J Natl Cancer Inst* 1996;88:716.
34. Joslyn SA. Racial differences in treatment and survival from early-stage breast carcinoma. *Cancer* 2002;95:1759.
35. Clark RM, Whelan T, Levine M, et al. Randomized clinical trial of breast irradiation following lumpectomy and axillary dissection for node-negative breast cancer: an update. Ontario Clinical Oncology Group. *J Natl Cancer Inst* 1996;88:1659.
36. Haynes MA, Smedley BD, eds. *Washington DC. The unequal burden of cancer: an assessment of NIH research and programs for ethnic minorities and the medically underserved.* Washington, DC: Institute of Medicine, National Academy Press, 1999.

37. Singh GK, Miller BA, Hankey BF, Edwards BK. Area socioeconomic variations in US cancer incidence, mortality, and survival, 1975–1999. Bethesda, MD: National Cancer Institute, 2003:137.

38. Armstrong B, Doll R. Environmental factors and cancer incidence and mortality in different countries, with special reference to dietary practices. *Int J Cancer* 1975;15:617.

39. Gray GE, Pike MC, Henderson BE. Breast-cancer incidence and mortality rates in different countries in relation to known risk factors and dietary practices. *Br J Cancer* 1979;39:1.

40. Buell P, Dunn J. Cancer mortality among Japanese Issei and Nisei of California. *Cancer* 1965;18:656.

41. Devesa SS, Grauman DJ, Blot WJ, et al. *Atlas of cancer mortality in the United States 1950–1994.* Bethesda: National Institutes of Health, 1999.

42. Blot WJ, Stone BJ, Fraumeni JF Jr, Morris LE. Cancer mortality in US counties with shipyard industries during world war II. *Environ Res* 1979;18:281.

43. *Centers for Disease Control and Prevention.* The National Breast and Cervical Cancer Early Detection Program—reducing mortality through screening. World Wide Web URL: http://www.cdc.gov/cancer/nbccedp/about.htm, 2004.

44. Jemal A, Cokkinides VE, Shafey O, Thun MJ. Lung cancer trends in young adults: an early indicator of progress in tobacco control (United States). *Cancer Causes Control* 2003;14:579.

45. Roche LM, Skinner R, Weinstein RB. Use of a geographic information system to identify and characterize areas with high proportions of distant stage breast cancer. *J Public Health Manag Pract* 2002;8:26.

46. Athas WF, Adams-Cameron M, Hunt WC, Amir-Fazli A, Key CR. Travel distance to radiation therapy and receipt of radiotherapy following breast-conserving surgery. *J Natl Cancer Inst* 2000;92:269.

47. Kim H, Feuer E, Midthune D. Permutation tests for joinpoint regression with applications to cancer rates. *Stat Med* 2000;19:335.

48. Clegg LX, Feuer EJ, Midthune DN, Fay MP, Hankey BF. Impact of reporting delay and reporting error on cancer incidence rates and trends. *J Natl Cancer Inst* 2002;94:1537.

49. Feuer EJ, Merrill RM, Hankey BF. Cancer surveillance series: interpreting trends in prostate cancer—part II: cause of death misclassification and the recent rise and fall in prostate cancer mortality. *J Natl Cancer Inst* 1999;91:1025.

50. Anderson RN, Minino AM, Hoyert DL, Rosenberg HM. Comparability of cause of death between ICD-9 and ICD-10: preliminary estimates. *Natl Vital Stat Rep* 2001;49:1.

51. Jemal A, Ward E, Anderson R, Thun M. The influence rules from the Tenth Revision of the International Classification of Diseases on U.S. cancer mortality trends. *J Natl Cancer Inst* 2003;95:1727.

52. Clayton D, Schifflers E. Models for temporal variation in cancer rates. I: age-period and age-cohort models. *Stat Med* 1987;6:449.

53. Clayton D, Schifflers E. Models for temporal variation in cancer rates. II: age-period-cohort models. *Stat Med* 1987;6:469.

CHAPTER 12

Principles of Surgical Oncology

SECTION 1

STEVEN A. ROSENBERG

General Issues

Surgery is the oldest treatment for cancer and, until recently, was the only treatment that could cure patients with cancer. The surgical treatment of cancer has changed dramatically over the last several decades. Advances in surgical techniques and a better understanding of the patterns of spread of individual cancers have allowed surgeons to perform successful resections for an increased number of patients. The development of alternate treatment strategies that can control microscopic disease has prompted surgeons to reassess the magnitude of surgery necessary.

The surgeon who treats cancer must be familiar with the natural history of individual cancers and with the principles and potentialities of surgery, radiation therapy, chemotherapy, immunotherapy, and other new treatment modalities. The surgeon has a central role in the prevention, diagnosis, and definitive treatment of the disease and in palliation and rehabilitation of the cancer patient. The principles underlying each of these roles of the surgical oncologist are discussed in this chapter.

HISTORICAL PERSPECTIVE

Although the earliest discussions of the surgical treatment of tumors are found in the Edwin Smith papyrus from the Egyp-

tian Middle Kingdom (circa 1600 BC), the modern era of elective surgery for visceral tumors began in frontier America in 1809.[1,2] Ephraim McDowell removed a 22-pound ovarian tumor from a patient, Mrs. Jane Todd Crawford, who survived for 30 years after the operation. This procedure, the first of 13 ovarian resections performed by McDowell, was the first elective abdominal operation and provided a great stimulus to the development of elective surgery.

The treatment of most tumors depended on two subsequent developments in surgery. The first of these was the introduction of general anesthesia by two dentists, Dr. William Morton and Dr. Crawford Long. The first major operation using general ether anesthesia was an excision of the submaxillary gland and part of the tongue, performed by Dr. John Collins Warren on October 16, 1846, at the Massachusetts General Hospital. The second major development stimulating the widespread application of surgery resulted from the introduction of the principles of antisepsis by Joseph Lister in 1867. Based on the concepts of Pasteur, Lister introduced carbolic acid in 1867 and described the principles of antisepsis in an article in the *Lancet* in that same year.

These developments freed surgery from pain and sepsis and greatly increased its use for the treatment of tumors. In the decade before the introduction of ether, only 385 operations were performed at the Massachusetts General Hospital. By the last decade of the nineteenth century, more than 20,000 operations per year were performed at that same hospital.[3]

Table 12.1-1 lists selected milestones in the history of surgical oncology. Although this list does not include all the important developments, it does indicate the tempo of the application of surgery to cancer treatment.[4] Major figures in the evolution of surgical oncology included Albert Theodore Billroth, who, in

TABLE 12.1-1. Selected Historical Milestones in Surgical Oncology

Year	Surgeon	Event
1809	Ephraim McDowell	Elective abdominal surgery (excised ovarian tumor)
1846	John Collins Warren	Use of ether anesthesia (excised submaxillary gland)
1867	Joseph Lister	Introduction of antisepsis
1860–1890	Albert Theodore Billroth	First gastrectomy, laryngectomy, and esophagectomy
1878	Richard von Volkmann	Excision of cancerous rectum
1880s	Theodore Kocher	Development of thyroid surgery
1890	William Stewart Halsted	Radical mastectomy
1896	G. T. Beatson	Oophorectomy for breast cancer
1904	Hugh H. Young	Radical prostatectomy
1906	Ernest Wertheim	Radical hysterectomy
1908	W. Ernest Miles	Abdominoperineal resection for rectal cancer
1912	E. Martin	Cordotomy for the treatment of pain
1910–1930	Harvey Cushing	Development of surgery for brain tumors
1913	Franz Torek	Successful resection of cancer of the thoracic esophagus
1927	G. Divis	Successful resection of pulmonary metastases
1933	Evarts Graham	Pneumonectomy
1935	A. O. Whipple	Pancreaticoduodenectomy
1945	Charles B. Huggins	Adrenalectomy for prostate cancer
1958	Bernard Fisher	Organization of NSABP to conduct prospective randomized trials

NSABP, National Surgical Adjuvant Breast and Bowel Project.

addition to developing meticulous surgical techniques, performed the first gastrectomy, laryngectomy, and esophagectomy. In the 1890s, William Stewart Halsted elucidated the principles of *en bloc* resections for cancer, as exemplified by the radical mastectomy. Examples of radical resections for cancers of individual organs include the radical prostatectomy performed by Hugh Young in 1904, the radical hysterectomy performed by Ernest Wertheim in 1906, the abdominoperineal resection for cancer of the rectum performed by W. Ernest Miles in 1908, and the first successful pneumonectomy performed for cancer by Evarts Graham in 1933. Modern technical innovations continue to extend the surgeon's capabilities. Recent examples include the development of microsurgical techniques that enable the performance of free graft procedures for reconstruction, automatic stapling devices, sophisticated endoscopic equipment that allows for a wide variety of "incisionless" surgery, and major improvements in postoperative management and critical care of patients that have improved the safety of major surgical therapy.

Critics who believe that the application of surgery has reached a plateau beyond which it will not progress should remember the words of a famous British surgeon, Sir John Erichsen, who, in his introductory address to the medical institutions at University College, said,

> There must be a final limit to the development of manipulative surgery, the knife cannot always have fresh fields for conquest and although methods of practice may be modified and varied and even improved to some extent, it must be within a certain limit. That this limit has nearly, if not quite, been reached will appear evident if we reflect on the great achievements of modern operative surgery. Very little remains for the boldest to devise or the most dextrous to perform.

These comments, published in *Lancet* in 1873, preceded most important developments in modern surgical oncology.

ANESTHESIA FOR ONCOLOGIC SURGERY

Modern anesthetic techniques have greatly increased the safety of major oncologic surgery. Regional and general anesthesia play important roles in a wide variety of diagnostic techniques, in local therapeutic maneuvers, and in major surgery.

Anesthetic techniques may be divided into those for regional and those for general anesthesia. Regional anesthesia involves a reversible blockade of pain perception by the application of local anesthetic drugs. These agents generally work by preventing the activation of pain receptors or by blocking nerve conduction. Agents commonly used for local and topical anesthesia for biopsy procedures in cancer patients are listed in Tables 12.1-2 and 12.1-3.[5] *Topical anesthesia* refers to the application of local anesthetics to the skin or mucous membranes. Good surface anesthesia of the conjunctiva and cornea, oropharynx and nasopharynx, esophagus, larynx, trachea, urethra, and anus can result from the application of these agents.

Local anesthesia involves injection of anesthetic agents directly into the operative field. *Field block* refers to injection of local anesthetic by circumscribing the operative field with a continuous wall of anesthetic agent. Lidocaine (Xylocaine) in concentrations from 0.5% to 1.0% is the most common anesthetic agent used for this purpose. Peripheral nerve block results from the deposition of a local anesthetic surrounding major nerve trunks. It can provide local anesthesia to entire anatomic areas.

Major surgical procedures in the lower portion of the body can be performed using epidural or spinal anesthesia. Epidural anesthesia results from the deposition of a local anesthetic agent into the extradural space within the vertebral canal. Catheters can be left in place in the epidural space, allowing the intermittent injection of local anesthetics for prolonged operations. The major advantage of epidural over spinal anes-

TABLE 12.1-2.   Infiltration Anesthesia

Drug	Concentration (%)	Plain Solution		Epinephrine-Containing Solution	
		Maximum Dose (mg)	Duration (min)	Maximum Dose (mg)	Duration (min)
SHORT DURATION					
Procaine					
Chloroprocaine	1.0–2.0	800	15–30	1000	30–90
MODERATE DURATION					
Lidocaine	0.5–1.0	300	30–60	500	120–360
Mepivacaine	0.5–1.0	300	45–90	500	120–360
Prilocaine	0.5–1.0	500	30–90	600	120–360
LONG DURATION					
Bupivacaine	0.25–0.5	175	120–240	225	180–420
Etidocaine	0.5–1.0	300	120–180	400	180–420

(From ref. 5, with permission.)

thesia is that it does not involve puncturing the dura, and the injection of foreign substances directly into the cerebrospinal fluid is avoided.

Spinal anesthesia involves the direct injection of a local anesthetic into the cerebrospinal fluid. Puncture of the dural sac generally is performed between the L-2 and L-4 vertebrae. Spinal anesthesia provides excellent anesthesia for intraabdominal operations, operations on the pelvis, or procedures involving the lower extremities. Because the patient is awake during spinal anesthesia

and is breathing spontaneously, it often has been thought that spinal anesthesia is safer than general anesthesia. There is no difference in the incidence of intraoperative hypotension with spinal anesthesia and with general anesthesia, and there is no clear benefit in using spinal anesthesia for patients with ischemic heart disease.[6] Because patients are awake during spinal anesthesia and can become agitated during the surgical procedure, spinal anesthesia actually can cause more myocardial stress than general anesthesia. The health status of patients with preoperative evi-

TABLE 12.1-3.   Various Preparations Intended for Topical Anesthesia

Anesthetic Ingredient	Concentration (%)	Pharmaceutical Application Form	Intended Area of Use
Benzocaine	1–5	Cream	Skin, mucous membrane
	20	Ointment	Skin, mucous membrane
	20	Aerosol	Skin, mucous membrane
Cocaine	4	Solution	Ear, nose, throat
Dibucaine	0.25–1.0	Cream	Skin
	0.25–1.0	Ointment	Skin
	0.25–1.0	Aerosol	Skin
	0.25	Solution	Ear
	2.5	Suppositories	Rectum
Cyclonine	0.5–1.0	Solution	Skin, oropharynx, tracheobronchial tree, urethra, rectum
Lidocaine	2–4	Solution	Oropharynx, tracheobronchial tree, nose
	2	Jelly	Urethra
	2.5–5.0	Ointment	Skin, mucous membrane, rectum
	2	Viscous	Oropharynx
	10	Suppositories	Rectum
	10	Aerosol	Gingival mucosa
Tetracaine	0.5–1.0	Ointment	Skin, rectum, mucous membrane
	0.5–1.0	Cream	Skin, rectum, mucous membrane
	0.25–1.0	Solution	Nose, tracheobronchial tree
EMLA	2.5	Cream	Skin
TAC	Tetracaine, 0.5 Epinephrine, 1:2000 Cocaine, 11.8	Solution	Skin

EMLA, eutectic mixture of lidocaine and prilocaine; TAC, tetracaine, epinephrine, and cocaine.
(From ref. 5, with permission.)

dence of congestive heart failure is more likely to be worsened by general anesthesia than by spinal anesthesia. Because of the local irritating effects of general anesthesia on the lung, it has been suggested that spinal anesthesia may be safer for patients with severe pulmonary disease.

General anesthesia refers to the reversible state of loss of consciousness produced by chemical agents that act directly on the brain. Most major oncologic procedures are performed using general anesthesia, which can be induced using intravenous or inhalational agents. The advantages of intravenous anesthesia are the extremely rapid onset of unconsciousness and improved patient comfort and acceptance.

A variety of inhalational anesthetic agents are in clinical use. Nitrous oxide is popular, usually in combination with narcotics and muscle relaxants. This technique provides a safe form of general anesthesia with the use of nonexplosive agents. Fluorinated hydrocarbons were introduced in the mid-1950s and represented a major improvement over other inhalational agents such as ether or chloroform because they facilitated more rapid induction and emergence than other inhalational agents. Halothane was widely used but has several significant side effects. Halothane depresses myocardial function, reduces cardiac output, causes significant vasodilatation, and sensitizes the myocardium to endogenous and administered catecholamines, which can lead to life-threatening cardiac arrhythmias. In rare instances, halothane also caused severe hepatotoxicity, which began 2 to 5 days after surgery. These side effects have largely led to the replacement of halothane by other agents. Isoflurane, approved in 1979, rapidly replaced halothane as the most commonly used inhalational agent. Isoflurane induces less reduction of cardiac output and less sensitization to the arrhythmia-inducing effects of catecholamines, although isoflurane-induced tachycardia continues to represent a clinical problem. The agent has a pungent odor and is therefore rarely used for inhalational induction. Sevoflurane and desflurane are other inhalational agents in common use.

Intravenous agents are often used to induce anesthesia, although they are rarely used to provide total anesthesia for surgical procedures. Intravenous induction is rapid, pleasant, and safe and is usually preferred over inhalational induction. The five most common intravenous agents used in the United States for induction of anesthesia are sodium thiopental, ketamine, propofol, etomidate, and midazolam.

Virtually all general anesthetics affect biochemical mechanisms, with actions, including depression of bone marrow, alteration of the phagocytic activity of macrophages, and immunosuppression. General anesthetic agents such as cyclopropane and diethyl ether rarely are used because of their explosive potential.

Intravenous neuromuscular blocking agents, called *muscle relaxants*, are commonly used during general anesthesia. These agents either are nondepolarizing (e.g., pancuronium), preventing access of acetylcholine to the receptor site of the myoneural junction, or are depolarizing (e.g., succinylcholine), acting in a manner similar to that of acetylcholine by depolarizing the motor endplate. These agents induce profound muscle relaxation during surgical procedures but have the disadvantage of inhibiting spontaneous respiration because of paralysis of respiratory muscles. Succinylcholine is short acting (3 to 5 minutes) with a rapid recovery phase, whereas nondepolarizing agents can cause more prolonged paralysis (30 to 40 minutes).

DETERMINATION OF OPERATIVE RISK

As with any treatment, the potential benefits of surgical intervention in cancer patients must be weighed against the risks of surgery. The incidence of operative mortality is of major importance in formulating therapeutic decisions and varies greatly in different patient situations (Table 12.1-4). The incidence of operative mortality is a complex function of the basic disease process that involves surgical factors, anesthetic technique, operative complications, and, most importantly, the general health status of patients and their ability to withstand operative trauma.

In an attempt to classify the physical status of patients and their surgical risks, the American Society of Anesthesiologists (ASA) has formulated a general classification of physical status that appears to correlate well with operative mortality.[7] Patients are classified into five groups depending on their general health status (as shown in Table 12.1-5).

Operative mortality usually is defined as mortality that occurs within 30 days of a major operative procedure. In oncologic patients, the basic disease process is a major determinant of operative mortality. Patients undergoing palliative surgery for widely metastatic disease have a high operative mortality rate even if the surgical procedure can alleviate the symptomatic problem. Examples of these situations include surgery for intestinal obstruction in patients with widespread ovarian cancer and surgery for gastric outlet obstruction in patients with cancer of the head of the pancreas. These simple palliative procedures are associated with mortality rates of approximately 20% in most series because of the debilitated state of the patient and the rapid progression of the basic disease.

Anesthesia-related mortality has decreased in the last four decades, largely because of the development of rigid practice standards and improved intraoperative monitoring techniques.[8–11] A summary of the specific intraoperative monitoring methods used to achieve improved anesthetic safety is presented in Table 12.1-6.[12] A study of 485,850 instances of anesthetic administration in 1986 in the United Kingdom revealed the risk of death from anesthesia alone to be approximately 1 in 185,000.[9] In a retrospective review encompassing cases from 1976 through 1988, Eichhorn[10] estimated anesthetic mortality in ASA class I and II patients to be 1 in 200,200. These are probably underestimates, because underreporting of anesthetic-related deaths is a problem in all studies. Most cancer patients undergoing elective surgery fall between physical status classes I and II; thus, an anesthetic mortality rate of 0.01% to 0.001% is a realistic estimate for this group.

Anesthesia-related mortality is rare, and factors related to the patient's preexisting general health status and disease are far more important indicators of surgical outcome. A study of

TABLE 12.1-4. Determinants of Operative Risk

General health status
Severity of underlying illness
Degree to which surgery disrupts normal physiologic functions
Technical complexity of the procedure (related to incidence of complications)
Type of anesthesia required
Experience of personnel

TABLE 12.1-5. American Society of Anesthesiologists Classification of Physical Status

Class I

A normal healthy patient with no organic, physiologic, biochemical, or psychiatric disturbance. The abnormal process for which operation is to be performed is localized and does not entail a systemic disturbance (i.e., a fit patient with inguinal hernia or a fibroid uterus in an otherwise healthy woman).

Class II

A patient with mild to moderate systemic disturbance caused either by the condition to be treated surgically or by other pathophysiologic processes (i.e., nonorganic or only slightly limiting organic heart disease, mild diabetes, essential hypertension, or anemia). Some might list the neonate or the octogenarian, even if no discernible systemic disease is present. Extreme obesity and chronic bronchitis may be included in this category.

Class III

A patient with severe systemic disease that limits activity but is not incapacitating, even though it may not be possible to define the degree of disability with finality (i.e., severely limiting organic heart disease; severe diabetes with vascular complications; moderate to severe degrees of pulmonary insufficiency; and angina pectoris or healed myocardial infarction).

Class IV

A patient with an incapacitating systemic disease that is a constant threat to life and not always correctable by operation (i.e., patients with organic heart disease showing marked signs of cardiac insufficiency, persistent anginal syndrome, or active myocarditis; and advanced degrees of pulmonary, hepatic, renal, or endocrine insufficiency).

Class V

A moribund patient who is not expected to survive 24 hours without operation or who has little chance of survival but is submitted to operation in desperation (i.e., the burst abdominal aneurysm with profound shock, major cerebral trauma with rapidly increasing intracranial pressure, and massive pulmonary embolus). Most of these patients require operation as a resuscitative measure with little, if any, anesthesia.

Status E

In the event of emergency operation, precede the number with an E. Any patient in one of the classes listed previously who is operated on as an emergency is considered to be in poorer physical condition. The letter E is placed beside the numeric classification. Thus, the patient with a hitherto uncomplicated hernia now incarcerated and associated with nausea and vomiting is classified as IE. By definition, class V always constitutes an emergency.

(From ref. 7, with permission.)

the factors contributing to the risk of 7-day operative mortality after 100,000 surgical procedures yielded the findings shown in Table 12.1-7.[13] The 7-day perioperative mortality in this study was 71.4 deaths per 10,000 cases, and the major determinants of death were the physical status of the patient, the emergent nature of the procedure, and the magnitude of the operation.

The five most common causes of death after surgery are bronchopneumonia, congestive heart failure, myocardial infarction, pulmonary embolism, and respiratory failure. Perioperative pulmonary complications therefore are a major threat, and the patient-related risk factors associated with postoperative pulmonary complications are shown in Table 12.1-8.

Patients with a recent myocardial infarction have a significantly higher incidence of reinfarction and cardiac death associated with surgery (Table 12.1-9). Significant improvements have occurred as new techniques of anesthetic monitoring and hemodynamic support have been developed.[14–16]

The impact of general health status on operative mortality is seen when operative mortality as a function of age is analyzed. In a study of the postoperative mortality of 17,199 patients undergoing general surgical procedures, the overall mortality rate for patients younger than age 70 was 0.25%, compared with 9.2% for patients older than age 70.[17] In these elderly patients, the operative mortality rate for emergency operations was 36.8%, compared with 7.8% for elective surgical procedures. The four leading causes of operative mortality that accounted for approximately 75% of all postoperative deaths in this age group were pulmonary embolism, pneumonia, cardiovascular collapse, and the primary illness itself.

More recently, Hoskings et al.[18] reviewed the outcome of surgery performed on 795 patients aged 90 years or older. Surgery was generally well tolerated. As with younger patients, the ASA classification was an important predictor of outcome.

Cancer is often a disease of the elderly, and there is sometimes a tendency to avoid even curative major surgery for can-

TABLE 12.1-6. Summary of Specific Intraoperative Monitoring Methods

Variable	Monitoring Methods
Inspired gas	Oxygen analyzer with a low oxygen concentration alarm
Blood oxygenation	A quantitative method, such as pulse oximetry; adequate illumination and exposure to assess color
Endotracheal tube position	Correct positioning in the trachea must be verified by clinical assessment and identification of CO_2 in the expired gas
Ventilation	Clinical assessment; monitoring of CO_2 content and volume of expired gas encouraged
Ventilator disconnect	A device with audible alarm, capable of detecting disconnection of components of the breathing system when a mechanical ventilator is used
Circulation	Continuous electrocardiography; blood pressure and heart rate determined every 5 min; continual evaluation of circulation by pulse palpation, heart auscultation, intraarterial pressure tracing, ultrasonographic pulse monitor, pulse plethysmography, or oximetry
Temperature	Measurement when changes in temperature are intended, anticipated, or suspected

(From ref. 12, with permission.)

TABLE 12.1-7.   Risk Factors Associated with 7-Day Operative Mortality

Variable	Description	Relative Odds of Dying
PATIENT FACTORS		
Age	>80 y vs. <60 y	3.29
Gender	Female vs. male	0.77
Physical status	ASA III–V vs. ASA I–II	10.65
SURGICAL FACTORS		
Operation type	Major vs. minor	3.82
Length	>2 h vs. <2 h	1.08
Urgency	Emergency vs. elective	4.44
ANESTHESIA FACTORS		
Techniques	Inhalation + narcotic vs. inhalation alone	0.76
	Narcotic alone vs. inhalation alone	1.41
	Narcotic + inhalation vs. inhalation alone	0.79
	Spinal vs. inhalation alone	0.53
	Number of anesthetic drugs: 1–2 vs. >3	2.94
Experience of anesthetist	>600 procedures/y for 8+ y vs. <600 procedures/y for <8 y	1.06

ASA, American Society of Anesthesiologists.
(From ref. 13, with permission.)

cer in patients of advanced age. In the United States and in most Western countries, life expectancies for the elderly have increased substantially. The life expectancy in years of patients between the ages of 62 and 104 in the United States is shown in Table 12.1-10. The average life expectancies for 80-year-old men and women in the United States are 8 and 10.5 years, respectively. The expected survival of 90-year-old men and women is 4.7 and 6.0 years, respectively. Thus, even in the very old cancer patient, aggressive curative surgery can be warranted.[19]

Reports of most surgical series include an account of operative mortality and operative complications. These results, combined with a consideration of the general health status of the

TABLE 12.1-8.   Patient-Related Risk Factors Associated with Postoperative Pulmonary Complications

Potential Risk Factor	Type of Surgery	Relative Risk Associated with Factor
Smoking	Coronary bypass	3.4
	Abdominal	1.4–4.3
ASA class higher than II	Unselected	1.7
	Thoracic or abdominal	1.5–3.2
Age older than 70 y	Unselected	1.9–2.4
	Thoracic or abdominal	0.9–1.9
Obesity	Unselected	1.3
	Thoracic or abdominal	0.8–1.7
Chronic obstructive pulmonary disease	Unselected	2.7–3.6
	Thoracic or abdominal	4.7

ASA, American Society of Anesthesiologists.
(From ref. 8, with permission.)

TABLE 12.1-9.   Incidence of Perioperative Myocardial Infarction in Patients with a Previous Myocardial Infarction

Time from MI to Operation (Mo)	Incidence of Reinfarction[a]		
	Topkins and Artusio[14] (1959–1963)	Tarhan et al.[15] (1975–1976)	Rao et al.[16] (1976–1982)
0–3	12/22 (55%)	3/8 (37%)	3/52 (6%)
4–6	12/22 (55%)	3/19 (16%)	2/36 (2%)
7–12	9/36 (25%)	2/24 (5%)	1/104 (1%)
>12	—	(5%)	(1%)

MI, myocardial infarction.
[a]The incidence of MI in patients with no previous evidence of an MI is approximately 0.3%.

TABLE 12.1-10.   Life Expectancy as a Function of Age

Male		Female	
Age (Y)	Life Expectancy (Y)	Age (Y)	Life Expectancy (Y)
62	19.2	62	23.6
63	18.4	63	22.7
64	17.6	64	21.9
65	16.9	65	21.0
66	16.1	66	20.2
67	15.4	67	19.4
68	14.7	68	18.6
69	14.0	69	17.9
70	13.3	70	17.1
71	12.7	71	16.4
72	12.1	72	15.6
73	11.5	73	14.9
74	10.9	74	14.3
75	10.4	75	13.6
76	9.9	76	12.9
77	9.4	77	12.3
78	8.9	78	11.7
79	8.4	79	11.1
80	8.0	80	10.5
81	7.5	81	10.0
82	7.1	82	9.5
83	6.8	83	9.0
84	6.4	84	8.5
85	6.1	85	8.0
86	5.8	86	7.6
87	5.5	87	7.1
88	5.2	88	6.7
89	4.9	89	6.4
90	4.7	90	6.0
91	4.4	91	5.6
92	4.2	92	5.3
93	4.0	93	5.0
94	3.8	94	4.7
95	3.6	95	4.4
96	3.4	96	4.4
97	3.2	97	4.1
98	3.0	98	3.8
99	2.8	99	3.5
100	2.6	100	3.3
101	2.4	101	3.0
102	2.2	102	2.8
103	2.0	103	2.6
104	1.9	104	2.4

patient, allow a reasonable estimate of the operative mortality for any given surgical intervention in the treatment of patients with cancer.

ROLES FOR SURGERY

PREVENTION OF CANCER

Because surgeons are often the primary providers of medical care, they are responsible for educating patients about carcinogenic hazards and direct surgical intervention for the prevention of cancer. All surgical oncologists should be aware of the high-risk situations that require surgery to prevent subsequent malignant disease.

Some underlying conditions or congenital or genetic traits are associated with an extremely high incidence of subsequent cancer. When these cancers are likely to occur in nonvital organs, it is necessary to remove the potentially involved organ to prevent subsequent malignancy.[20] Examples of diseases associated with a high incidence of cancer that can be prevented by prophylactic surgery are presented in Table 12.1-11 and are considered in more detail in Chapter 21. An excellent illustration is presented by patients with the genetic trait for multiple polyposis of the colon. If colectomy is not performed in these patients, approximately one-half will develop colon cancer by the age of 40. By age 70, virtually all patients with multiple polyposis will develop colon cancer.[20] It is therefore advisable for all patients containing the mutant gene for multiple polyposis to undergo prophylactic colectomy before age 20 to prevent these cancers. Approximately 40% of patients with ulcerative colitis who have total colonic involvement ultimately die of colon cancer if they survive the ulcerative colitis.[21] Three percent of children with ulcerative colitis develop cancer of the colon by the age of 10, and 20% develop cancer during each ensuing decade.[22] Colectomy is indicated for patients with ulcerative colitis if the chronicity of this disease is well established. Patients with multiple endocrine neoplasia type 2A can be screened using polymerase chain reaction–based direct DNA testing for mutations in the *RET* protooncogene. This is the preferred method for screening kindreds with multiple endocrine neoplasia type 2A to identify individuals in whom total thyroidectomy is indicated, regardless of the plasma calcitonin levels.[23] A more complex example of the role of surgery in cancer prevention involves women at high risk for breast cancer. Because the risk of cancer in some women is increased substantially over the normal risk (but does not approach 100%), counseling that explains the benefits and risks of prophylactic mastectomy is an important part of the care of these patients. Genetic tests for the presence of BRCA1 and BRCA2 mutations provide valuable information. Statistical techniques can provide approximations of the risk for patients, depending on the frequency of disease in the family history, the age at the first pregnancy, and the presence of fibrocystic disease.

DIAGNOSIS OF CANCER

The major role of surgery in the diagnosis of cancer lies in the acquisition of tissue for exact histologic diagnosis. The principles underlying the biopsy of malignant lesions vary, depending on the natural history of the tumor under consideration. Various techniques exist for obtaining tissues suspected of malignancy, including aspiration biopsy, needle biopsy, incisional biopsy, and excisional biopsy.

Aspiration biopsy involves the aspiration of cells and tissue fragments through a needle that has been guided into the suspect tissue.

In *needle biopsy*, a core of tissue is obtained through a specially designed needle introduced into the suspect tissue. The core of tissue provided by needle biopsy is sufficient for the diagnosis of most tumor types. Soft tissue and bony sarcomas often present major difficulties in differentiating benign and reparative lesions from malignancies and often cannot be diagnosed accurately. If these latter lesions are considered in the diagnosis, attempts should be made to obtain larger amounts of tissue than are possible from a needle biopsy.

Incisional biopsy refers to removal of a small wedge of tissue from a larger tumor mass. Incisional biopsies often are necessary for diagnosis of large masses that require major surgical procedures for even local excision. Incisional biopsies are the preferred method of diagnosing soft tissue and bony sarcomas because of the magnitude of the surgical procedures necessary to extirpate these lesions definitively.

In *excisional biopsy*, an excision of the entire suspected tumor tissue with little or no margin of surrounding normal tissue is performed. Excisional biopsy is the procedure of choice for most tumors if it can be performed without contaminating new tissue planes or further compromising the ultimate surgical procedure.

The following principles guide the performance of all surgical biopsies:

1. Needle tracks or scars should be placed carefully so that they can be conveniently removed as part of the subsequent definitive surgical procedure. Placement of biopsy incisions is extremely important, and misplacement often can compromise subsequent care. Incisions on the extremity generally should be placed longitudinally so as to make the removal of underlying tissue and subsequent closure easier.
2. Care should be taken to avoid contaminating new tissue planes during the biopsy procedure. The development of large hematomas after biopsy can lead to tumor spread and must be scrupulously avoided by securing excellent hemostasis during the biopsy. For biopsies on extremities, the use of a tourniquet may help to control bleeding. Instruments used in a biopsy procedure are

TABLE 12.1-11. Conditions in Which Prophylactic Surgery Can Prevent Cancer

Underlying Condition	Associated Cancer	Prophylactic Surgery
Cryptorchidism	Testicular	Orchiopexy
Polyposis coli	Colon	Colectomy
Familial colon cancer	Colon	Colectomy
Ulcerative colitis	Colon	Colectomy
Multiple endocrine neoplasia types 2 and 3	Medullary cancer of the thyroid	Thyroidectomy
Familial breast cancer	Breast	Mastectomy
Familial ovarian cancer	Ovary	Oophorectomy

another potential source of contamination of new tissue planes. It is not uncommon to take biopsy samples from several suspected lesions at one time. Care should be taken to avoid using instruments that may have come in contact with tumor when obtaining tissue from a potentially uncontaminated area.

3. Adequate tissue samples must be obtained to meet the needs of the pathologist. For the diagnosis of selected tumors, electron microscopy, tissue culture, or other techniques may be necessary. Sufficient tissue must be obtained for these purposes if diagnostic difficulties are anticipated.

4. When knowledge of the orientation of the biopsy specimen is important for subsequent treatment, the surgeon should mark distinctive areas of the tumor carefully to facilitate subsequent orientation of the specimen by the pathologist. Certain fixatives are best suited to specific types or sizes of tissue. If all biopsy specimens are placed in formalin immediately, the opportunity to perform valuable diagnostic tests may be lost. The handling of excised tissue is the surgeon's responsibility. Biopsy tissue obtained from breast cancer lesions, for example, should be saved for estrogen receptor studies and placed in cold storage until ready for processing.

5. Placement of radiopaque clips during biopsy and staging procedures is sometimes important to delineate areas of known tumor and to guide the subsequent delivery of radiation therapy to these areas.

TREATMENT OF CANCER

Surgery can be a simple, safe method to cure patients with solid tumors when the tumor is confined to the anatomic site of origin. The extension of the surgical resection to include areas of regional spread can cure some patients, although regional spread often is an indication of undetectable distant micrometastases.

The role of surgery in the treatment of cancer patients can be divided into six separate areas: (1) definitive surgical treatment for primary cancer, selection of appropriate local therapy, and integration of surgery with other adjuvant modalities; (2) surgery to reduce the bulk of disease (e.g., ovarian cancer); (3) surgical resection of metastatic disease with curative intent (e.g., pulmonary metastases in sarcoma patients, hepatic metastases from colorectal cancer); (4) surgery for the treatment of oncologic emergencies; (5) surgery for palliation; and (6) surgery for reconstruction and rehabilitation. In each area, integration with other treatment modalities can be essential for a successful outcome.

Resection of the Primary Cancer

Three major challenges confront the surgical oncologist in the definitive treatment of solid tumors: accurate identification of patients who can be cured by local treatment alone; development and selection of local treatments that provide the best balance between local cure and the impact of treatment morbidity on the quality of life; and development and application of adjuvant treatments that can improve the control of locally invasive and distant metastatic disease. The selection of the appropriate local therapy to be used in cancer treatment varies with the individual cancer type and the site of involvement. In

many instances, definitive surgical therapy that encompasses a sufficient margin of normal tissue is sufficient local therapy. The treatment of many solid tumors falls into this category, including the wide excision of primary melanomas in the skin, which can be cured locally by surgery alone in approximately 90% of cases. The resection of colon cancers with a 5-cm margin from the tumor results in anastomotic recurrences in fewer than 5% of cases.

In other instances, surgery is used to obtain histologic confirmation of diagnosis, but primary local therapy is achieved through the use of a nonsurgical modality, such as radiation therapy. Examples include the treatment of Ewing's sarcoma in long bones and the treatment of selected primary malignancies in the head and neck. In each instance, selection of the definitive local treatment involves careful consideration of the likelihood of cure balanced against the morbidity of the treatment modality.

The magnitude of surgical resection is modified in the treatment of many cancers by the use of adjuvant treatment modalities. Rationally integrating surgery with other treatments requires a careful consideration of all effective treatment options. It is knowledge of this rapidly changing field that separates the surgical oncologist from the general surgeon most distinctly.

In some instances, the availability of effective adjuvant modalities has led to a decrease in the magnitude of surgery. The evolution of treatment for childhood rhabdomyosarcoma is a striking example of the successful integration of adjuvant therapies with surgery in the treatment of cancer.[24,25] Childhood rhabdomyosarcoma is the most common soft tissue sarcoma in infants and children. Before 1970, surgery alone was used almost exclusively, and 5-year survival rates of 10% to 20% were commonly reported. Local surgery alone failed in patients with rhabdomyosarcomas of the prostate and extremities because of extensive invasion of surrounding tissues and the early development of metastatic disease. The failure of surgery alone to control local disease in patients with childhood rhabdomyosarcoma led to the introduction of adjuvant radiation therapy. This resulted in a marked improvement in local control rates that was further improved dramatically by the introduction of combination chemotherapy. Long-term cure rates are now in the range of 80%. Many other examples of the integration of surgery with other treatment modalities appear throughout this text.

Cytoreductive Surgery

In some instances, the extensive local spread of cancer precludes the removal of all gross disease by surgery. The partial surgical resection of bulk disease in the treatment of selected cancers improves the ability of other treatment modalities to control residual gross disease that has not been resected.[26,27] Studies that suggest the merit of this approach are discussed in the chapters dealing with Burkitt's lymphoma and ovarian cancer, respectively.

Enthusiasm for cytoreductive surgery has led to the inappropriate use of surgery to reduce the bulk of tumor in some cases. Clearly, cytoreductive surgery is of benefit only when other effective treatments are available to control the residual disease that is unresectable. Except in rare palliative settings, there is no role for cytoreductive surgery in patients for whom little other effective therapy exists.

Metastatic Disease

The value of surgery in the cure of patients with metastatic disease tends to be overlooked and is the subject of an entire section of this text (see Chapter 51). As a general principle, patients with a single site of metastatic disease that can be resected without major morbidity should undergo resection of that metastatic cancer. Some patients with limited metastases to lung or liver or brain can be cured by surgical resection. This approach is especially appropriate for cancers that do not respond well to systemic chemotherapy. The resection of pulmonary metastases from soft tissue and bony sarcomas can cure disease in as many as 30% of patients. As effective systemic therapy is developed for the treatment of these diseases, cure rates may increase. Studies have shown that similar cure rates occur in patients with adenocarcinomas when resected metastatic disease in the lung is the sole clinical site of metastases. Small numbers of pulmonary metastases often are the only clinically apparent metastatic disease in patients with sarcomas. However, this is rare in the natural history of most adenocarcinomas. If solitary metastases to the lung do occur in patients with carcinoma of the colon or other adenocarcinomas, surgical resection is indicated.

Similarly, resection of hepatic metastases, especially from colorectal cancer, in patients in whom the liver is the only site of known metastatic disease can lead to long-term cure in approximately 25%. This far exceeds the cure rates of any other available treatment.

Resection for cure of solitary brain metastases should also be considered when the brain is the only site of known metastatic disease. The exact location and functional sequelae of resection should be considered when making this treatment decision.

Oncologic Emergencies

As for all patients, emergencies arise for oncologic patients that require surgical intervention. These generally involve the treatment of exsanguinating hemorrhage, perforation, drainage of abscesses, or impending destruction of vital organs. Each category of surgical emergency is unique and requires an individual approach.

The oncologic patient often is neutropenic and thrombocytopenic and has a high risk of hemorrhage or sepsis. Perforations of an abdominal viscus can be caused by direct tumor invasion or by tumor lysis resulting from effective systemic treatments. Perforation of the gastrointestinal tract after effective treatment for lymphoma involving the intestine is not uncommon. Surgery to decompress cancer invading the central nervous system represents another emergency surgical procedure that can lead to preservation of function.

Palliation

Surgical resection often is required for the relief of pain or functional abnormalities. The appropriate use of surgery in these settings can improve the quality of life for cancer patients. Palliative surgery may include procedures to relieve mechanical problems, such as intestinal obstruction, or the removal of masses that are causing severe pain or disfigurement. A study by Krouse et al. has emphasized the role of surgery in the palliative treatment of cancer patients.[28]

Reconstruction and Rehabilitation

Surgical techniques are being refined that aid in the reconstruction and rehabilitation of cancer patients after definitive therapy. The ability to reconstruct anatomic defects can substantially improve function and cosmetic appearance. The development of free flaps using microvascular anastomotic techniques is having a profound impact on the ability to bring fresh tissue to resected or heavily irradiated areas. Lost function (especially of extremities) often can be restored by surgical approaches. These includes lysis of contractures or muscle transposition to restore muscular function that has been damaged by previous surgery or radiation therapy.

SURGICAL ONCOLOGIST

In the last decade, a substantial increase has been seen in the creation of separate sections of surgical oncology in departments of surgery within universities. This enthusiasm derives from the recognition that modern oncologic management requires levels of expertise in cancer surgery, chemotherapy, and radiation therapy that are not common in most general surgeons and from a desire to effectively use the resources being committed to cancer care and research by hospitals, private foundations, and the federal government. A sense of urgency has existed, because some surgical leaders believe that the surgeon is experiencing a declining intellectual role in modern cancer treatment and research and that steps must be taken to reassert the surgeon's role in modern oncology.

Within the next several decades, the United States will experience a dramatic growth in the number of older individuals. The 2000 Nationwide Inpatient Sample and the 1996 National Survey of Ambulatory Surgery estimated that by the year 2020

TABLE 12.1-12. World Federation of Surgical Oncology Societies

Austrian Society of Surgical Oncology
Brazilian Society of Surgical Oncology
British Association of Surgical Oncology
Canadian Society of Surgical Oncology
Dutch Society of Surgical Oncology
European Society of Surgical Oncology
French Cancer Centre Surgeons
Hellenic Society of Surgical Oncology
Hungarian Society of Surgical Oncology
Indian Society of Surgical Oncology
Indonesian Society of Surgical Oncology
Italian Society of Surgical Oncology
Korean Surgical Oncology Society
Portuguese Society of Surgical Oncology
Scandinavian Society of Surgical Oncology
Society of Surgical Oncology, United States
South African Society of Oncological Surgeons
Surgical Oncology Section, German Society of Surgeons
Surgical Oncology Section, Polish Surgeons Association
Surgical Oncology Section, Swiss Society of Surgeons

(From ref. 32, with permission.)

TABLE 12.1-13. Training Requirements for Specialists in Surgical Oncology

KNOWLEDGE, SKILLS, AND CLINICAL EXPERIENCES

Clinical and technical skills for providing comprehensive care to cancer patients. An essential component of the fellowship is training in new techniques to produce surgeons capable of providing state-of-the-art surgical care to cancer patients.

Skills in performing special and unusual operations for patients with complex or recurrent neoplasms.

Expertise in diagnosis and management of rare or unusual tumors, based on knowledge of the natural history of such cancers.

Knowledge and experience to determine disease stage and treatment options for individual cancer patients, at the time of diagnosis and throughout the disease course.

Broad knowledge of other cancer treatment modalities (including radiotherapy, chemotherapy, immunotherapy, and endocrine therapy). This requires an understanding of the fundamental biology of cancer, clinical pharmacology, tumor immunology, and endocrinology as well as an understanding of potential complications of multimodality therapy.

Expertise in the selection of patients for surgical therapy in combination with other forms of cancer treatment, as well as knowledge of the benefits and risks associated with a multidisciplinary approach.

Expertise in palliative techniques, including proper selection of patients, proper performance of appropriate palliative surgical procedures, and knowledge of nonsurgical palliative treatments.

Knowledge of tumor biology, carcinogenesis, epidemiology, tumor markers, and tumor pathology.

CANCER RESEARCH

Knowledge to design and implement a prospective database and to conduct clinical cancer research, especially prospective clinical trials.

Sufficient familiarity with statistical methods to properly evaluate results of published research studies.

Knowledge to guide a trainee or other personnel in laboratory or clinical oncology research.

Knowledge of the interface of basic science with clinical cancer care, to facilitate translational research.

CANCER EDUCATION

Educational knowledge and skills to train students and physicians in the multimodal management of cancer patients.

Knowledge and skills to train nonphysicians (physician assistants, oncology nurses, enterostomal therapists, etc.) in specialized cancer care.

Skills to organize and conduct cancer-related public education programs.

LEADERSHIP IN ONCOLOGY

Skills to develop and support the following:

Institutional programs relating to cancer, including a tumor registry

Institutional policies regarding cancer programs and problems

Interdisciplinary meetings and discussions on cancer topics, patient care, and oncology research program

Psychosocial and rehabilitative programs for cancer patients and their families

---

the number of patients undergoing oncologic procedures will increase by 24% and that these will include both outpatient and inpatient procedures.[29] The increase in the number of surgical oncology fellowships available is playing a valuable role in ensuring the supply of surgical oncologic specialists. In one study, 69% of all surgical oncology fellows trained at a major cancer center held "academic full-time" positions.

Further fueling the need for specialists in surgical oncology is a vast body of accumulating data that indicate that the number of difficult surgical procedures for cancer performed by the surgeon is directly related to patient outcome. Many studies have shown that increasing hospital volume for major cancer surgery also has positive impact on patient survival. In one

study of 5013 patients in the Surveillance, Epidemiology, and End Results registry of patients aged 65 years or older, high hospital volume was linked with lower mortality for patients undergoing pancreatectomy ($P = .004$), esophagectomy ($P < .001$), liver resection ($P = .04$), and pelvic exenteration ($P = .04$). In patients undergoing esophagectomy, for example, operative mortality was 17.3% in low-volume hospitals compared with 3.4% in high-volume hospitals. For patients undergoing pancreatectomy, the corresponding rates were 12.9% versus 5.8%.[30] In another study of 474,108 patients who underwent one of eight cardiovascular procedures or cancer resections, a highly significant inverse relationship was seen between surgeon volume and operative mortality for lung resection ($P = .003$) and for bladder cystectomy, esophagectomy, and pancreatic resection ($P < .001$).[31]

Surgical oncology is increasingly becoming an acknowledged specialty within surgery. The creation of a world federation of surgical oncology societies is helping to increase information exchange (Table 12.1-12).

Another positive development in this area was the creation of the American College of Surgeons Oncology Group to bring surgeons together in the performance of clinical trials in surgical oncology. This program has initiated multiple trials exploring the role of surgery in treatment of a variety of cancer types.[32]

The development of surgical oncology as a specialty area of surgery depends on a clear delineation of its role. The Society of Surgical Oncology in the United States has formalized training guidelines for surgeons intending to specialize in surgical oncology that fall in four broad areas, presented in Table 12.1-13.

REFERENCES

1. Brested JH. *The Edwin Smith surgical papyrus.* Chicago: University of Chicago Press, 1930.
2. Thorwald J. *Science and the secrets of early medicine.* New York: Harcourt, Brace, and World, 1962.
3. Wangensteen OH. Has medical history importance for surgeons? *Surg Gynecol Obstet* 1975;140:434.
4. Hill GJ. Historic milestones in cancer surgery. *Semin Oncol* 1979;6:409.
5. Strichartz GR, Berde CB. Local anesthetics. In: Miller RD, ed. *Anesthesia.* New York: Churchill Livingstone, 1994.
6. Goldman L, Caldera DL, Nussbaum SR, et al. Multifactorial index of cardiac risk in noncardiac surgical procedures. *N Engl J Med* 1977;297:845.
7. Dripps RD, Eckenhoff JE, Vandam LD. *Introduction to anesthesia,* 2nd ed. Philadelphia: WB Saunders, 1988.
8. Miller, RD, ed. *Anesthesia,* 5th ed. Philadelphia: Churchill Livingstone, 2000.
9. Buck N, Devlin HB, Lunn JN. *Report on the confidential enquiry into perioperative deaths.* London: Nuffield Provincial Hospitals Trust, The Kings Fund Publishing House, 1987.
10. Eichhorn JH. Prevention of intraoperative anesthesia accidents and related severe injury through safety monitoring. *Anesthesiology* 1989;70:572.
11. Eichhorn JH. Documenting improved anesthesia outcome. *J Clin Anesth* 1991;3:351.
12. Ross AF, Tinker JH. Anesthesia risk. In: Miller RD, ed. *Anesthesia.* New York: Churchill Livingstone, 1994.
13. Cohen MM, Duncan PG, Tate RB. Does anaesthesia contribute to operative mortality? *JAMA* 1988;260:2859.
14. Topkins MJ, Artusio JF. Myocardial infarction and surgery: a five year study. *Anesth Analg* 1964;43:715.
15. Tarhan S, Moffitt EA, Taylor WF, et al. Myocardial infarction after general anesthesia. *JAMA* 1972;199:318.
16. Rao TLK, Jacobs KH, El-Etr AA. Reinfarction following anesthesia in patients with myocardial infarction. *Anesthesiology* 1983;59:499.
17. Palmberg S, Hirsjarvi E. Mortality in geriatric surgery. *Gerontology* 1979;25:103.
18. Hoskings MP, Warner MA, Lobdell EM, et al. Outcomes of surgery in patients 90 years of age and older. *JAMA* 1989;261:1909.
19. Manton KC, Vaupel JW. Survival after the age of 80 in the United States, Sweden, France, England, and Japan. *N Engl J Med* 1995;333:1232.
20. Mulvihill JJ. Cancer control through genetics. In: Arrighi FE, Rao PN, Stubblefield E, eds. *Genes, chromosomes, and neoplasia.* New York: Raven Press, 1980.
21. MacDougall IPM. The cancer risk in ulcerative colitis. *Lancet* 1964;2:655.

22. Devroede GJ, Taylor WF, Sauer WG. Cancer risk and life expectancy of children with ulcerative colitis. *N Engl J Med* 1971;285:17.
23. Wells SA, Chi DD, Toshima K, et al. Predictive DNA testing and prophylactic thyroidectomy in patients at risk for multiple endocrine neoplasia type 2A. *Ann Surg* 1994;220:237.
24. Kilman JW, Clatworthy HW Jr, Newton WA, et al. Reasonable surgery for rhabdomyosarcoma: a study of 67 cases. *Ann Surg* 1973;3:346.
25. Heyn RM, Holland R, Newton WA, et al. The role of combined chemotherapy in the treatment of rhabdomyosarcoma in children. *Cancer* 1974;34:2128.
26. McCarter MD, Fong Y. Role for surgical cytoreduction in multimodality treatments for cancer. *Ann Surg Oncol* 2001;8:38.
27. Wong RJ, De Cosse JJ. Cytoreductive surgery. *Surg Gynecol Obstet* 1990;170:276.
28. Krouse RS, Nelson RA, Farrell BR, et al. Surgical palliation at a cancer center. *Arch Surg* 2001;136:773.
29. Etzioni DA, Liu JH, Maggard MA, et al. Workload projections for surgical oncology: will we need more surgeons? *Ann Surg Oncol* 2003;10:1112.
30. Begg CB, Cramer LD, Hoskins WJ, et al. Impact of hospital volume on operative mortality for major cancer surgery. *JAMA* 1998;280:1747.
31. Birkmeyer JD, Stukel TA, Siewers AE, et al. Surgeon volume and operative mortality in the United States. *N Engl J Med* 2003;349:2117.
32. Wells SA. The American college of surgeons oncology group: its genesis and future directions. *Bull Am Coll Surg* 1998;83:13.

SECTION 2

ALBERT S. KO
ALAN T. LEFOR

Laparoscopic Surgery

Over the past two decades, laparoscopy has emerged as a valuable tool in the diagnosis and management of many diseases. For some conditions, laparoscopy has rapidly become the gold standard in treatment, relegating open surgery to a second line of therapy. One such procedure is laparoscopic cholecystectomy, which has allowed a dramatic decrease in length of hospital stay, increased patient comfort, and rapid return to employment. Despite the widespread acceptance of laparoscopy for benign conditions, its role in oncology remains limited, somewhat undefined, and under investigation.

The development of laparoscopy spans over a century, and much of the early work is credited to Georg Kelling.[1] In 1901, in a canine model, Kelling insufflated the abdomen via a puncture and then placed a hollow tube through which a viewing laparoscope was inserted. This allowed direct visualization of the abdominal cavity. In the same year in Germany, a description was presented of the illumination of the abdominal cavity through a small vaginal incision using a head mirror and speculum. A decade later, a report of a series of 115 thoracoscopic and laparoscopic examinations for a wide variety of indications including malignancy was published, followed by description of a series of 2000 laparoscopic procedures performed without a death in 1951.[1]

The early adopters of this technology were gynecologists, and this was the field in which the first English-language textbook on the procedure, *Laparoscopy and Gynaecology*, was written in 1967.[1] Numerous reports of diagnostic laparoscopy and sterilization were subsequently published. However, widespread application of this technique remained elusive because of the inability to disseminate the technology widely. The teaching model was the surgeon and an assistant with a cumbersome optic lens system that allowed two people to view the procedure. In the 1980s, the development of high-quality video cameras and display systems opened laparoscopic procedures to viewing by larger groups, which allowed the current mentoring education process to be widely practiced.

In the last two decades, the role of laparoscopy has expanded to include diagnosing, staging, treating, monitoring, and palliating a long list of malignancies. The early role of laparoscopy in diagnosis was strictly visual. Intraabdominal masses were characterized visually, which gave a subjective impression as to their malignant potential. The invention of laparoscopic biopsy forceps allowed the verification of malignancy by providing tissue specimens. Recently, laparoscopic ultrasonographically guided biopsy techniques allow for the detection and biopsy of masses deep within solid organs such as the liver. Once a diagnosis is established, laparoscopic staging can identify unresectable disease, which often dramatically alters therapy. Originally used to determine the treatment course of lymphomas, laparoscopy now plays a role in excluding major abdominal resections when metastases are identified. For resectable disease, major laparoscopic resections ranging from splenectomy to complex pancreaticoduodenectomy have been described. After resection, tumor surveillance can be performed by direct observation, with carcinomatosis identified in second-look operations. In the case of unresectable disease or complications of advanced disease, laparoscopic procedures can provide palliation, for example, by relieving or bypassing bowel obstruction.

Although the list of procedures performed laparoscopically has grown exponentially, the body of evidence supporting their use remains limited. Further meticulous, well-designed clinical trials are needed before laparoscopic surgery can be designated as an oncologically safe treatment option. Surgical procedures should maximally benefit the patient and should not be performed simply because they can be.

PHYSIOLOGY OF LAPAROSCOPY

CELLULAR AND IMMUNE EFFECTS

Some of the benefits of laparoscopic surgery are the reduction in postoperative pain, decreased healing time, and decreased adhesion formation. These may easily be attributed to the use of smaller incisions and avoidance of the need for retractors to hold incisions open for hours. However, patients who undergo laparoscopic splenectomy and then require an incision for removal of the intact specimen also note decreased pain in their incisions. Implicated in the beneficial effects of laparoscopy is the CO_2 gas that is commonly used to insufflate the abdominal wall. West et al. investigated the effect of different insufflation gases on murine peritoneal macrophage intracellular pH and correlated their use with alterations in lipopolysaccharide-stimulated inflammatory cytokine release.[2] Peritoneal macrophages were incubated for 2 hours in air, helium, or CO_2, and the effect on tumor necrosis factor (TNF) level, interleukin-1 level, and cytosol pH was determined. Macrophages incubated in CO_2 produced significantly less tumor necrosis factor and interleukin-1 than those incubated in air or helium. In addition, exposure to CO_2, but not to air or helium, produced a marked acidification of the cytosol. These authors concluded that cellular acidification induced by peritoneal CO_2 insufflation contributes to the diminished local inflammatory response seen in laparoscopic surgery. In a human model, harvested peritoneal macrophages from volunteers were exposed to CO_2 under pressures similar to those used in laparoscopy and to a helium control environment.[3] The results show a decrease in intraabdominal polymorphonuclear leukocyte function as evidenced by a decrease in superoxide production. Also, the peritoneal macrophages secreted less TNF-α and interleukin-1, and the activity of mitochondrial dehydrogenase became significantly impaired for up to 12 hours after CO_2 exposure. It was also concluded that CO_2 was responsible for the decreased inflammation and pain after laparoscopy. In a randomized trial of laparoscopic versus conventional colon resections, Wu et al. measured levels of interleukin-6, interleukin-8, and TNF-α in patients undergoing colon resections for malignancy.[4] The laparoscopic group had significant reductions in serum interleukin-6 and interleukin-8 levels, whereas TNF-α was undetectable in both groups. These results confirm the attenuation of the acute-phase systemic response previously reported in clinical trials.

Despite the reduction in local peritoneal inflammatory response, systemic immunocompetence appears better preserved after laparoscopic surgery than after open procedures. Some studies have shown significant decreases in the CD4 and CD8 cell counts in patients undergoing open cholecystectomy, and others have shown a derangement in the ratios of the T-cell subsets.[5] Vallina and Velasco studied peripheral lymphocyte populations in 11 patients undergoing laparoscopic cholecystectomy and found a transient decrease in the CD4 to CD8 ratio, with no difference in absolute CD4 and CD8 cell counts, followed by a return to the preoperative ratio within 1 week of surgery.[6] In a study of delayed-type hypersensitivity in sepsis, death rate was 2.9% in patients with a normal delayed-type hypersensitivity response, whereas death rate was 20.9% in anergic patients.[7] In prospective animal and human studies comparing laparotomy and laparoscopy, the laparotomy group had a significantly sustained decrease in delayed-type hypersensitivity; the inference is thus that systemic cell-mediated immunity is better preserved with laparoscopy.[8] In animal studies, tumor inoculum implanted remotely from the abdomen showed greater growth after laparotomy than after laparoscopy. Further studies are needed to illuminate the complex factors that lead to attenuation of the local immune response while systemic immunocompetence is preserved.

CENTRAL NERVOUS SYSTEM EFFECTS

Much of what is known about the central nervous system effects of laparoscopy is derived from porcine models. In an intracranial pressure transduction study, CO_2, helium, and nitric oxide all increased intracranial pressure equally.[9] The rise in intracranial pressure was independent of changes in acid-base balance and was thought to be secondary to increased intraabdominal pressure from the pneumoperitoneum. Despite the low morbidity shown in a single small retrospective study of patients with ventriculoperitoneal shunts, caution is advised in patients with intracranial pathology.[10]

CARDIAC EFFECTS

As the population ages, it is not uncommon to operate on older patients with cancer who also have significant medical comorbidities such as heart disease. It becomes imperative that the physiologic cardiovascular consequences of laparoscopic surgery be understood to prevent adverse results. The documentation of these effects in humans has been aided by the use of invasive and noninvasive devices. In a hemodynamic study carried out during laparoscopic colectomy for carcinoma, patients were monitored with arterial and pulmonary artery catheters along with transesophageal echocardiography.[11] The mean arterial pressure, central venous pressure, mean pulmonary artery pressure, pulmonary capillary wedge pressure, and systemic vascular resistance all increased significantly. Cardiac index and ejection fraction decreased significantly, whereas heart rate remained relatively unchanged. To understand the physiologic consequences, Giebler et al. studied intraperitoneal laparoscopy and retroperitoneal laparoscopy in a pig model.[12] They found significant pressure gradients along the iliac veins and vena cava in the intraperitoneal group that were absent in the retroperitoneal group. Also, airway pressures increased in the intraperitoneal group. It is likely that the decrease in cardiac function is the direct result of an interaction between decreased venous return and increased transmitted intrathoracic pressure.

PULMONARY EFFECTS

In the usual clinical setting, the lungs remain a compliant organ. By manipulating ventilation, the anesthesiologist is able to prevent significant acid-base disturbances and keep the partial pressure of carbon dioxide (pCO_2) within the normal range. To understand the effects on an injured lung, a porcine adult respiratory distress syndrome model was used.[13] After adult respiratory distress syndrome was induced, animals were divided into two groups; one underwent laparoscopy and the other underwent conventional laparotomy. The laparoscopic group demonstrated significantly decreased pulmonary compliance compared with the laparotomy group, had a higher pCO_2, and was more acidotic. Despite the increase in pulmonary derangements caused by laparoscopy in animals with adult respiratory distress syndrome, overall cardiopulmonary function was preserved.

VISCERAL EFFECTS

That visceral organs have diminished blood flow during insufflation with a variety of gases is well accepted. The magnitude of reduction can be significant, with reductions in flow of more than 30%. Often the ischemia is mild, manifested by low urine output, but severe intestinal ischemia has also been observed in rare cases. The reduced blood flow has been attributed to a combination of factors, including direct vascular compression and reflexive neural pathways.

EFFECTS ON MALIGNANT CELLS

A common physiologic change during laparoscopy is the exposure of the abdominal contents to high intraabdominal pressures. Gutt et al. exposed cultures of two human tumor cell lines (CX-2 colon adenocarcinoma and DAN-G pancreatic adenocarcinoma) to 0-mm Hg, 6-mm Hg, and 12-mm Hg CO_2 pressures.[14] The proliferation of colon carcinoma cells increased significantly as pressure increased, whereas the pancreatic carcinoma cells proliferated with CO_2 exposure independently of ambient pressure. In a rat model, 36 anesthetized rats underwent laparoscopy under 0-mm Hg, 4-mm Hg, and 16-mm Hg pressure.[15] A 1-mL suspension of a moderately differentiated colon adenocarcinoma line was injected intraperitoneally and pneumoperitoneum was held for 60 minutes. On day 11, the rats were sacrificed and the volume of tumor was assessed by independent blinded observers. Rats that underwent higher pressure laparoscopy had a greater volume of tumor. In similar studies, other investigators have shown increased rates of metastases.

In a cellular study, an increase in ambient pressure increased tumor adherence to matrix proteins; this effect was mitigated by administration of antibodies to the β_1-integrin subunit.[16] In a matrix gel experiment, laparoscopic conditions created using both CO_2 and helium caused an increase in tumor invasiveness, which was abolished with matrix metalloproteinase blockade.[17] In addition to altering the biologic characteristics of tumors so that they adhere to and invade tissues more readily, increased pressure also adversely affects the host barrier of normal mesothelial cells and thus decreases the natural defenses to tumor growth. One hour after laparoscopy was performed on mice, electron microscopy of the normal peritoneal surfaces revealed retraction and condensation of mesothelial cells.[18] Over the next 12 hours, the intercellular clefts increased in size, exposing the basal membrane. In animals inoculated with tumor, the peritoneal surfaces rapidly became coated with malignant cells, which created widespread intraabdominal metastases mimicking the carcinomatosis reported in humans after laparoscopy. In the control group exposed to pressureless laparoscopy, tumor cells remained on top of intact mesothelial cells for a prolonged period before invading in a sporadic fashion. The growth of tumor remained localized to the port sites and lower abdomen, similar to the pattern of recurrences seen after open laparotomy. The effect of pressure is multifold: It induces tumor cells to grow larger, adhere better to cells, and penetrate more quickly. Not only does this lead to peritoneal host defense damage but it has been hypothesized to explain early carcinomatosis after laparoscopy.

Another component of routine laparoscopy is use of the insufflation gas CO_2. In tissue culture experiments, CO_2 (in comparison to helium and air) increased ovarian carcinoma cell growth by 52%; however, in *in vivo* studies, CO_2 had no impact on tumor growth and metastases.[19] In an elegant rat model, the cecal wall was inoculated via a 1-cm abdominal incision with 2 million viable tumor cells using a 30-gauge needle under microscopic vision.[19] Two weeks later, the rats were randomly assigned to laparoscopy or laparotomy. In the laparoscopy group, a standard 5-mm port was inserted, and the abdominal cavity was insufflated for 30 minutes with CO_2. The laparotomy group underwent a midline 4-cm incision, which was remained open for 30 minutes. Four weeks after the second procedure, tissues were examined histologically and grossly. There was no difference between groups in liver metastases, lung metastases, nodal metastases, wound/port metastases, or cecal tumor weight. A major criticism of the study is that the subjects underwent two operations, which confounds the results and conclusion. Because of the numerous conflicting results of *ex vivo* and *in vivo* studies, the effects of CO_2 on tumor cells still remain unknown.

The cause of the controversy concerning laparoscopic tumor cell biology is multifactorial. During laparoscopy, abdominal contents, including malignant cells, are exposed to changes in homeostasis. The effects of these changes have been studied mainly in animal models, and controversy exists regarding which species most represents human biology. Another common criticism is the lack of significant statistical power when a small number of subjects are included. Also, many models used tumor inocula far in excess of what would be found in humans and were placed in non–naturally occurring locations under extreme environmental conditions. Even the tumor cell lines used varied from study to study, ranging from melanoma to mesothelioma to uncommon lines of colonic adenocarcinoma. Despite a multitude of research, basic questions regarding tumor cell biology remain unanswered, and previous results should be analyzed with great caution.

PORT-SITE METASTASES

As the popularity of laparoscopic treatment of malignancies has risen, case reports of port-site metastases have increased in frequency since an early report in the 1970s. *Port-site metastasis*, broadly defined, is the recurrence of tumor at the small wounds created for the transabdominal placement of ports used to pass instruments or retrieve specimens. Before any large studies on the true incidence of port-site metastases were conducted, numerous anecdotal reports suggested that the rate of wound metastases after laparoscopic procedures far exceeded that after laparotomy. Small series indicated that port-site metastases occurred in up to 21% of patients.[20] Because of these early concerns, enthusiasm for minimally invasive surgery for malignancy became tempered. As a result, studies were initiated to determine the true incidence of metastasis at the same time that laboratory studies were conducted to try to explain the phenomena.

Before implicating the laparoscopic method itself, the incidence of wound recurrences after laparotomy had to be established. Hughes et al. reviewed data for 1603 patients with colon carcinoma and found a total recurrence rate of 0.8%. Recurrences consisted of 11 cases in the laparotomy scar and five in the stoma or drain site.[21] Reilly et al. reviewed 1711 laparotomy cases and found a 0.6% recurrence rate.[22] From these large retrospective studies, the wound recurrence in open cases is estimated to be less than 1%.

Early reports of port-site recurrences after laparoscopic surgery for colorectal carcinoma were discouraging; however, later reports showed such recurrences to be an uncommon phenomena. Results for a series of 480 patients in the American Society of Colon and Rectal Surgeons laparoscopic registry showed a port-site recurrence rate of 1.1%.[23] In 2001, Zmora and Weiss performed a metaanalysis of laparoscopic colorectal resections for carcinoma, including only studies that included more than 50 patients.[24] This step was taken to eliminate bias in reports from surgeons early on the learning curve. Of 1737 patients, they identified 17 (0.6%) with port-site metastases. Unfortunately, many of the early studies were nonprospective and nonrandomized, and had a short follow-up period. Despite these limitations, the results compare favorably with those of prospective randomized studies. Lacy et al. published the results of a randomized prospective trial involving 219 patients and found only one port-site metastasis in 106 colectomies.[25] Randomized studies with greater power are currently accruing patients or are in the observational phase. The Colon Carcinoma Laparoscopic or Open Resection (COLOR) trial was initiated in 1997 to evaluate oncologic outcomes; the trial involves a international group of participants and has a target accrual of 1200 patients.[26] The participation criteria are rigid, requiring surgeons to have experience with more than 20 laparoscopic procedures and to conform to set guidelines for resection. Other large trials in the United States (National Institutes of Health), Great Britain, and Germany are now under way. After the completion of these and other well-designed studies, the incidence of port-site metastases and the oncologic safety of laparoscopic surgery for colorectal carcinoma can be ascertained.

Large series have also shown low rates of port-site metastasis after laparoscopic surgery for upper gastrointestinal malignancies. In a prospective 1965 study of laparoscopic procedures involving placement of 4299 ports, 0.79% of port sites developed recurrences at times ranging from 15 days to 17 months after surgery.[27] Wound recurrence for open procedures was 0.86%. A preponderance of patients with port-site metastases and wound recurrences had an advanced stage of disease at initial presentation, which allowed the authors to conclude that port-site or wound recurrence is a marker of advanced disease. One particular upper gastrointestinal malignancy, gallbladder carcinoma, continues to be associated with a high incidence of port-site metastases. In an international survey of 117,840 cholecystectomies for presumed benign disease, 409 nonapparent gallbladder cancers were identified and wound recurrence occurred in 70 (17.1%) of the cases.[28] Currently, long-term data on the effects of laparoscopic surgery in treatment of gynecologic and urologic malignancies are pending.

Given the lack of knowledge about the true incidence of port-site metastases, it is even more difficult to analyze their significance. In the larger series, port-site metastases occurred in association with advanced disease at initial presentation; however, numerous cases have been reported in patients with early disease in a relatively short period of time after surgery. The occurrences in patients with early disease, such as stage I colon cancer, have been associated with carcinomatosis and adverse outcomes. This group of patients otherwise would have done well. Only through the use of protocols and diligent studies will the importance be known.

Soon after port-site metastases were reported, a number of laboratory studies attempted to explain the phenomenon. One theory is that the constant flow of gas used to create a pneumoperitoneum seeds the port site through the constant exposure to aerosolized tumor cells. Hewett et al., using an *in vivo* pig model, inserted radiolabeled tumor cells into the peritoneum. As observed by gamma camera, tumor cells traveled throughout the abdominal cavity faster with pneumoperitoneum.[29] In a later complex study, Hewett's group inserted radiolabeled human colon cancer cells into the peritoneal cavity of pigs. Ports were placed and pneumoperitoneum established. After 2 hours, the ports were removed, and the port sites were excised and examined.[30] The study examined the effects of two variables, tumor burden and insufflation pressure. The intraabdominal tumor inoculum ranged from 1.5×10^5 to 120×10^5 cells. Insufflation pressure was 0, 4, 8, or 12 mm Hg. With increased tumor burden (more than 2.5×10^6 cells), tumor became detectable at the port sites. In the second portion of the study, as insufflation pressure increased, less tumor was identified at the port sites. Caution is advised in interpreting the second portion of this study because

only eight animals were studied in this arm. To further test the significance of aerosolized tumor cells, Mathew et al. inserted adenocarcinoma cells into the peritoneum of primary rats, each of which had a venting peritoneal plastic tube connected to the abdominal cavity of a recipient secondary rat.[31] One group of primary rats underwent standard insufflation, whereas a second group of primary rats underwent gasless laparoscopy. Five of six secondary recipient rats in the insufflation group developed peritoneal metastases, whereas none of the secondary recipient rats in the gasless group did. These results show the clinical significance of aerosolized tumor cells. In a separate study, the intraoperative manipulation of tumor using laparoscopic instruments, thought to enhanced tumor dispersion, also led to increased rates of port-site metastases.[32] In humans, radiolabeled red blood cells injected into the bed of the gallbladder during standard laparoscopic cholecystectomy migrated to port sites, even though the specimen was removed using a protective bag.[33] In a group undergoing gasless laparoscopy, no radioactivity was detected at the port sites. In another human trial, laparoscopic surgery for benign and malignant disease was performed using a saline suction trap to filter the pneumoperitoneum effluent.[34] Normal mesothelial cells were identified in the trap in the benign group, whereas large numbers of malignant cells were collected in the trap for 2 of 15 patients with malignancies. Those two patients were found to have carcinomatosis during the initial laparoscopic procedure, and one went on to develop port-site metastasis. Despite some disagreement, it appears that aerosolization caused by pneumoperitoneum and tumor manipulation as well as tumor burden are important factors for port-site metastases. The amount of tumor required to cause port-site metastases in humans is currently unknown.

Other investigators looked at abdominal wall trauma as a factor promoting the development of port-site metastases. In a scanning electron microscopy study, tumor cells were injected into the abdomen of rats, followed by the placement of ports and 20 minutes of laparoscopy.[35] The rats were sacrificed on day 0, 3, or 8, and the port sites were examined under an electron microscope. Immediately after laparoscopy on day 0, the peritoneal lining was noted to have been peeled away, subperitoneal tissue was exposed, and inflammatory cells with tumor cells were present in the underlying damaged tissues. On day 3, the peritoneal wound was covered by regenerative and immature mesothelial cells with a scattering of malignant cells. The subperitoneal surfaces and muscular defects were replaced by granulation tissue. On day 8, a small macroscopic tumor nodule, completely covered by a layer of mesothelial cells and consisting of numerous cancer cells, was found to have invaded the damaged muscular layer of the port site. The peritoneum was completely intact in the surrounding areas of damage. Tissue trauma, whether by repeated insertions of a port or devitalization by crushing, appears to provide a medium for tumor adherence, invasion, and growth.

Port composition has also been implicated in the promotion of metastases. Brundell et al. studied the effects of different port compositions and the removal and replacement of ports to mimic typical laparoscopy.[36] Significantly more tumor adhered to metal ports than to plastic ports. The removal and replacement of a port resulted in significantly more tumor deposition in the wound than if the port was left *in situ* for the duration of the procedure. Brundell et al. concluded that, to minimize risks, the use of plastic ports that are secured to prevent dislodgement is mandatory.

Other investigators have put forward an immunosuppression theory of the development of port-site metastases. Local peritoneal inflammatory changes are clearly demonstrated with laparoscopy; however, there is no consensus as to the significance of these changes. The physiologic and immunologic changes that occur are discussed in Physiology of Laparoscopy, earlier in the chapter.

After the recognition of the problem, several investigators attempted to mitigate factors leading to the development of port-site metastases. A simple procedural change would be to use plastic bags to remove specimens; however, it has already been shown that aerosolized cells adhere to ports and port sites. To eliminate the effects of pneumoperitoneum, gasless laparoscopy has been recommended, but port-site metastases have been reported even under these conditions. The studies that investigated changing the insufflation gas to helium or some other agent often generated conflicting results. Wu et al. excised the wound during surgery, but this did not completely eliminate metastases.[37] Moreover, excising port sites enlarges the wound and thus eliminates one of the purported advantages of laparoscopy—small wounds. Some authors have irrigated the wound with a variety of agents, from lactated Ringer's solution or povidone iodine to chemotherapeutic agents, and have shown decreased metastasis in animal models.[38] Additional studies are recommended, however, before anything other than standard crystalloid irrigation is used. Table 12.2-1 briefly outlines the causes that have been suggested for port-site metastases and interventions to minimize these causes.

LAPAROSCOPY IN THE DIAGNOSIS OF MALIGNANCY

As technology has progressed, it has become a rare event that the diagnosis of malignancy is unknown before surgical intervention. Available tools include ultrasonography (US), spiral computed tomography (CT), magnetic resonance imaging (MRI), and positron emission tomography (PET), as well as various upper and lower endoscopic maneuvers. Further information is gained with imaging-guided core-needle biopsy techniques, which provide tissue for definitive diagnosis. In certain situations, such as retroperitoneal adenopathy, imaging and material gained from core biopsy may not reliably diagnose a lymphoma. Because this information determines which radiotherapeutic or chemotherapeutic regimen will be instituted, diagnostic laparoscopy becomes

TABLE 12.2-1. Possible Causes of Tumor Cell Dissemination in Laparoscopic Surgery for Cancer

Possible Cause	Intervention to Potentially Minimize This Cause
Adverse effects of CO_2 gas	Use helium, nitrogen, or ambient room air.
Dispersion of cells by insufflation gas	Avoid sudden loss of pneumoperitoneum.
Tumor spillage from manipulation and instrumentation	Avoid excessive manipulation of the tumor.
Tumor spillage at extraction site	Use protected tumor extraction (plastic bag).
Immunosuppressive effect of pneumoperitoneum	Irrigate the abdomen with tumoricidal solutions.

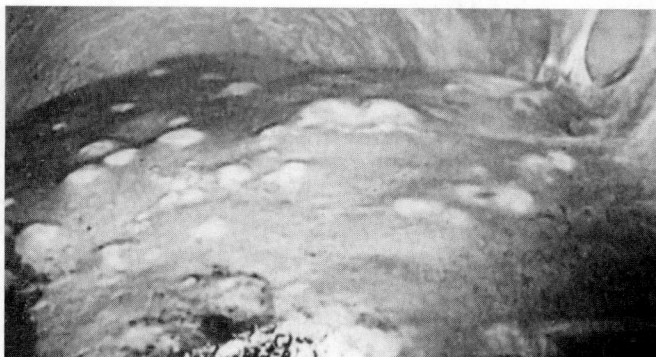

FIGURE 12.2-1. Laparoscopic view of carcinomatosis. (See Color Fig. 12.2-1 in the CD-ROM.)

an important tool. Similarly, a tumor in the mesentery is often not amenable to imaging-guided biopsy but is accessible to laparoscopic biopsy and extirpation. In the later situation, laparoscopy provides a diagnosis, stages the intraabdominal disease, and provides treatment in a single procedure.

Masses identified on preoperative imaging studies are often amenable to laparoscopic biopsy. Figure 12.2-1 shows carcinomatosis that was proven to be adenocarcinoma on biopsy. Some studies have evaluated the tactile sensation afforded by laparoscopic instruments and have found it to be almost comparable with that with open palpation.[39] Techniques available for the biopsy of masses under laparoscopic control include the following:

- Percutaneous insertion of a Tru-Cut biopsy needle with direct puncture of the mass. This is easily performed under the direct vision afforded by the laparoscope and provides a core of tissue for the pathologist.
- Wedge biopsy using the electrocautery. This method should be used cautiously to avoid thermal destruction of the specimen (Fig. 12.2-2).
- Cup forceps biopsy. Careful use of cup forceps allows removal of adequate tissue for histopathologic examination while avoiding destruction of the specimen. This technique is extremely useful for the biopsy of small lesions such as those present on peritoneal surfaces.

In addition to direct biopsy of visualized masses, laparoscopy allows for cytologic evaluation via washings. In a prospective study, laparoscopic peritoneal lavage was performed in patients without ascites with upper gastrointestinal malignancy; 100% of those patients with cytologic findings positive for malignancy died.[40] This study has been repeated with similar results in patients with other gastrointestinal malignancies such as pancreatic cancer.[41]

A previous limitation of laparoscopic diagnosis of abdominal malignancies was that the lesion had to be visualized through the laparoscope. The introduction of laparoscopic intracorporeal ultrasonography (LICU) has permitted the detection and biopsy of masses deep in solid organs such as the liver, which was not previously possible. The 1-cm size limitation for detection of malignancy by CT scanning does not apply to LICU, in which lesions smaller than 1 cm can be identified, subjected to biopsy, and even treated by adjunctive laparoscopic ablation techniques. Also, LICU permits real-time

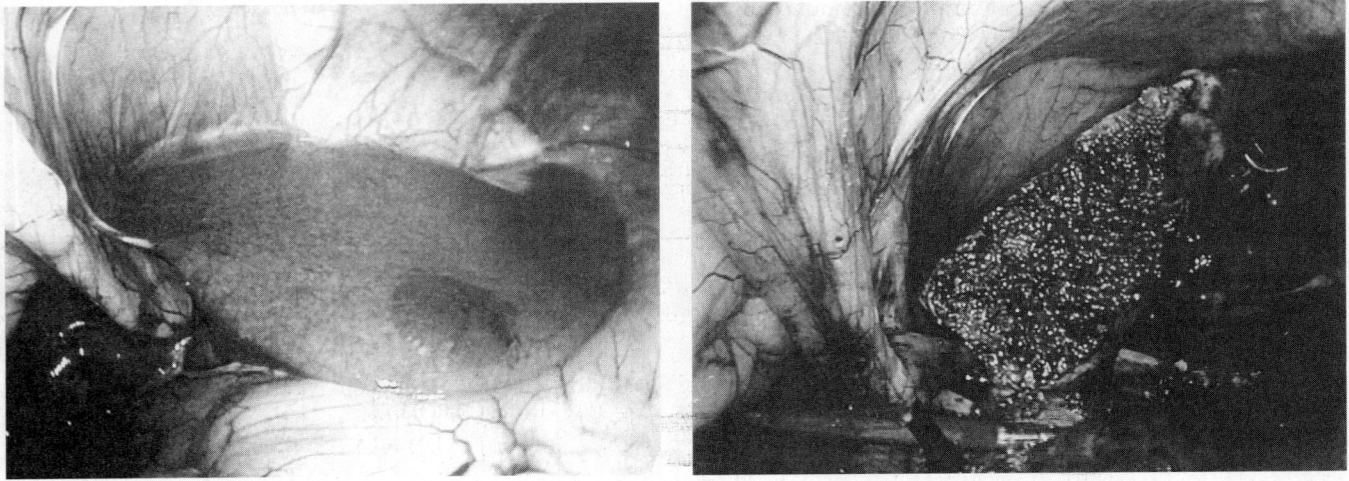

FIGURE 12.2-2.   A 40-year-old woman underwent multiple nondiagnostic computed tomography–guided core biopsies of a liver lesion. Laparoscopy was then used for diagnosis and treatment. **A:** Laparoscopic view of the left lobe of the liver. **B:** Completed resection.

retroperitoneal examination and focused exploration. The addition of Doppler US allows identification of vascular structures to be avoided intraoperatively. Because the laparoscopic ultrasound probe is placed directly on the tissue being examined, the acoustic interference from bowel gas and distance that limits transabdominal US is eliminated and a clearer picture is obtained.

One very common problem to which laparoscopy has been applied is diagnosis of adnexal masses in gynecologic surgery. The list of differential diagnoses is long and includes a wide variety of lesions, from benign cysts to endometriosis to ovarian malignancy, and occasionally the cause is totally unrelated to gynecology. There has been great controversy about whether this minimal surgical procedure is safe in diagnosing malignancy. In cases of nonmalignancy, outpatient bilateral oophorectomy can be performed easily using a laparoscope with minimal pain and discomfort, and the patient can return to work within a week. Unfortunately, there is no foolproof noninvasive gold standard for classifying an adnexal mass as benign, suspicious, or frankly malignant. Various scoring systems using menopausal status, level of CA 125 (cancer antigen 125), serologic findings, CT, and transvaginal US have been reported. A review showed that the actual malignancy rate for tumors judged to be malignant using such scoring systems ranged from less than 1% to 15%, depending on the criteria used to classify an adnexal mass as suspicious for malignancy.[42] During laparoscopy for suspicious masses, diagnostic maneuvers include visual inspection, mass or cyst aspiration, LICU, and resection, all of which can be performed as easily as in benign cases. For ovarian cysts, it is below the standard of care to aspirate the cyst if malignancy is suspected; however, such cysts are often ruptured during laparoscopic removal. If a malignancy is discovered at the time of diagnostic laparoscopy or on frozen section, a formal ovarian cancer operation can be performed. Although laparoscopic evaluation is technically feasible, outcomes have been alarming. Numerous case reports and series reveal port-site metastases, as have been identified with other aggressive tumors that disseminate via carcinomatosis. Port-site metastases have occurred not only with ovarian carcinoma that is advanced at the time of lap-

aroscopy, but also with early stage I disease. In an alarming series of 192 cases, when definitive ovarian cancer surgery was performed longer than 8 days after diagnostic laparoscopy, 56% of patients with stage IC or II disease and 47% of those with stage III cancer developed port-site metastasis.[43] Of the 72 cases of apparent stage IA ovarian cancer, 28 (39%) showed rapid progression to stage III identified at laparotomy. It is suspected that faulty technique resulted in the high dissemination rate, but the needless death of even a single patient with curable ovarian cancer is not tolerable. Additional studies of the oncologic safety of this procedure are needed before diagnostic laparoscopy can be recommended as the standard of care.

LAPAROSCOPY IN THE STAGING OF MALIGNANCY

GENERAL CONSIDERATIONS

One of the most important benefits of laparoscopic staging is the ability to exclude patients from undergoing a major operation by identifying metastatic disease or unresectable disease. One very clear advantage is the ability to identify peritoneal carcinomatosis, which is easily missed on imaging studies, and perform biopsy of the lesions. Lesions deeper than the peritoneal surfaces can also be identified using intraoperative US, and biopsy can then be performed. With increased accuracy in staging, many patients can be spared the pain of and hospitalization for a nontherapeutic laparotomy.

ESOPHAGEAL CANCER

Current staging of esophageal cancer is in flux because of differing opinions as to whether an esophagectomy should be performed if lymph node metastases are identified preoperatively. Generally, the presence of lymph node metastases far from the primary disease and carcinomatosis are considered to be contraindications for surgical resection with curative intent. Imaging modalities currently used to stage esophageal carcinoma include CT, MRI, PET, and endoscopic US (EUS). In a review of noninvasive imaging modalities, CT was found to have an accuracy of 45% to 60% in detecting lymph node involvement, whereas occult distant metastatic disease was missed in 15% to 20% of patients.[44] EUS was found to have an accuracy of 65% to 85%. Overstaging has also been noted to occur due to inflammation around the tumor that results in reactive enlargement of lymph nodes. Because of the inaccuracies of noninvasive staging methods, the use of laparoscopy for staging has generated interest. Krasna et al. reviewed results for 111 patients who underwent thoracoscopic/laparoscopic (Ts/Ls) staging along with CT, MRI, and EUS.[45] The staging accuracy for mediastinal and abdominal metastases was 58% and 68%, respectively, for imaging staging and 91% and 96% for Ts/Ls staging. After the publication of retrospective studies advocating Ts/Ls staging, the National Cancer Institute funded a prospective multi-institutional study in the United States to evaluate the feasibility of Ts/Ls staging.[46] Of 137 patients, 73% met the requirement for Ts/Ls staging. Among those for which both imaging and Ts/Ls staging were performed, 53% of patients were found to have positive nodes. CT, MRI, and EUS failed to detect 25% of cases of metastatic disease correctly identified by laparoscopy. EUS was also noted to overstage disease in 10 patients. Based on early prospective data, it appears that Ts/Ls staging is more accurate than imaging staging alone for patients with esophageal cancer. More importantly, noninvasive staging may incorrectly overstage disease and thus prevent an attempt at curative resection.

GASTRIC CANCER

In gastric cancer, as in esophageal cancer, carcinomatosis and metastatic disease are general contraindications for curative resection, whereas the implications of nodal involvement for resection remain controversial. Even after resection for presumed localized gastric cancer, locoregional and metastatic recurrences are common. The currently available diagnostic staging tools, CT and US, have high false-negative rates, which can result in nontherapeutic laparotomies with the associated morbidity and cost. To reduce unnecessary operations, laparoscopic staging systems have been advocated to improve staging and resection rates. Laparoscopic staging can be performed in the preoperative outpatient setting before a definitive resection is scheduled or during diagnostic laparoscopy immediately preceding laparotomy. The recent development of instruments to allow the laparoscopic collection of peritoneal washings for cytologic analysis permits additional prognostic information to be obtained that might indicate lower probability of survival.

In a detailed review of early work on laparoscopic staging, undetected metastatic disease was found in 13% to 57% of patients initially staged as having no metastatic disease using conventional imaging.[47] Because of the discovery of the unexpected metastatic disease, exploratory laparotomy was not performed in over 20% of the cases. In addition, prospective studies have shown accuracy rates of more than 90% for laparoscopy in detection of metastatic disease and carcinomatosis, whereas detection accuracy for imaging was between 70% and 80%.

The addition of the capability for cytologic analysis to laparoscopy has raised very important questions. As the stage of gastric cancer increases, the likelihood of cytologic findings that are positive for malignancy increases.[47] Positive cytologic findings are rare for T1 to 2, M0 cases, whereas the rate of positive findings approaches 10% for T3 to 4 disease and is much higher for M1 disease. In isolated cases showing positive cytologic findings, the prognosis is grim, and patients have the same survival as if overt carcinomatosis is identified. It is the authors' belief that, if preoperative diagnostic laparoscopy is to be performed, cytologic washings should be taken as part of a clinical study.

Because of the increased accuracy of staging with laparoscopy, many patients can be spared a nontherapeutic laparotomy. In addition, increased accuracy allows for improved design of clinical trials, especially those involving neoadjuvant therapy protocols based on precise preoperative staging. Despite its increased accuracy, laparoscopic staging has recently come under assault when conducted as a routine procedure. Authors have argued that, in patients with larger, often symptomatic lesions encountered in the United States and Europe, a palliative resection or procedure should be performed. In the case of smaller asymptomatic lesions, for which laparoscopy might have the greatest impact, the likelihood of finding metastatic disease diminishes rapidly. Its true value remains unknown, and laparoscopic staging for gastric cancer remains experimental and should be performed in a protocol setting.

PANCREATIC TUMORS

Laparoscopy has been used in the staging of carcinoma of the pancreas for some time. In fact, one of the first reports of the use of laparoscopy in the United States was in the evaluation of patients with carcinoma, including carcinoma of the pancreas.[1] The goal of laparoscopy in the staging of carcinoma of the pancreas is to avoid the need for laparotomy in those patients who, despite being deemed to have resectable disease by preoperative imaging studies, in fact have distant disease. Despite these conceptual goals, disagreement persists over what is considered resectable. Typical criteria used for resectability include the lack of metastatic disease, localization of disease to the pancreas without extension into the colonic mesentery, presence of a patent portal vein, and lack of involvement of the superior mesenteric/celiac artery. The presence of lymph node involvement has an adverse prognostic significance, and when it occurs outside of the resection field the disease is categorized as M1. Despite this, some groups have advocated major vascular resection and extended resection, quoting slightly prolonged survival time. Even after curative resection for localized resectable carcinoma, the survival rates remain dismal, and recurrence is the rule with very few cures. Because of this general lack of benefit of resection, various groups have attempted to improve the selection process for resection. It is difficult to determine with certainty who will benefit from surgery; however, it is clear that an "open and close" operation with discovery of unresectable disease does not provide any benefit to the patient, who on average has less than 1 year to live. Such a nontherapeutic laparotomy has been estimated to have occurred more than 20% of the time in the United States over the past decade. Initial early results of the use of laparoscopy to improve the selection process provided hope; however, enthusiasm has waned recently with improvement in imaging technology. Despite these advances in staging, improved cure rates have yet to be clearly seen.

From 1980 to the early 1990s, staging methods used nonhelical early-generation CT, transabdominal US, and mesenteric angiography to determine resectability. Major medical centers reported intraoperative detection of M1 disease during standard laparotomy in 20% to 40% of cases in which disease was initially staged as metastasis free (M0) using the imaging modalities available at the time.[48] Early studies comparing imaging to a combination of laparoscopy and LICU reported an approximately 20% rate of detection of M1 or unresectable disease that resulted in a change in the operative plan to either no resection or a palliative procedure. In a large study, Van Dijkum et al. examined laparoscopic and LICU staging in more than 400 patients with upper gastrointestinal malignancies from 1992 to 1996; 214 patient had periampullary tumors.[49] Laparoscopy correctly identified locally advanced periampullary carcinoma in 32 of 37 patients, but it also incorrectly overstaged disease in five patients who successfully underwent a curative resection. In the characterization of advanced tumor invasion, positive predictive value was 86%, specificity was 95%, and negative predictive value was 73%. Overall, 9% of M1 disease was missed with laparoscopy and 8 patients (2%) developed wound metastases exclusively in the port sites. There were no cases of laparotomy wound involvement. When the investigators examined the effect of time, preventable laparotomies decreased from 19% in the early period of the study to 14% during the later period. Some of this decrease is likely attributable to the incorporation of newer imaging modalities.

Between 1997 and 1999, a review of the Johns Hopkins experience identified 188 patients with periampullary or pancreatic carcinoma who underwent both CT and laparotomy.[50] Resectability rate was 67.5% for periampullary carcinoma and 17.6% for body and tail lesions. Excluding those patients who underwent surgical palliation, laparoscopy would have prevented only 2.3% of patients from undergoing a nontherapeutic laparotomy. Over the past several years, because of the increasing use of a combination of imaging modalities such as high-quality helical CT, MRI, and EUS, the intraoperative detection of occult unresectability has declined to 4% to 13% of cases.[48] Because laparoscopy has a relatively low yield compared with high-resolution imaging, because a false-positive finding excludes resection, and because a significant false-negative detection rate is seen, routine laparoscopy cannot be recommended as the standard of care.

One setting in which laparoscopy may still be useful is in the evaluation of pancreatic body and tail lesions. In the Johns Hopkins Hospital data, only 17.6% of these lesions were resectable; in the remainder disease was staged as M1 or was locally advanced.[50] This experience is similar to that of other institutions. Symptoms from pancreatic body and tail lesions are vague and can easily be misdiagnosed as gastritis or gallbladder disease. Jaundice is not a typical feature. By the time these lesions are discovered, they have reached a large size with a propensity to invade into the retroperitoneal tissues and metastasize. Also, intraperitoneal free cancer cell detection is greater with body and tail lesions. When such lesions are discovered, the prognosis is the same as in patients with carcinomatosis.

HEPATOBILIARY TUMORS

Unlike esophageal, gastric, and pancreatic cancers, hepatic tumors include primary and secondary (hepatic metastatic) malignancies, which have their own staging and treatment protocols. When lesions are isolated and treatment is indicated, con-

troversy exists regarding the optimal therapy and whether it should be resection, hepatic transplantation, cryoablation, radiofrequency ablation, ethanol injection, hepatic artery chemoperfusion, or microwave ablation, among other novel modalities. Traditionally, surgical resection has been the mainstay, but there is tremendous room for patient individualization.

Staging for primary hepatic cancer such as hepatocellular cancer (HCC) and cholangiocarcinoma remains very important, because there is no role for palliative hepatic resection in the event that the tumor is found to be unresectable or M1 disease is discovered. Other palliative procedures that require exploratory laparotomy remain very limited, which makes accurate staging crucial. In older studies, more than a 50% incidence of nontherapeutic laparotomy is reported. These studies used currently outdated imaging modalities, however, and some did not even use CT or MRI but relied solely on abdominal US. These older series are typically underpowered with fewer than 50 subjects. Despite the availability of newer modalities such as contrast-enhanced spiral CT with image acquisition in different phases of contrast delivery and MRI image reformatting, nontherapeutic laparotomy still remains a significant problem and approaches 50%. A nontherapeutic laparotomy adds cost, creates patient discomfort, and delays alternative therapy until healing has occurred.

In standard open surgery, exploration using manual palpation and intraoperative US is the gold standard. Palpation is somewhat limited in the often cirrhotic HCC patient, and, thus, US findings are weighted significantly. Because of their reliance on intraoperative imaging, laparoscopy and LICU are thought by some to mimic a standard exploration. Experience in the laparoscopic staging of primary hepatic malignancies is currently limited, and only a handful of studies have been published suggesting up to a 16% exclusion rate for open resection. In a prospective study from 1998 to 2000, 68 consecutively treated patients with HCC lesions suggested to be resectable by imaging underwent laparoscopic staging using LICU.[51] Of these, 55 patients had hepatitis C cirrhosis, 7 had hepatitis B cirrhosis, and 8 had alcoholic cirrhosis. The preoperative workup included US with either lipiodol contrast CT or dual-phase spiral CT. Exclusion criteria included a tumor size greater than 5 cm, more than three nodules, complete portal thrombosis, and Child's C cirrhosis. Fourteen percent of patients required complete lysis of adhesions to facilitate exploration. At the time of laparoscopy, 63 of 68 primary tumors were histologically proven to be HCC; the remainder included two cases of cholangiocarcinoma and three cases of high-grade dysplastic nodules. Thus diagnosis was changed in five cases (7%). In 14 cases (22%), new malignant HCC nodules were identified as well as a case of adrenal metastasis. The sizes of the new lesions were small, averaging 14 mm, and many were below the 10-mm limit of detection of CT. Laparoscopic staging changed the operative procedure in 12 of the 15 patients with additional tumor nodules. Four patients were excluded from laparotomy, seven patients underwent either ethanol injection or thermoablation, and a single patient underwent adrenalectomy. Ethanol injection, thermoablation, and adrenalectomy can be performed laparoscopically. This particular study highlights the problem with laparoscopic staging in HCC. In the cirrhotic patient, adhesions can develop between the liver and peritoneal surfaces. This creates a difficult environment for LICU and requires the skill of laparoscopic lysis of adhesions to facilitate hepatic surface exposure for the ultrasonic probe. When additional tumor nodules are identified, numerous treatment modalities are available; some are treatable by laparoscopy as a stand-alone procedure or in combination with resection. The question of how much liver can be removed or ablated in a cirrhotic patient is still an ongoing controversy. Only when metastatic disease is present or innumerable lesions are identified does laparoscopy provide a clear indication to avoid laparotomy. Until treatment becomes standardized, it is doubtful that sweeping conclusions can be drawn regarding the role of laparoscopic staging for primary hepatic malignancies.

Unlike in the case of primary hepatic malignancies, staging and treatment of secondary hepatic malignancies have been studied extensively for colorectal metastases to the liver. In the largest prospective study to date, D'Angelica et al. at Memorial Sloan-Kettering Cancer Center analyzed data for 401 patients who underwent staging laparoscopy for hepatobiliary malignancy.[52] The study incorporated primary and secondary malignancies from 1997 to 2001. Preoperative studies included CT, MRI, CT portography, and, for some patients, PET scanning. In the multidisciplinary conference, each case was assigned to a resectability likelihood category based on a surgeon's overall impression of the lesion as probably unresectable, equivocally resectable, probably resectable, and resectable. The exclusion criteria was narrow and included the following:

1. Cirrhosis with insufficient remnant function
2. Cholangiocarcinoma or gallbladder carcinoma with metastasis
3. Extensive biliary tract involvement precluding obtaining negative margins
4. Extensive biliary tract involvement precluding safe anatomic resection

The view of what was resectable was very aggressive and included portal vein resection for tumor involvement if it could be done safely. Patients with other intrahepatic malignancies, even those with bilobar or multiple metastases, underwent resection if all disease could be resected safely. In the 401 patients, there were 199 colorectal metastases (49.6%), 59 hilar cholangiocarcinomas (14.7%), 50 gallbladder carcinomas (12.5%), and 33 hepatocellular carcinomas (8.2%). Two hundred sixty-six patients (66.3%) had previously undergone a laparotomy. Eighty-four patients (20.9%) were found to have unresectable disease. Laparoscopy and LICU had the least yield in determining unresectability in metastatic colorectal carcinoma, detecting 10% of the total of 20% unresectable colorectal cases. In the preoperative setting, the surgeon's impression of resectability was statistically significant in determining outcomes. The authors of the study pointed out that in their experience, as time progressed, the ability to exclude laparotomy by laparoscopic staging decreased from approximately one-third in prior studies to the current level of 10% through the use of modern imaging methods. Although the yield in staging hepatic colorectal metastases with laparoscopy is low, for those going on to laparotomy, the procedure added only 30 minutes. To exclude one patient from exploratory laparotomy, 5 patient-hours of laparoscopy had to be performed. Caution is advised in the interpretation of these data, because the institution had very aggressive resection criteria. Some of these tumors may be lesions that surgeons at other institutions would

consider unresectable. In a community hospital with limited imaging resources, laparoscopic staging may exclude a significant portion of patients from undergoing a laparotomy. It remains the decision of each institution to develop a protocol based on its own data.

Apart from the staging of primary and secondary hepatic malignancies, extrahepatic proximal biliary cancer staging deserves special mention because of the high incidence of unresectable disease discovered at the time of operation. These malignancies, consisting of hilar cholangiocarcinoma and gallbladder carcinoma, are often detected when they are in the advanced stages, which results in very few cures. Only for early gallbladder carcinomas discovered incidentally in cholecystectomy specimens are any meaningful survival data expected. Data from the National Cancer Institute Surveillance, Epidemiology, and End Results (SEER) program, encompassing more than 1800 patients, showed that only 28% of patients presented with localized disease.[53] Even after extensive preoperative workup, fewer than half the patients undergoing exploratory laparotomy are candidates for curative resection. In a modern prospective study, 100 patients with gallbladder and hilar cholangiocarcinoma treated at Memorial Sloan-Kettering Cancer Center from 1997 to 2001 underwent laparoscopic staging.[54] Preoperative imaging was extensive and often was repeated at the tertiary referral center; only tumors considered resectable were included in the analysis. Of the 100 patients, 56 had hilar cholangiocarcinoma and 44 had gallbladder cancer. Of those with gallbladder malignancies, 10 patients had had a previous cholecystectomy and presented for re-resection. Laparoscopy with LICU excluded 35 of 100 patients from undergoing laparotomy. The reasons for exclusion were hepatic metastases, carcinomatosis, and nodal metastasis. Of those patients proceeding to laparotomy, an additional 34 had unresectable disease. Thus laparoscopy detected 35 of 69 cases of unresectable disease, an accuracy of 51% in gallbladder carcinoma. The reason for unresectability discovered at laparotomy was mainly the locally advanced nature of the tumor. When gallbladder carcinoma cases were subdivided, laparoscopy was found to detect 19 of 34 unresectable cases in which the gallbladder remained *in situ* (58% accuracy) but only 2 of 10 cases in patients who had previously undergone cholecystectomy. For hilar cholangiocarcinoma, the majority of unresectable cases were missed with laparoscopy because patients tended to have less carcinomatosis and more locally advanced tumors, which were difficult to evaluate with laparoscopy. However, 14 of 33 cases were correctly identified. Overall resectability rate for both malignancies was dismal, with 69 out of 100 patients found to have unresectable disease despite undergoing preoperative imaging. Although accuracy was low, the high incidence of unresectability yielded a positive result in just 3 patients; thus, the use of laparoscopic staging is a viable option for these aggressive tumors. Furthermore, the high incidence of port-site metastases seen after laparoscopy in gallbladder malignancy may provide a better marker of the cancer's virulence than a purely local wound phenomenon.

UROLOGIC TUMORS

Prostate cancer is a very common malignancy, with the incidence depending on the method of screening, whether by prostate-specific antigen (PSA) screening protocols or by autopsy studies, the latter of which reveals most older men to have the disease. With such a high incidence, one would have expected that detection, staging, and treatment would have become standardized by now. However, this has not occurred. For localized disease of the prostate, the general management modalities currently used include watchful waiting, some form of prostatectomy, hormonal manipulation, and conformal radiotherapy. Various schemes of prostate cancer staging and treatment have been developed in the last few years to determine who will benefit from therapy. A noninvasive method of selecting those at high risk considers Gleason score, PSA level, and MRI findings. As the Gleason score increases above 7 and the PSA level rises above 10 ng/mL, metastatic and local disease recurrence can be expected to occur in more than 25% of patients treated only locally. Those with lower scores and levels have a much better prognosis, which allows local treatment protocols of focused radiotherapy and prostatectomy. For prostatectomy to be considered an option, the life expectancy of the patient must typically be longer than 10 years, and no metastatic disease must be present. If lymph node involvement is documented, radical prostatectomy is aborted in favor of systemic treatment. Typically, the nodes retrieved include those in the iliac and obturator regions in a formal lymphadenectomy specimen. Recently, the procedure of node retrieval has come under criticism because patients at highest risk for lymph node involvement—those with high Gleason scores and high PSA levels—would be treated by systemic therapy regardless of nodal status, and those at low risk are found to have lymph node metastasis in fewer than 10% of dissections in contemporary studies. In a randomized prospective study examining the use of limited nodal dissection versus extended lymph node dissection, the detection rate for metastatic nodal disease in cases of presumed localized prostate cancer was only 6.5% overall, but the morbidity with the extended dissection was significant and included lymphoceles, bladder injuries, and vascular complications.[55] When nodal staging by laparoscopy is compared with staging by open laparotomy, there is no difference in the number of nodes retrieved or the complication rate. Laparoscopic staging is often combined with laparoscopic prostatectomy, which reduces morbidity, lowers costs, shortens hospital stays, and reduces the number of blood transfusions. It remains to be seen if laparoscopy will impact urologic surgery as much as it has impacted gallbladder surgery.

In addition to prostate cancer staging, laparoscopy has been used for staging of nonseminomatous testicular cancers, which have a 20% to 30% incidence of retroperitoneal spread of disease to paraaortic nodes at the time of diagnosis. As in other areas of oncology, the debate continues as to whether retroperitoneal node dissection is purely prognostic or is also therapeutic in this patient population. In surveillance studies, the surgical cure rate for patients with fewer than three small positive lymph nodes is 80% to 85% after orchiectomy without adjuvant therapy.[56] Recurrent disease outside the pelvis is found in 8% to 12% of patients who have negative lymph node findings. In those with less favorable pathologic findings who receive chemotherapy, the cure rate increases to 95%. The feasibility of treating patients with testicular cancers only by surgery and subsequent observation and without chemotherapy was confirmed in a large series of the German Testicular Cancer Study Group, which showed a surgical cure rate of 70% in patients with a maximum of three positive lymph nodes.[56] To

see whether laparoscopic nodal staging had the same outcomes, Bhayani et al. reviewed the long-term experience at Johns Hopkins Hospital.[57] Of those with stage I nonseminomatous germ cell tumor with vascular invasion or embryonal carcinoma, or both, who underwent laparoscopic node dissection, 17 of 29 patients had histologically negative lymph nodes and underwent observation. Of these 17, only two experienced recurrences, and these patients showed a complete response after adjuvant chemotherapy. Although large studies are lacking, it appears that laparoscopic staging may be an option for this malignancy, which has a generally favorable prognosis.

GYNECOLOGIC TUMORS

Cervical cancer remains a common gynecologic malignancy, and treatment relies on two modes of therapy, hysterectomy and radiotherapy, which have been shown to produce equivalent survival rates for localized disease. One advantage of radiotherapy is the ability to treat a wide age range of patients, even those with comorbidities. Also, patients with unsuspected locally advanced disease do better with initial radiation therapy than with incomplete surgery followed by radiation treatment. The disadvantages of radiotherapy are the loss of ovarian function, radiation-induced changes to the vagina, bowel irradiation, and possible inducement of pelvic sarcomas. For young patients, ovary-sparing hysterectomy may prevent menopause, and if postoperative radiotherapy is required, the ovaries can be fixed outside the radiation field. Also, in the case of very early lesions, resection of only the cervix with reanastomosis of the uterus to the vaginal cuff has preserved fertility. For patients undergoing surgery, the typical operation consists of pelvic and aortic lymphadenectomy followed by hysterectomy. If nodal disease is identified, surgical resection is usually aborted in favor of radiotherapy. The highest level of positive lymph node is noted, so the area of irradiation can be expanded. The problem with this surgical staging approach is that laparotomy induces small intestinal adhesions that prevent small bowel mobility, which results in a greater radiation dose to an isolated bowel loop leading to its injury.[42] For these often younger patients with early International Federation of Gynecology and Obstetrics (FIGO) stage I cervical cancer, the incidence of surgically staged nodal positivity is between 5% and 13%; this rate increases to 30% for stage III cancer. Thus, for later stages of cancer, a larger number of patients will undergo a nontherapeutic laparotomy. To reduce the morbidity of the procedure, laparoscopic staging has been advocated because of its theorized lower rate of adhesion formation. One prospective randomized controlled trial compared laparotomy staging, laparoscopic staging, and clinical staging in locally advanced cervical cancer.[58] For those patients undergoing surgical staging, no difference was seen in operating time, blood loss, lymph node yield, or survival with laparoscopic staging versus staging at laparotomy. Twenty-five percent of patients had lymph node metastasis. Compared with both surgical groups, the clinical staging group tended to have bulkier nodal disease on imaging, underwent radiotherapy much earlier after random assignment to the treatment arm, and had a higher rate of concurrent chemotherapy. Survival data at 3 months showed a significant difference in disease-free rate: 80% in the clinically staged arm versus 63% in the surgically staged arm. After an interim analysis, the study was closed for ethical reasons, because the number of patients who died from their disease in the clinical arm was half that in the surgically staged arm. The survival difference may have resulted from the fact that a larger number of patients received chemotherapy in the clinically staged group. It is difficult to draw any sound conclusions from only a single randomized study. It appears that open and laparoscopic staging are both effective in detecting unresectable disease and that those with nodal disease have a poor prognosis.

With increasing experience in the use of laparoscopy in patients with ovarian tumors, numerous case reports of wound metastasis and tumor cell dissemination are appearing. Of great concern is the potential induction of carcinomatosis in stage I ovarian cancers that otherwise would have been cured. In addition to laparoscopy for primary diagnosis and staging, laparoscopic second-look operations have been reported, but overall experience remains very limited and no firm recommendations can be made. At the current time, laparoscopic staging and evaluation of ovarian malignancies appears to affect outcome adversely and is not advised.

LYMPHOMA

Lymphomas are a diverse group of malignant disorders of the lymphatic system that arise in nodal tissues. Typically, they are categorized by histologic findings into Hodgkin's lymphoma (HL) and non-HL (NHL). To secure the diagnosis, a lymph node biopsy is usually required because of the high false-negative and false-positive rates with fine-needle aspiration. Also, a nodal biopsy specimen that preserves a significant portion of the architecture can provide tissue to subcategorize the type of lymphoma, which allows for a focused treatment plan.

Treatment for HL is typically based on the stage of the disease. Historically, staging was divided into clinical stage and pathologic stage determined via laparotomy. Using the imaging modalities of the time with what is now considered low-quality CT scanning, clinical staging frequently missed intraabdominal disease. One area of poor detection was the spleen, which can be normal in size and yet harbor an occult malignancy in one-third of cases.[59] In 1993, the author's (A. T. L.'s) group reported a case of complete laparoscopic staging followed by splenectomy, with the patient returning to work in 11 days.[60] If known disease is isolated to the cervical nodal basin, the knowledge of occult splenic involvement is critical, because its presence excludes the use of isolated radiotherapy to the head and neck region. To qualify for radiation monotherapy, patients underwent exploratory laparotomy with biopsy of the liver and multiple nodes along with splenectomy. If disease was found below the diaphragm, patients received multimodal therapy with the addition of chemotherapy. The toxic chemotherapy regimens of the time, such as MOPP [mechlorethamine (Mustargen), vincristine (Oncovin), procarbazine, prednisone], resulted in gonadal toxicity and leukemia and were typically reserved for patients with advanced disease. With the advent of nonleukemogenic gonad-sparing regimens such as ABVD [doxorubicin (Adriamycin), bleomycin, vinblastine, dacarbazine] and improved imaging, the roles of radiation therapy and staging laparotomy have been reassessed. A study of the European Organization for Research and Treatment of Cancer (EORTC) randomly assigned patients with stage I and II disease to undergo clinical staging or surgical staging with treatment based on the staging workup.[61] Disease-free survival

was 93% for clinical staging and 89% for staging by laparotomy. The authors reported that the decrease in survival from surgical staging was due to operative deaths. Among those receiving infradiaphragmatic radiation therapy, the EORTC study showed an almost fourfold increase in late-term radiation complications in patients who had undergone a staging laparotomy procedure. A single-institution study of the experience of M. D. Anderson in treating stage I HL for 30 years also showed a lack of improvement in survival with staging laparotomy.[62] Not only did staging laparotomy result in operative complications and increased radiation-induced toxicity, but the spleen was often removed during the procedure, which carried the associated risk of encapsulated organism septicemia, or "overwhelming postsplenectomy sepsis." Despite the diminishing role of staging laparotomy, various groups have reported favorable results with staging laparoscopy in detection of infradiaphragmatic disease. The procedure permits the assessment of the same abdominal organs and also allows for splenectomy, which can easily be performed with low immediate morbidity. Until a clear benefit is shown for surgical staging, laparoscopic staging should be performed only in a protocol setting.

For NHL, differences in histologic characteristics and prognosis make it difficult to evaluate the efficacy of a particular therapy. Despite the wide variation in disease behavior, the staging of NHL typically does not require a laparotomy.[59] The risk of abdominal compartment involvement is much higher in patients with NHL than in those with HL, and a combination of radiation therapy and chemotherapy remains the mainstay of treatment. In cases in which NHL is suspected to reside in the spleen and a tissue diagnosis is required, laparoscopic splenectomy is indicated for diagnostic purposes.

LAPAROSCOPY IN THE TREATMENT OF MALIGNANCY

GENERAL CONSIDERATIONS

Descriptions of laparoscopic resections have now been reported for practically every major intraabdominal organ system spanning different surgical subspecialties. Although some of the procedures were palliative, the vast majority had a curative intent. The three major concerns regarding laparoscopic surgery for the treatment of cancer are (1) maintenance of the integrity of the oncologic resection (e.g., margins of resection, lymph node harvest, evaluation of other intraabdominal organs), (2) demonstration of feasibility in improving outcome parameters for the resection without undue risk (e.g., decreased hospital stay, decreased pain, decreased cost, more rapid return to work), and (3) absence of any negative impact on survival (e.g., induction of carcinomatosis or metastasis by laparoscopy, port-site recurrences). At the current time, randomized trials are accruing patients or are in the observational phase of study with targeted completion in the next few years. Despite the lack of conclusive evidence of efficacy and safety, many laparoscopic resections for cancer are being performed routinely in many centers. Just because we *can*, however, does not mean we *should* without valid evidence. The cause of this phenomenon is a complex interaction between patients' preferences for a "minimally invasive procedure" and health care economics and marketing.

UPPER GASTROINTESTINAL CANCER

The debate on the optimal type of resection for esophageal and gastric cancer is ongoing. One group recommends radical resections for both lesions. In esophageal cancer, a radical resection includes cervical, thoracic, and abdominal *en bloc* lymphadenectomy with an esophagectomy via three incisions (laparotomy, thoracotomy, and cervical incision). In gastric cancer, a radical resection removes the spleen, celiac nodes, hepatic nodes, and infrapancreatic aortic nodes *en bloc* with the stomach. On the other end of the spectrum is the palliative approach. For the esophagus, a laparotomy is used for mobilization of the stomach, which is then pulled through the mediastinum into a cervical incision for a cervical gastroesophageal anastomosis. No effort is made to resect nodes or contiguous involved structures, and the majority of the mediastinal dissection is done blindly. In gastric cancer, a limited resection incorporates a 5-cm gastric margin free of tumor and a very limited perigastric nodal retrieval. To this existing wide range of open operations for upper gastrointestinal malignancies, laparoscopy adds more options. Minimally invasive procedures include complete resection via laparoscopy and/or thoracoscopy, hand-assisted resection, and mini-laparotomy–assisted resection. As of early 2004, no large randomized trial has been performed to evaluate the oncologic safety of any of these procedures. In small prospective studies, it appears that no significant difference exists in complication rate and that the blood transfusion rate may actually be lower with laparoscopy.[63] In addition, for gastric cancer, many of the reports of laparoscopic resection originated in Japan, and the cancer there may behave differently than those encountered in Western countries. Given the reports of port-site recurrences, caution is advised in performing such resections with curative intent.

PANCREATIC AND HEPATOBILIARY CANCER

Perhaps one of the most ambitious applications of laparoscopy in surgery is in pancreatic and hepatobiliary surgery. Although operating times are long, laparoscopic performance of pancreaticoduodenectomy (Whipple procedure) and major liver resections has been reported. It is unlikely that laparoscopic procedures will become commonly used for these major organ resections; however, less extensive procedures may become more frequent. Laparoscopic liver wedge resections and distal pancreatectomies can be performed rapidly with low morbidity. With no laparotomy incision, pain is substantially reduced, which permits rapid recovery and early hospital discharge. In addition, for liver malignancies, laparoscopic radiofrequency ablation and cryoablation under laparoscopic ultrasonographic guidance allow detection and treatment of small metastases that would be missed by conventional imaging. Figure 12.2-3 shows a CT scan of a patient with significant comorbidities and a colon metastasis to the confluence of the hepatic veins who was treated by laparoscopic radiofrequency ablation. The impact on survival of these nonresection procedures has yet to be determined.

COLON CANCER

Although colorectal carcinoma is one of the leading causes of death in the United States, it is a more commonly cured disease than many other gastrointestinal malignancies such as pancreatic cancer. Given the common occurrence of this cancer and the growing experience in laparoscopic appendectomy and colon resection for benign disease, laparoscopic colon resection for malignancy was thought be a natural extension of these procedures. The majority of standard open resections, such as total mesorectal resection and abdominoperineal resection, have now been reported to be performed laparoscopically. The resection margins and lymph node retrieval are no lower for laparoscopy than for laparotomy when attention to detail is maintained. The proposed advantages are decreased pain, shorter time for postoperative ileus, shorter hospital stay, decreased adhesions, and shorter convalescence with an earlier return to work so that the economic impact is lower. Although numerous uncontrolled nonrandomized prospective studies and small randomized prospective studies have shown substantial advantages for laparoscopic surgery over laparotomy, a large randomized study found otherwise. The National Cancer Institute funded the large randomized controlled colon cancer study Clinical Outcomes of Surgical Therapy (COST) to evaluate disease-free survival, overall survival, and quality of life (QOL) after open and laparoscopic colectomy.[64] The QOL component closed in 1999 after the random assignment of 449 patients to the various arms and results were subsequently reported in 2002; data on disease-free survival and overall survival continue to accrue. The QOL study examined scores on the Symptoms Distress Scale, Quality of Life Index, and a single-item global rating scale measured at 2 days, 2 weeks, and 2 months after surgery, as well as analgesic use and length of hospital stay. In the laparoscopic group, analgesic use was lower by a small amount ($P < .03$) and hospital stay was decreased by 0.8 days ($P < .001$). The only indicator for which open resection was superior to laparoscopy in the QOL measures was score on the global rating scale at the 2-week mark, which indicated a slight advantage for the open procedure. At 2 days and 2 months, there were no significant differences in the QOL indicators measured. Thus, the advantages of laparoscopy were limited to analgesia and hospital stay. This is the first report from a series of well-designed large colorectal trials. The oncologic outcomes of the COST study, the international COLOR study, and the British and German studies are anxiously awaited; until these results are known, laparoscopic surgery for colon cancer must be considered experimental.

UROLOGIC MALIGNANCY

As in colorectal surgery, laparoscopic approaches to surgery of the kidney and prostate have been reported. In 2003, results of a series of more than 1000 patients in Germany were reported; procedures included 450 radical prostatectomies, 558 nodal dissections, 45 radical nephrectomies, 22 radical nephroureterectomies, 12 partial nephrectomies, and 11 adrenalectomies.[65] At a median follow-up of 58 months, there were only eight local recurrences (0.73%) and two port-site metastases (0.18%). In the hands of these surgeons, the laparoscopic approach to surgery for urologic malignancy appears to be safe and feasible; however, no randomized trials have confirmed these data.

GYNECOLOGIC MALIGNANCY

Unlike for colorectal and urologic cancers, for gynecologic malignancies the role of laparoscopic surgery has been limited due largely to the experience with ovarian carcinoma. Results of oophorectomy for suspicious adnexal masses suggest that

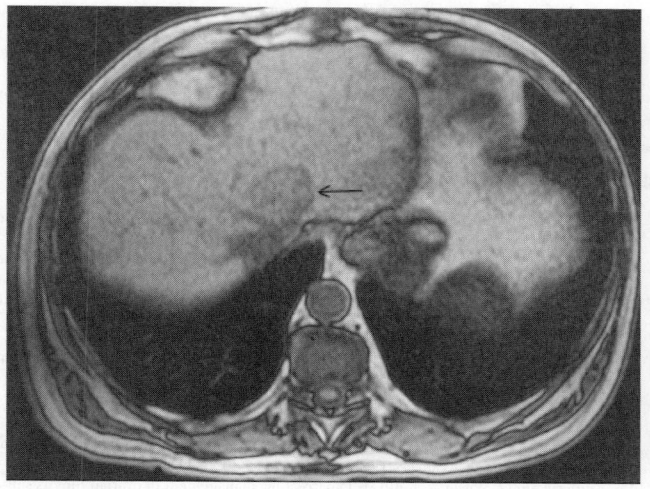

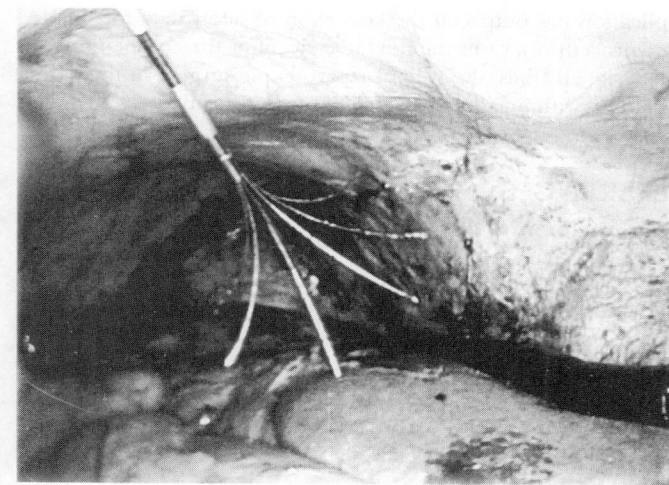

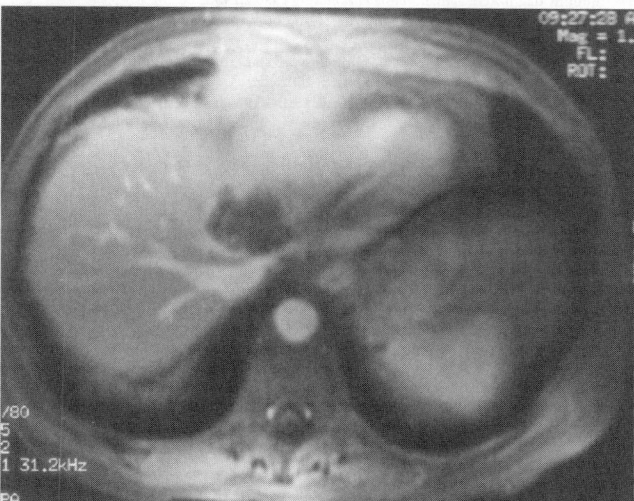

FIGURE 12.2-3. A 79-year-old man presented for treatment with colon cancer metastatic to the liver at the hepatic vein confluence. The lesion was treated by laparoscopic radiofrequency ablation. **A:** Preoperative magnetic resonance image (MRI) of the lesion. **B:** The radiofrequency probe. **C:** Postoperative MRI of the lesion. (See Color Fig. 12.2-3*C* in the CD-ROM.)

laparoscopy may induce wound metastasis and carcinomatosis in early curable disease. The role of laparoscopic hysterectomy for cervical and uterine cancer is under investigation; no large randomized trials have been completed.

LAPAROSCOPY IN THE PALLIATION OF MALIGNANCY

The role of laparoscopy extends beyond diagnosis and treatment. At times patients need palliation of the complications from their malignancy or from the therapy for their malignancy. A common scenario is gastric outlet obstruction or intestinal obstruction. When the gastric outlet is obstructed by a tumor such as an incurable gastric or pancreatic cancer, a laparoscopic stapled gastrojejunostomy can be performed quickly to provide pain relief and allow resumption of eating. Intestinal stomas can also be created when bowel loops are involved with tumor and intestinal bypass is not feasible. When small bowel loops are stuck into the pelvis after radiation therapy for cervical cancer, an intestinal bypass procedure can relieve the symptoms resulting from treatment of the malignancy. The biliary tree also lends itself to bypass procedures in the event of

distal obstruction as can occur with pancreatic cancer. The aforementioned palliative bypass or intestinal stoma creation procedures can be done as stand-alone procedures for a known malignancy or can be performed during the diagnostic laparoscopic phase when a cancer is first diagnosed and found to be unresectable. Other adjunct laparoscopic procedures for therapy and palliation include the placement of feeding tubes for alimentary nutrition or for decompression of obstruction.

CONCLUSION

Although each year advances in technology are introduced as revolutionary, many fall by the wayside never to be seen again. Laparoscopy is an old procedure that has sparked renewed interest because of the advances in video imaging, optics, and instrumentation. Its application has been profound. Laparoscopic surgery is now considered the gold standard in uncomplicated cholecystectomy and may soon be for the treatment of gastroesophageal reflux and other benign conditions as well. Pioneers have now applied this technique to all aspects of oncology, including diagnosis, staging, therapy, and palliation. Although its use is now relatively common in major medical centers, its application has outpaced the collection of safety data for oncologic procedures. Over the next decade, after the completion of well-designed trials, the role of laparoscopic surgery in the care of patients with malignancies will be further clarified.

REFERENCES

1. Stellato. History of laparoscopic surgery. *Surg Clin North Am* 2001;72:997.
2. West MA, Hackam DJ, Baker J, et al. Mechanism of decreased in vitro murine macrophage cytokine release after exposure to carbon dioxide. *Ann Surg* 1997;226:179.
3. Kopernik G, Avinoach E, Grossman Y, et al. The effect of a high partial pressure of carbon dioxide environment on metabolism and immune functions of human peritoneal cells—relevance to carbon dioxide pneumoperitoneum. *Am J Obstet Gynecol* 1998;179:1503.
4. Wu F, Sietses C, Blomberg B, et al. Systemic and peritoneal inflammatory response after laparoscopic or conventional colon resection in cancer patients. *Dis Colon Rectum* 2003;46:147.
5. Hansborough JF, Bender EM, Zapata-Sirvent R, et al. Altered helper and suppressor lymphocyte populations in surgical patients: a measure of postoperative immunosuppression. *Am J Surg* 1984;148:303.
6. Vallina VL, Velasco JM. The influence of laparoscopy on lymphocyte subpopulations in the surgical patient. *Surg Endosc* 1996;10:481.
7. Christou NV, Meakins JL, Gordon J, et al. The delayed hypersensitivity response and host resistance in surgical patients 20 years later. *Ann Surg* 1995;222:534.
8. Allendorf JD, Bessler M, Whelan RL, et al. Better preservation of immune function after laparoscopic assisted vs open bowel resection in a murine model. *Dis Colon Rectum* 1996;39:67.
9. Schob OM, Allen DC, Benzel E. A comparison of the pathophysiologic effects of carbon dioxide, nitrous oxide, and helium pneumoperitoneum on intracranial pressure. *Am J Surg* 1996;172:248.
10. Jackman SV, Weingart JD, Kinsman SL, et al. Laparoscopic surgery in patients with ventriculoperitoneal shunts: safety and monitoring. *J Urol* 2000;164:1352.
11. Harris SN, Ballantyne GH, Luther MA, et al. Alterations of cardiovascular performance during laparoscopic colectomy: a combined hemodynamic and echocardiographic analysis. *Anesth Analg* 1996;83:482.
12. Giebler RM, Kabatnik M, Stegan BH, et al. Retroperitoneal and intraperitoneal CO2 insufflation have markedly different cardiovascular effects. *J Surg Res* 1997;68:153.
13. Greif WM, Forse A. Cardiopulmonary effects of the laparoscopic pneumoperitoneum in a porcine model of ARDS. *Am J Surg* 1999;177:216.
14. Gutt NC, Kim ZG, Hollander D, et al. CO2 environment influences the growth of cultured human cancer cells dependent on insufflation pressure. *Surg Endosc* 2001;15:314.
15. Witich P, Steyerber EW, Simons SH, et al. Intraperitoneal tumor growth is influenced by pressure of carbon dioxide pneumoperitoneum. *Surg Endosc* 2000;14:817.
16. Basson MD, Yu CF, Herden-Kirchoff O, et al. Effects of increased ambient pressure on colon cancer cell adhesion. *J Cell Biochem* 2000;78:47.
17. Ridgway PF, Smith A, Ziprin P, et al. Pneumoperitoneum augmented tumor invasiveness is abolished by matrix metalloproteinase blockade. *Surg Endosc* 2002;16:533.
18. Volz J, Koster S, Spacek Z, et al. The influence of pneumoperitoneum used in laparoscopic surgery on an intraabdominal tumor growth. *Cancer* 1999;86:770.
19. Lecuru F, Agostini A, Camatte S, et al. Impact of pneumoperitoneum on tumor growth. *Surg Endosc* 2002;16:1170.
20. Berends FJ, Kazemier G, Bonjer HJ, et al. Subcutaneous metastases after laparoscopic colectomy. *Lancet* 1994;344:58.
21. Hughes ES, McDermontt FT, Poligless AL, et al. Tumor recurrence in the abdominal wall scar tissue after large bowel cancer surgery. *Dis Colon Rectum* 1983;26:571.
22. Reilly WT, Nelson H, Schroeder G, et al. Wound recurrence following conventional treatment of colorectal cancer. A rare but perhaps underestimated problem. *Dis Colon Rectum* 1996;39:200.
23. Vukasin P, Ortega AE, Greene FL, et al. Wound recurrence following laparoscopic colon cancer resection: results of the American Society of Colon and Rectal Surgeons laparoscopic registry. *Dis Colon Rectum* 1996;39:S20.
24. Zmora O, Weiss E. Trocar site recurrence in laparoscopic surgery for colorectal cancer, myth or real concern? *Surg Oncol Clin N Am* 2001;10:625.
25. Lacy AM, Garcia-Valdecasas JC, Delgado S, et al. Laparoscopy assisted colectomy versus open colectomy for treatment of non-metastatic colon cancer: a randomised trial. *Lancet* 2002;359:2224.
26. Hazebroek EJ. COLOR: a randomized clinical trial comparing laparoscopic and open resection for colon cancer. *Surg Endosc* 2002;16:949.
27. Shoup M, Brennan MF, Karpeh MS, et al. Port site metastasis after diagnostic laparoscopy for upper gastrointestinal tract malignancies: an uncommon entity. *Ann Surg Oncol* 2002;9:632.
28. Paolucci V, Schaeff B, Schneider M, et al. Tumor seeding following laparoscopy: international survey. *World J Surg* 1999;23:989.
29. Hewett PJ, Texler ML, Anderson D, et al. In vivo real time analysis of intraperitoneal radiolabeled tumor cell movement during laparoscopy. *Dis Colon Rectum* 1999;42:868.
30. Brundell SM, Tucker K, Brown B, et al. Variables in the spread of tumor cells to trocars and port sites during operative laparoscopy. *Surg Endosc* 2002;16:1413.
31. Mathew G, Watson DI, Ellis T, et al. The effect of laparoscopy on the movement of tumor cells and metastasis to surgical wounds. *Surg Endosc* 1997;11:1163.
32. Mathew G, Watson DI, Rofe AM, et al. Wound metastases following laparoscopic and open surgery for abdominal cancer. *Br J Surg* 1996;83:1087.
33. Cavina E, Goletti O, Molea N, et al. Trocar site tumor recurrences: may pneumoperitoneum be responsible? *Surg Endosc* 1998;12:1294.
34. Ikramuddin S, Lucas J, Ellison C, et al. Detection of aerosolized cells during carbon dioxide laparoscopy. *J Gastrointest Surg* 1998;2:580.
35. Hirabayashi Y, Yamaguchi K, Shiraishi N, et al. Development of port site metastasis after pneumoperitoneum: a scanning electron microscopy study. *Surg Endosc* 2002;16:864.
36. Brundell S, Tsopelas C, Chatterton B, et al. Effect of port composition on tumor cell adherence. *Dis Colon Rectum* 2003;46:637.
37. Wu JS, Guo LW, Ruiz MB, et al. Excision of trocar sites reduces tumor implantation in an animal model. *Dis Colon Rectum* 1998;41:1107.
38. Cannis M, Botchorishvili R, Wattiez A, et al. Cancer and laparoscopy, experimental studies: a review. *Eur J Obstet Gynecol* 2000;91:1.
39. Foley EF, Kolecki RV, Schirmer BD. The accuracy of laparoscopic ultrasound in the detection of colorectal cancer liver metastases. *Am J Surg* 1998;176:262.
40. Ribeiro U, Gama Rodriques JJ, Safatle-Ribeiro AV, et al. Prognostic significance of intraperitoneal free cancer cells obtained by laparoscopic peritoneal lavage in patients with gastric cancer. *J Gastrointest Surg* 1998;2:244.
41. Cuschieri A, Hall AW, Clark J. Value of laparoscopy in the diagnosis and management of pancreatic carcinoma. *Gut* 1978;19:672.
42. Manolitsas TP, Folwer JM. Role of laparoscopy in the management of adnexal mass and staging of gynecologic cancers. *Clin Obstet Gynaecol* 2001;44:495.
43. Kindermann G, Massen V, Kuhn W. Laparoscopic management of ovarian tumors subsequently diagnosed as malignant. *J Pelvic Surg* 1996;2:245.
44. Buenaventura, P, Luketich J. Surgical staging of esophageal cancer. *Chest Surg Clin N Am* 2000;10:487.
45. Krasna, MJ, Jiao X, Mao YS, et al. Thoracoscopy/laparoscopy in the staging of esophageal cancer. *Surg Laparosc Endosc Percutan Tech* 2002;12:213.
46. Krasna MJ, Reed CE, Nedzwiecki D, et al. CALGB 9380: a prospective trial of the feasibility of thoracoscopy/laparoscopy in staging esophageal cancer. *Ann Thorac Surg* 2001; 71:1073.
47. D'Ugo DM, Pende V, Persiani R, et al. Laparoscopic staging of gastric cancer: an overview. *J Am Coll Surg* 2003;196:965.
48. Pisters PW, Lee JE, Vauthey JN, et al. Laparoscopy in the staging of pancreatic cancer. *Br J Surg* 2001;88:325.
49. Van Dijkum EJ, de Wit LT, van Delden OM, et al. Staging laparoscopy and laparoscopic ultrasonography in more than 400 patients with upper gastrointestinal carcinoma. *J Am Coll Surg* 1999;189:459.
50. Barreiro CJ, Lillemoe KD, Koniaris LG, et al. Diagnostic laparoscopy for periampullary and pancreatic cancer: what is the true benefit? *J Gastrointest Surg* 2002;6:75.
51. Montorsi M, Santambrogio R, Bianchi P, et al. Laparoscopy with laparoscopic ultrasound for pretreatment staging of hepatocellular carcinoma: a prospective study. *J Gastroinest Surg* 2001;5:312.
52. D'Angelica M, Fong Y, Weber S, et al. The role of laparoscopy in hepatobiliary malignancy: prospective analysis of 401 cases. *Ann Surg Oncol* 2003;10:183.
53. Carriaga MT, Henson DE. Liver, gallbladder, extrahepatic bile ducts, and pancreas. *Cancer* 1995;75:171.
54. Weber SM, DeMatteo RP, Fong Y, et al. Staging laparoscopy in patients with extrahepatic biliary carcinoma. *Ann Surg* 2002;235:392.
55. Clark T, Parekh D, Cookson MS, et al. Randomized prospective evaluation of extended versus limited lymph node dissection in patients with clinically localized prostate cancer. *J Urol* 2003;169:145.
56. Heidenreich A, Albers P, Hartmann M, et al. Complications of primary nerve sparing retroperitoneal lymph node dissection for clinical stage I nonseminomatous germ cell tumors of the testis: experience of the German testicular cancer study group. *J Urol* 2003;169:1710.
57. Bhayani SB, Ong A, Oh WK, et al. Laparoscopic retroperitoneal lymph node dissection for clinical stage I nonseminomatous germ cell testicular cancer: a long term update. *Urology* 2003;62:324.
58. Lai CH, Huang KG, Hong JH, et al. Randomized trial of surgical staging (extraperitoneal or laparoscopic) versus clinical staging in locally advanced cervical cancer. *Gynecol Oncol* 2003;89:160.
59. Lefor AT. Laparoscopic interventions in lymphoma management. *Semin Laparosc Surg* 2000;7:129.
60. Lefor AT, Flowers JL, Heyman MR. Laparoscopic staging of Hodgkin's disease. *Surg Oncol* 1993;2:217.
61. Carde P, Hagenbeek A, Hayat M, et al. Clinical staging versus laparotomy and combined modality with MOPP versus ABVD in early-stage Hodgkin's disease: the H6 twin randomized trials from the European Organization for Research and Treatment of Cancer Lymphoma Cooperative Group. *J Clin Oncol* 1993;11:2258.
62. Vlachaki MT, Ha CS, Hagemeister FB, et al. Stage I: Hodgkin disease: radiation therapy and chemotherapy at the University of Texas MD Anderson Cancer Center, 1967–1997. *Radiology* 1998;208:739.
63. Pierre AF, Luketich JD. Technique and role of minimally invasive esophagectomy for premalignant and malignant diseases of the esophagus. *Surg Oncol Clin N Am* 2002;11:337.
64. Weeks JC, Nelson H, Belber S, et al. Short-term quality of life outcomes following laparoscopic assisted colectomy vs open colectomy for colon cancer: a randomized trial. *JAMA* 2002;287:321.
65. Rassweiller Jens, Tsivian A, Ravi Kumar AV, et al. Oncologic safety of laparoscopic surgery for urological malignancy: experience with more than 1,000 operations. *J Urol* 2003; 169:2072.

Philip P. Connell
Mary K. Martel
Samuel Hellman

CHAPTER **13**

Principles of Radiation Oncology

The history of radiation therapy for the treatment of cancer dates back to the late nineteenth century, after Wilhelm Roentgen's description of x-rays in 1895 and the discovery of radium by Marie and Pierre Curie in 1898. Within the first few decades of the twentieth century, ionizing radiation had been used to treat a variety of human malignancies, including inoperable testicular tumors and cancers of the uterine cervix. Technologic advances in the latter half of the twentieth century led to the development of cobalt 60 (^{60}Co) teletherapy units and linear accelerators. These were capable of producing higher-energy x-rays that could penetrate deeper into tissue and reduce dose to skin, and thus represented an enormous step forward in the ability to treat internal tumors. Over the past 20 years, much of the technologic progress has come in the form of treatment planning advances. In particular, three-dimensional treatment planning systems and intensity-modulated radiotherapy techniques have significantly improved the ability to localize radiation dose to difficult locations and unusual shapes. These "conformal" treatment planning tools allow for more effective treatment of tumors while better protecting the adjacent normal tissues.

In modern decades, radiotherapy has become a standard treatment option for a wide range of malignancies. Data from the U.S. Surveillance, Epidemiology, and End Results (SEER) program show that radiation treatment is commonly included in primary oncologic decisions. For example, radiotherapy was used in the initial management of 32.9% of prostate cancers and 44.1% of lung cancers in the United States between 1991 and 1996.[1] If subsequent palliative interventions are also included, more than half of cancer patients receive radiotherapy during at least one point in their care.

Although total body irradiation is occasionally administered, the primary use of radiation is for treatment of local and regional disease sites. Depending on the clinical situation, this can take the form of either palliative or potentially curative treatment. The radiation therapy process begins with an initial evaluation by a radiation oncologist. Because modern cancer treatments are increasingly multimodal, this initial planning period requires close collaboration with surgical and medical oncology colleagues. The patient then undergoes a radiation planning session, called a simulation. During the simulation, a custom immobilization is created and the patient is imaged to delineate the regions that require treatment and to identify the neighboring normal anatomic structures that must be protected. Once this planning process is completed, the treatment course commences.

To understand the practice and principles of radiation oncology, one must study the consequences of irradiating biologic material from three fundamental perspectives: biologic, physical, and clinical. Consequently, the discussion in this chapter has been divided into these areas.

BIOLOGIC ASPECTS OF RADIATION ONCOLOGY

RADIATION DEPOSITS ENERGY IN TISSUE AND PRODUCES IONIZATION EVENTS

Radiation can be considered as packets of energy in the form of photons (e.g., x-rays, ultraviolet light) or particles (e.g., protons, neutrons, α-particles, and electrons). As these packets of energy penetrate into tissue, they produce ionizations either directly or indirectly in biologically important molecules. The subatomic collisions caused by the particle types of radiation

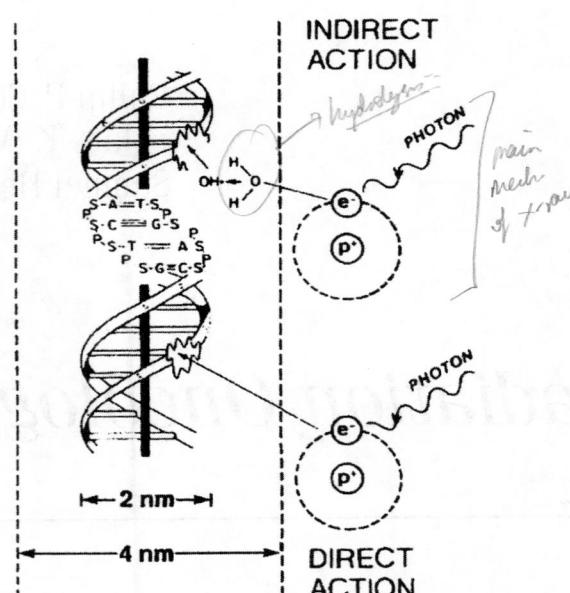

FIGURE 13-1. Photons collide with the orbiting electrons of biologic molecules, which leads to the ejection of fast electrons. The ejected electrons damage DNA either directly or indirectly via the production of hydroxyl radicals. (From ref. 2, with permission.)

can induce direct biologic damage within cells, which is termed *direct ionization.* X-rays, on the other hand, transfer their energy to chemical intermediates within tissue, and it is these intermediates that produce the actual biologic damage. This is called *indirect ionization.*

Ionization events occur as these packets of energy travel through tissue and deposit their energy. Radiation *dose* is the term that describes the quantity of energy deposited per mass of tissue. Radiation oncologists frequently express radiation using the International System unit *gray* (Gy), which equals 1 J/kg. An older unit of dose is the *rad*, which is equal to 1/100 Gy or 1 cGy.

In the case of electromagnetic radiation, high-energy x-ray photons collide with orbiting electrons of biologic molecules, which leads to the ejection of fast electrons (Fig. 13-1). These fast electrons can then directly damage biologic target (e.g., DNA) in a process called *direct action.* More commonly, however, the fast electrons collide with the plentiful water molecules in tissue. This results in the production of hydroxyl radicals (OH^-), which in turn can damage biologic targets (termed *indirect action*). This indirect action is thought to account for approximately two-thirds of the biologic damage that is produced by x-rays.[2]

Radiation can also be delivered directly in the form of electrons (or β-particles), and this produces events that are similar in principle to those of x-rays. Electron radiation can be thought of as the secondary fast electrons that are created by x-rays. However, these electrons are directly produced from a machine or a radioactive isotope (e.g., phosphorus 32), unlike the secondary fast electrons that are produced in tissue by x-rays.

LINEAR ENERGY TRANSFER AND RELATIVE BIOLOGIC EFFECTIVENESS

Other types of particulate radiation (neutrons, α-particles) result in more complex patterns of ionization. Because of their

large mass (relative to that of an electron), these particles carry greater energy. As these particles pass through tissue, they create a relatively large number of ionization events along the path traversed. This density of damage per unit of length is referred to as *linear energy transfer* (LET) and is reported as energy deposited per unit distance traversed (kiloelectron volts per micron). Fast neutrons, for example, are a high-LET form of radiation that produce both direct and indirect ionization events. Their action is quite different from that of x-rays and electrons, in that fast neutrons collide with the nuclei of atoms rather than with orbiting electrons. These collisions set into motion a variety of nuclear fragments, including α-particles, which are also high-LET forms of ionizing radiation. One fast neutron may elastically scatter off a large number of nuclei along its path through tissue.

Despite the relatively large mass of protons, these particles predominately interact with atomic electrons as they traverse through tissue. Their pattern of LET is unusual, in that LET increases as the particles pass through tissue and give up energy. The point of maximum LET, termed the *Bragg peak*, occurs immediately before the proton comes to rest. From a physics perspective, this phenomenon has potential applications for localizing dose delivery to specific depths in tissue (see Physical Aspects of Radiation Oncology, later in this chapter). Biologically, however, the typical sources of proton radiation used therapeutically can be considered as low-LET forms of radiation with tissue effects very similar to those of x-rays.

The dense path of ionization events created by high-LET radiation results in a relatively high probability of inducing damage at more than one site within a biologic target along its path (e.g., the creation of a double-strand DNA break). This clustered pattern of damage, in turn, results in a greater likelihood of inducing a lethal event within a cell (Fig. 13-2). Consequently, high-LET forms of radiation are associated with relatively higher biologic effects per unit of energy deposited. This biologic observation, termed *relative biologic effectiveness* (RBE), measures the ratio of doses required to yield an equal biologic effect. In addition to depending on the LET, RBE is also affected by the rate of dose delivery (*dose rate*), the dose delivered per treatment session (*fraction size*), and the total

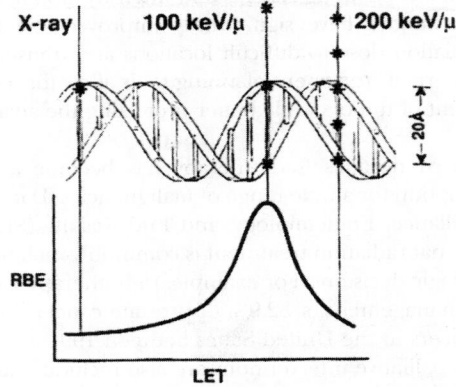

FIGURE 13-2. The relationship between relative biological effectiveness (RBE) and linear energy transfer (LET) for different forms of radiation. This phenomenon is explained by the pattern of ionization events (represented by stars) created along the traversed path. (From ref. 2, with permission.)

dose delivered. For simplicity, however, the RBE of photons, electrons, and protons can be considered to be approximately 1. Neutrons and α-particles have considerably higher RBEs.

INDUCTION AND REJOINING OF DNA DOUBLE-STRAND BREAKS

In terms of cellular lethality from ionizing radiation, DNA is generally considered to be a principal intracellular target. Although both single-strand breaks and double-strand breaks (DSBs) are observed, it is the DSBs that are thought to represent the lethal event.[3] Radiobiologists estimate that a 1-Gy x-ray dose results in approximately 10^5 ionization events per cell, producing 1000 to 2000 single-strand breaks and 40 DSBs.[2,4] The formation of radiation-induced DNA breaks has been well studied, and the resulting DNA fragments can been quantified by a number of techniques (reviewed by Prise et al.[5]). These techniques are often performed at cold temperatures to measure the amount of *initial DNA damage* after radiation (i.e., before any DNA repair). Levels of initial DSBs vary for different human cancer cell lines, which may be due to differences in chromatin compactness or varying levels of substances that interact with free radicals, or both. Such measurements, however, do not address the ultimate levels of unrepaired or incorrectly repaired damage (after repair), and hence the biologic significance of initial DNA damage remains debated.[6]

The rejoining of DSBs can also be directly measured, and this topic has been well studied. It is important to distinguish *DSB rejoining* from *DNA repair*, however, because the typical assays used to measure rejoining do not provide information as to whether the genetic code has been correctly repaired. The majority of radiation-induced DSBs are rejoined in cells within 2 hours, but the process can continue for up to 24 hours (Fig. 13-3). This rejoining of DSBs appears follow a biphasic kinetic pattern, consisting of an initial rapid phase (10 to 20 minutes) followed by a slow phase (several hours).[6,7] The relative proportions of these two phases are dose dependent, in that slower rates of DSB rejoining are observed after delivery of higher radiation doses. This kinetic dose dependency may represent a saturation of repair capabilities occurring with high levels of DNA damage.[7]

Numerous studies have demonstrated a direct correlation between cellular survival after irradiation and the efficiency of DSB rejoining (reviewed by Nunez et al.[6]). The efficiency of both the rapid[8] and slow components[9] of rejoining have been significantly correlated with the portion of cells surviving treat-ment with 2 Gy for a variety of cell lines. Other studies have investigated the rates of DSB rejoining in radiosensitive cell lines that are known to harbor mutations in genes required for DNA repair.[10–12] As expected, such cells have impaired rates of DSB rejoining.

CELLULAR DOSE RESPONSE TO RADIATION

Radiation effects are randomly distributed, which is an important principle in describing the general nature of cell killing. The biologically important effects of radiation therapy are those concerned with reproductive integrity. At least four possible consequences of radiation interaction with cells can affect long-term reproductive viability of the cell or its progeny: necrosis, apoptosis, accelerated senescence, and terminal differentiation. A cell that is damaged by radiation and loses its reproductive integrity may divide once or more before all the progeny are rendered reproductively sterile. Those colonies in which some reproductively viable progeny emerge may then regrow.[13]

Survival curves plot the fraction of cells surviving radiation against the dose given. Survival is determined by the ability to form a macroscopic colony. The simplest relation can be seen for bacteria, in which survival is a constant exponential function of dose. The importance of this exponential relation is that, for a given dose increment, a constant proportion (rather than a constant number) of cells is killed. Because of the randomness of radiation damage, if there is an average of one lethal lesion per cell, some cells have one lesion, some have more than one, and some have fewer than one. Under such circumstances, the proportion of cells that have fewer than one (i.e., no lethal events) is e^{-1}, or a survival fraction of 0.37. The dose required to reduce the survival fraction to 37% on the exponential curve is known as the D_o. This term is related to the slope of the exponential survival curve. If a smaller dose is required to reduce the survival fraction to 37%, then those cells are considered to be more sensitive to radiation.

Survival curves of most mammalian cells differ from those of bacterial cells by having a "shoulder" in the low-dose region and an exponential relation at higher doses. This shoulder indicates a reduced efficiency of cell killing per unit dose at low doses. Such an idealized curve is shown in Figure 13-4, with the shorthand terminology used to describe survival curves. The terminal exponential portion is described by the D_o, whereas the initial shoulder region can be described by the extrapolation number n or the D_q, the quasi-threshold dose. The former is the number on the ordinate found when the exponential portion is extrapolated to 0 dose, whereas D_q is the dose at which the straight portion of the survival curve extrapolated backward intersects the line where the survival fraction is unity. If any two of these are known, the third can be calculated. The survival curve is described as follows: $\log e^n = D_q/D_o$.

This survival curve is best described by a linear quadratic model[14] with the following formula: Survival $= e^{-(\alpha D + \beta D^2)}$. The α and β terms in this equation and the α/β ratio are used to describe survival curve characteristics and to classify cellular response to radiation. Survival curves have been determined for benign and neoplastic mammalian cells in culture. No general characteristics of tumor cells make them different from normal cells in culture. The survival curves for various human tumors

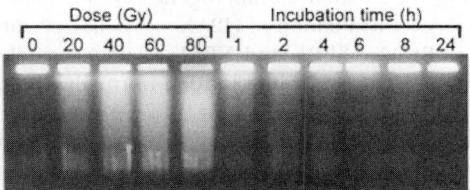

Dose (Gy)					Incubation time (h)					
0	20	40	60	80	1	2	4	6	8	24

FIGURE 13-3. The formation of double-strand DNA breaks in AA8 CHO cells and DNA rejoining over time. Ethidium bromide–stained pulsed-field electrophoretic gel showing DNA from cells irradiated with various doses (*left*) and then incubated to determine the rate of DNA rejoining after 80 Gy of irradiation (*right*). (Adapted from ref. 25, with permission.)

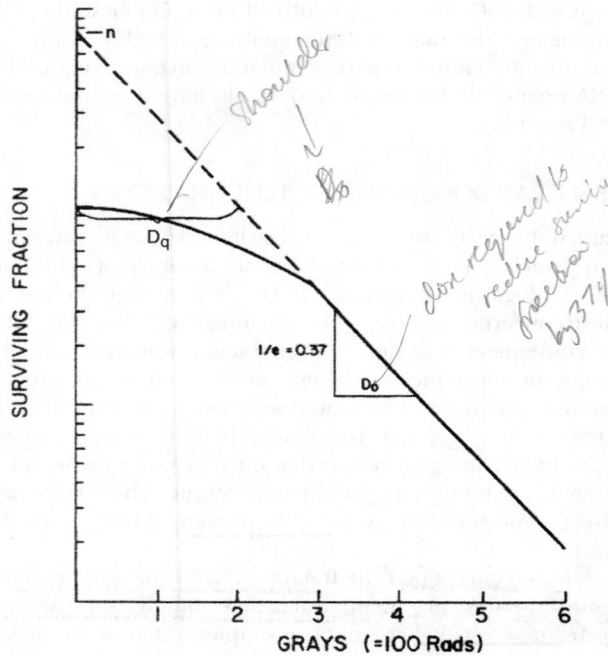

FIGURE 13-4. Idealized radiation survival curve. D_o is the dose required to reduce the surviving fraction to 37% on the exponential portion of the curve. D_q is the quasi-threshold dose.

thought to be sensitive or resistant to radiation were studied by Weichselbaum and colleagues, who did not find any survival curve characteristics that allow these two to be separated.[15] Therefore, the differences in clinical response cannot be explained by simple acute differences in survival curves, although recurrent tumors tend to have the radiobiologic characteristics of the more resistant subclones of the primary tumor.

Normal tissues also have been studied using clonogenic survival as an end point, with survival curves determined analogously to those for cells in tissue culture. An early clonal system, as originally described by Till and McCulloch, was used for murine bone marrow stem cells.[16] When bone marrow cells are injected into lethally irradiated recipient animals, colonies are formed in the animals' spleens. These can be used to assess the reproductive integrity of the injected cells. The viability of the small intestinal clonogenic mucosal cells can be assessed by looking at sections of the small intestine at various times after irradiation and determining the appearance of colonies derived from cells surviving this radiation.[17] When these and other techniques are used, the general properties describing normal and tumor cells are comparable. The survival curves for tumor cells generally resemble those of their normal tissue of origin.

Radiobiologic models used to describe clonogenic survival assays frequently refer to the concept of *potentially lethal damage repair*. Potentially lethal damage can be thought of as damage that leads to cell death under certain circumstances. If, however, the postirradiation conditions are modified to allow repair, cells that would have died can be salvaged. In general, postirradiation conditions that suppress cell division are the ones most favorable to repair of potentially lethal damage. The first and simplest example of this was the effect seen in bacteria subjected to ultraviolet irradiation and x-irradiation.[18] A simi-

lar effect was seen in mammalian cells, and this effect persists into the first few postirradiation generations. Potentially lethal damage repair is among the most important factors for relating cell culture studies of human tumors to their clinical responses. Weichselbaum and colleagues showed that osteogenic sarcoma, a tumor characteristically thought to be resistant to radiation, has a great capacity for potentially lethal damage repair compared with tumors that may be much more responsive to radiation.[19] In the clinical situation, irradiated tumor cells may not be faced with the necessity for rapid cell division and thus may have the opportunity for potentially lethal damage repair.

MOLECULAR RESPONSES TO RADIATION-INDUCED CELLULAR INJURY

Each cell undergoes a critical period after injury from radiation that determines whether the cell will die, repair the damage, or proceed through cellular division despite the damage. On the molecular level, radiation-induced damage initiates complex signaling cascades in cells, which results in a variety of responses that include cell-cycle arrest, induction of stress response genes, DNA repair, and apoptosis. The signaling and surveillance proteins ATM and ATR appear to have central roles in these response pathways and act via direct phosphorylation of downstream targets (Fig. 13-5). ATM and ATR have somewhat overlapping actions because they have overlapping substrate specificities[20] and because ATR overexpression can phenotypically complement ATM-deficient cells.[21] The two appear to differ primarily in terms of the types of damage that each protein recognizes. For example, phosphorylation of p53 is predominantly ATM dependent after radiation damage, whereas ATR performs this phosphorylation in response to ultraviolet radiation–induced damage.[22] The protein p53 has a key role in the activation of apoptosis and cell-cycle arrest after DNA damage. Treatment with a chemical inhibitor of p53 called α pifithrin was shown to rescue mice after doses of total body radiation that are normally lethal.[23]

One of the early phosphorylation targets of ATM is the chromatin protein histone H2AX.[24] Subnuclear focus formation by the phosphorylated version, γ-H2AX, can be microscopically visualized with fluorescent antibodies within minutes of DNA damage. Immunofluorescence detection of γ-H2AX foci has also been used as a surrogate for following unrepaired DNA breaks over time (Fig. 13-6).[25] The p53 binding protein 1 (53BP1) also localizes into radiation-induced foci rapidly, in contrast to BRCA1 protein and the RAD50-MRE11-NBS1 complex, which localize into foci much more slowly (45 minutes to hours).[26,27] Mice lacking H2AX survive embryogenesis but display genomic instability.[28] After irradiation of H2AX −/− cells, several proteins (including BRCA1, 53BP1, and NBS1) can successfully migrate to DSB regions, but they do not localize normally into radiation-induced foci.[28,29] This suggests that γ-H2AX is not the primary signal needed to recruit some repair proteins to the vicinity of DNA lesions, but that it functions by concentrating these repair proteins in the microenvironment of the DSB.[30] RAD51 focus formation, on the other hand, proceeds normally regardless of H2AX status,[28] which suggests that γ-H2AX may not be required for the initiation of homologous recombinational repair (discussed in detail in Specific Pathways for the Repair of Double-Strand DNA Breaks, later in this chapter).

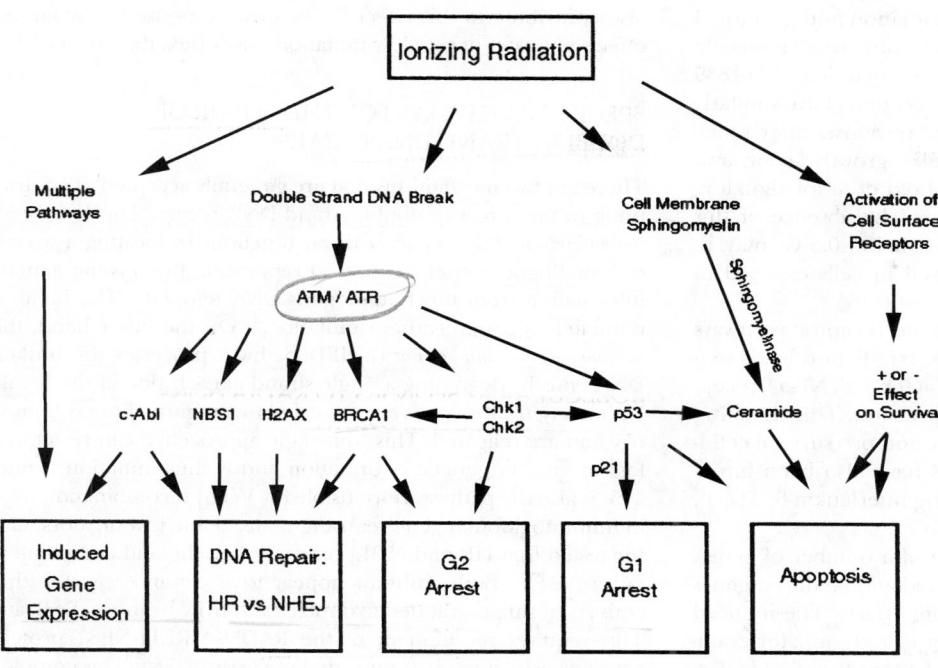

FIGURE 13-5. Partial and simplified summary of molecular events that occur in response to cellular irradiation. HR, homologous recombination; NHEJ, nonhomologous end joining.

Many of the downstream functions of radiation-induced signaling appear to be complementary. For example, cell-cycle arrest can allow extra time for DNA repair to be completed and thereby avoid the replication or segregation of damaged DNA. Targeted disruption of the checkpoint gene Chk1 leads to early embryonic lethality in mice, and embryonic stem cells conditionally lacking Chk1 proceed prematurely to mitosis after irradiation. Consistent with these genetic data, pharmacologic inhibition of the cell-cycle checkpoint machinery can sensitize cells to the lethal effects of DNA damage.[31] Tumor cells frequently have abnormal G_1 checkpoint functions but have intact G_2 checkpoint mechanisms. Therefore, targeted inhibition of G_2 checkpoint components can sensitize tumor cells to radiation, whereas the cells in normal tissue are preferentially protected due to their intact G_1 checkpoints.[32,33] This anticancer treatment strategy has been investigated further using several G_2 checkpoint inhibitors, which have included caffeine, pentoxifylline, UCN-01, and newer novel compounds such as PD0166285.

Ionizing radiation damage activates a number of stress response–signaling pathways that contribute to lethality, and many of these may be independent of DNA damage. For example, radiation can activate sphingomyelinase, which hydrolyzes plasma membrane–derived sphingomyelin and produces ceramide. Ceramide, in turn, can promote apoptosis.[34] Further evidence for this pathway stems from the radioresistance seen in cells that are sphingomyelinase deficient.[35] It should be noted, however, that radiation-induced ceramide production can also result from a DNA damage–dependent pathway that involves the enzyme ceramide synthase.[36] The precise mechanism for ceramide-induced apoptosis remains unclear at present, but it appears to involve the stress-activated protein kinase pathway.[4]

Radiation also activates many signaling pathways that promote cell survival, and many of these pathways are normally used by mitogens such as growth factors. Many of these effects depend on cell type. Several membrane-bound receptors have

been implicated in such signaling and act via downstream activation of multiple pathways, including the mitogen-activated protein kinase, phosphatidylinositol 3 kinase, K-/H-Ras, JAK/STAT, and c-Jun NH_2-terminal kinase pathways (reviewed by Dent et al.[37]). One example is the radiation-induced signaling of epidermal growth factor receptor (EGFR). Pharmacologic inhibition of EGFR signaling can be used to oppose this pro-survival effect. Huang et al. showed that treatment of cells with an EGFR-bind-

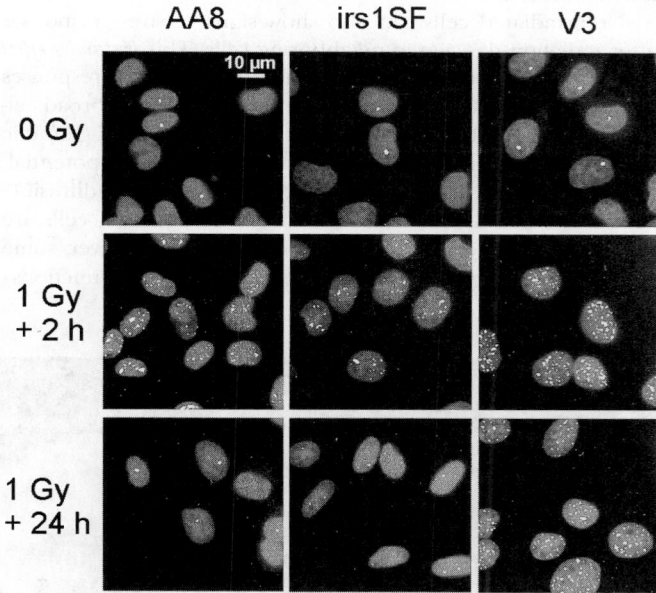

FIGURE 13-6. Immunofluorescence detection of γ-H2AX used as a surrogate for following unrepaired DNA breaks over time. The CHO cells used are the parental line (AA8) or DNA repair mutant cell lines irs1SF (deficient in the homologous recombination protein XRCC3) and V3 (deficient in the nonhomologous end-joining protein DNA-PKcs). (From ref. 25, with permission.)

ing antibody (C-225) sensitized cells to radiation and promoted apoptosis.[38] Similar effects have been seen using small-molecule inhibitors of the EGFR tyrosine kinase, including ZD-1839 (Iressa) and OSI-774. Other cell surface receptors have similarly been implicated in pro-survival–signaling responses after radiation, including HER2, vascular endothelial growth factor, and basic fibroblast growth factor. The threshold dose for signaling through EGFR is approximately 0.5 Gy.[39] The absence of this pro-survival–signaling observed with doses below 0.5 Gy may, in part, explain the hypersensitivity observed in cells exposed to very low doses (i.e., low-dose hyperradiosensitivity).[40]

Many other growth factor and cytokine receptor pathways are also involved in radiation responses. Irradiation leads to a rapid activation of the tumor necrosis factor-α (TNF-α) receptor and induction of TNF-α protein expression. This signaling appears to result in competing apoptotic and pro-survival cellular responses.[37] Several other cytokines have also been implicated in antiapoptotic signaling, including interleukin-6, TGF-β, and urokinase-type plasminogen activator.

Radiation also induces the expression of a number of genes. The members of this ever-growing list of radiation-induced genes produce a broad spectrum of downstream effects. The induced expression of early growth response 1 (Egr-1) and c-Jun, for example, may help cells survive after radiation damage.[41] This radiation inducibility depends on modifications of transcriptional factors by the protein kinase C pathway.[42] Targeted inhibition of Egr-1 and c-Jun proteins prevents the onset of S phase and reduces the survival of human cells after radiation damage.[43] Other radiation-inducible genes were reviewed[44] and include GADD45, β-actin, interleukin-1, protein kinase C, basic fibroblast growth factor, interleukin-1β, and tissue plasminogen activator. Identification of the promoter regions upstream of the Egr-1 gene has led to the development of radiation-inducible gene therapy technology[44] (discussed in detail in Clinical Aspects of Radiation Oncology later in this chapter).

Nonirradiated cells can also show signs of stress responses after radiation damage to neighboring cells. This *bystander effect* has been well described by several authors.[45,46] These responses appear to be cell-type dependent, and they consist of broad cellular changes including gene induction, induction of genomic instability, differentiation, and changes in apoptotic potential. These effects appear to be mediated, at least in part, by diffusible substances, because the effect occurs when bystander cells are physically separated from the irradiated cells[47]; however, some authors have suggested that cell-cell contacts (gap junctions) also contribute to this effect.[48] The dose response for bystander effects saturates at very low radiation doses (less than 0.1 Gy).

SPECIFIC PATHWAYS FOR THE REPAIR OF DOUBLE-STRAND DNA BREAKS

There are two mechanisms that are generally accepted as contributing to the repair of double-strand DNA breaks. The *homologous recombination* (HR) repair pathway functions by locating a stretch of homologous genetic code and replicating the missing genetic information from this homologous DNA template. The break is ultimately repaired without mutation.[49] On the other hand, the *nonhomologous end-joining* (NHEJ) pathway processes the broken DNA ends by degrading a single strand at each side of the break. Ultimately, the two ends are annealed in a region of microhomology and are religated. This "duct-tape approach"[50] can result in a loss or gain in genetic information and is thus mutation prone. This is also the pathway responsible for V(D)J recombination used in immunoglobulin gene rearrangments. Some investigators have suggested that HR and NHEJ have overlapping and complementary roles.[25,51] Both pathways appear to share an early step that consists of single-stranded exonuclease activity from the DSB site. This requires recruitment of the RAD50-MRE11-NBS1 protein complex, which has demonstrated nuclease activity. This complex appears to be essential for both HR[52] and NHEJ.[53] Petrini's group has microscopically visualized the recruitment of the RAD50-Mre11-Nbs1 complex to sites of nuclear damage after irradiation (Fig. 13-7).[54]

The NHEJ pathway is a dominant mechanism for repairing double-strand DNA breaks in mammalian cells (Fig. 13-8). The proposed model for this repair process begins with the binding of Ku to the DSB, followed by nuclease activity by the Artemis-DNA-PKcs complex to "trim" the DNA ends, and the final ligation is performed by the ligase IV/XRCC4 protein complex.[55] Several investigators have attempted to overcome resistance to DNA-damaging therapies by inhibiting the proteins required for NHEJ. For example, antisense DNA strategies have been used to down-regulate the gene expression of Ku70, Ku86, and DNA-PKcs. In all three cases, this down-regulation resulted in enhanced sensitivity to radiation in human cell lines.[56–58] Small interfering RNAs were similarly used to "knock down" expression of DNA-PKcs protein, which resulted in radiosensitization of human fibroblasts.[59] Two of the key proteins in the NHEJ pathway are ligase IV and XRCC4. In mice, gene-targeted mutations in either of these genes leads to early embryonic lethality,

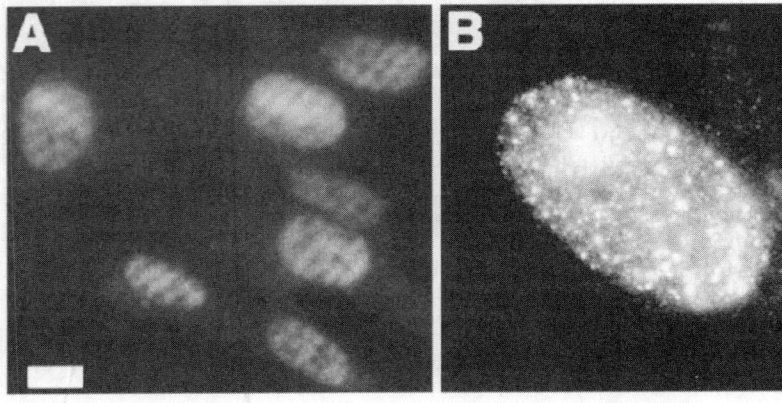

FIGURE 13-7. Localization of hMre11 to irradiated nuclear sites after partial volume irradiation with a striped pattern. The 37Lu cells were fixed after irradiation and stained for hMre11 or hRad51. **A:** Anti-hMre11, 30 minutes after irradiation. **B:** Anti-hRad51, 30 minutes after irradiation. Bar in **A** indicates 10 μm; bar in **B** indicates 5 μm. (Adapted from ref. 54, with permission.)

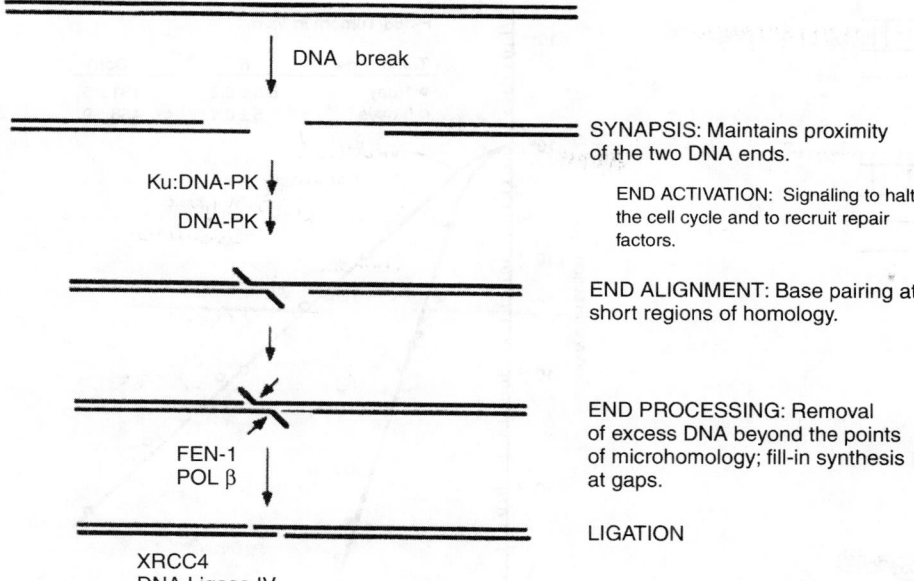

SYNAPSIS: Maintains proximity of the two DNA ends.

END ACTIVATION: Signaling to halt the cell cycle and to recruit repair factors.

END ALIGNMENT: Base pairing at short regions of homology.

END PROCESSING: Removal of excess DNA beyond the points of microhomology; fill-in synthesis at gaps.

LIGATION

FIGURE 13-8. Basic features of the nonhomologous DNA end-joining repair pathway. (From Lieber MR. The biochemistry and biological significance of nonhomologous DNA end joining: an essential repair process in multicellular eukaryotes. *Genes Cells* 1999;4:77, with permission.)

and the resulting embryonic cells are hypersensitive to ionizing radiatiom.[60] Likewise, hypersensitivity has been observed in a human cell line (180BR) that contains a mutation in ligase IV.[61] XRCC4 appears to stabilize and enhance the activity of ligase IV,[62] and the two readily form a heterodimer.[63] The ligase IV/XRCC4 complex binds specifically to duplex DNA ends and can act as a bridging factor, linking together duplex DNA molecules with complementary but nonligatable ends.[64]

HR is the other dominant pathway for repairing double-strand DNA breaks, and this pathway has a strong role in maintaining chromosomal stability (Fig. 13-9). The proposed mechanism for this pathway begins with 5' to 3' nuclease activity at the DSB, resulting in a 3' single-stranded tail. The tail is coated by replication protein A (RPA), which is subsequently replaced by a helical filament of RAD51 protein. This displacement of RPA by RAD51 appears to be mediated by a number of protein complexes, which include RAD52 and a family of RAD51 paralog proteins.[49,65] These RAD51 filaments can be microscopically visualized with fluorescent antibodies, and they appear as subnuclear foci (see Fig. 13-7).[66] The RAD51 coated 3' tail then invades a double-stranded stretch of homologous template DNA. The genetic code is essentially copied from this template by polymerase activity and branch migration, in a structure termed the Holiday junction. The Holiday junction is ultimately resolved by cleavage in one of two possible directions, which forms either crossover or noncrossover gene conversion products.[49] Although this model of HR is well accepted for meiotic recombination, the gene conversion events observed after mitotic recombination strongly favor noncrossover gene products.[67] For this reason, some investigators have suggested that a variant mechanism of HR exists, in which a single-stand re-annealing step follows the polymerase and branch migration activities.

Genetic studies have shown that HR requires RAD51 and all five RAD51 paralogs, which include XRCC2, XRCC3, RAD51B, RAD51C, and RAD51D.[68] Biochemical studies have revealed that XRCC3 forms a stable heterodimeric complex with RAD51C. A

second complex of RAD51 paralogs has also been described, comprised of RAD51B, RAD51C, RAD51D, and XRCC2.[69,70] Together, these two complexes are thought to function by promoting the assembly of RAD51 filaments at sites of DNA damage. This model is supported by biochemical analyses performed by Patrick Sung's group using a partial complex of paralogs that includes RAD51B and RAD51C. This RAD51B-RAD51C complex was shown to promote RAD51-mediated homologous DNA pairing and strand exchange. Importantly, this stimulatory effect occurred under conditions in which RAD51 needed to compete with RPA protein for sites of single-stranded DNA binding.[71] The importance of these proteins is underscored by the fact that they are required for embryonic survival. Transgenic knockout mice have been generated lacking RAD51, RAD51B, RAD51D, and XRCC2, and each of these knockouts has resulted in embryonic lethality. Other proteins thought to play roles in HR include BRCA1, BRCA2, RAD54, BLM, and ATM/ATR.

IMPORTANCE OF OXYGEN IN RADIATION EFFECTS

A primary modifier of the biologic effect of ionizing irradiation is molecular oxygen. Although the effect was first noted in the 1920s, its importance was not realized until Mottram studied it systematically.[72] Figure 13-10 shows survival curves for cells under oxygenated and hypoxic conditions. For equivalent cell killing at every level of survival, higher doses are required under hypoxic conditions than under oxygenated conditions. There is some disagreement in the literature as to whether the dose ratio is the same throughout the survival curve. Most data suggest a smaller difference when low doses are used. A shorthand term, the *oxygen enhancement ratio*, often is used. The oxygen enhancement ratio is the ratio of dose required for equivalent cell killing in the absence of oxygen compared with the dose required in the presence of oxygen. This term has most relevance for the exponential portion of the curve, because there appears to be a reduced shoulder on the survival curve of cells under hypoxic conditions. Tumor cells allowed to

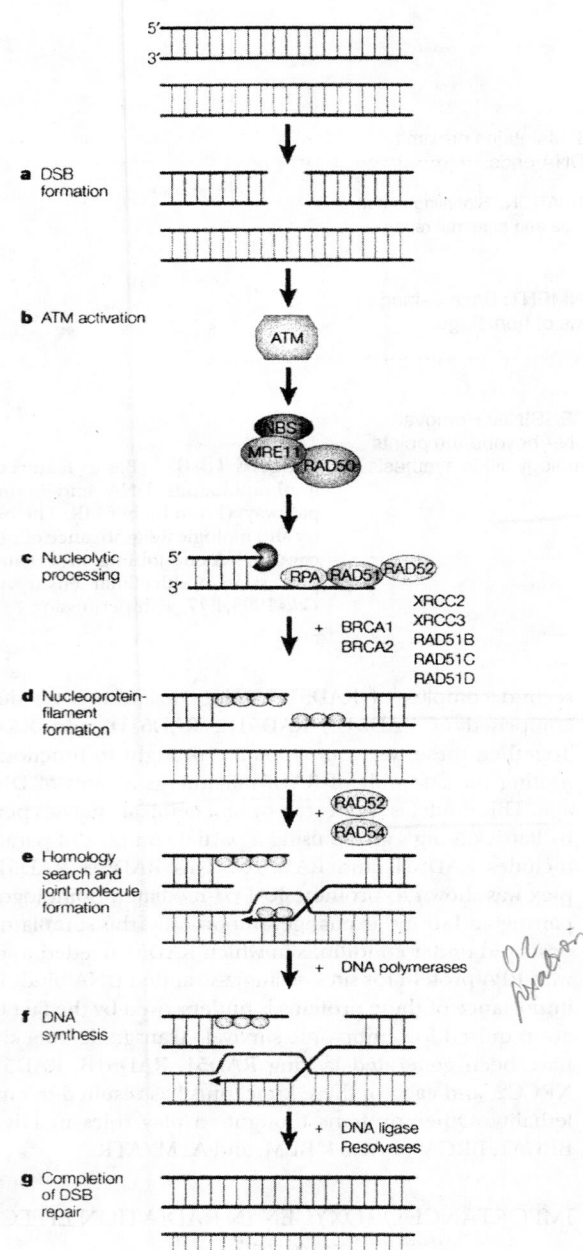

FIGURE 13-9. Basic features of the homologous recombinational DNA repair pathway. DSB, double-strand break; RPA, replication protein A. (From van Gent DC, Hoeijmakers JH, Kanaar R. Chromosomal stability and the DNA double-stranded break connection. *Nat Rev Genet* 2001;2:196, with permission.)

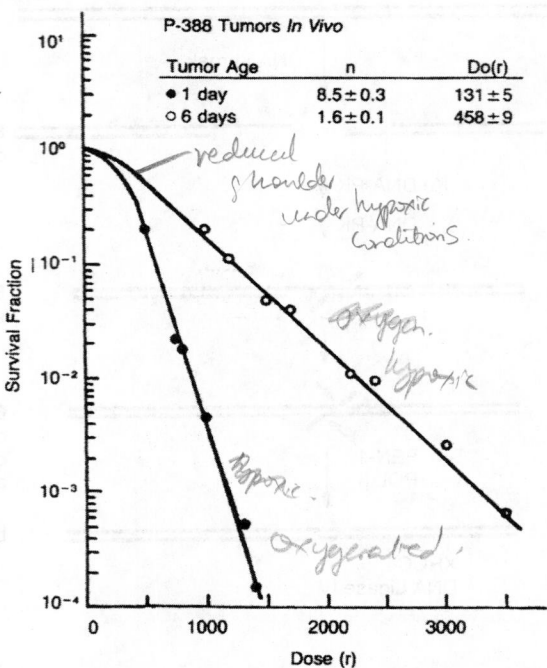

FIGURE 13-10. *In vivo* survival curves for oxygenated (*filled circles*) and hypoxic (*open circles*) cells. (From Belli JA, Dicus GJ, Bonte FJ. Radiation response of mammalian tumor cells. I. Repair of sublethal damage in vivo. *J Natl Cancer Inst* 1967;38:673, with permission.)

gen tension at the time of irradiation. A very low oxygen tension (approximately 30 mm Hg) must be reached before a protective effect of hypoxia is seen. The mechanism is commonly accepted to be that oxygen "fixes" free radical–induced damage into a permanent state and that this damage is otherwise short-lived. The effects of high-LET forms of radiation depend much less on oxygen,[73] presumably because their damage is predominantly via direct action, rather than via hydroxyl radical intermediates.

The clinical importance of the oxygen effect has led to clinical and laboratory experiments, including the use of high-pressure oxygen with radiation therapy. These studies have indicated that, when the number of radiation fractions is small, hyperbaric oxygen increases curability. If normal fractionation

grow into physiologic hypoxia have reduced capacity to repair sublethal damage. The oxygen enhancement ratios for different cells that have been studied vary from 2.5 to 3.5. This means that, for reduction to a given survival level, three times as much radiation is required under hypoxic conditions as under oxygenated conditions. Because the curves are exponential, the ratio of survival fractions increases with dose.

Furthermore, studies have shown that oxygen must be present at the time of irradiation for this effect to occur. Figure 13-11 shows the relative radiosensitivity of cells as a function of the oxy-

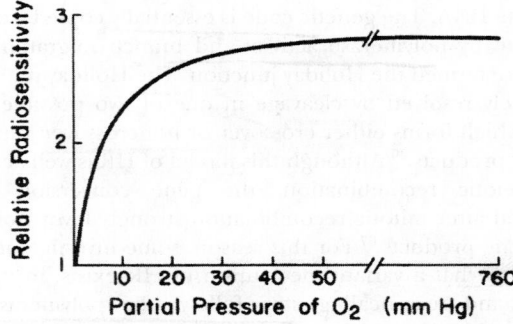

FIGURE 13-11. Radiation sensitivity as a function of ambient oxygen partial pressure. (Adapted from Deschner EE, Gray LH. Influence of oxygen tension of x-ray induced chromosomal damage in Ehrlich ascites tumor cells irradiated in vitro and in vivo. *Radiat Res* 1959;11:115, with permission.)

schemes are used, hyperbaric oxygen often does not show an advantage. However, some reports involving tumors of the head and neck and uterine cervix indicate that the use of hyperbaric oxygen with 10 fractions of radiation results in greater cure rates than conventional daily fractionation.[74,75] A metaanalysis showed that use of hyperbaric oxygen improves the local control of solid tumors treated with radiation by approximately 10%.[76] Although these studies appear promising, the hyperbaric oxygen technique is cumbersome and difficult to administer. A logistically easier approach is the use of inhaled carbogen, which is an unpressurized mixture of 95% oxygen and 5% carbon dioxide. This is often combined with nicotinamide to increase vascular perfusion. Such approaches are under investigation in clinical trials.

A practical clinical concern is whether the presence of anemia affects tumor response to radiation. Historic review and a prospective study at the Princess Margaret Hospital showed that anemic patients with carcinoma of the cervix have reduced curability by radiation and that correction of the anemia via transfusion improves the probability of pelvic control.[77] A more modern approach for improving hemoglobin levels is the use of recombinant human erythropoietin. Several studies have shown that recombinant human erythropoietin can improve hemoglobin levels in patients receiving chemotherapy and radiation.[78,79] However, a randomized trial examining radiotherapy for head and neck cancers showed that administration of epoetin β did not improve cancer control or survival. To the contrary, patients receiving epoetin β experienced worse locoregional progression–free survival rates, despite improvements in their hemoglobin levels.[80] Further studies are needed to further define the role of erythropoietin use with radiotherapy.

MODULATORS OF RADIATION OTHER THAN OXYGEN

Numerous drugs have been used to modulate the effects of radiation. The combined effects of drugs and radiation can be divided into the following types: (1) independent—the agents act independently, their mechanisms of action are independent, and their damage is independent; (2) additive—the agents act via related mechanisms, and therefore their sublethal damage and their lethal damage are additive; (3) synergistic—the two agents have a result that is more effective than pure additivity; (4) protective—combined treatment results in less lethal damage than either treatment alone.

Some of the earliest radiation-sensitizing agents came in the form of hypoxic cell sensitizers. In the 1960s, several investigators began searching for compounds that would mimic oxygen in its effect. They sought agents that would be metabolized slowly and reach all portions of the tumor. This is an important distinction, because high-pressure oxygen increases diffusion only slightly, whereas slowly metabolized sensitizers can reach all areas of the tumor. Nitroimidazoles are the most well-studied class of these agents, which include misonidazole, desmethylmisonidazole (DMM), etanidazole (SR-2508), and nimorazole. These agents appear to be toxic to hypoxic cells and may also sensitize cells to chemotherapeutic agents. Despite the encouraging preclinical data with these agents, few clinical trials to date have provided evidence of improved therapeutic index for radiation. A newer class of hypoxic cell sensitizers, which include tirapazamine and por-

firomycin, are presently under investigation. Preclinical studies demonstrated that these bioreductive alkylating drugs are preferentially toxic to hypoxic cells.[81] Early clinical results for use of these drugs plus radiation are encouraging.[82]

The modified nucleosides represent another large class of radiosensitizing drugs. Although these agents act via several mechanisms, they frequently sensitize cells to radiation by inhibiting the nucleoside synthesis machinery and by direct incorporation into newly synthesized strands of DNA, RNA, or both.[83] In the case of 5-fluorouracil, the radiosensitizing activity involves inhibition of thymidylate synthase and inappropriate progression of cells through S phase.[84] The actions of gemcitabine include an inhibition of ribonucleotide reductase with a resulting depletion in deoxyadenosine triphosphate pools.[85] Other examples of radiosensitizing nucleosides include fludarabine, bromodeoxyuridine, and iododeoxyuridine.

The majority of conventional chemotherapeutic drugs also sensitize cells to radiation, using mechanisms that are diverse and only partially understood. Combining cisplatin and other platinum analogs with radiation has enhanced radiation kill via numerous mechanisms. Radiation appears to increase the cellular uptake of platinum drugs[86] and increase the number of toxic platinum intermediates.[87] The level of kill from combined platinum and radiation may also be related to alterations in DNA repair and cell-cycle checkpoint functions. Hydroxyurea is a cytotoxic agent that preferentially kills cells in the most radioresistant phase of the cell cycle (S).[88] Conversely, paclitaxel is thought to synchronize tumor cells in G_2/M, which is a relatively radiosensitive phase. Other examples of chemotherapeutic agents that cooperate with radiation-induced cell killing include camptothecin compounds (topotecan, CPT-11), etoposide, doxorubicin, and dactinomycin. Classic studies showed that sublethal damage apparently is inhibited by dactinomycin but not by doxorubicin.[89] Strong evidence suggests that these drugs can and do modify radiation effects when given simultaneously. Furthermore, when given after radiation therapy, they can recall the irradiated volumes by erythema on the skin or by production of pulmonary reactions.

Free radical scavenger agents, such as sulfhydryl-containing compounds, act in the reverse fashion and tend to make cells more resistant.[90] They have also been shown to reduce chromosome abnormalities associated with radiation, which suggests a potential use in reducing treatment-induced cancers.[91] The thiol-containing drug amifostine (WR-2721) is the best-studied drug of this type. Randomized trials have shown that amifostine reduces treatment-related toxicities, including radiation-induced parotid damage (xerostomia)[92] and cisplatin-induced nephrotoxicity.[93] There is concern that thiol drugs might also protect tumor cells from the lethality of radiation treatment. Although no convincing evidence of tumor protection has been observed in the clinical trials to date, critics argue that these trials have been insufficiently powered to detect tumor protection if such effects do truly exist.

Another modality that can be considered a modulator of radiation is *hyperthermia*. Localized heat treatment can be delivered with external devices that produce microwave, ultrasonic, or radiofrequency energy. Cell culture–based assays have shown that temperatures above 41°C kill cells. In particular, the temperature 42.5°C appears to be critical; small increments in temperature above 42.5°C lead to steep increments in lethality.[94] This lethal effect is thought to result, at least in part, from the denaturation of proteins. In contrast to radiation-induced kill, lethality from heat is most pronounced when cells are in S phase.[95] Hyperthermia and radiation, when delivered simultaneously *in vitro*, have a greater than additive lethal effect.[96] This may result from heat-induced kill of the radioresistant S-phase cells or from denaturation of DNA repair proteins. In the clinical setting, however, the interaction between the two modalities appears to be only additive or independent. A number of randomized clinical trials have tested radiation with or without hyperthermia, and although some have shown a benefit to adding hyperthermia, others have not. One lingering limitation of hyperthermia is the technical difficulty of delivering homogeneous doses of heat to anatomically deep tissues. For this reason, treatment of melanoma and breast cancers remains among the most common applications.

IMPORTANCE OF HOST-DERIVED VASCULATURE AND ANGIOGENESIS IN RADIATION THERAPY

Historically, the DNA within tumor cells has been considered the principal target in radiation therapy. Newer research, however, has suggested that radiation-induced damage to blood vessels contributes significantly to both tumor control and normal tissue toxicity. Paris et al. studied normal tissue toxicity in mice after single doses of radiation. These data suggest that radiation preferentially damages the microvasculature of mouse intestines and that the adjacent epithelial cells within crypts subsequently die as a secondary event. Mice deficient in the sphingomyelinase gene were protected against this effect, which suggests that ceramide production within endothelial cells is involved in this mechanism.[97] In a subsequent study, xenograft tumors were induced in apoptosis-resistant mice (transgenic sphingomyelinase-deficient or Bax-deficient mice). Compared with tumors grown in wild-type mice, the tumors grew two to four times faster in the apoptosis-resistant host mice. After treatment with a single fraction of radiation, the tumors in apoptosis-resistant mice

exhibited reduced levels of endothelial apoptosis and progressive tumor growth.[98]

Tumor angiogenesis is now generally accepted as an important aspect of tumor formation and progression. Many inhibitors of angiogenesis have been developed as potential cancer treatments after the initial discoveries of angiostatin and endostatin by Michael O'Reilly and Judah Folkman.[99,100] Weichselbaum's group demonstrated that the combined treatment with angiostatin and radiation in a murine model containing human xenografts resulted in greater than additive antitumor effects (Fig. 13-12). Furthermore, histologic analysis of the treated tumors revealed a reduction in vascular density after this combined treatment.[101] A later study showed that concomitant radiation with angiogenesis inhibition was more effective than sequential treatment schedules.[102] This synergy may seem counterintuitive, because oxygen (and hence blood supply) is known to enhance the cellular kill induced by radiation. Surprisingly, however, several reports have shown that antiangiogenic agents actually elevate the intratumoral PO_2.[103,104] Therefore, the observed synergy may result from reoxygenation of tumor regions that were previously hypoxic. Alternatively, the synergy could simply represent a combination of radiation-induced and drug-induced blood vessel damage, which starves the tumor of oxygen and nutrients.

PHYSICAL ASPECTS OF RADIATION ONCOLOGY

Radiologic physics and dosimetry are the foundation for the physical aspects of radiotherapy.[105,106] The technologic developments for cancer treatment have built on basic physics principles of atomic and nuclear structure, electromagnetic and particle radiation, radioactivity and production of x-rays, interaction of radiation with matter, and determination of absorbed dose. The tissue interactions and dosimetric properties of radiation sources determine their suitability for given situations. To be useful for therapeutic treatment, ionizing radiation must penetrate sufficiently for adequate deposition of dose in targeted tissues. These basic principles are discussed in the context of two general types of treatment: (1) *teletherapy* (*tele* from New Latin meaning "at a distance"), also known as *external-beam therapy*, and (2) *brachytherapy* (*brachys* from Greek meaning "short"), which is usually administered with internal sources. The discussion in this section emphasizes the physical aspects of the production and delivery of commonly used therapeutic radiation sources.

CHARACTERISTICS OF SOURCES OF EXTERNAL-BEAM RADIATION

The first type of source used for external-beam irradiation was the x-ray machine. The x-ray source was a glass tube consisting of an *anode* (positive electrode) at one end and a *cathode* (negative electrode) at the other. The cathode is a filament that emits electrons when heated. When a high voltage is applied as a potential difference between the cathode and the anode, the electrons (which are negatively charged) accelerate toward the positive electrode and are stopped in a metallic target. X-rays are produced as the electrons collide with the metallic target, either via collisions with orbital electrons (forming *characteristic x-rays*) or when the electrons are decelerated by positively charged nuclei

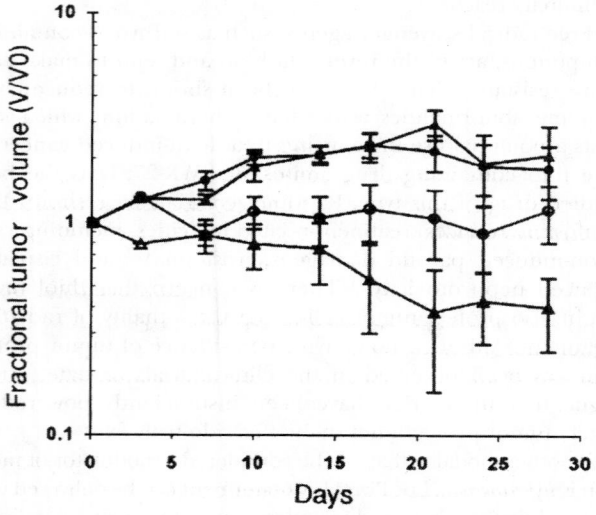

FIGURE 13-12. SQ-20B xenograft tumor growth in mice treated with combinations of human angiostatin and radiation. Filled triangles represent no treatment (controls); open circles represent treatment with radiation; filled circles represent treatment with angiostatin; open triangles represent treatment with angiostatin and radiation. (From ref. 101, with permission.)

A

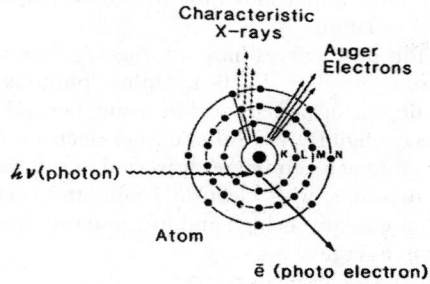

B

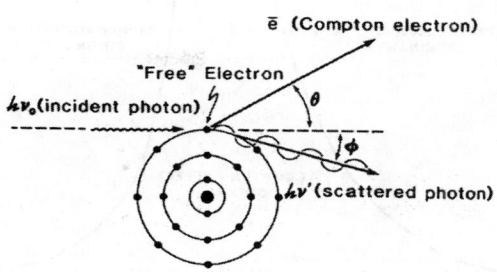

C

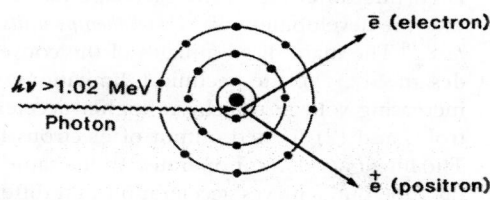

FIGURE 13-13. Diagram illustrating the photoelectric effect (**A**), Compton scatter effect (**B**), and pair production (**C**). (Adapted from ref. 7, with permission.)

within the target (*bremsstrahlung* effect). A *spectrum* of x-ray energies is produced, such that the maximum energy is equal to the energy of the incoming electrons. This energy is related to the applied tube voltage. For example, if 250 kVp (kilovoltage peak) is the applied voltage, the electrons from the cathode will reach the target with energy of 250 keV and produce x-rays with maximum energies of 250 kV.

X-rays are part of the electromagnetic spectrum, which also includes radio and television waves, radar, visible light, and ultraviolet radiation. X-rays have shorter wavelengths and higher frequencies than these other types of radiation, however, and as a result are more energetic. Consequently, x-rays exhibit the important properties of penetration and deposition of dose in matter.

ATTENUATION OF DOSE WITHIN BIOLOGIC MATERIAL

Attenuation is a combination of absorption and scatter of energy, which results from several types of physical interactions of x-rays with atoms.[107,108] The first is called the *photoelectric effect*, which is an absorption process shown schematically in Figure 13-13*A*. The incoming x-ray transfers all its energy to an inner-orbit electron, which is ejected from the atom. An outer-shell electron fills the vacant hole, which results in the production of a photon. This type of attenuation predominates when relatively low-energy photons collide with materials that have higher atomic numbers (like bone or metal). The second type of interaction is *Compton scattering* (see Fig. 13-13*B*), in which energy is both absorbed and scattered. The incoming photon interacts with a loosely bound electron in an atom's outer shell, knocking the electron out of the atom with part of the incoming energy. The photon emerges with reduced energy and a change in

direction, and either continues with further interactions or is transmitted without interaction. This type of interaction occurs with relatively higher-energy photons and depends much less on the atomic number of the material irradiated. The third interaction is called *pair production*, an absorption process (see Fig. 13-13*C*). The incoming photon interacts with the electric field of the nucleus, which depends on the atomic number of the material. An electron and a positive electron (positron) are produced, which then deposit energy through collisions with other electrons. Because the two particles created have a combined energy of 1.02 MeV, this interaction occurs only when incoming photons have energies of at least this threshold value. For photon energies above this threshold, the probability of pair production increases with increasing photon energy.

The relative probability of occurrence of these processes depends on (1) photon energy and (2) the atomic number of the irradiated material (Fig. 13-14). Because the photoelectric effect dominates in materials with higher atomic numbers and with low-energy photons, selective attenuation occurs in bone (Z = 11.6 to 13.8) as opposed to soft tissue (Z = 7.4).[108] With higher-energy photons (up to 10 MeV), the Compton effect dominates, and the dependence of attenuation on atomic number is much less. This explains why low-energy x-rays allow the contrast required for good diagnostic images (Fig. 13-15). From a therapeutic perspective, however, low-energy photons have the undesirable effect of greater dose deposition in bone than in soft tissue (or tumor).

DEPTH DOSE CHARACTERISTICS OF RADIATION

Low-energy x-rays in the diagnostic range are 20 to 120 kVp. Higher energies of 120 to 500 kVp are referred to as *orthovolt-*

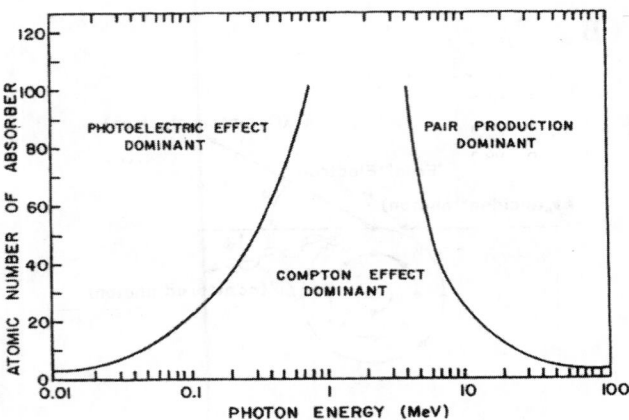

FIGURE 13-14. Relative contributions of the photoelectric, pair production, and Compton effects that occur as photons interact with tissue. (From ref. 8, with permission.)

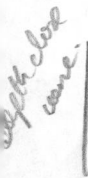

age. These higher-energy photons deposit dose deeper into tissue but still not deeply enough for centrally located tumors. Instead, the maximum dose is deposited close to the skin surface, with 90% of the maximum occurring at a depth of 2 cm and 50% or less at a depth of 10 cm. Accordingly, if dose is prescribed at a depth of 10 cm, then more than twice this dose will be given to the skin. This relative dose relationship between dose deposition and depth can be represented graphically by a *depth dose* curve. Figure 13-16A shows depth dose curves plotted for varying incident photon energies as they enter water.[109]

As discussed earlier in Biologic Aspects of Radiation Oncology, the deposition of dose within biologic materials results from the generation of secondary electrons. In the case of megavoltage photon energies, electrons are primarily set in forward motion by Compton interactions, which then penetrate deeper into tissue. Energy is deposited into tissue as these electrons slow down. The average distance that the electrons travel is called D_{max} (depth of maximum dose). This is the depth at which equal numbers of electrons are stopping and moving forward, termed *electronic equilibrium*. As the energy of the incident beam increases, the D_{max} increases. Higher values

of D_{max} allow for minimal deposition of dose at superficial depths (*skin sparing*) and increased dose at deeper depths (see Fig. 13-16A). Both of these characteristics of depth dose curves have critical implications for treatment planning in different clinical situations.

Depth dose curves have also been generated for beams of electrons (see Fig. 13-16B). Unlike photons, electrons have finite depths of penetration in tissue, beyond which absorbed dose is negligible. As a general rule, electrons deposit 2 MeV of energy for each centimeter traversed in soft tissue. Unlike with photon beams, with electron beams the surface doses (skin doses) are relatively high and increase with increasing incident electron energies.

EQUIPMENT FOR PRODUCING MEGAVOLTAGE PHOTONS AND ELECTRONS

High photon energies (megavoltage range) became available with the development of ^{60}Co *teletherapy units* and *linear accelerators*.[110] The main disadvantages of the conventional x-ray tube design are (1) the technical limitations to applying ever-increasing voltage to achieve higher acceleration of the electrons, and (2) limited output of electrons from the filament. The linear accelerator operates on the same principles as an x-ray tube but achieves acceleration in a different manner (Fig. 13-17). The electrons are emitted from a hot cathode (1000°C) and formed into a "pencil beam." This allows a large number of electrons to be accelerated and hence the resulting beam has a high intensity (or *dose rate*). The electrons then pass through a long tube composed of evacuated cavities, called a *waveguide* or *accelerating structure*. Within the accelerating structure an electric field (generated by microwave power) forms the electrons into bunches and accelerates them to 99% of the velocity of light. This increases their mass and penetration power. The electrons travel with the crest of the electric field wave as the field propagates in the cavities over time. Longer waveguides produce higher electron energies. As the energetic electrons exit the waveguide they reach the "head" of the machine, where they are redirected from a horizontal to a vertical position through a bending magnet and collide with a target. This thick metallic target absorbs most of the incident

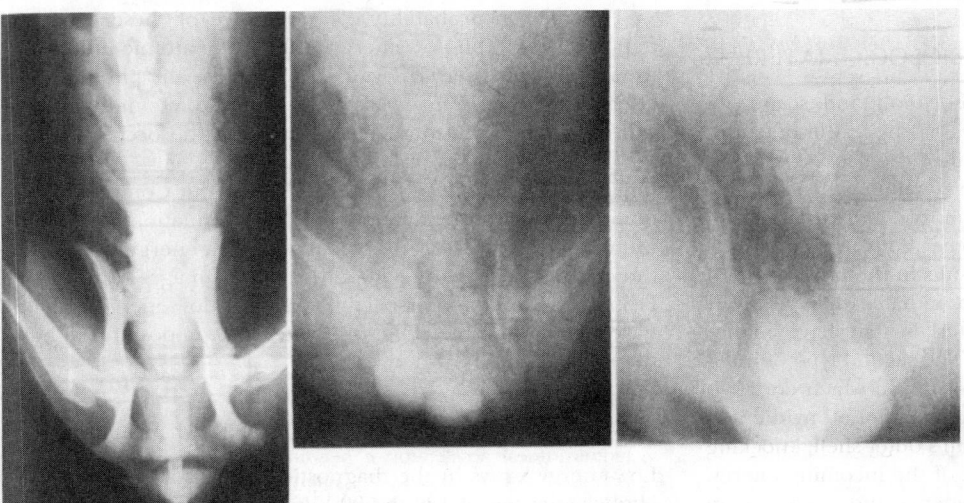

FIGURE 13-15. Radiographs taken at 70 kVp (kilovoltage peak), 250 kVp, and 1.25 MeV (cobalt 60), demonstrating the loss of radiographic contrast at higher photon energies. (From ref. 8, with permission.)

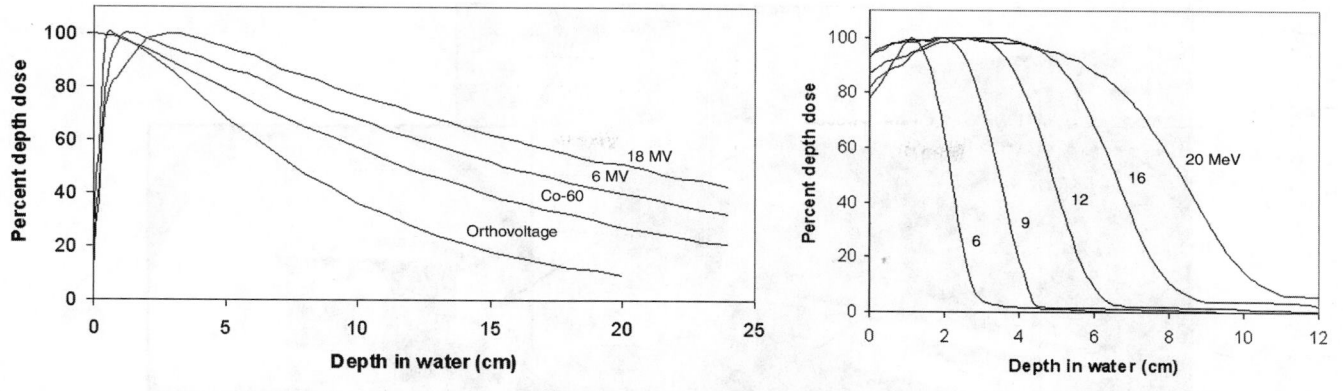

FIGURE 13-16. **A:** Depth dose curves for varying incident photon energies in water. **B:** Depth dose curves for a range of electron energies from 6 to 20 MeV.

electrons, and a resulting photon beam exits the target in the same direction as the incident electrons. These photon beams are more intense in the center than in the periphery of the beam, so a centrally thick filter is used to differentially absorb the photons or flatten the photon field. Next, the beam is shaped by large movable jaws (or *collimators*), which adjust the width and length of the beam (or *field size*). A *monitor chamber* measures the amount of radiation being produced by the machine and terminates the radiation when the desired dose is achieved. The machine head also contains other lead shielding to block radiation other than the intended beam. Furthermore, thick shielding lines the walls of the treatment room to protect patients and workers outside. The linear accelerator can also be operated in *electron mode* to produce beams of electrons, which are useful for treating tumors located close to the surface of the patient's body. In this mode, the pencil electron beam is spread over a wider area by allowing the beam to strike a scattering foil, thin enough so that x-ray production is kept to low levels. The linear accelerator design can reliably deliver photon beams with energies up to 25 MV, with good energy stability and high dose rates.

Modern linear accelerators are mounted as *gantries*, which allows them to be rotated 360 degrees in space around a treatment table (Fig. 13-18).[111] The focal point of the gantry's rotation is a point in space called the *isocenter*. This point is demarcated in the treatment room by red or green lasers mounted on the walls and ceiling, which intersect at the isocenter. Patients (or tumors) are aligned in the treatment room relative to the isocenter. This represents a basic but critically important step in treatment planning. As an illustrative example, consider a patient positioned on the table so that his tumor is located at the isocenter. The radiation beam can then be rotated around the tumor at preplanned angles. By aiming beams from multiple directions, one can create a region where beams overlap, resulting in a summation of dose in the tumor.

Photons with energies higher than 25 MV can be produced with a *racetrack microtron*. In this design, a linear accelerating structure is placed between two separated magnets. An accelerated electron beam takes oval orbits with 180-degree bends of increasing radii, which permits energy to be increased with each lap. The microtron has a compact design, and it requires a relatively low-power microwave source to produce electron energies up to 50 MeV.

The ^{60}Co teletherapy unit is a megavoltage machine that uses radioactive material as the photon source. The ^{60}Co is prepared by irradiating stable cobalt ^{59}Co with neutrons in a reactor. The ^{60}Co source decays to nickel 60 with the emission of a β-particle and two gamma rays of 1.17 and 1.33 MeV. The ^{60}Co sources used have high radiation activities, which lessen over time (see Physical Aspects of Brachytherapy, later in this chapter). Unlike radiation-generating machines, the ^{60}Co source is always on and must be kept in a shielded position until exposed for treatment purposes. ^{60}Co units are designed with beam collimation and isocentric gantries similar to those of linear accelerators.

PHYSICAL ASPECTS OF PROTONS AND NEUTRONS

Although photon and electron beams are the primary modalities in radiation oncology, two types of particle beams are also available. *Protons* can be produced by a *cyclotron, synchrocyclotron,* or *proton linear accelerator*. In a cyclotron charged particles are confined by two separated magnets to a circular orbit, are accelerated by an electric field in the gap between the magnets, and

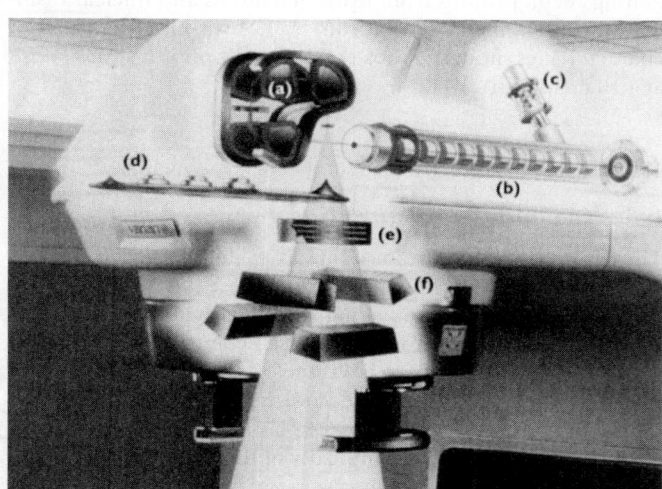

FIGURE 13-17. Schematic representation of the components within a modern linear accelerator: *a,* bending magnet; *b,* accelerating structure; *c,* energy switch; *d,* flattening filter, scattering foils; *e,* primary jaws; *f,* secondary jaws. (From ref. 110 and Varian Associates, with permission.)

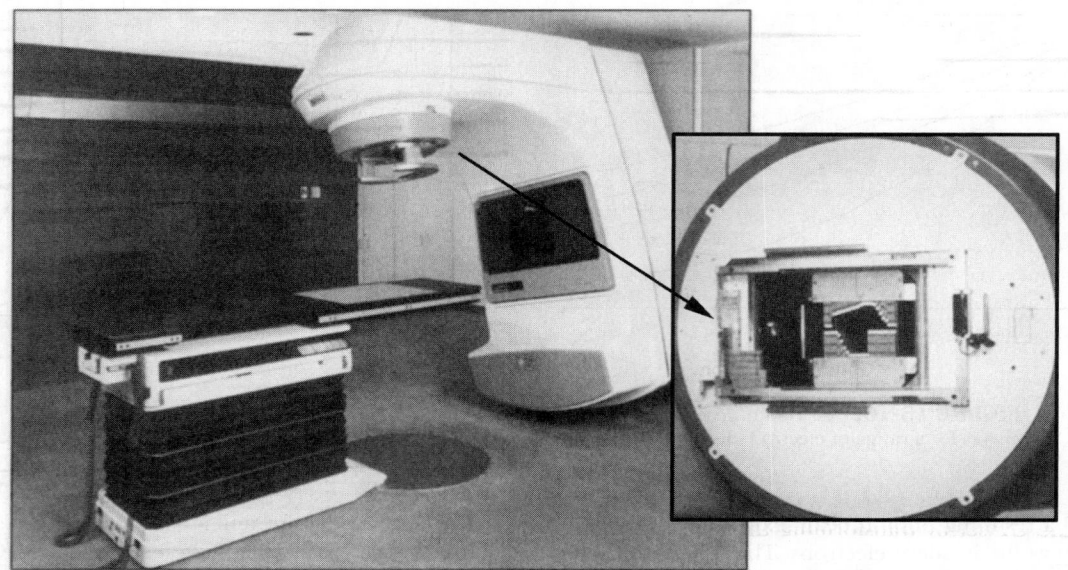

FIGURE 13-18.   Modern linear accelerator used for treatment and a view into the head (multileaf collimator) of the machine (*inset*).

are finally extracted at the desired energy. These positively charged particles deposit energy along a straight path in matter, with the rate of energy deposition constant with depth. At the end of the track, the rate of energy deposition rises sharply as the particle comes to a stop. This peak of dose deposition is called the *Bragg peak*. The energy of the proton beam can be modulated so that the Bragg peak occurs at a depth in tissue that corresponds to a tumor location. This is the primary physical advantage of protons over x-rays in cancer treatment. Proton beams in the energy range of 50 to 500 MeV have been used.

Neutron beams can be produced by accelerating a deuteron (a proton and a neutron) beam in a cyclotron. This beam collides with a target of low atomic number such as beryllium, which is converted into boron with a release of fast neutrons. Neutrons have no charge and interact in matter mainly by generating recoil protons from hydrogen atoms and nuclear disintegrations. High-energy neutrons (50 MeV) have penetration characteristics similar to those of 4 to 6 MV photons (63% dose at a 10 cm depth).

TREATMENT PLANNING

Imaging and Target Delineation

The ultimate goal of radiotherapy is to deliver a high dose to the target volume while minimizing dose to normal tissue. Advances in computers, imaging, and treatment machine technology has provided more sophisticated means to reach this goal. Planning and delivery is a multistep process that is patient specific. It consists of target and normal structure delineation, radiation beam design, delivery of planned treatment, and verification of delivery. The complexity of this process depends on the clinical objectives, which can range from simple (e.g., palliative treatments) to very complex (e.g., potentially curative treatments on a dose-escalation protocol).

The treatment planning phase is highly dependent on how target volumes and normal structures are determined for a given patient. If a target volume is defined so that it does not cover the full extent of disease, then geographic miss by the radiation beams will occur. If a defined target volume is too large and includes surrounding normal tissue, then the probability of complications increases. Consequently, a carefully constructed tumor target volume is the crucial first step in the treatment process. To encourage systematic target volume definition on an international basis, the International Commission on Radiation Units and Measurements (ICRU) published nomenclature and guidelines.[112,113] For tumor target volume delineation, several concentric volumes were described. First, the extent of the malignant tumor that is visible on imaging studies, including any involved nodes, is called the *gross tumor volume* (GTV). Next, a margin around the GTV is added to account for potential locoregional subclinical extension and is called the *clinical target volume* (CTV). The GTV and the CTV are based solely on anatomic and biologic considerations. The final volume is the *planning target volume* (PTV). This volumetric expansion accounts for the uncertainties in the geographic position of the CTV from day to day. Specifically, an internal margin is added to compensate for physiologic changes in the size, shape, and position of internal anatomy. An additional margin is added to account for patient movement (e.g., breathing) and differences in patient positioning from day to day (*setup uncertainty*).

Next, beams are designed to cover target volumes and avoid normal structures. The simplest method for localization of patient anatomy involves the use of the x-ray *simulator*. This machine has the same geometric features as a linear accelerator (identical isocentric gantry design and position of treatment table) but has a diagnostic x-ray generator in the head of the machine. It generates two-dimensional radiographs that visualize the intended anatomic area of treatment, primarily using bony landmarks to approximate the location of target volumes. The main limitation of the simulator is its lack of fine soft tissue detail and the lack of three-dimensional image acquisition. Computed tomography (CT) can image both soft tissue and bone for volume delineation (diagnostic imaging technologies are discussed in detail elsewhere in this book). Axial images are usually acquired with thin slices through the target area, and the scanned volume must encompass normal adjacent structures (e.g., lungs, kidneys). Computers are later used to reconstruct this data into a three-dimensional display of target volumes relative to normal anatomy.

It is now commonplace to use CT to obtain anatomic information for volume definition, but defining tumor as opposed to normal surrounding lung and soft tissue with CT is not always straightforward, even with the use of contrast agents during scanning. Imaging with magnetic resonance imaging (MRI) is also commonly used to delineate target volumes for some anatomic sites, because it has superior soft tissue resolution (particularly in brain, sarcoma, and prostate cases). In the prostate, for example, MRI can better differentiate between the gland and the surrounding muscle. MRI is generally not used by itself for treatment planning because of imaging distortion and dose calculation issues. For this reason, the MRI information must be correlated with CT scans through the use of image registration software. Image data in the MRI set is aligned with the CT set by transforming the MRI coordinate system to match that of the CT. Several types of algorithms exist to achieve this transformation. For example, anatomic landmarks can be identified in each data set and be used to tie the two images together. A more complex registration method uses the entire volume of image data (i.e., intensities of the image voxels) for matching. Once the different image series are registered, image fusion software is used to display the two modalities simultaneously.

After imaging data have been generated for a given patient, the radiation oncologist and other treatment planning personnel must define target volumes and normal anatomic structures. This is largely a manual process in which each structure is circled (or contoured) on individual axial images using image display work stations. The contouring process segments the image data into separate structures, each uniquely identified. Semiautomated algorithms are available that will contour structures that have the same density, which allows rapid definition of an entire three-dimensional region. For example, lungs have one-third of the density of soft tissue and can be easily distinguished from surrounding tissue. Surfaces for each structure are generated from the segmented contours and can be viewed in any plane that can be generated through the surface. For instance, prostate, rectal, and bladder volumes are shown in axial, coronal, and sagittal planes in Figure 13-19, which will be useful during treatment beam design. Anatomy can also be viewed and manipulated in three dimensions with software programs.

Often, it is difficult to identify tumor volumes based solely on anatomic imaging such as CT and MRI. As discussed earlier, the CTV is intended to include microscopic extensions of disease beyond the gross tumor. Imaging with functional information will aid in defining these volumes. Of the many types of functional imaging available, the most commonly used is positron emission tomography. Positron-emitting isotopes (carbon 11, nitrogen 13, oxygen 15) can be inserted into labeling compounds that are metabolically active to yield direct imaging studies of metabolism. When the positron annihilates with an electron in a patient, a pair of 511-keV photons are emitted traveling in opposite directions and are detected simultaneously by a ring of scintillation detectors. The distribution of the radioactivity can be represented as serial two-dimensional tomographic images. In general, the positron emission in

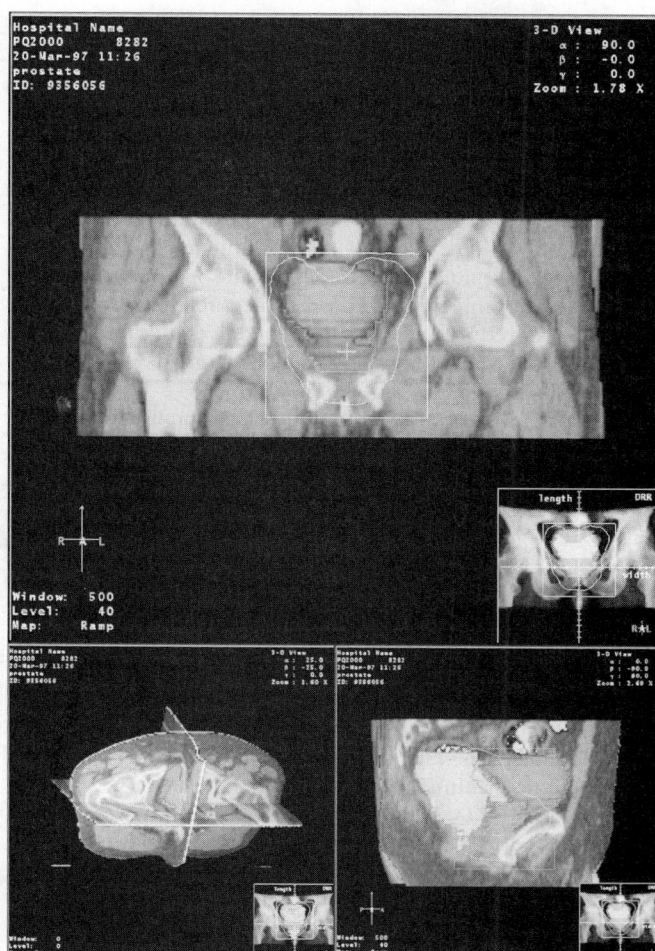

FIGURE 13-19. Prostate, rectal, and bladder volumes shown on computed tomographic slices in coronal plane (*upper panel*), three orthogonal planes with axial orientation (*lower left panel*), and sagittal plane (*lower right panel*). The beam's eye view (BEV) tool is shown in the lower right of each panel, with the beam shaped to expose the planning target volume to radiation but block the surrounding normal tissues. The BEV is overlaid on the digitally reconstructed radiograph. (Generated with a Philips AcQsim VoxelQ.) (See Color Fig. 13-19 in the CD-ROM.)

positron emission tomography images is considered to have more quantitative information than the photon emission in single photon emission CT, which relies on decaying radioisotopes. On the other hand, the variety of tracers available for single photon emission CT is larger, and single photon emission CT scanners are more widely available. Much like MRI scans, scans obtained using these functional imaging modalities can be directly correlated with CT scans using registration software.

Immobilization and Coordinate System

Imaging studies used for treatment planning must be performed with the patient in the *treatment position*. Before any imaging studies are done, the patient must be placed on the support couch in a position that can be easily reproduced during treatment setup. For nearly all patients, immobilization devices are used to help duplicate the same position on each

MLC

day of treatment. The simplest devices are standard head and knee pillows made of high-density foam. More commonly, custom devices are made to fit individual patients. Sheets of plastic made pliable with heat (called thermoplastic sheets) or quick-drying plaster bandages can be used to form a mask around the patient's head and neck area. Custom foam cradles are used for immobilization of thorax, pelvis, and extremities. A foam mixture is used to fill the space between a Styrofoam form and the patient, to conform the cradle to the body shape. These devices are attached with pegs to the treatment table, so that the positioning is very reproducible. Well-made immobilization devices reduce the magnitude of daily setup uncertainty. This, in turn, permits the use of smaller margins when the PTV is designed.

A consistent coordinate system must be established between the imaging studies and the treatment machine. This is accomplished through the use of an alignment system common to the simulator, CT scanner, and treatment rooms. Wall-mounted lasers project lines in three planes (axial, sagittal, and coronal) and intersect at the isocenter. In a conventional simulator or CT simulator (a CT scanner with a laser system and localization software), the patient is aligned so that the approximate center of the tumor is positioned at the isocenter. The intersection of the lasers with the patient's skin surface is then marked in the simulator. These reference marks are used to realign the patient when the patient returns for daily treatments.

At the time of the imaging, tumor motion due to respiration may also be determined. This can, in turn, help define the margin required for PTV delineation. On a conventional simulator, the tumor motion, diaphragm motion, or both can be observed with fluoroscopy. If a CT simulator is used, CT images may be acquired during different phases of the respiratory cycle (i.e., at maximum inhalation and exhalation positions). The observed tumor or organ motion can be accounted for in the treatment design. Alternatively, breath-control devices can be used to momentarily stop breathing at a chosen point of the respiratory cycle and a CT scan be performed. The patient is then treated with the device at the same respiration point.[114]

Beam Design and Dose Calculation

The next step in the treatment process is the design of radiation beam aperture. In the simplest case, the radiation field borders can be set in a rectangular fashion using radiographs generated by a conventional simulator. The shape of beams can be customized using shaped metallic blocks, which are placed in the head of the machine to block unwanted portions of the beam. With more complex treatments, the beam apertures are designed using three-dimensional treatment planning software, in a process called *virtual simulation*. Beam directions must be selected, and this is aided by the use of the beam's eye view tool. Target and normal structures can be viewed from different directions in planes perpendicular to the beam's central axis using the beam's eye view tool. Structures are distinguished from each other by the use of different colors. Manipulation of the beam direction can create separation of the tumor structure from normal volumes and will result in desirable treatment angles. The beam shape is modified by designing a block that will allow full dose to the PTV but minimal dose to surrounding normal tissue. Blocks consist of heavy material mounted on a tray that is placed in the head of the

machine, or a block substitute called a *multileaf collimator*. The multileaf collimator consists of a number of small leaves that move independently of each other to form the planned shape. The multileaf collimator is contained in the head of the machine and is shown in Figure 13-18.

Once beams are designed and optimized, dose calculations are performed. Because it is not possible to measure a three-dimensional dose distribution in each patient, a general dose calculation system must be used to predict the dose in the patient. These calculations incorporate basic dosimetric data, such as depth dose curves and isodose information. Computerized algorithms have been developed to calculate the dose distributions generated by more complicated combinations of beams using patient-specific information such as depth of the calculation point, external body shape, and varying densities of anatomic structures. Dose distributions are generally displayed with concentric curves that denote particular doses, termed *isodose curves*, which are overlaid on anatomic diagrams. These curves are often normalized to a reference dose, which is generally either the dose at isocenter or the lowest isodose curve that completely surrounds the PTV. All isodose curves are then reported as a percentage of this reference dose.

Treatment plans often use arrangements of multiple beams to concentrate the high isodose region at the isocenter and in the tumor target volume, to cover target volumes and avoid normal tissue. A practical example is shown in Figure 13-20. Two opposed beams produce a more uniform dose distribution throughout the volume than does a single beam. When four beams are used, the dose to normal tissues can be further reduced. When custom beams generated with planning software are used, the resulting plan shows further improvements in isodose distributions. An ideal treatment plan is both *conformal* (i.e., high isodoses wrap closely around the PTV) and *homogeneous* (i.e., there is little variability of dose within the PTV). It is often challenging to simultaneously optimize these two dosimetric features, because improvements in one feature often worsen the other. A set of criteria for normal tissue tolerances must be given to guide the treatment planner. The computerized treatment plan can be evaluated with regard to whether it meets the objectives of target coverage and normal tissue avoidance. Isodoses can be viewed in axial, sagittal, and coronal planes, and isodose surfaces can be viewed relative to three-dimensional anatomy. These dose distributions in three-dimensional volumes can be displayed graphically with *dose-volume histograms* in which a different curve is generated for each structure (GTV, CTV, PTV, and each normal organ). The dose-volume histogram is a plot of the volume of a given structure receiving a certain dose (Fig. 13-21). As with isodose curves, the data displayed in dose-volume histograms are usually reported as a percentage of the reference dose. Therefore, the *absolute doses* received by these organs depend on how much dose is prescribed to cover the PTV. If the treatment plan does not meet its objectives, beam arrangements or other parameters must be adjusted. Such adjustments can include a change of beam energy, beam angle, or beam intensity. Normally the beam intensity is relatively uniform across the beam width and length. The simplest modification of the intensity is the use of a wedge-shaped filter (or *wedge*) placed in the machine head. A more complex method is to break the field aperture into segments with varying beam-on times. Currently the most intricate form of intensity modulation achieves a

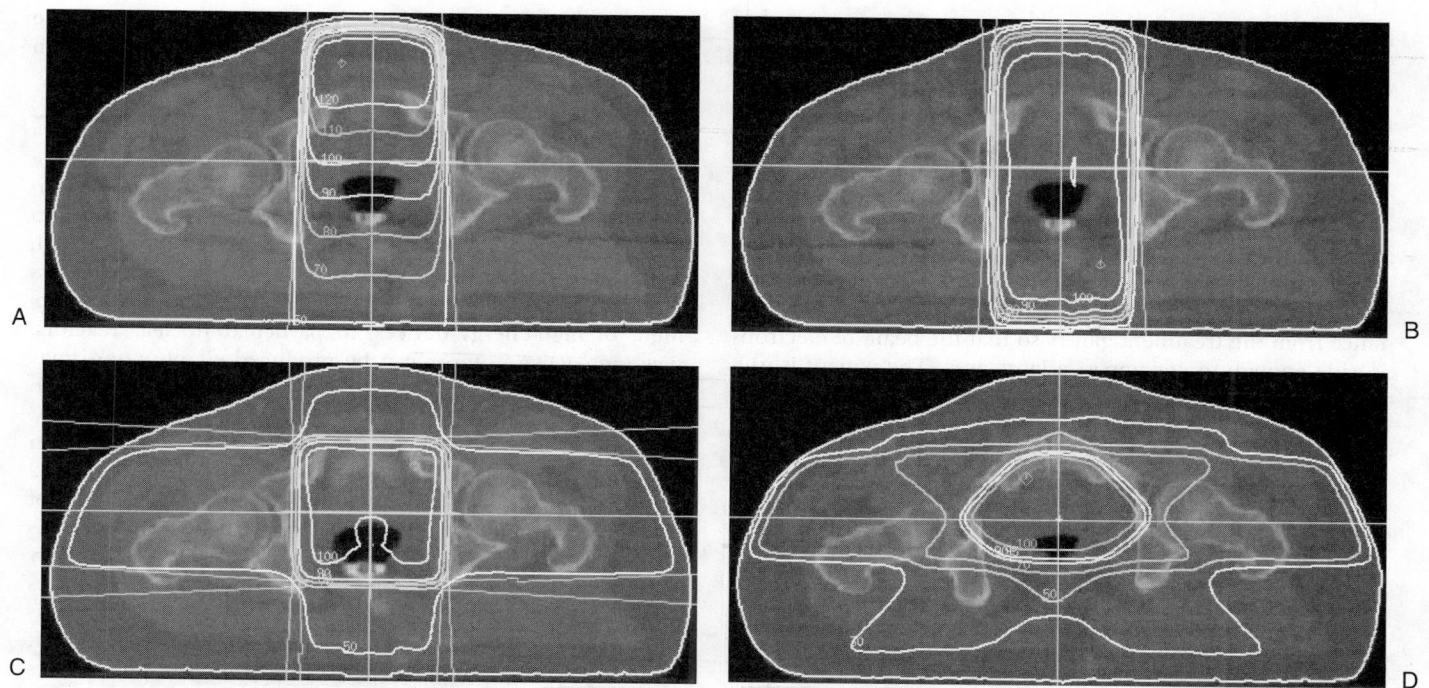

FIGURE 13-20. Sample isodose curves overlaid on an axial pelvic computed tomographic image, demonstrating dose distributions achieved using a single photon beam (**A**), two parallel opposed beams (**B**), a "four-field box" arrangement (**C**), and a six-field conformal beam arrangement (**D**). (See Color Fig. 13-20 in the CD-ROM.)

checkerboard pattern in which each square is a different intensity. This type of pattern is delivered by using a compensator or by moving the multileaf collimator under computer control. This is called *intensity-modulated radiotherapy*,[115] and this technique potentially allows a high degree of control over the shaping of the dose distribution. Because the intensity pattern is so complex, a different type of computerized treatment planning is used, called inverse planning. The treatment planner defines the dose to be delivered to a target volume, the acceptable dose to the surrounding normal tissues, and beam angles. The computer determines the corresponding intensity profiles to achieve the desired dose distribution.

Once final beam angles are chosen, x-ray images called *digitally reconstructed radiographs* are generated from the treatment planning CT in the beam's eye view plane (see Fig. 13-19). These are compared with portal images taken before treatment, which are either films placed in the beam that is exiting the patient or images made with an electronic portal device that uses fluoroscopy or ionization chamber arrays. The majority of linear accelerators are computer controlled, and often treatment beam parameters are transferred directly from the computer planning system to the computer operating the accelerator. Such a system is called a *record and verify system*. The patient must be properly positioned on the treatment table, but several sources of random and systematic errors do exist. Verification of the radiation beam placement is performed before treatment so that patient position can be adjusted accordingly. Beam delivery is carried out with the use of beam modifiers such as blocks, multileaf collimators, wedges, compensators, or intensity-modulated radiotherapy systems.

OTHER EXTERNAL-BEAM MODALITIES

Stereotactic radiosurgery is a single-day procedure for treating small intracranial lesions. The technique requires a metallic frame that is rigidly attached to the patient's head, providing a fixed coordinate system for treatment planning and delivery. The patient undergoes a CT scan with the head frame in place, and three-dimensional treatment planning is performed shortly thereafter. A number of small beams are designed to create a highly conformal treatment plan with very small margins. Because of the stereotactic ring apparatus, beam delivery has millimeter accuracy. The treatment is delivered as a single large fraction (15 to 20 Gy).

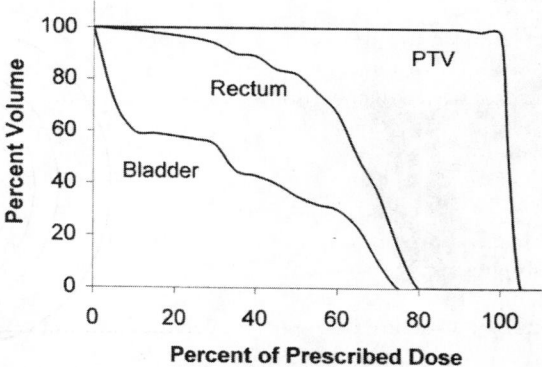

FIGURE 13-21. Sample dose-volume histogram reporting the dose distribution within different anatomic structures in a prostate cancer treatment plan. PTV, planning target volume.

Total body irradiation and *total skin electron irradiation* are two techniques for treating relatively large anatomic regions. Total body irradiation uses lower-energy megavoltage beams (6 MV) at an extended distance from the treatment gantry to achieve low dose rates of 5 to 10 cGy/min. Special tables and stands are often used to support the patient during treatment. These also enable special blocks to be placed to reduce dose to certain organs, such as the lungs. Total skin electron irradiation is performed with low-energy electrons (6 to 9 MeV) to treat superficial skin lesions that cover large areas of the body. As with total body irradiation, treatment is carried out at an extended distance from the treatment gantry so that the beam of electrons is wide enough to encompass a large area. The patient is usually repositioned several times during each treatment to ensure uniform dose coverage of all skin surfaces.

PHYSICAL ASPECTS OF BRACHYTHERAPY

Brachytherapy is radiation treatment delivered from close range to tumors that can be accessed by interstitial, intracavitary, or surface applicators. Inserted into the applicators are sources of radioactive material encapsulated in cylinder or seed form. Radioactive materials are unstable isotopes that return to a stable state by spontaneous emission of energetic particles or photons, or both, by a process called *decay* or *disintegration*. Relative to external-beam energies, the emitted spectra are of low energy. High doses can be delivered within a few centimeters of the source. With increasing distances away from the source, the absorbed dose drops off in inverse proportion to the distance squared (known as the inverse square law). The number of radioactive atoms decreases over time, which is quantified by the *activity* of the source (measured in becquerels, or disintegrations per second). The *half-life* is the time required for half of the initial number of nuclei to decay. The intensity of a radioactive source is commonly specified in terms of dose in air at 1 m from the source, called *air kerma rate* (measured in grays per second at 1 m per Bq).

The suitability of an isotope for a particular brachytherapy procedure depends mainly on the energy, half-life, air kerma rate, and other factors such as availability and radiation safety. The first radioisotope used for brachytherapy was the naturally

occurring radium 226 (^{226}Ra). ^{226}Ra eventually decays to stable lead, producing more than 40 gamma energies ranging from 0.184 to 2.45 MeV. The average energy is 0.83 MeV, which provides good penetration for large tumors. The other advantage of radium sources is the half-life of 1600 years, which ensures a good supply of activity for an extended period of time. The main disadvantage of the use of ^{226}Ra is that radon gas is generated during the decay process. Leakage of radon gas from a broken seal on a source container can be a significant hazard. Artificially produced sources that are equally effective but less hazardous than ^{226}Ra have become available. With the development of high-energy devices, in particular nuclear reactors, new radioactive isotopes can be produced. Stable nuclei may be transformed into radioactive species by bombardment with suitable particles or photons of sufficiently high energy. Cesium 137 (^{137}Cs) is a radioisotope produced by fission in nuclear reactors. It emits a gamma ray with energy of 0.662 MeV. ^{137}Cs has a long half-life of 30 years, with a decay rate of 2% per year. Radioisotopes with longer half-lives such as ^{137}Cs are suitable for temporary implants because a source inventory with high activities can be maintained for years, which makes reuse feasible. Another isotope used for temporary implants is iridium 192 (^{192}Ir). With an average energy of 0.38 MeV, it requires less shielding for personnel protection than does ^{137}Cs. ^{192}Ir has a short half-life of 74 days, a disadvantage because sources are useful only for several weeks. However, most temporary implantations last for 3 to 10 days, and ^{192}Ir source activity will vary by only a few percent during the implant time. Isotopes with properties of very short half-lives and low energy are used for permanent implants. Iodine 125 (^{125}I) emits characteristic x-rays in the range of 27 to 35 keV. Because of the low photon energy, little shielding is required for protection of workers before implantation and for family members after implantation. Palladium 103 (^{103}Pd) has a lower x-ray energy of 20 to 23 keV, but a much shorter half-life (17 days) than ^{125}I (59.4 days). Because of the shorter half-life, ^{103}Pd delivers the dose at a faster rate than ^{125}I.

The dose distribution around a hypothetical point source of radioactive material is isotropic; that is, it has a symmetric emission in all directions. Actual brachytherapy sources are not simply points in space, however, and instead can measure up to

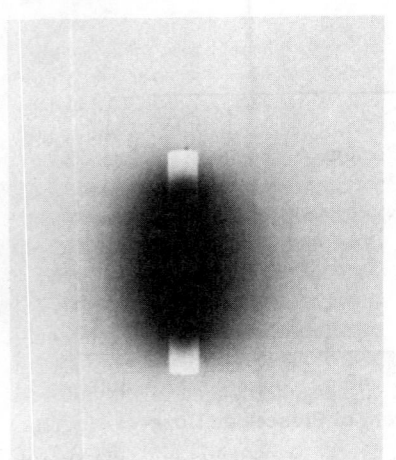

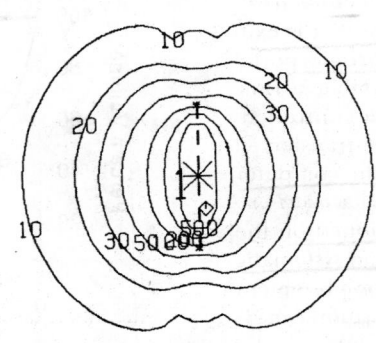

A   **B**

FIGURE 13-22. Autoradiograph demonstrating the asymmetric distribution of radiation (anisotropy) emitted from cesium 137 brachytherapy sources **(A).** This distribution is also shown graphically in the form of isodose curves **(B).** (From ref. 107, with permission.)

several centimeters. Furthermore, brachytherapy sources are encased in metal, often steel. These factors result in some asymmetry of emission (*anisotropy*), particularly at the ends of the sources (Fig. 13-22).[116]

The planning of brachytherapy implantation uses established rules based on clinical experience, including the Manchester system, Quimby method, Paris method, and nomograms developed at Memorial Sloan-Kettering Cancer Center. Computer calculations are also available that can optimize source positions and strengths using trial-and-error methods. For postimplantation dosimetry, x-ray films taken in two orthogonal directions are used to localize the sources (which are metal) and reference points. Dose is prescribed by overlaying the calculated radiation distributions on the x-ray films. In this method, the target size, shape, and location are approximated. Standard reference points are often used for dose prescription (e.g., *point A* in gynecologic applications). Doses are also calculated for normal organs, based on anatomic landmarks or objects with contrast (e.g., rectal tube or Foley balloon). Generally, a limited number of points is calculated and may not reflect the highest dose for that organ.

CT-based treatment planning is now often used in brachytherapy planning. Anatomy can be modeled in three dimensions, as previously described for external-beam planning in Treatment Planning. Normal organs and target volumes can be visualized in relation to applicator and source location. Preimplant planning is routinely facilitated by the use of axial imaging, for example, in transperineal prostate implantations.

CLINICAL ASPECTS OF RADIATION ONCOLOGY

TISSUE EFFECTS FROM RADIATION

Radiation effects in tissue are commonly categorized into one of two types, *early* or *late effects.* Early (or acute) effects typically occur within weeks after irradiation. They often occur in tissues that have rapid cell turnover, and these effects are thought to result from the depletion of the clonogenic or stem cells within that tissue. Examples include the shrinkage of malignant tumors, skin irritation and desquamation, and loss of hematopoietic tissue within irradiated bones. Late effects, on the other hand, occur months to years after irradiation. Examples of late effects include radiation-induced nerve injury, renal failure, bowel obstruction or perforation, and fibrosis. The frequencies of late effects depend very strongly on radiation fraction size (i.e., there are fewer late effects with smaller fraction sizes).

As discussed earlier in Cellular Dose Response to Radiation, dose response to radiation can be described by the linear quadratic formula $S = e^{-(\alpha D + \beta D^2)}$, where S represents survival and D represents dose. The α/β ratio represents the dose at which the quadratic (β) and linear (α) components of cell kill are equivalent. In other words, a cell type with a large α/β ratio has a large shoulder in the low-dose portion of its kill curve, even though it may be relatively sensitive to high radiation doses. As demonstrated in Figure 13-23, this survival advantage is considerably less significant or absent after treatment with high-LET radiation sources such as neutrons.[117] The α/β ratios for various tumors and normal tissues have been determined, and these are commonly used to describe dose-response character-

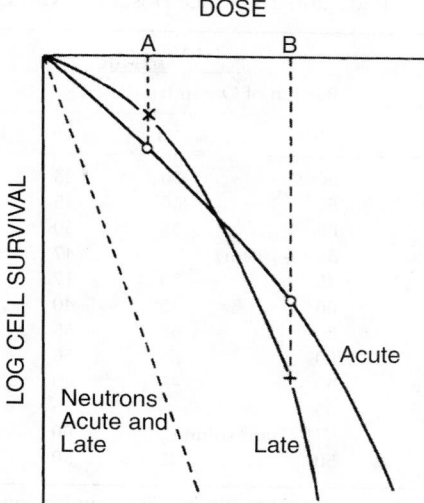

FIGURE 13-23. Hypothetical survival curves for clonogenic cells located within an early (acute)-responding tissue and a late-responding tissue. Small fractions of photon radiation (dose A) result in a survival advantage favoring late-responding tissues. With larger fraction sizes, this advantage is lost or even reversed (dose B). This differential effect is lost with high-linear-energy-transfer radiation sources like neutrons. (From ref. 117, with permission.)

istics. Typical human tumors and early-responding normal tissues (e.g., skin, small bowel, testis, bone marrow) have large α/β ratios (9 to 13 Gy), whereas late-responding tissues (e.g., brain, kidney, lung, bladder, liver, bone) have relatively small α/β ratios (1 to 5 Gy). Based on this model, an isoeffect formula was developed by Withers and coworkers[118]:

$$\frac{D_1}{D_{ref}} = \frac{\alpha/\beta + d_{ref}}{\alpha/\beta + d_1}$$

The symbols D_{ref} and d_{ref} represent a reference total dose and reference fraction size, respectively. Using the known α/β ratio for a given tissue type, the "biologically equivalent" total dose (D_1) can be calculated for different fraction sizes (d_1).

Late complications after fractionated radiotherapy have been well studied by many researchers. Radiation tolerance doses (TDs) for normal tissues are commonly reported as TD 5/5 (the average dose that results in a 5% complication risk within 5 years) or TD 50/5 (the average dose that results in a 50% complication risk within 5 years). The probability of developing late complications depends on many factors including fraction size, tissue type, total radiation dose, and the portion of an organ that receives radiation. In 1991, Emami and coworkers carried out an extensive literature search and reported average TDs for a variety of normal organs (Table 13-1).[119]

An anatomic-physiologic factor that affects the probability of normal tissue complications is the organization of functional subunits within a particular organ. Some organs—the small bowel, for example—can be thought of as a collection of serially arranged subunits. In this situation, a radiation-induced complication of one segment (e.g., bowel stricture) will result in an insult that affects the entire organ, and hence the patient. Other organs can be thought of as collections of subunits arranged in parallel. The kidney is an example of tissue

TABLE 13-1. Radiation Tolerance Doses for Normal Tissues

| | TD 5/5 (Gy) | | | TD 50/5 (Gy) | | | |
| | Portion of Organ Irradiated | | | Portion of Organ Irradiated | | | |
	$^1/_3$	$^2/_3$	$^3/_3$	$^1/_3$	$^2/_3$	$^3/_3$	Complication End Point(s)
Kidney	50	30	23	—	40	28	Nephritis
Brain	60	50	45	75	65	60	Necrosis, infarct
Brainstem	60	53	50	—	—	65	Necrosis, infarct
Spinal cord	50 (5–10 cm)	—	47 (20 cm)	70 (5–10 cm)	—	—	Myelitis, necrosis
Lung	45	30	17.5	65	40	24.5	Radiation pneumonitis
Heart	60	45	40	70	55	50	Pericarditis
Esophagus	60	58	55	72	70	68	Stricture, perforation
Stomach	60	55	50	70	67	65	Ulceration, perforation
Small intestine	50	—	40	60	—	55	Obstruction, perforation, fistula
Colon	55	—	45	65	—	55	Obstruction, perforation, fistula, ulceration
Rectum	(100 cm³ volume)		60	(100 cm³ volume)		80	Severe proctitis, necrosis, fistula
Liver	50	35	30	55	45	40	Liver failure

TD 5/5, the average dose that results in a 5% complication risk with 5 years; TD 50/5, the average dose that results in a 50% complication risk within 5 years.
(Adapted from ref. 119, with permission.)

organized in parallel, so that each subunit operates independently of other subunits. Consequently, radiation that inactivates only a portion of one kidney results in minimal, if any, adverse signs or symptoms.

PRINCIPLES UNDERLYING FRACTIONATION

A standard course of radiotherapy consists of multiple daily radiation fractions over weeks or months, with each fraction consisting of a relatively small dose (1.2 to 3.0 Gy). Such *fractionated* dose schedules appear to amplify the small survival advantage observed between normal organs and tumors when relatively small fraction sizes are used (see Fig. 13-23). This proposed survival difference in the shoulder of the survival curves, albeit small, becomes expanded when a dose of radiation is spread out over multiple smaller fractions (Fig. 13-24B). The basis for this effect is thought to result from four independent factors that occur dur-

ing the course of treatment: sublethal damage repair, redistribution of cell cycle, reoxygenation of tumors, and repopulation of cells in tissue.

1. Repair: A proposed explanation for the shoulder of radiation survival curves is that cells can repair some of the radiation damage, particularly the damage incurred with low doses of radiation. This radiobiologic concept is termed *sublethal damage repair*. Early studies by Elkind and Sutton helped to characterize this shoulder.[120] Their results showed that, if a dose of radiation is divided into two fractions separated by a few hours, the shoulder effect is seen with both fractions. Therefore, two or more fractions of radiation separated in time are less lethal than the same total dose given as a single dose (as demonstrated in Fig. 13-24A). The majority of sublethal damage repair occurs within 6 hours after irradiation.

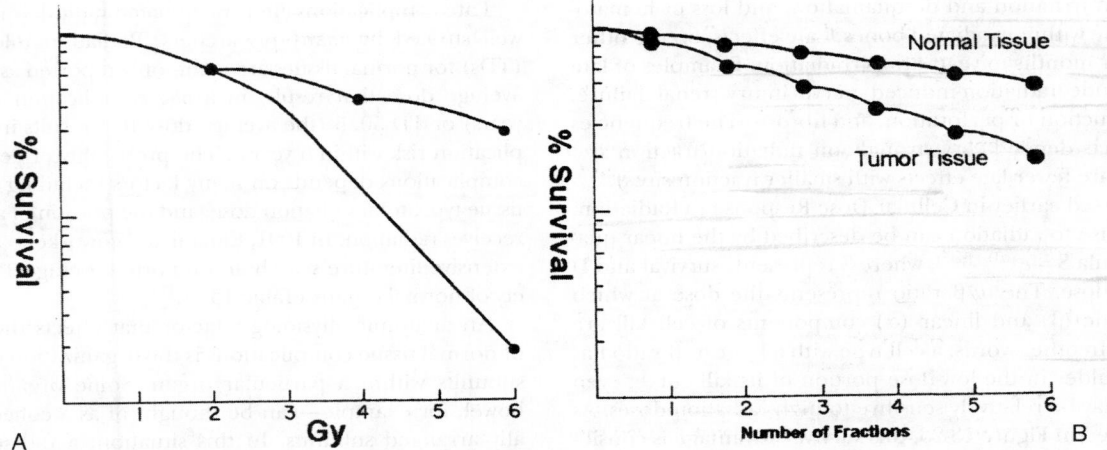

FIGURE 13-24. **A:** Idealized survival curve for 6-Gy radiation dose, delivered either in a single fraction or in daily fractions of 2 Gy. **B:** Idealized survival curve for fractionated course, comparing the survival of clonogens within either normal tissue or tumor tissue. The small differential in survival becomes amplified as the number of fractions increases.

2. Redistribution: Cells have a variable radiation response that depends on position within the cell cycle. The mitotic phase (M) is most sensitive and G_2 is almost as sensitive. G_1 is relatively sensitive in cells with a short G_1 phase. Cells gradually increase in resistance as they proceed through the late G_1 and S phases, reaching a maximum of resistance in the late S phase. In cells with a long G_1 phase, a peak of resistance is seen early in G_1. The clinical consequences of differential fractional survival after 2 Gy can be significant over a long course of fractionated therapy, because small differences in fractional survival, when repeated, have profound consequences in overall cumulative cell killing. A second consequence of differential cell killing and the mitotic delay induced by radiation is a tendency to partially synchronize the cells. The timing of the second dose of a fractionated scheme may be critical. This synchronization is short-lived because cells desynchronize rapidly and redistribute themselves according to the original cell age distribution. This phenomenon, which could present a clinical problem or a clinical advantage, does not seem to be important unless an incomplete redistribution between fractions exists.

3. Repopulation: During a course of fractionated radiation, the ultimate response of the tumor and normal tissue depends on whether cell proliferation has taken place between the fractions and thereby increased the number of cells exposed to radiation. This cell increase may be caused by cell proliferation within the irradiated volume (i.e., within the tumor or normal cell renewal tissue) or by migration of cells from unirradiated adjacent areas, as in seen in the skin and oral gastrointestinal mucosa, or from great distances, as found with bone marrow and lymph node repopulation. The balance between radiation-induced cell killing and repopulation is responsible for much of the clinical findings seen during fractionated radiotherapy treatment.[121] In addition to spontaneous repopulation, an induced cell proliferation, or recruitment of cells, may take place.[122,123] Physiologically, many tissues of the body respond to trauma by being recruited into rapid proliferation (e.g., after a wound in the skin, a break in bone, or a partial hepatectomy). The reparative process requires proliferation of the undamaged cells. Similarly, when the oral mucosa is irradiated, strong evidence indicates that the cell-cycle time is decreased and that net cell proliferation increases. This also may occur in some tumors but appears to be of less magnitude than in normal tissues.[124] Part of the differential effect of fractionated radiation may lie in differential recruitment of normal versus tumor cells. Finally, a phenomenon called *accelerated repopulation* can occur within the irradiated population of tumor cells, in which tumors regrow more rapidly after a sublethal dose of radiation.[125]

4. Reoxygenation: Thomlinson and Gray[126] recognized the importance of the oxygen effect in a classic paper in which they showed that tumors from humans frequently had anoxic regions. Calculations of oxygen diffusion from capillaries and metabolism predicted that the oxygen tension would decrease to zero at approximately 150 µm. They measured the width of tumor cords and showed that tumors can be modeled as shown in Figure 13-25. Those cells within approximately 100 µm of the capillary are well oxygenated, those beyond 150 µm are anoxic and necrotic, and those between 100 and 150 µm are hypoxic

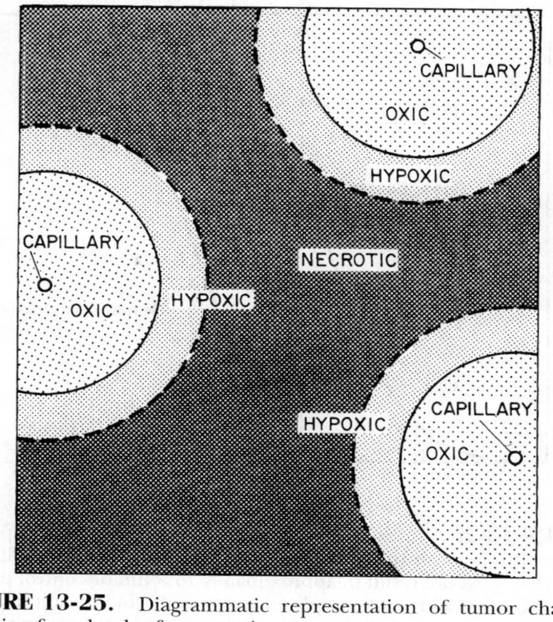

FIGURE 13-25. Diagrammatic representation of tumor changes resulting from levels of oxygenation.

at an oxygen tension that might protect cells from radiation. Laboratory experiments have indicated that immediately after a single dose of radiation, the surviving tumor cells are mainly the original hypoxic cells. After a period, the proportion of hypoxic cells returns to the preradiation level. This process has been called *reoxygenation*.[127] The term can be confusing, because these are indirect experiments and do not record the fate of individual cells. The results of these experiments can be explained by suggesting that tumor cells do reoxygenate for several reasons: (1) reduced total tumor cell population relative to the surface area of tumor blood vessels; (2) reduced separation of hypoxic cells from the blood vessels, which results from preferential cell kill of oxygenated cells; (3) increased oxygen diffusion; and (4) decreased intratumoral pressure, which opens blood vessels.

Research examining low doses of radiation has led to the discovery of a phenomenon called *low-dose hyperradiosensitivity*. This effect describes the higher than predicted sensitivity of certain cell lines to radiation doses lower than 0.5 to 1.0 Gy.[128–130] A proposed mechanistic explanation is that cells do not efficiently recognize such low levels of damage and that consequently the proper repair mechanisms are not triggered.[128] This is supported by a study using a pair of cell lines that differ in DNA repair capabilities (with or without DNA-PKcs), which have similar survival responses to low doses (0 to 0.3 Gy) but differ in radiosensitivities above 0.4 Gy.[131] If such low-dose exposures are fractionated, each fraction appears to elicit this hypersensitivity effect, which results in a *reverse fractionation* effect for fractions less than 1 Gy. For example, Joiner and coworkers delivered 6 Gy to cells in 0.4-Gy fractions (three times daily over 5 days), and this resulted in greater cell kill than delivery of the same total dose in 1.2-Gy daily fractions.[132] This may have important implications for continuous low dose-rate therapies, including interstitial or intracavitary implants. This may also have important implications regarding carcinogenic effects with low-dose radiation.

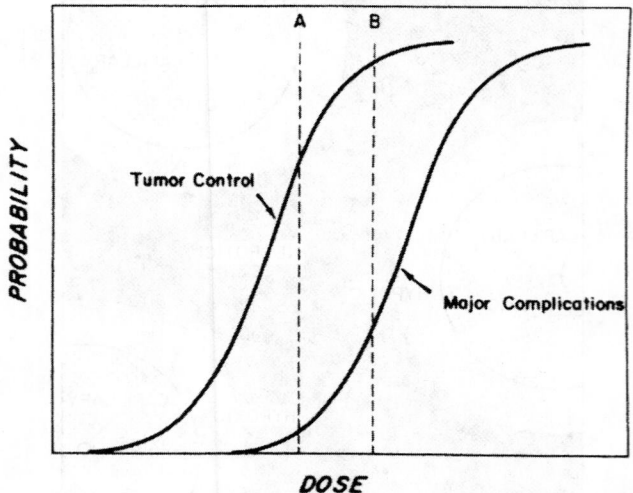

FIGURE 13-26. Idealized sigmoid curves representing the probabilities of tumor control and major complications, based on radiation dose. Dose A would result in approximately 75% tumor control probability with minimal risk of complications. Dose B would result in maximal tumor control probability with a significant risk of complications.

BALANCING OF TUMOR CONTROL PROBABILITY AND NORMAL TISSUE COMPLICATIONS

With increasing radiation dose, one can expect increasing probabilities of both tumor control and normal tissue complications. This relationship of tumor control probability (TCP) and complication probability can be represented by sigmoid curves, when plotted against radiation dose (Fig. 13-26). The shapes and relative locations of such curves depend on many factors. For tumors, the TCP depends on the sensitivity of tumor clonogens to radiation and the number of tumor cells within the treatment volume. Radiation damage to tumor cells follows a Poisson distribution, which can be described mathematically as follows:

$$TCP = e^{-(SF \times M)}$$

In this formula, SF is the surviving fraction of tumor cells and M is the initial number of tumor cells before treatment. The SF will be smaller when tumor cells are sensitive to radiation damage. A clinical example of this is treatment of Hodgkin's lymphoma with radiation alone, for which the steep portion of the sigmoid curve lies in the 20- to 40-Gy range.[133] In contrast, tumor cells within vocal cord carcinomas are less sensitive to radiation damage, and consequently the steep part of the sigmoid curve lies in the 60- to 70-Gy range.[134] The initial tumor burden (M) is also a central factor in determining TCP. For this reason, increasing doses are required to control subclinical microscopic disease versus small tumors versus large tumors.

In the realistic clinical situation, the sigmoid curves describing TCP and normal tissue complications are often less steep and are located closer together than those shown in Figure 13-26. The separation between the curves, or therapeutic index, varies widely depending on the tumor type and size and the tolerance of adjacent normal organs. When patients are treated with curative intent, it is often suggested that the goal is to pursue a treatment plan with the greatest probability of uncomplicated cure. Although this goal is desirable, circumstances actually may dictate a different policy. Consider Figure 13-26, in which the curve for complications is to the right of the sigmoid curve for tumor control. If tumor treatment failure can be salvaged by subsequent surgery but complications are severe, long-lived, and difficult to manage, then dose A is the optimal choice.[135] An example of this would be the treatment of T2 and T3 glottic cancer. On the other hand, if complications are not severe or are remediable but cancer treatment failure is fatal, then dose B would be appropriate. This is the case in advanced carcinomas of the uterine cervix. There is no simple answer. Often, the worst complication of treatment is tumor recurrence.

For symptomatic palliation rather than curative intention, there is often more flexibility in terms of radiation doses and schedules. Frequently, symptoms of tumors can be reduced or eliminated with relatively low radiation doses. With such treatments, the risk of major complications is low, because (1) doses are frequently below the TD 5/5 of adjacent normal organs, and (2) there is often an inadequate length of time for complications to develop in patients with metastatic disease and hence short life expectancy. Because lower doses are well tolerated by normal tissue, larger fraction sizes can be safely used. This, in turn, reduces the number of treatment days that a patient must endure, and it reduces the overall financial cost. Common palliative regimens include daily schedules of 2.5 Gy/d × 14 or 15 days, 3 Gy/d × 10 days, 4 Gy/d × 5 days, or 8 Gy × 1 day. A metaanalysis compared several common fractionation schedules used for palliation of painful bone metastases, and it showed no significant differences in terms of pain relief.[136] However, many clinicians contend that the treatment regimens using higher total doses result in longer-lasting palliation. Consistent with this view, the metaanalysis showed that patients treated with relatively low total doses (e.g., a single fraction of 8 Gy) were more likely to require subsequent reirradiation. This consideration may be particularly important for patients with long anticipated survival times.

ALTERED FRACTIONATION SCHEDULES

When tumors are irradiated with curative intent, standard fractionation schedules typically consist of daily (Monday through Friday) fractions of 1.8 to 2 Gy/d. As discussed earlier (see Balancing of Tumor Control Probability and Normal Tissue Complications, earlier in this chapter), however, it is often challenging to deliver tumoricidal doses while respecting normal tissue tolerances. For this reason, novel fractionation schedules have been developed to further amplify the differential responses of tumors and normal tissues, and thereby improve the therapeutic ratio of radiotherapy.

The term *hyperfractionation* refers to radiotherapy schedules that use multiple daily fractions with reduced fraction sizes and increased number of fractions. The underlying aim is to maximally exploit the differential effects observed between tumors and normal tissues after irradiation with small doses (see Fig. 13-23). Because most of the sublethal damage repair occurs within 6 hours, hyperfractionated schedules typically consist of twice-daily fractions separated by at least 6 hours. As discussed earlier in Tissue Effects from Radiation, late-responding normal tissues are relatively sensitive to fraction size, and the reduced fraction sizes allow for an increase in total dose while maintaining similar or reduced complication probabilities. Improved tumor control probabilities would be expected with the higher total doses. A large randomized trial performed by the European Organization for Research and Treatment of Cancer compared standard and hyperfractionated regimens in the treatment of oropharyngeal carcinomas.[137] The treatment arms underwent regimens of 80.5

Gy over 7 weeks (1.15 Gy delivered twice daily) versus 70 Gy over 7 weeks (2 Gy delivered once daily). The arm receiving hyperfractionated treatments showed a significantly improved 5-year locoregional control rate (59% vs. 40%, P = .02), and no differences were noted in late treatment-related complications between the two arms. However, worse acute mucosal reactions were seen in the hyperfractionated arm, which would be expected because the oral mucosa is an early-responding type of tissue.

Accelerated fractionation is another form of altered fractionation schedule. The underlying aim is to reduce the overall treatment time and thereby reduce the potential for tumor cell proliferation during the course of treatment. Overall treatment time is known to be an important factor in TCP, particularly because radiation itself can stimulate accelerated tumor cell repopulation during the course of treatment.[125] Late complication rates for normal tissue would not be expected to increase with such regimens, provided that (1) fraction size is not increased, and (2) the time interval between fractions is adequate for the repair of sublethal damage and repopulation. The simplest example of accelerated treatment is the delivery of radiation fractions 6 or 7 days a week, rather than just Monday through Friday. Researchers of the Danish Head and Neck Cancer Study Group randomly assigned patients to receive either five or six treatments per week, but the total doses and fraction sizes were kept identical. Patients receiving the accelerated regimen experienced greater local control rates, but this came at the expense of greater acute morbidity.[138] Turrisi and coworkers reported on a randomized comparison of standard and accelerated radiotherapy schedules, which were combined with chemotherapy for the treatment of limited-stage small cell lung cancers. Although the same total dose of 45 Gy was delivered in both treatment arms, the accelerated regimen (1.5 Gy twice daily over 3 weeks) was superior to a daily regimen (1.8 Gy once daily over 5 weeks) in terms of 5-year overall survival rate (26% vs. 16%).[139]

Many altered fractionation schedules combine together the hyperfractionation and accelerated fractionation concepts into novel regimens. Researchers at Mount Vernon Hospital in the United Kingdom developed a short intensive regimen called *continuous hyperfractionated accelerated radiation therapy*, which consists of 1.5-Gy fractions delivered three times daily for 12 consecutive days (54 Gy total dose).[140] Investigators at the University of Chicago have reported on several versions of a concomitant chemotherapy plus radiotherapy regimen in which a week of hyperfractionated accelerated radiation (1.5-Gy fractions delivered twice daily) is delivered on alternating weeks.[141] An *accelerated fractionation with concomitant boost* regimen was developed at the M. D. Anderson Cancer Center. In this regimen, the patient receives standard fractionated radiation at the beginning of the treatment course; the last 12 days of treatment consist of twice-daily radiation—wide-field radiation in the morning and boost treatment to gross disease in the afternoon.[142] A randomized trial (RTOG 9003) compared investigational fractionation schedules used for advanced head and neck squamous cell carcinomas (Fig. 13-27). This study reported better locoregional control rates with hyperfractionation and with accelerated fractionation with concomitant boost, compared to standard fractionation. However, this benefit came at the cost of increased acute toxicity.[143]

CLINICAL ASPECTS OF BRACHYTHERAPY

The term *brachytherapy* is derived from the Greek root *brachys*, which means close or short distance. It refers to the delivery of radiation

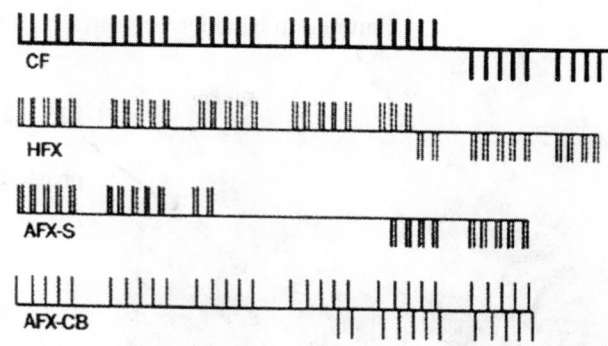

FIGURE 13-27. Schematic representation of the four fractionation schedules used in a randomized trial (RTOG 9003) of the treatment of advanced head and neck cancers. Upward tick marks represent treatments to initial treatment volumes; downward tick marks represent reduced-volume treatments to gross disease only. AFX-CB, accelerated fractionation with a concomitant boost strategy; AFX-S, accelerated split-course fractionation; CF, conventional fractionation; HFX, hyperfractionation. (From Nguyen LN, Ang KK. Radiotherapy for cancer of the head and neck: altered fractionation regimens. *Lancet Oncol* 2002;3:693, with permission.)

from sealed radioactive sources that are positioned in close proximity to tumor sites. This exploits the physical distribution of radiation surrounding radioactive sources, whereby radiation exposure decreases exponentially with increasing distances from a source. Thus brachytherapy can be used to deliver high radiation doses to nearby tumor tissue, while sparing normal tissues located at more distant locations. This is the major potential advantage of brachytherapy over external-beam delivery strategies. The main disadvantage of brachytherapy is its heterogeneous distribution of dose deposition within tissue, which could potentially lead to complications at "hot spots" or tumor recurrences at low-dose regions.

Brachytherapy is frequently performed using temporary intracavitary applicators. These devices are surgically positioned into a body cavity and then afterloaded with radioactive materials. The most common example is the tandem and colpostat applicator for the treatment of tumors of the uterine cervix (Fig. 13-28). The central tandem is inserted through the cervical os into the uterine cavity, and the two colpostats are positioned laterally in the upper vagina. This spacial positioning of sources allows the delivery of high doses to the cervix and parametrial tissues, while respecting the radiation tolerances of normal bladder and rectum. The treatment is customized depending on the geometry of the tandem and colpostats relative to the patient's anatomy. With use of low dose-rate ^{137}Cs sources, the physicist and physician can customize the number of sources to be used (four or five), the source strengths (10- to 30-mg radium equivalents), the positions of sources within the device, and the total time of treatment (typically 1 to 3 days). After this allotted time, the device and sources are removed. Several newer types of intracavitary devices are now under investigation in which balloons are inflated within a surgical cavity and afterloaded with radioactive material (e.g., ^{125}I-containing fluid or ^{192}Ir seed). Examples include the MammoSite Radiation Therapy System for local irradiation of breast cavities after lumpectomy and the GliaSite Radiation Therapy System for treatment of brain cavities after resection of intracranial tumors.[144,145]

Interstitial implantation represents another form of brachytherapy. This can be accomplished via surgical placement of temporary catheters, which are subsequently afterloaded with

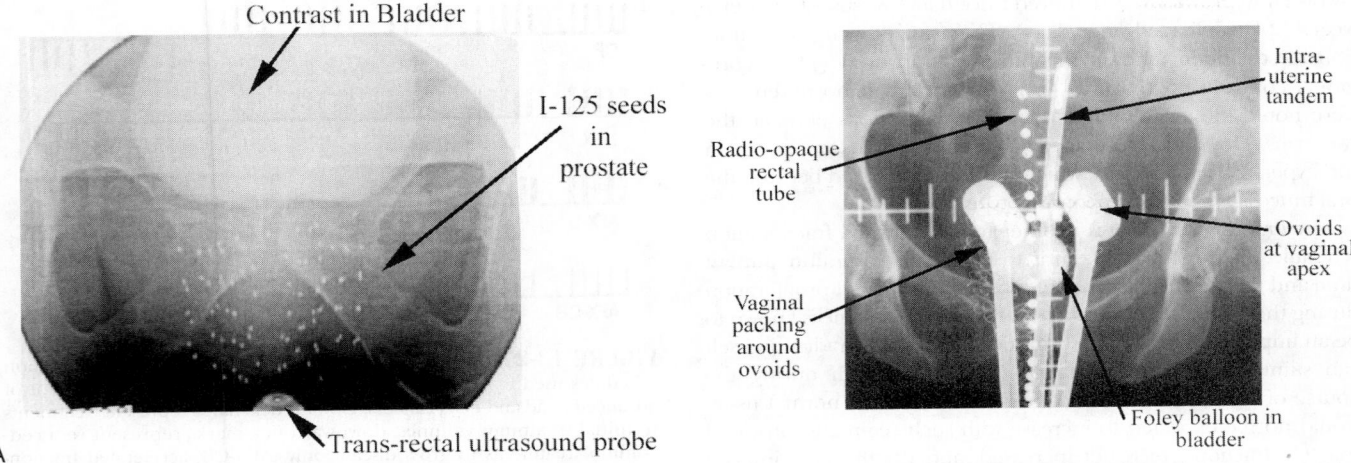

FIGURE 13-28. Clinical examples of brachytherapy. **A:** Prostate cancer treated via permanent interstitial implant with iodine 125 seeds. **B:** Radiograph demonstrating the temporary implantation of a tandem and ovoid–type applicator (Fletcher-Suit) for the treatment of a tumor of the uterine cervix.

radioactive sources. This method can be used to irradiate gross tumors (e.g., oral cavity, parametrial, and prostate tumors) or microscopic disease after surgical procedures like breast lumpectomy or soft tissue sarcoma resection. Implantation with permanent radioactive seeds is the other major type of interstitial brachytherapy. For the treatment of prostate cancer, transrectal ultrasonography is used to guide the placement of steel-encapsulated ^{125}I or ^{103}Pd seeds throughout the prostate gland (see Fig. 13-28). With ^{125}I seeds, the total treatment doses are relatively high (145 Gy); however, the rates of delivery (*dose rates*) are relatively low. Furthermore, the dose rate declines during the actual treatment period as the iodine within the implanted seed decays (the half-life of ^{125}I is 59.6 days). Because of these factors, it is difficult to speculate regarding the predicted biologic effects of permanent prostate implants versus fractionated external-beam regimens. One drawback of permanent implantation is the potential for underdosing a portion(s) of the tumor. This can possibly occur if seeds are misplaced during the procedure, or they move after placement. Furthermore, asymmetric radiation emissions are observed around cylindrical seeds (*anisotropy*; see Fig. 13-22), which further raises the potential for underdosing of some regions. That said, the clinical reports to date suggest that prostate tumors with favorable prognosis are equally well controlled with interstitial implants and fractionated external-beam treatments.[146]

The rate of dose delivery is an important factor in brachytherapy. Traditionally, temporary implants have been manually afterloaded with sources that deliver *low dose-rate* (LDR) radiation treatment. Typical treatments deliver 0.4 to 2.0 Gy/h and thus require inpatient admissions for several days. More recently, robotic afterloading machines have been developed to remotely transfer a source from a shielded vault into the intracavitary device and then back into the vault. This safe and automated design allows for the use of highly active sources that deliver *high dose-rates* (HDRs). The International Commission on Radiation Units and Measurements has defined HDR as any dose rate greater than 12 Gy/h. The rapid rate allows brachytherapy to be delivered in a matter of minutes in an outpatient setting. Some radiation oncologists have warned of the need for caution in changing from LDR to HDR treatment

schedules. This argument is based on the idea that slow, prolonged, continuous radiation approximates a fractionated course of radiotherapy and hence benefits from processes like sublethal damage repair, redistribution of cell cycle, reoxygenation of tumors, and repopulation of cells in normal tissue (see Principles Underlying Fractionation, earlier in this chapter). One might expect these differential tissue effects to be lost with HDR delivery. However, the reported clinical outcomes to date have shown essentially no differences in efficacy between HDR and LDR treatment schedules.

OTHER RADIATION MODALITIES AND FUTURE DEVELOPMENTS

Nonsealed injectable radionuclides represent another modality for irradiating malignant and benign diseases. Depending on the institution, treatment is administered by radiation oncology or nuclear medicine personnel, or both. The most commonly used isotope is iodine 131. Intravenously administered iodine is efficiently absorbed by the thyroid gland and hence is effective against hyperthyroidism and some histologic types of thyroid cancer. Strontium 29 and samarium 153 ethylene diamine tetramethylene phosphate (^{153}Sm-EDTMP) are bone-seeking compounds that emit β-radiation. After systemic administration they become concentrated at areas of osteoblastic bone activity. These radiopharmaceuticals can be used to palliate painful bone metastases and to treat osteogenic sarcomas.[147]

More recently, radiation-emitting isotopes have been conjugated with high-affinity antibodies to generate *radioimmunoglobulins*. This powerful combination of technologies concentrates radionuclides in the neighborhood of malignant cells. Yttrium 90 (^{90}Y) ibritumomab tiuxetan (Zevalin) was the first radioimmunotherapeutic agent approved for use by the U.S. Food and Drug Administration. The ibritumomab component is a chimeric murine-human monoclonal antibody that specifically binds to CD20, which is expressed on the majority of B-cell lymphomas. Tiuxetan is a modified metal chelator that links the antibody to ^{90}Y, which emits β-radiation. Clinical trials have demonstrated high response rates (70% to 80%) for patients with a variety of B-cell non-Hodgkin's lymphomas.[148,149]

Another promising recent development is the combination of gene therapy with radiotherapy. Weichselbaum and coworkers have developed an adenoviral vector containing the Egr-1 gene promoter, which is stimulated by ionizing radiation. The TNF-α gene was engineered upstream of this radiation-inducible promoter. The resulting replication-deficient virus (Ad.EGR-TNF) has been administered by direct injection into human tumors during the course of external-beam radiotherapy. The early phase I data have demonstrated striking antitumor effects, resulting in high rates of complete and partial responses. The mechanism of action appears to involve TNF-α–mediated destruction of tumor vasculature. This novel approach is currently being tested in a variety of sites and tumor types.[44]

REFERENCES

1. Virnig BA, Warren JL, Cooper GS, et al. Studying radiation therapy using SEER-Medicare-linked data. *Med Care* 2002;40:IV-49.
2. Hall EJ. *Radiobiology for the radiologist.* Philadelphia: Lippincott Williams and Wilkins, 2000:558.
3. Radford IR. The level of induced DNA double-strand breakage correlates with cell killing after X-irradiation. *Int J Radiat Biol Relat Stud Phys Chem Med* 1985;48:45.
4. Lewanski CR, Gullick WJ. Radiotherapy and cellular signaling. *Lancet Oncol* 2001;2:366.
5. Prise KM, Ahnstrom G, Belli M, et al. A review of dsb induction data for varying quality radiations. *Int J Radiat Biol* 1998;74:173.
6. Nunez MI, McMillan TJ, Valenzuela MT, et al. Relationship between DNA damage, rejoining and cell killing by radiation in mammalian cells. *Radiother Oncol* 1996;39:155.
7. Frankenberg-Schwager M, Frankenberg D. Shouldered survival curves in accordance with the unsaturated rejoining kinetics of DNA double-strand breaks. *BJR Suppl* 1992;24:23.
8. Nunez MI, Villalobos M, Olea N, et al. Radiation-induced DNA double-strand break rejoining in human tumour cells. *Br J Cancer* 1995;71:311.
9. Whitaker SJ, Ung YC, McMillan TJ. DNA double-strand break induction and rejoining as determinants of human tumour cell radiosensitivity. A pulsed-field gel electrophoresis study. *Int J Radiat Biol* 1995;67:7.
10. Jeggo PA, Hafezparast M, Thompson AF, et al. Localization of a DNA repair gene (XRCC5) involved in double-strand-break rejoining to human chromosome 2. *Proc Natl Acad Sci U S A* 1992;89:6423.
11. Ross GM, Eady JJ, Mithal NP, et al. DNA strand break rejoining defect in xrs-6 is complemented by transfection with the human Ku80 gene. *Cancer Res* 1995;55:1235.
12. Coquerelle TM, Weibezahn KF, Lucke-Huhle C. Rejoining of double strand breaks in normal human and ataxia-telangiectasia fibroblasts after exposure to 60Co gamma-rays, 241Am alpha-particles or bleomycin. *Int J Radiat Biol Relat Stud Phys Chem Med* 1987;51:209.
13. Thompson LH, Suit HD. Proliferation kinetics of x-irradiated mouse L cells studied WITH TIME-lapse photography. II. *Int J Radiat Biol Relat Stud Phys Chem Med* 1969;15:347.
14. Elkind MM. The initial part of the survival curve: does it predict the outcome of fractionated radiotherapy? *Radiat Res* 1988;114:425.
15. Weichselbaum RR, Nove J, Little JB. X-ray sensitivity of human tumor cells in vitro. *Int J Radiat Oncol Biol Phys* 1980;6:437.
16. Till JE, McCulloch EA. A direct measurement of the radiation sensitivity of normal mouse bone marrow cells. *Radiat Res* 1961;14:213.
17. Withers HR, Elkind MM. Microcolony survival assay for cells of mouse intestinal mucosa exposed to radiation. *Int J Radiat Biol Relat Stud Phys Chem Med* 1970;17:261.
18. Alper T, Gillies NE. Restoration of Escherichia coli strain B irradiation: its dependence on suboptimal growth conditions. *J Gen Microbiol* 1958;18:461.
19. Weichselbaum R, Little JB, Nove J. Response of human osteosarcoma in vitro to irradiation: evidence for unusual cellular repair activity. *Int J Radiat Biol Relat Stud Phys Chem Med* 1977;31:295.
20. Kim ST, Lim DS, Canman CE, et al. Substrate specificities and identification of putative substrates of ATM kinase family members. *J Biol Chem* 1999;274:37538.
21. Cliby WA, Roberts CJ, Cimprich KA, et al. Overexpression of a kinase-inactive ATR protein causes sensitivity to DNA-damaging agents and defects in cell cycle checkpoints. *EMBO J* 1998;17:159.
22. Tibbetts RS, Brumbaugh KM, Williams JM, et al. A role for ATR in the DNA damage-induced phosphorylation of p53. *Genes Dev* 1999;13:152.
23. Komarov PG, Komarova EA, Kondratov RV, et al. A chemical inhibitor of p53 that protects mice from the side effects of cancer therapy. *Science* 1999;285:1733.
24. Burma S, Chen BP, Murphy M, et al. ATM phosphorylates histone H2AX in response to DNA double-strand breaks. *J Biol Chem* 2001;276:42462.
25. Rothkamm K, Kruger I, Thompson LH, et al. Pathways of DNA double-strand break repair during the mammalian cell cycle. *Mol Cell Biol* 2003;23:5706.
26. Paull TT, Rogakou EP, Yamazaki V, et al. A critical role for histone H2AX in recruitment of repair factors to nuclear foci after DNA damage. *Curr Biol* 2000;10:886.
27. Maser RS, Monsen KJ, Nelms BE, et al. hMre11 and hRad50 nuclear foci are induced during the normal cellular response to DNA double-strand breaks. *Mol Cell Biol* 1997;17:6087.
28. Celeste A, Petersen S, Romanienko PJ, et al. Genomic instability in mice lacking histone H2AX. *Science* 2002;296:922.
29. Bassing CH, Chua KF, Sekiguchi J, et al. Increased ionizing radiation sensitivity and genomic instability in the absence of histone H2AX. *Proc Natl Acad Sci U S A* 2002;99:8173.
30. Celeste A, Fernandez-Capetillo O, Kruhlak MJ, et al. Histone H2AX phosphorylation is dispensable for the initial recognition of DNA breaks. *Nat Cell Biol* 2003;5:675.
31. Tenzer A, Pruschy M. Potentiation of DNA-damage-induced cytotoxicity by G2 checkpoint abrogators. *Curr Med Chem Anti-Canc Agents* 2003;3:35.
32. Walworth NC. DNA damage: Chk1 and Cdc25, more than meets the eye. *Curr Opin Genet Dev* 2001;11:78.
33. Sampath D, Plunkett W. Design of new anticancer therapies targeting cell cycle checkpoint pathways. *Curr Opin Oncol* 2001;13:484.
34. Haimovitz-Friedman A, Kan CC, Ehleiter D, et al. Ionizing radiation acts on cellular membranes to generate ceramide and initiate apoptosis. *J Exp Med* 1994;180:525.
35. Santana PR, Souza VH, Marquetti GP, et al. Acid sphingomyelinase-deficient human lymphoblasts and mice are defective in radiation-induced apoptosis. *Percept Mot Skills* 1996;82:1123.
36. Haimovitz-Friedman A. Radiation-induced signal transduction and stress response. *Radiat Res* 1998;150:S102.
37. Dent P, Yacoub A, Contessa J, et al. Stress and radiation-induced activation of multiple intracellular signaling pathways. *Radiat Res* 2003;159:283.
38. Huang SM, Bock JM, Harari PM. Epidermal growth factor receptor blockade with C225 modulates proliferation, apoptosis, and radiosensitivity in squamous cell carcinomas of the head and neck. *Cancer Res* 1999;59:1935.
39. Schmidt-Ullrich RK, Mikkelsen RB, Dent P, et al. Radiation-induced proliferation of the human A431 squamous carcinoma cells is dependent on EGFR tyrosine phosphorylation. *Oncogene* 1997;15:1191.
40. Mothersill C, Seymour CB, Joiner MC. Relationship between radiation-induced low-dose hypersensitivity and the bystander effect. *Radiat Res* 2002;157:526.
41. Dunphy E, Kuchibhotla J, Kraft A, et al. C-jun and Egr-1 participate in DNA synthesis and cell survival in response to ionizing radiation exposure. *Int J Radiat Oncol Biol Phys* 1996;36:355.
42. Hallahan DE, Virudachalam S, Schwartz JL, et al. Inhibition of protein kinases sensitizes human tumor cells to ionizing radiation. *Radiat Res* 1992;129:345.
43. Hallahan DE, Dunphy E, Virudachalam S, et al. C-jun and Egr-1 participate in DNA synthesis and cell survival in response to ionizing radiation exposure. *J Biol Chem* 1995;270:30303.
44. Weichselbaum RR, Kufe DW, Hellman S, et al. Radiation-induced tumour necrosis factor-alpha expression: clinical application of transcriptional and physical targeting of gene therapy. *Lancet Oncol* 2002;3:665.
45. Mothersill C, Seymour C. Radiation-induced bystander effects: past history and future directions. *Radiat Res* 2001;155:759.
46. Turesson I, Carlsson J, Brahme A, et al. Biological response to radiation therapy. *Acta Oncol* 2003;42:92.
47. Mothersill C, Seymour CB. Cell-cell contact during gamma irradiation is not required to induce a bystander effect in normal human keratinocytes: evidence for release during irradiation of a signal controlling survival into the medium. *Radiat Res* 1998;149:256.
48. Azzam EI, de Toledo SM, Little JB. Direct evidence for the participation of gap junction-mediated intercellular communication in the transmission of damage signals from alpha-particle irradiated to nonirradiated cells. *Proc Natl Acad Sci U S A* 2001;98:473.
49. Thompson LH, Schild D. Homologous recombinational repair of DNA ensures mammalian chromosome stability. *Mutat Res* 2001;477:131.
50. Thompson LH, Schild D. Recombinational DNA repair and human disease. *Mutat Res* 2002;509:49.
51. Takata M, Sasaki MS, Sonoda E, et al. Homologous recombination and non-homologous end-joining pathways of DNA double-strand break repair have overlapping roles in the maintenance of chromosomal integrity in vertebrate cells. *EMBO J* 1998;17:5497.
52. Tauchi H, Kobayashi J, Morishima K, et al. Nbs1 is essential for DNA repair by homologous recombination in higher vertebrate cells. *Nature* 2002;420:93.
53. Paull TT, Gellert M. The 3′ to 5′ exonuclease activity of Mre 11 facilitates repair of DNA double-strand breaks. *Mol Cell* 1998;1:969.
54. Nelms BE, Maser RS, MacKay JF, et al. In situ visualization of DNA double-strand break repair in human fibroblasts. *Science* 1998;280:590.
55. Ma Y, Pannicke U, Schwarz K, et al. Hairpin opening and overhang processing by an Artemis/DNA-dependent protein kinase complex in nonhomologous end joining and V(D)J recombination. *Cell* 2002;108:781.
56. Belenkov AI, Paiement JP, Panasci LC, et al. An antisense oligonucleotide targeted to human Ku86 messenger RNA sensitizes M059K malignant glioma cells to ionizing radiation, bleomycin, and etoposide but not DNA cross-linking agents. *Cancer Res* 2002;62:5888.
57. Omori S, Takiguchi Y, Suda A, et al. Suppression of a DNA double-strand break repair gene, Ku70, increases radio- and chemosensitivity in a human lung carcinoma cell line. *DNA Repair (Amst)* 2002;1:299.
58. Sak A, Stuschke M, Wurm R, et al. Selective inactivation of DNA-dependent protein kinase with antisense oligodeoxynucleotides: consequences for the rejoining of radiation-induced DNA double-strand breaks and radiosensitivity of human cancer cell lines. *Cancer Res* 2002;62:6621.
59. Peng Y, Zhang Q, Nagasawa H, et al. Silencing expression of the catalytic subunit of DNA-dependent protein kinase by small interfering RNA sensitizes human cells for radiation-induced chromosome damage, cell killing, and mutation. *Cancer Res* 2002; 62:6400.
60. Frank KM, Sekiguchi JM, Seidl KJ, et al. Late embryonic lethality and impaired V(D)J recombination in mice lacking DNA ligase IV. *Nature* 1998;396:173.
61. Riballo E, Critchlow SE, Teo SH, et al. Identification of a defect in DNA ligase IV in a radiosensitive leukaemia patient. *Curr Biol* 1999;9:699.

62. Grawunder U, Wilm M, Wu X, et al. Activity of DNA ligase IV stimulated by complex formation with XRCC4 protein in mammalian cells. *Nature* 1997;388:492.

63. Mizuta R, Cheng HL, Gao Y, et al. Molecular genetic characterization of XRCC4 function. *Int Immunol* 1997;9:1607.

64. Chen L, Trujillo K, Sung P, et al. Interactions of the DNA ligase IV-XRCC4 complex with DNA ends and the DNA-dependent protein kinase. *J Biol Chem* 2000;275:26196.

65. Gasior SL, Olivares H, Ear U, et al. Assembly of RecA-like recombinases: distinct roles for mediator proteins in mitosis and meiosis. *Proc Natl Acad Sci U S A* 2001;98:8411.

66. Bishop DK, Ear U, Bhattacharyya A, et al. Xrcc3 is required for assembly of Rad51 complexes in vivo. *J Biol Chem* 1998;273:21482.

67. Johnson RD, Jasin M. Sister chromatid gene conversion is a prominent double-strand break repair pathway in mammalian cells. *EMBO J* 2000;19:3398.

68. Takata M, Sasaki MS, Tachiiri S, et al. Chromosome instability and defective recombinational repair in knockout mutants of the five Rad51 paralogs. *Mol Cell Biol* 2001;21:2858.

69. Masson JY, Stasiak AZ, Stasiak A, et al. Complex formation by the human RAD51C and XRCC3 recombination repair proteins. *Proc Natl Acad Sci U S A* 2001;98:8440.

70. Liu N, Schild D, Thelen MP, et al. Involvement of Rad51C in two distinct protein complexes of Rad51 paralogs in human cells. *Nucleic Acids Res* 2002;30:1009.

71. Sigurdsson S, Van Komen S, Bussen W, et al. Mediator function of the human Rad51B-Rad51C complex in Rad51/RPA- catalyzed DNA strand exchange. *Genes Dev* 2001;15:3308.

72. Mottram JC. Factors of importance in radiosensitivity of tumors. *Br J Radiol* 1926;9:606.

73. Barendsen GW. Response of cultured cells, tumours, and normal tissues to radiations of different linear energy transfer. *Curr Top Radiat Res Q* 1968;4:293.

74. Henk JM, Smith CW. Radiotherapy and hyperbaric oxygen in head and neck cancer. Interim report of second clinical trial. *Lancet* 1977;2:104.

75. Watson ER, Halnan KE, Dische S, et al. Hyperbaric oxygen and radiotherapy: a Medical Research Council trial in carcinoma of the cervix. *Br J Radiol* 1978;51:879.

76. Overgaard J, Horsman MR. Modification of hypoxia-induced radioresistance in tumors by the use of oxygen and sensitizers. *Semin Radiat Oncol* 1996;6:10.

77. Bush RS, Jenkin RD, Allt WE, et al. Definitive evidence for hypoxic cells influencing cure in cancer therapy. *Br J Cancer Suppl* 1978;37:302.

78. Harrison LB, Chadha M, Hill RJ, et al. Impact of tumor hypoxia and anemia on radiation therapy outcomes. *Oncologist* 2002;7:492.

79. Rosen FR, Haraf DJ, Kies MS, et al. Multicenter randomized phase II study of paclitaxel (1-hour infusion), fluorouracil, hydroxyurea, and concomitant twice daily radiation with or without erythropoietin for advanced head and neck cancer. *Clin Cancer Res* 2003;9:1689.

80. Henke M, Laszig R, Rube C, et al. Erythropoietin to treat head and neck cancer patients with anaemia undergoing radiotherapy: randomised, double-blind, placebo-controlled trial. *Lancet* 2003; 362:1255.

81. Brown JM, Wang LH. Tirapazamine: laboratory data relevant to clinical activity. *Anticancer Drug Des* 1998;13:529.

82. Lee DJ, Trotti A, Spencer S, et al. Concurrent tirapazamine and radiotherapy for advanced head and neck carcinomas: a phase II study. *Int J Radiat Oncol Biol Phys* 1998;42:811.

83. Lawrence TS, Blackstock AW, McGinn C. The mechanism of action of radiosensitization of conventional chemotherapeutic agents. *Semin Radiat Oncol* 2003;13:13.

84. Lawrence TS, Tepper JE, Blackstock AW. Fluoropyrimidine-radiation interactions in cells and tumors. *Semin Radiat Oncol* 1997;7:260.

85. Lawrence TS, Chang EY, Hahn TM, et al. Radiosensitization of pancreatic cancer cells by 2′,2′-difluoro-2′-deoxycytidine. *Int J Radiat Oncol Biol Phys* 1996;34:867.

86. Yang LX, Douple EB, Wang HJ. Irradiation enhances cellular uptake of carboplatin. *Int J Radiat Oncol Biol Phys* 1995;33:641.

87. Richmond RC. Toxic variability and radiation sensitization by dichlorodiammineplatinum(II) complexes in Salmonella typhimurium cells. *Radiat Res* 1984;99:596.

88. Sinclair WK. Hydroxyurea: effects on Chinese hamster cells grown in culture. *Cancer Res* 1967;27:297.

89. Hellman S, Hannon E. Effects of adriamycin on the radiation response of murine hematopoietic stem cells [Letter]. *Radiat Res* 1976;67:162.

90. Yuhas JM, Yurconic M, Kligerman MM, et al. Combined use of radioprotective and radiosensitizing drugs in experimental radiotherapy. *Radiat Res* 1977;70:433.

91. Kataoka Y, Perrin J, Hunter N, et al. Antimutagenic effects of amifostine: clinical implications. *Semin Oncol* 1996;23:53.

92. Brizel DM, Wasserman TH, Henke M, et al. Phase III randomized trial of amifostine as a radioprotector in head and neck cancer. *J Clin Oncol* 2000;18:3339.

93. Kemp G, Rose P, Lurain J, et al. Amifostine pretreatment for protection against cyclophosphamide-induced and cisplatin-induced toxicities: results of a randomized control trial in patients with advanced ovarian cancer. *J Clin Oncol* 1996;14:2101.

94. Dewey WC, Hopwood LE, Sapareto SA, et al. Cellular responses to combinations of hyperthermia and radiation. *Radiology* 1977;123:463.

95. Westra A, Dewey WC. Variation in sensitivity to heat shock during the cell-cycle of Chinese hamster cells in vitro. *Int J Radiat Biol Relat Stud Phys Chem Med* 1971;19:467.

96. Sapareto SA, Hopwood LE, Dewey WC. Combined effects of X irradiation and hyperthermia on CHO cells for various temperatures and orders of application. *Radiat Res* 1978;73:221.

97. Paris F, Fuks Z, Kang A, et al. Endothelial apoptosis as the primary lesion initiating intestinal radiation damage in mice. *Science* 2001;293:293.

98. Garcia-Barros M, Paris F, Cordon-Cardo C, et al. Tumor response to radiotherapy regulated by endothelial cell apoptosis. *Science* 2003;300:1155.

99. O'Reilly MS, Holmgren L, Shing Y, et al. Angiostatin: a novel angiogenesis inhibitor that mediates the suppression of metastases by a Lewis lung carcinoma. *Cell* 1994;79:315.

100. O'Reilly MS, Boehm T, Shing Y, et al. Endostatin: an endogenous inhibitor of angiogenesis and tumor growth. *Cell* 1997;88:277.

101. Mauceri HJ, Hanna NN, Beckett MA, et al. Combined effects of angiostatin and ionizing radiation in antitumor therapy. *Nature* 1998;394:287.

102. Gorski DH, Mauceri HJ, Salloum RM, et al. Potentiation of the antitumor effect of ionizing radiation by brief concomitant exposures to angiostatin. *Cancer Res* 1998;58:5686.

103. Griffin RJ, Williams BW, Wild R, et al. Simultaneous inhibition of the receptor kinase activity of vascular endothelial, fibroblast, and platelet-derived growth factors suppresses tumor growth and enhances tumor radiation response. *Cancer Res* 2002;62:1702.

104. Lee CG, Heijn M, di Tomaso E, et al. Anti-vascular endothelial growth factor treatment augments tumor radiation response under normoxic or hypoxic conditions. *Cancer Res* 2000; 60:5565.

105. Attix FH. *Introduction to radiological physics and radiation dosimetry.* New York: Wiley, 1986; xxi:607.

106. Johns HE, Cunningham JR. *The physics of radiology.* Springfield, Il: CC Thomas, 1983;xix:796.

107. Khan FM. *The physics of radiation therapy.* Philadelphia: Lippincott Williams and Wilkins, 2003.

108. Hendee WR. *Radiation therapy physics.* Chicago: Year Book Medical Publishers, 1981;x:195.

109. Central axis depth dose data for use in radiotherapy. A survey of depth doses and related data measured in water or equivalent media. *Br J Radiol Suppl* 1983;17:1.

110. Metcalfe P, Kron T, Hoban P. The physics of radiotherapy X-rays from linear accelerators. Madison, WI: Medical Physics Pub, 1997;ix:493.

111. Karzmark CJ, Nunan CS, Tanabe E. *Medical electron accelerators.* New York: McGraw-Hill Inc., Health Professions Division, 1993;xiv:316.

112. International Commission on Radiation Units and Measurements. Prescribing, recording, and reporting photon beam therapy. ICRU report: 50. Bethesda, MD: International Commission on Radiation Units and Measurements, 1993;viii:72.

113. International Commission on Radiation Units and Measurements. Prescribing, recording, and reporting photon beam therapy. ICRU report: 62. Bethesda, MD: International Commission on Radiation Units and Measurements, 1999:52.

114. Wong JW, Sharpe MB, Jaffray DA, et al. The use of active breathing control (ABC) to reduce margin for breathing motion. *Int J Radiat Oncol Biol Phys* 1999;44:911.

115. Intensity-modulated radiation therapy: the state of the art. American association of physicists in medicine medical physics monograph. Madison, WI: Medical Physics Pub, 2003:29.

116. Ling CC, Yorke ED, Spiro IJ, et al. Physical dosimetry of 125I seeds of a new design for interstitial implant. *Int J Radiat Oncol Biol Phys* 1983;9:1747.

117. Withers HR, Thames HD Jr, Peters LJ. Biological bases for high RBE values for late effects of neutron irradiation. *Int J Radiat Oncol Biol Phys* 1982;8:2071.

118. Withers HR, Thames HD Jr, Peters LJ. A new isoeffect curve for change in dose per fraction. *Radiother Oncol* 1983;1:187.

119. Emami B, Lyman J, Brown A, et al. Tolerance of normal tissue to therapeutic irradiation. *Int J Radiat Oncol Biol Phys* 1991;21:109.

120. Elkind MM, Sutton H. Radiation response of mammalian cells grown in culture: part 1. Repair of x-ray damage in surviving Chinese hamster cells. *Radiat Res* 1960;13:556.

121. Hellman S. Cell kinetics, models, and cancer treatment—some principles for the radiation oncologist. *Radiology* 1975;114:219.

122. Chaffey JT, Hellman S. Studies on dose fractionation as measured by endogenous spleen colonies in the mouse. *Radiology* 1968;90:363.

123. Chaffey JT, Hellman S. Radiation fractionation as applied to murine colony-forming cells in differing proliferative states. *Radiology* 1969;93:1167.

124. Hermens AF, Barendson GW. Changes in cell proliferation characteristics in a rat rhabdomyosarcoma before and after x-irradiation. *Eur J Cancer Clin Oncol* 1969;5:173.

125. Withers HR, Taylor JM, Maciejewski B. The hazard of accelerated tumor clonogen repopulation during radiotherapy. *Acta Oncol* 1988;27:131.

126. Thomlinson RH, Gray LH. The histologic structure of some human lung cancers and possible implications for radiotherapy. *Br J Cancer* 1955;9:539.

127. Kallman RF. The phenomenon of reoxygenation and its implications for fractionated radiotherapy. *Radiology* 1972;105:135.

128. Joiner MC. Induced radioresistance: an overview and historical perspective. *Int J Radiat Biol* 1994;65:79.

129. Marples B, Joiner MC. The response of Chinese hamster V79 cells to low radiation doses: evidence of enhanced sensitivity of the whole cell population. *Radiat Res* 1993;133:41.

130. Wouters BG, Sy AM, Skarsgard LD. Low-dose hypersensitivity and increased radioresistance in a panel of human tumor cell lines with different radiosensitivity substructure in the radiation survival response at low dose in cells of human tumor cell lines. *Radiat Res* 1996;146:399.

131. Marples B, Cann NE, Mitchell CR, et al. Evidence for the involvement of DNA-dependent protein kinase in the phenomena of low dose hyper-radiosensitivity and increased radioresistance. *Int J Radiat Biol* 2002;78:1139.

132. Short SC, Kelly J, Mayes CR, et al. Low-dose hypersensitivity after fractionated low-dose irradiation in vitro. *Int J Radiat Biol* 2001;77:655.

133. Kaplan HS. Evidence for a tumoricidal dose level in the radiotherapy of Hodgkin's disease. *Cancer Res* 1966;26:1221.

134. Mendenhall WM, Parsons JT, Million RR, et al. T1-T2 squamous cell carcinoma of the glottic larynx treated with radiation therapy: relationship of dose-fractionation factors to local control and complications. *Int J Radiat Oncol Biol Phys* 1988;15:1267.

135. Bloomer WD, Hellman S. Normal tissue responses to radiation therapy. *N Engl J Med* 1975;293:80.

136. Wu JS, Wong R, Johnston M, et al. Meta-analysis of dose-fractionation radiotherapy trials for the palliation of painful bone metastases. *Int J Radiat Oncol Biol Phys* 2003;55:594.

137. Horiot JC, Le Fur R, N'Guyen T, et al. Hyperfractionation versus conventional fractionation in oropharyngeal carcinoma: final analysis of a randomized trial of the EORTC cooperative group of radiotherapy. *Radiother Oncol* 1992;25:231.

138. Overgaard J, Hansen HS, Specht L, et al. Five compared with six fractions per week of conventional radiotherapy of squamous-cell carcinoma of head and neck: DAHANCA 6 and 7 randomised controlled trial. *Lancet* 2003;362:933.

139. Turrisi AT 3rd, Kim K, Blum R, et al. Twice-daily compared with once-daily thoracic radiotherapy in limited small-cell lung cancer treated concurrently with cisplatin and etoposide. *N Engl J Med* 1999;340:265.

140. Saunders MI, Dische S, Grosch EJ, et al. Experience with CHART. *Int J Radiat Oncol Biol Phys* 1991;21:871.

141. Vokes EE, Stenson K, Rosen FR, et al. Weekly carboplatin and paclitaxel followed by concomitant paclitaxel, fluorouracil, and hydroxyurea chemoradiotherapy: curative and organ-preserving therapy for advanced head and neck cancer. *J Clin Oncol* 2003;21:320.

142. Ang KK, Peters LJ, Weber RS, et al. Concomitant boost radiotherapy schedules in the treatment of carcinoma of the oropharynx and nasopharynx. *Int J Radiat Oncol Biol Phys* 1990;19:1339.

143. Fu KK, Pajak TF, Trotti A, et al. A Radiation Therapy Oncology Group (RTOG) phase III randomized study to compare hyperfractionation and two variants of accelerated fractionation to standard fractionation radiotherapy for head and neck squamous cell carcinomas: first report of RTOG 9003. *Int J Radiat Oncol Biol Phys* 2000;48:7.

144. Keisch M, Vicini F, Kuske R, et al. Two-year outcome with the mammosite breast brachytherapy applicator: factors associated with optimal cosmetic results when performing partial breast irradiation. *Int J Radiat Oncol Biol Phys* 2003;57:S315.

145. Tatter SB, Shaw EG, Rosenblum ML, et al. An inflatable balloon catheter and liquid 125I radiation source (GliaSite Radiation Therapy System) for treatment of recurrent malignant glioma: multicenter safety and feasibility trial. *J Neurosurg* 2003;99:297.

146. D'Amico AV, Whittington R, Malkowicz SB, et al. Biochemical outcome after radical prostatectomy, external beam radiation therapy, or interstitial radiation therapy for clinically localized prostate cancer. *JAMA* 1998;280:969.

147. Anderson PM, Wiseman GA, Dispenzieri A, et al. High-dose samarium-153 ethylene diamine tetramethylene phosphonate: low toxicity of skeletal irradiation in patients with osteosarcoma and bone metastases. *J Clin Oncol* 2002;20:189.

148. Witzig TE, Gordon LI, Cabanillas F, et al. Randomized controlled trial of yttrium-90-labeled ibritumomab tiuxetan radioimmunotherapy versus rituximab immunotherapy for patients with relapsed or refractory low-grade, follicular, or transformed B-cell non-Hodgkin's lymphoma. *J Clin Oncol* 2002;20:2453.

149. Wiseman GA, Gordon LI, Multani PS, et al. Ibritumomab tiuxetan radioimmunotherapy for patients with relapsed or refractory non-Hodgkin lymphoma and mild thrombocytopenia: a phase II multicenter trial. *Blood* 2002;99:4336.

Edward Chu
Vincent T. DeVita, Jr.

CHAPTER **14**

Principles of Medical Oncology

The development of chemotherapy in the 1950s and 1960s resulted in the availability of curative therapeutic strategies for patients with hematologic malignancies and several types of advanced solid tumors. These advances confirmed the principle that chemotherapy could indeed cure cancer and provided the rationale for integrating chemotherapy into combined modality programs with surgery and radiation therapy in early stages of disease so as to provide clinical benefit. The principal obstacles to the clinical efficacy of chemotherapy have been toxicity to the normal tissues of the body and the development of cellular drug resistance. The development and application of molecular techniques to analyze gene expression of normal and malignant cells at the level of DNA, RNA, and protein has helped to identify some of the critical mechanisms through which chemotherapy exerts its antitumor effects and activates the program of cell death. This modern-day technology has also provided insights into the molecular and genetic events within cancer cells that can confer chemosensitivity to drug treatment. This enhanced understanding of the molecular pathways by which chemotherapy exerts its cytotoxic activity and by which genetic change can result in resistance to drug therapy has provided a rationale for the development of innovative therapeutic strategies in which molecular, genetic, and biologic therapies can be used in combination to directly attack these novel targets. As we now move forward in this new millennium, the implementation of such novel treatment approaches provides an important paradigm shift regarding which therapy is administered. The long-term goal of these intense research efforts is to improve the clinical outcome for cancer patients undergoing treatment, especially those with cancers that traditionally have been resistant to conventional chemotherapy.

HISTORICAL PERSPECTIVE

The systemic treatment of cancer has its roots in the initial work of Paul Ehrlich, who coined the term *chemotherapy*. The use of *in vivo* rodent model systems to develop antibiotics for treating infectious diseases led Clowes and colleagues at Roswell Park Memorial Institute, in the early 1900s, to develop inbred rodent lines bearing transplanted tumors to screen potential anticancer drugs. This *in vivo* system provided the foundation for mass screening of novel compounds.[1] Alkylating agents represent the first class of chemotherapeutic drugs to be used in the clinical setting. Of note, application of this class of compounds was a direct product of the secret gas program of the United States during both world wars, based on the astute observation that exposure to mustard gas in World War II resulted in bone marrow and lymphoid hypoplasia. This experience led to the first clinical use of nitrogen mustard in patients with hematologic malignancies, including Hodgkin's disease and lymphocytic lymphomas, at the Yale Cancer Center in 1943. Treatment with this alkylating agent resulted in dramatic regressions in advanced lymphomas and thereby generated significant excitement in the field of cancer pharmacology. At about this same time, Sidney Farber reported that folic acid had a significant proliferative effect on leukemic cell growth in children with lymphoblastic leukemia. These observations led to the development of folic acid analogs as cancer drugs to inhibit cellular folate metabolism and thus initiated the era of cancer chemotherapy. In fact, the entire class of antimetabolites, including the fluoropyrimidines, cytarabine, and gemcitabine, and the purine analogs were all designed with the expectation that they would inhibit the normal pathways involved in pyrimidine and purine metabolism, respectively, and thereby

295

inhibit cancer cell proliferation and growth. Indeed, these compounds represent the very first examples of targeted anticancer agents to be developed for clinical application.

CLINICAL APPLICATION OF CHEMOTHERAPY

Chemotherapy is presently used in four main clinical settings: (1) primary induction treatment for advanced disease or for cancers for which there are no other effective treatment approaches (Tables 14-1 and 14-2); (2) neoadjuvant treatment for patients with localized disease for whom local forms of therapy, such as surgery or radiation, or both, are inadequate by themselves (Table 14-3); (3) adjuvant treatment to local methods of treatment, including surgery or radiation therapy, or both (Table 14-4); and (4) direct instillation into sanctuary sites or site-directed perfusion of specific regions of the body directly affected by the cancer.

Primary induction chemotherapy refers to drug therapy administered as the primary treatment for patients who present with advanced cancer for which no alternative treatment exists.[2] This has been the mainstay approach to treating patients with advanced, metastatic disease, and in most cases, the goals of therapy are to palliate tumor-related symptoms, improve overall quality of life, and prolong time to tumor progression and survival. Studies involving a wide range of solid tumor types have clearly shown that in patients with advanced disease chemotherapy confers survival benefit when compared with supportive care, which provides sound rationale for the early initiation of drug treatment. Cancer chemotherapy can be curative in a relatively small subset of patients who present with advanced disease. In adults, these curable cancers include Hodgkin's and non-Hodgkin's lymphoma, germ cell cancer, and choriocarcinoma; curable childhood cancers include acute lymphoblastic leukemia, Burkitt's lymphoma, Wilms' tumor, and embryonal rhabdomyosarcoma.

Neoadjuvant chemotherapy refers to the use of chemotherapy in patients who present with localized cancer for which alternative local therapies, such as surgery, exist but are less than completely effective.[3] For chemotherapy to be used as the initial treatment for a cancer that would be partially curable by either surgery or radiation therapy, there must be documented evidence for its clinical efficacy in the advanced disease setting. At present, neoadjuvant therapy is most often administered in the treatment of anal cancer, bladder cancer, breast cancer, esophageal cancer, laryngeal cancer, locally advanced non–small cell lung cancer, and osteogenic sarcoma. For some of these dis-

TABLE 14-1. Primary Chemotherapy: Neoplasms for Which Chemotherapy Is the Primary Treatment Modality

Non-Hodgkin's lymphoma
Lymphoblastic lymphoma
Burkitt's lymphoma and non-Burkitt's, undifferentiated lymphoma
Hodgkin's lymphoma
Primary central nervous system lymphoma
Wilms' tumor
Embryonal rhabdomyosarcoma
Small cell lung cancer

TABLE 14-2. Primary Chemotherapy: Neoplasms for Which There Is an Expanding Role for Primary Chemotherapy of Advanced Disease

Bladder cancer
Breast cancer
Cervical cancer
Esophageal cancer
Gastric cancer
Head and neck cancer
Nasopharyngeal cancer
Non–small cell lung cancer
Ovarian cancer
Pancreatic cancer
Prostate cancer

eases, such as anal cancer, gastroesophageal cancer, laryngeal cancer, and non–small cell lung cancer, optimal clinical benefit is derived when chemotherapy is administered with radiation therapy, either concurrently or sequentially.

One of the most important roles for cancer chemotherapy is as an adjuvant to local treatment modalities such as surgery and radiation therapy, and this has been termed *adjuvant chemotherapy*.[4] The development of disease recurrence, either locally or systemically, after surgery or radiation or both is due mainly to the spread of occult micrometastases. Thus, the goal of adjuvant therapy is to reduce the incidence of both local and systemic recurrence and to improve the overall survival of patients. In general, chemotherapy regimens with clinical activity against advanced disease may have curative potential after surgical resection of the primary tumor, provided the appropriate dose and schedule are used. Several well-conducted randomized phase III clinical studies have documented the effectiveness of adjuvant chemotherapy in prolonging both disease-free and overall survival in patients with breast cancer, colorectal cancer, gastric cancer, non–small cell lung cancer, Wilms' tumor, and osteogenic sarcoma. There is also evidence to support the use of adjuvant chemotherapy in patients with anaplastic astrocytomas. Patients with primary malignant melanoma at high risk of metastases derive benefit in terms of improved disease-free survival and overall survival from adjuvant treatment with the biologic agent interferon-α, although this treatment must be given for 1 year for maximal clinical efficacy. Finally, the antiestrogen tamoxifen is an effective adjuvant drug in postmenopausal women whose breast tumors express the estrogen receptor. Because this agent is cytostatic

TABLE 14-3. Neoadjuvant Chemotherapy: Neoplasms for Which Neoadjuvant Chemotherapy Is Indicated for Locally Advanced Disease

Anal cancer
Bladder cancer
Breast cancer
Esophageal cancer
Head and neck cancer
Gastric cancer
Osteogenic sarcoma
Rectal cancer
Soft tissue sarcoma

TABLE 14-4. Adjuvant Chemotherapy: Neoplasms for Which Adjuvant Therapy Is Indicated after Surgery

---

Anaplastic astrocytoma
Breast cancer
Colorectal cancer
Gastric cancer
Malignant melanoma[a]
Non–small cell lung cancer
Osteogenic sarcoma

---

[a]See Chapter 38.2 for a complete discussion of the controversy over the interpretation of the data from the interferon adjuvant trials.

rather than cytocidal, however, adjuvant therapy with tamoxifen must be administered on a long-term basis, and the standard recommended treatment length is 5 years.

CLINICAL END POINTS IN EVALUATING RESPONSE TO CHEMOTHERAPY

PRIMARY INDUCTION CHEMOTHERAPY

In induction chemotherapy for patients with advanced cancer and measurable disease, it is possible to assess response to drugs on an individual basis. *Partial response rate* is defined as the fraction of patients who demonstrate at least a 50% reduction in measurable tumor mass. There is growing evidence to suggest that quality-of-life indices are higher in patients who show either a response to therapy or a minimal response than in those receiving supportive care, even when overall survival is not improved. However, partial responses are also useful in the evaluation of new drugs or new drug regimens, to determine whether a specific experimental approach is worthy of further clinical development.

Clearly, however, the most important indicator of the effectiveness of chemotherapy is the rate of complete response.[5] No patient with advanced cancer has ever been cured without first achieving a complete remission. In support of this concept is the fact that the recent advances in the treatment of advanced colorectal, breast, and non–small cell lung cancer have brought significant improvements in overall response rates and survival, yet have not translated into actual cure for these respective diseases. The reason is that the complete response rate for even these newer regimens has been uniformly lower than 10%. When new anticancer drugs alone or in combination with other agents consistently produce more than an occasional complete remission, they have invariably been proven to have significant clinical benefit in medical practice. Thus, in clinical trials, complete and partial responses should always be reported separately. The most important indicator of the quality of a complete remission is the relapse-free survival from the time treatment is discontinued. This criterion is the only clinical counterpart of the quantifiable cytoreductive effect of drugs in *in vivo* preclinical models. The use of freedom from progression as a measure in groups of patients who have shown a mixture of complete and partial responses can be misleading when a new treatment is evaluated. This method of analyzing clinical outcomes is a relatively simple indicator of the practical potential of a new treatment. For experimental treatments, however, it obscures the value of a

relapse-free survival in those showing complete response as the major determinant of the quality of remission and the potential for cure. Other clinical end points, such as median response duration and median survival, although used in clinical trial design, are also of little practical value until treatment results have been refined to the point at which complete response rates are higher than 50%.

NEOADJUVANT CHEMOTHERAPY

The unique feature of administering chemotherapy to cancer patients with localized disease before or in place of strictly local treatments such as surgery, radiation therapy, or both is the preservation of the presenting tumor mass as a biologic marker of chemosensitivity to the drugs. Moreover, this approach has allowed the sparing of vital normal organs, including the larynx, the anal sphincter, and the bladder, as the primary tumor is reduced in size and rendered easier to treat by traditional local modalities, such as surgery. As with induction chemotherapy for patients with advanced cancer, it is possible to determine the potential efficacy of a new treatment program on an individual basis. A good response to chemotherapy identifies a patient who may benefit from further treatment. In contrast, a poor response of the primary tumor to chemotherapy identifies a patient for whom alternative methods of treatment should be seriously considered. Another feature of primary neoadjuvant chemotherapy is the ability to differentiate those showing partial response who have varying prognoses.[5] Removal of residual tumor masses and histologic examination of the tissue allow determination of the viability and character of the remaining tumor cells. The response duration of those showing complete and partial responses must be catalogued separately. Such an approach could result in the development of treatment programs that are shorter, produce less morbidity, and are more effective. One of the other positive aspects of neoadjuvant chemotherapy is that it may be effective in killing micrometastatic disease that is present locally, systemically, or both. Given this fact, the complete extent of disease may not be entirely clear with respect to locoregional lymph node status when chemotherapy is administered in the preoperative setting, either alone or concurrently with radiation therapy. As in the case of locally advanced rectal cancer, additional cycles of chemotherapy are mandated to reduce the incidence of both local and systemic recurrence.

ADJUVANT CHEMOTHERAPY

The rationale for adjuvant chemotherapy is to treat micrometastatic disease at a time when tumor burden is at a minimum, which thereby enhances the potential efficacy of drug treatment. It was assumed that chemotherapy, when administered at such an early stage, would result in significantly higher cure rates.[6,7] Unfortunately, because the primary tumor has already been removed, the major indicator of clinical efficacy of a chemotherapy program—the complete remission rate—is absent in the adjuvant setting. Treatment is selected for individual patients based on response rates experienced in an entirely different population, namely that of patients with advanced disease of the same histologic type. In adjuvant programs, relapse-free survival and overall survival remain the major end points. The relapse-free survival in the adjuvant setting measures time to regrowth to clinically detectable levels of cells unresponsive, partially responsive, or exquisitely sensitive to chemotherapy, and this end point is the equivalent of the duration of remission of a combined group of those showing complete response, partial response, and nonresponse. Of note, an analysis of adjuvant clinical studies for early-stage colon cancer conducted in the United States and Europe has suggested that the vast majority of relapses occurs within the first 3 years after completion of adjuvant therapy. These findings provide a rationale for considering 3-year disease-free survival as the primary end point in adjuvant clinical trials of primary colon cancer.

CANCER CELL KINETICS AND RESPONSE TO CHEMOTHERAPY

The key principles of chemotherapy were initially defined by Skipper et al.[8,9] using the murine leukemia L1210 cells as their experimental model system. However, the drug treatment of human cancers requires a clear understanding of the differences between the growth characteristics of this rodent leukemia and those of human cancers, as well as an understanding of the differences in growth rates of normal target tissues in mice and in humans. For example, L1210 is a rapidly growing leukemia with a high percentage of cells synthesizing DNA, as measured by the uptake of tritiated thymidine (the labeling index). Because L1210 leukemia has a growth fraction of 100% (i.e., all its cells are actively progressing through the cell cycle), its life cycle is consistent and predictable.

Based on findings with the murine L1210 model, the cytotoxic effects of anticancer drugs follow logarithmic cell-kill kinetics. In general, a given agent would be predicted to kill a constant fraction of cells as opposed to a constant number. Thus, if an individual drug leads to a 3 log kill of cancer cells and reduces the tumor burden from 10^{10} to 10^7 cells, the same dose used at a tumor burden of 10^5 cells reduces the tumor mass to 10^2. Cell kill is therefore proportional, regardless of tumor burden. When treatment failed in sensitive cell lines, it was because the initial tumor burden was too high for even potentially curative doses of chemotherapy to eradicate the very last leukemia cell. The cardinal rule of chemotherapy—the invariable inverse relation between cell number and curability—was established with this model, and this relationship can be applied to other model systems, including both hematologic malignancies and solid tumors.

Although growth of murine leukemias simulates exponential cell kinetics, mathematical modeling data suggest that most human solid tumors do not grow in such an exponential manner. Taken together, the experimental data for human solid cancers support a Gompertzian model of tumor growth and regression. The critical distinction between Gompertzian and exponential growth is that in Gompertzian kinetics, the growth fraction of the tumor is not constant but decreases exponentially with time (exponential growth is matched by exponential retardation of growth). The growth fraction peaks when the tumor is approximately 37% of its maximum size. Under the Gompertzian model, when a patient with advanced cancer is treated, the tumor mass is larger, its growth fraction is low, and the fraction of cells killed is therefore small. An important feature of Gompertzian growth is that response to chemotherapy in drug-sensitive tumors depends, in large measure, on where the tumor is on its particular growth curve.

Predictions can be made about the behavior of small tumors, such as microscopic tumors present after primary surgical therapy. When the tumor is clinically undetectable, its growth fraction is at its highest level, and although the numerical reduction in cell number is small, the fractional cell kill from a known-to-be-effective therapeutic dose of a chemotherapy agent would be significantly higher than later in the tumor course. This observation was initially used to justify dose reductions at lower tumor volumes. However, such an unnecessary dose reduction may account for some of the disappointments in the outcomes of studies of adjuvant chemotherapy in early-stage breast cancer. The Gompertzian model for tumor growth is important because it can help to predict patterns of regrowth of residual tumor cells. Norton[10] analyzed the clinical data from multiple adjuvant studies for primary breast cancer and from available studies of untreated patients with localized disease. In each clinical study, the Gompertzian model precisely fit the growth curves of these tumors. In the adjuvant setting, the model predicted that relapse-free survival and overall survival curves will be unable to discriminate between a residual cell population of only 1 cell and a residual population of 1 million cells, because the regrowth of residual cell populations will be faster for smaller volumes than for larger volumes, and identical results will be produced sometimes at 5 years after diagnosis and treatment. These findings suggest that, unless total eradication of micrometastases (cure) is achieved, varying residual volumes will produce similar 5-year relapse-free survival rates and obscure the major differences in tumor reduction by different programs. This information has been especially useful in the design of new adjuvant treatment protocols for early-stage breast cancer, which is addressed next in Principles Governing the Use of Chemotherapy.

PRINCIPLES GOVERNING THE USE OF CHEMOTHERAPY

With rare exceptions (e.g., choriocarcinoma and Burkitt's lymphoma), single drugs at clinically tolerable dosages have been unable to cure cancer. In the 1960s and early 1970s, drug combination regimens were developed based on known biochemical actions of available anticancer drugs rather than on their clinical efficacy. Such regimens were largely ineffective, however.[11,12] The era of effective combination chemotherapy began when a number of active drugs from different classes became available for use in combination in the treatment of the acute leukemias and lymphomas. After this initial success with hematologic malignancies, combination chemotherapy was extended to the treatment of most solid tumors.

Combination chemotherapy using conventional cytotoxic agents accomplishes several important objectives not possible with single-agent therapy. First, it provides maximal cell kill within the range of toxicity tolerated by the host for each drug as long as dosing is not compromised. Second, it provides a broader range of interaction between drugs and tumor cells with different genetic abnormalities in a heterogeneous tumor population. Finally, it may prevent or slow the subsequent development of cellular drug resistance.

Certain principles have been useful in guiding the selection of drugs in the most effective drug combinations, and they provide a paradigm for the development of new drug therapeutic programs. First, only drugs known to be partially effective against the same tumor when used alone should be selected for use in combination. If available, drugs that produce some fraction of complete remission are preferred to those that produce only partial responses. Second, when several drugs of a class are available and are equally effective, a drug should be selected that has toxicity that does not overlap with the toxicity of other drugs to be used in the combination. Although such selection leads to a wider range of side effects, it minimizes the risk of a lethal effect caused by multiple insults to the same organ system by different drugs and allows dose intensity to be maximized. In addition, drugs should be used at their optimal dose and schedule, and drug combinations should be given at consistent intervals. Because long intervals between cycles negatively affect dose intensity, the treatment-free interval between cycles should be the shortest possible time necessary for recovery of the most sensitive normal target tissue, which is usually the bone marrow. Finally, there should be a clear understanding of the biochemical, molecular, and pharmacokinetic mechanisms of interaction between the individual drugs in a given combination, to allow for maximal effect. Omission of a drug from a combination may allow overgrowth by a cell line sensitive to that drug alone and resistant to other drugs in the combination. Finally, arbitrary reduction in the dosage of an effective drug to add other less effective drugs may dramatically reduce the dosage of the most effective agent below the threshold of effectiveness and destroy the capacity of the combination to cure disease in a given patient.

Most standard treatment programs were designed around the kinetics of recovery of the bone marrow in response to chemotherapy exposure. The introduction of the colony-stimulating factors, such as filgrastim and the long-acting molecule pegfilgrastim, has been a significant advance for cancer therapy, because they help to accelerate bone marrow recovery and prevent the onset of severe myelosuppression.[13] These cytokine growth factors have played an instrumental role in facilitating the delivery of dose-intense chemotherapy by reducing the incidence of infections and the need for hospitalizations. Without question, these agents have revolutionized the next generation of chemotherapy treatment.

No rigid schedule can accommodate all the variables assumed to be important for maximum effectiveness of combination chemotherapy. Physicians must often adjust doses at intervals to allow for the safe administration of drugs. The certainty that the therapeutic effect of a drug or drug combination can be lost if the dose or schedule is altered should temper these judgments. Reductions in dose rates also often result in only minimal decreases in toxicity but can lead to a major reduction in the capacity to attain a complete remission in patients with drug-responsive tumors.[14] The application of appropriate guidelines for dose reductions preserves the intervals between treatment cycles, preserves the integrity of each drug combination, and, finally, provides consistency across patients and various clinical studies.

For many years, clinical trial design was dominated by the use of alternating cycles of combination chemotherapy. The basis for this approach was the translation of preclinical experimental data into a model for clinical treatment. In 1943, Luria and Delbruck[15] observed that the bacterium *Escherichia coli* developed resistance to bacterial viruses (bacteriophages) not by surviving exposure but by expanding clones of bacteria that had

spontaneously mutated to a type inherently resistant to phage infection. This was a seminal principle in bacterial genetics that laid the framework for the understanding of the development of spontaneous resistance to cancer chemotherapy. In 1979, Goldie and Coldman[16] applied this principle to the development of resistance to anticancer drugs by cancer cells without prior exposure to these drugs. They proposed that the nonrandom cytogenetic changes now known to be associated with most human cancers probably were tightly associated with the development of the capacity to resist the action of certain types of anticancer drugs. They developed a mathematical model that predicted that tumor cells mutate to drug resistance at a rate intrinsic to the genetic instability of a particular tumor. Their model predicted that such events would begin to occur at population sizes between 10^3 and 10^6 tumor cells (1000 to 1 million cells), much lower than the mass of cells considered to be clinically detectable (10^9, or 1 billion, cells). The probability that a given tumor contains resistant clones when a patient's disease is newly diagnosed is a function of both tumor size and the inherent mutation rate. If the mutation rate is as infrequent as 10^{-6}, a tumor composed of 10^9 cells (a 1-cm mass) would be predicted to have at least one drug-resistant clone; however, the absolute number of resistant cells in a tumor composed of 10^9 cells would be relatively small. Therefore, in the clinical setting, such tumors should initially respond to treatment with a partial or complete remission but will recur as the resistance clone expands to repopulate the tumor mass. Such a pattern is commonly seen in the clinical setting with the use of chemotherapy, even in many drug-responsive tumors.

The Goldie-Coldman model predicts that cellular drug resistance should be present even with small tumors and that the maximal chance for cure occurs when all available effective drugs are given simultaneously. Because this involves using multiple drugs, perhaps up to eight to ten drugs, administered simultaneously, this approach has not generally been tested in the clinic for fear that the use of more than five cytotoxic drugs at full doses would not be possible. An alternative approach, using two programs of equally effective, non–cross-resistant drug combinations in alternating cycles, has been under evaluation since the mid-1980s. However, many studies purporting to test the Goldie-Coldman hypothesis have not been properly designed. First, in many instances, inadequate testing has been carried out to determine whether the alternate combination is truly non–cross-resistant and is as effective as the primary treatment. In most instances, these requirements are not met. Second, except in rare cases, dosing is usually not controlled properly. Doses of essential drugs are modified downward, *a priori*, without testing the potential impact of such dose reductions on outcome. Finally, the requirement for symmetry in biologic characteristics of tumors in different patients is unrealistic. The use of alternating cycles of combination chemotherapy has not yet proven to be more effective than full doses of a single effective combination program.

In the late 1980s and early 1990s, Norton and Day[17,18] reanalyzed the Goldie-Coldman hypothesis, and their mathematical model relaxed the requirement for symmetry. Although they confirmed the basic tenets of the Goldie-Coldman hypothesis, their model suggested a different approach to sequencing combinations. According to their work, the sequential use of drug combinations was predicted to outperform alternating cycles, because no two combinations were likely to be strictly non–cross-resistant or have equal cell-killing capacity, the symmetry assumed in the Goldie-Coldman model. There is now a growing list of clinical examples in which sequential therapies have outperformed alternating cyclic use of the same programs, when the dose intensity of the two regimens is carefully controlled.[19,20]

One final issue relating to chemotherapy relates to the optimal duration of drug administration. Several randomized trials of the adjuvant treatment of breast and colorectal cancer have shown that short-course treatment on the order of 6 months is as effective as long-course therapy (12 months).[21,22] Although progressive disease during chemotherapy is a clear indication to stop treatment in the advanced disease setting, the optimal duration of chemotherapy for patients without disease progression has not been well defined. With the development of novel and more potent drug regimens, the potential risk of cumulative adverse events, such as cardiotoxicity secondary to the anthracyclines and neurotoxicity secondary to the taxanes and the platinum analogs, must also be factored into the decision-making process. There is, however, no evidence of clinical benefit in continuing therapy indefinitely until disease progression. A randomized study of advanced colorectal cancer comparing continuous and intermittent palliative chemotherapy showed that a policy of stopping and rechallenging with the same chemotherapy provides a reasonable treatment option for patients.[23] Similar observations have been made in the treatment of advanced metastatic disease affecting other organ sites, including non–small cell lung cancer, breast cancer, germ cell cancer, ovarian cancer, and small cell lung cancer. Several requirements must be met, however, for such an intermittent treatment approach to be adopted into clinical practice. First, the induction chemotherapy regimen must be of sufficient clinical efficacy and duration to ensure that the majority of responses are achieved during the treatment period. Second, a good response must be shown to the reinitiation of the same chemotherapy or to the administration of an effective salvage chemotherapy regimen. Third, there should be a sufficient time interval between the termination of primary induction chemotherapy and the onset of progressive disease. Finally, patients who are taken off of active chemotherapy must be followed closely to ensure that treatment can be reinstituted at the first sign of disease progression.

CONCEPT OF DOSE INTENSITY

One of the main factors limiting the ability of chemotherapy and radiation therapy to achieve cure is effective dosing. The dose-response curve in biologic systems is usually sigmoidal, with a threshold, a lag phase, a linear phase, and a plateau phase. For chemotherapy and radiation therapy, therapeutic selectivity is significantly dependent on the differential between the dose-response curves of normal tissues and tumor tissues. In experimental *in vivo* models, the dose-response curve is usually steep in the linear phase, and a reduction in dose when the tumor is in the linear phase of the dose-response curve almost always results in a loss in the capacity to cure the tumor effectively before a reduction in the antitumor activity is observed. Thus, although complete remissions continue to be observed with dose reduction to as low as 20%, residual tumor cells may not be entirely eliminated, which thereby allows for eventual relapse to occur.

Using the transplantable Ridgway osteosarcoma tumor model, Skipper[9] showed that a reduction in the average dose intensity of the two-drug combination of L-phenylalanine mustard and cyclophosphamide resulted in a marked decrease in the cure rate before a significant reduction in the complete remission rate could occur. On average, a dose reduction of approximately 20% gave rise to a loss of 50% in the cure rate. Although *in vivo* systems may not represent the ideal model for human malignancies, the general principles may be applicable to the clinical setting. Because anticancer drugs are associated with toxicity, it is often appealing for clinicians to avoid acute toxicity by simply reducing the dose or by increasing the time interval between each cycle of treatment. Such empiric modifications in dose represent a major reason for treatment failure in patients with drug-sensitive tumors who are receiving chemotherapy in either the adjuvant or advanced disease setting.

As noted earlier, a major issue facing clinicians is the ability to deliver effective doses of chemotherapy in a dose-intense manner. The concept of dose intensity was put forth by Hryniuk et al.,[24–27] who defined *dose intensity* as the amount of drug delivered per unit of time. Specifically, this was expressed as milligrams per square meter per week, regardless of the schedule or route of administration. The dose intensity of each drug regimen is then determined based on the time period in which the treatment program is administered. Specific calculations can be made of the intended dose intensity, which is the dose intensity originally proposed in the treatment regimen, or of the received dose intensity. It is the received dose intensity, rather than the intended dose intensity, that is the more clinically relevant issue, because it reflects the direct impact of dose reductions and treatment delays imposed in actual practice. A positive relationship between dose intensity and response rate has been documented in treatment of several solid tumors, including advanced ovarian, breast, lung, and colon cancers, as well as in hematologic malignancies, including the lymphomas.[25–27]

Frei et al.[28] and Hryniuk et al.[29] have proposed the term *summation dose intensity* to reflect the close relationship between dose and combination chemotherapy. As part of this concept, they suggested that the final outcome of a combination treatment must be related in some manner to the sum of the dose intensities of all the agents used in that treatment. The intrinsic chemosensitivity of a given tumor is critical for treatment success. It has been established that, for nearly all malignancies, a combination regimen incorporating at least three active drugs is necessary for cure. In the case of childhood leukemia, the cure rate increases linearly when the number of active drugs increases from three to seven. The critical issue for this concept is that all active agents must be used at their full therapeutic doses. Although the concept of summation dose intensity is not new, it does offer a unified approach for the careful design and interpretation of clinical trials.

Calculations of the impact of dose intensity on outcome are particularly important in estimating the efficacy of adjuvant chemotherapy. The steep dose-response curve for most anticancer drugs indicates that dose reductions in adjuvant chemotherapy programs are likely to be associated with significantly less therapeutic effect. Historically, dose reduction has been the common practice in the design of adjuvant trials. One example is the standard CMF [cyclophosphamide, methotrexate, and 5-fluorouracil (5-FU)] regimen for breast cancer. The initial reports for this regimen revealed an impressive complete remission rate of approximately 30% in the advanced disease setting, albeit at the expense of considerable toxicity. When this regimen was advanced for use in the cooperative group setting, initially for advanced disease and later for adjuvant trials by Bonadonna et al.,[30] the doses of the respective agents were arbitrarily reduced without first testing the potential impact of such reductions on clinical outcome. In addition, further reduction was empirically made for patients older than 60 years, on the assumption that such a dose reduction would be required for age. Careful analysis of the data suggest that such dose reductions have had a negative impact on clinical outcome.[31] In premenopausal women, the differences in relapse-free survival at low and high doses of CMF are statistically significant. The importance of dose effect was further confirmed by a large study in which a survival benefit was observed as a result of increasing dose intensity in the adjuvant chemotherapy for women with stage II node-positive breast cancer.[32]

At present, there are three main approaches to delivery of chemotherapy in a dose-intense fashion. The first approach is through dose escalation in which the doses of the anticancer agents are increased. The second strategy is to administer anticancer agents in a dose-dense manner by reducing the interval between treatment cycles. The third approach involves sequential scheduling of either single agents or combination regimens. The use of sequential scheduling should also be considered as a means of delivering chemotherapy in a dose-dense approach.

As has already been discussed in Cancer Cell Kinetics and Response to Chemotherapy, the growth of most solid tumors follows a pattern of gompertzian kinetics. In this setting, the growth of cells is significantly faster in the early part of the growth curve than at any other stage in the growth kinetics. For this reason, the initiation of chemotherapy at an earlier stage would theoretically produce greater effects than initiation at a later stage. The log cell kill generated by chemotherapy would, therefore, be higher in tumors of small volume than in those of large volume. In such cases, the regrowth of cancer cells between chemotherapy cycles is more rapid. Thus, the more frequent administration of cytotoxic chemotherapy would represent an attractive strategy to minimize residual tumor burden. In computer simulations, this relatively simple maneuver has, indeed, achieved significantly higher benefit by minimizing the regrowth of cancer cells between cycles of treatment. The clinical relevance of dose density was supported by a landmark randomized phase III trial comparing dose-dense versus conventionally scheduled chemotherapy in the adjuvant treatment of node-positive primary breast cancer (INT C9741). In this study, Citron and colleagues[33] showed that a dose-dense schedule, in which the anticancer agents doxorubicin, cyclophosphamide, and paclitaxel were administered every 2 weeks rather than at the conventional 3-week intervals, resulted in significantly improved clinical outcomes with respect to disease-free survival and overall survival. Of note, because of the concomitant use of the colony-stimulating factor filgrastim (granulocyte colony-stimulating factor), dose-dense therapy was not accompanied by an increase in toxicity. Although a dose-dense approach may have its greatest application in the adjuvant setting, examples are growing of cases in which this strategy is also effective in the treatment of metastatic disease. Dose-dense regimens have shown superior clinical activity compared with standard chemotherapy in metastatic colorectal cancer, extensive-stage small cell lung cancer, and poor-prognosis germ cell cancer.

One of the potential limitations of modern combination chemotherapy is that dose levels of individual drugs are generally reduced in an effort to limit toxicity when the drugs are used in combination. To address this issue, investigators have administered drug combinations in an alternating sequence to deliver a greater number of different drugs per unit time. This strategy may not allow for enhanced dose intensity, however; in fact, it may actually compromise clinical benefit. A randomized clinical trial conducted by Bonadonna et al.[20] observed that four 3-week cycles of doxorubicin followed by eight 3-week cycles of CMF in women with high-risk primary breast cancer (four or more positive lymph nodes) was better in terms of disease-free survival and overall survival than an alternating schedule of doxorubicin and CMF. Sledge et al.[34] addressed the issue of sequential versus combination therapy in the Eastern Cooperative Oncology Group E1193 randomized phase III trial of sequential single-agent therapy with doxorubicin and paclitaxel versus a combination of the two agents as the first-line treatment for metastatic breast cancer. Although combination therapy yielded a superior response rate and time to disease progression, this improvement in clinical benefit did not translate into a survival benefit when compared with sequential single-agent therapy. Moreover, combination therapy did not improve patient quality of life. Thus, this clinical study provides support for the notion that sequential chemotherapy represents a reasonable treatment option in patients with metastatic breast cancer. Such sequential strategies are being developed for treatment of other solid tumors, including colorectal cancer and ovarian cancer. In advanced colorectal cancer, sequential treatment with single-agent 5-FU followed by 5-FU–based combination regimens has shown considerable promise, with improvements in median survival in the 8- to 10-month range.

APOPTOSIS, CELL-CYCLE CONTROL, AND RESISTANCE TO CHEMOTHERAPY

The kinetic models described are relevant only in the context of a tumor that is sensitive to chemotherapy. For more than 30 years, the classic view of anticancer drug action has involved the specific interaction between a given drug and its respective target. Cell death arises as a direct consequence of this drug-receptor interaction. However, the critical molecular mechanisms involved, from facilitation of the initial coupling of the stimulus to the final response of the cell, were never clearly elucidated. Because of the enhanced understanding of the molecular mechanisms underlying the control of the cell cycle and the process of programmed cell death (apoptosis), it is now clear that this simplistic model is insufficient to explain the cytotoxic effects of anticancer agents. In contrast to the view of the classic model that the drug–target interaction leads directly to cell death, it is now well appreciated that such an interaction acts as the initial stimulus that then sets off a cascade of events that eventually results in apoptosis. This pathway involves some type of sensor that detects a death-inducing signal, a signal transduction network, and an execution machinery that facilitates the process of cell death. Moreover, this entire process is exceedingly complex, because it is highly dependent on the specific cell type under study, the specific anticancer agent being tested, and the cellular context and environment in which the drug–target interaction is being considered.

In addition, the capacity of certain cancers to resist the cytotoxic effects of cancer chemotherapy may be more closely connected either to abnormalities in the genetic machinery of cancer cells or to alterations in the critical pathways of cell-cycle checkpoint control and apoptosis than to the specific mechanisms of resistance unique to each agent. This observation is underscored by the general failure to overcome resistance to chemotherapy in the clinic with approaches that attack only the classic biochemical or molecular mechanisms of resistance (or both). This section briefly reviews the complex interrelationship between products of cell-cycle checkpoint genes, oncogenic viruses, transcription factors, apoptosis, and chemotherapy as they relate to drug resistance. More detailed discussions of these topics are available elsewhere.[35–39]

One of the remarkable features of both radiation therapy and chemotherapy is that their cytotoxic effects initially may be greater in neoplastic cells than in normal host tissues, including the bone marrow and the gastrointestinal (GI) tract, when administered to sensitive tumors. Doses that eradicate some sensitive tumors will not ablate the bone marrow or destroy the capacity of the GI mucosa to regenerate. Until recently, no molecular basis for this therapeutic selectivity was known. Molecular genetic studies have revealed that, in contrast to malignant cells, normal cells such as those derived from the bone marrow and gut express an intact genetic machinery. As a result, the normal mechanisms for apoptosis and cell-cycle arrest after exposure to genotoxic and cytotoxic stresses remain present. Thus, normal bone marrow and GI precursor cells are able to effectively monitor and repair DNA damage after exposure to a genotoxic stress, as well as destroy cells with irreparable DNA, rather than allowing damaged cells to progress through the normal cell cycle and potentially replicate their damaged DNA. Because normal cells express an intact genetic machinery, they are able to recover from exposure to DNA-damaging anticancer agents, except in the case of high-dose chemotherapy as observed in transplantation programs. In the transplant setting, high doses of chemotherapy are able to overwhelm these protective mechanisms, which results in direct cellular necrosis.

p53

The protein p53 is a tumor suppressor protein and critical transcriptional activator that plays a key role in mediating G_1 and G_2 arrest of the cell cycle after exposure to DNA-damaging agents and other genotoxic stress.[35–39] This function is thought to be essential in preserving the integrity of the cellular genome in response to treatment with a cytotoxic agent. In addition to playing a role in preserving the cell-cycle checkpoint, p53 is a potent inducer of programmed cell death (apoptosis) of a cell in which DNA damage has occurred.[50] The basis for the cell's decision either to undergo growth arrest with subsequent repair of DNA damage or to induce apoptosis remains unclear. Significant research efforts are focused on elucidating the critical factors that determine the eventual cellular function of p53. This is undoubtedly a complex issue that must take into account the extent of DNA damage, the stage of the cell cycle at which the DNA damage occurs, the presence of other genetic abnormalities in either the cell-cycle regulatory

apparatus or the signaling machinery, the specific cellular environment within the cell, and exogenous factors within the cellular matrix. Of note, some cell types, such as germ cell tumors, lymphocytes, and the tumors derived from them, have a more rapid access to apoptotic mechanisms than the large majority of epithelial cancers.

Mutations in the p53 gene are among the most common genetic alterations observed in human tumor samples and have been estimated to occur in at least 50% of all human tumors.[40] The initial studies showing that loss of p53 function was associated with resistance to radiation therapy as well as chemotherapy came from *in vivo* model systems using p53 knockout mice.[41,42] Subsequent studies have confirmed that various malignant cell lines and tumors expressing mutant or deleted p53 are chemoresistant to a wide range of anticancer agents.[43,44] Loss of p53 function is not always associated with chemoresistance, however. Some studies suggest that cells with impaired p53 function can become sensitized to various anticancer agents. Thus, the relationship between p53 status and chemosensitivity is complex and is presumably dependent on a number of factors, including the specific cytotoxic stimuli, tissue-specific differences, and the specific cellular context that incorporates the overall genetic machinery and the various intracellular signaling pathways.

The specific cytotoxic treatment, the conditions of treatment, p53 status, and other cell-cycle regulatory elements may all contribute to the outcome of an exposure of a cell to DNA-damaging agents. If the dose of the treatment is exceedingly high, nonapoptotic cell death (e.g., necrotic cell death due to DNA or other damage) may occur. At an intermediate level of dose intensity, p53-dependent or p53-independent apoptotic cell death can occur. When p53 function is intact, the level of inhibitors of p53 is not high, and the regulatory environment of the cell is such that the cell circumvents the interruption of the cell-cycle progression that occurs after DNA damage, the cell will undergo p53-dependent apoptosis. However, in the setting of abnormal p53 function, whether through the acquisition of point mutations in the p53 gene, posttranslation inactivation of p53 through binding to other protein partners (e.g., MDM2) or enhancement of degradation (e.g., the E6 protein of the human papillomavirus), or decreased translation of wild-type p53 messenger RNA by the folate-dependent enzyme thymidylate synthase, the cell is unable to undergo cell-cycle arrest or apoptosis in response to DNA damage. In a tumor population, the functional inactivation of p53 through any of these regulatory mechanisms facilitates genomic instability and contributes to the development of cellular resistance. Normal hematopoietic and GI mucosa cells are genetically stable as a result of an intact p53 mechanism that provides them with the ability to undergo apoptosis after treatment with chemotherapy.

Some of the genes that are transcriptionally activated by p53 belong to a class of proteins known to inhibit the cyclin-dependent kinases.[45] One of these proteins, known as *p21* (Waf-1, Cip-1), can form a complex with proliferating cell nuclear antigen or inhibit the full activation of the cyclin-dependent kinase. When the cyclin kinase is fully active, it acts on another tumor suppressor, the retinoblastoma (RB) gene, to phosphorylate it. This causes the release of the E2F family of transcription factors, which then bind to the regulatory regions of a number of genes that participate in the synthesis of DNA. These genes include ribonucleotide reductase, dihydrofolate reductase, DNA-dependent RNA polymerase, thymidylate synthase, c-myc, c-fos, and c-myb.

Activation of this family of proteins promotes and supports cell entry from G_1 into the S phase of the cell cycle. The activation of cyclin-dependent kinases and the consequent turning on of the DNA synthetic machinery by release of E2F from RB occur in normal cells after growth factor stimulation, which probably provides the signal for the initiation of the cyclin clock. When normal p53 is activated after DNA damage, significant induction occurs in the levels of p21, p27, and other gene products, such as those of MDM2, an apparent feedback regulator of p53, and GADD45, a gene involved in DNA repair. When the expression of p21 is induced to high levels, it exerts an inhibitory effect on the formation of the fully active cyclin kinase complex. This critical checkpoint function of p53, which restricts the procession of the cell into the DNA-synthetic phase of the cell cycle, also prevents the E2F-dependent expression of gene products related to rapid cell growth.

One of the downstream genes potentially influenced by p53 is the mdr-1 gene, because it has been shown that wild-type p53 suppresses the promoter of the mdr-1 gene. In contrast, there is evidence in some systems that mutant p53 protein is able to stimulate the promoter.[46] The biologic basis for this action is not readily apparent, but when the foregoing effects are considered *in toto*, dysregulation of the p53 pathway, which would be expected to be associated with more rapid growth, might well be a prominent mechanism of drug resistance due to the overproduction of gene products responsible for entry into S phase and rapid cell growth. The activation or induction of these genes could theoretically increase the resistance of cells to a wide range of chemotherapeutic agents, including methotrexate, 2-chlorodeoxyadenosine, hydroxyurea, fludarabine, cytosine arabinoside, and 5-FU. Furthermore, the action of an entire array of the most effective natural product antitumor agents could be suppressed through stimulation of the mdr-1 promoter directly by a mutant form of p53. Thus, an active p53 in the setting of such DNA-damaging agents as chemotherapy or irradiation increases the levels of key gene products to levels that are sufficient to inhibit the phosphorylation of the RB gene by cyclin-dependent kinase. This, in turn, prevents the expression of the gene products necessary for DNA synthesis to occur.

It is conceivable that increasing growth rates may be associated with increasing levels of drug resistance through the increased transcription of genes involved in rapid cell growth and entry into the cell cycle. The high degree of resistance in more advanced tumors, including the spontaneous development of resistance, which was the basis of the Goldie-Coldman hypothesis, as well as the development of multidrug resistance appears more likely to be related to mutations in key genes in the cell-cycle regulatory system than to drug-specific spontaneous mutations, as was proposed in the past. Cell death in response to exposure to DNA-damaging agents may require an intact p53-dependent apoptotic mechanism under some experimental circumstances. However, it also may depend on the activation of alternative pathways of apoptosis or some degree of reregulation of the system that would ultimately lead to the reduced release of transcription factors from genes such as RB or a homologous gene, p107, and the production of lower levels of growth-related gene products, which thereby sensitizes cells to chemotherapeutic agents. An enhanced understanding of the complexities surrounding chemotherapy-induced cell death may shed new insights which would have profound implications for the design of future approaches to therapy that might couple standard cytotoxic agents with new biologic agents that attack specific molecular targets to reregulate the cell-cycle checkpoint.

ROLE OF BCL-2 FAMILY IN APOPTOSIS

Because apoptosis is a genetically programmed event, inactivation of genes that induce the apoptotic program or activation of antiapoptotic genes can result in the development of cellular drug resistance. Bcl-2 is a potent suppressor of apoptotic cell death, and a number of studies have shown that its expression leads to repression of cell death triggered by either gamma irradiation or a variety of anticancer agents.[47,48] Not only does it play a critical role in apoptosis, but Bcl-2 protein has been shown to be overexpressed in several human cancers, including non-Hodgkin's lymphoma, prostate cancer, melanoma, breast cancer, and non–small cell lung cancer. In further support of the role of Bcl-2 as an inhibitor of cell death are preclinical *in vitro* and *in vivo* studies demonstrating that treatment of certain human leukemia or non-Hodgkin's lymphoma cell lines with an antisense strategy directed against Bcl-2 leads to the reversal of chemoresistance.

In addition, the phosphorylation status of Bcl-2 may play an important role as a determinant of chemosensitivity.[49] There is growing evidence that the phosphorylated form of Bcl-2 interacts less efficiently with its heterodimer protein partner bax, which results in cell death. Bcl-x_l, a functional and structural homologue of Bcl-2, is also able to confer protection against radiation-induced apoptosis as well as against a wide number of anticancer agents, including bleomycin, cisplatin, etoposide, and vincristine. Recently, the antiapoptotic effects of Bcl-2 and Bcl-x_l were compared using FL5.12 lymphoid cells. These two proteins have a differential ability to protect against chemotherapy-induced cell death. This differential effect depends more on the molecular mechanism targeted than on the cell-cycle specificity of an individual drug. In contrast to Bcl-2 and Bcl-x_l, other family members, including Bax, Bcl-x_s, and Bak, have been shown to promote apoptosis in response to either radiation or various anticancer drugs (or both). The underlying mechanisms through which these Bcl-2 family members control apoptosis are complex, and this field remains an active area of investigation.

DEATH EXECUTIONER PATHWAY

The molecular mechanisms and intracellular signal transduction pathways initiated by a given cytotoxic or genotoxic stress may differ significantly. However, the final stage of these various death pathways is mediated through the activation of caspases,[50,51] which represent a highly conserved family of cysteine proteases. The specific caspases involved in apoptosis include 3, 6, 7, 8, and 9, and they exert their effects through cleavage of protein kinases and other signal transduction proteins, cytoskeletal proteins, chromatin-modifying protein, and DNA repair proteins.

The activation of caspases is determined by the intrinsic and extrinsic pathways of apoptosis. The intrinsic pathway is a mitochondrial-dependent pathway mediated by the Bcl-2 family of proteins. Exposure to cytotoxic stress results in disruption of the mitochondrial membrane, which then leads to release of cytochrome *c* and other protease activators. Cytochrome *c* binds with Apaf-1, which allows for interaction with procaspase 9 and other proteases. Caspase 9 is subsequently activated, setting off a cascade of events that commits the cell to undergo apoptosis. The extrinsic pathway is mediated by ligand binding to the tumor necrosis factor (TNF) family of receptors, which includes TNF receptor-1, Fas, DR3, DR4 [TNF-related apoptosis-inducing ligand (TRAIL) R1], DR5 (TRAILR2), or DR6, coupled with an intracytoplasmic death domain protein and certain essential adaptor proteins. These adaptor proteins recruit various proteases and then cleave the N-terminal domain of caspase 8, which leads to activation of the caspase cascade. There are important links between the intrinsic and extrinsic pathways, and caspase 3 plays the key role in this regard. Studies of several knockout mouse models expressing germline disruptions of Apaf-1, caspase 3, or caspase 9 have shown that these genetically engineered mice are resistant to gamma irradiation and chemotherapy.

CELL SURVIVAL PATHWAYS

The presence of several external stimuli, including various cytokines, TNF-α, chemotherapy, and radiation, leads to activation of the transcription factor nuclear factor κB (NFκB).[52] Paradoxically, activation of NFκB results in potent suppression of the apoptotic potential of these stimuli. Several studies have demonstrated that inhibition of NFκB *in vitro* leads to enhanced apoptosis in response to different stimuli.[53] There is preclinical *in vivo* evidence that the adenoviral delivery of a modified form of IκBα, an inhibitor of NFκB, results in inhibition of NFκB expression. Moreover, chemoresistant fibrosarcoma tumors derived from HT1080 cells become resensitized to the apoptotic potential of TNF-α and the topoisomerase I compound irinotecan, which leads to significant antitumor activity. These findings suggest that activation of NFκB expression in response to chemotherapy may represent an important mechanism of inducible tumor chemoresistance. Moreover, they suggest that strategies to inhibit NFκB may represent a rational approach to enhance chemosensitivity to antitumor therapy through increased apoptosis. Such an approach is discussed next in, Development of Novel Therapeutic Strategies.

DEVELOPMENT OF NOVEL THERAPEUTIC STRATEGIES

Significant focus continues to be placed on understanding the molecular events that are involved in the development of human cancers. Clearly, there is a wide range of signal transduction pathways critical for the growth and proliferation of individual tumors. In addition, evidence is growing that many of these signaling pathways are intimately involved with other key cellular events, including DNA repair, cell survival signals, invasion and metastasis, and the process of angiogenesis. It is also now being increasingly appreciated that many of these same signaling pathways may play a key role in mediating sensitivity to chemotherapy or radiation therapy. With this enhanced understanding of the pivotal events involved in cancer cell growth and proliferation, serious efforts are being made to translate this knowledge into the rational design and development of novel therapeutic approaches to improve the efficacy of chemotherapy.

The agent that ushered in this new era of targeted therapies is the signal transduction inhibitor imatinib. This anticancer agent was rationally designed based on the crystal structure of the Bcr-Abl tyrosine kinase, which had been found to be expressed solely in chronic myelogenous leukemia (CML), and this molecule binds to the adenosine triphosphate (ATP) pocket within the enzyme. In addition, imatinib inhibits other related tyrosine kinases, including platelet-derived growth factor, stem cell factor, and c-kit. In so doing, imatinib functions as a potent competitive inhibitor of ATP binding and inhibits substrate phosphorylation and downstream-signaling pathways. This agent is currently approved for the treatment of CML.[54] Of note, given its high level of specificity for CML, this agent has a favorable safety profile, and its associated side effects are usually mild. Not only is it used to treat CML, but treatment with imatinib is curative in patients with refractory GI stromal tumors that express the c-kit tyrosine kinase.[55]

The epidermal growth factor receptor (EGFR)–signaling pathway is presently one of the most actively investigated areas in cancer drug development.[56] Preclinical studies have shown that activation of EGFR and its downstream-signaling events plays a key role in regulating tumor cell growth and proliferation, DNA repair and survival, invasion and metastasis, and angiogenesis. Second, increased expression of EGFR is observed in a broad range of solid tumors, including colorectal cancer, non–small cell lung cancer, head and neck cancer, pancreatic cancer, and breast cancer. Finally, a number of clinical studies have correlated expression of EGFR with disease progression, poor treatment outcome, and poor patient survival. Several approaches have been devised to inhibit the EGFR pathway. These include development of small-molecule inhibitors of the tyrosine kinase (TKI) domain of the receptor, monoclonal antibodies directed against the cell surface receptor, and antisense molecules directed against the messenger RNA encoding the EGFR-associated tyrosine kinase. The first two strategies have been tested in the clinical setting, and there is evidence that both TKIs and monoclonal antibodies have clinical activity. Gefitinib (ZD1839, Iressa) is an orally active, highly selective, reversible inhibitor of the tyrosine kinase domain associated with the EGFR, and this agent was approved by the Food and Drug Administration in the spring of 2003 as monotherapy for the treatment of patients with locally advanced or metastatic non–small cell lung cancer after failure of platinum-based chemotherapy or second-line docetaxel chemotherapy (or both).[57] Patients with the bronchoalveolar pathologic subtype of non–small cell lung cancer appear to be more sensitive to therapy than those with other histologic subtypes. Several phase II and III studies are currently investigating the role of gefitinib as monotherapy and in combination regimens with standard chemotherapy for treatment of other solid tumors such as head and neck, breast, prostate, gastric, and colorectal cancers. With respect to antibody-directed therapy, three monoclonal antibodies currently are being investigated: cetuximab, EMD72000, and ABX-EGF. The chimeric immunoglobulin G1 antibody cetuximab is furthest along in clinical development, and it has shown promising clinical activity as monotherapy, with a 10% to 12% response rate in heavily pretreated patients with advanced colorectal cancer.[58] Perhaps of greater significance is the fact that in patients with irinotecan-resistant advanced colorectal cancer treated with cetuximab in combination with the topoisomerase I inhibitor irinotecan, sensitivity to irinotecan therapy is restored, which yields overall response rates in the 21% to 23% range.[59] Recent studies also suggest that the addition of cetuximab is able to restore chemosensitivity to chemotherapy regimens on which patients with advanced non–small cell lung cancer, head and neck cancer, and pancreatic cancer were already progressing.

A critical determinant for a cancer cell to undergo apoptosis or cell-cycle arrest with repair of DNA damage may be the presence or absence of essential growth factors within the cellular environment. Thus, in the absence of growth factor stimuli, the cell would become committed to the apoptotic pathway after exposure to a cytotoxic stress. Both preclinical and clinical studies suggest that this scenario may indeed be true. The positive clinical results with the anti-EGFR antibody cetuximab in combination with irinotecan certainly provide support for this concept. A similar enhancement has been observed when the anti–HER2-neu monoclonal antibody (trastuzumab), a member of the erbB family and closely related to the anti-EGFR antibodies, is used together with either paclitaxel or the combination of cyclophosphamide and doxorubicin for the treatment of advanced breast cancer.[60] Although this antibody has single-agent activity in Her2-neu–expressing breast cancer, significantly higher activity is observed when it is used in combination with chemotherapy. This agent is currently approved by the U.S. Food and Drug Administration for both monotherapy and combination treatment of women with advanced breast cancer.

The ras/raf-signaling cascade is a key step in growth factor–mediated signal transduction through the mitogen-activated protein kinase pathway.[61] There is considerable evidence that Raf-1 possesses oncogenic potential and that it plays an important role in tumorigenesis, which provides a rationale for novel therapies directed against Raf expression or activity. BAY 43-9006 is an orally active, small-molecule inhibitor of Raf kinase with broad-spectrum activity against colorectal cancer, non–small cell lung cancer, and pancreatic, ovarian, and hepatocellular tumors *in vivo*. Not only does it show an inhibitory effect on Raf kinase, but there is evidence that this molecule inhibits the vascular endothelial growth factor receptor-2, one of the main target receptors for a key proangiogenic factor, vascular endothelial growth factor. Phase I studies have documented clinical activity in cancers of the liver, kidney, colorectum, ovary, and cervix, and recent phase II studies have documented clinical responses in advanced renal cell cancer. These studies suggest that Raf inhibition is a rational target for cancer chemotherapy, and studies are now being extended to determine whether this molecule can be effectively combined with standard chemotherapy.

Because of the pivotal role of Bcl-2 as a mediator of apoptosis and its increased expression in a number of human solid tumors and hematologic malignancies, serious efforts have focused on Bcl-2 as a potential target for drug design and development.[62] An antisense phosphorothioate oligonucleotide (G3139) was designed to target the first 18 nucleotides of the human Bcl-2 protein-coding region. In the preclinical setting, treatment with this antisense molecule resulted in degradation of Bcl-2 messenger RNA with subsequent downregulation of Bcl-2 protein expression. Further *in vitro* and *in vivo* studies showed that Bcl-2 antisense treatment significantly enhanced the antitumor effects of various anticancer agents in a wide range of model systems, including melanoma, lymphoma, prostate cancer, and non–small cell lung cancer. This 18-nucleotide antisense oligonucleotide has shown documented activity in refractory, heavily pretreated non-Hodgkin's lymphoma and chronic lymphocytic leukemia in a phase I trial.[63] Several combination studies are now under way to investigate the ability of the Bcl-2 antisense treatment to enhance the clinical efficacy of standard chemotherapy for melanoma, chronic lymphocytic leukemia, non–small cell lung cancer, and multiple myeloma.

Inhibition of NFκB represents a rational approach to enhance or restore chemosensitivity in antitumor therapy. Bortezomib (PS-341) is a modified dipeptidyl boronic acid that is a reversible inhibitor of the chymotrypsin-like activity of the 26S proteasome in mammalian cells. The 26S proteasome is a large ATP-dependent multicatalytic protein complex that degrades ubiquitinated proteins. The ubiquitin-proteasome degrades several short-lived intracellular regulatory proteins that govern certain critical signaling pathways involved in cell cycle, transcription factor activation, apoptosis, angiogenesis, cell trafficking, invasion, and metastasis.[64] Of note, this system mediates proteolysis of IκB, the endogenous inhibitor of NFκB. Degradation of IκB by the proteasome leads to activation of NFκB, which results in stimulation of cell growth, inhibition of apoptosis, and induction of cellular drug resistance. Inhibition of proteasome multienzyme complex by bortezomib leads to inhibition of targeted proteolysis of multiple critical cellular proteins, and the end effect is cell-cycle arrest, induction of apoptosis, and restoration of chemosensitivity. In preclinical models of multiple myeloma, bortezomib was shown to induce apoptosis, reduce adherence of myeloma cells to bone marrow stromal cells, and block production and intracellular signaling of interleukin-6. This work was extended into the clinical setting, where this agent has shown promising clinical activity in patients with refractory multiple myeloma.[65] Based on these promising clinical results, bortezomib was approved by the U.S. Food and Drug Administration in 2003 for treatment of relapsing or refractory multiple myeloma. Several phase I and II clinical trials are currently evaluating the role of bortezomib in treatment of other tumor types, including CML, neuroendocrine tumors, renal cell carcinoma, melanoma, platinum-sensitive ovarian cancer, soft tissue sarcomas, colorectal cancer, breast cancer, low-grade lymphoproliferative disorders, and mantle cell lymphoma.

It is well established that a universal pathway allowing mitogenic and growth factor signals to promote progression from the S to G_1 phase requires the phosphorylation and inactivation of the retinoblastoma gene product (Rb), a key tumor suppressor gene product critical for G_1 control.[66] Rb inactivation results from its phosphorylation by serine/threonine kinases, known as *cyclin-dependent kinases*. At least nine different cyclin-dependent kinases have been identified to date, and they form complexes with proteins known as cyclins, of which 15 have been described. Most human cancers express aberrancy in some component of the Rb pathway, which can result from hyperactivation of cyclin-dependent kinase; amplification or overexpression of cyclins and other positive factors or downregulation of negative factors, or both; increased expression of cyclin-dependent kinase inhibitors; or a mutation in the Rb protein itself. Inhibition of cyclin-dependent kinases represents an attractive strategy to treat human cancer, and one such cyclin-dependent kinase modulator, flavopiridol, is presently in clinical development. Flavopiridol is a semisynthetic flavonoid derived from rohutukine, a plant indigenous to India, and it is a potent inhibitor of all cyclin-dependent kinases. Treatment with this agent also leads to a reduction in the expression of cyclin D1, an oncogene that is overexpressed in a broad range of human cancers. Finally, preclinical studies provide intriguing evidence that flavopiridol may also have antiangiogenic activity by promoting the degradation of vascular endothelial growth factor messenger RNA. Phase I and II clinical studies have shown clinical activity in renal cell cancer and non–small cell lung cancer, and further studies are now being designed to optimize the schedule of administration.[67]

REFERENCES

1. Marchall EK Jr. Historical perspectives in chemotherapy. *Adv Chemother* 1964;1:1.
2. DeVita VT. The evolution of therapeutic research in cancer. *N Engl J Med* 1978;298:907.
3. Frei A 3rd, Clark JR, Miller D. The concept of neoadjuvant chemotherapy. In: Salmon SE, ed. *Adjuvant therapy of cancer*, 5th ed. Orlando, FL: Grune and Stratton, 1987:67.
4. Muggia FM. Primary chemotherapy: concepts and issues. In: *Primary chemotherapy in cancer medicine*. New York: Alan R. Liss, 1985:377.
5. DeVita VT. On the value of response criteria in therapeutic research. *Bull Cancer* 1988;75:863.
6. Goldie JH, Coldman AJ. Theoretical considerations regarding the early use of adjuvant chemotherapy. *Recent Results Cancer Res* 1986;103:30.
7. Goldie JH. Scientific basis for adjuvant and primary (neoadjuvant) chemotherapy. *Semin Oncol* 1987;14:1.
8. Skipper HE, Schabel FM Jr, Mellet LB, et al. Implications of biochemical, cytokinetic, pharmacologic and toxicologic relationships in the design of optimal therapeutic schedules. *Cancer Chemother Rep* 1950;54:431.
9. Skipper HE. Kinetics of mammary tumor cell growth and implications for therapy. *Cancer* 1971;28:1479.
10. Norton LA. A Gompertzian model of human breast cancer growth. *Cancer Res* 1988;48:7067.
11. Nathanson L, Hall TC, Schilling AC, et al. Concurrent combination chemotherapy of human solid tumors: experience with three-drug regimen and review of the literature. *Cancer Res* 1969;29:419.
12. DeVita VT, Schein PS. The use of drugs in combination for the treatment of cancer: rationale and results. *N Engl J Med* 1973;288:998.
13. Glaspy JA. Hematopoietic management in oncology practice. Part I. Myeloid growth factors. *Oncology* 2003;17:1593.
14. DeVita VT. The influence of information on drug resistance on protocol design: the Harry Kaplan memorial lecture given at the fourth international conference on malignant lymphoma. *Ann Oncol* 1991;2:93.
15. Luria SE, Delbruck M. Mutations of bacteria from virus sensitivity to virus resistance. *Genetics* 1943;28:491.
16. Goldie JH, Coldman AJ. A mathematical model for relating the drug sensitivity of tumors to the spontaneous mutation rate. *Cancer Treat Rep* 1979;63:1727.
17. Day RS. Treatment sequencing, asymmetry, and uncertainty: protocol strategies for combination chemotherapy. *Cancer Res* 1986;46:3876.
18. Norton L, Day RS. Potential innovations in scheduling in cancer chemotherapy. In: DeVita VT Jr, Hellman S, Rosenberg SA, eds. *Important advances in oncology 1991*. Philadelphia: Lippincott-Raven Publishers, 1991:57.
19. Buzzoni R, Bonadonna G, Valagussa P, et al. Adjuvant chemotherapy with doxorubicin plus cyclophosphamide, methotrexate, and fluorouracil in the treatment of resectable breast cancer with more than three positive axillary nodes. *J Clin Oncol* 1991;9:2134.
20. Bonadonna G, Zambetti M. Sequential or alternating doxorubicin and CMF regimens in breast cancer with more than three positive nodes. *JAMA* 1995;273:542.
21. Fuchs CS, Mayer RJ. Adjuvant chemotherapy for colon and rectal cancer. *Semin Oncol* 1995;22:472.
22. Early Breast Cancer Trialists' Collaborative Group. Systemic treatment of early breast cancer by hormonal, cytotoxic, or immune therapy. *Lancet* 1992;339:71.
23. Maughan TS, James RD, Kerr DJ, et al. Comparison of intermittent and continuous palliative chemotherapy for advanced colorectal cancer: a multicenter randomized trial. *Lancet* 2003;361:457.
24. Hryniuk WM. Average relative dose intensity and the impact on design of clinical trials. *Semin Oncol* 1987;14:65.
25. Levin L, Hryniuk W. Dose intensity analysis of chemotherapy regimens in ovarian carcinoma. *J Clin Oncol* 1987;5:756.
26. Hryniuk W, Bush H. The importance of dose intensity in chemotherapy of metastatic breast cancer. *J Clin Oncol* 1984;2:1281.
27. Hryniuk W, Goodyear M. The calculation of received dose intensity. *J Clin Oncol* 1990;8:1935.
28. Frei E 3rd, Elias A, Wheeler C, et al. The relationship between high-dose treatment and combination chemotherapy: the concept of summation dose intensity. *Clin Cancer Res* 1998;4:2027.
29. Hryniuk W, Frei E 3rd, Wright FA. A single scale for comparing dose-intensity of all chemotherapy regimens in breast cancer: summation dose-intensity. *J Clin Oncol* 1998;16:3137.
30. Bonadonna G, Brusamalino MP, Valagussa R, et al. Combination chemotherapy as an adjuvant treatment in operable breast cancer. *N Engl J Med* 1976;298:405.
31. Bonadonna G, Calagussa R. Dose-response effect of adjuvant chemotherapy in breast cancer. *N Engl J Med* 1981;304:10.
32. Wood W, Korzan AH, Cooper R, et al. Dose and dose intensity of adjuvant chemotherapy for stage II node positive breast cancer. *N Engl J Med* 1994;330:1253.
33. Citron ML, Berry DA, Cirrincione C, et al. Randomized trial of dose-dense versus conventionally scheduled and sequential versus concurrent combination chemotherapy as postoperative adjuvant treatment of node-positive primary breast cancer: first report of intergroup trial C9741/Cancer and Leukemia Group B Trial 9741. *J Clin Oncol* 2003;12:1431.
34. Sledge GW, Neuberg D, Bernardo P, et al. Phase III trial of doxorubicin, paclitaxel, and the combination of doxorubicin and paclitaxel as front-line chemotherapy for metastatic breast cancer: an intergroup trial (E1193). *J Clin Oncol* 2003;21:588.
35. El-Deiry WS. The role of p53 in chemosensitivity and radiosensitivity. *Oncogene* 2003;22:7486.
36. Canman CE, Kastan MB. Role of p53 in apoptosis. *Adv Pharmacol* 1997;41:429.
37. Levine AJ. p53, the cellular gatekeeper for growth and division. *Cell* 1997;88:323.
38. Sax JK, El-Deiry WS. p53 downstream targets and chemosensitivity. *Cell Death Differ* 2003;10:413.
39. McGill G, Fisher DE. p53 and cancer therapy: a double-edged sword. *J Clin Invest* 1999;104:223.
40. Hollstein M, Sidransky DE, Vogelstein B, et al. p53 mutations in human cancers. *Science* 1991;253:49.
41. Lowe SW, Ruley HE, Jacks T, et al. p53-dependent apoptosis modulates the cytotoxicity of anticancer agents. *Cell* 1993;74:957.
42. Lowe SW, Bodis S, McClatchey A, et al. p53 status and the efficacy of cancer therapy in vivo. *Science* 1994;266:807.
43. Wu GS, El-Deiry WS. p53 and chemosensitivity. *Nat Med* 1996;2:255.
44. Wahl AF, Donaldson KL, Fairchild C, et al. Loss of normal p53 function confers sensitization to Taxol by increasing G2/M arrest and apoptosis. *Nat Med* 1996;2:72.
45. El-Deiry WS. Regulation of p53 downstream genes. *Cancer Biol* 1998;8:345.
46. Bush JA, Li G. Cancer chemoresistance: the relationship between p53 and multidrug transporters. *Int J Cancer* 2002;98:323.
47. Miyashita T, Reed JC. Bcl-2 oncoprotein blocks chemotherapy-induced apoptosis in a human leukemia cell line. *Blood* 1993;81:151.
48. Reed JC. Bcl-2 and the regulation of programmed cell death. *J Cell Biol* 1994;124:1.
49. Korsmeyer SJ. Regulators of cell death. *Trends Genet* 1995;11:101.
50. Green DR. Apoptotic pathways: the roads to ruin. *Cell* 1998;94:695.
51. Thornberry NA, Lazebnik Y. Caspases: enemies within. *Science* 1998;238:1312.
52. Wang CY, Mayo MW, Baldwin AS. TNF-α and cancer therapy-induced apoptosis: potentiation by inhibition of NF-κB. *Science* 1996;274:784.
53. Wang CY, Cusack JC Jr, Liu R, et al. Control of inducible chemoresistance: enhanced antitumor therapy through increased apoptosis by inhibition of NF-kappaB. *Nat Med* 1999;5:412.
54. Druker BJ, et al. Efficacy and safety of a specific inhibitor of the BCR-ABL tyrosine kinase in chronic myelogenous leukemia. *N Engl J Med* 2001;344:1031.
55. Demetri GD, et al. Efficacy and safety of imatinib mesylate in advanced gastrointestinal stromal tumors *N Engl J Med* 2002;347:472.
56. Baselga J. Targeting the epidermal growth factor receptor: a clinical reality. *J Clin Oncol* 2001;19[Suppl]:41S.
57. Herbst R, et al. Dose-comparative monotherapy trials of ZD1839 in previously treated non-small cell lung cancer patients. *Semin Oncol* 2003;30[Suppl 1]:30.
58. Saltz L, Meropol NJ, Loehrer PJ, et al. Single agent IMC-C225 has activity in CPT-11 refractory colorectal cancer (CRC) that expresses the epidermal growth factor receptor (EGFR). *Proc Am Soc Clin Oncol* 2002;21:127a(abst).
59. Cunningham D, Humblet Y, Siena S, et al. Cetuximab (IMC-C225) alone or in combination with irinotecan (CPT-11) in patients with epidermal growth factor receptor (EGFR)-positive, irinotecan-refractory metastatic colorectal cancer (MCRC). *Proc Am Soc Clin Oncol* 2003;22:252(abst).
60. Slamon DJ, et al. Use of chemotherapy plus a monoclonal antibody against HER2 for metastatic breast cancer that overexpresses HER2. *N Engl J Med* 2001;344:783.
61. Gelmon KA, Eisenhuer EA, Harris AL, et al. Anticancer agents targeting signaling molecules and cancer cell environment: challenges for drug development? *J Natl Cancer Inst* 1999;91:1281.
62. Tolcher AW. Regulators of apoptosis as anticancer targets. *Hematol Oncol Clin North Am* 2002;16:1255.
63. Kim R, Tanabe K, Emi M, et al. Potential roles of antisense therapy in the molecular targeting of genes involved in cancer. *Int J Oncol* 2004;24:5.
64. Takimoto CH, Diggikar S. Heat shock protein and proteosome targeting agents. *Hematol Oncol Clin North Am* 2002;16:1269.
65. Richardson P, et al. A phase II study of bortezomib in relapsed, refractory myeloma. *N Engl J Med* 2003;348:2609.
66. Senderowicz AM, Sausville EA. Preclinical and clinical development of cyclin-dependent kinase modulators. *J Natl Cancer Inst* 2000;92:376.
67. Senderowicz AM. Cyclin-dependent kinases as new targets for the prevention and treatment of cancer. *Hematol Oncol Clin North Am* 2002;16:1229.

CHAPTER 15

Pharmacology of Cancer Chemotherapy

SECTION **1**

EDWARD CHU

Drug Development

Since the 1950s, significant advances have been made in the chemotherapeutic management of cancer. Unfortunately, more than 50% of all cancer patients either do not respond to initial therapy or experience relapse after an initial response to treatment and ultimately die from progressive metastatic disease. Thus, the ongoing commitment to the design and discovery of new anticancer agents is critically important.[1-3] Chemotherapy, in its classic form, has been focused primarily on killing rapidly proliferating cancer cells by targeting general cellular metabolic processes, including DNA, RNA, and protein biosynthesis and, because of this, may not be entirely specific for malignant versus normal cells. The growing understanding of the molecular events underlying the etiology of the different cancers as well as the signaling events that are critical for the continued growth and proliferation of cancer cells has enhanced the opportunities to develop novel agents. This new type of chemotherapy has been termed *targeted therapy*, and the goal of this modern-day chemotherapy is to provide molecularly based agents that are more specific for cancer cells. Current research efforts are being driven by the rapid discoveries in the underlying biology of cancer to fully elucidate the development of the malignant process (e.g., factors controlling tumor angiogenesis, signal transduction and cellular signaling, and invasion and metastasis). The hope for improvements in treatment outcomes for the large majority of cancer patients with metastatic disease relies on these novel targeted therapies, used alone or in combination with standard chemotherapy and with other biologic agents and immunologically based therapies. Moreover, these novel strategies may find particular promise in treating cancer patients at an earlier stage in disease.

Considerable expenditures of money, time, and resources are required for the drug development process to move a new agent from initial discovery to its ultimate approval for clinical use in the treatment of a specific cancer. There are significant challenges that may threaten the development of a promising agent, such as excessive early toxicity, ineffective schedule or route of administration, inappropriate formulation, unpredictable acute or cumulative toxicities, and unpredictable and unavoidable delays in the actual conduct of clinical trials. The time to approval for anticancer agents varies but in general ranges from 6 to 12 years from drug discovery to the completion and analysis of the pivotal clinical trials. Considerable efforts are being made to accelerate both the preclinical and clinical components of drug development in the hopes of shortening the time required to get a drug approved for widespread use in clinical practice.

DRUG DISCOVERY

In establishing research programs for drug discovery, investigators must address two fundamental questions: Which screening system should be used to identify a compound of interest? Which compounds should be tested in this system? These issues are critical in defining whether the research effort is purely empiric or whether it focuses on a specific molecular target. The history of cancer drug discovery reflects an evolution from highly empiric approaches, based on testing of randomly selected compounds for activity against rapidly proliferating murine leukemia, to the current, more focused testing of natural products, rationally synthesized agents, and biologic products for activity against well-characterized human cancer cell lines or molecular targets or both. Two of the first rationally targeted therapies to be developed for the clinic were the antifolates and the fluoropyrimidines, because each of these classes of anticancer agent was designed to inhibit specific target enzymes, namely, dihydrofolate reductase and thymidylate synthase, respectively.

The history of the discovery of antifolates is especially instructive because it highlights the important interplay between cancer biology and drug discovery. Farber et al.[4] made the astute observation that the leukemic process was dramatically accelerated in patients being treated with folic acid. A series of folic acid antagonists was then provided to Farber and colleagues by the medicinal chemists at Lederle Laboratories. Although the precise structure-activity relationship of antifolates and the intracellular target of these compounds was unknown at that time, preclinical laboratory studies revealed that modified folate analogs were potent inhibitors of leukemia cell growth. The initial clinical trial involved the administration of the folic acid analog pteroylaspartic acid to a moribund patient with progressive acute myeloid leukemia, which resulted in a markedly hypocellular bone marrow but provided no clinical benefit. Investigators were sufficiently encouraged, however, to administer a more powerful folic acid antagonist, aminopterin (2,4-diaminopteroylglutamate), to children with advanced stages of acute leukemia. The substitution of an amino group at the 4 position of the folate pteridine ring created a tight-binding inhibitor of dihydrofolate reductase and yielded analogs with the potential to induce remissions. Approximately 10 of the first 16 patients treated with aminopterin demonstrated evidence of hematologic and clinical improvement. This early clinical experience provided the framework for medicinal chemists to synthesize a series of analog compounds, and these structure-activity studies identified agents with varying inhibitory activity on dihydrofolate reductase and with different growth-inhibitory effects on leukemia cells.

At present, rational design efforts have progressed to the use of computer modeling of drug–enzyme interactions as the basis for cancer drug discovery. Advances in x-ray crystallography and nuclear magnetic resonance have facilitated the structural characterization of ligands and their target molecules and have significantly enhanced the potential for rational drug design and the discovery and development of novel lead compounds. Such research efforts are identifying novel small molecules with activity against various human malignancies. The folate-dependent enzyme thymidylate synthase is one of the earliest molecular targets for cancer chemotherapy to have been identified. Based on the x-ray crystal structure of the thymidylate synthase enzyme, investigators designed a series of compounds that bound to the folate-binding pocket of the enzyme, which resulted in potent inhibition of catalytic activity.[5] One of these antifolate analogs, nolatrexed, displayed clinical activity against hepatocellular cancer and head and neck cancer in early phase I and II studies, and based on these promising results, this agent is presently in late-stage phase III clinical development for the treatment of unresectable hepatocellular cancer.[6]

In most current drug discovery programs, rational and empiric approaches are being used either in parallel or in combination with one another. Lead compounds are identified as inhibitors for molecular targets through molecular screening.[7] The lead compound is then modified or enhanced by chemical synthesis based on a variety of considerations, including a detailed analysis of target–inhibitor interaction. The complete characterization of the target and its interaction with the lead agent provides the basis for enhancing drug–target interaction. A key decision in this approach is the identification and selection of a suitable target, the manipulation of which is likely to have an impact on clinical outcome (enzyme, growth factor receptor, or oncogene product). Once a specific biologic target is identified, the next important challenge in this process is to develop an appropriate and practical assay that can then begin to identify active lead compounds.

Although the early efforts in cancer drug discovery focused on agents that came from the broad universe of synthetic chemicals, attention has focused increasingly on natural products as an important source of agents to treat patients with cancer.[8,9] The enormous diversity and complexity of chemical entities that have evolved as part of nature's chemical warfare cannot be readily duplicated by compounds synthesized in the laboratory. Moreover, such natural compounds are not easily available for screening. Approximately 30% of the effective anticancer drugs used in current clinical practice are derived from natural sources or are derivatives of a natural product.[14] Such examples include paclitaxel, isolated from the bark of the Pacific yew tree *Taxus brevifolia*; irinotecan, extracted from the bark of the *Camptotheca accuminata* tree; the vinca alkaloids, isolated from the periwinkle plant *Catharanthus roseus*; and etoposide, which comes from the mandrake plant *Podophyllum peltatum*. Certain themes run through the efforts to discover and develop natural products. Active compounds often have exceedingly complex structures that complicate efforts at total synthesis. The dependence on a natural resource, which could then affect material source supply, is another important issue to consider. Structure-activity relationships are sometimes difficult to characterize, given the difficulties presented by the unusual chemistry of these compounds and by the multiple chiral centers in these molecules. However, medicinal and synthetic organic chemists have been able to overcome many of these obstacles, and their efforts have resulted in the development of several anticancer agents that have entered the clinical arena.

The class of microbial antibiotics represents one of the most important natural product sources of cytotoxic agents. Because of the advances in the field of microbiology during the 1940s and the era of effective antibiotic therapy, potent anticancer drugs were sought in fermentation broths obtained from soil microbes, including bacteria, fungi, and related organisms. The discoveries of the actinomycins, anthracyclines, bleomycin, and deoxycoformycin have made important contributions to the repository of effective antineoplastic agents. Natural product drug discovery, however, must be complemented by efforts to improve leads through chemical modification and analog synthesis. The history of the discovery and subsequent clinical development of the anthracycline class of compounds highlights the importance of the collaborative interplay of chemistry, biology, and clinical pharmacology in the development of improved anticancer agents.

Daunorubicin was originally isolated from a colony of *Streptomyces* in 1957 and was shown to have significant activity in patients with acute myeloid leukemia.[10] Further research to induce mutant strains of *Streptomyces* resulted in the isolation of doxorubicin. Although the difference between these two anthracyclines is limited chemically to a single hydroxyl group, a marked difference exists in their clinical spectrum of activity. Doxorubicin is active in hematologic malignancies as well as in a broad range of solid tumors, whereas the activity of daunorubicin is limited strictly to treatment of acute leukemias.[11] The cardiac toxicity associated with the chronic administration of both these agents, however, led to efforts to design a new generation of anthracycline compounds with an improved safety profile. Although none of the newer anthracycline analogs is completely devoid of cumulative cardiotoxicity, these agents target different diseases. For example, the anthraquinone mitoxantrone is active in acute myeloid leukemia and other cancers, including non-Hodgkin's lymphoma and breast cancer.[11] Thus, modification of the chemical structure of a natural product may yield novel agents with differing spectra of clinical activity.

Several new plant-derived natural products have proven to be of significant benefit in the treatment of cancer. The taxane paclitaxel was originally isolated from the bark of the Pacific yew tree *Taxus brevifolia* in the early 1970s.[12] It has a unique mechanism of action in that it binds with high affinity to microtubules, thereby enhancing tubulin polymerization with resultant inhibition of the normal dynamics of microtubule formation.[13] Preclinical studies revealed that it was active against a number of human tumor xenografts, including breast cancer, ovarian cancer, and non–small cell lung cancer. Subsequent clinical studies confirmed the high degree of activity in patients with a wide range of solid tumors, including breast, bladder, ovary, head and neck, esophagus, stomach, testes, and non–small cell and small cell lung cancer. One of the initial obstacles to the clinical use of paclitaxel in cancer therapy was the extremely limited supply of source material present in the Pacific Northwest region of the United States. However, the supply issue was eventually resolved using new sources of drug from various nursery species, and, in addition, the total chemical synthesis of this complex molecule was eventually accomplished.[14,15] Advances in the chemistry of isoserines and taxoid anticancer agents have facilitated the synthesis of second-generation taxoid compounds with activity against drug-resistant cancer cells. Moreover, the epothilones, which are a class of macrolactone natural products from the myxobacterial species *Sorangium cellulosum*, have been shown to exert cytotoxic and antitumor activity in a manner identical to paclitaxel.[16] In sharp contrast to paclitaxel, the epothilones appear to be equally active against drug-sensitive and multidrug-resistant human cancer cell lines *in vitro*. Furthermore, studies suggest that epothilone B retains antitumor activity *in vivo* in paclitaxel-resistant human tumor models. BMS-247550 and EPO906 are two examples of epothilone B analogs that are undergoing clinical testing, and both have shown activity in patients with various solid tumors, including breast, ovarian, lung, and colorectal cancer.[17]

Another natural product with broad anticancer activity is derived from the bark of *C accuminata*, a tree valued for its medicinal properties in traditional Chinese medicine.[18] The camptothecin derivatives are unique because they inhibit topoisomerase I, a key enzyme that maintains DNA in a torsionally relaxed state. Irinotecan and topotecan are camptothecin analogs, and they display significant activity in patients with advanced malignancies, including colorectal cancer, gastroesophageal cancer, non–small cell and small cell lung cancer, and cervical cancer.[19] Considerable efforts are focused on developing novel analogs of camptothecin with enhanced biochemical, biophysical, molecular, and biologic activity. The agents 9-nitroaminocamptothecin, 9-aminocamptothecin, exatecan, karenitecin, edotecarin, and oral irinotecan are all

at various stages of clinical testing. With the discovery of topoisomerase I as a clinically relevant target for cancer chemotherapy, several noncamptothecin inhibitor compounds have been developed, including the indolocarbazoles (NB-506 and J-107088), and these agents are being tested in clinical trials.[20]

Marine organisms represent a largely unexplored and untapped source of unique toxic chemicals. These toxins are elaborated by sponges and other sessile saltwater organisms as defenses against their predators. The isolation of C-nucleosides from the Caribbean sponge *Cryptotheca crypta* provided the rational basis for the synthesis of the antimetabolite cytarabine, which represents the first marine-derived anticancer agent to be developed for clinical use. Significant advances have been made in the technology of deep-sea collection, extraction, and large-scale production, and these advances have facilitated the use of marine organisms as a source of new anticancer therapies. A number of novel, highly potent experimental agents derived from marine sources have been identified, and they have shown interesting antitumor activity against unique molecular targets in preclinical models as well as in clinical studies. These molecules include the bryostatins (which inhibit protein kinase C), the dolastatins and halichondrins (which bind to microtubules), and the tunicate-derived ecteinascidins (which bind to the minor groove of DNA).[21-23] Ecteinascidin-743 (ET-743) exerts its cytotoxic action through binding to the minor groove of DNA, and it also interferes with the action of DNA-binding proteins and several key transcription factors.[23,24] Clinical trials have shown that this novel agent has clinical efficacy against soft tissue sarcoma as well as melanoma and breast cancer.[25] Overall, it displays a favorable safety profile, with myelosuppression being dose limiting. Although the marine environment represents an untapped potential source for interesting new chemical entities, certain unique problems are associated with this biosphere. Scale-up procurement of bulk material from marine sources presents a special challenge in biomass collection. However, because of the potential clinical activity of agents derived from these sources, sophisticated chemistry technology is now well under way to synthesize the active element once novel therapeutic leads are identified from these natural products.[26]

COMBINATORIAL CHEMISTRY

The field of combinatorial chemistry represents a revolution in both the concepts and construction of chemical entities. This revolution not only has changed the fields of chemical catalysis, materials science, and methods development, but it has also influenced the field of drug development. The human genome has 50,000 to 150,000 unique genes, and each encodes a protein product that is potentially a therapeutic target.[27,28] For example, between 1000 and 3000 unique members are predicted to exist within the protein kinase family, which has now been shown to be an important class of therapeutic targets.[29] Because the average medicinal chemist can synthesize, at most, 100 molecules per year, it is difficult to envision the identification of unique inhibitors for thousands of proteins using traditional chemistry techniques.

The concept of chemical diversity has been recognized since the early days of drug development, when natural products (biologically active chemical entities found in nature) were the main focus of the pharmaceutical industry. At that point, the methods of achieving chemical diversity—in other words, the techniques required to synthesize 10^3 to 10^6 molecules—were unknown, and

TABLE 15.1-1. The Mathematics of Chemical Diversity[a]

Libraries	Number of Positions	Number of Compounds
SYNTHETIC LIBRARIES		
8^n, where n = number of positions		
	1	8
	2	64
	3	512
	4	4096
	5	32,768
	6	262,144
	7	2,097,152
	8	16,777,216
20^n, where n = number of positions		
	1	20
	2	400
	3	8000
	4	160,000
	5	3,200,000
	6	64,000,000
	7	1,280,000,000
$8 \times 12 \times n$, where n = number of plates	*Number of Plates*	*Number of Compounds*
	4	384
	48	4608
	480	46,080
	4800	460,800
	48,000	4,608,000
DNA/RNA LIBRARIES		
4^n, where n = number of positions	*Number of Positions*	*Number of Compounds*
	1	4
	2	16
	3	64
	4	256
	5	1024
	6	4096
	7	16,384
	8	65,536
	9	262,144
	10	1,048,576
	20	1.09×10^{12}
	30	1.15×10^{18}
	40	1.21×10^{24}
PHAGE-DISPLAY LIBRARIES		
64^n, where n = number of positions	*Number of Positions*	*Number of Phages*
	1	64
	2	4096
	3	262,144
	4	16,777,216
	5	1,073,741,824
	6	68,719,476,740
	7	4,398,046,511,000
32^n, where n = number of positions	*Number of Positions*	*Number of Phages*
	1	32
	2	1024
	3	32,768
	4	1,048,576
	5	33,554,432
	6	1,073,741,824
	7	34,359,738,370

[a]The way in which the number of molecules in a library relates to Avogadro's number, 6.0221×10^{23}.

researchers depended on nature for diversity. *Combinatorial chemistry* is a collective term referring to those techniques that are used to achieve chemical diversity. A collection of diverse molecules is referred to as a *chemical library* or, often, a *combinatorial library*.

One issue that must be addressed when designing a chemical library or evaluating a combinatorial phage peptide library is the total number of individual molecules in that library. Table 15.1-1 shows the diversity that one might expect from different chemical and biologic libraries. In any library, the formula for diversity can be described as the number of monomer units raised to the power of the number of variable positions. For example, if a heptapeptide library is synthesized using all 20 natural amino acids, the library will contain 20^7 or 1.28 billion different molecules. If phage display is used to create the same heptapeptide library, the diversity increases to 64^7, or 4.4×10^{12}, library members, which is clearly an unmanageable number of clones for sequencing and analysis. Proper design of the library and use of the wobble position can reduce the required number of codons to 32, which decreases the diversity to 32^7, or 3.4×10^{10}, library members, a number that is still quite large.

The size and chemical diversity of the library must be considered. Accumulating data suggest that it is more important for a library to be diverse than to be large. Permutational libraries, such as libraries of peptides, do not have to cover their diversity. In all likelihood, the epitope is likely to be smaller than the total positions varied. For example, a peptide sequence such as RGD, a common motif in integrin recognition, would come up many times in a heptapeptide library. Some phage-display libraries contain 12 randomized amino acids, with no hope of containing that diversity. These libraries, however, are useful for the identification of discontinuous epitopes within the same peptide. In summary, phage display offers the most accessible first entry into chemical diversity, but often it must be followed up with a synthetic library.

Modern drug development often begins with the screening of thousands of molecules to generate chemical "hits" against a therapeutic target or cell line. A *hit* is defined as a molecule that shows activity in an assay below a certain activity level. High-throughput screening of chemical compounds emerged in the early 1990s to aid the rapid evaluation of the large chemical stocks that were being amassed in the pharmaceutical industry. The high-throughput assay is usually an *in vitro* assay, although it is not necessarily cell free. Once a molecule has been identified as a hit, it is evaluated by a medicinal chemist, who then begins a synthetic effort to obtain a structure-activity relationship for the molecule. If the activity of the initial hit can be optimized for *in vitro* activity, the molecule becomes a *lead* molecule. This process is known as *"hit to lead" development*. Although each therapeutic target has different criteria for the categorization of a lead molecule, the development process is essentially the same. Once a lead is identified, a series of *in vivo* tests and further development take place to determine whether the chemical lead has the proper pharmacologic properties and *in vivo* efficacy to become an actual drug.

Combinatorial chemistry is presently in its adolescent stage with regard to cancer drug development. However, the technologic advances in combinatorial approaches for synthesizing large numbers of complex substances have already provided new sources for novel anticancer agents. For example, the enzyme farnesyltransferase is responsible for targeting the ras oncoprotein to the cellular membrane, and it was one of the first targets explored using combinatorial chemistry because of the well-defined CAAX sequence present at the farnesylation site.[30] The receptor tyrosine kinases and cellular kinases have been identified as therapeutic cancer targets, and the development of kinase inhibitors is an intense area of research with multiple combinatorial library approaches being taken.[31,32] In addition to the active site of kinases, the SH2 recognition and SH3 regulation domains, which are involved in kinase activation, have been identified as attractive targets of combinatorial drug design.[33,34]

DRUG SCREENING

In general, current screening efforts favor model systems that are relatively simple and that can accommodate high-volume testing of unknown compounds. The cancer screen may use as its main end point the activity against a biologic target (e.g., tumor cell cytotoxicity, growth inhibition, differentiation) or the activity against a biochemical-molecular target that is known to be important for the growth and proliferation of cancer cells.

The evolution of strategies at the National Cancer Institute (NCI) illustrates the marked changes in screening patterns that have resulted from the advances in cancer biology and cancer genetics. Early NCI cancer screening efforts used murine leukemias (L1210 and P388) as the index tumors in an *in vivo* screening effort.[35] The screen identified agents with activity in humans in the treatment of leukemias and lymphoproliferative malignancies. However, the failure of this screen to identify agents active against solid tumors resulted in a significant change in the approach of the NCI in the mid-1970s, when animal solid tumor and human tumor xenografts were incorporated as a secondary *in vivo* tumor panel. In 1985, a second important shift in focus occurred when the increasing availability of a number of cell lines derived from human solid tumors and well characterized with respect to drug response patterns, growth factor dependence, oncogene expression, and other biochemical-molecular features presented an opportunity to focus screening efforts on the unique biology of human solid tumors.[36]

A wide range of human solid tumor cell lines were selected to provide a disease-oriented approach to drug discovery in contrast with the previous compound-oriented drug discovery methods. A total of 60 human tumor cell lines derived from seven cancer types (e.g., lung, colon, melanoma, kidney, ovary, brain, and leukemia) formed the original cell line panel, with human breast cancer cell lines being subsequently added. The initial concept proposed that lead compounds demonstrating disease specificity would be identified with this screen and that antitumor activity could be further examined by *in vivo* testing in animal model systems using the most sensitive *in vitro* index tumor cell lines.

In the current NCI anticancer screen, each candidate agent is tested in a broad range of concentrations against every cell line in the panel.[2,3,37] Active compounds are selected for further testing based on several different criteria: disease-type specificity in the *in vitro* assay, unique structure, potency, and demonstration of a unique pattern of cellular cytotoxicity or cytostasis, indicating a unique mechanism of action or intracellular target. The agents selected for further investigation are then subjected to additional testing to assess their *in vivo* therapeutic index.[3,41] The current version of the cancer drug screening program of the NCI has been in use since 1990. This high-capacity screen was designed to accommodate testing of approximately 10,000 individual chemicals annually, with additional capacity for screening natural product extracts. Approximately 5% of the compounds tested in the initial screen show sufficient activity to warrant subsequent evaluation in *in vivo* screens or in biochemical-molecular assays. More than 60,000 agents have been screened against a panel of 60 human cancer cell lines. The tumors that are represented in this cell line panel include melanomas, leukemias, and cancers of the breast, prostate, colon, ovary, kidney, and central nervous system. To date, this approach has identified several novel agents (e.g., a tyrosine kinase inhibitor, a protein kinase C inhibitor, and several disease-specific agents) for further testing in clinical trials, and they include the proteosome inhibitor PS341, flavoperidol, UCN-01, the rapamycin analog CCI-779, and depsipeptide.

The central concept of cancer drug discovery is the acquisition of a large number of diverse materials for examination. In the case of the NCI, an extensive program for acquiring both defined chemical entities and diverse natural products has been pursued. The pharmaceutical industry is also actively engaged in the procurement of large numbers of interesting chemical agents and natural products for testing in their respective cancer screens, many of which focus on specific molecular targets. Difficult decisions must be made in selecting among the large number of unknown entities for initial testing and to facilitate the prioritization of known active compounds for further development. Sophisticated bioinformatics programs have been developed to assist in this effort and to enhance the diversity of potential chemical entries and crude natural products introduced into the screening process.

After an agent has been tested in the cancer screen, its unique response pattern can be compared with the results for all other agents within the database. A computer program called COMPARE uses a simple algorithm for aligning and contrasting the patterns for each compound with the patterns of other compounds in the database.[38,39] A compound is entered into the program as a seed, and the computer database elicits a list of those agents that have similar patterns of tumor cellular responsiveness. A correlation coefficient is also expressed, relating the closeness of the seed to those agents listed by the computer program. Close correlations between agents appear to have biologic and pharmacologic importance, implying a common intracellular target despite a dissimilarity in structure (e.g., tubulin-binding agents, topoisomerase-interactive agents). The COMPARE program has several important features. It can identify the intracellular target or mechanism of action of a new compound through a comparison of its fingerprint with that of known agents. It can search for compounds previously tested in the cancer screen that have a fingerprint similar to that of a lead compound known to inhibit a unique target. It also has the power to detect inhibition of integrated biochemical and molecular pathways that are not adequately represented by a single molecule or molecular interaction. The comparison also allows recognition of a new agent that does not match compounds having known mechanisms of action. Given the critical roles of an intact cell-cycle checkpoint and apoptotic pathways in determining chemosensitivity, such an algorithmic approach may help identify candidate anticancer drugs that are not dependent on an intact checkpoint and apoptosis function. Finally, this strategy provides the rational basis for future pharmacophore development.

Computer approaches to data analysis similar to that described by the NCI are being developed by academic centers and industry to search for agents interacting with specific molecular targets. In addition, the NCI has conducted an elaborate characterization of specific molecular targets expressed by the existing tumor cell lines within its screen.[40] For example, because certain cell lines are known to contain a mutated or overexpressed oncogene, such as k-ras or HER2-neu, it is possible to search the existing database for agents active against only those particular cell lines.[41] This process may ultimately combine the advantages of both cell line–based and molecular screens but will require separate validation to confirm that identified leads do indeed interact with the purported molecular target in specific assays directed at that entity. Although the NCI cell line screen represents a carefully constructed system for obtaining and analyzing voluminous data on diverse compounds, alternative screening systems in academic centers and industry increasingly rely on high-throughput assays based on specific molecular targets, against which combinatorial chemistry inventories are tested.

MOLECULARLY TARGETED SCREENING

With the rapid advances in defining the molecular pathology of neoplastic cells, specific oncogenes have been identified that are expressed uniquely in malignant tissue. The discovery of inappropriately expressed or mutated genes has provided rationale for establishing screens designed to detect specific inhibitors and modulators of these abnormal gene products. Intracellular signaling pathways that mediate the actions of growth factors and oncogenes on cell proliferation, such as protein tyrosine kinases, G proteins, and transcription activators, provide additional novel targets for anticancer drugs. However, given the considerable overlap of access to various growth factor–signaling pathways (many signals use the same distal steps), signal transduction inhibitors may lack the same type of specificity for malignant cells.[42]

The paradigm of a cancer-specific target is the oncofusion protein that results from the BCR-ABL translocation in chronic myeloid leukemia (CML). In patients with CML and in approximately 20% of adult patients with acute lymphocytic leukemia (ALL), a characteristic reciprocal translocation between chromosomes 9 and 22 is observed. The protooncogene (ABL) from chromosome 9 is translocated at the breakpoint cluster region (BCR) on chromosome 22. This translocation encodes the Bcr-Abl protein, which expresses constitutively activated tyrosine kinase function. It is a 210-kD oncoprotein, and expression of p210 Bcr-Abl induces a disease in mice resembling CML, which confirms the critical role of this oncoprotein in the development of CML.[43] The p210 Bcr-Abl protein is present in 95% of patients with CML and in 5% to 10% of adults with ALL in whom there is no evidence of CML. A second fusion protein of 185 kD is found in 10% of adult cases and in 5% to 10% of pediatric cases of ALL.

The expression of this genetic rearrangement is essential for maintaining the malignant phenotype. Of note, the aberrant tyrosine kinase resulting from this abnormal genetic rearrangement (BCR-ABL) within hematopoietic stem cells does not exist in normal host cells. This abnormal gene provides an ideal molecular target for therapeutic intervention. The crystal structure of several protein kinases has been solved, and a number of compounds were designed based on the structure of the adenosine triphosphate (ATP) binding site of the enzyme. In screening against the recombinant Bcr-Abl kinase protein, the 2-phenylaminopyrimidine derivative known as imatinib (STI 571) was found to be a potent and selective inhibitor, targeting the ATP-binding pocket.[44] This compound inhibits all Abl tyrosine kinases at submicromolar concentrations *in vitro*, and it has minimal to no inhibitory effect on the colony-forming potential of normal bone marrow cells. In addition, imatinib demonstrates potent activity against other related tyrosine kinases, including platelet-derived growth factor, stem cell factor, and c-kit.[45] This agent has a favorable safety profile, with its main toxicities being only mild nausea (grade 1), muscle cramps, and arthralgias. In newly diagnosed CML, hematologic responses are observed as early as 2 weeks after initiation of therapy, and the median time to complete hematologic responses is 4 weeks after the start of therapy. Complete hematologic responses are observed in nearly 95% of patients, and complete cytogenetic responses are reported in 74% of cases. Typically, cytogenetic responses are observed as early as 2 months and up to 10 months after starting therapy, and the median time to best cytogenetic response is approximately 5 months. This agent is currently approved as first-line therapy for the chronic phase of CML, as second-line therapy for the chronic phase of CML after failure of interferon-α therapy, for treatment of CML in the accelerated phase or in blast crisis, and for treatment of Philadelphia chromosome–positive ALL.[46] In addition, it has shown striking clinical activity against gastrointestinal stromal tumors expressing the c-kit tyrosine kinase, a disease for the treatment of which it has recently received U.S. Food and Drug Administration (FDA) approval.

Another attractive target for therapeutic intervention is the epidermal growth factor receptor (EGFR)–signaling pathway.[47] The EGFR is a transmembrane receptor involved in cell proliferation, growth, invasion, metastasis, angiogenesis, and survival. In addition, activation of this pathway renders cancer cells more resistant to the cytotoxic effects of chemotherapy and radiation therapy. Increased expression of the EGFR has been observed in a wide range of human solid tumors, including colorectal cancer, pancreatic cancer, non–small cell lung cancer, head and neck cancer, breast cancer, and ovarian cancer. Moreover, tumors that express high levels of EGFR are associated with advanced disease and poor clinical prognosis. For these reasons, EGFR represents an attractive target for the development of novel anticancer agents.

The EGFR is composed of three distinct domains, an extracellular ligand-binding domain, a transmembrane domain, and an intracellular domain with intrinsic tyrosine kinase activity. Binding of the activating ligands, epidermal growth factor and transforming growth factor-α, to the extracellular domain leads to autophosphorylation of the receptor, which then activates downstream-signaling pathways such as the phosphatidylinositol 3 kinase/Akt and Ras/Raf/mitogen-activated protein kinase pathways. Two main approaches have been taken to inhibit this pathway. Monoclonal antibodies directed against the cell surface receptor have been developed, including cetuximab, EMD72000, and ABX-EGF, and they competitively bind to the EGFR and inhibit subsequent tyrosine kinase activation.[48] Cetuximab has single-agent activity in advanced colorectal cancer and is active when used in combination with

irinotecan in a metastatic disease setting in which patients were documented to be irinotecan resistant. Small-molecule inhibitors of the tyrosine kinase domain (TKIs) bind to the ATP pocket of the tyrosine kinase enzyme and inhibit normal ATP binding.[49] Several TKIs are in clinical development, with gefitinib and erlotinib furthest along in development. Gefitinib was approved by the FDA in 2003 as monotherapy for chemotherapy-refractory patients with non–small cell lung cancer, and clinical trials are ongoing to determine whether gefitinib and other small-molecule TKIs can be used in combination with standard chemotherapy.

As an alternative to targeting intracellular signaling pathways, significant attention has focused on strategies to inhibit the process of angiogenesis.[50] This approach stems from the seminal work of Folkman and colleagues,[51] who first proposed that the growth of a tumor mass is dependent on the formation of a vascular network that supplies the tumor with essential nutrients. This dependence on vascular supply holds for the growth of both primary tumors and metastatic disease. The targeting of the tumor vasculature has two potential advantages over conventional biochemical-molecular targets. First, this approach does not require tailoring of therapy to the unique genetic makeup of the tumor, because it appears that all solid tumors are dependent, to some extent, on angiogenesis for growth. Second, the primary target of this approach is the normal vascular endothelial cells. In contrast to malignant cells, vascular endothelial cells are genetically stable, and they are therefore less likely to develop cellular drug resistance. At present, much attention has centered on inhibiting the pathway modulated by vascular endothelial growth factor (VEGF), which has been shown to play an important role in the growth and proliferation of several solid tumors, such as colorectal cancer, non–small cell lung cancer, and renal cell cancer. Several strategies have been taken to inhibit the VEGF-signaling pathway, and they include antibodies targeting the VEGF ligand, antibodies targeting the receptor (VEGFR) to which VEGF binds, small-molecule inhibitors of the VEGFR, chimeric decoy receptors that incorporate certain key aspects of VEGFR and bind with high affinity to VEGF, and catalytic RNAs targeting certain sequences on the VEGFR messenger RNA. Studies have shown that the anti-VEGF monoclonal antibody bevacizumab significantly enhanced the clinical activity of fluoropyrimidine-based chemotherapy alone or in combination with irinotecan in colorectal cancer patients with advanced disease.[52] This antibody is expected to receive approval by the FDA for this indication, which validates the role of the VEGF-signaling pathway as a key target for drug development.

PRECLINICAL PHARMACOLOGY

There is an urgent need to move promising new therapies into clinical trials. Before this is done, however, the *in vivo* antitumor activity, clinical pharmacology in animals, and toxicity profile of an investigational agent must be well characterized. Each of these issues must be carefully addressed in a timely manner to provide safe and reasonable starting dosages for the implementation of phase I trials in patients. The steps required in the development of a cancer agent and its introduction into clinical practice are complex and, as outlined in Figure 15.1-1, they are both time and resource intensive.

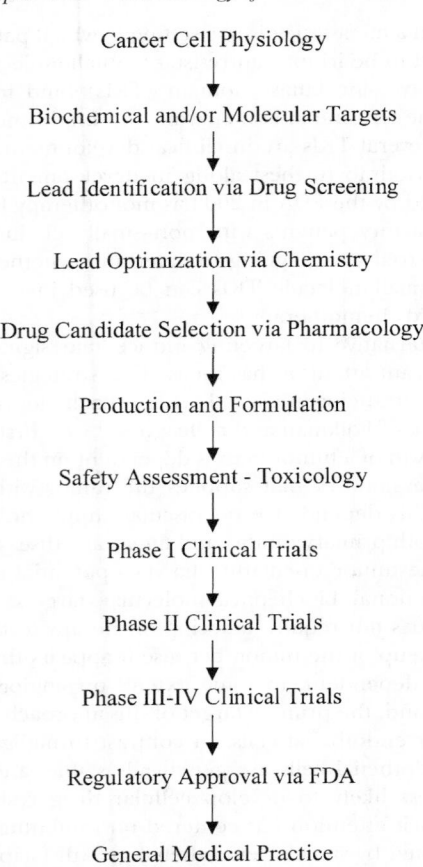

Cancer Cell Physiology

↓

Biochemical and/or Molecular Targets

↓

Lead Identification via Drug Screening

↓

Lead Optimization via Chemistry

↓

Drug Candidate Selection via Pharmacology

↓

Production and Formulation

↓

Safety Assessment - Toxicology

↓

Phase I Clinical Trials

↓

Phase II Clinical Trials

↓

Phase III-IV Clinical Trials

↓

Regulatory Approval via FDA

↓

General Medical Practice

FIGURE 15.1-1. Steps in cancer drug development. FDA, U.S. Food and Drug Administration.

Secondary *in vitro* studies to optimize the schedule of administration with respect to cytotoxic activity are important for investigators planning *in vivo* animal studies. Examination of the dose-response data for several human cancer cell lines should permit selection of the optimal model systems for evaluating *in vivo* efficacy. Furthermore, preliminary pharmacologic studies in non–tumor-bearing animals provide valuable information about the plasma concentrations potentially achievable and offer insights into the acute toxicity profile associated with a new agent. The successful identification of new therapies relies heavily on the expeditious, yet careful, conduct of *in vivo* animal studies.[53,54]

In the current NCI development schema, the human tumor cell line most sensitive to an active candidate *in vitro* is selected for testing as a xenograft in a subcutaneous implant site in a nude mouse. Compounds identified in molecular screens are then usually tested against human or murine tumors engineered to overexpress the specific drug target. Failure to demonstrate *in vivo* efficacy for agents that display strong *in vitro* evidence of cytotoxic activity should prompt further studies to determine whether the loss of antitumor activity might be related to unpredictable pharmacokinetics, drug metabolism or drug clearance, bioavailability, or some combination of these. The initial lead agent, discovered either through an empiric screen or as a result of rational drug design, is usually not the optimal chemical entity for clinical investigation. Lead optimization and an iterative process between chemists and

tumor biologists may be required to enhance the *in vivo* therapeutic index. Factors such as poor solubility and rapid *in vivo* metabolism may be improved through the process of analog development. In this manner, significantly more potent and less toxic compounds can often be subsequently developed.

Preclinical studies in mice, rats, and dogs provide essential information about pharmacokinetics and provide a basis for rational schedule development for the testing of new drugs in humans. Factors such as bioavailability (for agents administered by the oral route), metabolism, renal excretion, and penetration and distribution into the central nervous system and other sanctuary sites in the body contribute to the overall understanding of how best to test a new drug in humans. Although there is no firm guarantee that human subjects will metabolize a new drug in the exact same manner as the animal species, the major pathways for drug metabolism and excretion are qualitatively, if not quantitatively, the same across species.

FORMULATION STUDIES

Although preliminary pharmacologic and toxicologic studies may begin before a decision is made on the final formulation of a product, the investigational new drug–directed toxicology studies must be performed with the formulation that is to be used in clinical trials. In addition, other critical studies may be influenced by characteristics of the formulation (e.g., bioavailability of an oral formulation, insolubility of an agent demonstrating interesting antitumor activity in the cancer screen). Three important factors that have an impact on formulation studies include solubility, stability, and dosage requirements.[55]

Because drug administration for antineoplastic agents has been mainly through the intravenous route, the issue of solubility has been a major challenge for a number of agents with limited aqueous solubility. Efforts to improve the solubility of an agent have primarily involved physical measures, including the use of various mixed-solvent systems. Novel approaches, including the use of micronization, liposomal encapsulation, nanotechnology, and other unique delivery systems have been investigated in an attempt to improve methods of drug delivery to tissues. Major efforts are needed to expand the vehicles available for intravenous drug delivery of agents with limited aqueous solubility and stability.

The prodrug approach uses the process of chemical modification to resolve difficulties associated with drug insolubility and rapid degradation. One example of a simple prodrug approach is the synthesis of the monophosphate derivative of 2-fluoroadenine arabinoside (fludarabine). This halogenated nucleoside was observed to be poorly soluble in aqueous solution. In contrast, the monophosphate form of fludarabine was much more soluble and could be readily cleaved enzymatically *in vivo* to the respective 2-fluoroadenine arabinoside. Once transported within the cell by a specific nucleoside carrier system, the nucleoside could then be rapidly phosphorylated to the active cytotoxic metabolites and thus be effective as an anticancer agent. In the case of the oral fluoropyrimidine capecitabine, the carbamate moiety linked to the fluoropyrimidine allowed 5-fluorouracil to be completely and readily absorbed by the gut mucosa in contrast to the parent compound, 5-fluorouracil, which is readily inactivated by the enzyme dihydropyrimidine dehydrogenase. This relatively simple chemical modification allowed this agent to be administered orally. Clinical studies have now shown that oral capecitabine is equivalent to intravenous 5-fluorouracil in terms of clinical efficacy but has an improved safety profile.

PRECLINICAL TOXICOLOGY

Preclinical toxicologic assessment is the final step in moving a new anticancer drug into clinical testing in humans.[56] The major objectives of the preclinical toxicologic studies include (1) defining the qualitative and quantitative organ toxicities (including dose and schedule dependencies), (2) identifying the reversibility of these effects, and (3) determining the initial safe starting dosage for humans. In general, the ideal approach is to ensure that the preclinical toxicologic studies accurately reflect the intended clinical investigations in humans (i.e., identical formulation, schedules, and routes of drug administration, and dose levels anticipated to reflect the likely experience in patients).

The current toxicologic investigations accepted by the FDA involve a simplified two-step approach. The initial step focuses on acute toxicity in small animals (e.g., mice), with the primary end point being determination of the dosage level that is lethal in 10% of subjects. The second phase of preclinical toxicologic studies is more extensive. In this setting, emphasis is placed on a careful qualitative and quantitative characterization of the organ-specific toxicities in rodents associated with the schedule and route of administration that is to be used in the initial clinical trial. Attention is given to accurately defining those toxicities that are likely to be observed at dosages slightly higher than the highest nontoxic dose. Careful investigation of the dosages in animals that approximate the highest projected tolerable dosage in the model should provide data that are more relevant to the anticipated clinical experience in patients.

Historically, most new anticancer agents were tested clinically using two relatively fixed schedules of drug administration: single-bolus intravenous dose once every 3 to 4 weeks, and 5 consecutive days of treatment repeated at 3- to 4-week intervals. The most frequently used toxicology protocols reflect each of these schedules. However, other schedules of administration, including weekly intravenous infusion, intravenous infusion every 2 weeks, continuous intravenous infusion, and oral dosing, are now being developed in an effort to enhance the clinical activity and safety profile of various agents. With this in mind, it is critically important for the preclinical toxicologic protocols to be planned and implemented before their introduction in the clinical setting.

Because substantial variation may exist between species in tolerance to a given drug, the safety of a projected starting dosage in humans is confirmed by examining the preclinical toxicities in at least two species.[57,58] Both the qualitative and the quantitative toxicities are usually well defined after studies in a small-animal model (e.g., mouse) and a larger animal (e.g., dog). On occasion, additional testing is needed in a large-animal species (e.g., monkey).

Certain organ-specific toxicities are reliably detected with the current toxicologic models, such as myelosuppression and gastrointestinal toxicity.[59] In contrast, hepatic and renal toxicities are difficult to assess in animal testing. Toxicities involving the heart, lung, nervous system, pancreas, and skin are even less reliably characterized. Preclinical studies can help to establish a safe starting dosage for humans and may predict acute organ toxicity. However, the true safety profile of a new agent emerges only after it has been extensively investigated in the clinical setting.

CLINICAL DEVELOPMENT

The traditional development of a promising anticancer agent in the clinical setting involves the initiation of phase I trials. The primary end point of these studies is to identify the maximally tolerated dosage and the dose-limiting toxicities. As well, the overall safety profile, reversibility of toxicity, metabolism and clearance of the drug, bioavailability, and schedule of administration are evaluated in the phase I setting. Although therapeutic activity is assessed in this initial phase of clinical development, it is important to emphasize that clinical efficacy is only a secondary end point of phase I studies. Once the optimal dose and schedule have been identified and it has been documented that an investigational agent can be administered safely to patients, phase II studies are conducted. In this setting, the agent is tested in patients with specific tumor types at an advanced stage of disease. The main goal of these studies is to determine clinical efficacy as well as to further define the toxicity profile. Should the phase II trials reveal promising clinical efficacy against a certain tumor type combined with an acceptable safety profile, phase III randomized trials are then initiated to compare the clinical efficacy and safety profile of the investigational agent with those of an existing standard chemotherapy regimen. The patient sample in such a trial must be of sufficient size and uniformity so that appropriate conclusions can be made as to the true clinical benefit of the investigational agent. Overall survival has been the traditional primary end point of phase III studies, and it has been the measure on which the FDA has based its approval of new agents. However, there is growing appreciation that the survival end point may not be the ideal marker of antitumor activity because it also takes into account the effects of second-line salvage therapies. For this reason, there has been a recent shift toward considering time to disease progression as a more reliable indicator of the clinical activity of a given agent. In addition to clinical activity and toxicity, effects on quality of life, pharmacoeconomics, and patient satisfaction are being incorporated as important end points of phase III studies.

One of the potential challenges in the clinical development of novel targeted therapies is that their effects are usually cytostatic and not cytocidal. As a result, the classic end points used in clinical trials may not be directly applicable. Because of this, clinical trials with these targeted agents should not incorporate the maximally tolerated dose as the main end point in the phase I setting. Instead, the minimum dose of the agent that results in maximal inhibition of the molecular target should be considered. The traditional phase II study focused on treatment of a specific tumor; however, when a targeted therapy is being evaluated, therapy should be selected for an individual patient based on the presence of the specific target within that particular tumor type. To meet these challenges, it is essential that molecular tests be developed and validated to identify the status of expression or activity of a given target and to determine whether treatment with a targeted agent is indeed having a biologic effect. Finally, there is growing evidence that several

TABLE 15.1-2. Stages in Clinical Testing of New Anticancer Agents

Stage of Drug Testing	Objectives	Patient Population Studied

Phase I	Determine tolerance
	   Maximally tolerable dose
	   Limiting toxicity
	   Reversibility of toxicity
	   Proper schedule
	Pharmacology
	   Bioavailability
	   Plasma clearance
	   Biotransformation
	   Excretion
	Therapeutic effect
	Secondary
		Histologically confirmed advanced malignancies; no longer amenable to conventional therapy; physiologically well compensated.

Phase II	Therapeutic effect
	   Determine effectiveness in a panel of human tumors
	Dose-response relationships
	Nontherapeutic effects
	   Toxicity in relationship to therapeutic effect.
		Histologically confirmed advanced malignancy; measurable tumor masses; no longer amenable to conventional therapy; a variety of tumor types in groups of 15 to 30; physiologically well compensated.

Phase III	Therapeutic effectiveness
	   Compare experimental therapy to existing standard therapy
	Nontherapeutic effects
	   Are toxic effects tolerable in the context of observed therapeutic effect and in comparison with standard therapy?
		Histologically confirmed malignancy; patient sample must be of adequate size and uniformity; usually previously untreated; controls usually are selected randomly, but on occasion, historical controls are used.

Phase IV	Therapeutic effectiveness
	   Integration of drug therapy into primary treatment in combination with surgery or radiation therapy (e.g., postoperative drug treatment in breast cancer)
	Compare to concurrent standard program
	Nontherapeutic effects
	   Are toxic effects sufficiently minimal to risk giving drug to patients whose tumor might not necessarily recur?
	   Long-term toxic effects require monitoring (second tumors, sterility, marrow aplasia)
		Histologically confirmed malignancy; patient sample must be of adequate size and uniformity; controls usually randomized.

of the novel targeted therapies being developed do not have single-agent activity and are best used in combination with standard chemotherapy. The key challenge is to develop methods to determine how best to integrate these novel targeted agents with standard chemotherapy.

CONCLUSION

The discovery and development of novel anticancer agents involves substantial time, effort, and resources. The strategies used for drug discovery range from empiric screening (the source of most of the active drugs currently available) to rational drug design based on an enhanced understanding of the critical molecular and biochemical targets. As outlined in this chapter, an extensive series of preclinical investigations is necessary before the decision to enter clinical trials can be made. Significant efforts are then required for the successful completion of clinical testing, in which an individual agent is taken from the initial phase I trials through to the randomized phase III and IV settings (Table 15.1-2). The effective development of new cancer agents demands the close interaction of a multidisciplinary team that includes basic research scientists, clinical pharmacologists,

clinical research nurses, data managers, and clinical investigators. The combined resources of government, academic centers, and the pharmaceutical industry are required for successfully accomplishing the formidable task of identifying effective new therapeutic agents for cancer patients.

REFERENCES

1. Kaufman DC, Chabner BA. Clinical strategies for cancer treatment: the role of drugs. In: Chabner BA, Longo DL, eds. *Cancer chemotherapy and biotherapy*. New York: Lippincott–Raven, 2001:1.
2. Johnson JI, Monks A, Hollingshead MG, et al. Preclinical aspects of cancer drug discovery and development. In: Chabner BA, Longo DL, eds. *Cancer chemotherapy and biotherapy*. New York: Lippincott–Raven, 2001:17.
3. Grever MR, Schepartz S, Chabner BA. The National Cancer Institute: cancer drug discovery and development program. *Semin Oncol* 1992;19:622.
4. Farber S, Diamond LK, Mercer RD, et al. Temporary remissions in acute leukemia in children produced by folic acid antagonist, 4-aminopteroyl-glutamic acid (aminopterin). *N Engl J Med* 1948;238:787.
5. Appelt K, Baquet RJ, Bartlett CA, et al. Design of enzyme inhibitors using iterative protein crystallographic analysis. *J Med Chem* 1991;3:1925.
6. Chu E, Callender MA, Farrell MP, et al. Thymidylate synthase inhibitors as anticancer agents: from bench to bedside. *Cancer Chemother Pharmacol* 2003;52[Suppl]:S80.
7. Johnson RK. Screening methods in antineoplastic drug discovery. *J Natl Cancer Inst* 1990;82:1082.
8. Suffness M, Newman DJ, Snader K. Discovery and development of antineoplastic agents from natural sources. *Bioorg Med Chem* 1989;3:131.

9. Cragg GM, Newman DJ, Weiss RB. Coral reefs, forests, and thermal vents: the worldwide exploration of nature for novel antitumor agents. *Semin Oncol* 1997;24:156.

10. Weiss RB, Sarosy G, Clagett-Carr K, et al. Anthracycline analogs: the past, present, and future. *Cancer Chemother Pharmacol* 1986;18:185.

11. Bianschi M, Biglioni M, Cipollone A, et al. Anthracyclines: selected new developments. *Curr Med Chem Anti-Canc Agents* 2001;12:113.

12. Rowinsky EK, Donehower RC. Drug therapy: paclitaxel (Taxol). *N Engl J Med* 1995;332:1004.

13. Abal M, Andreu JM, Barasoain I. Taxanes: microtubule and centrosome targets, and cell cycle dependent mechanisms of action. *Curr Cancer Drug Targets* 2003;3:193.

14. Mann J. Steps to a successful synthesis. *Nature* 1994;367:594.

15. Gordon M. Taxol supply problem? What problem? *Nat Biotechnol* 1996;14:1635.

16. Wartmann M, Altmann KH. The biology and medicinal chemistry of epothilones. *Curr Med Chem Anti-Canc Agents* 2002;2:123.

17. Rothermal J, Wartmann M, Chen T, et al. EPO906 (epothilone B): a promising novel microtubule stabilizer. *Semin Oncol* 2003;30[Suppl 6]:51.

18. Garcia-Carbonero R, Supko JG. Current perspectives on the clinical experience, pharmacology, and continued development of the camptothecins. *Clin Cancer Res* 2002;8:641.

19. Pizxzolato JF, Saltz LB. The camptothecins. *Lancet* 2003;361:2235.

20. Meng LH, Liao ZY, Pommier Y. Non-camptothecin DNA topoisomerase I inhibitors in cancer therapy. *Curr Top Med Chem* 2003;3:305.

21. Clamp A, Jayson GC. The clinical development of the bryostatins. *Anticancer Drugs* 2002;13:673.

22. Schwartzmann G, Brondana AD, Berlinck RG, et al. Marine organisms as a source of new anticancer agents. *Lancet Oncol* 2001;2:221.

23. Schwartzmann G, Brondana AD, Mattei J, et al. Marine-derived anticancer agents in clinical trials. *Expert Opin Investig Drugs* 2003;12:1367.

24. Rinehart KL. Antitumor compounds from tunicates. *Med Res Rev* 2000;20:1.

25. D'Incalci M, Jimeno J. Preclinical and clinical results with the natural marine product ET-743. *Expert Opin Investig Drugs* 2003;12:1843.

26. Menchaca R, Martinez, V, Rodriguez A. et al. Synthesis of natural ecteinascidins (ET-729, ET-745, ET-759B, ET-736, ET-637, ET-594) from cyanosafracin B. *J Org Chem* 2003;68:8859.

27. Schuler GD, Boguski MS, Stewart EA, et al. A gene map of the human genome. *Science* 1996;274:540.

28. Hunter T. 1001 protein kinases redux—towards 2000. *Semin Cell Biol* 1994;5:367.

29. Veber DF, Drake FH, Gowen M. The new partnership of genomics and chemistry for accelerated drug development. *Curr Opin Chem Biol* 1997;1:151.

30. Ohkanda J, Knowles DB, Blaskovich MA, et al. Inhibitors of protein farnesyltransferase as novel anticancer agents. *Curr Top Med Chem* 2002;2:303.

31. Hoekstra WJ, Poulter BL. Combinatorial chemistry techniques applied to nonpeptide integrin antagonists. *Curr Med Chem* 1998;5:195.

32. Lloyd AW. Combinatorial chemistry-hydroxystilbene kinase inhibitor library. *Drug Discov Today* 1997;2:556.

33. Combs AP, Kapoor TM, Feng S, et al. Protein structure-based combinatorial chemistry: discovery of non-peptide binding elements to src SH3 domain. *J Am Chem Soc* 1996; 118:287.

34. Feng S, Kapoor TM, Shirai F, et al. Molecular basis for the binding of SH3 ligands with non-peptide elements identified by combinatorial synthesis. *Chem Biol* 1996;3:661.

35. Boyd MR. Status of the NCI preclinical antitumor drug discovery screen. *PPO Updates* 1989;3:1.

36. Skehan P, Storeng R, Scudiero D, et al. New colorimetric cytotoxicity assay for anticancer drug screening. *J Natl Cancer Inst* 1990;82:1107.

37. Chabner BA. In defense of cell-line screening. *J Natl Cancer Inst* 1990;82:1083.

38. Paull KD, Shoemaker RH, Hodes L, et al. Display and analysis of patterns of differential activity of drugs against human tumor cell lines: development of mean graph and COMPARE algorithm. *J Natl Cancer Inst* 1989;81:1088.

39. Weinstein JN, Myers TG, O'Connor PM, et al. An information-intensive approach to the molecular pharmacology of cancer. *Science* 1997;275:343.

40. Monks A, Scudiero DA, Johnson GS, et al. The NCI anti-cancer drug screen: a smart screen to identify effectors of novel targets. *Anticancer Drug Des* 1997;12:533.

41. Wosikowski K, Schuurhuis D, Johnson K, et al. Identification of epidermal growth factor receptor and c-erbB2 pathway inhibitors by correlation with gene expression patterns. *J Natl Cancer Inst* 1997;89:1505.

42. Gibbs JB. Anticancer drug targets: growth factors and growth factor signaling. *J Clin Invest* 2000;105:9.

43. Daley GQ, Van Etten RA, Baltimore D. Induction of chronic myelogenous leukemia by the P210bcr/abl gene of the Philadelphia chromosome. *Science* 1990;247:824.

44. Druker BJ, Tamura S, Buchdunger E, et al. Effects of a selective inhibitor of the ABL tyrosine kinase on the growth of BCR-ABL positive cells. *Nat Med* 1996;2:561.

45. Druker BJ, Lydon NB. Lessons learned from the development of an Abl tyrosine kinase inhibitor for chronic myelogenous leukemia. *J Clin Invest* 2000;105:3.

46. Druker BJ. STI571 (Gleevec) as a paradigm for cancer therapy. *Trends Mol Med* 2002;8:S14.

47. Mendelsohn J, Baselga J. The EGF receptor family as targets for cancer therapy. *Semin Cancer Biol* 1990;1:339.

48. Herbst RS, Shin DM. Monoclonal antibodies to target epidermal growth factor receptor-positive tumors: a new paradigm for cancer therapy. *Cancer* 2002;94:1593.

49. Mendolsohn J. Targeting the epidermal growth factor receptor for cancer therapy. *J Clin Oncol* 2002;20[Suppl 18]:1S.

50. Keshet E, Ben-Sasson SA. Anticancer drug targets: approaching angiogenesis. *J Clin Invest* 1999;104:1497.

51. Hanahan D, Folkman J. Patterns and emerging mechanisms of the angiogenic switch during tumorigenesis. *Cell* 1996;86:353.

52. Fernando NH, Hurwitz, HI. Inhibition of vascular endothelial growth factor in the treatment of colorectal cancer. *Semin Oncol* 2003;30[Suppl 6]:39.

53. Corbett TH, Wozniak A, Gerpheide S, et al. In vitro and in vivo models for detection of new antitumor drugs. In: Hanka IJ, Kondo T, White RJ, eds. *Proceedings of a workshop at the 14th International Congress of Chemotherapy at Kyoto.* Tokyo: University of Tokyo Press, 1985:5.

54. Grindey GB. Current status of cancer drug development: failure or limited success? *Cancer Cells* 1990;2:163.

55. Davignon JP, Craddock JC. The formulation of anticancer drugs. In: Hellman K, Carter SK, eds. *Fundamentals of cancer chemotherapy.* New York: McGraw-Hill, 1987:212.

56. Lowe MC, Davis RD. The current toxicology protocol of the National Cancer Institute. In: Hellman K, Carter SK, eds. *Fundamentals of cancer chemotherapy.* New York: McGraw-Hill, 1987:228.

57. Lowe M. Large animal toxicological studies of anticancer drugs. In: Hellman K, Carter SK, eds. *Fundamentals of cancer chemotherapy.* New York: McGraw-Hill, 1987:238.

58. Schurig JE, Bradner WT. Small animal toxicology of cancer drugs. In: Hellman K, Carter SK, eds. *Fundamentals of cancer chemotherapy.* New York: McGraw-Hill, 1987:248.

59. Schein P, Anderson T. The efficacy of animal studies in predicting clinical toxicity of cancer chemotherapeutic drugs. *Int J Clin Pharmacol* 1973;8:228.

SECTION **2**

CHRIS H. TAKIMOTO

Pharmacokinetics

INTRODUCTION

The pharmacologic treatment of human malignancies involves the clinical use of some of the most challenging therapeutic agents in all of medicine. The practicing medical oncologist must manage the risk of serious toxicities, optimize therapies with relatively narrow efficacy profiles, and adjust for high interpatient variability on a routine basis during the administration of cancer chemotherapy. Because the science of clinical pharmacology attempts to rationally explain and predict the sources of variability of drug action, it has great relevance for the field of medical oncology. Clinical pharmacology can be broadly defined as the study of drugs in humans, and it can be subdivided into two major disciplines: *pharmacokinetics* and *pharmacodynamics.*[1] Atkinson et al. have defined pharmacokinetics as "the quantitative analysis of the process of drug absorption, distribution and elimination that determine the time course of drug action."[1] Ratain and Mick have paraphrased this definition of pharmacokinetics as "what the body does to the drug."[2] Classically, pharmacokinetics involves the characterization of an agent's absorption, distribution, metabolism, and excretion through the measurement of drug concentrations in an accessible compartment over time. In contrast, *pharmacodynamics* is directly related to drug-induced clinical outcomes,[1] and, in a practical sense, it links drug dosing and kinetics to clinical drug effects, such as efficacy or toxicity. In simplified terms, pharmacodynamics is "what the drug does to the body."[2]

WHY STUDY PHARMACOKINETICS AND PHARMACODYNAMICS?

The clinical importance of pharmacokinetics and pharmacodynamics is predicated on the principle that concentration-response relationships are generally less variable than dose-response relationships for any specific agent.[1] Drug receptor theory predicts that drug concentrations in measurable compartments at equilibrium are directly proportional to the concentrations at the effective site of action. Understanding interpatient variability in drug kinetics allows for the implementation of strategies to reduce this variability and thereby achieve more consistent clinical results. The ultimate goal of the medical oncologist is to use pharmacokinetic and pharmacodynamic knowledge to maximize therapeutic benefits for individual patients. The clinical pharmacology of a new anticancer agent is typically characterized by careful integrated pharmacokinetic and pharmacodynamic studies initiated early in the drug development process. The data obtained from these analyses, when rationally applied to the clinical setting, allows the practicing oncologist to optimize treatment regimens for patients even before the first dose is administered. It also provides valuable information on how to adjust treatment doses and schedules when the initial treatment is unsatisfactory due to excessive toxicities or other complications.

Understanding a drug's pharmacokinetic properties provides the medical oncologist and drug development scientist with clinically useful descriptive, explanatory, and predictive information.[3] The descriptive power of pharmacokinetics is easily illustrated by summarizing a drug's behavior in a defined population using a specific pharmacokinetic model. For example, the characterization of a one-compartment, open, linear pharmacokinetic model with first-order elimination with mean values for the volume of distribution and the elimination rate constant can succinctly describe an extensive amount of concentration versus time data in a large number of cancer patients (Fig. 15.2-1). Furthermore, the relative standard deviations for the population estimates of the volume of distribution and elimination rate constant can provide insight into the degree of interpatient variability in drug kinetics within the study population.[2] This diversity may have great clinical relevance in understanding variability in clinical outcomes of drug therapy.

Pharmacokinetic analyses can also provide substantial explanatory information about the underlying physiologic processes affecting drug behavior.[3] This can lead to specific hypotheses about the underlying mechanisms responsible for the distribution, elimination, or metabolism of a specific agent. For example, if drug clearance correlates with creatinine clearance, then renal excretion may be hypothesized to be an important route of drug elimination (Fig. 15.2-2). Such findings suggest that caution is warranted during administration of the drug to patients with

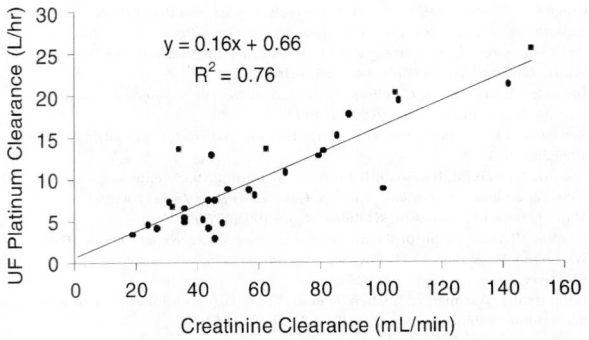

FIGURE 15.2-2. Correlation between the clearance of platinum species from plasma ultrafiltrates (UF) and the measured 24-hour urinary creatinine clearance in adult solid tumor patients with varying degrees of renal dysfunction after treatment with oxaliplatin. (Data are taken from a clinical trial described in ref. 32.)

impaired renal function. In addition, a strong correlation between renal function and drug clearance may lead to the development of individualized dosing strategies for patients based on estimations of the glomerular filtration rate (GFR). A common clinical example is the individualized dosing of carboplatin using estimates of the GFR to achieve a targeted area under the concentration curve (AUC).[4,5] Individual pharmacokinetic parameters may also correlate with other important covariate factors, including age, gender, hepatic dysfunction, pharmacogenetic polymorphisms in drug-metabolizing enzymes, use of concomitant medications, or differences in body surface area. These covariate relationships may further explain the degree of pharmacokinetic variability present within the study population. The ability to predict interpatient variability based on patient covariates obtained before drug administration can form the basis for tailored dosing guidelines for individual patients.

Finally, pharmacokinetic knowledge about a drug allows specific predictions to be made when different doses and schedules of administration are used.[3] For example, pharmacokinetic parameter estimates obtained after a single intravenous drug bolus can be used to calculate the time needed to achieve steady state as well as the magnitude of the steady-state concentration when the drug is given as a prolonged continuous infusion. This predictive function is also clinically important for making rational dose adjustments while treatments are ongoing. For drugs with dose-proportional pharmacokinetics, decreasing the dose will proportionally decrease systemic exposures in a highly predictable fashion. For agents with nonlinear, saturable pharmacokinetics, however, it may be difficult to accurately predict the exact consequences of standard dose adjustments on plasma drug concentrations. A classic example of an agent that is difficult to administer using a one-size-fits-all dosing scheme in the absence of therapeutic drug monitoring is phenytoin, a drug with well-defined, nonlinear Michaelis-Menten pharmacokinetic behavior.[6]

Because of their focus on clinical outcomes, pharmacodynamic studies have direct relevance to the practice of medical oncology.[7] Drug kinetics may account for only a portion of the variability seen in treatment outcomes. Patients with identical systemic exposures may experience very different clinical effects in terms of efficacy or, more commonly, toxicity, depending on the drug and the situation. For example, a patient who has been

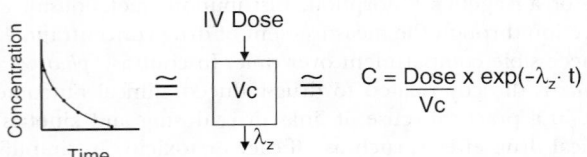

FIGURE 15.2-1. One-compartment, open pharmacokinetic model with intravenous bolus input is defined by two pharmacokinetic parameters: the apparent volume of distribution, Vc, and the elimination rate constant, λ_z. The raw pharmacokinetic concentration versus time data can be represented by a schematic box diagram or by a monoexponential mathematical formula with two unknown parameters, Vc and λ_z. In the mathematical representation of these data, time (t) is the independent variable, concentration (C) is the dependent variable, and *dose* is a known constant.

heavily pretreated with chemotherapy with a myelosuppressive alkylating agent or who has received extensive prior radiation therapy may experience substantially more bone marrow toxicity than a minimally pretreated patient treated at the same dose and systemic exposure. A well-defined pharmacodynamic model strips away the contribution of pharmacokinetic variability and allows the investigator to focus on inherent differences in the target tissues of interest. The understanding of pharmacodynamic variability in antitumor efficacy is still quite limited, compared with knowledge of drug toxicity end points; however, the molecular profiling of tumors using powerful genomic microarray technologies suggests that knowledge in this area will continue to evolve rapidly. Furthermore, the integration of pharmacodynamic studies into early clinical trials of novel anticancer agents has grown impressively, due to pioneering efforts by investigators such as Ratain and Egorin.[7]

WHY CANCER PATIENTS PRESENT A UNIQUE CHALLENGE

The medical oncologist involved in designing rational, pharmacologically sound treatment strategies must face some uniquely complex issues when treating patients with cancer. The relevant toxicity and efficacy profile of any anticancer agent is characterized by its therapeutic index, which is defined as the ratio between the systemic drug exposure associated with unacceptable toxicity and the exposure that maximizes the likelihood of inducing the intended drug response. The therapeutic index of anticancer drugs is probably the narrowest of any class of agents in common use. Furthermore, pharmacokinetic variability in cancer patients may be enhanced by a variety of factors, including prior gastrointestinal surgery, poor nutritional status, hypoalbuminemia, polypharmacy, advanced age, and altered renal or hepatic function. Factors that may alter pharmacodynamic drug effects include prior chemotherapy or radiation therapy, poor performance status, comorbid disease states, and bone marrow involvement by the underlying tumor. Finally, the pharmacodynamics of most anticancer agents are complex, in that long lag times exist between the times of drug exposure and clinically relevant outcomes, such as myelosuppressive toxicity or tumor response. All of these factors must be accounted for when designing pharmacologic strategies for treating patients with cancer. Despite these obstacles, the number of new, molecularly targeted agents with activity in the treatment of human malignancies is increasing at an unprecedented rate. Because of this growth, the challenge for the practicing oncologist is to assimilate the knowledge about the clinical pharmacology of these new therapies and to apply them in the most expeditious ways possible for the benefit of patients with cancer.

PHARMACOKINETIC CONCEPTS

A drug's pharmacokinetic properties can be readily described by defining a relatively few pharmacokinetic parameters in a specific population of patients. These pharmacokinetic parameters relate to fundamental processes affecting drug behavior over time, such as drug absorption, distribution, metabolism, and excretion. In the following sections, a few of the most basic pharmacokinetic and pharmacodynamic parameters are discussed, with an emphasis on their clinical relevance.

BIOAVAILABILITY

Historically, most anticancer therapies have been administered intravenously; however, the use of orally administered agents in oncology is growing.[8] The pharmacokinetic parameter most closely associated with oral absorption is bioavailability. Bioavailability (F) is defined as the fraction of an administered dose that reaches the systemic circulation for a given method of administration, compared with that for a reference method of administration, which, by convention, has been the intravenous route. For an oral agent, bioavailability is defined as the AUC after oral administration divided by the AUC observed after intravenous administration. The bioavailability of an oral drug can range from 0 to 1.0 and is defined using the following formula[9]:

$$F = dose(IV) \times AUC(oral)/[dose(oral) \times AUC(IV)] \quad \text{(Eq. 1)}$$

where *dose(IV)* and *dose(oral)* are the intravenous and oral doses, respectively, and *AUC(oral)* and *AUC(IV)* are the oral and intravenous AUC values, respectively. Because the actual extent of absorption from the gut into the systemic circulation may vary, the precise amount of drug entering the systemic circulation cannot be determined if only an oral formulation of an agent is available. However, kinetic parameters, such as clearance or volume of distribution, can still be determined using standard methods if the results are corrected for bioavailability.[9] Thus, apparent volume of distribution can be reported as V/F and clearance (CL) as CL/F, when bioavailability, F, is unmeasured. In many pharmacokinetic studies in oncology, it is not practical to administer both oral and intravenous drug formulations to cancer patients.

The absorption process is a complex series of events beginning with ingestion and followed by drug disintegration and dissolution, diffusion through gastrointestinal fluids, membrane permeation, uptake into the portal circulation, passage through the liver, and, finally, entry into the systemic circulation.[10] Oral bioavailability is influenced by many factors, including drug solubility, molecular size, degree of ionization, tissue binding, stability in the gastrointestinal tract, interaction with food products, lipophilicity, and the presence or absence of specific membrane transport systems. For example, the P glycoprotein drug efflux pump associated with pleiotropic drug resistance is also expressed on the apical membrane of intestinal cells and serves to pump drugs out of the cell back into the gut lumen. Thus, enhanced intestinal P glycoprotein expression can decrease oral bioavailability. Furthermore, after oral administration, extensive drug metabolism in the gut and liver or high biliary excretion can limit the amount of drug entering the systemic circulation, a process called the first-pass effect.[11] Finally, oral bioavailability may be altered in cancer patients due to changes in the integrity of the gastrointestinal tract arising from surgery, chemotherapy side effects, radiation therapy, or nausea and vomiting.

VOLUMES OF DISTRIBUTION

The volume of distribution relates the amount of drug in the body to the concentration observed in the measured compartment. As such, it represents a constant of proportionality that can be calculated under different conditions and at different times. The volume of distribution does not always correspond to an actual physiologic compartment, and several different volume of distribution terms are in common use. This situation is made more confusing because not all volume terms are directly representative of drug distribution processes. In oncology studies, commonly reported parameters include the apparent volume of distribution at steady state (V_{ss}), volume of distribution of the central compartment (V_c), and volume of distribution during the terminal elimination phase $(V_z$ or $V_{area})$.

The apparent volume of distribution at steady state (V_{ss}) is the constant of proportionality relating the amount of drug in the body to the steady–state plasma concentration.[12] This is the most clinically useful parameter of drug distribution because it directly reflects the anatomic space occupied by the drug and the relative amount of tissue penetration and binding at equilibrium.[11] The V_{ss} is independent of drug clearance and half-life, and its estimation does not require steady-state drug administration. However, estimations of V_{ss} inherently assume that drug elimination occurs only in the central compartment and that no drug is lost in the peripheral and more slowly equilibrating sites. In a multicompartment model, V_{ss} is defined by

$$V_{ss} = V_1 + V_2 + \ldots + V_n \qquad \text{(Eq. 2)}$$

where n is the number of compartments in the model. Using noncompartmental analytical methods based on statistical moment theory, the V_{ss} can be calculated after an intravenous drug bolus as follows[12]:

For a single-bolus dose: $V_{ss} = dose(AUMC)/(AUC)^2$ (Eq. 3)

where $AUMC$ is the area under the first moment curve (concentration multiplied by time versus time plot) and AUC is the area under the concentration versus time curve. After an infusion, V_{ss} can be calculated from the following[12]:

For a drug infusion: $V_{ss} = dose(AUMC)/(AUC)^2 - [R_0T^2/2(AUC)]$
$$\text{(Eq. 4)}$$

where T is the duration of the infusion and R_0 is the dose rate of infusion. In general, larger values for V_{ss} suggest more widespread tissue distribution, whereas a V_{ss} that approximates the plasma volume suggests an agent limited to the intravascular space.

The volume of distribution of the central compartment (V_c) is the constant of proportionality relating drug dose and the immediate postbolus infusion plasma drug concentration for a drug with monoexponential kinetics. In the simplest pharmacokinetic system consisting of a one-compartment, open, linear model, V_c corresponds to volume of distribution of the central compartment. This parameter is useful for the determination of the maximal drug concentration (C_{max}) immediately after intravenous drug bolus; however, it provides little or no information about the extent of drug distribution or tissue binding, which makes it much less useful as a fundamental pharmacokinetic parameter.[11] In a multicompartment model, V_c can be calculated using nonlinear regression methods; in a simple monoexponential model, it can be estimated by back extrapolation after a bolus dose to estimate the maximal plasma concentration at time zero (C_0):

For a single IV bolus: $V_c = dose/C_0$ (Eq. 5)

For multiple doses: $V_c = dose/(C_{postdose} - C_{predose})$ (Eq. 6)

where $C_{postdose}$ is the concentration immediately after the infusion and $C_{predose}$ is the drug concentration immediately before the infusion.

The terminal disposition volume of distribution $(V_z$ or $V_{area})$ is the constant of proportionality relating the amount of drug in the measured compartment during the terminal elimination phase. This volume of distribution term is useful for calculating the loading dose necessary to ensure that average plasma drug concentrations never fall below the targeted mean steady-state concentration. This volume term can be estimated from the following formula:

$$V_z = V_{area} = CL/\lambda_z = dose/(\lambda_z \times AUC) \qquad \text{(Eq. 7)}$$

where λ_z is the elimination rate constant and CL is clearance. The overall clinical utility of this volume term may vary because V_z does not always reflect changes in the drug distribution process.[11] Estimates of V_z are increased when drug clearance is enhanced, independent of any change in drug distribution (Eq. 7). Although V_z may approximate V_{ss} in some situations, for unstable agents or drugs with short half-lives and high clearance, estimates of V_z will be much larger than V_{ss}.[11]

The rate and extent to which a drug distributes into various tissues depends on a number of factors, including the drug lipophilicity, tissue permeability, tissue-binding constants, and local organ blood flow. Large apparent volumes of distribution are common for agents that are highly tissue bound or those that demonstrate high lipid solubility. Distribution into specific body compartments, such as the testes or central nervous system, may be limited by natural barriers, such as the blood–brain barrier. Poor drug penetration into these compartments may have important clinical consequences. For example, the treatment of carcinomatous meningitis or acute leukemia in the central nervous system typically requires direct administration of chemotherapy into the intrathecal space.[13]

PROTEIN BINDING AND FREE DRUG CONCENTRATIONS

Bioanalytic drug assays typically measure total plasma concentrations and often do not distinguish between the free and protein-bound drug fractions. Although at equilibrium free and bound drug vary in parallel, only the free fraction directly equilibrates with extravascular spaces and, thus, is more biologically relevant for predicting pharmacodynamic drug effects. Most drugs show some degree of binding to plasma proteins, such as human serum albumin for acidic drugs[14] and α_1-acid glycoprotein for basic drugs,[15] or to other blood components, such as erythrocytes. If a highly bound drug has substantial variability in protein binding, then clinical correlations based only on total plasma drug concentrations may be misleading. In such cases, measurement of free, unbound drug concentrations using specialized methods, such as ultrafiltration or equilibrium dialysis, may be preferable. The extent and variability of protein binding can directly affect a drug's pharmacokinetics,[15] and interspecies differences in drug protein binding may complicate animal scale-up experiments. Furthermore, protein biding may be altered in cancer patients due to concomitant factors, such as renal or hepatic dysfunction, altered levels of the acute-phase reactant α_1-acid glycoprotein, or hypoalbuminemia caused by malnutrition, poor biosynthetic reserve in the liver, or paraneoplastic nephrotic syndrome. Thus, protein binding may be an important source of interpatient variability in drug kinetics. Competitive drug displacement from plasma proteins was once thought to be a major mechanism for adverse drug interactions, such as those seen between warfarin and phenylbutazone.[16] However, most drug displacement protein-binding interactions are not clinically relevant, unless drug clearance is also inhibited.[16,17]

CLEARANCE

Of all the parameters in clinical pharmacology, total systemic clearance is probably the most relevant to the practice of medical oncology. Drug clearance reflects all processes in the body that contribute to the elimination of a drug over time. This includes metabolism in the liver forming inactive metabolites, urinary excretion in the kidneys, and hepatic excretion through the biliary system. Clearance is not a rate; instead, it is a volume of drug that is cleared per unit time. For a drug with dose-proportional kinetics, clearance is independent of concentration and dose, which makes it an extremely useful fundamental parameter. Total systemic drug clearance (CL) is the sum of all individual clearance processes occurring throughout the body and can be defined by the following equation:

$$CL = CL_{renal} + CL_{hepatic} + CL_{other} \qquad \text{(Eq. 8)}$$

where CL_{renal} is renal clearance, $CL_{hepatic}$ is hepatic clearance, and CL_{other} is all other clearance processes in the body.

Drug clearance is fundamentally important because it defines the relationship between drug dose as prescribed by the practicing physician and systemic drug exposures, as measured by the pharmacokineticist using *AUC*. If AUC_{0-INF} is the area under the concentration versus time curve extrapolated to infinity after a single dose of drug, then

$$CL = dose/AUC_{0-INF} \qquad \text{(Eq. 9a)}$$

or, rearranging,

$$AUC_{0-INF} = dose/CL \qquad \text{(Eq. 9b)}$$

As seen in Equation 9b, variability in clearance is the sole determinant of variation in systemic drug exposure at any fixed dose. In pharmacokinetic studies, interpatient variability in drug clearance can be approximated by the coefficient of variation (CV%), which is the relative standard deviation expressed as a percent of the mean clearance value. Many anticancer agents have CV% in the range of 20% to 40%. Clearance also determines the steady-state concentrations (C_{ss}) during continuous schedules of drug administration, such as during prolonged intravenous drug infusions, as defined by the formula

$$CL = infusion\ rate/C_{ss} \qquad \text{(Eq. 10)}$$

Whether consciously aware of it or not, the practicing medical oncologist makes an estimation of a patient's drug clearance every time cancer chemotherapy is prescribed on a milligram-per-square-meter basis. Dosing of cancer chemotherapy using body surface area (BSA) is justified only if the therapeutic intent is to achieve a uniform *AUC* in all sizes of patients and if *CL* is directly related to body size (Eq. 9b). However, the correlation between *CL* and BSA is often weak and frequently does not support the uncritical widespread implementation of this practice.[18] The routine use of BSA-based dosing of anticancer drugs has been heavily criticized, and the use of fixed doses of drugs for patients of different sizes may be a more rational approach for a large number of oncology agents.[18–23]

For many agents, drug metabolism represents a major route of systemic clearance. The liver is the predominant site for most drug-metabolizing reactions, although biotransformation can also occur in the gut, lung, kidneys, blood, tumors, and virtually anywhere else in the body. Traditionally, drug-metabolizing reactions have been divided into phase I and II reactions, both of which typically generate more polar, biologically inactive metabolites. Phase I reactions add a functional group through enzymatic oxidation or reduction, often converting the molecule into a substrate for subsequent phase II conjugation reactions. The cytochrome P-450 monooxygenase system is the best-characterized family of phase I drug-metabolizing enzymes. These enzymes are grouped into 17 families with numerous subgroups identified based on amino acid sequence homology. In humans, CYP1, CYP2, and CYP3 families are involved the vast majority of drug-metabolizing reactions, with two isoforms, CYP3A4 and CYP3A5, being responsible for approximately 50% of human drug metabolism. Individual cytochrome P-450 isoforms have characteristic induction and inhibition profiles, and their substrate specificity is typically well defined, although overlap between different isoforms is common. These enzymes are involved in the endogenous biosynthesis of fatty acids and steroids, and they are presumed to have an evolutionary role in protecting against xenobiotic toxins. In most circumstances, these phase I metabolic pathways are detoxifying reactions; however, cytochrome P-450–induced drug and carcinogen activation has been described.[24] Clinically significant drug interactions with agents such as ketoconazole, ritonavir, erythromycin and clarithromycin, and the macrolides due to inhibition of drug metabolism by enzymes such as CYP3A4 are well documented.[24]

Phase II reactions involve drug conjugation to glucuronic acid, amino acids, glutathione, or sulfate groups. The resulting water-soluble polar metabolites are usually substrates for subsequent drug excretion in urine or bile. Glucuronidation is principally mediated through uridine diphosphate glucuronosyltransferases found in the liver, intestines, kidney, and skin. Glucuronidation followed by biliary excretion is important for the elimination of endogenous compounds such as steroids, bile acids, and bilirubin, and it is a major rate-limiting pathway for the excretion of anticancer agents such as SN-38, the active metabolite of irinotecan. N-acetyltransferases and sulfotransferases found in the liver and other tissues are also responsible for drug transformation to more water-soluble species. Genetic polymorphisms in all types of drug-metabolizing enzymes are increasingly being recognized as an important source of variability in drug-metabolizing pathways.[25] The impact of hepatic dysfunction on liver drug-metabolizing pathways can be difficult to assess. Liver dysfunction can affect glucuronidation, and cirrhosis can reduce drug-metabolizing capacity by 30% to 50%.[26] Malnutrition has also been implicated in alterations in hepatic clearance of drugs.[27]

Drug clearance may also be mediated by excretion processes occurring in either the kidneys or the biliary system. The importance of assessing renal function before dosing renally excreted agents is well recognized.[4,5] Agents such as topotecan, etoposide, and carboplatin require dose adjustments in patients with impaired renal function. Usually, dosing decisions are based on estimations of the GFR; however, renal drug excretion is more complex, and it may also be influenced by other processes such as tubular secretion and reabsorption. In the proximal tubules, drugs are actively excreted via the action of P-glycoprotein and MRP2 (also known as the *canalicular multispecific organic anion transporter* or cMOAT) drug efflux pumps. In distal tubules and collecting ducts, passive reabsorption dominates, and these processes are often greatly affected by urinary pH. The excretion of weak acids is often enhanced by urinary alkalinization. Finally, because body size affects GFR, individual estimates of GFR should probably be scaled to BSA and expressed in term of milliliters per minute per 1.73 m² whenever BSA-adjusted drug dosing schemes are used.[22]

Biliary drug excretion pathways are less well characterized renal mechanisms, but cellular transporters, such as P glycoprotein and MRP2, in the biliary canaliculi are important in mediating these processes. P glycoprotein transports amphipathic lipid-soluble drugs, and MRP2 acts on conjugated metabolites, including drug glucuronides and sulfates and organic cations. Biliary excretion is an important route of drug clearance for anticancer agents such as irinotecan metabolites and for anthracyclines such as doxorubicin. The inducible activity of these biliary transport enzymes can lead to clinically significant changes in drug clearance. Cancer patients treated with enzyme-inducing antiepileptic drugs, such as phenytoin and carbamazepine, may have twofold to threefold higher drug clearance than control patients.[28,29] Biliary excretion pathways are also involved in enterohepatic circulation of some anticancer agents. Cleavage of glucuronidated metabolites of irinotecan by endogenous gut flora can lead to enterohepatic circulation and prolonged retention within the gastrointestinal tract.[30]

The clinical relevance of renal and hepatic clearance mechanisms in medical oncology is highlighted by the treatment of patients with end-organ dysfunction. Alterations in hepatic function are quite common in patients with hepatic metastases from colorectal cancer and can lead to significant diminutions in drug clearance. In other cancer patients, administration of nephrotoxic chemotherapeutic agents, such as cisplatin, or tumor-induced obstructive nephropathies may result in chronic renal impairment that complicates the use of renally excreted agents. Formal pharmacokinetic studies in cancer patients with abnormal renal and hepatic function are still relatively few; however, the importance of these studies in developing formal dosing guidelines to assist the clinician faced with the difficult dilemma of treating these patient populations cannot be overstated.[31,32]

ELIMINATION HALF-LIFE

The elimination half-life is the amount of time required for 50% of an administered drug dose to be eliminated.[1] The terminal elimination half-life ($t_{1/2}$) can be readily calculated from the elimination rate constant, λ_z, using the following formula:

$$t_{1/2} = ln\ (2)/\ \lambda_z,\ = 0.693/\lambda_z \qquad \text{(Eq. 11)}$$

The terminal elimination rate constant, λ_z, is expressed in units of 1/time and can be estimated by unweighted regression of the log-linear terminal elimination phase of the concentration versus time curve (Fig. 15.2-3).[9] The elimination rate constant is related to volume of distribution of the central compartment and clearance by the following formula:

$$CL = V_c \times \lambda_z \qquad \text{(Eq. 12)}$$

The terminal elimination half-life is not considered a fundamental pharmacokinetic parameter because it is derived from the terminal elimination rate constant (Eq. 11) and because it is a function of both clearance and the apparent volume of distribution (Eq. 12).[1] The time to reach steady state on a multi-

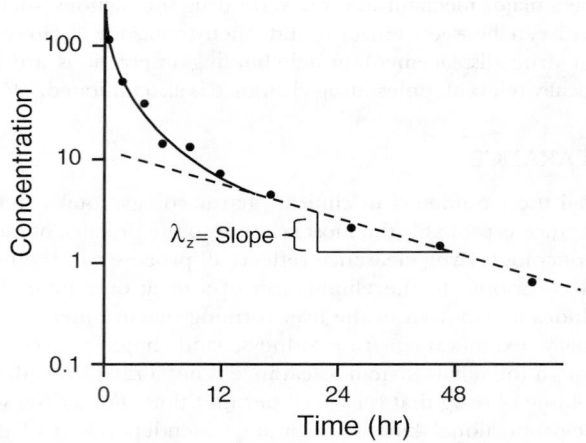

FIGURE 15.2-3. Estimation of the terminal elimination rate constant, λ_z, by regression analysis of the terminal portion of the log-linear concentration versus time plot.

dose schedule or during a continuous intravenous drug infusion is directly related to the terminal elimination half-life for a drug with dose-proportional kinetics. After an infusion period of four half-lives, the drug concentrations will be 94% of the steady-state value.

Because half-life is an easily visualized pharmacokinetic parameter, its clinical utility is often overemphasized. In actual practice, the terminal elimination half-life may not be relevant for determining the proper time interval for repeated drug dosing. For example, if an agent is converted into active metabolites, the biologically effective half-life may be much longer than the measured half-life. Furthermore, drugs with multicompartmental pharmacokinetic behavior may demonstrate several different half-lives, depending on the sensitivity of the analytical method used. For example, use of a highly sensitivity mass spectroscopic assay to measure plasma 5-fluorouracil (5-FU) concentrations detected extremely low plasma concentrations of this agent that persisted for prolonged times after drug administration. This previously unrecognized long terminal 5-FU elimination half-life was attributed to the slow efflux of drug from deep tissue compartments. However, these very low plasma drug concentrations did not relate to any clinical drug effects and, thus, were not felt to be biologically important.[33] In other situations, prolonged terminal drug elimination half-life may have great clinical relevance. For example, after distribution of methotrexate into large third-space fluid compartments, such as ascites or pleural effusions, the drug is slowly released back into the systemic circulation over time. The resulting prolongation of the terminal half-life can induce substantial drug toxicity.[34] Thus, the clinical relevance of the terminal elimination half-life may vary depending on the clinical situation.

DOSE PROPORTIONALITY

When measured drug concentrations are strictly proportional to the dose of drug administered, then the condition of dose proportionality holds. If doubling the drug dose results in a doubling of the plasma concentration, then fundamental pharmacokinetic parameters, such as rate constants, the apparent volume of distribution, and clearance, remain constant and are independent of changes in dose and concentration.[35,36] In contrast, parameters of drug exposure, such as AUC, steady-state plasma concentrations (C_{ss}), or maximum plasma concentrations (C_{max}), will change proportionally with drug dose. By strict definition, drugs with linear pharmacokinetics are dose proportional. Linear pharmacokinetics means that a drug's pharmacologic behavior can be described by a series of linear differential equations, such as those used to describe a multicompartmental model with first-order rate constants when elimination is restricted to the central compartment.

Dose proportionality is clinically important because it means that dose adjustments will generate predictable changes in systemic drug exposure. For drugs that lack dose proportionality, parameters such as clearance will demonstrate concentration or time dependence, or both, which makes it difficult to predict the effect of dose adjustments on the resulting plasma drug concentrations. Drugs with nonlinear pharmacokinetics have been well described in the literature. Some of the best examples are drugs with saturable Michaelis-Menten elimination processes, such as phenytoin.[6] Other physiologic factors that can cause deviations from dose proportionality include saturable oral absorption, capacity-limited distribution, saturable protein binding, or the autoinduction of drug-metabolizing enzymes. For example, all-*trans*-retinoic acid, which is used in the treatment of acute promyelocytic leukemia, can induce its own metabolism during prolonged drug administration.[37]

Multiple ways are available to test for dose proportionality.[9,35,36] The most robust method is to perform a comparative crossover pharmacokinetic study in which each patient received a series of different doses over time. However, such studies are rare in clinical oncology. More often, dose proportionality is assessed during dose escalation in phase I clinical trials in which small groups of patients are treated at a single dose level in parallel study design. The statistical power of these classic studies to detect deviations from dose proportionality is poor; however, phase I studies are often the only opportunity to examine anticancer drug kinetics over a wide range of doses. In these trials, dose proportionality can be assessed formally by plotting the weighted regression of the AUC or C_{max} against dose level to see if the resulting line passes through the origin.[9] If the result is a simple regression line that fits the AUC versus dose plot but does not pass through the origin, then there is no dose proportionality (doubling the dose does not exactly double the AUC), and the definition of linear pharmacokinetics is not met. More rigorous tests of dose proportionality include the application of the power model[35] or analysis-of-variance testing of the log-transformed CL or log-transformed dose-normalized AUC (AUC/dose) values examined across various dose levels.[9,35]

PHARMACODYNAMIC CONCEPTS

In a pharmacodynamic model, clinical drug effects are correlated with drug dose, concentrations, or other pharmacokinetic parameters.[2] For an anticancer agent, the ideal pharmacodynamic model defines the variation in clinical outcomes in subjects treated at a single uniform dose level that arises independent of changes in pharmacokinetics. Variability in pharmacodynamic response may also be heavily influenced by clinical covariates such as age, gender, prior chemotherapy, prior radiotherapy, concomi-

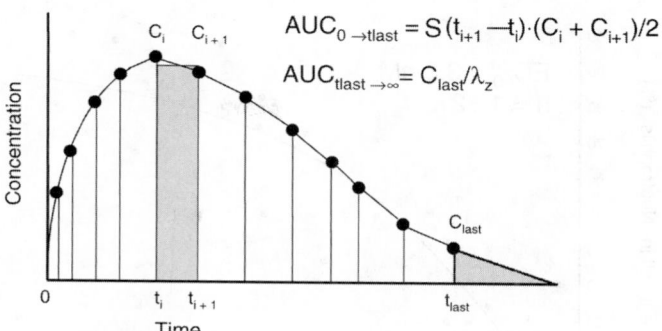

FIGURE 15.2-4. Estimation of the area under the concentration versus time curve (AUC) using the log-linear trapezoidal rule. The area under the curve from time zero to t_{last} is defined by $AUC_{0 \to tlast} = S(t_{i+1} - t_i) \times (C_i + C_{i+1})/2$, and the area under the curve from time t_{last} extrapolated to infinity is defined by $AUC_{tlast \to \infty} = C_{last}/\lambda_z$. The total extrapolated to infinity, $AUC_{0 \to \infty}$, is the sum of these two AUC terms. λ_z, elimination rate constant.

tant medications, or other variables.[38] The kinetic parameters that are most often correlated with drug effects are markers of drug exposure, such as AUC, or plasma drug concentrations, such as C_{max} or C_{ss}. However, other parameters may also have pharmacodynamic utility. For example, the toxic effects of highly schedule-dependent agents may be better explained by the duration that drug concentrations remain above a particular threshold value than by using the standard AUC. This approach has been successfully applied to pharmacodynamic studies of paclitaxel.[39] In general, which specific parameter is used as the independent variable in a pharmacodynamic analysis depends on the particular characteristics of the study drug.

The area under the concentration versus time curve is frequently used as a kinetic parameter to assess systemic drug exposure in formal pharmacodynamic studies of anticancer agents. Numerous pharmacodynamic studies have validated use of this parameter as a predictor of anticancer drug toxicity and efficacy in preclinical and clinical models.[7] As mentioned previously in Clearance, AUC is related to clearance by drug dose (Eq. 9a), and it is also useful for estimating other pharmacokinetic parameters such as clearance and volume of distribution at steady-state in a noncompartmental pharmacokinetic analyses (Eqs. 1, 4, 7, and 9a). Although the use of AUC in pharmacokinetic studies has been criticized,[17] it is still a useful parameter in oncology. The AUC can be directly estimated from concentration versus time data using relatively simple mathematical integration methods such as the linear trapezoidal rule or the log-linear trapezoidal rule with extrapolation to infinity (Fig. 15.2-4).[9]

In oncology, pharmacodynamic studies of drug effects have most often focused on toxicity end points. Continuous response variables, such as the percent fall in the absolute blood count from baseline, are easily analyzed using nonlinear regression methods. Dose-limiting neutropenia has been frequently analyzed using a sigmoid maximum effect model described by the modified Hill equation (Fig. 15.2-5)[40]:

Percent fall in blood counts = 100% $\times C^h/[C^h + (EC_{50})^h]$ (Eq. 13)

where C is the input parameter of drug exposure (often AUC or C_{ss}), EC_{50} is the value of C that produces a 50% fall in blood counts, and h is the Hill constant that is related to the degree of

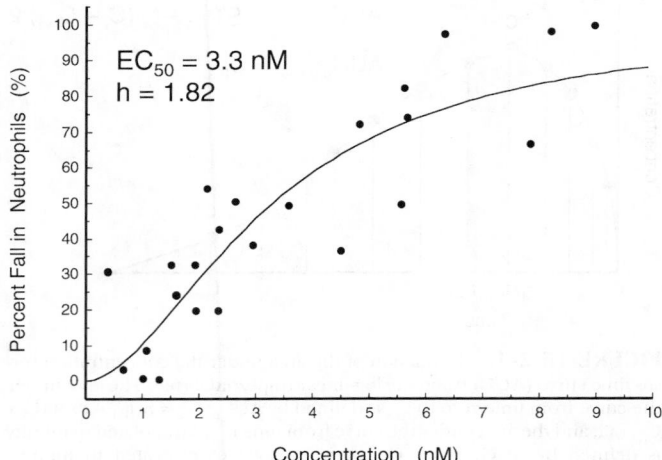

FIGURE 15.2-5. Pharmacodynamic sigmoid E_{max} model. The percent fall in the absolute neutrophil count from baseline in adult solid tumor patients treated with a 72-hour infusion of 9-aminocamptothecin (9-AC) is graphed as a function of the steady-state plasma drug concentration. The EC_{50} is the plasma concentration of 9-AC lactone associated with a 50% fall in neutrophil counts from baseline, and h is the Hill coefficient. (Data are taken from a clinical trial described in ref. 60.)

sigmoidicity of the exposure-effect curve. The pharmacodynamic analysis of subjectively graded clinical end points, such as common toxicity criteria scores that assess drug-related adverse events as mild (grade 1), moderate (grade 2), severe (grade 3), or life threatening (grade 4), may require more sophisticated statistical methods. Logistical regression methods have been used to model these types of categorical (ordinal) response or outcome variables.[2]

Several more complex mechanistic pharmacodynamic models of anticancer therapy–related myelosuppression have now been developed to describe the severity and time course of clinically important dose-limiting toxicities.[38,41–43] Models for neutropenia induced by paclitaxel[42,43] and etoposide[38,43] have been derived using indirect compartmental and population mixed-effect models. The ability of these models to predict both the severity and duration of drug-induced neutropenia substantially enhances their clinical usefulness and ultimately may lead to a better understanding of drug pharmacodynamics. Attempts to model objective tumor responses have been much less successful, perhaps due to the relatively limited efficacy seen in oncology trials that also incorporate pharmacokinetic monitoring. Nonetheless, the rapid advances in anticancer therapeutics raise the hope that pharmacodynamic analyses may ultimately be applied to the most important end points in clinical oncology: antitumor efficacy and prolonged survival.[44,45]

SPECIAL TOPICS IN PHARMACOKINETICS AND PHARMACODYNAMICS

THERAPEUTIC DRUG MONITORING AND ADAPTIVE CONTROL

For drugs with a narrow therapeutic index, high interpatient pharmacokinetic variability, and a well-defined pharmacodynamic profile, dosing patients to achieve a target concentra-

tion using only clinical judgment can be a major challenge. Under these circumstances, therapeutic drug monitoring and adaptive control may be of substantial clinical benefit.[1] However, the practical application of therapeutic drug monitoring also requires that intrapatient (within patient) kinetic variability be predictable and that an assay for drug concentrations be commercially available. Although such approaches are commonplace in other therapeutic areas in medicine, such as antibiotic and antiepileptic drug administration, examples of routine therapeutic drug monitoring in oncology are, unfortunately, rare. Notable exceptions include the use of high-dose methotrexate therapy with monitoring to guide leucovorin rescue[46] and the use of methotrexate in the treatment of pediatric acute lymphocytic leukemia.[45] In the investigational setting, adaptive control and therapeutic drug monitoring has been studied in the administration of 5-FU to patients with head and neck cancer[47] and of etoposide to patients with various solid tumors,[48] and in the clinical development of experimental anticancer agents such as suramin[49] and amonafide.[50] The present trend in oncologic developmental therapeutics toward the use of less toxic, molecularly targeted agents may ultimately lessen the need for precisely targeting a narrow range of drug concentrations in the clinical setting.

POPULATION PHARMACOKINETICS

Ultimately, the goal of pharmacokinetic studies is to define a drug's pharmacokinetic behavior and variability within a large population of patients.[51] Traditionally, this is performed using a classic "two-stage" pharmacokinetic analysis in which parameter estimates for individual patients are pooled and characterized using summary statistics, such as means, variances, and covariances. In these circumstances, the relative standard deviation or coefficient of variation (CV%) for each pharmacokinetic parameter is used as an indicator of the degree of interpatient variability within the population.[2] This approach has significant limitations, however, in that the true measures of interindividual variability are not defined separately from the random residual error. A more sophisticated and complex approach is to define a population pharmacostatistical model that simultaneously estimates interindividual and random residual variability within the population using a nonlinear mixed-effect model. This can be implemented using software programs such as NONMEM.[52] The power of this approach is the ability to incorporate key clinical covariates in the population pharmacokinetic model that help explain the variability of pharmacokinetic parameters. Population analysis with bayesian estimation is also a powerful method to estimate individual pharmacokinetic parameters for individual patients using a relatively few blood samples. Other population approaches include nonparametric population modeling, which requires fewer assumptions about the distribution of parameters within the population. Finally, an exciting area of drug development is the use of pharmacokinetic-pharmacodynamic population models of anticancer action as a tool for large-scale detailed clinical trial simulation of phase III studies.[53]

PHARMACOGENOMICS

A major goal of clinical pharmacology is to explain and understand variability in drug action. Pharmacogenomics is the scientific study of the variability in pharmacokinetics (involving drug absorption, distribution, metabolism, and elimination) and pharmacodynamics (involving drug effects in cells and tissues) at the most basic level of the human genome. McLeod and Evans define pharmacogenomics as the study of "the inherited nature of interindividual differences in drug disposition and effects."[25] The explosion of knowledge in the study of the human genome has allowed the identification of numerous single-nucleotide polymorphisms (genetic variants that occur with a frequency of 1% or higher) that can potentially alter gene function and influence response to drug therapy. Currently, most pharmacogenomic studies have focused on pharmacokinetically relevant polymorphisms in drug-metabolizing enzymes. For example, clinically significant polymorphisms have been identified in human CYP3A4, CYP2C9, and CYP2D6 cytochrome P-450 isoforms.[54] However, drug-metabolizing polymorphisms that have direct clinical relevance to medical oncology are still relatively few.[55] One well-characterized example is the inherited deficiency of thiopurine-S-methyltransferase that is associated with severe intolerance to thiopurine therapy.[56] Pretreatment recognition of thiopurine-S-methyltransferase deficiency in patients can lead to dosage adjustments that minimize the toxicities associated with thiopurine chemotherapy. Another example is the inherited variation in the activity of dihydropyrimidine dehydrogenase, the rate-limiting enzyme responsible for the catabolism of 5-FU.[57] Genetic alterations associated with dihydropyrimidine dehydrogenase deficiency have been identified in rare cases in which patients experienced severe and fatal toxicity after treatment with standard doses of 5-FU. Other relevant drug-metabolizing polymorphisms in clinical oncology include variations in the uridine diphosphate glucuronyltransferase 1A1 gene, which is responsible for the glucuronidation of SN-38, the active metabolite of irinotecan. The UGT1A1*28 allele is associated with reduced glucuronidating activity and an increased risk of irinotecan-induced diarrhea.[58]

Clinically relevant polymorphisms are not limited to drug-metabolizing enzymes; however, knowledge of pharmacodynamically relevant polymorphisms that affect drug targets such as receptors or specific enzymes is still quite limited. Polymorphisms in the promoter region of the thymidylate synthase gene have been correlated with tumor response to 5-FU–based chemotherapy.[59] In the near future, this understanding of pharmacogenomic variation in pharmacokinetics and pharmacodynamics will provide the ultimate method for individualizing pharmacotherapy.

PHARMACOKINETICS AND PHARMACODYNAMICS IN ONCOLOGY DRUG DEVELOPMENT

Carefully designed clinical pharmacology studies should be fully integrated into overall drug development plans. Ideally, the collection of pharmacokinetic and pharmacodynamic information should begin at the earliest stages of drug development. Preclinical laboratory studies can characterize potential risk of serious drug interactions by identifying important drug-metabolizing enzymes, such as CYP3A4, using *in vitro* test systems.[24] These studies can also suggest important pathways of drug clearance. At this stage, analytical assays can be developed

and validated with sufficient sensitivity and reliability to perform pharmacokinetic studies. Efforts should also be directed toward validating measurements of pharmacodynamic end points by characterizing suitable surrogate markers for molecular drug effects. Application of these assays to animal models provides the first information about pharmacokinetic-pharmacodynamic relationships in intact organisms. These experiments can provide valuable information for the design of first time in human studies.

The first time in a human phase I trial is the initial opportunity to obtain detailed clinical pharmacokinetic information about a new molecular entity. Summary descriptive pharmacokinetics allows an assessment of the degree of kinetic variability, and covariate analyses can highlight the important factors that underlie this variability. Because dose escalation is a hallmark of traditional phase I oncologic studies, an analysis of dose proportionality over the dose range studied can be implemented. Toxicity assessments are also important end points in phase I studies; thus, pharmacodynamic correlations between drug exposure and drug toxicity can also be initiated at this phase of drug development. However, the most clinically useful pharmacodynamic information is collected at the end of dose escalation when larger numbers of patients are being treated at the recommended phase II dose.[2] In an ideal program, phase I pharmacokinetic studies should also incorporate the collection of DNA samples for pharmacogenomic screening. Although important genetic polymorphisms may not be known before the initiation of these early trials, the ability to retrospectively analyze data is a valuable tool for any rational drug development program. Finally, the information obtained in these early, intensive pharmacokinetic studies can be used to develop optimal and limited sampling strategies that can readily be applied to pharmacokinetic monitoring in clinical studies during later stages of development.

In phase II studies, clinical efficacy trials are typically conducted at multiple institutions in multiple disease types. Thus, the total number of patients treated increases substantially from this point forward. Often, fiscal and logistical difficulties prohibit performing extensive pharmacokinetic sampling at this stage. However, the implementation of formal limited or sparse pharmacokinetic sampling strategies may allow for further expansion of the pharmacokinetic database. Pooled data from all the pharmacokinetic studies performed can be analyzed in population pharmacokinetic studies. Nonlinear mixed-effect modeling can further characterize the magnitude of kinetic variation within the population and can identify important covariates that may be used in selecting special subpopulations for further study. Finally, comprehensive population pharmacokinetic-pharmacodynamic models developed at this stage can serve as the basis for early clinical trial forecasting and simulations that assist in the design of larger, more resource-intense randomized phase III trials.[53]

Simultaneously with expanded phase II testing, combination phase I studies may be initiated at this stage. Coadministration of a new agent with standard anticancer therapies can be rationally planned based on synergistic antitumor activity or because the agent is being targeted for use in a specific disease type such as lung, colon, or breast cancer. A phase I trial of any new drug combination should always include pharmacokinetic monitoring to define potential drug interactions. Other specialized clinical trials include formal mass balance studies that define the total excretion of an experimental agent in urine and feces and other bodily fluids over time. Typically, these studies are performed in carefully controlled settings with radioactively labeled drug. The results of mass balance studies combined with information obtained from other early pharmacokinetic trials can precisely define the major routes of drug elimination and may highlight the need to perform additional specialized studies. For example, a drug that is largely excreted unchanged in the urine will need to be carefully examined in pharmacokinetic studies in patients with renal dysfunction. In contrast, a hepatically metabolized drug or one that undergoes biliary excretion should be examined in formal studies in patients with liver dysfunction. Finally, if the growing body of clinical information identifies potential drug interactions, then a formalized drug interaction study can be performed with the compound of interest. Other pharmacokinetic studies of potential importance include phase I trials in special populations such as pediatric cancer patients, patients with acute leukemia, or geriatric patients. This phase of drug development may temporally overlap with other phases of drug development and may even stretch into the postmarketing period.

The final and most resource-intense phase of drug development is the randomized phase III trial. Consequently, the growing field of clinical trial forecasting and simulation based on pharmacokinetic-pharmacodynamic modeling may offer the greatest benefit immediately before this stage of drug development. Ideally, this involves the maximal use of all pharmacologic information collected up to that time. Formalized simulations of various study designs and possible outcomes can then be explored in detail. If the results are favorable, then this stage culminates in the initiation of a randomized phase III clinical trial, most often the final step in a successful registration program.

CONCLUSION

The impact of advances in science and technology on the clinical practice of medicine has never been greater than in the current era. The sequencing of the human genome and the ability to profile thousands of genes simultaneously in tumor specimens and normal tissues has led to the proliferation of promising new and novel targets for anticancer therapeutics. These milestone achievements, coupled with advances in high-throughput drug screening and drug discovery, have caused the pipeline of new therapies for the treatment of cancer to overflow. Never before has the medical oncologist had this number and diversity of active therapeutic agents at his or her disposal, and because of the rapid pace of scientific progress, this growth will only continue to accelerate. In addition, these same scientific advances are providing tools for understanding drug action in individual patients with degrees of precision never before imagined. These developments are causing a revolution of change in all areas of medicine, and the field of clinical pharmacology and cancer therapeutics is no exception. Pharmacogenomic studies of drug-metabolizing pathways are completely altering the approach to clinical pharmacokinetics. Likewise, gene expression profiling of tumors means that the pharmacodynamics of drug action can now be examined at the molecular level. Because of these developments, the future of cancer chemotherapy has never been brighter. However, these remarkable advances also place an increasing burden on the practicing oncologist to apply this pharmacologic knowledge in the most rational way possible for the maximal benefit of patients with cancer.

REFERENCES

1. Atkinson AJ, Daniels CE, Dedrick RL, et al. *Principles of clinical pharmacology.* San Diego: Academic Press, 2001.
2. Ratain MJ, Mick R. Principles of pharmacokinetics and pharmacodynamics. In: Schilsky RL, Milano GA, Ratain MJ, eds. *Principles of antineoplastic drug development and pharmacology.* New York: Marcel Dekker, Inc., 1996:123.
3. Bourne DWA. *Mathematical modeling of pharmacokinetic data.* Lancaster: Technomic, 1995:95.
4. Calvert AH. Dose optimisation of carboplatin in adults. *Anticancer Res* 1994;14:2273.
5. Egorin MJ, Van Echo DA, Olman EA, et al. Prospective validation of a pharmacologically based dosing scheme for the cis-diamminedichloroplatinum(II) analogue diamminecyclobutanedicarboxylatoplatinum. *Cancer Res* 1985;45:6502.
6. Ludden TM. Nonlinear pharmacokinetics: clinical implications. *Clin Pharmacokinet* 1991;20:429.
7. Ratain MJ, Schilsky RL, Conley BA, et al. Pharmacodynamics in cancer therapy. *J Clin Oncol* 1990;8:1739.
8. Takimoto CH. The clinical pharmacology of the oral fluoropyrimidines. *Curr Probl Cancer* 2001;25:134.
9. Noe DA. Noncompartmental pharmacokinetic analysis. In: Grochow LB, Ames MM, eds. *A clinician's guide to chemotherapy: pharmacokinetics and pharmacodynamics.* Baltimore: Lippincott Williams & Wilkins, 1998:515.
10. Martinez MN, Amidon GL. A mechanistic approach to understanding the factors affecting drug absorption: a review of fundamentals. *J Clin Pharmacol* 2002;42:620.
11. Gibaldi M, Perrier D. *Pharmacokinetics,* 2nd ed. New York: Marcel Dekker, 1982:445.
12. Perrier D, Mayersohn M. Noncompartmental determination of the steady-state volume of distribution for any mode of administration. *J Pharm Sci* 1982;71:372.
13. Blaney SM, Balis FM, Poplack DG. Current pharmacological treatment approaches to central nervous system leukaemia. *Drugs* 1991;41:702.
14. Mick R, Ratain MJ. Modeling interpatient pharmacodynamic variability of etoposide. *J Natl Cancer Inst* 1991;83:1560.
15. Stewart CF, Zamboni WC. Plasma protein binding of chemotherapeutic agents. In: Grochow LB, Ames MM, eds. *A clinician's guide to chemotherapy: pharmacokinetics and pharmacodynamics.* Baltimore: Lippincott Williams & Wilkins, 1998:55.
16. Benet LZ, Hoener BA. Changes in plasma protein binding have little clinical relevance. *Clin Pharmacol Ther* 2002;71:115.
17. Holford NH. Input from the deep south compartment. A personal viewpoint. *Clin Pharmacokinet* 1995;29:139.
18. Sawyer M, Ratain MJ. Body surface area as a determinant of pharmacokinetics and drug dosing. *Invest New Drugs* 2001;19:171.
19. Grochow LB, Baraldi C, Noe D. Is dose normalization to weight or body surface area useful in adults? *J Natl Cancer Inst* 1990;82:323.
20. Gurney H. Dose calculation of anticancer drugs: a review of the current practice and introduction of an alternative. *J Clin Oncol* 1996;14:2590.
21. Felici A, Verweij J, Sparreboom A. Dosing strategies for anticancer drugs: the good, the bad and body-surface area. *Eur J Cancer* 2002;38:1677.
22. Ratain MJ. Dear doctor: we really are not sure what dose of capecitabine you should prescribe for your patient. *J Clin Oncol* 2002;20:1434.
23. Egorin MJ. Horseshoes, hand grenades, and body-surface area-based dosing: aiming for a target. *J Clin Oncol* 2003;21:182.
24. Hasler JA. Pharmacogenetics of cytochromes P450. *Mol Aspects Med* 1999;20:12.
25. McLeod HL, Evans WE. Pharmacogenomics: unlocking the human genome for better drug therapy. *Annu Rev Pharmacol Toxicol* 2001;41:101.
26. Hoyumpa AM, Schenker S. Is glucuronidation truly preserved in patients with liver disease? *Hepatology* 1991;13:786.
27. Murry DJ, Riva L, Poplack DG. Impact of nutrition on pharmacokinetics of anti-neoplastic agents. *Int J Cancer Suppl* 1998;11:48.
28. Kuhn JG. Influence of anticonvulsants on the metabolism and elimination of irinotecan. A North American Brain Tumor Consortium preliminary report. *Oncology (Huntingt)* 2002;16:33.
29. Relling MV, Pui CH, Sandlund JT, et al. Adverse effect of anticonvulsants on efficacy of chemotherapy for acute lymphoblastic leukaemia. *Lancet* 2000;356:285.
30. Gupta E, Lestingi TM, Mick R, et al. Metabolic fate of irinotecan in humans: correlation of glucuronidation with diarrhea. *Cancer Res* 1994;54:3723.
31. O'Reilly S, Rowinsky EK, Slichenmyer W, et al. Phase I and pharmacologic study of topotecan in patients with impaired renal function. *J Clin Oncol* 1996;14:3062.
32. Takimoto CH, Remick SC, Sharma S, et al. Dose-escalating and pharmacological study of oxaliplatin in adult cancer patients with impaired renal function: a National Cancer Institute Organ Dysfunction Working Group Study. *J Clin Oncol* 2003;21:2664.
33. van Groeningen CJ, Pinedo HM, Heddes J, et al. Pharmacokinetics of 5-fluorouracil assessed with a sensitive mass spectrometric method in patients on a dose escalation schedule. *Cancer Res* 1988;48:6956.
34. Chabner BA, Stoller RG, Hande K, et al. Methotrexate disposition in humans: case studies in ovarian cancer and following high-dose infusion. *Drug Metab Rev* 1978;8:107.
35. Gough K, Hutchison M, Keene O, et al. Assessment of dose proportionality: report from the statisticians in the pharmaceutical industry/pharmacokinetics UK joint working party. *Drug Inf J* 1995;29:1039.

36. Smith BP, Vandenhende FR, DeSante KA, et al. Confidence interval criteria for assessment of dose proportionality. *Pharm Res* 2000;17:1278.
37. Adamson PC. Clinical and pharmacokinetic studies of all-trans-retinoic acid in pediatric patients with cancer. *Leukemia* 1994;8:1813.
38. Karlsson MO, Port RE, Ratain MJ, et al. A population model for the leukopenic effect of etoposide. *Clin Pharmacol Ther* 1995;57:325.
39. Kearns CM, Gianni L, Egorin MJ. Paclitaxel pharmacokinetics and pharmacodynamics. *Semin Oncol* 1995;22:16.
40. Gabrielsson J, Weiner D. *Pharmacokinetic and pharmacodynamic data analysis, concepts and applications*, 2nd ed. Stockholm: Swedish Pharmaceutical Press, 1997.
41. Rosner GL, Muller P. Pharmacodynamic analysis of hematologic profiles. *J Pharmacokinet Biopharm* 1994;22:499.
42. Karlsson MO, Molnar V, Bergh J, et al. A general model for time-dissociated pharmacokinetic-pharmacodynamic relationship exemplified by paclitaxel myelosuppression. *Clin Pharmacol Ther* 1998;63:11.
43. Minami H, Sasaki Y, Saijo N, et al. Indirect-response model for the time course of leukopenia with anticancer drugs. *Clin Pharmacol Ther* 1998;64:511.
44. Evans WE, Crom WR, Abromowitch M, et al. Clinical pharmacodynamics of high-dose methotrexate in acute lymphocytic leukemia. Identification of a relation between concentration and effect. *N Engl J Med* 1986;314:471.
45. Evans WE, Relling MV, Rodman JH, et al. Conventional compared with individualized chemotherapy for childhood acute lymphoblastic leukemia. *N Engl J Med* 1998;338:499.
46. Ackland SP, Schilsky RL. High-dose methotrexate: a critical reappraisal. *J Clin Oncol* 1987;5:2017.
47. Santini J, Milano G, Thyss A, et al. 5-FU therapeutic monitoring with dose adjustment leads to an improved therapeutic index in head and neck cancer. *Br J Cancer* 1989;59:287.
48. Joel SP, Ellis P, O'Byrne K, et al. Therapeutic monitoring of continuous infusion etoposide in small-cell lung cancer. *J Clin Oncol* 1996;14:1903.
49. Cooper MR, Lieberman R, La Rocca RV, et al. Adaptive control with feedback strategies for suramin dosing. *Clin Pharmacol Ther* 1992;52:11.
50. Ratain MJ, Mick R, Janisch L, et al. Individualized dosing of amonafide based on a pharmacodynamic model incorporating acetylator phenotype and gender. *Pharmacogenetics* 1996;6:93.
51. Miller R. Population pharmacokinetics. In: Atkinson AJ, Daniels CE, Dedrick RL, et al., eds. *Principles of clinical pharmacology*. San Diego: Academic Press, 2001:113.
52. Beal SL, Sheiner LB. *NONMEM user's guides*. San Francisco: University of California, 1989.
53. Holford NH, Kimko HC, Monteleone JP, et al. Simulation of clinical trials. *Annu Rev Pharmacol Toxicol* 2000;40:209.
54. Flockhart DA. Clinical pharmacogenetics. In: Atkinson AJ, Daniels CE, Dedrick RL, et al., eds. *Principles of clinical pharmacology*. San Diego: Academic Press, 2001:158.
55. Krynetski EY, Evans WE. Pharmacogenetics of cancer therapy: getting personal. *Am J Hum Genet* 1998;63:11.
56. Relling MV, Hancock ML, Rivera GK, et al. Mercaptopurine therapy intolerance and heterozygosity at the thiopurine S-methyltransferase gene locus. *J Natl Cancer Inst* 1999; 91:2001.
57. Diasio RB, Johnson MR. The role of pharmacogenetics and pharmacogenomics in cancer chemotherapy with 5-fluorouracil. *Pharmacology* 2000;61:199.
58. Iyer L, Das S, Janisch L, et al. UGT1A1*28 polymorphism as a determinant of irinotecan disposition and toxicity. *Pharmacogenomics J* 2002;2:43.
59. Villafranca E, Okruzhnov Y, Dominguez MA, et al. Polymorphisms of the repeated sequences in the enhancer region of the thymidylate synthase gene promoter may predict downstaging after preoperative chemoradiation in rectal cancer. *J Clin Oncol* 2001; 19:1779.
60. Takimoto CH, Dahut W, Marino MT, et al. Pharmacodynamics and pharmacokinetics of a 72-hour infusion of 9-aminocamptothecin in adult cancer patients. *J Clin Oncol* 1997;15:1492.

SECTION **3**

HOWARD L. MCLEOD
BOON-CHER GOH

Pharmacogenomics

Uncertainty remains as to the use of cytotoxic agents to treat patients with cancer. We have accepted that a proportion of patients will experience toxicity and a certain proportion of patients will have response. This is because drug development in oncology traditionally uses a dosage for the average patient in a defined patient cohort, with an average incidence of toxicity and response. Further refinements of drug dose in accordance with patient factors (e.g., ability to degrade or transport a medicine) or genetic constitution of their cancers are currently not generally incorporated into the trial designs. With the growing number of agents with an apparently similar degree of antitumor activity for most cancers, we now need better tools for the selection of anticancer therapy.

For cancer chemotherapy, where cytotoxic agents are administered at doses close to their maximal tolerable dose and therapeutic windows are relatively narrow, minor differences in individual drug handling may lead to severe toxicities. Therefore, an understanding of the sources of this variability would lead to the possibility of individualizing dosages or influencing clinical decisions that can improve patient care.

A drug's disposition and pharmacodynamic effects can be influenced by a number of variables, including patient age, diet, concomitant medications, and underlying disease processes.[1] However, an individual's genetic constitution is an important regulator of variability in drug effect. Differences in drug effects are more pronounced between individuals compared to within an individual. Indeed, studies in monozygotic and dizygotic twins identified that 20% to 80% of the variation in drug disposition is mediated by inheritance.[2] Drug-metabolizing enzymes, cellular transporters, and tissue receptors are governed by genetic variation. These variations in the DNA sequences encoding these proteins may take the form of deletions, insertions, repeats, frameshift mutations, nonsense mutations, and missense mutations, resulting in an inactive, truncated, unstable, or otherwise dysfunctional protein. The most common change involves single-nucleotide substitutions, called *single-nucleotide polymorphisms* (SNPs), which occur at approximately 1 per 1000 base pairs on the human genome. Variability in toxicity or activity can also be mediated by postgenomic events, at the level of RNA, protein, or functional activity (Fig. 15.3-1).

Pharmacogenetics is the study of the hereditary basis of drug response and in practical terms is focused on DNA markers that are predictive for toxicity or therapeutic outcomes.[1] Pharmacogenomics refers to a broader field, encompassing the application of DNA, RNA, or protein information to understand the effect of a drug. Pharmacogenetics is based on our understanding of how predetermined genetic factors impact on each individual's response to treatment and how they can explain the interindividual and interethnic variability of drug response. Pharmacogenomics has putative utility in therapy selection and clinical study design and as a tool to improve understanding of the pharmacology of a medication (Table 15.3-1).

PHARMACOGENOMICS OF CHEMOTHERAPY DRUG TOXICITY

Advances in the treatment of most common malignancies have resulted in the availability of multiple distinct combination chemotherapy regimens with similar or equal anticancer efficacy. Therefore, differences in systemic toxicity have become a major determinant in the selection of therapy. The majority of pharmacogenomic examples affecting adverse events from cytotoxic drugs involve hepatic metabolizing enzymes that detoxify or biotransform xenobiotics (Table 15.3-2).[1–5] A contribution by

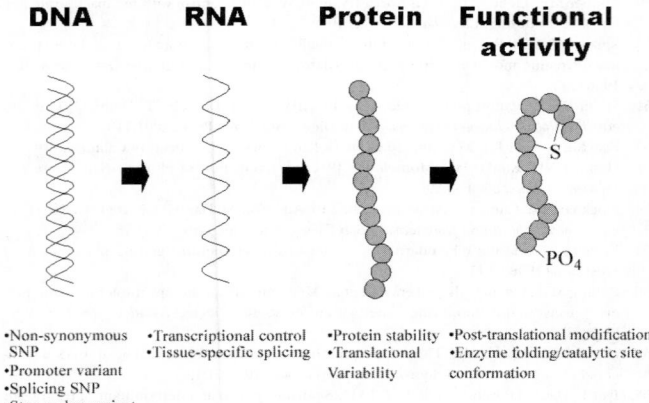

FIGURE 15.3-1. Sources of pharmacogenomic variability at the level of DNA, RNA, protein, and functional activity. SNP, single-nucleotide polymorphism.

other proteins relevant to cytotoxic drug pharmacology, such as cellular transporters or tissue targets, is also emerging.

THIOPURINE METHYLTRANSFERASE

One of the best-studied pharmacogenetic syndromes involves the metabolism of the thiopurine drugs 6-mercaptopurine (6-MP), 6-thioguanine, and azathioprine, which have wide applications, including maintenance therapy for childhood acute lymphocytic leukemia and adult leukemias.[6] These prodrugs must be activated to thioguanine nucleotides to have antiproliferative effects. However, most of the variability in the formation of active metabolites is mediated by methylation via thiopurine methyltransferase (TPMT).[7] TPMT is a cytosolic enzyme that catalyzes S-methylation of thiopurine agents, resulting in an inactive metabolite. Erythrocyte TPMT activity has a trimodal distribution, with 90% of patients having high activity, 10% intermediate activity, and 0.3% very low or no detectable activity. TPMT deficiency results in higher intracellular activation of 6-MP to form thioguanine nucleotides, resulting in severe or fatal hematologic toxicity from standard doses of therapy.[6] The variable activity results from polymorphism in the TPMT gene, located on chromosome locus 6p22.3. Genetic variants at codon 238 (TPMT*2), codon 719 (TPMT*3C), or codon 460 and 719 (TPMT*3A) are the most clinically significant, accounting for 95% of the patients with reduced TPMT activity.[8] Heterozygotes (one wild-type and one variant allele) are common (10% of patients) and have elevated

TABLE 15.3-1. Areas of Clinical Potential for Pharmacogenomics

THERAPY SELECTION
Toxicity avoidance
Efficacy optimization
CLINICAL TRIAL DESIGN
Population stratification
Genotype-specific phase II/III evaluation
Exclusion of patients with low chance of benefit
PHARMACOLOGIC DISCOVERY
Definition of mechanism of action
Identification of targets for modulation of activity

TABLE 15.3-2. Examples of Therapeutically Relevant Genetic Variation in Oncology

Genomic Aberration	Affected Agents	Consequence
GENE COPY		
Her-2 amplification	Trastuzumab	Tumor response
GENE REARRANGEMENT		
9:22 translocation	Imatinib	Tumor response
SOMATIC MUTATION		
c-kit exon 11 variant	Imatinib	Tumor response
GERMLINE POLYMORPHISM		
Thiopurine methyltransferase	6-Mercaptopurine	Severe neutropenia
Dihydropyrimidine dehydrogenase	5-Fluorouracil	Severe neutropenia, neurotoxicity
CYP2D6	Tamoxifen	Lower active metabolite levels
UGT1A1	Irinotecan	Severe neutropenia
Thymidylate synthase	5-Fluorouracil/capecitabine	Drug resistance

levels of active metabolites (two-fold more than homozygous wild-type); they required more cumulative dose reductions of 6-MP for maintenance acute lymphocytic leukemia chemotherapy compared to that for homozygous wild-type patients (Fig. 15.3-2).[9] Patients with a homozygous variant TPMT genotype are at four-fold risk of severe toxicity compared with wild-type patients.[8] TPMT genotype tests are now available commercially in a Clinical Laboratories Improvement Act–certified environment. To date, patients homozygous for TPMT variant alleles appear to tolerate 10%, and heterozygotes 65% of the recommended doses of 6-MP, with no apparent decrease in clinical efficacy (see Fig. 15.3-2).[9] This has formed the basis for prospective, TPMT genotype-guided dosing of 6-MP to avoid severe toxicity.

DIHYDROPYRIMIDINE DEHYDROGENASE

Although 5-fluorouracil (5-FU) has been available for more than 40 years, it remains one of the most commonly prescribed chemotherapy agents. 5-FU is a prodrug that is activated intracellularly to 5 fluoro-2-deoxyuridine monophosphate (5FdUMP), which inhibits thymidylate synthase (TS), among other mechanisms of action. TS inhibition results in impaired *de novo* pyrimidine synthesis and suppression of DNA synthesis. Approximately

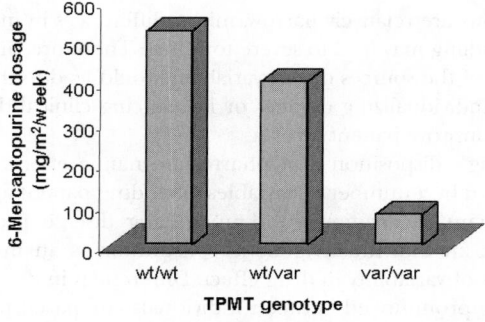

FIGURE 15.3-2. Thiopurine methyltransferase (TPMT) variants determine the tolerable dose of 6-mercaptopurine in children with acute lymphocytic leukemia. var, variant; wt, weight.

85% of a 5-FU dose is catabolized by dihydropyrimidine dehydrogenase (DPD) to inactive metabolites. Therefore, DPD is a primary regulator of 5-FU activity. DPD deficiency has been described, resulting in higher 5-FU blood levels, greater formation of active metabolites, and severe or fatal clinical toxicity, predominately myelosuppression, mucositis, and cerebellar toxicity.[10] In theory, this toxicity could be reduced or avoided by screening for DPD activity in surrogate tissues, such as peripheral mononuclear cells. However, the technical requirements for preparation of these samples make it impractical for many practice sites. Understanding the molecular basis for DPD deficiency will provide an approach for prospective identification of patients at high risk for severe 5-FU toxicity. The gene encoding DPD is composed of 23 exons, and at least 23 SNPs have been found.[11]

Studies in DPD-deficient patients have identified several distinct molecular variants associated with low enzyme activity. Many of these are rare, and base substitutions, splicing defects, and frameshift mutations have been described. The prevalent variation is the splice recognition site in intron 14 (DPYD*2A), in which a G to A substitution results in skipping of exon 14, producing an inactive enzyme.[12–14] This polymorphism has been associated with severe DPD deficiency in heterozygous patients, with a homozygous genotype associated with a mental retardation syndrome. Patients with severe 5-FU toxicity may harbor one or more variant alleles of DPD, and a study has shown that 61% of cancer patients experiencing severe 5-FU toxicities had decreased DPD activity in peripheral mononuclear cells, and DPYD*2A was commonly found.[15] In the patients with grade 4 neutropenia, 50% harbored at least one DPYD*2A. It is estimated that in the white population, homozygotes for the variant alleles have an incidence of 0.1% and heterozygotes occur at an incidence of 0.5% to 2.0%. Additional DPD mutations have been associated with impaired enzyme activity. However, many patients with severe 5-FU toxicity have normal DPD activity. This highlights the fact that many factors, including multiple genes, are potential causes of 5-FU toxicity and that there will not be one simple test to avoid this important clinical problem.

URIDINE DIPHOSPHATE GLUCURONOSYLTRANSFERASE

An important association is emerging between polymorphism in the UGT1A1 promoter and irinotecan toxicity. Clinical use of irinotecan produces variable plasma levels of irinotecan and SN-38 and unpredictable diarrhea and neutropenia.[16,17] Irinotecan pharmacokinetics correlates poorly with body surface area; thus, clinical dosing is largely empiric. Glucuronidation is a phase II reaction that conjugates an expansive range of endogenous substrates and exogenous xenobiotics. In humans, there are two families of glucuronosyltransferases, UGT1 and UGT2, which mediate glucuronidation. UGT1A1 is the main isoform that inactivates the potent topoisomerase I inhibitor SN-38, the active metabolite of irinotecan.[16]

Clinical syndromes of hyperbilirubinemia due to UGT1A1 deficiency are well described. Crigler-Najjar syndrome is the more serious due to coding region SNPs, whereas Gilbert's syndrome is an asymptomatic hyperbilirubinemia arising from a reduced UGT1A1 expression. The mechanistic basis for Gilbert's syndrome is a homozygous inheritance of a common promoter polymorphism consisting of seven TA repeats (UGT1A1*28), compared to the wild type of six repeats.[18] The function of UGT1A1 is inversely related to the number of TA repeats. UGT1A1*28 has a 70% reduction in transcription and has been associated with greater toxicity. The incidence of Gilbert's syndrome shows ethnic variability, with an incidence ranging from 10% to 13% in whites and up to 19% in Canadian Inuits.[18] In Asians, Gilbert's syndrome may occur as a result of heterozygous inheritance of missense mutations in the coding region of the UGT1A1 gene. Patients with Gilbert's syndrome have less ability to glucuronidate SN-38 and experience greater toxicity from irinotecan therapy (Fig. 15.3-3A).

A retrospective study in 118 Japanese cancer patients showed that having a UGT1A1*28 allele was significantly associated with severe toxicity from irinotecan treatment.[19] A prospective pilot clinical study of irinotecan pharmacokinetics and pharmacodynamics suggested higher SN-38 AUC (area under the concentration-time curve) and a lower absolute neutrophil count after a fixed dose of irinotecan higher toxicity in patients who harbored the UGT1A1*28 allele.[20] In a prospective study, irinotecan, 350 mg/m², was administered over 90 minutes to 66 patients with advanced disease.[21] Genetic variants in UGT1A1 were assessed, including an interesting novel promoter SNP at base −3156 and the previously mentioned TA repeat. UGT1A1 genotype and haplotype were then correlated with SN-38 pharmacology and incidence of severe toxicity. Patients with the 7/7 genotype (UGT1A1*28 homozygous) had 9.3-fold greater risk of developing grade 4 neutropenia compared to the patients with a 6/6 or 6/7 genotype (see Fig. 15.3-3B).[21] Avoiding irino-

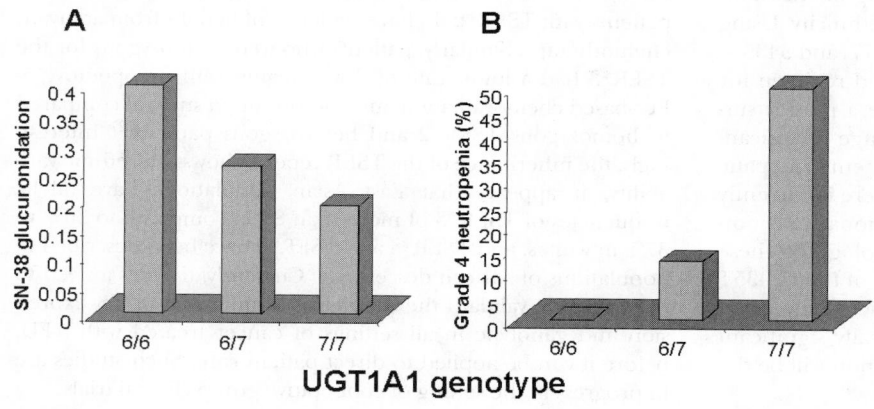

A **B**

UGT1A1 genotype

FIGURE 15.3-3. UGT1A1 promoter TA repeat is associated with inactivation of SN-38 (**A**) and severity of neutropenia (**B**).

tecan administration in the patients with a 7/7 genotype would have cut the incidence of severe neutropenia in half. Assessment of the presence of the UGT1A1*28 allele in patients before irinotecan treatment may predict individuals at risk for severe toxicity from irinotecan, allowing the selection of lower doses or alternative therapies.

CELLULAR TRANSPORTERS

Several large families of membrane-bound efflux pumps influence the disposition of anticancer drugs.[22] The most well characterized are the adenosine triphosphate–binding cassette (ABC) transmembrane efflux transporters. ABCB1 (also known as *MDR1* or *P glycoprotein*) was initially found in cancer cell lines resistant to multiple cytotoxic agents, including anthracyclines, taxanes, vinca alkaloids, and epipodophyllotoxins. Its distribution in the body tissues reflects its protective function against xenobiotics. These include the gastrointestinal tract, where it may limit drug absorption, as well as hepatocytes, biliary tract, and renal tubules, where it may affect drug clearance. Its expression at the capillary endothelium of the brain and the testes affects the disposition of chemotherapy. Therefore, the pharmacokinetics of many anticancer drugs may be affected by P glycoprotein function. Polymorphisms in the coding region of ABCB1 have been discovered, of which the C3435T polymorphism in exon 26 has been shown to affect the pharmacokinetics of digoxin, nelfinavir, fexofenadine, and anthracycline chemotherapy agents.[22] However, the association of this polymorphism and P glycoprotein expression, function, and influence on drug pharmacology is unclear, as conflicting results of the TT genotype on P glycoprotein expression and function have been found. Several investigators have shown that individuals homozygous for TT genotype have higher plasma AUC of digoxin, presumably because of reduced intestinal P glycoprotein expression leading to enhanced bioavailability. However, the opposite effect on digoxin has been found by other investigators.

The fact that the C3435T SNP does not result in amino acid substitution suggests that associations with phenotype occur as a result of a close linkage with another as yet undermined functional SNP. This silent polymorphism is in linkage disequilibrium with other polymorphisms, G2677T in exon 21 and the C1236T polymorphism in exon 12, and ethnic differences exist between whites and African Americans, where the TT genotype at the C3435T SNP is 25% in whites and only 6% in populations of African descent.[22] More importantly, these three polymorphisms could be studied in haplotype assignments, and these also demonstrate variability according to ethnicity. Using haplotype for these three nucleotides—1236, 2677, and 3435— homozygotes treated with an anthracycline-based regimen for acute myeloid leukemia were observed to have a poorer survival and higher relapse rates.[23] With a wide range of anticancer drug substrates and the potential to affect enterohepatic recirculation and biliary and renal clearance, there is currently great interest in studying the impact of functional polymorphisms of ABC transporters on the pharmacology of these agents. However, given the modest *in vitro* effect of the C3435T polymorphism on MDR1 expression (twofold lower P glycoprotein in homozygous TT), it is likely that clinically significant examples of this polymorphism on drug disposition will be difficult to detect.

PHARMACOGENOMICS OF TUMOR RESPONSE

Tumor response to chemotherapy is regulated by a complex, multigenic network of genes that encompasses inherent characteristics of the tumor, differentially activated pathways of cell signaling, proliferation and DNA repair, factors that control drug delivery to the tumor cells (e.g., metabolism, transport), and cell death. These may in turn be modulated by previously administered treatment or drug exposure, which may up-regulate target proteins or activate alternative pathways of drug resistance. The polygenic nature of drug response implies that a better understanding of genotype-phenotype associations would require more than the usual single-gene pharmacogenetic strategies used to date. However, there are instances in which the genomic context of a single gene within a cancer is of high impact for specific therapeutic agents (see Table 15.3-2). Patients with a 9:22 chromosomal translocation CML or a c-kit mutation in gastrointestinal stromal cell tumor have a high degree of tumor response from imatinib therapy compared to patients without these variants. An enhanced response to trastuzumab is seen in Her-2 overexpressing breast cancer. These single gene effect studies have also extended to cellular targets of currently used chemotherapy.

As mentioned earlier in Dihydropyrimidine Dehydrogenase, TS is a key intracellular target for 5-FU and other antifolate agents. Intratumoral levels of TS messenger RNA and protein have been correlated with response and survival to 5-FU therapy.[24] For most published studies high intratumoral TS activity is correlated with poorer response to 5-FU in metastatic cancer patients. However, the marker was most predictive when RNA profiling was conducted using biopsy material from the target metastatic lesion. Archival material from a previous resection was not consistently associated with outcome, likely due to differences in TS expression between primary and metastatic tumor.[25] Therefore, evaluation of TS genetic variants has been conducted.[26]

TS expression is regulated by a polymorphism in the 5' promoter region consisting of a 28-base-pair tandem repeat that exists in two (TSER*2), three (TSER*3), four (TSER*4), five (TSER*5), and nine (TSER*9) copies, with TSER*2 and *3 being the most common.[26] Expression of TS increases with more copies of the tandem repeat, with homozygous TSER*3 patients having the highest levels and the greatest resistance to 5-FU. In the adjuvant setting, stage III colon cancer patients with a homozygous TSER*3 genotype have similar outcome after adjuvant therapy to that seen in patients receiving surgery alone. The patients with TSER*2 do have evidence of benefit from adjuvant chemotherapy. Similarly, patients who were homozygous for the TSER*3 had a lower rate of down-staging with preoperative 5-FU–based chemoradiation and compromised survival compared to homozygous TSER*2 and heterozygous patients.[27] Interestingly, the inheritance of the TSER repeats shows interethnic variability; it appears that East Asian populations have allelic frequencies of TSER*3 of more than 80%, compared to 30% to 37% in whites, and TSER*4 and TSER*9 have been described in populations of African descent.[28,29] Currently, there is a need to prospectively validate the predictive significance of TS expression and genotype in all settings of cancer treated with 5-FU, before it can be applied to direct patient care. Such studies are in progress in the setting of cooperative group clinical trials.

Other examples of single-gene correlations with drug outcome have been observed with the platinum agents. Nucleotide excision repair is one of the many cellular defense mechanisms involved in the elimination of DNA damage caused by platinum agents. Polymorphisms in the xeroderma pigmentosum group D gene [official Human Genome Organisation (HUGO) name ERCC2] have been identified as being involved in platinum-based treatment outcome. An SNP at ERCC2 codon 751 was associated with a 24% objective response rate in wild-type [lysine/lysine (Lys/Lys)] patients with metastatic colorectal cancer treated with 5-FU/oxaliplatin, versus 10% in those with a genetic variant.[30] In addition, patients with the Lys/Lys genotype had a median survival of 17.4 months, versus 12.8 and 3.3 for Lys/glutamine (Lys/Gln) and Gln/Gln, respectively. Polymorphisms in XRCC1 have also been shown to be associated with platinum agent response. Although numerous studies report the role of XRCC1 in increasing the risk of cancer, a polymorphism in the *XRCC1* gene, leading to the amino acid change arginine (Arg) → Gln at codon 399, was significantly associated with response after 5-FU/oxaliplatin therapy for advanced colorectal cancer. Higher response (73%) was seen in the Arg/Arg patients, whereas 66% of the nonresponders have either Arg/Gln or Gln/Gln.[31]

APPLICATION OF GENOME-WIDE GENE EXPRESSION PROFILING TO GUIDE THERAPY

Single-gene approaches may not reflect the overall complexity of genetic regulation of chemotherapy responses. Genomic strategies using global gene expression data are able to provide a more complete picture of the tumor, through disease classification.[32] These strategies may identify subgroups of patients with early disease who need adjuvant chemotherapy or those who will not benefit from standard therapy or may help with the selection of chemotherapy from a menu of potentially active agents. The Netherlands Cancer Institute developed a 70-gene predictive panel that appears to segregate stages I and II breast cancer into favorable prognosis and poor prognosis. The predictor was found to be a good independent variable of prognosis, and 10-year metastatic disease–free survival was 50.6% in the group with a poor-prognosis signature and 85.2% in the group with a good-prognosis signature.[33,34] Prospective studies are needed to validate these findings but may reveal a patient subpopulation in need of more aggressive therapy.

In diffuse, large B-cell non-Hodgkin's lymphoma, application of gene expression profiling defined three subsets of patients, one expressing genes of an activated peripheral blood B cell (AB), those expressing genes of a normal germinal center B-cell phenotype, and a diffuse large B-cell lymphoma profile. The normal germinal center B-cell phenotype had a better survival at 5 years (60%) than the activated peripheral blood B-cell subtype (35%) and the diffuse, large B-cell lymphoma (39%) after treatment with chemotherapy.[35,36] The validation of this approach now opens the door to molecular profiling as an important component of medical decision making for this important disease. In pediatric acute lymphoblastic leukemia, it has been recognized for some time that subgroups of patients with defined genetic lesions have different prognostic outcome with conventional-dose chemotherapy. It would be beneficial to use a single platform to better define subgroups with favorable outcome who would receive conventional or even less intensive chemotherapy

(presumably with less long-term toxicity), and subgroups with poor prognosis who would benefit from more intensive treatment, such as bone marrow transplantation. A study of 327 diagnostic bone marrow samples interrogated using microarrays was shown to predict patients who would relapse after conventional treatment and, interestingly, identify patients who were at risk of developing secondary leukemia.[37]

The critical element of all approaches to predict tumor response to chemotherapy is validation of the ability of the marker to define a patient group that clearly benefits from the planned intervention. This is very difficult, as archived tissue was treated with "yesterday's" therapy and therefore is not as useful for determining whether a gene signature is predictive for response to modern treatment regimens. It is also necessary to have an adequate sample size to clearly ascertain the impact of a particular marker or panel, which is challenging with the current clinical trial structure in North America.

CONCLUSION

Cytotoxics have narrow therapeutic windows and wide interindividual variability in drug pharmacokinetics and pharmacodynamics. Better understanding of pharmacogenomics of these agents will help remove some of this variability and has the potential to influence patient care. It is expected that in the next few years, pharmacogenomics will be applied to optimize cancer chemotherapy to reduce toxicity and enhance response. Data are also emerging for a role of pharmacogenetics in the optimization of antiemetics, pain control, and infection prophylaxis.[38–40] The rapid advances in genomic and proteomic technology will allow application of high-throughput sequencing and expression profiling to be applied for these purposes. For the practicing oncologist, some knowledge of this field will be necessary, as therapeutic decisions of drug selection and dosage may eventually be based on more molecularly and genetically defined variables than the current phenotypic information of tumor type, immunohistochemistry, and body surface area. To realize this potential, it is essential for pharmacogenomic end points to be integrated into large cooperative randomized clinical trials that enroll large enough numbers of patients to enable robust genotype-phenotype correlations to be made. This will also allow the generation of treatment guidelines that quantitate the risk of toxicity or therapeutic success, or both, for individual patients.

REFERENCES

1. Evans W, McLeod H. Pharmacogenomics—drug disposition, drug targets, and side effects. *N Engl J Med* 2003;348:538.
2. Watters J, McLeod H. Cancer pharmacogenomics: current and future applications. *Biochim Biophys Acta* 2003;1603:99.
3. Evans W, Relling M. Pharmacogenomics: translating functional genomics into rational therapeutics. *Science* 1999;286:487.
4. Relling M, Dervieux T. Pharmacogenetics and cancer therapy. *Nat Rev Cancer* 2001;1:99.
5. Innocenti F, Ratain M. Update on pharmacogenetics in cancer chemotherapy. *Eur J Cancer* 2002;38:639.
6. McLeod H, Krynetsk E, Relling M, et al. Genetic polymorphism of thiopurine methyltransferase and its clinical relevance for childhood acute lymphoblastic leukemia. *Leukemia* 2000;14:567.
7. Krynetski E, Evans W. Drug methylation in cancer therapy: lessons from the TPMT polymorphism. *Oncogene* 2003;22:7403.
8. Evans W, Hon Y, Bomgaars L, et al. Preponderance of thiopurine S-methyltransferase deficiency and heterozygosity among patients intolerant to mercaptopurine or azathioprine. *J Clin Oncol* 2001;19:2293.

9. Relling M, Hancock M, Rivera G, et al. Mercaptopurine therapy intolerance and heterozygosity at the thiopurine S-methyltransferase gene locus. *J Natl Cancer Inst* 1999; 91:2001.

10. Mattison L, Soong R, Diasio R. Implications of dihydropyrimidine dehydrogenase on 5-fluorouracil pharmacogenetics and pharmacogenomics. *Pharmacogenomics* 2002;3:485.

11. McLeod H, Collie-Duguid E, Vreken P, et al. Nomenclature for human DPYD alleles. *Pharmacogenetics* 1998;8:455.

12. Wei X, Elizondo G, Sapone A, et al. Characterization of the human dihydropyrimidine dehydrogenase gene. *Genomics* 1998;51:391.

13. Ridge S, Sludden J, Wei X, et al. Dihydropyrimidine dehydrogenase pharmacogenetics in patients with colorectal cancer. *Br J Cancer* 1998;77:497.

14. Johnson M, Wang K, Diasio R. Profound dihydropyrimidine dehydrogenase deficiency resulting from a novel compound heterozygote genotype. *Clin Cancer Res* 2002;8:768.

15. Van Kuilenburg A, Meinsma R, Zoetekouw L, et al. Increased risk of grade IV neutropenia after administration of 5-fluorouracil due to a dihydropyrimidine dehydrogenase deficiency: high prevalence of the IVS14+1g>a mutation. *Int J Cancer* 2002;101:253.

16. Ratain M. Irinotecan dosing: does the CPT in CPT-11 stand for "can't predict toxicity"? *J Clin Oncol* 2002;20:7.

17. Mathijssen R, Marsh S, Karlsson M, et al. Irinotecan pathway genotype analysis to predict pharmacokinetics. *Clin Cancer Res* 2003;9:3246.

18. Beutler E, Gelbart T, Demina A. Racial variability in the UDP-glucuronosyltransferase 1 (UGT1A1) promoter: a balanced polymorphism for regulation of bilirubin metabolism? *Proc Natl Acad Sci U S A* 1998;95:8170.

19. Ando Y, Saka H, Ando M, et al. Polymorphisms of UDP-glucuronosyltransferase gene and irinotecan toxicity: a pharmacogenetic analysis. *Cancer Res* 2000;60:6921.

20. Iyer L, Das S, Janisch L, et al. UGT1A1*28 polymorphism as a determinant of irinotecan disposition and toxicity. *Pharmacogenomics J* 2002;2:43.

21. Innocenti F, Undevia SD, Iyer L, et al. Genetic variants in the UDP-glucuronosyltransferase 1A1 gene predict the risk of severe neutropenia of irinotecan. *J Clin Oncol* 2004;22:1382.

22. Marzolini C, Paus E, Buclin T, et al. Polymorphisms in human MDR1 (P-glycoprotein): recent advances and clinical relevance. *Clin Pharmacol Ther* 2004;75:13.

23. Illmer T, Schuler U, Thiede C, et al. MDR1 gene polymorphisms affect therapy outcome in acute myeloid leukemia patients. *Cancer Res* 2002;62:4955.

24. Popat S, Matakidou A, Houlston RS. Thymidylate synthase expression and prognosis in colorectal cancer: a systematic review and meta-analysis. *J Clin Oncol* 2004;22:529.

25. Marsh S, McKay JA, Curran S, et al. Primary colorectal tumour is not an accurate predictor of thymidylate synthase in lymph node metastasis. *Oncol Rep* 2002;9:231.

26. Marsh S, McLeod H. Thymidylate synthase pharmacogenetics in colorectal cancer. *Clin Colorectal Cancer* 2001;1:175.

27. Villafranca E, Okruzhnov Y, Dominguez M, et al. Polymorphisms of the repeated sequences in the enhancer region of the thymidylate synthase gene promoter may predict downstaging after preoperative chemoradiation in rectal cancer. *J Clin Oncol* 2001;19:1779.

28. Marsh S, Ameyaw MM, Githang'a J, et al. Novel thymidylate synthase enhancer region alleles in African populations. *Hum Mutat* 2000;16:528.

29. Marsh S, Collie-Duguid ES, Li T, et al. Ethnic variation in the thymidylate synthase enhancer region polymorphism among Caucasian and Asian populations. *Genomics* 1999;58:310.

30. Park D, Stoehlmacher J, Zhang W, et al. A Xeroderma pigmentosum group D gene polymorphism predicts clinical outcome to platinum-based chemotherapy in patients with advanced colorectal cancer. *Cancer Res* 2001;61:8654.

31. Stoehlmacher J, Ghaderi V, Iobal S, et al. A polymorphism of the XRCC1 gene predicts for response to platinum based treatment in advanced colorectal cancer. *Anticancer Res* 2001;21:3075.

32. Ramaswamy S, Golub T. DNA microarrays in clinical oncology. *J Clin Oncol* 2002;20:1932.

33. van de Vijver MJ, He YD, van't Veer LJ, et al. A gene-expression signature as a predictor of survival in breast cancer. *N Engl J Med* 2002;347:1999.

34. van't Veer LJ, Dai H, van de Vijver MJ, et al. Gene expression profiling predicts clinical outcome of breast cancer. *Nature* 2002;415:530.

35. Alizadeh AA, Eisen MB, Davis RE, et al. Distinct types of diffuse large B-cell lymphoma identified by gene expression profiling. *Nature* 2000;403:503.

36. Rosenwald A, Wright G, Chan W, et al. The use of molecular profiling to predict survival after chemotherapy for diffuse large-B-cell lymphoma. *N Engl J Med* 2002;346:1937.

37. Yeoh E, Ross M, Shurtleff S, et al. Classification, subtype discovery, and prediction of outcome in pediatric acute lymphoblastic leukemia by gene expression profiling. *Cancer Cell* 2002;1:133.

38. Kaiser R, Sezer O, Papies A, et al. Patient-tailored antiemetic treatment with 5-hydroxytryptamine type 3 receptor antagonists according to cytochrome P-450 2D6 genotypes. *J Clin Oncol* 2002;20:2805.

39. Sawyer M, Innocenti F, Das S, et al. A pharmacogenetic study of uridine diphosphate-glucuronosyltransferase 2B7 in patients receiving morphine. *Clin Pharmacol Ther* 2003;73:566.

40. Somech R, Amariglio N, Spirer Z, et al. Genetic predisposition to infectious pathogens: a review of less familiar variants. *Pediatr Infect Dis J* 2003;22:457.

SECTION 4

O. MICHAEL COLVIN
HENRY S. FRIEDMAN

Alkylating Agents

HISTORY OF THE ALKYLATING AGENTS

A nitrogen mustard alkylating agent was the first nonhormonal chemical that demonstrated significant clinical antitumor activity. The clinical evaluation of nitrogen mustards as antitumor agents evolved from the observed clinical effects of sulfur mustard gas used as a weapon in World War I. This gas was used because of its vesicant effect on the skin and mucous membranes, especially the eyes and respiratory tract. However, in addition to this deadly effect, depression of the hematopoietic and lymphoid systems was observed in victims and experimental animals.[1] These observations led to further studies that used the less volatile nitrogen mustards (Fig. 15.4-1). Studies published in 1946 demonstrated regression of tumors, especially lymphomas,[2-4] and led to the introduction of the compound nitrogen mustard (mechlorethamine or Mustargen) into clinical practice. Subsequently, less toxic and more clinically effective nitrogen mustard derivatives and other types of alkylating agents have been developed.

CHEMISTRY AND CYTOTOXICITY OF ALKYLATING AGENTS

The alkylating agents react with (or "alkylate") many electron-rich atoms in cells to form covalent bonds. The most important reactions with regard to their antitumor activities are reactions with DNA bases. Some alkylating agents are monofunctional and react with only one strand of DNA. Others are bifunctional and react with an atom on each of the two strands of DNA to produce a "cross-link" that covalently links the two strands of the DNA double helix. Unless repaired, this lesion will prevent the cell from replicating effectively. The lethality of the monofunctional alkylating agents results from the recognition of the DNA lesion by the cell and the response of the cell to that lesion. Analogous cellular reactions may occur to the interstrand cross-links, but such reactions have not been definitively established.

CLASSES OF ALKYLATING AGENTS AND THEIR PROPERTIES

NITROGEN MUSTARDS

Mustargen

Mustargen, the original nitrogen mustard, is currently used in the MOPP [Mustargen, vincristine (Oncovin), procarbazine, prednisone] regimen for the treatment of Hodgkin's disease but rarely for other purposes. The other nitrogen mustards in significant clinical use are cyclophosphamide, ifosfamide, melphalan, and chlorambucil (Fig. 15.4-2). All these compounds produce cytotoxicity by forming covalent interstrand cross-links in DNA. The nitrogen mustard cross-link has been demonstrated to occur in the G-X-C/C-Y-G configuration,[5] as opposed to the G-C/C-G cross-link that had previously been predicted.[6] The formation of the G-X-C/C-X-G cross-link has been postulated to occur on the basis of the greater frequency

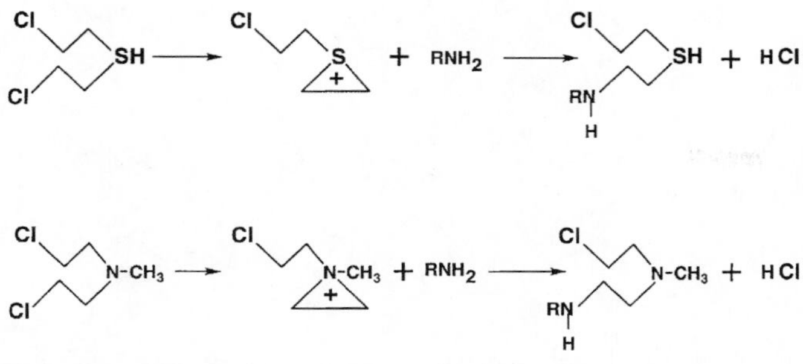

FIGURE 15.4-1. Structures and alkylation mechanisms for sulfur mustard and the nitrogen mustard, Mustargen (mechlorethamine).

of approximation of the N7 atoms of the two guanylates in the G-X-C/C-X-G configuration of the DNA helix, as opposed to the G-C/C-G configuration.[7]

Mustargen is available only as an intravenous preparation that can also be used topically for cutaneous malignancies. In the MOPP regimen, Mustargen is used at a dose of 6 mg/m^2 on days 1 and 8 of the monthly schedule. Toxicities unique to the agent are topical irritation and pain on injection if given too rapidly. The clearance of the drug is very rapid, but pharmacokinetics have not been performed using modern techniques.

Cyclophosphamide

The most frequently used alkylating agent, cyclophosphamide, is used for the treatment of breast cancer in combination with doxorubicin (Adriamycin)[8] or with methotrexate and 5-fluorouracil[9] and for the treatment of lymphomas,[10] childhood tumors, and many solid tumors. High doses of cyclophosphamide are frequently used in conjunction with bone marrow transplantation[11] and for the treatment of autoimmune diseases.[12,13]

Cyclophosphamide is inactive *in vitro* and is metabolized by P-450 enzymes in the liver to active species, as shown in Figure 15.4-3. The initial product is 4-hydroxycyclophosphamide (4-HOCy), which is released from the liver into the circulation.[14] This compound is in equilibrium with an open-ring tautomer, aldophosphamide. Aldophosphamide spontaneously eliminates acrolein to produce phosphoramide mustard,[15] which is an active bifunctional alkylating species.[16] Phosphoramide mustard is zwitterionic at physiologic pH[17] and enters cells poorly. 4-HOCy–aldophosphamide is not charged and enters cells facilely. Although phosphoramide mustard is toxic to cells *in vitro* at concentrations of 100 μM and higher, 4-HOCy is cytotoxic in the range of 10 μM.[18] Thus, 4-HOCy–aldophosphamide serves as an efficient delivery system for the polar phosphoramide mustard, which has been demonstrated to produce an interstrand DNA cross-link analogous to the cross-link produced by mechlorethamine.[16–18] Studies by Shulman-Roskes et al.[19] have demonstrated that phosphoramide mustard readily eliminates chloroethylaziridine, which probably also plays a role in the alkylation of DNA in cells exposed to 4-HOCy.

As shown in Figure 15.4-3, 4-HOCy is a substrate for the enzyme aldehyde dehydrogenase.[20] In cells that contain this

enzyme, the bulk of the 4-HOCy is oxidized to carboxyphosphamide, which is not an active alkylating or cytotoxic agent and is excreted in the urine. Consequently, cells with high aldehyde dehydrogenase content are resistant to the metabolites of cyclophosphamide.[20,21] Early hematopoietic stem cells[22] and megakaryocytes contain high levels of aldehyde dehydrogenase, as do the epithelial stem cells in the small intestine and mucous membranes.[23] These observations explain why cyclophosphamide administration produces a shorter period of hematopoietic depression, is relatively sparing of platelets, and is associated with less gastrointestinal toxicity and mucositis than the other alkylating agents.

4-HOCy is too unstable to be used as a reagent, but the compound 4-hydroperoxycyclophosphamide (see Fig. 15.4-3), commonly called *4HC*, is spontaneously converted in aqueous solution to 4-HOCy and can be used for *in vitro* studies of DNA cross-linking and cell sensitivity.[24,25]

Cyclophosphamide is available as tablets for oral administration or as an intravenous preparation. The drug is used at a variety of doses and schedules. Oral administration is particularly used for autoimmune diseases at a daily dose of approximately 100 mg. Because of its rapid absorption and high bioavailability, even very high doses can be given orally, but high intermittent doses are usually given intravenously. In moderate-dose combination chemotherapy, doses of cyclophosphamide in the range of 750 mg are usually used. For high-dose therapy in conjunction with hematopoietic cell transplantation, doses of up to 50 mg/kg for 2 or 4 days in combination with other agents are used.

Approximately 70% of a dose of cyclophosphamide is excreted in the urine as the inactive carboxyphosphamide metabolite.[26,27] At high doses (around 50 mg/kg), plasma concentrations of up to 400 μM of cyclophosphamide are achieved,[27] and clearance of the parent drug depends on renal clearance and the rate of microsomal metabolism in the liver.

With improved and more facile techniques to measure 4-HOCy concentrations accurately, the clinical pharmacology of cyclophosphamide and this critical transport intermediate are being more carefully defined. Studies of patients receiving high-dose therapy have demonstrated considerable variation in the rates of clearance of cyclophosphamide between patients, with consequent differences in the peak concentrations (1 to 15 μM) and total exposure of the patient to 4-HOCy (60 to 140 μM.hours).[27,28] The total systemic exposure to 4-HOCy is probably the major determinant of therapeutic effect and toxicities.

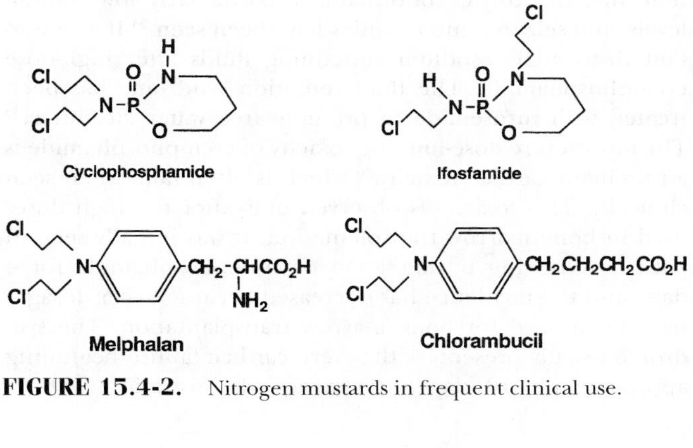

FIGURE 15.4-2. Nitrogen mustards in frequent clinical use.

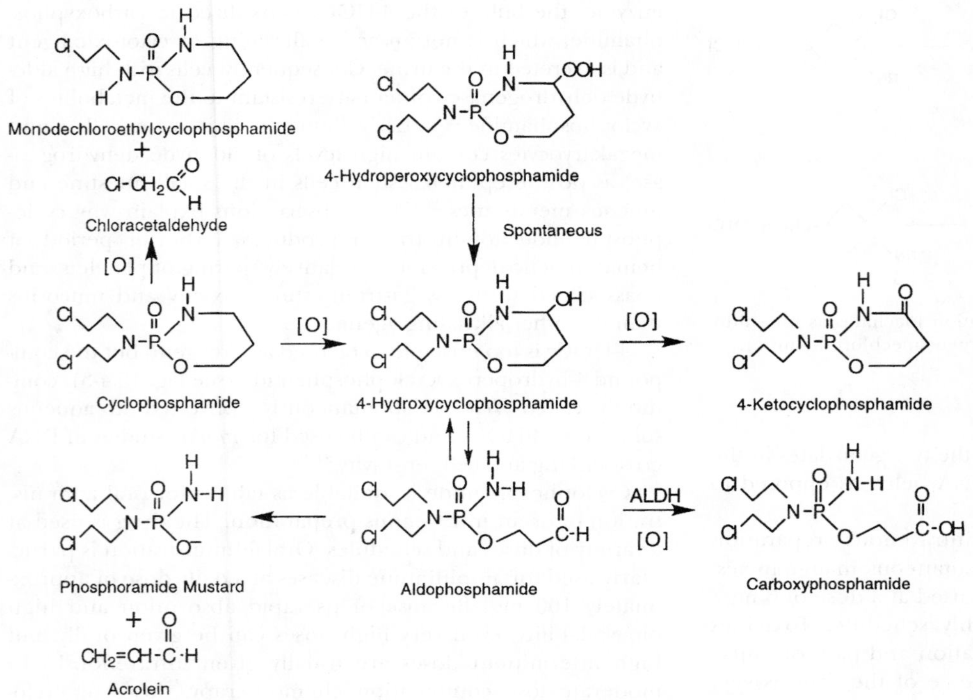

FIGURE 15.4-3. Metabolism of cyclophosphamide. ALDH, aldehyde dehydrogenase.

Currently, several programs are evaluating dose-adjustment regimens based on the initial pharmacokinetics of cyclophosphamide and 4-HOCy. Although it is known that substantial concentrations of phosphoramide mustard are present in plasma (up to 10 μM after 60 mg/kg of cyclophosphamide[28,29]), this concentration is below the concentrations needed for *in vitro* cytotoxicity of phosphoramide mustard.[14]

A unique toxicity of cyclophosphamide and other oxazaphosphorines is a characteristic hemorrhagic cystitis[30,31] due to irritation of the bladder mucosa by urinary metabolites. Acrolein has been identified as the metabolite most responsible for this effect,[32] but phosphoramide mustard and chloroacetaldehyde may contribute to this toxicity. Careful attention to hydration of patients and emptying of the bladder are crucial to avoiding this toxicity, which has produced massive and even fatal hemorrhage. Another toxicity that has been associated with cyclophosphamide administration is an antidiuretic effect, especially at high doses.[33]

This antidiuretic effect may produce marked fluid retention and electrolyte abnormalities, particularly low sodium levels, and seizures and fatalities have been seen.[34] It is important to avoid low-sodium–containing fluids after high-dose cyclophosphamide. The fluid retention syndrome has been treated with furosemide to promote free water clearance.[35] The most severe dose-limiting toxicity of cyclophosphamide is a fulminant cardiac toxicity,[36] which is often fatal when seen clinically. This toxicity is observed only after the high doses used in bone marrow transplantation. It was initially seen in patients receiving 60 mg/kg/d of cyclophosphamide for 4 days, and the incidence has decreased because lower dosages have been used for bone marrow transplantation. The syndrome usually presents with severe cardiac failure beginning approximately 10 days after drug administration, with a dilated heart and low electrocardiogram voltage. There is a characteristic pathologic picture of edema, interstitial hemorrhage, and cardiac necrosis.[36]

Ifosfamide

Ifosfamide is a structural isomer of cyclophosphamide that is often used in the treatment of sarcomas and pediatric tumors (see Fig. 15.4-2). There is more chloroethyl side-chain oxidation of ifosfamide (up to 50%) than of cyclophosphamide (less than 10%), and the degree of such metabolism is more variable than with cyclophosphamide.[37] Oxidation of the chloroethyl groups produces chloroacetaldehyde, which is probably responsible for the neurotoxicity[38] and renal toxicity[39] that have been seen with ifosfamide therapy. Because the oxidation of a chloroethyl side chain produces a much less toxic monofunctional agent, higher dosages of ifosfamide than of cyclophosphamide must be used clinically. The studies of the clinical pharmacology of ifosfamide have been more limited than those of cyclophosphamide but have demonstrated significant variability in the pharmacokinetics and metabolism of the agent between individuals and with repeated administrations to the same individual.[40,41]

Melphalan

Melphalan is now used principally for the treatment of multiple myeloma, for high-dose myeloablative therapy in conjunction with bone marrow transplantation, and for the isolated limb perfusion of localized tumors,[42] especially malignant melanoma and sarcomas. Melphalan (see Fig. 15.4-2) is an amino acid analogue and is actively transported into cells by amino acid transport systems.[43,44] It has been demonstrated that cellular uptake[45] and transport into the central nervous system

(CNS)[46] of melphalan can be modulated by the amino acid content in the extracellular fluid.

Melphalan is available both as tablets and as an intravenous preparation. For the treatment of multiple myeloma, melphalan is usually used orally at a dosage of 0.25 mg/kg for 4 days, with prednisone on the same schedule, every 4 to 6 weeks. At these dosages, peak plasma concentrations of 0.625 μM are found, but absorption is variable.[47] For bone marrow transplantation, doses of melphalan of 100 to 140 mg/m² are used.[48] At these doses, peak concentrations of melphalan of 40 to 50 μM are reached.[48,49]

Chlorambucil

Chlorambucil is used for the treatment of B-cell chronic lymphocytic leukemia and lymphomas and for immunosuppressive therapy for autoimmune diseases. It is administered orally and is well tolerated when given either by daily administration or intermittent high-pulse doses. Chlorambucil is well tolerated by most patients and can be used successfully by patients who have severe nausea and vomiting with cyclophosphamide or melphalan.[50]

Chlorambucil is available only in an oral formulation. For chronic leukemia and immunosuppression, daily doses of 3 to 6 mg are given for a number of weeks, or 12 mg/m² may be given monthly. Pulsed-dose chlorambucil for lymphoma is given orally at a dosage of 16 mg/m² daily for 5 consecutive days each month. Chlorambucil is metabolized to a less active derivative, phenylacetic acid mustard, and the clinical pharmacology of chlorambucil is similar to that of melphalan.[51]

AZIRIDINES AND EPOXIDES

The aziridine agents are related to the nitrogen mustards but contain uncharged aziridine rings that are less reactive than the aziridinium rings formed by most of the nitrogen mustards. The two aziridine agents that are frequently used clinically are thiotepa and mitomycin C (Fig. 15.4-4). The diepoxide dianhydrogalactitol reacts with DNA in a similar fashion to the aziridines but has been succeeded in clinical use by dibromodulcitol, which spontaneously generates dianhydrogalactitol *in situ*.

Thiotepa

Thiotepa is now used most frequently in combination with other alkylating agents in high-dose therapy with stem cell support.[28] Thiotepa has been demonstrated to react with the N7 position of guanylic acid in DNA[52] and to cross-link DNA,[53] which indicates that it is acting similarly to the nitrogen mustards. Thiotepa is desulfurated by cytochrome P-450 enzymes[54] to produce tepa. Tepa is less toxic than thiotepa and has been demonstrated to produce alkali-labile sites in DNA, rather than cross-links.[52,53] These findings indicate that tepa reacts differently from thiotepa and produces monofunctional alkylation of DNA.

In combination with cyclophosphamide for high-dose therapy, thiotepa has been given as a continuous infusion for 4 days, at a daily dose of 200 mg/m². Under these conditions, steady-state levels of 2 to 6 μM of thiotepa are rapidly achieved. Thiotepa is also used at a dose of 900 mg/m² in combination with high-dose cyclophosphamide and cisplatin.[55]

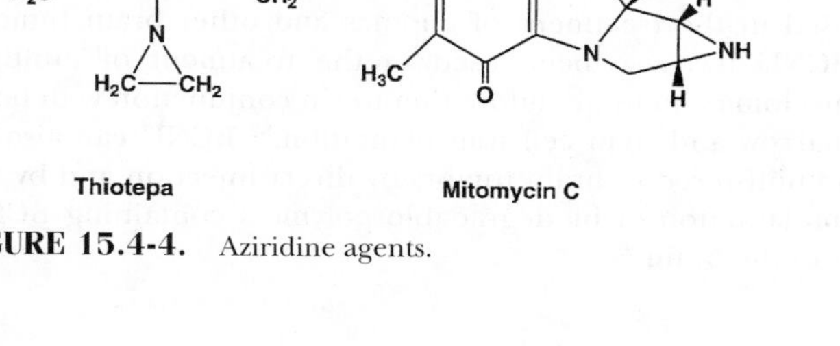

Mitomycin C

Mitomycin C is an antibiotic extracted from a *Streptomyces* species and is used for the treatment of breast cancer,[56] esophageal cancer, and gastrointestinal tumors. As seen in Figure 15.4-4, this compound contains an aziridine ring. Particularly under hypoxic conditions, mitomycin C is reduced, with activation of the C1 position of the aziridine ring. This carbon then reacts in the minor groove with the extracyclic N2 amino group of a guanylic acid,[57,58] positioning the 10 carbon of the carbamate moiety to react with the N2 of a guanylic acid residue in an adjacent base pair in the complementary DNA strand. Mitomycin C and its reduced metabolites can also produce intrastrand guanylic acid–guanylic acid cross-links that produce bending of the DNA.[59]

In combination regimens, mitomycin C is given at dosages of 10 to 15 mg/m² every 4 to 6 weeks. After a dose of 15 mg/m², peak plasma concentrations of 3 μM are seen.[60]

Dianhydrogalactitol

Dianhydrogalactitol is a hexitol derivative that contains two epoxide groups and cross-links DNA through the N7 atoms of guanylic acid,[61] presumably through the nucleophilic attack of the N7 atoms on the strained-ring epoxide groups. This compound was evaluated in clinical trials and demonstrated modest antitumor activity.[62,63] However, the structurally related dibromodulcitol has demonstrated better antitumor activity[64,65] and is used in combination chemotherapy for breast cancer, cervical cancer, and brain tumors. Dibromodulcitol is hydrolyzed to dianhydrogalactitol, and its better antitumor activity is presumably due to more effective localization of the reactive agent in tumor cells. Dibromodulcitol is usually administered at a dose of 1 g/m², which produces a maximum plasma concentration of approximately 50 μM.[66,67]

ALKYL SULFONATES: BUSULFAN

Busulfan (Myleran), other alkyl sulfonates, and the related sulfamates react with DNA by a direct displacement reaction (as shown in Fig. 15.4-5). Busulfan has been demonstrated to cross-link DNA,[68] but the structure of the cross-link has not been established. A chemically related agent, hepsulfam, with seven methylene units between the reactive groups, has been demonstrated to form a DNA G-X-C/C-X-G interstrand cross-link analogous to the cross-links formed by the nitrogen mustards.[69] Haddow and Timmis[70] reported in 1953 that busulfan

Thiotepa   **Mitomycin C**

FIGURE 15.4-4. Aziridine agents.

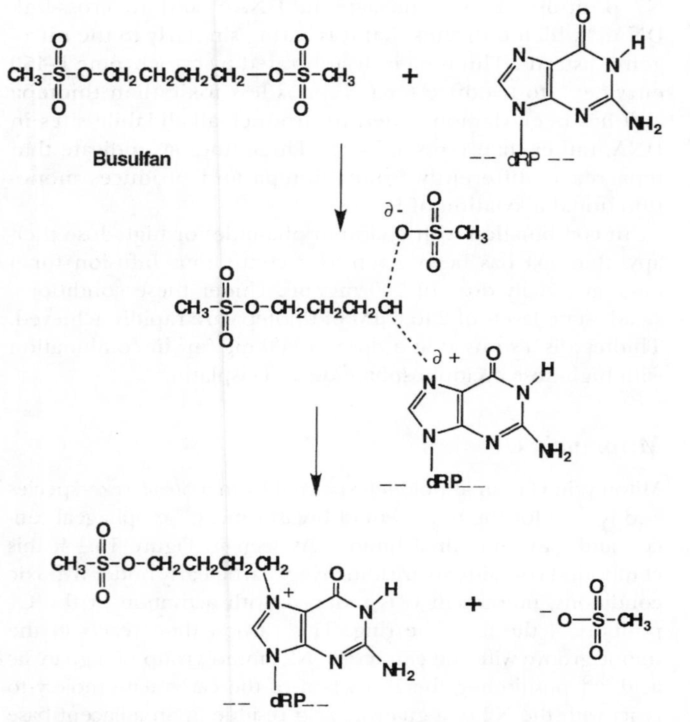

FIGURE 15.4-5. Alkylation of guanylate in DNA by busulfan through S_N2 alkylation. A second displacement reaction with the N7 of a guanylate in the complementary strand creates a G-X-C/C-X-G interstrand cross-link.

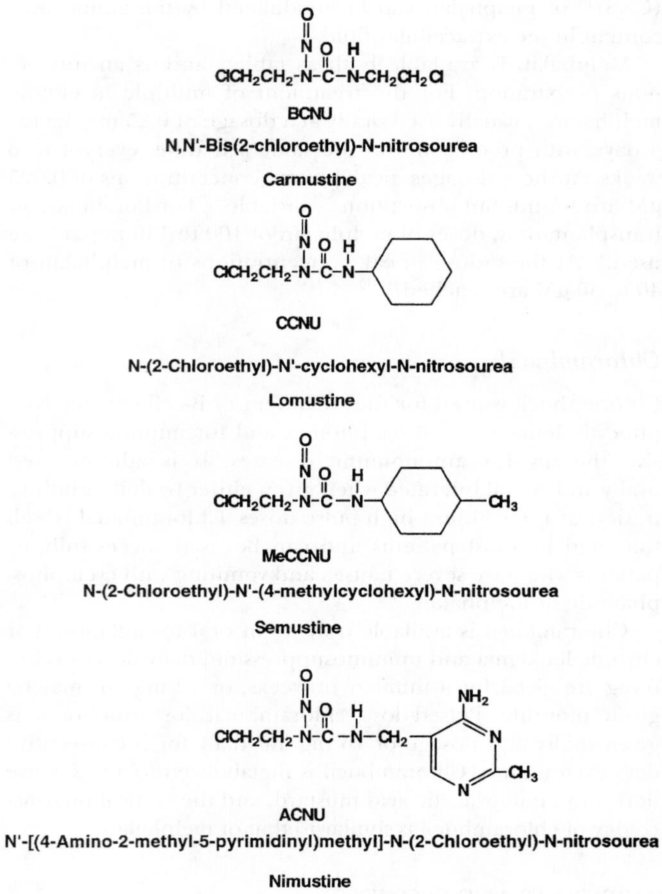

FIGURE 15.4-6. Nitrosoureas.

was active against chronic myelogenous leukemia. Busulfan was for many years the principal agent used to treat this disease, before being succeeded by the use of hydroxyurea and interferon-α, both of which have proved to be as effective and less toxic than busulfan. The most frequent use of busulfan in cancer therapy today is in high-dose therapy for many tumors, including refractory chronic myelogenous leukemia, in conjunction with bone marrow or stem cell transplantation. For this application, high doses of busulfan are combined with cyclophosphamide, total body irradiation, or other agents. The effectiveness of busulfan for this purpose is undoubtedly related to its marked myeloablative properties,[71] the mechanistic bases of which are not understood.

Until recently, busulfan was available only as an oral preparation, but an intravenous preparation is now available. For hematopoietic transplantation, busulfan is usually given as 1 mg/kg every 6 hours for 4 days, for a total dose of 16 mg/kg. Peak concentrations of busulfan after each dose are approximately 10 μM.[72] High exposure to busulfan has been associated with venoocclusive disease of the liver.[72] This syndrome consists of hepatomegaly, jaundice, ascites, and hepatic failure with a high mortality rate.[73] Grochow et al.[72] have demonstrated that pharmacokinetic monitoring and dose adjustment of the busulfan can markedly reduce the incidence of venoocclusive disease.

NITROSOUREAS

The members of the nitrosourea group of therapeutic alkylating agents are related to the alkylnitrosoamines and similar compounds that have long been known to be carcinogenic.

Methylnitrosoguanidine and methylnitrosourea are monofunctional alkylating agents and were found to have modest antitumor activity.[74] Montgomery[75] and Schabel[76] evaluated a number of analogues of these compounds and demonstrated the remarkable antitumor effects of bischloroethylnitrosourea (BCNU; Fig. 15.4-6) against mouse tumors, and particularly against intracerebral tumors, which had been refractory to most agents because of the blood–brain barrier. BCNU was found to produce interstrand cross-linking of DNA,[77] which has been demonstrated to occur through the spontaneous generation of a chloroethyl diazonium species[78] and the series of reactions. This interstrand cross-link occurs between a guanylate in DNA and the base-paired cytidylate in the other strand of the DNA.[79,80]

Bischloroethylnitrosourea

BCNU, or carmustine (see Fig. 15.4-6), demonstrated activity against brain tumors clinically[81] and has continued to be used in the treatment of gliomas and other brain tumors. BCNU has also been used in the treatment of multiple myeloma and in high-dose therapy in conjunction with bone marrow and stem cell transplantation.[82] BCNU can also be administered to brain tumors by direct injection and by the implantation of biodegradable polymers containing BCNU into the brain.[83]

Cyclohexylchloroethylnitrosourea

Cyclohexylchloroethylnitrosourea (CCNU or lomustine; see Fig. 15.4-6) is a more lipid-soluble DNA cross-linking nitrosourea. It is administered orally and is used in the treatment of brain tumors.[84]

Methylcyclohexylchloroethylnitrosourea

Methylcyclohexylchloroethylnitrosourea (semustine; see Fig. 15.4-6) is an oral investigational drug that has been used in the treatment of gastrointestinal tumors.[85]

N'-[(4-Amino-2-Methyl-5-Pyrimidinyl)Methyl]-N-(2-Chloroethyl)-N-Nitrosourea

N'-[(4-amino-2-methyl-5-pyrimidinyl)methyl]-N-(2-chloroethyl)-N-nitrosourea (nimustine; see Fig. 15.4-6) is more water soluble than the other chloroethylnitrosoureas and has been used for the treatment of CNS tumors by the intraarterial[86] and intrathecal routes.[87]

Clinical Pharmacology

As a single agent, BCNU is usually used in a dosage of 125 to 200 mg/m² every 6 to 8 weeks. In combination with doxorubicin for multiple myeloma, a dosage of 30 mg/m² every 3 to 4 weeks has been used.[88] After doses in the range of 100 mg/m², peak plasma concentrations are in the range of 5 µM.[89] For high-dose therapy of breast cancer, BCNU has been given at a dose of 600 mg/m² in combination with cyclophosphamide and cisplatin.[90] After this dose of BCNU, the peak plasma levels of BCNU have been shown to be approximately 5 µM.[91] Phenobarbital has been demonstrated to increase the clearance of BCNU[92] and to decrease the toxic and therapeutic effects. CCNU is administered in dosages similar to those of BCNU. The parent CCNU has not been detected, but the peak concentrations of the ring hydroxylated metabolites are approximately 3 µM after doses of 130 mg/m².[93]

Specific Toxicities

Hematopoietic toxicity of the nitrosoureas is severe and is delayed, with the nadir of the granulocytes occurring 5 to 6 weeks after administration.[94] This finding suggests that these agents selectively damage a very early hematopoietic precursor. In mice and other animals, the nadir is not delayed so dramatically, so that the mechanism of phenomenon has not been extensively explored.

HYDRAZINE AND TRIAZINE DERIVATIVES

The hydrazine and triazine derivative compounds are analogous to the nitrosoureas in that they decompose spontaneously or are metabolized to produce an alkyl carbonium ion, which alkylates DNA. Hydrazine and its substituted analogues are known carcinogens[95] that inhibit gluconeogenesis in cells[96] and have been promoted as antitumor agents.[97] However, objective preclinical and clinical studies have not supported a significant antitumor effect[98] for hydrazine analogues in general.

Procarbazine

Procarbazine is a phenylhydrazine derivative that was initially developed as an inhibitor of monoamine oxidase but was found to have significant antitumor activity in preclinical models and clinical testing. Procarbazine is one of the components of the first effective combination chemotherapy regimen, MOPP, for Hodgkin's disease. The agent is currently also used for the treatment of primary brain tumors.[100] Procarbazine has been demonstrated to be metabolized to a DNA-methylating agent,[101] which has been demonstrated to be methylazoxyprocarbazine.[102,103]

Because procarbazine is a monoamine oxidase inhibitor, patients can experience CNS depression[104] or stimulation[105] and acute hypertension, especially after the ingestion of tyramine-rich foods.

Dacarbazine

Dacarbazine, or DTIC [(dimethyltriazeno)imidazole-carboxamide], is a triazine derivative that is metabolized by microsomal N-demethylation, predominantly in the liver, to an intermediate that spontaneously decomposes to release a methyl diazonium that methylates DNA (Fig. 15.4-7).[106–108] Dacarbazine is used in the regimen of doxorubicin, bleomycin, vinblastine, and dacarbazine for the treatment of Hodgkin's disease[109] and for the treatment of malignant melanoma.[110]

Temozolomide

Temozolomide is a triazine analogue that spontaneously decomposes to produce a methyl diazonium ion,[111,112] as illustrated in Figure 15.4-7. This compound may produce a more homogeneous systemic distribution of the short-lived MTIC [(methyltriazeno)-imidazole-carboxamide], which is spontaneously generated from temozolomide at all sites, than does dacarbazine, which is metabolized to MTIC in the liver. The principal toxicities seen in phase I trials have been neutropenia and thrombocytopenia, and tumor responses were seen in those trials[113,114] in patients with glioma and melanoma. Phase II trials in patients with gliomas have shown response rates of 20% to 30%,[115,116] but phase II trials in patients with sarcomas[117] and pancreatic cancer did not demonstrate significant responses.

The methylating agents exert their cytotoxicity predominantly through the methylation of the O6 position of guanylic acid in DNA. Therefore, cells that contain significant O⁶-alkyltransferase or are deficient in mismatch repair[99] are resistant to them (as discussed in Mechanisms of Toxicity and Drug Resistance, later in this chapter). As discussed earlier, greater efficacy of temozolomide against brain tumors may derive from the fact that, in contrast to dacarbazine and procarbazine, temozolomide is spontaneously activated, instead of being enzymatically activated, and the more distributed production of the active methylating moiety may result in higher concentrations of the active compound within the brain and other tumor target tissues. Whether or not temozolomide will prove to be more effective than dacarbazine and procarbazine against other types of tumors remains to be seen, although this does not appear to be the case thus far.

Procarbazine is an oral preparation used in the MOPP regimen for Hodgkin's disease at a dosage of 100 mg/m²/d for 14

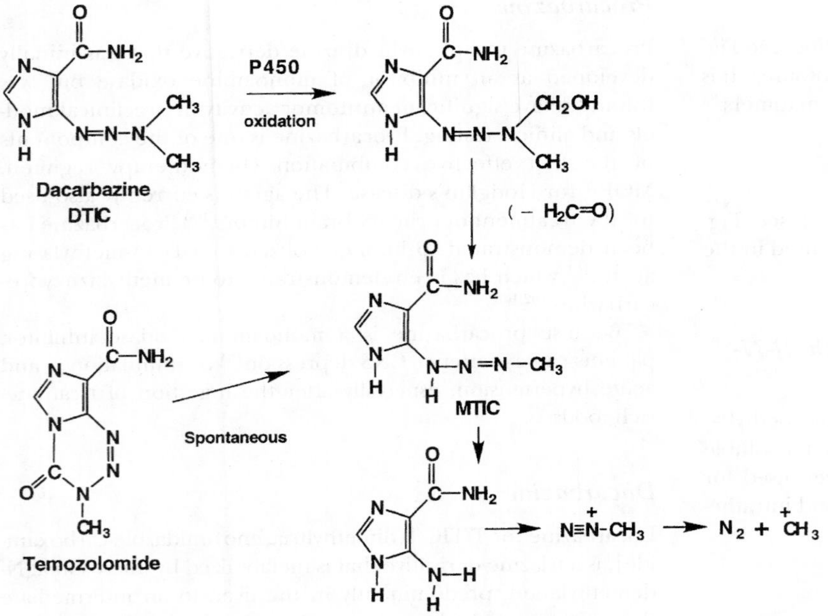

FIGURE 15.4-7. Generation of methyl diazonium from the triazines dacarbazine and temozolomide.

days.[109] Because of its complex metabolism, pharmacokinetic studies have been limited. Dacarbazine is an intravenous preparation and is used in the ABVD regimen of doxorubicin, bleomycin, vinblastine, and dacarbazine for Hodgkin's disease at a dosage of 375 mg/m²/d for 15 days.[109] For the treatment of malignant melanoma, a dosage of 200 to 250 mg/m²/d for 5 days is used. Breithaupt et al. measured concentrations of dacarbazine after the administration of different doses of 5 to 7 mg/kg, and peak concentrations of the agent of 1 to 6 µg/mL were observed.[118]

Temozolomide is usually given orally at 150 to 250 mg/m²/d for 5 days. Reid et al.[119] measured peak concentrations of MTIC of 0.5 to 5.0 µM after administration of these doses of temozolomide. Baker et al.[120] studied the pharmacokinetics of carbon 14–labeled temozolomide and found peak concentrations of temozolomide of approximately 30 µM and peak concentrations of MTIC of approximately 1 µM.

MECHANISMS OF TOXICITY AND DRUG RESISTANCE

REACTION WITH CELLULAR MOLECULES

The alkylating agents are potent electrophiles and react with many electron-rich molecules within the cell to be inactivated. The principal such molecule is glutathione (GSH), a tripeptide with a free cysteine sulfhydryl that is present at millimolar concentrations in cells (Fig. 15.4-8). This small nucleophile is known to react with and inactivate virtually all the therapeutic alkylating agents, and a correlation between elevated cellular GSH concentrations and resistance to nitrogen mustards has been demonstrated.[121] The GSH S-transferase enzymes catalyze the conjugation of GSH with electrophiles, and increased activity of this class of enzymes enhances GSH-mediated resistance.[122–124] The GSH conjugates of specific alkylating agents have been characterized,[125–127] and the specific isoenzymes of GST that catalyze their formation have been characterized.[128–132]

Buthionine sulfoximine is an inhibitor of γ-glutamylcysteine synthetase, the rate-limiting enzyme in the GSH synthesis pathway, and decreases the GSH concentration in cells.[133] Exposure to this compound sensitizes both normal and tumor cells to alkylating agents.[134,135] In a phase I clinical trial, buthionine sulfoxime has been shown to increase the hematologic toxicity of melphalan,[136] and it is currently in further clinical trials to determine whether this agent can increase the clinical antitumor efficacy of melphalan without significantly increasing toxicity.

Cells can also be sensitized to alkylating agents by exposure to inhibitors of GSH S-transferases,[137,138] and a clinical trial of the GSH S-transferase inhibitor sulfasalazine with melphalan demonstrated increased nausea and vomiting but no increase in hematopoietic toxicity.[139] The membrane transporter multidrug resistance protein is known to mediate the efflux of GSH conjugates from the cell,[140] and Barnouin et al.[141] have demonstrated that this system can transport the GSH conjugates of chlorambucil and melphalan from cells. These observations suggest that modulation of these systems could enhance the efficacy of alkylating agents.

Kelley et al.[142] demonstrated that transfection of metallothionein into cells produced increased resistance to chlorambucil and melphalan. Subsequently, Yu et al.[143] and others[144] have demonstrated that the thiol groups of metallothionein bind melphalan and phosphoramide mustard. It has also been demonstrated that exposure of cells to zinc increases metallothionein concentration in the cell and increases resistance of the cells to melphalan, doxorubicin, and cisplatin.[145]

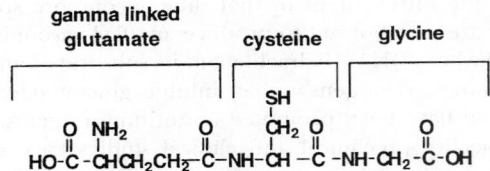

FIGURE 15.4-8. Structure of glutathione.

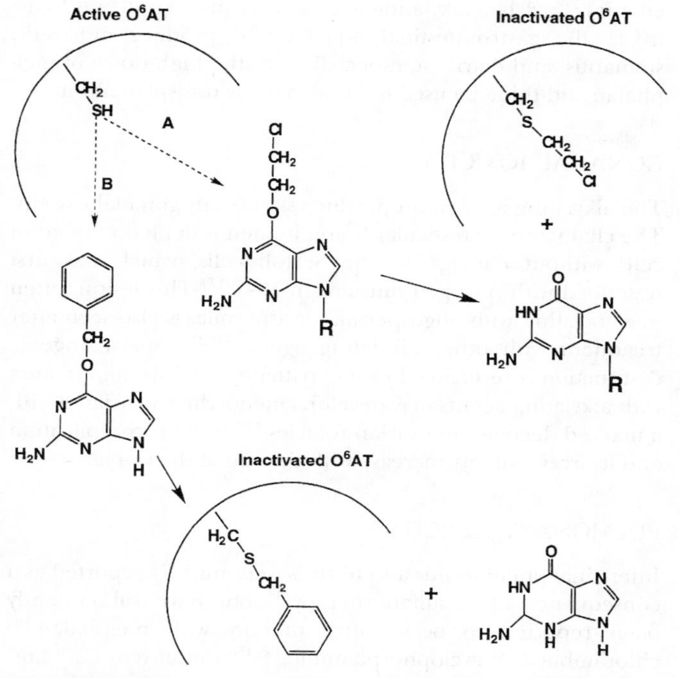

FIGURE 15.4-9. Interactions of O⁶-alkylguanine-DNA alkyltransferase. Pathway A: Repair of O⁶ alkylation by O⁶-alkylguanine-DNA alkyltransferase (O⁶AT). Pathway B: Inactivation of O⁶AT by benzylguanine.

ENHANCED DNA REPAIR: O⁶ ALKYLATION

Another mechanism of cellular resistance to alkylating agents is repair of the DNA damage that the agents produce. The most defined mechanism of cellular repair of alkylating agent damage is that of the enzyme O⁶-alkylguanine-alkyltransferase. As illustrated in Figure 15.4-9, this enzyme can remove an alkyl group from the O6 position of guanine, and the alkylated enzyme is then rapidly degraded.[146] This mechanism has been shown to be effective in protecting normal and tumor cells from the carcinogenic and toxic effects of DNA methylating agents, such as temozolomide and procarbazine.[147] Erickson et al.[148] demonstrated that this enzyme would also remove the 6-chloroethyl lesion produced by the alkylation of guanine by

the chloroethylnitrosoureas and produce resistance to these compounds, and this observation has been confirmed and extended.[149]

It has been shown that such compounds as O⁶-benzylguanine are acted on by O⁶-alkylguanine-DNA alkyltransferase (see Fig. 15.4-9) to remove the benzyl group[150] and that the enzyme is then rapidly degraded and depleted. Such compounds have been demonstrated to reverse tumor resistance due to O⁶-alkylguanine-DNA alkyltransferase (O⁶AT) to the O⁶ alkylating agents *in vitro* and *in vivo*,[151,152] and clinical trials of the combination of such agents and O⁶-methylguanine are currently in progress.[153,154] However, inhibitors of O⁶AT enhance the hematopoietic toxicity of O⁶ alkylating therapeutic agents. Hematopoietic stem cells have been successfully transfected with O⁶AT variants that are resistant to O⁶-benzylguanine and related compounds.[155] The hematopoietic systems of animals populated with these cells are resistant to the combination of O⁶-benzylguanine and BCNU, and clinical trials of this approach to improve the clinical efficacy of chloroethylnitrosoureas and methylating agents are planned.

CROSS-LINK REPAIR

The use of alkaline elution and other techniques (Fig. 15.4-10) has demonstrated that DNA interstrand cross-links produced by nitrogen mustards can be removed in bacteria[156] and mammalian cells.[157] The mechanism of such repair has not been elucidated, but nucleotide excision repair[158] and poly(adenosine diphosphate-ribose) polymerase[159] appear to play a role. Caffeine and related compounds have been demonstrated to enhance the cytotoxicity of nitrogen mustard.[160] This effect was associated with abrogation of G₂ arrest. O'Connor et al.[161,162] demonstrated that the G₂ arrest associated with nitrogen mustard resistance was associated with decreased activity of cdc2 kinase in the resistant cells. Caffeine has also been shown to inhibit nucleotide excision repair by binding to the subunit that recognizes the damage and helps to mediate this repair activity.[160–163] Elevated Bcl-2 has also been associated with nitrogen mustard resistance.[164]

A medulloblastoma cell line has been demonstrated to be resistant to activated cyclophosphamide (4-hydroperoxycyclophosphamide) on the basis of increased removal of DNA inter-

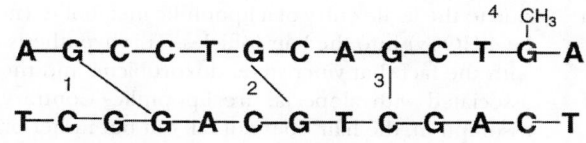

1. G-X-C/C-X-G interstrand crosslink	2. G-C/C-G interstrand crosslink	3. G/C interstrand crosslink	4. O⁶-G Methylation
Nitrogen mustards Thiotepa ? Busulfan ?	Mitomycin C	Chloroethylnitrosoureas	Procarbazine Temozolomide Dacarbazine
Must be repaired for cell survival. Mustard crosslink can be excised by some resistant cells	Must be repaired for cell survival. Excision of crosslink not demonstrated.	Must be repaired for cell survival. Initial chloroethyl alkylation can be removed by O-6-AT to prevent crosslink. Excision of crosslink not demonstrated.	Recognition by mismatch repair necessary for toxicity. O-6 methyl can be removed by O-6AT.

FIGURE 15.4-10. DNA lesions produced by alkylating agents.

strand cross-links.[24] This cell does not repair cross-links produced by BCNU and busulfan, which indicates that the recognition of the nitrogen mustard cross-link is different from that of the BCNU cross-link.[165]

IN VIVO RESISTANCE

Kobayashi et al.[166] and St. Croix et al.[167] have described resistance to alkylating agents and other antitumor agents that is associated with aggregation of tumor cells. This resistance is present when the tumor cells are growing *in vivo* or in three-dimensional *in vitro* culture with adherence between the cells but is not present when the cells are dispersed in two-dimensional culture. This type of resistance has also been associated with increased metastatic potential.[168]

COMMON TOXICITIES OF ALKYLATING AGENTS

Toxicities that are associated with specific alkylating agents are described in the discussions of the individual agents. The toxicities common to the alkylating agents as a class are described here.

HEMATOPOIETIC TOXICITY

The usual dose-limiting toxicity for an alkylating agent is hematopoietic toxicity. Cyclophosphamide produces a relatively short nadir of the granulocytes, with recovery within 3 weeks after a single dose or short course.[169] Cyclophosphamide is also relatively platelet sparing. The reason for the relative hematopoietic sparing properties of cyclophosphamide is the high concentrations of the enzyme aldehyde dehydrogenase in hematopoietic stem cells and megakaryocytes.[22]

The nitrosoureas produce an unusual delayed hematopoietic toxicity, with nadirs of both granulocytes and platelets at 5 to 6 weeks after administration, which indicates that these agents have a marked effect on very early hematopoietic stem cells, whose damage takes longer to become manifest. Severe granulocytopenia and thrombocytopenia are characteristic of busulfan.[169] An interesting characteristic of busulfan is its relative sparing of lymphocytes. The different hematopoietic effects of alkylating agents, except for the characteristics of cyclophosphamide, are not explained but suggest significant differences in selectivity of antitumor agents for the different hematopoietic precursors.

GASTROINTESTINAL TOXICITY

The alkylating agents frequently produce nausea and vomiting, although this effect is usually not as severe as with the platinum agents. Cyclophosphamide produces severe nausea and vomiting in some patients, but these patients usually tolerate chlorambucil, which is clinically less emetogenic. The nausea and vomiting produced by alkylating agents are known to be mediated significantly through the CNS[170,171] and are much better controlled with the new generation of antiemetics. With the higher doses of alkylating agents used in bone marrow transplantation, increased nausea and vomiting are seen but can usually be controlled by corticosteroids and the newer anti-emetics.[172,173] The alkylating agents can cause significant toxicity to the gastrointestinal mucosa and produce mucositis, stomatitis, and diarrhea, especially with the high doses of melphalan and thiotepa used in bone marrow transplantation.

GONADAL TOXICITY

The alkylating agents can produce significant gonadal toxicity. The characteristic testicular lesion in men is depletion of germ cells without damage to the Sertoli cells, which was first described with nitrogen mustard in 1948.[174] This lesion, often in association with oligospermia or aspermia, is also seen after treatment with other alkylating agents.[175,176] Spermatogenic dysfunction is reversible in some patients.[177,178] Women treated with alkylating agents may develop amenorrhea associated with a marked decrease in ovarian follicles.[179–181] This complication and its irreversibility increase with the age of the woman.

PULMONARY TOXICITY

Interstitial pneumonitis and fibrosis were initially reported as a consequence of busulfan therapy[182] but have subsequently been reported to occur after therapy with melphalan,[183] chlorambucil,[184] cyclophosphamide,[185,186] mitomycin C,[187] and BCNU.[188,189] The clinical manifestations of this toxicity are dyspnea and a nonproductive cough, which can progress to cyanosis, pulmonary insufficiency, and death. The syndrome has particularly been associated in frequency and severity with high doses of BCNU.[190,191] The greater pulmonary toxicity of BCNU may be due to the spontaneous decomposition of BCNU, which produces chloroethyl isocyanate[192] in addition to the alkylating chloroethyl diazonium moiety described in Nitrosoureas, earlier in this chapter. Chloroethyl isocyanate is an analogue of methyl isocyanate, a known pulmonary toxin that produced many deaths when released in an industrial accident in Bhopal, India.[193]

ALOPECIA

Alopecia from chemotherapy was first described after administration of dimethylmyeleran, an analogue of busulfan.[194] The alkylating agents now most associated with alopecia are cyclophosphamide and ifosfamide. Feil and Lamoureux[195] examined the alopecia-producing effects of metabolites and analogues of cyclophosphamide and proposed that the alopecic effect was due to the facile entry of a lipophilic metabolite (now known to be 4-HOCy) into the hair follicles. This hypothesis is consistent with the fact that vincristine, doxorubicin, and the taxanes, all associated with alopecia, are lipophilic. Contrary to popular assumption, the hair does not fall out but rather breaks off due to a nick in the hair produced at the time of exposure of the hair follicle to drug because of decreased synthesis. Thus, patients should be instructed not to brush the hair vigorously during and after the period of drug administration.

TERATOGENICITY

All the therapeutically used alkylating agents are teratogenic in animal studies.[196–199] A review of the literature in 1968 found that 4 of 25 children born to mothers who received alkylating agents during the first trimester of pregnancy had fetal malformations.[200] On the basis of the limited information available, women treated with an alkylating agent during the first trimester of pregnancy may have a risk as high as 15% of having a malformed infant. Administration of alkylating agents during the second and third trimesters has not been associated with increased fetal malformations.[201–204] One report cites 19 women treated during the first trimester with no infant malformations.[204]

CARCINOGENESIS

In the 1970s, there were reports of acute leukemia occurring in patients who had been treated with alkylating agents,[205–209] and subsequent experience has confirmed the occurrence of this complication. The incidence of leukemia is difficult to estimate because of the variety of agents, doses, and combinations used but is approximately 5%. In one group of 12 ovarian cancer patients receiving a high dose of melphalan, 4 developed acute leukemia.[208] In one report, the incidence of leukemia was found to be higher after melphalan treatment than after cyclophosphamide therapy.[210] This observation may be related to the stem cell–sparing properties of cyclophosphamide.[22] An increased frequency of solid tumors also occurs after alkylating agent therapy.[211,212]

IMMUNOSUPPRESSION

In 1921, Hektoen and Corper[213] reported an inhibitory effect of sulfur mustard on antibody production. Although all the alkylating agents produce some degree of immunosuppression, cyclophosphamide is the most immunosuppressive.[214] Cyclophosphamide and chlorambucil are the alkylating agents most commonly used for the treatment of autoimmune diseases.[215–218] Selective inhibition of immunosuppressor cells with low doses of an activated analogue of cyclophosphamide and with melphalan has been demonstrated *in vitro*[219–222] and *in vivo*,[223,224] and enhancement of this immune response with cyclophosphamide has been shown *in vivo*.[223] For this reason, low doses of cyclophosphamide have been used in conjunction with immunotherapy. Because of its potent immunosuppressive properties, cyclophosphamide has long been used in preparative regimens for allogeneic stem cell transplantation for malignancy.[11] The use of high doses of cyclophosphamide without stem cell support has now been reported to produce complete remissions in autoimmune diseases.[12,13,225]

REFERENCES

1. Adair CPJ, Bogg HJ. Experimental and clinical studies of the treatment of cancer by dichloroethylsulfide (mustard gas). *Ann Surg* 1931;93:190.
2. Rhoads C. Nitrogen mustards in treatment of neoplastic disease. *JAMA* 1946;131:6568.
3. Goodman LS, Wintrobe MM, Dameshek W, et al. Use of methyl-bis(beta-chlorethyl)amine hydrochloride for Hodgkin's disease lymphosarcoma, leukemia. *JAMA* 1946;132:126.
4. Jacobson LP, Spurr C, Barron E, et al. Studies of the effect of methyl-bis(beta-chloroethyl)amine hydrochloride on neoplastic diseases and allied disorders of the hematopoietic system. *JAMA* 1946;132:263.
5. Millard JT, Raucher S, Hopkins PB. Mechlorethamine cross links deoxyguanosine residues at 5' GNC sequences in duplex DNA sequences in duplex DNA fragments. *J Am Chem Soc* 1990;112:2459.
6. Brookes P, Lawley PD. The reaction of mono- and difunctional alkylating agents with nucleic acids. *Biochem J* 1961;80:486.
7. Dong Q, Barsky D, Colvin ME, et al. A structural basis for a phosphoramide mustard-induced DNA interstrand cross-link at 5'-d(GAC). *Proc Natl Acad Sci U S A* 1995;92:12170.
8. Fisher B, Anderson S, Wickerham DL, et al. Increased intensification and total dose of cyclophosphamide in a doxorubicin-cyclophosphamide regimen for the treatment of primary breast cancer: findings from National Surgical Adjuvant Breast and Bowel Project B-22. *J Clin Oncol* 1997;15:1858.
9. Weiss RB, Woolf SH, Demakos E. Natural history of more than 20 years of node-positive primary breast carcinoma treated with cyclophosphamide, methotrexate, and fluorouracil-based adjuvant chemotherapy: a study by the Cancer and Leukemia Group B. *J Clin Oncol* 2003;21:1825.
10. Chao NJ, Rosenberg SA, Horning SJ. CEPP(B): an effective and well-tolerated regimen in poor-risk, aggressive non-Hodgkin's lymphoma. *Blood* 1990;76:1293.
11. Santos GW, Sensenbrenner LL, Burke PJ, et al. Marrow transplantation in man following cyclophosphamide. *Transplant Proc* 1971;3:400.
12. Ferrara F, Copia C, Annunziata M, et al. Complete remission of refractory anemia following a single high dose of cyclophosphamide. *Ann Hematol* 1999;78:87.
13. Brodsky RA, Petri M, Smith BD, et al. Immunoablative high-dose cyclophosphamide without stem-cell rescue for refractory, severe autoimmune disease. *Ann Intern Med* 1998;129:1031.
14. Colvin M, Hilton J. Pharmacology of cyclophosphamide and metabolites. *Cancer Treat Rep* 1981;3:89.
15. Colvin M, Padgett CA, Fenselau C. A biologically active metabolite of cyclophosphamide. *Cancer Res* 1973;33:915.
16. Colvin M, Brundrett RB, Kan MN, Jardine I, Fenselau C. Alkylating properties of phosphoramide mustard. *Cancer Res* 1976;36:1121.
17. Gamcsik MP, Ludeman SM, Shulman-Roskes EM, et al. Protonation of phosphoramide mustard and other phosphoramides. *J Med Chem* 1993;36:3636.
18. Hilton J. Deoxyribonucleic acid cross-linking by 4-hydroperoxycyclophosphamide in cyclophosphamide-sensitive and -resistant L1210 cells. *Biochem Pharmacol* 1984;33:1867.
19. Shulman-Roskes EM, Noe DA, Gamcsik MP, et al. The partitioning of phosphoramide mustard and its aziridinium ions among alkylation and P-N bond hydrolysis reactions. *J Med Chem* 1998;41:515.
20. Hilton J. Role of aldehyde dehydrogenase in cyclophosphamide-resistant L1210 leukemia. *Cancer Res* 1984;44:5156.
21. Russo JE, Hilton J. Characterization of cytosolic aldehyde dehydrogenase from cyclophosphamide resistant L1210 cells. *Cancer Res* 1988;48:2963.
22. Kastan MB, Schlaffer E, Russo JE, et al. Direct demonstration of elevated aldehyde dehydrogenase in human hematopoietic progenitor cells. *Blood* 1990;75:1947.
23. Russo JE, Hilton J, Colvin OM. The role of aldehyde dehydrogenase isozymes in cellular resistance to the alkylating agent cyclophosphamide. *Prog Clin Biol Res* 1989;290:65.
24. Dong Q, Bullock N, Aliosman F, et al. Repair analysis of 4-hydroperoxycyclophosphamide induced DNA interstrand cross-linking in the C-Myc gene in 4-hydroperoxycyclophosphamide-sensitive and -resistant medulloblastoma cell lines. *Cancer Chemother Pharmacol* 1996;37:242.
25. Gamcsik MP, Millis KK, Colvin M. Noninvasive detection of elevated glutathione levels in Mcf-7 cells resistant to 4-hydroperoxycyclophosphamide. *Cancer Res* 1995;55:2012.
26. Bakke JE, Feil VJ, Fjelstul CE, Thacker EJ. Metabolism of cyclophosphamide by sheep. *J Agric Food Chem* 1972;20:384.
27. Jardine I, Fenselau C, Appler M, et al. Quantitation by gas chromatography-chemical ionization mass spectrometry of cyclophosphamide, phosphoramide mustard, and nornitrogen mustard in the plasma and urine of patients receiving cyclophosphamide therapy. *Cancer Res* 1978;38:408.
28. Chen TL, Kennedy MJ, Anderson LW, et al. Nonlinear pharmacokinetics of cyclophosphamide and 4-hydroxycyclophosphamide/aldophosphamide in patients with metastatic breast cancer receiving high-dose chemotherapy followed by autologous bone marrow transplantation. *Drug Metab Dispos* 1997;25:544.
29. Ren S, Kalhorn TF, McDonald GB, et al. Pharmacokinetics of cyclophosphamide and its metabolites in bone marrow transplantation patients. *Clin Pharmacol Ther* 1998;64:289.
30. Phillips FS, Sternberg SS, Cronin AP, Vidal PM. Cyclophosphamide and urinary bladder toxicity. *Cancer Res* 1961;21:1577.
31. Forni AM, Koss LG, Geller W. Cytological study of the effect of cyclophosphamide on the epithelium of the urinary bladder in man. *Cancer* 1964;17:1348.
32. Cox PJ. Cyclophosphamide cystitis—identification of acrolein as the causative agent. *Biochem Pharmacol* 1979;28:2045.
33. DeFronzo RA, Braine H, Colvin M, Davis PJ. Water intoxication in man after cyclophosphamide therapy. Time course and relation to drug activation. *Ann Intern Med* 1973;78:861.
34. Harlow PJ, DeClerck YA, Shore NA, et al. A fatal case of inappropriate ADH secretion induced by cyclophosphamide therapy. *Cancer* 1979;44:896.
35. Green TP, Mirkin BL. Prevention of cyclophosphamide-induced antidiuresis by furosemide infusion. *Clin Pharmacol Ther* 1981;29:634.
36. Slavin RE, Millan JC, Mullins GM. Pathology of high dose intermittent cyclophosphamide therapy. *Hum Pathol* 1975;6:693.
37. Colvin M. The comparative pharmacology of cyclophosphamide and ifosfamide. *Semin Oncol* 1982;9[Suppl 1]:2.
38. Pratt CB, Green AA, Horowitz ME, et al. Central nervous system toxicity following the treatment of pediatric patients with ifosfamide/mesna. *J Clin Oncol* 1986;4:1253.
39. Pratt CB, Meyer WH, Jenkins JJ, et al. Ifosfamide, Fanconi's syndrome, and rickets. *J Clin Oncol* 1991;9:1495.
40. Boddy AV, Yule SM, Wyllie R, et al. Intrasubject variation in children of ifosfamide pharmacokinetics and metabolism during repeated administration. *Cancer Chemother Pharmacol* 1996;38:147.
41. Boddy AV, Proctor M, Simmonds D, Lind MJ, Idle JR. Pharmacokinetics, metabolism and clinical effect of ifosfamide in breast cancer patients. *Eur J Cancer* 1995;1:69.
42. Norda A, Loos U, Sastry M, Goehl J, Hohenberger W. Pharmacokinetics of melphalan in isolated limb perfusion. *Cancer Chemother Pharmacol* 1999;43:35.
43. Goldenberg GJ, Lee M, Lam HY, Begleiter A. Evidence for carrier-mediated transport of melphalan by L5178Y lymphoblasts in vitro. *Cancer Res* 1977;37:755.

44. Begleiter A, Lam HY, Grover J, Froese E, Goldenberg GJ. Evidence for active transport of melphalan by two amino acid carriers in L5178Y lymphoblasts in vitro. *Cancer Res* 1979;39:353.
45. Vistica DT, Rabon A, Rabinovitz M. Amino acid conferred protection against melphalan: comparison of amino acids which reduce melphalan toxicity to murine bone marrow precursor cells (CFU-C) and murine L1210 leukemia cells. *Res Commun Chem Pathol Pharmacol* 1979;23:171.
46. Groothuis DR, Lippitz BE, Fekete I, et al. The effect of an amino acid-lowering diet on the rate of melphalan entry into brain and xenotransplanted glioma. *Cancer Res* 1992;52:5590.
47. Pallante SL, Fenselau C, Mennel RG, et al. Quantitation by gas chromatography-chemical ionization-mass spectrometry of phenylalanine mustard in plasma of patients. *Cancer Res* 1980;40:2268.
48. Hersh MR, Ludden TM, Kuhn JG, Knight WA 3rd. Pharmacokinetics of high-dose melphalan. *Invest New Drugs* 1983;1:331.
49. Pinguet F, Martel P, Fabbro M, et al. Pharmacokinetics of high-dose intravenous melphalan in patients undergoing peripheral blood hematopoietic progenitor-cell transplantation. *Anticancer Res* 1997;17:605.
50. Branten AJW, Reichert LJM, Koene RAP, Wetzels JFM. Oral cyclophosphamide versus chlorambucil in the treatment of patients with membranous nephropathy and renal insufficiency. *QJM* 1998;91:359.
51. Alberts DS, Chang SY, Chen H-SG, Larcom BJ, Evans TL. Comparative pharmacokinetics of chlorambucil and melphalan in man. *Recent Results Cancer Res* 1980;74:124.
52. Andrievsky GY, Sukhodub LF, Pyatigorskaya TL, et al. Direct observation of the alkylation products of deoxyguanosine and DNA by fast atom bombardment mass spectrometry. *Biol Mass Spectrom* 1991;20:665.
53. Cohen NA, Egorin MJ, Snyder SW, et al. Interaction of N,N',N''-triethylenethiophosphoramide and N,N',N''-triethylenephosphoramide with cellular DNA. *Cancer Res* 1991;51:4360.
54. Chang TK, Chen G, Waxman DJ. Modulation of thiotepa antitumor activity in vivo by alteration of liver cytochrome P450-catalyzed drug metabolism. *J Pharmacol Exp Ther* 1995;274:270.
55. Hussein AM, Petros WP, Ross M, et al. A phase I/II study of high dose cyclophosphamide, cisplatin, and thiotepa followed by autologous bone marrow and granulocyte colony stimulating factor-primed peripheral blood progenitor cells in patients with advanced malignancies. *Cancer Chemother Pharmacol* 1996;37:561.
56. Lyss AP, Luedke S, Einhorn L, Luedke DW, Raney M. Vindesine and mitomycin C in metastatic breast cancer: a Southeastern Cancer Study Group Trial. *Oncology* 1989;46:357.
57. Borowy-Borowski H, Lipman R, Chowdary D, Tomasz M. Duplex oligodeoxyribonucleotides cross-linked by mitomycin C at a single site: synthesis, properties, and cross-link reversibility. *Biochemistry* 1990;29:2992.
58. Tomasz M, Lipman R, Chowdary D, et al. Isolation and structure of a covalent cross-link adduct between mitomycin C and DNA. *Science* 1987;235:1204.
59. Rink SM, Lipman R, Alley SC, Hopkins PH, Tomasz M. Bending of DNA by the mitomycin C-induced, GpG intrastrand cross-link. *Chem Res Toxicol* 1996;9:382.
60. den Hartigh J, McVie JG, van Oort WJ, Pinedo HM. Pharmacokinetics of mitomycin C in humans. *Cancer Res* 1983;43:5017.
61. Institoris E, Tamas J. Alkylation by 1,2:5,6-dianhydrogalactitol of deoxyribonucleic acid and guanosine. *Biochem J* 1980;185:659.
62. Haas CD, Baker L, Thigpen T. Phase II evaluation of dianhydrogalactitol in lung cancer: a Southwest Oncology Group Study. *Cancer Treat Rep* 1981;65:115.
63. Edmonson JH, Frytak S, Letendre L, Kvols LK, Eagan RT. Phase II evaluation of dianhydrogalactitol in advanced head and neck carcinomas. *Cancer Treat Rep* 1979;63:2081.
64. Levin VA, Edwards MS, Gutin PH, et al. Phase II evaluation of dibromodulcitol in the treatment of recurrent medulloblastoma, ependymoma, and malignant astrocytoma. *J Neurosurg* 1984;61:1063.
65. Nguyen HN, Nordqvist SR. Chemotherapy of advanced and recurrent cervical carcinoma. *Semin Surg Oncol* 1999;16:247.
66. Horvath IP, Csetenyi J, Kerpel-Fronius S, et al. Pharmacokinetics and metabolism of dianhydrogalactitol DAG in patients: a comparison with the human disposition of dibromodulcitol DBD. *Eur J Cancer Clin Oncol* 1986;22:163.
67. Kelley SL, Peters WP, Andersen J, et al. Pharmacokinetics of dibromodulcitol in humans: a phase I study. *J Clin Oncol* 1986;4:753.
68. Hartley JA, Berardini MD, Souhami RL. An agarose gel method for the determination of DNA interstrand cross-linking applicable to the measurement of the rate of total and "second-arm" cross-link reactions. *Anal Biochem* 1991;193:131.
69. Streeper RT, Cotter RJ, Colvin ME, Hilton J, Colvin OM. Molecular pharmacology of hepsulfam, NSC 3296801: identification of alkylated nucleosides, alkylation site, and site of DNA cross-linking. *Cancer Res* 1995;55:1491.
70. Haddow A, Timmis GM. Myeleran in chronic myeloid leukemia—chemical constitution and biological action. *Lancet* 1953;1:207.
71. Elson LA. Hematologic effects of the alkylating agents. *Ann N Y Acad Sci* 1958;68:826.
72. Grochow LB, Jones RJ, Brundrett RB, et al. Pharmacokinetics of busulfan: correlation with veno-occlusive disease in patients undergoing bone marrow transplantation. *Cancer Chemother Pharmacol* 1989;25:55.
73. Jones RJ, Lee KS, Beschorner WE, et al. Venoocclusive disease of the liver following bone marrow transplantation. *Transplantation* 1987;44:778.
74. Johnston TP, McCaleb GS, Montgomery JA. The synthesis of antineoplastic agents: XXXII. N-nitrosoureas. *J Med Chem* 1963;6:669.
75. Montgomery JA. Chemistry and structure-activity studies of the nitrosoureas. *Cancer Treat Rep* 1976;60:651.
76. Schabel FM Jr. Nitrosoureas: a review of experimental antitumor activity. *Cancer Treat Rep* 1976;60:665.
77. Kohn KW. Interstrand cross-linking of DNA by 1,3-bis(2-chloroethyl)-1-nitrosourea and other 1-(2-haloethyl)-1-nitrosoureas. *Cancer Res* 1977;37:1450.
78. Colvin M, Brundrett RB, Cowens W, Jardine I, Ludlum DB. A chemical basis for the antitumor activity of chloroethylnitrosoureas. *Biochem Pharmacol* 1976;25:695.
79. Tong WP, Kirk MC, Ludlum DB. Mechanism of action of the nitrosoureas: V. Formation of O**6-(2-fluoroethyl)guanine and its probable role in the cross-linking of deoxyribonucleic acid. *Biochem Pharmacol* 1983;32:2011.
80. Fischhaber PL, Gall AS, Duncan JA, Hopkins PB. Direct demonstration in synthetic oligonucleotides that N,N'-bis(2-chloroethyl)-nitrosourea cross-links N-1 of deoxyguanosine to N-3 of deoxycytidine on opposite strands of duplex DNA. *Cancer Res* 1999;59:4363.
81. Walker MD, Alexander E Jr, Hunt WE, et al. Evaluation of BCNU and/or radiotherapy in the treatment of anaplastic gliomas. A cooperative clinical trial. *J Neurosurg* 1978;49:333.
82. Eder JP, Antman K, Peters W, et al. High-dose combination alkylating agent chemotherapy with autologous bone marrow support for metastatic breast cancer. *J Clin Oncol* 1986;4:1592.
83. Brem H, Piantadosi S, Burger PC, et al. Placebo-controlled trial of safety and efficacy of intraoperative controlled delivery by biodegradable polymers of chemotherapy for recurrent gliomas. *Lancet* 1995;345:1008.
84. Prados MD, Scott C, Curran WJ, et al. Procarbazine, lomustine, and vincristine (PCV) chemotherapy for anaplastic astrocytoma: a retrospective review of Radiation Therapy Oncology Group protocols comparing survival with carmustine or PCV adjuvant chemotherapy. *J Clin Oncol* 1999;17:3389.
85. Clark JL, Barcewicz P, Nava HR, Goodwin PS, Douglass HO Jr. Adjuvant 5-FU and MeCCNU improves survival following curative gastrectomy for adenocarcinoma. *Am Surg* 1990;56:423.
86. Paccapelo A, Piana C, Rychlicki F, et al. Treatment of malignant gliomas: a new approach. *Tumori* 1998;84:529.
87. Arita N, Ushio Y, Hayakawa T, et al. Intrathecal ACNU—a new therapeutic approach against malignant leptomeningeal tumors. *J Neurooncol* 1988;6:221.
88. Alberts DS, Durie BG, Salmon SE. Doxorubicin/B.C.N.U. chemotherapy for multiple myeloma in relapse. *Lancet* 1976;1:926.
89. Levin VA, Hoffman W, Weinkam RJ. Pharmacokinetics of BCNU in man: a preliminary study of 20 patients. *Cancer Treat Rep* 1978;62:1305.
90. Meisenberg BR, Ross M, Vredenburgh JJ, et al. Randomized trial of high-dose chemotherapy with autologous bone marrow support as adjuvant therapy for high-risk, multi-node-positive malignant melanoma. *J Natl Cancer Inst* 1993;85:1080.
91. Henner WD, Peters WP, Eder JP, et al. Pharmacokinetics and immediate effects of high-dose carmustine in man. *Cancer Treat Rep* 1986;70:877.
92. Levin VA, Stearns J, Byrd A, Finn A, Weinkam RJ. The effect of phenobarbital pretreatment on the antitumor activity of 1,3-bis(2-chloroethyl)-1-nitrosourea (BCNU), 1-(2-chloroethyl)-3-cyclohexyl-1-nitrosourea (CCNU) and 1-(2-chloroethyl)-3-(2,6-dioxo-3-piperidyl-1-nitrosourea (PCNU), and on the plasma pharmacokinetics and biotransformation of BCNU. *J Pharmacol Exp Ther* 1979;208:1.
93. Lee FY, Workman P, Roberts JT, Bleehen NM. Clinical pharmacokinetics of oral CCNU (lomustine). *Cancer Chemother Pharmacol* 1985;14:125.
94. DeVita VT, Carbone PP, Owens AH Jr, et al. Clinical trials with 1,3-Bis(2-chloroethyl)-1-nitrosourea, NSC-409962. *Cancer Res* 1965;25:1876.
95. Toth B. Synthetic and naturally occurring hydrazines as possible cancer causative agents. *Cancer Res* 1975;35:3693.
96. Silverstein R, Bhatia P, Svoboda DJ. Effect of hydrazine sulfate on glucose-regulating enzymes in the normal and cancerous rat. *Immunopharmacology* 1989;17:37.
97. Gold J. Use of hydrazine sulfate in terminal and preterminal cancer patients: results of investigational new drug (IND) study in 84 evaluable patients. *Oncology* 1975;32:1.
98. Kamradt JM, Pienta KJ. The effect of hydrazine sulfate on prostate cancer growth. *Oncol Rep* 1998;5:919.
99. Fink D, Aebi S, Howell SB. The role of DNA mismatch repair in drug resistance. *Clin Cancer Res* 1998;4:1.
100. Friedman HS, Johnson SP, Dong Q, et al. Methylator resistance mediated by mismatch repair deficiency in a glioblastoma multiforme xenograft. *Cancer Res* 1997;57:2933.
101. Bianchini F, Weiderpass E, Kyrtopoulos S, et al. Detection of DNA methylation adducts in Hodgkin's disease patients treated with procarbazine. *Biomarkers* 1996;1:226.
102. Erikson JM, Tweedie DJ, Ducore JM, Prough RA. Cytotoxicity and DNA damage caused by the azoxy metabolites of procarbazine in L1210 tumor cells. *Cancer Res* 1989;49:127.
103. Swaffar DS, Horstman MG, Jaw JY, et al. Methylazoxyprocarbazine, the active metabolite responsible for the anticancer activity of procarbazine against L1210 leukemia. *Cancer Res* 1989;49:2442.
104. Massie MJ, Holland JC. Diagnosis and treatment of depression in the cancer patient. *J Clin Psychiatry* 1984;45:25.
105. Pfefferbaum B, Pack R, van Eys J. Monoamine oxidase inhibitor toxicity. *J Am Acad Child Adolesc Psychiatry* 1989;28:954.
106. Farina P, Benfenati E, Reginato R, et al. Metabolism of the anticancer agent 1-(4-acetylphenyl)-3,3-dimethyltriazene. *Biomed Mass Spectrom* 1983;10:485.
107. Skibba JL, Beal DD, Ramirez G, Bryan GT. N-demethylation of the antineoplastic agent4(5)-(3,3-dimethyl-1-triazeno)imidazole-5(4)-carboxamide by rats and man. *Cancer Res* 1970;30:147.
108. Vaughan K, Tang Y, Llanos G, et al. Studies of the mode of action of antitumor triazenes and triazines: 6. 1-Aryl-3-(hydroxymethyl)-3-methyltriazenes: synthesis, chemistry, and antitumor properties. *J Med Chem* 1984;27:357.
109. DeVita VT, Mauch PM, Harris NL. Hodgkin's disease. In: DeVita VT Jr, Hellman S, Rosenberg S, eds. *Cancer: principles and practice of oncology.* Philadelphia: Lippincott–Raven, 1997:2268.
110. Falkson CI, Ibrahim J, Kirkwood JM, et al. Phase III trial of dacarbazine versus dacarbazine with interferon alpha-2b versus dacarbazine with tamoxifen versus dacarbazine with interferon alpha-2b and tamoxifen in patients with metastatic malignant melanoma: an Eastern Cooperative Oncology Group study. *J Clin Oncol* 1998;16:1743.

111. Lowe PR, Sansom CE, Schwalbe CH, Stevens MF, Clark AS. Antitumor imidazotetrazines: 25. Crystal structure of 8-carbamoyl-3-methylimidazo[5,1-d]-1,2,3,5-tetrazin-4(3H)-one (temozolomide) and structural comparisons with the related drugs mitozolomide and DTIC. *J Med Chem* 1992;35:3377.
112. Denny BJ, Wheelhouse RT, Stevens MF, Tsang LL, Slack JA. NMR and molecular modeling investigation of the mechanism of activation of the antitumor drug temozolomide and its interaction with DNA. *Biochemistry* 1994;33:9045.
113. Nicholson HS, Krailo M, Ames MM, et al. Phase I study of temozolomide in children and adolescents with recurrent solid tumors—a report from the Children's Cancer Group. *J Clin Oncol* 1998;16:3037.
114. Hammond LA, Eckardt JR, Baker SD, et al. Phase I and pharmacokinetic study of temozolomide on a daily-for-5-days schedule in patients with advanced solid malignancies. *J Clin Oncol* 1999;17:2604.
115. Paulsen F, Hoffmann W, Becker G, et al. Chemotherapy in the treatment of recurrent glioblastoma multiforme: ifosfamide versus temozolomide. *J Cancer Res Clin Oncol* 1999;125:411.
116. Newlands ES, Oreilly SM, Glaser MG, et al. The Charing Cross Hospital experience with temozolomide in patients with gliomas. *Eur J Cancer* 1996;13:2236.
117. Woll PJ, Judson I, Lee SM, et al. Temozolomide in adult patients with advanced soft tissue sarcoma: a phase II study of the EORTC Soft Tissue and Bone Sarcoma Group. *Eur J Cancer* 1999;35:410.
118. Breithaupt H, Dammann A, Aigner K. Pharmacokinetics of dacarbazine (DTIC) and its metabolite 5-aminoimidazole-4-carboxamide (AIC) following different dose schedules. *Cancer Chemother Pharmacol* 1982;9:103.
119. Reid JM, Stevens DC, Rubin J, Ames MM. Pharmacokinetics of 3-methyl-(triazen-1-yl)imidazole-4-carboximide following administration of temozolomide to patients with advanced cancer. *Clin Cancer Res* 1997;3:2393.
120. Baker SD, Wirth M, Statkevich P, et al. Absorption, metabolism, and excretion of 14C-temozolomide following oral administration to patients with advanced cancer. *Clin Cancer Res* 1999;5:309.
121. Suzukake K, Petro BJ, Vistica DT. Reduction in glutathione content of L-PAM resistant L1210 cells confers drug sensitivity. *Biochem Pharmacol* 1982;31:121.
122. Buller AL, Clapper ML, Tew KD. Glutathione S-transferases in nitrogen mustard-resistant and -sensitive cell lines. *Mol Pharmacol* 1987;31:575.
123. Puchalski RB, Fahl WE. Expression of recombinant glutathione S-transferase pi, Ya, or Yb1 confers resistance to alkylating agents. *Proc Natl Acad Sci U S A* 1990;87:2443.
124. Townsend AI, Fields WR, Haynes RL, et al. Chemoprotective functions of glutathione S-transferases in cell lines induced to express specific isozymes by stable transfection. *Chem Biol Interact* 1998;112:389.
125. Dulik DM, Colvin OM, Fenselau C. Characterization of glutathione conjugates of chlorambucil by fast atom bombardment and thermospray liquid chromatography/mass spectrometry. *Biomed Environ Mass Spectrom* 1990;19:248.
126. Dulik DM, Fenselau C, Hilton J. Characterization of melphalan-glutathione adducts whose formation is catalyzed by glutathione transferases. *Biochem Pharmacol* 1986;35:3405.
127. Yuan ZM, Fenselau C, Dulik DM, et al. Laser desorption electron impact: application to a study of the mechanism of conjugation of glutathione and cyclophosphamide. *Anal Chem* 1990;62:868.
128. Bolton MG, Colvin OM, Hilton J. Specificity of isozymes of murine hepatic glutathione S-transferase for the conjugation of glutathione with L-phenylalanine mustard. *Cancer Res* 1991;51:2410.
129. Ciaccio PI, Tew KD, LaCreta FP. The spontaneous and glutathione S-transferase-mediated reaction of chlorambucil with glutathione. *Cancer Commun* 1990;2:279.
130. Dirven HA, van Ommen B, van Bladeren PI. Involvement of human glutathione S-transferase isoenzymes in the conjugation of cyclophosphamide metabolites with glutathione. *Cancer Res* 1994;54:6215.
131. Pallante SL, Lisek CA, Dulik DM, Fenselau C. Glutathione conjugates. Immobilized enzyme synthesis and characterization by fast atom bombardment mass spectrometry. *Drug Metab Dispos* 1986;14:313.
132. Horton JK, Roy G, Piper JT, et al. Characterization of a chlorambucil-resistant human ovarian carcinoma cell line overexpressing glutathione S-transferase mu. *Biochem Pharmacol* 1999;58:693.
133. Anderson ME. Glutathione: an overview of biosynthesis and modulation. *Chem Biol Interact* 1998;112:1.
134. Smith AC, Liao JT, Page JG, Wientjes MG, Grieshaber CK. Pharmacokinetics of buthionine sulfoximine (NSC 326231) and its effect on melphalan-induced toxicity in mice. *Cancer Res* 1989;49:5385.
135. Friedman HS, Colvin OM, Griffith OW, et al. Increased melphalan activity in intracranial human medulloblastoma and glioma xenografts following buthionine sulfoximine-mediated glutathione depletion. *J Natl Cancer Inst* 1989;81:524.
136. Bailey HH, Ripple G, Tutsch KD, et al. Phase I study of continuous-infusion L-S,R-buthionine sulfoximine with intravenous melphalan. *J Natl Cancer Inst* 1997;89:1789.
137. Morgan AS, Ciaccio PI, Tew KD, Kauvar LN. Isozyme specific glutathione S-transferase inhibitors potentiate drug sensitivity in cultured human tumor cell lines. *Cancer Chemother Pharmacol* 1996;37:363.
138. Zhang K, Yang EB, Wong KP, Mack P. GSH, GSH-related enzymes and GS-X pump in relation to sensitivity of human tumor cell lines to chlorambucil and adriamycin. *Int J Oncol* 1999;14:861.
139. Gupta V, Jani JP, Jacobs S, et al. Activity of melphalan in combination with the glutathione transferase inhibitor sulfasalazine. *Cancer Chemother Pharmacol* 1995;36:3.
140. Keppler D, Leier I, Jedlitschky G, Konig J. Atp-dependent transport of glutathione S-conjugates by the multidrug resistance protein Mrp1 and its apical isoform Mrp2. *Chem Biol Interact* 1998;112:153.
141. Barnouin K, Leier I, Jedlitschky G, et al. Multidrug resistance protein-mediated transport of chlorambucil and melphalan conjugated to glutathione. *Br J Cancer* 1998;77:201.
142. Kelley S, Basu A, Teicher BA, et al. Overexpression of metallothionein confers resistance to anticancer drugs. *Science* 1988;241:1813.
143. Yu X, Wu Z, Fenselau C. Covalent sequestration of melphalan by metallothionein and selective alkylation of cysteines. *Biochemistry* 1995;34:3377.
144. Wei D, Fabris D, Fenselau C. Covalent sequestration of phosphoramide mustard by metallothionein—an in vitro study. *Drug Metab Dispos* 1999;27:786.
145. Satoh M, Cherian MG, Imura N, Shimizu H. Modulation of resistance to anticancer drugs by inhibition of metallothionein synthesis. *Cancer Res* 1994;54:5255.
146. Pegg AE, Boosalis M, Samson L, et al. Mechanism of inactivation of human O^6-alkylguanine-DNA alkyltransferase by O^6-benzylguanine. *Biochemistry* 1993;32:11998.
147. Pegg AE. Mammalian O^6-alkylguanine-DNA alkyltransferase: regulation and importance in response to alkylating carcinogenic and therapeutic agents. *Cancer Res* 1990;50:6119.
148. Erickson LC, Laurent G, Sharkey NA, Kohn KW. DNA cross-linking and monoadduct repair in nitrosourea-treated human tumour cells. *Nature* 1980;288:727.
149. Bodell WJ, Tokuda K, Ludlum DB. Differences in DNA alkylation products formed in sensitive and resistant human glioma cells treated with N-(2-chloroethyl)-N-nitrosourea. *Cancer Res* 1988;48:4489.
150. Dolan ME, Moschel RC, Pegg AE. Depletion of mammalian O^6-alkylguanine-DNA alkyltransferase activity by O**6-benzylguanine provides a means to evaluate the role of this protein in protection against carcinogenic and therapeutic alkylating agents. *Proc Natl Acad Sci U S A* 1990;87:5368.
151. Gerson SL, Berger SI, Varnes ME, Donovan C. Combined depletion of O^6-alkylguanine-DNA alkyltransferase and glutathione to modulate nitrosourea resistance in breast cancer. *Biochem Pharmacol* 1994;48:543.
152. Cussac C, Rapp M, Mounetou E, et al. Enhancement by O^6-benzyl-N-acetylguanosine derivatives of chloroethylnitrosourea antitumor action in chloroethylnitrosourea-resistant human malignant melanocytes. *J Pharmacol Exp Ther* 1994;271:1353.
153. Friedman HS, Kokkinakis DM, Pluda J, et al. Phase I trial of O-6-benzylguanine for patients undergoing surgery for malignant glioma. *J Clin Oncol* 1998;16:3570.
154. Spiro TP, Gerson SL, Liu LL, et al. O-6-benzylguanine: a clinical trial establishing the biochemical modulatory dose in tumor tissue for alkyltransferase-directed DNA repair. *Cancer Res* 1999;59:2402.
155. Allay JA, Dumenco LL, Koc ON, Liu L, Gerson SL. Retroviral transduction and expression of the human alkyltransferase cDNA provides nitrosourea resistance to hematopoietic cells. *Blood* 1995;85:3342.
156. Kohn KW, Steigbigel NH, Spears CL. Cross-linking and repair of DNA in sensitive and resistant strains of *E. coli* treated with nitrogen mustard. *Proc Natl Acad Sci U S A* 1154;53:1154.
157. Crathorn AR, Roberts JJ. Mechanism of the cytotoxic action of alkylating agents in mammalian cells and evidence for the removal of alkylated groups from deoxyribonucleic acid. *Nature* 1966;211:150.
158. Sancar A. Mechanisms of DNA excision repair. *Science* 1994;266:1954.
159. Stevnsner T, Ding R, Smulson M, Bohr VA. Inhibition of gene-specific repair of alkylation damage in cells depleted of poly(ADP- ribose) polymerase. *Nucleic Acids Res* 1994;22:4620.
160. Das SK, Lau CC, Pardee A. Comparative analysis of caffeine and 3-aminobenzamide as DNA repair inhibitors in Syrian baby hamster kidney cells. *Mutat Res* 1984;131:71.
161. O'Connor PM, Ferris DK, White GA, et al. Relationships between cdc2 kinase, DNA cross-linking, and cell cycle perturbations induced by nitrogen mustard. *Cell Growth Differ* 1992;3:43.
162. O'Connor PM, Ferris DK, Hoffmann I, et al. Role of the cdc25C phosphatase in G2 arrest induced by nitrogen mustard. *Proc Natl Acad Sci U S A* 1994;91:9480.
163. Selby CP, Sancar A. Molecular mechanisms of DNA repair inhibition by caffeine. *Proc Natl Acad Sci U S A* 1990;87:3522.
164. Walton MI, Whysong D, O'Connor PM, et al. Constitutive expression of human Bcl-2 modulates nitrogen mustard and camptothecin induced apoptosis. *Cancer Res* 1993;53:1853.
165. Dong Q, Johnson SP, Colvin OM, et al. Multiple DNA repair mechanisms and alkylator resistance in the human medulloblastoma cell line D-283 Med (4-HCR). *Cancer Chemother Pharmacol* 1999;43:73.
166. Kobayashi H, Man S, Graham CH, et al. Acquired multicellular-mediated resistance to alkylating agents in cancer. *Proc Natl Acad Sci U S A* 1993;90:3294.
167. St Croix B, Man S, Kerbel RS. Reversal of intrinsic and acquired forms of drug resistance by hyaluronidase treatment of solid tumors. *Cancer Lett* 1998;131:35.
168. Kerbel RS, Kobayashi H, Graham CH. Intrinsic or acquired drug resistance and metastasis: are they linked phenotypes? *J Cell Biochem* 1994;56:37.
169. Fried W, Kedo A, Barone J. Effects of cyclophosphamide and of busulfan on spleen colony-forming units and on hematopoietic stroma. *Cancer Res* 1977;37:1205.
170. Borison HL, Brand ED, Orland RK. Emetic action of nitrogen mustard in dogs and cats. *Am J Physiol* 1968;192:410.
171. Fetting JH, McCarthy LE, Borison HL, Colvin M. Vomiting induced by cyclophosphamide and phosphoramide mustard in cats. *Cancer Treat Rep* 1982;66:1625.
172. Spitzer TR, Grunberg SM, Dicato MA. Antiemetic strategies for high-dose chemoradiotherapy-induced nausea and vomiting. *Support Care Cancer* 1998;6:233.
173. Bauduer F, Coiffier B, Desablens B. Granisetron plus or minus alprazolam for emesis prevention in chemotherapy of lymphomas: a randomized multicenter trial. *Leuk Lymphoma* 1999;34:341.
174. Spitz S. The histological effects of nitrogen mustards on human tumors and tissues. *Cancer* 1948;1:383.
175. Miller DG. Alkylating agents and human spermatogenesis. *JAMA* 1971;217:1662.
176. Sherins RJ, DeVita VT Jr. Effect of drug treatment for lymphoma on male reproductive capacity. Studies of men in remission after therapy. *Ann Intern Med* 1973;79:216.
177. Blake DA, Heller RH, Hsu SH, Schacter BZ. Return of fertility in a patient with cyclophosphamide-induced azoospermia. *Johns Hopkins Med J* 1976;139:20.
178. Hinkes E, Plotkin D. Reversible drug-induced sterility in a patient with acute leukemia. *JAMA* 1490;223:1490.

179. Galton DAG, Till M, Wiltshaw E. Busulfan (1,4-dimethanesulfonyloxybutane, Myeleran): summary of clinical results. *Ann N Y Acad Sci* 1958;68:967.

180. Rose DP, Davis TE. Ovarian function in patients receiving adjuvant chemotherapy for breast cancer. *Lancet* 1977;1:1174.

181. Koyama H, Wada T, Nishizawa Y, Iwanaga T, Aoki Y. Cyclophosphamide-induced ovarian failure and its therapeutic significance in patients with breast cancer. *Cancer* 1403;39:1403.

182. Oliner H, Schwartz R, Rubio FJ. Interstitial pulmonary fibrosis following busulfan therapy. *Am J Med* 1961;31:134.

183. Codling BW, Chakera TM. Pulmonary fibrosis following therapy with melphalan for multiple myeloma. *J Clin Pathol* 1972;25:668.

184. Cole SR, Myers TJ, Klatsky AU. Pulmonary disease with chlorambucil therapy. *Cancer* 1978;41:455.

185. Mark GJ, Lehimgar-Zadeh A, Ragsdale BD. Cyclophosphamide pneumonitis. *Thorax* 1978;33:89.

186. Patel AR, Shah PC, Rhee HL, Sassoon H, Rao KP. Cyclophosphamide therapy and interstitial pulmonary fibrosis. *Cancer* 1976;38:1542.

187. Orwoll ES, Kiessling PJ, Patterson JR. Interstitial pneumonia from mitomycin. *Ann Intern Med* 1978;89(3):352.

188. Bailey CC, Marsden HB, Jones PH. Fatal pulmonary fibrosis following 1,3-bis(2-chloroethyl)-1-nitrosourea (BCNU) therapy. *Cancer* 1978;42:74.

189. Holoye PY, Jenkins DE, Greenberg SD. Pulmonary toxicity in long-term administration of BCNU. *Cancer Treat Rep* 1976;60:1691.

190. Litam JP, Dail DH, Spitzer G, et al. Early pulmonary toxicity after administration of high-dose BCNU. *Cancer Treat Rep* 1981;65:39.

191. Wilczynski SW, Erasmus JJ, Petros WP, Vredenburgh JJ, Folz RJ. Delayed pulmonary toxicity syndrome following high-dose chemotherapy and bone marrow transplantation for breast cancer. *Am J Respir Crit Care Med* 1998;157:565.

192. Colvin M, Cowens JW, Brundrett RB, Kramer BS, Ludlum DB. Decomposition of BCNU (1,3-bis(2-chloroethyl)-1-nitrosourea) in aqueous solution. *Biochem Biophys Res Commun* 1974;60:515.

193. Vijayan VK, Sankaran K. Relationship between lung inflammation, changes in lung function and severity of exposure in victims of the Bhopal tragedy. *Eur Respir J* 1977;9:1977.

194. Bierman HR, Kelly KH, Knudson AG Jr, Maekawa T, Timmis GM. The influence of 1,4-dimethylsulfonoxy-1,4-dimethylbutane (CB 2348, dimethylmyeleran) in neoplastic disease. *Ann N Y Acad Sci* 1968;68:1211.

195. Feil VJ, Lamoureux CH. Alopecia activity of cyclophosphamide metabolites and related compounds in sheep. *Cancer Res* 1974;34:2596.

196. Bodenstein D, Goldin A. A comparison of the effects of various nitrogen mustard compounds on embryonic cells. *J Exp Zool* 1948;108:75.

197. Murphy ML, Del Moro A, Lacon C. The comparative effects of five polyfunctional alkylating agents on the rat fetus, with additional notes on the chick embryo. *Ann N Y Acad Sci* 1958;68:762.

198. Hales BF. Effects of phosphoramide mustard and acrolein, cytotoxic metabolites of cyclophosphamide, on mouse limb development in vitro. *Teratology* 1989;40:11.

199. Mirkes PE. Cyclophosphamide teratogenesis: a review. *Teratog Carcinog Mutagen* 1985;5:75.

200. Nicholson HO. Cytotoxic drugs in pregnancy. Review of reported cases. *J Obstet Gynaecol Br Comm* 1968;75:307.

201. Lergier JE, Jimenez E, Maldonado N, Veray F. Normal pregnancy in multiple myeloma treated with cyclophosphamide. *Cancer* 1974;34:1018.

202. Ortega J. Multiple agent chemotherapy including bleomycin of non-Hodgkin's lymphoma during pregnancy. *Cancer* 1977;40:2829.

203. Reichman BS, Green KB. Breast cancer in young women: effect of chemotherapy on ovarian function, fertility, and birth defects. *J Natl Cancer Inst Monogr* 1994;16:125.

204. Aviles A, Diaz-Maqueo JC, Talavera A, Guzman R, Garcia EL. Growth and development of children of mothers treated with chemotherapy during pregnancy: current status of 43 children. *Am J Hematol* 1991;36:243.

205. Hochberg MC, Shulman LE. Acute leukemia following cyclophosphamide therapy for Sjögren's syndrome. *Johns Hopkins Med J* 1978;142:211.

206. Rosner F, Grunwald H. Multiple myeloma terminating in acute leukemia. Report of 12 cases and review of the literature. *Am J Med* 1974;57:927.

207. Rosner F, Grunwald H. Hodgkin's disease and acute leukemia. Report of eight cases and review of the literature. *Am J Med* 1975;58:339.

208. Einhorn N. Acute leukemia after chemotherapy (melphalan). *Cancer* 1978;41:444.

209. Reimer RR, Hoover R, Fraumeni JF Jr, Young RC. Acute leukemia after alkylating-agent therapy of ovarian cancer. *N Engl J Med* 1977;297:177.

210. Greene MH, Harris EL, Gershenson DM, et al. Melphalan may be a more potent leukemogen than cyclophosphamide. *Ann Intern Med* 1986;105:360.

211. Einhorn N, Eklund G, Lambert B. Solid tumours and chromosome aberrations as late side effects of melphalan therapy in ovarian carcinoma. *Acta Oncol* 1988;27:215.

212. Tucker MA, Coleman CN, Cox RS, Varghese A, Rosenberg SA. Risk of second cancers after treatment for Hodgkin's disease. *N Engl J Med* 1988;318:76.

213. Hektoen L, Corper HJ. The effect of mustard gas (dichloroethylsulphide) on antibody formation. *J Infect Dis* 1921;28:279.

214. Makinodan T, Santos GW, Quinn RP. Immunosuppressive drugs. *Pharmacol Rev* 1970;22:189.

215. Barratt TM, Soothill JF. Controlled trial of cyclophosphamide in steroid-sensitive relapsing nephrotic syndrome of childhood. *Lancet* 1970;2:479.

216. Laros RKJ, Penner JA. "Refractory" thrombocytopenic purpura treated successfully with cyclophosphamide. *JAMA* 1971;215:445.

217. Kleta R. Cyclophosphamide and mercaptoethane sulfonate therapy for minimal lesion glomerulonephritis. *Kidney Int* 1999;56:2312.

218. Bargman JM. Management of minimal lesion glomerulonephritis: evidence-based recommendations. *Kidney Int* 1999;55[Suppl 70]:S3.

219. Ozer H, Cowens JW, Colvin M, Nussbaum-Blumenson A, Sheedy D. In vitro effects of 4-hydroperoxycyclophosphamide on human immunoregulatory T subset function: I. Selective effects on lymphocyte function in T-B cell collaboration. *J Exp Med* 1982;155:276.

220. Smith JJ, Mihich E, Ozer H. In vitro effects of 4-hydroperoxycyclophosphamide on human immunoregulatory T subset function. *Methods Find Exp Clin Pharmacol* 1987;9(9):555.

221. Mokyr MB, Colvin M, Dray S. Cyclophosphamide-mediated enhancement of antitumor immune potential of immunosuppressed spleen cells from mice bearing a large MOPC-315 tumor. *Int J Immunopharmacol* 1985;7:111.

222. Dray S, Mokyr MB. Cyclophosphamide and melphalan as immunopotentiating agents in cancer therapy. *Med Oncol Tumor Pharmacother* 1989;6:77.

223. Berd D, Mastrangelo MJ. Effect of low dose cyclophosphamide on the immune system of cancer patients: depletion of CD4+, 2H4+ suppressor-inducer T-cells. *Cancer Res* 1988;48:1671.

224. Berd D, Mastrangelo MJ. Active immunotherapy of human melanoma exploiting the immunopotentiating effects of cyclophosphamide. *Cancer Invest* 1988;6:337.

225. Nousari HC, Brodsky RA, Jones RJ, Grever MR, Anhalt GJ. Immunoablative high-dose cyclophosphamide without stem cell rescue in paraneoplastic pemphigus: report of a case and review of this new therapy for severe autoimmune disease. *J Am Acad Dermatol* 1999;40:750.

STEVEN W. JOHNSON
PETER J. O'DWYER

SECTION 5

Cisplatin and Its Analogues

The platinum drugs represent a unique and important class of antitumor compounds. Alone or in combination with other chemotherapeutic agents, *cis*-diamminedichloroplatinum (II) (cisplatin) and its analogues have made a significant impact on the treatment of a variety of solid tumors for nearly 30 years. The unique activity and toxicity profile observed with cisplatin in early clinical trials fueled the development of platinum analogues that are less toxic and more active against a variety of tumor types, including those that have developed resistance to cisplatin. In addition to cisplatin, two other platinum complexes are currently approved for use in the United States: *cis*-diam-

minecyclobutanedicarboxylato platinum (II) (carboplatin) and 1,2-diaminocyclohexaneoxalato platinum (II) (oxaliplatin). In addition to these, several other analogues with unique activities are in various stages of clinical development. Continued progress in the development of superior analogues requires a thorough understanding of the chemical, biologic, pharmacokinetic, and pharmacodynamic properties of this important class of drugs. A review of these properties is the focus of this chapter.

HISTORY

The realization that platinum complexes exhibited antitumor activity began somewhat serendipitously in a series of experiments carried out by Dr. Barnett Rosenberg and colleagues beginning in 1961.[1] These studies involved determining the effect of electromagnetic radiation on the growth of bacteria in a chamber equipped with a set of platinum electrodes. Exposure of the bacteria to an electric field resulted in a profound change in their morphology, in particular, the appearance of long filaments that were several hundred times longer than that of their unexposed counterparts. This effect was not due directly to the electric field, but to the electrolysis products produced by the platinum electrodes. An analysis of these products revealed that the predominant species was ammonium chloroplatinate $[NH_4]_2[PtCl_6]$. This compound was inactive in reproducing the filamentous growth originally observed; however, Rosenberg and colleagues soon discovered that the conversion of this complex to a neutral species by ultraviolet light resulted in an active species. Attempts to synthesize the active neutral platinum complex failed. They realized, however, that the neutral compound could exist in two isomeric forms, *cis* or *trans*, and the latter species is the one that they had synthesized. Subsequently, the *cis* isomer was synthesized and shown to be the active compound.

The observation that *cis*-diamminedichloroplatinum (II) and *cis*-diamminetetrachloroplatinum (IV) inhibited bacterial growth led to the testing of four neutral platinum compounds for antineoplastic activity in mice bearing the Sarcoma-180 solid tumor and L1210 leukemia cells.[2] All four compounds showed significant antitumor activity, with *cis*-diamminedichloroplatinum (II) exhibiting the most efficacy. Further studies in other tumor models confirmed these results and indicated that cisplatin exhibited a broad spectrum of activity. Although early clinical trials demonstrated significant activity against several tumor types, particularly testicular cancers, the severe renal and gastrointestinal toxicity caused by the drug nearly led to its abandonment. Cvitkovic and colleagues[3,4] showed that these effects could be ameliorated, in part, by aggressive prehydration, which rekindled interest in its clinical use. Currently, cisplatin is curative in testicular cancer and significantly prolongs survival in combination regimens for ovarian cancer. The drug also has therapeutic benefit in head and neck, bladder, and lung cancer.[5] Continued study is demonstrating activity in other tumors as well.

PLATINUM CHEMISTRY

Platinum exists primarily in either a 2+ or 4+ oxidation state. These oxidation states dictate the stereochemistry of the carrier ligands and leaving groups surrounding the platinum atom. Platinum (II) compounds exhibit a square planar geometry, whereas platinum (IV) compounds exhibit an octahedral geometry. Interconversion of the two oxidation states may readily occur; however, the kinetics of this reaction depend on the nature of the bound ligands. The nature of the ligands also determines the stability of the complex and the rate of substitution. For platinum (II) compounds, the rate of substitution of a ligand is strongly influenced by the type of ligand located opposite to it. Therefore, ligands that are bound more strongly will stabilize the moieties that are situated *trans* to it. For *cis*-diamminedichloroplatinum (II), the two chloride ligands are prone to substitution, whereas substitution of the amino groups is thermodynamically unfavorable.[6] The stereochemistry of platinum complexes is critical to their antitumor activity as evidenced by the significantly reduced efficacy observed with *trans*-diamminedichloroplatinum (II).

In aqueous solution, the chloride leaving groups of cisplatin are subject to mono- and diaqua substitution, particularly at chloride concentrations below 100 mmol, which exist intracellularly. The equilibria may be described by the following two equations:

$$cis\text{-}(NH_3)_2PtCl_2 + H_2O \leftrightarrows Cl^- + cis\text{-}(NH_3)_2PtCl(H_2O)^+$$

$$cis\text{-}(NH_3)_2PtCl(H_2O)^+ + H_2O \leftrightarrows Cl^- + cis\text{-}(NH_3)_2Pt(H_2O)_2^{2+}$$

where equilibrium constants for each reaction may be written:

$$K_1 = \frac{[Cl^-][cis\text{-}(NH_3)_2PtCl(H_2O)^+]}{[cis\text{-}(NH_3)_2PtCl_2]} \text{ and}$$

$$K_2 = \frac{[Cl^-][cis\text{-}(NH_3)_2Pt(H_2O)_2^{2+}]}{[cis\text{-}(NH_3)_2PtCl(H_2O)^+]}$$

These descriptions illustrate the key role of ambient chloride concentrations in determining aquation rates. In weakly acidic solutions, the monochloromonoaqua and diaqua complexes become deprotonated to form the neutral dihydroxo species. The monohydroxo and dihydroxo complexes are the predominant species present in low chloride-containing environments such as the nucleus. A detailed analysis of the equations and rate constants that govern these reactions has now been published.[7] Based on studies of the reaction of cisplatin metabolites with inosine, the predominant cisplatin species that react with DNA are likely to be the chloroaqua and hydroxoaqua species.[7]

NOVEL PLATINUM COMPLEXES

Early in the clinical development of cisplatin it became clear that its toxicity was a barrier to widespread acceptance and that its activity, although striking in certain diseases, did not extend to all cancers. These observations simultaneously gave rise to approaches to modifying toxicity and to the search for structural analogues with activity in cisplatin-resistant tumor models. In addition to stimulation of the development of antiemetics and other supportive care measures for use with cisplatin, structural modifications in the molecule were sought to alter the tissue distribution. Progress in understanding the chemistry and pharmacokinetics of cisplatin has guided the development of new analogues. In general, modification of the chloride leaving groups of cisplatin results in compounds with different pharmacokinetics, whereas modification of the carrier ligands alters the activity of the resulting complex. This section summarizes the features of the more important platinum analogues that have been developed, which are shown in Figure 15.5-1.

CARBOPLATIN

Substitution of the chloride leaving groups of cisplatin resulted in compounds with diminished nephrotoxicity but equivalent activity. Using a murine screen for nephrotoxicity, it was discovered that substituting a cyclobutanedicarboxylate moiety for the two chloride ligands of cisplatin resulted in a complex with reduced renal toxicity. This observation was translated to the clinic in the form of carboplatin, a more stable and pharmacokinetically predictable analogue.[8,9] The results in humans were accurately predicted by the animal models, and marrow toxicity rather than nephrotoxicity was the principal side effect. At effective doses,

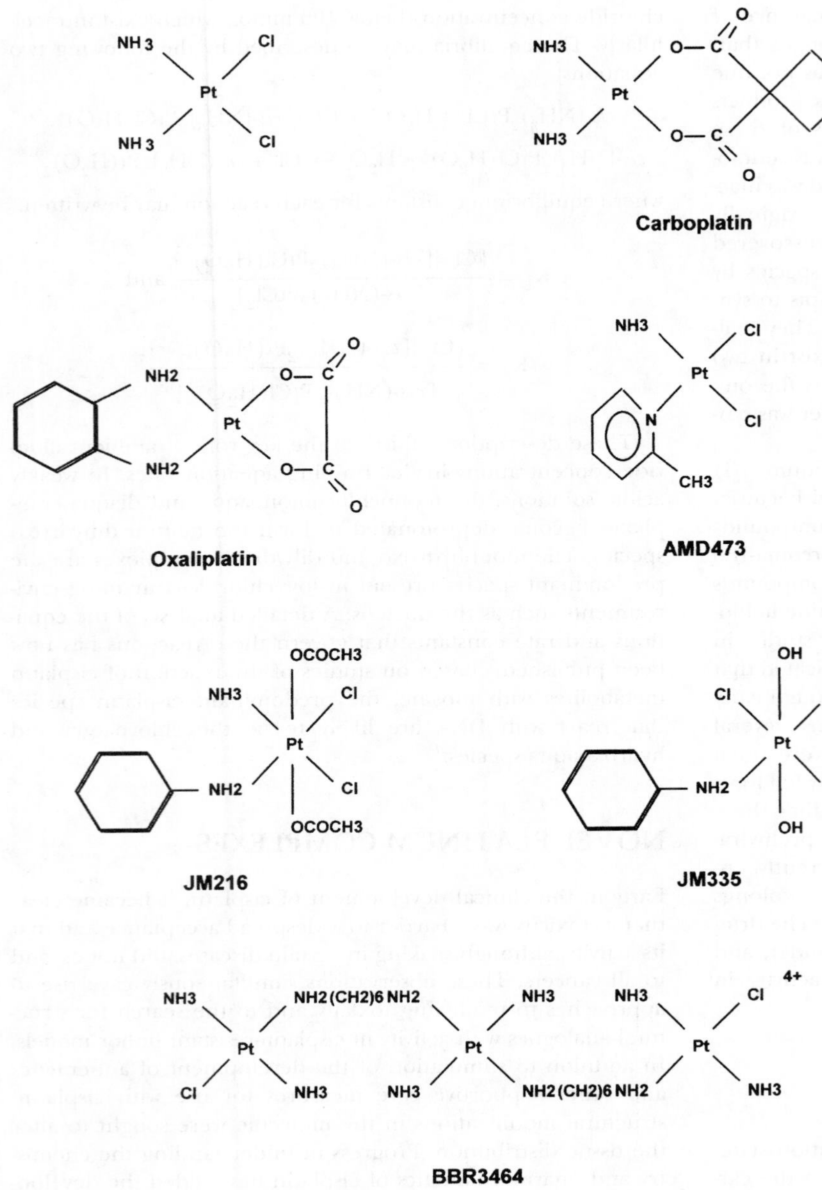

FIGURE 15.5-1. Structures of cisplatin and analogues.

carboplatin produced less nausea, vomiting, nephrotoxicity, and neurotoxicity than cisplatin. Furthermore, the myelosuppression was closely associated with the pharmacokinetics. The work of Calvert et al.[10] and Egorin and colleagues[11] showed that toxicity can be made more predictable and dose intensity less variable by dosing strategies based on the exposure. Carboplatin was shown to be indistinguishable from cisplatin in its clinical activity in all but a handful of tumor types and is the most frequently used form of platinum in current use.

1,2-DIAMINOCYCLOHEXANE DERIVATIVES

Compounds with activity in cisplatin-resistant models emerged from modifications to the carrier group (left side of the analogues in Fig. 15.5-1). The pioneer in this field was Dr. Tom Connors, who in the late 1960s synthesized platinum coordination compounds with varying physicochemical characteristics and found

that the series that possessed a diaminocyclohexane (DACH) carrier group was active in cell culture models of cancer.[12] Burchenal et al. provided *in vivo* confirmation that these structures were indeed active in solid tumors and leukemias in which cisplatin had little or no activity.[13] Subsequent *in vitro* studies supported the idea that DACH-based platinum complexes were non–cross-resistant in cisplatin-resistant cell lines.[14,15] In support of these studies, Rixe et al.[16] showed that DACH derivatives exhibited a unique cytotoxicity profile compared to cisplatin and carboplatin using the National Cancer Institute 60 cell line screen.

An early analogue that was developed out of this work was tetraplatin (ormaplatin), which underwent a relatively slow development over the next 20 years, culminating in phase I trials in the early 1990s. The severe neurotoxicity of the agent led to its abandonment. Attention had already focused, however, on another DACH analogue that had been synthesized by Kidani and colleagues in the early 1970s and had undergone a similarly slow gestation into the clinic. Oxaliplatin, a coordination compound of a DACH carrier group and an oxalato leaving group, is substantially less lipophilic than tetraplatin but retains the latter's spectrum of activity in cisplatin-resistant tumor models. Like cisplatin, oxaliplatin preferentially forms adducts at the N7 position of guanine and to a lesser extent adenine. However, there is evidence that the three-dimensional structure of the DNA adducts and biologic response(s) they elicit are different from those of cisplatin. Oxaliplatin was first studied in two phase I trials in which suitable doses and schedules were determined, and an early hint of colorectal cancer activity was identified.[17,18] Oxaliplatin demonstrated activity in combination with 5-fluorouracil and leucovorin in colon cancer, a disease that was previously considered to be unresponsive to platinum drugs.[19] There followed a series of consistent phase II and III clinical trial results showing the activity of oxaliplatin in colorectal cancer. Oxaliplatin is now approved for the first-line treatment of advanced colorectal cancer, and preliminary data indicate that it improves the survival of patients with stage II and III disease when used in the adjuvant setting. The potential of oxaliplatin in other diseases is at an early stage of exploration, and additional therapeutic applications may emerge.

PLATINUM (IV) STRUCTURES

The octahedral stereochemistry adopted by platinum (IV) compounds has led investigators to speculate that they may exhibit a different spectrum of activity than that of platinum (II) drugs. Two compounds that have been tested clinically without much success are ormaplatin and iproplatin. Ormaplatin was neurotoxic in phase I trials, and iproplatin failed to demonstrate activity in phase II trials.[20–22] More recently, two platinum (IV) compounds, JM216 [bis(acetato)amminedichloro(cyclohexylamine) platinum (IV)] and JM335 [*trans*-ammine(cyclohexylamine)dichlorodihydroxo platinum (IV)], have been developed and contain several unique features.[23] These compounds may also be classified as mixed amines or ammine-amine platinum (IV) complexes. JM216 is the first orally active platinum compound; it has undergone extensive clinical testing in phase II and III trials.[24,25] Some activity has been noted in lung cancer (small cell and non–small cell) and in ovarian cancer, but more marked activity has been associated with its use in prostate cancer. A small, randomized trial involving 50 patients suggested a benefit for the combination of JM216 (now called satraplatin) and prednisone over prednisone alone in hormone-resistant disease.[26] A definitive phase III trial is under way for this indication.

Based on the lack of antitumor activity of transplatin [*trans*-diamminedichloroplatinum (II)], it has been generally believed that most, if not all, *trans* platinum compounds were inactive. Renewed interest in *trans* compounds has occurred, however, with the observation that JM335 and a related group of complexes exhibited significant antitumor activity in murine ADJ/PC6 and human ovarian cancer models.[23] Siddik and colleagues[27] have also produced *trans* platinum (IV) compounds containing the DACH moiety, which they demonstrated to be non–cross-resistant to cisplatin.

MULTINUCLEAR PLATINUM COMPLEXES

An approach based on the chemistry of the platinum-DNA interaction led to design and synthesis by Farrell et al.[28] of a novel class of compounds containing multiple platinum atoms (see Fig. 15.5-1). These bi- and trinuclear structures form adducts that span greater distances across the minor groove of DNA and have a profile of cell kill that differs from that of the small molecules. These compounds are unique in that their interaction with DNA is considerably different from that of cisplatin, particularly in the abundance of interstrand cross-links formed. Also, the observation that multinuclear platinum complexes containing the *trans* geometry exhibit antitumor activity contradicts the original dogma that platinum drugs containing the *trans* geometry are inactive. Currently, the lead compound in this class of drugs is BBR3464. Its structure is described as two *trans*-$[PtCl(NH_3)_2]^+$ units linked together by a noncovalent tetraamine $\{Pt(NH_3)_2[H_2N(CH_2)_6NH_2]_2\}^{2+}$ unit. Preclinical testing of BBR3464 shows it to be significantly more potent than cisplatin and to be active in cisplatin-resistant xenografts and p53 mutant tumors. Information on the clinical activity of BBR3464 awaits the completion of phase II trials.

OTHER PLATINUM COMPLEXES

Efforts have been made to design novel platinum analogues that can circumvent known cisplatin resistance mechanisms. An example of this is *cis*-amminedichloro(2-methylpyridine) platinum (II) (also known as *AMD473* and *ZD0473*). This compound is a sterically hindered platinum complex that was designed to have minimal reactivity with thiols and thus avoid inactivation by molecules such as glutathione.[29,30] A number of platinum drugs are in clinical trials, and there is interest in defining a profile different from that of the currently approved agents. ZD0473 was studied in phase I and had but brief phase II trials.[31,32] Responses were identified with its use, and myelosuppression was dose limiting. Other toxicities were mild with this agent. Continuing clinical research is likely. A major goal of current research is to identify the molecular characteristics of tumors that predispose them to response to one or another of the analogues. This information can then be used to refine and individualize treatment.

MECHANISM OF ACTION

DNA ADDUCT FORMATION

The observation by Rosenberg[1] that cisplatin induces filamentous growth in bacteria without affecting RNA and protein synthesis implicated DNA as the cytotoxic target of the drug. Evidence from several subsequent experiments supported this idea.[33–37] The differential cytotoxic effects observed with platinum drugs are determined, in part, by the structure and relative amount of DNA adducts formed. Cisplatin and its analogues react preferentially at the N7 position of guanine and adenine residues to form a variety of monofunctional and bifunctional adducts.[38] The first step of the reaction involves the formation of monoadducts. These monoadducts may then react further to form intrastrand or interstrand cross-links. The predominate bidentate lesions that are formed with DNA *in vitro* or in cultured cells are the d(GpG)Pt, d(ApG)Pt, and d(GpNpG)Pt intrastrand cross-links. Cisplatin also forms interstrand cross-links between guanine residues located on opposite strands that account for fewer than 5% of the total DNA-bound platinum.

These adducts may contribute to the drug's cytotoxicity because they impede certain cellular processes that require the separation of both DNA strands, such as replication and transcription.

The adducts that are formed in the reaction between carboplatin and DNA in cultured cells are essentially the same as those of cisplatin; however, higher concentrations of carboplatin are required (20- to 40-fold for cells) to obtain equivalent total platinum-DNA adduct levels due to its slower rate of aquation.[39] As with cisplatin, a relatively low number of monoadducts and interstrand cross-links are observed. The relative amounts and frequencies of the DNA adducts formed in cultured cells by oxaliplatin has also been examined. Oxaliplatin intrastrand adducts form more slowly due to a slower rate of conversion from monoadducts; however, they are formed at similar DNA sequences and regions as cisplatin adducts. Saris et al.[40] reported that oxaliplatin forms predominantly d(GpG)Pt and d(ApG)Pt intrastrand cross-links *in vitro* and in cultured cells; however, at equitoxic doses, oxaliplatin forms fewer DNA adducts than does cisplatin. This suggests that oxaliplatin lesions are more cytotoxic than those formed by cisplatin.

The differences observed in cytotoxicity between the diammine (e.g., cisplatin, carboplatin) and DACH platinum compounds does not appear to depend on the type and relative amounts of the adducts formed but is more likely due to the overall three-dimensional structure of the adduct and its recognition by various cellular proteins. Structural analysis of the cisplatin d(GpG)Pt intrastrand cross-link has been accomplished by both x-ray crystallography and nuclear magnetic resonance spectroscopy. These studies revealed that the binding of platinum to DNA causes a variety of perturbations in the double helix, including a roll of 26 to 50 degrees between the cross-linked guanine bases, displacement of platinum from the planes of the guanine rings, a bend of the helical axis toward the major groove, and an unwinding of the DNA.[41] Scheeff et al.[42] used computer modeling to demonstrate that oxaliplatin produces a similar DNA bend, base rotation, and base propeller as cisplatin. The major difference, however, is the protrusion of the DACH moiety of oxaliplatin into the major groove of DNA, which thus produces a bulkier adduct than that of cisplatin. This bulkier, more hydrophobic adduct may be recognized differently by a host of cellular proteins involved in sensing DNA damage.[43] The functional consequences of these effects are twofold: Proteins such as polymerases that recognize and participate in reactions on DNA under normal circumstances may be perturbed, whereas processes that are controlled by proteins that recognize damaged DNA may become activated. The latter group of proteins may function in the DNA repair process or in the initiation of programmed cell death.

DAMAGE RECOGNITION, SURVIVAL, AND APOPTOSIS

The sequence of events that leads to cell death after the formation of platinum-DNA adducts has not yet been elucidated; however, cells treated with platinum drugs display the biochemical and morphologic features of apoptosis.[44] These features are common to cells treated with other cytotoxic and biologic agents. Therefore, understanding the pathway(s) that are involved in the early stages of programmed cell death, including the detection-initiation and decision-commitment phases, is important for understanding the unique activities of platinum

drugs. The sensitivity of a cell to a platinum drug depends, in part, on cell cycle. For example, proliferating cells are relatively sensitive, whereas quiescent cells or cells in G_0 or G_1 are relatively insensitive.[45] Thus, it is possible that programmed cell death initiated at various cell-cycle checkpoints is governed by different proteins and signal transduction pathways.

A model for cisplatin-induced cell death has been provided by Sorenson and Eastman.[46] using DNA repair-deficient Chinese hamster ovary (CHO) cells. In these studies, cisplatin-treated CHO/AA8 cells experienced slow progression through S phase and accumulated in G_2. At low drug concentrations, the cells recovered and continued to cycle. At high drug concentrations, the cells died after a protracted G_2 arrest. An aberrant mitosis was observed before apoptosis. Further studies with G_2-synchronized cells revealed that passage through S phase is necessary for G_2 arrest and cell death, which suggests that DNA replication on a damaged template may result in the accumulation of further damage, causing the cells to ultimately die. Abrogating the G_2 checkpoint with pharmacologic agents such as caffeine or 7-hydroxystaurosporine was shown to enhance the cytotoxicity of cisplatin.[47] It is not yet clear how these events specifically transduce a proapoptotic signal; however, the observations provide a valuable framework to begin to elucidate the initial steps.

Dissecting the initiation events that ultimately result in platinum drug-induced apoptosis has proven difficult. One area of investigation that has produced some insight into this process has been the discovery of platinum-DNA damage recognition proteins. The idea that a specific protein or protein complex can bind to a platinum-DNA adduct and transmit a cell death signal has intrigued researchers. Furthermore, mutation or down-regulation of such a protein could result in or lead to the development of platinum drug resistance. Efforts to identify such molecules have resulted in the discovery of several candidates. The first of these were the high-mobility group proteins HMG1 and HMG2.[48-50] These proteins are capable of bending DNA as well as recognizing bent DNA structures, such as that produced by cisplatin. Interestingly, HMG1 has an affinity for adducts formed by cisplatin but not by the inactive transplatin isomer. The HMG domain, which consists of a highly basic 80–amino acid motif, has been found in other proteins, most of which are involved in gene expression.[51] Although a functional role for these proteins in platinum sensitivity and resistance has yet to be conclusively demonstrated, a number of theories have emerged. It has been suggested that HMG domain proteins are responsible for communicating the presence of DNA damage to either the repair machinery or to programmed cell death pathways. Alternatively, the presence of platinum-DNA adducts could sequester HMG domain proteins and thus prevent their normal function or even shield DNA adducts from being properly recognized by other cellular proteins. A definitive role for this class of molecules awaits further study.

A number of other platinum-DNA damage recognition proteins have been identified, including histone H1, RNA polymerase I transcription upstream binding factor (hUBF), the TATA binding protein (TBP), and proteins involved in mismatch repair (MMR). The latter have received significant interest, because the recognition of platinum-DNA adducts by the MMR complex has been implicated in cisplatin sensitivity.[52] Studies have shown that the MSH2 and MLH1 proteins participate in the recognition of DNA adducts formed by cisplatin.[53,54] The presence of a platinum lesion may result in the continuous futile cycle of repair synthesis on the DNA strand opposite the lesion. This could result in the accumulation of DNA strand breaks and ultimately lead to cell death. Interestingly, oxaliplatin adducts are not well recognized by the MMR protein complex, which could account for differences in the cytotoxicity profiles observed between these two platinum complexes.

Although the specific proteins involved in platinum-DNA adduct recognition remain undefined, a number of signaling events have been shown to occur after treatment of a cell with cisplatin.[55] For example, the ATM- and Rad3-related protein (ATR), which is involved in cell-cycle checkpoint activation, is activated by cisplatin. This kinase, in turn, phosphorylates and activates several downstream effectors that regulate cell cycle, DNA repair, cell survival, and apoptosis. These include p53, CHK2, and members of the mitogen-activated protein kinase (MAPK) pathway [extracellular signal-related kinase (ERK), c-Jun amino-terminal kinase (JNK), p38 kinase]. The pleiotropic nature of this stress response only grows, because each of these molecules subsequently controls the activity and expression of many more proteins. As a result of this complexity, it is not surprising that a lack of consistency exists in conclusions drawn by investigators as to the role of these pathways in cell survival and apoptosis. This is also due to the various experimental conditions used, including differences in cell type, treatment, selection of end points, and duration of the effect. As an example, the role of p53 activation in the fate of platinum-treated cells has been a subject of debate. It is well known that p53 function is required for the activation of proapoptotic proteins such as the Bcl-2 family member Bax. However, disruption of p53 function has not always led to an observed decrease in cisplatin sensitivity. Two studies have shown that disrupting p53 function sensitizes cells to cisplatin, rather than causing them to be resistant.[56,57] One explanation for the increased sensitivity in p53-deficient cells is that a concomitant reduction in the cell-cycle inhibitor $p21^{Waf1/Cip1}$ causes cells to progress through G_2 and M unregulated. A premature mitosis may then occur in the presence of DNA damage, which results in cell death.

From these studies, it is apparent that the inherent sensitivity of a cell to any drug is influenced by a variety of factors. With respect to DNA-damaging agents such as cisplatin, the magnitude and duration of an apoptotic signal may be either enhanced or suppressed by the activity of other cellular signaling pathways. Thus, a damage or DNA adduct threshold may exist that is unique to each tumor cell and reflects the overall balance of prosurvival and proapoptotic signals. As the field of signal transduction has grown, so has the number of candidate effectors and pathways that may influence platinum drug sensitivity. The list is large and includes cytokines, growth factors, kinases, phosphatases, second messengers, transcription factors, redox proteins, and extracellular matrix proteins. Some of these molecules attenuate sensitivity only to platinum drugs and DNA-damaging agents, whereas others influence cellular sensitivity to a variety of unrelated chemotherapeutic drugs.

Some insight into the role of signaling in platinum drug sensitivity has been provided in studies using activators or inhibitors of known signal transduction pathways. For example, treatment of various cell lines with tamoxifen, epidermal growth factor, interleukin-1α, tumor necrosis factor-α, bombesin, and rapamycin enhances cisplatin cytotoxicity.[58–62] Also, the expression of certain protooncogenes, including *Ha-Ras*, *v-abl*, and *Her2/neu*, has been shown in some instances to promote cell survival after cisplatin exposure.[63–66] As mentioned earlier, members of the ERK/MAPK family as well as their upstream activators have been implicated in these events. The JNK/stress-activated protein kinase (SAPK) and p38 kinase pathways have been shown to be activated by a variety of environmental stimuli and inflammatory cytokines.[67] JNK/SAPK and p38 phosphorylate and regulate the activity of the ATF2 and Elk-1 transcription factors. JNK/SAPK also phosphorylates c-Jun, a component of the AP-1 transcription factor complex, on serine residues 63 and 73. There is considerable evidence to suggest that these protein kinases are involved in transmitting a drug-induced cell death signal. For example, Zanke et al.[68] demonstrated that in mouse fibroblasts, the inhibition of JNK phosphorylation by the stable transfection of a dominant-negative complementary DNA encoding SEK1, the protein kinase responsible for activating JNK, resulted in reduced sensitivity to cisplatin. Sanchez-Perez et al.[69] observed a prolonged activation of JNK by cisplatin that was related to cell death. Modulating the activity of kinases upstream of JNK, including c-Abl, MKK3/MKK6, MEKK1, and ASK1, also influences cellular drug sensitivity.[70] For example, Chen et al.[71] demonstrated that overexpression of a dominant-negative ASK1, which inhibits activation of JNK, resulted in an inhibition of cisplatin-induced apoptosis. Clearly, activation of these pathways occurs after drug exposure in some cells, and it is important to understand the contribution of these intracellular signaling events to overall platinum drug sensitivity.

MECHANISMS OF RESISTANCE

The major limitation to the successful treatment of solid tumors with platinum-based chemotherapy is the emergence of drug-resistant tumor cells.[55,72] Platinum drug resistance may be intrinsic or acquired and may occur through multiple mechanisms (Fig. 15.5-2). These mechanisms may be classified into two major groups: (1) those that limit the formation of cytotoxic platinum-DNA adducts, and (2) those that prevent cell death from occurring after platinum-DNA adduct formation. The first group of mechanisms includes decreased drug accumulation and increased drug inactivation by cellular protein and nonprotein thiols. The second group of mechanisms includes increased platinum-DNA adduct repair and increased platinum-DNA damage tolerance. Despite progress in the identification of specific proteins that are involved in platinum drug resistance, their relevance to clinical resistance remains to be defined. This is an important area of investigation, because the understanding of the molecular basis of the drug-resistant phenotype will lead to the development of reversal strategies.

REDUCED ACCUMULATION

The majority of cell lines that have been selected for cisplatin resistance *in vitro* exhibit a decreased platinum accumulation phenotype, and it is generally believed that this is due to decreased drug uptake rather than enhanced drug efflux. Cisplatin and its analogues may accumulate within cells by passive diffusion or facilitated transport.[73] Cisplatin uptake has been shown to be nonsaturable, even up to its solubility limit, and

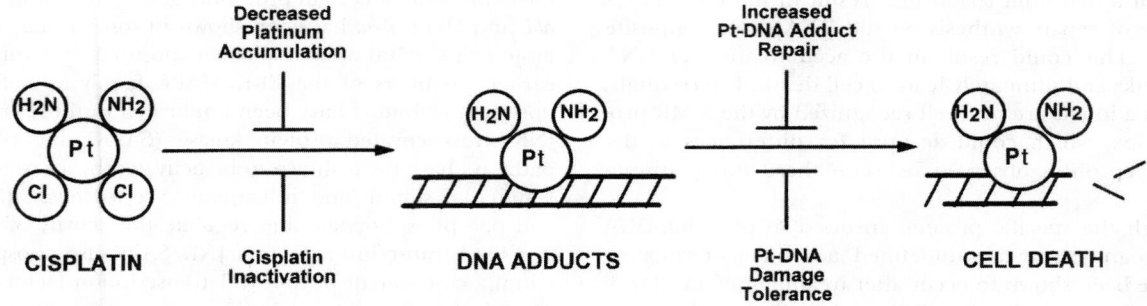

FIGURE 15.5-2. Cellular mechanisms of cisplatin resistance.

not inhibited by structural analogues. Carrier-mediated transport is supported by the observation that uptake is partially energy dependent, ouabain inhibitable, sodium dependent, and influenced by membrane potential and cyclic adenosine monophosphate levels. Although a specific human transporter has yet to be identified, progress has been made with respect to the identification of a copper transporter that can shuttle cisplatin into cells. In a study by Lin et al.[74] using a yeast model, the copper transporter CTR1 was shown to regulate the influx of cisplatin, carboplatin, oxaliplatin, and AMD473. Comparison of the wild-type and ctr-1 knockout strains revealed an eightfold reduction in cisplatin uptake after 1 hour. These ctr-1–deficient yeast cells were also twofold more resistant to cisplatin. These results increase the likelihood that analogous carrier-mediated transport pathways exist in human cells.

The prospect of an active efflux mechanism for platinum drugs has emerged after the discovery of a group of MRP-related transport proteins. MRP is a member of the ABC (adenosine triphosphate–binding cassette) family of transport proteins that participates in the extrusion of glutathione-coupled and unmodified anticancer drugs from cells.[75] Overexpression of MRP confers resistance to a variety of drugs, but not to cisplatin. For platinum complexes, the formation of a glutathione-platinum drug conjugate may be the rate-limiting step for producing an MRP substrate. The MRP homologue cMOAT (cannalicular multispecific organic anion transporter) shares 49% amino acid sequence identity and a similar substrate specificity with MRP. Taniguchi et al.[76] showed that cMOAT (MRP2) is overexpressed in some cisplatin-resistant human cancer cell lines exhibiting a decreased platinum accumulation phenotype. This group also demonstrated that transfection of an antisense cMOAT complementary DNA into HepG2 cells results in decreased cMOAT protein levels and a five-fold increase in cisplatin sensitivity.[77] Kool et al.[78] examined the expression of MRP, cMOAT, and three other MRP homologues (MRP3, MRP4, and MRP5) in a set of cell lines selected for cisplatin resistance *in vitro*. MRP1 and MRP4 messenger RNA levels were not increased in any of the cisplatin-resistant sublines. MRP3 and MRP5 were overexpressed in a few cell lines, but the messenger RNA levels were not associated with cisplatin resistance. In contrast, cMOAT was significantly overexpressed in some of the cisplatin-resistant cell lines. With respect to clinical relevance, an immunohistochemical analysis of the expression of P glycoprotein, MRP1, and MRP2 revealed that none of these transporters was associated with response to platinum-based chemotherapy in ovarian cancer.[79] Another class of proteins that is involved in the sequestration and efflux of platinum drugs is the copper-trans-

porting P-type adenosine triphosphatases 7A and 7B (ATP7A, ATP7B). Transfection of epidermoid carcinoma cells with ATP7B led to a ninefold decrease in cisplatin sensitivity.[80] Howell's group has confirmed this and demonstrated that acquired cisplatin resistance is accompanied by increased expression of these export pumps.[81,82] This group also found that increased expression of ATP7A is associated with poor survival in ovarian cancer patients treated with platinum-based regimens.[83]

INACTIVATION

The formation of conjugates between glutathione and platinum drugs may be an important step in their inactivation and elimination from the cell. For many years, investigators have attempted to make positive correlations between platinum drug sensitivity, glutathione levels, and the relative expression of the enzymes involved in glutathione metabolism. There have been many reports showing a strong association between platinum drug sensitivity and glutathione levels[84–87]; however, reducing intracellular glutathione levels with drugs such as buthionine sulfoximine has resulted in only low to modest potentiation of cisplatin sensitivity.[88,89] Part of the reason for this may be due to the fact that the formation of glutathione-platinum conjugates is a slow process.[90] The formation of a glutathione-platinum complex, however, has been reported to occur in cultured cells, and glutathione has been shown to quench platinum-DNA monoadducts *in vitro*, preventing them from being converted to potentially cytotoxic cross-links.[91–93] Another nonprotein thiol that has been implicated in cisplatin resistance is cysteinylglycine. This product is generated during glutathione catabolism by γ-glutamyltransferase. The affinity of cysteinylglycine for cisplatin is significantly higher than that of glutathione, and transfection studies have demonstrated that overexpression of γ-glutamyltransferase confers resistance to cisplatin.[94] One unresolved question is whether the intracellular reaction of platinum drugs with glutathione is catalyzed by glutathione S-transferases (GSTs). In support of this, a three-fold increase in cisplatin resistance was reported in CHO cells transfected with the GSTπ isoenzyme.[95] In contrast, transfection of NIH3T3 cells with GSTπ resulted in hypersensitivity to cisplatin.[96] Studies attempting to associate GST activity with cisplatin sensitivity in cell lines and tumor biopsy specimens have failed to consistently show a positive correlation between GST expression or activity and cisplatin sensitivity.[86–88,97]

Inactivation of the platinum drugs may also occur through binding to the metallothionein (MT) proteins. The MTs are a family of sulfhydryl-rich, low-molecular-weight proteins that participate in heavy metal binding and detoxification. *In vitro*, cisplatin binds stoichiometrically to MT, and up to ten molecules of cisplatin can be bound to one molecule of MT.[98] Kelley et al.[99] demonstrated that overexpression of the full-length MT-II$_A$ in mouse C127 cells conferred a fourfold resistance to cisplatin. Furthermore, this group showed that embryonic fibroblasts isolated from MT-null mice were hypersensitive to cisplatin.[100] These studies clearly show that modulating MT levels can alter cisplatin sensitivity; however, the contribution of MT to clinical platinum drug resistance is unclear. In some cell lines, elevated MT levels have been shown to be associated with cisplatin resistance, whereas in others, they have not.[86,101] Studies with human tumors has shown that, in some instances, MT expression level is associated with response to chemotherapy. For example, a significant correlation between MT overexpression, and response and survival was reported in urothelial transitional cell carcinoma patients.[102] Overexpression of MT has also been observed in bladder tumors from patients for whom cisplatin chemotherapy failed.[103]

INCREASED DNA REPAIR

Once platinum-DNA adducts are formed, cells must either repair or tolerate the damage to survive. The capacity to rapidly and efficiently repair DNA damage clearly plays a role in determining a tumor cell's sensitivity to platinum drugs and other DNA-damaging agents. There is evidence to suggest that cell lines derived from tumors that are unusually sensitive to cisplatin, such as testicular nonseminomatous germ cell tumors, are deficient in their ability to repair platinum-DNA adducts.[104] Increased repair of platinum-DNA lesions in cisplatin-resistant cell lines as compared to their sensitive counterparts has been shown in several human cancer cell lines, including ovarian,[105,106] breast,[107] and glioma,[108] as well as murine leukemia cell lines.[109] Evidence for increased repair of cisplatin interstrand cross-links in specific gene and nongene regions in cisplatin-resistant cell lines has also been demonstrated. These studies have been done using a variety of *in vivo* methods, including unscheduled DNA synthesis, host cell reactivation of cisplatin-damaged plasmid DNA, atomic absorption spectrometry, quantitative polymerase chain reaction, and renaturing agarose gel electrophoresis.

The repair of platinum-DNA adducts occurs predominantly by nucleotide excision repair (NER); however, the molecular basis for the increased repair activity observed in cisplatin-resistant cells is unknown.[110] Because the rate-limiting step in this process is platinum adduct recognition and incision, increased expression of the proteins that control this step are likely to enhance NER activity. Using an *in vitro* assay, Ferry et al.[111] demonstrated that the addition of the ERCC1/XPF protein complex increased the platinum-DNA adduct excision activity of an ovarian cancer cell extract. There is also circumstantial evidence that implicates *ERCC1* expression in increased NER and cisplatin resistance. For example, expression levels of the *ERCC1* and *XPA* genes have been shown to be higher in malignant tissue from ovarian cancer patients resistant to platinum-based therapy than in tissue from those responsive to treatment.[112] *ERCC1* expression has also been shown to correlate with NER activity and cisplatin resistance in human ovarian cancer cells.[111] Increased levels of XPE, a putative DNA repair protein

that recognizes many DNA lesions including platinum-DNA adducts, has been observed in tumor cell lines resistant to cisplatin.[113] It should be noted, however, that XPE is not a necessary component for the *in vitro* reconstitution of NER.[112,114] Increased expression of alpha-DNA polymerase and beta-DNA polymerase has been observed in cisplatin-resistant cell lines, and increased expression of these polymerases, as well as of DNA ligase, has been described in human tumors after cisplatin exposure *in vivo*.[108] The possible significance of these findings is unclear, because the primary polymerases involved in NER are thought to be delta-DNA polymerase or epsilon-DNA polymerase.[110] Although it is probably not involved in NER, beta-DNA polymerase may be involved in translesion DNA synthesis.[115]

Inhibiting DNA repair activity to enhance platinum drug sensitivity has been an active area of investigation. Selvakumaran et al.[116] showed that down-regulation of ERCC-1 using an antisense approach sensitized a platinum-resistant cell line to cisplatin both *in vitro* and *in vivo*. Pharmacologic agents have also been used, including nucleoside analogues such as gemcitabine, fludarabine, and cytarabine; the ribonucleotide reductase inhibitor hydroxyurea; and the inhibitor of alpha- and gamma-DNA polymerases aphidicolin. All of these agents interfere with the repair synthesis stage of various repair processes, including NER. It should be noted that these compounds are also likely to affect DNA replication, and as such should not be strictly characterized as repair inhibitors. The potentiation of cisplatin cytotoxicity by treatment with aphidicolin has been studied extensively in human ovarian cancer cell lines. Although some studies have demonstrated a clear synergism with this drug combination,[117,118] others have not.[119] In an *in vivo* mouse model of human ovarian cancer, the combined treatment of cisplatin and aphidicolin glycinate, a water-soluble form of the drug, was found to be significantly more effective than cisplatin alone.[120] The combination of cytarabine and hydroxyurea was found to demonstrate cytotoxic synergy with cisplatin in a human colon cancer cell line[121] and in rat mammary carcinoma cell lines.[122] Moreover, the modulatory effect of cytarabine and hydroxyurea on cisplatin was associated with an increase in DNA interstrand cross-links in both cellular systems. Similarly, the drugs gemcitabine[123] and fludarabine[124] have both been shown to synergize with cisplatin in causing cell death in *in vitro* systems, and both of these drugs have been shown to interfere with the removal of cisplatin-DNA adducts. The likelihood of a significant improvement in the therapeutic index of cisplatin in refractory patients by the coadministration of a repair inhibitor is limited, however, by the typically multifactorial nature of resistance in tumor cells. Combining an inhibitor of the repair process with other modulators of resistance may be a more viable avenue in treating patients with recurrent disease. Furthermore, a modest change in drug sensitivity may bring some refractory tumors into a range that is treatable with conventional chemotherapy.

INCREASED DNA DAMAGE TOLERANCE

After platinum-DNA adduct formation, the sensitivity of a cell depends on the efficiency with which DNA adducts are recognized and transmittal of a damage signal to the apoptotic machinery. Thus, any disruption, loss, or reduced activity of the components of this pathway(s) can result in a platinum-DNA damage tolerance or multidrug resistance phenotype or both. Platinum-DNA damage tolerance has been observed in both cisplatin-resistant cells derived from chemotherapy-refractory patients and cells selected for primary cisplatin resistance *in vitro*. The contribution of this mechanism to resistance is significant, and it has been shown to correlate strongly with cisplatin resistance as well as resistance to other drugs in two ovarian cancer model systems.[106,125] Like other cisplatin resistance mechanisms, this phenotype may result from alterations in a variety of cellular pathways. Some of these individual mechanisms may confer resistance only to platinum drugs, whereas others may be responsible for multidrug resistance.

One component of DNA damage tolerance that has been observed in cisplatin-resistant cells involves the loss of function of the DNA MMR system. The main function of the MMR system is to scan newly synthesized DNA and remove mismatches that result from nucleotide incorporation errors made by the DNA polymerases. In addition to causing genomic instability, it has been reported that loss of MMR is associated with low-level cisplatin resistance and that the selection of cells in culture for resistance to this drug often yields cell lines that have lost a functional MMR system.[126] MMR deficiency may create an environment that promotes the accumulation of mutations in drug sensitivity genes. Another hypothesis is that the MMR system serves as a detector of platinum-DNA adducts. MSH2 alone, and in combination with MSH6, has been shown to bind to cisplatin 1,2-d(GpG)Pt intrastrand adducts with high efficiency.[54,127] In addition, MSH2- and MLH1-containing protein-DNA complexes have been observed when nuclear extracts of MMR-proficient cell lines are incubated with DNA preincubated with cisplatin, but not with oxaliplatin. These data suggest that MMR recognition of damage may trigger a programmed cell death pathway rendering cells with intact MMR more sensitive to DNA damage.[53] Another possibility is that the cytotoxicity involves repeated rounds of synthesis past the platinum-DNA lesions followed by recognition and subsequent removal of the newly synthesized strand by the MMR system. This futile cycling may generate DNA strand gaps and breaks that trigger programmed cell death.[128] Loss of MMR would thus increase the cell's ability to tolerate platinum-DNA lesions.

Another possible tolerance mechanism related to MMR is enhanced replicative bypass. This is defined as the ability of the replication complex to synthesize DNA past a platinum adduct.[115,129] Increased replicative bypass has been shown to occur in cisplatin-resistant human ovarian cancer cells.[129] These cells are also MMR deficient, and it was shown that in steady-state chain elongation assays, a 2.5- to 6.0-fold increase in replicative bypass of cisplatin adducts occurred. Oxaliplatin adducts are not recognized by the MMR complex, and no significant differences in bypass of oxaliplatin adducts in MMR-proficient and MMR-defective cells were observed. Beta-DNA polymerase, the most inaccurate of the DNA polymerases, may also function in this process.[115] The activity of this enzyme was found to be significantly increased in cells derived from a human malignant glioma resistant to cisplatin compared to its drug-sensitive counterpart.[108]

The tolerance mechanisms just described are related primarily to cisplatin resistance. Because the platinum-DNA damage tolerance phenotype is often associated with cross-resistance to other unrelated chemotherapeutic drugs,[125] the existence of a more general resistance mechanism must be considered. One possible explanation is that the platinum-DNA damage toler-

ance phenotype is the result of decreased expression or inactivation of one or more components of the programmed cell death pathway. As mentioned previously, a number of proapoptotic and antiapoptotic signaling pathways have been implicated in cisplatin sensitivity. The possibility exists that cells containing defective or constitutively down-regulated stress signaling pathways such as SAPK/JNK may exhibit resistance to cisplatin. The weight of the evidence favors a proapoptotic role for both JNK and p38 in tumor cells, whereas their role in normal cells is more equivocal.[68,69,130,131] Paradoxically, c-Jun, a target of JNK, may contribute to cisplatin resistance,[132,133] which speaks to the importance of characterizing dimers in the MAPK pathway, the composition of which may determine the balance of proapoptotic and antiapoptotic signaling.[130] Signaling for apoptosis in oxaliplatin-treated cells appears qualitatively different from that in cisplatin-treated cells. Variation in the activity of the JNK and p38 pathways is not a determinant of cell death signaling in colon cancer cells, whereas resistance to oxaliplatin is influenced very markedly by the activity of the NFκB pathway.[134] In other cells the activity of ATF2, a substrate for JNK and p38, is also a determinant of resistance.[135] The activity of these signaling pathways on mediators of apoptosis cannot easily be separated from effects on transcription of many of the mediators of detoxification, DNA repair, and DNA damage tolerance discussed earlier in this chapter, and active research is in progress to test their role in the clinic.

Cell death may also be influenced by expression of members of the bcl-2 gene family. This group of proapoptotic and antiapoptotic proteins regulates mitochondrial function and functions as a cell survival and cell death rheostat by forming homodimers and heterodimers with one another. The antiapoptotic bcl-2 and bcl-X_L proteins are localized in the outer mitochondrial membrane and may be involved in the formation of transmembrane channels. Overexpression of bcl-2 or bcl-X_L has been shown to prevent disruption of the mitochondrial transmembrane potential and to prolong cell survival in some cells after exposure to cisplatin and other anticancer drugs.[136,137] The activity of these proteins is negated, however, in the presence of high levels of the proapoptotic protein Bax, another bcl-2 family member. Therefore, the relative intracellular levels of these proteins may also confer resistance to platinum drugs.

CLINICAL PHARMACOLOGY

PHARMACOKINETICS

The pharmacokinetic differences observed between platinum drugs may be attributed to the structure of their leaving groups. Platinum complexes containing leaving groups that are less easily displaced exhibit reduced plasma protein binding, longer plasma half-lives, and higher rates of renal clearance. These features are evident in the pharmacokinetic properties of cisplatin, carboplatin, and oxaliplatin, which are summarized in Table 15.5-1. Platinum drug pharmacokinetics have also been reviewed elsewhere.[138,139]

Cisplatin

After intravenous infusion, cisplatin rapidly diffuses into tissues and is covalently bound to plasma protein. More than 90% of

TABLE 15.5-1. Comparative Pharmacokinetics of Platinum Analogues after Bolus or Short Intravenous Infusion

	Cisplatin	*Carboplatin*	*Oxaliplatin*
$T_{1/2}\alpha$ (min)			
Total platinum	14–49	12–98	26
Ultrafiltrate	9–30	8–87	21
$T_{1/2}\beta$ (h)			
Total platinum	0.7–4.6	1.3–1.7	—
Ultrafiltrate	0.7–0.8	1.7–5.9	—
$T_{1/2}\gamma$ (h)			
Total platinum	24–127	8.2–40.0	38–47
Ultrafiltrate	—	—	24–27
Protein binding	>90%	24–50%	85%
Urinary excretion	23–50%	54–82%	>50%

$T_{1/2}\alpha$, half-life of first phase; $T_{1/2}\beta$, half-life of second phase; $T_{1/2}\gamma$, half-life of terminal phase.
(Data adapted from refs. 10 and 130–139.)

platinum is bound to plasma protein at 4 hours after infusion.[140] The disappearance of ultrafiltrable platinum is rapid and occurs in a biphasic fashion. Half-lives of 10 to 30 minutes and 0.7 to 0.8 hours have been reported for the initial and terminal phases, respectively.[141,142] Cisplatin excretion is dependent on renal function, which accounts for the majority of its elimination. The percentage of platinum excreted in the urine has been reported to be between 23% and 40% at 24 hours after infusion.[143,144] Only a small percentage of the total platinum is excreted in the bile.[145]

Carboplatin

The differences in pharmacokinetics observed between cisplatin and carboplatin depend primarily on the slower rate of conversion of carboplatin to a reactive species. Thus, the stability of carboplatin results in a low incidence of nephrotoxicity. Carboplatin diffuses rapidly into tissues after infusion; however, it is considerably more stable in plasma. Only 24% of a dose was bound to plasma protein at 4 hours after infusion.[146] The disappearance of platinum from plasma after short intravenous infusions of carboplatin has been reported to occur in a biphasic or triphasic manner. The initial half-lives for total platinum, which vary considerably among several studies, are listed in Table 15.5-1. The half-lives for total platinum range from 12 to 98 minutes during the first phase ($T_{1/2}\alpha$) and from 1.3 to 1.7 hours during the second phase ($T_{1/2}\beta$). Half-lives reported for the terminal phase range from 8.2 to 40 hours. The disappearance of ultrafiltrable platinum is biphasic with $T_{1/2}\alpha$ and $T_{1/2}\beta$ values ranging from 7.6 to 87 minutes and 1.7 to 5.9 hours, respectively. Carboplatin is excreted predominantly by the kidneys, and cumulative urinary excretion of platinum is 54% to 82%, most as unmodified carboplatin. The renal clearance of carboplatin is closely correlated with the glomerular filtration rate (GFR).[147] This observation enabled Calvert et al.[10] to design a carboplatin dosing formula based on the individual patient's GFR.

Oxaliplatin

After oxaliplatin infusion, platinum accumulates into three compartments: plasma bound platinum, ultrafiltrable platinum, and platinum associated with erythrocytes. When specific and sensitive mass spectrometric techniques are used, oxaliplatin itself is undetectable in plasma, even at end infusion.[148] The active forms of the drug have not been extensively characterized. Approximately 85% of the total platinum is bound to plasma protein at 2 to 5 hours after infusion.[149] Plasma elimination of total platinum and ultrafiltrates is biphasic. The half-lives for the initial and terminal phases are 26 minutes and 38.7 hours, respectively, for total platinum and 21 minutes and 24.2 hours, respectively, for ultrafiltrable platinum (see Table 15.5-1).[140] Thus, as with carboplatin, substantial differences between total and free platinum kinetics are not observed. As with cisplatin, a prolonged retention of oxaliplatin is observed in red blood cells. However, unlike cisplatin, oxaliplatin does not accumulate to any significant level after multiple courses of treatment.[149] This may explain why neurotoxicity associated with oxaliplatin is reversible. Oxaliplatin is eliminated predominantly by the kidneys, with more than 50% of the platinum being excreted in the urine at 48 hours.

PHARMACODYNAMICS

Pharmacodynamics relates pharmacokinetic indices of drug exposure to biologic measures of drug effect, usually toxicity to normal tissues or tumor cell kill. Two issues to be addressed in such studies are whether the effectiveness of the drug can be enhanced and whether the toxicity can be attenuated by knowledge of the platinum pharmacokinetics in an individual. These questions are appropriate to the use of cytotoxic agents with relatively narrow therapeutic indices. Toxicity to normal tissues can be quantitated as a continuous variable when the drug causes myelosuppression. Thus, the early studies of carboplatin demonstrated a close relationship of changes in platelet counts to the area under the concentration-time curve (AUC) in the individual. The AUC was itself closely related to renal function, which was determined as creatinine clearance. Based on these observations, Egorin et al.[11] and Calvert et al.[10] derived formulas based on creatinine clearance to predict either the percentage change in platelet count or a target AUC. More recently, Chatelut and colleagues[150] have derived a formula that relies on serum creatinine levels as well as morphometric determinants of renal function. Application of pharmacodynamically guided dosing algorithms for carboplatin has been widely adopted as a means of avoiding overdosage (by producing acceptable nadir platelet counts) and of maximizing dose intensity in the individual. There is good evidence that this approach can decrease the risk of unacceptable toxicity. Accordingly, a dosing strategy based on renal function is recommended for the use of carboplatin.

A key question is whether maximizing carboplatin exposure in an individual can measurably increase the probability of tumor regression or survival. In an analysis by Jodrell et al.,[151] carboplatin AUC was a predictor of response, thrombocytopenia, and leukopenia. The likelihood of a tumor response increased with increasing AUC up to a level of 5 to 7 mg × h/mL, after which a plateau was reached. Similar results were obtained with carboplatin in combination with cyclophosphamide, and neither response rate nor survival was determined by the carboplatin AUC in a cohort of ovarian cancer patients.[152]

The relationship of pharmacokinetics to response may also be explored by investigating the cellular pharmacology of these agents.[153] As discussed in DNA Adduct Formation, earlier in this chapter, platinum compounds form various types of DNA adducts. The formation and repair of these adducts in human cells are not easily measured. One approach is to measure specific DNA adducts (using antibody-based assays), whereas another is to measure total platinum bound to DNA. The formation and repair of platinum-DNA adducts has been studied in white blood cells obtained from various groups of patients. Schellens and colleagues[154,155] have reevaluated the pharmacokinetic and pharmacodynamic interactions of cisplatin administered as a single agent. In a series of patients with head and neck cancer, they found that cisplatin exposure (measured as the AUC) closely correlated with both the peak DNA adduct content in leukocytes and the area under the DNA-adduct-time curve. These measures were important predictors of response, both individually and in logistic regression analysis.

PHARMACOGENOMICS

Variability in pharmacokinetics and pharmacodynamics of cytotoxic drugs is an important determinant of therapeutic index. This interindividual variation may be attributed in part to genetic differences among patients. For platinum drugs, genetic differences underlying pharmacokinetic variation have not been described. Several groups are actively investigating the basis of pharmacodynamic variation, and the initial work has focused on proteins that are involved in some of the mechanisms described in Mechanism of Action, earlier in this chapter. Detoxification pathways and DNA repair have been studied in several clinical trials. Single nucleotide polymorphisms in genes related to glutathione metabolism and in ERCC genes have been identified in small studies,[156] but larger scale studies have not confirmed early findings. These early studies have much promise, however, both to identify patients with greater or lesser toxicity from standard dosages and to determine subgroups of patients with differing probabilities of response.

FORMULATION AND ADMINISTRATION

CISPLATIN (PLATINOL)

Cisplatin is administered in a chloride-containing solution intravenously over 0.5 to 2.0 hours. To minimize the risk of nephrotoxicity, patients are prehydrated with at least 500 mL of salt-containing fluid. Immediately before cisplatin administration, mannitol (12.5 to 25.0 g) is given parenterally to maximize urine flow. A diuretic such as furosemide may be used also, along with parenteral antiemetics. These currently include dexamethasone together with a 5-hydroxytryptamine (5-HT$_3$) antagonist. A minimum of 1 L of posthydration fluid is usually given.[157] The intensity of hydration varies somewhat with the dose of cisplatin. High-dose cisplatin (up to 200 mg/m^2/course) may be administered in a formulation containing 3% sodium chloride, but this method is no longer widely used. Cisplatin may also be administered regionally to increase local drug exposure and diminish side effects. Its intraperitoneal use was defined by Ozols et al.[158] and by Howell and colleagues.[159] Measured drug exposure in the peritoneal cavity is some 50-fold higher compared to

levels achieved with intravenous administration.[159] At standard dosages in ovarian cancer patients with low-volume disease, a randomized intergroup trial suggested that intraperitoneal administration is superior to intravenous cisplatin in combination with intravenous cyclophosphamide.[160] The development of combinations of carboplatin and paclitaxel has, however, superseded this technique in treatment of ovarian cancer, and the intraperitoneal route is now infrequently used. Regional uses also include intra-arterial delivery (as for hepatic tumors, melanoma, and glioblastoma), but none has been adopted as a standard method of treatment. There is growing interest in chemoembolization for the treatment of tumors confined to the liver, and cisplatin is a component of many popular regimens.[161]

CARBOPLATIN (PARAPLATIN)

Cisplatin treatment over 3 to 6 hours is burdensome for clinical resources and tiring for cancer patients. Previously given as in-hospital treatment, it is now usually administered in the outpatient setting. The exigencies of the modern health care environment have contributed to the expanding use of carboplatin as an alternative to cisplatin except in circumstances in which cisplatin is clearly the superior agent. Carboplatin is substantially easier to administer. Extensive hydration is not required because of the lack of nephrotoxicity at standard dosages.[162] Carboplatin is reconstituted in chloride-free solutions (unlike cisplatin, because chloride can displace the leaving groups) and administered over 30 minutes as a rapid intravenous infusion. Carboplatin has been incorporated in high-dose chemotherapy regimens at dosages over threefold higher than those of the standard regimens.[163] In some regimens, continuous infusion has been substituted for a rapid intravenous infusion; however, it is doubtful that there is an advantage to this approach. Carboplatin dosages up to 20 mg × min/mL may be safely administered in 200 mL of dextrose 5% in water over 2 hours.[164]

OXALIPLATIN (ELOXATIN)

Oxaliplatin is also uncomplicated in its clinical administration. For bolus infusion, the required dose is administered in 500 mL of chloride-free diluent over a period of 2 hours. In studies of colorectal cancer, oxaliplatin has been administered as a 5-day continuous infusion, during which the dosage rate has been modified to observe principles of chronopharmacologic administration.[165] Oxaliplatin is more frequently given as a single dose every 2 weeks (85 mg/m^2) or every 3 weeks (130 mg/m^2), alone or with other active agents. It is common to pretreat patients with active antiemetics, such as a 5-HT$_3$ antagonist, but the nausea is not as severe as with cisplatin. No prehydration is required. The predominant toxicity of oxaliplatin is neurotoxicity: The development of an oropharyngeal dysesthesia, often precipitated by exposure to cold, requires prolongation of the duration of administration to 6 hours. On occasion, the occurrence of hypersensitivity requires slowing of the infusion also.

TOXICITY

A substantial body of literature documents the side effects of platinum compounds. The nephrotoxicity of cisplatin almost

TABLE 15.5-2. Toxicity Profiles of Platinum Analogues in Clinical Use

Toxicity	Cisplatin	Carboplatin	Oxaliplatin
Myelosuppression		X	
Nephrotoxicity	X		
Neurotoxicity	X		X
Ototoxicity	X		
Nausea and vomiting	X	X	X

led to its abandonment, until Cvitkovic and colleagues introduced aggressive hydration, which prevented the development of acute renal failure.[3,4] As noted in History, earlier in this chapter, the toxicity of cisplatin was a driving force both in the search for less toxic analogues and for more effective treatments for its side effects, especially nausea and vomiting. The toxicities associated with cisplatin, carboplatin, and oxaliplatin are described in detail in the following sections and summarized in Table 15.5-2.

CISPLATIN

The side effects associated with cisplatin (at single doses of more than 50 mg/m²) include nausea and vomiting, nephrotoxicity, ototoxicity, neuropathy, and myelosuppression. Rare effects include visual impairment, seizures, arrhythmias, acute ischemic vascular events, glucose intolerance, and pancreatitis.[157] The nausea and vomiting stimulated a search for new antiemetics. These effects are currently best managed with 5-HT_3 antagonists, usually given with a glucocorticoid, although other combinations of agents are still widely used. In the weeks after treatment, continuous antiemetic therapy may be required. Nephrotoxicity is ameliorated but not completely prevented by hydration. The renal damage to both glomeruli and tubules is cumulative, and after cisplatin treatment, serum creatinine level is no longer a reliable guide to GFR. An acute elevation of serum creatinine level may follow a cisplatin dose, but this index returns to normal with time. Tubule damage may be reflected in a salt-losing syndrome that also resolves with time.

Ototoxicity is a cumulative and irreversible side effect of cisplatin treatment that results from damage to the inner ear. Therefore, audiograms are recommended every two to three cycles.[157] The initial audiographic manifestation is loss of high-frequency acuity (4000 to 8000 Hz). When acuity is affected in the range of speech, cisplatin should be discontinued under most circumstances and carboplatin substituted where appropriate. Peripheral neuropathy is also cumulative, although less common than with agents such as vinca alkaloids. This neuropathy is usually reversible, although recovery is often slow. A number of agents with the potential for protection from neuropathy have been developed, but none is yet used widely.[166]

CARBOPLATIN

Myelosuppression, which is not usually severe with cisplatin, is the dose-limiting toxicity of carboplatin.[162] The drug is most toxic to the platelet precursors, but neutropenia and anemia are frequently observed. The lowest platelet counts after a single dose of carboplatin are observed 17 to 21 days later, and recovery usually occurs by day 28. The effect is dose dependent, but individuals vary widely in their susceptibility. As shown by Egorin et al.[11] and Calvert et al.,[10] the severity of platelet toxicity is best accounted for by a measure of the drug exposure in an individual, the AUC. Both groups derived pharmacologically based formulas to predict toxicity and guide carboplatin dosing. That of Calvert and colleagues targets a particular exposure to carboplatin:

$$\text{Dose (mg)} = \text{target AUC (mg} \cdot \text{min/mL)} \times (\text{GFR mL/min} + 25)$$

This formula has been widely used to individualize carboplatin dosing and permits targeting at an acceptable level of toxicity. Patients who are elderly or have a poor performance status, or have a history of extensive pretreatment have a higher risk of toxicity even when dosage is calculated with these methods,[10,11] but the safety of drug administration has been enhanced. In the combination of carboplatin and paclitaxel, AUC-based dosing has helped to maximize the dose intensity of carboplatin.[167] Dosages some 30% higher than those using a dosing strategy based solely on body surface area may safely be used. A determination of whether this approach to dosing improves outcome will require a randomized trial.

The other toxicities of carboplatin are generally milder and better tolerated than those of cisplatin. Nausea and vomiting, although frequent, are less severe, shorter in duration, and more easily controlled with standard antiemetics [i.e., prochlorperazine (Compazine)], dexamethasone, lorazepam) than that after cisplatin treatment. Renal impairment is infrequent, although alopecia is common, especially with the paclitaxel-containing combinations. Neurotoxicity is also less common than with cisplatin, although it is observed more frequently with the increasing use of high-dose regimens. Ototoxicity is also less common.

OXALIPLATIN

The dose-limiting toxicity of oxaliplatin is sensory neuropathy, a characteristic of all DACH-containing platinum derivatives. The severity of the toxicity is dramatically less than that observed with another DACH-containing analogue, ormaplatin. This side effect takes two forms. First, a tingling of the extremities, which may also involve the perioral region, that occurs early and usually resolves within a few days. With repeated dosing, symptoms may last longer between cycles, but do not appear to be of long duration or cumulative. Laryngopharyngeal spasm and cold dysesthesias have also been reported but are not associated with significant respiratory symptoms and can be prevented by prolonging the duration of infusion. A second neuropathy, more typical of that seen with cisplatin, affects the extremities and increases with repeated doses. Definitive physiologic characterization of oxaliplatin-induced neuropathy has proven difficult in large studies. Electromyograms performed in six patients treated by Extra et al.[18] revealed an axonal sensory neuropathy, but nerve conduction velocities were unchanged. Specimens from peripheral nerve biopsies performed in this study showed decreased myelinization and replacement with collagen pockets. The neurologic effects of oxaliplatin appear to be cumulative in that they become more pronounced and of greater duration with successive cycles; however, unlike those of cisplatin, they are reversible with drug cessation. In a review of 682 patient experiences, Brienza et al.[168] reported that 82% of patients who experienced grade 2 neurotoxicity or higher had their symptoms regress within 4 to 6 months. In a larger adjuvant trial, de Gramont et al.[169] reported that 12% of patients had grade 3 toxicity at the end of a 6-month treatment period and that the majority of these patients had relief, but not always complete resolution of the symptoms, by 1 year later. The persistence of the neurotoxicity has led to approaches to ameliorate it, including the use of protective agents (calcium and magnesium salts intravenously before and after each infusion)[149] or a more intensive schedule initially, followed by interruption of the oxaliplatin component of the chemotherapy for a few cycles.[169] Ototoxicity is not observed with oxaliplatin. Nausea and vomiting do occur and generally respond to 5-HT$_3$ antagonists. Myelosuppression is uncommon and is not severe with oxaliplatin as a single agent, but it is a feature of combinations including this drug. Oxaliplatin therapy is not associated with nephrotoxicity.

REFERENCES

1. Rosenberg B, VanCamp L, Trosko J, et al. Platinum compounds: a new class of potent antitumor agents. *Nature* 1969;222:385.
2. Rosenberg B. Platinum complexes for the treatment of cancer: why the search goes on. In: Lippert B, ed. *Cisplatin: chemistry and biochemistry of a leading anticancer drug.* Zurich: Verlag Helvetica Chimica Acta, 1999:3.
3. Cvitkovic E, Spaulding J, Bethune V, et al. Improvement of cis-dichlorodiammineplatinum (NSC 119875): therapeutic index in an animal model. *Cancer* 1977;39:1357.
4. Hayes D, Cvitkovic E, Golbey R, et al. High dose cis-platinum diamine dichloride: amelioration of renal toxicity by mannitol diuresis. *Cancer* 1977;39:1372.
5. O'Dwyer P, Stevenson J, Johnson S. Clinical status of cisplatin, carboplatin and other platinum-based antitumor drugs. In: Lippert B, ed. *Cisplatin: chemistry and biochemistry of a leading anticancer drug.* Zurich: Verlag Helvetica Chimica Acta, 1999:31.
6. Roberts J, Thomson A. The mechanism of action of antitumor platinum compounds. *Nucleic Acids Res* 1979;22:71.
7. Martin R. Platinum complexes: hydrolysis and binding to N(7) and N(1) of purines. In: Lippert B, ed. *Cisplatin: chemistry and biochemistry of a leading anticancer drug.* Zurich: Verlag Helvetica Chimica Acta, 1999:183.
8. Harrap K. Preclinical studies identifying carboplatin as a viable cisplatin alternative. *Cancer Treat Rev* 1985;12:A21.
9. Harrap K. Initiatives with platinum- and quinazoline-based antitumor molecules—fourteenth Bruce F. Cain memorial award lecture. *Cancer Res* 1995;55:2761.
10. Calvert A, Newell D, Gumbrell L, et al. Carboplatin dosage: prospective evaluation of a simple formula based on renal function. *J Clin Oncol* 1989;7:1748.
11. Egorin M, Echo DV, Olman E, et al. Prospective validation of a pharmacologically based dosing scheme for the cis-diamminedichloroplatinum(II) analogue diamminecyclobutanedicarboxylatoplatinum. *Cancer Res* 1985;45:6502.
12. Connors T, Jones M, Ross W, et al. New platinum complexes with anti-tumour activity. *Chem Biol Interact* 1972;5:415.
13. Burchenal J, Kalaker K, Dew K, et al. Rationale for development of platinum analogs. *Cancer Treat Rep* 1979;63:1493.
14. Kidani Y, Inagaki K, Tsukagoshi S. Examination of antitumor activities of platinum complexes of 1,2-diaminocyclohexane isomers and their related complexes. *Gann* 1976;67:921.
15. Burchenal J, Irani G, Kern K, et al. 1,2-Diaminocyclohexane platinum derivatives of potential clinical value. *Rec Res Cancer Res* 1980;74:146.
16. Rixe O, Ortuzar W, Alvarez M, et al. Oxaliplatin, tetraplatin, cisplatin, and carboplatin: spectrum of activity in drug-resistant cell lines and in the cell lines of the National Cancer Institute's anticancer drug screen panel. *Biochem Pharmacol* 1996;52:1855.
17. Mathe G, Kidani Y, Triana K, et al. A phase I trial of trans-l-diaminocyclohexane oxalatoplatinum (l-OHP). *Biomed Pharmacother* 1986;40:372.
18. Extra J, Espie M, Calvo F, et al. Phase I study of oxaliplatin in patients with advanced cancer. *Cancer Chemother Pharmacol* 1990;25:299.
19. Cvitkovic E, Bekradda M. Oxaliplatin: a new therapeutic option in colorectal cancer. *Semin Oncol* 1999;26:647.
20. Hubbard K, Pazdur R, Ajani J, et al. Phase II evaluation of iproplatin in patients with advanced gastric and pancreatic cancer. *Am J Clin Oncol* 1992;15:524.
21. Murphy D, Lind M, Prendiville J, et al. Phase I/II study of intraperitoneal iproplatin in patients with minimal residual disease following platinum-based systemic therapy for epithelial ovarian carcinoma. *Eur J Cancer* 1992;28A:870.
22. Schilder R, LaCreta F, Perez R, et al. Phase I and pharmacokinetic study of ormaplatin (tetraplatin, NSC 363812) administered on a day 1 and day 8 schedule. *Cancer Res* 1994;54:709.
23. Kelland L. The development of orally active platinum drugs. In: Lippert B, ed. *Cisplatin: chemistry and biochemistry of a leading anticancer drug.* Zurich: Verlag Helvetica Chimica Acta 1999:497.
24. Fokkema E, Groen HJ, Bauer J. Phase II study of oral platinum drug JM216 as first-line treatment in patients with small-cell lung cancer. *J Clin Oncol* 1999;17:3822.
25. Judson I, Cerny T, Epelbaum R, et al. Phase II trial of the oral platinum complex JM216 in non-small-cell lung cancer: an EORTC early clinical studies group investigation. *Ann Oncol* 1997;8:604.
26. Sternberg CN, Hetherington J, Paluchowska B, et al. Randomized phase III trial of a new oral platinum, satraplatin (JM-216) plus prednisone or prednisone alone in patients with hormone refractory prostate cancer. *Proc Am Soc Clin Oncol* 2003;22:395.
27. Khokhar A, al-Baker S, Shamsuddin S, et al. Chemical and biological studies on a series of novel (trans-(1R, 2R)-, trans-(1S, 2S)-, and cis-1, 2-diaminocyclohexane) platinum (IV) carboxylate complexes. *J Med Chem* 1997;40:112.
28. Farrell N, Qu Y, Bierbach U, et al. Structure-activity relationships within di- and trinuclear platinum phase-I clinical anticancer agents. In: Lippert B, ed. *Cisplatin: chemistry and biochemistry of a leading anticancer drug.* Zurich: Verlag Helvetica Chimica Acta, 1999.
29. Holford J, Sharp S, Murrer B, et al. In vitro circumvention of cisplatin resistance by the novel sterically hindered platinum complex AMD473. *Br J Cancer* 1998;77:366.
30. Raynaud F, Boxall F, Goddard P, et al. cis-Amminedichloro(2-methylpyridine) platinum(II) (AMD473), a novel sterically hindered platinum complex: in vivo activity, toxicology, and pharmacokinetics in mice. *Clin Cancer Res* 1997;3:2063.
31. Beale P, Judson I, O'Donnell A, et al A Phase I clinical and pharmacological study of cis-diamminedichloro(2-methylpyridine) platinum II (AMD473). *Br J Cancer* 2003;88:1128.
32. Flaherty K, Stevenson J, Redlinger M, et al. A phase I, dose-escalation trial of ZD0473, a novel platinum analogue, in combination with gemcitabine. *Cancer Chemother Pharmacol* 2004 (in press).
33. Harder H, Rosenberg B. Inhibitory effects of anti-tumor platinum compounds on DNA, RNA and protein syntheses in mammalian cells in vitro. *Int J Cancer* 1970;6:207.
34. Howle J, Gale G. Cis-dichlorodiammineplatinum (II). Persistent and selective inhibition of deoxyribonucleic acid synthesis in vivo. *Biochem Pharmacol* 1970;19:2757.
35. Reslova S. The induction of lysogenic strains of Escherichia coli by cis-dichloro-diammineplatinum (II). *Chem Biol Interact* 1971;4:66.
36. Poll EHA, Abrahams PJ, Arwert F, et al. Host cell reactivation of cis-diamminedichloroplatinum (II)-treated SV40 DNA in normal human, Fanconi anaemia and xeroderma pigmentosum fibroblasts. *Mutation Res* 1984;132:181.
37. Fraval HNA, Rawlings CJ, Roberts JJ. Increased sensitivity of UV-repair deficient human cells to DNA bound platinum products which unlike thymine dimers are not recognized by an endonuclease extracted from Micrococcus luteus. *Mutation Res* 1978;51:121.
38. Eastman A. The formation, isolation and characterization of DNA adducts produced by anticancer platinum complexes. *Pharmacol Ther* 1987;34:155.
39. Blommaert F, van Kijk-Knijnenburg H, Dijt F, et al. Formation of DNA adducts by the anticancer drug carboplatin: different nucleotide sequence preferences in vitro and in cells. *Biochemistry* 1995;34:8474.
40. Saris C, van de Vaart P, Rietbroek R, et al. In vitro formation of DNA adducts by cisplatin, lobaplatin and oxaliplatin in calf thymus DNA in solution and in cultured cells. *Carcinogenesis* 1996;17:2763.
41. Zamble D, Lippard S. The response of cellular proteins to cisplatin-damaged DNA. In: Lippert B, ed. *Cisplatin: chemistry and biochemistry of a leading anticancer drug.* Zurich: Verlag Helvetica Chimica Acta, 1999:73.
42. Scheef E, Briggs J, Howell S. Molecular modeling of the intrastrand guanine-guanine DNA adducts produced by cisplatin and oxaliplatin. *Mol Pharmacol* 1999;56:633.
43. Raymond E, Faivre S, Woynarowski J, et al. Oxaliplatin: mechanism of action and antineoplastic activity. *Semin Oncol* 1998;25:4.
44. Sorenson C, Eastman A. Mechanism of cis-diamminedichloroplatinum (II)-induced cytotoxicity: role of G2 arrest and DNA double-strand breaks. *Cancer Res* 1988;48:4484.
45. Evans D, Dive C. Effects of cisplatin on the induction of apoptosis in proliferating hepatoma cells and nonproliferating immature thymocytes. *Cancer Res* 1993;53:2133.
46. Sorenson C, Barry M, Eastman A. Analysis of events associated with cell cycle arrest at G2 phase and cell death induced by cisplatin. *J Natl Cancer Inst* 1990;82:749.
47. Bunch R, Eastman A. 7-Hydroxystaurosporine (UCN-01) causes redistribution of proliferating cell nuclear antigen and abrogates cisplatin-induced S-phase arrest in Chinese hamster ovary cells. *Cell Growth Differ* 1997;8:779.
48. Toney J, Donahue B, Kellett P, et al. Isolation of cDNAs encoding a human protein that binds selectively to DNA modified by the anticancer drug cis-diamminedichloroplatinum. *Proc Natl Acad Sci U S A* 1989;86:8328.
49. Bruhn S, Pil P, Essigmann J, et al. Isolation and characterization of human cDNA clones encoding a high mobility group box protein that recognizes structural distortions to DNA caused by binding of the anticancer agent cisplatin. *Proc Natl Acad Sci U S A* 1989;89:2307.
50. Hughes EN, Engelsberg BN, Billings PC. Purification of nuclear proteins that bind to cisplatin-damaged DNA. Identity with high mobility group proteins 1 and 2. *J Biol Chem* 1992;267:13520.
51. Grosschedl R, Giese K, Pagel J. HMG domain proteins: architectural elements in the assembly of nucleoprotein structures. *Trends Genet* 1994;10:94.
52. Fink D, Zheng H, Nebel S, et al. In vitro and in vivo resistance to cisplatin in cells that have lost DNA mismatch repair. *Cancer Res* 1997;57:1841.
53. Fink D, Nebel S, Aebi S, et al. The role of DNA mismatch repair in platinum drug resistance. *Cancer Res* 1996;56:4881.
54. Mello J, Acharya S, Fishel R, et al. The mismatch-repair protein hMSH2 binds selectively to DNA adducts of the anticancer drug cisplatin. *Chem Biol* 1996;3:579.
55. Siddik ZH. Cisplatin: mode of cytotoxic action and molecular basis or resistance. *Oncogene* 2003;22:7265.

56. Fan S, Smith ML, Rivet DJ, et al. Disruption of p53 function sensitizes breast cancer MCF-7 cells to cisplatin and pentoxifylline. *Cancer Res* 1995;55:1649.

57. Hawkins DS, Demers GW, Galloway DA. Inactivation of p53 enhances sensitivity to multiple chemotherapeutic agents. *Cancer Res* 1996;56:892.

58. McClay EF, Albright KD, Jones JA, et al. Modulation of cisplatin resistance in human malignant melanoma cells. *Cancer Res* 1992;52:6790.

59. Kroning R, Jones JA, Hom DK, et al. Enhancement of drug sensitivity of human malignancies by epidermal growth factor. *Br J Cancer* 1995;72:615.

60. Chang MJ, Yu WD, Reyno LM, et al. Potentiation by interleukin 1 alpha of cisplatin and carboplatin antitumor activity: schedule-dependent and pharmacokinetic effects in the RIF-1 tumor model. *Cancer Res* 1994;54:5380.

61. Isonishi S, Jekunen AP, Hom DK, et al Modulation of cisplatin sensitivity and growth rate of an ovarian carcinoma cell line by bombesin and tumor necrosis factor-alpha. *J Clin Invest* 1992;90:1436.

62. Shi Y, Frankel A, Radvanyi L, et al. Rapamycin enhances apoptosis and increases sensitivity to cisplatin in vitro. *Cancer Res* 1995;55:1982.

63. Sklar M. Increased resistance to cis-diamminedichloro platinum (II) in NIH3T3 cells transformed by RAS oncogenes. *Cancer Res* 1988;48:793.

64. Isonishi S, Hom DK, Thiebaut FB, et al. Expression of the c-Ha-ras oncogene in mouse NIH 3T3 cells induces resistance to cisplatin. *Cancer Res* 1991;51:5903.

65. Chapman RS, Whetton AD, et al. Characterization of drug resistance mediated via the suppression of apoptosis by Abelson protein tyrosine kinase. *Mol Pharmacol* 1995;48:334.

66. Benz CC, Scott GK, Sarup JC, et al. Estrogen-dependent, tamoxifen-resistant tumorigenic growth of MCF-7 cells transfected with HER2/neu. *Breast Cancer Res Treat* 1993;24:85.

67. Ip Y, Davis R. Signal transduction by the c-Jun N-terminal kinase (JNK)—from inflammation to development. *Curr Opin Cell Biol* 1998;10:205.

68. Zanke B, Boudreau K, Rubie E, et al. The stress-activated protein kinase pathway mediates cell death following injury induced by cis-platinum, UV irradiation or heat. *Curr Biol* 1996;6:606.

69. Sanchez-Perez I, Murguia J, Perona R. Cisplatin induces a persistent activation of JNK that is related to cell death. *Oncogene* 1998;16:533.

70. Jarpe M, Widmann C, Knall C, et al. Anti-apoptotic versus pro-apoptotic signal transduction: checkpoints and stop signs along the road to death. *Oncogene* 1998;17:1475.

71. Chen Z, Seimiya H, Naito M, et al. ASK1 mediates apoptotic cell death induced by genotoxic stress. *Oncogene* 1999;18:173.

72. Johnson S, Ferry K, Hamilton T. Recent insights into platinum drug resistance in cancer. *Drug Resist Updates* 1998;1:243.

73. Gately DP, Howell SB. Cellular accumulation of the anticancer agent cisplatin: a review. *Br J Cancer* 1993;67:1171.

74. Lin X, Okuda T, Holzer A, et al. The copper transporter CTR1 regulates cisplatin uptake in Saccharomyces cerevisiae. *Mol Pharmacol* 2002;62:1154.

75. Borst P, Kool M, Evers R. Do cMOAT (MRP2), other MRP homologues, and LRP play a role in MDR? *Semin Cancer Biol* 1997;8:205.

76. Taniguchi K, Wada M, Kohno K, et al. A human canalicular multispecific organic anion transporter (cMOAT) gene is overexpressed in cisplatin-resistant human cancer cell lines with decreased drug accumulation. *Cancer Res* 1996;56:4124.

77. Koike K, Kawabe T, Tanaka T, et al. A canalicular multispecific organic anion transporter (cMOAT) antisense cDNA enhances drug sensitivity in human hepatic cancer cells. *Cancer Res* 1997;57:5475.

78. Kool M, de Haas M, Scheffer G, et al. Analysis of expression of cMOAT (MRP2), MRP3, MRP4, and MRP5, homologues of the multidrug resistance-associated protein gene (MRP1), in human cancer cell lines. *Cancer Res* 1997;57:3537.

79. Arts H, Katsaros D, Vries ED, Massobrio M, et al. Drug resistance-associated markers P-glycoprotein, multidrug resistance-associated protein 1, multidrug resistance-associated protein 2, and lung resistance protein as prognostic factors in ovarian carcinoma. *Clin Cancer Res* 1999;5:2798.

80. Komatsu M, Sumizawa T, Mutoh M, et al. Copper-transporting P-type adenosine triphosphatase (ATP7B) is associated with cisplatin resistance. *Cancer Res* 2000;60:1312.

81. Katano K, Safaei R, Samimi G, et al. The copper export pump ATP7B modulates the cellular pharmacology of carboplatin in ovarian carcinoma cells. *Mol Pharmacol* 2003;64:466.

82. Katano K, Kondo A, Safaei R, et al. Acquisition of resistance to cisplatin is accompanied by changes in the cellular pharmacology of copper. *Cancer Res* 2002;62:6559.

83. Samimi G, Varki NM, Wilczynski S, Safaei R, et al. Increase in the expression of the copper transporter ATP7A during platinum drug-based treatment is associated with poor survival in ovarian cancer patients. *Clin Cancer Res* 2003;9:5853.

84. Godwin A, Meister A, O'Dwyer P, et al. High resistance to cisplatin in human ovarian cancer cell lines is associated with marked increase in glutathione synthesis. *Proc Natl Acad Sci U S A* 1992;89:3070.

85. Hosking LK, Whelan RDH, Shellard SA, et al. An evaluation of the role of glutathione and its associated enzymes in the expression of differential sensitivities to antitumor agents shown by a range of human tumour cell lines. *Biochem Pharmacol* 1990;40:1833.

86. Mistry P, Kelland L, Abel G, et al. The relationships between glutathione, glutathione-S-transferase and cytotoxicity of platinum drugs and melphalan in eight human ovarian carcinoma cell lines. *Br J Cancer* 1991;64:215.

87. Britten RA, Green JA, Broughton C, et al. The relationship between nuclear glutathione levels and resistance to melphalan in human ovarian tumour cells. *Biochem Pharmacol* 1991;41:647.

88. Hamilton T, Winker M, Louie K, et al. Augmentation of adriamycin, melphalan and cisplatin cytotoxicity in drug-resistant and -sensitive human ovarian cancer cell lines by buthionine sulfoximine mediated glutathione depletion. *Biochem Pharmacol* 1985;34:2583.

89. Smith E, Brock AP. An in vitro study comparing the cytotoxicity of three platinum complexes with regard to the effect of thiol depletion. *Br J Cancer* 1988;57:548.

90. Dedon P, Borch R. Characterization of the reactions of platinum antitumor agents with biologic and nonbiologic sulfur-containing nucleophiles. *Biochem Pharmacol* 1987;36:1955.

91. Ishikawa T, Ali-Osman F. Glutathione-associated cis-diamminedichloroplatinum (II) metabolism and ATP-dependent efflux from leukemia cells. *J Biol Chem* 1993;268:20116.

92. Mistry P, Loh S, Kelland L, et al. Effect of buthionine sulfoximine on PtII and PtIV drug accumulation and the formation of glutathione conjugates in human ovarian carcinoma cell lines. *Int J Cancer* 1993;55:848.

93. Eastman A. Cross-linking of glutathione to DNA by cancer chemotherapeutic platinum coordination complexes. *Chem Biol Interact* 1987;61:241.

94. Daubeuf S, Leroy P, Paolicchi A, et al. Enhanced resistance of HeLa cells to cisplatin by overexpression of gamma-glutamyltransferase. *Biochem Pharmacol* 2002;15:207.

95. Miyazaki M, Kohno K, Saburi Y, et al. Drug resistance to cis-diamminedichloroplatinum (II) in Chinese hamster ovary cell lines by transfection with glutathione S-transferase gene. *Biochem Biophys Res Commun* 1990;166:1358.

96. Nakagawa K, Saijo N, Tsuchida S, et al. Glutathione S-transferase pi as a determinant of drug resistance in transfectant cell lines. *J Biol Chem* 1990;265:4296.

97. Hrubisko M, McGown AT, Fox BW. The role of metallothionein, glutathione, glutathione S-transferases and DNA repair in resistance to platinum drugs in a series of L1210 cell lines made resistant to anticancer platinum agents. *Biochem Pharmacol* 1993;45:253.

98. Pattanaik A, Bachowski G, Laib J, et al. Properties of the reaction of cis-dichlorodiammineplatinum(II) with metallothionein. *J Biol Chem* 1992;267:16121.

99. Kelley S, Basu A, Teicher B, et al. Overexpression of metallothionein confers resistance to anticancer drugs. *Science* 1988;241:1813.

100. Kondo Y, Woo ES, Michalska AE, et al. Metallothionein null cells have increased sensitivity to anticancer drugs. *Cancer Res* 1995;55:2021.

101. Kojima M, Kikkawa F, Oguchi H, et al. Sensitization of human ovarian carcinoma cells to cis-diamminedichloroplatinum (II) by amphotericin B in vitro and in vivo. *Eur J Cancer* 1994;30A:773.

102. Siu L, Banerjee D, Khurana F, et al. The prognostic role of p53, metallothionein, P-glycoprotein, and MIB-1 in muscle-invasive urothelial transitional cell carcinoma. *Clin Cancer Res* 1998;4:559.

103. Wood D, Klein E, Fair W, et al. Metallothionein gene expression in bladder cancer exposed to cisplatin. *Mod Pathol* 1993;6:33.

104. Koberle B, Grimaldi K, Sunters A, et al. DNA repair capacity and cisplatin sensitivity of human testis tumour cells. *Int J Cancer* 1997;70:551.

105. Johnson S, Perez R, Godwin A, et al. Role of platinum-DNA adduct formation and removal in cisplatin resistance in human ovarian cancer cell lines. *Biochem Pharmacol* 1994;47:689.

106. Johnson S, Swiggard P, Handel L, et al. Relationship between platinum-DNA adduct formation and removal and cisplatin cytotoxicity in cisplatin-sensitive and -resistant human ovarian cancer cells. *Cancer Res* 1994;54:5911.

107. Yen L, Woo A, Christopoulopoulos G, et al. Enhanced host cell reactivation capacity and expression of DNA repair genes in human breast cancer cells resistant to bi-functional alkylating agents. *Mutat Res* 1995;337:179.

108. Ali-Osman F, Berger M, Rairkar A, et al. Enhanced repair of a cisplatin-damaged reporter chloramphenicol-O-acetyltransferase gene and altered activities of DNA polymerases α and β, and DNA ligase in cells of a human malignant glioma following in vivo cisplatin therapy. *J Cell Biochem* 1994;54:11.

109. Eastman A, Schulte N. Enhanced DNA repair as a mechanism of resistance to cis-diamminedichloroplatinum(II). *Biochemistry* 1988;27:4730.

110. Wood R. Nucleotide excision repair in mammalian cells. *J Biol Chem* 1997;272:23465.

111. Ferry K, Hamilton T, Johnson S. Increased nucleotide excision repair in cisplatin-resistant ovarian cancer cells: role of ERCC1-XPF *Biochem Pharmacol* 2000;60:1305.

112. Dabholkar M, Vionnet J, Bostick-Bruton F, et al. Messenger RNA levels of XPAC and ERCC1 in ovarian cancer tissue correlate with response to platinum-based chemotherapy. *J Clin Invest* 1994;94:703.

113. Chu G, Chang E. Cisplatin-resistant cells express increased levels of a factor that recognizes damaged DNA. *Proc Natl Acad Sci U S A* 1990;87:3324.

114. Mu D, Park C-H, Matsunaga T, et al. Reconstitution of human DNA repairs excision nuclease in a highly defined system. *J Biol Chem* 1995;270:2415.

115. Hoffmann JS, Pillaire MJ, Maga G, et al. DNA polymerase beta bypasses in vitro a single d(GpG)-cisplatin adduct placed on codon 13 of the HRAS gene. *Proc Natl Acad Sci U S A* 1995;92:5356.

116. Selvakumaran M, Piscarcik DA, Bao R, et al. Enhanced cisplatin cytotoxicity by disturbing the nucleotide excision repair pathway in ovarian cancer cell lines. *Cancer Res* 2003;63:1311.

117. Masuda H, Tanaka T, Matsuda H, et al. Increased removal of DNA-bound platinum in a human ovarian cancer cell line resistant to cis-diamminedichloroplatinum (II). *Cancer Res* 1990;50:1863.

118. Katz E, Andrews P, Howell S. The effect of DNA polymerase inhibitors on the cytotoxicity of cisplatin in human ovarian carcinoma cells. *Cancer Commun* 1990;2:159.

119. Dempke WC, Shellard M, Fichtinger-Schepman SA, et al. Lack of significant modulation of the formation and removal of platinum-DNA adducts by aphidicolin glycinate in two logarithmically growing ovarian tumour cell lines in vitro. *Carcinogenesis* 1991;12:525.

120. O'Dwyer P, Moyer J, Suffness M, et al. Antitumor activity and biochemical effects of aphidicolin glycinate (NSC 303812) alone and in combination with cisplatin in vivo. *Cancer Res* 1994;54:724.

121. Albain K, Swinnen L, Erickson L, et al. Cytotoxic synergy of cisplatin with concurrent hydroxyurea and cytarabine: summary of an in vitro model and initial clinical pilot experience. *Semin Oncol* 1992;19:102.

122. Alaoui-Jamali M, Loubaba B-B, Robyn S, et al. Effect of DNA-repair-enzyme modulators on cytotoxicity of L-phenylalanine mustard and cis-diamminedichloroplatinum (II) in mammary carcinoma cells resistant to alkylating agents. *Cancer Chemother Pharmacol* 1994;34:153.

123. Peters G J, Bergman AM, Ruiz van Haperen VW, et al. Interaction between cisplatin and gemcitabine in vitro and in vivo. *Semin Oncol* 1995;22:72.

124. Li L, Keatin M, Plunkett W, et al. Fludarabine-mediated repair inhibition of cisplatin-induced DNA lesions in human chronic myelogenous leukemia-blast crisis K562 cells: induction of synergistic cytotoxicity independent of reversal of apoptosis resistance. *Mol Pharmacol* 1997;52:798.

125. Johnson S, Laub P, Beesley J, et al. Increased platinum-DNA damage tolerance is associated with cisplatin resistance and cross-resistance to various chemotherapeutic agents in unrelated human ovarian cancer cell lines. *Cancer Res* 1997;57:850.

126. Aebi S, Kurdi-Haidar B, Gordon R, et al. Loss of DNA mismatch repair in acquired resistance to cisplatin. *Cancer Res* 1996;56:3087.

127. Duckett D, Drummond J, Murchie A, et al. Human MutSa recognizes damaged DNA base pairs containing O6-methylguanine, O4-methylthymine, or the cisplatin-d(GpG) adduct. *Proc Natl Acad Sci U S A* 1996;93:6443.

128. Karran P, Bignami M. DNA damage tolerance, mismatch repair and genome instability. *BioEssays* 1994;16:833.

129. Mamenta E, Poma E, Kaufmann W, et al. Enhanced replicative bypass of platinum-DNA adducts in cisplatin-resistant human ovarian carcinoma cell lines. *Cancer Res* 1994;54:3500.

130. Vasilevskaya I, O'Dwyer PJ. Role of Jun and Jun kinase in resistance of cancer cells to therapy. *Drug Resist Updates* 2003;6:147.

131. Vasilevskaya IA, Rakitinam TV, O'Dwyer PJ. Quantitative effects on c-Jun N-terminal protein kinase signaling determine synergistic interaction of cisplatin and 17-allylamino-17-demethoxygeldanamycin in colon cancer cell lines. *Mol Pharmacol* 2004;65:235.

132. Pan B, Yao K-S, Monia BP, et al. Reversal of cisplatin resistance by a c-jun antisense oligodeoxynucleotide (ISIS 10582): evidence for the role of transcription factor overexpression in determining resistant phenotype. *Biochem Pharmacol* 2002;63:1699.

133. Hayakawa J, Ohmichi M, Kurachi H, et al. Inhibition of extracellular signal-regulated protein kinase or c-Jun N-terminal protein kinase cascade, differentially activated by cisplatin, sensitizes human ovarian cancer cell line. *J Biol Chem* 1999;274:31648.

134. Rakitina TV, Vasilevskaya IA, O'Dwyer PJ. Additive interaction of oxaliplatin and 17-allyl-amino-17-demethoxygeldanamycin in colon cancer cell lines results from inhibition of nuclear factor kappa B signaling. *Cancer Res* 2003;63:8600.

135. Hayakawa J, Depatie C, Ohmichi M, et al. The activation of c-Jun NH2-terminal kinase (JNK) by DNA-damaging agents serves to promote drug resistance via activating transcription factor 2 (ATF2)-dependent enhanced DNA repair. *J Biol Chem* 2003;278:20582.

136. Miyashita T, Reed JC. Bcl-2 oncoprotein blocks chemotherapy-induced apoptosis in a human leukemia cell line. *Blood* 1993;81:151.

137. Minn A, Rudin C, Boise L, Thompson C. Expression of Bcl-xL can confer a multidrug resistance phenotype. *Blood* 1995;86:1903.

138. Duffull S, Robinson B. Clinical pharmacokinetics and dose optimization of carboplatin. *Clin Pharmacokinet* 1997;33:161.

139. VanderVijgh W. Clinical pharmacokinetics of carboplatin. *Clin Pharmacokinet* 1991;21:242.

140. Extra J, Marty M, Brienza S, et al. Pharmacokinetics and safety profile of oxaliplatin. *Semin Oncol* 1998;25:13.

141. DeConti R, Toftness B, Lange R, et al. Clinical and pharmacological studies with cis-diam-minedichloroplatinum (II). *Cancer Res* 1973;33:1310.

142. Himmelstein K, Patton T, Belt R, et al. Clinical kinetics on intact cisplatin and some related species. *Clin Pharmacol Ther* 1981;29:658.

143. Vermorken J, Vijgh W, Klein VD, et al. Pharmacokinetics of free and total platinum species after short-term infusion of cisplatin. *Cancer Treat Rep* 1984;68:505.

144. Gormley P, Bull J, LeRoy A, et al. Kinetics of cis-dichlorodiammineplatinum. *Clin Pharmacol Ther* 1979;25:351.

145. Belt R, Himmelstein K, Patton T, et al. Pharmacokinetics of non-protein-bound platinum species following administration of cis-dichlorodiammineplatinum (II). *Cancer Treat Rep* 1979;63:1515.

146. Casper E, Kelsen D, Alcock N, et al. Platinum concentrations in bile and plasma following rapid and 6-hour infusions of cis-dichlorodiammineplatinum (II). *Cancer Treat Rep* 1979;63:2023.

147. Harland S, Newell D, Siddik Z, et al. Pharmacokinetics of cis-diammine-1,1-cyclobutane dicarboxylate platinum (II) in patients with normal and impaired renal function. *Cancer Res* 1984;44:1693.

148. Graham MA, Lockwood GF, Greenslade D, et al. Clinical pharmacokinetics of oxaliplatin: a critical review. *Clin Cancer Res* 2000;6:1205.

149. Gamelin E, Bouil A, Boisdron-Celle M, et al. Cumulative pharmacokinetic study of oxaliplatin, administered every three weeks, combined with 5-fluorouracil in colorectal cancer patients. *Clin Cancer Res* 1997;3:891.

150. Chatelut E, Canal P, Brunner V, et al. Prediction of carboplatin clearance from standard morphological and biological patient characteristics. *J Natl Cancer Inst* 1995;87:573.

151. Jodrell D, Egorin M, Canetta R, et al. Relationships between carboplatin exposure and tumor response and toxicity in patients with ovarian cancer. *J Clin Oncol* 1992;10:520.

152. Reyno L, Egorin M, Canetta R, et al. Impact of cyclophosphamide on relationships between carboplatin exposure and response or toxicity when used in the treatment of advanced ovarian cancer. *J Clin Oncol* 1993;11:1156.

153. O'Dwyer P, Hamilton T, Yao K, et al. Cellular pharmacodynamics of anticancer drugs. In: Schilsky R, Milano G, Ratain M, eds. *Cancer pharmacology*. New York: Dekker, 1996:329.

154. Ma J, Verweij J, Planting A, et al. Current sample handling methods for measurement of platinum-DNA adducts in leucocytes in man lead to discrepant results in DNA adduct levels and DNA repair. *Br J Cancer* 1995;71:512.

155. Schellens J, Ma J, Planting A, et al. Relationship between the exposure to cisplatin, DNA-adduct formation in leucocytes and tumour response in patients with solid tumours. *Br J Cancer* 1996;73:1569.

156. Stoehlmacher J, Goekkurt E, Lenz HJ. Pharmacogenetic aspects in treatment of colorectal cancer—an update. *Pharmacogenomics* 2003;4:767.

157. Loehrer P, Einhorn L. Drugs five years later. Cisplatin. *Ann Intern Med* 1984;100:704.

158. Ozols R, Corden B, Jacob J, et al. High-dose cisplatin in hypertonic saline. *Ann Intern Med* 1984;100:19.

159. Howell S, Pfeifle C, Wung W, et al. Intraperitoneal cis-diamminedichloroplatinum with systemic thiosulfate protection. *Cancer Res* 1983;43:1426.

160. Alberts D, Liu P, Hannigan E, et al. Intraperitoneal cisplatin plus intravenous cyclophosphamide versus intravenous cisplatin plus intravenous cyclophosphamide for stage III ovarian cancer. *N Engl J Med* 1996;335:1950.

161. Solomon B, Soulen M, Baum R, et al. Chemoembolization of hepatocellular carcinoma with cisplatin, doxorubicin, mitomycin-C, Ethiodol, and polyvinyl alcohol: prospective evaluation of response and survival in a US population. *J Vasc Interv Radiol* 1999;10:793.

162. Evans B, Raju K, Calvert A, et al. Phase II study of JM8, a new platinum analog, in advanced ovarian carcinoma. *Cancer Treat Rep* 1983;67:997.

163. Ozols R, Behrens B, Ostchega Y, et al. High dose cisplatin and high dose carboplatin in refractory ovarian cancer. *Cancer Treat Rev* 1985;12:59.

164. Schilder R, Johnson S, Gallo J, et al. Phase I trial of multiple cycles of high-dose chemotherapy supported by autologous peripheral-blood stem cells. *J Clin Oncol* 1999;17:2198.

165. Levi F, Giacchetti S, Adam R, et al. Chronomodulation of chemotherapy against metastatic colorectal cancer. International Organization for Cancer Chronotherapy. *Eur J Cancer* 1995;31A:1264.

166. McMahon S, Priestley J. Peripheral neuropathies and neurotrophic factors: animal models and clinical perspectives. *Curr Opin Neurobiol* 1995;5:616.

167. Langer C, Leighton J, Comis R, et al. Paclitaxel and carboplatin in combination in the treatment of advanced non-small-cell lung cancer: a phase II toxicity, response, and survival analysis. *J Clin Oncol* 1995;13:1860.

168. Brienza S, Vignoud J, Itzhaki M, et al. Oxaliplatin (L-OHP): global safety in 682 patients. *Proc Am Soc Clin Oncol* 1995;14:209.

169. de Gramont A, Banzi M, Navarro M, et al. Oxaliplatin/5-FU/LV in adjuvant colon cancer: results of the International Randomized Mosaic Trial. *Proc Am Soc Clin Oncol* 2003;22:253.

SHIVAANI KUMMAR
VANITA NORONHA
EDWARD CHU

SECTION **6**

Antimetabolites

METHOTREXATE

Aminopterin was the first antimetabolite to demonstrate clinical activity in the treatment of patients with malignancy. This antifolate analogue was used to induce remissions in children with acute leukemia in the 1940s. Aminopterin was subsequently replaced by methotrexate (MTX), the 4-amino, 10-methyl analogue of folic acid. MTX remains the most widely used antifolate in cancer chemotherapy, with documented activity against a wide range of human malignancies, including many solid tumors and hematologic malignancies. Antifolates have also been used to treat a host of nonmalignant disorders, including psoriasis, rheumatoid arthritis, graft-versus-host disease, bacterial and plasmodial infections, and parasitic infections associated with acquired immunodeficiency syndrome. This class of agents represents the best-characterized and most versatile of all chemotherapeutic drugs in current clinical use.

MECHANISM OF ACTION

MTX is a tight-binding inhibitor of dihydrofolate reductase (DHFR), a critical enzyme in folate metabolism (Fig. 15.6-1).[1]

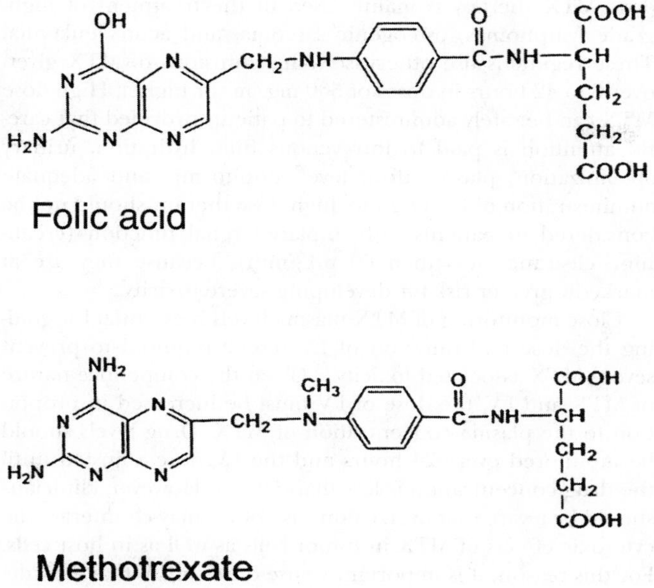

Folic acid

Methotrexate

FIGURE 15.6-1. Structures of methotrexate and folic acid.

The importance of DHFR stems from its role in maintaining the intracellular folate pool in its fully reduced form as tetrahydrofolates. These compounds serve as one-carbon carriers required for the synthesis of thymidine-5'-monophosphate (thymidylate), purine nucleotides, and certain amino acids. Thymidylate synthase (TS) catalyzes the formation of thymidine-5'-monophosphate from 2'-deoxyuridine-5'-monophosphate (deoxyuridylate, or dUMP). This reaction uses 5,10-methylenetetrahydrofolate as a methyl donor and results in the oxidation of the reduced folate to dihydrofolate. The reduced folate, 10-formyltetrahydrofolate, serves as a substrate for two folate-dependent enzymes of *de novo* purine synthesis, glycinamide ribonucleotide transformylase and aminoimidazole carboxamide ribonucleotide transformylase. An intact DHFR pathway is therefore necessary for *de novo* thymidylate and purine nucleotide biosynthesis.[1]

The precise mechanism by which MTX produces metabolic inhibition remains a subject of ongoing debate. The long-held view has been that inhibition of DHFR depletes the intracellular pool of reduced folates, which results in inhibition of *de novo* thymidylate and purine biosynthesis as well as inhibition of protein synthesis. However, several studies have demonstrated that intracellular reduced folates are depleted by only 50% to 70% after exposure of malignant cells to inhibitory concentrations of MTX, a level presumably insufficient to account for the observed inhibition of DNA synthesis.

The cytotoxic effects of MTX are mediated by their metabolism to polyglutamate forms. MTX polyglutamates are formed by the enzyme folylpolyglutamyl synthetase, which adds up to five to seven glutamyl groups in a γ-peptide linkage. Polyglutamation is a time- and concentration-dependent process that occurs in tumor cells and, to a lesser extent, in normal tissues. These polyglutamate metabolites have a prolonged intracellular half-life and allow for prolonged drug action in malignant cells. The relative difference in polyglutamate formation in normal versus malignant cells may account for the

selective activity of the drug. As much as 80% of MTX present in malignant tissues is in the polyglutamated forms, and these metabolites are potent, direct inhibitors of several folate-dependent enzymes, including DHFR, TS, and aminoimidazole carboxamide ribonucleotide and glycinamide ribonucleotide transformylases.[1]

MTX enters cells by the same active transport mechanisms used by physiologic reduced folates. Folate transport is a complex process with at least two carrier-mediated, energy-dependent mechanisms existing in mammalian cells. The first is the classic reduced folate carrier (RFC) system that exhibits a relatively low affinity for MTX and reduced folates such as leucovorin (LV), with affinity constants in the micromolar range.[2,3] The RFC system is primarily responsible for transport of MTX into cells at pharmacologic drug concentrations. A second folate transport system involves a high-affinity, membrane-bound folate receptor–binding protein with affinity constants for reduced folates and folic acid in the nanomolar range. The human folate receptor protein (FR) is expressed on the surface of various normal tissues, including human placenta, choroid plexus, renal tubules, and fallopian tubes.[4] Of note, this receptor is also highly expressed on the surface of a number of epithelial tumors, including ovarian cancer, but not on normal ovarian tissue, which makes it an attractive target for antigen-directed anticancer therapies. At least three different isoforms of the human FR have been described to date, and they are classified as FR-α, FR-β, and FR-γ.[2]

MECHANISMS OF RESISTANCE

The development of cellular resistance to MTX remains a major obstacle to its clinical efficacy. In experimental systems, resistance to antifolates may result from several mechanisms, including an alteration in antifolate transport due to either a defect in the RFC or FR systems, decreased capacity to polyglutamate MTX through either decreased expression of folylpolyglutamyl synthetase, or increased expression of the catabolic enzyme γ-glutamyl hydrolase, and alterations in the target enzyme DHFR through either increased expression of the wild-type protein or overexpression of a mutant protein with reduced binding affinity for MTX.[5-7] Amplification of the DHFR gene is one of the most common forms of MTX resistance observed in experimental systems. The amplified gene may be stably integrated into chromosomal DNA in the form of a homogeneously staining region or it may exist in extrachromosomal pieces of DNA known as *double-minute chromosomes*.[8] An alternative mechanism of resistance has been ascribed to mutations that result in a DHFR protein product with an altered binding affinity for MTX. There is evidence that naturally occurring DHFR alleles with differing affinities to MTX may exist in cells and provide a mechanism for the rapid emergence of MTX resistance.[9] In several *in vitro* experimental model systems, the levels of DHFR enzyme activity acutely increase after exposure to MTX and other antifolate compounds. This acute induction of DHFR in response to drug exposure is mediated, in part, by a translational regulatory mechanism. DHFR protein, in its unbound or free state, is capable of specifically repressing the translation of its own messenger RNA (mRNA). However, when DHFR protein is bound to an antifolate inhibitor, it is unable to repress DHFR mRNA translation, and the rate of new DHFR protein synthesis increases. Thus, induction of DHFR may represent a clinically relevant mechanism for the acute development of cellular drug resistance.[10]

Despite many years of active investigation, the relative contribution of each of these different mechanisms to the development of cellular resistance to MTX remains unclear. There is growing evidence, however, to support the concept that the emergence of MTX resistance in the clinical setting is a multifactorial process. DHFR gene amplification, defective transport, and decreased polyglutamate formation have all been observed in clinical specimens taken from MTX-resistant patients.

CLINICAL PHARMACOLOGY AND PHARMACOKINETICS

The absorption of oral MTX is saturable and erratic at doses greater than 25 mg/m^2. As a result, MTX is usually administered intravenously. Although plasma pharmacokinetics are variable, MTX metabolism generally follows a three-phase pattern. The initial distribution phase lasts for only a few minutes and is followed by a second phase lasting 12 to 24 hours, during which time the drug is eliminated with a half-life of 2 to 3 hours. The final phase of drug clearance has a half-life of 8 to 10 hours. The last two phases of drug elimination are considerably lengthened in patients with renal dysfunction.

The distribution of MTX into third-space fluid collections, such as pleural effusions and ascitic fluid, can substantially alter MTX pharmacokinetics. The slow release of accumulated MTX from these third spaces over time prolongs the terminal half-life of the drug, leading to potentially increased clinical toxicity.[1] Although no strict guidelines exist for the treatment of patients with ascites or pleural effusions, it is advisable to evacuate these fluid collections before treatment and monitor plasma drug concentrations closely. In addition, patients with bladder cancer who have undergone cystectomy and ileal conduit loop diversion may experience increased toxicity secondary to MTX treatment.[11] Thus, caution should be used when treating this particular subset of patients with MTX.

Elimination of MTX occurs primarily through renal excretion. MTX is filtered by the glomerulus and is actively secreted in the proximal tubule. Renal excretion of MTX is inhibited by probenecid, penicillins, cephalosporins, aspirin, and nonsteroidal antiinflammatory drugs. Patients with impaired renal function (creatinine clearance less than 60 mL/min) should not be treated with high-dose MTX. Moreover, standard dosages of MTX should be reduced in proportion to reductions in creatinine clearance.

Biliary excretion of MTX represents approximately 10% of overall MTX drug clearance. However, in the presence of renal dysfunction, enterohepatic circulation may assume a more important role in drug elimination. The majority of MTX excreted in bile is reabsorbed as intact drug, but an undefined fraction is converted by intestinal flora to the inactive metabolite 2,4-diamino-N^{10}-methyl pteroic acid (DAMPA). Intestinal binding of drug with oral charcoal or the anion-exchange resin cholestyramine enhances nonrenal drug excretion. Given the relatively minor role of biliary excretion in drug elimination, no adjustments in MTX dosage are necessary for patients with hepatic dysfunction.

The safe use of high-dose MTX with LV rescue requires a thorough understanding of MTX pharmacokinetics.[12] High-dose MTX therapy is mainly used in the treatment of high-grade lymphomas, osteogenic sarcoma, and acute leukemia. These regimens use otherwise lethal infusions of MTX given over 6 to 42 hours in doses of 500 mg/m^2 or higher. High-dose MTX can be safely administered to patients provided that careful attention is paid to intravenous fluid hydration, urinary alkalinization, plasma drug level monitoring, and adequate administration of LV. Of note, high-dose therapy should not be considered in patients with impaired renal function (creatinine clearance less than 60 mL/min), because they are at markedly greater risk for developing severe toxicity.

Close monitoring of MTX plasma levels is essential for guiding the dose and duration of LV rescue required to prevent severe MTX-associated toxicity.[13] Given the competitive nature of MTX and LV, the dose of LV must be increased in proportion to the plasma concentration of MTX. Drug levels should be monitored every 24 hours and the LV dose adjusted until the drug concentration is less than 50 nM. However, clinicians should be aware that overzealous use of LV may counteract the cytotoxic effects of MTX in tumor cells as well as in host cells. For this reason, it is important to use doses of LV that are adequate but not excessive, so that normal but not tumor cells are rescued. In patients with delayed MTX excretion, LV is usually given intravenously, because its oral bioavailability is decreased at total doses higher than 40 mg.

MTX penetrates poorly into the cerebrospinal fluid (CSF), and CSF levels are 30-fold lower than plasma levels at equilibrium.[14] However, after high-dose MTX therapy, peak CSF levels greater than the therapeutic threshold of 1 μmol can be achieved. Systemic high-dose MTX therapy has been used to prevent meningeal leukemia and lymphoma. Intrathecal injection of MTX can also be used for prophylaxis. For treatment of meningeal carcinomatosis, injection of MTX through an indwelling Ommaya reservoir is recommended, because drug administered into the CSF via the lumbar space circulates poorly into the ventricles, which results in inadequate CSF drug levels.

TOXICITY

The main side effects of MTX therapy are myelosuppression and gastrointestinal toxicity (Table 15.6-1). The occurrence of these adverse effects depends on the dose, schedule, and route of drug administration. Mucositis usually appears 3 to 7 days after MTX therapy and precedes the decrease in granulocyte and platelet count by several days. Myelosuppression and mucositis are usually completely reversed within 14 days, unless drug elimination mechanisms are impaired. In patients with compromised renal function, even small doses of MTX may result in serious toxicity. MTX-induced nephrotoxicity is thought to result from the intratubular precipitation of MTX and its metabolites in acidic urine. Antifolates may also exert a direct toxic effect on the renal tubules. Vigorous hydration and urinary alkalinization have greatly reduced the incidence of renal failure in patients on high-dose regimens.[1]

MTX is associated with both acute and chronic hepatotoxicity. Acute elevations in hepatic enzyme levels, as well as hyperbilirubinemia, are often observed during high-dose therapy, but these levels usually return to normal within 10 days. Chronic administration of daily oral MTX, as has been used in the treatment of psoriasis, is associated with the development of hepatic fibrosis in as

TABLE 15.6-1. Antimetabolites: Dosages and Toxicities

Chemotherapeutic Agent	Dosage	Indications	Common Toxicities
Methotrexate	Low dose: 25 mg/m² IV weekly Moderate dose: 40 mg/m² IV every 3 wk High dose: 1–12 g/m² IV every 3 wk Intrathecal: 10–15 mg/m² once or twice a week	Breast cancer, ALL, lymphoma, meningeal carcinomatosis	Myelosuppression, mucositis, acute cerebral dysfunction, pneumonitis
5-Fluorouracil	Mayo Clinic regimen: 425 mg/m² IV on d 1–5 every 28 d Roswell Park regimen: 500 mg/m² IV weekly for 6 wk every 8 wk	Colorectal, breast, head and neck, gastrointestinal malignancies	Myelosuppression, mucositis, diarrhea, hand-foot syndrome, neurotoxicity, photosensitivity
Capecitabine	1250 mg/m² b.i.d. orally for 14 d followed by 1 wk of rest; repeat every 3 wk; may reduce dosage to 900–1000 mg/m² b.i.d. to reduce toxicity with no reduction in activity	Metastatic breast and colorectal cancer	Hand-foot syndrome, diarrhea, nausea, vomiting
Cytarabine	Standard dose: 100 mg/m²/d IV on d 1–7 as a continuous infusion High dose: 1.5–3.0 g/m² IV every 12 h for 3 d Intrathecal: 10–30 mg IT up to 3 times weekly	AML	Myelosuppression, nausea, vomiting, cerebellar toxicity
Gemcitabine	Pancreatic cancer: 1000 mg/m² IV every week for 7 wk with 1 wk rest Bladder cancer: 1000 mg/m² IV on d 1, 8, 15 Lung cancer: 1200 mg/m² IV on d 1, 8, 15	Non–small cell lung, pancreatic, bladder cancer	Myelosuppression, nausea, vomiting, flu-like syndrome, infusion reaction
6-Mercaptopurine	2.5 mg/kg PO daily	ALL	Myelosuppression, hepatotoxicity, mucositis
6-Thioguanine	1–3 mg/kg PO daily	ALL, AML	Myelosuppression, nausea, vomiting, hepatotoxicity
Fludarabine	25 mg/m²/d for 5 d every 28 d (administered IV over 30 min)	CLL, lymphoproliferative disorders	Myelosuppression, immunosuppression, hemolytic anemia, myalgias, arthralgias, fever
Cladribine	0.09 mg/kg/d IV continuous infusion for 7 d	Hairy cell leukemia, lymphoproliferative disorders	Myelosuppression, immunosuppression, fever, nausea, vomiting

ALL, acute lymphoblastic leukemia; AML, acute myeloid leukemia; CLL, acute lymphocytic leukemia.

many as 25% of patients. Cirrhosis of the liver has also been described in this group. MTX causes a poorly defined, self-limited pneumonitis characterized by fever, cough, and interstitial pulmonary infiltrates. Lung biopsy studies have not revealed consistent pathologic findings. Although a hypersensitivity reaction has been proposed as a possible explanation, rechallenge with MTX does not uniformly result in a return of symptoms.

Three distinct neurotoxic syndromes are associated with intrathecal MTX therapy.[15] The most common syndrome is an acute chemical arachnoiditis that arises immediately after intrathecal drug administration. This syndrome is characterized by severe headaches, nuchal rigidity, vomiting, fever, and an inflammatory cell infiltrate in the CSF. A subacute form of neurotoxicity is seen in approximately 10% of patients and usually occurs after the third or fourth course of intrathecal therapy. It is most common in adults with active meningeal leukemia and consists of motor paralysis, cranial nerve palsies, and seizures or coma, or both. A change in therapy is absolutely indicated, because continued intrathecal MTX therapy may result in death. The third syndrome is a chronic demyelinating encephalopathy, typically occurring in children months to years after receiving intrathecal MTX. Patients present with dementia, limb spasticity, and, in advanced cases, coma. Computed tomographic scan reveals ventricular enlargement, cortical thinning, and diffuse intracerebral calcifications.

High-dose systemic MTX therapy is occasionally associated with an acute, transient cerebral dysfunction with symptoms of paresis, aphasia, and behavioral abnormalities, and seizures have also been described in 4% to 15% of patients receiving high-dose MTX. Symptoms occur within 6 days of MTX treatment and usually completely resolve within 48 to 72 hours. In addition, a chronic form of neurotoxicity is manifested as an encephalopathy with dementia and motor paresis developing in the second or third month after treatment. At present, the underlying mechanism of CNS toxicity from MTX remains unknown. There is no evidence to support the therapeutic use of LV in patients who develop neurotoxic symptoms.

NEW ANTIFOLATES

RALTITREXED

Raltitrexed (ZD1694, Tomudex) is a quinazoline antifolate that is a potent and specific inhibitor of TS. Like MTX, raltitrexed is actively transported into the cell via the RFC and undergoes polyglutamation to higher polyglutamate forms, which are 100-fold more potent at inhibiting TS than the parent compound. Several mechanisms of resistance to raltitrexed have been identified, including reduced transport, decreased polyglutamation, and overexpression of the target enzyme, TS.[16,17]

This antifolate analogue is eliminated mainly via renal excretion, with a terminal half-life of 10 to 22 hours. The major toxicities include an anorexia and fatigue syndrome, diarrhea, myelosuppression, and reversible transaminasemia. This agent has shown clinical activity against a wide spectrum of solid tumors, including advanced colorectal, breast, hepatocellular, platinum-resistant ovarian, non–small cell lung, gastric, and pancreatic cancers, and malignant pleural mesothelioma.[18] At present, it is approved as first-line therapy for patients with advanced colorectal cancer in Australia, Canada, and several European countries, but it remains an investigational agent in the United States. Recently, focus has been placed on developing novel combination regimens incorporating raltitrexed, and the combination of raltitrexed with oxaliplatin appears especially promising for the treatment of advanced colorectal cancer and malignant mesothelioma.

PEMETREXED

Pemetrexed (LY231514) is a pyrrolopyrimidine, multitargeted antifolate analogue that targets multiple enzymes involved in folate metabolism, including TS, DHFR, glycinamide ribonucleotide formyltransferase, and aminoimidazole carboxamide formyl transferase.[19] It enters the cell via the RFC system and to a lesser extent via the FR system. It undergoes polyglutamation within the cell to the pentaglutamate form, which is at least 60-fold more potent than the parent compound. Pemetrexed exerts its cytotoxic activity by arresting cells in the G_1-S phase of the cell cycle. Phase I studies identified the optimal dose and schedule to be 500 to 600 mg/m^2 intravenously administered every 3 weeks. The mean half-life is 3.1 hours, and it is primarily cleared by renal excretion, with as much as 90% of the parent drug in the urine during the first 24 hours after administration. For this reason, this drug must be used with caution in patients with renal dysfunction, and dosage reduction should be considered.

The main toxicities of this agent include dose-limiting myelosuppression, mucositis, and skin rash. Other toxicities include reversible transaminasemia, anorexia and fatigue syndrome, and gastrointestinal toxicity. These toxicities are markedly decreased by supplementation with folic acid (350 µg orally daily) and vitamin B_{12} (1000 µg intramuscularly given 1 to 3 weeks before starting therapy, then repeated every 3 weeks). The clinical evidence to date suggests that this vitamin supplementation does not reduce the clinical efficacy of pemetrexed.[20]

This novel antifolate has shown activity in a broad range of solid tumors, including malignant mesothelioma and breast, pancreatic, head and neck, non–small cell lung, colon, gastric, cervical, and bladder cancers. A published phase III study compared single-agent cisplatin with the combination of cisplatin and pemetrexed in patients with malignant pleural mesothelioma. The addition of pemetrexed to cisplatin therapy significantly improved the clinical efficacy in terms of response rate, progression-free survival, and overall survival. Based on these findings, the U.S. Food and Drug Administration (FDA) has approved this combination for treatment of malignant pleural mesothelioma.[21]

5-FLUOROPYRIMIDINES

The fluoropyrimidine 5-fluorouracil (5-FU) was synthesized by Dr. Charles Heidelberger in 1957 based on the seminal observation that rat hepatoma cells used uracil more effi-

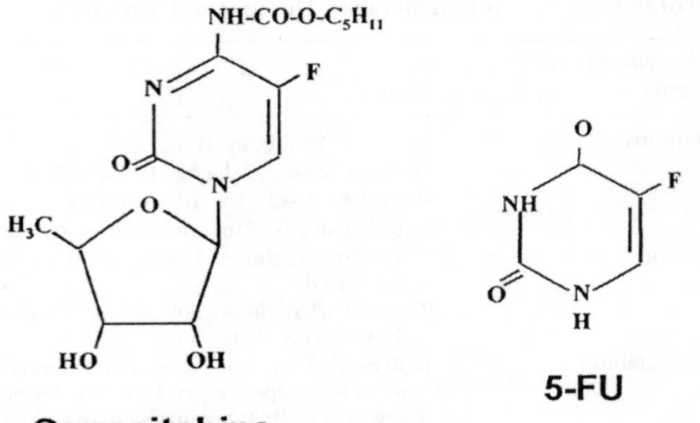

FIGURE 15.6-2. Structures of fluoropyrimidines of clinical interest. 5-FU, 5-fluorouracil.

ciently than normal rat intestinal mucosa. This finding suggested that uracil metabolism might represent a potential target for cancer chemotherapy. The fluoropyrimidines are active in a wide range of solid tumors, including gastrointestinal malignancies (esophageal, gastric, pancreatic, colorectal, anal, and hepatocellular cancers), and breast, head and neck, and ovarian carcinomas.

The chemical structures of the fluoropyrimidines commonly used in clinical practice are shown in Figure 15.6-2. 5-FU has a fluorine atom substituted in place of hydrogen at the C5 position of the pyrimidine ring. The deoxyribonucleoside derivative 5-fluoro-2'-deoxyuridine (FUdR) is limited in its clinical use given its rapid degradation in normal and tumor tissues. For this reason, it is not administered systemically, but rather its use has been strictly limited to hepatic arterial infusions. Tegafur and 5'-deoxyfluorouridine are oral prodrug fluoropyrimidine analogues that are widely used in Asia for the treatment of colorectal cancer and other gastrointestinal malignancies but remain under investigation in the United States.

Mechanism of Action

In its parent form, 5-FU is inactive and requires intracellular activation to exert cytotoxic effects. 5-FU readily enters cells via the facilitated uracil transport mechanism, whereas FUdR is a substrate for the facilitated nucleoside transport system. These compounds are anabolized to cytotoxic forms by several biochemical pathways. 5-FU is converted to FUdR by thymidine phosphorylase. Subsequent phosphorylation of FUdR by thymidine kinase results in formation of the active metabolite 5-fluoro-2'-deoxyuridine monophosphate (FdUMP). In the presence of the reduced folate cofactor 5,10-methylenetetrahydrofolate, FdUMP forms a stable covalent complex with TS. TS catalyzes the sole intracellular *de novo* formation of thymidine-5'-monophosphate from dUMP. Inhibition of TS leads to depletion of deoxythymidine triphosphate (dTTP), thus interfering with DNA biosynthesis and repair. 5-FU is metabolized to fluorouridine monophosphate through the sequential action of uridine phosphorylase and uridine kinase. In the presence of 5'-phosphoribosyl-1-pyrophosphate, orotic acid phosphoribosyltransferase directly converts 5-FU to fluorouridine monophosphate. This metabolite is further metabolized to fluorouridine diphosphate and then to the triphosphate form (FUTP), which is subsequently incorporated into RNA.[22,23]

Inhibition of TS by FdUMP is considered one of the principal mechanisms of 5-FU action. The TS-FdUMP-folate ternary complex is slowly dissociable, and the intracellular level of 5,10-methylenetetrahydrofolate is critical for ternary complex formation as well as for maintaining enzyme inhibition. Depletion of intracellular reduced folate pools prevents ternary complex formation in various tissue culture systems.[24] Pharmacologic concentrations of LV (5-formyltetrahydrofolate) enhance the cytotoxicity of 5-FU by expanding the intracellular pools of 5,10-methylenetetrahydrofolate and thereby increasing the extent and duration of TS inhibition. Randomized clinical trials in advanced colorectal cancer indicate that the addition of LV to bolus 5-FU significantly improves the response rate compared with bolus 5-FU alone.[25] However, the actual benefit in patient survival is marginal and on the order of only 2 to 3 months.

The 5-FU metabolite FUTP is incorporated into both nuclear and cytoplasmic RNA species. Incorporation into RNA interferes with normal RNA processing and function.[26] The extent of RNA incorporation correlates with cytotoxicity in some *in vitro* tissue culture and *in vivo* models. Inhibition of TS leads not only to depletion of dTTP but to accumulation of dUMP. Both FdUMP and dUMP may be subsequently metabolized to their respective triphosphate forms. Incorporation of deoxyuridine triphosphate (dUTP) and fluorodeoxyuridine triphosphate (FdUTP) into cellular DNA, with resultant inhibition of DNA synthesis and function, may represent another mechanism of cytotoxicity. dUTP nucleotidehydrolase degrades triphosphate nucleotides and limits the intracellular accumulation of (F)dUTP. The nucleotide excision repair enzyme uracil-DNA glycosylase attempts to repair DNA that contains uracil and 5-FU; however, this is unsuccessful if the intracellular nucleotide ratio favors (F)dUTP over dTTP. The combined effects of dTTP depletion and (F)dUTP-DNA incorporation result in inhibition of nascent DNA chain elongation, altered DNA stability, production of DNA single-strand breaks, and interference with DNA repair. The genotoxic stress resulting from TS inhibition may also activate programmed cell death pathways in susceptible cells, which leads to induction of parental DNA fragmentation. Factors operating downstream from TS (e.g., Bcl-2 and p53 status) may influence the cellular response to such genotoxic stress.[27,28] Studies suggest that 5-FU cytotoxicity in some human colon cancer cells is related to activation of Fas-mediated pathways.[29]

Mechanisms of Resistance

Given the multiple sites of cytotoxic action of 5-FU and the various metabolic pathways required for its activation, it is not surprising that several mechanisms of resistance have been identified in experimental and clinical settings. In human and murine tumor cells selected *in vitro* for resistance to 5-FU, a variety of mechanisms have been described. Deletion or diminished activity of thymidine or uridine kinase, thymidine or uridine phosphorylase, and orotate phosphoribosyl transferase interferes with metabolic activation. Decreased accumulation of FUTP, FdUMP, and (F)dUTP may result from increased activity of catabolic enzymes [acid and alkaline phosphatases, dUTP hydrolase, and dihydropyrimidine dehydrogenase (DPD)]. Decreased incorporation of 5-FU into both RNA and DNA may result in decreased sensitivity. A relative deficiency of the reduced folate substrate 5,10-methylenetetrahydrofolate may also compromise the cytotoxic action of FdUMP on TS. This may result from low extracellular levels of reduced folates, decreased membrane transport of reduced folates, or reduced activity of folylpolyglutamate synthase, which thereby prevents its polyglutamation.[22] However, the relative contribution of each of these mechanisms in the development of cellular resistance to 5-FU in the actual clinical setting remains unclear.

Alterations in the target enzyme TS represent the most commonly described mechanism of resistance to 5-FU. Point mutations in the protein-coding region of the TS gene A give rise to a decrease in binding affinity of the 5-FU metabolite FdUMP to the TS target. *In vitro*, *in vivo*, and clinical model systems have shown a strong correlation between the levels of TS enzyme activity and TS protein and chemosensitivity to 5-FU. In this regard, cell lines and tumors with higher levels of TS are relatively more resistant to 5-FU. This increase in TS protein content is usually associated with amplification of the TS gene.[22] In several *in vitro* and *in vivo* model systems, the levels of TS enzyme activity and TS protein acutely increase after exposure to 5-FU, other specific TS inhibitor compounds, or both. Moreover, acute increases in the expression of TS protein have been identified in the clinical setting in paired tumor tissue biopsy specimens obtained from patients before and during therapy with 5-FU. This acute induction of TS protein in response to drug exposure is mediated by two different mechanisms. The first relates to enhanced stability of the protein via a posttranslational event. The second is controlled by a translational regulatory mechanism. TS protein, in its unbound or free state, is capable of specifically repressing the translation of its own mRNA. However, when TS protein is bound to either nucleotide, antifolate inhibitors, or both, it is unable to repress TS mRNA translation, and the rate of new TS protein synthesis increases. Thus, induction of TS may represent an efficient and clinically relevant mechanism for the acute development of drug resistance.

Clinical Pharmacology

5-FU is normally given intravenously, and it has a short metabolic half-life on the order of 15 minutes. It is not administered by the oral route because its bioavailability is erratic given the high levels of the breakdown enzyme DPD present in the gut mucosa. Floxuridine (FUdR) exerts its cytotoxic activity in a manner similar to that of 5-FU, and it is only used for hepatic artery infusions. A cream incorporating 5-FU is used topically for treating basal cell cancers of the skin.

5-FU is administered by either intravenous bolus or continuous infusion. The volume of distribution is slightly larger than the extracellular space, and 5-FU readily penetrates into tissues, CSF, and extracellular third-space accumulations such as ascites or pleural effusions. After intravenous bolus doses, metabolic elimination is rapid, with a primary half-life of 8 to 14 minutes. Plasma levels of 5-FU fall below 1 μmol within 2 hours, an approximate threshold for cytotoxic effects. More than 85% of an administered dose of 5-FU is enzymatically inactivated by DPD.[30,31] Although the liver expresses the highest levels of DPD in the body, this enzyme is widely distributed in other tissues, including gastrointestinal mucosa and peripheral lymphocytes. Rare patients with inherited DPD deficiency may experience life-threatening or fatal toxicity when treated with fluoropyrimidine-based chemotherapy.[32,33] Because affected individuals are in otherwise good health, the first indication of the presence of this inborn error of metabolism usually follows an unexpectedly severe reaction to 5-FU chemotherapy. Careful testing of DPD-deficient patients has revealed an autosomal recessive pattern of inheritance. It is now estimated that as many as 3% to 5% of adult cancer patients may exhibit this pharmacogenetic syndrome. Several molecular defects, including point mutations and deletions due to exon skipping, have been identified in DPD-deficient patients who experience severe toxicity in response to 5-FU.

Toxicity

The primary effects of 5-FU are exerted on rapidly dividing tissues, specifically gastrointestinal mucosa and bone marrow (see Table 15.6-1). The spectrum of toxicities associated with 5-FU varies considerably according to the dose, schedule, and route of administration. Epithelial ulceration may occur throughout the gastrointestinal tract and is manifested as mucositis or diarrhea or both. The diarrhea associated with 5-FU therapy may be watery or bloody, and the combination of nausea, vomiting, and profuse diarrhea can lead, in some cases, to profound dehydration and orthostatic hypotension. Disruption of the integrity of the gut lining may permit access of enteric organisms into the blood stream, with the potential for overwhelming sepsis, particularly if the granulocyte nadir coincides with diarrhea. 5-FU should be withheld in the face of ongoing mucositis or diarrhea, even if mild, and subsequent doses should be reduced when the patient has fully recovered. If diarrhea occurs, supportive care and vigorous hydration should be given. Antidiarrheal agents such as diphenoxylate and loperamide may help control mild to moderate diarrhea, but they are generally ineffective in controlling diarrhea of greater severity. In this setting, the somatostatin analogue octreotide has been effective. Mouth cooling (oral cryotherapy) with oral ice chips for 30 minutes starting immediately before bolus 5-FU reduces the severity of mucositis. Nausea and vomiting may occur but are usually controlled with antiemetics. Myelosuppression may also be observed, with granulocytopenia occurring more than thrombocytopenia. With the schedule of a daily dose for 5 days, the granulocyte and platelet nadirs tend to occur during the second or third week of treatment. In contrast, myelosuppression generally occurs after the fourth weekly dose on the weekly bolus 5-FU schedule.

Other dermatologic toxicities associated with 5-FU therapy include alopecia, changes in the fingernails, and dermatitis that varies from a pruritic erythematous rash followed by scaling to more severe cases with vesicle formation. 5-FU enhances the cutaneous toxicity of radiation, and reactions usually occur within 7 days of radiation. Photosensitivity reactions, increased pigmentation over the veins into which 5-FU has been administered as well as more generalized hyperpigmentation, and atrophy are possible. Hand-foot syndrome most often occurs with protracted infusion schedules of 5-FU but may also be seen in patients receiving bolus schedules of 5-FU. Ocular toxicity includes blepharitis, epiphora, tear duct stenosis, and acute and chronic conjunctivitis. Acute neurologic symptoms have also been reported, and they include somnolence, cerebellar ataxia, and upper motor signs. A syndrome of chest pain, cardiac enzyme elevations, and electrocardiographic changes consistent with myocardial ischemia may be seen in temporal

association with 5-FU administration. In some patients, coronary angiography reveals no abnormalities, which suggests vasospasm as a possible mechanism.

Intrahepatic administration of FUdR is complicated mainly by cholestatic jaundice and biliary sclerosis. These adverse side effects result from direct perfusion of the blood supply to the gallbladder and upper bile duct with high local drug concentrations. Of note, this complication occurs much less frequently with hepatic arterial infusion of 5-FU.[34] Addition of dexamethasone to the infusion mixture reduces the incidence of hepatotoxicity from 30% to 9%, and this combination yields improved clinical activity in patients with liver-limited disease. Biliary sclerosis typically occurs by the third cycle of treatment. Catheter-related complications include thrombosis of the catheterized vessel, hemorrhage or infection at the site of insertion, and slippage of the catheter into the gastroduodenal artery with resultant necrosis of the intestinal epithelium, hemorrhage, and perforation.

Drug Interactions

Significant efforts have focused on enhancing the antitumor activity of 5-FU through the process of biochemical modulation whereby 5-FU is combined with various agents, including LV, MTX, N-phosphonoacetyl-L-aspartic acid, interferon-α, interferon-γ, and a whole host of other agents.[35] For the past 20 to 25 years, the reduced folate LV has been used as the main biochemical modulator of 5-FU. However, although all of the randomized studies have shown a significant improvement in overall response rate, use of this combination has not translated into a meaningful survival benefit. Moreover, the toxicity of 5-FU appears to be increased on addition of LV. An alternative approach has been to alter the schedule of 5-FU administration. Given the S-phase specificity of this agent, it was proposed that prolonged exposures of tumor cells to 5-FU would increase the fraction of cells being exposed to drug. With this in mind, protracted continuous infusion schedules were developed. Overall response rates are significantly higher in patients treated with infusional schedules of 5-FU than in those treated with bolus 5-FU, and this improvement in response rate has translated into a survival benefit, albeit of only 1 month. Moreover, the overall safety profile is improved with infusional regimens, specifically as it relates to the reduced incidence of grade 3 or 4 myelosuppression. A hybrid schedule of bolus and infusional 5-FU in combination with LV was developed by de Gramont and colleagues[35a] in France and has shown superior clinical activity compared to bolus 5-FU plus LV schedules. This infusional de Gramont regimen now serves as a main backbone for combination therapy for advanced colorectal cancer.

Preclinical studies demonstrate that 5-FU significantly enhances the cytotoxicity of ionizing radiation. Both preclinical and clinical studies have revealed that the cytotoxic and antitumor effects of radiation therapy are enhanced in the presence of prolonged exposure to 5-FU.[36,37] The underlying mechanisms for this synergistic interaction include increased DNA damage, inhibition of DNA repair, and accumulation of cells in S phase. Some work suggests that the G_1-S checkpoint may play a critical role in determining the ability of 5-FU to enhance the cytotoxic effects of radiation therapy. One example highlighting the successful clinical application of this

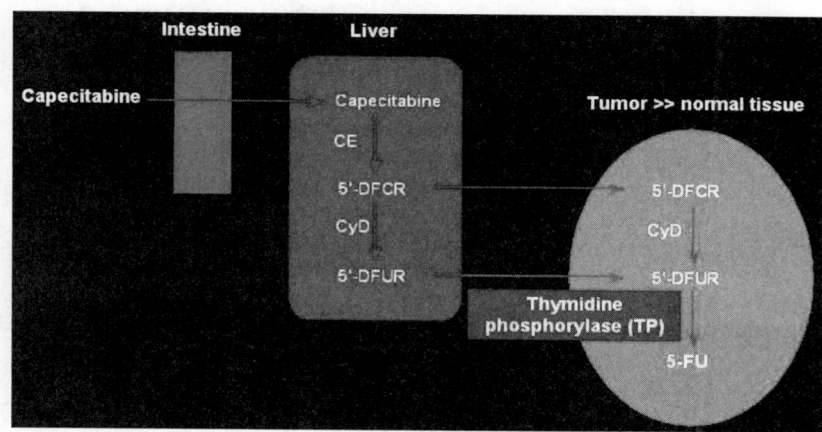

FIGURE 15.6-3. Mechanism of activation of capecitabine. CE, carboxylesterase; CyD, cytidine deaminase; 5'-DFCR, 5'-deoxy-5-fluorocytidine; 5'-DFUR, 5'-deoxy-5-fluorouridine; 5-FU, 5-fluorouracil. (See Color Fig. 15.6-3 in the CD-ROM.)

approach is the use of protracted infusional 5-FU during pelvic radiation in the neoadjuvant treatment of locally advanced rectal cancer.

ORAL FLUOROPYRIMIDINES

An alternative strategy to modulating 5-FU–based chemotherapy has been the development of oral fluoropyrimidine analogues.[38,39] The initial rationale for oral therapy was to provide treatment that would more closely mimic infusional schedules of 5-FU but avoid the complications associated with intravenous infusional therapy. In addition, oral therapy would certainly be more convenient for patients and allow patients to maintain their normal activities of daily living by being able to take their treatment at home. The initial attempts at developing oral 5-FU were largely unsuccessful, mainly due to the fact that 5-FU is poorly and erratically absorbed and rapidly degraded in the intestinal mucosa by the catabolic enzyme DPD. Efforts were then focused on developing prodrug forms of 5-FU that could overcome the rapid breakdown by DPD.

Capecitabine

Capecitabine (N^4-pentoxycarbonyl-5'-deoxy-5-fluorocytidine, Xeloda) is a novel oral fluoropyrimidine carbamate that was rationally designed to allow for selective 5-FU activation in tumor tissue (see Fig. 15.6-2).[40] In contrast to 5-FU, it is rapidly and extensively absorbed by the gut mucosa, with nearly 80% oral bioavailability. It is inactive in its parent form and must undergo enzymatic conversion via three successive steps (Fig. 15.6-3). It is first hydrolyzed in the liver by a hepatic carboxylesterase to an intermediate, 5'-deoxy-5-fluorocytidine, which in turn is converted to 5'-deoxy-5-fluorouridine by the enzyme cytidine deaminase. The third and final step occurs in tumor tissue and involves the conversion of 5'-deoxy-5-fluorouridine to 5-FU by the enzyme thymidine phosphorylase. Of particular interest is the fact that thymidine phosphorylase is expressed at significantly higher concentrations in tumors, including cancers of the breast, colon and rectum, cervix, head and neck, and stomach, than in surrounding normal tissue. Clinical studies have shown that 5-FU concentrations are nearly 3.5-fold higher in tumor tissue than in normal tissue and are more than 20-fold higher in tumor than in serum. After ingestion of capecitabine, peak plasma levels are attained in 1.5 hours, with peak 5-FU blood levels occurring at 2 hours.

Capecitabine and capecitabine metabolites are primarily excreted by the kidneys, and caution must be taken in the presence of renal dysfunction, with formal recommendations for dosage reduction. The dosage selected from trials is 1250 mg/m^2 orally twice a day for 2 weeks followed by a 1-week rest (see Table 15.6-1). Dose-limiting toxicities include nausea, vomiting, diarrhea, and hand-foot syndrome. Uncommon side effects include myelosuppression and hyperbilirubinemia.

Capecitabine is most active in breast and colorectal cancer, but it is also active in many other solid tumors, including pancreatic, gastroesophageal, ovarian, and head and neck cancers. It was initially approved by the FDA in 1998 as salvage therapy in anthracycline- and taxane-resistant breast cancer, after phase II studies that demonstrated a 20% to 30% response rate to capecitabine in this heavily pretreated subset of patients.[41] Preclinical studies demonstrated that docetaxel up-regulates thymidine phosphorylase and that the combination of docetaxel and capecitabine showed striking synergy.[41a] Based on these findings, a large international phase III trial was conducted comparing the combination of docetaxel and capecitabine with single-agent docetaxel in women with anthracycline-resistant breast cancer. There was significantly improved clinical benefit in terms of response rate, time to tumor progression, and median survival in favor of capecitabine and docetaxel compared to single-agent docetaxel.[42] This regimen was subsequently approved by the FDA as second-line therapy in metastatic breast cancer. This oral agent is also FDA-approved for use in the first-line treatment of metastatic colorectal cancer when fluoropyrimidine therapy alone is preferred. This approval was based on results of two large randomized phase III trials in patients with metastatic colorectal cancer that compared capecitabine to bolus 5-FU plus LV and showed that capecitabine was equivalent in terms of clinical efficacy but clearly superior with regard to safety profile and patient convenience.[43] Currently, efforts are focused on investigating the efficacy of capecitabine in combination with irinotecan or oxaliplatin, or both, in the treatment of advanced colorectal cancer; on determining the role of capecitabine in adjuvant therapy for early-stage colon cancer; and on incorporating capecitabine in combination with radiation therapy as part of neoadjuvant therapy for locally advanced rectal cancer. In addition, the role of capecitabine as monotherapy and in combination regimens for the treatment of other solid tumors is being actively investigated.

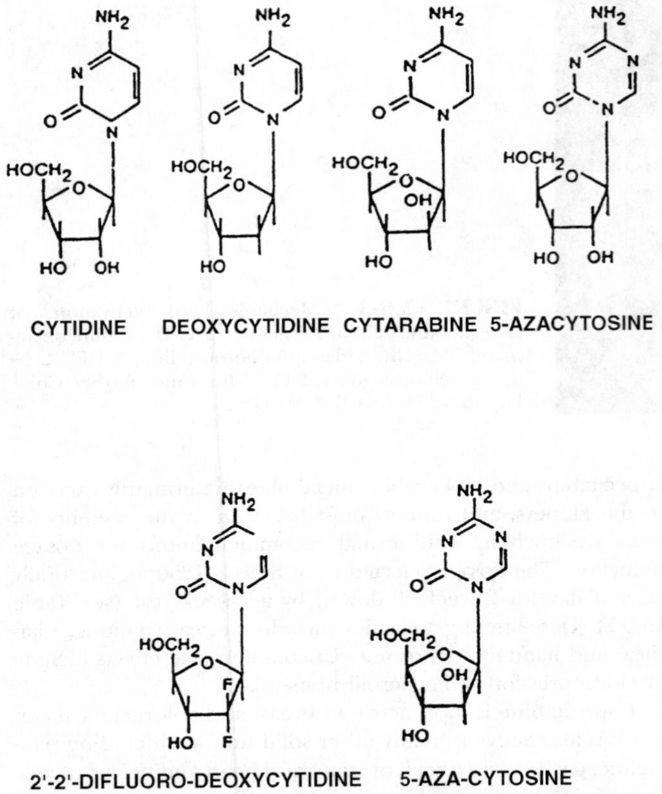

CYTIDINE   DEOXYCYTIDINE   CYTARABINE   5-AZACYTOSINE

2'-2'-DIFLUORO-DEOXYCYTIDINE   5-AZA-CYTOSINE
                                 ARABINOSIDE

FIGURE 15.6-4. Structures of deoxycytidine analogues of clinical interest.

Cytarabine

Cytarabine (1-β-D-arabinofuranosylcytosine, cytarabine, Ara-C) is one of several arabinose nucleosides isolated from the sponge *Cryptothethya crypta*, differing from its physiologic counterpart by virtue of a stereotypic inversion of the 2'-hydroxyl group of the sugar moiety (Fig. 15.6-4). It is one of the critical agents for the treatment of acute myelogenous leukemia (AML). A regimen of Ara-C combined with an anthracycline, given as a 5- or 7-day continuous infusion, is considered the standard induction treatment for AML. Furthermore, Ara-C is used in the treatment of other hematologic malignancies, such as non-Hodgkin's lymphoma, chronic myelogenous leukemia, and acute lymphocytic leukemia.

MECHANISM OF ACTION. As with other nucleoside analogues and their physiologic counterparts, Ara-C enters cells via nucleoside transport proteins, the most important one being the es (equilibrative inhibitor-sensitive) receptor. Once within the cytoplasm, Ara-C requires activation for its cytotoxic effects. The first metabolic step is the conversion of Ara-C to ara-cytidine monophosphate (Ara-CMP) by the enzyme deoxycytidine kinase (dCK). This enzyme is the rate-limiting step in intracellular anabolism of Ara-C. Ara-CMP is subsequently phosphorylated to ara-cytidine diphosphate (Ara-CDP) and ara-cytidine triphosphate (Ara-CTP) by the enzymes pyrimidine monophosphate kinase and pyrimidine diphosphate kinase, respectively. Ara-CTP competes with the native substrate deoxycytidine triphosphate

(dCTP) for DNA incorporation by DNA-directed DNA polymerase. The incorporated Ara-CTP residue is a potent inhibitor of DNA polymerase, delta-DNA polymerase, and beta-DNA polymerase. Inhibition of DNA polymerases, in turn, interferes with DNA chain elongation during both semiconservative DNA replication and DNA repair. In addition, Ara-CTP is incorporated into DNA and functions as a DNA chain terminator, interfering with chain elongation.[44,45] In some human leukemic cell lines, Ara-C–mediated DNA damage is accompanied by a pattern of internucleosomal DNA fragmentation typical of apoptosis (programmed cell death).[46] There is evidence suggesting that Ara-C metabolism in AML blasts differs from that in normal bone marrow mononuclear cells and CD34+ hematopoietic stem cells.[47] The total levels of phosphorylated Ara-C metabolites, including Ara-CMP, Ara-CDP, Ara-CTP, Ara-CDP–choline, and Ara–uridine monophosphate (Ara-UMP), were twofold to fourfold higher in leukemic blast cells than in normal bone marrow cells, both at standard and high doses of Ara-C.

Ara-C is most active in the S phase of the cell cycle. The rate of DNA synthesis influences Ara-C cytotoxicity, with maximum effects observed when cells are exposed to Ara-C during periods of rapid DNA synthesis. Prolonged exposures allow a greater proportion of cells to enter S phase, and such a schedule provides for enhanced incorporation of Ara-CTP into DNA. Thus, the duration of Ara-C exposure is a critical determinant of its cytotoxicity.[48,49]

Catabolism of Ara-C involves two key enzymes, cytidine deaminase and deoxycytidylate deaminase.[44] They convert Ara-C and Ara-CMP into the inactive metabolites, Ara-U and Ara-UMP, respectively. Other catabolic enzymes that may affect Ara-C metabolism include dCTP pyrophosphatase, 5'-nucleotidase, and alkaline and acid phosphatases. The balance between intracellular activation and degradation is critical in determining the amount of drug that is ultimately converted to Ara-CTP and, thus, its subsequent cytotoxic and antitumor activity.[50]

MECHANISMS OF RESISTANCE. Several mechanisms of resistance to Ara-C have been described. Impaired transmembrane transport, decreased rate of anabolism, and increased rate of catabolism may result in the development of Ara-C resistance. *In vitro* studies have demonstrated that amplification of the cytidine deaminase gene with resultant overexpression of the corresponding protein product leads to Ara-C resistance.[51] The level of cytidine deaminase enzyme activity has been shown to correlate with clinical response in patients with AML undergoing induction chemotherapy with Ara-C–containing regimens.[52] Blasts from patients who attained complete remission and from those with previously untreated leukemia had significantly lower levels of cytidine deaminase than blasts from patients with refractory disease.

Deletion of the gene encoding dCK, expansion of CTP and dCTP pools, overexpression of Bcl-2, and decreased intracellular half-life of Ara-CTP after drug removal are additional mechanisms that have been implicated in Ara-C resistance. The cytotoxicity of Ara-C in leukemic cells isolated from patients correlates well with both the extent of DNA incorporation and the intracellular retention of Ara-CTP after drug exposure.

CLINICAL PHARMACOLOGY AND PHARMACOKINETICS. Ara-C has poor oral bioavailability (approximately 20%) due to extensive deamination within the gastrointestinal tract. As a result, Ara-C is administered via the intravenous route. The drug can also be given subcutaneously. After intravenous bolus administration, Ara-C is rapidly cleared with biphasic elimination. The initial half-life is approximately 12 minutes, whereas the terminal half-life is approximately 2 hours. Within 24 hours, 78% of a bolus dose is excreted in the urine (71% as Ara-U, 7% as Ara-C). With continuous infusion of doses of 100 to 200 mg/m^2/d, steady-state plasma levels range from 0.2 to 1.0 μmol, and CSF levels are approximately 50% of the plasma levels.[53] Ara-C crosses the blood–brain barrier when used at high doses, with CSF levels between 7% and 14% of plasma levels and reaching peak levels of up to 10 μmol. Because cytidine deaminase enzyme activity is nearly completely absent in CSF, the drug displays a longer half-life in the CSF (2 to 4 hours).[54] Ara-C can also be given intrathecally to provide prophylaxis against CNS tumor involvement and to treat leptomeningeal disease of both hematologic and solid malignancies. The usual dose is 10 to 30 mg, administered twice weekly until documentation of three consecutive negative CSF cytologic results. Intrathecal administration of 50 mg/m^2 Ara-C yields peak concentrations of 1 mmol, and cytotoxic concentrations (0.4 μmol or above) are maintained for 24 hours.[44] Finally, Ara-C can also be administered via the intraperitoneal route. This approach is considered as salvage therapy for ovarian cancer patients presenting primarily with intraperitoneal disease, and the drug is usually given in combination with cisplatin.

A depot formulation has been developed (DTD 101, Depo-Cyt) in which Ara-C is encapsulated in multivesicular liposomes for sustained release into the CSF. This formulation increases the elimination half-life of free ara-C in the CSF from 3.4 hours for native ara-C to 130 to 277 hours.[55] Cytotoxic concentrations of drug are maintained in the CSF for up to 14 days or more. The usual dosage is 50 mg every 2 weeks, and the dose-limiting toxicities are headache and arachnoiditis.

TOXICITY. The toxicity profile of Ara-C is highly dependent on the dose and schedule of administration (see Table 15.6-1). Myelosuppression is the dose-limiting toxicity with a standard regimen of 100 to 200 mg/m^2/d for 7 days. Leukopenia and thrombocytopenia are observed most frequently, with nadirs occurring between days 7 and 14 after drug administration. However, the duration of the nadir can be significantly influenced by the concomitant use of other cytotoxic agents and also by previous treatment with chemotherapy.

Gastrointestinal toxicity commonly manifests as a mild to moderate degree of anorexia, nausea, and vomiting. Mucositis, diarrhea, ileus, and abdominal pain can also be observed. Less commonly, epithelial ulceration can occur, ranging from superficial ulceration to intramural hematoma formation and perforation. Transient hepatic dysfunction, manifested as elevation of liver enzyme levels, may also occur with Ara-C given at conventional doses. Acute pancreatitis has been associated with Ara-C, mostly when given as a continuous infusion. The Ara-C syndrome has been described in pediatric patients receiving Ara-C for hematologic malignancies and is characterized by fever, myalgia, bone pain, maculopapular rash, conjunctivitis, malaise, and occasional chest pain. These symptoms usually begin within 12 hours after Ara-C infusion. This syndrome most likely represents an allergic reaction to Ara-C, because patients usually develop symptoms months after the first dose, and corticosteroids can prevent its onset.

Administration of Ara-C at high doses (2 to 3 g/m^2 intravenously over 1 to 3 hours, every 12 hours) produces severe myelosuppression, sometimes with prolonged nadirs. Severe gastrointestinal toxicity in the form of mucositis, diarrhea, or both, is also frequently observed. Neurologic toxicity is significantly more common with high-dose Ara-C than with standard doses.[56] The clinical manifestations of neurologic toxicity are diverse and include seizures, cerebral and cerebellar dysfunction, peripheral neuropathy, bilateral rectus muscle palsy, aphasia, and parkinsonian symptoms. Clinical signs of cerebellar dysfunction occur in up to 15% of patients within 8 days and include dysarthria, dysdiadochokinesia, dysmetria, and ataxia. Change in alertness and cognitive ability, memory loss, and frontal lobe release signs reflect cerebral toxicity. Despite discontinuation of therapy, clinical recovery is incomplete in up to 30% of affected patients. The severity of peripheral neuropathy increases with higher cumulative Ara-C doses. Neurotoxicity may also be reduced by prolonged intravenous administration (over 3 hours or more). Patients older than 50 years and patients with elevated serum creatinine levels are particularly susceptible to neurologic toxicity. Intrathecal administration of Ara-C is usually uneventful. However, it may produce fever, seizures, and alterations in mental status within the first 24 hours of administration.

Pulmonary complications may include noncardiogenic pulmonary edema, acute respiratory distress, and pneumonia, resulting from *Streptococcus viridans* infection. Other side effects associated with high-dose Ara-C include conjunctivitis (often responsive to topical corticosteroids), a painful hand-foot syndrome, and, rarely, anaphylactic reactions. Neutrophilic eccrine hydradenitis, an unusual cutaneous reaction manifested as plaques or nodules, can occur during the second week after high-dose Ara-C. Although Ara-C is teratogenic in animals, it has not yet been established to be a carcinogen in humans.

GEMCITABINE

Gemcitabine (2',2'-difluorodeoxycytidine, dFdC, Gemzar) is a difluorinated analogue of deoxycytidine (see Fig. 15.6-4). This compound has shown significant clinical activity against several human solid tumors, including pancreatic, small cell and non–small cell lung, bladder, ovary, and breast cancers. In contrast to Ara-C, the spectrum of antitumor activity of gemcitabine is much broader, despite its similarities in structure, metabolism, and mechanism of action.[44]

Mechanism of Action

Transport of gemcitabine into cells requires the nucleoside transporter system.[57] Nucleoside transport–deficient cells are highly resistant to gemcitabine. The intracellular concentration of adenosine triphosphate (ATP) may affect the sensitivity of a tumor cell to gemcitabine, and ATP-replete cells accumulate significantly less drug, which suggests the existence of an active efflux mechanism for gemcitabine. Gemcitabine is five-fold more lipophilic than Ara-C, a feature that is thought to contribute to the 65% greater rate of accumulation of gemcitabine in cells when compared with Ara-C on a molar basis. Gemcitabine is inactive in its parent form and requires intracellular activation for its cytotoxic effects. The steps involved in the metabolic activation of gemcitabine are similar to those observed with Ara-C, with both drugs being activated by the same enzymatic machinery. The enzyme dCK converts dFdC into difluorodeoxycytidine monophosphate (dFdCMP). The drug is subsequently phosphorylated by nucleoside monophosphate and diphosphate kinases to the respective 5'-diphosphate (dFdCDP) and 5'-triphosphate (dFdCTP) derivatives. The intracellular concentration of dFdCTP determines to a large extent its subsequent metabolism. In cells with lower concentrations of this metabolite (less than 100 μmol) the main route of elimination is via deamination, whereas in cells with higher concentrations (more than 100 μmol), dephosphorylation and urinary excretion predominate. Furthermore, dFdCTP, by inhibiting dCMP deaminase, establishes a mechanism of self-potentiation, with a marked prolongation of its terminal half-life from 3.6 hours to 19.0 hours. This phenomenon may explain, at least in part, the differences observed between the spectrum of clinical activity of Ara-C and gemcitabine.[58-60]

Mechanisms of Resistance

Several mechanisms of resistance to gemcitabine in preclinical experimental models have been described. Nucleoside transport–deficient cells are highly resistant to gemcitabine. Furthermore, the efficiency of gemcitabine uptake can vary significantly according to the specific nucleoside transporter expressed on the cell surface.[44] Several enzymes involved in the intracellular metabolism of gemcitabine have been implicated in the development of resistance to this drug, including dCK enzyme activity deficiency and overexpression of ribonucleotide reductase.[61]

Clinical Pharmacology and Pharmacokinetics

Gemcitabine is administered via the intravenous route, and after a 30-minute intravenous infusion at doses ranging up to 1000 mg/m², the plasma concentration–versus–time curve (area under the concentration-time curve) increases in a linear fashion. The renal clearance of parent drug is less than 10% of the systemic clearance. The main catabolic metabolite, difluorodeoxyuridine (dFdU), is eliminated by biphasic kinetics and is characterized by a long terminal-phase half-life of 14 hours. The Cancer and Leukemia Group B conducted a phase I pharmacokinetic study to characterize the appropriate dosing of gemcitabine in patients with renal or hepatic impairment.[62] They found that patients with elevated levels of transaminases could be safely treated with full-dose gemcitabine; however, when serum bilirubin levels were higher than 1.6 mg/dL, an increased risk of hepatotoxicity was observed. These findings promoted a recommendation for dosage reduction in the setting of liver dysfunction. Patients with renal dysfunction presented with unusual side effects in response to gemcitabine, especially skin toxicity in the form of diffuse erythema and desquamation. Unfortunately, there is insufficient clinical evidence at this time to provide specific dosing recommendations for patients with renal insufficiency.

The dosing schedule of gemcitabine is dependent on the specific tumor type being treated (see Table 15.6-1). Until recently, the most commonly used schedule for pancreatic cancer was 1000 mg/m² intravenously administered weekly for 7 weeks with a 1-week rest, followed by weekly for 3 weeks with a 1-week rest.[63] In a randomized phase II study in patients with advanced pancreatic cancer, Tempero et al. demonstrated that

a dose of 1500 mg/m² administered as a fixed rate of 10 mg/m²/min produced an optimal plasma drug concentration of 20 μmol with a twofold increase in the intracellular formation of the cytotoxic active metabolite dFdCTP. A total of 92 patients were randomly assigned to receive the usual dose and schedule of gemcitabine and the fixed-dose infusion. Although the time to tumor progression was comparable in both arms, there was a significant prolongation of 1-year survival (9% vs. 29%; *P* = .014) and 2-year survival (2% vs. 18%; *P* = .007) in favor of the fixed-dose infusional schedule. Hematologic toxicity was the most significant adverse event, with 37% of patients experiencing grade 3 or 4 thrombocytopenia, 49% experiencing neutropenia, and 9% experiencing grade 4 anemia.[64]

Toxicity

In general, gemcitabine is a relatively well tolerated drug when used as a single agent. The main dose-limiting toxicity is myelosuppression, with all three cell lines affected. Toxicity is schedule dependent, with longer infusions producing greater hematologic toxicity. With regard to nonhematologic toxicities, transient flu-like symptoms including fever, headache, arthralgias, and myalgias occur in 45% of patients. Asthenia and transient transaminasemia may occur.

Dyspnea is a relatively uncommon side effect of gemcitabine and in certain instances may require discontinuation of the drug. Patients usually present with a clinical picture consistent with acute respiratory distress syndrome, with hypoxemia, pulmonary infiltrates, and no evidence of left ventricular failure. The onset of pulmonary symptoms is usually 2 to 40 days after the first dose of gemcitabine. Thus, close monitoring of patients for any change in baseline respiratory status is crucial. Continuation of treatment once dyspnea develops may lead to a fatal outcome.[65]

A rare yet potentially fatal complication of gemcitabine is hemolytic-uremic syndrome (HUS).[66] The incidence of this complication has been estimated to be 0.015%. Early recognition of HUS is important and should prompt the immediate discontinuation of therapy to prevent death from HUS-related complications.

Drug Interactions

Gemcitabine has been combined with various chemotherapeutic agents in the treatment of several solid tumors. Preclinical *in vitro* studies have provided evidence for synergism between gemcitabine and various other anticancer agents. Cisplatin is one of the agents most commonly used in combination with gemcitabine. *In vitro* studies with different human cancer cell lines have shown synergistic interaction between gemcitabine and cisplatin resulting from increased formation of platinum-DNA adducts, with incorporation of dFdC into DNA. Oxaliplatin, a diaminocyclohexane-platinum compound, has also demonstrated synergy with gemcitabine. In human leukemia and colorectal cancer cell lines, a schedule-dependent supraadditive effect was obtained when tumor cells were first exposed to gemcitabine followed 24 hours later by oxaliplatin. In addition, the gemcitabine-oxaliplatin combination was shown to be more potent than the gemcitabine-cisplatin combination in mismatch repair–deficient HCT116 human colon cancer cells. Such combinations have been extended to the clinical setting, and these two gemcitabine-platinum regimens show promising activity in the treatment of advanced pancreatic cancer.[67]

Gemcitabine is a potent radiosensitizer. Preclinical studies have suggested that this effect may be mediated via gemcitabine-induced deoxyadenosine triphosphate depletion and cell-cycle redistribution into the S phase. Maximal cytotoxicity occurs when gemcitabine is administered before radiation. The extent of dFdCMP incorporation into DNA does not appear to correlate with the radiosensitizing effect of gemcitabine, which suggests that ribonucleotide reductase plays a key role. A phase II study of gemcitabine 300 mg/m^2 intravenously weekly with concurrent radiation (40 Gy in a split course) after curative resection of pancreatic head cancer has shown that this regimen is feasible and relatively well tolerated.[68]

6-THIOPURINES

The development of the purine analogues in cancer chemotherapy began in the early 1950s with the synthesis of the thiopurines (Fig. 15.6-5). For this seminal work, Hitchings and Elion received the Nobel Prize in Medicine in 1988. The purine analogues 6-mercaptopurine (6-MP) and 6-thioguanine (6-TG) continue to be used principally in the management of acute leukemia. 6-MP has an important role in maintenance therapy for acute lymphoblastic leukemia (ALL), whereas 6-TG is active in remission induction and in maintenance therapy for AML. These analogues have a single substitution of a thiol group in place of the 6-hydroxyl group of the purine base. 6-MP is a structural analogue of hypoxanthine, whereas 6-TG is an analogue of guanine. Azathioprine is a derivative of 6-MP and acts as a prodrug to provide sustained release of 6-MP.

Mechanism of Action

6-MP and 6-TG act similarly with regard to their cellular biochemistry. In their respective monophosphate nucleotide forms, they inhibit *de novo* purine synthesis and purine interconversion reactions, whereas the nucleotide triphosphate metabolites are incorporated directly into nucleic acids. The relative contribution of each of these actions to the mechanism of cytotoxicity of these agents is unclear. Both 6-MP and 6-TG are converted to their respective monophosphate forms by hypoxanthine-guanine phosphoribosyl transferase (HGPRT).[69] These ribonucleotide monophosphates inhibit the first step of *de novo* purine synthesis catalyzed by glutamine phosphoribosylpyrophosphate aminotransferase and block the conversion of inosinic acid to adenylic acid or to guanylic acid. Inhibition of purine nucleotide synthesis leads to the buildup of 5'-phosphoribosyl-1-pyrophosphate, which facilitates the activation of 6-MP and 6-TG to their active nucleotide forms by HGPRT. Both thiopurine ribonucleotide and deoxyribonucleotide metabolites are formed, which can then be incorporated into cellular RNA and DNA, respectively. In some experimental model systems, incorporation of thiopurine nucleotides into DNA correlates with cytotoxicity.[70]

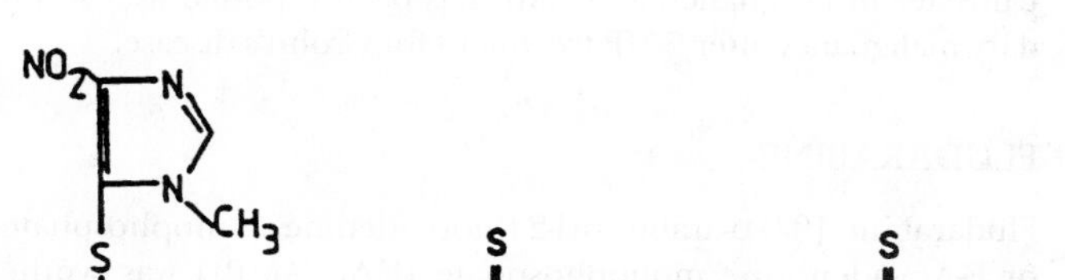

Mechanisms of Resistance

Biochemical resistance to 6-thiopurines results from a decreased ability to form cytotoxic nucleotide metabolites. In experimental systems, resistant cells express either a complete or partial deficiency of HGPRT. An alteration in the affinity of HGPRT for 6-thiopurines has also been described.[71] Studies have shown that decreased transmembrane transport of 6-TG can also result in drug resistance. Mismatch repair–defective cells exhibited higher levels of drug resistance and increased mutagenic response at the HGPRT locus to 6-TG compared with their mismatch repair–proficient counterparts.[72] In clinical samples derived from patients with AML, drug resistance has been associated with either increased concentrations of a membrane-bound alkaline phosphatase or a conjugating enzyme, 6-thiopurine methyltransferase (TPMT).[73] Patients who express high levels of TPMT activity are unable to form sufficiently high levels of active nucleotide metabolites after treatment with 6-MP.

Clinical Pharmacology and Pharmacokinetics

6-MERCAPTOPURINE. Oral dosages of 6-MP of 70 to 100 mg/m^2/d are commonly used in the maintenance therapy for ALL (see Table 15.6-1). Oral absorption of 6-MP is highly erratic, with only 16% to 50% of the administered dose reaching the systemic circulation. This effect is mainly due to rapid first-pass metabolism in the liver.[69] Food intake and coadministration with the antibiotic co-trimoxazole significantly reduce drug absorption. The variable bioavailability of oral 6-MP may be an important determinant of therapeutic outcome, because low plasma drug concentrations over time correlate with an increased risk of relapse in children with ALL.[74]

6-MP is usually administered at a dosage of 25 to 100 mg/m^2/d orally for several weeks. Oral 6-MP is well distributed into most body compartments, with the exception of the CSF. With high-dose intravenous 6-MP (200 mg/m^2 bolus followed by 800 mg/m^2 over 8 hours), a CSF to plasma ratio of 0.15 is achieved. This schedule is currently being used to prevent CNS relapse in ALL.[75] Approximately 30% of the drug binds weakly to plasma proteins. The plasma half-life is approximately 50 minutes after intravenous injection and 90 minutes after oral administration. Renal excretion of 6-MP is minimal, but at high doses, as much as 20% to 40% of the drug is removed by the kidneys. Exceed-

FIGURE 15.6-5. Purine analogues and their physiologic counterparts, hypoxanthine and guanine.

ingly high doses of 6-MP (more than 1 g/m^2) in children may cause renal precipitation of drug with hematuria and crystalluria. In patients with renal dysfunction, dosage reductions of 6-MP should be considered.[69]

The major route of drug elimination is via metabolism by several enzymatic pathways. 6-MP is oxidized to the inactive metabolite 6-thiouric acid by xanthine oxidase. Enhanced 6-MP toxicity may result from the concomitant administration of both oral and intravenous 6-MP and the xanthine oxidase inhibitor allopurinol. In patients receiving both 6-MP and allopurinol, the 6-MP dose should be reduced by at least 50% to 75%.[76] 6-MP also undergoes S-methylation by the enzyme TPMT to yield 6-methylmercaptopurine. After further phosphorylation, 6-methylmercaptopurine nucleotides are themselves capable of inhibiting *de novo* purine biosynthesis, but to a lesser extent than thioguanine nucleotides (TGNs). TPMT plays a similar role in 6-TG and azathioprine metabolism.

It has been shown that TPMT enzyme activity may vary considerably among patients. Moreover, the levels of TPMT enzyme activity correlate inversely with intracellular levels of TGNs and with the duration of 6-MP–induced cytopenia, which suggests that the level of inherited TPMT activity may directly affect 6-MP cytotoxicity and host toxicity. Due to an autosomal codominant genetic polymorphism, a series of TPMT phenotypes with alleles of differing enzymatic activity are present in the general population. Point mutations or loss of alleles of TPMT resulting in altered enzyme activity correlate with a defect in thiopurine metabolism, thus defining a true pharmacogenetic syndrome.[77] A polymerase chain reaction–based method is widely used for the genetic detection of these TPMT mutations. Approximately 0.3% of the white population expresses either a homozygous deletion or mutation of both alleles of the TPMT gene. In these patients, grossly elevated TGN concentrations, profound myelotoxicity with pancytopenia, and extensive gastrointestinal symptoms are seen after only a brief course of thiopurine treatment.[78,79] An estimated 10% of patients may be at increased risk for toxicity due to heterozygous loss of the gene or a mutant allele coding for a less enzymatically active TPMT.

6-THIOGUANINE. The main intracellular pathway for 6-TG activation is catalyzed by HGPRT, with resultant formation of ribonucleotide monophosphates. Although the main metabolites of 6-TG are TGNs, thioinosine nucleotides are formed as well. However, the clinical significance of these respective metabolites as determinants of 6-TG cytotoxicity remains unclear. Although higher erythrocyte levels of TGNs are detected after treatment with maximum tolerated dose levels of 6-TG than of 6-MP, this pharmacodynamic parameter does not clearly correlate with the myelosuppression associated with 6-TG.[80]

6-TG is administered orally in dosages of 75 to 200 mg/m^2/d for 5 to 7 days in the treatment of AML (see Table 15.6-1). Its oral bioavailability is erratic, with peak plasma levels occurring 2 to 4 hours after ingestion. The median plasma half-life of 6-TG is approximately 90 minutes. The catabolism of 6-TG differs from that of 6-MP in that S-methylation with subsequent removal of the sulfur atom is an important pathway of drug elimination. In a second catabolic pathway, 6-TG undergoes deamination by the enzyme guanine deaminase (guanase); this results in 6-thioxanthene, which is then oxidized by xanthine oxidase to 6-thiouric acid. In contrast to 6-MP, 6-TG is not a direct substrate for xanthine oxidase. Because the inhibition of xanthine oxidase results in the accumulation of 6-thioxanthene, an inactive metabolite, adjustments in 6-TG dosage are not required for patients receiving allopurinol.

Toxicity

The major dose-related toxicities of 6-MP are myelosuppression and gastrointestinal toxicity. Leukopenia and thrombocytopenia are maximal 7 days after treatment. Full hematologic recovery usually occurs after 14 days. In TPMT-deficient patients, dosage reduction to 5% to 25% of the standard dosage (75 mg/m^2/d) is necessary to prevent excessive toxicity. Gastrointestinal toxicities include nausea and vomiting, anorexia, diarrhea, and stomatitis. 6-MP hepatotoxicity occurs in up to 30% of adult patients and is manifested mainly as cholestatic jaundice, although elevations of hepatic transaminases may also be seen. Hepatotoxicity is usually mild and reversible after discontinuation of 6-MP, but frank hepatic necrosis can occur after high doses of the drug. Combinations of 6-MP with other known hepatotoxic agents should be avoided, and liver function test results should be closely monitored. The mechanism of liver toxicity is not known but may relate to the cytochrome P-450–dependent metabolism of 6-MP to a hepatotoxic metabolite or accumulation of 6-MP metabolites in the liver. 6-TG also causes dose-limiting bone marrow suppression but is associated with fewer gastrointestinal side effects and less hepatotoxicity than 6-MP.[81]

As a class of drugs, the 6-thiopurine analogues are potent suppressors of cell-mediated immunity. Because of this, prolonged therapy results in an increased predisposition to bacterial and parasitic infections. Given their immunosuppressive effects, these agents have been used to prevent rejection of transplanted organs and to treat autoimmune diseases, such as Crohn's disease, ulcerative colitis, and rheumatoid arthritis. Therapeutic immunosuppression occurs at 100 mg/d, a dosage associated with only mild leukopenia. Long-term immunosuppressive therapy with azathioprine increases the risk of squamous carcinoma of the skin, non-Hodgkin's lymphoma, and Kaposi's sarcoma. Chronic 6-MP treatment is associated with teratogenic effects during the first trimester of pregnancy, and AML has been reported as a secondary malignancy after 6-MP treatment for Crohn's disease.

FLUDARABINE

Fludarabine [9-β-D-arabinosyl-2-fluoroadenine monophosphate, or F-Ara-adenosine monophosphate (F-Ara-AMP)] was synthesized as part of a rational process to develop more active analogues of cytarabine (Fig. 15.6-6). The first compound in this series was adenine arabinoside (vidarabine, Ara-A). However, because this compound was inactivated via extensive deamination, its clinical use was limited. The 2'-fluoro derivative of Ara-A was subsequently found to be relatively resistant to deamination, but was difficult to formulate and poorly soluble. Addition of a 5'-monophosphate moiety to the sugar group yielded fludarabine, a compound that is relatively resistant to deamination and displays enhanced solubility.

Mechanism of Action

After intravenous administration, F-Ara-AMP is rapidly dephosphorylated to F-Ara-A, which enters cells by nucleoside-specific

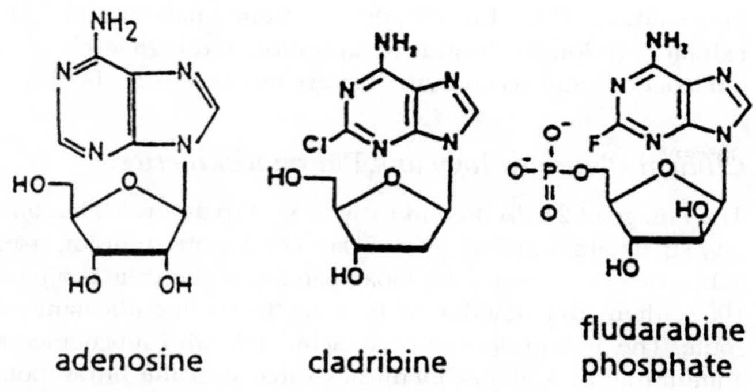

FIGURE 15.6-6. Structures of purine analogues, fludarabine and cladribine.

membrane transport mechanisms.[82] F-Ara-A is then rephosphorylated by dCK to F-Ara-AMP, which is subsequently metabolized to the triphosphate form (F-ara-ATP), which is the cytotoxic metabolite. F-ara-ATP competes with deoxyadenosine triphosphate (dATP) for incorporation into DNA and serves as a highly effective chain terminator. In addition, F-Ara-ATP directly inhibits enzymes involved in DNA replication, including DNA polymerases, DNA primase, DNA ligase I, and ribonucleotide reductase.[83] F-ara-ATP is also incorporated into RNA, causing inhibition of RNA function, processing, and mRNA translation. In contrast to other antimetabolites, fludarabine is active against nondividing cells. In fact, the primary effect of fludarabine may result from activation of apoptosis, as evidenced by the presence of typical apoptotic fragmentation of DNA into high-molecular-weight fragments after drug treatment.[84] This finding may explain the activity of fludarabine in indolent lymphoproliferative diseases with relatively low growth fractions.[85]

Mechanisms of Resistance

A number of fludarabine-resistant cell lines have been established. In these resistant lines, nucleoside transport of F-Ara-AMP is intact, and no alterations in intracellular drug accumulation have been observed. However, decreased dCK activity with diminished intracellular formation of F-Ara-ATP is the principal mechanism of resistance in each of these cell lines.[86] Subsequent work has shown that deletion of one allele of dCK is sufficient to result in decreased expression of dCK. Of note, a high degree of cross-resistance develops to multiple nucleoside analogues requiring activation by dCK, including Ara-C, gemcitabine, and cladribine.[69]

Clinical Pharmacology and Pharmacokinetics

Peak concentrations of F-Ara-A are reached 3 to 4 hours after intravenous administration. After intravenous administration, the decline in plasma levels has been reported to be bi-exponential, with a distribution half-life of 0.6 to 2.0 hours and a terminal half-life of 6.9 to 19.7 hours.[69] However, other reports describe a three-compartment model with a terminal half-life between 10 and 30 hours.[87] The rate-limiting step in elimination is release from tissues and renal function. Caution should be used in the setting of renal dysfunction, and dosage reduction should be considered.

Clinical Activity

Fludarabine is the most active single agent in the treatment of chronic lymphocytic leukemia (CLL).[88] It is also active against indolent non-Hodgkin's lymphoma, prolymphocytic leukemia, cutaneous T-cell lymphoma, and Waldenström's macroglobulinemia. This agent has shown promising activity in approximately one-third of patients with mantle cell lymphoma, albeit with relatively brief response. There is emerging data that fludarabine may have some activity when added to standard therapy for multiple myeloma. In contrast to its activity in hematologic malignancies, this compound displays minimal activity against solid tumors.

Toxicity

Myelosuppression and immunosuppression are the major side effects of fludarabine (see Table 15.6-1). Dose-limiting and possibly cumulative lymphopenia and thrombocytopenia are well established. Suppression of the immune system affects T-cell more than B-cell function. Fevers, often in the setting of neutropenia, occur in 20% to 30% of patients. Lymphocyte counts, particularly of CD4+ cells, decrease rapidly after initiation of therapy, and levels can drop to as low as $150/\mu L$ by approximately 6 months. CD4+ cell recovery is slow, and restoration of normal levels may take longer than 1 year. Common opportunistic pathogens include varicella-zoster virus, *Candida*, and *Pneumocystis carinii*. The addition of prednisone to fludarabine does not improve the response rate or survival, but significantly increases the risk of opportunistic infections, notably listeriosis and *P carinii* infection.[89] If concurrent corticosteroid treatment is necessary, such as in patients with autoimmune anemia or thrombocytopenia, long-term prophylaxis against *P carinii* is mandatory. Hemolytic anemia has been observed and, in some instances, has resulted in death on rechallenge with fludarabine. Thrombocytopenia, precipitation of Evans' syndrome, and fulminant fatal myelofibrosis have also been reported. The prolonged immunosuppression experienced with fludarabine has raised the possibility of an increased incidence of secondary malignancies.[89] However, this increased risk is now thought to be due to the underlying immune defects of the malignancy and not to the carcinogenic effects of the nucleoside analogue.

Tumor lysis syndrome occurs in fewer than 1% of patients, but in some cases, it can be fatal. Prophylaxis is not uniformly effective.[88] Other uncommon toxicities include rash, nausea, vomiting, diarrhea, stomatitis, anorexia, increased salivation, abdominal cramps, a metallic taste, transient elevations in levels of hepatic enzymes, and renal dysfunction. Treatment-associated disseminated skin rash, progressing to pemphigus-like epidermal necrolysis, has been described. Pulmonary toxicity, in the form of interstitial pneumonitis, can develop after multiple courses of treatment. At times, the pulmonary sequelae may be difficult to distinguish from those associated with opportunistic infections. This toxicity usually responds to corticosteroids and does not tend to recur on retreatment.

Drug Interactions

Purine analogues achieve significant clinical activity in low-grade lymphomas, presumably due to their ability to induce apoptosis in these otherwise drug-resistant malignancies. The responses seen, however, are mostly partial and of short duration. This has generated interest in identifying drug regimens incorporating fludarabine with enhanced activity. Fludarabine inhibits the nucleotide excision repair used by cells to remove the DNA cross-links induced by alkylating agents (cyclophosphamide, cisplatin).[90] Response rates of nearly 90% have been observed when fludarabine and cyclophosphamide are used in combination in patients with previously untreated low-grade lymphomas. The combination of fludarabine with the anthracycline analogue mitoxantrone with or without dexamethasone (FN and FND regimens) has been successfully developed to treat indolent non-Hodgkin's lymphomas.[91]

CLADRIBINE

Cladribine [2-chlorodeoxyadenosine (2-CdA)] is a deoxyadenosine purine nucleoside analogue. A single substitution of a chlorine atom for a hydrogen atom at the 2 position of the purine ring of deoxyadenosine renders this compound resistant to adenosine deaminase (ADA) (see Fig. 15.6-6). It was developed initially as an immunosuppressive agent. 2-CdA exhibits a dose-dependent *in vitro* inhibition of lymphoid neoplasms and human leukemic cell lines but has no activity against solid tumors. At present, it is the drug of choice in hairy cell leukemia (HCL) with activity in low-grade lymphoproliferative disorders as well.[92]

Mechanism of Action

Deoxyadenosine is cleaved within cells by ADA to the deoxyinosine form. A deficiency of this enzyme leads to toxic accumulation of deoxyadenosine in lymphocytes, manifesting as the severe combined immunodeficiency clinical syndrome. 2-CdA enters cells via the nucleoside transporter system. Given its resistance to deamination by ADA, an ADA-deficiency–like state develops, in which 2-CdA accumulates within cells, eventually reaching lymphotoxic levels.[93] On entry into the cell, it first undergoes conversion to cladribine-monophosphate (Cd-AMP), which is then metabolized to the active metabolite, cladribine-triphosphate (Cd-ATP). The rate-limiting step is catalyzed by dCK. In contrast, catabolism of 2-CdA is mediated by a 5'-nucleotidase. The greatest accumulation of Cd-ATP is observed in cells with high levels of dCK and low 5'-nucleotidase activity. Cd-ATP competitively inhibits incorporation of the normal nucleotide dATP into DNA, a process that results in termination of chain elongation.[69] Progressive accumulation of Cd-ATP leads to an imbalance in deoxyribonucleotide pools, thereby inhibiting further DNA synthesis and repair. The accumulation of unrepaired DNA breaks over time may initiate the apoptosis of quiescent, nondividing lymphocytes. Activation of the caspase 3 proteolytic cascade has been implicated as a potential mechanism for the onset of apoptosis.

Mechanisms of Resistance

Resistance to 2-CdA has been attributed to altered intracellular metabolism of the drug. A reduction in the activity of dCK, the enzyme responsible for generating cytotoxic nucleotide metabolites, is a major determinant of acquired resistance. Cd-AMP and Cd-ATP are dephosphorylated by the cytoplasmic enzyme 5'-nucleotidase. WSU-CLL cells, derived from a patient with CLL, exhibit both low levels of dCK expression and high-levels of 5'-nucleotidase, and accordingly, they are resistant to 2-CdA.[69]

Clinical Pharmacology and Pharmacokinetics

The dosage of 2-CdA used in early clinical trials was 0.09 to 0.10 mg/kg/d administered as a 7-day continuous infusion (see Table 15.6-1). Of note, the bioavailability of the drug is almost 100% when given at a dose of 0.14 mg/kg via the subcutaneous route. The area under the curve achievable with subcutaneous administration is almost identical to that with the intravenous route.[94] 2-CdA pharmacokinetics follows a two-compartment model, with mean α and β half-lives of 35 ± 12 minutes and 6.5 ± 2.5 hours, respectively. Although there seems to be a close relationship between dose and plasma steady-state concentrations, the relationship between dose and clinical activity remains to be defined. 2-CdA has also been tested as a 2-hour infusion of 0.09 to 0.10 mg/kg/d for 5 to 7 days and a 1-hour infusion at 6 mg/m² for 5 days of a 28-day cycle.[95,96] A dose-escalation study of bolus daily cladribine established no dose-limiting nonhematologic toxicity up to 21.5 mg/m²/d, given in a daily 1-hour intravenous bolus infusion for 5 days to patients with advanced hematologic malignancies. At higher dose levels, prolonged cytopenias and severe infections define the upper dose limit of the drug. In a small series of patients with HCL, no significant difference in response rate or toxicity was observed between a 7-day continuous infusion and a daily 2-hour bolus for 5 days. Although the daily dose for 5 days appears to be more convenient as an outpatient regimen, the standard administration schedule remains the 7-day continuous infusion.

2-CdA is eliminated via renal excretion. Renal clearance is approximately 50%, whereas 20% to 35% of the drug is excreted unchanged in the urine.[96] 2-CdA is able to cross the blood–brain barrier and penetrates into the CSF. Although CSF concentrations reach only 25% of detected plasma levels in the absence of meningeal disease, CSF levels exceed plasma levels in patients with meningeal involvement.

Clinical Activity

A single course of 2-CdA achieves durable complete remissions in 65% to 91% of patients with HCL.[97,98] Salvage treatment of patients previously treated with interferon-α or splenectomy is as effective as first-line treatment. Although minimal residual disease is often found on reexamination of bone marrow specimens of HCL patients in clinical complete response, relapse rates are low. Retreatment with cladribine results in complete response in up to 60% of relapsing patients.[98] Responses in patients with CLL and non-Hodgkin's lymphoma tend to be brief, and salvage of relapsed or refractory disease is less efficacious than in HCL. Although 2-CdA achieves high response rates in pediatric patients with AML, its activity in adult patients is much lower.

Toxicity

At conventional doses, myelosuppression is dose-limiting and all three cell lines are equally affected. Recovery from thrombocytopenia usually occurs within 2 to 4 weeks, and recovery from neutropenia in 3 to 5 weeks, after a single course of the drug. Severe autoimmune hemolytic anemia with fatal bone marrow aplasia has been described in CLL patients receiving repeated cycles of the drug, because 2-CdA–induced lymphopenia may exacerbate autoimmune hemolysis. Of note, foci of bone marrow hypoplasia are seen in 2-CdA–treated patients, although the long-term clinical significance of this effect remains unclear.

Immunosuppression accounts for the late morbidity observed in 2-CdA–treated patients. Lymphocyte counts, particularly CD4+ cells, decrease within 1 to 4 weeks of drug administration and may remain depressed for several years. After discontinuation of 2-CdA, a median time of up to 40 months may be required for complete recovery of normal CD4+ counts.[99] Fevers occur in 40% to 50% of patients, typically correlating with the duration of granulocytopenia. These episodes may be profound, prolonged, and cumulative. Opportunistic infections are common, although usually seen less frequently than with fludarabine. Herpes zoster is most typical, and infections with a variety of other pathogens are also seen, including *Candida, Pneumocystis, Pseudomonas aeruginosa, Listeria monocytogenes, Cryptococcus neoformans, Aspergillus, P carinii,* cytomegalovirus, and common bacteria. Infectious complications correlate with decreases in CD4+ count, and they are more frequent with repeated courses of therapy.

In patients with HCL and CLL, long-term studies have failed to identify an increase in drug-related mortality. Specifically, initial concerns about an increased risk for secondary malignancies have not been confirmed, because the incidence of second cancers is no higher than would be expected from the underlying hematologic disorder. However, lymphoid neoplasms occur significantly more commonly than expected.

Tumor lysis syndrome is rare, tends to occur after the first course, and is generally mild and reversible. However, in rare instances, this process may be fatal, even in patients with prior therapy. Cardiotoxicity is uncommon, but cardiac deaths have been reported, mainly in patients with a prior history of cardiac disease. Pulmonary complications of 2-CdA therapy are uncommon, but in some cases, they have been fatal. Rashes, although uncommon, may be severe and can present as fatal toxic epidermal necrolysis. Mild to severe gastrointestinal toxicities occur in 15% of patients, with nausea, vomiting, and diarrhea, and there have been rare reports of anorexia, severe mucositis, or both. Transient elevations in levels of hepatic enzymes occur but are usually clinically asymptomatic. Renal failure occurs only at high doses. Mild to moderate neurotoxicity occurs in 15% of patients and is at least partly reversible with discontinuation of the drug.[100]

REFERENCES

1. Messmann RA, Allegra CJ. Antifolates. In: Chabner BA, Longo DL, eds. *Cancer chemotherapy and biotherapy: principles and practice,* 3rd ed. Philadelphia: Lippincott–Raven, 2001:139.
2. Antony AC. The biological chemistry of folate receptors. *Blood* 1992;79:2807.
3. Shen F, Ross JF, Wang X, et al. Identification of a novel folate receptor, a truncated receptor, and receptor type b in hematopoietic cells: cDNA cloning, expression, immunoreactivity, and tissue specificity. *Biochemistry* 1994;33:1209.
4. Weitman SD, Lark RH, Coney LR, et al. Distribution of the folate receptor GP38 in normal and malignant cell lines and tissues. *Cancer Res* 1992;52:3396.
5. Jansen G, Mauritz RM, Assaraf YG, et al. Regulation of carrier-mediated transport of folates and antifolates in methotrexate-sensitive and resistant leukemia cells. *Adv Enzyme Regul* 1997;37:59.
6. Flintoff WF, Bertino JR. Defective transport is a common mechanism of acquired methotrexate resistance in acute lymphocytic leukemia and is associated with decreased reduced folate carrier expression. *Blood* 1997;89:1013.
7. Galpin AJ, Schuetz JD, Mason E, et al. Differences in folylpolyglutamate synthetase and dihydrofolate reductase expression in human B-lineage versus T-lineage leukemic lymphoblasts: mechanisms for lineage differences in methotrexate polyglutamylation and cytotoxicity. *Mol Pharmacol* 1997;52:155.
8. Haber DA, Schimke RT. Unstable amplification of an altered dihydrofolate reductase gene associated with double-minute chromosomes. *Cell* 1981;26:355.
9. Chu E, Takimoto CH, Voeller D, et al. Specific binding of human dihydrofolate reductase protein to dihydrofolate reductase messenger RNA in vitro. *Biochemistry* 1993;32:4756.
10. Matherly LH, Taub JW, Wong SC, et al. Increased frequency of expression of elevated dihydrofolate reductase in T-cell versus B-precursor acute lymphoblastic leukemia in children. *Blood* 1997;90:578.
11. Fossa SD, Heilo A, Bormer O. Unexpectedly high serum methotrexate levels in cystectomized bladder cancer patients with an ileal conduit treated with intermediate doses of the drug. *J Urol* 1990;143:498.
12. Pinedo HM, Zaharko DS, Bull JM, et al. The reversal of methotrexate cytotoxicity to mouse bone marrow cells by leucovorin and nucleosides. *Cancer Res* 1976;36:4418.
13. Widemann BC, Balis FM, Murphy RF, et al. Carboxypeptidase-G2, thymidine, and leucovorin rescue in cancer patients with methotrexate-induced renal dysfunction. *J Clin Oncol* 1997;15:2125.
14. Shapiro WR, Young D, Mehta BM. Methotrexate distribution in cerebrospinal fluid after intravenous ventricular and lumbar injections. *N Engl J Med* 1975;293:161.
15. Walker RW, Allen JC, Rosen G, et al. Transient cerebral dysfunction secondary to high-dose methotrexate. *Cancer* 1984;53:1849.
16. Takimoto CH. Antifolates in clinical development. *Semin Oncol* 1997;24[Suppl 18]:S18.
17. Van Custem E, Cunningham D, Maroun J, et al. Raltitrexed: current clinical status and future directions. *Ann Oncol* 2002;13:513.
18. Baas P, Ardizzoni A, Grossi F, et al. The activity of raltitrexed in malignant pleural mesothelioma, an EORTC phase II study (08992). *Eur J Cancer* 2003;39:353.
19. Paz-Ares L, Bezares S, Tabernero J, et al. Review of a promising new agent pemetrexed disodium. *Cancer* 2003;97:2056.
20. Scagliotti GV, Shin DM, Kindler HL, et al. Phase II study of pemetrexed with and without folic acid and vitamin B12 as front-line therapy in malignant pleural mesothelioma. *J Clin Oncol* 2003;21:1556.
21. Vogelzang N, Rusthoven J, Symanowski J, et al. Phase III study of pemetrexed in combination with cisplatin versus cisplatin alone in patients with malignant pleural mesothelioma. *J Clin Oncol* 2003;21:2636.
22. Grem JL. 5-Fluoropyrimidines. In: Chabner BA, Longo DL, eds. *Cancer chemotherapy and biotherapy: principles and practice,* 3rd ed. Philadelphia: Lippincott–Raven, 2001:185.
23. Longley D, Harkin P, Johnston P. 5-Fluorouracil: mechanisms of action and clinical strategies. *Nat Rev Cancer* 2003;3:330.
24. Sotos GA, Grogan L, Allegra CJ. Preclinical and clinical aspects of biomodulation of 5-fluorouracil. *Cancer Treat Rev* 1994;20:11.
25. Piedbois P, Buyse M, Rustum Y, et al. For the advanced colorectal cancer meta-analysis project. Modulation of fluorouracil by leucovorin in patients with advanced colorectal cancer: evidence in terms of response rate. *J Clin Oncol* 1992;10:896.
26. Chu E, Allegra CJ. The role of thymidylate synthase as an RNA binding protein. *BioEssays* 1996;18:191.
27. Lowe SW, Ruley HE, Jacks T, et al. p53-Dependent apoptosis modulates the cytotoxicity of anticancer agents. *Cell* 1993;74:957.
28. Fisher TC, Milner AE, Gregory CD, et al. Bcl-2 modulation of apoptosis induced by anticancer drugs: resistance to thymidylate stress is independent of classical resistance pathways. *Cancer Res* 1993;53:3321.
29. Houghton JA, Harwood FG, Tillman DM. Thymineless death in colon carcinoma cells is mediated via Fas signaling. *Proc Natl Acad Sci U S A* 1997;94:8144.
30. Diasio RB, Lu ZH. Dihydropyrimidine dehydrogenase activity and fluorouracil chemotherapy. *J Clin Oncol* 1994;12:2239.
31. DiPaolo A, Danesi R, Falcone A, et al. Relationship between 5-fluorouracil disposition, toxicity, and dihydropyrimidine dehydrogenase activity in cancer patients. *Ann Oncol* 2001;12:1301.
32. Harris BE, Carpenter JT, Diasio RB. Severe 5-fluorouracil toxicity secondary to dihydropyrimidine dehydrogenase deficiency as a potentially more common pharmacogenetic syndrome. *Cancer* 1993;68:499.
33. Takimoto CH, Lu ZH, Zhang R, et al. Severe neurotoxicity following 5-fluorouracil-based chemotherapy in a patient with dihydropyrimidine dehydrogenase activity. *Clin Cancer Res* 1995;2:477.
34. Kemeny N, Fata F. Hepatic-arterial chemotherapy. *Lancet Oncol* 2001;2:418.
35. Marsh JC, Bertino JR, Katz KH, et al. The influence of drug interval on the effect of methotrexate and fluorouracil in the treatment of advanced colorectal cancer. *J Clin Oncol* 1991;9:371.
35a. de Gramont A, Bosset JF, Milan C, et al. Randomized trial comparing monthly low-dose leucovorin and fluorouracil bolus with bi-monthly high-dose leucovorin and fluorouracil bolus plus continuous infusion for advanced colorectal cancer: a French intergroup study. *J Clin Oncol* 1997;15:808.
36. Rich TA. Irradiation plus 5-fluorouracil: cellular mechanisms of action and treatment schedules. *Semin Radiat Oncol* 1997;7:267.
37. O'Connell MJ, Martenson JA, Wieand HS, et al. Improving adjuvant therapy for rectal cancer by combining protracted infusion fluorouracil with radiation therapy after curative surgery. *N Engl J Med* 1994;331:502.
38. Lamont EB, Schilsky RL. The oral fluoropyrimidines in cancer chemotherapy. *Clin Cancer Res* 1999;5:2289.
39. de Bono JS, Twelves CJ. The oral fluorinated pyrimidines. *Invest New Drugs* 2001;19:41.
40. Shimma N, Umeda I, Arasaki M, et al. The design and synthesis of a new tumor-selective fluoropyrimidine carbamate, capecitabine. *Bioorg Med Chem* 2000;8:1697.
41. Blum JL, Jones SC, Buzdar SC, et al. Multicenter phase II trial of capecitabine in paclitaxel-refractory metastatic breast cancer. *J Clin Oncol* 1999;17:485.

42. O'Shaughnessy J, Miles D, Vukelja S, et al. Superior survival with capecitabine plus docetaxel combination therapy in anthracycline-pretreated patients with advanced breast cancer: phase III trial results. *J Clin Oncol* 2002;20:2812.

42a. Sawada N, Ishikawa T, Fukase Y, et al. Induction of thymidine phosphorylase activity and enhancement of capecitabine efficacy by taxol/taxotere in human cancer xenografts. *Clin Cancer Res* 1998;4:1013.

43. Hoff PM, Ansari R, Batist G, et al. Comparison of oral capecitabine versus intravenous fluorouracil plus leucovorin as first line treatment in 605 patients with metastatic colorectal cancer: results of a randomized phase III study. *J Clin Oncol* 2001;19:2282.

44. Garcia-Carbonero R, Ryan DP, Chabner BA. Cytidine analogs. In: Chabner BA, Longo DL, eds. *Cancer chemotherapy and biotherapy: principles and practice*, 3rd ed. Philadelphia: Lippincott-Raven, 2001:265.

45. Mikita T, Beardsley GP. Functional consequences of the arabinosylcytosine structural lesion in DNA. *Biochemistry* 1988;27:4698.

46. Nakamura T, Takauji R, Kamiya K, et al. Intracellular pharmacodynamics of ara-C and flow cytometric analysis of cell cycle progression in leukemia chemotherapy. *Leukemia* 1997;11[Suppl 3]:548.

47. Braess J, Wegendt C, Feuring-Buske M, et al. Leukemic blasts differ from normal bone marrow mononuclear cells and CD34+ hematopoietic stem cells in their metabolism of cytosine arabinoside. *Br J Haematol* 1999;105:388.

48. Capizzi RL, White JC, Powell BL, et al. Effect of dose on the pharmacokinetic and pharmacodynamic effects of cytarabine. *Semin Hematol* 1991;28[Suppl 4]:54.

49. Donehower RC, Karp JE, Burke PJ. Pharmacology and toxicity of high-dose cytarabine by 72-hour continuous infusion. *Cancer Treat Rep* 1986;70:1059.

50. Plunkett W, Liliemark JO, Estey E, et al. Saturation of ara-CTP accumulation during high-dose ara-C therapy: pharmacologic rationale for intermediate-dose ara-C. *Semin Oncol* 1987;14[Suppl 1]:159.

51. Momparler RL, Laliberte J, Eliopoulos N, et al. Transfection of murine fibroblast cells with human cytidine deaminase cDNA confers resistance to cytosine arabinoside. *Anticancer Drugs* 1996;7:266.

52. Plunkett W, Iacoboni S, Estey E, et al. Pharmacologically directed ara-C therapy for refractory leukemia. *Semin Oncol* 1985;12[Suppl 3]:20.

53. Capizzi RL, Yang J-L, Cheng E, et al. Alteration of the pharmacokinetics of high-dose ara-C by its metabolite ara-U in patients with acute leukemia. *J Clin Oncol* 1983;12:763.

54. Damon LE, Plunkett W, Linker CA. Plasma and cerebrospinal fluid pharmacokinetics of 1-β-arabinofuranosylcytosine and 1-β-D-arabino-furanosyluracil following the repeated intravenous administration of high- and intermediate dose 1-β-D-arabinofuranosylcytosine. *Cancer Res* 1991;51:4141.

55. Glantz MJ, LaFollette S, Jaeckle KA, et al. Randomized trial of a slow release versus a standard formulation of cytarabine for the intrathecal treatment of lymphomatous meningitis. *J Clin Oncol* 1999;17:3110.

56. Baker WJ, Royer GL, Weiss RB. Cytarabine and neurologic toxicity. *J Clin Oncol* 1991;9:679.

57. Plunkett W, Huang P, Searcy CE, et al. Gemcitabine: preclinical pharmacology and mechanisms of action. *Semin Oncol* 1996;23[Suppl 10]:3.

58. Heinemann V, Hertel LW, Grindey GB, et al. Comparison of the cellular pharmacokinetics and toxicity of 2',2'-difluorodeoxycytidine and 1-β-D-arabinofuranosylcytosine. *Cancer Res* 1988;48:4024.

59. Cappella P, Tomasoni D, Faretta M, et al. Cell cycle effects of gemcitabine. *Int J Cancer* 2001;93:401.

60. Csoka K, Liliemark J, Larsson R, et al. Evaluation of the cytotoxic activity of gemcitabine in primary cultures of tumor cells from patients with hematologic or solid tumors. *Semin Oncol* 1995;22:47.

61. Goan YG, Zhou B, Hu E, et al. Overexpression of ribonucleotide reductase as a mechanism of resistance to 2,2-difluorodeoxycytidine in the human KB cancer cell line. *Cancer Res* 1999;59:4204.

62. Venook A, Egorin M, Rosner G, et al. Phase I and pharmacokinetic trial of gemcitabine in patients with renal or hepatic dysfunction: Cancer and Leukemia Group B 9565. *J Clin Oncol* 2000;18:2780.

63. Storniolo AM, Enas NH, Brown CA, et al. An investigational new drug treatment program for patients with gemcitabine. Results for over 3000 patients with pancreatic carcinoma. *Cancer* 1999;85:1261.

64. Tempero M, Plunkett W, Ruiz van Halperen V, et al. Randomized phase II comparison of dose-intense gemcitabine: thirty-minute infusion and fixed dose rate in patients with pancreatic adenocarcinoma. *J Clin Oncol* 2003;21:3402.

65. Pavlakis N, Bell DR, Millward MJ, et al. Fatal pulmonary toxicity resulting from treatment with gemcitabine. *Cancer* 1997;80:286.

66. Fung MC, Storniolo AM, Nguyen B, et al. A review of hemolytic uremic syndrome in patients treated with gemcitabine therapy. *Cancer* 1999;85:2023.

67. Louvet C, André T, Lledo G, et al. Gemcitabine combined with oxaliplatin in advanced pancreatic adenocarcinoma: final results of a GERCOR multicenter phase II study. *J Clin Oncol* 2002;20:1512.

68. Van Laethem J, Demols A, Gay F, et al. Postoperative adjuvant gemcitabine and concurrent radiation after curative resection of pancreatic head carcinoma: a phase II study. *Int J Radiat Oncol Biol Phys* 2003;56:974.

69. Hande KR. Purine antimetabolites. In: Chabner BA, Longo DL, eds. *Cancer chemotherapy and biotherapy: principles and practice*, 3rd ed. Philadelphia: Lippincott–Raven, 2001:295.

70. Christie NT, Drake S, Meyn RE, et al. 6-Thiopurine-induced DNA damage as a determinant of cytotoxicity in cultured Chinese hamster ovary cells. *Cancer Res* 1984;44:3665.

71. Bemi V, Turchi G, Margotti E, et al. 6-Thioguanine resistance in a human colon carcinoma cell line with unaltered levels of hypoxanthine guanine phosphoribosyltransferase activity. *Int J Cancer* 1999;82:556.

72. Glaab WE, Risinger JI, Umar A, et al. Resistance to 6-thioguanine in mismatch-repair deficient human cancer cell lines correlates with an increase in induced mutations at the HPRT locus. *Carcinogenesis* 1998;19:1931.

73. Lennard L, Lilleyman JS. Individualizing therapy with 6-mercaptopurine and 6-thioguanine related to the thiopurine methyltransferase genetic polymorphism. *Ther Drug Monit* 1996;18:328.

74. Balis FM, Holcenberg JS, Poplack DG, et al. Pharmacokinetics and pharmacodynamics of oral methotrexate and mercaptopurine in children with lower risk acute lymphoblastic leukemia: a Joint Children's Cancer Group and Pediatric Oncology Branch Study. *Blood* 1998;92:3569.

75. Jacqz-Aigrain E, Nafa S, Medard Y, et al. Pharmacokinetics and distribution of 6-mercaptopurine administered intravenously in children with lymphoblastic leukemia. *Eur J Clin Pharm* 1997;53:71.

76. Keuzenkamp-Jansen CW, DeAbreu RA, Bokkerink JP, et al. Metabolism of intravenously administered high-dose 6-mercaptopurine with and without allopurinol treatment in patients with non-Hodgkin's lymphoma. *J Pediatr Hematol Oncol* 1996;18:145.

77. Krynetski EY, Evans WE. Pharmacogenetics as a molecular basis for individualized drug therapy: the thiopurine S-methyltransferase paradigm. *Pharm Res* 1999;16:342.

78. Yates CR, Krynetski EY, Loennechen T, et al. Molecular diagnosis of thiopurine S-methyltransferase deficiency: genetic basis for azathioprine and mercaptopurine intolerance. *Ann Intern Med* 1997;126:608.

79. Andersen JB, Szumlanski C, Weinshilboum RM, et al. Pharmacokinetics, dose adjustments, and 6-mercaptopurine/methotrexate drug interactions in two patients with thiopurine methyltransferase deficiency. *Acta Pediatr* 1998;87:108.

80. Erb N, Harms DO, Janka-Schaub G. Pharmacokinetics and metabolism of thiopurines in children with acute lymphoblastic leukemia receiving 6-thioguanine versus 6-mercaptopurine. *Cancer Chemother Pharmacol* 1998;42:266.

81. Lancaster DL, Lennard L, Rowland K, et al. Thioguanine versus mercaptopurine for therapy of childhood lymphoblastic leukemia: a comparison of haematological toxicity and drug metabolite concentrations. *Br J Haematol* 1998;102:439.

82. Belt JA. Heterogeneity of nucleoside transport in mammalian cells. Two types of activity in L1210 and other cultured neoplastic cells. *Mol Pharmacol* 1983;24:479.

83. Kamiya K, Huang P, Plunkett W. Inhibition of the 3'→ 5' exonuclease of human DNA polymerase epsilon by fludarabine-terminated DNA. *J Biol Chem* 1996;271:19428.

84. Huang P, Robertson LE, Wright S, et al. High molecular weight DNA fragmentation: a critical event in nucleoside analog-induced apoptosis in leukemia cells. *Clin Cancer Res* 1995;1:1005.

85. Plunkett W, Gandhi V. Cellular metabolism of nucleoside analogs in CLL: implications for drug development. In: Cheson BD, ed. *Chronic lymphocytic leukemia: scientific advances and clinical developments*. New York: Marcel Dekker, 1993:197.

86. Dumontet C, Fabianowska-Majewska K, Mantincic D, et al. Common resistance mechanisms to deoxynucleoside analogs in variants of the human erythroleukemic line K562. *Br J Haematol* 1999;106:78.

87. Malspeis L, Grever MR, Staubus AE, et al. Pharmacokinetics of 2-F-ara-A (9-b-D-arabinofuranosyl-2-fluoroadenine) in cancer patients during the phase I clinical investigation of fludarabine phosphate. *Semin Oncol* 1990;17[Suppl 8]:18.

88. Hussain K, Mazza JJ, Clouse LH, et al. Tumor lysis syndrome following fludarabine therapy for chronic lymphocytic leukemia (CLL): case report and review of the literature. *Am J Hematol* 2003;72:212.

89. Cheson B. Immunologic and immunosuppressive complications of purine analogue therapy. *J Clin Oncol* 1995;13:2431.

90. Li L, Liu X, Glassman AB, et al. Fludarabine triphosphate inhibits nucleotide excision repair of cisplatin-induced DNA adducts in vitro. *Cancer Res* 1997;57:1487.

91. Tsimberidou AM, McLaughlin P, Younes A, et al. Fludarabine, mitoxantrone, dexamethasone (FND) compared with an alternating triple therapy (ATT) regimen in patients with stage IV indolent lymphoma. *Blood* 2002;100:4351.

92. Robak T. Purine nucleoside analogues in the treatment of myeloid leukemias. *Leuk Lymphoma* 2003;44:391.

93. Seto S, Carrera CJ, Kubota M, et al. Mechanism of deoxyadenosine and 2-chlorodeoxyadenosine toxicity to nondividing human lymphocytes. *J Clin Invest* 1985;75:377.

94. Liliemark J, Juliusson G. Cellular pharmacokinetics of 2-chloro-2'-deoxyadenosine nucleotides: comparison of intermittent and continuous intravenous infusion and subcutaneous and oral administration in leukemia patients. *Clin Cancer Res* 1995;1:385.

95. Liliemark J. The clinical pharmacokinetics of cladribine. *Clin Pharmacokinet* 1997;32:120.

96. Albertioni F, Lindemalm S, Reichelova V, et al. Pharmacokinetics of cladribine in plasma and its 5'-monophosphate and 5'-triphosphate in leukemic cells of patients with chronic lymphocytic leukemia. *Clin Cancer Res* 1998;4:653.

97. Mey U, Strehl J, Gorschluter M, et al. Advances in the treatment of hairy cell leukemia. *Lancet Oncol* 2003;4:86.

98. Goodman GR, Burian C, Koziol JA, et al. Extended followup of patients with hairy cell leukemia after treatment with cladribine. *J Clin Oncol* 2003;21:891.

99. Carson DA, Wasson DB, Beutler E. Antileukemic and immunosuppressive activity of 2-chloro-2'-deoxyadenosine. *Proc Natl Acad Sci U S A* 1984;81:2252.

100. Cheson BD, Vena D, Foss F, et al. Neurotoxicity of purine analogs: a review. *J Clin Oncol* 1994;12:2216.

CHRIS H. TAKIMOTO

SECTION **7**

Topoisomerase Interactive Agents

The sheer size and complexity of the human genome present formidable challenges to proliferating cells engaged in the constant manipulation of the DNA double helix. Essential cellular functions such as DNA replication, transcription, and cell division require the frequent packaging and unpackaging of the DNA genome on a regular basis. As key facilitators of these cellular transactions, the DNA topoisomerase enzymes have the unique ability to relax and untangle large strands of intertwined DNA, thereby maintaining order within the cell and preserving the structural integrity of the genetic code. The topoisomerases literally prevent the cell from becoming embroiled in a tangled mess. The fundamental importance of the DNA topoisomerases is highlighted by their stringent conservation across prokaryotic and eukaryotic species and by their absolute necessity for cell proliferation. Because of these functions, the DNA topoisomerases also represent important molecular targets for cancer chemotherapy.

MAMMALIAN TOPOISOMERASES

The DNA topoisomerases modulate the topology of DNA by modifying the tertiary structure of the double helix without altering the primary nucleotide sequence.[1-3] They are responsible for relaxing the torsional stress that accumulates when the DNA double helix unwinds to allow DNA or RNA polymerases access to the genetic code. In the absence of topoisomerases, the accumulation of torsionally strained supercoiled DNA would ultimately interfere with vital cellular functions. During cell division, DNA topoisomerases also function to untangle and physically separate the replicated DNA by facilitating the passage of an intact DNA strand through a double-strand nick in the DNA helix. Thus, two linked circular DNA molecules can be physically separated (decatenated) by the action of specific DNA topoisomerases.

All DNA topoisomerases act by forming temporary single- or double-strand breaks in the double helix in which the enzyme is covalently bound via a tyrosine residue to one of the nicked ends of the phosphodiester DNA backbone. This normally transient intermediate, called the *cleavable complex*, allows for the passage of an intact single or double strand of DNA through this break, resulting in the unwinding or untangling of the DNA molecule. Subsequent religation and release of the enzyme restore the integrity of the DNA double helix.

The first DNA topoisomerase was discovered in *Escherichia coli* by James Wang in 1971.[4] All subsequently characterized DNA topoisomerases can be categorized into two broad families, types I and II, based on structure and function.[1] Type I DNA topoisomerases generate transient single-strand breaks in DNA, and these are further divided into subfamilies type IA or IB, depending on whether they form a covalent bond to the 5' or 3' phosphate group, respectively (Table 15.7-1). In contrast, type II DNA topoisomerases generate transient double-strand breaks in DNA, and these are also further subdivided into subfamilies type IIA and type IIB based on differences in protein structure. In higher eukaryotes and humans, three groups of topoisomerases have been identified. One group includes human topoisomerase I and the mitochondrial DNA topoisomerase, which are both type IB enzymes. The second group includes human DNA topoisomerases IIα and IIβ, which are type II enzymes, and the final group consists of human topoisomerases IIIα and IIIβ, which are both type IA enzymes. The human enzymes with the greatest relevance for cancer chemotherapy are DNA topoisomerase I and DNA topoisomerases IIα and IIβ (see Table 15.7-1).

Human DNA topoisomerase I is a monomeric, 91-kD protein composed of 765 amino acids[2] that is encoded for by the TOP1 gene on chromosome 20. The large human TOP1 gene contains 21 exons extending over 85 kb of DNA.[3] The topoisomerase I protein can be divided into four distinct structural domains. The most highly conserved regions include amino acid residues 198 to 651, which form the proteolytically resistant central core of the protein, and amino acids 713 to 765 at the C-terminal end that encompass the DNA-binding tyrosine residue 723. The x-ray crystallographic structure of human topoisomerase I bound to DNA suggests that the intact protein forms a V-shaped hinged clamp that opens and closes around the DNA double helix.[2]

Human DNA topoisomerase I preferentially binds to positively or negatively supercoiled double-stranded DNA and relaxes the torsional strain via an adenosine triphosphate–independent reaction. In the process, the DNA phosphodiester bond is cleaved and the enzyme forms a covalent link at tyrosine 723 with the 3' end of the nicked single strand of DNA (Fig. 15.7-1). This cleavable complex intermediate allows for relaxation of the DNA torsional strain either by passage of the opposite intact strand through the gap in the nicked DNA,

TABLE 15.7-1. Human Topoisomerases

Human Topoisomerase	Subfamily	Structure	Size (Amino Acids)	Gene Location
DNA topoisomerase I	IB	Monomer	765	20q12-13.1
Mitochondrial topoisomerase I	IB	Monomer	601	8q24.3
DNA topoisomerase IIα	IIA	Homodimer	1531	17q21-22
DNA topoisomerase IIβ	IIA	Homodimer	1626	3q24
DNA topoisomerase IIIα	IA	Monomer	1001	17p11.2-12
DNA topoisomerase IIIβ	IA	Monomer	862	22q11

(Modified from ref. 2.)

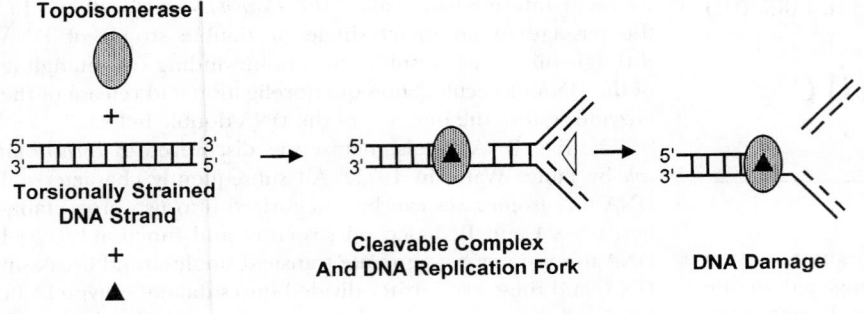

FIGURE 15.7-1. Topoisomerase I and camptothecin mechanism of action.

thereby decreasing the DNA linking number by one, or by free rotation of the DNA about the noncleaved strand. Finally, religation of the strand break restores the integrity of the DNA double helix, followed by enzyme dissociation from the now relaxed molecule. Topoisomerase I catalysis is rapid, and the transient protein binding to the DNA molecule cannot be isolated under normal conditions. Topoisomerase I–induced cleavable complexes do not form randomly throughout the genomic DNA; instead, they occur at weak consensus sequences, with preferential binding occurring at sites that contain thymidine nucleotides.

Human topoisomerase I is uniformly expressed throughout the cell cycle, even in nondividing cells. In mammalian cells, DNA topoisomerase I is essential for cell viability; however, yeast mutants that completely lack topoisomerase I have been identified. In comparative studies topoisomerase I protein and messenger RNA expression are higher in malignant tissues, including human ovarian, colon, and prostate cancers, compared to their normal tissue counterparts. This initially raised expectations that topoisomerase interactive agents may selec-

tively target tumors over normal tissues; however, the relative expression of topoisomerase I has not reliably predicted drug sensitivity.[3]

In contrast to topoisomerase I, two homologous but distinct isoforms of type II human topoisomerases have been characterized, DNA topoisomerase IIα and IIβ.[5] Human topoisomerase IIα is a 170-kD protein encoded for by a gene on chromosome 17q21-22, whereas the human topoisomerase IIβ gene is located on chromosome 3q24 and is associated with a 180-kD protein.[6] Both proteins exist as homodimers, although heterodimerization of IIα and IIβ topoisomerases can occur. These homodimers bind to DNA, forming an energy-independent double-strand DNA break in which the proteins are covalently bound to the 5' end of the broken DNA strands to form the topoisomerase II cleavable complex. In this state, the protein dimer is stabilized by bridging disulfide bonds that literally form a gate in the DNA through which a second intact DNA double-helix strand can pass in an energy-dependent reaction (Fig. 15.7-2). After strand passage is complete, religation and protein dissociation restore the intact DNA double

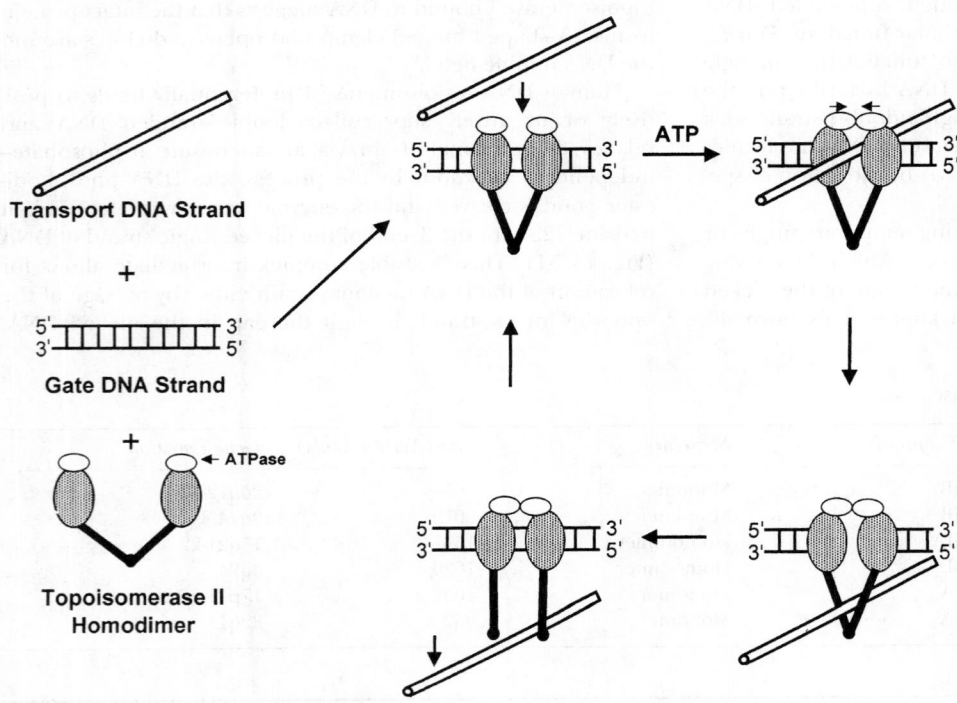

FIGURE 15.7-2. Topoisomerase II catalytic mechanism. ATP, adenosine triphosphate; ATPase, adenosine triphosphatase.

helix. Topoisomerase I and II can relax positively or negatively supercoiled DNA; however, only topoisomerase II enzymes can decatenate intertwined DNA strands.

In proliferating cells, the expression of topoisomerase IIα varies in different phases of the cell cycle, with maximum expression occurring during the G_2/M phase.[5] In contrast, quiescent cells express low levels of topoisomerase IIα. The ability of topoisomerase IIα to decatenate DNA during cell proliferation suggests that it may be important for the higher-order organization and segregation of newly replicated DNA in chromosomes.[1] Increased topoisomerase IIα activity is associated with transformed malignant cells, and overexpression of topoisomerase IIα is associated with increased tumor aggressiveness in some cancers, such as soft tissue sarcomas.[5] In contrast, topoisomerase IIβ expression is relatively constant throughout the cell cycle, suggesting that these two isoforms have distinct but as yet unidentified functions. However, some overlap in activity is present, as overexpression of topoisomerase IIβ can rescue proliferating cells that express low levels of topoisomerase IIα.

MECHANISM OF ACTION OF TOPOISOMERASE INTERACTIVE AGENTS

The precise mechanism by which pharmacologic modulation of topoisomerases is converted into cytotoxic drug effects has not been fully characterized. However, the initial interaction between topoisomerase targeting agents and these enzymes is well defined. The majority of topoisomerase interactive agents cause the accumulation of DNA cleavable complexes composed of protein-linked DNA strand breaks. The persistence of these lesions in the presence of ongoing DNA replication or RNA transcription leads to cytotoxic DNA damage, ultimately causing cell-cycle arrest and death by apoptosis or cell necrosis.

The best-characterized agents that interfere with topoisomerase I function are the camptothecin analogues. These natural product derivatives bind noncovalently to the topoisomerase I enzyme in the presence of DNA and stabilize the topoisomerase I–DNA cleavable complex. Camptothecins inhibit DNA religation (see Fig. 15.7-1) and trap the topoisomerase I enzyme in a covalent linkage to DNA at the site of a single-strand nick. The accumulation of these topoisomerase I–DNA cleavable complexes alone is not toxic to cells, because if the drug is removed, these lesions are highly reversible and they rapidly disappear. However, according to the "fork collision model," when a DNA replication fork encounters a stabilized cleavable complex, more lethal DNA damage occurs.[7] As a consequence, the camptothecins are relatively S phase cell cycle–specific cytotoxic agents, and inhibitors of DNA synthesis, such as aphidicolin or hydroxyurea, can decrease camptothecin-induced cytotoxicity.[3] These observations have substantial clinical relevance because cell-cycle–specific cytotoxicity generally requires prolonged exposure times to maximize the fractional cell kill.[8] Furthermore, the presence of topoisomerase I is absolutely essential for the generation of camptothecin-induced cytotoxicity. For example, mutant yeast cells that lack functional topoisomerase I are completely resistant to the camptothecins; however, when topoisomerase I is transfected into these mutants, drug sensitivity is restored.[9]

Camptothecin derivatives are sometime erroneously referred to as *topoisomerase I inhibitors*. Although these agents can inhibit topoisomerase I enzyme activity at high concentrations, their cytotoxic mechanism of action does not involve the loss of an essential enzyme activity. Instead, the camptothecins convert an endogenous protein, DNA topoisomerase I, into a cellular poison by trapping it in a covalent complex with DNA. For this reason, the camptothecin derivatives are more correctly referred to as *topoisomerase I interactive agents* or *topoisomerase poisons* rather than classic inhibitors.

In contrast to topoisomerase I, a large number of diverse chemical compounds have been identified that affect topoisomerase II enzymes. These include agents such as the anthracyclines and epipodophyllotoxins with a long history of clinical use in oncology. In the 1970s, Ross et al.[10] found that these agents caused the accumulation of protein-linked double-strand breaks in DNA; however, the involvement of topoisomerase II was not recognized until the 1980s.[6] Most of these drugs act by stabilizing human DNA topoisomerase IIα cleavable complexes, which are ultimately converted into cytotoxic DNA damage. Many of these agents, such as the anthracyclines and anthracenediones, are flat, planar molecules that intercalate into the double helix to alter DNA structure and function. However, the precise mechanism by which these compounds affect topoisomerase II function may differ. For example, compounds with strong intercalating activity, such as the quinolones, can inhibit topoisomerase II catalytic activity without trapping cleavable complexes, and other non-DNA binding agents can directly suppress topoisomerase II function by preventing cleavable complex formation.[6] The multiplicity of these interactions, many of which are still poorly understood at the molecular level, may partially explain the wide diversity of chemical structures that interact with topoisomerase II in cancer chemotherapy.

CAMPTOTHECINS

Camptothecin is a naturally occurring alkaloid isolated from the bark and wood of the Chinese plant, *Camptotheca acuminata*. Cytotoxic extracts from the Camptotheca tree were first discovered in the 1950s, and in 1966, Wall et al. identified camptothecin as the active ingredient.[3] However, the poor aqueous solubility camptothecin required its formulation for initial clinical testing in the 1970s as the less active carboxylate sodium salt. In early studies, camptothecin generated objective tumor responses; however, severe and unpredictable toxicities, such as hemorrhagic cystitis, halted its further clinical development. Interest in the camptothecins was renewed in 1985 by the discovery that their molecular target was the novel nuclear enzyme topoisomerase I.[11] At approximately the same time, several new water-soluble camptothecin analogues were synthesized, including irinotecan (CPT-11) and topotecan, and these subsequently demonstrated predictable clinical toxicity profiles and meaningful antitumor activity (Table 15.7-2).[3] In 1996, topotecan was approved as second-line chemotherapy for advanced ovarian cancer, and it later gained an indication for treating patients with refractory small cell lung cancer. Also in 1996, irinotecan was registered for the treatment of 5-fluorouracil–refractory advanced colorectal cancer. This represented the first new agent approved for treating this disease in the United States in nearly 40 years. Newer camptothecin analogues still in clinical development include rubitecan (9-nitrocamptothecin), lurtotecan (GI47211), exatecan mesylate (DX-8951f), and karenitecin (BNP-1350).

TABLE 15.7-2. Camptothecin Clinical Characteristics

Features	Topotecan	Irinotecan
Mechanism of action	Topoisomerase I poison, stabilizes cleavable complexes	Prodrug, active metabolite, SN-38 released by irinotecan-converting enzyme, predominantly in the liver; SN-38 is a potent topoisomerase I poison
Route of administration	Intravenous	Intravenous
Elimination/excretion	Renal excretion predominates	Hepatic metabolism by CYP3A to APC and NPC metabolites, biliary excretion and glucuronidation of SN-38 by UGT1A1
Toxicities	Myelosuppression, predominantly neutropenia; nausea and vomiting, mild; diarrhea, mild; fatigue; alopecia; skin rashes; mild transaminitis	Early-onset diarrhea with cholinergic symptoms (flushing, diaphoresis, cramping, and vomiting); late-onset diarrhea, can be severe; myelosuppression, predominantly neutropenia; alopecia; nausea and vomiting; mucositis; fatigue; mild transaminitis
Dosing in organ dysfunction	Dose adjustments required in renal dysfunction	Dose adjustments required in hepatic dysfunction, especially hyperbilirubinemia

APC, 7-ethyl-10-[4-N-(5-aminopentanoic acid)-1-piperidino]carbonyloxy-camptothecin; CYP3A, cytochrome P-450 3A; NPC, 7-ethyl-10-(4-amino-1-piperidino)carbonyloxycamptothecin; SN-38, 7-ethyl-10-hydroxycamptothecin; UGT1A1, uridine diphosphate glucuronosyltransferase. (Modified from ref. 3.)

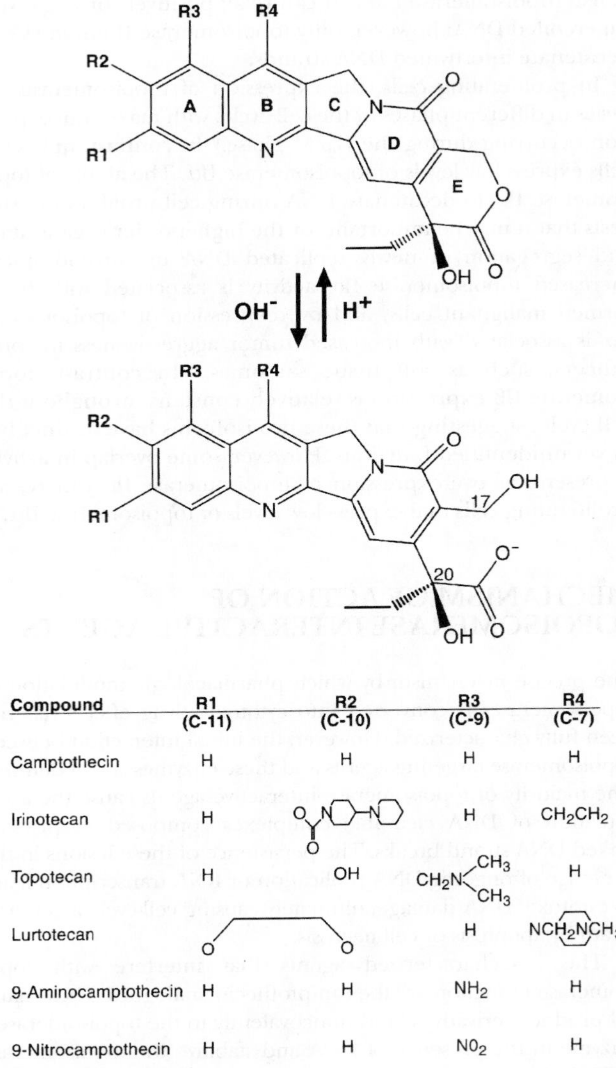

Compound	R1 (C-11)	R2 (C-10)	R3 (C-9)	R4 (C-7)
Camptothecin	H	H	H	H
Irinotecan	H	(dipiperidino carbonyloxy)	H	CH₂CH₃
Topotecan	H	OH	CH₂N(CH₃)₂	H
Lurtotecan	(dioxyethylene)		H	NCH₂N·CH₃
9-Aminocamptothecin	H	H	NH₂	H
9-Nitrocamptothecin	H	H	NO₂	H

FIGURE 15.7-3. Camptothecin structures.

STRUCTURE

All the camptothecins share a central five-ring structure with a chiral center at C-20 and a terminal α-hydroxy-δ-lactone E ring (Fig. 15.7-3). The naturally occurring (S)-isomer of camptothecin is 10 to 100 times more biologically active than the (R)-isomer.[3] In aqueous solutions, the terminal lactone ring can undergo rapid hydrolysis via a nonenzymatic, reversible, pH-dependent reaction to form the open-ring hydroxy carboxylic acid (see Fig. 15.7-3). At equilibrium in physiologic or alkaline pH, the less active open-ring carboxylate species predominates; however, acidic environments favor ring closure forming the biologically active lactone. This equilibrium explains the severe toxicities seen in the early development of camptothecin, because excretion of the carboxylate sodium salt in to the low-pH environment of the bladder led to closure of the lactone ring, ultimately causing the severe hemorrhagic cystitis. Topotecan contains a stable basic side chain at position C-9 that enhances its water solubility but does not interfere with interactions with topoisomerase I (see Fig. 15.7-3). In contrast, the prodrug irinotecan contains a bulky dipiperidino side chain at C-10 that must be cleaved by a carboxylesterase-converting

enzyme in the liver and other tissues to generate the active metabolite, SN-38 (7-ethyl-10-hydroxy camptothecin) (see Fig. 15.7-3). The unmetabolized parent drug is inactive as a topoisomerase I targeting agent; however, irinotecan is a weak inhibitor of acetylcholinesterases, and it can cause acute cholinergic symptoms in some patients.

MECHANISMS OF ACTION AND RESISTANCE

The camptothecins are the best-characterized agents that interfere with mammalian DNA topoisomerase I function. All the camptothecins in clinical development are potent stabilizers of topoisomerase I cleavable complexes, with the exception of irinotecan, which must first be enzymatically converted to SN-38 for biologic activity. Although little is known about clinical resistance in patients, *in vitro* studies have identified a number of different mechanisms of camptothecin resistance in cell lines.[12] Mutant forms of topoisomerase I have been characterized *in vitro* that confer a relative resistance to the camptothecins without abolishing its catalytic activity. Many are single point mutations that span large portions of the protein; however, the identification of topoisomerase I mutations in clinical specimens has been exceedingly rare.[12] Camptothecin resistance can also result from down-regulation of topoisomerase I due to chromosomal deletions or hypermethylation of the TOP1 gene. However, the absolute level of topoisomerase I expression in tumor tissues has not been highly predictive of drug efficacy in experimental studies.[3]

Another important potential mechanism of camptothecin resistance is decreased intracellular drug accumulation mediated by various drug efflux pumps. The precise role of the P-glycoprotein–associated multidrug resistance (MDR) phenotype in camptothecin resistance is controversial. Irinotecan and its metabolite SN-38 do not appear to be substrates for the MDR drug efflux pump,[3] and cross-resistance to irinotecan is not seen in MDR-overexpressing cell lines that are highly resistant to vincristine and doxorubicin. In contrast, topotecan is a modest P-glycoprotein substrate; MDR-expressing cells are ninefold more resistant to topotecan than parental wild-type cells. This magnitude of MDR-associated resistance to topotecan is much less than the 200-fold change in sensitivity typically described for classic MDR substrates, such as doxorubicin or etoposide. Other drug efflux pumps may be even more important in modulating camptothecin resistance. The MDR–associated protein-2 (MRP2) has been associated with resistance to SN-38 and 9-aminocamptothecin.[12] More recently, a new transporter called the *breast cancer resistance protein* (BCRP) has also been implicated in resistance to camptothecins.[13] Other factors that can affect camptothecin sensitivity include a reduction in the number of cells in S phase or the decreased intratumoral production of SN-38 by the irinotecan carboxyl-esterase-converting enzyme. Finally, double-strand DNA break repair activity, cell-cycle checkpoint integrity, and the sensitivity of cells to triggering apoptosis may also modulate camptothecin-induced cytotoxicity.[3] Whether any of these multiple mechanisms is responsible for clinical drug resistance must still be defined.

CLINICAL USE AND TOXICITY

The most commonly used dose of topotecan is 1.5 mg/m^2 given as a 30-minute intravenous infusion daily for 5 days every 3 weeks.[14] Because of its schedule-dependent cytotoxicity,[8] topotecan has also been administered via prolonged infusions for up to 21 days; however, clear superiority over shorter infusions has not been generated.[14] Interest has grown in exploring weekly topotecan infusions as a means to enhance patient convenience and reduce myelosuppressive toxicities while preserving antitumor activity.[15] Preliminary evidence suggests that weekly schedules are clinically promising, and further studies are in progress. Oral and intraperitoneal topotecan administration have been studied, but neither of these routes of drug administration is in common clinical use.

As a class, the camptothecins have a broad spectrum of antitumor activity. Topotecan is indicated in the second-line treatment of advanced refractory ovarian[16] and small cell lung cancer,[17,18] and it also has activity in the treatment of hematologic malignancies, including myelodysplastic syndromes and multiple myeloma.[14] Tumor responses have also been reported in patients with pediatric malignancies, such as neuroblastoma, and central nervous system gliomas. Although topotecan has

been combined with a variety of other therapies, including radiation, cisplatin, paclitaxel, and doxorubicin in clinical trials, none of these combinations has achieved any routine use in clinical oncology. This may be due, in part, to the frequent myelosuppressive toxicity of topotecan that has made it difficult to combine in high doses with other bone marrow–suppressive agents.[19]

The most common dose-limiting toxicity for topotecan is reversible, noncumulative myelosuppression, especially neutropenia, which is seen on all schedules of drug administration. On the daily-for-5-days administration schedule, the mean onset of grade 3 or 4 neutropenia is on day 9 and persists for approximately 14 days, with recovery in most cases by day 21.[14] Grade 4 neutropenia is very common, with a reported incidence of 79% in previously treated ovarian cancer patients.[16] Thrombocytopenia and moderate to severe anemia are somewhat less common, although blood transfusions are often required. Extensive prior radiation or previously bone marrow–suppressive chemotherapy increases the risk of topotecan-induced myelosuppression, and extensive prior carboplatin treatment specifically increases the risk of subsequent thrombocytopenia.[20] Supportive administration of colony-stimulating factors may ameliorate topotecan-induced neutropenia to some extent; however, these agents should not be given concurrently with topotecan. Other less frequent and typically mild toxicities include nausea and vomiting, diarrhea, low-grade fevers, fatigue, alopecia, skin rash, and transient hepatic transaminitis; however, hemorrhagic cystitis has not been seen. In leukemia patients treated with 5-day continuous topotecan infusions, mucositis and diarrhea are dose limiting. In patients receiving topotecan chemotherapy, blood counts should be monitored closely with periodic evaluation of renal and liver function tests. All patients should be instructed about the risks of febrile neutropenia.

In contrast to topotecan, irinotecan has been routinely administered intravenously on more infrequent dosing schedules. The most commonly administered schedules of irinotecan are a 90-minute intravenous infusion of 125 mg/m^2 given weekly for 4 of every 6 weeks or 350 mg/m^2 given every 3 weeks. None of these regimens shows clear superiority, although irinotecan-associated diarrhea may be somewhat less on the every-3-week schedule.[21] In combination therapy, irinotecan has been given weekly with bolus fluorouracil and leucovorin[22] or every 2 weeks with infusional fluorouracil.[23] Prolonged drug infusion schedules have been well tolerated in phase I trials and are associated with more efficient enzymatic conversion of irinotecan to the active metabolite, SN-38, than shorter infusions. However, whether infusional irinotecan produces any greater clinical benefit than standard schedule is still unknown. Oral dosing of irinotecan has been tested but remains investigational.

Irinotecan is indicated as a single agent or in combination with fluorouracil and leucovorin in treating patients with colorectal cancer.[22,23] It also has substantial activity in small cell lung cancer when given in combination with cisplatin, and this combination is active in non–small cell lung cancer as well.[14] Antitumor responses have also been reported in ovarian, esophageal, cervical, and gastric cancer and malignant gliomas, and lesser degrees of antitumor activity have been reported in breast cancer, non-Hodgkin's lymphoma, and acute leukemias. Despite irinotecan's association with frequent gastrointestinal side effects, combination regimens have been developed with other therapies, including fluorouracil, etoposide, oxaliplatin, cisplatin, and radiation.[22,23]

Irinotecan's dose-limiting toxicities are neutropenia and delayed-onset diarrhea. Irinotecan is also associated with an acute diarrhea seen immediately after drug administration that results from its cholinergic properties. This early-onset diarrhea and any associated cholinergic-type symptoms can be easily treated by administering atropine premedication to those patients who experience this adverse reaction. Irinotecan's delayed-onset diarrhea is generally defined as occurring at least 24 hours after drug administration and can be potentially life threatening, especially in combination chemotherapy regimens with bolus intravenous fluorouracil and leucovorin.[24] Patients should be instructed to take high-dose loperamide at the first onset of any irinotecan-associated delayed diarrhea, and antidiarrheal therapy should be administered continuously until all diarrhea has stopped for at least 12 hours. The mechanism of irinotecan-induced delayed diarrhea is not known, but it is believed to result from the direct toxic effects of the active metabolite, SN-38, on the intestinal epithelium.[3] Irinotecan should not be administered to patients with any degree of ongoing diarrhea above their baseline, and it should be used with caution in frail patients with borderline performance status. Irinotecan neutropenia should be managed aggressively with antibiotics, especially when associated with gastrointestinal symptoms.[24] Other toxicities associated with irinotecan chemotherapy include a cholinergic syndrome (flushing, bradycardia, tearing, diaphoresis, and visual accommodation symptoms), abdominal cramping, fatigue, alopecia, nausea, and vomiting. Routine antiemetic premedication is recommended before irinotecan administration.

CLINICAL PHARMACOLOGY

After intravenous administration, topotecan plasma concentrations decrease in a biphasic pattern with a short terminal half-life of 2.0 to 3.5 hours.[25] Because of its rapid hydrolysis, hydroxyl carboxylic acid accounts for 65% to 80% of the total circulating topotecan in plasma.[3] Topotecan penetration into the central nervous system is greater than that of other camptothecins, resulting in cerebrospinal fluid drug concentrations that are approximately 30% of plasma levels.[25] Only 25% to 40% of topotecan is bound to plasma proteins, and drug concentrations increase dose proportionally, although at high dose levels drug clearance may be nonlinear.[3] Topotecan's pharmacokinetics do not change with repeated dosing cycles; its kinetics in pediatric patients are similar to those in adult patients. Renal excretion of topotecan hydroxy carboxylic acid is the predominant route of drug elimination, and glomerular filtration rates (GFRs) strongly correlate with total drug clearance. Approximately 25% to 40% of the total administered dose is excreted into the urine over the initial 24 hours after drug administration, and after prolonged urine collections, the percent of drug excreted renally may reach as high as 90%.[3] Small amounts of topotecan are also excreted into the bile; however, the importance of this elimination pathway is thought to be minimal. Topotecan is also hepatically metabolized to N-desmethyl metabolites that are detectable at low concentrations in human plasma, urine, and feces. The clinical importance of this metabolic pathway has not been defined.

Because it is a prodrug, irinotecan's pharmacokinetics are more complex. After drug administration, the lactone and carboxylate forms of irinotecan and its active metabolite, SN-38, are detectable in plasma.[25] SN-38 is generated from irinotecan by the action of irinotecan-converting enzyme, predominantly in the liver.[3] Irinotecan peak concentrations occur at the end of a 90-minute infusion, but SN-38 concentrations peak 2 to 3 hours later and are approximately 50 to 100 times lower than the irinotecan. Irinotecan plasma concentrations increase proportionally with dose, but SN-38 concentrations do not, consistent with possible saturation of the irinotecan-converting enzyme.[3] In primates, irinotecan penetration into the central nervous system is low. The presence of large volumes of pleural fluid or ascites is not associated with increased clinical toxicity due to third-space effects. Irinotecan is approximately 30% to 68% plasma protein bound; however, it is the lactone species that is preferentially bound (95%) to plasma albumin. This interaction may help explain why more than 50% of SN-38 circulates in plasma as the biologically active lactone form, in contrast to most other camptothecins, in which the inactive carboxylate species predominates. The mean terminal elimination half-life for irinotecan lactone is approximately 6 hours (range, 5.0 to 9.6 hours); however, the apparent SN-38 half-life is approximately 11.5 hours due to its slow generation from irinotecan metabolism.[3] Renal excretion of irinotecan accounts for 14% to 37% of the administered dose, with the remainder being eliminated by hepatic metabolism and biliary excretion. However, clinical drug effects may be more closely related to SN-38 pharmacokinetics, and only approximately 0.26% of the administered dose is renally excreted as SN-38.[3]

Two well-characterized inactive hepatic metabolites of irinotecan are APC (7-ethyl-10-[4-N-(5-aminopentanoic acid)-1-piperidino]carbonyloxycamptothecin) and NPC (7-ethyl-10-(4-amino-1-piperidino)carbonyloxycamptothecin). Both are generated by cytochrome P-450 (CYP) 3A metabolism.[25] In contrast, SN-38 is predominantly cleared via conjugation by liver uridine diphosphate glucuronosyltransferase (UGT) to form the inactive β-glucuronidated derivative, SN-38G (10-O-glucuronyl-SN-38). SN-38G plasma concentrations peak rapidly within 10 to 20 minutes after the end of the irinotecan infusion, and they exceed the plasma concentrations of SN-38 by four- or five-fold.[3] SN-38G plasma concentrations decrease in parallel with SN-38 over time, consistent with UGT being the rate-limiting step responsible for SN-38 elimination. Direct biliary excretion of irinotecan and its multiple metabolites is a major route of drug clearance. Biliary excretion is modulated by the canalicular multispecific organic anion transporter (cMOAT), also know as *MRP2*, a membrane transporter identified in drug-resistant cells. Finally, enterohepatic circulation of SN-38 can occur and may be enhanced by the hydrolysis of SN-38G in the bile by gut microbial flora, leading to reabsorption of free SN-38. Some strategies for reducing irinotecan-associated diarrhea include the administration of antibiotics or bacterial β-glucuronidase inhibitors to reduce the production of free SN-38 in the intestinal lumen.[3] Other strategies include blocking direct biliary excretion of these agents using drugs such as cyclosporin A, which reduces bile flow and inhibits bile canalicular active transport. Finally, a substantial number of biliary metabolites of irinotecan have yet to be fully characterized.[26]

ADJUSTMENTS IN ORGAN DYSFUNCTION

Because of its extensive renal clearance, topotecan dose adjustments are required in patients with renal dysfunction.[20,27] Any patient with a creatinine clearance (CrCL) greater than 60 mL/min can be treated with standard topotecan doses of 1.5 mg/m^2/d. For minimally pretreated patients with an estimated CrCL of 40 to 59 mL/min, full doses of topotecan can be administered; however, if the CrCL is 20 to 39 mL/min, these patients should be dose reduced to 0.75 mg/m^2/d. Patients with extensive prior chemotherapy or radiation therapy can receive full doses of topotecan if their CrCL is greater than 60 mL/min; however, heavily pretreated patients should receive a reduced topotecan dose of 1.0 mg/m^2/d for a CrCL of 40 to 59 mL/min, and further decreases to 0.5 mg/m^2/d should be instituted for a CrCL of 20 to 39 mL/min.[20] Guidelines for any patient with an estimated CrCL below 20 mL/min have not been established. Renal hemodialysis quickly reduces topotecan plasma concentrations, but in a study of one patient, postdialysis topotecan plasma concentrations rapidly rebounded, presumably because of equilibration with tissue compartments.[28] No topotecan dose adjustments are required in patients with hepatic dysfunction as defined by an elevation of total serum bilirubin levels greater than 1.2 mg/dL; however, only a limited number of patients have been studied with hyperbilirubinemia exceeding 3.5 mg/dL.[29]

In contrast to topotecan, the extensive hepatic metabolism of irinotecan and its metabolites mandates careful dosing in the face of liver dysfunction, especially hyperbilirubinemia.[30] In a formal study of irinotecan administered every 3 weeks to patients with varying degrees of hyperbilirubinemia, full doses of 350 mg/m^2 were well tolerated by patients with total bilirubin levels less than 1.50 times the upper limit of normal (ULN).[31] In contrast, patients with bilirubin levels 1.51 to 3.0 times the ULN required dose reductions to 200 g/m^2. No treatment recommendations were established for patients with more severe levels of hyperbilirubinemia. Interestingly, hepatic dysfunction was associated with increased exposures to irinotecan and SN-38; however, metabolic conversion to APC and SN-38G, respectively, remained intact, suggesting the importance of biliary secretion over enzymatic transformation as the major route of hepatic elimination.[31] In pharmacokinetic studies, changes in irinotecan dosing in patients with renal dysfunction do not appear to be necessary; however, clinical data are limited in patients with severe elevations of serum creatinine greater than 3.5 mg/dL.[32,33]

DRUG INTERACTIONS

In a clinical study examining sequential administration of topotecan and cisplatin, a potential drug interaction was observed when cisplatin was administered before topotecan, resulting in substantially greater hematologic toxicity than the reverse sequence.[34] Pharmacokinetic analyses revealed that cisplatin causes a transient reduction in topotecan clearance that was attributed to platinum-induced subclinical renal tubular toxicity induced by the platinum analogue.[34] In another combination study, administration of topotecan before docetaxel chemotherapy decreases docetaxel clearance by 50% and increases the incidence of neutropenia compared to the reverse drug administration sequence.[35] Although the mechanism of this interaction was not defined, alterations in docetaxel's hepatic metabolism and excretion were proposed. When topotecan is administered to patients treated with antiepileptic drugs that can induce hepatic metabolism and drug transporters, such as phenobarbital and phenytoin, an enhancement of topotecan clearance is seen. Furthermore, low topotecan clearance was observed in another patient simultaneously treated

with terfenadine, suggesting a potential topotecan interaction involving CYP3A metabolism.[25] Hepatic CYP3A metabolism is also important in the metabolism of irinotecan. Coadministration of irinotecan with inhibitors of CYP3A4, such as ketoconazole, erythromycin, St. John's wort, and cyclosporine, has demonstrated altered clearance and increased drug activation and, thus, should be approached cautiously. For example, when irinotecan was administered concomitantly with ketoconazole, up to fourfold dose reductions were recommended.[36] Because of the large number of drugs that are substrates or inhibitors of CYP3A4, practicing clinicians need to be aware of the potential for clinically relevant pharmacokinetic interactions when using topotecan or irinotecan.

PHARMACOGENETICS

Because of the complexity of irinotecan metabolism, it is a prime target for studying the effects of genetic polymorphisms in cancer chemotherapy. Although the clinical relevance of pharmacogenomics is currently limited to a few examples, the explosion of knowledge in this area is likely to substantially change the way cancer chemotherapy is administered in the future. Because UGT-mediated glucuronidation is the rate-limiting step in SN-38 clearance, variability in its activity may contribute to interpatient differences in drug toxicity during irinotecan chemotherapy.[25] The UGT1A1 isoform that catalyzes bilirubin glucuronidation is also the major enzyme responsible for glucuronidation of SN-38. Genetic abnormalities associated with decreased UGT1A1 activity have been well characterized in conditions as common as Gilbert's syndrome, which is present in 3% to 7% of individuals in the United States, and the highly rare Crigler-Najjar syndrome of familial hyperbilirubinemia. Patients with these genetic alterations may be at risk for severe irinotecan-induced diarrhea due to an inability to conjugate and detoxify SN-38. Severe diarrhea was observed in two patients with Gilbert's syndrome treated with standard doses of irinotecan.[25] Genetic testing for the UGT1A1*28 promoter region polymorphism associated with decreased glucuronidating activity is undergoing prospective evaluation in larger clinical studies of irinotecan-based therapy.[37]

In another pharmacogenetic study, the impact of a panel of genes on irinotecan pharmacokinetics was analyzed in patients receiving irinotecan chemotherapy.[38] These genes included MDR1 (ABCB1), *MRP1* (ABCC1) and *MRP2* (cMOAT, ABCC2), BCRP (ABCC2), human carboxyl esterases 1 and 2 (CES1, CES2), UGT1A1, and XRCC1, a DNA repair enzyme. Although 18 genetic variants were identified in 65 cancer patients, only a single polymorphism in the *MDR1* gene significantly correlated with increased exposures to irinotecan. Nonetheless, although the clinical impact of pharmacogenetic profiling is currently modest, this approach still has great potential to optimize irinotecan chemotherapy as important new polymorphisms are identified in drug-metabolizing genes in the future.

EPIPODOPHYLLOTOXINS

The indigenous peoples of North America have a long history of using extracts of the mandrake (mayapple) plant, *Podophyllum peltatum*, for medicinal purposes as a cathartic, emetic, and anthelmintic.[6] However, formal pharmaceutical use of the

TABLE 15.7-3. Epipodophyllotoxin Clinical Characteristics

Features	Etoposide/Etoposide Phosphate	Teniposide
Mechanism of action	Nonintercalating topoisomerase II poison	Nonintercalating topoisomerase II poison
Route of administration	Intravenous, oral	Intravenous
Elimination/excretion	Hepatic metabolism ~33%, renal excretion 35–40%	Hepatic metabolism predominates
Toxicity	Myelosuppression, predominantly neutropenia, mild thrombocytopenia; alopecia, hypersensitivity; mucositis	Similar to etoposide
Dosing in organ dysfunction	Dose reduction recommended in renal dysfunction; no consensus for dosing in hepatic dysfunction, but reductions may be necessary for severe cases	Dose reduction may be necessary for hepatic dysfunction; no formal guidelines available

(Modified from ref. 6.)

podophyllotoxins in the United States did not begin until 1820, and clinical studies in oncology were not initiated until 1946.[39] Initially, severe systemic toxicities limited the use of podophyllotoxins to the topical treatment of condylomata acuminata. Subsequent efforts in the 1960s to develop less toxic podophyllotoxins led to the synthesis of the glycoside derivatives etoposide (VP-16-213) and teniposide (VP-26; Table 15.7-3). Clinical testing of these newer epipodophyllotoxins in the 1970s demonstrated predictable toxicity profiles and meaningful antitumor activity in diseases such as acute myelocytic leukemia, non-Hodgkin's lymphomas, and breast, ovarian, gastric, and lung cancers. In 1983, etoposide (VePesid) was approved for the treatment of testicular and small cell lung cancer, and in 1993, teniposide was approved for treating pediatric leukemias and lymphomas. Currently, etoposide is commonly used in cancer chemotherapy, with meaningful clinical activity in diseases such as germ cell tumors, ovarian cancer, small and non–small cell lung cancer, non-Hodgkin's lymphoma, acute leukemia, Ewing's sarcoma, Kaposi's sarcoma, and neuroblastoma. Teniposide has a less broad spectrum of clinical use, but it has been used in the treatment of pediatric acute leukemia, neuroblastoma, and small cell lung, bladder, and central nervous system cancers.

Etoposide and teniposide are large-molecular-weight glycosidic podophyllotoxin derivatives with poor aqueous solubility (Fig. 15.7-4). They are structurally similar, with teniposide differing from etoposide only by the presence of a sulfur-containing thenylidine group on the glycosidic sugar moiety. Due to enhanced cellular uptake, teniposide is tenfold more potent than etoposide; but it is also less water soluble. Etoposide phosphate is a recently developed water-soluble prodrug of etoposide with similar pharmacokinetic and pharmacodynamic profiles.[40] It requires lower fluid volumes for intravenous

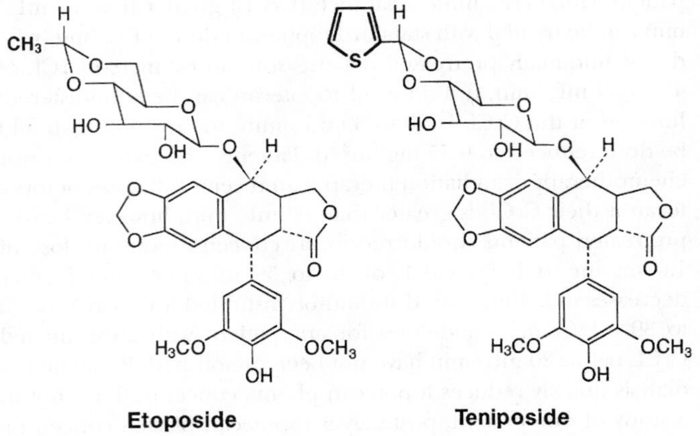

Etoposide   **Teniposide**

FIGURE 15.7-4. Epipodophyllotoxin structures.

administration, and this has facilitated the use of high-dose etoposide in stem cell transplantation regimens.

BIOCHEMICAL AND MOLECULAR PHARMACOLOGY

The earliest pharmacologic studies of the podophyllotoxins demonstrated their ability to inhibit microtubule formation and block mitosis in rapidly dividing cells. However, subsequent studies revealed that etoposide's growth-inhibitory properties occurred at drug concentrations lower than those required to inhibit with microtubule assembly. Further studies subsequently revealed that the epipodophyllotoxin's mechanism of action was mediated through its interaction with topoisomerase II. In 1984, the epipodophyllotoxins were among the first agents recognized as targeting human DNA topoisomerase II.[41] Etoposide and teniposide block the religation reaction of topoisomerase IIα by a mechanism independent of DNA binding, leading to the accumulation of protein-linked single- and double-strand DNA breaks (cleavable complexes). Cells in the S and G$_2$ phases of the cell cycle show the greatest sensitivity to these agents; however, unlike topoisomerase I poisons, inhibition of DNA synthesis only partially protects against etoposide-induced cytotoxicity.[42] This may be due, in part, to the cytotoxic interaction between the cell's RNA transcriptional machinery and the drug-stabilized, topoisomerase II DNA cleavable complexes. The ensuing accumulation of DNA damage, especially in the presence of altered cell-cycle checkpoint controls, ultimately becomes incompatible with cell survival.[6]

Resistance to the epipodophyllotoxins may be mediated by a number of diverse mechanisms. Similar to other topoisomerase II targeting agents, the epipodophyllotoxins are substrates for the 170-kD P-glycoprotein drug efflux pump that is encoded for by the MDR-1 gene. Tumor cell lines that overexpress P-glycoprotein are generally resistant to etoposide and teniposide because of reduced intracellular drug accumulation.[6] Another potential mechanism of resistance is the down-regulation of topoisomerase IIα enzyme activity. Decreased cellular expression of topoisomerase IIα enzyme activity has been associated with resistance to the epipodophyllotoxins in some experimental systems. Finally, *in vitro* experiments have identified cell lines resistant to the epipodophyllotoxins due to point mutations in topoisomerase IIα.[6] However, the clinical relevance of these observations is uncertain because drug-resistant topoisomerase II mutations have not been frequently observed in resistant clinical tumor samples.[43]

CLINICAL USE AND TOXICITIES

Etoposide and teniposide are commonly administered intravenously to cancer patients; however, their poor solubility requires their formulation with complex vehicles such as Cremophor EL or polysorbate (Tween) 80. The prodrug, etoposide phosphate, does not require specialized vehicles for intravenous administration, and it is associated with a lower incidence of infusion-related reactions than earlier etoposide formulations.[40] Intravenous etoposide infusions are often administered at doses of 50 to 100 mg/m^2/d for 3 or 5 days every 3 weeks. Repeated daily treatments administered intermittently are more effective than more infrequent administration schedules.[39] High-dose etoposide at 2 to 13 g/m^2 has been administered with autologous stem cell support. An oral etoposide gelatin capsule formulation has facilitated the testing of prolonged drug exposure regimens.[40] The oral daily dose of etoposide is typically twice the intravenous dose; however, the therapeutic profile of this agent administered orally is unchanged.

Etoposide and etoposide phosphate are indicated in the treatment of small cell lung cancer and germ cell neoplasms. Combination chemotherapy with platinum agents is a commonly used first-line therapy for limited- and extensive-stage small cell lung cancer. Platinum, bleomycin, and etoposide combinations are standard treatments for germ cell tumors that are capable of inducing high cure rates, even in advanced disease. Etoposide is also active in a variety of tumor types, including acute leukemia, non-Hodgkin's lymphoma, pediatric tumors, unknown primary tumors, Ewing's sarcoma, osteosarcoma, and ovarian, gastric, esophageal, and non–small cell lung cancers. Teniposide's use is predominantly limited to the treatment of acute pediatric lymphoblastic leukemia as a component of combination chemotherapy.

The major dose-limiting toxicity for etoposide and for teniposide is myelosuppression, especially leukopenia, with thrombocytopenia being less common. Nadir leukocyte counts occur on days 10 to 14, with recovery typically occurring after 21 days. Other toxicities associated with etoposide and teniposide therapy include mild to moderate nausea and vomiting, mucositis, diarrhea, and alopecia. Hypotension, hypersensitivity reactions, and thrombophlebitis have also been reported, although some of these reactions may be caused by the solubilizing agents required for infusional therapy such as Cremophor EL.[44] An acute autoimmune hemolytic anemia has been associated with teniposide therapy.[45] When etoposide is administered as a component of high-dose chemotherapy with stem cell support, the major dose-limiting toxicity is mucositis.[39]

CLINICAL PHARMACOLOGY

After intravenous administration, etoposide plasma concentrations decrease in a biphasic pattern, with a final terminal elimination half-life of approximately 4 to 11 hours.[46] Etoposide plasma concentrations increase proportionally, with increasing dose levels up to 800 mg/m^2.[39] More than 96% of etoposide in plasma is protein bound, mostly to albumin; however, in cancer patients the unbound free drug fraction is highly variable and can range from 5% to 45%.[46] Alterations in protein binding

have clinical relevance, because the pharmacodynamic effects of etoposide are strongly correlated with the unbound free fraction in plasma. Bilirubin can displace etoposide from albumin-binding sites, and as a consequence, the free unbound etoposide fraction in plasma is increased by high bilirubin concentrations and by low serum albumin levels. Etoposide poorly penetrates into the central nervous system, with equilibrium drug concentrations in cerebrospinal fluid reaching less than 5% of plasma drug concentrations. After oral administration, etoposide is rapidly absorbed, with a relative bioavailability of 50% (range, 24% to 137%) with high interpatient variability.[46] Oral etoposide's bioavailability tends to decrease at absolute doses greater than 300 mg.[39] Variability in etoposide absorption may be due in part to intestinal P-glycoprotein expression. After oral absorption is complete, etoposide's pharmacokinetics mirror those seen after intravenous administration, and the oral route of administration has not altered the therapeutic profile of this agent. Teniposide also has a biphasic pattern of elimination after intravenous administration, although its terminal half-life is longer than etoposide's, ranging from 5 to 40 hours. It is more than 99% plasma protein bound, and its penetration into the central nervous system is also low, but clinical activity in treating lung cancer metastatic to the brain has been reported, possibly due to teniposide's increased lipophilicity and greater potency than etoposide.[46]

Etoposide is cleared via renal and hepatic mechanisms. Nonrenal clearance pathways are responsible for the majority of etoposide's elimination, but the precise clinically relevant metabolic pathways in humans have not been fully elucidated. Typically, renal excretion accounts for 35% to 45% of etoposide elimination,[47] and biliary excretion is minor. Known hepatic metabolism accounts for approximately another third of drug clearance. In the liver, etoposide undergoes phase II conjugation reactions to form inactive glucuronide and sulfate derivatives. In addition, it is a substrate for CYP3A4 demethylation reactions. Some of the O-demethylation etoposide and teniposide reaction products are reactive orthoquinone derivatives that can potentially damage DNA via oxidation reactions.[46] However, the clinical relevance of these toxic epipodophyllotoxin metabolites have yet to be determined. Teniposide has less renal clearance (10% to 21%) and is more hepatically metabolized than etoposide; however, little is known about teniposide's metabolic pathways in humans.

Because etoposide clearance is linearly related to CrCL, dose reductions are uniformly recommended in patients with substantial renal impairment.[48] Although validated guidelines for etoposide dose adjustments in renal failure are lacking, some investigators have recommended a 25% decrease in dose for patients with GFRs ranging from 10 to 50 mL/min and 50% dose reductions for patients with GFRs less than 10 mL/min.[39] No dosage adjustments appear to be necessary for patients with GFRs greater than 50 mL/min. In patients with hepatic dysfunction, hypoalbuminemia and hyperbilirubinemia have been associated with increased etoposide toxicities. However, no consensus guidelines exist for etoposide dosing in patients with hepatic failure. Most clinical studies have used lower doses of etoposide in the presence of severe hepatic failure, such as a 50% dose reduction when the bilirubin is between 1.5 and 3.0 mg/dL or the aspartate transaminase is between 60 and 180 units[49]; however, dose reductions were not recommended in patients with acute jaundice and normal renal function in two formal studies.[48,50] Nonetheless, etoposide should be used cautiously in patients with severe hepatic impairment, and it should probably be held when the serum bilirubin is greater than 3.1 mg/dL.[49] Guidelines for dosing teniposide in patients with organ dysfunction are even more limited. Compared with etoposide, teniposide has greater hepatic metabolism and less renal excretion, and dose reductions in the presence of organ dysfunction have not been formally recommended.

Clinically significant drug interactions have been reported when etoposide and teniposide are coadministered with anticonvulsants such as phenytoin and phenobarbital. In a pediatric study, concurrent treatment with anticonvulsants increased teniposide clearance by two- to threefold.[46] In similar studies with etoposide, concurrent administration of phenytoin or phenobarbital increased drug clearance by 37% in adults and 77% in children.[46] Thus, anticonvulsant therapy can lead to underdosing of epipodophyllotoxin chemotherapy. A pharmacokinetic interaction between etoposide and cisplatin has also been reported. Administration of etoposide 1 to 2 days after an infusion of cisplatin was associated with a 34% decrease in etoposide clearance, and similar findings were seen after carboplatin administration. Although the exact mechanism of interaction has not been characterized, it may be related to a platinum effect on decreasing etoposide's renal clearance. Finally, drugs such as cyclosporine that interfere with CYP3A4 metabolism can decrease etoposide's metabolic clearance. St. John's wort may interfere with etoposide via a dual mechanism. The active ingredient in St. John's wort, hypericin, is an inhibitor of topoisomerase II that can antagonize the formation of etoposide-induced cleavable complexes, and St. John's wort is also an inducer of CYP3A4.[51]

ANTHRACYCLINES AND RELATED COMPOUNDS

The anthracycline antibiotics are natural products derived from the actinobacteria *Streptomyces peucetius* var. *caesius*. After its initial isolation, daunorubicin was quickly discovered to induce tumor shrinkage in murine models, and it subsequently demonstrated impressive clinical activity in the treatment of pediatric acute leukemia (Table 15.7-4).[52] Further research in the 1970s led to the discovery of doxorubicin, a hydroxylated daunorubicin derivative with an extremely broad range of therapeutic activity. Doxorubicin is commonly used in the treatment of a number of diverse tumor types, including non-Hodgkin's and Hodgkin's lymphoma, multiple myeloma, and lung, ovarian, gastric, thyroid, breast, sarcoma, and pediatric cancers. In contrast, daunorubicin's use is generally limited to the induction treatment of acute leukemia. Several newer anthracyclines have been developed, including epirubicin, a less cardiotoxic doxorubicin analogue with activity in gastric and breast cancer, and idarubicin, a daunorubicin analogue with improved activity as induction therapy for acute myelogenous leukemia (AML). Finally, valrubicin is an anthracycline indicated for the intravesicular treatment of early bladder cancer. The anthracyclines have the widest range of clinical use of any class of drugs in all of oncology. In spite of their well-defined toxicity profile that includes cardiac toxicity and myelosuppression, they remain rela-

TABLE 15.7-4. Anthracycline Clinical Characteristics

Features	Doxorubicin	Epirubicin	Daunorubicin	Idarubicin
Mechanism of action	Stabilization of topoisomerase IIα cleavable complexes, inhibition of TOP2 catalytic activity, stimulation of apoptosis, generation of reactive oxygen intermediates, activation of signal transduction pathways	Same	Same	Same
Route of administration	Intravenous	Intravenous	Intravenous	Intravenous
Elimination/excretion	Formation of active alcohol metabolites by aldoketoreductases, aglycone formation, biliary excretion	Formation of active alcohol metabolites by aldoketoreductases, only anthracycline to be glucuronidated	Avid substrate for aldoketoreductases to form daunorubicinol, which is renally excreted; aglycone formation and biliary metabolism	Avid substrate for aldoketoreductases, aglycone to form idarubicinol, which is renally excreted; formation and biliary metabolism
Toxicity	Myelosuppression; cardiotoxicity, acute and chronic; mucositis; alopecia; extravasation risk; cumulative dose limit of 400 to 550 mg/m²	Same; less cardiotoxic than doxorubicin; cumulative dose limit of 900 mg/m²	Same; cumulative dose limit of 400–550 mg/m²	Same; less cardiotoxic than doxorubicin
Dosing in organ dysfunction	Dose reduce in hepatic dysfunction	Dose reduce in hepatic dysfunction	Dose reduce for hyperbilirubinemia and severe renal dysfunction	Dose reduce for hepatic dysfunction and severe renal dysfunction

(Modified from ref. 52.)

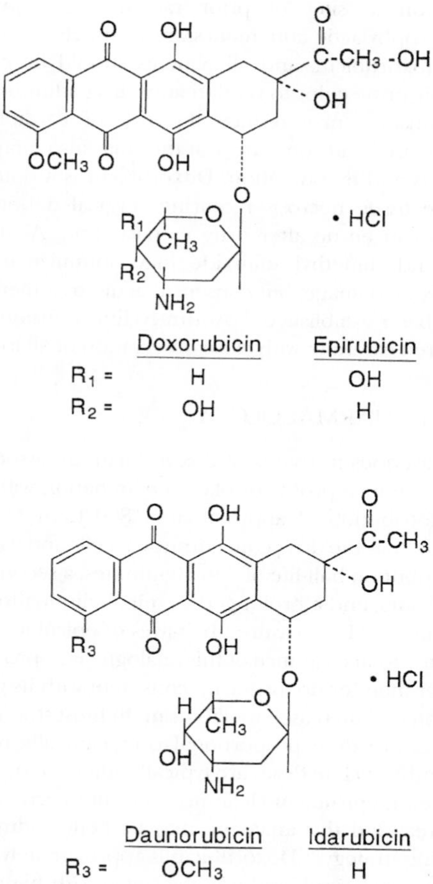

FIGURE 15.7-5. Anthracycline structures.

tively easy to combine with other agents and are frequently used in combination chemotherapy regimens (Fig. 15.7-5).

All anthracyclines share a quinone-containing rigid planar aromatic ring structure bound by a glycosidic bond to an amino sugar, daunosamine.[53] Doxorubicin (hydroxyl daunorubicin) differs from daunorubicin only by the presence of a C-14 hydroxyl group, and epirubicin is an epimer of doxorubicin differing only in the orientation of the C-4 hydroxyl group on the sugar. This modest structural change reduces epirubicin's cardiac toxicity but preserves its broad anticancer activity. Idarubicin is a daunorubicin analogue that lacks a C-4 methoxy group resulting in enhanced lipophilicity. Because of their complex aromatic structures, the anthracyclines absorb ultraviolet and visible light, giving them all a deep orange-red color. Because of their photosensitivity, shielding the drug from ambient light is recommended during preparation and administration. Furthermore, the presence of a common quinone moiety in anthracycline ring structure has substantial clinical importance. This chemical group can readily participate in oxidation-reduction reactions that ultimately generate highly reactive chemical species thought to be responsible for anthracycline-induced cardiotoxicity.

BIOCHEMICAL AND MOLECULAR PHARMACOLOGY

Although rapidly recognized as potent anticancer agents, the anthracycline's precise mechanism of action initially remained obscure because of their complex pharmacology. Early studies demonstrated that daunorubicin inhibits DNA and RNA synthesis by mechanisms originally attributed to the physical intercalation of these flat, planar molecules into the DNA double helix. Later studies suggested that the anthracycline's quinone structure enhanced the catalysis of reduction-oxidation reactions, promoting the generation of oxygen free radicals that also contributed to antitumor effects. However, only in 1984 were the anthracyclines recognized as targeting topoisomerase IIα.[54] Anthracycline-induced inhibition of topoisomerase IIα's religation reaction causes the accumulation of protein-linked double- and single-strand DNA breaks (cleavable complexes), which are ultimately converted into cytotoxic DNA damage and cell death. These seminal observations subsequently led to the general acceptance of this molecular mechanism as being most important for anthracycline-induced antitumor activity. However, the precise steps by which the anthracyclines stabilize DNA topoisomerase IIα cleavable complexes has not been fully defined and may in fact be independent of DNA intercalation. Furthermore, the pattern of cleavable complex formation in DNA induced by specific anthracyclines can vary, suggesting that differences may exist between these drugs at the molecular level.[52] Anthracyclines such as daunorubicin and doxorubicin can also directly inhibit cellular helicases, the enzymes that unwind DNA into single strands, and they may also have direct inhibitory effects on topoisomerase IIα independent of cleavable complex stabilization. Thus, some of the anthracyclines may act in part as true topoisomerase enzyme inhibitors.[52] As a consequence of their diverse molecular effects, the ultimate mechanism of cytotoxic action of the anthracyclines may involve multiple different pathways.

Anthracyclines enter cells via passive diffusion, and intracellular accumulation can result in concentrations that are 10- to 500-fold greater than extracellular drug levels.[53] The efficiency of their cellular uptake depends on their lipophilicity, with equilibration occurring more rapidly for daunorubicin than for doxorubicin, and the polar metabolites of both drugs enter cells even more slowly. Because they are weak alkaloids, daunorubicin, doxorubicin, and idarubicin become polar, charged molecules at low pH, which can contribute to their selective retention in acidic, hypoxic environments. All anthracyclines are substrates for the P-glycoprotein–mediated drug efflux pump, and MDR-1–associated pleiotropic drug resistance may be an important determinant of clinical drug sensitivity in the treatment of hematologic cancers and in pediatric, breast, and other tumors. Idarubicin is a less avid substrate for P-glycoprotein than other anthracyclines, and this may enhance its clinical activity. Other drug efflux pumps such as BCRP can also reduce intracellular anthracycline accumulation and may contribute to clinical drug resistance.[13] In addition, drug resistance resulting from topoisomerase IIα point mutations or from down-regulation of this enzyme has been characterized in laboratory studies. However, the relevance of these mechanisms to clinical drug resistance is not clear. In general, the absolute expression of topoisomerase IIα in tumors does not correlate well with drug efficacy. Finally, evidence suggests that topoisomerase IIβ expression may also influence anthracycline responsiveness. In cell lines in which anthracyclines act by targeting topoisomerase IIα activity, enhanced expression of topoisomerase IIβ may compensate and protect cells. For example, leukemia cells deficient in topoisomerase IIβ are much more sensitive to anthracyclines independent of their relative topoisomerase IIα expression.[55]

CLINICAL USE AND TOXICITIES

The anthracyclines are most often administered intravenously, typically as bolus or short-term infusions. Doxorubicin infusions of 30 to 75 mg/m² given intravenously every 3 weeks have been extensively studied in a wide variety of tumors; however, prolonged administration schedules, including weekly, daily for 3 days, and 4 days, or longer, infusions, have also been examined.[53] Protracted infusions may have favorable toxicity profiles with a reduced incidence of congestive heart failure. Doxorubicin can be administered as a single agent, or more frequently as a component of combination chemotherapy. Epirubicin is also most often given as a short, intermittent bolus infusion, whereas daunorubicin and idarubicin are typically administered on a fractionated schedule given daily for 3 or 5 days. Intraarterial doxorubicin has been examined in sarcoma patients, and intraperitoneal administration has been used in ovarian cancer; however, both approaches remain investigational. Idarubicin is the only anthracycline that has been extensively tested as an oral agent, although intravenous use remains most common. Finally, valrubicin is predominantly administered as intravesicular therapy for localized bladder tumors.

Doxorubicin is formally indicated in a wide range of human malignancies, including tumors of the bladder, stomach, ovary, lung, and thyroid.[52] It is one of the most active agents available for the treatment of breast cancer, and other indications include acute lymphoblastic and myelogenous leukemias, Hodgkin's and non-Hodgkin's lymphomas, Ewing's and osteogenic bone tumors, soft tissue sarcomas, and pediatric cancers such as neuroblastoma and Wilms' tumors. Doxorubicin also has activity in the treatment of multiple myeloma, chronic lymphocytic leukemia, cutaneous T-cell lymphomas, and uterine, urothelial, carcinoid, cervical, endometrial, esophageal, islet cell, and hepatocellular cancers. Epirubicin is indicated for the treatment of breast cancer, but it also has activity in combination chemotherapy for the treatment of gastric, carcinoid, endometrial, lung, ovarian, esophageal, and prostate cancers and soft tissue sarcomas. Use of daunorubicin and idarubicin is predominantly limited to the induction treatment of adult acute myelogenous and lymphocytic leukemia.

The major dose-limiting toxicities of doxorubicin are cardiotoxicity and myelosuppression, predominantly neutropenia and leukopenia, with thrombocytopenia and anemia being less severe. Anthracycline-induced myelosuppression is characterized by leukocyte count nadirs occurring 7 to 10 days after drug administration, with recovery occurring by day 21. All anthracyclines can induce cardiac toxicity, which is characterized by acute and chronic effects. Cumulative exposures to anthracyclines are associated with an increased risk of cardiomyopathy and congestive heart failure. Total doses of bolus doxorubicin greater than 400 to 550 mg/m² should not be exceeded during a patient's lifetime, especially if the drug is coadministered with other cardiotoxic agents such as radiation therapy or concomitant cyclophosphamide. Epirubicin may have a decreased risk of cardiotoxicity compared to doxorubicin, but serious cardiac dysfunction can occur with any anthracycline. Other common anthracycline-induced side effects include mucositis, alopecia, moderate nausea and vomiting, diarrhea, anorexia, and localized skin reactions, such as pigmentation changes, local irritation, radiation sensitization, and inflammation at sites of prior radiation therapy (radiation recall).[52] Prophylactic antiemetics are routinely given with bolus doses of doxorubicin, and all patients should be cautioned to expect their urine color to redden after drug administration. Prolonged infusions may reduce the risk of cardiotoxicity and decrease nausea and vomiting, but they may also increase the risk of mucositis and extravasation. Doxorubicin is a potent vesicant, and severe tissue necrosis requiring surgical débridement and skin grafts can ensue after drug extravasation. Acute treatment with ice and dimethyl sulfoxide may minimize extravasation-induced tissue damage, but consensus acute treatment guidelines have not been established.[56] Anthracycline infusions should be administered carefully, with close observation of all infusion sites.

CLINICAL PHARMACOLOGY

Short intravenous infusions of doxorubicin are associated with a triphasic clearance profile of plasma elimination with a large volume of distribution of approximately 800 L/m².[53] Distribution occurs rapidly as the drug concentrates in cells and tissues, with an initial distribution half-life of 5 to 10 minutes, a secondary half-life of 1 to 3 hours, and a prolonged terminal elimination half-life of 24 to 50 hours. The measured half-lives of epirubicin are similar; however, the total clearance of this analogue is approximately twofold higher than for doxorubicin, consistent with its greater tissue penetration and increased metabolism. In most studies, doxorubicin kinetics are dose proportional over clinically relevant dose ranges. Anthracycline doses are typically adjusted for body surface area; however, epirubicin clearance does not correlate with body surface area, and this analogue may be better administered via fixed dosing strategy.[57] Doxorubicin is approximately 75% to 80% plasma protein bound, and it is associated with high tissue penetration and retention in nucleated cells, due to its lipophilicity and DNA binding. Drug penetration into the central nervous system is low. Daunorubicin and idarubicin show similar plasma clearance profiles, with terminal elimination half-lives of approximately 20 hours.[53]

Anthracycline drug clearance is predominately mediated by hepatic metabolism and biliary excretion. For doxorubicin, 80% of the administered dose is excreted in the bile and feces. A common metabolic pathway is the reduction of the anthracycline ketone group by aldoketoreductases to form polar alcoholic metabolites, such as doxorubicinol and daunorubicinol. Typically, the biologic activity of these 13(S)-dihydro-derivatives is slightly less than the parental compounds because of reduced lipophilicity and decreased cellular penetration. However, idarubicinol is an exception. Its biologic activity is similar to that of idarubicin, which may contribute to its greater efficacy over daunorubicin in the treatment of acute leukemia. Aldoketoreductases are widely distributed throughout the body, with high activity found in the liver and in erythrocytes. Daunorubicin and idarubicin are avid substrates for this enzyme, rapidly forming daunorubicinol and idarubicinol, both of which have extended half-lives and circulate in plasma at concentrations that exceed those of the parental compounds. For these agents, these alcohol derivatives may contribute substantially toward their biologic activity. In contrast, doxorubicin and epirubicin are less avidly metabolized by this route, and as a consequence, their metabolites, doxorubicinol and epirubicinol, are much less important. Anthracyclines can also undergo enzymatic deglycosylation to form inactive aglycones, which can contribute to overall drug clearance. Epirubicin has a unique steric orientation of the C-4 hydroxyl group, making it the only anthracycline substrate for conjugation reactions mediated by glucuronyltransferases and sulfatases. Finally, urinary excretion of doxorubicin and other anthracylines is low, comprising less than 10% of the administered dose; however, this is enough to redden the patient's urine color.

All anthracyclines should be dose reduced in patients with hepatic dysfunction. Historically, dose adjustments have been recommended based on the degree of hyperbilirubinemia. For example, the dose of doxorubicin has traditionally been reduced by 50% for plasma bilirubin concentrations ranging from 1.2 to 3.0 mg/dL and by 75% for values of 3.1 to 5.0 mg/dL, and the dose held altogether for values greater than 5 mg/dL.[58] More modest dose reductions have been recommended for daunorubicin in patients with similar degrees of hyperbilirubinemia. These anthracycline guidelines have been criticized. For example, a pharmacokinetic study of doxorubicin in patients with liver dysfunction found that other liver function parameters such as the degree of aspartate aminotransferase (AST) elevation and indocyanine green clearance also correlated with doxorubicin exposure, suggesting that bilirubin alone was a poor predictor of drug clearance.[59] In addition, patients with Gilbert's syndrome and elevated total bilirubin levels due to decreased UGT glucuronidation activity may not require doxorubicin dose reductions.[60] Doxorubicin conjugation is not a major route of drug elimination, and clearance may not be impaired in these patients. Further studies to establish more precise doxorubicin dosing guidelines are warranted. Epirubicin should also be dose reduced for hyperbilirubinemia; however, formal recommendations also suggest a 50% epirubicin dose reduction for AST values two to five times the ULN and reductions of 75% for AST values greater than five times the ULN.[61] Renal adjustments are not recommended for doxorubicin; however, the situation is more complex for other anthracycline analogues. For example, daunorubicinol undergoes substantial elimination by the kidneys, and formal daunorubicin dose reductions of 50% are recommended for patients with serum creatinine greater than 3 mg/dL.[62] Idarubicin and epirubicin should also be dose reduced in patients with renal failure, but precise guidelines do not exist.

Caution is warranted when doxorubicin is coadministered with paclitaxel. Sequential administration of paclitaxel followed by doxorubicin in breast cancer patients is associated with cardiomyopathy at total doxorubicin doses above 340 to 380 mg/m². This increased risk was attributed to a pharmacokinetic drug interaction that increased the relative doxorubicin exposure by 30% when paclitaxel was administered before the anthracycline.[63] Systemic toxicities and changes in drug clearance were not observed when the reverse sequence of drug administration was used. The mechanism underlying this pharmacokinetic interaction is not known. Another potentially serious drug interaction is enhanced cardiotoxicity of trastuzumab, when coadministered with doxorubicin. Trastuzumab by itself is associated with left ventricular dysfunction and congestive heart failure, and these risks are enhanced when it is combined with anthracycline therapy. Concomitant use of these potentially cardiotoxic agents is generally contraindicated.

ANTHRACYCLINE CARDIOTOXICITY

Anthracycline-induced cardiotoxicity may be either acute or chronic. Acute effects include electrocardiographic changes such as sinus tachycardia, ectopic contractions, nonspecific ST and T-wave changes, decreased QRS voltage, prolonged QT intervals, and heart block. These acute toxicities are generally reversible and clinically insignificant, and they do not predict future cumulative drug-related cardiac complications. A potentially more severe acute pericarditis-myocarditis syndrome can also occur within 1 or 2 days after anthracycline administration.[64] In contrast, chronic anthracycline-induced cardiotoxicity is characterized by myocardial dysfunction and congestive heart failure, most often starting after 1 year of treatment. It is typically irreversible and is associated with cumulative drug exposure. However, the risk of chronic cardiotoxicity may vary, and it is heavily influenced by other factors, including a history of chest irradiation or coadministration of additional agents, such as paclitaxel, cyclophosphamide, or trastuzumab.[52] Other potential risk factors include female gender, treatment at a young age, and any prior or concomitant heart disease. The medical management of anthracycline-induced cardiomyopathy includes standard treatments for congestive heart failure, but the overall prognosis is generally poor. Characteristic histopathologic changes typical of anthracycline-induced damage are seen in endomyocardial biopsies, and anthracycline-specific grading criteria for assessing myocardial damage have been developed. Prolonged infusions may decrease the risk of subsequent cardiotoxicity. Late-onset anthracycline-induced cardiotoxicity occurring up to 15 years after treatment has been described, and this represents a major problem for treating pediatric patients with potentially curative malignancies.

Because of their quinone structure, the anthracyclines can facilitate cyclic reduction and oxidation reactions, ultimately generating a diverse array of highly reactive oxidative chemical species. The chelating ability of the anthracycline's hydroxyquinone structure greatly enhances these redox reactions in the presence of iron.[52] One-electron reduction reactions within cells are catalyzed by a number of different enzymes, including xanthine oxidase, CYP reductase, cytochrome b5 reductase, and NADH (nicotinamide adenine dinucleotide) dehydrogenase. Anthracyclines interact with these reductive enzymes to generate semiquinone radicals that react with oxygen to form superoxide anions. These reactive intermediates are further converted into hydrogen peroxide and other highly reactive hydroxyl free radicals, which can damage a variety of different cellular structures, including lipid membranes, DNA bases, and chromatin proteins. Ultimately, the cell's endogenous defenses, such as superoxide dismutase, catalase, and glutathione peroxidase, that normally protect against free radical formation are overwhelmed leading to cellular necrosis. Catalase and glutathione levels are normally high in the liver; however, catalase levels are low in cardiac muscle. Furthermore, cardiac tissues also have high oxygen tension, plentiful mitochondria, and large amounts of iron-containing myoglobin and hemoglobin. All of these factors may help to explain the relative sensitivity of the heart to the toxic effects of the anthracyclines. Oxidative damage may also contribute to anthracycline-induced antitumor activity. High glutathione concentrations and elevated superoxide dismutase and glutathione peroxidase activity are all associated with increased doxorubicin sensitivity in tumor cell lines studied *in vitro*.

The total cumulative lifetime dose of doxorubicin should be limited to 400 to 550 mg/m².[53] For example, when total doses of doxorubicin are less than 400 mg/m² the risk of cardiomyopathy is only 0.14%, but this increases to 7% at doses of 550 mg/m² and to 18% at a total dose of 700 mg/m^2.[64] Infusional drug administration may be associated with less cardiotoxicity, and cumulative doxorubicin doses exceeding these guidelines have been administered to some patients using prolonged infusion schedules. However, extreme caution should be used in applying these guidelines to individual patients because severe congestive heart failure can occur after only a single dose of doxorubicin and other factors may substantially increase these risks. Clinical monitoring of left ventricular function (LVEF) using radionuclide angiocardiography or echocardiography has been proposed as a noninvasive way to assess the cardiotoxic risk of further doxorubicin chemotherapy. Cardiac monitoring should be initiated at a cumulative dose of doxorubicin of 400 mg/m^2 and periodically thereafter. Baseline cardiac evaluations are recommended for any patient with preexisting cardiac risk factors. During therapy, an absolute LVEF below 45%, a 10% decline in LVEF to below the lower limit of normal, or an absolute decline of 20% at any level is suggestive of a significant deterioration in cardiac function and should lead to a reevaluation of anthracycline therapy.[64] On the electrocardiogram, a greater than 30% decrease in QRS voltage in limb leads from baseline may also herald an increased risk of drug-induced cardiomyopathy. Nonetheless, caution is warranted in applying these guidelines because prospective studies are lacking and it is not clear that strict adherence to these recommendations will uniformly identify or prevent the development of clinical congestive heart failure. For daunorubicin, recommended cumulative dose limit is 400 to 550 mg/m^2,[62] and for epirubicin it is 900 mg/m^2.[61]

Because of the importance of iron in enhancing anthracycline-mediated redox reactions, iron chelator agents have been explored as a means to reduce cardiac toxicity. In clinical studies, the iron chelator dexrazoxane (ICRF-187) reduced the incidence of doxorubicin-induced cardiac toxicity in breast cancer patients without affecting antitumor efficacy.[52] Dexrazoxane, an intravenous prodrug, is hydrolyzed to release an active iron chelator that increases urinary iron clearance by tenfold. Dexrazoxane is approved for patients treated with more than 300 mg/m^2 doxorubicin as a means to prevent cardiac toxicity. The agent is given at ten times the doxorubicin dose (milligram to milligram), and it is administered within 30 minutes of the anthracycline.

Liposomal encapsulation of doxorubicin and daunorubicin appears to improve the therapeutic index of these agents. Liposomal doxorubicin is indicated for the treatment of ovarian cancer and human immunodeficiency virus–related Kaposi's sarcoma, and daunorubicin citrate liposome is approved for treating Kaposi's sarcoma. Drug encapsulation within liposomes alters their pharmacokinetic properties and results in the selective delivery of drug to the reticuloendothelial system and other tissues. More than 90% of drug circulating in plasma is liposome encapsulated. For example, liposomal doxorubicin's overall clearance is approximately 300-fold lower than free drug, and its volume of distribution is substantially reduced. The clinical toxicity profile is also altered by liposomal encapsulation. Common side effects associated with liposomal doxorubicin include palmar-plantar erythrodysesthesia, relatively mild myelosuppression, mild nausea and vomiting, and an acute infusion reaction manifested by flushing, dyspnea, edema, fever, chills, rash, bronchospasm, and hypertension. These infusion-related events appear to be related to the rate of drug infusion; they have generally not been seen with conventional doxorubicin administration and may represent a reaction to the liposomal component. Clinical use also suggests that liposomal formulations reduce anthracycline cardiac toxicity; however, because formal comparisons are lacking, adherence to cardiac monitoring guidelines established for free anthracycline therapy still seems prudent.

OTHER TOPOISOMERASE INTERACTIVE AGENTS

Mitoxantrone is an anthracenedione derivative that was originally synthesized in the 1970s during efforts to develop noncardiotoxic anthracycline-like compounds. In preclinical studies, it is highly potent against a variety of murine tumor models, and in clinical studies, it has demonstrated decreased cardiotoxicity compared to doxorubicin.[52] Mitoxantrone is indicated in the treatment of acute leukemias and hormone-refractory prostate cancer, and it also has activity in breast cancer and non-Hodgkin's lymphomas and in the treatment of multiple sclerosis. Its major dose-limiting toxicity is potent myelosuppression, especially leukopenia. Although less cardiotoxic than doxorubicin, anthracycline-like congestive heart failure has been associated with total cumulative mitoxantrone doses greater than 120 mg/m^2. Other acute toxicities include local reactions, nausea and vomiting, and alopecia. Mitoxantrone is less of an extravasation risk than doxorubicin, and its bluish color can cause discoloration of the sclera, fingernails, and urine. Overall, mitoxantrone is less toxic than doxorubicin; however, its spectrum activity is also more limited, which has restricted its more widespread clinical use.[65]

Because of its rigid flat structure, mitoxantrone's initial proposed mechanism of action was via DNA intercalation. However, it is now recognized as a potent agent that stabilizes topoisomerase IIα DNA cleavable complexes.[66] It is less likely to undergo reduction-oxidation–type reactions than the anthracyclines, and this may account for its decreased cardiotoxicity. Mitoxantrone is a modest substrate for the P-glycoprotein–mediated drug resistance pump, but other membrane transporters, such as BCRP, encoded for by the mitoxantrone resistance gene, MXR, are associated with drug resistance.[67] Mitoxantrone is typically administered as a short intravenous infusion at doses of 12 mg/m^2 infused over 30 minutes, and its pharmacokinetics resemble those of the anthracyclines. Its plasma elimination profile is triphasic, with a long terminal elimination half-life of 75 hours. Mitoxantrone is highly concentrated in tissues, and only a small amount of drug is excreted in the urine. Clearance is substantially decreased in hepatic dysfunction, but formal dosing guidelines are not available.

Dactinomycin was the first actinomycin antibiotic isolated from a *Streptomyces* species in the 1940s. The only derivative presently in clinical use is dactinomycin. Structurally, it contains two cyclic polypeptides attached to a phenoxazone ring that can intercalate into DNA. Dactinomycin inhibits DNA and especially RNA synthesis, and it can intercalate into DNA, with some preference for insertion between two G-C pairs. Its major mechanism of action is the generation of DNA strand breaks through an interaction with topoisomerase II; however, the precise molecular steps involved are not well characterized. Resistance to dactinomycin is associated with decreased drug accumulation within cells and overexpression of the MDR gene. Dactinomycin is commonly used in combination with other chemotherapy in the treatment of pediatric tumors such as Ewing's sarcoma, rhabdomyosarcoma, and Wilms' tumors. It is also a potent radiation sensitizer. After intravenous administration, dactinomycin has a rapid distribution phase with a prolonged plasma half-life of 1.5 days. Approximately 20% of the drug is excreted in the urine and 13% in the feces.[68] Formal dosing recommendations in patients with organ dysfunction are not available. Dactinomycin's major dose-limiting toxicity is myelosuppression, which can include severe neutropenia and thrombocytopenia. Other common side effects include gastrointestinal pains, nausea and vomiting, stomatitis, diarrhea, alopecia, skin rash, and extravasation reactions.

Amsacrine is a planar acridine derivative with weak DNA intercalating properties that is now recognized as a topoisomerase II interactive agent.[69] Etoposide-resistant cell lines have been characterized that are not cross-resistant to amsacrine, suggesting that it has molecular effects that are distinct from other topoisomerase II targeting agents. Amsacrine is commonly used in the treatment of refractory AML. It is less cardiotoxic than the anthracyclines, and its major dose-limiting toxicity is bone marrow suppression, especially leucopenia.[70] Other common side effects include nausea and vomiting, mucositis, ventricular arrhythmias, localized phlebitis, and hepatotoxicity. In contrast to the anthracyclines, it is less cardiotoxic and may be better tolerated when this is a concern.[70] The drug is predominantly cleared in the liver via conjugation with glutathione and via biliary excretion. Approximately 10% to 20% of an administered dose is created in the urine.[6] Dose reductions are recommended for patients with liver dysfunction or severe renal dysfunction.

SECONDARY MALIGNANCIES AND TOPOISOMERASE TARGETING THERAPIES

Because of their propensity to damage DNA, the topoisomerase targeting agents are associated with an increased risk of secondary malignancies, especially AML. Furthermore, the wide use of these agents as adjuvant therapies and their use in the treatment of potentially curative malignancies mean that their carcinogenic risk is a long-term clinical problem. Treatment with epipodophyllotoxins, such as etoposide or teniposide, is associated with an incidence of secondary AML approaching 6% over 4 years after therapy in patients with pediatric acute lymphocytic leukemia. The classic features of epipodophyllotoxin-induced secondary acute leukemias include a monocytic subtype (FAB M-4 or M-5 classification) with a relatively acute onset occurring 2 to 3 years after treatment and an associated translocation of the MLL gene on chromosome 11q23.[71] In contrast, alkylating agent–associated secondary leukemias have a longer time to onset, are frequently preceded by a preliminary myelodysplastic syndrome, and commonly have deletions of chromosome 5 or 7. The risk of developing a secondary leukemia after etoposide chemotherapy increased by higher cumulative drug exposures[72] and by the use of more frequent schedules of drug administration.[73] In older patients with testicular cancer, the use of etoposide combination chemotherapy is associated with less than a 1% risk of secondary AML. Other topoisomerase II targeting agents, such as doxorubicin, are also associated with an increased risk of secondary leukemia, but the incidence is lower than with epipodophyllotoxins.[73] Studies of the carcinogenic potential of these agents are complicated by their frequent use with alkylating agents and radiation therapy, treatments that also increase the risk of secondary malignancies.

Finally, the absolute risk of second malignancies after treatment with topoisomerase I targeting agents requires further study. Because of their ability to cause double-strand DNA damage, the camptothecins are mutagenic and can produce chromosomal damage, including increased sister chromatid exchanges, gene deletions, and chromosomal rearrangements.[74] These lesions are similar to those generated by other DNA-damaging agents that are also associated with an increased risk of secondary malignancies. Thus, camptothecins may also have carcinogenic potential; however, clinical information on the long-term follow-up of patients treated with topoisomerase I targeted therapy is still limited.[74]

REFERENCES

1. Wang JC. Cellular roles of DNA topoisomerases: a molecular perspective. *Nat Rev Mol Cell Biol* 2002;3:430.
2. Champoux JJ. DNA topoisomerases: structure, function, and mechanism. *Annu Rev Biochem* 2001;70:369.
3. Takimoto CH, Arbuck SG. Topoisomerase I targeting agents: the camptothecins. In: Chabner BA, Longo DL, eds., *Cancer chemotherapy & biotherapy: principles and practice*, 3rd ed. Philadelphia: Lippincott Williams & Wilkins, 2001:579.
4. Wang JC. Interaction between DNA and an *Escherichia coli* protein omega. *J Mol Biol* 1971;55:523.
5. Kellner U, Sehested M, Jensen PB, et al. Culprit and victim—DNA topoisomerase II. *Lancet Oncol* 2003;3:235.
6. Pommier YG, Goldwasser F, Strumberg D. Topoisomerase II inhibitors: epipodophyllotoxins, acridines, ellipticines, and bisdioxopiperazines. In: Chabner BA, Longo DL, eds., *Cancer chemotherapy & biotherapy: principles and practice*, 3rd ed. Philadelphia: Lippincott Williams & Wilkins, 2001:538.
7. Hsiang YH, Lihou MG, Liu LF. Arrest of replication forks by drug-stabilized topoisomerase I-DNA cleavable complexes as a mechanism of cell killing by camptothecin. *Cancer Res* 1989;49:5077.
8. Gerrits CJ, de Jonge MJ, Schellens JH, et al. Topoisomerase I inhibitors: the relevance of prolonged exposure for present clinical development. *Br J Cancer* 1997;76:952.
9. Bjornsti MA, Benedetti P, Viglianti GA, et al. Expression of human DNA topoisomerase I in yeast cells lacking yeast DNA topoisomerase I: restoration of sensitivity of the cells to the antitumor drug camptothecin. *Cancer Res* 1989;49:6318.
10. Ross WE, Glaubiger D, Kohn KW. Qualitative and quantitative aspects of intercalator-induced DNA strand breaks. *Biochim Biophys Acta* 1979;562:41.
11. Hsiang YH, Liu LF. Identification of mammalian DNA topoisomerase I as an intracellular target of the anticancer drug camptothecin. *Cancer Res* 1988;48:1722.
12. Rasheed ZA, Rubin EH. Mechanisms of resistance to topoisomerase I-targeting drugs. *Oncogene* 2003;22:7296.
13. Doyle LA, Ross DD. Multidrug resistance mediated by the breast cancer resistance protein BCRP (ABCG2). *Oncogene* 2003;22:7340.
14. Pizzolato JF, Saltz LB. The camptothecins. *Lancet* 2003;361:2235.
15. Rowinsky EK. Weekly topotecan: an alternative to topotecan's standard daily x 5 schedule? *Oncologist* 2002;7:324.
16. ten Bokkel Huinink W, Gore M, Carmichael J, et al. Topotecan versus paclitaxel for the treatment of recurrent epithelial ovarian cancer. *J Clin Oncol* 1997;15:2183.
17. Schiller JH, Adak S, Cella D, et al. Topotecan versus observation after cisplatin plus etoposide in extensive-stage small-cell lung cancer: E7593—a phase III trial of the Eastern Cooperative Oncology Group. *J Clin Oncol* 2001;19:2114.
18. von Pawel J, Schiller JH, Shepherd FA, et al. Topotecan versus cyclophosphamide, doxorubicin, and vincristine for the treatment of recurrent small-cell lung cancer. *J Clin Oncol* 1999;17:658.
19. Miller AA, Lilenbaum RC, Lynch TJ, et al. Treatment-related fatal sepsis from topotecan/cisplatin and topotecan/paclitaxel [Letter]. *J Clin Oncol* 1996;14:1964.
20. Armstrong D, O'Reilly S. Clinical guidelines for managing topotecan-related hematologic toxicity. *Oncologist* 1998;3:4.
21. Fuchs CS, Moore MR, Harker G, et al. Phase III comparison of two irinotecan dosing regimens in second-line therapy of metastatic colorectal cancer. *J Clin Oncol* 2003;21:807.
22. Saltz LB, Cox JV, Blanke C, et al. Irinotecan plus fluorouracil and leucovorin for metastatic colorectal cancer. Irinotecan Study Group. *N Engl J Med* 2002;343:905.
23. Douillard JY, Cunningham D, Roth AD, et al. Irinotecan combined with fluorouracil compared with fluorouracil alone as first-line treatment for metastatic colorectal cancer: a multicentre randomized trial. *Lancet* 2000;355:1041.
24. Rothenberg ML, Meropol NJ, Poplin EA, et al. Mortality associated with irinotecan plus bolus fluorouracil/leucovorin: summary findings of an independent panel. *J Clin Oncol* 2001;19:3801.
25. Garcia-Carbonero R, Supko JG. Current perspectives on the clinical experience, pharmacology, and continued development of the camptothecins. *Clin Cancer Res* 2002;8:641.
26. Chabot GG. Clinical pharmacokinetics of irinotecan. *Clin Pharmacokinet* 1997;33:245.

27. O'Reilly S, Rowinsky EK, Slichenmyer W, et al. Phase I and pharmacologic study of topotecan in patients with impaired renal function. *J Clin Oncol* 1996;14:3062.

28. Herrington JD, Figueroa JA, Kirstein MN, et al. Effect of hemodialysis on topotecan disposition in a patient with severe renal dysfunction. *Cancer Chemother Pharmacol* 2001;47:89.

29. O'Reilly S, Rowinsky E, Slichenmyer W, et al. Phase I and pharmacologic study of topotecan in patients with impaired hepatic function. *J Natl Cancer Inst* 1996;88:817.

30. van Groeningen CJ, Van der Vijgh WJ, Baars JJ, et al. Altered pharmacokinetics and metabolism of CPT-11 in liver dysfunction: a need for guidelines. *Clin Cancer Res* 2000;6:1342.

31. Raymond E, Boige V, Faivre S, et al. Dosage adjustment and pharmacokinetic profile of irinotecan in cancer patients with hepatic dysfunction. *J Clin Oncol* 2002;20:4303.

32. Chabot GG, Abigerges D, Catimel G, et al. Population pharmacokinetics and pharmacodynamics of irinotecan (CPT-11) and active metabolite SN-38 during phase I trials. *Ann Oncol* 1995;6:141.

33. Venook AP, Enders Klein C, Fleming G, et al. A phase I and pharmacokinetic study of irinotecan in patients with hepatic or renal dysfunction or with prior pelvic radiation: CALGB 9863. *Ann Oncol* 2003;14:1783.

34. Rowinsky EK, Kaufman SH, Baker SD, et al. Sequences of topotecan and cisplatin: phase I, pharmacologic, and in vitro studies to examine sequence dependence [see comments]. *J Clin Oncol* 1996;14:3074.

35. Zamboni WC, Egorin MJ, Van Echo DA, et al. Pharmacokinetic and pharmacodynamic study of the combination of docetaxel and topotecan in patients with solid tumors. *J Clin Oncol* 2000;18:3288.

36. Kehrer DF, Mathijssen RH, Verweij J, et al. Modulation of irinotecan metabolism by ketoconazole. *J Clin Oncol* 2002;20:3122.

37. Iyer L, Das S, Janisch L, et al. UGT1A1*28 polymorphism as a determinant of irinotecan disposition and toxicity. *Pharmacogenomics* 2002;2:43.

38. Mathijssen RH, Marsh S, Karlsson MO, et al. Irinotecan pathway genotype analysis to predict pharmacokinetics. *Clin Cancer Res* 2003;9:3246.

39. Hande KR. Etoposide: four decades of development of a topoisomerase II inhibitor. *Eur J Cancer* 1998;34:1514.

40. Budman DR. Early studies of etoposide phosphate, a water-soluble prodrug. *Semin Oncol* 1996;23:8.

41. Ross W, Rowe T, Glisson B, et al. Role of topoisomerase II in mediating epipodophyllotoxin-induced DNA cleavage. *Cancer Res* 1984;44:5857.

42. Holm C, Covey JM, Kerrigan D, et al. Differential requirement of DNA replication for the cytotoxicity of DNA topoisomerase I and II inhibitors in Chinese hamster DC3F cells. *Cancer Res* 1989;49:6365.

43. Kubo A, Yoshikawa A, Hirashima T, et al. Point mutations of the topoisomerase IIalpha gene in patients with small cell lung cancer treated with etoposide. *Cancer Res* 1996;56:1232.

44. Weiss RB. Hypersensitivity reactions. *Semin Oncol* 1992;19:458.

45. Habibi B, Lopez M, Serdaru M, et al. Immune hemolytic anemia and renal failure due to teniposide. *N Engl J Med* 1982;306:1091.

46. McLeod HL, Evans WE. Epipodophyllotoxins. In: Grochow LB, Ames MM. eds. *A clinician's guide to chemotherapy pharmacokinetics and pharmacodynamics*, 3rd ed. Baltimore: Williams & Wilkins, 1998:259.

47. D'Incalci M, Rossi C, Zucchetti M, et al. Pharmacokinetics of etoposide in patients with abnormal renal and hepatic function. *Cancer Res* 1986;46:2566.

48. Arbuck SG, Douglass HO, Crom WR, et al. Etoposide pharmacokinetics in patients with normal and abnormal organ function. *J Clin Oncol* 1986;4:1690.

49. Perry MC. Hepatotoxicity of chemotherapeutic agents. *Semin Oncol* 1982;9:65.

50. Hande KR, Wolff SN, Greco FA, et al. Etoposide kinetics in patients with obstructive jaundice. *J Clin Oncol* 1990;8:1101.

51. Peebles KA, Baker RK, Kurz EU, et al. Catalytic inhibition of human DNA topoisomerase IIalpha by hypericin, a naphthodianthrone from St. John's wort (*Hypericum perforatum*). *Biochem Pharmacol* 2001;62:1059.

52. Doroshow JH. Anthracyclines and anthracenediones. In: Chabner BA, Longo DL, eds. *Cancer chemotherapy and biotherapy: principles and practice*, 3rd ed. Philadelphia: Lippincott Williams & Wilkins, 2001:500.

53. Robert J. Anthracyclines. In: Grochow LB, Ames MM, eds. *A clinician's guide to chemotherapy pharmacokinetics and pharmacodynamics*, 3rd ed. Baltimore: Williams & Wilkins, 1998:93.

54. Tewey KM, Rowe TC, Yang L, et al. Adriamycin-induced DNA damage mediated by mammalian DNA topoisomerase II. *Science* 1984;226:466.

55. Gieseler F, Glasmacher A, Kampfe D, et al. Topoisomerase II activities in AML blasts and their correlation with cellular sensitivity to anthracyclines and epipodophyllotoxins. *Leukemia* 1996;10[Suppl 3]:S46.

56. Bertelli G, Gozza A, Forno GB, et al. Topical dimethylsulfoxide for the prevention of soft tissue injury after extravasation of vesicant cytotoxic drugs: a prospective clinical study. *J Clin Oncol* 1995;13:2851.

57. Dobbs NA, Twelves CJ. What is the effect of adjusting epirubicin doses for body surface area? *Br J Cancer* 1998;78:662.

58. Adriamycin RDF(R). In: *Physicians' Desk Reference*, 56th ed. Montvale: Medical Economics, Inc., 2002:2767.

59. Twelves CJ, Dobbs NA, Gillies HC, et al. Doxorubicin pharmacokinetics: the effect of abnormal liver biochemistry tests. *Cancer Chemother Pharmacol* 1998;42:229.

60. Cupp MJ, Higa GM. Doxorubicin dosage guidelines in a patient with hyperbilirubinemia of Gilbert's syndrome. *Ann Pharmacother* 1998;32:1026.

61. Ellence. In: *Physicians' Desk Reference*, 56th ed. Montvale: Medical Economics, Inc., 2002:2806.

62. Cerubidine. In: *Physicians' Desk Reference*, 56th ed. Montvale: Medical Economics, Inc., 2002:947.

63. Perez EA. Doxorubicin and paclitaxel in the treatment of advanced breast cancer: efficacy and cardiac considerations. *Cancer Invest* 2001;19:155.

64. Shan K, Lincoff AM, Young JB. Anthracycline-induced cardiotoxicity. *Ann Intern Med* 1996;125:47.

65. Wiseman LR, Spencer CM. Mitoxantrone. A review of its pharmacology and clinical efficacy in the management of hormone-resistant advanced prostate cancer. *Drugs Aging* 1997;10:473.

66. Crespi MD, Ivanier SE, Genovese J, et al. Mitoxantrone affects topoisomerase activities in human breast cancer cells. *Biochem Biophys Res Commun* 1986;136:521.

67. Litman T, Brangi M, Hudson E, et al. The multidrug-resistant phenotype associated with overexpression of the new ABC half-transporter, MXR (ABCG2). *J Cell Sci* 2000;113(Pt 11):2011.

68. Verweij J, Sparreboom A, Nooter K. Antitumor antibiotics. In: Chabner BA, Longo DL, eds. *Cancer chemotherapy & biotherapy: principles and practice*, 3rd ed. Philadelphia: Lippincott Williams & Wilkins, 2001:482.

69. Zwelling LA. Topoisomerase II as a target of antileukemia drugs: a review of controversial areas. *Hematol Pathol* 1989;3:101.

70. Cassileth PA, Gale RP. Amsacrine: a review. *Leuk Res* 1986;10:1257.

71. Pui CH, Ribeiro RC, Hancock ML, et al. Acute myeloid leukemia in children treated with epipodophyllotoxins for acute lymphoblastic leukemia. *N Engl J Med* 1991;325:1682.

72. Smith MA, Rubinstein L, Anderson JR, et al. Secondary leukemia or myelodysplastic syndrome after treatment with epipodophyllotoxins. *J Clin Oncol* 1999;17:569.

73. Erlichman C, Moore M. Carcinogenesis: a late complication of cancer chemotherapy. In: Chabner BA, Longo DL, eds. *Cancer chemotherapy and biotherapy: principles and practice*, 3rd ed. Philadelphia: Lippincott Williams & Wilkins, 2001:67.

74. Hashimoto H, Chatterjee S, Berger NA. Mutagenic activity of topoisomerase I inhibitors. *Clin Cancer Res* 1995;1:369.

SECTION 8

ERIC K. ROWINSKY
ANTHONY W. TOLCHER

Antimicrotubule Agents

Microtubules are the principal target of a large and diverse group of natural product anticancer drugs. Given the widespread success of antimicrotubule therapeutics in curative and palliative cancer treatment, the microtubule is perhaps the single best cancer target identified to date and continues to be recognized as a strategic subcellular target against which to direct developmental therapeutic efforts. This chapter reviews the structure and function of microtubules, as well as the two major classes of antimicrotubule agents, the vinca alkaloids and the taxanes. In addition, estramustine and other novel antimicrotubule and antimitotic agents in early development are discussed.

MICROTUBULES

Microtubules are vital and dynamic cellular organelles, which can be disrupted by a broad range of anticancer agents, most of which are derived from natural products, most notably the vinca alkaloids and taxanes. Over the last several decades, an increasing number of novel natural products and synthetic compounds that disrupt microtubules have also been identified.[1,2] Although the antiproliferative effects of these agents are largely due to their disruptive actions on the dynamics of microtubules that constitute the mitotic spindle, thereby interfering with cell division and proliferation, microtubules are also integrally involved in many nonmitotic functions, such as chemotaxis, membrane

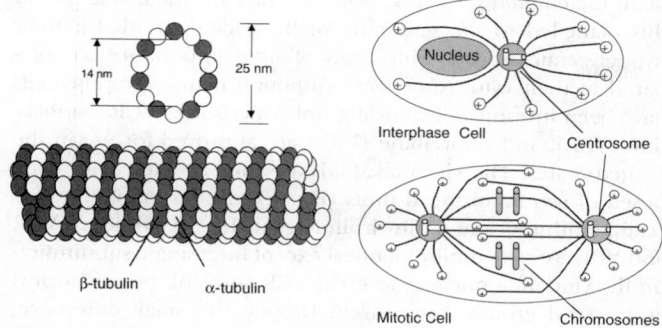

FIGURE 15.8-1. Dimers of α- and β-tubulin polymerize to form microtubules, which are composed of 13 protofilaments assembled around a hollow core. The minus ends of the microtubules are anchored in the centrosomes. In interphase cells, the centrosome is located near the nucleus and microtubules extend outward to the cell periphery. During mitosis, duplicated centrosomes separate and microtubules reorganize to form the mitotic spindle.

and intracellular scaffolding, transport, secretion, anchorage of organelles and receptors, adhesion, locomotion, and mitogenic signaling, and antimicrotubule agents may critically disrupt many of these nonmitotic functions.[3–6] Microtubules are composed of polymers of heterodimers that consist of two closely related 55,000-kD polypeptides, α-tubulin and β-tubulin, which consist of approximately 450 amino acids. α- and β-tubulin are encoded by small families of related genes. α- and β-tubulins are of at least six isotypes, which are distinguished by slightly different amino acid sequences and encoded by different genes.[4,7] Equivalent isotype profiles that are expressed in the same tissues of different species are highly conserved, suggesting that tubulin isotypes confer functional specificity.[4,7,8] However, the intrinsic dynamicity of microtubules is also influenced by the isotypic composition of tubulin, and the sensitivity of microtubules to depolymerizing and polymerizing agents is related, in part, to the composition of tubulin isotypes and microtubule-associated proteins (MAPs).[4,8,9] A third member of the tubulin superfamily, γ-tubulin, which is less abundant than the α and β forms, comprises the microtubule-organizing center or centrosome.

Microtubules are composed of 13 linear protofilaments of polymerized αβ-tubulin heterodimers arranged in parallel around a cylindrical axis, as shown in Figure 15.8-1. The dimers are aligned side by side around a hollow core with the β subunit of one dimer in contact with the α-tubulin subunit of the next. The specific biologic functions of microtubules are due to their unique polymerization dynamics.[3–5] Tubulin polymerization occurs by a nucleation-elongation mechanism, in which the formation of a short microtubule "nucleus" is followed by elongation of the microtubule at its ends, which involves the reversible, noncovalent addition of αβ-tubulin heterodimers. In essence, the microtubule polymer is in a complex and dynamic equilibrium with the intracellular pool of αβ-tubulin heterodimers, resulting in the incorporation of free heterodimers into the polymerized structures and the simultaneous release of heterodimers into the soluble tubulin pool. The process uses energy provided by the hydrolysis of guanosine triphosphate (GTP). Tubulin binds GTP with high affinity, and as tubulin-GTP is added to the end of a growing microtubule, the GTP is gradually hydrolyzed to guanosine diphosphate (GDP) and P_i. The P_i ultimately dissociates from

the microtubule, leaving a microtubule core that consists of tubulin bound to GDP. The two ends of microtubules are not equivalent; one end, termed the *plus end*, is kinetically more dynamic than the other end, termed the *minus end*. Although tubulin polymerization and dissociation, and consequently microtubule elongation and shortening, occur simultaneously at each end, the net changes in length at the plus end are much larger over time than the changes at the minus end. Microtubules undergo long periods of slow lengthening, short periods of rapid shortening, and periods of pause of attenuated dynamics.

Microtubule dynamics are governed by two principal processes. The first, known as *treadmilling*, is the net growth at one end of the microtubule and the net shortening at the opposite end.[10] Treadmilling plays a role in many microtubule functions, most notably the polar movement of the chromosomes during the anaphase stage of mitosis. The second dynamic behavior, termed *dynamic instability*, is a process in which the microtubule ends switch spontaneously between states of slow sustained growth and rapid shortening.[11] The transition between microtubule growth and shortening is regulated, in part, by the presence or absence of the region of GTP-containing tubulin at the microtubule end. A microtubule can grow as long as it maintains a stabilizing cap of tubulin-GTP or tubulin-GDP-P_i. The loss of the cap induces microtubule depolymerization.[12] The rate of dynamic instability is accelerated during some processes, such as mitosis, resulting in the formation and attachment of the mitotic spindles to the chromosomes. Dynamic instability and treadmilling are regulated by MAPs and other cellular effectors and are adversely affected by antimicrotubule agents.[3,10]

In the nonmitotic phases of the cell cycle, microtubules radiate from the microtubule-organizing center, which is located centrally near the nucleus and consists of a centrosome, a lattice of MAPs, γ-tubulin, and a pair of centrioles. The minus ends of the microtubules are positioned in or near the centrosome, whereas the plus ends extend out toward the cell periphery, as shown in Figure 15.8-1. The centrosome duplicates before mitosis, and the two centrosomes then separate into the poles of the forming mitotic spindle. The microtubules of the interphase array depolymerize and, as the nuclear envelope breaks down and releases the now condensed chromosomes, a spindle-shaped array of newly assembled microtubules is organized. In essence, the interphase microtubule network disassembles at the onset of mitosis and is replaced by a new population of spindle microtubules that are much more dynamic than the microtubules that constitute the interphase cytoskeleton.[13] In fact, the rapid dynamics of spindle microtubules render them sensitive to the vinca alkaloids, taxanes, and other antimicrotubule agents.[14] Dynamic instability and treadmilling are vital to the assembly and function of the mitotic spindle, and the high dynamicity of mitotic spindle microtubules is required for the precise attachment of the chromosomes to the spindle and their proper alignment at metaphase and separation during anaphase. These processes enable the microtubules of the forming mitotic spindles to make vast growing and shortening excursions, essentially probing the cytoplasm, until becoming attached to a chromosome at the kinetochore in prometaphase. If even a single chromosome is unable to achieve a bipolar attachment to the spindle, perhaps due to drug-induced suppression of microtubule dynamics, the cell cannot traverse beyond a prometaphase/metaphase-like state, which eventually triggers programmed cell death or apoptosis. The mitotic spindle can form in the presence of low concentrations of antimicrotubule agents, but mitosis cannot progress beyond the mitotic cell-cycle checkpoint at the metaphase/anaphase transition or is delayed in this stage, which can also trigger apoptosis.[12,15]

Dynamic instability gives rise to a dynamically changing cytoplasm. At any instant, cytoplasmic microtubules are either rapidly growing or catastrophically dissociating. Because of their dynamaticity, several mechanisms for stabilizing cytoplasmic microtubules have evolved. One adaptation that results in microtubule stability is capping of the plus end of the microtubule. Microtubule capping by the kinetochore of the chromosomes selectively stabilizes mitotic spindle microtubules that emanate from the centrosomes. Other molecular and biochemical modifications that can regulate the behavior and stability of cytoplasmic microtubules include posttranslational modifications of tubulin and the interaction of microtubules with MAPs. The principal posttranslation modifications of tubulin in cellular microtubules are detyrosination and acetylation, which occur after polymerization and enhance microtubule stability.[1,3–5] The amino acid composition and posttranslational modifications of tubulin may also account for the functional diversity of microtubules.[3,7] MAPs, which differ from species to species and cell type to cell type, also regulate the dynamic behavior and stability of cytoplasmic microtubules.[3–5] Among the best-characterized MAPs are those found in the mammalian brain, such as the tau proteins, MAP1, MAP1c (an adenosine triphosphatase), MAP2, MAP4, and dynein (a guanosine triphosphatase), which promote tubulin polymerization and microtubule stability. Some MAPs, such as the dyneins and kinesins, function as microtubule motors, transmitting chemical energy to mechanical sliding force and moving various solutes and subcellular organelles along the microtubule.[3–5,16] Motor proteins function in many types of cellular events, such as mitosis, premeiotic events, and organelle transport.

VINCA ALKALOIDS

The vinca alkaloids are naturally occurring or semisynthetic compounds that are found in minute quantities in the periwinkle plant *Catharanthus roseus G. Don*.[17–25] The early medicinal uses of this plant led to the screening of these compounds for their hypoglycemic activity, which was of little importance as compared to their cytotoxic effects. Although many vinca alkaloids have been investigated clinically, only vincristine (VCR), vinblastine (VBL), and vinorelbine (VRL) are approved for use in the United States. The vinca alkaloids are dimeric molecules composed of two multiringed units (Fig. 15.8-2): an indole nucleus (catharanthine) and a dihydroindole nucleus (vindoline). VCR and VBL are structurally identical except for a single substitution on the vindoline nucleus, whereas VCR and VBL possess formyl and methyl groups, respectively. Despite this small difference, these two agents significantly differ in their antitumor and toxicologic profiles. VCR is used more commonly to treat pediatric than adult cancers, owing to the greater sensitivity of pediatric malignancies to VCR and to the better tolerance of therapeutic VCR doses in children. VCR is an essential part of the combination chemotherapeutic regimens used for acute lymphocytic leukemia and lymphoid blast crisis of chronic myeloid leukemia and plays an important role in the treatment of Hodgkin's and non-Hodgkin's lymphomas. More recently, VCR-based combination regimens, in which VCR as a protracted infusion or daily bolus injections of VCR are administered in combination with doxorubicin and dexamethasone and occasionally other agents, have become a mainstay of systemic therapy to treat multiple myeloma. VCR also plays a role in the multimodality therapy of Wilms' tumor, Ewing's sarcoma, neuroblastoma, oligodendroglioma, medulloblastoma, and rhabdomyosarcoma in children, as well as in the treatment of multiple myeloma in adults and small cell lung cancer to a lesser extent. VBL has been an integral component of chemotherapeutic regimens for germ cell malignancies and advanced lymphoma and has been used in combination with other agents to treat Kaposi's sarcoma and bladder, brain (similar to those mentioned previously for children), and non–small cell lung and breast cancers.[17–20]

Deacetyl VBL (vindesine, or VDS), initially identified as a metabolite of VBL, was introduced in the 1970s.[20,21] VDS is registered in many countries but is available for investigational use in the United States. It has been used in combination with other

Vindoline nucleus

Catharanthine nucleus

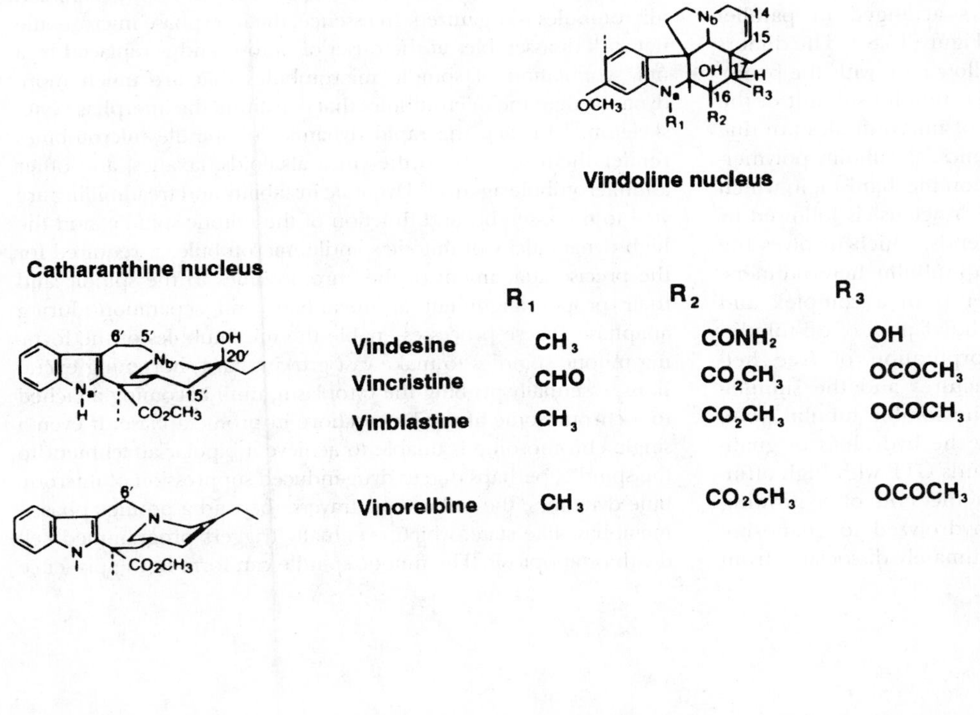

	R₁	R₂	R₃
Vindesine	CH_3	$CONH_2$	OH
Vincristine	CHO	CO_2CH_3	$OCOCH_3$
Vinblastine	CH_3	CO_2CH_3	$OCOCH_3$
Vinorelbine	CH_3	CO_2CH_3	$OCOCH_3$

FIGURE 15.8-2. Structural modifications of the vindoline and catharanthine rings in various vinca alkaloids.

agents, particularly the platinating agents or mitomycin C (or both), to treat non–small cell lung cancer, but it is also active in hematologic and other solid neoplasms.[20,21] The semisynthetic VBL derivative VRL (5'-norhydro-VBL), which is structurally modified on its catharanthine nucleus, is approved in the United States for treating non–small cell lung cancer as either a single agent or in combination with cisplatin and has also been registered for advanced breast cancer in many other countries.[22,23] VRL has been reported to confer notable therapeutic indices in the treatment of elderly patients with advanced breast and lung cancers. The agent has also demonstrated anticancer activity in advanced ovarian carcinoma and lymphoma; however, a unique role in the therapy of these malignancies has not been defined.

MECHANISM OF ACTION

The principal mechanism of cytotoxicity of the vinca alkaloids is by interacting with tubulin and disrupting microtubule function, particularly that of microtubules comprising the mitotic spindle apparatus.[1,6,25–29] However, the vinca alkaloids are also capable of many other disruptive actions that may or may not be related to their effects on microtubules.[29] In support of antimicrotubule activities as the principal cytotoxic actions of the vinca alkaloids, the dissolution of the mitotic spindle apparatus, appearance of mitotic figures, and cytotoxicity strongly correlate with drug concentration and the duration of treatment.[28] Nevertheless, the vinca alkaloids and other antimicrotubule agents also affect non-malignant and malignant cells in the nonmitotic phases of the cell cycle.

In contrast to colchicine, the vinca alkaloids bind directly to microtubules without first forming a complex with soluble tubulin and do not copolymerize with the tubulin lattice of the microtubule.[1,6,30,31] Two vinca alkaloid–binding sites, which have different binding affinities and are distinct from those of the taxanes, colchicine, podophyllotoxin, and GTP, have been characterized.[1,6,23–27] The vinca alkaloids bind to tubulin at the microtubule ends with high affinity (K_d, 1 to 2 µmol) and bind with considerably lower affinity (K_d, 0.25 to 0.30 mmol) to tubulin sites located along the sides of the microtubule surface.[1,27] Approximately 16 to 17 high-affinity binding sites per microtubule are located at the ends of each microtubule. The binding of the vinca alkaloids to high-affinity sites is responsible for the potent suppression of tubulin exchange that occurs at low drug concentrations (less than 1 µmol). At low concentrations, treadmilling dynamics are inhibited, but microtubule mass is not affected. Furthermore, low concentrations of the vinca alkaloids affect dynamic instability in an "end-dependent" fashion. Dynamic instability is strongly enhanced at the minus ends (kinetic destabilization), whereas dynamic instability is inhibited at the plus end (kinetic stabilization). In essence, these actions increase the time that microtubules spend in a state of attenuated activity, neither growing nor shortening, and contribute to the potent mitotic block at the metaphase/anaphase transition in a number of cell types. At higher concentrations, these effects are accompanied by microtubule depolymerization. Binding of the vinca alkaloids to the low-affinity sites at higher concentrations induces tubulin to self-associate into nonmicrotubule polymers and ordered aggregates through a self-propagation pathway. Self-propagation occurs as vinca alkaloid binding progressively weakens the lateral interactions between protofila-

ments, induces conformation changes in tubulin, and exposes new sites. The exposure of new sites further increases the binding affinity of the vinca alkaloids and may be responsible for the formation of vinca alkaloid–tubulin spiral aggregates, protofilaments, and paracrystalline structures at high (µmol) concentrations, ultimately leading to microtubule disintegration.[32]

The vinca alkaloids potently block mitosis at the metaphase/anaphase transition. After nuclear envelope breakdown, the agents block mitotic spindle formation. Although the chromosomes may condense, they remain scattered in the cells. Despite the fact that the chromosomes separate along their lengths, they remain attached at their centromeres. Cyclin B concentrations may remain high, and cell-cycle progression to interphase in the absence of anaphase or cytokinesis may occur, resulting in chromatin decondensation and formation of multilobed nuclei. At low concentration, the vinca alkaloids may induce mitotic arrest, which does not involve microtubule depolymerization. Nevertheless, the disruption of spindle microtubule dynamics without microtubule depolymerization may ultimately lead to cell death by apoptosis (see Mechanism of Action and Mechanisms of Resistance sections under Vinca Alkaloids and Taxanes, earlier and later in this chapter, respectively).[24]

The naturally occurring vinca alkaloids VCR and VBL, the semisynthetic analogue VRL, and a novel bifluorinated analogue vinflunine, which is currently in early clinical investigations, have similar mechanisms of action; however, they possess distinct differences as well.[33,34] For example, vinflunine appears to be more active than the other vinca alkaloids against several murine and human tumor xenografts even though it has a significantly lower affinity to tubulin and a lower potential to induce vinca alkaloid–tubulin spiral polymers.[35] However, the effects of vinflunine and VRL on microtubule dynamics are distinct from those induced by VBL and VCR in that they decrease the growth rate and duration of time growing but greatly decrease the total time spent in attenuation. In contrast, VBL and VCR decrease the shortening rate and increase the time spent in attenuation.

Tissue and tumor sensitivities to the vinca alkaloids, which relate in part to differences in drug transport and accumulation, are widely disparate. Intracellular/extracellular concentration ratios range from 5- to 500-fold depending on the cell type.[36–40] Although the vinca alkaloids are retained in cells for long periods of time and thus may have prolonged cellular effects, intracellular retention is markedly different among the various vinca alkaloids.[38–42] The results of early studies suggested that the vinca alkaloids entered cells by energy-dependent and temperature-dependent transport processes, but it now appears that temperature-independent, nonsaturable mechanisms, analogous to simple diffusion, account for the majority of drug transport and that temperature-dependent saturable processes are less important.[27–29,38] Another important determinant of drug accumulation and retention is lipophilicity, and VBL appears to be retained to a much greater degree than either VCR or VDS.[38–40] Drug uptake and retention are also influenced by tissue-specific factors, as illustrated by studies demonstrating that the accumulation and retention of VRL in neurons are less than those of other vinca alkaloids.[42,43] One important tissue-specific factor is tubulin isotype composition, which may influence the intracellular accumulation of the vinca alkaloids and other antimicrotubule agents that avidly bind tubulin.[3,7–9] Tubulin isotypes confer variable drug-binding characteristics, involve different drug uptake and efflux pump mechanisms, and determine the magnitude of the intracellular reservoir for drug accumulation.[25] In addition, differences in the type and quantity of MAPs and GTP, which may influence drug interactions with tubulin, and variability in cellular permeation and retention, may influence the formation and stability of complexes formed between the vinca alkaloids and tubulin.[28,29,33,42–44] Differences in the pharmacokinetics between the vinca alkaloids may account in part for differential tissue sensitivity. In addition, the drug concentration and duration of treatment are important determinants of drug accumulation and cytotoxicity, but the duration of drug exposure above a critical threshold concentration appears to be the most important determinant.[39–41]

MECHANISMS OF RESISTANCE

Two basic mechanisms of resistance to the vinca alkaloids have been described *in vitro*. The first is pleiotropic or multidrug resistance (MDR), which can be either innate or acquired. Although a large number of proteins mediate MDR, the adenosine triphosphate (ATP)-binding cassette (ABC) transporters, which belong to the largest known transporter gene family and translocate a variety of substrates across cellular compartments, are the best characterized. These intracellular and extracellular membrane-spanning proteins transport endobiotics and xenobiotics and confer resistance to the vinca alkaloids and other structurally bulky, natural product chemotherapeutic agents *in vitro*.[45] The most important ABC transporters that confer resistance to the vinca alkaloids are the permeability glycoprotein (P-gp) or the *MDR1*-encoded gene product MDR1 (ABC subfamily B1; ABCB1) and the MDR protein (MRP; ABC subfamily C2; ABCB1).[45–50] MDR1 is a 170-kD P-gp transmembrane that regulates the efflux of a large range of amphiphatic hydrophobic substances, resulting in decreased drug accumulation. MDR1 confers varying degrees of cross-resistance to other structurally bulky natural products, such as the taxanes, anthracyclines, epipodophyllotoxins, and colchicine.[46–50] The amino acid sequence of the specific P-gp associated with resistance to the vinca alkaloids differs slightly from P-gp of cells selected for resistance to other agents.[47,48] These proteins also undergo posttranslational modifications, resulting in further structural diversity, which may explain the greater degree of resistance for the specific agent, in which resistance was selected against, and the variable degrees of resistance to agents aside from that specific agent. The composition of membrane gangliosides in cancer cells resistant to the vinca alkaloids has also been shown to differ from that of wild-type cells. The clinical ramifications of these mechanisms are not known. In one study in childhood acute lymphoblastic leukemia, VCR resistance measured *in vitro* did not correlate with P-gp overexpression.[50] MRP1 is a 190-kD membrane-spanning protein that shares 15% amino acid homology with MDR1.[45,51] MRP1 expression has been demonstrated in multiple tumor types and has been implicated as a component of the MDR phenotype in cancers of the lung, colon, breast, bladder, and prostate, as well as leukemia.[45,51] MRP1 has been shown to transport glutathione conjugates of several types of compounds, including alkylating agents, as well as etoposide and doxorubicin, but only confers resistance to the latter agents. The MRP1 resistance profile also includes the vinca alkaloids and methotrexate.[40,51] The clinical significance of MRP1's role in transporting conjugated forms of certain chemotherapy agents has not been determined. Although many other ABC transporters have been characterized *in vitro* and several enhance cellular resistance to the vinca alkaloids, their roles in conferring inherent or acquired resistance to the vinca alkaloids in the clinic are even less clear than those of MDR1 and MRP1.

A wide range of structurally distinct agents reverse resistance conferred by MDR1 and MRP *in vitro*, and the role of MDR modulators has been a source of great contemporary interest. However, the interpretation of clinical studies of resistance modulation has been confounded by the fact that MDR modulators, particularly MDR1 reversal agents, also enhance drug uptake in normal cells, decrease biliary elimination and drug clearance, and lead to enhanced toxicity.[52–54] Overall, strategies aimed at reversing resistance to the vinca alkaloids in the clinic with pharmacologic modulators of MDR, principally MDR1 and MRP to a lesser extent, have been disappointing, perhaps due to the inherent aspects of the therapeutic agents but more likely due to the plasticity of the MDR phenotype with regard to the cells' capability of producing a large number of alternate resistance proteins in response to environmental stress.[45] Nevertheless, the characterization of the genetics and role of the ABC transporters in normal organ function and the disposition of chemotherapeutic agents have led to the delineation of genetic polyporphisms that may have an impact on pharmacokinetics and drug toxicity.

Structural and functional alterations in α- or β-tubulin, resulting from either genetic mutations and consequential amino acid substitutions or posttranslational modifications, have been identified in tumor cells with acquired resistance to the vinca alkaloids.[6–9,55–58] The consequences of functionally significant differences in α- and β-tubulins are "hyperstable" microtubules that are collaterally sensitive to the taxanes and similar tubulin-stabilizing natural products (discussed later in Taxanes, Mechanisms of Resistance). Although the means by which tubulin alterations confer resistance to the vinca alkaloids is not entirely clear, an increasing body of experimental evidence suggests that this phenomenon is not due to decreased drug-binding affinity of the altered tubulin. Instead, it is becoming apparent that the alterations in α- and β-tubulins promote resistance to agents that inhibit microtubule assembly by increasing microtubule stability, perhaps by promoting longitudinal interdimer and intradimer interactions or lateral interactions between protofilaments, or both, which increase resistance.[58]

PHARMACOLOGY

The vinca alkaloids are usually administered intravenously as a brief infusion, and their pharmacokinetic behavior in plasma has generally been fit by three-compartment models. Table 15.8-1 displays several pertinent pharmacokinetic features of these agents. At conventional adult doses, peak plasma concentrations range from 100 to 500 nmol, but levels of this magnitude are sustained in plasma for only short periods (α half-lives less than 5 minutes).[18–22,39,59–67] The vinca alkaloids share many pharmacokinetic characteristics, including large volumes of distribution, high clearance rates, and long terminal half-lives, which reflect the high magnitude and avidity of drug binding in peripheral tissues as discussed in the previous sections. Large interindividual and intraindividual variability is present in their pharmacologic behavior, which has been attributed to differences in protein and tissue binding, hepatic metabolism, and biliary clearance.[62]

TABLE 15.8-1. Vinca Alkaloids: Comparative Pharmacokinetic and Toxicologic Characteristics

	Vincristine	*Vinblastine*	*Vindesine*	*Vinorelbine*
Standard adult dose (range, mg/m²/wk)	1–2	6–8	3–4	15–30
Pharmacokinetic behavior	Triphasic	Triphasic	Triphasic	Triphasic
Plasma half-lives				
α (min)	<5	<5	<5	<5
β (min)	50–155	53–99	55–99	49–168
γ (h)	23–85	20–64	20–24	18–49
Clearance (L/kg/h)	0.16	0.74	0.25	0.40–1.29
Primary route	Hepatic metabolism and biliary elimination	Hepatic metabolism and biliary elimination	Hepatic metabolism and biliary elimination	Hepatic metabolism and biliary elimination
Principal toxicity	Neurotoxicity	Neutropenia	Neutropenia	Neutropenia
Other toxicities	Constipation, SIADH	Alopecia, neurotoxicity, mucositis	Alopecia, neurotoxicity	Neurotoxicity, vomiting, constipation, mucositis

SIADH, syndrome of inappropriate secretion of antidiuretic hormone.

Although prolonged infusion schedules may avoid excessively toxic peak concentrations and increase the duration of drug exposure in plasma above biologically relevant threshold concentrations for any given tumor, there is little, if any, evidence to support the notion that prolonged infusion schedules are more effective than bolus schedules. This approach has primarily been directed at achieving plasma concentrations for relevant periods, because the duration of exposure to relevant concentrations is a principal determinant of cytotoxicity *in vitro;* however, rapid, high, and avid distribution and binding of the vinca alkaloids to peripheral tissues, owing to the ubiquitous nature of tubulin, is likely responsible for the efficacy of short administration schedules.

In comparative studies of the vinca alkaloids, VCR had the longest terminal half-life and the lowest clearance rate, VBL had the shortest terminal half-life and the highest clearance rate, and VDS had intermediate characteristics.[18,20–23,60] Comparable values for VLR overlap with those of VDS and VBL. The longest half-life and lowest clearance rate of VCR may account for its greater propensity to induce neurotoxicity,[60] but there are many other nonpharmacokinetic determinants of tissue sensitivity, as discussed earlier in Mechanism of Action.

Vincristine

After conventional doses of VCR (1.4 mg/m²) given as brief infusions, peak plasma levels approach 0.4 μmol.[18,20,21,59–64] VCR binds extensively to plasma proteins (reported values, 48% to 75%) and formed blood elements, particularly platelets, which contain high concentrations of tubulin and led, in the past, to the use of VCR-loaded platelets for treating disorders of platelet consumption, such as idiopathic thrombocytopenic purpura.[20] The platelet count has been demonstrated to inversely influence drug exposure.[20,42] Penetration of VCR and other vinca alkaloids across the blood–brain barrier and other tumor sanctuary sites is poor, probably because of its large size and the fact that it is an avid substrate for the ABC transporters, as discussed in Mechanisms of Resistance, earlier in this section, that maintain the integrity of these blood–tissue barriers.[18,20,21,64–67] Plasma clearance is slow, and terminal half-lives ranging from 23 to 85 hours have been reported.[18,20,21,39,59,62–64]

VCR is metabolized and excreted primarily by the hepatobiliary system. Seventy-two hours after the administration of radiolabeled VCR, approximately 12% of the radiolabel is excreted in the urine (at least 50% of which consists of metabolites), and approximately 70% to 80% is excreted in the feces (40% of which consists of metabolites).[18,21,39,59–67] The nature of the VCR metabolites identified to date, as well as the results of metabolic studies *in vitro,* indicate that VCR metabolism is mediated principally by hepatic cytochrome P-450 CYP3A.[18,21,39] Conflicting evidence, albeit sparse, indicates that peak VCR plasma concentration or systemic exposure correlates positively with the degree of neurotoxicity.[19]

Vinblastine

The clinical pharmacology of VBL is similar to that of VCR. Binding of VBL to plasma proteins and formed elements of blood is extensive.[32,59,63,65,68,69] Peak plasma drug concentrations are approximately 0.4 μmol after rapid intravenous injections of VBL at standard doses. Distribution is rapid, and terminal half-lives range from 20 to 24 hours.[21,39,59,63,65,68,69] Tissue sequestration appears to be greater for VBL than VCR; 73% of radioactivity remained in the body 6 days after treatment with radiolabeled drug in one study.[39,68] Like VCR, VBL disposition is principally through the hepatobiliary system and into the feces (approximately 95%); however, fecal excretion of the parent compound is low, indicating that hepatic metabolism is extensive.[39] *In vitro* studies indicate that the cytochrome P-450 CYP3A isoform is primarily responsible for the drug biotransformation.[39,69] Although the metabolic fate of VBL has not been fully characterized, 4-deacetyl-VBL, or VDS, which appears to be as active as the parent compound, is the principal metabolite of VBL.[39,69]

Vindesine

VDS is rapidly distributed to tissues, and terminal half-lives range from 20 to 24 hours.[21,39,59,66,70–74] Its large volume of distribution, low renal clearance, and long terminal half-life suggest that VDS undergoes extensive tissue binding and delayed elimination and that drug accumulation may occur with repeated administration at short intervals. Although peak VDS concentrations ranging from 0.1 to 1.0 μmol are achieved with rapid intravenous administration, plasma levels typically decline to less than 0.1 μmol in 1 to 2 hours after treatment. Plasma levels achieved with rapid injections are approximately 16-fold higher than those achieved with protracted infusions; however, prolonged periods of exposure above concentrations resulting in cytotoxicity *in vitro* (0.01 to 0.10 μmol) are readily achieved using protracted infusions (1.2 to 2.0 mg/m^2/d for 2 to 5 days).[21,39,62,72,74] Nevertheless, the overall merits of protracted administration schedules have not been established. Renal clearance is negligible, accounting for 1% to 12% of drug disposition.[31,39,73] Similar to the other vinca alkaloids, VDS disposition is primarily by hepatic metabolism and biliary clearance, and the cytochrome P-450 isoform CYP3A plays a major role in drug metabolism.[31,39,75]

Vinorelbine

The pharmacologic behavior of VRL is essentially similar to that of the other vinca alkaloids, and plasma concentrations after rapid intravenous administration have been reported to decline in either a biexponential or triexponential manner.[31,33,39,76–78] After intravenous administration, there is a rapid decay of VRL concentrations followed by a much slower elimination phase (terminal half-life, 18 to 49 hours). Plasma protein binding, principally to α_1-acid glycoprotein, albumin, and lipoproteins, has been reported to range from 80% to 91%, and drug binding to platelets is extensive.[23,25,39]

VRL is widely distributed, and high concentrations are found in virtually all tissues, except the central nervous system.[23,24,39,79] VRL's wide distribution reflects its lipophilicity, which is among the highest of the vinca alkaloids. In fact, drug concentrations in human lung have been shown to be 300-fold greater than plasma levels and 3.4- to 13.8-fold higher than lung concentrations achieved with VDS and VCR, respectively. As with other vinca alkaloids, the liver is the principal excretory organ, and 33% to 80% of VRL is excreted in the feces, whereas urinary excretion represents only 16% to 30% of total drug disposition, the bulk of which is unmetabolized VLR.[22,23,39,80,81] Studies in humans indicate that 4-O-deacetyl-VRL and 3,6-epoxy-VRL are the principal metabolites, and several minor hydroxy-VRL isomer metabolites have been identified.[23,24,81] Although most metabolites are inactive, the deacetyl-VRL metabolite may be as active as VRL. The cytochrome P-450 CYP3A isoenzyme appears to be principally involved in biotransformation.[23,24,39] Human studies of powder- and liquid-filled gelatin capsules have shown that bioavailability of the parent compound is 43% for the powder-filled and 27% for the liquid-filled capsules.[78] Plasma concentrations peak within 1 to 2 hours after oral treatment, and interindividual variability is moderate.

DRUG INTERACTIONS

Methotrexate accumulation in tumor cells is enhanced *in vitro* by the presence of VCR or VBL, an effect mediated by a vinca alkaloid–induced blockade of drug efflux; however, the minimal concentrations of VCR required to achieve this effect occur only transiently *in vivo*.[82,83] The vinca alkaloids also inhibit the cellular influx of the epipodophyllotoxins *in vitro*, resulting in less cytotoxicity, but the clinical implications of this potential interaction are unknown.[84] L-Asparaginase may reduce the hepatic clearance of the vinca alkaloids, which may

result in increased toxicity. To minimize the possibility of this interaction, the vinca alkaloids should be given 12 to 24 hours before L-asparaginase. The combined use of mitomycin C and the vinca alkaloids has been associated with acute dyspnea and bronchospasm. The onset of these pulmonary toxicities has ranged from within minutes to hours after treatment with the vinca alkaloids or up to 2 weeks after mitomycin C.

Treatment with the vinca alkaloids has precipitated seizures associated with subtherapeutic plasma phenytoin concentrations.[83,85] Reduced plasma phenytoin levels have been noted from 24 hours to 10 days after treatment with VCR and VBL. Because of the importance of the cytochrome P-450 CYP3A isoenzyme in vinca alkaloid metabolism, administration of the vinca alkaloids with erythromycin and other inhibitors of CYP3A may lead to severe toxicity.[86] Concomitantly administered drugs, such as pentobarbital and H$_2$-receptor antagonists, may also influence VCR clearance by modulating hepatic cytochrome P-450 metabolic processes.[83,87] Another potential drug interaction may occur in patients who have Kaposi's sarcoma associated with the acquired immunodeficiency syndrome and are receiving concurrent treatment with 3'-azido-3'-deoxythymidine (AZT) and the vinca alkaloids, as the vinca alkaloids may impede glucuronidation of AZT to its 5'-O-glucuronide metabolite.[88] Based on a report of a constellation of severe toxicities, including syndrome of inappropriate secretion of antidiuretic hormone (SIADH), bilateral cranial nerve palsies, peripheral neuropathy in upper and lower extremities, cranial nerve palsies, heart failure, and cardiovascular effects after VCR treatment in children with acute lymphocytic leukemia who had been receiving treatment with nifedipine and itraconazole, these medications may potentially enhance the neurologic and cardiovascular effects of the vinca alkaloids.[89]

TOXICITY

Despite close similarities in structure, the vinca alkaloids differ significantly in their toxicologic profiles. VCR principally induces neurotoxicity characterized by a peripheral, symmetric mixed sensory-motor, and autonomic polyneuropathy.[19,21–23,90–92] Its primary neuropathologic effects are axonal degeneration and decreased axonal transport due to interference with axonal microtubule function. Initially, only symmetric sensory impairment and paresthesias in a length-dependent manner (distal extremities first) usually are encountered. Neuritic pain and loss of deep tendon reflexes may develop with continued treatment, which may be followed by foot drop, wrist drop, motor dysfunction, ataxia, and paralysis. Back, bone, and limb pains occasionally occur. Nerve conduction velocities are usually normal, although diminished amplitude of sensory and motor nerve action potentials and prolonged distal latencies, suggesting axonal degeneration, may be noted.[19,90–92] Cranial nerves may be affected rarely, resulting in hoarseness, diplopia, jaw pain, and facial palsies. The uptake of VCR into the central nervous system is low, and although manifestations of central neurotoxicity, including confusion, mental status changes, depression, hallucinations, agitation, insomnia, seizures, coma, SIADH, and visual disturbances, have been reported, these toxicities are rare.[19,65,93] Acute, severe autonomic neurotoxicity is uncommon but may arise as a consequence of high-dose therapy (greater than 2 mg/m^2) or in patients with altered hepatic function. Toxic manifestations include constipation, abdominal cramps, paralytic ileus, urinary retention, orthostatic hypotension, and hypertension.[94-96] Laryngeal paralysis has also been reported.[97]

In adults, neurotoxicity may occur after treatment with cumulative doses as little as 5 to 6 mg, and manifestations may be profound after cumulative doses of 15 to 20 mg. Children appear to be less susceptible than adults, but the elderly are particularly prone. However, the apparent influence of age may, in fact, be due to previously inadequate dose calculation by body weight in children and adults and by body surface area (BSA) in infants.[98,99] In infants, VCR doses are calculated now according to body weight. Patients with antecedent neurologic disorders, such as Charcot-Marie-Tooth disease, hereditary and sensory neuropathy type 1, Guillain-Barré syndrome, and childhood poliomyelitis, are highly predisposed.[100] Impaired drug metabolism and delayed biliary excretion in patients with hepatic dysfunction or obstructive liver disease are associated with increased risk of neurotoxicity.

The only known treatment for VCR neurotoxicity is discontinuation of the drug or reduction of the dose or frequency of treatment.[92,101,102] Although a number of antidotes, including thiamine, vitamin B_{12}, folinic acid, and pyridoxine, have been used, these treatments have not been clearly shown to be effective.[19-21,92,101-103] However, results with several other protective agents appear promising. In one randomized, double-blind trial, coadministration of glutamic acid and VCR has been demonstrated to decrease neurotoxicity.[19,103] The adrenocorticotropic hormone (4-9) analogue ORG 2766 has also been shown to protect against VCR-induced neuropathy in an animal model and in cancer patients in a double-blind, placebo-controlled pilot study, but the younger ages of patients receiving ORG 2766 compared to those receiving placebo may have accounted for this result. Experimental results suggest that several other agents, such as nerve growth factor, insulin-like growth factor-1, and amifostine, might alter the natural course of drug-induced neurotoxicity.[19]

The manifestations of neurotoxicity are similar for the other vinca alkaloids; however, they are typically less common and severe.[18-23] Severe neurotoxicity is observed infrequently with VBL and VDS. VRL has been shown to have a lower affinity for axonal microtubules than either VCR or VBL, which seems to be confirmed by clinical observations.[46,104] Mild to moderate peripheral neuropathy, principally characterized by sensory effects, occurs in 7% to 31% of patients, and constipation and other autonomic effects are noted in 30% of subjects, whereas severe toxicity occurs in 2% to 3%. Muscle weakness, jaw pain, and discomfort at tumor sites may also occur. In a study in patients with non–small cell lung cancer randomly assigned to treatment with either VRL alone, VRL plus cisplatin, or VDS plus cisplatin, the rate of severe neurotoxicity was lower in the single-agent VRL and VRL plus cisplatin arms than in the VDS plus cisplatin arm.[105] Furthermore, the addition of cisplatin did not significantly increase the incidence of severe toxicity in excess of that observed with VRL alone.

Neutropenia is the principal dose-limiting toxicity of VBL, VDS, and VRL. Thrombocytopenia and anemia occur less commonly. The onset of neutropenia is usually 7 to 11 days after treatment, and recovery is generally by days 14 to 21. Myelosuppression is not typically cumulative. Clinically relevant hematologic effects are uncommon after VCR treatment, but may be observed after inadvertent administration of high dosages or in the presence of hepatic dysfunction. Gastrointestinal effects, aside from those caused by autonomic dysfunction, may be caused by all vinca alkaloids.[18-23,106] Gastrointestinal autonomic dysfunction, as manifested by bloating, constipation, ileus, and abdominal pain, occur most commonly with VCR or high doses of the other vinca alkaloids. Mucositis occurs more frequently with VBL than with VRL or VDS and is least common with VCR. Nausea, vomiting, and diarrhea may also occur to a lesser extent. Pancreatitis has been reported with VRL.[107]

The vinca alkaloids are potent vesicants and may cause tissue damage if extravasation occurs. If extravasation is suspected, treatment should be discontinued, and aspiration of any residual drug remaining in the tissues should be attempted.[108-110] In animal models, cold appears to increase toxicity, whereas heat limits tissue damage. Therefore, the immediate application of heat for 1 hour four times daily for 3 to 5 days and the injection of hyaluronidase, 150 to 1500 U (15 U/mL in 6 mL 0.9% sodium chloride solution) subcutaneously, through six clockwise injections in a circumferential manner using a 25-gauge needle (changing the needle with each new injection) into the surrounding tissues, is the treatment of choice for minimizing discomfort and latent cellulitis. The use of calcium leucovorin, diphenydramine, hydrocortisone, isoproterenol, sodium bicarbonate, and vitamin A cream has been ineffective in animal models.[109] A surgical consultation to consider early débridement is also recommended. Discomfort, signs of phlebitis, and latent sclerosis may also occur along the course of an injected vein. The risk of phlebitis is increased if the vein is not adequately flushed after treatment.

Mild and reversible alopecia occurs in approximately 10% and 20% of patients treated with VLR and VCR, respectively. Acute cardiac ischemia, chest pains without evidence of ischemia, fever without an obvious source, Raynaud's phenomenon, hand-foot syndrome, and pulmonary and liver toxicity (transaminitis and hyperbilirubinemia, to a lesser extent) have also been reported with the vinca alkaloids.[111-116] All of the vinca alkaloids can cause SIADH, and patients who are receiving intensive hydration are particularly prone to severe hyponatremia secondary to SIADH.[19-23] This entity has been associated with elevated plasma levels of antidiuretic hormone and usually remits within 2 to 3 days. Hyponatremia generally responds to fluid restriction, as with hyponatremia associated with SIADH due to other causes. Tumor pain, rash, photosensitivity, and dermatitis are uncommon.

ADMINISTRATION

VCR is commonly administered to children weighing more than 10 kg (BSA of 1 m^2 or greater) as a rapid intravenous injection at a dosage of 1.5 to 2.0 mg/m^2 weekly, whereas 0.05 to 0.065 mg/kg weekly is commonly used in smaller children (less than 10 kg or BSA less than 1 m^2). For adults, the conventional weekly dose is 1.4 mg/m^2 weekly. A restriction of the absolute single dose of VCR to 2.0 to 2.5 mg in children and 2 mg in adults (often called *capping*) has been adopted based on early reports of substantial gastrointestinal toxicity in small numbers of patients treated at higher doses. However, this practice may be unfounded on toxicokinetic grounds, and available evidence suggests that it should be reconsidered, particularly in light of the wide interpatient variability in pharmacokinetic behavior and tolerance.[117] Significant interpatient variability is found in the clearance of VCR (as much as 11-fold), and some patients are able to tolerate much higher doses with little or no toxicity. Moreover, the safety and efficacy of treatment regimens that do not use capping at 2.0 mg have been documented in adults.[117] In any case, doses should not be reduced for mild peripheral neurotoxicity, particularly if the agent is being used in a potentially curative setting. Instead, doses should be modified for manifestations indicative of more serious neurotoxicity, including severe symptomatic sensory changes, motor and cranial nerve deficits, and ileus, until toxicity resolves. In clearly palliative situations, dose reductions, lengthened dosing intervals, or selection of an alternative agent may be justified in the event of moderate neurotoxicity. A routine prophylactic regimen, consisting of stool softeners, dietary bulk, and laxatives, to prevent the consequences of severe autonomic toxicity, particularly severe constipation, is also recommended.

The most common schedule for VBL in combination chemotherapy regimens uses a rapid intravenous injection at a dosage of 6 mg/m^2 weekly. Approved recommendations for weekly dosing are 2.5 and 3.7 mg/m^2 for children and adults, respectively, followed by gradual escalation in increments of 1.8 and 1.25 mg/m^2 weekly based on hematologic tolerance. It is recommended that weekly VBL doses of 18.5 mg/m^2 in adults and 12.5 mg/m^2 in children not be exceeded as a single agent; however, these doses are much higher than most patients can tolerate because of myelosuppression, even on less frequent schedules of administration. Doses in the range of 1.5 to 2.0 mg/m^2/d are recommended for patients receiving VBL as a 5-day continuous intravenous infusion. Because the severity of leukopenia that may occur with identical VBL doses varies widely, VBL should probably not be given more frequently than once each week. Intralesional injections have also been used to treat oral Kaposi's sarcoma.[118]

VDS has been administered intravenously on many schedules, including as a weekly or biweekly bolus. VDS has also been given in fractionated doses as either an intermittent or a continuous infusion over 1 to 5 days. However, VDS is most commonly administered as a single intravenous dose of 2 to 4 mg/m^2 every 7 to 14 days. Intermittent or continuous infusion schedules have used VDS doses of 1 to 2 mg/m^2/d for 1 to 2 days every 2 to 4 weeks or 1.2 mg/m^2/d for 5 days every 3 to 4 weeks.[62]

VRL is usually administered at a dose of 30 mg/m^2 on a weekly or biweekly schedule as a 6- to 10-minute intravenous injection through a sidearm port into a running infusion (alternatively, a slow bolus injection followed by flushing the vein with 5% dextrose or 0.9% sodium chloride solutions) or as a short infusion over 20 minutes.[22] It appears that the more rapid infusions result in less local venous toxicity. Oral dosages of 80 to 100 mg/m^2 given weekly are generally well tolerated, but an acceptable oral formulation has not yet been approved. Other dosing schedules that have been evaluated include chronic oral administration of low doses, intermittent high dose, and prolonged intravenous infusion schedules.

The vinca alkaloids are potent vesicants and should not be administered intramuscularly, subcutaneously, intravesically, or intraperitoneally. Direct intrathecal injection of VCR and other vinca alkaloids, which has occurred as an inadvertent clinical mishap, induces a severe myeloencephalopathy characterized by ascending motor and sensory neuropathies, encephalopathy, and rapid death. These serious consequences of intrathecal injections necessitate distinct labeling of vinca alkaloid injection syringes to avoid inadvertent intrathecal injections. Diluting the vinca alkaloids for intravenous bolus dosing into a small-volume intravenous bag, rather than in a syringe, is another simple method for eradicating the risk of catastrophic inadvertent intrathecal administration.

Although it has not been carefully evaluated, the major role of the liver in the disposition of the vinca alkaloids implies that dose modifications should be strongly considered for patients with hepatic dysfunction, particularly hepatic excretory insufficiency.[119] However, firm guidelines have not been established, particularly for VCR, VBL, and VDS. A 50% dose reduction is often recommended for patients with total bilirubin levels between 1.5 and 3.0 mg/dL (50% dose reduction for bilirubin levels between 2 and 3 mg/dL is recommended for VRL) and at least a 75% dose reduction for plasma total bilirubin levels greater than 3 mg/dL. Dose reduction for renal dysfunction is not indicated.

TAXANES

The unique chemical structure and mechanism of action of the taxanes, coupled with their broad antitumor activities, has rendered the taxanes one of the most important classes of anticancer agents. Interest in the taxanes began in 1963, when a crude extract of the bark of the Pacific yew tree, *Taxus brevifolia*, was shown to have impressive activity in preclinical tumor models. In 1971, paclitaxel was identified as the active constituent of the bark extract.[120,121] Although the early development of paclitaxel was hampered by the limited supply of its primary source; the difficulties inherent in large-scale isolation, extraction, and preparation of bulk compound for a natural product; and its poor aqueous solubility, interest was maintained after characterization of its novel mechanism of cytotoxic action and the availability of an adequate drug supply for requisite preclinical and limited clinical evaluations. The early search for taxanes derived from more abundant and renewable resources led to the development of docetaxel, which is synthesized by the addition of a side chain to 10-deacetylbaccatin III, an inactive taxane precursor found in the needles and other components of more abundant yew species.[122] The supply of paclitaxel is no longer a limiting issue because the agent is also produced semisynthetically and in large scale from 10-deacetylbaccatin III and other abundant, albeit inactive, taxane precursors.

The structures of paclitaxel, docetaxel, and their precursor, 10-deacetylbaccatin III, which is a complex ester consisting of a 15-member taxane ring system linked to an unusual four-member oxetan ring, are shown in Figure 15.8-3. The taxane rings of paclitaxel and docetaxel (but not 10-deacetylbaccatin III) are linked to an ester side chain attached to the C13 position of the ring, which is essential for antimicrotubule and antitumor activity. The structures of paclitaxel and docetaxel differ in substitutions at the C10 taxane ring position and on the ester side chain attached at C13.

The most impressive clinical activity of the taxanes has been in patients with ovarian and breast cancers.[120-125] Paclitaxel initially received regulatory approval in the United States and many other countries for the treatment of patients with ovarian cancer after failure of first-line or subsequent chemotherapy.[120,121] It

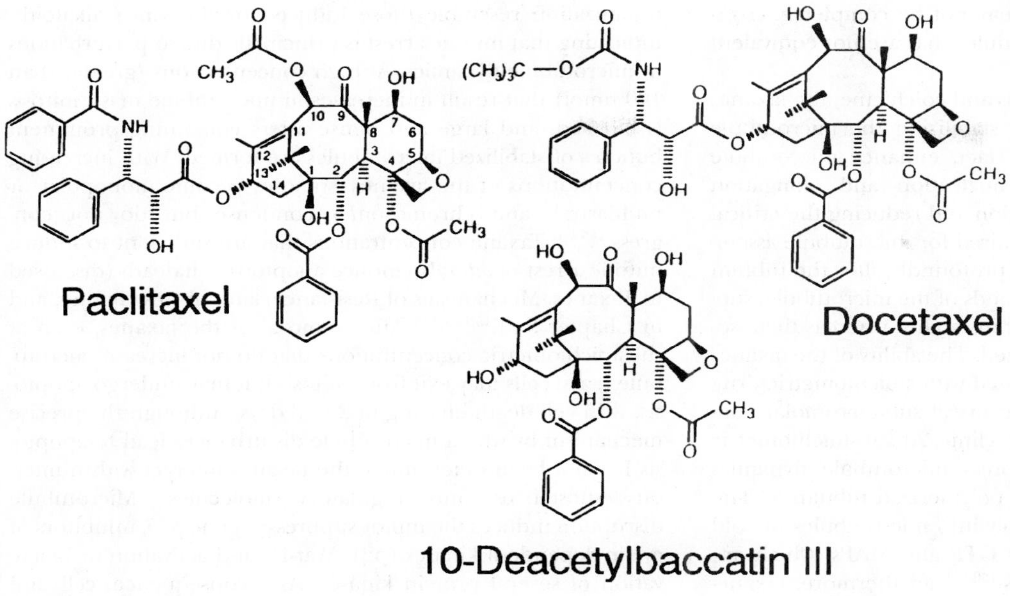

FIGURE 15.8-3. Structures of paclitaxel, docetaxel, and a precursor, 10-deacetylbaccatin III.

later received regulatory approval for patients with advanced breast cancer after failure of combination chemotherapy or at relapse within 6 months of adjuvant chemotherapy.[121,124] Subsequently, paclitaxel was determined to be indicated in combination with a platinum compound as primary induction therapy in suboptimally debulked stage III or IV ovarian cancer, which demonstrated a clear survival advantage in randomized phase III evaluations.[123] It also received regulatory approval for treating patients with lymph node–positive breast cancer when administered sequentially after standard doxorubicin-based adjuvant combination chemotherapy subsequent to the early results of a phase III study showing superior progression-free survival; however, an overall survival advantage was not apparent with longer-follow-up, and the optimal use of the taxanes and whether they affect overall survival in the adjuvant setting are not entirely clear at this time.[125] Intriguing results have been observed after treatment of patients with lymph node–positive breast cancer with alternative adjuvant regimens, particularly "dose-dense" regimens, consisting of sequential or concurrent treatment with doxorubicin, cyclophosphamide, and paclitaxel with hematopoietic growth factor support, but more robust evaluations of the merits of these approaches are being carried out.[126] Paclitaxel has also received regulatory approval in the United States for second-line treatment of Kaposi's sarcoma associated with AIDS, in combination with cisplatin as primary treatment of non–small cell lung cancer.[127,128]

Docetaxel initially received regulatory approval in the United States for patients with metastatic breast cancer that progressed or relapsed after anthracycline-based chemotherapy, which was later broadened to a general second-line indication.[122,124] Its role as a component of adjuvant and neoadjuvant chemotherapy after local treatment of early-stage breast cancer and first-line chemotherapy for locally advanced or metastatic breast cancer is being evaluated. Similar to the situation with paclitaxel, benefit conferred appears intriguing, but longer patient follow-up is required to discern the merits of docetaxel with regard to its impact on overall survival in the adjuvant setting. In non–small cell lung cancer, docetaxel initially received regulatory approval

in the United States and many other countries for treatment of nonresectable, locally advanced, or metastatic disease after consistently demonstrating increased survival after failure of cisplatin-based therapy, and, more recently, regulatory approval was granted for docetaxel in combination with cisplatin as first-line treatment for such patients.[129] The clinical antitumor spectra for paclitaxel and docetaxel are similar, with activity noted in many other diverse tumor types that are generally refractory to conventional therapies, including head and neck, esophageal, prostate, gastric, endometrial, bladder, small cell lung, and germ cell carcinomas and lymphomas. The extent to which apparent differences in response rates and other end points between docetaxel and paclitaxel reflect differences in study design, experience, dose, schedule, or inherent drug activities cannot be determined at this juncture.

MECHANISMS OF ACTION

The unique mechanism of action for paclitaxel was initially defined by Horwitz and colleagues in 1979.[130,131] The taxanes bind to the interior surface of the microtubule lumen at binding sites that are distinct from those of exchangeable GTP, colchicine, podophyllotoxin, and the vinca alkaloids and does not inhibit the binding of these agents to their respective sites. Paclitaxel binds to the N-terminal 1 to 31 amino acids and residues 217 to 233 of the β-tubulin subunit, and the paclitaxel pharmacophore is now well characterized.[132,133] Paclitaxel binds reversibly to microtubules reassembled *in vitro* with high affinity (K_d, 10 nmol).[1,2,6,15,131–135] Docetaxel, which is slightly more water soluble than paclitaxel, appears to share the same tubulin-binding site as paclitaxel but has a slightly higher affinity (approximately 1.9-fold) than paclitaxel for the site.[190] Tubulin assembly induced by docetaxel also proceeds with a critical protein concentration that is 2.1-fold lower than that of paclitaxel.[134] However, these differences may not confer greater therapeutic indices to docetaxel because greater potency may also portend more severe toxicity at identical drug concentrations *in vivo*. Nevertheless, the results of preclinical and clinical studies suggest that the taxanes may not be completely cross-resistant, but the use of dose schedules that are not equivalent may explain such observations.[136–138]

In contrast to the vinca alkaloids and colchicine, the taxanes disrupt microtubule dynamics by stabilizing the microtubule against depolymerization and, in fact, enhance microtubule polymerization, promoting the nucleation and elongation phases of the polymerization reaction and reducing the critical tubulin subunit concentration required for microtubule assembly.[1,2,6,14,15,27,131,139–141] The taxanes profoundly alter the tubulin dissociation rate constants at both ends of the microtubule, suppressing treadmilling and dynamic instability, whereas the association rate constants are not affected. The ability of the taxanes to induce polymerization is associated with stoichiometric drug binding to microtubules, which occurs at submicromolar concentrations readily achieved in the clinic. At substoichiometric concentrations, the taxanes suppress microtubule dynamics without increasing the amount of polymerized tubulin.[139] The taxanes induce tubulin self-assembly into microtubules in cold and in the absence of exogenous GTP and MAPs, which are normally required for this process.[130,131] Furthermore, taxane-treated microtubules are highly stable, resisting depolymerization by cold, calcium ions, dilution, and other antimicrotubule agents. This stability inhibits the dynamic reorganization of the microtubule network, which is essential for many vital cellular functions in mitosis and interphase.

The specific effects of the taxanes on tubulin dynamics *in vitro* are complex and depend in part on the stoichiometry of drug binding to the microtubule. Stoichiometric and substoichiometric binding inhibit the proliferation of cells, principally by inducing a sustained mitotic block at the metaphase/anaphase boundary. At low concentrations (10 to 50 nmol), the binding of a small number of paclitaxel molecules to microtubules reduces the rate and extent of shortening at microtubule plus ends.[142] Low paclitaxel concentrations (10 to 100 nmol), which are readily achieved in cancer patients, preferentially suppress tubulin dynamics and induce a modest increase in microtubule length at the plus ends but have little effect on dynamics at the minus ends.[143] At intermediate concentrations (100 nmol to 1 μmol), growing and shortening rates are suppressed to the same extent, and microtubules remain in a state of attenuation. At very high concentrations (1 to 20 μmol), which are barely achieved in plasma but likely achieved intracellularly after administration of standard doses, the binding of paclitaxel to microtubules saturates at stoichiometry of 1 mole drug per mole tubulin, and the mass of microtubule polymer increases sharply as tubulin is recruited into microtubules. Tubulin dissociation is inhibited at both microtubule ends, but the ends remain free for tubulin addition.[142,143] The taxanes also inhibit treadmilling.[1,144] Docetaxel suppresses tubulin dynamics in a manner similar to that of paclitaxel; however, the structural aspects of abnormal microtubules induced by paclitaxel and docetaxel may differ in that paclitaxel appears to induce the formation of microtubules with predominantly 12 protofilaments instead of 13, whereas 13 protofilaments are usually evident after docetaxel treatment.[134]

The taxanes result in delay or blockage of mitosis at the metaphase/anaphase, similar to the vinca alkaloids. At low concentrations (less than 10 nmol), mitosis is blocked, with no concomitant increase in microtubule mass. Alterations in spindle organization resemble those induced by the vinca alkaloids, indicating that mitotic arrest is principally due to perturbations in microtubule dynamics. At high concentrations (greater than 100 nmol) that result in increases in microtubule mass, mitosis is blocked, and large and dense asters containing prominent bundles of stabilized microtubules are formed. With increasing concentrations of the taxanes, spindles become monopolar or multiastral, and chromosomes condense but do not congress.[145,146] Taxane concentrations that are sufficient to induce mitotic arrest *in vitro* also induce apoptotic cell death (discussed in Taxanes, Mechanisms of Resistance, later in this chapter, and in Chapter 3.3).[15,146–156] After removal of the taxanes, even at substoichiometric concentrations that do not increase microtubule mass, cells may exit from mitosis but may undergo apoptosis, with cell death ensuing in 2 to 3 days. Although the precise mechanism by which microtubule disturbances lead to apoptosis has not been determined, the taxanes interact with numerous substances and regulatory molecules. Microtubule disruption induces the tumor suppressor gene *p53*, inhibitors of cyclin-dependent kinases (p21/Waf-1), and activation or inactivation of several protein kinases. As a consequence, cells are arrested in G_2/M, after which time they may either undergo apoptosis or traverse through G_2/M and divide.[156] Taxane-induced apoptosis is associated with the phosphorylation (inactivation) of the antiapoptotic Bcl-x_L/Bcl-2 family members.[156] The taxanes also affect interphase microtubules in nonproliferating cells. The agents can induce the formation of morphologically altered tubulin polymers, a phenomenon of as yet undetermined significance.[141] These structures, which often resemble hoops and ribbons, consist of bundles of microtubules. Paclitaxel has also been reported to induce transcription factors and enzymes that govern proliferation, apoptosis, and inflammation, and, interestingly, some of these effects, such as the induction of tumor necrosis factor-α.[147,157]

Paclitaxel and docetaxel have been shown to enhance the effects of ionizing radiation *in vitro* at clinically achievable concentrations (less than 50 nmol) and *in vivo*, which may be related to the inhibition of cell-cycle progression in the G_2 phase, which is the most radiosensitive phase of the cell cycle.[158–160] The taxanes also inhibit angiogenic activity at concentrations below those that induce cytotoxicity, but the contribution of these effects on malignant angiogenesis to the overall antitumor effects is not clear.[160–162]

MECHANISMS OF RESISTANCE

The MDR phenotype that is mediated by several members of the ABC transporter family and confers cross-resistance to a wide range of xenobiotics (discussed in Vinca Alkaloids, Mechanisms of Resistance, earlier in this chapter) is the best-characterized mechanism of taxane resistance *in vitro*, and the best-characterized ABC transporter with respect to conferring drug resistance is the P-gp or the *MDR1*-encoded gene product MDR1 (ABC subfamily B1; ABCB1) and MDR2 (ABC subfamily ABCB4).[45,161] Although the ABCC family of transporter proteins, particularly ABCC1 (MRP1) and ABCC2 (MRP2), confer cellular resistance to the vinca alkaloids, they do not appear to be involved in taxane transport.[45,51,162,163] Low-level taxane resistance also appears to be conferred by the bile salt export protein (also known as *ABCC11*).[45] Cross-resistance to the taxanes and anthracycline is incomplete, which has had significant clinical ramifications in developing the taxanes for women with advanced breast cancer after treatment with the anthracyclines. However, the role of MDR as a cause of anthracycline resistance in those patients is unclear. Similar to the vinca alkaloids, MDR encompassing taxane resistance can be reversed by many classes of drugs, including the calcium channel blockers, tamoxifen, cyclosporin A, and antiarrhythmic agents. In fact, plasma concentrations of the principal component of the vehicles used to formulate paclitaxel and docetaxel (polyoxyethylated castor oil and polysorbate 80, respectively) can reverse taxane resistance *in vitro*. Plasma concentrations of polyoxyethylated castor oil achieved with paclitaxel on clinically relevant dose schedules are sufficient to reverse MDR, but sufficient modulatory concentrations of polysorbate 80 are not achieved with docetaxel in the clinic. Strategies aimed at reversing taxane resistance in the clinic by using various classes of drug transport inhibitors have resulted in minimally positive results, at best, but the interpretation of these studies is confounded by the effects of early MDR transporter modulators (e.g., verapamil, cyclosporin A, and nonimmunomodulatory cyclosporin A analogues) on taxane clearance and toxicity.[66] However, the feasibility of administering the taxanes with novel MDR modulators that do not affect taxane pharmacokinetics and toxicity, thereby not confounding the interpretation of the inherent effects of these agents on MDR modulation, is being evaluated.[164,165]

Several taxane-resistant mutant cell lines that have structurally altered α- and β-tubulin proteins and an impaired ability to polymerize into microtubules also have been identified (discussed in Vinca Alkaloids, Mechanisms of Resistance, earlier in this chapter).[7–9,56,147,166,167] These mutants lack normal interpolar mitotic spindles and have an inherently slow rate of microtubule assembly, which is normalized in the presence of the drug. Mutants with "hypostable" microtubules exhibit collateral sensitivity to the vinca alkaloids. Furthermore, cells that are resistant to the taxanes and other tubulin-binding agents have tubulin content, tubulin isotype expression, and tubulin polymerization dynamics.[168–170] Mutations of tubulin isotype genes, gene amplifications, and isotype switching have also been reported in taxane-resistant cell lines.[56,147,171–173] Although early clinical data from patients with non–small cell lung cancer suggested that β-tubulin mutations may confer taxane resistance, these data have not been confirmed, and the results may have been due to the amplification of pseudogenes.[171,172] Higher levels of class III β-tubulin RNA levels have also been reported in non–small cell

lung cancers of patients who did not respond to taxane treatment, which is in line with *in vitro* findings.

The regulation and integrity of genes that regulate apoptosis, such as *p53*, *bcl-2*, *bcl-x*, and their gene products have been implicated as determinants of taxane sensitivity.[56,146,147,151–155,174–181] The taxanes have also been shown to modulate the function of genes involved in apoptotic regulation, and the disruption of microtubule dynamics by the taxanes and other antimicrotubule drugs results in the phosphorylation of such regulatory proteins as Bcl-x$_L$ and Bcl-2, thereby annulling the antiapoptotic functions of these regulators. MAPs are also likely to be involved in these mechanisms of resistance to drug-induced apoptosis, as illustrated by the fact that MAP4, which is negatively regulated by wild-type *p53*, has been shown to increase the sensitivity to paclitaxel.[178] It has been proposed that paclitaxel induces apoptosis through two different mechanisms—a *p53*-independent pathway in cells blocked in prophase and a *p53*-dependent mechanism in cells that accumulate in the G$_1$ cell-cycle phase—and requires functional *p53*.[147,179] However, several lines of experimental evidence suggest that *p53* induction by paclitaxel represents a mechanism of drug resistance; cumulative experimental data pertaining to the role of *p53* as a determinant of cell sensitivity to paclitaxel are conflictory.[180]

PHARMACOLOGY

The taxanes are commonly administered by intravenous infusion at dosages ranging from 175 to 225 mg/m² over 3 hours (for paclitaxel; indicated dose, 175 mg/m²) or 75 to 100 mg/m² over 1 hour (for docetaxel) every 3 weeks. Various other schedules have been evaluated (discussed later in Administration, Dose, and Schedule). The oral bioavailability of paclitaxel and docetaxel is poor, owing in part to the constitutive overexpression of P-gp and other ABC transporters by enterocytes or first-pass metabolism in the liver or intestines, or both. However, biologically relevant plasma concentrations are transiently achieved if the taxanes are administered orally with oral modulators of ABC transporters or cytochrome P-450 mixed-function oxidases such as cyclosporin A, or both.[182,183] As shown in Table 15.8-2, paclitaxel and docetaxel share the following pharmacologic characteristics: large volumes of distribution; rapid, avid, and protracted binding to all tissues except for the unperturbed central nervous system; long terminal half-lives; and substantial hepatic metabolism and biliary excretion.

TABLE 15.8-2. Taxanes: Comparative Pharmacokinetic and Toxicologic Characteristics

Characteristic	Paclitaxel	Docetaxel
Standard adult dose range (mg/m²/3 wk)	135 (24-h infusion), 175–225 (3-h infusion)	75–100 (1-h infusion)
Pharmacokinetic behavior	Saturable elimination and distribution	Triphasic
Plasma half-lives (terminal)	10–20 h	10–20 h
Clearance	20–25 L/h[a]	36 L/h
Primary route	Hepatic metabolism and biliary elimination	Hepatic metabolism and biliary elimination
Principal toxicity	Neutropenia	Neutropenia
Other toxicities	Alopecia, neurotoxicity, myalgia, hypersensitivity reactions, asthenia	Alopecia, skin and nail toxicity, asthenia, myalgia, fluid retention, neurotoxicity, hypersensitivity reactions

[a]Dose schedule: 175 mg/m² over 3 hours.

Paclitaxel

Pharmacologic studies of paclitaxel on long and short administration schedules have been performed (discussed in Administration, Dose, and Schedule, later in this chapter). In early studies that principally evaluated prolonged (6- and 24-hour) schedules, substantial interpatient variability was noted, and nonlinear, dose-dependent behavior was not observed.[121,122,182,184] In these studies, drug disposition was characterized as a biphasic process, with values for alpha and beta half-lives averaging approximately 20 minutes and 6 hours, respectively. However, subsequent studies of paclitaxel administered on shorter schedules, particularly as a 3-hour infusion, indicate that its pharmacokinetic behavior is nonlinear.[182,184,185] Nonlinearity occurs with all administration schedules, but it is more apparent with shorter infusions resulting in higher plasma paclitaxel concentrations that more effectively saturate drug elimination and tissue distribution processes. Saturable distribution and elimination processes may, in part, be responsible for paclitaxel's nonlinear behavior, with tissue distribution becoming saturated at lower drug concentrations (achieved with doses less than 175 mg/m² over 3 hours) compared to elimination processes that are effectively saturated at higher concentrations (achieved with doses greater than 175 mg/m² over 3 hours). Shorter infusion schedules may also result in higher plasma concentrations of paclitaxel's polyoxyethylated castor oil vehicle, which may also be responsible for nonlinearity or pseudononlinearity.[186] True nonlinear pharmacokinetics may have important clinical implications, particularly regarding dose modifications, because a small increase in dose may result in a disproportionate increase in drug exposure and hence toxicity, whereas a small dose reduction may result in a disproportionate decrease in drug exposure, thereby decreasing antitumor activity. Interestingly, shorter paclitaxel infusions are associated with reduced clearance of the polyoxyethylated castor oil vehicle and reduced exposure to unbound paclitaxel, which may explain the lower incidence of hematologic toxicity and higher incidence of hypersensitivity reactions with shorter schedules.[187]

Paclitaxel's volume of distribution is much larger than the volume of total body water, indicating extensive drug binding to plasma proteins or other tissue elements, probably tubulin. Plasma protein binding is high (greater than 95%) and readily reversible.[182] Drug binding to platelets is extensive and saturable, and animal distribution studies indicate extensive drug uptake and retention by virtually all tissues, except classic "tumor sanctuary sites" such as the central nervous system and testes.[182] In addition, paclitaxel disposition is related to BSA, providing a rationale for dosing based on this parameter.[188] In humans, peak plasma concentrations achieved with 3- to 96-hour infusions (greater than 0.05 to 10.0 μmol) and concentrations in third-space fluid collections, such as ascites (greater than 0.1 μmol), are sufficient to induce relevant biologic effects *in vitro*, but drug penetration into the normal central nervous system is negligible.[182,184–191]

The liver, which is the principal organ involved with paclitaxel clearance, metabolizes and excretes paclitaxel and metabolites into the bile.[183,191–194] Ninety-eight percent of radioactivity is recovered from feces collected for 6 days after rats are treated with radiolabeled paclitaxel, and approximately 71% of an administered dose of paclitaxel is excreted in the feces over 5 days as either parent compound or metabolites in humans, with the principal metabolite, 6α-hydroxypaclitaxel, accounting for

26% of the dose. Only 5% is unchanged paclitaxel. Renal clearance of paclitaxel and metabolites is minimal, accounting for 14% of the administered dose.[182] In humans, the bulk of drug disposition is metabolism by cytochrome P-450 mixed-function oxidases, specifically the isoenzymes CYP2C8 and CYP3A4, which metabolize paclitaxel to hydroxylated 3'p-hydroxypaclitaxel (minor) and 6α-hydroxypaclitaxel (major), as well as dihydroxylated metabolites, all of which are inactive.

Pharmacodynamic studies as part of individual phase I and II trials indicated that several pharmacokinetic indices of drug exposure can be related to the various toxicities of paclitaxel, the most important and consistent of which is the relationship between the severity of neutropenia and the duration of drug exposure above biologically relevant plasma concentrations ranging from 0.05 to 0.1 μmol.[182,184,185,189] However, a prospective analysis of pharmacokinetic determinants of outcome in several hundred patients with advanced non–small cell lung cancer treated with the combination of cisplatin and paclitaxel at either 135 or 250 mg/m² over 24 hours showed that the magnitude of the steady-state plasma concentration correlated poorly with antitumor activity, disease-free survival, and overall survival.[195] In randomized trials evaluating the effects of paclitaxel dose on relevant clinical end points in patients with advanced ovarian, non–small cell lung, breast, and head and neck cancer, neither progression-free nor overall survival was significantly increased by administering doses above 175 mg/m².

Docetaxel

The pharmacokinetics of docetaxel on a 1-hour schedule are triexponential and linear at doses of 115 mg/m² or less.[122,196–200] Terminal half-lives ranging from 11.1 to 18.5 hours have been reported. In one population study, plasma concentration data were optimally fit by a three-compartment model, and the following pharmacokinetic parameters were generated: $T_{1/2}\gamma$ of 12.4 hours, clearance of 1 L/h/m², and steady-state volume of distribution of 74 L/m².[197,198] The most important determinants of docetaxel clearance were the BSA, hepatic function, and plasma α_1-acid glycoprotein concentration, whereas age and albumin level had significant (albeit minor) influences on clearance. As with paclitaxel, plasma protein binding is high (greater than 80% to 90%), and binding is primarily to α_1-acid glycoprotein, albumin, and lipoproteins.[196–199] Docetaxel is distributed to all tissues except the central nervous system.[281,282] In dogs and mice treated with radiolabeled drug, fecal excretion accounts for 70% to 80% of total radioactivity, whereas urinary excretion accounts for 10% or less.[200] The hepatic cytochrome P-450 mixed-function oxidases, particularly isoforms CYP3A4 and CYP3A5, are principally involved in biotransformation that, in contrast to paclitaxel, affects the C13 side chain and not the taxane ring.[200–202]

The principal pharmacokinetic determinants of toxicity, particularly neutropenia, are drug exposure and the time that plasma concentrations exceed biologically relevant concentrations.[200–202] A population pharmacodynamic analysis of determinants of outcome in phase II trials of docetaxel revealed that the strongest determinants of the time to progression in patients with metastatic breast cancer are the pretreatment plasma α_1-acid glycoprotein concentration, number of prior chemotherapy regimens, and number of disease sites, whereas drug exposure and the pretreatment α_1-acid glycoprotein concentration were determinants of time to progression in patients with advanced lung cancer.[197] Conversely, the pretreatment plasma α_1-acid glycoprotein concentration negatively, albeit significantly, related to the probability of experiencing severe neutropenia and febrile neutropenia.

DRUG INTERACTIONS

Sequence-dependent pharmacokinetic and toxicologic interactions between paclitaxel and several other chemotherapy agents have been noted.[182,203] The sequence of cisplatin followed by paclitaxel (24-hour schedule) induces more profound neutropenia than the reverse sequence, which is explained by a 33% reduction in the clearance of paclitaxel after cisplatin.[203–205] The least toxic sequence—paclitaxel before cisplatin—was demonstrated to induce more cytotoxicity *in vitro*; therefore, this drug sequence was selected for further clinical development.[203–205] As expected, however, sequence dependence does not appear to be a clinically relevant phenomenon on shorter schedules. Treatment with paclitaxel on either a 3- or 24-hour schedule followed by carboplatin has been demonstrated to produce equivalent neutropenia and less thrombocytopenia as compared to carboplatin as a single agent, which is not explained by pharmacokinetic interactions.[200,206] Although sequence dependence has not been demonstrated between carboplatin and paclitaxel, which has been consistently noted to induce less thrombocytopenia than comparable doses of carboplatin alone, the phenomenon of sequence dependence has been noted with other paclitaxel-based chemotherapy combinations, the most important of which involve the anthracyclines.[203,206] Neutropenia and mucositis are more severe when paclitaxel is administered on a 24-hour schedule before doxorubicin, compared to the reverse sequence, which is most likely due to an approximately 32% reduction in the clearance rates of doxorubicin and doxorubicinol when doxorubicin is administered after paclitaxel.[207] Although neither sequence-dependent pharmacologic nor toxicologic interactions between doxorubicin and paclitaxel (3-hour schedule) have been noted, pharmacologic interactions occur with both sequences, and combined treatment with paclitaxel (3-hour schedule) and doxorubicin as a bolus infusion is associated with a higher incidence of congestive cardiotoxicity than would have been expected from an equivalent cumulative doxorubicin dose given without paclitaxel (discussed later in Toxicity).[203,208,209] The etiology for these interactions is unclear. The pharmacokinetic interactions may not be of sufficient magnitude to account for the enhanced cardiotoxicity of the combination and experimental data, indicating that paclitaxel accelerates the metabolism of doxorubicin to doxorubicinol and other cardiotoxic metabolites in cardiomyocytes. Docetaxel does not appear to influence doxorubicin pharmacokinetics, but experimental data suggest that docetaxel also enhances the metabolism of doxorubicin to toxic species in the human heart. Similar decrements in the clearance of epirubicin and its metabolites have been noted in studies of paclitaxel combined with epirubicin, but cardiotoxicity does not appear to be enhanced.[210] Competition for the hepatic or biliary P-gp transport of the anthracyclines with paclitaxel or its polyoxyethylated castor oil vehicle, or both, is another explanation.[203,208] The vehicle is suspected because similar effects have not been noted with docetaxel, which is not formulated in polyoxyethylated cas-

tor oil. Hematologic toxicity has been more severe with the sequence of cyclophosphamide before paclitaxel (24-hour schedule) than the reverse sequence.[211] In human tumor xenografts, paclitaxel and docetaxel have been demonstrated to induce thymidine phosphorylase activity, which may increase the metabolic activation of the oral fluoropyrimidine prodrug capecitabine.[212]

Drug interactions may also result from the effects of other classes of drugs on the cytochrome P-450–dependent metabolism of the taxanes. Various inducers of cytochrome P-450 mixed-function oxidases, such as the anticonvulsants phenytoin and phenobarbital, accelerate the metabolism of paclitaxel and docetaxel in human microsomes and in children and adults who are concurrently receiving treatment with these anticonvulsants, as manifested by rapid drug clearance and tolerance of high drug doses.[182,192–194,202,203,213,214] Conversely, many types of agents that inhibit cytochrome P-450 mixed-function oxidases, such as orphenadrine, erythromycin, cimetidine, testosterone, ketoconazole, fluconazole, midazolam, polyoxyethylated castor oil, and corticosteroids, interfere with the metabolism of paclitaxel and docetaxel in human microsomes *in vitro*; however, the inhibitory concentrations of these agents exceed those achieved in clinical practice, and the clinical relevance of these findings is not known.[182,192–194,202,203,213–215] Although there has been concern that the use of corticosteroids and different H_2-receptor antagonists with variable cytochrome P-450 inhibitory activities as components of premedication regimens may differentially affect drug clearance and hence toxicity, neither toxicologic nor pharmacologic differences between the agents were noted in a randomized clinical trial.

TOXICITY

Myelosuppression is the principal toxicity of paclitaxel and docetaxel. However, despite similar structures, these agents differ modestly in their toxicity spectra.

Paclitaxel

Neutropenia is the principal toxicity of paclitaxel. The onset is usually on days 8 to 10, and recovery is generally complete by days 15 to 21 on every-3-week dosing regimens. The main clinical determinant of the severity of neutropenia is the extent of prior myelosuppressive therapy. Neutropenia is noncumulative, and the duration of severe neutropenia, even in heavily pretreated patients, is usually brief. The most important pharmacologic determinant of the severity of neutropenia is the duration that plasma concentrations are maintained above biologically relevant levels (0.05 to 0.10 μmol; discussed earlier in Pharmacology), which may explain why neutropenia is more severe with longer infusion schedules.[216] This does not necessarily mean that longer schedules portend superior antitumor activity in the clinic. Instead, the results of randomized clinical studies do not indicate that there is an optimal schedule for any particular tumor, although treatment with higher doses or "equitoxic doses" should be considered if shorter schedules are used.[217] At paclitaxel doses exceeding 175 mg/m^2 on a 24-hour schedule and 225 mg/m^2 on a 3-hour schedule, nadir neutrophil counts are typically less than 500/μL for fewer than 5 days, even in untreated patients. Even patients who have received extensive prior therapy can usually tolerate paclitaxel doses of 175 to 200 mg/m^2 over 3 or 24 hours. More frequent administration schedules, particularly weekly treatment with doses of 80 to 100 mg/m^2, are associated with less severe neutropenia and at least equivalent antitumor activity in a number of cancers, as compared to single-dose schedules (discussed in Administration, Dose, and Schedule, later in this chapter). Severe thrombocytopenia and anemia are unusual, except in heavily pretreated patients.

Although the incidence of major hypersensitivity reactions in early phase I trials was approximately 30%, it decreased to 1% to 3% after development of effective prophylaxis.[120,121,182,216–219] Major reactions, which are characterized by dyspnea, bronchospasm, urticaria, hypotension, chest, and abdominal and back pain, usually occur within the first 10 minutes after the first (and less frequently after the second) treatment and resolve completely after stopping treatment; they occasionally occur after treatment with antihistamines, fluids, and vasopressors. Patients who have major reactions have been rechallenged successfully after receiving high doses of corticosteroids, but this approach is not always successful.[220] Rechallenge appears to be most successful in patients who experience severe hypersensitivity reactions within minutes of starting treatment, if the infusion is immediately discontinued, and if treatment resumes within 30 minutes. This observation is likely due to profound and persistent depletion of histamines and other mediators at the time of the rechallenge. Although minor reactions, such as flushing and rash, occur in as many as 40% of patients, minor hypersensitivity reactions do not portend the development of major reactions. Hypersensitivity reactions are probably caused by a nonimmunologically mediated release of histamine-like substances, owing to the taxane moiety or, more likely, its polyoxyethylated castor oil vehicle, possibly through complement activation. Although the rate of major hypersensitivity reactions is reduced with lower administration rates and longer infusion durations, the rates of major reactions are low on 3- and 24-hour schedules when patients are premedicated with corticosteroids and H$_1$- and H$_2$-receptor antagonists (discussed later in Administration, Dose, and Schedule).[216] In an assessment of the relative safety of two different paclitaxel schedules (3 vs. 24 hours), the rates of major reactions were low and similar (2.1% vs. 1.0%) in patients receiving paclitaxel for 3 or 24 hours, respectively, with premedication.[216]

Paclitaxel induces a peripheral neuropathy characterized by sensory symptoms, such as numbness in a symmetric glove-and-stocking distribution.[221,222] Neurologic examination reveals sensory loss and loss of deep tendon reflexes. Neurophysiologic studies support a primary disruption of neuronal microtubules resulting in axonal degeneration and demyelination as the primary pathogenic mechanism; however, manifestations suggestive of microtubule disruption, resulting in a neuronopathy, may be noted, particularly at higher doses or when combined with other neurotoxic agents, such as cisplatin.[222] Severe neurotoxicity is uncommon when paclitaxel is given alone at dosages below 200 mg/m^2 on a 3- or 24-hour schedule every 3 weeks or below 100 mg/m^2 on a continuous weekly schedule, but almost all "low-risk" patients experience mild or moderate effects. Patients with preexisting neuropathy due to prior exposure to other neurotoxic agents, diabetes mellitus, congenital conditions, or alcoholism, even when manifestations are subclinical, are more prone to development of paclitaxel-induced neuropathy. Symptoms may begin as soon as 24 to 72 hours

after treatment with higher doses (250 mg/m^2 or greater) but usually occur only after multiple courses at 135 to 250 mg/m^2 every 3 weeks. Neurotoxicity is generally more pronounced when paclitaxel is administered on short infusion schedules, indicating that peak plasma concentration is a principal determinant. The combination of paclitaxel on a 3-hour schedule and cisplatin is particularly neurotoxic, and regimens consisting of paclitaxel and carboplatin, albeit still neurotoxic, produce less neurotoxicity relative to paclitaxel-cisplatin regimens. Motor and autonomic dysfunction may occur, especially at high doses and in patients with preexisting neuropathies due to diabetes mellitus and alcoholism. Although several measures, such as the administration of amifostine, sulfhydryl group scavenger drugs, glutamate, pyridoxine, and anticonvulsants, have been reported to reduce the neurotoxic effects of paclitaxel in some experimental models, anecdotal reports, or insufficiently powered randomized trials, there is no convincing evidence that any specific measure is effective at ameliorating existing manifestations or preventing the development or worsening of neurotoxicity.[219,222–224] Transient myalgia and arthralgia of uncertain etiology, usually noted 24 to 48 hours after therapy and apparently dose related, are also common, and a myopathy has been described in patients receiving high doses with cisplatin. Several investigators have reported that treatment with corticosteroids, specifically prednisone, 10 mg twice daily for 5 days beginning 24 hours after treatment, is effective at reducing myalgia and arthralgia.[218,224] Optic nerve disturbances, manifested by scintillating scotoma, may also occur.[225] Acute encephalopathy, which can progress to coma and death, has been reported after treatment with high doses (600 mg/m^2 or greater).[226]

Paclitaxel treatment has been associated with cardiac rhythm disturbances, but the clinical relevance of these effects is not known.[218,223,227–229] The most common rhythm disturbance, a transient bradycardia, was noted in 29% of patients in one trial.[218,228,229] Isolated asymptomatic bradycardia without hemodynamic effects should not be considered an indication for discontinuing paclitaxel. More important bradyarrhythmias, including Mobitz type I (Wenckebach syndrome), Mobitz type II, and third-degree heart block, have been noted, but the incidence in a large National Cancer Institute database was only 0.1%.[228] Most documented episodes have been asymptomatic, and almost all documented events involved patients enrolled in early trials that required continuous cardiac monitoring, indicating that second- and third-degree heart block are likely underreported because such monitoring is not usually performed. However, these bradyarrhythmias are probably caused by paclitaxel, as related taxanes affect cardiac automaticity and conduction, and similar disturbances have occurred in humans and animals after ingesting various species of yew plants. Myocardial infarction, cardiac ischemia, atrial arrhythmias, and ventricular tachycardia have been noted, but whether there is a causal relationship between paclitaxel and these events is uncertain. No evidence has been shown that chronic, long-term treatment with paclitaxel causes progressive cardiac dysfunction. Routine cardiac monitoring during paclitaxel therapy is not necessary but is advisable for patients who may not be able to tolerate bradyarrhythmias, such as those with atrioventricular conduction disturbances or ventricular dysfunction. Although patients with a wide range of cardiac abnormalities and cardiac histories were broadly and empirically restricted from participating in early clinical trials, paclitaxel treatment has been reported to be well tolerated in a small series of gynecologic cancer patients with major cardiac risk factors.[229] On the other hand, repetitive treatment of patients with the combined regimen of paclitaxel on a 3-hour schedule and doxorubicin as a brief infusion is associated with a higher frequency of congestive cardiotoxicity than would be expected to occur with the same cumulative doxorubicin dose given without paclitaxel (discussed previously in Drug Interactions).[208,209] In one study of previously untreated women with advanced breast cancer treated with paclitaxel (3-hour infusion) and doxorubicin, 60 mg/m^2 to a cumulative dose of 480 mg/m^2, which would be predicted to result in a less than 5% incidence of congestive cardiotoxicity in patients treated with doxorubicin alone, the incidence of congestive cardiotoxicity was approximately 25%.[209] However, the incidence of cardiotoxicity was less than 5% when similar patients received identical schedules of paclitaxel and doxorubicin, but the cumulative doxorubicin dose did not exceed 360 mg/m^2. Experimental and early clinical results suggest that dexrazoxane may reduce the cardiotoxicity of the doxorubicin and paclitaxel combination.[230] The rate of congestive heart failure was also higher in breast cancer patients treated with the combination of trastuzumab and paclitaxel than paclitaxel alone in a phase III trial; therefore, careful monitoring of patients receiving this combination is warranted.[231]

Drug-related gastrointestinal effects, such as vomiting and diarrhea, are uncommon. Higher paclitaxel doses or protracted (96-hour) infusional administration may cause mucositis.[232,233] Rare cases of neutropenic enterocolitis and gastrointestinal necrosis have been noted, particularly in patients given high doses of paclitaxel in combination with doxorubicin or cyclophosphamide.[234] Severe hepatotoxicity and pancreatitis have also been noted rarely.[235,236] Acute bilateral pneumonitis has been reported in fewer than 1% of patients treated on a 3-hour schedule in one series, and interstitial and parenchymal pulmonary toxicity have been reported, but clinically significant pulmonary effects are uncommon.[237] Paclitaxel also induces reversible alopecia of the scalp, but all body hair is usually lost with cumulative therapy. Although the agent is often not considered a potent vesicant, in contrast to the vinca alkaloids, extravasation of large volumes can cause moderate soft tissue injury. Inflammation at the injection site and along the course of an injected vein may occur. Paclitaxel also induces reversible alopecia of the scalp in a dose-related fashion, and loss of all facial and body hair is usually lost with cumulative therapy. Alopecia appears to be less profound on weekly schedules, generally occurring after repeated weekly administration. Nail disorders have been reported, particularly in patients treated on weekly schedules.[238] Recall reactions in previously irradiated sites have also been noted.

Docetaxel

Neutropenia is the main toxicity of docetaxel.[122,239] After treatment with docetaxel administered over 1 hour every 3 weeks, the onset of neutropenia is usually noted on day 8 and complete resolution typically occurs by days 15 to 21. At a dose of 100 mg/m^2 administered over 1 hour, neutrophil counts are commonly below 500/μL and the rate of neutropenic sequelae is high. Although the incidence of severe neutropenia at 75 mg/m^2 is also high, the duration of neutropenia and incidence of neutropenic complications are lower than the higher dose. As with paclitaxel, neutropenia is significantly less when low doses are administered frequently (i.e., weekly, as discussed in Administration, Dose, and Schedule). The most important determinant of neutropenia is the extent of prior treatment. Significant effects on platelets and red blood cells are uncommon in patients treated with docetaxel alone.

Despite the fact that docetaxel is not formulated in polyoxyethylated castor oil, hypersensitivity reactions were noted in approximately 31% of patients receiving the drug without premedications in early studies.[122,239] As with paclitaxel, major reactions characterized by dyspnea, bronchospasm, and hypotension typically occur during the first two courses and within minutes after the start of treatment. Signs and symptoms generally resolve within 15 minutes after cessation of treatment, and docetaxel can usually be reinstituted without sequelae after treatment with an H$_1$-receptor antagonist. Fortunately, most events are minor and rarely result in discontinuation of treatment.[223] The incidence and severity of hypersensitivity reactions appear to be reduced by premedication with corticosteroids and H$_1$- and H$_2$-receptor antagonists (discussed later in Administration, Dose, and Schedule), but the corticosteroid premedication regimen is principally administered to prevent fluid retention. As with paclitaxel, patients who experience major reactions have been re-treated successfully after the resolution of symptoms and after treatment with corticosteroids and H$_1$-receptor antagonists. Furthermore, there are several anecdotal reports of patients treated successfully with docetaxel after severe hypersensitivity reactions due to paclitaxel, but it is not known whether these reactions would have occurred if the patients had been re-treated with paclitaxel.[223,240] Docetaxel induces a unique fluid retention syndrome characterized by edema, weight gain, and third-space fluid collection.[122,223,241–243] Fluid retention is cumulative and does not appear to be due to hypoalbuminemia or cardiac, renal, or hepatic dysfunction. Instead, several lines of evidence indicate that it is due to increased capillary permeability.[241] Capillary filtration studies in patients who were not receiving corticosteroid premedication have revealed a two-stage process, with progressive congestion of the interstitial space by proteins and water starting between the second and fourth course and followed by insufficient lymphatic drainage.[241] In early studies, in which prophylactic medication was not used, fluid retention was not usually significant at cumulative docetaxel doses below 400 mg/m^2; however, the incidence and severity of fluid retention increased sharply at cumulative doses of 400 mg/m^2 or greater and often resulted in the delay or termination of treatment. Prophylactic treatment with corticosteroids with or without H$_1$- and H$_2$-receptor antagonists has been demonstrated to reduce the incidence of fluid retention and increase the number of courses and cumulative docetaxel dose before the onset of this toxicity (discussed in Administration, Dose, and Schedule).[242] Fluid retention typically resolves slowly after docetaxel is stopped, with complete resolution occurring several months after treatment in patients with severe toxicity. Aggressive and early treatment with progressively more potent diuretics starting with potassium-sparing diuretics has been successfully used to manage fluid retention.[223,241,242] The incidence of fluid retention has been lower in studies using lower docetaxel doses (60 to 75 mg/m^2) during each course, but this may be due to the administration of lower overall cumulative doses, and the effects of lower doses on antitumor activity are unknown.

Skin toxicity may occur in as many as 50% to 75% of patients[122,223,243,244]; however, premedication may reduce the overall incidence of this effect. An erythematous, pruritic maculopapular rash that affects the forearms, hands, or feet is typical. Other cutaneous effects include desquamation of the hands and feet, palmar-plantar erythrodysesthesia that may respond to pyridoxine or cooling,[242] and onychodystrophy characterized by brown discoloration, ridging, onycholysis, soreness, and brittleness and loss of the nail plate. Skin and nail changes appear to be most prominent in patients treated with high cumulative doses over long periods, particularly on weekly administration schedules.[245]

Docetaxel produces neurotoxicity, which is qualitatively similar to that of paclitaxel.[122,223,244] Patients typically complain of paresthesia and numbness, but peripheral motor effects may also occur. Neurosensory and neuromuscular effects are generally less frequent and less severe with docetaxel as compared to paclitaxel, and preferential use of docetaxel should be considered in high-risk patients in whom taxane treatment is indicated.[223,246,247] Nevertheless, mild to moderate peripheral neurotoxicity occurs in approximately 40% of untreated patients,[122,223,240,248] and patients who had received prior cisplatin appear to be particularly susceptible, with the incidence approaching 74% in one trial.[224,248] Severe toxicity has been unusual after repetitive treatment with docetaxel doses less than 100 mg/m^2, except in patients with antecedent neurotoxicity and relevant disorders, such as alcohol abuse and diabetes mellitus. Transient arthralgia and myalgia are occasionally noted within days after treatment. Asthenia has been a prominent complaint in patients who have been treated with large cumulative doses, particularly when docetaxel is administered on a continuous weekly schedule.[122,223,245,246,249]

Although major cardiovascular events, including angina, arrhythmia, conduction disturbances, congestive heart failure, hypertension, and hypotension, have been noted rarely in the peritreatment period, there is no convincing evidence that directly links docetaxel to these events. Stomatitis appears to occur more frequently with docetaxel than paclitaxel, particularly with prolonged infusions, which are rarely used. Nausea, vomiting, and diarrhea have also been observed infrequently, but severe manifestations are rare. Empiric use of antiemetic premedication does not appear to be warranted. Mild to moderate conjunctivitis, which is responsive to topical corticosteroids, and canalicular stenosis causing lacrimation may also occur, particularly with weekly administration.[250] Nausea, vomiting, and diarrhea have also been observed, but severe gastrointestinal toxicity is rare. Similar to paclitaxel, docetaxel is not a potent vesicant and infusion site reactions are uncommon and generally mild to moderate in severity. Other rare events reported that may or may not be drug related included arrythmias, confusion, erythema multiforme, neutropenic enterocolitis, hepatitis, ileus, interstitial pneumonia, seizures, pulmonary fibrosis, hepatitis, radiation recall, and visual disturbances.[245,249]

ADMINISTRATION, DOSE, AND SCHEDULE

Paclitaxel

Although early clinical evaluation studies were limited to the 24-hour schedule, largely owing to an apparent increased rate of severe hypersensitivity reactions on shorter schedules, the development of effective premedication regimens led to evaluations of a broad range of dosing schedules. Paclitaxel, 135 mg/m^2 on a 24-hour every-3-week schedule, was initially approved for patients with refractory and recurrent ovarian cancer, but regulatory approval was later obtained for paclitaxel, 175 mg/m^2 as a 3-hour infusion. In patients with advanced breast and ovarian cancers, the cumulative body of randomized study results indicates that the schedules are equivalent, particularly with regard to event-free and overall survival, although response rates have occasionally been higher with the 24-hour infusion.[234,251-253,317]

Intriguing results were initially obtained with more protracted infusion schedules, such as a 96-hour infusion in patients with advanced breast cancer.[217,233,254] The development of such schedules was based on the observation that duration of exposure above a biologically relevant threshold is one of the most important determinants of cytotoxicity *in vitro* (discussed earlier in Pharmacology), but there has been no clear evidence that protracted infusions are superior to shorter schedules with regard to clinical efficacy or toxicity.[217,253-256] The extensive and rapid distribution of the taxanes to peripheral tissues and, more importantly, the avid and protracted tissue binding of these agents may explain the lack of differences in antitumor activity between short and more protracted administration schedules despite substantial differences in tissue culture experiments in which the agents are washed out. Considerable interest has also been shown in intermittent schedules, particularly those in which paclitaxel is administered as a 1-hour infusion weekly, which results in substantially less myelosuppression than every-3-week schedules.[245,249,257,258] Although there have been preliminary reports of impressive activity and efficacy of paclitaxel administered weekly in some disease settings,[259] no convincing evidence has been shown that weekly administration results in relevant activity in tumors unresponsive to taxane on every-3-week schedules. Nevertheless, the weekly schedule may offer advantages for patients who are at high risk for development of severe myelosuppression, but there appears to be a higher incidence of neuromuscular effects. Paclitaxel is generally administered every 3 weeks at a dosage of 175 mg/m^2 over 3 hours or 135 to 175 mg/m^2 over 24 hours. Several phase III studies in patients with advanced lung, head and neck, and ovarian cancers have consistently failed to show that paclitaxel doses greater than 135 to 175 mg/m^2 on a 24-hour schedule confer superior efficacy than conventional doses.[217,253,260] Nearly identical results have been obtained in a phase III study in patients with metastatic breast cancer, in which efficacy was not increased in patients treated with paclitaxel doses greater than 175 mg/m^2 on a 3-hour schedule.[353] The following doses have been recommended on less conventional schedules: 200 mg/m^2 over 1 hour as either a single dose or three divided doses every 3 weeks, 140 mg/m^2 over 96 hours every 3 weeks, and 80 to 100 mg/m^2 weekly. The most common schedules evaluated in patients with AIDS-associated Kaposi's sarcoma are paclitaxel, 135 mg/m^2 over 3 or 24 hours every 3 weeks, and 100 mg/m^2 every 2 weeks.[127] Paclitaxel has also been administered into the pleural and peritoneal cavities.[361-363] Biologically relevant plasma concentrations have also been achieved with intraperitoneal administration, and concentrations in the peritoneal cavity are several orders of magnitude greater than plasma concentrations; the results of a single randomized trial indicate that the administration of intraperitoneal paclitaxel in conjunction with carboplatin and paclitaxel administered intravenously confers a survival advantage in previously untreated women with optimally debulked advanced ovarian cancer.[261–263]

The following premedication is recommended to prevent major hypersensitivity reactions: dexamethasone, 20 mg orally or intravenously, 12 and 6 hours before treatment; an H_1-receptor antagonist (e.g., diphenhydramine, 50 mg intravenously) 30 minutes before treatment; and an H_2-receptor antagonist (e.g., cimetidine, 300 mg; famotidine, 20 mg; or ranitidine, 150 mg intravenously) 30 minutes before treatment. A single dose of a corticosteroid (dexamethasone, 20 mg intravenously) administered 30 minutes before treatment also appears to confer effective prophylaxis against major hypersensitivity reactions.[264] Contact of paclitaxel with plasticized polyvinyl chloride equipment or devices must be avoided because of the risk of exposure to plasticizers that may be leached from polyvinyl chloride infusion bags or sets. Paclitaxel solutions should be diluted and stored in glass or polypropylene bottles or suitable plastic bags (polypropylene or polyolefin) and administered through polyethylene-lined administration sets that include an in-line filter with a microporous membrane not greater than 0.22 µm.

The extensive involvement of hepatic metabolism and biliary excretion in the disposition of paclitaxel—similar to that of other anticancer drugs, such as the vinca alkaloids—in which dose modifications are required indicates that doses should be modified in patients with hepatic dysfunction. Official recommendations have not been formulated, but prospective evaluations indicate that patients with moderate to severe elevations in serum concentrations of hepatocellular enzymes or bilirubin (or both) are more likely to develop severe toxicity than patients without hepatic dysfunction.[265] Therefore, it would be prudent to reduce paclitaxel doses by at least 50% in patients with moderate or severe hepatic excretory dysfunction (hyperbilirubinemia) or significant elevations in hepatic transaminases. Renal clearance contributes minimally to overall clearance (5% to 10%), and even patients with severe renal dysfunction do not appear to require dose modification.[266] Based on the pharmacologic behavior, particularly the wide distributive properties of the taxanes, dose modifications are not required solely for peripheral edema and third-space fluid collections.

Docetaxel

In the United States, docetaxel is indicated in a dose range of 60 to 100 mg/m² and 75 mg/m² over 1 hour in patients with breast and non–small cell lung cancers, respectively, but most early trials in patients with advanced breast, ovarian, and non–small cell lung cancers evaluated doses of 75 to 100 mg/m².[173,268] The most common dose schedule used as a single agent or in combination is 75 mg/m² over 1 hour. Although some untreated or minimally pretreated patients generally tolerate docetaxel at a dose of 100 mg/m² without severe toxicity, tolerance is poorer in more heavily pretreated patients, in whom 75 mg/m² is much more reasonable from a toxicologic perspective.[267] Like paclitaxel, docetaxel has also been administered as a 1-hour infusion weekly. Although there are no clear benefits of chronic weekly drug administration in terms of antitumor activity, hematologic effects are much less than conventional dose schedules. Weekly schedules have been associated with higher incidences of cumulative asthenia and neurotoxicity, particularly with docetaxel doses exceeding 36 mg/m²/wk.[223,249] Despite the use of a polysorbate 80 formulation instead of polyoxyethylated castor oil, which is used to formulate paclitaxel, higher rates of hypersensitivity reactions and profound fluid retention than in patients who did not receive premedication led to the use of several effective premedication regimens, the most popular of which is dexamethasone, 8 mg orally twice daily for 3 or 5 days starting 1 or 2 days, respectively, before docetaxel, with or without H_1- and H_2-receptor antagonists given 30 minutes before docetaxel.[223,242]

A retrospective review of docetaxel pharmacokinetics in patients without hyperbilirubinemia demonstrated that docetaxel clearance is reduced by approximately 25% in patients with elevations in serum concentrations of both hepatic transaminases (1.5-fold or greater) and alkaline phosphatase (2.5-fold or greater), regardless of whether the elevations are due to hepatic metastases.[198,199] Therefore, dose reductions by at least 25% are recommended for such individuals. More substantial reductions (50% or greater) may be required in patients who have moderate or severe hepatic excretory dysfunction (hyperbilirubinemia). As with paclitaxel (discussed previously in Administration, Dose, and Schedule, Paclitaxel), there is no rationale for dose modification solely for renal deficiency or third-space fluid accumulation (or both). Also similar to the case with paclitaxel, glass bottles or polypropylene or polyolefin plastic products should be used for preparation and storage, and docetaxel should be administered through polyethylene-lined administration sets.

ESTRAMUSTINE PHOSPHATE

Estramustine (Fig. 15.8-4), a conjugate of the alkylating agent nor-nitrogen mustard linked to 17β-estradiol by a carbamate

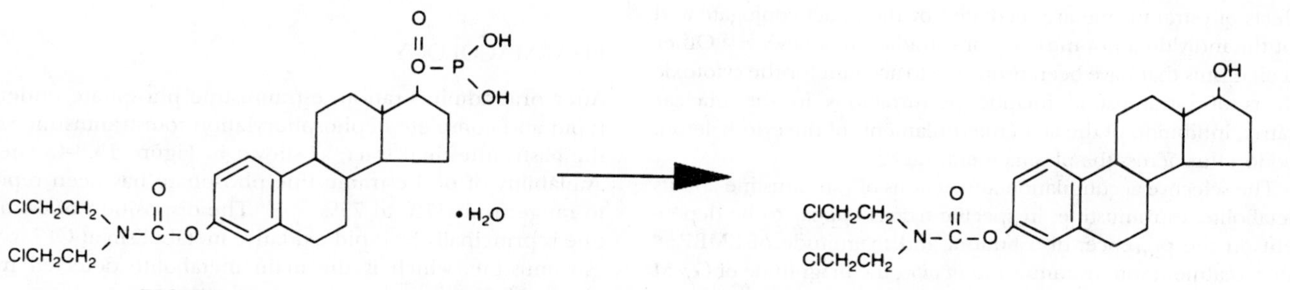

FIGURE 15.8-4. Structure of estramustine phosphate undergoing dephosphorylation to estramustine.

ester bridge, is administered as the prodrug estramustine phosphate, which is rapidly dephosphorylated after oral administration by gastrointestinal tract phosphatases to produce estramustine. Estramustine was originally synthesized so that the 17β-estradiol component would specifically bind to, and accumulate in, estrogen receptor–bearing breast cancer cells and selectively deliver the nor-nitrogen mustard alkylating moiety, after degradation of the carbamate ester. However, the agent did not demonstrate significant anticancer activity in clinical trials in patients with breast cancer and, thereafter, it was determined that alkylation of DNA did not occur.[268] Further studies in rats treated with radiolabeled estramustine phosphate established that the agent preferentially accumulated in the ventral prostate in a manner that was not related to the estrogen receptor.[269] This selective accumulation was mediated by a specific protein in prostate tissue termed the *estramustine-binding protein* (EMBP).[269,270] Clinical studies of estramustine phosphate were then initiated in patients with prostate cancer based on estramustine's unique pattern of distribution, and anticancer activity was demonstrated in patients with prostate cancers refractory to the estrogen analogue diethylstilbestrol.[271]

MECHANISM OF ACTION

Although several mechanisms have been proposed to account for the principal cytotoxic actions of estramustine, the preponderance of experimental data indicate that the agent perturbs microtubule dynamics. Estramustine depolymerizes microtubules and microfilaments, binds to and disrupt MAPs, and inhibits cell growth at high concentrations, resulting in mitotic arrest and apoptosis in tumor cells.[272,273] In the prostate cancer cell line DU145, for example, the IC_{50} (inhibitory concentration) for estramustine is 16 μmol, whereas the IC_{50} value for VBL (3 nmol) is 5000-fold lower.[1] Estramustine binds to β-tubulin (K_d approximately equal to 23 μmol) at a site distinct from the colchicine and vinca alkaloid binding sites, and its binding affinity to β-tubulin is tubulin isotype dependent.[1,273,275] Although the phosphorylated form binds to MAPs and estramustine itself binds to other cellular proteins besides tubulin, the drug's interaction with tubulin appears to be principally responsible for its anticancer activity.[273–276] Estramustine reduces the rates of microtubule lengthening and shortening, inhibits dynamic instability and polymerization of MAP-free microtubules, and modestly increases microtubule mass.[273,277–279] Although estramustine may affect microtubules that comprise the interphase cytoskeleton, it principally affects microtubules of the mitotic spindle apparatus and induces arrest in G_2/M. Similar to the vinca alkaloids and taxanes, estramustine-induced mitotic arrest is often followed by the induction of apoptosis. The aforementioned antimicrotubule effects of estramustine are mediated by the intact conjugate and not the individual nor-nitrogen or estradiol moieties.[273,274] Other mechanisms that have been proposed to account for the cytotoxic effects of estramustine include perturbations in the nuclear matrix, inhibition of the actin microfilaments of the cytoskeleton, and ion flux across the plasma membrane.[280,281]

The selective accumulation and actions of estramustine and its metabolite, estromustine, in specific tissues appear to be dependent on the presence, distribution, and magnitude of EMBP.[279] After treatment with estramustine *in vitro*, the magnitude of G_2/M phase arrest appears to be directly related to intracellular concentrations of EMBP.[279,280] In addition to prostate cancer, EMBP and related binding proteins have been identified in malignant brain tumors.[281–284] Because estramustine phosphate blocks cell-cycle traverse in G_2/M, crosses the blood–brain barrier, and accumulates in gliomas and astrocytomas, its potential to selectively sensitize brain tumors to irradiation is being evaluated.[285]

MECHANISMS OF RESISTANCE

Three distinct mechanisms of resistance have been characterized in experimental cell lines that have been selected for resistance to estramustine and include alterations in β-tubulin isotype expression, alterations in MAP expression, and ATP-dependent drug efflux. As previously discussed in this chapter in the section Microtubules, tissues and tumors have distinct compositions of β-tubulin isotypes, which may influence drug sensitivity. Prostate cancer cell lines with acquired resistance to estramustine have been shown to possess higher ratios of $β_{III}$- and $β_{IVa}$-tubulin isotypes relative to other β-tubulin isotypes in drug-sensitive parental cells.[276,286] Microtubules containing the $β_{III}$-tubulin isotype appear to bind estramustine less avidly than other β-tubulin isotypes, and tumor cells with high levels of $β_{III}$-tubulin have been reported to be less prone to the inhibitory and destabilizing effects of estramustine on microtubule dynamics.[276,286–288] However, the transfection of the gene encoding $β_{III}$-tubulin into DU145 prostate cancer cells with resultant overexpression of $β_{III}$-tubulin protein has neither conferred resistance to estramustine nor to other antimicrotubule agents.[288] These results suggest that estramustine resistance in experimental cell lines that overexpress $β_{III}$-tubulin is multifactorial, including the aggregate expression of multiple tubulin isotypes ($β_{II}$, $β_{III}$, and $β_{IVb}$), not necessarily overexpression of a single isotype.[288]

Some prostate cancer cell lines with acquired resistance to estramustine overexpress the MAP tau.[289] Exposure to estramustine induces quantitative and qualitative changes in tau, leading to a sevenfold increase in estramustine resistance in some cancer cell lines.[289] However, the extent to which alterations in tau or other altered MAPs contribute to clinical estramustine resistance is not known.

Although estramustine is a substrate for the drug efflux pump characterized by the MDR phenotype, P-gp does not necessarily confer resistance to estramustine.[290,291] Evidence has indicated that estramustine may, in fact, competitively inhibit P-gp function, reducing the efflux of cytotoxic agents that are substrates for P-gp.[290,291] Another drug efflux mechanism, distinct from MDR1, that can mediate estramustine resistance has also been described.[291] Cells that exhibit this mechanism of resistance have amplifications of the ABC2 transporter gene and demonstrate a magnitude of estramustine resistance that is proportional to the level of ABC2 gene amplification.[292]

PHARMACOLOGY

After oral administration, estramustine phosphate undergoes rapid and complete dephosphorylation to estramustine within the gastrointestinal tract, as shown in Figure 15.8-4. The bioavailability of oral estramustine phosphate has been reported to range from 37% to 75%.[293,294] The disposition of estramustine is principally by rapid oxidative metabolism at C17 to yield estromustine, which is the main metabolite detected in the plasma.[295] Estromustine concentrations in plasma are maximal within 2 to 4 hours after oral administration, and the mean elimination half-life of estromustine is 14 hours.[293] The pharmacokinetic behavior of estromustine in plasma is linear after oral administration of estramustine phosphate in its therapeutic dosing range. In patients treated orally with estramustine phosphate, 560 mg/d, peak plasma concentrations average 227 ng/mL for estromustine, 23 ng/mL for estramustine, 95 ng/mL for estrone, and 9.3 ng/mL for estradiol.[295]

Significant first-pass hepatic metabolism occurs after oral administration of estramustine phosphate, resulting in marked interpatient variability in drug metabolism. Further hydrolysis of estromustine and its carbamate linker in the liver results in the formation of estrone and the release of the alkylating group. After oral and intravenous administration of radiolabeled estramustine phosphate in humans, estromustine and estramustine are principally excreted in the feces, with only small amounts of conjugated estrone and estradiol detected in the urine (less than 1%).[293–296] Although the pathways responsible for hepatic metabolism of estramustine, estromustine, and the estrogen metabolites have not been fully elucidated, hepatic CYP1A2 and CYP3A4 enzymes are largely responsible for oxidative metabolism of estradiol- and estrone-like steroids in hepatic microsome studies.[297]

An intravenous formulation of estramustine phosphate, which is available only for investigational use in the United States, results in 10- to 15-fold higher peak plasma concentrations of estramustine phosphate, estramustine, and estromustine than those achieved after oral administration.[293–298] The parenteral formulation is also associated with markedly less interpatient variability in pharmacokinetics.[293–298] The absence of first-pass hepatic metabolism with parenteral administration results in lower clearance rates; the terminal half-lives of elimination for estramustine phosphate, estromustine, and estramustine average 3.7, 110.0, and 64.0 hours, respectively, after intravenous administration.[296] The reduced clearance of intravenous estramustine results in the accumulation of estromustine, estramustine, estradiol, and estrone in the plasma of patients treated on weekly intravenous dosing regimens.[298]

DRUG INTERACTIONS

Coadministration of food, particularly dairy products, significantly impairs the gastrointestinal absorption of estramustine phosphate.[299] Calcium-rich foods appear to result in the formation of poorly absorbable calcium complexes. Therefore, it is recommended that patients fast for at least 2 hours before oral administration of estramustine phosphate and avoid calcium-rich food and antacids.

Estramustine phosphate reduces the systemic clearance of docetaxel and paclitaxel, most likely by inhibiting the effects of estramustine on the P-450 CYP3A4 isoenzyme, which is principally responsible for taxane clearance.[297,300,301] Therefore, the recommended doses of docetaxel and paclitaxel in combination with estramustine phosphate are less than single-agent doses, despite the fact that the taxanes and estramustine phosphate do not have common toxicities.

Toxicity

Nausea and vomiting, which are the principal toxicities encountered with oral estramustine phosphate, may occasionally require modification of dose schedule or termination of treatment. On conventional dose schedules, nausea and vomiting are readily managed with standard antiemetic medications. Diarrhea has also been observed in patients treated with estramustine phosphate for protracted periods. Myelosuppression is rarely clinically relevant in patients treated with estramustine phosphate as a single agent. Common estrogenic side effects of treatment with estramustine phosphate include gynecomastia, nipple tenderness, and fluid retention. Caution should be exercised in prescribing estramustine phosphate to patients with a history of congestive heart failure because of the risk for fluid retention and edema, which can result in a decompensated cardiac state. Thromboembolic complications, including venous thrombosis, pulmonary emboli, and cerebrovascular and coronary thrombotic events, which may occur in up to 10% of patients, represent the most serious toxicities of estramustine phosphate. The cardiovascular effects of oral estramustine phosphate have been attributed to high intrahepatic concentrations of estrogenic metabolites, which result in reduced antithrombin III levels and hypercoagulability.[302] Transient elevations in hepatic transaminases have been reported in approximately 33% of patients. In a phase III study, in which patients with advanced prostate carcinoma were randomized to treatment with either estramustine phosphate or diethylstilbestrol, the rates of hepatic toxicity were similar on both treatment arms. Clinically relevant hypocalcemia is an uncommon toxicity of estramustine phosphate.[303] Pathogenic mechanisms that have been proposed to explain this toxicity, which is often acute, include uptake of calcium by osteoblastic metastases, increased uptake of calcium by healing bone lesions, or, alternatively, the unmasking of a subclinical vitamin D–deficient state. Asymptomatic reductions in serum calcium concentrations occur in up to 20% of patients.

Acute perianal and/or perineal pain A toxicity has been noted in patients receiving estramustine phosphate by the intravenous route. This toxicity can be minimized by administering the agent over a more protracted infusion duration (60 to 90 minutes).[297]

ADMINISTRATION, DOSE, AND SCHEDULE

Estramustine phosphate has received regulatory approval for treating patients with hormone-refractory prostate cancer (HRPC). The recommended daily dose of estramustine phosphate, which is available as a 140-mg capsule, is 14 mg/kg body weight in three to four divided daily doses; however, patients are usually treated in the daily dosing range of 10 to 16 mg/kg. Estramustine phosphate should be administered with water at least 1 hour before or 2 hours after meals. Patients are generally treated for 30 to 90 days before assessment of therapeutic benefit. Chronic oral therapy can be maintained for months or even years. Abbreviated 1-, 3-, and 5-day courses of oral estramustine phosphate have been proposed for use in combination with other chemotherapeutic agents, particularly paclitaxel and docetaxel.[300,304,305] These schedules permit the concurrent administration of estramustine phosphate with intravenous therapeutics, while minimizing protracted nausea, vomiting, and diarrhea associated with chronic oral administration. In studies with docetaxel using this abbreviated schedule, the recommended dose of estramustine phosphate is 280 mg three times daily (approximately 600 mg/m^2/d) for 5 days.[301]

Although therapy with estramustine mediates the cytotoxic effects principally by disrupting microtubules, encouraging antitumor activity has been noted in patients with HRPC who have been treated with estramustine phosphate in combination with other antimicrotubule targeting agents. In a randomized trial, in which patients with HRPC were treated with either estramustine phosphate plus weekly intravenous VBL or VBL alone, overall and progression-free survival were superior in patients treated with combined therapy.[306] Furthermore, single- and multicenter phase II studies of the combination of estramustine phosphate and docetaxel have demonstrated decrements in prostate-specific antigen in 50% of patients, as well as encouraging survival data.[301,307] These results were the impetus for an ongoing pivotal phase III study comparing treatment with estramustine plus docetaxel to mitoxantrone plus prednisone in patients with HRPC.

NOVEL COMPOUNDS TARGETING MICROTUBULES

The success with the taxanes has provided the impetus to discover new chemotypes that have similar mechanisms of action but yet evade mechanisms of taxane resistance and confer less toxicity, thereby conferring higher therapeutic indices. Several classes of natural products, including the epothilones, eleutherobins, discodermolides, sarcodictyins, and laulimalides (Fig. 15.8-5) that promote tubulin polymerization, have been identified.[1,2] The epothilones were isolated from the myxobacterium *Sorangium cellulosum*, eleutherobins from the soft coral *Eleutherobia* species, sarcodictyins from the Mediterranean stoloniferan coral *Sarcodictyon roseum*, and laulimalides from the marine sponge *Cacospongia mycofijiensis*. Eleutherobin, discodermolide, and laulimalide are especially potent, with K_i values in the 5 to 40 nM range.[1,2] All of the aforementioned compounds possess either low-level or no substrate affinity for P-gp and other ABC transporters and retain various degrees of activity against taxane-resistant cells *in vitro*, but the clinical significance of these characteristics is not clear.[1,2]

Not only do the epothilones promote tubulin polymerization and induce mitotic arrest, but many epothilones possess significantly greater cytotoxic potency than either paclitaxel or docetaxel.[308–310] The epothilones, like the taxanes, induce tubulin polymerization in the absence of GTP or MAPs, or both, resulting in microtubules that are relatively long, rigid, and resistant to destabilization. However, the epothilones are generally more potent than the taxanes, possessing IC_{50} values in the sub- or low nanomolar range.[1,2,308–310] In contrast to the taxanes and vinca alkaloids, overexpression of P-gp minimally affects the cytotoxicity of epothilones A and B.[1,2,308–310] In addition, various point mutations in β-tubulin, which confer resistance to the taxanes *in vitro*, are not necessarily responsible for resistance to the epothilones, but the significance of β-tubulin isotypes in conferring clinical resistance to tubulin-polymerizing agents is not clear. Epothilone B (EPO906) and the epothilone B analogue BMS-247550 are currently undergoing clinical evaluations.[311,312] BMS-247550 is metabolized by cytochrome P-450 systems, whereas EPO906 is metabolized by carboxyesterases.[311,312] These differences may be responsible for their different principal toxicities, namely diarrhea (EPO906) and myelosuppression and neurotoxicity (BMS-247550).[311,312] In early clinical trials, antitumor responses have been noted in patients with breast, lung, and ovarian cancers, some of which recurred after or during treatment with the taxanes.[311,312] Antitumor activity has also been observed with EPO906 in patients with colorectal and renal cancers, which are almost always unresponsive to antimicrotubule agents, but the magnitude of appreciable activity in cancers with primary or acquired taxane resistance is negligible.[311,312] Epothilone D (desoxyepothilone B; KOS862), which possesses equivalent potency and less toxicity than the taxane and epothilone B analogues in preclinical studies, is also undergoing clinical development.[313]

Similar to the epothilones A and B, discodermolide-induced tubulin polymers are very stable to treatment with calcium and composed of short microtubules instead of tubulin spirals.[1,2,314] In addition to complete cross-resistance to P-gp–overexpressing cancer cells, paclitaxel and epothilone-resistant human tumor cells that express mutant β-tubulin retain sensitivity to discodermolide.[1,2,314] Furthermore, discodermolide and paclitaxel have demonstrated synergistic cytotoxicity *in vitro*, suggesting that their tubulin-binding sites may not be identical.[315] Early clinical evaluations with discodermolide (XAA296) have begun in patients with advanced solid malignancies. The marine soft coral–derived natural products—sarcodictyins A and B and eleutherobin—also promote tubulin polymerization in a manner analogous to that of paclitaxel.[1,2,316] The marine-derived, microtubule-stabilizing cytotoxins laulimalide and isolaulimalide appear to be poor substrates for ABC transporters such as P-gp.[1,2,317] Because eleutherobin, epothilones A and B, and discodermolide competitively inhibit paclitaxel binding to microtubules, a common pharmacophore was sought and identified, which may enable the development of hybrid constructs with more desirable biologic characteristics.[318]

Other natural products and semisynthetic antimicrotubule compounds under evaluation interact with tubulin in the vinca alkaloid– or colchicine-binding domains. Among the most potent are the cryptophycin depsipeptides, which are a family of cyanobacterial macrolides that deplete microtubules in intact cells, including cells with the MDR phenotype.[1,2,319] The cryptophycins compete for the binding of VBL and inhibit GTP hydrolysis by isolated tubulin. Picomolar concentrations induce cytotoxicity in preclinical studies, which may be attrib-

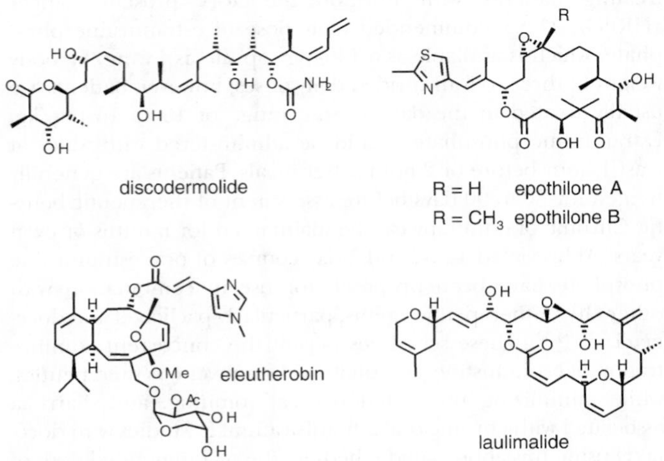

discodermolide

R = H   epothilone A
R = CH₃ epothilone B

eleutherobin

laulimalide

FIGURE 15.8-5. Structures of discodermolide, epothilones A and B, eleutherobin, and laulimalide.

uted to their high affinity for tubulin and low reversibility after binding. The cryptophycins also have impressive activity against a wide array of human tumor xenografts, including those resistant to the vinca alkaloids. However, the clinical development of one semisynthetic analogue, cryptophycin-52, was terminated after an unacceptably low level of antitumor activity and significant toxicity, particularly neurotoxicity, were noted in clinical studies. The dolastatins constitute a series of oligopeptides isolated from the sea hare, *Dolabela auricularia*.[1,2,320] Two of the most potent dolastatins, dolastatin-10 and -15, noncompetitively inhibit the binding of the vinca alkaloids to tubulin, inhibit tubulin polymerization and tubulin-dependent GTP hydrolysis, stabilize the colchicine-binding activity of tubulin, and possess cytotoxic activity in the picomolar to low nanomolar range. Dolastatin-10 and semisynthetic dolastatin analogues are undergoing clinical evaluations.[1,2] Phomopsin A, halichondrin B, homohalichondrin B, and spongistatin 1, which competitively inhibit vinca alkaloid binding to tubulin, are also in various stages of development.[1,2,320,321] Halichondrin B, a large polyether macrolide originally isolated from the marine sponge *Halicondrin okadai*, and less complex synthetic marocyclic ketone analogues (ER-076349 and ER-086526) are undergoing clinical development. These compounds bind to tubulin, inhibit tubulin polymerization, disrupt mitotic spindle formation, induce mitotic arrest, and inhibit the growth of tumors at subnanomolar concentrations.

NOVEL COMPOUNDS TARGETING MITOTIC MOTOR PROTEINS

Although tubulin is the most abundant protein component of the mitotic spindle apparatus, many additional proteins, such as mitotic kinesins, play critical roles in the mechanics of mitosis and in progression through the premitotic cell-cycle checkpoint. Kinesins are motor proteins that convert chemical energy released by the hydrolysis of ATP into mechanical force for movement of a wide variety of cellular organelles and cargoes, depending on the particular kinesin and cell type.[23,322] The mitotic kinesins are a subgroup of kinesin motor proteins that function exclusively in mitosis.[23,322] During mitosis, different, highly specialized mitotic kinesins play critical roles in various aspects of mitotic spindle assembly, including the establishment of spindle bipolarity, spindle pole organization, chromosome alignment and segregation, and regulation of microtubule dynamics. The establishment of mitotic spindle bipolarity is among the earliest events in spindle assembly, and it requires the function of the kinesin motor protein KSP (also known as *Eg5*), which has no known role outside of mitosis. The expression profiles of KSP messenger RNA in normal tissues are consistent with preferential expression of KSP in proliferating cells relative to normal adjacent tissue. As essential elements in mitotic spindle assembly and function, KSP and mitotic kinesins provide attractive targets for intervention into the cell cycle. A therapeutic targeting KSP may also be devoid of the potential for neurotoxicity or other side effects caused by the disruption of tubulin dynamics in nondividing cells. A polycyclic, nitrogen-containing heterocycle, SB-715992, is the first KSP-targeting therapeutic to enter clinical trials.[323,324] The compound, which is 10,000-fold more selective for KSP than other kines-

ins, blocks assembly of a functional mitotic spindle, thereby causing cell-cycle arrest in mitosis followed by apoptosis.

REFERENCES

1. Jordan MA. Mechanism of action of antitumor drugs that interact with microtubules and tubulin. *Curr Med Chem Anti-Canc Agents* 2002;2:1.
2. Kavallaris M, Verrills NM, Hill BT. Anticancer therapy with novel tubulin-interacting drugs. *Drug Resist Updates* 2001;4:392.
3. Gelfand VI, Bershadsky AD. Microtubule dynamics: mechanism, regulation, and function. *Annu Rev Cell Biol* 1991;7:93.
4. Hyams JF, Lloyd CW. *Microtubules.* New York: Wiley-Liss, 1993.
5. Nogales E, Whittaker M, Milligan RA, Downing KH. High-resolution model of the microtubule. *Cell* 1999;96:78.
6. Correia JJ, Lobert S. Physiochemical aspects of tubulin-interacting antimitotic drugs. *Curr Pharm Des* 2001;7:1213.
7. Luduena RF. Multiple forms of tubulin: different gene products and covalent modifications. *Int Rev Cytol* 1998;178:207.
8. Khan A, Luduena F. Different effects of vinblastine on the polymerization of isotypically purified tubulins from bovine brain. *Invest New Drugs* 2003;21:3.
9. Druckman S, Kavallaris M. Microtubule alterations and resistance to tubulin-binding agents. *Int J Oncol* 2002;21:621.
10. Margolis RL, Wilson L. Microtubule treadmilling: what goes around comes around. *Bioessays* 1998;20:830.
11. Mitchison T, Kirchner M. Dynamic instability of microtubule growth. *Nature* 1984;312:237.
12. Wilson L, Jordan MA. Microtubule dynamics: taking aim at a moving target *Chem Biol* 1995;2:569.
13. Rusan NM, Fagerstrom CJ, Yvon A, Wadsworth P. Cell cycle-dependent changes in microtubule dynamics in living cells expressing green fluorescent protein-alpha tubulin. *Mol Biol* 2001;111:3003.
14. Yvon A-M, Wadsworth P, Jordan MA. Taxol suppresses dynamics of individual microtubules in living human tumor cells. *Mol Biol Cell* 1999;10:947.
15. Jordan MA, Wendell KL, Gardiner S, et al. Mitotic block induced in HeLa cells by low concentrations of paclitaxel (Taxol) results in abnormal mitotic exit and apoptotic cell death. *Cancer Res* 1996;56:816.
16. Schliwa M, Woehlke G. Molecular motors. *Nature* 2003;422:759.
17. Johnson IS. Historical background of vinca alkaloid research and areas of future interest. *Cancer Chemother Rep* 1968;52:455.
18. Gidding CE, Kellie SJ, Kamps WA, de Graaf SS. Vincristine revisited. *Crit Rev Oncol Hematol* 1999;29:267.
19. Johnson IS, Armstrong JG, Gorman M, et al. The vinca alkaloids: a new class of oncolytic agents. *Cancer Res* 1963;23:1390.
20. Rowinsky EK, Donehower RC. The clinical pharmacology and use of antimicrotubule agents in cancer chemotherapeutics. *Pharmacol Ther* 1992;52:35.
21. Joel S. The comparative clinical pharmacology of vincristine and vindesine: does vindesine offer any advantage in clinical use? *Cancer Treat Rev* 1995;21:513.
22. Budman DR. Vinorelbine (Navelbine): a third-generation vinca alkaloid. *Cancer Invest* 1997;15:475.
23. Johnson SA, Harper P, Hortobagyi GN, Pouillart P. Vinorelbine: an overview. *Cancer Treat Rev* 1996;22:127.
24. Himes RH. Interactions of the catharanthus (vinca) alkaloids with tubulin and microtubules. *Pharmacol Ther* 1991;51:256.
25. Jordan MA, Thrower D, Wilson L. Mechanism of inhibition of cell proliferation by the vinca alkaloids. *Cancer Res* 1991;51:2212.
26. Jordan MA, Thrower D, Wilson L. Effects of vinblastine, podophyllotoxin and nocodazole on mitotic spindles. Implications for the role of microtubule dynamics in mitosis. *J Cell Sci* 1992;102:401.
27. Wilson L, Jordan MA. Pharmacological probes of microtubule function. In: Hyams JF, Lloyd CD, eds. *Microtubules.* New York: Wiley-Liss, 1993:59.
28. Howard SMH, Theologides A, Sheppard JR. Comparative effects of vindesine, vinblastine, and vincristine on mitotic arrest and hormone response of L1210 leukemia cells. *Cancer Res* 1980;40:2695.
29. Beck WT. Alkaloids. In: Fox BW, Fox M, eds. *Antitumor drug resistance.* Berlin: Springer-Verlag, 1984:589.
30. Jordan MA, Margolis RL, Himes RH, Wilson LJ. Identification of a distinct class of vinblastine binding sites on microtubules. *J Mol Biol* 1986;187:61.
31. Jordan MA, Wilson L. Kinetic analysis of tubulin exchange at microtubule ends at low vinblastine concentrations. *Biochemistry* 1990;29:2730.
32. Lobert S, Fahy J, Hill BT, et al. Vinca alkaloid-induced tubulin spiral formation correlates with cytotoxicity in the leukemic L1210 cell line. *Biochemistry* 2000;39:12053.
33. Ngan V, Bellman K, Hill B, Wilson L, Jordan M. Novel actions of the antitumor drugs vinflunine and vinorelbine on microtubules. *Mol Pharmacol* 2001;60:225.
34. Jordan MA, Himes RH, Wilson L. Comparison of the effects of vinblastine, vincristine, indesine, and vinepidine on microtubule dynamics and cell proliferation in vitro. *Cancer Res* 1985;45:2741.
35. Lobert S, Correia JJ. Energetics of vinca alkaloid interactions with tubulin. *Methods Enzymol* 2000;323:77.
36. Lengfeld AM, Dietrich J, Schultze-Maurer B. Accumulation and release of vinblastine and vincristine in HeLa cells: light microscopic, cinematographic, and biochemical study. *Cancer Res* 1982;42:3798.

37. Bleyer WA, Frisby SA, Oliverio VT. Uptake and binding of vincristine by murine leukemia cells. *Biochem Pharmacol* 1975;24:633.
38. Zhou XJ, Placidi M, Rahmani R. Uptake and metabolism of vinca alkaloids by freshly isolated human hepatocytes in suspension. *Anticancer Res* 1994;14:1017.
39. Rahmani R, Zhou XJ. Pharmacokinetics and metabolism of vinca alkaloids. In: Workman P, Graham, M, eds. *Cancer surveys, vol 17: pharmacokinetics and cancer chemotherapy.* Plainview, NY: Cold Spring Harbor Laboratory Press, 1993:269.
40. Ferguson PJ, Cass CE. Differential cellular retention of vincristine and vinblastine by cultured human promyelocytic leukemia HL-60/C-1 cells: the basis of differential toxicity. *Cancer Res* 1985;45:5480.
41. Jackson DV, Bender RA. Cytotoxic thresholds of vincristine in a murine and human leukemia cell line in vitro. *Cancer Res* 1979;39:4346.
42. Ferguson PJ, Philips JR, Seiner M, Cass CE. Biochemical effects of Navelbine on tubulin and associated proteins. *Cancer Res* 1984;44:3307.
43. Himes RH, Kersey RN, Heller-Bettinger I, Sampson FE. Action of the vinca alkaloids, vincristine and vinblastine, and desacetyl vinblastine amide on microtubules in vitro. *Cancer Res* 1976;36:3798.
44. Lobert S, Vulevic B, Correria JJ. Interaction of vinca alkaloids with tubulin: a comparison of vinblastine, vincristine, and vinorelbine. *Biochemistry* 1996;35:6806.
45. Lockhart A, Tirona G, Kim B. Pharmacogenetics of ATP-binding cassette transporters in cancer and chemotherapy. *Mol Ther* 2003;2:695.
46. Safa AR, Glover CJ, Meyers MB, et al. Vinblastine photoaffinity labeling of a high molecular weight surface membrane glycoprotein specific for multidrug-resistant cells. *Biochemistry* 1987;262:13685.
47. Greenberger LM, Williams SS, Horwitz SB. Biosynthesis of heterogeneous forms of multidrug resistance associated glycoproteins. *J Biol Chem* 1987;262:13685.
48. Choi K, Chen C, Kriegler M, Roninson IB. An altered pattern of cross-resistance in multidrug-resistant human cells results from spontaneous mutations in the mdr1 (P-glycoprotein) gene. *Cell* 1988;53:519.
49. Peterson RHF, Meyers MB, Spengler BA. Alterations of plasma membrane glycopeptides and gangliosides of Chinese hamster cells accompanying development of resistance to daunorubicin and vincristine. *Cancer Res* 1983;43:222.
50. Pieters R, Hongo T, Loonen AH, et al. Different types of non-P-glycoprotein mediated multiple drug resistance in children with relapsed acute lymphoblastic leukemia. *Br J Cancer* 1992;65:691.
51. Zaman GJ, Floens JM, van Leusden MR, et al. The human multidrug resistance-protein MRP is a plasma membrane drug-efflux pump. *Proc Natl Acad Sci U S A* 1994;91:8822.
52. Betrand Y, Capdeville R, Balduck N, et al. Cyclosporin A used to reverse drug resistance increases vincristine neurotoxicity. *Am J Hematol* 1992;40:158.
53. Pinkerton CR. Multidrug resistance reversal in childhood malignancies potential for a real step forward? *Eur J Cancer* 1996;32A:641.
54. List AF, Kopecky KJ, Willman CL, et al. Benefit of cyclosporine modulation of drug resistance in patients with poor-risk acute myeloid leukemia: a Southwest Oncology Group Study. *Blood* 2001;98:3212.
55. Houghton JA, Houghton PJ, Hazelton BJ, Douglas EC. In situ selection of a human rhabdomyosarcoma resistant to vincristine with altered α-tubulins. *Cancer Res* 1985;45:2706.
56. Cabral FR, Barlow SB. Resistance to the antimitotic agents as genetic probes of microtubule structure and function. *Pharmacol Ther* 1991;52:159.
57. Reichle A, Diddens H, Altmayr F, et al. Beta-tubulin and P-glycoprotein: major determinants of vincristine accumulation in B-CLL cells. *Leuk Res* 1995:19:823.
58. Hari M, Wang Y, Veeraraghavan S. Mutations in alpha- and beta-tubulin that stabilize microtubules and confer resistance to colcemid and vinblastine. *Mol Cancer Ther* 2003;2:597.
59. Nelson RL, Dyke RW, Root MA. Comparative pharmacokinetics of vindesine, vincristine, and vinblastine in patients with cancer. *Cancer Treat Rev* 1980;7[Suppl]:17.
60. Rahmani R, Bruno R, Iliadis A, et al. Clinical pharmacokinetics of the antitumor drug Navelbine (5'-noranhydrovinblastine). *Cancer Res* 1987;47:5796.
61. Jehl F, Quoix E, Leveque D, et al. Pharmacokinetic and preliminary metabolic fate of Navelbine in humans as determined by high performance liquid chromatography. *Cancer Res* 1991;51:2073.
62. Jackson DV Jr. The periwinkle alkaloids. In: Lokich JJ, ed. *Cancer chemotherapy by infusion.* Chicago: Precept Press Inc, 1990:155.
63. Bender RA, Castle MC, Margileth DA, Oliverio VT. The pharmacokinetics of [3H]-vincristine in man. *Clin Pharmacol Ther* 1977;22:430.
64. Sethi VS, Jackson DV, White CT, et al. Pharmacokinetics of vincristine sulfate in adult cancer patients. *Cancer Res* 1981;41:3551.
65. Zhou XJ, Martin M, Placidi M, et al. In vivo and in vitro pharmacokinetics and metabolism of vinca alkaloids: II. Vinblastine and vincristine. *Eur J Drug Metab Pharmacokinet* 1990;15:323.
66. Owellen RJ, Root MA, Hains FO. Pharmacokinetic of vindesine and vincristine in humans. *Cancer Res* 1977;37:2603.
67. Jackson DV, Castle MC, Bender RA. Biliary excretion of vincristine. *Clin Pharmacol Ther* 1978;24:101.
68. Owellen RJ, Hartke CA, Hains FO. Pharmacokinetics and metabolism of vinblastine in humans. *Cancer Res* 1977;37:2597.
69. Zhou-Pan XR, Seree E, Zhou XJ, et al. Involvement of human liver cytochrome P450 3A in vinblastine metabolism: drug interactions. *Cancer Res* 1993;53:5121.
70. Rahmani R, Zhou XJ, Placidi M, et al. In vivo and in vitro pharmacokinetics and metabolism of vinca alkaloids in rat. I. Vindesine (4-deacetyl-vinblastine 3-carboxyamide). *Eur J Drug Metab Pharmacokinet* 1990;15:49.
71. Hande K, Gay J, Gober J, Greco FA. Toxicity and pharmacology of bolus vindesine injection and prolonged vindesine infusion. *Cancer Treat Rev* 1980;7:25.
72. Jackson DV Jr, Sethi VS, Long TR, et al. Pharmacokinetics of vindesine bolus and infusion. *Cancer Chemother Pharmacol* 1994;13:114.
73. Ohnuma T, Norton L, Andrejczuk A, Holland JF. Pharmacokinetics of vindesine given as an intravenous bolus and 24-hour infusion in humans. *Cancer Res* 1985;45:464.
74. Rahmani R, Martin M, Favre R, et al. Clinical pharmacokinetics of vindesine: repeated treatments by intravenous bolus injections. *Eur J Cancer Clin Oncol* 1984;20:1409.
75. Zhou XJ, Zhou-Pan XR, Gauthier T, et al. Human liver microsomal cytochrome P450 3A isoenzymes mediated vindesine biotransformation: metabolic drug interactions. *Biomed Pharmacol* 1993;4:853.
76. Levêque D, Jehl F. Clinical pharmacokinetics of vinorelbine. *Clin Pharmacokinet* 1996;31:184.
77. Jehl F, Quoix E, Levêque D, et al. Pharmacokinetic and preliminary metabolic fate of Navelbine in humans as determined by high performance liquid chromatography. *Cancer Res* 1991;51:2073.
78. Rowinsky EK, Noe DA, Lucas VS, et al. A phase I, pharmacokinetic and absolute bioavailability study of oral vinorelbine (Navelbine) in solid tumor patients. *J Clin Oncol* 1994;12:1754.
79. Rahmani R, Gueritte F, Martin M, et al. Comparative pharmacokinetics of antitumor vinca alkaloids: intravenous bolus injections of Navelbine and related alkaloids to cancer patients and rats. *Cancer Chemother Pharmacol* 1986;16:223.
80. Levêque D, Merle-Melet M, Bresler L, et al. Biliary elimination and pharmacokinetics of vinorelbine in micropigs. *Cancer Chemother Pharmacol* 1993;32:487.
81. Krikorian A, Rahmani R, Bromet M, et al. Pharmacokinetics and metabolism of Navelbine. *Semin Oncol* 1989;16[Suppl 4]:21.
82. Bender RA, Bleyer WA, Frisby SA. Alteration of methotrexate uptake in human leukemia cells by other agents. *Cancer Res* 1975;35:1305.
83. Chan JD. Pharmacokinetic drug interactions of vinca alkaloids. Summary of case reports. *Pharmacotherapy* 1998;18:1304.
84. Yalowich JC. Effect of microtubule inhibition on etoposide accumulation and DNA damage in human K562 cells in vitro. *Cancer Res* 1987;47:1010.
85. Jarosinski PF, Moscow JA, Alexander MS, et al. Altered phenytoin clearance during intensive chemotherapy for acute lymphoblastic leukemia. *J Pediatr* 1988;112:996.
86. Tobe SW, Siu LL, Jamal SA, et al. Vinblastine and erythromycin: an unrecognized serious drug interaction. *Cancer Chemother Pharmacol* 1995;35:188.
87. Crom WR, De Graaf SSN, Synold T, et al. Pharmacokinetics of vincristine in children and adolescents with acute lymphocytic leukemia. *J Pediatr* 1994;125:642.
88. Rajaonarison JF, Lacarelle B, Catalin J, et al. Effect of anticancer drugs on the glucuronidation of 3'azido-3'-deoxythymidine in human liver microsomes. *Drug Metab Dispos* 1993;21:823.
89. Sathiapalan RK, El-Soth H. Enhanced vincristine neurotoxicity from drug interactions: case report and review of literature. *Pediatr Hematol Oncol* 2001;18:543.
90. Casey EB, Jellife AM, Le Quesne PM, Millett YL. Vincristine neuropathy, clinical and electrophysiological observations. *Brain* 1973;96:69.
91. Quasthoff S, Hartung HP. Chemotherapy-induced peripheral neuropathy. *J Neurol* 2002; 249:9.
92. Peltier AC, Russell JW. Recent advances in drug-induced neuropathies. *Curr Opin Neurol* 2002;15:633.
93. Greig NH, Soncrant TT, Shetty HU, et al. Brain uptake and anticancer activities of vincristine and vinblastine are restricted by their low cerebrovascular permeability and binding to plasma constituents in rat. *Cancer Chemother Pharmacol* 1990;26:263.
94. Hironen HE, Saknu TT, Heinonen E, et al. Vincristine treatment of acute lymphoblastic leukemia induces transient autonomic cardioneuropathy. *Cancer* 1988;64:801.
95. Gottlieb RJ, Cuttner J. Vincristine-induced bladder atony. *Cancer* 1971;28:674.
96. Carmichael SM, Eagleton L, Ayers CR, Mohler D. Orthostatic hypotension during vincristine therapy. *Arch Intern Med* 1970;126:290.
97. Burns BV, Shotton JC. Vocal fold palsy following vinca alkaloid treatment. *J Laryngol Otol* 1998;112:485.
98. Morgan E, Baum E, Breslow N, et al. Chemotherapy-related toxicity in infants treated according to the second national Wilms' tumor study. *J Clin Oncol* 1988;6:51.
99. Woods WG, O'Leary M, Nesbit ME. Life-threatening neuropathy and hepatotoxicity in infants during induction therapy for acute lymphoblastic leukemia. *J Pediatr* 1981;98:642.
100. Trobaugh-Lotrario AD, Smith AA, Odom LF. Vincristine neurotoxicity in the presence of hereditary neuropathy. *Med Pediatr Oncol* 2003;40:39.
101. Desai ZR, Van den Berg HW, Bridges JM, et al. Can severe vincristine neurotoxicity be prevented? *Cancer Chemother Pharmacol* 1982;8:211.
102. Boyle FM, Wheeler HR, Shenfield GM. Glutamate ameliorates experimental vincristine neuropathy. *J Pharmacol Exp Ther* 1996;279:410.
103. Jackson DV, Wells HB, Atkins JN, et al. Amelioration of vincristine neurotoxicity by glutamic acid. *Am J Med* 1988;84:1016.
104. Binet S, Fellous A, Lataste H, et al. In situ analysis of the action of Navelbine on various types of microtubules using immunofluorescence. *Semin Oncol* 1989;16[Suppl 4]:5.
105. Le Chevalier T, Brisgand D, Douillard J-Y, et al. Randomized study of vinorelbine and cisplatin versus vindesine and cisplatin versus vindesine and cisplatin versus vinorelbine alone in non-small cell lung cancer: results of a European multicenter trial including 612 patients. *J Clin Oncol* 1994;12:360
106. Sharma RK. Vincristine and gastrointestinal transit. *Gastroenterology* 1988;95:1435.
107. Tester W, Forbes W, Leighton J. Vinorelbine-induced pancreatitis: a case report. *J Natl Cancer Inst* 1997;89:1631.
108. Dorr RT, Alberts DS. Vinca alkaloid skin toxicity: antidote and drug disposition studies in the mouse. *J Natl Cancer Inst* 1985;74:113.
109. Dorr T. Antidotes to vesicant chemotherapy extravasation. *Blood Rev* 1990;4:41.
110. Schrijvers DL. Extravasation: a dreaded complication of chemotherapy. *Ann Oncol* 2003;14[Suppl 3]:iii26.
111. Hoff PM, Valero V, Ibrahim N, Willey, Hortobagyi GN. Hand-foot syndrome following prolonged infusion of high doses of vinorelbine. *Cancer* 1998;85:965.

112. Karminsky N, Merimsky O, Kovner F, Inbar M. Vinorelbine-related acute cardiopulmonary toxicity. *Cancer Chemother Pharmacol* 1999;43:180.
113. Tassinari D, Sartori S, Gianni L, Pasguini E, Ravaioli A. Is acute dyspnea a rare side effect of vinorelbine? *Ann Oncol* 1997;8:503.
114. Subar M, Muggia FM. Apparent myocardial ischemia associated with vinblastine administration. *Cancer Treat Rep* 1986;70:690.
115. Hantel A, Rowinsky EK, Donehower RC. Nifedipine and oncologic Raynaud's phenomenon. *Ann Intern Med* 1988;108:767.
116. Israel RH, Olson JP. Pulmonary edema associated with intravenous vinblastine. *JAMA* 1978;240:1585.
117. Sulkes A, Collins JM. Reappraisal of some dosage adjustment guidelines. *Cancer Treat Rep* 1987;71:229.
118. Ramirez-Amador V, Esquivel-Pedraza L, Lozada-Nur F. Intralesional vinblastine vs. 3% sodium tetradecyl sulfate for the treatment of the oral Kaposi's sarcoma. A double blind, randomized clinical trial. *Oral Oncol* 2002;38:460.
119. Shibata SI, Synold TW, Carroll M, et al. A pilot study of the tolerability and pharmacokinetics of vinorelbine in patients with varying degrees of liver dysfunction. *Proc Am Soc Clin Oncol* 1999;18:190a(abst).
120. Rowinsky EK, Cazenave LA, Donehower RC. Taxol: a novel investigational antineoplastic agent. *J Natl Cancer Inst* 1990;82:1247.
121. Rowinsky EK, Donehower RC. Drug therapy: paclitaxel (Taxol). *N Engl J Med* 1995;332:1004.
122. Cortes JE, Pazdur R. Docetaxel. *J Clin Oncol* 1995;13:2643.
123. McGuire WP, Hoskins WJ, Brady MF, et al. Cyclophosphamide and cisplatin compared with paclitaxel and cisplatin in patients with stage III and IV ovarian cancer. *N Engl J Med* 1996;334:1.
124. Sparano JA. Taxanes for breast cancer: an evidence-based review of randomized phase II and phase III trials. *Clin Breast Cancer* 2000;1:32, discussion 41.
125. Henderson IC, Berry D, Demetri G, et al. Improved outcomes from adding sequential Paclitaxel but not from escalating Doxorubicin dose in an adjuvant chemotherapy regimen for patients with node-positive primary breast cancer. *J Clin Oncol* 2003;21:976.
126. Citron ML, Berry DA, Cirrincione C, et al. Randomized trial of dose-dense versus conventionally scheduled and sequential versus concurrent combination chemotherapy as postoperative adjuvant treatment of node-positive primary breast cancer: first report of Intergroup Trial C9741/Cancer and Leukemia Group B Trial 9741. *J Clin Oncol* 2003;21:1431.
127. Jie C, Tulpule A, Zheng T, et al. Treatment of epidemic AIDS-related Kaposi's sarcoma. *Curr Opin Oncol* 1997;9:433.
128. Bonomi P, Kim K, Fariclough D, et al. Comparison of survival and quality of life in advanced non-small cell lung cancer patients treated with two dose levels of paclitaxel combined with cisplatin versus etoposide with cisplatin: results from an Eastern Cooperative Oncology Group trial. *J Clin Oncol* 2000;18:623.
129. Simon GR, Bunn PA Jr. Taxanes in the treatment of advanced (stages III and IV) non-small cell lung cancer (NSCLC): recent developments. *Cancer Invest* 2003;21:87.
130. Schiff PB, Fant J, Horwitz SB. Promotion of microtubule assembly in vitro by taxol. *Nature* 1979;22:665.
131. Manfredi JJ, Parness J, Horwitz SB. Taxol binds to cellular microtubules. *J Cell Biol* 1982;94:688.
132. Rao S, Krauss NE, Heerding JM, et al. 3'-(p-Azidobenzamido)taxol photolabels the N-terminal 31 amino acids of β-tubulin. *J Biol Chem* 1994;269:3132.
133. Rao S, Orr GA, Chaudhary AG, et al. Characterization of the Taxol binding site on the microtubule: 2-(m-azidobenzoyl)taxol photolabels a peptide (amino acids 217-231) of beta tubulin. *J Biol Chem* 1995;270:20235.
134. Diaz JF, Andreu JM. Assembly of purified GDP-tubulin into microtubules induced by taxol and taxotere: reversibility, ligand stoichiometry and competition. *Biochemistry* 1993;32:2747.
135. Caplow M, Shanks J, Ruhlen R. How taxol modulates microtubule disassembly. *J Biol Chem* 1994;269:23399.
136. Vanhoerfer U, Cao S, Harstrict A, Seeber S, Rustum YM. Comparative antitumor efficacy of docetaxel and paclitaxel in nude mice bearing human tumor xenografts that overexpress the multidrug resistant protein. *Ann Oncol* 1997;8:1221.
137. Valero V, Jones SE, Von Hoff DD, et al. A phase II study of docetaxel in patients with paclitaxel-resistant metastatic breast cancer. *J Clin Oncol* 1998;16:3362.
138. Ravdin P, Erban J, Overmoyer B, et al. Phase III comparison of docetaxel (D) and paclitaxel (P) in patients with metastatic breast cancer (MBC). *Proc Eur Cancer Conf* 2003;12:670.
139. Jordan MA, Toso RJ, Thrower D, Wilson L. Mechanism of mitotic block and inhibition of cell proliferation by taxol at low concentrations. *Proc Natl Acad Sci U S A* 1993;90:9552.
140. Ringel I, Horwitz SB. Studies with RP56976 (Taxotere): a semisynthetic analogue of taxol. *J Natl Cancer Inst* 1991;83:288.
141. Rowinsky EK, Donehower RC, Jones RJ, Tucker RW. Microtubule changes and cytotoxicity in leukemic cell lines treated with taxol. *Cancer Res* 1988;48:4093.
142. Derry WB, Wilson L, Jordan MA. Substoichiometric binding of taxol suppresses microtubule dynamics. *Biochemistry* 1995;34:2203.
143. Derry WB, Wilson L, Jordan MA. Low potency of taxol at microtubule minus ends: implications for its antimitotic and therapeutic mechanism. *Cancer Res* 1998;58:1177.
144. Wilson L, Miller HP, Farrell KW, et al. Taxol stabilization of microtubules in vitro: dynamics of tubulin addition and loss at opposite microtubule ends. *Biochemistry* 1985;24:5254.
145. DeBrabander M, Geuens G, Nuydens R, et al. Taxol induces the assembly of free microtubules in living cells and blocks the organizing capacity of the centrosomes and kinetochores. *Proc Natl Acad Sci U S A* 1981;78:5608.
146. Poruchynsky MS, Wang EE, Rudin CM, Blagosklonny MV, Fojo T. Bcl-xL is phosphorylated in malignant cells following microtubule disruption. *Cancer Res* 1998;58:3331.
147. Dumontet C, Sikic B. Mechanism of action and resistance to antitubulin agents: microtubule dynamics, drug transport, and cell death. *J Clin Oncol* 1999;17:1061.
148. Bhalla K, Ibrado AM, Tourkina E, et al. Taxol induces internucleosomal DNA fragmentation associated with programmed cell death in human myeloid leukemia cells. *Leukemia* 1993;7:563.
149. Strobel T, Swanson L, Korsmeyer S, Cannistra SA. BAX enhances paclitaxel-induced apoptosis through a p53-independent pathway. *Proc Natl Acad Sci U S A* 1996;93:14094.
150. Strobel T, Kraeft SK, Chen LB, Cannistra SA. BAX expression is associated with enhanced intracellular accumulation of paclitaxel: a novel role for BAX during chemotherapy-induced cell death. *Cancer Res* 1998;58:4776.
151. Scatena CD, Stewart ZA, Mays D, et al. Mitotic phosphorylation of Bcl-2 during normal cell cycle progression and Taxol-induced cell growth arrest. *J Biol Chem* 1998;273:30777.
152. Torres K, Horwitz SB. Mechanisms of Taxol-induced cell death are concentration dependent. *Cancer Res* 1998;58:3620.
153. Fernlini C, Raspaglio G, Mozzetti S. Bcl-2 down-regulation is a novel mechanism of paclitaxel resistance. *Mol Pharmacol* 2003;64:51.
154. Griffon-Etienne G, Boucher Y, Brekken C, et al. Taxane-induced apoptosis decompresses blood vessels and lowers interstitial fluid pressure in solid tumors: clinical implications. *Cancer Res* 1999;59:776.
155. Moos PJ, Fitzpatrick FA. Taxane-mediated gene induction is independent of microtubule stabilization: induction of transcription regulators and enzymes that modulate inflammation and apoptosis. *Proc Natl Acad Sci U S A* 1998;95:3896.
156. Ganansia-Leymarie V, Bischoff P, Bergerat JP. Signal transduction pathways of taxanes-induced apoptosis. *Curr Med Chem Anti-Canc Agents* 2003;3:291.
157. Burkhart CA, Berman JW, Cwindell CS, et al. Relationship between taxol and other taxanes on induction of tumor necrosis factor-α gene expression and cytotoxicity. *Cancer Res* 1994;54:5779.
158. Tishler RB, Geard CR, Hall EJ, Schiff PB. Taxol sensitizes human astrocytoma cells to radiation. *Cancer Res* 1992;52:3595.
159. Creane M, Seymour CB, Colucci S. Radiobiological effects of docetaxel (Taxotere): a potential radiation sensitizer. *Int J Radiat Biol* 1999;75:731.
160. Belotti D, Vergani V, Drudis T, et al. The microtubule-affecting drug paclitaxel has anti-angiogenic activity. *Clin Cancer Res* 1996;2:1843.
161. Horwitz SB, Cohen D, Rao S, et al. Taxol: mechanisms of action and resistance. *J Natl Cancer Inst Monogr* 1993;15:63.
162. Cole SPC, Sparks KE, Fraser K, et al. Pharmacological characterization of multidrug resistant MRP-transfected human tumor cells. *Cancer Res* 1994;54:5902.
163. Lorico A, Rappa G, Flavell RA, et al. Double knockout of the MRP gene leads to increased drug sensitivity in vitro. *Cancer Res* 1996;56:5351.
164. Rowinsky EK, Smith L, Chaturvedi P, et al. Pharmacokinetic and toxicologic interactions between the multidrug resistance reversal agent VX-710 and paclitaxel in cancer patients. *J Clin Oncol* 1998;16:2964.
165. Patnaik A, Oza AM, Warner E, et al. A phase I dose-finding and pharmacokinetic study of paclitaxel and carboplatin with oral valspodar in patients with advanced solid tumors. *J Clin Oncol* 2000;18:3677.
166. Cabral F, Wible L, Brenner S, Brinkley BR. Taxol-requiring mutants of Chinese hamster ovary cells with impaired mitotic spindle activity. *J Cell Biol* 1983;97:30.
167. Kavallaris M, Kuo DYS, Burkhart CA, et al. Taxol-resistant ovarian tumors are associated with altered expression of specific beta-tubulin isotypes. *J Clin Invest* 1997;100:1282.
168. Blade K, Menick DR, Cabral F. Overexpression of class I, II, or IVb beta-tubulin isotypes in CHO cells is insufficient to confer resistance to paclitaxel. *J Cell Sci* 1999;112:2213.
169. Kavallaris M, Burkhart CA, Horwitz SB. Antisense oligonucleotides to class III beta-tubulin sensitize drug resistant cells to Taxol. *Br J Cancer* 1999;80:1020.
170. Giannakakou P, Sackett DL, Kang YK, et al. Paclitaxel-resistant human ovarian cancer cells have mutant beta-tubulins that exhibit impaired paclitaxel-driven polymerization. *J Biol Chem* 1997;272:17118.
171. Monzo M, Rosell R, Sánchez JJ, et al. Paclitaxel resistance in nonsmall cell lung cancer associated with beta tubulin gene mutations. *J Clin Oncol* 1999;17:1786.
172. Kelley MJ, Li S, Harpole DH. Genetic analysis of the β-tubulin gene, TUBB, in non-small cell lung cancer. *J Natl Cancer Inst* 2001;93:1886.
173. Gonzalez-Garay ML, Chang L, Blade K, Menick DR, Cabral F. A β-tubulin leucine cluster involved in microtubule assembly and paclitaxel resistance. *J Biol Chem* 1999;274:23875.
174. Liu Q-Y, Stein CA. Taxol and estramustine-induced modulation of human prostate cancer cell apoptosis via alteration in bcl-xL and bax expression. *Clin Cancer Res* 1997;3:2039.
175. Tang C, Willingham MC, Reed JC, et al. High levels of p26BCL-2 oncoprotein related Taxol-induced apoptosis in human pre-B leukemia cells. *Leukemia* 1994;8:1960.
176. Yusuf RZ, Duan Z, Lamendola DE. Paclitaxel resistance: molecular mechanisms and pharmacologic manipulation. *Curr Cancer Drug Targets* 2003;3:1.
177. Kolfschoten GM, Hulscher TM, Duyndam MC. Variation in the kinetics of caspase-3 activation, Bcl-2 phosphorylation and apoptotic morphology in unselected human ovarian cancer cell lines as a response to docetaxel. *Biochem Pharmacol* 2002;63:733.
178. Zhang CC, Yang JM, White E, et al. The role of MAP4 expression in the sensitivity to paclitaxel and resistance to vinca alkaloids in p53 mutant cells. *Oncogene* 1998;16:1617.
179. Woods CM, Zhu J, McQueney PA, et al. Taxol-induced mitotic block triggers rapid onset of a p53-independent apoptotic pathway. *Mol Med* 1995;1:506.
180. Tisher RB, Lamppu DM, Park S, et al. Microtubule-active drugs Taxol, vinblastine, and nocodazole increase the level of transcriptionally active p53. *Cancer Res* 1995;55:6021.
181. Srivastava RK, Srivastava AR, Korsmeyer SJ, et al. Involvement of microtubules in the regulation of Bcl2 phosphorylation and apoptosis through cyclic AMP-dependent protein kinase. *Mol Cell Biol* 1998;18:3509.
182. Rowinsky EK. Pharmacology and metabolism. In: McGuire WG, Rowinsky EK, eds. *Paclitaxel in cancer treatment.* New York: Marcel Dekker, 1995:91.
183. Malingre MM, Beijnen JH, Schellens JHM. Oral delivery of the taxanes. *Invest New Drugs* 2001;19:155.
184. Huizing MT, Keung ACF, Rosing H, et al. Pharmacokinetics of paclitaxel and metabolites

in a randomized comparative study in platinum-pretreated ovarian cancer patients. *J Clin Oncol* 1993;11:2127.

185. Gianni L, Kearns C, Gianni A. et al. Nonlinear pharmacokinetics and metabolism of paclitaxel and its pharmacokinetic/pharmacodynamic relationships in humans. *J Clin Oncol* 1995;13:180.
186. Sparreboom A, van Zuylen L, Brouwer E, et al. Cremophor EL-mediated alterations of paclitaxel distribution in human blood: clinical pharmacokinetic implications. *Cancer Res* 1999;59:1454.
187. Gelderblom H, Mross K, ten Tije AJ, et al. Comparative pharmacokinetics of unbound paclitaxel during 1- and 3-hour infusions. *J Clin Oncol* 2002;20:574.
188. Smorenburg CH, Sparreboom A, Bontenbal M, Stoter G, Nooter K, Verweij J. Randomized cross-over evaluation of body-surface area-based dosing versus flat-fixed dosing of paclitaxel. *J Clin Oncol* 2003;21:197.
189. Ohtsu T, Sasaki Y, Tamura T, et al. Clinical pharmacokinetics and pharmacodynamics of paclitaxel: a 3-hour infusion versus a 24-hour infusion. *Clin Cancer Res* 1995;1:599.
190. Lesser G, Grossman SA, Eller S, Rowinsky EK. The neural and extra-neural distribution of systemically administered [3H]paclitaxel in rats: a quantitative autoradiographic study. *Cancer Chemother Pharmacol* 1995;34:173.
191. Glantz MJ, Choy H, Kearns CM, et al. Paclitaxel disposition in plasma and central nervous systems of humans and rats with brain tumors. *J Natl Cancer Inst* 1995;87:1077.
192. Monsarrat B, Alvinerie P, Dubois J, et al. Hepatic metabolism and biliary clearance of taxol in rats and humans. *Natl Cancer Inst Monogr* 1993;15:39.
193. Cresteil T, Monsarrat B, Alvinerie P, et al. Taxol metabolism by human liver microsomes: identification of cytochrome P450 isoenzymes involved in its biotransformation. *Cancer Res* 1994;54:386.
194. Walle T, Walle UK, Kumar GN, Bhalla KN. Taxol metabolism and disposition in cancer patients. *Drug Metab Dispos* 1995;23:506.
195. Rowinsky EK, Bonomi P, Jiroutek M, et al. Paclitaxel steady-state plasma concentration as a determinant of disease outcome and toxicity in lung cancer patients treated with paclitaxel and cisplatin. *Clin Cancer Res* 1999;5:767.
196. Clarke SJ, Rivory LP. Clinical pharmacokinetics of docetaxel. *Clin Pharmacokinet* 1999;36:99.
197. Bruno R, Hille D, Riva A, et al. Population pharmacokinetic/pharmacodynamics of docetaxel in phase II studies in patients with cancer. *J Clin Oncol* 1998;16:186.
198. Bruno R, Vivier N, Veyrat-Follet C, et al. Population pharmacokinetics and pharmacokinetic-pharmacodynamic relationships for docetaxel. *Invest New Drugs* 2001;19:163.
199. McLeod HL, Kearns CM, Kuhn JG, Bruno R. Evaluation of the linearity of docetaxel pharmacokinetics. *Cancer Chemother Pharmacol* 1998;42:155.
200. Marland M, Gaillard C, Sanderink G, et al. Kinetics, distribution, metabolism and excretion of radiolabeled Taxotere (14C-RPR 56976) in mice and dogs. *Proc Am Assoc Cancer Res* 1993;34:393(abst).
201. Sparreboom A, Van Tellingen O, Scherrenburg EJ, et al. Isolation, purification and biological activity of major docetaxel metabolites from human feces. *Drug Metab Dispos* 1996;24:655.
202. Royer I, Bonsarrat B, Sonnier M, Wright M, Cresteil T. Metabolism of docetaxel by human cytochromes P450: interactions with paclitaxel and other antineoplastic agents. *Cancer Res* 1996;56:58.
203. Vigano L, Locatelli A, Grasselli G, Gianni L. Drug interactions of paclitaxel and docetaxel and their relevance for the design of combination therapy. *Invest New Drugs* 2001;19:197.
204. Rowinsky EK, Gilbert M, McGuire WP, et al. Sequences of taxol and cisplatin: a phase I and pharmacologic study. *J Clin Oncol* 1991;9:1692.
205. Rowinsky EK, Citardi M, Noe DA, Donehower RC. Sequence-dependent cytotoxicity between cisplatin and the antimicrotubule agents taxol and vincristine. *J Cancer Res Clin Oncol* 1993;119:737.
206. Belani CP, Kearns CM, Zuhowski EG, et al. Phase I trial, including pharmacokinetic and pharmacodynamic correlations, of combination paclitaxel and carboplatin in patients with metastatic non-small-cell lung cancer. *J Clin Oncol* 1999;17:676.
207. Holmes FA, Madden T, Newman RA, et al. Sequence-dependent alteration of doxorubicin pharmacokinetics by paclitaxel in a phase I study of paclitaxel and doxorubicin in patients with metastatic breast cancer. *J Clin Oncol* 1996;14:2713.
208. Gianni L, Vigano L, Locatelli A, et al. Human pharmacokinetic characterization and in vitro study of the interactions between doxorubicin and paclitaxel in patients with breast cancer. *J Clin Oncol* 1997;15:1906.
209. Gianni L, Munzone E, Capri G, et al. Paclitaxel by 3-hour infusion in combination with bolus doxorubicin in women with untreated metastatic breast cancer: high antitumor efficacy and cardiac effects in a dose-finding and sequence-finding study. *J Clin Oncol* 1995;13:2688.
210. Gennari A, Salvadori B, Donati S, et al. Cardiotoxicity of epirubicin/paclitaxel-containing regimens: role of cardiac risk factors. *J Clin Oncol* 1999;11:3596.
211. Kennedy MJ, Zahurak ML, Donehower RC, et al. Phase I and pharmacologic study of sequences of paclitaxel and cyclophosphamide supported by granulocyte colony-stimulating factor in women with previously treated metastatic breast cancer. *J Clin Oncol* 1995;14:783.
212. Sarvada N, Ishikawa T, Fukase Y, et al. Induction of thymidine phosphorylase activity and enhancement of capecitabine efficacy by taxol/taxotere in human cancer xenografts. *Clin Cancer Res* 1998;4:1013.
213. Fettel MR, Grossman SA, Fisher J, et al. Pre-irradiation paclitaxel in glioblastoma multiforme (GBM): efficacy, pharmacology, and drug interactions. *J Clin Oncol* 1997;15:3121.
214. Monsarrat B, Chatelut E, Royer I, et al. Modification of paclitaxel metabolism in a cancer patient by induction of cytochrome P450 3A4. *Drug Metab Dispos* 1998;26:229.
215. Bun SS, Ciccolini J, Bun H. Drug interactions of paclitaxel metabolism in human liver microsomes. *J Chemother* 2003;15:266.
216. Eisenhower E, ten Bokkel Huinink W, Swenerton KD, et al. European-Canadian randomized trial of taxol in relapsed ovarian cancer: high vs. low dose and long vs. short infusion. *J Clin Oncol* 1994;12:2654.
217. Rowinsky EK. The taxanes: dosing and scheduling considerations. *Oncology* 1997;11[Suppl 2]:1.
218. Rowinsky EK, Eisenhauer EA, Chaudhry V, Arbuck SA, Donehower RC. Clinical toxicities encountered with taxol. *Semin Oncol* 1993;20[Suppl 3]:1.
219. Weiss R, Donehower RC, Wiernik PH, et al. Hypersensitivity reactions from taxol. *J Clin Oncol* 1990;8:1263.
220. Peereboom D, Donehower RC, Eisenhauer EA, et al. Successful retreatment with taxol after major hypersensitivity reactions. *J Clin Oncol* 1993;11:885.
221. Rowinsky EK, Chaudhry V, Cornblath DR, Donehower RC. The neurotoxicity of taxol. *J Natl Cancer Inst Monogr* 1993;15:107.
222. Chaudhry V, Rowinsky EK, Sartorious SE, Donehower RC, Cornblath DR. Peripheral neuropathy from taxol and cisplatin combination chemotherapy: clinical and electrophysiological studies. *Ann Neurol* 1994;35:490.
223. Markman M. Managing taxane toxicities. *Support Care Cancer* 2003;11:144.
224. Garrison JA, McCune JS, Livingston RB. Myalgias and arthralagias associated with paclitaxel. *Oncology* 2003;17:271.
225. Capri G, Munzone E, Tarenzi E, Fulgaro F, Gianni L. Optic nerve disturbances: a new form of paclitaxel neurotoxicity. *J Natl Cancer Inst* 1994;86:1099.
226. Nieto Y, Cagnoni PJ, Bearman SI, Shpall EJ. Acute encephalopathy: a new toxicity associated with high-dose paclitaxel. *Clin Cancer Res* 1999;5:501.
227. Rowinsky EK, McGuire WP, Guarnieri T, Christian MA, Donehower RC. Cardiac disturbances during the administration of taxol. *J Clin Oncol* 1991;9:1704.
228. Arbuck SG, Strauss H, Rowinsky EK, et al. A reassessment of the cardiac toxicity associated with taxol. *J Natl Cancer Inst Monogr* 1993;15:117.
229. Markman M, Kennedy A, Webser K, et al. Paclitaxel administration to gynecologic cancer patients with major cardiac risk factors. *J Clin Oncol* 1998;16:3483.
230. Sparano JA, Speyer J, Gradishar WJ, et al. Phase I trial of escalating doses of paclitaxel plus doxorubicin and dexrazoxane in patients with advanced breast cancer. *J Clin Oncol* 1999;17:880.
231. Jeriah S, Keegan P. Cardiotoxicity associated with paclitaxel/trastuzumab combination chemotherapy. *J Clin Oncol* 1999;17:1647.
232. Rowinsky EK, Burke PJ, Karp JE, et al. Phase I and pharmacodynamic study of taxol in refractory adult acute leukemia. *Cancer Res* 1989;49:4640.
233. Wilson WH, Berg S, Bryant G, et al. Paclitaxel in doxorubicin-refractory or mitoxantrone-refractory breast cancer: a phase I/II trial of 96 hour infusion. *J Clin Oncol* 1994;12:1621.
234. Pestalozzi BC, Sotos GA, Choyke PL, et al. Typhlitis resulting from treatment with taxol and doxorubicin in patients with metastatic breast cancer. *Cancer* 1993;71:1797.
235. Feenstra J, Vermeer RJ, Stricker BH. Fatal hepatic coma attributed to paclitaxel. *J Natl Cancer Inst* 1997;16;582.
236. Hoff PM, Valero V, Homes FA, et al. Paclitaxel-induced pancreatitis: a case report. *J Natl Cancer Inst* 1997;89:91.
237. Ramanathan RK, Belani CP. Transient pulmonary infiltrates: a hypersensitivity reaction to paclitaxel. *Ann Intern Med* 1996;124:278.
238. Luftner D, Flath B, Akrivakis C, et al. Dose-intensified weekly paclitaxel induces multiple nail disorders. *Ann Oncol* 1998;9:1139.
239. Schrijvers D, Wanders J, Dirix L, et al. Coping with toxicities of docetaxel (Taxotere). *Ann Oncol* 1993;4:610.
240. Bernstein BJ. Docetaxel as an alternative to paclitaxel after acute hypersensitivity reactions. *Ann Pharmacother* 2000;34:1332.
241. Semb KA, Aamdal S, Oian P. Capillary protein leak syndrome appears to explain fluid retention in cancer patients who receive docetaxel treatment. *J Clin Oncol* 1998;16:3426.
242. Piccart MJ, Klijn J, Paridaens R, et al. Corticosteroids significantly delay the onset of docetaxel-induced fluid retention: final results of a randomized study of the European Organization for Research and Treatment of Cancer, Investigational Drug Branch for Breast Cancer. *J Clin Oncol* 1997;15:149.
243. Zimmerman GC, Keeling JH, Barris HA, et al. Acute cutaneous reactions to docetaxel, a new chemotherapeutic agent. *Arch Dermatol* 1995;131:202.
244. Vukeljia SJ, Baker WJ, Burris HA III, Keeling JH, Von Hoff DD. Pyridoxine therapy for palmar-plantar erythrodysesthesia associated with Taxotere. *J Natl Cancer Inst* 1993;85:1432.
245. Hainsworth JD, Burris HA, Greco FA. Weekly administration of docetaxel (Taxotere): summary of clinical data. *Semin Oncol* 1999;26[Suppl 10]:19.
246. Hilkens PH, Verweij J, Stoter G, et al. Peripheral neurotoxicity induced by docetaxel. *Neurology* 1996;46:104.
247. Vasey PA. Survival and long-term toxicity results of the SCOTROC study: docetaxel-carboplatin (DC) vs. paclitaxel-carboplatin (PC) in epithelial ovarian cancer. *Proc Am Soc Clin Oncol* 1992;21:202a.
248. Frances P, Schneider J, Hann L, et al. Phase II trial of docetaxel in patients with platinum-refractory advanced ovarian cancer. *J Clin Oncol* 1994;12:2201.
249. Hainsworth JD, Burris HA, Greco FA. Weekly administration of docetaxel (Taxotere): summary of clinical data. *Semin Oncol* 1999;26[Suppl 10]:19.
250. Esamaeli B, Hortobagyi G, Esteva F. Canalicular stenosis secondary to weekly docetaxel: a potentially preventable side effect. *Ann Oncol* 2002;13:218.
251. Smith RE, Brown AM, Mamounas EP, et al. Randomized trial of 3-hour versus 24-hour infusion of high-dose paclitaxel in patients with metastatic or locally advanced breast cancer: National Surgical Adjuvant Breast and Bowel Project Protocol B-26. *J Clin Oncol* 1999;17:3403.
252. Omura GA, Brady MF, Look KY, et al. Phase III trial of paclitaxel at two dose levels, the higher dose accompanied by filgrastim at two dose levels in platinum-pretreated epithelial ovarian cancer: an intergroup study. *J Clin Oncol* 2003;21:2843.
253. Takimoto CH, Rowinsky EK. Dose-intense paclitaxel: deja vu all over again? *J Clin Oncol* 2003;21:2810.
254. Seidman AD, Hochhauser D, Gollub M, et al. Ninety-six-hour paclitaxel infusion after progression during short taxane exposure: a phase II pharmacokinetic and pharmacodynamic study in metastatic breast cancer. *J Clin Oncol* 1996;14:1877.

255. Markman M, Rose PG, Jones E, et al. Ninety-six-hour infusional paclitaxel as salvage therapy of ovarian cancer patients previously failing treatment with 3-hour or 24-hour paclitaxel infusion. *J Clin Oncol* 1998;16:1849.

256. Holmes FA, Valero V, Buzdar AU, et al. Final results: randomized phase III trial of paclitaxel by 3-hr versus 96-hr infusion in patients with metastatic breast cancer. *Proc Am Soc Clin Oncol* 1999;18:110a(abst).

257. Seidman AD, Hudis CA, Albanel J, et al. Dose-dense therapy with weekly 1-hour paclitaxel infusions in the treatment of metastatic breast cancer. *J Clin Oncol* 1998;16:3353.

258. Greco FA, Thomas M, Hainsworth JD. One-hour paclitaxel infusions: review of the safety and efficacy. *Cancer J Sci Am* 1999;5:179.

259. Green MC, Buzdar AU, Smith T, et al. Weekly paclitaxel followed by FAC as primary systemic chemotherapy of operable breast cancer improves pathologic complete remission rates when compared to every 3-week paclitaxel therapy followed by FAC—final results of a prospective randomized phase III study. *Proc Am Soc Clin Oncol* 2002;21:35a(abst).

260. Winer E, Berry D, Duggan D, et al. Failure of higher dose paclitaxel to improve outcome in patients with metastatic breast cancer results from CALGB 9342. *Proc Am Soc Clin Oncol* 1998;17:101a(abst).

261. Francis P, Rowinsky E, Schneider J, et al. Phase I feasibility and pharmacologic study of intraperitoneal paclitaxel: a Gynecologic Oncology Group study. *J Clin Oncol* 1995;13:2961.

262. Markman M, Brady MF, Spirtos NM, Hanjani P, Rubin SC. Phase II trial of intraperitoneal paclitaxel in carcinoma of the ovary, tube, and peritoneum: a Gynecologic Oncology Group study. *J Clin Oncol* 1998;16:2620.

263. Armstrong DK, Bundy BN, Baergen R, et al. Randomized phase III study of intravenous (IV) paclitaxel and cisplatin versus IV paclitaxel, intraperitoneal (IP) cisplatin and IP paclitaxel in optimal stage III epithelial ovarian cancer (OC): a Gynecologic Oncology Group trial (GOG 172). *Proc Am Soc Clin Oncol* 2002;21:201a(abst).

264. Bookman MA, Kloth DD, Kover PE, Smolinski S, Ozols RF. Short-course intravenous prophylaxis for paclitaxel-related hypersensitivity reactions. *Ann Oncol* 1997;8:611.

265. Venock AP, Egorin MJ, Rosner GL, et al. Phase I and pharmacokinetic trial of paclitaxel in patients with hepatic dysfunction. Cancer and leukemia group B 9264. *J Clin Oncol* 1998;16:1811.

266. Woo MH, Gregornik D, Shearer PD, Meyer WH, Relling MV. Pharmacokinetics of paclitaxel in an anephric patient. *Cancer Chemother Pharmacol* 1999;43:92.

267. Salminen E, Bergman M, Huhtala S, et al. Docetaxel: standard recommended dose of 100 mg/m² is effective but not feasible for some metastatic breast cancer patients heavily pretreated with chemotherapy—a phase II single-center study. *J Clin Oncol* 1999;17:1127.

268. Fex H, Hogberg B, Konyves I. Estramustine phosphate—historical overview. *Urology* 1984;23:4.

269. Forsberg JG, Hoisaeter PA. Effects of hormone-cytostatic complexes on the rat ventral prostate in vivo and in vitro. *Vitam Horm* 1975;33:137.

270. Forsgren B, Bjork P, Carlstrom K, et al. Purification and distribution of a major protein in rat prostate that binds estramustine, a nitrogen mustard derivative of estradiol-17 beta. *Proc Natl Acad Sci U S A* 1979;76:3149.

271. Nilsson T, Muntzing J. Initial clinical studies with estramustine phosphate. *Urology* 1984;23:49.

272. Hartley-Asp B. Estramustine-induced mitotic arrest in two human prostatic carcinoma cell lines DU 145 and PC-3. *Prostate* 1984;5:93.

273. Stearns ME, Tew KD. Antimicrotubule effects of estramustine, an antiprostatic tumor drug. *Cancer Res* 1985;45:3891.

274. Dahllof B, Billstrom A, Cabral F, Hartley-Asp B. Estramustine depolymerizes microtubules by binding to tubulin. *Cancer Res* 1993;53:4573.

275. Stearns ME, Wang M, Tew KD, Binder LI. Estramustine binds a MAP-1-like protein to inhibit microtubule assembly in vitro and disrupt microtubule organization in DU 145 cells. *J Cell Biol* 1988;107:2647.

276. Stearns ME, Tew KD. Estramustine binds MAP-2 to inhibit microtubule assembly in vitro. *J Cell Sci* 1988;89:331.

277. Panda D, Miller HP, Islam K, Wilson L. Stabilization of microtubule dynamics by estramustine by binding to a novel site in tubulin: a possible mechanistic basis for its antitumor action. *Proc Natl Acad Sci U S A* 1997;94:10560.

278. Laing N, Dahllof B, Hartley-Asp B, Ranganathan S, Tew KD. Interaction of estramustine with tubulin isotypes. *Biochemistry* 1997;36:871.

279. Walz PH, Bjork P, Gunnarsson PO, Edman K, Hartley-Asp B. Differential uptake of estramustine phosphate metabolites and its correlation with the levels of estramustine binding protein in prostate tumor tissue. *Clin Cancer Res* 1998;4:2079.

280. Pienta KJ, Lehr JE. Inhibition of prostate cancer growth by estramustine and etoposide: evidence for interaction at the nuclear matrix. *J Urol* 1993;149:1622.

281. Stearns ME, Jenkins DP, Tew KD. Dansylated estramustine, a fluorescent probe for studies of estramustine uptake and identification of intracellular targets. *Proc Natl Acad Sci U S A* 1985;82:8483.

282. Yoshida D, Cornell-Bell A, Piepmeier JM. Selective antimitotic effects of estramustine correlate with its antimicrotubule properties on glioblastoma and astrocytes. *Neurosurgery* 1994;34:863.

283. Bjork P, Borg A, Ferno M, Nilsson S. Expression and partial characterization of estramustine-binding protein (EMBP) in human breast cancer and malignant melanoma. *Anticancer Res* 1991;11:1173.

284. Vallbo C, Bergenheim AT, Bergstrom P, Gunnarsson PO, Henriksson R. Apoptotic tumor cell death induced by estramustine in patients with malignant glioma. *Clin Cancer Res* 1998;4:87.

285. Yoshida D, Piepmeier J, Weinstein M. Estramustine sensitizes human glioblastoma cells to irradiation. *Cancer Res* 1994;54:1415.

286. Ranganathan S, Dexter DW, Benetatos CA, et al. Increase of beta(III)- and beta(IVa)-tubulin isotopes in human prostate carcinoma cells as a result of estramustine resistance. *Cancer Res* 1996;56:2584.

287. Ranganathan S, Dexter DW, Benetatos CA, Hudes GR. Cloning and sequencing of human betaIII-tubulin cDNA: induction of betaIII isotype in human prostate carcinoma cells by acute exposure to antimicrotubule agents. *Biochim Biophys Acta* 1998;1395:237.

288. Ranganathan S, Dexter DW, Hudes GR. Modulation of endogenous β-tubulin isotype expression as a result of human βIII cDNA transfection into prostate carcinoma cells. *Br J Cancer* 2001;85:735.

289. Sangrajrang S, Denoulet P, Millot G, et al. Estramustine resistance correlates with tau over-expression in human prostatic carcinoma cells. *Int J Cancer* 1998;77:626.

290. Yang CP, Shen HJ, Horwitz SB. Modulation of the function of P-glycoprotein by estramustine. *J Natl Cancer Inst* 1994;86:723.

291. Speicher LA, Barone LR, Chapman AE, et al. P-glycoprotein binding and modulation of the multidrug-resistant phenotype by estramustine. *J Natl Cancer Inst* 1994;86:688.

292. Laing NM, Belinsky MG, Kruh GD, et al. Amplification of the ATP-binding cassette 2 transporter gene is functionally linked with enhanced efflux of estramustine in ovarian carcinoma cells. *Cancer Res* 1998;58:1332.

293. Gunnarsson PO, Andersson SB, Johansson SA, Nilsson T, Plym-Forshell G. Pharmacokinetics of estramustine phosphate (Estracyt) in prostatic cancer patients. *Eur J Clin Pharmacol* 1984;26:113.

294. Forshell GP, Muntzing J, Ek A, Lindstedt E, Dencker H. The absorption, metabolism, and excretion of Estracyt (NSC 89199) in patients with prostatic cancer. *Invest Urol* 1976; 14:128.

295. Dixon R, Brooks M, Gill G. Estramustine phosphate: plasma concentrations of its metabolites following oral administration to man, rat and dog. *Res Commun Chem Pathol Pharmacol* 1980;27:17.

296. Gunnarsson PO, Forshell GP. Clinical pharmacokinetics of estramustine phosphate. *Urology* 1984;23:22.

297. Yamazaki H, Shaw PM, Guengerich FP, Shimada T. Roles of cytochromes P450 1A2 and 3A4 in the oxidation of estradiol and estrone in human liver microsomes. *Chem Res Toxicol* 1998;11:659.

298. Hudes G, Haas N, Yeslow G, et al. Phase I clinical and pharmacologic trial of intravenous estramustine phosphate. *J Clin Oncol* 2002;20:1115.

299. Gunnarsson PO, Davidsson T, Andersson SB, Backman C, Johansson SA. Impairment of estramustine phosphate absorption by concurrent intake of milk and food. *Eur J Clin Pharmacol* 1990;38:189.

300. Petrylak DP, Macarthur RB, O'Connor J, et al. Phase I trial of docetaxel with estramustine in androgen-independent prostate cancer. *J Clin Oncol* 1999;17:958.

301. Kelly WK, Zhu AX, Scher H, et al. Dose escalation study of intravenous estramustine phosphate in combination with paclitaxel and carboplatin in patients with advanced prostate cancer. *Clin Cancer Res* 2003;9:2098.

302. Von Schoultz B, Carlstrom K, Collste L, et al. Estrogen therapy and liver function-metabolic effects of oral and parenteral administration. *Prostate* 1989;14:389.

303. Park DS, Vassilopoulou R, Tu S-M. Estramustine-related hypocalcemia in patients with prostate carcinoma and osteoblastic metastases. *Urology* 2001;58:105.

304. Sinibaldi VJ, Carducci MA, Moore-Cooper S, et al. Phase II evaluation of docetaxel plus one-day oral estramustine phosphate in the treatment of patients with androgen independent prostate carcinoma. *Cancer* 2002;94:1457.

305. Ferrari AC, Chachoua A, Singh H, et al. A phase I/II study of weekly paclitaxel and 3 days of high dose oral estramustine in patients with hormone-refractory prostate carcinoma. *Cancer* 2001;91:2039.

306. Hudes G, Ross E, Roth B, et al. Improved survival for patients with hormone refractory prostate cancer receiving estramustine-based antimicrotubule therapy: final report of a Hoosier oncology group and Fox Chase Network phase III trial comparing vinblastine and vinblastine plus oral estramustine. *Proc Am Soc Clin Oncol* 2002:21:177a(abst).

307. Savarese DM, Halabi VH, Akerley WL, et al. Phase II study of docetaxel, estramustine and low-dose hydrocortisone in men with hormone-refractory prostate cancer: a final report of CALGB 9780. *J Clin Oncol* 2001;19:2509.

308. Wartmann M, Altmann KH. The biology and medicinal chemistry of epothilones. *Curr Med Chem Anti-Canc Agent* 2002;2:123.

309. Kamath K, Jordan MA. Suppression of microtubule dynamics by epothilone B is associated with mitotic arrest. *Cancer Res* 2003;63:6026.

310. Kowalski RJ, Giannakakou P, Hamel E. Activities of the microtubule-stabilizing agents epothilones A and B with purified tubulin and in cells resistant to paclitaxel (Taxol). *J Biol Chem* 1997;272:2534.

311. Rothermel J, Wartmann M, Chen T, Hohneker J. EPO906 (epothilone B): a promising novel microtubule stabilizer. *Semin Oncol* 2003;3[Suppl 6]:51.

312. Lee FY, Borzilleri R, Fairchild CR, et al. BMS-247550: a novel epothilone analog with a mode of action similar to paclitaxel but possessing superior antitumor efficacy. *Clin Cancer Res* 2001;7:1429.

313. Chou TC, Zhang XG, Harris CR, et al. Desoxyepothilone B is curative against human tumor xenografts that are refractory to paclitaxel. *Proc Natl Acad Sci U S A* 1998;95:15798.

314. ter Haar E, Kowalski RJ, Hamel E, et al. Discodermolide, a cytotoxic marine agent that stabilizes microtubules more potently than taxol. *Biochemistry* 1996;35:243.

315. Martello LA, McDaid HM, Regl DL, et al. Taxol and discodermolide represent a synergistic drug combination in human carcinoma cell lines. *Clin Cancer Res* 2000;6:1978.

316. Hamel E, Sackett DL, Vourloumis D, Nicolaou KC. The coral-derived natural products eleutherobin and sarcodictyins A and B: effects on the assembly of purified tubulin with and without microtubule-associated proteins and binding at the polymer taxoid site. *Biochemistry* 1999;38:5490.

317. Mooberry SL, Tien G, Hernandez AH, et al. Laulimalide and isolaulimalide, new paclitaxel-like microtubule-stabilizing agents. *Cancer Res* 1999;59:653.

318. Ojima I, Chakravarty S, Inoue T, et al. A common pharmacophore for cytotoxic natural products that stabilize microtubules. *Proc Natl Acad Sci U S A* 1999;96:4256.

319. Panda D, DeLuca K, Williams D, Jordan MA, Wilson L. Antiproliferative mechanism of action of cryptophycin-52: kinetic stabilization of microtubule dynamics of high-affinity binding to microtubule ends. *Proc Natl Acad Sci U S A* 1998;95:9313.
320. Hamel E. Natural products which interact with tubulins in the vinca domain: maytansine, rhizoxin, phomopsin A, dolastatin 10-15 and halicondrin B. *Pharmacol Ther* 1992;55:31.
321. Towle MJ, Salvato KA, Budrow J, et al. In vitro and in vivo anticancer activities of synthetic macrocyclic ketone analogues of halichondrin B. *Cancer Res* 2001;61:1013.
322. Wood KW, Cornwell WD, Jackson JR. Past and future of the mitotic spindle as an oncology target. *Curr Opin Pharmacol* 2001;4:370.
323. Chu Q, Holen KD, Rowinsky EK, et al. A phase I study to determine the safety and pharmacokinetics of IV administered SB-715992, a novel kinesin spindle protein (KSP) inhibitor, in patients (pts) with solid tumors. *Proc Am Soc Clin Oncol* 2003;22:131(abst).
324. Sakowicz R, Finer JJ, Berard C, et al. Antitumor activity of a kinesin inhibitor. *Cancer Res* 2004;64:3276.

MEHMET SITKI COPUR
MICHAL G. ROSE
EDWARD CHU

SECTION 9

Miscellaneous Chemotherapeutic Agents

L-ASPARAGINASE

L-Asparaginase (L-asparagine aminohydrolase, EC 3.5.1.1) is a naturally occurring enzyme found in a variety of plants and microorganisms. Highly purified enzyme has been derived from the bacterial species *Escherichia coli* and *Erwinia chrysanthemi*, and these preparations demonstrate significant activity against acute lymphoblastic leukemia (ALL). This enzyme exerts its antitumor activity by depleting circulating pools of L-asparagine. Although normal cells are able to synthesize asparagine from aspartic acid through a reaction catalyzed by asparagine synthase, malignant cells lack this enzyme and are thus dependent on exogenous sources of L-asparagine for survival. Depletion of the essential amino acid L-asparagine results in rapid inhibition of protein synthesis, and studies have confirmed that cytotoxicity of this agent correlates well with inhibition of protein synthesis. The inhibitory activity of this agent appears to be maximal in the G_1 phase of the cell-cycle studies. In addition to depletion of L-asparagine, L-asparaginase may exert its antitumor activity through a glutaminase effect, whereby depletion of essential glutamine stores leads to inhibition of DNA biosynthesis.[1]

The development of cellular resistance to L-asparaginase has been attributed to increased expression of L-asparaginase synthetase via amplification of the gene copy number in tumor cells. The increased synthesis of the synthetase enzyme facilitates the cellular production of L-asparagine from endogenous sources. A second resistance mechanism has been identified in which there is formation of antibodies against L-asparaginase, resulting in inhibition of function. Preferential use by leukemic cells of asparagine produced by normal cells and preferential regrowth of resting leukemic cells not affected by L-asparaginase may also contribute to resistance.[2,3]

L-Asparaginase is not absorbed by the gastrointestinal tract, and it must be administered via the intravenous (IV) or intramuscular (IM) route. After IV administration, plasma levels correlate closely with a given dose. After IM injection, peak plasma levels are reached within 14 to 24 hours, and they are approximately one-half those achieved with IV administration. Plasma protein binding is on the order of 30%. L-Asparaginase diffuses poorly out of the capillaries, and the apparent volume of distribution is approximately 70% to 80% of the total plasma volume. The pharmacokinetics of L-asparaginase vary depending on the particular source of the enzyme.[4] Pharmacokinetic studies in newly diagnosed children with ALL have shown peak serum concentrations in the range of 1 to 10 IU/mL, which are observed 24 to 48 hours after a single injection of 2500 to 25,000 IU/m² of the enzyme derived from *E coli*. After a dose of 25,000 IU/m² of the enzyme derived from *Erwinia* species, peak serum levels are achieved within 24 hours; however, the half-life is significantly shorter (15 hours) than that observed for *E coli* L-asparaginase (40 to 50 hours). In contrast, a polyethylene glycol (PEG) modified form of L-asparaginase (PEG–L-asparaginase), when administered at a dose of 2500 IU/m², achieves peak drug levels at 72 to 96 hours and has a significantly longer half-life (5.7 days) than for the *E coli* L-asparaginase preparation.[5] The metabolism of L-asparaginase has not been well characterized, although there appears to be minimal hepatobiliary or urinary excretion.

With regard to drug interactions, L-asparaginase has been shown to antagonize the antineoplastic effects of methotrexate when administered either together with it or when given immediately before. For this reason, these two drugs should be administered at least 24 hours apart. L-Asparaginase has also been shown to inhibit the metabolic clearance of vincristine, and this interaction can result in increased toxicity, especially as it relates to neurotoxicity. Toxicity is less pronounced when L-asparaginase is administered after vincristine, and for this reason, vincristine is normally administered at least 12 to 24 hours before L-asparaginase.

Hypersensitivity reactions occur in up to 25% of patients, and a mild form is usually manifested as skin rash and urticaria. Life-threatening anaphylactic reactions present as facial edema, hypotension, bronchospasm, and respiratory distress. These hypersensitivity reactions generally occur on repeated exposure, and the risk is increased when L-asparaginase is used as a single agent without the concurrent use of steroids or methotrexate. Although PEG–L-asparaginase has less immunogenic potential than the native nonpegylated forms of the enzyme, hypersensitivity reactions can still occur.[6] A number of other side effects are observed that are secondary to the inhibitory effects of L-asparaginase on cellular protein synthesis. Decreased serum levels of insulin, key lipoproteins, and albumin have been reported. L-Asparaginase can cause alterations in thyroid function tests as early as 2 days after an administered dose, and this effect is believed to be secondary to a reduction in the serum levels of thyroxine-binding globulin. Alterations in coagulation parameters with prolonged thrombin time, prothrombin (PT) time, and partial thromboplastin time have been observed. In addition, decreased levels of vitamin K–dependent clotting factors, including factors V, VII, VIII, and IX, and a reduction in fibrinogen levels have been observed.

Reductions in serum antithrombin III, protein C, protein S, plasminogen, and α_2-antiplasmin can also be caused by treatment. As a result, patients treated with L-asparaginase are at increased risk for bleeding and for thromboembolic events.[7] L-Asparaginase is contraindicated in patients with a prior history of pancreatitis, as there is a 10% incidence of acute pancreatitis. Neurologic toxicity includes lethargy, confusion, agitation, hallucinations, and/or coma, and in many instances, the severe form of neurotoxicity resembles ammonia toxicity. In contrast to the other anticancer agents used to treat ALL, myelosuppression is rarely seen with L-asparaginase therapy.

BLEOMYCIN

Bleomycin sulfate is composed of a mixture of cytotoxic glycopeptide antineoplastic antibiotics (bleomycin A_2 and bleomycin B_2) isolated from the culture broths of the fungus *Streptomyces verticillus*. The bleomycins constitute a family of peptides with a molecular weight of approximately 1500 daltons. A DNA-binding region and an iron-binding region are present at opposite ends of the molecule. The cytotoxic effects of bleomycin result from the formation of oxygen free radicals, which then cause single- and double-strand DNA breaks.[8] Bleomycin-mediated DNA damage requires the presence of a redox-active Fe^{2+} metal ion in the presence of oxygen to generate the activated free radical species. Within the last several years, it has also become apparent that bleomycin mediates the oxidative degradation of all major classes of cellular RNAs.[9,10] The effects of bleomycin are cell cycle specific, as its major effects are mediated in the G_2 and M phases of the cell cycle. With regard to determinants of cytotoxic and antitumor activity, three mechanisms of cellular resistance have been identified.[8] They include increased drug inactivation through increased expression of the catabolic enzyme bleomycin hydrolase, increased expression of DNA repair enzymes resulting in enhanced repair of DNA damage, and decreased drug accumulation through altered cellular uptake. At present, bleomycin is mainly used as part of combination regimens for the treatment of Hodgkin's and non-Hodgkin's lymphoma, germ cell tumors, squamous cell cancer of the head and neck, and squamous cell carcinomas of the skin, cervix, vulva, and penis. As a single agent, it is used as a sclerosing agent to control malignant pleural effusions and ascites.

The oral bioavailability of bleomycin is poor, and for this reason, it is administered via the IV or IM routes. After IV administration of 15 U/m^2 bleomycin, there is a rapid biphasic disappearance from the circulation. The initial distribution half-life is on the order of 10 to 20 minutes, whereas the terminal half-life is in the range of 3 hours. Bleomycin is absorbed rapidly after IM injection, and peak blood levels approximately one-third to one-half those achieved after an IV dose are usually reached in 30 to 60 minutes. In contrast to nearly all other anticancer agents, bleomycin can also be administered via the intracavitary route to control malignant pleural effusions or ascites, or both. Approximately 45% to 55% of an administered intracavitary dose of bleomycin is absorbed into the systemic circulation after intrapleural or intraperitoneal administration. Elimination of bleomycin is primarily via the kidneys, and approximately 60% to 70% of an administered dose is excreted unchanged in the urine. In patients with a creatinine clearance

of less than 25 to 35 mL/min, the terminal elimination half-life is increased significantly. For this reason, dose reductions are required in the setting of renal dysfunction.[8]

The dose-limiting toxicity of bleomycin is the induction of pulmonary toxicity.[11] The central event is endothelial cell damage to the lung vasculature that results from the induction of various cytokines and the formation of oxygen free radicals. Bleomycin-induced pneumonitis occurs in approximately 10% of patients, and this side effect is dose and age related. The risk is increased in patients older than 70 years of age and in those who receive a total cumulative dose greater than 400 units. In addition, patients with underlying lung disease; prior irradiation to the chest or mediastinum, or both; and exposure to high concentrations of inspired oxygen are also at increased risk for development of pulmonary toxicity. The clinical presentation includes cough, dyspnea, dry inspiratory crackles, and infiltrates on chest x-ray. Pulmonary function testing is the most sensitive approach to monitor patients, with specific focus on the carbon monoxide diffusion capacity in the lung and vital capacity. Pulmonary function tests should be obtained at baseline before the start of therapy and before each cycle of therapy. A decrease of greater than 15% in either diffusion capacity of carbon dioxide or vital capacity should mandate immediate discontinuation of bleomycin. Idiosyncratic hypersensitivity reactions in the form of fever, chills, urticaria, periorbital edema, and wheezing are observed in up to 25% of patients. Of note, these allergic-type reactions are more commonly seen in patients with lymphoma. These reactions may be immediate or delayed for several hours and usually occur after the first or second dose. A test dose of 1 mg bleomycin may be helpful before administration of the first dose of bleomycin in patients with lymphoma. Mucocutaneous toxicity is a relatively late but common manifestation that appears to be dose dependent. This toxicity presents as mucositis, erythema, hyperpigmentation, induration, hyperkeratosis, and skin peeling that may progress to ulceration, usually developing in the second and third week of treatment and after a cumulative dose of 150 to 200 units of the drug. It is interesting to note that the levels of bleomycin hydrolase are relatively low in lung and skin tissue, perhaps offering an explanation as to why these normal tissues are more adversely affected by bleomycin. Myelosuppression and immunosuppression are relatively mild. In rare cases, vascular events, including myocardial infarction, stroke, and Raynaud's phenomenon, have been reported.

IMATINIB MESYLATE

Imatinib mesylate (STI 571, Gleevec) is a rationally developed anticancer agent that functions as a signal transduction inhibitor. It is a phenylaminopyrimidinemethanesulfonate analogue and occupies the adenosine triphosphate (ATP) binding site of the Bcr-Abl tyrosine kinase and other related tyrosine kinases, including platelet-derived growth factor, stem cell factor, and c-kit. Imatinib functions as a potent competitive inhibitor of ATP binding and, in so doing, inhibits substrate phosphorylation and downstream signaling pathways. Induction of apoptosis through as yet not well-characterized mechanisms is another mechanism by which this agent exerts its antitumor activity.[12-14] This agent is currently approved as first-line therapy for the chronic phase of chronic myeloid leukemia (CML); as second-line therapy for the chronic phase of CML after failure on interferon-alpha therapy; for CML in the accelerated phase or blast crisis, or both; for Philadelphia chromosome–positive ALL; and for gastrointestinal stromal tumors expressing the c-kit tyrosine kinase.[15-20] In newly diagnosed CML, hematologic responses are observed as early as 2 weeks after initiation of therapy, and the median time to complete hematologic responses is 4 weeks after the start of therapy. Complete hematologic responses are observed in nearly 95% of patients, and complete cytogenetic responses are reported in 74% of cases. Typically, cytogenetic responses are observed as early as 2 months and up to 10 months after starting therapy, and the median time to best cytogenetic response is approximately 5 months.

Although imatinib has only gained widespread use in the clinic over the past 2 to 3 years, the development of cellular drug resistance has already been described. The most common mechanism of resistance relates to increased expression of Bcr-Abl tyrosine kinase protein through gene amplification or increased transcription, or both. Mutations in the kinase domain have been identified that result in alterations in the binding affinity of the enzyme to drug. Increased expression of the multidrug resistance P170 protein gives rise to enhanced drug efflux, with subsequent decreased intracellular drug accumulation. In addition, increased degradation or metabolism of the drug, or both, through as yet not well-defined mechanisms have also been reported. Finally, there are cases in which no specific mechanism of resistance has been identified. In this group of patients, the process of clonal evolution has resulted in intracellular signaling pathways other than that controlled by the Bcr-Abl tyrosine kinase taking over with respect to the ongoing growth and proliferation of the tumor cells.

Imatinib is well absorbed after oral administration, with maximal serum concentrations being achieved within 2 to 4 hours. The oral bioavailability for the capsule form is nearly 100%. With once-daily dosing, median peak serum concentrations at steady state are 5.4 μM, and median trough levels are 1.43 μM. These concentrations are several-fold higher than that required to inhibit the tyrosine kinase enzyme, at least as determined by preclinical *in vitro* assays measuring enzyme activity.[21] Steady-state drug concentrations are reached in 2 to 3 days. Binding to plasma proteins is extensive, on the order of 95%, and binding is mainly to albumin and α_1-acid glycoprotein. Imatinib is metabolized in the liver, primarily by the CYP3A4 microsomal enzyme. After oral administration, the elimination half-lives of imatinib and its major metabolite, the N-desmethyl piperazine derivative, are approximately 18 and 40 hours, respectively.[22]

With regard to drug interactions, caution must be used when imatinib is administered in the presence of phenytoin (Dilantin) and other drugs that stimulate the liver microsomal CYP3A4 enzyme, including dexamethasone, carbamazepine, rifampicin, phenobarbital, and St. John's wort. These drugs increase the rate of metabolism of imatinib, thereby resulting in its inactivation. Drugs that inhibit the liver microsomal CYP3A4 system, such as ketoconazole, itraconazole, erythromycin, and clarithromycin, decrease the rate of metabolism of imatinib and give rise to increased drug levels and potentially increased toxicity. Thus, dose adjustments of imatinib should be considered with the concurrent use of inhibitors and inducers of the liver microsomal system. Finally, patients receiving oral anticoagulants such as warfarin need to be closely monitored with respect to their coagulation parameters, as imatinib inhibits the metabolism of warfarin by the liver P-450 system. As such, the dose of warfarin requires careful adjustment, depending on the PT/international normalized ratio values.

Imatinib has a favorable safety profile, and side effects are usually mild.[15,19] Nonhematologic toxicities include peripheral edema, fluid retention, mild nausea, muscle cramps, abdominal pain, mild diarrhea, skin rashes, arthralgias, myalgias, bone pain, and mild transient elevations in serum transaminases. Myelosuppression with neutropenia and thrombocytopenia is usually a reflection of clinical efficacy, but in some cases, it may represent the toxic effects of imatinib on normal hematopoietic cells. In general, severe neutropenia and thrombocytopenia are more common in patients with advanced disease, particularly those in blast crisis. In patients with chronic-phase CML, discontinuation of therapy may be advisable in the setting of myelosuppression during imatinib therapy. However, in patients with advanced disease or those in blast crisis, or both, continuation of therapy with or without myeloid growth factors may be justified.

GEFITINIB

Gefitinib (ZD1839, Iressa) is an orally active, highly selective, reversible inhibitor of the tyrosine kinase domain associated with the epidermal growth factor receptor (EGFR). This agent blocks the EGFR signaling pathway, which has been shown to be expressed in a wide range of solid tumors. It is a low-molecular-weight (447-dalton) synthetic anilinoquinazoline [4-(3-chloro-4-fluoroanilino)-7-methoxy-6-(3-morpholinopropoxy) quinazoline] (Fig. 15.9-1) that was originally developed from a lead series of 4-anilinoquinazoline compounds. Gefitinib was identified as a lead candidate based on its good oral bioavailability and its ability to yield sustained blood levels over a 24-hour period.[23,24]

The mechanism by which gefitinib exerts its cytotoxic and antitumor action is not fully characterized. It inhibits the intracellular phosphorylation and signaling of EGFR–tyrosine kinase through competitive binding of the ATP-binding domain of the receptor (Fig. 15.9-2). Although EGFR is a member of the erb-B receptor family, gefitinib is approximately 100-fold less effective in inhibiting HER-2 tyrosine kinase activity than the EGFR-associated enzyme. In preclinical experimental studies, treatment with gefitinib was associated with cell-cycle arrest at the G_0/G_1 boundary in a dose- and time-dependent manner involving up-regulation of p27 and p21 cyclin-dependent kinase inhibitors.[25,26] It has now been well established that inhibition of the EGFR signaling pathway initiates a cascade of events that results in inhibition of critical mitogenic and antiapoptotic signals involved in cell proliferation and growth, metastasis and invasion, angiogenesis, and response to chemotherapy or radiation therapy, or both.[25,27]

Gefitinib is slowly absorbed by the gastrointestinal tract, and its oral bioavailability approaches 60%. Ingestion of food does not appear to impair drug absorption. Peak plasma levels are achieved in 3 to 7 hours, whereas steady-state drug concentrations are observed in 7 to 10 days. The terminal half-life of the drug is 48 hours. Gefitinib undergoes extensive metabolism by the liver, predominantly by the CYP3A4 microsomal enzyme. Metabolism of gefitinib involves three sites of biotransforma-

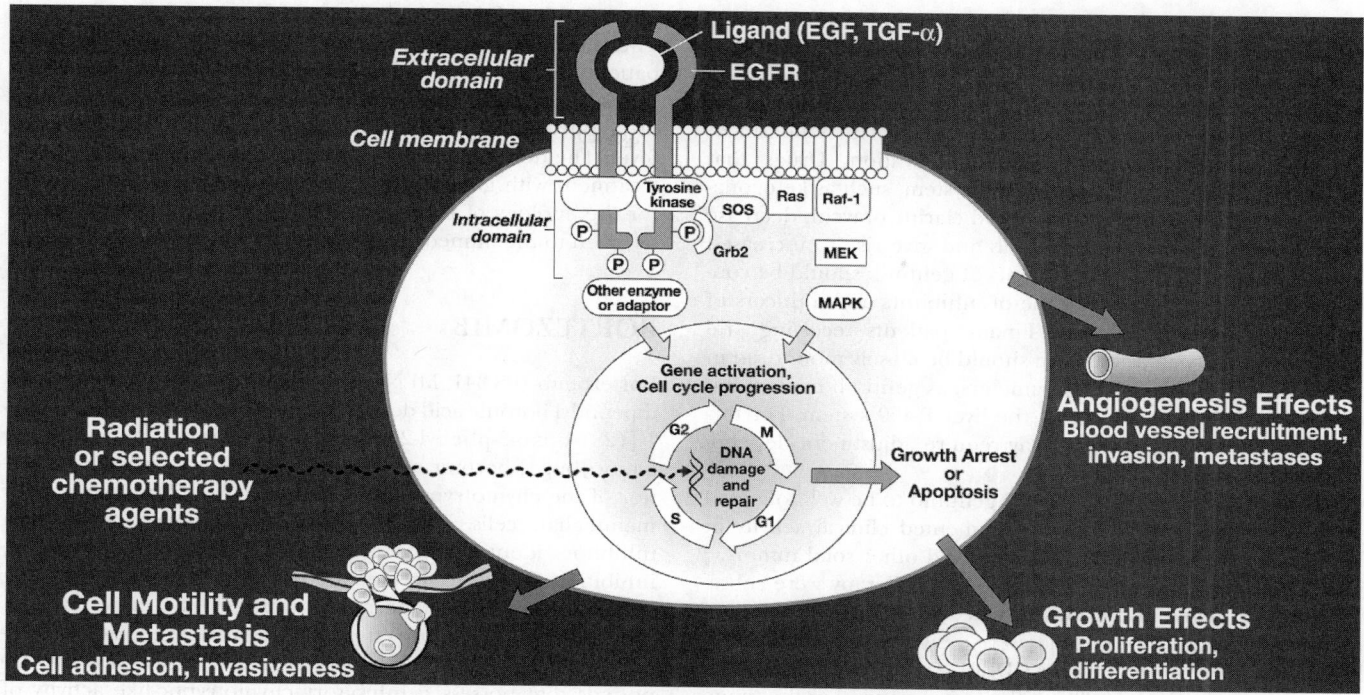

FIGURE 15.9-1. Role of the epidermal growth factor receptor (EGFR) pathway in signal transduction and tumor progression. MAPK, mitogen-activated protein kinase; SOS, son of sevenless; TGF-α, transforming growth factor-α. (From Harari PM, Huang S-M. Modulation of molecular targets to enhance radiation. *Clin Cancer Res* 2000;6:323, with permission.) (See Color Fig. 15.9-1 in the CD-ROM.)

tion: metabolism of the N-propoxymorpholino group, demethylation of the methoxy substituent on the quinazoline, and oxidative defluorination of the halogenated phenyl group. The main metabolite is the O-desmethyl piperazine derivative, which is significantly less potent than the parent drug. Gefitinib is eliminated primarily by hepatobiliary excretion. Renal elimination of parent drug and its metabolites accounts for less than 4% of an administered dose.

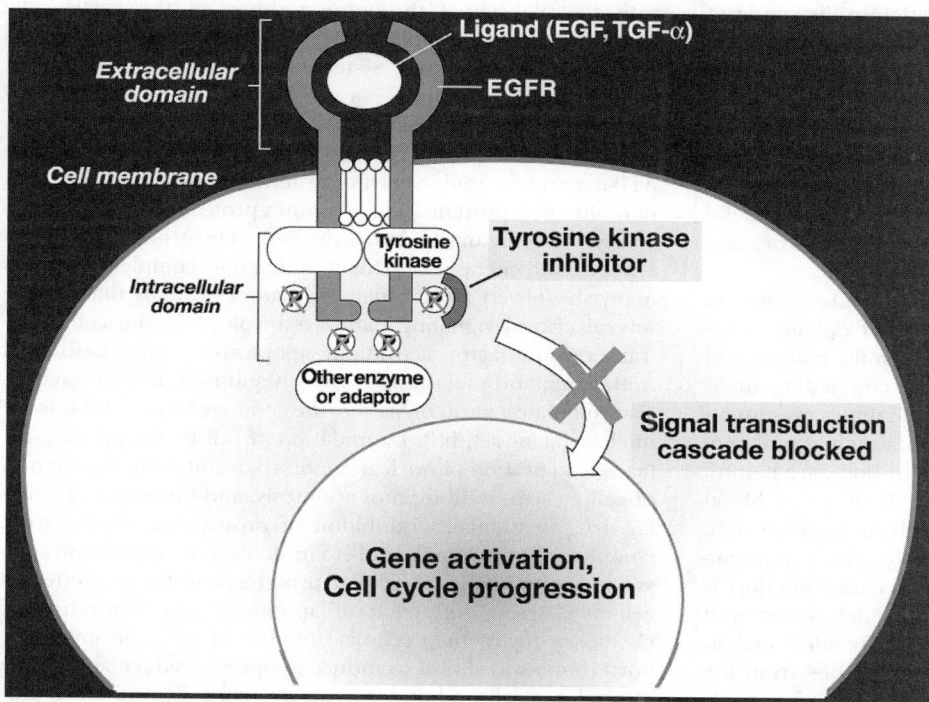

FIGURE 15.9-2. Inhibition of epidermal growth factor receptor (EGFR) via tyrosine kinase inhibitors, including gefitinib. TGF-α, transforming growth factor-α. (See Color Fig. 15.9-2 in the CD-ROM.)

With regard to drug interactions, caution must be used when gefitinib is administered in the presence of drugs that stimulate the liver microsomal CYP3A4 enzyme, including phenytoin, carbamazepine, rifampicin, phenobarbital, and St. John's wort. These drugs increase the rate of metabolism of gefitinib, thereby resulting in its inactivation. Drugs that inhibit the liver microsomal CYP3A4 system, such as ketoconazole, itraconazole, erythromycin, and clarithromycin, decrease the rate of metabolism of gefitinib and give rise to increased drug levels. Thus, dose adjustments of gefitinib should be considered with the concurrent use of inhibitors and inducers of the liver microsomal system. Finally, patients receiving oral anticoagulants such as warfarin should be closely monitored in terms of their coagulation parameters, as gefitinib may inhibit the metabolism of warfarin by the liver P-450 system. For this reason, the dose of warfarin may require adjustment depending on the PT/INR values.

A phase I study initially showed gefitinib to be well tolerated as a single agent and to have documented clinical activity in non–small cell lung cancer (NSCLC) and other solid tumors.[28] Two large phase II trials of gefitinib monotherapy were subsequently conducted in previously treated patients with refractory recurrent NSCLC. These studies were designated *Iressa Dose Evaluation in Advanced Lung Cancer* (IDEAL) I and II, and objective response rates of 10% to 20% with median survival in the range of 6 to 8 months were reported.[29,30] Randomized phase III trials were subsequently performed in Europe and North America investigating the combination of gefitinib and standard first-line chemotherapy regimens. These clinical studies, designated as *Iressa NSCLC Trial Assessing Combination Treatment* (INTACT) I and II trials combined gefitinib and chemotherapy in previously untreated advanced NSCLC patients. Unfortunately, the addition of gefitinib to standard platinum-based chemotherapy regimens failed to demonstrate a survival advantage over the chemotherapy regimens alone.[31,32] Despite these negative results with combination therapy, gefitinib was approved as monotherapy by the U.S. Food and Drug Administration in the spring of 2003 for the treatment of patients with locally advanced or metastatic NSCLC after failure of platinum-based chemotherapy or second-line docetaxel chemotherapy, or both. Patients with the bronchoalveolar pathologic subtype of NSCLC may be more sensitive to therapy than other histologic subtypes. Several phase II/III studies are currently investigating the role of gefitinib as monotherapy as well as in combination regimens for other solid tumors, such as head and neck, breast, prostate, gastric, and colorectal cancers.[33]

In general, gefitinib is well tolerated. The most common adverse events reported with the recommended 250-mg monotherapy dose are diarrhea, mucositis, and mild nausea and vomiting.[28] A common side effect of EGFR-targeted agents is skin rash, which typically is an acneiform rash that is present on the face and upper trunk. Topical antibiotics such as oral clindamycin or minocycline clindamycin gel, or both, are helpful in reducing the severity of the skin rash. Elevations in blood pressure, especially in patients with underlying hypertension, and mild to moderate transient elevations in serum transaminases are also observed. A potentially serious adverse effect is the onset of interstitial lung disease (ILD), which occurs with an overall incidence of approximately 1%. A detailed analysis identified 408 cases of ILD (324 from Japan and 84 from the United States/rest of the world) out of a total 50,005 patients treated with gefitinib (including 18,960 patients from Japan).[34] The median time to onset of ILD was 24 days in Japanese patients and 42 days in U.S. patients. Approximately one-third of cases were fatal. Patients often presented with an acute onset of dyspnea in the absence or presence of cough or low-grade fever. The development of dyspnea, cough, and fever while on treatment with gefitinib should prompt immediate evaluation for the etiology of these symptoms, and consideration should be given to the immediate discontinuation of drug therapy.[34]

BORTEZOMIB

Bortezomib (PS-341, MLN341, LDP-341, Velcade) is a modified dipeptidyl boronic acid designated chemically as [(1R)-3-methyl-1-[(2S)-1-oxo-3-phenyl-2-[(pyrazinyl-carbonyl) amino]propyl] amino]butyl] boronic acid (Fig. 15.9-3). It is a reversible inhibitor of the chymotrypsin-like activity of the 26S proteasome in mammalian cells. The initial investigations of proteasome inhibitors identified the proapoptotic effects of proteasome inhibition. Efforts to develop a proteasome inhibitor with therapeutic potential resulted in the synthesis of a large series of compounds with varying efficacy. The earliest reported proteasome inhibitors included tripeptidyl aldehydes, a class of compounds that possessed inhibitory chymotryptic-like activity of the proteasome complex. However, these compounds were relatively nonspecific in their cytotoxic effects as they inhibited other thiol proteases, including cathepsin B and calpains. In addition, they displayed poor stability and limited bioavailability. The initial breakthrough came with the synthesis of peptidyl boronic acids, with a 100-fold enhancement in potency eventually leading to the discovery of bortezomib, a more potent and selective proteasome inhibitor. Bortezomib is highly specific for the chymotryptic activity of the proteasome, and the empty p-orbital of the boron atom within the molecule presumably allows it to form a stable tetrahedral intermediate with the N-terminal threonine residues of the catalytically active proteasome β-subunits.[35,36] In a broad range of preclinical experimental model systems, bortezomib demonstrated antitumor activity as either a single agent or in combination with other cytotoxic agents.[37–39]

Bortezomib inhibits the 26S proteasome, which is a large ATP-dependent multicatalytic protein complex that degrades ubiquitinated proteins. The ubiquitin-proteasome system plays an essential role in regulating the cell cycle, growth and proliferation, and metastasis. This multienzyme complex degrades many short-lived intracellular regulatory proteins that govern several critical signaling pathways involved in the cell cycle, transcription factor activation, apoptosis, angiogenesis, cell trafficking, and metastasis.[40] The ubiquitin-proteasome system also mediates proteolysis of the endogenous inhibitor of nuclear factor κB, IκB. Degradation of IκB by the proteasome leads to activation of nuclear factor κB, resulting in stimulation of cell growth, inhibition of apoptosis, and induction of cellular drug resistance.[41] Inhibition of proteasome multienzyme complex by bortezomib leads to inhibition of targeted proteolysis of multiple critical cellular proteins, and the end effect is cell-cycle arrest, induction of apoptosis, and restoration of chemosensitivity. In preclinical models of multiple myeloma, bortezomib was shown to induce apoptosis, reduce adherence of myeloma cells to bone marrow stromal cells, and block pro-

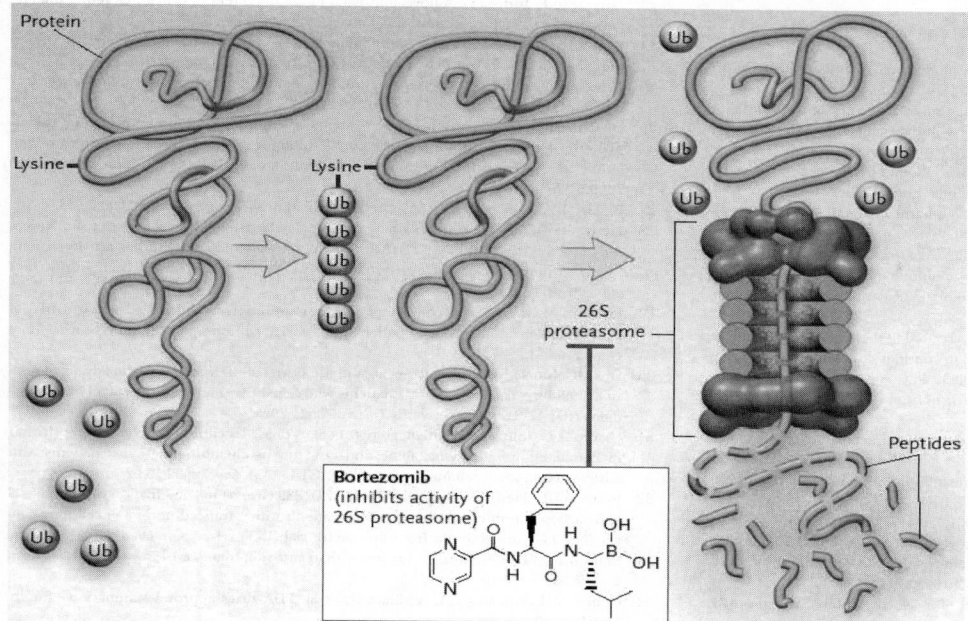

FIGURE 15.9-3. Mechanism of activation of bortezomib. Proteins are targeted to the 26S proteasome for degradation by a process of polyubiquitination. Bortezomib inhibits the catalytic activity of the proteasome. Ub, ubiquitin. (See Color Fig. 15.9-3 in the CD-ROM.)

duction and intracellular signaling of interleukin-6. Restoration of apoptotic response, blockage of the production of several essential angiogenic factors, and enhancement of the cytotoxic effects of dexamethasone and other chemotherapeutic agents are other effects mediated by bortezomib.[40]

This agent is not orally bioavailable, and as such, it is administered via the IV route. It is rapidly cleared from the vascular compartment in a biphasic manner characterized by a rapid distribution phase followed by a prolonged terminal elimination phase. The mean elimination half-life ranges from 9 to 15 hours. The volume of distribution is not yet well characterized. Nearly 80% of the drug is bound to plasma proteins. Bortezomib is primarily metabolized by the liver microsomal system, and the main cytochrome enzymes involved are CYP3A4, 2D6, 2C19, 2C9, and 1A2. The major metabolic pathway is deboronation to form two deboronated metabolites, and both of these metabolites are inactive as proteasome inhibitors. The effects of renal or hepatic impairment have not been fully evaluated.

Inhibition of proteasome activity can be measured in whole blood or isolated peripheral blood mononuclear cells. After IV administration of bortezomib, 26S proteasome activity is inhibited in a dose-dependent and reversible manner, and this inhibitory effect can be used to monitor the biologic activity of the drug. Initial clinical trials were designed to target a plasma concentration of bortezomib that resulted in greater than 70% proteasome inhibition (1.3 to 1.6 mg/m^2). Unfortunately, clinical efficacy and the levels of proteasome inhibition measured in peripheral blood mononuclear cells did not correlate with one another. Intense efforts are ongoing to identify specific molecular biomarkers that can help to better identify response to this agent.

A multicenter, open-label, nonrandomized, phase II trial enrolled 202 patients with multiple myeloma who had received at least two prior therapies and who had evidence of disease progression while on their most recent therapy.[42] After 24 weeks, the overall tumor response rate with bortezomib alone (1.3 mg/m^2 two times each week) was 35%. Seven patients (4%) had a complete response with no evidence of detectable myeloma protein. The median duration of response was 1 year, and the median overall survival was 16 months. A small, phase II, open-label multicenter randomized dose-ranging study evaluated 54 patients with refractory or relapsed multiple myeloma. In this study, the overall response rates were 33% and 50% at the 1.0 and 1.3-mg/m^2 dose levels, respectively. Based on these promising clinical results, bortezomib was approved by the U.S. Food and Drug Administration for relapsing or refractory multiple myeloma. Several phase I and II clinical trials are currently evaluating the role of bortezomib in other tumor types, including CML, neuroendocrine tumors, renal cell carcinoma, melanoma, platinum-sensitive ovarian cancer, soft tissue sarcomas, colorectal cancer, breast cancer, low-grade lymphoproliferative disorders, and mantle cell lymphoma.[43]

With regard to toxicity, the most frequently reported adverse events include fatigue, malaise, and generalized weakness. The initial onset of fatigue is usually observed during the first or second cycles of therapy. Gastrointestinal side effects in the form of nausea/vomiting and diarrhea occur in up to 55% of patients, although grade 3/4 toxicity is unusual. Fever in the absence of infection has been reported in 20% to 40% of patients. Myelosuppression with thrombocytopenia and neutropenia is observed in up to 40% of patients. Peripheral sensory neuropathy is the most clinically significant adverse event and is reported in approximately 30% of patients. The neurologic symptoms generally improve and return to baseline on discontinuation of the drug. Orthostatic hypotension occurs in 12% of patients, and for this reason, this agent must be used with caution in patients with a prior history of syncope and in those who are receiving antihypertensive medications. In addition, patients should be well hydrated before starting therapy with bortezomib to reduce the risk of orthostatic hypotension.

REFERENCES

1. Asselin BL. The three asparaginases. Comparative pharmacology and optimal use in childhood leukemia. *Adv Exp Med Biol* 1999;457:621.

2. Aslanian AM, Kilberg MS. Multiple adaptive mechanisms affect asparaginase synthase substrate availability in asparaginase-resistant MOLT-4 human leukemia cells. *Biochem J* 2001;358:59.

3. Woo MH, Hak LJ, Storm MC, et al. Anti-asparaginase antibodies following E. coli asparaginase therapy in pediatric acute lymphoblastic leukemia. *Leukemia* 1998;10:1527.

4. Asselin BL, Whitin JC, Coppola DJ, et al. Comparative pharmacokinetic studies of three asparaginase preparations. *J Clin Oncol* 1993;11:1780.

5. Graham ML. Pegasparagase: a review of clinical studies. *Adv Drug Deliv Rev* 2003;55:1293.

6. Wang B, Relling MV, Storm MC, et al. Evaluation of immunologic cross reaction of anti-asparaginase antibodies in acute lymphoblastic leukemia (ALL) and lymphoma patients. *Leukemia* 2003;17:1583.

7. Alberts SR, Bretscher M, Wiltsie JC, et al. Thrombosis related to the use of L-asparaginase in adults with acute lymphoblastic leukemia: a need to consider coagulation monitoring and clotting factor replacement. *Leuk Lymphoma* 1999;32:489.

8. Dorr RT. Bleomycin pharmacology: mechanism of action and resistance, and clinical pharmacokinetics. *Semin Oncol* 1992;19(2S):3.

9. Hecht SM. Bleomycin: new perspectives on the mechanism of action. *J Nat Prod* 2000; 63:158.

10. Abraham AT, Lin JJ, Newton DL, et al. RNA cleavage and inhibition of protein synthesis by bleomycin. *Chem Biol* 2003;10:45.

11. Sleijfer S. Bleomycin-induced pneumonitis. *Chest* 2001;120:617.

12. Buchdunger E, Zimmermann J, Mett H, et al. Selective inhibition of the platelet-derived growth factor signal transduction pathway by a protein-tyrosine kinase inhibitor of the 2-phenylaminopyrimidine class. *Proc Natl Acad Sci U S A* 1995;92:2558.

13. Druker BJ, Tamura S, Buchdunger E, et al. Effects of a selective inhibitor of the ABL tyrosine kinase on the growth of BCR-ABL positive cells. *Nat Med* 1996;2:561.

14. Druker BJ, Lydon NB. Lessons learned from the development of an ABL tyrosine kinase inhibitor for chronic myelogenous leukemia. *J Clin Invest* 2000;105:3.

15. Druker BJ, Talpaz M, Resta DJ, et al. Efficacy and safety of a specific inhibitor of the BCR-ABL tyrosine kinase in chronic myeloid leukemia. *N Engl J Med* 2001;344:1031.

16. Kantarjian H, Sawyers C, Hochaus A, et al. Hematologic and cytogenetic responses to imatinib mesylate in chronic myelogenous leukemia. *N Engl J Med* 2002;346:645.

17. Talpaz M, Silver RT, Druker BJ, et al. Imatinib induces durable hematologic and cytogenetic responses in patients with accelerated phase chronic myeloid leukemia: results of a phase 2 study. *Blood* 2002;99:1928.

18. Druker BJ, Sawyers CL, Kantarjian H et al. Activity of a specific of the BCR-ABL tyrosine kinase in the blast crisis of chronic myeloid leukemia and acute lymphoblastic leukemia with the Philadelphia chromosome. *N Engl J Med* 2001;344:1038.

19. Demetri GD, von Mehren M, Blanke CD, et al. Efficacy and safety of imatinib mesylate in advanced gastrointestinal stromal tumors. *N Engl J Med* 2002;347:472.

20. O'Brien SG, Guilhot F, Larson RA, et al. Imatinib compared with interferon and low-dose cytarabine for newly diagnosed chronic-phase chronic myeloid leukemia. *N Engl J Med* 2003;348;11:994.

21. Deininger MW, Druker BJ, et al. Specific targeted therapy of chronic myelogenous leukemia with imatinib. *Pharmacol Rev* 2003;55:401.

22. Druker BJ. Imatinib mesylate in the treatment of chronic myeloid leukemia. *Expert Opin Pharmacother* 2003;6:963.

23. Ciaardello F, Tortora G. A novel approach in the treatment of cancer: targeting the epidermal growth factor receptor. *Clin Cancer Res* 2001;7:2958.

24. Woodburn JR, Barker AJ. 4-Anilinoquiazolines—a potential new therapy for major human solid tumors overexpressing the EGF receptor. *Br J Cancer* 1996;74:18.

25. Grunwald V, Hidalgo M. Developing inhibitors of the epidermal growth factor receptor for cancer treatment. *J Natl Cancer Inst* 2003;95:851.

26. DiGennaro E, Marcella B, Bruzzese F, et al. Growth inhibition of tumor cells by epidermal growth factor receptor tyrosine kinase inhibitor ZD1839 is associated with upregulation of p27 and p21 cyclin-dependent kinase inhibitors. *Clin Cancer Res* 1999;5:3753s(abst118).

27. Baselga J, Averbuch SD. ZD1839 (Iressa) as an anticancer agent. *Drugs* 2000;60:33.

28. Herbst RS, Maddox AM, Rothenberg ML, et al. Selective epidermal growth factor receptor tyrosine kinase inhibitor ZD1839 is generally well-tolerated and has activity in non-small-cell lung cancer and other solid tumors: results of a phase I trial. *J Clin Oncol* 2002;20:3815.

29. Fukuoka M, Yano S, Giaccone G, et al. Multi-institutional randomized phase II trial of gefitinib for previously treated patients with advanced non-small cell lung cancer. *J Clin Oncol* 2003;21:2237.

30. Kris MG, Natale RB, Herbst RS, et al. A phase II trial of ZD1839 (Iressa) in advanced non-small cell lung cancer (NSCLC) patients who failed platinum and docetaxel based regimens (IDEAL 2). *Proc Am Soc Clin Oncol* 2002;21:292a.

31. Giaccone G, Johnson DH, Manegold C, et al. A phase III clinical trial of ZD1839 (Iressa) in combination with gemcitabine and cisplatin in chemotherapy-naive patients with advanced non-small cell lung cancer (INTACT-1). *Ann Oncol* 2002;13S:2.

32. Johnson DH, Herbst R, Giaccone G, et al. ZD1839 (Iressa) in combination with paclitaxel and carboplatin in chemotherapy-naïve patients with advanced non-small cell lung cancer (NSCLC): initial results from a phase III trial (INTACT-2). *Ann Oncol* 2002;13S:127.

33. Ranson M. ZD1839 (Iressa): for more than just non-small cell lung cancer. *Oncologist* 2002;7:16.

34. Cohen MH, Williams GA, Sridhara R, et al. FDA drug approval summary: Gefitinib. *Oncologist* 2003;8:303.

35. Adams J. Proteasome inhibition in cancer: development of PS-341. *Semin Oncol* 2001; 28:535.

36. Adams J, Behnke M, Chen S, et al. Potent and selective inhibitors of the proteasome dipeptidylboronic acids. *Bioorg Med Chem Lett* 1998;8:333.

37. Adams J, Palombella VJ, Sauswille EA, et al. Proteasome inhibitors: a novel class of potent and effective antitumor agents. *Cancer Res* 1999;59:2615.

38. Cusack JC Jr, Liu R, Houston M, et al. Enhanced chemosensitivity to CPT-11 with proteasome inhibitor PS-341: implications for systemic nuclear factor-κb inhibition. *Cancer Res* 2001;61:3535.

39. Hideshima T, Richardson P, Chauhan D, et al. The proteasome inhibitor PS-341 inhibits growth, induces apoptosis, and overcomes drug resistance in human multiple myeloma cells. *Cancer Res* 2001;61:3071.

40. Adams J. The proteasome: structure, function and role in the cell. *Cancer Treat Rev* 2003;29:3.

41. Sunwoo JB, Chen Z, Dong G, et al. Novel proteasome inhibitors PS-341 inhibits activation of nuclear factor-κb, cell survival, tumor growth, and angiogenesis in squamous cell carcinoma. *Clin Cancer Res* 2001;7:1419.

42. Richardson PG, Barlogie B, Berenson J, et al. A phase 2 study of bortezomib in relapsed refractory myeloma. *N Engl J Med* 2003;348:2609.

43. Wright JJ, Zerivitz K, Schoenfeldt M. Clinical trials referral resource. Current clinical trials for bortezomib. *Oncology* 2003;17:677.

CHAPTER 16

Pharmacology of Cancer Biotherapeutics

VERNON K. SONDAK
BRUCE G. REDMAN

SECTION 1

Interferons

The compounds known as *interferons* are among the most powerful immunomodulatory substances available for therapeutic use. Interferons are highly pleiotropic: In addition to affecting the immune system, they also have direct cytostatic and cytotoxic properties. Both the desired and the adverse effects of interferons can vary dramatically based on the dose, schedule, and route of administration, as well as pharmacologic manipulations of the interferon molecule. In this chapter, the biologic properties of interferons are examined; the dose, schedule, and route dependencies of their effects are discussed; and examples of the therapeutic use of interferons are provided.

Interferons were initially discovered based on their ability to prevent the replication of the influenza virus in the chick embryo. Subsequently the replication of other viruses was shown to be due to "interference factors." These initial reports led to the eventual isolation, characterization, and ultimate cloning of the interferon genes. In humans, the interferons are made up of two classes referred to as *type I* and *type II interferons.* Both types induce a state in which viral replication is impaired by the synthesis of a number of enzymes that interfere with cellular and viral processes. In addition, processes involved in the development of an antiviral state have the capability to induce antiproliferative as well as immunomodulatory activities. These additional activities induced by interferons can be looked on as an extension or enhancement of their antiviral activities. It is these additional functions induced by interferons that resulted in their evaluation as anticancer agents.

The type I family is composed of α (by convention, the pharmacologic forms of interferon-α are referred to as *interferon alfa*), β, and ω subtypes. The type II interferon family is composed entirely of the γ interferon subtype. The various subtypes are further subdivided for pharmaceutical preparations (e.g., interferon alfa-2a, interferon gamma-1b). Although related, the two interferon families are distinct. The genes for type I interferons are located on the short arm of chromosome 9, and all bind to the same receptor. Type I interferons are induced primarily in response to a viral infection of a cell. There are at least 12 natural interferon-α protein products but only one each of interferon-β and interferon-ω. Interferon-α and interferon-ω are produced predominantly from leukocytes, but interferon-β can be produced by most cell types, especially fibroblasts.

Interferon-γ is composed of a single subtype. It is produced predominantly by T lymphocytes and natural killer (NK) cells in response to immune and inflammatory stimuli. Interferon-γ binds to its own unique receptor. The distinct receptors and the downstream signaling that is initiated by ligand-receptor interactions are responsible for the biologic effects of the individual type I and type II interferons.

INTERFERON INDUCTION

The induction of interferon-β production by fibroblasts during viral infection has been well studied and is mediated by nuclear factor κB (NFκB).[1,2] Viral double-stranded RNA (dsRNA) activates dsRNA-dependent protein kinase R (PKR), which then activates the IκKβ subunit of the multicomponent inhibitor of κB (IκB) kinase. Once phosphorylated, IκB releases its inhibition on NFκB, and the latter then enters the nucleus and activates transcription of a variety of proteins, including interferon-β. The viral induction of interferon-α in leukocytes is less well understood but is distinct from its induction in fibroblasts. Although viral infection is the classical means by which interferon-α and interferon-β production is stimulated, it is clearly not the sole stimulus. Treatment of cells with proteins or DNA constructs of microbial derivation, such as bacterial endotoxins or CpG dinucleotide repeats, also stimulates production of type I interferons.[3]

Interferon-γ is produced by T cells and NK cells in response to antigen-presenting cells and inflammatory cytokines. NK cells are part of the innate immune response; their activation is not dependent on antigen recognition. Both activating and inhibitory receptors and ligands have been defined that regulate NK cell function and proliferation.[4,5] Major histocompatibility complex (MHC) class I proteins are the classic inhibitory signal for NK cells. When signals from activating receptors are greater than those from inhibitory receptors, NK cells produce interferon-γ. NK cells are also stimulated to produce interferon-γ when exposed to inflammatory cytokines from macrophages. Tumor necrosis factor-α and interleukin-12 (IL-12) produced by macrophages act together to stimulate interferon-γ production from NK cells.[6] In a positive amplification loop, the interferon-γ from NK cells then stimulates the secretion of tumor necrosis factor-α and IL-12 from macrophages.

T cells are part of the adaptive immune response, requiring stimulation of an antigen-specific receptor for activation. Stimulation of the T-cell receptor by specific antigen or nonspecific mitogens induces transcriptional activation of the interferon-γ gene.[7] Mature T cells express one of two cell surface markers, CD8 or CD4, which serve to restrict antigen binding based on the MHC molecules expressed by the antigen-presenting cell. Specifically, CD8+ and CD4+ T cells are MHC class I and class II restricted, respectively. CD4+ T cells are further divided into T helper 1 (Th1) and T helper 2 (Th2) subsets based on their cytokine secretion repertoire. On antigen stimulation, Th1 CD4+ T cells secrete interferon-γ and IL-2, whereas Th2 CD4+ T cells secrete IL-4 and IL-10. Interferon-γ can also be produced by T cells via an antigen-independent pathway involving IL-12 and IL-18.[8] These two cytokines act synergistically to induce interferon-γ by T cells.

BIOLOGIC EFFECTS OF INTERFERONS

Once induced, type I and type II interferons must bind to their respective receptors to exert their biologic effects. Interferons α and β bind to the same receptor, which is composed of two subunits (Fig. 16.1-1).[9] The binding of either interferon-α or interferon-β to this receptor results in the activation of Janus tyrosine kinases Jak1 and Tyk2, which results in the phosphorylation of signal transducers and activators of transcription 1 and 2 (STAT1 and STAT2). The phosphorylation of STAT1 and STAT2 results in their heterodimerization, dissociation from the interferon receptor, and resultant translocation to the nucleus. In the nucleus, the STAT complex associates with DNA-binding protein p48. This complex, called *interferon-stimulated gene factor 3* (ISGF3), binds to the interferon-stimulated response element of

α- and β-responsive genes. Binding to the interferon-stimulated response element results in the induction of interferon target genes, which are ultimately responsible for the biologic effects of interferons α and β.

Interferon-γ binds as a homodimer to the specific interferon-γ receptor.[10] The interferon-γ receptor is similar to the type I interferon receptor in that it also is composed of two subunits that dimerize on interferon-γ binding (see Fig. 16.1-1). Dimerization of the receptor activates the Janus tyrosine kinases Jak1 and Jak2, which ultimately results in the phosphorylation of STAT proteins. Instead of activating STAT1 and STAT2 as with the type I interferon receptor, interferon-γ activates two separate STAT1 molecules. These two STAT1 molecules then form a homodimer. The STAT1 homodimer is referred to as the γ-activated factor (GAF), which translocates to the nucleus and binds to γ-activating sequences (GAS), elements of interferon-γ inducible genes.

The antiviral activity of interferons is mediated by three pathways. These are the 2'-5' oligoadenylate synthetases, dsRNA-dependent PKR, and Mx pathways.[1] The group of 2'-5' oligoadenylate synthetases catalyzes the formation of adenosine oligomers (2'-5'A) from adenosine triphosphate. The 2'-5'A molecules bind to and activate endoribonuclease L. Activated endoribonuclease L cleaves single-stranded RNA, including messenger RNA, which leads to the inhibition of protein synthesis and hence cellular proliferation. PKR is activated by binding to dsRNA. Once activated, PKR phosphorylates the translation initiation factor eIF2, which inhibits messenger RNA translation. PKR also can activate NFκB, which can lead to increased cytokine and chemokine levels. Increased PKR activity can also induce apoptosis by a Bcl2- and caspase-dependent mechanism. Another group of proteins induced by interferon that exhibits antiviral properties is the Mx family of glutamyl transpeptidases.[11] MxA is produced during viral infections and inhibits viral replication at the level of transcription. MxA binds to susceptible viral nucleocapsids in the cytoplasm and prevents their movement into the nucleus.

Interferons induce hundreds of specific gene products, most of which are important in regulation of cell proliferation and apoptosis. Type I interferons up-regulate the cyclin-dependent kinase inhibitor p21, which results in the inhibition of the transition in the cell cycle from G_1 to S phase.[12] Interferon-γ has been shown to down-regulate the transcription of c-myc that is essential in driving cell-cycle progression.[13] Interferon-γ also induces Fas and Fas ligand, both of which can increase cell sensitivity to apoptosis.[14] Interferon-α in concert with anti-CD3 induces the surface expression of tumor necrosis–related apoptosis-inducing ligand on peripheral T cells.[15] In several malignant cell lines, interferons induce apoptosis by activation of several members of the caspase pathway.[16]

The biologic effects of interferons on the immune system are extensive and involve both innate and adaptive responses (Table 16.1-1).[17] Both type I and type II interferons can enhance the activity of the cellular components of the innate immune response, which is composed of NK cells, natural killer T cells (NKT) cells, and macrophages. The innate immune system represents the front-line defense against viral and microbial invasion, and also serves to signal the adaptive immune response. All interferons increase the cytotoxic activity of NK cells. Interferon-γ also increases the antimicrobial activity of macrophages by increasing the production of reactive oxygen and nitrogen intermediates through stimulation of

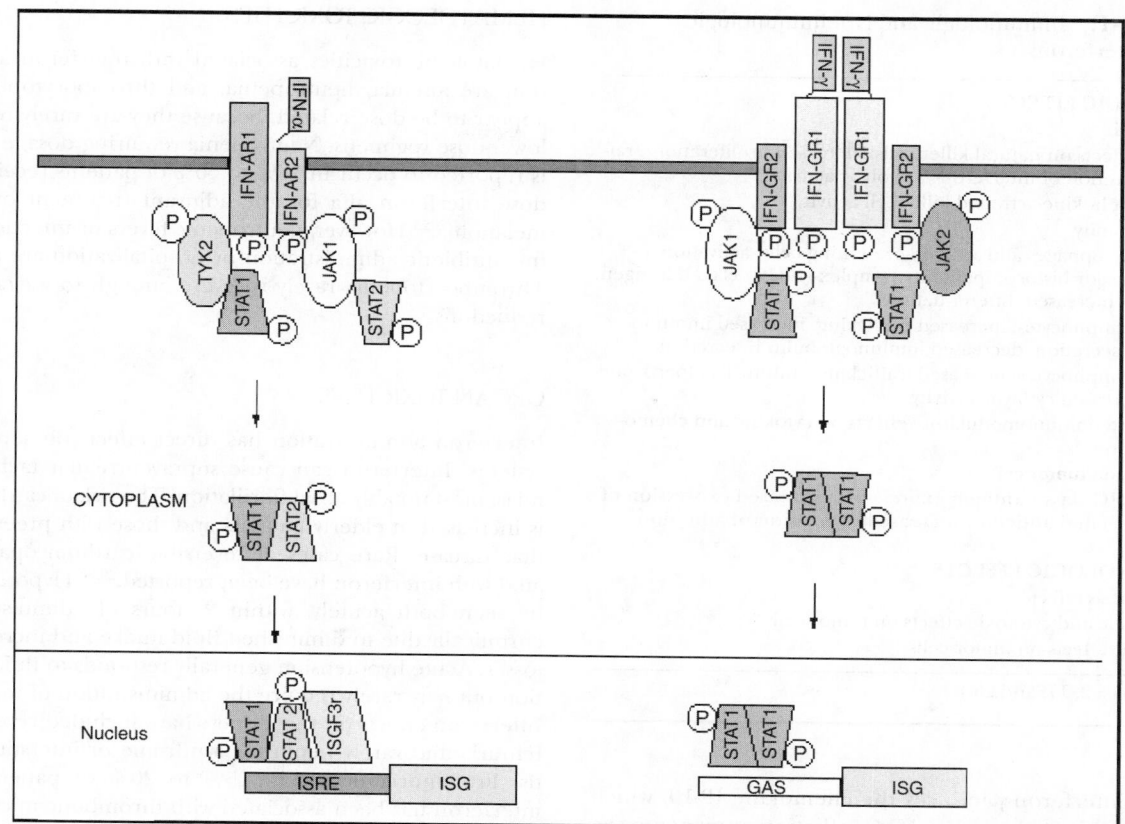

FIGURE 16.1-1. The effects of interferon (IFN) are mediated by receptors on the cell surface. Different receptors bind type I interferons (α and β, left side of figure) and type II interferons (γ, right side of figure). For both types of interferons, binding to their respective receptor initiates phosphorylation of cytoplasmic proteins (indicated by P) that results in nuclear translocation and binding to interferon-stimulated response elements (ISRE) or γ-activating sequences (GAS), which leads to regulation of interferon-stimulated genes (ISG). IFN-AR, interferon-α receptor; IFN-GR, interferon-γ receptor; ISGF, interferon-stimulated gene factor; JAK, janus kinase; STAT, signal transduction and activators of transcription; TYK, tyrosine kinase. (From ref. 26, with permission.)

inducible nitric oxide synthetase.[18] In addition, interferon-γ induces the production of chemokines that are selective for the recruitment of lymphocytes and macrophages. These chemokines include inducible protein-10 (IP-10) and macrophage inflammatory protein-1α (MIP-1α).[18]

Both type I and type II interferons enhance the MHC class I antigen presentation pathway. They do this by increasing the expression of MHC class I and β₂-microglobulin, as well as by increasing essential elements of the class I antigen-processing pathway. Essential proteins in this pathway that are up-regulated include transporter associated with antigen processing 1 and 2 (TAP1, TAP2) and low-molecular-mass polypeptide 2 (LMP-2).[19]

Interferons also interact with the adaptive immune response through their effect on dendritic cells. Dendritic cells are unique antigen-presenting cells that are able to stimulate a naive T-cell response to antigen. In their immature state dendritic cells take up antigen, and after maturation they are able to present antigen to T cells. Type I and II interferons can induce the *in vitro* maturation of dendritic cells.[20] In the presence of granulocyte-macrophage colony-stimulating factor, type I interferons can up-regulate the expression of the chemokine receptor CCR7, which is integral to dendritic cell trafficking to lymph nodes.[21] In this regard, interferons are one of several

molecules that regulate the relationship between the innate and the adaptive immune responses.

Interferon-γ also has unique effects on the immune system not shared with type I interferons. Interferon-γ regulates the MHC class II antigen-processing pathway, which is constitutively expressed on "professional" antigen-presenting cells: dendritic cells and B lymphocytes. This pathway is regulated by a single interferon-γ–inducible transcription factor called class II transactivator.[22] Paradoxically, type I interferons antagonize the induction of the MHC class II antigen-processing pathway by interferon-γ.[18] Another unique effect of interferon-γ is the ability to inhibit the expression of IL-4. By inhibiting IL-4, interferon-γ plays an integral role in the skewing of the immune response to a Th1 (cellular) response and away from a Th2 (antibody-mediated) response.[18]

Interferons, either directly or indirectly, may exhibit antiangiogenic properties. Type I interferons inhibit the synthesis of basic fibroblast growth factor, IL-8, and collagenase type IV, which are proangiogenic factors.[23] This has been shown to have clinical significance in the treatment of infantile hemangiomas.[24] Interferons have also been shown to inhibit endothelial cell migration, an essential mechanism in new blood vessel development. In addition, as previously

TABLE 16.1-1. Immunologic and Nonimmunologic Effects of Interferons

IMMUNOLOGIC EFFECTS

Innate immunity

Stimulatory effects on natural killer cells: increased proliferation, trafficking, secretion of interferon-γ, cytolytic activity

Increased lymphokine-activated killer cell activity

Adaptive immunity

Effects on macrophages and antigen-presenting cells: activation, increased major histocompatibility complex (MHC) class II antigen expression, increased differentiation

Effects on B lymphocytes: increased trafficking, increased immunoglobulin G secretion, decreased immunoglobulin E secretion

Effects on T lymphocytes: increased trafficking, shift to T helper 1 phenotype, increased cytolytic activity

Regulatory and immunomodulatory effects on cytokine and chemokine secretion

Direct effects on tumor cells

Increased MHC class I antigen expression, increased expression of tumor-associated antigens, increased expression of adhesion molecules

NONIMMUNOLOGIC EFFECTS

Antiangiogenesis effects

Direct cytostatic and cytotoxic effects on tumor cells

Antimetastatic effects on tumor cells

(Data from refs. 2, 17, and 26.)

described, interferon-γ induces the chemokine IP-10, which is another angiogenic molecule. Conflicting angiogenic signals are also possible from proteins induced by type I interferons. The gene for hypoxia-inducible factor 1α is induced by interferon-α, which in turn activates transcription of vascular endothelial growth factor.

CLINICAL TOXICITY OF INTERFERON ADMINISTRATION

CONSTITUTIONAL TOXICITIES

The most extensive toxicity analysis of interferon in an oncology patient population is from trials of the use of recombinant interferon alfa in the adjuvant treatment of high-risk melanoma.[25,26] There is also an extensive literature on the toxicity profile of interferon alfa in the treatment of hepatitis C.[27] Clinical trials with recombinant interferon-gamma have also been reported.[28] The clinical toxicities associated with interferon administration are schedule and dose dependent as well as highly variable in type and degree across individuals. The most common toxicities seen with all interferons are constitutional. Acute administration can result in fever, chills, myalgias, arthralgias, headache, nausea, vomiting, and fatigue. With repetitive dosing, tachyphylaxis occurs in relation to fever and chills. Rigors can occur with interferon treatment but are not common. Fatigue usually increases with repetitive dosing until a baseline level of fatigue is reached at a stable dosage of interferon. For many patients, appropriate timing of interferon administration (e.g., at or just before bedtime) can limit the impact of symptoms. Anorexia and weight loss are commonly seen with higher-dose regimens and can be related to nausea or can occur independently of any gastrointestinal symptoms.

HEMATOLOGIC TOXICITIES

Hematologic toxicities associated with interferon administration are anemia, neutropenia, and thrombocytopenia. They appear to be dose related, because they are rarely reported in lower-dose regimens. Neutropenia requiring dosage reduction is reported to occur in 26% to 60% of patients receiving high-dose interferon alfa for the adjuvant treatment of high-risk melanoma.[25] However, neutropenic fevers or infections requiring antibiotic administration or hospitalization are quite rare. Thrombocytopenia rarely is severe enough to warrant dosage reductions.

ORGAN TOXICITIES

Interferon administration has direct effects on several organ systems. Interferon can cause supraventricular tachydysrhythmias, most notably atrial fibrillation. The risk of cardiac toxicity is increased in elderly patients and those with preexisting cardiac disease. Rare cases of reversible cardiomyopathy associated with interferon have been reported.[29,30] Hypotension may be seen both acutely, within 2 hours of administration, or chronically due to diminished fluid intake and increased fluid losses. Acute hypotension generally responds to fluid resuscitation but may rarely require the administration of vasopressors. Interferon effects on the kidneys have included reversible proteinuria and rarely nephrotic syndrome or interstitial nephritis. Proteinuria occurs in 15% to 20% of patients. Rarely, interferon has been associated with thrombotic microangiopathy in patients with chronic myelogenous leukemia treated for several years.[31] This is in contrast to other nephropathies associated with interferon, which usually manifest after only several months of treatment. The skin can also be a target of interferon toxicity with occasional macular rashes and reports of psoriatic-type skin reactions that require treatment and resolve with discontinuation of therapy.[32,33]

High-dose interferon regimens can cause acute hepatic toxicity. This toxicity is manifested as an increase in serum levels of alanine aminotransferase and aspartate aminotransferase, and can result in fatal hepatotoxicity.[25] This serious complication was identified early in the initial trial of high-dose interferon alfa for adjuvant therapy of melanoma. Once careful monitoring was instituted with requirements for dosage reduction tied to serum transaminase elevations, there were no further cases of fatal hepatotoxicity on this trial or on subsequent cooperative group trials using the same dose and schedule. Hence, with careful monitoring and appropriate dosage modification, fatal complications can be avoided and therapy can continue for patients who develop transaminase elevations during high-dose therapy.

Type I interferon administration has been associated with retinopathy.[34] The retinopathy includes retinal hemorrhages and cotton-wool spots, either alone or together. The retinopathy can be unilateral or bilateral. The retinal hemorrhages occur mainly around the optic disc and can be linear or patchy. The incidence of interferon retinopathy has been reported to range from 18% to 86% in different series. The different rates may reflect a dosage effect, may be related to surveillance intensity, or both. Diabetes mellitus may be an associated risk factor for the development as well as the progression of interferon retinopathy. The retinopathy rarely results in any visual disturbance and disappears spontaneously during treatment or resolves after interferon is discontinued.

NEUROPSYCHIATRIC TOXICITIES

The neuropsychiatric or neurocognitive toxicities associated with interferon therapy can manifest as subtle changes that are detected only by formal testing or can be overt with depression, hypomania, or suicidal ideation requiring discontinuation of interferon and active intervention.[35–37] Acute neuropsychiatric changes include impaired memory, difficulty in concentration, and decreased initiative. With the continued administration of interferon, subacute and chronic changes are manifest. These consist of behavioral (personality), mood, and affect changes. The prophylactic use of the selective serotonin reuptake inhibitor (SSRI) paroxetine has been suggested to ameliorate depressive symptoms by results of a small, placebo-controlled trial involving patients receiving high-dose interferon for high-risk melanoma.[38] Changes in tryptophan metabolism were observed in untreated depressed patients, and it appeared that paroxetine attenuated the consequences of these changes.[39] In this study, however, the placebo group had a higher rate of discontinuation of interferon therapy due to depression (35%) than previously reported. In previous trials of adjuvant interferon for high-risk melanoma, fewer than 10% of patients were reported as having grade 3 or 4 depression.[25,26] In patients with a past history of clinical depression or psychiatric disorders, the benefits and risks of interferon use should be considered carefully. Whether SSRIs such as paroxetine should be used routinely or selectively in patients receiving high-dose interferon alfa remains an unresolved issue. Other strategies for ameliorating the constitutional and neuropsychiatric effects of high-dose interferon, such as the use of methylphenidate or exercise or both, are the subject of active investigation.

ENDOCRINE AND METABOLIC TOXICITIES

Thyroid abnormalities have been reported in 5% to 31% of patients receiving interferon therapy.[37] Although up to 70% to 80% of patients exhibiting thyroid disorders while on interferon have detectable thyroid autoantibodies, the exact mechanism of thyroid toxicity is unknown. It may be a direct effect of the action of interferon on the thyroid gland or an indirect effect due to suppression of thyroid-stimulating hormone release. Autoimmune thyroiditis may be a manifestation of an increased risk of autoimmune disorders in general that has been seen in patients taking interferon. A high degree of clinical suspicion for thyroid dysfunction must be maintained because of the similarities between hypothyroidism and the clinical spectrum of fatigue and hair loss that can be seen from interferon administration in the euthyroid patient.

Metabolic alterations in the blood lipid profile associated with interferon include hypertriglyceridemia and elevated levels of low-density lipoprotein, secondary to inhibition of lipoprotein lipase.[40] Interferon may depress the plasma cholesterol level in 15% to 40% of patients.

OTHER REPORTED COMPLICATIONS ASSOCIATED WITH INTERFERON THERAPY

As mentioned previously in Endocrine and Metabolic Toxicities, interferon therapy is associated with the risk of autoim-

mune phenomena. In addition to thyroid disorders, other autoimmune alterations that have been reported include rheumatoid arthritis and Raynaud's and Sjögren's syndromes.[41–43] Associations between female gender and longer duration of therapy with interferon have been reported for autoimmune disorders. Whether interferon is causing the autoimmune disorder or unmasking a preexisting disorder is unclear.

Rhabdomyolysis has been reported with high-dose interferon therapy.[44]

Another unusual but potentially serious association is the occurrence of sarcoidosis in patients receiving interferon.[45,46] Both pulmonary and cutaneous manifestations of sarcoidosis have been reported. If it is symptomatic, the manifestations of sarcoid usually regress after the discontinuation of interferon. The pulmonary manifestations of sarcoid can be misinterpreted to represent progressive cancer. A diagnosis of sarcoid is a contraindication to interferon administration, as is a preexisting autoimmune disease.

POTENTIAL DRUG INTERACTIONS

Potential interactions between interferons and other drugs have not been extensively examined, particularly for the high-dose interferon alfa-2b regimen used for adjuvant therapy. In a study of 17 patients, treatment with high-dose interferon alfa resulted in inhibition of the activity of cytochrome P-450 isozymes CYP1A2 and CYP2D within 24 hours of the first intravenous dose.[47] After 26 days of treatment, significant inhibition of CYP2C19 was found. The implication of these findings is that the activity of drugs metabolized by these enzymes could be expected to be diminished after interferon therapy. Such drugs include tricyclic antidepressants, SSRIs, theophylline, phenytoin, and many others. However, clinically significant drug-interferon interactions have not been reported.

ONCOLOGIC APPLICATIONS OF INTERFERONS

PHARMACOLOGY AND DOSAGE

Interferons are available for clinical usage in both natural and recombinant forms, with the latter used most commonly for oncologic applications.[48] Commercially available interferon formulations include human leukocyte–derived interferon alfa-n3 (Alferon N); recombinant "consensus" interferon (produced from a 166-amino acid sequence derived by sequencing several natural interferon-α subtypes and assigning the most frequent amino acid in each corresponding position), alfacon-1 (Infergen); recombinant interferon alfa-2a (Roferon-A); recombinant interferon alfa-2b (Intron A); recombinant interferon beta-1a (Avonex, Rebif); recombinant interferon beta-1b (Betaseron); and recombinant interferon gamma-1b (Actimmune, InterMune). Most of the oncologic experience has been accumulated with interferon alfa-2a and alfa-2b, which are approved by the U.S. Food and Drug Administration for use in hairy cell leukemia, acquired immunodeficiency syndrome–related Kaposi's sarcoma, and Philadelphia chromosome–positive chronic myelogenous leukemia (interferon alfa-2a), and hairy cell leukemia, acquired immunodeficiency syndrome–

TABLE 16.1-2. Oncologic Applications of Interferons

TUMOR TYPES WITH ESTABLISHED INDICATIONS
Chronic myelogenous leukemia
Hairy cell leukemia
Non-Hodgkin's lymphoma
Acquired immunodeficiency–related Kaposi's sarcoma
Malignant melanoma
TUMOR TYPES FOR WHICH INTERFERONS ARE COMMONLY USED
Renal cell carcinoma
Bladder carcinoma (intravesical therapy)
OTHER TUMOR TYPES FOR WHICH INTERFERONS HAVE SHOWN SOME EVIDENCE OF ACTIVITY
Colorectal carcinoma (with 5-fluorouracil)
Carcinoid tumor
Desmoid tumor (aggressive fibromatosis)

(Data from refs. 2 and 26.)

related Kaposi's sarcoma, follicular lymphoma, and malignant melanoma (interferon alfa-2b). Experience has been accumulated with interferons of various types in a host of other tumor types as well (Table 16.1-2).

The half-life of recombinant interferon alfa-2 varies between 2 and 8 hours in the blood after subcutaneous or intramuscular administration, and is probably somewhat shorter after intravenous administration. Oral delivery is impractical due to proteolytic degradation. Peak plasma concentrations are highest after intravenous administration.[47] Generally speaking, intravenous administration of interferon alfa is performed daily (5 days per week in the most commonly used regimen for adjuvant therapy of interferon), whereas subcutaneous or intramuscular administration is performed thrice weekly. Other dose schedules have been explored in the hopes of maximizing certain properties of interferons while minimizing toxicities (e.g., low-dose, twice-daily schedules of subcutaneous interferon alfa in "antiangiogenesis" trials).

NEUTRALIZING ANTIBODIES

The development of neutralizing antibodies can alter the pharmacology and efficacy of recombinant cytokines after repeated administration. Neutralizing antibodies have been observed in 25% to 30% of patients treated with interferon alfa-2a, but fewer than 3% of patients treated with interferon alfa-2b.[49,50] Neutralizing antibodies are also frequently encountered after administration of interferon beta.[51] The development of neutralizing antibodies has been associated with a loss of clinical efficacy.[52]

EFFECTS OF DOSE AND SCHEDULE ON EFFICACY AND TOXICITY

A great variety of doses, schedules, and routes of administration of interferon have been tested in clinical trials, particularly in the setting of adjuvant therapy for melanoma patients at risk of recurrence after complete surgical resection. Interferon alfa has been shown to have detectable but low levels of antitumor activity in melanoma patients with metastatic disease, resulting in objective regressions in approximately 10% of patients treated

using any of several dose and schedule regimens.[53] There has been no consistent observation that responses are linked to a specific dose or schedule of administration. Responses are more common in patients with small, generally soft tissue or lung nodules. Interferon gamma in immunologically active doses has failed to demonstrate any but the most minimal activity in metastatic melanoma[54] and was likewise ineffective in two randomized trials evaluating similar dosages in the adjuvant setting.[28,55]

The remarkable variety of doses, schedules, and routes of administration of interferon alfa that have been tested in clinical trials is, in part, due to a lack of knowledge regarding the specific mechanisms responsible for interferon's antitumor activity. To date, surrogate markers of immunologic or other parameters have not been informative in determining what constitutes a sufficient dose and route of delivery.[56–58] Clinical trials have clearly established a greater incidence of grade 3 and 4 toxicity for high-dose regimens than for lower doses.[59–61] The results of the E1690 trial, a three-arm U.S. Intergroup trial that compared high-dose and low-dose interferon alfa-2b to observation after surgery for high-risk stage II and stage III (thick node-negative or node-positive) melanoma, are representative (Table 16.1-3).[59]

The effect of dose and schedule of adjuvant interferon therapy on overall survival has been more controversial.[62,63] When three randomized phase III trials of high-dose interferon alfa-2b were included in a metaanalysis, there was a 15 ± 8% reduction in deaths associated with high-dose interferon treatment, more of an impact than was seen in the low-dose trials, but this did not reach statistical significance ($P = .06$).[64]

INTERFERON ALFA-2A VERSUS ALFA-2B

No direct comparative data exist to allow any conclusions regarding the relative efficacy of equitoxic doses or the relative toxicity of equally effective doses of recombinant interferon alfa-2a and alfa-2b. All adjuvant therapy trials to date involving intravenous administration have used interferon alfa-2b. Because of uncertainty regarding the equivalent dosing for intravenous administration of interferon alfa-2a, its substitution for interferon alfa-2b in high-dose adjuvant therapy cannot be recommended.[65]

PHARMACOLOGIC MODIFICATION OF INTERFERONS

As is the case with many cytokines, the relatively short half-life of interferons requires repetitive dosing to maintain exposure to biologically effective concentrations. Toxicity may well be related to peak plasma concentrations, whereas efficacy may be more closely linked to duration of exposure (area under the curve). A pharmacologic approach to improving interferon efficacy and decreasing toxicity has been to couple the recombinant interferon molecule with a polyethylene glycol moiety ("pegylation"). This slows metabolism of the interferon, providing more sustained levels of exposure, but also diminishes the specific activity of the interferon, because steric interference decreases binding affinity with its receptor. Two pegylated interferons are commercially available, each using a different form of polyethylene glycol: branched-chain pegylated interferon alfa-2a (Pegasys) and succinimidyl carbonate–polyethylene glycol 12000 (straight-chain pegylated) interferon alfa-2b (PEG-Intron). When used in comparable concentrations, each pegylated interferon formulation appears to have biologic activity identical to that of the unmodified recombinant molecule.[66,67]

TABLE 16.1-3. Toxicity of High- versus Low-Dose Interferon Alfa in a Randomized Clinical Trial

| | HDI | | | | LDI | | | |
| | Grade 3 | | Grade 4 | | Grade 3 | | Grade 4 | |
Toxicity Type	*No. of Events*	*%*	*No. of Events*	*%*	*No. of Events*	*%*	*No. of Events*	*%*
Granulocytopenia	85	40	9	4	12	6	—	—
Liver toxicity	61	29	—	—	8	4	1	0.05
Fatigue	49	23	2	1	7	3	—	—
Neuroclinical effects	42	20	—	—	14	6	—	—
Myalgia	35	16	2	1	18	8	—	—
Leukopenia	30	14	—	—	2	1	—	—
Nausea	19	9	—	—	5	2	—	—
Neuropsychiatric effects	18	8	2	1	5	2	—	—
Neuromotor effects	12	6	1	0.05	2	1	—	—
Vomiting	11	5	1	0.05	3	1	—	—

HDI, high-dose interferon; LDI, low-dose interferon.
(From ref. 59, with permission.)

Although only limited experience has been accumulated in oncologic applications to date with pegylated interferons, their efficacy in treating hepatitis C appears to be as good as or better than standard recombinant interferon when used at equitoxic doses.[27] In a phase I-II trial involving 35 patients with advanced solid tumors of a variety of histologic types, the maximum tolerated dose of pegylated interferon alfa-2b for long-term treatment was found to be 6 µg/kg/wk.[68] This was the same maximum tolerated dose as determined in a phase I trial in patients with chronic-phase chronic myelogenous leukemia.[69] In the chronic myelogenous leukemia study, a complete hematologic or improved cytogenetic response was observed in 48% of patients who were intolerant to or did not respond to prior interferon alfa therapy. In the solid tumor trial, 9 of 69 patients (13%) experienced objective remissions, including four complete responses, with responses predominantly seen with dosages at or above 6 µg/kg/wk. Responses were seen in both visceral and nonvisceral sites. Results for previously untreated patients with renal cell carcinoma were encouraging: Objective responses were seen in 6 of 14 patients (44%), including two complete responses. Two of six melanoma patients also had complete responses. These clinical results certainly appear to be at least comparable to those achieved with recombinant interferon alfa, with equal or less toxicity. Moreover, pegylated interferons seem better suited to chronic administration because they allow once-a-week dosing, which has prompted a randomized trial of very long term (5 years), low-dose pegylated interferon alfa therapy versus observation for patients with stage III melanoma. Pegylated interferons may also be better choices for investigating the antiangiogenic properties of interferon therapy.

COMBINATIONS OF INTERFERON AND OTHER AGENTS

The activity and toxicity profiles of interferons make them logical candidates for combination with other immunologic and cytotoxic therapies. To date, combination therapy including interferon has been evaluated in a multitude of clinical trials, but no studies have established a definitive role for combination regimens. Randomized trials have established that high-dose interferon therapy does not diminish the ability to respond to a ganglioside vaccine[70] and may augment or maintain the immune response to vaccines.[71,72]

Nonetheless, specific evidence for synergy between interferon and immunologic or cytotoxic therapy is lacking.[73]

CONCLUSION

Interferons are the most commonly used immunomodulatory cytokines in contemporary oncologic practice, with applicability in the treatment of both solid tumors and hematologic malignancies. Recent years have seen an enormous increase in the understanding of the basic biology of interferon effects, but this has not yet been matched by comparable increases of the understanding of the mechanisms of antitumor activity. Because of this, it is highly likely that interferons are not yet being used in manners that maximize their antitumor effects while minimizing toxicity. Opportunities exist for well-designed clinical trials using immunologic and other intermediate biologic end points to increase both the knowledge of and success with interferon therapy for cancer.

REFERENCES

1. Goodbourn S, Didcock L, Randall RE. Interferons: cell signaling, immune modulation, antiviral responses and virus countermeasures. *J Gen Virol* 2000;81:2341.
2. Pfeffer LM, Dinarello CA, Herberman RB, et al. Biologic properties of recombinant alpha-interferons: 40th anniversary of the discovery of interferons. *Cancer Res* 1998;58:2489.
3. Sung S, Zhang X, Tough DF, Sprent J. Type I interferon-mediated stimulation of T cells by CpG DNA. *J Exp Med* 1998;188:2335.
4. Bakker AB, Wu J, Phillips JH, et al. NK cell activation: distinct stimulatory pathways counter balancing inhibitory signals. *Hum Immunol* 2000;61:18.
5. Pende D, Rivera P, Marcenaro S, et al. Major histocompatibility complex class I-related chain A and UL16-binding protein expression on tumor cell lines of different histotypes: analysis of tumor susceptibility to NKG2D-dependent natural killer cell cytotoxicity. *Cancer Res* 2002;62:6178.
6. Trinchieri G. Interleukin 12: a proinflammatory cytokine with immunoregulatory functions that bridge innate resistance and antigen-specific adaptive immunity. *Annu Rev Immunol* 1995;13:251.
7. Young HA. Regulation of interferon-gamma gene expression. *J Interferon Cytokine Res* 1996;16:563.
8. Tominaga K, Yoshimoto T, Torigoe K, et al. IL-12 synergizes with IL-18 or IL-1β for IFN-γ production from human T cells. *Int Immunol* 2000;12:151.
9. Brierley MM, Fish EN. IFN-α/β receptor interactions to biologic outcomes: understanding the circuitry. *J Interferon Cytokine Res* 2002;22:835.
10. Stark GR, Kerr IM, Williams BR, et al. How cells respond to interferons. *Annu Rev Biochem* 1998;67:227.

11. Haller O, Kochs G. Interferon-induced Mx proteins: dynamin-like GTPases with antiviral activity. *Traffic* 2002;3:710.

12. Subramaniam PS, Johnson HM. A role for the cyclindependent kinase inhibitor p21 in the G1 cell cycle arrest mediated by the type I interferons. *J Interferon Cytokine Res* 1997;17:11.

13. Ramana CV, Grammatikakis N, Chernov M, et al. Regulation of C-myc expression by IFN-gamma through Stat1-dependent and -independent pathways. *EMBO J* 2000;19:263.

14. Xu X, Fu XY, Plate J, et al. IFN-gamma induces cell growth inhibition by Fas-mediated apoptosis: requirement of Stat1 protein for up-regulation of Fas and FasL expression. *Cancer Res* 1998;58:2832.

15. Kayagaki N, Yamaguchi N, Nakayama M, et al. Type I interferons (IFNs) regulate tumor necrosis factor-related apoptosis-inducing ligand (TRAIL) expression on human T cells: a novel mechanism for the antitumor effects of type I IFNs. *J Exp Med* 1999;189:1451.

16. Thyrell L, Erickson S, Zhivotovsky B, et al. Mechanisms of interferon-alpha induced apoptosis in malignant cells. *Oncogene* 2002;21:1251.

17. Brassard DL, Grace MJ, Bordens R. Interferon-α as an immunotherapeutic protein. *J Leukoc Biol* 2002;71:565.

18. Boehm U, Klamp T, Groot M, et al. Cellular responses to interferon-γ. *Annu Rev Immunol* 1997;15:749.

19. Chatterjee-Kishore M, Kishore R, Hicklin DJ, et al. Different requirements for signal transducer and activator of transcription 1α and interferon regulatory factor 1 in the regulation of low molecular mass polypeptide 2 and transporter associated with antigen processing 1 gene expression. *J Biol Chem* 1998;273:16177.

20. Ito T, Amakawa R, Inaba M, et al. Differential regulation of human blood dendritic cell subsets by IFNs. *J Immunol* 2001;166:2961.

21. Parlato S, Santini SM, Lapenta C, et al. Expression of CCR-7, MIP-3β, and Th-1 chemokines in type I IFN-induced monocyte-derived dendritic cells: importance for the rapid acquisition of potent migratory and functional activities. *Blood* 2001;98:3022.

22. Chang CH, Flavell RA. Class II transactivator regulates the expression of multiple genes involved in antigen presentation. *J Exp Med* 1995;181:765.

23. Fidler IJ. Regulation of neoplastic angiogenesis. *J Natl Cancer Inst Monogr* 2000;28:10.

24. Chang E, Boyd A, Nelson CC, et al. Successful treatment of infantile hemangiomas with interferon-alpha-2b. *J Pediatr Hematol Oncol* 1997;19:237.

25. Kirkwood JM, Bender C, Agarwala S, et al. Mechanisms and management of toxicities associated with high-dose interferon alfa-2b therapy. *J Clin Oncol* 2002;20:3703.

26. Jonasch E, Kumar UN, Linette GP, et al. Adjuvant high-dose interferon alfa-2b in patients with high-risk melanoma. *Cancer J Sci Am* 2000;6:139.

27. National Institutes of Health Consensus Development Conference Statement: management of hepatitis C 2002 (June 10–12, 2002). *Gastroenterology* 2002;123:2082.

28. Sondak VK, Kopecky KJ, Smith JW II, et al. Is interferon-γ detrimental? Results of a Southwest Oncology Group randomized trial of adjuvant human interferon-γ versus observation in malignant melanoma. In: Salmon SE, ed. Adjuvant therapy of cancer VIII. Philadelphia, PA: Lippincott–Raven, 1997:259.

29. Sonnenblick M, Rosin A. Cardiotoxicity of interferon: a review of 44 cases. *Chest* 1991; 99:557.

30. Cohen MC, Huberman MS, Nesto RW. Recombinant alpha2 interferon-related cardiomyopathy. *Am J Med* 1988;85:549.

31. Zuber J, Martinez F, Droz D, et al. Alpha-interferon-associated thrombotic microangiopathy: a clinicopathologic study of 8 patients and review of the literature. *Medicine* 2002;81:321.

32. Georgetson MJ, Yarze JC, Lalos AT, et al. Exacerbation of psoriasis due to interferon-alpha treatment of chronic active hepatitis. *Am J Gastroenterol* 1993;88:1756.

33. Funk J, Langeland T, Schrumpf E, et al. Psoriasis induced by interferon-alpha. *Br J Dermatol* 1991;125:463.

34. Hayasaka S, Nagaki Y, Matsumoto M, et al. Interferon associated retinopathy. *Br J Ophthalmol* 1998;82:323.

35. Trask PC, Esper P, Riba M, et al. Psychiatric side effects of interferon therapy: prevalence, proposed mechanisms, and future directions. *J Clin Oncol* 2000;18:2316.

36. Vial T, Choquet-Kastylevsky G, Liautard C, et al. Endocrine and neurological adverse effects of the therapeutic interferons. *Toxicology* 2000;142:161.

37. VanGool AR, Kruit WH, Engels FK, et al. Neuropsychiatric side effects of interferon-alfa therapy. *Pharm World Sci* 2003;25:11.

38. Musselman DL, Lawson DH, Gumnick JF, et al. Paroxetine for the prevention of depression induced by high-dose interferon alfa. *N Engl J Med* 2001;344:961.

39. Capuron L, Neurauter G, Musselman DL, et al. Interferon-alpha–induced changes in tryptophan metabolism: relationship to depression and paroxetine treatment. *Biol Psychiatry* 2003;54:906.

40. Massaro ER, Borden EC, Hawkins MJ, et al. Effects of recombinant interferon-alpha 2 treatment upon lipid concentrations and lipoprotein composition. *J Interferon Res* 1986;6:655.

41. Steegmann JL, Requena MJ, Martin-Requeira P, et al. High incidence of autoimmune alterations in chronic myeloid leukemia patients treated with interferon-α. *Am J Hematol* 2003;72:170.

42. Schapira D, Nahir AM, Hadad N. Interferon-induced Raynaud's syndrome. *Semin Arthritis Rheum* 2002;32:157.

43. Wilson LE, Widman D, Dikman SH, et al. Autoimmune disease complicating antiviral therapy for hepatitis C virus infection. *Semin Arthritis Rheum* 2002;32:163.

44. Reinhold N, Hartl C, Hering R, et al. Fatal rhabdomyolysis and multiple organ failure associated with adjuvant high-dose interferon alfa in malignant melanoma. *Lancet* 1997; 349(9051):540.

45. Li SD, Yong S, Srinivas D, et al. Reactivation of sarcoidosis during interferon therapy. *J Gastroenterol* 2002;37:50.

46. Rubinowitz AN, Naidich DP, Alinsonorin C. Interferon-induced sarcoidosis. *J Comput Assist Tomogr* 2003;27:279.

47. Islam M, Frye RF, Richards TJ. Differential effect of IFN α-2b on the cytochrome P450 enzyme system: a potential basis of IFN toxicity and its modulation by other drugs. *Clin Cancer Res* 2002;8:2480.

48. Jonasch E, Haluska FG. Interferon in oncologic practice: review of interferon biology, clinical applications, and toxicities. *Oncologist* 2002;6:34.

49. Itri LM, Sherman MI, Palleroni AV, et al. Incidence and clinical significance of neutralizing antibodies in patients receiving recombinant interferon-alpha 2a. *J Interferon Res* 1989;9:S9.

50. Speigel RJ, Jacobs SL, Treuhaft MS. Anti-interferon antibodies to interferon-alpha 2b: results of comparative assays and clinical perspective. *J Interferon Res* 1989;9:S17.

51. Rudick RA. Biologic impact of interferon antibodies, and complexities in assessing their clinical significance. *Neurology* 2003;61:31S.

52. Wussow PV, Jakschies D, Freund M, et al. Treatment of anti-recombinant interferon-alpha 2 antibody positive CML patients with natural interferon-alpha. *Br J Haematol* 1991;78:210.

53. Steiner A, Wolf CH, Pehamberger H. Comparison of the effects of three different treatment regimens of recombinant interferons (r-IFN alpha, r-IFN gamma and r-IFN alpha + cimetidine) in disseminated malignant melanoma. *J Cancer Res Clin Oncol* 1987;113:459.

54. Schiller JH, Pugh M, Kirkwood JM, et al. Eastern cooperative group trial of interferon gamma in metastatic melanoma: an innovative study design. *Clin Cancer Res* 1996;2:29.

55. Kleeborg U, Broecker EB, Chartier C, et al. EORTC 18871 adjuvant trial in high risk melanoma patients: IFNα vs IFNγ vs Iscador vs observation. *Eur J Cancer* 1999;35:[Suppl 4]264(abst).

56. Kirkwood JM, Bryant J, Schiller JH, et al. Immunomodulatory function of interferon-gamma in patients with metastatic melanoma: results of a phase II-B trial in subjects with metastatic melanoma, ECOG study E 4987. *J Immunother* 1997;20:146.

57. Kirkwood JM, Richards T, Zarour HM, et al. Immunomodulatory effects of high-dose and low-dose interferon alpha2b in patients with high-risk resected melanoma: the E2690 laboratory corollary of intergroup adjuvant trial E1690. *Cancer* 2002;95:1101.

58. Sondak VK. How does interferon work? Does it even matter? *Cancer* 2002;95:947.

59. Kirkwood JM, Ibrahim JG, Sondak VK, et al. High- and low-dose interferon alfa-2b in high-risk melanoma: first analysis of Intergroup trial E1690/S9111/C9190. *J Clin Oncol* 2000;18:2444.

60. Cascinelli N, Belli F, Mackie RM, et al. Effect of long-term adjuvant therapy with interferon alpha-2a in patients with regional node metastases from cutaneous melanoma: a randomised trial. *Lancet* 2001;358:866.

61. Hancock BW, Wheatley K, Harris S, et al. Adjuvant interferon in high-risk melanoma: the AIM HIGH study—United Kingdom Coordinating Committee on Cancer Research randomized study of adjuvant low-dose extended-duration interferon alfa-2a in high-risk resected malignant melanoma. *J Clin Oncol* 2004;22:53.

62. Schucter LM. Adjuvant interferon therapy for melanoma: high-dose, low-dose, no dose, which dose? *J Clin Oncol* 2004;22:7.

63. Moschos SJ, Kirkwood JM, Konstantinopoulos PA. Present status and future prospects for adjuvant therapy of melanoma: time to build upon the foundation of high-dose interferon alfa-2b. *J Clin Oncol* 2004;22:11.

64. Wheatley KM, Ives N, Hancock B, et al. Does adjuvant interferon-α for high-risk melanoma provide a worthwhile benefit? A meta-analysis of the randomised trials. *Cancer Treat Rev* 2003;29:241.

65. Hanson DS, Leggette CT. Severe hypotension following inadvertent intravenous administration of interferon alfa-2a (letter). *Ann Pharmacother* 1997;31:371.

66. Certa U, Wilhelm-Seiler M, Foser S, et al. Expression modes of interferon-α inducible genes in sensitive and resistant melanoma cells stimulated with regular and pegylated interferon-α. *Gene* 2003;315:79.

67. Vyas K, Brassard DL, DeLorenzo MM, et al. Biologic activity of polyethylene glycol12000—interferon-α2b compared with interferon-α2b: gene modulatory and antigrowth effects in tumor cells. *J Immunother* 2003;26:202.

68. Bukowski R, Ernstoff MS, Gore ME, et al. Pegylated interferon alfa-2b treatment for patients with solid tumors: a phase I/II study. *J Clin Oncol* 2002;20:3841.

69. Talpaz M, O'Brien S, Rose E, et al. Phase I study of polyethylene glycol formulation of interferon alpha-2b (Schering 54031) in Philadelphia chromosome-positive chronic myelogenous leukemia. *Blood* 2001;98:1708.

70. Kirkwood JM, Ibrahim J, Lawson DH, et al. High-dose interferon alfa-2b does not diminish antibody response to GM2 vaccination in patients with resected melanoma: results of the multicenter Eastern Cooperative Oncology Group phase II trial E2696. *J Clin Oncol* 2001;19:1430.

71. Mitchell MS. Immunotherapy as part of combinations for the treatment of cancer. *Int Immunopharmacol* 2003;3:1051.

72. Astaturov I, Petrella T, Bagriacik EU, et al. Amplification of virus-induced antimelanoma T-cell reactivity by high-dose interferon-α2b: implications for cancer vaccines. *Clin Cancer Res* 2003;9:4347.

73. Falkson CI, Ibrahim J, Kirkwood JM, et al. Phase III trial of dacarbazine versus dacarbazine with interferon alpha-2b versus dacarbazine with tamoxifen versus dacarbazine with interferon alpha-2b and tamoxifen in patients with metastatic malignant melanoma: an Eastern Cooperative Oncology Group study. *J Clin Oncol* 1998;16:1743.

JAMES W. MIER
MICHAEL B. ATKINS

SECTION **2**

Interleukin-2

Interleukin-2 (IL-2) was the first agent available for the treatment of metastatic cancer that functions solely through the activation of the immune system. Originally described as a growth factor for activated T cells, IL-2 was later found to exert multiple effects on cellular immune function and to induce tumor regression in mice. Subsequent clinical trials involving patients with renal cell carcinoma and malignant melanoma have demonstrated sufficient efficacy to establish IL-2 as a U.S. Food and Drug Administration (FDA)–approved treatment for both of these malignancies.

ISOLATION, CHARACTERIZATION, AND CLONING OF INTERLEUKIN-2

In 1976, Morgan et al. demonstrated the existence of a growth factor present in the conditioned medium of lectin-stimulated human peripheral blood mononuclear cells that could sustain indefinitely the *ex vivo* proliferation of human T cells.[1] This initial report was followed in short order by the isolation, biochemical characterization, and, ultimately, the cloning of what was then termed *T-cell growth factor.*[2] Subsequently designated *interleukin-2*, this factor was shown to be a 15-kD polypeptide made up of 153 amino acids, the first 20 of which form a signal sequence that is proteolytically cleaved during secretion. Natural IL-2 is glycosylated, although the attachment of sugar moieties is not essential for biologic activity. The molecule has cysteine residues at positions 58, 105, and 125, the first two of which form an intramolecular disulfide bridge. The third cysteine is not essential for biologic activity and can be replaced with alternative amino acids to minimize polymerization and increase shelf life. Crystallographic analysis indicates that IL-2 is a spherical molecule comprised of six α-helical regions.

INTERLEUKIN-2 RECEPTOR

The various biologic effects of IL-2 are the result of the binding of the lymphokine to specific surface receptors (reviewed in ref. 3). As with IL-2 itself, the expression of high-affinity IL-2 receptors is induced as a result of signaling through the T-cell antigen receptor. With the exception of a minor population of memory T cells that presumably were activated *in vivo* by a prior antigen exposure, freshly isolated peripheral blood T cells do not constitutively express high-affinity IL-2 receptors.

The high-affinity IL-2 receptor consists of three distinct subunits designated the α, β, and γ chains (Fig. 16.2-1). The α chain[4] is a 251–amino acid polypeptide with a large extracellular domain, a transmembrane span, and a short 13-residue cytoplasmic tail. The extracellular domain of this protein binds IL-2 with low affinity. The cytoplasmic domain of this receptor has no known biologic function and is dispensable for IL-2–induced signaling.

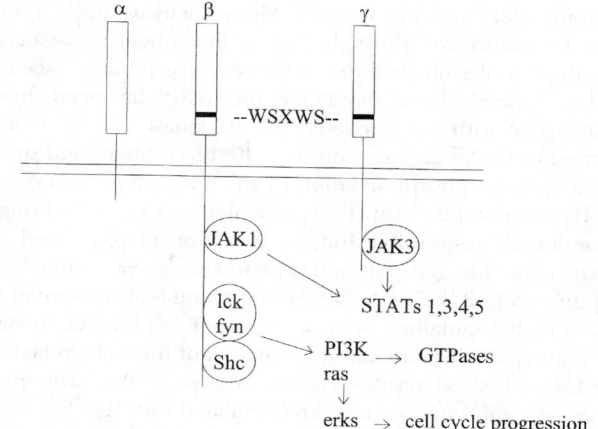

FIGURE 16.2-1.   The high-affinity interleukin-2 (IL-2) receptor and associated signaling pathways. The cytoplasmic domains of the β and γ chains contain several tyrosines that, when phosphorylated, provide docking and activation sites for numerous downstream kinases that affect cell proliferation, gene expression, and cell motility. GTPases, guanosine triphosphatases; JAK, janus kinase; PI3K, phosphoinositide 3 kinase; STAT, signal transduction and activators of transcription.

The IL-2 receptor β chain has a 214–amino acid extracellular domain, a transmembrane motif, and a large 286-residue cytoplasmic tail.[5] In contrast to the cytoplasmic domain of the α chain, that of the β chain is essential for IL-2 signaling. The IL-2 receptor β chain has paired cysteines at two sites within the extracellular domain and a perimembrane WSXWS motif characteristic of the members of an enlarging cytokine receptor superfamily that includes the receptors for IL-3, IL-4, IL-6, IL-7, granulocyte-macrophage colony-stimulating factor, prolactin, erythropoietin, and growth hormone.

The γ chain is a novel 64-kD protein that physically associates with the β chain. Like the β chain, the γ chain is a member of the cytokine receptor superfamily.[6] These two together bind IL-2 with intermediate affinity. When cotransfected along with the complementary DNAs of the α and β chains, the complementary DNA encoding the γ chain yields a high-affinity IL-2 receptor that transduces signals and is internalized in response to IL-2 binding. More recent studies have demonstrated that this receptor chain is shared by the receptors for several lymphokines, including IL-4, IL-7, IL-9, and IL-15, as well as IL-2.[7] Mutations in the gene encoding this receptor chain account for most, if not all, cases of X-linked severe combined immunodeficiency.[8] When antibodies against these receptor chains were used, resting T cells were found to constitutively express low levels of the IL-2 receptor γ chain but not the α or β chains. All three chains are up-regulated as a result of antigenic stimulation. Resting natural killer (NK) cells constitutively express the β chain, and both the α and γ chains are induced in these cells by exposure to IL-2 or IL-12.[9]

INTERLEUKIN-2–ACTIVATED SIGNALING PATHWAYS

The binding of IL-2 to its receptor induces the tyrosine phosphorylation of numerous cellular proteins, including the IL-2 receptor β chain itself. Because all three chains of the IL-2 receptor lack intrinsic tyrosine kinase activity, these events must be transduced through kinases that physically associate with the cytoplasmic domains of the receptor subunits (see Fig. 16.2-1). Indeed, the *src* family member p56[lck] has been shown to associate with the β chain, and its kinase activity is augmented by IL-2.[10] IL-2 also induces the recruitment and subsequent tyrosine phosphorylation of the adaptor protein *Shc* to the IL-2 receptor β chain. This particular association is thought to be largely responsible for the activation of p21[ras] and the downstream mitogen-activated protein kinases *erk-1* and *erk-2* in response to IL-2.[11] The IL-2 receptor γ chain is also essential for IL-2–induced signaling, because mutant T-cell lines expressing the α and β chains and a mutant version of the γ chain lacking the C-terminal 68 residues failed to express the protooncogenes *c-fos, c-jun,* and *c-myc* when stimulated with IL-2.[12]

In addition to associating with *src* family tyrosine kinases, both the β and γ receptor chains associate with members of the Janus kinase family of tyrosine kinases.[13] Janus kinase family member JAK3 associates with the C-terminal of the IL-2 receptor γ chain and both JAK1 and JAK2 associate with the β chain. JAK1 has been shown to bind to a specific serine-rich domain present in the membrane proximal region of the β chain. Janus kinases activate various members of the signal transduction and activators of transcription (STAT) family of transcription factors. The binding of IL-2 to its receptor results in the activation of STAT1, STAT3, and STAT5 in T cells and of an additional member, STAT4, in NK cells.[14]

IN VITRO EFFECTS OF INTERLEUKIN-2

As mentioned earlier in Isolation, Characterization, and Cloning of Interleukin-2, IL-2 was originally isolated based on its ability to induce the growth of previously activated T cells.[1] In addition to having proliferative effects, IL-2 induces the synthesis of an array of secondary cytokines such as IL-1, tumor necrosis factor (TNF), IL-6, and lymphotoxin.[11] Several of these secondary cytokines are detectable in the circulation of cancer patients receiving IL-2 immunotherapy (see Toxicity of High-Dose Interleukin-2, later in this chapter) and are thought by many investigators to contribute to the side effects of IL-2 therapy.[15]

The biologic effect of IL-2 arguably most pertinent to its use as an antitumor agent is its ability to enhance the cytolytic activity of antigen-specific cytotoxic T lymphocytes and NK cells.[16] The biochemical basis for this enhanced cytolytic function is currently unclear, but it is thought to be due in part to the increased expression of genes encoding the lytic components of cytotoxic granules (e.g., perforin, granzymes) as well as adhesion molecules (LFA-1) that facilitate the binding of activated leukocytes to tumor endothelium and the tumor cells themselves. In addition to increasing the HLA-restricted cytolytic activity of cytotoxic T lymphocytes for cells expressing a particular antigen and that of NK cells for susceptible tumor cell targets, IL-2 markedly diversifies the range of target cells susceptible to killing by these effectors. Indeed, human peripheral blood lymphocytes exposed only to high concentrations of IL-2 without prior exposure to tumor cells are able to kill virtually all tumor cell lines and most freshly isolated tumor cells *in vitro* regardless of the particular HLA class I alleles expressed by the target cell. Some nontransformed cells, in particular cul-

tured endothelial cells, are similarly susceptible to IL-2–primed peripheral blood lymphocytes in isotope release assays. The cells responsible for this HLA-unrestricted killing in response to IL-2 have been termed *lymphokine-activated killer* (LAK) *cells.*[17] LAK cells appear to be a mixture of activated NK cells and CD3+/CD8+ cytotoxic T cells, the relative contributions of which depend on the duration of culture in IL-2 and whether human peripheral blood lymphocytes or murine spleen suspensions are used as an LAK cell source. As described in Clinical Investigations Involving High-Dose Interleukin-2, these *ex vivo*–activated LAK cells featured prominently in the early clinical trials carried out with IL-2 in cancer patients.

PRECLINICAL STUDIES WITH INTERLEUKIN-2 IN TUMOR-BEARING MICE

The results of the *in vitro* studies cited earlier in *In Vitro* Effects of Interleukin-2 demonstrating that IL-2 could enhance the cytolytic activity of NK cells and tumor-specific cytotoxic T lymphocytes suggested that systemically administered IL-2 might induce tumor regression in tumor-bearing mice. IL-2 has since undergone extensive evaluation as an antitumor agent in a variety of murine tumor models. IL-2 has been used alone, in combination with other cytokines, and in conjunction with the adoptive transfer of various *ex vivo*–activated lymphoid preparations to eradicate a wide range of local and metastatic tumors. Early studies demonstrated that IL-2 used alone could reduce or eliminate pulmonary metastases from methylcholanthrene-induced sarcoma and melanoma cell lines and that this antitumor effect was strictly dependent on the dose of IL-2 administered.[18] In some animal models, tumor eradication by IL-2 administration resulted in immunization against the tumor. In other studies in which mice were immunized with dendritic cells pulsed with tumor lysates, the concurrent systemic administration of IL-2 was shown to enhance the efficacy of the vaccine.[19]

In several studies, the effects of IL-2 could be enhanced by the concurrent administration of LAK cells generated by culturing splenocytes *ex vivo* in IL-2–containing media.[20] Mice bearing hepatic micrometastases from poorly immunogenic MCA-105 or MCA-102 sarcomas or MCA-38 adenocarcinoma cells, for example, were highly responsive to treatment with the combination of IL-2 and LAK cells but unresponsive to LAK cells alone and only partially responsive to IL-2.

Lymphocytes present within tumor infiltrates are often enriched for effector cells capable of killing tumor cells. When isolated and tested *in vitro* for cytolytic activity against autologous tumor cells, these tumor-infiltrating lymphocytes (TILs) are 50- to 100-fold more potent than IL-2–activated splenocytes (LAK cells). This apparent superiority was also evident *in vivo*. The infusion of 2×10^6 TILs with IL-2, for example, completely eradicated the pulmonary metastases of mice previously inoculated with MCA-105 sarcoma cells.[21] As many as 2×10^8 LAK cells were required for a comparable antitumor effect.

CLINICAL APPLICATIONS OF INTERLEUKIN-2

The potent immunomodulatory and antitumor effects of IL-2 in the *in vitro* experiments and preclinical animal tumor models described earlier prompted the rapid movement of IL-2 into the clinical setting. Early clinical trials involving the brief administration of modest doses of purified, cell-derived IL-2 produced only transient fever and lymphopenia, but no sustained ill effects or tumor responses. Because preclinical trials had shown that tumor responses were dose dependent and maximal when IL-2 was combined with LAK cells, the advent of recombinant IL-2 led quickly to a series of trials using higher doses of IL-2 with and without LAK cells.

CLINICAL INVESTIGATIONS INVOLVING HIGH-DOSE INTERLEUKIN-2

Investigators at the National Cancer Institute (NCI) Surgery Branch developed a regimen that involved the administration of high-dose intravenous (IV) bolus IL-2.[22] In this regimen, IL-2 was administered at 600,000 to 720,000 IU/kg IV every 8 hours on days 1 to 5 and 15 to 19 of a treatment course. A maximum of 28 to 30 doses per course was administered; however, doses were frequently withheld because of excessive toxicity. Treatment courses were repeated at 8- to 12-week intervals in responding patients. During initial studies, patients underwent daily leukapheresis on days 8 to 12 during which large numbers of lymphocytes were obtained to be cultured in IL-2 for 3 or 4 days to generate LAK cells; these LAK cells were then reinfused into the patient during the second 5-day period of IL-2 administration.

This high-dose IL-2 regimen with or without LAK cells produced overall tumor responses in 15% to 20% of patients with metastatic melanoma or renal cell cancer in clinical trials conducted at either the NCI Surgery Branch or within the Cytokine Working Group (formerly the Extramural IL-2 and LAK Working Group).[23] Complete responses were noted in 4% to 6% of patients with each disease and were frequently durable. Rare responses, usually partial and of shorter duration, were also noted in patients with either Hodgkin's or non-Hodgkin's lymphoma, or non–small cell lung, colorectal, or ovarian carcinoma.[24] Randomized and sequential clinical trials comparing IL-2 plus LAK cells with high-dose IL-2 alone failed to show sufficient benefit for the addition of LAK cells to justify their continued use.[25] Because of the quality and durability of tumor responses to this high-dose IL-2 regimen, IL-2 received FDA approval for the treatment of metastatic renal cell carcinoma in 1992 and for treatment of metastatic melanoma in 1998.[26,27] Long-term follow-up data for patients with melanoma and renal cell cancer treated in the initial high-dose bolus IL-2 trials presented to the FDA[28,29] have confirmed the earlier findings of response durability, with median duration for complete responses yet to be reached and few, if any, relapses observed in patients free of disease for longer than 30 months. In fact, several patients have remained free of disease in excess of 10 years since initiating treatment. These data suggest that high-dose IL-2 treatment may actually have led to the cure of some patients with these advanced malignancies previously considered incurable.

TOXICITY OF HIGH-DOSE INTERLEUKIN-2

The usefulness of high-dose IL-2 therapy has been limited by toxicity, many features of which resemble bacterial sepsis. Side effects are dose dependent and, fortunately, largely predictable and rapidly reversible. Common side effects include fever, chills, lethargy, diarrhea, nausea, anemia, thrombocytopenia, eosin-

TABLE 16.2-1.   Safety of High-Dose Intravenous Bolus Recombinant Interleukin-2 Therapy[a]: The National Cancer Institute Experience

Adverse Event	1985 Incidence (%)	1997 Incidence (%)
Hypotension	81	31
Diarrhea	92	12
Neuropsychiatric toxicity	19	8
Line sepsis	18	4
Pulmonary complications	12	3

Note: With patient selection and experience in managing side effects, high-dose recombinant interleukin-2 is safe. No treatment-related deaths in 809 consecutive patients. Incidence of grade 3–4 adverse events has been greatly reduced.
[a]720,000 IU/kg every 8 hours.
(Adapted from ref. 32, with permission.)

ophilia, diffuse erythroderma, hepatic dysfunction, and confusion.[30] Myocarditis also occurs in approximately 5% of patients. IL-2 therapy also commonly produces a "capillary leak syndrome," leading to fluid retention, hypotension, early adult respiratory distress syndrome, prerenal azotemia, and occasionally myocardial infarction. As a consequence of these side effects, few patients are able to receive all of the proposed therapy. IL-2 has also been shown to produce a neutrophil chemotactic defect that predisposes patients to infection with gram-positive and occasionally gram-negative bacteria.[31] Early high-dose IL-2 studies were associated with 2% to 4% mortality, largely related to infection or cardiac toxicity.[27,30] The routine use of antibiotic prophylaxis, more extensive cardiac screening, and more judicious IL-2 administration have greatly enhanced the safety of this therapy; since 1990 the mortality rates at experienced treatment centers have been less than 1%[32] (Table 16.2-1). Nonetheless, the considerable toxicity of the high-dose IL-2 regimen has continued to limit its application to highly selected patients with excellent performance status and adequate organ function treated at medical centers with considerable experience with this approach.

Laboratory studies have suggested that the toxicity of IL-2 is in part mediated by the release of secondary cytokines such as TNF-α, IL-1, and IL-6.[15] Nonetheless, attempts to block the toxicity of IL-2 by the coadministration of soluble receptors of IL-1 or TNF, or CNI-1493, an inhibitor of IL-1 and TNF signaling, have yielded only a modest reduction in the hypotension, vascular leak, and other serious side effects routinely observed in patients receiving high-dose IL-2.[33–35] The hypotension associated with IL-2 is in part due to the overproduction of the vasodilator nitric oxide. This diffusible gas is generated from the deamination of the amino acid arginine, and its production can be inhibited with various arginine analogs. Kilbourn et al. were able to demonstrate that the administration of NG-monomethyl-L-arginine to patients with renal cell carcinoma reversed the hypotension associated with IL-2 treatment.[36] The concurrent administration of M40403, a superoxide dismutase mimetic, has also been shown to reduce IL-2–associated hypotension in tumor-bearing mice.[37] This particular agent also appeared to enhance the antitumor activity of IL-2, presumably through the inhibition of superoxide production by macrophages. Whether or not any of these new agents will find widespread applicability and prove capable of converting the highly toxic high-dose IL-2 regimen into one that can be safely administered on the open ward in community hospitals remains to be seen.

MANAGEMENT OF PATIENTS RECEIVING HIGH-DOSE INTERLEUKIN-2

The safe administration of high-dose IL-2 requires first of all a careful selection of patients capable of tolerating the fever, hypotension, and edema that often develop during treatment. Because of this, high-dose IL-2 should be considered a reasonable treatment option only in patients without significant cardiac disease (i.e., angina, congestive heart failure, arrhythmia, or prior myocardial infarction). Patients older than 40 years of age should undergo stress testing and those found to have exercise-induced ischemia should be excluded. Patients should be specifically screened for central nervous system metastases, and those with positive findings on head computed tomographic scan or magnetic resonance image should not be given high-dose IL-2. Patients should also have adequate renal, hepatic, and pulmonary function with a serum creatinine level of less than 1.6 mg/dL, bilirubin level of less than 1.5 mg/dL, and a forced expiratory volume in 1 second of more than 2 L. They should also have a performance score on the Eastern Cooperative Oncology Group scale of less than 2.

Once a decision is made to offer high-dose IL-2 to a patient, the various treatment-associated side effects[30] can be ameliorated by the concomitant administration of acetaminophen and indomethacin to reduce fever and chills, H_2 blockers to prevent gastritis, and prophylactic antibiotics to prevent central line–associated infections. Patients should receive antiemetics and antidiarrheals as needed. IL-2–induced pruritus and dermatitis can be minimized with diphenhydramine and various skin creams. Steroids should be avoided because they antagonize the immunostimulatory properties of IL-2. Hypotension is best managed initially with fluid replacement, but many patients require IV dopamine and, in some instances, both dopamine and phenylephrine. Most patients require supplemental IV sodium bicarbonate to prevent acidosis. In the event of life-threatening toxicity (e.g., hypotension refractory to pressors), the IL-2 is discontinued but may be resumed after the resolution of the problem. Generally, doses of IL-2 withheld because of toxicity are not made up at the end of a treatment cycle. With careful patient selection and the appropriate use of concurrent medications, most patients can safely receive high-dose IL-2; however, the unusual array and severity of treatment side effects mandate that this form of immunotherapy be administered by a team of physicians and nurses experienced in the use of this agent.

LOWER-DOSE OR ALTERNATIVE INTERLEUKIN-2 REGIMENS

Because of the significant toxicity associated with the high-dose IV bolus IL-2 regimen and the expense involved with the necessary hospitalization and intensive monitoring, various investigators have attempted to establish active regimens using lower doses of IL-2. In these regimens, IL-2 was administered either by lower-dose IV bolus, continuous IV infusion, or subcutaneous injection in an effort to reduce toxicity without compromising antitumor efficacy. The more commonly used lower-dose regimens are listed in Table 16.2-2.

TABLE 16.2-2. Commonly Used Treatment Regimens of Interleukin-2 (IL-2) Alone

Regimen	IL-2 Dose	IL-2 Schedule	Clinical Setting
High-dose IV bolus IL-2	600,000–720,000 IU/kg	IV q8h d 1–5, 15–19	ICU-like
Continuous infusion IL-2	18 MIU/m²/d	CIV infusion d 1–5, 15–19	ICU-like
Low-dose IV bolus IL-2	72,000 IU/kg	IV q8h d 1–5, 15–19	Ward
Subcutaneous IL-2	250,000 IU/kg/d	SC d 1–5, wk 1	Outpatient
	125,000 IU/kg/d	SC d 1–5, wk 2–6	
Decrescendo IL-2	18 MIU/m²/6 h	CIV infusion × 1 d	Ward
	18 MIU/m²/12 h	CIV infusion × 1 d	
	18 MIU/m²/24 h	CIV infusion × 1 d	
	4.5 MIU/m²/24 h	CIV infusion × 3 d	
Ultra-low-dose IL-2	≤1 MIU/d	CIV infusion × 14–42 d	Outpatient

CIV, continuous intravenous; ICU-like, intensive care unit or specialized unit capable of providing blood pressure support.

The maximum tolerated dose of IL-2 when administered by a 5-day (120-hour) continuous infusion was shown to be 18 MIU/m²/d or approximately one-fifth the total amount of IL-2 tolerated by IV bolus IL-2 regimens.[38] Although continuous infusion IL-2 regimens were shown to produce response rates similar to those of the high-dose IV bolus IL-2 regimen, the toxicity was also generally comparable. Other regimens, such as those using lower doses of IL-2 administered either by IV bolus or subcutaneous injections, are better tolerated and enable patients to be treated on a conventional inpatient hospital ward or even as outpatients. Side effects associated with these regimens are generally limited to flu-like or constitutional symptoms, which allows even patients with limited cardiopulmonary reserve to receive this agent. However, it remains to be seen whether or not a less toxic, lower-dose regimen can be devised that duplicates the benefits of high-dose IL-2.

The question of whether high-dose regimens are more effective than those using lower doses remains controversial. In the case of metastatic melanoma, low-dose regimens consistently yield response rates below 5% and are regarded as clearly inferior to high-dose IL-2.[39] In contrast, studies of low-dose IL-2 in treatment of patients with renal cancer have consistently shown tumor regression in 10% to 20% of patients, comparable to the rate achieved with high-dose IL-2 in some studies. However, a phase III randomized trial assigning patients with renal cancer to either high-dose IL-2 or one of two lower-dose regimens (one IV and one subcutaneous) yielded a 21% response rate in the high-dose limb,[40] but only 13% and 10% response rates for the low-dose IV and subcutaneous regimens, respectively. Although no survival difference between the treatment groups was discernible, more durable responses were seen in patients receiving high-dose IL-2, which suggests an advantage to the high-dose regimens.

As part of this trial, investigators examined the pharmacokinetics of IL-2 in an effort to explain differences in biologic and

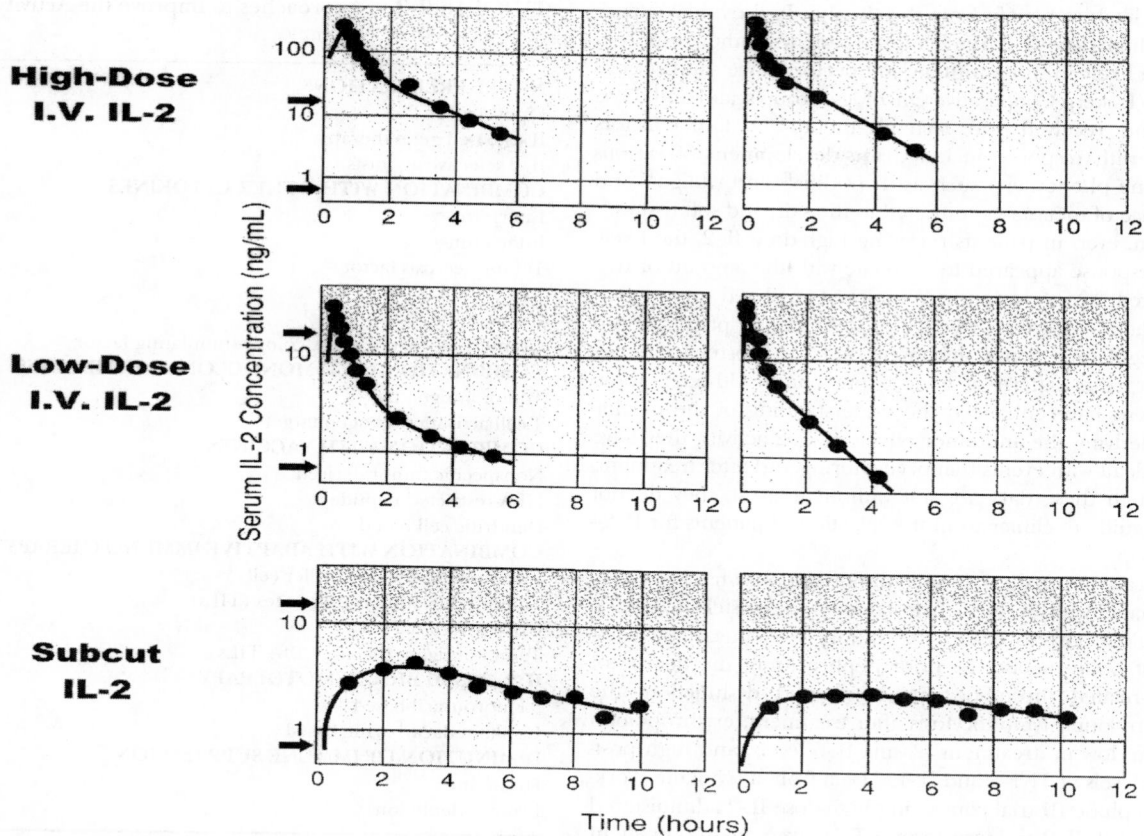

FIGURE 16.2-2. Examples of pharmacokinetic studies on representative patients with metastatic renal cell carcinoma measuring biologically active interleukin-2 (IL-2) levels after the first administration of recombinant IL-2 at 720,000 IU/kg by intravenous bolus, 72,000 IU/kg by intravenous bolus, or 250,000 IU/kg by subcutaneous injection. For each graph, the upper arrow indicates the K_d for the low-affinity IL-2 receptor, and the lower arrow indicates the K_d for the high-affinity IL-2 receptor. Potential target for serum IL-2 level is the area between the two K_d values to minimize secondary cytokine toxicity from natural killer cells while supporting specific T-cell expansion. Levels must be much higher to sustain an IL-2 target level in the extravascular compartment. (Adapted from ref. 41, with permission.)

clinical effects of the various administration schedules[41] (Fig. 16.2-2). Peak concentrations of 4680 ± 1188 IU/mL were achieved after the first injection of high-dose IL-2. Subsequent clearance was biphasic with an initial half-life of 12.6 ± 5.4 minutes and a terminal half-life of 1.6 ± 0.4 hours. Patients receiving IV low-dose IL-2 had peak serum levels of 486 ± 198 IU/mL with a similar clearance pattern and rate. Those receiving IL-2 by subcutaneous injection had peak levels of 61 ± 34 IU/mL 2 to 3 hours after the injection with a half-life of 5.3 ± 1.9 hours. Levels in excess of 18 IU/mL were maintained in those treated with either the high-dose IV or subcutaneous regimen. The inability of lower-dose regimens to produce sustained blood levels above the K_d of the low-affinity IL-2 receptor has been proposed as a potential explanation for their apparent diminished efficacy.

In addition to simply lowering the IL-2 dose, there have been several other attempts at improving the therapeutic index of IL-2. One example is the use of BAY 50-4798, a selective IL-2 receptor agonist engineered to bind preferentially to the high-affinity IL-2 receptor on T cells and less well to the lower-affinity IL-2 receptor present on NK cells. The rationale for the development of this agent rested on the unproven assumption that cytotoxic T cells expressing high-affinity IL-2 receptors were responsible for IL-2–

induced tumor regression, whereas NK cells expressing only the β- and γ-receptor chains were responsible for the production of pyrogenic cytokines and much of the toxicity of IL-2. This novel version of IL-2 was expected to enhance T-cell–mediated tumor killing while minimizing toxicity. Although clinical investigations with this agent appeared to show some reduction in toxicity, the antitumor activity of the cytokine has not yet been shown to be comparable to that of conventional IL-2.[42] Other approaches still under investigation include the formulation of IL-2 into liposomes and the direct intratumoral administration of a plasmid DNA–lipid complex containing the IL-2 gene.[43,44]

Although these alternative IL-2 regimens and formulations may eventually show benefits, at the present time the high-dose bolus IL-2 regimen remains the treatment of choice for appropriate patients with access to such treatment and is the gold standard to which other IL-2–based regimens should be compared.

PREDICTORS OF RESPONSE TO INTERLEUKIN-2–BASED THERAPY

Because of the toxicity and expense of high-dose IL-2 treatment, considerable effort has been expended to identify patient populations most likely to benefit from this therapy. In the initial experience with high-dose IL-2 in melanoma patients, tumor responses were more likely in those with a good performance status (score of 0 on the Eastern Cooperative Oncology Group scale) and those who had not received prior systemic therapy.[26,27] Other factors associated with response included the development of various autoimmune phenomena such as thyroiditis[45] and vitiligo[46] and the presence of metastases restricted to the skin and soft tissues.[47] In addition, even in patients receiving high-dose IL-2, the likelihood of response appeared to correlate with the amount of IL-2 administered.[48] More recently, Wang et al. analyzed tumors during IL-2 therapy for the presence of RNA transcripts of various immunoregulatory genes and were able to correlate tumor response to the pattern of gene expression.[49] Although these investigations have enhanced the understanding of the mechanisms underlying the antitumor effects of IL-2 activity, they have generally dealt with events that occur during and after treatment, and although these data are not without interest, they do not serve as a guide to clinicians in the selection of patients for IL-2–based therapy.

In the case of renal carcinoma, tumor response has been variably associated with performance status on the Eastern Cooperative Oncology Group scale, the number of metastatic sites, absence of bone metastases, prior nephrectomy, the degree of treatment-related thrombocytopenia, thyroid dysfunction, the extent of rebound lymphocytosis after treatment, erythropoietin production, low pretreatment plasma IL-6 levels, and high post-treatment levels of TNF-α and IL-1.[50] Data from a Cytokine Working Group phase III trial comparing high-dose IL-2 administered in hospital with IL-2 and interferon (IFN) given on an outpatient basis (see Combination Interleukin-2–Based Therapy, later in this chapter) suggested that in those receiving outpatient treatment, disease site factors such as an unresected primary tumor or the presence of hepatic or skeletal metastases correlated with poor treatment outcome.[51] These factors were less predictive of response in patients receiving high-dose IL-2. Additional retrospective studies suggested that the histologic pattern of the renal cancer also correlates with the probability of response to IL-2.[52] Response rates as high as 40% have been seen in patients whose primary tumors possessed favorable histologic features, such as clear cell histologic type with alveolar but no papillary or granular cell components. Conversely, those whose tumors displayed papillary or more than 50% granular features were unlikely to show a response. These correlations have been independently confirmed for metastatic lesions. Immunohistochemical studies have suggested that the expression of the G250 antigen (carbonic anhydrase IX) on a large percentage of renal cancer cells is also associated with an increased likelihood of benefit from IL-2 treatment.[53,54] Although these findings are intriguing, they all need to be independently validated in large prospective trials before any of these biochemical or histologic parameters can be used in the clinic to select patients for treatment with high-dose IL-2. However, it is likely that in the near future RNA microarray and other studies currently under way in several laboratories will lead to the generation of a molecular profile of tumors for which use of this toxic, but sometimes highly effective, therapy is justified.

COMBINATION INTERLEUKIN-2–BASED THERAPY

A number of agents have been combined with IL-2 in an effort to improve the activity of IL-2–based therapy. These are listed in

TABLE 16.2-3. Approaches to Improve the Activity of Interleukin-2 (IL-2)

NOVEL PREPARATIONS
Liposomal IL-2
IL-2–based gene therapy
IL-2 selective agonists
COMBINATION WITH OTHER CYTOKINES
Interferon-α
Interferon-γ
Tumor necrosis factor
IL-4
IL-12
Granulocyte-macrophage colony-stimulating factor
COMBINATION WITH MONOCLONAL ANTIBODIES
Tumor antigen target
T-cell activation antigen target
COMBINATION WITH VACCINES
Nonspecific tumor derived
HLA-restricted peptide
Dendritic cell based
COMBINATION WITH ADAPTIVE IMMUNOTHERAPY
Lymphokine-activated killer cell
Tumor-infiltrating lymphocytes (TILs)
CD8+ selected TILs
Tumor antigen–specific CD8+ TILs
IL-2–BASED BIOCHEMOTHERAPY
5-Fluorouracil based
Cisplatin-dacarbazine based
DIMINUTION OF IMMUNE SUPPRESSION
Histamine
Lymphodepletion

Table 16.2-3. Although preclinical laboratory and animal studies may have provided a strong rationale for these combinations, for the most part, the subsequent clinical trials have failed to demonstrate any advantage of these combinations over high-dose IL-2 monotherapy.[55]

A major focus of this line of investigation has involved combinations of IL-2 and IFN-α. Despite promising laboratory studies suggesting synergy, early clinical studies with high-dose IL-2 and IFN have not demonstrated any benefit over high-dose IL-2 alone.[56,57] On the other hand, a number of regimens involving combinations of low-dose IL-2 and IFN appeared promising. These regimens can be administered safely in an outpatient setting and appear to possess sufficient antitumor activity to be considered by many as an alternative to high-dose IL-2.[58,59] In addition, these low-dose IL-2 and IFN combinations can be modified to include other potentially active agents such as chemotherapeutic drugs.

Phase III investigations of low-dose IL-2 and IFN combinations have, however, prompted a reconsideration of these apparent advantages. For example, the Cytokine Working Group completed a phase III trial comparing high-dose IL-2 therapy with IL-2 and IFN therapy given in an outpatient setting in patients with metastatic renal cancer. This study demonstrated a higher response rate in those randomly selected to receive the high-dose bolus IL-2 regimen (23% vs. 9%), with more patients progression free at 3 years (10 vs. 3).[60] In addition, despite the greater acute toxicity associated with high-dose IL-2, the overall quality of life appeared to be at least equivalent to that of patients receiving the more protracted lower-dose regimen.[61]

As previously mentioned in Lower-Dose or Alternative Interleukin-2 Regimens, low-dose IL-2 regimens are generally ineffective in melanoma,[39] and it remains to be seen whether the addition of IFN and other agents (e.g., chemotherapeutic drugs) appreciably extends the survival of patients with advanced metastatic disease. Despite promising phase II data, several phase III studies have failed to show any advantage for biochemotherapy (the addition of cisplatin and dacarbazine–based chemotherapy to IL-2 and IFN) relative to chemotherapy or immunotherapy alone.[62–64] Preliminary data suggest that the addition of maintenance low-dose IL-2 after an initial course of biochemotherapy may improve overall responses. If this proves true in large prospective studies, a modified form of biochemotherapy featuring long-term low-dose IL-2 administration may yet revive the interest of clinicians in complicated multiagent regimens of this sort.

Efforts to combine IL-2 with other potentially active cytokines such as IFN-γ, TNF, IL-4, and granulocyte-macrophage colony-stimulating factor were largely unsuccessful and have been abandoned.[55] One study has suggested that IL-2 can restore and maintain the biologic activity of IL-12 when it is administered chronically and that such restoration may enhance the clinical efficacy of this agent; however, overall response rates for this combination were still modest at best.[65] Combinations of IL-2 with a variety of monoclonal antibodies directed either against tumor antigens (GD2 or GD3 gangliosides or CD20) or T-cell activation antigens (CD3) have also been disappointing.[40,66,67] Histamine has been administered in association with IL-2 in an effort to block immune dysfunction associated with superoxide production by macrophages. Although a randomized phase III trial comparing low-dose IL-2 plus histamine to low-dose IL-2 alone in patients with metastatic melanoma produced few tumor responses, improved survival was noted for those receiving the combination, particularly in the subset of patients with hepatic metastases.[68] A confirmatory trial restricted to patients with hepatic metastases has recently been completed and results should be available shortly.

Investigators have also continued to pursue the use of IL-2 together with cellular therapy approaches. IL-2 and TIL combinations were extremely promising in animal tumor models,[69] and preliminary studies involving administration of IL-2 and TILs to patients with melanoma or IL-2 plus IFN and selected CD8+ TILs to patients with renal cell carcinoma yielded encouraging results; however, selection bias could not be excluded as an explanation for the unusually high response rates reported.[70] A subsequent randomized trial of low-dose IL-2 with or without CD8+ TILs in patients with metastatic renal cell carcinoma produced such a disappointingly low response rate for both treatment arms[71] that no definite conclusion could be drawn regarding the potential role of TILs in the treatment of this disease. Interest in adoptive immunotherapy has been revived by an NCI Surgery Branch study involving the administration of clonally expanded, tumor antigen–specific CD8+ lymphocytes and IL-2 after fludarabine-induced lymphodepletion that showed encouraging antitumor activity in patients with refractory melanoma.[72] The extent to which this approach can be streamlined and exported outside the National Institutes of Health remains to be determined.

TILs have also proven to be a valuable tool for identifying melanoma-associated tumor regression antigens.[73] Extensive research at the NCI Surgery Branch and elsewhere has identified HLA-restricted melanocyte lineage–specific antigens that are recognized by the cellular immune system in patients exhibiting a response to IL-2–based therapy. Active immunization trials with immunodominant peptides derived from these tumor regression antigens have produced some encouraging results.[74] For example, vaccination with a mutated version of the GP100 peptide antigen together with high-dose IL-2 produced tumor responses in more than 40% of patients.[75] Unfortunately, these promising results could not be confirmed by the Cytokine Working Group, which found that only 10% of patients exhibited tumor responses.[76] Evaluation of different schedules of IL-2 administration and different peptide antigens, and a randomized trial of high-dose IL-2 with or with the GP100 peptide vaccine are still ongoing. In addition, trials examining combinations of similarly HLA-restricted antigens or antigen-presenting cells pulsed with these peptides together with IL-2 have been be initiated with generally mixed results.

CONCLUSION

Although the clinical application of IL-2 has benefited only a small portion of patients with either melanoma or renal cancer to date, it remains the only treatment that can produce durable benefit in more than an occasional patient with one of these diseases. Unfortunately, efforts to build on the successes seen with high-dose IL-2 alone have been largely disappointing. However, as more information is gained about the mechanism of action of IL-2 and the workings of the immune system in general, it is likely that IL-2–based treatment regimens will be refined and the appropriate patient populations to receive IL-2 will be better defined, which will lead ultimately to improved therapeutic results.

REFERENCES

1. Morgan D, Ruscetti FW, Gallo R. Selective in vitro growth of T-lymphocytes from normal bone marrows. *Science* 1976;193:1007.
2. Taniguchi T, Matsui H, Fujita T, et al. Structure and expression of a cloned cDNA for human interleukin-2. *Nature* 1983;302:305.
3. Taniguchi T, Minami Y. The IL-2/IL-2 receptor system: a current overview. *Cell* 1993;73:5.
4. Leonard WJ, Depper J, Uchiyama T, et al. A monoclonal antibody that appears to recognize the receptor for T cell growth factor: partial purification of the receptor. *Nature* 1982;300:267.
5. Hatakeyama M, Tsudo M, Minamoto S, et al. Interleukin-2 receptor beta chain gene: generation of three receptor forms by cloned human alpha and beta chain cDNAs. *Science* 1989;244:551.
6. Takeshita T, Asao H, Ohtani K, et al. Cloning of the gamma-chain of the human IL-2 receptor. *Science* 1992;257:379.
7. Lodolce JP, Boone DL, Chai S, et al. IL-15 receptor maintains lymphoid homeostasis by supporting lymphocyte homing and proliferation. *Immunity* 1998;9:669.
8. Noguchi M, Yi H, Rosenblatt HM, et al. Interleukin-2 receptor gamma chain mutation results in X-linked severe combined immunodeficiency in humans. *Cell* 1983;73:147.
9. Nakarai T, Robertson MJ, Streuli M, et al. Interleukin-2 receptor gamma chain expression on resting and activated lymphoid cells. *J Exp Med* 1994;180:241.
10. Hatakeyama M, Kono T, Kobayashi N, et al. Interaction of the IL-2 receptor with the family kinase p56lck: identification of novel intermolecular association. *Science* 1991;252:1523.
11. Friedmann MC, Migone TS, Russell SM, Leonard WJ. Different interleukin-2 receptor beta chain tyrosines couple to at least two signaling pathways and synergistically mediate interleukin-2-induced proliferation. *Proc Natl Acad Sci U S A* 1996;93:2077.
12. Asao H, Takeshita T, Ishii N, et al. Reconstitution of functional interleukin 2 receptor complexes on fibroblastoid cells: involvement of the cytoplasmic domain of the gamma chain in two distinct signaling pathways. *Proc Natl Acad Sci U S A* 1993;90:4127.
13. Russell SM, Johnston JA, Noguchi M, et al. Interaction of IL-2 receptor beta and gamma c chains with JAK1 and JAK3: implications for XSCID and XCID. *Science* 1994;266:1042.
14. Wang KS, Ritz J, Frank DA. IL-2 induces STAT4 activation in primary NK cells and NK cell lines, but not in T cells. *J Immunol* 1999;162:299.
15. Gemlo BT, Palladino MA, Jaffe HS, Espevik TP, Rayner AA. Circulating cytokines in patients with metastatic cancer treated with recombinant interleukin-2 and lymphokine-activated killer cells. *Cancer Res* 1988;48:5864.

16. Lotze MT, Grimm EA, Mazumder A, Strausser JL, Rosenberg SA. Lysis of fresh and cultured autologous tumor by human lymphocytes cultured in T-cell growth factor. *Cancer Res* 1981;41:4420.

17. Grimm EA, Mazumder A, Zhang HZ, Rosenberg SA. Lymphokine-activated killing phenomenon: lysis of natural killer resistant fresh solid tumor cells by interleukin-2 activated autologous human peripheral blood lymphocytes. *J Exp Med* 1982;155:1823.

18. Rosenberg SA, Mule JJ, Spiess PJ, Reichert CM, Schwarz SL. Regression of established pulmonary metastases and subcutaneous tumors mediated by the systemic administration of high-dose recombinant interleukin-2. *J Exp Med* 1985;161:1169.

19. Shimizu K, Fields RC, Giedlin M, Mule JJ. Systemic administration of interleukin-2 enhances the therapeutic efficacy of dendritic cell-based tumor vaccines. *Proc Natl Acad Sci U S A* 1999;96:2268.

20. Lafreniere R, Rosenberg SA. Adoptive immunotherapy of murine hepatic metastases with lymphokine activated killer (LAK) cells and recombinant interleukin-2 (RIL-2) can mediate the regression of both immunogenic and nonimmunogenic sarcomas and an adenocarcinoma. *J Immunol* 1985;135:4273.

21. Spiess PJ, Yang JC, Rosenberg SA. In vivo antitumor activity of tumor-infiltrating lymphocytes expanded in recombinant interleukin-2. *J Natl Cancer Inst* 1987;79:1067.

22. Rosenberg SA, Lotze MT, Muul LM, et al. Observations on the systemic administration of autologous lymphokine-activated killer cells and recombinant interleukin-2 to patients with metastatic cancer. *N Engl J Med* 1985;313:1485.

23. Rosenberg SA, Yang JC, Topalian SL, et al. Treatment of 283 consecutive patients with metastatic melanoma or renal cell cancer using high-dose bolus interleukin-2. *JAMA* 1994;271:907.

24. Sznol M, Hawkins MJ. Interleukin-2 in malignancies other than melanoma and renal cell carcinoma. In: Atkins MB, Mier JW, eds. *Therapeutic applications of interleukin-2.* New York: Marcel Dekker, 1993:177.

25. Rosenberg SA, Lotze MT, Yang JC, et al. Prospective randomized trial of high-dose interleukin-2 alone or in conjunction with lymphokine-activated killer cells for the treatment of patients with advanced cancer. *J Natl Cancer Inst* 1993;8:622.

26. Fyfe G, Fisher RI, Rosenberg SA, et al. Results of treatment of 255 patients with metastatic renal cell carcinoma who received high-dose recombinant interleukin-2 therapy. *J Clin Oncol* 1995;13:688.

27. Atkins MB, Lotze MT, Dutcher JP, et al. High-dose recombinant interleukin-2 therapy for patients with metastatic melanoma: analysis of 270 patients treated between 1985 and 1993. *J Clin Oncol* 1999;17:2105.

28. Fisher RI, Rosenberg SA, Fyfe G. Long-term survival update for high-dose recombinant interleukin-2 in patients with renal cell carcinoma. *Cancer J Sci Am* 2000;6[Suppl 1]:S55.

29. Atkins MB, Kunkel L, Sznol M, Rosenberg SA. High-dose Aldesleukin therapy in metastatic melanoma: long-term survival update. *Cancer J Sci Am* 2000;6[Suppl 1]:S11.

30. Margolin K. The clinical toxicities of high-dose interleukin-2. In: Atkins MB, Mier JW, eds. *Therapeutic applications of interleukin-2.* New York: Marcel Dekker, 1993:331.

31. Klempner M, Noring R, Mier J, Atkins MB. An acquired neutrophil chemotactic defect in patients receiving immunotherapy with interleukin-2. *N Engl J Med* 1990;322:959.

32. Kammula US, White DE, Rosenberg SA. Trends in the safety of high dose bolus interleukin-2 administration in patients with metastatic cancer. *Cancer* 1998;83:797.

33. DuBois J, Trehu EG, Mier JW, et al. Randomized placebo-controlled clinical trial of high-dose interleukin-2 (IL-2) in combination with the soluble TNF receptor IgG chimera (TNFR: Fc). *J Clin Oncol* 1997;15:1052.

34. McDermott D, Trehu E, DuBois J, et al. Phase I clinical trial of the soluble IL-1 receptor either alone or in combination with high-dose IL-2 in patients with advanced malignancies. *Clin Cancer Res* 1998;5:1203.

35. Atkins MB, Redman B, Mier J, et al. A Phase I study of CNI-1493, an inhibitor of cytokine release, in combination with high dose interleukin-2 in patients with renal cancer and melanoma. *Clin Cancer Res* 2002;7:486.

36. Kilbourn RG, Fonseca GA, Trissel LA, Griffith OW. Strategies to reduce side effects of interleukin-2: evaluation of the antihypotensive agent NG-monomethyl-L-arginine. *Cancer J Sci Am* 2000;6:S21.

37. Samlowski WE, Petersen R, Cuzzocrea S, et al. A nonpeptidyl mimic of superoxide dismutase, M40403, inhibits dose-limiting hypotension associated with interleukin-2 and increases its antitumor effects. *Nat Med* 2003;9:750.

38. West WH, Tauer KW, Yannelli JR, et al. Constant-infusion recombinant interleukin-2 in adoptive immunotherapy of advanced cancer. *N Engl J Med* 1987;16:898.

39. Atkins MB, Shet A, Sosman JA. IL-2 clinical applications: melanoma. In: DeVita VT Jr, Hellman S, Rosenberg SA, et al. *Biologic therapy of cancer principles and practice,* 3rd ed. Philadelphia: JB Lippincott, 2000:50.

40. Yang JC, Sherry RM, Steinberg SM, et al. Randomized study of high-dose and low-dose interleukin-2 in patients with metastatic renal cancer. *J Clin Oncol* 2003;21:3127.

41. Yang JC, Rosenberg SA. An ongoing prospective randomized comparison of interleukin-2 regimens for the treatment of metastatic renal cell cancer. *Cancer J Sci Am* 1997;3:S79.

42. Margolin KA, Atkins MB, Weber J, et al. Phase I study of interleukin-2 (IL-2) selective agonist BAY-50-4798 (BAY) in patients (pts.) with advanced melanoma (Mel) and renal cell carcinoma (RCC). *Proc Am Soc Clin Oncol* 2002;21:12a.

43. Neville ME, Boni LT, Pflug LE, Popescu MC, Robb RJ. Biopharmaceutics of liposomal interleukin 2, oncolipin. *Cytokine* 2000;12:1691.

44. Figlin RA, Parker SE, Horton HM. Technology evaluation: interleukin-2 gene therapy for the treatment of renal cell carcinoma. *Curr Opin Mol Ther* 1999;1:271.

45. Atkins MB. Autoimmune disorders induced by interleukin-2 therapy. In: Atkins MB, Mier JW, eds. *Therapeutic applications of interleukin-2.* New York: Marcel Dekker, 1993:389.

46. Rosenberg SA, White DE. Vitiligo in patients with melanoma: normal tissue antigens can be targets for cancer immunotherapy. *J Immunother* 1996;19:81.

47. Phan GQ, Attia P, Steinberg SM, et al. Factors associated with response to high-dose interleukin-2 in patients with metastatic melanoma. *J Clin Oncol* 2001;19:3477.

48. Royal RE, Steinberg SM, Krouse RS, et al. Correlates of response to IL-2 therapy in patients treated for metastatic renal cancer and melanoma. *Cancer J Sci Am* 1996;2:91.

49. Wang E, Miller LD, Ohnmacht GA, et al. Prospective molecular profiling of melanoma metastases suggests classifiers of immune responsiveness. *Cancer Res* 2002;62:3581.

50. Atkins MB, Garnick M. Renal neoplasia. In: Brenner BM, ed. *The kidney,* 6th ed. Philadelphia: WB Saunders, 2000:1844.

51. Atkins MB, McDermott DF. Results of the cytokine working group phase III trial of high dose IL-2 vs low dose IL-2 and IFN therapy in patients with metastatic renal cell carcinoma. Chemotherapy Foundation Symposium XX Innovative Cancer Therapy for Tomorrow 2002;72:87.

52. Upton MP, Parker RA, Youmans A, Connolly C, Atkins MB. Histologic predictors of renal cell carcinoma (RCC) response to interleukin-2-based therapy. *Proc Am Soc Clin Oncol* 2003;22:851.

53. Bui MH, Seligson D, Han KR, et al. Carbonic anhydrase IX is an independent predictor of survival I advanced renal clear cell carcinoma: implications for prognosis and therapy. *Clin Cancer Res* 2003;9:802.

54. Atkins M, Mcdermott D, Mier J, et al. High carbonic anhydrase IX (CAIX) expression predicts for renal cell carcinoma (RCC) response to IL-2 therapy. *J Immunother* 2003 (*in press*).

55. Atkins MB, Trehu EG, Mier JW. Combination cytokine therapy. In: DeVita VT Jr, Hellman S, Rosenberg SA, eds. *Biologic therapy of cancer principles and practice,* 2nd ed. Philadelphia: JB Lippincott, 1995:443.

56. Atkins MB, Sparano J, Fisher RI, et al. A randomized phase II trial of high dose IL-2 either alone or in combination with interferon alpha 2B in advanced renal cell carcinoma. *J Clin Oncol* 1993;11:661.

57. Sparano JA, Fisher RI, Sunderland M, et al. Randomized phase III trial of treatment with high-dose interleukin-2 either alone or in combination with alfa-2A in patients with advanced melanoma. *J Clin Oncol* 1993;11:1969.

58. Keilholz U, Scheibenbogen C, Tilgen W, et al. Interferon-α and interleukin-2 in the treatment of metastatic melanoma: comparison of two phase II trials. *Cancer* 1993;72:607.

59. Atzpodien J, Lopez HE, Kirchner H, et al. Multi-institutional home therapy trial of recombinant human interleukin-2 and interferon alfa-2 in progressive metastatic renal cell carcinoma. *J Clin Oncol* 1995;13:497.

60. McDermott D, Flaherty L, Clark J, et al. A randomized phase III trial of high-dose interleukin-2 (HD IL2) versus subcutaneous (SC) IL2/interferon (IFN) in patients with metastatic renal cell carcinoma (RCC). *Proc Am Soc Clin Oncol* 2001;20:172a.

61. Cole B, McDermott D, Parker R, et al. The impact of treatment with high-dose interleukin-2 (HD IL-2) or subcutaneous (SC) IL-2/interferon alfa-2b (IFN) on quality of life (QOL) in patients with metastatic renal cell carcinoma (mRCC). *Proc Am Soc Clin Oncol* 2003;22:387a.

62. Atkins MB, Lee S, Flaherty LE, Sondak VK, Kirkwood JM. A prospective randomized phase III trial of concurrent biochemotherapy (BCT) with cisplatin, vinblastine, dacarbazine (CVD), IL-2 and interferon α-2b (IFN) versus CVD alone in patients with metastatic malignant melanoma (E3695): an ECOG-coordinated Intergroup Trial. *Proc Am Soc Clin Oncol* 2003;22:708a.

63. Keilholz U, Goey SH, Punt CJ, et al. Interferon alfa-2a and interleukin-2 with or without cisplatin in metastatic melanoma: a randomized trial of the European Organization for Research and Treatment of Cancer Melanoma Cooperative Group. *J Clin Oncol* 1997;15:2579.

64. Keilholz U, Punt CJ, Gore M, et al. Dacarbazine, cisplatin and IFN-α2b with or without IL-2 in advanced melanoma: final analysis of EORTC randomized phase III trial. *Proc Am Soc Clin Oncol* 2003;22:708.

65. Gollob JA, Veenstra KG, Parker RA, et al. Phase I trial of concurrent twice-weekly rhIL-12 plus low-dose IL-2 in patients with melanoma or renal cell carcinoma. *J Clin Oncol* 2003;21:2564.

66. Sosman J, Weiss G, Margolin K, et al. Phase 1B clinical trial of anti-CD3 followed by high dose interleukin-2 in patients with metastatic melanoma and advanced renal cell carcinoma: clinical and immunologic effects. *J Clin Oncol* 1993;11:1496.

67. Friedberg JW, Neuberg D, Gribben JG, et al. Combination immunotherapy with rituximab and interleukin 2 patients with relapsed or refractory follicular non-Hodgkin's lymphoma. *Br J Haematol* 2002;117:828.

68. Agarwala SS, Glaspy J, O'Day SJ, et al. Results from a randomized phase III study comparing combined treatment with histamine dihydrochloride plus interleukin-2 versus interleukin-2 alone in patients with metastatic melanoma. *J Clin Oncol* 2002;20:125.

69. Rosenberg SA, Schwartz SL, Spiess PJ. Combination immunotherapy for cancer: synergistic antitumor interactions of interleukin-2, alfa interferon, and tumor-infiltrating lymphocytes. *J Natl Cancer Inst* 1988;80:1393.

70. Figlin RA, Pierce WC, Kaboo R, et al. Treatment of metastatic renal cell carcinoma with nephrectomy, interleukin-2 and cytokine-primed or CD8(+) selected tumor infiltrating lymphocytes from primary tumor. *J Urology* 1997;158:740.

71. Figlin RA, Thompson JA, Bukowski RM, et al. Multicenter, randomized, phase III trial of CD8+ tumor-infiltrating lymphocytes in combination with recombinant interleukin-2 in metastatic renal cell carcinoma. *J Clin Oncol* 1999;17:2521.

72. Dudley ME, Wunderlich JR, Robbins PF, et al. Cancer regression and autoimmunity in patients after clonal repopulation of with antitumor lymphocytes. *Science* 2002;298:850.

73. Kawakami Y, Eliejahu S, Jennings C, et al. Recognition of multiple epitopes in the human melanoma antigen gp100 by tumor infiltrating T-lymphocytes associated with tumor regression. *J Immunol* 1995;154:3461.

74. Parkhurst MR, Salgaller ML, Southwood S, et al. Improved induction of melanoma-reactive CTL with peptides from the melanoma antigen gp100 modified at HLA-A* 0201-binding residues. *J Immunol* 1996;157:2539.

75. Rosenberg SA, Yang JC, Schwartzentruber DJ, et al. Immunologic and therapeutic evaluation of a synthetic peptide vaccine for the treatment of patients with metastatic melanoma. *Nat Med* 1998;4:321.

76. Gollob J, Flaherty L, Smith J, et al. A cytokine working group (CWG) phase II trial of a modified gp100 melanoma peptide (gp100 (209M)) and high dose interleukin-2 (HD IL-2) administered q3 weeks in patients with stage IV melanoma: limited antitumor activity. *Proc Am Soc Clin Oncol* 2001;20:357a.

PAUL A. MARKS
VICTORIA M. RICHON
THOMAS A. MILLER
WM. KEVIN KELLY

SECTION 3

Histone Deacetylase Inhibitors: New Targeted Anticancer Drugs

The base sequence of DNA provides the genetic code for proteins. The regulation of expression or suppression of genes is largely determined by the structure of the chromatin associated with the DNA—referred to as epigenetic gene regulation.[1–5] It is now understood that posttranslation modifications of the histones of chromatin have a fundamental role in regulating gene expression. Enzymes involved in these epigenetic events include histone deacetylases (HDACs) and histone acetyltransferases (HATs). Alterations in the structure or expression of HATs and HDACs occur in many cancers.[6–10] A structurally diverse group of small molecules has been developed that can inhibit HDACs.[8,10–12] These inhibitors induce growth arrest, differentiation, or apoptosis of cancer cells *in vitro* and *in vivo*. Clinical trials with several of these agents have shown that they have antitumor activity against various cancers at doses that are well tolerated by patients.

CHROMATIN STRUCTURE

DNA is packaged into chromatin, which is structurally complex and dynamic, and consists of DNA, histones, and nonhistone proteins.[1–5] Nucleosomes are repeating units in chromatin composed of approximately 146 base pairs of two superhelical turns of DNA wrapped around an octamer core of pairs of histones H4, H3, H2A, and H2B. The amino-terminal tails of the histones are subject to posttranslational modification by acetylation of lysine, methylation of lysine and arginine, phosphorylation of serine, and ubiquitination of lysine. HDACs and HATs determine the pattern of histone acetylation (Fig. 16.3-1). It has been hypothesized that histone modifications acting alone, sequentially, or in combination represent a "code" that can be recognized by nonhistone proteins forming complexes involved in the regulation of gene expression.

It is probably an oversimplification, but suppression of gene expression is generally considered to be mediated by a condensation of chromatin structure, whereas neutralization of the positive charge of histones, primarily by acetylation of histone lysines, leads to a more open structure of the chromatin that provides for greater access to promoter regions of genes for transcription factor complexes.

HISTONE DEACETYLASES AND HISTONE ACETYL TRANSFERASES

The acetylation status of chromatin that is associated with particular genes is dependent on both HAT and HDAC activities. As suggested in Chromatin Structure, earlier in this chapter, HDACs are involved primarily in the repression of gene transcription by virtue of the compaction of chromatin structure that accompanies the removal of charge-neutralizing acetyl groups from the histone lysine tails.

There are three classes of human HDAC enzymes.[10–13] Class I includes HDACs 1, 2, 3, and 8, which are related to yeast RPD3 deacetylase and have molecular weights of 22 to 55 kD. Class II deacetylases includes HDACs 4, 5, 6, 7, 9, and 10, which are larger molecules with molecular weights between 120 and 130 kD and are related to yeast Hda1 deacetylase. HDAC11 contains conserved residues in the catalytic core region shared by both class I and II enzymes. A third class of HDACs has been identified that are in the nicotinamide adenine dinucleotide–dependent Sir 2 family of deacetylases, which are not inhibited by compounds that inhibit class I and II HDACs. This third class of HDACs appears not to act on histones.

There is now abundant evidence that HDACs are not redundant in function.[14–16] For example, class I HDACs are found almost exclusively in the cell nucleus, whereas class II HDACs shuttle between the nucleus and cytoplasm on certain cellular signals. Mutation of HDAC1 results in embryonic lethality despite increased expression of HDAC2 and HDAC3. Class II HDACs block myocyte enhancer factor 2 activation of cardiac hypertrophy.[17] HDAC7 appears to have selectivity in regulating T-cell differentiation in the thymus. HDAC6 has a unique deacetylase activity toward microtubules.

Although class I and II HDACs are present in most cells, the level of the different HDACs does vary among the types of tissue. The level of class I HDACs, particularly HDAC1, has been found to be high in many transformed cells. Studies with short interfering RNA that selectively inhibited HDAC1 and HDAC3 suggested that inhibition of these class I HDACs inhibited cervical cancer cell proliferation.

HDACs and HATs do not bind directly to DNA but are recruited to DNA by transcription factor protein complexes that differ in their subunit composition. For example, HDAC1 and -2 have been found in complexes with Sir3, NuRD (nucleosome remodeling and deacetylation), and N-CoR (nuclear receptor corepressor). HATs are found in complexes with other HATs, for example, p300 and corepressor binding protein (CBP), as well as with various factors involved in regulating gene expression.

HISTONE ACETYLTRANSFERASES AND HISTONE DEACETYLASE INHIBITORS AND HUMAN CANCERS

Disruption of HAT or HDAC activity has been found in many human cancers. Genes that encode HAT enzymes are translocated, amplified, overexpressed, or mutated in various cancers, both hematologic and epithelial.[6–8,12–16,18] Two closely related HATs, CBP and p300, are altered in some tumors by either mutation or translocation. Missense mutations in p300 and mutations associated with truncated p300 have been identified in colorectal and gastric primary tumors and in other epithelial cancers. In these cases, the second allele was frequently deleted. Individuals with the Rubinstein-Taybi syndrome, a developmental disorder, carry a mutation in CBP that inactivates its HAT activity, and these individuals have an increased risk of cancer. Loss of heterozygosity of p300 has been described in 80% of glioblastomas, and loss of heterozygosity around the CBP locus has been observed in hepatocellular carcinomas.

Translocations of CBP and p300, resulting in in-frame fusion with a number of genes, have been identified in several hematologic malignancies. MOZ (monocyte–leukemia zinc fin-

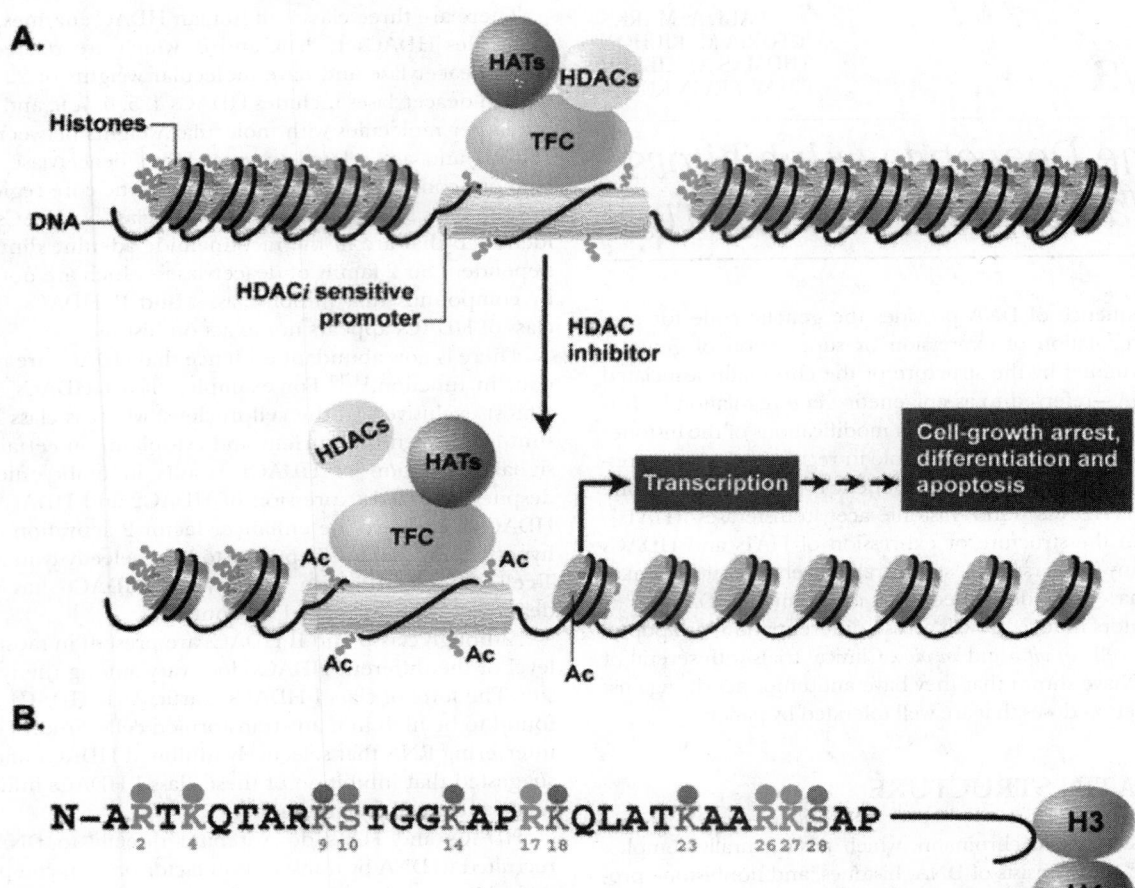

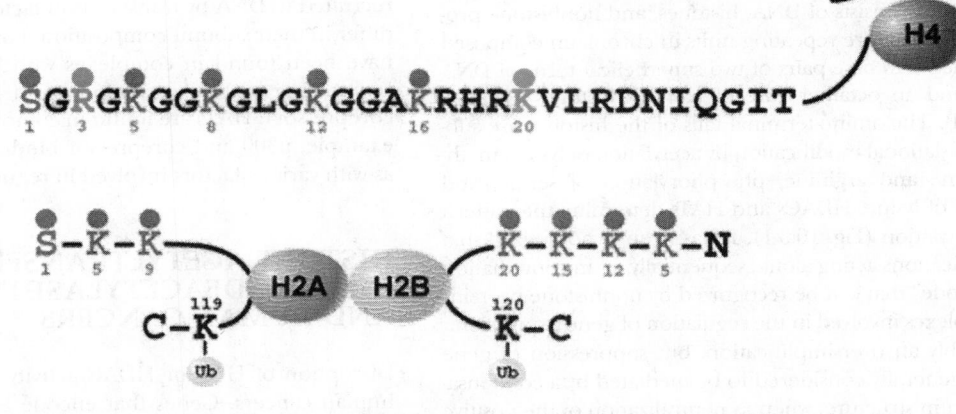

FIGURE 16.3-1. Schematic representation of the proposed mechanism of action of histone deacetylase (HDAC) inhibitors. **A:** HDAC inhibitor directly interacts with HDACs that are recruited to the transcription factor complex (TFC) of proteins, which includes histone acetyltransferases (HATs) (corepressor binding protein and p300). This complex binds to the promoter region of genes. The DNA (*black line*) is wrapped around the core histones (*blue*) consisting of dimers of histones H3, H4, H2A, and H2B. HDAC inhibitor–sensitive gene promoter region associated histones (*lime green*). The amino-terminal tails (*red*) of histones are subject to posttranslational modification. The HDAC inhibitor causes HDACs to dissociate from the TFC, causing an accumulation of acetylated histones and active transcription of the gene(s), which, through downstream effects, leads to cell growth arrest, differentiation, and apoptosis. **B:** Schematic representation of the possible modifications of the amino acid sequence of amino-terminal tails of histones H3, H4, H2A, and H2B. The color-coded dots indicate acetylation (*gray*), methylation (*red*), or phosphorylation (*blue*) of the amino acid. A, alanine; Ac, acetyl; C, cysteine; D, aspartic acid; H, histidine; G, glycine; I, isoleucine; K, lysine; L, leucine; N, asparagine; P, proline; Q, glutamine; R, arginine; S, serine; T, threonine; V, valine; Ub, ubiquitin. (Adapted from ref. 3.) (See Color Fig. 16.3-1 in the CD-ROM.)

ger protein) has been found fused to TIF1 (transcriptional mediator/intermediary factor 1) in a leukemia-associated chromosome 8 inversion [inv(8)(p11;q13)] and to transcripts of CBP in a subtype of acute myeloid leukemia. Translocations of CBP and p300 have also been described in treatment-related leukemias and myelodysplastic syndromes.

HDACs are involved in mediating the function of oncogenic translocation products in specific forms of leukemia and lymphoma. For example, the oncoprotein that is encoded by one of the translocation-generated fusion genes in acute promyelocytic leukemia, PML-RAR-α, represses transcription by associating with a corepressor complex that contains HDAC activity. In non-Hodgkin's lymphoma, the transcriptional repressor LAZ3/BCL6 (lymphoma-associated zinc finger 3/B-cell lymphoma) is inappropriately overexpressed and associated with aberrant transcriptional repression through recruitment of HDACs, which leads to lymphoid oncogenic transformation. Acute myeloid leukemia M2 subtype is associated with the t(8;21) chromosomal translocation, which produces an AML1-ETO fusion protein—a potent dominant transcriptional repressor—through its recruitment of HDAC activity.

In these examples, transcriptional repression seems to be mediated by the recruitment of HDACs and provides a mechanistic rational for the treatment of these leukemias and other neoplasms with inhibitors of HDAC activity.

Imbalance in histone acetylation can lead to changes in chromatin structure and transcriptional dysregulation of genes as reviewed in Chromatin Structure, earlier in this chapter, and, in addition, can alter the structure and activity of proteins involved in regulation of cell-cycle progression, including p53 and Rb proteins. Furthermore, altered HDAC or HAT activity may disrupt normal mitosis and cytokinesis. In sum, altered HDAC or HAT function, or both, can affect gene transcription, cell-cycle progression, and cell division.

HISTONE DEACETYLASE INHIBITORS

HDAC inhibitors reported to date can be divided into several structural classes, including hydroxamates, cyclic peptides, aliphatic acids, benzamides, and electrophilic ketones (Table 16.3-1). Trichostatin A (TSA)[19] was the first natural product hydroxamate discovered to inhibit HDACs directly. Suberoylanilide hydroxamic acid (SAHA), which contains relatively less structural complexity, was found to be a nanomolar inhibitor of partially purified HDAC.[20] LAQ824 is another hydroxamic acid–based analog that is a nanomolar inhibitor of HDACs.[15] Cyclic tetrapeptides, which constitute the most structurally complex class of HDAC inhibitors, include depsipeptide, apicidin, and the CHAPs molecules and are active at nanomolar levels.[21-23]

The aliphatic acids, the least potent class of HDAC inhibitors, possess millimolar levels of activity and include valproic acid and phenyl butyrate.[24,25] The benzamide class, MS-275 and CI-994, is in general less potent than the corresponding hydroxamates and cyclic tetrapeptides.[26,27]

Electrophilic ketones are a new class of HDAC inhibitors.[28] These agents include various trifluoromethyl ketones and α-ketoamides and, like the benzamides, possess micromolar-level inhibitory activities of HDAC.

The structural details of HDAC inhibitor-enzyme interactions have been elucidated by Finnin et al.[29] The crystal structure of a

TABLE 16.3-1. Histone Deacetylase Inhibitors

Class	Compound	Structure
Hydroxamate	Trichostatin A (TSA)	
	Suberoylanilide hydroxamic acid (SAHA)	
Cyclic peptide	Depsipeptide (FK-228)	
Aliphatic acid	Valproic acid	
	Phenyl butyrate	
Benzamide	MS-275	
	CI-994	
Electrophilic ketone	Trifluoromethyl ketones	
	α-Ketoamides	

Note: For references, see text.

histone deacetylase-like protein (HDLP), a homologue of mammalian HDAC, was solved with the HDAC inhibitors TSA and SAHA (Fig. 16.3-2A). The structure-activity relationships of the HDAC inhibitor classes validate key features found in the x-ray crystal structure. Particularly, the direct interaction of the inhibitor with the active-site zinc appears to be a prerequisite to optimal inhibitory activity. The structural characteristics of most HDAC inhibitors reported to date can be summarized as depicted in Figure 16.3-2B.

ACTIVITY OF HISTONE DEACETYLASE INHIBITORS

EFFECT ON GENE EXPRESSION

A model for the antitumor activity of HDAC inhibitors is that they cause an accumulation of acetylated histones, which leads to the

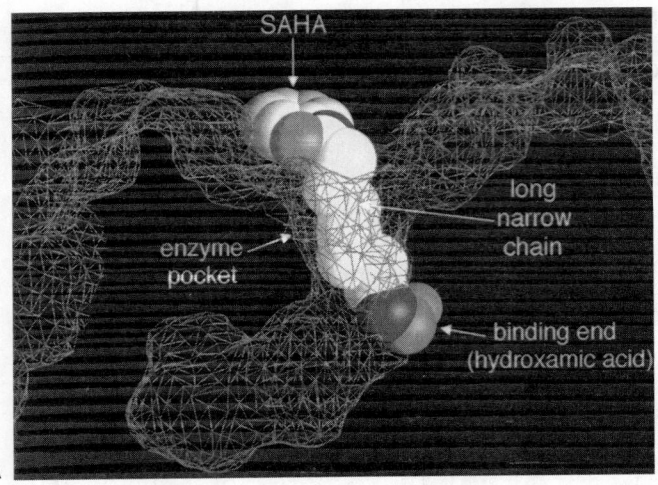

B

| Surface Recognition | Linker | Metal Binding |

FIGURE 16.3-2. **A:** Schematic representation of the crystal structure of the histone deacetylase (HDAC)–like protein with suberoylanilide hydroxamic acid (SAHA) that inserts into the pocket-like catalytic site of the enzyme. At the base of the catalytic pocket is a zinc molecule with which the hydroxamic moiety of SAHA binds.[29] **B:** Structural features of hydroxamic acid–based inhibitors of HDAC. (See Color Fig. 16.3-2 in the CD-ROM.)

activation of transcription of genes whose expression causes inhibition of tumor cell proliferation (see Fig. 16.3-1). Expression profiling of cells cultured with HDAC inhibitors support this model, at least in part. Expression profiling studies demonstrate that the expression of a finite number of genes (2% to 5% of the expressed genes) is regulated after exposure to HDAC inhibitors.[30–32] Although the model predicts that accumulation of acetylated histones leads to activation of gene expression, the expression profiling studies reveal that the transcription of many genes is repressed. The mechanism of repression is currently not well understood and may result from either direct or indirect effects on histone acetylation or, alternatively, from the increase in acetylation of proteins other than histones, such as transcription factors. Thus, it has been shown that HDAC is required for the transcriptional activity mediated by the STAT (signal transduction and activators of transcription) proteins.[33] Inhibiting HDAC activity can prevent expression of genes for which STATs are required. The subsequent changes in protein expression cause inhibition of tumor cell growth. This inhibition is not due to effects on histone H3 or H4 acetylation or chromatin remodeling within the promoter region.

One of the genes most commonly induced by HDAC inhibitors is the cell-cycle kinase inhibitor p21[WAF1]. The increase in p21[WAF1] protein can lead to arrest of cells in G$_1$. It has been shown that the HDAC inhibitor–induced expression of p21[WAF1] correlates with an increase in the acetylation of histones associated with the p21[WAF1] promoter region.[34,35] This suggests that p21[WAF1] is a direct target gene for HDAC inhibitors. Moreover, a link between HDAC1 and p21[WAF1] expression has now been demonstrated.[36] HDAC1-deficient embryonic stem cells show reduced proliferation rates, which correlate, in part, with elevated levels of p21[WAF1].

Although the induction of p21[WAF1] may play an important role in the antiproliferative effects caused by HDAC inhibitors, it is not required for HDAC inhibitor–induced apoptosis. In fact, blocking SAHA-induced p21[WAF1] expression leads to increased apoptosis.[37] In addition to p21[WAF1], several other genes are commonly induced or repressed by HDAC inhibitors, and their induction or repression may also play an important role in the HDAC inhibitor–induced antiproliferative response.[31] The elucidation of the downstream pathways of HDAC inhibition should provide a mechanistic rationale for therapies to be administered in combination with HDAC inhibitors.

In addition to the effects on gene expression, HDAC inhibitor–induced accumulation of acetylated histones may affect cell-cycle progression by altering the ability of tumor cells to undergo mitosis.[12,38] Histone acetylation may be important for proper deposition of histones during DNA synthesis and chromosome segregation during mitosis. An increase in acetylated histones during the S (DNA synthesis) and G$_2$ (premitosis) phase of the cell cycle can activate a G$_2$ checkpoint, resulting in arrest of cells in the G$_2$ phase. Loss of the G$_2$ checkpoint is a frequent event in cancer cells.

EFFECT ON NONHISTONE PROTEINS

In addition to histones, many other proteins have been shown to be reversibly acetylated on lysine residues.[39,40] The acetylation state of several of these proteins is increased after exposure to class I and class II HDAC inhibitors, including p53, Rb, α-tubulin, and Hsp90 (heat-shock protein 90). Acetylation of certain of these proteins leads to their activation and antiproliferative effects. Thus, in addition to histones, SAHA and TSA cause the accumulation of acetylated α-tubulin (but MS-275 does not).[37] A small molecule, tubacin, has been discovered that is a selective inhibitor of HDAC6 activity and causes an accumulation of acetylated α-tubulin, but does not affect acetylation of histones and does not inhibit cell-cycle progression.[41] Therefore, it appears that only a subset of acetylated nonhistone proteins play a role in the antiproliferative effects of HDAC inhibitors.

In addition to effects on gene transcription and mitosis, it is clear that HDAC inhibitors can cause changes in the activity of proteins regulating cell-cycle progression by acetylation. For example, depsipeptide causes an increase in acetylation of the chaperone protein Hsp90.[42] Acetylation of Hsp90 inhibits the binding of the chaperone protein to client proteins, which results in the degradation of the client proteins. Further studies are required to determine the relative roles of inhibition of gene transcription and enhanced protein degradation in causing a decrease of the levels of critical proteins after treatment with HDAC inhibitors. In certain cases, it may be a combination of both transcriptional and posttranslational effects that leads to the decrease in protein expression. Considered as a whole, HDAC inhibition can lead to changes in both gene transcriptional activity and protein stability through the increased acetylation of proteins such as histones and Hsp90.

ACTIVITY OF HISTONE DEACETYLASE INHIBITORS WITH OTHER AGENTS

HDAC inhibitors have been found to be synergistic or additive with a number of anticancer agents, including radiation, anthracyclines, flavopiridol, imatinib mesylate (Gleevec), and all-*trans*-retinoic acid (ATRA)[8,10,12] in tumor cells in culture. HDAC inhibitors may act synergistically or additively with agents that act on DNA (e.g., radiation and anthracyclines) by altering the conformation of chromatin, which results in a more open structure that allows access to DNA and increases the ability to cause damage to DNA. HDAC inhibitors may alter gene expression, which then causes cells to become more sensitive to agents such as imatinib and flavopiridol. The combination of an HDAC inhibitor and an inhibitor of protein regulation cell-cycle progression, such as flavopiridol, may be synergistic because multiple sites of aberrant function in cancer cells are targeted.

EFFECTS OF HISTONE DEACETYLASE INHIBITORS IN TUMOR-BEARING ANIMALS

Animal studies show that HDAC inhibitors cause growth arrest of a wide variety of tumors *in vivo* with little or no toxicity.[8,43] Several HDAC inhibitors—including TSA, CHAP1 and CHAP31, SAHA, pyroxamide, m-carboxy cinnamic acid bishydroxamic acid (CBHA), and oxamflatin—administered intravenously or intraperitoneally, inhibit tumor growth in animal models of breast, prostate, lung, and stomach cancers, neuroblastoma, and leukemia, with little toxicity. SAHA and MS-275, administered orally to rats or mice that have solid tumors, could suppress tumor growth. HDAC inhibitors cause an accumulation of acetylated histones in tumor and normal tissues [spleen, liver, and peripheral mononuclear (PMN) cells]. Increased accumulation of acetylated histones is a useful marker of HDAC biologic activity and has been used to monitor dosing in clinical trials involving cancer patients (see Clinical Trials with Histone Deacetylase Inhibitors).

Hydroxamic acid–based HDAC inhibitors—SAHA, CBHA, and pyroxamide, in particular—have been tested extensively in animal studies. For example, in nude mice that have transplanted androgen-dependent human prostate tumors, treatment with SAHA suppressed tumor growth by as much as 97% compared with untreated animals. Acetylation of histones H3 and H4 increased in the prostate tumor cells within 6 hours after injection of SAHA. Pyroxamide had similar effects in this model, as did CBHA on the growth of human neuroblastoma xenografts in nude mice. At dosages that markedly inhibit tumor growth, SAHA, pyroxamide, and CBHA cause little or no toxicity as evaluated by weight gain, histologic studies, and examination of multiple tissues at autopsy.

TSA, SAHA, and depsipeptide are reported to block angiogenesis *in vivo*. These HDAC inhibitors block hypoxia-induced angiogenesis in different carcinoma models. Hypoxia induces HDAC1 and angiogenesis, so inhibition of HDACs might have a role in blocking new tumor blood vessel formation. HDAC inhibitors could, therefore, inhibit tumor growth both directly by causing growth arrest, terminal differentiation, and apoptosis of cancer cells, and indirectly by inhibiting neovascularization of tumors.

In studies with transformed cells in culture, tumor cell lines were tenfold more sensitive to HDAC inhibitors than were normal fibroblasts. Although the selective inhibitory effects on transformed cells compared to normal cells are not completely understood, they do not appear to be due to a difference in the ability to inhibit HDAC activity. Accumulation of acetylated histones occurs in both normal and transformed cells.[15,35,44]

HDAC inhibitors fall into a class of agents that target an activity (reversible protein acetylation) that occurs in all cells rather than targeting an abnormal process in the cancer cell. The favorable therapeutic index observed in tumor-bearing animal studies and in clinical trials (see Clinical Trials with Histone Deacetylase Inhibitors) may result from the differential response of the cancer cells and normal cells to inhibition of HDAC activity. This type of selectivity that takes advantage of the contextual differences between normal and cancer cells has been described for the proteosome inhibitor MLN341 and the heat-shock inhibitor geldanamycin.[45]

CLINICAL TRIALS WITH HISTONE DEACETYLASE INHIBITORS

A number of HDAC inhibitors are in clinical trials. Only phenylacetate is approved for human use in the treatment of urea cycle disorders in children, portal encephalopathy, and chemotherapy-induced hyperammonemia. In patients with malignant diseases, phenylacetate demonstrated modest palliative benefits and produced limited objective tumor regression; dose-limiting toxicities were reversible confusion and lethargy.[46] Phenylbutyrate (PB) is a precursor of phenylacetate after β-oxidization in the liver and kidney. PB has been shown to inhibit histone acetylation, modify lipid metabolism, and activate peroxisome proliferation activator receptor. Studies using a prolonged intravenous infusion of PB have resulted in the occurrence of somnolence and confusion at the highest dosage levels.[47] Modest clinical activity was documented in patients with leukemia, myelodysplastic syndrome, and several solid tumors. An oral formulation of PB has been tested that showed good bioavailability and was able to reach biologically active plasma concentrations (0.5 mM). Nausea, vomiting, dyspepsia, confusion, peripheral edema, fatigue, and hypocalcemia were the principal adverse effects of the oral preparation of PB. Clinical studies of PB have been disappointing, with few objective tumor regressions; however, prolonged stabilization of the disease was seen in several patients, which suggests cytostatic effects. In one report, PB was combined with ATRA, which restored the sensitivity to ATRA in patients with acute promyelocytic leukemia that progressed after ATRA treatment alone.[43] It is postulated that PB inhibits the corepressor complex containing HDAC for the oncoprotein that is encoded by one of the translocation-generated fusion genes in acute promyelocytic leukemia, *PML-RAR-α*. Other trials using retinoic acid and demethylation agents are ongoing to exploit the cell-modulating effects of PB.

Valproic acid is a short-chain fatty acid that is a well-tolerated antiepileptic agent and that has been shown to be an inhibitor of HDACs.[48] In a clinical trial in a patient with acute myelogenous leukemia, valproic acid induced a transient partial remission. Ongoing clinical trials are further evaluating the use of valproic acid in patients with hematologic and solid cancers.

Other investigational HDAC inhibitors are undergoing clinical evaluation. These include the cyclic peptide depsipeptide; the hydroxamic acid–based HDAC inhibitor SAHA; pyroxamide and LAQ824; the benzamide MS-275; and N-acetyl amide (CI-994), which inhibits HDAC by an undetermined mechanism.

Depsipeptide is isolated from *Chromobacterium violaceum* and inhibits HDACs at nanomolar concentrations. Fatigue, nausea, vomiting, and thrombocytopenia were the dose-limiting toxicities in a phase I study in which depsipeptide was administered as a 4-hour intravenous infusion on days 1 and 5 of a 21-day cycle. Although preclinical models suggested that cardiac toxicity was a concern, few cardiac events were seen in the initial phase I study. These trials established the biologic activity of depsipeptide by showing an increased accumulation of acetylated histones in posttreatment samples of PMN cells. An antitumor effect was seen in patients with renal cell carcinoma and in a patient with T-cell lymphomas. A phase II clinical trial is ongoing with depsipeptide.[49]

SAHA and pyroxamide are two potent hydroxamic acid–based inhibitors of HDACs. Phase I studies with intravenously administered SAHA showed that this novel agent causes the accumulation of acetylated histones in normal and malignant cells, and antitumor effects were seen in patients with solid and hematologic cancers.[50] An oral formulation of SAHA has been under clinical development that has shown good oral bioavailability and favorable pharmacokinetic profile.[51] After a single oral dose of SAHA, accumulation of acetylated histones in PMN cells can persist for up to 10 hours. Patients with renal cell carcinoma, squamous cell carcinoma of the head and neck, papillary thyroid cancer, mesothelioma, B- and T-cell lymphomas, and Hodgkin's disease have shown clinical improvement with oral SAHA therapy. There have been durable responses, with the longest duration of therapy extending to over 18 months. There have been no drug-related deaths. The dose-limiting toxicities have been nonhematologic, including dehydration, anemia, fatigue, and diarrhea. All toxicities have been reversible on cessation of drug administration. SAHA is under evaluation in phase II clinical trials.

MS-275 is a potent inhibitor of HDAC that has entered into phase I clinical trials. Initial daily dosing schedules was poorly tolerated, probably due to the longer than expected half-life of the drug. Alternative dosing schedules have been better tolerated, and preliminary results suggest an *in vivo* effect, with an increase in acetylated histones in PMN cells and an induction of apoptosis in leukemic cells.

CI-994 (N-acetyl amide) is an orally bioavailable compound that has been shown to cause phosphorylation and degradation of nuclear proteins with subsequent accumulation of acetylated histones in malignant cell lines. CI-994 is a weak inhibitor of HDAC. Cytostatic effects are seen in multiple solid tumor cell lines. The oral preparation is well tolerated; nausea, vomiting, diarrhea, fatigue, neutropenia, and anemia are the most common adverse events, and all are reversible on cessation of drug administration. Phase II studies involving patients with non–small cell lung cancer showed minimal clinical activity, with 2 out of 32 patients (7%) showing a partial response to therapy and 28% of the patients having stable disease for over 8 weeks.[52] In phase II studies involving patients with metastatic renal cell carcinoma, stable disease for longer than 8 weeks was documented in 58% of patients. CI-994 was combined with capecitabine, which led to significant thrombocytopenia and hand-foot syndrome at the highest doses with partial response reported in one patient with colorectal cancer. A randomized trial of gemcitabine versus gemcitabine plus CI-994 involving patients with advanced relapsed non–small cell lung cancer failed to show any survival difference between the two treatment arms.

CONCLUSION AND PERSPECTIVES

HDAC inhibitors are promising new targeted anticancer agents. In clinical phase I and II trials, orally administered agents such as depsipeptide and SAHA have shown significant activity against both hematologic and solid tumors at dosages well tolerated by patients. These agents inhibit class I and class II HDACs and lead to acetylation of histone in normal and tumor cells. The accumulation of acetylated histones in PMN cells can be used as a marker of biologic activity. HDAC inhibitors attack cancer cells at several molecular levels, selectively altering gene transcription and probably the activity of transcription factors and proteins involved in cell-cycle regulation by leading to accumulation of acetylated forms of these proteins. HDAC inhibitors induce cancer cell growth arrest, differentiation, and apoptosis. Normal cells are much less sensitive to HDAC inhibitors than are transformed cells. The molecular basis for this favorable differential sensitivity is not yet understood. Furthermore, the activities of the individual HDACs remain to be more fully defined. Discovery of more potent HDAC inhibitors and agents that are selective inhibitors of one or another HDAC is needed to help answer these questions. Clinically, further trials are required to define the optimal dosage, range of responsive neoplasms, long-term adverse effect profile, and use of HDAC inhibitors in combination with other anticancer therapeutic modalities.

REFERENCES

1. Jenuwein T, Allis CD. Translating the histone code. *Science* 2001;293(5532):1074.
2. Spotswood HT, Turner BM. An increasingly complex code. *J Clin Invest* 2002;110(5):577.
3. Zhang Y, Reinberg D. Transcription regulation by histone methylation: interplay between different covalent modifications of the core histone tails. *Genes Dev* 2001;15(18):2343.
4. Agalioti T, Chen G, Thanos D. Deciphering the transcriptional histone acetylation code for a human gene. *Cell* 2002;111(3):381.
5. Richards EJ, Elgin SC. Epigenetic codes for heterochromatin formation and silencing: rounding up the usual suspects. *Cell* 2002;108(4):489.
6. Timmermann S, Lehrmann H, Polesskaya A, Harel-Bellan A. Histone acetylation and disease. *Cell Mol Life Sci* 2001;58(5–6):728.
7. Wang C, Fu M, Mani S, et al. Histone acetylation and the cell-cycle in cancer. *Front Biosci* 2001;6:D610.
8. Marks P, Rifkind RA, Richon VM, et al. Histone deacetylases and cancer: causes and therapies. *Nat Rev Cancer* 2001;1(3):194.
9. Jones PA, Baylin SB. The fundamental role of epigenetic events in cancer. *Nat Rev Genet* 2002;3(6):415.
10. Marks P, Miller T, Richon V. Histone deacetylases. *Curr Opin Pharmacol* 2003;3(4):344.
11. Grozinger CM, Schreiber SL. Deacetylase enzymes: biological functions and the use of small-molecule inhibitors. *Chem Biol* 2002;9(1):3.
12. Johnstone RW, Licht JD. Histone deacetylase inhibitors in cancer therapy: is transcription the primary target? *Cancer Cell* 2003;4(1):13.
13. de Ruijter AJ, van Gennip AH, Caron HN, Kemp S, van Kuilenburg AB. Histone deacetylases (HDACs): characterization of the classical HDAC family. *Biochem J* 2003;370(Pt 3):737.
14. Khochbin S, Verdel A, Lemercier C, Seigneurin-Berny D. Functional significance of histone deacetylase diversity. *Curr Opin Genet Dev* 2001;11(2):162.
15. Verdin E. *Proceedings Novartis Foundation Symposium* 2003;259.
16. Cress WD, Seto E. Histone deacetylases, transcriptional control, and cancer. *J Cell Physiol* 2000;184(1):1.
17. McKinsey TA, Zhang CL, Olson EN. Control of muscle development by dueling HATs and HDACs. *Curr Opin Genet Dev* 2001;11(5):497.
18. Urnov FD, Yee J, Sachs L, et al. Targeting of N-CoR and histone deacetylase 3 by the oncoprotein v-erbA yields a chromatin infrastructure-dependent transcriptional repression pathway. *EMBO J* 2000;19(15):4074.
19. Yoshida M, Kijima M, Akita M, Beppu T. Potent and specific inhibition of mammalian histone deacetylase both in vivo and in vitro by trichostatin A. *J Biol Chem* 1990;265(28):17174.
20. Richon VM, Emiliani S, Verdin E, et al. A class of hybrid polar inducers of transformed cell differentiation inhibits histone deacetylases. *Proc Natl Acad Sci U S A* 1998;95(6):3003.
21. Furumai R, Matsuyama A, Kobashi N, et al. FK228 (depsipeptide) as a natural prodrug that inhibits class I histone deacetylases. *Cancer Res* 2002;62(17):4916.
22. Singh SB, Zink DL, Liesch JM, et al. Structure and chemistry of apicidins, a class of novel cyclic tetrapeptides without a terminal alpha-keto epoxide as inhibitors of histone deacetylase with potent antiprotozoal activities. *J Org Chem* 2002;67(3):815.

23. Furumai R, Komatsu Y, Nishino N, et al. Potent histone deacetylase inhibitors built from trichostatin A and cyclic tetrapeptide antibiotics including trapoxin. *Proc Natl Acad Sci U S A* 2001;98(1):87.

24. Phiel CJ, Zhang F, Huang EY, et al. Histone deacetylase is a direct target of valproic acid, a potent anticonvulsant, mood stabilizer, and teratogen. *J Biol Chem* 2001;276(39):36734.

25. Boivin AJ, Momparler LF, Hurtubise A, Momparler RL. Antineoplastic action of 5-aza-2'-deoxycytidine and phenylbutyrate on human lung carcinoma cells. *Anticancer Drugs* 2002;13(8):869.

26. Prakash S, Foster BJ, Meyer M, et al. Chronic oral administration of CI-994: a phase 1 study. *Invest New Drugs* 2001;19(1):1.

27. Saito A, Yamashita T, Mariko Y, et al. A synthetic inhibitor of histone deacetylase, MS-27-275, with marked in vivo antitumor activity against human tumors. *Proc Natl Acad Sci U S A* 1999;96(8):4592.

28. Frey RR, Wada CK, Garland RB, et al. Trifluoroethyl ketones as inhibitors of histone deacetylase. *Bioorg Med Chem Lett* 2002;12(23):3443.

29. Finnin MS, Donigian JR, Cohen A, et al. Structures of a histone deacetylase homologue bound to the TSA and SAHA inhibitors. *Nature* 1999;401(6749):188.

30. Butler LM, Zhou X, Xu W-S, et al. The histone deacetylase inhibitor SAHA arrests cancer cell growth, up-regulates thioredoxin-binding protein-2, and down-regulates thioredoxin. *Proc Natl Acad Sci U S A* 2002;99(18):11700.

31. Glaser KB, Staver MJ, Waring JF, et al. Gene expression profiling of multiple histone deacetylase (HDAC) inhibitors: defining a common gene set produced by HDAC inhibition in T24 and MDA carcinoma cell lines. *Mol Cancer Ther* 2003;2(2):151.

32. Van Lint C, Emiliani S, Verdin E. The expression of a small fraction of cellular gene is changed in response to histone hyperacetylation. *Gene Expr* 1996;5:245.

33. Rascle A, Johnston JA, Amati B. Deacetylase activity is required for recruitment of the basal transcription machinery and transactivation by STAT5. *Mol Cell Biol* 2003;23(12):4162.

34. Sambucetti LC, Fischer DD, Zabludoff S, et al. Histone deacetylase inhibition selectively alters the activity and expression of cell cycle proteins leading to specific chromatin acetylation and antiproliferative effects. *J Biol Chem* 1999;274(49):34940.

35. Richon VM, Sandhoff TW, Rifkind RA, Marks PA. Histone deacetylase inhibitor selectively induces p21WAF1 expression and gene-associated histone acetylation. *Proc Natl Acad Sci U S A* 2000;97(18):10014.

36. Lagger G, O'Carroll D, Rembold M, et al. Essential function of histone deacetylase 1 in proliferation control and CDK inhibitor repression. *EMBO J* 2002;21(11):2672.

37. Vrana JA, Decker RH, Johnson CR, et al. Induction of apoptosis in U937 human leukemia cells by suberoylanilide hydroxamic acid (SAHA) proceeds through pathways that are regulated by Bcl-2/Bcl-XL, c-Jun, and p21CIP1, but independent of p53. *Oncogene* 1999;18(50):7016.

38. Warrener R, Beamish H, Burgess A, et al. Tumor cell-selective cytotoxicity by targeting cell cycle checkpoints. *FASEB J* 2003;17(11):1550.

39. Kouzarides T. Acetylation: a regulatory modification to rival phosphorylation? *EMBO J* 2000;19(6):1176.

40. Polevoda B, Sherman F. The diversity of acetylated proteins. *Genome Biol* 2002;3(5):reviews0006.

41. Haggarty SJ, Koeller KM, Wong JC, Grozinger CM, Schreiber SL. Domain-selective small-molecule inhibitor of histone deacetylase 6 (HDAC6)-mediated tubulin deacetylation. *Proc Natl Acad Sci U S A* 2003;100(8):4389.

42. Yu X, Guo ZS, Marcu MG, et al. Modulation of p53, ErbB1, ErbB2, and Raf-1 expression in lung cancer cells by depsipeptide FR901228. *J Natl Cancer Inst* 2002;94(7):504.

43. Kelly WK, O'Connor OA, Marks PA. Histone deacetylase inhibitors: from target to clinical trials. *Expert Opin Investig Drugs* 2002;11(12):1695.

44. Qiu L, Kelso MJ, Hansen C, et al. Anti-tumour activity in vitro and in vivo of selective differentiating agents containing hydroxamate. *Br J Cancer* 1999;80(8):1252.

45. Reddy A, Kaelin WG Jr. Using cancer genetics to guide the selection of anticancer drug targets. *Curr Opin Pharmacol* 2002;2(4):366.

46. Chang SM, Kuhn JG, Robins HI, et al. Phase II study of phenylacetate in patients with recurrent malignant glioma: a North American Brain Tumor Consortium report. *J Clin Oncol* 1999;17(3):984.

47. Gilbert J, Baker SD, Bowling MK, et al. A phase I dose escalation and bioavailability study of oral sodium phenylbutyrate in patients with refractory solid tumor malignancies. *Clin Cancer Res* 2001;7(8):2292.

48. Gottlicher M, Minucci S, Zhu P, et al. Valproic acid defines a novel class of HDAC inhibitors inducing differentiation of transformed cells. *EMBO J* 2001;20(24):6969.

49. Piekarz RL, Robey R, Bakke S, et al. Histone deacetylase inhibitor for the treatment of peripheral or cutaneous T-cell lymphoma. *Am Soc Clin Oncol* 2001:232b.

50. Kelly WK, Richon VM, O'Connor O, et al. Phase I clinical trial of histone deacetylase inhibitor: suberoylanilide hydroxamic acid (SAHA) administered intravenously. *Clin Cancer Res* 2003;9:3578.

51. Kelly WK, O'Connor O, Richon VM, et al. A phase I clinical trial of an oral formulation of the histone deacetylase inhibitor of suberoylanilide hydroxamic acid (SAHA). 14th EORTC-NCI-AACR, Frankfurt, 2002.

52. Wozniak A, O'Shaughnessy J, Fiorica J, Grove W. Phase II trial of CI-994 in patients with advanced nonsmall cell lung cancer. *Am Soc Clin Oncol* 1999:487a.

JONATHAN D. CHENG
GREGORY PAUL ADAMS
MATTHEW K. ROBINSON
LOUIS M. WEINER

SECTION **4**

Monoclonal Antibodies

Antibody-based therapeutics have come of age. Early antibody therapy studies attempted to explicitly target cancers based on the structural and biologic properties that distinguish neoplastic cells from their normal counterparts. The first generation of monoclonal antibodies (MAbs) that was evaluated in clinical trials demonstrated a limited effectiveness. To a large degree, this was due to their immunogenicity and inefficient effector function.[1-3] Initial MAbs used in clinical trials were murine in origin, and it became clear early on that patients developed human antimouse antibody (HAMA) responses against the therapeutic agents that limited both the efficacy of the MAb by rapidly clearing it from the body and the number of times the therapy could be administered. Although these early clinical studies yielded inconsistent and often disappointing clinical results, more recent work has identified a number of important and useful applications for antibody-based cancer therapy. Currently, the U.S. Food and Drug Administration (FDA) has approved six antibodies for the treatment of cancer (Table 16.4-1) and ten more are in late-stage clinical trials.[4,5] Five of these MAbs, such as rituximab, used for the treatment of non-Hodgkin's lymphoma, are approved for the treatment of blood-borne cancers. Radioimmunoconjugates directed against CD20 and chemoimmunoconjugate containing an anti-CD33 antibody and calicheamicin also demonstrate significant clinical activity.[6-8] The sixth, trastuzumab, is approved for the treatment of metastatic breast cancer and is the only antibody-based therapy currently approved for the treatment of solid tumors, although a number of other antibodies show promise in treatment of colorectal carcinomas. These results provide ample evidence that strategies using unconjugated antibodies or antibody conjugates carrying toxic payloads such as radiation or chemotherapy agents have clinical benefits. Antibodies thus provide an important means by which to exploit the capacity of the immune system to specifically recognize and direct antitumor responses.

Antibodies are produced by B cells and arise in response to exposure to a variety of structures, termed *antigens*, as a result of a series of recombinations of V, D, and J germline genes. Somatic hypermutation occurs with each subsequent exposure to the antigen and introduces further variation that can increase binding affinity or alter target antigen specificity. The resulting proteins exhibit selective targeting of a variety of potential antigens and can direct the clearance or immune recognition of such antigens. Immunoglobulin G (IgG) molecules are most commonly used as the working backbones of current therapeutic MAbs, although various other isotypes of antibodies have specialized functions (e.g., IgA molecules play important roles in mucosal immunity and IgE molecules are involved in anaphylaxis).

Before 1975, the ability of antibodies to specifically target immunogens for therapeutic applications was hindered by the

TABLE 16.4-1. U.S. Food and Drug Administration–Approved Antibodies for the Treatment of Cancer

Monoclonal Antibody	Trade Name	Indication	Antibody Category	Year Approved
Rituximab	Rituxan	Non-Hodgkin's lymphoma	Unconjugated antibody	1997
Trastuzumab	Herceptin	Breast cancer	Unconjugated antibody	1998
Gemtuzumab ozogamicin	Mylotarg	Acute myelogenous leukemia	Immunotoxin	2000
Alemtuzumab	Campath	Chronic lymphocytic leukemia	Unconjugated antibody	2001
Ibritumomab tiuxetan	Zevalin	Non-Hodgkin's lymphoma	Radiolabeled antibody	2002
Tositumomab	Bexxar	Non-Hodgkin's lymphoma	Radiolabeled antibody	2003

necessity for antibody preparations to be derived from poly-clonal antisera obtained from immunized animals. The development of hybridoma technology by Kohler and Milstein made it possible to produce large quantities of antibodies with high purity and monospecificity for a single binding region (epitope) on an antigen.[9] This led to the speculation that MAbs would provide a "magic bullet" for the treatment of diseases such as cancer.

The mechanisms that antibody-based therapeutics use to elicit antitumor effects can be broadly divided into two categories. The first category encompasses the mechanisms carried out by unconjugated antibodies, such as altering signal transduction,[10] blocking ligand-receptor interactions,[11] and preventing enzymatic cleavage of cell surface proteins.[12] Unconjugated MAbs can also evoke an immune response against targeted cells by activating processes such as antibody-dependent cellular cytotoxicity[13] (ADCC) or complement-mediated lysis.[14] The second category encompasses the mechanisms by which antibodies deliver toxic compounds such as radionuclides or chemotherapeutic agents specifically to the tumor sites.

IMMUNOGLOBULIN STRUCTURE

STRUCTURAL AND FUNCTIONAL DOMAINS

An IgG molecule is typically divided into three domains consisting of two identical antigen-binding (Fab) domains connected to an effector or Fc domain by a flexible hinge sequence. Figure 16.4-1 shows the structure of an IgG molecule as well as enzymatically derived or recombinantly prepared antibody fragments. IgG antibodies are comprised of two identical light chains and two identical heavy chains, with the chains joined by disulfide bonds, which results in a bilaterally symmetrical complex. The Fab domains mediate the binding of IgG molecules to their cognate antigens and are composed of an intact light chain and half of a heavy chain. Each chain in the Fab domain is further divided into variable and constant regions with the variable region containing hypervariable, or complementarity-determining, regions (CDRs) in which the antigen-contact residues reside. The light- and heavy-chain variable regions each contain three CDRs (CDR1, CDR2, and CDR3). All six CDRs combine to form the antigen-binding pocket and are collectively defined in immunologic terms as the idiotype of the antibody. Although each of the six CDRs contributes to the binding process, in the majority of cases the variable heavy-chain CDR3 plays a dominant role.[15] Antibodies achieve diversity by varying the amino acid sequences of the CDRs from V, D, and J recombinations and somatic hypermutations as a consequence of antigen exposure.

The different isotypes of immunoglobulins are defined by the structure and function of their Fc domains. The Fc domain, composed of the C_H2 and C_H3 regions of the antibody's heavy chains, is the critical determinant of how an antibody mediates effector functions, transports across cellular barriers, and persists in circulation. Immunologic effector functions such as targeted cellular killing and immune complex clearance are regulated by interactions between cellular Fc receptors and sequences in the Fc domain.[13] For example, human IgG1, murine IgG2a, and murine IgG3 can trigger the classic complement cascade after their binding to tumor cell surfaces and are also most efficient in promoting ADCC. Another class of Fc receptor, the neonatal Fc receptor (FcRn), binds to the Fc domain at the interface between the C_H2 and C_H3 regions. These receptors are involved in maternal-fetal transfer of IgG across the placenta and have been found to be present on endothelial cells, where they serve as an IgG salvage receptor that mediates its long serum persistence.[16]

MODIFIED ANTIBODY-BASED MOLECULES

Advances in antibody engineering and molecular biology have facilitated the development of many novel antibody-based structures with unique physical and pharmacokinetic properties (see Fig. 16.4-1). These include chimeric human-murine antibodies with human constant regions and murine variable regions,[17] humanized antibodies in which murine CDR sequences have been grafted into human IgG molecules, and entirely human anti-

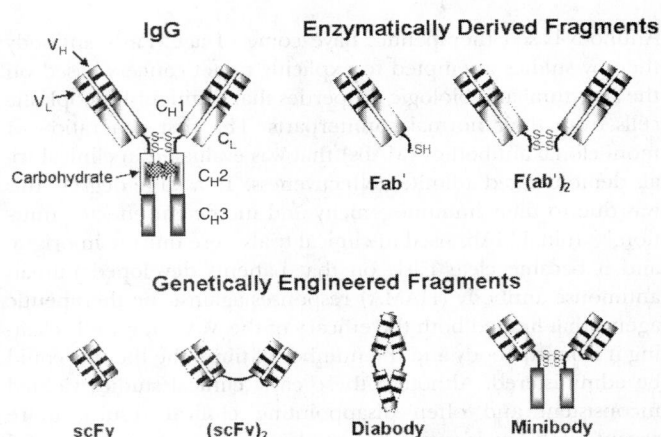

FIGURE 16.4-1. Structures of common enzymatically derived and genetically engineered antibody-based molecules. C, constant; Fab', fragment of immunoglobulin G; F(ab')$_2$, fragment of IgG after pepsin digestion; H, heavy chain; IgG, immunoglobulin G; L, light chain; S, sulfur; SH, sulfhydryl; scFv, single-chain Fv; (scFv)$_2$, dimeric scFv.; V, variable. (See Color Fig. 16.4-1 in the CD-ROM.)

bodies derived from human hybridomas and more recently from transgenic mice expressing human immunoglobulin genes.[18] The basic building block for these molecules is the 25-kD, monovalent single-chain Fv (scFv) that is comprised of the variable domains (V_H and V_L) of an antibody fused together with a short peptide linker. This has led to a plethora of promising structures that include monovalent scFv derived from murine hybridomas[19–21] or phage-display libraries[22,23] and multivalent dimeric Fv [(scFv)$_2$],[24] diabodies,[25,26] triabodies,[27] and minibodies.[28]

Two proteolytic enzymes originally used to digest antibodies to identify their functional domains are also commonly used to create smaller antibody fragments that retain antigen-binding properties. The enzyme papain cleaves IgG molecules in the hinge region, which results in the production of two identical Fab fragments and an intact Fc fragment. A second enzyme, pepsin, cleaves IgG at the amino-terminal end of the hinge region, yielding an F(ab')$_2$ fragment composed of the two Fab domains linked via disulfide bonds in the remaining section of the hinge. Examining the behavior of these engineered molecules has allowed the identification of many critical properties that affect the uptake of the antibodies into solid tumors.

FACTORS REGULATING ANTIBODY-BASED TUMOR TARGETING

A number of obstacles to treatment efficacy have been identified in preclinical studies and in clinical trials (Table 16.4-2).

ANTIBODY SIZE

One of the main obstacles to effective targeting of antibody-based therapies to solid tumors is the physiology of the tumor itself. IgG molecules are large proteins of approximately 150-kD mass, whereas most chemotherapy agents have a molecular weight of less than 1 kD. Thus, MAbs have significantly slower kinetics of distribution and are more limited in their tissue penetration properties than are smaller molecules. Nonuniform distribution of systemically administered antibody is generally observed in biopsied specimens of solid tumors. Although heterogeneous tumor antigen expression is an important factor, physiologic barriers to MAb penetration bear the greatest responsibility for their limited distribution within a tumor mass. Heterogeneous tumor blood supply limits uniform antibody delivery to tumors, and elevated interstitial pressures in the centers of tumors oppose inward diffusion.[29] This high interstitial pressure leads to a net outward gradient from the tumor center and slows the diffusion of IgG molecules from their vascular extravasation site. Thus, high interstitial pressure present within solid tumors differentially inhibits the diffusion of larger molecules in comparison to smaller molecules, because smaller molecules are more effective in penetrating solid tumors.[30,31] This is supported experimentally by studies of LS-174T human colon carcinoma xenografts injected with iodine 125–labeled CC49 anti–TAG-72 antibodies of different sizes, such as its scFv, Fab', F(ab')$_2$, and IgG forms.[32] Tumor penetration was directly related to the size of the antibody molecules, with approximately tenfold greater tumor retention of scFv than of IgG. This inverse relationship between molecular size and tumor penetration supports Jain's model that smaller fragments are better at penetrating solid tumors.

The relatively large transport distances in the tumor interstitium substantially increase the time required for large IgG macromolecules to reach target cells. The previously described model suggests that diffusion of an intact IgG molecule into a solid tumor is limited to 100 µm in 1 hour, 1 mm in 2 days, and 1 cm in 7 to 8 months.[33] These physiologic barriers pose substantial obstacles to antibody penetration in the majority of solid tumors and bulky lymphomas, potentially compromising MAb treatment of patients with large tumors.

Smaller antibody-based constructs and fragments such as F(ab')$_2$, Fab, and scFv molecules have been used to improve the poor tumor penetration of IgG MAb. These derivative structures generally exhibit target antigen-binding affinities on the same order of magnitude as the intact parental immunoglobulin, with the advantage of more rapid tumor penetration. However, their small size also mediates their rapid clearance from solid tumors and from the tumor-bearing host. In general, the smaller molecules have the advantages of improved tumor penetration, rapid systemic clearance, and improved specificity of tumor targeting during the terminal phases of elimination. These advantages are counterbalanced by decreased quantitative tumor targeting and their rapid clearance from solid tumors.[34,35] The inability of small molecules like scFv to be retained in solid tumors is directly related to the rate of systemic clearance [β half-life ($T_{1/2}\beta$)] of the protein. To a first approximation, the pharmacokinetic behavior of a protein correlates with its size relative to the renal threshold; proteins less than approximately 65 kD are small enough to pass through the glomeruli of the kidney and undergo rapid, first-pass renal clearance.[36] In the case of the antibody-based molecules described in Figure 16.4-1, only the scFv, (scFv')$_2$, and diabody are small enough to be eliminated in this manner. A good depiction of this comes from an examination of the clearance rates of different forms of the CC49 anti–TAG-72 IgG.[37,38] The pharmacokinetic properties of the examined molecules were directly related to their sizes, because the larger fragments were retained in circulation significantly longer than the smaller fragments. The slower $T_{1/2}\beta$ was not due solely to the natural recycling process because F(ab')$_2$ and Fab' lacking Fc domains had slower blood clearance rates than the scFv.

Therefore, optimal tumor penetration requires that the antibody-based fragment be large enough to be maintained in circulation so that it can accumulate in the tumor but small enough to successfully diffuse throughout the tumor. The proper size of tumor-targeting antibodies thus depends on the intended therapeutic application. For therapeutic applications that are benefited by a long $T_{1/2}\beta$, IgG and larger engineered fragments can obtain a higher percent injected dose per gram tumor than smaller fragments due to increased opportunity to come in contact with tumor antigens from a slower clearance.

TABLE 16.4-2. Obstacles to Successful Monoclonal Antibody Therapy

Impaired antibody distribution and delivery to tumor sites
Inadequate trafficking of effector cells to tumor
Intratumoral and intertumoral antigenic heterogeneity
Shed or internalized targets
Insufficient tumor specificity of target antigens
Human antimouse antibody responses

In contrast, the faster clearance rates of small molecules may make them better suited for applications such as imaging or therapeutic strategies involving toxic payloads or immunotoxins in which high tumor to organ ratios are required to increase efficacy without compromising host safety by being rapidly cleared from normal organs.

TUMOR ANTIGENS

The distribution of antigen expression may be a critical determinant of therapeutic effect for a variety of antibody-based applications. Heterogeneity of antigen expression by tumor cells is manifested not only as the presence or absence of antigen on a cell, but also by the density of its expression on a given cell. For example, large concentrations of shed antigen in the tumor microenvironment may saturate the antibody's binding sites and prevent binding to the cell surface. In contrast, rapid internalization of antigen may deplete the quantity of cell surface MAb capable of initiating ADCC or cytotoxic signal transduction events. Antibody targets may also be *tumor associated* or *tumor specific*. Tumor-associated targets have been most frequently identified and are typically oncofetal antigens or overexpressed growth factor receptors with extracellular membrane domains. Tumor-associated antigens are usually relatively overexpressed on tumor cells but are found to a lesser extent on normal cellular counterparts and on other normal cells. Potential consequences of targeting this class of antigens with toxic immunoconjugates can include decreased targeting specificity and unacceptable normal tissue cytotoxicity. Tumor-specific antigens that exhibit high levels of expression limited to malignant tissue are both highly desirable and rare. Typically these antigens arise as a result of unique genetic recombinations that are the cause or consequence of oncogenic transformation, such as clonal immunoglobulin idiotypes expressed on the surface of B-cell lymphomas.[39]

Although effective tumor targeting requires that the antibody have an affinity for its tumor antigen, extremely high affinity may in fact be detrimental. Weinstein and others put forth the "binding-site barrier" hypothesis which postulated that antibodies with extremely high affinity for target antigen would bind irreversibly to the first antigen encountered on entering the tumor[40,41]; this would limit the diffusion of antibody into the tumor and it would accumulate instead in regions surrounding the tumor vasculature. The effect of antibody affinity on tumor retention and penetration was described in more detail in a set of experiments using a series of anti-HER2/*neu* scFv with affinities ranging from 1.6×10^{-6} M to 1.5×10^{-11} M.[42,43] In direct support of Weinstein's binding-site barrier hypothesis, a low-affinity scFv (C6G98A, 3.2×10^{-7} M) distributed diffusely throughout the vascularized regions of the tumors within 24 hours after injection, whereas the high-affinity scFv (C6B1D-2, 1.5×10^{-11} M) was only detected within several cell diameters of the blood vessels. These results suggest that the affinity for therapeutic antibodies must be finely balanced to be high enough to mediate prolonged tumor retention but not so high as to limit the ability of the antibody to penetrate into the tumor.

VALENCE AND CHARGE

The presence of additional antigen-binding sites, or increased valence, on an antibody molecule can increase the functional affinity of the antibody through an avidity effect. Divalent anti-HER2/*neu* (scFv')$_2$ retention in HER2/*neu* overexpressing tumors is 3.5- to 4.0-fold higher percent injected dose per gram tumor than the monovalent scFv'. Tetravalent IgG homodimers exhibited increased ability to slow tumor growth compared with the parent IgG,[44] and trivalent F(ab')$_3$ complexes showed increased tumor uptake compared to divalent F(ab')$_2$.[45]

A number of reports have investigated the role of protein charge on accumulation of antibody-based fragments in nontarget tissues. As stated in Antibody Size, earlier in this chapter, antibody-based fragments below approximately 65-kD are cleared from the blood pool primarily by glomeruli filtration. This method of clearance leads to significant renal accumulation and potential problems with renal toxicity if the antibody-based fragments are conjugated to toxic compounds such as radionuclides. Renal accumulation of radiolabeled antibody-based fragments was significantly decreased in animal models by blocking the negative charge of the renal tubules by infusing the animals with positively charged lysine and arginine before antibody injection.[46]

UNCONJUGATED ANTIBODIES

CELL-MEDIATED CYTOTOXICITY

As components of the immune system, effector cells such as natural killer cells and monocytes-macrophages represent a natural line of defense against oncologically transformed cells. Effector cells express Fcγ receptors (FcγRs) on their cell surfaces that interact with the Fc domain of IgG molecules. This receptor family is comprised of three classes (types I, II, and III) that are further divided into subclasses (IIa and IIb, IIIa and IIIb). Each of these family members has a characteristic subunit composition, pattern of expression, and binding specificity for the Fc domain of different IgG isotypes.[47] Recognition of transformed cells by immune effector cells leads to cell-mediated killing through processes such as ADCC and phagocytosis as shown in Figure 16.4-2. For example, FcγRI is a

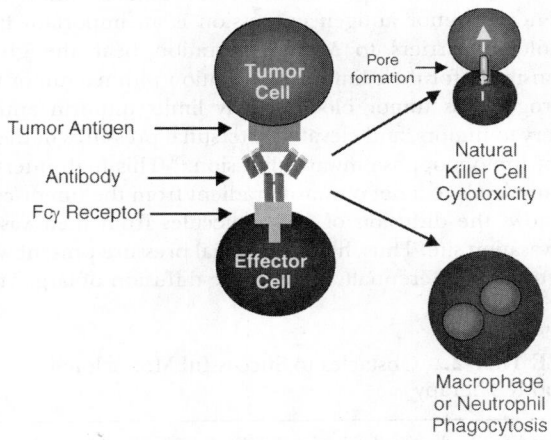

FIGURE 16.4-2. Antibody-dependent cellular cytotoxicity. The antibody engages the tumor antigen, and the Fc domain binds to cellular Fcγ receptors to bridge effector and target cells. This bridging induces effector cell activation, resulting in natural killer cell cytotoxicity or phagocytosis by neutrophils, monocytes, or macrophages. (See Color Fig. 16.4-2 in the CD-ROM.)

high-affinity receptor capable of binding to monomeric IgG, whereas FcγRII and FcγRIII are low-affinity receptors that preferentially bind multimeric complexes of IgG. In addition, engagement of different members of the FcγR family results in disparate signaling outcomes. Signaling through type I, IIa, and IIIa receptors results in activation of effector cells due to associated immunoreceptor tyrosine-based activation motifs (ITAMs), whereas engagement of type IIb receptors inhibits cell activation through associated immunoreceptor tyrosine-based inhibitory motifs (ITIMs).[47,48]

Development of transgenic mice that lack the type I and type III FcγRs due to deletion of the gene encoding for the common γ subunit[49] led to direct evidence that antibodies are capable of targeting of immune effector cells against cancer cells in the *in vivo* setting.[50] Fc receptor γ[-/-] mice, unlike congenic C57BL/6 mice, failed to demonstrate protective immunity in a B16F10 melanoma model. Wild-type and γ[-/-] mice were injected intravenously with B16 melanoma cells and then received a series of injections (200 µg per injection) of the anti-gp75 TA99 MAb or an isotype control MAb (UPC10). Wild-type animals injected with TA99 showed roughly a fivefold decrease in the number of lung metastases (50 vs. 250) compared with UPC10-injected animals. This protective effect was lost in γ[-/-] animals, which implies a role for the type I and type III activating FcγRs in eliciting this protective effect. Deletion of the inhibitory type II FcγR (FcγRIIb) led to an increase in the protective effect of TA99, which suggests that FcγRIIb acts to modulate ADCC activity *in vivo*.[51] A low dose of TA99 injected into either wild-type or γ[-/-] mice at 20 µg per injection failed to provide a protective effect against lung metastases in the B16F10 model system. However, this lower dose provided complete protection when injected into *FcγRIIB[-/-]* mice that lack the inhibitory FcγRIIb receptor. Effector cell engagement through Fc-FcγR interactions appears to be an important component of the therapeutic effect of clinical antibodies. The antitumor activities of trastuzumab (anti-HER2/*neu*) and rituximab (anti-CD20) were lost in γ[-/-] mice injected with BT474M1 and Raji B cells, respectively. In addition, subtherapeutic doses of trastuzumab provided complete inhibition of tumor growth in *FcγRIIB[-/-]* mice but had no effect in wild-type animals.[51]

These results suggest that modulating the ability of MAbs to bind to effector cells may increase the efficacy of new therapeutic molecules. A number of strategies have been developed to exploit this concept. One strategy is to select the appropriate IgG subclass during MAb construction. Each class of FcγR exhibits a characteristic specificity for IgG subclasses.[52] For example, the activating FcγRIII binds preferentially to IgG1 and IgG3, whereas the inhibitory FcγRIIb binds with somewhat less affinity to IgG1, which suggests that IgG1 may be the best backbone to elicit effector function. Presta's group[53] performed a series of mutagenetic experiments to map the residues required for IgG1-FcγR interaction. They identified a number of mutations that increased binding to FcγRIIIa but had either no effect on FcγRIIb (E333A, K334A, A339T) or lowered binding to it (S298A). As predicted, in the context of an anti-p[185]HER2 IgG1 these mutants exhibited higher ADCC activity against the SK-BR-3 cell line that overexpresses HER2 than the parent IgG1 molecule. Although *in vivo* testing was not performed, the lack of effect on FcγRIIb binding *in vitro* and the increase in ADCC activity suggests that these variants of IgG1 may increase the efficacy of trastuzumab and rituximab, as was seen in *FcγRIIB[-/-]* mice.

An alternative to modifying the Fc region of MAbs is to create bispecific antibodies (bsAbs) capable of eliciting immune effector function.[54-56] As the name suggests, bsAbs bind two distinct antigens. When engineered to recognize a tumor-associated antigen and a "trigger antigen" present on the surface of an immune effector cell, bsAbs can redirect the cytotoxic potential of the effector cell against the tumor.[57-59] Traditionally, bsAbs are produced by coexpressing two IgGs with different specificity in a quadroma and then isolating the IgG of proper specificity from the ten possible combinations.[60] An example of such a molecule is the anti-HER2/FcγRIII antibody 2B1. Alternatively, bsAbs are made by chemically fusing Fab' fragments made either by enzymatic digestion of MAbs as was done for the anti-HER2/FcγRI antibody MDX-H210[58] or in bacteria as exemplified by the anti-HER2/CD3 molecule described by Shalaby and coworkers.[61] Each of the aforementioned antibodies is capable of eliciting effector function against HER2-expressing cell lines *in vitro* and in animal models. In the case of 2B1 and MDX-H210, the efficacy in animal models resulted in phase I clinical trials.[62,63] However, isolation of useful amounts of bsAb by these techniques is challenging, and new strategies have been developed based on antibody engineering techniques.

The bsAbs have a number of possible advantages over IgG molecules. First, varying the specificity of the antieffector arm of the antibody allows the cytotoxic potential of any immune effector cell population to be directed against the tumor cell target, including that of cells not normally recruited by IgG molecules. For example, cytotoxic T cells can be recruited by targeting the T-cell receptor (CD3) present on their surfaces.[64,65] Second, bsAbs can be selected to bind epitopes on FcγR not required for Fc interaction. This allows recruitment of effector function in the presence of excess IgG,[59] the situation predicted to occur *in vivo*. Third, recent advances in affinity maturation of scFv molecules allow custom tailoring of the affinity of the bsAb to match effector cell characteristics. These advantages may allow more effective recruiting of effector cells.

COMPLEMENT-DEPENDENT CYTOTOXICITY

In addition to promoting cell-mediated killing (see Cell-Mediated Cytotoxicity, earlier in this chapter), MAbs can recruit the complement cascade to kill cells via complement-dependent cytotoxicity (CDC). CDC occurs when MAb complexed with antigen on the surface of a cell binds to C1q, a constituent of the first component of complement. When engaged by multiple MAbs, C1q activates a cascade of serum proteases, which results in killing of the antibody-bound cells.[66,67] The ability of an MAb therapeutic agent to elicit CDC can be modified by several different mechanisms. First, as with ADCC, the human IgG subclass used to construct a therapeutic MAb dictates its ability to elicit CDC. For example, IgG1 is extremely efficient at fixing complement, IgG2 is relatively inefficient, and IgG4 is incapable of mediating this type of effect.[68] Second, mutations in the C_H2 domain of the Fc region have been identified that either suppress or enhance the ability of MAb to bind C1q and activate CDC.[69,70] In these studies mutagenesis of the C_H2 domain of rituximab, a chimeric MAb with a human IgG1 Fc region, resulted in the identification of four residues (D270, K322, P329, and P331) that reduce C1q binding and CDC activity when mutated to alanine. Some mutations such as K322A and P329A inhibited CDC activity, reducing the ability of the MAbs to recruit complement but not its ability to elicit ADCC. Other mutations (K326 and E333) increased C1q binding by MAb and enhanced complement activation. This ability to manipulate complement fixation through engineering approaches warrants *in vivo* testing to determine the impact of these changes on the efficacy and toxicity of rituximab.

HALF-LIFE AND CLEARANCE RATE

The concentration of intact IgG in mammalian serum is maintained at constant levels with half-lives of IgGs measured in days. This homeostasis is regulated in part by the major histocompatibility complex (MHC) class I–related Fc receptor FcRn. FcRn is a dimer comprised of a 50-kD protein with homology to the MHC α chains and the 15-kD nonpolymorphic β_2-microglobulin, an invariant component of MHC class I. This homology to the MHC family of proteins makes FcRn distinct from all other members of the Fc receptor family discussed earlier. FcRn was originally identified based on its ability to transcytose maternal IgGs across the neonatal gut endothelium and has subsequently been shown to act as a salvage receptor for intact IgGs. Several lines of evidence related both to the FcRn and to IgGs are consistent with FcRn's acting to regulate IgG homeostasis. C57BL/6 mice that lack β_2-microglobulin have lower serum IgG levels than wild-type mice. Mutations in the Fc domain of IgGs that increase the affinity for FcRn lead to a significantly increased IgG half-life in serum. Finally, the increased serum half-life of those IgGs is dependent on a functional FcRn; IgG mutations that increase serum half-life in a wild-type mouse fail to do so in C57BL/6 mice that lack a functional FcRn.[71]

FcRn is expressed in endothelial cells, the predominant cell type in the body and one with close proximity to the vasculature. FcRn binds to the C_H2–C_H3 domain interface in the Fc region of IgG molecules. Site-directed mutagenesis studies using both rodent and human model systems have implicated a number of residues within this region of the Fc domain, including His[310] and His[434], as being important for the FcRn-IgG interaction.[53,71] Together with His[250] and His[251] of FcRn, these Fc domain residues impart a pH dependence to the FcRn-IgG interaction. In the case of the mouse, the IgG1-FcRn interaction occurs with a K_d of 2 to 7 nM at pH 6.0 but fails to occur at pH 7.4.[16,47] This pH dependence supports a model in which endothelial cells take up IgG by fluid-phase pinocytosis and traffic the proteins into acidic intracellular vesicles. The drop in pH results in the association of intact IgG with the FcRn receptors and facilitates their recycling to the cell membrane. This is consistent with the role that endothelial cells are known to play in receptor-mediated transcytosis involving the endosomal system and bidirectional transcellular movement of vesicles. Intact IgGs bound to the FcRn in the acidic environment of the intracellular vesicles are recycled to the cell membrane, whereas IgGs incapable of binding to FcRn due to damage or subclass are trafficked to the lysosome for degradation. As was shown in the mouse system, manipulation of the FcRn-IgG interaction could modulate the half-life of therapeutic IgGs. Using alanine-scanning mutagenesis, Shields et al.[53] identified a mutation (N434A) that alone, and in combination with other mutations in the region, preferentially affected increased binding at pH 6.0. This is very similar to the situation that led to increased serum persistence in the mouse model.

The pharmacokinetics of full-length IgG molecules makes them particularly well suited for antitumor mechanisms that require prolonged IgG retention in the body. However, the increase in serum half-life imparted by the Fc region is countered by the limited ability of full-length IgGs to penetrate solid tumors compared with smaller antibody-based fragments. As discussed earlier in Antibody Size, one of the major determinants of a protein's pharmacokinetics is whether its molecular weight is above or below the renal threshold for first-pass clearance. Therefore, multiple strategies have been developed to increase the serum persistence of antibody-based fragments, and other classes of protein therapeutic agents, by increasing their size. This has been accomplished by creating gene fusions with normal serum proteins such as serum albumin[72,73] or by conjugating the protein therapeutic agent to polyethylene glycol.[74] Increases in molecular weight, and therefore increased blood retention, also have been achieved by introducing mutations that result in increased glycosylation *in vivo*.[75] Although favorable with regards to pharmacokinetics, an increase in size may be detrimental to tumor penetration of antibody-based fragments. Dennis et al.[76] have developed an approach to increase the serum persistence of a Fab molecule without significantly altering its molecular weight. This was accomplished by fusing the D3H44 antitissue factor Fab fragment to a small albumin-binding peptide. The peptide-fused Fab fragment exhibited 37- and 26-fold increases in serum half-life in rabbits and mice, respectively, compared with the original D3H44 Fab fragment. These clearance rates were similar to those of a D3H44 F(ab')$_2$ fragment that was twice their size. Importantly, the Fab fragment was capable of simultaneous binding to both serum albumin and its target antigen, tissue factor. This approach has a number of possible advantages over the strategies mentioned earlier. First, the noncovalent interaction between the Fab fragment and serum albumin allows for dissociation of the complex and penetration of the Fab based on its native properties. This approach should also be applicable to smaller fragments such as scFv or diabodies and may provide a means of taking advantage of the excellent tumor-penetration properties of these small molecules. Second, altering the affinity of the peptide for albumin may provide a means of tailoring the serum half-life of the antibody. Alternatively, it may be possible to alter the serum half-life by using a peptide that binds to a different serum protein.

GLYCOSYLATION

IgGs undergo N-linked glycosylation at the conserved Asn residue at position 297 within the C_H2 domain of the constant region. Glycosylation status of the residue has long been known to impact the ability of IgGs to bind effector ligands such as FcγR and C1q and in turn affects their ability to participate in Fc-mediated functions such as ADCC and CDC.[77–79] The biantennary core oligosaccharide initially attached at Asn[297] is subsequently elaborated with a mixture of galactose and galactose-sialic acid residues and varying degrees of bisecting N-acetylglucosamine (GlcNAc) and fucose moieties, which leads to a heterogeneous population of IgGs with respect to carbohydrate content. Multiple factors influence the nature of the final glycosylation pattern including interactions between the sugars and the peptide backbone as well as the cell line used to produce the MAb.[80]

The production of MAbs for therapeutic purposes often uses nonhuman cell lines. The glycosylation pattern associated with production in these cells is similar to that seen in serum but often lacks the bisecting GlcNAc. When produced in a rat myeloma cell line capable of adding the bisecting sugar, the anti-CD52 IgG1, Campath, exhibited similar levels of ADCC *in vitro* with or without the bisecting sugar. However, antibodies containing the bisecting sugar were capable of eliciting ADCC at much lower concentrations, which indicate that this sugar plays a role in enhancing effector function.[81] Modification of standard production cell lines to express different glycosyltransferases has been one approach to produce MAbs with glycosylation patterns that better mimic the natural pattern of glycosylation. By engineering Chinese hamster ovary (CHO) cells to express the $\beta(1,4)$-N-acetylglucosaminyltransferase III (GnTIII) enzyme required to add the bisecting sugar under control of a tetracycline-regulated promoter, Bailey's group[79] was able to alter the glycosylation of the chimeric IgG1, chCE7. The chCE7 recognizes a 190-kD membrane-bound antigen on neuroblastoma with a K_d of 10^{-10} M and elicits limited amounts of ADCC when produced in SP2/0 mouse myeloma cells that fail to add the bisecting GlcNAc. Moderate levels of GnTIII expression led to an increase in the percentage of chCE7 that contained the bisecting GlcNAc and correlated with an increase in ADCC activity against IMR-32 neuroblastoma cells mediated by human lymphocytes. At high levels of GnTIII expression there was a decrease in bisected GlcNAc addition and ADCC activity, which suggests an optimal level of GnTIII expression for appropriate levels of bisected GlcNAc.

IMMUNOCONJUGATES

MAbs that are not capable of directly eliciting antitumor effects, either by altering signal transduction or directing immune system cells, can still be effective against tumors by delivering cytotoxic payloads (Table 16.4-3). MAbs have been used to deliver a wide variety of agents, including chemotherapeutic drugs, toxins, radioisotopes, and cytokines.[82] When the appropriate combination of toxic agent and MAb is selected, this therapeutic approach can also lead to synergistic effects. For example, an antibody that delivers a therapeutic radioisotope would be significantly more effective if by binding to its target antigen it also

TABLE 16.4-3. Advantages of Different Immunoconjugate Strategies

---

IMMUNOTOXINS
Exceedingly potent
Catalytic action
Well-defined biology and chemistry
DRUG IMMUNOCONJUGATES
Proven efficacy of antineoplastic components in cancer medicine
Well-defined spectra of efficacy and toxicity
Possibility of bystander effect
Internalization of immunoconjugate not required
RADIOIMMUNOCONJUGATES
Multiple available isotopes permit customized approaches
Multiple cell radius of action to address antigenic heterogeneity
Internalization not usually required
Predictable toxicity based on dosimetry

---

activated a signaling cascade that increased the target cell's sensitivity to ionizing radiation. MAbs can be modified either chemically or genetically to incorporate a toxic moiety. Chemotherapeutic drugs, toxins, cytokines, and chelates that capture radionuclides can be conjugated directly onto amino groups on lysine residues,[83,84] exposed free sulfhydryl groups on cysteine residues,[85] or carbohydrates in the cleft between the two C_H2 domains.[86] Cleavable linkages have also been developed to facilitate the release of cytotoxic agents from sites of immunoconjugate catabolism, such as the liver and kidneys.[87] More recently, antibody-engineering techniques have been used to create novel fusion proteins that incorporate a cytotoxic agent (e.g., a toxin) or a radionuclide "pocket"[88] directly into the antibody molecule. Genetic manipulation of the antibody can also be used to support chemical conjugation procedures, such as the removal of an undesirable conjugation site from a sensitive region of the antibody.[89]

IMMUNODRUG CONJUGATES

Although chemotherapeutic drugs are often effective in the treatment of many types of malignancies, systemic toxicity typically limits their dosages so that tumor is incompletely eradicated. Conjugating chemotherapeutic agents to tumor-specific antibodies focuses the delivery of a drug to the tumor and thus allows increased dosages with limited normal tissue toxicity. A number of groups have pursued this strategy in both preclinical and clinical trials.[90] Much has been learned from the development of the immunodrug conjugate BR-96–doxorubicin that targeted the Lewis[y] antigen. Although this conjugate was associated with compelling preclinical efficacy in a rat model that expressed a cross-reactive antigen on normal tissues,[91] it was associated with unacceptable dose-related gastrointestinal toxicity when evaluated in a clinical trial.[92] This illustrates the limited ability of even the best preclinical models to predict clinical efficacy and toxicity.

Antibodies can also be used to target liposome-encapsulated drugs[93] and other cytotoxic agents such as antisense RNA[94] or even radionuclides to tumors. These complexes, termed *immunoliposomes*, are composed of an antibody-studded phospholipid bilayer vesicle containing the cytotoxic agent. They offer the distinct advantage of delivering multiple molecules of the agent to the tumor while physically separating the compound from its environment and thus potentially limiting nontargeted toxicities and degradation. In preclinical studies, anti-HER2 scFv immunoliposomes containing doxorubicin displayed prolonged retention in circulation and were associated with therapeutic efficacy that was superior to that of free doxorubicin, nonantibody conjugated liposomal doxorubicin, and anti-HER2 MAb (trastuzumab).[93] A report by Koning et al. indicates that immunoliposomes produced with intact IgG molecules are subjected to increased liver macrophage–based degradation mediated by Fc receptor interactions.[95] This suggests that it may be beneficial to use scFv or Fab molecules in constructing immunoliposomes. A potential drawback of immunoliposomes is that their large size may limit their ability to penetrate into tumor tissue from the vasculature.

IMMUNOTOXINS

The highly specific tumor localization of antibodies that target internalized antigens has led to their use for the targeting of a variety of toxins.[96] These toxic agents are very potent due to their catalytic nature, which allows as few as one toxin molecule to kill a cell. The most commonly used toxins are derived from plants (e.g., ricin) or microorganisms (e.g., *Pseudomonas*). In construction of an immunotoxin, the toxin's natural translocation domain is replaced by an antibody to limit its internalization to cells that express the target antigen. Additional modifications, such as the endoplasmic reticulum retention sequence KDEL, have been incorporated to facilitate the transfer of the toxin from the endosomal compartment to the cytoplasm of the target cell.[97] Immunotoxins have demonstrated significant antitumor effects in preclinical models. For example, Kreitman et al. have reported complete regressions of human Burkitt's lymphoma xenografts in mice that were treated with a recombinant anti-CD22 immunotoxin, RFB4(dsFv)-PE38, at relevant doses based on those tolerated by cynomolgus monkeys.[98] However, in clinical trials the use of immunotoxins has been associated with unacceptable neurotoxicity[99] and life-threatening vascular leak syndrome.[100] The latter effect has been linked to a conserved $(x)D(y)$ sequence found on a number of toxins and on interleukin-2 (IL-2).[101] In a mouse model, removal of this sequence from ricin A chain appeared to decrease the degree of vascular leak.[102] Planned clinical evaluation of these compounds will clarify the role played by this sequence and may reinvigorate the immunotoxin field.

RADIOIMMUNOCONJUGATES

Radionuclide-antibody conjugates have been associated with effective treatment of human tumor xenografts in immunodeficient mouse models for many years.[103] Although scientists have long been adept at treating tumors in mice, progress in the clinical setting has been significantly slower. The FDA approval of ibritumomab (Zevalin), the first therapeutic radioimmunoconjugate for human use, represents a milestone in this field, and it is expected to be the first of many clinically effective radioimmunoconjugates. Ibritumomab is an yttrium 90 (^{90}Y)–labeled anti-CD20 MAb that has demonstrated effectiveness for the treatment of non-Hodgkin's lymphoma. A second anti-CD20 radioimmunoconjugate, tositumomab (Bexxar), which has also now been FDA approved, uses iodine 131 (^{131}I) in place of ^{90}Y and has been associated with equally impressive efficacy in clinical trials.[104] In clinical trials, the overall response rate of lymphoma patients treated with ibritumomab was 67% (25% complete responses and 41% partial responses). Patients with low-grade disease exhibited an even better overall response rate of 82% (27% complete responses and 56% partial responses).[105] Significantly, therapeutic efficacy was seen even in the presence of bulky disease and splenomegaly. Besides targeting the same tumor-associated antigen, both ibritumomab and tositumomab share other important similarities. Both are full-length murine MAbs that incorporate β-emitting radioisotopes. Although using MAbs of nonhuman origin in a clinical setting can lead to a HAMA response, this has not been observed frequently with these two radioimmunoconjugates.[106] This lack of immune rejection is believed to result from both the immunosuppressed nature of the non-Hodgkin's lymphoma patient population and the targeted destruction of the CD20+ B-cell population that elicits the HAMA response. The two β-emitting radionuclides used in these therapeutic agents, ^{90}Y and ^{131}I, are the most commonly used therapeutic radioisotopes for radioimmunotherapy. The β-particles emitted by ^{90}Y and ^{131}I have a moderate linear

energy transfer on the order of approximately 0.2 keV/μm and therefore require up to thousands of "hits" to kill a cell.[107] This is balanced by their long mean track length (approximately 4000 μm for ^{90}Y). This broad field of impact leads to a "crossfire" effect that can kill tumor cells that lack the targeted antigen or lie beyond the diffusion radius of the radioimmunoconjugate.

More recently, investigators have begun to examine the usefulness of α-particle–emitting radioisotopes in radioimmunotherapy applications. These isotopes include bismuth 213, bismuth 212, astatine 211, lead 212, and actinium 225. In contrast to β-particles, α-particles have such a high linear energy transfer (approximately 100 keV/μm) that only a few hits are required to kill a cell.[107] However, these large particles have a very limited track length of one to two cell diameters. This property has made them particularly appealing for radioimmunotherapy for leukemia, because their range focuses their effects on the cells to which the antibody has bound and limits the bystander killing of healthy cells. Still, their limited track length, combined with the very short half-lives (minutes to hours) of most α-emitters, has left in doubt their ability to treat solid tumors. The α-emitters that have half-lives of less than 1 hour, such as bismuth 213 ($T_{1/2}$ = 46 minutes) have proven to be ineffective for the treatment of solid tumors even when directly conjugated to small scFv and diabody molecules.[89] Their greatest use is likely for locoregional radioimmunotherapy (e.g., peritoneal cavity) or pretargeted radioimmunotherapy (PRIT).

Although radioimmunoconjugates have been associated with efficacy in the setting of hematologic neoplasms, they have yet to achieve significant effect in solid malignancies. This is thought to be due to a number of the factors discussed earlier that ultimately lead to inadequate tumor penetration and incomplete targeting of the tumor cells.[108] A possible solution to this hurdle is described in a report by Pedley et al., which cited significant improvements in preclinical efficacy using a combination of ^{131}I-A5B7–anti–carcinoembryonic antigen (CEA) MAb and the antivascular agent combretastatin A-4 3-0-phosphate compared with the use of either therapeutic agent alone.[109] In this study, the median survivals were approximately 20 days for the control animals and those that only received 200 mg/kg combretastatin A-4 3-0-phosphate and 60 days for the mice that received ^{131}I-A5B7–anti-CEA antibody at 7.4 MBq/40 μg antibody. In contrast, 85% of the animals that received a combination of both of the described treatments were alive when the study was terminated at 9 months after treatment. A macroscopic examination of the tumor regions affected by each therapeutic agent alone revealed complementary cytotoxic effects, which supports the enhanced efficacy of the combination of both agents.

IMMUNOCYTOKINE CONJUGATES

Immunocytokine fusions have been the focus of intense efforts to use antibodies to direct the patient's immune response to his or her own tumor.[110] A number of cytokines have been incorporated into antibody-based constructs, including IL-2,[111,112] interferon-γ,[113] tumor necrosis factor-α,[113] vascular endothelial growth factor (VEGF),[114] and IL-12.[115] Many of these strategies have failed to demonstrate enhanced targeting of the cytokine or enhanced therapeutic efficacy over that seen with the cytokine alone. For example, because VEGF has been associated with the induction of vascular permeability, it was believed that use of a fusion protein of VEGF and L19, an scFv specific for the oncofetal ED-B domain of fibronectin that is expressed in angiogenic tissue, could enhance the tumor delivery of the construct. However, the tumor localization of the fusion protein was no better that that of the unconjugated L19 scFv.[114]

Some immunocytokine constructs have been associated with promising preclinical results. For example, IL-2 has been effectively used both to enhance T-cell–mediated immune responses[112] and to elicit a vascular leak syndrome in the tumor with the goal of enhancing the localization of subsequently administered MAb.[111] A fusion protein containing a tumor-specific recombinant anti–ganglioside GD$_2$ antibody and IL-2, termed *ch14.18-IL-2*, effectively prevented liver and marrow metastases after a lethal challenge with NXS2 wild-type cells (a poorly immunogenic murine neuroblastoma model) in mice that were previously vaccinated with single-chain IL-12–producing NXS2 cells and given a booster injection of low-dose ch14.18-IL-2 fusion protein. In contrast, control animals treated with a nonspecific fusion protein or an equivalent mixture of antibody and IL-2 developed metastases.[112] The observation of a sequential increase in the usage of T-cell receptor chains Vβ11 and Vβ13 in CD8+ T cells in the mice suggested that the initial polyclonal CD8+ T-cell response was effectively boosted by targeted IL-2.

A fusion protein consisting of IL-12 and L19 was found to be superior to IL-12 alone in the treatment of metastatic tumors in mouse lung.[115] In these studies, the metastatic load in the lungs at 22 days after treatment in the mice treated with the fusion protein was five times lower than that in mice receiving a saline control and four times lower than that in mice treated with IL-12 alone. Additional improvements have been incorporated into the design of immunocytokine conjugates based on intact IgG molecules. Because these molecules often suffer from accelerated systemic clearance, site-directed mutagenesis of the FcRn site on the Fc domain has been successfully used to prolong their retention in circulation.[116]

PRETARGETED ANTIBODY CONJUGATES

Multistep pretargeted immunotherapy strategies have been developed to take advantage of the specificity of antibody-based targeting without subjecting the host to the potentially considerable toxic side effects associated with the systemic delivery of an active chemotherapeutic drug or the relatively slow delivery of a radioimmunoconjugate. In pretargeted antibody therapy, an antibody-enzyme or antibody-ligand conjugate is administered and allowed to localize in the tumor. After it has cleared from the circulation and normal tissues or has been actively removed through the use of a clearing agent, a cytotoxic agent is administered that can only be activated or retained by the pretargeted antibody in the tumor. In this manner, the cytotoxic effects are further focused on the tumor.

ANTIBODY-DIRECTED ENZYME-PRODRUG THERAPY

In antibody-directed enzyme-prodrug therapy (ADEPT), the pretargeted antibody is conjugated to an enzyme that is capable of activating a subsequently administered inactive form of a drug (prodrug).[117] A number of enzymes have been used in preclinical trials of ADEPT, including β-lactamase (which can activate prodrug forms of doxorubicin and paclitaxel), cytosine deaminase (which can activate a prodrug form of 5-fluorouracil), and carboxypepti-

dase G2 (which can be used to produce nitrogen mustards).[82] In animal models, ADEPT has been associated with highly specific tumor localization of active chemotherapeutic drugs. In an immunodeficient mouse model, Bhatia et al. reported remarkable tumor to tissue ratios of enzymatic activity (371:1, tumor to liver; 450:1, tumor to lung; 562:1, tumor to kidney; 1477:1, tumor to colon; and 1618:1, tumor to spleen) 48 hours after the administration of the recombinant fusion protein MFE-23::CPG2, composed of MFE-23, an anti-CEA scFv antibody, fused to the amino-terminal of the enzyme carboxypeptidase G2 (CPG2).[118]

In human clinical trials, treatment with CPG2 chemically conjugated to an F(ab)$_2$ fragment of the A5B7–anti-CEA mouse MAb followed by the prodrug bis-iodo phenol mustard (ZD2767P) led to observations of stable disease.[119] However, the ability to treat patients with additional cycles of ADEPT was limited by a human antienzyme antibody and HAMA responses. Efforts are currently being made to decrease the immunogenicity of the pretargeted enzyme by modifying the dominant epitopes that were recognized by the immune systems of the treated patients.[120] Other groups have focused their efforts on identifying human enzymes that could be used in ADEPT strategies. However, the use of human enzymes, even those that are normally only present in the intracellular environment, is always associated with the possibility of untargeted and unwelcome prodrug activation.

PRETARGETED RADIOIMMUNOTHERAPY

Multistep strategies also have been used to deliver therapeutic radioisotopes to tumors with the similar goal of separating the delivery of the highly toxic radioisotope from the prolonged circulation of the MAb molecule. In the most commonly applied PRIT approaches, antitumor MAb-streptavidin or MAb-biotin conjugates are administered systemically and allowed to localize to the tumor over a period of days.[121–123] A clearing agent (e.g., biotin–galactose–human serum albumin or streptavidin) is then administered to direct hepatic clearance of the MAb conjugate remaining in circulation. A biotin-chelate-^{90}Y complex is then administered that binds specifically to the MAb conjugate prelocalized in the tumor. To date, a number of PRIT clinical trials have been performed involving patients with solid and diffuse malignancies.[124] Although the best responses were observed in patients with non-Hodgkin's lymphoma (objective responses in six of seven patients treated),[125] clinical responses also have been observed in patients with solid tumors.[126] More recently, a number of groups have begun to develop bsAb-based molecules as vehicles for PRIT. In this strategy, one arm of the antibody binds to the tumor, whereas the second arm binds to a subsequently administered radiolabeled ligand.[127,128] A particularly innovative modification used a bivalent hapten as a ligand to mediate cross-linking of two bsAbs on the tumor surface to increase the binding avidity and prolong tumor retention of the complex.[129,130]

UNCONJUGATED ANTIBODIES WITH CLINICAL ACTIVITY IN SOLID TUMORS

RhuMAb HER2,[131] also known as trastuzumab or Herceptin, is a humanized antibody derived from 4D5, a murine MAb that recognizes HER-2/*neu*. HER-2/*neu* (c-erbB-2), a member of the epidermal growth factor receptor (EGFR) family, has been targeted for antibody therapy because it is overexpressed due to gene amplification on 25% of breast cancers. In a phase II trial involving women with metastatic breast cancer, Baselga et al. reported an objective response rate of 11.6% with responses seen in the liver, mediastinum, lymph nodes, and chest wall metastases,[157] and Cobleigh et al. treated 222 women with metastatic breast cancer, finding an objective response rate of 16%.[132] Thus, trastuzumab clearly has single-agent activity in breast cancer patients who overexpress HER-2/*neu* and was the first FDA-approved antibody targeting solid tumors. Furthermore, trastuzumab in combination with cytotoxic chemotherapy demonstrates improved response rates compared to chemotherapy alone, from 25.0% to 57.3% with a taxane regimen.[133] Myocardial dysfunction seen with anthracycline therapy was observed with increased frequency in patients receiving antibody alone[134] or with doxorubicin or epirubicin, and therefore trastuzumab is not recommended in combination with anthracyclines.

EPIDERMAL GROWTH FACTOR RECEPTOR SIGNALING PERTURBATION

Antibodies directed against selected growth factor receptors, such as EGFR, directly inhibit the growth of receptor-bearing tumors *in vitro* and *in vivo*, and synergize with a number of antineoplastic agents. The receptor and its ligands epidermal growth factor and transforming growth factor-α act in an autocrine loop to stimulate cancer growth. Antibodies that block the binding of EGFR ligands limit receptor activation by tyrosine kinases and inhibit growth of normal fibroblasts[135] as well as tumor cells in culture.[136] The anti-EGFR antibody C225 (ERBITUX) is an IgG1 MAb targeting the extracellular domain of EGFR with a K_d of 0.5 nM. C225 blocks *in vitro* phosphorylation of the EGFR and induces receptor internalization as occurs with binding of the natural ligand.[137] Smaller bivalent $F(ab')_2$ and univalent Fab' forms of this antibody also inhibit growth and decrease receptor phosphorylation, although the bivalent form is superior to the monovalent form.[138] The antibody is thought to inhibit binding of the natural ligand, limit receptor phosphorylation and thus downstream signals, and induce receptor internalization.

Evidence confirms the activity of C225 in colorectal cancers both as a single agent and in combination with chemotherapy. Single-agent responses to C225 of 10.5% are roughly doubled to 19.2% when C225 is given in combination with irinotecan.[139] These response rates are similar even for patients who have previously progressed on irinotecan, with single-agent C225 activity of 10.8% and combination irinotecan plus C225 responses of 22.9%. Therefore, C225 has shown significant clinical activity even in heavily pretreated patients and is an active agent. Other anti-EGFR antibodies have similar antitumor properties.

VASCULAR ENDOTHELIAL GROWTH FACTOR SIGNALING

Tumor angiogenesis is a critical component of tumor invasion, growth, and metastasis. VEGF is a critical determinant of tumor angiogenesis and is an endothelial cell–specific mitogen[140] and vascular permeability factor produced by a large variety of human tumors.[141] Expression of VEGF by invasive tumors has been shown to correlate with vascularity and cellular proliferation, and is prognostic for several human cancers.[142–144] Quantitative immunohistochemical analyses of VEGF in human tumor xenograft models have been reported.[145] In these systems, VEGF expression was directly associated with tumor aggressiveness, which suggests that it plays a critical role in progression to a

more aggressive phenotype. High-affinity endothelial-specific VEGF receptors have included KDR (kinase insert domain–containing receptor)[146,147] and Flt-1 (fms-like tyrosine kinase).[148] *In situ* hybridization has shown that KDR and Flt-1 are expressed on endothelial cells.[147,149] *In vitro* transformation of resting vascular endothelium to an angiogenic phenotype is associated with up-regulation of the VEGF-specific receptor *kdr* gene.[150] In addition, studies of tumor angiogenesis have shown that expression of KDR on endothelial cells correlates with vascularity, metastasis, and proliferation of human colon cancer,[151] the growth of human gliomas,[152] and human hepatic tumorigenesis.[153] These studies provide strong evidence that KDR is critical for the transformation to an angiogenic phenotype. The critical role of Flk-1 in tumor angiogenesis has been demonstrated in different studies in which the receptor pathway has been disrupted using dominant-negative strategies or neutralizing antibodies.[154,155]

Bevacizumab, also known as Avastin or rhuMAb VEGF, is a humanized MAb targeting the VEGF with broad activity in preclinical models. Bevacizumab, when given in combination with cytotoxic chemotherapeutic agents such as 5-fluorouracil and irinotecan as front-line therapy for patients with metastatic colorectal cancer, improved response rates from 35% to 45% compared with chemotherapy alone, with enhanced response durations.[156] More importantly, it improved survival in patients receiving chemotherapy plus bevacizumab by approximately 5 months. Therefore, adding a MAb targeting VEGF to standard chemotherapy can result in a clinically meaningful improvement in survival. This clinical benefit has implications for the fields of colorectal cancer therapy and angiogenesis inhibition.

CONCLUSION

In the little more than a quarter-century since Kohler and Milstein first developed the hybridoma technology that enabled antibody-based therapeutics, the field has made remarkable progress. Numerous antibody-based molecules are currently in clinical trials, and many more are under development. Multiple therapeutic antibodies have established their clinical benefit and have been licensed by the FDA. The thoughtful application of advances in cancer biology and antibody engineering suggest that this progress will continue.

REFERENCES

1. Badger CC, Anasetti C, Davis J, et al. Treatment of malignancy with unmodified antibody. *Pathol Immunopathol Res* 1987;6:419.
2. Khazaeli MB, Conry RM, LoBuglio AF. Human immune response to monoclonal antibodies. *J Immunother* 1994;15:42.
3. Lee J, Fenton BM, Koch CJ, et al. Interleukin 2 expression by tumor cells alters both the immune response and the tumor microenvironment. *Cancer Res* 1998;58:1478.
4. Carter P. Improving the efficacy of antibody-based cancer therapies. *Nat Rev Cancer* 2001;1:118.
5. Hudson PJ, Souriau C. Engineered antibodies. *Nat Med* 2003;9:129.
6. Press OW, Eary JF, Appelbaum FR, et al. Radiolabeled-antibody therapy of B-cell lymphoma with autologous bone marrow support. *N Engl J Med* 1993;329:1219.
7. Kaminski MS, Zasadny KR, Francis IR, et al. Radioimmunotherapy of B-cell lymphoma with 131I-anti-B1 (anti-CD20) antibody. *N Engl J Med* 1993;329:459.
8. Sievers EL, Bernstein ID, Spielberger RT, et al. Dose escalation phase I study of recombinant engineered human anti-CD33 antibody-calicheamicin drug conjugate (CMA-676) in patients with relapsed or refractory acute myeloid leukemia (AML). *Proc Am Soc Clin Oncol* 1997;16:A8.
9. Kohler G, Milstein C. Continuous cultures of fused cells secreting antibody of predefined specificity. *Nature* 1975;256:495.
10. Trauth BC, Klas C, Peters AM, et al. Monoclonal antibody-mediated tumor regression by induction of apoptosis. *Science* 1989;245:301.
11. Yang XD, Jia XC, Corvalan JR, et al. Eradication of established tumors by a fully human monoclonal antibody to the epidermal growth factor receptor without concomitant chemotherapy. *Cancer Res* 1999;59:1236.

12. Baselga J, Albanell J, Molina MA, et al. Mechanism of action of trastuzumab and scientific update. *Semin Oncol* 2001;28:4.
13. Steplewski Z, Lubeck MD, Koprowski H. Human macrophages armed with murine immunoglobulin G2a antibodies to tumors destroy human cancer cells. *Science* 1983;221:865.
14. Houghton AN, Mintzer D, Cordon-Cardo C, et al. Mouse monoclonal IgG3 antibody detecting GD3 ganglioside: a phase I trial in patients with malignant melanoma. *Proc Natl Acad Sci U S A* 1985;82:1242.
15. Komissarov AA, Calcutt MJ, Marchbank MT, et al. Equilibrium binding studies of recombinant anti-single-stranded DNA Fab. Role of heavy chain complementarity-determining regions. *J Biol Chem* 1996;271:12241.
16. Ghetie V, Ward ES. FcRn: the MHC class I-related receptor that is more than an IgG transporter. *Immunol Today* 1997;18:592.
17. LoBuglio AF, Wheeler RH, Trang J, et al. Mouse/human chimeric monoclonal antibody in man: kinetics and immune response. *Proc Natl Acad Sci U S A* 1989;86:4220.
18. Kudo T, Saeki H, Tachibana T. A simple and improved method to generate human hybridomas. *J Immunol Methods* 1991;145:119.
19. Huston JS, Levinson D, Mudgett-Hunter M, et al. Protein engineering of antibody binding sites: recovery of specific activity in an anti-digoxin single-chain Fv analogue produced in Escherichia coli. *Proc Natl Acad Sci U S A* 1988;85:5879.
20. Begent RH, Verhaar MJ, Chester KA, et al. Clinical evidence of efficient tumor targeting based on single-chain Fv antibody selected from a combinatorial library. *Nat Med* 1996;2:979.
21. Mack M, Riethmuller G, Kufer P. A small bispecific antibody construct expressed as a functional single-chain molecule with high tumor cell cytotoxicity. *Proc Natl Acad Sci U S A* 1995;92:7021.
22. Schier R, Marks JD, Wolf EJ, et al. In vitro and in vivo characterization of a human anti-c-erbB-2 single-chain Fv isolated from a filamentous phage antibody library. *Immunotechnology* 1995;1:73.
23. Clackson T, Hoogenboom HR, Griffiths AD, et al. Making antibody fragments using phage display libraries. *Nature* 1991;352:624.
24. Pluckthun A, Pack P. New protein engineering approaches to multivalent and bispecific antibody fragments. *Immunotechnology* 1997;3:83.
25. Holliger P, Prospero T, Winter G. "Diabodies": small bivalent and bispecific antibody fragments. *Proc Natl Acad Sci U S A* 1993;90:6444.
26. Adams GP, Schier R, McCall AM, et al. Prolonged in vivo tumour retention of a human diabody targeting the extracellular domain of human HER2/neu. *Br J Cancer* 1998;77:1405.
27. Iliades P, Kortt AA, Hudson PJ. Triabodies: single chain Fv fragments without a linker form trivalent trimers. *FEBS Lett* 1997;409:437.
28. Hu S, Shively L, Raubitschek A, et al. Minibody: a novel engineered anti-carcinoembryonic antigen antibody fragment (single-chain Fv-CH3) which exhibits rapid, high-level targeting of xenografts. *Cancer Res* 1996;56:3055.
29. Jain RK. Transport of molecules in the tumor interstitium: a review. *Cancer Res* 1987;47:3039.
30. Jain RK. Physiological barriers to delivery of monoclonal antibodies and other macromolecules in tumors. *Cancer Res* 1990;50:814s.
31. Jain RK, Baxter LT. Mechanisms of heterogeneous distribution of monoclonal antibodies and other macromolecules in tumors: significance of elevated interstitial pressure. *Cancer Res* 1988;48:7022.
32. Yokota T, Milenic DE, Whitlow M, et al. Rapid tumor penetration of a single-chain Fv and comparison with other immunoglobulin forms. *Cancer Res* 1992;52:3402.
33. Jain RK. Transport of molecules across tumor vasculature. *Cancer Metastasis Rev* 1987;6:559.
34. Colcher D, Bird R, Roselli M, et al. In vivo tumor targeting of a recombinant single-chain antigen-binding protein. *J Natl Cancer Inst* 1990;82:1191.
35. Adams GP, McCartney JE, Tai MS, et al. Highly specific in vivo tumor targeting by monovalent and divalent forms of 741F8 anti-c-erbB-2 single-chain Fv. *Cancer Res* 1993;53:4026.
36. Wochner RD, Strober W, Waldmann TA. The role of the kidney in the catabolism of Bence Jones proteins and immunoglobulin fragments. *J Exp Med* 1967;126:207.
37. Milenic DE, Yokota T, Filpula DR, et al. Construction, binding properties, metabolism, and tumor targeting of a single-chain Fv derived from the pancarcinoma monoclonal antibody CC49. *Cancer Res* 1991;51:6363.
38. Pavlinkova G, Beresford GW, Booth BJ, et al. Pharmacokinetics and biodistribution of engineered single-chain antibody constructs of MAb CC49 in colon carcinoma xenografts. *J Nucl Med* 1999;40:1536.
39. Miller RA, Maloney DG, Warnke R, et al. Treatment of B-cell lymphoma with monoclonal anti-idiotype antibody. *N Engl J Med* 1982;306:517.
40. Fujimori K, Covell DG, Fletcher JE, et al. A modeling analysis of monoclonal antibody percolation through tumors: a binding-site barrier. *J Nucl Med* 1990;31:1191.
41. Weinstein JN, van Osdol W. The macroscopic and microscopic pharmacology of monoclonal antibodies. *Int J Immunopharmacol* 1992;14:457.
42. Adams GP, Schier R, Marshall K, et al. Increased affinity leads to improved selective tumor delivery of single-chain Fv antibodies. *Cancer Res* 1998;58:485.
43. Adams GP, Schier R, McCall AM, et al. High affinity restricts the localization and tumor penetration of single-chain Fv antibody molecules. *Cancer Res* 2001;61:4750.
44. Wolff EA, Schreiber GJ, Cosand WL, et al. Monoclonal antibody homodimers: enhanced antitumor activity in nude mice. *Cancer Res* 1993;53:2560.
45. Werlen RC, Lankinen M, Offord RE, et al. Preparation of a trivalent antigen-binding construct using polyoxime chemistry: improved biodistribution and potential for therapeutic application. *Cancer Res* 1996;56:809.
46. Behr TM, Sharkey RM, Juweid ME, et al. Reduction of the renal uptake of radiolabeled monoclonal antibody fragments by cationic amino acids and their derivatives. *Cancer Res* 1995;55:3825.
47. Raghavan M, Bjorkman PJ. Fc receptors and their interactions with immunoglobulins. *Annu Rev Cell Dev Biol* 1996;12:181.
48. Daeron M. Fc receptor biology. *Annu Rev Immunol* 1997;15:203.
49. Takai T, Li M, Sylvestre D, et al. FcR gamma chain deletion results in pleiotropic effector cell defects. *Cell* 1994;76:519.
50. Clynes R, Takechi Y, Moroi Y, et al. Fc receptors are required in passive and active immunity to melanoma. *Proc Natl Acad Sci U S A* 1998;95:652.
51. Clynes RA, Towers TL, Presta LG, et al. Inhibitory Fc receptors modulate in vivo cytotoxicity against tumor targets. *Nat Med* 2000;6:443.
52. Gessner JE, Heiken H, Tamm A, et al. The IgG Fc receptor family. *Ann Hematol* 1998;76:231.
53. Shields RL, Namenuk AK, Hong K, et al. High resolution mapping of the binding site on human IgG1 for Fc gamma RI, Fc gamma RII, Fc gamma RIII, and FcRn and design of IgG1 variants with improved binding to the Fc gamma R. *J Biol Chem* 2001;276:6591.
54. Carter P. Bispecific human IgG by design. *J Immunol Methods* 2001;248:7.
55. Peipp M, Valerius T. Bispecific antibodies targeting cancer cells. *Biochem Soc Trans* 2002;30:507.
56. Segal DM, Weiner GJ, Weiner LM. Bispecific antibodies in cancer therapy. *Curr Opin Immunol* 1999;11:558.
57. Akewanlop C, Watanabe M, Singh B, et al. Phagocytosis of breast cancer cells mediated by anti-MUC-1 monoclonal antibody, DF3, and its bispecific antibody. *Cancer Res* 2001;61:4061.
58. Keler T, Graziano RF, Mandal A, et al. Bispecific antibody-dependent cellular cytotoxicity of HER2/neu-overexpressing tumor cells by Fc gamma receptor type I-expressing effector cells. *Cancer Res* 1997;57:4008.
59. Weiner LM, Holmes M, Richeson A, et al. Binding and cytotoxicity characteristics of the bispecific murine monoclonal antibody 2B1. *J Immunol* 1993;151:2877.
60. Milstein C, Cuello AC. Hybrid hybridomas and their use in immunohistochemistry. *Nature* 1983;305:537.
61. Shalaby MR, Shepard HM, Presta L, et al. Development of humanized bispecific antibodies reactive with cytotoxic lymphocytes and tumor cells overexpressing the HER2 protooncogene. *J Exp Med* 1992;175:217.
62. Valone FH, Kaufman PA, Guyre PM, et al. Phase Ia/Ib trial of bispecific antibody MDX-210 in patients with advanced breast or ovarian cancer that overexpresses the proto-oncogene HER-2/neu. *J Clin Oncol* 1995;13:2281.
63. Weiner LM, Clark JI, Davey M, et al. Phase I trial of 2B1, a bispecific monoclonal antibody targeting c-erbB-2 and Fc gamma RIII. *Cancer Res* 1995;55:4586.
64. Lanzavecchia A, Scheidegger D. The use of hybrid hybridomas to target human cytotoxic T lymphocytes. *Eur J Immunol* 1987;17:105.
65. Liu MA, Kranz DM, Kurnick JT, et al. Heteroantibody duplexes target cells for lysis by cytotoxic T lymphocytes. *Proc Natl Acad Sci U S A* 1985;82:8648.
66. Makrides SC. Therapeutic inhibition of the complement system. *Pharmacol Rev* 1998;50:59.
67. Walport MJ. Complement. First of two parts. *N Engl J Med* 2001;344:1058.
68. Presta LG. Engineering antibodies for therapy. *Curr Pharm Biotechnol* 2002;3:237.
69. Idusogie EE, Presta LG, Gazzano-Santoro H, et al. Mapping of the C1q binding site on rituxan, a chimeric antibody with a human IgG1 Fc. *J Immunol* 2000;164:4178.
70. Idusogie EE, Wong PY, Presta LG, et al. Engineered antibodies with increased activity to recruit complement. *J Immunol* 2001;166:2571.
71. Ghetie V, Popov S, Borvak J, et al. Increasing the serum persistence of an IgG fragment by random mutagenesis. *Nat Biotechnol* 1997;15:637.
72. Syed S, Schuyler PD, Kulczycky M, et al. Potent antithrombin activity and delayed clearance from the circulation characterize recombinant hirudin genetically fused to albumin. *Blood* 1997;89:3243.
73. Yeh P, Landais D, Lemaitre M, et al. Design of yeast-secreted albumin derivatives for human therapy: biological and antiviral properties of a serum albumin-CD4 genetic conjugate. *Proc Natl Acad Sci U S A* 1992;89:1904.
74. Lee LS, Conover C, Shi C, et al. Prolonged circulating lives of single-chain Fv proteins conjugated with polyethylene glycol: a comparison of conjugation chemistries and compounds. *Bioconjug Chem* 1999;10:973.
75. Keyt BA, Paoni NF, Refino CJ, et al. A faster-acting and more potent form of tissue plasminogen activator. *Proc Natl Acad Sci U S A* 1994;91:3670.
76. Dennis MS, Zhang M, Meng YG, et al. Albumin binding as a general strategy for improving the pharmacokinetics of proteins. *J Biol Chem* 2002;277:35035.
77. Lund J, Takahashi N, Pound JD, et al. Multiple interactions of IgG with its core oligosaccharide can modulate recognition by complement and human Fc gamma receptor I and influence the synthesis of its oligosaccharide chains. *J Immunol* 1996;157:4963.
78. Shields RL, Lai J, Keck R, et al. Lack of fucose on human IgG1 N-linked oligosaccharide improves binding to human Fcgamma RIII and antibody-dependent cellular toxicity. *J Biol Chem* 2002;277:26733.
79. Umana P, Jean-Mairet J, Moudry R, et al. Engineered glycoforms of an antineuroblastoma IgG1 with optimized antibody-dependent cellular cytotoxic activity. *Nat Biotechnol* 1999;17:176.
80. Wright A, Morrison SL. Effect of glycosylation on antibody function: implications for genetic engineering. *Trends Biotechnol* 1997;15:26.
81. Lifely MR, Hale C, Boyce S, et al. Glycosylation and biological activity of CAMPATH-1H expressed in different cell lines and grown under different culture conditions. *Glycobiology* 1995;5:813.
82. Allen TM. Ligand-targeted therapeutics in anticancer therapy. *Nat Rev Cancer* 2002;2:750.
83. Shankar S, Vaidyanathan G, Affleck D, et al. N-Succinimidyl 3-[(131)I]Iodo-4-phosphonomethylbenzoate ([(131)I]SIPMB), a negatively charged substituent-bearing acylation agent for the radioiodination of peptides and mAbs. *Bioconjug Chem* 2003;14:331.
84. Wilbur DS, Hadley SW, Hylarides MD, et al. Development of a stable radioiodinating reagent to label monoclonal antibodies for radiotherapy of cancer. *J Nucl Med* 1989;30:216.
85. Willner D, Trail PA, Hofstead SJ, et al. (6-Maleimidocaproyl)hydrazone of doxorubicin—a new derivative for the preparation of immunoconjugates of doxorubicin. *Bioconjug Chem* 1993;4:521.
86. Johnson DA, Baker AL, Laguzza BC, et al. Antitumor activity of L/1C2-4-desacetylvinblastine-3-carboxhydrazide immunoconjugate in xenografts. *Cancer Res* 1990;50:1790.
87. Kukis DL, Novak-Hofer I, DeNardo SJ. Cleavable linkers to enhance selectivity of antibody-targeted therapy of cancer. *Cancer Biother Radiopharm* 2001;16:457.
88. George AJ, Jamar F, Tai MS, et al. Radiometal labeling of recombinant proteins by a genetically engineered minimal chelation site: technetium-99m coordination by single-chain Fv antibody fusion proteins through a C-terminal cysteinyl peptide. *Proc Natl Acad Sci U S A* 1995;92:8358.
89. Adams GP, Shaller CC, Chappell LL, et al. Delivery of the alpha-emitting radioisotope bismuth-213 to solid tumors via single-chain Fv and diabody molecules. *Nucl Med Biol* 2000;27:339.
90. Trail PA, Bianchi AB. Monoclonal antibody drug conjugates in the treatment of cancer. *Curr Opin Immunol* 1999;11:584.

91. Trail PA, Willner D, Lasch SJ, et al. Cure of xenografted human carcinomas by BR96-doxorubicin immunoconjugates. *Science* 1993;261:212.
92. Saleh MN, LoBuglio AF, Trail PA. Immunoconjugate therapy of solid tumors: studies with BR96-doxorubicin. In: Grossbard M, ed. *Antibody-based therapy of cancer.* New York: Marcel Dekker, 1998:397.
93. Park JW, Hong K, Kirpotin DB, et al. Anti-HER2 immunoliposomes: enhanced efficacy attributable to targeted delivery. *Clin Cancer Res* 2002;8:1172.
94. Rodriguez M, Coma S, Noe V, et al. Development and effects of immunoliposomes carrying an antisense oligonucleotide against DHFR RNA and directed toward human breast cancer cells overexpressing HER2. *Antisense Nucleic Acid Drug Dev* 2002;12:311.
95. Koning GA, Kamps JA, Scherphof GL. Interference of macrophages with immunotargeting of liposomes. *J Liposome Res* 2002;12:107.
96. Reiter Y, Pastan I. Recombinant Fv immunotoxins and Fv fragments as novel agents for cancer therapy and diagnosis. *Trends Biotechnol* 1998;16:513.
97. Kreitman RJ, Pastan I. Importance of the glutamate residue of KDEL in increasing the cytotoxicity of Pseudomonas exotoxin derivatives and for increased binding to the KDEL receptor. *Biochem J* 1995;307(Pt 1):29.
98. Kreitman RJ, Wang QC, FitzGerald DJ, et al. Complete regression of human B-cell lymphoma xenografts in mice treated with recombinant anti-CD22 immunotoxin RFB4(dsFv)-PE38 at doses tolerated by cynomolgus monkeys. *Int J Cancer* 1999;81:148.
99. Pai LH, Bookman MA, Ozols RF, et al. Clinical evaluation of intraperitoneal Pseudomonas exotoxin immunoconjugate OVB3-PE in patients with ovarian cancer. *J Clin Oncol* 1991;9:2095.
100. Baluna R, Vitetta ES. Vascular leak syndrome: a side effect of immunotherapy. *Immunopharmacology* 1997;37:117.
101. Baluna R, Rizo J, Gordon BE, et al. Evidence for a structural motif in toxins and interleukin-2 that may be responsible for binding to endothelial cells and initiating vascular leak syndrome. *Proc Natl Acad Sci U S A* 1999;96:3957.
102. Smallshaw JE, Ghetie V, Rizo J, et al. Genetic engineering of an immunotoxin to eliminate pulmonary vascular leak in mice. *Nat Biotechnol* 2003;21:387.
103. Behr TM, Goldenberg DM, Becker WS. Radioimmunotherapy of solid tumors: a review "of mice and men." *Hybridoma* 1997;16:101.
104. Juweid ME. Radioimmunotherapy of B-cell non-Hodgkin's lymphoma: from clinical trials to clinical practice. *J Nucl Med* 2002;43:1507.
105. Witzig TE, White CA, Wiseman GA, et al. Phase I/II trial of IDEC-Y2B8 radioimmunotherapy for treatment of relapsed or refractory CD20(+) B-cell non-Hodgkin's lymphoma. *J Clin Oncol* 1999;17:3793.
106. White CA, Weaver RL, Grillo-Lopez AJ. Antibody-targeted immunotherapy for treatment of malignancy. *Annu Rev Med* 2001;52:125.
107. McDevitt MR, Sgouros G, Finn RD, et al. Radioimmunotherapy with alpha-emitting nuclides. *Eur J Nucl Med* 1998;25:1341.
108. Carlsson J, Forssell Aronsson E, Hietala SO, et al. Tumour therapy with radionuclides: assessment of progress and problems. *Radiother Oncol* 2003;66:107.
109. Pedley RB, El-Emir E, Flynn AA, et al. Synergy between vascular targeting agents and antibody-directed therapy. *Int J Radiat Oncol Biol Phys* 2002;54:1524.
110. Lode HN, Xiang R, Becker JC, et al. Immunocytokines: a promising approach to cancer immunotherapy. *Pharmacol Ther* 1998;80:277.
111. Hornick JL, Khawli LA, Hu P, et al. Pretreatment with a monoclonal antibody/interleukin-2 fusion protein directed against DNA enhances the delivery of therapeutic molecules to solid tumors. *Clin Cancer Res* 1999;5:51.
112. Lode HN, Xiang R, Duncan SR, et al. Tumor-targeted IL-2 amplifies T cell-mediated immune response induced by gene therapy with single-chain IL-12. *Proc Natl Acad Sci U S A* 1999;96:8591.
113. Sharifi J, Khawli LA, Hu P, et al. Generation of human interferon gamma and tumor necrosis factor alpha chimeric TNT-3 fusion proteins. *Hybrid Hybridomics* 2002;21:421.
114. Halin C, Niesner U, Villani ME, et al. Tumor-targeting properties of antibody-vascular endothelial growth factor fusion proteins. *Int J Cancer* 2002;102:109.
115. Halin C, Rondini S, Nilsson F, et al. Enhancement of the antitumor activity of interleukin-12 by targeted delivery to neovasculature. *Nat Biotechnol* 2002;20:264.
116. Gillies SD, Lo KM, Burger C, et al. Improved circulating half-life and efficacy of an antibody-interleukin 2 immunocytokine based on reduced intracellular proteolysis. *Clin Cancer Res* 2002;8:210.
117. Senter PD, Springer CJ. Selective activation of anticancer prodrugs by monoclonal antibody-enzyme conjugates. *Adv Drug Deliv Rev* 2001;53:247.
118. Bhatia J, Sharma SK, Chester KA, et al. Catalytic activity of an in vivo tumor targeted anti-CEA scFv: carboxypeptidase G2 fusion protein. *Int J Cancer* 2000;85:571.
119. Francis RJ, Sharma SK, Springer C, et al. A phase I trial of antibody directed enzyme prodrug therapy (ADEPT) in patients with advanced colorectal carcinoma or other CEA producing tumours. *Br J Cancer* 2002;87:600.
120. Spencer DI, Robson L, Purdy D, et al. A strategy for mapping and neutralizing conformational immunogenic sites on protein therapeutics. *Proteomics* 2002;2:271.
121. Axworthy DB, Beaumier PL, Bottino BJ, et al. Preclinical optimization of pretargeted radioimmunotherapy components: high efficiency curative 90Y delivery to mouse tumor xenografts. *Tumor Targeting* 1996;2:156.
122. Goodwin DA, Meares CF, McCall MJ, et al. Pre-targeted immunoscintigraphy of murine tumors with indium-111-labeled bifunctional haptens. *J Nucl Med* 1988;29:226.
123. Paganelli G, Riva P, Deleide G, et al. In vivo labelling of biotinylated monoclonal antibodies by radioactive avidin: a strategy to increase tumor radiolocalization. *Int J Cancer Suppl* 1988;2:121.
124. von Mehren M, Adams GP, Weiner LM. Monoclonal antibody therapy for cancer. *Annu Rev Med* 2003;54:343.
125. Weiden PL, Breitz HB, Press O, et al. Pretargeted radioimmunotherapy (PRIT) for treatment of non-Hodgkin's lymphoma (NHL): initial phase I/II study results. *Cancer Biother Radiopharm* 2000;15:15.
126. Knox SJ, Goris ML, Tempero M, et al. Phase II trial of yttrium-90-DOTA-biotin pretargeted by NR-LU-10 antibody/streptavidin in patients with metastatic colon cancer. *Clin Cancer Res* 2000;6:406.
127. Feng X, Pak RH, Kroger LA, et al. New anti-Cu-TETA and anti-Y-DOTA monoclonal antibodies for potential use in the pre-targeted delivery of radiopharmaceuticals to tumor. *Hybridoma* 1998;17:125.
128. Kraeber-Bodere F, Faibre-Chauvet A, Sai-Maurel C, et al. Bispecific antibody and bivalent hapten radioimmunotherapy in CEA-producing medullary thyroid cancer xenograft. *J Nucl Med* 1999;40:198.
129. Janevik-Ivanovska E, Gautherot E, Hillairet de Boisferon M, et al. Bivalent hapten-bearing peptides designed for iodine-131 pretargeted radioimmunotherapy. *Bioconjug Chem* 1997;8:526.
130. Karacay H, Sharkey RM, McBride WJ, et al. Pretargeting for cancer radioimmunotherapy with bispecific antibodies: role of the bispecific antibody's valency for the tumor target antigen. *Bioconjug Chem* 2002;13:1054.
131. Carter P, Presta L, Gorman CM, et al. Humanization of an anti-p185HER2 antibody for human cancer therapy. *Proc Natl Acad Sci U S A* 1992;89:4285.
132. Cobleigh MA, Vogel CL, Tripathy D, et al. Efficacy and safety of Herceptin™(humanized anti-HER2 antibody) as a single agent in 222 women with HER2 overexpression who relapsed following chemotherapy for metastatic breast cancer. *Proc Am Soc Clin Oncol* 1998;17:A376.
133. Slamon D, Leyland-Jones B, Shak S, et al. Addition of Herceptin™ (humanized anti-HER2 antibody) to first line chemotherapy for HER2 overexpressing metastatic breast cancer (HER2+/MBC) markedly increases anticancer activity: a randomized multinational controlled phase III trial. *Proc Am Soc Clin Oncol* 1998;17:A377.
134. Ewer MS, Gibbs HR, Swafford J, et al. Cardiotoxicity in patients receiving trastuzumab (Herceptin): primary toxicity, synergistic or sequential stress, or surveillance artifact? *Semin Oncol* 1999;26:96.
135. Sato JD, Kawamoto T, Le AD, et al. Biological effects in vitro of monoclonal antibodies to human epidermal growth factor receptors. *Mol Biol Med* 1983;1:511.
136. Arteaga CL, Coronado E, Osborne CK. Blockade of the epidermal growth factor receptor inhibits transforming growth factor α-induced but not estrogen-induced growth of hormone-dependent human breast cancer. *Mol Endocrinol* 1988;2:1064.
137. Sunada H, Magun BE, Mendelsohn J, et al. Monoclonal antibody against epidermal growth factor receptor is internalized without stimulating receptor phosphorylation. *Proc Natl Acad Sci U S A* 1986;83:3825.
138. Fan Z, Masui H, Altas I, et al. Blockade of epidermal growth factor receptor function by bivalent and monovalent fragments of 225 anti-epidermal growth factor receptor monoclonal antibodies. *Cancer Res* 1993;53:4322.
139. Cunningham D, Humblet Y, Siena S, et al. Cetuximab (C225) alone or in combination with irinotecan (CPT-11) in patients with epidermal growth factor receptor (EGFR)-positive, irinotecan-refractory metastatic colorectal cancer (MCRC). *Proc Am Soc Clin Oncol* 2003;22:A1012.
140. Zetter BR. Migration of capillary endothelial cells is stimulated by tumour-derived factors. *Nature* 1980;285:41.
141. Berse B, Brown LF, Van de Water L, et al. Vascular permeability factor (vascular endothelial growth factor) gene is expressed differentially in normal tissues, macrophages, and tumors. *Mol Biol Cell* 1992;3:211.
142. Takahashi Y, Tucker SL, Kitadai Y, et al. Vessel counts and expression of vascular endothelial growth factor as prognostic factors in node-negative colon cancer. *Arch Surg* 1997;132:541.
143. Brown LF, Berse B, Jackman RW, et al. Expression of vascular permeability factor (vascular endothelial growth factor) and its receptors in breast cancer. *Hum Pathol* 1995;26:86.
144. Obermair A, Kohlberger P, Bancher-Todesca D, et al. Influence of microvessel density and vascular permeability factor/vascular endothelial growth factor expression on prognosis in vulvar cancer. *Gynecol Oncol* 1996;63:204.
145. Ma J, Fei ZL, Klein-Szanto A, et al. Modulation of angiogenesis by human glioma xenograft models that differentially express vascular endothelial growth factor. *Clin Exp Metastasis* 1998;16:559.
146. Terman BI, Dougher-Vermazen M, Carrion ME, et al. Identification of the KDR tyrosine kinase as a receptor for vascular endothelial cell growth factor. *Biochem Biophys Res Commun* 1992;187:1579.
147. Millauer B, Wizigmann-Voos S, Schnurch H, et al. High affinity VEGF binding and developmental expression suggest Flk-1 as a major regulator of vasculogenesis and angiogenesis. *Cell* 1993;72:835.
148. de Vries C, Escobedo JA, Ueno H, et al. The fms-like tyrosine kinase, a receptor for vascular endothelial growth factor. *Science* 1992;255:989.
149. Peters KG, De Vries C, Williams LT. Vascular endothelial growth factor receptor expression during embryogenesis and tissue repair suggests a role in endothelial differentiation and blood vessel growth. *Proc Natl Acad Sci U S A* 1993;90:8915.
150. Watson JC, Alperin-Lea RC, Redmann JG, et al. Initiation of KDR gene transcription is associated with conversion of human vascular endothelium to an angiogenic phenotype. *Owen H. Wangensteen Surgical Forum* 1996;47:462.
151. Takahashi Y, Kitadai Y, Bucana CD, et al. Expression of vascular endothelial growth factor and its receptor, KDR, correlates with vascularity, metastasis, and proliferation of human colon cancer. *Cancer Res* 1995;55:3964.
152. Plate KH, Breier G, Weich HA, et al. Vascular endothelial growth factor is a potential tumour angiogenesis factor in human gliomas in vivo. *Nature* 1992;359:845.
153. Warren RS, Yuan H, Matli MR, et al. Regulation by vascular endothelial growth factor of human colon cancer tumorigenesis in a mouse model of experimental liver metastasis. *J Clin Invest* 1995;95:1789.
154. Rockwell P, Witte L, Hicklin D, et al. Antitumor activity of anti-Flk-1 monoclonal antibodies. *Proc Am Assoc Cancer Res* 1997;38:266.
155. Angelov L, Salhia B, Roncari L, et al. Inhibition of angiogenesis by blocking activation of the vascular endothelial growth factor receptor 2 leads to decreased growth of neurogenic sarcomas. *Cancer Res* 1999;59:5536.
156. Hurwitz H, Fehrenbacher L, Cartwright T, et al. Bevacizumab (a monoclonal antibody vascular endothelial growth factor) prolongs survival in first-line colorectal cancer (CRC): results of a phase III trial of Bevacizumab in combination with bolus IFL (irinotecan, 5-fluorouracil, leucovorin) as first-line therapy in subjects with metastatic CRC. *Proc Am Soc Clin Oncol* 2003;22:A3646.
157. Baselga J, Tripathy D, Mendelsohn J, et al. Phase II study of weekly intravenous recombinant humanized anti-p185HER2 monoclonal antibody in patients with HER2/neu-overexpressing metastatic breast cancer. *J Clin Oncol* 1996;14:737.

Matthew P. Goetz
Charles Erlichman
Charles L. Loprinzi

CHAPTER **17**

Pharmacology of Endocrine Manipulation

There are many hormonal agents used in the treatment of patients with cancer. The primary use of these agents is in the treatment of hormonally responsive cancers, such as breast, prostate, or endometrial carcinomas. Other uses for some hormonal therapies include the treatment of paraneoplastic syndromes, such as carcinoid syndrome, and symptoms caused by cancer, including anorexia. This chapter discusses the major hormonal agents for such therapy, first with a general overview of their use in practice, then with more detailed pharmacologic information regarding them.

SELECTIVE ESTROGEN RECEPTOR MODULATORS

TAMOXIFEN

Tamoxifen is most frequently used in the adjuvant treatment of women with resected breast cancer. There is a general consensus, at present, that tamoxifen use should be continued for 5 years. In the setting of hormone-responsive metastatic breast cancer, tamoxifen has generally been replaced by the aromatase inhibitors[1,2]; however, patients who progress after using aromatase inhibitors may still benefit from tamoxifen. In addition, tamoxifen has undergone prospective evaluation as a potential breast cancer chemoprevention drug in multiple studies.[3–6] An overview of these studies that compared tamoxifen to placebo demonstrated a 38% reduction in breast cancer incidence, with no effect in estrogen receptor (ER)-negative cancers but a 48% reduction in ER-positive breast cancers.[7] However, neither in the individual studies nor in the overview has a survival advantage been demonstrated for the tamoxifen group.

The standard dose of tamoxifen is 20 mg. The long terminal half-life of the drug indicates that this dose can be given once daily. Tamoxifen is among the least toxic antineoplastic agents. Randomized, placebo-controlled trials have demonstrated that it does not cause any more gastrointestinal symptoms than placebo causes. The most prominent toxicity from tamoxifen is hot flashes, which affect approximately 50% of women who are treated. These hot flashes are of varying intensity and duration. Tamoxifen-induced hot flashes appear to increase over the first 3 months of therapy and then plateau.[8] They appear to be more prominent in women with a history of hot flashes or estrogen replacement use. They can be ameliorated by the concurrent use of low doses of megestrol[9,10] or antidepressants such as venlafaxine, paroxetine, or fluoexetine.[11–13]

The estrogenic properties of tamoxifen are responsible for both beneficial and deleterious side effects. Although the incidence of endometrial cancer in patients receiving tamoxifen is increased, the absolute risk is small. The annual incidence rate of endometrial cancer in the United States is 1 per 1000.[14] For women receiving tamoxifen, the increase in the incidence of endometrial cancer is approximately 2.58 (ratio of incidence rates).[15] The incidence of a rarer form of uterine cancer, uterine sarcoma, is also increased after tamoxifen use.[16] This form of endometrial cancer comprises approximately 15% of all uterine malignancies that develop after tamoxifen use.[16] Beneficial estrogenic effects from tamoxifen include a decrease in total cholesterol,[9,17] the preservation of bone density in postmenopausal women,[19] and possibly decreased cardiovascular disease.[18] In premenopausal women, tamoxifen has a negative effect on bone density.[20] Although most patients do not complain of vaginal symptoms, a few complain of vaginal dryness, whereas others

457

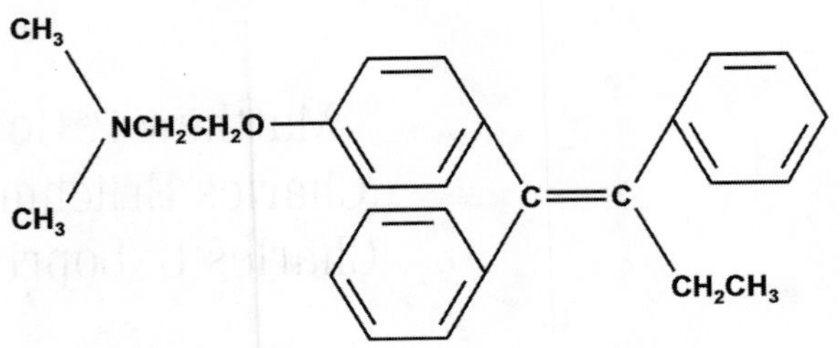

FIGURE 17-1. Structure of tamoxifen.

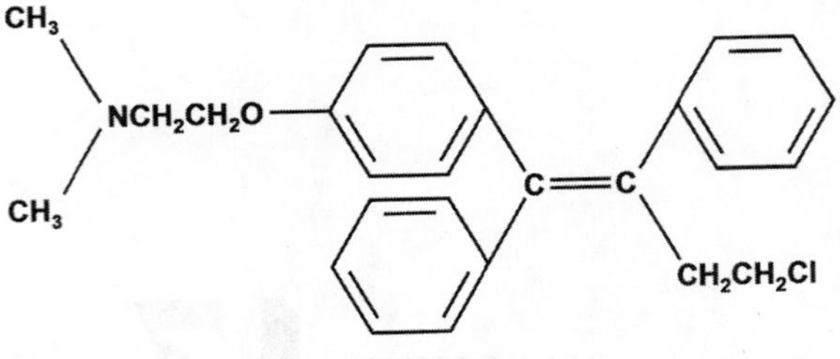

FIGURE 17-2. Tamoxifen metabolism.

have increased vaginal secretions with a resultant vaginal discharge. An uncommon effect from tamoxifen is retinal toxicity. However, no difference in the rate of vision-threatening ocular toxicity has been seen among prospectively treated tamoxifen patients.[21] Tamoxifen may predispose patients to thromboembolic phenomena, especially if used with concomitant chemotherapy. Depression has also been described, but this association with tamoxifen is not clear. Although liver cancers have been noted in laboratory animals, there is no clear-cut association between tamoxifen and liver cancers in humans.

Pharmacology

The chemical structure of tamoxifen is shown in Figure 17-1. It acts by blocking estrogen stimulation of breast cancer cells, inhibiting both translocation and nuclear binding of the ER. This alters transcriptional and posttranscriptional events mediated by this receptor.[22,23] *In vivo*, tamoxifen activity is complicated by the potential actions of the metabolite *trans*-4-hydroxy-tamoxifen, which is a potent antiestrogen. Tamoxifen has agonistic, partial agonistic, or antagonistic effects, depending on the species, target, or end points that have been assessed.

Resistance to tamoxifen can be intrinsic or acquired, and several mechanisms for this resistance have been proposed. At each step of the signal transduction pathway with which tamoxifen interferes, there is potential for an alteration in response. Tamoxifen binds to the ER, and subsequent translocation of this complex to the nucleus and binding to the estrogen response element occur. This binding prevents transcriptional activation of estrogen-responsive genes. Laboratory and clinical data have suggested that ER-positive breast cancers that overexpress HER-2 may be associated with tamoxifen resistance.[24-27] In these tumors, ligand-independent activation of the ER by mitogen-activated protein kinase (MAPK) pathways may contribute to resistance.[28-30] In addition, expression of AIB1, an estrogen-receptor coactivator, may be associated with tamoxifen resistance in patients whose breast cancers overexpress HER-2.[31] Tamoxifen resistance may also be explained by the fact that breast cancers with higher levels of HER-2 expression or with amplification of HER-2 have significantly lower levels of ER/progesterone receptor (PgR) than tumors with lower levels of HER-2 overexpression or amplification.[32]

In some cases, resistance occurs after loss of ER-positive cells.[33,34] Although ER mutation has been suggested as a mechanism of resistance, little evidence for such changes in the ER have been demonstrated.[35] Phosphorylation of the ER can mediate the hormone binding, DNA binding, and ultimately transcriptional activation. Alterations in this phosphorylation mediated by changes in protein kinases A and C could lead to

resistance. Finally, modifications of the estrogen-response element, such as sequence alteration and element duplication, may lead to binding of the tamoxifen-ER complex with increased transcription of the estrogen-response genes.

The carcinogenic potential of tamoxifen has been recognized in rat studies[36-38] and in humans.[39] Although the mechanism of these carcinogenic effects is not understood, it has been proposed that generation of reactive intermediates that bind covalently to macromolecules underlies the process. Such reactive intermediates have been demonstrated *in vitro*.[40-42] In addition, induction of covalent DNA adducts in rat livers treated with tamoxifen has been reported.[43] Both constitutive and inducible cytochrome P-450 (CYP) enzymes have been implicated in the formation of metabolites with tamoxifen,[44,45] and the flavone-containing monooxygenase has been implicated in the formation of the N-oxide of tamoxifen. Reactive intermediates from such metabolic steps are being evaluated for their carcinogenic potential *in vitro* and *in vivo*.

The pharmacokinetics of tamoxifen have not been fully elucidated, despite clinical use of the drug for more than 20 years. The oral bioavailability in humans is not known, but results from animal studies suggest that the drug is well absorbed.[46] Oral administration of [^{14}C]tamoxifen results in only 30% of radioactive material detectable in feces and approximately 11% in urine.[47] Whereas oral absorption may be good, first-pass metabolism may significantly alter exposure *in vivo*. The metabolic pathway of tamoxifen, outlined in Figure 17-2, is dependent on CYP2D6 and -2C9, with a minor contribution from CYP2B6.[48] CYP3A may also play an additional role,[49] as both tamoxifen and 4-hydroxy-tamoxifen significantly increase CYP3A4 expression and activity, most likely as a result of activation of the human pregnane X receptor (hPXR), a key regulator of CYP3A4 expression.[49] 4-Hydroxy-tamoxifen, which exists as two stereoisomers, is a potent antiestrogen[50] as the *trans*-isomer but is much less potent as the *cis*-isomer.[51,52] The predominant species in serum are N-desmethyl-tamoxifen and N-desdimethyl-tamoxifen, whereas 4-hydroxy-tamoxifen, 4-hydroxy-N-desmethyl-tamoxifen, and metabolite Y, which are more hydrophilic, are found in lower concentrations. Metabolism affects the actions of tamoxifen because the hydroxylated metabolites have a higher affinity for the ER than the parent compound.[51] The polymorphic expression of SULT1A1, known to be the predominant SULT isoform involved in the *trans*-selective sulfation of 4-OH-tamoxifen isomers,[53] may also be responsible for some of the differences seen in the outcome of women treated with tamoxifen. In one retrospective study, women treated with tamoxifen as adjuvant therapy for breast cancer who were homozygous for the SULT1A1*2 polymorphism (corresponding to a tenfold lower phenol sulfotransferase activity) had a threefold increased risk of death, compared with those either homozygous for the common allele or heterozygous (SULT1A1*1/*2). This finding was not seen in patients who did not receive tamoxifen.[54] Tamoxifen is 98% bound to human serum albumin.[55,56] α_1-acid glycoprotein binding by tamoxifen may have an impact on its clinical activity because the presence of α_1-acid glycoprotein in tissue cultures abolishes the inhibitory effect of tamoxifen and toremifene on P glycoprotein.[48]

Peak plasma levels of tamoxifen (C_{max}) are seen 3 to 7 hours after oral administration. Assuming an oral bioavailability of 30%, the volume of distribution has been calculated to be 20 L/kg, and plasma clearance ranges from 1.2 to 5.1 L/h.[57] The terminal half-life of tamoxifen has been reported to range between 4 and 11 days.[58,59] The elimination half-life of tamoxifen increases with successive doses.[58,207] This finding is consistent with tamoxifen inhibition of its own metabolism. The drug's distribution in tissues is extensive. Levels of the parent drug and metabolites have been reported to be higher in tissue than in plasma in animal studies.[199,200] Reports of tamoxifen concentrations ten- to 60-fold higher than plasma concentrations in liver, lung, brain, pancreas, skin, and bone have appeared.[201,202] Concentrations of tamoxifen in pleural, pericardial, and peritoneal effusions approach those in plasma, with effusion to serum ratios ranging between 0.2 and 1.0. These findings are consistent with the large calculated volume of distribution. Elevated levels of tamoxifen with biliary obstruction have been reported.[203]

Tamoxifen has been reported to interact with coumadin,[204–207] digitoxin, phenytoin,[208] and medroxyprogesterone.[207] Lien et al.[57] have reported that tamoxifen serum concentrations and those of metabolites Y, 4-hydroxy-tamoxifen, 4-hydrox-N-desmethyl-tamoxifen, N-desmethyl-tamoxifen, and N-desdimethyl-tamoxifen are markedly reduced after aminoglutethimide administration. The mean increase in tamoxifen clearance was 249% when administered with aminoglutethimide. In addition, tamoxifen has been shown to interact with the aromatase inhibitor anastrozole. In the ATAC trial, which compared anastrozole alone and tamoxifen alone with the combination as 5-year adjuvant treatment in postmenopausal women with early breast cancer, patients who received the combination had anastrozole levels that were 27% lower (90% Cl, 20% to 33%; $P < .001$) in the presence of tamoxifen than with anastrozole alone.[60] Although significant, this observed fall in blood anastrozole levels did not seem to have a significant effect on estradiol (E_2) suppression by anastrozole and therefore was thought not to be of clinical significance. Each of these clinical drug interactions is consistent with an effect at the level of CYP3A. Inasmuch as progestational agents, such as megestrol acetate, are CYP3A substrates, these agents may also alter tamoxifen metabolism and, ultimately, elimination. Conversely, tamoxifen-induced activation of hPXR, resulting in induction of CYP3A4, may increase elimination of concomitantly administered CYP3A substrates.[61] This indicates that administration of tamoxifen to individuals taking medication dependent on CYP3A metabolism may alter drug levels extensively, and careful consideration of this should be made when prescribing tamoxifen.

TOREMIFENE

Toremifene, an agent similar to tamoxifen, is thought to be a more pure antiestrogen. It is available in the United States for the treatment of patients with metastatic breast cancer. A randomized comparison of toremifene and tamoxifen in metastatic breast cancer suggested that these two medications were equivalent.[62] Clinical trials in postmenopausal women with metastatic breast cancer concluded that there is major cross-resistance between tamoxifen and toremifene.[63,64]

Pharmacology

Toremifene is an antiestrogen with a chemical structure that differs from that of tamoxifen by the substitution of a chlorine for a hydrogen atom that is retained when toremifene undergoes metabolism.[65] Like tamoxifen, toremifene is metabolized by CYP3A.[66] Toremifene and its 4-hydroxylated metabolite both bind to the ER.[67] Although the oral bioavailability has not been defined, toremifene's oral absorption appears to be good. The time to peak plasma concentrations after oral administration ranges from 1.5 to 6.0 hours,[68] with the terminal half-lives for toremifene and one metabolite, 4-hydroxy toremifene, being 5 to 6 days.[69,70] The apparent clearance is 5.1 L/h. The terminal half-life for the major metabolite, N-desmethyl-toremifene, is 21 days.[71] Time to reach plasma steady-state concentrations is 1 to 5 weeks. Plasma protein binding is more than 99%. As with tamoxifen, toremifene tissue distribution in rats has been studied and found to be extensive and in high concentrations. Consistent with this is the high apparent volume of distribution, 958 L. Seventy percent of the drug is excreted in feces as metabolites. Studies in patients with impaired liver function secondary to alcoholic cirrhosis and in patients on anticonvulsants known to induce CYP3A have been undertaken.[71] Those patients with hepatic dysfunction had decreased clearance of toremifene and N-desmethyl-toremifene, whereas those patients on anticonvulsants had an increased clearance. Interestingly, toremifene appears to be less carcinogenic than tamoxifen in preclinical models.[42,72,73]

RALOXIFENE

Raloxifene is an estrogen agonist and antagonist that was initially developed as an anti–breast cancer agent. Initial studies were not promising regarding this approach, but large placebo-controlled randomized studies have reported that this drug does retard osteoporosis in women at risk for such. These studies demonstrated an apparent reduction in breast cancer in treated women, leading to the development of a second-generation breast cancer chemoprevention trial in which raloxifene is being compared with tamoxifen in high-risk postmenopausal women. Although this drug is relatively well tolerated, it can produce hot flashes. A potential advantage for raloxifene over tamoxifen is that it does not appear to induce endometrial cancer.

Pharmacology

Raloxifene is partially estrogenic in bone[74] and lowers cholesterol.[75] It is antiestrogenic in mammary tissue[76,77] and uterine tissue.[78] The mechanism whereby raloxifene exerts tissue-selective effects is not clear. Several hypotheses have been proposed. Coactivators and corepressor proteins are involved in the transcription complex when ER is bound. There may be differential distribution of these coactivators or corepressors, which are responsible for the changes in estrogenicity seen in tissue. The discovery of a second estrogen, ER-β, with 55% homology between it and ER-α raises the possibility that there is a differential expression of these two ERs in different tissue.[79] This presence of two forms of the receptor also raises the possibility that there are different downstream effectors when one or the other ER is activated.[80,81]

The pharmacokinetics of raloxifene have been studied principally in postmenopausal women.[82-85] Pharmacokinetic parameters of raloxifene show considerable interindividual variation. Limited information is available on the pharmacokinetics of raloxifene in individuals with hepatic impairment, renal impairment, or both.

Raloxifene is rapidly absorbed from the gastrointestinal tract. Because raloxifene undergoes extensive first-pass glucuronidation, oral bioavailability of unchanged drug is low. Although approximately 60% of an oral dose is absorbed, absolute bioavailability as unchanged raloxifene is only 2%. However, systemic availability of raloxifene may be greater than that indicated in bioavailability studies because circulating glucuronide conjugates are converted back to the parent drug in various tissues.

After oral administration of a single 120- or 150-mg dose of raloxifene hydrochloride, peak plasma concentrations of raloxifene and its glucuronide conjugates are achieved at 6 and 1 hour(s), respectively. Plasma concentrations of raloxifene's glucuronide conjugates exceed those of the parent drug, and the time to achieve maximum concentrations of the drug and glucuronide metabolites depends on the extent and rate of systemic interconversion and enterohepatic circulation. After oral administration of radiolabeled raloxifene, less than 1% of total circulating radiolabeled material in plasma represents parent drug.

The area under the curve (AUC) for plasma concentration and time after a single dose of raloxifene is the same as the AUC after multiple doses of the drug. Increasing the dose of raloxifene hydrochloride over a range of 30 to 150 mg results in a slightly less-than-proportional increase in the AUC of raloxifene. Administration of raloxifene with a standardized high-fat meal increases the raloxifene peak plasma concentration by 28% and the AUC by 16% when compared with administration on an empty stomach but does not result in clinically important changes in systemic exposure.

Results of a single-dose study in patients with cirrhosis of the liver (Child-Pugh class A) and total serum bilirubin concentrations of 0.6 to 2.0 mg/dL indicate that plasma raloxifene concentrations correlate with serum bilirubin concentrations and are 2.5 times higher in such individuals than in individuals with normal hepatic function. In postmenopausal women receiving raloxifene in clinical trials, plasma concentrations of raloxifene and the glucuronide conjugates in those with renal impairment (i.e., estimated creatinine clearance values as low as 23 mL/min) were similar to values in women with normal renal function.

Distribution of raloxifene into body tissues and fluids has not been fully characterized. Raloxifene and raloxifene 4'-glucuronide have been detected in saliva after oral administration of radiolabeled drug. In studies in rats given radiolabeled raloxifene 6-glucuronide, the liver contained the highest concentration of radioactivity, followed by serum, lung, and kidney. Although bone and the uterus contained relatively low concentrations of radiolabeled metabolite, 24% of the radioactivity in bone, 14% in the uterus, and 23% in the liver represented raloxifene. Results of this study indicate that the conversion of metabolite to parent drug occurs readily in a variety of tissues, including the liver, lung, spleen, kidney, bone, and uterus. The apparent volume of distribution after

oral administration of single doses of raloxifene hydrochloride, 30 to 150 mg, is 2348 L/kg, suggesting extensive tissue distribution. The volume of distribution is not dose dependent over a dosage range of 30 to 150 mg daily.

Raloxifene and its monoglucuronide conjugates are more than 95% bound to plasma proteins. Raloxifene binds to albumin and α_1-acid glycoprotein.

Raloxifene undergoes extensive first-pass metabolism to the glucuronide conjugates raloxifene 4'-glucuronide, 6-glucuronide, and 6,4'-diglucuronide. UGT1A1 and -1A8 have been found to catalyze the formation of both the 6-β-and 4'-β-glucuronides, whereas UGT1A10 formed only the 4'-β-glucuronide.[86] Metabolism of raloxifene does not appear to be mediated by CYP enzymes, as metabolites other than glucuronide conjugates have not been identified.

The plasma elimination half-life of raloxifene at steady state averages 32.5 hours (range, 15.8 to 86.6 hours).

Raloxifene is excreted principally in feces as unabsorbed drug and via biliary elimination as glucuronide conjugates, which, subsequently, are metabolized by bacteria in the gastrointestinal tract to the parent drug. After oral administration, less than 0.2% of a raloxifene dose is excreted as parent compound and less than 6% as glucuronide conjugates in urine.

FULVESTRANT

An alternative endocrine treatment to tamoxifen is fulvestrant (previously known as ICI 182,780). Fulvestrant is an ER antagonist that has no known agonist activity and results in ER down-regulation.[87-90] Like tamoxifen, fulvestrant competitively binds to the ER but with a much stronger affinity—approximately 100 times greater than that of tamoxifen[91-93]—thus preventing endogenous estrogen from exerting its effect in target cells.

Results from two phase III clinical trials have shown fulvestrant to be as effective as anastrozole in the treatment of postmenopausal women with advanced hormone receptor–positive breast cancer previously treated with antiestrogen therapy (mainly tamoxifen).[94,95] Based on these data, fulvestrant has been approved in the United States for the treatment of postmenopausal women with hormone receptor–positive metastatic breast cancer after progression on antiestrogen therapy.

Fulvestrant is well tolerated. The most common drug-related events (greater than 10% incidence) from the randomized phase III studies were injection-site reactions and hot flashes. Common events (1% to 10% incidence) included asthenia, headache, and gastrointestinal disturbances such as nausea, vomiting, and diarrhea, with minor gastrointestinal disturbances being the most commonly described adverse event.

Pharmacology

Fulvestrant is a steroidal molecule derived from E_2 with an alkylsulphinyl side chain in the 7-alpha position (Fig. 17-3). Because fulvestrant is poorly soluble and has low and unpredictable oral bioavailability, a parenteral formulation of fulvestrant was developed in an attempt to maximize delivery of the drug.[87] The intramuscular formulation provides prolonged release of the drug over several weeks. The pharmacokinetics of three different single doses of fulvestrant (50, 125, and 250 mg) have been published.[87] In this phase I/II multicenter study, postmenopausal women with primary breast cancer who

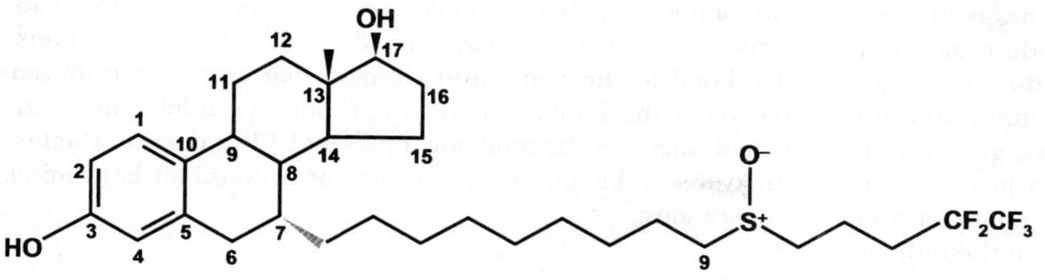

FIGURE 17-3. Structure of fulvestrant.

were awaiting curative surgery received either fulvestrant, tamoxifen, or placebo. After single intramuscular injections of fulvestrant, the time of maximal concentration (t_{max}) ranged from 2 to 19 days, with the median being 7 days for each dose group. At the interval of 28 days, C_{min} values were two- to five-fold lower than the C_{max} values. For most patients in the 125- and 250-mg dose groups, significant levels of fulvestrant were still measurable 84 days after administration. Pharmacokinetic modeling of the pooled data from the 250-mg cohort was best described by a two-compartment model in which a longer terminal phase began approximately 3 weeks after administration.

Pharmacodynamic data from the same study[96] demonstrated that in the primary breast tumors, fulvestrant produced dose-dependent reductions in ER and PgR content and in the Ki-67 labeling index assessed immunohistochemically. The reductions in ER expression were statistically significant at all doses of fulvestrant compared with placebo and for the 250-mg dose compared with tamoxifen ($P = .024$). For PgR, there were statistically significant reductions after treatment with the 125-mg ($P = .003$) and 250-mg doses ($P = .0002$) compared with placebo.

MEDROXYPROGESTERONE AND MEGESTROL

Medroxyprogesterone and megestrol are 17-OH-progesterone derivatives differing in a double bond between C6 and C7 positions in megestrol. Megestrol has been most commonly used as a hormonal agent for patients with advanced breast cancer, usually at a total daily dose of 160 mg. It has also been used frequently for the treatment of hormonally responsive metastatic endometrial cancer, at a dosage of 320 mg/d. In addition, dosages of 160 mg/d are occasionally used as a hormonal therapy for prostate cancer.[97] Megestrol has also been extensively evaluated for the treatment of anorexia-cachexia related to cancer or acquired immunodeficiency syndrome.[98–101] Various dosages ranging from 160 to 1600 mg/d have been used. Prospective studies have demonstrated a dose-response relationship with dosages up to 800 mg/d.[102] Low dosages of megestrol (40 mg/d) have been shown to be an effective means of reducing hot flashes in women with breast cancer and in men who have undergone androgen ablation therapy.[10] Although megestrol has historically been commonly administered four times per day, the long terminal half-life supports that once-per-day dosing is reasonable.

Megestrol is a relatively well-tolerated medication, with its most prominent side effects being appetite stimulation and resultant weight gain. Although these may be beneficial effects in patients with anorexia-cachexia, they can be important problems in patients with breast or endometrial cancers. Another side effect of megestrol acetate is the marked suppression of adrenal steroid production by suppression of the pituitary-adrenal axis.[103] Although this appears to be an asymptomatic state in the majority of patients, reports suggest that this adrenal suppression can cause clinical problems in some patients.[104] This drug has been abruptly stopped for decades without the recognition of untoward sequelae in patients, and it seems reasonable to continue this practice. Nonetheless, if Addisonian signs or symptoms develop after drug discontinuation, corticosteroids should be administered. Furthermore, if patients receiving megestrol have a significant infection, experience trauma, or undergo surgery, then corticosteroid coverage should be administered. There may be a slightly increased incidence of thromboembolic phenomena in patients receiving megestrol alone.[102] This risk appears to be higher if megestrol is administered with concomitant cytotoxic therapy.[105] There are conflicting reports regarding megestrol causing edema.[106] If it does, the edema is generally minimal and easily handled with a mild diuretic. Megestrol may cause impotence in some men.[107] The incidence of this is controversial, although it is generally agreed that this is a reversible situation. Megestrol can cause menstrual irregularities, the most prominent of which is withdrawal menstrual bleeding within a few weeks of drug discontinuation.[10] Although nausea and vomiting have been attributed as a toxicity, there are data to demonstrate that this drug has antiemetic properties.[98,101,105] In terms of magnitude, megestrol appears to decrease both nausea and vomiting in advanced-stage cancer patients by approximately two-thirds.

Medroxyprogesterone has many of the same properties, clinical uses, and toxicities as megestrol acetate. It is not used commonly in the United States but has been used more in Europe. Medroxyprogesterone is available in 2.5- and 10.0-mg tablets and in injectable formulations of 100 and 400 mg/L. Dosing for the treatment of metastatic breast or prostate cancer is 400 mg/wk or more and 1000 mg/wk or more for metastatic endometrial cancer. Injectable or daily oral doses have been used for controlling hot flashes.

PHARMACOLOGY

The exact mechanism of antitumor effect of medroxyprogesterone and megestrol is unclear. These drugs have been reported to suppress adrenal steroid synthesis,[108] suppress ER levels,[109] alter tumor hormone metabolism,[110] enhance steroid metabolism,[111] and directly kill tumor cells.[112] In addition, progestins may influence some growth factors,[113] suppress plasma estrone sulfate formation, and, at high concentrations, inhibit P glycoprotein.

The oral bioavailability of these progestational agents is unknown, although absorption appears to be poor for medroxyprogesterone relative to megestrol.

The terminal half-life for megestrol is approximately 14 hours[114,115], with a t_{max} of 2 to 5 hours after oral ingestion.[116]

The AUC for a single megestrol dose of 160 mg is between 2.5- and eightfold higher than that for single-dose medroxyprogesterone at 1000 mg. Of the radioactive dose of megestrol, 50% to 78% is found in the urine after oral administration, and 8% to 30% is found in the feces. Three glucuronide metabolites of megestrol have been identified in the urine: megestrol hydroxylated in the 2 position, the 6-methyl position, or both. They account for only 5% to 8% of the radioactive dose administered.

Metabolism and excretion of medroxyprogesterone have been incompletely characterized. In humans, 20% to 50% of a [³H]medroxyprogesterone dose is excreted in the urine and 5% to 10% in the stool after intravenous administration.[117-119] Metabolism of medroxyprogesterone occurs via hydroxylation, reduction, demethylation, and combinations of these different reactions.[120] The major urinary metabolite is a glucuronide. Less than 3% of the dose is excreted as unconjugated medroxyprogesterone in humans. Clearance of medroxyprogesterone has been reported to range between 27 and 70 L/h.[119] The initial volume of distribution is between 4 and 8 L in humans. The mean terminal half-life is 60 hours. The t_{max} for medroxyprogesterone occurs 2 to 5 hours after oral administration. Medroxyprogesterone appears to be concentrated in small intestine, colon, and adipose tissue in human autopsy studies.[121] Drug interactions of medroxyprogesterone have been reported with aminoglutethimide, which decreases plasma medroxyprogesterone levels.[122] Medroxyprogesterone may reduce the concentration of the N-desmethyl-tamoxifen metabolite concentration. Progestational agents also may increase plasma coumadin levels.[123] These reports are consistent with CYP3A being the site of interaction.

AROMATASE INHIBITORS

At menopause, the synthesis of ovarian hormones ceases. However, estrogen continues to be converted from androgen (produced by the adrenal glands) by aromatase, an enzyme of the CYP superfamily. Aromatase is the enzyme complex responsible for the final step in estrogen synthesis via the conversion of the androgens androstenedione and testosterone to the estrogens estrone (E_1) and E_2. This biologic pathway served as the basis for the development of the antiaromatase class of compounds. Both nonsteroidal and steroidal antiaromatase compounds have been developed and are now widely used as breast cancer therapy in postmenopausal women.

Aromatase inhibitors have been classified in a number of different ways, including first, second, and third generation; steroidal and nonsteroidal; and reversible (ionic binding) and irreversible (suicide inhibitor, covalent binding).[124] The nonsteroidal aromatase inhibitors include aminoglutethimide (first generation), rogletimide and fadrozole (second generation), and anastrozole, letrozole, and vorozole (third generation). The steroidal aromatase inhibitors include formestane (second generation) and exemestane (third generation).

Steroidal and nonsteroidal aromatase inhibitors differ in their modes of interaction with, and their inactivation of, the aromatase enzyme. Steroidal inhibitors compete with the endogenous substrates androstenedione and testosterone for the active site of the enzyme and are processed into intermediates that bind irreversibly to the active site, causing irreversible enzyme inhibition.[125]

Nonsteroidal inhibitors also compete with the endogenous substrates for access to the active site, where they then form a reversible bond to the heme iron atom so that enzyme activity can recover if the inhibitor is removed; however, inhibition is sustained whenever the inhibitor is present.[125] It is unclear whether the type of inhibition (i.e., reversible or irreversible) has clinical implications.

AMINOGLUTETHIMIDE

Aminoglutethimide was the first clinically used aromatase inhibitor. When it became available, it was used to cause a *medical adrenalectomy*. A 32% response rate in metastatic breast cancer[126] has been reported. However, because of the lack of selectivity for aromatase and the resultant suppression of aldosterone and cortisol, administration of aminoglutethimide necessitated the coadministration of a corticosteroid, such as hydrocortisone. Because of the development of more selective and less toxic aromatase inhibitors, aminoglutethimide is now rarely used for treating metastatic breast cancer. Aminoglutethimide has also occasionally been used to try to reverse excess hormone production by adrenocortical cancers.[127]

LETROZOLE AND ANASTROZOLE

Both letrozole and anastrozole are indicated as first-line therapy for women with receptor-positive metastatic breast cancer. These recommendations are based on two separate phase III studies, one of which compared anastrozole with tamoxifen and the other of which compared letrozole with tamoxifen.[1,2] In both trials, the median time to progression for patients who received either anastrozole or letrozole was significantly longer when compared with tamoxifen. Furthermore, in patients receiving letrozole, a trend toward improvement in overall survival was seen, compared to those receiving tamoxifen.

In the second-line treatment of metastatic breast cancer in women for whom tamoxifen therapy has been unsuccessful, randomized trials have demonstrated improved clinical efficacy of letrozole and anastrozole over megestrol acetate.

In the adjuvant setting, results from the Arimidex, Tamoxifen, Alone or in Combination (ATAC) trial led to the approval of anastrozole for the adjuvant treatment of postmenopausal breast cancer.[128] In this study, which compared anastrozole, tamoxifen, and a combination of tamoxifen and anastrozole, patients receiving anastrozole had significant improvements in disease-free survival, time to treatment failure, and tolerability. However, no differences in overall survival were seen. In contrast, the combination arm showed no benefit over tamoxifen alone.

Side effects of both anastrozole and letrozole appear to be similar. These include arthralgias as well as decreases in bone mineral density. The preliminary data of the ATAC trial suggest that anastrozole therapy is associated with a higher incidence of bone-related events (i.e., fractures) compared with the tamoxifen arm of the study.[128] At the present time, long-term (longer than 5 years) clinical data regarding the effect of aromatase inhibitors on bones are lacking. When offering anastrozole for extended periods of time to patients with early breast cancer, physicians should consider a baseline bone density. Those patients with documented development of bone loss should be offered bisphosphonate therapy. Prospective studies are being conducted to define the benefit of bisphosphonates in this subset of patients.[129]

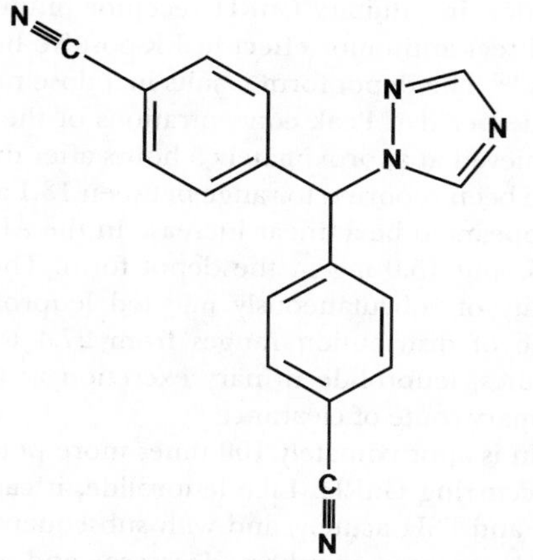

FIGURE 17-4. Structure of letrozole.

No impact has been seen with anastrozole on adrenal steroidogenesis at up to ten times the clinically recommended dose.[130] Conversely, letrozole studies showed a decrease in basal and adrenocorticotropic hormone–stimulated cortisol synthesis. In one study, patients with advanced breast cancer showed a significant decrease in adrenocorticotropic hormone–stimulated aldosterone levels after 3 months of letrozole treatment.[129,131] Aromatase inhibitors may have differential effects on lipids as well. In a large study of over 900 patients at study entry with metastatic disease, anastrozole showed no marked effect on lipid profile, compared with baseline.[132] Conversely, administration of letrozole in women with advanced breast cancer resulted in a significant increase in total cholesterol and low-density lipoprotein from baseline after 8 and 16 weeks of therapy.[133]

Letrozole (Fig. 17-4) is a nonsteroidal aromatase inhibitor with a high specificity for the inhibition of estrogen production. Letrozole is 180 times more potent than aminoglutethimide as an inhibitor of aromatase *in vitro*. Aldosterone production *in vitro* is inhibited by concentrations 10,000 times higher than those required for inhibition of estrogen synthesis.[134,135] In a normal male volunteer study, letrozole was shown to decrease E_2 and serum E_1 levels to 10% of baseline with a single 3-mg dose. In phase I studies,[136,137] letrozole caused a significant decline in plasma E_1 and E_2 within 24 hours of a single oral dose of 0.1 mg. After 2 weeks of treatment, the blood levels of E_2, E_1, and estrone sulfate were suppressed 95% or more from baseline. This continued over the 12 weeks of therapy. There was no apparent alteration in plasma levels of cortisol and aldosterone with letrozole or after corticotropin stimulation.[136] In postmenopausal women with advanced breast cancer, the drug did not have any effect on follicle-stimulating hormone (FSH), luteinizing hormone (LH), thyrotropin (previously *thyroid-stimulating hormone*), cortisol, 17-α-hydroxyprogesterone, androstenedione, or aldosterone blood levels.[138,139]

Anastrozole is a nonsteroidal aromatase inhibitor that is 200-fold more potent than aminoglutethimide.[140] No effect on the adrenal glands has been detected. In human studies, the t_{max} is 2 to 3 hours after oral ingestion.[141] Elimination is primarily via hepatic metabolism, with 85% excreted by that route and only 10% excreted unchanged in urine. The main circulating metabolite is triazole after cleavage of the two rings in anastrozole by N-dealkylation. Linear pharmacokinetics have been observed in the dose range of 1 to 20 mg and do not change with repeat dosing. The terminal half-life is approximately 50 hours, and steady-state concentrations are achieved in approximately 10 days with once-a-day dosing and are three to four times higher than peak concentrations after a single dose. Plasma protein binding is approximately 40%.[142] In one study, anastrozole, 1 mg and 10 mg daily, inhibited *in vivo* aromatization by 96.7% and 98.1%, respectively, and plasma E_1 and E_2 levels were suppressed 86.5% and 83.5%, regardless of dose.[143] Thus, 1 mg of anastrozole achieves near maximal aromatase inhibition and plasma estrogen suppression in breast cancer patients.

EXEMESTANE

In the setting of tamoxifen-refractory metastatic breast cancer, exemestane is superior to megestrol acetate, as demonstrated in a phase III trial in which improvements in both median time to tumor progression and median survival were observed.[144] Although phase III data comparing exemestane to tamoxifen in the first-line therapy of metastatic breast cancer have yet to be published, results of a randomized phase II study comparing exemestane with tamoxifen suggests that exemestane may be superior.[145]

Exemestane has a steroidal structure and is classified as a type I aromatase inhibitor, also known as an *aromatase inactivator* because it irreversibly binds with and permanently inactivates the enzyme.[129]

Side Effects of Exemestane

Unlike anastrozole and letrozole, exemestane appears to favorably affect bone density. In the preclinical setting, exemestane as well as the metabolite 17-hydroexemestane have been evaluated and shown to significantly prevent bone loss in ovariectomized rats.[146,147] Furthermore, significant reductions in both total cholesterol and low-density lipoprotein–cholesterol levels were also seen in this system. In regard to steroidogenesis, no impact on either cortisol or aldosterone levels was seen in a small study after the administration of exemestane for 7 days.[148] Finally, exemestane has weak androgenic properties, and its use at higher doses has been associated with steroidal-like side effects, such as weight gain and acne.[149,150]

Pharmacology

Exemestane is administered once daily by mouth, and the recommended daily dose is 25 mg. The time needed to reach maximal E_2 suppression is 7 days,[151] and its half-life is 27 hours.[152] At daily doses of 10 to 25 mg, exemestane suppresses estrogen concentrations to 6% to 15% of pretreatment levels. This activity is more pronounced than that produced by formestane and comparable to that produced by the nonsteroidal aromatase inhibitors anastrozole and letrozole.[125,153,154] Exemestane does not appear to affect cortisol or aldosterone levels when evaluated after 7 days of treatment, based on dose-ranging studies including doses from 0.5 to 800 mg.[148] Exemestane is metabolized by CYP3A4.[129] Although drug–drug interactions have not been formally reported for exemestane, there is the potential for interactions with drugs that affect CYP3A4.[129]

GONADOTROPIN-RELEASING HORMONE ANALOGUES

Gonadotropin-releasing hormone (GnRH) analogues result in a *medical orchiectomy* in men and are used as a means of providing androgen ablation for metastatic prostate cancer.[155] Because the initial agonist activity of GnRH analogues can cause a *tumor flare* from temporarily increased androgen levels, concomitant use of the antiandrogen flutamide has been used to prevent this effect. GnRH analogues can also cause tumor regressions in hormonally responsive breast cancers[156] and have received U.S. Food and Drug Administration approval for the treatment of metastatic breast cancer in premenopausal women. Data suggest that these drugs may be useful as adjuvant therapy of premenopausal women with resected breast cancer.[157] The use of these drugs in combination with adjuvant chemotherapy for premenopausal women with primary breast cancer is the subject of large, ongoing, international clinical trials. The primary toxicities of GnRH analogues are secondary to the ablation of sex steroid concentrations and include hot flashes, sweating, and nausea.[158] These symptoms can be reversed with low doses of progestational analogues.[10]

GnRH analogues available for clinical use include goserelin[159,160] and leuprolide.[161] Both are available in depot intramuscular preparations to be given at monthly intervals. The recommended monthly dose of leuprolide is 7.5 mg and of goserelin is 3.6 mg. There are also longer-acting depot preparations that are only administered every 3 months.

PHARMACOLOGY

Analogues of the decapeptide GnRH[160–162] have been synthesized by modifications of position 6 in which the L-glycine has been exchanged for a D-amino acid and the C-terminal amino acid has been either replaced by an ethylamide or substituted for a modified amino acid. These changes increase the affinity of the analogue for the GnRH receptor and decrease the susceptibility to enzymatic degradation. There is an amino acid structure of GnRH with the substitutions for leuprolide and goserelin. Initial administration of these compounds results in stimulation of gonadotropin release. However, prolonged administration has led to profound inhibition of the pituitary-gonadal axis.[163] Plasma E_2 and progesterone are consistently suppressed to postmenopausal or castrate levels after 2 to 4 weeks of treatment with goserelin or leuprolide.[164,165] These drugs are administered intramuscularly or subcutaneously in a parenteral sustained-release microcapsule preparation, because parenteral administration of the parent drug otherwise is associated with rapid clearance. The GnRH analogues are metabolized in the liver, kidney, hypothalamus, and pituitary gland by neutral peptidase cleavage of the peptide bond between the tyrosine in the 5 position and the amino acid in position 6 and by a postproline cleaving enzyme that cleaves the peptide bond between proline in the 9 position and the glycine-NH_2 in the 10 position. Substitutions at the glycine 6 position and modification of the C-terminal make these analogues more resistant to this enzymatic cleavage.

Leuprolide is approximately 80 to 100 times more potent than endogenous GnRH. It induces castrate levels of testosterone in men with prostate cancer within 3 to 4 weeks of drug administration after an initial sharp increase in LH and FSH. The mechanisms of action include pituitary desensitization after reduction in pituitary GnRH receptor binding sites and possibly a direct antitumor effect in ER-positive human breast cancer cells.[161] The depot form results in a dose rate of 210 µg of leuprolide per day. Peak concentrations of the depot form that are achieved at approximately 3 hours after drug administration have been reported to range between 13.1 and 54.5 µg/L. There appears to be a linear increase in the AUC for doses of 3.75, 7.5, and 15.0 mg in the depot form. The parenteral bioavailability of subcutaneously injected leuprolide is 94%. The volume of distribution ranges from 27.4 to 37.1 L. In human studies, leuprolide urinary excretion as a metabolite was the primary route of clearance.

Goserelin is approximately 100 times more potent than the naturally occurring GnRH. Like leuprolide, it causes stimulation of LH and FSH acutely, and with subsequent administration, GnRH receptor numbers decrease, and the pituitary becomes desensitized with decreasing LH and FSH levels. Castrate levels of testosterone are achieved within 1 month. In women, goserelin inhibits ovarian androgen production, but serum levels of dihydroepiandrosterone sulfate and, to a lesser extent, androstenedione, are preserved. *In vitro*, goserelin has demonstrated antitumor activity in estrogen-dependent MCF-7 human breast cancer cells and LNCaP-2 prostate cancer cells. The drug is released at a continuous mean rate of 120 µg/d in the depo form, with peak concentrations in the range of 2 to 3 µg/L achieved. The mean volume of distribution in six patients has been reported to be 13.7 L,[166] consistent with extracellular fluid volume. Goserelin is principally excreted in the urine, with a mean total body clearance of 8 L/h in patients with normal renal function. The total body clearance is reduced by approximately 75%, with renal dysfunction and the elimination half-life increased two- or threefold. However, dose adjustment for renal insufficiency does not appear to be necessary. The 5 to 10 hexapeptide and the 4 to 10 hexapeptide were detected in urine in animal studies.[167] The terminal half-life of goserelin is approximately 5 hours after subcutaneous injection. Protein binding is low, and no known drug interactions have been documented.

ANTIANDROGENS

FLUTAMIDE

The antiandrogen flutamide is used in men with metastatic prostate cancer either as initial therapy, combined with GnRH analogue administration, or when the metastatic prostate cancer is unresponsive, despite androgen ablation therapy. The recommended dosage is 250 mg PO three times a day. In patients whose prostate cancer is growing despite flutamide use, stopping flutamide can clearly cause a flutamide-withdrawal response.

The most common toxicity seen with flutamide is diarrhea, with or without abdominal discomfort. Gynecomastia, which can be tender, frequently occurs in men who are not receiving concomitant androgen ablation therapy.[168] Flutamide can rarely cause hepatotoxicity, a condition that is reversible if detected early but can also be fatal.[169] There is no accepted, clinically recommended testing schedule to screen for flutamide-induced hepatotoxicity other than being aware of this phenomenon and testing for liver function if hepatic symptoms develop.

Pharmacology

Flutamide is a pure antiandrogen with no intrinsic steroidal activity.[170] Flutamide's mechanism of action is as an androgen-receptor antagonist. This binding prevents the dihydrotestosterone binding and subsequent translocation of the androgen-receptor complex into the nuclei of cells. Because it is a pure antiandrogen, it acts only at the cellular level, with no progestational effects. Administration of flutamide alone leads to increased LH and FSH production and a concomitant increase in plasma testosterone and E_2 levels. Plasma protein binding ranges between 94% and 96% for flutamide and between 92% and 94% for 2-hydroxy-flutamide, its major metabolite. When the drug is administered three times a day, steady-state levels are achieved by day 6. The steady-state C_{max} is 112.7 ng/L and occurs at approximately 1.13 hours after drug administration. The steady-state C_{max} is between three and five times higher than after the first dose. The elimination half-life at steady state is 7.8 hours. 2-Hydroxy-flutamide achieves concentrations 50 times higher than the parent drug at steady state and has a potency equal to or greater than that of flutamide.[170] The mean C_{max} averaged 1719 ng/mL at steady state and was achieved 1.9 hours after drug administration. The elimination half-life for the metabolite is 9.6 hours. The high plasma concentrations of 2-hydroxy-flutamide, as compared with flutamide, suggest that the therapeutic benefits of flutamide are mediated primarily through its active metabolite.[171]

BICALUTAMIDE (CASODEX)

Casodex is another nonsteroidal antiandrogen that has been approved by the U.S. Food and Drug Administration for use in the United States. The recommended dose is one 50-mg tablet per day. One randomized trial reported that Casodex compared favorably with flutamide in patients with advanced prostate cancer.[172] Casodex appears to be relatively well tolerated and is associated with a lower incidence of diarrhea than is flutamide.

Pharmacology

Casodex[173,174] has a binding affinity to the androgen receptor in the rat prostate that is four times greater than that of 2-hydroxy-flutamide. *In vivo*, Casodex caused marked inhibition of growth of accessory sex organs in rats, with a potency five to ten times greater than that of flutamide. Unlike flutamide, Casodex did not cause a significant increase in LH or testosterone in rats. Casodex bioavailability in humans has not been defined. The drug has a long plasma half-life of 5 to 7 days, so the drug may be administered on a weekly schedule. Pharmacokinetics of the drug showed a dose-dependent increase in mean peak plasma concentrations, and the AUC increased linearly with dose. The half-life of Casodex in humans was approximately 6 days, and the drug clearance was not saturable at plasma concentrations up to 1000 ng/mL. Daily dosing of the drug led to an approximately tenfold accumulation after 12 weeks of administration. In contrast to results in rats, serum concentrations of testosterone and LH increased significantly from baseline at all dose levels tested in humans. Whereas serum FSH concentrations remained essentially unchanged, the median serum E_2 concentrations increased significantly.[175]

NILUTAMIDE

Nilutamide represents the third variation of antiandrogens available for use in patients with prostate cancer. Although it may be less expensive than the other antiandrogens, it has two unique toxicities, night blindness and pulmonary toxicity, that limit its use.

Pharmacology

Nilutamide[176,177] is a newer nonsteroidal antiandrogen that has a high bioavailability with moderate plasma protein binding. It is extensively metabolized, with less than 2% of parent drug administered isolated in urine over 5 days. Oxidation of a methyl group forms two stereoisomeric metabolites whose pharmacokinetics and pharmacodynamics are not characterized. Sixty-two percent of oral drug is eliminated in the urine as metabolites. The terminal half-life varies from 38 to 59 hours. Steady-state levels are achieved in 2 to 4 weeks with 150 mg given twice a day, with approximately a twofold accumulation of drug over that time.

FLUOXYMESTERONE

Fluoxymesterone is an androgen that has been used in women with metastatic breast cancer who have hormonally responsive cancers and who have progressed on other hormonal therapies such as tamoxifen, an aromatase inhibitor, or megestrol acetate. The usual dose is 10 mg given twice daily. Although the overall response rate is low for fluoxymesterone used in this clinical situation,[178] there are some patients who have substantial antitumor responses lasting for months or even years.

Toxicities associated with fluoxymesterone are those that would be expected with an androgen: hirsutism, male-pattern baldness, voice lowering (hoarseness), acne, enhanced libido, and erythrocytosis. Fluoxymesterone can also cause elevated liver function test results in some patients and, rarely, has been associated with hepatic neoplasms.

PHARMACOLOGY

Fluoxymesterone is a chlorinated synthetic analogue of testosterone with potent androgenic and anabolic activity in humans. Limited pharmacologic information is available on this agent. Colburn,[179] using a radioimmunoassay, studied two subjects after a single oral administration of a 50-mg dose. Peak serum concentrations were achieved between 1 and 3 hours after administration, with the average peak concentrations being 335 ng/mL. By 5 hours after drug administration, serum levels had declined to approximately 50% of the peak concentration. Urinary excretion of a 10-mg dose can be detected for 24 hours, and at least 6-hydroxy, 4 ene, 3 β, and 11-hydroxy metabolites of fluoxymesterone have been detected.[180]

DIETHYLSTILBESTROL AND ESTRADIOL (ESTRACE)

Diethylstilbestrol (DES) used to be the primary hormonal therapy for postmenopausal metastatic breast cancer. Randomized comparative trials demonstrated that it had a similar response rate to that for tamoxifen.[181,182] However, based on these trials, DES use was supplanted by tamoxifen primarily because DES has more toxicity. DES is occasionally used in metastatic breast cancer patients who have hormonally sensitive cancers that have failed to respond to multiple other hormonal therapies. The usual dose in this situation is 15 mg/d (either as a single dose or as divided doses). DES was also used as androgen ablation therapy in men with metastatic prostate cancer.[183] Doses of approximately 3 mg/d result in testosterone levels that are seen in an anorchid state.

In women, DES may cause a number of toxicities. One of the most common is nausea and vomiting. It also can cause breast tenderness and a darkening of the nipple-areolar complex. DES increases the risk of thromboembolic phenomenon, and this may result in life-threatening complications. In men, DES results in increased thromboembolic events and mortality, thus, limiting its use. It also causes painful gynecomastia. Although breast irradiation before DES administration appears to prevent this toxicity, it does not appear to help if it is given after the toxicity develops.

DES has not been clinically available in the United States in recent years, but similar antitumor effects and toxicities are seen with Estrace, 1 mg PO three times a day.

PHARMACOLOGY

DES disposition studies in humans have been limited.[184] In animal studies, the oral absorption is approximately 20%. The drug undergoes hepatic metabolism and is excreted as dienestrol and hydroxydienestrol in urine.[185] The parent compound has been detected in feces. After administration of a radioactive dose of DES, approximately 40% of the drug was found in urine in the first 24 hours, with 87% of this being in the form of glucuronides. The peak plasma concentrations were achieved approximately 20 hours after ingestion, and the terminal half-life for the radioactivity ranged between 2 and 3 days.

Estrace is a micronized form of E_2. The pharmacology of E_2 has been extensively described elsewhere.[186]

OCTREOTIDE

Octreotide is a somatostatin analogue that has revolutionized the therapy of carcinoid syndrome and other hormonal excess syndromes associated with some pancreatic islet cell cancers and acromegaly. Response rates are high and, on average, last for several months, sometimes for years. Occasionally, antitumor responses temporarily related to octreotide are seen with these tumors. Octreotide has been investigated as a potential therapy in breast cancer. Results of a randomized study in women with metastatic breast cancer demonstrated no benefit for the addition of octreotide to tamoxifen.[187] Finally, octreotide can also alleviate severe diarrhea caused by 5-fluorouracil–based chemotherapy and also pelvic irradiation.[188–194]

Octreotide can be administered intravenously or subcutaneously. Initial doses of 50 μg are given two to three times on the first day. The dose is titrated upward, with a usual daily dose of 300 to 450 μg/d for most patients. At times, doses up to 1500 μg/d have been given. A depot preparation is available, allowing doses to be administered at monthly intervals. Octreotide is generally well tolerated overall. It appears to cause more toxic-ity in acromegalic patients, with such problems as bradycardia, diarrhea, hypoglycemia, hyperglycemia, hypothyroidism, and cholelithiasis.

PHARMACOLOGY

Octreotide is an 8-amino acid synthetic analogue of the 14-amino acid peptide somatostatin.[195] Octreotide has a similar high affinity for somatostatin receptors, as does its parent, with a concentration that inhibits the receptor by 50% in the subnanomolar range. Octreotide inhibits insulin, glucagon, pancreatic polypeptide, gastric inhibitory polypeptide, and gastrin secretion. It has a much longer duration of action than the parent compound because of its greater resistance to enzymatic degradation. Its absorption after subcutaneous administration is rapid, and bioavailability is 100% after subcutaneous injection. Peak concentrations of 4 μg/L after a 100-μg dose occur within 20 to 30 minutes of subcutaneous injection and are 20% to 40% of the corresponding intravenous injection. Both peak concentration and AUC for octreotide increase linearly with dose. The total body clearance in healthy volunteers is 9.6 L/h. Hepatic metabolism of octreotide accounts for 30% to 40% of the drug's disposition, and 11% to 20% is excreted unchanged in the urine. The volume of distribution ranges between 18 and 30 L, and the terminal half-life is reported to be between 72 and 98 minutes. Sixty-five percent of the drug is protein bound primarily to the lipoprotein fraction.[195,196] Because of the short half-life, classic octreotide is administered subcutaneously two or three times per day.[197] A slow-release form of octreotide, designed for once-per-month administration, controls the symptoms of carcinoid syndrome at least as well as three-times-per-day octreotide.[198]

REFERENCES

1. Nabholtz JM, Buzdar A, Pollak M, et al. Anastrozole is superior to tamoxifen as first-line therapy for advanced breast cancer in postmenopausal women: results of a North American multicenter randomized trial. Arimidex Study Group. *J Clin Oncol* 2000;18:3758.
2. Mouridsen H, Gershanovich M, Sun Y, et al. Phase III study of letrozole versus tamoxifen as first-line therapy of advanced breast cancer in postmenopausal women: analysis of survival and update of efficacy from the International Letrozole Breast Cancer Group. *J Clin Oncol* 2003;21:2101.
3. Cuzick J, Forbes J, Edwards R, et al. First results from the International Breast Cancer Intervention Study (IBIS-I): a randomized prevention trial. *Lancet* 2002;360:817.
4. Fisher B, Costantino JP, Wickerham DL, et al. Tamoxifen for prevention of breast cancer: report of the National Surgical Adjuvant Breast and Bowel Project P-1 Study. *J Natl Cancer Inst* 1998;90:1371.
5. Powles T, Eeles R, Ashley S, et al. Interim analysis of the incidence of breast cancer in the Royal Marsden Hospital tamoxifen randomised chemoprevention trial. *Lancet* 1998;352:98.
6. Veronesi U, Maisonneuve P, Sacchini V, et al. Tamoxifen for breast cancer among hysterectomized women. *Lancet* 2002;359:1122.
7. Cuzick J, Powles T, Veronesi U, et al. Overview of the main outcomes in breast-cancer prevention trials. *Lancet* 2003;361:296.
8. Kiang DT, Kennedy BJ. Tamoxifen (antiestrogen) therapy in advanced breast cancer. *Ann Intern Med* 1977;87:687.
9. Love RR, Cameron L, Connell BL, et al. Symptoms associated with tamoxifen treatment in postmenopausal women. *Arch Intern Med* 1991;151:1842.
10. Loprinzi CL, Michalak JC, Quella SK, et al. Megestrol acetate for the prevention of hot flashes. *N Engl J Med* 1994;331:347.
11. Loprinzi CL, Kugler JW, Sloan JA, et al. Venlafaxine in management of hot flashes in survivors of breast cancer: a randomised controlled trial. *Lancet* 2000;356:2059.
12. Loprinzi CL, Sloan JA, Perez EA, et al. Phase III evaluation of fluoxetine for treatment of hot flashes. *J Clin Oncol* 2002;20:1578.
13. Stearns V, Beebe KL, Iyengar M, et al. Paroxetine controlled release in the treatment of menopausal hot flashes: a randomized controlled trial. *JAMA* 2003;289:2827.
14. Parkin DM, Muir CS. Cancer incidence in five continents. Comparability and quality of data. *IARC Sci Publ* 1992;45.
15. Tamoxifen for early breast cancer: an overview of the randomised trials. Early Breast Cancer Trialists' Collaborative Group. *Lancet* 1998;351:1451.
16. Wickerham DL, Fisher B, Wolmark N, et al. Association of tamoxifen and uterine sarcoma. *J Clin Oncol* 2002;20:2758.

17. Dewar JA, Horobin JM, Preece PE, et al. Long term effects of tamoxifen on blood lipid values in breast cancer. *BMJ* 1992;305:225.
18. McDonald CC, Stewart HJ. Fatal myocardial infarction in the Scottish adjuvant tamoxifen trial. The Scottish Breast Cancer Committee. *BMJ* 1991;303:435.
19. Love RR, Mazess RB, Barden HS, et al. Effects of tamoxifen on bone mineral density in postmenopausal women with breast cancer. *N Engl J Med* 1992;326:852.
20. Powles TJ, Hickish T, Kanis JA, et al. Effect of tamoxifen on bone mineral density measured by dual-energy x-ray absorptiometry in healthy premenopausal and postmenopausal women. *J Clin Oncol* 1996;14:78.
21. Gorin MB, Day R, Costantino JP, et al. Long-term tamoxifen citrate use and potential ocular toxicity. *Am J Ophthalmol* 1998;125:493.
22. Jaiyesimi IA, Buzdar AU, Decker DA, et al. Use of tamoxifen for breast cancer: twenty-eight years later. *J Clin Oncol* 1995;13:513.
23. Tonetti DA, Jordan VC. Possible mechanisms in the emergence of tamoxifen-resistant breast cancer. *Anticancer Drugs* 1995;6:498.
24. Benz CC, Scott GK, Sarup JC, et al. Estrogen-dependent, tamoxifen-resistant tumorigenic growth of MCF-7 cells transfected with HER2/neu. *Breast Cancer Res Treat* 1993;24:85.
25. Borg A, Baldetorp B, Ferno M, et al. ERBB2 amplification is associated with tamoxifen resistance in steroid-receptor positive breast cancer. *Cancer Lett* 1994;81:137.
26. Houston SJ, Plunkett TA, Barnes DM, et al. Overexpression of c-erbB2 is an independent marker of resistance to endocrine therapy in advanced breast cancer. *Br J Cancer* 1999;79:1220.
27. Lipton A, Ali SM, Leitzel K, et al. Serum HER-2/neu and response to the aromatase inhibitor letrozole versus tamoxifen. *J Clin Oncol* 2003;21:1967.
28. Kato S, Endoh H, Masuhiro Y, et al. Activation of the estrogen receptor through phosphorylation by mitogen-activated protein kinase. *Science* 1995;270:1491.
29. Bunone G, Briand PA, Miksicek RJ, et al. Activation of the unliganded estrogen receptor by EGF involves the MAP kinase pathway and direct phosphorylation. *EMBO J* 1996;15:2174.
30. Pietras RJ, Arboleda J, Reese DM, et al. HER-2 tyrosine kinase pathway targets estrogen receptor and promotes hormone-independent growth in human breast cancer cells. *Oncogene* 1995;10:2435.
31. Osborne CK, Bardou V, Hopp TA, et al. Role of the estrogen receptor coactivator AIB1 (SRC-3) and HER-2/neu in tamoxifen resistance in breast cancer. *J Natl Cancer Inst* 2003;95:353.
32. Konecny G, Pauletti G, Pegram M, et al. Quantitative association between HER-2/neu and steroid hormone receptors in hormone receptor-positive primary breast cancer. *J Natl Cancer Inst* 2003;95:142.
33. Encarnacion CA, Ciocca DR, McGuire WL, et al. Measurement of steroid hormone receptors in breast cancer patients on tamoxifen. *Breast Cancer Res Treat* 1993;26:237.
34. Watts CK, Handel ML, King RJ, et al. Oestrogen receptor gene structure and function in breast cancer. *J Steroid Biochem Mol Biol* 1992;41:529.
35. Karnik PS, Kulkarni S, Liu XP, et al. Estrogen receptor mutations in tamoxifen-resistant breast cancer. *Cancer Res* 1994;54:349.
36. Williams GM, Iatropoulos MJ, Djordjevic MV, et al. The triphenylethylene drug tamoxifen is a strong liver carcinogen in the rat. *Carcinogenesis* 1993:315.
37. Williams GM. Tamoxifen experimental carcinogenicity studies: implications for human effects. *Proc Soc Exp Biol Med* 1995;208:141.
38. Fendl KC, Zimniski SJ. Role of tamoxifen in the induction of hormone-independent rat mammary tumors. *Cancer Res* 1992;52:235.
39. Rutqvist LE, Johansson H, Signomklao T, et al. Adjuvant tamoxifen therapy for early stage breast cancer and second primary malignancies. Stockholm Breast Cancer Study Group. *J Natl Cancer Inst* 1995;87:645.
40. Mani C, Kupfer D. Cytochrome P-450-mediated activation and irreversible binding of the antiestrogen tamoxifen to proteins in rat and human liver: possible involvement of flavin-containing monooxygenases in tamoxifen activation. *Cancer Res* 1991;51:6052.
41. Mani C, Pearce R, Parkinson A, et al. Involvement of cytochrome P4503A in catalysis of tamoxifen activation and covalent binding to rat and human liver microsomes. *Carcinogenesis* 1994;15:2715.
42. Styles JA, Davies A, Lim CK, et al. Genotoxicity of tamoxifen, tamoxifen epoxide and toremifene in human lymphoblastoid cells containing human cytochrome P450s. *Carcinogenesis* 1994;15:5.
43. Han XL, Liehr JG. Induction of covalent DNA adducts in rodents by tamoxifen. *Cancer Res* 1992;52:1360.
44. Mani C, Gelboin HV, Park SS, et al. Metabolism of the antimammary cancer antiestrogenic agent tamoxifen. I. Cytochrome P-450-catalyzed N-demethylation and 4-hydroxylation. *Drug Metab Dispos* 1993;21:645.
45. Mani C, Hodgson E, Kupfer D. Metabolism of the antimammary cancer antiestrogenic agent tamoxifen. II. Flavin-containing monooxygenase-mediated N-oxidation. *Drug Metab Dispos* 1993;21:657.
46. Fromson JM, Pearson S, Bramah S. The metabolism of tamoxifen (I.C.I. 46,474). I. In laboratory animals. *Xenobiotica* 1973;3:693.
47. Fromson JM, Pearson S, Bramah S. The metabolism of tamoxifen (I.C.I. 46,474). II. In female patients. *Xenobiotica* 1973;3:711.
48. Coller JK, Krebsfaenger N, Klein K, et al. The influence of CYP2B6, CYP2C9 and CYP2D6 genotypes on the formation of the potent antioestrogen Z-4-hydroxy-tamoxifen in human liver. *Br J Clin Pharmacol* 2002;54:157.
49. Crewe HK, Ellis SW, Lennard MS, et al. Variable contribution of cytochromes P450 2D6, 2C9 and 3A4 to the 4-hydroxylation of tamoxifen by human liver microsomes. *Biochem Pharmacol* 1997;53:171.
50. Jordan VC, Collins MM, Rowsby L, et al. A monohydroxylated metabolite of tamoxifen with potent antiestrogenic activity. *J Endocrinol* 1977;75:305.
51. Robertson DW, Katzenellenbogen JA, Long DJ, et al. Tamoxifen antiestrogens. A comparison of the activity, pharmacokinetics, and metabolic activation of the cis and trans isomers of tamoxifen. *J Steroid Biochem* 1982;16:1.
52. Katzenellenbogen JA, Carlson KE, Katzenellenbogen BS. Facile geometric isomerization of phenolic non-steroidal estrogens and antiestrogens: limitations to the interpretation of experiments characterizing the activity of individual isomers. *J Steroid Biochem* 1985;22:589.
53. Nishiyama T, Ogura K, Nakano H, et al. Reverse geometrical selectivity in glucuronidation and sulfation of cis- and trans-4-hydroxytamoxifens by human liver UDP- glucuronosyltransferases and sulfotransferases. *Biochem Pharmacol* 2002;63:1817.
54. Nowell S, Sweeney C, Winters M, et al. Association between sulfotransferase 1A1 genotype and survival of breast cancer patients receiving tamoxifen therapy. *J Natl Cancer Inst* 2002;94:1635.
55. Lien EA, Solheim E, Lea OA, et al. Distribution of 4-hydroxy-N-desmethyltamoxifen and other tamoxifen metabolites in human biological fluids during tamoxifen treatment. *Cancer Res* 1989;49:2175.
56. Shah IG, Parsons DL. Human albumin binding of tamoxifen in the presence of a perfluorochemical erythrocyte substitute. *J Pharm Pharmacol* 1991;43:790.
57. Lien EA, Anker G, Lonning PE, et al. Decreased serum concentrations of tamoxifen and its metabolites induced by aminoglutethimide. *Cancer Res* 1990;50:5851.
58. Adam HK, Patterson JS, Kemp JV. Studies on the metabolism and pharmacokinetics of tamoxifen in normal volunteers. *Cancer Treat Rep* 1980;64:761.
59. Patterson JS, Settatree RS, Adam HK, et al. Serum concentrations of tamoxifen and major metabolite during long-term Nolvadex therapy, correlated with clinical response. *Eur J Cancer* 1980;[Suppl 1]1:89.
60. Dowsett M, Cuzick J, Howell A, et al. Pharmacokinetics of anastrozole and tamoxifen alone, and in combination, during adjuvant endocrine therapy for early breast cancer in postmenopausal women: a sub-protocol of the arimidex and tamoxifen alone or in combination (ATAC) trial. *Br J Cancer* 2001;85:317.
61. Desai PB, Nallani SC, Sane RS, et al. Induction of cytochrome P450 3A4 in primary human hepatocytes and activation of the human pregnane X receptor by tamoxifen and 4-hydroxytamoxifen. *Drug Metab Dispos* 2002;30:608.
62. Hayes DF, Van Zyl JA, Hacking A, et al. Randomized comparison of tamoxifen and two separate doses of toremifene in postmenopausal patients with metastatic breast cancer. *J Clin Oncol* 1995;13:2556.
63. Stenbygaard LE, Herrstedt J, Thomsen JF, et al. Toremifene and tamoxifen in advanced breast cancer—a double-blind cross-over trial. *Breast Cancer Res Treat* 1993;25:57.
64. Vogel CL, Shemano I, Schoenfelder J, et al. Multicenter phase II efficacy trial of toremifene in tamoxifen-refractory patients with advanced breast cancer. *J Clin Oncol* 1993;11:345.
65. Kangas L. Review of the pharmacological properties of toremifene. *J Steroid Biochem* 1990;36:191.
66. Berthou F, Dreano Y, Belloc C, et al. Involvement of cytochrome P450 3A enzyme family in the major metabolic pathways of toremifene in human liver microsomes. *Biochem Pharmacol* 1994;47:1883.
67. Simberg NH, Murai JT, Siiteri PK. In vitro and in vivo binding of toremifene and its metabolites in rat uterus. *J Steroid Biochem* 1990;36:197.
68. Kohler PC, Hamm JT, Wiebe VJ, et al. Phase I study of the tolerance and pharmacokinetics of toremifene in patients with cancer. *Breast Cancer Res Treat* 1990;16[Suppl]:S19.
69. Wiebe VJ, Benz CC, Shemano I, et al. Pharmacokinetics of toremifene and its metabolites in patients with advanced breast cancer. *Cancer Chemother Pharmacol* 1990;25:247.
70. Tominaga T, Abe O, Izuo M. A phase I study of toremifene. *Breast Cancer Res Treat* 1990;16[Suppl]:27.
71. Anttila M, Laakso S, Nylanden P, et al. Pharmacokinetics of the novel antiestrogenic agent toremifene in subjects with altered liver and kidney function. *Clin Pharmacol Ther* 1995;57:628.
72. Montandon F, Williams GM. Comparison of DNA reactivity of the polyphenylethylene hormonal agents diethylstilbestrol, tamoxifen and toremifene in rat and hamster liver. *Arch Toxicol* 1994;68:272.
73. Hard GC, Iatropoulos MJ, Jordan K, et al. Major difference in the hepatocarcinogenicity and DNA adduct forming ability between toremifene and tamoxifen in female Crl:CD(BR) rats. *Cancer Res* 1993;53:4534.
74. Delmas PD, Bjarnason NH, Mitlak BH, et al. Effects of raloxifene on bone mineral density, serum cholesterol concentrations, and uterine endometrium in postmenopausal women. *N Engl J Med* 1997;337:1641.
75. Draper MW, Flowers DE, Huster WJ, et al. A controlled trial of raloxifene (LY139481) HCl: impact on bone turnover and serum lipid profile in healthy postmenopausal women. *J Bone Miner Res* 1996;11:835.
76. Gottardis MM, Jordan VC. Antitumor actions of keoxifene and tamoxifen in the N-nitrosomethylurea-induced rat mammary carcinoma model. *Cancer Res* 1987;47:4020.
77. Anzano MA, Peer CW, Smith JM, et al. Chemoprevention of mammary carcinogenesis in the rat: combined use of raloxifene and 9-cis-retinoic acid. *J Natl Cancer Inst* 1996;88:123.
78. Black LJ, Jones CD, Falcone JF. Antagonism of estrogen action with a new benzothiophene derived antiestrogen. *Life Sci* 1983;32:1031.
79. Kuiper GG, Carlsson B, Grandien K, et al. Comparison of the ligand binding specificity and transcript tissue distribution of estrogen receptors alpha and beta. *Endocrinology* 1997;138:863.
80. Paech K, Webb P, Kuiper GG, et al. Differential ligand activation of estrogen receptors ERalpha and ERbeta at AP1 sites. *Science* 1997;277:1508.
81. Webb P, Lopez GN, Uht RM, et al. Tamoxifen activation of the estrogen receptor/AP-1 pathway: potential origin for the cell-specific estrogen-like effects of antiestrogens. *Mol Endocrinol* 1995;9:443.
82. Forgue ST, Rudy AC, Knadler MP. Raloxifene pharmacokinetics in healthy postmenopausal women. *Pharmaceut Res* 1996;13:S430.
83. Ni L, Allerheiligen S, Basson R. Pharmacokinetics of raloxifene in men and postmenopausal women volunteers. *Pharmaceut Res* 1996;13:S430.
84. Allerheiligen S, Geiser J, Knadler M. Raloxifen (RAL) pharmacokinetics and the associated endocrine effects in premenopausal women treated during the follicular, ovulatory, and luteal phases of the menstrual cycle. *Pharmaceut Res* 1996;13:S430.

85. Hochner-Celnikier D. Pharmacokinetics of raloxifene and its clinical application. *Eur J Obstet Gynecol Reprod Biol* 1999;85:23.
86. Kemp DC, Fan PW, Stevens JC. Characterization of raloxifene glucuronidation in vitro: contribution of intestinal metabolism to presystemic clearance. *Drug Metab Dispos* 2002;30:694.
87. Robertson JF, Odling-Smee W, Holcombe C, et al. Pharmacokinetics of a single dose of fulvestrant prolonged-release intramuscular injection in postmenopausal women awaiting surgery for primary breast cancer. *Clin Ther* 2003;25:1440.
88. Howell A, Osborne CK, Morris C, et al. ICI 182,780 (Faslodex): development of a novel, "pure" antiestrogen. *Cancer* 2000;89:817.
89. Howell A, DeFriend DJ, Robertson JF, et al. Pharmacokinetics, pharmacological and anti-tumour effects of the specific anti-oestrogen ICI 182780 in women with advanced breast cancer. *Br J Cancer* 1996;74:300.
90. Coopman P, Garcia M, Brunner N, et al. Anti-proliferative and anti-estrogenic effects of ICI 164,384 and ICI 182,780 in 4-OH-tamoxifen-resistant human breast-cancer cells. *Int J Cancer* 1994;56:295.
91. Wakeling AE, Bowler J. Steroidal pure antioestrogens. *J Endocrinol* 1987;112:R7.
92. Wakeling AE, Dukes M, Bowler J. A potent specific pure antiestrogen with clinical potential. *Cancer Res* 1991;51:3867.
93. Piccart M, Parker LM, Pritchard KI. Oestrogen receptor downregulation: an opportunity for extending the window of endocrine therapy in advanced breast cancer. *Ann Oncol* 2003;14:1017.
94. Howell A, Robertson JF, Quaresma Albano J, et al. Fulvestrant, formerly ICI 182,780, is as effective as anastrozole in postmenopausal women with advanced breast cancer progressing after prior endocrine treatment. *J Clin Oncol* 2002;20:3396.
95. Osborne CK, Pippen J, Jones SE, et al. Double-blind, randomized trial comparing the efficacy and tolerability of fulvestrant versus anastrozole in postmenopausal women with advanced breast cancer progressing on prior endocrine therapy: results of a North American trial. *J Clin Oncol* 2002;20:3386.
96. Robertson JF, Nicholson RI, Bundred NJ, et al. Comparison of the short-term biological effects of 7alpha-[9-(4,4,5,5,5-pentafluoropentylsulfinyl)-nonyl]estra-1,3,5, (10)-triene-3,17beta-diol (Faslodex) versus tamoxifen in postmenopausal women with primary breast cancer. *Cancer Res* 2001;61:6739.
97. Bonomi P, Pessis D, Bunting N, et al. Megestrol acetate used as primary hormonal therapy in stage D prostatic cancer. *Semin Oncol* 1985;12:36.
98. Loprinzi CL, Ellison NM, Schaid DJ, et al. Controlled trial of megestrol acetate for the treatment of cancer anorexia and cachexia. *J Natl Cancer Inst* 1990;82:1127.
99. Bruera E, Macmillan K, Kuehn N, et al. A controlled trial of megestrol acetate on appetite, caloric intake, nutritional status, and other symptoms in patients with advanced cancer. *Cancer* 1990;66:1279.
100. Feliu J, Gonzalez-Baron M, Berrocal A, et al. Usefulness of megestrol acetate in cancer cachexia and anorexia. A placebo-controlled study. *Am J Clin Oncol* 1992;15:436.
101. Tchekmedyian NS, Hickman M, Siau J, et al. Megestrol acetate in cancer anorexia and weight loss. *Cancer* 1992;69:1268.
102. Loprinzi CL, Michalak JC, Schaid DJ, et al. Phase III evaluation of four doses of megestrol acetate as therapy for patients with cancer anorexia and/or cachexia. *J Clin Oncol* 1993;11:762.
103. Loprinzi CL, Jensen MD, Jiang NS, et al. Effect of megestrol acetate on the human pituitary-adrenal axis. *Mayo Clin Proc* 1992;67:1160.
104. Leinung MC, Liporace R, Miller CH. Induction of adrenal suppression by megestrol acetate in patients with AIDS. *Ann Intern Med* 1995;122:843.
105. Rowland KM Jr, Loprinzi CL, Shaw EG, et al. Randomized double-blind placebo-controlled trial of cisplatin and etoposide plus megestrol acetate/placebo in extensive-stage small-cell lung cancer: a North Central Cancer Treatment Group study. *J Clin Oncol* 1996;14:135.
106. Loprinzi CL, Johnson PA, Jensen M. Megestrol acetate for anorexia and cachexia. *Oncology* 1992;49[Suppl 2]:46.
107. Von Roenn JH, Armstrong D, Kotler DP, et al. Megestrol acetate in patients with AIDS-related cachexia. *Ann Intern Med* 1994;121:393.
108. Alexieva-Figusch J, Blankenstein MA, Hop WC, et al. Treatment of metastatic breast cancer patients with different dosages of megestrol acetate; dose relations, metabolic and endocrine effects. *Eur J Cancer Clin Oncol* 1984;20:33.
109. Tseng L, Gurpide E. Effects of progestins on estradiol receptor levels in human endometrium. *J Clin Endocrinol Metab* 1975;41:402.
110. Gurpide E, Tseng L, Gusberg SB. Estrogen metabolism in normal and neoplastic endometrium. *Am J Obstet Gynecol* 1977;129:809.
111. Gordon GG, Altman K, Southren AL, et al. Human hepatic testosterone A-ring reductase activity: effect of medroxyprogesterone acetate. *J Clin Endocrinol Metab* 1971;32:457.
112. Allegra JC, Kiefer SM. Mechanisms of action of progestational agents. *Semin Oncol* 1985;12:3.
113. Ewing TM, Murphy LJ, Ng ML, et al. Regulation of epidermal growth factor receptor by progestins and glucocorticoids in human breast cancer cell lines. *Int J Cancer* 1989;44:744.
114. Martin F, Adlercreutz H. Aspects of megestrol acetate and medroxyprogesterone acetate metabolism. In: Garattini S, Berendes HW, eds. *Pharmacology of steroid contraceptive drugs.* New York: Raven Press, 1977:99.
115. Adlercreutz H, Eriksen PB, Christensen MS. Plasma concentration of megestrol acetate and medroxyprogesterone acetate after single oral administration to healthy subjects. *J Pharm Biomed Anal* 1983;1:153.
116. Gaver RC, Pittman KA, Reilly CM, et al. Bioequivalence evaluation of new megestrol acetate formulations in humans. *Semin Oncol* 1985;12:17.
117. Fotherby K, Kamyab S, Littleton P. Metabolism of synthetic progestational compounds in humans. *J Reprod Fertil* 1968;5[Suppl]:51.
118. Fukushima DK, Levin J, Liang JS, et al. Isolation and partial synthesis of a new metabolite of medroxyrogesterone acetate. *Steroids* 1979;34:57.
119. Utaaker E, Lundgren S, Kvinnsland S, et al. Pharmacokinetics and metabolism of medroxyprogesterone acetate in patients with advanced breast cancer. *J Steroid Biochem* 1988;31:437.
120. Sturm G, Haberlein H, Bauer T, et al. Mass spectrometric and high-performance liquid chromatographic studies of medroxyprogesterone acetate metabolites in human plasma. *J Chromatogr* 1991;562:351.
121. Pannuti F, Camaggi CM, Strocchi E. Medroxyprogesterone acetate pharmacokinetics. In: Pelligrini A, ed. *Role of medroxyprogesterone in endocrine related tumors.* New York: Raven Press, 1984:43.
122. Lundgren S, Lonning PE, Aakvaag A, et al. Influence of aminoglutethimide on the metabolism of medroxyprogesterone acetate and megestrol acetate in postmenopausal patients with advanced breast cancer. *Cancer Chemother Pharmacol* 1990;27:101.
123. Lundgren S, Kvinnsland S, Utaaker E, et al. Effect of oral high-dose progestins on the disposition of antipyrine, digitoxin, and warfarin in patients with advanced breast cancer. *Cancer Chemother Pharmacol* 1986;18:270.
124. Goss PE, Strasser K. Aromatase inhibitors in the treatment and prevention of breast cancer. *J Clin Oncol* 2001;19:881.
125. Buzdar A, Howell A. Advances in aromatase inhibition: clinical efficacy and tolerability in the treatment of breast cancer. *Clin Cancer Res* 2001;7:2620.
126. Santen RJ. Suppression of estrogens with aminoglutethimide and hydrocortisone (medical adrenalectomy) as treatment of advanced breast carcinoma: a review. *Breast Cancer Res Treat* 1981;1:183.
127. Schteingart DE, Cash R, Conn JW. Amino-glutethimide and metastatic adrenal cancer. Maintained reversal (six months) of Cushing's syndrome. *JAMA* 1966;198:1007.
128. Baum M, Budzar AU, Cuzick J, et al. Anastrozole alone or in combination with tamoxifen versus tamoxifen alone for adjuvant treatment of postmenopausal women with early breast cancer: first results of the ATAC randomised trial. *Lancet* 2002;359:2131.
129. Buzdar AU. Pharmacology and pharmacokinetics of the newer generation aromatase inhibitors. *Clin Cancer Res* 2003;9:468S.
130. Plourde PV, Dyroff M, Dukes M. Arimidex: a potent and selective fourth-generation aromatase inhibitor. *Breast Cancer Res Treat* 1994;30:103.
131. Bisagni G, Cocconi G, Scaglione F, et al. Letrozole, a new oral non-steroidal aromatase inhibitor in treating postmenopausal patients with advanced breast cancer. A pilot study. *Ann Oncol* 1996;7:99.
132. Dewar JA, Nabholtz JM, Bonneterre J, et al. The effect of anastrozole (Arimidex) on serum lipids: data from a randomized comparison of anastrozole (AN) versus tamoxifen (TAM) in postmenopausal (PM) women with advanced breast cancer (ABC). *Breast Cancer Res Treat* 2000;64:51.
133. Elisaf MS, Bairaktari ET, Nicolaides C, et al. Effect of letrozole on the lipid profile in postmenopausal women with breast cancer. *Eur J Cancer* 2001;37:1510.
134. Bhatnagar AS, Hausler A, Schieweck K, et al. Highly selective inhibition of estrogen biosynthesis by CGS 20267, a new non-steroidal aromatase inhibitor. *J Steroid Biochem Mol Biol* 1990;37:1021.
135. Bhatnagar AS, Hausler A, Schieweck K. Inhibition of aromatase in vitro and in vivo by aromatase inhibitors. *J Enzyme Inhib* 1990;4:179.
136. Demers LM. Effects of fadrozole (CGS 16949A) and letrozole (CGS 20267) on the inhibition of aromatase activity in breast cancer patients. *Breast Cancer Res Treat* 1994;30:95.
137. Lipton A, Demers LM, Harvey HA, et al. Letrozole (CGS 20267). A phase I study of a new potent oral aromatase inhibitor of breast cancer. *Cancer* 1995;75:2132.
138. Iveson TJ, Smith IE, Ahern J, et al. Phase I study of the oral nonsteroidal aromatase inhibitor CGS 20267 in postmenopausal patients with advanced breast cancer. *Cancer Res* 1993;53:266.
139. Trunet PF, Muller PH, Bhatnagar A. Phase I study in healthy male volunteers with the non-steroidal aromatase inhibitor GCS 20267. *Eur J Cancer* 1990;26:173.
140. Dukes M, Edwards PN, Large M, et al. The preclinical pharmacology of "Arimidex" (anastrozole; ZD1033)—a potent, selective aromatase inhibitor. *J Steroid Biochem Mol Biol* 1996;58:439.
141. Yates RA, Dowsett M, Fisher GV, et al. Arimidex (ZD1033): a selective, potent inhibitor of aromatase in postmenopausal female volunteers. *Br J Cancer* 1996;73:543.
142. Lonning PE, Geisler J, Dowsett M. Pharmacological and clinical profile of anastrozole. *Breast Cancer Res Treat* 1998;49[Suppl 1]:S53.
143. Geisler J, King N, Dowsett M, et al. Influence of anastrozole (Arimidex), a selective, non-steroidal aromatase inhibitor, on in vivo aromatisation and plasma oestrogen levels in postmenopausal women with breast cancer. *Br J Cancer* 1996;74:1286.
144. Kaufmann M, Bajetta E, Dirix LY, et al. Exemestane is superior to megestrol acetate after tamoxifen failure in postmenopausal women with advanced breast cancer: results of a phase III randomized double-blind trial. The Exemestane Study Group. *J Clin Oncol* 2000;18:1399.
145. Paridaens R, Dirix L, Lohrisch C, et al. Mature results of a randomized phase II multicenter study of exemestane versus tamoxifen as first-line hormone therapy for postmenopausal women with metastatic breast cancer. *Ann Oncol* 2003;14:1391.
146. Goss PE, Grynpas M, Qi S, et al. The effects of exemestane on bone and lipids in the ovariectomized rat. *Breast Cancer Res Treat* 2001;69:224.
147. Goss PE, C AM, Lowery C, et al. Comparison of the effects of exemestane, 17-hydroexemestane and letrozole on bone and lipid metabolism in the ovariectomized rat. *Breast Cancer Res Treat* 2002;76[Suppl 1]:S107.
148. Evans TR, Di Salle E, Ornati G, et al. Phase I and endocrine study of exemestane (FCE 24304), a new aromatase inhibitor, in postmenopausal women. *Cancer Res* 1992;52:5933.
149. Bajetta E, Zilembo N, Noberasco C, et al. The minimal effective exemestane dose for endocrine activity in advanced breast cancer. *Eur J Cancer* 1997;33:587.
150. Michaud LB, Buzdar AU. Risks and benefits of aromatase inhibitors in postmenopausal breast cancer. *Drug Saf* 1999;21:297.
151. Demers LM, Lipton A, Harvey HA, et al. The efficacy of CGS 20267 in suppressing estrogen biosynthesis in patients with advanced stage breast cancer. *J Steroid Biochem Mol Biol* 1993;44:687.

152. Spinelli R, Jannuzzo MG, Poggesi I, et al. Pharmacokinetics (PK) of Aromasin (Exemestane, EXE) after single and repeated doses in healthy postmenopausal volunteers (HPV). *Eur J Cancer* 1999;35[Suppl 4]:S295.

153. Johannessen DC, Engan T, Di Salle E, et al. Endocrine and clinical effects of exemestane (PNU 155971), a novel steroidal aromatase inhibitor, in postmenopausal breast cancer patients: a phase I study. *Clin Cancer Res* 1997;3:1101.

154. Jones S, Vogel C, Arkhipov A, et al. Multicenter, phase II trial of exemestane as third-line hormonal therapy of postmenopausal women with metastatic breast cancer. Aromasin Study Group. *J Clin Oncol* 1999;17:3418.

155. Ahmann FR, Citrin DL, deHaan HA, et al. Zoladex: a sustained-release, monthly luteinizing hormone-releasing hormone analogue for the treatment of advanced prostate cancer. *J Clin Oncol* 1987;5:912.

156. Corbin A. From contraception to cancer: a review of the therapeutic applications of LHRH analogues as antitumor agents. *Yale J Biol Med* 1982;55:27.

157. Kaufmann M, Jonat W, Blamey R, et al. Survival analyses from the ZEBRA study. Goserelin (Zoladex) versus CMF in premenopausal women with node-positive breast cancer. *Eur J Cancer* 2003;39:1711.

158. Harvey HA, Lipton A, Max DT, et al. Medical castration produced by the GnRH analogue leuprolide to treat metastatic breast cancer. *J Clin Oncol* 1985;3:1068.

159. Vogelzang NJ, Chodak GW, Soloway MS, et al. Goserelin versus orchiectomy in the treatment of advanced prostate cancer: final results of a randomized trial. Zoladex Prostate Study Group. *Urology* 1995;46:220.

160. Brogden RN, Faulds D. Goserelin. A review of its pharmacodynamic and pharmacokinetic properties and therapeutic efficacy in prostate cancer. *Drugs Aging* 1995;6:324.

161. Plosker GL, Brogden RN. Leuprorelin. A review of its pharmacology and therapeutic use in prostatic cancer, endometriosis and other sex hormone-related disorders. *Drugs* 1994;48:930.

162. Brogden RN, Buckley MM, Ward A. Buserelin. A review of its pharmacodynamic and pharmacokinetic properties, and clinical profile. *Drugs* 1990;39:399.

163. Nillius SJ. The therapeutic uses of gonadotropin-releasing hormone and its analogues. In: Beardwell C, Robertson GL, eds. *Clinical endocrinology 1: the pituitary.* London: Butterworth, 1981:211.

164. Harvey HA, Lipton A, Max DT. LH-RH agonist treatment breast cancer: a phase II study in the USA. In: Klijn JG, ed. *Hormonal manipulation of cancer.* New York: Raven Press, 1987:321.

165. Klijn JG, DeJong FH, Blankenstein MA. Anti-tumor and endocrine effects of chronic LHRH agonist treatment (buserelin) with or without tamoxifen in premenopausal metastatic breast cancer. *Breast Cancer Res Treat* 1984;4:209.

166. Clayton RN, Bailey LC, Cottam J, et al. A radioimmunoassay for GnRH agonist analogue in serum of patients with prostate cancer treated with D-Ser (tBu)6 AZA Gly10 GnRH. *Clin Endocrinol (Oxf)* 1985;22:453.

167. Chrisp P, Goa KL. Goserelin. A review of its pharmacodynamic and pharmacokinetic properties, and clinical use in sex hormone-related conditions. *Drugs* 1991;41:254.

168. Brogden RN, Clissold SP. Flutamide. A preliminary review of its pharmacodynamic and pharmacokinetic properties, and therapeutic efficacy in advanced prostatic cancer. *Drugs* 1989;38:185.

169. Wysowski DK, Freiman JP, Tourtelot JB, et al. Fatal and nonfatal hepatotoxicity associated with flutamide. *Ann Intern Med* 1993;118:860.

170. Brogden RN, Chrisp P. Flutamide. A review of its pharmacodynamic and pharmacokinetic properties, and therapeutic use in advanced prostatic cancer. *Drugs Aging* 1991;1:104.

171. Radwanski E, Perentesis G, Symchowicz S, et al. Single and multiple dose pharmacokinetic evaluation of flutamide in normal geriatric volunteers. *J Clin Pharmacol* 1989;29:554.

172. Schellhammer PF, Sharifi R, Block NL, et al. A controlled trial of bicalutamide versus flutamide, each in combination with luteinizing hormone-releasing hormone analogue therapy, in patients with advanced prostate carcinoma. Analysis of time to progression. CASODEX Combination Study Group. *Cancer* 1996;78:2164.

173. Furr BJ. Casodex (ICI 176,334)—a new, pure, peripherally-selective anti-androgen: preclinical studies. *Horm Res* 1989;32[Suppl 1]:69.

174. Furr BJ. Casodex: preclinical studies. *Eur Urol* 1990;18[Suppl 3]:2.

175. Kennealey GT, Furr BJ. Use of the nonsteroidal anti-androgen Casodex in advanced prostatic carcinoma. *Urol Clin North Am* 1991;18:99.

176. Mahler C, Verhelst J, Denis L. Clinical pharmacokinetics of the antiandrogens and their efficacy in prostate cancer. *Clin Pharmacokinet* 1998;34:405.

177. Dole EJ, Holdsworth MT. Nilutamide: an antiandrogen for the treatment of prostate cancer. *Ann Pharmacother* 1997;31:65-75.

178. Kennedy BJ. Hormonal therapies in breast cancer. *Semin Oncol* 1974;1:119.

179. Colburn WA. Radioimmunoassay for fluoxymesterone (Halotestin). *Steroids* 1975;25:43.

180. Kammerer RC, Merdink JL, Jagels M, et al. Testing for fluoxymesterone (Halotestin) administration to man: identification of urinary metabolites by gas chromatography-mass spectrometry. *J Steroid Biochem* 1990;36:659.

181. Ingle JN, Ahmann DL, Green SJ, et al. Randomized clinical trial of diethylstilbestrol versus tamoxifen in postmenopausal women with advanced breast cancer. *N Engl J Med* 1981;304:16.

182. Stewart HJ, Forrest AP, Gunn JM, et al. The tamoxifen trial—a double-blind comparison with stilboestrol in postmenopausal women with advanced breast cancer. *Eur J Cancer* 1980;[Suppl 1]1:83.

183. Byar DP. Proceedings: The Veterans Administration Cooperative Urological Research Group's studies of cancer of the prostate. *Cancer* 1973;32:1126.

184. Marselos M, Tomatis L. Diethylstilboestrol: I, pharmacology, toxicology and carcinogenicity in humans. *Eur J Cancer* 1992;28A:1182.

185. Metzler M. Metabolic activation of carcinogenic diethylstilbestrol in rodents and humans. *J Toxicol Environ Health* 1976;[Suppl 1]:21.

186. Loose-Mitchell DS, Stancel GM. Estrogens and progestins. In: Hardman JG, Limbird LE, Goodman Gilman A, eds. *The pharmacological basis of therapeutics.* New York: McGraw-Hill, 2001.

187. Bajetta E, Procopio G, Ferrari L, et al. A randomized, multicenter prospective trial assessing long-acting release octreotide pamoate plus tamoxifen as a first line therapy for advanced breast carcinoma. *Cancer* 2002;94:299.

188. Cascinu S, Fedeli A, Fedeli SL, et al. Control of chemotherapy-induced diarrhea with octreotide in patients receiving 5-fluorouracil. *Eur J Cancer* 1992;28:482.

189. Cascinu S, Fedeli A, Fedeli SL, et al. Octreotide versus loperamide in the treatment of fluorouracil-induced diarrhea: a randomized trial. *J Clin Oncol* 1993;11:148.

190. Gebbia V, Carreca I, Testa A, et al. Subcutaneous octreotide versus oral loperamide in the treatment of diarrhea following chemotherapy. *Anticancer Drugs* 1993;4:443.

191. Cascinu S, Fedeli A, Fedeli SL, et al. Control of chemotherapy-induced diarrhea with octreotide. A randomized trial with placebo in patients receiving cisplatin. *Oncology* 1994;51:70.

192. Wasserman E, Hidalgo M, Hornedo J, et al. Octreotide (SMS 201-995) for hematopoietic support-dependent high-dose chemotherapy (HSD-HDC)-related diarrhea: dose finding study and evaluation of efficacy. *Bone Marrow Transplant* 1997;20:711.

193. Yavuz MN, Yavuz AA, Ilis E, et al. A randomized study of the efficacy of octreotide versus diphenoxylate on radiation-induced diarrhea. *Proc Am Soc Clin Oncol* 2000;19:2370.

194. Wadler S, Benson AB 3rd, Engelking C, et al. Recommended guidelines for the treatment of chemotherapy-induced diarrhea. *J Clin Oncol* 1998;16:3169.

195. Harris AG. Somatostatin and somatostatin analogues: pharmacokinetics and pharmacodynamic effects. *Gut* 1994;35:S1.

196. Chanson P, Timsit J, Harris AG. Clinical pharmacokinetics of octreotide. Therapeutic applications in patients with pituitary tumours. *Clin Pharmacokinet* 1993;25:375.

197. Marbach P, Briner U, Lemaire M. From somatostatin to Sandostatin: pharmacodynamics and pharmacokinetics. *Digestion* 1993;54[Suppl 1]:9.

198. Rubin J, Ajani J, Schirmer W, et al. Octreotide acetate long-acting formulation versus open-label subcutaneous octreotide acetate in malignant carcinoid syndrome. *J Clin Oncol* 1999;17:600.

199. Lien EA, Solheim E, Ueland PM. Distribution of tamoxifen and its metabolites in rat and human tissues during steady-state treatment. *Cancer Res* 1991;51:4837.

200. Lien EA, Wester K, Lonning PE, Solheim E, Ueland PM. Distribution of tamoxifen and its metabolites into brain tissue and brain metastases in breast cancer patients. *Br J Cancer* 1991;63:641.

201. Daniel P, Gaskell SJ, Bishop H, Campbell C, Nicholson RI. Determination of tamoxifen and biologically active metabolites in human breast tumours and plasma. *Eur J Cancer Clin Oncol* 1981;17:1183.

202. Robinson SP, Langan-Fahey SM, Johnson DA, Jordan VC. Metabolites, pharmacodynamics, and pharmacokinetics of tamoxifen in rats and mice compared to the breast cancer patient. *Drug Metab Dispos* 1991;19:36.

203. DeGregorio MW, Wiebe VJ, Venook AP, Holleran WM. Elevated plasma tamoxifen levels in a patient with liver obstruction. *Cancer Chemother Pharmacol* 1989;23:194.

204. Lodwick R, McConkey B, Brown AM. Life threatening interaction between tamoxifen and warfarin. *Br Med J (Clin Res Ed)* 1987;295:1141.

205. Ritchie LD, Grant SM. Tamoxifen-warfarin interaction: the Aberdeen hospitals drug file. *BMJ* 1989;298:1253.

206. Tenni P, Lalich DL, Byrne MJ. Life threatening interaction between tamoxifen and warfarin. *BMJ* 1989;298:93.

207. Camaggi CM, Strocchi E, Canova N, Costanti B, Pannuti F. Medroxyprogesterone acetate (MAP) and tamoxifen (TMX) plasma levels after simultaneous treatment with 'low' TMX and 'high' MAP doses. *Cancer Chemother Pharmacol* 1985;14:229.

208. Rabinowicz AL, Hinton DR, Dyck P, Couldwell WT. High-dose tamoxifen in treatment of brain tumors: interaction with antiepileptic drugs. *Epilepsia* 1995;36:513.

Richard M. Simon

CHAPTER **18**

Design and Analysis of Clinical Trials

Clinical trials are experiments to determine the value of treatments. There are two key components to the experimental approach. First, results rather than plausible reasoning are required to support conclusions. Second, experiments should be prospectively planned and conducted under controlled conditions to provide definitive answers to well-defined questions. Comparing the survival rates (based on tumor registry data) of prostate cancer patients treated with surgery to those of patients receiving radiotherapy is an example of an *observational study*, not a clinical trial. In an observational study, the investigators are passive observers. Treatment assignments, staging workup, and follow-up procedures are out of the control of the investigators and are conducted with no considerations about the validity of the subsequent attempt at comparison. The statistical associations resulting from such studies are, consequently, a weak basis for causal inferences about relationships between the treatments administered and the outcomes observed. Treatments are usually selected on the basis of subjective assessment of the prognosis of the patient, specialties of the physician, and various diagnostic evaluations. Unknown patient selection factors generally are more important determinants of patient outcome than are differences between treatments.

Clinical trials require careful planning. The first result of the planning process is a written protocol. Typical subject headings for the protocol are shown in Table 18-1, and the protocol development process is discussed in more detail by McFadden[1] and by Green et al.[2] The protocol should define treatment and evaluation policies for a well-defined set of patients. It also should define the specific questions to be answered by the study and should directly justify that the number of patients and the nature of the controls are adequate to answer these questions. Some clinical trials are really only guidelines for clinical management supplemented by lofty objectives with no scientific

meaning and no realistic chance of providing a reliable answer to a well-defined medical question. Such studies do not warrant the expenditure of limited clinical research dollars and represent a disservice to the patients who may be willing to undergo some inconvenience to contribute to the welfare of future patients. In this chapter, the author attempts to provide information that will help to avoid such clinical trials.

PHASE I CLINICAL TRIALS

The objective of a phase I trial is to determine a dose that is appropriate for use in phase II and III trials. Patients with advanced disease that is resistant to standard therapy are usually included in such trials, but it is important that the patients have normal organ function.

Phase I trials of a new cytotoxic drug are designed to determine the maximal tolerated dose. Such studies are usually performed by starting with a low dose that is not expected to produce serious toxicity in any patients. A starting dose of one-tenth the lethal dose (expressed as milligrams per square meter of body surface area) in the most sensitive species usually is used.[3] This dose is increased for subsequent patients according to a series of preplanned steps. Dose escalation for subsequent patients occurs only after sufficient time has passed to observe acute toxic effects for patients treated at lower doses. Cohorts of three to six patients are treated at each dose level. Usually, if no dose-limiting toxicity (DLT) is seen at a given dose level, the dose is escalated for the next cohort. If the incidence of DLT is 33%, then three more patients are treated at the same level. If no further cases of DLT are seen in the additional patients, then the dose level is escalated for the next cohort. Otherwise, dose escalation stops. If the incidence of DLT is greater than

TABLE 18-1. Subject Headings for a Protocol

Introduction and scientific background
Objectives
Selection of patients
Design of study (including schematic diagram)
Treatment plan
Drug information
Toxicities to be monitored and dosage modifications
Required clinical and laboratory data and study calendar
Criteria for evaluating the effect of treatment and end point definition
Statistical considerations
Informed consent and regulatory considerations
Data forms
References
Study chairperson, collaborating participants, addresses, and telephone numbers

33% at a given level, then dose escalation also stops. The phase II recommended dose often is taken as the highest dose for which the incidence of DLT is less than 33%. Usually, six or more patients are treated at the recommended dose.

The dose levels themselves are commonly based on a modified Fibonacci series. The second level is twice the starting dose, the third level is 67% greater than the second, the fourth level is 50% greater than the third, the fifth is 40% greater than the fourth, and each subsequent step is 33% greater than that preceding it. Escalating doses for subsequent courses in the same patient are generally not done, except at low doses before any DLT has been encountered.

ACCELERATED TITRATION DESIGNS

There is no compelling scientific basis for the approach just outlined, except that experience has shown it to be safe. Traditional phase I trials have three limitations:

1. They sometimes expose too many patients to subtherapeutic doses of the new drug.
2. The trials may take a long time to complete.
3. They provide very limited information about interpatient variability and cumulative toxicity.

New trial designs have been developed to address these problems.[4] One new class of designs, *accelerated titration designs*,[5] permit within-patient dose escalation and use only one patient per dose level until grade 2 or greater toxicity is seen. Doses are titrated within patients to achieve grade 2 toxicity. The analysis consists of fitting a statistical model to the full set of data that includes all grades of toxicity for all courses of a patient's treatment. The model includes parameters that represent the steepness of the dose-toxicity curve, the degree of interpatient variability in the location of the dose-toxicity curve, and the degree (if any) of cumulative toxicity. All these parameters are estimated from the data.

In developing the accelerated titration designs, Simon et al.[5] fit a stochastic model to data from 20 phase I trials of nine different drugs. New data were then simulated using the model with the parameters estimated from the actual trials, and the performance of alternative phase I designs on this simulated data was evaluated. Design 1 was a conventional design using cohorts of three to six patients with 40% dose-step increments

and no intrapatient dose escalation. Designs 2 through 4 included only one patient per cohort until one patient experienced DLT or two patients experienced grade 2 toxicity. Designs 3 and 4 use 100% dose steps during this initial accelerated phase. After the initial accelerated phase, designs 2 through 4 resort to standard cohorts of three to six patients with 40% dose-step increments. Designs 2 through 4 use intrapatient dose escalation if the worst toxicity is grade 0 to 1 in the previous course for that patient.

Only three of the actual trials showed any evidence of cumulative toxicity. The average number of patients required was reduced from 39.9 for design 1 to 24.4, 20.7, and 21.2 for designs 2, 3, and 4, respectively. The average number of patients who had grade 0 to 1 toxicity as their worst toxicity grade over three cycles of treatment was 23.3 for design 1 but only 7.9, 3.9, and 4.8 for designs 2, 3, and 4, respectively. The average number of patients with a worst toxicity grade of 3 increased from 5.5 for design 1 to 6.2, 6.8, and 6.2 for designs 2, 3, and 4, respectively. The average number of patients with a worst toxicity grade of 4 increased from 1.9 for design 1 to 3.0, 4.3, and 3.2 for designs 2, 3, and 4, respectively. Accelerated titration designs appear to be effective in reducing the number of patients who are undertreated, speeding the completion of phase I trials, and providing increased information.

CONTINUAL REASSESSMENT METHODS

O'Quigley et al.[6] used a dose-toxicity model to guide the dose escalation, as well as to determine the maximum tolerated dose. The model used contains a parameter α that reflects the steepness of the dose-toxicity curve.[6] A Bayesian prior distribution is established for the parameter and the distribution is updated after each patient is treated. The model is based on using only first-course treatment data and whether the patient experiences DLT. This approach is called the *continual reassessment method*. For each new patient, the model is used to determine the dose predicted to cause DLT to a specified percentage of the patients. That dose is assigned to the next patient. Many modifications of the original continual reassessment method have been subsequently proposed by O'Quigley[7] and others.[8-11] The continual reassessment method approach has two objectives: to reduce the number of undertreated patients and to provide a better estimate of the maximum tolerated dose.

Today, there are phase I trials other than the traditional single-agent cytotoxic phase I study. Some phase I trials involve the simultaneous escalation of two or more drugs. The design of such trials has been discussed by Korn and Simon.[12]

VACCINES AND MOLECULARLY TARGETED DRUGS

There is an increasing need to identify the dose for therapeutics expected to be nontoxic. Some molecularly targeted drugs and therapeutic vaccines are of this type. Simon et al.[13] suggested that many therapeutic vaccines do not require a toxicity trial because they are based on DNA constructs, viral vectors, and cytokines that have been determined as safe from previous clinical trials. They also pointed out that end-stage patients without intact immune systems have little likelihood of benefit or toxicity from a tumor vaccine. Feasibility issues limit the maximum doses of certain recombinant proteins, viruses, or whole tumor cell vaccines that can be produced for administration to patients. Hence, in many cases, the dose selected will be based on preclinical findings or on practical considerations.

For many molecularly targeted therapeutics, preclinical studies provide a target serum concentration of the active moiety necessary to maximally inhibit the target. In such cases, the phase I trial can be designed to estimate the relationship between the dose administered and serum concentration. In some cases, drug administration can be titrated for each patient to the targeted serum concentration. In others, a cohort of patients are treated at each of several dose levels without intrapatient dose titration. If small cohorts at many dose levels are used, then it may be best to fit a statistical model to the dose versus concentration data. In many cases, the target concentration is a steady-state level or a concentration integrated over time ($C \times T$). Rubinstein and Simon[14] provide a formula for determining the sample size per dose level for this approach. In some cases, phase I studies of the pharmacokinetics of a molecularly targeted drug have been carried out in healthy volunteers.

If a target serum concentration of a nontoxic molecularly targeted drug is not known, the design of a meaningful phase I trial becomes more difficult. Often, low doses have no effect—there is an approximately linear dose region and then saturation of effect at high dose. For molecularly targeted therapeutics, the biologic effect might be a measure of the degree of inhibition of the target. Because it can be very difficult to obtain tumor samples before and after treatment, biologic effect is sometimes measured in an accessible surrogate tissue, such as peripheral blood lymphocytes or skin, or by using functional imaging.[15] For therapeutic vaccines, the biologic effect might be a measure of stimulation of tumor reactive T cells.

Ideally, a trial design should provide the smallest dose that gives maximum biologic effect. This is rarely practical in a phase I trial, as it requires a large number of patients. In comparing the mean response between two doses, the number of patients per dose is $2(k_\alpha + k_\beta)^2 / (\delta/\sigma)^2$, where k_α and k_β are percentiles of the standard gaussian distribution, α is the significance level for the comparison, 1-β is the statistical power for detecting a difference in means between the two doses of size δ, and σ is the standard deviation of biologic responses among different patients in the same dose group. For example, suppose we have a phase I trial of k dose levels and we wish to select the level for which the biologic response is significantly greater than the next lower level and not significantly less than the next higher level. If the significance tests are performed at the one-sided 0.10 level (α) and the statistical power is 0.90 (1-β) for detecting a 1 standard deviation difference in means, then $k_\alpha = k_\beta = 1.28$, $\delta/\sigma = 1$, and n = 13.1. Consequently, 14 patients per dose level are required. σ Incorporates both interpatient biologic variability and assay variability. For $\delta/\sigma = 0.75$, the resulting sample size increases to n = 24 per dose level.

A more limited objective is to identify a dose that is biologically active. Korn et al.[16] developed a sequential procedure for finding such a dose when the measure of biologic response is binary. During an initial accelerated phase they treat one patient per dose level until a biologic response is seen. Then,

they treat cohorts of three to six patients per dose level. With 0 to 1 biologic responses among three patients at a dose level, they escalate to the next level. With 2 to 3 responses among three patients, they expand the cohort to six patients. With 5 to 6 biologic responses from the six patients, they declare that dose to be the biologically active level and terminate the trial. With 4 or fewer biologic responses at a level, they continue to escalate.

PHASE II CLINICAL TRIALS

PATIENT SELECTION

Whereas phase I trials need not be performed separately by tumor type, this is not usually the case for phase II trials, because the biologic response of interest is that of the tumor itself. When a drug enters phase II trials, it should be tested in the patient group that is most likely to show a favorable effect but for whom no effective therapy is available. This is best accomplished by patients with maximum performance status and a minimum amount of prior chemotherapy. Full-dose chemotherapy is often impossible in patients debilitated by prior treatment, and lack of chemotherapeutic activity in previously treated patients may not indicate lack of clinical usefulness in earlier disease. This issue was well illustrated by etoposide in small cell lung carcinoma. For the less chemosensitive cancers, chemotherapy offers little or no palliative benefit, and initial phase II trials should be conducted in patients with no prior chemotherapy. For very chemosensitive tumors, the "window-of-opportunity design" sometimes is used; non–previously treated patients are given one or two courses of a phase II drug and then are switched to a standard combination. In general, agents should be shown to be active in a favorable population of patients before they are given to a less favorable group. Adherence to this principle saves patients with advanced disease from exposure to inactive agents for which the likelihood of toxicity is much greater than the likelihood of benefit.

Molecularly targeted drugs should be studied in an adequate number of patients whose tumors express the target. Consequently, it is important to develop an adequate assay for the target and have the assay available at the time that phase II development begins.[15]

TRIALS OF SINGLE AGENTS

There is some confusion about the appropriate objectives of phase II trials. For most single-agent phase II trials, the objective is simply to determine whether the drug has activity against the tumor type in question. For this objective, response rate is an appropriate end point. It is important to recognize, however, that tumor response is not a direct measure of patient benefit, and, hence, it cannot be assumed that response rate is an appropriate end point for drawing conclusions about treatment efficacy. A treatment that causes partial responses is not necessarily beneficial to the patient, and analyses that demonstrate that responders live longer than nonresponders are invalid for concluding that a treatment extended survival.[17,18] First, *responders*, by definition, have lived long enough to achieve that status. Second, responders may have more favorable prognostic factors. Finally, treatment may shorten survival of nonresponders while not influencing survival of responders. To demonstrate that treatment extends survival, it must be demonstrated that the treated group as a whole lives longer than an appropriate control group. Phase II trials do not have an internal control group and, hence, drawing conclusions about survival from such trials is very problematic.

A variety of statistical accrual plans and sample size methods have been developed for phase II trials. One of the most popular approaches is the optimal two-stage design.[19] A number (n_1) of evaluable patients is entered into study in the first stage of the trial. If no more than than a specified r_1 responses are obtained among these n_1 patients, then accrual terminates and the drug is rejected as being of little interest. Otherwise, accrual continues to a total of n evaluable patients. At the end of the second stage, the drug is rejected if the observed response rate is less than or equal to r/n, where r and n are determined by the design used.

Tables 18-2 and 18-3 illustrate some of these optimized designs. To select a design, researchers must specify a target activity level of interest, p_1, and also a lower activity level, p_0. The first row of each triplet of optimal designs provides designs with probability $\leq .10$ of accepting drugs worse than p_0 and probability $\leq .10$ of rejecting drugs better than p_1. Subject to these two constraints, the optimal designs minimize the average sample size. The average sample size is calculated at the lower activity level p_0 to optimize protection of patients from exposure to inactive drugs. The tables show for each design the optimal values of r_1, n_1, r, and n; the average sample size; and the probability of stopping after the first stage for a drug with activity level p_0.

These tables also show the "minimax" designs, which provide the smallest maximum sample size n that satisfies the two constraints just described. Although minimax designs have somewhat larger average sample sizes than do optimal designs, in some instances, they are preferable because the small increase in average sample size is more than compensated for by a large reduction in maximum sample size.

The designs shown in Tables 18-2 and 18-3 are two-stage designs with the potential for early stopping for lack of activity. Optimized three-stage designs have been described by Ensign et al.[20] Others have developed methods to include toxicity[21,22] or progression information[23] explicitly into the design.

When sufficient numbers of patients and several treatments are available to test, there are advantages to randomized phase II trials.[24] Although phase II trials are not comparative, in selecting the most promising treatment or schedule to pursue, it is advantageous to evaluate the candidates on comparable patients. Table

TABLE 18-2.   Simon Two-Stage Phase II Designs for $p_1 - p_0 = .20^a$

		Optimal Design				Minimax Design			
		Reject Drug if Response Rate				Reject Drug if Response Rate			
p_0	p_1	$\leq r_1/n_1$	$\leq r/n$	EN (p_0)	PET (p_0)	$\leq r_1/n_1$	$\leq r/n$	EN (p_0)	PET (p_0)
.05	.25	0/9	2/24	14.5	.63	0/13	2/20	16.4	.51
		0/9	2/17	12.0	.63	0/12	2/16	13.8	.54
		0/9	3/30	16.8	.63	0/15	3/25	20.4	.46
.10	.30	1/12	5/35	19.8	.65	1/16	4/25	20.4	.51
		1/10	5/29	15.0	.74	1/15	5/25	19.5	.55
		2/18	6/36	22.5	.71	2/22	6/23	26.2	.62
.20	.40	3/17	10/37	26.0	.55	3/19	10/36	28.2	.46
		3/13	12/43	20.6	.75	4/18	10/33	22.3	.50
		4/19	15/54	30.4	.67	5/24	13/45	31.2	.66
.30	.50	7/22	17/46	29.9	.67	7/28	15/39	35.0	.36
		5/15	18/46	23.6	.72	6/19	16/39	25.7	.48
		8/24	24/63	34.7	.73	7/24	21/53	36.6	.56
.40	.60	7/18	22/46	30.2	.56	11/28	20/41	33.8	.55
		7/16	23/46	24.5	.72	17/34	20/39	34.4	.91
		11/25	32/66	36.0	.73	12/29	27/54	38.1	.64
.50	.70	11/21	26/45	29.0	.67	11/23	23/39	31.0	.50
		8/15	26/43	23.5	.70	12/23	23/37	27.7	.66
		13/24	36/61	34.0	.73	14/27	32/53	36.1	.65
.60	.80	6/11	26/38	25.4	.47	18/27	24/35	28.5	.82
		7/11	30/43	20.5	.70	8/13	25/35	20.8	.65
		12/19	37/53	29.5	.69	15/26	32/45	35.9	.48
.70	.90	6/9	22/28	17.8	.54	11/16	20/25	20.1	.55
		4/6	22/27	14.8	.58	19/23	21/26	23.2	.95
		11/15	29/36	21.2	.70	13/18	26/32	22.7	.67

^{a}For each value of (p_0, p_1), designs are given for three sets of error probabilities (α, β). The first, second, and third rows correspond to error probability limits (.10, .10), (.05, .20), and (.05, .10), respectively. α is the probability of accepting a drug with response probability p_0. β is the probability of rejecting a drug with response probability p_1. For each design, EN (p_0) and PET (p_0) denote the expected sample size and the probability of early termination when the true response probability is p_0.

TABLE 18-3. Simon Two-Stage Phase II Designs for $p_1 - p_0 = .15$[a]

		Optimal Design				Minimax Design			
		Reject Drug if Response Rate				Reject Drug if Response Rate			
p_0	p_1	$\leq r_1/n_1$	$\leq r/n$	EN (p_0)	PET (p_0)	$\leq r_1/n_1$	$\leq r/n$	EN (p_0)	PET (p_0)
.05	.20	0/12	3/37	23.5	.54	0/18	3/32	26.4	.40
		0/10	3/29	17.6	.60	0/13	3/27	19.8	.51
		1/21	4/41	26.7	.72	1/29	4/38	32.9	.57
.10	.25	2/21	7/50	31.2	.65	2/27	6/40	33.7	.48
		2/18	7/43	24.7	.73	2/22	7/40	28.8	.62
		2/21	10/66	36.8	.65	3/31	9/55	40.0	.62
.20	.35	5/27	16/63	43.6	.54	6/33	15/58	45.5	.50
		5/22	19/72	35.4	.73	6/31	15/53	40.4	.57
		8/37	22/83	51.4	.69	8/42	21/77	58.4	.53
.30	.45	9/30	29/82	51.4	.59	16/50	25/69	56.0	.68
		9/27	30/81	41.7	.73	16/46	25/65	49.6	.81
		13/40	40/110	60.8	.70	27/77	33/88	78.5	.86
.40	.55	16/38	40/88	54.5	.67	18/45	34/73	57.2	.56
		11/26	40/84	44.9	.67	28/59	34/70	60.1	.90
		19/45	49/104	64.0	.68	24/62	45/94	78.9	.47
.50	.65	18/35	47/84	53.0	.63	19/40	41/72	58.0	.44
		15/28	48/83	43.7	.71	39/66	40/68	66.1	.95
		22/42	60/105	62.3	.68	28/57	54/93	75.0	.50
.60	.75	21/34	47/71	47.1	.65	25/43	43/64	54.4	.46
		17/27	46/67	39.4	.69	18/30	43/62	43.8	.57
		21/34	64/95	55.6	.65	48/72	57/84	73.2	.90
.70	.85	14/20	45/59	36.2	.58	15/22	40/52	36.8	.51
		14/19	46/59	30.3	.72	16/23	39/49	34.4	.56
		18/25	61/79	43.4	.66	33/44	53/68	48.5	.81
.80	.95	5/7	27/31	20.8	.42	5/7	27/31	20.8	.42
		7/9	26/29	17.7	.56	7/9	26/29	17.7	.56
		16/19	37/42	24.4	.76	31/35	35/40	35.3	.94

[a]For each value of (p_0, p_1), designs are given for three sets of error probabilities (α, β). The first, second, and third rows correspond to error probability limits (.10, .10), (.05, .20), and (.05, .10), respectively. α is the probability of accepting a drug with response probability p_0. β is the probability of rejecting a drug with response probability p_1. For each design, EN (p_0) and PET (p_0) denote the expected sample size and the probability of early termination when the true response probability is p_0.

18-4 shows the number of patients per treatment arm required to ensure that the best treatment will have the highest observed response rate. This calculation assumes that the true response probability for the best treatment is 10 percentage points better than for the others. Simon et al.[24] provide similar tables for 15% differences. This selection approach is useful when one treatment will be carried forward and the treatments are similar with regard to cost and toxicity. Steinberg and Venzon[25] developed two-stage randomized phase II selection designs.

TRIALS OF COMBINATION REGIMENS

Many so-called phase II trials of combination regimens are conducted. The objectives of such trials are often unclear. One reasonable objective is sometimes merely to ensure that the combination is feasible and tolerable when used in a multicenter setting before embarking on a phase III trial. Achieving this objective does not require many patients. An alternative objective is to determine whether the new regimen is promising enough to warrant a phase

TABLE 18-4. Number of Patients per Treatment Group for Selecting Better Treatment When True Response Probabilities Differ by 10 Percentage Points[a]

Baseline Response Probability	85% Probability of Correct Selection	90% Probability of Correct Selection
.05	20	29
.10	28	42
.15	35	53
.20	41	62
.30	49	75
.40	54	82
.50	54	82
.60	49	75
.70	41	62
.80	28	53

[a]Assumes that investigator is indifferent to treatment selected when true response probabilities differ by less than 10 percentage points.

TABLE 18-5. Number of Patients Needed in an Experimental Group for 80% Power to Detect (One-Sided $\alpha = 0.05$) a Specified Difference in Success Rates

Proportion of Success for Historical Controls	No. of Historical Controls (Patients)						
	20	30	40	50	75	100	200
0.10	a	223[b]	108	80	58	50	42
	116	53[c]	40	35	29	27	24
	39	27[d]	23	21	18	18	16
	22	17[e]	15	14	13	13	12
0.20	a	a	285	167	101	83	65
	385	98	67	55	44	40	35
	67	40	33	30	26	24	22
	31	23	21	19	18	17	16
0.30	a	a	554	259	137	108	80
	882	137	87	69	54	48	42
	86	49	39	35	30	29	26
	31	27	24	22	20	19	18
0.40	a	a	699	303	153	120	88
	913	147	92	74	58	52	44
	85	50	41	36	32	30	27
	36	27	24	22	21	20	19
0.50	a	a	538	267	145	115	86
	455	122	83	68	55	50	43
	67	44	37	34	30	28	26
	30	24	22	20	18	18	17
0.60	a	a	295	185	117	97	76
	179	83	63	55	46	42	38
	45	33	29	27	25	24	22
	22	19	17	17	15	15	15

[a]Required sample size >1000.
[b]Number of patients needed for the new treatment to detect a difference in success rate of 15 percentage points.
[c]Number of patients needed to detect a difference in success rate of 20 percentage points.
[d]Number of patients needed to detect a difference in success rate of 25 percentage points.
[e]Number of patients needed to detect a difference in success rate of 30 percentage points.

III trial. If an optimal two-stage design or minimax design is used, the response probability of no interest (p_0) should represent the level of activity of the most active single-agent component or the level of activity of previously studied combination regimens (as presumably the new regimen would be considered promising only if it is promising relative to other existing regimens).

Although Tables 18-2 and 18-3 can be used for the design of phase II trials of combination regimens, one should take into account the sizes of the studies on which the specification of p_0 was based, and these studies should be prospectively identified so that a specific group of patients can be evaluated for prognostic comparability. Although such historical control comparisons are not considered reliable enough to eliminate the need for phase III trials, if done carefully, they will provide better decisions about which new regimens are worthy of phase III evaluation. For comparative trials of response rates using historical controls, appropriate tables for sample size planning are given by Makuch and Simon[26] and are summarized in Table 18-5. This table is for achieving 80% power with a one-sided 5% significance level. If the historical control group of 50 patients showed a response rate of 30%, and the target level of improvement is a 50% response rate, then 69 patients should be treated with the experimental regimen. If there were 100 appropriate historical control patients, then only 48 new patients are required. If there were only 30 historical control patients, then 137 new patients are needed for the experimental treatment. If the uncertainty in the level of response

achievable with standard treatment is substantial because of the limited number of appropriate historical controls, then it is not efficient to conduct a phase II trial of the new regimen. It would be more efficient to conduct a randomized phase II or phase III trial of the new regimen and the standard treatment.

Thall et al.[27] have developed Bayesian methods for planning and conducting trials in which the precision in the response probability p_0 is quantified by a "prior probability distribution." These Bayesian designs provide for continual analysis of results after evaluation of response for each patient. This is difficult logistically for multicenter trials but provides a valid statistical basis for the intensive monitoring of cancer center or pharmaceutical industry trials in which patients may be limited or time may be critical. One begins with a prior probability distribution for p_1 that is flat over the range 0 to 1. After each patient is evaluated on the experimental regimen, the "posterior probability distribution" for p_1 is updated. This permits calculation of the posterior probability distribution for $p_1 - p_0$.

Let δ denote the difference in response probabilities that is of interest. If, at some point during the trial, the posterior probability that $p_1 - p_0 \geq \delta$ becomes small—say less than 0.05—one might terminate the trial and conclude that the new regimen is not promising. If, at some point during the trial, the posterior probability that $p_1 - p_0 \geq 0$ becomes large—say greater than 0.95—one might terminate the trial and conclude that the new regimen appears better than the historical control. In this case, one could

TABLE 18-6. Thall-Simon Bayesian Phase II Design

| p_1 | Sample Size Percentiles | | | Probability Reject Regimen | Probability Accept Regimen |
	25%	50%	75%		
.20	10	12	20	.92	.07
.40	10	13	22	.15	.83

continue entry of patients if it were desirable to study the regimen further in a phase II setting.

With this Bayesian approach, the trial is designed with a maximum number of patients, n_{max}, that limits sample size even if neither early termination condition occurs. Table 18-6 shows an example of the operating characteristics of a design of this type. In this example, the historical data indicate that the expected response probability for the control regimen is .20 and that the width of the 90% confidence interval is around .20 for the true value is approximately 0.20. The table also represents targeting a 20–percentage point improvement in response probability ($\delta = 0.20$). The maximum sample size is set at 65, and it is assumed that the trial is arbitrarily not terminated before ten patients are evaluated. As can be seen from the table, the median number of patients required is 12 under the null hypothesis that the response probability for the experimental regimen is .20 and is only 13 under the alternative hypothesis. The table also indicates that 75% of the time the trial will terminate by the evaluation of 20 to 22 patients. Bayesian continuing-monitoring phase II designs have also been developed for simultaneously monitoring multiple end points, including efficacy and toxicity. Designs of this type used in actual clinical trials have been illustrated in the work of Thall et al.[27]

Some investigators and statisticians do not like to use approaches based on explicit comparison to historical controls. Phase II trials of combinations are inherently comparative, however. Going through the exercise of explicitly quantifying the basis of comparison, which these methods require, clarifies beforehand whether the uncertainty in outcome for the control group is so great that a phase II trial is not useful. Phase II trials of combinations are problematic. Only by using methods that provide more careful statistical planning of such trials can we streamline the drug development process.

Many reports in the literature of phase II trials of combination regimens conclude that the treatment is effective. As noted, response rates generally are not a measure of patient benefit. Such reports generally fail to make any meaningful attempt at determining outcome on standard treatment for a prognostically comparable set of patients. Often, these trials are not conducted as a prelude to a phase III evaluation, and, hence, their value to clinical therapeutics is difficult to identify.

CYTOSTATIC DRUGS

Standard phase II designs cannot be used for the evaluation of drugs that are not expected to cause tumor shrinkage. Time until tumor progression is usually the end point of interest for such studies. Unfortunately, however, time till progression is inherently a comparative end point that requires either a concurrent or historical control group for evaluation. Mick et al.[28] proposed that the time to progression of a patient on a phase II

trial be compared to the time to progression of the same patient on his/her previous trial. The ratio of these time to progressions was called a *growth modulation index*, and the agent was considered active if the index was greater than 1.3 on average. In practice, however, there are several limitations to this design. Because the follow-up intervals on different protocols are different, there may be substantial variability and bias in computing the ratio of progression times. In cases for which progression intervals get shorter with subsequent treatments, the design may have a substantial chance of missing active agents. As tumors grow larger, the doubling time may increase and hence in some cases the chance of false-positive findings may be inflated.[29]

Rosner et al.[30] describe a "randomized discontinuation design" for phase II studies of therapeutically targeted drugs. All eligible patients are started on the drug and given two to four courses of treatment. Patients are then evaluated: Those with progression are removed from study, those with objective tumor response are continued on treatment, and the remaining patients are randomized to either continue or discontinue the drug. The continued and discontinued groups of randomized patients are compared with regard to time to progression. Whereas this may be a viable approach to phase II screening, it is problematic if viewed as a phase III design. It addresses the question of whether prolonged treatment extends time to progression compared to short-term treatment for patients who have stable disease on short-term treatment. It does not establish which patients, if any, benefit from the treatment.

Simon et al.[13] described a *phase 2.5 design* for evaluating cancer vaccines and molecularly targeted drugs. Patients are randomized to the drug or to no further treatment, and the randomization groups are compared with regard to time to progression. It differs from a phase III design in that the significance level α of the design may be set above the conventional 5% level, a large difference may be targeted, and no claim is made that time to progression necessarily represents patient benefit. This design was also discussed by Korn et al.[31]

Simon et al.[13] showed that one can take advantage of the nontoxic nature of some molecularly targeted drugs to efficiently evaluate multiple drugs in the same study. They propose using a factorial design in which concurrent randomizations are made for each drugs. For example, if there are three drugs (A, B, C) being evaluated, then some patients will receive all three, some will receive pairs (AB, AC, or BC), some will receive single drugs (A, B, C), and one group will receive none of the drugs. In evaluating each drug, the time to progressions for all patients receiving that drug are compared to the times for all patients not receiving that drug. The trial can be sized as if it were a single two-arm trial. The design is effective as long as there are not negative interactions. Most negative interactions result from the toxicity of one drug interfering with the full dose administration of other drugs, which may not be a problem for many molecularly targeted drugs.

The randomized phase II screening designs of Simon et al.[24] were generalized by Liu et al.[32] for use with time to progression or survival data. Such a design can be used to select the best regimen for phase III evaluation. Without a control arm, however, one will not know whether the selected regimen is really promising. Liu et al.[32] cautioned against using a control arm in a randomized phase II design because the design may be mistaken for a phase III design, although the sample size is not sufficient for a phase III comparison. Sher and

Heller[33] have argued that phase II designs are generally misleading even for cytotoxics, leading so often to negative phase III trials. They propose conducting phase III trials with multiple experimental regimens, a control arm, and early termination of all experimental arms that are not promising. They used the statistical design of Schaid et al.[34] for time to event data. Thall et al.[35] had studied such designs when the end point was binary.

Some studies use time till progression as end point with a historical control group. It is very difficult, however, to identify a historical control group that is prognostically comparable to the new study group and for whom time to progression is measured in a comparable manner. Nevertheless, Dixon and Simon[36] have developed tables for planning historically controlled phase II comparative studies with a survival or time-to-progression end point.

DESIGN OF PHASE III CLINICAL TRIALS

Good therapeutic research requires asking important questions and getting reliable answers. As noted earlier in Trials of Combination Regimens, many phase II trials of combination regimens do not provide reliable answers. Some phase III trials, however, do not ask important questions. The most important clinical trials are often the most difficult to conduct.[37] They may involve withholding a treatment established by tradition, potentially transferring patient management responsibility across specialties, standardizing procedures among physicians who believe that their way is best, and sharing recognition with a large group of collaborators.

Phase III trials attempt to provide guidance to practicing physicians to help them make treatment decisions with their patients. Consequently, the trials should provide reliable information concerning end points of relevance to the patients. The major end points for evaluating the effectiveness of a treatment should be direct measures of patient welfare. Survival and symptom control are two such end points. The latter is not routinely used because of the difficulty of measuring it reliably and because it may be influenced by concomitant treatments. As stated, tumor shrinkage usually is not an appropriate end point for phase III trials because it may have little or no relation to patient benefit. Torri et al.[38] performed a metaanalysis of the relationship between difference in response rates and difference in median survivals for randomized clinical trials of advanced ovarian carcinoma. They found that large improvements in response rates corresponded to very small improvements in median survival. Hence, use of response rate as an end point results in giving patients increasingly intensive and toxic therapy with little or no net benefit to them.

It is usually important that the results of phase III trials be applicable to patients seen in the community outside of clinical research settings. This is accomplished by conducting the trials in multi-institution settings that include community physician participation. The eligibility criteria established for the trial also has a bearing on the generalizability of the conclusions; trials conducted with narrow eligibility criteria tend to be less generalizable. Narrow eligibility criteria also complicate trials logistically. Narrow eligibility criteria tend to require extensive and expensive patient workups and, thereby, do not facilitate

broad participation, especially in an era of closely monitored medical costs. For these and other reasons, there is a trend toward broadened eligibility criteria for phase III clinical trials. In the United Kingdom, many trials are designed using the *uncertainty principle,* an approach that leaves much of the decision making about eligibility to the treating physician. There may be guidelines for eligibility, but the ultimate decision is made by the treating physician; if he or she is uncertain about which treatment is more appropriate for the patient, then the patient is eligible.

RANDOMIZATION

To determine whether a new treatment cures any patients with a disease that is uniformly and rapidly fatal, history is a satisfactory control. Once we leave this setting of complete determinism, however, the definition of an adequate nonrandomized control group becomes problematic. In studies using nonrandomized controls, often diagnostic and staging procedures, supportive care, secondary treatments, and methods of evaluation and follow-up are different for the controls and for the new patients. There is generally differential bias in the selection of patients to be treated resulting from judgments by the physicians, self-selection by the patients, and differences in referral patterns. There may be bias in treatment ineligibility rates. Current patients sometimes are excluded from analysis for not meeting eligibility criteria, not receiving "adequate" treatment, refusing treatment, or committing a major protocol violation. The control group, on the other hand, generally contains all the patients. There may be differences in the distribution of known and unknown prognostic factors between the controls and the current treatment group. Often, there is inadequate information to determine whether such differences are present, and current known prognostic factors may not have been measured for the controls. It generally is difficult or impossible to determine whether the controls would have been eligible for the current study and in what way they represent a selection of all eligible patients.

Formation of the control group by random treatment assignment as an integral part of the planned study can avoid most of the systematic biases just mentioned.[39–42] Randomization does not ensure that the study will include a representative sample of all patients with the disease, but it does help to ensure an unbiased evaluation of the relative merits of the two treatments for the types of patients entered.

It is sometimes said that randomization is unnecessary because matched historical or concurrent controls can be selected. However, matching can be done only with regard to known prognostic factors, and these generally are not sufficient for the construction of prognostically homogeneous groups of patients. Matching with regard to known factors gives no assurance that the distributions of unknown factors are similar between the groups. It also is sometimes said that randomization is not effective in ensuring that the treatment groups are similar with regard to unknown prognostic factors unless the number of patients is large. This is true but reflects a misunderstanding of the purpose of randomization. Randomization does not ensure that the groups are medically equivalent, but it distributes the unknown biasing factors according to a known random distribution so that their effects can be rigorously allowed for in significance tests and confidence intervals. This is true regardless of the study size. A significance level represents the probability that differences in outcome can be the result of random fluctuations. Without a randomized treatment allocation, a "statistically significant difference" may be the result of a nonrandom difference in the distribution of unknown prognostic factors.

Many investigators see a useful role for both nonrandomized and randomized clinical trials. The nonrandomized format is used for determining which regimens are sufficiently promising for randomized phase III evaluation and for use in clinical settings in which outcome is uniformly poor. For major questions of public health importance, unless the treatment effects are huge, the need for reliable answers dictates the use of randomized phase III trials.

Randomization of a patient should be performed after the patient has been found eligible and has consented to participate in the trial and to accept either of the randomized options. A truly random and nondecipherable randomization procedure should be used and implemented by calling a central randomization office staffed by individuals who are independent of participating physicians.

STRATIFICATION

When important prognostic factors are known for patients in a randomized trial, it is often advisable to stratify the randomization to ensure equal distribution of these factors. This is usually accomplished by preparing a separate randomization list (or set of cards in sealed envelopes) for each stratum of patients. Each list must be balanced so that after each block of four to ten patients within the stratum, the treatment groups contain equal numbers of patients. Within the blocks, the sequence of treatment assignments is random. The stratification factors must be known for each patient at the time of randomization.

It is generally best to limit stratification to those factors definitely known to have important independent effects on outcome. If two factors are closely correlated, only one needs to be included. Peto and colleagues[43,44] believe that stratification is an unnecessary complication because adjustment for imbalances of known factors can be made in the analysis. This is true for large trials. Stratification helps to ensure balance for interim analyses when the sample sizes may be limited and provides the medical audience with confidence in the results, which often is not available when depending on complex adjustment methods to deal with prognostic imbalances. Stratification also is a convenient way of specifying *a priori* what are considered the important prognostic factors. Subsequent "subset analyses" can then be limited to the patient subsets determined by the stratification factors.

Many clinical trials use adaptive stratification methods. The most popular such method is that conceived by Pocock and Simon,[45] which permits effective balancing with regard to many prognostic factors. Kalish and Begg[46] have also studied analytic aspects of adaptive stratification methods.

SAMPLE SIZE

The protocol for a phase III trial should specify the number of patients to be accrued and the duration of follow-up after the close of accrual when the final analysis will be performed.

Methods of sample size planning are usually based on the assumption that at the conclusion of the follow-up period, a statistical significance test will be performed comparing the experimental treatment to the control treatment with regard to a single primary end point. A statistical significance level of .05 has the following meaning: If there is no true difference in treatment effectiveness, the probability of obtaining a difference in outcomes as extreme as that observed in the data is .05. The significance level does not represent the probability that the null hypothesis is true; it represents a probability of an observed difference, assuming that the null hypothesis is true. Conventional statistical theory ascribes no probabilities to hypotheses, only to data.

A one-sided significance level represents the probability, by chance alone, of obtaining a difference as large as and in the same direction as that actually observed. A two-sided significance level represents the probability of obtaining by chance a difference in either direction as large in absolute magnitude as that actually observed. The two-sided significance level is usually twice the one-sided significance level. Controversy exists over the appropriateness of one-sided or two-sided significance levels. Although this is a somewhat trivial issue, a two-sided significance level of .05 has become widely accepted as a standard level of evidence.

With few patients in the trial, the difference in observed outcomes must be extreme to obtain statistical significance. Consequently, the probability of obtaining a statistically significant result may be low even when a substantial true difference in effectiveness exists. The probability of obtaining a statistically significant result when the treatments differ in effectiveness is called the *power* of the trial. As the sample size and extent of follow-up increases, the power increases. The power depends critically, however, on the size of the true difference in effectiveness of the two treatments. Generally, one sizes the trial so that the power is either .80 or .90 when the true difference in effectiveness is the smallest size that is considered medically important to detect.

Statisticians have developed useful methods for planning sample size to compare survival curves or disease-free survival curves in phase III trials. Table 18-7 demonstrates results that are valid whenever the *hazard ratio*—the ratio of forces of mortality for the two treatment groups—is constant over time.[47] The table shows the total number of deaths that must occur in a given cohort to reflect 90% power for detecting a specified reduction in the hazard for the experimental treatment rela-

TABLE 18-7. Number of Events Needed for Comparing Survival Curves

Percentage Reduction in Hazard of Death	Ratio of Median Survival for Exponential Distributions	No. of Total Deaths to Observe[a]
20	1.25	846
30	1.43	330
33	1.50	257
40	1.67	162
50	2.0	88

[a]Total number of deaths in both groups to have power .90 for detecting ratio of median survival. Type I error α = .05 (two-sided).

TABLE 18-8. Number of Patients in Each of Two Treatment Groups (One-Sided Test)

Smaller Success Rate	Larger Minus Smaller Success Rate									
	0.05	0.10	0.15	0.20	0.25	0.30	0.35	0.40	0.45	0.50
0.05	512[a]	172	94	62	45	35	28	23	19	16
	381[b]	129	72	48	35	27	22	18	15	13
0.10	786	236	121	76	54	40	31	25	21	17
	579	176	91	58	41	31	24	20	16	14
0.15	1026	292	144	88	60	44	34	27	22	18
	752	216	108	66	46	34	26	21	17	14
0.20	1231	339	163	98	66	48	36	29	23	19
	900	250	121	73	50	37	28	22	18	15
0.25	1402	377	178	105	70	50	38	29	23	19
	1024	278	132	79	53	38	29	23	18	15
0.30	1539	407	189	111	73	52	38	30	23	19
	1122	300	141	83	55	39	30	23	18	15
0.35	1642	429	197	114	74	52	38	29	23	18
	1196	315	146	85	56	40	30	23	18	14
0.40	1711	441	201	115	74	52	38	29	22	17
	1246	324	149	86	56	39	29	22	17	14
0.45	1745	446	201	114	73	50	36	27	21	16
	1271	327	149	85	55	38	28	21	16	13
0.50	1745	441	197	111	70	48	34	25	19	15
	1271	324	146	83	53	37	26	20	15	12

[a]Upper figure: significance level = .05, power = .90.
[b]Lower figure: significance level = .05, power = .80.

tive to the control treatment. For exponential distributions, the percentage reduction in hazard of death can be expressed as a ratio of median survivals, which is displayed in the second column of Table 18-7. For comparing disease-free survival curves, *deaths* should be replaced by *events*, wherein death, disease recurrence, or development of a second cancer are considered events. The translation of the number of deaths or events required to the number of patients required depends on the actual shape of the survival distributions, the rate of accrual, and the duration of follow-up after close of accrual. Generally, however, it is best to specify the time of the final analysis as the time when the specified number of deaths or events is obtained—not in terms of absolute calendar time.

In some cases, it may be convenient to think in terms of the proportion of patients who survive beyond some landmark time, such as 5 years. Tables 18-8 and 18-9 provide required numbers of patients for clinical trials planned on this basis. This approach is less flexible for studies in which survival or disease-free survival is the end point, as it presumes that all patients will be followed for the landmark time as a minimum. These tables can, however, be used generally for detecting differences in a binary end point, denoted *success rate* in the tables. Table 18-8 is for one-sided significance tests, and Table 18-9 is for two-sided tests. For comparing treatments, differences of more than 15 percentage points usually are unrealistic.

Establishing a sample size that provides good statistical power for detecting realistically expected treatment improvements is important. Many published "negative" results are actually uninterpretable because the sample sizes are too small.[48] For trials comparing a standard treatment to a more conservative or less invasive therapy, small reductions in effectiveness will be medically important because survival time or cure probability is being traded for convenience or cosmesis. High statistical power for detecting small differences requires large trials. False acceptance of the null hypothesis of equivalence may result in erroneous adoption of a new, more conservative, and less effective therapy. The burden of proof for therapeutic equivalence trials should generally be on showing that results are similar, not on demonstrating that they are different. These trials should be planned using the specialized methods described later in Therapeutic Equivalence Trials. If standard frequency methods are used to analyze such trials, rather than the Bayesian methods described in Therapeutic Equivalence Trials, confidence intervals rather than statistical significance tests should be used. The confidence interval for the true difference of effectiveness gives a much clearer picture of which differences are consistent with the data. Makuch and Simon[49] and Durrleman and Simon[50] discuss this approach for planning and monitoring therapeutic equivalence trials.

FACTORIAL DESIGNS

In a two-by-two factorial design, there are actually four treatment groups. The first factor represents two alternative interventions, such as amputation and resection. The second factor represents two other alternatives superimposed on the first factor, such as adjuvant chemotherapy and no chemotherapy. In another example, the first factor might be chemotherapy regimen A or B, and the second factor might be the duration of treatment, 6 or 12 months. Although there are actually four treatment groups, the average effect of each treatment factor can be evaluated using all of the patients and pooling with regard to the other factor (or by accounting for the influence of the other factor in the analysis by stratification but not by separate analyses for each level of the other factor). Usually, the sample size for a two-by-two factorial trial is computed

TABLE 18-9. Number of Patients in Each of Two Treatment Groups (Two-Sided Test)

Smaller Success Rate	Larger Minus Smaller Success Rate									
	0.05	0.10	0.15	0.20	0.25	0.30	0.35	0.40	0.45	0.50
0.05	620[a]	206	113	74	54	42	33	27	23	19
	473[b]	159	88	58	43	33	27	22	18	16
0.10	956	285	146	92	64	48	38	30	25	21
	724	218	112	71	50	38	30	24	20	17
0.15	1250	354	174	106	73	53	41	33	26	22
	944	269	133	82	57	42	32	26	21	18
0.20	1502	411	197	118	79	57	44	34	27	22
	1132	313	151	91	62	45	34	27	22	18
0.25	1712	459	216	127	84	60	45	35	28	23
	1289	348	165	98	65	47	36	28	22	18
0.30	1880	495	230	134	88	62	46	36	28	22
	1414	375	175	103	68	48	36	28	22	18
0.35	2006	522	239	138	89	63	46	35	27	22
	1509	395	182	106	69	49	36	28	22	18
0.40	2090	537	244	139	89	62	45	34	26	21
	1571	407	186	107	69	48	36	27	21	17
0.45	2132	543	244	138	88	60	44	33	25	19
	1603	411	186	106	68	47	34	26	20	16
0.50	2132	537	239	134	84	57	41	30	23	17
	1603	407	182	103	65	45	32	24	18	14

[a]Upper figure: significance level = .05, power = .90.
[b]Lower figure: significance level = .05, power = .80.

assuming that there is no interaction between the effects of the factors. The sample size is approximately the same as for a simple two-arm trial. This sample size will not provide enough patients to test adequately the assumption of no interaction between the factors. The factorial design offers the possibility of answering two questions for the cost of one, but there is a risk of ambiguity in the interpretation of results.[51] For situations in which negative interactions are unlikely or in which it is unlikely that both factors will have substantial effects, the factorial design can provide a substantial improvement in the efficiency of clinical trials.

The use of a factorial design for a clinical trial is sometimes controversial.[2] Proponents sometimes indicate that factorial designs are ideal for studying interactions. Others have questioned how factorial trials can provide meaningful information about interactions when the trials are sized only to detect main effects. Brittain and Wittes[51] noted that the power for detecting an effect of treatment A is substantially impaired by a negative interaction. Consequently, factorial designs often are used only when one can assume with confidence that there will be no interactions between the effects of the factors and can determine sample size on the basis of that assumption.

Simon and Freedman[52] developed a Bayesian method for the design and analysis of factorial trials. Their approach avoids the need to dichotomize one's assumptions that interactions either do or do not exist and provides a flexible approach to the design and analysis of such clinical trials. The Bayesian method encourages the quantification of prior belief about the size of interactions that may exist. Rather than forcing the investigator to adopt one of two extreme positions regarding interactions, it provides for the specification of intermediate positions. The Bayesian approach also avoids a preliminary test of interaction having poor power. The Bayesian model suggests

that in planning a factorial trial in which interactions are unlikely but cannot be excluded, the sample size should be increased by approximately 30%, as compared to a simple two-arm clinical trial for detecting the same size of treatment effect. This is less extreme than doubling the sample size but is a recommendation that differs greatly from current usage. The 30% figure allows for a 5% prior probability of a medically important, qualitative interaction between the treatment effects.

Factorial designs can also be useful in phase II trials when an internal control is needed.[13] For example, consider the investigation of non-toxic drugs A and B for patients in partial remission after induction chemotherapy. With a factorial design, there would be four treatment groups. One group would receive neither agent, one would receive A, one group would receive B, and one group would receive both A and B. Patients are randomized to the four groups. For analyzing the effect of A, the time to progressive disease for the two arms that received A are compared to the time to progressive distribution for the two arms that did not receive A. Analyzing the effect of B is performed analogously. The single-arm phase II trial is problematic when the end point is disease stabilization or time to progression. It is easy to come up with a definition of disease stabilization, but just defining it does not make it valid for measurement of treatment effect. Data are needed that demonstrate that such stabilization does not occur in the absence of treatment in a comparable group of patients. This is difficult to do reliably because of the usual difficulties of identifying comparable historical controls and because of special difficulties involved with documenting stabilization or measuring time to disease progression in a consistent manner, comparable to the way it was done with historical controls. Consequently, the use of disease stabilization or time to progression as an end point in single-arm phase II trials is particularly problematic. The factorial design is internally controlled for evaluating the effects of the factors and, hence, the use of time to progression is not problematic.

THERAPEUTIC EQUIVALENCE TRIALS

Therapeutic equivalence trials are also called *noninferiority trials* and attempt to determine whether a new treatment is equivalent to a standard therapy with regard to a specified clinical end point. This is contrasted to bioequivalence trials in which the objective is to demonstrate equivalence of serum concentrations of the active moiety. In some cases, investigators would like to demonstrate that the new treatment is effective as compared to no treatment but, because use of a no-treatment arm is not feasible, they attempt to demonstrate therapeutic equivalence to a treatment that is considered effective.

Therapeutic equivalence trials are problematic because it is impossible to demonstrate equivalence. If the outcomes for the two treatments are similar, one can only conclude that results are consistent with differences within specified limits. In superiority trials, rejection of the null hypothesis leads to change in the treatment of future patients. The implications of failure to reject the null hypothesis are more difficult to interpret. In an equivalence trial, failure to reject the null hypothesis often is interpreted as a demonstration of therapeutic equivalence and grounds for adoption of the new regimen but may merely reflect inadequate sample size or ineffectiveness of the standard treatment for the patients in the clinical trial.

Large sample sizes are often needed for meaningful therapeutic equivalence trials. For example, consider a cancer trial evaluating tumor resection as an alternative to amputation of the organ containing the tumor in a setting in which amputation is the standard therapy known to be curative in a large number of cases. Tumor resection may have clear advantages with regard to quality of life, but few patients would be interested in these advantages unless they were assured that any reduction in the chance of cure would be very small. Hence, the appropriate trial should focus on distinguishing the null hypothesis in which the difference in efficacy is expressed as $\Delta = 0$ from that in which the difference in efficacy is expressed as $\Delta = \delta$, where δ is very small. Consequently, this trial would have to be very large.

In a therapeutic equivalence trial, there is no internal validation of the assumption that the control treatment C is actually effective for the patient population at hand. It is not enough for the experimental treatment E to be therapeutically equivalent to C; what is wanted is equivalence coupled with the effectiveness of E and C relative to no treatment or to whatever was standard before the adoption of C.

None of the conventional approaches to the design and analysis of therapeutic equivalence trials is satisfactory. These approaches depend on the specification of a minimal difference (δ) in efficacy that one is willing to tolerate but do not address how δ should be determined. Simon[53] developed a Bayesian approach to the use of information from previous trials in the design and analysis of therapeutic equivalence trials. The effectiveness of the control treatment C relative to no treatment or to the previous standard before C was adopted is represented by a parameter β. The previous standard is denoted by P. The effectiveness of C relative to P will not be known with certainty and may vary among trials. The information about β is summarized by a prior distribution, which is normal with mean μ_β and standard deviation σ_β and these values are obtained from a metaanalysis of the previously conducted randomized trials comparing C to P.

The result of the therapeutic equivalence trial is summarized by a value y, which estimates the effectiveness of E relative to C.

With some simplifying assumptions, the posterior distribution of the effectiveness of E relative to P is a normal distribution with mean $\mu_\beta + y$. This is the expected effectiveness of C relative to P plus the estimate of the effectiveness of E relative to C based on the therapeutic equivalence trial. The variance of this posterior distribution is $\sigma_\beta^2 + \sigma^2$, where σ_β^2 is the variance of the prior distribution of β and σ is the standard error of y. Simon[53] also shows how the sample size of the therapeutic equivalence trial may be planned and how the size depends critically on the strength and consistency of the evidence that the active control C is superior to P and the size of that difference in effectiveness.

BAYESIAN METHODS

Conventional statistical methods regard the data collected in an experiment as being randomly sampled to test hypotheses about parameters that represent fixed but unknown quantities such as treatment effects. Conventional methods, also called *frequentist methods*, derive probability statements about the data under assumed hypotheses about the fixed parameters. *Bayesian* statistical methods consider the parameters, as well as the data, as being randomly drawn from distributions. The distributions that the parameters are drawn from are called *prior distributions*. Bayesian methods use Bayes' theorem to update the prior distributions of the parameters using the data from the study to produce the posterior distribution of the parameters. Using the posterior distribution, hypotheses can be tested. Consequently, Bayesian methods can derive direct probability statements about the parameters, such as, "the probability that the treatment effect is zero is .04." The probability statements about the parameters seem to tell us what we want to know, but their meaningfulness depends on the meaningfulness of the assumption that the parameters are randomly drawn from the specified prior distributions.

In some cases, the prior distribution of a parameter can be interpreted as being determined by previous studies. For example, a study may be evaluating a device and several other devices of the same class have previously been evaluated. For some parameters, there may be a general consensus that large values are unlikely, and this may be incorporated into a widely acceptable prior distribution. For example, there is generally broad consensus that large treatment-effect by patient-subset interactions are unlikely. Generally, however, there is no meaningful consensus about the average effect of treatment. Randomized clinical trials are done because the opinions of experts are often wrong. Generally, therefore, the prior distribution is a theoretical construct representing a subjective view of the parameter before the current trial under consideration. The subjective nature of the prior distribution is problematic for the interpretation of phase III clinical trials, because different individuals will have different prior distributions. It is not surprising that, although the results of a clinical trial should be objectively reported, different individuals have different interpretations of the results. Bayesian methods, however, intermingle the data with the prior distributions in producing the posterior distributions and the conclusions.

There are several important misconceptions about the use of Bayesian methods for clinical trials. First, some people believe that Bayes' theorem is somehow a substitute for randomization. In fact, however, randomization is just as important for the validity of Bayesian methods as for frequentist methods. Second, some people mistakenly believe that Bayesian clinical trials require fewer patients than frequentist trials. Bayesian sample size calculations depend on the prior distribution used. If the prior distribution for the treatment effect is a *skeptical prior*—that is, a prior that represents skepticism about the new treatment—then the sample size needed with Bayesian methods may be much larger than the conventional sample size. Third, some statisticians believe that the main impediment to use of Bayesian methods in clinical trials has been the difficulty of computing posterior distributions. The main limitation has been the fact that subjectivity of analysis is problematic for phase III clinical trials. Bayesian methods are applicable to phases I and II designs in which the prior distribution need only be appropriate for the investigator or company developing the regimen. For phase III trials, the subjective opinion of the investigator or company sponsoring the trial is of no interest to the regulatory body, physicians, or patients who are consumers of the results of the trial. Bayesian methods are most easily applicable to phase III trials for problems in which a prior can be defined that is widely acceptable to all of the consumers of the research. Such priors are possible for parameters representing interaction effects,[52,54] for the effectiveness of active controls in noninferiority trials,[55] and for unexpected findings with multiple safety end points.[56] Spiegelhalter et al.[57] have defined the concept of skeptical prior, which may serve as a consensus prior for primary treatment effects. In general, however, the conflict between the need for objectivity in phase III trials and the subjectivity of prior distributions limits the applicability of Bayesian methods in clinical trials.

ANALYSIS OF PHASE III CLINICAL TRIALS

INTENTION-TO-TREAT ANALYSIS

One of the important principles in the analysis of phase III trials is called the *intention-to-treat* principle. This indicates that all randomized patients should be included in the primary analysis of the trial. For cancer trials, this has often been interpreted to mean all "eligible" randomized patients. Because eligibility requirements sometimes are vague and unverifiable by an external auditor, excluding "ineligible" patients can itself result in bias. However, excluding patients from analysis because of treatment deviations, early death, or patient withdrawal can severely distort the results.[44,58,59] Often, excluded patients have poorer outcomes than do those who are not excluded. Investigators frequently rationalize that the poor outcome experienced by a patient was due to lack of compliance to treatment, but the direction of causality may be the reverse. For example, in the Coronary Drug Project, the 5-year mortality for poor adherents to the placebo regimen was 28.3%, significantly greater than the 15.1% experienced by good adherents to the placebo regimen.[60] In randomized trials, there may be poorer compliance in one

treatment group than the other, or the reasons for poor compliance may differ. Excluding patients, or analyzing them separately (which is equivalent to excluding them), for reasons other than eligibility is generally considered unacceptable. The intention-to-treat analysis with all eligible randomized patients should be the primary analysis. If the conclusions of a study depend on exclusions, then these conclusions are suspect. The treatment plan should be viewed as a policy to be evaluated. The treatment intended cannot be delivered uniformly to all patients, but all eligible patients should generally be evaluable in phase III trials.

INTERIM ANALYSES

If statistical significance tests are performed repeatedly, the probability that the difference in outcomes will be found to be statistically significant (at the .05 level) at some point may be considerably greater than 5%. This probability is called the *type I error* of the analysis plan. Fleming et al.[61] have shown that the type I error can be as great as 26% if a statistical significance test is performed every 3 months of a 3-year trial that compares two identical treatments. Many trials are published without stating the target sample size, without indicating whether a target sample size was stated in the protocol, and without describing whether the published analysis represented a planned final analysis or was one of multiple analyses performed during the course of the trial. In such cases, one must suspect that the investigators were not aware of good statistical practices and of the dangers of informal multiple analyses. Consequently, the statistical significance reported in such trials must be discounted as uninterpretable.

Interim analyses can be very misleading, and the significance levels of interim analyses cannot be taken at face value.[2] Nevertheless, the random trends often seen in interim analyses can destroy accrual to a clinical trial and interfere with a physician's attempt to state honestly to the patient that there is no reliable evidence indicating that one treatment option or the other is preferable. For these reasons, it has become standard in multicenter clinical trials to have a data-monitoring committee review interim results, rather than having the monitoring done by participating physicians. This approach helps to protect patients by having interim results carefully evaluated by an experienced group of individuals and helps to protect the study from damage that ensues from misinterpretation of interim results.[62,63] Generally, interim outcome information is available to only the data-monitoring committee. The study leaders are not part of the data-monitoring committee, because they may have a perceived conflict of interest in continuing the trial. The data-monitoring committee determines when results are mature and should be released. These procedures are used only for phase III trials.

A number of useful statistical designs have been developed for monitoring interim results. The simplest is owing to Haybittle et al.[44] Interim differences are discounted unless the difference is statistically significant at the two-sided $P<.0025$ level. If the interim differences are not significant at that level, the trial continues until its originally intended size. The final analysis is performed without regard to the interim analyses, and the type I error is almost unaffected by the monitoring.

Others have developed group-sequential methods for interim monitoring based on a prespecified number of planned interim analyses.[64–67] The critical P value for determining whether an interim difference should be judged statistically significant depends on the number of analyses that will be performed dur-

TABLE 18-10. Nominal Two-Sided Significance Levels for Early Stopping in Interim Monitoring Methods That Maintain an Overall Type I Error Level of .05

Analysis Number	Pocock[65]	Haybittle[44]	O'Brien and Fleming[64]	Fleming et al.[66]
1	.016	.0027	.00001	.0051
2	.016	.0027	.0013	.0061
3	.016	.0027	.008	.0073
4	.016	.0027	.023	.0089
Final	.016	.049	.041	.0402

ing the trial. For a five-stage trial—four interim analyses and one final analysis—the critical *P* values are shown in Table 18-10.

Extreme treatment differences at an interim analysis are unusual in cancer clinical trials. It is more common to find that interim results do not support the hypothesis that the experimental treatment is substantially better than the control. The method of stochastic curtailment[68] was developed for evaluating such a circumstance. At any interim analysis, the probability of rejecting the null hypothesis at the end of the trial is computed. This probability is calculated as being conditional on the data already obtained and on the assumption that the alternative hypothesis of superiority of the experimental treatment used initially in planning the sample size for the trial is true. If this conditional power is less than approximately 0.20, then the trial may be terminated with acceptance of the null hypothesis. The 0.20 cutoff can be raised substantially to at least 0.40 if this type of interim analysis is performed only a few times during the course of the trial. With stochastic curtailment, interim analyses need not be equally spaced, and the number of interim analyses need not be specified in advance.

Several other investigators have developed other designs for early termination of the clinical trial if results are not promising for the experimental treatment.[69,70] Schaid et al.[34] and Wieand et al.[71] developed designs for early termination when results are not promising in survival studies. Such designs have been reviewed by Simon.[72] Jennison and Turnbull[67] developed methods for calculating confidence intervals for treatment differences at interim analyses. Such confidence intervals can be useful in deciding when to terminate the trial.

Stopping trials when the experimental regimen *E* is not appearing more effective than *C* but is not statistically significantly worse than *C* is sometimes controversial. Statisticians tend to want data as definitively as possible. One must also be cautious with survival or disease-free survival end points, as early parts of the survival curve may not reflect latter parts. Another argument for continuing such trials even if it is clear that *E* will not be found to be significantly better than *C* is that additional data will provide narrower confidence intervals for the true difference. The alternative point of view is that it is not appropriate to continue to expose patients to a more toxic and debilitating treatment *E* if the essential outcome of the trial is well assured. Data-monitoring committees are charged with helping to make these difficult judgments.

SIGNIFICANCE LEVELS, HYPOTHESIS TESTS, AND CONFIDENCE INTERVALS

Medical decision making is complicated, and clinicians frequently misinterpret statistical significance tests in search of clear-cut answers from ambiguous data. A statistical significance level for comparing outcomes represents the probability of obtaining a difference as large as that actually observed if the treatments were actually of equal efficacy and differences occur merely by chance. If differences in either direction as large in absolute value as the one actually obtained are included, the significance level is called *two-sided*. If the probability is calculated only for differences in the same direction as that actually obtained, the significance level is called *one-sided*. Generally, the two-sided significance level is twice the one-sided level.

After significance tests had been used for many years, Neyman and Pearson formalized a mathematical theory of hypothesis testing. In this theory, a study must prespecify a null hypothesis, an alternative hypothesis, and a decision rule for accepting one hypothesis and rejecting the other based on the data obtained. The theory has appealed to clinicians because it simplifies complex medical decision making by providing yes or no answers; either the difference is statistically significant or it is not. The distinction between one- and two-sided decision rules becomes crucial because a one-sided *P* = .05 is simply nonsignificant if a type I error of .05 based on a two-sided decision rule is prespecified.

The concept of prespecification of hypotheses is important for medical experimentation. However, the accept–reject nomenclature of the Neyman-Pearson theory provides an oversimplified and sometimes misleading interpretation of the data. Significance levels can serve as useful aids to interpretation of results, but quibbling about whether a one-sided *P* = .04 is significant makes little sense. Significance levels are influenced by sample sizes, and failure to reject the null hypothesis does not mean that the treatments are equivalent. There is no simple index of truth for interpreting results. Some attempt to use the notion of statistical significance in this way, but thorough presentation, skeptical evaluation, and cautious interpretation of results always are required.

Confidence intervals are generally much more informative than are significance levels. A confidence interval for the size of the treatment difference provides a range of effects consistent with the data. The significance level tells nothing about the size of the treatment effect because it depends on the sample size. However, it is the size of the treatment effect, as communicated by a confidence interval, that should be used in weighing the costs and benefits of clinical decision making. Many so-called negative results are actually noninformative, and confidence intervals help to determine when this is the case. Simon[73] has presented a nontechnical discussion of how to calculate confidence intervals for treatment differences with the types of end points commonly used in cancer clinical trials.

CALCULATION OF SURVIVAL CURVES

Most cancer clinical trials display results by showing survival curves or disease-free survival curves. Survival curves display the probability of surviving beyond any specified time, with time shown on the horizontal axis. In disease-free survival curves, it is the time until recurrence or death that is shown. Other time-to-event distributions can be similarly represented using the same methods. The usual statistical methods are not appropriate for analyzing survival because they ignore the fact that surviving patients have a limited follow-up period after which their survivals are "censored."

TABLE 18-11. Life-Table Method for Estimating a Survival Distribution

Years after Randomization	No. Alive at Beginning of Interval l_x	No. Lost to Follow-Up or Withdrawn Alive during Interval w_x	No. Died during Interval d_x	At Risk during Interval (Col 2 − $^1/_2$ Col 3)	Proportion Dying (Col 4/Col 5) q_x	Proportion Surviving (Col 1 − Col 6) p_x	Cumulative Proportion Surviving (S_x) ($p_1 \times p_2 \times \ldots \times p_x$)
0–1	252	38	94	233	0.40	0.60	0.60
1–2	120	34	10	103	0.10	0.90	0.54
2–3	76	30	4	61	0.07	0.93	0.50
3–4	42	18	4	33	0.12	0.88	0.44
4–5	20	12	0	14	0.00	1.00	0.44
5–6	8	8	0	4	0.00	1.00	0.44

Col, column.

The most satisfactory way of representing such data is to estimate the survival function $S(t)$. This function represents the probability of surviving more than t time units. Time t is measured from diagnosis, start of treatment, or some other meaningful time point. For randomized studies, it is best to measure time from the date of randomization. There are basically two satisfactory methods for estimating $S(t)$. The first is the life-table or actuarial method. It frequently is attributed to Berkson and Gage[74] or Cutler and Ederer[75] and is appropriate when the number of patients is large. The other method is the product limit method of Kaplan and Meier.[76] This method is appropriate for any number of patients, but it involves more effort than the life-table method when the number of patients is large.

The first step in the application of either method is the calculation of survival time for all patients. Survival is the duration from the chosen baseline (e.g., date of randomization) until death or date last known to be alive for patients who are not known to have died. To use the life-table method, intervals for the grouping of survival times are determined. The life table, shown in Table 18-11, is then filled out. This sample life table is prepared with yearly intervals in the first column. The number of patients alive at the beginning of the interval is entered in column 2. The number who died in the interval is entered in column 4. Patients dying exactly at a time that represents a boundary between two intervals (e.g., 365 days) are considered to have died in the preceding interval (e.g., 0 to 1 year). Column 3 contains the number of patients who are lost to follow-up during the interval or who are alive with maximum follow-up duration included in the interval. These latter patients are referred to as *withdrawn alive* in the conventional life-table terminology. The life-table method assumes that patients lost to follow-up or withdrawn alive during the interval are at risk of death for one-half of the interval. Hence, column 5—the number alive at the start of the interval minus half the number lost or withdrawn during the interval—represents an approximate number of patients at risk of death during the interval. Column 6 gives the ratio of the number of patients who died during the interval to the number at risk during the interval. Column 7 gives the estimated probability of surviving the interval for patients alive at the start of the interval.

Column 8 should be studied carefully, because it provides the life-table estimate of the survival distribution and indicates the logic behind the method. The probability of surviving more than 3 years after randomization, for example, equals the

entry in the third row of column 8 (0.50). The logic is as follows: To survive 3 full years, the patients must survive through the first year; and given that they have survived the first year, they must survive the second year; and given that they have survived the second year, they must survive the third year. Consequently, the probability of surviving for at least 3 years is estimated by the product $p_1 \times p_2 \times p_3$ of factors in column 7. By using this product, the life-table method takes maximal advantage of the mortality experience of patients with limited follow-up. The entry S_x in column 8, row x, represents the life-table estimate of the probability of surviving more than x years from randomization. Computational shortcuts to observe are those for column 8: $S_x = p_x \times S_{x-1}$ and for column 2: $l_{x+1} = l_x - w_x - d_x$.

The product limit method of Kaplan and Meier is similar in concept to the life-table method. With the Kaplan-Meier approach, however, the intervals are defined by the actual survival times of patients who have died. Suppose, for example, that the survivals are 3, 3, 3+, 5, 6, 8+, 8+, 10, 10, and 12+ months, where a plus sign follows survivals for patients still alive. Then the intervals are 0 to 3, 3 to 5, 5 to 6, and 6 to 10 months, as shown in Table 18-12. With the Kaplan-Meier method, deaths occur only at the ends of intervals. The entry in column 5 equals $l_x - w_x$ rather than $l_x - 2w_x$ for the life-table method. This is because deaths occur only at the ends of intervals here, and the number of patients at risk of death just before the interval end is $l_x - w_x$. In the entry w_x in column 3 for the Kaplan-Meier method, patients who are lost to follow-up or withdrawn alive at the end of an interval are considered not lost or withdrawn until the following interval. These differences between the Kaplan-Meier and life-table methods render the former more appropriate for studies with fewer patients.

Once the values S_x have been calculated for the Kaplan-Meier method, they may be graphed with time on the horizontal axis. The graph is a step function that starts at time zero and ordinate 1.0. It drops to value S_x at time x, where x is the time at the right end of an interval. The survival curve corresponding to Table 18-12 is shown in Figure 18-1. The tic marks are placed on the curve at 3, 8, and 12 months to represent the follow-up times of living patients. The step function can be extended horizontally out to 12 months to represent follow-up of the last patient, but the right-hand end of the curve usually is very imprecisely estimated, and concluding that a plateau exists at the level shown on the curve is often erroneous.

For any time t, the Kaplan-Meier curve is an estimator of the true unknown value of $S(t)$. The estimator is approximately

TABLE 18-12. Kaplan-Meier Method for Estimating a Survival Distribution

Months after Randomization	No. Alive at Beginning of Interval l_x	No. Lost to Follow-Up or Withdrawn Alive during Interval w_x	No. Died during Interval d_x	Effective No. Exposed to Risk of Dying Just Before End of Interval (Col 2 – Col 3)	Proportion Dying (Col 4/Col 5) q_x	Proportion Surviving (Col 1 – Col 6) p_x	Cumulative Proportion Surviving $(p_1 \times p_2 \times \ldots \times p_x)$ S_x
0–3	10	0	2	10	0.2	0.8	0.8
3–5	8	1	1	7	0.14	0.86	0.68
5–6	6	0	1	6	0.17	0.83	0.57
6–10	5	2	2	3	0.67	0.33	0.19

Col, column.

normally distributed in large samples. If m patients remain alive at time x, the standard error of the estimate can be conservatively estimated[44] as

$$S_x\sqrt{(1 - S_x)/m}$$

The Kaplan-Meier estimate of a survival distribution is based on the assumption that censoring is noninformative, which means that the censoring time is independent of the prognosis of the patient. Most censoring in a randomized clinical trial results from the fact that some patients are alive and still being followed at the time of analysis. This is noninformative censoring. However, if patients are lost to follow-up—if they fail to return to clinic when they are too sick to travel—then the censoring is informative and all the usual methods of survival analysis are invalidated. Consequently, it is essential to obtain follow-up information actively on *all* patients before analysis. If some patients have not been contacted for many months and their status is unknown, that information should be obtained before any analysis is performed. Examining the distribution of time since the last contact for patients not known to have died is a good way to examine the adequacy of follow-up.

The issue of informative censoring also arises in considering end points other than death. For example, one may be attempting to estimate the distribution of time until tumor recurrence in the central nervous system (CNS) in a pediatric leukemia trial. How should one handle patients whose disease recurs in the marrow without evidence of CNS recurrence? One may be tempted to censor the time to CNS recurrence of such patients at their time of marrow recurrence, but that implicitly assumes that the censoring is noninformative. Because CNS and marrow recurrence may be biologically linked, the assumption of noninformative censoring may not be valid. Other issues of informative censoring can be similarly problematic. Clearly, one should never censor patients because of lack of compliance with therapy, as this can severely bias results. More extensive discussions of statistical methods for the analysis of clinical trial data are given by Marubini and Valsecchi.[77]

MULTIPLE COMPARISONS

Table 18-13 shows the probability of obtaining one statistically significant ($P < .05$) difference by chance alone as a function of the number of independent comparisons of two equivalent treatments. With only five comparisons, the chance of at least one false-positive conclusion is 22.6%. When the number of end points, interim analyses, and patient subsets are considered in the analysis of clinical trials, these results are disturbing.[78] The comparisons performed in clinical trials are not entirely independent, but this does not have much effect on ameliorating the problem. Fleming and Watelet[79] performed a computer simulation to determine the chance of obtaining a statistically significant treatment difference when two equivalent treatments in six subsets determined by three dichotomous variables are compared. The chance of a statistically significant difference between treatments in at least one subset was 20% at the final analysis and 39% in the final or one of the three interim analyses. Subset analysis, comparison of treatments with regard to multiple end points, and multiple interim analyses are common sources of erroneous conclusions. The primary end point should be defined in the protocol. Subset analyses and analyses with regard to secondary end points should be specified in advance, and statistical significance should be declared only for significance levels much more extreme than the conventional .05. The simplest approach to multiple comparisons is to declare statistical significance only if the P value is $<.05/n$, where n denotes the number of comparisons to be made. For example if $n = 10$, then .005 should be the threshold for declaring significance for a secondary analysis. The number of comparisons planned in the protocol is represented by n. Comparisons that are not preplanned should not be considered significant in any case and represent hypothesis generation to be tested in subsequent trials.

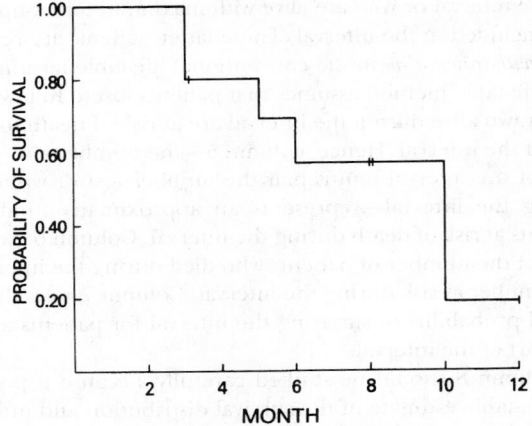

FIGURE 18-1. Example of estimated survival distribution.

TABLE 18-13. Probability of Obtaining at Least One Statistically Significant ($P<.05$) Difference by Chance Alone in Multiple Comparisons of Two Equivalent Treatments

Comparisons	Probability of at Least One "Significant" Difference (%)
1	5
2	9.7
3	14.3
4	18.5
5	22.6
10	40
20	64.1

Interaction tests are statistical procedures that test for lack of homogeneity of treatment effect across subsets of patients. A statistically significant interaction should be documented before claiming that treatment effects vary among subsets. Such tests are described by Gail and Simon.[80]

Generally, it is not valid to adjust the analysis by characteristics measured after the start of treatment (e.g., compliance, dose delivered, toxicity). New approaches to subset analysis and multiple end point analysis using Bayesian methods have been described by Simon et al.[54,81]

REPORTING RESULTS OF CLINICAL TRIALS

Effective reporting of results is an integral part of good research. Unfortunately, numerous reviews have indicated that the quality of reporting of clinical trial results is poor.[59,82,83] Pocock et al.[82] concluded that "overall, the reporting of clinical trials appears to be biased toward an exaggeration of treatment differences." Tannock and colleagues[58,78] have given clear illustration of how this is easily done. Simon and Wittes[84] developed a set of methodologic guidelines for reports of clinical trials, and these guidelines have been adopted by several cancer journals. These nine guidelines are summarized below:

1. Authors should discuss briefly the quality control methods used to ensure that the data (including response assessments) are complete and accurate.
2. All patients registered on study should be accounted for.
3. The study should not have an inevaluability rate of greater than 15% for major end points.
4. In randomized trials, the report should include a comparison of survival and other major end points for all eligible patients as randomized, with no exclusions other than those not meeting eligibility criteria.
5. The sample size should be sufficient to establish or conclusively rule out the existence of effects of clinically important magnitude. For "negative" conclusions in therapeutic comparisons, the adequacy of sample size should be demonstrated by presenting confidence limits for the true treatment differences.
6. The report should indicate the initial target sample size. It should specify how many interim analyses were performed and how the decisions to stop accrual and report results were made.
7. Claims of therapeutic efficacy should not be made based on nonrandomized phase II trials, unless the disease is so rare or the prognosis so poor that properly controlled randomized trials are not possible. In the latter case, nonrandomized trials should use explicit historical controls for which comparability of patients can be thoroughly evaluated. Comparison of survival between responders and nonresponders is not a valid way of establishing therapeutic efficacy.
8. The patients studied should be adequately described. Applicability of conclusions to the general population of patients should be carefully discussed. Claims of subset-specific treatment differences should be carefully documented statistically as more than the random result of multiple significance testing.
9. The methods of statistical analysis should be described in detail sufficient that a knowledgeable reader could reproduce the analyses if the data were available.

FALSE DISCOVERY RATE

Many of the positive results reported from small trials are expected to be false-positive results.[85] In 100 trials, suppose that there are ten in which the experimental treatment is sufficiently better than the control such that there is an 80% chance of the difference being detected in a small or moderate-sized clinical trial. Of these ten trials, obtaining a statistically significant difference in eight cases is expected. Of the remaining 90 trials, it is assumed that the treatments are approximately equivalent to the control. A statistically significant difference could be expected in 5% (4.5) of these cases. Hence, of the 12.5 (8.0 + 4.5) trials that yield statistically significant results, the finding is false-positive in 4.5 or 36% of the cases (4.5/12.5). The 36% false discovery rate is striking. It depends on the assumption that only 10% of the trials represent important advances, but this assumption does not seem overly pessimistic.

An additional factor to consider is that of publication bias,[86] which denotes the preference of journals to publish positive rather than negative results. A negative result may not be published at all, particularly from a small trial. If it is published, it is likely to appear in a less widely read journal than it would if the result were positive.

These observations emphasize that results in the medical literature often cannot be accepted at face value. It is essential to recognize that "positive" results need confirmation, particularly positive results of small studies, before they can be believed and applied to the general population. A more complete Bayesian analysis of the implication of these results is described by Simon.[87]

METAANALYSIS

A *metaanalysis* is a quantitative summary of research in a particular area. It is distinguished from the traditional literature review by its emphasis on quantifying results of individual studies and combining results across studies. Key components of this approach are to include only randomized clinical trials, to include all relevant randomized clinical trials that have been initiated, regardless of whether they have been published, to exclude no randomized patients from the analysis, and to assess therapeutic effectiveness based on the average results pooled across trials.[88]

Attention is restricted to randomized trials, because the bias from nonrandomized comparisons may be larger than the small to moderate therapeutic effects likely to be present. Including all relevant randomized trials that have been initiated in a geographic area (e.g., the world, or the Americas and Europe) represents an attempt to avoid publication bias. Avoiding exclusion of any randomized patients also functions to avoid bias. Assessing therapeutic effectiveness based on average pooled results is an attempt to make the evaluation on the totality of evidence rather than on extreme isolated reports. In calculating average treatment effects, a measure of difference in outcome between treatments is calculated separately for each trial. For example, an estimate of the logarithm of the hazard ratio can be computed for each trial. A weighted average of these study-specific differences then is computed, and the statistical significance of this average is evaluated. This approach to metaanalysis requires access to individual patient data for all randomized patients in each trial. It also requires collaboration of the leaders of all the relevant trials and is very labor-intensive. Nevertheless, it represents the gold standard for metaanalysis methodology.

A major issue of concern in metaanalyses is whether the individual trials are sufficiently similar to make calculation of average effects medically meaningful. If the therapeutic interventions or control treatments differ too greatly or if the patient populations are too different, then the results may not be medically meaningful as a basis for making treatment decisions for individual patients. Often in cancer therapeutics, the studies will not be identical in their treatment regimens or their patient populations, but they will not be so different as to make the results meaningless. In this case, the metaanalysis may be useful for answering important questions about a class of treatments that the individual trials cannot address reliably. For example, trials evaluating adjuvant treatment of primary breast cancer often are designed to detect differences in disease-free survival, and a metaanalysis is often required to evaluate survival. Similarly, subset analysis can usually be meaningfully evaluated only in the context of a metaanalysis, because individual trials are not sized for this objective.

Metaanalysis is not an alternative to properly designed and sized randomized clinical trials. Some have suggested that one need not be concerned about computing sample size in the traditional ways, as small, randomized trials can be pooled for metaanalysis. Because most investigators would prefer to "do their own thing," this would lead to a proliferation of diverse trials of inconsequential individual size that were too heterogeneous to permit a meaningful metaanalysis. Given that sufficient large, randomized clinical trials of very similar treatment regimens have been conducted, metaanalysis can provide supplemental information about a given class of treatments that is not available from the individual trials.

REFERENCES

1. McFadden E. *Management of data in clinical trials.* Wiley, 1997.
2. Green S, Benedetti J, Crowley J. *Clinical trials in oncology*, 2nd ed. Chapman and Hall/CRC, 2003.
3. Leventhal BG, Wittes RE. *Research methods in clinical oncology.* New York: Raven Press, 1988.
4. Eisenhauer EA, O'Dwyer PJ, Christian M, et al. Phase I clinical trial design in cancer drug development. *J Clin Oncol* 2000;18:684.
5. Simon R, Freidlin B, Rubinstein L. Accelerated titration designs for phase I clinical trials in oncology. *J Natl Cancer Inst* 1997;89:1138.
6. O'Quigley J, Pepe M, Fisher L. Continual reassessment method: a practical design for phase I clinical trials. *Biometrics* 1990;46:33.
7. O'Quigley J. Dose finding designs using continual reassessment methods. In: Crowley J, ed. *Handbook of statistics in clinical trials.* New York: Marcel Dekker, 2001:35.
8. Goodman SN, Zahurak ML, Piantadosi S. Some practical improvements in the continual reassessment method for phase I studies. *Stat Med* 1995;14:1149.
9. Moller S. An extension of the continual reassessment methods using a preliminary up-and-down design in a dose finding study in cancer patients, in order to investigate a greater range of doses. *Stat Med* 1995;14:911.
10. Babb J, Rogatko A, Zacks S. Cancer phase I clinical trials: efficient dose escalation with overdose control. *Stat Med* 1998;17:1103.
11. Potter DM. Adaptive dose finding for phase I clinical trials of drugs used for the chemotherapy of cancer. *Stat Med* 2002;21:1805.
12. Korn EL, Simon R. Using the tolerable-dose diagram in the design of phase I combination chemotherapy trials. *J Clin Oncol* 1993;11:794.
13. Simon RM, Steinberg SM, Hamilton M, et al. Clinical trial designs for the early clinical development of therapeutic cancer vaccines. *J Clin Oncol* 2001;19:1848.
14. Rubinstein LV, Simon RM. Phase I clinical trial design. In: Budman DR, Calvert AH, Rowinsky EK, eds. *Handbook of anticancer drug development.* Philadelphia: Lippincott Williams & Wilkins, 2003:297.
15. Fox E, Curt GA, Balis FM. Clinical trial design for target-based therapy. *Oncologist* 2002;7:401.
16. Korn EL, Rubinstein LV, Hunsberger SA, et al. Clinical trial designs for cytostatic agents and agents directed at novel molecular targets. In: Adei AA, Buolamwini JK, eds. *Strategies for discovery and clinical testing of novel anticancer agents.* Amsterdam: Elsevier, 2004.
17. Anderson JR, Cain KC, Gelber RD. Analysis of survival by tumor response. *J Clin Oncol* 1983;1:710.
18. Simon R, Makuch RW. A nonparametric graphical representation of the relationship between survival and the occurrence of an event: application to responder versus nonresponder bias. *Stat Med* 1984;3:1.
19. Simon R. Optimal two-stage design for phase II clinical trials. *Control Clin Trials* 1989;10:1.
20. Ensign LG, Gehan EA, Kamen DS, et al. An optimal three-stage design for phase II clinical trials. *Stat Med* 1994;13:1727.
21. Bryant J, Day R. Incorporating toxicity considerations into the design of two-stage phase II clinical trials. *Biometrics* 1995;51:1372.
22. Conaway M, Petroni G. Designs for phase II trials allowing for a trade-off between response and toxicity. *Biometrics* 1996;52:1375.
23. Zee B, Melnychuk D, Dancey J, et al. Multinomial phase II cancer trials incorporating response and early progression. *J Biopharm Stat* 1999;9:351.
24. Simon R, Wittes RE, Ellenberg SS. Randomized phase II clinical trials. *Cancer Treat Rep* 1994;69:1375.
25. Steinberg SM, Venzon DJ. Early selection in a randomized phase II clinical trial. *Stat Med* 2002;21:1711.
26. Makuch RW, Simon R. Sample size considerations for nonrandomized comparative studies. *J Chronic Dis* 1980;33:171.
27. Thall PF, Simon R, Estey E. New statistical strategy for monitoring safety and efficacy in single-arm clinical trials. *J Clin Oncol* 1996;14:296.
28. Mick R, Crowley JJ, Carroll RJ. Phase II clinical trial design for nontoxic anticancer agents for which time to disease progression is the primary endpoint. *Control Clin Trials* 2000;21:343.
29. Seymour L. The design of clinical trials for new molecularly targeted compounds: progress and new initiatives. *Curr Pharm Des* 2002;8:2279.
30. Rosner G, Stadler W, Ratain M. Randomized discontinuation design: application to cytostatic antineoplastic agents. *J Clin Oncol* 2002;20:4478.
31. Korn EL, Arbuck SG, Pluda JM, et al. Clinical trial designs for cytostatic agents: are new approaches needed? *J Clin Oncol* 2001;19:265.
32. Liu PY, Dahlberg S, Crowley J. Selection designs for pilot studies based on survival. *Biometrics* 1993;49:391.
33. Sher HI, Heller G. Picking the winners in a sea of plenty. *Clin Cancer Res* 2002;8:400.
34. Schaid DJ, Wieand S, Therneau TM. Optimal two-stage screening designs for survival comparisons. *Biometrika* 1990;77:507.
35. Thall PF, Simon R, Ellenberg SS. Two-stage selection and testing designs for comparative clinical trials. *Biometrika* 1988;75:303.
36. Dixon DO, Simon R. Sample size considerations for studies comparing survival curves using historical controls. *J Clin Epidemiol* 1988;41:1209.
37. Simon R. Randomized clinical trials in oncology: principles and obstacles. *Cancer* 1994;74:2614.
38. Torri V, Simon R, Russek-Cohen E, et al. Relationship of response and survival in advanced ovarian cancer patients treated with chemotherapy. *J Natl Cancer Inst* 1992;84:407.
39. Hill A. The clinical trial. *BMJ* 1951;7:278.
40. Byar DP, Simon R, Friedewald WT, et al. Randomized clinical trials: perspectives on some recent ideas. *N Engl J Med* 1976;295:74.
41. Chalmers TC, Block JB, Lee S. Controlled studies in clinical cancer research. *N Engl J Med* 1972;287:75.
42. Pocoock SJ. Randomized clinical trials. *BMJ* 1977;1:1161.
43. Peto R, Pike MC, Armitage P, et al. Design and analysis of randomized clinical trials requiring prolonged observation of each patient: I. Introduction and design. *Br J Cancer* 1976;34:585.
44. Peto R, Pike MC, Armitage P, et al. Design and analysis of randomized clinical trials requiring prolonged observation of each patient: II. Analysis and examples. *Br J Cancer* 1977;35:1.
45. Pocock S, Simon R. Sequential treatment assignment with balancing for prognostic factors in the controlled clinical trial. *Biometrics* 1975;31:103.
46. Kalish LA, Begg CB. The impact of treatment allocation procedures on nominal significance levels and bias. *Control Clin Trials* 1987;27:15.

47. Rubinstein L, Gail M, Santner T. Planning the duration of a comparative clinical trial with loss to follow-up and a period of continued observation. *J Chronic Dis* 1981;34:469.

48. Frieman JA, Chalmers TC, Smith HJ. The importance of beta, the type II error, and sample size in the design and interpretation of the randomized control trial: survey of 71 "negative" trials. *Cancer Treat Rep* 1978;62.

49. Makuch R, Simon R. Sample size requirements for evaluating a conservative therapy. *Cancer Treat Rep* 1978;62:1037.

50. Durrleman S, Simon R. Planning and monitoring of equivalence studies. *Biometrics* 1990;69:1055.

51. Brittain E, Wittes J. Factorial designs in clinical trials: the effects of non-compliance and subadditivity. *Biometrics* 1989;8:161.

52. Simon R, Freedman LS. Bayesian design and analysis of 2 by 2 factorial clinical trials. *Biometrics* 1997;53:456.

53. Simon R. Bayesian design and analysis of active control clinical trials. *Biometrics* 1999;66:484.

54. Simon R. Bayesian subset analysis: application to studying treatment-by-gender interactions. *Stat Med* 2002;21:2909.

55. Simon R. Bayesian design and analysis of active control clinical trials. *Biometrics* 1999;55:484.

56. Simon R. Discovering the truth about tamoxifen: problems of multiplicity in the evaluation of biomedical data. *J Natl Cancer Inst* 1995;87:627.

57. Spiegelhalter DJ, Freedman LS, Parmar MKB. Bayesian approaches to randomized trials. *J R Stat Soc [Ser A]* 1994;157:357.

58. Barr J, Tannock I. Analyzing the same data two ways: a demonstration model illustrate the reporting and misreporting of clinical trials. *J Clin Oncol* 1989;7:969.

59. Tannock I, Murphy K. Reflections on medical oncology: an appeal for better clinical trials and improved reporting of their results. *J Clin Oncol* 1983;1:66.

60. Group C. Influence of adherence to treatment and response of cholesterol on mortality in the coronary drug project. *New Engl J Med* 1980;302:1038.

61. Fleming TR, Green SJ, Harrington DP. Considerations of monitoring and evaluation treatment effects in clinical trials. *Control Clin Trials* 1984;5:55.

62. Smith M, Ungerleider R, Korn E, et al. The role of independent data monitoring committees in randomized clinical trials sponsored by the national cancer institute. *J Clin Oncol* 1997;15:2736.

63. Ellenberg S, Fleming TR, DeMets D. *Data monitoring committees in clinical trials: a practical perspective.* Wiley, 2002.

64. O'Brien PC, Fleming TR. A multiple testing procedure for clinical trials. *Biometrics* 1979;35:549.

65. Pocock SJ. Interim analyses for randomized clinical trials. *Biometrics* 1982;39:153.

66. Fleming TR, O'Brien PC, Harrington DP. Designs for group sequential tests. *Control Clin Trials* 1984;5:348.

67. Jennison C, Turnbull BW. *Group sequential methods with applications to clinical trials.* Chapman and Hall, 1999.

68. Lan KKG, Simon R, Halperin M. Stochastically curtailed test in long-term clinical trials. *Commun Stat Seqen Anal* 1982;1:207.

69. Storer BE. A sequential phase II/III trial for binary outcomes. *Stat Med* 1990;9:229.

70. Thall PF, Simon R, Ellenberg SS, et al. Optimal two-stage design for clinical trials with binary response. *Stat Med* 1988;7:571.

71. Wieand S, Schroeder G, O'Fallon JR. Stopping when the experimental regimen does not appear to help. *Stat Med* 1994;13:1453.

72. Simon R. Designs for efficient clinical trials. *Oncology* 1989;3:34.

73. Simon R. Confidence intervals for reporting results from clinical trials. *Ann Intern Med* 1986;105:429.

74. Berkson J, Gage RP. Calculation of survival rates for cancer. *Mayo Clinic Proc* 1950;25:270.

75. Cutler SJ, Ederer F. Maximum utilization of the life table method in analyzing survival. *J Chronic Dis* 1958;8:699.

76. Kaplan EI, Meier P. Nonparametric estimation from incomplete observations. *J Am Stat Assoc* 1958;53:457.

77. Marubini E, Valsecchi MG. *Analyzing survival data from clinical trials and observational studies.* New York: Wiley, 1995.

78. Tannock IF. False-positive results in clinical trials: multiple significance tests and the problem of unreported comparisons. *J Natl Cancer Inst* 1996;88:206.

79. Fleming TR, Watelet L. Approaches to monitoring clinical trials. *J Natl Cancer Inst* 1989;81:188.

80. Gail M, Simon R. Testing for qualitative interactions between treatment effects and patient subsets. *Biometrics* 1985;41:361.

81. Dixon DO, Simon R. Bayesian subset analysis. *Biometrics* 1991;47:871.

82. Pocock SJ, Hughes MD, Lee RJ. Statistical problems in the reporting of clinical trials: a survey of three medical journals. *New Engl J Med* 1987;317:426.

83. Begg CB. Quality of clinical trials. *Ann Oncol* 1990;1:319.

84. Simon R, Wittes RE. Methodologic guidelines for reports of clinical trials. *Cancer Treat Rep* 1985;69:1.

85. Simon R. Randomized clinical trials and research strategy. *Cancer Treat Rep* 1982;66:1083.

86. Begg CB, Berlin JA. Publication bias and dissemination of clinical research. *J Natl Cancer Inst* 1989;81:107.

87. Simon R. Clinical trials and sample size considerations: another perspective. *Stat Sci* 2000;15:95.

88. Collins R, Gray R, Godwin J, et al. Avoidance of large biases and large random errors in the assessment of moderate treatment effects: the need for systematic overviews. *Stat Med* 1987;6:245.

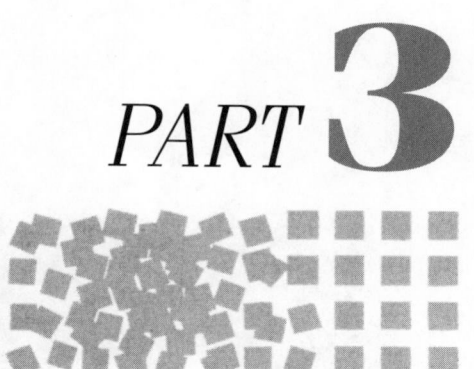

PART **3**

PRACTICE OF ONCOLOGY

Howard K. Koh
Alan C. Geller

CHAPTER **19**

Cancer Prevention: Preventing Tobacco-Related Cancers

Tobacco addiction ranks as the greatest public health catastrophe of our time. The practice of inhaling cigarette smoke, which gained widespread acceptance only during the twentieth century, has generated devastating cancer outcomes for our society. Specifically, lung cancer, previously rare, ranks as the leading cancer killer in American men and women.[1,2] Worldwide estimates suggest that the annual deaths attributable to smoking, currently 4.83 million, will rise to 12 million by the year 2050.[3-5] Future medical historians undoubtedly will recall the 1900s as the Tobacco and Cancer Century.[2]

A healthier twenty-first century requires a societal commitment to reducing and eradicating tobacco addiction. This chapter reviews the impact of tobacco on cancer and explores individual and societal strategies for tobacco control.

TOBACCO AND NICOTINE ADDICTION

Tobacco and tobacco smoke contain at least 4000 chemicals, of which 55 are known carcinogens identified by the International Agency for Research on Cancer.[6] The most notable carcinogen classes include polycyclic aromatic hydrocarbons, N-nitrosamines, and miscellaneous organic compounds. Of the polycyclic aromatic hydrocarbons, benzo[a]pyrene (BaP) is the most extensively studied lung carcinogen. Of the N-nitrosamines, 4-(methylnitrosamino)-1-(3-pyridyl)-1-butanone (NNK) is best known. Metabolic activation of these agents can incite DNA adduct formation, gene mutations, and a sequence of events that can lead to cancer. The balance between detoxification and metabolic activation determines, in part, the susceptibility of smokers to cancer.[6]

Although nicotine does not cause cancer, addiction to nicotine exposes the user to carcinogens. Nicotine addiction fulfills the physiologic, behavioral, and social characteristics of a dependence syndrome.[7] The American Psychiatric Association's *Diagnostic and Statistical Manual of Mental Disorders* (3rd ed) requires a minimum of three of seven diagnostic symptoms for drug dependency: (1) tolerance, (2) withdrawal, (3) greater use than intended, (4) persistent desire to quit, (5) great amounts of time spent smoking, (6) activities given up or reduced due to smoking, and (7) continued smoking despite knowledge of having persistent physical or psychological problems with the substance.[7] The 1988 Surgeon General's report focused on the concept of nicotine addiction and its clinical ability to produce brief, pleasurable psychoactive effects; its continued use despite known adverse health outcomes; development of tolerance during early usage; and occurrence of withdrawal symptoms on cessation of use.[8] Withdrawal symptoms include nervousness, restlessness, anxiety, impaired cognition, headache, drowsiness, gastrointestinal disturbances, nicotine cravings, increased appetite and weight gain, and anxiety.[7-9]

HEALTH EFFECTS

As early as 1928, Lombard and Doering[10] reported higher smoking rates among patients with cancer than among controls. Later, the pioneering epidemiologic work of Doll and Hill,[11] Wynder and Graham,[12] and Hammond and Horn[13] led to further investigations, which culminated in the 1964 U.S. Surgeon General's report on smoking and health.[14] This report concluded that cigarette smoking was the major cause of lung

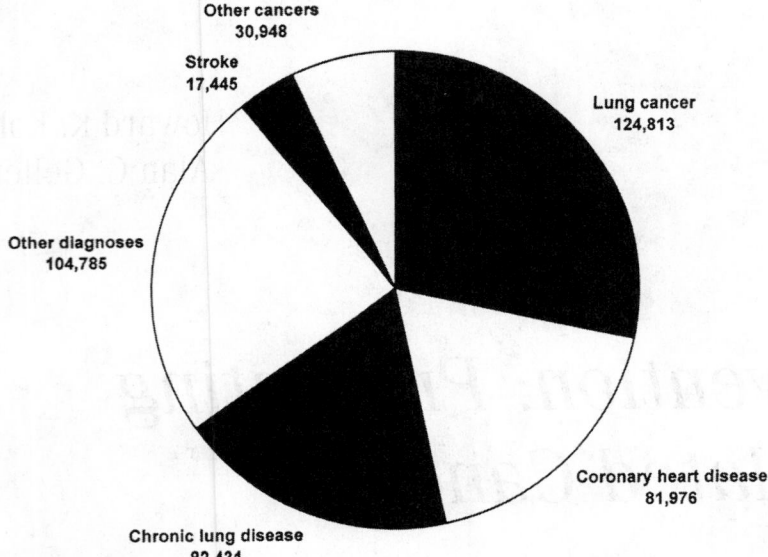

FIGURE 19-1. Each year, 442,398 U.S. deaths are attributable to cigarette smoking. (From ref. 15, with permission.)

cancer in men and was causally related to laryngeal cancer and oral cancer in men.[14]

In total, more than 60,000 studies and two dozen additional reports of the Surgeon General have confirmed the devastating impact of tobacco use on human health. Tobacco use, causing approximately 30% of all deaths and more than 440,000 deaths annually, is the leading cause of preventable death in the United States[1,15,16] (Fig. 19-1). Tobacco use kills more Americans each year than do alcohol, cocaine, heroin, homicide, suicide, car accidents, firearms, and AIDS combined.[17]

Smoking causes more than 85% to 90% of lung cancers, with a clear dose-response relationship between risk and daily cigarette consumption.[18] People who smoke more than a pack of cigarettes per day have a risk that is as much as 20 times that of nonsmokers.[18] In smokers exposed to other carcinogens in the workplace (e.g., pipefitters exposed to asbestos; uranium workers exposed to radon), the risk for lung cancer is raised in a synergistic fashion.[19–22]

Lung cancer is the leading cause of cancer mortality in men and in women. U.S. estimates for 2003 include approximately 171,900 lung cancer deaths. Male lung cancer mortality peaked in 1990 at 90.6 per 100,000 and has now dropped to 76.9.[23] Among U.S. women, however, lung cancer surpassed breast cancer as the leading cause of cancer death in the 1980s, and mortality has not declined.[1,23]

Lung cancer incidence also varies by subpopulation. Female lung cancer incidence rose from a low of 24.5 per 100,000 in 1975 to 52.8 per 100,000 in 1998, although rates dropped to 49.8 per 100,000 in 2000. Lung cancer incidence in men dropped from a high of 102.1 per 100,000 (1984) to a low of 79.8 per 100,000 in 2000, the lowest level since the National Cancer Institute's Surveillance, Epidemiology, and End Results program began recording rates in 1975.[23] Variations occur by race and ethnicity, from a high of 82.6 per 100,000 in African Americans to a low of 31.5 among Hispanics.[1,23]

Smoking is accepted as the major cause of cancers of the larynx, pharynx, oral cavity, and esophagus and is a contributory factor in cancers of the pancreas, bladder, kidney, stomach, colon, and uterine cervix and in acute leukemia.[24,25] Oral cavity

cancers are also caused by the use of pipes, cigars, and spit tobacco in its various forms (plug tobacco, loose-leaf tobacco, twist tobacco, and moist snuff).[18,24–28] Tobacco use is responsible for more than 90% of tumors of the oral cavity among men and 60% among women.[27]

The disease burden induced by tobacco comes at a tremendous cost. Americans spend an estimated $75.5 billion annually on direct medical care for smoking-related illnesses.[29] Lost productivity and forfeited earnings due to smoking-related mortality account for an additional $81.9 billion per year.[29]

SMOKING RATES AND TRENDS

With the vigorous promotion of the blended cigarette in the twentieth century, the annual adult per capita consumption of cigarettes skyrocketed from 54 cigarettes (1900) to a peak of 4345 cigarettes (1963).[30] Although per capita consumption has since declined, approximately 500 billion cigarettes were sold in the United States in 1995.[6] Historically, smoking rates in men have far exceeded those in women, but the gender difference has narrowed as male rates declined and female rates rose.[1,30] The tobacco industry's attempts to recruit women range from the American Tobacco Company's advertising campaign, "To keep a slender figure, reach for a Lucky Strike instead of a sweet" (1920s) to Philip Morris's Virginia Slims slogan, "You've come a long way, baby."[31] Rates for most races and ethnic groups have decreased since 1978, although the rate of decrease has ebbed[32] (Fig. 19-2).

ADULTS

Approximately 1.2 billion smokers are found worldwide.[33] According to the 2000 National Health Interview Study, in the United States, nearly 46.5 million adults (23.3%) currently smoke, either daily (19.1%) or on some days (4.1%).[32] Currently, men (25.7%) are more likely to smoke than are women (21.0%). Among racial and ethnic groups, American Indians

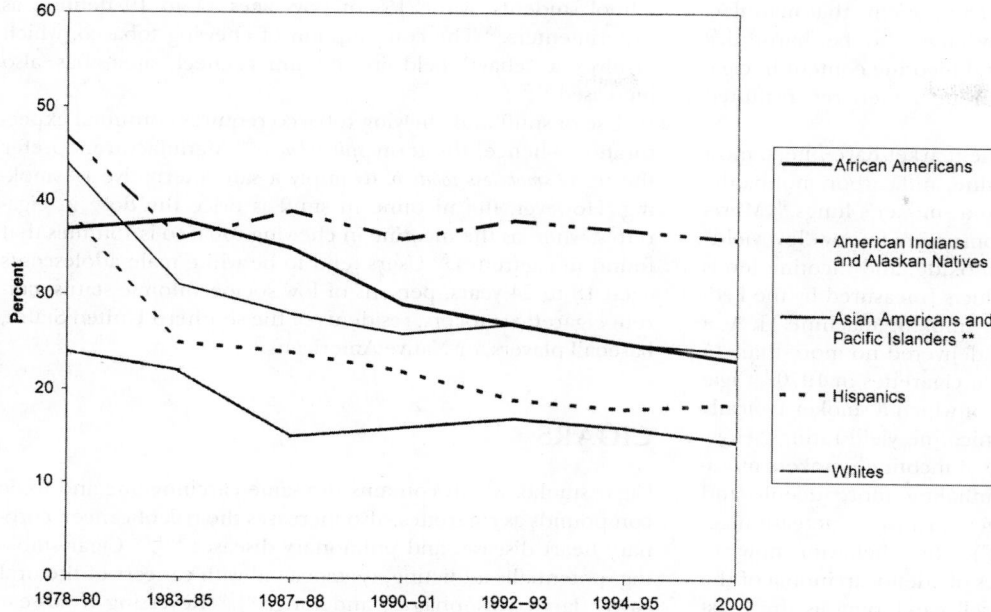

FIGURE 19-2. Current cigarette smoking among adults, National Health Interview Surveys, U.S. 1978 to 2000 aggregate data. **2000 data do not include Native Hawaiians and other Pacific Islanders. (From ref. 32, with permission.)

and Alaskan natives have the highest prevalence (36.0%), whereas Asian Americans and Pacific Islanders have the lowest (14.4%).[32] Educational level is the most important predictor of smoking prevalence.[9]

Since the landmark 1964 Surgeon General's report, overall U.S. smoking prevalence has declined by one-half, from 50.2% (1965) to 25% (1998), although adult smoking rates reached a plateau in the 1990s.[1] Declines in smoking prevalence were greater among African American, Hispanic, and white men who were high school graduates than among those with less education.[1]

CHILDREN, ADOLESCENTS, AND COLLEGE STUDENTS

Tobacco use qualifies as a pediatric disease.[34] The 2001 Youth Risk Behavior Survey indicated smoking rates for girls and boys as 61.6% and 66.3%, respectively, for lifetime cigarette use and 27.7% and 29.2%, respectively, for current cigarette use.[35] Nearly 90% of adult smokers begin smoking by the age of 18 years. Even by grade 9, 58.4% of children have experimented with cigarettes.[35] It is estimated that of nearly 3000 young people who start smoking each day, 1 in 3 will die prematurely.[36,37] At least three million American teenagers smoke regularly.[9]

The national 2001 Youth Risk Behavior Survey indicated that cigarette smoking prevalence among U.S. high school students increased from 27.5% in 1991 to 36.4% in 1997 but then fell to 28.5% in 2001.[35] This trend occurred in all racial and ethnic groups [e.g., whites (30.9% to 39.7% to 31.9%), African Americans (12.6% to 22.7% to 14.7%), and Hispanics (25.3% to 34.0% to 26.6%)]. Monitoring the Future Project data (an analysis of high school seniors from 1976 to 2002) shows that the current smoking rate among high school seniors (defined as smoking in the past 30 days) rose from 28.3% in 1991 to 34% in 1996, then fell to 26.7% in 2003.[38] Rates for grades 8 and 10 show a similar trend.[39]

Of concern, the age of smoking initiation has declined over the past four decades, for whites (by 2.4 years) and for African Americans (by 1 to 3 years).[9] The decline is particularly striking for girls (5.4 years and 4.6 years for whites and African Americans, respectively).[9] Twenty-five percent of students have smoked a whole cigarette before age 13.[40] Also, half of the nation's six million smokeless tobacco users were younger than 21 years, and several national surveys show an increase in prevalence, especially among boys.[9]

Tobacco use in children is linked to alcohol and illegal drug use.[41,42] Among boys especially, aggressive or disruptive classroom behavior as early as first grade has been found to predict later tobacco and other heavy drug use, as well as antisocial behavior and criminality.[41] The National Household Study on Drug Abuse from 1985 showed that children who smoke are 3 times more likely to drink alcohol, 8 times more likely to smoke marijuana, and 22 times more likely to use cocaine.[42] Children's tobacco and alcohol use also were associated with less effective parenting behaviors in the children's families and with parental use of tobacco and alcohol.[43]

Newer data point to increasing smoking rates among college students.[44] In serial surveys of nearly 15,000 randomly selected college students, Wechsler et al.[44] found that the prevalence of current cigarette smoking rose by 27.8% (from 22.3% to 28.5% during the period 1993 to 1997). Defying earlier trends, 11% of college smokers had their first cigarette and 28% began to smoke regularly at or after age 19. Half of current college smokers tried to quit in the previous year; 18% had made five or more attempts to quit.[44]

CIGARETTE PRODUCT MODIFICATION

For years, the tobacco industry has tried to design less toxic cigarette products. For example, in the 1950s, confronted with declining cigarette sales after studies linked smoking to lung cancer, tobacco companies began producing filter-tip brands designed to remove certain smoke components that manufacturers had not heretofore acknowledged to be harmful.[45] Methods used to decrease the tar and nicotine content in cigarettes were filter tips, porous cigarette paper, reconstituted tobacco, and filter-tip ventilation.[45]

Today, almost all cigarettes on the market have filters, most with perforations to dilute tar, nicotine, and carbon monoxide, thereby decreasing their delivery to a smoker's lungs.[46] Moreover, active promotion led many consumers to buy "low yield" cigarettes that emit tar, carbon monoxide, and nicotine levels that were lower than standard products [measured by the Federal Trade Commission's assay ("the smoking machine")]. As a result, by 1995, 72.7% of cigarettes delivered no more than 15 mg tar, as compared to only 3.6% of cigarettes in 1970.[1] Cigarettes contain 6 to 11 mg nicotine, of which a smoker typically absorbs 1 to 3 mg, irrespective of nicotine yield ratings. However, to maintain the desired intake of nicotine, smokers modified their smoking behavior by inhaling more deeply and blocking filter vents with their fingers or lips to increase nicotine yield ("compensatory smoking"). These behaviors now are suspected to be linked to rising rates of adenocarcinoma of the lung, which surpassed squamous cell carcinoma as the most common type of lung cancer in the United States.[24]

For years, the tobacco industry has continued to suggest health benefits to consumers through promotion of "light," "ultralight," "mild," "medium," "slim," and "superslim" cigarettes.[26] However, a monograph from the National Cancer Institute has concluded that evidence does not indicate a benefit to public health from low-tar cigarettes. In fact, reduced-yield products might, in fact, impede public health by helping to delay genuine attempts to quit.[47]

Most recently, a series of products have been developed that potentially could be applied toward the goal of "harm reduction" (use of products that lower tobacco-related mortality and morbidity even though such use may involve continued exposure to tobacco-related toxicants). These potential reduced-exposure products include modified tobacco products with reportedly reduced yield of selected toxicants and cigarette-like agents with less combustion than cigarettes. An Institute of Medicine report concluded that potential reduced-exposure products have not been subjected to the comprehensive rigorous scientific evaluation required to demonstrate a reduced risk of disease compared to conventional tobacco use. Such research must be a high public health priority for the future. In addition, the Institute of Medicine also concluded that, although harm reduction could serve as a justifiable and feasible component of a comprehensive national tobacco control program that emphasizes abstinence-oriented prevention and treatment, its possible implementation would require firm regulation of product promotion, advertising, and labeling, as well as the supply of full and accurate information for the public.[48]

SPIT TOBACCO

Spit tobacco (smokeless tobacco), available as snuff or chewing tobacco, has gained great popularity over the last few decades.[49-53] Snuff dipping, the practice of sucking on a pinch of powdered, flavored tobacco in the cavity between gum and cheek, has increased. The 2001 Youth Risk Behavior Survey documented an 8.2% prevalence of current spit tobacco use among high school students, with 21% of boys ages 11 to 19 defined as experimenters.[35] The consumption of chewing tobacco, which involves a "chaw" held in the inner cheek area, has also increased.[51,53]

Use of snuff and chewing tobacco requires continual expectoration—hence, the term *spit tobacco*.[50] Manufacturers prefer the term *smokeless tobacco*, to imply a safe alternative to smoking. However, the nicotine in snuff is twice the dose in cigarettes, whereas the nicotine in chewing tobacco is 15 times that found in cigarettes.[53] Users tend to be white male adolescents aged 18 to 24 years, persons of low socioeconomic status, current cigarette smokers, residents of the southern United States, baseball players, or Native Americans.[52]

CIGARS

Cigar smoke, which contains the same carcinogenic and toxic compounds as cigarettes, also increases the risk of cancer, coronary heart disease, and pulmonary diseases.[8,54-56] Cigar smoking, potentially addicting, is associated with cancers of the oral cavity, larynx, esophagus, and lung.[8,54,56] Reversing a 20-year decline, cigar sales increased by 50% from 1993 to 1997,[56] prompted by industry marketing and the belief that cigars are less dangerous than cigarettes. Young to middle-aged men of high socioeconomic status, teenagers, and women are the groups responsible for the increased consumption of cigars.[55] The overall prevalence of current cigar use among high school students was 15.2% in 2001, with males most at risk.[35]

ENVIRONMENTAL TOBACCO SMOKE

The 1986 U.S. Surgeon General's report defined environmental tobacco smoke (ETS), also called *secondhand smoke*, as the combination of sidestream smoke (released from a burning cigarette between puffs) and the fraction of mainstream smoke exhaled by the smoker.[57] The more hazardous sidestream smoke has double the amount of nicotine than mainstream smoke and a higher concentration of carcinogens.[57] Most people spend 90% of their time in the two microenvironments of home and work, where ETS exposure usually occurs.[58] Those at greatest risk for harm from ETS are those who live with smokers in homes. Levels of serum cotinine, a nicotine metabolite, are increased in nonsmokers who live with smokers and are correlated to the number of cigarettes smoked.[59]

An increasing number of studies have documented the health risks of the nonsmoker exposed to ETS.[57-63] Case-control studies first noted that nonsmoking wives of smoking husbands had an increased risk of lung cancer.[59] In 1992, the U.S. Environmental Protection Agency (EPA), in the most thoroughly documented analysis ever undertaken of the effects of exposure to ETS, concluded that secondhand smoke can cause lung cancer in nonsmoking adults and can impair the respiratory systems of children. The EPA classified ETS as a group A carcinogen, a designation reserved for agents such as asbestos. Of 30 studies analyzed in the EPA report, 24 found an increased risk of lung cancer for nonsmoking wives of husbands who smoked, and each of the 17 studies that examined risk based on exposure level reported increased lung cancer among those most exposed.[62]

The EPA report and other ETS studies now attribute approximately 3000 deaths a year in the United States to lung cancer, up to 62,000 deaths to ischemic heart disease, and up to 2700 deaths to sudden infant death syndrome.[62] The 1997 California EPA report also notes that ETS is responsible for new cases of low-birth-weight infants (up to 18,600 per year), new cases of childhood asthma (up to 26,000 per year), exacerbation of childhood asthma (up to 1 million new cases per year), and bronchitis or pneumonia in children aged 18 months and younger (up to 300,000 cases per year). Workers at great risk for harm from ETS include flight attendants, casino workers, and restaurant and bar workers, among others.[63]

TOBACCO INDUSTRY ADVERTISING STRATEGIES

Tobacco companies have dedicated considerable resources to corner new markets and to replace the loss of an estimated 3500 Americans who quit smoking and an additional 1200 customers who die of smoking-related illness each day. During the last three decades, the tobacco industry has increased its marketing expenditures nearly eightfold[64,65] (Fig. 19-3). The 1994 U.S. Surgeon General's report, *Preventing Tobacco Use among Young People*,[66] summarized:

Young people constitute a highly strategic market for the tobacco industry.

Young people are continuously exposed to cigarette messages through print media and promotional activities.

Cigarette advertising uses images, not information, to portray the attractiveness of smoking.

Cigarette advertisements capitalize on the disparity between an ideal and actual self-image, implying that smoking may close the gap.

Cigarette advertising appears to affect young people's perceptions of the pervasiveness, image, and function of smoking. Such misperceptions increase young people's risk of smoking.

Many adolescents now experiment with tobacco almost as a rite of passage and have high recollection of tobacco industry promotional messages. Nearly 70% of children aged 13 reported at least moderate receptivity to marketing materials, indicating susceptibility.[67] Adolescents and youth are susceptible to image advertising and promotional themes as they seek to find their own identities.[68] One study found that 6-year-old children were as likely to identify Joe Camel as they were Mickey Mouse.[69]

In addition, adolescents smoke the most heavily advertised brands.[68] Pierce et al.[68] provided the first longitudinal evidence that tobacco promotional activities are causally related to the onset of smoking. A total of 1752 adolescents who had never smoked and who were not susceptible to smoking (when first interviewed in 1993) were reinterviewed in 1996. Nearly 50% progressed toward smoking (by becoming susceptible, by experimenting, or by consuming at least 100 cigarettes). The authors attributed 34% of all adolescent tobacco experimentation in California (from 1993 through 1996) to industry promotional activities.[68] Tobacco marketing strategies include magazine and newspaper advertising, sponsorship of sporting events and public entertainment, and distribution of free samples of cigarettes in public places. Promotions and specialty items include mailings and giveaways of multiple packs (buy one, get one free) and coupon reductions for attractive specialty items (such as T-shirts,

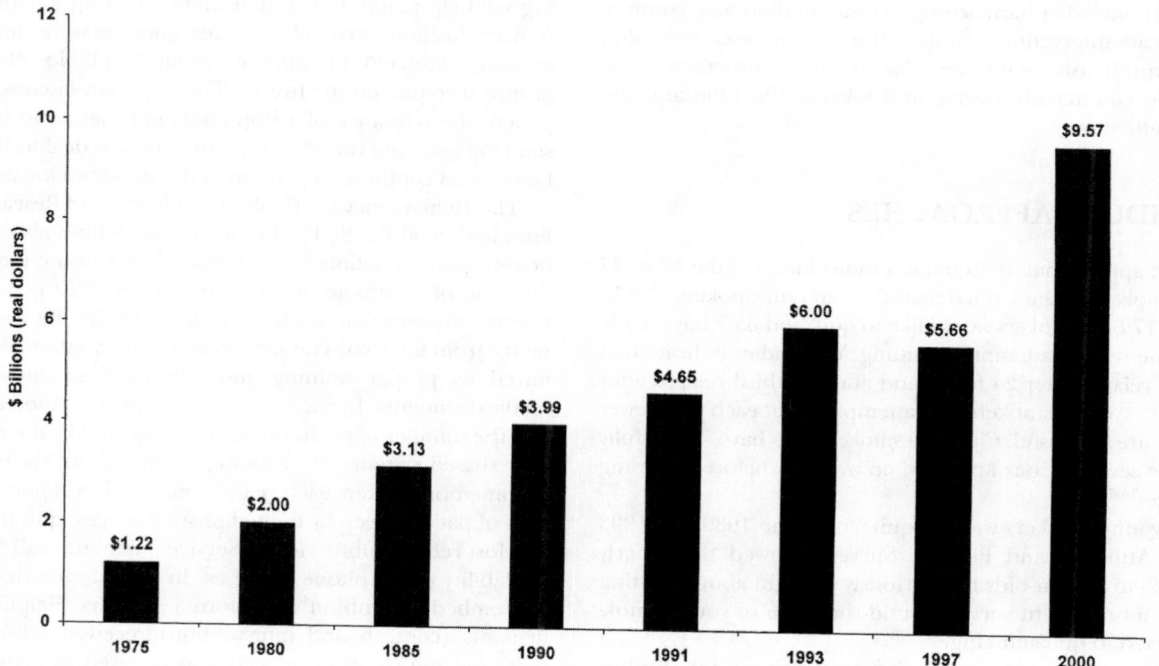

FIGURE 19-3. Cigarette advertising and promotion expenditures in the United States have increased nearly eightfold in 25 years. (From ref. 64, with permission.)

caps, calendars, and sporting goods).[9,36,70] Surveys have found that half of all adolescent smokers and one-fourth of adolescent nonsmokers own at least one tobacco promotional item.[36] Tobacco companies also pay retailers for shelf space and engage them to promote point-of-sale advertising, a technique that places the tobacco products in convenient visible racks and in point-of-purchase displays.[9,36]

The tobacco industry also uses its considerable financial and legal resources to influence local and national policy.[30,71–73] The industry frames the public debate about smoking regulations around rights and liberty rather than health, portrays adversaries as extremists, and invests millions of dollars in campaign contributions to the leading political parties.[30,71–74] They successfully solicit allies (including advertisers, civil libertarians, and restaurant owners) to help lobby or advance arguments that oppose regulation.[72]

The tobacco industry has generally escaped strong government legislation. Federal legislation, including the Controlled Substances Act (1970), Consumer Product Safety Act (1972), and Toxic Substances Control Act (1976) all excluded tobacco from regulation.[73] The landmark 1965 Federal Cigarette Labeling and Advertising Act, the first federal statute enacting labeling requirements for cigarette packages, contained a federal preemption clause preventing individual states from making laws to regulate tobacco advertising.[73]

STRATEGIES FOR TOBACCO CONTROL

For decades, the concept of tobacco control focused solely on cessation strategies for individual smokers. More recently, the emphasis has broadened to encompass prevention strategies that stress denormalization of tobacco use for the entire community. Hence, key dimensions now include individual approaches that expand the role of the clinician in smoking cessation services, which include pharmacologic cessation therapies, community and state interventions, policy strategies, tobacco taxes that fund comprehensive statewide tobacco control programs, mass media and counter-advertising, and tobacco litigation and the tobacco settlement.[73]

INDIVIDUAL APPROACHES

Each year, approximately 20 million individuals (of the 46 to 47 million smokers in the United States) try to quit smoking.[74–76] In addition, 77% of smokers would like to quit, and 65% have made at least one serious attempt at quitting. Yet, studies indicate that one-third relapse after 24 hours and another third relapse after 48 hours.[74–76] Of all smokers who attempt to quit each year, fewer than 10% are successful. Cigarette smokers who have successfully quit made seven serious attempts, on average, before achieving abstinence.[74–76]

Even young smokers want to quit.[36,77,78] The 1989 and 1993 Teenage Attitudes and Practice Surveys showed that nearly 75% of 12- to 18-year-olds had seriously thought about quitting smoking; more recent surveys found that 73% of young smokers had tried to quit smoking.[36,77,78]

Smoking cessation restores a chance of living a full, healthy life.[79] Quitting smoking reduces the risk of lung cancer by 50% at 5 years; by 10 years, lung cancer risk drops almost to the rate for nonsmokers.[30] After a year, mortality from heart disease decreases by half, and by 5 years it equals the rate for nonsmokers.

CLINICIAN'S ROLE

Physicians and health professionals should view smoking cessation as a cornerstone of their practice.[80] Providing a brief physician intervention to all smokers could more than double annual quit rates.[81] Seventy percent of smokers see their doctors at least once annually, thereby granting physicians ample opportunity for smoking cessation counseling.[82] If only one-half of all U.S. physicians gave brief advice to their patients regarding smoking cessation, leading to success in 10%, clinician intervention would account for two million new nonsmokers in the United States each year.[83,84]

Treating Tobacco Use and Dependence (2000), a Public Health Service–sponsored clinical practice guideline, updates new, effective treatments for tobacco dependence. The key recommendations stress that "clinicians and health care delivery systems institutionalize the consistent identification, documentation, and treatment of every tobacco user in a health care setting." The guideline also recommends use of effective pharmacotherapies for smoking cessation, including sustained-release buproprion as well as nicotine replacement therapy (NRT; patch, gum, inhaler, nasal spray, lozenge), in all patients who are attempting to quit (except in the presence of contraindications).[85]

Smoking cessation guidelines incorporate the National Cancer Institute's five As: ask, advise, assess, assist, and arrange.[80] The physician should ask each patient about his or her smoking status as part of a routine patient vital sign assessment[86]; advise the patient to stop and educate him or her regarding the long-term health consequences of smoking; assess whether the patient is willing to make a quit attempt; assist by helping the patient to set a stop date, prescribing pharmacologic interventions, and supplying self-help pamphlets; and arrange follow-up.[87] This National Cancer Institute manual provides good reasons for quitting smoking, targeted to different groups[88] (Table 19-1). Other groups recommend the five Rs: The physician discusses with the patient the relevance of a stop-smoking program to health, the smoking risks, the rewards of quitting, how to deal with the roadblocks, and continues repetition of the stop-smoking message.[80]

The 1996 Agency for Health Care Policy and Research guidelines and 2000 Public Health Service guidelines also describe a dose-response relationship that exists between the intensity and duration of treatment and its effectiveness.[80] In general, more intense intervention leads to more effective long-term abstinence from tobacco. The success of an intervention also is maximized by proper training and education of physicians and medical students, by increasing the number of modalities used and the number of professionals involved, and by the creation of office-based systems.[86–89] Although only 2% to 3% of smokers become nonsmokers each year,[81] some studies report that up to 15% of patients seen by trained physicians have quit smoking.[90]

Most recent Public Health Service guidelines call for greater availability of telephone quitlines. In a randomized, controlled trial embedded within the California Smokers' Helpline, all participants (controls and intervention) received self-help materials, and intervention subjects also received as many as seven counseling sessions. Among participants who had made at least one attempt to quit during the year, Zhu et al.[91] found stronger

TABLE 19-1. Good Reasons to Stop Smoking

FOR TEENAGERS
Bad breath
Stained teeth
Cost
Lack of independence, controlled by cigarettes
Sore throats
Cough
Dyspnea (might affect participation in sports)
Frequent respiratory infections
FOR PREGNANT WOMEN
Increased rate of spontaneous abortion and fetal death
Increased risk of low birth weight
FOR PARENTS
Increased coughing and respiratory infections among children of smokers
Poor role model for child
FOR NEW SMOKERS
Easier to stop now
FOR LONG-TERM SMOKERS
Decreased risk of heart disease and cancer if you stop
FOR MEMBERS OF A FAMILY WITH HISTORY OF HEART DISEASE, CANCER, ETC.
Risk of death increased even more by smoking
FOR ASYMPTOMATIC ADULTS
Twice the risk of heart disease
Six times the risk of emphysema
Ten times the risk of lung cancer
Shortened life span by 5–8 y
Cost of cigarettes
Cost of sick time
Bad breath
Socially unacceptable
Wrinkles
FOR SYMPTOMATIC ADULTS (CORRELATE CURRENT SYMPTOMS WITH):
Upper respiratory infections, cough
Sore throats
Dyspnea
Ulcers
Angina
Claudication
Osteoporosis
Esophagitis
Gum disease
FOR ANY SMOKER
Money saved by stopping
Improved health (feel better)
Improved ability to exercise
May live long enough to enjoy retirement, grandchildren, etc.
May be able to work more, with less illness

(From ref. 88, with permission.)

12-month abstinence rates in intervention subjects compared with control group subjects (23.3 vs. 18.4, $P<.001$).

Three particularly effective elements of smoking cessation treatment are (1) NRT, (2) social support (clinician-provided encouragement and assistance), and (3) skills training and problem-solving techniques for achieving and maintaining abstinence.[85] Individualizing the message to the patient increases the likelihood for success.[26] Studies have shown that 3 minutes or less of advice increased quit rates from 7.9% to 10.2%.[90] For example, quit rates of 50% to 63% 6 months after a myocardial infarction

can increase to 65% to 75% for those patients who received other interventions in addition to physician contact. Blum[26] recommends that physicians ask nonthreatening questions, such as "What brand do you buy?" and "How much do you spend on cigarettes?" The term *inhalation count* can remind a pack-a-day patient that he or she will breathe in as many as one million doses of cyanide, ammonia, carcinogens, and carbon monoxide in less than 15 years. To the construction worker, the physician could link smoking cessation to the likelihood of fewer lost paydays, greater physical strength, and greater ability to work. A high school student, unresponsive to discussions of future emphysema and lung cancer, might be more receptive to the cosmetic unattractiveness of yellow teeth, bad breath, loss of athletic ability, or the financial drain of cigarettes.[26]

Also, the physician needs to tailor the message to the patient's readiness to change, according to the Prochaska et al.[92] model: precontemplation, contemplation, preparation, action, and maintenance. During precontemplation, the patient has not considered quitting. During the contemplation phase, the patient is thinking about quitting. In the preparation stage, the patient states that he or she intends to quit smoking in the next month. In the action phase, the patient is preparing and attempting to quit, and, during maintenance, the patient is avoiding relapse. Patients do not necessarily pass through each stage in orderly fashion; they may skip a stage or regress.[92]

NICOTINE REPLACEMENT THERAPY

Hundreds of cessation methods are reported in the literature, ranging from group therapy, hypnosis, and self-help manuals to acupuncture.[26] The introduction of nicotine-based medications in the form of chewing gum or a transdermal patch, combined with counseling, now provides cessation rates roughly double that of a control group (a factor of 1.4 to 2.6) as compared to placebo treatments. However, 70% to 80% of smokers who use these therapies still start to smoke again.[85,93,94]

By providing a substitute source of nicotine, NRT lessens the withdrawal symptoms associated with quitting and improves the cessation process. As dozens of published studies have demonstrated its efficacy, safety, and utility, the Smoking Cessation Clinical Practice Guideline of the Agency for Health Care Policy and Research recommends NRT as a first-line treatment for tobacco dependence "except in the presence of special circumstances."[80,85] Most commonly, NRT is used in the form of nicotine (polacrilex) gum [first approved by the U.S. Food and Drug Administration (FDA) in 1984] or the transdermal nicotine patch (FDA approved in 1991). In 1996, both of these medications became available as over-the-counter products,[74,75] greatly increasing access. In a metaanalysis, Fiore et al.[94] studied 42 randomized controlled trials of nicotine gum, as well as trials with fewer subjects using a transdermal patch and nasal spray inhaled nicotine. From their studies of nearly 18,000 persons, the authors concluded that NRT was effective, either as sole therapy or as an adjunct to other therapeutic approaches.[94,95] Dosing of nicotine gum should initially be titrated by the level of nicotine dependence and then adjusted if withdrawal symptoms are not relieved. The Fagerstrom Test for Nicotine Dependence (which features such questions as "How soon after you wake up do you smoke your first cigarette?") helps guide dosing decisions.[76]

Other agents also show promising results. Attention has focused on bupropion, an antidepressant, in combination with the nicotine patch. A double-blind, placebo-controlled smoking cessation trial found 12-month abstinence rates of 15.6% for placebo, 16.4% for the nicotine patch alone, 30.3% for sustained-release bupropion (Zyban) alone, and 35.5% for bupropion in conjunction with the nicotine patch. Treatment consisted of 9 weeks of bupropion (150 mg/d) for the first 3 days and then 150 mg twice a day.[93]

SPECIAL POPULATIONS

Targeting cessation efforts to persons of low socioeconomic status and to those with a recent history of mental illness may improve strategies for tobacco control. Adults who earned a high school equivalency diploma had the highest smoking prevalence (50.1% and 44.3% for men and women, respectively), whereas persons with graduate degrees had the lowest (9.1% and 7.5%, respectively).[32]

Wong et al.[96] estimated cause-specific risks of death from data from the National Health Interview Survey conducted from 1986 through 1994 and from linked vital statistics. Persons without a high school education lost 12.8 potential life-years per person, and smoking was one of the few conditions found to account for most of this disparity.[96]

Lasser et al.[97] analyzed data from 4411 respondents aged 15 to 54 years from the National Comorbidity Survey. Current smoking rates for respondents with no mental illness, lifetime mental illness, and past-month mental illness were 22.5%, 34.8%, and 41%, respectively. Odds ratios for current and lifetime smoking in respondents with mental illness in the past month versus respondents without mental illness (adjusted for age, sex, and region of the country) were 2.7 and 2.7, respectively. Persons with a mental disorder in the past month consumed approximately 44% of cigarettes smoked by this nationally representative sample.[97]

NATIONAL ACTION PLAN FOR TOBACCO CESSATION

A special national Subcommittee on Cessation of the United States Interagency Committee on Smoking and Health released a national plan designed to help five million smokers quit in its first year of implementation and thereby prevent three million premature deaths. The plan included a nationwide Tobacco Cessation Quitline, a national media campaign to encourage cessation, insurance coverage for all 100 million federally covered individuals, a new tobacco research and training infrastructure, and a Smokers' Health Fund, created by increasing the federal excise tax on cigarettes by $2 a pack (from $0.39 to $2.39 a pack).[98] Federal officials are weighing the recommendations of this plan.

TOBACCO RESTRICTIONS AT THE POLICY LEVEL

RESTRICTING YOUTH ACCESS

Preventing youth access to tobacco products should affect youth smoking rates.[99–101] All states prohibit the sale and distribution of tobacco products to minors under the age of 18. In several dozen states, additional laws prevent youth access by designating enforcement authorities, enforcing license suspension or revo-

cation for sales to minors, banning vending machines in areas accessible to minors, or restricting advertising. In just 2002 alone, 11 states passed measures related to youth access to tobacco products. Laws focused on enforcement and penalties, tobacco product packaging, product samples and displays, vending machines, age and identification requirements, and bidis.[102]

However, one study found that even when 82% of merchants complied with laws banning sales to minors, teenagers reported only a small decrease in their ability to purchase tobacco and no decline in its use.[101] More data are needed to verify the effectiveness of reducing sales to minors in actually limiting adolescents' access.

RESTRICTING SMOKING IN PUBLIC PLACES

Restricting smoking in workplaces has the potential to decrease greatly human exposure to ETS. Data show that in 1994, of 122 million full-time workers in the United States, nearly 100 million worked indoors.[102] The 1994 National Health Interview Survey showed that smoking prevalence of indoor workers was 26%, and 59% of workers (59 million) worked in buildings where smoking was not permitted.[102] A review of 19 studies of the impact of smoke-free workplaces found that almost all reported declines in daily smoking rates and smoking prevalence. Approximately 13% of the national decline in cigarette consumption in the United States between 1988 and 1994 was attributed to smoke-free workplaces.[102] An ongoing challenge is to guarantee that local smoke-free policies are not subject to preemption (i.e., legislation that prevents any local jurisdiction from enacting restrictions that are more stringent than the state law).

As of 2004, six states (California, New York, Delaware, Connecticut, Maine, and Massachusetts) had enacted comprehensive statewide smoke-free policies covering indoor public places. Because other jurisdictions, such as Boston and Dallas, also have enacted strong smoke-free policies, such laws now protect about one-fourth of the U.S. population.[103]

TOBACCO TAXES THAT FUND DEDICATED, COMPREHENSIVE STATEWIDE TOBACCO CONTROL PROGRAMS

Most public health experts regard tobacco taxes to be the single most effective measure for decreasing tobacco consumption.[73] Economic research documents price elasticity (i.e., a 10% increase in cigarette price generally reduces overall consumption by 4%).[104] Studies show that youth, lower-income smokers, young adults, and minority smokers are more likely than others to be encouraged to quit smoking by a price increase.[105] Government has traditionally taxed tobacco to fund government services, but public health professionals support increased taxes on tobacco products to deter consumption. The Canadian tobacco tax experience in the 1980s and early 1990s demonstrated the potential health impact. The combined average federal and provincial tax reached close to $3, pushing the average price per pack to more than $4. As a result, per capita cigarette consumption (adjusted for estimates of tobacco smuggling) dropped by 38% (1982 to 1992).[104,106]

In the United States, the current federal cigarette tax is 39 cents per pack; the average state cigarette tax is 73 cents per pack. Currently, 15 states have cigarette taxes of $1 or higher, with New

Jersey's the highest at $2.05.[107] The current national budget crisis has prompted many states to raise their excise taxes.

In general, the public has demonstrated willingness to increase tobacco taxes if those extra revenues are earmarked for specific purposes such as health programs.[108] The Centers for Disease Control and Prevention studied state experiences and disseminated best practices for comprehensive tobacco control programs.[109]

California has served as a model. In 1988, voters approved a ballot initiative that increased the state cigarette tax by 25 cents, allocating 20% of the revenue to establish a comprehensive statewide tobacco education and prevention program.[110,111] The initiative also funded mass media antitobacco campaigns, assistance to local health agencies for providing technical support and monitoring adherence to antismoking laws, community-based interventions, smoking cessation services (including a statewide quit-smoking telephone hotline), and enhancement of school-based prevention programs.[110,111] As a result, the efforts of the California Tobacco Control Program resulted in a rate of decline in cigarette consumption that was 50% more rapid than that seen in the rest of the country. The tax increase and the funded tobacco control program contributed to this decline. In multiple surveys (1990 to 1999) conducted to evaluate the California Tobacco Control Program, adult daily smoking prevalence dropped from 15.9% to 13.0%. Moderate to heavy daily smoking (15 or more cigarettes per day) decreased from 10.3 to 7.4 and heavy daily smoking (25 or more cigarettes per day) from 3.4 to 1.9 in 1999. The percentage of light smokers, who are more likely to quit than heavy smokers, increased (between 1996 and 1999) to 60%.[112,113]

The California Tobacco Control Program was associated with 33,300 fewer deaths from heart disease (between 1989 and 1997) than would have been expected. Such gains were made despite cutbacks to the program 3 years into its inception in 1989.[114]

In 1992, Massachusetts became the second state to approve a special cigarette tax (25 cents per pack) to fund a statewide tobacco control program.[108] The Massachusetts Tobacco Control Program had three major goals: to prevent onset of tobacco use by children, to assist smokers in quitting, and to guard against the harm of ETS.[115] Like California's program, the Massachusetts Tobacco Control Program consisted of funding for local cessation efforts and local coalitions, a statewide quit-smoking telephone hotline, funding of local boards of health, a statewide public awareness and counter-advertising campaign, and comprehensive school-based programs.[116] Adult per capita tobacco consumption in Massachusetts declined by 20% from the program's inception in 1992 through 1996, reflecting a threefold increase over the reduction observed at the national level.[117] Weintraub and Hamilton[118] documented a statewide drop in smoking prevalence to 19.4% in 1999. Other states have since launched tobacco control programs through ballot initiatives or other legislative measures. After passage of a 1996 ballot measure in Oregon that increased the excise tax by 30 cents per pack of cigarettes, per capita consumption declined 11.3% in Oregon, or the equivalent of 200 cigarettes per capita.[119] Arizona's ballot initiative in 1994 raised cigarette prices by 40 cents.[119]

The question has arisen whether declining consumption in states with comprehensive tobacco control programs is attributable solely to increased cigarette prices and not the program itself. A landmark economic analysis by Farrelly et al.[120] used multivariate analyses to control for other possible explanations of smoking declines and demonstrated clearly that statewide programs work. Specifically, the study found that states with the best-funded, most sustained programs through the 1990s (California, Massachusetts, Oregon, and Arizona) had reduced cigarette sales more than twice that of the country at large (43% vs. 20%).[120] Such results highlighted the negative public health impact of state funding cuts that have reduced tobacco control budgets in California by a third, in Oregon by 75%, and in Massachusetts by 95%.[120]

MASS MEDIA AND COUNTER-ADVERTISING

All the statewide tobacco control programs just cited have incorporated (dependent on funding) counter-advertising efforts through mass media. Minnesota (1986) and Michigan (1994) also have initiated limited tax-funded media campaigns.[119] Such efforts counter the tobacco industry's efforts to normalize a lethal product through advertising and promotional cigarette sales. A counter-advertising public health approach aims to reduce tobacco use by deglamorizing and denormalizing use of the product. To be effective, such mass media antismoking campaigns should provide consistent messages from multiple sources, repeatedly and over a long period, and should work in concert with other interventions and policies, with the goal of changing societal norms.[70]

The effects of these counter-advertising media campaigns, especially those in California and Massachusetts, have been striking. Of the California Tobacco Control Program's decline in cigarette consumption, approximately 20% was estimated to be attributable to the media campaign.[70,121,122] One study of California adults who successfully quit smoking (1990 and 1991) found that for 41% of residents, the media counter-advertising campaign had influenced their decision to stop.[123]

The effectiveness of counter-advertising first emerged in 1967, when the Federal Communications Commission invoked the Fairness Doctrine to require broadcasters to air one antismoking message for every three cigarette commercials aired.[70] When such antismoking advertising prompted a decline in per capita cigarette consumption of at least 5%, the tobacco industry then agreed (in 1970) to Congressional legislation to ban all tobacco advertising on television and radio, thereby eliminating the need for free antismoking ads.[70]

Later, research in Vermont and Minnesota showed that community- and school-based interventions highlighted by prominent mass media campaigns could reduce smoking in young persons by up to 40%.[74,124,125] However, such mass media campaigns before 1988 usually occurred on a sporadic basis. Also, institutionalizing counter-advertising campaigns has posed a public health challenge, as funding for such campaigns can be subjected to legislative diversion.[70] Typically, public service announcements on television did not air during prime time and therefore reached smaller audiences.[70]

Goldman and Glantz[126] have concluded that messages challenging social norms are more successful than are those aimed at changing individual behavior to improve health. Focus groups analysis by these researchers found that the most effective themes stressed the tobacco industry's manipulation of young persons, the negative impact of secondhand smoke, and the burden of cigarette addiction. Such advertisements can be controversial yet memorable and, ultimately, effective.[74,126]

TOBACCO LITIGATION, TOBACCO SETTLEMENT, AND INTERNATIONAL TREATIES

Public health lawyers have advocated bringing suits against tobacco companies as a cancer prevention strategy.[127] The last half century of tobacco litigation can be divided into three waves. Wave 1 (1954 through 1973) featured a number of individual lawsuits against an industry that maintained that tobacco products had never been proven to cause disease. The industry claimed that smokers chose to smoke, hence assuming risk for themselves. In essence, the 1965 Federal Cigarette Labeling and Advertising Act, which requires warning labels on all cigarette packaging and labeling, ironically served as a shield from liability. Wave 2 (1983 through 1992) featured *Cipollone vs. Liggett Group, Inc.*, a suit brought by a smoker and continued by her husband after her death. Although the original jury verdict of $400,000 favored the plaintiff, it was reversed on appeal, and the case finally was dropped after years of litigation.

Wave 3 (1994 to the present) capitalizes on the release of internal industry documents and subsequent industry concessions that tobacco is addictive and causes cancer and that tobacco companies had consciously marketed their products to children. From this ensued an increasing number of individual lawsuits and class action suits. Among the class action suits is *Broin vs. Philip Morris*, brought on behalf of flight attendants injured by ETS and settled for $349 million. The money realized from this suit established a foundation for the study of diseases associated with tobacco.[127–131] In 2000, the tobacco industry suffered its largest punitive damage award ever in *Engle vs. R. J. Reynolds*, brought on behalf of addicted and sick smokers in Florida. In this massive class action suit, the industry was initially found liable for punitive damages in the range of $145 billion dollars. However, in May 2003, a Florida appeals court voided the award.[132] Meanwhile, in 1999, the U.S Justice Department filed lawsuit against the nation's tobacco companies seeking $289 billion dollars to recover federal costs of treating smoking-related illness.

The most notable litigation to date has been lawsuits brought by states' attorneys general against the tobacco industry to recoup Medicaid costs for the treatment of ill smokers.[133] First, the major tobacco manufacturers settled individually with Mississippi, Texas, Minnesota, and Florida at a cost of $40 billion over 25 years. Then, the industry signed a Master Settlement Agreement (MSA) with 46 state attorneys general in November 1998, agreeing to pay $206 billion over 25 years in exchange for no future state litigation and other conditions including some advertising restrictions (e.g., bans on billboard advertisements).

The MSA expressly states that parties

> "...have agreed to settle their respective lawsuits and potential claims pursuant to terms which will achieve for the Settling States and their citizens significant funding for the advancement of public health, the implementation of important tobacco-related public health measures, including the enforcement of mandates and restrictions related to such measures, as well as funding for a national foundation dedicated to significantly reducing the use of tobacco products by youth...."[133]

Yet, challenges to implementing the MSA have been notable. Gross et al.[134] evaluated state expenditures for tobacco-control programs in 2001 in the context of the amount of tobacco settlement funds received and allocated to tobacco control programs. The average state received $28.35 per capita from settlement funds but allocated only 6% to tobacco control programs.[134] Also, despite the MSA prohibition of tobacco advertising that targets people younger than 18 years of age, King and Siegel[135] found that, in 2000, magazine advertisements for youth brands of cigarettes reached more than 80% of young people in the United States.

The Framework Convention on Tobacco Control, adopted in May 2003 by the World Health Organization, seeks to curtail the use of tobacco throughout the world. Members of the Framework Convention Alliance made a number of recommendations, including a ban on direct and indirect tobacco advertising, promotion, and sponsorship within 5 years of ratifying the treaty; large health warnings to cover 30% to 50% of a standard cigarette pack; the requirement that all parties implement effective measures to protect nonsmokers in public places; the recognition of, and the need for, increased tobacco taxes as a public health strategy; the consideration of litigation approaches; and prohibition of the words *light* and *mild* to describe cigarettes.[136]

The European Union Commission, a participant of the World Health Organization's Framework Convention on Tobacco Control, has already begun implementing a "Tobacco Products Directive," which became law in May 2001. It imposes maximum limits on tar (10 mg per cigarette), nicotine (1 mg per cigarette), and carbon monoxide (10 mg per cigarette). In addition, it requires larger warning labels (at least 30% of the front and 40% of the back) on all tobacco products and bans any descriptors that may be misleading, such as "light" or "mild." Finally, this law requires tobacco companies to disclose details of any additives and their purpose.

In addition, the European Union Commission has promoted the "Directive on Tobacco Advertising," which became law in May 2003. It bans tobacco advertising in the press and on the Internet, as well as via radio. The sponsorship of radio programs by tobacco companies is also banned (sponsorship of television programs has been outlawed already by the Television without Frontiers Directive).[137–139]

PROPOSED U.S. FOOD AND DRUG ADMINISTRATION REGULATIONS

The Federal Food, Drug and Cosmetic Act defines a drug as "an article (except for food) intended to affect the structure and function of the body."[127] Universal scientific consensus indicates that nicotine is an addictive drug. Evidence of the intent of the industry had been supported by the release of internal documents showing that tobacco manufacturers knew that nicotine caused significant pharmacologic effects and designed their products to provide pharmacologically active doses.[127] For these reasons, in 1996, the FDA proposed strategies to restrict access to tobacco products and advertising to youth. The first step, effected in part in 1997, involved stricter enforcement of laws affecting minors. The remaining proposed steps included banning free samples, restricting advertising within 1000 feet of schools and playgrounds, and limiting to black-and-white text print advertising in youth publications.[128] In 2000, the U.S. Supreme Court rejected these proposals, saying that the FDA had never received authority from Congress to regulate tobacco products.[140]

In the fall of 2003, the push for FDA regulation of tobacco regained momentum. Senator Judd Gregg from the Senate

Committee on Health, Education, Labor and Pensions drafted a bill that would give the FDA the power to regulate tobacco products. The bill proposed to give the agency the authority to eliminate nicotine and other toxins from cigarettes as well as provide consumers details about cigarette brands. Furthermore, as part of the bill, farmers are pressing for a buyout of tobacco quotas by the industry, which could possibly end a seven-decade-old program of government crop limits and price supports.[141]

CONCLUSION

The dawn of the twenty-first century offers a new opportunity to achieve a smoke-free society. All health care professionals can work to achieve this goal and prevent cancer. At the individual level, we must maximize access to cessation services for all smokers and promote further research into improving nicotine replacement therapies and other pharmacologic approaches. Health care professionals can raise awareness and promote cessation with every clinical opportunity. Reducing and even eliminating nicotine from cigarettes are also technically feasible and may hold the future to eradicating the potential for addiction.

On a broader societal level, communities can commit to achieving a nonsmoking social norm. Internationally, the adoption of the Framework Convention for Tobacco Control has set a universal standard. Efforts to restrict tobacco advertising and promotion to children, prohibit tobacco access by youth and teenagers, enhance public education, raise tobacco excise taxes, and control tobacco exports can save lives. In the United States, dedication of tobacco settlement funds to state-wide tobacco control programs can reduce cigarette consumption and promote prevention. Key to such comprehensive programs are broad-scale counter-advertising programs that deglamorize tobacco use. The proposed National Action Plan for Tobacco Cessation has the potential to prevent three million premature deaths.

On the legal and regulatory front, multiple individual and class action suits ultimately may change the tobacco industry's ability to conduct business as usual. Congressional movement to allow the FDA to regulate tobacco would be seismic and historic. Vigorous research on the possible adoption of products that promote harm reduction for smokers is critical.

In summary, on all fronts domestic and international, tobacco control is at a crossroads. It is hoped that all these combined efforts will cause the decline and prevention of tobacco-related cancers in the new millennium. Medical historians can then officially mark the end of the so-called Tobacco and Cancer Century and celebrate the beginning of a new smoke-free chapter in public health.[2]

REFERENCES

1. Wingo PA, Ries LA, Giovino GA, et al. The annual report to the nation on the status of cancer 1973–1996 with a special section on lung cancer and tobacco smoking. *J Natl Cancer Inst* 1999;91:675.
2. Koh HK. The end of the tobacco and cancer century. *J Natl Cancer Inst* 1999;91:60.
3. Peto R, Lopez AD, Boreham J, et al. Mortality from tobacco in developed countries: indirect estimation from national vital statistics. *Lancet* 1996;39:1268.
4. Peto R. Smoking and death: the past 40 years and the next 40. *BMJ* 1994;309:937.
5. Ezzati M, Lopez AD. Estimates of global mortality attributable to smoking in 2000. *Lancet* 2003;362:847.
6. Hecht SS. Tobacco smoke carcinogens and lung cancer. *J Natl Cancer Inst* 1999;91:1194.
7. Bergen AW, Caporaso N. Cigarette smoking. *J Natl Cancer Inst* 1999;91:1365.
8. Report of the surgeon general: the health consequences of smoking: nicotine addiction; 1988; publication no (CDC) 88-8406. Available from: Department of Health and Human Services, Washington, DC.
9. Novotny TE, Shane P, Daynard RA, et al. Tobacco use as a sociologic carcinogen: the case for a public health approach. *Cancer Prev* 1992:1.
10. Lombard HL, Doering CR. Cancer studies in Massachusetts: habits, characteristics, and environment of individuals with and without cancer. *N Engl J Med* 1928;198:481.
11. Doll R, Hill AB. Lung cancer and other causes of death in relation to smoking: second report on mortality of British doctors. *BMJ* 1956;2:1071.
12. Wynder EL, Graham EA. Tobacco smoking as a possible etiologic factor in bronchogenic carcinoma. *JAMA* 1950;143:329.
13. Hammond EL, Horn D. Smoking and death rates: report on forty-four months of follow-up of 187,783 men. *JAMA* 1958;166:1294.
14. US Department of Health, Education, and Welfare. Smoking and health: a report of the Advisory Committee to the Surgeon General. Atlanta: Centers for Disease Control and Prevention, 1964.
15. Centers for Disease Control and Prevention. Annual smoking-attributable mortality, years of potential life lost, and economic costs—United States, 1995–1999. *MMWR Morb Mortal Wkly Rep* 2002;51:300.
16. Cigarette brand use among adult smokers—United States, 1986. *MMWR Morb Mortal Wkly Rep* 1990;39:665.
17. Epps RP, Manley MW, Glynn TJ. Tobacco use among adolescents. *Pediatr Clin North Am* 1995;42:389.
18. US Department of Health and Human Services. The health consequences of smoking: cancer. A report of the surgeon general; 1982; DHHS publication no (PHS)82-50179. Available from: US Department of Health and Human Services, Public Health Service, Office of Smoking and Health, Rockville, MD.
19. Steenland K. Age specific interactions between smoking and radon among United States uranium miners. *Occup Environ Med* 1994;51:192.
20. Berry G, Newhouse ML, Antonis P. Combined effect of asbestos and smoking on mortality from lung cancer and mesothelioma in factory workers. *BMJ* 1985;42:12.
21. Selikoff IJ, Seidman H, Hammond EC. Mortality effects of cigarette smoking among amosite asbestos factory workers. *J Natl Cancer Inst* 1980;65:507.
22. US Department of Health and Human Services. The health consequences of smoking: cancer and chronic lung disease in the workplace. A report of the surgeon general; 1985; DHHS publication no (PHS)85-50207. Available from: US Department of Health and Human Services, Public Health Service, Centers for Disease Control and Prevention, Office of Smoking and Health, Washington, DC.
23. Ries LAG, Eisner MP, Kosary CL, et al, eds. *SEER Cancer Statistics Review, 1975–2000, National Cancer Institute.* Bethesda, MD, 2003. Available at: http://seer.cancer.gov/csr/1975_2000, 2004.
24. Thun M, Lally C, Flannery J, et al. Cigarette smoking and changes in the histopathology of lung cancer. *J Natl Cancer Inst* 1997;89:1580.
25. US Department of Health, Education, and Welfare. Smoking and health: a report of the surgeon general; 1979; DHEW publication no(PHS) 79-50066. Available from: Public Health Service, Office of the Assistant Secretary for Health, Office of Smoking and Health, Washington, DC.
26. Blum A. Cancer prevention: preventing tobacco-related cancers. In: DeVita C, Hellman S, Rosenberg S, eds. *Cancer: principles and practice of oncology*, 5th ed. Philadelphia: Lippincott–Raven Publishers, 1997.
27. Flanders WD, Rothman KJ. Interaction of alcohol and tobacco in laryngeal cancer. *Am J Epidemiol* 1982;115:371.
28. US Department of Health and Human Services. The health consequences of smokeless tobacco: a report of the Advisory Committee to the Surgeon General; 1986; (NIH) publication no 86-2874. Available from: US Department of Health and Human Services, Public Health Service, Washington, DC.
29. Annual Smoking-Attributable Mortality, Years of Potential Life Lost, and Economic Costs—United States, 1995–1999. *MMWR Morb Mortal Wkly Rep* 2002;51.
30. Bartecchi CE, MacKenzie TD, Schrier RW. The global tobacco epidemic. *Sci Am* 1995;5.
31. Ernster VL. Mixed messages for women: a social history of cigarette smoking and advertising. *N Y State J Med* 1985;85:335.
32. Centers for Disease Control and Prevention. Cigarette smoking among adults—United States, 2000. *MMWR Morb Mortal Wkly Rep* 2002;51:642.
33. American Cancer Society. *Facts and Figures*, 2003.
34. Kessler DA, Natanblut SL, Wilkenfield JP, et al. Nicotine addiction: a pediatric disease. *J Pediatr* 1997;130:518.
35. Centers for Disease Control and Prevention. Youth risk behavior surveillance—United States, 2001. *Morb Mortal Wkly Rep Surveill Summ* 2002;4:1.
36. *Growing up tobacco-free: preventing nicotine addiction in children and youths.* Washington, DC: Institute of Medicine, National Academy Press, 1994.
37. An LC, O'Malley PM, Schulenberg JE, et al. Changes at the high end of risk in cigarette smoking among US high school seniors, 1976–1995. *Am J Public Health* 1999;89:699.
38. Johnston LD, O'Malley PM, Bachman JG. Monitoring the future: national results on adolescent drug use: overview of key findings; 2003; (NIH) publication no 03-5374. National Institute on Drug Abuse, Bethesda, MD.
39. Centers for Disease Control and Prevention. Trends in cigarette smoking among high school students—United States, 1991–2001. *MMWR Morb Mortl Wkly Rep* 2002;51:409.
40. CDC, Youth Risk Behavior Surveillance—United States, 1995. *MMWR Morb Mortl Wkly Rep* 1996;45:1.
41. Kellam SG, Anthony JC. Targeting early antecedents to prevent tobacco smoking: findings from an epidemiologically based randomized field trial. *Am J Public Health* 1998;88:1490.

42. Jackson C, Henriksen L, Dickinson D, et al. The early use of alcohol and tobacco: its relation to children's competence and parents' behavior. *Am J Public Health* 1997;87:59.

43. Bachman JG, Wallace JM, O'Malley PM, et al. Racial/ethnic differences in smoking, drinking, and illicit drug use among American high school seniors, 1976–1989. *Am J Public Health* 1991;81:372.

44. Wechsler H, Rigotti NA, Gledhill-Hoyt J, et al. Increased levels of cigarette use among college students. *JAMA* 1998;280:1673.

45. Miller GH. The less hazardous cigarette: a deadly delusion. *N Y State J Med* 1985;85:313.

46. Filter ventilation levels in selected US cigarettes, 1997. *MMWR Morb Mortal Wkly Rep* 1997;46:1043.

47. National Cancer Institute Monograph 13. *Risks associated with smoking cigarettes with low machine-measured yields of tar and nicotine.* United States Department of Health and Human Services, National Institutes of Health, National Cancer Institute, November 2001.

48. Institute of Medicine. *Clearing the smoke: assessing the science base for tobacco harm reduction 2001.* Washington, DC: National Academy Press, 2001.

49. State-specific prevalence among adults of current cigarette smoking and smokeless tobacco use and per capita tax-paid sales of cigarettes—United States, 1997. *MMWR Morb Mortal Wkly Rep* 1998;47:922.

50. Blum A. Smokeless tobacco. *JAMA* 1980;244:192.

51. Spangler J, Salisbury P. Smokeless tobacco: epidemiology, health effects and cessation strategies. *Am Fam Physician* 1995;52:1421.

52. Tomar S, Giovino G. Incidence and predictors of smokeless tobacco use among US youth. *Am J Public Health* 1998;88:20.

53. Smokeless (spit) tobacco: a review of the state of the science. Proceedings of a symposium during the seventy-fourth general session of the International Association for Dental Research, San Francisco, CA, March 13, 1996. *Adv Dent Res* 1997;11:305.

54. Iribarren C, Tekaiva I, Sidney S, et al. Effect of cigar smoking on the risk of cardiovascular disease, chronic obstructive pulmonary disease and cancer in men. *N Engl J Med* 1999;340:1773.

55. Cigar smoking among teenagers—United States, Massachusetts, and New York, 1996. *MMWR Morb Mortal Wkly Rep* 1997;46:433.

56. Satcher D. Cigars and public health. *N Engl J Med* 1999;340:1829.

57. US Department of Health and Human Services. The health consequences of involuntary smoking: a report of the surgeon general; 1986; publication no (CDC)87-8398. Available from: Public Health Service, Centers for Disease Control and Prevention, Office on Smoking and Health, Department of Health and Human Services, Washington, DC.

58. Davis RM. Exposure to environmental tobacco smoke: identifying and protecting those at risk. *JAMA* 1998;280:1947.

59. Brownson RC, Eriksen MP, Davis RM, et al. Environmental tobacco smoke: health effects and policies to reduce exposure. *Annu Rev Public Health* 1997;18:163.

60. National Research Council, National Academy of Sciences. *Environmental tobacco smoke: measuring exposures and assessing health effects.* Washington, DC: National Academy Press, 1986.

61. California Environmental Protection Agency. Health effects of exposure to environmental tobacco smoke. *Tob Control* 1997;6:346.

62. US Environmental Protection Agency. Respiratory health effects of passive smoking: lung cancer and other disorders; 1992; Environmental Protection Agency publication no (EPA)600/6-90/006F. Available from: Environmental Protection Agency, Office of Air and Radiation, Washington, DC.

63. California Environmental Protection Agency. Health effects of exposure to environmental tobacco smoke. Sacramento: California Environmental Protection Agency, Office of Environmental Health Hazard Assessment, 1997.

64. Federal Trade Commission. *Cigarette report for 2000.* Washington, DC: Federal Trade Commission, 2002.

65. Federal Trade Commission. *Pursuant to the Comprehensive Smokeless Tobacco Health Education Act of 1986.* Washington, DC: Federal Trade Commission, 1993.

66. Centers for Disease Control and Prevention. Preventing tobacco use among young people: a report of the surgeon general, 1994. S/N 017-001-004901-0. Washington, DC: US Government Printing Office, 1994:175.

67. Feighery E, Borzekowski DL, Schooler C, et al. Seeing, wanting, owning: the relationship between receptivity to tobacco marketing and smoking susceptibility in young people. *Tob Control* 1998;7:123.

68. Pierce JP, Choi WS, Gilpin EA, et al. Tobacco industry promotion of cigarettes and adolescent smoking. *JAMA* 1998;279:511.

69. Difranza JR, Richards JW, Paulman PM, et al. RJR Nabisco's cartoon camel promotes Camel cigarettes to children. *JAMA* 1991;266:3149.

70. Siegel M. Mass media antismoking campaigns: a powerful tool for health promotion. *Ann Intern Med* 1998;129:128.

71. Bloch M, Daynard R, Roemer R. A year of living dangerously: the tobacco control community meets the global settlement. *Public Health Rep* 1998;113:488.

72. Arno PS, Brandt AM, Gostin LO, et al. Tobacco industry strategies to oppose federal regulation. *JAMA* 1996;275:1258.

73. Emmons KM, Kawachi I, Barclay G. Tobacco control: a brief review of its history and prospects for the future. *Hematol Oncol Clin North Am* 1997;11:177.

74. Cinciripini PM, McClure JB. Smoking cessation: recent developments in behavioral and pharmacologic interventions. *Oncology* 1998;12:249.

75. Cinciripini PM, Hecht SS, Henningfield JE, et al. Tobacco addiction: implications for treatment and cancer prevention. *J Natl Cancer Inst* 1997;89:1852.

76. Henningfield J. Nicotine medication for smoking cessation. *N Engl J Med* 1995;333:1196.

77. Zhu SH, Sun J, Billings S, et al. Predictors of smoking cessation in US adolescents. *Am J Prev Med* 1999;16:202.

78. Selected cigarette smoking initiation and quitting behaviors among high school students—United States, 1997. *MMWR Morb Mortal Wkly Rep* 1998;47:386.

79. Skaar K, Tsoh J, Cinciripini P, et al. Current approaches in smoking cessation. *Curr Opin Oncol* 1996;8:434.

80. Agency for Health Care Policy and Research, Smoking Cessation Clinical Practice Guideline Panel and Staff. Smoking cessation clinical practice guideline. *JAMA* 1996;275:1270.

81. Fiore MC, Bailey WC, Cohen SC, et al. Smoking cessation: clinical practice guideline no 18. AHCPR publication no 96-0692. Available from: Agency for Health Care Policy and Research, Rockville, MD, April 1996.

82. Sherin K. Smoking cessation: the physician's role. *Postgrad Med* 1982;11:71.

83. Fiore MC, Novotny TE, Pierce JP, et al. Methods used to quit smoking in the United States. *JAMA* 1990;263:2760.

84. Glynn TJ. Methods of smoking cessation—finally, some answers. *JAMA* 1990;263:2795.

85. Fiore MC. US public health service clinical practice guideline: treating tobacco use and dependence. *Respir Care* 2000;45(10):1200.

86. Fiore MC. The new vital sign. Assessing and documenting smoking status. *JAMA* 1991;266:3183.

87. Ferry LH, Grissino LM, Runfola PS. Tobacco dependence curricula in US undergraduate medical education. *JAMA* 1999;282:825.

88. Glynn TJ, Manley MW. How to help your patients stop smoking: a National Cancer Institute manual for physicians. Washington, DC: US Department of Health and Human Services, Public Health Service, National Institutes of Health, 1993.

89. US Department of Health and Human Services, Public Health Service, Agency for Health Care Policy and Research. Smoking cessation: a systems approach. A guide for health care administrators, insurers, managed care organizations, and purchasers. AHCPR Pub. No. 97-0698. Washington, DC: US Department of Health and Human Services, Public Health Service, April 1997.

90. Ockene JK, Zapka JG. Physician-based smoking intervention: a rededication to a five-step strategy to smoking research. *Addict Behav* 1997;22:835.

91. Zhu SH, Anderson CM, Tedeschi GJ, et al. *N Engl J Med* 2002;347:1087.

92. Prochaska JO, DiClemente CC, Norcross JC. In search of how people change. Applications to addictive behaviors. *Am Psychol* 1992;47:1102.

93. Jorenby DE, Leischow SJ, Nides MA, et al. A controlled trial of sustained-release bupropion, a nicotine patch, or both for smoking cessation. *N Engl J Med* 1999;340:685.

94. Fiore MC, Bailey WC, Cohen SJ, et al. Smoking cessation. Clinical practice guideline no. 18. Rockville, MD: AHCPR Pub. No. 96-0692.

95. Shiffman S, Mason KM, Henningfield JE. Tobacco dependence treatments: review and prospects. *Annu Rev Public Health* 1998;19:335.

96. Wong MD, Shapiro MF, Boscardin WJ, et al. Contribution of major diseases to disparities in mortality. *N Engl J Med* 2002;347:1585.

97. Smoking and mental illness: a population-based prevalence study. *JAMA* 2000;284:2606.

98. Fiore M, Croyle R, Curry S, et al. *Am J Public Health* 2004 (in press).

99. Fishman JA, Allison H, Knowles SB, et al. State laws on tobacco control—United States, 1998. *MMWR Morb Mortal Wkly Rep* 1999;48:22.

100. Forster JL, Wolfson M. Youth access to tobacco: policies and politics. *Annu Rev Public Health* 1998;19:203.

101. Rigotti N, DiFranza J, Chang Y, et al. The effect of enforcing tobacco-sales laws on adolescents: access to tobacco and smoking behavior. *N Engl J Med* 1997;337:1044.

102. Chapman S, Borland R, Scollo M, et al. The impact of smoke-free workplaces on declining cigarette consumption in Australia and the US. *Am J Public Health* 1999;89:1018.

103. National Cancer Institute. *State cancer legislative database. Special report: 2002 year in review.* United States Department of Health and Human Services, National Institutes of Health. Issue 52, Winter 2003.

104. Grossman M, Chaloupka FJ. Cigarette taxes. The straw to break the camel's back. *Public Health Rep* 1997;112:290.

105. Farrelly M, Bray J. Response to increases in cigarette prices by race/ethnicity, income and age groups, United States 1976–1993. *MMWR Morb Mortal Wkly Rep* 1998;47:605.

106. Kaiserman MJ, Rogers B. Tobacco consumption declining faster in Canada than in the US. *Am J Public Health* 1991;81:902.

107. Tobacco Free Kids. Available at: http://www.tobaccofreekids.org. Accessed: September 28, 2003.

108. Koh HK. An analysis of the successful 1992 Massachusetts tobacco tax initiative. *Tob Control* 1996;5:220.

109. *Best practices for comprehensive tobacco control programs.* Atlanta: Centers for Disease Control and Prevention, Office of Smoking and Health, August 1999.

110. Bal DG, Kizer KW, Felten PG, et al. Reducing tobacco consumption in California. Development of a statewide anti-tobacco use campaign. *JAMA* 1990;264:1570.

111. Flewelling RL, Kenney E, Elder JP, et al. First-year impact of the 1989 California cigarette tax increase on cigarette consumption. *Am J Public Health* 1992;82:867.

112. Gilpin EA, Pierce JP. The California Tobacco Control Program and potential harm reduction through reduced cigarette consumption in continuing smokers. *Nicotine Tob Res* 2002;[Suppl 4]2:S157.

113. Tobacco Control Section. California tobacco control update. Sacramento: California Department of Health Services, 2000.

114. Fichtenberg CM, Glanz SA. Association of the California Tobacco Control Program with declines in cigarette consumption and mortality from heart disease. *N Engl J Med* 2000;343:1772.

115. Koh HK. Accomplishments of the Massachusetts Tobacco Control Program. *Tob Control* 2002;2:[Suppl 11]ii1.

116. Connolly G, Robbins H. Designing an effective statewide tobacco control program—Massachusetts. *Cancer* 1998;83[Suppl]:2722.

117. Cigarette smoking before and after an excise tax increase and an antismoking campaign—Massachusetts, 1990–1996. *MMWR Morb Mortal Wkly Rep* 1996;45:966.

118. Weintraub JM, Hamilton WL. Trends in prevalence of current smoking, Massachusetts and states without tobacco control programmes, 1990–1999. *Tob Control* 2002;11:[Suppl 2]:ii8.

119. Nicholl J. Tobacco tax initiatives to prevent tobacco use. A study of eight statewide campaigns. *Cancer* 1998;83[Suppl]:2666.

120 Farrelly MC, Pechacek TF, Chaloupka FJ. The impact of tobacco control program expenditures on aggregate cigarette sales: 1981–2000. *J Health Econ* 2003;22:843.

121. Hu T, Keeler TE, Sung H, et al. The impact of California anti-smoking legislation on cigarette sales, consumption, and prices. *Tob Control* 1995;4[Suppl 1]:S34.

122. Hu T, Sung HY, Keeler TE. Reducing cigarette consumption in California: tobacco taxes versus an anti-smoking media campaign. *Am J Public Health* 1995;85:1218.

123. Popham WJ, Potter LD, Bal DG, et al. Do anti-smoking media campaigns help smokers quit? *Public Health Rep* 1993;108:510.

124. Secker-Walker RH, Worden JK, Holland RR, et al. A mass media program to prevent smoking among adolescents: costs and cost effectiveness. *Tob Control* 1997;6:207.

125. Flynn BS, Worden JK, Secker-Walker RH, et al. Mass media and school interventions for cigarette smoking prevention: effects 2 years after completion. *Am J Public Health* 1994;84:1148.

126. Goldman LK, Glantz SA. Evaluation of antismoking advertising campaigns. *JAMA* 1998;279:772.

127. Hurt R, Robertson CR. Prying open the door to the tobacco industry's secrets about nicotine: the Minnesota tobacco trial. *JAMA* 1998;280:1173.

128. Kessler DA, Barnett PS, Witt A, et al. The legal and scientific basis for FDA's assertion of jurisdiction over cigarettes and smokeless tobacco. *JAMA* 1997;277:405.

129. Broder J. Cigarette maker concedes smoking can cause cancer. *New York Times* 1998 Nov 14:1.

130. Kelder GE, Daynard RA. Tobacco litigation as a public health and cancer control strategy. *J Am Med Womens Assoc* 1996;51:57.

131. Meier B. Tobacco windfall begins tug-of-war among lawmakers. *New York Times* 1999 Jan 10:1.

132. Langley A. World Health meeting approves treaty to discourage smoking. *New York Times* 2003 May 22.

133. Multistate Master Settlement Agreement, November 23, 1998. National Association of Attorneys General Web site. World Wide Web URL: http://www.naag.org/cigna.rtf, 1998.

134. Gross CP, Soffer B, Bach PB, et al. State expenditures for tobacco-control programs and the tobacco settlement. *N Engl J Med* 2002;347:1080.

135. King C 3rd, Siegel M. The Master Settlement Agreement with the tobacco industry and cigarette advertising in magazines. *N Engl J Med* 2001;345:504.

136. Framework Convention Alliance. Available at: http://fctc.org. Accessed on September 6, 2003.

137. Collin J, Gilmore AB. Tobacco control, the European Union and WHO. Two conventions provide opportunities to advance public health. *Eur J Public Health* 2002;12:242.

138. McCarthy M. European Union continues negotiations on tobacco control. *Lancet* 2002;35:504.

139. European Union Smoking and Tobacco Policy. World Wide Web URL: http://www.eurunion.org/legislat/smoking/smoking.htm, 2003.

140. Greenhouse L. High court holds FDA can't impose rules on tobacco. *New York Times* 2000 March 22:1.

141. Hulse C. In hard times, tobacco growers consider giving up price supports. *New York Times* 2003 Aug.

CHAPTER 20

Cancer Prevention: Diet and Chemopreventive Agents

SECTION **1**

WALTER C. WILLETT

Dietary Fat

In recent years, reduction in dietary fat has been at the center of cancer prevention efforts. In the landmark 1982 National Academy of Sciences review of diet, nutrition, and cancer,[1] reduction in fat intake to 30% of calories was the primary recommendation. This objective has been echoed in subsequent dietary recommendations as well.[2–4]

Interest in dietary fat as a cause of cancer began in the first half of the twentieth century, when studies by Tannenbaum and colleagues[5,6] indicated that diets high in fat could promote tumor growth in animal models. In this early work, energy (caloric) restriction also profoundly reduced the incidence of tumors. A vast literature on dietary fat and cancer in animals has subsequently accumulated (reviewed elsewhere[1,7–11]). Dietary fat has a clear effect on tumor incidence in many models, although not in all[12,13]; however, a central issue has been whether this is independent of the effect of energy intake. An independent effect of fat consumption has been seen in some animal models,[7,9,14] but this relationship has been either weak[15] or nonexistent[16] in some studies designed specifically to address this issue.

In the 1970s, the possible relation of dietary fat intake to cancer incidence gained greater attention as the large international differences in rates of many cancers were noted to be strongly correlated with apparent per capita fat consumption.[17,18] Particularly strong associations were seen with cancers of the breast, colon, prostate, and endometrium, which include the most important cancers not due to smoking in affluent countries.[19] These correlations were observed to be limited to animal, not vegetable, fat.[20] Complementing these correlational observations, studies of populations migrating from low- to high-incidence areas indicated that the migrating groups adopted the cancer rates of the new environment.[11,21] This provided powerful evidence that the large international differences in cancer incidence were not due to genetic factors and therefore that the high rates of specific cancers in affluent countries were potentially avoidable. Although such evidence did not directly implicate dietary factors, the animal studies noted earlier made the area of diet a strong suspect.

A principal limitation of both the international correlational studies and the migrant studies is the potential for confounding. Many other differences besides dietary fat exist between the countries with low fat consumption (less affluent) and high fat consumption (more affluent). Indeed, the correlations with gross national product are similar to those for fat intake.[18] Among the many factors that differ between countries with low fat consumption and those with high fat consumption, reproductive behaviors, physical activity level, and body fatness are particularly notable and are strongly associated with specific cancers.[22,23] The quality of dietary data used in the international correlations has also been problematic; this information is not based on actual intakes but rather on estimated production figures.

Despite their limitations, the suggestive findings of at least some studies of animal models as well as the international correlations and migrant studies have clearly indicated the need for more detailed studies in humans. In particular, studies that can control for the confounding influences of lifestyle factors other than fat intake are particularly important. Two general approaches, discussed elsewhere in detail,[24] are available: case-control or cohort epidemiologic studies and randomized trials. Both case-control and cohort studies depend on a reasonably valid assessment of dietary intake. Although, for some nutrients, biochemical measurements can be used to assess intake, for total fat consumption a useful biochemical indicator does not exist. Since 1980, considerable effort has been directed at the development of standardized questionnaires for measuring intake of fat and other dietary components, and numerous studies have been conducted to assess the validity of these methods.[25–28] These investigations have clearly demonstrated that an informative range of fat consumption exists within the populations of the United States and other countries and that standardized food frequency questionnaires can reasonably measure differences among subjects. Although the range of fat intake that can be studied is restricted to the range of diets in the study population, this typically includes both the levels that have often been recommended (less than 30% of energy) as well as more traditional U.S. levels (more than 40% of energy).[29] Moreover, by combining the data from multiple large prospective studies, the range of fat has been extended from less than 20% of energy to more than 45% of energy, which is similar to the current range observed internationally.[30]

In principle, the most definitive approach to evaluate the relation between fat intake and cancer is to conduct a large randomized trial. Many practical problems exist in conducting such a trial, however, the most important being the need to maintain a difference in fat intake between the intervention and control groups for many years. The experience of the pilot studies for the Women's Health Initiative[31] and the Multiple Risk Factor Intervention Trial heart disease prevention study[32] indicate that this may be difficult. Moreover, the necessary duration for such a trial is not known. Much evidence suggests that factors acting from childhood through postmenopausal years can influence breast cancer risk. Because trials of cancer prevention require tens of thousands of subjects to be randomly assigned to treatment conditions and the costs of instruction in dietary change is high, such studies are extremely expensive; for example, the Women's Health Initiative will cost on the order of a billion dollars.[31]

Since 1985 information on fat intake and cancer has grown rapidly and will continue to accrue exponentially as the populations of ongoing cohort studies age and as recently started cohort studies begin to report their findings. In the following sections, current data on the relation of fat intake to cancers of the breast, colon, and prostate are briefly reviewed because these are the cancers for which the current evidence is most abundant.

FAT AND BREAST CANCER

Breast cancer is the most frequent malignancy among women in Western countries, and incidence rates have been increasing for decades.[33,34] Rates in most parts of Asia, South America, and Africa have been only approximately one-fifth as high as that in the United States,[35,36] but in almost all these areas rates of breast cancer are also increasing. Populations that migrate from low- to high-incidence countries develop breast cancer rates that approximate those of the new host country.[37,38] Among Japanese immigrants to the United States, however, rates do not approach those of the general U.S. population until the second or third genera-

tion.[11,39] This slower rate of change for Japanese immigrants may indicate delayed acculturation, although a similar delay in rate increase is not observed for colon cancer.

A major rationale for the dietary fat hypothesis has been the international correlation between fat consumption and national breast cancer mortality.[18] However, in a study of 65 Chinese counties,[40] in which both dietary assessment and mortality rates were measured using standardized methods and per capita fat intake varied from 6% to approximately 30% of energy, only a weak positive association was seen between fat intake and breast cancer mortality. Notably, inhabitants of four counties consumed approximately 25% of energy from fat, yet experienced rates of breast cancer far below those of U.S. women with similar fat intake,[29] a finding which provides strong evidence that factors other than fat intake account for the large international differences.

Breast cancer incidence rates have increased substantially in the United States during the twentieth century, as have the estimates of per capita fat consumption based on food disappearance data. Surveys based on reports of individual actual intake, rather than food disappearance, however, indicate that consumption of energy from fat, either as absolute intake or as a percentage of energy, has actually declined in the last several decades,[41,42] a time during which breast cancer incidence has increased.[43]

CASE-CONTROL STUDIES

A number of case-control studies have been performed to investigate the effect of dietary fat on breast cancer risk. A large study by Graham et al.[44] used a food frequency questionnaire to compare the fat intake of 2024 women with breast cancer to that reported by 1463 women control subjects entering the hospital with benign conditions. Both animal fat intake and total fat intake were essentially identical in the two groups. The results from 12 smaller case-control studies have been summarized in a metaanalysis by Howe et al.,[45] which included 4312 cases and 5978 controls. The pooled relative risk (RR) was 1.35 (P <.0001) for a 100-g increase in daily total fat intake, although the risk was somewhat stronger for postmenopausal women (RR, 1.48; P <.001). This magnitude of association, however, could potentially be compatible with biases due to recall of diet or the selection of controls.[46]

COHORT STUDIES

A substantial body of data from cohort studies is now available to assess the relation between dietary fat intake and breast cancer in developed countries. Because of the prospective design, most of the methodologic biases of case-control studies are avoided. In a pooled analysis of the seven prospective studies with more than 200 cases of breast cancer, which included 337,000 women who developed 4980 incident cases of breast cancer,[30] no overall association was seen for fat intake over the range of less than 20% to more than 45% of energy. A similar lack of association was seen among postmenopausal women only and for specific types of fat. Only among the small number of women consuming less than 15% of energy from fat was a significant association seen; breast cancer risk was elevated twofold in this group. This lack of association with total fat intake was confirmed in a subsequent analysis of the pooled prospective studies of diet and breast cancer that included over 7000 cases.[47] An updated analysis of the Nurses' Health Study included 14 years of follow-up, during which time 2956 women developed breast cancer.[48] Because repeated assessments of diet were obtained at 2- to 4-year intervals, this analysis provided a particularly detailed evaluation of the fat intake over an extended period in relation to breast cancer risk. For total fat intake, the overall association was weakly inverse and statistically significant. No suggestion of any reduction in risk was seen at intakes below 25% of energy. These cohort findings therefore do not support the hypothesis that dietary fat is an important cause of breast cancer.

Estrogen level in blood has now been established as a risk factor for breast cancer.[49] Thus, the effects of fat and other dietary factors on estrogen levels are of potential interest. Vegetarian women, who consume higher amounts of fiber and lower amounts of fat, have lower blood levels and reduced urinary excretion of estrogens, apparently due to increased fecal excretion.[50] A metaanalysis has suggested that reduction in dietary fat may reduce plasma estrogen levels,[51] but the studies included were plagued by the lack of concurrent controls, short duration, and confounding by negative energy balance.[52] In a large randomized trial among postmenopausal women with a previous diagnosis of breast cancer, reduction in dietary fat did not affect estradiol levels when the data were appropriately analyzed.[53,54]

DIFFERENT TYPES OF FAT

In animal mammary tumor models, the tumor-promoting effect of fat intake has been observed primarily for polyunsaturated fats when fed in the presence of high-fat diets containing approximately 45% of energy.[8,55,56] In a metaanalysis of animal studies, monounsaturated fat had no significant effect on mammary carcinogenesis and the effect of saturated fat was weak.[8]

In several prospective cohort studies, an inverse association has been found between monounsaturated fat and breast cancer.[29,57] This is an intriguing observation because of the relatively low rates of breast cancer in Southern European countries with high intakes of monounsaturated fats due to the use of olive oil as the primary fat. In case-control studies in Spain, Greece, and Italy, women who used more olive oil had reduced risks of breast cancer.[58–60] Also, olive oil has been protective relative to other sources of fats in several animal studies.[7,8] Further examination is needed of the hypothesis that monounsaturated fats, and perhaps olive oil in particular, may protect against breast cancer.

In a report of findings for the Nurses' Health Study cohort of premenopausal women, higher intake of animal fat was associated with an approximately 50% greater risk of breast cancer, but no association was seen with intake of vegetable fat.[61] This suggests that factors in foods containing animal fats (e.g., hormones in milk), rather than fat per se, may account for the findings. Also, diet during early adult life may be particularly important, because positive associations with animal fat generally were not been seen in earlier cohort studies, which primarily assessed intake during midlife or later.

FAT AND AGE AT PUBERTY

An earlier age at menarche is an established risk factor for breast cancer. Although the RRs associated with early menarche are generally modest, usually lower than approximately 1.5 for the earliest compared with the latest age groups within a population,

this is likely to be due to the limited range of age at menarche within a given population. For example, in the United States the average age is between 12 and 13 years,[62] but in rural China the typical age is approximately 17 to 18 years.[63] Furthermore, the average age at menarche has been declining worldwide for the last 200 years,[62] which suggests that the rising breast cancer rates that occur with increased industrialization are caused in part by a decreasing average age at menarche.

For this reason, dietary factors that influence age at menarche are of particular interest. Nutritional factors have been examined as potential predictors of age at menarche in several prospective cohort studies. Body mass index, height, and weight have consistently been strong determinants of age at menstruation.[64–66] In the U.S.[64] as well as in the Canadian cohorts,[66] no association was found between the fat composition of the diet and time of occurrence of menarche, but a suggestion of earlier onset with higher fat intake was seen in a German study.[65] Collectively, these studies provide strong evidence that rapid growth rates before puberty play an important role in determining future risk of breast cancer, but that overall energy balance rather than fat intake is most important.

FAT AND BREAST CANCER SURVIVAL

High intake of dietary fat has been hypothesized to affect survival adversely in patients with breast cancer, in part because of observations that, with appropriate adjustments for cancer stage, survival is lower in the United States than in Japan.[67] However, obesity has often been associated with lower breast cancer survival rates. This provides an alternative hypothesis, because Japanese women tend to be substantially leaner than U.S. women, and other dietary and lifestyle factors differed substantially between the United States and Japan.

At present, studies of the relation between dietary fat intake and breast cancer survival are few and have substantial limitations. Most were not specifically designed for this purpose but instead are based on findings from the follow-up of the control series of case-control or cohort studies examining breast cancer incidence. Thus, they usually refer to premorbid diet assessed either before or at about the time of diagnosis rather than to diet after diagnosis. Moreover, most studies have been small in terms of the failure end points. Mixed results have been seen in the published work; positive associations have been found in several studies[68–73] but not in others.[74–77] In an analysis of data from the Nurses' Health Study,[78] fat intake after diagnosis was not significantly associated with survival, but a modest effect could not be excluded. Unexpectedly, higher protein intake was associated with improved survival. A randomized trial has been started to evaluate the effect of a diet low in fat (15% of energy from fat is the dietary goal) on survival of breast cancer patients.[79]

FAT AND COLON CANCER

In comparisons among countries, rates of colon cancer are strongly correlated with national per capita disappearance of animal fat and meat, with correlation coefficients ranging between 0.8 and 0.9.[18,20] Rates of colon cancer rose sharply in Japan after World War II, paralleling a 2.5-fold increase in fat.[36] Based on these epidemiologic investigations and animal studies, a hypothe-

TABLE 20.1-1. Large Prospective Studies of the Effects of Energy, Fat, and Meat Intake on Colon Cancer

			Relative Risk for High vs. Low Intake		
Study	Population	No. of Cases	Energy	Total Fat	Meat
Willett et al., 1990[107]	88,751 U.S. women	150	0.94	2.0	2.52 beef, main dish 1.21 processed
Bostick et al., 1994[109]	35,215 U.S. women	212	0.60	0.88	1.21 beef, main dish 1.51 processed
Goldbohm et al., 1994[108]	120,852 Dutch women and men	215	0.74	1.07	1.17 (per SD) processed
Giovannucci et al., 1994[110]	47,949 U.S. men	205	0.94	1.19	3.57 beef, main dish
Thun et al., 1992[111]	764,343 U.S. men and women	1150 (deaths)	—	1.14 (M)	—
			—	0.85 (F)	—
Gaard et al., 1996[145]	50,535 Norwegian men and women	143	1.13 (M)	1.16 (M)	0.80 all (M)
			1.49 (F)	0.47 (F)	1.87 all (F)
Kato et al., 1997[146]	14,727 New York women	100	1.20	1.05	1.23 red
Hsing et al., 1998[147]	17,633 Minnesota men	120	—	—	1.8 red
Singh and Fraser, 1998[148]	32,051 Adventist men and women	157	—	—	1.85 all 1.41 red
Terry et al., 2001[149]	61,463 Swedish women	460	—	NS	—
Flood et al., 2001[150]	45,496 U.S. women	487	—	1.14	1.04 red 0.97 processed
Jarvinen et al., 2001[151]	9959 Finnish men and women	109	NS	1.86	1.34 red
Pietinen et al., 1999[152]	27,111 Finnish men	185	1.7	0.9	1.1 red

F, female; M, male; NS, not significant; SD, standard deviation.

sis has developed that higher dietary fat increases excretion of bile acids, which can be converted to carcinogens or promoters.[80] However, evidence from many studies that obesity and low levels of physical activity increase the risk of colon cancer[81] means that at least part of the high rates in affluent countries previously attributed to fat intake is probably due to sedentary lifestyle.

With some exceptions,[82–85] case-control studies have generally shown an association between risk of colon cancer and intake of fat[86–93] or red meat.[94–99] In many of these studies, however, a positive association between total energy intake and risk of colon cancer has also been observed,[86–90,92,93] which raises the question of whether it is general overconsumption of food or the fat composition of the diet that is etiologically important. A metaanalysis by Howe of 13 case-control studies found a significant association between total energy intake and colon cancer, but amounts of saturated, monounsaturated, and polyunsaturated fat were not associated with colon cancer independently of total energy.[100]

Prospective cohort studies of colon cancer are less prone to selection and recall bias. Earlier prospective data showed positive,[101,102] inverse,[103,104] and null associations[105,106] with fat or meat consumption. These studies were limited by a small number of cases or crude assessments of diet. More recent cohort studies have largely avoided these limitations (Table 20.1-1). The Nurses' Health Study showed an approximately twofold higher risk of colon cancer among women in the highest quintile of animal fat intake compared to those in the lowest quintile.[107] In a multivariate analysis of these data, which included red meat intake and animal fat intake in the same model, red meat intake remained significantly predictive of risk of colon cancer, whereas the association with animal fat was eliminated. A cohort study in the Netherlands showed a significant direct association between intake of processed meats and risk of colon cancer, but no relationship was observed for fresh meats or overall fat intake.[108] A cohort study in Iowa women also found a direct association with intake of processed meats, although this was not statistically significant.[109] In a large cohort study of men, a direct association

between red meat consumption and risk of colon cancer was seen, but no association was observed with other sources of fat.[110] In this study, no overall relationship existed between consumption of total or saturated fat and colon cancer despite a substantial range in fat intake. A similar association between red meat consumption and cancer risk was noted for colorectal adenomas in the same cohort of men.[80] In the large American Cancer Society study cohort,[111] little relation was seen between either meat or fat intake and mortality due to colon cancer, but the dietary questionnaire was brief and of uncertain validity. As can be seen in Table 20.1-1, other cohort studies have also failed to support an association with fat intake, even though positive associations with red meat consumption were often observed. In a metaanalysis of prospective studies,[112] red meat consumption was associated with risk of colon cancer (RR, 1.24; 95% confidence interval, 1.09 to 1.41 for an increment of 120 g/d). The association with consumption of processed meats was particularly strong (RR, 1.36; 95% confidence interval, 1.15 to 1.61 for an increment of 30 g/d).

The apparently stronger association with red meat consumption than with fat intake in most large cohort studies needs further confirmation, but such an association could result if the fatty acids or nonfat components of meat (e.g., the heme iron or carcinogens created by cooking) were the primary etiologic factors. This issue has major practical implications, because current dietary recommendations[113] support the daily consumption of red meat as long as it is lean. Virtually no data exist on the relation of dietary fat to survival of colon cancer.

FAT AND PROSTATE CANCER

Consumption of animal fat, but not vegetable fat, is strongly correlated with prostate cancer mortality internationally.[18] Associations with fat intake have been seen in many case-control studies[114–123] but sometimes only in subgroups. In a large case-

TABLE 20.1-2.   Prospective Studies of Dietary Fat and Prostate Cancer Risk

Study	Population	No. of Cases	Relative Risk for High vs. Low Intake	
			Total Fat	Saturated Fat
Severson et al., 1989[125]	8000	174	0.9	1.0
Mills et al., 1989[126]	14,000	180	—	1.4 animal fat
Giovannucci et al., 1993[127]	52,000	126 (aggressive cases)	1.8	1.6
Le Marchand et al., 1994[129]	20,316	198	—	1.6 animal fat
Schuurman et al., 1999[130]	58,279	642	1.1	1.19

control study encompassing various ethnic groups within the United States,[124] consistent associations with prostate cancer risk were seen for saturated fat but not for other types of fat.

The association between fat intake and prostate cancer risk has been assessed in only a few cohort studies (Table 20.1-2). In a cohort of 8000 Japanese men living in Hawaii, no association was seen between total fat intake or intake of unsaturated fat.[125] Diet was assessed with a single 24-hour recall in this study, however, so the lack of association may not be informative. In a study of 14,000 Seventh-Day Adventist men living in California, a positive association between the percentage of calories from animal fat and prostate cancer risk was seen, but this was not statistically significant.[126] In the Health Professionals Follow-up Study of 51,000 men, a positive association was seen between cancer risk and red meat, total fat, and animal fat intake; the association was largely limited to aggressive prostate cancers.[127] No association was seen with intake of vegetable fats, but intake of n-3 fatty acids from fish was inversely related to risk.[128] In another cohort in Hawaii, increased risks of prostate cancer were seen with consumption of beef and animal fat.[129] In contrast, no relation was seen between either total fat intake or intake of saturated fat and incidence of prostate cancer in a large Dutch cohort.[130]

Although further data are desirable, the evidence from international correlations, case-control, and cohort studies provides some support for an association between consumption of fat-containing animal products and prostate cancer incidence. This evidence does not generally support a relation with intake of vegetable fat, which suggests that either the type of fat or other components of animal products are responsible. Some evidence also indicates that animal fat consumption may be most strongly associated with the incidence of aggressive prostate cancer, which suggests an influence on the transition from the widespread indolent form to the more lethal form of this malignancy. Data are limited on the relation of fat intake to the probability of survival after the diagnosis of prostate cancer.

FAT AND OTHER CANCERS

Rates of other cancers that are common in affluent countries, including those of the endometrium and ovary, are, of course, also correlated with fat intake internationally. Although these have been studied in a small number of case-control investigations, consistent associations with fat intake have not been seen.[131–140] In prospective studies among Iowa and Canadian women,[141,142] no evidence of a relation between fat intake and risk of endometrial cancer was found. Positive associations between dietary fat and lung cancer were observed in many

case-control studies. However, in a pooled analysis of large prospective studies that included over 3000 incident cases, no association was seen.[143] These findings provide further evidence that the results of case-control studies of diet and cancer are likely to be misleading.

CONCLUSION

Largely on the basis of the results of animal studies, international correlations, and a few case-control studies, great enthusiasm developed in the 1980s that modest reductions in total fat intake would have a major impact on breast cancer incidence. As the findings from large prospective studies have become available, however, support for this relationship has greatly weakened. Although evidence suggests that high intake of animal fat early in adult life may increase the risk of premenopausal breast cancer, this is not likely to be due to fat per se because vegetable fat intake was not related to risk. For colon cancer, the associations seen with animal fat intake internationally have been supported in numerous case-control and cohort studies, but this also appears to be explained by factors in red meat other than simply its fat content. Further, the importance of physical activity and leanness as protective factors against colon cancer indicates that international correlations probably overstate the contribution of diet to differences in colon cancer incidence. At present the available evidence most strongly suggests an association between animal fat consumption and risk of prostate cancer, particularly the aggressive form of this disease. As with colon cancer, the possibility remains that other factors in animal products contribute to risk.

Despite the large body of data on dietary fat and cancer that has accumulated since 1985, any conclusions should be regarded as tentative, because these are disease processes that are poorly understood and that are likely to take many decades to develop. Because almost all of the reported literature from prospective studies is based on fewer than 20 years of follow-up, further evaluation of the effects of diet earlier in life and at longer intervals of observation are needed to understand fully these complex relationships. Nevertheless, persons interested in reducing their risk of cancer could be advised, as a prudent measure, to minimize their intake of foods high in animal fat, particularly red meat. Such a dietary pattern is also likely to be beneficial from the standpoint of cardiovascular disease. On the other hand, unsaturated fats (with the exception of *trans* fatty acids) reduce blood low-density lipoprotein cholesterol levels and risk of cardiovascular disease,[144] and little evidence suggests that they adversely affect cancer risk. Thus, efforts to reduce unsaturated fat intake are not warranted at this time and are likely to have adverse effects on cardiovascular disease. Because excess adiposity increases risks of several cancers and cardiovascular disease, balancing calories from any source with adequate physical activity is extremely important.

REFERENCES

1. Committee on Diet Nutrition and Cancer, Assembly of Life Sciences, National Research Council. *Diet, nutrition, and cancer*. National Academy Press, 1982.
2. US Department of Agriculture, US Department of Health and Human Services. *Nutrition and your health: dietary guidelines for Americans*, 4th ed. 1995.
3. National Research Council-Committee on Diet and Health. *Diet and health: implications for reducing chronic disease risk*. Washington, DC: National Academy Press, 1989.
4. US Department of Agriculture, US Department of Health and Human Services. *Nutrition and your health: dietary guidelines for Americans*, 5th ed. 2000.
5. Tannenbaum A. The genesis and growth of tumors. III. Effects of a high fat diet. *Cancer Res* 1942;2:468.
6. Tannenbaum A, Silverstone H. Nutrition in relation to cancer. *Adv Cancer Res* 1953;1:451.
7. Welsch CW. Relationship between dietary fat and experimental mammary tumorigenesis: a review and critique. *Cancer Res* 1992;52[Suppl 7]:2040S.
8. Fay MP, Freedman LS. Meta-analyses of dietary fats and mammary neoplasms in rodent experiments. *Breast Cancer Res Treat* 1997;46:215.
9. Birt DF. Dietary fat and experimental carcinogenesis: a summary of recent in vivo studies. *Adv Exp Med Biol* 1986;206:69.
10. Albanes D. Total calories, body weight, and tumor incidence in mice. *Cancer Res* 1987;47:1987.
11. World Cancer Research Fund, American Institute for Cancer Research. *Food, nutrition and the prevention of cancer: a global perspective*. Washington, DC: American Institute for Cancer Research, 1997.
12. Sonnenschein E, Glickman L, Goldschmidt M, et al. Body conformation, diet, and risk of breast cancer in pet dogs: a case-control study. *Am J Epidemiol* 1991;133:694.
13. Appleton BS, Landers RE. Oil gavage effects on tumor incidence in the National Toxicology Program's 2-year carcinogenesis bioassay. *Adv Exp Med Biol* 1986;206:99.
14. Freedman LS, Clifford C, Messina M. Analysis of dietary fat, calories, body weight, and the development of mammary tumors in rats and mice: a review. *Cancer Res* 1990;50:5710.
15. Ip C. Quantitative assessment of fat and calorie as risk factors in mammary carcinogenesis in an experimental model. In: Mettlin CJ, Aoki K, eds. *Recent Progress in Research on Nutrition and Cancer: proceedings of a workshop sponsored by the International Union Against Cancer, held in Nagoya, Japan, November 1–3, 1989*. New York, NY: Wiley-Liss, Inc, 1990:107.
16. Boissonneault GA, Elson CE, Pariza MW. Net energy effects of dietary fat on chemically induced mammary carcinogenesis in F344 rats. *J Natl Cancer Inst* 1986;76:335.
17. Carroll MD, Abraham S, Dresser CM, for the National Center for Health Statistics. *Dietary intake source data: United States, 1976–1980*, Series 11. 1983.
18. Armstrong B, Doll R. Environmental factors and cancer incidence and mortality in different countries, with special reference to dietary practices. *Int J Cancer* 1975;15:617.
19. Prentice RL, Sheppard L. Dietary fat and cancer. Consistency of the epidemiologic data, and disease prevention that may follow from a practical reduction in fat consumption. *Cancer Causes Control* 1990;1:81.
20. Rose DP, Boyar AP, Wynder EL. International comparisons of mortality rates for cancer of the breast, ovary, prostate, and colon, and per capita food consumption. *Cancer* 1986;58:2263.
21. Ziegler RG, Hoover RN, Pike MC, et al. Migration patterns and breast cancer risk in Asian-American women. *J Natl Cancer Inst* 1993;85:1819.
22. Giovannucci E, Ascherio A, Rimm EB, et al. Physical activity, obesity, and risk for colon cancer and adenoma in men. *Ann Intern Med* 1995;122:327.
23. Harris JR, Lippman ME, Veronesi U, et al. Breast cancer. *N Engl J Med* 1992;327:319.
24. Willett WC. Nutritional epidemiology. In: Rothman KJ, Greenland S, eds. *Modern epidemiology*, 2nd ed. Philadelphia: Lippincott–Raven Publishers, 1998:623.
25. Willett WC. *Nutritional epidemiology*. New York, NY: Oxford University Press, 1990.
26. Rimm EB, Giovannucci EL, Stampfer MJ, et al. Reproducibility and validity of an expanded self-administered semiquantitative food frequency questionnaire among male health professionals. *Am J Epidemiol* 1992;135:1114.
27. Pietinen P, Hartman AM, Haapa E, et al. Reproducibility and validity of dietary assessment instruments. I. A self-administered food use questionnaire with a portion size picture booklet. *Am J Epidemiol* 1988;128:655.
28. Block G. A review of validations of dietary assessment methods. *Am J Epidemiol* 1982;115:492.
29. Willett WC, Hunter DJ, Stampfer MJ, et al. Dietary fat and fiber in relation to risk of breast cancer: an 8-year follow-up. *JAMA* 1992;268:2037.
30. Hunter DJ, Spiegelman D, Adami HO, et al. Cohort studies of fat intake and the risk of breast cancer: a pooled analysis. *N Engl J Med* 1996;334:356.
31. Michels KB, Willett WC. The Women's Health Initiative: daughter of politics or science? *Principles and Practices of Oncology* 1992;6:1.
32. Multiple Risk Factor Intervention Trial Research Group. Multiple risk factor intervention trial: risk factor changes and mortality results. *JAMA* 1982;248:1465.
33. Sondik EJ. Breast cancer trends—incidence, mortality, and survival. *Cancer* 1994;74[Suppl S]:995.
34. Garfinkel L, Boring CC, Heater CW. Changing trends—an overview of breast cancer incidence and mortality. *Cancer* 1994;74[Suppl S]:222.
35. Anonymous. *Cancer incidence on five continents*. International Agency for Research on Cancer. IARC Scientific, 1987;5:882.
36. Aoki K, Hayakawa N, Kurihara M, et al. *Death rates for malignant neoplasms for selected sites by sex and five-year age group in 33 countries, 1953–1957 to 1983–1987. International Union Against Cancer*. Nagoya, Japan: University of Nagoya Coop Press, 1992.
37. Staszewski J, Haenszel W. Cancer mortality among the Polish-born in the United States. *J Natl Cancer Inst* 1965;35:291.
38. Adelstein AM, Staszewski J, Muir CS. Cancer mortality in 1970–1972 among Polish-born migrants to England and Wales. *Br J Cancer* 1979;40:464.
39. Buell P. Changing incidence of breast cancer in Japanese-American women. *J Natl Cancer Inst* 1973;51:1479.
40. Marshall JR, Qu Y, Chen J, et al. Additional ecological evidence: lipids and breast cancer mortality among women aged 55 and over in China. *Eur J Cancer* 1992;28A:1720.
41. Stephen AM, Wald NJ. Trends in individual consumption of dietary fat in the United States, 1920–1984. *Am J Clin Nutr* 1990;52:457.
42. McDowell MA, Briefel RR, Alaimo K, et al., National Center for Health Statistics, Centers for Disease Control and Prevention, Public Health Service, US Department of Health and Human Services, Hyattsville, MD. Energy and macronutrient intakes of persons ages 2 months and over in the United States: third national health and nutrition examination survey, phase I 1988–1991;1994; DHHS Publication no (PHS) 95-1250.
43. American Cancer Society. *Cancer facts and figures*. Atlanta, GA: American Cancer Society, Inc., 1994.
44. Graham S, Marshall J, Mettlin C, et al. Diet in the epidemiology of breast cancer. *Am J Epidemiol* 1982;116:68.
45. Howe GR, Hirohata T, Hislop TG, et al. Dietary factors and risk of breast cancer: combined analysis of 12 case-control studies. *J Natl Cancer Inst* 1990;82:561.
46. Giovannucci E, Stampfer MJ, Colditz GA, et al. A comparison of prospective and retrospective assessments of diet in the study of breast cancer. *Am J Epidemiol* 1993;137:502.
47. Smith-Warner SA, Spiegelman D, Adami HO, et al. Types of dietary fat and breast cancer: a pooled analysis of cohort studies. *Int J Cancer* 2001;92:767.
48. Holmes MD, Hunter DJ, Colditz GA, et al. Association of dietary intake of fat and fatty acids with risk of breast cancer. *JAMA* 1999;281:914.
49. Hankinson SE, Willett WC, Manson JE, et al. Plasma sex steroid hormone levels and risk of breast cancer in postmenopausal women. *J Natl Cancer Inst* 1998;90:1292.
50. Goldin BR, Aldercreutz H, Gorbach SL, et al. Estrogen excretion patterns and plasma levels in vegetarian and omnivorous women. *N Engl J Med* 1982;307:1542.
51. Wu AH, Pike MC, Stram DO. Meta-analysis: dietary fat intake, serum estrogen levels, and the risk of breast cancer. *J Natl Cancer Inst* 1999;91:529.
52. Holmes MD, Schisterman EF, Spiegelman D, et al. Meta-analysis: dietary fat intake, serum estrogen levels, and the risk of breast cancer [Letter]. *J Natl Cancer Inst* 1999;91:1511.
53. Rose DP, Connolly JM, Chlebowski RT, et al. The effects of a low-fat dietary intervention and tamoxifen adjuvant therapy on the serum estrogen and sex hormone-binding globulin concentrations of postmenopausal breast cancer patients. *Breast Cancer Res Treat* 1993;27:253.
54. Willett WC. Dietary fat and breast cancer. *Nutritional epidemiology*, 2nd ed. New York: Oxford Press, 1998.
55. Hopkins GJ, Carroll KK. Relationship between amount and type of dietary fat in promotion of mammary carcinogenesis induced by 7,12-dimethylbenz(a)anthracene. *J Natl Cancer Inst* 1979;62:1009.
56. Hopkins GJ, Kennedy TG, Carroll KK. Polyunsaturated fatty acids as promoters of mammary carcinogenesis induced Sprague-Dawley rats by 7,12-dimethylbenz[a]anthracene. *J Natl Cancer Inst* 1981;66:517.
57. Wolk A, Bergstrom R, Hunter D, et al. A prospective study of association of monounsaturated and other types of fat with risk of breast cancer. *Arch Intern Med* 1998;158:41.
58. Martin-Moreno JM, Willett WC, Gorgojo L, et al. Dietary fat, olive oil intake and breast cancer risk. *Int J Cancer* 1994;58:774.
59. Trichopoulou A, Katsouyanni K, Stuver S, et al. Consumption of olive oil and specific food groups in relation to breast cancer risk in Greece. *J Natl Cancer Inst* 1995;87:110.
60. La Vecchia C, Negri E, Franceschi S, et al. Olive oil, other dietary fats, and the risk of breast cancer (Italy). *Cancer Causes Control* 1995;6:545.
61. Cho E, Spiegelman D, Hunter DJ, et al. Premenopausal fat intake and risk of breast cancer. *J Natl Cancer Inst* 2003;95:1079.
62. Wyshak G, Frisch RE. Evidence for a secular trend in age of menarche. *N Engl J Med* 1982;306:1033.
63. Chen J, Campbell TC, Junyao L, et al. *Diet, life-style, and mortality in China: a study of the characteristics of 65 Chinese counties*. Oxford, England: Oxford University Press, 1990.
64. Maclure M, Travis LB, Willett WC, et al. A prospective cohort study of nutrient intake and age at menarche. *Am J Clin Nutr* 1991;54:649.
65. Merzenich H, Boeing H, Wahrendorf J. Dietary fat and sports activity as determinants for age at menarche. *Am J Epidemiol* 1993;138:217.
66. Moisan J, Meyer F, Gingras S. Diet and age at menarche. *Cancer Causes Control* 1990;1:149.
67. Chlebowski RT, Rose D, Buzzard IM, et al. Adjuvant dietary fat intake reduction in postmenopausal breast cancer patient management. The Women's Intervention Nutrition Study (WINS). *Breast Cancer Res Treat* 1992;20:73.
68. Nomura AMY, Marchand LL, Kolonel LN, et al. The effect of dietary fat on breast cancer survival among Caucasian and Japanese women in Hawaii. *Breast Cancer Res Treat* 1991;18:S135.

69. Gregorio DI, Emrich LJ, Graham S, et al. Dietary fat consumption and survival among women with breast cancer. *J Natl Cancer Inst* 1985;75:37.

70. Verreault R, Brisson J, Deschenes L, et al. Dietary fat in relation to prognostic indicators in breast cancer. *J Natl Cancer Inst* 1988;80:819.

71. Holm LE, Nordevang E, Hjalmar ML, et al. Treatment failure and dietary habits in women with breast cancer. *J Natl Cancer Inst* 1993;85:32.

72. Jain M, Miller AB, To T. Premorbid diet and the prognosis of women with breast cancer. *J Natl Cancer Inst* 1994;86:1390.

73. Zhang S, Folsom AR, Sellers TA, et al. Better breast cancer survival for postmenopausal women who are less overweight and eat less fat. *Cancer* 1995;76:275.

74. Newman SC, Miller AB, Howe GR. A study of the effect of weight and dietary fat on breast cancer survival time. *Am J Epidemiol* 1986;123:767.

75. Rohan TE, Hiller JE, McMichael AJ. Dietary factors and survival from breast cancer. *Nutr Cancer* 1993;20:167.

76. Ewertz M, Gillanders S, Meyer L et al. Survival of breast cancer patients in relation to factors which affect the risk of developing breast cancer. *Int J Cancer* 1991;49:526.

77. Kyogoku S, Hirohata T, Nomura Y, et al. Diet and prognosis of breast cancer. *Nutr Cancer* 1992;17:271.

78. Holmes MD, Stampfer MJ, Colditz GA, et al. Dietary factors and the survival of women with breast carcinoma. *Cancer* 1999;86:826.

79. Chlebowski RT, Blackburn GL, Buzzard IM, et al. Adherence to a dietary fat intake reduction program in postmenopausal women receiving therapy for early breast cancer—the Women's Intervention Nutrition Study. *J Clin Oncol* 1993;11:2072.

80. Giovannucci E, Stampfer MJ, Colditz GA, et al. Relationship of diet to risk of colorectal adenoma in men. *J Natl Cancer Inst* 1992;84:91.

81. Vainio H, Bianchini F, eds. Weight control and physical activity. IARC handbooks of cancer prevention / International Agency for Research on Cancer, World Health Organization, Vol. 6. Lyon: IARC Press, 2002.

82. Macquart-Moulin G, Riboli E, Cornee J, et al. Case-control study on colorectal cancer and diet in Marseilles. *Int J Cancer* 1986;38:183.

83. Berta JL, Coste T, Rautureau J, et al. Diet and rectocolonic cancers. Results of a case-control study. *Gastroenterol Clin Biol* 1985;9:348.

84. Tuyns AJ, Haelterman M, Kaaks R. Colorectal cancer and the intake of nutrients: oligosaccharides are a risk factor, fats are not. A case-control study in Belgium. *Nutr Cancer* 1987;10:181.

85. Meyer F, White E. Alcohol and nutrients in relation to colon cancer in middle-aged adults. *Am J Epidemiol* 1993;138:225.

86. Jain M, Cook GM, Davis FG, et al. A case-control study of diet and colon-rectal cancer. *Int J Cancer* 1980;26:757.

87. Potter JD, McMichael AJ. Diet and cancer of the colon and rectum: a case-control study. *J Natl Cancer Inst* 1986;76:557.

88. Lyon JL, Mahoney AW, West DW, et al. Energy intake: its relationship to colon cancer risk. *J Natl Cancer Inst* 1987;78:853.

89. Graham S, Marshall J, Haughey B, et al. Dietary epidemiology of cancer of the colon in western New York. *Am J Epidemiol* 1988;128:490.

90. Bristol JB, Emmett PM, Heaton KW, et al. Sugar, fat, and the risk of colorectal cancer. *Br Med J (Clin Res Ed)* 1985;291:1467.

91. Kune GA, Kune S, Watson LF. The nutritional causes of colorectal cancer: an introduction to the Melbourne Study. *Nutr Cancer* 1987;9:5.

92. West DW, Slattery ML, Robison LM, et al. Dietary intake and colon cancer: sex- and anatomic site-specific associations. *Am J Epidemiol* 1989;130:883.

93. Peters RK, Pike MC, Garabrandt D, et al. Diet and colon cancer in Los Angeles County, California. *Cancer Causes Control* 1992;3:457.

94. Manousos O, Day NE, Trichopoulos D, et al. Diet and colorectal cancer: a case-control study in Greece. *Int J Cancer* 1983;32:1.

95. La Vecchia C, Negri E, Decarli A, et al. A case-control study of diet and colorectal cancer in northern Italy. *Int J Cancer* 1988;41:492.

96. Miller AB, Howe GR, Jain M, et al. Food items and food groups as risk factors in a case-control study of diet and colo-rectal cancer. *Int J Cancer* 1983;32:155.

97. Young TB, Wolf DA. Case-control study of proximal and distal colon cancer and diet in Wisconsin. *Int J Cancer* 1988;42:167.

98. Benito E, Obrador A, Stiggelbout A, et al. A population-based case-control study of colorectal cancer in Majorca. I. Dietary factors. *Int J Cancer* 1990;45:69.

99. Lee HP, Gourley L, Duffy SW, et al. Colorectal cancer and diet in an Asian population—a case-control study among Singapore Chinese. *Int J Cancer* 1989;43:1007.

100. Howe GR. Meeting presentation. Advances in the biology and therapy of colorectal cancer. M.D. Anderson's Thirty-Seventh Annual Clinical Conference. M.D. Anderson Cancer Center, Houston, Texas, 1993.

101. Gerhardsson M, Floderus B, Norell SE. Physical activity and colon cancer risk. *Int J Epidemiol* 1988;17:743.

102. Bjelke E. Epidemiology of colorectal cancer, with emphasis on diet. In: Davis W, Harrup KR, Stathopoulos G, eds. *Human cancer. Its characterization and treatment.* Congress Series No. 484. Amsterdam, Exerpta Medica, Int., 1980:158–174.

103. Stemmermann GN, Nomura AM, Heilbrun LK. Dietary fat and the risk of colorectal cancer. *Cancer Res* 1984;44:4633.

104. Hirayama T. A large-scale study on cancer risks by diet—with special reference to the risk reducing effects of green-yellow vegetable consumption. In: Hayashi Y, Magao M, Sugimura T, et al., eds. *Diet, nutrition, and cancer.* Tokyo: Japan Scientific Societies Press, 1986:41.

105. Garland C, Shekelle RB, Barrett-Conner E, et al. Dietary vitamin D and calcium and risk of colorectal cancer: a 19-year prospective study in men. *Lancet* 1985;1:307.

106. Phillips RL, Snowdon DA. Association of meat and coffee use with cancers of the large bowel, breast, and prostate among Seventh-Day Adventists: preliminary results. *Cancer Res* 1983;43[Suppl]:2403S.

107. Willett WC, Stampfer MJ, Colditz GA, et al. Relation of meat, fat, and fiber intake to the risk of colon cancer in a prospective study among women. *N Engl J Med* 1990;323:1664.

108. Goldbohm RA, van den Brandt PA, van't Veer P, et al. A prospective cohort study on the relation between meat consumption and the risk of colon cancer. *Cancer Res* 1994;54:718.

109. Bostick RM, Potter JD, Kushi LH, et al. Sugar, meat, and fat intake, and non-dietary risk factors for colon cancer incidence in Iowa women (United States). *Cancer Causes Control* 1994;5:38.

110. Giovannucci E, Rimm EB, Stampfer MJ, et al. Intake of fat, meat, and fiber in relation to risk of colon cancer in men. *Cancer Res* 1994;54:2390.

111. Thun MJ, Calle EE, Namboodiri MM, et al. Risk factors for fatal colon cancer in a large prospective study. *J Natl Cancer Inst* 1992;84:1491.

112. Norat T, Lukanova A, Ferrari P, et al. Meat consumption and colorectal cancer risk: dose-response meta-analysis of epidemiological studies. *Int J Cancer* 2002;98:241.

113. US Department of Agriculture. *The food guide pyramid.* Washington, DC: Governmental Printing Office, 1992:30.

114. Talamini R, La Vecchia C, Decarli A, et al. Nutrition, social factors, and prostatic cancer in a northern Italian population. *Br J Cancer* 1986;53:817.

115. Rotkin ID. Studies in the epidemiology of prostatic cancer: expanded sampling. *Cancer Treat Rep* 1977;61:173.

116. Mishina T, Watanabe H, Araki H, et al. Epidemiological study of prostate cancer by matched-pair analysis. *Prostate* 1985;6:423.

117. Talamini R, Franceschi S, La Vecchia C, et al. Diet and prostatic cancer: a case-control study in northern Italy. *Nutr Cancer* 1992;18:277.

118. Schuman LM, Mandel JS, Radke A, et al. Some selected features of the epidemiology of prostatic cancer: Minneapolis-St. Paul, Minnesota case-control study, 1976–1979. In: Magnus K, ed. *Trends in cancer incidence: causes and practical implications.* Washington, DC: Hemisphere Publishing Corp, 1982:345.

119. Graham S, Haughey B, Marshall J, et al. Diet in the epidemiology of carcinoma of the prostate gland. *J Natl Cancer Inst* 1983;70:687.

120. Ross RK, Shimizu H, Paganini-Hill A, et al. Case-control studies of prostate cancer in blacks and whites in southern California. *J Natl Cancer Inst* 1987;78:869.

121. West DW, Slattery ML, Robison LM, et al. Adult dietary intake and prostate cancer risk in Utah: a case-control study with special emphasis on aggressive tumors. *Cancer Causes Control* 1991;2:85.

122. Kolonel LN, Yoshizawa CN, Hankin JH. Diet and prostatic cancer: a case-control study in Hawaii. *Am J Epidemiol* 1988;127:999.

123. Heshmat MY, Kaul L, Kovi J, et al. Nutrition and prostate cancer: a case-control study. *Prostate* 1985;6:7.

124. Whittemore AS, Kolonel LN, Wu AH, et al. Prostate cancer in relation to diet, physical activity, and body size in blacks, whites, and Asians in the United States and Canada. *J Natl Cancer Inst* 1995;87:652.

125. Severson RK, Nomura AMY, Grove JS, et al. A prospective study of demographics, diet, and prostate cancer among men of Japanese ancestry in Hawaii. *Cancer Res* 1989;49:1857.

126. Mills PK, Beeson WL, Phillips RL, et al. Cohort study of diet, lifestyle, and prostate cancer in Adventist men. *Cancer* 1989;64:598.

127. Giovannucci E, Rimm EB, Colditz GA, et al. A prospective study of dietary fat and risk of prostate cancer. *J Natl Cancer Inst* 1993;85:1571.

128. Augustsson K, Michaud DS, Rimm EB, et al. A prospective study of intake of fish and marine fatty acids and prostate cancer. *Cancer Epidemiol Biomarkers Prev* 2003;12:64.

129. Le Marchand L, Kolonel LN, Wilkens LR, et al. Animal fat consumption and prostate cancer: a prospective study in Hawaii. *Epidemiology* 1994;5:276.

130. Schuurman AG, van den Brandt PA, Dorant E, et al. Association of energy and fat intake with prostate carcinoma risk. *Cancer* 1999;86:1019.

131. Cramer DW, Welch WR, Hutchison GB, et al. Dietary animal fat in relation to ovarian cancer risks. *Obstet Gynecol* 1984;63:833.

132. La Vecchia C, Decarli A, Negri E, et al. Dietary factors and the risk of epithelial ovarian cancer. *J Natl Cancer Inst* 1987;79:663.

133. Shu XO, Gao YT, Yuan JM, et al. Dietary factors and epithelial ovarian cancer. *Br J Cancer* 1989;59:92.

134. Byers T, Marshall J, Graham S, et al. A case-control study of dietary and nondietary factors in ovarian cancer. *J Natl Cancer Inst* 1983;71:681.

135. Slattery ML, Schuman KL, West DW, et al. Nutrient intake and ovarian cancer. *Am J Epidemiol* 1989;130:497.

136. Risch HA, Jain M, Marrett LD, et al. Dietary fat intake and risk of epithelial ovarian cancer. *J Natl Cancer Inst* 1994;86:1409.

137. Levi F, Franceschi S, Negri E, et al. Dietary factors and the risk of endometrial cancer. *Cancer* 1993;71:3575.

138. Barbone F, Austin H, Partridge EE. Diet and endometrial cancer: a case-control study. *Am J Epidemiol* 1993;137:393.

139. Potischman N, Swanson CA, Brinton LA, et al. Dietary associations in a case-control study of endometrial cancer. *Cancer Causes Control* 1993;4:239.

140. Shu XO, Zheng W, Potischamn N, et al. A population based case-control of dietary factors and endometrial cancer in Shanghai, People's Republic of China. *Am J Epidemiol* 1993;137:155.

141. Zheng W, Kushi LH, Potter JD, et al. Dietary intake of energy and animals foods and endometrial cancer incidence. *Am J Epidemiol* 1995;142:388.

142. Jain MG, Rohan TE, Howe GR, et al. A cohort study of nutritional factors and endometrial cancer. *Eur J Epidemiol* 2000;16:899.

143. Smith-Warner SA, Ritz J, Hunter DJ, et al. Dietary fat and risk of lung cancer in a pooled analysis of prospective studies. *Cancer Epidemiol Biomarkers Prev* 2002;11:987.

144. Willett WC. Diet and coronary heart disease. In: Willett WC, ed. *Nutritional epidemiology*, 2nd ed. New York: Oxford University Press, 1998.

145. Gaard M, Tretli S, Loken EB. Dietary factors and risk of colon cancer: a prospective study of 50,535 young Norwegian men and women. *Eur J Cancer Prev* 1996;5:445.

146. Kato I, Akhmedkhanov A, Koenig K, et al. Prospective study of diet and female colorectal cancer: the New York University Women's Health Study. *Nutr Cancer* 1997;28:276.

147. Hsing AW, McLaughlin JK, Chow W-H, et al. Risk factors for colorectal cancer in a prospective study among US white men. *Int J Cancer* 1998;77:549.

148. Singh PN, Fraser GE. Dietary risk factors for colon cancer in a low-risk population. *Am J Epidemiol* 1998;148:761.

149. Terry P, Bergkvist L, Holmberg L, et al. No association between fat and fatty acids intake and risk of colorectal cancer. *Cancer Epidemiol Biomarkers Prev* 2001;10:913.

150. Flood A, Velie EM, Sinha R, et al. Meat, fat, and their subtypes as risk factors for colorectal cancer in a prospective cohort of women. *Am J Epidemiol* 2003;158:59.

151. Jarvinen R, Knekt P, Hakulinen T, et al. Dietary fat, cholesterol and colorectal cancer in a prospective study. *Br J Cancer* 2001;85:357.

152. Pietinen P, Malila N, Virtanen M, et al. Diet and risk of colorectal cancer in a cohort of Finnish men. *Cancer Causes Control* 1999;10:387.1.Committee on Diet Nutrition and Cancer, Assembly of Life Sciences, National Research Council. *Diet, nutrition, and cancer.* National Academy Press, 1982.

SECTION 2

KARIN B. MICHELS

Dietary Fiber

DIET AND CANCER ETIOLOGY

Cancer is caused by hereditary, genetic, and environmental factors. Studies of cancer incidence among populations migrating to a country with different lifestyle factors have indicated that cancer etiology likely has a large environmental component. Although the contribution of environmental influences differs by cancer type, the incidence of most cancers changes considerably among migrants over time, approaching that of the host country. The age at migration affects the degree of adaptation among first-generation migrants, which indicates that the susceptibility to environmental carcinogenic influences varies with age. Identifying the environmental and lifestyle factors most important to cancer etiology, however, has proven difficult.

Cancer is characterized by an excess of cells beyond the number necessary for normal organ function. Mutation of DNA induces malignant cell transformation. Cancerous cells have escaped their own self-repair mechanisms, which usually protect them from malfunctioning. Given the large number of cells, such failure of self-repair is rare. DNA can be altered by environmental influences to adapt, to change, and to allow natural selection. This potential for change of the DNA makes it also more susceptible to damage.

Environmental influences such as diet may increase the likelihood of DNA mutation but may also protect DNA, either by aiding DNA repair or by supporting apoptosis (the death of a cell) in cells whose DNA is damaged beyond repair.

PROPERTIES OF DIETARY FIBER

Dietary fiber is defined as "all plant polysaccharides and lignin which are resistant to hydrolysis by the digestive enzymes of men."[1] Fiber, both soluble and insoluble, is fermented by the luminal bacteria of the colon. Among the properties of fiber that make it a candidate for cancer prevention are its "bulking" effect, which reduces colonic transit time, and the binding of potentially carcinogenic luminal chemicals. Fiber may also aid in producing short-chain fatty acids that may be directly anticarcinogenic, and fiber may induce apoptosis.

OBSERVATIONAL STUDIES AND CLINICAL TRIALS

The association between dietary fiber and the risk of cancer has been the subject of a number of epidemiologic studies. When exploring the relation between diet and cancer outcomes, epidemiologists use a variety of study designs, the most common of which are the case-control study, the cohort study, and the randomized clinical trial.

CASE-CONTROL STUDIES

Case-control studies of diet may be affected by recall bias and control selection bias. Diet is a particularly difficult exposure to measure in observational research, because people generally do not accurately remember what they ate. In a case-control study, participants affected by the disease under study (cases) and healthy controls are asked to recall their past diet. It is possible that the cases overestimate their consumption of foods that are commonly considered "unhealthy" and underestimate their consumption of foods considered "healthy." Unfortunately, the validity of recalled diet is almost impossible to determine. Giovannucci and colleagues have documented differential reporting of fat intake before and after disease occurrence.[2] Thus, the possibility of recall bias in a case-control study poses a real threat to the validity of the observed associations.

As is the case with any observational study, confounding by other factors may distort the association of interest. Individuals maintaining a healthy diet often have other health-seeking behaviors: They are more physically active, maintain a lower body weight, smoke less, drink less alcohol, and are more likely to take vitamin supplements. Even if the influence of these confounding variables is analytically controlled, residual confounding likely remains, because all variables are measured with error. In addition, it is probably not possible to assess all indicators of a healthy lifestyle, which leaves unmeasured confounding.

COHORT STUDIES

Prospective cohort studies of the effects of diet are likely to have a much higher validity than retrospective case-control studies, because diet is recorded by participants before disease occurrence. Cohort studies are still affected by measurement error, because diet consists of a large number of foods, and it is almost impossible to estimate one's own intake of individual foods correctly. Accurate individual food recording is even more difficult, given the increasing tendency to consume meals prepared away from home that may contain a variety of ingredients of which the consumer may not be aware. Confounding by other lifestyle factors is also a problem in cohort studies.

RANDOMIZED CLINICAL TRIALS

The gold standard in medical research is the randomized clinical trial (RCT). In an RCT, diet is randomly assigned to participants; hence, the association between diet and the cancer of interest should not be confounded by other factors, and misclassification of diet will be low if participants maintain the assigned diet. The difficulty with RCTs of diet is that it is likely an unreasonable burden for participants to maintain the assigned diet strictly over many years, as would be necessary for diet to have an impact on cancer incidence. Hence, randomized trials are rarely used to examine the effect of diet on cancer but have better promise for the study of diet and adenoma recurrence, which requires considerably shorter follow-up time. The randomized design also lends itself to the study of the effects of dietary supplements such as multivitamin supplements or fiber supplements.

TYPES OF DIETARY FIBER

Fiber is designated *soluble* or *insoluble* according to its degree of solubility in water. Soluble fiber absorbs water and is fermentable; insoluble fiber is insoluble in water and usually nonfermentable. Sources of soluble fiber are fruits and vegetables, beans, barley, and oat bran. Sources of insoluble fiber are whole grains, in particular whole wheat, cereals, beans, and the skins of fruits and vegetables. Soluble fiber includes pectins, gums, starches, some hemicelluloses, and other polysaccharides. Insoluble fiber includes cellulose, most hemicelluloses, and lignins. Fiber is also subcategorized by its source as cereal, fruit, or vegetable fiber.

CALCULATION OF FIBER INTAKE

Fiber intake is estimated from foods consumed. In observational studies, common diet assessment methods are the food frequency questionnaire, the 7-day diet record, and the 24-hour recall. Fiber intake is derived from these dietary questionnaires using nutrient composition tables, which specify the fiber content of each individual food. Different methods have been established to define fiber intake: Association of Official Analytical Chemists (AOAC) method (accepted by the U.S. Food and Drug Administration and the Food and Agriculture Organization of the World Health Organization for nutrition labeling purposes),[3] Southgate,[4] and Englyst nonstarch polysaccharides fiber[5,6] (used primarily in the United Kingdom). Although the AOAC definition includes some starch as dietary fiber, Southgate and Englyst distinguish nonstarch polysaccharides from starch. The Englyst nonstarch polysaccharides definition is a refinement of the Southgate method that allows subdivision into several subcomponents such as cellulose and noncellulose.

DIETARY FIBER AND COLORECTAL CANCER

In 1969, Dennis Burkitt hypothesized that dietary fiber may play a role in colon carcinogenesis.[7] While working as a physician in Africa, Burkitt noticed the low incidence of colon cancer among African populations whose diet was high in fiber. Burkitt concluded that a link might exist between the fiber-rich diet and the low incidence of colon cancer. Burkitt's observations were followed by numerous case-control studies that seemed to confirm his theories. A combined analysis of 13 case-control studies[8] as well as a metaanalysis of 16 case-control studies[9] indicated an inverse association between fiber intake and colorectal cancer. Inclusion of studies was selective, however, and effect estimates unadjusted for potential confounders were used for most studies. Moreover, recall bias is a severe threat to the validity of retrospective case-control studies of fiber intake and any disease outcome.

Data from prospective cohort studies have largely failed to support the inverse association between dietary fiber and colorectal cancer incidence found in retrospective studies. Evidence from at least ten prospective studies is currently available[10–21] (Table 20.2-1). Initial analyses from the Nurses' Health Study[16] and the Health Professionals Follow-up Study[13] found no important association between dietary fiber and colorectal cancer. These studies of two large cohorts of women and men followed at Harvard University in Boston may provide the most comprehensive data on fiber intake and colorectal cancer, because they include repeated assessments of fiber intake. The Nurses' Health Study, initiated in 1976, includes 121,700 U.S. female registered nurses aged 30 to 55 years at baseline. In an analysis of data from 1980 through 1996, encompassing 1,408,232 person-years of follow-up and 787 cases of colorectal cancer, no important association was observed between fiber intake and colorectal cancer.[16] Similarly, in the Health Professionals Follow-up Study initiated in 1986, which included 51,529 male health professionals aged 40 to 75 years at baseline, a 4-year follow-up encompassing 55,561 person-years and 205 colon cancer cases did not indicate any important relation between fiber intake and colorectal cancer.[13] A significant inverse association between fiber intake and incidence of colorectal cancer was reported by the European Prospective Investigation into Nutrition and Cancer (EPIC) study. EPIC, coordinated by the International Agency for Research on Cancer, Lyon, France, includes 22 centers in ten countries in Europe. The analysis presented on dietary fiber and colorectal cancer encompassed 434,209 women and men from eight European countries, 1,939,011 person-years of follow-up, and 1065 cases of colorectal cancer.[19] The analytic model used by the EPIC investigators included adjustments for age, height, weight, total caloric intake, sex, and center assessed at baseline, and identified a significant inverse association between fiber intake and colorectal cancer. In an updated analysis including participants of the Nurses' Health Study and the Health Professionals Follow-up Study and encompassing 1.8 million person-years of follow-up and 1572 cases of colorectal cancer, analyses adjusting for age or simulating the EPIC analytic model revealed associations similar to those found in the EPIC study.[21] After more complete adjustment for potential confounding variables, however, the association vanished[21] (see Table 20.2-1).

The association between dietary fiber and colorectal cancer appears to be confounded by a number of other dietary and nondietary factors. These methodologic considerations must be taken into account when interpreting the available evidence. It is possible that other dietary factors such as folate intake are more important for colorectal cancer pathogenesis than dietary fiber.

TABLE 20.2-1. Prospective Studies of Dietary Fiber and Colorectal Cancer Incidence

Study	No. of Participants	Follow-Up (Y)	Cancer Site	No. of Cases	Comparison	Covariate-Adjusted RR (95% CI)[a]	P for Trend across Quantiles
Hawaiian Japanese cohort[10]	8006 men	16	Colon	102	Lowest vs. highest quartile	1.40	0.35
			Rectal	60	Lowest vs. highest quartile	0.83	0.19
Iowa Women's Study[11]	41,837 women	5	Colon	212	Highest vs. lowest quartile	0.80 (0.49–1.31)	NS
Family history[12]	4239 women	10	Colon	65	>22.6 g/d vs. 16.2 g/d	1.2 (0.6–2.6)	0.6
No family history[12]	22,698 women	10	Colon	180	>22.6 g/d vs. 16.2 g/d	0.8 (0.5–1.2)	0.3
New York University Women's Health Study[14]	14,727 women	7.1	Colorectal	100	Highest vs. lowest quartile	1.51 (0.85–2.68)	0.14
Alpha-Tocopherol, Beta-Carotene Cancer Prevention Study[15]	27,111 male smokers	8	Colorectal	185	Highest vs. lowest quartile	1.0 (0.6–1.5)	0.79
Swedish Mammography Screening Cohort[17]	61,463 women	9.6	Colorectal	460	Highest vs. lowest quartile	0.96 (0.70–1.33)	0.98
Breast Cancer Detection Demonstration Project[18]	45,491 women	8.5	Colorectal	487	Highest vs. lowest quintile	0.94 (0.70–1.26)	—
European Prospective Investigation into Nutrition and Cancer[19]	300,197 women 134,012 men	4.5	Colorectal	1065	Highest vs. lowest quintile	0.75 (0.59–0.95)	0.005
Cancer Prevention Study II Nutrition Cohort[20]	70,554 women 62,609 men	5	Colon	210 298	Highest vs. lowest quintile Highest vs. lowest quintile	1.09 (0.58–2.05) 1.01 (0.62–1.65)	0.65 0.59
Nurses' Health Study[21]	76,228 women	16	Colorectal	904	>14 g/1000 cal/d vs. <8 g/1000 cal/d	0.97 (0.69–1.37)	0.81
Health Professionals Follow-up Study[21]	47,202 men	14	Colorectal	668	>14 g/1000 cal/d vs. <8 g/1000 cal/d	0.90 (0.64–1.26)	0.71

NS, not significant.
[a]Covariate-adjusted relative risk (RR) estimate and 95% confidence interval (CI); covariates adjusted differ in each study.

FIBER INTAKE AND COLORECTAL ADENOMAS

In a few prospective cohort studies, the primary occurrence of colorectal polyps was investigated. Although no consistent relation was found in the Nurses' Health Study, the Health Professionals Follow-up Study, and the Wheat Bran Fiber Trial, a report from the Prostate, Lung, Colorectal and Ovarian Cancer Screening Trial described an inverse association between high dietary fiber and colorectal adenomas.

The study of fiber intake and colorectal adenoma recurrence lends itself to a randomized clinical trial design because of the relatively short follow-up necessary. A number of RCTs have explored the effect of fiber supplementation on colorectal adenoma recurrence.[22-27] Evidence has consistently indicated no effect of fiber intake. In one RCT, an increase in adenoma recurrence was observed among participants randomly assigned to use fiber supplementation, which was stronger among those with high dietary calcium.[26]

FIBER INTAKE AND BREAST CANCER

It has been speculated that dietary fiber reduces the risk of breast cancer through reduction in intestinal absorption of estrogens excreted via the biliary system.[28] A diet low in fat and high in fiber has been associated with reduced serum estrogen levels.[29] Fiber may also lower insulin sensitivity, which may play a role in breast cancer pathogenesis.

Relatively few epidemiologic studies have examined the association between fiber intake and breast cancer. In a metaanalysis of ten case-control studies, a significant inverse association was observed.[30] However, these retrospective studies were likely affected by the aforementioned biases—recall bias, in particular.

Results from at least six prospective cohort studies of the association between fiber intake and breast cancer incidence have been reported.[31-37] In the Nurses' Health Study, no important association between dietary fiber intake and subsequent incidence of breast cancer was observed.[31] A lack of association was also found in the New York State Cohort, which included 344 breast cancer cases.[32] In an early analysis of the Canadian National Breast Screening Study (519 breast cancer cases), an inverse association with dietary fiber was found.[33] An updated analysis of data for this cohort, however, which encompassed 16.2 years of follow-up and 2536 incident cases of breast cancer, did not reveal any association between breast cancer incidence and total dietary fiber or intake of any of the specific fiber fractions.[34] Similarly, dietary fiber was not found to be related to incidence of breast cancer in the Netherlands Cohort Study,[35] a study conducted in Finland,[36] and the California Teachers Study.[37]

DIETARY FIBER AND STOMACH CANCER

The association between fiber intake and stomach cancer has been considered in at least one prospective cohort study. The results from retrospective case-control studies of fiber intake and gastric cancer risk are inconsistent. In the Netherlands Cohort Study, dietary fiber was not associated with incidence of gastric carcinoma.[38] Further investigation through prospective cohort studies must be completed before conclusions about the relation between fiber intake and stomach cancer incidence can be drawn.

TIMING OF DIET

Most epidemiologic studies of diet and cancer have assessed dietary intake among adults. Dietary habits likely take decades to affect cancer development. Given the long latency between dietary intake and the onset of cancer, it is possible that data on diet during childhood or early adolescence are more relevant for carcinogenesis and cancer prevention. Such data are difficult to collect prospectively, however. Data from migrant studies suggest that the age of migration affects the change in rates of incidence for several cancers, which indicates that environmental influences earlier in life may affect incidence of at least some cancer types. Because diet is an important environmental factor, diet in early life may play an important role in carcinogenesis. Similarly, markers of early-life diet such as height and age at menarche are associated with cancer incidence. Although the evidence for a link between fiber intake and cancer risk is currently weak, it cannot be concluded from the available data that high fiber intake early in life does not affect risk of colorectal, breast, stomach, or any other cancer type.

CONCLUSION

The observational data presently available do not indicate an important role for dietary fiber in the prevention of cancer. The long-held perception that a high intake of fiber conveys protection originated largely from retrospectively conducted studies, which are affected by a number of biases, in particular, the potential for differential recall of diet, and from studies that were not well controlled for potential confounding variables.

REFERENCES

1. Trowell H, Southgate DA, Wolever TM, et al. Dietary fiber redefined [Letter]. *Lancet* 1976;1:967.
2. Giovannucci E, Stampfer MJ, Colditz GA, et al. A comparison of prospective and retrospective assessments of diet in the study of breast cancer. *Am J Epidemiol* 1993;137:502.
3. Prosky L, Asp NG, Furda I, et al. Determination of total dietary fiber in foods and food products: collaborative study. *J Assoc Anal Chem* 1985;68:677.
4. Southgate DA. Determination of carbohydrates in foods. II. Unavailable carbohydrates. *J Sci Food Agric* 1969;20:331.
5. Englyst HN, Bingham SA, Runswick SA, et al. Dietary fibre (non-starch polysaccharides) in fruit, vegetables and nuts. *J Hum Nutr Diet* 1988;1:247.
6. Englyst HN, Bingham SA, Runswick SA, et al. Dietary fibre (non-starch polysaccharides) in cereal. *J Hum Nutr Diet* 1989;2:253.
7. Burkitt DP. Related disease—related cause? *Lancet* 1969;2:1229.
8. Howe GR, Benito E, Castelleto R, et al. Dietary intake of fiber and decreased risk of cancers of the colon and rectum: evidence from the combined analysis of 13 case-control studies. *J Natl Cancer Inst* 1992;84:1887.
9. Trock B, Lanza E, Greenwald P. Dietary fiber, vegetables, and colon cancer: critical review and meta-analyses of the epidemiologic evidence. *J Natl Cancer Inst* 1990;82:650.
10. Heilbrun LK, Nomura A, Hankin JH, et al. Diet and colorectal cancer with special reference to fiber intake. *Int J Cancer* 1989;44:1.
11. Steinmetz KA, Kushi LH, Bostick RM, et al. Vegetables, fruit, and colon cancer in the Iowa Women's Health Study. *Am J Epidemiol* 1994;139:1.
12. Sellers TA, Bazyk AE, Bostick RM, et al. Diet and risk of colon cancer in a large prospective study of older women: an analysis stratified on family history (Iowa, United States). *Cancer Causes Control* 1998;9:357.
13. Giovannucci E, Rimm EB, Stampfer MJ, et al. Intake of fat, meat, and fiber in relation to risk of colon cancer in men. *Cancer Res* 1994;54:2390.
14. Kato I, Akhmedkhanov A, Koenig K, et al. Prospective study of diet and female colorectal cancer: The New York University Women's Health Study. *Nutr Cancer* 1997;28:276.
15. Pietinen P, Malila N, Virtanen M, et al. Diet and risk of colorectal cancer in a cohort of Finnish men. *Cancer Causes Control* 1999;10:387.
16. Fuchs CS, Giovannucci EL, Colditz GA, et al. Dietary fiber and the risk of colorectal cancer and adenoma in women. *N Engl J Med* 1999;340:169.
17. Terry P, Giovannucci E, Michels KB, et al. Fruit, vegetables, dietary fiber, and risk of colorectal cancer. *J Natl Cancer Inst* 2001a;93:525.
18. Mai V, Flood A, Peters U, et al. Dietary fibre and risk of colorectal cancer in the Breast Cancer Detection Demonstration Project (BCDDP) follow-up cohort. *Int J Epidemiol* 2003;32:234.
19. Bingham SA, Day NE, Luben R, et al. Dietary fibre in food and protection against colorectal cancer in the European Prospective Investigation into Cancer and Nutrition (EPIC): an observational study. *Lancet* 2003;361:1496.
20. McCullough ML, Robertson AS, Chao A, et al. A prospective study of whole grains, fruits, vegetables and colon cancer risk. *Cancer Causes Control* 2004 *(in press).*
21. Michels KB, Fuchs CS, Giovannucci E, et al. Fiber intake and colorectal cancer incidence in the Nurses' Health Study and the Health Professionals Follow-up Study *(submitted for publication).*
22. McKeown-Eyssen GE, Bright-See E, Bruce WR, et al. A randomized trial of a low fat high fibre diet in the recurrence of colorectal polyps. Toronto Polyp Prevention Group. *J Clin Epidemiol* 1994;47:525.
23. MacLennan R, Macrae F, Bain C, et al. Randomized trial of intake of fat, fiber, and beta carotene to prevent colorectal adenomas. The Australian Polyp Prevention Project. *J Natl Cancer Inst* 1995;87:1760.
24. Schatzkin A, Lanza E, Corle D, et al. Lack of effect of a low-fat, high-fiber diet on the recurrence of colorectal adenomas. Polyp Prevention Trial Study Group. *N Engl J Med* 2000;342:1149.
25. Alberts DS, Martinez ME, Roe DJ, et al. Lack of effect of a high-fiber cereal supplement on the recurrence of colorectal adenomas. Phoenix Colon Cancer Prevention Physicians' Network. *N Engl J Med* 2000;342:1156.
26. Bonithon-Kopp C, Kronborg O, Giacosa A, et al. Calcium and fibre supplementation in prevention of colorectal adenoma recurrence: a randomised intervention trial. European Cancer Prevention Organisation Study Group. *Lancet* 2000;356:1300.
27. Jacobs ET, Giuliano AR, Roe DJ, et al. Intake of supplemental and total fiber and risk of colorectal adenoma recurrence in the wheat bran fiber trial. *Cancer Epidemiol Biomarkers Prev* 2002;11:906.
28. Goldin BR, Adlercreutz H, Gorbach SL, et al. Estrogen excretion patterns and plasma levels in vegetarian and omnivorous women. *N Engl J Med* 1982;307:1542.
29. Woods MN, Gorbach SL, Longcope C, et al. Low-fat, high-fiber diet and serum estrone sulfate in premenopausal women. *Am J Clin Nutr* 1989;49:1179.
30. Howe GR, Hirohata T, Hislop TG, et al. Dietary factors and risk of breast cancer: combined analysis of 12 case-control studies. *J Natl Cancer Inst* 1990; 82:561.
31. Willett WC, Hunter DJ, Stampfer MJ, et al. Dietary fat and fiber in relation to risk of breast cancer. An 8-year follow-up. *JAMA* 1992;268:2037.
32. Graham S, Zielezny M, Marshall J, et al. Diet in the epidemiology of postmenopausal breast cancer in the New York State Cohort. *Am J Epidemiol* 1992;136:1327.
33. Rohan TE, Howe GR, Friedenreich CM, et al. Dietary fiber, vitamins A, C, and E, and risk of breast cancer: a cohort study. *Cancer Causes Control* 1993;4:29.
34. Terry P, Jain M, Miller AB, et al. No association among total dietary fiber, fiber fractions, and risk of breast cancer. *Cancer Epidemiol Biomarkers Prev* 2002;11:1507.
35. Verhoeven DT, Assen N, Goldbohm RA, et al. Vitamins C and E, retinol, beta-carotene and dietary fibre in relation to breast cancer risk: a prospective cohort study. *Br J Cancer* 1997;75:149.
36. Jarvinen R, Knekt P, Seppanen R, et al. Diet and breast cancer risk in a cohort of Finnish women. *Cancer Lett* 1997;19:114:251.
37. Horn-Ross PL, Hoggatt KJ, West DW, et al. Recent diet and breast cancer risk: the California Teachers Study (USA). *Cancer Causes Control* 2002;13:407.
38. Botterweck AA, van den Brandt PA, Goldbohm RA. Vitamins, carotenoids, dietary fiber, and the risk of gastric carcinoma: results from a prospective study after 6.3 years of follow-up. *Cancer* 2000;88:737.

SECTION 3   KARIN B. MICHELS

Fruit and Vegetable Consumption

FRUITS AND VEGETABLES

Two decades ago, Doll and Peto speculated that 35% (range, 10% to 70%) of all cancer deaths in the United States may be preventable by alterations in diet.[1] Fruits and vegetables may be major dietary contributors to cancer prevention, because they are rich in potential anticarcinogenic substances. Fruits and vegetables contain antioxidants and minerals and are good sources of fiber, potassium, carotenoids, vitamin C, folate, and other vitamins. Although fruits and vegetables supply less than 5% of total energy intake in most countries worldwide on a population basis, the concentration of micronutrients in these foods is greater than in most others.

The comprehensive report of the World Cancer Research Fund and the American Institute for Cancer Research entitled *Food, Nutrition and the Prevention of Cancer: A Global Perspective* reached the consensus based on the available evidence that "there is a strong and consistent pattern showing that diets high in vegetables and fruits decrease the risk of many cancers, and perhaps cancer in general."[2] However, with additional evidence accumulating from prospective cohort studies, which had previously been scarce, doubts have been cast on the protective association between fruit and vegetable consumption and cancer.

The majority of available data on the association between fruit and vegetable intake and cancer risk comes from case-control studies. Case-control studies, in which diet is assessed retrospectively in individuals with and without cancer, are prone to recall bias. Participants with cancer may underreport their consumption of foods that are considered "healthy" and overestimate consumption of foods that are considered "unhealthy," as they try to find the reasons for their malignancy.

DIET ASSESSMENT INSTRUMENTS

In population-based studies, diet is generally assessed with a self-administered instrument. The most widely used diet assessment instruments are the food frequency questionnaire, the 7-day diet record, and the 24-hour recall. Although the 7-day diet record may provide the most accurate documentation of intake during the week the participant keeps a diet diary, the burden of computerizing the information and extracting foods and nutrients has made the use of the 7-day diet record prohibitive in most large-scale studies. The 24-hour recall provides only a snapshot of diet on 1 day, which may or may not be representative of the participant's usual diet and is thus affected by both within-person variation and seasonal variation. The food frequency questionnaire, the most widely used instrument in large population-based studies, asks participants to report their average intake of a large number of foods during the previous year. Participants tend to overreport their fruit and vegetable consumption on the food frequency questionnaire, to the

extent of reporting almost double their true intake.[3] This may reflect "social desirability bias," which leads to overreporting of healthy foods and underreporting of less healthy foods. In case-control studies, this misclassification of true intake may be different for cases and controls, and the resulting bias could distort the risk estimate in either direction, that is, the association between diet and cancer incidence could be underestimated or overestimated. In prospective cohort studies, the misclassification would be nondifferential, because at the time participants report their dietary intake, they do not know whether or not they will develop the disease during follow-up. Therefore, the association would be underestimated.

CONFOUNDING

When the results from epidemiologic studies are interpreted, the potential for confounding must be considered. Confounding can affect case-control and cohort studies alike. Individuals with a high consumption of fruits and vegetables are likely to exhibit other indicators of a healthy lifestyle, including regular physical activity, use of multivitamin supplements, lower smoking rates, lower alcohol consumption, and lower red meat consumption.[4] If all potential confounding factors are not adequately adjusted for in the analytic model, residual or unmeasured confounding is likely to remain, creating a spurious inverse association between fruit and vegetable consumption and cancer outcomes.

FRUIT AND VEGETABLE CONSUMPTION AND COLORECTAL CANCER

The association between fruit and vegetable consumption and the incidence of colon or rectal cancer has been examined prospectively in at least six studies. In some of these prospective cohorts, inverse associations were observed for individual foods or particular subgroups of fruits or vegetables, whereas many comparisons revealed no such links. The results from the largest studies, the Nurses' Health Study and the Health Professionals Follow-up Study, indicated no important association between consumption of fruits and vegetables and incidence of cancers of the colon or rectum.[4] In these two large cohorts, diet was assessed repeatedly during follow-up with a detailed food frequency questionnaire. No overall association was found during 1,743,645 person-years of follow-up, during which 937 cases of colon cancer and 244 cases of rectal cancer occurred (Fig. 20.3-1).

FRUIT AND VEGETABLE CONSUMPTION AND STOMACH CANCER

At least 11 prospective cohort studies have examined consumption of some fruits and vegetables and incidence of stomach cancer.[5–15] Six of these studies considered total vegetable intake. Three found a significant protection from stomach cancer,[8,12,14] whereas three did not.[6,13,15] All other comparisons were made for subgroups of vegetables and produced inconsistent results. Eight prospective cohort studies investigated the association between fruit consumption and stomach cancer

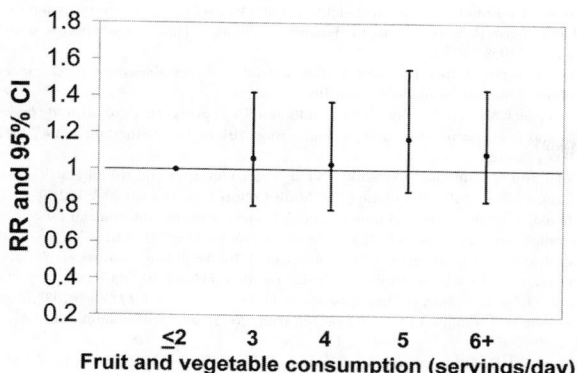

FIGURE 20.3-1. Fruit and vegetable consumption and relative risk (RR) of colorectal cancer in the Nurses' Health Study and the Health Professionals Follow-up Study. CI, confidence interval.

risk.[6-8,11-15] Four studies found an inverse association of borderline statistical significance.[8,11,12,14]

FRUIT AND VEGETABLE CONSUMPTION AND BREAST CANCER

The most comprehensive evaluation of fruit and vegetable consumption and the incidence of breast cancer was provided by a pooled analysis of all cohort studies.[16] Data were pooled from eight prospective studies that included 351,825 women, 7377 of whom developed incident invasive breast cancer during follow-up. The pooled relative risk adjusted for potential confounding variables was 0.93 (95% confidence interval, 0.86 to 1.0; *P* for trend, .08) for the highest versus the lowest quartile of fruit consumption, 0.96 (95% confidence interval, 0.89 to 1.04; *P* for trend, .54) for vegetable intake, and 0.93 (95% confidence interval, 0.86 to 1.0; *P* for trend, .12) for total consumption of fruits and vegetables combined. The authors concluded that fruit and vegetable consumption during adulthood is not significantly associated with reduced risk of breast cancer.

FRUIT AND VEGETABLE CONSUMPTION AND LUNG CANCER

The relation between fruit and vegetable consumption and the incidence of lung cancer has been considered in at least 11 prospective cohort studies.[17-27] Most studies indicated an inverse association of lung cancer with fruit or with fruit and vegetable consumption. Because of the powerful effect of smoking on lung cancer incidence and its correlation with low consumption of fruits and vegetables, smoking is a strong confounder of the association between fruit and vegetable intake and risk of lung cancer. Although all studies included adjustments for smoking characteristics, residual confounding by smoking is likely. In the Nurses' Health Study, the Health Professionals Follow-up Study, and a study conducted among members of a California retirement community, the inverse association was restricted to women, which possibly indicates that residual confounding by unmeasured smoking characteristics remained.[21,25] In the two large Harvard cohorts, however,

high consumption of fruits and vegetables was protective for both men and women who never smoked.[25]

MICRONUTRIENT COMPONENTS OF FRUITS AND VEGETABLES AND CANCER

FOLATE

Folate is a micronutrient commonly found in fruits and vegetables, particularly oranges, orange juice, asparagus, beets, and peas. Folate may reduce carcinogenesis through various mechanisms: DNA methylation, DNA synthesis, and DNA repair. In the animal model, folate deficiency enhances intestinal carcinogenesis.[28] Folate deficiency is related to incorporation of uracil into human DNA and to an increased frequency of chromosomal breaks. A number of epidemiologic studies indicate that a diet rich in folate may lower risk of colorectal adenoma and colorectal cancer.[2] Because folate intake from dietary sources is generally relatively low, dietary folate is highly susceptible to oxidative destruction by cooking and food processing, and folate is not well absorbed, folate intake from supplements plays an important role. Although the optimal dose of folate supplementation to minimize colorectal cancer risk has not been established, preliminary evidence based on pooled results from nine prospective studies suggests that intake of 400 to 500 μg/d may be required to minimize risk.[29]

Potential interactions between alcohol consumption, folate intake, and methionine intake have been described. Although alcohol consumption has been fairly consistently related to an increase in colorectal cancer, this elevated risk has not been found among individuals with a high intake of folate and methionine.[28] A similar folate-alcohol interaction has been observed for breast cancer risk. Although the incidence of breast cancer has been positively correlated with alcohol intake, the potential detrimental effect of alcohol seems to be eliminated in women with high folate intake.[30]

Genetic susceptibility may explain this effect modification. A polymorphism of the MTHFR gene (cytosine to thymine transition at position 677) may result in a relative deficiency of methionine. Homozygotes for this allele experience the greatest protection from high folate or methionine intake and low alcohol consumption.[31] The evidence is inconclusive, however, due to the present scarcity of data.

CAROTENOIDS

Carotenoids, prevalent in fruits and vegetables, are antioxidants, enhance cell-to-cell communication, promote cell differentiation, and modulate immune response. In 1981, Peto and colleagues speculated that β-carotene may be a major player in cancer prevention and encouraged testing of its anticarcinogenic properties.[32] Indeed, subsequent observational studies supported a reduced cancer risk—in particular, of lung cancer—with high intake of carotenoids.[2] Clinical trials randomizing intake of β-carotene supplements, in contrast, have not revealed evidence of a protective effect of β-carotene.[33-37] In fact, β-carotene was found to increase the risk of lung cancer and total mortality among smokers in the Finnish Alpha-Tocopherol, Beta-Carotene Cancer Prevention Study.[33] These adverse affects disappeared during longer periods of follow-up, however.[37] The discrepancy in evidence between epidemiologic studies and randomized clinical trials has been attributed to recall bias in case-control studies and to residual confounding.[38,39]

CONCLUSION

Consumption of fruits and vegetables and some of their main micronutrients appears to be less important in cancer prevention than previously assumed. With accumulation of data from prospective cohort studies and randomized trials, a lack of association of these foods and nutrients with cancer outcomes has become apparent. Folate intake, however, holds promise for cancer prevention.

One possible explanation for the lack of associations observed is the measurement error associated with self-reported dietary intake. This misclassification can easily obscure a true decrease in cancer risk of 10% to 30%. Thus, a diet rich in fruits and vegetables may be associated with a modest decrease in the risk of cancer that might not be detected in observational studies. Possibly, high consumption of fruits and vegetables during childhood and adolescence is more effective in reducing cancer risk than consumption in adult life due to the long latency of cancer manifestation. Few data are available on diet during earlier periods of life and adult cancer risk.

Conversely, it is possible that, with the fortification of breakfast cereal, flour, and other foods, the frequent consumption of fruits and vegetables has become less essential for cancer prevention. Nevertheless, an abundance of fruits and vegetables as part of a healthy diet is recommended, because evidence consistently shows that it lowers the incidence of heart disease, diabetes, and obesity.

REFERENCES

1. Doll R, Peto R. The causes of cancer. *J Natl Cancer Inst* 1981;66:1191.
2. World Cancer Research Fund and American Institute for Cancer Research. Food, nutrition and prevention of cancer: a global perspective. Washington: American Institute for Cancer Research, 1997:216.
3. Michels KB, Bingham SA, Luben R, et al. The effect of correlated measurement error in multivariate models of diet. *Am J Epidemiol* 2004 (in press).
4. Michels KB, Giovannucci E, Joshipura KJ, et al. A prospective study of fruit and vegetable consumption and colorectal cancer incidence. *J Natl Cancer Inst* 2000;92:1740.
5. Hirayama T. A large-scale study on cancer risks by diet—with special reference to the risk reducing effects of green-yellow vegetable consumption. In: Hayashi Y, Magao M, Sugimura T, et al., eds. *Diet, nutrition, and cancer.* Tokyo: Japan Scientific Societies Press, 1986:41.
6. Kneller RW, McLaughlin JK, Bjelke E, et al. A cohort study of stomach cancer in a high-risk American population. *Cancer* 1991;68:672.
7. Kato I, Tominaga S, Ito Y, et al. A prospective study of atrophic gastritis and stomach cancer risk. *Jpn J Cancer Res* 1992;83:1137.
8. Nomura AM, Stemmermann GN, Chyou PH. Gastric cancer among the Japanese in Hawaii. *Jpn J Cancer Res* 1995;86:916.
9. Chyou PH, Nomura AMY, Hankin JH, et al. A case-control study of diet and stomach cancer. *Cancer Res* 1990;50:7501.
10. Dorant E, van den Brandt PA, Goldbohm RA, et al. Consumption of onions and a reduced risk of stomach carcinoma. *Gastroenterology* 1996;110:12.
11. Galanis DJ, Kolonel LN, Lee J, et al. Intakes of selected foods and beverages and the incidence of gastric cancer among the Japanese residents of Hawaii: a prospective study. *Int J Epidemiol* 1998;27:173.
12. Terry P, Nyren O, Yuen J. Protective effect of fruits and vegetables on stomach cancer in a cohort of Swedish twins. *Int J Cancer* 1998;76:35.
13. Botterweck AA, van den Brandt PA, Goldbohm RA. A prospective cohort study on vegetable and fruit consumption and stomach cancer risk in The Netherlands. *Am J Epidemiol* 1998;148:842.
14. Kobayashi M, Tsubono Y, Sasazuki S, et al. Vegetables, fruit and risk of gastric cancer in Japan: a 10-year follow-up of the JPHC Study Cohort I. *Int J Cancer* 2002;102:39.
15. Masaki M, Sugimori H, Nakamura K, et al. Dietary patterns and stomach cancer among middle-aged male workers in Tokyo. *Asian Pac J Cancer Prev* 2003;4:61.
16. Smith-Warner SA, Spiegelman D, Yaun SS, et al. Intake of fruits and vegetables and risk of breast cancer: a pooled analysis of cohort studies. *JAMA* 2001;285:769.
17. Kvale G, Bjelke E, Gart JJ. Dietary habits and lung cancer risk. *Int J Cancer* 1983;31:397.
18. Long-de W, Hammond EC. Lung cancer, fruit, green salad and vitamin pills. *Chin Med J* 1985;98:206.
19. Kromhout D. Essential micronutrients in relation to carcinogenesis. *Am J Clin Nutr* 1987;45:1361.
20. SGE, Beeson WL, Phillips RL. Diet and lung cancer in California Seventh-Day Adventists. *Am J Epidemiol* 1991;133:683.
21. Shibata A, Paganini-Hill A, Ross RK, et al. Intake of vegetables, fruits, beta-carotene, vitamin C and vitamin supplements and cancer incidence among the elderly: a prospective study. *Br J Cancer* 1992;66:673.
22. Steinmetz KA, Potter JD, Folsom AR. Vegetables, fruit, and lung cancer in the Iowa Women's Health Study. *Cancer Res* 1993;53:536.
23. Ocke MC, Bueno-de-Mesquita HB, Feskens EJ, et al. Repeated measurements of vegetables, fruits, beta-carotene, and vitamins C and E in relation to lung cancer. The Zutphen Study. *Am J Epidemiol* 1997;145:358.
24. Voorrips LE, Goldbohm RA, Verhoeven DT, et al. Vegetable and fruit consumption and lung cancer risk in the Netherlands Cohort Study on diet and cancer. *Cancer Causes Control* 2000;11:101.
25. Feskanich D, Ziegler RG, Michaud DS, et al. Prospective study of fruit and vegetable consumption and risk of lung cancer among men and women. *J Natl Cancer Inst* 2000;92:1812.
26. Holick CN, Michaud DS, Stolzenberg-Solomon R, et al. Dietary carotenoids, serum beta-carotene, and retinol and risk of lung cancer in the Alpha-Tocopherol, Beta-Carotene Cohort Study. *Am J Epidemiol* 2002;156:536.
27. Neuhouser ML, Patterson RE, Thornquist MD. Fruits and vegetables are associated with lower lung cancer risk only in the placebo arm of the beta-carotene and retinol efficacy trial (CARET). *Cancer Epidemiol Biomarkers Prev* 2003;12:350.
28. Giovannucci E. Epidemiologic studies of folate and colorectal neoplasia: a review. *J Nutr* 2002;132:2350S.
29. Kim DH, Smith-Warner SA, Hunter DJ, et al. Pooled analysis of prospective cohort studies on folate and colorectal cancer. Pooling Project of Diet and Cancer Investigators. *Am J Epidemiol* 2001;[Suppl 153]:S118.
30. Zhang S, Hunter DJ, Hankinson SE, et al. A prospective study of folate intake and the risk of breast cancer. *JAMA* 1999;281:1632.
31. Chen J, Giovannucci E, Kelsey K, et al. A methylenetetrahydrofolate reductase polymorphism and the risk of colorectal cancer. *Cancer Res* 1996;56:4862.
32. Peto R, Doll R, Buckley JD, et al. Can dietary beta-carotene materially reduce human cancer rates? *Nature* 1981;290:201.
33. Alpha-Tocopherol, Beta-Carotene Prevention Study Group. The effect of vitamin E and beta carotene on the incidence of lung cancer and other cancers in male smokers. *N Engl J Med* 1994;330:1029.
34. Omenn GS, Goodman GE, Thornquist MD, et al. Effects of a combination of beta carotene and vitamin A on lung cancer and cardiovascular disease. *N Engl J Med* 1996;334:1150.
35. Hennekens CH, Buring JE, Manson JE, et al. Lack of effect of long-term supplementation with beta carotene on the incidence of malignant neoplasms and cardiovascular disease. *N Engl J Med* 1996;334:1145.
36. Lee IM, Cook NR, Manson JE, et al. Beta-carotene supplementation and incidence of cancer and cardiovascular disease: the Women's Health Study. *J Natl Cancer Inst* 1999;91:2102.
37. Virtamo J, Pietinen P, Huttunen JK, et al. ATBC Study Group. Incidence of cancer and mortality following alpha-tocopherol and beta-carotene supplementation: a postintervention follow-up. *JAMA* 2003;290:476.
38. Marshall JR. Beta-carotene: a miss for epidemiology. *J Natl Cancer Inst* 1999;91:2068.
39. Stram DO, Huberman M, Wu AH. Is residual confounding a reasonable explanation for the apparent protective effects of beta-carotene found in epidemiologic studies of lung cancer in smokers? *Am J Epidemiol* 2002;155:622.

SECTION **4**

SUSAN T. MAYNE
SCOTT M. LIPPMAN

Retinoids, Carotenoids, and Micronutrients

Cancer chemoprevention can be defined as pharmacologic intervention with specific nutrients or other chemicals to suppress or reverse carcinogenesis and to prevent the development of invasive cancer.[1] Two basic concepts underlie this cancer control strategy—multistep carcinogenesis and field carcinogenesis. Carcinogenesis is a chronic, multistep process characterized by the accumulation of specific genetic and phenotypic alterations that can evolve over a 10- to 20-year period from the first initiating event. The premise of human chemoprevention is that one can intervene (and suppress) at many steps in the carcinogenic process and over a many-year period. A wave of new technology (e.g., high-resolution endoscopy, laser capture microdissection, multiplex gene/expression/protein arrays, and small interfering RNA) is rapidly increasing the understanding of neoplastic evolution. It is now understood that this process can involve mutations in key tumor suppressor genes or oncogenes or both, epigenetic changes via aberrations of histone acetylation or DNA methylation, genetic instability, and defects in signal transduction, with clonal expansion and, remarkably, intraepithelial spread of premalignant cells.[2] Field carcinogenesis was first described in the early 1950s as "field cancerization" in the head and neck and subsequently was ascribed to many epithelial sites. The field concept is that patients at high risk for an epithelial cancer have a wide surface area of carcinogenic tissue change that can be detected at the gross level (oral premalignant lesions, polyps), microscopic level (metaplasia, dysplasia), and molecular level (gene loss or amplification). Molecular studies detecting profound genetic alterations in histologically normal tissue from high-risk individuals have provided strong support for the field carcinogenesis concept. The implication of the field effect is that multifocal, genetically distinct, and clonally related premalignant lesions can progress over a broad tissue region. The clinical importance of this effect is best illustrated in head and neck squamous cancer, for which both synchronous and metachronous "second" primary tumors (SPTs) are common. The latter develop at an annual rate of 5% to 7% in prospective studies and are the principal cause of cancer death in early-stage disease and in long-term survivors of head and neck cancer, regardless of the stage of the first cancer at diagnosis. The essence of chemoprevention, then, is intervention within the multistep carcinogenic process and throughout a wide field.

To date, retinoids (the natural derivatives and synthetic analogues of vitamin A) and one member of the carotenoid class, β-carotene, are among the best-studied agents in human chemoprevention (Fig. 20.4-1). This review focuses on these compounds, with brief discussion of other selected micronutrients that have also been evaluated in randomized trials for chemopreventive efficacy, specifically vitamins E and C and the trace mineral selenium.

HISTORICAL PERSPECTIVE

Vitamin A was first recognized as an essential nutrient in 1913. In 1925, Wolbach and Howe described the histopathologic

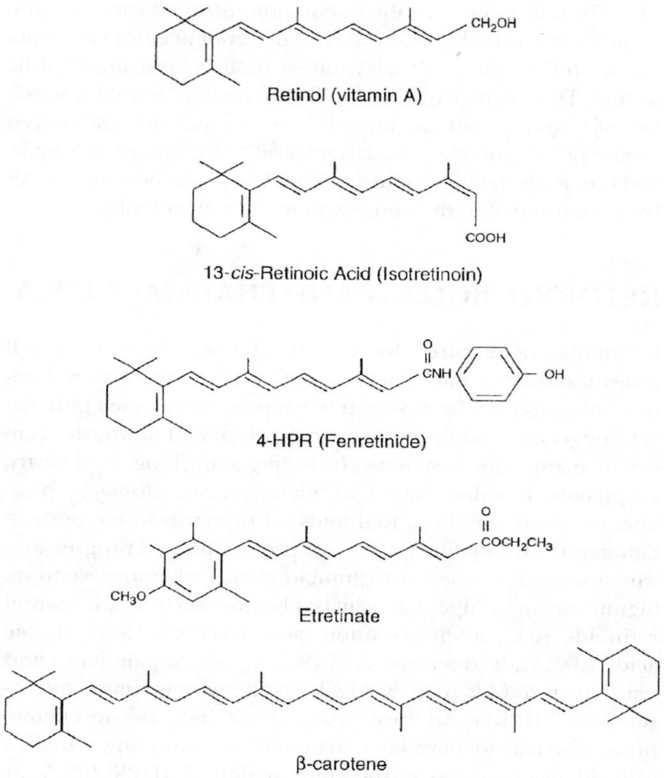

FIGURE 20.4-1. Structure of selected retinoids and the carotenoid β-carotene. Retinol, 13-*cis*-retinoic acid, and β-carotene are naturally occurring; 4HPR and etretinate are synthetic retinoids.

changes in epithelia associated with vitamin A deficiency.[3] This led to the identification of retinol and some of its naturally occurring retinoid derivatives (see Fig. 20.4-1) and production of a large body of research aimed at understanding the role of vitamin A and retinoids in cellular differentiation and in neoplastic transformation. Epidemiologic studies of vitamin A and cancer incidence began to emerge in the 1970s, in which it was shown that computed indices of total vitamin A intake were associated significantly with lower cancer risk, particularly for lung cancer.[4]

Vitamin A is a nonspecific term embracing two families of dietary factors: preformed vitamin A (chiefly retinyl esters, but also retinol and retinal) and another family consisting of the various provitamin A carotenoids (β-carotene and those other carotenoids that can be metabolic precursors of retinol). Preformed vitamin A is found predominantly in foods of animal origin, whereas provitamin A carotenoids are found predominantly in fruits and vegetables.

Epidemiologic studies conducted in the 1980s and 1990s evaluated the independent associations of preformed retinol and provitamin A carotenoids with cancer risk in humans. Dietary intake of provitamin A carotenoids, such as β-carotene, but not of retinol, was associated with a lower risk of cancer.[4] Interpretation of observational epidemiologic studies is difficult because carotenoids are consumed in the form of fruits and vegetables, which contain numerous other substances, many of which may have cancer preventive properties.[5] In contrast, the primary dietary sources of retinol are animal products, consumption of which tends to be associated positively with cancer risk. Thus, in evaluating the chemopreventive efficacy of carotenoids and retinoids, one must consider evidence from epidemiologic studies, clinical trials, animal models, and mechanistic factors. This chapter reviews briefly the biology and pharmacology of retinoids and carotenoids, then focuses on randomized cancer prevention clinical trials involving carotenoids, retinoids, and other selected micronutrients, and discusses how these trials have contributed to the understanding of cancer biology.

RETINOID BIOLOGY AND PHARMACOLOGY

Retinoids are required for the maintenance of normal cell growth, differentiation, and loss within epithelial tissues. Various retinoids have been shown to suppress or reverse epithelial carcinogenesis and to prevent the development of invasive cancer in many animal systems, including skin, lung, oral cavity, esophagus, bladder, mammary gland, cervix, stomach, prostate, pancreas, and liver. Retinoids act primarily in the postcarcinogen (postinitiation) phases of promotion and progression, which are most relevant to human cancer chemoprevention. Significant single-agent activity has been observed with natural retinoids [e.g., all-*trans*-retinoic acid (ATRA), 13-*cis*-retinoic acid (13cRA), 9-*cis*-retinoic acid (9cRA), retinyl palmitate] and synthetic retinoids [e.g., N-4-hydroxyphenyl retinamide or fenretinide (4HPR)]. Additive to synergistic increases in chemopreventive activity have been achieved by combining retinoids with other agents,[6] as in the combination of 4HPR, 9cRA, or retinoid X receptor (RXR)–selective retinoids with tamoxifen in mammary carcinogenesis systems.

The term *retinoid* was redefined in 1985 by Sporn and Roberts[7] to include a substance that binds and activates one or more specific receptors, the latter producing a biologic response. Much has been learned about the specific receptors and mechanisms of action for the retinoids. The retinoid molecular mechanism of action is similar to that of steroid and thyroid hormones in that retinoid nuclear receptors are members of the steroid receptor superfamily.[8,9] These elusive nuclear receptors were discovered simultaneously by two groups of investigators and reported in 1987. Subsequent studies indicate that retinoid receptors are different from other members of the steroid receptor family in that two receptor classes exist: retinoic acid receptors (RARs) and RXRs. Each receptor contains α, β, and γ subtypes, and several of these subclasses have multiple isoforms. These receptors are DNA-binding transcription factors that can activate or suppress the expression of many genes, the products of which mediate retinoid effects on cell growth, differentiation, and apoptosis. Different retinoids bind to the different receptor classes and subclasses with different affinities. This receptor complexity and great diversity in ligand-binding, activation, and receptor function have important preventive and therapeutic implications.

As with other members of the steroid family, retinoid receptors are active only as dimers. Two retinoid receptor dimer types have been identified: RAR/RXR heterodimers and RXR/RXR homodimers (RAR/RAR homodimers have not been identified). Part of the retinoid receptor binds to the ligand and part binds to specific DNA sequences (RARE or RXRE), and either induces or suppresses gene transcription. The best-characterized pathway involves RAR/RXR heterodimers. RXRs have been shown to form heterodimers with other members of the steroid receptor family, including the vitamin D receptor and thyroid hormone receptor. RXRs and their ligands, therefore, can modulate the activities of other steroid hormones.[10] The different ligand-binding patterns can be illustrated with the three major natural retinoic acid derivatives, 13cRA, ATRA, and 9cRA, which are found endogenously in human plasma, albeit at very low physiologic levels. RARs bind ATRA, and 9cRA and RXRs bind only 9cRA. The retinoid 13cRA does not bind directly to nuclear receptors but is rapidly isomerized to ATRA. Ligand binding stabilizes the receptor dimers and activates gene transcription.[8,9]

The retinoid receptor distribution pattern in normal and neoplastic human tissue is under intense study. The tissue distribution of these receptor classes, subclasses, and isoforms varies greatly in normal and pathologic conditions and in different sites within the human body. In normal conditions, RAR-α is expressed in most tissues, RAR-β has more limited expression (e.g., it is not expressed in the skin), and RAR-γ is expressed predominantly in the skin. In cancer, these normal tissue patterns can change (e.g., RAR-β is lost in aerodigestive tract carcinogenic progression).

More than 1000 retinoids have been synthesized.[7,11–13] Current intensive efforts to develop more active and less toxic retinoids for cancer prevention and therapy are directed toward the study of which retinoid receptors mediate retinoid effects on cell growth, differentiation, and apoptosis in different systems and the synthesis of new receptor-selective ligands to obtain the desired retinoid pharmacologic effect.[12,13] An exciting development for chemoprevention is the finding that certain retinoids can interfere with the activity of certain transcription factors such as AP-1 and therefore inhibit neoplastic cell proliferation.[12] Mechanistic studies of retinoid pharmacology provide a basis for rational retinoid development programs for chemoprevention.[13]

CAROTENOID BIOLOGY AND ACTIONS

As described by Krinsky,[14] carotenoids have both biologic functions and biologic actions. Carotenoids function as accessory pigments in photosynthesis via singlet excited carotenoid; they offer protection against photosensitization via triplet excited carotenoid; and some carotenoids serve as provitamin A compounds via central and excentric cleavage. Mechanisms for these functions have been reasonably well characterized. Carotenoids also have been reported to have a number of biologic actions, including antioxidant activity, immunoenhancement, inhibition of mutagenesis and transformation, and regression of premalignant lesions. In contrast to the mechanisms of carotenoid functions, mechanisms of carotenoid action are far from clear. Some of the actions of carotenoids, such as regression of premalignant lesions, are shared by the retinoids, so the potential exists for a similar mechanism of action. The identification of retinoid cleavage products from carotenoids[15] certainly suggests that retinoids and carotenoids may share not only structural similarities and "vitamin A" activity, but perhaps other mechanisms of action that are not fully appreciated at present. However, carotenoids and retinoids also have distinct differences in action, the most notable of which is in antioxidant activity.

Many carotenoids including β-carotene have the ability to quench singlet oxygen, a highly reactive form of oxygen. The quenching involves a physical reaction in which the energy of the excited oxygen is transferred to the carotenoid and an excited-state molecule is formed.[14] Quenching of singlet oxygen is the basis for β-carotene's well-known therapeutic efficacy in erythropoietic protoporphyria, a photosensitivity disorder.[16] The ability of β-carotene and other carotenoids to quench excited oxygen is limited, however, because the carotenoid itself can be oxidized during the process (auto-oxidation). Burton and Ingold,[17] and others, have shown that β-carotene auto-oxidation *in vitro* is dose dependent and dependent on oxygen concentrations.

In addition to singlet oxygen, carotenoids are also thought to quench oxygen free radicals. A relatively large body of literature has linked oxygen free radicals with carcinogenesis; thus, there is considerable interest in antioxidant compounds and antioxidant activity as a mechanism for cancer prevention. Despite the focus on antioxidants and cancer, and the clear evidence of chemopreventive efficacy of β-carotene in some animal carcinogenesis models,[18] it is not clear that antioxidant activity is responsible for the chemoprotective effects observed in the animal studies. For example, β-carotene–induced immunologic enhancement could play a significant role in tumor inhibition by increasing levels of natural killer cells and activating immunoregulatory lymphocytes important in host defense.[19] Various carotenoids have been reported to affect gap junctional communication, related to their ability to up-regulate the expression of the connexin43 gene.[20] This activity was not related to the antioxidant activities of the various carotenoids. Lycopene, at physiologic concentrations, has been reported to inhibit human cancer cell growth by interfering with growth factor receptor signaling and cell-cycle progression.[21] These and other potential mechanisms suggest that it is biologically plausible that carotenoids may have chemopreventive activity, although far less is known about mechanisms of action for the carotenoids than for the retinoids.

Given the interest in antioxidant activity as a potential mechanism for chemopreventive effects, it is not surprising that other dietary antioxidants have been studied for chemopreventive efficacy, particularly vitamins E and C and selenium. These agents are often evaluated in combination. However, as is the case with β-carotene, these micronutrients may have biologic actions independent of antioxidant activity. For example, vitamin E is known to inhibit protein kinase C activity and modulate gene transcription,[22] and selenium has many possible anticarcinogenic effects depending on dose, with some mechanisms mediated through functions of selenium-dependent enzymes, and others through selenium metabolites that are produced at higher dosages.[23] The biochemical complexities of the retinoids, carotenoids, and other micronutrients make it difficult to predict potential chemopreventive efficacy based on mechanistic considerations alone; careful evaluations of efficacy in human clinical studies are required.

CLINICAL TRIALS

A number of randomized cancer prevention trials involving carotenoids and retinoids and a few other micronutrients are ongoing or have been completed. Completed trials involving retinoids are summarized in Table 20.4-1 and those involv-

TABLE 20.4-1. Randomized Trials of the Use of Retinoids for Human Cancer Chemoprevention[a]

Study	Population	Intervention	n	End Point	Result	P Value
Hong et al., 1986[32]	U.S.—oral leukoplakia	13cRA (2 mg/kg/d) Placebo	24 20	Regression	67% (response) 10%	.0002
Stich et al., 1988[36]	India—oral leukoplakia	Vitamin A (200,000 IU/d) Placebo	21 33	Regression	57% (CR) 3%	<.05
Han et al., 1990[37]	China—oral leukoplakia	4HCR (40 mg/d) Placebo	31 30	Regression	87% (CR) 17%	<.01
Lippman et al., 1993[33]	U.S.—oral leukoplakia	13cRA (0.5 mg/kg/d) β-carotene (30 mg/d)	24 29	Progression after 13cRA induction	8% 55%	<.001
Chiesa et al., 1993[34,b]	Italy—oral leukoplakia	4HPR (200 mg/d) No treatment (control)	74 79	Recurrence and new lesion	6% (failure) 30%	<.05
Hong et al., 1990[38]; Benner et al., 1994[39]	U.S.—prior HNSCC	13cRA (50–100 mg/m²/d) Placebo	49 51	Second primary tumor	4% (32 mo); 14% (55 mo)[c] 24% (32 mo); 31% (55 mo)	.005 (32 mo) .042 (55 mo)
Bolla et al., 1994[42]	France—prior HNSCC	Etretinate (50/25 mg/d) Placebo	156 160	Second primary tumor	18% (41 mo)[c] 18%	NS
Khuri et al., 2003[40,b]	U.S.—prior HNSCC	13cRA (30 mg/d) Placebo	590 600	Second primary tumor	4.7% 4.7%	NS
van Zandwijk et al., 2000[61]	Europe—prior HNSCC, NSCLC	Vitamin A (300,000/150,000 IU/d) ± N-acetylcysteine Placebo	2592 total	Second primary tumor	NS	NS
Arnold et al., 1992[46]	Canada—bronchial metaplasia	Etretinate (25 mg/d) Placebo	75 75	Improvement	32% 30%	NS
Lee et al., 1994[47]	U.S.—bronchial metaplasia	13cRA (1 mg/kg/d) Placebo	41 45	Improvement	54% 59%	NS

(*continued*)

TABLE 20.4-1.   (Continued)

Study	Population	Intervention	n	End Point	Result	P Value
Kurie et al., 2000[48]	U.S.—bronchial metaplasia	4HPR, 200 mg/d Placebo	33 35	Improvement	42% 51%	NS
Pastorino et al., 1993[60]	Italy—prior NSCLC	Retinol palmitate (300,000 IU/d) No treatment (control)	150 157	Second primary tumor	Longer time to second primary tumor	.045
Lippman et al., 2001[62]	U.S.—prior NSCLC	13cRA (30 mg/d) Placebo	589 577	Second primary tumor	HR = 1.08	NS
Veronesi et al., 1999[67]	Italy—prior breast cancer	4HPR (200 mg/d) No treatment	1432 1435	Contralateral breast cancer	RR = 0.92 (0.66–1.29)	NS
Moriarty et al., 1982[73]	Ireland—actinic keratosis	Etretinate (75 mg/d) Placebo	44 42	Regression	84% 5%	<.05
Watson, 1986[74]	Australia—actinic keratosis	Etretinate (75 mg/d) Placebo (crossover)	15 total	Regression	93% 13%	<.05
Kligman et al., 1991[72]	U.S.—actinic keratosis	Topical ATRA (0.05%) Vehicle control	266 261	Regression	42% 34%	NS
Kligman et al., 1991[72]	U.S.—actinic keratosis	Topical ATRA (0.10%) Vehicle control	226 229	Regression	55% 41%	<.001
Tangrea et al., 1992[82]	U.S.—prior BCC	13cRA (10 mg/d) Placebo	490 491	Second BCC	0.94 tumor/patient/y 0.96 tumor/patient/y	NS
Moon et al., 1997[84]	U.S.—prior actinic keratosis	Retinol (25,000 IU/d) Placebo	2298 total	Skin cancer	— —	<.05 (SCC) NS (BCC)
Levine et al., 1997[83]	U.S.—prior BCC/SCC of the skin	13cRA (5–10 mg/d) Retinol (25,000 IU/d) Placebo	525 total	Second skin cancer	n = 40 SCC, n = 103 BCC n = 41 SCC, n = 106 BCC n = 41 SCC, n = 110 BCC	NS (both arms)
Bouwes Bavinck et al., 1995[78]	Netherlands—renal transplantation	Acitretin (30 mg/d) Placebo	19 19	Skin cancer	Two patients Nine patients	.01
George et al., 2002[79]	Australia—renal transplantation	Acitretin (25 mg/d, y 1 or y 2, crossover design) No treatment	23 total	Skin cancer	Decreased SCC Decreased BCC	.002 NS (small numbers)
de Sevaux et al., 2003[80]	Netherlands—renal transplantation	Acitretin (0.4 mg/kg/d) Acitretin (0.2 mg/kg/d)	14 12	Skin cancer, actinic keratosis	NS = SCC, BCC Reduced actinic keratosis	NS <.0001
Lamm et al., 1994[92]	U.S.—prior bladder TCC	Megadose vitamins (40,000 IU retinol/d) RDA vitamins	35 30	Recurrence	41% 91%	.0014
Alfthan et al., 1983[90]	Finland—prior bladder cancer	Etretinate (25–50 mg/d) Placebo	15 15	Preventive rate (complete and partial) of recurrence	73% 27%	<.01
Pederson et al., 1984[89]	Denmark—prior bladder cancer	Etretinate (50 mg/d) Placebo	33 40	Freedom from recurrence at 8 mo	27% 37%	NS
Studer et al., 1984[91]	Switzerland—prior bladder cancer	Etretinate (25–50 mg/d) Placebo	38 40	Recurrence	29%/35%/29% (recurrence)[d] 40%/55%/56%[e]	<.02[e]
Meyskens et al., 1994[94]	U.S.—CIN 2,3	Topical ATRA (0.372%) Placebo	150 151	Complete response	43% (CIN 2); 25% (CIN 3) 27% (CIN 2); 31% (CIN 3)	.041 (CIN 2) NS (CIN 3)
Alvarez et al., 2003[98]	U.S.—CIN 2,3	Aliretinoin (50 mg/d) Aliretinoin (25 mg/d) Placebo	33 34 37	Histologically determined regression	36% 32% 32%	NS
Robinson et al., 2002[97]	U.S.—low-grade SIL (HIV+)	13cRA (0.5 mg/kg/d) Observation	56 58	Histologically determined progression	14% 22%	NS
Follen et al., 2001[96]	U.S.—CIN 2,3	4HPR (200 mg/d) Placebo	22 17	Histologically determined regression	23% 41%	NS

(continued)

TABLE 20.4-1. (*Continued*)

Study	Population	Intervention	n	End Point	Result	P Value
Ruffin et al., 2003[95,b]	U.S.—CIN 2,3	Topical ATRA (0.37%)	48	Complete response	40%	NS
		Topical ATRA (0.28%)	44		50%	
		Topical ATRA (0.16%)	45		56%	
		Placebo	38		47%	
Munoz et al., 1985[103]	Huixian, China—high risk	Retinol (50,000 IU/wk) + riboflavin (200 mg/wk) + zinc (50 mg/wk)	610 total	Precancerous esophageal lesions	48.9%	NS (dysplasia)
		Placebo			45.3%	

ATRA, all-*trans*-retinoic acid; BCC, basal cell carcinoma; CIN, cervical intraepithelial neoplasia; CR, complete response; 13cRA, 13-*cis*-retinoic acid; 4HCR, N-4-hydroxycarbophenyl retinamide; HIV+, positive for human immunodeficiency virus infection; HNSCC, head and neck squamous cell carcinoma; 4HPR, N-4-hydroxyphenyl retinamide; HR, hazard ratio; NS, not significant; NSCLC, non–small cell lung cancer; RR, relative risk; SCC, squamous cell carcinoma; SIL, squamous intraepithelial lesion; TCC, transitional cell carcinoma.

[a]Trials of retinoids that also included β-carotene are listed in Table 20.4-2 only.
[b]Ongoing or reported in abstract only.
[c]Median study follow-up in months.
[d]Tumor recurrence at 3 mo/12 mo/24 mo.
[e]P value is for 12-mo rates of multifocal recurrence (more than three tumors).

ing β-carotene are summarized in Table 20.4-2. Retinoid trials have tested efficacy of several retinoids, including retinol, retinyl palmitate, ATRA, 13cRA, etretinate, and 4HPR. Cancer prevention trials examining carotenoids, however, are limited to β-carotene at present, with the exception of some short-term intermediate end point studies involving lycopene, which are discussed in Prostate Trials, later in this chapter.

TABLE 20.4-2. Randomized Trials of the Use of β-Carotene for Human Cancer Chemoprevention

Study	Population	Intervention	n	End Point	Result	P Value
Stich et al., 1988[28]	India—betel nut chewers	BC (180 mg/wk)	27	Oral leukoplakia (complete remission)	14.8%	NS
		BC + retinol (100,000 IU/wk)	51		27.5%	<.05
		Placebo	33		3%	
Sankaranarayanan et al., 1997[30]	India—tobacco chewers	Vitamin A (300,000 IU/wk)	50	Oral leukoplakia (complete regression)	52%	<.0001
		BC (360 mg/wk)	55		33%	
		Placebo	55		10%	
Zaridze et al., 1993[31]	Uzbekistan—oral leukoplakia, esophagitis	BC (40 mg/d) + retinol (100,000 IU/wk) + vitamin E (80 mg/wk)	384	Leukoplakia prevalence	OR = 0.62 (0.39–0.98)	<.05
		Placebo	291	Progression/stability vs. regression	OR = 0.66 (0.37–1.16)	NS
Mayne et al., 2001[43]	U.S.—prior head/neck cancer	BC (50 mg/d)	135	Second head/neck cancer	OR = 0.69 (0.39–1.25)	NS
		Placebo	129	Lung cancer	OR = 1.44 (0.62–3.39)	NS
McLarty et al., 1995[44]	U.S.—male asbestos workers	Retinol (25,000 IU q.o.d.) + BC (50 mg/d)	755 total	Sputum atypia	OR = 1.24 (0.78–1.96)	NS
		Placebo				
ATBC Group, 1994[50]	Finland—male smokers	BC (20 mg/d) ± vitamin E (50 mg/d)	29,133 total	Lung cancer	BC: RR = 1.18 (1.03–1.36)	<.05
		Placebo				
Omenn et al., 1996[52]	U.S.—smokers and asbestos workers	BC (30 mg/d) + retinol (25,000 IU/d)	18,314 total	Lung cancer	RR = 1.28 (1.04–1.57)	<.05
		Placebo				
Hennekens et al., 1996[53]	U.S.—male physicians	BC (50 mg q.o.d.) Placebo	22,071 total	Total cancers	RR = 0.98 (0.91–1.06)	NS
Lee et al., 1999[54]	U.S.—female health professionals	BC (50 mg q.o.d.) Placebo	19,939 19,937	All cancers	RR = 1.03 (0.89–1.18)	NS

(continued)

TABLE 20.4-2. *(Continued)*

Study	Population	Intervention	n	End Point	Result	P Value
Heart Protection Study Group, 2002[55]	U.K.—adults at risk for CHD	BC (20 mg/d) + vitamin E (600 mg/d) + vitamin C (250 mg/d)	20,536 total	Total cancers	7.8%	NS
		Placebo			8%	
Greenberg et al., 1990[85]	U.S.—prior skin cancer	BC (50 mg/d) Placebo	1805 total	Second skin cancer	RR = 1.05 (0.91–1.22)	NS
Green et al., 1999[86]	Australia—general population	BC (30 mg/d)	1383 total	Incidence of squamous cell skin cancer	RR = 1.35 (0.84–2.19)	NS
		Placebo		Incidence of basal cell skin cancer	RR = 1.04 (0.73–1.27)	
DeVet et al., 1991[99]	Netherlands—CIN	BC (10 mg/d) Placebo	278 total	Regression	OR = 0.68 (0.28–1.60)	NS
Romney et al., 1997[100]	U.S.—cervical dysplasia	BC (30 mg/d) Placebo	69 total	Persistent CIN	OR = 1.53 (0.38–6.18)	NS
Mackerras et al., 1999[101]	Australia—cervical atypia/CIN	BC (30 mg/d) ± vitamin C (500 mg/d) Placebo	141 total	Regression	HR = 1.58 (0.86–2.93)	NS
Keefe et al., 2001[102]	U.S.—CIN 2,3	BC (30 mg/d) Placebo	103 total	Regression	25% 38%	NS
Blot et al., 1993[104]	Linxian County, China—general population	BC (15 mg/d) + vitamin E (30 mg/d) + selenium (50 μg/d)	29,584 total	Stomach cancer death	RR = 0.79 (0.64–0.99)	<.05
		Placebo		Esophageal cancer death	RR = 0.96 (0.78–1.18)	NS
Li et al., 1993[105]	Linxian County, China—esophageal dysplasia	Multivitamin/multimineral + BC (15 mg/d)	3318 total	Stomach cancer death	RR = 1.18 (0.76–1.85)	NS
		Placebo		Esophageal cancer death	RR = 0.84 (0.54–1.29)	NS
Greenberg et al., 1994[109]	U.S.—resected adenoma	BC (25 mg/d) ± vitamin C (1 g/d) + vitamin E (400 mg/d) Placebo	751 total	Recurrent adenoma	BC: RR = 1.01 (0.85–1.20)	NS
Kikendall et al., 1991[108]	U.S.—resected adenoma	BC (15 mg/d) Placebo	132 125	Recurrent polyps	29% 24%	NS
MacLennan et al., 1995[107]	Australia—resected adenoma	BC (20 mg/d) ± wheat bran ± low-fat diet Placebo	390 total	Recurrent adenoma	OR = 1.4 (0.8–2.3)	NS
Correa et al., 2000[106]	Columbia—gastric dysplasia	BC (30 mg/d) ± vitamin C, triple therapy	852 total	Regression: subjects with atrophy	RR = 5.1 (1.7–15.0)	<.05
		Placebo	631	Regression: subjects with intestinal metaplasia	RR = 3.4 (1.1–9.8)	<.05

ATBC, Alpha-Tocopherol, Beta-Carotene Cancer Prevention Study; BC, β-carotene; CHD, coronary heart disease; CIN, cervical intraepithelial neoplasia; HR, hazard ratio; NS, not significant; OR, odds ratio; RR, relative risk.

HEAD AND NECK TRIALS

Premalignancy

Oral premalignant lesions include leukoplakias and erythroplakias. Small hyperplastic leukoplakia lesions have a 30% to 40% spontaneous regression rate and less than a 5% risk of malignant transformation. Erythroleukoplakia and dysplastic leukoplakia lesions, however, are associated with a low rate of spontaneous regression and a 30% to 40% long-term risk of oral cancer.[2,24] Molecular markers (e.g., aneuploidy and loss of heterozygosity) have been shown to potently predict cancer risk.[25] High-risk, diffuse, and multifocal disease, accounting for 10% to 15% of all oral premalignant lesions, often is not controlled adequately by local therapy. Oral premalignant lesions are markers of field carcinogenesis, because patients with oral premalignancy develop squamous cancers at the site of the lesions, as well as in distant sites within the upper aerodigestive tract. Thus, regression of oral premalignant lesions has been used to screen agents that may have utility in the prevention of upper aerodigestive tract cancers.

Studies in the 1980s in populations at high risk for oral cancer (tobacco chewers, betel quid chewers) demonstrated that supplemental β-carotene and retinol significantly reduced the frequency of oral micronuclei.[26–28] As for premalignant lesions, many trials have investigated the effects of supplemental β-carotene, alone or in combination with other agents, on regression of oral leukoplakia. Nonrandomized studies (reviewed in ref. 29) have reported response rates ranging from 44% to 97%. Response rates in uncontrolled studies must be interpreted cautiously, however, because leukoplakias are known to regress spontaneously. Few placebo-controlled trials of β-carotene supplementation in patients with oral leukoplakia are available. Stich et al.[28] reported that the combination of β-carotene plus retinol produced complete remissions in 27.5%; β-carotene alone, in 14.8%; and placebo, in 3.0% of subjects (partial remissions were not reported) with a 6-month intervention. Sankaranarayanan et al.[30] reported higher response rates with a longer duration of intervention (12 months): complete regression in 33% given β-carotene and in 52% given retinyl palmitate versus in 10% in the placebo arm. In a trial in Uzbekistan,[31] 6 months of treatment with the combination of retinol, β-carotene, and vitamin E led to a significant reduction in the prevalence odds ratio (OR) of oral leukoplakia [OR, 0.62; 95% confidence interval (CI), 0.39 to 0.98].

The effect of retinoids on the reversal of oral premalignant lesions also has been studied extensively.[2,24] One of the first such trials, reported in 1986,[32] was a 3-month placebo-controlled study of 13cRA (2 mg/kg/d). The complete plus partial response rate in the 44 evaluable patients was 67% in the retinoid arm and 10% in the placebo arm ($P = .0002$). The rate of histopathologic improvement (i.e., reversal of dysplasia) was also higher in the retinoid arm (54% vs. 10%; $P = .01$). Two major problems were seen with this high-dose, short-term approach, however. First, high-dose 13cRA toxicity was substantial and not acceptable in this clinical setting. Second, over half of those showing a response experienced recurrence or developed new lesions within 3 months after stopping the intervention.

Based on the results of this placebo-controlled trial, a randomized maintenance trial was designed.[33] In this trial, patients initially received a 3-month induction course of high-dose 13cRA (1.5 mg/kg/d), followed by a 9-month maintenance course with low-dose 13cRA (0.5 mg/kg/d) or β-carotene (30 mg/d) in patients who had responding or stable lesions during the high-dose induction phase. The induction-phase response rate was 55% (95% CI, 42% to 67%). During the maintenance phase, 2 (8%) of the patients in the retinoid group showed lesion progression versus 16 (55%) in the β-carotene group ($P < .001$). Toxic effects of low-dose 13cRA maintenance therapy were mild, although greater than for β-carotene, and no patients discontinued therapy because of toxicity.

Fenretinide (4HPR) is also being evaluated in oral premalignancy. A randomized study was begun in 1988 at the Milan Cancer Institute to evaluate the efficacy of 52 weeks of systemic 4HPR maintenance therapy (vs. no intervention) after complete laser resection of oral premalignant lesions. Reports of this ongoing study in the mid-1990s included data from 153 patients randomly assigned to treatment groups.[34,35] The rate of treatment failure (recurrence plus new lesions) among those patients who completed the 12-month intervention was 6% in the 4HPR group and 30% in the control group. A 3-day drug holiday at the end of each month was prescribed to avoid the adverse effects (night blindness) of lowering serum retinol level by 4HPR treatment.

Other trials investigating the use of retinoids in oral premalignancy include two randomized studies involving retinol[30,36] and another involving N-4-hydroxycarbophenyl retinamide.[37] All observed significant retinoid chemopreventive activity.

Malignancy

Phase III trials examining the use of retinoids or β-carotene for adjuvant chemoprevention in head and neck cancer have been completed. The first, reported by Hong et al., tested the use of high-dose 13cRA in 103 head and neck cancer patients.[38] After definitive local treatment of stage I to IV (M0) disease with surgery or radiotherapy or both, patients were assigned randomly to 12 months of high-dose 13cRA (50 to 100 mg/m^2/d) or placebo. At a median follow-up of 32 months, no significant differences were seen in primary disease recurrence (local, regional, or distant) or survival. The rate of SPTs, however, was significantly lower in the retinoid arm than in the placebo group. Such tumors developed in two (4%) of the 13cRA-treated patients compared with 12 (24%) of the placebo-treated patients ($P = .005$). Side effects were substantial and included skin dryness and peeling, cheilitis, conjunctivitis, and hypertriglyceridemia. Approximately 30% of the retinoid-treated patients required dose reduction and 18% did not complete the 12-month intervention because of toxicity.

Data from this trial have been reanalyzed with a longer median follow-up of 55 months.[39] With the additional follow-up, each group had one more SPT in the aerodigestive tract, which resulted in a cumulative total of 3 in the retinoid group and 13 in the placebo group ($P = .008$).

Based on this high-dose adjuvant trial, a large-scale National Cancer Institute (NCI) Intergroup phase III trial of low-dose, long-term 13cRA administration was launched in 1991 and recruited patients with stage I or II head and neck squamous cell carcinoma who had been definitively treated with radiation therapy or surgery. Of 1384 registered patients, 1191 were eligible for the study, and these individuals were randomly assigned to receive either 13cRA or placebo for 3 years and were followed for 4 more years. Patients were stratified by cancer stage (I or II), smoking status (currently smoking vs. formerly smoked vs. never smoked), and primary tumor site (larynx, oral cavity, or oral pharynx). No significant differences were seen between the treatment and placebo arms in overall survival or SPT- or recurrence-free survival,[40] although recurrences were decreased in the 13cRA arm (vs. placebo). This provocative nonsignificant effect was lost after treatment stopped, which suggests its association with 13cRA. This phase III trial supports current laboratory analyses designed to better distinguish between SPTs and recurrences on the basis of molecular characteristics. Data from this phase III trial and a related clinical trial[41] also support further study of the administration of retinoids in combination with other agents (currently being tested clinically and mechanistically, e.g., with regard to cyclin D1 polymorphisms) in this setting.

The third randomized trial studied use of the synthetic retinoid etretinate in 316 patients after definitive treatment of stage I to III (T1,2; N0,1) squamous cell carcinoma of the oral cavity and oropharynx.[42] In this French trial, the etretinate dosage was 50 mg/d for 1 month and then 25 mg/d for 2 years. The etretinate was well tolerated. At a median follow-up of 41 months, the rate of SPT development in the two arms was not significantly different.

The EUROSCAN trial included SPTs associated with both head and neck and lung cancer and is discussed in the Malignancy section under Lung Trials, later in this chapter.

As of 2003, only one chemoprevention trial of supplemental β-carotene for prevention of SPTs of the mouth and throat is available.[43] After definitive local therapy, 264 patients with stage I or II head and neck cancer were randomly assigned to receive either supplemental β-carotene (50 mg/d) or identical-appearing placebo. The median follow-up was 51.1 months from the date of randomization. Persons randomly assigned to receive supplemental β-carotene had a 31% decrease in second head and neck cancer risk [relative risk (RR), 0.69; 95% CI, 0.39 to 1.25], but a 44% increase in lung cancer risk (RR, 1.44; 95% CI, 0.62 to 3.39). A smaller Italian trial of β-carotene involving this patient population has been completed but not yet reported as of 2003.

LUNG TRIALS

Premalignancy

The Tyler (Texas) Chemoprevention Trial randomly assigned 755 asbestos workers to receive β-carotene (50 mg/d) and retinol (25,000 IU every other day) or placebo to see if the nutrient combination could reduce the prevalence of atypical cells in sputum. After a mean intervention period of 58 months, there was no significant difference in the two groups in the prevalence of sputum atypia.[44]

In a French trial, chronic smokers with squamous metaplasia of the bronchial epithelium detected in initial bronchoscopy specimens were treated with etretinate (25 mg/d) for 6 months.[45] In this uncontrolled trial, a decline in the extent of squamous metaplasia was observed in most treated patients. The positive result of this French study led to the initiation of three randomized trials—one of etretinate in Canada, and one of 13cRA and one of 4HPR in the United States. The Canadian study evaluated the ability of a course of 25 mg/d of etretinate for 6 months to reverse sputum atypia in chronic smokers.[46] Toxicity was mild, and the number of subjects who required dosage reductions or dropped out was very small and similar in both arms. No difference in the degree of atypia was seen between the etretinate and placebo groups. In the U.S. 13cRA study, chronic smokers underwent bronchoscopy, with endobronchial biopsy specimens taken from six specific anatomic sites within the proximal lung field,[47] as reported in the earlier single-arm French study.[45] Ninety-three of the 152 chronic smokers who underwent bronchoscopic biopsy had squamous metaplasia or dysplasia. Eligible smokers with metaplasia or dysplasia were randomly assigned to receive 6 months of 13cRA or placebo. The extent of metaplasia decreased similarly (in approximately 50% of subjects) in both study arms. Only smoking cessation was associated significantly with a reduction in the metaplasia index during the 6-month intervention. Use of 4HPR was studied in a more recent trial.[48] This study was similar to the earlier 13cRA study with regard to overall design (except for the drug used) and lack of treatment effect.[47] Subsequent retinoid studies have focused on high-risk former smokers, with some promising early results using intermediate end points.[49]

Malignancy

Some major large trials of micronutrient administration for primary prevention of lung cancer have been completed. The earliest involved 29,133 men aged 50 to 69 years in Finland,[50] who were heavy cigarette smokers at entry. The study used a two-by-two factorial design with participants randomly assigned to receive either supplemental β-carotene (20 mg/d), α-tocopherol (50 mg/d), a combination of the two, or placebo for 5 to 8 years. Unexpectedly, participants receiving β-carotene (alone or in combination with α-tocopherol) showed a statistically significant 18% increase in lung cancer incidence (RR, 1.18; 95% CI, 1.03 to 1.36) and 8% increase in total mor-

tality (RR, 1.08; 95% CI, 1.01 to 1.16) relative to participants receiving placebo. Supplemental β-carotene did not appear to affect the incidence of other major cancers occurring in this population. Although it was not the primary outcome of this trial, an interesting observation was made with regard to vitamin E and prostate cancer. Men randomly assigned to receive α-tocopherol had a 32% decrease in prostate cancer incidence and a 41% decrease in prostate cancer mortality.[51] This promising finding will be followed up in future trials (see Prostate Trials, later in this chapter).

The finding of an increased incidence of lung cancer in smokers who took β-carotene supplements was replicated in another major trial. The Carotene and Retinol Efficacy Trial (CARET) was a multicenter lung cancer prevention trial in which supplemental β-carotene (30 mg/d) plus retinol (25,000 IU/d), or placebo, was given to asbestos workers and smokers.[52] CARET was terminated early because interim analyses of the data indicated that, were the trial to have continued for its planned duration, it was highly unlikely that the intervention would have been found to be beneficial. Furthermore, the interim results indicated that the group receiving the supplements was developing more lung cancer, not less, consistent with the results of the Finnish trial. Overall, lung cancer incidence was increased by 28% in the subjects given supplements (RR, 1.28; 95% CI, 1.04 to 1.57) and total mortality was also increased (RR, 1.17; 95% CI, 1.03 to 1.33). The increase in lung cancer after supplementation with β-carotene and retinol was observed for current but not former smokers. In contrast, the Physicians' Health Study examining supplemental β-carotene versus placebo in 22,071 male U.S. physicians reported no significant effect—positive or negative—of 12 years of supplementation with β-carotene (50 mg every other day) on total cancer, lung cancer, or cardiovascular disease.[53] The RR for lung cancer in current smokers randomly assigned to receive β-carotene was 0.90 (95% CI, 0.58 to 1.40). Among nonsmokers, the RR was 0.78 (95% CI, 0.34 to 1.79). A similar lack of effect of supplemental β-carotene on overall cancer incidence was seen in the Women's Health Study, although the duration of intervention was short (median, 2.1 years)[54] and in the Medical Research Council/British Heart Foundation (MRC/BHF) Heart Protection Study of antioxidant vitamin supplementation, although a combination intervention was used (600 mg vitamin E, 250 mg vitamin C, and 20 mg β-carotene daily).[55]

A clear mechanism to explain the apparent enhancement of lung carcinogenesis in smokers by supplemental β-carotene, alone or in combination with retinol, has yet to emerge. As detailed elsewhere,[56] it should be noted that the two trials that observed this enhancing effect had higher median plasma β-carotene concentrations in their intervention groups than did the trials that did not observe an enhancing effect. Thus, it is possible that high tissue concentrations of β-carotene in the presence of strongly oxidative tobacco smoke cause an interaction that affects carcinogenesis. Wang et al. have used the ferret to model β-carotene and tobacco interactions in lung and noted a relative lack of both retinoic acid and RAR-β expression in the lungs of smoke-exposed ferrets given high-dose β-carotene.[57] The authors suggested that oxidative metabolites of β-carotene might cause diminished retinoid signaling and thus increase tumorigenesis. In contrast with a pharmacologic dose of β-carotene, a physiologic dose of β-carotene in smoke-exposed ferrets had no potentially detrimental effects and may have afforded weak protection against lung damage induced by cigarette smoke.[58] Other groups are also studying β-carotene oxidation products. For example, Salgo et al.[59] reported that under some conditions β-carotene oxidation products, but not β-carotene, enhanced binding of cytochrome P-450–catalyzed metabolites of benzo[a]pyrene to DNA. Although mechanistic studies continue, it is prudent to recommend that heavy smokers, particularly those from well-nourished populations, avoid high-dose supplements of β-carotene for lung cancer chemoprevention.

Encouraging data suggesting that retinoid chemoprevention may help control SPTs, recurrence, and mortality in patients with stage I non–small cell lung cancer[60] and showing retinoid activity in related carcinogenic systems led to large-scale phase III retinoid trials in the setting of SPT prevention. One of these was a European trial called EUROSCAN,[61] which was an open-label multicenter trial using a two-by-two factorial design to test the efficacy of 2 years of administration of retinyl palmitate and N-acetylcysteine in preventing second primary tumors in 2592 patients. Patients had completed definitive treatment of early-stage head and neck cancer (larynx, Tis, T1 to 3, N0 to 1; oral cavity, T1 to 2, N0 to 1) and non–small cell lung cancer (T1 to 2, N0 to 1, and T3N0). Treatment with retinyl palmitate or N-acetylcysteine or both produced no improvement in event-free survival, survival, or incidence of SPTs.

The other large SPT trial, called the Lung Intergroup Trial, was a multicenter U.S. NCI Intergroup phase III trial (NCI No. I91-0001) involving 1166 patients with pathologic stage I non–small cell lung cancer (6 weeks to 3 years from definitive resection and no prior radiotherapy or chemotherapy), who were randomly assigned to receive placebo or 13cRA (30 mg/d) for 3 years in a double-blind fashion. Patients were stratified at randomization by tumor (T) stage, histologic classification, and smoking status. The primary end point was time to SPT and the secondary end points were times to recurrence and death. After a median follow-up of 3.5 years, no statistically significant differences were seen between the placebo and 13cRA arms with respect to the time to SPTs, recurrences, or mortality.[62] The unadjusted hazard ratio (HR) of treatment versus placebo was 1.08 (95% CI, 0.78 to 1.49) for SPTs, 0.99 (95% CI, 0.76 to 1.29) for recurrences, and 1.07 (95% CI, 0.84 to 1.35) for mortality. Multivariate analyses showed that occurrence of SPTs was not affected by any stratification factor. Recurrence was affected by T stage (HR for T2 vs. T1, 1.77; 95% CI, 1.35 to 2.31) and treatment-by-smoking interaction (HR for treatment by currently smoking vs. never smoked status, 3.11; 95% CI, 1.0 to 9.71). Mortality was affected by T stage (HR for T2 vs. T1, 1.39; 95% CI, 1.10 to 1.77), histologic classification (HR for squamous vs. nonsquamous, 1.31; 95% CI, 1.03 to 1.68), and treatment-by-smoking interaction (HR for treatment by currently smoking vs. never smoked status, 4.39; 95% CI, 1.11 to 17.29). Mucocutaneous toxicity ($P < .001$) was higher in the 13cRA arm than in the placebo arm, as was noncompliance (40% vs. 25% at 3 years). Secondary multivariate and subset analyses suggested that 13cRA was harmful in current smokers and beneficial in those who had never smoked. The carotenoid and retinoid trials thus indicate that chemoprevention in current smokers may be particularly challenging. Despite the generally negative findings to date, new retinoid formulations and delivery systems (e.g., aerosolization) and potential secondary lung benefits using this agent class are under active study.[63,64]

BREAST TRIALS

The retinamide fenretinide (4HPR) is a potent apoptosis-inducing retinoid with retinoid receptor–dependent and retinoid receptor–independent activities and accumulates in human breast tissue.[65] Moon and colleagues first showed that 4HPR was among the most active cancer chemopreventive agents for the breast, having a high therapeutic index and synergistic interaction with tamoxifen in mammary carcinogenesis model studies.[66] This laboratory work led to a large-scale randomized trial of the use of 4HPR (vs. no treatment) for 5 years to prevent contralateral breast cancer in women aged 30 to 70 years with a history of resected early breast cancer and no prior adjuvant therapy.[67] The intervention produced no significant overall effect. Subset analyses suggested that reduced contralateral and ipsilateral breast cancer rates occurred in premenopausal women and that an opposite trend occurred in postmenopausal women.[67] Secondary analyses also indicated a 4HPR-related decrease in ovarian cancer.[68] Promising new retinoids for breast cancer prevention include other potent apoptosis-inducing retinoids and RAR-subtype-selective, RXR-selective, and anti–AP-1 retinoids.[69]

As for β-carotene, observational data have suggested that higher intake of β-carotene from foods is an important prognostic factor in breast cancer.[70] Given this, randomized trials aimed at increasing vegetable intake to prevent breast cancer recurrence are under way.[71] These interventions clearly influence circulating carotenoid concentrations and illustrate a food-based approach to investigate potential chemopreventive efficacy.

SKIN TRIALS

Data suggest that topical ATRA has significant dose-related activity in reversing premalignant skin lesions (e.g., actinic keratoses, which undergo malignant transformation at a rate of 5%).[72] Systemic retinoid therapy has produced significant activity in two reported randomized trials.[73,74] Several small, single-arm studies have found that systemic retinoids can reduce skin cancer incidence significantly in very high risk patients with xeroderma pigmentosum (XP) and in renal and heart transplant recipients.[75–77]

The XP trial, published in 1988, was a landmark trial in the field of chemoprevention in general in that it was the first human trial to establish a significant reduction in tumor development.[75] Although it included only five XP patients, the extremely high rate of skin cancer development and rigorous documentation of skin tumor rates before, during, and after the 2-year high-dose (2 mg/kg/d) 13cRA intervention provided statistically valid results. The overall average reduction in skin cancer incidence during therapy was 63% ($P = .019$). Two major problems were evident from this trial: severe, acute mucocutaneous toxicity occurred with this very high 13cRA dosage, and the preventive effect of the retinoid was lost after retinoid therapy was stopped, as indicated by a mean 8.5-fold increase in the annual rate of skin tumor development ($P = .007$). The retinoid chemopreventive effect in this study was greatest in the XP patients with the highest frequency of *de novo* skin tumor development and, in subsequent studies, was found to be dose related.

Based on positive findings of a single-arm retinoid study,[76] a randomized, placebo-controlled trial of the retinoid acitretin (30 mg/d for 6 months) was conducted in 38 renal transplant recipients.[78] The retinoid group had significant reductions in (1) the number of premalignant lesions ($P = .008$); (2) the number of patients with skin cancer ($P = .01$), and (3) the cumulative number of skin cancers ($P = .009$). Nine of the 19 patients in the placebo group developed a total of 18 skin cancers, and 2 of the 19 patients in the retinoid group developed skin cancer, one cancer each. After the intervention was completed, the rate of skin cancer development in the retinoid arm increased and became similar to that in the placebo arm. Toxicity in the retinoid group was frequent but mild, and the retinoid had no adverse effect on renal function. Two other randomized trials examined the use of acitretin in this setting; in one, skin squamous cell carcinoma was significantly reduced[79] and in the other actinic keratoses were significantly reduced.[80] A nested cohort study suggested that administration of oral retinoids can reduce the high risk of skin squamous cell carcinoma associated with psoralen–ultraviolet A light treatment of psoriasis.[81]

Some large-scale randomized phase III trials of the use of retinoids to prevent skin cancer have been reported. A trial of very low-dose 13cRA (10 mg/d)[82] and a trial of retinol (25,000 IU/d) or 13cRA (5 to 10 mg/d) versus placebo in patients with prior skin cancers[83] found no chemopreventive effects. The third trial, in which retinol was given to patients with prior actinic keratoses, did see a significant reduction of squamous but not of basal skin cancers in the retinoid arm.[84] The contrasting results of the phase III trials of retinoids in skin cancer chemoprevention suggest the importance of retinoid dose, biologic timing of intervention, and target histopathologic type.

Greenberg and colleagues[85] conducted a large randomized clinical trial of supplemental β-carotene (50 mg/d for 5 years) encompassing 1805 persons with a previous nonmelanoma skin cancer. No difference was observed between the two groups in the rate of occurrence of the first new nonmelanoma skin cancer (relative rate, 1.05; 95% CI, 0.91 to 1.22). Use of supplemental β-carotene (30 mg/d) also failed to prevent either basal cell carcinoma or squamous cell carcinoma of the skin in an Australian trial.[86]

Selenium is another nutrient that has been evaluated for efficacy in the prevention of second skin cancers. Clark et al.[87] randomly assigned a total of 1312 patients with a history of nonmelanoma skin cancer to receive either 200 μg/d of selenium or placebo. Selenium supplementation did not affect the incidence of second skin cancers (RR, 1.10 for basal cell carcinoma; RR, 1.14 for squamous cell carcinoma). However, a significant reduction was seen in total cancer mortality (RR, 0.50; 95% CI, 0.31 to 0.80), due mainly to reductions in the incidence of lung, colorectal, and prostate cancers. Other selenium trials are now being initiated (see Prostate Trials, later in this chapter), given these promising results. One should note, however, that additional follow-up in this trial for the primary skin cancer end points indicated that selenium supplementation remained ineffective in preventing basal cell carcinoma but that it significantly increased the risk of squamous cell carcinoma of the skin (HR, 1.25) and total nonmelanoma skin cancer (HR, 1.17).[88]

BLADDER TRIALS

Data from *in vivo* animal, *in vitro*, and epidemiologic studies have suggested efficacy of retinoids for bladder cancer prevention. Three randomized clinical trials tested the use of the retinoid etretinate in patients after resection of their superficial (noninvasive) bladder tumors, which recur in 40% to 90% of cases. All three studies were limited substantially because of mucocutaneous toxicity.[89–91] In two of these three trials, however, prolonged

(longer than 1 year) low-dose etretinate (25 mg/d) apparently was effective. These positive results require a cautious reading, because of the small number of patients and short-term follow-up.

Another chemoprevention trial randomly assigned 65 patients with biopsy-confirmed transitional cell carcinoma of the bladder to receive a multivitamin (recommended daily allowance levels) alone or supplemented with 40,000 IU retinol, 100 mg pyridoxine, 2000 mg ascorbic acid, 400 U α-tocopherol, and 90 mg zinc.[92] The 5-year estimate of tumor recurrence was 91% in the arm receiving the recommended daily allowances versus 41% in the arm given the megadoses ($P = .0014$). These results are promising because the intervention was essentially nontoxic, with only one patient (3%) requiring dosage reduction for mild stomach upset. Further research is needed to replicate this finding and to identify which vitamin(s) were responsible for chemopreventive effect.

Bladder cancer chemoprevention studies of newer synthetic retinoids with better therapeutic ratios are also anticipated. One such leading candidate is 4HPR, which tests as one of the strongest anticarcinogenic retinoids in the rodent bladder, is less toxic than either etretinate or 13cRA in humans, and has produced promising results in a phase IIa trial.[93]

CERVICAL TRIALS

Many randomized and nonrandomized studies of chemoprevention in cervical dysplasia have been conducted. Randomized trials include studies of folic acid, of interferons, of β-carotene, and of retinoids. Only one of these trials, using topical ATRA,[94] found a significant treatment effect. Three hundred and one patients with moderate cervical intraepithelial neoplasia (CIN) 2 and severe dysplasia (CIN 3) were randomly assigned to receive topical ATRA or placebo. This trial administered a 0.372% β-ATRA solution by collagen sponge in a cervical cap delivery system for 4 days initially, then for 2 days at months 3 and 6. The major finding was a higher complete response rate in the ATRA group (43%) than in the placebo group (27%; $P = .041$) among the 141 patients with moderate dysplasia. No significant differences in dysplasia regression rates between the two study arms were detected in patients with severe dysplasia. Acute toxicity was infrequent, mild, and reversible, consisting primarily of local (vaginal and vulvar) irritation, and occurred in fewer than 5% of treated subjects. Major problems with compliance (e.g., 52 patients were lost to follow-up) suggest a cautious interpretation of the findings of this trial. More recent randomized retinoid studies involving topical ATRA[95] and oral 4HPR,[96] 13cRA,[97] and 9cRA[98] have all yielded no significant results.

Randomized trials involving β-carotene have also been published. The first was a trial in the Netherlands in which women with a histologic diagnosis of cervical dysplasia were randomly assigned to receive either 10 mg/d of β-carotene for 3 months or placebo. After 3 months of intervention, no detectable effect of supplemental β-carotene on the regression and progression of cervical dysplasia was observed.[99] Romney et al.[100] randomly assigned women with cervical dysplasia to receive 30 mg β-carotene/d (n = 39) or placebo (n = 30). After 9 months of intervention, no beneficial effect of β-carotene supplementation was seen. An Australian trial used a factorial design to investigate the effects of supplemental β-carotene (30 mg/d) or vitamin C (500 mg/d) in 141 women with minor cervical abnormalities.[101] There was no significant effect of either agent in this trial. A more recently reported trial randomly assigned 101 women with high-grade CIN to receive β-carotene (30 mg/d) or placebo; regression rates were similar in both arms when stratified by CIN grade.[102]

ESOPHAGUS AND STOMACH TRIALS

Certain regions of China (Huixian and Linxian) have strikingly high incidence rates of esophageal and gastric cancers; moreover, intake and blood levels of various micronutrients are consistently low in these populations. These observations have led to several trials examining prevention of esophageal or gastric cancer or both in China.[103–105] The first involved high-risk Chinese subjects from Huixian and tested the combination of retinol, riboflavin, and zinc for 13.5 months. After the intervention, no overall difference was seen between the two arms in the occurrence of premalignant lesions or the prevalence or severity of dysplasia.[103]

Other trials were performed in Linxian County. One trial was conducted among residents from the general population.[104] Nearly 30,000 men and women aged 40 to 69 years took part in the study, which tested the efficacy of four different nutrient combinations in inhibiting the development of esophageal and gastric cancers. The nutrient combinations included retinol plus zinc, riboflavin plus niacin, ascorbic acid plus molybdenum, and the combination of β-carotene, selenium, and vitamin E. After a 5-year intervention period, the group given the combination of β-carotene, vitamin E, and selenium had 13% fewer total cancer deaths (RR, 0.87; 95% CI, 0.75 to 1.00), 4% fewer esophageal cancer deaths (RR, 0.96; 95% CI, 0.78 to 1.18), and 21% fewer gastric cancer deaths (RR, 0.79; 95% CI, 0.64 to 0.99). None of the other nutrient combinations reduced gastric or esophageal cancer deaths significantly in this trial. The finding that vitamin supplements reduced cancer deaths in this population provides compelling evidence in support of the concept of cancer prevention through the use of nutrients; however, the applicability of these results to populations with adequate nutritional status and to tumors at other sites may be limited. Also, it is unclear which nutrient (β-carotene, vitamin E, selenium, or some combination of these) was responsible for the observed protection. It is perhaps of interest that selenium levels were not deficient in this population.

Another Linxian trial was performed to determine whether a multivitamin and multimineral preparation plus β-carotene (15 mg) reduced esophageal and gastric cardia cancers in 3318 residents with esophageal dysplasia.[105] In the group receiving the supplements, cumulative esophageal and gastric cardia death rates after the 6-year intervention period were 8% lower (RR, 0.92; 95% CI, 0.67 to 1.28), esophageal cancer mortality was 16% lower (RR, 0.84; 95% CI, 0.54 to 1.29), and total cancer mortality was 4% lower (RR, 0.96; 95% CI, 0.71 to 1.29). Surprisingly, stomach cancer mortality was 18% higher (RR, 1.18; 95% CI, 0.76 to 1.85) in the supplemented group. None of the results was statistically significant.

Intermediate end point trials have also been performed in other parts of the world. A trial in Uzbekistan used a factorial design to study the combination of β-carotene, retinol, and α-tocopherol, with and without riboflavin, in subjects with chronic esophagitis.[31] The risk of progression or no change versus regression was nonsignificantly decreased by 34% in those receiving retinol, β-carotene, and α-tocopherol (OR, 0.66; 95% CI, 0.37 to 1.16) compared with those who did not receive these agents. Correa et al. investigated the use of sup-

plemental antioxidant nutrients (β-carotene, vitamin C) and anti–*Helicobacter pylori* therapy in participants with gastric dysplasia in Columbia.[106] All three basic interventions resulted in statistically significant increases in the rates of regression.

COLORECTAL TRIALS

Several randomized trials aimed at the prevention of recurrent colorectal adenomas with supplemental β-carotene have been completed. The Australian Polyp Prevention Project evaluated the efficacy of reducing dietary fat to 25% of total calories and supplementing the diet daily with 25 g of wheat bran, 20 mg of β-carotene, or both, in a factorial design.[107] Use of β-carotene did not reduce the incidence of adenomas. At 24 months, 50 patients on the β-carotene arm had adenomas versus 36 patients on the placebo arm. Patients taking β-carotene had a statistically significantly lower proportion of positive nuclei in the upper rectal crypt compartments than those taking placebo, however, which suggests that β-carotene modified preneoplastic mucosal proliferation rather than adenoma growth. Another trial (n = 291) in which a lower dose of 15 mg/d of β-carotene was used also failed to find a reduction in adenomas with supplementation.[108] The largest trial studied 751 patients who had had an adenoma diagnosed and removed within the previous 3 months.[109] Participants were randomly assigned to treatment groups using a two-by-two factorial design, with the active treatments being β-carotene (25 mg/d), and the combination of 1 g of vitamin C plus 400 mg vitamin E. No evidence was seen that either β-carotene or vitamins C and E reduced the incidence of adenomas in this 4-year trial. The RR for β-carotene supplementation was 1.01 (95% CI, 0.85 to 1.20); for supplementation with vitamins C and E, it was 1.08 (95% CI, 0.91 to 1.29). A subsequent report from this trial[110] noted that alcohol intake and cigarette smoking modified the efficacy of β-carotene supplementation. Among nonsmokers and nondrinkers, supplemental β-carotene was associated with a significant decrease in the risk for one or more recurrent adenomas (RR, 0.56); however, among persons who smoked and also drank more than one alcoholic drink per day, β-carotene supplementation significantly increased the risk of recurrent adenoma (RR, 2.07).

PROSTATE TRIALS

Evidence suggests that oxidative stress may play a role in the pathogenesis of prostate cancer,[111] and several antioxidant nutrients, including lycopene, vitamin E, and selenium, are under investigation for chemopreventive efficacy in prostate cancer. As described earlier, provocative secondary analyses of the data of prior phase III NCI trials (test of selenium supplementation for skin cancer prevention[87] and test of vitamin E supplementation for lung cancer prevention[51]) indicated that men randomly assigned to receive vitamin E or selenium experienced fewer incident prostate cancers. In response, the NCI has initiated the Selenium Vitamin E Chemoprevention Trial (SELECT), a phase III trial testing selenium and vitamin E in a two-by-two factorial design. The SELECT accrual goal is 32,400 men (African Americans, 50 years of age or older; other men, 55 years of age or older) with an age-related risk of developing prostate cancer. SELECT is translational, with prospectively collected data and a biorepository for ancillary molecular epidemiologic and other biologic studies of prostate carcinogenesis and agent effects.[112] The study was activated in July 2001, and study accrual was over 80% complete in early November 2003 and is expected to be completed well ahead of the originally estimated completion date in 2006.

In addition to this large primary prevention trial, a number of smaller trials using intermediate end points for prostate carcinogenesis are under way or completed. For example, several smaller trials involving selenium supplementation are under way at the University of Arizona.[113] Intermediate end point studies involving lycopene are also being conducted. Kucuk et al. evaluated 3 weeks of supplementation with lycopene versus placebo in 26 men scheduled for radical prostatectomy and noted a possible decrease in biomarkers of prostate cancer progression.[114] Bowen et al. are studying a tomato sauce intervention and noted that the intervention reduced markers of DNA damage and concentrations of prostate-specific antigen.[115] The use of a tomato sauce–based intervention is supported by animal data indicating that tomato powder (which includes lycopene along with other phytochemicals) but not lycopene alone was effective in inhibiting prostate carcinogenesis.[116]

TRANSLATIONAL AND INTERMEDIATE END POINT STUDIES IN RETINOID CHEMOPREVENTION

Retinoids and carotenoids have not yet shown efficacy in the prevention of invasive cancer in phase III trials; however, translational research conducted within these same trials has greatly contributed to the understanding of epithelial carcinogenesis. Translational research is critical for developing new and better chemopreventive agents and for moving their use more quickly into standard care. Study of the effect of retinoids on head and neck carcinogenesis (oral premalignancy) has proven to be a valuable model for translational research.[24,117,118] Advanced oral lesions can be visualized, biopsied, and monitored prospectively; they are linked to carcinogenesis throughout the aerodigestive tract; and these lesions clearly respond to the use of retinoids and β-carotene in randomized trials. Work in the retinoid–oral premalignancy system offers a paradigm for translational collaborations involving other tumor sites and other agents. This work has provided useful methods for understanding the value of biomarker modulation for predicting clinical outcome and for correlating various markers within the same system; has increased knowledge of the biology of epithelial carcinogenesis and agent mechanisms; and relates to work in validating intermediate end point biomarkers in many sites.

The discovery and early descriptions of nuclear receptors came from molecular *in vitro* studies in several systems (reviewed in Retinoid Biology and Pharmacology, earlier in this chapter). These receptors are also being studied intensively in clinical specimens from many cancer types and sites. The best-studied site with regard to chemoprevention is the head and neck. Xu and colleagues used a nonradioactive RNA *in situ* hybridization method to study the expression of all six human retinoid receptors in squamous cell carcinoma and surrounding premalignant and normal tissue contained in surgical resection specimens.[119] All six receptors were strongly expressed in 100% of oral tissue from healthy nonsmoking volunteers. In premalignant and malignant specimens, however, there was a selective, histopathologic stage–dependent loss of RAR-β messenger RNA expression, with expression detected in 72% of histologically normal and hyperplastic tissue adjacent

to squamous cell carcinomas, 56% of dysplastic tissue, and 35% of squamous cell carcinomas ($P < .05$).

This finding, which suggests an apparent tumor suppressor function in carcinogenic progression, led to a translational study of RAR-β that had three major findings.[120] First, in contrast to the 100% expression seen in healthy controls, RAR-β messenger RNA was detected in only 40% (21 of 52) of oral premalignant lesions ($P = .003$). The expression of the other five receptors, detected in 70% (RXR-β) to 100% (RXR-α) of oral premalignant lesions, did not differ significantly from that in healthy controls. The loss of RAR-β in oral premalignant lesions was not associated significantly with tobacco use. Second, a striking retinoid up-regulation of RAR-β expression was seen after 3 months of high-dose 13cRA, from 40% to 90%. Third, RAR-β up-regulation was associated with clinical response—receptor up-regulation was observed in 82% of responding lesions (including all four complete responses) and 47% of nonresponding lesions ($P = .039$). The early and progressive loss of RAR-β in premalignant tissues and significant 13cRA up-regulation (in association with lesion response) meets several major criteria for a potential intermediate end point. Similar findings have been reported in the lung in three randomized trials.[49,121,122] Future long-term validation trials will determine if early RAR-β up-regulation is associated with late lesion response and a reduction in cancer incidence.

These translational RAR-β findings in the retinoid–oral premalignant system are consistent with *in vitro* data.[123] The RAR-β promoter has a DR5 response element and is the most tightly retinoid-regulated receptor. Mutations, deletions, or structural changes in the RAR-β gene or its promoter, however, have not been identified. Data suggested that loss of RAR-β expression in oral premalignant lesions is related to a defect in intracellular vitamin A metabolism (and reduced levels of retinoic acid in premalignant cells), which can be corrected by pharmacologic doses of retinoic acid.[124] These translational findings are consistent with preclinical data in vitamin A–deficient animals.

The available *in vitro* and *in vivo* data suggest a molecular model of retinoid action (Fig. 20.4-2). *In vitro* transfection studies in lung cancer and other experimental systems suggest that RAR-β, which is located on chromosome 3p, may have tumor suppressor activity,[125,126] contributing to suppression of the premalignant phenotype. Loss of RAR-β may enhance the progression of carcinogenesis by rendering the epithelium resistant to physiologic retinoic acid levels. Pharmacologic doses of retinoic acid, administered systemically, can enter premalignant cells and, by means of residual RARs (e.g., RAR-γ), induce the synthesis of RAR-β via heterodimer binding to the RAR-β promoter and subsequent activation of RAR-β gene transcription. Although 13cRA does not bind directly to RARs, it is isomer-

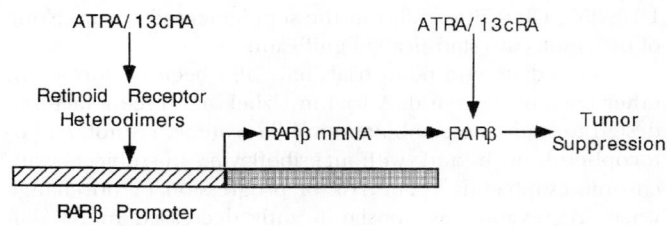

FIGURE 20.4-2. Molecular model of retinoid chemoprevention. ATRA, all-*trans*-retinoic acid; mRNA, messenger RNA; 13cRA, 13-*cis*-retinoic acid; RARβ, retinoic acid receptor beta.

ized to ATRA. The 13cRA can activate RAR-β RARE transcription *in vitro* at levels comparable to those for ATRA. This model of RAR-β up-regulation and tumor suppressor activity may represent the basis of retinoid action.

Earlier and recent advances in the retinoid–head and neck carcinogenesis model are helping to advance the entire field of chemoprevention. Studies in this model of p53, genetic instability, RAR-β, loss of heterozygosity, and cyclin D1 have helped advance the understanding of chemopreventive molecular targets and markers for developing drugs, monitoring interventions, and assessing cancer risk and pharmacogenomics.[127–129] For example, a study suggested that a 13cRA-based regimen may have preventive activity against development of head and neck cancer in persons with a certain *cyclin D1* genotype.[130] Studies of retinoid chemoprevention in head and neck cancer also have shown that chemopreventive agents can delay the onset of clinically detected cancer. Mechanisms of cancer delay may involve suppressing genetic instability and detouring multistep carcinogenesis down alternate molecular pathways.[131] For example, retinoic acid may produce head and neck cancer delay via a molecular detour at 11q13 involving cyclin D1.[130,131] After the substantive contributions to the biology of epithelial carcinogenesis and to molecular monitoring of drug activity, one of the most promising new directions of study in the oral premalignancy model is work in characterizing molecular risk.[132] The ability to select the highest-risk subsets of oral premalignancy patients for preventive interventions—for example, using retinoid combinations—will allow the monitoring of potentially meaningful molecular and clinical responses in the highest-risk lesions and will make it possible to conduct cost-efficient cancer end point trials because control-arm event-rate estimates will be sufficiently high.[133]

OTHER RETINOIDS AND CAROTENOIDS

The retinamide 4HPR is a promising retinoid now in clinical trials for human chemoprevention.[1,2,34,35,67,93] It has a unique mechanism of action and favorable toxicity profile, and has already generated significant chemopreventive activity in several animal carcinogenesis systems, including mammary and bladder models. Several clinical chemoprevention trials targeting cervix, skin, bladder, and lung are currently in progress.

The retinamide 4HPR has potent apoptosis-inducing activity in several neoplastic systems (including leukemia, neuroblastoma, melanoma, small cell lung cancer, and cervical and head and neck squamous cell carcinoma), including those resistant to ATRA and 9cRA. The finding that 4HPR is a potent inducer of apoptosis has exciting clinical implications.[134] Eliminating premalignant, genetically damaged cells by apoptosis may be more effective in cancer prevention than suppressing proliferation. The clinical effects of current chemopreventive agents, most of which primarily suppress proliferation, cease on stopping the drug. Apoptosis-inducing agents such as 4HPR, on the other hand, could allow shorter-term effective chemoprevention with less toxicity. The mechanism(s) by which 4HPR induces apoptosis is not yet understood, but such knowledge would facilitate the design of future preventive approaches using rational combinations of 4HPR and other agents.

Clinical and translational study of other new retinoids is focused on ligands that are selective for RAR subtypes, RXRs, or the downstream target AP-1.[69,135,136] Data support the use of

RXR-selective ligands in cancer prevention. RXRs have a unique role in the control of apoptosis and as obligate heterodimer partners for RARs and many other intracellular receptors (e.g., vitamin D receptor and peroxisome proliferator–activated receptors). Via versatile dimer-partnering behavior and other complex effects, RXR agonists can modulate other endocrine signaling pathways. The potential importance of RXRs in breast carcinogenesis was first illustrated by mammary carcinogenesis studies suggesting that the RAR/RXR panagonist 9cRA is more active than RAR agonists. Subsequent prevention studies of selective RXR agonists in a rat mammary carcinoma model produced the following findings: These agents were less toxic and more active than 9cRA; they inhibited estrogen- and tamoxifen-stimulated uterine proliferation; they showed activity in tamoxifen-resistant disease and activity similar to that of tamoxifen; and they had supraadditive effects when combined with tamoxifen. This study of RXR agonists has led to intensive study of their combination with selective estrogen receptor modulators.[69]

Several carotenoids also appear to have promising chemopreventive activity in animal studies, and intake of others has been inversely associated with human cancer risk in observational epidemiologic studies. Lycopene was previously mentioned with regard to prostate cancer; however, in a review, 57 of 72 studies examined reported inverse associations between tomato intake or blood lycopene level and the risk of various cancers. Thirty-five of these inverse associations were statistically significant.[137] Other carotenoids, including crocetin, canthaxanthin, fucoxanthin, and α-carotene, have been found to inhibit tumorigenesis in animal models.[14] Although considerable interest has been shown in the use of these and other carotenoids for cancer prevention, large-scale human trials should be undertaken with great caution, particularly in smokers, given the lack of a clear understanding of the apparent mechanism of β-carotene in promoting lung carcinogenesis. Of note, lycopene, unlike β-carotene, did not produce squamous metaplasia of the lung in lycopene-supplemented ferrets exposed to cigarette smoke.[138]

CONCLUSION

A number of chemoprevention trials involving retinoids, β-carotene, and other micronutrients are ongoing or have been completed. Although many of the trials have reported chemopreventive efficacy with various retinoids and β-carotene, especially in oral premalignancy, other trials, such as the Alpha-Tocopherol, Beta-Carotene Cancer Prevention Study and CARET involving β-carotene and two large SPT prevention trials involving 13cRA, have found no preventive effects or even suggestions of promotional effects. These dichotomous results suggest that the patient population and lifestyle habits (e.g., smoking, drinking), tumor site, histopathologic characteristics, choice of agent(s), dose, duration, and timing of intervention may be critical in determining efficacy. The last decade has witnessed a dramatic increase in the understanding of retinoid mechanisms but not of carotenoid mechanisms, which need further study. Nonrandomized phase I and II trials provide useful information regarding toxicity, feasibility, and potential drug activity. For a rigorous evaluation of efficacy, however, randomized phase IIb and III trials are clearly necessary, especially in assessment of intermediate end points, which are very difficult to interpret and may produce spurious findings in uncontrolled trials. The completion of ongoing trials of retinoids (e.g., in combination with other agents such as interferon), carotenoids (alone or in combination with other agents such as vitamins E and C and selenium), and other promising micronutrients (e.g., the SELECT trial of selenium and vitamin E) will increase the clinical and translational understanding of these prevention agents alone and in combinations. In the meantime, retinoids, carotenoids, vitamins E and C, and selenium remain investigational agents for cancer prevention.

REFERENCES

1. Lippman SM, Benner SE, Hong WK. Cancer chemoprevention. *J Clin Oncol* 1994;12:851.
2. Lippman SM, Hong WK. Cancer prevention science and practice. *Cancer Res* 2002;62:5119.
3. Wolbach SB, Howe PR. Tissue changes following deprivation of fat soluble A vitamin. *J Exp Med* 1925;42:753.
4. Ziegler RG, Mayne ST, Swanson CA. Diet and lung cancer. *Cancer Causes Control* 1996;7:157.
5. Dragsted LO, Strube M, Larsen JC. Cancer protective factors in fruits and vegetables: biochemical and biological background. *Pharmacol Toxicol* 1993;72[Suppl]:s116.
6. Anzano MA, Byers SW, Smith JM, et al. Prevention of breast cancer in the rat with 9-cis-retinoic acid as a single agent and in combination with tamoxifen. *Cancer Res* 1994;54:4614.
7. Sporn MB, Roberts AB. What is a retinoid? *CIBA Found Symp* 1985;113:1.
8. Mangelsdorf DJ, Umesono K, Evans RM. The retinoid receptors. In: Sporn MB, Roberts AB, Goodman DS, eds. *The retinoids*, 2nd ed. New York: Raven Press, 1994:319.
9. Chambon P. The retinoid signaling pathway: molecular and genetic analyses. *Semin Cell Biol* 1994;5:115.
10. Demirpence E, Balaguer P, Trousse F, et al. Antiestrogenic effects of all-trans-retinoic acid and 1,25-dihydroxyvitamin D3 in breast cancer cells occur at the estrogen response element level but through different molecular mechanisms. *Cancer Res* 1994;54:1458.
11. Lippman SM, Kessler JF, Meyskens FL Jr. Retinoids as preventive and therapeutic anticancer agents. *Cancer Treat Rep* 1987;71:391, 493.
12. Fanjul A, Dawson MI, Hobbs PD, et al. A new class of retinoids with selective inhibition of AP-1 inhibits proliferation. *Nature* 1994;372:107.
13. Freemantle SJ, Spinella MJ, Dmitrovsky E. Retinoids in cancer therapy and chemoprevention: promise meets resistance. *Oncogene* 2003;22:7305.
14. Krinsky NI. Actions of carotenoids in biological systems. In: Olsen RE, Bier DM, McCormick DB, eds. *Annual review of nutrition*. Palo Alto: Annual Reviews, Inc., 1993;13:561.
15. Wang X-D, Krinsky NI. Identification and quantification of retinoic acid and other metabolites from beta-carotene excentric cleavage in human intestine in vitro and ferret intestine in vivo. *Methods Enzymol* 1997;282:117.
16. Mathews-Roth MM. Carotenoids in erythropoietic protoporphyria and other photosensitivity diseases. *Ann N Y Acad Sci* 1993;691:127.
17. Burton GW, Ingold KU. Beta-carotene: an unusual type of lipid antioxidant. *Science* 1984;224:569.
18. International Agency for Research on Cancer (IARC). *IARC Handbooks of Cancer Prevention: Carotenoids*. North Carolina: Oxford University Press, 1998:2.
19. Watson RR, Rybski J. Immunomodulation by retinoids and carotenoids. In: Chandra RK, ed. *Nutrition and immunology*. New York: Alan R. Liss, 1988:87.
20. Zhang LX, Cooney RV, Bertram JS. Carotenoids up-regulate connexin43 gene expression independent of their provitamin A or antioxidant properties. *Cancer Res* 1992;52:5707.
21. Heber D, Lu Q-Y. Overview of mechanisms of action of lycopene. *Exp Biol Med* 2002;227:920.
22. Ricciarelli R, Zingg JM, Azzi A. Vitamin E: protective role of a Janus molecule. *FASEB J* 2001;15:2314.
23. Combs GF Jr, Gray WP. Chemopreventive agents: selenium. *Pharmacol Ther* 1998;79:179.
24. Vokes EE, Weichselbaum RR, Lippman SM, et al. Head and neck cancer. *N Engl J Med* 1993;328:184.
25. Lippman SM, Hong WK. Molecular markers of the risk of oral cancer. *N Engl J Med* 2001;344:1323.
26. Stich HF, Rosin MP, Vallejera MO. Reduction with vitamin A and beta-carotene administration of proportion of micronucleated buccal mucosal cells in Asian betel nut and tobacco chewers. *Lancet* 1984;1:1204.
27. Stich HF, Hornby AP, Dunn BP. A pilot beta-carotene intervention trial with Inuits using smokeless tobacco. *Int J Cancer* 1985;36:321.
28. Stich HF, Rosin MP, Hornby P, et al. Remission of oral leukoplakias and micronuclei in tobacco/betel quid chewers treated with beta-carotene and with beta-carotene plus vitamin A. *Int J Cancer* 1988;42:195.
29. Mayne ST, Cartmel B, Morse DE. Chemoprevention of oral premalignant lesions. In: Ensley JF, Gutkind JS, Jacobs JR, et al., eds. *Head and neck cancer: emerging perspectives*. New York: Academic Press, 2003:261.
30. Sankaranarayanan R, Mathew B, Varghese C, et al. Chemoprevention of oral leukoplakia with vitamin A and beta carotene: an assessment. *Oral Oncol* 1997;33:231.
31. Zaridze D, Evstifeeva T, Boyle P. Chemoprevention of oral leukoplakia and chronic esophagitis in an area of high incidence of oral and esophageal cancer. *Ann Epidemiol* 1993;3:225.
32. Hong W, Endicott J, Itri LM, et al. 13-cis retinoic acid in the treatment of oral leukoplakia. *N Engl J Med* 1986;315:1501.
33. Lippman SM, Batsakis JG, Toth BB, et al. Comparison of low-dose isotretinoin with beta carotene to prevent oral carcinogenesis. *N Engl J Med* 1993;328:15.
34. Chiesa F, Tradati N, Marazza M, et al. 4HPR in chemoprevention of oral leukoplakia. *J Cell Biochem Suppl* 1993;17F:255.
35. Costa A, Formelli F, Chiesa F, et al. Prospects of chemoprevention of human cancers with the synthetic retinoid fenretinide. *Cancer Res* 1994;54:2032s.
36. Stich HF, Hornby AP, Mathew B, et al. Response of oral leukoplakias to the administration of vitamin A. *Cancer Lett* 1988;40:93.
37. Han J, Lu Y, Sun Z, et al. Evaluation of N-4-(hydroxycarbophenyl) retinamide as a cancer prevention agent and as a cancer chemotherapeutic agent. *In Vivo* 1990;4:153.
38. Hong WK, Lippman SM, Itri LM, et al. Prevention of second primary tumors with 13cRA in squamous-cell carcinoma of the head and neck. *N Engl J Med* 1990;323:795.
39. Benner SE, Pajak TF, Lippman SM, et al. Prevention of second primary tumors with isotretinoin in patients with squamous cell carcinoma of the head and neck: long term follow-up. *J Natl Cancer Inst* 1994;86:140.
40. Khuri F, Lee JJ, Lippman SM, et al. Isotretinoin effects on head and neck cancer recurrence and second primary tumors. *Proc Am Soc Clin Oncol* 2003;22:90(abst).
41. Shin DM, Khuri FR, Murphy B, et al. Combined interferon-α, 13-cis-retinoic acid and α-tocopherol in locally advanced head and neck squamous cell carcinoma: novel bioadjuvant phase II trial. *J Clin Oncol* 2001;19:3010.
42. Bolla M, Lefur R, Ton Van J, et al. Prevention of second primary tumours with etretinate in squamous cell carcinoma of the oral cavity and oropharynx. Results of a multicentric double-blind randomised study. *Eur J Cancer* 1994;30A:767.
43. Mayne ST, Cartmel B, Baum M, et al. Randomized trial of supplemental beta-carotene to prevent second head and neck cancer. *Cancer Res* 2001;61:1457.
44. McLarty JW, Holiday DB, Girard WM, et al. Beta-carotene, vitamin A and lung cancer chemoprevention: results of an intermediate endpoint study. *Am J Clin Nutr* 1995;62:1431S.
45. Misset JL, Mathe G, Santelli G, et al. Regression of bronchial epidermoid metaplasia in heavy smokers with etretinate treatment. *Cancer Detect Prev* 1986;9:167.
46. Arnold AM, Browman GP, Levine MN, et al. The effect of the synthetic retinoid etretinate on sputum cytology: results from a randomized trial. *Br J Cancer* 1992;65:737.
47. Lee JS, Lippman SM, Benner SE, et al. Randomized placebo-controlled trial of isotretinoin in chemoprevention of bronchial squamous metaplasia. *J Clin Oncol* 1994;12:937.
48. Kurie JM, Lee JS, Khuri FR, et al. N(4-hydroxyphenyl) retinamide in the chemoprevention of squamous metaplasia and dysplasia of the bronchial epithelium. *Clin Cancer Res* 2000;6:2973.
49. Kurie JM, Lotan R, Lee JJ, et al. Treatment of former smokers with 9-cis-retinoic acid reverses loss of retinoic acid receptor-beta expression in the bronchial epithelium: results from a randomized placebo-controlled trial. *J Natl Cancer Inst* 2003;95:206.
50. The Alpha-Tocopherol, Beta Carotene Cancer Prevention Study Group. The effect of vitamin E and beta carotene on the incidence of lung cancer and other cancers in male smokers. *N Engl J Med* 1994;330:1029.
51. Heinonen OP, Albanes D, Virtamo J, et al. Prostate cancer and supplementation with alpha-tocopherol and beta-carotene: incidence and mortality in a controlled trial. *J Natl Cancer Inst* 1998;90:440.
52. Omenn GS, Goodman GE, Thornquist MD, et al. Effects of a combination of beta carotene and vitamin A on lung cancer and cardiovascular disease. *N Engl J Med* 1996;334:1150.
53. Hennekens CH, Buring JE, Manson JE, et al. Lack of effect of long-term supplementation with beta carotene on the incidence of malignant neoplasms and cardiovascular disease. *N Engl J Med* 1996;334:1145.
54. Lee IM, Cook NR, Manson JE, et al. Beta-carotene supplementation and incidence of cancer and cardiovascular disease: the Women's Health Study. *J Natl Cancer Inst* 1999;91:2102.
55. Heart Protection Study Collaborative Group. MRC/BHF Heart Protection Study of antioxidant vitamin supplementation in 20,536 high-risk individuals: a randomised placebo-controlled trial. *Lancet* 2002;360:23.
56. Mayne ST. Beta-carotene, carotenoids, and cancer prevention. *Principles and Practice of Oncology Updates* 1998;12:1.
57. Wang XD, Liu C, Bronson RT, et al. Retinoid signaling and activator protein-1 expression in ferrets given beta-carotene supplements and exposed to tobacco smoke. *J Natl Cancer Inst* 1999;91:60.
58. Liu C, Wang XD, Bronson RT, et al. Effects of physiological versus pharmacological beta-carotene supplementation on cell proliferation and histopathological changes in the lungs of cigarette smoke-exposed ferrets. *Carcinogenesis* 2000;21:2245.
59. Salgo MG, Cueto R, Winston GW, et al. Beta carotene and its oxidation products have different effects on microsome mediated binding of benzo[a]pyrene to DNA. *Free Radic Biol Med* 1998;26:162.
60. Pastorino U, Infante M, Maioli M, et al. Adjuvant treatment of stage I lung cancer with high-dose vitamin A. *J Clin Oncol* 1993;11:1216.
61. van Zandwijk N, Dalesio O, Pastorino U, et al. EUROSCAN, a randomized trial of vitamin A and N-acetylcysteine in patients with head and neck cancer or lung cancer. For the European Organization for Research and Treatment of Cancer Head and Neck and Lung Cancer Cooperative Groups. *J Natl Cancer Inst* 2000;92:977.
62. Lippman SM, Lee JJ, Karp DD, et al. Randomized phase III intergroup trial of isotretinoin to prevent second primary tumors in stage I non-small-cell lung cancer. *J Natl Cancer Inst* 2001;93:605.
63. Parthasarathy R, Gilbert B, Mehta K. Aerosol delivery of liposomal all-trans-retinoic acid to the lungs. *Cancer Chemother Pharmacol* 1999;43:277.
64. Massaro GD, Massaro D. Retinoic acid treatment abrogates elastase-induced pulmonary emphysema in rats. *Nat Med* 1997;3:675.
65. Sabichi AL, Modiano MR, Lee JJ, et al. Breast tissue accumulation of retinamides in a randomized short-term study of fenretinide. *Clin Cancer Res* 2003;9:2400.

66. Moon RC, Mehta RG, Rao KV. Retinoids and cancer in experimental animals. In: Sporn MB, Roberts AB, Goodman DS, eds. *The retinoids*, 2nd ed. New York: Raven Press, 1994:573.

67. Veronesi U, De Palo G, Marubini E, et al. Randomized trial of fenretinide to prevent second breast malignancy in women with early breast cancer. *J Natl Cancer Inst* 1999;91:1847.

68. De Palo G, Mariani L, Camerini T, et al. Effect of fenretinide on ovarian carcinoma occurrence. *Gynecol Oncol* 2002;86:24.

69. Lippman M, Brown PH. Tamoxifen prevention of breast cancer: an instance of the fingerpost. *J Natl Cancer Inst* 1999;91:1809.

70. Jain M, Miller AB, To T. Premorbid diet and the prognosis of women with breast cancer. *J Natl Cancer Inst* 1994;86:1390.

71. Pierce JP, Faerber S, Wright FA, et al. Feasibility of a randomized trial of a high-vegetable diet to prevent breast cancer recurrence. *Nutr Cancer* 1997;28:282.

72. Kligman AM, Thorne EG. Topical therapy of actinic keratosis with tretinoin. In: Marks R, ed. *Retinoids in cutaneous malignancy*. Cambridge, MA: Blackwell Scientific, 1991:66.

73. Moriarty M, Dunn J, Darragh A, et al. Etretinate in treatment of actinic keratosis: a double blind crossover study. *Lancet* 1982;1:364.

74. Watson AB. Preventative effect of etretinate therapy on multiple actinic keratoses. *Cancer Detect Prev* 1986;9:161.

75. Kraemer KH, DiGiovanna JJ, Moshell AN, et al. Prevention of skin cancer in xeroderma pigmentosum with the use of oral isotretinoin. *N Engl J Med* 1988;318:1633.

76. Kelly JW, Sabto J, Gurr FW, et al. Retinoids to prevent skin cancer in organ transplant recipients. *Lancet* 1991;338:1407.

77. McNamara IR, Muir J, Galbraith AJ. Acitretin for prophylaxis of cutaneous malignancies after cardiac transplantation. *J Heart Lung Transplant* 2002;21:1201.

78. Bouwes Bavinck JN, Tieben LM, Van Der Woude FJ, et al. Prevention of skin cancer and reduction of keratotic skin lesions during acitretin therapy in renal transplant recipients: a double-blind, placebo-controlled study. *J Clin Oncol* 1995;13:1933.

79. George R, Weightman W, Russ GR, et al. Acitretin for chemoprevention of non-melanoma skin cancers in renal transplant recipients. *Australas J Dermatol* 2002;43:269.

80. de Sevaux RG, Smit JV, de Jong EM, et al. Acitretin treatment of premalignant and malignant skin disorders in renal transplant recipients: clinical effects of a randomized trial comparing two doses of acitretin. *J Am Acad Dermatol* 2003;49:407.

81. Nijsten TE, Stern RS. Oral retinoid use reduces cutaneous squamous cell carcinoma risk in patients with psoriasis treated with psoralen-UVA: a nested cohort study. *J Am Acad Dermatol* 2003;49:644.

82. Tangrea JA, Edwards BK, Taylor PR, et al. Long-term therapy with low-dose isotretinoin for prevention of basal cell carcinoma: a multicenter clinical trial. *J Natl Cancer Inst* 1992;84:328.

83. Levine N, Moon TE, Cartmel B, et al. Trial of retinol and isotretinoin in skin cancer prevention: a randomized, double-blind, controlled trial. Southwest Skin Cancer Prevention Study Group. *Cancer Epidemiol Biomarkers Prev* 1997;6:957.

84. Moon TE, Levine N, Cartmel B, et al. Effect of retinol in preventing squamous cell skin cancer in moderate-risk subjects: a randomized, double-blind, controlled trial. *Cancer Epidemiol Biomarkers Prev* 1997;6:949.

85. Greenberg ER, Baron JA, Stukel TA, et al. and the Skin Cancer Prevention Study Group. A clinical trial of beta carotene to prevent basal cell and squamous cell cancers of the skin. *N Engl J Med* 1990;323:789.

86. Green A, Williams G, Neale R, et al. Daily sunscreen application and beta-carotene supplementation in prevention of basal-cell and squamous-cell carcinomas of the skin: a randomized controlled trial. *Lancet* 1999;354:723.

87. Clark LC, Combs GF Jr, Turnbull BW, et al. Effects of selenium supplementation for cancer prevention in patients with carcinoma of the skin. A randomized controlled trial. Nutritional Prevention of Cancer Study Group. *JAMA* 1996;276:1957.

88. Duffield-Lillico AJ, Slate EH, Reid ME, et al. Selenium supplementation and secondary prevention of nonmelanoma skin cancer in a randomized trial. *J Natl Cancer Inst* 2003;95:1477.

89. Pedersen H, Wolf H, Jensen SK, et al. Administration of a retinoid as prophylaxis of recurrent non-invasive bladder tumors. *Scand J Urol Nephrol* 1984;18:121.

90. Alfthan O, Tarkkanen J, Grohn P, et al. Tigason (etretinate) in prevention of recurrence of superficial bladder tumors. *Eur Urol* 1983;9:6.

91. Studer UE, Biedermann C, Chollet D, et al. Prevention of recurrent superficial bladder tumors by oral etretinate: preliminary results of a randomized, double blind multicenter trial in Switzerland. *J Urol* 1984;131:47.

92. Lamm DL, Riggs DR, Shriver JS, et al. Megadose vitamins in bladder cancer: a double-blind clinical trial. *J Urol* 1994;151:21.

93. Decensi A, Bruno S, Costantini M, et al. Phase IIa study of fenretinide in superficial bladder cancer, using DNA flow cytometry as an intermediate end point. *J Natl Cancer Inst* 1994;86:138.

94. Meyskens FL, Surwit E, Moon TE, et al. Enhancement of regression of cervical intraepithelial neoplasia II (moderate dysplasia) with topically applied all-trans-retinoic acid: a randomized trial. *J Natl Cancer Inst* 1994;86:539.

95. Ruffin IV MT, Bailey JM, Normolle DP, et al. Topical all-trans retinoic acid in high grade squamous intraepithelial lesions. *Proc Am Assoc Cancer Res* 2003;44:1301(abst).

96. Follen M, Atkinson EN, Schottenfeld D, et al. A randomized clinical trial of 4-hydroxyphenylretinamide for high-grade squamous intraepithelial lesions of the cervix. *Clin Cancer Res* 2001;7:3356.

97. Robinson WR, Andersen J, Darragh TM, et al. Isotretinoin for low-grade cervical dysplasia in human immunodeficiency virus-infected women. *Obstet Gynecol* 2002;99:777.

98. Alvarez RD, Conner MG, Weiss H, et al. The efficacy of 9-cis-retinoic acid (aliretinoin) as a chemopreventive agent for cervical dysplasia: results of a randomized double-blind clinical trial. *Cancer Epidemiol Biomarkers Prev* 2003;12:114.

99. DeVet HCW, Knipschild PG, Willebrand D, et al. The effect of beta-carotene on the regression and progression of cervical dysplasia: a clinical experiment. *J Clin Epidemiol* 1991;44:273.

100. Romney SL, Ho GYF, Palan PR, et al. Effects of beta-carotene and other factors on outcome of cervical dysplasia and human papillomavirus infection. *Gynecol Oncol* 1997;65:483.

101. Mackerras D, Irwig L, Simpson JM, et al. Randomized double-blind trial of beta-carotene and vitamin C in women with minor cervical abnormalities. *Br J Cancer* 1999;79:1448.

102. Keefe KA, Schell MJ, Brewer C, et al. A randomized, double blind, phase III trial using oral beta-carotene supplementation for women with high-grade cervical intraepithelial neoplasia. *Cancer Epidemiol Biomarkers Prev* 2001;10:1029.

103. Munoz N, Wahrendorf J, Bang LJ, et al. No effect of riboflavin, retinol and zinc on prevalence of precancerous lesions of esophagus: randomized double-blind intervention study in high-risk population of China. *Lancet* 1985;2:111.

104. Blot WJ, Li J-Y, Taylor PR, et al. Nutrition intervention trials in Linxian, China: supplementation with specific vitamin/mineral combinations, cancer incidence, and disease-specific mortality in the general population. *J Natl Cancer Inst* 1993;85:1483.

105. Li J-Y, Taylor PR, Li B, et al. Nutrition intervention trials in Linxian, China: multiple vitamin/mineral supplementation, cancer incidence, and disease-specific mortality among adults with esophageal dysplasia. *J Natl Cancer Inst* 1993;85:1492.

106. Correa P, Fontham ET, Bravo JC, et al. Chemoprevention of gastric dysplasia: randomized trial of antioxidant supplements and anti-*Helicobacter pylori* therapy. *J Natl Cancer Inst* 2000;92:1881.

107. MacLennan R, Macrae F, Bain C, et al. Randomized trial of intake of fat, fiber and beta carotene to prevent colorectal adenomas. *J Natl Cancer Inst* 1995;87:1760.

108. Kikendall JW, Mobarhan S, Nelson R, et al. Oral beta carotene does not reduce the recurrence of colorectal adenomas. *Am J Gastroenterol* 1991;36:1356(abst).

109. Greenberg ER, Baron JA, Tosteson TD, et al. and the Polyp Prevention Study Group. A clinical trial of antioxidant vitamins to prevent colorectal adenoma. *N Engl J Med* 1994;331:141.

110. Baron JA, Cole BF, Mott L, et al. Neoplastic and antineoplastic effects of beta-carotene on colorectal adenoma recurrence: results of a randomized trial. *J Natl Cancer Inst* 2003;95:717.

111. Fleshner NE, Klotz LH. Diet, androgens, oxidative stress and prostate cancer susceptibility. *Cancer Metastasis Rev* 1998–99;17:325.

112. Hoque A, Albanes D, Lippman SM, et al. Molecular epidemiologic studies within the Selenium and vitamin E Cancer Prevention Trial (SELECT). *Cancer Causes Control* 2001;12:627.

113. Marshall JR. Larry Clark's legacy: randomized controlled, selenium-based prostate cancer chemoprevention trials. *Nutr Cancer* 2001;40:74.

114. Kucuk O, Sarkar FH, Sakr W, et al. Phase II randomized clinical trial of lycopene supplementation before radical prostatectomy. *Cancer Epidemiol Biomarker Prev* 2001;10:861.

115. Bowen P, Chen L, Stacewicz-Sapuntzakis M. Tomato sauce supplementation and prostate cancer: lycopene accumulation and modulation of biomarkers of carcinogenesis. *Exp Biol Med* 2002;227:886.

116. Boileau TW, Liao Z, Kim S, et al. Prostate carcinogenesis in N-methyl-N-nitrosourea (NMU)-testosterone-treated rats fed tomato powder, lycopene, or energy-restricted diets. *J Natl Cancer Inst* 2003;95:1578.

117. Lippman SM, Lee JS, Lotan R, et al. Biomarkers as intermediate end points in chemoprevention trials. *J Natl Cancer Inst* 1990;82:555.

118. Hong WK, Lippman SM, Wolf GT. Recent advances in head and neck cancer—larynx preservation and cancer chemoprevention. *Cancer Res* 1993;53:5113.

119. Xu X-C, Ro JY, Lee JS, et al. Differential expression of nuclear retinoic acid receptors in normal, premalignant, and malignant head and neck tissues. *Cancer Res* 1994;54:3580.

120. Lotan R, Xu X-C, Lippman SM, et al. Suppression of retinoic acid receptor-β in premalignant oral lesions and its upregulation by isotretinoin. *N Engl J Med* 1995;332:1405.

121. Xu XC, Lee JS, Lee JJ, et al. Nuclear retinoid receptor beta in bronchial epithelium of smokers before and during chemoprevention. *J Natl Cancer Inst* 1999;91:1317.

122. Ayoub J, Jean-Francois R, Cormier Y, et al. Placebo-controlled trial of 13-cis-retinoic acid activity on retinoic acid receptor-beta expression in a population at high risk: implications for chemoprevention of lung cancer. *J Clin Oncol* 1999;17:3546.

123. D'Ambrosio SM, Gibson-D'Ambrosio RE, Wani G, et al. Modulation of Ki67, p53 and RARbeta expression in normal, premalignant and malignant human oral epithelial cells by chemopreventive agents. *Anticancer Res* 2001;21:3229.

124. Xu X-C, Zile MH, Lippman SM, et al. Anti-retinoic acid (RA) antibody binding to human premalignant oral lesions, which occurs less frequently than binding to normal tissue, increases after 13-cis-RA treatment in vivo and is related to RA receptor beta expression. *Cancer Res* 1995;55:5507.

125. Houle B, Rochette-Egly C, Bradley WE. Tumor-suppressive effect of the retinoic acid receptor beta in human epidermoid lung cancer cells. *Proc Natl Acad Sci U S A* 1993;90:985.

126. Frangioni JV, Moghal N, Stuart-Tilley A, et al. The DNA binding domain of retinoic acid receptor β is required for ligand-dependent suppression of proliferation: application of general purpose mammalian co-expression vectors. *J Cell Sci* 1994;107:827.

127. Lippman SM, Shin DM, Lee JJ, et al. p53 and retinoid chemoprevention of oral carcinogenesis. *Cancer Res* 1995;55:16.

128. Mao L, Lee JS, Fan YH, et al. Frequent microsatellite alterations at chromosome 9p21 and 3p14 in oral premalignant lesions and its value in cancer risk assessment. *Nat Med* 1996;2:682.

129. Mao L, Lee JS, Kurie JM, et al. Clonal genetic alterations in the lungs of current and former smokers. *J Natl Cancer Inst* 1997;89:857.

130. Izzo JG, Papadimitrakopoulou VA, Liu DD, et al. Cyclin D1 genotype, response to bio-

chemoprevention, and progression rate to upper aerodigestive tract cancer. *J Natl Cancer Inst* 2003;95:198.

131. Lippman SM, Hong WK. Cancer prevention by delay. *Clin Cancer Res* 2002;8:305.

132. Sudbo J, Kildal W, Risberg B, et al. DNA content as a prognostic marker in patients with oral leukoplakia. *N Engl J Med* 2001;344:1270.

133. Lee JJ, Hong WK, Hittelman WN, et al. Predicting cancer development in oral leukoplakia: ten years of translational research. *Clin Cancer Res* 2000;6:1702.

134. Lotan R. Retinoids and apoptosis: implications for cancer chemoprevention and therapy. *J Natl Cancer Inst* 1995;87:1655.

135. Lippman SM, Lee JJ, Sabichi AL. Cancer chemoprevention: progress and promise. *J Natl Cancer Inst* 1998;90:1514.

136. Hong WK, Sporn MB. Recent advances in chemoprevention of cancer. *Science* 1997;278:1073.

137. Giovannucci E. Tomatoes, tomato-based products, lycopene, and cancer: review of the epidemiologic literature. *J Natl Cancer Inst* 1999;91:317.

138. Liu C, Lian F, Smith DE, et al. Lycopene supplementation inhibits lung squamous metaplasia and induces apoptosis via up-regulating insulin-like growth factor-binding protein 3 in cigarette smoke-exposed ferrets. *Cancer Res* 2003;63:3138.

SECTION 5

PETER GREENWALD

Dietary Carcinogens

The human diet is a highly complex and variable mixture of naturally occurring and synthetic compounds, including compounds that have been identified as carcinogens. Although chemicals such as food additives, synthetic pesticides, and environmental contaminants have received considerable research and public attention, these agents comprise less than 1% of all carcinogens found in food.[1] The majority of dietary carcinogens are "natural pesticides," toxins produced by plants for protection; mycotoxins produced by molds in foods; or substances produced during food preparation. This section discusses dietary carcinogens in each group, reviewing common food sources, mechanisms of action, human exposure, and degree of human risk. It also provides a brief overview of issues concerning synthetic carcinogens in the diet.

In many cases, current knowledge is incomplete and does not allow reliable estimates of risk. For many potentially carcinogenic constituents of foods, concentration data do not exist. In addition, determination of human exposure levels is difficult and sometimes inconclusive. Dietary assessment tools are subjective and often biased. The food levels of some substances can vary widely, and exposure to mixtures of substances at low doses might be more important than exposure to single agents.

Determination of carcinogenic potential and potency is based on information obtained from epidemiologic observations, animal models, and *in vitro* systems. The Carcinogenic Potency Database (http://potency.berkeley.edu) describes chemicals that have been tested for mutagenicity, carcinogenicity, carcinogenic potency (median toxic dose), and target sites in a range of animal carcinogenicity studies and experiments. Approximately 50% of all chemicals tested thus far have been shown to be carcinogenic in animals. As extensive as this database is, however, most food constituents have not undergone carcinogenic or toxicity testing. Furthermore, extrapolation of the effects of the near-toxic doses used in animals to risk to humans consuming low concentrations of the same dietary constituents is difficult, particularly without a more complete understanding of the mechanisms of action of these compounds and of the level of human exposure.

Food mutagens may act directly through the formation of adducts with cellular macromolecules such as DNA.[2] Dietary constituents also may act indirectly, causing cellular or genetic

damage or interfering with programmed cell death (apoptosis) by modulating epigenetic factors such as DNA methylation patterns.[2] Mutagenic compounds can cause DNA damage at low doses, and the carcinogenic risk associated with mutagens in animal testing may be relevant to assessing risk in humans.

To increase the reliability of exposure estimates, biomarkers are being developed to indicate internal dose, putative early response, and susceptibility. For example, DNA-carcinogen adducts have been used as measurable end points in laboratory studies and, to a more limited extent, in humans to assess dietary carcinogen exposure, carcinogen metabolism, mutagenesis, and tumorigenesis.[2] In addition, genetic and acquired susceptibility traits have been shown to affect carcinogen metabolism, DNA damage, and DNA repair.[2] More than a dozen polymorphic genes or phenotypes related to the metabolism of dietary carcinogens are possible actors in the complex process of carcinogenesis at many sites.[3] Perhaps the most appropriate means of evaluating risk is through a panel of biomarkers.[2] No single biomarker has been validated for this purpose, however, and the use of these markers to indicate target organ risk has yet to be determined. Furthermore, most biomarkers of exposure, including carcinogen-DNA adducts and carcinogen metabolites, are studied using surrogate tissues such as blood and urine rather than samples from target organs.

NATURALLY OCCURRING DIETARY CARCINOGENS

Most naturally occurring dietary carcinogens are either natural pesticides (produced by plants for protection against fungi, insects, and animal predators) or mycotoxins (secondary metabolites produced by molds in foods). Table 20.5-1 lists some of the most common substances in both categories.

NATURAL PESTICIDES

Animal studies have provided evidence for the carcinogenicity of a large number of individual plant constituents when fed at high doses. However, no firm conclusions can be drawn about the overall effects of most of these substances on human health. Plant foods contain thousands of phytochemicals representing various chemical classes and exhibiting diverse molecular structures, and only a small fraction of potential carcinogens produced by plant foods have been tested systematically.[1] For example, cabbage contains approximately 50 naturally occurring pesticides, including glucosinolates, indoles, isothiocyanates, cyanides, alcohols, ketols,

TABLE 20.5-1. Food Sources of Naturally Occurring Dietary Carcinogens

NATURAL PESTICIDES

Caffeic acid	Apples, pears, plums, cherries, carrots, celery, lettuce, potatoes, endive, grapes, eggplant, thyme, basil, anise, sage, dill, caraway, rosemary, tarragon, coffee beans
Allyl isothiocyanate	Cabbage, cauliflower, Brussels sprouts, mustard, horseradish
Saffrole	Nutmeg, mace, pepper, cinnamon, natural root beer
Estragole	Basil, fennel, tarragon
Carvacrol	Marjoram
Furocoumarins	Lime, citrus oils, carrots, celery, parsley, parsnips
Hydrazines	Mushrooms
Pyrrolizidine	Herbal teas (comfrey)
MYCOTOXINS	
Aflatoxins	Corn, peanuts, seed nuts, peanut butter
Ochratoxin A	Grains, green coffee beans
T-2 toxin	Barley, maize, safflower seeds, cereals
Zearalenone	Feed grains, soybean, maize, wheat
Fumonisins	Corn
Deoxynivalenol	Wheat, maize
Nivalenol	Wheat, maize, barley

phenols, and tannins; however, only a few have been tested for carcinogenicity.[1]

The difficulties described earlier in assessing human risk are well illustrated by naturally occurring pesticides. Caffeic acid, a common plant polyphenol that has been shown to cause cancer in animal studies, is a good example, although the relevance of animal studies to humans is uncertain. In addition, *in vitro*, caffeic acid may act either as a pro-oxidant or antioxidant, and it has been observed to be both protective and enhancing when administered orally in combination with known carcinogens. Studies show that dietary or oral exposure to caffeic acid phenethyl ester inhibits the development of chemically induced colon tumors, aberrant crypt foci, and metastatic lung disease derived from colon carcinoma cells.[4] Caffeic acid phenethyl ester may act through both p53-mediated and p53-independent pathways.

Another dietary constituent that appears to possess both cancer-preventive and cancer-promoting activities is capsaicin, found in peppers. Epidemiologic evidence suggests an increased risk for stomach and liver cancers in populations consuming large amounts of capsaicin and in countries where people have high intakes of this spice. Capsaicin alters the metabolism of chemical carcinogens, and at high doses it may promote tumorigenesis. However, *in vitro* experiments also show that capsaicinoids inhibit cell growth and induce apoptosis in various transformed cell lines. Despite many challenges, researchers can make inferences about human risk from natural pesticides with additional information on factors such as exposure levels, concentration levels, mechanisms of action, and human clinical experience. For example, studies of coumarin—a substance found in many foods, including cinnamon, that has been found to be carcinogenic in rats and mice—have concluded that it poses no health risk to humans.

From a public health perspective, dietary exposure to natural pesticides can generally be controlled by selecting genetic strains of plants that produce lower pesticide concentrations and by reducing plant stress during the growing season. The occurrence of certain natural pesticides that are carcinogenic in animals might be minimized through crop breeding or engineering of crops if research indicates they could be hazardous to humans.

MYCOTOXINS

Mycotoxins are structurally diverse, toxic, fungal metabolites that are common contaminants of ingredients in animal feed and human food. To date, more than 300 mycotoxins have been identified.[5] The mycotoxins listed in Table 20.5-1 are among those shown to have carcinogenic potential in animals. However, only aflatoxin B_1 (AFB_1) and naturally occurring mixtures of aflatoxins are known to be genotoxic and carcinogenic in humans.[5] The weight of evidence suggests that another mycotoxin, fumonisin B1, is possibly carcinogenic to humans.[6]

AFLATOXINS

AFB_1 is a potent carcinogen in many species of animals, including rodents, nonhuman primates, and fish.[5] Epidemiologic studies show a direct association between AFB_1 intake in Africa and China and the risk for primary liver and lung cancer in humans.[7] AFB_1-associated risk for hepatocellular carcinoma is synergistic with both viral hepatitis B and alcohol consumption in humans. In some regions of China, the combination of hepatitis B and aflatoxin increased the risk of liver cancer by 60-fold compared to the risk in unexposed populations. High levels of AFB_1, produced by the *Aspergillus* species, are found in regions of Africa, Southeast Asia, and southern China, where the foods contaminated with aflatoxins are dietary staples for humans and animals.

Aflatoxins have been extensively characterized with respect to chemistry, biology, and toxicology. Like most other mycotoxins, with the exception of fumonisins, aflatoxins are genotoxic agents, and substantial research has been conducted on the genetic damage created by AFB_1 in liver and lung tumors. A key biomarker, the predominant AFB_1-DNA adduct (AFB_1-7-Gua), has been identified and correlated with the incidence of hepatic tumor in trout and rats.[8] Formation of the AFB_1-DNA adduct requires metabolic activation of AFB_1 to its carcinogenic form, the 8,9-epoxide. A prospective study of more than 18,000 men in Shanghai, China, demonstrated a significant increase in risk (relative risk, 3.4) for liver cancer in individuals in whom aflatoxin-DNA adducts were detected in urine.[7]

Chemopreventive agents may modulate the expression of enzymes that activate aflatoxins and subsequent DNA-adduct formation. Induction of both phase 1 and phase 2 enzymes may contribute to protection against aflatoxin exposure. Chemopreventive agents also may be effective in ameliorating the impact of coinfection with the hepatitis B virus, which may, in turn, increase aflatoxin metabolism. For example, liver injury in hepatitis B virus–transgenic mice is associated with increased expression of cytochrome P-450 enzymes, whereas in humans infected with hepatitis B virus, hepatic glutathione S-transferase activity is reduced.[5]

Striking species differences exist in the oncogenic mutations involving AFB_1. For example, a considerable amount of evidence shows that dietary AFB_1 exposure can produce codon

249 (AGG to AGT) p53 tumor suppressor gene mutations during human liver carcinogenesis.[9] A study of residents in Fusui, China, and neighboring areas of the Guangxi region showed that 57% of hepatocellular carcinoma cases (20 of 35 cases) had a G to T transversion at codon 249 of the p53 tumor suppressor gene, comparable to the rate in other parts of the world with high levels of aflatoxin contamination.[10] Although these mutations are associated with exposure, their significance in terms of mechanistic involvement in tumorigenesis needs further elucidation.

Elimination of exposure to aflatoxins is not possible given the ubiquitous nature of the molds that produce them. Primary prevention methods include development of aflatoxin-resistant plants, improved processing and handling of crops before storage, the construction of better storage facilities for grains to reduce humidity, and the establishment of worldwide regulatory and testing programs.[11] Implementation of hepatitis B vaccination programs globally, or the use of chemopreventive agents such as oltipraz in selected areas, could markedly lower the risk of liver cancer, particularly in regions where aflatoxin food contamination and consumption of contaminated food are high.[11]

FUMONISINS

Fumonisins are naturally occurring toxins produced by the molds *Fusarium moniliforme, Fusarium proliferatum,* and other *Fusarium* species that are common natural contaminants of corn. Fumonisin B1, the most toxic of this group of compounds, is carcinogenic in rats and mice at high doses, although its target sites vary by species and gender.[12] Epidemiologic evidence of an association between cancer risk and exposure in humans is inconclusive, but some data from Africa and China suggest a link between dietary fumonisin exposure and esophageal cancer in regions where high amounts of contaminated corn are consumed. Although evidence in humans for the carcinogenicity of fumonisins is insufficient, the majority of the evidence from animal studies suggests that fumonisin B1 may be carcinogenic to humans.[6]

Fumonisin B1 is inactive in bacterial mutation assays, but it induces DNA damage, such as micronuclei damage, in both *in vitro* and *in vivo* experiments.[6] Research suggests that the addition of antioxidants reduces the DNA-damaging effects of fumonisin B1 and that fumonisin toxicity also may be mediated through the inhibition of ceramide synthase, a key enzyme in the sphingolipid biosynthetic pathway.[12] Further evidence demonstrates that fumonisin-related hepatotoxicity is ameliorated in mice lacking either the TNFR1 or TNFR2 tumor necrosis factor-α receptors. The disruption of various aspects of lipid metabolism, membrane structure, and signal transduction pathways—pathways mediated by lipid second messengers—appears to be an important aspect of the various proposed mechanisms of action of fumonisin B1, including its mechanism of carcinogenicity. Fumonisins in urine, and altered sphingolipid metabolism (sphinganine/sphingosine ratio) in urine and blood, are being investigated as possible cancer markers.[12]

The growing body of evidence on fumonisins and other mycotoxins as possible human carcinogens indicates that additional investigation of these agents is needed to clearly define their risk to public health.

PRODUCTS OF FOOD PREPARATION AND PROCESSING

Food preparation and preservation are major sources of dietary carcinogens, including heterocyclic aromatic amines (HAAs), formed during frying, broiling, and grilling of high-protein foods (more prevalent in well-done meats); polycyclic aromatic hydrocarbons (PAHs), formed during broiling and smoking of food; acrylamide, formed during high-temperature cooking of starchy foods such as potato chips and French fries; and N-nitroso compounds (NOCs), formed in smoked, salted, and pickled foods cured with nitrate or nitrite. NOCs also form endogenously at sites such as the stomach from nitrites and amines in the diet. Table 20.5-2 lists common carcinogens produced during food preparation and related food sources and cooking methods. Although human risk from these compounds is not always well understood, it may be prudent to minimize exposure by modifying meat cooking methods and eating fewer fried starchy foods and fewer foods containing NOCs.

HETEROCYCLIC AROMATIC AMINES

HAAs are potent mutagens and animal carcinogens, causing cancers of the liver, colon, mammary gland, skin, Zymbal gland, large intestine, prostate, lymphoid tissues, oral cavity, lung, and clitoral gland in rodent models.[13] More than 20 HAAs have been isolated, of which four are possibly carcinogenic in humans: 2-amino-3-methylimidazo[4,5-*f*]quinoline (IQ); 2-amino-3,4-dimethylimidazo[4,5-*f*]quinoline (MeIQ); 2-amino-3,8-dimethylimidazo[4,5-*f*]quinoxaline (8-MeIQx); and 2-amino-1-methyl-6-phenylimidazo[4,5-*b*]pyridine (PhIP).[13]

Estimation of the human cancer risk of HAAs is confounded in part by a lack of information on the effect of typical cooking methods and degree of doneness on concentrations of HAAs, as well as on variations in exposure.[13] Assessment of human dietary exposure to HAAs is complicated further by difficulties in recovering and accurately determining the very small amounts of HAAs present in the diet (usually at nanogram per gram levels) and the need for several isolation steps to quantify individual HAAs.[14] These challenges are exemplified by the results of a review of epidemiologic studies which indicates that daily intake of HAAs varies considerably, ranging from 0 to approximately 15 μg/person/d.[14]

Obtaining additional information on meat cooking methods, portion size, and intake frequency improves estimates,[14] and a database for HAAs has been developed. The database is now being used in conjunction with a validated meat cooking food frequency questionnaire in controlled clinical studies and in assessment of epidemiologic evidence.[15] Linking the food frequency questionnaire information to the HAA database showed that the increased risk for colorectal adenomas in one case-control study was due to consumption of red meat, cooked until well or very well done, or cooked by high-temperature methods such as grilling. Increased risk was further associated with high intake of MeIQx and possibly PhIP.[15] Studies suggest that components of the diet, including fat, dairy products, and certain flavors extracted from thyme, marjoram, and rosemary, act as promotional factors in HAA-related carcinogenesis in animal studies, but these data remain difficult to interpret.

Adduct formation is also used to estimate HAA exposure and related cancer risk. Studies of animal tumors relate amino-

TABLE 20.5-2. Dietary Carcinogens Produced during Food Preparation: Sources and Cooking Methods

URETHANE	All fermented and yeast-leavened foods: wines, yogurt, soy sauce, sake, ale, beer, bread
HETEROCYCLIC AROMATIC AMINES	
2-amino-3-methylimidazo[4,5 *f*]quinoline (IQ)	Broiled beef, salmon; fried ground beef, fish
2-amino-3,8-dimethylimidazo[4,5-*f*]quinoxaline (8-MeIQx)	Barbecued chicken, fish, pork; broiled beef, chicken, mutton, pork; fried bacon, ground beef, fish
2-amino-3,4-dimethylimidazo[4,5-*f*]quinoline (MeIQ)	Barbecued chicken, pork; broiled chicken, mutton; fried bacon, fish; smoked mackerel
2-amino-1-methyl-6-phenylimidazo[4,5-*b*]pyridine (PhIP)	Barbecued pork, fish; broiled beef, chicken, mutton, fish; fried bacon, fish, ground beef, ground pork
2-amino-9H-pyrido[2,3-*b*]indole	Barbecued fish; broiled beef, chicken, mutton
POLYCYCLIC AROMATIC HYDROCARBONS	
Pyrene	Charcoal-broiled/grilled steak, beef patties, chicken, frankfurters, pork; bacon; liquid smoke; smoked fish
Benz[a]anthracene	Charcoal-broiled/grilled steak, beef patties, chicken, frankfurters, pork; liquid smoke; smoked fish
Chrysene	Charcoal-broiled/grilled steak, beef patties, chicken, frankfurters, pork; bacon; smoked fish
Benzo[a]pyrene	Charcoal-broiled/grilled steak, beef patties, chicken, frankfurters, pork; liquid smoke; smoked fish
ACRYLAMIDE	Starchy foods cooked at very high temperatures: potato chips, French fries
N-NITROSO COMPOUNDS	
N-Nitrosomethylamine	Cured meats; fried bacon; millet flour, grain products; dairy, cheese products; pickled/fermented vegetables; beer; whiskey
N-Nitrosoethylamine	Cured meats, salami; millet flour; grain products
N-Nitrosobutylamine	Cured meats; smoked chicken; dried fish
N-Nitrosopyrrolidine	Cured meats; fried bacon; broiled squid; pickled vegetables; mixed spices; dried chilies
N-Nitrosopiperidine	Cured meats; fried bacon; peppered salami; pepper; mixed spices; pickled vegetables

midazoazaarenes (AIA)-DNA adduct–induced mutagenic events with the mutations found in critical genes associated with oncogenesis, and AIA-DNA adduct levels in target tissues are strongly related to tumor incidence.[13] Although HAA-DNA adducts can be useful biomarkers, their detection in humans has proved difficult.

Metabolic activation is necessary for the formation of HAA-DNA adducts in animals and humans and is critical to the mutagenicity and carcinogenicity of HAAs.[13] The metabolic activation of HAAs varies among species, but activation in humans occurs via N-oxidation to form N-hydroxy metabolites, followed by phase II esterification (O-acetylation) to form N-acetoxy arylamines that bind to DNA.[13] These steps are catalyzed by hepatic cytochrome P-4501A2 (CYP1A2), and N-acetyltransferase-1 or N-acetyltransferase-2, respectively.

There is wide interindividual variation in the capacity of human tissues to activate HAAs, and polymorphisms of related enzymes in humans have been investigated for their potential relationship to cancer risk. For example, a polymorphism in the GSTA1 proximal promoter, the variant GSTA1*B allele, lowers expression of GSTA1 and thereby reduces its detoxifying capability.[16] A case-control study found the GSTA1*B/*B genotype to be associated with increased risk of colorectal cancer, with the greatest risk in persons consuming well-done meat.[16] In some but not all studies, individuals who are both rapid N-oxidizers and rapid acetylators have a greater risk of colon cancer than those who are both slow N-oxidizers and slow acetylators.

POLYCYCLIC AROMATIC HYDROCARBONS

PAHs, several of which have been found to be carcinogenic in animal studies, are ubiquitous in the environment, as a by-product of cooking meats over an open flame and as a contaminant in animal and human foods. Charcoal broiling of beef or chicken releases three to five times more PAHs than grilling. Despite widespread distribution of PAHs, available exposure and carcinogenicity data are insufficient to allow a reliable estimate of dietary PAH risk in humans. Fat dripping onto coals, and the subsequent deposition of PAHs that rise with smoke onto the meat being grilled, contribute significantly to PAH exposure. Benzo[a]pyrene, the most carcinogenic PAH, has been reported at levels of up to 50 μg/kg in charcoal-broiled steaks and ground beef, five times greater than levels in some less fatty pork cuts and chicken.

Several studies demonstrate a consistent association between recent consumption of charcoal-broiled foods and increased PAH-DNA adduct concentrations in peripheral white blood cells and excretion of 1-hydroxypyrene in urine. One review suggests a correlation between PAH-DNA adducts and *ras* oncogene mutations.[17] Some evidence suggests that an antioxidant response element plays a significant role in PAH carcinogenesis. There may be genetic factors, such as the polymorphic hGSTP1 gene, that are influenced by diet and exposure to tobacco smoke, and that account for the carcinogenic properties of PAHs.

ACRYLAMIDE

In 2002, studies in Sweden and the United States reported elevated acrylamide levels in cooked and heat-processed carbohydrate-rich foods.[18] The discovery of acrylamide in foods is of concern because it is classified as a probable human carcinogen based on animal studies and *in vitro* testing. Acrylamide also has adverse effects on the nervous system when administered orally or inhaled (e.g., through cigarette smoke). When administered by gavage or intraperitoneal injection, acrylamide increases the incidence and multiplicity of mouse lung adenomas.[19]

Few studies have examined dietary exposure in humans, and no clear association exists between dietary acrylamide and cancer risk.[18] No excess risk or trend toward cancer is seen among persons consuming foods containing moderate (30 to 299 μg/kg) or high (300 to 1200 μg/kg) levels of acrylamide.[18]

One study estimates that U.S. adults consume 0.5 to 0.7 µg acrylamide per kilogram of body weight per day; for children and teens, average exposure is estimated to be 0.60 to 1.62 µg acrylamide per kilogram of body weight per day.[20] However, adults whose diets favor the most heavily tainted foods may consume as much as 6.2 µg/kg daily, with their children consuming up to 1.8 µg/kg. These levels are still significantly lower than the U.S. Food and Drug Administration's acceptable daily intake recommendation of 12 µg per person. Other studies found the lifetime cancer risk for men related to mean daily intake of acrylamide to be 0.6×10^{-3}, which suggests that 6 out of 10,000 males may develop cancer from dietary acrylamide.[18]

Additional studies are under way to determine whether a link exists between dietary acrylamide and cancer risk in humans. Until more is known, the U.S. Food and Drug Administration is not recommending that consumers change their diet or cooking methods. Consumers are advised to eat a balanced diet, choosing a variety of foods that are low in fat and rich in high-fiber grains, fruits, and vegetables.

N-NITROSO COMPOUNDS

Individuals consume NOCs by eating smoked, salted, and pickled foods cured with nitrate or nitrite. NOCs administered orally to animals, including nonhuman primates, consistently elicit carcinogenic responses. These compounds also may be a significant risk factor for human cancers of the stomach, esophagus, colon and rectum, nasopharynx, urinary bladder, and liver.[21] Although a review of epidemiologic evidence found the available data on dietary exposures and cancer risk inconclusive, an association between NOCs and human cancer cannot be ruled out. The author postulated that inadequate available data may be obscuring a small to moderate carcinogenic effect of NOCs.[21]

Many NOCs undergo α-hydroxylation by CYP2E1 to form DNA adducts. In one study, individuals with a polymorphism (a 96-bp 5' insert) in CYP2E1 had a 60% greater risk for colorectal cancer than persons without this insert.[22] Rectal cancer risk among CYP2E1 insert carriers was twofold to threefold higher among those with the highest intake of red meat or processed meat, respectively, compared with noncarriers.

The formation of endogenous NOCs by bacterial decarboxylation of amino acids in the large gut is exacerbated by consumption of red meat, as evidenced by dose-dependent increases in total NOCs in the feces. In contrast, consumption of the same amount of white meat has no effect on fecal excretion of nitrogenous compounds.[23] Naturally occurring compounds in foods, such as ascorbic acid, tocopherols, retinoids, phenolic compounds, and sulfhydryl compounds, as well as tea, orange peel, and certain fruits and vegetables may inhibit endogenous formation of NOCs. This may in part explain the generally protective effect of vegetables and fruits consistently observed in epidemiologic studies.[24]

SYNTHETIC CARCINOGENS IN THE DIET

Animals and humans also are exposed to a variety of synthetic chemicals in their foods from food additives. Direct (intentional) synthetic additives include antioxidants, colorants, flavor ingredients, artificial sweeteners, solvents, and humectants.

Regulation of synthetic or natural chemicals intentionally added to food has led to extensive data on exposure. Indirect (unintentional) synthetic additives include pesticides, solvents, and packaging-derived chemicals that enter the food supply during production, processing, packaging, and storage from a variety of sources. Very little data exist on exposure to these chemicals.

Pesticides are of most concern to the public and regulatory agencies compared with other indirect food additives. Most, if not all, pesticides have possible human toxicity, including carcinogenic potential. In general, levels encountered are below allowable tolerances, although actual estimates of risk are problematic.[25] Studies of one widely used fungicide, *ortho*-phenylphenol, considered by the Environmental Protection Agency to be a probable human carcinogen, suggests that *ortho*-phenylphenol in the diet of male rats causes hyperplastic lesions in the bladder and tumors of the urinary bladder and renal pelvis. Packaging materials, including vinyl chloride, and several phthalate esters used as plasticizers have gained attention from researchers as yet other unintentional additions to packaged foods with potential risks to human health.

The metabolic pathways involved in the biotransformation of both synthetic and naturally occurring chemicals are similar, and evidence to date also suggests that the processes of carcinogenesis are similar, if not identical. Not surprisingly, the difficulties that complicate risk prediction for naturally occurring dietary carcinogens also apply to the synthetic carcinogens.[25]

FUTURE RESEARCH NEEDS

Human epidemiologic data demonstrate that diet contributes to an appreciable portion of cancer. However, continuing research is needed for better identification of the risk to humans from specific carcinogens in the diet. Although we have begun to understand some of the key factors affecting risk estimation for some of the phytochemicals in plant foods, both naturally occurring and synthetic chemicals are numerous and diverse. A multidisciplinary research paradigm that integrates nutrition, molecular biology, epidemiology, genetics, and chemistry will provide a clearer picture in identifying and characterizing gene-nutrient interactions that contribute to cancer risk and in identifying groups of individuals who may benefit from targeted interventions to counter the effects of dietary carcinogens. Such investigations will assist in uncovering the molecular targets responsible for regulating the complex physiologic events that maintain homeostasis, induce or inhibit cellular proliferation and differentiation, induce apoptosis, and ultimately trigger the carcinogenic process. The identification of polymorphisms that determine an individual's response to specific dietary cancer-protective factors, such as folate, or cancer-inducing dietary carcinogens, such as heterocyclic amines that arise from high-temperature grilling of meats, will provide key insights into vulnerable subpopulations.

Such an approach holds promise for greatly advancing the understanding of the complex interactions between dietary constituents and individual genetic variations as they influence the many pathways that contribute to the carcinogenic process.

Several emerging technologies show promise in expanding the knowledge and understanding of the substances discussed in this chapter and their impact on human cancer risk. High-throughput screening methods for mechanistic and toxicologic end points are under development for use in experimental systems and epidemiologic studies. These methods include large-scale genomic screens based on microarrays and proteomic screens that use two-dimensional gel electrophoresis with mass-spectrometry or surface-enhanced laser desorption/ionization. Such methods will allow investigators to identify a large number of cellular or genetic effects in multiple subjects and experiments.

REFERENCES

1. Ames BN, Gold LS. Dietary carcinogens, environmental pollution, and cancer: some misconceptions. *Med Oncol Tumor Pharmacother* 1990;7:69.
2. Goldman R, Shields PG. Food mutagens. *J Nutr* 2003;133[Suppl 3]:965S.
3. Sinha R, Caporaso N. Diet, genetic susceptibility and human cancer etiology. *J Nutr* 1999;129:556S.
4. Nagaoka T, Banskota AH, Tezuka Y, et al. Selective antiproliferative activity of caffeic acid phenethyl ester analogues on highly liver-metastatic murine colon 26-L5 carcinoma cell line. *Bioorg Med Chem* 2002;10:3351.
5. International Agency for Cancer Research. *Aflatoxins.* IARC Monograph 2002a;82:171. World Wide Web URL: http://www-cie.iarc.fr/htdocs/monographs/vol82/82-04.html, 2004.
6. International Agency for Cancer Research. *Fumonisin B1.* IARC Monograph 2002b;82:301. World Wide Web URL: http://www-cie.iarc.fr/htdocs/monographs/vol82/82-05.html, 2004.
7. Wang J-S, Huang T, Su J, et al. Hepatocellular carcinoma and aflatoxin exposure in Zhuqing Village, Fusui County, People's Republic of China. *Cancer Epidemiol Biomarkers Prev* 2001;10:143.
8. Wang J-S, Groopman JD. DNA damage by mycotoxins. *Mutation Res* 1999;424:167.
9. Hussain SP, Harris CC. Molecular epidemiology of human cancer. *Toxicol Lett* 1998; 102:219.
10. Deng Z, Ma Y. Aflatoxin sufferer and p53 gene mutation in hepatocellular carcinoma. *World J Gastroenterol* 1998;4:28.
11. Hall AJ, Wild CP. Liver cancer in low and middle income countries. *BMJ* 2003;326:994.
12. Voss KA, Howard PC, Riley RT, et al. Carcinogenicity and mechanism of action of fumonisin B1: a mycotoxin produced by *Fusarium moniliforme (F. verticillioides). Cancer Detect Prev* 2002;26:1.
13. Turesky RJ. Heterocyclic aromatic amine metabolism, DNA adduct formation, mutagenesis, and carcinogenesis. *Drug Metab Rev* 2002;34:625.
14. Skog K. Problems associated with the determination of heterocyclic amines in cooked foods and human exposure. *Food Chem Toxicol* 2002;40:1197.
15. Sinha R. An epidemiologic approach to studying heterocyclic amines. *Mutat Res* 2002;506:197.
16. Sweeney C, Coles BF, Nowell S, et al. Novel markers of susceptibility to carcinogens in diet: associations with colorectal cancer. *Toxicology* 2002;181:83.
17. Ross JA, Nesnow S. Polycyclic aromatic hydrocarbons: correlations between DNA adducts and *ras* oncogene mutations. *Mutat Res* 1999;424:155.
18. Dybing E, Sanner T. Risk assessment of acrylamide in foods. *Toxicol Sci* 2003;75:7.
19. Paulsson B, Kotova N, Grawe J, et al. Induction of micronuclei in mouse and rat by glycidamide, genotoxic metabolite of acrylamide. *Mutat Res* 2003;535:15.
20. Storey ML, Forshee RA. Acrylamide in the food supply. Letter dated October 30, 2002, to the FDA regarding 67 FR 57827 (September 12, 2002), Docket No. 02N-0393, 2002.
21. Eichholzer M, Gutzwiller F. Dietary nitrates, nitrites, and n-nitroso compounds and cancer risk: a review of the epidemiologic evidence. *Nutr Rev* 1998;56:95.
22. Le Marchand L, Donlon T, Seifried A, et al. Red meat intake, CYP2E1 genetic polymorphisms, and colorectal cancer risk. *Cancer Epidemiol Biomarkers Prev* 2002;11:1019.
23. Bingham SA, Hughes R, Cross AJ. Effect of white versus red meat on endogenous N-nitrosation in the human colon and further evidence of a dose response. *J Nutr* 2002; 132[Suppl 11]:3522S.
24. World Cancer Research Fund. *Food, nutrition and the prevention of cancer: a global perspective.* Washington, DC: American Institute for Cancer Research, 1997.
25. Committee on Comparative Toxicity of Naturally Occurring Carcinogens, Board of Environmental Studies and Toxicology, Commission of Life Sciences, National Research Council. *Carcinogens and anticarcinogens in the human diet.* Washington, DC: National Academy Press, 1996.

SECTION **6**

MICHAEL J. THUN
S. JANE HENLEY

Cyclooxygenase Inhibitors

Nonsteroidal antiinflammatory drugs (NSAIDs), especially highly selective cyclooxygenase-2 (COX-2) inhibitors, show promise as anticancer agents.[1] NSAIDs inhibit the development of a variety of cancers in animal models, restore apoptosis in cells that have lost function of the adenomatous polyposis coli (APC) gene,[1,2] and inhibit angiogenesis in cell culture and animal models.[3,4] Numerous epidemiologic studies report lower risk of colorectal cancer and, to some extent, of other cancers, in persons who take NSAIDs long term compared with nonusers (reviewed in refs. 1, 5). Randomized trials demonstrate that aspirin use inhibits the development of colorectal adenomas in patients with a previous adenoma or cancer and that sulindac and celecoxib inhibit polyp growth in patients with familial adenomatous polyposis (FAP) or previous adenoma. Despite these encouraging results, questions about the safety of long-term NSAID prophylaxis and the efficacy of NSAIDs against cancers other than colon and rectal cancer currently limit their clinical application to FAP patients. This chapter summarizes the literature regarding NSAIDs and cancer, and identifies barriers that must be overcome before there can be broader clinical application of NSAIDs for the prevention or treatment of cancer.

PHARMACOLOGY OF NONSTEROIDAL ANTIINFLAMMATORY DRUGS

The characteristic that defines NSAIDs as a class is their ability to inhibit COX activity of the enzyme prostaglandin H-synthase[6] (Fig. 20.6-1). COX inhibition prevents the formation of prostaglandin H, the first committed step in the metabolism of arachidonic acid into a complex cascade of signaling lipids termed *prostanoids*. Prostaglandins and other prostanoids are released from cells immediately after synthesis. They coordinate signaling to both the cell of origin (autocrine) and neighboring cells (paracrine) by binding with transmembrane G protein–coupled receptors.[7] Conventional wisdom holds that all of the established pharmacologic effects of NSAIDs result from modulation of the production of prostanoids. However, there is continuing controversy about whether the effects of NSAIDs can be explained entirely by COX inhibition or also involve non-COX pathways.

Two distinct isoforms of prostaglandin H-synthase have been recognized since 1991, conventionally designated COX-1 and COX-2.[8,9] COX-1 is expressed constitutively in many tissues of the body and plays a central role in platelet aggregation and gastric cytoprotection.[10,11] COX-2 is induced during inflammation, wound healing, and neoplasia, although it is expressed constitutively in the human kidney, brain, and spinal cord. NSAIDs vary in their ability to inhibit COX-1 or COX-2 at different concentrations and in different tissues. Aspirin at dosages of 50 to 100 mg daily is a relatively selective inhibitor of COX-1. Aspirin is the only NSAID that covalently and irreversibly inactivates COX-1 in

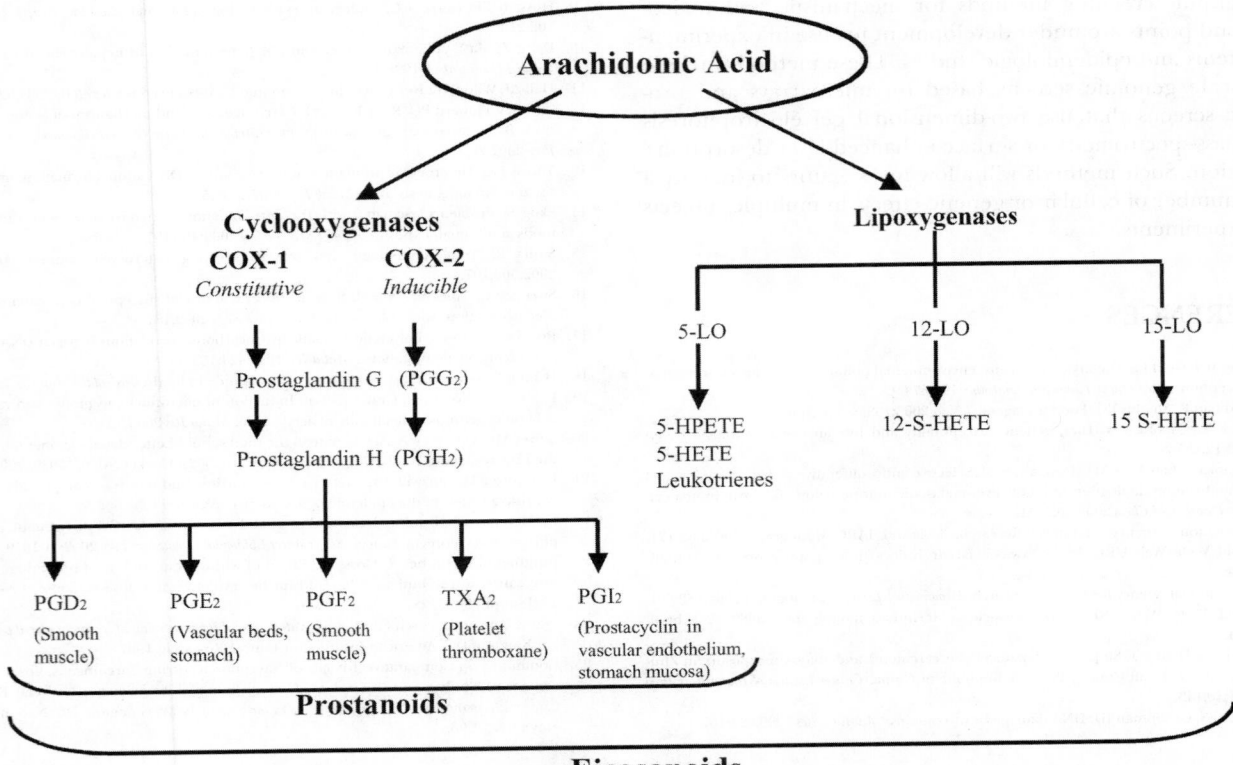

FIGURE 20.6-1. Major metabolites of arachidonic acid produced by the cyclooxygenase (COX) and lipoxygenase (LO) pathways. Indicated in parentheses are examples of tissues in which individual prostanoids exert prominent effects. HETE, hydroxyeicosatetraenoic acid; HPETE, hydroperoxyeicosatetraenoic acid; PG, prostaglandin; TX, thromboxane. (From ref. 1, with permission.) (See Color Fig. 20.6-1 in the CD-ROM.)

platelets. Because platelets lack a nucleus and cannot synthesize new enzyme, daily use of low-dose aspirin (100 mg or less) provides full protection against platelet aggregation despite its having a half-life of approximately 20 minutes in the systemic circulation. Higher concentrations (usually in the low micromolar range) of aspirin and other conventional NSAIDs, such as ibuprofen, indomethacin, and piroxicam, inhibit both COX-1 and COX-2. A new class of NSAIDs designated coxibs by the World Health Organization selectively inhibits COX-2.[12,13] Drugs such as celecoxib and rofecoxib were developed to spare the cytoprotective effects of COX-1 on the gastric epithelium. The availability of coxibs has stimulated research on the role of COX-2 in neoplasia and the potential efficacy and safety of selective COX-2 inhibition against cancer.

TOXICITY OF NONSTEROIDAL ANTIINFLAMMATORY DRUGS

Potentially deleterious effects of aspirin and other nonselective NSAIDs include serious gastrointestinal or intracranial bleeding and impaired renal hemodynamics. Aspirin inhibits platelet aggregation, even at dosages of 30 to 100 mg/d. This reduces the risk of thrombosis and embolism but increases the risk of bleeding. Nonaspirin NSAIDs can inhibit the cardiovascular benefit of low-dose aspirin and, at antiinflammatory concentrations, can suppress formation of prostacyclin (prostaglandin I_2)

in vascular endothelial cells. Coxibs have substantially less serious gastrointestinal toxicity than conventional nonselective NSAIDs but decrease urinary excretion of prostacyclin metabolites in normal subjects. Widespread clinical use of coxibs is still too recent to determine whether prolonged treatment or more complete suppression of COX-2 will have unexpected adverse effects.[14,15] Given the biologic complexity of prostanoid metabolism, however, it is not surprising that drugs that inhibit the activity of COX isoenzymes can have adverse as well as desirable effects on human health.

HISTORY OF THE INFLAMMATION HYPOTHESIS

The theory that chronic inflammation may predispose to certain cancers dates at least to Virchow in the mid–nineteenth century.[16] Virchow's theory, prompted by a North African patient who developed bladder cancer after prolonged infection with *Schistosoma haematobium*, was that chronic irritation or injury could promote tumor development. Other conditions in which chronic inflammation predisposes to malignant transformation of the affected organ include inflammatory bowel disease, reflux esophagitis, gallstones, infection with *Helicobacter pylori* or liver flukes, pneumoconioses, and surgical implants (reviewed in ref. 17). Because NSAIDs inhibit inflammation mediated by prostaglandins, the hypothesis that NSAIDs inhibit the development of certain cancers is closely linked to the more general hypothesis that chronic inflammation promotes tumorigenesis.

NONSTEROIDAL ANTIINFLAMMATORY DRUGS IN COLORECTAL CANCER

Evidence that inflammatory mediators might contribute to tumorigenesis, even in the absence of clinically evident inflammation, emerged in the mid-1970s when Bennett and others observed that many tumors overproduce prostaglandins.[18,19] The concentration of prostaglandin E_2 was higher in human colorectal tumor tissue than in surrounding tumor tissue. This finding, and the knowledge that NSAIDs inhibit the production of prostaglandins, stimulated over 40 experimental studies to assess the potential of NSAIDs to inhibit the growth of chemically induced intestinal cancer in rats or mice (reviewed in ref. 1). These experiments involved administration of NSAIDs to rodents injected with azoxymethane or other carcinogens that induce intestinal cancer. Virtually all NSAIDs tested suppressed chemically induced colon cancer in this model. The highest tolerated dosage typically reduced tumor incidence by 40% to 60% but did not eliminate all tumors. Treatment had to be continued without interruption to prevent resumption of tumor growth.

The earliest clinical studies of NSAIDs and cancer risk were a series of uncontrolled interventions to assess whether the pro-NSAID sulindac inhibits the growth of adenomatous polyps in patients with the rare hereditary condition FAP (studies reviewed in ref. 20). FAP carriers inherit a germline mutation inactivating one allele of the APC gene. Loss of the remaining functional APC allele results in the growth of hundreds to thousands of adenomatous polyps by the second or third decade of life. Although FAP accounts for only 1% of human colorectal cancers, it provides a model of APC inactivation as an early genetic event for the approximately 85% of cancers that develop from sporadic adenomatous polyps. In uncontrolled case studies, FAP patients treated with sulindac were reported to develop fewer adenomatous polyps and to experience regression of some existing adenoma and extracolonic desmoid tumors. Sulindac is a pro-NSAID that is reputedly metabolized by intestinal flora to the active sulindac sulfide and then concentrated in the enterohepatic circulation.

The hypothesis that aspirin or other NSAIDs might inhibit the development of cancer in humans received strong support from two epidemiologic studies[21,22] published in 1991. These studies reported approximately 40% lower incidence and death rates from colorectal cancer among people who regularly used aspirin than among those who did not. By relating these findings to the previously published studies of NSAIDs in rodents and clinical observations in FAP patients, these studies drew widespread interest and research funding to the NSAID hypothesis. Most of the nearly 40 epidemiologic (nonrandomized) studies that have now examined this issue have also found a 30% to 50% lower risk of colorectal adenoma or cancer among people who regularly use NSAIDs (reviewed in refs. 1, 5). This finding is one of the strongest and most consistent associations seen in epidemiologic studies of colorectal cancer. Like the animal experiments, the epidemiologic studies suggest that the duration and continuity of NSAID use may be more critical than the daily dose and that tumors resume growth after termination of NSAID treatment.

Numerous mechanistic studies have subsequently been conducted in mouse models of FAP to determine the efficacy of nonselective NSAIDs and selective COX-2 inhibitors in suppressing spontaneous intestinal adenomas (reviewed in ref. 1). Both nonselective NSAIDs, such as piroxicam, sulindac, and aspirin, and selective COX-2 inhibitors, such as celecoxib and rofecoxib, inhibit tumor development in Apc-deficient mice. These models mimic the rapid development of adenomatous polyps in FAP patients except that the mouse tumors occur predominantly in the small intestine.

RANDOMIZED CLINICAL TRIALS OF COLORECTAL ADENOMA OR CANCER

Several phase II or III randomized clinical trials have now established that two NSAIDs, the pro-NSAID sulindac[23-25] and the selective COX-2 inhibitor celecoxib,[26] effectively suppress the development of adenomatous polyps and cause regression of existing adenomas in FAP patients (Table 20.6-1). Celecoxib has been formally approved by the U.S. Food and Drug Administration as adjuvant therapy for patients with FAP. In the only trial involving carriers of APC mutations who had not yet developed polyposis, sulindac was not effective in suppressing adenoma development.[27]

Randomized, double-blind, placebo-controlled trials have also confirmed that aspirin treatment suppresses adenoma recurrence in patients previously treated for an adenomatous polyp or cancer (see Table 20.6-1). Baron et al.[28] observed polyp suppression at an aspirin dosage of 80 mg/d but not at 325 mg/d. Sandler et al.[29] observed suppression of recurrent adenomas in patients with a previous cancer at a dosage of 325 mg/d of aspirin. Sample et al.[30] found that the lowest dosage of aspirin that reduced prostaglandin E_2 levels in rectal epithelium was 81 mg/d. In contrast, two other studies of subjects with previous sporadic adenoma have found no evidence that sulindac suppresses adenoma recurrence[31] or that acceptable dosages of piroxicam suppress prostaglandin E_2 levels in rectal mucosa[32] (see Table 20.6-1). Although randomized trials have now confirmed the efficacy of aspirin use in preventing recurrent adenoma, they have not resolved questions about the optimal treatment regimen or the risk/benefit balance of administering prolonged treatment with NSAIDs prophylactically to healthy people.

Only one randomized trial of aspirin use in the primary prevention of cardiovascular end points has been sufficiently large to measure incidence or death rates from colorectal cancer, although the aspirin arm of this trial was terminated after 5 years.[33] The Physicians' Health Study showed no reduction in either invasive or *in situ* colorectal cancer incidence nor a reduction in colorectal cancer mortality among 22,071 male physicians who were randomly assigned to receive 325 mg aspirin or placebo every other day for 5 years and who were followed for 12 years.[33] The short duration of randomized treatment, the lack of systematic screening for adenomatous polyps or colorectal cancer at the beginning and end of the trial, and the relatively low dose of aspirin limit the interpretability of these results.

NONSTEROIDAL ANTIINFLAMMATORY DRUGS IN RELATION TO OTHER CANCERS

Animal experiments and epidemiologic studies suggest that NSAIDs may inhibit the onset or progression of cancers at a variety of other sites, although the evidence is more limited

TABLE 20.6-1.   Published Phase II and III Randomized Clinical Trials of Nonsteroidal Antiinflammatory Drugs and Adenomatous Colorectal Polyps

Study	Population (Total No.)	Drug (Dose), Duration	Phase	Results
PATIENTS WITH FAP				
Labayle et al., 1991[23]	FAP (10)	Sulindac (100 mg t.i.d.), 4 mo	III	Polyps regressed completely in six patients, partly in three.
Giardiello et al., 1993[79]	FAP (22)	Sulindac (150 mg b.i.d.), 9 mo	III	Sulindac decreased number of polyps by 56% and size by 65%.
Nugent et al., 1993[25]	FAP (24)	Sulindac (400 mg), 6 mo	III	Duodenal polyps <2 mm regressed in 9 of 11 patients treated with sulindac.
Steinbach et al., 2000[26]	FAP (77)	Celecoxib (100 mg b.i.d. or 400 mg b.i.d.), 6 mo	II	Celecoxib significantly decreased the number of colon polyps.
Giardiello et al., 2002[27]	Carriers of APC gene mutations (41)	Sulindac (75 or 150 mg b.i.d.), 48 mo	III	Sulindac is not recommended as primary treatment for FAP.
OTHER PATIENT POPULATIONS				
Ladenheim et al., 1995[31]	Previous adenomatous polyps (44)	Sulindac (300 mg), 4 mo	III	Sulindac did not significantly decrease number or size of polyps.
Calaluce et al., 2000[32]	Previous adenomatous polyps (96)	Piroxicam (7.5 mg), 2 y	IIB	The toxicity of piroxicam treatment may outweigh its benefit.
Sample et al., 2002[30]	Previous adenomatous polyps (60)	Aspirin (81, 325, or 650 mg q.d.), 4 wk	II	The lowest effective dose of aspirin to suppress rectal prostaglandin E_2 levels was 81 mg.
Sandler et al., 2003[29]	History of colorectal cancer (635)	Aspirin (325 mg q.d.), 3 y	III	Daily aspirin use was associated with delayed development of adenomas.
Baron et al., 2003[28]	Previous adenomatous polyps (1121)	Aspirin (81 mg q.d. or 325 mg q.d.) and/or folate, 3 y	III	Low-dose aspirin reduced the recurrence of colon polyps.

APC, adenomatous polyposis coli; FAP, familial adenomatous polyposis.

than for colorectal cancer. In animal models, NSAIDs have been shown to inhibit induced or transplanted tumors of the esophagus, stomach, skin, breast, lung, prostate, and urinary bladder (reviewed in ref. 1). In humans, COX-2 production is induced during the development of tumors of the esophagus, stomach, colorectum, pancreas, breast, prostate, skin, lung, urinary bladder, and uterine cervix.[34]

Results from epidemiologic studies pertaining to nine cancers other than colon or rectal cancer are summarized in Figure 20.6-2. These results derive from cohort and case-control studies of NSAID use in the general population but do not include studies of rheumatoid arthritis[35–38] or analgesic abuse.[39] The cancers investigated in these studies include cancers of the esophagus,[40–43] stomach,[42–44] pancreas,[41–43,45,46] lung,[42,43,47,48] breast,[5,42,43,49,50] ovary,[5,42,43] prostate,[5,42,43,51–53] urinary bladder,[39,42,43,54–59] and kidney.[42,43,54–56]

An inverse relationship with NSAID use is seen consistently with cancers of the esophagus and stomach. A metaanalysis of the epidemiologic studies of esophageal cancer found a relative risk (RR) of 0.57 [95% confidence interval (CI), 0.47 to 0.71] associated with regular NSAID use.[40] In the few studies that examined this relationship by subsite, the association was similar for squamous cell carcinoma (RR, 0.58; 95%CI, 0.43 to 0.78) and adenocarcinoma (RR, 0.67; 95% CI, 0.51 to 0.87). A metaanalysis of the studies of NSAID use and gastric cancer[44] found a summary RR of 0.78 (95% CI, 0.69 to 0.87) associated with regular use of aspirin or other NSAIDs. The association was similar for aspirin and for nonaspirin NSAIDs and for cardia and noncardia cancers.

The results for breast and ovarian cancer could be compatible with a small reduction in risk among women who use NSAIDs, although two large prospective studies have not found an inverse association between NSAID use and either breast cancer incidence[60] or mortality.[55] Questions about residual bias

or confounding or an effect on survival after diagnosis with breast cancer remain unresolved. Several of the cohort studies of NSAID use in relation to bladder and kidney cancer[42,43,57] suggest that NSAID use may be associated with a small increase in the risk of these cancers, although the evidence is limited.

In contrast, the relationship between NSAID use and cancers of the pancreas, lung, and prostate is inconsistent across epidemiologic studies (see Fig. 20.6-2), with little evidence of an association or gradient in risk with dosage (data not shown). Studies that have reported strong inverse associations between NSAID use and cancers of the lung or pancreas have been small or of case-control design. Some studies have observed increased risk of these cancers in association with NSAID use.[42,51,57]

Relatively few studies have examined the relationship between NSAID use and incidence or mortality from all cancers combined.[42,43,55–57] One study[56] has reported significantly lower risk in people who use NSAIDs than in those who do not, whereas two population-based studies in Denmark[42,43] found higher cancer risk among persons receiving one or more prescriptions for NSAIDs over the previous 6 years. The published data are limited in terms of the number of studies and lack of control for other risk factors for cancer besides age. However, the lack of an inverse association between NSAID use and overall cancer risk in these studies underscores the need for caution in postulating a broad anticancer effect of NSAIDs.

MECHANISMS OF CANCER INHIBITION

Two cellular processes by which NSAIDs may inhibit clonal proliferation and tumor development are restoration of normal apoptosis in APC-deficient cells (reviewed in refs. 1, 2) and

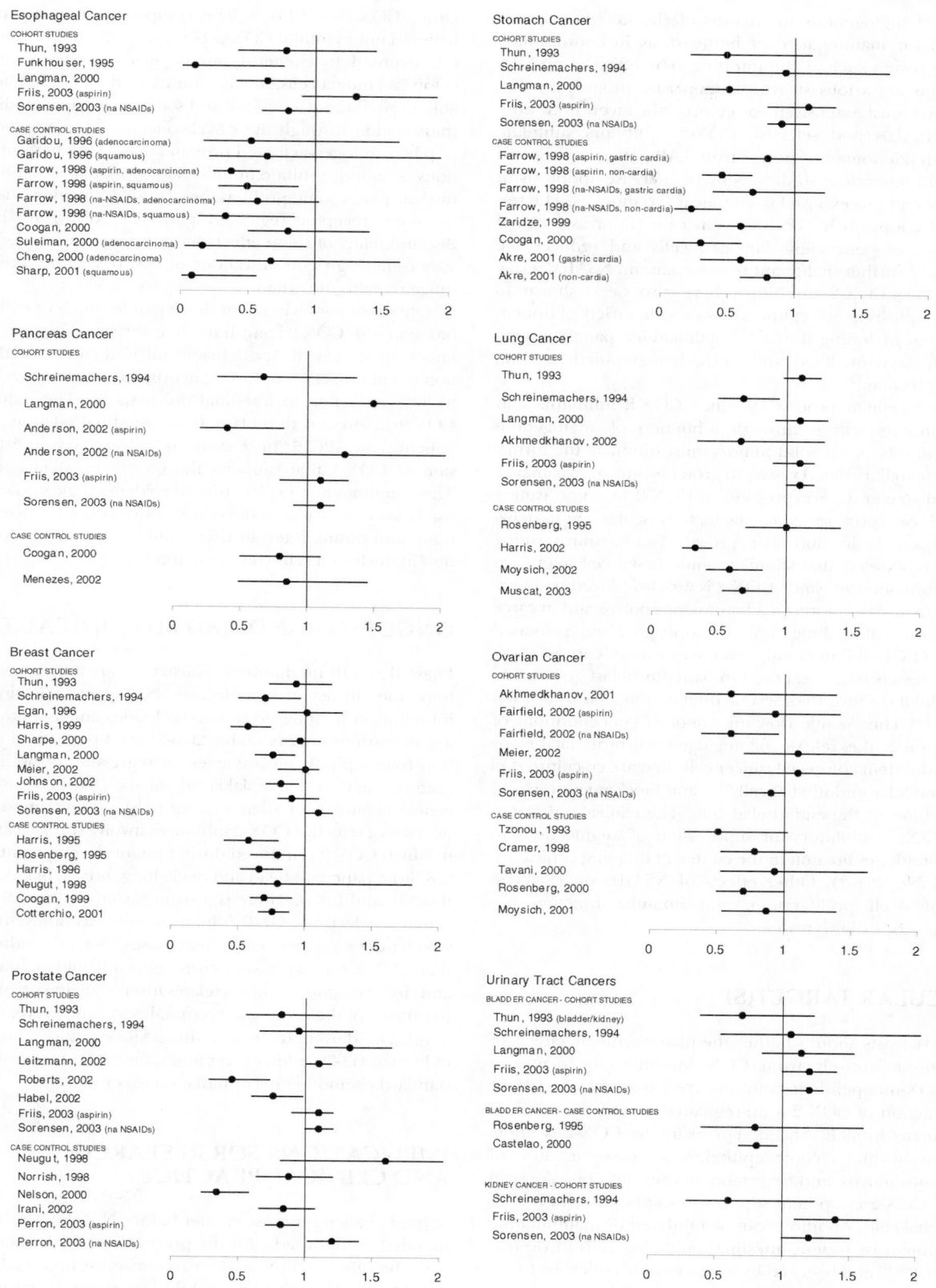

FIGURE 20.6-2. Relative risk estimates (*circles*) and 95% confidence intervals (*bars*) for cancer incidence or death rate among regular users of nonsteroidal antiinflammatory drugs (NSAIDs) compared to nonusers. Citations for the individual studies are provided from the following reviews and references: esophagus: 40–43; stomach: 42–44; pancreas: 41–43,45,46; lung: 42,43,47,48; breast: 5,42,43,49,50; ovary: 5,42,43; prostate: 5,42,43,51–53; urinary bladder: 39,42,43,54–59; and kidney: 42,43,54–56. na NSAIDs, nonaspirin NSAIDs.

inhibition of angiogenesis and neovascularization.[3,4] Apoptosis is essential for maintenance of homeostasis in continuously replicating tissues such as the intestine. The effect of NSAIDs on apoptosis at various stages of neoplastic progression has been studied most extensively for colorectal cancer. Both non-selective NSAIDs and selective COX-2 inhibitors stimulate apoptosis in adenomatous polyps from FAP patients (reviewed in 1, 80). In laboratory studies, NSAIDs increase apoptosis in Apc^{Min} mice and rats exposed to chemical carcinogens. The restoration of apoptosis in APC-deficient cells suppresses clonal proliferation of genetically damaged cells and reduces the probability of further malignant transformation. NSAIDs, especially selective COX-2 inhibitors, have also been shown to increase apoptosis in cell cultures from a wide variety of human malignancies, including stomach,[61] gallbladder, pancreas, central nervous system, head and neck, hematopoietic system, lung, and prostate.[62]

A second cellular process by which COX-2 inhibitors may inhibit tumor growth is through inhibition of angiogenesis (reviewed in refs. 3, 4). Solid tumors must stimulate the formation of new capillary blood vessels to grow beyond approximately 2 mm in diameter. Overexpression of COX-2 by colon cancer cells produces proangiogenic factors (vascular endothelial growth factor, basic fibroblast growth factor, transforming growth factor-β, etc.) that stimulate endothelial cell migration and tube formation *in vitro*.[63] COX-2 is widely induced in angiogenic vasculature in colorectal adenomatous polyps and in carcinomas of the colon, lung, breast, esophagus, and prostate.[4] Selective COX-2 inhibitors suppress the growth of corneal capillary blood vessels in rats exposed to basic fibroblast growth factor and inhibit the growth of several human tumors transplanted into mice.[4,64] Therapeutic (low micromolar) concentrations of coxibs suppress the release of angiogenic growth factors by human and rodent colorectal cancer cells that are co-cultured *in vitro* with vascular endothelial cells[63,65] and block migration and tube formation by the endothelial cells. The clinical efficacy of selective COX-2 inhibitors for suppression of angiogenesis in humans is under evaluation in the contex of ongoing clinical trials (see Table 20.6-2). Other effects of NSAIDs on cell-cycle checkpoints, cell proliferation, and immune function are beyond the scope of this review.

MOLECULAR TARGET(S)

Controversy exists about whether the pharmacologic effects of NSAIDs result entirely from COX inhibition or may also involve COX-independent pathways (reviewed in refs. 1, 66). The production of COX-2 is up-regulated during the development of many human cancers. For example, COX-2 is undetectable in normal colonic epithelium, present in 40% of adenomatous polyps, and detectable in over 80% of colorectal cancers.[67] COX-2 is a potent suppressor of apoptosis in intestinal epithelial cells. Apoptosis can be inhibited by manipulating normal human or rodent intestinal epithelial cells to overexpress COX-2[68,69] and restored by treatment with selective COX-2 inhibitors.

However, other experimental studies suggest that some of the effects of NSAIDs may involve COX-independent pathways. At high concentrations, the selective COX-2 inhibitors celecoxib and NS-398 stimulate apoptosis in cells that do not express either COX-1 or COX-2. The compound sulindac sulfone is believed not to inhibit COX activity, yet it stimulates apoptosis in rats exposed to chemical carcinogens and in human HT-29 colon carcinoma cells. At concentrations that may not be achievable *in vivo*, sulindac sulfone and sodium salicylate modify signal transduction through the c-MYC oncogene, nuclear factor κB, or p38, a mitogen-activated protein kinase. Very high concentrations of sulindac sulfide inhibit transcriptional activation by the nuclear peroxisome proliferator–activated receptor δ, a nuclear hormone receptor regulated partly by APC gene function. Because many of these effects have been demonstrated only *in vitro* using high concentrations of NSAIDs, their clinical relevance remains uncertain.

Questions also exist about the extent to which COX-1 in combination with COX-2 contributes to colorectal neoplasia. Genetic knockout studies of Apc-deficient mice demonstrate that deletion of either COX-1 or COX-2 activity causes an equivalent 70% to 80% reduction in intestinal polyposis.[70,71] The induction of COX-2 in stromal fibroblasts from intestinal adenoma in FAP patients and APC$^{\Delta716}$ mice seems to require constitutive expression of COX-1 that supports the growth of small adenoma.[72] These findings may explain why, in epidemiologic studies, aspirin use is associated with reduced risk of colorectal cancer even at doses and dosing intervals that could not sustain COX-2 inhibition in nucleated cells (reviewed in ref. 1).

ONGOING RANDOMIZED CLINICAL TRIALS

Phase II and III randomized clinical trials are under way to determine the efficacy of nonselective NSAIDs and selective COX-2 inhibitors in treating precancerous lesions and as adjuvant therapy for various tumors (Table 20.6-2). End points in the prevention trials typically involve arrest or regression of premalignant lesions such as leukoplakia, dysplasia, Barrett's esophagus, actinic keratoses, or adenomatous polyps.[73] Ongoing therapeutic trials of selective COX-2 inhibitors involve diverse cancer sites in which COX-2 is induced during tumor development: esophagus, liver, pancreas, head and neck, lung, breast, bladder, cervix, thyroid, and brain. There is a strong scientific basis for testing whether selective COX-2 inhibitors given as adjuvant therapy affect tumor recurrence or metastases. Several studies report that COX-2 overexpression correlates with higher tumor stage and size at diagnosis and correlates inversely with patient survival in cancers of the colon and rectum, breast, and cervix (reviewed in ref. 1). Adjuvant treatment with coxibs enhances the response of human HT-29 colon cancer and mouse sarcoma transplants to standard chemotherapy or radiation therapy.

IMPLICATIONS FOR RESEARCH AND CLINICAL PRACTICE

Several challenges must be met before NSAIDs can be recommended more broadly for the prevention or treatment of cancer. The efficacy of NSAID treatment must be established for indications other than the inhibition of colorectal adenoma. Furthermore, the "safety" of NSAID treatment (favorable balance of benefits to risks) must be demonstrated for specific treatment regimens in well-defined patient populations. These issues may be addressed more easily in therapeutic trials than

TABLE 20.6-2. Clinical Trials of Selective Cyclo-Oxygenase-2 Inhibitors and Diseases Other Than Colorectal

Lead Investigator (Protocol No.)	Cancer (n)	Phase	Type
HEAD AND NECK			
Boyle (NCI-G01-1930)[a]	Oral premalignant lesions (84)	II	P
Mulshine (NCI-98-C-0118)[a]	Oropharyngeal leukoplakia (57)	IIB	P
Posner (DFCI-02024)[a]	Head/neck cancer (20)	II pilot	P
DIGESTIVE			
Forastiere (NCI-P00-0145)[a]	Barrett's esophagus (200)	II	P
Dawsey (NCI-OH95-C-N026)[a]	Esophageal dysplasia (240–600)	II pilot	P
Altorki (NYH-CMC-0902-463)[a]	Esophagus cancer (25)	II	T
Mulcahy (NU-0216)[a]	Hepatocellular carcinoma (52)	I/II	T
Xiong (MDA-2003-0288)[a]	Pancreas cancer (40)	II	T
Argiris (NU-02V2)[a]	Head/neck or lung cancer (121)	II pilot	T
RESPIRATORY			
Mao (NCI-G01-1966)[a]	Lung cancer (20)	II pilot	P
Argiris (NU-01L2)[a]	Lung cancer (70)	I/II	T
Gore (RTOG-0213)[a]	Lung cancer (116)	I/II	T
Bonomi (NCI-5416)[a]	Lung cancer (80)	II	T
Figlin (UCLA-0208074)[a]	Lung cancer (110)	II	T
Gadgeel (NCI-V01-1687)[a]	Lung cancer (39)	II	T
Gadgeel (NCI-V01-1688)[a]	Lung cancer (39)	II	T
Gadgeel (WSU-C-2563)[a]	Lung cancer (27)	II	T
BREAST			
Fabian (KUMC-HSC-8919-02)[a]	Breast cancer (110)	II	P
Dang (NCI-G00-1869)[a]	Breast cancer (12–37)	II	T
Shapiro (CLB-40105)[a]	Breast cancer (132)	II	T
Goss (CAN-NCIC-MA27)[a]	Breast cancer (6830)	III	T
GENITOURINARY			
Sabichi (NCI-P00-0165)[a]	Bladder cancer (200)	IIB/III	P
Gaffney (RTOG-C-0128)[a]	Cervical cancer (83)	I/II	T
Carducci (NCI-P01-0186)[a]	Prostate cancer (60–70)	I	T
OTHER			
Bickers (NCI-P01-0191)[a]	Skin cancer (36)	II	P
Epstein (NCI-P01-0190)[a]	Skin cancer (60)	II	P
Elmets (NCI-P00-0161)[a]	Actinic keratoses (300)	II/III	P
Shah (OSU-0239)[a]	Thyroid cancer (35)	II	T
Grossman (NABTT-2100)[a]	Glioma (44)	II	T
Wen (NCI-G02-2117)[a]	Glioma (48)	II	T
Chang (ID01-460)[b]	Glioma (30)	I	T
Wen (NCI-G02-2118)[a]	Glioblastoma (55)	II	T
Felgenhauerp (COG-AEWS02P1)[a]	Ewing's sarcoma (36)	II pilot	T
Basche (NCI-3858)[a]	Solid tumors (41)	I	T

P, preventive; T, therapeutic.
[a]PDQ® Clinical Trials Database, National Cancer Institute (http://cancer.gov/search/clinical_trials).
[b]Clinical Trials.gov, National Institutes of Health (http://clinicaltrials.gov/ct/gui/c/r).

in studies of cancer prevention.[1] Therapeutic trials can be much smaller and have shorter follow-up than prevention trials and are thus easier to conduct and more cost effective.[4] They can directly measure clinical end points such as tumor recurrence and survival as well as surrogate end points. The high risk of cancer recurrence or progression in therapeutic settings offsets some of the constraints on toxicity that limit prevention.

Currently, the known benefits of aspirin and other NSAIDs for the suppression of colorectal adenoma do not justify their prophylactic use in healthy populations because of the potential risk of serious bleeding complications. *Safety* is a relative term. The balance of benefits to risks may be favorable in high-risk populations in which the event that motivates treatment is common, but precarious or unfavorable in average- or low-risk populations. In general, tolerance for toxicity is low when prophylactic treatment

must be administered long term to healthy people. For example, in the case of colorectal cancer, only 3% of women and 4% of men in the United States will develop colorectal cancer by age 79. The cumulative probability increases to 5.6% in both sexes over full life expectancy.[74] Thus, in the general population, over 94% of people treated prophylactically to prevent colorectal cancer will not benefit from treatment unless the benefits of treatment extend to other health end points. In contrast, the risk of colorectal cancer is considerably higher in certain genetically susceptible subgroups. Estimates of lifetime risk, based on studies of high-risk families, are approximately 17% for persons with two affected first-degree relatives, 70% among those with hereditary, nonpolyposis colon cancer (HNPCC) mutations, and over 95% in persons with FAP.[75] These high-risk groups account for a small fraction of all cases of colorectal cancer, however.

Strategies that can improve the balance of benefits to risks include restricting treatment to high-risk populations in which the benefits are more likely to outweigh any attendant toxicity, identifying the lowest effective dosage and critical time period when the drug must be given to achieve a specific pharmacologic effect, and identifying combinations of drugs that are effective at very low dosages.[76,77] Some studies suggest that simultaneous use of NSAIDs and cholesterol-lowering statin drugs may be more effective and require lower dosages than when either drug is given alone.[78] Other drugs that are being studied in combination with NSAIDs are ornithine decarboxylase inhibitors, the spice curcumin, and EKI-785, an irreversible inhibitor of the epidermal growth factor receptor kinase (reviewed in ref. 1).

CONCLUSION

It is now established that both nonselective NSAIDs and selective COX-2 inhibitors suppress the development of colorectal adenoma in FAP patients and that aspirin suppresses the recurrence of sporadic polyps in high-risk populations. Despite these encouraging results, the clinical application of NSAIDs as anticancer agents is still limited to suppression of polyposis in FAP patients. Fundamental questions must still be resolved concerning the safety of long-term NSAID prophylaxis, the efficacy of NSAIDs against cancers other than those of the colon and rectum, and the indications or contraindications for preventive therapy.

REFERENCES

1. Thun M, Henley S, Patrono C. Nonsteroidal anti-inflammatory drugs as anticancer agents: mechanistic, pharmacologic, and clinical issues. *J Natl Cancer Inst* 2002;94:252.
2. Chan TA. Nonsteroidal anti-inflammatory drugs, apoptosis, and colon-cancer chemoprevention. *Lancet Oncol* 2002;3:166.
3. Nie D, Honn KV. Cyclooxygenase, lipoxygenase and tumor angiogenesis. *Cell Mol Life Sci* 2002;59:799.
4. Masferrer J, Leahy K, Koki A, et al. Antiangiogenic and antitumor activities of cyclooxygenase-2 inhibitors. *Cancer Res* 2000;60:1306.
5. Baron JA. Epidemiology of non-steroidal anti-inflammatory drugs and cancer. *Prog Exp Tumor Res* 2003;37:1.
6. Vane J, Flower R, Botting R. History of aspirin and its mechanism of action. *Stroke* 1990;21[Suppl 4]:12.
7. Morrow J, Roberts L. Lipid-derived autacoids. In: Hardman J, Limbird L, eds. *The pharmacological basis of therapeutics*. New York: McGraw-Hill, 2001:669.
8. Smith W, Garavito R, DeWitt D. Prostaglandin endoperoxide H synthases (cyclooxygenases)-1 and -2. *J Biol Chem* 1996;271:33157.
9. Xie W, Robertson D, Simmons D. Mitogen-inducible prostaglandin G/H synthase: a new target for nonsteroidal antiinflammatory drugs. *Drug Dev Res* 1992;25:249.
10. Campbell W. Lipid-derived autacoids: eicosanoids and platelet-activating factor. In: Goodman L, Gilman A, eds. *Pharmacological basis of therapeutics*, 4th ed. London: Macmillan Company, 1995:600.
11. Lipsky P, Abramson S, Crofford S, et al. The classification of cyclooxygenase inhibitors. *J Rheumatol* 1998;25:2298.
12. Peterson W, Cryer B. COX-1-sparing NSAIDs—is the enthusiasm justified? *JAMA* 1999;282: 1961.
13. Willoughby DA, Moore AR, Coville-Nash PR. COX-1, COX-2, and COX-3 and the future treatment of chronic inflammatory disease. *Lancet* 2000;355:646.
14. FitzGerald G, Patrono C. The coxibs, selective inhibitors of cyclooxygenase. *N Engl J Med* 2001;345:433.
15. Bombardier C, Laine L, Reicin A, et al. Comparison of upper gastrointestinal toxicity of rofecoxib and naproxen in patients with rheumatoid arthritis. VIGOR Study Group. *N Engl J Med* 2000;343:1520.
16. Parsonnet J. Introduction. In: Parsonnet J, ed. *Microbes and malignancy—infection as a cause of human cancers.* New York: Oxford University Press, 1999:3.
17. Thun M, Henley S, Gansler T. Inflammation and cancer: an epidemiological perspective. In: Novartis Symposium Foundation 256, eds. *Cancer and inflammation.* Chichester: Wiley, 2004:56.
18. Bennett A, del Tacca M. Proceedings: prostaglandins in human colonic carcinoma. *Gut* 1975;16:409.
19. Jaffe B. Prostaglandins and cancer: an update. *Prostaglandins* 1974;6:453.
20. Thun M. NSAIDS use and decreased risk of gastrointestinal cancers. *Gastroenterol Clin North Am* 1996;25:333.
21. Rosenberg L, Palmer J, Zauber A, et al. A hypothesis: nonsteroidal anti-inflammatory drugs reduce the incidence of large-bowel cancer. *J Natl Cancer Inst* 1991;83;355.
22. Thun M, Namboodiri M, Heath CJ. Aspirin use and reduced risk of fatal colon cancer. *N Engl J Med* 1991;325:1593.
23. Labayle D, Fischer D, Vielh P, et al. Sulindac causes regression of rectal polyps in familial adenomatous polyposis. *Gastroenterology* 1991;101:635.
24. Giardiello FM. NSAID-induced polyp regression in familial adenomatous polyposis patients. *Gastroenterol Clin North Am* 1996;25:349.
25. Nugent K, Farmer K, Spigelman A, et al. Randomized controlled trial of the effect of sulindac on duodenal and rectal polyposis and cell proliferation in patients with familial adenomatous polyposis. *Br J Surg* 1993;80:1618.
26. Steinbach G, Lynch P, Phillips R, et al. The effect of celecoxib, a cyclooxygenase-2 inhibitor, in familial adenomatous polyposis. *N Engl J Med* 2000;342:1946.
27. Giardiello FM, Yang VW, Hylind LM, et al. Primary chemoprevention of familial adenomatous polyposis with sulindac. *N Engl J Med* 2002;346:1054.
28. Baron JA, Cole BF, Sandler RS, et al. A randomized trial of aspirin to prevent colorectal adenomas. *N Engl J Med* 2003;348:891.
29. Sandler RS, Halabi S, Baron JA, et al. A randomized trial of aspirin to prevent colorectal adenomas in patients with previous colorectal cancer. *N Engl J Med* 2003;348:883.
30. Sample D, Wargovich M, Fischer SM, et al. A dose-finding study of aspirin for chemoprevention utilizing rectal mucosal prostaglandin E(2) levels as a biomarker. *Cancer Epidemiol Biomarkers Prev* 2002;11:275.
31. Ladenheim J, Garcia G, Titzer D, et al. Effect of sulindac on sporadic colonic polyps. *Gastroenterology* 1995;108:1083.
32. Calaluce R, Earnest D, Heddens D, et al. Effects of piroxicam on prostaglandin E_2 levels in rectal mucosa of adenomatous polyp patients: a randomized phase IIb trial. *J Cancer Epidemiol Prev* 2000;9:1287.
33. Gann P, Manson J, Glynn R, et al. Low-dose aspirin and incidence of colorectal tumors in a randomized trial. *J Natl Cancer Inst* 1993;85:1220.
34. Koki A, Khan NK, Woerner BM, et al. Cyclooxygenase-2 in human pathological disease. *Adv Exp Med Biol* 2002;507:177.
35. Isomaki H, Hakulinen T, Joutsenlahti U. Excess risk of lymphomas, leukemia and myeloma in patients with rheumatoid arthritis. *J Chronic Dis* 1978;31:691.
36. Gridley G, McLaughlin J, Ekbom A. Incidence of cancer among patients with rheumatoid arthritis. *J Natl Cancer Inst* 1993;85:307.
37. Cibere J, Sibley J, Haga M. Rheumatoid arthritis and the risk of malignancy. *Arthritis Rheum* 1997;40:1580.
38. Thomas E, Brewster DH, Black RJ, et al. Risk of malignancy among patients with rheumatic conditions. *Int J Cancer* 2000;88:497.
39. Bucher C, Jordan P, Nickeleit V, et al. Relative risk of malignant tumors in analgesic abusers. Effects of long-term intake of aspirin. *Clin Nephrol* 1999;51:67.
40. Corley DA, Kerlikowske K, Verma R, et al. Protective association of aspirin/NSAIDs and esophageal cancer: a systematic review and meta-analysis. *Gastroenterology* 2003;124:47.
41. Shaheen NJ, Straus WL, Sandler RS. Chemoprevention of gastrointestinal malignancies with nonsteroidal antiinflammatory drugs. *Cancer* 2002;94:950.
42. Sorensen HT, Friis S, Norgard B, et al. Risk of cancer in a large cohort of nonaspirin NSAID users: a population-based study. *Br J Cancer* 2003;88:1687.
43. Friis S, Sorensen HT, McLaughlin JK, et al. A population-based cohort study of the risk of colorectal and other cancers among users of low-dose aspirin. *Br J Cancer* 2003;88:684.
44. Wang W, Huang J, Zheng G, et al. Non-steroidal anti-inflammatory drug use and the risk of gastric cancer: a systematic review and metaanalysis. *J Natl Cancer Inst* 2003;95:1784.
45. Anderson K, Johnson T, Lazovitch D, et al. Association between nonsteroidal anti-inflammatory drug use and the incidence of pancreatic cancer. *J Natl Cancer Inst* 2002;94:1168.
46. Menezes RJ, Huber KR, Mahoney MC, et al. Regular use of aspirin and pancreatic cancer risk. *BMC Public Health* 2002;2:18.
47. Moysich KB, Menezes RJ, Ronsani A, et al. Regular aspirin use and lung cancer risk. *BMC Cancer* 2002;2:31.
48. Muscat J, Chen S, Richie J, et al. Risk of lung cancer among users of nonsteroidal antiinflammatory drugs. *Cancer* 2003;97:1732.
49. Khuder S, Mutgi A. Breast cancer and NSAID use: a meta-analysis. *Br J Cancer* 2001; 84:1188.
50. Johnson TW, Anderson KE, Lazovich D, et al. Association of aspirin and nonsteroidal anti-inflammatory drug use with breast cancer. *Cancer Epidemiol Biomarkers Prev* 2002;11: 1586.
51. Leitzmann MF, Stampfer MJ, Ma J, et al. Aspirin use in relation to risk of prostate cancer. *Cancer Epidemiol Biomarkers Prev* 2002;11:1108.
52. Irani J, Ravery V, Pariente JL, et al. Effect of nonsteroidal anti-inflammatory agents and finasteride on prostate cancer risk. *J Urol* 2002;168:1985.
53. Perron L, Bairati I, Moore L, et al. Dosage, duration and timing of nonsteroidal antiinflammatory drug use and risk of prostate cancer. *Int J Cancer* 2003;106:409.
54. Paganini-Hill A, Chao A, Ross R, et al. Aspirin use and chronic diseases: a cohort study of the elderly. *BMJ* 1989;299:1247.
55. Thun M, Namboodiri M, Calle E, et al. Aspirin use and risk of fatal cancer. *Cancer Res* 1993;53:1322.
56. Schreinemachers D, Everson R. Aspirin use and lung, colon, and breast cancer incidence in a prospective study. *Epidemiology* 1994;5:138.
57. Langman MJS, Cheng KK, Gilman EA, et al. Effect of anti-inflammatory drugs on overall risk of common cancer: case-control study in general practice research database. *BMJ* 2000;320:1642.
58. Rosenberg L. Nonsteroidal anti-inflammatory drugs and cancer. *Prev Med* 1995;24:107.

59. Castelao J, Yuan J-M, Gago-Dominguez M, et al. Non-steroidal anti-inflammatory drugs and bladder cancer prevention. *Br J Cancer* 2000;82:1364.
60. Egan K, Stampfer M, Giovannucci E, et al. Prospective study of regular aspirin use and the risk of breast cancer. *J Natl Cancer Inst* 1996;88:988.
61. Uefuji K, Ichikura T, Shinomiya N, et al. Induction of apoptosis by JTE-522, a specific cyclo-oxygenase-2 inhibitor, in human gastric cancer cell lines. *Anticancer Res* 2000;20: 4279.
62. Umar A, Viner JL, Anderson WF, et al. Development of COX inhibitors in cancer prevention and therapy. *Am J Clin Oncol* 2003;26:S48.
63. Tsujii M, Kawano S, Tsuji S, et al. Cyclooxygenase regulates angiogenesis induced by colon cancer cells. *Cell* 1998;93:705.
64. Williams CS, Tsujii M, Reese J, et al. Host cyclooxygenase-2 modulates carcinoma growth. *J Clin Invest* 2000;105:1589.
65. Jones M, Wang H, Peskar BM, et al. Inhibition of angiogenesis by nonsteroidal anti-inflammatory drugs: insights into mechanisms and implications for cancer growth and ulcer healing. *Nat Med* 1999;5:1418.
66. Hawk E, Viner J, Dannenberg A, et al. COX-2 in cancer—a player that's defining the rules. *J Natl Cancer Inst* 2002;94:545.
67. Eberhart C, Coffey R, Radhika A, et al. Up-regulation of cyclooxygenase 2 gene expression in human colorectal adenomas and adenocarcinomas. *Gastroenterology* 1994;107: 1183.
68. Tsujii M, DuBois R. Alterations in cellular adhesion and apoptosis in epithelial cells over-expressing prostaglandin endoperoxide synthase 2. *Cell* 1995;83:493.
69. DuBois R, Shao J, Tsujii M, et al. G1 delay in cells overexpressing prostaglandin endoper-oxide synthase-2. *Cancer Res* 1996;56:733.
70. Langenbach R, Loftin C, Lee C, et al. Cyclooxygenase knockout mice: models for eluci-dating isoform-specific functions. *Biochem Pharm* 1999;58:1237.
71. Langenbach R, Morham S, Tiano H, et al. Prostaglandin synthase 1 gene disruption in mice reduces arachidonic acid-induced inflammation and indomethacin-induced gastric ulceration. *Cell* 1995;83:483.
72. Takeda H, Sonoshita M, Oshima H, et al. Cooperation of cyclooxygenase 1 and cyclooxy-genase 2 in intestinal polyposis. *Cancer Res* 2003;63:4872.
73. Hawk E, Viner J, Umar A. Nonsteroidal anti-inflammatory and cyclooxygenase-2-selective inhibitors in clinical cancer prevention trials. In: Dannenberg A, DuBois R, eds. *COX-2: a new target for cancer prevention and treatment*. New York: Karger, 2003;37:210.
74. Jemal A, Murray T, Samuels A, et al. Cancer statistics, 2003. *CA Cancer J Clin* 2003;53:5.
75. American Society of Clinical Oncology. *Hereditary colorectal cancer syndromes. Cancer genetics & cancer predisposition testing: an ASCO curriculum.* Vol. II. American Society of Clinical Oncology, 1998.
76. Torrance CJ, Jackson PE, Montgomery E, et al. Combinatorial chemoprevention of intes-tinal neoplasia. *Nat Med* 2000;6:1024.
77. Gupta R, DuBois R. Combinations for cancer prevention. *Nat Med* 2000;6:974.
78. Agarwal B, Rao C, Bhendwal S, et al. Lovastatin augments sulindac-induced apoptosis in colon cancer cells and potentiates chemopreventive effect of sulindac. *Gastroenterology* 1999;117:838.
79. Giardiello FM, Hamilton SR, Krush AJ, et al. Treatment of colonic and rectal adenomas with sulindac in familial adenomatous polyposis. *N Engl J Med* 1993;328:1313.
80. Chan AT. Aspirin, non-steroidal anti-inflammatory drugs and colorectal neoplasia: future challenges in chemoprevention. *Cancer Causes Control* 2003;14:413.

SECTION 7

GRAHAM A. COLDITZ
KATHLEEN YAUS WOLIN

Physical Activity and Body Weight

PHYSICAL ACTIVITY

The 1994 report of the U.S. Surgeon General concludes that lack of physical activity is causally related to increased risk for coronary heart disease, diabetes, and colon cancer.[1,2] The relation with some other cancers is listed as suggestive. In 2002, the International Agency for Research on Cancer published an updated report on weight control and physical activity that concluded that the evidence for colon and breast cancer was convincing and that associations are suggested for endometrial, prostate, and lung cancers.[3] Other researchers reviewing the evidence have reached similar, although not identical, conclusions regarding the strength of the evidence.[4,5] The evidence is summarized in the following sections.

MEASURES

Epidemiologic studies have measured activity in two ways: by occupation and by leisure time activities. These measures may represent somewhat different patterns of energy expenditure. Activity demanded by employment in a certain occupation may be relatively constant from week to week and year to year, whereas leisure time activity is far more labile, changing from week to week, season to season, and year to year. Over the past century, occupational energy expenditure within any class of occupation has declined steadily as mechanization has increased. Leisure time activity, on the other hand, varies substantially from season to season, reaching a high in the summer months and a low during winter.

In the epidemiologic study of chronic diseases like colon cancer, long-term patterns of activity may be the relevant factor in determining disease risk. Therefore, occupational activity may be a better marker of cancer-determining activity level than is self-reported leisure time activity. Both the methods used to measure activity and the validity or accuracy of the methods vary considerably. Similar methodologic issues arose in the study of heart disease[6]: When poor measures of activity were used, studies tended to underestimate the true impact of activity on health. In other words, studies using poor measures of physical activity failed to measure true activity levels and then failed to provide data showing a strong association with activity, even though physical activity is, in truth, protective against heart disease.[1]

The same is true for colon cancer: When less accurate measures of physical activity are used, the estimated benefit from this activity is smaller than its probable true benefit. Thus, the protection offered by physical activity is underestimated. Nonetheless, as summarized later in this chapter, the most precise studies using validated measures of physical activity have shown, overall, that higher levels of physical activity are related to lower levels of certain cancers.

VALIDITY OF ACTIVITY MEASURES

The validity of activity measures has been assessed and is quite variable.[3] For the better measures, one observes a correlation between the self-reported measure of activity and an independent gold standard (such as a diary of 28 days of activity) in the range of 0.5 to 0.7.[7-9] Thus, the epidemiologic associations observed using these measures of activity and disease outcome are considerably attenuated and perhaps underestimate a true association by as much as half. For example, Giovannucci et al. reported a relative risk that was 0.88 [95% confidence interval (CI), 0.81 to 0.95] per 10-MET increase in physical activity per week, which is approximately equivalent to 3 hours of walking per week.[10] A MET is a "metabolic equivalent of task" that accounts for both the duration and intensity of activity. After correction was made for measurement error, the relative risk was strengthened to 0.65 (95% CI, 0.48 to 0.88). In general, questionnaires are better at measuring higher-intensity activities.[4,11]

COLON CANCER

Numerous studies have illustrated a relation between physical activity and colon cancer. Higher levels of physical activity are associated with lower rates of colon cancer.[1,3,12]

The rates of colon cancer vary considerably among countries. During the 1960s and 1970s, a gradual increase in colon cancer was seen in most industrialized countries, and in European countries with low rates there was an increase to the rates observed in high-risk countries such as the United States and England. Reported incidence is higher in the United States, Australia, and Western Europe than in most Asian countries, although rates in Japan have now risen to be closer to those of North America and Europe.[13] Numerous lifestyle factors have been proposed to explain this large international variation.[14]

Several reviews of the literature have been published.[2,3,12] These present detailed summary data for each study, including the relative risk for each level of activity. In addition, studies published through July 2003 are reviewed here.

Case-Control Studies

Overall, the published case-control studies suggest a consistent inverse relation between both occupational and leisure time activity and colon cancer risk among men and women. These results have been replicated in a wide range of countries including China, Japan, New Zealand, Spain, Sweden, Turkey, and the United States.

Cohort Studies

Cohort studies generally enroll healthy individuals to assess elements of lifestyle, behavior, environment, and occupation that are thought to influence later development of disease. The initial follow-up of college athletes by Polednak failed to show any protective effect of activity on colon cancer risk, although data were not available on lifestyle characteristics (including family history, diet, smoking, etc.).[15] Other cohort studies show a reduction in risk similar to that observed in the case-control studies. Higher activity in adult life is generally related to reduced risk of colon cancer, although the cohort results are less consistent than are the results of the case-control studies. Inconsistency in the findings of cohort studies may be attributed in part to that fact that some studies focused on college activity and cancer risk many years later[15,16] or included both colon and rectal cancer in a single outcome category.[16–18] (An inverse association between activity and rectal cancer is generally not seen when rectal cancer is analyzed as a separate outcome variable.) When occupation was used to categorize activity in a study of Swedish men, those with higher activity had a lower risk of colon cancer (relative risk, 0.8).[19] In that study, the strongest contrast was based on a joint classification of occupation and recreational activity. Men in the highest activity group with regard to both occupation and recreation had a relative risk of 0.3 (95% CI, 0.1 to 0.8), which represented a 70% reduction in risk compared with men who were inactive at work and engaged in little recreational activity.

Leisure time activity is addressed separately in the Harvard Alumni Study, in which a cohort of graduates of Harvard College was followed starting in 1960 to study the relation between activity level and chronic diseases. Lee and colleagues observed a strong inverse association between activity level and disease risk among men who were active both in the 1960s and in 1977 when surveys were administered.[20] Men expending more than 2500 kcal per week in leisure activity had a 50% reduction in risk of colon cancer compared with those expending less than 1000 kcal per week.

Overall, the cohort studies conducted in Denmark, Norway, Sweden, Switzerland, and the United States support a dose-response relationship across increasing activity levels: Higher activity levels are related to lower levels of colon cancer risk. A dose-response effect was found in nearly all studies that examined trends in risk.[12] Those in the highest activity category have approximately a 40% to 50% reduction in risk of colon cancer compared with those in the least active category.[2]

Although historically data have suggested that the association between physical activity and reduced risk of colon cancer is stronger in men than in women, this finding may, in part, reflect the small number of women in the high-activity category. More recently, one study found men and women to have similar risks,[21] another found a stronger effect in women,[22] and a third supported early findings of a stronger effect in men.[23]

Site-Specific Risk

Studies that examined activity in relation to site of cancer in the colon have suggested that the relation between higher activity and lower risk of cancer may be stronger for the left than for the right colon.[2,24] One large case-control study showed no difference in the strength of association between vigorous activity and proximal or distal colon cancer.[25] In a more recent analysis, however, a lifestyle characterized by high levels of physical activity had a stronger effect on cancer risk in the proximal than the distal colon in men and women.[26] Studies consistently show the association to be stronger for the colon than for the rectum; activity level is at best associated only very weakly with risk for rectal cancer.

Adenomas

A case-control study examined the impact of exercise on risk of large and small adenomas, as well as colon cancer, and found the strongest effect for colon cancer. Total and occupational activity had an effect on risk for large adenomas but no effect was seen on risk for small adenomas.[27] Similar results were found in two U.S.-based cohorts.[3] A limited number of studies have looked at the effect of activity on adenoma development and most have found a protective effect. However, Colbert and colleagues examined the effect of activity on polyp recurrence and found no effect for recent physical activity.[28]

Interpretation

Despite the use of variable and often poor measures of activity, a consistent reduction in risk associated with activity is observed across different study designs and different populations, and for both occupational and leisure time activity. A consistent dose-response relationship emerges, so that those with higher levels of activity are at reduced risk of colon cancer. Across studies, the evidence suggests that the relation is stronger for cancer of the left colon and weaker or absent for rectal cancer. Few studies have addressed the relation between specific activities and cancer risk (e.g., is swimming less protective than jogging?) or the importance of the age at which a person is active in determining the likelihood of cancer (e.g., is activity more protective in youth, middle age, or the years immediately before the diagnosis of cancer?). Three studies that address physical activity during early adulthood show no relation with cancer risk.[15,16,29] Although these studies failed to control for several colon cancer risk factors, the results are consistent with the view that activity has an effect later in the pathway to cancer. Findings of a study by Lee and colleagues also support a role for activity later in the pathway to cancer. For men who had increased their level of activity during follow-up of the cohort, a suggestion was seen of lower risk of colon cancer during subsequent follow-up,[20] but in a later analysis of the data with longer follow-up, no effect was found.[30] More data are needed, however, to refine the understanding of the temporal relation between change in physical activity and change in risk of cancer. In general, the studies based on classification of activity by occupation show a stronger dose-response relationship than those based on leisure time activity and support a protective effect across the wide range of activities encompassed by high-activity occupations.

How does one know that physical activity is actually protecting individuals from developing colon cancer? Is it possible that active men and women are also healthier in other ways (e.g., consume less red meat and ingest more folate) and that these factors are the real reason for the observed protective effect of physical activity? Several studies have reported analyses that address the independent relation between activity and colon cancer risk; that is, they control for other lifestyle factors (body mass index or BMI, alcohol consumption, and diet) that may be related to higher levels of physical activity and could therefore bias or distort the protection attributed to physical activity. Activity has effects independent of dietary fat and fiber intake in these studies and also independent of BMI, a measure of adiposity. Although not all studies examined for the independence of activity from other lifestyle factors, the magnitude of the inverse relation has not been materially altered when investigators have controlled for diet, BMI, and other factors. The one exception is the study by Whittemore et al., who saw a shift in the magnitude of association after controlling for diet in analyzing the case-control data from the People's Republic of China but no substantial change in effect after controlling for diet in analyzing data from the United States.[31] In a detailed analysis of data from the Health Professionals Follow-up Study, which followed a cohort of some 50,000 men to study the relation between diet and chronic diseases, Giovannucci et al. showed that individuals with higher physical activity levels were more likely to use multivitamins, had a lower intake of saturated fat and a higher intake of fiber, had a lower prevalence of cigarette smoking, and had a lower BMI (men were leaner).[10] After controlling for these risk factors, as well as use of aspirin and family history, they found that the protection for those in the top quintile of activity was reduced from 56% to 47% [the relative risk changed from 0.4 (95% CI, 0.3 to 0.7) to 0.5 (95% CI, 0.3 to 0.9)]. In other words, the protection remained at almost 50% despite controlling for all the other factors known to relate to colon cancer risk. The inverse trend in risk with increasing activity remained statistically significant. Thus, the conclusion is that activity is not merely a marker of a healthier lifestyle but exerts an independent protective effect.

Mechanisms

Several biologic mechanisms for the protective effect of physical activity have been proposed reflecting changes in physiologic measures after physical activity. The role of insulin is increasingly viewed as important because abdominal obesity and low physical activity are independently related to insulin resistance. A review by Giovannucci outlines the evidence and possible mechanisms in detail.[32] Across a range of physical activity levels, insulin sensitivity improves with exercise. Further, insulin is a strong growth factor for colon mucosal cells in laboratory studies and in an animal model of colon cancer. Thus, activity may exert its protective effect through reduced insulin levels.

Another proposed mechanism is the effect of prostaglandins on colon cell proliferation. Physical activity produces an increase in the level of prostaglandin $F_{2\alpha}$, which increases intestinal motility and inhibits colonic cell proliferation. Activity also results in a decrease in prostaglandin E_2 levels, which in cell culture can act to stimulate colon cell proliferation.

Changes in adiposity may also help explain the connection between activity and colon cancer, although the effect of physical activity remains after control for BMI or weight, which indicates a separate, independent, effect of activity.

With this large body of epidemiologic data and supporting laboratory studies, it is apparent that low levels of physical activity are causally related to increased risk of colon cancer. Causal considerations include a consistent decrease in risk with higher levels of physical activity, measured as either occupational activity or leisure time activity, a dose-response relationship with hours of activity per week or level of occupational physical activity, specificity for the relation with colon cancer and not rectal cancer, and a temporal relation in which activity measures precede the onset of colon cancer by years, although relationships are stronger for more recent activity than for distant past activity.

BREAST CANCER

Regular physical activity has been hypothesized to prevent breast cancer, largely by reducing circulating levels of sex hormones. The mechanisms by which physical activity reduces exposure to hormones vary by period of life. Young girls participating in strenuous athletic training such as running and ballet dancing have delayed menarche,[33–35] which is known to reduce risk of breast cancer, and even moderate-intensity physical activity may also delay menstruation.[36] A later menarche is associated with a later onset of regular ovulatory cycles as well as lower serum estrogen concentrations during adolescence. Once menstruation has been established, anovulatory and irregular menstrual cycles may be more frequent among moderately and strenuously active women than among inactive women,[35,3,37] although there is disagreement regarding the degree to which the intensity of physical activity influences menstrual abnormalities.[38] Among older women, levels of past and current physical activity influence fat stores,[33,34,39,40] which after menopause are the locus of conversion of androstenedione to estrogen.[41,42] The suggestion has also been made that immune mechanisms, like the actions of natural killer cells or macrophages, may mediate relationship between the breast cancer and physical activity.[3]

Reviews of the evidence that higher levels of physical activity are associated with reduced risk of breast cancer have considered that this evidence is now convincing[3,4] or that such an associated is probable.[5] The majority of studies have found a reduction in risk; the average decrease in risk is 20% to 40% but has reached as high as 70% in some studies.[3,41]

Reduction in risk has been shown to be greater in some subgroups but is seen across certain factors, including menopausal status and type of activity (recreational vs. occupational). Evidence exists for a trend of decreasing risk with increasing activity, although this trend is clearer for frequency and duration of activity than for intensity of activity.[3]

Indirect evidence has suggested that physical activity may be more important in decreasing the risk of postmenopausal breast cancer because of the significant role of activity in controlling weight gain, an important cause of postmenopausal breast cancer. This, in addition to many other benefits of staying lean and fit, provides additional justification for including regular physical activity in daily life.

PROSTATE CANCER

Based on available evidence, an association between physical activity and reduced risk of prostate cancer has been considered probable[4] or possible,[3,5] although one review concluded that the evidence for a protective effect of activity was inconsistent.[43] The greatest risk reduction in a cohort study was seen in a prospective cohort of 7570 men.[44] Men in the highest quartile of fitness had a 70% lower risk for prostate cancer than men in the lowest quartile of fitness. An assessment of occupational activity in a case-control study found an 80% lower risk in the most active group compared to the least active group.[45] More recently, results from a British heart study found that men in the vigorous activity group had an 80% lower risk of prostate cancer than men in the group with no to moderate activity, even after control for known risk factors, although men in the moderate to vigorous activity group experienced no decrease in risk of prostate cancer.[18] Most studies, however, have found risk reductions of 20% to 50%. Of the 14 studies that reported a risk reduction as cited in Friedenreich and Thune's review,[43] over half observed a significant reduction. Six studies found no association between activity level and prostate cancer, and four found an increased risk with higher activity. The results of case-control studies are more inconsistent. Of 18 studies that looked for a dose-response relationship, only 7 found such a trend to exist. In general, the majority of studies have found an association between activity and cancer risk, with moderate risk reductions suggested.

Methodology

As in the studies of breast and colon cancer, a wide range of methods was used to assess physical activity in the prostate cancer analyses, and a range of study designs was used.

Mechanism

Understanding the mechanisms by which physical activity reduces prostate cancer risk is made difficult by the fact that the biology of prostate cancer is relatively poorly understood.[43] In general, physical activity is known to enhance immune func-

tioning. Strenuous exercise has been shown to alter hormone levels, although its influence on testosterone levels is less clear. Physically active men have been found to have lower serum testosterone levels. However, results of studies relating hormone levels to prostate cancer risk have been mixed.[46]

OBESITY

A strong and consistent relation has been reported between obesity and mortality from all cancers among men and women.[47,48] Because of the association with postmenopausal breast cancer and endometrial cancer, the relation is stronger among women than among men, with obesity and overweight accounting for 14% of cancer deaths among men and 20% of cancer deaths among women.[48]

BREAST CANCER

Attained weight and weight change in adults provide sensitive measures of the balance between long-term energy intake and expenditure. Although the relation between these variables and breast cancer risk has been complex and confusing, findings for postmenopausal women provide a more coherent picture and indicate a major contribution of weight gain to risk of postmenopausal breast cancer. The two main results of this research seem contradictory: (1) In affluent Western populations with high rates of breast cancer, measures of body fatness have been inversely related to risk of premenopausal breast cancer and (2) body fatness has been consistently related to increased risk of postmenopausal breast cancer.

An inverse relation between body weight (typically measured as BMI, calculated as weight in kilograms divided by height in square meters, to account for variation in height) and incidence of premenopausal breast cancer has been consistently seen in prospective studies[3,49] and has also been found in a metaanalysis of both case-control and cohort studies,[50] although the risk reductions noted have been modest. Little association between BMI and breast cancer mortality has been observed in premenopausal women, probably because delayed detection and diagnosis in heavier women counterbalance the lower incidence among these women. Heavier premenopausal women, even those at the upper limits of what are considered to be healthy weights, have more irregular menstrual cycles and increased rates of anovulatory infertility,[51] which suggests that their lower risk may be due to a lower number of ovulatory cycles and decreased exposure to ovarian hormones. Increased rates of menstrual irregularity and anovulatory infertility are also seen among very lean women, but such women are uncommon in Western populations. In case-control studies, a consistent relation between menstrual cycle regularity and breast cancer risk has not emerged, which could cast doubt on this explanation, but this may be due to the indirect relation between menstrual regularity and ovulation and to difficulties in remote recall. In a prospective study of younger women, compared with regular cycles of approximately 28 days, both shorter and longer or irregular cycles were associated with reduced risk of breast cancer.[52] This finding lends support to the view that irregular anovulation is responsible for the lower risk in heavier women.

Among postmenopausal women, in contrast, higher BMIs are associated with increased risk of breast cancer. In analyses of data from the Pooling Project (which combined data from eight cohort studies in four countries), women with a BMI above 20 and up to 28 had an increased risk of breast cancer. The association was found to be stronger in women who had never used hormone replacement therapy.[53] A case-control analysis suggested that risk is also modified by family history of breast cancer: Women without a family history have only a modestly increased risk, but BMI is strongly associated with risk in women with a positive family history.[54] Although the majority of studies have found an increased risk, the magnitude of the effect is generally modest and increases linearly with increasing age after menopause.[3]

Thus, an elevated BMI in a postmenopausal woman represents two opposing risks: a protective effect due to the correlation between early weight and postmenopausal weight, and an adverse effect due to elevated estrogen levels after menopause. For this reason, weight *gain* from early adult life to postmenopause should be more strongly related to postmenopausal breast cancer risk than attained weight. Indeed, an association between weight gain and risk of postmenopausal breast cancer has been consistently supported by both case-control and prospective studies.[3] Among women who never used postmenopausal hormones in the Women's Health Initiative, a change in BMI from age 18 was associated with a nearly twofold increase in risk of breast cancer compared with a women whose BMI remained unchanged.[55] Similar results were found in the Nurses' Health Study in which the combination of either using postmenopausal hormones or gaining weight after age 18 years accounted for one-third of postmenopausal breast cancer cases.[49]

In summary, as in animal studies, energy balance appears to play an important but complex role in the etiology of human breast cancer. During early adult life, overweight is associated with a lower incidence of breast cancer but no reduction in breast cancer mortality. However, weight gain after age 18 years and overweight or obesity are associated with a graded and substantial increase in postmenopausal breast cancer that is seen most clearly in the absence of hormone replacement therapy.

OTHER CANCERS

The relation between obesity and risk of endometrial cancer follows from the excess exposure to estrogen that is associated with adiposity. This direct relation has been long observed. A review by Kaaks et al. summarizes the current state of knowledge of the relationship between obesity, sex hormones, and endometrial cancer.[56] Obesity or overweight appears to incur a twofold to threefold increased risk of endometrial cancer.[3]

An association between obesity and colon cancer has been observed among both women and men, and persists even after control for physical activity and dietary patterns.[3] It is postulated that excess weight gain may act through increased insulin resistance and hyperinsulinemia to promote colon carcinogenesis.[57,58] Activity also decreases abdominal fat mass, which is the most metabolically active fat depot.[4] Research has also suggested that estrogen plays a role in colon cancer pathogenesis by influencing insulin-like growth factor-1 receptors and thus increasing susceptibility to the higher levels of insulin associated with obesity.[59]

Although only a few studies have examined the relation between obesity and esophageal cancer risk, those that do exist consistently find a twofold or higher increased risk of esophageal cancer among those with a BMI over 25 kg/m^2.[3]

Obesity is consistently associated with increased risk of kidney cancer. Nearly all studies have found that both obese men and obese women have nearly two times the risk of renal cell cancer of normal-weight individuals.[3]

CONCLUSION

Lack of physical activity and adult weight gain are marks of our Western culture, and both act to increase risk of major malignancies. Through numerous mechanisms these two lifestyle factors contribute substantially to the risk of colon and breast cancer. The evidence is strong for a link between obesity and endometrial cancer, but less consistent for an effect of obesity on risk for other major malignancies.

REFERENCES

1. U.S. Department of Health and Human Services. *Physical activity and health: a report of the Surgeon General.* Atlanta, Georgia: US Department of Health and Human Services, Centers for Disease Control and Prevention, National Center for Chronic Disease Prevention and Health Promotion; 1996.
2. Colditz GA, Cannuscio CC, Frazier AL. Physical activity and reduced risk of colon cancer: implications for prevention. *Cancer Causes Control* 1997;8:649.
3. International Agency for Research on Cancer, WHO, IARC Handbooks of Cancer Prevention. *Weight control and physical activity.* Lyon, France: International Agency for Research on Cancer, 2002:6.
4. McTiernan A, Ulrich C, Slate S, et al. Physical activity and cancer etiology: associations and mechanisms. *Cancer Causes Control* 1998;9:487.
5. Marrett LD, Theis B, Ashbury FD. Workshop report: physical activity and cancer prevention. *Chronic Dis Can* 2000;21:143.
6. Berlin JA, Colditz GA. A meta-analysis of physical activity in the prevention of coronary heart disease. *Am J Epidemiol* 1990;132:612.
7. Chasan-Taber S, Rimm EB, Stampfer MJ, et al. Reproducibility and validity of a self-administered physical activity questionnaire for male health professionals. *Epidemiology* 1996;7:81.
8. Lee IM, Sesso HD, Paffenbarger RS Jr. Physical activity and risk of lung cancer. *Int J Epidemiol* 1999;28:620.
9. Wolf AM, Hunter DJ, Colditz GA, et al. Reproducibility and validity of a self-administered physical activity questionnaire. *Int J Epidemiol* 1994;23:991.
10. Giovannucci E, Ascherio A, Rimm EB, et al. Physical activity, obesity, and risk for colon cancer and adenoma in men. *Ann Intern Med* 1995;122:327.
11. Ainsworth BE, Sternfeld B, Slattery ML, et al. Physical activity and breast cancer: evaluation of physical activity assessment methods. *Cancer* 1998;83[Suppl 3]:611.
12. Friedenreich CM. Physical activity and cancer prevention: from observational to intervention research. *Cancer Epidemiol Biomarkers Prev* 2001;10:287.
13. Parkin DM, Whelan S, Ferlay J, et al. *Cancer incidence in five continents.* Lyon, France: International Agency for Research on Cancer, 2002:8.
14. Potter, JD, Slattery ML, Bostick RM, et al. Colon cancer: a review of the epidemiology. *Epidemiol Rev* 1993;15:499.
15. Polednak AP. College athletics, body size, and cancer mortality. *Cancer* 1976;38:382.
16. Paffenbarger RS Jr, Hyde RT, Wing AL. Physical activity and incidence of cancer in diverse populations: a preliminary report. *Am J Clin Nutr* 1987;45[Suppl 1]:312.
17. Albanes D, Blair A, Taylor PR. Physical activity and risk of cancer in the NHANES I population. *Am J Public Health* 1989;79:744.
18. Wannamethee SG, Shaper AG, Walker M. Physical activity and risk of cancer in middle-aged men. *Br J Cancer* 2001;85:131.
19. Gerhardsson M, Floderus B, Norell SE, et al. Physical activity and colon cancer risk. *Int J Epidemiol* 1988;17:743.
20. Lee IM, Paffenbarger RS Jr, Hsieh C. Physical activity and risk of developing colorectal cancer among college alumni. *J Natl Cancer Inst* 1991;83:1324.
21. Martinez ME, Giovannucci E, Spiegelman D, et al. Leisure-time physical activity, body size, and colon cancer in women. Nurses' Health Study Research Group. *J Natl Cancer Inst* 1997;89:948.
22. Thune I, Lund E. Physical activity and risk of colorectal cancer in men and women. *Br J Cancer* 1996;73:1134.
23. Nilsen TI, Vatten LJ. Prospective study of colorectal cancer risk and physical activity, diabetes, blood glucose and BMI: exploring the hyperinsulinaemia hypothesis. *Br J Cancer* 2001;84:417.
24. Colbert LH, Hartman TJ, Malila N, et al. Physical activity in relation to cancer of the colon and rectum in a cohort of male smokers. *Cancer Epidemiol Biomarkers Prev* 2001;10:265.
25. Slattery ML, Potter J, Caan B, et al. Energy balance and colon cancer—beyond physical activity. *Cancer Res* 1997;57:75.
26. Slattery ML, Edwards SL, Boucher KM, et al. Lifestyle and colon cancer: an assessment of factors associated with risk. *Am J Epidemiol* 1999;150:869.

27. Boutron-Ruault MC, Senesse P, Meance S, et al. Energy intake, body mass index, physical activity, and the colorectal adenoma-carcinoma sequence. *Nutr Cancer* 2001;39:50.

28. Colbert, LH, Lanza E, Ballard-Barbash R, et al. Adenomatous polyp recurrence and physical activity in the Polyp Prevention Trial (United States). *Cancer Causes Control* 2002;13:445.

29. Marcus PM, Newcomb PA, Storer BE, et al. Early adulthood physical activity and colon cancer risk among Wisconsin women. *Cancer Epidemiol Biomarkers Prev* 1994;3:641.

30. Lee IM, Paffenbarger RS Jr. Physical activity and its relation to cancer risk: a prospective study of college alumni. *Med Sci Sports Exerc* 1994;26:831.

31. Whittemore AS, AH Wu-Williams, Lee M, et al. Diet, physical activity, and colorectal cancer among Chinese in North America and China. *J Natl Cancer Inst* 1990;82:915.

32. Giovannucci E. Insulin, insulin-like growth factors and colon cancer: a review of the evidence. *J Nutr* 2001;131[Suppl 11]:3109S.

33. Frisch RE, Gotz-Welbergen AV, McArthur JW, et al. Delayed menarche and amenorrhea of college athletes in relation to age of onset of training. *JAMA* 1981;246:1559.

34. Frisch RE, Wyshak G, Vincent L. Delayed menarche and amenorrhea in ballet dancers. *N Engl J Med* 1980;303:17.

35. Malina RM, Spirduso WW, Tate C, et al. Age at menarche and selected menstrual characteristics in athletes at different competitive levels and in different sports. *Med Sci Sports* 1978;10:218.

36. Merzenich H, Boeing H, Wahrendorf J. Dietary fat and sports activity as determinants for age at menarche. *Am J Epidemiol* 1993;138:217.

37. Harlow SD, Matanoski GM. The association between weight, physical activity, and stress and variation in the length of the menstrual cycle. *Am J Epidemiol* 1991;133:38.

38. Cumming DC, Wheeler GD, Harber VJ. Physical activity, nutrition, and reproduction. *Ann N Y Acad Sci* 1994;709:55.

39. Russell JB, Mitchell D, Musey PI, et al. The relationship of exercise to anovulatory cycles in female athletes: hormonal and physical characteristics. *Obstet Gynecol* 1984;63:452.

40. Broocks A, Pirke KM, Schweiger U, et al. Cyclic ovarian function in recreational athletes. *J Appl Physiol* 1990;68:2083.

41. Brinton LA, Bernstein L, Colditz GA. Summary of the workshop: workshop on physical activity and breast cancer. *Cancer* 1998;83[Suppl 3]:595.

42. Siiteri PK. Adipose tissue as a source of hormones. *Am J Clin Nutr* 1987;45[Suppl 1]:277.

43. Friedenreich CM, Thune I. A review of physical activity and prostate cancer risk. *Cancer Causes Control* 2001;12:461.

44. Oliveria SA, Kohl HW 3rd, Trichopoulos D, et al. The association between cardiorespiratory fitness and prostate cancer. *Med Sci Sports Exerc* 1996;28:97.

45. Bairati I, Larouche R, Meyer F, et al. Lifetime occupational physical activity and incidental prostate cancer. *Cancer Causes Control* 2000;11:759.

46. Hartman TJ, Albanes D, Rautalahti M, et al. Physical activity and prostate cancer in the Alpha-Tocopherol, Beta-Carotene (ATBC) Cancer Prevention Study (Finland). *Cancer Causes Control* 1998;9:11.

47. Lew EA, Garfinkel L. Variations in mortality by weight among 750,000 men and women. *J Chronic Dis* 1979;32:563.

48. Calle EE, Rodriguez C, Walker-Thurmond K, et al. Overweight, obesity, and mortality from cancer in a prospectively studied cohort of U.S. adults. *N Engl J Med* 2003;348:1625.

49. Huang Z, Hankinson SE, Colditz GA, et al. Dual effects of weight and weight gain on breast cancer risk. *JAMA* 1997;278:1407.

50. Ursin G, Longnecker MP, Haile RW, et al. A meta-analysis of body mass index and risk of premenopausal breast cancer. *Epidemiology* 1995;6:137.

51. Rich-Edwards JW, Goldman MB, Willett WC, et al. Adolescent body mass index and infertility caused by ovulatory disorder. *Am J Obstet Gynecol* 1994;171:171.

52. Garland M, Hunter DJ, Colditz GA, et al. Menstrual cycle characteristics and history of ovulatory infertility in relation to breast cancer risk in a large cohort of U.S. women. *Am J Epidemiol* 1998;147:636.

53. van den Brandt PA, Spiegelman D, Yaun SS, et al. Pooled analysis of prospective cohort studies on height, weight, and breast cancer risk. *Am J Epidemiol* 2000;152:514.

54. Carpenter CL, Ross RK, Paganini-Hill A, et al. Effect of family history, obesity and exercise on breast cancer risk among postmenopausal women. *Int J Cancer* 2003;106:96.

55. Morimoto LM, White E, Chen Z, et al. Obesity, body size, and risk of postmenopausal breast cancer: the Women's Health Initiative (United States). *Cancer Causes Control* 2002; 13:741.

56. Kaaks R, Lukanova A, Kurzer MS. Obesity, endogenous hormones, and endometrial cancer risk: a synthetic review. *Cancer Epidemiol Biomarkers Prev* 2002;11:1531.

57. Giovannucci E. Insulin and colon cancer. *Cancer Causes Control* 1995;6:164.

58. McKeown-Eyssen G. Epidemiology of colorectal cancer revisited: are serum triglycerides and/or plasma glucose associated with risk? *Cancer Epidemiol Biomarkers Prev* 1994;3:687.

59. Slattery ML, Ballard-Barbash R, Edwards S, et al. Body mass index and colon cancer: an evaluation of the modifying effects of estrogen (United States). *Cancer Causes Control* 2003;14:75.

Richard M. Sherry

CHAPTER **21**

Cancer Prevention: Role of Surgery in Cancer Prevention

Prophylactic surgery, when performed properly in appropriate patients, can be extraordinarily effective in reducing the risk of cancer. It has long been recognized that certain conditions, such as inflammatory bowel disease and cryptorchidism, confer on patients an increased risk of developing fatal organ-specific malignancies. Rapid advances in molecular biology coupled with an increased appreciation that cancer is a genetic disorder have made accurate risk evaluation with genetic screening a reality for certain malignancies. As the understanding of cancer susceptibility has advanced, so too has the appreciation of the complexity of the associated social and clinical issues. Genetic evaluation for cancer susceptibility requires informed consent, sophisticated laboratory analysis, accurate risk assessment, knowledge of effective and investigational prevention strategies, and emotional support for affected patients and families.

That surgery can and should be used to prevent cancer is obvious (Table 21-1). The fact that colonoscopy can help to prevent colorectal cancer is now largely taken for granted.[1] Unfortunately, the evidence to support the use of other procedures is not as convincing. A critical challenge facing surgeons is to clearly define the role of prophylactic surgery in patients with organ-specific cancer susceptibility. This chapter focuses on the current use of surgery to prevent cancer.

MULTIPLE ENDOCRINE NEOPLASIA TYPE 2 AND FAMILIAL MEDULLARY THYROID CARCINOMA

Multiple endocrine neoplasia (MEN) is characterized by the development of multiple tumors in endocrine organs in a patient and close relatives. The syndrome is divided into MEN 1, MEN 2A, and MEN 2B. MEN 2 is defined by the combination of tissues affected and the presence of developmental abnormalities and has been the focus of extensive genetic analysis. MEN 2A is associated with medullary carcinoma of the thyroid and hyperparathyroidism. Individuals with MEN 2B have medullary carcinoma of the thyroid, pheochromocytoma, and developmental abnormalities involving hyperplasia of intestinal autonomic nerve plexuses and growth of nerve axons in the lips, oral mucosa, and conjunctiva, which gives rise to the characteristic facies. A syndrome related to MEN 2 is familial medullary thyroid carcinoma, in which patients have only medullary carcinoma of the thyroid. MEN 2A, MEN 2B, and familial medullary thyroid carcinoma have an autosomal dominant pattern of inheritance and account for approximately 25% of all cases of medullary carcinoma of the thyroid.[2]

In 1993, it was established that mutations in the RET protooncogene were responsible for the hereditary predisposition to medullary thyroid cancer.[3,4] This genetic breakthrough has allowed accurate identification of kindreds at high risk for developing medullary carcinoma of the thyroid and has permitted families to consider the risks and benefit of prophylactic thyroidectomy.

In 1994, Wells et al. reported the first experience with prophylactic thyroidectomy based on identification of RET protooncogene mutations.[5] Thirteen patients were confirmed to carry a mutation in the RET protooncogene in association with MEN 2A and underwent immediate thyroidectomy. In each patient, the resected thyroid gland demonstrated C-cell hyperplasia. There were no metastases found in regional nodes and all patients had normal postoperative stimulated plasma calcito-

TABLE 21-1. Prophylactic Surgery for the Prevention of Cancer

Clinical Condition	Associated Malignancy	Recommendations for Prophylactic Surgery
Multiple endocrine neoplasia 2A, 2B Familial medullary thyroid cancer	Medullary thyroid cancer	Timing of total thyroidectomy is based on specific RET protooncogene mutation.
Barrett's esophagus	Adenocarcinoma of the esophagus	Esophagectomy should be considered for healthy patients with high-grade dysplasia.
Hereditary diffuse gastric cancer	Gastric cancer	Rare. Surveillance may not be effective. Gastrectomy appears to be effective but has high long-term morbidity.
BRCA1 gene mutation BRCA2 gene mutation	Breast cancer	Bilateral total mastectomy is a reasonable option in selected patients.
	Ovarian cancer	Bilateral oophorectomy is recommended after childbearing or after age 35 y.
Ulcerative colitis	Colon cancer	Colectomy should be considered if dysplasia is present, at 10 y for patients with pancolitis, and at 20 y for most patients.
Familial adenomatous polyposis	Colon cancer	Colectomy is recommended in teenage years or earlier if polyps detected on endoscopy.
Hereditary non-polyposis colorectal cancer	Colon cancer	Surveillance colonoscopy and polypectomy reduces the risk of cancer. The role of prophylactic colectomy is controversial.
Cryptorchidism	Testicular cancer	Orchiectomy is recommended for a *nonpalpable* undescended testicle. Orchiopexy is recommended for most patients.

TABLE 21-2. RET Protooncogene Mutations and the Timing of Thyroid Surgery

Risk Stratification Level	Codon Mutations	Prophylactic Thyroidectomy
I	609, 630, 768, 790, 791, 768, 804, 891	Thyroidectomy by 5–10 y (incomplete consensus)
II	611, 618, 620, 634[a]	Thyroidectomy by 5 y Consideration of central node dissection
III	883, 918, 922, 634[a] All children with multiple endocrine neoplasia 2B	Thyroidectomy by 6 mo Central node dissection indicated

[a]Codon mutation associated with high risk of hyperthyroidism.

nin levels. Subsequent reports have confirmed the validity of this approach, and prophylactic thyroidectomy is now recommended for these patients at approximately age 6. Kebebew et al. reported a review of ten published series of patients who had prophylactic thyroidectomy for RET protooncogene germline mutations.[6] Two hundred nine patients were included in this review and only 3.4% of these patients had normal thyroid histologic findings. A central node dissection was performed on 139 of these patients, and 12 individuals (8.6%) were found to have cervical node metastases. These 12 patients ranged in age from 14 to 70 years. Overall, the morbidity from total thyroidectomy was low. These investigators have recommended that a central node dissection be included when prophylactic total thyroidectomy is performed for patients with RET protooncogene mutations.

Over the last decade, the molecular genetics of this disorder have been delineated, and it is now clear that specific codon muta-

tions of RET correlate with the aggressiveness of the thyroid malignancy. This fact has important implications for the timing and extent of prophylactic thyroid surgery. In 2001, the Seventh International Workshop published a consensus statement on the relevance of specific RET protooncogene mutations.[7] Based largely on the age at which patients showed malignant changes and the risk of associated nodal metastasis, patients with specific mutations were assigned to one of three risk levels as identified in Table 21-2. The recommendation was that children at risk level III undergo a thyroidectomy with a central node dissection within the first 6 months and preferably within the first month of life. Children at risk level II should undergo thyroidectomy by age 5, and most surgeons recommended that a central node dissection be included in the procedure. No consensus was reached on the management of children at risk level I; some experts recommended thyroidectomy for these patients by age 5 to 10 years, whereas others recommended surgery only after abnormal results on pentagastrin-stimulated computed tomographic testing.[7] The Seventh International Workshop on MEN classified patients with mutations in codon 634 at risk level II, whereas other investigators have reported it to be a more aggressive phenotype. Specific RET protooncogenes can also be used to assess the risk of developing the other manifestations associated with this syndrome, including hyperparathyroidism and pheochromocytoma.[8]

Thyroidectomy has rapidly become the treatment of choice for patients with RET protooncocogene mutations, and if it is performed at an appropriate age, the cure rate should be 100%. The identification and management of patients with a RET protooncocogene is perhaps the best example of prophylactic surgery in patients known to be at risk for an inherited malignancy. Genetic testing allows the accurate identification of patients at high risk of developing invasive cancer. The organ at risk can be surgically removed with low morbidity.

BARRETT'S ESOPHAGUS AND ESOPHAGEAL CANCER

Barrett's esophagus is a premalignant condition in which the stratified squamous epithelium in the distal esophagus is replaced to a variable extent by metaplastic columnar epithelium. This is significant from an oncologic perspective because of the close association between Barrett's esophagus and the development of adenocarcinoma of the esophagus. This association has taken on increased significance because of the recent and rapid rise in the incidence of this malignancy and because survival in advanced stages is poor.[9,10]

Barrett's esophagus develops as a sequela of chronic inflammation caused by reflux of gastric contents, including acid, pepsin, and bile acids. Esophageal motility studies and pH monitoring suggest that these patients exhibit weak lower esophageal sphincter tone and slow clearance of gastric acid.[11–15] Although Barrett's esophagus can be recognized or suspected based on the appearance of the esophagus on endoscopy, a definitive diagnosis must be based on biopsy and histologic analysis. The histologic features of Barrett's esophagus include a demonstration of goblet cells interspersed among mucin-type columnar cells. This represents the so-called specialized columnar epithelium and is pathognomonic of the process.[16]

The incidence of Barrett's esophagus is difficult to determine. The majority of individuals with Barrett's esophagus in the general population are probably asymptomatic and therefore do not seek medical attention.[17]

Historically, Barrett's esophagus has been taken to mean the presence of specialized columnar epithelium that was determined to be over 3 cm in length, and consequently much of the published information regarding the incidence and natural history was generated by analysis of the data from patients with long segments of diseased tissue. It is now recognized that intestinal metaplasia of less than 3 cm should be classified as Barrett's syndrome. It has been reported that up to 33% of all patients undergoing upper endoscopy may have histologic evidence of Barrett's esophagus.[18–21] Approximately 10% of patients with frequent reflux symptoms are identified as having a long segment of Barrett's esophagus.[22]

Numerous reports have confirmed that patients with Barrett's esophagus are at increased risk for developing adenocarcinoma of the esophagus.[10,23–25] Intestinal metaplasia can be detected in the mucosa adjacent to virtually all adenocarcinomas of the esophagus and in most adenocarcinomas of the gastric cardia.[26] In a review of 18 published series, Tytgat estimated the median incidence of esophageal adenocarcinoma in patients with Barrett's esophagus to be approximately one cancer per 100 patient-years of follow-up. The overall risk was approximately 40 times higher than that in the general population.[24] The annual rate of cancer development in these patients is low and is estimated to be approximately 0.8%.[23] Information on the risk of developing adenocarcinoma in short segments (less than 3 cm) of Barrett's esophagus is more limited, but data suggest that the presence of such segments is associated with significant potential for malignant degeneration.[10,23]

Epithelial dysplasia is the best indicator of the risk of cancer and is an important clinical factor used to stratify patients with Barrett's esophagus. The Practice Parameters Committee of the American College of Gastroenterology reviewed the collective experience of 783 patients from one registry and the five centers that have performed prospective studies on the natural history of dysplasia. Patients were followed for 2.7 to 7.3 years. Nine of 382 (2%) were followed from no dysplasia to cancer and 5 of 72 patients (7%) were followed from low-grade dysplasia to cancer.[27] Dent et al. reviewed eight published series and reported the outcome of 50 patients with high-grade dysplasia in Barrett's esophagus. These individuals were followed for up to 5 years, and adenocarcinoma developed in 16 patients

(32%). Eleven patients had a resection for dysplasia with no malignancy found in the specimen.[28]

Several factors must be considered before this information is incorporated into clinical decisions for patients with Barrett's esophagus. First, it is clear that not all high-grade dysplasia will progress to cancer, and regression of a short segment of Barrett's esophagus that contained high-grade dysplasia has been reported.[29,30] Second, sampling errors are always a concern in this situation. Finally, the pathologic analysis for these cases can be problematic because of observer variation in the grading of dysplasia.

EFFECT OF TREATMENT ON CANCER RISK

Most patients with reflux are treated medically with weight reduction, elevation of the head of the bed, and administration of H_2-receptor antagonists or proton pump inhibitors. The goal of therapy is symptomatic relief of gastroesophageal reflux. Although symptoms of reflux often improve with therapy, there is no evidence to suggest that medical therapy will consistently induce regression of the metaplastic columnar epithelium.[31–33] Evidence is conflicting regarding the efficacy of antireflux surgery to reverse or prevent malignant transformations in patients with Barrett's esophagus. Two small prospective randomized trials have been reported that showed no differences between medical and surgical therapy with respect to preventing Barrett's esophagus from progressing to dysplasia or cancer.[34,35] Unfortunately, given the natural history of Barrett's esophagus, these studies were not sufficiently powered to detect realistic differences in the rate of malignant transformation. Several retrospective studies have documented that Barrett's esophagus can regress after antireflux surgery. Gurski et al. reported on 77 patients with Barrett's who underwent antireflux surgery and noted that 17 of 25 patients (68%) demonstrated regression from low-grade dysplasia to nondysplastic Barrett's esophagus and that 11 of 52 patients (21.2%) showed regression from intestinal metaplasia to normal. Eight patients (10%) progressed to low- or high-grade dysplasia.[36] Oelschlager et al. reported that 30 of 54 patients (55%) with short segment Barrett's esophagus and 0 of 36 patients with long segment Barrett's esophagus demonstrated complete resolution of intestinal metaplasia after laparoscopic antireflux surgery.[37] The long-term impact of these procedures has yet to be determined. The role for antireflux procedures in preventing adenocarcinoma of the esophagus remains controversial. The optimal management of Barrett's esophagus has not been established. Although no complete agreement exists regarding the best approach for these patients, most experts rely on the degree of dysplasia associated with Barrett's esophagus to guide treatment recommendations.

BARRETT'S ESOPHAGUS WITHOUT DYSPLASIA

Esophagectomy has no role in the management of patients who have Barrett's esophagus and no evidence of dysplasia. The clinical issues for these patients concern the efficacy of screening and the role of antireflux surgery. Most patients who are healthy enough to be considered surgical candidates are enrolled into surveillance programs. The current recommendation for patients with Barrett's esophagus without dysplasia is to perform endoscopic surveillance and biopsy every 3 years.[27]

BARRETT'S ESOPHAGUS WITH LOW-GRADE DYSPLASIA

Esophagectomy has no role in the treatment of patients with low-grade dysplasia associated with Barrett's esophagus. Clearly the risks of developing severe dysplasia or adenocarcinoma of the esophagus are significant. The current recommendation for healthy patients with low-grade dysplasia associated with Barrett's esophagus is to undergo histologic surveillance every 6 to 12 months. The role of antireflux surgery is controversial. Innovative techniques such as mucosal ablation, photodynamic therapy, and chemoprevention are under active investigation.[27]

BARRETT'S ESOPHAGUS WITH HIGH-GRADE DYSPLASIA

Most experts recommend that healthy patients with high-grade dysplasia undergo esophagectomy by an experienced surgeon. The pathologic diagnosis should be independently confirmed.[25,28,38] Because there is a wide spectrum of reported mortality after esophagectomy (1.4% to 21.0%) and because not all patients with high-grade dysplasia develop adenocarcinoma, some experts have made a case for aggressive surveillance for these patients. Levine et al. described and reported on an aggressive biopsy protocol in which up to 12 biopsy specimens were collected per centimeter of Barrett's mucosa in patients with high-grade dysplasia. Seventy patients with high-grade dysplasia were followed, and 12 were found to have early-stage adenocarcinoma of the esophagus within an average of 2 months after the diagnosis. Of the remaining 58 patients, 15 (23%) progressed to early-stage cancer after an average of 1.1 years of follow-up. None of the remaining 43 patients (74%) developed cancer when followed an average of 2.5 years.[39,40] These results have not been confirmed at other institutions. It should be noted that over 25% of these patients developed esophageal adenocarcinoma. In addition, the described surveillance protocol may be impractical for most physicians to follow.

The recommendation for surgery or surveillance must weigh the mortality and morbidity of esophagectomy against the risk and expected prognosis associated with invasive cancer. Most surgical series report an operative mortality of less than 10% when esophagectomy is performed for malignant disease. The mortality for prophylactic esophagectomy may be lower than the mortality associated with surgery for malignant disease because many patients with malignant disease are debilitated. In addition, prophylactic esophagectomy does not require an extensive nodal dissection. Either a transhiatal or multi-incisional approach with cervical anastomosis appears to be appropriate. The 5-year survival for patients undergoing esophagectomy for known invasive cancer is estimated to be 18% to 32%.[41] The survival of patients with invasive adenocarcinoma detected during a rigorous surveillance program is likely higher.

HEREDITARY DIFFUSE GASTRIC CANCER

In 1998, Guilford et al. reported that three germline mutations in the E-cadherin gene (CDH1) were found in kindreds of Maori families from New Zealand who had early onset of poorly differentiated diffuse gastric cancer.[42] The E-cadherin gene is located on chromosome band 16q22.1, and its normal protein product is an adhesion molecule involved in the differentiation and architecture of epithelial tissues.[43] Since then, other CDH1 mutations have been found in other families with diffuse gastric cancer. It has become clear that a small percentage of gastric cancers (1% to 3%) arise as a result of this inherited syndrome.

Germline mutations in the E-cadherin gene are inherited as autosomal dominant traits with high penetrance. Estimates are that affected individuals have a lifetime risk of developing gastric cancer of approximately 70%, and patients with this syndrome have developed gastric cancer as early as age 18. In 1999, the International Gastric Cancer Linkage Consortium published guidelines to facilitate the diagnosis and management of this syndrome.[44] Diagnosis of the clinical syndrome requires that two or more cases of diffuse gastric cancer be identified in first- or second-degree relatives with at least one case diagnosed before age 50, or that three or more confirmed cases of diffuse gastric cancer be identified in first- or second-degree relatives. Oliveira reported that 36% of families that met the clinical criteria for hereditary diffuse gastric cancer syndrome in fact had documented CDH1 germline mutations.[148]

The optimal management of patients with hereditary diffuse gastric cancer has not been defined. Endoscopic screening for diffuse gastric cancer is problematic because early abnormalities may not be visible as masses and these tumors tend to spread along the submucosa. Multiple reports suggest that prophylactic total gastrectomy may be effective in preventing gastric cancer. However, the estimated mortality of total gastrectomy is 1% to 2%, and acute morbidity rates are 10% to 20% with 100% long-term morbidity related to weight loss and abnormalities in intestinal transit, including dumping and diarrhea. That patients may develop gastric cancer by age 18 suggests that prophylactic surgery may be indicated at an early age. It is recommended that patients electing not to have prophylactic gastrectomy undergo endoscopy every 6 to 12 months.

COLORECTAL CANCER

Approximately 75% of all colorectal cancers occur in patients with no known risk factors for colon cancer. Individuals with ulcerative colitis, familial polyposis, and hereditary nonpolyposis colon cancer are at increased risk for developing the disease, but these patients probably account for fewer than 10% of all colorectal cancer cases. Despite the low incidence of these conditions in the general population, understanding and managing these patients has provided insights into the etiology of cancer and the potential role of surgery in the prevention of cancer.

ULCERATIVE COLITIS

Ulcerative colitis is a nonspecific inflammatory bowel disease of unknown etiology that involves the rectum, usually all or part of the colon, and frequently the distal terminal ileum as a result of colonic reflux. The clinical course of ulcerative colitis is variable, ranging from intermittent to chronic, and the severity of attacks also varies widely from mild to fulminant. The incidence of ulcerative colitis is relatively low at approximately 8 to 15 cases per 100,000 people.[45–48] From an oncologic perspective ulcerative colitis is important because of its association with colorectal cancer. Although only a small fraction of colon cancer occurs in the setting of ulcerative colitis, colorectal cancer is the major cause of the increased morbidity and mortality of patients with this inflammatory disease.[48-50]

It is difficult to precisely determine the risk of colorectal cancer in patients with ulcerative colitis. Most studies, but not all,[51,52] have noted a significant increase in the risk of colorectal cancer in this population. The duration of disease and the extent of colonic involvement at the time of diagnosis are the most important clinical factors that determine the degree of increased cancer risk. In patients with pancolitis, the cancer risk is approximately 0.5% to 1% per year after 10 years of disease.[53] Disease duration of 20 years in patients with pancolitis is associated with an estimated cumulative incidence of malignancy of between 5% and 35%.[48,54,55] The cumulative risk of malignancy increases over time and is reported to be as high as 75% after 40 years of disease.[56]

Patients with pancolitis are known to be at higher risk for cancer development than patients with left-sided colitis. Ulcerative colitis limited to the left colon is associated with an estimated cumulative incidence of cancer of between 1% and 5% at 20 years.[48,55,57] Patients with only proctitis appear to be at only average risk for colorectal cancer compared with the general population.[55] There is evidence that the risk of developing colon cancer is higher for patients with both ulcerative colitis and primary sclerosing cholangitis and for those with a family history of colon cancer.[58,59]

Treatment recommendations for patients with long-standing ulcerative colitis vary from prophylactic colectomy after 10 to 20 years of disease to vigilant surveillance with colonoscopic examination and multiple random biopsies to exclude dysplasia. In the latter strategy colectomy is recommended based on the presence and degree of dysplasia. The differences in management strategies are not surprising given the heterogeneous nature of inflammatory bowel disease and the patient population and the absence of randomized clinical trials to support one strategy over another.

Agreement is widespread that colonic dysplasia is a strong but imperfect marker for identifying patients likely to develop colorectal cancer. Colonic surveillance is performed on the assumption that a dysplastic lesion can be detected before invasive cancer has developed. Invasive cancer can be found in approximately 10% of patients with ulcerative colitis at initial screening. Patients with no dysplasia identified in a biopsy specimen have a 3% cumulative risk of developing cancer when followed over time. Patients found to have indefinite or low-grade dysplasia are thought to progress to invasive cancer or severe dysplasia between 16% and 54% of the time. Forty percent to 45% of patients with ulcerative colitis identified as having high-grade dysplasia or dysplasia associated with a mucosal mass develop colorectal cancer. Many of these patients already have evidence of nodal metastasis.[60-62] One must also recognize that, although the risk of developing colorectal cancer in the absence of histologic evidence of dysplasia appears to be low, up to 25% of patients with ulcerative colitis–associated invasive cancer demonstrate no dysplasia in the resected specimens.[61,63,64]

There are no well-controlled trials that confirm the efficacy of colonic surveillance in reducing the mortality of ulcerative colitis–associated colorectal cancer. Lennard-Jones reviewed four published series that included 423 patients who were screened regularly by colonoscopy over a period of 12 to 15 years. Eleven patients underwent surgery for precancerous lesions, and only three Dukes' A lesions and one Dukes' B lesion were found. No cancer deaths occurred during the surveillance period. The author suggested that surveillance colonoscopy should be performed only in individuals with long-standing ulcerative colitis involving the entire colon.[64]

Despite the limitations and lack of data to support surveillance for colonic dysplasia, physicians appear reluctant to recommend prophylactic colectomy for patients with long-standing ulcerative colitis. The fact that surgery can eliminate the symptoms of ulcerative colitis, including bleeding, diarrhea, anemia, steroid dependence, and the need for cyclosporin therapy, as well as eliminate the risk of colorectal cancer, may be underappreciated. Several surgical alternatives are available for patients undergoing colectomy, and the operation should be tailored to the individual as well as the clinical situation. For example, in the setting of acute colitis, most surgeons recommend a subtotal colectomy and ileostomy. In the elective surgical setting, many options are available, including proctocolectomy and ileostomy, colectomy and ileorectal anastomosis (assuming the rectum is free of inflammation), proctocolectomy and Kock continent ileostomy, and ileal pouch–anal anastomosis. Each procedure is associated with reported complications; however, surgery for ulcerative colitis is extremely safe for most patients, and the reported operative mortality is less than 1% even in the emergency setting.[65] Although comparison of the outcomes of each procedure is difficult and controlled studies do not exist, most patients report a high quality of life regardless of the procedure performed. Obviously surgical options should be tailored to the individual patient.

It is evident that some consideration should be given to colectomy 10 years after the diagnosis of ulcerative colitis in patients with pancolitis. After a 20-year disease interval, a stronger case can be made for prophylactic colectomy even in the absence of dysplasia. Colonic surveillance for dysplasia is an option favored by many clinicians and is most appropriate for patients with disease limited to the left colon or rectum and for patients with a short duration of disease. Any surveillance strategy that recommends colectomy based solely on histologic evidence of dysplasia will miss some patients with invasive cancer. The precise number of patients in this situation is unknown. If surveillance is the strategy adopted, then the recommendation is that in the absence of dysplasia colonoscopy and multiple biopsies be performed every 2 years until the patient has had the disease for 20 years. After 20 years of disease, surveillance colonoscopy should be performed annually.[62]

HEREDITARY COLORECTAL CANCER

Estimates are that up to 20% of patients with colorectal cancer may have some form of inherited susceptibility.[66] Hereditary colon cancer currently includes familial adenomatous polyposis (FAP) and hereditary nonpolyposis colorectal cancer (HNPCC).

FAMILIAL ADENOMATOUS POLYPOSIS

FAP is a rare disease with an autosomal dominant mode of inheritance, in which patients develop hundreds to thousands of adenomatous polyps. The clinical diagnosis is based on the histologic confirmation of at least 100 adenomas. These polyps are similar on histologic examination to sporadic adenomatous polyps and usually appear during the second or third decade of life.[67] The genetic cause of FAP is a mutation of the adenomatous polyposis coli (APC) gene located on chromosome 5 (5q21).[68] The genetic alterations found in patients with FAP are similar to those identified in sporadic colon cancer except that an APC mutation is present as a germline mutation.[69] Approximately 25% of all cases have been attributed to new sporadic mutations in the APC gene and thus show no family history of colon cancer.[70] Genetic tests for APC mutations are commercially available.

The obvious phenotypic appearance of FAP, coupled with the fact that over 90% of patients with FAP will develop colon cancer by age 40, has helped to establish standard treatment for this disease.[71] Elective prophylactic colectomy is the current mainstay of therapy and has been performed for FAP since the 1930s. There are no trials that compare surgery with surveillance. The current recommendations for treatment of this genetic disorder include annual sigmoidoscopy beginning by age 10 and prophylactic colectomy in the teenage years or when colonic polyps are detected at endoscopy.[72]

The choice of operations for patients with FAP includes proctocolectomy with ileostomy, proctocolectomy with ileal distal rectal anastomosis, and proctocolectomy with ileal-anal anastomosis. Each of these operations has strengths and weaknesses. Overall these procedures are performed with low morbidity. The operation of choice is proctocolectomy and ileoanal pouch. Patients with relatively few polyps may elect to have colectomy and ileorectal anastomosis. Estimates of the risk of rectal cancer after subtotal colectomy vary widely and have been reported to be as high as 55% at 30 years. Patients with ileorectal anastomosis require lifelong endoscopic surveillance. The choice of operation should be based on patient preference and the experience of the operating surgeon.

FAP is associated with extracolonic manifestations of disease. These can include desmoid tumors and osteomas. Polyps occur at other intestinal locations, and carcinomas of the upper intestine have been reported as the most common fatal malignancy in patients after prophylactic colectomy.[73] It is recommended that these patients undergo upper endoscopy every 6 months to 3 years starting by age 20.[72] Many agents, including sulindac, vitamin C, and indomethacin, have been investigated as chemopreventive agents. Although some agents have shown promise, none has been proven to be effective in reducing the number of polyps or the risk of cancer in these patients.[74]

HEREDITARY NONPOLYPOSIS COLORECTAL CANCER

HNPCC is a clinical syndrome of colorectal cancer that occurs with early onset and in multiple family members. This syndrome is the most common form of hereditary colorectal cancer, accounting for up to 5% of all colorectal cancers. In contrast to FAP, HNPCC has no antecedent phenotype, and malignancy develops in the absence of adenomatosis of the colon and rectum. The expression of disease may be limited to the colorectum (Lynch's syndrome type I) or coexist with extracolonic tumors, typically endometrial cancer (Lynch's syndrome type II). Other associated malignancies include stomach, small intestine, hepatobiliary, pancreas, breast, ovary, brain, and skin cancers.[75–78]

In 1991, the International Collaborative Group on Hereditary Non-Polyposis Colorectal Cancer established the minimum clinical criteria required to identify families with HNPCC. The Amsterdam criteria are: (1) colorectal cancer in three or more relatives, one of whom is the first-degree relative of the other two; (2) at least two generations of individuals affected with colorectal cancer; and (3) diagnosis of one or more of the cancers before the age of 50. FAP must be excluded.[79] When the predisposition for extracolonic cancers was fully appreciated, these criteria were expanded to include the occurrence of colorectal cancer in at least two family members and endometrial cancer in one family member over at least two generations.[80] The genetic basis of HNPCC has been identified as a germline mutation in one of a set of genes responsible for DNA mismatch repair.[81–85] More than 90% of the identified mutations are in two genes, hMSH2 and hMLH1, located on chromosome arms 2p and 3p, respectively, but multiple additional loci have since been identified.[86] These genes are dominantly inherited with a penetrance of approximately 90%. Consequently, gene carriers have a 90% likelihood of developing colorectal cancer.[87]

Another consequence of defects in mismatch repair genes is the accumulation of mutations in the microsatellite regions of DNA. Microsatellites are tandemly repeated DNA sequences located in noncoding regions of DNA. Mutations in mismatch repair genes lead to variability in the lengths of microsatellite regions. Microsatellite instability is a consequence of defects in mismatch repair genes and thus can be used as a screening tool for HNPCC.[89] This test can be performed on paraffin-embedded tissue or blood, and many experts recommend that initial screening for HNPCC be done with microsatellite instability testing. Patients suspected of carrying an APC mutation can also be tested for mismatch repair gene mutations by commercial laboratories.

HNPCC gene carriers develop colorectal cancer at an average of age 45 years. These tumors occur more commonly in the right colon and tend to be poorly differentiated.[90,91] Synchronous and metachronous cancers are frequent, and should a segmental colectomy be performed for a primary cancer, there is a 45% risk for a new primary cancer within 10 years.[87] Lynch and Smyrk have reported that colonic polyps can be identified in up to 17% of first-degree relatives of cancer patients during colonoscopic screening.[92] Adenomas are more likely to grow and progress to invasive cancer in this patient population than in the general population.[93,94]

Substantial evidence from uncontrolled studies suggests that surveillance colonoscopy and polypectomy is effective in reducing the risk of invasive cancer in these patients. Jarvinen et al. reported a 62% decrease in the diagnosis of colorectal cancer in HNPCC patients followed in a screening program at a medium follow-up of 117 months compared with patients not followed by colonoscopy at 10 years.[94] It has been recommended that surveillance colonoscopy be performed on gene carriers starting at age 20 and be repeated every 1 to 2 years.[95] Patients older than 35 years of age should have annual colonoscopy.[87,96]

Currently, no consensus exists among experts regarding the role of prophylactic subtotal colectomy for patients with HNPCC.[87,97] Given the high penetrance of the disorder and the high rate of synchronous and metachronous disease among mutation carriers, a strong case can be made for prophylactic surgery in patients with this disease. A subtotal colectomy is currently the procedure of choice, and this can be performed with minimal morbidity and mortality. Patients who elect to undergo a subtotal colectomy require colonoscopic surveillance of the remaining rectum. Patients undergoing prophylactic surgery may still face the risk of extracolonic cancers. Patients electing not to undergo prophylactic surgery must commit to lifelong surveillance, and should a colon cancer be detected, a subtotal colectomy is then indicated. There are no prospective clinical trials comparing different treatment strategies in patients with HNPCC. Given the current understanding of the increased risk of colorectal and extracolonic malignancy in these patients, the suggested benefit of surveillance colonoscopy, and the low morbidity of prophylactic subtotal colectomy, either vigilant surveillance or prophylactic surgery is a reasonable management option.

BREAST CANCER

Estimates are that 5% to 10% of women with breast cancer have hereditary breast cancer.[98–101] BRCA1 was identified on the long arm of chromosome 17 (17q21) in 1990, and over 500 different mutations in this gene have been identified.[99–101] BRCA1 is transmitted as an autosomal dominant gene with high penetrance, so that 50% of the children of carriers inherit the trait. It has been estimated that women with a BRCA1 gene mutation have a 56% to 85% lifetime risk of developing breast cancer.[101,102] Frequently these patients develop invasive cancer before the age of 50.[103] A second breast cancer susceptibility gene, BRCA2, has been identified and localized to the long arm of chromosome 13 (13q12-13).[104–106] Women with BRCA2 germline mutations are estimated to have a lifetime risk of breast cancer that is similar to that of BRCA1 carriers.

The management strategy for patients with BRCA1 and BRCA2 mutations must be individualized. The clinical options for these patients are obvious and include increased surveillance, chemoprevention, and prophylactic bilateral total mastectomy. There are no prospective trials that compare these options. Clearly, counseling regarding any option must take into account the uncertainties associated with the estimation of cancer risk, the lack of definitive research regarding risk, and the social, medical, and psychological status of the patient. Ideally these factors should be reviewed during counseling that occurs before genetic screening.

The most obvious management strategy and one that appears currently to be most popular among clinicians is to depend on increased surveillance of patients with BRCA1 or BRCA2 mutations. This approach is based on the assumption that an invasive cancer will be detected at an early stage that is associated with a good prognosis. The current recommendation for surveillance in these women includes monthly self-examination beginning by age 18, annual or semiannual clinician breast examination, and annual mammography beginning at age 25 to 35.[107]

These recommendations reflect a common-sense approach to attempt to reduce the risk of breast cancer–related mortality. Unfortunately, evidence to support such a strategy is limited. A randomized trial that assessed the efficacy of breast self-examination showed no difference in the stage of detected cancers and no reduction in mortality from breast cancer in the cohort

trained in self-examination.[108] The sensitivity of breast cancer examination by a clinician varies widely based on tumor size, breast density, and the experience of the examiner.[109,110] Palpation of a breast mass smaller than 10 mm is problematic even for the most experienced clinician.

Mammography has been firmly established to reduce breast cancer mortality by up to 30% to 40% for women aged 50 to 70 years.[111] For women 40 to 49 years of age, findings on the benefit of mammography have been inconsistent.[112–114] Screening mammography has not been effective in younger women because the density of their breast tissue limits the quality of the radiograph. The sensitivity and specificity of mammography for detecting nonpalpable breast cancers in young women with BRCA1 or BRCA2 mutations are unknown. Breast magnetic resonance imaging has shown promise in detecting abnormalities not detected by mammography, but its use as a screening tool remains investigational.

Tamoxifen therapy is effective for women with breast cancer in the adjuvant and metastatic settings and has been shown to reduce the incidence of breast cancer in women considered to be at high risk. The evidence that tamoxifen is of benefit to women with BRCA1 and BRCA2 mutations is less clear. Narod et al. reported a matched case-control study that compared cancer risk in 209 women with BRCA1 and BRCA2 mutations and with bilateral breast cancer to that in 384 mutation carriers with unilateral disease. The use of tamoxifen was associated with a 50% decrease in the risk of developing cancer in the contralateral breast. Interestingly, chemotherapy and oophorectomy were also associated with a reduced risk of contralateral breast cancer.[115] The National Surgical Adjuvant Breast and Bowel Project Breast Cancer Prevention Trial found that tamoxifen treatment reduced the incidence of breast cancer in healthy BRCA2 carriers by 62% but was of no benefit for women with BRCA1 mutations.[116] Despite this uncertainty, most physicians recommend tamoxifen to women with both BRCA1 and BRCA2 mutations.[117]

Because breast tumors are sensitive to hormone manipulation and women with BRCA1 and BRCA2 mutations are at risk for both breast and ovarian malignancy, the relationship between prophylactic oophorectomy and breast cancer has generated considerable interest. As part of a study of 259 BRCA1 and BRCA2 carriers who had undergone bilateral prophylactic oophorectomy, the Prevention and Observation of Surgical End Points Study Group analyzed cancer incidence in a subset of 99 women with BRCA1 or BRCA2 mutations with no history of breast cancer or prophylactic mastectomy who had undergone bilateral prophylactic oophorectomy and compared it with the incidence in 142 matched control mutation carriers with no history of breast cancer or oophorectomy (Table 21-3). After an average follow-up of more than 10 years, there was a 21.2% incidence of breast cancer in the prophylactic oophorectomy group and a 42.3% incidence in the control group (hazard ratio, 0.47; 95% confidence interval, 0.29 to 0.77). Only the first primary breast cancer was considered in calculating the risk reduction.[118]

Prophylactic mastectomy is another option for reducing breast cancer risk. This procedure had fallen out of favor because of multiple case reports of breast cancer after prophylactic mastectomy combined with a lack of credible evidence to support the efficacy of the intervention. Breast tissue can be detected in the areas of the chest wall, axilla, and abdomen that are distant to the typical surgical field during subcutane-

TABLE 21-3. Bilateral Prophylactic Oophorectomy in BRCA1 and BRCA2 Mutation Carriers

	Total Patients: 551		
	S/P Oophorectomy Group	*Matched Control Group*	*Risk Reduction*
No. of patients	259	292	—
Observed cases of ovarian cancer	8 (3.08%)	58 (19.9%)	—
Diagnosed at surgery	6 (2.3%)	—	Hazard ratio, 0.04
Diagnosed on follow-up	2 (0.8%)	—	(95% CI, 0.01–0.16)

	Total Patients: 241 (Subset Analysis of Patients with No History of Breast Cancer or Prophylactic Mastectomy)		
	S/P Oophorectomy Group	*Matched Control Group*	*Risk Reduction*
No. of patients	99	142	—
Observed cases of breast cancer	21 (21%)	60 (42.3%)	Hazard ratio, 0.47
			(95% CI, 0.29–0.77)

CI, confidence interval; S/P, status post.

ous or total mastectomy. Residual breast tissue remains after mastectomy, with larger amounts of breast tissue presumed to be present after subcutaneous mastectomy than after total mastectomy.[119–121]

Hartmann et al. published a retrospective study based on the Mayo Clinic experience with prophylactic mastectomy that strongly suggested that prophylactic mastectomy reduces the incidence of breast cancer in women at high risk for developing invasive cancer[122] (Table 21-4). The study included 639 women who had undergone prophylactic mastectomy between 1960 and 1993. Patients were categorized into either a high-risk or moderate-risk group based on family history. The high-risk cohort had a family history that suggested an autosomal dominant predisposition to breast cancer. All other women were considered to be at moderate risk for developing breast cancer. A control study group of sisters was used for the analysis of the high-risk probands. The Gail model was used to predict the expected number of breast cancers and breast cancer–related deaths for women in the moderate-risk group. The authors found that 4 breast cancers developed in the 425 patients with moderate risk, whereas the Gail model predicted 37.4 cases of cancer. In the high-risk group, 3 of 214 women developed breast cancer after prophylactic mastectomy. Among their 403 sisters who had not undergone a prophylactic mastectomy, 115 cases of breast cancer were diagnosed before their sibling's decision to undergo prophylactic surgery, 38 cases were diagnosed after their sibling's decision to have prophylactic surgery, and the time of diagnosis was unknown in 3 cases. The authors concluded that bilateral prophylactic mastectomy was associated with at least a 90% reduction in the incidence of breast cancer in these women. Women in both the high-risk cohort and moderate-risk cohort appeared to have a significant reduction in the risk of dying from breast cancer after prophylactic surgery.

TABLE 21-4. Efficacy of Bilateral Prophylactic Mastectomy in Women with a Family History of Breast Cancer: Mayo Clinic Experience, 1960 to 1993

	Patients at High Risk for Breast Cancer (Family History Suggesting Inherited Breast Cancer)		
	Patients Undergoing BPM	*Female Sibling Controls*	*Reduction in Risk*
No. of patients	214	403	—
Observed cases of breast cancer	3 (1.4%)	156 (38%)	90%
		115 before sibling's BPM	
		38 after sibling's BPM	
		3 diagnosis date unknown	
Observed deaths from breast cancer	2	10.5–19.4[a]	81–94%

	Patients at Moderate Risk for Breast Cancer (All Other Patients Electing BPM)		
	Patients Undergoing BPM	*Gail Model Prediction[b]*	*Reduction in Risk*
No. of patients	425		—
Observed cases of breast cancer	4 (0.9%)	Expected cases 37.4	89.5%
Observed deaths from breast cancer	0	Expected deaths 10.4	70–100%

BPM, bilateral prophylactic mastectomy.
[a]Adjusted for ascertainment bias.
[b]The Gail model was used to predict the incidence and risk of death from breast cancer.

Interestingly, all seven women who developed breast cancer after prophylactic surgery had undergone bilateral subcutaneous mastectomy. No patient who had bilateral total mastectomy developed breast cancer (7 of 575 vs. 0 of 64; *P* = .38). Most experts recommend bilateral total mastectomy as the procedure of choice for patients who choose prophylactic mastectomy.

A report by Robson et al. provides additional support for preventive surgery.[123] These investigators followed women of Ashkenazi Jewish descent who underwent lumpectomy and radiation therapy for invasive breast cancer. Outcomes were compared for women with and without a BRCA1 or BRCA2 mutation. Women with BRCA1 or BRCA2 mutations were more likely to develop ipsilateral local cancer recurrence, although this difference was not statistically significant. Women with mutations were also significantly more likely to have cancer before the age of 50, were more likely to develop contralateral breast cancer, and were more likely to have metastatic nodal involvement. Distant disease-free survival and breast cancer–specific survival was shorter for women with a BRCA1 or BRCA2 mutation (fewer women alive at 10 years).

Reconstructive surgical techniques that include autologous tissue transfer have dramatically improved the cosmetic results of breast surgery. Although the surgical morbidity associated with bilateral mastectomy is low, it is inevitably increased when breast reconstruction is added. The psychological effects of prophylactic surgery in patients have not been completely evaluated. There is evidence that women receive a psychological benefit because of a reduced fear of developing breast cancer but that body image and sexual relationships are adversely affected.[124]

Bilateral prophylactic mastectomy is currently the most effective risk reduction strategy for women with BRCA1 and BRCA2 mutations. Although prophylactic oophorectomy dramatically reduces the incidence of breast cancer in mutation carriers, over 20% of these patients are likely to develop a breast malignancy. There is a clear need to define and then to improve the efficacy of surveillance strategies and chemoprevention. Until more accurate clinical information is available, women must be counseled based on the limited information at hand.

LOBULAR CARCINOMA *IN SITU*

Lobular carcinoma *in situ* (LCIS) is a histopathologic entity characterized by cellular proliferation originating in the lobules and terminal ducts of the breast. Women found to have LCIS on analysis of breast biopsy specimens are known to be at increased risk of developing invasive ductal and lobular carcinoma of the breast. The critical clinical features of LCIS are that it is a noninvasive process, it is frequently found to be multifocal and bilateral, and it generally lacks clinical and mammographic signs. The precise incidence of LCIS is unknown, but it is estimated to be identifiable in approximately 0.5% to 1.5% of all benign breast biopsy specimens and approximately 2% of breast specimens obtained because of mammographic abnormalities.[125–127]

Women with LCIS are clearly at increased risk for developing subsequent invasive carcinoma. There are six published series of women with LCIS who were followed for an average of at least 15 years. These series reported that between 12.5% and 34.5% of women with LCIS developed invasive breast cancers.[125–130] A metaanalysis of 389 women with LCIS followed for

a mean of 10.9 years noted that invasive breast cancers developed in 16.4% of these women and the breast cancer mortality rate was 2.8%.[131]

Treatment options for patients with LCIS remain controversial. Close observation with or without tamoxifen therapy is the most popular current choice. Evidence from the National Surgical Adjuvant Breast and Bowel Project tamoxifen prevention trial noted that women with LCIS treated with tamoxifen demonstrated a decrease in the incidence of invasive cancer compared to the control group (5.69 per 1000 vs. 12.99 per 1000).[132] Bilateral prophylactic mastectomy is an appropriate choice for healthy women who are unwilling to accept the risks associated with LCIS or with tamoxifen chemoprevention.

OVARIAN CANCER

Women who carry a mutation in BRCA1 and BRCA2 are at high risk for developing ovarian cancer as well as breast cancer. The lifetime risk of developing ovarian cancer for a woman with a BRCA1 mutation is approximately 30% to 60%, although some estimates are as high as 85%.[10,103,133] Patients with BRCA2 mutations have an estimated lifetime risk of ovarian cancer of approximately 10% to 20%.[104,134]

The National Institutes of Health Consensus Panel on Ovarian Cancer[135] and the American College of Obstetricians and Gynecologists[136] have concluded that prophylactic bilateral oophorectomy should be recommended to women older than 35 years of age or after childbearing is completed if there is an inherited predisposition for ovarian cancer. This recommendation is not new and is based largely on the fact that ovarian cancer is an aggressive malignancy without effective surveillance strategies. Screening for ovarian carcinoma has been hampered by the low sensitivity and specificity of the available techniques, which include pelvic examination, determinations of serum CA 125 (cancer antigen 125) levels, and transvaginal ultrasonography. The low incidence in the general population of approximately 1 in 70 women makes surveillance difficult.[135] In addition, a laparoscopy or laparotomy is required to make the diagnosis of ovarian cancer. Currently, routine screening in the general population has not been shown to affect the morbidity and mortality associated with ovarian cancer and is not recommended. The usefulness of increased surveillance in patients with BRCA1 and BRCA2 mutations has not been thoroughly investigated. It is known, however, that approximately 70% of patients diagnosed with ovarian cancer have stage III or stage IV disease and that 5-year median survival is generally poor for these patients.

Faced with a lack of effective screening methods for ovarian cancer and the poor prognosis of advanced disease, prophylactic oophorectomy has been suggested as a reasonable alternative for women considered to be at high risk for invasive cancer. The Prevention and Observation of Surgical End Points Study Group reported the most convincing evidence that bilateral prophylactic oophorectomy reduces the risk of ovarian cancer in patients with BRCA1 and BRCA2 mutations (see Table 21-3).[118] The clinical outcomes of 552 women from North American and European registries with BRCA1 or BRCA2 mutations were analyzed. The incidence of ovarian cancer was determined in 259 women who had undergone prophylactic oophorectomy and compared to that in 292 matched controls who had not had the procedure. The length of follow-up for both groups was at least 8 years. Six women in the study group (2.8%) were found to have stage I ovarian cancer at surgery and two women (0.8%) were diagnosed with papillary serous carcinoma 3.8 and 8.6 years after surgery. Fifty-eight women in the control group (19.9%) were diagnosed with ovarian cancer. Prophylactic oophorectomy significantly reduced the incidence of ovarian cancer in BRCA1 and BRCA2 carriers (hazard ratio, 0.04; 95% confidence interval, 0.01 to 0.16).

The fact that patients in the control arm of this study who developed ovarian cancer tended to have more advanced disease is reflected by the fact that only 11% presented with stage I disease and over 74% presented with stage II or IV disease. It is also worth noting that prophylactic oophorectomy did not totally eliminate the risk of developing abdominal carcinomatosis that histologically resembled ovarian cancer. This is likely due to the fact that the peritoneum has the same embryologic origin as the ovarian epithelium, and the entire peritoneum may be at risk for malignant degeneration. Also, it is not clear whether the surgical procedures included both tube and ovary.

Although consensus is growing that bilateral prophylactic oophorectomy is the recommended strategy for women with an inherited predisposition for ovarian cancer, many unanswered questions remain. Little is known about the long-term effects of this surgery on the risk for coronary and vascular disease, osteoporosis, sexual function, and mental health. What the timing of surgery should be and whether hormone replacement is dangerous remain uncertain. The management of these patients remains a difficult challenge.

TESTICULAR CANCER AND CRYPTORCHIDISM

Cryptorchidism or undescended testis is characterized by the absence of at least one testis in the scrotum and is the most common genitourinary disorder of childhood. Approximately 3% of children born at full term and up to 30% of children born prematurely have an undescended testis.[137] There is a well known but poorly understood association between cryptorchidism and testicular cancer. In 1929, Cooper noted that the longer a testis remained cryptorchid and the higher the testis lay from the scrotum, the more likely it was to be histologically abnormal.[138] The reported risk for malignancy in cryptorchidism is 48.9 cases per 100,000, which is more than 20 times the risk of testicular cancer in the general population.[139] It has been estimated that approximately 10% of testicular tumors arise from an undescended testis.[140]

Either orchiopexy in association with observation or observation alone is recommended for patients with cryptorchidism. Multiple reasons exist for correcting an undescended testis in a child, including the desire to eliminate a visible defect, to prevent psychological problems associated with the defect, to enhance the possibility of future fertility, and to place the testis in a site in which it can be easily examined. Correction of an undescended testicle may be achieved using hormonal therapy or surgery. Most experts agree that this should be accomplished as early as 12 months of age.[141]

Whether correction of an undescended testicle alters the risk of developing testicular cancer is not clear. There are conflicting reports in the literature regarding the protective effects of correcting cryptorchidism, and virtually no information is available on patients in whom an undescended testicle was corrected at less than 2 years of age.[142–144] Most reports are population-based case-control studies. It is known that patients with unilateral cryptorchidism have an increased risk of testicular cancer in both the undescended and normally descended testis.[145,146]

Farrer et al. extensively addressed the management of an undescended testis in a postpubertal population. These authors completed a statistical analysis that compared the estimated risk of death from a germ cell testis tumor in patients with cryptorchidism to the risk of death from an orchiectomy. They concluded that the risk of death from orchiectomy is greater than the risk of death from testicular cancer in patients older than 32 years of age. The authors recommended that orchiectomy be considered only for patients younger than 32 years of age who have postpubertal unilateral cryptorchidism.[146] Other experts recommend orchiopexy or observation for older patients depending on patient preference and assuming that the testicle is palpable.[147] There is general agreement that a nonpalpable undescended testicle should be removed.

REFERENCES

1. Winawer SJ, Zauber AG, Ho MN, et al. Prevention of colorectal cancer by colonoscopic polypectomy. *N Engl J Med* 1993;329:1977.
2. Marsh DJ, Leagroyd DL, Robinson BG. Medullary thyroid carcinoma: recent advances and management update. *Thyroid* 1995;5:407.
3. Mulligan LM, Kwok JBJ, Healey CS, et al. *Nature* 1993;363:458.
4. Donis-Keller H, Dou S, Chi D, et al. Mutations in the RET proto-oncogene are associated with Men2A and FMTC. *Hum Mol Genet* 1993;2:851.
5. Wells SA Jr, Chi DD, Toshima K, et al. Predictive DNA testing and prophylactic thyroidectomy in patients at risk for multiple endocrine neoplasia type 2A. *Ann Surg* 1994;220:237.
6. Kebebew E, Tresler PA, Siperstein AE, et al. Normal thyroid pathology in patients undergoing thyroidectomy for finding a RET gene germ line mutation: a report of three cases and review of the literature. *Thyroid* 1999;9:127.
7. Brandi ML, Gagel RF, Angeli A, et al. Consensus: guidelines for diagnosis and therapy of MEN type 1 and type 2. *J Clin Endocrinol Metab* 2001;86:5658.
8. Machens A, Niccoli-Sire P, Hoeel J, et al. Early malignant progression of hereditary medullary thyroid cancer. *N Engl J Med* 2003;349:1517.
9. Devesa SS, Blot WJ, Fraumeni J. Changing patterns in the incidence of esophageal and gastric cancer in the United States. *Cancer* 1998;83:2049.
10. Rudolf RE, Vaughn TL, Storer BE, et al. Effect of segment length on risk for neoplastic progression in patients with Barrett's esophagus. *Ann Intern Med* 2000;132:612.
11. Iascone C, DeMeester TR, Little AG, et al. Barrett's esophagus functional assessments, proposed pathogenesis and surgical therapy. *Arch Surg* 1983;118:543.
12. Gillen P, Keeling P, Byrne PJ, et al. Barrett's esophagus: profile. *Br J Surg* 1987;74:774.
13. Vaaezi MF, Richter JC. Role of acid and duodenal-gastroesophageal reflux in gastroesophageal reflux disease. *Gastroenterology* 1996;111:1192.
14. Fiorucli S, Santucci L, Farroni F, et al. Effect of omeprazole on gastroesophageal reflux in Barrett's esophagus. *Am J Gastroenterol* 1989;84:1263.
15. Dent J, Holloway RH, Toouli J, et al. Mechanism of lower esophageal sphincter incompetence in patients with symptomatic gastroesophageal reflux. *Gut* 1988;29:1020.
16. Antonioli DA, Wang HH. Morphology of Barrett's esophagus and Barrett's associated dysplasia and adenocarcinoma. *Gastroenterol Clin North Am* 1997;26:495.
17. Cameron AJ, Zinsmeister AR, Ballard DJ, et al. Prevalence of columnar-lined esophagus, comparison of population-based clinical and autopsy findings. *Gastroenterology* 1990;99:918.
18. Cameron AJ, Kamath PS, Carpenter HE. Barrett's esophagus: the prevalence of short and long segments in reflux patients. *Gastroenterology* 1996;108:A65.
19. Johnston MH, Hammond AS, Lasker W, et al. The prevalence and clinical characteristics of short segments of specialized intestinal metaplasia in the distal esophagus on routine endoscopy. *Am J Gastroenterol* 1996;91:1507.
20. Nandurkar S, Ng T, Adams S, et al. Short segment Barrett's esophagus: prevalence, diagnosis and association. *Gastroenterology* 1996;110:A27.
21. Heies SK, Seif F, Webber S, et al. Short segment Barrett's esophagus: clinical and histologic findings. *Gastroenterology* 1996;99:110:A132.
22. Cameron AJ. Management of Barrett's esophagus. *Mayo Clin Proc* 1998;73:457.
23. Sharma P, Movales TG, Samplings RE. Short segment Barrett's esophagus—the need for standardization of the definition of endoscopic criteria. *Am J Gastroenterol* 1998;93:1033.
24. Tytgat GN. Does endoscopic surveillance in esophageal columnar metaplasia have any real value? *Endoscopy* 1995;27:19.
25. Spechler SJ. Barrett's esophagus. *Semin Oncol* 1994;21:431.
26. Ruol A, Porentia A, Zantnotto G, et al. Intestinal metaplasia if the probable precursor of

adenocarcinoma in Barrett's esophagus and adenocarcinoma of the gastric cardia. *Cancer* 2000;88:2052.

27. Sampliner R, Practice Parameters Committee. Updated guidelines for the diagnosis, surveillance, and therapy of Barrett's esophagus. *Am J Gastroenterol* 2002;97:1888.

28. Dent J, Bremner CG, Collon MJ, et al. Working party report to the world congress of gastroenterology: Barrett's esophagus. *J Gastroenterol Hepatol* 1991;6:1.

29. Levine DS, Haggitt RC, Irvine S, et al. Natural history of high grade dysplasia in Barrett's esophagus. *Gastroenterology* 1996;110:A550.

30. Levine DS, Haggin RC, Radinovitch PS, et al. Complete regression of high grade dysplasia, DNA content abnormalities, and Barrett's esophagus. *Gastroenterology* 1995;108:A496.

31. Provenzale D, Kemp A, Arora S, et al. A guide for surveillance of patients with Barrett's esophagus. *Am J Gastroenterol* 1994;89:670.

32. Gore S, Healey CJ, Sutton R, et al. Regression of columnar-lined esophagus with continuous omeprazole therapy. *Aliment Pharmacol Ther* 1993;7:623.

33. Galmiche JP, Dumas R, Boyer J, et al. Long-term omeprazole effects on Barrett's mucosa. *Gastroenterology* 1993;104:A85.

34. Spechler JS, Lee E, Ahnen D, et al. Long term outcome of medical and surgical therapies for gastroesophageal reflux disease. *JAMA* 2001;285:2331.

35. Parrilla P, Martinez de Haro LF, Ortiz A, et al. Long term results of a randomized prospective study comparing medical and surgical treatment of Barrett's esophagus. *Arch Surg* 2003;237:291.

36. Gurski RR, Peters JH, Demeester SR, et al. Barrett's esophagus can and does regress after antireflux surgery: a study of prevalence and predictive features. *J Am Coll Surg* 2003;196:706.

37. Oelschlager BK, Barreca M, Chang L, et al. Clinical and pathologic responses of Barrett's esophagus to laparoscopic antireflux surgery. *Ann Surg* 2003;238:458.

38. DeMeester TR. The surgical treatment of dysplasia and adenocarcinoma. *Gastroenterol Clin North Am* 1997;26:669.

39. Levine DS, Hagg HRC, Blount PL, et al. An endoscopic biopsy protocol can differentiate high grade dysplasia from early adenocarcinoma in Barrett's esophagus. *Gastroenterology* 1993;105:40.

40. Levine DS. Management of dysplasia in the columnar-lined esophagus. *Gastroenterol Clin North Am* 1997;26:613.

41. Naunheim KS. Barrett's esophagus. In: Cameron JL, ed. *Current surgical therapy*. St. Louis: Mosby Inc., 1998:62.

42. Guilford P, Hopkins J, Harraway J, et al. E-cadherin germline mutations in familial gastric cancer. *Nature* 1998;392:402.

43. Graziano F, Humar B, Guilford P. The role of the E-cadherin gene (CDH1) in diffuse gastric cancer: from laboratory to clinical practice. *Ann Oncol* 2003;14:1705.

44. Carlos C, Fatima C, Lynch HT, et al. Familial gastric cancer: overview and guidelines for management. *J Med Genet* 1999;36:873.

45. Stonnington CM, Phillips SF, Melton LJ III, et al. Chronic ulcerative colitis: incidence and prevalence in a community. *Gut* 1997;28:402.

46. Langhel B, Munlcholm P, Neilsen GH, et al. Incidence and prevalence of ulcerative colitis in Copenhagen county from 1962 to 1987. *Scand J Gastroenterol* 1991;26:1247.

47. Kitalosa T, Ulsunomiya Y, Yakota A. Epidemiological study of ulcerative colitis in Japan: incidence and familial occurrence. *J Gastroenterol* 1995;30[Suppl 8]:5.

48. Devroede GJ, Taylor UF, Saucer WG, et al. Cancer risk and life expectancy of children with ulcerative colitis. *N Engl J Med* 1971;285:17.

49. Ekbom A, Helmick CG, Zack M, et al. Extra colonic malignancies in inflammatory bowel disease. *Cancer* 1991;67:2015.

50. Eekbom A, Helmick CG, Zack M, et al. Survival and causes of death in patients with inflammatory bowel disease. A population based study. *Gastroenterology* 1992;103:954.

51. Bonnevie O, Binder V, Anthonisen P, et al. The prognoses of ulcerative colitis. *Scand J Gastroenterol* 1974;9:81.

52. Langholtz E, Munkholm P, Davidsen M, et al. Colorectal cancer and mortality in patients with ulcerative colitis. *Gastroenterology* 1992;103:1444.

53. Kornlluth A, Sachar DB. Ulcerative colitis practice guidelines in adults. *Am J Gastroenterol* 1997;92:204.

54. Lennard-Jones JE, Melville DM, Moison BC, et al. Precancer and cancer in extensive colitis: findings among 401 patients over 22 years. *Gut* 1990;31:800.

55. Ekbom A, Helmick C, Zack M, et al. Ulcerative colitis and colorectal cancer: a population-based study. *N Engl J Med* 1990;323:1228.

56. Devroede G. Risk of cancer in inflammatory bowel disease. In: Winawer SJ, Schottenfeld D, Sherlock P, eds. *Colorectal cancer: prevention, epidemiology, and screening*. New York: Raven Press, 1980:325.

57. Gyde S, Privr P, Dew MJ, et al. Mortality in ulcerative colitis. *Gastroenterology* 1982;83:36.

58. Shetty K, Rybickil L, Brzezinski A, et al. The risk for cancer or dysplasia in ulcerative colitis in patients with primary sclerosing cholangitis. *Am J Gastroenterol* 1999;94:1643.

59. Nuako KW, Ahiquist DA, Mahoney DW, et al. Familial predisposition for colorectal cancer in chronic ulcerative colitis: a case controlled study. *Gastroenterology* 1998;115:1079.

60. Connell UR, Lennard-Jones JE, William CB, et al. Factory affecting the outcome of endoscopic surveillance for cancer in ulcerative colitis. *Gastroenterology* 1994;107:934.

61. Bernstein CN. How do we assess the values of surveillance techniques in ulcerative colitis. *J Gastrointest Surg* 1998;2:318.

62. Ranshoff DF, Riddell RH, Levin B. Ulcerative colitis and colonic cancer problems in assessing the diagnostic usefulness of mucosal dysplasia. *Dis Colon Rectum* 1985;28:383.

63. Taylor BA, Pembertory JH, Carpenter HA, et al. Dysplasia in chronic ulcerative colitis. Implications for surveillance. *Dis Colon Rectum* 1992;35:950.

64. Lennard-Jones JE. Is colonoscopic cancer surveillance in ulcerative colitis essential for every patient? *Eur J Cancer* 1995; 31A:1178.

65. Mcleod RS. Chronic colitis. In: Cameron JL, ed. *Current surgical therapy*. St. Louis: Mosby Inc., 1998:179.

66. Peterson SM, Brensinger JD, Johnson KA, et al. Genetic testing and counseling for hereditary form of colorectal cancer. *Cancer* 1999;86[Suppl]:2540.

67. Kinzler KW, Vogelstein B. Colorectal tumors. In: Vogelstein B, Kunzler KW, eds. *The genetic bases of human cancers*. New York: McGraw-Hill, 1998:565.

68. Kinzler KW, Nildert MC, Su LK, et al. Identification of FAP locus genes from chromosome 5q21. *Science* 1991;253:662.

69. Powell SM. Clinical application of molecular genetics in colorectal cancer. *Semin Colon Rectal Surg* 1995;6:2.

70. Bisgard ML, Fenger K, Bulow S, et al. Familial adenomatous polyposis: frequency penetrance, and mutation rate. *Hum Mutat* 1994;3:121.

71. Lindor NM, Greene MH. The cancer handbook of family cancer syndromes. Mayo familial cancer program. *J Natl Cancer Inst* 1998;90:1039.

72. Tzrdiman JP, Conrad PG, Sleisenger MH. Gastric testing in hereditary colorectal cancer: indication and procedures. *Am J Gastroenterol* 1999;94:2344.

73. Spigelman AD, Talbot IC, Williams CB, et al. Upper gastrointestinal cancer in patients with familial adenomatous polyposes. *Lancet* 1989;783.

74. Hawk E, Lubet R, Limburg P. Chemoprevention in hereditary colorectal cancer syndromes. *Cancer* 1999;86:[Suppl]2551.

75. Lynch HT, Lynch PM, Pestar J, et al. The cancer family syndrome: rare cutaneous phenotypic linkage of Toss's syndrome. *Arch Intern Med* 1981;141:607.

76. Vasen HFA, Offerhaus GJA, den Hartog Jager FCA, et al. The tumor spectrum in hereditary nonpolyposis colorectal cancer: a study of 24 kindreds in the Netherlands. *Int J Cancer* 1990;46:31.

77. Lynch HT, Smyrk TC, Watson P, et al. Genetics, natural history, tumor spectrum, and pathology of hereditary nonpolyposis colorectal cancer: an updated review. *Gastroenterology* 1993;104:1535.

78. Watson P, Lynch HT. Extracolonic cancer in hereditary nonpolyposis colorectal cancer. *Cancer* 1993;71:677.

79. Vasen HF, Mecklin JP, Khan PM, et al. The international collaborative group on hereditary nonpolyposis colorectal cancer: an international cooperative study of 165 families. *Dis Colon Rectum* 1993;36:1.

80. Lynch HT, de al Chapelle A. Hereditary colorectal cancer. *N Engl J Med* 2003;348:919.

81. Fishel R, Lescoe MK, Rao MR, et al. The human mutator gene homolog MSH2 and its association with hereditary nonpolyposis colon cancer. *Cell* 1993;75:1027.

82. Leach FS, Nicolaides NC, Papadopoolos N, et al. Mutation of a mut S homolog in hereditary nonpolyposis colorectal cancers. *Cell* 1993;75:215.

83. Bronner CE, Baker SM, Mossison PT, et al. Mutation in the DNA mismatched repair gene homologous hMLH1 is associated with hereditary nonpolyposis colon cancer. *Nature* 1994;368:258.

84. Nicolaides NC, Papadopoulos N, Liu B, et al. Mutation of two PMS homologous in hereditary nonpolyposis colon cancer. *Nature* 1994;371:75.

85. Miyaki M, Konishi M, Tanaka K, et al. Germline mutations of MSH6 on the cancer of hereditary nonpolyposis colorectal cancer. *Nat Genet* 1997;17:271.

86. Peltomaki P, Vasen HF. Mutations predisposing to hereditary nonpolyposis colorectal cancer. Data and results of a collaborative study. The International Collaborative Group of Hereditary Nonpolyposis Colorectal Cancer. *Gastroenterology* 1997;113:140.

87. Lynch HT. Is there a role for prophylactic subtotal colectomy among hereditary nonpolyposis colorectal cancer germ line mutation carriers? *Dis Colon Rectum* 1996; 39:109.

88. Reference deleted.

89. Yu HA, Lin KM, Ota DM, et al. Hereditary nonpolyposis colorectal cancer: preventive management. *Cancer Treat Rev* 2003;29:461.

90. Jass JR, Smyrk TC, Stewart SM, et al. Pathology of hereditary nonpolyposis colorectal cancers. *Anticancer Res* 1994;14:1631.

91. Merklin JT, Jarvinzn H. Treatment and follow-up strategies in hereditary nonpolyposis colorectal carcinomas. *Dis Colon Rectum* 1993;36:927.

92. Lynch HT, Smyrk T. Hereditary nonpolyposis colorectal cancer (Lynch syndrome) an updated review. *Cancer* 1996;78:1149.

93. Kinzler KW, Vogelstein B. Lesions from hereditary colorectal cancer. *Cell* 1996;87:159.

94. Jarvinen HJ, Mecklin JP, Sistonen P. Screening reduces colorectal cancer in hereditary nonpolyposis colorectal cancer families. *Gastroenterology* 1995;108:1405.

95. Bulow S, Bulow C, Nielson TF, et al. Centralized registration results in improved prognosis in familial adenomatosis polyposis. *Scand J Gastroenterol* 1995;30:989.

96. Burtz W, Peterson D, Lynch HT, et al. Recommendation for follow-up care for individuals with an inherited predisposition to cancer. Hereditary nonpolyposis colon cancer. *JAMA* 1997;277:915.

97. Rodriquez-Bigas MA. Prophylactic colectomy for gene carriers in hereditary nonpolyposis colorectal cancer. Has the time come? *Cancer* 1996;78:199.

98. Newman B, Austin MA, Lee M. Inheritance of breast cancer: evidence for autosomal dominant transmission in high risk families. *Proc Natl Acad Sci U S A* 1988;85:3011.

99. Hall JM, Lee MK, Newana B, et al. Linkage of early asset breast cancer to chromosome 17q21. *Science* 1990;250:1684.

100. Miki Y, Swensen J, Sshattuck E, et al. A strong candidate for the breast and ovarian cancer susceptibility gene BRCA1. *Science* 1994;226:66.

101. Ford D, Easton DF, Stratton M, et al. Genetic heterogenicity and penetrance analysis of the BRCA1 and BRCA2 genes in breast cancer families. *Am J Hum Genet* 1998;62:676.

102. Strauewing JP, Hartge P, Waholder S, et al. The risk of cancer associated with specific mutation of BRCA1 and BRCA2 among Ashkenazic Jews. *N Engl J Med* 1997;336:1401.

103. Easton DF, Ford D, Bishop DT, et al. Breast and ovarian cancer incidence in BRCA1 mutation carriers. *Am J Hum Genet* 1995;56:265.

104. Wooster R, Bignell G, Lancaster J, et al. Identification of the breast cancer susceptibility gene BRCA2. *Nature* 1995;378.

105. Phelan CM, Lancaster JM, Tonin P, et al. Mutational analysis of BRCA2 gene in 49 site specific breast cancer families. *Nat Genet* 1996;13:120.

106. Tavtigan SV, Simnd J, Romans J, et al. The BRCA2 gene and mutation in chromosome 12q-linked kindreds. *Nat Genet* 1996;12:333.

107. Bburle W, Paly M, Garber J, et al. Recommendations for follow-up care of individuals with an ulcerated predisposition to cancer. Consensus statement of the cancer genetics studies consortium. *JAMA* 1997;277:997.

108. Thomas DB, Gao DE, Self SQ, et al. Randomized trial of breast self examination in Shanghai: methodology and preliminary results. *J Natl Cancer Inst* 1997;89:355.

109. Miller AB, Baines CJ, Turnball C. The role of the nurse examiner in the national breast screening study. *Can J Public Health* 1991;82:162.

110. Campbell HS, Fletcher SW, Liu S, et al. Improving physicians and nurses clinical breast examination. *Am J Prev Med* 1991;7:1.

111. Kerlikoowske E, Grady D, Aukin SM, et al. Efficacy of screening mammography: a meta-analysis. *JAMA* 1995;273:149.

112. Elwood JM, Cox B, Richardson AK. The effectiveness of breast cancer screening by mammography in younger women. *Online J Curr Clin Trials* 1993;32:93.

113. Eckhardt S, Badellino F, Murphy GP. Breast cancer screening in premenopausal women in developed countries. *Int J Cancer* 1994;56:1.

114. Smart CR, Hendrick RE, Rutldege JH, et al. Benefit of mammography in women ages 40 to 49 years: current evidence from randomized trials. *Cancer* 1995;75:1619.

115. Narod SA, Brunet J-S, Ghadirian P, et al. Tamoxifen and the risk of contralateral breast cancer in BRCA-1 and BRCA-2 mutation carriers. *Lancet* 2000;356:1876.

116. King MC, Wieand S, Hale K, et al. Tamoxifen and breast cancer incidence among women with inherited mutations in BRCA-1 and BRCA-2. *JAMA* 2001;286:2251.

117. Peshkin BN, Isaacs C, Finch C, et al. Tamoxifen and chemoprevention in BRCA-1 and BRCA-2 mutation carriers with breast cancer: a pilot study of physicians. *J Clin Oncol* 2003;21:9322.

118. Rebbeck TR, Lynch HT, Neuhausen SL, et al. Prophylactic oophorectomy in carriers of BRCA-1 and BRCA-2 mutations. *N Engl J Med* 2002;346:1616.

119. Eldar S, Mequio MM, Beztty JD. Cancer of the breast after prophylactic subcutaneous mastectomy. *Am J Surg* 1984;148:6932.

120. Goodnight JE, Quagliana JM, Monton DL. Failure of subcutaneous mastectomy to prevent the development of breast cancer. *J Surg Oncol* 1984;26:198.

121. Ziegler LD, Kroll SS. Primary breast cancer after prophylactic mastectomy. *Am J Clin Oncol* 1991;14:451.

122. Hartmann LC, Scharo DJ, Woods JE, et al. Efficacy of bilateral prophylactic mastectomy in women with a family history of breast cancer. *N Engl J Med* 1999;340:77.

123. Robson M, Levin D, Federic M, et al. Breast conservation therapy for invasive breast cancer in Ashkenazi women with BRCA gene founder mutations. *J Natl Cancer Inst* 1999;91:2112.

124. Van Oostrom I, Meijers-Heijboer H, Lodder LN, et al. Long term psychological impact of carrying a BRCA-1 or BRCA-2 and prophylactic surgery: a 5 year follow up study. *J Clin Oncol* 2003;20:3867.

125. Anderson JA. Lobular carcinoma in situ of the breast: an approach to rational treatment. *Cancer* 1977;39:2597.

126. Page SL, Kidd TE Jr, Puport UD, et al. Lobular neoplasia of the breast: higher risk for subsequent invasive cancer predicted by more extensive disease. *Hum Pathol* 1991;22:1232.

127. Fryberg ER, Bland KI. In situ breast carcinoma. *Adv Surg* 1993;26:29.

128. Wheeler JE, Enterline HT, Roreman JM, et al. Lobular carcinoma in situ of the breast: long term follow up. *Cancer* 1974;34:554.

129. Rosen PP, Kosloff C, Lieberman PH, et al. Lobular carcinoma in situ of the breast. Detailed analysis of 99 patients with average follow up of 24 years. *Am J Surg Pathol* 1978;3:225.

130. Bodian CA, Perizin KH, Luttes R. Lobular neoplasia long-term risk of breast cancer and related to other forms. *Cancer* 1996;78:1024.

131. Bradley SJ, Weaver DW, Bouwman DE. Alternatives on the surgical management of in situ breast cancer. A meta analysis of outcome. *Am Surg* 1990;56:428.

132. Fisher B, Costantino JP, Wickerham DE, et al. Tamoxifen for the prevention of breast cancer: report of the National Surgical Adjuvant Breast and Bowel Project P-1 study. *J Natl Cancer Inst* 1998;90:1271.

133. Ford D, Easton DF, Bishop DT, et al. Risks of cancer in BRCA1 mutation carriers. Breast cancer linkage consortium. *Lancet* 1994;363:692.

134. Ford D, Easton DF. The genetics of breast and ovarian cancer. *Br J Cancer* 1995;72:805.

135. NIH Consensus development panel on ovarian cancer. Ovarian cancer: screening, treatment, and follow up. *JAMA* 1995;273:491.

136. American college of obstetricians and gynecologists committee on quality assessment: ACOQ criteria set for prophylactic bilateral oophorectomy to prevent epithelial carcinoma. *Int J Gynaecol Obstet* 199;52:101.

137. Scorer CG. The descent of the testis. *Arch Dis Child* 1964;39:605.

138. Cooper ER. The histology of the retained testis in the human subject at different sizes and its comparison with the testis. *J Anat* 1929;64:5.

139. Gill B, Kogan S. Cryptorchidism: current concepts. *Pediatr Clin North Am* 1997;44:1211.

140. Abratt RP, Reddi VB, Sarembock LA. Testicular cancer and cryptorchidism. *Br J Urol* 1992;70:656.

141. Action Committee Report of the Urology Section, American Academy of Pediatrics: timing of elective surgery on the genitalia of male children with particular reference to the risks, benefits and psychological effects of surgery and anesthesia. *Pediatrics* 1997;97:590.

142. United Kingdom Testicular Cancer Study Group. A etiology of testicular cancer association with congenital abnormalities, age of puberty, infertility and exercise. *BMJ* 1994;308:1393.

143. Pike MC, Chiluers C, Peckham MHJ. Effects of age at orchiopexy on risk of testicular cancer. *Lancet* 1986;1:1246.

144. Depue RH, Pike MC, Henderson BE. Cryptorchidism and testicular cancer. *J Natl Cancer Inst* 1986;77:830

145. Chilvers C, Pike MC. Epidemiology of undescended testis. In: Oliver RTD, Blandy JP, Hope-Stone HF, eds. *Urological and genital cancer.* Oxford: Blackwell Scientific Publications, 1989;306.

146. Farrer JH, Walker AH, Rajfer J. Management of the post-pubertal cryptorchid testis: a statistical review. *J Urol* 1985;134:1071.

147. Rajfer J. Congenital anomalies or the testis and scrotum. In: Walsh PC, Retik AB, Vaughan ED, et al., eds. *Campbell's urology.* Philadelphia: WB Saunders, 1998:2172.

148. Oliveira C, Bordin MC, Grehan N, et al. Screening E-cadherin in gastric cancer families reveals germline mutations only in hereditary diffuse gastric cancer kindred. *Hum Mutat* 2002;19(5):510.

Barbara K. Rimer
Joellen M. Schildkraut
Robert A. Hiatt

CHAPTER **22**

Cancer Screening

The goal of cancer screening is a very practical one—to detect cancer at an early stage when it is treatable and curable. However, the reality is quite complex. For a screening test to be useful, the test or procedure should detect cancer earlier than would occur otherwise, *and* there should be evidence that earlier diagnosis results in improved outcomes.[1] Advances in genetics and molecular biology undoubtedly will make it possible to detect cancer at earlier and earlier stages along the carcinogenesis pathway. Thus, the line between prevention and screening may narrow further, as it has for colorectal and cervical cancers. In spite of the potential of molecular diagnostics, screening must be evaluated according to its present reality, which is to detect asymptomatic disease when it is potentially curable and can reduce deaths from cancers. The potential of screening still has not been fully realized. A report by the National Cancer Policy Board and the Institute of Medicine[2] estimated that a 19% decline in the rate at which new cancers occur and a 29% decline in the rate of cancer deaths could be achieved by 2015 through changes in behavior and greater dissemination of proven technologies, including cancer screening. The National Cancer Policy Board also estimated that appropriate use of screening among persons aged 50 and older could reduce the mortality from colorectal cancer by 30% to 80%; screening among women aged 50 and older could reduce mortality from breast cancer by 25% to 30%, and screening women aged 18 and older could reduce the rate of cervical cancer mortality by 20% to 60%.

The purpose of this chapter is to provide an overview of cancer screening—what it is, key terms, measures of effectiveness, and consequences. We also review briefly the status of screening for several prevalent cancers (breast, cervical, skin, prostate, colorectal, and lung). The recommendations are for the general population, and not for people with identified mutations in cancer susceptibility genes. High-risk populations are the subject of other chapters. Generally, it is recommended that people with cancer susceptibility mutations be screened at earlier ages and more frequently for the cancers to which they are predisposed.

This chapter cannot provide comprehensive information on any of the cancer sites reviewed, because the literature for each is vast. Rather, the chapter provides a succinct summary of the field and a perspective for clinicians to use in determining the efficacy of particular screening tests. Several texts and on-line resources provide good overviews of the issues related to screening for specific kinds of cancer.[1] The National Cancer Institute's (NCI) Physician Data Query (PDQ; http://www.cancer.gov/cancerinfo/pdq/cancerdatabase) is an excellent source for the latest data on the specific screening tests discussed here. Similarly, the American Cancer Society (ACS) Web site (http://www.cancer.org) provides current information on cancer rates and ACS screening guidelines. Many other good sites are available as well.

WHAT IS CANCER SCREENING?

Appropriate cancer screening should lead to early detection of asymptomatic or unrecognized disease by the application of acceptable, inexpensive tests or examinations in a large number of persons.[1] The results of a screening test then should be applied expeditiously to separate apparently well persons who probably have disease from those who probably do not. The main objective of cancer screening is to reduce morbidity and mortality from a particular cancer among persons screened (Table 22-1).

Several characteristics make particular cancers suitable for screening. These include substantial morbidity and mortality,

TABLE 22-1. Characteristics of Screening Tests versus Diagnostic Tests

Screening	Diagnosis
Applied to asymptomatic groups	Applied to symptomatic individuals
Lower cost per test	Higher cost; all necessary tests applied to identify disease
Lower yield per test	Higher probability of case detection
Lower adverse consequences of error	Failure to identify true positives can delay treatment and worsen prognosis

TABLE 22-2. Definitions of Criteria for Evaluating a Screening Test

Screening Test Results	Truth (Diagnostic Classification)	
	Cancer Present	Cancer Absent
Positive	TP	FP
Negative	FN	TN

Sensitivity = TP/TP + FN × 100
Specificity = TN/FP + TN × 100
PV+ = TP/TP + FP × 100
PV− = TN/TN + FN × 100
Accuracy = TP + TN/TP + TN + FP + FN × 100

FN, false-negative (number of subjects with cancer who are incorrectly classified as cancer-free by the test); FP, false-positive (number of cancer-free subjects who are incorrectly classified as having cancer by the test); PV, predictive value; TN, true-negative (number of cancer-free subjects who are correctly classified by the test); TP, true-positive (number of subjects with cancer who are correctly classified by the test).

high prevalence in a detectable preclinical state, possibility of effective and improved treatment because of early detection, and availability of a good screening test with high sensitivity and specificity, low cost, and little inconvenience and discomfort. Only breast, cervical, and colorectal screening have met the rigorous criteria of the U.S. Preventive Services Task Force and have sufficient high-quality evidence to justify population-based screening.[3]

EVALUATION OF A SCREENING TEST

In evaluating a screening test, it is essential to answer questions concerning its ability to accurately predict the presence or absence of disease. If the test is *abnormal*, what are the chances that disease is present? If the test result is *normal*, what are the chances that disease is absent? The validity of a screening test is measured by whether it correctly classifies those persons who have disease as test-positive and those without it as test-negative.

Sensitivity and *specificity* address the validity of screening tests. Sensitivity is the probability of testing positive if the disease is truly present. As sensitivity increases, the number of persons with the disease who are classified as test-negative (false-negative) decreases. Specificity is the probability of screening negative if the disease is truly absent. A highly specific test rarely is positive in the absence of disease and therefore results in a lower proportion of persons without disease who are incorrectly classified as test-positive (false-positive). PV+ is an estimate of test accuracy in predicting presence of disease; PV− is an estimate of the accuracy of the test in predicting absence of disease. Predictive value is a function of sensitivity, specificity, and prevalence of disease. *Accuracy* is a measure of the percent of all results that are true results, whether positive or negative, that is, total correct test results. A screening test that results in many false-positive findings is inefficient and potentially dangerous, because it subjects people to follow-up procedures that are often costly, with a range of risks. Similarly, false-negative results can be life threatening, because they miss cancers that could possibly be identified and treated. Every organized screening program must balance the potential for false-positives and false-negatives when establishing criteria for follow-up (Table 22-2).

Sources of bias are of particular importance in evaluating screening programs. People who choose to participate in screening programs (volunteers) are likely to be different from the general population in ways that affect survival; thus, *volunteer bias* is a concern.[1] *Lead-time bias* is defined as the interval between diagnosis of disease at screening and when it would have been detected due to the development of symptoms.[1] If lead-time bias is not taken into account, survival erroneously may appear to be increased among screen-detected cases as compared to unscreened cases. Finally, *length bias* is the over-representation among screen-detected cases of those with a long preclinical period (thus, less rapidly fatal), leading to the incorrect conclusion that screening was beneficial.[1]

MEASURES OF EFFECTIVENESS

Several measures have been used to judge the effectiveness of screening. As Goldie and Kuntz[4] discussed, biologic characteristics of cancers and their precursor lesions may affect test efficacy. In addition, we make assumptions about the heterogeneity of risk factors in screened and unscreened populations; measures of effectiveness tend to minimize true differences within populations. The most definitive measure of efficacy and least subject to bias is breast cancer mortality as determined by the comparison of screened and unscreened groups in a randomized clinical trial (RCT).[1] Other outcome measures have been proposed, including case finding and survival. Each has limitations.

Another potential outcome is improved quality of life.[5] Unfortunately, few trials have collected such data. These data are being collected as part of the NCI's Prostate, Lung, Colorectal, Ovarian (PLCO) cancer screening trial and the newer NCI-funded trial to compare special computed tomography (CT) for lung cancer screening versus chest x-rays.

Increasingly, reports include the number needed to treat to convey the size of the populations that do and do not benefit.[2] The number is usually very small for cancer screening—often in the range of five or fewer people benefiting per 5000 people screened.

In assessing effectiveness of screening technologies, the RCT has been the gold standard. It is the most powerful methodology for demonstrating the value of screening in comparison to an unscreened group. RCTs minimize biases inherent in other designs, especially lead time, length bias,[6] selection bias, and overdiagnosis.[7] Case-control studies also can provide useful information, and at less cost than RCTs. In addition, increasingly sophisticated statistical modeling techniques may be helpful in assessing the impact of screening, especially in situations in which large RCTs cannot be conducted. The U.S. Preventive Services Task Force,[3] PDQ,[8] and others have rated levels of evidence; the RCT is uniformly regarded as the highest level of evidence.

POSITIVE AND NEGATIVE CONSEQUENCES OF SCREENING

Every medical activity has positive and negative consequences, and screening is no exception. Potential benefits include improved prognosis for those with screen-detected cancers, the possibility of less radical treatment, reassurance for those with negative test results, and resource savings if treatment costs are reduced because of less radical treatments. The optimal outcome is a reduction in cancer mortality. Potential negative effects of screening include physical, economic, and psychological consequences of false-positives and false-negatives, the potential for overdiagnosis, the potential carcinogenic effects of screening, and the labeling phenomenon.[9–13] The last refers to the fact that telling individuals that they have cancer may change how they see themselves or how others see them. In addition, Baines[14] has noted the largely unexplained increase in cancer among the unscreened group as a negative consequence of screening.

Physicians should engage patients in discussions of the risks and benefits of cancer screening. Because most people overestimate the risks for certain types of cancers (e.g., breast),[15] they may inflate the need for screening and the potential benefits.[16] For some cancers, such as colorectal cancer, people may underestimate their personal susceptibility and may need encouragement to consider screening, with positive as well as negative consequences. In the case of prostate cancer, for which the evidence is still equivocal and population-based screening is not recommended, it is especially important that men understand the limitations of screening and make informed decisions with full understanding of the potential downstream effects of positive and negative test results.[17] Informed decision making increasingly is becoming a paradigm with the potential to be achieved in contemporary clinical practice. Informed decision making occurs when an individual understands the disease or condition being addressed and also comprehends what the clinical service involves, including its benefits, risks, limitations, alternatives, and uncertainties; has considered his or her own preferences, as appropriate; believes he or she has participated in decision making at a level that he or she desires; and makes a decision consistent with his or her preferences.[18] Decision aids are tools used to help patients examine the nature of screening tests and their benefits and limitations.

Austoker[19] outlined topics that should be included when helping patients to make informed decisions about cancer screening. These include the purpose of screening; the likelihood of positive and negative findings and the possibility of false-positive or false-negative results; the uncertainties and risks involved; any significant medical, social, or financial implications of screening; and follow-up plans.

BREAST CANCER SCREENING

In 2003, approximately 211,300 new invasive cases of breast cancer (and 55,700 new ductal carcinoma *in situ* cases) and approximately 39,800 deaths due to the disease were estimated to have occurred in the United States.[20] For a woman of average risk, lifetime breast cancer incidence is 7.8%, and mortality is 2.3%.[21] Widely accepted techniques for breast cancer screening, but with differing levels of evidence, include mammography, clinical breast examination (CBE), and breast self-examination (BSE). No cancer screening test has been studied more than mammography (with or without CBE).

RANDOMIZED CLINICAL TRIALS

Eight randomized trials have been conducted over more than 40 years to assess the impact of mammography. Together, these trials have included more than 500,000 women, with 180,000 women aged 40 to 49. The eight international RCTs have varied greatly[22] (Table 22-3). Most trials have included women in their 40s, although two trials began accrual at age 45. One of the Canadian trials [the first National Breast Cancer Screening Study (NBSS1)] was designed to examine mammography and CBE versus usual care for women in their 40s,[23] with a separate study (NBSS2) to assess mammography plus CBE versus CBE alone for women aged 50 to 59.[24] The international studies have varied in key ways, as shown in Table 22-3.

MAMMOGRAPHY

It was not until 1963 that the first RCT—and the only RCT conducted within the United States—commenced at the Health Insurance Plan of New York. Women were aged 40 to 64 at entry; nearly 62,000 women were randomized to the study (two-view mammography and CBE) or control group (usual care). Two-view mammography and physical examination were offered every 12 months for 3 years, and follow-up was continued for 18 years.[25]

The Swedish Two-County Trial in Kopparberg and Ostergotland began in 1977 to 1978; 135,000 women were randomized to one-view mammography every 24 (younger than age 50 years) or 33 months (older than age 50 years). Within those geographic areas, all women were invited to enroll by letters of invitation, using the population registry list. Screening continued for four rounds for younger women and three rounds for older women.[26,27]

The Malmö Trial was begun in 1976 in one city in Sweden. It was one of only two trials that began screening at age 45 years, and it stopped entry at age 69 years. It used two-view mammography every 18 to 24 months for five rounds; randomization was by cluster based on birth cohort. Approximately 68,000 women were enrolled in this trial.[28]

The Stockholm Study began in 1981 and enrolled approximately 59,000 women aged 40 to 64 years, who received single-view mammography every 28 months. Like the Malmö trial, randomization was by birth cohort within clusters.[29]

The final Swedish study was conducted in Gothenburg, starting in 1982. The trial began with nearly 50,000 women aged 40 to 59 years, who received two-view mammography every 18 months. Randomization of women aged 40 to 49 years was by individual, whereas clustered randomization was used for women aged 50 to 59 years. Verified results have not yet been published,[26] but additional data were provided in 1997 for the National Institutes of Health Consensus Conference on Breast Cancer Screening in women aged 40 to 49 years.[30]

The Edinburgh trial began in 1976 as a randomized component of the larger, nonrandomized United Kingdom trial

TABLE 22-3. Selected Characteristics of Eight Randomized Controlled Trials of Breast Cancer Screening

Study (Year Begun)	Age at Entry (Y)	Screening Modality	Periodicity (Mo)	Randomization	Sample Size Study	Control	Screened at First Examination (%)	Follow-Up (Y)	Reduction in Mortality Screen vs Control/Comparison Group[133]
HIP (1963)	40–64	2-view annual MM and CBE	12	Individual	30,239	30,756	67	18	0.71 (0.62–1.07) at 15 y
Sweden, 2-county: Ostergot-land and Koppar-berg (1977)	40–74	1-view MM	24 (age <50 y) 33 (age ≥50 y)	Cluster: geographic	~78,085	56,782	89	12 12	0.82 (0.64–1.05) 0.68 (0.52–0.89)
Malmö[a] (1976)	45–69	2-view MM	18–24	Individual within birth cohort	34,616	33,437	74	12	0.82 (0.64–1.05)
Stockholm (1981)	40–64	1-view MM	28	Cluster: birth cohort	39,164	19,943	81	8	0.80 (0.53–1.22)
Gothenburg (1982)	40–59	2-view MM	18	Individual (age 40–49 y); cluster (age 50–59 y)	20,724	28,809	84	12	0.86 (0.54–1.37)
Edinburgh (1976)	45–64	2-view MM initially (later, usually 1-view MM)	12 (CBE), 24 (MM)	Cluster: by physician practices	23,226	21,904	61	10	0.84 (0.63–1.12)
Canada NBSS1 (1980)	40–49	2-view MM and CBE	12	Individual: volunteers	25,214	25,216	~100[b]	11–16	0.97 (0.74–1.27)
Canada NBSS2 (1980)	50–59	2-view MM and CBE vs. CBE only	12	Individual: volunteers	19,711	19,694	~100[b]	13	1.02 (0.78–1.33)

CBE, clinical breast examination; HIP, Health Insurance Plan of New York; MM, mammography; NBSS1 and -2, first and second Canadian National Breast Cancer Screening Study.
[a]Different reports use different numbers for this trial.
[b]Study design included randomization of volunteers after CBE; accordingly, virtually 100% had their first screening examination.

for the Early Detection of Breast Cancer. Approximately 45,000 women aged 45 to 64 years were randomized to two-view mammography plus CBE on either a 12- or 24-month schedule. The purpose was to assess the impact of mammography and CBE in reducing mortality from breast cancer.[31]

The NBSS1 was designed to examine the value of two-view mammography and CBE compared to usual care in women aged 40 to 49. Approximately 50,000 women were enrolled, starting in 1980, and received follow-up yearly for 5 years. Unlike the other trials, the women were recruited as volunteers and then randomized. As Miller et al.[23] have reported, these women were different from the rest of the Canadian population in several ways—for example, they were less likely to smoke, and they had higher levels of education.

The second Canadian study, the NBSS2, also begun in 1980, enrolled nearly 40,000 women aged 50 to 59 years, and was designed to compare two-view mammography and CBE against CBE only. In other words, the question was whether mammography has benefits over and above CBE in this age group. This is the only trial planned to assess the additive impact of mammography in addition to CBE.[24] Critiques of this trial have appeared by several authors.[32,33] The

criticisms are probably overstated, and the results should not be discounted.

NONRANDOMIZED CLINICAL TRIALS

A number of nonrandomized trials have been conducted around the world. Much can be learned from these studies. However, because of a number of design limitations, their results alone should not be used in establishing screening guidelines and policies.[34] The largest study of mammography and CBE was the U.S. Breast Cancer Detection Demonstration Project (BCDDP): 280,000 women aged 35 and older were recruited and screened in 28 centers annually with mammograms and CBE during the 1970s.[35] The BCDDP was sponsored jointly by the NCI and the ACS. Because BCDDP participants were not a random sample of the population, there were some important differences from women in the general population. Most notably, the BCDDP population was at much higher risk, with a substantially higher incidence of breast cancer. A subset of women were followed as part of a case-control study conducted by Morrison et al.[36] to examine case fatality rates within the BCDDP. Breast cancer mortality was approximately 20%

TABLE 22-4.   Metaanalyses of Trials for Women Aged 40 to 49 Years

Description	Authors	Relative Risk	Confidence Interval (%)	Reduction in Mortality (%)
Without NBSS	Miller et al., 1992[134]	0.85	0.68–1.08	15[a]
With NBSS	Eckhardt et al., 1994[135]	0.93	0.76–1.15	7[a]
With NBSS	Elwood et al., 1993[6]	0.93	0.77–1.11	7
Without NBSS	Smart et al., 1995[35]	0.76	0.62–0.95	24[b]
With NBSS	Hendrick et al., 1997[30]	0.82	0.71–0.95	18[b]
With NBSS	Berry, 1998[22]	0.82	0.49–1.17	18[b]
Without Edinburgh	Humphrey et al., 2002[29]	0.85	0.73–0.99	15
Without NBSS	Humphrey et al., 2002[29]	0.80	0.67–0.96	20

NBSS, National Breast Cancer Screening Study (Canada).
[a]Nonsignificant.
[b]Significant.

less than expected from national data. A benefit was seen for younger women, but it was less than for older women.

EVIDENCE FOR MAMMOGRAPHY

More than 3.5 million women-years of observation have been recorded for women of all ages, and more than 2.7 million women-years for women aged 40 to 49 years at entry from the breast cancer screening RCTs.[30] One of the challenging aspects of tracking these trials is the constantly shifting nature of the data.[22] The trialists provide updates at different points in time, and some reports use nonverified data. Thus, at any given point, review articles may vary substantially in the numbers they report (see Table 22-3). Now, several years later, with most of the international RCTs having more than 10 years of follow-up, trends are clearer: Six of the trials show reductions in mortality for women who were in their 40s at entry. However, a large variability remains in the relative risk of dying from breast cancer for women younger than 50 years. Also, significant controversy surrounds many of the reported numbers.

Although the randomized trials have included too few women older than age 70 years to offer guidance about screening for older women, the Forum on Breast Cancer Screening[37] recommended regular mammograms for women aged 70 years who are otherwise healthy. A case-control analysis in the Nijmegen study[38] confirmed the benefit of mammography for women older than 70 years.

Seven particularly important published metaanalyses, including the two mentioned earlier, provide assessments regarding the impact of breast cancer screening, especially mammography (Table 22-4). They generally have examined results separately for women aged 40 to 49 years and those aged 50 years and older. (Few women are in the older categories.) For women in their 50s and 60s, there is general agreement about the benefits of mammography. The most recent review done by the U.S. Preventive Services Task Force shows a modest benefit for women aged 40 years and older.[29] Thus, there is now general consistency in the evidence reviews.

BREAST CANCER SCREENING GUIDELINES

The question, "At what age should women begin getting regular mammograms?," has been one of the most contentious in science and medicine. In 1993, the International Workshop on Screening for Breast Cancer[13] created considerable controversy when it concluded that for women aged 40 to 49 years, random-

ized controlled trials consistently demonstrated no benefit from screening in the first 5 to 7 years after entry and a marginal benefit after that. The issue became even more inflamed after a 1997 National Institutes of Health Consensus Conference on Breast Cancer Screening for Women Ages 40 to 49.[39] The report, contrary to expectations, found insufficient data to recommend that women in their 40s get regular mammograms. Disagreement still exists over whether the modest reduction in mortality warrants a recommendation that all women in their 40s be screened.[40] The argument turns primarily on the small population benefit achieved and the fact that most of the benefit occurs when screened women are in their 50s. Only 1 to 2 women's lives would be extended per 1000 women of 40 to 50 years of age who are screened annually for 10 years. However, in agreeing on a reduction in breast cancer mortality of 18%, the ACS and the NCI changed their screening recommendations, with the ACS now advising annual mammograms for women aged 40 years and older. Annual screening for women in their 40s is based on the assumption of a shorter lead time for younger women.[41]

Controversy flared again in 2000, when Gotzsche and Olsen[42] published another metaanalysis of the world's mammography trials and found most of the trials methodologically flawed. They concluded that mammography did not show a statistically significant benefit for women in any group.

Over the past several years, there has been a convergence of opinion across most medical organizations, including those that are grounded in evidence-based decision making, that mammography benefits women aged 40 years and older. Current controversies focus on the net benefits and optimal screening schedule. The benefit is modest. Because no trials have included sufficient numbers of older women to permit separate analyses by age, there are no good data on the upper limit of benefit. Most informed sources (e.g., ACS) now recommend regular screening for women aged 40 years and over, with some organizations recommending annual and some biennial screening (Table 22-5).

The evidence suggests that a 5% to 20% additional benefit in mortality reduction can be achieved by adding a high-quality CBE.[6,13] The U.S. Preventive Services Task Force reviewed the data regarding CBE and concluded that they were insufficient to reach conclusions about efficacy or to issue population-based recommendations. No evidence has shown that BSE reduces mortality from breast cancer. Large trials conducted in China and Russia did not result in the hoped-for reduction of cancer mortality as a result of careful BSE instruction. In its 2002 report,

TABLE 22-5. Screening Guidelines for Breast, Colorectal, Prostate, and Cervical Cancers for Selected Health Care Organizations

Type of Cancer	American Cancer Society[20]	U.S. Preventive Services Task Force[3]	National Cancer Institute's Physician Data Query (PDQ) System[1]
Breast cancer	Annual mammography for women aged 40–69 y. No age cutoff. To the extent possible, a CBE should be performed at the time of mammography. Monthly BSE.[136] Women aged 20–39 y should have a CBE from a health professional every 3 y and should perform BSE monthly.[20]	Recommends screening mammogram, with or without CBE, every 1–2 y.	Mammography every 1–2 y for women age 40 y and older. Women at higher risk should talk with their physicians about schedule.
Cervical cancer	For all women who are, or have been, sexually active or who have reached age 21 y, Pap test and pelvic examination yearly with Pap tests or every 3 y with liquid-based tests. At or after age 30 y, women who have had 3 normal tests can be screened every 2–3 y. Women with risk factors (e.g., HPV infection) may require more frequent screening. Screening is not necessary for women who have had total hysterectomies unless the surgery was for treatment of cervical cancer.	Pap test every 1–3 y for all women who are sexually active and/or have a cervix. No evidence to support an upper limit, but age 65 y can be defended in women with a history of normal and regular Pap tests.	Evidence strongly suggests a decrease in mortality for regular screening with Pap tests in women who are sexually active or who have reached age 18 y. The upper limit at which such screening ceases to be effective is unknown.
Colorectal cancer	One of the following schedules for men and women aged 50 y and over at average risk: FOBT yearly; sigmoidoscopy every 5 y; FOBT + sigmoidoscopy every 5 y; colonoscopy every 10 y; DCBE every 5 y. Those at high risk for colorectal cancer should begin screening earlier and/or more frequently.	Screening for colorectal cancer is strongly recommended for men and women aged 50 y and over. Several screening modalities are effective. Good evidence has been shown that periodic FOBT reduces mortality from colorectal cancer, and there is fair evidence that sigmoidoscopy alone or in combination with FOBT reduces mortality. No direct evidence has been shown for either colonoscopy or DCBE.	FOBT either annually or biennially using rehydrated or nonrehydrated stool specimens in people aged 50 y and over decreases mortality for colorectal cancer. Regular screening by sigmoidoscopy in people over age 50 y may decrease mortality from colorectal cancer. Evidence is insufficient to determine the optimal interval for such screening.
Prostate cancer	PSA test and DRE should be offered annually, beginning at age 50 y, to men who have a life expectancy of at least 10 y. Men at high risk for cancer should start screening at 45 y. Men should be given the information needed to make informed decisions about prostate cancer screening.	Evidence is insufficient to recommend for or against routine screening for prostate cancer using PSA testing or DRE.	Evidence is insufficient to establish that a decrease in mortality occurs with screening by DRE, transrectal ultrasound, or PSA.

BSE, breast self-examination; CBE, clinical breast examination; DCBE, double-contrast barium enema; DRE, digital rectal examination; FOBT, fecal occult blood test; HPV, human papillomavirus; Pap, Papanicolaou; PSA, prostate-specific antigen.

the U.S. Preventive Services Task Force concluded that the data also are insufficient to reach conclusions about BSE.[29] Green and Taplin[21] recommended that if women want to perform BSE, they be taught to do it correctly. Given the small windows of time physicians have to counsel and teach, time probably is best spent giving strong messages about the importance of mammography and performing a thorough CBE. Data from a large-scale service delivery program suggest that CBE may be most useful for women in their 40s where mammography may be somewhat less efficacious.[43] Although the recommendations of different medical organizations vary, most encourage women to have a CBE yearly (see Table 22-5).

CERVICAL CANCER SCREENING

A steady 70% decline in mortality from cervical cancer has been observed since the mid-century after the introduction of widespread Papanicolaou (Pap) cytologic screening.[20] This is a major success story for cancer control in the United States. In 2003, there were an estimated 12,200 new cases of invasive cervical cancer and 4100 deaths.[20] Although mortality from this cancer is no longer as common as in the past in the United States, cervical cancer is still the second most common cancer worldwide.[44] In developed countries, fatalities from this disease should be entirely avoidable with currently available technology. Incidence and mortality are higher in women with no prior screening, those with concurrent human papillomavirus (HPV) infection, and women of lower socioeconomic status.

Newer methods of screening make use of increased understanding of the essential etiologic role of approximately 15 oncogenic types of HPV.[45] Various combinations of HPV DNA testing; newer cytologic methods, especially liquid-based cytology; and traditional Pap smears offer opportunities to improve sensitivity and specificity of cervical cancer screening.[46] However, traditional cytologic screening with Pap smears remains the primary method of screening.

The value of Pap smear screening is of little doubt, even though there has never been an RCT to confirm its efficacy. In the absence of an RCT, evidence for the effectiveness of cytologic screening has come from observed trends in countries with large national screening programs[47,48] and case-control studies in varied geographic areas.[49–52] When to start, when to stop, and the interval between tests have been important questions within the context of traditional cytologic screening.

Current U.S. recommendations are that screening should start approximately 3 years after the onset of sexual activity, at least by age 21 years.[53,54] This is based on the observed high prevalence of HPV infection in young, sexually active women and the frequency of low- and high-grade squamous intraepithelial lesions. However, up to 70% of high-risk HPV infections are transient in young women in their 20s, and 90% of low-grade squamous intraepithelial lesions regress in this age group.[55] Furthermore, incidence is not measurable until 20 to 24 years of age, when it is still only 1.7 per 100,000 per year.[56] Given the low incidence of serious disease and the high likelihood of regression of early dysplastic lesions in younger women, there is concern that screening adolescents and women in their 20s could lead to overdiagnosis, aggressive treatment, and unnecessary harm from ablative surgical procedures.[54,57] To address this reality, some European countries (e.g., Denmark) do not start screening until age 30 years.

More than one-half of invasive cervical cancers occur in women who have never been screened, or at least not within the previous 5 years.[58,59] Progress toward further reductions in death from this cancer could be made by concerted efforts to reach and screen such women. However, evidence is limited on the question of the optimal interval between screening tests. After its review of evidence, the U.S. Preventive Services Task Force left the interval variable from 1 to 3 years.[53] The principal study on which this judgment was based was a comprehensive analysis of large-scale screening programs and case-control studies that used various designs and methods but which showed increased efficacy with shorter intervals up to annual testing. Sample size, even in this large analysis, was insufficient to distinguish efficacy between intervals of every 2 versus every 3 years.[60] A case-control study in a large, stable health plan population confirmed that annual screening is more likely to pick up invasive cervical cancers than is using an interval of every 2 years, and likewise for 2- versus 3-year intervals. The advantage was very small, and cost-effectiveness studies are needed.[61] For women who have had hysterectomies for benign conditions, the likelihood of detecting vaginal dysplasia is extremely low and the false-positive rate high.[62] The continued practice of screening at any interval in this group is inappropriate.

Data are also inadequate on which to base recommendations for an upper age limit for regular screening. Although there is concern that Pap testing is less sensitive in older women because of a receded squamocolumnar junction of the cervix, the primary reason for invasive cervical cancer in older women is still lack of any screening.[63]

International studies using DNA testing have demonstrated that almost all cervical cancers are associated with infection by sexually transmitted HPV.[44,64] However, HPV infection is highly transient in young women, and screening protocols that use HPV testing are still being evaluated. Protocols that add HPV

DNA testing to the traditional Pap test for cytologic results of atypical squamous cells of undetermined significance (ASCUS) have demonstrated increased sensitivity over repeated Pap smear testing.[65] Among 3488 women with ASCUS followed for 2 years in the ASCUS/LSIL (low-grade squamous intraepithelial lesion) Triage Study, HPV DNA testing was more sensitive for detecting cervical intraepithelial neoplasia 3 or invasive cancer and just as specific as repeat cytology.[66] Comparisons of the multiple strategies now available, including visual screening, conventional cytology, liquid-based cytology, and HPV DNA testing, have found that either liquid-based cytology or HPV DNA testing provides a better balance between sensitivity and specificity for cervical intraepithelial neoplasia 3+ than conventional methods.[46] However, although these new technologies are promising, the results are highly dependent on local resources and prevalence of disease. In most situations, clinicians are still likely to have their greatest effect by ensuring full coverage and follow-up for women who receive traditional cytologic screening. The challenge for the future may be less of a technical nature and more dependent on local finances and screening policies.[46]

COLORECTAL CANCER SCREENING

The importance of screening for colorectal cancer is based on the high incidence and mortality from this cancer and the availability of screening methods of demonstrated efficacy. Cancers of the colon and rectum account for the third largest number of new cancer cases after lung cancer, with 105,500 colon and 42,000 rectum cases estimated, respectively, in 2003; approximately 57,100 deaths were predicted for colon and rectum cancers combined.[20] Whereas declining incidence rates have stabilized since 1995, the steady decline in death rates has accelerated since the mid-1980s, especially for whites.[67]

Four procedures are currently in use for colon cancer screening: fecal occult blood test (FOBT), sigmoidoscopy, colonoscopy, and high-contrast barium enema. All professional organizations that have published guidelines recommend screening for adults 50 years and older with some combination of these four modalities.[68–72] For the general population, age 50 years was chosen, because that is when the incidence of colorectal cancer begins to increase and where efficacy is supported by evidence. For individuals at high risk, age 40 years is generally recommended as the starting age.[68]

1. *Fecal occult blood test.* Direct support for use of FOBT comes from three large randomized controlled trials, including a Minnesota trial of 46,501 participants between the ages of 50 and 80 years of age.[73] This study found that annual FOBT with rehydration of the samples decreased 13-year cumulative mortality from colorectal cancer by 33% and biennial screening by 21%.[73] Most (75% to 84%) of this reduction resulted from the test itself rather than from incidental discovery of cancers by follow-up colonoscopy.[74] Data from case-control studies are generally consistent with the conclusions of these trials.[75–77] The main limitation of the FOBT is its limited specificity.[2]

2. *Flexible sigmoidoscopy.* The advantage of sigmoidoscopy screening over FOBT is that it frequently includes the

actual removal of cancer or a precancerous lesion in a biopsied polyp, thus combining screening and treatment in one step.[78] Another advantage is that it needs to be performed only infrequently, perhaps every 5 to 10 years.[79] At least two large randomized trials of flexible sigmoidoscopy screening are in progress. In the first of these randomized trials, the PLCO trial is evaluating the efficacy of examinations every 3 years in 74,000 men and women, 55 to 74 years of age, and an equal number of controls.[80] In the United Kingdom, a trial of 200,000 men and women, 55 to 64 years of age, is evaluating one sigmoidoscopy delivered to approximately 65,000 adults randomized for screening.[81] Meanwhile, supporting evidence for efficacy comes from several case-control studies in health plans in northern California and Wisconsin and from American veterans.[79,82,83]

3. *Colonoscopy and double-contrast barium enema.* No direct evidence supports the efficacy of either colonoscopy or double-contrast barium enema. A strong rationale for the use of colonoscopy is based on its superior sensitivity and specificity.[84] Because there may never be a randomized trial mounted to evaluate the efficacy of colonoscopy directly,[85] choices about its use will depend more on concerns about its safety, the capacity of the health care system to make it available, and its cost effectiveness.[69] Colonoscopy has risks: Approximately 1 in 1000 patients experience perforation, 3 in 1000 have major hemorrhage, and 1 to 3 in 10,000 die as a result of the procedure.[2] Double-contrast barium enema is an alternative for examining the entire colon and finds its usefulness in situations in which individuals cannot tolerate endoscopic procedures and in which the relevant expertise exists.[68]

Multiple studies of the cost effectiveness of colorectal cancer screening are consistent in concluding that the cost per year of a life saved is within the limits accepted for most preventive procedures from a societal perspective (approximately $50,000). However, no one modality stands out as superior.[69]

Alternatives to current methods are being investigated and have been reviewed.[86] Immunohistochemical screening tests of stool may offer more sensitive and specific alternatives to guaiac-based testing.[87] The molecular detection of DNA mutations in cells exfoliated from neoplasms in the stool may be a highly sensitive and specific approach that is noninvasive and thus more acceptable to patients.[88]

Newer detection techniques include "virtual" colonoscopy that uses CT of the prepared colon and avoids the invasiveness and discomfort of conventional optical colonoscopy. Fenlon et al.[89] provided data on a study in which a crossover design was used; 100 patients were given virtual colonoscopies immediately before conventional colonoscopies. Test performance was compared and was similar, with a threshold of detection for virtual colonoscopy at approximately 5 mm. Pickhardt et al.[90] reported on test performance using a similar design but with a much larger population (1233 asymptomatic patients) and one that offers more potential for generalizing findings to average-risk patients. They showed that a three-dimensional endoluminal display can achieve 93.8% sensitivity and a specificity of 96.0% for polyps at least 10 mm in diameter compared to optical colonoscopy on the

same asymptomatic average-risk subjects.[90] These and other studies of newer technology will be commanding much attention in the near future.

Meanwhile, despite the evidence supporting the value and cost effectiveness of traditional colorectal cancer screening procedures, compliance with guidelines remains low, at approximately 30% of the population; disparities in screening rates between race and ethnic groups are increasing.[91] Access to screening varies greatly by region of the country and the availability of trained personnel. However, the primary barriers to increased compliance are behavioral for physicians and for patients and associated with the complexity of and perceptions about the nature of the recommended procedures.[69] Efforts to improve compliance should focus on getting individuals over 50 years screened at least once by any modality, rather than on the superiority of any one test.[92] Choices among individuals vary consistently regarding which test is preferred.[2]

SKIN CANCER SCREENING

The incidence of skin cancer has increased worldwide, with U.S. incidence data mirroring this trend.[20] In the United States, the incidence rate for melanoma has increased approximately 4% per year since the early 1970s, with a 162% increase in male melanoma cases and 95% in women.[20] It is unclear whether this increase is due to actual changes in prevalence or is partly a function of increased awareness, with subsequent diagnosis, improved reporting by tumor registries, or both. In 2003, 63,400 new cases of skin cancer and 12,000 deaths were projected, with 54,200 new cases of melanoma (skin) and 7600 deaths.[20] Melanoma now ranks sixth in incidence among cancers in males and seventh in incidence among cancers in females. Approximately 800,000 nonmelanoma skin cancers are diagnosed each year.[20] The United States lags behind many other countries in the creative application of interventions to reduce the incidence of and mortality from melanoma and other skin cancers. Australia, which has the highest reported incidence of melanoma anywhere, has mounted successful population-based programs that have had dramatic effects.[93]

Experts have not agreed about screening guidelines for skin cancer. The U.S. Preventive Services Task Force recommends routine screening for individuals at high risk (e.g., those who have a family or personal history of skin cancer, clinical evidence of precursor lesions, and increased exposure to sunlight). The Task Force neither defines what is meant by routine screening nor reports on the specific recommendations for skin self-examination.[3,94] The ACS recommends a cancer-related checkup, including a skin examination, every 3 years, and more frequently for persons at risk.[72] The NCI also recognizes the benefits of skin cancer screening but offers no specific guidelines for such screening.[95] Only one study demonstrates evidence regarding skin self-examination. Although it showed a decrease in mortality, there were limitations that preclude making recommendations on the basis of this study alone.[96,97]

PROSTATE CANCER SCREENING

Prostate cancer is the most commonly diagnosed cancer among men in the United States and is the second leading cause of male cancer deaths. It is estimated that in 2003, 220,900 new cases of prostate cancer were identified, with 28,900 deaths.[20] However, consensus is lacking about recommendations for prostate cancer screening. The controversy has been raised for several reasons. First, there is no definitive evidence that prostate cancer screening results in improved clinical outcomes, especially a reduction in mortality from the disease.[98,99] Second, the rise in the incidence of prostate cancer from 1989 to 1992 (see http://www.seer.cancer.gov) was due largely to detection of latent, asymptomatic cases with uncertain clinical relevance, thus putting the value of screening in doubt.[98,99]

SCREENING TESTS FOR PROSTATE CANCER

The two main screening modalities for prostate cancer include digital rectal examination (DRE) and serum prostate-specific antigen (PSA; concentration more than 4 ng/dL) and endorectal (transrectal) ultrasonography (TRUS). The most widely used and oldest technique for detection of prostate cancer is the DRE; ranges in estimates of sensitivity and specificity are reported. Estimates suggest a PPV of 15% to 30% and a sensitivity of approximately 60%.[2] Ultimately, only one in three patients with a positive DRE has prostate cancer.[100] With the development and application of intraluminal (rectal) probes with high resolution, studies have shown that small, nonpalpable malignant lesions of the prostate could be detected.[101] TRUS has fallen short of expectations, with large variation in reports of sensitivity and specificity, both ranging from 41% to 79%.[101,102] Despite this, TRUS is considered an excellent ancillary modality to increase accuracy of biopsy over the digital guidance alone.

PSA is a blood test that allows for earlier detection of many prostate cancers, with sensitivity of up to 80% to 85%. Unfortunately, PSA tests have low specificity, resulting in high rates of false-positives.[2] Interest in the PSA grew in the late 1980s as PSA levels were shown to drop to undetectable levels after prostatectomy.[103,104] However, normal PSA values are found in approximately one-third of men with localized cancers, and PSA levels are often elevated in men with noncancerous conditions, such as benign prostatic hyperplasia.[104,105] Only approximately 7% of prostate cancers detected by screening are microfocal and low grade.[106]

Some investigators have argued that integration of DRE with determination of PSA levels and the use of TRUS in selected cases should improve prostate cancer detection.[104,107] Using age-specific PSA ranges may be a promising strategy for increasing PSA sensitivity.[108] Prostate cancer screening is more controversial in older men; concerns about quality of life outweigh potential benefit of screening.[109] Several reports indicate that men over age 70 years are unlikely to benefit from PSA testing.[100]

Nonrandomized Studies

Two nonrandomized studies are ongoing to evaluate screening tests for prostate cancer [the ACS National Prostate Cancer Detection Project (ACS-NPCDP)[110,111] and a multicenter study headquartered at Washington University[112] involving 6 university medical centers]. Results of the ACS-NPCDP trial indicate that a combined modality approach (DRE, TRUS, and PSA) to prostate cancer detection yields high levels of early detection. Data from the Washington

University study also indicate that screening with PSA or PSA in combination with DRE, or both, is reasonable for detecting carcinomas at an early stage.[113] Continued follow-up to evaluate longer-term morbidity and mortality data from these studies will not be available until the end of the first decade of the twenty-first century. Thus, clinicians and patients must make decisions in the absence of RCT data. Table 22-6 summarizes the sensitivity, specificity, and predictive value of available data.

Randomized Clinical Trials

The NCI-funded PLCO trial is a 16-year randomized control study that began in 1993.[80] It is accruing 74,000 men aged 60 to 74 years and has a design power of 90% to determine 20% reduction of prostate cancer mortality. PLCO will provide important information about the efficacy of screening. A second large randomized trial, the European Randomized Study of Screening for Prostate Cancer, is being conducted in eight European countries[114] with men aged 55 to 74 years at entry; there are approximately 180,000 participants. Investigators in the European Randomized Study of Screening for Prostate Cancer and PLCO trials are collaborating to share data to increase statistical power. Results from these trials are expected in 2005 to 2008. Finally, based on a randomized study in Sweden of 9972 men aged 50 to 65 years, it was concluded that it is safe to screen biennially in men with PSA of less than 2 ng/mL, with different screening intervals determined based on baseline PSA.[115] Further confirmation of appropriate screening intervals for PSA screening is needed.

As is the case for other kinds of cancer screening, there is concern about overdiagnosis for prostate cancer. In fact, it is an even greater potential problem for prostate than for some other kinds of cancer screening because of studies showing that many men die of prostate cancer without ever having known they had the disease. Draisma et al.[116] attempted to provide some insight into the potential overdiagnosis problem using models to simulate lead time. They estimated that annual screening from age 55 to 67 years would result in an overdetection rate of 50%, and the lifetime prostate cancer risk was increased to 80%. People will argue whether the model is correct, and all models have imprecision. Nevertheless, this is further caution about the limitations of screening for prostate cancer, the need for better understanding of the biology of the disease, and the parallel need for better screening tests.

Trends and What They Mean

National data from 1990 to 1996 show that prostate cancer incidence peaked in 1992 at 190.8 per 100,000 and declined at an average rate of 8.5% from 1992 to 1996.[117] A series of related reports in the *Journal of the National Cancer Institute*, based on data from the Surveillance, Epidemiology, and End Results Cancer Registry program show a decline in incidence of regional stage disease,[117] as well as a decline in incidence-based mortality of distant stage disease and flat incidence-based mortality trends for localized and distant stage disease.[99] Statistical methods were applied to consider the effect of screening by limiting some analyses to the contribution from cases diagnosed since 1987, when

TABLE 22-6. Estimates of Screening Test Performance for Prostate Cancer

Investigation	Screening Test	Sample Size	Ages (Y)	Sensitivity (%)	Specificity (%)	Positive Predictive Value (%)	Detection Rate (%)
Cancer Detection Study; Jenson et al., 1960[137]	DRE	4367	>50	NA	NA	94	0.8
Cancer Detection Study; Gilbertsen, 1971[138]	DRE	5856	>45	NA	NA	NA	1.3
Chodak and Schoenberg, 1984[139]	DRE	811	41–85	NA	NA	29	1.7
Thompson et al., 1984[140]	DRE	2005	40–70	NA	NA	26	0.8
Mueller et al., 1988[141]	DRE	4843	40–79	NA	NA	39	2.5
Lee et al., 1988[142]	DRE			45	97	34	1.3
	TRUS	784	60–86	91	94	31	2.6
Cooner et al., 1990[105]	DRE			77	53	43	14.6 (overall)
	TRUS	1807	50–89	NA	NA	32	
	PSA			80	61	48	
	DRE/PSA			90	64	62	
Catalona et al., 1991[104]	DRE			84	51	37	2.2 (overall)
	TRUS	1653	≥50	90	27	30	
	PSA			79	60	33	
Mettlin et al., 1991[143]	DRE	2425	55–70	58	96	28	4.6
Babaian et al., 1992[111]	TRUS	2425	55–70	77	89	15	2.4 (overall)
	PSA			67	82	43	
Catalona et al., 1994[112]	DRE	6630	≥50	55	45	21	3.2
Smith et al., 1997[113]	PSA	30,000	>50	82	48	32	
	PSA and/ or DRE			NA	NA	25–33	3–10
Mettlin et al., 1997[110]	DRE	2999	55–70	39	96	NA	2.0
	TRUS			66	92		
	PSA			69	90		

DRE, digital rectal examination; NA, not available; PSA, prostate-specific antigen; TRUS, transrectal ultrasonography.

widespread screening using the PSA test had occurred. In a review of published data from five prospective trials, treatment of localized disease was associated with a marked decrease in prostate cancer deaths.[106] Thus, some evidence shows improved prognosis for screen-detected cases. However, alternative interpretations, such as the possibility that cause-of-death misclassification could explain these findings, cannot be ruled out.

PROSTATE CANCER SCREENING RECOMMENDATIONS

In light of the limitations of evidence regarding prostate cancer screening, it is important to consider the natural history of this disease and subgroups of men at high risk for developing prostate cancer. These considerations are critical for determining public health policy.[100] Men's preferences regarding testing vary, and these preferences also are important in deciding on screening. Most medical organizations now stress the importance of individualizing screening decisions based on factors such as patients' preference, health history, and health status (see Table 22-5).

LUNG CANCER SCREENING

Lung cancer screening is not recommended on a population basis due to lack of evidence that any available screening procedure, even for smokers, can identify tumors early enough to reduce mortality.[118] This remains a major challenge to research

and technology because of the tremendous burden caused by this cancer, including among ex-smokers. In 2003, there were an estimated 171,900 new cases and 157,200 deaths, making it by far the most common killer from cancer in men and in women.[20]

None of four randomized trials conducted during the 1960s and 1970s reduced mortality significantly over no screening.[119–122] The Mayo Lung Project, the primary trial contributing to this evidence, demonstrated that screening with either chest x-rays or chest x-rays plus sputum cytology lowered the stage at presentation and increased survival, but neither approach had any effect on lung cancer mortality.[122] Although lack of connection between improved survival and the absence of a mortality benefit can be attributed to lead-time and length biases, these studies have been criticized for other methodologic reasons.[123,124] Extended mortality follow-up of participants in the Mayo Lung Project suggested that overdiagnosis, the identification of clinically unimportant lung cancer lesions, may have occurred.[125]

Low-dose CT scanning is a new and potentially efficacious method for early detection of lung cancer.[126] This noninvasive technique, which creates an image of the entire thorax during a single held breath with a low radiation dose, is being offered by an increasing number of imaging facilities for older smokers and former smokers. However, to date, evidence of high sensitivity comes only from observational studies that are susceptible to lead-time and length-time bias. The possibility of overdiagnosis and concerns of harm from CT screening have also been raised,[124] and there is, as yet, insufficient evidence to support mass lung cancer screening with this procedure.[125] Nevertheless, the potential of this technology and the enormous societal burden imposed by lung cancer motivated the NCI to begin a large, randomized controlled trial to assess the effect of low-dose CT screening compared to standard chest x-ray on lung cancer mortality. Other observational studies of low-dose CT screening are ongoing and may add to the evidence produced by the NCI-supported trial, which will take approximately 10 years to produce results.[124] Meanwhile, decisions about use of CT scans for lung cancer screening remain a matter of individual judgment between physicians and patients.[123] Several reports suggest the need for caution in adopting lung CT screening, especially in view of aggressive direct-to-consumer marketing of the procedure.[127,128] In a detailed decision analysis, Mahadevia et al.[128] showed that even if efficacy of helical CT is shown, it is unlikely to be cost effective. Like many tests, helical CT may be able to identify small lesions. However, questions remain about the mortality impact and cost effectiveness. Thus, the ongoing trial is of critical import.[129] Efforts to prevent initiation, especially by youth, and cessation of tobacco use remain the physician's best tool for combating lung cancer.

ADHERENCE TO CANCER SCREENING

Over the years, substantial research has been conducted to understand people's barriers to cancer screening.[2] Several lessons are clear. First, physician recommendations are the most important factor in motivating people to be screened. Even then, however, many people will not get necessary tests. Several reviews show that simple reminders and letters, delivered in print or by telephone, can double or triple the odds that people will attain needed tests. This is true even among vulnerable populations.[130–132] Interventions often are needed at several levels: individual, provider, and health system. The Centers for Disease Control and Prevention's Task Force on Community Preventive Services has reviewed interventions to promote screening and publishes regular updates (http://www.cdc.gov).

Some people are at risk for being un- or underscreened. These include recent immigrants, people without health insurance, people with no usual source of health care, and people with very low incomes. Although age and ethnicity are important determinants for some cancers, this is not the case for others.[91]

The best source of U.S. data on cancer screening practices is the National Health Interview Survey. In the 2000 National Health Interview Survey, 70% of women aged 40 years and older reported having recent mammograms, 82% of women aged 25 and older reported having recent Pap tests, 41% of men and 37.5% of women reported having either an FOBT within the past year or colorectal endoscopy within the past 5 years, and 41% of men aged 50 years and over had a PSA test within the past 5 years.[91] Rates of regular screening for all these tests are considerably lower than reports of recent screening.

FUTURE OF SCREENING

Many challenges lie ahead for cancer screening. Better detection methods are urgently needed, and molecular detection methods may surpass current techniques. At the same time,

more effort is required to encourage adherence to proven cancer screening modalities. Adherence to screening is less than optimal for all the major recommended screening techniques.[91] With discovery of mutations in susceptibility genes that predispose to cancer, new challenges in cancer screening arise with the need for appropriate screening recommendations and programs for high-risk subgroups. Not only are those who have inherited mutations for cancer susceptibility at higher risk for developing some cancers, but, often, the age at onset among such individuals is younger than age at onset in the general population. This creates challenges for those who recommend and promote screening regimens. The example of the *BRCA1* susceptibility gene for breast cancer illustrates a perplexing situation in which recommendations for screening with mammography do not address the early age at onset of this disease. Moreover, there are no good population data on which to base guidelines. Further study is needed to establish efficacious screening protocols for those who are genetically predisposed to cancer.

Among the challenges of the future is how to evaluate new screening technologies in a world where large RCTs may be increasingly difficult to conduct. In screening, as in other areas of medicine and public health, the inclination to recommend screening tests on the basis of an intriguing and promising study must be balanced by a careful assessment of the evidence.

REFERENCES

1. Kramer BS, Gohagan JK, Prorok PC. *Cancer screening: theory and practice.* New York: Marcel Dekker, Inc., 1999.
2. National Cancer Policy Board and IOM. *Fulfilling the potential of cancer prevention and early detection.* Washington, DC: National Research Council, Institute of Medicine, 2003.
3. US Preventive Services Task Force. *Guide to clinical preventive services.* International Medical Publishing, 1996.
4. Goldie SJ, Kuntz KM. A potential error in evaluating cancer screening: a comparison of 2 approaches for modeling underlying disease progression. *Med Decis Making* 2003;23:232.
5. Kaplan RM. The significance of quality of life in health care. *Qual Life Res* 2003;12[Suppl 1]:3.
6. Elwood JM, Cox B, Richardson AK. The effectiveness of breast cancer screening by mammography in younger women. *Online J Curr Clin Trials* 1993;32:23.
7. Miller AB. Mammography: reviewing the evidence. Epidemiology aspect. *Can Fam Physician* 1993;39:85.
8. National Cancer Institute. What is randomization? World Wide Web URL: http://cancer.gov/clinicaltrials/understanding/what-is-randomization, 2004.
9. Lerman C, Trock B, Rimer BK, et al. Psychological and behavioral implications of abnormal mammograms. *Ann Intern Med* 1991;114:657.
10. Elmore JG, Barton MB, Moceri VM, et al. Ten-year risk of false positive screening mammograms and clinical breast examinations. *N Engl J Med* 1998;338:1089.
11. Fletcher SW. False-positive screening mammograms: good news, but more to do. *Ann Intern Med* 1999;131:60.
12. Paskett E, Rimer BK. Psychosocial effects of abnormal Pap tests and mammograms: a review. *J Womens Health* 1995;4:73.
13. Fletcher SW, Black W, Harris R, et al. Report of the International Workshop on Screening for Breast Cancer. *J Natl Cancer Inst* 1993;85:1644.
14. Baines CJ. Mammography screening: are women really giving informed consent? *J Natl Cancer Inst* 2003;95:1508.
15. Lipkus IM, Rimer BK, Strigo TS. Relationships among objective and subjective risk for breast cancer and mammography stages of change. *Cancer Epidemiol Biomarkers Prev* 1996;5:1005.
16. Harris R. Decision-making about screening individual and policy levels. In: Kramer BS, Gohagan JK, Prorok PC, eds. *Cancer screening: theory and practice.* Marcel Dekker, Inc., 1999.
17. Volk RJ, Cass AR, Spann SJ. A randomized controlled trial of shared decision making for prostate cancer screening. *Arch Fam Med* 1999;8:333.
18. Briss PA, Rimer BK, Reilley B, et al. Promoting informed decisions about cancer screening in communities and healthcare systems. *Am J Prev Med* 2004;26:67.
19. Austoker J. Gaining informed consent for screening. Is difficult—but many misconceptions need not be undone. *BMJ* 1999;319:722.
20. American Cancer Society. *Cancer facts and figures, 2003.* Atlanta: American Cancer Society, 2003.
21. Green BB, Taplin SH. Breast cancer screening controversies. *J Am Board Fam Pract* 2003;16:233.

22. Berry DA. Benefits and risks of screening mammography for women in their forties: a statistical appraisal. *J Natl Cancer Inst* 1998;90:1431.

23. Miller AB, To T, Baines CJ, et al. The Canadian National Breast Screening Study-1: breast cancer mortality after 11 to 16 years of follow-up. A randomized screening trial of mammography in women age 40 to 49 years. *Ann Intern Med* 2002;137:305.

24. Miller AB, To T, Baines CJ, et al. Canadian National Breast Screening Study-2: 13-year results of a randomized trial in women aged 50–59 years. *J Natl Cancer Inst* 2000;92:1490.

25. Shapiro S. Periodic screening for breast cancer: the HIP Randomized Controlled Trial. Health Insurance Plan. *J Natl Cancer Inst Monogr* 1997:27.

26. Tabar L, Fagerberg G, Duffy SW, et al. Update of the Swedish two-county program of mammographic screening for breast cancer. *Radiol Clin North Am* 1992;30:187.

27. Tabar L, Vitak B, Chen HH, et al. The Swedish Two-County Trial twenty years later. Updated mortality results and new insights from long-term follow-up. *Radiol Clin North Am* 2000;38:625.

28. Andersson I, Aspegren K, Janzon L, et al. Mammographic screening and mortality from breast cancer: the Malmö mammographic screening trial. *BMJ* 1988;297:943.

29. Humphrey LL, Helfand M, Chan BK, et al. Breast cancer screening: a summary of the evidence for the US Preventive Services Task Force. *Ann Intern Med* 2002;137:347.

30. Hendrick RE, Smith RA, Rutledge JH 3rd, et al. Benefit of screening mammography in women aged 40–49: a new meta-analysis of randomized controlled trials. *J Natl Cancer Inst Monogr* 1997:87.

31. Alexander FE, Anderson TJ, Brown HK, et al. 14 Years of follow-up from the Edinburgh randomised trial of breast-cancer screening. *Lancet* 1999;353:1903.

32. Burhenne LJ, Burhenne HJ. The Canadian National Breast Screening Study: a Canadian critique. *AJR Am J Roentgenol* 1993;161:761.

33. Kopans DB. The Canadian screening program: a different prospective [Commentary]. *AJR Am J Roentgenol* 1990;155:748.

34. Prorok PC, Kramer BS, Gohagan JK. Screening theory and study design: the basics. In: *Cancer screening: theory and practice*. New York: Marcel Dekker, Inc., 1999.

35. Smart CR, Hendrick RE, Rutledge JH 3rd, et al. Benefit of mammography screening in women ages 40 to 49 years. Current evidence from randomized controlled trials. *Cancer* 1995;75:1619.

36. Morrison AS, Brisson J, Khalid N. Breast cancer incidence and mortality in the Breast Cancer Detection Demonstration Project [published erratum appears in *J Natl Cancer Inst* 1989;81(19):1513]. *J Natl Cancer Inst* 1988;80:1540.

37. Costanza ME. The extent of breast cancer screening in older women. *Cancer* 1994; 74[Suppl 7]:2046.

38. van Dijck JA, Holland R, Verbeek AL, et al. Efficacy of mammographic screening of the elderly: a case-referent study in the Nijmegen program in The Netherlands. *J Natl Cancer Inst* 1994;86:934.

39. National Institutes of Health. Proceedings of the National Institutes of Health Consensus Conference on Breast Cancer Screening for Women Ages 40–49. Bethesda, MD, 21–23 January 1997. *J Natl Cancer Inst Monogr* 1997;22:vii.

40. Ransohoff DF, Harris RP. Lessons from the mammography screening controversy: can we improve the debate? *Ann Intern Med* 1997;127:1029.

41. Tabar L, Duffy SW, Vitak B, et al. The natural history of breast carcinoma: what have we learned from screening? *Cancer* 1999;86:449.

42. Gotzsche PC, Olsen O. Is screening for breast cancer with mammography justifiable? *Lancet* 2000;355:129.

43. Bobo JK, Lawson HW, Lee NC. Risk factors for failure to detect a cancer during clinical breast examinations (United States). *Cancer Causes Control* 2003;14:461.

44. Bosch FX, Manos MM, Munoz N, et al. Prevalence of human papillomavirus in cervical cancer: a worldwide perspective. International Biological Study on Cervical Cancer (IBSCC) Study Group. *J Natl Cancer Inst* 1995;87:796.

45. Bosch FX, Lorincz A, Munoz N, et al. The causal relation between human papillomavirus and cervical cancer. *J Clin Pathol* 2002;55:244.

46. Ferreccio C, Bratti MC, Sherman ME, et al. A comparison of single and combined visual, cytologic, and virologic tests as screening strategies in a region at high risk of cervical cancer. *Cancer Epidemiol Biomarkers Prev* 2003;12:815.

47. Laara E, Day NE, Hakama M. Trends in mortality from cervical cancer in the Nordic countries: association with organised screening programmes. *Lancet* 1987;1:1247.

48. Miller AB, Lindsay J, Hill GB. Mortality from cancer of the uterus in Canada and its relationship to screening for cancer of the cervix. *Int J Cancer* 1976;17:602.

49. Clarke EA, Anderson TW. Does screening by "Pap" smears help prevent cervical cancer? A case-control study. *Lancet* 1979;2:1.

50. Aristizabal N, Cuello C, Correa P, et al. The impact of vaginal cytology on cervical cancer risks in Cali, Colombia. *Int J Cancer* 1984;34:5.

51. La Vecchia C, Franceschi S, Decarli A, et al. "Pap" smear and the risk of cervical neoplasia: quantitative estimates from a case-control study. *Lancet* 1984;2:779.

52. Herrero R, Brinton LA, Reeves WC, et al. Screening for cervical cancer in Latin America: a case-control study. *Int J Epidemiol* 1992;21:1050.

53. US Preventive Services Task Force. Screening for cervical cancer: recommendations and rationale. World Wide Web URL: http://www.ahcpr.gov/clinic/3rduspstf/cervcan/cerv-canrr.htm, 2004.

54. Saslow D, Runowicz CD, Solomon D, et al. American Cancer Society guideline for the early detection of cervical neoplasia and cancer. *CA Cancer J Clin* 2002;52:342.

55. Moscicki AB, Shiboski S, Broering J, et al. The natural history of human papillomavirus infection as measured by repeated DNA testing in adolescent and young women. *J Pediatr* 1998;132:277.

56. Reis LA, Eisner MP, Kosary CL, et al. *SEER cancer statistics review, 1973–1999*. Bethesda, MD: National Cancer Institute, 2002.

57. Chan PG, Sung HY, Sawaya GF. Changes in cervical cancer incidence after three decades of screening US women less than 30 years old. *Obstet Gynecol* 2003;102:765.

58. National Institutes of Health. Cervical cancer. *NIH Consens Statement* 2003;14:1.

59. Kinney W, Sung HY, Kearney KA, et al. Missed opportunities for cervical cancer screening of HMO members developing invasive cervical cancer (ICC). *Gynecol Oncol* 1998;71:428.

60. International Agency for Research on Cancer. Working Group on Evaluation of Cervical Cancer Screening Programmes: screening for squamous cervical cancer: duration of low risk after negative results of cervical cytology and its implications for screening policies. *BMJ* 1986;293:6599.

61. Miller MG, Sung HY, Sawaya GF, et al. Screening interval and risk of invasive squamous cell cervical cancer. *Obstet Gynecol* 2003;101:29.

62. Pearce KF, Haefner HK, Sarwar SF, et al. Cytopathological findings on vaginal Papanicolaou smears after hysterectomy for benign gynecologic disease. *N Engl J Med* 1996;335:1559.

63. Sawaya GF, Sung HY, Kearney K, et al. Advancing age and cervical cancer screening and prognosis. *J Am Geriatr Soc* 2002;49:1499.

64. Wallboomers JM, Jacobs MV, Manos MM. Human papillomavirus is a necessary cause of invasive cervical cancer worldwide. *J Pathol* 1999;189:12.

65. Manos MM, Kinney WK, Hurley LB, et al. Identifying women with cervical neoplasia: using human papillomavirus DNA testing for equivocal Papanicolaou results. *JAMA* 1999;281:1605.

66. Schiffman M, Solomon D. Findings to date from the ASCUS-LSIL Triage Study (ALTS). *Arch Pathol Lab Med* 2003;127:946.

67. Weir HK, Thun MJ, Hankey BF, et al. Annual report to the nation on the status of cancer, 1975–2000, featuring the uses of surveillance data for cancer prevention and control. *J Natl Cancer Inst* 2003;95:1276.

68. Winawer S, Fletcher R, Rex D, et al. Colorectal cancer screening and surveillance: clinical guidelines and rationale—update based on new evidence. *Gastroenterology* 2003;124:544.

69. Walsh JM, Terdiman JP. Colorectal cancer screening: clinical applications. *JAMA* 2003;289:1297.

70. Rex DK, Johnson DA, Lieberman DA, et al. Colorectal cancer prevention 2000: screening recommendations of the American College of Gastroenterology. American College of Gastroenterology. *Am J Gastroenterol* 2000;95:868.

71. US Preventive Services Task Force. Screening for colorectal cancer: recommendations and rationale. World Wide Web URL: http://www.ahcpr.gov/clinic/3rduspstf/colorec-tal/colorr.htm, 2004.

72. Smith RA, von Eschenbach AC, Wender R, et al. American Cancer Society guidelines for the early detection of cancer: update of early detection guidelines for prostate, colorectal, and endometrial cancers. Also: update 2001—testing for early lung cancer detection. *CA Cancer J Clin* 2001;51:38.

73. Mandel JS, Church TR, Ederer F, et al. Colorectal cancer mortality: effectiveness of biennial screening for fecal occult blood. *J Natl Cancer Inst* 1999;91:434.

74. Ederer F, Church TR, Mandel JS. Fecal occult blood screening in the Minnesota study: role of chance detection of lesions. *J Natl Cancer Inst* 1997;89:1423.

75. Selby JV, Friedman GD, Quesenberry CP Jr, et al. Effect of fecal occult blood testing on mortality from colorectal cancer. A case-control study. *Ann Intern Med* 1993;118:1.

76. Saito H, Soma Y, Koeda J, et al. Reduction in risk of mortality from colorectal cancer by fecal occult blood screening with immunochemical hemagglutination test. A case-control study. *Int J Cancer* 1995;61:465.

77. Lazovich D, Weiss NS, Stevens NG, et al. A case-control study to evaluate efficacy of screening for faecal occult blood. *J Med Screen* 1995;2:84.

78. Winawer SJ, Flehinger BJ, Schottenfeld D, et al. Screening for colorectal cancer with fecal occult blood testing and sigmoidoscopy. *J Natl Cancer Inst* 1993;85:1311.

79. Selby JV, Friedman GD, Quesenberry CP Jr, et al. A case-control study of screening sigmoidoscopy and mortality from colorectal cancer. *N Engl J Med* 1992;326:653.

80. Gohagan JK, Prorok PC, Kramer BS, et al. Prostate cancer screening in the prostate, lung, colorectal and ovarian cancer screening trial of the National Cancer Institute. *J Urol* 1994;152:1905.

81. Atkin WS, Hart A, Edwards R, et al. Uptake, yield of neoplasia, and adverse effects of flexible sigmoidoscopy screening. *Gut* 1998;42:560.

82. Newcomb PA, Norfleet RG, Storer BE, et al. Screening sigmoidoscopy and colorectal cancer mortality. *J Natl Cancer Inst* 1992;84:1572.

83. Muller AD, Sonnenberg A. Protection by endoscopy against death from colorectal cancer. A case-control study among veterans. *Arch Intern Med* 1995;155:1741.

84. Lieberman DA, Weiss DG, Bond JH, et al. Use of colonoscopy to screen asymptomatic adults for colorectal cancer. Veterans Affairs Cooperative Study Group 380. *N Engl J Med* 2000;343:162.

85. Anderson WF, Guyton KZ, Hiatt RA, et al. Colorectal cancer screening for persons at average risk. *J Natl Cancer Inst* 2002;94:1126.

86. Levin B, Brooks D, Smith RA, et al. Emerging technologies in screening for colorectal cancer: CT colonography, immunochemical fecal occult blood tests, and stool screening using molecular markers. *CA Cancer J Clin* 2003;53:44.

87. Allison JE, Tekawa IS, Ransom LJ, et al. A comparison of fecal occult-blood tests for colorectal-cancer screening. *N Engl J Med* 1996;334:155.

88. Ahlquist DA, Shuber AP. Stool screening for colorectal cancer: evolution from occult blood to molecular markers. *Clin Chim Acta* 2002;315:157.

89. Fenlon HM, Nunes DP, Schroy PC 3rd, et al. A comparison of virtual and conventional colonoscopy for the detection of colorectal polyps. *N Engl J Med* 1999;341:1496.

90. Pickhardt PJ, Choi JR, Hwang I, et al. Computed tomographic virtual colonoscopy to screen for colorectal neoplasia in asymptomatic adults. *N Engl J Med* 2003;349:2191.

91. Swan J, Breen N, Coates RJ, et al. Progress in cancer screening practices in the United States: results from the 2000 National Health Interview Survey. *Cancer* 2003;97:1528.

92. Ransohoff DF, Sandler RS. Clinical practice. Screening for colorectal cancer. *N Engl J Med* 2002;346:40.

93. Marks R. Two decades of the public health approach to skin cancer control in Australia: why, how and where are we now? *Australas J Dermatol* 1999;40:1.

94. Hill L, Ferrini RL. Skin cancer prevention and screening: summary of the American College of Preventive Medicine's practice policy statements. *CA Cancer J Clin* 1998;48:232.

95. National Cancer Institute. *PDQ cancer screening/prevention summary: skin cancer screening.* Bethesda, MD: National Cancer Institute, 1994.

96. Berwick M, Begg CB, Fine JA, et al. Screening for cutaneous melanoma by skin self-examination. *J Natl Cancer Inst* 1996;88:17.

97. US Preventive Services Task Force. Counseling to prevent skin cancer: recommendations and rationale of the US Preventive Services Task Force. *MMWR Recomm Rep* 2003;52:13.

98. Etzioni R, Legler JM, Feuer EJ, et al. Cancer surveillance series: interpreting trends in prostate cancer—part III: quantifying the link between population prostate-specific antigen testing and recent declines in prostate cancer mortality. *J Natl Cancer Inst* 1999;91:1033.

99. Feuer EJ, Merrill RM, Hankey BF. Cancer surveillance series: interpreting trends in prostate cancer—part II: cause of death misclassification and the recent rise and fall in prostate cancer mortality. *J Natl Cancer Inst* 1999;91:1025.

100. Harris R, Lohr KN. Screening for prostate cancer: an update of the evidence for the US Preventive Services Task Force. *Ann Intern Med* 2002;137:917.

101. Cupp MR, Oesterling JE. Prostate-specific antigen, digital rectal examination, and transrectal ultrasonography: their roles in diagnosing early prostate cancer. *Mayo Clin Proc* 1993;68:297.

102. Stamey TA, Yang N, Hay AR, et al. Prostate-specific antigen as a serum marker for adenocarcinoma of the prostate. *N Engl J Med* 1987;317:909.

103. Lange PH, Ercole CJ, Lightner DJ, et al. The value of serum prostate specific antigen determinations before and after radical prostatectomy. *J Urol* 1989;141:873.

104. Catalona WJ, Smith DS, Ratliff TL, et al. Measurement of prostate-specific antigen in serum as a screening test for prostate cancer. *N Engl J Med* 1991;324:1156.

105. Cooner WH, Mosley BR, Rutherford CL Jr, et al. Prostate cancer detection in a clinical urological practice by ultrasonography, digital rectal examination and prostate specific antigen. *J Urol* 1990;143:1146.

106. Labrie F. Screening and early hormonal treatment of prostate cancer are accumulating strong evidence and support. *Prostate* 2000;43:215.

107. Mettlin C, Murphy GP, Lee F, et al. Characteristics of prostate cancer detected in the American Cancer Society—National Prostate Cancer Detection Project. *J Urol* 1994;152:1737.

108. Linton KD, Hamdy FC. Early diagnosis and surgical management of prostate cancer. *Cancer Treat Rev* 2003;29:151.

109. Ko YJ, Bubley GJ. Prostate cancer in the older man. *Oncology* 2001;15:1113.

110. Mettlin C, Murphy GP, Babaian RJ, et al. Observations on the early detection of prostate cancer from the American Cancer Society National Prostate Cancer Detection Project. *Cancer* 1997;80:1814.

111. Babaian RJ, Mettlin C, Kane R, et al. The relationship of prostate-specific antigen to digital rectal examination and transrectal ultrasonography. Findings of the American Cancer Society National Prostate Cancer Detection Project. *Cancer* 1992;69:1195.

112. Catalona WJ, Richie JP, Ahmann FR, et al. Comparison of digital rectal examination and serum prostate specific antigen in the early detection of prostate cancer: results of a multicenter clinical trial of 6,630 men. *J Urol* 1994;151:1283.

113. Smith DS, Humphrey PA, Catalona WJ. The early detection of prostate carcinoma with prostate specific antigen: the Washington University experience. *Cancer* 1997;80:1852.

114. Schroder FH. Screening for prostate cancer. *Urol Clin North Am* 2003;30:239.

115. Hugosson J, Aus G, Lilja H, et al. Prostate specific antigen based biennial screening is sufficient to detect almost all prostate cancers while still curable. *J Urol* 2003;169:1720.

116. Draisma G, Boer R, Otto SJ, et al. Lead times and over detection due to prostate-specific antigen screening: estimates from the European Randomized Study of Screening for Prostate Cancer. *J Natl Cancer Inst* 2003;95:868.

117. Hankey BF, Feuer EJ, Clegg LX, et al. Cancer surveillance series: interpreting trends in prostate cancer—part I: evidence of the effects of screening in recent prostate cancer incidence, mortality, and survival rates. *J Natl Cancer Inst* 1999;91:1017.

118. Bach PB, Niewoehner DE, Black WC. Screening for lung cancer: the guidelines. *Chest* 2003;123[Suppl 1]:83S.

119. Brett GZ. The value of lung cancer detection by six-monthly chest radiographs. *Thorax* 1968;23:414.

120. Melamed MR, Flehinger BJ, Zaman MB, et al. Screening for early lung cancer. Results of the Memorial Sloan-Kettering study in New York. *Chest* 1984;86:44.

121. Kubik A, Parkin DM, Khlat M, et al. Lack of benefit from semi-annual screening for cancer of the lung: follow-up report of a randomized controlled trial on a population of high-risk males in Czechoslovakia. *Int J Cancer* 1990;45:26.

122. Fontana RS, Sanderson DR, Woolner LB, et al. Lung cancer screening: the Mayo program. *J Occup Med* 1986;28:746.

123. Mulshine JL, Smith RA. Lung cancer. 2: Screening and early diagnosis of lung cancer. *Thorax* 2002;57:1071.

124. Bach PB, Kelley MJ, Tate RC, et al. Screening for lung cancer: a review of the current literature. *Chest* 2003;123[Suppl 1]:72S.

125. Marcus PM. Lung cancer screening: an update. *J Clin Oncol* 2001;19[Suppl 18]:83S.

126. Henschke CI, McCauley DI, Yankelevitz DF, et al. Early Lung Cancer Action Project: overall design and findings from baseline screening. *Lancet* 1999;354:99.

127. Banerjee S. Multi-slice/helical computed tomography for lung cancer screening. *Issues Emerg Health Technol* 2003:1.

128. Mahadevia PJ, Fleisher LA, Frick KD, et al. Lung cancer screening with helical computed tomography in older adult smokers: a decision and cost-effectiveness analysis. *JAMA* 2003;289:313.

129. Truong MT, Munden RF. Lung cancer screening. *Curr Oncol Rep* 2003;5:309.

130. Wagner TH. The effectiveness of mailed patient reminders on mammography screening: a meta-analysis. *Am J Prev Med* 1998;14:64.

131. Legler J, Meissner HI, Coyne C, et al. The effectiveness of interventions to promote mammography among women with historically lower rates of screening. *Cancer Epidemiol Biomarkers Prev* 2002;11:59.

132. Yabroff KR, Mandelblatt JS. Interventions targeted toward patients to increase mammography use. *Cancer Epidemiol Biomarkers Prev* 1999;8:749.

133. National Cancer Institute. Screening for breast cancer (PDQ): screening. World Wide Web URL: http://cancer.gov/cancerinfo/pdq/screening/breast/healthprofessional, 2004.

134. Miller AB, Baines CJ, To T, et al. Canadian National Breast Screening Study: 1. Breast cancer detection and death rates among women aged 40 to 49 years. *CMAJ* 1992;147:1459.

135. Eckhardt S, Badellino F, Murphy GP. UICC meeting on breast-cancer screening in premenopausal women in developed countries. Geneva, 29 September–1 October 1993. *Int J Cancer* 1994;56:1.

136. National Guideline Clearinghouse Guideline Synthesis. Screening for breast cancer. World Wide Web URL: http://www.guideline.gov/, 2004.

137. Jenson CB, Shahon DB, Wangensteen OH. Evaluation of annual examinations in the detection of cancer. Special reference to cancer of the gastrointestinal tract, prostate, breast, and female generative tract. *JAMA* 1960;174:1783.

138. Gilbertsen VA. Cancer of the prostate gland. Results of early diagnosis and therapy undertaken for cure of the disease. *JAMA* 1971;215:81.

139. Chodak GW, Schoenberg HW. Early detection of prostate cancer by routine screening. *JAMA* 1984;252:3261.

140. Thompson IM, Ernst JJ, Gangai MP, et al. Adenocarcinoma of the prostate: results of routine urological screening. *J Urol* 1984;132:690.

141. Mueller EJ, Crain TW, Thompson IM, et al. An evaluation of serial digital rectal examinations in screening for prostate cancer. *J Urol* 1988;140:1445.

142. Lee F, Littrup PJ, Torp-Pedersen ST, et al. Prostate cancer: comparison of transrectal US and digital rectal examination for screening. *Radiology* 1988;168:389.

143. Mettlin C, Lee F, Drago J, et al. The American Cancer Society National Prostate Cancer Detection Project. Findings on the detection of early prostate cancer in 2425 men. *Cancer* 1991;67:2949.

José C. Costa
Paul M. Lizardi

CHAPTER **23**

Advanced Molecular Diagnostics

In the last decades of the twentieth century, the success of the reductionistic program of research has yielded unprecedented advances in the understanding of the basic mechanisms of cancer at the molecular and cell biologic level.[1] This progress, together with technologic breakthroughs and the development of information technology, provides a platform that can be readily applied to the diagnostics of cancer. For the purposes of this chapter, we define advanced diagnostics as the integrated and quantitative evaluation of the molecular characteristics of the tumor and its host that leads to an optimal therapeutic intervention or to an accurate prognosis, or both. The ultimate goal of advanced diagnostics in a specific clinical setting is to arrive at the best personalized and predictive medical decision by integrating comprehensive information on the tumor and the constitutive characteristics of the host to epidemiologic and outcomes knowledge. Advanced diagnostics goes beyond the morphologic and biochemical characteristics of the lesion and its host to integrate as broad an array of data as it is possible to conceive. The goal is to accurately predict the fate of a patient.

Although the interpretation of diagnostic tests has always been integrative in nature and has sought coherence between diverse bodies of information (clinical presentation, laboratory values, histopathology, imaging, epidemiology), the invention and adoption of computational biology tools adapted to clinical practice have changed the domains of information that can be integrated during the diagnostic process. With the aid of decision-support systems, the data from different diagnostic modalities discussed in this chapter can be integrated with multiple knowledge bases to derive an optimal therapeutic decision. In other words the product of this process is an outcomes-based recommendation rationalized on the basis of statistical methodologies applied to a broad-based data set (Fig. 23-1). The final therapeutic recommendation, tempered by the joint wisdom of the diagnostician and the therapist, is not only based on the characteristics of the tumor and the patient but also incorporates the detailed experiential knowledge stored in databases derived from treating large groups of patients in a similar situation.[2]

Using a broad array of technologies to characterize patients and their diseases will change the way we classify tumors (Table 23-1). The phenotypic classification of tumors by site of origin and histopathology remains one of the most powerful determinants of therapy, but new knowledge has already brought the need for complementary nosologies. Next to the etiologic classifications, relevant to population science because of their importance in prevention, mechanistic classifications are emerging as practical tools in the practice of oncology. Detailed knowledge of the molecular basis of cancer (see Chapters 1.3 and 2) provides the opportunity for molecular intervention. This knowledge identifies structural or functional molecular abnormalities (targets), or both, that underlie the neoplastic behavior of the tumor cells and enable the design of means to correct the dysfunction by molecular intervention. This scenario significantly modifies the process of drug design clinical development and practical use of molecular therapeutics. Of particular relevance here is the consideration that molecular therapy requires diagnostic tests that identify the target and that predict and assess the response to therapy. As molecular drugs come on line, therapy will be governed to a much lesser extent by the tumor type, grading, and staging and to a much greater extent by the mechanistic category of the tumor. Mechanistic classifications group tumor types that are unrelated in the phenotypic classification but emerge as closely linked by a common defect that can be corrected by molecular intervention. Drugs that inhibit a family of protein kinases can be presumed to have an effect in most if not all lesions characterized by hyperfunction of these enzymes. The quintessential example is the effectiveness of imatinib mesylate

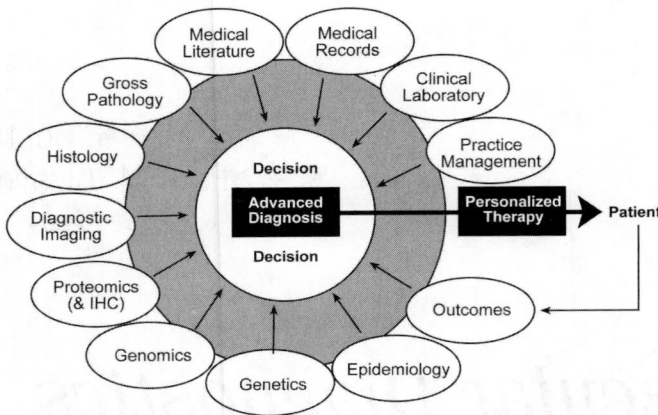

FIGURE 23-1. Integrated advanced diagnostics of cancer. A series of data streams (periphery) are processed with the help of computer-aided support (*inner circle*) to arrive at an integrated advanced diagnosis that serves as a base for a rational therapy and prognosis. IHC, immunohistochemistry. (Modified from ref. 2.)

(Gleevec) in chronic myelogenous leukemia and gastrointestinal stromal tumors, two unrelated entities except for hyperfunction of the tyrosine kinase part of signal transduction pathways. As our knowledge of what is wrong with the circuitry controlling cell function increases, mechanistic classifications will grow in complexity. It is intuitively evident that if we want to achieve maximum efficiency and to avoid the development of resistance to molecular intervention we will have to target dysfunctional pathways at several points and simultaneously address several pathways or networks. It follows that the diagnostic modalities providing the classifiers for mechanistic categories will have to evolve and be adapted to this increasingly complex task. Mechanistic classifications are likely to be complemented by predictive taxonomies. Detailed knowledge of the physiopathology of a tumor in a specific patient will not only tell us what pathways to target with what drug combinations but will also enable us to predict treatment success or failures.

If the practice of advanced diagnostics as presented here is successfully implemented, it is likely that the present nosology of cancer, based on site, histotype, grading, and staging, will be

superseded by an integrative classification of tumors in which tumor site and type will be annotated by a set of personalized and predictive characteristics relevant to therapy and prognosis.

PRESENT IMPACT OF NOVEL TECHNOLOGIES ON CLINICAL PRACTICE

The critical assessment of the practical impact of new technologies is still in flux, but enough evidence is available to draw preliminary conclusions about the contributions of advanced diagnostics to the clinical practice of oncology. Widespread adoption of new methods and tests will not only be shaped by the substance of their contribution to patient management but also by economic factors, accessibility, training, and regulatory issues.

In the not so distant days of the "one gene–one protein–one biomarker" paradigm, the pace of progress was relatively slow. Today, the implementation of comprehensive modalities of analysis is taking place at such speed that by the time novel strategies are validated and integrated into established patterns of medical practice they may be obsolete. This circumstance calls for a codification and streamlining of the validation pathways to facilitate the organization of large-scale cooperative studies designed to validate new diagnostic tools (Fig. 23-2). The establishment standards and common protocols to cleanse, report, and analyze data will be of critical importance in the dissemination of new technologies.

Are the new technologies advancing practical patient care? At the closing of 2003, the answer appeared to be yes. We do indeed have proof of concept that the application of high-throughput comprehensive technologies to the characterization of tumors improves patient care. Preliminary evidence indicates that expression profiling may contribute to clarify disease categories that are difficult to define using morphology even when combined with a few molecular traits. For example, expression profiling studies show that malignant fibrous histiocytoma, a controversial category of soft tissue sarcoma whose existence has been questioned, exhibits an expression signature that clusters a subgroup of cases into one category.[3] Whether the category is due to a specific cell of origin or to a pathway of tumor

TABLE 23-1. Classification of Tumors

Classification	Technology	Application
Phenotypic	Histopathology	Dx and class
	Morphometry	Conventional Rx
Mechanistic	Genomics	Rx and classification
	Proteomics	Rx and classification
Prognostic	Histologic grade	Per-pred of response
	Morphometry	
	Genomics	
	Proteomics	
Etiologic	History of exposure	Dx and prevention
	Serology	
	Xenobiot sequences	
	Mutational signatures	

Dx, diagnosis; per-pred, personalized and predictive; Rx, therapy.

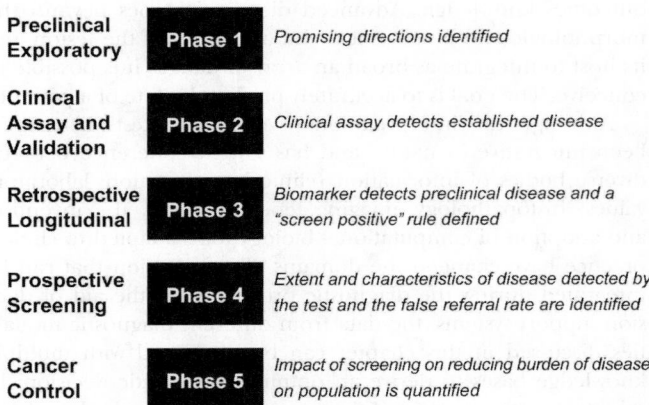

FIGURE 23-2. Progress toward goals—phases of discovery and validation. The interpretation of data obtained from tissues that are not accurately characterized is vulnerable to the variable composition of the tissue sampled. *In situ* and microdissection of tissue avoids this pitfall.

progression remains to be established, but the existence of such a category (cluster) of malignant fibrous histiocytomas provides a rationale for implementing therapies directed at the molecular defects present in this class of tumors.

In a similar fashion, expression profiling studies enhance the risk stratification of pediatric acute lymphoblastic leukemia (ALL) patients. They do so by discovering new and clinically relevant subtypes of this disease and by predicting in which patients therapy will eventually fail.[4,5] These hallmark studies indicate that expression profiling of leukemic cells in pediatric ALL is key in refining the tailoring of the treatment intensity to the specific patients. In addition, the profile of expression predicts which patients experiencing B-cell ALL are at high risk for the development of secondary AML. Not only is this information of prognostic relevance for the individual patient, but it also suggests that a subset of ALL patients may have an underlying molecular defect in a hematopoietic stem cell that predisposes them to AML and that this hypothetical defect is also reflected in the expression profile found in their B-cell ALL blasts. Another example of how comprehensive data sets provide biologic and pathogenetic insights can be found in mixed-lineage leukemia. Comprehensive expression profiling studies of patients harboring mixed-lineage leukemia gene rearrangements in the tumor cells led to the identification of a tyrosine kinase receptor FLT3 as a therapeutic target,[6] and trials using inhibitors of FLT3 are in progress. This cycle of discovery and immediate clinical application demonstrates the potential of advanced diagnostics to accelerate improvements in the management of patients with cancer.

The use of arrays containing probes for a set of genes tailored to provide information concerning a specific group of diseases or clinical setting, as opposed to generic arrays, is likely to facilitate the integration of comprehensive technologies into clinical practice. The "lymphochip"[7] provides a good case study illustrating how an array can be designed based on knowledge of the biology of disease and the diseased cell (e.g., activated vs. quiescent lymphocytes). Such an array has uncovered distinct, clinically relevant, groups within diffuse large B-cell lymphoma (DLBCL). The studies not only define three groups within DLBCL but indicate that using the expression profiles of the tumor cells in combination with major histocompatibility complex class II, proliferation index, expression of BMP6, and the International Prognostic Index significantly improves the risk stratification of patients.[8] This series of studies focusing on DLBCL underscores the power of the highly integrated use of diagnostic data and also suggests that we will witness an increasing use of specialized chips or arrays tailored to specific clinical questions.

Application of comprehensive analytic techniques to common epithelial cancer types is also providing valuable information capable of transforming the practice of oncology. The initial studies of gene expression in breast cancer suggested that ductal carcinomas may be derived from two distinct cell types, a basal cell and a luminal type, and unsupervised analysis divided the cases in five subgroups with differences in survival.[9,10] Subsequent work by other investigators suggests a signature of 70 genes that identifies the subset of node-negative patients in whom metastases will develop 5 years after initial therapy.[11] The same set of genes is effective in assigning patients with lymph node involvement at the time of diagnosis to good- and poor-prognosis groups.[12] Validation of these studies is required, but

they are a clear indication that we soon will have means for a more refined prognosis and risk stratification of patients with breast cancer. At present it appears safe to predict that DNA microarray technology will represent a viable alternative to cytogenetics, conventional molecular diagnostics, and fluorescence *in situ* hybridization (FISH), particularly when assays become robust and easily implemented in routine clinical reference laboratories.[13] A clear indication of the trend is the relatively recent changes in the regulatory stance of the U.S. Food and Drug Administration vis-à-vis the approval of DNA-based multiplex technology for commercial diagnostic testing.[14] Out of very large data sets that are correlated with the natural history of the disease and the response to treatments will come specialized chips tailored to the specific decision points of a practice algorithm. Implementation of this new paradigm will require adapting the present laboratory practices, particularly in anatomic pathology, to the routine use of genomic and proteomic characterization of cytologic and histologic samples. Procurement of tissue in the operating room and protocols for rapid freeze, fixation, and storage of samples will have to be integrated in the routine diagnostic operation of a surgical pathology laboratory.

Comprehensive analysis of the protein profiles found in tissue or biologic fluids is also coming of age, and examples of practical applications are beginning to appear in the literature (see Chapter 2). The interest in exploiting the proteome for predictive-personalized oncology and advanced diagnostics resides in the fact that posttranslational modification of proteins is key in regulating many of their functions. Detailed information about the functional state of a molecule and, perhaps more importantly, information about the proportion of molecules that are modified (e.g., activated) can only be captured by direct analysis of the proteome. This introduces a double challenge: the need for exquisite sensitivity and the difficulty of distinguishing minor differences in a molecular species (e.g., phosphorylation at a specific tyrosine) in a complex mixture of proteins. Nevertheless, advances in instrumentation and computational methods are bringing proteomics to the clinic and can be expected to continue to support the application of comprehensive protein analysis to clinical questions. Proteomics laboratories require expensive instrumentation and highly trained staff,[15] but automation is a powerful force placing proteomics within the reach of the clinical oncologist. One approach that is likely to see increasing clinical application is the "protein chip." Microspots of antibodies can be arrayed on a solid support and used to interrogate plasma. The value of the protein chip technology is demonstrated by the ability to simultaneously measure the plasma levels of 75 different cytokines with a sensitivity ranging from 1 to 1000 pg/mL.[16] This indicates that future proteomic spectra may also involve the use of assays that report information regarding a patient's immune status, as well as transient inflammatory responses. The information provided by the cytokine assays is likely to be useful in assessing the patient's progress in cases in which immune status is crucial for cancer treatment.

The investigation of proteomic signatures in plasma, serum, or other biologic fluids promises to revolutionize the diagnosis and therapeutic monitoring in the oncology clinic. Plasma contains all tissue proteins plus the classic plasma proteins and immunoglobulins. Theoretically, such a repository is likely to contain proteins whose abundance and structural changes reflect many if not all human diseases. Translating the plasma or serum proteome into practical diagnostics has to overcome daunting barriers,[17] but recent developments suggest that those impediments are not insurmountable. A powerful force speeding up the application of serum proteomics to the clinic is knowledge engineering and machine learning technology. Statistical techniques first tested by cosmologists and astronomers can be applied to any large data set to identify diagnostic patterns masked by noise. Enabling learning machines to examine large data sets in an agnostic fashion, in other words, free of any preconceived hypothesis, may indeed uncover signatures that will classify and predict outcome of subgroups of patients in specific clinical settings. An interesting quality of learning machines is their ability to base a decision or classification on accumulated experience and to constantly refine their ability to correctly diagnose a case. Clearly, it is this characteristic that drives their application to integrative advanced diagnostics as defined in the first paragraphs of this chapter. Accumulating experience derived from very large and diverse data sets can be harnessed to augment the predictive power that underlies personalized medicine.

As with traditional laboratory tests, it is important to remember that the performance characteristics of a diagnostic is in part dictated by the characteristics of the clinical question addressed by the test. Highly reproducible diagnostic signatures defined in artificially constructed training sets for ovarian cancer suffer significant erosion of their performance when put to work in the real-world clinical environment.[18–20] This serves as a clear reminder of the need to tailor the use of technologies to specific clinical scenarios, as the resolutive and predictive power of the methods depend as much on the clinicobiologic context of the question asked as on the intrinsic technical parameters of the technology. The contributions that proteomics can bring to clinical practice are illustrated by the predictive power of proteomic profiles in non–small cell lung cancer. Applying MALDI-TOF-MS (matrix-assisted laser desorption/ionization–time-of-flight mass spectrometry) to proteins extracted from frozen sections of lung tumors, it is possible to classify the tumor correctly in terms of histologic type (including primary vs. metastatic) and to predict nodal involvement and survival.[21] This study clearly shows how fresh frozen tumor readily collectable in a conventional clinical setting can be used to correctly classify tumors and to predict their stage and prognosis.

A common characteristic of the comprehensive analytic approaches we have so far discussed is that they analyze tissue homogenates or biologic fluids. Thus, the information obtained cannot be related to the spatial distribution of the biologic elements from which they derive. Yet, we have always known that the precise ways that parts are put together is crucial to understanding the functioning of the whole. Furthermore, *in situ* approaches that reveal the precise location of a molecular lesion are helpful in interpreting results derived from genomics and proteomic analysis of tissue extracts, as they serve to sort out differences caused by variation in the composition of the sample (Fig. 23-3). Therefore, there is value in attempting to precisely map complex data sets on the spatial and architectural elements that make up a tumor. Two avenues that have been explored to achieve this goal are (1) acquiring defined cell populations through microdissection and then submitting the samples to comprehensive analysis and (2) multiplex *in situ* approaches. Of the two strategies, the one that has been developed furthest is micro-

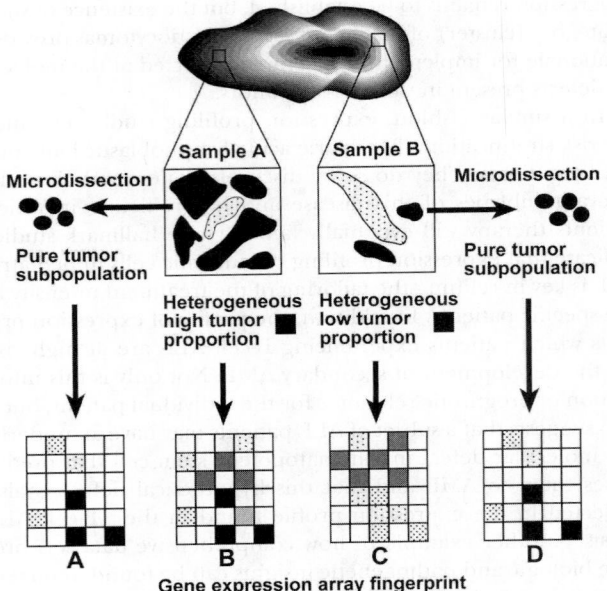

FIGURE 23-3. Heterogeneous tissue samples. Codification of the pathway from discovery to clinical use of diagnostic technology will facilitate the large cooperative studies necessary to speed up validation at a time when technologies move forward at a rapid pace.

acquisition followed by comprehensive analysis. Proteomic and expression profiling can be applied to microdissected cell populations with success, whereas multiplex *in situ* techniques lag behind in their applicability. *In situ* multiplex protein measurements using fluorescence, *in situ* analysis of transcriptional activity (FISH&CHIPS),[22] and *in situ* demonstration of structural genetic abnormalities by FISH[23] have not yet found widespread clinical applications, and they remain discovery technologies better suited to hypothesis-driven inquiry or validation of discoveries reached through agnostic approaches. Only FISH is used as a routine test to detect amplification of Her2/neu in breast cancer.

The efforts to extract topologic information coupled to advances in imaging and data analysis have revitalized morphometric approaches in an attempt to unlock the information contained in the phenotype and put it to use as a predictive tool. Feature extraction from conventional images can be automated and subjected to machine learning. Other modalities such as spectral analysis of light microscopy can provide information that can be correlated to the biologic properties of the cells or tissues analyzed and to the outcome of therapies. The role of these image-based techniques when integrated to the technologies discussed is still being tested, but it is likely that they will complement and perhaps enhance predictive applications.

CHARTING THE FUTURE

In recent years it has become apparent that several advanced diagnostics-driven clinical care strategies are beginning to play out simultaneously in an integrated fashion. One of these strategies involves diagnostics-guided therapeutics (DGT) for personalized cancer treatment. Another consists of prognostics-guided preventive intervention for the evaluation of relative cancer risk and the implementation and periodic monitoring of personalized cancer prevention strategies.

DIAGNOSTICS-GUIDED THERAPEUTICS

Pharmacogenomics of the host is already guiding therapeutic intervention. The AmpliChip CYP450, a product introduced by Roche Diagnostics (Indianapolis, IN), is a diagnostic device based on Affymetrix DNA microarray technology. The Ampli-Chip is intended to identify naturally occurring genetic variations or common mutations in cytochrome P-450 genes that play a crucial role in determining how a person can process or metabolize a variety of drugs. The microarray is a multisignal device composed of probes for 33 different mutations in two genes, CYP2D6 and CYP2C19. The chip can determine if a person is a poor metabolizer (PM) or an ultra-rapid metabolizer. PMs have trouble inactivating certain drugs and eliminating them from the body. Generally, a PM is at increased risk for experiencing adverse drug reactions, toxicities, and even dangerous side effects of therapies. Ultra-rapid metabolizers, on the other hand, with additional functional copies of the genes, have an increased risk of being nonresponders because they can inactivate and eliminate a drug before it has had a chance to achieve its therapeutic effect. During regulatory review of the device by the Food and Drug Administration, the agency pointed out that the AmpliChip CYP450 can be classified as a medical device, as defined by Section 201(h) of the Federal Food, Drug, and Cosmetic Act. This reflects an ongoing trend of technology convergence in which the diagnostic device requires medical device approval as it becomes more and more an integral part of the therapeutic regimen.

The Human Haplotype Project initiated by the Human Genome Research Institute has as a goal the establishment of a database of human single-nucleotide polymorphisms that can be used, on a continuing basis, to assemble and refine a knowledge base of human haplotypes and their relationships to disease susceptibility. The set of relationships linking haplotypes and cancer susceptibility can be readily translated to DGT-driven clinical practice, assuming that low-cost technology to obtain individual patient haplotypes will become available in less than a decade. Some of the genetic information required for DGT-based practice is acquired at birth, and this would include haplotypes as well as structural alterations present in the germline, such as mutations in cancer susceptibility genes. Information on acquired structural alterations present in specific somatic tissue patches is harder to obtain, but developments in mutation detection technologies suggest that progress in this area will be rapid. For example, a method has been reported[24] that permits the detection of specific somatic point mutations in total genomic DNA in less than 15 minutes, without using polymerase chain reaction amplification. The method is based on single-pair fluorescence resonance energy transfer in combination with optics and avalanche photodiode detectors that enable single-photon counting. As these and other advanced mutation detection methods are improved and incorporated into commercial products, it may become possible to acquire a large amount of somatic mutation data in a clinical setting, enabling DGT-driven clinical practice. Evidence that tumors are composed of genetically diverse cell populations[25] indicates that therapies will be selected specifically targeting the populations. Because therapy is an agent of

disturbance (it kills cell populations), we will be capable of driving the selection of defined populations in ways that avoid resistance to drugs. We should hope that we can follow the dynamics of the evolving pharmacogenomics of the tumor cell (somatic pharmacogenomics).

The power of microarray technologies to generate gene expression profiles of diseased tissue is summarized above and discussed in great detail in Chapter 1.3, in which new microarray technologies that permit the measurement of copy number changes in individual genes occurring in tumors are presented. A related suite of microarray technologies is emerging that permits the measurement of changes in the epigenetic status of genes (that is, the presence of the DNA encoding a gene product in an open or closed "chromosomal packaging" state that either facilitates or inhibits expression). All of these microarray technologies are evolving at a rapid pace, and some of the most advanced formats use amperometric (electrical current) readout, which offers great potential for future cost reductions. We envision the emergence of future DGT devices analogous to the AmpliChip 450 but capable of providing additional information on gene expression, gene copy number, and epigenetic status for a highly informative subset of cancer gene loci. Likewise, future DGT devices may be designed to generate proteomic and metabolomic spectra (see Chapter 2). The DGT devices will be capable of generating spectra from tissues or body fluids, and learning algorithms will be used to generate a diagnostic call by integrating information from thousands of peaks present in a mass spectrum. This type of DGT device will provide information enabling precise diagnosis of cancer subtype and stage, as well as optimal personalized therapeutic decisions.

We have already alluded to the importance of mapping functional alterations to tissue or tumor architecture. New reagents for fluorescence-based immunodiagnostics and imaging applications are being developed rapidly and are likely to enable significant progress in this area.

An important advance in imaging reagents is the development of "fluorobodies."[26] These reagents have been generated by inserting diverse binding loops derived from antibody protein sequences into four of the exposed loops at one end of green fluorescent protein. Libraries of these proteins, comprising millions of binding loops of different sequence, can be screened to select molecules capable of binding with high specificity to any biologic molecule of interest. The resulting fluorobody reagents combine the advantages of antibodies (high binding specificity) with the fluorescence emission capabilities of green fluorescent protein. Because there exist at least five flavors of fluorescent proteins (yellow, blue, green, etc.), the production of fluorobodies in several colors will not take long to materialize. In parallel, advances in nanotechnology have produced a new generation of extremely stable fluorescent reagents based on semiconductor quantum dots.[27] Luminescent quantum dots are semiconductor nanocrystals that represent a promising alternative to organic dyes for fluorescence-based applications. These nanometer-sized particles can be excited at a single wavelength and emit light of different wavelengths, depending on the molecular dimensions of the semiconductor layers. They are being used for a variety of imaging applications, including cell imaging, by coupling of quantum dots to specific antibodies for specific cell surface proteins.[28] An important issue that may hinder the clinical use of quantum dot or fluorobody imaging reagents and modalities is the possibility of undesired immune responses in the patients.

Nonetheless, these reagents are likely to lead to the implementation of more advanced forms of multicolor immunohistochemistry in standard pathology practice.

Yet another interesting new class of imaging agents consists of quenched fluorophore-polymer conjugates that become fluorescent on activation by matrix metalloproteinases and intracellular enzymes present in tumors.[29] This report showed that it is feasible to image matrix metalloproteinase 2 (MMP-2) enzyme activity *in vivo* by using near-infrared optical imaging technology and matrix metalloproteinase-sensitive probes. The quenched fluorophore-polymer conjugate was highly activatable by means of MMP-2–induced conversion. The MMP-2–sensitive probe was activated by MMP-2 *in vitro*, producing up to an 850% increase in near-infrared fluorescent signal intensity. MMP-2–positive tumors in mice were easily identified as high-signal-intensity regions as early as 1 hour after intravenous injection of the MMP-2 probe, whereas contralateral MMP-2–negative tumors showed little to no signal intensity.

Further diagnostic progress will come from tissue-homing devices combining tissue-specific drug delivery and real-time reporting of exact anatomic localization of drugs or immune cells. The molecular diversity of the tumor-associated vasculature provides a basis for the development of advanced tumor-targeted diagnostics.[30] By injection into mice of phage libraries comprising millions of different short amino acid sequences, specific peptide sequences have been discovered that are capable of homing to specific organ sites harboring a unique tumor vasculature composition. These peptides will expand the repertoire of specific tissue homing reagents available for directing diagnostics and therapeutic molecules to tumors. Because peptides are small, nonimmunogenic, and readily attached to proteins or nanoparticles, they can be used as generic homing moieties for advanced diagnostics.

In the emerging field of medical nanotechnology, a significant development is the synthesis of various configurations of dendritic polymer macromolecular carriers.[31] Dendrimers are synthetic, highly branched, mono-disperse macromolecules of nanometer dimensions. Desirable properties of dendrimers are uniform size, water solubility, modifiable surface functionality, and presence of internal cavities. Current dendrimer technology development efforts include multifunction nanodevices that combine targeting molecules (such as the aforementioned homing peptides),[30] imaging moieties, and drug delivery functions in a single macromolecular entity. Efforts are under way to assess the potential animal toxicity of these exciting imaging-therapeutic nanodevices.

Cell-based DGT strategies can be designed using specially modified T cells that report their exact location in tissues. Kircher et al.[32] reported novel, biocompatible, and physiologically inert nanoparticles made of cross-linked iron oxide for highly efficient intracellular labeling of a variety of cell types that allow *in vivo* magnetic resonance imaging tracking of systemically injected cells at near single-cell resolution. CD8+ cytotoxic T lymphocytes labeled with CLIO-HD were detectable via magnetic resonance imaging with a detection threshold of approximately three cells/voxel *in vivo* in live mice. Using B16-OVA melanoma and nanoparticle-labeled OVA-specific CD8+ T cells, they demonstrated high-resolution imaging of T-cell recruitment to intact tumors *in vivo*. The images reveal the extensive three-dimensional spatial heterogeneity of T-cell recruitment to target tumors and demonstrate a temporal regulation of T-cell recruitment within the tumor. The Kircher data indicate that serial administrations of CD8+ T cells are capable of homing to different intratumoral locations.

Receptor-based DGT strategies are also feasible, whereby the diagnostic reagent is capable of homing to a specific receptor molecule. Epidermal growth factor (EGF) is an attractive model for this paradigm, because it is overexpressed in many cancers. The specificity of a novel EGF-Cy5.5 fluorescent optical probe in the detection of EGF receptor (EGFR) has been reported.[33] *In vivo* imaging was performed in mice with MDA-MB-468 and MDA-MB-435 tumors. Monitoring of the time-fluorescence intensity in mice confirmed that indocyanine green dye and Cy5.5 had no favorable binding to tumor regardless of EGFR expression level. In contrast, EGF-Cy5.5 accumulated only in MDA-MB-468 tumors. Their data suggest that EGF-Cy5.5 can be used as a specific near-infrared contrast agent for noninvasive imaging of EGFR expression and monitoring of responses to molecularly targeted therapy.

PROGNOSTICS-GUIDED PREVENTIVE INTERVENTION

One of the major goals of advanced diagnostics is to enable *in vivo* diagnostics by visualizing functional parameters of tumors and tumor cells. First tested *ex vivo*, advanced technologies should move to *in vivo* applications. It is not unrealistic to think that molecular probes will report discernible signals that can be acquired quantified and interpreted with enough accuracy to guide surgical intervention in real time or to evaluate tumor dosage and response to medical intervention. It is to be expected that many of the data now obtained *ex vivo* will be obtainable *in vivo*. The identification of cells with dysfunctional physiology in growth survival and interaction with matrix and other cellular constituents of their milieu and the ability to monitor lesions *in vivo* holds great promise for the continuing surveillance of preneoplastic lesions and for implementing an integrated strategy of prognostics-guided preventive intervention. The future ability to implement functional imaging of preneoplastic lesions suggests that the effects of chemopreventive intervention, modification of exposure, and/or change in habits could be monitored by *in vivo* analysis of the target tissues. A clinical cancer preventive consultation one decade from today may comprise (1) germline haplotype, cytochrome P-450 genotype, and disease susceptibility genotype; (2) somatic structural alterations as assessed from fluids or surrogate tissue samples (breast lavage, colonoscopy lavage, etc.); (3) DNA epigenetic profiles; (4) serum proteomic profiles; (5) patient environmental exposure data; and (6) integration of all data sets using a learning machine knowledge base. It is hoped that the outcome of such a consultation will be the personalized prediction of risk for specific organs, the institution of adequate preventive intervention, and the periodic monitoring of its efficacy. The desired result of this futuristic clinical consultation is to stratify patients into high-risk, as opposed to low-risk, profiles and to institute the appropriate PGIP or DGT clinical interventions, as indicated.

CONCLUSION

Little doubt remains that the technologies discussed in this chapter will become routine in the management of cancer patients once their indications have been sharply defined and once the cost and complexity of conducting the analysis have been simplified. The accurate prediction of response and outcome will not only benefit individual patients but will also change the conduct of clinical trials by discriminating groups of patients who are very likely to be responders or resistant to the effect of a drug.

One of the major goals of advanced diagnostics is to move *ex vivo* tests to *in vivo* diagnostics by visualizing functional parameters of tumors and tumor cells. Molecular probes will report discernible signals that can be acquired quantified and interpreted with enough accuracy to guide surgery in real time or to evaluate response to medical targeted intervention. The identification of cells with dysfunctional physiology in growth survival and interaction with matrix and other cellular constituents of their milieu and the ability to monitor lesions *in vivo* holds great promise for the study of preneoplastic lesions and preventive intervention.

REFERENCES

1. Hahn WC, Weinberg RA. Modeling the molecular circuitry of cancer. *Nat Rev Cancer* 2002;2:331.
2. Sinard JH, Morrow JS. Informatics and anatomic pathology: meeting challenges and charting the future. [Letter] *Hum Pathol* 2001;32:143.
3. Segal NH, Pavlidis P, Antonescu CR, et al. Classification and subtype prediction of soft tissue sarcoma by functional genomics and support vector machine analysis. *Am J Pathol* 2003;163:691.
4. Yeoh EJ, Ross ME, Shurtleff SA, et al. Classification, subtype discovery, and prediction of outcome in pediatric acute lymphoblastic leukemia by gene expression profiling. *Cancer Cell* 2002;1:133.
5. Armstrong, SA, Staunton JE, Silverman LB, et al. MLL translocations specify a distinct gene expression profile that distinguishes a unique leukemia. *Nat Genet* 2002;30:41.
6. Armstrong SA, Kung AL, Mabon ME, et al. Inhibition of FLT3 in MLL. Validation of a therapeutic target identified by gene expression based classification. *Cancer Cell* 2003;3:173.
7. Alizadeh AA, Eisen MB, Davis RE, et al. Distinct types of diffuse large B-cell lymphoma identified by gene expression profiling. *Nature* 2000;403:503.
8. Rosenwald A, Wright G, Chan WC, et al. The use of molecular profiling to predict survival after chemotherapy for diffuse large-B-cell lymphoma. *N Engl J Med* 2002;346:1937.
9. Perou CM, Sorlie T, Eisen MB, et al. Molecular portraits of human breast tumours. *Nature* 2000;406:747.
10. Sorlie T, Perou CM, Tibshirani R, et al. Gene expression patterns of breast carcinomas distinguish tumor subclasses with clinical implications. *Proc Natl Acad Sci U S A* 2001;98:10869.
11. van't Veer LJ, Dai H, van de Vijver MJ, et al. Gene expression profiling predicts clinical outcome of breast cancer. *Nature* 2002;415:530.
12. van de Vijver MJ, He YD, van't Veer LJ, et al. A gene-expression signature as a predictor of survival in breast cancer. *N Engl J Med* 2002;347:1999.
13. Staudt LM. It's ALL in the diagnosis. *Cancer Cell* 2002;1:109.
14. US Department of Health and Human Services. *Multiplex tests for heritable DNA markers, mutations and expression patterns; draft guidance for industry and FDA reviewers.* FDA, Center for Devices and Radiological Health. February 2003.
15. Dillon D, Stone K, Williams K. Potential application for proteomics in oncology. In: DeVita VT, Rosenberg SA, Hellman S, eds. *Progress in oncology 2002.* Boston: Jones & Bartlett 2002:1.
16. Schweitzer B, Roberts S, Grimwade B, et al. Multiplexed protein profiling on microarrays by rolling-circle amplification. *Nat Biotechnol* 2002;20:359.
17. Anderson NL, Anderson NG. The human plasma proteome. *Mol Cell Proteomics* 2002;1:845.
18. Petricoin EF 3rd, Ardekani AM, Hitt BA, et al. Use of proteomic patterns in serum to identify ovarian cancer. *Lancet* 2002;359:572.
19. Rockhill B. Correspondence: proteomic patterns in serum and identification of ovarian cancer. *Lancet* 2002;360:169.
20. Daly MB, Ozols RF. The search for predictive patterns in ovarian cancer: proteomics meets bioinformatics. *Cancer Cell* 2002:111.
21. Yanagisawa K, Shyr Y, Xu BJ, et al. Proteomic patterns of tumour subsets in non-small-cell lung cancer. *Lancet* 2003:433.
22. Levsky JM, Shenoy SM, Pezo RC, Singer RH. Single-cell gene expression profiling. *Science* 2002;297:836.
23. Walch A, Bink K, Hutzler P, Bowerling K, Letsiou I. Sequential multilocus fluorescence in situ hybridization can detect complex patterns of increased gene dosage at the single cell level in tissue sections. *Lab Invest* 2001;81:1457.
24. Wabuyele MB, Farquar H, Stryjewski W, et al. Approaching real-time molecular diagnostics: single-pair fluorescence resonance energy transfer (spFRET) detection for the analysis of low abundant point mutations in K-ras oncogenes. *J Am Chem Soc* 2003;125:6937.
25. Gonzalez-Garcia I, Sole RV, Costa J. Metapopulation dynamics and spatial heterogeneity in cancer. *Proc Natl Acad Sci U S A* 2002;99:13085.
26. Zeytun A, Jeromin A, Scalettar BA, Waldo GS, Bradbury AR. Fluorobodies combine GFP fluorescence with the binding characteristics of antibodies. *Nat Biotechnol* 2003;21:1473.
27. West JL, Halas NJ. Engineered nanomaterials for biophotonics applications: improving sensing, imaging, and therapeutics. *Annu Rev Biomed Eng* 2003;5:285.
28. Jaiswal JK, Mattoussi H, Maruo JM, Simon SM. Long-term multiple color imaging of live cells using quantum dot bioconjugates. *Nat Biotechnol* 2003;2:47.
29. Bremer C, Bredow S, Mahmood U, Weissleder R, Tung CH. Optical imaging of matrix metalloproteinase-2 activity in tumors: feasibility study in a mouse model. *Radiology* 2001;221:523.
30. Zurita A, Arap W, Pasqualini R. Mapping tumor vascular diversity by screening phage display libraries. *J Control Release* 2003;91:183.
31. Quintana A, Raczka E, Piehler L, et al. Design and function of a dendrimer-based therapeutic nanodevice targeted to tumor cells through the folate receptor. *Pharm Res* 2002;19:1310.
32. Kircher MF, Allport JR, Graves EE, et al. In vivo high resolution three-dimensional imaging of antigen-specific cytotoxic T-lymphocyte trafficking to tumors. *Cancer Res* 2003;63:6838.
33. Ke S, Wen X, Gurfinkel M, et al. Near-infrared optical imaging of epidermal growth factor receptor in breast cancer xenografts. *Cancer Res* 2003;63:7870.

CHAPTER **24**

Advanced Imaging Methods

HEDVIG HRICAK
OGUZ AKIN
MICHELLE S. BRADBURY
LAURA LIBERMAN
LAWRENCE H. SCHWARTZ
STEVEN M. LARSON

SECTION **1**

Functional and Metabolic Imaging

Since the introduction of cross-sectional modalities [ultrasound (US), computed tomography (CT), magnetic resonance imaging (MRI)], imaging has become a much more integral part of cancer care, playing a role in every phase, from screening and diagnosis, to staging, and to treatment planning and follow-up. Breast cancer screening mammography was the first attempt at early cancer detection by imaging. Today, although still controversial, CT screening for lung cancer and CT virtual colonography for colon cancer are emerging as valuable methods for early detection in select populations. Such techniques are likely only the forerunners of an imminent, broad expansion of oncologic imaging applications, as the development of molecular imaging promises to open up new horizons in preclinical cancer detection and imaging assessment of tumor biology. Molecular imaging is already facilitating the development of new drugs and providing novel insights into cancer biology and phenotypic behavior. In the future, molecular imaging will also be an integral part of individualized treatment decisions and earlier and more accurate detection of cancer recurrence.

By almost completely replacing exploratory laparotomy, imaging has already markedly changed treatment planning, and as a result, patient triage between surgery, radiation therapy, and medical therapy has improved notably. Oncologic imaging above all requires a clinically relevant approach. Although a number of imaging modalities are now available, it is essential to use imaging prudently, to choose the modality that has the best chance of giving a definitive answer while avoiding repetitive "fishing expeditions." Imaging efficacy is specific to each cancer type and site. For some cancers, imaging offers a definitive diagnosis, accurate staging, and accurate and sensitive detection of recurrent disease. At times, however, imaging results are indeterminate. It is important to recognize the limitations of imaging and not to try to use every modality available when, in the end, invasive biopsy or surgical exploration still cannot be avoided.

This chapter presents recent advances in imaging, emphasizing the combined use of anatomic and functional imaging and describing the potential of molecular imaging. Discussions of specific technologies focus only on the latest developments; the sections on major individual cancer sites describe practical, site-specific imaging approaches and provide best-practice guidelines. For each type of cancer, the five basic functions of imaging—detection of primary tumor (in screening), characterization, staging, assessment of therapeutic efficacy, and detection of recurrence—are emphasized.

IMAGING MODALITIES

RADIOGRAPHY

Radiography was the first radiologic technique, born in 1895 with the discovery of the x-ray by Wilhelm Conrad Roentgen. It is based on the simple physical principle that the degree to which an x-ray beam is weakened, or attenuated, as it passes through a substance is determined by the density and electronic composition of that substance as well as by its thickness. Dense materials (such as the metals calcium and barium) extensively attenuate an x-ray beam, whereas, at the other extreme, air only minimally attenuates such a beam. A thick amount of a tissue attenuates an x-ray beam more than does a thinner amount of the same tissue. Most soft tissues attenuate an x-ray beam to a similar degree, resulting in the markedly limited ability of radiography to distinguish various tissues (such as liver metastases from normal liver tissue).

Since the advent of cross-sectional imaging techniques, the role of radiography in cancer care has steadily declined. Chest radiography is still commonly used to provide a quick, inexpensive, general overview of the chest, but CT is rapidly becoming the first-line examination of the chest to evaluate for metastases and tumor treatment response and to assess for complications such as pulmonary embolus. Abdominal radiography is similarly limited due to its suboptimal ability to detect such complications of cancer as bowel obstruction and to determine its cause (e.g., tumor vs. postsurgical adhesion). The various contrast-enhanced radiographic studies, such as barium enema, intravenous urography, and percutaneous transhepatic cholangiopancreatography, are decreasing in importance in oncology, and lymphangiography is no longer used in most centers. Bone radiographs, however, remain a vital element in characterizing many bone lesions by demonstrating characteristic calcified cartilaginous or osseous matrix within a bone lesion. Also, information provided by bone radiographs can help prevent misdiagnosis of various bony abnormalities (e.g., stress fracture or fibrous dysplasia) detected on other modalities (e.g., MRI or bone scintigraphy).

Newer implementations of radiography, such as computed radiography and digital radiography, offer an array of basic and advanced image manipulation functions, as well as a direct means for transferring radiographic images into a picture archive and communications system. For example, dual-energy radiography can be used to evaluate the calcium content of a pulmonary nodule and thus help assess its likelihood of being malignant.

ULTRASOUND

US is an effective and commonly used diagnostic imaging technique that has been applied in clinical practice for more than half a century. US uses high-frequency US waves to create grayscale images (B-mode US) and to provide information about vascular flow (pulsed-wave Doppler US and color flow imaging). In cancer patients, US is most commonly used to image superficial structures (e.g., thyroid, breast, testis), the thorax (pleural or pericardial effusions, chest-wall masses), the abdomen (especially liver, biliary system, and kidneys), the pelvis (pelvic genitourinary organs), and the vascular system. In addition, US can be used to guide interventional radiology procedures, such as biopsy, tumor ablation, and drainage.

The major advantage of US is that it renders "real-time" tomographic images. In addition, US is relatively inexpensive and portable compared with MRI and CT, and it has no proven harmful effects to the patient at the power levels used for diagnostic examinations. Its major limitation is that US waves cannot propagate through bone and air (e.g., bowel gas and lung parenchyma). The soft tissue resolution of US is relatively low compared to that of CT and MRI; US is also more operator dependent and less reproducible than other imaging modalities.

Several innovations in US technology have become available in clinical practice and have improved image quality and expanded the applications of US.[1,2] Such new developments include tissue harmonic imaging, which significantly augments image quality; extended field-of-view imaging, which allows visualization of large anatomic regions in a single image and simplifies evaluation and measurement of large lesions; and three-dimensional (3D) US imaging, which allows traditional two-dimensional (2D) images to be registered in various image planes, creating a 3D display. In addition, several novel US contrast agents that show potential in lesion detection and characterization are currently under investigation.[3]

COMPUTED TOMOGRAPHY

Since its introduction in the 1970s, CT has become one of the most widely used radiologic modalities. In CT, ionizing radiation beams passed through the patient from multiple different angles and subsequent computer analysis of the attenuated radiation coming out the other side of the patient are used to produce a cross-sectional image showing even subtle differences in x-ray absorption by specific tissues. CT is effective in the detection and characterization of many types of diseases in almost all body parts, including the head, neck, chest, abdomen, pelvis, and musculoskeletal system. In many types of cancers, CT can accurately show the extent of local and distant spread of tumor. CT can also be used to guide interventional procedures, such as biopsy and drainage, and to facilitate the targeting of radiation treatment.

The major advantage of CT is that it provides very high-quality images of many different organ systems with no anatomic overlap, while distinguishing various normal and abnormal tissues from each other. It can easily allow imaging of large body areas, such as the chest, abdomen, and pelvis, in one examination, and with the latest generation of multidetector scanners, the entire body can be scanned in less than 1 minute. CT is helpful in the evaluation of body parts composed of various tissue densities, such as air (lung, visceral organs), fat, soft tissue, and bone. It is also a cost-efficient, widely available, and easily reproducible technique. The major limitations of CT are that it delivers substantial doses of ionizing radiation to the imaged tissues and that the iodinated intravenous contrast materials used are potentially nephrotoxic and can cause severe adverse reactions (including renal failure or death). In addition, CT cannot be performed portably.

Recent years have witnessed amazing improvements in CT technology, which has evolved from conventional CT to helical (spiral) CT, and most recently to multidetector CT.[4] These technologic advances have dramatically increased the sensitivity and specificity of CT for many pathologic conditions. In addition, modern CT scanners are able to perform whole body examinations in a very short time and with excellent image resolution. In the past, a CT study was composed of multiple contiguous sections obtained through the body part of interest. Today, CT produces a volume of data that can be analyzed in a 2D axial display or in multiplanar reformations and 3D imaging. One major advantage of helical CT is that it virtually eliminates the previously common discontinuous sections caused by inconsistent breath-holding.

One exciting application of multidetector CT is virtual colonography. By providing conventional axial views, endoluminal views, and various 2D and 3D reformations of the entire colon, CT colonography can depict even subcentimeter-sized colonic polyps, and unlike conventional endoscopic colonoscopy, this technique can visualize those portions of the colon located beyond a stricture or constricting mass. Based on recent reports, if no polyp or mass is detected at CT colonography, the patient can safely be spared conventional colonoscopy. This noninvasive "virtual" technique thus has the potential to substantially improve patient compliance with recommendations for colon cancer screening. Other forms of "virtual endoscopy," such as CT bronchoscopy and CT urography, have some uses in cancer staging but are still under development and evaluation.

Multidetector CT enables us to evaluate multiple physiologic features simultaneously. For example, information regarding the vascular and the parenchymal phases of contrast enhancement can be obtained to provide angiographic and organ-directed imaging during the same examination, thus significantly improving lesion detection and characterization.[5] The availability of computer programs that can perform quantitative analyses of perfusion, blood volume, and capillary permeability has led to the introduction of functional imaging with CT. The quantitative analysis of physiologic parameters to assess tumor angiogenesis *in vivo* will not only assist with diagnosis, staging, and therapy monitoring for patients with cancer but will also facilitate the development of better antineoplastic chemotherapeutic agents.[6]

MAGNETIC RESONANCE IMAGING

MRI is a cross-sectional imaging technique that uses strong magnetic fields and multiple radiofrequency pulses to generate images with outstanding spatial resolution and tissue contrast. MRI is based on the principles of nuclear magnetic resonance (NMR), a nondestructive technique used in physical chemistry to analyze the composition of substances. Certain nuclei have a magnetic moment because they are composed of an odd number of protons and neutrons. When placed in a magnetic field, these nuclei attempt to align with the field and rotate, or spin (precess), about the axis of the magnetic field.

The most commonly imaged nucleus is hydrogen (^{1}H) because of its abundance in the body and its high gyromagnetic ratio compared with other nuclei with a magnetic moment, such as phosphorus (^{31}P), sodium (^{23}Na), and carbon (^{13}C). When nuclei, such as hydrogen, are placed in a strong magnetic field and excited by the addition of a radiofrequency pulse transmitted at their Larmor frequency, they momentarily gain energy. When the radiofrequency pulse is turned off, the nuclei return to their resting state and emit the previously absorbed energy at the same frequency. The magnitude of the emitted signal and the time it takes for the nuclei to return to the resting state are dependent on certain intrinsic properties of the nuclei, including the nuclear spin density (or proton density), longitudinal (T1) relaxation time, transverse (T2) relaxation time, and flow.

Localizing within the patient the precise position of the signal emitted from a specific nucleus is known as *spatial encoding*. Magnetic field gradients are used to accomplish this encoding by changing the gyromagnetic ratio along the gradient. Gradients applied perpendicularly to the magnetic field are generally used to localize an image slice and determine the slice thickness; the stronger the gradient applied, the thinner the

slice. Gradients are also applied to two dimensions within a given slice to localize the nuclei within the slice. Because application and magnitude of the gradients are electronically controlled, image slices can be obtained in the axial, coronal, sagittal, or any oblique imaging plane.

The versatility of MR technology is evident not only in the many options it offers for obtaining anatomic information but in its capacity to obtain functional MRI (fMRI), MR perfusion, or MR spectroscopic information as well. Many extrinsic parameters or variables can be manipulated to change the tissue contrast, and thus the appearance, of an image. For instance, fMRI, obtained by asking the patient in the MRI scanner to perform a task (such as finger tapping) may demonstrate regions of increased cerebral blood flow associated with the task being performed. Functional data may be superimposed on an anatomic MRI image, thus providing information about function and anatomy that is very helpful in preoperative neurosurgical planning.

Rapid imaging techniques such as echoplanar imaging, by which images can be obtained in a fraction of a second, have also ushered in fMRI of brain function. fMRI studies are performed either as contrast-enhanced functional imaging with gadolinium-diethylenetriamine pentaacetic acid (e.g., to study the visual cortex, based on the increase of blood flow with task activation) or as fMRI (based on the different magnetic properties of oxy- and deoxyhemoglobin). Deoxyhemoglobin is paramagnetic, induces local magnetic field inhomogeneities within the blood vessels, enhances the relaxation of water molecules, and decreases the signal in T2-weighted images. Stimulation of the brain by task activation increases blood flow to the stimulated region, resulting in increased oxyhemoglobin and increased signal in T2-weighted images. This blood oxygenation level–dependent method has been used in a variety of functional and physiologic studies, including sensory stimulation, motor function, language, and vision. fMRI is being used increasingly for treatment planning in radiation oncology and surgical planning for intracranial tumors. The typical battery of tasks for neurosurgical planning includes hand tactile stimulation, hand-motor activity (finger-thumb tapping), picture naming (internal speech), and listening to the spoken word (language comprehension). An important application of this noninvasive procedure for radiation oncology is in conformal avoidance of critical areas of the brain to minimize the possibility of loss of essential functions.

Perfusion MRI is another imaging technique that is useful for measuring blood flow through an organ or tumor. MRI signal data are acquired continuously after injection of a contrast agent. The properties of the contrast agent are such that the MRI signal changes relative to the amount of contrast material present. MRI perfusion techniques have been used extensively to assess tumor angiogenesis and the response to therapy.[7,8] In addition to perfusion, dynamic contrast-enhanced imaging can also be used to measure or extract parameters such as cerebral blood volume, blood–brain barrier permeability, necrotic fraction, extracellular space volume, and permeability–surface area product. The use of dynamic techniques to assess tumor grade and type, treatment efficacy, and possibly long-term prognosis as applied to brain, breast, sarcoma, and other sites is being studied.

Another MRI technique is diffusion imaging. The *in vivo* mobility of water molecules depends on the properties of the diffusing medium and the presence of physical barriers. Therefore, diffusion-weighted imaging (DWI) can provide information on the cellular milieu, for example, viscosity due to proteins that bind to water molecules and slow their motion and barriers such as cell membranes that limit motion. By obtaining multiple images with different diffusion "weighting" factors, the apparent diffusion coefficient (ADC) of *in vivo* water can be measured. The measured ADC values can be displayed as a parametric image, and the ADC may differ for the milieus of normal and pathologic states. Compared with T1- or T2-weighted images, diffusion-weighted images provide excellent tissue discrimination in certain diseases. In preliminary studies, DWI was tested in patients with a variety of hepatic tumors and was used in individuals with glioma to differentiate between cystic and necrotic regions; the technique was also used in assessing tumor response to therapy.

Using magnetic resonance spectroscopy (MRS), the presence and concentration of various metabolites at micromolar levels can be measured. This technique exploits the phenomenon of "chemical shift" in the NMR spectrum. Specifically, after the nuclei of a particular nuclide (e.g., ^{31}P) are excited with a radiofrequency pulse, their relaxation time depends on the surrounding electron clouds and adjacent nuclei and therefore on the structure of the parent molecule. Thus, the ^{31}P in adenosine triphosphate can be distinguished from the ^{31}P in adenosine diphosphate. This chemical shift, or small changes in resonant frequency due to molecular structure, can yield the "molecular signature" of the sample in question. MRS provides information about the presence and amount of hydrogen protons attached to different molecules. These protons possess intrinsic differences in resonant frequencies because of their differing molecular environments. A spectrum can be generated that corresponds to a scale of resonant frequencies. MRS is useful in characterization of certain tumors. For instance, compared to benign prostate processes, prostate cancers have increased levels of choline.[9] MRS may also permit noninvasive monitoring to assess the response of residual tumor to therapy or to differentiate tumor necrosis from recurrence.

^1H SPECTROSCOPY

^1H-MRS imaging [MRS(I)] combines the advantages of obtaining biochemical data by water-suppressed ^1H spectroscopy with the spatial localization of those data. Relative to spectroscopy of other nuclei, ^1H-MRS has the advantage of better sensitivity than all the other nuclides, which results in better spatial resolution and signal-to-noise ratio and decreased acquisition time. In addition, detection of proton metabolites requires no hardware additional to standard clinical scanners, although pulse sequences to suppress water and lipids are necessary. Therefore ^1H-MRS(I) has been used extensively. Voxel (volume element) sizes as small as 0.24 cm^3 (6 mm^3 × 6 mm^3 × 6 mm^3) have been studied in the brain and prostate. Metabolic data from a single voxel can be spatially selected with specific radiofrequency pulses and magnetic field gradients using techniques such as point-resolved spectroscopy (PRESS) or stimulated echo acquisition mode (STEAM). Multivoxel data can be obtained by combining single-voxel or slice selection techniques with chemical shift imaging methods.

A large number of compounds have been detected *in vivo* using water-suppressed ^1H-NMR spectroscopy. Chemicals commonly detected in many tissues include choline, lactate, and creatine. Certain metabolites observed in the proton spectrum are characteristic of particular normal tissues, such as N-acetylaspar-

tate in the brain and citrate in the peripheral zone of the prostate. N-acetylaspartate is thought to be a neuronal marker, whereas citrate is produced and secreted by the glandular tissue of the peripheral zone of the prostate. The choline peak in proton spectra may contain not only choline but phosphocholine, glycerophosphocholine, and taurine. Increased choline in tumors is regarded as an indicator of enhanced cell membrane phospholipid turnover due to tumor cell proliferation and increased cellularity and/or growth. A decreased choline level in tumor has been associated with response to radiation therapy.

NUCLEAR MEDICINE METHODOLOGIES

Nuclear medicine is widely used in oncology to detect cancer recurrence and to stage malignancy. Nuclear medicine is an example of a functional imaging technique because it uses tracers of the body's own normal or abnormal biochemistry or physiology. The technique involves two parts: injecting a radioactive tracer and detecting the distribution of the tracer within the body using a radioactivity detector system, such as the Anger camera, single-photon emission CT (SPECT), or positron emission tomography (PET). Table 24.1-1 lists commonly used tracers and indications.

Technetium 99m (^{99m}Tc) phosphate bone scanning is a useful example. After intravenous injection of the tracer, there is rapid deposition of radioactivity in the bones. The mechanism of action is based on the physical accretion of phosphonates into the hydroxyapatite crystal of living bone, a process that occurs within minutes. After allowing a couple of hours for unreacted radioactivity to be cleared from the blood and surrounding tissues, an image of the radioactivity distribution is obtained with a gamma or Anger camera. The presence of a tumor or other damage to the bone shows up as a "hot spot" superimposed on a background of normal bone uptake (Fig. 24.1-1).

The ^{99m}Tc bone scan is used to stage patients with tumors that have a propensity to spread to bones, such as lung, prostate, breast, and renal tumors; neuroblastoma; and sarcoma. In general, the bone scan is used when there is a reasonable likelihood that the tumor has spread. For instance, in prostate cancer, bone scanning is recommended when prostate-specific antigen (PSA) is greater than 10. In breast cancer, bone scanning should be used when local disease is T2 or greater or when there is clinical evidence of local or axillary metastases.

The Anger, or gamma, camera, invented by H. Anger in the 1950s, has evolved into a high-resolution instrument that uses robotics to fetch components and facilitate automated operations. The radioactive detector is sensitive to individual gamma rays, and focusing is done with a lead collimator (a 2-in. lead sheet with straight holes punched in it to permit entry of gamma rays into the region of the crystal).

SPECT is used to create 3D images of the distribution of radioactivity in the human body. It is performed by rotating a gamma camera over 360 degrees around the patient to collect projection information. A computer is then used to reconstruct the distribution of radioactivity into a 3D image. Many tens of thousands of nuclear medicine procedures are performed in the United States each day, primarily in cardiac and oncologic imaging. SPECT and planar gamma camera imaging are used for the bulk of these procedures. Within the last 5 years, CT has been added to SPECT, with reported benefits analogous to those described for PET/CT imaging.[10]

TABLE 24.1-1. Commonly Used Diagnostic and Therapeutic Radiopharmaceuticals

Nuclide	Pharmaceutical	Pharmacology	Dosage	Patient Preparation	Use
^{18}F	FDG	Glycolysis	10 mCi	Fasting	Tumor viability
^{67}Ga	Citrate	Transferrin receptor	10 mCi	Laxatives	Lymphoma, inflammation
^{131}I	MIBG	Catecholamine uptake	0.5 mCi	Off α, β blockers	Neuroendocrine tumor
^{123}I	Sodium iodide	Thyroid hormone	25 μCi	Off thyroid hormone, iodides	Thyroid dysfunction
^{111}In	Leukocytes	Target inflammation	5 mCi	None	Phlegmon
^{111}In	Pentetreotide	Somatostatin receptors	5 mCi	Off steroids and octreotide; laxatives	Endocrine malignancy
^{111}In	Prostascint	Anti-PSMA MoAb	6 mCi	Laxatives, enema	Prostate cancer recurrence
^{99m}Tc	Phosphonates	Bone mineralization	25 mCi	None	Bone disease
^{99m}Tc	Sulfur colloid	Lymphatic clearance	0.2–0.5 mCi	None	Identify sentinel node
^{99m}Tc	Aggregated albumin	Capillary blockade	5 mCi	None	Pulmonary emboli
^{99m}Tc	Erythrocytes	Vascular marker	30 mCi	Off β blockers	Measure LVEF
^{99m}Tc	Pertechnetate	Thyroid iodine trap	10 mCi	Off thyroxine, iodide	Thyroid nodule
^{99m}Tc	MIBI	Lipophilicity and intra-cellular binding	20 mCi	Fasting; stop xanthines	Tumor viability, cardiac perfusion
^{99m}Tc	CEA scan	Anti-CEA MoAb	20–30 mCi	Laxatives	Colorectal cancer
^{201}Tl	Chloride	Na$^+$, K$^+$ pump	5 mCi	None	Tumor viability

CEA, carcinoembryonic antigen; FDG, fluorodeoxyglucose; LVEF, left ventricular ejection fraction; MIBG, metaiodobenzylguanidine; MIBI, methoxyisobutyl isonitrile; MoAb, monoclonal antibody; PSMA, prostate-specific membrane antigen.
(Modified from Divgi CR, Larson SM. Nuclear medicine. In: Casciato D, ed. *Manual of clinical oncology*, 5th ed. Philadelphia: Lippincott Williams & Wilkins, 2004:29.)

Lymphoscintigraphy has become a common nuclear medicine technique in the last few years as a result of improved techniques and the recognition that common human tumors, particularly breast and melanoma, spread from their primary site to a "sentinel" lymph node at an early stage of metastasis. Sampling of the sentinel lymph node is a highly accurate technique for determining regional metastases,[11,12] and in a patient with breast cancer it has become the standard of care for primary lesions less than 5 cm in size. Studies have also shown that sentinel lymph node dissection can have excellent results for melanoma, provided that great care is taken in the pathologic assessment of the sentinel node.[13,14]

POSITRON EMISSION TOMOGRAPHY/ COMPUTED TOMOGRAPHY

PET takes advantage of the unique physics of positron decay to produce high-resolution, quantitative 3D images of the distribution of radioactivity in the human body. In PET, a positron-labeled form of a biologically relevant molecule is injected into the body and used to trace the biochemical behavior of that molecule through noninvasive imaging. Thus, every PET study requires prior injection of a specific radiolabeled PET tracer to create the PET images of a distinct molecular distribution or tissue function. For example, the biochemistry of glucose use can be quantitatively imaged using the positron-emitting glucose analog, ^{18}F-2-fluoro-2-deoxy, 2-D-glucose, known as *FDG*. To image a different tissue function, such as blood flow, a different tracer would be required, such as 15O-H2O. As a tool for "molecular imaging" in oncology, PET has superb versatility, because it can be used in combination with literally thousands of radiotracers to image many key molecules and molecularly based events that are important to normal tissue physiology and pathophysiology.

PET-FDG imaging is increasingly becoming an essential component of the management of oncology patients. The

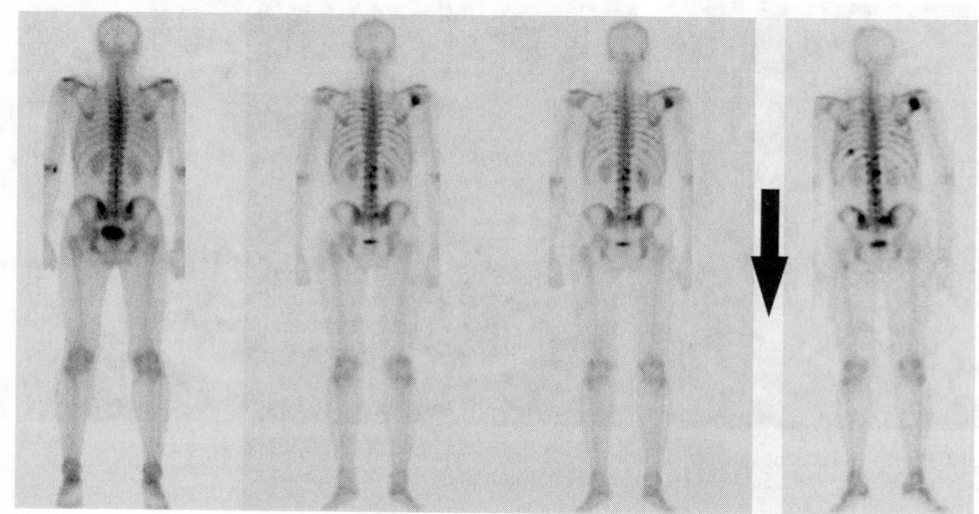

FIGURE 24.1-1. Technetium 99m methylene diphosphonate image in a patient with metastatic prostate cancer involving the spine and pelvis.

accelerated glycolysis of malignancy has proven to be a shared feature of most common tumors, and PET-FDG imaging can provide information regarding tumor detection, staging, and treatment response. Recognizing the benefits of PET-FDG to the oncology patient, the Centers for Medicare and Medicaid Services has recommended a growing list of common tumors for PET reimbursement. At present, recognized applications for PET-FDG imaging include the following tumor sites: non–small cell lung cancer, colorectal cancer, head and neck cancer, esophageal cancer, breast cancer, thyroid cancer, and lymphoma.

The PET/CT unit combines a high-resolution PET unit with a high-resolution spiral CT unit. The resulting images depict tissue function and biochemistry in a high-resolution, anatomic context. Combination with CT has proven to be a major enhancement for PET, creating images that are easier to interpret and more rapidly produced.[15] Additional advantages of PET/CT include improved diagnostic resolution through respiratory gating[16] and improved radiation oncology treatment planning.

THERAPEUTIC RESPONSE ASSESSMENT

The response of tumors to therapeutic agents such as chemotherapy and radiotherapy is commonly assessed on radiologic images. Serial radiologic examinations performed before, during, and after chemotherapy or radiation therapy regimens provide critical information about changes in tumor size. Such assessment, which in most cases cannot reliably be obtained from physical examination, is essential for determining whether a particular therapy or experimental therapeutic agent is beneficial to the patient or effective against a specific tumor.

The World Health Organization (WHO) first established response assessment criteria in 1979 to standardize the recording and reporting of response assessment for solid tumors so that response outcomes could be compared between various research organizations, trials, and therapies.[17,18] The WHO criteria require that the response assessment be performed on the basis of measurements in two dimensions. After therapy, the percentage reduction or percentage increase in the corresponding measurements is used for calculating treatment response. According to the WHO criteria, a partial response (PR) is achieved with a 50% reduction in the sum of the tumor cross products. Disease progression is considered a 25% increase in the sum of one or more of the tumor deposits.

The WHO criteria were used as the standard for many years. Over time, researchers, cooperative groups, and industrial sponsors modified the criteria such that the standards were no longer comparable among different research organizations and studies. Variabilities were introduced in the definitions of "measurable" and "evaluable" lesions, the minimum lesion size and the number of lesions to be recorded for patients with multiple lesions, the definition of progressive disease, and the processing and analysis of imaging data from relatively new technologies, such as CT/MRI.

In 1994, several organizations, including the European Organization for Research and Treatment of Cancer, Belgium, and the National Cancer Institute, USA, began to review the response assessment criteria with the intent of revising them. Their goal was to create a modified set of criteria that (1) continued to use the four categories of responses defined as complete response (CR; total disappearance), PR (Fig. 24.1-2), stable disease, and progressive disease; (2) maintained the meaning and concept of PR so that it would be possible to compare favorable results from experimental therapies with those already in use, even though the measurement criteria would be different; (3) modified the concept of disease progression; and (4) used unidimensional measurements, which are believed to be easier to obtain and calculate.

Under these principles, response evaluation criteria in solid tumors (RECIST) guidelines have been published.[18] Response data from several trials were reanalyzed using both sets of criteria to assess the extent of agreement between them. James et al.[19] analyzed 569 patients accrued on eight phase II and phase III studies of various cancers and reported a kappa coefficient of 0.95 as a demonstration of excellent agreement between the response and nonresponse categories as assigned by WHO and RECIST criteria. Therasse et al.[18] also analyzed 4000 patients' data from 14 trials and reported a difference in (CR + PR) rate for WHO and RECIST ranging from 1% to 3% and a differ-

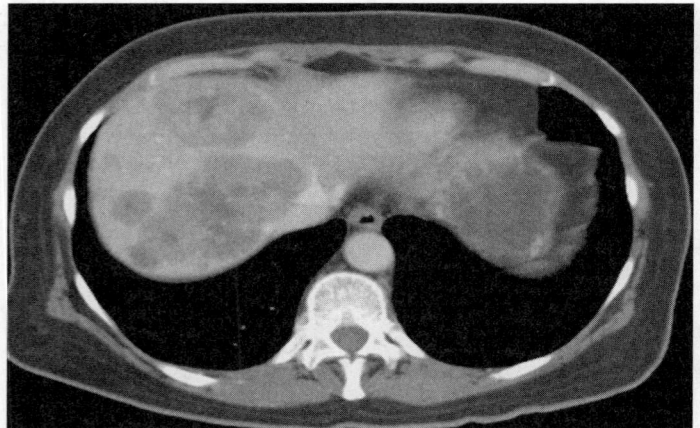
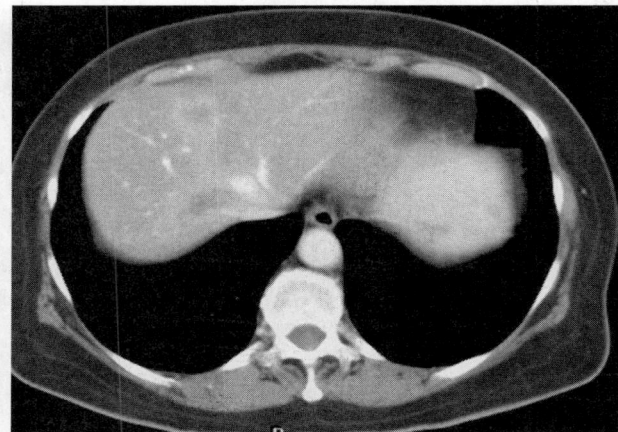

FIGURE 24.1-2. Axial CT scans in a patient with metastatic colorectal cancer. At baseline, before therapy (**A**), multiple hepatic metastases are present, which at follow-up (**B**) are smaller, indicating a partial response.

ence in progression rate ranging from 1% to 18%, reinforcing the above conclusion.

Controversy has surrounded the implementation of RECIST with concern about the differences in response assessment between the two methodologies, especially in measuring time to tumor progression. It is recognized that some tumor shapes are less well estimated with a unidimensional measurement than others. Also, the RECIST criteria do not address important areas of tumor involvement including bones and bone marrow.

Other techniques and modalities have been used to assess response. PET and MRI have been used in early clinical trials and have demonstrated the ability to detect changes in tumor metabolism earlier than changes in the actual size of the tumor. Similarly rapid CT perfusion techniques have been developed for use with the newer multidetector CT scans to measure perfusion changes in tissues. These techniques are gaining acceptance in smaller and early-stage clinical trials as early predictors of response.

BRAIN AND HEAD/NECK CANCERS

Technologic advances in neuroradiology during the past 15 years have vastly improved our ability to detect, diagnose, stage, and assess the therapeutic response of brain or head/neck tumors after radiotherapy, with or without adjunctive chemotherapy. Although the vast majority of imaging studies have focused on the morphologic evaluation of tumors for accurate lesion mapping, there has been steadily increasing interest in the application of newer, functional imaging strategies for probing tumor physiology and metabolism. The evolution of these techniques has been fueled, in part, by the need for prompt and accurate recognition of malignant progression or posttherapeutic tumor recurrence, the desire to tailor treatment plans to individual patients, and the ongoing effort to develop highly specific and effective antitumor therapies. Early results from the application of these techniques suggest that they may offer improvements over cross-sectional imaging with regard to identifying recurrent tumor, monitoring treatment success or failure, and detecting metastatic nodal disease.

DETECTION AND DIAGNOSIS

An ever-increasing array of diagnostic imaging tools has become commercially available for evaluation and improved characterization of brain tumors, as well as head and neck lesions. Conventional cross-sectional imaging (i.e., multidetector CT and MRI) is highly sensitive but lacks specificity for predicting histologic tumor grade and for distinguishing tumor recurrence from posttreatment tumor necrosis. To improve tissue specificity, a number of promising approaches have been developed. These include the implementation of novel MRI pulse sequences (fast fluid attenuated inversion recovery) and the application of physiologic and metabolic techniques (^{1}H-MRS, fMRI, and perfusion/DWI).

Brain

Approximately 17,000 new cases of primary central nervous system tumors are diagnosed each year,[20] excluding patients with benign brain tumors or metastatic disease to the brain. MRI is

generally recognized as the noninvasive imaging study of choice for diagnosis and presurgical planning of suspected primary brain tumors and metabolic disease. MRI is especially useful in identifying tumors of the pituitary region, brainstem, and posterior fossa, including the cerebellopontine angle. Due to issues of cost containment and scanner availability, however, CT continues to play a limited role in lesion detection. Occasionally, CT scans may be used to provide supplemental information relating to osseous destruction in skull-based lesions or to tumor calcification, thus helping to limit differential possibilities.

The inherently high sensitivity of MRI for lesion detection, its completeness of lesion delineation, multiplanar capabilities, high spatial resolution (less than 2-mm slices), and ability to accurately define the extent of surrounding peritumoral edema, mass effect, cyst formation, and intratumoral hemorrhage have made this modality indispensable for lesion characterization. The resolution, however, is not high enough to detect distant tumor infiltration. Several imaging findings, specifically the extent of peritumoral edema and the presence of necrosis, have been found to roughly correlate with histologic grading of cerebral gliomas. Routinely available imaging techniques include fast-spin echo sequences to decrease imaging time, heavily T2-weighted fast fluid attenuated inversion recovery sequences to increase intraparenchymal lesion conspicuity, and fat saturation pulses to improve tissue visualization. Postcontrast T1-weighted images facilitate identification of the tumor nidus, as well as improve visualization of dural-based masses, leptomeningeal deposits, and the ependymal spread of tumor.

To minimize the morbidity of surgery for tumors in eloquent areas of the brain, physiologic imaging techniques such as fMRI are increasingly being used in preoperative planning. In addition, 3D multivoxel ^{1}H-MRS has been added to routine clinical sequences to complement information obtained from conventional MRI. Noninvasive measurements of brain tumor metabolites, such as choline and N-acetylaspartate, are used to guide lesion biopsy but are deemed unreliable for lesions smaller than 2.0 cm or those adjacent to bone, fat, or cerebrospinal fluid secondary to signal contamination.[21] Perfusion-weighted imaging (PWI) provides information about tumor tissue perfusion and is useful in the preoperative planning and grading of gliomas.[22] These perfusion measurements, given in terms of a relative cerebral blood volume, vary roughly according to tumor grade, with maximum relative cerebral blood values of high-grade gliomas being significantly larger than those of low-grade gliomas.[23] However, PWI cannot sensitively discriminate between grade I and II tumors, II and III tumors, or III and IV tumors.[24] DWI techniques have been used largely for tumor characterization, enabling differentiation of densely packed cellular tumors, such as lymphoma (hyperintense on DWI), from cerebral gliomas (hypointense on DWI). DWI has low specificity, as the diffusion values of low- and high-grade tumors partially overlap. In addition, tumor infiltration cannot be distinguished from vasogenic edema. DWI can usually distinguish necrotic tumors (central hypointensity) from abscesses (central hyperintensity), not often possible using conventional sequences.[25]

Head and Neck

The majority of all malignant head and neck tumors are squamous cell carcinomas, primarily involving the nasopharynx, oral cavity, oropharynx, and larynx. Metastatic lymph node involvement is the most important prognostic factor affecting patient survival. Five percent to 10% of patients with squamous cell carcinoma may present with cervical metastases, although no primary tumor of the upper aerodigestive tract may be apparent on head and neck exmination.[26] Important sites to consider that may harbor small, occult primaries are the nasopharynx, tonsil, piriform sinus, and the tongue base. The initial complete head and neck examination should include an examination of the oral cavity, oropharynx, nasopharynx, and larynx by fiberoptic endoscopy, palpation of the oral cavity and tongue base, and examination of the salivary glands, scalp, external ear, orbits, and thyroid gland.

A number of imaging techniques can subsequently be used to image the soft tissues of the head and neck, primarily CT, MRI, and PET. The choice of a particular imaging modality and the timing of the examination vary among institutions, reflecting the expertise and preferences of interpreting neuroradiologists. Many institutions subscribe to contrast-enhanced CT imaging from the skull base to the clavicles, often as the primary and sole imaging examination for evaluating the soft tissues of the head and neck. Although either CT or MRI can be used, the radiologist may often arrive at a correct diagnosis more rapidly and confidently when interpreting a CT study.[27] In addition, CT is more readily available than MRI, and the examination takes less time and is less expensive. MRI is generally favored when the suspected lesion is located near the skull base or when the mass is situated within the upper aerodigestive tract, including the parapharyngeal space, masticator space, parotid gland, and tongue.[27] MRI offers superior soft tissue delineation, multiplanar capabilities, and the ability to sensitively detect perineural tumor spread, tumor invasion, and marrow involvement. CT, on the other hand, is believed to better demonstrate metastatic nodal disease as well as more sensitively and accurately detect early cortical skull base erosion and invasion of the walls of the orbits and sinonasal cavities. Because they complement each other, CT and MRI studies are frequently acquired together, particularly for evaluation of sinonasal, nasopharyngeal, and oropharyngeal tumors.

In patients harboring head and neck metastases with no identifiable primary lesion, PET has been shown to be more beneficial than cross-sectional imaging for tumor detection. In one reported series, PET successfully localized unknown primary lesions in 40% of cases for which conventional anatomic imaging found no obvious lesion.[28] A promising technique that has shown particular utility in the head and neck is combined PET/CT, with preliminary studies suggesting that this new modality increases the accuracy of PET interpretations, reduces the number of equivocal PET interpretations, improves patient management, and reduces the imaging time per patient (Fig. 24.1-3).[15,29]

STAGING

Accurate pretreatment lymph node staging for resectable lesions is critical for optimizing the surgical strategy. For nonresectable lesions, prescribing individualized radiation treatment mandates precise definition of metastatic nodal involvement. Staging of the head and neck is based on a combination of physical examination (i.e., palpation) and cross-sectional imaging. Classification of nodal levels by cross-sectional imaging has eliminated areas of confusion that arise from previously adopted, clinically based classification schemes.[30] Clinically relevant nodal groups commonly affected in patients with head and neck cancers are the subman-

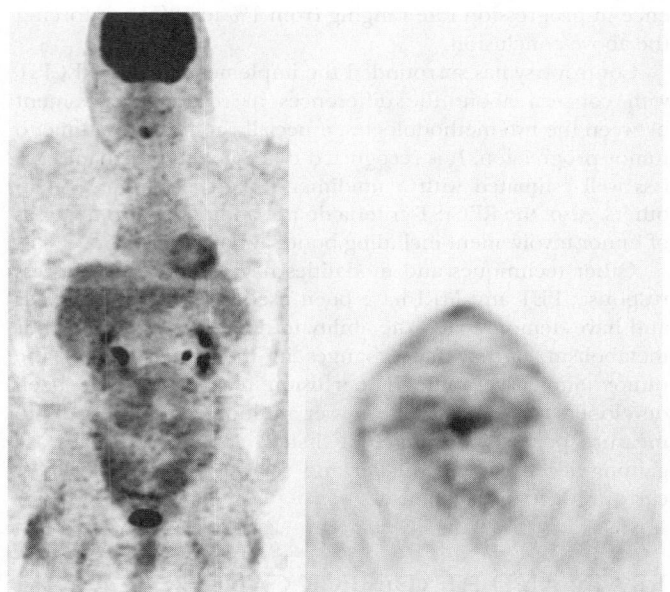

A

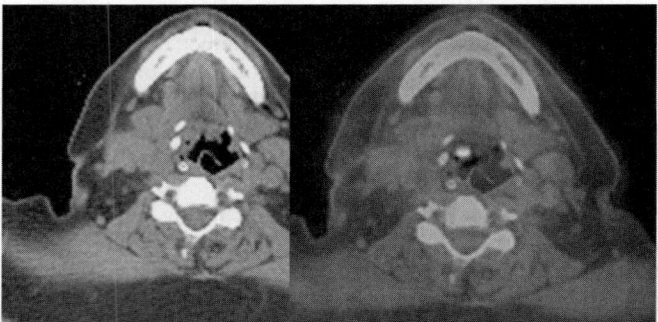

B

FIGURE 24.1-3.   A 74-year-old man with a history of melanoma who recently presented with right cervical lymphadenopathy. The patient underwent a right selective neck dissection (level II and III), with histopathology showing a poorly differentiated squamous cell carcinoma, suggestive of a primary carcinoma in the aerodigestive tract. An initial contrast computed tomography (CT) demonstrated mild, symmetric fullness of the tongue base without a discrete mass to suggest a primary tumor (not shown). A positron emission tomography (PET)/CT study with ¹⁸FDG was performed 2 weeks later and showed the following: **A:** Coronal and corresponding transaxial PET images, obtained 2 weeks after the contrast CT study, reveal a focal area of increased activity within the upper aerodigestive tract on the right. **B:** Companion low-dose CT image (*left*), which is acquired as part of the PET/CT, and PET/CT fusion image (*right*). Mild symmetric fullness in the region of the tongue base on the axial CT image (*left*) may represent lymphoid tissue; however, the corresponding PET/CT fusion image (*right*) clearly defines the exact location and extent of focally increased activity at the right tongue base. Subsequent histopathology revealed the primary squamous cell carcinoma at the base of the tongue. (Courtesy of Heiko Schöder, MD, New York, New York.) (See Color Fig. 24.1-3*B* in the CD-ROM.)

dibular, submental, retropharyngeal, and lateral cervical nodes (including the deep internal jugular chain, posterior triangle, and supraclavicular regions). Locoregional nodal spread of tumor decreases the 5-year survival to nearly 50%. Additional radiographic evaluation for staging purposes depends on the exact location of the tumor, although a chest x-ray, Panorex views, or barium swallow may be acquired to evaluate for synchronous lesions or metastatic involvement of the chest, mandible, or esophagus, respectively.

The two major imaging criteria used to determine the presence of nodal metastases on CT or MR imaging are central focal necrosis or nodal inhomogeneity and nodal size.[31] As a result of their dependence on size criteria, CT and MRI have been found to lack sensitivity and specificity. Proposed size criteria recommendations have commonly been based on the maximum longitudinal diameter of the node (although criteria also exist for the minimum axial diameter and longitudinal length/transaxial width); a node measuring greater than 1.5 cm in the jugulodigastric (level II) or submandibular regions (level I), as well as a node measuring greater than 1.0 cm elsewhere in the neck, is considered suspicious for metastatic disease.[31] These size criteria are inaccurate in 20% to 28% of tumors,[31] as normal-sized, nonnecrotic nodes may harbor small tumor deposits, whereas enlarged nodes may simply be reactive. The shape of the node is also important, as a more spherical-appearing node (vs. the typically elongated node), particularly without an identifiable fatty hilum, is suspicious for harboring metastases. Tumor penetration through the nodal capsule (i.e., thickened, enhancing rim with adjacent tissue infiltration) suggests extranodal tumor spread and is associated with a decrease in survival.[31]

To date, clinical studies suggest that lymph node staging with PET is more sensitive and accurate than with CT or MRI.[32,33] PET scans can detect tumor-harboring lymph nodes down to 4 mm, potentially missing lesions below this level.[26] A study examined lymph node staging in head and neck cancer, prospectively comparing PET with conventional imaging modalities (CT, MRI). PET was found to have a sensitivity and specificity of 90% and 94%, respectively, compared to 82% and 85% for CT and 88% and 79% for MRI.[32] PET has also proven beneficial in cases of clinical N0 disease (no pathologic lymphadenopathy by clinical examination or imaging), as 20% to 30% of patients are found to have occult lymph node metastases.[26]

POSTTREATMENT EVALUATION AND TUMOR RECURRENCE

Brain

A postoperative MRI study is typically obtained 4 to 6 weeks after surgery, serving as a baseline for the evaluation of recurrent tumor on subsequent serial scans. However, MRI cannot reliably differentiate residual or recurrent tumor from late radiation necrosis (i.e., 6 months to 2 years after therapy), as the latter preferentially occurs in the immediate vicinity of the original tumor. Problematically, radiation necrosis and recurrent tumor can frequently coexist. An enhancing mass lesion associated with edema may be seen on CT or MRI, mimicking the imaging appearance of residual or recurrent tumor. Radiation necrosis is a strong consideration given the appropriate time interval relative to treatment. Although the diagnosis is made by surgical biopsy, several functional imaging studies may also suggest the diagnosis, including 3D multivoxel ^{1}H-MRS, PET, thallium 201 SPECT, or PWI.[34]

3D multivoxel (or single-voxel) ^{1}H-MRS is commonly used to differentiate tumor recurrence from radiation necrosis as part of the standard MRI protocol (Fig. 24.1-4). After tumor debulking, areas of radiation necrosis reveal markedly reduced levels of choline, whereas choline is significantly elevated in areas of tumor recurrence. Alternatively, PET imaging, with a reported accuracy of 85%, demonstrates decreases in ^{18}F-FDG activity for radiation necrosis compared with increases in activity for recurrent or residual tumor.

Head and Neck

A number of imaging modalities, including CT, MRI, and PET, have been used for the differentiation of recurrent tumor from posttreatment changes. More recently, combined PET/CT, ^{1}H-MRS, and MR/CT perfusion have emerged as promising diagnostic tools for evaluating early recurrent tumor and for monitoring treatment response during therapy.[15] The choice of the most appropriate imaging modality for differentiating tumor recurrence from posttreatment changes remains controversial within the neuroradiology community. Increasingly, metabolic imaging has become the accepted technique for this determination, as distortion of anatomic structures after surgery and radiation therapy renders CT and MRI less reliable. However, MRI is the preferred technique for detecting early intracranial extension or perineural spread as a posttreatment baseline study, particularly in patients with nasopharyngeal, sinonasal, and skull base tumors.

PET has been found to have a higher diagnostic accuracy than cross-sectional imaging with regard to detecting residual/recurrent tumors.[33,35] It accurately detects residual or recurrent tumor, resulting in patient management changes.[33] Although the sensitivity of PET in detecting residual/recurrent disease (88% to 100%) is comparable to conventional CT and MRI (70% to 92%), the specificity is significantly higher (75% to 100% vs. 50% to 57%).[33] PET can detect residual or recurrent nodal metastases with greater specificity than CT or MRI.[33]

In the larynx, PET differentiates tumor recurrence from postradiation fibrotic changes more accurately than CT or MRI (85% vs. 42%),[33] maintaining salvage laryngectomy as a viable option. When endoscopic evaluation and conventional imaging studies were inconclusive, PET imaging was able to accurately discriminate these findings.[36]

Mukherji and Wolf[37] have made several recommendations regarding selection of the appropriate modality for assessment of the postoperative neck based on clinical suspicion of disease. Briefly, PET should be the imaging study of choice in instances in which (1) no clinically obvious mass is present in a patient with nonspecific symptoms suggestive of recurrence or (2) low clinical suspicion of recurrence is favored in a patient with advanced head and neck cancer. Cross-sectional imaging should be performed when there is a positive or equivocal PET study or to evaluate tumor extent in cases of biopsy-proven recurrence or a suspicious palpable mass. Early-stage disease and low clinical suspicion or recurrence precludes an imaging study.

LUNG CANCER

Lung cancer is the most common cancer in men and women, and its global incidence is increasing. Consequently, a great deal of biologic and clinical research has focused on various aspects of lung cancer. The role of radiologic methods in the evaluation of lung cancer is discussed briefly in this section.

SCREENING

The use of chest radiography to screen high-risk individuals has been reported to identify tumors at a more favorable stage,

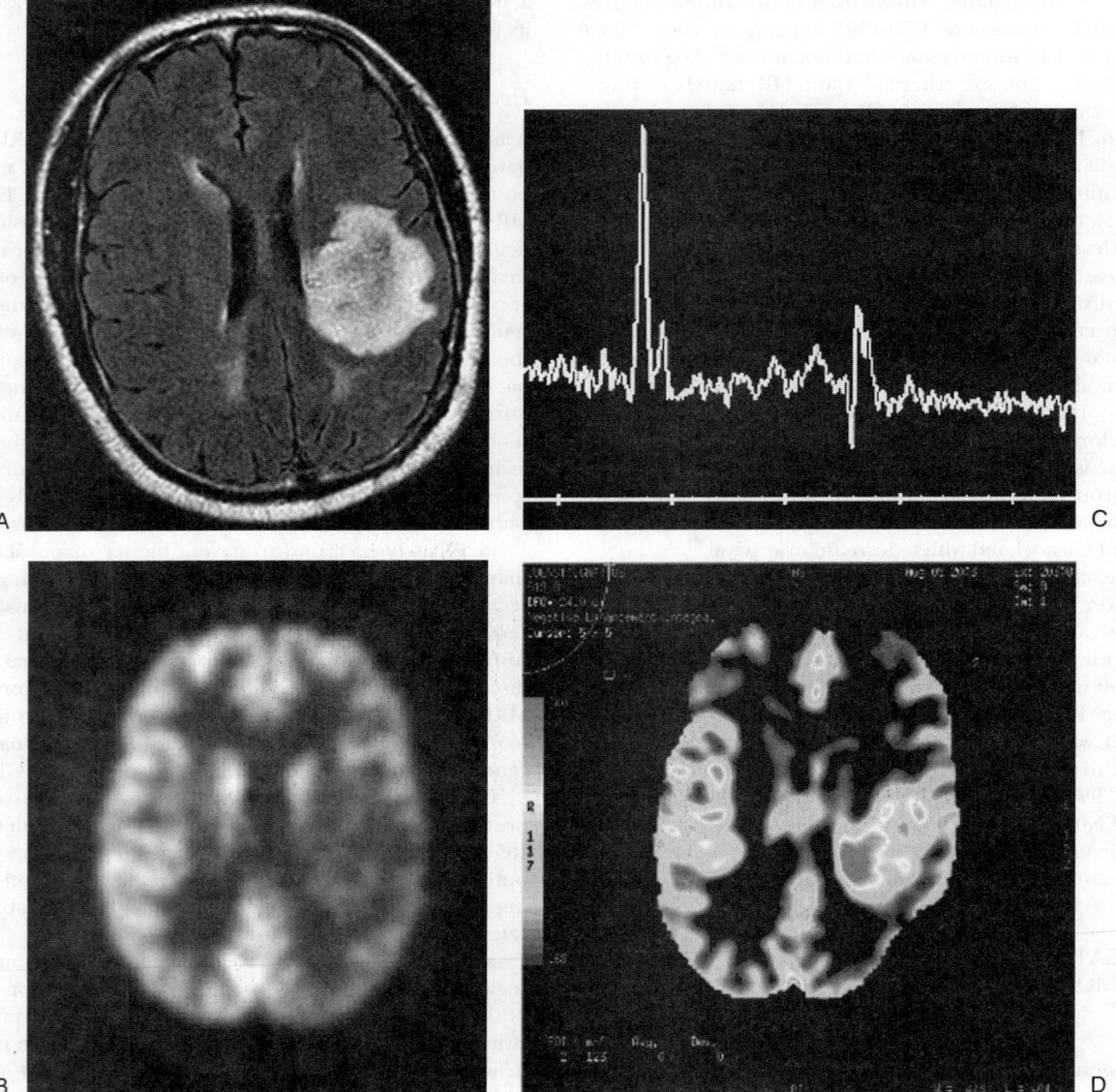

FIGURE 24.1-4. Forty-year-old man after resection of a left anaplastic pleomorphic astrocytoma in March 2002. He was initially treated with Gliadel wafer placement and subsequently followed by external-beam radiotherapy and concomitant temozolomide (chemotherapy) until May 2003. **A:** Axial T2-weighted fast fluid attenuated inversion recovery (FLAIR) magnetic resonance imaging of the brain after termination of chemotherapy reveals a 6.7-cm × 5.4-cm left posterior frontal/parietal mass extending medially to the ependymal surface of the left lateral ventricle, worrisome for tumor recurrence. Associated subtle left-to-right midline shift is present. Additional involvement of the left basal ganglia, genu/body of the corpus callosum, right caudate head, and medial aspect of the right thalamus was noted on axial FLAIR and postcontrast T1-weighted imaging (not shown), proven to be carcinoma. **B:** Subsequent positron emission tomography imaging reveals heterogeneous, mild to moderate increased activity at the corresponding site of the lesion within the left posterior frontal/parietal lobe, consistent with recurrent disease. **C:** Single-voxel magnetic resonance spectroscopy, performed on a selected region of interest within the lesion, demonstrates a markedly increased choline peak (left of spectrum) as well as a smaller lactate peak to the right of the choline peak, suggesting tumor recurrence. The expected peak for N-acetylaspartate (i.e., between the choline and lactate peaks) is markedly diminished. **D:** Perfusion imaging at the site of the left frontoparietal mass demonstrates a heterogeneous perfusion pattern, with sites of maximum perfusion (i.e., relative cerebral blood volume), depicted in red, along the medial and anterior aspects of the mass, suspicious for high-grade tumor recurrence. Histopathology revealed a pleomorphic xanthoastrocytoma with anaplastic features. (See Color Fig. 24.1-4*D* in the CD-ROM.)

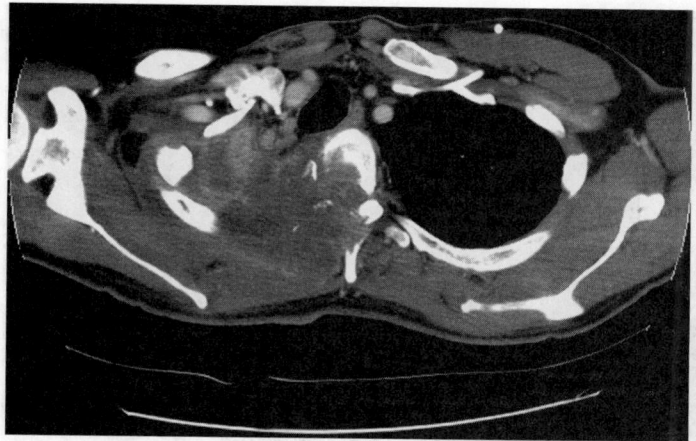
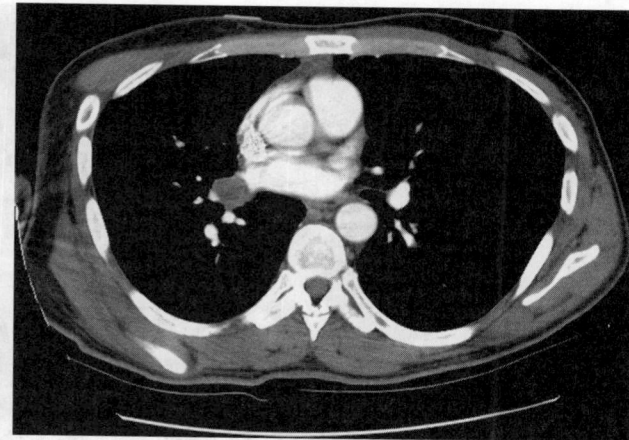

A

B

FIGURE 24.1-5. A 46-year-old man with lung cancer. Axial computed tomography (CT) image demonstrates a large right Pancoast tumor that invades the ribs and vertebrae and extends to paraspinal muscles posteriorly and spinal canal medially (**A**). Right hilar lymphadenopathy is also seen on a more caudal CT image (**B**).

with better 5-year survival rates. However, overall mortality was not improved by such screening.[38–40] Current research on lung cancer screening is focused on the use of low-dose CT,[40,41] but it is still too early to tell whether detecting tumors on CT that are smaller than those discovered on chest radiography will decrease mortality. To answer this question, large, randomized controlled trials with a follow-up of at least 10 years are needed. Besides, the biologic behavior of lung cancer is variable and the relationship between tumor size, survival, and stage at presentation is not clear-cut.[42] Another issue that remains to be analyzed is the burden of such mass screening on financial and human resources.

STAGING

Although chest radiography is used commonly in the detection of lung cancer, it is usually not sufficient for staging unless an obvious bone metastasis or bulky contralateral mediastinal lymphadenopathy is evident. CT is the most commonly used and cost-effective imaging modality in the evaluation of lung cancer. Newer multidetector CT systems allow the whole chest and abdomen to be scanned in a single breath hold and provide high-quality images (Fig. 24.1-5). However, there are discrepancies between preoperative staging with CT and operative findings in 35% to 45% of patients, primarily because of limitations in the detection of hilar (N1) or mediastinal (N2/N3) lymph node metastases and chest wall (T3) or mediastinal invasion (T4).[43,44] These are the critical stages of the disease that dictate the decision between surgical and nonsurgical management options. Yet CT is still widely used because it provides very important information that can, for example, guide mediastinoscopy and surgery.[45]

Due to its multiplanar imaging capability and better soft tissue resolution, MRI has advantages over CT in the evaluation of tumor invasion. MRI is superior to CT in the detection of mediastinal or chest wall invasion and in the evaluation of superior sulcus tumors with neurovascular invasion. For the evaluation of mediastinal lymphadenopathy, MRI and CT are equally sensitive.[46–48]

PET is not only sensitive and specific for the detection of malignant lung nodules, it is also very promising in the staging of lung cancer, especially if combined with CT. PET is significantly superior to CT in the detection of mediastinal nodal metastases. The negative predictive value of PET is as high as that of mediastinoscopy for mediastinal nodal disease, suggesting that a negative PET may obviate mediastinoscopy. PET is also very sensitive for bone and adrenal metastases, but it is not suitable for the detection of brain metastases due to the high glucose uptake of the normal brain. In the staging of lung cancer, PET, with its 83% accuracy, is superior to conventional imaging (chest CT, bone scintigraphy, and brain CT or MRI), which has an accuracy of 65%. Despite being a promising imaging tool, PET is expensive and not yet widely available.[49–51]

TREATMENT PLANNING

The imaging modalities discussed above play important roles in treatment planning for lung carcinoma. The first question to be answered by imaging is whether the primary tumor is resectable. Unless indicated by clinical signs or symptoms, it is unnecessary to search routinely for extrathoracic metastatic disease.

Adrenals are the most common metastatic site for lung cancer in the abdomen. Staging CT of the chest routinely includes CT of the upper abdomen to detect adrenal metastases, because this does not increase radiation dose significantly. The majority of adrenal masses in patients with lung cancer are benign. Adrenal adenomas are the most common adrenal tumors and often can be recognized on unenhanced CT by their low attenuation, which is due to their lipid content. New advances in chemical shift imaging with MRI and metabolic information obtained with PET may also allow distinction of adrenal adenomas from metastases. Both tests have a high rate of false-positives, necessitating the performance of biopsy for any suspicious adrenal mass.[52,53]

Routine imaging of liver, brain, and bones is not warranted, because the likelihood of metastatic disease is low in the absence of clinical suspicion. In patients with abnormal clinical

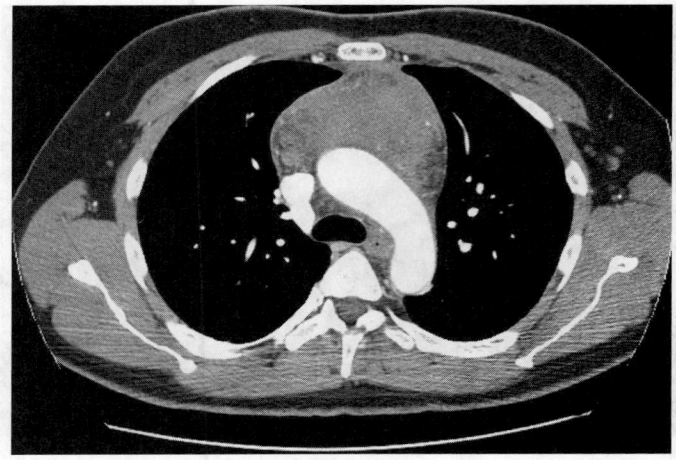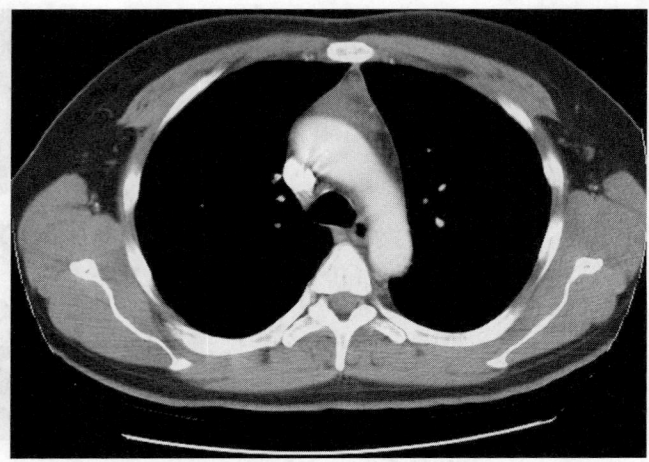

FIGURE 24.1-6. A 49-year-old man with lymphoma. Axial computed tomography (CT) image through the chest shows a large mediastinal lymphomatous mass (**A**). After treatment, CT reveals a significant decrease in the size of the previously seen lymphomatous mass in the mediastinum (**B**).

findings, further evaluation is indicated, because approximately 50% of these patients have metastatic disease. Dedicated imaging modalities can be used in these cases. Any abnormality seen on CT, MRI, bone scan, or PET must be carefully analyzed, because false-positives are common. In cases in which there is any doubt, biopsy should be performed to ensure accurate staging and treatment.[54]

TREATMENT FOLLOW-UP

Accurate imaging is essential for assessing the response to treatment and the recurrence of lung cancer. CT and MRI provide important anatomic information, and a sequential increase in the size of a lesion or a change in its morphology may suggest progression or recurrence. However, on CT and MRI, it can be difficult to differentiate recurrent disease from posttreatment changes. PET appears promising in this regard, because it provides metabolic information. It has been shown that PET is superior to CT in the assessment of treatment response.[55,56]

LYMPHOMA

Lymphoma is a common neoplasm, with non-Hodgkin's lymphomas more common than Hodgkin's disease. In this section, the role of imaging in the evaluation of patients with lymphoma is discussed.

STAGING

Lymphangiography can demonstrate abnormal lymph nodes in pelvic and paraaortic groups. However, it is not useful in the evaluation of celiac, portal, splenic hilar, and mesenteric chains. In the era of helical CT, the use of lymphangiography in lymphoma has nearly vanished.[57]

In lymphoma patients, CT is the modality used most often for initial staging and treatment follow-up (Fig. 24.1-6). CT is very efficient in the detection of involved lymph node groups in the chest, abdomen, and pelvis. In addition it can detect pul-

monary parenchymal involvement and the involvement of abdominal organs, such as the liver and spleen. However, in some cases splenic involvement may be inapparent at CT. CT evaluation of bone marrow is limited.

MRI is an effective alternative to CT in patients with lymphoma. It is as sensitive as CT in the detection of lymphadenopathy and the demonstration of focal organ lesions. However, MRI does not use ionizing radiation, and there is no need for intravenous contrast administration to differentiate lymph nodes from vessels. In addition, MRI is sensitive for detecting bone marrow involvement in lymphoma.[58,59] The use of iron oxide particles as a contrast agent in MRI of lymph nodes is a recent area of research. Unlike normal lymph nodes, lymph nodes containing tumor do not demonstrate uptake of iron oxide, and thus the use of iron oxide as a contrast agent increases the sensitivity of MRI in the detection of metastatic lymph nodes.[60]

PET is highly accurate in the staging of lymphoma. It detects more disease sites above and below the diaphragm than does gallium scintigraphy. Current imaging modalities use size criteria in the detection of involved lymph nodes. However, PET provides metabolic information that helps in the detection of small lymph nodes with lymphomatous involvement and in showing that some enlarged lymph nodes are reactive and are not involved by lymphoma.[61,62] PET detection of bone marrow involvement is limited by physiologic bone marrow uptake. Moreover, diffusely increased uptake in the bone marrow is not specific and is commonly seen in reactive bone marrow, particularly after chemotherapy and administration of marrow-stimulating drugs. In addition, in patients with limited involvement of the bone marrow, FDG-PET findings may be false-negative.[63]

TREATMENT PLANNING

Both types of lymphoma are potentially curable. Treatment options are based on the initial stage and grade of the disease, which are determined by noninvasive imaging modalities and invasive procedures such as node and bone marrow biopsy and, occasionally, laparotomy.

The remarkable cure rate in lymphoma patients is due to the improvement of combination chemotherapy and radiotherapy. However, it has been recognized that late side effects of treatment such as infertility and secondary malignancies are common among long-term survivors. Therapy must therefore be tailored to decrease complications and provide better quality of life. As a noninvasive staging tool, imaging provides crucial information in the initial management of lymphoma patients. Accurate evaluation of the extent of disease with imaging allows modification of radiation therapy ports and chemotherapy.

In the detection of disease below the diaphragm, imaging modalities may be falsely positive or negative in 25% to 33% of patients. Therefore, staging laparotomy (including splenectomy), biopsy of mesenteric and retroperitoneal lymph nodes, and core biopsy of the bone marrow and liver are indicated when therapeutic decisions may be substantially altered. Even in these cases, however, imaging is useful in providing a road map for areas to biopsy.

TREATMENT FOLLOW-UP

Imaging modalities are frequently used to monitor treatment response in lymphoma patients. After therapy, residual masses are seen in a significant number of patients. CT is effective in the detection of residual disease, with a sensitivity of 84%. However, the specificity of CT for residual disease is only 31%, because CT cannot distinguish residual lymphoma within treated lymph nodes that remain enlarged. PET is slightly more sensitive (88%) but significantly more specific (83%) than CT for the detection of residual disease.[64] Furthermore, PET can be used as a prognostic tool, because a positive PET scan after therapy is associated with a poorer survival rate than a negative PET scan after therapy.

BREAST CANCER

Although mammography remains the standard of care for breast cancer screening, recent improvements in MRI and other non-mammographic imaging techniques as well as percutaneous biopsy methods are revolutionizing the detection, diagnosis, staging, and posttreatment follow-up of breast cancer.

DETECTION AND DIAGNOSIS

The American Cancer Society[65] recommends that women begin monthly breast self-examination at age 20 years. From age 20 to 39 years, women should have a clinical breast examination by a health care professional every 3 years. Annual clinical breast examination and annual mammography should begin at age 40 years. Women with specific risk factors (e.g., personal or strong family history of breast cancer, prior atypia or lobular carcinoma *in situ*, or prior mantle irradiation for Hodgkin's disease) should consult their physicians about earlier screening and use of supplementary modalities such as sonography or MRI.

Mammography

Screening mammography reduces breast cancer mortality and may enable breast conservation rather than mastectomy.[65] The most common mammographic patterns of breast cancer are masses and calcifications. Most malignant masses are invasive; most malignant calcifications are ductal carcinoma *in situ*

(DCIS).[66] On mammogram reports, a final assessment category is assigned; the categories are defined by the American College of Radiology (ACR) Breast Imaging Reporting and Data System lexicon as follows: 0, needs additional imaging evaluation; 1, normal; 2, benign; 3, probably benign; 4, suspicious; 5, highly suggestive of malignancy; 6, proven malignancy.[67] Carcinoma is present in 23% to 34% of category 4 lesions and in 81% to 97% of category 5 lesions.[66]

Biopsy options for nonpalpable lesions include needle localization for surgical biopsy or percutaneous image-guided needle biopsy.[68] Percutaneous biopsy is faster, less invasive, and less expensive than surgery.[68] The likelihood of undergoing a single definitive operation instead of two or more surgeries is higher in women with cancers diagnosed percutaneously rather than by surgical biopsy.[68] In women with large areas of malignant calcifications attempting conservation, preoperative localization with bracketing wires facilitates complete excision of calcifications but does not ensure clear margins.[69]

Sonography

Breast sonography assists in distinguishing cystic from solid, characterizing solid masses, and guiding interventional procedures. A lexicon has been developed by the ACR to describe lesions detected by sonography.[67] Sonography may detect otherwise occult breast cancers, especially in dense breasts, but is not the standard of care for breast cancer screening.[70] Breast sonography is observer dependent, has limited sensitivity in detecting DCIS, and has false-positives. In prior reports, screening breast sonography led to biopsy in 2% to 4% of women; of these biopsies, carcinoma was found in 10% to 16%, of which 83% to 100% were invasive and 0% to 17% were DCIS.[70] The prevalence of cancer detected by screening breast sonography was approximately 3 per 1000. The ACR Imaging Network trial 6666 is evaluating screening sonography in high-risk women.[70]

Magnetic Resonance Imaging

Breast MRI is also being evaluated as a screening technique in high-risk women. Cancers are generally hypervascular and enhance with intravenous contrast (gadolinium).[71] Features defined by the breast MRI lexicon include type of enhancement (focus, mass, or nonmass), morphology, and kinetic pattern (time course of enhancement).[67] Work is ongoing to quantify the positive predictive value of specific MRI features.[72]

In women at high risk of developing breast cancer, MRI led to biopsy in 13% (range, 7% to 18%). Cancer was found by MRI in 33% (range, 24% to 88%) of women who had biopsy and in 4% (range, 2% to 7%) of high-risk women who had MRI screening (Fig. 24.1-7). Of MRI-detected cancers, histology was invasive in 67% (range, 43% to 100%) and DCIS in 33% (range, 0% to 57%).[73] MRI spectroscopy, which can detect the choline content of breast cancers, may improve specificity in diagnosis.[74]

Among nonpalpable, mammographically occult, MRI-detected lesions warranting biopsy, up to 77% cannot be identified with sonography and therefore require biopsy under MRI guidance.[75] Biopsy of MRI-detected lesions can be performed with MRI-guided needle localization[76] or with MRI-guided needle biopsy, using a fine-needle, core-needle, or vacuum-assisted probe.[75] Advantages of vacuum-assisted biopsy include speed, ability to acquire large volumes of tis-

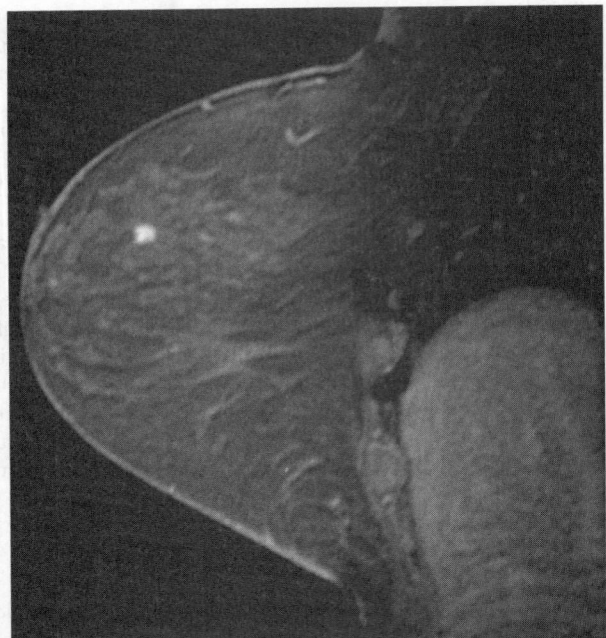

FIGURE 24.1-7. A 62-year-old asymptomatic woman with a family history of breast cancer in two first-degree relatives (daughter and sister) who had heterogeneously dense breasts without suspicious findings at mammography (not shown). T1-weighted, contrast-enhanced image from high-risk screening magnetic resonance imaging (MRI) examination shows a 0.7-cm irregularly shaped, irregularly marginated, heterogeneously enhancing mass in the right upper inner quadrant retroareolar region, not identified at mammography or sonography. MRI-guided vacuum-assisted biopsy yielded infiltrating ductal carcinoma, moderately differentiated. Subsequent lumpectomy showed a 0.5-cm infiltrating ductal carcinoma, histologic and nuclear grade 2, with negative sentinel lymph nodes.

sue, better characterization of lesions with atypia or DCIS, and ability to place a localizing clip.[75]

STAGING

Breast imaging is valuable in defining extent of local disease. In a woman with one proven site of cancer, the radiologist scrutinizes the mammogram for other sites of disease in the same quadrant (multifocal cancer), which may warrant wider excision, or in different quadrants (multicentric cancer), which may require mastectomy.[77] The radiologist also looks for mammographic evidence of disease in the axilla or contralateral breast. Sonography can identify additional ipsilateral disease, but observer dependence and low sensitivity in detecting DCIS limit sonography in this regard.[78]

MRI is sensitive in evaluating the ipsilateral and contralateral breast in women with breast cancer (Fig. 24.1-8). In women with one proven site of cancer, breast MRI detects an additional site of ipsilateral cancer in 6% to 34%[77] and contralateral cancer in 3% to 24%[79] and is particularly useful in women with infiltrating lobular carcinoma.[77] MRI identifies the primary tumor in 70% to 75% of women presenting with occult breast carcinoma metastatic to the axilla.[80]

Nuclear medicine techniques are useful in breast cancer staging. PET scanning can identify nodal and distant metastases and may assist in monitoring treatment response.[81] Lymphoscintigraphy can identify sentinel lymph nodes (the first nodes draining the tumor) for breast cancer surgery.[82] Sentinel node biopsy has

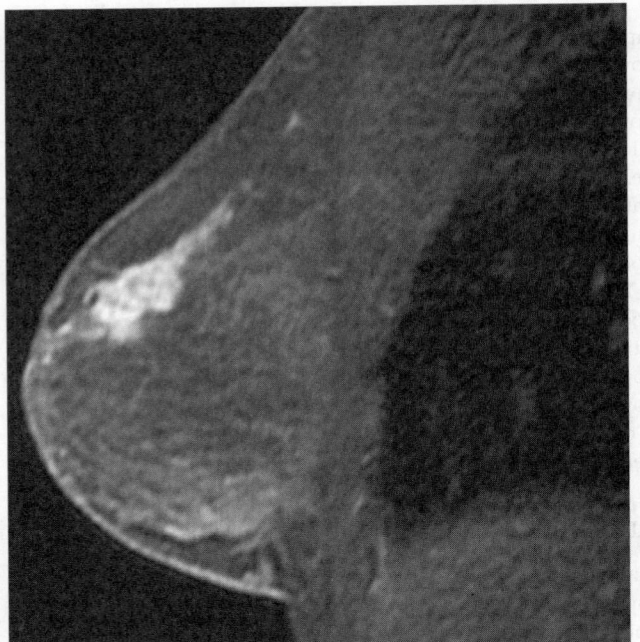

A

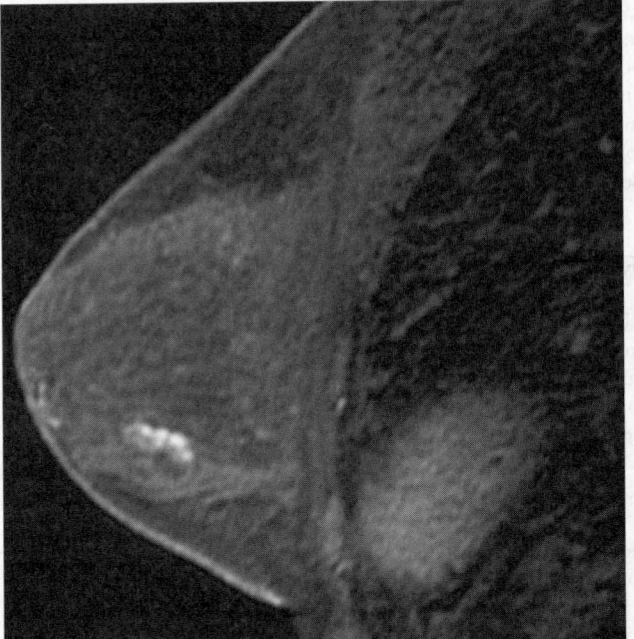

B

FIGURE 24.1-8. A 38-year-old woman with a strong family history of breast cancer and dense breasts on mammography (not shown), who had a palpable lump in the right breast upper outer quadrant for which needle core biopsy under the guidance of palpation yielded infiltrating ductal carcinoma. **A:** T1-weighted, contrast-enhanced magnetic resonance imaging (MRI) of the right breast shows lobulated, irregularly marginated, heterogeneously enhancing 2.5-cm mass in the right breast upper outer quadrant, corresponding to the palpable biopsy-proven cancer. Additional clumped ductal enhancement is noted posterior to the mass, spanning at least 2 cm. The patient chose to undergo mastectomy, revealing infiltrating ductal carcinoma, 2.6 cm, and extensive ductal carcinoma *in situ* (DCIS). **B:** T1-weighted, contrast-enhanced MRI of the left (contralateral) breast shows clumped ductal enhancement spanning more than 2 cm. MRI-guided vacuum-assisted biopsy yielded DCIS, solid and cribriform types, intermediate nuclear grade. Residual DCIS was found adjacent to the biopsy site at mastectomy.

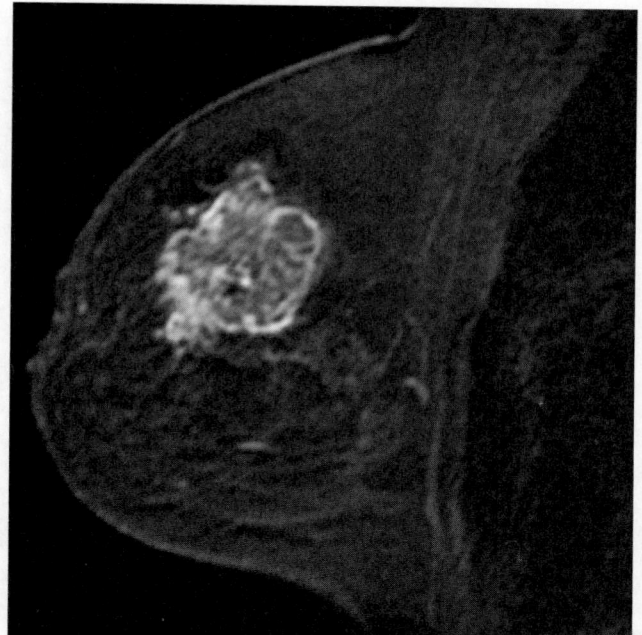

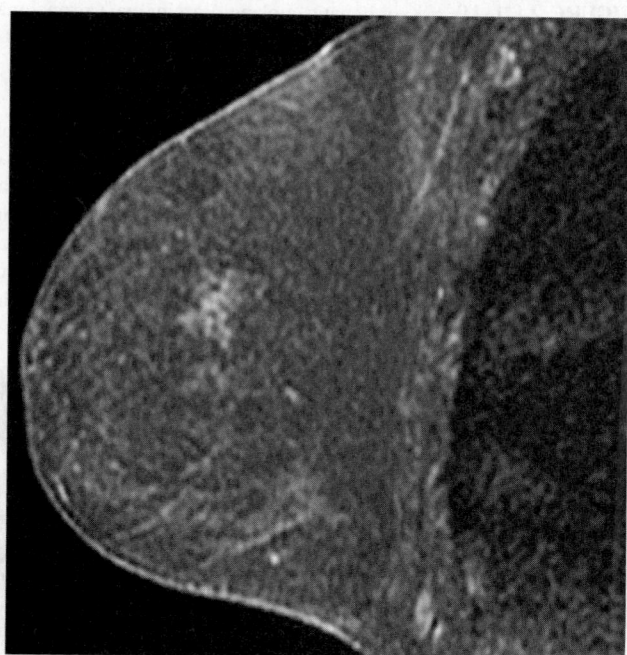

FIGURE 24.1-9. A 39-year-old woman who presented with a large palpable lump in the left breast upper outer quadrant for which core-needle biopsy yielded infiltrating ductal carcinoma, poorly differentiated. **A:** T1-weighted, contrast-enhanced magnetic resonance imaging (MRI) of the left breast before treatment shows a large irregularly shaped, irregularly marginated, heterogeneous, and rim-enhancing mass spanning greater than 4.4 cm in the left breast upper outer quadrant, corresponding to the palpable cancer. **B:** T1-weighted, contrast-enhanced MRI of the left breast performed 7 weeks later, after completion of chemotherapy, shows almost complete resolution of enhancement. Subsequent mastectomy yielded a localized area with prominent fibroinflammatory changes and foamy histiocytes, consistent with tumor treatment response. A few scattered atypical cells were present, but no definite residual tumor was identified.

become the standard of care for primary lesions less than 5 cm in size. It has a technical success rate of 88%, sensitivity of 93%, and accuracy of 97%; accuracy is highest when radioisotope and blue dye are used together.[82] Lymphoscintigraphy is reproducible, shows lymphatic drainage pathways, and predicts technical success of sentinel node biopsy.[82]

A variety of techniques have been used for sentinel lymph node mapping. At the authors' institution, unfiltered ^{99m}Tc sulfur colloid is injected intradermally adjacent to the tumor site in the breast, and intraoperative monitoring is performed with a radioactivity probe to identify the sentinel node, usually 4 to 24 hours after injection. The surgeon also injects blue dye into the parenchyma of the breast, adjacent to the tumor site in the operating room before surgery and then performs biopsy of the sentinel nodes. If no tumor is present in the sentinel nodes and if intraoperative physical examination of the axilla is negative, then no additional lymph nodes are removed; if tumor is present in sentinel nodes, completion axillary dissection is often performed. In this way, patients with negative sentinal nodes are spared additional axillary surgery. More recently, a nomogram has been developed that defines a low-risk subgroup of patients with positive sentinel nodes who may not require a complete axillary dissection.[83]

TREATMENT FOLLOW-UP

Mammography is the standard of care for follow-up after breast cancer treatment.[84] After excision of malignant calcifications, postoperative mammography is necessary to assess for residual calcifications that may require needle localization and excision before radiation therapy. In long-term follow-up after breast conservation, mammography can detect nonpalpable ipsilateral or contralateral breast cancers.[84]

MRI complements mammography in posttreatment follow-up. In women with locally advanced breast cancer treated with preoperative chemotherapy, MRI may assess treatment response more accurately than mammography or physical examination (Fig. 24.1-9).[71] MRI may help assess for residual disease after lumpectomy.[71] In long-term follow-up after breast conservation, MRI may detect local recurrences, particularly more than 18 months after surgery, when postoperative enhancement has generally resolved.[71]

BREAST MAGNETIC RESONANCE IMAGING: CAVEATS

Although MRI is emerging as a valuable adjunct to mammography, several caveats should be remembered. MRI is less specific than it is sensitive; it is also expensive and requires intravenous contrast. Some women may not be able to have breast MRI due to limited access to facilities or factors such as pacemakers or claustrophobia. Breast MRI requires the capacity to perform MRI-guided biopsy. Finally, the impact of breast MRI on mortality has not yet been determined.

CONCLUSION

Mammography is the only imaging study shown to reduce breast cancer mortality. Sonography, a valuable adjunct to mammography in distinguishing cystic from solid, characterizing solid masses, and guiding interventional procedures, is being studied as a tool to screen high-risk women. Breast MRI complements mammography in the evaluation of women with known or suspected breast cancer. Percutaneous biopsy enables preoperative diagnosis of breast cancer, streamlining subsequent therapy. PET and lymphoscintigraphy are useful in breast cancer staging. Further work is needed to establish evidence-based guidelines for use of non-mammographic imaging in high-risk screening, extent of disease assessment, and follow-up after treatment of breast cancer.

HEPATOBILIARY CANCER

In the past few years, advances in imaging have provided hepatobiliary clinicians with a number of new or enhanced diagnostic imaging strategies to assess focal and diffuse liver disease. The initial approach to evaluation of the liver, despite all the improved imaging modalities, still consists of a complete history, physical examination, and laboratory assessment of the liver. One of the most common indications for imaging evaluation of the liver is the need for detection and characterization of a liver mass. Two of the main roles of imaging are to detect clinically significant disease within the liver and to characterize focal hepatic masses as benign or malignant.

The detection of focal hepatic lesions is of critical importance. A number of imaging modalities can be used, but multidetector CT is being chosen increasingly often. Multidetector CT of the liver can be performed in a multiphase fashion, such as during the early arterial, late arterial or portal venous, and equilibrium phases of imaging.[85] The detection rates achieved with various modalities depend not only on the precise equipment used but on the radiologist's clinical experience and the precise scanning techniques used. CT has demonstrated an overall detection rate of between 80% and 90%.[86] Multidetector CT also allows for accurate preoperative mapping of hepatic arterial, portal venous, and hepatic venous anatomy. Traditionally, catheter-based angiography has been used for this evaluation, but CT angiography has become an effective noninvasive alternative. The goal for imaging is to provide a vascular map of the liver and to identify the position of tumors relative to the major vascular structures. Additionally, it is important to identify arterial and venous variant anatomy so that an appropriate surgical approach can be undertaken. Another alternative therapy, intraarterial chemotherapy, also relies on accurate mapping of hepatic anatomy.[87]

Another major goal of hepatic imaging is in the accurate characterization of hepatic masses. Masses can be characterized as benign or malignant, and further attempts can be made to characterize them based on possible pathologic entities. Common benign liver tumors that are well characterized at CT or MRI include hepatic cysts, hemangioma, hepatocellular adenoma, and focal nodular hyperplasia. Because of the ability to show various patterns of lesion enhancement after administration of contrast media, contrast-enhanced MRI is generally preferred for focal hepatic lesion characterization.

Evaluation of the bile ducts is frequently performed in patients who present with jaundice. Possible causes of jaundice include choledocholithiasis, cholangiocarcinoma, pancreatic carcinoma, duodenal or ampullary carcinoma, or metastatic disease to the liver or bile ducts. US is generally the preferred initial diagnostic test to evaluate for obstruction. Subsequently, MR cholangiopancreatography is often performed to further evaluate the level and cause of obstruction. Endoscopic retrograde cholangiopancreatography and transhepatic cholangiography can also be performed but are increasingly being reserved for therapeutic purposes because of their invasive nature and associated potential

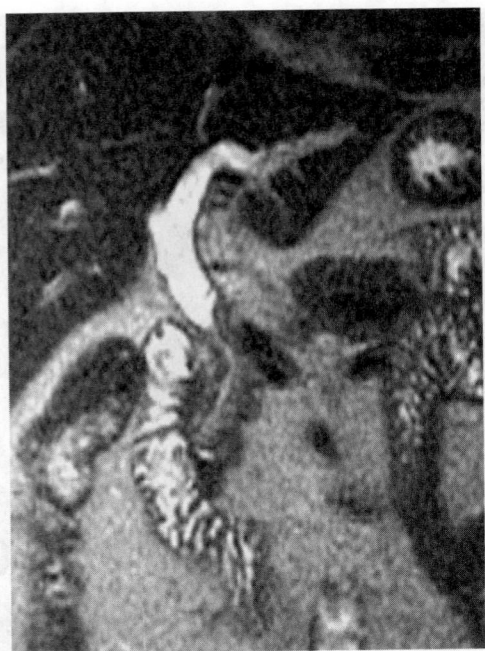

FIGURE 24.1-10. Extrahepatic cholangiocarcinoma. Coronal magnetic resonance cholangiogram demonstrating concentric narrowing of the distal common bile duct with proximal biliary dilatation.

complications. Magnetic resonance cholangiopancreatography (MRCP) uses special MRI sequences to visualize fluid in the biliary and pancreatic ducts. MRCP is of proven use in a variety of biliary and pancreatic diseases, including choledocholithiasis, congenital anatomic variants (such as pancreas divisum), chronic pancreatitis, postcholecystectomy disorders, and neoplastic duct obstruction (Figs. 24.1-10 and 24.1-11).[88–90] MRCP is an evolving

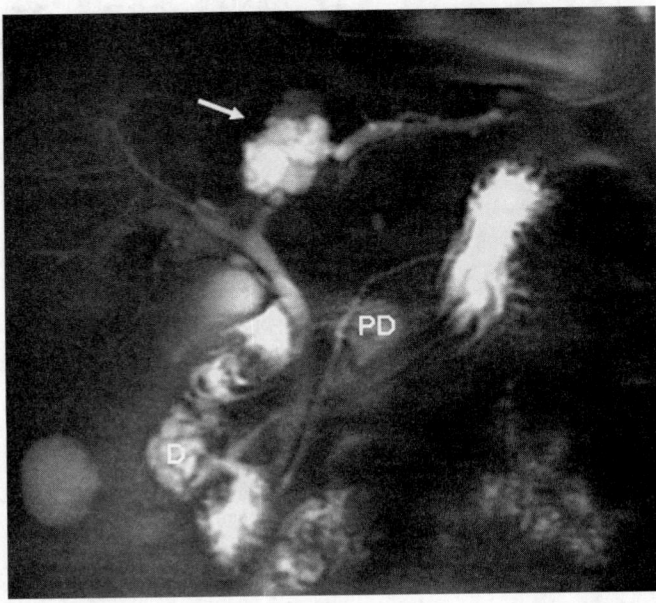

FIGURE 24.1-11. Biliary cystadenoma. T2-weighted, fat-suppressed magnetic resonance imaging scan demonstrating a lobulated mass (*arrow*) in the left lobe of the liver with continuity with the left bile duct. Note also the pancreatic duct (PD) and duodenum (D).

technique but is clinically useful and of comparable accuracy to conventional cholangiography. With further progress, it is likely that MRCP will replace diagnostic endoscopic retrograde cholangiopancreatography as the modality of choice for imaging the biliary and pancreatic ducts.[91]

With increasing acceptance of hepatic resection as a viable treatment option (especially for hepatic colorectal metastasis), the importance of accurate hepatic imaging is critical. Defining the anatomy of the liver in terms of segmental region localization using the Couinaud nomenclature is important. Within this system, the liver is anatomically divided by vertical and horizontal planes along the three main hepatic veins and the transverse plane along the right and left portal veins, resulting in eight segments. The segmental anatomy provides boundaries for potential hepatic resection.

COLORECTAL CANCER

Colorectal cancer is the most common gastrointestinal cancer and the second most common cause of cancer death. This section provides a brief overview of the role of imaging in the evaluation of colorectal cancer.

SCREENING

The screening and removal of the adenomas (which are the precursors of most colorectal cancers) should result in a decrease in the incidence of, and in the mortality from, colorectal cancer. Common screening modalities include fecal occult blood testing, flexible sigmoidoscopy, barium enema radiography, and colonoscopy. However, none of these methods is optimal in terms of performance, safety, and patient acceptance. Currently, there is interest in CT colonography as a noninvasive and accurate tool for colorectal cancer screening. This technique is basically a CT

examination of the fully prepared and air-distended colon. Volumetric CT data in the entire colon are acquired in only a few seconds or minutes of scanning, during approximately 15 minutes or less of total examination time. By examining these data with advanced imaging software, 2D and 3D images can be generated to evaluate the colon as well as the extracolonic tissues.

CT colonography has a reported sensitivity of 90% for polyps greater than 10 mm.[92] It has some advantages over barium enema radiography, such as better detection of polyps, the ability to evaluate extracolonic tissues, and better toleration by patients. In comparison with colonoscopy, CT colonography has the advantages of depicting colonic anatomy from an endoluminal perspective and in multiple cross sections (Fig. 24.1-12). Blind spots are eliminated, and the entire colon is almost always evaluated. The characterization of many filling defects is possible, without the risks associated with sedation and biopsy. A major disadvantage of CT colonography compared with colonoscopy is that a tissue sample cannot be obtained.

MR colonography is another new technique that, unlike CT colonography, uses no ionizing radiation and allows for direct imaging of the colon in multiple planes. Potential disadvantages of this technique, however, are its higher cost and the gadolinium-based enema that must be retained during the imaging procedure.[93] MR colonography is still under investigation and is not yet routinely available.

STAGING AND TREATMENT PLANNING

Most patients with colon cancer undergo surgery either for cure or palliation, with radiation treatment and chemotherapy as adjunctive therapeutic options. Treatment decisions are mainly based on the stage of the disease at the time of diagnosis.

CT, MRI, and/or transrectal US (TRUS) are commonly used in the initial staging of colorectal cancer. All of these modalities have

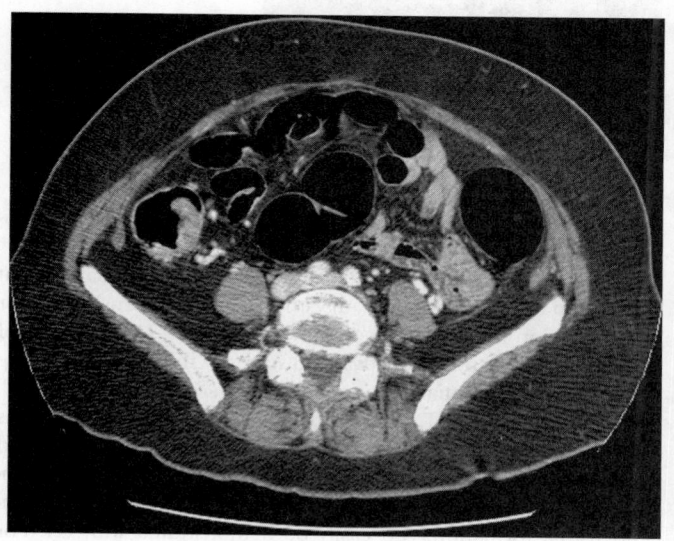

A

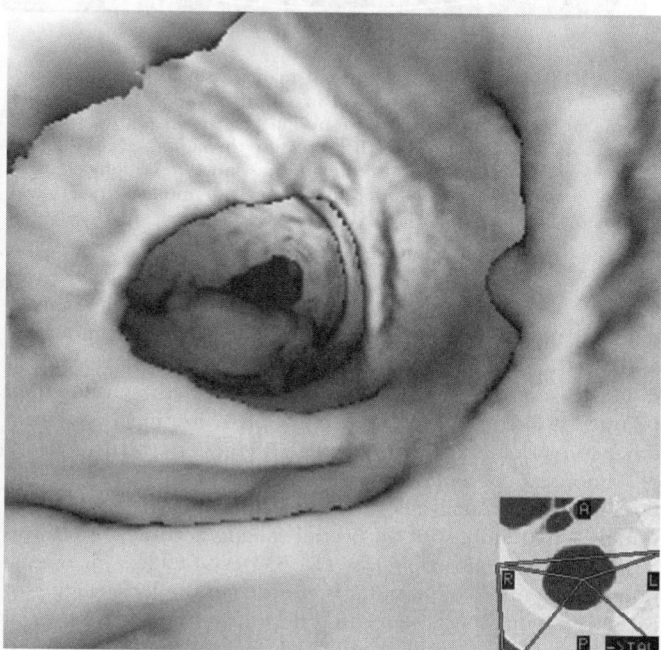

B

FIGURE 24.1-12. A 71-year-old woman with colon cancer. A mass is seen in the ascending colon on axial computed tomography image **(A)** and virtual colonoscopic image at the corresponding level **(B)**.

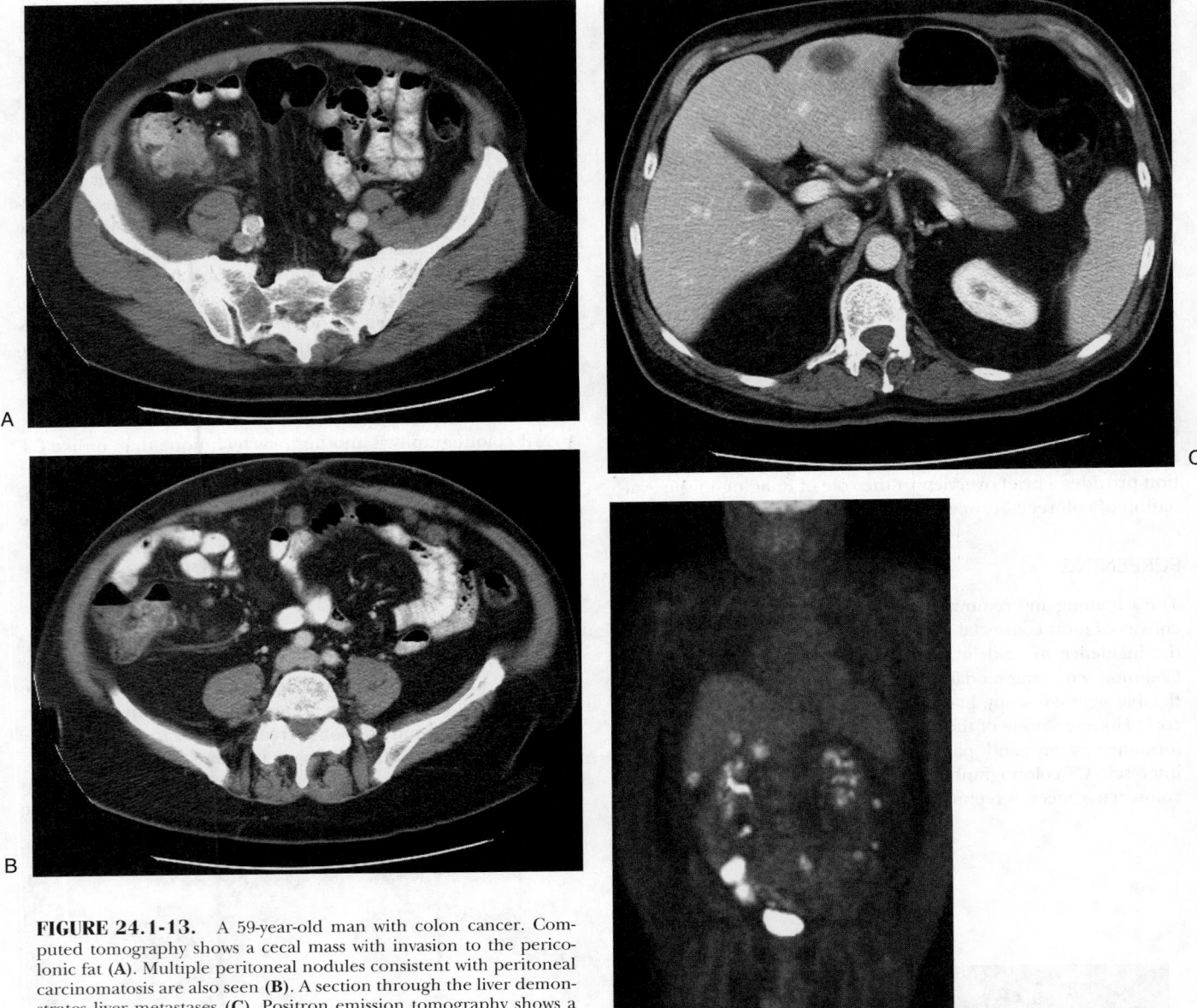

FIGURE 24.1-13. A 59-year-old man with colon cancer. Computed tomography shows a cecal mass with invasion to the pericolonic fat (**A**). Multiple peritoneal nodules consistent with peritoneal carcinomatosis are also seen (**B**). A section through the liver demonstrates liver metastases (**C**). Positron emission tomography shows a cecal mass in the right lower quadrant, with multiple peritoneal implants and liver metastases (**D**).

limitations, with most staging errors resulting from an inability to differentiate tumor from peritumoral edema and desmoplastic reaction. Imaging plays a very important role in the detection of distant metastases, particularly in the liver. US is less sensitive than CT and MRI in this regard. Differentiation of liver metastases from other commonly encountered benign liver lesions is crucial.

Endorectal or endoscopic US can show the layers of the bowel wall and usually allows for determination of the depth of tumor penetration, with an overall staging accuracy of 80% to 85%.[94] Unlike endoscopic US, TRUS does not allow for evaluation of the entire colon, but it is effective in the local staging of rectal carcinoma because it can differentiate the layers of rectal wall. The reported accuracy of TRUS for determining the local stage of rectal cancer is between 83% and 94%.[95,96] However, the accuracy of TRUS decreases in patients with advanced, large can-

cers and remote lymph node metastases, because penetration by US waves is limited. Therefore, TRUS is more useful for superficial rectal cancers.

Helical CT scans obtained during the mural enhancement phase can depict tumor and adjacent spread, with sensitivities for local invasion ranging between 50% and 70%.[94] The accuracy of staging by CT increases in advanced stages of the disease, because CT cannot differentiate the individual layers of the bowel wall. The specificity of CT for detecting lymph node metastasis is approximately 50%. However, CT has a very high sensitivity and specificity for the detection of liver metastases. In addition, complications of colorectal cancer, such as perforation, obstruction, and fistula formation, can easily be demonstrated with CT. For these reasons, CT is very commonly used in the initial evaluation of colorectal cancer (Fig. 24.1-13).[97]

MRI offers advantages over CT in the local staging of colorectal cancer because of its better soft tissue resolution. The reported accuracy of this method for local staging of colorectal cancer ranges from 71% to 91%.[95,98] Especially with the use of endorectal coils, individual layers of rectal wall can be differentiated, thus improving local staging. MRI is also better than CT in the evaluation of invasion of adjacent organs and pelvic musculature. For nodal involvement, the sensitivity and specificity of MRI are similar to those of CT. MRI can be safely used in patients in whom the use of iodinated contrast material is contraindicated. In addition, although CT is sufficient to characterize most liver lesions, MRI is superior to CT in this regard and can be used in indeterminate cases.

No reliable imaging criteria are available for the detection of metastatic lymph nodes. Size (short axis diameter greater than 1 cm) remains the primary criterion for predicting nodal metastasis using any cross-sectional modality, although it is well known that benign nodes may be enlarged and that subcentimeter nodes may contain metastatic disease.

TREATMENT FOLLOW-UP

Posttreatment follow-up in colorectal cancer includes laboratory, endoscopic, and imaging surveillance. Imaging may show locally recurrent tumor or distant metastases. CT and MRI are commonly used for posttreatment assessments of the patients. Both modalities are limited in differentiating recurrent tumor from scarring in the operative bed. Immunoscintigraphy and PET have shown promise in distinguishing recurrence from scar, and they can demonstrate distant metastases as well. If the recurrent tumor is detected and surgery is contemplated, the imaging modality of choice is MRI due to its superior soft tissue resolution and multiplanar capabilities.[99]

GYNECOLOGIC CANCER

Imaging plays an important role in tumor detection, characterization, staging, treatment planning, and follow-up for gynecologic cancer. The pretreatment evaluation of uterine (endometrial and cervical) and ovarian cancer has traditionally consisted of clinical evaluation, laboratory tests, and conventional radiographic studies (e.g., barium enema, intravenous pyelography, etc.). Advances in cross-sectional imaging by US, CT, MRI, and PET have expanded the role of imaging, making it a necessary component of clinical assessment. The choice of imaging modality is not only cancer site specific but depends on local gynecologic practice, radiologic expertise, and equipment availability. It should be tailored to answer specific clinical questions relevant to the individual patient.

ENDOMETRIAL CANCER

In the staging workup of endometrial cancer, imaging studies are requested only after a histologic diagnosis has been established. The main role of imaging in the evaluation of endometrial cancer is the assessment of the three main morphologic prognostic factors: the depth of myometrial invasion, endocervical tumor extension, and lymph node status.

STAGING

Transabdominal US is not recommended in the staging of endometrial cancer. Reports on the use of transvaginal US in the evaluation of myometrial invasion have shown promise, with accuracy rates varying between 68% and 99%.[100] However, the disparity in the range of reported accuracy limits its widespread use.[101] Furthermore, transvaginal US is inadequate for the assessment of cervical extension, lymph node status, or overall staging. Soft tissue contrast resolution of US is not sufficient to differentiate the tumor from the normal myometrium, cervical stroma, or coexisting benign pathology (e.g., uterine leiomyoma). Assessment of a large tumor is usually not permitted by the small field of view of transvaginal US.

CT, including multidetector CT, can also be used in the evaluation of endometrial carcinoma to assess the extent of disease and lymph node status. Helical CT has a sensitivity of 83% and a specificity of 42% for the detection of deep myometrial invasion and a sensitivity of 25% and a specificity of 70% for the detection of cervical invasion.[102] The main disadvantage of CT is its limitation in the assessment of cervical extension and overall staging. The performance of CT in the assessment of lymph node status is similar to that of MRI; both modalities suffer from the inability to differentiate enlarged metastatic from hyperplastic nodes and the inability to detect metastasis in normal-sized nodes.[103]

MRI is the most accurate and consistent imaging modality in the pretreatment evaluation of patients with endometrial cancer.[104] A comparison study showed that the accuracy of MRI in the detection of myometrial invasion is 89%, significantly higher than the accuracy of transvaginal US (69%) or CT (61%).[105] Contrast enhancement is essential in the evaluation of myometrial invasion, because the accuracy of dynamic contrast-enhanced MRI is significantly superior (91%) compared with that of T2-weighted images only (77%) (Fig. 24.1-14).[106] Cervical invasion is also better evaluated by MRI compared with US and CT. A study with metaanalysis showed that MRI has a sensitivity of 86% (range, 66% to 100%) and a specificity of 97% (range, 92% to 100%).[107] MRI and CT have similar accuracies for the evaluation of lymph node metastasis, and both modalities rely on size criteria.

TREATMENT FOLLOW-UP

Routine use of imaging is not recommended, because no difference in survival was seen when subclinical recurrence was found by CT.[103] However, when clinically warranted, imaging is an important adjunct in the assessment of endometrial cancer recurrence and its resectability. The choice of imaging modality depends on individual patient and clinical questions. CT is usually the first imaging modality. MRI is often a problem-solving imaging modality in cases with equivocal CT findings. The usefulness of PET in the follow-up of endometrial cancer is under investigation and has promising reported accuracy. In detecting recurrent lesions and evaluating treatment responses, FDG-PET, with the help of anatomic information from CT/MRI, showed better diagnostic ability (sensitivity, 100%; specificity, 88.2%; accuracy, 93.3%) compared with combined conventional imaging (sensitivity, 84.6%; specificity, 85.7%; accuracy, 85.0%) and tumor markers (sensitivity, 100%; specificity,

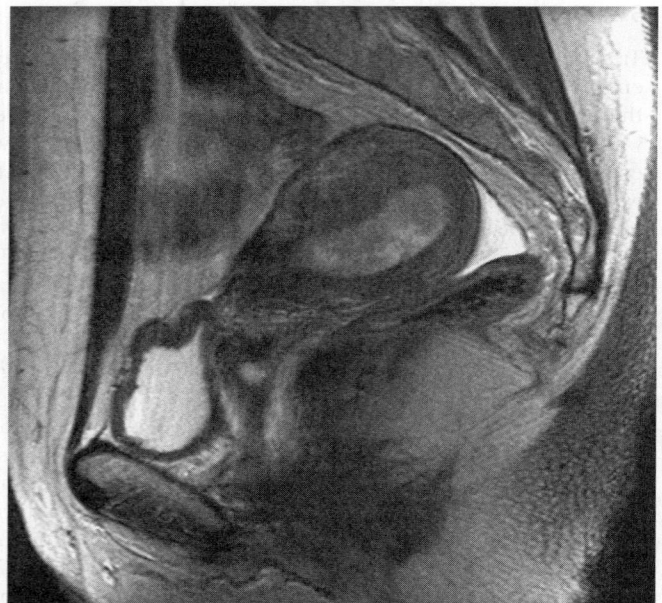

A

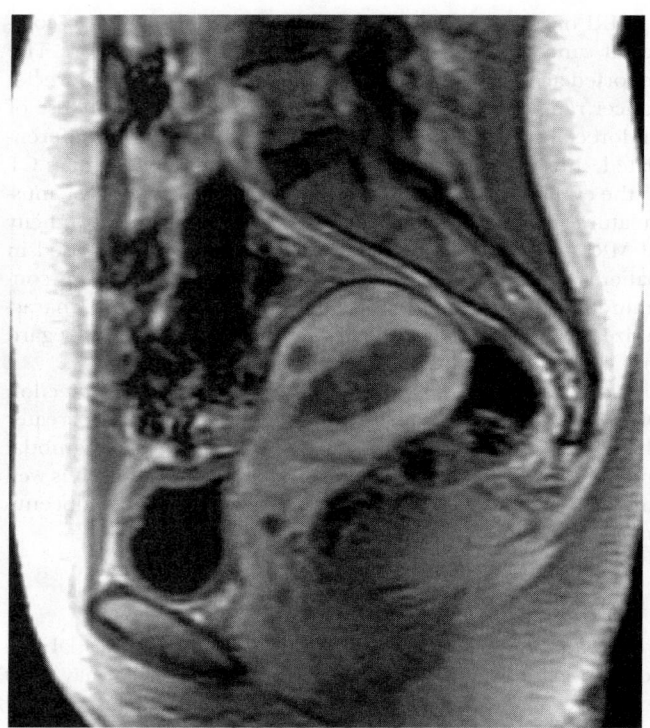

B

FIGURE 24.1-14. A 45-year-old woman with endometrial cancer. Sagittal T2-weighted **(A)** and postcontrast T1-weighted **(B)** magnetic resonance images demonstrate an endometrial mass with minimal myometrial invasion anteriorly.

70.6%; accuracy, 83.3%).[108] Furthermore, negative PET results correlate well with disease-free outcomes.

CERVICAL CANCER

The conventional imaging studies (chest x-ray, barium enema, intravenous urogram) recommended for clinical International Federation of Gynecology and Obstetrics (FIGO) staging are less commonly used in the current evaluation of cervical cancer. CT, MRI, and PET/CT are becoming the main imaging modalities in patients with cervical cancer.

STAGING

Staging of cervical cancer is based on clinical FIGO criteria. When compared to surgical staging, FIGO clinical staging results in errors in 17% to 32% of cases of stage IB disease and in 65% to 90% of cases of stage III to IV disease.[108] The greatest difficulties in the clinical evaluation of patients with cervical cancer are the assessment of parametrial and pelvic sidewall invasion; the estimation of tumor size, especially if the tumor is primarily endocervical in location; and the evaluation of lymph node and distant metastases. Nevertheless, tumor size, parametrial invasion, and lymph node status are all critical prognostic factors in staging and treatment planning.[110]

The most important issue in the staging of cervical cancer is to distinguish early disease (stages IA and IB) that can be treated with surgery from advanced disease that must be treated with radiation, alone or combined with chemotherapy. Imaging modalities are directed to solve this clinically important question.[109]

Although US can be used to reveal hydronephrosis, neither transabdominal nor endovaginal US is recommended for the staging of cervical cancer due to their poor soft tissue resolution.

CT can be used effectively for suspected advanced disease, mostly for the evaluation of lymph node metastasis. MRI is superior to CT and to clinical evaluation in the assessment of cervical cancer prognostic factors, including tumor size,[111,112] parametrial invasion (for which MR accuracy ranges from 77% to 96%),[113–115] and overall staging (90% for MRI compared with 65% for CT); MRI is also slightly more accurate than CT in the detection of lymph node metastases (88% to 89% for MRI vs. 83% to 85% for CT) (Fig. 24.1-15).[116,117] Although PET is more commonly used for the evaluation of recurrent disease, it can also be used in the initial staging of cervical cancer, mainly for the assessment of lymph node metastases. In detection of lymph node metastases in cervical cancer, the reported value of PET is greater than that of either CT or MRI (PET sensitivity and specificity of 100%/83% vs. MRI sensitivity and specificity of 96%/73%).[118]

TREATMENT FOLLOW-UP

CT and MRI play an important role in the assessment of recurrent cancer resectability. CT is widely available; however, MRI provides better assessment of local extent of recurrent tumor. For the evaluation of distant recurrences, CT is preferred. It is critical to distinguish postradiation changes from recurrent tumor. CT remains limited in this regard. MRI, especially with dynamic contrast enhancement, is more accurate in the detection of recurrent disease. Compared with T2-weighted images, dynamic MR imaging increases accuracy, from 64% to 74%, to 82% to 83% and increases specificity, from 22% to 38%, to 67%.[119–121] However, early postradiation change remains a problem. PET is helpful to increase the specificity and sensitivity of detection of recurrent disease and may obviate unnecessary biopsies or surgical interventions. In detecting recurrent cervical cancer, the sensitivity, specificity, and accuracy of PET were reported to be 100%, 94.4%, and 97.2%, respectively.[122]

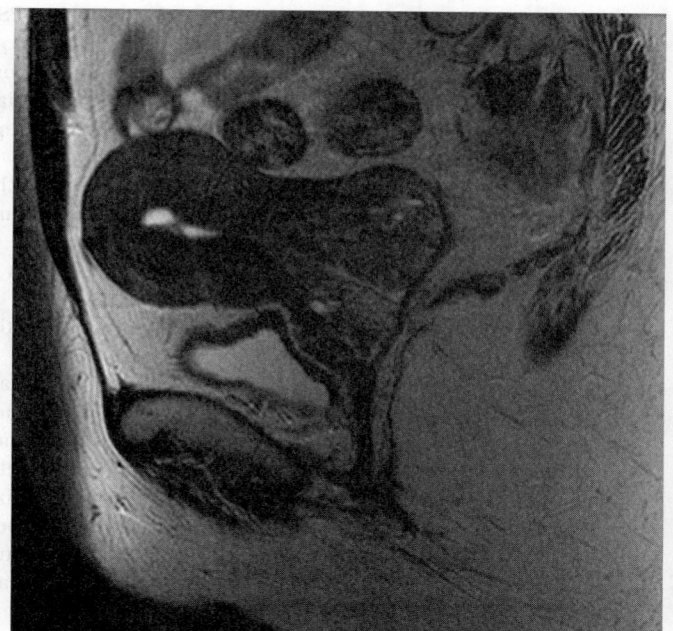
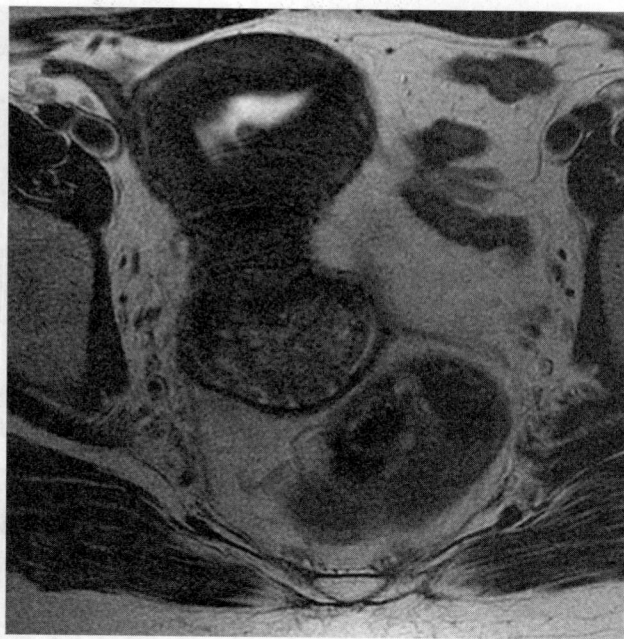

FIGURE 24.1-15. A 44-year-old woman with cervical cancer. Sagittal (**A**) and axial (**B**) T2-weighted magnetic resonance images show a bulky cervical mass bulging into the vagina. Invasion to the anterior vaginal wall is present, but the posterior vaginal wall is intact (**A**). Full-thickness cervical stromal invasion is seen, but no parametrial extension (**B**).

OVARIAN CANCER

Imaging plays several important roles in the management of patients with adnexal masses, including lesion detection, characterization of the primary tumor, staging, and detection of recurrence. In each category are a number of clinical challenges for which imaging information can be used as an adjunct to clinical and laboratory evaluation. Lesion characterization (benign vs. malignant) is important for treatment planning and subspecialty referral. Evaluation of extent of primary or recurrent ovarian cancer has a substantial impact on the modification of treatment, which may include surgery, neoadjuvant chemotherapy, or primary chemotherapy.

LESION CHARACTERIZATION

US is very effective in showing tumor location (e.g., differentiation of uterine from adnexal masses), as well as in distinguishing between a benign and malignant adnexal lesion. Analysis of morphologic findings on US combined with Doppler findings allows better lesion characterization.[123,124] When US is inconclusive, CT or MRI can be used to obtain additional information. The accuracy of MRI for diagnosing the malignancy of an adnexal mass is 93% and is superior to that of US or CT.[125,126]

STAGING

Ovarian cancer is staged surgically in accordance with the recommendations of FIGO. However, preoperative imaging has an important role to play and, in depicting the extent of disease, helps determine the sites at which biopsy will be performed at surgery. Furthermore, imaging can facilitate subspecialty referral and treatment planning.

Chest x-ray is no longer used routinely to demonstrate pulmonary metastases and pleural effusions. The use of excretory urography and barium enema has declined as a result of the increasing use of cross-sectional imaging, such as US, CT, and MRI.

Overall staging accuracy for CT and MRI is similar (77% vs. 78%, respectively).[127] A comparison study showed that MRI and CT were more accurate than US in the detection of peritoneal disease, especially in the subdiaphragmatic spaces and hepatic surfaces (Fig. 24.1-16).[128] For the detection of peritoneal disease, the sensitivity and specificity of US, CT, and MRI were 69%/93%, 92%/82%, and 95%/80%, respectively.[128] However, implants measuring 1 cm or less in diameter remain difficult to detect. In the evaluation of nodal disease, the sensitivity and specificity of US, CT, and MRI were 32%/93%, 43%/89%, and 38%/84%, respectively.[128] In the evaluation of liver metastases, the sensitivity and specificity of US, CT, and MRI were 57%/98%, 40%/96%, and 40%/96%, respectively.[128]

TREATMENT FOLLOW-UP

Imaging is recommended only when CA 125 is elevated or when there are new clinical symptoms (e.g., to rule out bowel obstruction). CT is the primary imaging modality. It accurately demonstrates macroscopic disease recurrence and can spare these patients from invasive restaging, second-look laparotomy. MRI can provide additional information in patients with questionable CT findings.[129] PET/CT is also promising in detecting recurrent disease, with a sensitivity of 83.3% in patients with clinically suspected recurrence but with negative or equivocal CT findings.[130]

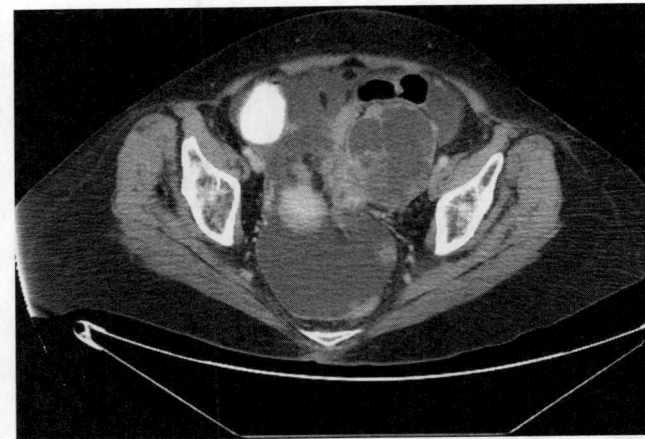

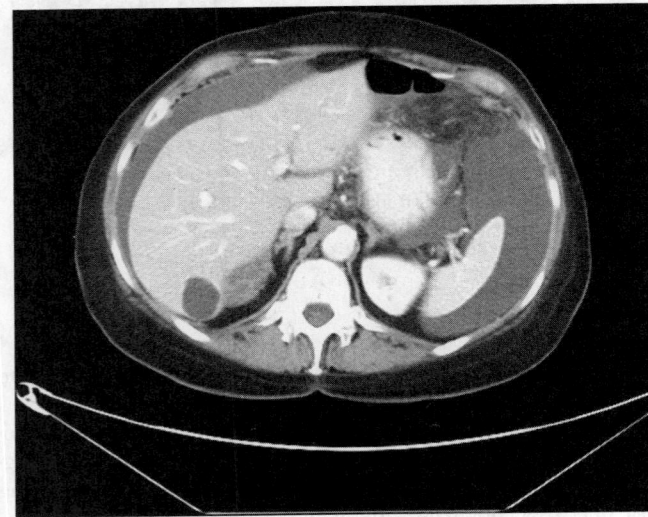

FIGURE 24.1-16. A 76-year-old woman with ovarian cancer. Axial computed tomography (CT) image through the pelvis shows a large cystic mass with solid nodular components in the left adnexa **(A)**. Ascites and peritoneal nodules are also seen **(A)**. CT image through the liver demonstrates a capsular implant in the posterior right lobe **(B)**. An incidental simple cyst is also seen adjacent to the capsular implant **(B)**.

In recurrent ovarian cancer, treatment choice depends on tumor bulk and extent and includes chemotherapy, surgical debulking, or palliative and supportive care. In this patient group, benefit from surgery is possible only when cytoreduction is optimal. Therefore, pretreatment identification of unresectable recurrent cancer is clinically relevant, assisting in patient management and outcome.

PROSTATE CANCER

Digital rectal examination and serum PSA level are very effective means for detecting prostate cancer. Definitive diagnosis is made by histopathologic examination of biopsy specimens obtained from the prostate in patients with clinical suspicion. Imaging has no role in screening, early detection, or diagnosis of prostate cancer. However, it is used in biopsy guidance and disease staging.[131]

TRUS allows examination of the prostate in multiple planes and provides accurate measurements of the size of the prostate gland, the finding necessary for calculating PSA density (PSA divided by the gland volume). Up to 40% of histologically confirmed prostate cancers are not seen with TRUS, and therefore TRUS is not recommended for cancer detection.[132,133] Today, TRUS is mostly used for biopsy guidance and brachytherapy seed placement in patients with prostate cancer.

CT does not provide adequate soft tissue resolution for the detection/visualization of prostate cancer within the normal prostate. Furthermore, CT has no advantages over TRUS in biopsy guidance. CT is, however, very useful in the detection of distant and lymph node metastases.[131]

MRI, especially with the use of endorectal coil, provides the highest-quality images in depicting normal zonal anatomy of the prostate.[131] The role of MRI in the evaluation of prostate cancer is mainly to determine whether the disease is confined to the prostate. MRS is a new technique used in prostate imaging; it provides metabolic information by detecting the cellular metabolites citrate, creatinine, and choline. In tumor localization, combined use of MRI and MRS provides the highest specificity (91%) among noninvasive methods.[134,135] Combined use of MRI and spectroscopy also improves detection of extracapsular extension.[136]

STAGING

The primary goal of local staging is to differentiate patients with tumors confined to the prostate (stages 1 and 2) from patients with tumor extracapsular extension, seminal vesicle invasion, or distant metastasis (stages 3 and 4). Clinical staging is inexpensive and simple. However, clinical staging alone is not accurate enough to be the basis for treatment decisions. Imaging has important roles in the staging of prostate cancer and in surgical and/or radiation treatment planning.[131]

TRUS was reported to have sensitivity in the range of 80% for detecting extracapsular extension and seminal vesicle invasion in the studies performed in the 1980s, when many cancers were large and of an advanced stage.[137] However, prostate cancer is now most commonly detected at an early stage, and TRUS is less effective.

The role of CT in local staging is limited due to its inadequate soft tissue resolution. However, CT is useful in the staging of locally advanced disease with gross invasion of adjacent structures, lymph node status, or distant metastases. The sensitivity of CT is approximately 36% for the detection of lymph node metastases,[138] as the nodal metastases are often microscopic and the nodes are not enlarged. Although CT can show bone metastases, bone scan and MRI are superior to CT in the detection of bone metastasis.

Reports of the accuracy of MRI in the local staging of prostate cancer range from 75% to 93% (Fig. 24.1-17).[139–141] These accuracy levels are higher than those of CT and TRUS. The combined use of MRI with MRS, although currently available only in a few centers, significantly improves tumor localization, tumor volume estimates, and evaluation of extracapsular extension. Data also show that ^{1}H-MRS(I) allows noninvasive assessment of tumor aggressiveness and improves detection of tumors located in the transition zone. Furthermore, the combined use of MRI and MRS(I) decreases interobserver variability, enhancing the value of MRI in the evaluation of prostate cancer.[138] For the detection of lymph node metastasis, MRI, like CT, has low sensitivity, because both modalities depend on size criteria. However,

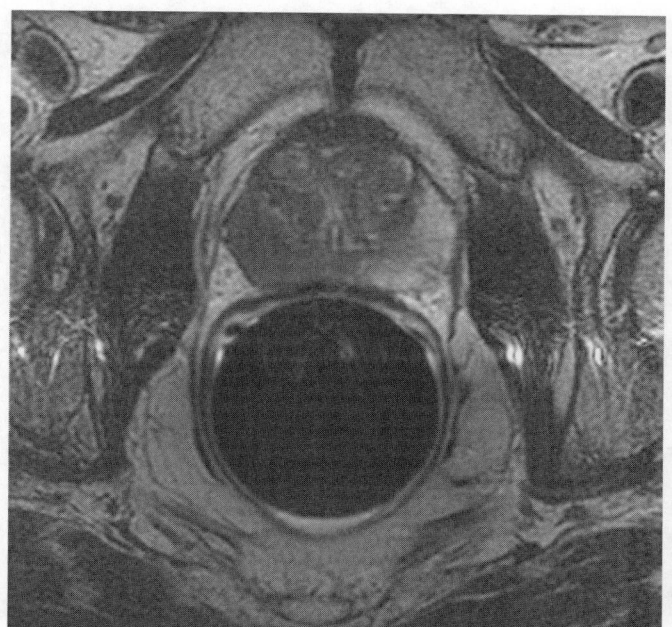
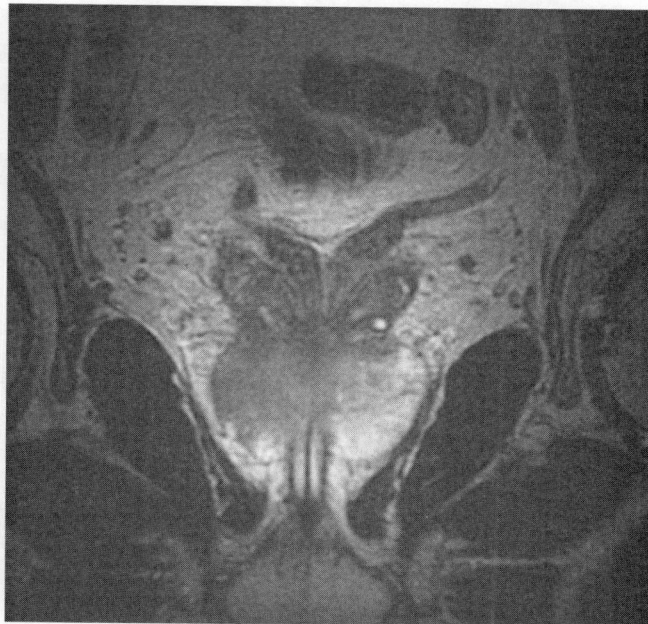

FIGURE 24.1-17. A 78-year-old man with prostate cancer. Axial T2-weighted endorectal magnetic resonance image shows bulky low-signal-intensity tumor in the right peripheral zone (**A**). Coronal T2-weighted image depicts bilateral seminal vesicle invasion (**B**).

use of ultrasmall, superparamagnetic iron oxide particles was reported to increase the sensitivity of MRI to 90.5%, because these agents provide tissue contrast.[142]

TREATMENT FOLLOW-UP

The standard means of posttreatment follow-up in prostate cancer are serial measurements of PSA and digital rectal examination. The first indication of recurrent cancer is a rising serum PSA level. Routine imaging is not needed unless the PSA is detectable or there are new clinical findings. In a patient with suspected recurrence, the question is whether the recurrence is local or distant.

For the assessment of local recurrence after prostatectomy, TRUS, CT, and MRI can be used. TRUS is more sensitive than digital rectal examination (76% and 44%, respectively) but less specific (67% and 91%, respectively) in the detection of local recurrence.[143] For the detection of local recurrence after radical prostatectomy, CT has a sensitivity of 36%.[144] MRI has the highest efficacy for the detection of local recurrence, with reported sensitivity and specificity of as high as 100%.[145]

Imaging also has an important role in patients with distant recurrence. Bone scan is the gold standard for detecting osseous metastases. Equivocal findings on a bone scan can be further evaluated for dedicated imaging studies, such as plain films, CT, or MRI. PET/CT, which can provide information about anatomy and metabolism, is controversial in the assessment of recurrent disease. However, the role of this technique is still being studied.[146]

MOLECULAR IMAGING IN ONCOLOGY

Molecular imaging in oncology is the noninvasive imaging of the key molecules and molecularly based events that are

responsible for the characteristic phenotype of human malignancy. Molecular imaging takes advantage of the latest developments in imaging science and molecular biology to image cancer in living animal models of human cancer and in humans.[147]

The ability to image a series of molecular events has powerful implications for diagnostic imaging. In principle, we can now image molecules and biochemical pathways that are at the heart of why the cancer cell metastasizes, whether it is hypoxic, how fast it is proliferating, and whether it contains molecules that are the targets for cancer therapy or that resist cancer therapy. Also, we can follow up to view how such molecules may be modulated during treatment.

Although we did not always recognize it as such, molecular imaging has been practiced for decades in conventional diagnosis, using nuclear medicine techniques. For example, iodine 131 is used as a tracer for the natural metabolism of elemental iodine by thyroid-like tissue, including thyroid cancer. Iodine 131 uptake by thyroid cancer, as imaged by the Anger gamma camera, has been a mainstay of nuclear medicine for decades. The degree of uptake of radioiodine in the cancer determines whether a given tumor can be treated effectively with iodine 131, and it was long thought that the "iodine trap" was responsible for the uptake. More recently, advances in cancer biology have resulted in a much improved understanding of the mechanism of iodine 131 uptake in thyroid cancer. Iodine 131 uptake is dependent on the expression of the sodium iodine symporter, or "NIS," a membrane-adapted glycoprotein. In addition, greatly improved imaging of radioactive iodine uptake, in terms of resolution and quantitation, is made possible by modern PET, using iodine 124 as a surrogate marker for iodine 131 (Figs. 24.1-18 and 24.1-19).

Clearly, the growing availability of high-resolution imaging techniques that are well suited to molecular imaging (e.g.,

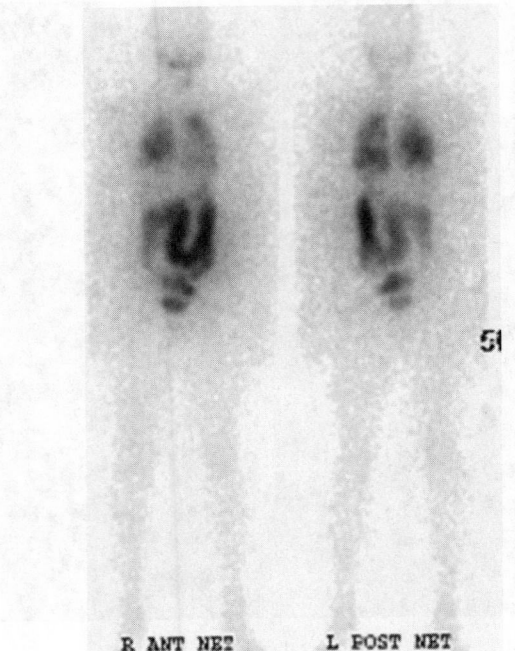

FIGURE 24.1-18.   A 20-year-old woman with metastatic papillary thyroid carcinoma TG2300, TSH 74 after thyroid hormone withdrawal. Posttherapy image 5 days after 139 mCi iodine 131.

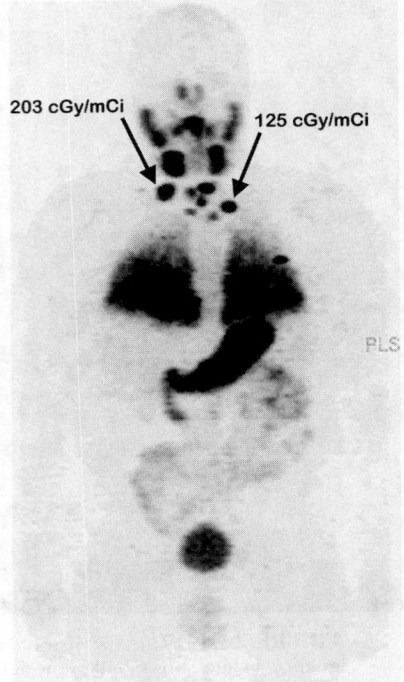

FIGURE 24.1-19.   Iodine 124 in thyroid cancer. (From Larson SM, Robbins R. Positron emission tomography in thyroid cancer management. *Semin Roentgenol* 202;37:169, with permission of Elsevier.)

PET/CT[15] and MRI/MRS[148]) provides increasing opportunities for translation of important laboratory discoveries into clinical imaging based on molecular imaging. It is important to recognize that molecular imaging is multimodal in nature, with important niche applications for fluorescence,[149] bioluminescence,[150] magnetic resonance,[151] and nuclear-based image detection. In general, the optically detected methodologies are most useful at the cellular and subcellular level, the bioluminescence methods for mouse-sized objects, and the magnetic resonance and nuclear methods for imaging larger animals, including humans.

In summary, molecular imaging is an old idea that is represented by time-tested tracer methodology in nuclear medicine. As is described below through examples, the reason for the current excitement about molecular imaging in cancer is its broadly expanding applicability to many facets that are relevant to patient care, including many more molecules and processes that can be imaged with modern high-resolution imaging technologies. Thus, progress in molecular imaging is based on advances in our knowledge of cancer biology on the one hand, coupled to advances in imaging technology on the other. This "new" molecular imaging is increasingly capable of disclosing the critical composition and physiology of the cancer cell noninvasively. The main areas of molecular imaging research are outlined in Table 24.1-2.

GENE EXPRESSION IMAGING

Blasberg and Gelovani-Tjuvajev developed a system of transgene expression imaging based on the presence of a reporter gene and a reporter substrate.[152–155] The initial work was based on radiotracers for 2'-fluoro-2'deoxy-1-b-D-arabinofuranysl-5-iodo-uracil (FIAU), as reporter substrate, and herpes simplex virus 1 thymidine kinase (HSV1-TK), as reporter enzyme. FIAU is a thymidine analog but is not a substrate for the prevalent form of mammalian thymidine kinase. For this reason, FIAU is taken up and retained only in cells that have been transfected with the herpes viral enzyme HSV1-TK. Many subsequent refinements have served to increase the versatility of this methodology, including the use of alternative reporter systems for detection,[156] the development of more sensitive reporter gene/substrate systems,[157,158] and the imaging of the interaction of key molecules at the subcellular level.[159]

The reporter substrate/reporter gene methodology can also be used for imaging the expression of specific genes, by having a promoter region for a gene of interest, such as p53, be the driver for the expression of the reporter gene (Fig. 24.1-20).[160] Using this methodology, the expression of a number of key regulatory and system control genes that are targets for drug treatment can be readily imaged. These gene imaging methods will likely aid in the development of novel cancer therapeutics.[155]

TABLE 24.1-2.   Molecular Imaging Themes

CANCER BIOLOGY
Gene expression imaging
Characteristic phenotype
DRUG DISCOVERY
Antibody and peptide based
Small molecules
Treatment selection and response
CELLULAR TRACERS
Cancer immunology
Stem cell physiology
Physiology of metastases

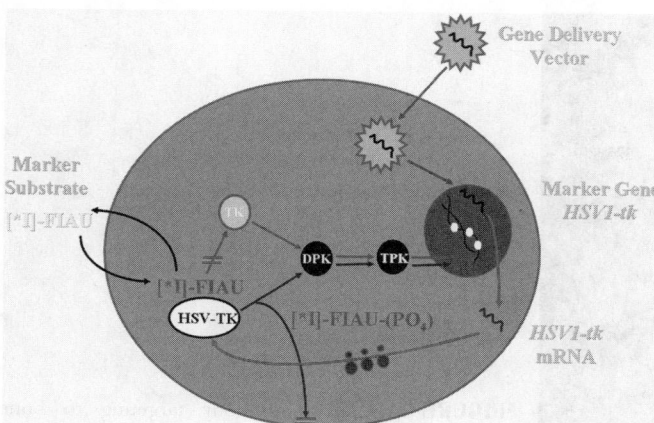

FIGURE 24.1-20. Principle of gene expression imaging. The reporter gene herpes-type thymidine kinase is transfected into a target cell. The system is designed so that the reporter substrate, in this case fluoro-iodo-arabinosyluridine containing a radiolabeled iodine, is taken up only in the transfected cells. The method allows for imaging of genes that are expressed in the transfected cells. mRNA, messenger RNA. (See Color Fig. 24.1-20 in the CD-ROM.)

CANCER PHENOTYPE IMAGING

Molecular alterations that are associated with the cancer phenotype, such as angiogenesis, hypoxia, altered apoptosis, unchecked growth, insensitivity to growth signals, invasion, and metastases, can be imaged. In this regard, the cancer's own biochemistry can be used as a basis for "functional" tumor imaging. The characteristic biochemical alterations of malignancy, such as accelerated glycolysis and amino acid transport, accompany the increased proliferation of the malignant state.

Functional imaging is performed by PET, SPECT, and MRI/MRS. The biochemistry imaged has included glycolysis, amino acid transport, thymidine analogs as a measure of nucleoside transport, choline as an indicator of membrane synthesis, and phosphorus 31 as an indicator of energy metabolism. In large part, human studies have been directed toward improving diagnostic imaging of human cancer. In addition, quantitative methods for imaging of key molecules have been developed using PET, and an example is shown in Figure 24.1-21. In this example, an androgen radiotracer, fluoro-dihydrotestosterone, is injected intravenously and is bound to the androgen receptor expressed in metastatic prostate cancer. A list of representative animal and human imaging applications is provided in Table 24.1-3.[161–165]

DRUG DISCOVERY BASED ON ANTIBODIES AND SMALL MOLECULES

Imaging techniques are playing an increasingly important role in the development of anticancer agents. In antibody-based drugs, for example, tracer studies demonstrated the degree of targeting to tumors and provided direct information about therapeutic index *in vivo* (Fig. 24.1-22). The favorable biodistribution of this radiopharmaceutical led to the development of active new therapies for acute myeloid leukemia, which has failed to respond to conventional treatments.[166,167]

Now that the human genome has been sequenced, there are many potential targets for development of cancer drugs. Imag-

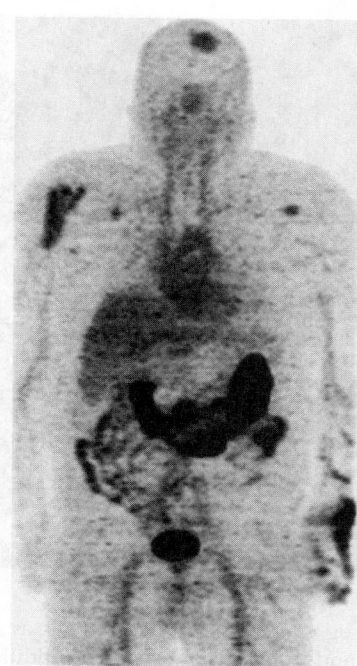

FIGURE 24.1-21. Imaging of the expression of androgen expression in a patient with progressing prostate cancer after castration. The image is taken 1 hour after the intravenous administration of the ^{18}F-fluoro-dihydrotestosterone (FDHT). Uptake is present in the skull, right upper humerus, and ribs, and the metabolites are seen in the blood pool gut and urine. (From Larsen SM, Morris M, Gunther I, et al. Tumor localization of 16beta-18F-fluoro-5alpha-dihydrotestosterone versus 18F-FDG in patients with progressive metastatic prostate cancer. *J Nucl Med* 2004;45:366, with permission of the Society of Nuclear Medicine.)

ing could be used to noninvasively detect the presence of the target and to determine the quantity of expression *in vivo* in the tumor tissue. Such studies can be done as a baseline before therapy and then again during therapy to determine if the drug is having the desired effect on the target *in vivo*. A review of applications of PET in drug discovery notes examples of imaging of a

TABLE 24.1-3. Imaging the Malignant Phenotype: Examples

Function	Substrate/Measure	Novel Findings
Membrane synthesis (Zakian et al., 2003)[161]	Choline and citrate ratio	Increased choline/citrate Ca metabolic signature
Glycolysis (Morris et al., 2002)[162]	FDG	FDG uptake precedes invasion
AA transport (Macapinlac et al., 1999)[163]	^{11}C methionine (CMET)	CMET>FDG in metastases
Angiogenesis (Santimaria et al., 2003)[164]	^{123}I-L19 antibody for extra domain of fibronectin	Extra domain of fibronectin is targeted in rapidly growing lung and colon cancer
Hypoxia (Zanzonico et al., 2004)[165]	^{124}I IAZG	Late imaging correlates best with {O$_2$}
Androgen receptor (see Fig. 24.1-21)	FDHT	Active expression in castrate failure

AA, amino acid; FDG, fluorodeoxyglucose; FDHT, ^{18}F-fluoro-dihydrotestosterone; IAZG, iodo-azomycin-galactoside.

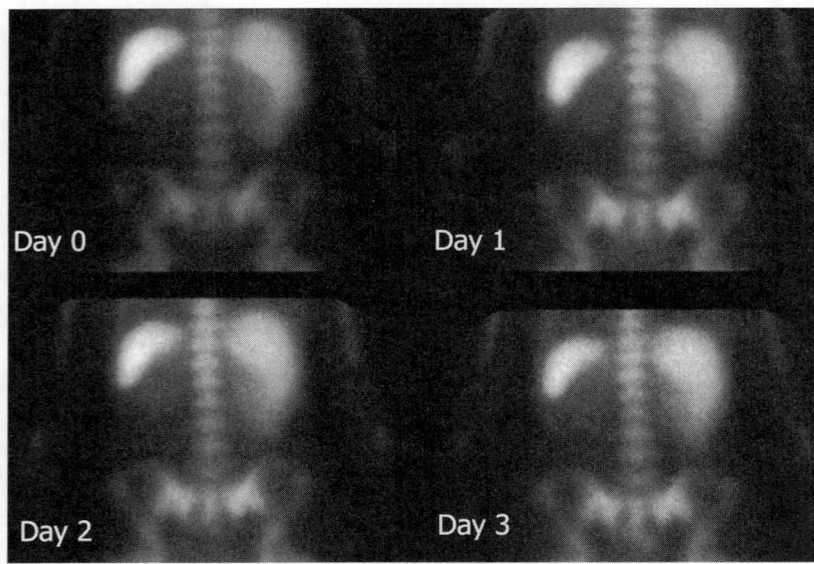

FIGURE 24.1-22. Antibody targeting to bone marrow of a patient with acute myelogenous leukemia. Indium 111 is used to label a chelated form of antibody M195, an anti-CD33 antibody. The differential antigen, CD33, is expressed in malignant cells and early hematopoietic precursors but not in the marrow stem cells. (See Color Fig. 24.1-22 in the CD-ROM.)

radiolabeled drug, such as [^{18}F]5-fluorouracil, as an aid to pharmacokinetics and pharmacodynamics. Additional benefits include the demonstration on imaging of a target for therapy, such as key receptors or a target protein.[168] Radiolabeled estradiol has been used to demonstrate the presence of estrogen receptor in human tumors and to show the effect of tamoxifen therapy.[169] It is likely that PET methods will be widely used to monitor response to therapy through functional imaging of metabolism.[170] MRI and MRS have also been exploited to study drug metabolism and effects *in vivo*, and with high field strength magnets being introduced into the clinic, these applications are likely to increase.[171] Thus, parallel developments in imaging technology and knowledge of cancer biology offer the possibility of an important partnership between imaging sciences on the one hand and drug development on the other.

CELLULAR IMAGING

Gene-directed labeling of human, immune-specific T cells *in vitro* was based on the transgene approach, and studies were performed to demonstrate immune selective targeting of T cells to Epstein-Barr virus human tumors as xenografts in immune-deficient mice. Subsequent refinements of the technique developed by Ponomarev and Gelovani allow for repeated *in vivo* imaging of the transfected T cells as a basis for more detailed assessment of immune properties, including *in vivo* proliferation and graft-versus-host disease (Fig. 24.1-23).[172–174] A similar approach can be used to transfect stem cells, and we may expect extensive applications of this technology in the future, using a variety of imaging methodologies.[172] Bioluminescence methodologies have already had a large impact on monitoring drug response in animal models of human tumors.[175] The fundamental principle is that the tumor that is part of the testing strategy is transfected with luciferase, a gene from the firefly, and transplanted as a xenograft into a mouse or rat. Luciferin, the substrate, is injected intravenously, and the tumor literally lights up. The light is collected by a sensitive camera system. The bioluminescence monitoring is repeated as necessary, with the light output being proportional to the number of cells present. Under the right circumstances, tumor response over a large, dynamic range can be studied, from many millions down to approximately 5000 tumor cells.

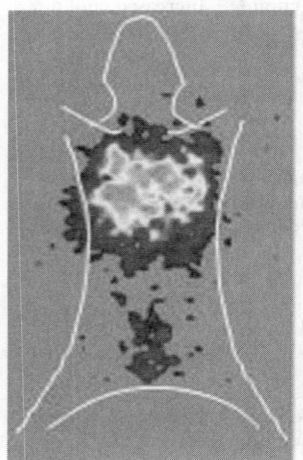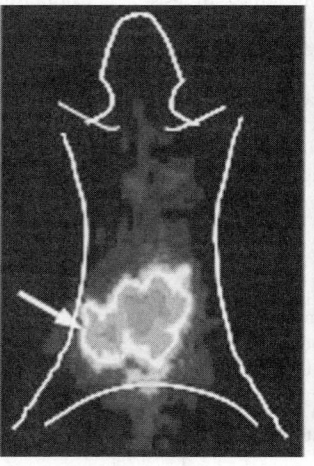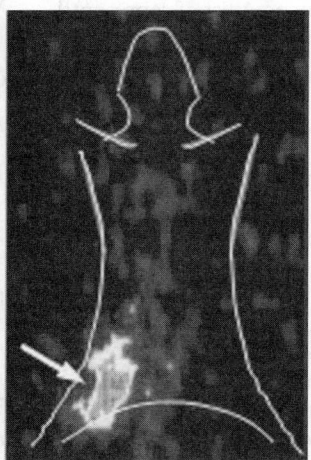

FIGURE 24.1-23. Selective targeting of Epstein-Barr virus (EBV) lymphoma. Immune T cells were transfected with herpes simplex virus 1 thymidine kinase; they were then radiolabeled with ^{131}I-FIAU (iodine 131–fluoro-iodo-arabinosyluridine) *in vitro* and imaged with a gamma camera over the next week. Remarkable selectivity of targeting to the tumor occurred, which was based on immune specificity to antigen determinants on the EBV lymphoma. (Adapted from Koehne G, Doubrovin M, Doubrovina E, et al. Serial in vivo imaging of the targeted migration of human HSV-TK-transduced antigen-specific lymphocytes. *Nat Biotechnol* 2003;21:405.) (See Color Fig. 24.1-23 in the CD-ROM.)

REFERENCES

1. Hangiandreou NJ. Topics in US: B-mode US: basic concepts and new technology. *Radiographics* 2003;23:1019.
2. Boote EJ. Topics in US: Doppler US techniques: concepts of blood flow detection and flow dynamics. *Radiographics* 2003;23:1315.
3. Correas JM, Bridal L, Lesavre A, et al. Ultrasound contrast agents: properties, principles of action, tolerance, and artifacts. *Eur Radiol* 2001;11:1316.
4. Hu H, He HD, Foley WD, et al. Four multidetector-row helical CT: image quality and volume coverage speed. *Radiology* 2000;215:55.
5. Foley WD. Special focus session: multidetector CT: abdominal visceral imaging. *Radiographics* 2002;22:701.
6. Miles KA. Functional computed tomography in oncology. *Eur J Cancer* 2002;38:2079.
7. Stevenson JP, Rosen M, Sun W, et al. Phase I trial of the antivascular agent combretastatin A4 phosphate on a 5-day schedule to patients with cancer: magnetic resonance imaging evidence for altered tumor blood flow. *J Clin Oncol* 2003;21:4428.
8. Morgan B, Thomas AL, Drevs J, et al. Dynamic contrast-enhanced magnetic resonance imaging as a biomarker for the pharmacological response of PTK787/ZK 222584, an inhibitor of the vascular endothelial growth factor receptor tyrosine kinases, in patients with advanced colorectal cancer and liver metastases: results from two phase I studies. *J Clin Oncol* 2003;21:3955.
9. Mueller-Lisse UG, Vigneron DB, Hricak H, et al. Localized prostate cancer: effect of hormone deprivation therapy measured by using combined three-dimensional 1H MR spectroscopy and MR imaging: clinicopathologic case-controlled study. *Radiology* 2001;221:380.
10. Keidar Z, Israel O, Krausz Y. SPECT/CT in tumor imaging: technical aspects and clinical applications. *Semin Nucl Med* 2003;33:205.
11. Martin RC, Derossis AM, Fey J, et al. Intradermal isotope injection is superior to intramammary in sentinel node biopsy for breast cancer. *Surgery* 2001;130:432.
12. McCarter MD, Yeung H, Yeh S, et al. Localization of the sentinel node in breast cancer: identical results with same-day and day-before isotope injection. *Ann Surg Oncol* 2001;8:682.
13. Clary BM, Brady MS, Lewis JJ, et al. Sentinel lymph node biopsy in the management of patients with primary cutaneous melanoma: review of a large single-institutional experience with an emphasis on recurrence. *Ann Surg* 2001;233:250.
14. McMasters KM, Reintgen DS, Ross MI, et al. Sentinel lymph node biopsy for melanoma: controversy despite widespread agreement. *J Clin Oncol* 2001;19:2851.
15. Schoder H, Erdi YE, Larson SM, et al. PET/CT: a new imaging technology in nuclear medicine. *Eur J Nucl Med Mol Imaging* 2003;30:1419.
16. Nehmeh SA, Erdi YE, Rosenzweig KE, et al. Reduction of respiratory motion artifacts in PET imaging of lung cancer by respiratory correlated dynamic PET: methodology and comparison with respiratory gated PET. *J Nucl Med* 2003;44:1644.
17. Miller AB, Hoogstraten B, Staquet M, et al. Reporting results of cancer treatment. *Cancer* 1981;47:207.
18. Therasse P, Arbuck SG, Eisenhauer EA, et al. New guidelines to evaluate the response to treatment in solid tumors. *J Natl Cancer Inst* 2000;92:205.
19. James K, Eisenhauer E, Christian M, et al. Measuring response in solid tumors: unidimensional versus bidimensional measurement. *J Natl Cancer Inst* 1999;91:523.
20. Ries LAG, Kosary CL, Hankey BF, et al. *SEER cancer statistics review, 1973–1996.* Bethesda: National Cancer Institute, 1999.
21. Rees J. Advances in magnetic resonance imaging of brain tumors. *Curr Opin Neurol* 2003;16:643.
22. Aronen HJ, Perkio J. Dynamic susceptibility contrast MRI of gliomas. *Neuroimag Clin N Am* 2002;12:501.
23. Knopp EA, Cha S, Johnson G, et al. Glial neoplasms: dynamic contrast-enhanced T2*-weighted MR imaging. *Radiology* 1999;211:791.
24. Lam W-W, Chan K-W, Wong W-L, et al. Preoperative grading of intracranial gliomas. Comparison of MR-determined cerebral blood volume maps with thallium-201 SPECT. *Acta Radiol* 2001;42:548.
25. Kim YJ, Chang KH, Song IC, et al. Brain abscess and necrotic or cystic brain tumor: discrimination with signal intensity on diffusion-weighted MR imaging. *AJR Am J Roentgenol* 1998;171:1487.
26. Mukherji SK, Fischbein JK, Castelijns JA. New imaging techniques. In: Som PM, Curtin HD, eds. *Head and neck imaging.* St. Louis: Mosby, 2003:2294.
27. Som PM. The present controversy over the imaging method of choice for evaluating the soft tissues of the neck. *Am J Neuroradiol* 1997;18:1869.
28. Aassar OS, Fischbein NJ, Caputo GR, et al. Metastatic head and neck cancer: role and usefulness of FDG PET in localizing occult primary tumors. *Radiology* 1999;210:177.
29. Kluetz P, Villemagne VV, Meltzer C, et al. The case for PET/CT. Experience at the University of Pittsburgh. *Clin Positron Imaging* 2000;3:174.
30. Ishikawa M, Yoshimi A. MR imaging of lymph nodes in the head and neck. *Magn Reson Imaging Clin N Am* 2002;10:527.
31. Som PM, Brandwein MS. Lymph nodes. In: Som PM, Curtin HD, eds. *Head and neck imaging.* St. Louis: Mosby, 2003:1865.
32. Adams S, Baum RP, Stuckensen T, et al. Prospective comparison of 18F-FDG PET with conventional imaging modalities (CT, MR, US) in lymph node staging of head and neck cancer. *Eur J Nucl Med* 1998;25:1255.
33. Kostakoglu L, Agress H, Goldsmith SJ. Clinical role of FDG-PET in evaluation of cancer patients. *Radiographics* 2003;23:315.
34. Atlas SW, Lavi E, Fisher PG. Intraaxial brain tumors. In: Atlas SW, ed. *Magnetic resonance imaging of the brain and spine,* 3rd ed. Philadelphia: Lippincott Williams & Wilkins, 2002:627.
35. Hanasono MM, Kunda LD, Segall GM, et al. Uses and limitations of FDG positron emission tomography in patients with head and neck cancer. *Laryngoscope* 1999;109:880.
36. Greven KM, Williams DW, Keyes JW Jr, et al. Positron emission tomography in patients with head and neck carcinoma before and after high dose irradiation. *Cancer* 1994;74:1355.
37. Mukherji SK, Wolf GT. Evaluation of head and neck squamous cell carcinoma after treatment. *Am J Neuroradiol* 2003;24:1743.
38. Fontana RS, Sanderson DR, Taylor WF, et al. Early lung cancer detection: results of the initial (prevalence) radiologic and cytologic screening in the Mayo Clinic Study. *Am Rev Respir Dis* 1984;130:561.
39. Frost JK, Ball WC, Levin ML, et al. Early lung cancer detection: results of the initial (prevalence) radiologic and cytologic screening in the Johns Hopkins Study. *Am Rev Respir Dis* 1984;130:549.
40. Melamed MR, Flehinger BJ, Zaman MB, et al. Screening for early lung cancer: results of the Memorial Sloan-Kettering Study in New York. *Chest* 1984;86:44.
41. Kaneko M, Eguchi K, Ohmatsu H, et al. Peripheral lung cancer: screening and detection with low-dose spiral CT versus radiography. *Radiology* 1996;201:798.
42. Patz EF Jr, Rossi S, Harpole DH Jr, et al. Correlation of tumor size and survival in patients with stage IA non–small cell lung cancer. *Chest* 2000;117:1568.
43. Lewis JW Jr, Pearlberg JL, Beute GH, et al. Can computed tomography of the chest stage lung cancer? Yes and no. *Ann Thorac Surg* 1990;49:591.
44. Gdeedo A, Van Schil P, Corthouts B, et al. Comparison of imaging TNM [(i)TNM] and pathological TNM [pTNM] in staging of bronchogenic carcinoma. *Eur J Cardiothorac Surg* 1997;12:224.
45. Quint LE, Francis IR. Radiologic staging of lung cancer. *J Thorac Imaging* 1999;14:235.
46. Manfredi R, Pirronti T, Bonomo L, et al. Accuracy of computed tomography and magnetic resonance imaging in staging bronchogenic carcinoma. *MAGMA* 1996;4:257.
47. Heelan RT, Demas BE, Caravelli JF, et al. Superior sulcus tumors: CT and MR imaging. *Radiology* 1989;170:637.
48. Thompson BH, Stanford W. MR imaging of pulmonary and mediastinal malignancies. *Magn Reson Imaging Clin N Am* 2000;8:729.
49. Erasmus JJ, McAdams HP, Patz EF Jr. Non–small cell lung cancer: FDG-PET imaging. *J Thorac Imaging* 1999;14:247.
50. Marom EM, McAdams HP, Erasmus JJ, et al. Staging non–small cell lung cancer with whole-body PET. *Radiology* 1999;212:803.
51. Pieterman RM, van Putten JW, Meuzelaar JJ, et al. Preoperative staging of non–small cell lung cancer with positron-emission tomography. *N Engl J Med* 2000;343:254.
52. Burt M, Heelan RT, Coit D, et al. Prospective evaluation of unilateral adrenal masses in patients with operable non–small cell lung cancer: impact of magnetic resonance imaging. *J Thorac Cardiovasc Surg* 1994;107:584.
53. Erasmus JJ, Patz EF Jr, McAdams HP, et al. Evaluation of adrenal masses in patients with bronchogenic carcinoma using ^{18}F-fluorodeoxyglucose positron emission tomography. *AJR Am J Roentgenol* 1997;168:1357.
54. Silvestri GA, Littenberg B, Colice GL. The clinical evaluation for detecting metastatic lung cancer: a meta-analysis. *Am J Respir Crit Care Med* 1995;152:225.
55. Patz EF, Connolly J, Herndon J. Prognostic value of thoracic FDG PET imaging after treatment for non-small cell lung cancer. *AJR Am J Roentgenol* 2000;174:769.
56. Mac Manus MP, Hicks RJ, Matthews JP, et al. Positron emission tomography is superior to computed tomography scanning for response-assessment after radical radiotherapy or chemoradiotherapy in patients with non-small-cell lung cancer. *J Clin Oncol* 2003;21:1285.
57. North LB, Wallace S, Lindell MM Jr, et al. Lymphography for staging lymphomas: is it still a useful procedure? *AJR Am J Roentgenol* 1993;161:867.
58. Jung G, Heindel W, von Bergwelt-Baildon M, et al. Abdominal lymphoma staging: is MR imaging with T2-weighted turbo-spin-echo sequence a diagnostic alternative to contrast-enhanced spiral CT? *J Comput Assist Tomogr* 2000;24:783.
59. Hoane BR, Shields AF, Porter BA, et al. Comparison of initial lymphoma staging using computed tomography (CT) and magnetic resonance (MR) imaging. *Am J Hematol* 1994;47:100.
60. Harisinghani MG, Saini S, Weissleder R, et al. MR lymphangiography using ultrasmall superparamagnetic iron oxide in patients with primary abdominal and pelvic malignancies: radiographic-pathologic correlation. *AJR Am J Roentgenol* 1999;172:1347.
61. Newman JS, Francis IR, Kaminski MS, et al. Imaging of lymphoma with PET with 2-[F-18]-fluoro-2-deoxy-D-glucose: correlation with CT. *Radiology* 1994;190:111.
62. Friedberg JW, Chengazi V. PET scans in the staging of lymphoma: current status. *Oncologist* 2003;8:438.
63. Kostakoglu L, Agress H, Goldsmith SJ. Clinical role of FDG PET in evaluation of cancer patients. *Radiographics* 2003;23:315.
64. Romer W, Hanauske A, Ziegler S, et al. Positron emission tomography in non-Hodgkin's lymphoma: assessment of chemotherapy with fluorodeoxyglucose. *Blood* 1998;91:4464.
65. Smith RA, Saslow D, Sawyer KA, et al. American Cancer Society guidelines for breast cancer screening: update 2003. *CA Cancer J Clin* 2003;53:141.
66. Liberman L, Menell JH. Breast imaging reporting and data system (BI-RADS). *Radiol Clin North Am* 2002;40:409.
67. American College of Radiology (ACR). *ACR Breast Imaging Reporting and Data System, Breast Imaging Atlas.* Reston, VA: American College of Radiology, 2003.
68. Liberman L. Percutaneous image-guided core breast biopsy: state of the art at the millennium. *AJR Am J Roentgenol* 2000;174:1191.
69. Liberman L, Kaplan J, Van Zee KJ, et al. Bracketing wires for preoperative breast needle localization. *AJR Am J Roentgenol* 2001;177:565.
70. Berg WA. Rationale for a trial of screening breast ultrasound: American College of Radiology Imaging Network (ACRIN) 6666. *AJR Am J Roentgenol* 2003;180:1225.
71. Orel SG, Schnall MD. MR imaging of the breast for the detection, diagnosis, and staging of breast cancer. *Radiology* 2001;220:13.
72. Liberman L, Morris EA, Lee MJY, et al. Breast lesions detected by MR imaging: features and positive predictive value. *AJR Am J Roentgenol* 2002;179:171.
73. Morris EA, Liberman L, Ballon DJ, et al. MRI of occult breast carcinoma in a high-risk population. *AJR Am J Roentgenol* 2003;181:619.

74. Katz-Brull R, Lavin PT, Lenkinski RE. Clinical utility of proton magnetic resonance spectroscopy in characterizing breast lesions. *J Natl Cancer Inst* 2002;94:1197.

75. Liberman L, Morris EA, Dershaw DD, et al. Fast MRI-guided vacuum-assisted breast biopsy: initial experience. *AJR Am J Roentgenol* 2003;181:1283.

76. Morris EA, Liberman L, Dershaw DD, et al. Preoperative MR imaging—guided needle localization of breast lesions. *AJR Am J Roentgenol* 2002;178:1211.

77. Liberman L, Morris EA, Dershaw DD, et al. MR imaging of the ipsilateral breast in women with percutaneously proven breast cancer. *AJR Am J Roentgenol* 2003;180:901.

78. Berg WA, Gilbreath PL. Multicentric and multifocal cancer: whole-breast US in preoperative evaluation. *Radiology* 2000;214:59.

79. Liberman L, Morris EA, Kim CM, et al. MR imaging findings in the contralateral breast in women with recently diagnosed breast cancer. *AJR Am J Roentgenol* 2003;180:333.

80. Olson JA Jr, Morris EA, Van Zee KJ, et al. Magnetic resonance imaging facilitates breast conservation for occult breast cancer. *Ann Surg Oncol* 2000;7:411.

81. Leung JWT. New modalities in breast imaging: digital mammography, positron emission tomography, and sestamibi scintimammography. *Radiol Clin North Am* 2002;40:467.

82. Liberman L. Lymphoscintigraphy for lymphatic mapping in breast carcinoma. *Radiology* 2003;228:313.

83. Van Zee KJ, Manasseh DM, Bevilacqua JL, et al. A nomogram for predicting the likelihood of additional nodal metastases in breast cancer patients with a positive sentinel node biopsy. *Ann Surg Oncol* 2003;10:1140.

84. Dershaw DD. Breast imaging and the conservative treatment of breast cancer. *Radiol Clin North* 2002;40:501.

85. Kopp AF, Heuschmid M, Claussen CD. Multidetector helical CT of the liver for tumor detection and characterization. *Eur Radiol* 2002;12:745.

86. Valls C, Andía E, Sánchez A, et al. Hepatic metastases from colorectal cancer: preoperative detection and assessment of resectability with helical CT. *Radiology* 2001;218:55.

87. Venook AP, Althaus B, Warren RS. Hepatic arterial infusion of chemotherapy for metastatic colorectal cancer. *N Engl J Med* 2000;342:1524.

88. Guibaud L, Bret PM, Reinhold C, et al. Bile duct obstruction and choledocholithiasis: diagnosis with MR cholangiography. *Radiology* 1995;197:109.

89. Coakley FV, Schwartz LH. Magnetic resonance cholangiopancreatography. *J Magn Reson Imaging* 1999;9:157.

90. Schwartz LH, Coakley FV, Sun Y, et al. Neoplastic pancreaticobiliary duct obstruction: evaluation with breathhold MR cholangiopancreatography. *AJR Am J Roentgenol* 1998;170:1491.

91. Taylor AC, Little AF, Hennessy OF, et al. Prospective assessment of magnetic resonance cholangiopancreatography for noninvasive imaging of the biliary tree. *Gastrointest Endosc* 2002;55:17.

92. Yee J, Akerkar GA, Hung RK, et al. Colorectal neoplasia: performance characteristics of CT colonography for detection in 300 patients. *Radiology* 2001;219:685.

93. Johnson CD, Dachman AH. CT colonography: the next colon screening examination? *Radiology* 2000;216:331.

94. Thoeni RF. Colorectal cancer: radiologic staging. *Radiol Clin North Am* 1997;35:457.

95. Maier A, Fuchsjager M. Preoperative staging of rectal cancer. *Eur J Radiol* 2003;47:89.

96. Kwok H, Bissett IP, Hill GL. Preoperative staging of rectal cancer. *Int J Colorectal Dis* 2000;15:9.

97. Zerhouni EA, Rutter C, Hamilton SR, et al. CT and MR imaging in the staging of colorectal carcinoma: report of the Radiology Diagnostic Oncology Group II. *Radiology* 1996;200:443.

98. Maldjian C, Smith R, Kilger A, et al. Endorectal surface coil MR imaging as a staging technique for rectal carcinoma: a comparison study to rectal endosonography. *Abdom Imaging* 2000;25:75.

99. Iyer RB, Silverman PM, DuBrow RA, et al. Imaging in the diagnosis, staging, and follow-up of colorectal cancer. *AJR Am J Roentgenol* 2002;179:3.

100. Ascher SM, Reinhold C. Imaging of cancer of the endometrium. *Radiol Clin North Am* 2002;40:563.

101. Artner A, Bosze P, Gonda G. The value of ultrasound in preoperative assessment of the myometrial and cervical invasion in endometrial carcinoma. *Gynecol Oncol* 1994;54:147.

102. Hardesty LA, Sumkin JH, Hakim C, et al. The ability of helical CT to preoperatively stage endometrial carcinoma. *AJR Am J Roentgenol* 2001;176:603.

103. Connor JP, Andrews JI, Anderson B, et al. Computed tomography in endometrial carcinoma. *Obstet Gynecol* 2000;95:692.

104. Kinkel K, Kaji Y, Yu KK, et al. Radiologic staging in patients with endometrial cancer: a meta-analysis. *Radiology* 1999;212:711.

105. Kim SH, Kim HD, Song YS, et al. Detection of deep myometrial invasion in endometrial carcinoma: comparison of transvaginal ultrasound, CT, and MRI. *J Comput Assist Tomogr* 1995;19:766.

106. Ito K, Matsumoto T, Nakada T, et al. Assessing myometrial invasion by endometrial carcinoma with dynamic MRI. *J Comput Assist Tomogr* 1994;18:77.

107. Seki H, Takano T, Sakai K. Value of dynamic MR imaging in assessing endometrial carcinoma involvement of the cervix. *AJR Am J Roentgenol* 2000;175:171.

108. Saga T, Higashi T, Ishimori T, et al. Clinical value of FDG-PET in the follow up of postoperative patients with endometrial cancer. *Ann Nucl Med* 2003;17:197.

109. Pannu HK, Corl FM, Fishman EK. CT evaluation of cervical cancer: spectrum of disease. *Radiographics* 2001;21:1155.

110. Kamura T, Tsukamoto N, Tsuruchi N, et al. Multivariate analysis of the histopathologic prognostic factors of cervical cancer in patients undergoing radical hysterectomy. *Cancer* 1992;69:181.

111. Hricak H, Lacey CG, Sandles LG, et al. Invasive cervical carcinoma: comparison of MR imaging and surgical findings. *Radiology* 1998;166:623.

112. Subak LL, Hricak H, Powell CB, et al. Cervical carcinoma: computed tomography and magnetic resonance imaging for preoperative staging. *Obstet Gynecol* 1995;86:43.

113. Kim SH, Choi BI, Lee HP, et al. Uterine cervical carcinoma: comparison of CT and MR findings. *Radiology* 1990;175:45.

114. Sheu M, Chang C, Wang J, et al. MR staging of clinical stage I and IIa cervical carcinoma: a reappraisal of efficacy and pitfalls. *Eur J Radiol* 2001;38:225.

115. Hawighorst H, Knapstein PG, Weikel W, et al. Cervical carcinoma: comparison of standard and pharmokinetic MR imaging. *Radiology* 1996;201:531.

116. Kim SH, Choi BI, Kim JK, et al. Preoperative staging of uterine cervical carcinoma: comparison of CT and MRI in 99 patients. *J Comput Assist Tomogr* 1993;17:633.

117. Yang WT, Lam WW, Yu MY, et al. Comparison of dynamic helical CT and dynamic MR imaging in the evaluation of pelvic lymph nodes in cervical carcinoma. *AJR Am J Roentgenol* 2000;175:759.

118. Reinhardt MJ, Ehritt-Braun C, Vogelgesang D, et al. Metastatic lymph nodes in patients with cervical cancer: detection with MR imaging and FDG PET. *Radiology* 2001;218:776.

119. Hawighorst H, Knapstein PG, Schaeffer U, et al. Pelvic lesions in patients with treated cervical carcinoma: efficacy of pharmacokinetic analysis of dynamic MR images in distinguishing recurrent tumors from benign conditions. *AJR Am J Roentgenol* 1996;166:401.

120. Kinkel K, Ariche M, Tardivon AA, et al. Differentiation between recurrent tumor and benign conditions after treatment of gynecologic pelvic carcinoma: value of dynamic contrast-enhanced subtraction MR imaging. *Radiology* 1997;204:55.

121. Yamashita Y, Harada M, Torashima M, et al. Dynamic MR imaging of recurrent postoperative cervical cancer. *J Magn Reson Imaging* 1996;6:167.

122. Park DH, Kim KH, Park SY, et al. Diagnosis of recurrent uterine cervical cancer: computed tomography versus positron emission tomography. *Korean J Radiol* 2000;1:51.

123. Kinkel K, Hricak H, Lu Y, et al. US characterization of ovarian masses: a meta-analysis. *Radiology* 2000;217:803.

124. Cohen LS, Escobar PF, Scharm C, et al. Three-dimensional power Doppler ultrasound improves the diagnostic accuracy for ovarian cancer prediction. *Gynecol Oncol* 2001;82:40.

125. Hricak H, Chen M, Coakley FV, et al. Complex adnexal masses: detection and characterization by MR imaging—multivariate analysis. *Radiology* 2000;214:39.

126. Brown DL, Zou KH, Tempany CM, et al. Primary versus secondary ovarian malignancy: imaging findings of adnexal masses in the Radiology Diagnostic Oncology Group Study. *Radiology* 2001;219:213.

127. Forstner R, Hricak H, Occhipinti KA, et al. Ovarian cancer: staging with CT and MR imaging. *Radiology* 1995;197:619.

128. Tempany CM, Zou KH, Silverman SG, et al. Staging of advanced ovarian cancer: comparison of imaging modalities—report from the Radiological Diagnostic Oncology Group. *Radiology* 2000;215:761.

129. Prayer L, Kainz C, Kramer J, et al. CT and MR accuracy in the detection of tumor recurrence in patients treated for ovarian cancer. *J Comput Assist Tomogr* 1993;17:626.

130. Bristow RE, del Carmen MG, Pannu HK, et al. Clinically occult recurrent ovarian cancer: patient selection for secondary cytoreductive surgery using combined PET/CT. *Gynecol Oncol* 2003;90:519.

131. Yu KK, Hricak H. Imaging prostate cancer. *Radiol Clin North Am* 2000;38:59.

132. Shinohara K, Wheeler TM, Scardino PT. The appearance of prostate cancer on transrectal ultrasonography: correlation of imaging and pathological examinations. *J Urol* 1989;142:76.

133. Shinohara K, Scardino PT, Carter SS, et al. Pathologic basis of the sonographic appearance of the normal and malignant prostate. *Urol Clin North Am* 1989;16:675.

134. Scheidler J, Hricak H, Vigneron DB, et al. Prostate cancer: localization with three-dimensional proton MR spectroscopic imaging—clinicopathologic study. *Radiology* 1999;213:473.

135. Wefer AE, Hricak H, Vigneron DB, et al. Sextant localization of prostate cancer: comparison of sextant biopsy, magnetic resonance imaging and magnetic resonance spectroscopic imaging with step-section histology. *J Urol* 2000;164:400.

136. Yu KK, Scheidler J, Hricak H, et al. Prostate cancer: prediction of extracapsular extension with endorectal MR imaging and three-dimensional proton MR spectroscopic imaging. *Radiology* 1999;213:481.

137. Scardino PT, Shinohara K, Wheeler TM, et al. Staging of prostate cancer. Value of ultrasonography. *Urol Clin North Am* 1989;16:713.

138. Wolf JS Jr, Cher M, Dall'era M, et al. The use and accuracy of cross-sectional imaging and fine needle aspiration cytology for detection of pelvic lymph node metastases before radical prostatectomy. *J Urol* 1995;153:993.

139. Bernstein MR, Cangiano T, D'Amico A, et al. Endorectal coil magnetic resonance imaging and clinicopathologic findings in T1c adenocarcinoma of the prostate. *Urol Oncol* 2000;5:104.

140. Cornud F, Flam T, Chauveinc L, et al. Extraprostatic spread of clinically localized prostate cancer: factors predictive of pT3 tumor and of positive endorectal MR imaging examination results. *Radiology* 2002;224:203.

141. May F, Treumann T, Dettmar P, et al. Limited value of endorectal magnetic resonance imaging and transrectal ultrasonography in the staging of clinically localized prostate cancer. *BJU Int* 2001;87:66.

142. Harisinghani MG, Barentsz J, Hahn PF, et al. Noninvasive detection of clinically occult lymph-node metastases in prostate cancer. *N Engl J Med* 2003;348:2491.

143. Leventis AK, Shariat SF, Slawin KM. Local recurrence after radical prostatectomy: correlation of US features with prostatic fossa biopsy findings. *Radiology* 2001;219:432.

144. Kramer S, Gorich J, Gottfried HW, et al. Sensitivity of computed tomography in detecting local recurrence of prostatic carcinoma following radical prostatectomy. *Br J Radiol* 1997;70:995.

145. Silverman JM, Krebs TL. MR imaging evaluation with a transrectal surface coil of local recurrence of prostatic cancer in men who have undergone radical prostatectomy. *AJR Am J Roentgenol* 1997;168:379.

146. Hricak H, Schoder H, Pucar D, et al. Advances in imaging in the postoperative patient with a rising prostate-specific antigen level. *Semin Oncol* 2003;30:616.

147. Gambhir SS, Herschman HR, Cherry SR, et al. Imaging transgene expression with radionuclide imaging technologies. *Neoplasia* 2000;2:118.

148. Nelson JB, Lepor H. Prostate cancer: radical prostatectomy. *Urol Clin North Am* 2003;30:703.

149. Mahmood U, Weissleder R. Near-infrared optical imaging of proteases in cancer. *Mol Cancer Ther* 2003;2:489.

150. Contag CH, Bachmann MH. Advances in in vivo bioluminescence imaging of gene expression. *Annu Rev Biomed Eng* 2002;4:235.

151. Rudin M, Weissleder R. Molecular imaging in drug discovery and development. *Nat Rev Drug Discov* 2003;2:123.

152. Tjuvajev JG, Stockhammer G, Desai R, et al. Imaging the expression of transfected genes in vivo. *Cancer Res* 1995;55:6126.

153. Blasberg RG, Gelovani J. Molecular-genetic imaging: a nuclear medicine-based perspective. *Mol Imaging* 2002;1:280.

154. Blasberg RG. Molecular imaging and cancer. *Mol Cancer Ther* 2003;2:335.

155. Gelovani Tjuvajev J, Blasberg RG. In vivo imaging of molecular-genetic targets for cancer therapy. *Cancer Cell* 2003;3:327.

156. Gambhir SS, Barrio JR, Wu L, et al. Imaging of adenoviral-directed herpes simplex virus type 1 thymidine kinase reporter gene expression in mice with radiolabeled ganciclovir. *J Nucl Med* 1998;39:2003.

157. Doubrovin M, Ponomarev V, Serganova I, et al. Development of a new reporter gene system—dsRed/xanthine phosphoribosyltransferase-xanthine for molecular imaging of processes behind the intact blood-brain barrier. *Mol Imaging* 2003;2:93.

158. Ponomarev V, Doubrovin M, Serganova I, et al. Cytoplasmically retargeted HSV1-tk/GFP reporter gene mutants for optimization of noninvasive molecular-genetic imaging. *Neoplasia* 2003;5:245.

159. Luker GD, Sharma V, Pica CM, et al. Noninvasive imaging of protein-protein interactions in living animals. *Proc Natl Acad Sci U S A* 2002;99:6961.

160. Doubrovin M, Ponomarev V, Beresten T, et al. Imaging transcriptional regulation of p53-dependent genes with positron emission tomography in vivo. *Proc Natl Acad Sci U S A* 2001;98:9300.

161. Zakian KL, Eberhardt S, Hricak H, et al. Transition zone prostate cancer: metabolic characteristics at 1H MR spectroscopic imaging—initial results. *Radiology* 2003;229:241.

162. Morris MJ, Akhurst T, Osman I et al. Fluorinated deoxyglucose positron emission tomography imaging in progressive metastatic prostate cancer. *Urology* 2002;59:913.

163. Macapinlac HA, Humm JL, Akhurst T, et al. Differential metabolism and pharmacokinetics of L-[1-(11)C]-Methionine and 2-[(18)F] fluoro-2-deoxy-D-glucose (FDG) in androgen independent prostate cancer. *Clin Positron Imaging* 1999;2:173.

164. Santimaria M, Moscatelli G, Viale GL, et al. Immunoscintigraphic detection of the ED-B domain of fibronectin, a marker of angiogenesis, in patients with cancer. *Clin Cancer Res* 2003;9:571.

165. Zanzonico P, O'Donoghue J, Chapman JD, et al. Iodine-124-labeled iodo-azomycin-galactoside imaging of tumor hypoxia in mice with serial microPET scanning. *Eur J Nucl Med Mol Imaging* 2004;31:117.

166. Jurcic JG, Larson SM, Sgouros G, et al. Targeted alpha particle immunotherapy for myeloid leukemia. *Blood* 2002;100:1233.

167. Burke JM, Caron PC, Papadopoulos EB, et al. Cytoreduction with iodine-131-anti-CD33 antibodies before bone marrow transplantation for advanced myeloid leukemias. *Bone Marrow Transplant* 2003;32:549.

168. Aboagye EO, Price PM. Use of positron emission tomography in anticancer drug development. *Invest New Drugs* 2003;21:169.

169. Dehdashti F, Siegel BA. Evaluation of breast and gynecologic cancers by positron emission tomography. *Semin Roentgenol* 2002;37:151.

170. Downey RJ, Akhurst T, Ilson D, et al. Whole body 18FDG-PET and the response of esophageal cancer to induction therapy: results of a prospective trial. *J Clin Oncol* 2003;21:428.

171. Spees WM, Yang G, Veach D, et al. A fluorine-labeled methotrexate as a probe for monitoring tumor antifolate pharmacokinetics: synthesis, in vitro cytotoxicity, and pilot in vivo 19F magnetic resonance spectra. *Mol Cancer Ther* 2003;2:933.

172. Kircher MF, Allport JR, Graves EE, et al. In vivo high resolution three-dimensional imaging of antigen-specific cytotoxic T-lymphocyte trafficking to tumors. *Cancer Res* 2003;63:6838.

173. Koehne G, Doubrovin M, Doubrovina E, et al. Serial in vivo imaging of the targeted migration of human HSV-TK-transduced antigen-specific lymphocytes. *Nat Biotechnol* 2003;21:405.

174. Hardy J, Edinger M, Bachmann MH, et al. Bioluminescence imaging of lymphocyte trafficking in vivo. *Exp Hematol* 2001;29:1353.

175. McCaffrey A, Kay MA, Contag CH. Advancing molecular therapies through in vivo bioluminescent imaging. *Mol Imaging* 2003;2:75.

SECTION 2

ANNE M. COVEY
KAREN T. BROWN

Interventional Radiology

Interventional radiology is playing an increasingly important role in the diagnosis and treatment of patients with malignant disease. Minimally invasive techniques come into play early for some patients, when imaging-guided needle biopsy results transform them from "well" patients into cancer patients. Although the procedure itself may seem trivial, it represents a huge breakthrough when compared to the way that cancer was diagnosed 20 years ago. Some patients go on to be treated for cure, in which case interventional radiology plays an adjunctive, but important, role. Patients receiving chemotherapy often require long-term venous access, which can be performed on an outpatient basis using ultrasound and fluoroscopy. Furthermore, interventional techniques offer the promise of palliation of symptoms or extension of survival with less time in the hospital.

What follows is a compendium of available solutions to common problems. The advances in image-guided intervention, including robotics, navigation, and virtual reality, make the field ever more exciting and offer new choices in less invasive cancer treatment.

PERCUTANEOUS BIOPSY

Percutaneous, imaging-guided needle biopsy has become a mainstay in the diagnosis of lesions almost anywhere in the body. Needle biopsy is indicated for tissue diagnosis when a preoperative diagnosis of a mass is considered essential, in patients who are not surgical candidates, to evaluate organ dysfunction (typically of the liver or kidney), or for special studies.

Needles ranging in size from 25 to 14 gauge are typically used and, outside the central nervous system, almost any abnormality that can be imaged can be biopsied. Smaller needles (25 to 20 gauge) are used to obtain cytologic specimens or to diagnose infection. Larger needles (19 to 14 gauge) are used to obtain tissue cores when histologic material is required for pathologic diagnosis or when special studies are to be performed. Common malignancies in which core specimens may be useful include lymphoma, sarcoma, thymoma, and mesothelioma. Tissue cores are rarely needed for other tumors because sophisticated cytologic methods are available for doing many immunohistochemical stains. Many immunohistochemical stains can be performed on cytologic smears, allowing for more accurate tissue typing and the ability to differentiate a metastasis from breast cancer, for example, from a metastasis from colon cancer in the case of a patient with lung nodules and a history of two primary malignancies.

In non-Hodgkin's lymphomas, flow cytometry is performed on cell suspensions; however, the cells are suspended in a culture medium, not the fixative used for a cell block. Cells placed in saline eventually undergo cell lysis related to osmotic shifts of saline into the cell. For this reason, a biopsy specimen placed in saline needs to be fixed or frozen within a few hours to avoid deterioration of the tissue sample that might preclude a diagnosis.

To increase the likelihood of a diagnostic biopsy and minimize complications, a well-performed imaging study should be available for review when the biopsy is being planned. This facilitates the procedure, assisting in biopsy planning so that the specimen is obtained with an appropriate needle and is handled properly. Additional information on how to position the patient, any anticipated difficulties (potential need to traverse lung or bowel) will also be evident and will need to be included in the discussion of relevant risks in the informed consent.

Contrast-enhanced computed tomography (CT) also allows for targeting the most viable area of the mass. As large masses outgrow their blood supply, they become necrotic, and diagnostic material will not be obtained from a necrotic area. Contrast-enhanced CT allows for targeting the areas that are most likely to yield a diagnostic specimen. Therefore, the biopsy should be planned with attention to avoiding unusual or unsustainable positions, complex needle angulation, and difficult breathing instructions.

Biopsies are generally divided into several anatomic areas. Although the basic principles remain the same, a few considerations are location specific.

LUNG/MEDIASTINUM BIOPSY

Lung biopsies can be performed with either CT or fluoroscopy but are much easier and faster with fluoroscopy when possible. The size, location, and nature of the target lesion determine which modality is used. Mediastinal biopsies are usually performed with CT guidance.

The two most common complications after lung biopsy include hemoptysis and pneumothorax.[1] Hemoptysis occurs in approximately 30% of lung biopsies and is generally self-limited, but can be frightening to the patient. Pneumothorax occurs in 20% to 30% of patients after biopsy but requires treatment in only 5% of cases. The risk of pneumothorax is typically patient related, not technique related. Patients of increased age or with underlying chronic obstructive pulmonary disease are more prone to development of a pneumothorax requiring treatment. A symptomatic or enlarging pneumothorax is treated with tube thoracostomy and rarely necessitates hospital admission.

Hemorrhagic pericardial tamponade is a rare, potentially life-threatening complication after mediastinal biopsy. Although hypoxemia may be a feature, this complication can be distinguished from iatrogenic pneumothorax clinically by the development of hypotension with narrowing of the pulse pressure, as well as diminished amplitude of the electrocardiographic complex on the monitor. It can be confirmed by scanning the heart/pericardium and can be treated by simply placing a drainage catheter into the pericardial space.

ADRENAL BIOPSY

The adrenal gland is a common site of metastatic disease. This gland is also the site of many benign neoplasms; adenomas occur in up to 10% of patients. Appropriately performed magnetic resonance imaging can often distinguish between an adenoma and a metastasis, eliminating the need for many adrenal biopsies.[2] In some cases, however, the mass remains indeterminate, and biopsy is indicated. It is often necessary to traverse the lung when performing a needle biopsy of the adrenal gland, introducing the possibility of a pneumothorax.

LIVER BIOPSY

Liver biopsy is one of the most commonly requested biopsy procedures. If the diagnosis of hemangioma, focal nodular hyperplasia, or adenoma is entertained, it should be excluded by an appropriately performed contrast-enhanced CT or magnetic resonance imaging before the procedure. These diagnoses should be entertained in solitary liver lesions (unless they are known to be new), lesions in otherwise healthy women on birth control pills or other similar hormones, and lesions with characteristics of hemangioma, focal nodular hyperplasia, or adenoma on a previously performed, but suboptimal, imaging study. Although these lesions can be biopsied, it is unusual to make a definitive diagnosis because they contain "normal site tissue."

In patients with a liver mass in the background of cirrhosis, an α-fetoprotein of 500 ng/mL or greater is diagnostic of hepatocellular carcinoma (HCC), and biopsy is not necessary. When the diagnosis of HCC is considered and the patient does not meet these criteria, percutaneous biopsy can often be established based on cytology alone. Smaller, encapsulated tumors are more likely to be well differentiated, and tissue cores may be required to distinguish a well-differentiated tumor from normal, or cirrhotic, liver.

PANCREAS BIOPSY

Despite our best efforts, and advances in imaging, most patients with pancreatic cancer still present with unresectable disease. Needle biopsy may be requested for tissue diagnosis so that treatment can be initiated. Pancreatic cancer often incites a scirrhous reaction, and abundant fibrous tissue is often admixed with tumor.[3] For this reason, several needle passes may be required to obtain diagnostic material. Therefore, the diagnosis is often obtained by biopsy of metastatic deposits in the liver, adjacent adenopathy, or even regions of infiltration around the celiac axis or superior mesenteric artery. If the pancreatic mass is the only potential biopsy site, we do not hesitate to traverse the lateral segment of the liver or perform the biopsy posteriorly, through a transcaval approach, because the pancreas is typically surrounded by other organs or structures, such as the colon, spleen, and mesenteric vessels.

RETROPERITONEAL AND PELVIS BIOPSY

Most retroperitoneal and pelvic biopsies are performed to diagnose the cause of lymphadenopathy. When the patient has a known malignancy with the proclivity to spread via retroperitoneal lymphatics, fine-needle aspiration is easily and simply performed. When lymphoma is a consideration, material should be obtained either for flow cytometry or tissue cores submitted for pathologic examination, depending on local practice and expertise.

Occasionally, a biopsy is performed to diagnose a soft tissue mass suspected to be a sarcoma. For primary diagnosis, histologic material is very useful for classifying the sarcoma. If recurrence is the issue, the diagnosis can usually be established on the basis of cytology alone. Needle biopsy in women with pelvic masses that might be adnexal should be performed only after the diagnosis of ovarian cancer has been excluded or an oncologic gynecologist consulted. The biopsy procedure itself may result in peritoneal contamination, relegating the patient to intraperitoneal chemotherapy where a simpler treatment regimen might have been possible.

BIOPSY FOR "ORGAN DYSFUNCTION"

The liver and kidney are the two most common sites from which tissue is requested to evaluate for "organ dysfunction." Most liver biopsies are performed by gastroenterologists without imaging guidance; however, unusual anatomy or a coagulopathy occasionally makes imaging-guided biopsy more appropriate. All kidney biopsies are performed with imaging guidance, and in some centers this has come to lie solely within the province of interventional radiology. Adequate tissue cores can be obtained with needles of 19 gauge and larger. If the patient has an underlying coagulopathy, it is often possible to correct the abnormality and perform the biopsy percutaneously. If the coagulopathy is severe or difficult to correct, either biopsy can be performed using a transjugular approach. With this technique there is very little risk of clinically significant bleeding, as the biopsy is performed endovascularly and any bleeding would occur back along the needle track, reentering the systemic venous circulation.

ENDOLUMINAL BIOPSY

Many malignancies arise within the mucosa of a tubular organ. When arising in the upper or lower gastrointestinal (GI) tract, these lesions are amenable to endoscopic biopsy. When arising in the bile duct or ureter, they also can be sampled endoluminally. Patients who present with a stricture in the bile duct or ureter frequently undergo operation for definitive treatment, and a diagnosis is obtained at surgery. In cases in which the patient is not a surgical candidate, or to distinguish recurrent tumor from an anastomotic stricture, biopsy of the stricture is indicated and can be performed with a brush, forceps, atherectomy device, or even percutaneously with a needle.[4]

RESULTS

Needle biopsy is a useful tool for diagnosing neoplasms, the cause of organ dysfunction, and staging metastatic disease. A specific diagnosis should be made in 80% to 95% of biopsies. Complications may occur, but most are either easily treated or self-limited. Tract seeding has been reported but occurs infrequently. It is important to recognize that there is no such thing as a "negative" biopsy.[5] If a diagnosis of malignancy is not made, a specific benign diagnosis should be determined. If nonspecific findings are evident on cytology (including inflammatory or reactive changes, fibrous tissue, or normal site tissue), or if atypical cells are present, the lesion should either be rebiopsied or closely followed up, depending on the pretest probability of disease.

CENTRAL VENOUS ACCESS

Central venous access is vital in the treatment of patients with cancer, and the role of interventional radiology in placing venous access devices has increased dramatically in the last decade. With the use of ultrasound and fluoroscopy, intravenous contrast, and specialized catheters and guidewires, interventional radiologists can place central venous catheters more safely and reliably than physicians relying on landmarks alone.[6] Access requirements vary from patient to patient, and as a result, many different types of catheters are available (Fig. 24.2-1).

Internal jugular access for catheter placement and proper catheter tip positioning minimize the risk of symptomatic venous thrombosis, and with ultrasound guidance the risk of pneumothorax is essentially eliminated. In addition, internal jugular catheters can be placed safely in patients who have undergone ipsilateral axillary lymph node dissections for breast cancer or melanoma surgery.[7] Subclavian access is associated with a higher risk of pneumothorax, development of venous stenosis, and pericatheter thrombosis causing symptomatic upper extremity edema. Access via the right internal jugular vein is preferred, because of a shorter intravascular route to the right atrium.

In patients who have had multiple prior catheters, conventional access sites may not be patent. Interventional radiology techniques are especially important in such cases, as central venous access can often be achieved by recanalizing an occluded vein or using collateral neck veins. Alternative access sites include the femoral vein, translumbar inferior vena cava (IVC), and transhepatic catheter placement.

GASTROINTESTINAL PROCEDURES

GASTROSTOMY/GASTROJEJUNOSTOMY

Enteral feeding via gastrostomy or transgastric jejunostomy is the preferred method of nutrition in patients with a functional GI tract who are unable to consume adequate nutrition by mouth. Gastrostomy catheters can also be used for gastric decompression in patients with chronic bowel obstruction, most commonly patients with advanced ovarian cancer. In these individuals, placement of a gastrostomy tube can alleviate symptoms of distention and nausea and, in some cases, allow patients to eat.

Gastrostomy or gastrojejunostomy catheters are commonly placed at the time of surgery or endoscopically, but percutaneous placement is a safe and effective technique that is gaining acceptance. In fact, it was only 1 year after the description of the endoscopic technique for gastrostomy placement in 1980 that Preshaw[8,9] described a percutaneous fluoroscopic technique. Percutaneous gastrostomy or gastrojejunostomy can be performed with less sedation than is typically used for endoscopic placement.

Contraindications to gastrostomy include previous gastrectomy, gastric varices, and uncorrectable coagulopathy. Percutaneous gastrostomy placement in the presence of ascites can be performed safely with the use of gastropexy to fix the stomach to the anterior abdominal wall. In fact, ascites is a common feature in patients referred to interventional radiologists for gastrostomy placement, because even moderate ascites makes endoscopic transillumination difficult.

Gastrostomy catheters can be placed by "push" or "pull-through" techniques; in the former, a tract is serially dilated and a gastrostomy tube is advanced through the abdominal wall into the stomach and held in position by an inflatable balloon or locking loop. In the pull-through type, a directional catheter is advanced from the stomach out the mouth and a snare is used to pull the gastrostomy catheter out the dermatotomy in the anterior abdominal wall, similar to endoscopic percutaneous endoscopic gastrostomy placement. The latter technique is increasingly popular, as larger catheters can be placed, long-term patency rates are higher, and complications (including intraperitoneal catheter place-

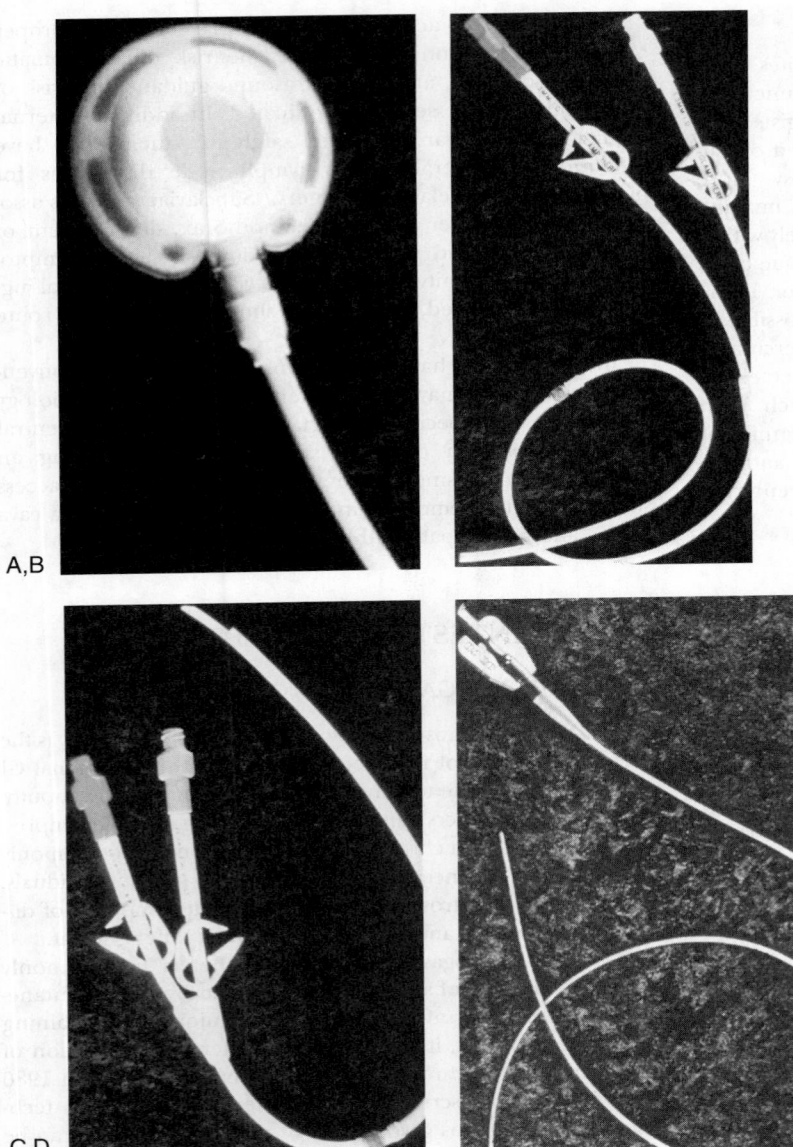

A,B

C,D

FIGURE 24.2-1. Central venous access catheters. **A:** Implantable port. **B:** Broviac. **C:** Leukapheresis/dialysis catheter. **D:** Peripherally inserted central catheter. (Used with permission from CR Bard Access Systems, Salt Lake City, UT.) (See Color Fig. 24.2-1 in the CD-ROM.)

ment) are low.[10,11] Several catheters in different sizes (No. 10 to 28 French) and with different locking mechanisms (pigtail, mushroom, inflatable balloon) are available. Larger catheters (No. 24 to 28 French) are preferred for decompression, especially in obstructed patients who want to eat.

Complications include site infection, peritonitis, tube malfunction, and dislodgment.[12] When gastropexy is performed or after a tract has been established (2 to 4 weeks), catheter replacement can be performed without imaging guidance.

GASTROINTESTINAL STENTS

Covered endoluminal stents can be delivered per oral into the esophagus or per rectum into the colon to palliate patients with malignant obstruction and to treat malignant fistulas (Fig. 24.2-2). These stents are most often self-expanding metallic stents covered with silicone or polytetrafluoroethylene to prevent tumor ingrowth in malignant obstruction and to seal fistulas or perforations. Most patients are able to resume a near

normal diet following esophageal stenting for malignant obstruction.[13] When used to seal fistulas, esophageal stents offer an immediate success of 73% to 100% with 20% to 39% recurrence rate, most often due to new fistula formation or stent migration.[14] Left-sided colonic stents have been used to reestablish luminal patency and palliate bowel obstruction (as occurs in 10% to 30% of cases of colorectal cancer). It has also been proposed as a preoperative adjunct in patients with obstruction as a bridge to definitive one-stage laparoscopic resection to avoid the increased mortality of emergent surgery[15] and the need to create, and then close, a colostomy.

GENITOURINARY PROCEDURES

Obstruction of the urinary tract is a common problem in patients with pelvic malignancies or metastases. Hydronephrosis may be caused by intraluminal or extrinsic masses, blood clot, or fibrosis. Placement of percutaneous nephrostomy,

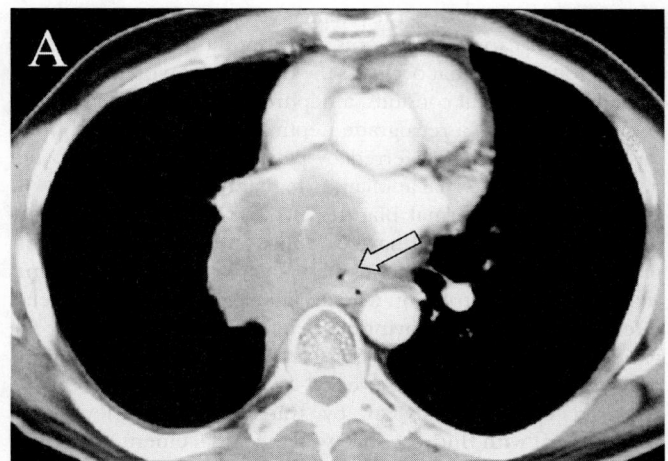
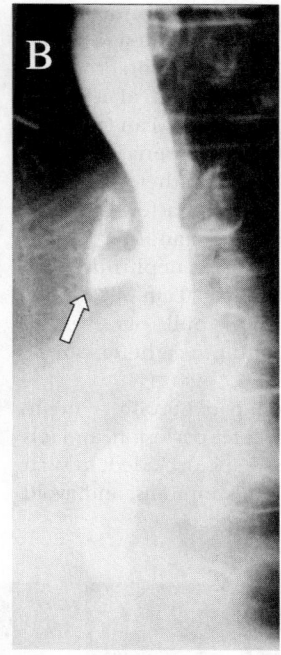
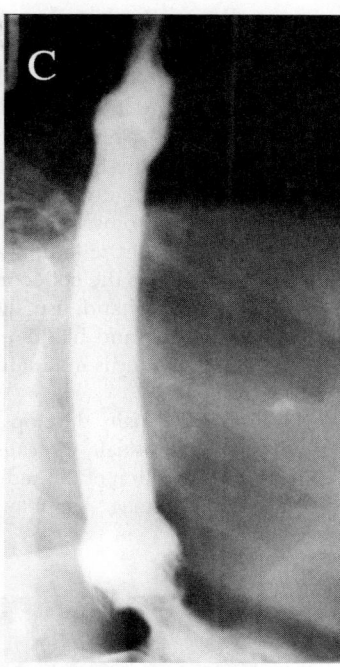

FIGURE 24.2-2. Esophageal stent. **A:** Computed tomography shows subcarinal mass compressing the esophagus with small air bubbles outside the lumen of the esophagus (*arrow*). **B:** Prestent esophagogram shows narrowing of the distal esophagus and ulceration into the mass (*arrow*). **C:** After stent placement, the esophagus is patent with rapid emptying into the stomach, and the ulcer is no longer seen.

nephroureterostomy, or ureteral stenting can be performed to preserve renal function and minimize damage to the kidney, or to treat pyonephrosis. Less commonly, patients present with urine leaks postoperatively or as a result of malignant fistulas (vesicovaginal, colovesical) and require urinary diversion. In these cases, percutaneous nephrostomy, alone or in combination with ureteral embolization, can be performed.

Preprocedure imaging is very important and is used to identify the cause and level of obstruction. It is also useful in defining the relevant anatomy of the kidney (e.g., duplicated systems) and the perirenal space (e.g., retrorenal colon, perinephric abscess) to allow for proper preprocedure planning, as well as triage of patients into those who should be treated percutaneously and those who should be approached from the bladder. Patients with normal bladders, who do not have large pelvic masses or obvious involvement of the trigone on the side to be treated, should have an attempt at retrograde stenting. Cystoscopic stent placement is the procedure of choice in these patients because it does not require external catheter placement.

Percutaneous nephrostomy tubes are placed via a flank approach, with the locking loop of the catheter positioned in the renal pelvis. Antibiotic prophylaxis targeting skin organisms is administered before the procedure.[16] After the procedure no antibiotics are necessary, even though virtually all of these catheters are colonized within 48 hours. In cases of known pyonephrosis or urinary sepsis, however, the choice and duration of antibiotic therapy should be tailored to the organism(s) most likely responsible. Antibiotic coverage is again indicated at the time of routine catheter change, usually every 3 months, as there is typically a transient bacteremia due to catheter manipulation.

Nephroureteral catheters, sometimes called *nephroureteral stents,* are catheters that enter the collecting system via an ipsilateral flank approach, like nephrostomy tubes. These catheters have a locking loop that is positioned in the renal pelvis

and then extend down the ureter, across the site of obstruction, and terminate in the bladder. These catheters can be converted to ureteral stents or can be capped to allow internal drainage into the bladder. Sometimes patients with bladder outlet obstruction elect to have a chronic indwelling nephroureterostomy catheter that can decompress their bladder, rather than a chronic Foley catheter. Common indications for the placement of nephroureteral catheters include malignant obstruction from transitional cell carcinoma or retroperitoneal/pelvic metastases and ureteral strictures, which may develop after pelvic or retroperitoneal surgery or radiotherapy. Nephroureterostomy catheters can also be placed in patients who are stent candidates but for some reason cannot have stents changed cystoscopically. These catheters can usually be capped within 24 hours of placement, allowing the patient to void normally and eliminating the need for drainage bags.

Ureterointestinal anastomotic strictures occur in 4% to 8% of patients who have undergone cystectomy and creation of a neobladder or ileal conduit. In these patients, open ureteral implantation has traditionally been the treatment of choice. Balloon dilation (cutting/angiographic), however, now offers a minimally invasive treatment option and is successful in approximately 50% of cases, obviating the need for long-term catheter drainage.[19,20] Another option for patients with an ileal conduit is to use antegrade access to the kidney to allow for crossing the obstruction into the conduit and then retrograde placement of a nephrostomy tube. The end of this catheter then protrudes from the patient's stoma and is placed in the stoma bag. Therefore, the lumen of the catheter does not become obstructed from mucus produced by the conduit, and the catheter can easily be changed from below.

Access to the kidney can be performed using ultrasound or fluoroscopic guidance. A needle is advanced into a posterior calyx to minimize the risk of bleeding, and an antegrade pyelogram is performed to define the nature and level of obstruction. If urinary diversion is the primary goal of percutaneous intervention, a locking loop (pigtail) nephrostomy catheter can then be placed. Alternatively, if internal drainage is the goal, a catheter and guidewire can be manipulated across the obstruction and into the bladder for placement of a nephroureteral catheter. Nephroureteral catheters can provide either internal (into the bladder) or external drainage (into a bag). Another advantage of nephroureteral catheters is their stability; if a nephrostomy tube pulls out even a few centimeters, it may be "out" of the kidney and require another needle stick to regain access to the collecting system. A nephroureteral catheter, on the other hand, usually has 24 to 30 cm of catheter in the kidney, ureter, and bladder, and if it pulls out even 20 cm, access to the kidney is maintained and the catheter can be easily replaced.

If fever or flank pain develops in a patient with a nephroureteral catheter, it usually indicates catheter occlusion, and it is typically the distal portion of the catheter that is occluded. In such cases, attaching a drainage bag may relieve symptoms, and avoid

urosepsis, before catheter exchange. Nephroureteral catheters should not be capped in patients with conduits or neobladders, as they secrete mucus that occludes the distal portion of the catheter. In patients with ileal conduits, a nephroureteral catheter can easily be converted to a retrograde nephrostomy, as discussed previously. This option is preferred by patients because they do not have additional external appliances to maintain (Fig. 24.2-3).

Patients with normal bladders who tolerate capped nephroureteral catheters can have double-J internal ureteral stents placed. Ureteral stents can also be placed primarily in patients with unilateral obstruction who are able to void. Ureteral stents offer the advantage of having no external portion, relieving the patient of catheter care and lifestyle limitations. Ureteral stents require routine exchange every 4 to 6 months, which can be achieved cystoscopically or by transurethral retrieval and replacement with fluoroscopic guidance. Placement of double-J stents is indicated when long-term drainage of the urinary system is required in patients with functioning bladders.

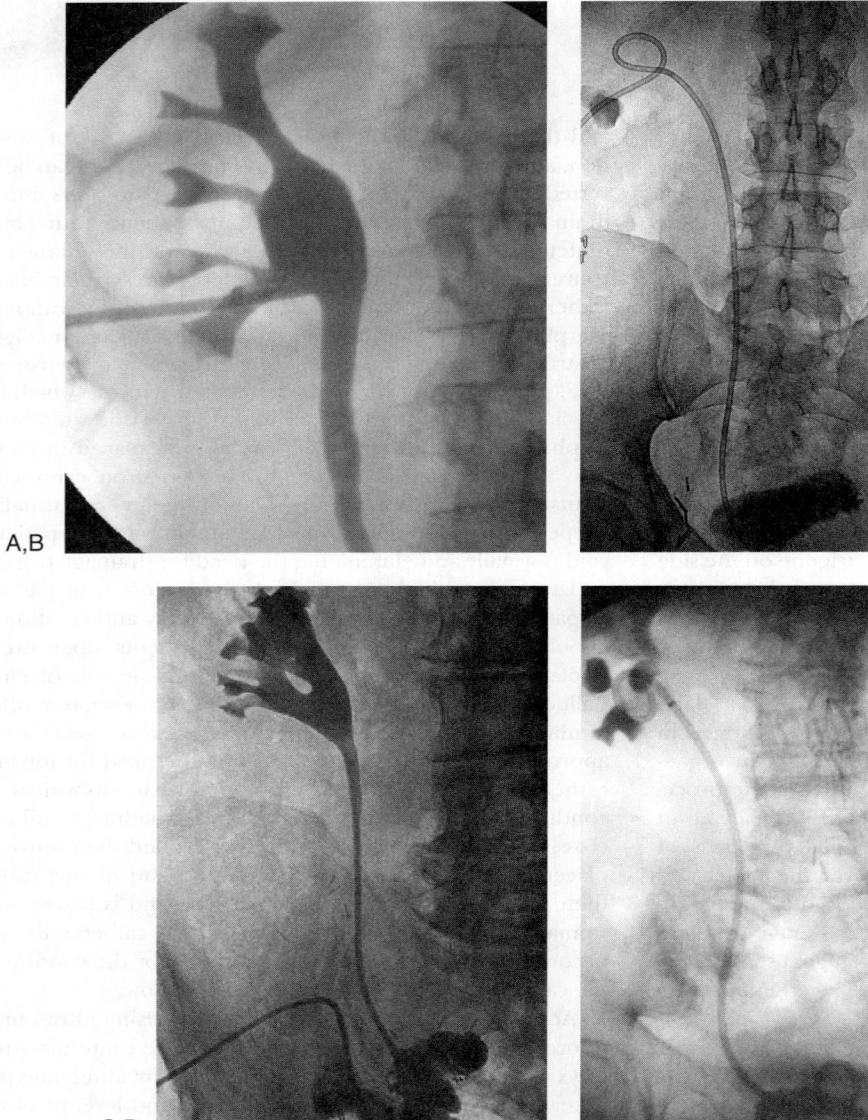

FIGURE 24.2-3. Urinary drainage catheters. **A:** Nephrostomy placed for urinary diversion in a patient with a postoperative urinoma (not shown). **B:** Nephroureteral catheter in a patient with retroperitoneal fibrosis associated with pancreatic cancer. Notice the medial deviation of the ureter. **C:** Retrograde nephrostomy catheter in a patient with ureteroenteric anastomotic stricture after cystectomy for bladder cancer. The locking loop of the catheter is positioned in the kidney, and the catheter drains into the urostomy bag. **D:** Ureteral stent in a patient with malignant ureteral obstruction from ovarian carcinoma.

In patients with malignant bladder fistulas or postoperative leaks, urinary diversion may be indicated to control leakage. Percutaneous nephrostomy catheters can be placed for urinary diversion, but in some cases this may not completely divert the urine. In such cases, as in chronic malignant bladder fistulas, ureteral embolization can be considered. Ureteral occlusion can be accomplished by placement of coils, gelatin sponge pledgets, or detachable latex balloons using the percutaneous nephrostomy site for access.[17,18]

Percutaneous urinary diversion is performed successfully in nearly all cases and is associated with a low incidence of major complications. The most common complications are due to hemorrhage, pneumothorax, and peritonitis. Transient hematuria occurs in most patients but usually clears within 24 to 48 hours. Minor complications include retroperitoneal or perirenal hematoma, extravasation of urine, and infection. Finally, if the catheter is inadvertently removed after an epithelialized tract has formed (more than 4 weeks), the track can be recanalized, allowing successful replacement without the need for a new puncture.

BILIARY PROCEDURES

BILIARY DRAINAGE

Interventional radiology plays an important role in the diagnosis and treatment of biliary obstruction. Biliary obstruction may be caused by primary or metastatic tumors to liver, bile ducts, or pancreas, as well as benign causes including strictures and stones. Bile duct obstruction can be divided into "high" and "low" obstruction. This is an important distinction, because low obstruction of the common bile duct or ampulla is best treated endoscopically, whereas high bile duct obstruction, commonly associated with isolated bile ducts, is best managed by interventional radiology. The term *isolated bile ducts* refers to the situation in which the centrally located obstruction obstructs the right- and left-sided bile ducts not only from the common bile duct but from each other as well. Because the right hepatic duct is shorter than the left, the obstruction can also extend to separate the right anterior and posterior divisions, or even the segmental bile ducts. In this situation, a percutaneously placed catheter may only drain a portion of the liver.

Primary biliary cancers include gallbladder and cholangiocarcinoma, but metastases to the bile ducts also occur, most often from melanoma or GI carcinomas. The diagnosis of primary bile duct tumors can be challenging, as they are often more desmoplastic than mass-like and may be difficult to characterize on cross-sectional imaging. Cholangiocarcinoma arises from the epithelial lining of the bile duct and is more common in men, whereas gallbladder carcinoma is seen more frequently in women. Risk factors include primary sclerosing cholangitis, choledochal cysts, Asiatic cholangiohepatitis, and chronic lithiasis.[21]

Cholangiocarcinoma is a slow-growing, infiltrating tumor with a peak incidence in the sixth and seventh decades. Local tumor invasion often renders surgical resection impossible, or at least very difficult. Patients with hilar (Klatskin) or more peripheral cholangiocarcinoma usually present late in the disease with symptoms of jaundice, pruritus, altered taste/appetite, new light-colored stools, and dark urine. When the tumor involves the common hepatic duct or the common bile duct, symptoms generally occur earlier. Complete surgical resection is the only curative option in these patients and is associated with a 3-year survival of 40% to 60%. Unfortunately, most patients present with unresectable disease.[21] A small minority of these patients, however, may benefit from preoperative chemoradiation and liver transplantation; data from the Mayo Clinic report 80% 5-year survival in patients with early-stage, unresectable hilar cholangiocarcinoma.[22] To date, no adjuvant therapy for cholangiocarcinoma has been shown to improve survival,[23] and therefore, palliative therapy plays a major role in the management of these patients.

Pancreatic cancer, another common malignancy that causes biliary obstruction, has a median survival of 6 months from diagnosis and little, if any, survival benefit from chemotherapy and radiation. Surgery is an option in only 10% to 20% of patients and does not increase survival in most. Thus, as for cholangiocarcinoma, the need for effective palliation is critical.

Because biliary drainage is a palliative procedure for this patient population, its goals should be clear from the outset and dictate management. Biliary dilation in and of itself is not an indication for drainage in asymptomatic patients. Palliation should be directly targeted toward relieving a symptom or prolonging life. A patient with multiple isolated ducts has the potential for multiple lifelong drainage catheters, and the catheter care and lifestyle limitations associated with multiple catheters should be discussed at the outset.

Effective biliary decompression can be achieved by endoscopic stenting or percutaneous transhepatic drainage. Low bile duct obstruction should be treated endoscopically when possible, because stents placed using this technique do not require external tubes or needle punctures. High bile duct obstruction is best treated by percutaneous transhepatic drainage because the operator can choose which ductal system to target to maximize the amount of parenchyma drained while attempting to avoid contamination of nontarget segments.

Palliation in patients with high bile duct obstruction and isolated ducts is challenging. Pruritus can be relieved with drainage of even one biliary segment, but drainage of more liver (which may require more catheters) is usually required to lower serum bilirubin to levels that allow for chemotherapy. When the patient presents with cholangitis, multiple catheters may be required to resolve sepsis.

Endoscopic drainage can be achieved by placing plastic stents that require routine exchange every 3 to 6 months to maintain patency. Plastic stents are useful in patients with long life expectancy, treatable biliary occlusions (lymphoma), or benign disease. Because they are easily removed, plastic stents are also useful for preoperative drainage. Self-expanding metallic stents can also be placed endoscopically and have the advantage of a wider lumen (8 to 10 mm) and intrinsic radial force, but once placed they cannot be removed in most cases. The expected patency of metal stents is 6 to 9 months, and therefore they are generally only indicated for malignant bile duct obstruction when the patient's life expectancy is such that they are unlikely to outlive the stent patency.

Percutaneous transhepatic biliary drainage is the procedure of choice in cases of unsuccessful endoscopic stent placement, prior biliary-enteric surgical reconstruction, or high bile duct obstruction (i.e., at or above the common hepatic duct). The role of preoperative biliary drainage is controversial, but some surgeons believe it facilitates reconstruction of the biliary tract and lowers postoperative morbidity.

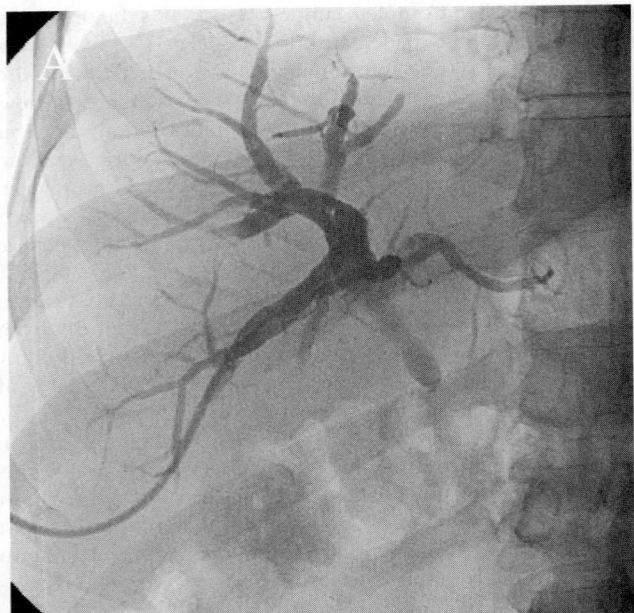
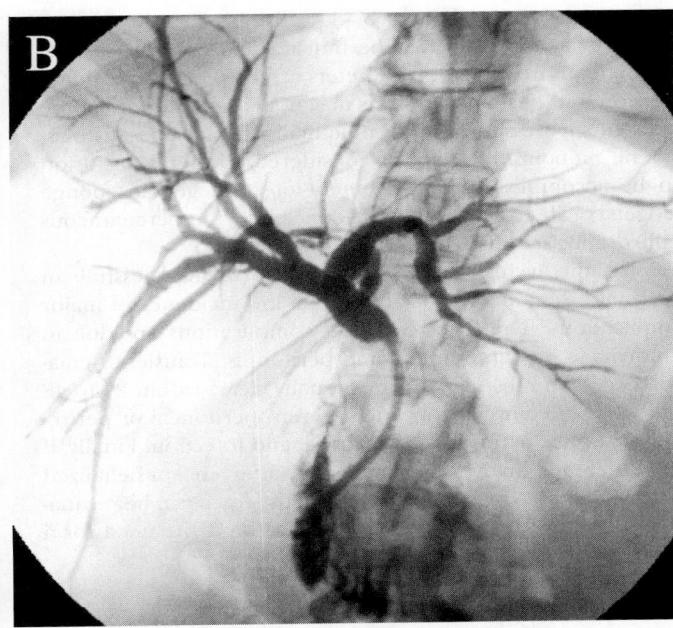

FIGURE 24.2-4. Biliary drainage catheters. **A:** Cholangiogram through an external drainage catheter placed at the hepatic hilus in a patient with distal cholangiocarcinoma. **B:** Internal/external drainage catheter in a different patient with occlusion of the distal common bile duct by pancreatic carcinoma. These catheters allow for preservation of bioenteric circulation and provide added stability based on the length of the catheter within the duct.

Patients scheduled to undergo percutaneous biliary drainage receive prophylactic broad-spectrum antibiotic coverage, and any coagulopathy should be corrected. Percutaneous transhepatic cholangiography is performed via a 21-gauge needle inserted into the target duct chosen on the basis of preprocedure imaging study. Contrast opacification of the biliary tree provides invaluable information about the nature, location, and extent of the obstruction. Steerable guidewires are then used to cross the obstruction and gain access into the duodenum. A multi-side-hole drainage catheter is placed across the obstruction, with side holes above and below the obstruction to maintain normal biliary-enteric flow (Fig. 24.2-4*B*). This catheter is referred to as an *internal/external drainage catheter*, as it allows for drainage internally into the small bowel via the catheter or externally into a bag, or both. The catheter is typically left to external drainage for 12 to 24 hours before it is capped to function as an internal drainage catheter.

If access into the small bowel cannot be achieved, an external catheter is placed in the bile ducts above the obstruction, and the catheter is connected to an external drainage bag (see Fig. 24.2-4*A*). A second or even third attempt to cross the obstruction in these patients is warranted and often successful after the ducts have decompressed. This provides a more stable catheter and preserves the bilioenteric flow of bile. In the face of duodenal obstruction, internal drainage options are limited, and catheters must be connected to a drainage bag indefinitely.

Occasionally, patients who have internal/external catheters are dependent on external drainage. High outputs can have metabolic consequences requiring oral replenishment of electrolytes and hydration. In the majority, however, reestablishment of bile flow usually causes rapid recovery of hepatic function, with decrease in liver enzymes and bilirubin, which in turn leads to relief of symptoms. Patients with external or internal/external catheters flush their catheters daily and undergo routine biliary tube exchange with antibiotic coverage approximately every 10 to 12 weeks to maintain patency and biliary-enteric flow.

Percutaneous biliary drainage is occasionally performed in patients with occluded endoscopic stents that either cannot be exchanged or have failed as a result of proximal tumor overgrowth, converting a low obstruction to a high obstruction. Endoscopic stents can be pushed into the small bowel and eliminated in the feces, or they can be removed percutaneously at the time of drainage by using a snare and pulling the stent through a sheath.

Self-expanding metallic stents are recommended for patients with malignant biliary obstruction and limited life expectancy who are not surgical candidates. Additionally, debilitated or nursing home patients who cannot care for their internal/external biliary tubes can also be treated with stents when possible. Placement of metallic stents improves quality of life because of the absence of external tubes and their associated maintenance and risks, which include skin infection, bile leakage, and catheter obstruction or dislodgment. Even patients with longer life expectancies should be considered for metal stent placement when they agree with the concept that several months of catheter-free existence is worth the price of a potential repeat drainage.

Metallic stents are deployed through the same tract established for biliary drainage using small delivery systems. These stents have an intrinsic radial force and, once released from the delivery device, expand to the stated diameter, ranging from 6 mm in the intrahepatic ducts to 10 mm in the common bile duct. With a larger lumen and intrinsic radial force, these

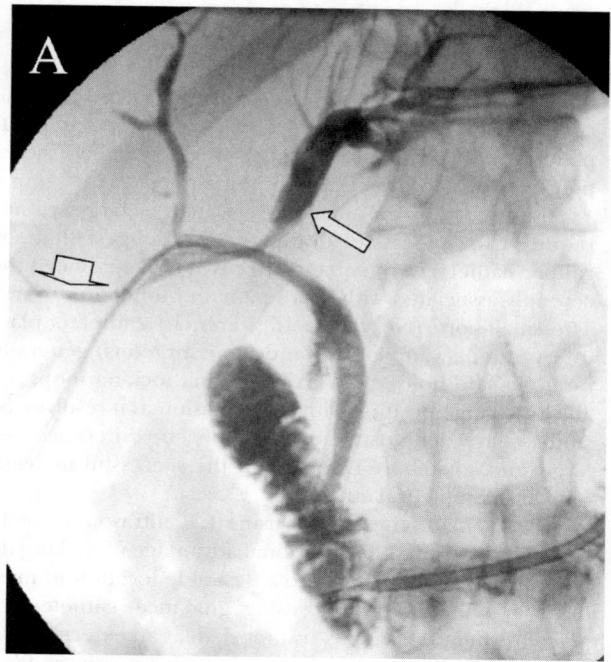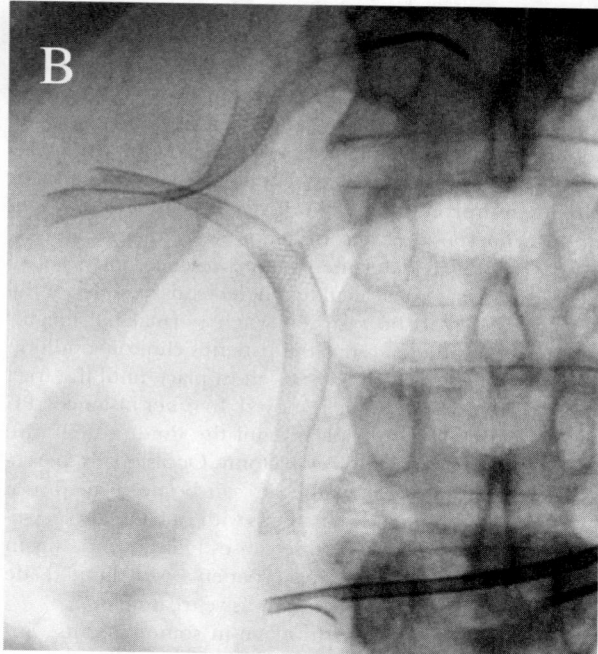

FIGURE 24.2-5. Biliary stent. **A:** Isolated left ducts (*arrow*) were catheterized from the right-sided puncture (*arrowhead*). **B:** Two wall stents were placed to drain bile internally in this patient with cholangiocarcinoma.

stents have a longer primary patency than plastic stents, with a median patency of 6 months. Self-expanding metallic stents are very flexible and remain patent despite relatively acute angulation. This is a useful feature when the tumor involves the confluence of hepatic ducts (Fig. 24.2-5).

In addition to biliary drainage, percutaneous access to the bile ducts provides a means for additional diagnostic and therapeutic procedures, including biopsy of bile duct masses, stone retrieval, percutaneous choledochoscopy, and placement of catheters for novel techniques such as local radiation (brachytherapy) or photodynamic therapy.

When the diagnosis of a bile duct occlusion is uncertain, bile duct biopsy can be performed through the tract created for biliary drainage. It is most effective for intraductal lesions, including cholangiocarcinoma and intraductal metastases, and is less effective in diagnosing extraductal lesions, including pancreatic cancer and extrinsic compression from liver or nodal metastases, because the specimens obtained are from the mucosa and superficial portion of the fibromuscular layer of the duct.[24] After cholangiography is performed, a forceps, brush, or atherectomy device is advanced to the obstruction and a specimen is obtained. Reported sensitivities of forceps biopsy range from 30% to 100% for malignancy, but in most studies a high false-negative rate effectively makes a "negative" biopsy nondiagnostic in most cases.

Biliary stone disease is surprisingly common in cancer patients, due to concurrent gallstone disease or biliary stasis. Small stones may pass from the gallbladder through the cystic duct into the common bile duct. When large, these are apparent preoperatively and can be removed endoscopically. Smaller stones, however, can be missed during surgery and identified by cholangiography in patients with persistent symptoms or hyperbilirubinemia. After maturation of a T-tube or biliary drainage tract, these stones can be safely treated in the majority of cases

using either a basket or snare to remove them percutaneously, a balloon to push them through the papilla into the small bowel, or a laser lithotripsy device to disintegrate them.[27] When associated with papillary stenosis or anastomotic strictures, balloon sphincterotomy is performed to allow stone fragments to pass. In contradistinction to endoscopic sphincterotomy, in which there is a high incidence of sepsis and pancreatitis, such complications after balloon sphincterotomy are uncommon.[25]

Percutaneous choledochoscopy is a technique adapted from the operating room, in which a fiberoptic scope similar to a bronchoscope is advanced percutaneously along the course of a biliary drainage catheter and used to visualize bile ducts, intraluminal masses, and stones in exquisite detail. Currently, the most common applications are intrahepatic stone retrieval and intraductal biopsy. Choledochoscopy is performed after the maturation of a percutaneous tract following biliary drainage, which usually takes 2 to 4 weeks. When used in concert with fluoroscopic cholangiography, the choledochoscope can be easily manipulated into the duct of interest. Once a stone is visualized through the scope, a basket, snare, or balloon catheter can be advanced through the instrument channel and used to remove the stone percutaneously or to push the stone across the papilla in the small bowel.

PERCUTANEOUS CHOLECYSTOSTOMY

Percutaneous cholecystostomy (PC) is indicated in patients with acute calculus or acalculous cholecystitis who are unable to undergo urgent cholecystectomy due to comorbid disease or debilitated condition. Because of the low procedure-related morbidity, in addition to its therapeutic role, PC is commonly used as a diagnostic tool in patients with unexplained sepsis.[26]

PC is performed using ultrasound or CT guidance. A transhepatic approach is generally preferred to minimize the risk of bile peritonitis and leakage during catheter placement and catheter exchanges. PC allows for rapid decompression of the diseased gallbladder as well as access for cholecystography and potential further intervention. Overdistention of the gallbladder at the time of placement is avoided because bile in diseased gallbladders is often infected, and overdistention may increase translocation across the gallbladder wall and worsen sepsis in these already compromised patients.[25]

After the acute sepsis has resolved, however, cholecystography can be very helpful in determining the presence and level of obstruction. In the case of acalculous cholecystitis, patency of the cystic duct is known to be restored when normal bile begins draining from the catheter. Once the patient's clinical condition improves, the catheter is capped and left in place until the tract matures, at which point it can be removed. In other instances, PC catheters are generally left in place until the time of definitive treatment, which is usually cholecystectomy. Occasionally, percutaneous stone removal through the PC can be performed as a definitive procedure in high-risk patients with calculus cholecystitis. Although recurrent stone disease causes biliary symptoms in 20% to 50% of cases within 5 years, patients with limited life expectancy may benefit from the less invasive treatment.

PC is also useful for biliary drainage in some patients with low bile duct occlusion. The gallbladder is a capacious organ, and in some cases it can enlarge to completely decompress the intrahepatic bile ducts, making percutaneous biliary drainage quite difficult. In the presence of low bile duct occlusion and a distended gallbladder, PC is technically simple and provides drainage of all bile segments. Alternatively, the gallbladder can be accessed with a needle and cholecystography performed to delineate the intrahepatic bile ducts, facilitating percutaneous transhepatic biliary drainage.

Complications of PC include bleeding, sepsis, bile peritonitis, gallbladder perforation, and catheter dislodgment. Removal of a PC before the formation of an epithelialized tract can also cause bile peritonitis. Tract maturation usually occurs within 4 weeks, even in debilitated patients, but may take longer in individuals who are receiving immunosuppressive drugs.[25]

CHEST INTERVENTIONS

PLEURAL EFFUSIONS

Malignant pleural effusions are common in patients with cancer, most frequently in breast carcinoma, lung carcinoma, and lymphoma. These effusions are exudates and result from weeping of fluid from pleural metastasis or lymphatic obstruction by tumor. The accumulation on fluid in the pleural space is often associated with dyspnea, cough, or chest pain.

Malignant effusions in patients with lymphoma or small cell lung cancer may have significant improvement or resolve with systemic therapy, but the majority of symptomatic patients with malignant pleural effusions require some form of drainage for relief. Treatment options include repeated thoracentesis, tube thoracostomy, video-assisted thoracic surgery, and pleurodesis. Thoracentesis can be performed on an outpatient basis or at bedside, but because malignant effusions recur in the vast majority, it does not represent a definitive treatment option.

Several different chest tubes, made of polyurethane or silicone, are available for drainage of pleural effusions, ranging in size from No. 8 to 36 French. Surgical chest tubes, placed at the bedside or in the operating room, are usually No. 24 to 36 French drainage catheters. When placed at the bedside, chest tube placement is a "blind" procedure relying on landmarks to access the effusion. Therefore, this technique is limited to patients with moderate to large free-flowing effusions, and poor catheter position is a common sequela.

Although surgical teaching is that a large catheter is required for successful drainage, data suggest that smaller-caliber catheters are equally effective. Large-caliber tubes are certainly associated with more pain and limitation of mobility. The small-bore (No. 8.0 to 15.5 French) catheters placed by interventional radiologists (and some surgeons) generally have multiple side holes and flexible pigtail locking loops and are able to change position within an effusion as it resolves. Several studies have demonstrated no significant difference between large- and small-bore catheters in the successful management of malignant pleural effusions.[29,30]

Placement of chest tubes using CT, ultrasound, or fluoroscopic imaging has the additional advantage of making it possible to place the catheter into a desirable location to maximize drainage. In other words, using guidance, catheters can be placed "where the fluid is" rather than at an external anatomic landmark. This is most important in patients with small or loculated effusions (Fig. 24.2-6).

Using imaging guidance, an appropriate puncture site is marked. The pleural space is accessed with an 18- to 21-gauge needle, and fluid is aspirated. A guidewire is advanced into the pleural space, and this guidewire can be used to disrupt septations in multiloculated effusions. The tract is then dilated, and a catheter is advanced over the wire into a dependent portion of the pleural space. Aspiration of 1.0 to 1.5 L can be performed immediately, after which the catheter is attached to a closed-system water-seal device (Pleur-evac). Gravity drainage is usually sufficient, but suction may improve drainage in a minority of patients.

A chest radiograph is obtained immediately after drainage to provide a new baseline and to evaluate for lung reexpansion. In chronic effusions, the lung may not be compliant and an *ex vacuo* air collection may be seen in the pleural space after drainage of pleural fluid. This usually resolves over days to weeks but may persist in some cases.

Daily outputs are measured and are critical in the tube management decision-making process. Low catheter output (less than 25 mL/d) indicates either tube malfunction or resolution, and a chest radiograph can differentiate between the two. If the catheter is malpositioned or malfunctioning, it can be exchanged over a guidewire. If the effusion has resolved, as happens in a significant minority of patients with malignant pleural effusions, the catheter can be removed without further intervention.

The majority of patients with malignant pleural effusions, however, do not have a durable, long-term response to thoracentesis or catheter placement alone. In this group of patients, mechanical or chemical pleurodesis can be performed. Mechanical pleurodesis or chemical pleurodesis, or both, can be performed during video-assisted thoracoscopy, whereas chemical pleurodesis can be performed at the bedside via a chest tube. Although surgical pleurodesis offers a slightly higher success rate and shorter hospital stay, it is more expensive, more invasive, and associated with higher morbidity.[33,34]

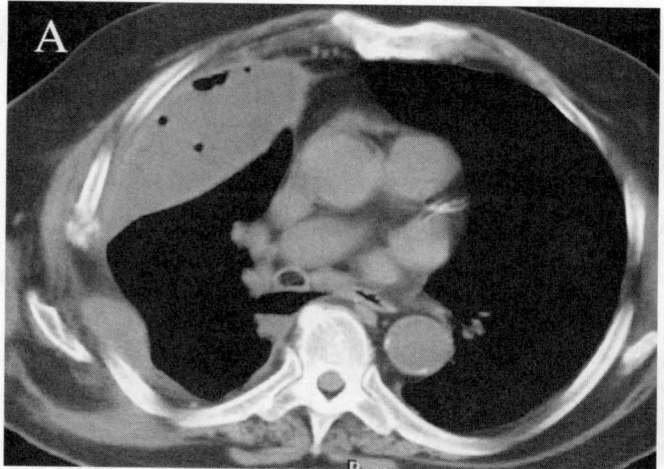 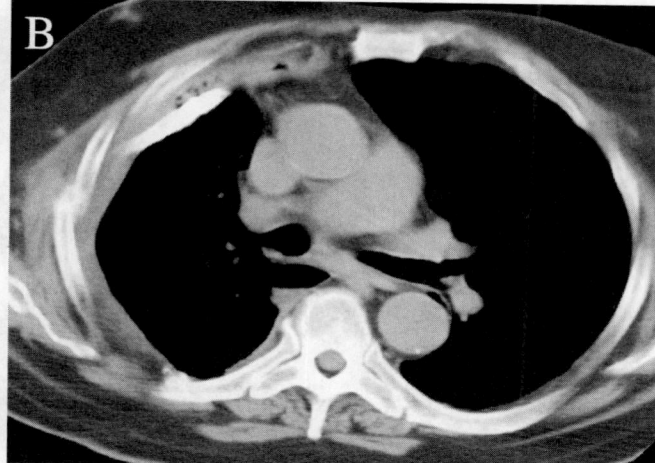

FIGURE 24.2-6. Tube thoracostomy. **A:** Loculated anterior empyema in a patient after lobectomy for lung cancer. (Surgically placed chest tube, not shown, is in the lower hemithorax remote from the collection.) **B:** Computed tomography–guided chest tube placement completely drained collection yielding 100 mL frank pus.

Chemical pleurodesis is achieved by instilling a sclerosing agent (asbestos-free talc, bleomycin, doxycycline) into the pleural space to incite an inflammatory reaction that ultimately causes the visceral pleura to adhere to the parietal pleura, thereby eliminating the potential space in which fluid can accumulate. The choice of agents is operator dependent, as each has pros and cons. Talc is inexpensive and readily available but has been associated with acute respiratory distress syndrome. Talc also forms a thick slurry and can occlude smaller-bore (No. 8 to 10 French) catheters. Bleomycin is slightly less effective and quite expensive. Doxycycline is relatively effective, inexpensive and available, and has therefore been the authors' agent of choice.[35]

For pleurodesis to be successful, the pleural space should be completely drained. Injecting a sclerosant into a persistent effusion can turn a simple effusion into a multiloculated effusion, often necessitating further intervention. Once adequate drainage is documented by imaging, 1% lidocaine is injected into the pleural space and intravenous analgesics administered before pleurodesis. The sclerosant (5 g talc in 100 mL normal saline, 500 mg doxycycline in 100 mL normal saline, 60 IU bleomycin in 100 mL 5% dextrose in water) is injected into the pleural space, the catheter is clamped, and the patient is instructed to change position every 15 minutes for 2 hours to distribute the agent in the pleural space. The tube is then reopened and removed when drainage is less than 100 mL/d.

Chemical pleurodesis is effective in 61% to 90% of patients but often requires prolonged hospitalization of 5 to 12 days to adequately drain the pleural space.[28,33,35] In a patient population with a median life expectancy of 6 to 12 months[28] and a 30-day mortality of 29% to 50%,[35] this may not be acceptable.

An alternate approach is to treat malignant pleural effusions with a long-term tunneled chest catheter (PleurX, Denver Biomedical, Golden, CO). This is a No. 15.5 French Silastic catheter with an airtight valve in the hub, allowing the catheter to remain in place indefinitely and be accessed for intermittent drainage using a vacuum bottle. These catheters can be placed on an outpatient basis with appropriate teaching, and intermittent drainage can be performed by the patient at home.

Mechanical pleurodesis is "spontaneously" achieved by almost 50% of patients at 30 days.[28]

To improve drainage of complex pleural collections, intrapleural lytic agents, including pharmacologic thrombolysis and urokinase, can be instilled into the pleural space. Thrombolytic agents promote enzymatic débridement of fibrinous septae in the pleural space and, when injected through a chest tube, can reestablish catheter patency and improve drainage of complex, multiloculated effusions and even empyema.[31,32]

BRONCHIAL STENTS

Patients with occlusion of the central airways by intrinsic tumor or extrinsic compression present with dyspnea and obstructive pneumonia and often have the sensation of impending suffocation.[36] When not amenable to resection, intraluminal malignant lesions can be effectively palliated bronchoscopically with laser ablation, electrocautery, brachytherapy, or photodynamic therapy. Placement of plastic or metallic stents is a useful adjuvant to reestablish and maintain airway patency in these cases, and it is the treatment of choice for endobronchial obstruction due to extrinsic compression.[36–38] In fact, 78% to 98% of patients stented can be expected to have immediate relief of respiratory symptoms related to central airway obstruction.[37]

As in the biliary tract, plastic stents have the advantage of being removable and replaceable but require rigid bronchoscopy for placement and are subject to occlusion by inspissated mucus or granulation tissue. Self-expanding metallic stents provide a larger lumen and can be placed via flexible bronchoscopy, but they are permanent.

Successful stent deployment requires a coordinated effort by a multidisciplinary team. CT with three-dimensional reconstruction is useful in determining the length and level of obstruction, as well as the anatomy of the airway. Flexible or rigid bronchoscopy is then performed (usually by a surgeon or pulmonologist) to confirm the imaging findings and provide access to the lesion. The scope is then removed over a guidewire in the side port and an angiographic catheter advanced central to the obstructing lesion. A self-expanding metallic stent is then advanced over the

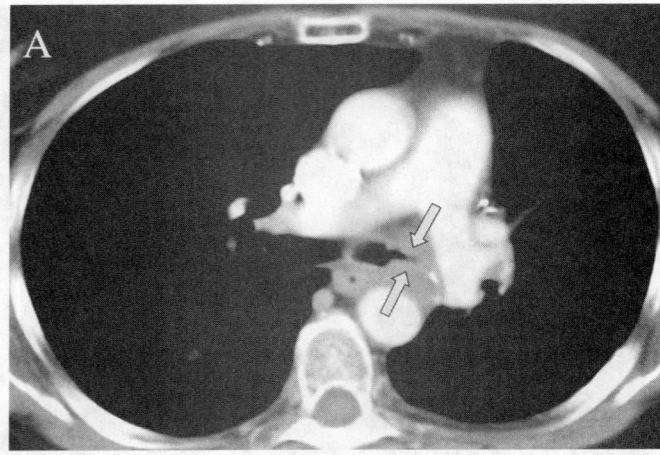

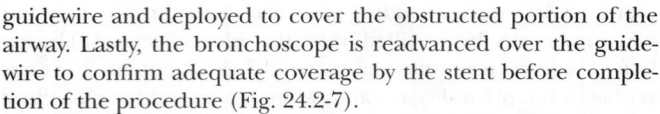

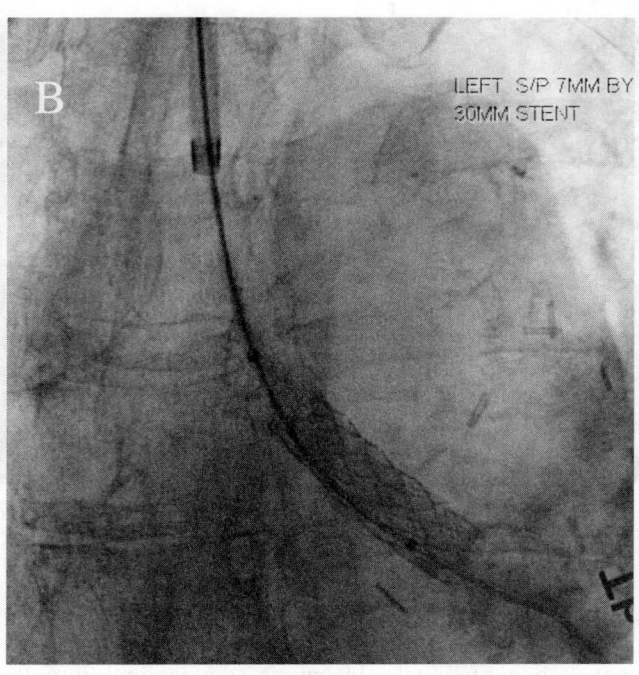

FIGURE 24.2-7. Bronchial stent. **A:** Short-segment obstruction of the left main-stem bronchus by metastatic lymph nodes from non–small cell lung carcinoma (*arrows*). **B:** Successful deployment of a stent across the obstruction performed in using a combination of flexible bronchoscopy and fluoroscopy. At last follow-up 4 months after stent placement, the patient remains asymptomatic from dyspnea.

guidewire and deployed to cover the obstructed portion of the airway. Lastly, the bronchoscope is readvanced over the guidewire to confirm adequate coverage by the stent before completion of the procedure (Fig. 24.2-7).

Long-term follow-up data are limited because the life expectancy of these patients is measured in weeks. Wood et al.[38] published Washington University's series of 53 patients stented for malignant disease, in whom 85% had adequate palliation with a mean follow-up of 4 months, with 28% requiring additional bronchoscopic procedures to reestablish stent patency. A study from Norway in which 14 patients were treated with endobronchial stents for malignant obstruction had a median survival of 11 weeks, with a range of 0.5 to 34.0 weeks.[35]

SUPERIOR VENA CAVA STENT

Malignant occlusion of the superior vena cava (SVC) is a common consequence of thoracic malignancies, most commonly lung cancer. Obstruction may be due to direct tumor involvement, extrinsic compression by tumor, or lymphadenopathy. Benign causes of SVC occlusion in cancer patients occur as well, most commonly as a result of malpositioned venous access devices.

Radiographic occlusion is often seen in patients with no clinical symptoms, due to abundant thoracic collateral channels predominantly draining into the azygous system or IVC. In such cases no treatment is indicated. In some patients, however, SVC obstruction is associated with the SVC syndrome, consisting of upper extremity and head and neck swelling, headache, mental status changes, and dyspnea.

In symptomatic patients, radiation for radiosensitive tumors has been the treatment of choice. Although this is often successful, it requires daily therapy for several weeks, and improvement occurs slowly over days to weeks. Recanalization of the SVC with balloon angioplasty or metallic stent, on the other hand, offers rapid and often dramatic relief of symptoms, typi-

cally within 24 hours. Although some success has been reported with angioplasty alone, the recurrence or failure rate after percutaneous transluminal angioplasty, particularly in patients with malignant obstruction, is quite high because of the elastic recoil that takes place secondary to the compressing tumor or fibrosis. Stent placement is the most durable method of reestablishing blood flow.

Contrast-enhanced chest CT is critical for procedure planning to define the level and length of obstruction. CT may also suggest the presence of acute thrombus, which may require thrombolysis before stenting. When venous access is also required (as is often the case in patients with cancer), an approach via the subclavian or internal jugular vein is preferred, and a venous access device is placed through the stent at the end the procedure. Alternatively, a transfemoral approach can be used. Once venography is performed the occlusion is crossed with a catheter and guidewire. If acute thrombus is present, pharmacologic thrombolysis (tPA, urokinase) is indicated before balloon dilation or stent placement to minimize the risk of procedure-related pulmonary embolism (PE) and stent occlusion by thrombus.

It is the authors' practice to place unilateral stents from the brachiocephalic vein of the punctured side to the high right atrium (Fig. 24.2-8). This is supported by a study by Dinkel et al.,[40] in which 84 patients with SVC syndrome underwent either unilateral or bilateral stenting (i.e., double-barreled stents into the SVC from both brachiocephalic veins) for malignant SVC syndrome. They found no difference in technical success or clinical response but a trend toward longer primary patency in the unilaterally stented group.[40]

Prestent angioplasty can be performed, and a self-expanding stent of appropriate diameter is then deployed across the occlusion. Technical success approaches 100%, and symptomatic relief is seen in 80% to 99%. Peri- and postprocedure anticoagulation is controversial and ranges from baby aspirin to full warfarin (Coumadin) anticoagulation for life.[39]

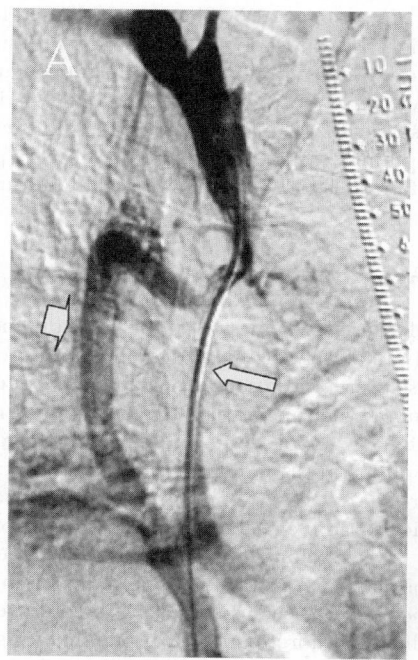

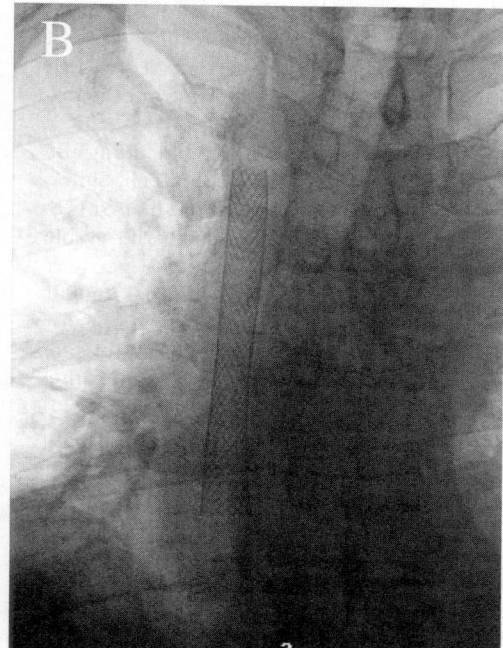

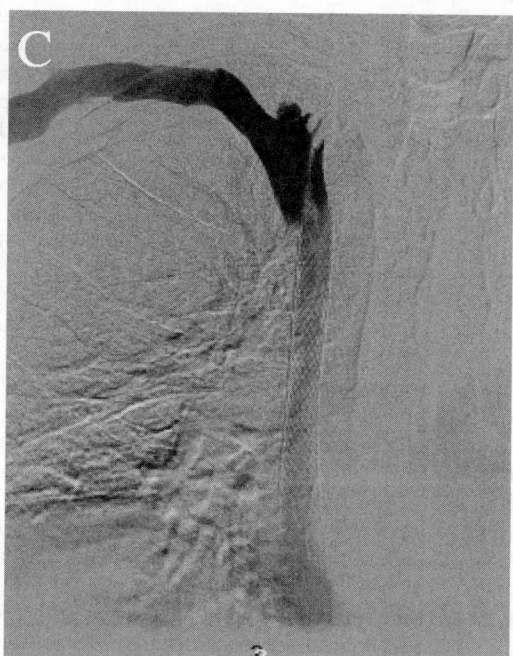

FIGURE 24.2-8. Superior vena cava (SVC) stent. **A:** Oblique venogram demonstrates an occluded SVC (*arrow*) and prominent azygos vein (*arrowhead*). **B:** Wall stent bridging SVC occlusion. **C:** Completion venography demonstrates recanalized SVC with no residual filling of the azygos vein.

Recurrent symptoms after successful stent placement suggest stent occlusion and should be evaluated with contrast chest CT. Common causes include tumor overgrowth, neointimal hyperplasia, and, rarely, stent migration. Recurrent obstruction can be treated with thrombolysis, balloon angioplasty, or repeat stenting.

INFERIOR VENA CAVA FILTERS

The association between venous thrombosis and malignancy has been known for more than a century. When venous thrombosis involves the deep system of the lower extremities anywhere from the IVC to the popliteal vein, the risk of PE is markedly increased.[41] Deep venous thrombosis (DVT) in the calves is not associated with PE and need not be treated unless symptomatic or propagating centrally.

In the United States, 550,000 cases of PE are diagnosed annually, nearly one-third of which are fatal. The incidence of PE in cancer patients is three times that of the general population. First-line treatment for DVT or PE is systemic anticoagulation. Indications for IVC filter placement include contraindication to anticoagulation (cerebrovascular accident, GI bleed, brain metastases), propagating thrombus or recurrent pulmonary thromboemboli despite anticoagulation, planned surgery, recent hemorrhage or stroke, and poor nutritional status. Free-floating IVC thrombus seen on CT or ultrasound is also a relative indication, as these types of thrombi have a high likelihood of becoming emboli. In such patients, mechanical filtration of the venous return from the pelvis and lower extremities is required to prevent PE.

Several IVC filters are commercially available, including the Greenfield stainless steel and titanium filters, Vena-Tech, Simon Nitinol, Bird's Nest, Trap-Ease, and Gunther Tulip. The first U.S. Food and Drug Administration–approved optionally retrievable filter, Recovery, has been introduced in the United States.

Filters can be deployed from a femoral or internal jugular approach. A jugular approach is preferred in most patients for several reasons. The vast majority (greater than 90%) of pulmonary emboli arise from lower extremity thrombi, and catheterization of the femoral vein not only risks dislodging a clot that is already present, but local thrombus develops after manual compression in 2% to 35%.[41] Also, after internal jugular puncture, patients remain in bed with the head elevated rather than flat for 4 hours, and they generally prefer this. Finally, if a venous access device is desired, it can be placed concurrently using the same puncture site.

A venogram is first performed to evaluate IVC anatomy, measure the diameter of the IVC, determine the location of the renal veins, and detect the presence of IVC thrombus. IVC anomalies occur uncommonly and include duplication (persistence of a left IVC draining into the left renal vein), interruption of the IVC, and left-sided IVC. In patients with extensive retroperitoneal tumor, the IVC may be occluded or too narrow for filter placement. In these patients, this effective interruption of the IVC serves as an "auto-filter," and no filter placement is indicated. Ideally, filters are placed immediately below the most caudal renal vein, but they can be placed in a suprarenal portion of the IVC if thrombus extends more centrally. Most filters are designed to be placed in vessels of 20 to 28 mm, and in the unusual case of a "mega-IVC," a Bird's Nest filter can be placed safely. Each filter has advantages and disadvantages, and selection of a specific filter often depends on the experience of the radiologist.

Complications of filter placement include nontarget placement, recurrent PE, IVC occlusion, migration, and access complications. The frequency of complications reported in the literature is difficult to interpret, as ranges of 3% to 69% for filter migration, 2% to 28% access site thrombosis, and 6% to 30% IVC occlusion are reported.[41,43] For more realistic numbers, a study of 1765 filters placed in 1731 patients over 26 years at the Massachusetts General Hospital was reported in 2000. In this large cohort, symptomatic IVC thrombosis occurred in 2.7% and recurrent PE in 5.6% (fatal in 3.7%).

An optionally retrievable IVC filter has been approved for use in the United States.[42] The term *optionally retrievable* refers to the fact that this filter can be removed up to 161 days after placement but also may function as a permanent filter if the contraindication to anticoagulation unexpectedly persists. This filter can provide short-term mechanical filtration for patients at high risk for PE and prevent the long-term complications associated with permanent filter placement. Indications include preoperative prophylaxis in high-risk patients who have no long-term contraindication to anticoagulation, protection during lower extremity or IVC thrombolysis, DVT in pregnancy, and trauma. An additional advantage is the ability to retrieve and reposition malpositioned filters after deployment. Currently, the Recovery is the only U.S. Food and Drug Administration–approved retrievable filter.

In summary, IVC filters are indicated for patients with, or at high risk for, DVT or PE and a contraindication to anticoagulation, propagation of DVT while anticoagulated, or free-floating IVC thrombosis. IVC filters reduce the risk of PE, but with an associated risk of IVC occlusion. With the recent addition of an optionally retrievable filter, the subset of patients who may benefit from short-term mechanical filtration will likely broaden.

ASCITES

Most ascites is due to liver disease, and medical management is the mainstay of therapy for this group of patients. Malignant ascites represents approximately 10% of cases and is most commonly seen in ovarian cancer. Because malignant ascites usually does not respond to chemotherapy, other treatment options must be considered. Many procedures aimed at controlling ascites are now in the armamentarium of the interventional radiologist, and more are no doubt forthcoming.

Large-volume paracentesis (LVP) is the most common means of managing refractory ascites. Safe drainage of up to 4 to 6 L per session seems relatively uncontroversial, and reports of draining more than 20 L at one time exist.[44,45] Although LVP is good for symptomatic relief, it requires patients to return repeatedly for the procedure, and each puncture is associated with a small but real risk of bleeding and infection. Concerns also exist regarding the loss of protein from the ascitic fluid.

Control of malignant ascites using percutaneously placed exteriorized catheters has been reported by several authors.[46–48] Nontunneled catheters are easily placed but have been reported to be associated with a high rate of infection and catheter-related sepsis. Tunneled catheters have been advocated by several authors and appear to provide effective relief for most patients.[48] The catheters are likely to be successfully managed by the patients and their families, although they do carry the psychosocial issues and physical constraints associated with other types of exteriorized catheters. As an alternative method for drainage, some authors advocate placement of subcutaneous peritoneal ports to provide access for intermittent drainage. Complications of catheter placement include infection, malfunction/occlusion, dislodgment, and loss of protein (as in repeated LVP).

The role of peritoneovenous shunting in the management of malignant ascites remains unclear. Potential benefits of shunting include the lack of repeated trips to a health care provider, lack of an exteriorized device, and reintroduction of the ascites volume and proteins into the circulation. Reports on the success and complications associated with the procedure are quite varied. A few reports have been published describing percutaneous placement of Denver (Denver Biomedical, Golden, CO) peritoneovenous shunts by interventional radiologists.[49] However, most reports come from the surgical literature. Reported complications include shunt malfunction from occlusion and disseminated intravascular coagulation. The occurrence of the latter appears to be reduced by completely draining the ascites at the time of shunt placement. Theoretical concern of decreasing survival by disseminating tumor cells in cases of malignant ascites has not been supported by the literature.

Transjugular intrahepatic portosystemic shunts (TIPS) have also been used to control ascites in patients with portal hypertension. TIPS is contraindicated in patients with encephalopathy or heart failure and is not well tolerated in poorly compensated cirrhosis. TIPS, in addition to medical therapy for ascites, has been shown to be superior to medical management alone. Compared with LVP, TIPS has been shown to lower the rate of ascites recurrence and the risk of developing hepatorenal syndrome, but with an increased incidence of encephalopathy due to portosystemic diversion of blood flow.

ABSCESS DRAINAGE

Percutaneous techniques have revolutionized the management of abdominal collections, and the "cure" rate is greater than 80% (where "cure" indicated complete drainage without the need for reoperation).[50] Postoperative collections may arise because of leaks (urinoma, biloma, bowel perforation, pancreatic leak), infection, and lymphatic obstruction (lymphocele, seroma). Indications for drainage include suspected infection, leak, symptoms from mass effect, and characterization of the fluid.

Abscesses almost always occur in the postoperative setting and are suspected clinically based on white cell count, fever, and pain. CT with oral and intravenous contrast is usually performed for diagnosis. Percutaneous drainage, when the collection is accessible, is the treatment of choice. However, it may not be possible in cases in which the collection is surrounded by bone or bowel, as in deep pelvic abscesses. Drainage catheters can be removed when output is less than 20 mL/24 hours and the collection has resolved, as demonstrated on CT or abscessogram, performed to exclude catheter malfunction.[51]

Postoperative urinomas result from injury to the renal collecting system from the kidney to the bladder or disrupted uretero-conduit anastomoses. Urine leaks are usually diagnosed by CT, and delayed images may clinch the diagnosis when high-density contrast is seen within the collection. Urinomas may be focal and mimic abscesses or diffuse, presenting as urinary ascites. They can be definitively diagnosed by sending a specimen from the collection for creatinine. Small urinomas often resorb spontaneously, but large or symptomatic collections usually require therapeutic drainage. Diversion of the urine upstream of the leak is often required in these cases, to allow the leak to seal. In the case of a renal collecting system, bladder, or conduit leak, nephrostomy catheters to external drainage are sufficient. In ureteral leaks, placement of a ureteral stent or nephroureterostomy (see Fig. 24.2-3) with side holes only in the renal pelvis and bladder can effectively divert the leak while allowing internal drainage and providing a mechanical scaffold around which the ureter can heal.

Bilomas are in the differential diagnosis of patients who have fever and rising bilirubin after hepatobiliary surgery. Like urinomas, they usually respond to catheter drainage. Diversion of bile may be necessary when leaking persists and may be accomplished with percutaneous biliary drainage or drainage through the biloma if the bile ducts can be visualized with contrast injection.

Drainage of collections resulting from injury to small or large bowel is often successful in resolving relatively small leaks. Once well drained, contrast injection is performed to demonstrate the site and size of the leak, as well as the residual cavity size. Small leaks from small bowel are more likely to heal without further surgical intervention, but the catheter may be required for several weeks.

Pancreatic leaks often result after partial pancreatectomy or ovarian cancer debulking and are more complicated to manage. Pancreatic leaks are often suspected before drainage and are confirmed by the presence of amylase in the aspirate more than three to five times serum amylase.[52] Before catheter removal in pancreatic leaks or pseudocysts, an abscessogram is performed to confirm resolution of the cavity, to evaluate for communication with the pancreatic duct, and, when present, to confirm adequate drainage into the duodenum.

EMBOLOTHERAPY FOR HEPATIC NEOPLASMS

The dual blood supply of the liver can be exploited to treat patients with either primary or secondary hepatic malignancies or, rarely, benign tumors. The hepatic artery provides very little blood flow to hepatic parenchyma, whereas it is the main source of blood supply for most hepatic tumors, even those that are "hypovascular." This allows a variety of agents to be injected into the hepatic artery to cause *in situ* tumor cell death. Some practitioners inject a combination of chemotherapeutic agent(s), ethiodized oil, and particles. For chemotherapy-responsive tumors, administering the chemotherapeutic agent directly into the liver may result in prolonged contact and higher concentrations of drug, with little to no systemic effect. Even in the case of HCC, for which there is no effective systemic chemotherapeutic agent, the higher concentration and prolonged contact might render HCC responsive to an agent that might be ineffective systemically. Early studies demonstrating higher concentration of doxorubicin within chemoembolized tumors were conducted on only a few patients.[53] More recent biodistribution studies suggest that the combination of doxorubicin, ethiodized oil, and an embolic agent results in the highest concentration of doxorubicin in the treated tumor, compared to infusing doxorubicin alone, or in combination with ethiodized oil.[55] *In vivo* and *in vitro* laboratory studies also suggest that ischemia promotes cellular uptake of a radiolabeled doxorubicin analogue, most likely secondary to reduced active transport of the analogue out of the cell.[54]

Hypervascular hepatic tumors are known to be sensitive to ischemia, and early treatment of such tumors was often by hepatic artery ligation alone. This has given rise to the practice of treating such tumors as HCC, metastatic neuroendocrine tumor, and other vascular metastases with particle embolization alone, relying on ischemia to effect cell death.[56,57] To this end, very small particles of polyvinyl alcohol are injected into the vessel supplying the tumor as selectively as possible, to cause terminal vessel blockade and cell death (Fig. 24.2-9). If the entire liver is to be treated for hypervascular metastases, a hemiliver is treated in each of two procedures. In the case of HCC and some vascular metastases for which there is no other treatment, the goal is to prolong survival. For patients with neuroendocrine tumor, control of symptoms is more commonly the end point. Embolotherapy may also be indicated for the control of pain in patients with bulky tumors.

A randomized controlled study from Spain demonstrated that chemoembolization combined with Gelfoam provided a significant survival benefit compared to conservative treatment.[58] The same study failed to demonstrate any significant difference between patients treated with chemoembolization and Gelfoam versus those embolized with Gelfoam alone at the time the study was stopped. To date there has been no study conclusively demonstrating a difference between any method of chemoembolization compared to particle embolization alone for prolonging survival in patients with HCC or for symptomatic treatment of

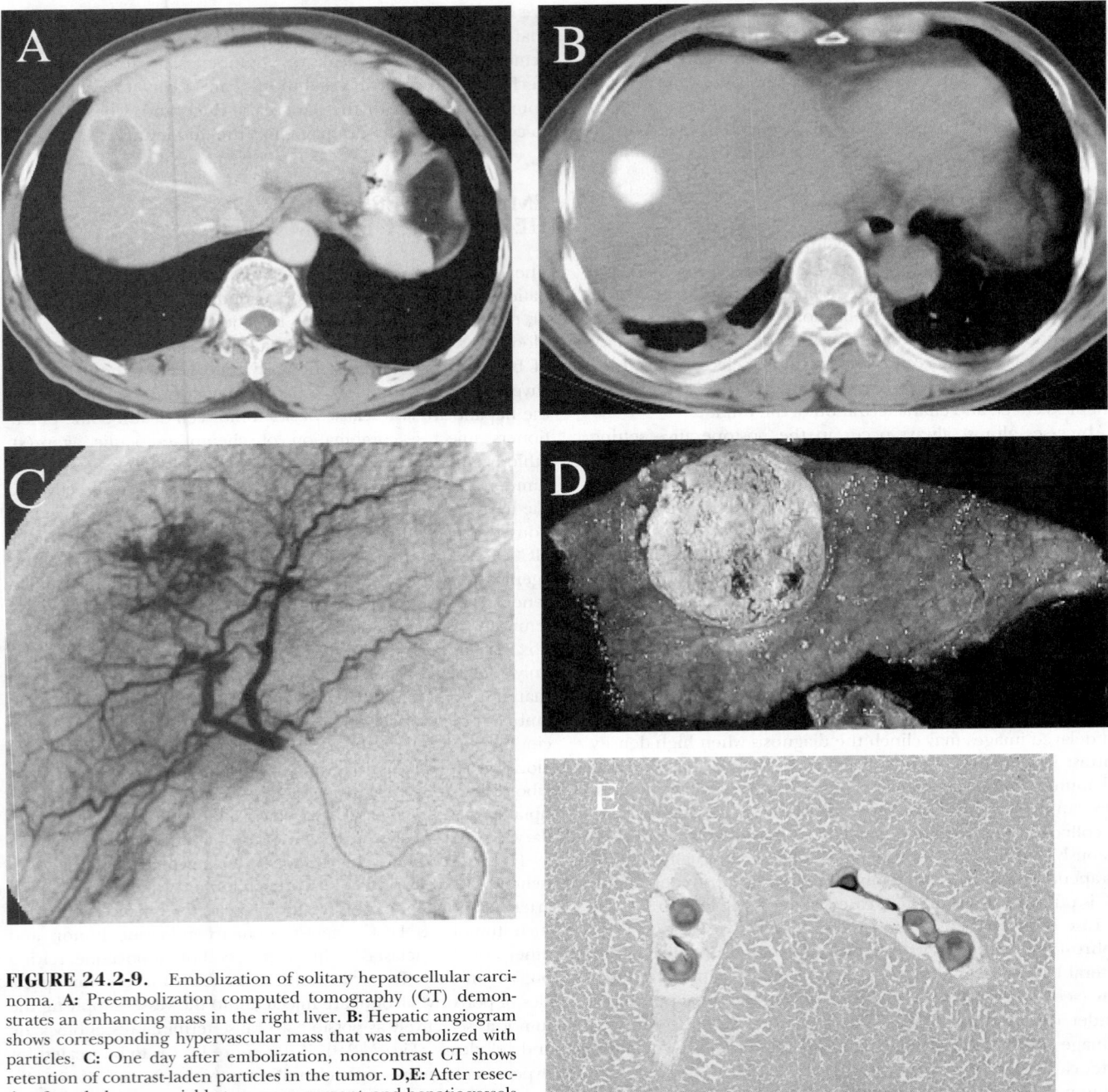

FIGURE 24.2-9. Embolization of solitary hepatocellular carcinoma. **A:** Preembolization computed tomography (CT) demonstrates an enhancing mass in the right liver. **B:** Hepatic angiogram shows corresponding hypervascular mass that was embolized with particles. **C:** One day after embolization, noncontrast CT shows retention of contrast-laden particles in the tumor. **D,E:** After resection 6 weeks later, no viable tumor was present, and hepatic vessels containing embospheres were identified in the background of necrosis. (See Color Figs. 24.2-9D and 24.2-9E in the CD-ROM.)

patients with metastatic neuroendocrine tumor. Particle embolization does not require the addition of chemotherapeutic agents or ethiodized oil and is therefore easier to perform, is less expensive, and does not expose the patient to any systemic side effects from chemotherapy. Of the two methods, chemoembolization would be expected to be more effective than particle embolization for patients with the more typical "hypovascular" metastatic lesions as seen with colorectal cancer and pancreatic cancer, for example. Postembolization syndrome consisting of pain, fever, nausea, and vomiting is seen to some degree with all methods and is usually self-limited.

TUMOR ABLATION

Although surgical resection is the treatment of choice for HCC, many tumors are either too advanced when diagnosed or occur in a background of cirrhosis that might be severe enough to preclude surgical resection. In areas where hepatitis B and C are endemic, the incidence of disease is quite high, so that even if the percentage of resectable patients were increased by screening, the costs of surgical resection would severely strain the health care system. Combining these facts with the understanding that, although the 5-year survival after resection is approximately 50%, the dis-

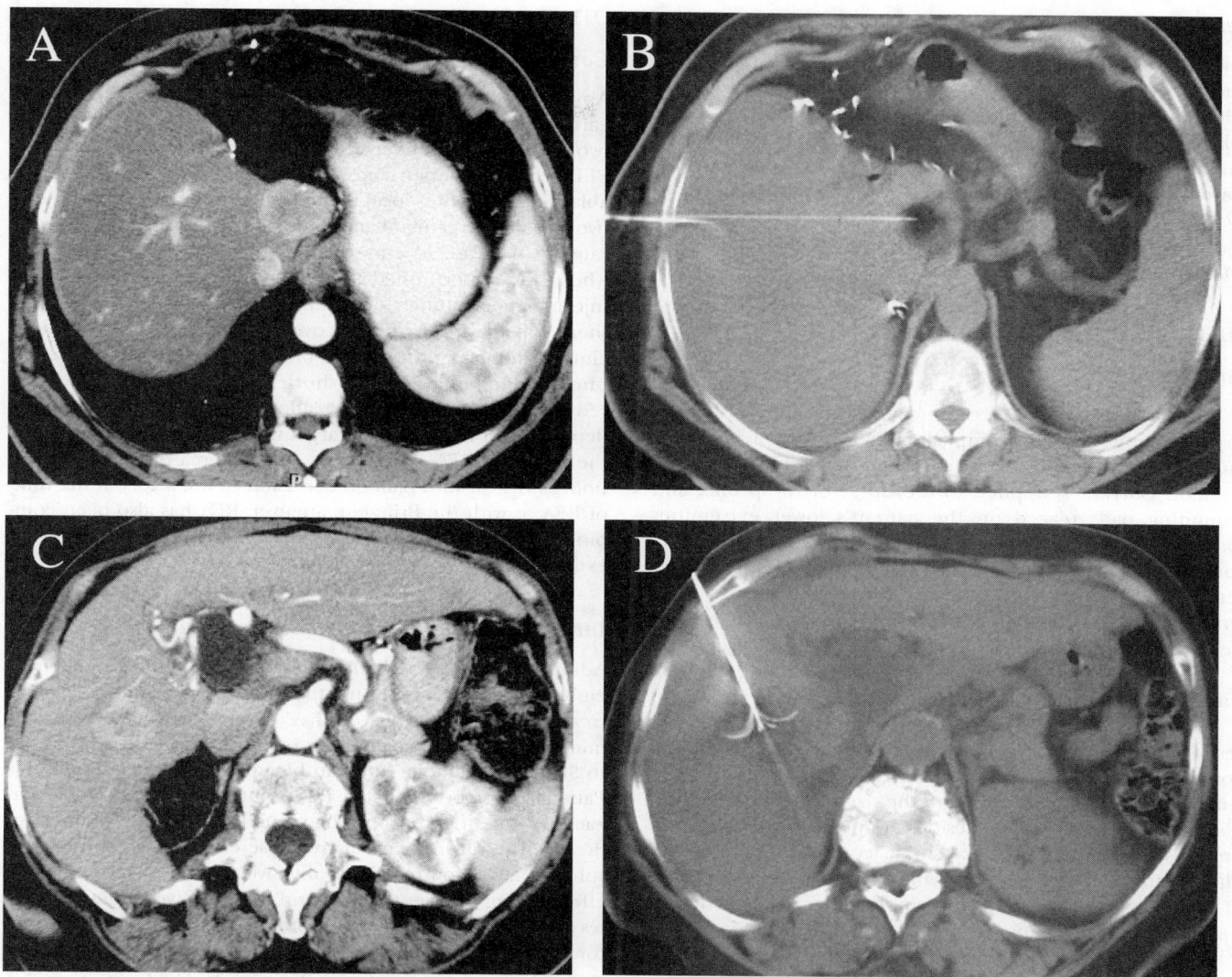

FIGURE 24.2-10. Tumor ablation. **A:** Hepatocellular carcinoma (HCC) recurrence in the caudate after left hepatectomy. **B:** Ethanol injection into the tumor shows good dispersion within the lesion but not in the surrounding liver. **C:** Solitary focus of HCC in a patient with Child's B cirrhosis. **D:** Radiofrequency probe centered in lesion.

ease-free 5-year survival is only approximately 20%, it is appropriate to think of HCC as a chronic disease that may require treatment other than surgical resection. Embolotherapy is the mainstay in patients with high-volume disease. For patients with one to three small lesions (less than 5 cm), percutaneous ablative therapies have been devised. Some of these ablative treatments can be applied to other hepatic neoplasms or, in the case of thermal ablation, even be used outside of the liver.

CHEMICAL ABLATION

Percutaneous Ethanol Injection Treatment

Absolute ethanol causes cell dehydration and denaturation as well as small vessel occlusion, presumably because of endothelial damage. Percutaneous ethanol injection (PEI) gained popularity in 1995, when Livraghi et al.[59] published a study of 746 patients with HCC that demonstrated survival results comparable to those of surgical resection. Small HCC tumors are particu-

larly well suited to PEI, as the typical HCC is a "soft" tumor occurring in the background of cirrhosis that results in a "hard" liver. This, coupled with the fact that many small HCC tumors are encapsulated, promotes the containment and uniform distribution of ethanol throughout the lesion.[60]

PEI is indicated for the treatment of HCC in patients with one to three tumors that are less than 5 cm in diameter. Ethanol toxicity may occur in the case of patients with larger tumors, as the intent is to inject a volume of ethanol equal to the volume of the tumor. In larger tumors, it is often difficult to effect uniform distribution of ethanol, and it is likely that the larger tumors have less favorable biology of disease. Ethanol is not effective for most metastatic liver lesions, as these tend to be hard tumors occurring in normal, noncirrhotic or soft livers, and the ethanol leaks back along the needle tract rather than penetrating the tumor. Radiofrequency ablation (RFA) has been shown to be more effective than PEI for small HCC and requires fewer treatments; however, PEI may still be indicated for tumors in locations that might not be amenable to thermal ablation (Fig. 24.2-10).

Percutaneous Acetic Acid Treatment

Several limitations of ethanol injection have prompted the study of other agents for chemical ablation. A variety of direct cellular toxins as well as more sophisticated chemotherapeutic gels have been investigated. Acetic acid was believed to be an attractive alternative to ethanol because of its ability to break down collagen, potentially allowing for better penetration into the tumor and thereby reducing the volume and the number of treatment sessions required to effect complete necrosis.[61] This agent is in use in many centers today.

THERMAL ABLATION

Radiofrequency Ablation

RFA involves using heat to cause coagulation necrosis in the target tissue.[62] This is accomplished by inserting a 17- to 15-gauge probe with an insulated shaft and noninsulated tip into a tumor. Current is applied to the tip(s) of the probe, and grounding pads placed on the patient's lower extremities complete the electrical circuit. Ionic agitation causes frictional heating at the probe tip(s), and with temperatures between 60°C and 90°C, coagulation necrosis ensues. Currently, the largest diameter necrotic lesion that can be created with a single probe is approximately 7 cm. Larger areas of necrosis can theoretically be created by heating overlapping spheres of tissue.

The main problem with the application of RFA is the limited size of coagulation necrosis that is achievable, presuming from the application of surgical experience that our goal is to cause an area of necrosis equal to the size of the lesion, plus a 0.5- to 1.0-cm margin. Some lesions are positioned adjacent to large vessels that serve as "heat sinks," continually cooling the adjacent tumor as RF energy is being applied, precluding cellular death along the "cooled" margin. In other cases the lesion might be adjacent to another structure that we do not wish to damage, such as the pancreas, colon, heart, or a major nerve (see Fig. 24.2-10).

Not only has RF ablation been used to treat tumors within the liver,[63] it has also been used to treat tumors in the lung, adrenal gland, kidney, and pelvis, as well as metastatic lesions in bone. Lung tumors are particularly well suited to RFA because the surrounding lung acts as an insulator and concentrates the RF energy within the tumor. The majority of patients with primary and secondary lung tumors are not operative candidates, and RF may play an important cytoreductive role in these patients. As adrenalectomy is being considered for some patients with metastatic lung cancer, one might consider using RFA instead, if indeed some benefit is found from surgical adrenalectomy.

With the increasing use of cross-sectional imaging for medical care as well as screening, the kidney has been found to be the site of many incidentally discovered masses. In older patients, or patients with comorbidities, the standard of care, which is total or partial nephrectomy, may not be warranted. Although treating centrally located tumors can be problematic, lesions that are peripheral or exophytic are amenable to RFA. Recurrent malignancy within the pelvis is not uncommon, and RFA may have a palliative role here, in selected patients, for local control of tumor.

OTHER ABLATIVE METHODS

Combination Therapy

Any of the minimally invasive treatment methods described earlier can be used conjunctively with one another.[64–66] The two methods we routinely use together are embolotherapy with PEI or embolotherapy and RFA. The biggest problem with any ablative treatment is local recurrence. It follows that the use of two different treatment methods may reduce the recurrence rate. In the case of embolotherapy and PEI, we found that when PEI was performed after embolotherapy it was possible to inject higher volumes of ethanol into the target tumor, and there appeared to be better coverage than when PEI was used alone. Embolizing the arterial blood supply to a hypervascular tumor might be expected to shorten treatment time for RFA by reducing the heat sink and allowing for immediate direct deposition of heat into the target tissue. It might also enhance the effects of RFA, resulting in a larger area of tissue destruction, as is seen with balloon occlusion of the artery at the time of RFA or with the Pringle maneuver. RFA has also been combined with PEI in a rat model, resulting in an increase in the extent of coagulation necrosis.[67]

Intraarterial Delivery of Radiopharmaceutical

Administering local radiation therapy by injecting radiolabeled embolic agent is another treatment option that can be used to treat virtually any type of liver tumor. Yttrium 90–labeled microspheres are beta-emitting microspheres that measure 20 to 30 μm in diameter and can be administered intraarterially. Patients must be evaluated for shunting to the lungs before each treatment and cannot be treated if their total pulmonary dose will result in a cumulative dose exceeding 30 Gy. These spheres have a low toxicity profile, with the most common side effects being transient nausea and fatigue. Liver function studies are transiently elevated, as with embolization, and GI symptoms may occur if there is inadvertent deposition of particles into the gastric or gastroduodenal arteries. The response rate is approximately 20%, with mean duration of response of 127 weeks and median time to progression of 44 weeks. Outpatient treatment is feasible, because beta radiation does not require medical confinement.

EMERGING THERAPIES AND FUTURE DIRECTIONS

The field of interventional radiology has undergone several metamorphoses since its inception almost 30 years ago, when Charles Dotter performed the first percutaneous dilation of a superficial femoral stenosis in a patient who had refused amputation. Minimally invasive image-guided techniques have replaced many open surgical procedures and provide new options for patients with previously untreatable diseases.

Progress continues, and many new and exciting techniques are emerging. Gene therapy is a promising new tool based on the transfer of genetic material to a target cell population. Preclinical and clinical studies in the treatment of liver metastases in which viral vectors containing either a "suicide gene" or corrective copies of a defective gene are injected directly into the hepatic artery or portal vein to reverse the malignant phenotype and induce apoptosis or growth arrest of tumor cells are being investigated.[68] The role of interventional radiology is not only to provide access for local delivery but in the development of maximally effective delivery systems.

Chemotherapy containing liposomes, including new "stealth" liposomes that evade destruction by the immune system, are currently in clinical trials for the treatment of melanoma, breast carcinoma, ovarian carcinoma, and acquired immunodeficiency syndrome–related Kaposi's sarcoma. Currently delivered systemically, catheter-directed delivery has the potential to maximize pharmacokinetics and minimize systemic toxicity.

In addition to novel treatment strategies, future trends in interventional radiology promise to include more effective and efficient ways to perform current procedures. Robots with arms and wrists have allowed complex open surgical procedures, including coronary artery bypass graft and hepatic resection, to be performed through tiny incisions and have facilitated surgical procedures on newborns and fetuses. The development of robotics has promised to revolutionize the field of surgery in replacing open surgical procedures with minimally invasive ones and developing entirely new procedures to treat disease. In the arena of interventional radiology, where essentially all procedures are "minimally invasive," robotics can be used to improve accuracy of needle placement when performing a biopsy, RFA, or targeted access to an organ or vessel.

A precursor to robotics includes an electromagnetic targeting system based on the global positioning system, which is commercially available for CT and for ultrasound. Using a sensor on a needle in a weak magnetic field, the exact position and orientation of a needle with respect to the target are displayed on a monitor in multiple planes, facilitating and optimizing needle placement.

REFERENCES

1. Westcott JL, Rao N, Colley DP. Transthoracic needle biopsy of small pulmonary nodules. *Radiology* 1997;202:97.
2. Schwartz LH, Ginsberg MS, Burt BE, et al. MRI as an alternative to CT-guided biopsy of adrenal masses in patients with lung cancer. *Ann Thorac Surg* 1998;65:193.
3. Dodd LG, Mooney EE, Layfield LJ, et al. Fine-needle aspiration of the liver and pancreas: a cytology primer for radiologists [Review]. *Radiology* 1997;203:1.
4. Savader SJ, Prescott CA, Lund GB, et al. Intraductal biliary biopsy: comparison of three techniques. *J Vasc Interv Radiol* 1996;7:743.
5. Phillips MS, Silverman SG, Cibas ES, et al. Negative predictive value of imaging-guided abdominal biopsy results: cytologic classification and implications for patient management. *AJR Am J Roentgenol* 1998;171:693.
6. Reeves AR, Shashadri R, Terotola SO. Recent trends in central venous catheter placement: a comparison of interventional radiology with other specialties. *J Vasc Interv Radiol* 2001;12:1211.
7. Gandhi RT, Getrajdman GI, Brown KT, et al. Placement of subcutaneous chest wall ports ipsilateral to axillary lymph node dissection. *J Vasc Interv Radiol* 2003;14:1063.
8. Gauderer MW, Ponsky JL, Izant RJ. Gastrostomy without laparotomy: a percutaneous endoscopic technique. *J Pediatr Surg* 1980;15:872.
9. Preshaw RM. A percutaneous method for inserting a feeding gastrostomy tube. *Surg Gynecol Obstet* 1981;152:659.
10. Trost DW, Titton R, Khilnani NM, et al. Radiologic placement of pull-type gastrostomies. *Cardiovasc Intervent Radiol* 2001;24:s175.
11. Jones VW. Percutaneous gastrostomy: is it a time to change direction? *Cardiovasc Intervent Radiol* 2001;24:s175.
12. Ozmen MN, Akhan O. Percutaneous radiologic gastrostomy [Review]. *Eur J Radiol* 2002;43:186.
13. Lee SH. The role of oesophageal stenting in the non-surgical management of oesophageal strictures [Review]. *Br J Radiol* 2001;74:891.
14. Abadal JM, Echenagusia A, Simo G, et al. Treatment of malignant esophagorespiratory fistulas with covered stents [Review]. *Abdom Imaging* 2001;26:565.
15. Morino M, Bertello A, Garbarini A, et al. Malignant colonic obstruction managed by endoscopic stent decompression followed by laparoscopic resections. *Surg Endosc* 2002;16:1483.
16. Spies JB, Rosen RJ, Lebowitz AS. Antibiotic prophylaxis in vascular and interventional radiology: a rational approach. *Radiology* 1988;166:381.
17. Farrell TA, Wallace M, Hicks ME. Long-term results of transrenal ureteral occlusion with use of Gianturco coils and gelatin sponge pledgets. *J Vasc Interv Radiol* 1997;8:449.
18. Schild HH, Gunther R, Thelen M. Transrenal ureteral occlusion: results and problems. *J Vasc Interv Radiol* 1994;5:321.
19. Yagi S, Goto T, Lee SU, et al. Long-term results of percutaneous balloon dilation for ureterointestinal anastomotic strictures. *Int J Urol* 2002;9:241.
20. Bierkens AF, Oosterhof GO, Meuleman EJ, et al. Anterograde percutaneous treatment of ureterointestinal strictures following urinary diversion. *Eur Urol* 1996;30:363.
21. Gores GJ. Cholangiocarcinoma: current concepts and insights. *Hepatology* 2003;37:961.
22. Sudan D, DeRoover A, Chinnakotla S, et al. Radiochemotherapy and transplantation allow long-term survival for unresectable hilar cholangiocarcinoma. *Am J Transplant* 2002;2:774.
23. Khan SA, Davidson BR, Goldin R, et al. Guidelines for the diagnosis and treatment of cholangiocarcinoma: consensus document. *Gut* 2002;51:VII-9.
24. Jung GS, Huh JD, Lee SU, et al. Bile duct: analysis of percutaneous transluminal forceps biopsy in 130 patients suspected of having malignant biliary obstruction. *Radiology* 2002;224:725.
25. Cope C. Percutaneous cholecystostomy. In: Baum S, Pentecost MA, eds. *Abrams' angiography: vol 3. Interventional radiology*, 4th ed. Boston: Little, Brown and Company, 1997:485.
26. Byrne MF, Suhocki P, Mitchell RM, et al. Percutaneous cholecystostomy in patients with acute cholecystitis: experience of 45 patients at a US referral center. *J Am Coll Surg* 2003;197:206.
27. Blumgart LH, Fong Y, eds. *Surgery of the liver and biliary tract*. New York: Saunders; 2002.
28. Pollak JS, Burdge CM, Rosenblatt M, et al. Treatment of malignant pleural effusions with tunneled long-term drainage catheters. *J Vasc Interv Radiol* 2001;12:201.
29. Parulekar W, DiPrimio G, Matzinger F, et al. Use of small-bore vs. large-bore chest tubes for treatment of malignant pleural effusions. *Chest* 2001;120:19.
30. Tattersall DJ, Traill C, Gleeson FV. Chest drains: does size matter? *Clin Radiol* 2000;55:415.
31. Jerjes-Sanchez C, Ramirez-Rivera A, Elizalde JJ, et al. Intrapleural fibrinolysis with streptokinase as an adjunctive treatment in hemothorax and empyema: a multicenter trial. *Chest* 1996;109:1514.
32. Erickson KV, Wost M, Bynoe R, et al. Primary treatment of malignant pleural effusions: video-assisted thoracoscopic surgery poudrage vs. tube thoracostomy. *Am Surg* 2002;68:955.
33. Colt HG. Thoracoscopic management of malignant pleural effusions [Review]. *Clin Chest Med* 1995;16:505.
34. Patz EF, McAdams P, Erasmus JJ, et al. Sclerotherapy for malignant pleural effusions: a prospective randomized trial of bleomycin vs. doxycycline with small-bore catheter drainage. *Chest* 1998;113:1305.
35. Vonk-Noordegraaf A, Postmus PE, Sutedja TG. Tracheobronchial stenting in the terminal care of cancer patients with central airways obstruction. *Chest* 2001;120:1811.
36. Monnier P, Mudry A, Stanzel F, et al. The use of the covered Wallstent for the palliative treatment of inoperable tracheobronchial cancers: a prospective, multicenter study. *Chest* 1996;110:1161.
37. Seijo LM, Sterman DH. Interventional pulmonology. *N Engl J Med* 2001;344:740.
38. Wood DE, Liu YH, Vallieres E. Airway stenting for malignant and benign tracheobronchial stenosis. *Ann Thorac Surg* 2003;76:167.
39. Chatziioannou A, Mourikis AD, Dardoufas K, et al. Stent therapy for malignant superior vena cava syndrome: should be first line therapy or simple adjunct to radiotherapy? *Eur J Radiol* 2003;47:247.
40. Dinkel HP, Mettke B, Schmid F, et al. Endovascular treatment of malignant superior vena cava syndrome: is bilateral wallstent placement superior to unilateral placement? *J Endovasc Ther* 2003;10:788.
41. Kinney TB. Update on inferior vena cava filters. *J Vasc Interv Radiol* 2003;14:425.
42. Brountzos EN, Kaufman JA, Venbrux AC, et al. A new optional vena cava filter: retrieval at 12 weeks in an animal model. *J Vasc Interv Radiol* 2003;14:763.
43. Kercher K, Sing RF. Overview of current inferior vena cava filters. *Am Surg* 2003;69:643.
44. Yu AS, Hu K. Management of ascites [Review]. *Clin Liver Dis* 2001;5:541.
45. Zervos EE, Rosemurgy AS. Management of medically refractory ascites [Review]. *Am J Surg* 2001;181:256.
46. Barnett TD, Rubins J. Placement of a permanent tunneled peritoneal drainage catheter for palliation in malignant ascites: a simplified approach. *J Vasc Interv Radiol* 2002;13:379.
47. O'Neill MJ, Weissleder R, Gervais DA, et al. Tunneled peritoneal catheter placement under sonographic and fluoroscopic guidance in the palliative treatment of malignant ascites. *AJR Am J Roentgenol* 2001;177:615.
48. Richard HM, Coldwell DM, Boyd-Kranis RL, et al. Pleurx tunneled catheter in the management of malignant ascites. *J Vasc Interv Radiol* 2001;12:373.
49. Park JS, Won JY, Park SI, et al. Percutaneous peritoneovenous shunt creation for the treatment of benign and malignant refractory ascites. *J Vasc Interv Radiol* 2001;12:1445.
50. Bakal CW, Sacks D, Burke DR, et al. Quality improvement guidelines for adult percutaneous abscess and fluid drainage. *J Vasc Interv Radiol* 2003;14:S223.
51. Maher MM, Kealey S, McNamara A, et al. Management of visceral interventional radiology catheters: a troubleshooting guide for interventional radiologists [Review]. *Radiographics* 2002;22:305.
52. Hashimoto N, Ohyanagi H. Pancreatic juice output and amylase level in the drainage fluid after pancreatoduodenectomy in relation to leakage. *Hepatogastroenterology* 2002;49:553.

53. Nakamura H, Hashimoto T, Oi H, et al. Transcatheter oily chemoembolization of hepatocellular carcinoma. *Radiology* 1989;170:783.

54. Kruskal JB, Hlatky L, Hahnfeldt P, et al. In vivo and in vitro analysis of the effectiveness of doxorubicin combined with temporary arterial occlusion in liver tumors. *J Vasc Interv Radiol* 1993;4:741.

55. Raoul JL, Heresbach D, Bretagne JF, et al. Chemoembolization of hepatocellular carcinomas. A study of the biodistribution and pharmacokinetics of doxorubicin. *Cancer* 1992;70:585.

56. Brown KT, Nevins AB, Getrajdman GI, et al. Particle embolization for hepatocellular carcinoma. *J Vasc Interv Radiol* 1998;9:822.

57. Brown KT, Koh BY, Brody LA, et al. Particle embolization of hepatic metastases for control of pain and hormonal symptoms. *J Vasc Interv Radiol* 1999;10:397.

58. Llovet JM, Real MI, Montana X, et al. Arterial embolization or chemoembolization versus symptomatic treatment in patients with unresectable hepatocellular carcinoma: a randomized controlled trial. *Lancet* 2002;359:1734.

59. Livraghi T, Giorgio A, Marin G, et al. Hepatocellular carcinoma and cirrhosis in 746 patients: long-term results of percutaneous ethanol injection. *Radiology* 1995;197:101.

60. Livraghi T, Goldberg SN, Lazzaroni S, et al. Small hepatocellular carcinoma: treatment with radio-frequency ablation versus ethanol injection. *Radiology* 1999;210:655.

61. Ohnishi K, Nomura F, Ito S, et al. Prognosis of small hepatocellular carcinoma (less than 3 cm) after percutaneous acetic acid injection: study of 91 cases. *Hepatology* 1996;23:994.

62. Goldberg SN, Dupuy DE. Image-guided radiofrequency tumor ablation: challenges and opportunities—Part I[Review]. *J Vasc Interv Radiol* 2001;12:1021.

63. Giorgio A, Tarantino L, de Stefano G, et al. Percutaneous sonographically guided saline-enhanced radiofrequency ablation of hepatocellular carcinoma. *AJR Am J Roentgenol* 2003;181:479.

64. Kitamoto M, Imagawa M, Yamada H, et al. Radiofrequency ablation in the treatment of small hepatocellular carcinomas: comparison of the radiofrequency effect with and without chemoembolization. *AJR Am J Roentgenol* 2003;181:997.

65. Dupuy DE, Goldberg SN. Image-guided radiofrequency tumor ablation: challenges and opportunities—Part II. *J Vasc Interv Radiol* 2001;12:1135.

66. Tanaka K, Nakamura S, Numata K, et al. The long term efficacy of combined transcatheter arterial embolization and percutaneous ethanol injection in the treatment of patients with large hepatocellular carcinoma and cirrhosis. *Cancer* 1998;82:78.

67. Goldberg SN, Kruskal JB, Oliver BS, et al. Percutaneous tumor ablation: increased coagulation by combining radio-frequency ablation and ethanol instillation in a rat breast model. *Radiology* 2000;217:827.

68. Prieto J, Herraiz M, Sangro B, et al. The promise of gene therapy in gastrointestinal and liver diseases[Review]. *Gut* 2003;52 [Suppl 2]:ii49.

CHAPTER 25

Cancer Diagnosis: Endoscopy

SECTION **1**   IRVING WAXMAN

Gastrointestinal Endoscopy

Recent advances in endoscopic technology and devices have led to a wide variety of new and exciting applications for endoscopy and minimally invasive endoscopic surgical procedures. Endoscopic ultrasound (EUS) has become the most accurate imaging modality for local-regional cancer staging of the gastrointestinal (GI) tract. Reorientation of the ultrasound transducer on the echoendoscope now allows for fine-needle aspiration (FNA) capabilities, leading to increased diagnostic accuracy in cancer staging. Self-expandable metal stents (SEMSs) are now available for endoscopic palliation of GI or biliary obstruction due to cancer. Endoscopic mucosal resection offers the potential for an exciting alternative to surgery in the treatment of early neoplastic lesions of the luminal GI tract as well as difficult colonic sessile lesions. In the pancreaticobiliary arena, EUS and magnetic resonance cholangiopancreatography offer noninvasive, minimal-risk alternatives to diagnostic endoscopic retrograde cholangiopancreatography (ERCP).

UPPER ENDOSCOPY

Upper esophagogastroduodenoscopy (EGD) remains today the best diagnostic method to evaluate pathology of the upper GI (UGI) tract. In addition to providing high-quality luminal and mucosal video imaging, its strength over any other noninvasive imaging modalities remains in its tissue-sampling capabilities, providing a tissue diagnosis either by forceps biopsy, brush cytology, or in combination. Upper endoscopy requires only mild sedation, is safe, and is well tolerated by the majority of patients. Recent advances in endoscope technology, and in particular in miniaturization of the charge couple device has led to the development of ultra-thin endoscopes (5 mm), allowing for unsedated transnasal or oral endoscopy.[1]

EGD remains the procedure of choice when suspecting a UGI malignancy, evaluating iron deficiency anemia after a negative colonoscopy, follow-up of an abnormal radiologic finding, or screening individuals at high risk for a UGI neoplastic process, that is, Barrett's esophagus, familial adenomatous polyposis (FAP), pernicious anemia, or partial gastrectomy and alarm signs (pain, weight loss, iron deficiency anemia, early satiety). It is also indicated in combination with EUS to document response to a particular treatment regimen, as in the case of *Helicobacter pylori*–associated mucosa-associated lymphoid tissue lymphoma.[2] Although controversy remains about the effectiveness and economic impact of screening and surveillance for preneoplastic or neoplastic changes in high-risk individuals, the current recommendations from the American Society of Gastrointestinal Endoscopy[3] are as stated in the following sections.

CAUSTIC INGESTION

The risk of developing esophageal cancer in patients with a history of caustic ingestion is well documented and is estimated to be approximately 1000 times greater than that of the general population.[4] The mean age at onset is the mid-40s, with a mean of 40 years after the ingestion.[4,5] The American Society of Gastrointestinal Endoscopy recommends endoscopic surveillance 15 to 20 years after caustic ingestion. The frequency and interval after the first examination are not well studied.

TYLOSIS

Patients with tylosis, a rare autosomal dominant condition characterized by yellow hyperkeratosis or thickening of palms and soles, carry a greater than 90% risk of developing squamous cell carcinoma of the esophagus by age 65.[6] Current recommendations suggest starting endoscopic surveillance at age 30. The frequency of subsequent examinations is not well studied. Intervals of up to 3 years are probably adequate.

BARRETT'S ESOPHAGUS

Although the true incidence of adenocarcinoma in Barrett's esophagus remains controversial, the fact that it is a major risk factor remains uncontested. Lack of accurate surrogate markers makes endoscopic surveillance with a biopsy protocol the procedure of choice. Because high-grade dysplasia and cancer in Barrett's esophagus can be multifocal and microinvasive, extensive random biopsies should be performed during surveillance endoscopy.[7] Currently, the most accepted protocol involves four-quadrant biopsies taken at 2-cm intervals, starting 1 cm below the esophagogastric junction and extending 1 cm above the squamocolumnar junction.[8] Patients over the age of 40 with long-standing gastroesophageal reflux disease should have a once-in-a-lifetime EGD to rule out Barrett's esophagus. If it is present, manifested by the presence of specialized intestinal metaplasia, surveillance should be performed every 3 to 5 years. In patients with low-grade dysplasia, EGD should be performed every 6 months for a year and, if the patient's condition is stable, every year. For high-grade dysplasia, two alternatives are proposed: intensive endoscopic surveillance until intramucosal carcinoma is detected or esophagectomy.[9] The finding of dysplasia in Barrett's epithelium should always be corroborated by a second experienced GI pathologist.[10]

FAMILIAL ADENOMATOUS POLYPOSIS AND OTHER VARIANTS OF POLYPOSIS SYNDROMES

Duodenal and gastric polyps may occur in 33% to 100% of patients with FAP.[11,12] Although the risk of malignancy in colonic adenomas is well established, the natural history of UGI adenomas is less well understood. However, the most common cause of death in FAP patients after colon cancer is excluded is adenocarcinoma from a UGI adenoma, in particular in the periampullary area.[13] Current recommendations for surveillance, although its efficacy remains to be demonstrated, involve an index upper endoscopy with a forward and side-viewing endoscope (which allows *en face* visualization of the periampullary region) at the time of colectomy to detect the presence of UGI adenomas. If negative, the examination should be repeated in 3 to 5 years. In patients with periampullary adenomas, surveillance should be performed at 1- to 3-year intervals. Lesions with low-grade dysplasia should have more frequent surveillance and, if disease is stable, be returned to "standard" surveillance. In patients with high-grade dysplasia of the periampullary region, surgical consultation should be obtained.[3]

Gastric Polyps

The majority of gastric polyps are incidentally found and are hyperplastic in nature. Gastric adenomatous polyps are premalignant, and the risk of cancer transformation is size dependent.[14,15] Some studies have suggested that the gastric mucosa in patients with ade-

nomatous polyps is at an increased risk for gastric cancer.[16] Current recommendations include sampling of small polyps and performing polypectomy in symptomatic polyps or lesions of 2 cm in size. If adenomas are present, sampling any surface abnormalities of the remaining gastric mucosa is indicated. One-year follow-up endoscopy is indicated after adenoma resection to rule out recurrence. If negative, surveillance at 3- to 5-year intervals is justified.

Pernicious Anemia

The standardized incidence of gastric cancer is approximately three times normal in patients with autoimmune pernicious anemia.[17] Nevertheless, the role of surveillance endoscopy remains controversial because of the lack of evidence-based data. The American Society of Gastrointestinal Endoscopy recommends a single index endoscopy to identify prevalent lesions (carcinoid tumors, gastric cancer), but there are insufficient data to support subsequent surveillance.[3]

Partial Gastrectomy

A history of a partial gastrectomy, whether for benign or malignant disease, is definitively associated with an increased risk of developing cancer in the remaining gastric stump. The risk increases at approximately 10- to 15-year intervals from the time of surgery.[18,19] The cost effectiveness of a surveillance program for these patient populations has not been analyzed, and hence there are no solid recommendations for it.

In spite of the advances in imaging technology, the quest for an "optical biopsy device" that will allow us to make a diagnosis without removing tissue remains elusive. A variety of enhanced endoscopic imaging modalities, including magnification endoscopy, fluorescence and light-scattering spectroscopy, and optical coherence tomography, to name a few, are currently being evaluated, and, if proven effective, one or more could be available in the foreseeable future.[20]

In addition to endoscopy being the modality of choice in the diagnosis of upper and lower GI pathology, the last decade has seen a dramatic evolution in the therapeutic capabilities of the technique. Therapeutic endoscopy today is an essential minimally invasive tool in the management and treatment of GI malignancies.

THERAPEUTIC APPLICATIONS OF ENDOSCOPY

Dilatation

Dilatation of benign and malignant strictures is performed either by using through-the-scope balloon dilators or by placing a guidewire for wire-guided dilatation. Esophageal dilatation can provide temporary relief of dysphagia until more definitive treatment can be accomplished. Most malignant strictures can be safely dilated to 16 or 17 mm over several sessions.[21] However, repeat dilatation is usually required every 3 to 4 weeks. Esophageal dilation is also associated with a small risk of perforation, especially if performed during radiotherapy.[22]

Endoscopic Mucosal Resection

Endoscopic mucosal resection was developed by the Japanese for resection of superficial cancers, with the advantage of providing a

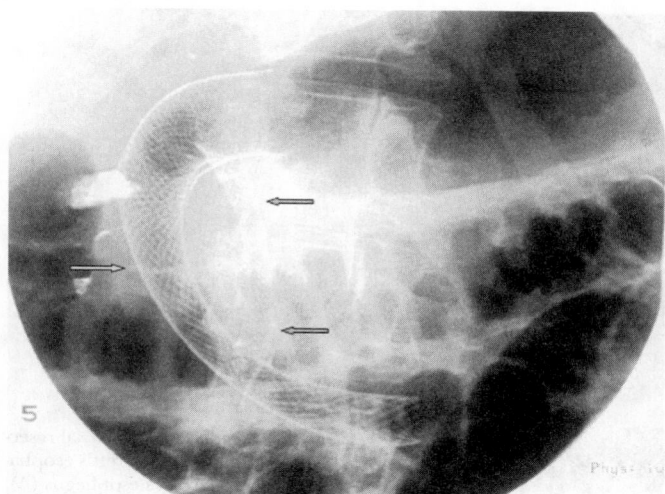

FIGURE 25.1-1. Fluoroscopic still image demonstrating a double biliary (*dark arrows*) and duodenal (*white arrow*) stent placement. (See Color Fig. 25.1-1 in the CD-ROM.)

complete specimen for histologic analysis. The first step is to stage and identify the whole extent of the lesion, using EUS and then chromoendoscopy or fluorescence. Next, the lesion is raised with a submucosal injection of saline. Section through the submucosa is then performed in one of various ways: using the lift and cut technique, a transparent cap, an endoscopic esophageal mucosal resection tube, or a two-channel endoscopic system.[23] Complications, including bleeding, perforation, and emphysema, have been reported to range from 3% to 13%.[24] Fortunately, they can usually be treated endoscopically. Main applications of this exciting technique in the United States and the Western world have been focused on treatment of Barrett's esophagus with high-grade dysplasia and early adenocarcinoma, as well as early gastric and colonic malignancies (Fig. 25.1-1).[25–27]

Enteral Stent Placement

Enteral stent placement is used for the palliation of esophageal, gastric, duodenal, biliary, or colonic malignant obstruction. The Food and Drug Administration has approved SEMSs for the palliation of malignant biliary and enteral obstruction. Although prospective randomized data are still being collected on enteral stenting, it has become apparent that in selected cases it offers a minimally invasive option for the treatment of esophageal, gastroduodenal, and colonic malignant obstruction and is the modality of choice for malignant tracheoesophageal fistulas. SEMSs were developed in 1990 to decrease the rate of complications and increase the ease of insertion.[28]

The technology was borrowed and modified from the vascular and coronary applications. Initial experience with SEMSs was reported for dysphagia due to esophageal malignancies. This metal-mesh stent was compared to a plastic prosthesis in a randomized prospective study involving 42 patients.[29]

The results demonstrated that, although dysphagia scores improved significantly in both groups, complications occurred in nine patients with the plastic prosthesis and in none with the metal stents. Hospital length of stay was significantly shorter in patients receiving the metal stent; therefore, placement of SEMSs was cost effective despite a higher stent cost. Additionally, a higher rate of stent migration was noted with the plastic stents. SEMSs are easier to place, require less degree of dilation (hence, less risk of perforation), and can be placed in the outpatient setting. Since the time of this report, multiple studies have reproduced similar results, and today SEMSs have replaced plastic prostheses and are the most common form of endoscopic palliation for malignant dysphagia and the device of choice for malignant tracheoesophageal fistula.[30–32]

Based on the success with malignant dysphagia, modified SEMSs were developed for malignant gastric outlet and duodenal obstruction. Although the data collected to date are from case series rather than controlled trials, SEMSs appear to achieve a similar success rate as surgical palliation (with approximately 90% of patients improving clinically) but are associated with less morbidity, procedure-related mortality, and cost (Fig. 25.1-2). Nevertheless, up to 40% of patients require reintervention for recurrent symptoms, and late complications, including distal stent migration, bleeding, and perforation, as well as fistula formation, have been reported.[33,34]

In malignant colonic obstruction, colonic stenting is a reasonable option for patients who require decompression as a bridging strategy to elective surgical intervention.[35,36] The technical success rate in such patients is greater than 90%, with most patients achieving adequate decompression. The major risk is perforation, which occurs in approximately 5% of patients when placed by experienced endoscopists. Colonic stenting has also been described for long-term palliation in patients who are not operative candidates. More than 75% of such patients can achieve adequate palliation with a stent; nevertheless, a significant proportion may require endoscopic reintervention.[37,38] Data are insufficient regarding the effects of radiation therapy on colonic stents.

Tumor Therapy by Laser Vaporization or Photocoagulation and Photodynamic Therapy

Laser therapy with neodymium:yttrium aluminum garnet (Nd:YAG) has been the traditional form of palliative treatment for esophageal cancer. However, studies suggest that photodynamic therapy (PDT) or placement of SEMSs might offer better palliation of dysphagia.[39] Nowadays, as a result of the development of safer and less expensive alternative technologies, the role of Nd:YAG laser in GI therapy has significantly decreased.

PDT is based on the ability of chemical agents, known as *photosensitizers*, to produce cytotoxicity in the presence of oxygen after stimulation by light of an appropriate wavelength. Patients are first orally or intravenously given a light-sensitizing agent that is incorporated into cells, resulting in intracellular free radical formation when exposed to light. The photosensitizer has a relative affinity for cancer cells; the mechanism is poorly understood. Next, a laser probe that emits a low-frequency laser light beam and activates the drug by light of a specific wavelength matched to its absorption spectrum is inserted, causing cellular destruction of the sensitized tissue. Hematoporphyrin derivative was the first photosensitizer tested. It is administered intravenously 2 to 3 days before endoscopy, when the concentration of the dye between tumoral and healthy tissue is believed to be at its peak. Photofrin, a more purified form, is the only photosensitizer that has received U.S. Food and Drug Administration approval for use in the esophagus. The major problem is the

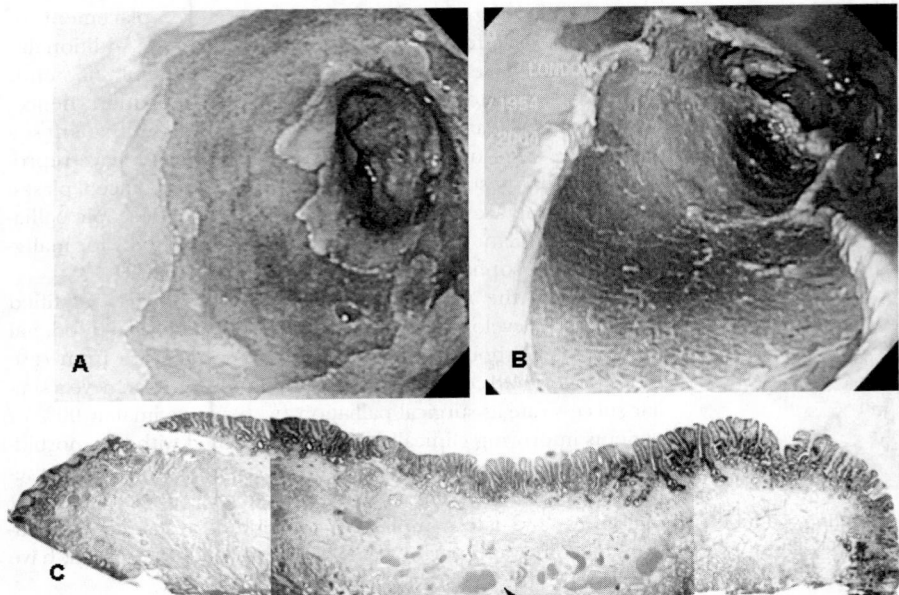

FIGURE 25.1-2.   Endoscopic mucosal resection for high-grade dysplasia in Barrett's esophagus. Endoscopic view of Barrett's esophagus (**A**); endoscopic view of the mucosectomy site (**B**); low-magnification photomicrograph of the resected pathology specimen (**C**; hematoxylin and eosin, 40×; *arrow* marks the submucosa). (See Color Fig. 25.1-2 in the CD-ROM.)

long-term skin photosensitization of 60 to 90 days. A new second-generation photosensitizer being used in trials is 5-aminolevulinic acid. It is administered orally 4 to 6 hours before endoscopy and has the advantage of limiting skin photosensitization to 2 days. Tetra (m-hydroxyphenyl) chlorine is a potent new agent that is administered in lower dosage and requires shorter irradiation times.[40]

A large amount of experience has been reported with PDT for palliation of malignant dysphagia.[41] PDT has been shown to be superior to Nd:YAG laser in patients with proximal esophageal tumors, providing longer luminal patency and less frequency of complications.[42,43] PDT has also been applied as experimental treatment in early superficial squamous cell esophageal cancer and in premalignant changes associated with Barrett's esophagus.[44,45] PDT provides a viable alternative to surgery in the treatment of Barrett's esophagus with high-grade dysplasia in patients who are poor surgical candidates. Advantages include its ease of use, the need for fewer endoscopic sessions compared to other endoscopic thermal ablative techniques, and reduced morbidity, mortality, and cost when compared to surgery. Limitations of PDT include the fact that it only reduces but does not eliminate the risk of progression to adenocarcinoma and has a significant risk of stricture formation and routine; close endoscopic surveillance is still necessary in these patients.[46,47]

ENDOSCOPIC HEMOSTASIS

New endoscopic accessories and coagulation devices are available to address complex GI bleeding. Endoscopic clips and loops are now commercially available, increasing the number of hemostatic tools when managing visible vessels, postpolypectomy bleeding, or mucosal gap defects spontaneous or secondary to resections. Hemostatic devices available only for surgical use, such as the argon plasma coagulator, have become part of the day-to-day endoscopic tools for the management of diffuse GI bleeding disorders such as arteriovenous malformations or radiation-induced proctitis.[48]

Most tumors that cause severe UGI bleeding are of a malignant histologic type and are already at an advanced stage. Endoscopic hemostasis of bleeding UGI tumors is safe and initially effective and may provide time for elective surgical palliation. Nevertheless, recurrence of bleeding is high and usually in the setting of advanced disease and poor performance status. Regardless of therapy, UGI tumors with severe bleeding have a poor 1-year survival.[49]

COLONOSCOPY

Up to the time of this writing, colonoscopy appears to have the greatest potential of reducing the incidence of colorectal cancer as well as the mortality associated with this disease. The technique offers the capability to biopsy suspicious lesions for colorectal cancer as well as remove by endoscopic polypectomy the majority of adenomatous lesions, the precursors for colorectal cancer. Evidence-based guidelines in the United States recommend screening for colorectal cancer in all asymptomatic, average-risk individuals beginning at the age of 50 years.[50,51] Of all screening strategies available, only fecal occult blood testing has been shown in a randomized control trial to be effective in reducing the incidence and mortality from colorectal cancer.[52] Nevertheless, many professional groups are presently recommending colonoscopy as the preferred screening method based on several lines of evidence. Colonoscopy was an integral part of the clinical trials with fecal occult blood testing screening that demonstrated this strategy for reduced colorectal cancer mortality.[52] Colonoscopy provides equal or better visualization of neoplasms as sigmoidoscopy, with the benefit that the whole colon is examined rather than a third and supported by direct evidence showing that sigmoidoscopy reduces colorectal cancer mortality.[53] In two large prospective studies of screening colonoscopy, approximately half of patients with advanced proximal neoplasms had no distal colonic neoplasms.[54,55] Screening

TABLE 25.1-1. Colon Cancer Screening Recommendations for People with Familial or Inherited Risk

Familial Risk Category	Screening Recommendation
First-degree relative affected with colorectal cancer or an adenomatous polyp at age ≥60 y or two second-degree relatives affected with colorectal cancer	Same as average risk but starting at age 40 y
Two or more first-degree relatives[a] with colon cancer or a single first-degree relative with colon cancer or adenomatous polyps diagnosed at age <60 y	Colonoscopy every 5 y, beginning at age 40 y or 10 y younger than the earliest diagnosis in the family, whichever comes first
One second-degree or any third-degree relative[b,c] with colorectal cancer	Same as average risk
Gene carrier or at risk for familial adenomatous polyposis[d]	Sigmoidoscopy annually, beginning at age 10–12 y[e]
Gene carrier or at risk for HNPCC	Colonoscopy every 1–2 y, beginning at age 20–25 y or 10 y younger than the earliest case in the family, whichever comes first

HNPCC, hereditary nonpolyposis colorectal cancer.
[a]First-degree relatives include patients, siblings, and children.
[b]Second-degree relatives include grandparents, aunts, and uncles.
[c]Third-degree relatives include great-grandparents and cousins.
[d]Included in the subcategories of familial adenomatous polyposis are Gardner's syndrome, some Turcot's syndrome families, and antibiotic-associated pseudomembranous colitis (AAPC).
[e]In AAPC, colonoscopy should be used instead of sigmoidoscopy because of the preponderance of proximal colonic adenomas. Colonoscopy screening in AAPC should probably begin in the late teens or early 20s. (From ref. 51, with permission.)

colonoscopy should be started for people of average risk for colorectal cancer at age 50 and, if negative, at 10-year intervals. This interval is based on the rate at which advanced adenomas develop and an estimate of the time from the development of an adenoma to its transformation into cancer.[56,57] The recommendations for screening in people of higher risk are described in Table 25.1-1. For patients with a personal history of colon cancer, a colonoscopy should be performed at the time of initial diagnosis to rule out synchronous lesions. If this or the preoperative examination is normal, subsequent colonoscopy should be offered after 3 years and then, if normal, every 5 years.[51]

ENDOSCOPIC ULTRASONOGRAPHY

EUS is currently the most accurate local-regional imaging modality for staging GI, retroperitoneal, and mediastinal malignancies. The strength of the technology lies in its capabilities of imaging the GI wall as a five acoustic layer structure that correlates to the histologic layers of the luminal GI tract. At low frequencies, EUS depth of penetration increases, allowing one to visualize the GI tract as a window to evaluate the mediastinum and retroperitoneum, making it a powerful staging tool in lung cancer and pancreaticobiliary neoplasms.[58] Although available now for almost 20 years, new endoscope and transducer designs leading to the development of the electronic curvilinear array endoscope have revolutionized and expanded its applications, mainly due to the ability to perform real-time EUS-guided FNA. Another important factor that has popularized this technology has been the demand from oncology centers for more accurate information for stage-oriented cancer treatment protocols.[59] With EUS-guided FNA capabilities for tissue diagnosis, endosonographers can provide the oncology team with accuracies of greater than 90% in nodal staging for luminal and pancreaticobiliary cancers.[58,59] Data are emerging on its clinical impact in esophageal, rectal, and pancreatic cancer.[60–64] In addition, new non-GI applications are being evaluated, such as the role of EUS-FNA for non–small cell lung carcinoma and evaluation of the posterior mediastinum (Fig. 25.1-3). EUS-FNA is a less invasive option that may eliminate the need for more invasive and costly staging procedures.[65–67] Overall, EUS improved accuracy in staging leads to more effective and efficient medical and surgical management.[58,59] Furthermore, the same capabilities that allow for safe tissue sampling are being explored for interventional applications, such as EUS-guided celiac plexus neurolysis for patients with pancreatic cancer and refractory pain as well as fine-needle injection, delivering immunotherapeutic and antitumor agents for locally advanced pancreatic cancer.[68–70]

SMALL BOWEL ENDOSCOPY AND CAPSULE ENDOSCOPY

Neoplasms located distal to the ligament of Treitz pose a diagnostic challenge to the endoscopist. "Push" enteroscopy (endoscopy using a pediatric colonoscope or specialized enteroscope) may allow visualization of the proximal 60 cm of jejunum.[71]

The introduction of the Given M2A (Given Imaging, Inc., Norcross, GA) video capsule endoscope (VCE) into clinical prac-

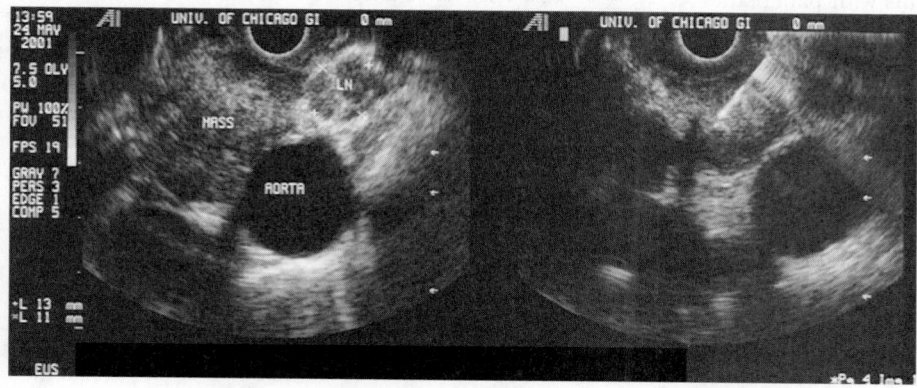

FIGURE 25.1-3. Endosonographic image of a mediastinal mass undergoing endoscopic ultrasound–fine-needle aspiration (EUS-FNA). Cytology reveals non–small cell lung cancer.

tice has, for the first time, permitted complete examination of the entire small intestinal mucosa.[72] The 11 mm × 26 mm video capsule is swallowed with water. The capsule takes two images per second, which are transmitted as JPEG files to the recorder. The recorder acquires up to 50,000 images over approximately 7 hours. Recorded images are downloaded to a workstation. Image management software then creates a video that can be viewed. Review of the video, selection of representative images, and generation of a report can take 30 to 90 minutes. VCE has been shown to be of clinical utility in diagnosing the etiology of obscure GI bleeding and is well tolerated by patients.[72–75] The role for VCE in the diagnosis of small bowel neoplasms is currently being defined. In a retrospective analysis[76] of 562 patients undergoing VCE for a variety of indications (most commonly obscure GI bleeding) at a single center, 50 (8.9%) small bowel tumors were diagnosed. Nineteen (53%) of the 36 patients for whom pathology was available had malignant neoplasms. The malignant diagnoses included adenocarcinoma, carcinoid, GI stromal tumor, and lymphoma. Interestingly, these 50 patients had undergone a total of 138 negative diagnostic tests before VCE. In another retrospective analysis[77] of 257 patients who underwent VCE, 16 (6.2%) were found to have tumors, 9 of which were malignant. Radiographic studies performed in 13 of the 16 patients identified the tumors in only 5 (38%) cases. Although prospective trials comparing VCE to conventional diagnostic techniques are needed in patients with suspected small bowel malignancies, it appears as though VCE will provide an important imaging tool in the workup of such patients.

ENDOSCOPIC RETROGRADE CHOLANGIOPANCREATOGRAPHY

ERCP has been an important tool in the diagnosis and management of pancreaticobiliary disorders since its initial description in 1968.[78] However, it is the most complex endoscopic procedure, requiring specialized equipment, and has a long learning curve to develop proficiency. Its benefits in the minimally invasive management of biliary and pancreatic disorders are offset by a higher potential for serious complications than any other endoscopic procedure.[79]

A National Institutes of Health Consensus Conference on ERCP concluded that, with newer diagnostic imaging technologies emerging, ERCP is evolving into a predominantly therapeutic procedure. In patients with pancreatic or biliary cancer, the principal advantage of ERCP is palliation of biliary obstruction when surgery is not elected. ERCP is still the best means to diagnose ampullary cancers.[80] Regarding the role of ERCP in tissue sampling for patients with pancreatic or biliary cancer not undergoing surgery, the diagnostic yield is low, 62% for cholangiocarcinoma and 37% for pancreatic carcinoma, as compared to 75% reported for EUS, a less invasive technique.[64,81]

Therapeutic ERCP with stent insertion, either plastic or metal, is safe and effective in relieving jaundice and pruritus and may improve quality of life in patients with malignant biliary obstruction.[82] In addition, endoscopic stent placement may offer lower morbidity and mortality, shorter hospitalization, and diminished overall cost as compared with surgical or radiologic approaches.[83] In a report using evidence-based medicine to look at endoscopic stent palliation for malignant biliary obstruction, Levy et al.[84] concluded that there is direct evidence to support the insertion of an SEMS for patients with biopsy-proven unresectable malignant obstruction or poor surgical candidates with a greater than 6-month expected survival. For patients in whom survival is expected to be less than 6 months, a plastic stent is the best cost-effective strategy.[84]

REFERENCES

1. Saeian K. Unsedated transnasal endoscopy: a safe and less costly alternative. *Curr Gastroenterol Rep* 2002;4:213.
2. Sackman M, Morgner A, Rudolph B, et al. Regression of gastric MALT lymphoma after eradication of Helicobacter pylori is predicted by endosonographic staging. MALT Lymphoma Study Group. *Gastroenterology* 1997;113:1087.
3. The role of endoscopy in the surveillance of premalignant conditions of the upper gastrointestinal tract. *Gastrointest Endosc* 1998;48:663.
4. Bigelow NH. Carcinoma of the esophagus developing at the site of lye stricture. *Cancer* 1953;6:1159.
5. Leape LL, Ashcraft KW, Scarpelli DG, et al. Hazard to health—liquid lye. *N Engl J Med* 1971;248:232.
6. Marger RS, Marger D. Carcinoma of the esophagus and tylosis. A lethal genetic combination. *Cancer* 1993;72:17.
7. Falk GW. Barrett's esophagus. *Gastroenterology* 2002;122:1569.
8. Levine DS, Haggitt RC, Blount PL, et al. An endoscopic biopsy protocol can differentiate high-grade dysplasia from early adenocarcinoma in Barrett's esophagus. *Gastroenterology* 1993;105:40.
9. Schnell TG, Sontag SJ, Chejfec G, et al. Long-term nonsurgical management of Barrett's esophagus with high-grade dysplasia. *Gastroenterology* 2001;120:1607.
10. Sampliner RE. Practice guidelines on the diagnosis, surveillance and therapy of Barrett's esophagus. The practice parameters committee of the American College of Gastroenterology. *Am J Gastroenterol* 1998;93;1028.
11. McGannon E. Gastric and duodenal polyps in familial adenomatous polyposis: a prospective study of the nature and prevalence of upper gastrointestinal polyps. *Gut* 1987;28:306.
12. Rustgi AK. Hereditary gastrointestinal polyposis and nonpolyposis syndromes. *N Engl J Med* 1994;331:1694.
13. Johan G, Offerhaus A, Giardiello M, et al. The risk of upper gastrointestinal cancer in familial adenomatous polyposis. *Gastroenterology* 1992;102:1980.
14. Nakamura T, Nakano G. Histopathological classification and malignant change in gastric polyps. *J Clin Pathol* 1985;38:754.
15. Kamiya T, Morishita T, Haakora H, et al. Histoclinical long-standing follow-up study of hyperplastic polyps of the stomach. *Am J Gastroenterol* 1981;75:275.
16. Harju E. Gastric polyposis and malignancy. *Br J Surg* 1986;73:632.
17. Hsing AW, Hansson LE, McLaughlin JK, et al. Pernicious anemia and subsequent cancer: a population-based cohort study. *Cancer* 1993;71:745.
18. Safatle-Ribeiro AV, Ribeiro U Jr, Reynolds JC. Gastric stump cancer: what is the risk? *Dig Dis* 1998;16:159.
19. Tersmette AC, Giardello FM, Tytgat GN, Hofferhaus GJA. Carcinogenesis after remote peptic ulcer surgery: the long term prognosis of partial gastrectomy. *Scan J Gastroenterol* 1995;30[suppl 212]:96.
20. Van Dam J. Novel methods of enhanced endoscopic imaging. *Gut* 2003;52[suppl IV]:iv12.
21. Boyce HW Jr. Palliation of dysphagia of esophageal cancer by endoscopic lumen restoration techniques. *Cancer Control* 1999;6:73.
22. Lundell L, Leth R, Lind T, et al. Palliative endoscopic dilatation in carcinoma of the esophagus and esophagogastric junction. *Acta Chir Scand* 1989;155:179.
23. Soetikno RM, Gotoda T, Nakanishi Y, et al. Endoscopic mucosal resection. *Gastrointest Endosc* 2003;57:567.
24. Ahmad NA, Kochman ML, Long WB, et al. Efficacy, safety, and clinical outcomes of endoscopic mucosal resection: a study of 101 cases. *Gastrointest Endosc* 2002;55:390.
25. Ell C, May A, Gossner L, et al. Endoscopic mucosal resection of early cancer and high-grade dysplasia in Barrett's esophagus. *Gastroenterology* 2000;118:670.
26. May A, Gossner L, Behrens A, et al. A prospective randomized trial of two different endoscopic resection techniques for early stage cancer of the esophagus. *Gastrointest Endosc* 2003;58:167.
27. Waxman I, Saitoh Y. Clinical outcome of endoscopic mucosal resection for superficial GI lesions and the role of high-frequency US probe sonography in an American population. *Gastrointest Endosc* 2000;52:322.
28. Baron TH. Expandable metal stents for the treatment of cancerous obstruction of the gastrointestinal tract. *N Engl J Med* 2001;344:1681.
29. Knyrim K, Wagner HJ, Bethge N, Keymling M, Vakil N. A controlled trial of an expansile metal stent for palliation of esophageal obstruction due to inoperable cancer. *N Engl J Med* 1993;329:1302.
30. De Palma GD, di Matteo E, Romano G, et al. Plastic prosthesis versus expandable metal stents for palliation of inoperable esophageal thoracic carcinoma: a controlled prospective study. *Gastrointest Endosc* 1996;43:478.
31. Cowling MG, Hale H, Grundy A. Management of malignant oesophageal obstruction with self-expanding stents. *Br J Surg* 1998;85:264.
32. Kozarek RA, Raltz S, Brugge W, et al. Prospective multi-center trial of esophageal Z-stent placement for malignant dysphagia and tracheoesophageal fistula. *Gastrointest Endosc* 1996;44:562.

33. Adler D, Baron TH. Endoscopic palliation of malignant gastric outlet obstruction using expanding metal stents: experience in thirty-six patients. *Am J Gastroenterol* 2002;97:72.
34. Yim HB, Jacobson BC, Saltzman JR, et al. Clinical outcome of the use of enteral stents for palliation of patients with malignant upper GI obstruction. *Gastrointest Endosc* 2001;53:329.
35. Mainar A, De Gregorio Ariza MA, Tejero E, Tobio R. Acute colorectal obstruction: treatment with self-expandable metallic stents before scheduled surgery—results of a multicenter study. *Radiology* 1999;210:65.
36. Law WL, Choi HK, Chu KW. Comparison of stenting with emergency surgery as palliative treatment for obstructing primary left-sided colorectal cancer. *Br J Surg* 2003;90:1429.
37. Spinelli P, Mancini A. Use of self-expanding metal stents for palliation of rectosigmoid cancer. *Gastrointest Endosc* 2001;53:203.
38. Binkert CA, Ledermann H. Acute colonic obstruction: clinical aspects and cost effectiveness of preoperative and palliative treatment with self-expanding metallic stents. *Radiology* 1998;206:199.
39. Adam A, Ellul J, Watkinson AF, et al. Palliation of inoperable esophageal carcinoma: a prospective randomized trial of laser therapy and stent placement. *Radiology* 1997;202:344.
40. Waxman I, Shami VM. Endoscopic treatment of early gastroesophageal malignancy. *Curr Opin Gastroenterol* 2002;18,587.
41. Lightdale CJ, Meier S, Marcon N, et al. A multicenter phase II trial of PDT versus Nd:YAG laser in the treatment of malignant dysphagia. *Gastrointest Endosc* 1993;3:283.
42. McCaughan JS Jr, Ellison EC, Guy JT, et al. Photodynamic therapy for esophageal malignancy: a prospective twelve-year study. *Ann Thorac Surg* 1996;62:1005.
43. Lightdale CJ, Heier SK, Marcon NE, et al. Photodynamic therapy with porfimer sodium versus thermal ablation therapy with Nd:YAG laser for palliation of esophageal cancer: a multicenter randomized trial. *Gastrointest Endosc* 1995;42:507.
44. Radu A, Wagnieres G, van den Bergh H, et al. Photodynamic therapy in early squamous cell cancers of the esophagus. *Gastrointest Endosc Clin North Am* 2000;10:439.
45. Buttar NS, Wang KK, Lutzke LS, et al. Combined endoscopic mucosal resection and photodynamic therapy for esophageal neoplasia within Barrett's esophagus. *Gastrointest Endosc* 2001;54:682.
46. Ackroyd R, Brown NJ, Davis MF, et al. Photodynamic therapy for dysplastic Barrett's oesophagus: a prospective, double blind, randomized, placebo controlled trial. *Gut* 2000;47:612.
47. Overholt BF, Panjehpour M, Halberg DL. Photodynamic therapy for Barrett's esophagus with dysplasia and/or early stage carcinoma: long-term results. *Gastrointest Endosc* 2003;58:183.
48. Canard JM, Vedrenne B. Clinical application of argon plasma coagulation in gastrointestinal endoscopy: has the time come to replace the laser? *Endoscopy* 2001;33:353.
49. Savides TJ, Jensen DM, Cohen J, et al. Severe upper gastrointestinal tumor bleeding: endoscopic findings, treatment, and outcome. *Endoscopy* 1996;28:244.
50. U.S. Preventive Services Task Force. Screening for colorectal cancer: recommendation and rationale. *Ann Intern Med* 2002;137:129.
51. Winawer S, Fletcher R, Rex D, et al. Colorectal cancer screening and surveillance: clinical guidelines and rationale-updated based new evidence. *Gastroenterology* 2003;124:544.
52. Mandel JS, Bond JH, Church TR, et al. Reducing mortality from colorectal cancer by screening for fecal occult blood. Minnesota Colon Cancer Control Study. *N Engl J Med* 1993;328:1365.
53. Selby JV, Freidman GD, Quesenberry CP Jr, et al. A case control study of screening sigmoidoscopy and mortality for colorectal cancer. *N Engl J Med* 1992;326:653.
54. Lieberman DA, Weiss DG, Bond JH, et al. Use of colonoscopy to screen asymptomatic adults for colorectal cancer. Veterans Affairs Cooperative Study Group 380. *N Engl J Med* 2000;343:162.
55. Imperiale TF, Wagner DR, Lin CY, et al. Risk of advanced proximal neoplasms in asymptomatic adults according to the distal colorectal findings. *N Engl J Med* 2000;343:169.
56. Winawer SJ, Zauber AG, Ho MN, et al. Prevention of colorectal cancer by colonoscopic polypectomy. The National Polyp Study Workgroup. *N Engl J Med* 1993;329:1977.
57. Hofstad B, Vatn M. Growth rate of colon polyps and cancer. *Gastrointest Endosc Clin N Am* 1997;7:345.
58. Byrne MF, Jowell PS. Gastrointestinal imaging: endoscopic ultrasound. *Gastroenterology* 2002;122:1631.
59. Waxman I, Dye C. Interventional endosonography. *Cancer J* 2002;8:S113.
60. Vazquez-Sequeiros E, Wiersema JM, Clain JE, et al. Impact of lymph node staging on therapy of esophageal carcinoma. *Gastroenterology* 2003;125:1626.
61. Wallace MB, Nietert PJ, Earle C, et al. An analysis of multiple staging management strategies for carcinoma of the esophagus: computed tomography, endoscopic ultrasound, positron emission tomography, and thoracoscopy/laparoscopy. *Ann Thorac Surg* 2002;74:1026.
62. Shami VM, Parmar K, Waxman I. Clinical impact of EUS and EUS-guided FNA in the management of rectal carcinoma. *Dis Colon Rectum* 2004;47:59.
63. Harewood GC, Wiersema MJ. A cost analysis of endoscopic ultrasound in the evaluation of pancreatic head adenocarcinoma. *Am J Gastroenterol* 2001;96:2651.
64. Hunt GC, Faigel DO. Assessment of EUS for diagnosing, staging, and determining resectability of pancreatic cancer: a review. *Gastrointest Endosc* 2002;55:232.
65. Gress FG, Savides TJ, Sandler A, et al. A comparison of endoscopic ultrasound (EUS), EUS directed fine-needle aspiration, and computed tomography of the mediastinum in the pre-operative staging of non-small cell lung cancer. *Ann Intern Med* 1997;127:604.
66. Fritscher-Ravens A, Bohuslavizki KH, Brandt L, et al. Mediastinal lymph node involvement in potentially resectable lung cancer. Comparison of CT, positron emission tomography, and endoscopic ultrasonography with and without fine-needle aspiration. *Chest* 2003;123:442.
67. Larsen SS, Krasnik M, Vilmann P, et al. Endoscopic ultrasound guided biopsy of mediastinal lesions has a major impact on patient management. *Thorax* 2002;57:98.
68. Gunaratnam NT, Sarma AV, Norton ID, Wiersema MJ. A prospective study of EUS-guided celiac plexus neurolysis for pancreatic cancer pain. *Gastrointest Endosc* 2001;54:316.
69. Chang KJ, Nguyen PT, Thompson JA, et al. Phase I clinical trial of allogeneic mixed lymphocyte culture (cytoimplant) delivered by endoscopic ultrasound-guided fine-needle-injection in patients with advanced pancreatic carcinoma. *Cancer* 2000;88:1325.
70. Terayama A, Chang KJ, Senzer N, et al. A novel gene transfer therapy against pancreatic cancer (TNFerade) delivered by endoscopic ultrasound (EUS) and percutaneous guided fine needle injection (FNI). *Gastrointest Endosc* 2004.
71. Lewis BS, Kornbluth A, Waye JD. Small bowel tumours: yield of enteroscopy. *Gut* 1991;32:763.
72. Iddan G, Meron G, Glukhovsky A, Swain P. Wireless capsule endoscopy. *Nature* 2000;405:417.
73. Pennazio M, Santucci R, Rondonotti E, et al. Outcome of patients with obscure gastrointestinal bleeding after capsule endoscopy: report of 100 consecutive cases. *Gastroenterology* 2004;126:643.
74. Costamagna G, Shah SK, Riccioni ME, et al. A prospective trial comparing small bowel radiographs and video capsule endoscopy for suspected small bowel disease. *Gastroenterology* 2002;123:1385.
75. Ell C, Remke S, May A, et al. The first prospective controlled trial comparing wireless capsule endoscopy with push enteroscopy in chronic gastrointestinal bleeding. *Endoscopy* 2002;34:685.
76. Corbin GM, Pittman RH, Lewis BS. Diagnosing small bowel tumors with capsule endoscopy. Abstract presented at the 3rd International Conference on Capsule Endoscopy, Miami, FL, 2003.
77. Keuchel M, Thaler C, Caselitz J, Hangenmller F. Diagnosis of small bowel tumors with video capsule endoscopy—report of 16 cases. Abstract presented at the 3rd International Conference on Capsule Endoscopy, Miami, FL, 2003.
78. McCune WS, Short PE, Moscovitz H. Endoscopic cannulation of the ampulla of Vater. *Ann Surg* 1968;167:752.
79. Freeman ML, Nelson DB, Sherman S, et al. Complications of endoscopic biliary sphincterotomy. *N Engl J Med* 1996;335:909.
80. Cohen S, Bacon BR, Berlin JA, et al. National Institutes of Health State-of-the-Science Conference Statement: ERCP for diagnosis and therapy, January 14–16, 2002. *Gastrointest Endosc* 2002;56:803.
81. De Bellis M, Sherman S, Fogel EL, et al. Tissue sampling at ERCP in suspected malignant biliary strictures (Part 1). *Gastrointest Endosc* 2002;56:552.
82. Abraham NS, Barkun JS, Barkun AN, et al. Palliation of malignant biliary obstruction: a prospective trial examining impact on quality of life. *Gastrointest Endosc* 2002;56:835.
83. Parmar K, Waxman I. Endoscopic palliation for locally advanced and metastatic disease: biliary and duodenal stents. In: Evans DB, Pisters PWT, Abbruzzese JL, eds. *MD Anderson solid tumor oncology series 3rd edition.* New York: Springer-Verlag, 2002;213.
84. Levy MJ, Baron TH, Gostout CJ, et al. Palliation of malignant extrahepatic biliary obstruction with plastic versus expandable metal stents: an evidence based approach. *Clin Gastroenterol Hepatol* 2004;2:273.

SECTION 2

DAO M. NGUYEN
RONALD M. SUMMERS
STEVEN E. FINKELSTEIN

Respiratory Tract

Benign or malignant disease of the chest is routinely evaluated, subsequent to a detailed medical history and physical examination, with noninvasive imaging modalities [plain radiography, computed tomography (CT) scan, magnetic resonance imaging, or sonography] and, when indicated, by invasive procedures (transthoracic needle biopsy or endoscopies, particularly flexible bronchoscopy) before definitive therapeutic interventions. The oncologists have at their disposal the following endoscopic modalities for expeditious and appropriate management of patients with malignant disease involving the thoracic cavity (Table 25.2-1).

BRONCHOSCOPY

Flexible fiberoptic bronchoscopy (FB) is used to evaluate and to treat endobronchial or lung parenchymal diseases. It

TABLE 25.2-1. Indications for Thoracic Endoscopies

Modality	Diagnostic	Therapeutic
Bronchoscopy	Endobronchial lesion Lung cancer staging and screening Hemoptysis Interstitial lung disease	Airway control (FB-assisted intubation), pulmonary toilet, ablation of endobronchial lesion (laser, PDT, cryotherapy, brachytherapy), stenting, balloon dilatation
Mediastinoscopy	Mediastinal mass Staging lung cancer	—
VATS	Pleural disease Parenchymal disease Staging lung or esophageal cancer	Pleural disease Resection of primary or secondary cancer of the lung

FB, fiberoptic bronchoscopy; PDT, photodynamic therapy; VATS, video-assisted thoracoscopic surgery.

can be performed at the bedside or in a dedicated endoscopy suite with intravenous sedation and topical local anesthesia or in the operating room with general anesthesia and endotracheal intubation using the standard endotracheal tube or the laryngeal mask airway. Rigid bronchoscopy, on the other hand, is much less frequently used and should only be performed by properly trained clinicians in the operating room under general anesthesia. The indications for rigid bronchoscopy are limited to management of massive hemoptysis, endobronchial tumors, foreign body, or placement of endoluminal stents.

DIAGNOSTIC BRONCHOSCOPY

FB is an essential component of preoperative evaluation of patients with primary or metastatic cancers of the lung. Diagnosis of malignancy can be obtained by biopsy of endobronchial tumor or cytologic examination of bronchial brushing and washing specimen. FB, aided by endobronchial ultrasound, is used to obtain transbronchial biopsy of paratracheal or subcarinal lymph nodes or lung masses with excellent yield and accuracy.[1–3] FB is routinely performed before lung resection, especially in cases of centrally located tumor in which the nature and the exact anatomic location of the endobronchial tumor dictate the magnitude of lung resection or the feasibility of bronchoplastic maneuvers. Interstitial lung disease in cancer patients is initially investigated with FB and bronchoalveolar lavage/transbronchial biopsy for microbiologic and cyto-/histopathologic diagnosis of the underlying etiology. Autofluorescence bronchoscopy [FB equipped with laser-induced fluorescence emission (LIFE system; Xillix Technologies, Vancouver, Canada)] is being extensively evaluated and developed to improve the sensitivity of white-light FB to detect premalignant endobronchial lesions in patients at high risk for lung cancer (ex- or current smokers, history of lung cancer or head/neck cancer).[4–10] The autofluorescence spectra of dysplasia and carcinoma *in situ* are reported to be substantially different from those of normal bronchial tissues when excited by violet (405 nm) or blue (442 nm) light.[4,5] LIFE system was approved by the U.S. Food and Drug Administration as an adjunct to white-light FB for the detection of moderate/severe dysplasia and carcinoma in patients with known or suspected lung cancer.[4]

THERAPEUTIC BRONCHOSCOPY

Flexible bronchoscopy is an essential adjunct in the management of difficult airways in the operating room or in the intensive care unit. The endotracheal tube is placed over the FB, which then is inserted nasally or orally to the upper airway for visualization of the vocal cords. Intubation is performed by sliding the endotracheal tube over the FB into the trachea under direct vision. Flexible bronchoscopy is routinely used in the postoperative period to clear retained bronchial secretions (bronchopulmonary toilet) in thoracic patients after major lung resection for cancer.[11] Either flexible or rigid bronchoscopy is used to manage endobronchial tumors causing airway obstruction or hemoptysis. They are frequently treated endoscopically by a combination of mechanical débridement using the tip of the rigid bronchoscope (core-out) or a large biopsy forceps followed by hemostasis and ablation of residual tumors with electrocautery, laser, or cryotherapy. Neodymium:yttrium aluminum garnet (Nd:YAG) laser is the most widely used modality to treat obstructing endobronchial tumors because it has deeper penetration and produces better hemostasis (Fig. 25.2-1).

Photodynamic therapy (PDT) is based on the specific photosensitization of malignant tissue containing hematoporphyrin or its derivative after exposure to a visible activating light (630 nm). PDT of obstructing endobronchial tumor is a two-step process involving intravenous administration of the U.S. Food and Drug Administration–approved photosensitizer porfimer sodium (Photofrin) and, after a 2-day delay, exposure of the endobronchial tumor to bronchoscopic illumination with a 630-nm wavelength of laser light. A follow-up bronchoscopy is then performed a few days later for débridement of necrotic tumor tissues. PDT is used for curative (carcinoma *in situ*) and palliative (inoperable obstructing cancers of central airways) intents to treat endobronchial tumors.[12–14] Brachytherapy for obstructing endobronchial cancers involves placement of the catheter next to the tumor by FB and, after withdrawal of the endoscope, loading of the catheter with radioactive seeds. This procedure is performed under intravenous sedation and topical anesthesia and lasts approximately 15 minutes. Endobronchial brachytherapy showed a symptomatic response rate of 90% for dyspnea, 82% for cough, 94% for hemoptysis, and 90% for obstructive pneumonia.[15]

Airway obstruction caused by extrinsic compression either by the primary tumor or by mediastinal lymphadenopathy requires placement of endobronchial stents (Fig. 25.2-2). A variety of Silastic and metallic self-expanding stents have been devised. The two most commonly used metal stents are the Wallstent and the Ultraflex. These are self-expandable stents with or without silicone coating (to reduce tumor or granulation tissue ingrowth). These stents are resistant to migration (a common problem of Silastic stents), readily conformable to airway anatomy, and easily inserted by FB; however, they are expensive.[16] Every oncologic patient presented with hemoptysis is subjected to bronchoscopic examination after appropriate clinical evaluation and imaging studies. FB is most frequently used to visualize the bleeding site. Rigid bronchoscopy is needed for massive hemoptysis to quickly clear the airway of blood and large, adherent clots. Once identified, the bleeding site is managed with combinations of topical 1:10,000 epinephrine, laser therapy, or electrocautery. Endobron-

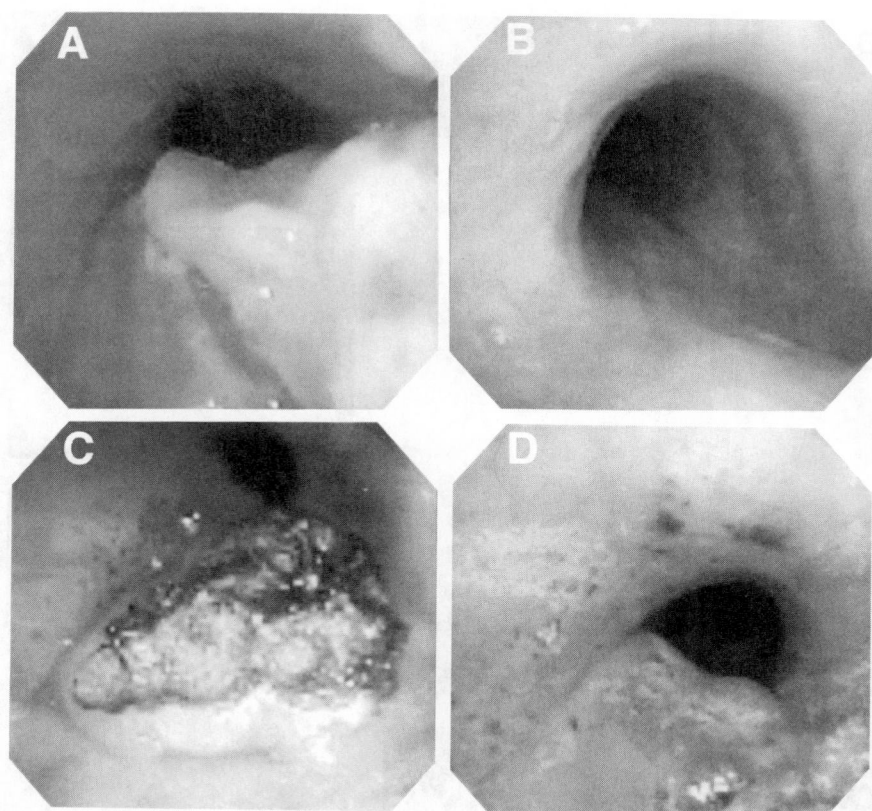

FIGURE 25.2-1. Ablation of an endobronchial tumor with neodymium:yttrium aluminum garnet (Nd:YAG) laser by fiberoptic bronchoscopy. **A:** Endobronchial recurrence of renal cell carcinoma at the orifice of the left main-stem bronchus causing partial airway obstruction and expiratory stridor on auscultation. **B:** Endoscopic examination revealing normal left main bronchus beyond the endobronchial tumor. **C:** Nd:YAG laser ablation of the tumor with the residual tumor base covered with eschar and debris. **D:** Follow-up bronchoscopy showing restoration of the luminal patency of the left main-stem bronchus. (See Color Fig. 25.2-1 in the CD-ROM.)

chial tamponade of a bleeding subsegmental bronchus can be achieved by using a Fogarty balloon-tipped catheter.

Complications of flexible and rigid bronchoscopy, such as hemorrhage or pneumothorax, are minimal. In one large series, 58 episodes of bleeding occurred, none fatal, in almost 7000 bronchoscopies, with transbronchial biopsy carrying the highest risk of hemorrhage.[17] Mortality due to interventional bronchoscopies was reported to range from 0.1% to 0.3%.[18,19] In a series of 4000 patients, major complications (pneumothorax, pulmonary hemorrhage, respiratory failure), occurred in 0.53% of flexible bronchoscopic procedures. Transbronchial biopsy was associated with a higher incidence of adverse events, with 6.8% of patients experiencing either hemorrhage (2.8%) or pneumothorax (4.0%).[20]

VIRTUAL BRONCHOSCOPY

In current clinical practice, patients with suspected airway stenosis may undergo a diagnostic workup consisting of chest x-ray, conventional helical CT of the chest, and FB.[21] With the advent of CT, two-dimensional cross-sectional images of the thorax have been increasingly used to provide information regarding peribronchial anatomy. CT is a useful tool to visualize intra- and extraluminal pathology; standard CT scans have been reported to have a sensitivity of 63% to 100% for detecting obstructive lesions and a specificity of 61% to 99%.[22–24] CT does have drawbacks caused by suboptimal scanning techniques, inappropriate slice thickness, and other artifacts that can decrease the accurate analysis of airway anatomy.[25] As such, oncologists use FB as an essential tool for evaluation and treatment of endoluminal and mucosal lesions. Nevertheless, FB yields no information about extent of extraluminal

disease or airway patency beyond a high-grade stenosis.[26] This modality is invasive and does carry some risks, particularly in patients with significant airway obstruction. Novel imaging modalities, such as virtual bronchoscopy (VB), are becoming increasingly

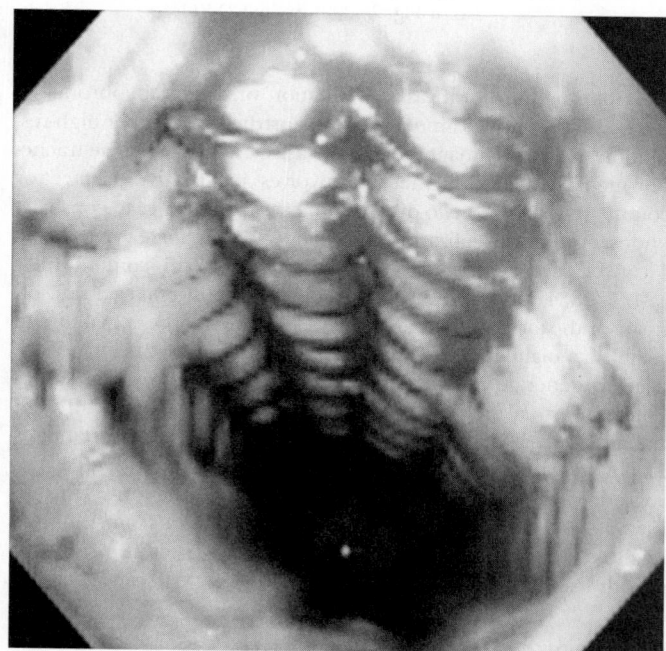

FIGURE 25.2-2. Endoscopic view of an endotracheal stent placed for malignant stricture due to extra- and intraluminal growth of metastatic renal cell cancer. (See Color Fig. 25.2-2 in the CD-ROM.)

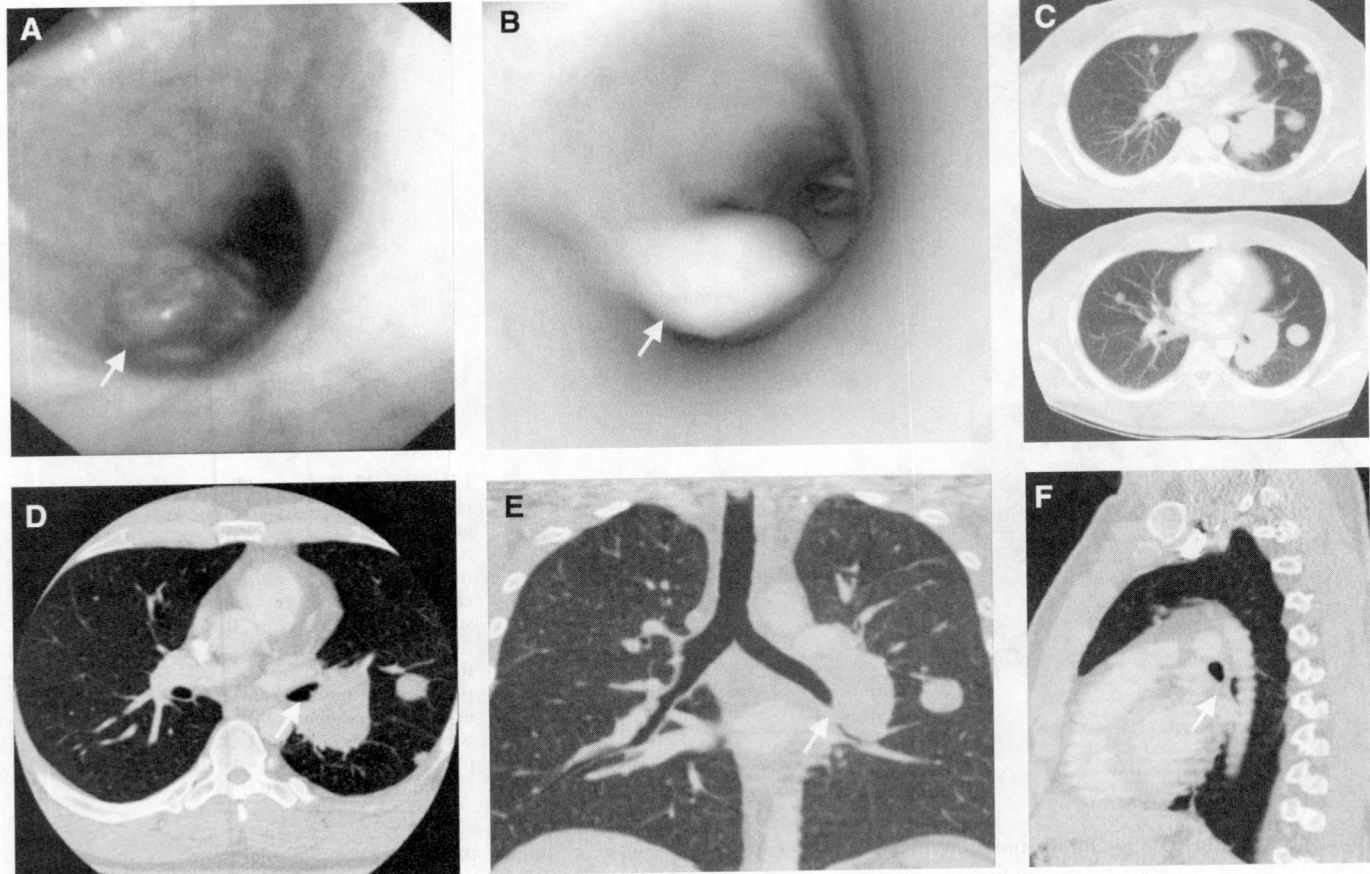

FIGURE 25.2-3.   Endoluminal lesion obstructing superior segment of left lower lobe in a 30-year-old man diagnosed with metastatic melanoma. Fiberoptic bronchoscopy (**A**), virtual bronchoscopy (**B**), and super high-resolution computed tomography (axial, coronal, and sagittal sections) (**D–F**) visualized this lesion (*white arrow*). However, this lesion was not appreciated on conventional computed tomography sections (**C**). (See Color Fig. 25.2-3*A* in the CD-ROM.)

available for the noninvasive evaluation of the tracheobronchial tree.[27] VB uses three-dimensional reconstruction of super high-resolution helical CT images for noninvasive evaluation of the tracheobronchial tree. This method involves perspective surface or volume rendering of two-dimensional CT scan images to construct endoscopic-like visualization of the airway (Fig. 25.2-3; web movie 1 can be seen at http://www.chestjournal.org/cgi/content/full/124/5/1834/DC1). VB uses the natural contrast between the soft tissue of the airway wall and the air in the tracheobronchial tree to establish a plane for generating the virtual airway[24]; the images are used to generate a three-dimensional model of airway anatomy. Once the virtual airway is created, the viewer can navigate through the airway in a three-dimensional manner analogous to standard FB. In addition, VB allows for unconventional images such as retrograde views of endoluminal and extraluminal anatomy[26]; the airway can be manipulated in space and evaluated from multiple angles. The radiation dose with this technique is the same or slightly less than that of a conventional thoracic CT scan.

TECHNIQUE

To generate a VB, 200 to 300 contiguous 1.25-mm images of the thorax are obtained using a multislice helical CT scanner.[28] The

authors' standard approach has been 1.25 collimation, high-speed mode [helical pitch 6; 7.5-mm table motion per rotation, 120 kilovolt peak (kVp), 100 mA, 0.8-second tube rotation], nonoverlapping reconstructions with a section interval of 1.25 mm, and an effective z-axis resolution of approximately 1.6 mm. With respect to the use of contrast, a study initiated for malignancy should use intravenous contrast to improve the identification of lesions. If a postinflammatory stricture is suspected, however, intravenous contrast is generally not necessary. In addition, oral contrast is not required for this imaging procedure. Two-dimensional CT images can then be reconstructed to three-dimensional VB endoscopic views using commercial software.

VIRTUAL BRONCHOSCOPY FOR THORACIC MALIGNANCIES

A review of the current literature suggests that VB can be important for the detection of partial or complete bronchial obstructions caused by endoluminal tumors and extrinsic compression. Fleiter et al.[29] reported a series of patients with thoracic malignancies who underwent VB using a double-detector CT unit and correlative FB. In this study VB images were successfully created in 19 of 20 patients. However, a strong heart pulsation produced motion artifact that prevented accurate reconstruction in one patient. Areas of high-grade stenosis were accurately detected using both techniques. VB accurately visualized areas beyond stenoses. Discrete malignant infiltration and extraluminal compression were not visualized by VB in five patients. Liewald et al.[30] evaluated 30 lung cancer patients with VB and FB. Three-dimensional images were created in all patients. Thirteen obstructive lesions were seen equally well by VB and FB. VB delineated tracheobronchial anatomy beyond high-grade stenosis in two patients. However, mucosal lesions were not visualized by VB. Rapp-Bernhardt et al.[31] compared VB with FB in 21 patients with esophageal carcinoma infiltrating the tracheobronchial tree. These authors found no statistically significant difference in the location or grading of stenoses when comparing VB with FB. These same authors also evaluated 18 patients with bronchogenic carcinoma. CT and VB were used to evaluate tracheobronchial stenoses that had been detected by FB. CT of the chest was found to have a sensitivity of 92.9% and a specificity of 100%. VB was found to have a sensitivity of 93.8% and a specificity of 99.7%.[32] Hoppe et al.[33] compared the efficacy of noninvasive multidetector CT, which included VB images, axial CT, coronal reformatted images, and sagittal reformatted images, with that of FB. In their examination of 200 bronchial sections obtained from 20 patients, 15 with bronchial carcinoma and 5 without central airway disease, they determined that VB findings were highly accurate for the grading of tracheobronchial stenosis. Indeed, images from VB correlated closely (r = 0.91) with those of FB. In addition, the authors suggest that interpretation of axial CT scan images and multiplanar reformatted images may be useful for evaluation of surrounding structures and optimal spatial orientation.[33]

The authors' extensive experience with respect to VB confirms that of other investigators who have evaluated the feasibility and utility of novel imaging in patients with primary or metastatic cancers involving the lungs and mediastinum.[34,35] By using the same commercial software (G.E. Navigator on a G.E. Advantage Windows workstation, Milwaukee, WI) that ships with most CT scanners, the authors prospectively compared the diagnostic potential of conventional CT, super high-resolution CT (SHR-CT), and VB to FB for the detection of tracheobronchial neoplasms.[35] Thirty-two patients who completed SHR-CT and VB had correlative FB within 1 month. In all patients with normal anatomy, SHR-CT and VB accurately correlated with the FB findings. However, CT demonstrated two false-positive obstructive lesions in one patient. Twenty-three patients were noted to have a total of 35 abnormal FB findings. The sensitivities of SHR-CT and VB for detection of endoluminal, obstructive, or mucosal lesions were 90%, 100%, and 16%, respectively. The overall sensitivities and specificities of SHR-CT and VB were 83% and 100%. In contrast, CT had sensitivities of 50%, 72%, and 0% for detection of endoluminal, obstructive, or mucosal lesions, with an overall sensitivity and specificity of 59% and 85%, respectively. In no case was conventional CT better at detecting lesions than either SHR-CT or VB. Thus, these data suggest that VB and SHR-CT can be used as accurate, noninvasive methods for identifying obstructions and endoluminal lesions. These novel imaging techniques are most valuable complementary modalities to FB for the detection and management of airway malignancies.

ADVANTAGES AND DISADVANTAGES OF VIRTUAL BRONCHOSCOPY IN PATIENTS WITH CANCER

The expanding body of literature suggests that VB has several advantages. It is noninvasive with no additional radiation expo-

sure relative to standard CT scans of the chest. The ability to examine two- and three-dimensional anatomic detail from countless directions yields an important advantage for extraluminal and intraluminal detection. VB can highlight anatomic detail beyond stenoses and the reach of FB secondary to size limitations of endoscopy. As VB provides accurate anatomic information before invasive scheduled procedures, these techniques may become invaluable for simulating various treatment options, including FB and surgical and laser dilations. VB may have similar uses for pediatric patients diagnosed with thoracic malignancies, although this population has not been studied with great detail. Accurate and reproducible assessment of airway wall and luminal areas may be vital follow-up assessment of conventional and experimental nontreatment options.

VB has some limitations with respect to the management of patients with cancer. The main limitations pertain to the inability to reliably evaluate the mucosal surface of the tracheobronchial tree. Although form can be detected, mucosal color, irregularity, or friability cannot be assessed. Although there exists the continual attempt to improve acquisition capabilities and image display techniques, our inability to recognize the mucosal surface remains a significant concern. Finally, noninvasive radiologic imaging does not enable acquisition of tissue samples for histologic or microbiologic analysis. However, the answer to these problems will most likely involve use of FB and VB as complementary modalities.

CERVICAL MEDIASTINOSCOPY AND ANTERIOR MEDIASTINOTOMY

Cervical mediastinoscopy (CM) is considered the gold standard staging modality to evaluate mediastinal lymph nodes for metastasis (N2 or N3 disease) in lung cancer patients before institution of appropriate stage-specific therapies.[36] Mediastinal lymph nodes located along the trachea (pretracheal nodal stations 1 and 3, paratracheal nodal stations 2 right/left and 4 right/left, precarinal or subcarinal nodal station 7) are readily accessible by CM. On the other hand, nodal stations 5 and 6 (pre-/paraaortic and aortopulmonary window/subaortic nodes) are best accessed by anterior mediastinotomy or by thoracoscopy. Some advocated extended CM to sample these nodal stations or to perform biopsy tumors in the anterior mediastinum.[37,38]

In certain centers, CM is routinely performed on every patient with potentially resectable lung cancer, whereas in others a more selective approach is adopted, taking into account factors such as size of lymph nodes on CT scan (greater than 10 mm short diameter), size and location of the primary tumors (central or superior sulcus), and positive positron emission tomography (PET) finding. Collective review of multiple large series comprising more than 5000 patients indicates that CM has 81% sensitivity, 91% negative predictive value, and 100% specificity and positive predictive value.[3] More recently, [18F]fluorodeoxyglucose (FDG)-PET scan has been extensively evaluated as a noninvasive imaging modality for preoperative staging of the mediastinum in lung cancer patients. The overall values for sensitivity, specificity, and positive and negative predictive values of FDG-PET for regional lymph node metastasis are 89% (range, 67 to 100), 92% (range, 79 to 100), 60% (range, 47 to 92), and 97% (range, 91 to 100).[39–44] A very high negative predictive value of FDG-PET suggests that CM can be omitted in patients with negative FDG-PET imaging of the mediastinum. On the other hand, positive mediastinal FDG-PET imaging requires histologic confirmation because of the low positive predictive value (high incidence of false-positive due to inflammatory lymphadenopathy) of the test.[41,44] In addition to its utility as a staging modality for lung cancer, CM is a very accurate and safe diagnostic procedure to evaluate mediastinal lymphadenopathy due to other conditions such as sarcoidosis or lymphoma.

CM can be performed as either an inpatient or outpatient procedure under general anesthesia. The patient is positioned supine with the neck extended. A small transverse skin incision is made approximately 2 cm above the sternal notch, and dissection is carried out to expose the pretracheal fascia. Blunt finger dissection of the pretracheal and paratracheal space is performed before the mediastinoscope is inserted. The areolar connective tissue in the paratracheal space is dissected by the tip of the metal suction catheter to isolate lymph nodes of the pretracheal stations (1 and 3), paratracheal stations (2R, 2L, 4R, 4L), and pre-/subcarinal stations.[7] Visualization of the operative field and the mediastinal lymph nodes before biopsy is limited by the narrow lumen of the scope and to the operating surgeon, making this a difficult procedure to teach. To avoid inadvertent biopsy of the major vessels (superior vena cava, azygos vein, pulmonary artery), which can have a dark-blue hue similar to that of anthracotic lymph nodes, fine-needle aspiration of the target lymph node is performed before the biopsy is taken by a forceps. As for extended CM, a small area between the innominate artery and left carotid artery is initially bluntly dissected and the mediastinoscope is then inserted. The areas over the aortic arch and aortopulmonary window are examined, and stations 5 and 6 lymph nodes can be sampled. This procedure, even though described to be safe, is difficult to master and therefore not frequently performed.

CM is an extremely safe procedure with morbidity rates of 0.6% to 3.7% and mortality rates of 0.0% to 0.3% reported in several large series totaling more than 25,000 procedures,[2] even in the presence of superior vena cava obstruction.[45] Surgical complications of CM include hemorrhage (due to injury of pulmonary artery, azygos vein, superior vena cava), pneumothorax, recurrent or phrenic nerve injury, tracheal or esophageal injury, wound infection, and other complications inherent to general anesthesia.

Anterior mediastinotomy[46] allows direct access to the anterior/superior mediastinum for biopsy of tumors (thymoma, germ cell tumor, lymphoma) or sampling of stations 5 and 6 lymph nodes (left side) or those anterior to the superior vena cava (right). Under general anesthesia and with the patient position supine, a parasternal transverse skin incision is made over the second intercostal space. The intercostal muscle is divided with or without resection of a small segment of the costal cartilage for added exposure; the internal thoracic veins and artery can either be divided or dissected free and retracted medially to allow access to the anterior mediastinum. The lung is packed laterally to expose the lymph nodes or the mediastinal tumor for incisional biopsy. The pleural cavity is then evacuated of residual air at the end of the procedure by simply closing the muscle and subcutaneous layers over a red rubber catheter that is placed in the chest and fully expanding the lung while rapidly removing the catheter, thus avoiding placement of a small chest tube.

VIDEO-ASSISTED THORACOSCOPY

Video-assisted thoracoscopy has evolved from a simple diagnostic procedure pleuroscopy to a sophisticated and indispensable

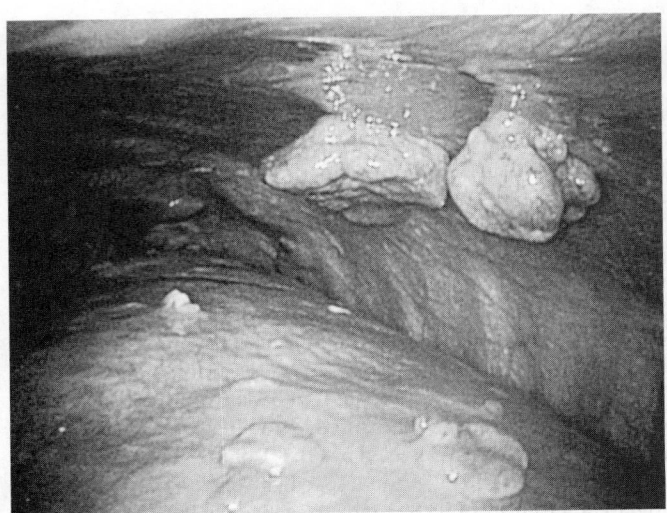

FIGURE 25.2-4. Thoracoscopic view of pleural metastasis of a patient with malignant melanoma. (See Color Fig. 25.2-4 in the CD-ROM.)

diagnostic/therapeutic modality in the armamentarium of the thoracic surgeon. This is made possible by the tremendous advances in videoendoscopic technologies and endosurgical techniques. Video-assisted thoracoscopic surgery (VATS) is most frequently performed for diagnosis and treatment of diseases involving the pleura or the lung parenchyma.

DIAGNOSTIC VIDEO-ASSISTED THORACOSCOPIC SURGERY

VATS is particularly useful in patients with recurrent pleural effusion whose etiology remains obscure despite exhaustive noninvasive diagnostic maneuvers. Loculated effusions can be drained adequately after lysis of adhesions. A large amount of pleural fluid can be collected for cytologic blocks. Biopsy of visually suspicious regions of the parietal pleura using large biopsy forceps and retrieval of adequate tissue samples allows accurate histopathologic diagnosis. VATS is particularly useful in the setting of pleural effusion or pleural mass due to malignant pleural mesothelioma in which a large biopsy specimen is essential for proper diagnosis and differentiation of mesothelioma from metastatic adenocarcinoma (Fig. 25.2-4). VATS is also indicated to evaluate the nature of pleural effusion in patients with potentially resectable lung cancer or esophageal cancer before resection if a diagnosis of malignant pleural effusion cannot be reliably excluded before thoracotomy.

Diffuse interstitial changes of the lung, particularly in the oncologic patient population, present a major diagnostic challenge for treating physicians. Interstitial changes may represent pulmonary carcinomatosis or opportunistic infection (in patients immunocompromised secondary to cytotoxic chemotherapy or bone marrow transplantation) or pulmonary fibrosis secondary to chemotherapy or thoracic irradiation. Before the advent of modern VATS, there was a great deal of reluctance to subject patients to invasive open lung biopsy by thoracotomy. Bronchoalveolar lavage, transthoracic needle aspirate, or transbronchial biopsy is less sensitive than open lung biopsy in providing an accurate diagnosis.[47] VATS is an ideal modality to provide a minimally invasive way to obtain adequate lung tissue for diagnosis

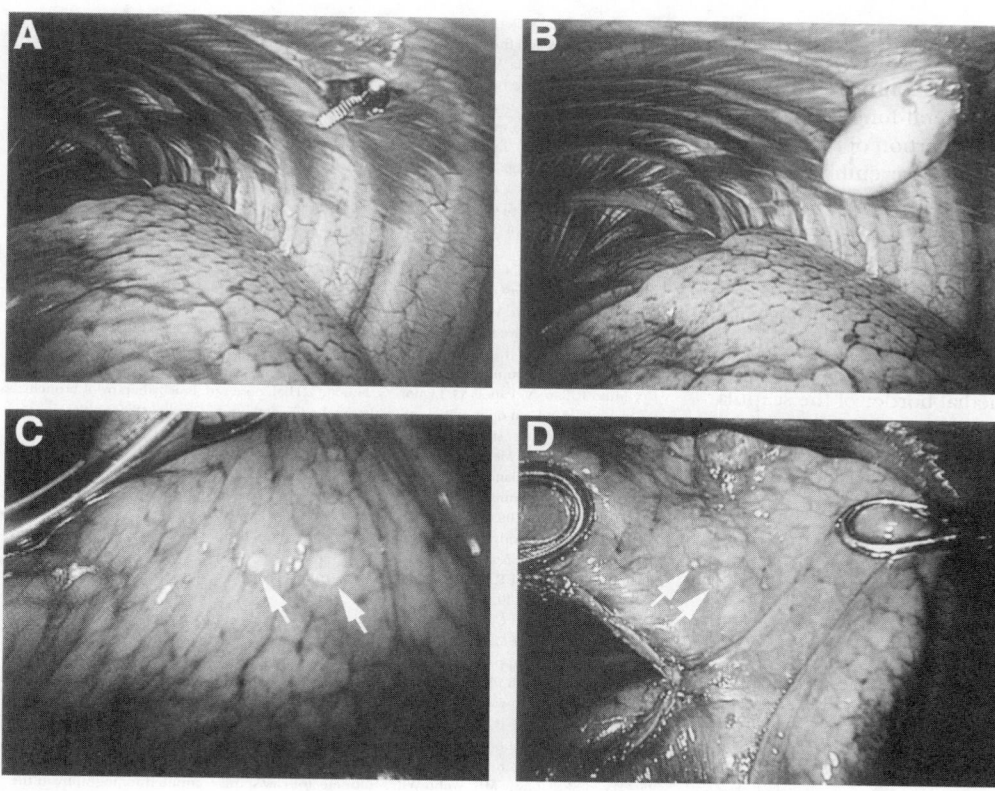

FIGURE 25.2-5. Sequence of video-assisted thoracoscopic surgery wedge lung biopsy of indeterminate lung nodules: thoracoscopic view of the pleural cavity with the lung deflated and the creation of a trocar site and digital exploration of the pleural cavity (**A,B**); identification of the subpleural nodules (*white arrows*) (**C**); and wedge excisional biopsy of the lung lesions using endoscopic stapling device (**D**). (See Color Fig. 25.2-5 in the CD-ROM.)

(Fig. 25.2-5). Increasing use of high-resolution CT scan of the thorax for lung cancer screening and other medical conditions unrelated to the chest results in the detection of subcentimeter parenchymal lung lesions that are asymptomatic and of indeterminate etiology. Excisional biopsy of anatomically favorable lesions is easily and safely performed by VATS.

Biopsy of the mediastinal lymph node stations 5 and 6 (pre-/paraaortic and aortopulmonary window/subaortic nodes) is frequently performed by anterior mediastinotomy or by VATS as part of the preoperative staging of lung cancer patients. VATS has also been extensively evaluated as a minimally invasive modality for more accurate preoperative staging of esophageal cancer. This method allows direct examination of the primary tumor for proper assignment of T status and biopsy of mediastinal lymph nodes or other suspicious intrathoracic lesions.[48–51] Mediastinal tumors, particularly those located in the middle or posterior compartments, which are not accessible by CM or anterior mediastinotomy, can be approached by VATS for incisional biopsy. VATS pericardial window is another treatment option for pericardial effusion, particularly recurrent or complicated effusion not amenable to a subxiphoid pericardiostomy.

THERAPEUTIC VIDEO-ASSISTED THORACOSCOPIC SURGERY

VATS is particularly useful in treating recalcitrant malignant pleural effusion. Drainage of loculated effusion, removal of pleural peel on the visceral pleura for proper lung expansion, mechanical abrasion of the parietal pleura, and insufflation of talc into the pleural space promote successful pleurodesis. In selected cases in which repeated talc poudrage fails to produce a satisfactory result, parietal pleurectomy may be required for adequate pleurodesis. Hemothorax due to bleeding from pleural metastatic deposits secondary to tumor necrosis or thrombocytopenia can be adequately managed with VATS by complete evacuation of hematoma and control of bleeding source by resection or coagulation using laser, argon beam, or electrocautery. Primary or secondary spontaneous pneumothorax is routinely treated with VATS blebectomy in conjunction with localized apical pleurectomy.[52,53]

VATS has been increasingly used as a therapeutic modality for solitary lung nodule. Excisional biopsy of benign lesions (e.g., granuloma, hamartoma) is diagnostic and therapeutic. Selected cases of solitary pulmonary metastasis can be managed by complete wedge resection via VATS.[54,55] The diagnosis of primary lung cancer on VATS specimen dictates pulmonary lobectomy and mediastinal lymph node resection. Although thoracotomy is the procedure of choice for lung cancer operation, lobectomy and mediastinal lymph node resection have successfully been performed by VATS in selected cases.[56–62] Similarly, laparoscopy and thoracoscopy have been used by a few specialized centers to perform minimally invasive esophagectomy for cancer of the esophagus.[63–65] The long-term results and oncologic values of such a minimally invasive approach to lung or esophageal cancers remain to be determined. Thymectomy for myasthenia gravis by VATS has been reported by a few centers,[66,67] but the experience is very limited and this approach is not yet considered a standard of care.

TECHNIQUES

The procedure is performed under general anesthesia and single lung ventilation using either a double-lumen endotracheal tube or an endotracheal tube with an endobronchial blocker.

The patient is placed in the full lateral decubitus position with the operating table flexed to lower the hip and to widen the intercostal space. Selective ventilation of the contralateral lung is instituted to allow deflation of the ipsilateral lung while a skin incision is made to create a port site for insertion of the thoracoscope. This is usually placed at the sixth or seventh intercostal space at the midaxillary line. This entrance is above the diaphragm and provides a panoramic view of the entire pleural cavity. The number and locations of the other ports are chosen based on intrathoracic findings and the procedure to be performed. Frequently, one is placed at the fourth intercostal space along the anterior axillary line and the other at the fifth intercostal space either at the posterior axillary line or even more posteriorly at the level between the medial border of the scapula and the thoracic spinous processes. The locations of these extratrocar sites are also chosen so that they can be incorporated into a thoracotomy incision if one needs to be performed. VATS for pleural biopsy or for pleurodesis can easily be performed through a single port using an operating thoracoscope that has a working channel for passage of instruments and a 5-mm viewing port. Intrathoracic manipulation is then performed by specially designed thoracoscopic instruments, including lung retractors, graspers, clip applicators, and endoscopic staplers. Once the procedure is completed, one or two chest tubes are inserted via the trocar sites and secured in place. Contraindications to VATS include dense pleural symphysis, ventilator dependence, noncompliant lung, small (less than 1 cm) deep-seated lesion, large (greater than 3 cm) lesion, chest wall invasion by tumor, inability to tolerate single ventilation or to obtain total collapse of the lung, hemodynamic instability, coagulopathy, and inability to adequately visualize operating instruments.

Complications of VATS include prolonged (greater than 7 days) air leak (1.0% to 6.7%), bleeding requiring transfusion or conversion to open thoracotomy (0.4% to 1.9%), respiratory failure requiring prolonged mechanical ventilation (0.01% to 1.0%), intercostal neuritis due to excessive manipulation of the intercostal track by bulky instrument causing nerve injury, stapling device failure, or inadvertent introduction of foreign body into the pleural cavity. More importantly, deposition and dissemination of tumor cells during VATS with subsequent tumor recurrence, particularly at the trocar sites, is a serious complication. Increased risk of pleural seeding leading to local recurrence was associated with pulling the neoplastic tissue through the narrow trocar sites when VATS is performed for malignant disease. Moreover, increased incidence of trocar site seedings is noted after thoracoscopic procedures for malignant pleural mesothelioma, metastatic sarcoma, or melanoma.[68–73]

REFERENCES

1. Falcone F, Fois F, Grosso D. Endobronchial ultrasound. *Respiration* 2003;70:179.
2. Herth FJ, Becker HD, Ernst A. Ultrasound-guided transbronchial needle aspiration: an experience in 242 patients. *Chest* 2003;123:604.
3. Toloza EM, Harpole L, Detterbeck F, McCrory DC. Invasive staging of non-small cell lung cancer: a review of the current evidence. *Chest* 2003;123:157S.
4. Kurie JM, Lee JS, Morice RC, et al. Autofluorescence bronchoscopy in the detection of squamous metaplasia and dysplasia in current and former smokers. *J Natl Cancer Inst* 1998;90:991.
5. Lam S, Kennedy T, Unger M, et al. Localization of bronchial intraepithelial neoplastic lesions by fluorescence bronchoscopy. *Chest* 1998;113:696.
6. van Rens MT, Schramel FM, Elbers JR, Lammers JW. The clinical value of lung imaging fluorescence endoscopy for detecting synchronous lung cancer. *Lung Cancer* 2001; 32:13.
7. Kennedy TC, Miller Y, Prindiville S. Screening for lung cancer revisited and the role of sputum cytology and fluorescence bronchoscopy in a high-risk group. *Chest* 2000;117:72S.
8. Sato M, Sakurada A, Sagawa M, et al. Diagnostic results before and after introduction of autofluorescence bronchoscopy in patients suspected of having lung cancer detected by sputum cytology in lung cancer mass screening. *Lung Cancer* 2001;32:247.
9. Shibuya K, Fujisawa T, Hoshino H, et al. Fluorescence bronchoscopy in the detection of preinvasive bronchial lesions in patients with sputum cytology suspicious or positive for malignancy. *Lung Cancer* 2001;32:19.
10. Weigel TL, Kosco PJ, Dacic S, et al. Postoperative fluorescence bronchoscopic surveillance in non-small cell lung cancer patients. *Ann Thorac Surg* 2001;71:967.
11. Mehrishi S, Raoof S, Mehta AC. Therapeutic flexible bronchoscopy. *Chest Surg Clin N Am* 2001;11:657.
12. Kato H, Okunaka T, Shimatani H. Photodynamic therapy for early stage bronchogenic carcinoma. *J Clin Laser Med Surg* 1996;14:235.
13. McCaughan JS Jr, Williams TE. Photodynamic therapy for endobronchial malignant disease: a prospective fourteen-year study. *J Thorac Cardiovasc Surg* 1997;114:940.
14. McCaughan JS Jr. Survival after photodynamic therapy to non-pulmonary metastatic endobronchial tumors. *Lasers Surg Med* 1999;24:194.
15. Muto P, Ravo V, Panelli G, Liguori G, Fraioli G. High-dose rate brachytherapy of bronchial cancer: treatment optimization using three schemes of therapy. *Oncologist* 2000;5:209.
16. Wood DE. Airway stenting. *Chest Surg Clin N Am* 2001;11:841.
17. Cordasco EM Jr, Mehta AC, Ahmad M. Bronchoscopically induced bleeding. A summary of nine years' Cleveland clinic experience and review of the literature. *Chest* 1991;100:1141.
18. Credle WF Jr, Smiddy JF, Elliott RC. Complications of fiberoptic bronchoscopy. *Am Rev Respir Dis* 1974;109:67.
19. Suratt PM, Smiddy JF, Gruber B. Deaths and complications associated with fiberoptic bronchoscopy. *Chest* 1976;69:747.
20. Pue CA, Pacht ER. Complications of fiberoptic bronchoscopy at a university hospital. *Chest* 1995;107:430.
21. Schaefer-Prokop C, Prokop M. New imaging techniques in the treatment guidelines for lung cancer. *Eur Respir J* 2002;35[Suppl]:71s.
22. Colice GL, Chappel GJ, Frenchman SM, Solomon DA. Comparison of computerized tomography with fiberoptic bronchoscopy in identifying endobronchial abnormalities in patients with known or suspected lung cancer. *Am Rev Respir Dis* 1985;131:397.
23. Naidich DP, Lee JJ, Garay SM, et al. Comparison of CT and fiberoptic bronchoscopy in the evaluation of bronchial disease. *AJR Am J Roentgenol* 1987;148:1.
24. Haponik EF, Aquino SL, Vining DJ. Virtual bronchoscopy. *Clin Chest Med* 1999;20:201.
25. Dawn SK, Gotway MB, Webb WR. Multidetector-row spiral computed tomography in the diagnosis of thoracic diseases. *Respir Care* 2001;46:912.
26. Aquino SL, Vining DJ. Virtual bronchoscopy. *Clin Chest Med* 1999;20:725.
27. McWilliams A, MacAulay C, Gazdar AF, Lam S. Innovative molecular and imaging approaches for the detection of lung cancer and its precursor lesions. *Oncogene* 2002; 21:6949.
28. Summers R, Sneller M, Langford C, et al. Improved virtual bronchoscopy using a multislice helical CT scanner. In: Chen CT, Clough A. eds. *Medical imaging 2000: physiology and function from multidimensional images* Vol. 3978. Bellingham, Washington: American Association of Physicists in Medicine, 2000:117.
29. Fleiter T, Merkle EM, Aschoff AJ, et al. Comparison of real-time virtual and fiberoptic bronchoscopy in patients with bronchial carcinoma: opportunities and limitations. *AJR Am J Roentgenol* 1997;169:1591.
30. Liewald F, Lang G, Fleiter, T, et al. Comparison of virtual and fiberoptic bronchoscopy. *Thorac Cardiovasc Surg* 1998;46:361.
31. Rapp-Bernhardt U, Welte T, Budinger M, Bernhardt TM. Comparison of three-dimensional virtual endoscopy with bronchoscopy in patients with oesophageal carcinoma infiltrating the tracheobronchial tree. *Br J Radiol* 1998;71:1271.
32. Rapp-Bernhardt U, Welte T, Doehring W, Kropf S, Bernhardt TM. Diagnostic potential of virtual bronchoscopy: advantages in comparison with axial CT slices, MPR and mIP? *Eur Radiol* 2000;10:981.
33. Hoppe H, Walder B, Sonnenschein M, Vock P, Dinkel HP. Multidetector CT virtual bronchoscopy to grade tracheobronchial stenosis. *AJR Am J Roentgenol* 2002;178:1195.
34. Finkelstein SE, Summers RM, Nguyen DM, et al. Virtual bronchoscopy for evaluation of malignant tumors of the thorax. *J Thorac Cardiovasc Surg* 2002;123:967.
35. Finkelstein SE, Schrump DS, Nguyen DM, et al. Comparative evaluation of super-high resolution CT and virtual bronchoscopy for thoracic malignancies. *Chest* 2003;124:1834.
36. Ginsberg RJ. Evaluation of the mediastinum by invasive techniques. *Surg Clin North Am* 1987;67:1025.
37. Ginsberg RJ, Rice TW, Goldberg M, Waters PF, Schmocker BJ. Extended cervical mediastinoscopy. A single staging procedure for bronchogenic carcinoma of the left upper lobe. *J Thorac Cardiovasc Surg* 1987;94:673.
38. Metin M, Sayar A, Turna A, Gurses A. Extended cervical mediastinoscopy in the diagnosis of anterior mediastinal masses. *Ann Thorac Surg* 2002;73:250.
39. Chang MY, Sugarbaker DJ. Surgery for early stage non-small cell lung cancer. *Semin Surg Oncol* 2003;21:74.
40. Cerfolio RJ, Ojha B, Bryant AS, et al. The role of FDG-PET scan in staging patients with nonsmall cell carcinoma. *Ann Thorac Surg* 2003;76:861.
41. Vansteenkiste JF, Stroobants SG, Dupont PJ, et al. Prognostic importance of the standardized uptake value on (18)F-fluoro-2-deoxy-glucose-positron emission tomography scan in non-small-cell lung cancer: An analysis of 125 cases. Leuven Lung Cancer Group. *J Clin Oncol* 1999;17:3201.
42. Vansteenkiste JF. PET scan in the staging of non-small cell lung cancer. *Lung Cancer* 2003;42:S27.
43. Pieterman RM, van Putten JW, Meuzelaar JJ, et al. Preoperative staging of non-small-cell lung cancer with positron-emission tomography. *N Engl J Med* 2000;343:254.

44. Farrell MA, McAdams HP, Herndon JE, Patz EF Jr. Non-small cell lung cancer: FDG PET for nodal staging in patients with stage I disease. *Radiology* 2000;215:886.

45. Jahangiri M, Goldstraw P. The role of mediastinoscopy in superior vena caval obstruction. *Ann Thorac Surg* 1995;59:453.

46. McNeill TM, Chamberlain JM. Diagnostic anterior mediastinotomy. *Ann Thorac Surg* 1966;2:532.

47. Burt ME, Flye MW, Webber BL, Wesley RA. Prospective evaluation of aspiration needle, cutting needle, transbronchial, and open lung biopsy in patients with pulmonary infiltrates. *Ann Thorac Surg* 1981;32:146.

48. Hazelrigg SR, Nunchuck SK, LoCicero J III. Video Assisted Thoracic Surgery Study Group data. *Ann Thorac Surg* 1993;56:1039.

49. Kirby TJ, Mack MJ, Landreneau RJ, Rice TW. Initial experience with video-assisted thoracoscopic lobectomy. *Ann Thorac Surg* 1993;56:1248.

50. Krasna MJ, Reed CE, Nedzwiecki D, et al. CALGB 9380: a prospective trial of the feasibility of thoracoscopy/laparoscopy in staging esophageal cancer. *Ann Thorac Surg* 2001;71:1073.

51. Krasna MJ, Jiao X, Mao YS, et al. Thoracoscopy/laparoscopy in the staging of esophageal cancer: Maryland experience. *Surg Laparosc Endosc Percutan Tech* 2002;12:213.

52. Yim AP, Liu HP. Video assisted thoracoscopic management of primary spontaneous pneumothorax. *Surg Laparosc Endosc* 1997;7:236.

53. Torresini G, Vaccarili M, Divisi D, Crisci R. Is video-assisted thoracic surgery justified at first spontaneous pneumothorax? *Eur J Cardiothorac Surg* 2001;20:42.

54. Lin JC, Wiechmann RJ, Szwerc MF, et al. Diagnostic and therapeutic video-assisted thoracic surgery resection of pulmonary metastases. *Surgery* 1999;126:636.

55. Mutsaerts EL, Zoetmulder FA, Meijer S, et al. Outcome of thoracoscopic pulmonary metastasectomy evaluated by confirmatory thoracotomy. *Ann Thorac Surg* 2001;72:230.

56. Nomori H, Horio H, Naruke T, Suemasu K. What is the advantage of a thoracoscopic lobectomy over a limited thoracotomy procedure for lung cancer surgery? *Ann Thorac Surg* 2001;72:879.

57. Sagawa M, Sato M, Sakurada A, et al. A prospective trial of systematic nodal dissection for lung cancer by video-assisted thoracic surgery: can it be perfect? *Ann Thorac Surg* 2002;73:900.

58. Yim AP. VATS major pulmonary resection revisited—controversies, techniques, and results. *Ann Thorac Surg* 2002;74:615.

59. Gharagozloo F, Tempesta B, Margolis M, Alexander EP. Video-assisted thoracic surgery lobectomy for stage I lung cancer. *Ann Thorac Surg* 2003;76:1009.

60. Walker WS, Codispoti M, Soon SY, et al. Long-term outcomes following VATS lobectomy for non-small cell bronchogenic carcinoma. *Eur J Cardiothorac Surg* 2003;23:397.

61. Nomori H, Ohtsuka T, Horio H, Naruke T, Suemasu K. Thoracoscopic lobectomy for lung cancer with a largely fused fissure. *Chest* 2003;123:619.

62. Koizumi K, Haraguchi S, Hirata T, et al. Lobectomy by video-assisted thoracic surgery for lung cancer patients aged 80 years or more. *Ann Thorac Cardiovasc Surg* 2003;9:14.

63. Luketich JD, Alvelo-Rivera M, Buenaventura PO, et al. Minimally invasive esophagectomy: outcomes in 222 patients. *Ann Surg* 2003;238:486.

64. Osugi H, Takemura M, Higashino M, et al. Video-assisted thoracoscopic esophagectomy and radical lymph node dissection for esophageal cancer. A series of 75 cases. *Surg Endosc* 2002;16:1588.

65. Fernando HC, Luketich JD, Buenaventura PO, Perry Y, Christie NA. Outcomes of minimally invasive esophagectomy (MIE) for high-grade dysplasia of the esophagus. *Eur J Cardiothorac Surg* 2002;22:1.

66. Savcenko M, Wendt GK, Prince SL, Mack MJ. Video-assisted thymectomy for myasthenia gravis: an update of a single institution experience. *Eur J Cardiothorac Surg* 2002;22:978.

67. Wright GM, Barnett S, Clarke CP. Video-assisted thoracoscopic thymectomy for myasthenia gravis. *Intern Med J* 2002;32:367.

68. Walsh GL, Nesbitt JC. Tumor implants after thoracoscopic resection of a metastatic sarcoma. *Ann Thorac Surg* 1995;59:215.

69. Collard JM, Reymond MA. Video-assisted thoracic surgery (VATS) for cancer. Risk of parietal seeding and of early local recurrence. *Int Surg* 1996;81:343.

70. Jancovici R, Lang-Lazdunski L, Pons F, et al. Complications of video-assisted thoracic surgery: a five-year experience. *Ann Thorac Surg* 1996;61:533.

71. Krasna MJ, Deshmukh S, McLaughlin JS. Complications of thoracoscopy. *Ann Thorac Surg* 1996;61:1066.

72. Yim AP, Liu HP. Complications and failures of video-assisted thoracic surgery: experience from two centers in Asia. *Ann Thorac Surg* 1996;61:538.

73. Downey RJ, McCormack P, LoCicero J III. Dissemination of malignant tumors after video-assisted thoracic surgery: a report of twenty-one cases. The Video-Assisted Thoracic Surgery Study Group. *J Thorac Cardiovasc Surg* 1996;111:954.

CHAPTER 26

Cancer of the Head and Neck

SECTION **1**

DAVID SIDRANSKY

Molecular Biology of Head and Neck Tumors

Cancer is a complex genetic disease derived from the accumulation of various genetic changes. These genetic alterations include activation of protooncogenes and inactivation of tumor suppressor genes. Moreover, inactivation of tumor suppressor gene function requires inactivation of both parental alleles, usually by point mutation and a chromosomal deletion. The correlation of these specific genetic changes with the various lesions depicted in the histopathologic progression of colorectal cancer has led to the development of a molecular progression model for this disease.[1] This molecular model now serves as a paradigm for the molecular progression of many other solid neoplasms.

A number of specific genetic events have been identified in the progression of head and neck squamous cell carcinoma (HNSCC). Primary tumor DNA can now be isolated and assessed directly for the presence of chromosomal deletions and amplification, as well as direct characterization of candidate oncogenes. Identification of the critical genetic changes that drive the neoplastic process has provided a molecular progression model for head and neck cancer. This model now delineates appropriate genetic targets for novel diagnostic, prognostic, and therapeutic strategies.

GENETIC SUSCEPTIBILITY

It has been estimated that up to 10% of all cancers have a strong hereditary component. Generally, familial clustering of cancer has suggested the possibility of genetic predisposing factors. A clustering of oral cancer has been seen in certain ethnic groups, and an increased risk of cancer has been noted among relatives of patients with one head and neck cancer.[2,3] Several studies have suggested a threefold higher risk of developing an oropharyngeal cancer in populations that have a first-degree relative with HNSCC.[4] Some suggestions have also been made of a remarkable increase in the relative risk of cancer in relatives of individuals with multiple primary tumors. Except for the finding of head and neck cancer in some rare cancer syndromes such as Li-Fraumeni syndrome and Fanconi's anemia, the basis of this genetic susceptibility has yet to be determined.[5,6]

An emerging area of study centers on the prevalence of specific polymorphisms in enzymes that are involved in the detoxification of several tobacco smoke–derived carcinogens. One larger study of 162 patients with head and neck cancer and 315 healthy controls suggested that certain glutathione S-transferase (GST) genotypes represented independent risk factors for head and neck cancer.[7] Some studies also have shown a two- to threefold risk for the GSTM1 and GSTT1 null genotypes, whereas others have shown no increase in HNSCC risk.[8–13] In all these studies, although it is difficult to exclude other important risk factors, such as smoking, there appears to be a consistent susceptibility based on certain metabolic genotypes. Others also have found that the repair capacity of peripheral lymphocytes or their ability to repair carcinogen-induced chromatic breaks may also define a certain risk for head and neck cancer.[14–16] A more precise contribution of these polymorphisms and other risk factors to the development of head and neck cancer needs to be elucidated in larger studies.

CYTOGENETIC ALTERATIONS

Statistical analysis based on the age-specific incidence of head and neck cancer suggests that HNSCC tumors arise after the accumulation of six to ten independent genetic events.[17] Cytogenetic approaches have given us some insights into potential areas of deletion and amplification involved in the progression of head and neck cancer. Previously, karyotypic studies concentrated on established cell lines with complex chromosomal abnormalities. Unfortunately, different cell culture conditions added substantial variation to these observed chromosomal alterations.[18] Moreover, cultured cells from the primary tumor may represent only a small clone derived from *in vitro* selection pressure that is not representative of the entire cell population. Short-term cultures of primary tumors have proven more reliable for the assessment of complex[19] chromosome abnormalities and rearrangements. These studies have already demonstrated consistent chromosomal abnormalities and the presence of important alterations.[19] Loss of chromosomes 3p, 5q, 8p, 9p, 18q, and 21q has been commonly identified. Preliminary data also suggest that loss of 18q may indicate the presence of a tumor with a poor prognosis.[19] Additionally, multiple chromosomal breakpoints, including those on 1p22, 3p21, 8p11, and distal 14q, have correlated with decreased radiosensitivity.[20] Fluorescence *in situ* hybridization potentially represents a more sensitive approach for recognizing chromosomal deletions and amplifications.[21] For example, genomic amplification at the 11q13 region can be detected in preneoplastic lesions and should allow its placement directly into a molecular progression model.

Comparative genomic hybridization has emerged as a comprehensive method for genome-wide evaluation to detect deletions or amplification. In this approach, tumor-normal DNA is mixed and hybridized to metaphase spreads from normal cells. Labeling of tumor-normal DNA by different fluorescent colors allows direct visualization of increased or decreased chromosomal material in neoplastic tissue by fluorescence detection. This approach is complementary to other methods for assessment of tissue culture and primary tumor material. In addition to the chromosomal areas previously noted, comparative genomic hybridization has demonstrated amplification of 3q, 5p, 11q13, and 19q.[22]

PROTOONCOGENES

Protooncogenes were initially identified as activated cellular genes specifically altered in some human neoplasms.[23] Despite the cloning of dozens of putative protooncogenes involved in the development of human neoplasms, few were found to be altered directly in the progression of primary tumors and cell lines. In addition to activation of oncogenes such as ras by point mutation, amplification is also a mechanism for activation of a protooncogene locus. Definitive studies suggested that the 11q13 amplification was associated with amplification of a critical protooncogene termed *cyclin D1* (PRAD1; CCND1). Although other genes were also coamplified in the same region, only cyclin D1 was consistently amplified in approximately 30% of HNSCC and most other neoplasms.[24,25] Moreover, amplification of this region correlated with increased expression of the cyclin D1 gene and may indicate a likelihood of progression in primary HNSCC.[26]

The role of cyclin D1 in the progression of human cancer is now well established.[27] Other tumor suppressor genes, including Rb and p16, are negative regulators of the cyclin D1 pathway and often are inactivated in human neoplasms. In head and neck cancer, p16 appears to be a major target of inactivation. Thus, abnormal cycling through this critical G_1/S check-

point may be a consistent genetic alteration in a majority of primary HNSCCs. Although p16 and Rb inactivation are almost always exclusive, cyclin D1 amplification is independent of p16 inactivation in head and neck cancers.[28]

As mentioned earlier, amplification of 3q has been noted in many SCCs, including head and neck cancer. A p53 homologue (p40/p51/p63) has been cloned and localized to the distal arm of 3q.[29] Although homologous to p53, this genetic locus was found to be amplified in a high frequency of squamous cell cancers, and this amplification correlated with increased expression at the RNA and protein level.[30] Although there has been no evidence of activating point mutations in squamous cell cancers, functional evidence suggests that p63 may in fact be a true oncogene in squamous cell cancers.[30] Interestingly, dominant negative mutations of p63 are responsible for a specific hereditary syndrome called *ectrodactyly–ectodermal dysplasia–clefting syndrome*.[31] Knockout mice display a lack of epithelial development consistent with the role of this gene in epithelial renewal.[32]

p63 encodes multiple proteins with transactivating, apoptosis-inducing, and oncogenic activities. Studies have shown that p63 is amplified and that ΔNp63 isotypes are overexpressed in HNSCC and enhance oncogenic growth *in vitro* and *in vivo*. p53 appears to regulate its family member by physically binding with ΔNp63α and mediating its degradation. A report has demonstrated that ΔNp63 associates with the B56α regulatory subunit of protein phosphatase 2A and glycogen synthase kinase-3β (GSK3β), leading to a dramatic inhibition of protein phosphatase 2A–mediated GSK3β reactivation. The inhibitory effect of ΔNp63 on GSK3β mediated a decrease in phosphorylation levels of β-catenin, which induces intranuclear accumulation of β-catenin and activates β-catenin–dependent transcription. These results suggest that ΔNp63 isotypes act as positive regulators of the β-catenin signaling pathway, providing a basis for their oncogenic properties in SCC.[33]

Like other epithelial neoplasms, the role of other protooncogenes has been much less definitive. Few mutations in ras have been identified in primary head and neck tumors. Although epidermal growth factor receptor has been an interesting candidate, increased levels of the receptor at the RNA or protein level rarely correlate with primary DNA amplification.[34] New evidence suggests that activation of signaling through Stat-3 leads to epidermal growth factor receptor–mediated cell growth and that antisense suppression of epidermal growth factor receptor protein leads to apoptosis (programmed cell death).[35,36] The protein eukaryotic initiation factor (eIF4E) binds to messenger RNA during initial protein synthesis, and its overexpression can result in the up-regulation of proteins essential for cell growth and division. Overexpression of eIF4E has been found in HNSCC, and there has been some evidence of gene amplification and protein overexpression in these tumors.[37,38] Overexpression of the protein in cells can lead to oncogenic transformation and may facilitate the synthesis of angiogenic factors such as vascular epidermal growth factor by enhancing their translation. In at least one study, there was a correlation between increasing eIF4E and vascular epidermal growth factor levels, suggesting its possible role in angiogenesis.[39]

Additionally, several other genes or gene products have been found to be overexpressed in head and neck tumors. High levels of cyclooxygenase-2 have been seen in SCCs by a competitive reverse transcription assay.[40] GSTP1 messenger RNA levels are found to be high in most moderately and poorly differentiated tumors,[41] but only a fraction of these had specific gene amplification. Newer microarray techniques (see Tumor Suppressor Genes, later in this chapter) may lead to the identification of important protooncogenes more commonly involved in the progression of HNSCC.

SUPPRESSIVE GROWTH REGULATION

In addition to growth factors with "positive" regulation and augmentation of tumor growth, other growth factor pathways may suppress cell growth. Transforming growth factor-β (TGF-β) is among these growth factors that have been implicated almost universally with suppression of tumor growth. Alterations of the type II TGF-β receptor, one target of TGF-β, were noted in primary colorectal cancers potentially involved in abrogation of this negative regulatory pathway.[42] Initially, some head and neck cancer cell lines were also found to harbor TGF-β receptor mutations, and mutations in the conserved serine-threonine kinase domain were found in 6 of 28 primary tumors.[43,44] The interaction of TGF-β with this critical receptor normally leads to an increase of negative regulators of the cell cycle (e.g., p15, INK4B) and G_1/S arrest; thus, normal negative regulation may be abrogated by mutations in the type II TGF-β receptor.

Through a different mechanism, retinoic acid receptors (RARs) have been implicated in the negative growth regulation of HNSCC. This negative regulation has been the cornerstone of successful chemopreventive approaches to diminish the incidence of second primary tumors by administration of *cis*-retinoic acid to patients with a primary HNSCC tumor.[45] Well-designed studies have demonstrated a significant reduction in the occurrence of second primary tumors in patients who receive retinoic acid. Although the regulation of retinoids is complex, one critical end point may be down-regulation of RAR-β. Studies in patients with premalignant disease (leukoplakia) have suggested that RAR-β levels are suppressed during immortalization and are closely associated with response to retinoic acid.[46,47] In particular, those patients with tumors that demonstrate low RAR-β levels, perhaps through promoter hypermethylation,[48] did not respond to retinoic acid. Further functional studies into the role of retinoic acid and RAR-β may yield important information regarding the role of this pathway in the progression of HNSCC and successful treatment of premalignant lesions.

TUMOR SUPPRESSOR GENES

Molecular analysis has now revolutionized the ability to look at primary neoplasms. Methods that required large amounts of DNA (e.g., Southern blot analysis) have now been supplemented by polymerase chain reaction (PCR)–based approaches that allow access to limited DNA samples. Minute primary specimens from paraffin can be evaluated by rapid and accurate techniques. DNA extracted from these samples can be amplified by PCR to reveal the presence of allelic losses. In practice, maternal and paternal alleles can be distinguished by testing highly polymorphic markers that occur naturally among DNA sequences.[49]

It is now generally believed that these allelic losses (or chromosomal deletions) are markers for inactivation of critical tumor suppressor genes contained within the regions of loss.[50]

Testing of highly polymorphic microsatellite markers (small 2- to 4-base-pair repeats) from a specific chromosomal region allows rapid assessment of allelic loss by comparing the alleles in tumor DNA to normal DNA. Perhaps the best example of this association is derived from loss of chromosome 17p. These losses led to characterization of p53 as a candidate gene within the deleted area and subsequent identification of point mutations within the remaining allele. Inactivation of p53 now represents the best-described and most common genetic change in all of human cancer.[51] More than 50% of all primary HNSCCs harbor p53 mutations in the conserved regions of the gene.[52,53]

A comprehensive allelotype of head and neck cancer has now been completed and refined.[54,55] The most commonly deleted region in head and neck cancer is located at chromosome 9p21-22.[54] Loss of chromosome 9p21 occurs in the majority of invasive tumors and is also present at a high frequency in the earliest definable lesions, including dysplasia and carcinoma *in situ*.[56] Furthermore, homozygous deletions in this region are frequent in HNSCC and represent one of the most common genetic changes identified in all human neoplasms. p16 (*CDKN2*) is contained within this critically deleted region and is a potent inhibitor of cyclin D1/*CDK4* complexes. Thus, p16 has emerged as an excellent candidate tumor suppressor gene within the deleted area.[57] Indeed, germline point mutations of p16 predispose to familial melanoma,[58] and loss of p16 may be necessary for immortalization of keratinocytes.[59]

Although initial enthusiasm for p16 as a target gene in head and neck cancer was diminished when sequence analysis revealed rare point mutation (approximately 10% to 15% of HNSCC tumors),[60,61] alternative mechanisms of inactivation were identified, suggesting that abrogation of p16 function may be a common occurrence in head and neck cancer. Homozygous deletion (deletion of both gene copies) and methylation of the 5' CpG region of p16 have been identified, each detected in approximately one-fourth of primary head and neck cancers.[62,63] This methylation is associated with complete block of p16 transcription and appears to be a common mechanism for p16 inactivation. The notion that p16 inactivation is directly involved in the progression of primary tumors has been strengthened. Lack of p16 protein was detected by immunostaining in most primary invasive lesions, and tumors with absent p16 protein contained a homozygous deletion, methylation, or point mutation of p16.[64] Loss of p16 protein has been observed in most advanced premalignant lesions.[65]

It is also possible that a second critical tumor suppressor gene resides at 9p21. The author's group and others have identified an alternative RNA transcript for p16 termed *alternative rating frame* (ARF; or p16β).[66] This unique transcript originates from an upstream initiating site in a novel exon 1 and codes for a protein through an ARF. Introduction of p16 or p16ARF into head and neck cancer cell lines results in potent growth suppression.[67] Although the human transcript is somewhat shorter than the murine protein, functional studies have suggested that ARF binds to MDM-2 (murine double-minute gene-2), leading to a decrease in p53 degradation and a subsequent increase in p53 levels.[68,69] Moreover, certain tumors develop in a knockout ARF mouse at an increased frequency.[70] In human tumors, homozygous deletion of the p16 locus concomitantly leads to knockout of ARF, and thus approximately 30% of HNSCCs have no ARF protein. Evidence in SCC of the lung suggests that p53 mutations and p16 inactivation are not exclusive, suggesting that, at least at the genetic level, they do not function in the same pathway.[71] Continuing studies in primary tumors and human models will help establish the precise role of ARF inactivation in SCC.

A second commonly deleted locus occurs on chromosome 3p. Several studies have suggested that this region of loss is complex in head and neck cancer and may in fact be composed of three distinct suppressor regions juxtaposed to one another.[72,73] As for 9p21, analysis of 3p21 losses in HNSCC has revealed frequent loss in early lesions. The 3p21 region is also frequently lost in lung cancer and has been the target of an intensive search for the critical tumor suppressor gene. The *FHIT* gene was found in a critical area of homozygous deletion and was evaluated as a possible tumor suppressor gene in many cancers. Although altered transcripts have been detected in primary tumors and cell lines, specific inactivating mutations of the second allele have not been forthcoming.[74,75] Promoter methylation of RASSF1A, a gene on 3p implicated in the *ras* pathway, was detected in 15% of primary tumors but not in the normal control DNA.[76,77] Moreover, an inverse correlation between RASSF1A and human papillomavirus (HPV) supports a biologic mechanism in which RASSF1A promoter methylation and HPV infection abrogate the same pathway in tumorigenesis. Thus, several candidate genes have been isolated on chromosomal arm 3p but await further characterization in the progression of these cancers.

Loss of chromosome 17p is a frequent occurrence in most human cancers, and head and neck cancer is no exception (occurring in 60% of invasive lesions).[52] Although p53 inactivation correlates closely with loss of 17p in invasive lesions, p53 mutations are quite rare in early lesions that contain 17p loss. Some evidence from cell lines also suggests that a distal breakpoint to p53 occurs in head and neck cancer. Together, these data suggest that a second tumor suppressor gene on 17p may be involved early in the progression of this neoplasm. p53 mutations, as in most tumors, generally rise in frequency between the preinvasive to the invasive state. This is consistent with a critical function for p53 in response to DNA damage.[78,79] This model is certain to become more complex but offers an important insight into the role of p53 in the progression of head and neck cancer and many other tumors.

Loss of chromosomal arm 10q is not uncommon in HNSCC and lung cancer. The *PTEN* gene was cloned and found to be homozygously deleted and inactivated in a variety of different cancers. Homozygous deletion and rare point mutation inactivation have been seen in HNSCC.[79–81] Although only 10% of these cancers have inactivated gene, it seems to be more common in advanced tumors and may harbor a poor prognosis.[82,83]

Loss of 13q also occurs in approximately 60% of primary tumors, and the minimal area of loss includes the tumor suppressor gene Rb. However, immunohistochemical analysis of Rb (which detects most Rb alterations) revealed inactivation of Rb in only small percentages of tumors with loss of 13q.[84] Again, as in many other chromosomal regions, there appears to be another tumor suppressor gene near Rb, putatively inactivated in the progression of head and neck cancer.

More recent work has suggested that there may be one or more regions of specific loss on the short arm of chromosome 8 and on 7q31.[85–88] Loss of 18q has been seen, and one of these minimally deleted regions harbors two tumor suppressor genes.[89,90] Homozygous deletions of *DCC* and *DPC4* have been noted in cell lines but have rarely been seen in primary tumors.[91] Many other areas of chromosomal loss have been seen in head and neck cancer consistent with the occurrence of multiple genetic events in the progression of these neoplasms. Except for those previously noted, critical tumor suppressor genes have not been identified from these loci and remain to be isolated and characterized. In addition to p16 and RASSF1A, promoter hypermethylation of MGMT (approximately 30% of primary tumors), death-associated protein kinase (approximately 20%), and E-cadherin (approximately 40%) were described in primary tumors.[92–95] Further fine mapping of these deletions, amplifications, and translocations with characterization of critical genes within these areas may provide important information about the biology and clinical behavior of these neoplasms.

MOLECULAR PROGRESSION MODELS

We have tested the ten most common allelic loss events in a large number of primary preinvasive lesions and invasive HNSCC to develop a molecular progression model.[96] As seen in Figure 26.1-1, the progression of head and neck cancer involves inactivation of many putative suppressor gene loci. Chromosomes 9p and 3p appear to be lost early, closely followed by loss of 17p. p53 mutations are seen in the progression of the preinvasive to invasive lesions, and many other genetic events occur later in progression. Other specific genetic events, such as amplification of cyclin D1 and inactivation of p16, have been tested predominantly in invasive lesions, and their precise order in the model cannot yet be determined. As noted in the molecular model for colorectal cancer, it is the accumulation and not necessarily the precise order of these genetic events that determines histopathologic progression. This is best exemplified by some early lesions that demonstrated a "late" event as the sole genetic alteration.

To test this model directly, the author's group was able to analyze lesions that demonstrated histologic progression from one area to another. In each of the cases, they confirmed that 9p and 3p loss were early events, with other genetic changes occurring in the more advanced histopathologic lesion. Moreover, lesions biopsied in the same area over time in a few critical patients also demonstrated the same general order of these events. Molecular progression models such as this one allow direct characterization of early genetic events that might be important in diagnos-

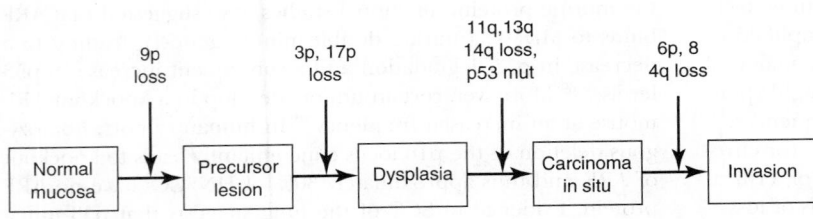

FIGURE 26.1-1. Preliminary progression model for head and neck squamous cell carcinoma. Genetic alterations have been ordered by testing a variety of preinvasive and invasive lesions and determining the frequency of these events at each stage in progression. Inactivation of p16 (chromosome 9p21) and amplification of cyclin D1 (chromosome 11q13q) have not been directly tested in preinvasive lesions. It is the accumulation and not necessarily the order of these genetic changes that determines progression.

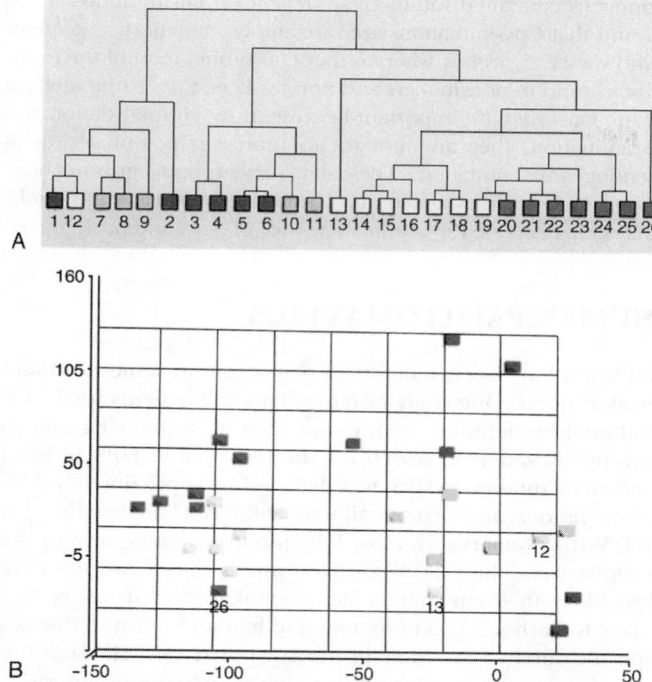

A

B

FIGURE 26.1-2. Clustering of histologic groups after microarray expression analysis. **A:** Hierarchic clustering analysis graphic in 26 samples demonstrating the separation of the four groups based solely on gene expression data. The segregation of the groups demonstrates that global expression differences that occur as head and neck lesions develop a malignant phenotype. Blue, normal; green, matched normal; yellow, premalignant; red, malignant. **B:** Principal components analysis graphic depicting a two-dimensional representation of the four histologic groups. The distance in space between the colored boxes represents the degree of relatedness between the samples. Close proximity of malignant and premalignant groups is noted, with separation from normal and matched normal samples. Blue, normal; green, matched normal; yellow, premalignant; red, malignant. (See Color Fig. 26.1-2 in the CD-ROM.)

tic strategies. Critical events that occur in the progression from the preinvasive state to the invasive state (e.g., p53 mutations) may be useful as prognostic indicators in primary lesions. Losses occurring later in progression, such as 11q, 13q, 14q, and 18q, and loss of p27 protein (another cyclin-dependent kinase inhibitor) have been found to correlate with a decrease in survival.[97–101] p53 mutations may correlate with response to chemotherapy and local regional failure after radiation therapy.[79,102]

Early losses at 3p14 and 9p21 may persist in premalignant lesions exposed to chemoprevention agents and may predict those likely to relapse despite apparent histologic remissions.[103,104] Several studies of head and neck cancer suggest that early genetic changes do not necessarily correlate with observable changes in morphology. Pivotal studies on prospectively collected oral cavity lesions with longitudinal follow-up have shown that virtually all (approximately 100%) progressive (within 3 to 5 years) lesions harbor 3p or 9p loss.[105–107] Moreover, the chance of an individual lesion progressing if 3p or 9p loss is present ranges from 44% to 71% in patients without a history of prior cancer. As predicted by the progression model, if 17p loss or p53 mutation is present in these early lesions, the chance of progression to cancer within 10 years

approaches 80% (33-fold relative risk). In patients with previous cancer, 3p or 9p loss, or both, in posttreatment leukoplakia was associated with a 26.3-fold increase in risk of developing second oral malignancy compared with those who retained both of these arms, with 60% of patients with loss of heterozygosity developing second oral malignancy in 2 years.[105] In contrast, histologic diagnosis (moderate or severe dysplasia vs. hyperplasia or mild dysplasia) without genetic changes had only a 1.7-fold increase in risk. One method to detect lesions that are not clinically evident is to use a toluidine blue stain. Studies have suggested that 80% of all lesions identified by this staining method harbor clonal genetic changes.[108,109] Thus, early detection of such lesions and testing for these genetic alterations or ploidy may identify patients who are at the greatest risk for progression or relapse.

Using complementary DNA microarrays, similar preneoplastic and malignant lesions have been tested for variations at the RNA level. One larger analysis revealed 965 up-regulated and 1106 down-regulated genes in malignant lesions relative to normal mucosa. The preneoplastic group of lesions demonstrated 108 up-regulated and 226 down-regulated genes relative to normal mucosa. Only a few genes were up-regulated or down-regulated genes between preneoplasia and malignancy. Hierarchic cluster analysis and principal components analysis revealed a consistent separation between the three groups but confirmed a closer association between preneoplasia and malignancy (Fig. 26.1-2). Similarly to the genetic progression model of HNSCC, transcriptional modeling revealed that the majority of alterations occurred before the development of clinical malignancy and identified key targets of transcriptional dysregulation during the histopathologic progression to the malignant state.[110] All of these genetic and transcriptional changes may one day provide the basis for appropriate targets and novel therapeutic approaches.

FIELD CANCERIZATION

Patients with head and neck cancer often present with second metachronous and synchronous tumors of the aerodigestive tract. Moreover, patients with primary lesions often have skip areas that are characterized by preinvasive lesions throughout the field. Slaughter et al.[111] originally coined the term *field cancerization* and attributed this to a field defect that allowed independent transformation of epithelial cells at a number of sites. Previous studies in bladder cancer demonstrated that multiple tumors arising in a single patient were derived from the uncontrolled spread of a single transformed cell.[112] These tumors then grew independently, with variable subsequent genetic alterations. For head and neck cancer, the author and colleague's working progression model allowed direct assessment of the genetic changes in surrounding areas of histopathologic abnormality. In every case, surrounding lesions appeared to share the same genetic events (e.g., critical breakpoints at chromosomes 9p21 and 3p21) present in the primary tumor, suggesting that a single transformed cell gave rise to the independent and apparently geographically distinct skip areas seen in these patients. Thus, Slaughter's original observations can be explained as follows: A cell is transformed by a critical genetic event and begins to migrate through or repopulate the normal mucosa. Additional genetic events in one critical lesion eventually give rise to the clinical tumor that is seen on presentation. However, direct molecular assessment of surrounding regions confirms the presence of clonal cell populations that are not yet fully transformed. Given time, these lesions arise as other preinvasive or invasive lesions in the same patient.

Although investigators have reported a confirmation of this field cancerization effect in head and neck cancer by detection of discordant p53 mutations in multiple tumors,[113] the author and colleague's working model suggests that this conclusion may be premature. Other genetic events, including loss of 9p and 3p, precede inactivation of p53. Thus, one of these early events probably leads to initial cell transformation and replacement of surrounding mucosa, whereas subsequent genetic events including p53 appear to arise independently. Thus, these investigators identified the diversity of subsequent genetic events rather than establish the distinct clonal origin of these clinically independent lesions. By examining the pattern of X chromosome inactivation (in female patients) and loss of chromosome 9p21 and other genetic changes in multiple tumors, the author's group and others demonstrated a common clonal origin in most of these cases.[114–118] Cytogenetic evidence in at least one patient identified the presence of a specific chromosomal marker in both primary neoplasms.[119] More recently, apparent second primary tumors of the lung and even rare esophageal tumors were found to be clonally related to the initial primary HNSCC.[120,121]

If minimally abnormal or benign-appearing premalignant lesions show clonal genetic changes adjacent to a primary HNSCC, it is conceivable that normal-appearing mucosal areas could harbor an occult neoplasm. Clinically detectable cervical lymph node metastases without identification of the primary tumor were assessed by molecular analysis of multiple surveillance biopsies. The author and colleagues investigated whether the site of origin of the primary tumor could be localized by detection of specific losses on some of the key chromosomes described in the molecular progression model.[122] In 10 of 18 patients, at least one pathologically benign biopsy demonstrated a pattern of genetic alterations identical to that present in cervical lymph node metastases. Three of these patients went on to develop primary tumors in the identical or adjacent mucosal region between 1 and 13 years later.[122] These data further support the notion that histopathologically benign mucosa may harbor patches of clonal preneoplastic cells that are genetically related to the metastatic HNSCC and that such mucosal sites are the sites of origin of unknown primary HNSCC.

MOLECULAR EPIDEMIOLOGY

The pattern of specific mutations within a given gene sequence may provide important information concerning the etiology (e.g., effect of a carcinogen) of that particular cancer.[123] The p53 gene can be inactivated by a large variety of distinct mutations and is frequently inactivated in many human cancers, providing an excellent candidate for this type of survey. Analysis of the pattern of the p53 gene mutation in 129 HNSCC patients has demonstrated that the incidence of p53 mutations is much higher among patients exposed to tobacco and alcohol than among those patients who abstained from both.[53] Moreover, the author's group found that the alcohol appeared to augment the effect of smoking, consistent with models in which alcohol is not a carcinogen per se but might lead to an increase in the absorbance of car-

cinogens contained within cigarette smoke. Furthermore, it was found that CpG mutations are rare among mutations in patients who smoke cigarettes, whereas they constituted most of the mutations found in nonsmokers and nondrinkers. C to T mutations at these CpG sites are important because, through methylation and deamination, they are thought to represent potential sites of "endogenous" mutations. These data thus support a growing body of epidemiologic evidence that abstinence from cigarette smoke may help decrease the overall incidence of head and neck cancer.

HUMAN PAPILLOMAVIRUS

HPV has long been thought to play a role in some head and neck cancers. One study of more than 250 patients used PCR followed by definitive techniques such as sequencing and *in situ* hybridization to search for the presence of HPV in head and neck tumors.[124] HPV was detected in approximately 25% of the lesions, and virtually all were "high-risk" oncogenic types (HPV-16). Remarkably, most HPV-positive tumors were in the oropharynx. These HPV-positive oropharyngeal cancers were less likely to occur among heavy smokers and drinkers, less likely to harbor a p53 mutation, and had an improved disease-specific survival. Another group suggested that HPV-positive tumors may also inactivate Rb and harbor a better prognosis.[125] These new data are consistent with previous studies of a smaller number of patients[126] or those that used less definitive techniques. It appears that HPV-positive oropharyngeal tumors compose a distinct clinical and pathologic disease entity causally associated with HPV.

DIAGNOSTICS

Clonal genetic alterations can be identified in clinical samples including bodily fluids. These clonal genetic alterations are generally considered to represent specific markers for the presence of neoplastic cells. In many clinical samples, however, the number of neoplastic cells are greatly outnumbered by normal cells within the same specimen. Therefore, the author's group and others have developed very sensitive and specific techniques to detect these rare clonal genetic alterations among many "normal" or wild-type DNA molecules. Clonal ras gene mutations have been detected in the stool of patients with colorectal cancer and p53 mutations in the urine of patients with bladder cancer.[127,128] Moreover, ras and p53 oncogene mutations were used as targets to detect neoplastic cells in the sputum of patients with lung cancer. In one case, the same clonal cell population containing the identical mutation eventually identified in the primary tumor was detected 1 year before clinical diagnosis in a patient with lung cancer.[129] Analysis of p53 mutations also confirmed the ability to detect neoplastic clones in the saliva of patients with head and neck cancer.[130]

Telomerase is a ribonuclear protein that maintains telomere length, and reactivation of its activity is associated with escape from cellular senescence. Using a modified PCR-based assay for telomerase activity, 80% to 100% of primary head and neck cancers were found to display telomerase activity.[131,132] Some authors have suggested that most dysplastic lesions and preneoplastic lesions also display telomerase activation.[132] Interestingly, 14 of 44 (32%) oral rinses from HNSCC patients were found to harbor

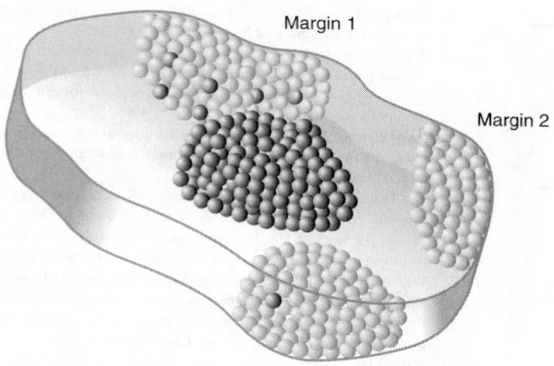

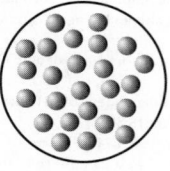 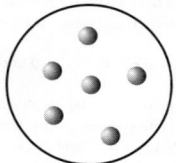 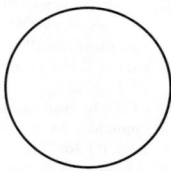 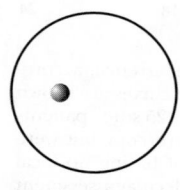

CULTURE PLATES

Tumor

Margin 1
Extensive
tumor infiltration

Margin 2
No cancer
infiltration

Margin 3
Molecular evidence
of tumor infiltration

FIGURE 26.1-3. Schematic representation of molecular staging. DNA is extracted from primary clinical (e.g., margin) material and then tested for the presence of infiltrating tumor cells that harbor the identical p53 mutations detected in the primary tumor. This polymerase chain reaction–based approach is much more sensitive than morphologic analysis by standard light microscopy. Patients positive by molecular analysis are at high risk for local regional occurrence.

telomerase activity, but a small percentage of normal controls also exhibited this telomerase activity.[131] Using a panel of 21 microsatellite markers, clonal genetic changes (loss of heterozygosity or microsatellite instability) were detected in 80% of the saliva samples from the patients with head and neck cancer.[133] Moreover, exfoliative cell samples were subjected to microsatellite analysis and found to contain the identical changes observed in the primary tumors.[134,135] Testing saliva with a panel of three methylation markers detected with high specificity approximately 60% of cancer patients.[93] Mitochondrial DNA mutations were also found in preneoplastic lesions and cancers and were readily detected in paired saliva DNA.[136,137] It is still unknown if these genetic or epigenetic changes can be identified in early lesions or if they can detect recurrence, as has been seen in bladder cancer through urinalysis. Clearly, the continued identification of molecular markers will lead to improved diagnostic techniques for SCC.

A more pressing problem in HNSCC is the high incidence of local-regional recurrence despite aggressive surgical therapy. A similar molecular approach was used to probe surgical margins and lymph nodes from patients with primary head and neck cancer after surgical resection.[138] A segment of the p53 gene is amplified by PCR from DNA extracted from the clinical sample. The PCR products are then cloned into phage, transferred to nylon membranes, and probed with a specific oligomer (small DNA strand) that is able to recognize the same mutation initially identified in the primary tumor. Thus, a unique DNA probe was synthesized and used to test the resected surgical margins and lymph nodes from affected patients. Perhaps not surprisingly, many of the apparently normal margins and lymph nodes by light microscopy were found to contain infiltrating tumor cells by this sensitive molecular analysis (Fig. 26.1-3).

In an initial pilot trial that contained 30 patients, thought to be completely negative by light microscopy, final pathology revealed at least one positive margin in 5 patients.[138] These 5 patients had markedly positive margins by molecular analysis and were further excluded from this study; the 25 remaining patients were still completely negative by light microscopy. Of these, 13 were positive by molecular analysis and 5 have recurred within 2 years (average, 9 to 12 months). Of the 12 patients who were completely negative by molecular assessment, none had recurred at 2-year follow-up. As expected, a significant improvement in survival occurred for those patients who were initially negative by molecular analysis (Fig. 26.1-4). In another study of 18 patients, locoregional recurrence developed in all 5 patients who harbored a molecular positive surgical margin or molecular evidence of field cancerization.[139] In a prospective study of 76 patients, mutated p53 margins predicted a sevenfold greater risk of local regional recurrence. Moreover, further analysis demonstrated that part of the local recurrences originated from residual precursor lesions.[140] The use of other markers to detect residual disease including eIF4E protein overexpression and increased E48 RNA levels has also been described.[141] Real-time assays have now brought the possibility of molecular staging directly into the operating room.

Although the above study must be confirmed by larger prospective trials, the results are already intriguing. Perhaps patients with negative molecular assessment may be spared adjuvant radiation therapy. Moreover, patients with positive margins will benefit from more aggressive chemotherapeutic approaches and perhaps novel approaches, including gene therapy. Microsatellites and promoter methylation have also been described in the serum DNA of patients with head and neck cancers, providing further prediction on possible systematic spread.[92,142,143] Because staging is so critical for many types of cancer, these approaches will be important for other tumors in addition to head and neck cancer.

The identification of new genes and other molecular markers will help in the early detection of head and neck cancer

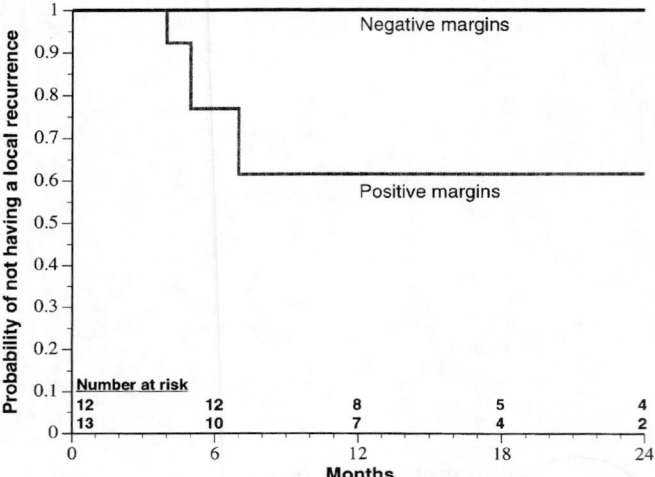

FIGURE 26.1-4. Probability of having no local recurrence, according to the results of the molecular assay. Kaplan-Meier curves are shown for the probability of having no local recurrence in the 25 study patients with surgical margins that were negative by light microscopy but were reevaluated with molecular probes. The probability of having no local recurrence in patients with positive margins by the molecular assessment was significantly lower than that in patients with negative margins (*P* = .02 by the log-rank test).

and may already provide useful prognostic information regarding clinical tumor behavior. As more is understood about critical pathways in the genesis of these tumors, chemotherapeutic, pharmacologic, and genetic approaches may all be useful in either reestablishing or abrogating newly established pathways that lead to tumor growth. These discoveries will eventually lead to improved surgical techniques, chemoprevention strategies, and novel therapeutic approaches.

REFERENCES

1. Fearon ER, Vogelstein B. A genetic model of colorectal tumorigenesis. *Cell* 1990;61:759.
2. Ankathil R, Mathew A, Joseph F. Is oral cancer susceptibility inherited? *Eur J Cancer B Oral Oncol* 1996;32B:63.
3. Gorsky M, Littner M, Sukman Y. The prevalence of oral cancer in relation to the ethnic origin of the Jewish population. *Oral Surg Oral Med Oral Pathol* 1994;78:408.
4. Foulkes WD, Brunet JS, Kowalski LP. Family history is a risk factor for squamous cell carcinoma of the head and neck in Brazil: a case control study. *Int J Cancer* 1995;63:769.
5. Jeffries S, Eeles R, Goldgar D, et al. The role of genetic factors in predisposition to squamous cell cancer of the head and neck. *Br J Cancer* 1999;79:865.
6. Rosnberg PS, Greene MH, Alter BP. Cancer incidence in persons with Fanconi anemia. *Blood* 2003;101:2136.
7. Cheng L, Sturgis EM, Eicher SA, et al. Glutathione S-transferase polymorphisms and risk of squamous-cell carcinoma of the head and neck. *Int J Cancer* 1999;84:220.
8. Morita S, Yano M, Tsujinaka T, et al. Genetic polymorphisms of drug-metabolizing enzymes and susceptibility to head-and-neck squamous-cell carcinoma. *Int J Cancer* 1999;80:685.
9. Jourenkova-Mironova N, Voho A, Bouchardy C, et al. Glutathione S-transferase GSTM3 and GSTP1 genotypes and larynx cancer risk. *Cancer Epidemiol Biomarkers Prev* 1999;8:185.
10. Nazar-Stewart V, Vaughan TL, Burt RD, et al. Glutathione S-transferase M1 and susceptibility to nasopharyngeal carcinoma. *Cancer Epidemiol Biomarkers Prev* 1999;8:547.
11. Lazarus P, Sheikh SN, Ren Q, et al. p53, but not p16 mutations in oral squamous cell carcinomas are associated with specific CYP1A1 and GSTM1 polymorphic genotypes and patient use. *Carcinogenesis* 1998;19:509.
12. Jourenkova N, Reinikainen M, Bouchardy C, et al. Larynx cancer risk in relation to glutathione S-transferase M1 and T1 genotypes and tobacco smoking. *Cancer Epidemiol Biomarkers Prev* 1998;7:19.
13. Park JY, Muscat JE, Ren Q, et al. CYP1A1 and GSTM1 polymorphisms and oral cancer risk. *Cancer Epidemiol Biomarkers Prev* 1997;6:791.
14. Cloos J, Nieuwenhuis EJ, Boomsma DI, et al. Inherited susceptibility to bleomycin-induced chromatid breaks in cultured peripheral blood lymphocytes. *J Natl Cancer Inst* 1999;91:1125.
15. Cheng L, Eicher SA, Guo Z, et al. Reduced DNA repair capacity in head and neck cancer patients. *Cancer Epidemiol Biomarkers Prev* 1998;7:465.
16. Wang LE, Sturgis EM, Eicher SA, et al. Mutagen sensitivity to benzo(a)pyrene diol epoxide and the risk of squamous cell carcinoma of the head and neck. *Clin Cancer Res* 1998;4:1773.
17. Renan MJ. How many mutations are required for tumorigenesis? Implications from human cancer data. *Mol Carcinog* 1993;7:139.
18. Jin Y, Mertens F, Mandahl N, et al. Chromosome abnormalities in eighty-three head and neck squamous cell carcinomas: influence of culture conditions on karyotypic pattern. *Cancer Res* 1993;53:2140.
19. Van Dyke DL, Worsham MJ, Benninger MS, et al. Recurrent cytogenetic abnormalities in squamous cell carcinomas of the head and neck region. *Genes Chromosomes Cancer* 1994;9:192.
20. Cowan JM, Beckett MA, Weichselbaum RR. Chromosome changes characterizing in vitro response to radiation in human squamous cell carcinoma lines. *Cancer Res* 1993;53:5542.
21. Visakorpi T, Hyytinen E, Koivisto P, et al. In vivo amplification of the androgen receptor gene and progression of human prostate cancer. *Nat Genet* 1995;9:401.
22. Brzoska PM, Levin NA, Fu KK, et al. Frequent novel DNA copy number increase in squamous cell head and neck tumors. *Cancer Res* 1995;55:3055.
23. Bishop JM. Molecular themes in oncogenes. *Cell* 1991;64:235.
24. Berenson JR, Yan J, Micke RA. Frequent amplification of the bcl-1 locus in head and neck squamous cell carcinomas. *Oncogene* 1989;4:1111.
25. Callender T, El-Nagger AK, Lee MS, et al. PRAD-1 (CCND1)/cyclin D1 oncogene amplification in primary head and neck squamous cell carcinomas. *Cancer* 1994;74:152.
26. Jares P, Fernández PL, Campo E, et al. PRAD-1/cyclin D1 gene amplification correlates with messenger RNA overexpression and tumor progression in human laryngeal carcinomas. *Cancer Res* 1994;54:4813.
27. Hunter T, Pines J. Cyclins and cancer. II. Cyclin D and CDK inhibitors come of age. *Cell* 1994;79:573.
28. Okami K, Reed AL, Cairns P, et al. Cyclin D1 amplification is independent of p16 inactivation in head and neck squamous cell carcinoma. *Oncogene* 1999;18:3541.
29. Trink B, Okami K, Wu L, et al. A new p53 homologue. *Nat Med* 1998;4:747.
30. Hibi K, Trink B, Patturajan M, et al. AIS is an oncogene amplified in squamous cell carcinoma. *Proc Natl Acad Sci U S A* 2000;97:5462.
31. Celli J, Dujif P, Hamel B, et al. Heterozygous germline mutations in the p53 homologue p63 are the cause of EEC syndrome. *Cell* 1999;99:143.
32. Yang A, Schweitzer R, Sun D, et al. p63 is essential for regenerative proliferation in limb, craniofacial and epithelial development. *Nature* 1999;398:714.
33. Patturajan M, Nomoto S, Sommer M, et al. DeltaNp63 induces beta-catenin nuclear accumulation and signaling. *Cancer Cell* 2000;1:369.
34. Grandis JR, Tweardy DJ. Elevated levels of transforming growth factor alpha and epidermal growth factor receptor messenger RNA are early markers of carcinogenesis in head and neck cancer. *Cancer Res* 1993;53:3579.
35. He Y, Zeng Q, Drenning SD, et al. Inhibition of human squamous cell carcinoma growth in vivo by epidermal growth factor receptor antisense RNA transcribed from the U6 promoter. *J Natl Cancer Inst* 1998;90:1080.
36. Grandis JR, Drenning SD, Chakraborty A, et al. Requirement of Stat3 but not Stat1 activation for epidermal growth factor receptor-mediated cell growth in vitro. *J Clin Invest* 1998;102:1385.
37. Sorrells DL, Ghali GE, Meschonat C, et al. Competitive PCR to detect eIF4E gene amplification in head and neck cancer. *Head Neck* 1999;21:60.
38. Sorrells DL, Meschonat C, Black D, et al. Pattern of amplification and overexpression of the eukaryotic initiation factor 4E gene in solid tumor. *J Surg Res* 1999;85:37.
39. Nathan CA, Franklin S, Abreo FW, et al. Expression of eIF4E during head and neck tumorigenesis: possible role in angiogenesis. *Laryngoscope* 1999;109:1253.
40. Chan G, Boyle JO, Yang EK, et al. Cyclooxygenase-2 expression is up-regulated in squamous cell carcinoma of the head and neck. *Cancer Res* 1999;59:991.
41. Wang X, Pavelic ZP, Li Y, et al. Overexpression and amplification of glutathione S-transferase pi gene in head and neck squamous cell carcinomas. *Clin Cancer Res* 1997;3;111.
42. Markowitz S, Wang J, Myeroff L, et al. Inactivation of the type II TGF-beta receptor in colon cancer cells with microsatellite instability. *Science* 1995;268:1336.
43. Garrigueantar L, Munozantonia T, Antonia SJ, et al. Missense mutations of the transforming growth factor beta type II receptor in human head and neck squamous cell carcinoma cells. *Cancer Res* 1995;55:3982.
44. Wang D, Song H, Evans JA, et al. Mutation and downregulation of the transforming growth factor beta type II receptor gene in primary squamous cell carcinomas of the head and neck. *Carcinogenesis* 1997;18:2285.
45. Lippman SM, Spitz MR, Huber MH, et al. Strategies for chemoprevention study of premalignancy and second primary tumors in the head and neck. *Curr Opin Oncol* 1995;7:234.
46. Lotan R, Xu XC, Lippman SM, et al. Suppression of retinoic acid receptor-beta in premalignant oral lesions and its up-regulation by isotretinoin. *N Engl J Med* 1995;332:1405.
47. McGregor F, Muntoni A, Fleming J, et al. Molecular changes associated with oral dysplasia progression and acquisition of immortality: potential for its reversal by 5-azacytidine. *Cancer Res* 2002;62:4757.
48. Kwong J, Lo KW, To KF, et al. Promoter hypermethylation of multiple genes in nasopharyngeal carcinoma. *Clin Cancer Res* 2002;8:131.
49. Weber JL, May PE. Abundant class of human DNA polymorphisms which can be typed using the polymerase chain reaction. *Am J Hum Genet* 1989;44:388.
50. Knudson AG Jr. Mutation and cancer: statistical study of retinoblastoma. *Proc Natl Acad Sci U S A* 1971;68:820.
51. Hollstein M, Sidransky D, Vogelstein B, et al. p53 mutations in human cancer. *Science* 1991;253:49.
52. Boyle JO, Koch W, Hruban RH, et al. The incidence of p53 mutations increases with progression of head and neck cancer. *Cancer Res* 1993;53:4477.

53. Brennan JA, Boyle JO, Koch WM, et al. Association between cigarette smoking and mutation of the p53 gene in head and neck squamous carcinoma. *N Engl J Med* 1995;332:712.
54. Nawroz H, van der Riet P, Hruban RH, et al. Allelotype of head and neck squamous cell carcinoma. *Cancer Res* 1994;54:1152.
55. Ahsee KW, Cooke TG, Pickford IR, et al. An allelotype of squamous carcinoma of the head and neck using microsatellite markers. *Cancer Res* 1994;54:1617.
56. van der Riet P, Nawroz H, Hruban RH, et al. Frequent loss of chromosome 9p21-22 early in head and neck cancer progression. *Cancer Res* 1994;54:1156.
57. Kamb A, Gruis NA, Weaver-Feldhaus J, et al. A cell cycle regulator potentially involved in genesis of many tumor types. *Science* 1994;264:436.
58. Hussussian CJ, Struewing JP, Goldstein AM, et al. Germline p16 mutations in familial melanoma. *Nat Genet* 1994;8:15.
59. Munro J, Stott FJ, Vousden KH, et al. Role of the alternative INK4A proteins in human keratinocyte senescence: evidence for the specific inactivation of p16INK4A upon immortalization. *Cancer Res* 1999;59:2516.
60. Zhang SY, Kleinszanto AJP, Sauter ER, et al. Higher frequency of alterations in the p16/CDKN2 gene in squamous cell carcinoma cell lines than in primary tumors of the head and neck. *Cancer Res* 1994;54:5050.
61. Cairns P, Mao L, Merlo A, et al. Low rate of p16 (MTS1) mutations in primary tumors with 9p loss. *Science* 1994;265:415.
62. Merlo A, Herman JG, Mao L, et al. 5′ CpG island methylation is associated with transcriptional silencing of the tumour suppressor p16/CDKN2/MTS1 in human cancers. *Nat Med* 1995;7:686.
63. Cairns P, Polascik TJ, Eby Y, et al. Frequency of homozygous deletion at p16/CDKN2 in primary human tumors. *Nat Genet* 1995;11:210.
64. Reed A, Califano J, Cairns P, et al. High frequency of p16CDKN2/MTS-1/INK4A inactivation in head and neck squamous cell carcinoma. *Cancer Res* 1996;56:3630.
65. Papadimitrakopoulou V, Izzo J, Lippman SM, et al. Frequent inactivation of p16INK4a in oral premalignant lesions. *Oncogene* 1997;14:1799.
66. Mao L, Merlo A, Bedi G, et al. A novel p16INK4A transcript. *Cancer Res* 1995;55:2995.
67. Liggett WH Jr, Sewell DA, Rocco J, et al. p16 and p16 β are potent growth suppressors of head and neck squamous carcinoma cells in vitro. *Cancer Res* 1996;56:4119.
68. Zhang Y, Xiong Y, Yarbrough WG. ARF promotes MDM2 degradation and stabilizes p53: ARF-INK4a locus deletion impairs both the Rb and p53 tumor suppression pathways. *Cell* 1998;92:725.
69. Pomerantz J, Schreiber-Agus N, Liegeois NJ, et al. The INK4a tumor suppressor gene product, p19ARF, interacts with MDM2 and neutralizes MDM2's inhibition of p53. *Cell* 1998;92:713.
70. Kamijo T, Zindy F, Roussel MF, et al. Tumor suppression at the mouse INK4a locus mediated by the alternative reading frame product p19ARF. *Cell* 1997;91:649.
71. Sanchez-Cespedes M, Reed AL, Buta M, et al. Inactivation of the INK4A/ARF locus frequently coexists with TP53 mutations in non-small cell lung cancer. *Oncogene* 1999;18:5843.
72. Maestro R, Gasparotto D, Vuksavljevic T, et al. Three discrete regions of deletion in head and neck cancers. *Cancer Res* 1993;53:5775.
73. Wu CL, Sloan P, Read AP, et al. Deletion mapping on the short arm of chromosome 3 in squamous cell carcinoma of the oral cavity. *Cancer Res* 1994;54:6484.
74. Chen YJ, Chen PH, Lee MD, et al. Aberrant FHIT transcripts in cancerous and corresponding non-cancerous lesions of the digestive tract. *Int J Cancer* 1997;72:955.
75. Mao L, Fan YH, Lotan R, et al. Frequent abnormalities of FHIT, a candidate tumor suppressor gene, in head and neck cancer cell lines. *Cancer Res* 1996;56:5128.
76. Dong SM, Sun DI, Benoit NE, et al. Epigenetic inactivation of RASSF1A in head and neck cancer. *Clin Cancer Res* 2003;9:3635.
77. Hogg RP, Honorio S, Martinez A, et al. Frequent 3p allele loss and epigenetic inactivation of the RASSF1A tumour suppressor gene from region 3p21.3 in head and neck squamous cell carcinoma. *Eur J Cancer* 2002;38:1585.
78. Hartwell LH, Kastan MB. Cell cycle control and cancer. *Science* 1994;266:1821.
79. Koch WM, Brennan JA, Zahurak M, et al. p53 mutation and locoregional treatment failure in head and neck squamous cell carcinoma. *J Natl Cancer Inst* 1996;88:1580.
80. Okami K, Wu L, Riggins G, et al. Analysis of PTEN/MMAC1 alterations in aerodigestive tract tumors. *Cancer Res* 1998;58:509.
81. Shao X, Tandon R, Samara G, et al. Mutational analysis of the PTEN gene in head and neck squamous cell carcinoma. *Int J Cancer* 1998;77:684.
82. Gasparotto D, Vukosavljevic T, Piccinin S, et al. Loss of heterozygosity at 10q in tumors of the upper respiratory tract is associated with poor prognosis. *Int J Cancer* 1999;84:432.
83. Poetsch M, Lorenz G, Kleist B. Detection of new PTEN/MMAC1 mutations in head and neck squamous cell carcinomas with loss of chromosome 10. *Cancer Genet Cytogenet* 2002;132:20.
84. Yoo GH, Xu HJ, Brennan JA, et al. Infrequent inactivation of the retinoblastoma gene despite frequent loss of chromosome 13q in head and neck squamous cell carcinoma. *Cancer Res* 1994;54:4603.
85. Wu CL, Roz L, Sloan P, et al. Deletion mapping defines three discrete areas of allelic imbalance on chromosome arm 8p in oral and oropharyngeal squamous cell carcinomas. *Genes Chromosomes Cancer* 1997;20:347.
86. Sunwoo JB, Sun PC, Gupta VK, et al. Localization of a putative tumor suppressor gene in the sub-telomeric region of chromosome 8p. *Oncogene* 1999;18:2651.
87. Ishwad CS, Shuster M, Bockmuhl U, et al. Frequent allelic loss and homozygous deletion in chromosome band 8p23 in oral cancer. *Int J Cancer* 1999;80:25.
88. Wang XL, Uzawa K, Miyakawa A, et al. Localization of a tumour-suppressor gene associated with human oral cancer on 7q31.1. *Int J Cancer* 1998;75:671.
89. Papadimitrakopoulou VA, Oh Y, El-Naggar A, et al. Presence of multiple incontiguous deleted regions at the long arm of chromosome 18 in head and neck cancer. *Clin Cancer Res* 1998;4:539.
90. Pearlstein RP, Benninger MS, Carey TE, et al. Loss of 18q predicts poor survival of patients with squamous cell carcinoma of the head and neck. *Genes Chromosomes Cancer* 1998;21:333.
91. Kim SK, Fan Y, Papadimitrakopoulou V, et al. DPC4, a candidate tumor suppressor gene, is altered infrequently in head and neck squamous cell carcinoma. *Cancer Res* 1996;56:2519.
92. Sanchez-Cespedes M, Esteller M, Wu L, et al. Gene promoter hypermethylation in tumors and serum of head and neck cancer patients. *Cancer Res* 2000;60:892.
93. Rosas SL, Koch W, daCosta Carvalho MG, et al. Promoter hypermethylation patterns of p16, O6-methylguanine-DNA-methyltransferase, and death-associated protein kinase in tumors and saliva of head and neck cancer patients. *Cancer Res* 2001;61:939.
94. Viswanathan M, Tsuchida N, Shanmugam G. Promoter hypermethylation profile of tumor-associated genes p16, p15, hMLH1, MGMT and E-cadherin in oral squamous cell carcinoma. *Int J Cancer* 2003;105:41.
95. Tsao SW, Liu Y, Wang X, et al. The association of E-cadherin expression and the methylation status of the E-cadherin gene in nasopharyngeal carcinoma cells. *Eur J Cancer* 2003;39:413.
96. Califano J, van der Riet P, Westra W, et al. A genetic progression model for head and neck cancer: implications for field cancerization. *Cancer Res* 1996;56:2488.
97. Ogawara K, Miyakawa A, Shiba M, et al. Allelic loss of chromosome 13q14.3 in human oral cancer: correlation with lymph node metastasis. *Int J Cancer* 1998;79:312.
98. Lee DJ, Koch WM, Yoo G, et al. Impact of chromosome 14q loss on survival in primary head and neck squamous cell carcinoma. *Clin Cancer Res* 1997;3:501.
99. Lazar AD, Winter MR, Nogueira CP, et al. Loss of heterozygosity at 11q23 in squamous cell carcinoma of the head and neck is associated with recurrent disease. *Clin Cancer Res* 1998;4:2787.
100. Mineta H, Miura K, Suzuki I, et al. Low p27 expression correlates with poor prognosis for patients with oral tongue squamous cell carcinoma. *Cancer* 1999;85:1011.
101. Venkatesan TK, Kuropkat C, Caldarelli DD, et al. Prognostic significance of p27 expression in carcinoma of the oral cavity and oropharynx. *Laryngoscope* 1999;109:1329.
102. Temam S, Flahault A, Perie S, et al. p53 gene status as a predictor of tumor response to induction chemotherapy of patients with locoregionally advanced squamous cell carcinomas of the head and neck. *J Clin Oncol* 2000;20:385.
103. Mao L, Lee JS, Fan YH, et al. Frequent microsatellite alterations at chromosomes 9p21 and 3p14 in oral premalignant lesions and their value in cancer risk assessment. *Nat Med* 1996;2:682.
104. Mao L, El-Naggar AK, Papadimitrakopoulou V, et al. Phenotype and genotype of advanced premalignant head and neck lesions after chemopreventive therapy. *J Natl Cancer Inst* 1998;90:1545.
105. Rosin MP, Lam WL, Poh C, et al. 3p14 and 9p21 loss is a simple tool for predicting second oral malignancy at previously treated oral cancer sites. *Cancer Res* 2002;62:6447.
106. Rosin MP, Cheng X, Poh C, et al. Use of allelic loss to predict malignant risk for low-grade oral epithelial dysplasia. *Clin Cancer Res* 2000;6:357.
107. Partridge M, Emilion G, Pateromichelakis S, et al. Allelic imbalance at chromosomal loci implicated in the pathogenesis of oral precancer, cumulative loss and its relationship with progression to cancer. *Oral Oncol* 1998;34:77.
108. Guo Z, Yamguchi K, Sanchez-Cespedes M, et al. Allelic losses in OraTest-directed biopsies of patients with prior upper aerodigestive tract malignancy. *Clin Cancer Res* 2001;7:1963.
109. Epstein JB, Zhang L, Poh C, et al. Increased allelic loss in toluidine blue-positive oral premalignant lesions. *Oral Surg Oral Med Oral Pathol Oral Radiol Endod* 2003;95:45.
110. Ha PK, Benoit NE, Yochem R, et al. A transcriptional progression model for head and neck cancer. *Clin Cancer Res* 2003;9:3058.
111. Slaughter DL, Southwick HW, Smejkal W. "Field cancerization" in oral stratified squamous epithelium: clinical implications of multicentric origin. *Cancer* 1953;6:963.
112. Sidransky D, Preisinger AC, Frost P, et al. Clonal origin of metachronous tumors of the bladder. *N Engl J Med* 1992;326:737.
113. Chung KY, Mukhopadhyay T, Kim J, et al. Discordant p53 gene mutations in primary head and neck cancers and corresponding second primary cancers of the upper aerodigestive tract. *Cancer Res* 1993;53:1676.
114. Bedi GC, Westra WH, Gabrielson E, et al. Multiple head and neck tumors: evidence for a common clonal origin. *Cancer Res* 1996;56:2484.
115. Partridge M, Pateromichelakis S, Phillips E, et al. A case-control study confirms that microsatellite assay can identify patients at risk of developing oral squamous cell carcinoma within a field of cancerization. *Cancer Res* 2000;60:3893.
116. Partridge M, Pateromicelakis S, Phillips E, et al. Profiling clonality and progression in multiple premalignant and malignant oral lesions identifies a subgroup of cases with a distinct presentation of squamous cell carcinoma. *Clin Cancer Res* 2001;7:1860.
117. Tabor MP, Brakenhoff RH, van Houten VM, et al. Persistence of genetically altered fields in head and neck cancer patients: biological and clinical implications. *Clin Cancer Res* 2001;7:1523.
118. Braakhuis BJ, Tabor MP, Kummer JA, et al. A genetic explanation of Slaughter's concept of field cancerization: evidence and clinical implications. *Cancer Res* 2003;63:1727.
119. Worsham MJ, Wolman SR, Carey TE, et al. Common clonal origin of synchronous primary head and neck squamous cell carcinomas. *Hum Pathol* 1995;26:251.
120. Leong PP, Rezai B, Koch WM, et al. Distinguishing second primary tumors from lung metastases in patients with head and neck squamous cell carcinoma. *J Natl Cancer Inst* 1998;90:972.
121. Califano J, Leong PL, Koch WM, et al. Second esophageal tumors in patients with head and neck squamous cell carcinoma: an assessment of clonal relationships. *Clin Cancer Res* 1999;5:1862.
122. Califano J, Westra WH, Meininger G, et al. Unknown primary head and neck squamous cell carcinoma: molecular identification of the site of origin. *J Natl Cancer Inst* 1999;91:599.

123. Harris CC, Hollstein M. Clinical implication of the p53 tumor-suppressor gene. *N Engl J Med* 1993;329:1318.
124. Gillison ML, Koch WM, Capone RB, et al. Evidence for a causal association between human papillomavirus and a subset of head and neck cancers. *J Natl Cancer Inst* 2000;92:709.
125. Andl T, Kahn T, Pfuhl A, et al. Etiological involvement of oncogenic human papillomavirus in tonsillar squamous cell carcinomas lacking retinoblastoma cell cycle control. *Cancer Res* 1998;58:5.
126. Haraf DJ, Nodzenski E, Brachman D, et al. Human papilloma virus and p53 in head and neck cancer: clinical correlates and survival. *Clin Cancer Res* 1996;2:755.
127. Sidransky D, Tokino T, Frost P, et al. Identification of ras oncogene mutations in the stool of patients with curable colorectal tumors. *Science* 1992;256:102.
128. Sidransky D, Von Eschenbach A, Tsai YC, et al. Identification of p53 gene mutations in bladder cancers and urine samples. *Science* 1991;252:706.
129. Mao L, Hruban RH, Boyle JO, et al. Detection of oncogene mutations in sputum precedes diagnosis of lung cancer. *Cancer Res* 1994;54:1634.
130. Boyle JB, Mao L, Brennan JA, et al. Gene mutations in saliva as molecular markers for head and neck squamous cell carcinomas. *Am J Surg* 1994;168:429.
131. Califano JA, Ahrendt S, Meininger G, et al. Detection of telomerase activity in oral rinses from head and neck squamous cell cancer patients. *Cancer Res* 1996;56:5720.
132. Mao L, El-Naggar AK, Fan YH, et al. Telomerase activity in head and neck squamous cell carcinoma and adjacent tissues. *Cancer Res* 1996;56:5600.
133. Spafford MF, Koch WM, Reed AL, et al. Detection of head and neck squamous cell carcinoma among exfoliated oral mucosal cells by microsatellite analysis. *Clin Cancer Res* 2001;7:607.
134. Rosin MP, Epstein JB, Berean K, et al. The use of exfoliative cell samples to map clonal genetic alterations in the oral epithelium of high-risk patients. *Cancer Res* 1997;57:5258.
135. Temam S, Trassard M, Leroux G, et al. Cytology vs molecular analysis for the detection of head and neck squamous cell carcinoma in oesopharyngeal brush samples: a prospective study in 56 patients. *Br J Cancer* 2003;88:1740.
136. Ha PK, Tong BC, Westra WH, et al. Mitochondrial C-tract alteration in premalignant lesions of the head and neck: a marker for progression and clonal proliferation. *Clin Cancer Res* 2002;8:2260.
137. Fliss MS, Usadel H, Caballero OL, et al. Facile detection of mitochondrial DNA mutations in tumors and bodily fluids. *Science* 2000;287:2017.
138. Brennan JA, Mao L, Hruban RH, et al. Molecular assessment of histopathologic staging. *N Engl J Med* 1995;332:429.
139. Patridge M, Li SR, Pateromichelakis S, et al. Detection of minimal residual cancer to investigate why oral tumors recur despite seemingly adequate treatment. *Clin Cancer Res* 2000;6:2718.
140. Tabor MP, van Houten VMM, Leemans CR, et al. Molecular explanation for locally recurrent head and neck cancer despite seemingly radical surgery. *J Natl Cancer Inst* (submitted for publication).
141. Nieuwenhuis EJ, Jaspars LH, Castelijns JA, et al. Quantitative molecular detection of minimal residual head and neck cancer in lymph node aspirates. *Clin Cancer Res* 2003;9:755.
142. Nawroz H, Koch W, Anker P, et al. Microsatellite alterations in serum DNA of head and neck cancer patients. *Nat Med* 1996;2:1035.
143. Nawroz-Danish H, Eisenberger CF, Yoo GH, et al. Microsatellite analysis of serum DNA in patients with head and neck cancer. *Int J Cancer* 2003 (in press).

WILLIAM M. MENDENHALL
CHARLES E. RIGGS, JR.
NICHOLAS J. CASSISI

SECTION 2

Treatment of Head and Neck Cancers

EPIDEMIOLOGY OF HEAD AND NECK CANCER

The estimated number of new head and neck cancer cases (excluding skin cancer) in the United States in 2003 is 37,200; this represents 2.8% of the total new cancer cases.[1] Approximately one-third of these patients are women.[1] The usual time of diagnosis is after the age of 40, except for salivary gland and nasopharyngeal tumors, which may occur in younger age groups. Cigarette smokers have an increased risk for multiple head and neck primary cancers as well as for lung cancer. Alcohol use has also been implicated as a causative factor for certain head and neck cancers, and the effects of alcohol and tobacco use seem to be additive. Patients with head and neck cancer have an increased risk for developing esophageal and lung cancer.[2]

ANATOMY

The following is a description of the anatomy of the head and neck lymph system; the anatomy pertaining to a particular primary site is described separately.

There are no capillary lymphatics in the epithelium. The tumor must penetrate the lamina propria before lymphatic invasion can occur. One can predict the richness of the capillary network in any given head and neck site by the relative incidence of lymph node metastases at presentation. The nasopharynx and pyriform sinus have the most profuse networks of capillary lymphatics. The paranasal sinuses, middle ear, and vocal cords have few or no capillary lymphatics. Muscle and fat contain few capillary lymphatics. Bone and cartilage are thought to have a few capillary lymphatics in the periosteum or perichondrium. There are no capillary lymphatics in the eye, and few in the orbit. The arrangement of the important lymph nodes in the head and neck is shown in Figure 26.2-1.[3]

PATHOLOGY

The vast majority of head and neck malignant neoplasms arise from the surface epithelium and are therefore squamous cell carcinoma or one of its variants, including lymphoepithelioma, spindle cell carcinoma, verrucous carcinoma, and undifferentiated carcinoma. Lymphomas and a wide variety of other malignant and benign neoplasms make up the remaining cases.[4,5]

Lymphoepithelioma is a carcinoma with a lymphoid stroma. Lymphoepithelioma occurs at anatomic sites with lymphoid aggregates in the submucosa, namely, the nasopharynx, tonsil, and base of the tongue. It may also occur in the major salivary glands.

In the spindle cell variant, found in 2% to 5% of upper aerodigestive tract malignancies, there is a component of spindle cells that resembles sarcoma intermixed with squamous cell carcinoma. For the most part, these lesions cannot be distinguished grossly from the usual squamous cell carcinoma. It is the authors' policy to consider the spindle cell variant as a high-grade carcinoma, but otherwise to disregard the spindle cell element in treatment decisions.

Verrucous carcinoma is a low-grade squamous cell carcinoma found most often in the oral cavity, particularly on the gingiva and buccal mucosa. It usually has an indolent growth pattern and is often associated with the chronic use of snuff or chewing tobacco. A verrucous tumor resembles a wart: distinct margins and a roughened, cobblestone surface. The patient with verrucous carcinoma very often has multiple biopsies of an obvious lesion, but the pathologist returns a diagnosis of hyperkeratosis or pseudoepitheliomatous hyperplasia. *De novo* verrucous carcinomas rarely develop lymph node metastases.

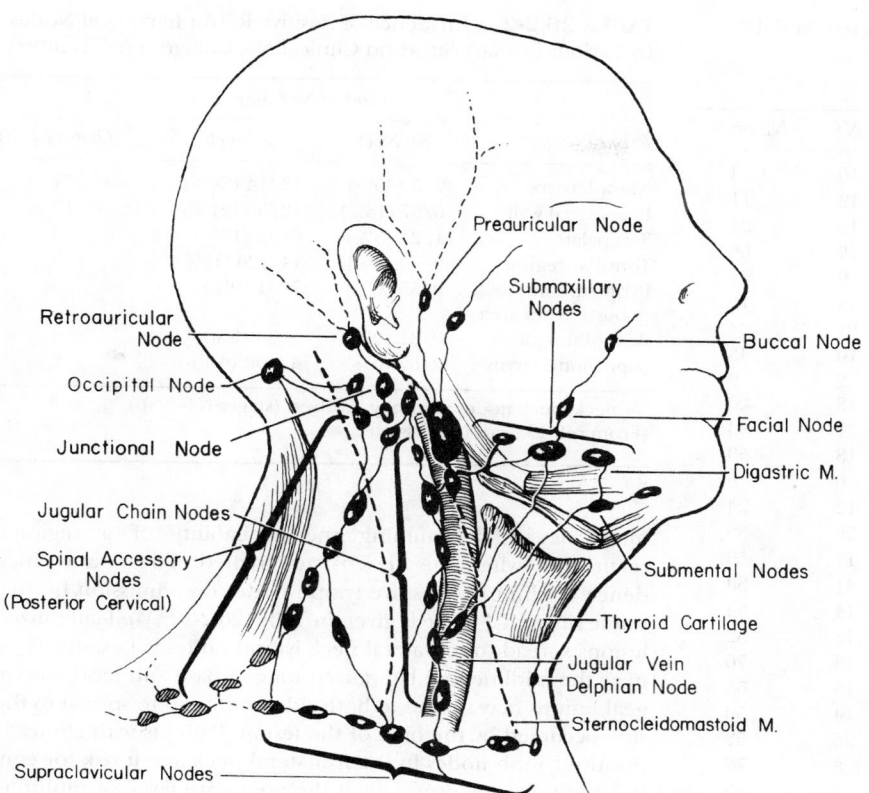

FIGURE 26.2-1. The cervical lymphatics. (Redrawn from Rouviere H. *Anatomy of the human lymphatic system.* Ann Arbor, MI: Edwards Brothers, 1938:27.)

Small cell neuroendocrine carcinoma occurs rarely throughout the head and neck region and is usually managed by radiation therapy and chemotherapy.

Lymphoma occurring in the upper aerodigestive tract almost always shows a diffuse non-Hodgkin's histologic pattern.[4] Nodular non-Hodgkin's lymphoma and Hodgkin's disease rarely involve mucosal sites.

NATURAL HISTORY AND PATTERNS OF SPREAD OF SQUAMOUS CELL CARCINOMA

PRIMARY LESION

Epidermoid carcinomas usually begin as surface lesions, but occasionally arise from ducts of minor salivary glands and therefore originate below the surface of the visible mucosa; this latter phenomenon is more likely to occur in the floor of the mouth, base of the tongue, and nasopharynx. In addition, superficial tumors arising in Waldeyer's ring may be difficult to distinguish from normal lymphatic tissue. The very early surface lesions may show only erythema and a slightly elevated, slightly roughened mucosa.

Spread is dictated by local anatomy, and each anatomic site has its own peculiar spread patterns. Muscle invasion is a common feature, and tumor may spread along muscle or fascial planes for a surprising distance from the palpable or visible lesion. Tumor may attach early to the periosteum or perichondrium, but actual bone or cartilage invasion is usually a late event.

Bone and cartilage usually act as a barrier to spread, and these structures generally are spared until the neoplasm has explored easier avenues of growth. Tumor that encounters cartilage or bone in its path is often diverted and spread along a path of less resistance. Slow-growing neoplasms of the gingiva may produce a smooth pressure defect of the underlying bone without actual bone invasion.

Entrance of tumor into the parapharyngeal space allows superior or inferior spread from the base of the skull to the root of the neck.

Spread inside the lumen of the sublingual, submandibular, and parotid gland ducts is not a prevalent pattern. The nasolacrimal duct, however, frequently is invaded in ethmoid sinus and nasal carcinoma.

Perineural spread is an important pathway for tumor spread and is observed in squamous cell carcinomas as well as minor salivary gland tumors, especially adenoid cystic carcinomas. The presence of perineural invasion predicts a poorer rate of local control when managed by surgery[6]; there are no specific data for definitive radiation therapy. Local recurrence increases the likelihood of perineural involvement, and tumors may track along a nerve to the base of the skull and the central nervous system (CNS). Peripheral perineural spread (growth away from the CNS) is also observed. Patients with perineural invasion often develop neurologic symptoms secondary to nerve invasion or, less frequently, entrapment of the nerve.

Vascular space invasion is associated with an increased risk for regional and distant metastases.

LYMPHATIC SPREAD

The differentiation of the tumor, the size of the primary lesion, the presence of vascular space invasion, and the density of cap-

TABLE 26.2-1. Percentage of Clinically Detected Nodal Metastasis in Admission by T Stage: M. D. Anderson Hospital, 1948–1965 (2044 Patients)

Primary Site	T Stage	N0	N1	N2 or N3
Oral tongue	T1	86	10	4
	T2	70	19	11
	T3	52	16	31
	T4	24	10	66
Floor of mouth	T1	89	9	2
	T2	71	18	10
	T3	56	21	24
	T4	46	10	43
Retromolar trigone and anterior tonsillar pillar	T1	88	2	9
	T2	62	18	20
	T3	46	21	33
	T4	32	18	50
Soft palate	T1	92	0	8
	T2	64	12	24
	T3	35	26	39
	T4	33	11	56
Tonsillar fossa	T1	30	41	30
	T2	32	14	54
	T3	30	18	52
	T4	10	13	76
Base of tongue	T1	30	15	55
	T2	29	14	56
	T3	26	23	52
	T4	16	8	76
Oropharyngeal walls	T1	75	0	25
	T2	70	10	20
	T3	33	22	44
	T4	24	24	52
Supraglottic larynx	T1	61	10	29
	T2	58	16	26
	T3	36	25	40
	T4	41	18	41
Hypopharynx	T1	37	21	42
	T2	30	20	49
	T3	21	26	54
	T4	26	15	58
Nasopharynx	T1	8	11	82
	T2	16	12	72
	T3	12	9	80
	T4	17	6	78

(Modified from ref. 10.)

TABLE 26.2-2. Incidence of Positive Retropharyngeal Nodes by Various Primary Sites and Clinical Neck Stages (794 Tumors)

Primary Site	Clinical Neck Stage		Overall (%)
	N0 Neck	N+ Neck	
Nasopharynx	2/5 (40%)	12/14 (86%)	74
Pharyngeal wall	6/37 (16%)	12/56 (21%)	19
Soft palate	1/21 (5%)	6/32 (19%)	13
Tonsillar region	2/56 (4%)	14/120 (12%)	9
Pyriform sinus or postcricoid area	0/55 (0%)	7/81 (9%)	5
Base of tongue	0/31 (0%)	5/90 (6%)	4
Supraglottic larynx	0/87 (0%)	4/109 (4%)	2

N+ neck, neck nodes clinically involved (stages N1–N3b).
(From ref. 13, with permission.)

illary lymphatics may predict the risk of lymph node metastasis. Recurrent lesions have an increased risk.

Although access to the capillary lymphatics determines the opportunity, histologic features also impact the likelihood of lymphatic spread. Low-grade minor salivary gland tumors and sarcomas have a lower risk of lymph node metastases than squamous cell carcinomas arising in similar mucosal sites.

A patient may present with squamous cell carcinoma in a cervical lymph node, and despite an extensive workup, the site of origin remains undetermined in approximately 60% of patients.[7,8] If only the neck is treated, a primary lesion may appear at a later date, but some may never show a primary site.[9]

The risk of subclinical disease in the patient with a clinically negative neck may be obtained either by studying the incidence of positive nodes found in elective neck dissection speci-

mens or by determining the probability of a regional recurrence when the neck is not treated. The relative incidence of clinically positive lymph nodes on admission by anatomic site and T stage is given in Table 26.2-1.[10] Well-lateralized lesions spread to ipsilateral neck lymph nodes.[11] Lesions on or near the midline and lateralized tongue base and nasopharyngeal lesions may spread to both sides, but tend to spread to the side occupied by the bulk of the lesion. Patients with clinically positive lymph nodes in the ipsilateral neck are at risk for contralateral disease, especially if the nodes are large or multiple. Obstruction of the lymphatic pathways by surgery or radiation therapy also shunts the lymphatic flow to the opposite neck. This shunting is mainly through anastomotic channels that cross through the submental space.[12]

When contralateral metastases occur from well-lateralized lesions, the subdigastric node (level II) is the most commonly involved but may be bypassed, with the midjugular (level III) or low jugular (level IV) next affected. Although there is usually an orderly progression of lymph node involvement, there are examples of skips. When lymph node metastases appear at an unusual site, a careful search must be made for a second primary. Rarely one sees retrograde lymph node metastases in the ipsilateral axilla associated with involvement of the lower neck nodes.

Before the availability of computed tomography (CT) and magnetic resonance imaging (MRI), the presence of metastatic disease in the retropharyngeal nodes was difficult to detect.[13] The likelihood of retropharyngeal adenopathy is related to the presence of clinically involved lymph nodes and primary site (Table 26.2-2). The percentage of patients with positive nodes reflects the incidence of radiographically positive nodes; the likelihood of occult disease is probably higher.

DISTANT SPREAD

Stage for stage, the risk of distant metastases is the same for patients treated by radiation therapy alone as for those treated by surgery alone. The risk of distant metastasis is related more to neck stage and location of involved nodes in the low neck than to primary stage.[14] The risk is less than 10% for N0 or N1 disease and rises to approximately 30% for N3 disease as well as N1 or N2 nodes with disease below the level of the thyroid notch. The lung is the most common site, accounting for half of the first recognized sites. Almost one-half of the metastases are recognized by 9 months, 80% by 2 years, and 90% by 3 years.[14,15] The risk of distant metastasis doubles in patients developing a recurrence above the clavicles.[15]

DIAGNOSTIC EVALUATION

The initial evaluation includes a thorough head and neck examination by one or more physicians. The location and extent of the primary tumor and any clinically positive cervical lymph nodes is documented. Almost all patients undergo contrast-enhanced CT or MRI or both to further delineate the extent of local-regional disease. The authors' preference is to use CT and reserve MRI for situations in which further information is required. The scan(s) should be obtained before biopsy so that changes from the biopsy are not confused with tumor. A chest radiograph is obtained to determine the presence of distant metastases or a synchronous primary lung cancer. Patients with N3 neck disease, as well as those with N2 adenopathy with adenopathy below the level of the thyroid notch, have a 20% to 30% risk of developing distant metastases and should be considered for chest CT. Positron emission tomography (PET) may be useful to determine whether a peripheral noncalcified pulmonary nodule is benign or malignant.

For tumors amenable to transoral biopsy, such as those in the oral cavity, biopsy may be performed using local anesthetics in the clinic. Otherwise direct laryngoscopy is performed to determine the extent of the tumor and to obtain a tissue diagnosis. Patients presenting with a metastatic node from an unknown primary site undergo fine-needle aspiration (FNA) of the node. Occasionally the diagnosis may be made by clinical and radiographic evaluation and biopsy avoided in situations in which the treatment is definitive radiation therapy and obtaining tissue is risky (i.e., paragangliomas or acoustic schwannomas).

Before initial treatment, the patient should be evaluated by all members of the team who may be involved in the initial management as well as possible salvage therapy. Cases treated at the University of Florida are presented at a weekly head and neck tumor conference attended by head and neck surgeons, radiation oncologists, medical oncologists, diagnostic radiologists, plastic surgeons, pathologists, and dentists. The treatment options are discussed and recommendations are presented to the patient, who makes the final decision.

STAGING

The staging for the primary lesions (T) is given in the site-specific section Oral Cavity. The American Joint Committee on Cancer (AJCC) (2002) neck staging (N) is common to all head and neck sites, except the nasopharynx.[16] Lesions may be clinically or pathologically staged; the latter is designated by pN.

Regional Lymph Nodes (N)

NX Regional lymph nodes cannot be assessed
N0 No regional lymph node metastasis
N1 Metastasis in a single ipsilateral lymph node, 3 cm or less in greatest dimension
N2a Metastasis in single ipsilateral lymph node more than 3 cm, but no more than 6 cm, in greatest dimension

N2b Metastasis in multiple ipsilateral lymph nodes, none more than 6 cm in greatest dimension
N2c Metastasis in bilateral or contralateral lymph nodes, none more than 6 cm in greatest dimension
N3 Metastasis in a lymph node more than 6 cm in greatest dimension

The format for combining T and N stages into an overall stage is as follows[16]:

Stage Grouping

Stage 0	Tis	N0	M0
Stage I	T1	N0	M0
Stage II	T2	N0	M0
Stage III	T3	N0	M0
	T1–T3	N1	M0
Stage IVA	T4a	N0–N1	M0
	T1–T4a	N2	M0
Stage IVB	Any T	N3	M0
	T4b	Any N	M0
Stage IVC	Any T	Any N	M1

Stage IV represents a wide spectrum of disease. One patient may have a T1, T2, or T3 lesion with treatable N2 neck disease and be a reasonable candidate for curative therapy, whereas another may have either advanced primary cancer (T4b) or far-advanced neck disease (N3) or both, and have a relatively low chance of cure.[17] Depending on primary site, the 5-year disease-free survival rate is significantly higher for patients with stage IVA cancers than for those with stage IVB malignancies.

GENERAL PRINCIPLES FOR SELECTION OF TREATMENT

Surgery and radiation therapy are the only curative treatments for carcinoma arising in the head and neck. Chemotherapy is useful in the adjuvant setting; used alone, it is not curative.

The advantages of an operation compared with radiation therapy, assuming similar cure rates, may include the following: (1) a limited amount of tissue is exposed to treatment, (2) treatment time is shorter, (3) the risk of immediate and late radiation sequelae is avoided, and (4) irradiation is reserved for a subsequent head and neck primary tumor, which may not be as suitable for an operation.

The advantages of irradiation may include the following: (1) the risk of a major postoperative complication is avoided, (2) no tissues are removed so that the probability of a functional or cosmetic defect may be reduced, (3) elective irradiation of the lymph nodes can be included with little added morbidity, whereas the surgeon must either observe the neck or proceed with an elective neck dissection (sometimes bilateral depending on the primary site), and (4) the surgical salvage of irradiation failure is probably more likely than the salvage of a surgical failure.

Rescue of a surgical failure may be attempted by operation, radiation therapy, or both. Surgical recurrences usually develop at the margins of the resection, in or near the suture line. It is difficult to distinguish the normal surgical scarring from recurrent disease, and diagnosis of recurrence is often delayed. Tumor response to radiation therapy under these circumstances is poor. An operation, radiation therapy, or both, however, may salvage small mucosal recurrences and some neck recurrences.

MANAGEMENT

PRIMARY SITE

The management of the primary cancer is considered separately for each anatomic site. Patients who are in poor nutritional condition may require a percutaneous gastrostomy before initiating irradiation, particularly if concomitant chemotherapy is used. If external-beam radiation therapy is selected, it may be given with either conventional once-daily fractionation to 66 to 70 Gy at 2 Gy/fraction, 5 days a week in a continuous course, or with an altered fractionation schedule. Whether an altered fractionation schedule is better than conventional fractionation depends on the altered fractionation technique that is selected. Two altered fractionation schedules shown to result in improved local-regional control rates are the University of Florida hyperfractionation technique and the M. D. Anderson concomitant boost technique.[18] The results of a prospective randomized Radiation Therapy Oncology Group trial comparing these altered fractionation schedules with conventional fractionation and the Massachusetts General Hospital accelerated split-course schedule are shown in Table 26.2-3. Acute toxicity is increased with altered fractionation; late toxicity is comparable with that for conventional fractionation.

Conventional external-beam techniques and brachytherapy are discussed in the following site-specific sections. External-beam radiation therapy may also be delivered with intensity-modulated radiation therapy (IMRT) to reduce the dose to the normal tissues.[19]

The disadvantages of IMRT are that it is much more time consuming to plan and treat the patient, the dose distribution is often less homogeneous so that "hot spots" may increase the risk of late complications, the risk of a marginal miss may be increased because the fields are more conformal, the total body irradiation dose is higher because of increased "beam on" time and scatter irradiation, and it is more costly. Therefore, it is essential that a clear reason for using IMRT versus conventional radiation therapy be identified. The usual indication for IMRT is to reduce the dose to the contralateral parotid gland and thus limit long-term xerostomia. Another indication is to reduce the temporal lobe dose in patients with nasopharyngeal cancer. Although IMRT can be used to treat patients who are suitable for conventional ipsilateral field arrangements, such as a wedge pair technique for a well-lateralized tonsillar cancer, it does not make sense to do so because of the disadvantages previously discussed.

NECK

Management of the neck is closely tied to management of the primary site, but certain general principles may be outlined. Death due only to failure to control neck disease, with the primary tumor controlled, should be an uncommon event if surgery and radiation therapy are used optimally.

In a standard *radical neck dissection*, the superficial and deep cervical fascia with its enclosed lymph nodes (levels I to V) is removed in continuity with the sternocleidomastoid muscle, the omohyoid muscle, the internal and external jugular veins, the spinal accessory nerve, and the submandibular gland. The incisions used by the surgeon are governed largely by the primary lesion. Proper physical therapy may minimize the functional changes associated with the loss of the spinal accessory nerve and sternocleidomastoid muscle.

The term *modified neck dissection* refers to any neck node resection that is less than the radical neck dissection. A modified neck dissection is tailored to remove those groups of lymph nodes at highest risk for metastatic disease while also attempting to reduce the sequelae by selectively preserving certain muscles, nerves, and vessels. A modified neck dissection sparing normal tissues (e.g., the functional neck dissection) is usually recommended for a clinically negative neck, for selected clinically positive necks (mobile, 1- to 3-cm lymph nodes), and for removal of residual disease after radiation therapy when there has been excellent regression of N2 or N3 disease.[20]

Complications after radical neck dissection include hematoma, seroma, lymphedema, wound infections and dehiscence, damage to the seventh, tenth, eleventh, and twelfth cranial nerves, carotid exposure, and carotid rupture. The last-mentioned can be minimized by covering the carotid artery with a dermal graft at the time of surgery.[20]

Clinically Negative Neck Lymph Nodes

The risk for subclinical disease for any particular patient may be estimated based on the primary site, the T stage of the primary

TABLE 26.2-3. Altered Fractionation: 2-Year Outcomes from the Radiation Therapy Oncology Group 90-03 Trial

	Fractionation Schedule			
Parameter	Conventional (70 Gy/35 Fx/7 wk)	Hyperfractionation (81.6 Gy/68 Fx/7 wk)	Accelerated Split Course (67.2 Gy/42 Fx/6 wk)	Accelerated Concomitant Boost (72 Gy/42 Fx/6 wk)
Number of patients	268	263	274	268
Local-regional control	46%	54% ($P = .045$)	48% ($P = .55$)	55% ($P = .050$)
Disease-free survival	32%	38% ($P = .067$)	33% ($P = .26$)	39% ($P = .054$)
Overall survival	46%	55% ($P = .13$)	46% ($P = .86$)	51% ($P = .40$)
Grade 3+ acute toxicity	35%	55% ($P < .0001$)	51% ($P = .0002$)	59% ($P < .0001$)
Grade 3+ late toxicity	28%	28% (NS)	28% (NS)	38% ($P = .011$)
Grade 3+ late toxicity at 2 y	6%	13% (NS)	8% (NS)	8% (NS)

Fx, fractions; NS, nonsignificant.
Note. *P* values reflect comparison of the experimental arms with standard fractionation.
(Data from ref. 18.)

TABLE 26.2-4. Definition of Risk Groups for the Clinically N0 Neck

Group	Estimated Risk of Subclinical Neck Disease (%)	T Stage	Site
I Low risk	<20	T1	Floor of mouth, oral tongue, retromolar trigone, gingiva, hard palate, buccal mucosa
II Intermediate risk	20–30	T1	Soft palate, pharyngeal wall, supraglottic larynx, tonsil
		T2	Floor of mouth, oral tongue, retromolar trigone, gingiva, hard palate, buccal mucosa
III High risk	>30	T1–T4	Nasopharynx, pyriform sinus, base of tongue
		T2–T4	Soft palate, pharyngeal wall, supraglottic larynx, tonsil
		T3–T4	Floor of mouth, oral tongue, retromolar trigone, gingiva, hard palate, buccal mucosa

(From ref. 21, with permission.)

TABLE 26.2-5. Control of Disease in the Clinically Negative Neck with Elective Neck Irradiation (Number Controlled/Number Treated)

Risk Group	No ENI	Partial ENI	Total ENI
I (<20%)	13/15 (87%)	16/17 (94%)	1/1 (100%)
II (20–30%)	6/9 (67%)	34/38 (89%)	10/11 (91%)
III (>30%)	3/4 (75%)	32/33 (97%)	61/62 (98%)
Total	22/28 (79%)	82/88 (93%)	72/74 (97%)

ENI, elective neck irradiation.
(From ref. 21, with permission.)

lesion, the differentiation of the neoplasm, and the presence of lymphatic invasion.[21–23] The estimated incidence of subclinical disease in the regional lymphatics when the neck lymph nodes are clinically negative is presented in Table 26.2-4.[21,22] Both irradiation and neck dissection are approximately 90% efficient in eradicating subclinical disease in the neck lymph nodes.[23] Alternatively, a policy of "wait and see" may be adopted for the clinically negative neck to avoid unnecessary treatment, and the neck may then be managed by surgery, radiation therapy, or both only if cervical metastases develop. The physician and patient must adhere to a schedule of very close observation and examination if they choose the policy of observation. Even though the salvage neck treatment may be regionally successful, these patients are at an increased risk to develop distant metastasis and therefore have a poorer prognosis compared with patients in whom the neck remains continuously disease-free. The salvage rate for patients developing clinically positive lymph nodes with the primary lesion controlled is only 50% to 60%.[21]

The relative effectiveness of irradiation and surgery in the management of the N0 neck is shown in Tables 26.2-5, 26.2-6, and 26.2-7.[21,24] Partial neck treatment is inefficient for primary lesions of the base of the tongue, soft palate, supraglottic larynx, or hypopharynx (see Tables 26.2-6 and 26.2-7), and treatment of the entire neck is advised for sites with a high rate of subclinical disease. Patients with lateralized T1 or T2 tonsillar cancers do not require elective treatment for the contralateral N0 neck.[11] Those with significant extension into the tongue or soft palate or both, as well as those with T3 or T4 cancers, should receive treatment to the entire neck.

When the primary tumor is to be treated surgically, an elective neck dissection should be performed when the risk of regional lymph node metastasis is 10% to 15% or greater. Modified neck dissection is used for the clinically negative neck so that there are few cosmetic or functional problems. Modified neck dissection has as good a rate of disease control as does radical neck dissection if patients who are found to have multiple positive nodes or disease extending through the capsule are then referred for postoperative irradiation.[25,26] If the primary lesion is to be treated with external-beam irradiation, then elective neck irradiation adds no cost and, if properly done, little additional morbidity. Radiation therapy occasionally fails to eradicate subclinical disease due to geographic miss, low dose, selection of the wrong beam energy (which results in low dose), and failure to detect a clinically positive node.

Clinically Positive Neck Lymph Nodes

The rates of neck failure by N stage and therapeutic category reported by the M. D. Anderson Hospital and the University of

TABLE 26.2-6. Failure of Initial Neck Treatment (596 Patients with Carcinoma of the Tonsillar Fossa, Base of Tongue, Supraglottic Larynx, or Hypopharynx, M. D. Anderson Hospital, 1948–1967)

	Stage							
	N0							
Treatment	No Treatment	Partial	Complete	N1	N2a	N2b	N3a	N3b
Radiation		15%	2%	15%	27%	27%	38%	34%
Surgery	55% (16/29)	35%	7%	11%	8%	42%	42%	41%
Combined		1/5	0/6	0	0	23%	23%	25%

(Adapted from ref. 24.)

TABLE 26.2-7. Cervical Metastasis Appearing in the Contralateral Neck (596 Patients with Carcinoma of the Tonsillar Fossa, Base of Tongue, Supraglottic Larynx, or Hypopharynx, M. D. Anderson Hospital, 1948–1967)

Treatment	N0 (%)	N1 (%)	N2a (%)	N2b (%)	N3a (%)
Radiation	4	2	9	7	0
Surgery	25	17	23	43	33
Combined	0	0	0	11	0

(Adapted from ref. 24.)

TABLE 26.2-9. Clinical Complete Response and Radiographic Complete Response versus Residual Disease in the Neck (n = 113 patients)

Clinical Complete Response	Radiographic Complete Response[a]	Proportion of Pathologically Positive Hemineck Specimens
Yes	No	6/13 (46%)
Yes	Yes	0/27 (0%)
No	No	31/73 (43%)

Note: Specificity = 36.8%; sensitivity = 97.3%; negative predictive value = 96.6%; positive predictive value = 42.9%.
[a]When a lymph node in a hemineck was seen on postoperative computed tomography to be 15 mm or less and free of significant internal defects or evidence of capsular rupture (rated less than grade 3 or 4 for both findings).
(Data from ref. 210.)

Florida are shown in Tables 26.2-6 and 26.2-8, respectively. In general, the irradiation precedes the operation if the primary site is to be treated by radiation therapy or if the node is fixed. The operation precedes the irradiation if the primary site is to be treated surgically.

Modified neck dissection is sufficient treatment for the ipsilateral neck for patients with N1 or N2a disease without extracapsular extension. Radiation therapy is added for N2b and N3 stages, for control of contralateral subclinical disease (see Table 26.2-7), for invasion through the capsule of the node, and for multiple positive nodes.[26]

When the primary lesion is to be managed by irradiation, then radiation therapy alone is sufficient for patients with N1 (1- to 3-cm) disease. Neck dissection may be added in selected cases in which the 3-cm node is fixed or fails to regress completely. Radiation therapy is followed by a neck dissection for most N2a and nearly all N3 disease. The decision to add a neck dissection for N2b and N2c disease is individualized based on the diameter of the largest node, the multiplicity of palpable nodes, and response to radiation therapy (Table 26.2-9). Large, fixed nodes require 60 to 80 Gy before neck dissection; some of the specimens will show "no viable tumor," and a substantial number of patients will have the disease controlled in the neck.

Many have condemned excisional or incisional biopsy of a neck mass for diagnosis. McGuirt and McCabe[27] compared results

of definitive surgery with and without a prior open biopsy and concluded that the risks of neck failure, distant metastases, and complications were all increased.

Ellis and coworkers[28] studied the results of therapy after open biopsy of a lymph node before treatment. Patients received definitive irradiation to the primary site and neck; a subset of patients underwent a postradiation therapy neck dissection. Open biopsy had no adverse impact on these patients compared with those who did not undergo an open biopsy[28] (Table 26.2-10).

Therefore, after open biopsy of the neck, radiation therapy is recommended as the initial treatment. If the primary tumor is to be managed by radiation therapy, no further neck treatment is needed if the neck node has been removed. If there is

TABLE 26.2-8. Five-Year Rate of Neck Control According to the 1983 American Joint Committee on Cancer[208] Stage and Treatment (459 Patients, 593 Heminecks[a])

Stage	RT Alone		RT + Neck Dissection		Significance (P)
	No. of Heminecks	Control (%)	No. of Heminecks	Control (%)	
N1	215	86	38	93	.28
N2a	29	79	24	68	.6
N2b	138	70	80	91	<.01
N3a	29	33	40	69	<.01

Note: The University of Florida data; patients were treated October 1964 to October 1985; analysis, December 1988, by Eric R. Ellis, MD. RT, radiation therapy.
[a]Excludes 67 heminecks that underwent incisional or excisional biopsy before treatment.
(From ref. 209, with permission.)

TABLE 26.2-10. Prognostic Factors in Order of Importance for Predicting the Time to Occurrence of Various Events

Event	Rank Order	Factor	Level of Significance (P)
Recurrence in neck (n = 660 heminecks)	1	Increasing N stage	.0001
	2	Treatment of neck with RT alone	.0001
	3	Fixed nodes	.0001
	4	T stage[a]	.0350
Death with disease present (n = 508)	1	Recurrence above the clavicles	.0001
	2	Increasing N stage	.0003
	3	Fixed nodes	.0053
	4	Treatment of neck with RT alone	.0121
Occurrence of distant metastasis (n = 508)	1	Recurrence above the clavicles	.0001
	2	Increasing N stage	.0003
	3	Fixed nodes	.0704
	4	Positive nodes below thyroid notch	.1023

RT, radiation therapy.
[a]This factor is thought to be correlated with the censoring pattern.
(From ref. 28, with permission.)

residual gross tumor in the neck after open biopsy, a planned neck dissection is added, depending on the results of a restaging CT scan 3 to 4 weeks after radiation therapy.[20] If the primary tumor is to be managed by operation, preoperative radiation therapy is recommended, followed by removal of the primary lesion in addition to an appropriate neck dissection.

Once the normal lymphatic pathways have been surgically interrupted by the open biopsy procedure, shunting of lymph nodes to the contralateral side of the neck may occur, placing it at risk for lymph node spread when the opposite neck would not normally be at risk.[12,29]

Chemotherapy

Chemotherapy may be administered to palliate symptoms in patients with incurable head and neck cancer or as an adjuvant to radiation therapy or surgery, or both, to improve the probability of cure. Adjuvant chemotherapy may be administered before definitive treatment (induction), simultaneously with radiation therapy (concomitant), or after radiation therapy or surgery (maintenance). In addition, chemoprevention implies the administration of natural or synthetic agents to reduce the risk of developing second primary tumors of the upper aerodigestive tract. This section addresses palliative chemotherapy and chemoprevention. Adjuvant chemotherapy is discussed in General Principles of Combining Modalities, in which combined modality treatment is addressed.

PALLIATIVE CHEMOTHERAPY. Patients with recurrent squamous cell carcinomas of the head and neck have a 6-month median survival and a 1-year survival rate of approximately 20%.[30] Chemotherapy may be administered to achieve tumor regression and, hopefully, palliate symptoms caused by the cancer. The response rates to various chemotherapeutic agents are reasonably well defined; whether tumor regression translates into meaningful palliation when weighed against the toxicity of treatment is less clear.[30,31] Some of the goals of palliative treatment are pain relief, improved swallowing, improved energy, return to "normal" activities, preservation of laryngeal speech, maintenance of understandable speech, and retention of normal taste and smell.[31]

Approximate response rates to single chemotherapeutic agents are as follows: methotrexate, 31%; bleomycin, 21%; cisplatin, 28%; carboplatin, 22%; fluorouracil, 15%; ifosfamide, 23%; paclitaxel, 15% to 40%, depending on dose; docetaxel, 30% to 33%, depending on dose; vinorelbine, 18%; gemcitabine, 13%; and topotecan, 14%.[30] Cisplatin is one of the most effective single agents and is usually administered at 80 to 100 mg/m^2 every 3 to 4 weeks.[30] Carboplatin has less renal, otologic, neurologic, and gastrointestinal toxicity and is usually reserved for patients who have renal dysfunction or a peripheral neuropathy that contraindicates the use of cisplatin.[30] Single-agent chemotherapy is often used for patients with relatively marginal performance status and those who are unwilling to accept the additional toxicity of combination chemotherapy.

The gold standard combination chemotherapeutic regimen is cisplatin 100 mg/m^2 on day 1 only and fluorouracil 1000 mg/m^2 daily for a 96-hour infusion, administered every 3 to 4 weeks.[30–32] The average response rate is approximately 50% with approximately 16% complete responses.[30] The combination of paclitaxel or docetaxel with either cisplatin or carboplatin

results in response rates of 30% to 40% with complete responses observed in 10% or fewer.[30,32–34] The median duration of response is approximately 4 months and the median survival remains approximately 6 months or a little better.[30,33,34] The toxicities of the taxane-based regimens are probably similar to those of the older drug combinations.

CHEMOPREVENTION. Patients who have a squamous cell carcinoma of the head and neck have an increased risk of developing a second primary tumor of the upper aerodigestive tract because of a combination of exposure to carcinogens and genetic predisposition.[35] The carcinogens thought to be responsible for induction of a significant proportion of head and neck cancers are tobacco and alcohol. The risk of developing a second primary tumor is 2.7% to 4% per year.[35–37] The high risk of developing a second cancer means that any increased probability of curing the index malignancy is offset, in part, by the chance of dying from a subsequent tumor. Natural and synthetic compounds may be used to reduce the probability of developing a second malignancy; the retinoids and β-carotene have been studied in prospective trials. The following summary is based on reviews by Munro[31] and Papadmitrakopoulou.[36]

Retinoids and β-carotene may cause regression of oral leukoplakia, but the lesions are likely to recur after cessation of the drug. Patients with oral leukoplakia have a lower risk of developing cancer after treatment with retinoids than after treatment with β-carotene. Administration of chemoprevention agents does not reduce the risk of recurrence of the index cancer. Reversal of moderate to severe dysplasia is unlikely with single-agent chemoprevention.

Cis-retinoic acid has been shown to reduce the risk of second primary tumors in patients previously treated for head and neck cancer. In contrast, etretinate has not been shown to be effective. The use of retinoids is associated with toxicity that precludes their use outside of prospective clinical trials and limits their usefulness for maintenance therapy. The impact of chemoprevention agents diminishes after cessation of the drug. Insufficient data exist pertaining to agents such as vitamin E and selenium.

In summary, although promising results have been obtained with some chemoprevention agents, they should not be used outside of controlled clinical trials.

General Principles of Combining Modalities

SURGERY PLUS RADIATION THERAPY. Either preoperative or postoperative radiation therapy may be used; there are advocates of each. Analysis of available data suggests there is no difference in local-regional control or survival rates for the two sequences.[26]

Combined modality therapy should be avoided for lesions with a high cure rate (70% or greater) by either surgery or radiation therapy alone. The increased morbidity from combined treatment is not associated with a significantly improved control rate, and many patients with local or regional failure can be treated successfully by secondary procedures.

The advantages of postoperative compared with preoperative radiation therapy include less operative morbidity,[38] more meaningful margin checks at the time of the operation, a knowledge of tumor spread for radiation treatment planning, safe use of a higher radiation dose, and no chance the patient will refuse surgery. The disadvantages of postoperative radiation therapy include the larger treatment volume necessary to cover surgical dissections and scars, a delay in the start of radiation therapy with possible growth (especially in contralateral neck nodes), and the higher dose required to accomplish the same rates of local-regional control.

Preoperative Radiation Therapy. Preoperative radiation therapy is recommended for the following situations: (1) fixed neck nodes, (2) initiation of postoperative radiation therapy delayed by more than 8 weeks due to reconstruction, (3) use of the gastric pull-up for reconstruction, and (4) open biopsy of a positive neck node.

Postoperative Radiation Therapy. Postoperative radiation therapy is considered when the risk of recurrence above the clavicles exceeds 20%. The operative procedure should be one stage and of such magnitude that irradiation is started no later than 6 to 8 weeks after surgery. The operation should be undertaken only if it is believed to be highly likely that all gross disease will be removed and margins will be negative. Partial removal of gross disease should be avoided; it is a maneuver that probably reduces the chance of control by radiation therapy rather than enhancing it.

Although no randomized trials have addressed the efficacy of postoperative adjuvant radiation therapy in the treatment of the head and neck cancer, excellent data that have bearing on this issue are available from the Medical College of Virginia. Two groups of surgeons operated on patients with head and neck cancer—general surgical oncologists who used surgery alone and reserved radiation therapy for treatment of recurrent disease, and otolaryngologists who routinely sent patients with locally advanced disease for postoperative irradiation.[39] One hundred twenty-five of 441 patients treated surgically between 1982 and 1988 had extracapsular extension or positive margins or both; 71 were treated with surgery alone, and 54 received postoperative radiation therapy. Patients were irradiated once daily at 1.8 to 2.0 Gy/fraction with cobalt 60 or 4-MV x-rays to doses of 50 to 50.99 Gy in 26 patients and to 60 Gy or more in the remainder. Local control rates at 3 years after surgery alone compared with surgery and radiation therapy were as follows: extracapsular extension, 31% and 66% (P = .03); positive margins, 41% and 49% (P = .04); and extracapsular extension and positive margins, 0% and 68% (P = .001). A multivariate analysis of local control was performed evaluating the impact of T stage, N stage, use of postoperative irradiation, number of positive nodes, number of nodes with extracapsular extension, primary site, microscopic and macroscopic extracapsular extension, and margin status. For the end point of local control, use of postoperative radiation therapy (P = .0001), macroscopic extracapsular extension (P = .0001), and margin status (P = .09) were of independent significance. Disease-free survival at 3 years was 25% after surgery alone and 45% after combined modality treatment (P = .0001). Cause-specific survival rates at 3 years were 41% for surgery alone and 72% for surgery and postoperative radiation therapy (P = .0003). Multivariate analysis of cause-specific survival showed that postoperative radiation therapy (P = .0001) and the number of nodes with extracapsular extension (P = .0001) significantly influenced this end point. Two irradiated patients experienced mandibular necrosis; one was treated with hyperbaric oxygen and the other with conservative management.

In another series, Lundahl et al.[40] reported on 95 patients with node-positive squamous cell carcinoma who were treated with a neck dissection and postoperative radiation therapy at the Mayo Clinic. A matched-pair analysis was performed using a series of patients treated with surgery alone; 56 matched pairs of patients were identified. The results showed that the rates of recurrence in the dissected neck [relative risk (RR) = 5.82; P = .0002], recurrence in either side of the neck (RR = 2.21; P = .0052), and death from any cause (RR = 1.67; P = .0182) were significantly higher for patients treated with neck dissection alone.

Thus, it appears that postoperative radiation therapy may significantly improve both local-regional disease control and survival for patients who are at high risk for failure after surgery.

Indications for postoperative radiation therapy include close (less than 5-mm) or positive margins, extracapsular extension, multiple positive nodes, invasion of the soft tissues of the neck, endothelial-lined space invasion, perineural invasion, and more than 5 mm of subglottic invasion.[26] The authors currently recommend 60 Gy in 6 weeks to 65 Gy in 7 weeks for patients with negative margins and fewer than three indications for radiation therapy. For patients with close (less than 5-mm) or positive margins, the authors recommend 70 Gy in 7 to 7.5 weeks or 74.4 Gy at 1.2 Gy twice a day. In the authors' experience, oral cavity lesions have a higher failure rate and may receive the higher doses even with negative margins.

ADJUVANT CHEMOTHERAPY AND DEFINITIVE RADIATION THERAPY. Chemotherapy may be combined with definitive radiation therapy to (1) improve the likelihood of cure, and (2) select patients who may be cured with definitive radiation therapy and thus avoid ablative surgery. Although it has been postulated that nasopharyngeal cancer may be more sensitive to cytotoxic drugs than other head and neck cancers, the response rates are similar and there are no convincing data to support this contention.[31] It is likely that the following observations that apply to head and neck cancers in general apply to nasopharyngeal carcinomas as well. The Veterans Administration Laryngeal Cancer Study Group trial showed that induction chemotherapy could be used to select patients who are likely to be cured with definitive radiation therapy, based on a complete or partial response to chemotherapy, without a survival decrement compared with survival after the initial surgery and postoperative irradiation.[41] A subsequent European Organization for Research and Treatment of Cancer randomized trial including patients with advanced squamous cell carcinoma of the pyriform sinus and aryepiglottic fold confirmed these findings.[42] Patients who were randomly assigned to receive induction chemotherapy and had a complete response were treated with definitive irradiation. Their survival rate was similar to that of patients who underwent initial surgery and postoperative radiation therapy. A recent metaanalysis of 63 randomized trials published between 1965 and 1993 encompassing 10,741 patients revealed an overall 5-year survival advantage of 4 percentage points (P <.0001) for patients who received adjuvant chemotherapy compared with those who did not receive chemotherapy.[43] The improvement in absolute survival at 5 years was limited to those who received concomitant chemotherapy (8%; P <.0001) and was not seen in patients who received induction chemotherapy (2%; P = .10) or maintenance chemotherapy (1%; P = .74). Thus, it appears that induction chemotherapy may be used to select patients likely to be cured with radiation therapy, but may not improve survival.

Parenthetically, primary tumor volume calculated on pretreatment CT or MRI may also predict the likelihood of local control after definitive irradiation.[44,45] The influence of tumor volume on local control varies with primary site and treatment.[44,46,47] It appears to be most useful for patients with moderately advanced cancers of the supraglottis and glottis. Mancuso et al.[45] calculated the primary tumor volumes for 63 patients treated with definitive irradiation for supraglottic carcinomas and found that local control was 89% for tumors less than 6 cm compared with 52% when volumes were 6 cm or larger ($P = .0012$). Similarly, the probability of maintaining a functional larynx after radiation therapy was significantly related to primary tumor volume ($P = .00004$). In contrast, a multivariate analysis of local control after definitive irradiation in a series of 114 patients treated for oropharyngeal carcinoma showed that primary tumor volume had a marginal impact ($P = .10$) on this end point.[46] For patients with laryngeal tumors, determination of primary tumor volume is less costly and morbid than several cycles of induction chemotherapy.

In contrast to induction chemotherapy, concomitant chemotherapy appears to result in improved survival. However, the optimal combination of chemotherapy and radiation therapy is unclear, particularly in light of the recent altered fractionation trials. A number of important randomized trials pertaining to concomitant chemotherapy and radiation therapy have been published in recent years.

Calais et al.[48] recently reported a study conducted by Groupe d'Oncologie Radiothérapie Tête et Cou in which 222 patients with stage III and IV squamous cell carcinoma of the oropharynx were randomly assigned to receive 70 Gy in 35 fractions over 7 weeks, alone or combined with three cycles of concomitant fluorouracil and carboplatin. The 3-year rates of local-regional control (66% vs. 42%; $P = .03$), disease-free survival (42% vs. 20%; $P = .04$), and survival (51% vs. 31%; $P = .02$) were significantly improved for patients who received concomitant chemotherapy. Patients in the combined radiation therapy-chemotherapy arm experienced higher rates of grade 3 and 4 mucositis (71% vs. 39%; $P = .005$), feeding tube placement (33% vs. 13%; $P = .02$), and severe cervical fibrosis (11% vs. 3%; $P = .08$).

Adelstein et al.[49] reported a single-institution trial in which 100 patients with stage III or IV squamous cell carcinoma were randomly assigned to receive to 66 to 72 Gy at 1.8 to 2 Gy/fraction once daily, alone or with two cycles of concomitant fluorouracil and cisplatin. Patients were evaluated after receiving 55 Gy, and those thought to be nonresponders were referred for surgery. A planned neck dissection followed radiation therapy or radiation therapy plus chemotherapy for patients with N2 and N3 neck disease. There was improvement in the rates of local control (77% vs. 45%; $P <.001$), distant metastasis–free survival (84% vs. 75%; $P = .09$), and 5-year recurrence-free survival (62% vs. 51%; $P = .04$) after radiation therapy with concomitant chemotherapy. There was no significant difference in the 5-year survival rates (50% vs. 48%; $P = .55$). Patients who received concomitant chemotherapy were significantly more likely to require a feeding tube (58% vs. 32%; $P <.01$).

Adelstein and coworkers[50] reported a prospective trial conducted by the Head and Neck Intergroup between 1992 and 1999 in which 295 patients with unresectable stage III or IV carcinomas were randomly assigned to arm A, 70 Gy in 35 fractions; arm B, 70 Gy in 35 fractions plus concomitant cisplatin on days 1, 22, and 43; or arm C, 60 to 70 Gy in 35 fractions, split course, with three cycles of concomitant fluorouracil and cis-

platin. Grade 3 or worse toxicity was significantly increased in arms B ($P <.0001$) and C ($P <.001$) compared with arm A. Incidence of distant metastases as the first site of relapse was essentially the same in all three arms of the study: arm A, 18%; arm B, 22%; and arm C, 19%. The 3-year survival rates were as follows: arm A, 23%; arm B, 37% ($P = .014$); and arm C, 27% (not significant). Although the addition of cisplatin to once-daily radiation therapy improved efficacy, the potential benefit of combination chemotherapy was offset by reducing the radiation therapy dose and prolonging the overall time.

The Radiation Therapy Oncology Group reported the results of their 91-11 trial. Patients with laryngeal squamous cell carcinomas were randomly assigned to receive three cycles of induction fluorouracil and cisplatin followed by irradiation in complete and partial responders, three cycles of cisplatin and concomitant radiation therapy, or radiation therapy alone.[51] The irradiation consisted of 70 Gy in 35 fractions over 7 weeks in all three arms. There were no significant differences in laryngectomy-free survival or overall survival between the three treatment arms. Time to laryngectomy for patients who received concomitant cisplatin was significantly improved compared with those receiving induction chemotherapy ($P = .009$) or radiation therapy alone ($P = .0004$). Thus, the addition of concomitant chemotherapy to once-daily irradiation improves the likelihood of local-regional control and, depending on primary site and stage, survival compared with radiation therapy alone.[43]

The question that follows is whether concomitant chemotherapy improves the likelihood of cure for patients treated with altered fractionation. A single-institution study reported by Brizel et al.[52] compared a more aggressive hyperfractionated irradiation schedule with radiation therapy, concomitant fluorouracil and cisplatin. Patients who underwent irradiation alone received 75 Gy in 60 twice-daily fractions; those who underwent concomitant chemotherapy received 70 Gy in 56 twice-daily fractions with a 7-day split. Adjuvant chemotherapy consisted of two cycles of concomitant cisplatin, 12 mg/m^2 and fluorouracil, 600 mg/m^2/d for 5 days, followed by two cycles of maintenance chemotherapy. There were 116 patients included in the study. Patients who received adjuvant chemotherapy had improved 3-year rates of local-regional control (70% vs. 40%; $P = .01$), relapse-free survival (61% vs. 41%; $P = .08$), and overall survival (55% vs. 34%; $P = .07$). Late osteonecrosis or soft tissue necrosis or both occurred in 20% of those who received hyperfractionated radiation therapy and chemotherapy, and 15% of those treated with irradiation alone ($P >.05$).

Jeremic et al.[53] reported on 130 patients who were randomly assigned to receive hyperfractionated radiation therapy (77 Gy at 1.1 Gy/fraction, twice daily, in a continuous course) alone or combined with concomitant daily cisplatin, 6 mg/m^2. Patients who received concomitant chemotherapy had significantly improved 5-year rates of local-regional control (50% vs. 36%; $P = .041$), distant metastasis–free survival (86% vs. 57%; $P = .001$), and survival (46% vs. 25%; $P = .008$). Treatment splits and hospitalization for acute toxicity occurred in 11% and 9%, respectively, of patients who received chemotherapy compared with 9% and 6%, respectively, of those who received irradiation alone ($P = .99$ and $P = .74$, respectively). The rates of myelotoxicity were significantly higher in those who received concomitant cisplatin: grade 3 or 4 leukopenia (12% vs. 0%, $P = .006$) and grade 3 or 4 thrombocytopenia (8% vs. 0%, $P = .058$).

Olmi and colleagues[54] reported a multicenter prospective randomized trial in which 192 patients with stage III and IV oropharyngeal carcinomas (excluding T1 to 2N1) were randomly assigned to arm A, 66 to 70 Gy in 33 to 35 fractions; arm B, 64 to 67.2 Gy at 1.6 Gy/fraction twice daily with a planned split; and arm C, 66 to 70 Gy in 33 to 35 fractions with three cycles of concomitant fluorouracil and carboplatin. Grade 3 or worse toxicity in any arm justified a treatment split or, in arm B, a prolongation of the planned break. Treatment splits occurred as follows: arm A, 61%; arm B, 52%; and arm C, 65%. There was no significant difference in the 2-year survival rates for the three treatment arms: arm A, 40%; arm B, 37%; and arm C, 51%. The 2-year disease-free survival rate was significantly improved for arm C compared with arm A (42% vs. 23%, $P = .022$). The 2-year disease-free survival rate for arm B was 20%. This trial shows that split-course radiation therapy results in poor outcomes, and concomitant chemotherapy can compensate, at least in part, for suboptimal irradiation.

A multicenter German trial reported by Staar et al.[55] randomly assigned 240 patients with stage III and IV squamous cell carcinoma of the oropharynx and hypopharynx to receive accelerated concomitant boost radiation therapy, alone or combined with two cycles of fluorouracil and carboplatin. A secondary randomization occurred in both treatment groups to receive or not receive granulocyte colony-stimulating factor to reduce mucositis. Patients who received concomitant chemotherapy had marginally improved rates of local-regional control ($P = .112$) and survival ($P = .092$); the improvement was observed primarily in patients with oropharyngeal cancers. The administration of granulocyte colony-stimulating factor significantly reduced the probability of local-regional control in both treatment arms. Thus, depending on the altered fractionation schedule that is used, the addition of concomitant chemotherapy may improve the likelihood of local-regional control and survival for patients with advanced head and neck cancer.

Thus, patients with advanced head and neck cancer treated with definitive radiation therapy appear to benefit from concomitant chemotherapy. However, the extent of disease in patients with stage III and IV malignancies is heterogeneous. Patients with low-volume, favorable stage III and IV cancers have an excellent prognosis after conservative surgery or radiation therapy, or both, and are unlikely to benefit from more aggressive organ preservation strategies.[17,44,45,56-59]

The optimal combination of radiation therapy and concomitant chemotherapy remains unclear and must be defined by future prospective randomized trials. The spectrum of combinations includes protracted split-course irradiation and very aggressive chemotherapy,[60] conventional continuous-course radiation therapy and moderately aggressive chemotherapy,[48] hyperfractionated or accelerated concomitant boost radiation therapy and less aggressive chemotherapy,[53] and radiation therapy combined with targeted intraarterial cisplatin.[61,62] The authors' current bias is to give the best radiation therapy combined with less aggressive chemotherapy consisting of weekly cisplatin or carboplatin plus paclitaxel (Taxol).[63] The disadvantage of the latter chemotherapy regimen is that acute toxicity appears to be more pronounced than that with weekly cisplatin. Weekly cisplatin is preferred in patients treated with hyperfractionated or accelerated concomitant boost radiation therapy. The latter is used if IMRT is employed because of logistical considerations. Otherwise, patients are treated with hyperfractionated irradiation.[64]

A caveat relating to organ preservation therapy is that, depending on the primary site, the likelihood of local control without preservation of function increases with tumor volume.[45] As the acute toxicity of treatment escalates and the proportion of patients requiring a feeding tube increases, there may be a higher likelihood of long-term swallowing disability. Patients who are cured with organ preservation in conjunction with a permanent tracheostomy and gastrostomy would have probably been better off had they been treated surgically.

Less toxic adjuvant therapies that may prove to be efficacious include carbogen breathing alone or combined with nicotinamide,[65,66] and vascular targeting agents.[67]

Surgery and Adjuvant Chemotherapy

Adjuvant chemotherapy may be used in conjunction with surgery to improve the chance of cure or as induction therapy to reduce the extent of resection. Licitra and coworkers[68] reported on 195 patients with T2 to T4 (larger than 3 cm) N0 to N2 resectable squamous cell carcinomas of the oral cavity who were randomly assigned to receive three cycles of induction fluorouracil and cisplatin followed by surgery, or surgery alone. Although there was no improvement in local-regional control, distant relapse, or survival, patients who received induction chemotherapy were less likely to undergo mandibular resection (31% vs. 52%) and to require postoperative radiation therapy (33% vs. 46%).

Follow-Up

Patients are seen for follow-up head and neck examination every 1 to 2 months for 2 years, every 3 months for the third year, every 6 months for the fourth and fifth years, and annually thereafter. Chest radiography and thyroid function tests are performed annually. Additional studies such as CT, MRI, and PET may be necessary to determine whether a patient has a recurrence or a complication.

ORAL CAVITY

The oral cavity consists of the lip, floor of the mouth, oral tongue (the anterior two-thirds of the tongue), buccal mucosa, upper and lower gingiva, hard palate, and retromolar trigone. Squamous cell carcinomas of the oral cavity mostly occur after the age of 45 and are associated with the use of tobacco and alcohol.

The AJCC staging system for all primary tumors of the oral cavity is as follows[16]:

Primary Tumor (T)

TX   Primary tumor cannot be assessed
T0   No evidence of primary tumor
Tis Carcinoma *in situ*
T1   Tumor 2 cm or less in greatest dimension
T2   Tumor more than 2 cm but no more than 4 cm in greatest dimension
T3   Tumor more than 4 cm in greatest dimension
T4   (Lip-vermilion border) Tumor invades through cortical bone, inferior alveolar nerve, floor of the mouth, or skin of face (i.e., chin or nose)
T4a (Oral cavity) Tumor invades adjacent structures [e.g., through cortical bone, into deep (extrinsic) muscle of tongue (genioglossus, hyoglossus, palatoglossus, and styloglossus), maxillary sinus, skin of face]

T4b Tumor invades masticator space, pterygoid plates, or skull base and/or encases internal carotid artery
Note: Superficial erosion alone of bone or tooth socket by gingiva primary is not sufficient to classify a tumor as T4.

Lip

The ratio between men and women with cancer of the lip is approximately 15:1.[69] Persons with light-colored skin or with prolonged exposure to sunlight are most prone to develop lip carcinoma.

ANATOMY. The lips are composed of the orbicular muscle with skin on the external surface and mucous membrane on the internal surface. The transition from skin to mucous membrane of the oral cavity is the lip vermilion. The blood supply is by way of the labial artery, a branch of the facial artery. The motor nerves are branches of the seventh cranial nerve. The sensory nerve to the upper lip is the infraorbital branch of the maxillary nerve, and the mental nerve supplies the lower lip.

PATHOLOGY. The most common neoplasms are squamous cell carcinomas. Basal cell carcinomas start on the skin of the lip and may secondarily invade the vermilion. Benign lesions such as hemangiomas, fibromas, and cysts may involve the lips. Keratoacanthoma occurs on the skin of the lips and may be mistaken grossly and histologically for squamous cell carcinoma.

Leukoplakia and carcinoma *in situ* are common problems on the lower lip and may precede the appearance of carcinoma by many years. Primary lesions arising from the moist mucosa of the lip are considered under the section Buccal Mucosa.

PATTERNS OF SPREAD. Squamous cell carcinoma starts on the vermilion of the lip and invades adjacent skin and the orbicular muscle. Advanced lesions invade the adjacent commissures of the lip, the buccal mucosa, the skin and wet mucosa of the lip, the adjacent mandible, and eventually the mental nerve. Perineural invasion occurred in 2% of the cases reported by Byers and coworkers[70] and was related to recurrent lesions, large tumor size, mandibular invasion, and poorly differentiated histology. Lymphatic spread moves to the submental and submandibular lymph nodes and then to the jugular chain. The risk for lymph node metastases is approximately 5% on admission. Bilateral involvement may occur.[71] The risk of lymphatic involvement is increased by high-grade histology, large lesions, invasion of the wet mucosa of the lip and buccal mucosa, and recurrent disease.

CLINICAL PICTURE. The vermilion is the most common site of origin. Squamous cell carcinoma may present as an enlarging discrete lesion that is not tender until it ulcerates. There is occasional minor bleeding. Some lesions develop very slowly on a background of leukoplakia and present as superficially ulcerated lesions with little or no bulk and a history of repeated episodes of scab formation without complete healing. An obvious carcinoma is often accompanied by leukoplakia or carcinoma *in situ* of the remaining lower lip.

Erythema of the adjacent skin suggests dermal lymphatic invasion. Palpation of the lip reveals the extent of induration. Anesthesia or paresthesia of the skin of the lip indicates nerve invasion.

TREATMENT

Selection of Treatment Modality. Early lesions may be cured equally well with surgery or radiation. The length of the relaxed lower lip is approximately 5 cm but tends to be shorter in edentulous patients. Surgical excision is preferred for the majority of lower lip lesions up to 2.0 cm in diameter that do not involve the commissure; the treatment is simple and the cosmetic result is satisfactory. Removal of more of the lip with simple closure usually results in a poor cosmetic and functional result and therefore requires reconstructive procedures. Irradiation is often preferred for lesions involving the commissure, for lesions over 2.0 cm in length, and for high-grade carcinomas. Upper lip carcinomas may require complex reconstruction, and radiation therapy may be preferred. Advanced lesions with bone, nerve, or node involvement frequently require a combined approach. Surgery is preferred for the younger patient who will have years of climatic exposure and for previously irradiated persons.

The regional lymphatics are not treated electively for early cases. Advanced lesions, high-grade lesions, and recurrent lesions should be considered for elective neck treatment. Clinically positive nodes are managed as previously discussed in Clinically Positive Neck Lymph Nodes, earlier in this chapter.

Surgical Treatment. Surgical treatment for early lesions (0.5 to 1.5 cm) involves a W or V excision (Fig. 26.2-2). V excisions may be used for very small lesions but do not give as good a margin for the lower lip defect. If the vermilion is diffusely involved with little or no involvement of the muscle, then the vermilionectomy (lip shave) may be done and the mucosa from the oral cavity advanced to cover the defect. Excision of a carcinoma may be combined with a vermilionectomy. If the commissure must be sacrificed, it must be reconstructed to prevent microstomia and to allow the denture patient to continue to wear dentures.

Irradiation Technique. Lip cancer may be successfully treated by external-beam radiation therapy, interstitial brachytherapy, or a combination of both. Interstitial brachytherapy may be accomplished with removable sources such as cesium needles or iridium 192 (^{192}Ir). External-beam techniques use orthovoltage or electrons with lead shields behind the lip to limit exit irradiation. The dose schemes are similar to those used for skin cancer. Fractionation schemes of 4 to 6 weeks are preferred over the shorter regimens for the larger lesions to decrease the effects on normal tissue.

RESULTS OF TREATMENT. MacKay and Sellers[71] reviewed 2864 patients with all stages of lip cancer, of whom 92% were managed initially by radiation therapy. The primary lesion was controlled by the initial treatment in 84% of cases; an additional 8% were salvaged by later treatment, for an overall local control rate of 92%. Fifty-eight percent of those who presented with clinically involved nodes had control of disease, but only 35% had control of disease when positive neck nodes appeared later. The 5-year cause-specific survival rate was 89%; the 5-year absolute survival rate was 65%. Death resulting from intercurrent disease occurred in 17% of patients.

Fitzpatrick[69] reviewed the Princess Margaret Hospital results for 361 lip carcinomas seen between 1971 and 1976. Surgery alone (85 patients) controlled the cancer in 89%, surgery with postoperative radiation therapy (70 patients) controlled the can-

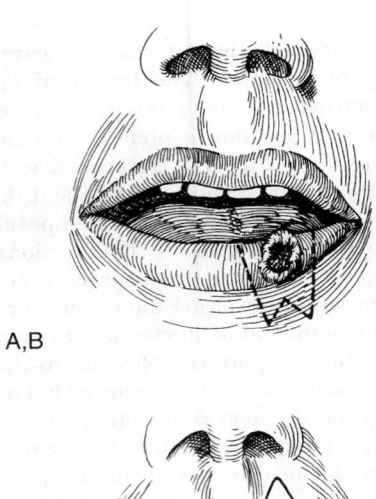
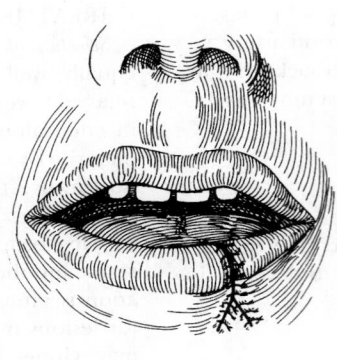

A,B

FIGURE 26.2-2. Small lip lesions that do not involve the oral commissure can be removed using a W excision (**A**) and can be closed primarily (**B**). Larger lesions of the lip may be removed in a V fashion (**C**), and the defect can be closed using an Abbe flap from the upper lip (**D,E**). A second procedure to release the flap also can be performed 2 weeks later. (From Million RR, Cassisi NJ, Clark JR. Cancer of the head and neck. In: DeVita VT Jr, Hellman S, Rosenberg SA, eds. *Cancer: principles and practice of oncology*, 3rd ed. Philadelphia: JB Lippincott, 1989:504, with permission.)

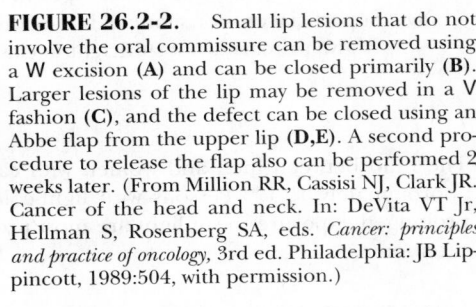

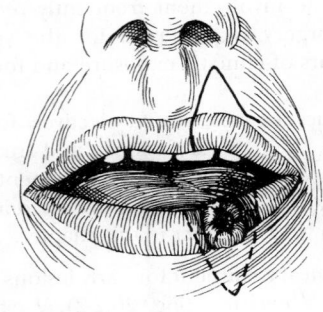
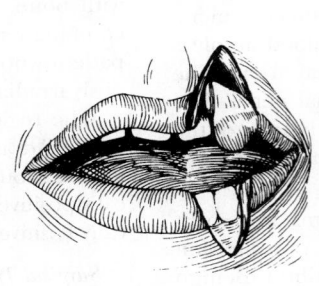
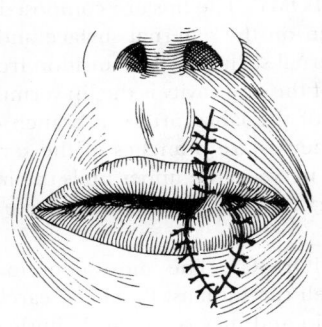

C–E

cer in 93%, and radiation therapy alone (206 patients) controlled the cancer in 94%. Regional node metastasis occurred in only 7%. Only 3% of the entire group died of lip cancer. Radiation necrosis of soft tissues requiring surgical intervention occurred in 3%. There were no cases of osteoradionecrosis.

Hendricks and coworkers[72] reviewed the Mayo Clinic surgical results for 613 patients seen between 1950 and 1969. The local recurrence rate was 5% for lesions less than 1 cm, 4% for lesions 1 to 3 cm, and 17% for lesions larger than 3 cm. Mohs and Snow[73] reported the results for 1448 patients treated with microscopically controlled surgery for squamous cell carcinomas of the lower lip between 1936 and 1976. Eighty-three percent had cancers less than 3 cm in diameter, with a 5-year cure rate of 96.6%. For 192 patients with cancers that measured 2 cm or more, the cure rate dropped to 60%. For patients with grade I or II carcinoma, the 5-year cure rate was 96%, as contrasted with 67% for 81 patients with grade III or IV carcinoma.

COMPLICATIONS OF TREATMENT. Microstomia and drooling secondary to oral incompetence may occur when a large flap reconstruction is necessary. If the oral opening is too small, the patient may not be able to insert a denture. Speech is not often affected.

There will be some atrophy of the irradiated tissues; this progresses with time. Continued soft tissue necrosis may occur; this problem is reduced by schemes that prolong the treatment. The irradiated lip must be protected from sun exposure by use of hats and ultraviolet protectants.

Floor of the Mouth

ANATOMY. The floor of the mouth is a U-shaped area bounded by the lower gum and the oral tongue; it terminates posteriorly at the insertion of the anterior tonsillar pillar into the tongue. The paired sublingual glands lie immediately below the mucous membrane; the paired genioglossus and geniohyoid muscles separate them. Bony protuberances, the genial tubercles, occur at the point of insertion of these two muscle groups at the symphysis and may interfere with the placement of interstitial sources. The mylohyoid muscle arises from the mylohyoid ridge of the mandible and is the muscular floor for the oral cavity; it ends posteriorly at approximately the level of the third molars. The normal submandibular gland is approximately the size of a walnut and rests on the external surface of the mylohyoid muscle between the mandible and the insertion of the mylohyoid. A tongue-like process wraps around the posterior border of the mylohyoid muscle and extends forward on the internal surface of the mylohyoid; this is absent in 10% to 20% of cases. The submandibular duct (Wharton's duct) is approximately 5 cm long. It courses between the sublingual gland and the genioglossus muscle and exits in the anterior floor of the mouth near the midline. The relationships of the lingual nerve, hypoglossal nerve, and submandibular duct are shown in Figure 26.2-3.

PATHOLOGY. Most neoplasms are squamous cell carcinomas, usually of moderate grade. Adenoid cystic and mucoepidermoid carcinomas account for approximately 5% of malignant tumors in this area.

PATTERNS OF SPREAD

Primary. Approximately 90% of neoplasms originate within 2 cm of the anterior midline floor of the mouth, penetrating early beneath the mucosa into the sublingual gland and eventually into the genioglossus and geniohyoid muscles. The mylohyoid muscle acts as an effective barrier until the lesion becomes very advanced. Extension toward the gingiva and periosteum of the mandible occurs early and frequently. Even small lesions may become attached to the periosteum. The periosteum is an effec-

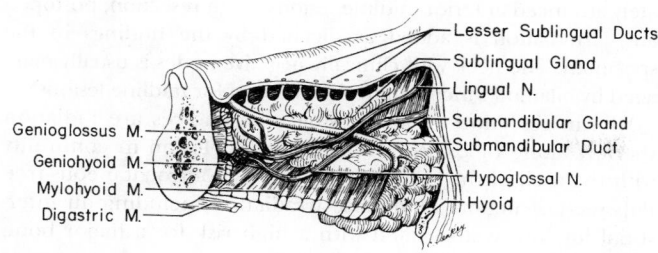

FIGURE 26.2-3.   Anatomic relationships of the floor of the oral cavity. (From Million RR, Cassisi NJ, Clark JR. Cancer of the head and neck. In: DeVita VT Jr, Hellman S, Rosenberg SA, eds. *Cancer: principles and practice of oncology,* 3rd ed. Philadelphia: JB Lippincott, 1989:506, with permission.)

tive barrier to mandibular invasion; when tumor reaches the periosteum, the tumor usually spreads along the periosteum rather than through it. Mandible invasion is usually a late manifestation. Tumors sometimes grow over the alveolar ridge before grossly invading the bone. The skin of the lower lip may be involved in advanced cases. Posterior extension occurs into the muscles of the root of the tongue. One or both submandibular ducts are frequently obstructed by tumor or after biopsy. An enlarged duct may be palpated through the floor of the mouth, and it may be difficult to distinguish between tumor extension and low-grade infection in an obstructed duct. Tumor rarely grows inside the duct but may grow along the path of the duct. The submandibular gland frequently enlarges, becoming firm and occasionally painful when the duct is obstructed. It is difficult to distinguish between tumor directly invading the gland and chronic infection related to obstruction. CT is very useful in making this distinction.

Tumors arising in the lateral floor of the mouth have the same general spread patterns. Extensive lesions may escape the oral cavity by following the anatomic plane of the mylohyoid muscle to its posterior extremity, emerging in the submandibular space of the neck.

Lymphatic.   Approximately 30% of patients have clinically positive nodes on admission; 4% have bilateral positive nodes. The reported incidence of conversion from N0 to N+ with no neck

treatment varies from 20% to 35%.[21,22] For T1 or superficial T2 lesions, the risk for occult metastasis is probably 10% to 15%.[21,22]

The first nodes involved are the submandibular (level I) and the subdigastric (level II) nodes (Fig. 26.2-4). The midline submental nodes are bypassed. Lindberg[10] reported 2% clinically positive submental nodes in 258 cases. Because most lesions either approach or cross the midline, the risk for bilateral spread is fairly high.[74]

CLINICAL PICTURE.   The earliest carcinomas are asymptomatic, red, slightly elevated mucosal lesions with ill-defined borders. A background of leukoplakia may be present. White lesions (leukoplakia) are less likely to be malignant, but 10% eventually become cancer. As the carcinoma progresses, the tumor is first noticed when the patient feels a lump in the floor of the mouth with the tip of the tongue. There is mild soreness when eating or drinking. Dentures may not fit properly. Advanced lesions produce pain, bleeding, foul breath, loose teeth, change in speech owing to fixation of the root of the tongue, and a submandibular mass that is often painful.

On physical examination, the earliest lesion appears as a red area, slightly elevated, with ill-defined borders and very little induration. As the lesion enlarges, the edges of the tumor become distinct, elevated, and "rolled," with a central ulceration and induration. Some lesions start with a background of leukoplakia. If the leukoplakia is extensive, it is difficult to know where or when to biopsy. Bimanual palpation determines the extent of the induration and the degree of fixation to the periosteum. Large lesions bulge into the submental space and rarely grow through the mylohyoid muscle into the soft tissue spaces of the neck, even through the skin. Gross invasion of the mandible may be detected, especially when the anterior teeth have been removed. A tumor may be seen growing through the mandible to involve the gingivolabial sulcus and lip.

The submandibular duct and gland are evaluated by bimanual palpation.

TREATMENT
Selection of Treatment Modality
LEUKOPLAKIA.   Patches of thin leukoplakia usually are observed. Biopsy is done if the area becomes symptomatic or if

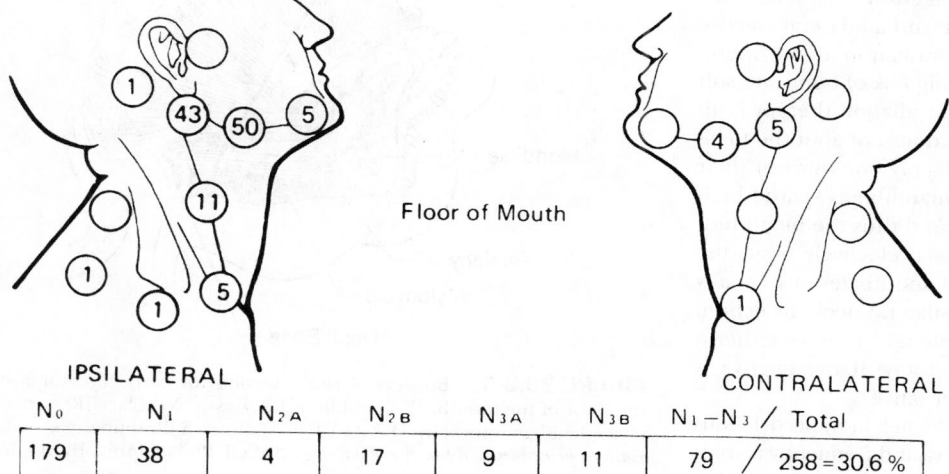

FIGURE 26.2-4.   Floor of mouth cancer: nodal distribution on admission, M. D. Anderson Hospital, 1948 to 1965. The circled numbers indicate the number of times the particular lymph node was involved. (From ref. 10, with permission.)

the appearance changes and malignancy is suspected. Localized areas of leukoplakia may be excised, but many patients have extensive or scattered areas of leukoplakia that preclude complete excision. Cryotherapy or laser therapy may be tried in these cases. Radiation therapy is not recommended for treatment of leukoplakia; however, when leukoplakia is inadvertently irradiated along with an adjacent carcinoma, the leukoplakia may disappear. In most cases, it will reappear at a later time.

EARLY LESIONS. Operation and radiation therapy are equally effective treatment for T1 or T2 lesions; therefore, treatment decisions are based on differences in the expected functional result, the management of the neck, and the risk of late complications. The status of the teeth and mandible and the age of the patient are considered.

A few patients are seen after excisional biopsy of a tiny lesion, and the only finding is a surgical scar with varying degrees of induration or nodularity under the scar (TX). The margins are often equivocal. If the excisional biopsy is judged inadequate, these patients are sometimes treated with an interstitial implant or intraoral cone, because the surgeon has difficulty knowing where to start and stop the reexcision. The radiation therapist can be generous with the treatment volume and cover potential spread without functional loss. The neck is usually observed. A review of six patients treated in this manner at the M. D. Anderson Hospital revealed a 100% local control rate; similar patients treated at the University of Florida also had a 100% local control rate.[75] None of the patients developed positive neck nodes. If the margins of the excisional biopsy are free and there is little or no induration or nodularity, 55 Gy is delivered. If the margins are positive or if there is slight induration or nodularity, the dose is raised to 65 Gy. In cases in which gross cut-through is suspected, one may wish to use external-beam radiation to a dose of 50 Gy to include the regional nodes before the interstitial implant. An alternative to radiation therapy for these patients is resection, if the surgeon is comfortable with the extent of the operation that is necessary.

Small lesions (less than 1 cm) may be excised transorally if there is a margin between the lesion and the gingiva. If the submandibular duct is surgically obstructed, then the submandibular gland must also be removed. A common presentation is an anterior midline lesion, 2 to 3 cm in diameter, which abuts the gingiva, with a clinically negative neck; there is a risk for subclinical disease in one or both sides of the neck in 10% to 30% of cases. Most of these lesions are managed by wide local excision with rim resection of the mandible and a bilateral elective functional neck dissection. Although radiation therapy produces similar cure rates, there is a lifelong risk of bone and soft tissue necrosis. The ideal candidate for radiation therapy is an edentulous patient in whom the lesion does not abut the mandible. These patients receive approximately one-third of their dose by an intraoral cone so that the mandible is spared high doses. The primary site and the neck (and thus the mandible) receive 45 Gy from external beam, which electively treats the lymph nodes. Well-lateralized floor of mouth lesions usually are treated by an operation with an ipsilateral neck dissection. These lesions usually abut the mandible and require either a rim resection or a partial mandibulectomy. If the gingiva is uninvolved, radiation therapy is an alternative.

MODERATELY ADVANCED LESIONS. Moderately advanced lesions usually involve the periosteum and gingiva and frequently involve the root of the tongue. The usual recommendation for moder-

ately advanced anterior midline lesions is rim resection; postoperative irradiation is added as dictated by the findings in the specimen. The neck with clinically negative nodes is usually managed by bilateral functional neck dissection for midline lesions.

If rim resection is not possible, the choices are radiation therapy alone or excision of the primary lesion in continuity with the arch of the mandible and an osteomyocutaneous free flap reconstruction. High-dose irradiation including an interstitial implant is associated with a high risk for a major bone necrosis. Surgery is usually preferred.

ADVANCED LESIONS. Massive lesions are usually associated with bone invasion and extension into the root of the tongue and have a small chance of cure with combined surgery and radiation therapy. The entire arch of the mandible must usually be removed. Only palliation can be offered in some cases.

SURGICAL TREATMENT

WIDE LOCAL EXCISION. Small lesions (5 mm or less in size) may be excised transorally with a 1-cm margin with primary closure or a skin graft. If the duct is involved, the submandibular gland and duct are removed in continuity.

RIM RESECTION. Rim (coronal) resection of the mandible in continuity with excision of the primary lesion preserves the arch and usually gives an adequate surgical margin; the procedure may be combined with postoperative radiation therapy (Fig. 26.2-5). Invasion of the periosteum is often an indication for this procedure. Patients who have been edentulous for a long time may have a thin, atrophic mandible and are not suitable for a rim resection because the mandible is likely to fracture. Rim resection is not recommended for patients with radiation treatment failures because of the risk of bone necrosis and pathologic fracture. If rim resection is attempted for radiation treatment failure, hyperbaric oxygen should be added before and after the operation.

MANDIBULECTOMY ("JAW-NECK")

LATERAL FLOOR OF THE MOUTH. For lesions of the lateral floor of the mouth, a modified radical neck dissection is performed and the specimen remains attached to the mandible. Partial mandibulectomy with resection of the floor of the mouth is

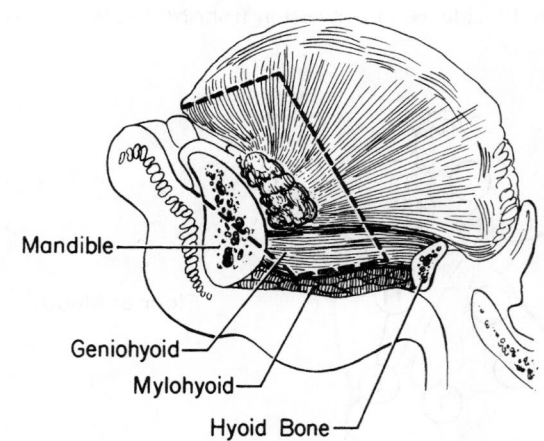

FIGURE 26.2-5.   Borders of rim resection for early carcinoma of the floor of the mouth. (From Million RR, Cassisi NJ, Clark JR. Cancer of the head and neck. In: DeVita VT Jr, Hellman S, Rosenberg SA, eds. *Cancer: principles and practice of oncology,* 3rd ed. Philadelphia: JB Lippincott, 1989:509, with permission.)

TABLE 26.2-11. Floor of Mouth Cancer: Cancer Control after Primary Radiation Therapy (RT)

Institution	RT Technique	Stage T1		Stage T2		Stage T3	
		RT Alone	Ultimate Control (%)[a]	RT Alone	Ultimate Control (%)[a]	RT Alone	Ultimate Control (%)[a]
M. D. Anderson Hospital[76]	Mixed[b]	48/49 (98%)	100	68/77 (88%)	93	46/60 (73%)	95
University of Florida[78]	Mixed	14/16 (88%)	88	13/17 (76%)	94	12/25 (48%)	68
University of California (San Francisco)[77]	External beam	29/38 (76%)	~90	21/39 (54%)	~70	8/32 (25%)	41

[a]Ultimate control includes successful salvage after a local recurrence.
[b]Mixed, external-beam irradiation and interstitial implant.

done through a lip-splitting incision or by using a visor flap. A cheek flap is elevated to the level of the mandibular condyle to provide exposure. The mandible is separated at the mental foramen anteriorly and the neck of the condyle posteriorly. The primary lesion and neck specimen are then removed in continuity. Primary closure is usually feasible, unless a sizable portion of the oral tongue must be removed, in which case use of a myocutaneous flap is necessary to repair the defect.

The cosmetic and functional result is acceptable to patients, and few request a mandibular reconstruction. The mandible shifts to the opposite side, and if the patient has teeth, chewing may be impaired but can be corrected with a glide plane. Edentulous patients cannot wear a lower denture. Alternatively, an osteomyocutaneous flap may be used to reconstruct the defect.

ANTERIOR FLOOR OF THE MOUTH. For lesions of the anterior floor of the mouth, a full-thickness resection of the anterior mandible (arch) is required. This operation results in major cosmetic and functional loss and is usually reserved for advanced lesions with bone invasion or for irradiation treatment failures. Techniques for reconstruction include the use of trapezius myocutaneous flap with a portion of the scapular spine to bridge the bony gap, or the use of a free flap such as the tibial free flap.

Irradiation Technique. Superficial T1 cancers are treated with either brachytherapy or intraoral cone irradiation to approximately 65 Gy and the neck is observed. Larger lesions are treated with external-beam irradiation to 45 to 50 Gy over 5 weeks followed by an interstitial implant for an additional 20 to 30 Gy. Lesions that are suitable for intraoral cone irradiation may be boosted with this technique before external-beam irradiation of the primary lesion and upper neck. Use of external-beam irradiation alone results in suboptimal cure rates and is discouraged (Table 26.2-11).[76–78] Prominent geniohyoid tubercles and tori as well as undesirable teeth should be removed if present before radiation therapy. A minimum of 3 weeks for healing is needed before starting treatment.

EXTERNAL-BEAM IRRADIATION. Opposed lateral external-beam portals are used to treat anterior floor of mouth carcinomas. The entire width of the mandibular arch is included and the superior border is shaped to spare part of the parotid gland. The submandibular and subdigastric nodes are included to the level of the thyroid notch if the neck is clinically negative; the lower neck may be electively irradiated on an individual basis. If the neck is clinically positive, the portals are enlarged to include all of the upper neck nodes, and *en face* neck field is added.

INTERSTITIAL IRRADIATION. The availability of interstitial brachytherapy (or intraoral cone therapy) is essential if maximum local control rates are to be obtained (see Table 26.2-11).[76–78]

Implantation of small lesions confined to the floor of the mouth with minimal extension to the mucosa of the tongue or minimal extension to the gingiva or periosteum can be accomplished with cesium needles or iridium in the form of ribbons using the plastic tube technique. A preloaded, custom-designed implant device for radium needles has been in use at the University of Florida since 1976.[79] It holds the cesium needles in a fixed position and is used only for T1 or T2 lesions. The arrangement of the needles for early lesions is usually a modified, curved, teardrop, two-plane implant with a single needle crossing the top of the implant. The arrangement of the needles for treatment of an early T2 lesion is shown in Figure 26.2-6.[79] Implants for late T2 and T3 lesions are usually modified volume implants. Iridium using the plastic tube technique is usually employed.

INTRAORAL CONE IRRADIATION. Intraoral cone therapy is preferable to interstitial irradiation because there is little or no irradiation of the mandible. An intraoral cone can be used for

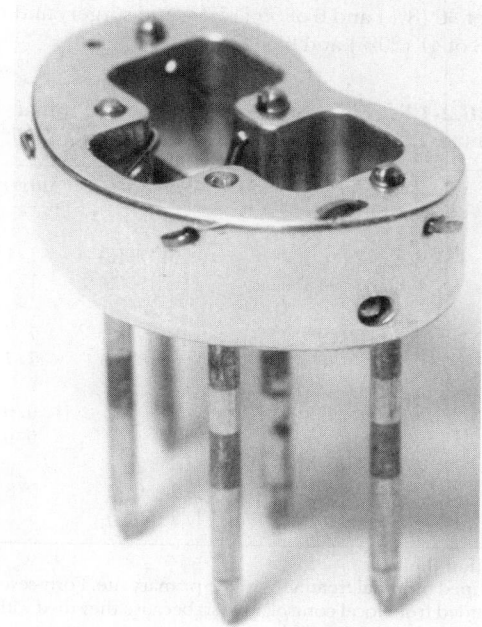

FIGURE 26.2-6. Custom-made implant device for stage T1 or T2 carcinoma of the floor of the mouth. (Modified from ref. 79.)

well-circumscribed anterior superficial lesions and is easiest to use in the edentulous patient. Minimal extension to the gingiva can sometimes be encompassed with the cone as well as early extension to the undersurface of the tongue. The orthovoltage cones in use at the University of Florida are 2 to 6 cm in diameter; they are poured from lead and can be trimmed individually to adapt the cone to the anatomy. Electron-beam cones can be fabricated individually as described by Tapley.[80] Intraoral cone therapy requires daily positioning by the physician.

Combined Treatment Policies. The results of combined surgery and irradiation may be better than those for single-modality therapy for large, infiltrative, ulcerative lesions. If rim resection is possible, postoperative irradiation is preferred, because the risk of bone complications and fistulas is higher with preoperative irradiation. Preoperative irradiation may be used if the patient has a large fixed node.

Management of Recurrence. Radiation treatment failures are treated by an operation. The salvage rate is good for patients with early lesions and moderately good for those with more advanced lesions.

Surgical treatment failures may be treated by a repeat operation, radiation therapy, or both on an individual basis. Radiation therapy alone is not likely to succeed.

RESULTS OF TREATMENT. Rodgers et al.[81] reported on 194 patients treated with surgery or radiation therapy or both at the University of Florida between 1964 and 1987. Initial and ultimate local control rates varied according to treatment group and are depicted in Table 26.2-12. The local control rates are similar for T1 and T2 tumors for the various treatment groups; those with T3 and T4 cancers have better local control after surgery and radiation therapy than after irradiation alone. The 5-year cause-specific survival rates were comparable for the treatment groups.[81] Mild to moderate and severe complications were observed as follows: radiation therapy alone, 49 of 117 (42%) and 6 of 117 (5%); surgery alone, 3 of 36 (8%) and 6 of 35 (17%); and surgery and radiation therapy, 8 of 41 (20%) and 6 of 41 (15%).[81]

TABLE 26.2-12. Floor of Mouth Carcinoma: Initial and Ultimate Local Control

Stage	RT	Surgery	Surgery and RT
T1			
Initial	32/37 (86%)	9/10 (90%)	1/1 (100%)
Ultimate	35/37 (94%)	9/10 (90%)	1/1 (100%)
T2			
Initial	25/36 (69%)	9/12 (75%)	7/7 (100%)
Ultimate	31/36 (86%)	10/12 (83%)	7/7 (100%)
T3			
Initial	11/20 (55%)	a	9/9 (100%)
Ultimate	13/20 (65%)	a	9/9 (100%)
T4			
Initial	2/5 (40%)	1/2 (50%)	5/8 (63%)
Ultimate	2/5 (40%)	1/2 (50%)	5/8 (63%)

RT, radiation therapy.
Note: Grouped by initial treatment to the primary site. Forty-seven patients were excluded from local control analysis because they died within 2 years of treatment with the primary site continuously disease-free.
[a]No patients in category.
(From ref. 81, with permission.)

Sessions et al.[82] reported on 280 patients treated with surgery or radiation therapy or both at Washington University between 1960 and 1994. The 5-year cause-specific and overall survival rates were as follows: stage I, 72% and 54%; stage II, 63% and 52%; stage III, 44% and 39%; and stage IV, 47% and 39%, respectively. There was no significant difference in cause-specific survival for the various treatment groups. Recurrence at the primary site (41%) was the predominant site of treatment failure.

Two hundred and seven patients treated with irradiation alone at the Centre Alexis Vautrin between 1976 and 1992 were reviewed by Pernot and colleagues.[83] Local control and cause-specific survival rates at 5 years were as follows: T1, 97% and 88%; T2, 72% and 47%; and T3, 51% and 36%, respectively. Six percent of patients developed complications necessitating surgical intervention and one patient experienced a fatal complication.

Intraoral cone electron-beam radiation therapy in conjunction with external-beam irradiation was used to treat 43 patients with T1N0 (18 patients) and T2N0 (25 patients) carcinomas at the Massachusetts General Hospital.[84] The 5-year local control rates were 93% for T1 cancers compared with 83% for T2 lesions. Five patients experienced some degree of soft tissue necrosis and two developed osteoradionecrosis.

FOLLOW-UP. There are two major difficulties in follow-up after irradiation: soft tissue ulcers and enlarged submandibular glands. An ulcer in the floor of the mouth within 2 years of treatment can be either recurrence or necrosis. If the lesion appears to be soft tissue necrosis, a trial of conservative therapy and observation at close intervals is adequate. The soft tissue necroses are notoriously slow to heal. Failure to stabilize or show some indication of healing is an indication for biopsy. A negative biopsy result does not rule out recurrence, and if the lesion remains suspicious, repeat deep biopsies are necessary.

An enlarged submandibular gland(s) may be a sequel to obstruction of the submandibular duct. The gland may be enlarged on initial examination, or it may enlarge during or after treatment. It is difficult to distinguish between an enlarged submandibular gland and tumor in a lymph node. A CT scan with contrast and needle biopsy are useful.

Follow-up of surgical cases may be difficult if skin grafts or flaps have been used because of the associated induration and thickness of the flaps. If the submandibular ducts have been reimplanted, stenosis may occur with subsequent enlargement of the submandibular glands, which must be distinguished from recurrence in a neck node.

COMPLICATIONS OF TREATMENT
Radiation Therapy. A small soft tissue necrosis may develop in the floor of the mouth, usually in the site of the original lesion where the dose is highest. These ulcers are moderately painful and respond to local anesthetics, antibiotics, and the tincture of time. Treatment with pentoxifylline 400 mg three times daily may be beneficial.

If the ulceration develops on the adjacent gingiva, then the underlying mandible is exposed. These areas are mildly painful. They are managed by discontinuance of denture wear, local anesthetics, antibiotics, and smoothing of the bone by filing if needed. These small bone exposures do not often progress to full-blown osteonecrosis. They either sequestrate a small piece of bone or are simply re-covered by mucous mem-

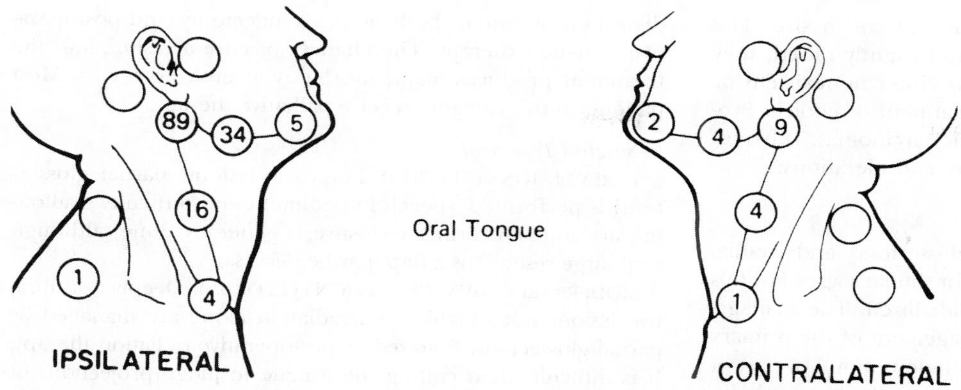

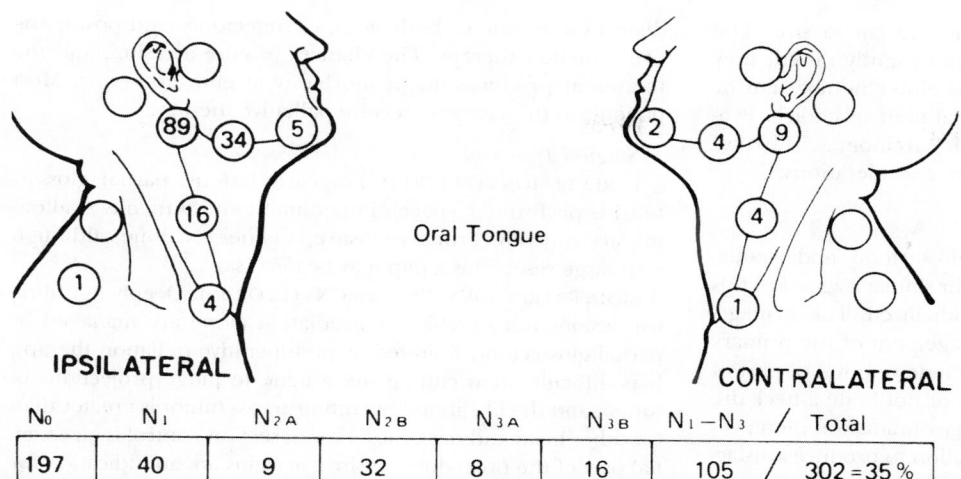

N0	N1	N2A	N2B	N3A	N3B	N1–N3 / Total
197	40	9	32	8	16	105 / 302 = 35 %

FIGURE 26.2-7. Oral tongue: nodal distribution at admission, M. D. Anderson Hospital, 1948 to 1965. The circled numbers indicate the number of times the particular lymph node was involved. (From ref. 10, with permission.)

brane. Healing is slow. Severe necrosis may require daily hyperbaric oxygen treatments for 4 to 6 weeks, either alone or in conjunction with surgical intervention.

Surgery. Surgical complications include bone exposure, orocutaneous fistula, and failure of osteomyocutaneous flaps. Salvage procedures after radiation therapy are associated with an increased risk of complications.

Oral Tongue

ANATOMY. The circumvallate papillae locate the division between the oral tongue and base of the tongue. The arterial supply is mainly by way of paired lingual arteries that are branches of the external carotid. One lingual artery may be sacrificed without danger of necrosis, but sacrifice of both lingual arteries results in an increased risk for loss of the oral tongue and almost certain loss of the base of the tongue. The sensory pathway is by way of the lingual nerve to the gasserian ganglion.

PATHOLOGY. More than 95% of oral tongue lesions are squamous cell carcinomas. Coexisting leukoplakia is common. Verrucous carcinoma and minor salivary gland tumors are quite uncommon. Granular cell myoblastoma is a benign tumor of uncertain origin that commonly occurs on the dorsum of the tongue and may be confused histologically with carcinoma because of the associated pseudoepitheliomatous hyperplasia.

PATTERNS OF SPREAD

Primary. Nearly all oral tongue squamous cell carcinomas occur on the lateral and undersurfaces of the tongue. A few lesions appear on the dorsum. Most of the carcinomas occur on the middle and posterior thirds of the oral tongue. Oral tongue carcinomas tend to remain in the tongue until large, unless they originate near the junction with the floor of the mouth. Perineural invasion and vascular space invasion may occur.

Anterior third (tip) lesions usually are diagnosed early. Advanced lesions invade the floor of the mouth and root of the tongue, producing ulceration and fixation. Middle third lesions invade the musculature of the tongue and later invade the lateral floor of the mouth.

Posterior third lesions grow into the musculature of the tongue, the floor of the mouth, anterior tonsillar pillar, base of the tongue, and glossotonsillar sulcus. Posterior third lesions behave more like base of tongue cancer with a higher incidence of lymph node metastasis compared to those in the anterior two-thirds of the oral tongue.

Lymphatic. The first-echelon nodes are the subdigastric and submandibular nodes (Fig. 26.2-7).[10] The submental and spinal accessory lymph nodes are seldom involved. Rouviere[3] describes lymphatic trunks that bypass the subdigastric and submandibular nodes and terminate in the midjugular lymph nodes. Byers et al.[85] evaluated nodal spread pattern in 277 patients treated surgically at the M. D. Anderson Hospital and observed skip metastases to the level III or IV nodes without involvement of levels I and II in 16% of patients. The lymphatic vessels of the tongue anastomose freely, allowing contralateral lymph flow. Thirty-five percent of patients with oral tongue cancer have clinically positive nodes on admission; 5% have bilateral positive nodes. The incidence of occult disease is approximately 30%. The incidence of positive nodes increases with T stage. Patients with N1 or N2 ipsilateral nodes have a significant risk of developing node metastasis in the opposite neck.

CLINICAL PICTURE. Mild irritation of the tongue is the most frequent complaint. The pain may occur only during eating or drinking. As ulceration develops, the pain becomes progressively worse and is referred to the external ear canal. Extensive infiltration of the muscles of the tongue affects speech and deglutition. Patients with advanced lesions have a foul mouth odor.

The extent of disease is determined by visual examination and palpation. The tongue protrudes incompletely and toward the side of the lesion as fixation develops. Posterior oral tongue lesions may grow inferiorly, behind the mylohyoid, and present as a mass in the neck at the angle of the mandible. The mass may be confused with an enlarged lymph node. Invasion of the hypoglossal nerve is rare and may cause atrophy. Posterolateral lesions may be difficult to evaluate because of pain; examination with the patient under anesthesia may be required.

DIFFERENTIAL DIAGNOSIS. The differential diagnosis includes granular cell myoblastomas, which are usually slow-growing, nontender masses, and 0.5 to 2.0 cm in size. The lesions are well circumscribed, firm, and slightly raised; they may be multiple. Malignant behavior is either nonexistent or rare, and wide local excision is the treatment of choice. Pyogenic granulomas mimic small exophytic carcinomas. Tuberculous ulcer and syphilitic chancre are rare considerations.

TREATMENT

Selection of Treatment Modality. Both glossectomy and irradiation result in cure rates that are similar for similar stages. For this reason, selection of treatment is individualized. The management of the neck may dictate the management of the primary lesion. The disadvantages of surgery include removal of part of the tongue and the decision of whether or not to do a neck dissection for the N0 neck. The disadvantage of radiation therapy is the risk of radiation necrosis. For irradiation to produce satisfactory control rates, the use of interstitial or intraoral cone therapy is essential. When hemiglossectomy is predicted to produce a significant degree of speech impediment and difficulty in swallowing, irradiation may be selected as the initial treatment, with glossectomy reserved for recurrence. Surgical salvage of irradiation treatment failures is fairly successful for early lesions, but is relatively low for larger lesions. Irradiation is not often successful in curing surgical failures. For this reason, glossectomy and radiation therapy are often combined as initial therapy for the more advanced lesions.

EXCISIONAL BIOPSY (TX). Excisional biopsy of a small lesion may show inadequate or equivocal margins.[75] An interstitial implant will produce a high rate of local control. An alternative is reexcision if the extent of the operation can be adequately defined.

EARLY LESIONS (T1 OR T2). For early lesions, operation and irradiation produce similar local control rates, and treatment decisions are based on anticipated functional loss, management of the neck, and patient preference. A limited glossectomy with primary closure or a skin graft may be done transorally and is usually the preferred therapy. Depending on the depth of invasion, an elective neck dissection may be indicated. Postoperative radiation therapy would only be added for indications previously discussed in Selection of Treatment Modality.

Glossectomy is the treatment of choice for small, well-circumscribed, well to moderately differentiated lesions that can be excised transorally; small lesions on the tip of the tongue; and the rare lesion on the dorsum of the tongue. Irradiation may be selected for larger T1 and T2 lesions to preserve speech and swallowing for poorly differentiated carcinomas, and for lesions that have a high risk for bilateral lymph node metastases. Currently the initial step in treatment for most patients at the authors' institution is surgery.

MODERATELY ADVANCED LESIONS (T2 OR T3). Lesions that have a large surface involvement but minimal infiltration are favorable lesions and may be managed with radiation therapy alone or surgery. Those deeply infiltrative lesions have a higher control rate with combined surgery and radiation therapy. Definitive radiation therapy with surgery reserved for salvage is a reasonable alternative; concomitant chemotherapy should be considered.

ADVANCED LESIONS (T4). For advanced lesions, combined treatment with surgery and radiation therapy cures very few patients, especially those with minimal neck disease. Operation usually implies total glossectomy, mandibulectomy, neck node dissection on one or both sides, laryngectomy, and postoperative radiation therapy. The chances of cure are slim, and the treatment produces major morbidity at enormous cost. Most patients in this category receive palliative therapy.

Surgical Treatment
EARLY LESIONS (T1 OR T2). For early lesions, partial glossectomy is performed; speech impediment and difficulty swallowing are unlikely. Primary closure is generally done, although with large resections a flap may be necessary.

MODERATELY ADVANCED LESIONS (T2 OR T3). Deeply infiltrative lesions not suitable for irradiation alone are managed by partial glossectomy followed by postoperative radiation therapy. It is difficult when cutting the tongue to judge projections of tumor, and the likelihood of cutting across tumor is greater than for other head and neck sites. Frozen-section control is an essential part of the procedure; positive margins are an indication for excision of additional tissue. Finally, if a mandibulotomy or mandibulectomy is done after preoperative radiation therapy, the likelihood of exposed bone, nonunion, and radionecrosis is increased.

ADVANCED LESIONS (T4). Advanced lesions require a total glossectomy and sometimes a laryngectomy combined with postoperative radiation therapy. The procedure would only be offered to patients in good general condition and with minimal neck disease.

Irradiation Technique. The ability to control the primary lesion is enhanced by giving all or part of the treatment by interstitial radiation therapy or by intraoral cone.[78,86,87] Superficial T1 tumors may be treated with ^{192}Ir brachytherapy alone using the plastic tube technique. Larger lesions that have an increased risk for subclinical neck disease may be treated with external-beam radiation therapy and a brachytherapy boost or with brachytherapy combined with an elective neck dissection. The time factor is critical for oral tongue cancer, and the external-beam portion of the treatment is shortened to 30 Gy in 10 daily fractions over 2 weeks to increase the proportion of the therapy given by either interstitial or intraoral cone therapy. An alternative is 38.4 Gy at 1.6 Gy twice daily combined with a boost. The interstitial therapy is given after the external-beam treatment; the intraoral cone therapy should be done before the external-beam treatment. The major advantage of intraoral cone therapy is avoidance of the trauma of the implant. The disadvantage of intraoral cone therapy is the technical difficulty in avoiding a geographic miss due to tongue mobility. Treatment of the neck is an integral part of the treatment plan. The authors favor elective neck irradiation for nearly all lesions.

Combined Treatment Policies. When glossectomy is selected for the treatment, postoperative irradiation is administered for indications previously outlined in Selection of Treatment Modality. If the indication for postoperative radiation therapy is neck node metastases, the area of primary resection should be included in the fields of irradiation.

Preoperative radiation therapy is advised only when fixed nodes are present.

Management of Recurrence. Most recurrences appear in the first 2 years. Local recurrence after radiation therapy or surgery is heralded by ulceration, pain, or increased induration. Recurrences have a slightly elevated or rolled border, whereas necroses do not. The induration associated with necrosis is usu-

TABLE 26.2-13. Oral Tongue: Probability of Local Control at 2 Years According to T Stage and Treatment Method

T Stage	Local Control			Ultimate Local Control		
	RT Alone[a]	Surgery Alone or Combined with RT	P Value	RT Alone[a]	Surgery Alone or Combined with RT	P Value
T1	79% (18)	76% (17)	.76	93%	82%	.34
T2	72% (48)	76% (19)	.86	83%	82%	.91
T3	45% (29)	82% (24)	.03	57%	91%	.01
T4	0% (10)	67% (5)	.08	0%	67%	.08

RT, radiation therapy.
Note: Numbers in parentheses indicate number of patients in each subset.
[a]Radiation therapy alone or followed by a neck dissection.
(From ref. 88, with permission.)

ally less than with recurrence. Biopsy should be done as soon as ulceration appears, if the ulcer is within the original tumor site. Ulcers that appear on adjacent normal tissues (e.g., the gingiva) are likely due to radiation effect and not cancer.

Radiation treatment failure is managed by glossectomy. Surgical treatment failure occasionally is salvaged by radiation therapy or an operation, if the recurrence is limited to the mucosa. Recurrence in the soft tissues of the neck is rarely eradicated by any procedure.

Nodes appearing in a previously untreated neck are managed by neck dissection with or without postoperative radiation therapy.

RESULTS OF TREATMENT. The local control rates for 170 patients treated with radiation therapy or surgery or both between 1964 and 1990 at the University of Florida are depicted in Table 26.2-13.[88] Local control rates for T1 or T2 cancers are comparable after radiation therapy versus surgery; patients with T3 or T4 lesions have improved local control if surgery is part of the treatment. The 5-year survival rates are depicted in Table 26.2-14; the differences in survival between the two treatment groups are not statistically significant.

Sessions et al.[89] reported on 332 patients treated with surgery or radiation therapy or both at Washington University between 1957 and 1996. Five-year overall and cause-specific survival rates were as follows: stage I, 67% and 76%; stage II, 56% and 64%; stage III, 29% and 39%; and stage IV, 21% and 27%, respectively.

There were no significant differences in the 5-year cause-specific survival rates for the various treatment modalities when the outcomes were stratified according to the stage of disease.

The results of brachytherapy alone or combined with external-beam radiation therapy for 448 patients treated at the Centre Alexis Vautrin were reported by Pernot et al.[90] and revealed the following 5-year local control and survival rates: T1, 93% and 69%; T2, 65% and 41%; and T3, 49% and 25%, respectively. The time interval between brachytherapy and external-beam radiation therapy significantly influenced local control and survival for those who received both modalities. Shorter intervals were associated with better outcomes.

COMPLICATIONS OF TREATMENT
Surgery. Orocutaneous fistula, flap necrosis, and dysphagia are the three most common complications of surgery of the tongue. Damage to the lingual nerve or the hypoglossal nerve during the course of surgery, although rare, increases the possibility that the patient may have difficulty in swallowing and in speaking. Fistula and flap necrosis must be handled judiciously, because the danger of carotid artery hemorrhage increases with either of these complications. Enunciation difficulties occur whenever the tongue is bound down by scarring. The incidence of complications increases for surgical salvage attempts after radiation failure, and multiple procedures may be necessary to obtain satisfactory healing. Thirteen of 65 patients (20%) treated with surgery alone or surgery combined with radiation

TABLE 26.2-14. Oral Tongue: Probability of Survival at 5 Years According to Treatment Method and AJCC Stage

AJCC Stage	Absolute Survival			Cause-Specific Survival			Relapse-Free Survival		
	RT Alone[a]	Surgery Alone or Combined with RT	P Value	RT Alone[a]	Surgery Alone or Combined with RT	P Value	RT Alone[a]	Surgery Alone or Combined with RT	P Value
I	50% (14)	49% (13)	.25	88%	63%	.18	65%	68%	.90
II	64% (31)	68% (15)	.71	82%	82%	.63	61%	37%	.16
III	39% (31)	50% (12)	.22	55%	74%	.36	43%	65%	.16
IVA	0% (15)	26% (17)	.41	0%	33%	.34	0%	40%	.18
IVB	14% (14)	29% (8)	.70	24%	50%	.68	27%	30%	.90

AJCC, American Joint Committee on Cancer; RT, radiation therapy.
Note: Numbers in parentheses indicate number of patients in each subset.
[a]Radiation therapy alone or followed by planned neck dissection.
(From ref. 88, with permission.)

therapy at the University of Florida developed significant complications.[88] Sessions et al.[89] observed major complications in 21 of 270 patients (8%) treated surgically at Washington University.

Radiation Therapy. Many patients complain of a sensitive tongue for many months after completion of treatment, even when the mucosa is well healed. The effect disappears with time. Taste reappears within several months after treatment and may return to normal, but often is "not quite as keen" as before. Return of saliva secretion is variable, depending on the treatment volume and the dose to the salivary glands. Patients treated with interstitial therapy alone eventually have nearly normal saliva secretion. Patients treated with 45 Gy external-beam therapy plus interstitial therapy eventually have significant return of saliva secretion if one parotid receives 26 Gy or less.

SOFT TISSUE NECROSIS. A minor soft tissue necrosis is fairly common. Once recurrence has been ruled out, considerable patience is required for healing. The treatment plan is mainly to rule out recurrent cancer, provide local anesthesia, and reduce local infection. The patient is followed closely. Broad-spectrum antibiotics (e.g., tetracycline, 1 g/d), local anesthetics such as viscous lidocaine (Xylocaine), and analgesics are prescribed as needed. Pentoxifylline 400 mg three times daily may be beneficial. Hyperbaric oxygen treatment may be tried in difficult cases. When all else fails, however, and necrosis is persistent and pain uncontrollable, the necrosis must be resected.

RADIATION-INDUCED BONE DISEASE. The edentulous person is less likely to develop serious radiation-induced disease of the mandible than a person with teeth. There are several ways in which the mandible may be affected.

The most frequent problem involving the mandible is termed *bone exposure.* The gingiva disappears, exposing the underlying bone, with the exposed area or areas usually varying from 2 mm to 2 cm in diameter. If the exposed area is small, the patient is often unaware of the problem. There may be modest discomfort; the bone appears intact. Biopsy is not needed unless there was tumor at that location on the gingiva before treatment. If the patient has dentures, their use should be discontinued or they should be altered by the dentist to relieve the pressure over the exposed bone. If sharp bony edges appear, they are filed to a smooth contour and the bone edge lowered to speed healing. The bone exposure may become more or less stationary at this point. Healing may require months or even years. Healing occurs when the gingiva regrows over the exposed area. A small superficial piece of bone may sequestrate first, and then the gingiva regrows to cover the exposed area. Patience is the major requirement; aggressive intervention may actually increase the likelihood of progression to osteoradionecrosis.

In some cases, the bone becomes frankly necrotic with intermittent sequestration. Hyperbaric oxygen treatment has been used with some success. It is a matter of individualization when surgical intervention should be instituted. Conservative measures should be given a fair trial, but if pain becomes a problem, an operative procedure must be considered. The dead bone is removed and replaced with tissue such as a myocutaneous flap carrying its own blood supply.

Severe complications were observed in 9 of 105 patients (9%) treated with radiation therapy at the University of Florida.[88] Pernot and colleagues[90] observed the following soft tissue or bone complications (or both) in a series of 448 patients: grade 1, 19%; grade 2, 6%; and grade 3, 3%.

Buccal Mucosa

EPIDEMIOLOGY. Squamous cell carcinoma is relatively uncommon in the United States. In southern India it is common and is related to chewing tobacco mixed with betel leaves, areca nut, and lime shell.[91]

ANATOMY. The buccal mucosa is the mucous membrane covering the inner surface of the cheeks and lips, ending above and below with a transition to the gingiva. It ends posteriorly at the retromolar trigone. The parotid duct opens into the buccal mucosa opposite the second upper molar. The blood supply is a branch of the facial artery. The long buccal nerve, a branch of the mandibular, is sensory to the buccal mucosa and the skin of the cheek, which overlies the buccinator muscle. The facial nerve is the motor nerve to the buccinator muscle.

PATHOLOGY. Most malignant tumors are low-grade squamous cell carcinomas, frequently appearing on a background of leukoplakia or lichen planus. Verrucous carcinoma occurs and may be particularly difficult to diagnose histologically. Minor salivary gland tumors and malignant melanoma occur rarely.

PATTERNS OF SPREAD. Almost all squamous cell carcinomas originate on the mucosa lining the cheeks; primary lesions seldom originate from the wet mucosa of the lips. Early lesions are usually discrete and exophytic. As they enlarge, they penetrate the underlying muscles and eventually extend to the skin. Peripheral growth occurs into the gingivobuccal gutters and eventually onto the gingiva and underlying bone.

The lymphatic spread is first to the submandibular and subdigastric nodes. The incidence of positive nodes on admission is 9% to 31%, and the risk of occult disease is 16%.[10,22]

CLINICAL PICTURE. Small lesions produce the sensation of a lump that is felt with the tongue. A background of leukoplakia is common and sometimes quite extensive. Pain is minimal even when the lesion becomes large, unless there is posterior extension to involve the lingual and dental nerves. Pain may be referred to the ear. Obstruction of Stensen's duct produces parotid enlargement. Extension posteriorly, behind the pterygomandibular raphe or into the buccinator and masseter muscles, eventually causes trismus.

DIFFERENTIAL DIAGNOSIS. The differential diagnosis includes lues and tuberculosis, both of which are quite uncommon. If the first biopsy report is chronic inflammation or pseudoepitheliomatous hyperplasia and there is an obvious neoplasm present, repeat biopsy is necessary.

TREATMENT

Selection of Treatment Modality. Small lesions (1 cm or less) may simply be excised with primary closure. Small lesions that involve the anterior commissure are sometimes treated by radiation therapy. Lesions 2 to 3 cm in size can be treated with surgery or radiation therapy, usually the former. Larger lesions are usually treated with surgery and postoperative radiation therapy.

Surgical Treatment. Lesions that invade the mandible or maxilla require resection of an appropriate amount of bone along with the soft tissues. Repair may require a maxillary prosthesis. A myocutaneous flap repairs full-thickness removal of the cheek.

Irradiation Technique. Buccal mucosa lesions are suited for treatment with electron, intraoral cone, and interstitial techniques to spare the contralateral normal tissues. When tumors extend into one of the gingivobuccal gutters or onto bone, treatment must be entirely by external beam.

RESULTS OF TREATMENT. Diaz et al.[92] reported the M. D. Anderson experience for 119 patients treated with surgery alone (84 patients) or surgery combined with adjuvant radiation therapy (35 patients) between 1974 and 1993. Tumor recurrence developed in 54 patients (45%), local recurrence in 27 patients (23%), regional recurrence in 13 patients (11%), local and regional recurrence in 11 patients (9%), and distant metastases in 3 patients (3%). The 5-year survival rates by stage were stage I, 78%; stage II, 66%; stage III, 62%; stage IV, 50%; and overall, 63%.

Ash[93] reported 35% absolute 5-year survival for 374 patients with carcinoma of the buccal mucosa for all stages. The primary lesion was controlled initially in 53% of patients with early lesions and in 25% with advanced lesions; salvage raised the ultimate control rates to 69% and 34%. The initial treatment to the primary lesion was radiation therapy in 97% of the patients.

Nair and coworkers[91] reported the radiation therapy results for 234 cases of buccal mucosa cancer treated in southern India by radical radiation therapy during the 1982 calendar year. The disease-free survival rate at 3 years by stage was as follows: stage I, 85%; stage II, 63%; stage III, 41%; and stage IV, 15%. Thirty-two patients had verrucous carcinoma; the 3-year disease-free survival rate was 47%, similar to that for other grades of squamous cell carcinoma.

COMPLICATIONS OF TREATMENT. The buccal mucosa is tolerant of high-dose radiation therapy, and complications are uncommon. Bone exposure may appear on the mandible or maxilla. Trismus may develop if the muscles of mastication receive high doses.

Surgical injury of Stensen's duct may cause obstruction and parotitis. Injury to branches of cranial nerve VII may occur. Split-thickness skin grafts may shrink and produce partial trismus. Resection of the lip commissure may produce oral incompetence.

Gingiva and Hard Palate (Including Retromolar Trigone)

Carcinomas arising from the upper and lower gingiva have a similar clinical picture and require a similar approach to diagnosis. Primary squamous cell carcinoma of the hard palate is uncommon because the majority of hard palate neoplasms are minor salivary gland tumors. Some authors include the retromolar trigone with the anterior tonsillar pillar, but in their natural history and management, these lesions are more similar to lesions of the lower gingiva.

ANATOMY. The lower gingiva includes the mucosa covering the mandible from the gingivobuccal gutter to the origin of the mobile mucosa on the floor of the mouth. Behind the third molar is a small triangular surface called the retromolar trigone; it is contiguous above with the maxillary tuberosity. Beneath the mucosa

of the retromolar trigone is the tendinous pterygomandibular raphe, which is attached to the pterygoid hamulus and the posterior mylohyoid ridge of the mandible and serves as the insertion of the buccinator, orbicular oris, and superior pharyngeal constrictor muscles. Just behind the pterygomandibular raphe and between the medial pterygoid muscle and the ascending ramus is the pterygomandibular space, which contains the lingual and dental nerves. The pterygomandibular space is related posteriorly to the deep lobe of the parotid and the contents of the parapharyngeal space. There are no minor salivary glands in the attached mucous membrane over the alveolar ridges.

PATHOLOGY. Most neoplasms of the lower gum and retromolar trigone are squamous cell carcinoma. Squamous cell carcinoma is relatively uncommon on the upper gum and hard palate, where minor salivary gland tumors, usually adenoid cystic carcinoma, are more frequent. Verrucous lesions occur, usually on the lower gingiva. Melanoma is reported. Metastatic lesions to the underlying bone may be confused with primary mucosal tumors.

Epidermoid carcinoma may arise within the body of the mandible or maxilla either from odontogenic epithelium or from epithelium trapped during embryonic development. It is more frequent in the mandible than the maxilla and is most common in the molar regions. It must be distinguished from metastatic squamous cell carcinoma and ameloblastoma.

Ameloblastoma is a rare tumor with an incidence of approximately 1% of all tumors of the maxilla and mandible. Most patients are in the age range of 20 to 50 years. Some 80% of cases of ameloblastoma occur in the mandible with the molar-ramus region most commonly involved. No appreciable differences are found by sex or race.[94] Histologically, the ameloblastoma is an epithelial tumor similar to basal cell carcinoma [95] and should be considered a low-grade malignancy.[96]

PATTERNS OF SPREAD

Lower Gum. Squamous cell carcinoma invades the periosteum and the adjacent buccal mucosa and floor of the mouth. Slow-growing, low-grade lesions tend to produce a smooth, saucerized defect before invading the mandible. Moderate-grade to high-grade lesions invade the bone directly or through recently opened dental sockets and produce a lytic defect.

Lymphatic spread is to the submandibular and subdigastric nodes. Eighteen percent to 52% have clinically positive nodes on admission. Occult disease occurs in 17% to 19%.[10,22]

Ameloblastoma is an indolent tumor usually arising in bone, expanding and destroying the bone, and extending to adjacent areas by contiguous growth. Regional and even distant metastasis may occasionally occur.

Upper Gum and Hard Palate. Most squamous cell carcinomas originate on the gingiva and spread secondarily to the hard palate, soft palate, buccal mucosa, and underlying bone. The maxillary antrum is invaded late unless there are recent extractions providing access. Primary carcinoma of the maxillary antrum must be excluded because it frequently presents in the upper gum and hard palate. The risk for positive lymph nodes is 13% to 24% on admission, and the incidence of occult disease is 22%.[10,22]

Retromolar Trigone. Carcinoma of the retromolar trigone spreads to adjacent buccal mucosa, anterior tonsillar pillar, and maxilla early. Posterior spread occurs into the pterygomandibular space and the medial pterygoid muscle. Posterolateral spread occurs into the buccinator muscle and fat pad. The first-echelon lymphatics are the submandibular and subdigastric nodes. The incidence of clinically positive nodes on presentation is approximately 30% and the risk for occult disease is 15% to 25%.[97]

CLINICAL PICTURE. The patient with squamous cell carcinoma may present to the dentist first with ill-fitting dentures, dental pain, loose teeth, or a sore that will not heal. A history of inappropriate dental extractions or root canal therapy is common. Intermittent bleeding and mild pain occur when the lesion is traumatized. Invasion into the mandible may involve the inferior dental nerve and produce paresthesia or anesthesia of the lower lip. A background of leukoplakia is frequently present.

Retromolar trigone lesions have pain referred to the external auditory canal and preauricular area. Invasion of the pterygoid muscle produces trismus.

Intraalveolar epidermoid carcinoma presents with a submucosal mass and dental symptoms. Radiographs show a lytic lesion in the mandible.

Ameloblastoma exhibits few symptoms in the early stages. Patients may notice a gradually increasing facial deformity or loosening of teeth. An intraoral submucosal mass may be present initially; ulceration occurs as the mass increases in size. On radiographs, a radiolucent area is seen with some of the following features: expansion of the overlying cortical plate, a scalloped margin, a multilocular appearance, or resorption of the roots of adjacent teeth.[98]

Minor salivary gland tumors start as a submucosal mass, enlarge slowly, and may present with a central ulceration.

DIFFERENTIAL DIAGNOSIS. The differential diagnosis includes dental disease and underlying bony cysts or tumors, including metastatic tumors.

TREATMENT
Selection of Treatment Modality
LOWER GUM. The majority of lesions of the lower gum are managed by operation. Early lesions may be resected intraorally, with removal of only soft tissue or a margin of bone (i.e., rim resection), and closed primarily or with a split-thickness graft. When bone invasion is present, removal of a segment of mandible is required; a neck dissection is usually included. Irradiation may be used for small lesions and for those with only a pressure defect in the bone, but the functional results are generally better after an operation. Postoperative irradiation may be indicated depending on pathologic findings.

AMELOBLASTOMA. The treatment for ameloblastoma is an operation; however, local recurrence is a problem. Sehdev and coworkers[99] reported that curettage was followed by local recurrence in 90% of mandibular and in all maxillary ameloblastomas. Subsequent resection controlled 80% of the mandibular but only 40% of the maxillary tumors. The initial use of segmental mandibular resection controlled 78% of cases (18 of 23) with subsequent resection controlling those that recurred. The use of partial maxillectomy as the first treatment controlled 100% of maxillary ameloblastomas (7 of 7) as opposed to only 40% when partial maxillectomy was performed for

recurrence. Hemimandibulectomy controlled 100% of curettage failures in one series.[100]

The lesions respond readily to irradiation. However, because radiation therapy has generally been applied to patients only after multiple operative failures and in cases of advanced disease, the curative ability is not clear.

RETROMOLAR TRIGONE. Small retromolar trigone lesions may appear innocuous and easily cured, but often are more extensive than they seem. For early, well-localized lesions without detectable bone invasion, a rim or marginal resection of the mandible may be performed. If rim resection is not feasible, radiation therapy should be considered for initial treatment, with partial mandibulectomy reserved for recurrence. Radiation therapy is recommended for lesions involving a rather large surface area, such as those with superficial extension to the anterior tonsillar pillar, soft palate, and buccal mucosa.[29] Evidence of bone invasion is an indication for partial mandibulectomy. Preference is given to surgical treatment unless the cosmetic and functional result would be unacceptable to the patient, in which case operation is reserved for radiation therapy failure. Moderately advanced lesions usually are managed by resection followed by postoperative radiation therapy.

UPPER GUM AND HARD PALATE. Surgical resection is the usual treatment for most lesions of the upper gum. Postoperative radiation therapy is added as needed. However, if the lesion is superficial and extensively involves the hard palate or involves a significant portion of the soft palate, then radiation should be considered for the initial therapy. If the lesion is small and discrete and there is no bone involvement, the resection includes the periosteum or occasionally some underlying bone. Bone invasion requires a partial maxillectomy. The defect usually is repaired with a prosthesis.

Surgical Treatment
RIM RESECTION (CORONAL). See Surgical Treatment in the section Floor of the Mouth, earlier in this chapter.
SEGMENTAL MANDIBULECTOMY. For small lesions with minimal bone invasion, a short section of mandible is removed in continuity with the tumor (e.g., removal of the mandible from the angle to the mental foramen).
PARTIAL MANDIBULEGTOMY. In partial mandibulectomy the mandible and tumor are usually resected from the mental foramen to the coronoid process, generally leaving the head of the condyle. Reconstruction of the mandible is usually accomplished with an osteomyocutaneous flap.
HEMIMANDIBULECTOMY. Extensive lesions may require removal of the mandible symphysis to the condyle on one side. Massive anterior lesions require removal of the mandible from angle to angle. This produces a major cosmetic and functional loss, and reconstruction is performed with a composite osteomyocutaneous flap.

Irradiation Technique. Small lesions of the lower gum and retromolar trigone may be treated by intraoral cone for all or part of their therapy. Well-lateralized lesions of the retromolar trigone and posterior gum may be treated by either an ipsilateral mixed-beam or angled wedge pair technique; the latter is preferred. Parallel-opposed portals treat anterior gum lesions.

The usual indication for irradiation of hard palate lesions is a carcinoma that involves nearly the entire hard palate and upper gums with little or no bone invasion. These lesions may be treated by external-beam radiation. An intraoral surface brachytherapy applicator is an option.

The dose for T1 retromolar trigone lesions is usually from 60 Gy in 6 weeks to 65 Gy in 7 weeks. Larger tumors are treated with altered fractionation, often combined with concomitant chemotherapy. Continuous-course hyperfractionation is used at the authors' institution: T2, 74.4 Gy in 62 fractions; and T3 or T4, 76.8 Gy in 64 fractions. The dose for gum lesions is similar.

Management of Recurrence. Radiation therapy failures are managed by operation. Surgical treatment failures may be managed by surgery, radiation therapy, or a combination of both.[29] Salvage procedures frequently are not attempted, however, because of the advanced nature of the recurrence and the low chance of cure.

RESULTS OF TREATMENT

Mandibular Gingiva. Overholt and coworkers[101] reported on 155 patients with squamous cell carcinomas of the lower gum treated at M. D. Anderson Hospital between 1970 and 1990. Surgery alone was used for 131 patients and the remainder received surgery and radiation therapy. Five-year survival for patients with T1 and T2 cancers was 85% and 84%, respectively, compared with 66% and 64% for those with T3 and T4 malignancies, respectively. Local control at 2 years was impacted by tumor size ($P = .021$) and margin status ($P = .027$), whereas 5-year cause-specific survival was influenced by tumor size ($P = .001$), margin status ($P = .011$), mandibular invasion ($P = <.05$), and the presence of lymph node metastases ($P<.001$).

Twenty-six patients were treated at the University of Florida for carcinoma of the lower gum with radiation therapy alone or surgery with or without adjuvant radiation therapy and had the following local control rates: T1, 1 of 1 and 2 of 2; T2, 1 of 5 and 3 of 5; T3, no data; and T4, 1 of 2 and 7 of 11, respectively.[29] Nine patients were treated for carcinoma of the upper gum, which was locally controlled in 0 of 3 patients after radiation therapy versus 4 of 6 patients after surgery alone or in combination with irradiation.[29]

Retromolar Trigone. Huang and coworkers[102] reported on 65 patients treated for cancer of the retromolar trigone at Washington University between 1971 and 1994. Patients received preoperative irradiation and surgery (10 patients), surgery and postoperative radiation therapy (39 patients), or radiation therapy alone (16 patients). Local-regional control rates after treatment were as follows: preoperative irradiation, 90%; postoperative radiation therapy, 77%; and radiation therapy alone, 56%. Multivariate analysis revealed that treatment group significantly influenced local-regional control ($P = .046$) and disease-free survival ($P = .002$).

Byers and coworkers[97] reported the M. D. Anderson Hospital results for 110 previously untreated patients with squamous cell carcinoma of the retromolar trigone treated between 1965 and 1977, with a minimum 5-year follow-up. Surgery was often selected for patients with leukoplakia, poor teeth, mandible invasion, large neck nodes, or trismus. Radiation therapy was selected for poorly differentiated tumors, for mainly exophytic lesions, for lesions involving the faucial arch or soft palate or lesions having ill-defined borders, and for poor surgical risk cases. The local control rates were as follows: T1, 12 of 13 (92%); T2, 50 of 57 (88%); T3, 18 of 20 (90%); and T4, 15 of 20 (75%). Local control was similar after surgery, radiation therapy, and both. In spite of the high local-regional control rates, the absolute 5-year survival rate was only 26% due to a high incidence of death due to intercurrent disease, with a 33% risk for second cancers.

Hard Palate. Shibuya and coworkers[103] reported the results for 38 cases of carcinoma of the hard palate and 82 cases of carcinoma of the upper gum treated between 1953 and 1982 in Japan. Sixty-six patients were managed initially by radiation therapy alone to the primary lesion, and 54 patients were managed by radiation therapy and surgery. The 5-year actuarial survival rate by stage was the following: stage I, 56%; stage II, 41%; stage III, 32%; and stage IV, 12%. There was no difference in survival when comparing hard palate versus upper gum, squamous cell carcinoma versus minor salivary gland tumor, or radiation therapy alone versus radiation therapy plus surgery as the initial therapy. The overall risk for metastatic lymph nodes was 47% for hard palate lesions and 49% for upper gum lesions. Thirty patients recorded as having "slight bone invasion" and no metastases had a 5-year survival rate of 75% when treated by radiation therapy. Major bone involvement was an indication for partial maxillectomy.

COMPLICATIONS OF TREATMENT. Surgical complications include orocutaneous fistula, bone exposure with sequestration, extrusion of a metal tray, and loss of graft or flap. After hemimandibulectomy, the edentulous patient usually cannot wear dentures and the patient with teeth cannot chew because of shifting of the remaining mandible.

The complications of radiation therapy include soft tissue necrosis with bone exposure and subsequent osteoradionecrosis. The risk is greatest for patients with advanced lesions of the lower gum and retromolar trigone. Byers and coworkers[97] reported that 14% of patients treated by radiation therapy for retromolar trigone lesions required a partial mandibulectomy for mandible necrosis. The risk was greatest for patients having preirradiation extractions for poor dentition or impacted molars. Huang and colleagues[102] reported the following rates of grade 3 bone and soft tissue complications in 65 patients treated for retromolar trigone carcinomas: preoperative irradiation, 0 of 10 patients (0%); surgery and postoperative radiation therapy, 5 of 39 patients (13%); and radiation therapy alone, 2 of 16 patients (13%).

OROPHARYNX

The oropharynx includes the base of the tongue, the tonsillar region (tonsillar fossa and tonsillar pillars), the soft palate, and the pharyngeal wall between the pharyngoepiglottic fold and the nasopharynx. The pharyngeal walls are considered in Hypopharynx: Pharyngeal Walls, Pyriform Sinus, and Postcricoid Pharynx, later in this chapter.

Anatomy

The base of the tongue is bounded anteriorly by the circumvallate papillae, laterally by the glossotonsillar sulci, and posteriorly by the epiglottis. The vallecula is a strip of mucosa that is the transition from the base of the tongue to the epiglottis; it is considered part of the base of the tongue. The surface of the base of the tongue appears irregular due to scattered submucosal lymphoid follicles. The musculature of the base of the tongue is continuous with that of the oral tongue. A midsagittal section through the oropharynx showing important relationships with neighboring sites is presented in Figure 26.2-8. A cross section through the oropharynx (Fig. 26.2-9) shows relationships to the lateral pharyngeal space.

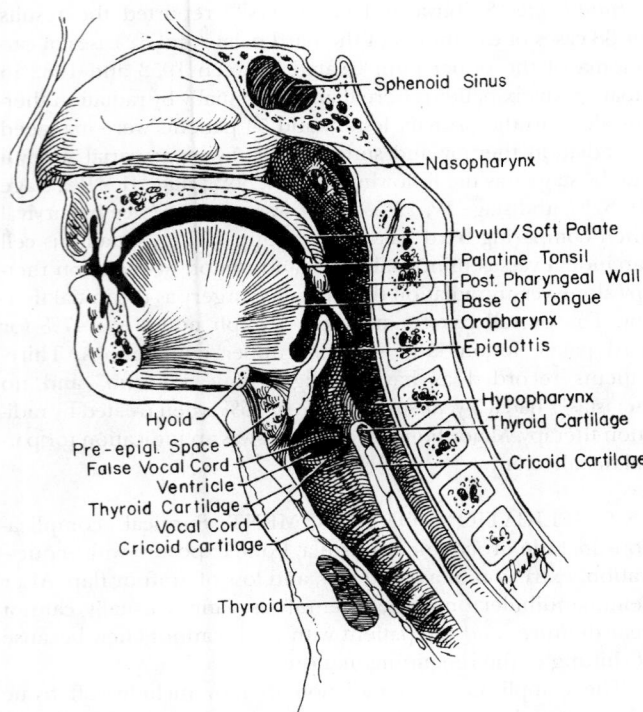

FIGURE 26.2-8. Sagittal section of the upper aerodigestive tract. (Redrawn from Sabbotta drawings in Clemente CD: *Anatomy: a regional atlas of the human body*. Philadelphia: Lea & Febiger, 1975, with permission. Copyright 1975, Urban & Schwarzenberg München, Berlin, Vienna.)

The tonsillar area is a triangular region bounded anteriorly by the anterior tonsillar pillar (palatopharyngeal muscle), posteriorly by the posterior tonsillar pillar (palatopharyngeal muscle), and inferiorly by the glossotonsillar sulcus and pharyngoepiglottic fold. The palatine tonsil lies within the triangle. The pharyngeal constrictor muscle and its fascia, the mandible, and the lateral pharyngeal space bound the tonsillar region laterally. The

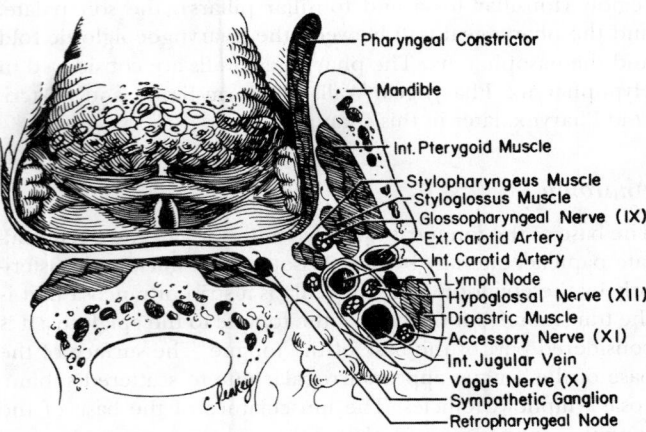

FIGURE 26.2-9. Section at the level of the mid-oropharynx, depicting relationships in the parapharyngeal area. (From Million RR, Cassisi NJ, Clark JR. Cancer of the head and neck. In: DeVita VT Jr, Hellman S, Rosenberg SA, eds. *Cancer: principles and practice of oncology*, 3rd ed. Philadelphia: JB Lippincott, 1989:523, with permission.)

tonsillar area is separated from the base of the tongue by the glossotonsillar sulcus, which extends from the anterior tonsillar pillar to the pharyngoepiglottic fold. Beneath the mucous membrane of the sulcus are the styloglossal muscle and the stylohyoid ligament.

The soft palate is a thin, mobile muscle complex separating the nasopharynx from the oral cavity and oropharynx. The epithelium of the oral side of the soft palate is squamous and the epithelium of the nasopharyngeal surface is respiratory. The soft palate is contiguous laterally with the tonsillar pillars.

Pathology

Squamous cell carcinoma or one of its variants accounts for 95% of malignant lesions. Lymphoepitheliomas occur in the tonsil and base of the tongue. Verrucous carcinomas occur rarely. Malignant lymphomas account for approximately 5% of tonsillar and 1% to 2% of base of tongue malignancies. Minor salivary gland malignancies, plasmacytomas, and other rare tumors make up the remainder of the malignancies.

Patterns of Spread

BASE OF THE TONGUE

Primary. Squamous cell carcinoma of the base of the tongue tends to develop early, silent, deep infiltration. The tumor usually remains in the tongue unless it begins at the very peripheral margin. Vallecular lesions spread along the mucosa to the lingual surface of the epiglottis, laterally along the pharyngoepiglottic fold, and then to the lateral pharyngeal wall and anterior wall of the pyriform sinus. Vallecular lesions frequently penetrate through the thin mucous membrane of the vallecula; tumor spread is contained for a while by the hyoepiglottic ligament, but this thin, often incomplete structure is eventually breached and cancer enters the preepiglottic space.

Lesions beginning on the lateral base of the tongue may invade the glossotonsillar sulcus. Deep penetration in the glossotonsillar sulcus allows tumor to escape into the neck, because there is no effective musculature barrier at this point. Although the mylohyoid muscle is an effective barrier for oral tongue lesions, it terminates near the angle of the mandible. The primary tumor mass may be palpable below the angle of the mandible and may be confused with an involved lymph node. Advanced lesions tend to spread toward the larynx, oral tongue, and parapharyngeal space. There is a tendency to underestimate the extent of disease.

Lymphatic. The first-echelon nodes are the subdigastric (level II); the path of spread is then along the jugular chain to the midjugular (level III) and lower jugular (level IV) nodes. The submandibular (level I) nodes may become involved if the tumor extends anteriorly into the oral tongue or if massive upper neck disease is present. The posterior cervical (level V) nodes are involved often enough to be included in treatment plans.

Approximately 75% of patients with base of tongue cancer have clinically positive neck nodes on admission; 30% have bilateral positive nodes (Fig. 26.2-10).[10] The risk of occult disease in the clinically negative neck is probably 40% to 50%.

TONSILLAR AREA

Anterior Tonsillar Pillar. Almost all malignant tumors arising on the anterior tonsillar pillar are squamous cell carcinomas.

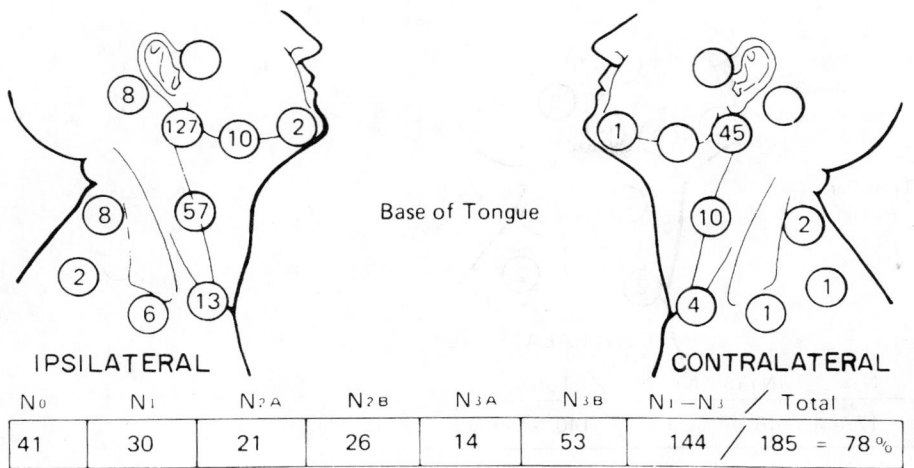

Base of Tongue

N₀	N₁	N₂A	N₂B	N₃A	N₃B	N₁–N₃ / Total
41	30	21	26	14	53	144 / 185 = 78%

FIGURE 26.2-10. Base of tongue carcinoma: nodal distribution on admission at M. D. Anderson Hospital, 1948 to 1965. The circled numbers indicate the number of times the particular lymph node was involved. (From ref. 10, with permission.)

The lesions tend to be diagnosed early and have relatively little bulk or infiltration. Asymptomatic lesions are common and may be red lesions, white lesions, or a mixture of both. Their borders are usually indistinct. As the lesions progress, they may develop a central ulcer with a rolled margin and infiltrate the palatoglossus. Superior medial spread occurs onto the soft palate, the most posterior hard palate, and the maxillary gingiva. Anterolateral spread to the retromolar trigone is frequent, with later spread to the posterior gingivobuccal sulcus. Once the tumor gains access to the buccal mucosa there is a threat for considerable occult anterior extension in the buccal pouch. Invasion of the tongue is frequent; careful palpation is necessary to detect the early submucosal nodule at the junction of the anterior tonsillar pillar and tongue. As these lesions advance, they adhere to the mandible and eventually invade the bone. Extension toward the base of the skull and nasopharynx is a late phenomenon, often associated with infiltration of the medial pterygoid muscle and erosion of the medial pterygoid plate. Such lesions produce trismus and marked temporal pain.

Tonsillar Fossa. Tonsillar fossa lesions arise either from the remnants of the palatine tonsil or from the mucous membrane within the triangle. There are differences in the early development and spread patterns for squamous cell carcinoma of the tonsillar fossa compared with anterior tonsillar pillar lesions. Leukoplakia rarely occurs within the fossa, and asymptomatic red mucosal lesions are seen infrequently. The initial lesions tend to be exophytic with central ulceration plus an infiltrative component. However, some lesions develop submucosally and present with neck nodes and no obvious tonsillar lesion. Extension to the posterior tonsillar pillar and the oropharyngeal wall occurs early. Invasion into the glossotonsillar sulcus and base of the tongue occurs in approximately 25% of cases. As the lesions advance, they penetrate to the parapharyngeal space and gain access to the base of the skull superiorly. Cranial nerve involvement is uncommon, however. Advanced lesions invade the mandible, nasopharynx, and base of the tongue and may extend below the pharyngoepiglottic fold into the pyriform sinus.

Posterior Tonsillar Pillar. Early lesions arising from the posterior tonsillar pillar are uncommon. There are two major differences in their potential spread patterns. They may spread inferiorly along the palatopharyngeal muscle to its insertions into the middle pharyngeal constrictor, the pharyngoepiglottic fold, and the posterior border of the thyroid cartilage. Also, the lymphatic trunks of the posterior tonsillar pillar are theoretically more likely to spread to the junctional (parapharyngeal) and spinal accessory lymph nodes.

Lymphatic. The distribution and N staging at diagnosis for previously untreated patients with retromolar trigone–anterior tonsillar pillar and tonsillar fossa squamous cell carcinomas are shown in Figure 26.2-11.[10]

Retromolar trigone–anterior tonsillar pillar lesions have a lower risk of clinically positive lymph nodes (45%) compared with lesions of the tonsillar fossa (76%). The distribution for the retromolar trigone–anterior tonsillar pillar on the ipsilateral side is to the jugular and submandibular lymph nodes, with a very low risk for junctional and spinal accessory lymph nodes. Contralateral spread is uncommon (5%) and is confined to the jugular chain. The risk of occult disease in the clinically negative neck (N0) is 10% to 15%. The incidence of positive nodes increases with T stage.

Tonsillar fossa lesions have a high risk of clinically positive lymph nodes on admission (76%). The lymph node distribution for tonsillar fossa lesions on the ipsilateral side includes the jugular, junctional, spinal accessory, and more posterior submandibular lymph nodes. Contralateral spread occurs in only 11% of patients and is mainly to the jugular chain lymph nodes, but there is some risk for spinal accessory and submandibular involvement. The risk of contralateral spread is related to invasion of the tongue, spread near or across the midline of the soft palate, and large lymph nodes in the ipsilateral neck that produce lymphatic obstruction; when these features are present, treatment of the opposite neck must be considered. The incidence of occult disease is probably 50% to 60%.

There is no information about lymphatic spread for posterior tonsillar pillar lesions.

SOFT PALATE

Primary. Nearly all soft palate squamous cell carcinomas occur on the oral side of the palate; the nasopharyngeal side is rarely involved. The earliest tumors are red lesions with ill-defined borders. White lesions are common on the soft palate and may be leukoplakia, carcinoma *in situ*, or early invasive car-

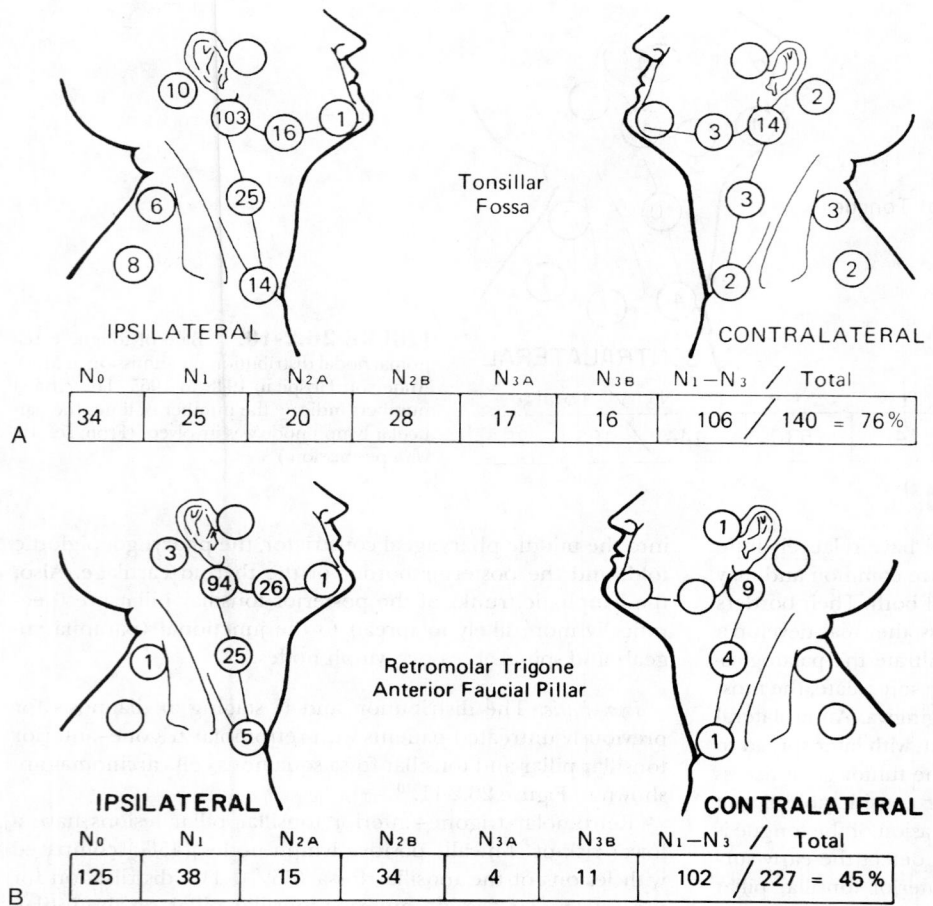

A

N$_0$	N$_1$	N$_{2A}$	N$_{2B}$	N$_{3A}$	N$_{3B}$	N$_1$–N$_3$	/ Total
34	25	20	28	17	16	106	/ 140 = 76%

B

N$_0$	N$_1$	N$_{2A}$	N$_{2B}$	N$_{3A}$	N$_{3B}$	N$_1$–N$_3$	/ Total
125	38	15	34	4	11	102	/ 227 = 45%

FIGURE 26.2-11. Nodal distribution on admission at M. D. Anderson Hospital, 1948 to 1965. The circled numbers indicate the number of times the particular lymph node was involved. **A:** Carcinoma of the retromolar trigone and anterior tonsillar pillar. **B:** Carcinoma of the tonsillar pillar. (From ref. 10, with permission.)

cinoma. Multiple sites of involvement with normal-appearing intervening mucosa are common, dramatically demonstrated during the first week of radiation therapy when a tumoritis "lights up" the tumor sites, some of which are unsuspected. The majority of soft palate carcinomas are diagnosed while still confined to the soft palate. Spread occurs first to the tonsillar pillars and hard palate. Lateral spread may eventually penetrate the superior constrictor muscle and base of the skull, and may rarely compress or invade cranial nerves in the parapha-

ryngeal space. Involvement of the lateral wall(s) of the nasopharynx is common in advanced lesions.

Lymphatic. The spread pattern is first to the subdigastric node and then along the jugular chain. The submandibular, submental, and spinal accessory nodes are less commonly involved.

Approximately 56% of patients have clinically positive nodes on admission; 16% have bilateral positive nodes (Fig. 26.2-12).[10] The incidence of occult disease is not well estab-

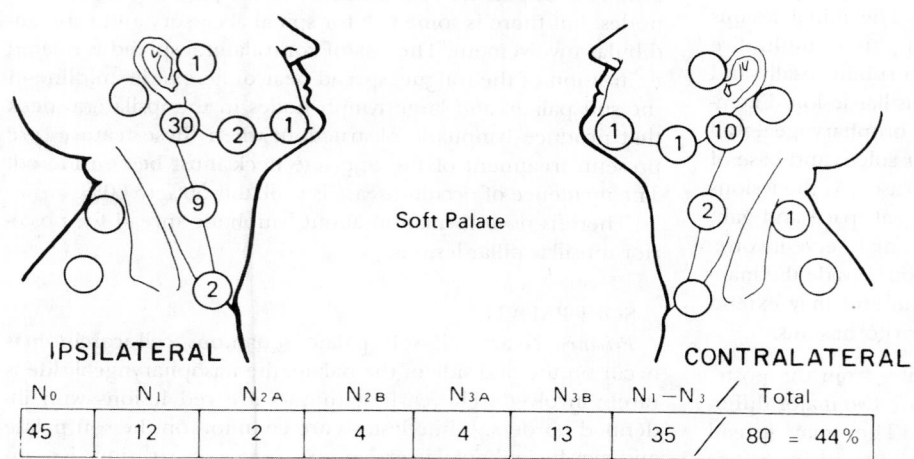

N$_0$	N$_1$	N$_{2A}$	N$_{2B}$	N$_{3A}$	N$_{3B}$	N$_1$–N$_3$	/ Total
45	12	2	4	4	13	35	/ 80 = 44%

FIGURE 26.2-12. Soft palate carcinoma: nodal distribution on admission at M. D. Anderson Hospital, 1948 to 1965. The circled numbers indicate the number of times the particular lymph node was involved. (From ref. 10, with permission.)

lished because the first-echelon nodes are usually irradiated in all but the earliest lesions. Lindberg and coworkers[104] noted an approximate 20% incidence of occult disease after either no or partial neck irradiation with the primary lesion controlled. The incidence of clinically positive nodes increases with T stage.[10]

Clinical Picture

BASE OF THE TONGUE. Asymptomatic lesions are rarely diagnosed, because the base of the tongue is visualized only by indirect mirror examination. Often, the earliest symptom is a mild sore throat. The patient may sense a lump in the back of the tongue and actually feel it by digital palpation. Because many of the early lesions are relatively silent, a subdigastric neck mass, often quite large, is often the first sign. Difficulty swallowing, a nasal voice quality, and deep-seated ear pain occur as the lesion enlarges. Far-advanced lesions fix the tongue. Deep ulceration and necrosis result in foul breath.

Indirect mirror examination, digital palpation, and a high level of suspicion are necessary for diagnosis of early lesions of the base of the tongue. Flexible fiberoptic endoscopy allows examination in some patients not easily examined by the indirect mirror method. A small lesion originating in the glossotonsillar sulcus area may ulcerate and produce symptoms quite early.

Lymphomas are usually large, mostly submucosal masses, and the diagnosis can be suspected by their appearance. Minor salivary gland tumors are also usually submucosal, but more discrete and firm than lymphomas.

TONSILLAR AREA

Anterior Tonsillar Pillar. Early symptoms of anterior tonsillar pillar lesions include sore throat, usually aggravated by food or drink. Pain is referred to the ear as soon as ulceration takes place. If the lesion involves the hard palate or posterior upper gum, dentures may fit improperly or cause irritation. Advanced lesions invade the pterygoid or buccinator muscle and produce trismus and temporal pain. Invasion of the tongue will eventually limit tongue mobility and, when accompanied by ulceration at the junction of the anterior tonsillar pillar and oral tongue, cause pain.

Tonsillar Fossa. Signs and symptoms of tonsillar fossa lesions are similar to those of the anterior tonsillar pillar, except that lesions tend to be larger before symptoms develop. Ipsilateral sore throat is the hallmark of these lesions. Detection by visual examination with a tongue depressor is sufficient for most lesions; however, a few cancers arise near the glossotonsillar sulcus or lower pole of the tonsil and are only visible by indirect examination. A few patients present with a node in the neck. Lymphomas of the tonsil tend to be large submucosal masses, but may ulcerate and appear similar to carcinomas.

SOFT PALATE. The earliest symptom of soft palate lesions is usually a mild sore throat, often aggravated by food or drink. The sore throat is not well localized. Discomfort may improve temporarily if antibiotics are given. Advanced lesions interfere with swallowing and may cause a voice change. Regurgitation of food and liquid into the nasopharynx and nose occurs with destruction, perforation, or fixation of the soft palate. Lateral and superior spread to the nasopharynx and parapharyngeal space is associated with trismus, otitis media, temporal headache, and, rarely, cranial nerve involvement.

Early lesions appear as red, white, or mixed changes in the mucosa. The mucosa may appear roughened with ill-defined margins. Multiple foci on the soft palate and anterior tonsillar pillars are common. Moderately advanced lesions have rolled edges with central ulceration, or they may be mainly exophytic, particularly around the uvula. The nasopharynx should be inspected and palpated for submucosal extension along the lateral wall. Extension along the nasopharyngeal surface of the soft palate is uncommon. Extension to the posterior nasal cavity is seen only in advanced lesions that erode the posterior hard palate.

AJCC Staging

The AJCC staging system for primary tumors of the oropharynx is as follows[16]:

T1 Tumor 2 cm or less in greatest dimension
T2 Tumor more than 2 cm but not more than 4 cm in greatest dimension
T3 Tumor more than 4 cm in greatest dimension
T4a Tumor invades the larynx, deep/extrinsic muscles of the tongue, medial pterygoid, hard palate, or mandible
T4b Tumor invades lateral pterygoid muscle, pterygoid plates, lateral nasopharynx, or skull base or encases the carotid artery

There is a tendency to overestimate the size of lesions in the oropharynx. The difference between T3 and T4 is not so easily determined. Bone involvement is uncommon and may be seen on radiographic studies. Invasion of soft tissues of the neck is best assessed by CT or MRI or both. Invasion of the root or deep musculature of the tongue is diagnosed if the tongue is partially fixed. Lesions that produce trismus or cranial nerve palsy are classified as T4. Pathologic staging usually results in up-staging. This stage migration renders a meaningful comparison of outcomes for clinically staged and pathologically staged lesions nearly impossible.

Treatment: Base of the Tongue

SELECTION OF TREATMENT MODALITY. Operation and irradiation produce similar cure rates for base of tongue lesions. However, because excision of the base of the tongue generally causes greater disability and because of the high risk for bilateral lymphatic involvement, radiation therapy is the treatment of choice for the majority of lesions, with operation reserved for salvage of radiation therapy failures and help in control of the neck disease. Radiation therapy automatically encompasses the neck nodes on both sides of the neck. Extended supraglottic laryngectomy may be used for limited vallecular lesions and lateralized base of tongue lesions, but anatomic criteria must be satisfied, and this selection limits its usefulness. The following conditions must be met: no gross involvement of the pharyngoepiglottic fold, preservation of one lingual artery, resection of less than 80% of the base of the tongue, and pulmonary and medical function suitable for supraglottic laryngectomy. At least an ipsilateral neck dissection is indicated, but with the high risk of bilateral neck disease even in the N0 patient, this represents incomplete treatment. Postoperative irradiation is often indicated in any event. Therefore, radiation therapy is usually the treatment of choice for the primary lesion, with neck dissection added as needed.

SURGICAL TREATMENT. The occasional patient with a low-volume T1 or early T2 cancer may be suitable for transoral laser excision in conjunction with a neck dissection.[105] The majority of patients present with disease too advanced for this alternative. Otherwise, the surgical approach for neoplasms of the base of the tongue is either by splitting the lip, mandible, and tongue in the midline to reach the base of the tongue, or by dividing the horizontal mandible and swinging it outward to expose the tongue base. Suprahyoid, transhyoid, and infrahyoid approaches also can be used to resect small lesions of the base of the tongue. After the tumor has been removed, the mandible is wired together. Only one lingual artery may be sacrificed. A neck dissection is done in continuity with excision of the base of tongue lesion. Removal of a large base of tongue tumor requires simultaneous removal of part of or the entire larynx.

IRRADIATION TECHNIQUE. Parallel opposed external-beam portals that also encompass the regional nodes on both sides are used to irradiate base of tongue cancer. Interstitial brachytherapy with flexible sources, such as ^{192}Ir ribbons, may be used for part of the treatment if the lesion is relatively small and discrete. In contrast to oral tongue cancer, there is no proven advantage in local control for interstitial boosts as opposed to external-beam treatment alone. The base of the tongue has a good vascular supply and tolerates high doses of radiation without soft tissue necrosis. Concomitant chemotherapy is usually considered for patients with endophytic T3 and T4 tumors as well as those associated with advanced N2 or N3 neck disease.

One of the common errors in planning external-beam portals is failure to recognize anterior growth of neoplasms as measured by palpation through the lateral floor of the mouth. Anterior extension is usually appreciated on CT or MRI. The inferior border of the lateral portals is usually the thyroid notch unless tumor has extended into the upper pyriform sinus, lateral pharyngeal wall, or preepiglottic space. The skin and subcutaneous fat in the submental area should be shielded if possible, because high-dose radiation therapy to this area produces considerable fibrosis. Shielding this area may not be possible if the patient is thin or if tumor is bulging into the mylohyoid muscle. Management of the lymphatics is critical. One of the major advantages of radiation therapy is the ease of irradiating all the nodes at risk. Even small, well-lateralized base of tongue lesions will spread to the opposite neck, and both sides are always treated.

The primary portals include the upper jugular, posterior submandibular, and posterior upper cervical node(s) when the neck is clinically negative. The superior border is approximately 2 cm above the tip of the mastoid even with clinically negative nodes to ensure coverage of the nodes near the base of the skull.

The lower neck nodes on both sides are always treated with a separate anterior portal. If the upper neck is clinically negative, the lower neck portals are carefully tailored to exclude as much normal tissue as possible; the midjugular nodes are the major risk area in this situation. If the upper neck is clinically positive, the lower neck portals become more generous.

The dose for T1 lesions is usually 60 to 66 Gy over 6 to 6.5 weeks. Since 1978, T2 to T4 lesions have been treated with 1.2 Gy twice daily with a minimum of 6 hours between fractions to a total dose of 74.4 to 79.2 Gy. Currently, T1 cancers are also treated with hyperfractionation to 74.4 Gy. Since 2001, IMRT has been used to treat selected patients with head and neck cancers in cases in which it is possible to adequately irradiate the cancer and spare enough salivary tissue to reduce the severity of long-term xerostomia. The M. D. Anderson concomitant boost technique is selected if IMRT is used.

COMBINED TREATMENT POLICIES. Combined treatment is seldom selected because an operation for moderately advanced lesions usually implies major functional loss, and few patients are willing to accept the morbidity and possible immediate mortality. There is also no convincing evidence that such treatment improves the likelihood of cure.[106]

MANAGEMENT OF RECURRENCE. Radiation treatment failures are treated surgically, but salvage is infrequent except for T1 and early T2 lesions. Surgical treatment failures are rarely salvaged by either an operation or radiation therapy, except for the early lesion with a discrete local recurrence in the base of the tongue. Recurrence of a small, discrete primary tumor may be managed by a wide local excision. The remaining recurrences require either a jaw-tongue-neck resection or glossectomy-laryngectomy. Palliative chemotherapy may be considered.

Results of Treatment: Base of the Tongue

The results of treatment with either surgery or radiation therapy are depicted in Tables 26.2-15 to 26.2-18. It is apparent that the likelihood of a cure is the same for either surgery or radiation therapy. The risk of severe complications is higher after surgery than after radiation therapy.

Follow-Up: Base of the Tongue

Surgical or radiation therapy, or both, occasionally salvages the treatment failure of an early lesion. Radiation treatment failures may present as an ulcer and must be distinguished from radiation necrosis. Most radiation ulcers appear in the vallecula or glossotonsillar sulcus, not on the base of the tongue proper. Deep biopsies usually must be done with the patient under general anesthesia to obtain adequate tissue and control bleeding.

Complications of Treatment: Base of the Tongue

SURGICAL COMPLICATIONS. The complications of surgery include an operative mortality of approximately 5%; fistula, mandibular necrosis, dysphagia, hoarseness, trismus, and carotid rupture are nonfatal complications (see Table 26.2-18). Pneumonia is frequent, due to aspiration when the glottis is preserved. The risk of complications is increased for patients who receive adjuvant radiation therapy.

COMPLICATIONS OF IRRADIATION. Bone exposure and osteoradionecrosis are uncommon. Soft tissue necrosis of mild to moderate degree occurs in approximately 10%, and bone exposure of mild to moderate degree occurs in 5% of patients treated solely by external-beam irradiation. Many necroses persist several months and may respond to pentoxifylline. Serious hemorrhage is uncommon. Hypoglossal nerve palsy occurs rarely. It is usually associated with an ulcer in the posterior glossotonsillar sulcus.

Occasionally a patient cured of advanced base of tongue cancer by radiation therapy may have difficulty swallowing solid

TABLE 26.2-15. Base of Tongue: Local Control According to Stage

Series	No. of Patients	% T4	Boost Technique	T1	T2	T3	T4	Overall
				*Local Control (%)*				
SURGERY ± ADJUVANT RADIATION THERAPY								
Mayo Clinic, Rochester, MN[211]	79	0	NA	84	87	76	ND	82
University of Pennsylvania, Philadelphia[212]	17	41	NA	ND	ND	ND	ND	77
Memorial Sloan-Kettering Cancer Center, New York, NY[213]	100	19	NA	ND	ND	ND	ND	82[a]
Washington University, St. Louis, MO[214]	101	9	NA	ND	ND	ND	ND	74
RADIATION THERAPY								
Memorial Sloan-Kettering Cancer Center, New York, NY[215,b]	68	3	[192]Ir	87	93	82	100[c]	89
Institut Gustave Roussy, Villejuif, France[216,b]	108	0	[192]Ir	85	50	69	ND	64
Hôpital Henri Mondor, Creteil, France[217,b]	48	0	[192]Ir	85	71	ND	ND	ND
M. D. Anderson Cancer Center, Houston, TX[218,d]	174	17	EBRT	91	71	78	52	74
M. D. Anderson Cancer Center, Houston, TX[219,b]	54	2	EBRT	100	96	67	ND	85
Institut Curie, Paris, France[220,b]	166	20	EBRT	96	57	45	23	44
University of Florida, Gainesville[221,b]	217	19	EBRT	96	91	81	38	79

EBRT, external-beam radiation therapy; ^{192}Ir, iridium 192 interstitial brachytherapy boost; NA, not applicable; ND, no data.
[a]First site of failure.
[b]Two patients.
[c]Crude local control rates.
[d]Actuarial.
(From ref. 221, with permission.)

foods. The action of the base of the tongue is to force the bolus of food into the hypopharynx, and loss of full motion impedes swallowing. This is probably a result of some fibrosis of the base of the tongue compounded by xerostomia. The addition of a radical neck dissection to radiation therapy increases the risk of this problem. Significant aspiration is unusual. It is rare for a patient to develop severe swallowing disability requiring feeding tube support.[107]

TABLE 26.2-16. Base of Tongue: Local-Regional Control According to American Joint Committee on Cancer Stage

Series	No. of Patients	% Stage IV	I	II	III	IV	Overall
			*Local-Regional Recurrence (%)*				
SURGERY ± ADJUVANT RADIATION THERAPY							
M. D. Anderson Cancer Center, Houston, TX[222,a]	34	76	ND	ND	ND	ND	56
Mayo Clinic, Rochester, MN[211,a]	79	33	56	79	55	54	59
Memorial Sloan-Kettering Cancer Center, New York, NY[213,a]	100	36	ND	ND	ND	ND	72[b]
Washington University, St. Louis, MO[214,c]	101	45	100	75	67	40	57
University of Pennsylvania, Philadelphia[212,c]	17	59	ND	ND	ND	ND	68
RADIATION THERAPY							
M. D. Anderson Cancer Center, Houston, TX[219,c]	54	63	ND	100	79	72	76
Memorial Medical Center, Long Beach, CA[223,a]	70	57	ND	100	75	73	77
University of Florida, Gainesville[221,c]	217	71	100	100	83	~65[d]	72

ND, no data.
[a]Crude local-regional control rate.
[b]First site of failure.
[c]Actuarial local-regional control rates.
[d]IVA, 64%; IVB, 66%.
(From ref. 221, with permission.)

TABLE 26.2-17.   Base of Tongue: Survival

Series	No. of Patients	% T4	% Stage IV	Overall (FU) (%)	Cause-Specific (FU) (%)
SURGERY ± ADJUVANT RADIATION THERAPY					
Mayo Clinic, Rochester, MN[211]	79	0	33	51 (5 y)	65 (5 y)
Memorial Sloan-Kettering Cancer Center, New York, NY[213]	100	19	36	55 (5 y)	65 (5 y)
Washington University, St. Louis, MO[214]	101	9	45	45 (5 y)	ND
University of Pennsylvania, Philadelphia[212]	17	41	59	46 (3 y)	ND
RADIATION THERAPY					
M. D. Anderson Cancer Center, Houston, TX[219]	54	2	63	59 (5 y)	65 (5 y)
Memorial Sloan-Kettering Cancer Center, New York, NY[215]	68	3	51	87 (5 y)	ND
Institut Curie, Paris, France[220]	166	20	57	27 (5 y)	ND
Institut Gustave Roussy, Villejuif, France[216]	108	0	30	26 (5 y)	ND
Memorial Medical Center, Long Beach, CA[223]	70	17	57	35 (5 y)	60 (5 y)
University of Florida, Gainesville[221]	217	19	71	50 (5 y)	64 (5 y)

FU, follow-up; ND, no data.
(From ref. 221, with permission.)

Treatment: Tonsillar Area

SELECTION OF TREATMENT MODALITY

Early (T1 or T2). Early lesions are generally treated by irradiation with a high rate of success and relatively low morbidity. A small lesion may be cured by wide local excision or tonsillectomy. A surgical approach for larger lesions usually implies removal of the mandible, the tonsillar area including both pillars, part of the soft palate, and part of the tongue; in addition, an ipsilateral neck dissection is performed even with a clinically negative neck. The functional loss from this operation is not justified in view of the high success rate with irradiation, which leaves the patient intact. Even a dry mouth may be avoided when well-lateralized lesions are treated by techniques that allow at least partial salivary recovery.[11] An operation often salvages the few radiation treatment failures. The local control rate is better for T1 or T2 tonsillar fossa lesions than for anterior tonsillar pillar lesions.[108] The cure rates after surgery alone or surgery combined with radiation therapy are similar (Tables 26.2-19 to 26.2-21). Therefore, primary radiation therapy is the preferred treatment for essentially all patients with tonsillar cancer.

Moderately Advanced (Late T2 or T3). For treatment of moderately advanced lesions, there are advocates of combining surgery and radiation therapy as the initial therapy and advocates of definitive radiation therapy with or without neck dissection, with surgery reserved for radiation therapy failure. Definitive radiation therapy is preferred at the University of Florida.

Advanced (Late T3 or T4). The preferred treatment for patients with unfavorable endophytic T3 and T4 carcinomas is radiation therapy and concomitant chemotherapy. There is no advantage

TABLE 26.2-18.   Base of Tongue: Severe Complications

Series	No. of Patients	% T4	Boost Technique	% Severe Complications	% Fatal
SURGERY ± ADJUVANT RADIATION THERAPY					
M. D. Anderson Cancer Center, Houston, TX[222]	34	41	NA	26	18
University of Pennsylvania, Philadelphia[212]	17	41	NA	29	0
Memorial Sloan-Kettering Cancer Center, New York, NY[213]	100	19	NA	ND[a]	0
Washington University, St. Louis, MO[214]	101	9	NA	28	4
M. D. Anderson Cancer Center, Houston, TX[224]	51	ND	NA	ND[a]	2
RADIATION THERAPY					
Memorial Sloan-Kettering Cancer Center, New York, NY[215]	68	3	192Ir	0	0
Hôpital Henri Mondor, Creteil, France[217]	48	0	192Ir	0	0
Institut Gustave Roussy, Villejuif, France[216]	108	0	192Ir	0	0
Memorial Medical Center, Long Beach, CA[223]	70	17	192Ir	0	0
M. D. Anderson Cancer Center, Houston, TX[218]	174	17	EBRT	3	0
M. D. Anderson Cancer Center, Houston, TX[219]	54	2	EBRT	0	0
University of Florida, Gainesville[221]	217	19	EBRT	4	1[b]

EBRT, external-beam radiation therapy; 192Ir, iridium 192; NA, not applicable; ND, no data.
[a]Postoperative complications were not graded according to severity.
[b]One patient died of myocardial infarction after neck dissection; one patient had fatal radiation-induced sarcoma.
(From ref. 221, with permission.)

TABLE 26.2-19. Tonsillar Squamous Cell Carcinoma: Local Control

Institution	Treatment	No. of Patients	% T4	Local Control (%)				
				T1	T2	T3	T4	Overall
Washington University Medical Center, St. Louis, MO[225]	Surgery + RT	230	14	80[a]	71[a]	65[a]	58[a]	68
Mayo Clinic, Rochester, MN[226]	Surgery ± RT	72	3	78[a]	76[a]	44[a]	0/2	71
Roswell Park Cancer Institute, Buffalo, NY[227]	Surgery	56	ND	ND	ND	ND	ND	75[a]
Memorial Medical Center, Long Beach, CA[228]	RT-[192]Ir	80	24	ND	ND	ND	ND	84[a]
Centre Alexis Vautrin, Vandoeu-vre-les-Nancy, France[229]	RT-[192]Ir	361	1	89[b]	85[b]	67[b]	ND	80[b]
Institut Curie, Paris, France[230]	RT	465	35	90[b]	84[b]	64[b]	47[b]	64[b]
M. D. Anderson Cancer Center, Houston, TX[231]	RT	150	5	94[a]	81[a]	67[a]	63[a]	75[a]
Washington University Medical Center, St. Louis, MO[225]	RT	154	23	76[a]	63[a]	59[a]	33[a]	56[a]
University of Maryland Hospital, Baltimore[232]	RT	185	14	94[c]	80[c]	51[c]	19[c]	58[c]
University of Florida, Gainesville[108]	RT	400	17	83[b]	81[b]	74[b]	60[b]	76[b]

[192]Ir, iridium 192 boost; ND, no data; RT, radiation therapy.
[a]Crude local control rates.
[b]Actuarial local control rates.
[c]Patients who died with intercurrent disease less than 2 y after treatment were excluded.
(From ref. 108, with permission.)

or improvement in either local-regional control or survival for patients treated with combined surgery and irradiation, and the risk of complications is higher (Table 26.2-22). Patients with an incomplete response in the neck are evaluated for a neck dissection 4 to 6 weeks after chemoradiation.

SURGICAL TREATMENT. Surgical treatment for early cancers of the tonsillar pillars consists of a wide local excision, including tonsillectomy, through a transoral approach. Larger lesions may require removal of the adjacent mandible as well as a portion of the tongue and soft palate. Depending on the size of the defect, a tongue, deltopectoral, or osteomyocutaneous flap may be required to close the defect. Flaps are usually necessary for extensive lesions or after radiation therapy failure. Deglutition is not generally a problem, but some patients remain on liquid diets. Chewing is difficult because a portion of the mandible has been removed, and the patient will be unable to wear dentures. Speech may be impaired if a signifi-

TABLE 26.2-20. Tonsillar Squamous Cell Carcinoma: Local-Regional Control

Institution	Treatment	No. of Patients	% Stage IV	Local-Regional Control (%)				
				I	II	III	IV	Overall
Mayo Clinic, Rochester, MN[226]	Surgery ± RT	72	25	73[a]	69[a]	53[a]	56[a]	63[a]
University of California School of Medicine, San Francisco[233]	Surgery ± RT	40	ND	ND	ND	ND	ND	73[a]
Roswell Park Cancer Institute, Buffalo, NY[227]	Surgery	56	29	78[a]		43[a]		48[a]
Memorial Medical Center, Long Beach, CA[228]	RT-[192]Ir	80	49	3/3	100[a]	85[a]	56[a]	75[a]
Centre Alexis Vautrin, Vandoeuvre-les-Nancy, France[229]	RT-[192]Ir	361	8	ND	ND	ND	ND	75[b]
Institut Curie, Paris, France[230]	RT	465	37	ND	ND	ND	ND	58[a]
M. D. Anderson Cancer Center, Houston, TX[234]	RT	83	53	ND	76[b]	65[b]	87[b]	77[b]
University of Florida, Gainesville[108]	RT	400	56	63[b]	73[b]	85[b]	IVA, 65 IVB, 52	70[b]

[192]Ir, iridium 192 boost; ND, no data; RT, radiation therapy.
[a]Crude local-regional control rates.
[b]Actuarial local-regional control rates.
(From ref. 108, with permission.)

TABLE 26.2-21. Tonsillar Squamous Cell Carcinoma: Survival

Institution	Treatment	No. of Patients	% Stage IV	5-Y Survival Rates (%)	
				Absolute	Cause-Specific
Roswell Park Cancer Institute, Buffalo, NY[227]	Surgery	56	29	ND	61
University of Cincinnati Medical Center, Cincinnati[235]	Surgery + RT	82	39	ND	56
University of Virginia Medical Center, Charlottesville[236]	Surgery + RT	22	68	ND	32
Upstate Medical Center, Syracuse, NY[237]	Surgery + RT	47	45	ND	57
University of Iowa, Iowa City[238]	Surgery + RT	20	20	ND	20
Centre Alexis Vautrin, Vandoeuvre-les-Nancy, France[229]	RT-[192]Ir	361	8	53	63
M. D. Anderson Cancer Center, Houston, TX[231]	RT	150	ND	ND	70
M. D. Anderson Cancer Center, Houston, TX[234]	RT	83	53	60	71
Princess Margaret Hospital, Toronto, Ontario[239]	RT	372	~54	38	54
University of Maryland Medical Center, Baltimore[232]	RT	185	46	30	42
University of Florida, Gainesville[108]	RT	400	56	49	70

[192]Ir, iridium 192 boost; ND, no data; RT, radiation therapy.
(From ref. 108, with permission.)

cant portion of the tongue or palate has been removed. A prosthesis may be needed for the palatal defect.

IRRADIATION TECHNIQUE. The basic portal arrangement depends on the extent of the local lesion and presence or absence of positive lymph nodes. The risk for contralateral lymph node metastases is low unless there is tongue invasion, invasion of the soft palate within 1 cm of the midline, or extensive clinically positive nodes in the ipsilateral neck.[11] If these risk features are absent, a wedge pair technique using 4 or 6 MV x-ray beams is used. An alternative is an *en face* combination of photon and electron beams to reduce the dose to the contralateral mucosa and salivary glands, if the medial extent of the primary lesion is no more than 4 cm from the ipsilateral skin surface. The major advantage of these techniques is a lower incidence of xerostomia secondary to partial preservation of minor and major salivary gland function on the contralateral side.

Lesions with extension 1 cm or more into the tongue or within 1 cm of the midline on the soft palate, as well as those with N3 neck disease, have a higher risk for positive nodes in the contralateral side of the neck and are treated with parallel opposed photon portals, usually weighted 2 to 1 or 3 to 2 to the involved side. If there are positive contralateral nodes or extension across the midline, the portals usually are equally weighted. The inferior border is placed 2 cm below the primary tumor. Depending on tumor extent, IMRT may be an option. The low neck is treated with a separate anterior field with a thin midline block over the larynx. Small, discrete lesions of the anterior tonsillar pillar may receive part of the treatment by intraoral cone.

The dose for tonsillar lesions is 74.4 to 76.8 Gy (1.2 Gy twice daily) for T1 to T3 lesions, and 76.8 Gy for T4 lesions.

MANAGEMENT OF RECURRENCE. An operation will salvage a good portion of T1 or T2 radiation therapy failures, but only an occasional advanced lesion is salvaged.

Results of Treatment: Tonsillar Area

The results and the complications after surgery alone or surgery combined with adjuvant irradiation are compared with those for radiation therapy alone in Tables 26.2-19 to 26.2-22.

TABLE 26.2-22. Tonsillar Squamous Cell Carcinoma: Severe Complications

Institution	Treatment	No. of Patients	Severe Complications (%)	Fatal Complications (%)
Washington University Medical Center, St. Louis, MO[225]	Preop RT + surgery	144	24	5
	Surgery + postop RT	86	24	2
Mayo Clinic, Rochester, MN[226]	Surgery ± RT	72	21	0
Memorial Medical Center, Long Beach, CA[228]	RT-[192]Ir	80	3	0
Centre Alexis Vautrin, Vandoeuvre-les-Nancy, France[229]	RT-[192]Ir	361	2	0.2
M. D. Anderson Cancer Center, Houston, TX[234]	RT	83	2	0
Princess Margaret Hospital, Toronto, Ontario[239]	RT	372	3	0
Washington University Medical Center, St. Louis, MO[225]	RT	154	10	1
Institut Gustave Roussy, Villejuif, France[240]	RT	193	6	0
University of Florida, Gainesville[108]	RT	400	8[a]	1[a]

[192]Ir, iridium 192 boost; preop, preoperative; postop, postoperative; RT, radiation therapy.
[a]Includes complications after planned neck dissection (8 patients) and salvage surgery (5 patients), and late treatment complications (19 patients).
(From ref. 108, with permission.)

There is no improvement in local-regional control or survival for patients who are treated surgically.[106]

Complications of Treatment: Tonsillar Area

RADIATION THERAPY. The risk for a severe complication, usually a bone or soft tissue necrosis, requiring surgical intervention is very low. The probability of a fatal complication is remote. An occasional patient, usually one treated for advanced disease, may have long-term swallowing problems. Other complications include trismus, hypoglossal nerve entrapment, and a remote risk of a radiation-induced malignancy or myelitis or both.

SURGERY. Complications of operation include oropharyngeal dysfunction (limited or no ability to swallow, and drooling), fistula, failure of flaps, complications of neck dissection, and aspiration occasionally leading to laryngectomy. The risk of severe or fatal complications is higher after surgery than after radiation therapy (see Table 26.2-22).

Treatment: Soft Palate

SELECTION OF TREATMENT MODALITY. Recommendations for management of soft palate cancer must consider the primary lesion and both sides of the neck. Although small, well-defined lesions may be excised and the neck observed, the risk of subclinical disease in the retropharyngeal or cervical nodes is high. Therefore, irradiation is the modality most often selected for all soft palate carcinomas. Neck dissection is added as needed. Concomitant chemotherapy should be considered for patients with T3 or T4 or advanced N2 or N3 disease (or both).

SURGICAL TREATMENT. Small, discrete lesions can be managed by transoral excision and repaired by a pharyngeal flap to prevent any velopharyngeal incompetence. Tonsillectomy may also be necessary to obtain an adequate margin. If full-thickness resection is necessary, however, then a prosthesis generally is required to restore velopharyngeal competence. Operations for salvage after failure of radiation therapy should generally include full-thickness removal of the soft palate.

IRRADIATION TECHNIQUE. The irradiation technique for early and advanced lesions involves equally weighted parallel opposed external-beam portals that include the primary lesion and the first-echelon upper neck nodes on both sides. A separate anterior portal is used to treat the low neck. If the primary lesion is discrete and the neck is clinically negative, a portion of the treatment may be given with an intraoral cone

before external-beam radiation when the lesion is clearly visible and the mouth is not yet sore from the radiation reaction.

Patients are treated with 4-MV to 6-MV photons to 74.4 to 76.8 Gy at 1.2 Gy/fraction, twice daily, in a continuous course.

COMBINED TREATMENT POLICIES. Combined therapy is seldom planned because of the success rate with radiation therapy and the morbidity associated with resection of the soft palate.

MANAGEMENT OF RECURRENCE. Soft tissue necrosis is uncommon after radiation therapy; thus, a persistent ulcer is the hallmark of recurrent disease after irradiation. Recurrence after irradiation is treated by surgical removal when feasible, and salvage is successful in a few patients.

Results of Treatment: Soft Palate

SURGICAL RESULTS. Ratzer and coworkers[109] reported the Memorial Sloan-Kettering Cancer Center results for 299 patients with squamous cell carcinoma of the soft palate; 112 were treated by surgery, 139 by radiation therapy, and 22 by combined treatment. The 5-year absolute survival rate was 21% and the cause-specific survival rate for the group treated by surgery alone was 38%. The main cause of failure was recurrence at the primary site.

IRRADIATION RESULTS. Erkal and coworkers[110] reported on 107 patients treated with radiation therapy alone or radiation therapy combined with a planned neck dissection at the University of Florida between 1965 and 1996. Local control rates at 5 years after radiation therapy were as follows: T1, 86%; T2, 91%; T3, 67%; and T4, 36%. Two patients received induction chemotherapy; no patient received concomitant chemotherapy. Local-regional control, distant metastasis–free survival, and survival rates are depicted in Table 26.2-23.

Complications of Treatment: Soft Palate

SURGICAL COMPLICATIONS. Nasal speech and regurgitation of food into the nasopharynx are sequelae of full-thickness resection of the soft palate. A prosthesis is only partially successful in correcting the functional defect when the defect is large. Oropharyngeal dysfunction may occur.

COMPLICATIONS OF IRRADIATION. Complications of irradiation are few. Soft tissue necrosis of the soft palate is uncommon; an ulcer must be considered to be a possible recurrence. The soft palate may become retracted after successful

TABLE 26.2-23. Soft Palate: 5-Year Outcomes after Radiation Therapy in 107 Patients

1983 AJCC Stage	No. of Patients	LR Control (%)	Ultimate LR Control (%)	DMFS (%)	CSS (%)	Survival (%)
I	14	82	90	93	84	40
II	25	83	92	100	91	66
III	26	68	84	92	74	52
IV	42	51	60	85	48	21

AJCC, American Joint Committee on Cancer; CSS, cause-specific survival; DMFS, distant metastases–free survival; LR, local-regional.
(Data from ref. 110.)

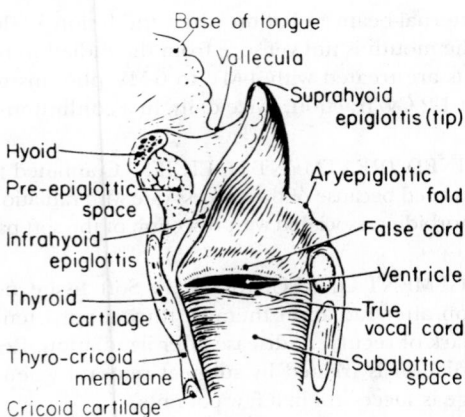

FIGURE 26.2-13. Diagrammatic sagittal section of the larynx. (Redrawn from Sabbotta drawings in Clemente CD: *Anatomy: a regional atlas of the human body.* Philadelphia: Lea & Febiger, 1975, with permission. Copyright 1975, Urban & Schwarzenberg München, Berlin, Vienna.)

treatment of advanced lesions; this may result in regurgitation into the nasopharynx and slight alteration in speech. Small perforations may persist after successful treatment at sites where tumor has grown through the soft palate. Bone necrosis requiring surgical management is relatively rare. Severe late complications were observed in 3 of 107 patients (3%) treated with definitive radiation therapy at the University of Florida.[110]

LARYNX

Cancer of the larynx is related primarily to cigarette smoking. The risk of tobacco-related cancers of the upper alimentary and respiratory tracts declines among ex-smokers after 5 years and is said to approach the risk of nonsmokers after 10 years of abstention.[111]

The importance of alcohol use in the etiology of laryngeal cancer remains unclear, but it is probably less important than in cancers of the other head and neck sites, for which alcohol use can be shown to be synergistic with tobacco use.[112]

Anatomy

The larynx is composed of several cartilages connected by ligaments and muscles, divided anatomically into the supraglottic, glottic, and subglottic regions. The supraglottic larynx consists of the epiglottis, false vocal cords, ventricles, aryepiglottic folds, and arytenoids; the arytenoids are cartilages that articulate on the cricoid (Fig. 26.2-13). The glottis includes the true vocal cords and the anterior commissure. The subglottic area is 2 cm long and extends from 5 mm below the free edge of the true vocal cords to the upper margin of the first tracheal ring.

The preepiglottic space is an important anatomic region because of frequent direct extension to this area. It is bounded by the epiglottis posteriorly, the hyoepiglottic ligament and vallecula superiorly, and the thyroid cartilage and thyrohyoid membrane anteriorly and laterally. It can be seen as a low-density area on a CT scan.

The supraglottic structures have a moderately rich capillary lymphatic plexus. The lymphatic trunks pass through the preepiglottic space and the thyrohyoid membrane to the subdi-

gastric nodes. A few trunks drain directly to the middle or lower jugular chain. There are essentially no capillary lymphatics of the true vocal cords. As a result, lymphatic spread from glottic cancer rarely occurs unless tumor extends to supraglottic or subglottic areas. The subglottic area has relatively few capillary lymphatics. The lymphatic trunks pass through the thyrocricoid membrane to the pretracheal (delphian) node(s) in the region of the thyroid isthmus, or the trunks may carry the tumor to the lower jugular nodes. The pretracheal nodes are midline in position and even when clinically positive are small (1 to 5 mm to rarely more than 1 to 2 cm). The subglottic area also drains posteriorly through the cricotracheal membrane, with some trunks going to the paratracheal (level VI) nodes whereas others pass to the inferior jugular chain.

Pathology

The laryngeal surfaces of the epiglottis and vocal cords are lined with stratified squamous epithelium and the remainder of the larynx is lined with pseudostratified ciliated columnar epithelium. Nearly all malignant tumors of the larynx arise from the surface epithelium and therefore are squamous cell carcinoma or one of its variants.

Minor salivary gland tumors arise from the mucous glands, but are rare; even more rare is the appearance of a soft tissue sarcoma, malignant lymphoma, small cell neuroendocrine carcinoma, or plasmacytoma. Benign hemangiomas, chondromas, and osteochondromas are reported, but their malignant counterparts are rare.

Carcinoma *in situ* is common on the vocal cords. Distinction between dysplasia, carcinoma *in situ*, squamous cell carcinoma with microinvasion, and true invasive carcinoma is often a problem. In patients with minimal lesions, biopsy of the cord is performed by stripping the mucosa; the specimen tends to curl or fold, which creates difficulty in orientation of the basement membrane. However, the precise distinction among carcinoma *in situ*, microinvasion, and invasive carcinoma is a bit academic. The authors recommend treatment, usually irradiation, for most patients. The local recurrence rate after irradiation for carcinoma *in situ* or microinvasive or invasive carcinoma is, surprisingly, approximately the same within the T1 category; the recurrences are almost always invasive carcinoma.

Most of the vocal cord carcinomas are either well differentiated or moderately well differentiated. In a few cases, there are an apparent carcinoma and sarcoma occurring together, but most of these are, in reality, a carcinoma with spindle cell stroma. The term *pseudosarcoma* is applied to a rare laryngeal lesion, usually polypoid or pedunculated with a string-like umbilical cord. It has a favorable prognosis. Verrucous carcinoma occurs on the vocal cords in 1% to 2% of patients with carcinoma.

Supraglottic carcinomas are less differentiated than those of the vocal cord; verrucous lesions are rare. Carcinoma *in situ* is rarely diagnosed as a distinct entity in the supraglottis, although a zone *in situ* may be seen at the margin between invasive tumor and normal mucosa.

Patterns of Spread

SUPRAGLOTTIC LARYNX

Suprahyoid Epiglottis. Some lesions of the suprahyoid epiglottis may grow like a mushroom, producing a huge exophytic mass with little tendency to destruction of cartilage or spread to adjacent structures. Others may infiltrate the tip and produce destruction of cartilage and eventual amputation of the tip. The latter lesions tend to invade the vallecula and preepiglottic space, the lateral pharyngeal walls, and the remainder of the supraglottic larynx.

Infrahyoid Epiglottis. Lesions of the infrahyoid epiglottis tend to produce irregular outgrowths of tumor nodules with simultaneous invasion through the porous epiglottic cartilage into the preepiglottic space. They grow circumferentially to involve the false cords, aryepiglottic folds, and eventually the medial wall of the pyriform sinus and the pharyngoepiglottic fold. Invasion of the anterior commissure and cords is usually a late phenomenon, and subglottic extension occurs only in advanced lesions. Lesions that extend onto or below the vocal cords are at a high risk for cartilage invasion, even if the cords are mobile.[113] Tumor may burrow through the epiglottic cartilage and preepiglottic fat space and present in the vallecula and base of the tongue without involving the suprahyoid epiglottis.

False Cord. Early false cord carcinomas usually have the appearance of a submucosal mass and are difficult to delineate accurately by indirect examination. They extend toward the thyroid cartilage and medial wall of the pyriform sinus. Extension to the infrahyoid epiglottis is common. Initial invasion of the vocal cord may occur submucosally and may be difficult to detect. Gross invasion of the vocal cord is often associated with thyroid cartilage invasion. Subglottic extension is uncommon until the lesion is advanced.

Aryepiglottic Fold and Arytenoid. Early lesions are usually exophytic. It is often difficult to decide whether they start on the medial wall of the pyriform sinus or the aryepiglottic fold. As the lesions advance, they extend to adjacent sites and eventually cause fixation of the larynx due to involvement of the cricoarytenoid muscle and joint. Advanced lesions invade the base of the tongue, pharyngeal wall, and postcricoid pharynx.

VOCAL CORD. The majority of lesions begin on the free margin and upper surface of the vocal cord and are easily visible. When diagnosed, approximately two-thirds are confined to one cord. The anterior two-thirds of the cord is the most common site, and extension to the anterior commissure is frequent. As vocal cord lesions enlarge, they extend to the ventricle, false cord, vocal process of the arytenoids, and subglottic region. Infiltrative lesions invade the vocal ligament and thyroarytenoid muscles, eventually reaching the thyroid cartilage. As cancers reach the cartilage, they tend at first to grow up or down along the paraglottic fat space rather than invading the cartilage. The conus elasticus acts initially as a barrier to subglottic penetration. Advanced glottic lesions eventually penetrate through the thyroid cartilage or thyrocricoid membrane to enter the neck and invade the thyroid gland.

SUBGLOTTIC LARYNX. Subglottic cancers are uncommon. It is difficult to determine whether a tumor started on the undersurface of the vocal cord or in the true subglottic larynx with extension to the cord. These lesions involve the cricoid cartilage quite early, because there is no intervening muscle layer. Fixation of a cord is common.

LYMPHATIC SPREAD

Supraglottic. The incidence of clinically positive nodes is 55% at the time of diagnosis; 16% are bilateral (Fig. 26.2-14).[10] Elective neck dissection shows pathologically positive nodes in 16% to 26% of cases. Observation of the neck is followed by the appearance of positive nodes in approximately 33% of cases. Extralaryngeal spread to the pyriform sinus and vallecula or base of the tongue increases the risk of node metastases. Delphian node involvement is rare and associated with extension to the anterior commissure or subglottic area.

Glottic. The incidence of clinically positive nodes at diagnosis approaches zero for lesions confined to the cords (T1) and is 2% and 5% for T2 lesions.[114] The incidence of neck metastases increases to 20% to 30% for T3 and T4 lesions. Supraglottic spread is associated with metastasis to the jugulodigastric nodes. Anterior commissure and anterior subglottic invasion is associated with midjugular, lower jugular, and midline pretracheal (delphian) node involvement. Delphian node involvement is associated with spread to the lower neck nodes on both sides and a high rate of neck failure when treated by surgery alone.[115]

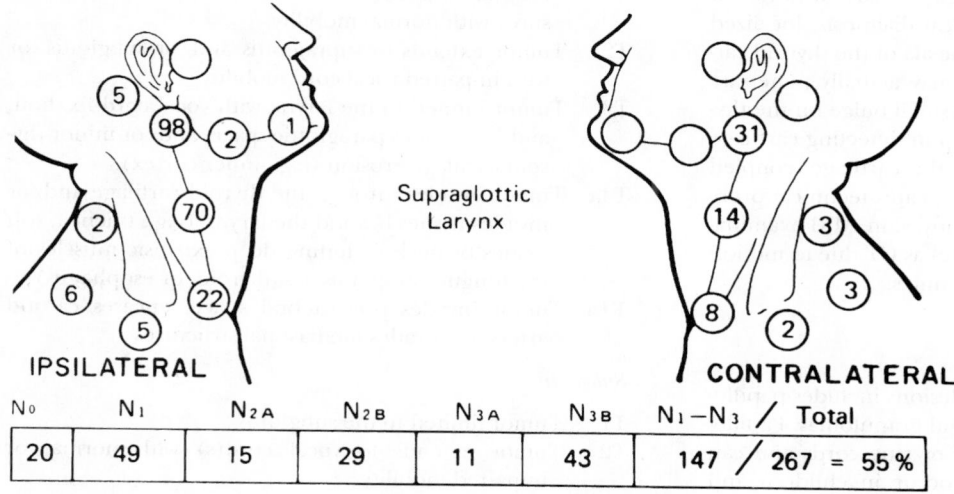

N0	N1	N2A	N2B	N3A	N3B	N1–N3 / Total
20	49	15	29	11	43	147 / 267 = 55%

FIGURE 26.2-14. Supraglottic laryngeal carcinoma: nodal distribution on admission at M. D. Anderson Hospital, 1948 to 1965. The circled numbers indicate the number of times the particular lymph node was involved. (From ref. 10, with permission.)

Subglottic. Lederman[116] reported a 10% incidence of clinically positive lymph nodes on admission. Spread is primarily to the delphian nodes and the lower jugular chain.

Clinical Picture

PRESENTING SYMPTOMS

Vocal Cords. Carcinoma arising on the true vocal cords produces hoarseness at a very early stage. Pain or sore throat is a symptom of advanced lesions. Dysphagia and airway obstruction producing respiratory distress are features of advanced lesions and are rarely seen even with bulky early-stage tumors.

Supraglottic Larynx. Hoarseness is not a prominent symptom for cancer of the supraglottis until the lesion becomes extensive. Pain on swallowing is the most frequent initial symptom and is often described as a mild, persistent irritation or sore throat. Often the patient can point to the area with one finger. Cancer of the epiglottis may be quite large before symptoms are produced. Pain is referred to the ear by way of the vagus nerve and auricular nerve of Arnold. A mass in the neck may be the first sign of a supraglottic cancer. Late symptoms include weight loss, foul breath, dysphagia, and aspiration.

PHYSICAL EXAMINATION. In addition to the laryngeal mirror, flexible fiberoptic endoscopes are routinely used to complement the mirror examination. Determination of the mobility of the larynx frequently requires multiple examinations because the subtle distinctions between mobile, partially fixed, and fixed cords are often difficult to make. A cord that appeared mobile before direct laryngoscopy may show sluggish motion or even a fixation after biopsy.

Invasion of the preepiglottic space occurs more frequently than one can diagnose clinically. Ulceration of the infrahyoid epiglottis or fullness of the vallecula is an indirect sign of preepiglottic space invasion. Palpation of diffuse, firm fullness above the thyroid notch with widening of the space between the hyoid and thyroid cartilages signifies invasion of the preepiglottic space. Lateral soft tissue radiographs of the neck may show irregular air cavities in patients with lesions of the suprahyoid epiglottis that invade into the preepiglottic space. CT scan is excellent in showing involvement of the preepiglottic space.

Postcricoid extension may be suspected when the laryngeal "click" disappears on physical examination. Early invasion of the thyroid cartilage is a difficult clinical diagnosis; localized pain or tenderness to palpation over one ala of the thyroid cartilage is suggestive. Advanced tumors may actually penetrate through the thyroid ala and be felt as a small bulge on the thyroid ala. CT scan of the larynx is of help in detecting cartilage invasion, but irregular calcification of the cartilage, coupled with volume averaging of the CT slice, creates technical problems in interpretation of early cartilage invasion. MRI examination of the larynx has not been as helpful as CT due to motion artifact associated with longer scanning times.

Differential Diagnosis

The differential diagnosis of laryngeal lesions includes papillomas, polyps, vocal nodules, fibromas, and granulomas. Papillomas can involve the epiglottis or false or true cords and can extend subglottically. They generally occur in children and young adults, possibly persisting into adulthood. Vocal polyps and nodules occur at the junction of the middle and anterior one-third of the true vocal cords. There is usually a history of voice abuse followed by hoarseness.

Granulomas of the larynx usually occur as a result of intubation and are located on the posterior one-third of the vocal cords, near the posterior commissure. Endoscopic removal is the definitive treatment. Tuberculosis of the larynx, although rare, still occurs. Generally, the lesion is destructive and occurs at the posterior commissure of the glottis, but the epiglottis and false cords may be involved. The appearance mimics that of cancer; pulmonary tuberculosis is usually present.

AJCC Staging

The AJCC staging system for primary tumors of the larynx is as follows[16]:

Primary Tumor (T)

TX	Primary tumor cannot be assessed
T0	No evidence of primary tumor
Tis	Carcinoma *in situ*

Supraglottis

T1	Tumor limited to one subsite of supraglottis with normal vocal cord mobility
T2	Tumor invades mucosa of more than one adjacent subsite of supraglottis or region outside the supraglottis (e.g., mucosa of base of the tongue, vallecula, medial wall of pyriform sinus) without fixation of the larynx
T3	Tumor limited to larynx with vocal cord fixation and/or invades any of the following: postcricoid area, preepiglottic tissues, paraglottic space, and/or minor thyroid cartilage erosion (e.g., inner cortex)
T4a	Tumor invades through the thyroid cartilage and/or invades tissues beyond the larynx (e.g., trachea, soft tissues of neck including deep extrinsic muscles of the tongue, strap muscles, thyroid, or esophagus)
T4b	Tumor invades prevertebral space, encases carotid artery, or invades mediastinal structures

Glottis

T1	Tumor limited to one (T1a) or both (T1b) vocal cord(s) (may involve anterior or posterior commissure) with normal mobility
T2	Tumor extends to supraglottis and/or subglottis, or with impaired vocal cord mobility
T3	Tumor limited to the larynx with vocal cord fixation, and/or invades paraglottic space, and/or minor thyroid cartilage erosion (e.g., inner cortex)
T4a	Tumor invades through the thyroid cartilage and/or invades tissues beyond the larynx (e.g., trachea, soft tissues of neck including deep extrinsic muscles of the tongue, strap muscles, thyroid, or esophagus)
T4b	Tumor invades prevertebral space, encases carotid artery, or invades mediastinal structures

Subglottis

T1	Tumor limited to the subglottis
T2	Tumor extends to vocal cord(s) with normal or impaired mobility

T3	Tumor limited to larynx with vocal cord fixation
T4a	Tumor invades cricoid or thyroid cartilage and/or tissues beyond the larynx (e.g., trachea, soft tissues of neck including deep extrinsic muscles of the tongue, strap muscles, thyroid, or esophagus)
T4b	Tumor invades prevertebral space, encases carotid artery, or invades mediastinal structures

Treatment

VOCAL CORD CARCINOMA

Selection of Treatment Modality. The goal is cure with the best functional result and the least risk of a serious complication.

DYSPLASIA, HYPERKERATOSIS, LEUKOPLAKIA. Complete stripping of the mucosa of the cord is often curative for lesions classified as leukoplakia, hyperkeratosis, or dysplasia. Careful observation is essential because regrowth often occurs. Although repeated stripping may seem a satisfactory plan of management, the cords may become thickened and the voice harsh, and it becomes increasingly difficult to tell whether invasive tumor is present. Irradiation may be recommended when there are repeated recurrences at short intervals.[117]

CARCINOMA *IN SITU.* Stripping the cord may sometimes control lesions diagnosed as carcinoma *in situ.* However, it is difficult to exclude the possibility of microinvasion in these specimens. Recurrence is frequent, and the cord may become thickened and the voice hoarse with repeated stripping. The authors recommend irradiation for carcinoma *in situ* in patients with multiple recurrences appearing in rapid succession.[117] Many of the patients diagnosed in the past as having carcinoma *in situ* had obvious residual gross lesions that probably contained invasive carcinoma. The authors have sometimes proceeded with radiation therapy rather than put the patient through a repeat biopsy.

EARLY VOCAL CORD LESION (T1, T2). In most centers, irradiation is the initial treatment prescribed for early lesions, with operation reserved for salvage of irradiation treatment failure. Although cordectomy or hemilaryngectomy produces comparable cure rates for selected T1 or T2 vocal cord lesions, irradiation is generally preferred. The major advantages of irradiation compared to cordectomy or hemilaryngectomy are that a major operation is avoided and the voice quality is likely to be better. The voice after hemilaryngectomy remains hoarse. After successful irradiation, the voice is usually better than before therapy, but occasional cases are seen in which there is no improvement or, uncommonly, a worsening of voice quality. Hemilaryngectomy may be used as a salvage operation in suitable cases after irradiation failure. Even if the patient has a local recurrence after a salvage hemilaryngectomy, there is a third chance with total laryngectomy, which may still be successful. Hemilaryngectomy is also used for patients who have had prior head and neck irradiation and patients who cannot afford 6 weeks away from home or job for the irradiation series. Although there have been reports that anterior commissure involvement predicts radiation therapy failure or necrosis, the authors' data do not support this finding.[114]

Currently, there is an increasing use of the carbon dioxide laser in removing early carcinomas involving the true vocal cords. If the laser is used, it should be used as a cutting instrument rather than for vaporization of the tumor. Using this technique, small midcord lesions may be treated with the laser. Voice quality depends on how much tissue is removed and is not as good as expected after radiation therapy if the tumor involves more than the middle third of one true cord.

Verrucous lesions have the reputation of being unresponsive to irradiation and in some instances of losing their indolent nature to convert into invasive, often anaplastic, metastasizing lesions after unsuccessful treatment. The authors, however, have observed typical verrucous lesions that have disappeared with radiation therapy and not recurred. Burns and coworkers[118] have also made this observation. The authors select partial laryngectomy for early verrucous carcinoma of the glottis, but favor radiation therapy if the alternative is total laryngectomy.

ADVANCED VOCAL CORD LESIONS (T3, T4). The mainstay of treatment for advanced lesions in most centers is total laryngectomy with or without postoperative irradiation. In some centers, radiation therapy is the initial modality for T3 lesions, with surgery reserved for the treatment failures. The most frequent sites of local failure after total laryngectomy are around the tracheal stoma, in the base of the tongue, and in the neck nodes. If the neck is clinically negative before operation and if postoperative irradiation is planned, neck dissection may be withheld and irradiation may be used to treat both sides of the neck. If nodes are clinically positive, a neck dissection is done with total laryngectomy.

Patients with fixed cord lesions (T3) treated by irradiation fall into two groups. One group consists of patients with high-volume, bilateral, advanced lesions who either refuse laryngectomy or are medically inoperable. Irradiation of lesions is seldom successful in these patients; 10% to 20% are cured. The second group includes patients with a fixed cord but minimal total tumor bulk.[119–121] They usually have subglottic extension and minor supraglottic extension confined to one side of the larynx; the airway is adequate and the larynx relatively easy to visualize. An attempt at irradiation in this group is worthwhile and results in a relatively high rate of local control. Concomitant chemotherapy should be considered, particularly if there is evidence of cartilage sclerosis on CT.[44,122] Patients must be followed closely and understand that total laryngectomy may be recommended purely on clinical grounds without biopsy-proven recurrence.

The major difficulty in the use of irradiation for advanced lesions is in distinguishing between radiation edema and local recurrence during follow-up examinations. Progressive edema, increased hoarseness, pain, and immobility of a formerly mobile cord are signs of recurrence. If the edema is stable or limited to the arytenoids, the patient may be watched, especially if there is no pain. The detection of recurrence is difficult because the surface epithelium may be intact, with tumor growing submucosally. Serial CT scans may aid in distinguishing necrosis from recurrent cancer; PET scan may also be useful. Deep biopsies are necessary, but may aggravate the radiation damage if no tumor is found.

Surgical Treatment. Stripping of the cord implies transoral removal of the mucosa of the edge of the cord. The operating microscope assists the surgeon in total stripping of the mucosa.

Cordectomy is an excision of the vocal cord and is usually performed via transoral laser. Its use is generally confined to well-defined lesions involving the middle third of the vocal cord. Although more extensive lesions may be excised, the probability of poor voice quality is related to the amount of tissue removed. The major advantages of laser excision are that it requires a day, as opposed to the 5.5 to 6.0 weeks necessary for radiation therapy, and that irradiation may be reserved in the event the patient develops a metachronous head and neck cancer.

Hemilaryngectomy is a partial, "vertical" laryngectomy allowing removal of limited cord lesions with voice preservation. There are restrictions with this operation. One entire cord plus 5 mm of the opposite cord is the maximum cordal involvement suitable for the operation in men; generally, the operation is reserved for lesions involving one cord. Partial fixation of one cord is not a contraindication to hemilaryngectomy; however, few surgeons attempt hemilaryngectomy for fixed cord lesions. The maximum subglottic extension allowable is 9 to 10 mm anteriorly and 5 mm posteriorly, because the cricoid cartilage must be preserved. Extension to the epiglottis, false cord, or interarytenoid area is a contraindication to hemilaryngectomy. One arytenoid may be sacrificed, but the vocal cord must be fixed in the midline or postoperative aspiration is a possibility, and therefore the patient must have satisfactory pulmonary function. More extensive partial laryngectomies have been described and are associated with a high probability of local control.[123] However, open partial laryngectomies are associated with poor voice quality and are more expensive than a course of radiation therapy; they are usually reserved for salvage of local recurrences after irradiation.

The last surgical alternative is total laryngectomy with or without a neck dissection. Total laryngectomy is used as a salvage procedure for radiation treatment failure in the early lesions that are not suited for conservative operations. It is the operation of choice for advanced lesions. The entire larynx is removed, the pharynx is reconstituted, and a permanent tracheostomy is required.

There have been numerous attempts to re-create the larynx after total laryngectomy, with very few producing predictable results. Prosthetic devices (e.g., the Singer-Blom valve) have been developed for insertion into a tracheoesophageal fistula; the prosthesis allows the patient to speak without the problem of aspiration.[124] Voice rehabilitation was evaluated in 173 patients who underwent a total laryngectomy and postoperative irradiation at the University of Florida; 118 patients were evaluable 2 to 3 years after treatment and 69 patients were evaluated for 5 years or longer.[124] Methods of voice rehabilitation at 2 to 3 years and 5 years or more after surgery were tracheoesophageal speech, 27% and 19%; artificial ("electric") larynx, 50% and 57%; esophageal speech, 1% and 3%; nonvocal, 17% and 14%; and no data, 5% and 7%, respectively.[124]

Irradiation Technique. Irradiation for early vocal cord cancer is delivered by small portals including only the primary lesion. Radiation portals for T1 lesions usually extend from the thyroid notch superiorly to the inferior border of the cricoid; the posterior border depends on posterior extension of the tumor. The field size ranges from 4 × 4 cm to 5 × 5 cm. Portals larger than this increase the risk of edema without increasing the cure rate. Because the portals are small and the skin of the neck is mobile, it is desirable to have the physician check the location of the portal on the treatment table each day by palpation of the anatomic landmarks. The portals for T2 lesions are slightly larger, depending on the anatomic extent of the lesion. Patients receive 2.25 Gy/fraction once daily to 63 Gy (T1 and T2a) or 65.25 Gy (T2b).

Treatment plans for T3 and T4 lesions include the primary lesion and the subdigastric, midjugular, low jugular, and delphian lymph nodes. The initial treatment with twice-a-day fractionation is delivered at 1.2 Gy/fraction to a total of 45.6 Gy. The portal then is reduced to include only the primary lesion; the final tumor dose is 74.4 Gy. The low neck is treated through a separate anterior portal.

Management of Recurrence. With careful follow-up, recurrence often is detected before the patient notices return of hoarseness. Edema of the larynx, particularly the false cords and arytenoids, suggests recurrence. Fixation of the cord usually implies local recurrence; rarely, fixation develops in an otherwise normal appearing cord in the absence of recurrent disease. A paralyzed left vocal cord should also suggest the possibility of lung cancer.

Irradiation treatment failures (T1 or T2) are almost always salvaged by cordectomy, hemilaryngectomy, or total laryngectomy. The salvage rate for T3 lesions recurring after radiation therapy is approximately 60%.[120]

Salvage by radiation therapy for recurrences or new tumors appearing after hemilaryngectomy is approximately 50%. Isolated tracheal stoma recurrences may be managed by radiation therapy or surgery; the chance of cure is relatively low. A multi-institutional surgical experience in the management of stomal recurrence for the years between 1970 and 1985 was reported by Gluckman and coworkers.[125] Forty-one came to operation. The 2-year determinate survival was 24%. Patients with localized recurrences had a 45% 5-year survival rate.

SUPRAGLOTTIC LARYNGEAL CARCINOMA

Selection of Treatment Modality. For purposes of treatment planning, patients may be considered to be in either a favorable group suitable for radiation therapy or supraglottic laryngectomy, or an unfavorable group managed either by total laryngectomy (with or without radiation therapy) or by radiation therapy with laryngectomy reserved for recurrence at the primary site. Patients with unfavorable lesions who are treated with definitive radiation therapy should be considered for concomitant chemotherapy.

EARLY SUPRAGLOTTIC LESIONS. T1 and T2 lesions are favorable cases. Low-volume lesions can be staged T3 without fixation and can be very suitable for definitive radiation therapy or supraglottic laryngectomy. Total laryngectomy is rarely indicated as the initial treatment for this group of patients and is reserved for those in whom the initial treatment fails.

Irradiation and supraglottic laryngectomy are both highly successful modes of therapy for the early lesions, and for this reason it is seldom necessary to combine radiation therapy and surgery for initial management of the primary lesions; however, combined treatment may be indicated to control the neck disease. Approximately 50% of patients having a supraglottic laryngectomy at the University of Florida have received postoperative radiation therapy.

Following are the authors' guidelines for selection of either supraglottic laryngectomy or radiation therapy. The patient and family are often instrumental in making the decision and should be apprised of the alternative modes of therapy. Approximately one-half of the patients seen in the authors' clinic whose lesions are anatomically suitable for treatment by a supraglottic laryngectomy are not suitable for medical reasons (e.g., inadequate pulmonary status or other major medical problems) and are managed by radiation therapy. The only contraindication to radiation therapy is prior radiation therapy to the laryngeal area. Analysis of local disease control by anatomic subsite within the supraglottic larynx shows no obvious differences in local control by radiation therapy when comparing similar stages.[126,127] Similarly, analysis of local control by anatomic subsite shows no obvious difference in local control by supraglottic laryngectomy when comparing similar stages. Transglottic lesions are not suitable for conventional supraglottic laryngectomy, but they may be managed by radiation therapy. Invasion of the preepiglottic space is not a contraindication to supraglottic laryngectomy or radiation therapy.

Mainly exophytic lesions are usually suitable for radiation therapy. Extensive submucosal disease predicts a less favorable result. The likelihood of local control after radiation therapy is related to primary tumor volume calculated from pretreatment CT scan.[45,128]

The status of the neck often determines the selection of treatment for the primary lesion. Patients with clinically negative neck nodes and a high risk for occult bilateral neck disease may be treated by radiation therapy because of the ease of bilateral elective neck irradiation. Alternatively, supraglottic laryngectomy and bilateral conservative neck dissections may be done.

When a patient presents with an early-stage primary lesion and advanced neck disease (N2b or N3), combined treatment is frequently necessary to produce a high rate of control of the neck disease. In these cases, the primary lesion is preferably treated for cure by irradiation, with neck dissection(s) added to the involved side(s) of the neck. If such a patient is managed with supraglottic laryngectomy followed by a neck dissection and postoperative radiation therapy, the functional result is likely to be poorer.

If the patient has early, resectable neck disease (N1 or N2a) and surgery is elected for the primary site, postoperative irradiation is only added because of unexpected findings (e.g., positive margins, multiple positive nodes, or extracapsular spread). The authors prefer to avoid routine high-dose preoperative or postoperative irradiation in conjunction with a supraglottic laryngectomy because the lymphedema of the remaining larynx may be considerable, although it tends to subside with time. The probability of a good functional result is improved if the dose to the remaining larynx is limited to 55 Gy at 1.8 Gy/fraction administered once daily.

ADVANCED SUPRAGLOTTIC LESIONS (UNFAVORABLE T3, T4). Selected T3 and T4 lesions of the upper supraglottic larynx that are mainly exophytic can be treated by irradiation, because the control rate is fairly high. Concomitant chemotherapy should be considered.

Lesions unsuitable for irradiation are endophytic, high-volume cancers often associated with vocal cord fixation and are managed by total laryngectomy. If the neck disease is resectable, then operation is the initial treatment, and postoperative irradiation is added if needed. If the neck disease is unresectable or borderline, preoperative irradiation is used.

Surgical Treatment

SUPRAGLOTTIC LARYNGECTOMY. Supraglottic laryngectomy is a voice-sparing operation that can be tailored to the individual supraglottic lesion. Because the patient has an increased tendency to aspirate, it is essential that adequate pulmonary reserves be present, as determined by blood gas levels, pulmo-

nary function tests, chest radiograph, and a work test (walking the patient up two flights of stairs to determine tolerance to pulmonary stress). The voice quality is generally good after supraglottic laryngectomy. All patients have some difficulty swallowing in the immediate postoperative period, but almost all learn to swallow in a short time; motivation is the key factor.

Supraglottic laryngectomy can be used successfully for lesions involving the epiglottis, a single arytenoid, the aryepiglottic fold, and false vocal cords. Extension of the tumor to the true vocal cords, anterior commissure, or either arytenoids; fixation; or cartilage invasion excludes supraglottic laryngectomy. The extended supraglottic laryngectomy may be used to include the base of the tongue to the level of the circumvallate papillae as long as one lingual artery is preserved. A neck dissection on one or both sides may be added; approximately 35% of patients have histologically positive nodes even when the neck is clinically negative. Postoperative irradiation is added only as needed, based on the surgical and pathologic findings. The incision is usually an apron flap. The neck dissection is completed and left attached to the thyrohyoid membrane. The perichondrium of the larynx is then elevated in continuity with the strap muscles; this is important because it will be used to close the surgical defect. Saw cuts are made through the thyroid cartilage and the hyoid bone so the preepiglottic space is included in the specimen. The pharynx is entered above the hyoid through the vallecula. The specimen is removed, with only the arytenoids and true vocal cords left. If one arytenoid has to be sacrificed, the cord must be fixed in the midline to prevent aspiration. Suturing the previously saved perichondrium and muscle into the base of the tongue closes the defect. After the tracheostomy tube is removed, usually within 7 days, the patient is retrained in the act of swallowing.

TOTAL LARYNGECTOMY. In total laryngectomy the entire larynx and preepiglottic space are resected *en bloc* and a permanent tracheostomy is fashioned. A portion of the thyroid gland usually is included with the specimen. The pharynx is sutured to the base of the tongue.

Irradiation Technique. In radiation treatment the primary lesion and both sides of the neck are included with opposed lateral portals. The inferior border of the portals depends on the inferior extent of the primary tumor; it is usually at the inferior border of the cricoid. The dose for T1 or T2 lesions is 74.4 Gy in 62 fractions twice daily in a continuous course. T3 or T4 cancers receive 74.4 to 76.8 Gy. The skin of the anterior neck is excluded if possible, to reduce the skin reaction and lymphedema. Patients with suitable lesions may be treated with IMRT. The lower neck nodes are irradiated through a separate anterior portal.

Patients develop a sore throat, loss of taste, and moderate dryness during irradiation. Edema of the arytenoids may occur and produce the sensation of a lump in the throat. Tracheostomy is seldom necessary before the start of therapy, even for bulky lesions. Edema of the larynx may persist for several months to a year. Neck dissection increases the degree of lymphedema on the side of the operation; bilateral neck dissection should be avoided if possible.[129] The lymphedema of the larynx and submental space resolve together. Patients who continue to smoke and drink heighten the side effects of dryness, dysphagia, and hoarseness.

Combined Treatment Policies. Either surgery or irradiation alone is preferred for the early primary lesions. If total laryn-

TABLE 26.2-24.   T1–2N0 Glottic Larynx: 5-Year Outcomes after Radiation Therapy in 519 Patients

Stage	No. of Patients	LC (%)	Ultimate LC (%)	LC with Larynx Preservation (%)	CSS (%)	Survival (%)
T1a	230	94	98	95	98	82
T1b	61	93	98	95	98	79
T2a	146	80	96	82	95	77
T2b	82	72	96	76	90	77

CSS, cause-specific survival; LC, local control.
(Data from ref. 114.)

gectomy is required and the lesion is resectable, postoperative irradiation is preferred, because there is no evidence that preoperative irradiation produces any better local-regional control or survival rates. Radiation therapy is added for indications previously discussed in General Principles of Combining Modalities, earlier in this chapter. The high-risk areas are usually the base of the tongue and neck. The stomal area is at risk only when subglottic extension is present or there is tumor in the low neck lymph nodes. Complications related to postoperative irradiation are relatively uncommon.

Irradiation is used before total laryngectomy when patients have technically unresectable neck nodes or when scheduling problems require a long delay to operation.

A number of patients either refuse laryngectomy or are medically unsuitable for the operation; hence, irradiation is the treatment by default.

Management of Recurrence. Treatment failures after supraglottic laryngectomy or irradiation frequently can be salvaged by further treatment; recognition of recurrence should be pursued vigorously. Salvage of recurrences that develop after total laryngectomy and preoperative or postoperative irradiation is quite uncommon.

SUBGLOTTIC LARYNGEAL CARCINOMA. Early lesions are treated with radiation therapy, and advanced lesions are usually managed by total laryngectomy and postoperative radiation therapy.

Results of Treatment

VOCAL CORD CANCER

Surgical Results. Garcia-Serra et al.[117] reviewed ten series containing 269 patients with carcinoma *in situ* of the vocal cord treated with stripping. The weighted average 5-year local control and ultimate local control rates were 71.9% and 92.4%, respectively. Similarly, ten series containing 177 patients treated with carbon dioxide laser revealed the following weighted average 5-year local control and ultimate local control rates: 82.5% and 98.1%, respectively.[117]

Thomas and coworkers[130] reported on 159 patients who underwent an open partial laryngectomy at the Mayo Clinic between 1976 and 1986. Seventeen of 159 patients had *in situ* lesions; the remaining were T1 invasive carcinomas. Local recurrence developed in 11 patients (7%), and 9 eventually required laryngectomy. Ten patients developed recurrent cancer in the neck, and distant metastases were observed in ten patients.

Hemilaryngectomy including the ipsilateral arytenoid was reported by Som[131] for 130 cases of vocal cord carcinoma extending to the vocal process and face of the arytenoid. The cure rate was 74% for 104 patients with T2 lesions, and 58% for 26 patients with T3 cancers.

Foote and coworkers[132] reported on 81 patients who underwent a laryngectomy for T3 cancers at the Mayo Clinic between 1970 and 1981. Seventy-five patients underwent a total laryngectomy and six underwent a near-total laryngectomy; 53 received a neck dissection. No patient underwent adjuvant radiation therapy or chemotherapy. The 5-year rates of local-regional control, cause-specific survival, and absolute survival were 74%, 74%, and 54%, respectively.

Radiation Therapy Results. Garcia-Serra et al.[117] reviewed 22 series containing 705 patients with carcinoma *in situ* of the vocal cord treated with radiation therapy and observed that the weighted average 5-year local control and ultimate local control rates were 87.4% and 98.4%, respectively.

The results of irradiation for 519 patients with T1–2N0 squamous cell carcinoma of the vocal cord treated by irradiation are presented in Table 26.2-24. The 5-year rates of neck control for 506 patients who received no elective neck treatment for the overall groups and for the subsets of patients who remained continuously disease free at the primary site were as follows: T1, 99% and 100%; T2a, 95% and 97%; and T2b, 87% and 92%, respectively.[114]

Harwood et al.[133] reported on 112 patients with T3 glottic carcinomas treated with definitive radiation therapy at the Princess Margaret Hospital. The local control and ultimate local control rates were 51% and 77%, respectively. The results of definitive radiation therapy for patients with T3 glottic carcinomas are compared with those for surgery alone or with adjuvant radiation therapy in a series of 118 patients treated at the University of Florida in Table 26.2-25. Irradiation was generally selected for fixed lesions with involvement of one vocal cord and with an adequate airway. The likelihood of local control after radiation therapy is related to primary tumor volume and cartilage sclerosis.[44]

Treatment results for T4 glottic carcinomas are shown in Table 26.2-26.

SUPRAGLOTTIC LARYNGEAL CANCER. The results of treatment after various treatment modalities are depicted in Tables 26.2-27 to 26.2-30.[127]

Complications of Treatment

SURGERY. Repeated stripping of the cord may result in a thickened cord and hoarse voice. Neel and coworkers[134] reported a 26% incidence of nonfatal complications for cordectomy. Immediate postoperative complications included atelectasis and pneumonia, severe subcutaneous emphysema in the neck, bleeding from the tracheotomy site or larynx, wound com-

TABLE 26.2-25. T3 Glottic Larynx—University of Florida (n = 118 Patients)

5-Year Outcomes	Definitive Radiation Therapy (%) (n = 53)	Surgery Alone or with Adjuvant Radiation Therapy (%) (n = 65)	Significance Level (P)
Local-regional control	62	75	.10
Ultimate local-regional control	84	82	.95
Cause-specific survival	75	71	.26
Survival	55	45	.119
Severe complications[a]	16	15	.558

[a]Includes complications after initial treatment and salvage treatment.
(Data from ref. 119.)

TABLE 26.2-26. T4 Glottic Cancer: Results of Treatment

Series	Stage	No. of Patients	Method of Treatment	Results (NED)
Jesse[241]	T4N0–N+	48	Laryngectomy	54% at 4 y
Ogura et al.[242]	T4N0	11	Laryngectomy	45% at 3 y
Skolnick et al.[243]	T4N0	7	Laryngectomy	30% at 5 y
Vermund[244]	T4N0	31	Laryngectomy	35% at 5 y
Stewart and Jackson[245]	T4N0	13	RT with surgery for salvage	38% at 5 y
Harwood et al.[246]	T4N0	56	RT with surgery for salvage	49% at 5 y[a]

NED, no evidence of disease; RT, radiation therapy.
[a]Actuarial survival, uncorrected for deaths due to intercurrent disease.
(Modified from ref. 246.)

TABLE 26.2-27. Supraglottic Larynx: Local Control after Transoral Laser Excision

Series	Staging	No. of Patients	% of Patients with T1 or T2 Tumors	T1 (%)	T2 (%)	T3 (%)	T4 (%)
Davis et al., 1991[247]	P	14 R	57	100	100	50	—
Steiner, 1993[248,a]	P	81 R	72	—	76	77	100
Zeitels et al., 1994[249]	ND	22	100	100	100	—	—
Zeitels et al., 1994[249]	ND	23 R	65	100	92	63	—
Csanády et al., 1999[250]	ND	23	100	70[b]		—	—
Rudert et al., 1999[251]	P	34 R	50	100	75	78	38

ND, type of staging not provided; P, pathologic staging; R, plus or minus radiation therapy.
Note. Some figures were estimated as closely as possible to fit table format if the information was not specifically stated in the cited reference.
[a]51 glottic and 30 supraglottic.
[b]Overall local control rates for T1 and T2.
(From ref. 127, with permission.)

TABLE 26.2-28. Supraglottic Larynx: Local Control after Radiation Therapy

Series	Institution	No. of Patients	T1 (%)	T2 (%)	T3 (%)	T4 (%)
Fletcher and Hamberger, 1974[252]	M. D. Anderson Hospital	173	88	79	62	47
Ghossein et al., 1974[253]	Fondation Curie	203	94	73	46[a]	52
Wang and Montgomery, 1991[254]	Massachusetts General Hospital	229 q.d.	73	60	54	26
		209 b.i.d.	89	89	71	91
Nakfoor et al., 1998[255]	Massachusetts General Hospital	164	96	86	76	43
Sykes et al., 2000[256]	Christie Hospital	331[b]	92[c]	81[c]	67[c]	73[c]
Hinerman et al., 2002[127]	University of Florida[d]	274	100	86	62	62

Note. Some figures were estimated as closely as possible to fit table format if the information was not specifically stated in the cited reference.
[a]All had cord fixation.
[b]All N0.
[c]After 17 underwent salvage by total laryngectomy.
[d]1998 American Joint Committee on Cancer staging.
(From ref. 127, with permission.)

TABLE 26.2-29. Supraglottic Larynx: Local Control after Supraglottic Laryngectomy

Series	Institution	No. of Patients	% of Patients with T1 or T2 Tumors	T1 (%)	T2 (%)	T3 (%)	T4 (%)
Ogura et al., 1975[257]	Washington University	177	78			94^a	
Bocca, 1991[258]	Milan University						
Stage I		47	100	94			
Stage II		252	100		82		
Stage III		205	53		80^b		
Stage IV		33				67^c	
Lee et al., 1990[259]	M. D. Anderson Cancer Center	60	58	100	100	100	100
DeSanto, 1990[260]	Mayo Clinic	70	100	100	100		
Steiniger et al., 1997[261]	Albany Medical Center	29	83			97^a	
Spriano et al., 1997[262]	Varese, Italy	54	100		96^d		
Burstein and Calcattera, 1985[263]	University of California, Los Angeles	40	58	100	85	94	100
Isaacs et al., 1998[264]	University of Florida	33	76	100	78	71	100
Lutz et al., 1990[265]	University of Pittsburgh	72	No data			99^e	

Note: Some figures were estimated as closely as possible to fit table format if the information was not specifically stated in the cited reference.
^a Overall local control rates for T1–T4.
^b Overall local control rates for T1–T3.
^c Overall local control rates for T2 and T3.
^d Overall local control rates for T1 and T2.
^e T stages were not specified.
(From ref. 127, with permission.)

plications, and airway obstruction requiring tracheotomy. Late complications included need for removal of granulation tissue by direct laryngoscopy to exclude recurrence, extrusion of cartilage, laryngeal stenosis, and obstructing laryngeal web.

The postoperative complications of hemilaryngectomy include aspiration, chondritis, wound slough, inadequate glottic closure, and anterior commissure webs.

The postoperative complications of total laryngectomy include operative death, hemorrhage, fistula, chondritis, wound slough, carotid rupture, dysphagia, and pharyngeal or esophageal stenosis.

The complication rate after supraglottic laryngectomy is approximately 10%, including fistula formation, aspiration, chondritis, dysphagia, dyspnea, and carotid rupture.[127]

RADIATION THERAPY. After irradiation, the quality and volume of the voice tend to diminish at the end of the day. Edema of the larynx is the most common sequela after irradiation for glottic or supraglottic lesions. The rate of clearance of the edema is related to dose of radiation, volume of tissue irradiated, addition of a neck dissection, continued use of alcohol and tobacco, and size and extent of the original lesion. Steroids (e.g., Decadron) have been used to reduce edema secondary to radiation effect after recurrence has been ruled out by biopsy. If ulceration and pain occur, antibiotics are used.

Soft tissue necrosis leading to chondritis occurs in approximately 1% of patients. Soft tissue and cartilage necroses mimic recurrence with hoarseness, pain, and edema; a laryngectomy may be recommended in desperation for fear of recurrent cancer, even though biopsy findings show only necrosis. Mendenhall et al.[114] recorded serious complications after definitive radiation therapy in 1 of 291 patients with T1 true cord cancers and 3 of 228 with T2 glottic malignancies.

COMBINED TREATMENT. Preoperative irradiation is associated with an increased risk of an operative complication and prolonged hospitalization. Overall complication rates are reduced by the use of postoperative radiation therapy. The major late effects of combined treatment are an increased fibrosis of soft tissues, stomal stenosis, and pharyngeal stricture.

HYPOPHARYNX: PHARYNGEAL WALLS, PYRIFORM SINUS, AND POSTCRICOID PHARYNX

Both the oropharyngeal and hypopharyngeal walls are considered together because there is no distinct difference in the presentation or treatment. The majority of hypopharyngeal lesions originate in the pyriform sinus. Postcricoid carcinomas are uncommon.

Anatomy

The epithelium of the pharyngeal mucous membrane is squamous; it is continuous with the mucous membrane of the nasopharynx. The dividing point between the nasopharynx and posterior pharyngeal wall is Passavant's ridge, a musculature ring that contracts to close the nasopharynx during swallowing. The thin constrictor muscles surround the posterior and lateral walls. Between the constrictor muscle and the prevertebral fascia covering the longitudinal spine muscles (longus colli and longus capitis) is a thin layer of loose areolar tissue, the retropharyngeal space. The entire thickness of the posterior pharyngeal wall from the mucous membrane to the anterior vertebral body is no more than 1 cm in the midline. Lateral to the pharyngeal wall are the vessels, nerves, and muscles of the parapharyngeal space. The constrictor muscles are

TABLE 26.2-30. Supraglottic Larynx: Severe Complications According to Treatment Modality

Series	Institution	No. of Severe Complications
RADIATION THERAPY		
Fletcher and Hamberger, 1974[252]	M. D. Anderson Cancer Center	10/173 (6%)
Ghossein et al., 1974[253]	Fondation Curie	8/117 (7%)
Nakfoor et al., 1998[255]	Massachusetts General Hospital	12/169 (7%)
Sykes et al., 2000[256]	Christie Hospital	7/331 (2%)
Hinerman et al., 2002[127]	University of Florida	12/274 (4%)
SUPRAGLOTTIC LARYNGECTOMY		
Lee et al., 1990[259]	M. D. Anderson Cancer Center	9/63 (14%)
Isaacs et al., 1998[264]	University of Florida	14/34 (41%)
Burstein and Calcaterra, 1985[263]	University of California, Los Angeles	14/41 (34%)
Steiniger et al., 1997[261]	Albany Medical College	12/29 (41%)
Spriano et al., 1997[262]	Varese, Italy	13/54 (24%)
Gall et al., 1977[266]	Washington University	20/133 (15%)
Weber et al., 1993[267]	University of Pittsburgh	12/69 (17%)
Beckhardt et al., 1994[268]	University of Wisconsin	15/50 (30%)
TRANSORAL LASER EXCISION		
Rudert et al., 1999[251]	University of Kiel, Germany	3/34 (9%)
Zeitels et al., 1994[249]	Massachusetts Eye and Ear Infirmary	2/45 (4%)
Steiner et al., 1993[248,a]	University of Göttingen, Germany	7/240 (3%)
Davis et al., 1991[247]	University of Utah, Salt Lake City	0/14 (0%)
Csanády et al., 1999[250]	Albert Szent Gyorgyi Medical University, Szeged, Hungary	0/23 (0%)

Note: Some figures were estimated as closely as possible to fit table format if the information was not specifically stated in the cited reference.
[a]Includes patients with glottic cancer.
(From ref. 127, with permission.)

relatively thin, especially the superior constrictor, and do not present much of an obstacle to tumor penetration. There is a variable weak spot in the lateral pharyngeal wall just below the hyoid where the middle and the inferior constrictor muscles fail to overlap. The lateral wall in this area is composed of the thin thyrohyoid membrane, which is penetrated by the vessels, nerves, and lymphatics of the laryngopharynx.

The pharyngeal walls are continuous with the cervical esophagus below. The hypopharyngeal walls are visible by indirect mirror examination; the transition to cervical esophagus is below the arytenoids (C-4) and is not visualized on mirror examination. The transition zone, 3 to 4 cm in length, is the postcricoid pharynx and is dealt with separately, because tumors of this area present a special clinical picture.

The lateral pharyngeal wall is a narrow strip of mucosa that lies behind the posterior tonsillar pillar in the oropharynx, is partially interrupted by the pharyngoepiglottic fold, and then continues into the hypopharynx, where it becomes the lateral wall of the pyriform sinus. The lateral pharyngeal wall has a max-

imum width of no more than 2 cm. The posterior cornu of the hyoid bone occasionally protrudes into the lateral pharyngeal wall on one or both sides, producing a submucosal bulge. The posterior pharyngeal wall is 4 to 5 cm wide and 6 to 7 cm in height. Submucosal bulges, caused by osteophytes on the anterior lips of the cervical vertebrae, may be mistaken for tumor.

The pyriform sinus is created by the intrusion of the larynx into the anterior aspect of the pharynx, which creates pharyngeal grooves lateral to the larynx. The superior margin of the pyriform sinus is the pharyngoepiglottic fold and the free margin of the aryepiglottic fold. The superolateral margin of the pyriform sinus is considered to be an oblique line along the lateral pharyngeal wall just opposite the aryepiglottic fold. The pyriform sinus is therefore made up of three walls: the anterior, lateral, and medial (there is no posterior wall). The pyriform sinus tapers inferiorly to the apex and usually terminates variably at a level between the superior and inferior borders of the cricoid cartilage. The superior limit of the pyriform sinus is opposite the hyoid. The thyrohyoid membrane is lateral to the upper portion of the pyriform sinus, and the thyroid cartilage, cricothyroid membrane, and cricoid cartilage are lateral to the lower portion. The internal branch of the superior laryngeal nerve, a branch of the vagus, lies under the mucous membrane on the anterolateral wall of the pyriform sinus. The auricular branch is sensory to the skin of the back of the pinna and the posterior wall of the external auditory canal.

The postcricoid pharynx is funnel-shaped to direct food into the gullet. The superior margin begins just below the arytenoids. The anterior wall lies behind the cricoid cartilage and is the posterior wall of the lower larynx. The posterior wall is a continuation of the hypopharyngeal walls. The recurrent laryngeal nerve lies between the lateral wall and the deep surface of the thyroid gland.

Pathology

More than 95% of malignant tumors are squamous cell carcinoma or one of its variants. Carcinoma *in situ* is commonly seen in surgical specimens at the edge of neoplasms of the pharyngeal wall, and multifocal skip areas of carcinoma *in situ* may make it difficult to obtain clear margins if excision is done. Minor salivary gland tumors are rare.

Patterns of Spread

POSTERIOR PHARYNGEAL WALL. Carcinomas of the posterior wall have a tendency to remain on the posterior wall, grow up or down the wall, and infiltrate posteriorly; they seldom spread circumferentially to the lateral walls, even when advanced. Early lesions are red, sometimes with white areas sprinkled over the involved area. As the lesion progresses, the tumor bulges into the pharyngeal cavity and a linear midline ulceration appears. The posterior tonsillar pillars may become involved, and tumor may spread up the pillars, eventually reaching the palate. Advanced lesions tend to terminate inferiorly at the level of the arytenoids without growing into the postcricoid region. Superiorly, they may extend into the nasopharynx. Direct invasion of the cervical vertebrae or base of the skull is uncommon.

LATERAL PHARYNGEAL WALL. Early tumors of the lateral wall may be well-defined exophytic lesions. As they advance, they have a tendency for lateral penetration through the constrictor muscle, thus entering the lateral pharyngeal space or the soft tissues of the neck. A mass may become palpable in the neck just below the hyoid and be confused with a lymph node.

The muscles of the pharynx originate from the base of the skull, eustachian tube, styloid process, pterygomandibular raphe, and hyoid bone; tumor may spread along muscle and fascial planes to all muscular points of origin.[135] Tumor also follows a course along cranial nerves IX and X and the sympathetic chain. The thyroid gland is adjacent to the lower walls and often is invaded. Tumor secondarily invades the pharyngoepiglottic fold, the vallecula, and the anterior and lateral walls of the pyriform sinus.

PYRIFORM SINUS. Early lesions of the pyriform sinus usually appear as nodular mucosal irregularities. Medial wall lesions may grow superficially along the aryepiglottic fold and arytenoids, or invade directly into the false cord and aryepiglottic fold. Medial wall lesions also extend posteriorly to the postcricoid region. Extensive submucosal spread is a characteristic feature. There is frequently an area of central ulceration for lesions larger than 1 to 2 cm.

Large bulky exophytic lesions may arise on the upper medial wall and appear similar to primary lesions of the aryepiglottic fold. The vocal cord becomes fixed because of infiltration of the intrinsic muscles of the larynx, the cricoarytenoid joint or muscle, or, less commonly, the recurrent laryngeal nerve. These lesions grow posteriorly to involve the postcricoid pharynx and cricoid cartilage and may extend to the opposite pyriform sinus. Spread into the cervical esophagus is a late event.

Lesions arising on the lateral wall tend toward early invasion of the posterior thyroid cartilage and the posterior superior cricoid cartilage. The ipsilateral superior lobe of the thyroid gland may be invaded after tumor penetrates the cartilage, but thyroid invasion can occur in cases with no cartilage invasion when tumor penetrates behind the thyroid cartilage or through the cricothyroid membrane. Kirchner[136] reported that thyroid cartilage invasion was associated with involvement of the apex of the pyriform sinus, and the extent of invasion could not be predicted from the extent of visible disease. Lesions of the lateral walls tend to spread submucosally to the posterior pharyngeal wall. It is often difficult to estimate the extent of posterior pharyngeal wall or postcricoid invasion except at direct laryngoscopy, because these areas are often difficult to visualize indirectly.

Advanced lesions of the pyriform sinus invade all three walls, fix the larynx, involve the ipsilateral posterior pharyngeal wall, invade the thyroid cartilage and thyroid gland, and often escape into the soft tissues of the neck. The preepiglottic space often is involved. Perineural invasion of the recurrent laryngeal nerve may be seen in whole organ sections.

POSTCRICOID PHARYNX. Early postcricoid lesions are rarely diagnosed. Lesions arising from the posterior wall tend to remain on the posterior wall. Lesions arising from the anterior wall tend to invade the posterior cricoarytenoid muscle and the cricoid and arytenoid cartilages. Advanced tumors eventually encircle the lumen. Because the apex of the pyriform sinus terminates in the postcricoid area, some lesions secondarily invade the apex of the pyriform sinus early.

LYMPHATICS

Pharyngeal Walls. The lymphatics of the pharyngeal walls terminate primarily in the jugular chain and secondarily in the spinal accessory chain. The jugulodigastric node is the most commonly involved node. Lindberg[10] reported that 59% of patients have clinically positive nodes on admission; 17% had bilateral positive nodes (Fig. 26.2-15). Retropharyngeal lymph node involvement is frequent.

Pyriform Sinus. The capillary lymphatics of the pyriform sinus are profuse. The distribution of lymph node metastases is mainly to the jugular chain with a relatively small proportion to the spinal accessory chain. The subdigastric node is the most commonly involved, but midjugular involvement occurs without subdigastric node involvement. On admission, 75% of patients have clinically positive nodes and at least 10% have bilateral positive nodes (see Fig. 26.2-15). There is no difference in the risk of lymph node metastases by T stage. Ogura and coworkers[137] reported a 62% incidence of subclinical disease; some of the patients had 15 to 30 Gy of preoperative irradiation. Retropharyngeal lymph node involvement occurs and is diagnosed by CT or MRI scan.

Clinical Picture

Tumors that are lateralized to the lateral pharyngeal wall or pyriform sinus produce a unilateral sore throat, a symptom rather specific for cancer because infectious sore throat is bilateral. Dysphagia, sensation of foreign body, ear pain, blood-streaked saliva, and voice change occur later. A neck mass may be the presenting complaint.

Lesions of the posterior pharyngeal wall are often overlooked even by competent physicians because of failure to examine the posterior pharyngeal wall routinely during indirect laryngoscopy. Small lesions of the pyriform sinus are easily missed unless very careful examinations are done. Many of these patients have active gag reflexes, and examination with a flexible endoscope is necessary. Lesions of the apex of the pyriform sinus or postcricoid area produce indirect findings that are clues to tumor not visible by indirect laryngoscopy. Pooling of secretions in the pyriform sinus indicates obstruction of the upper gullet. Edema of the arytenoids and inability to see into the apex of the pyriform sinus are clues to postcricoid or low-lying pyriform sinus tumors. Invasion of the palatopharyngeal muscle at its insertion into the inferior constrictor can cause shortening of the muscle and asymmetry of the posterior tonsillar pillars. As the postcricoid tumor enlarges it pushes the larynx anteriorly, producing a full, expanded neck appearance. The thyroid click is produced by the superior thyroid cornu's hitting against the spine while rocking the thyroid cartilage back and forth; this is lost when the larynx is displaced anteriorly.

AJCC Staging

The AJCC staging system for primary tumors of the hypopharynx is as follows[16]:

T1　Tumor limited to one subsite of hypopharynx and 2 cm or less in greatest dimension

T2　Tumor invades more than one subsite of hypopharynx or an adjacent site, or measures more than 2 cm but

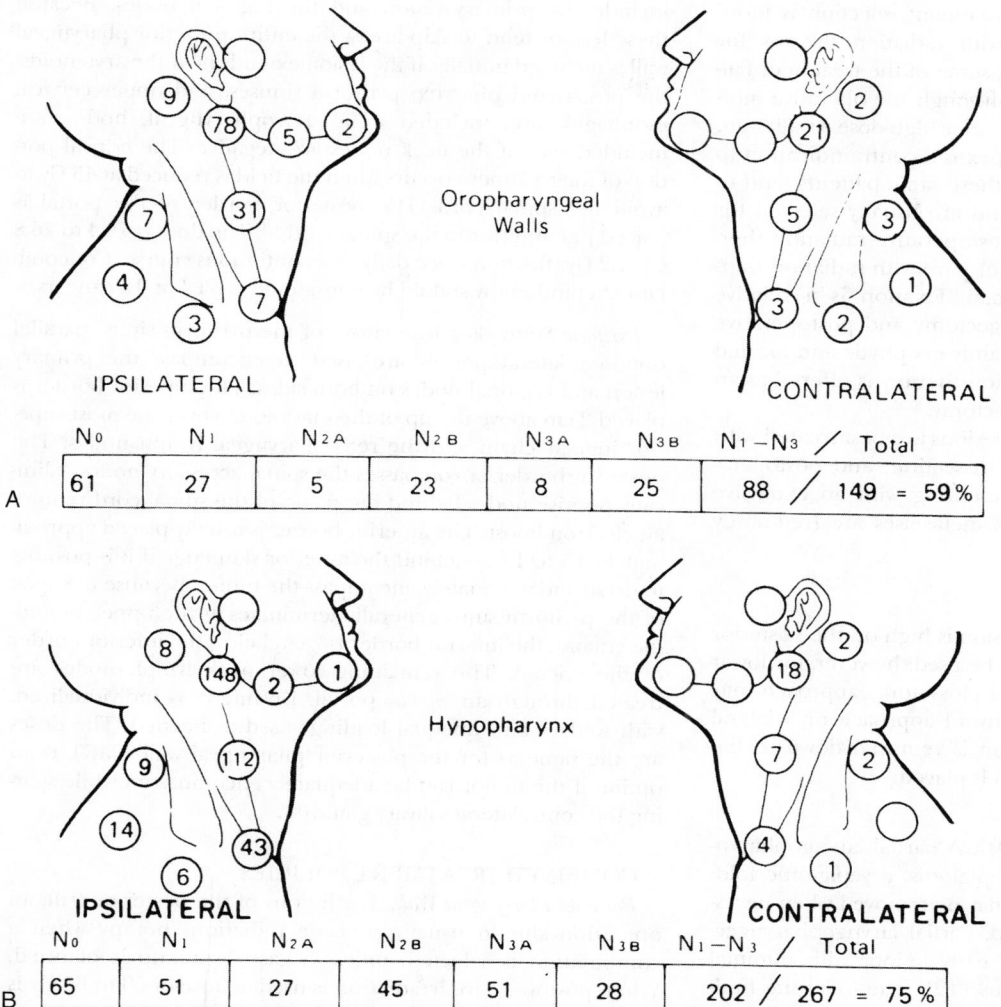

FIGURE 26.2-15. Nodal distribution on admission at M. D. Anderson Hospital, 1948 to 1965. The circled numbers indicate the number of times the particular lymph node was involved. **A:** Oropharyngeal walls. **B:** Hypopharynx. (From ref. 10, with permission.)

Oropharyngeal Walls

N₀	N₁	N₂ₐ	N₂ᵦ	N₃ₐ	N₃ᵦ	N₁–N₃ / Total
61	27	5	23	8	25	88 / 149 = 59%

A

Hypopharynx

N₀	N₁	N₂ₐ	N₂ᵦ	N₃ₐ	N₃ᵦ	N₁–N₃ / Total
65	51	27	45	51	28	202 / 267 = 75%

B

not more than 4 cm in greatest diameter without fixation of the hemilarynx

T3 Tumor more than 4 cm in greatest dimension or with fixation of the hemilarynx

T4a Tumor invades thyroid/cricoid cartilage, hyoid bone, thyroid gland, esophagus, or central compartment soft tissue[a]

T4b Tumor invades the prevertebral fascia, encases the carotid artery, or involves mediastinal structures

[a]Central compartment soft tissue includes the prelaryngeal strap muscles and subcutaneous fat.

Treatment

SELECTION OF TREATMENT MODALITY

Posterior Pharyngeal Wall. Most lesions on the posterior pharyngeal wall are treated by radiation therapy. Surgery and adjuvant radiation therapy have been used for selected, moderately advanced lesions, with limited success. All aspects considered, high-dose radiation therapy will produce cure rates similar to those produced by either surgery alone or combined surgery plus radiation therapy, and with less morbidity. For a few selected patients whose lesions fail to respond to radiation therapy or whose lesions recur after irradiation, salvage by pharyngectomy will be successful.

Lateral Pharyngeal Wall. There is very little local control information specifically related to the lateral walls. Small lesions (1 to 2 cm) are often exophytic and are usually managed by irradiation. Larger lesions tend to be deeply infiltrative, and the control rate by irradiation, surgery, or both is modest. An operation for a large lesion usually implies a laryngectomy in combination with pharyngectomy. Therefore, most of these patients are treated with definitive radiation therapy.

Pyriform Sinus. Lesions confined to the pyriform sinus with normal mobility (T1 and low-volume, favorable T2) are locally controlled in 80% to 90% of cases by irradiation or partial laryngopharyngectomy.[138,139] Irradiation is the preferred choice of the authors because it leaves the patient with nearly normal swallowing and speech, while permitting wider coverage of the regional lymphatics. Irradiation is more generally applicable, whereas there are certain anatomic and medical restraints on the use of partial laryngopharyngectomy.

High-volume endophytic lesions extending outside the pyriform sinus with normal or reduced mobility (T2 or T3) represent the group of cases in which treatment selection is more complex. The local control rate with radiation therapy for selected cases is approximately 60%; some of the treatment failures can be rescued by operation, although the operative mortality and morbidity are considerable after high-dose irradiation.

Invasion of the pyriform sinus apex is a contraindication to partial laryngopharyngectomy, but these same patients tend to do poorly with radiation therapy and are usually selected for total laryngopharyngectomy plus postoperative radiation therapy. However, they may be treated for cure with radiation therapy if apex involvement is minimal. Fixation is a relative indication for total laryngopharyngectomy and postoperative radiation therapy. If the lesion is mainly exophytic and located in the upper pyriform sinus, radiation therapy is offered as an alternative to total laryngopharyngectomy.

The more advanced, infiltrative lesions are best treated with total laryngopharyngectomy, neck dissection, and postoperative radiation therapy. Patients presenting with an extensive primary lesion and extensive neck metastases are frequently offered palliative therapy.

SURGICAL TREATMENT

Posterior Pharyngeal Wall. If the lesion is high on the posterior wall, then a transoral approach can be used; however, for lower lesions the midline mandibulolabial glossotomy approach may be used. Alternatives are the transhyoid approach or a lateral pharyngotomy approach. The lesion is removed down to the prevertebral fascia, and no skin graft is placed.

Pyriform Sinus

PARTIAL LARYNGOPHARYNGECTOMY. A partial laryngopharyngectomy removes the false cords, epiglottis, aryepiglottic fold, and pyriform sinus; one arytenoid may be removed when necessary. The vocal cords are preserved. Partial laryngopharyngectomy can be used successfully for early lesions with minimal extension beyond the pyriform sinus (T2). The following findings contraindicate partial laryngopharyngectomy: extension to apex of the pyriform sinus, fixed cord, extension to contralateral arytenoid, poor pulmonary function, and large, fixed lymph nodes. The apex of the pyriform sinus lies opposite the cricoid cartilage, and because the cricoid is the only cartilage forming a complete ring about the airway, it must remain intact to prevent collapse. There is a greater tendency to aspiration after partial laryngopharyngectomy compared with supraglottic laryngectomy, and the patient must be motivated to relearn to swallow.

TOTAL LARYNGOPHARYNGECTOMY. Total laryngopharyngectomy removes the larynx and varying amounts of pharyngeal wall. Advanced lesions require excision of nearly the entire circumference. The pharynx is reestablished by primary closure after a partial pharyngectomy. Reconstruction using a myocutaneous flap or gut graft (jejunal interposition or gastric transposition) is required after a total pharyngectomy.

Postcricoid Pharynx. Postcricoid carcinoma generally requires a total laryngopharyngectomy with immediate reconstruction, generally using a pectoralis major myocutaneous flap. If the lesion extends into the cervical esophagus, a gastric pull-up or jejunal free flap may be necessary for reconstruction.

IRRADIATION TECHNIQUE

Posterior Pharyngeal Wall. The irradiation technique for lesions of the posterior pharyngeal wall is opposed lateral fields to include the primary lesion and the regional nodes. Because these lesions tend to skip areas, the entire posterior pharyngeal wall is included initially. If the lesion extends near the arytenoids, the postcricoid pharynx, pyriform sinuses, and upper cervical esophagus are included. The retropharyngeal nodes are included even if the neck nodes are negative. The critical portion of the treatment occurs when the field is reduced at 45 Gy to avoid the spinal cord. The posterior border of the portal is placed just anterior to the spinal cord.[140] The dose is 74.4 to 76.8 Gy, 1.2 Gy/fraction twice daily in a continuous course. Concomitant chemotherapy should be considered for T3 or T4 cancers.

Pyriform Sinus. For irradiation of the pyriform sinus, parallel opposed lateral portals are used to encompass the primary lesion and regional nodes on both sides. The superior border is placed 2 cm above the tip of the mastoid to cover the most superior jugular chain and the retropharyngeal lymph nodes. The posterior border encompasses the spinal accessory nodes. Clinically positive nodes behind the plane of the spinal cord require an electron boost. The anterior border is usually placed approximately 0.5 to 1 cm behind the anterior skin edge if it is possible to do so and adequately encompass the tumor. Because the apex of the pyriform sinus generally terminates at the upper to middle cricoid, the inferior border is 2 cm below the inferior border of the cricoid. The remaining lower neck lymph nodes are treated through an *en face* portal. Dosimetry is individualized, with wedges and unequal loadings used as needed. The doses are the same as for the posterior pharyngeal wall. IMRT is an option if the tumor can be adequately encompassed while sparing the contralateral salivary gland(s).

COMBINED TREATMENT POLICIES

Posterior Pharyngeal Wall. For lesions of the posterior wall, an operation should usually precede radiation therapy when a combination is selected, unless a gastric pull-up is planned. When postoperative irradiation is used, a dose of 60 to 65 Gy is given with negative margins.

Pyriform Sinus. For lesions of the pyriform sinus, after total laryngopharyngectomy with or without neck dissection, radiation therapy is usually recommended for indications previously outlined in General Principles of Combining Modalities, earlier in this chapter. Irradiation is used before operation for patients with a large fixed node to reduce the size of the mass and to help obtain surgical margins. The preoperative dose to the node may be 60 to 75 Gy, although the dose to the primary mass will be only 45 to 50 Gy.

MANAGEMENT OF RECURRENCE

Posterior Pharyngeal Wall. Recurrence after radiation therapy may be limited to the posterior pharyngeal wall and suitable for surgical excision, with occasional salvage. There is frequently a persistent ulcer at the completion of radiation therapy for the more advanced lesions. If the ulcer does not heal in short order, it should be considered evidence of persistent disease. Surgical excision is limited posteriorly by the prevertebral fascia. Irradiation salvage of a surgical failure would be unusual.

Pyriform Sinus. The hallmark of local recurrence after radical irradiation of a pyriform sinus lesion is persistent edema with inability to visualize the pyriform sinus, pain, and fixation of laryngeal structures. Direct laryngoscopy is required, but biopsy findings may be negative and misleading. CT is often helpful for distinguishing local recurrence from necrosis. Eventually a decision may be made to recommend total laryngopharyngectomy for salvage without a positive biopsy result.

Recurrence after total laryngopharyngectomy is usually in the soft tissues of the neck, the untreated opposite neck, the base of the tongue, or stoma. Surgical treatment failures after partial laryngopharyngectomy for early lesions may be salvaged by total laryngopharyngectomy. Surgical treatment failures after total laryngopharyngectomy are rarely salvaged.

Results of Treatment

PHARYNGEAL WALL. For lesions of the pharyngeal wall, the treatment policy at the University of Florida primarily has been definitive irradiation with neck dissection added as necessary. The 5-year local control rates and ultimate local control rates for 148 patients treated between 1964 and 1990 were as follows: T1 (n = 15), 93% and 93%; T2 (n = 45), 82% and 87%; T3 (n = 76), 59% and 61%; and T4 (n = 12), 50% and 50%, respectively.[140] Local control rates have improved with the use of twice-daily fractionation and placement of the posterior of the "off-cord" reduced portals at the posterior border of the vertebral bodies.[140] The 5-year local-regional control, cause-specific survival, and survival rates are shown in Table 26.2-31.

Marks and coworkers[141] compared low-dose preoperative radiation therapy (25 to 30 Gy) followed by operation with radiation therapy alone. The local control was slightly better for the combined group, but the 3-year actuarial survival rate was 17%, and the 3-year absolute survival rate was 14%. An operative mortality of 14% and a high risk of major surgical complications offset any gain in local control. M. D. Anderson Hospital reported on a group of 25 patients (15 with stage T2 lesions, 10 with stage T3 or T4 lesions) treated by a combination of surgery and radiation therapy.[142] Nineteen patients received postoperative radiation therapy; seven had positive margins, and three had close margins. Fifteen patients were dead at 5 years: Six died of local recurrence or neck recurrence, five of distant metastasis, one of intercurrent disease, and three of uncertain causes. The 5-year absolute survival was 4 of 19 patients (21%).

PYRIFORM SINUS. The results of treatment for 80 patients with carcinoma of the pyriform sinus treated at Washington University, St. Louis, by preoperative radiation therapy followed

TABLE 26.2-31. Pharyngeal Wall Carcinoma: 5-Year Outcomes after Definitive Radiation Therapy (n = 148 Patients)

AJCC Stage	No. of Patients	Local-Regional Control (%)	Cause-Specific Survival (%)	Absolute Survival (%)
I	9	89	89	56
II	27	83	88	52
III	36	58	44	24
IV	76	47	34	22

AJCC, American Joint Committee on Cancer.
(Data from ref. 140.)

TABLE 26.2-32. Carcinoma of the Pyriform Sinus: Results of Treatment by Low-Dose Radiation Therapy plus Partial Laryngopharyngectomy or Total Laryngectomy and Partial Pharyngectomy (Washington University, St. Louis, 1964–1974)

Result	PLP (%) (80 Patients)[a]	TLP (%) (57 Patients)[b]
Local recurrence ± neck recurrence	14[c]	14
Neck recurrence ± distant metastases (primary controlled)	9	23
Distant metastases alone	11	21
5-y actuarial survival (no evidence of disease)	40	22

PLP, partial laryngopharyngectomy; TLP, total laryngopharyngectomy and partial pharyngectomy.
[a]T1, 70 patients; T2–T4, 10 patients [American Joint Committee on Cancer (AJCC) staging].
[b]T1, 35 patients; T2–T4, 22 patients (AJCC staging).
[c]Four patients underwent salvage treatment.
(Data from ref. 143.)

by partial laryngopharyngectomy are given in Table 26.2-32.[143] Seventy patients had the equivalent of AJCC T1 lesions (disease limited to the pyriform sinus) and 10 patients had disease extending beyond the pyriform sinus; none had invasion of the apex of the pyriform sinus. The cause of death was cancer in 26%, complications of treatment in 14%, and intercurrent disease in 20%. The 2-year absolute survival rate was 45 of 80 patients (56%) and the 5-year absolute survival was 25 of 66 patients (38%) (J. E. Marks, personal communication, 1979).

The results of treatment for 57 patients from the same institution who were treated by preoperative radiation therapy followed by total laryngectomy and partial pharyngectomy are shown in Table 26.2-32.[143] Thirty-five patients had lesions confined to the pyriform sinus (AJCC T1) and the remainder had extension beyond the pyriform sinus (AJCC T2 to T4). The cause of death was cancer in 56% of patients, complications of treatment in 11% of patients, and intercurrent disease in 18% of patients.

The 5-year rates of local control and ultimate local control for 101 patients treated with definitive radiation therapy for T1 (22 patients) and T2 (79 patients) pyriform sinus carcinomas were as follows: T1, 90% and 95%; and T2, 80% and 91%, respectively.[138] The 5-year rates of local-regional control, distant metastasis–free survival, and survival are shown in Table 26.2-33.

El-Badawi and coworkers[144] compared results for 203 patients treated by surgery alone and 125 patients treated by surgery (total laryngopharyngectomy) followed by 60 Gy of postoperative irradiation or preceded by 45 to 50 Gy of preoperative irradiation. The tumor stages for the three groups were comparable. There was a minimum follow-up of 4 years. The patients treated with combined therapy showed approximately a 15% improvement in survival at 5 years.

Complications of Treatment

POSTERIOR PHARYNGEAL WALL

Surgical Complications. Marks and coworkers[141] reported a 14% operative mortality plus major complications including pharyngocutaneous fistula (31%) and carotid rupture (14%) in patients treated with preoperative radiation therapy, 25 to 30 Gy.

TABLE 26.2-33.   T1–T2 Pyriform Sinus Carcinoma Treated with Definitive Radiation Therapy at the University of Florida (n = 101): 5-Year Outcomes

AJCC Stage	No. of Patients	Local-Regional Control (%)	Ultimate Local-Regional Control (%)	Distant Metastasis–Free Survival (%)	Cause-Specific Survival (%)	Survival (%)
I	7	100	96[a]	91[b]	96[a]	57
II	18	87				61
III	20	57	77		62	41
IVA	44	65	74	63	49	29
IVB	12	51	61	69	33	25

AJCC, American Joint Committee on Cancer.
[a]Stages I and II = 96%.
[b]Stages I and III = 91%.
(Data from ref. 138.)

Radiation Therapy Complications. Hull and coworkers[140] observed eight fatal complications (5%) in 148 patients who were treated at the University of Florida. These included aspiration pneumonia (four patients), soft tissue or cartilage necrosis (three patients), and laryngeal edema (one patient). Twenty-three patients (16%) experienced nonfatal severe complications including need for a permanent gastrostomy tube (15 patients); soft tissue or bone necrosis or both (7 patients); and carotid rupture, orocutaneous fistula, and need for tracheostomy, brachial plexopathy (1 patient).

PYRIFORM SINUS

Surgical Complications. The complications of partial laryngopharyngectomy included a 12% operative mortality, fistula, aspiration, and dysphagia.[143] The complications of total laryngopharyngectomy include a treatment-related mortality of 11%, fistula, and pharyngeal stenosis.[143] The complication rate is increased by the addition of radiation therapy.

Radiation Therapy Complications. The major radiation therapy complication is laryngeal necrosis. Laryngeal edema occurs temporarily in most cases and is increased by neck dissection. Late complications related to radiation therapy or salvage surgery (or both) occurred in 12 of 101 patients (12%) described by Amdur et al.[138] Three of 12 patients experienced fatal complications.

Complications of Salvage Treatment. Attempted surgical salvage of radiation therapy failures has a significant operative morbidity and mortality even in the best of hands, but few cures are produced.

NASOPHARYNX

Malignant tumors of the nasopharynx are uncommon in the United States. The Chinese have a high frequency; American-born second-generation Chinese maintain the risk of nasopharyngeal cancer. Nasopharyngeal cancer has also been shown to have an association with elevated titers of Epstein-Barr virus; this finding is independent of geography.[145] There is a 3:1 ratio of predominance in men. The age distribution for carcinoma is much younger than that for other head and neck sites; approximately 20% of patients are younger than 30 years of age.

Anatomy

The nasopharynx is roughly cuboidal. It is in direct continuity with the nasal cavity, and is connected inferiorly with the oropharynx and laterally with the middle ears by way of the eustachian tubes.

The mucosa of the roof and posterior wall is often irregular because of the pharyngeal bursa, pharyngeal tonsil (adenoids), and pharyngeal hypophysis. The mucosa tends to become smoother with age, but many folds may remain in the later years of life.

The lateral walls include the eustachian openings with the fossa of Rosenmüller (pharyngeal recess) located behind the torus tubarius. The superolateral muscular wall of the nasopharynx is incomplete and provides a meager barrier to tumor spread. Once tumor has penetrated the lateral wall, it enters the lateral pharyngeal space and its contents. The floor of the nasopharynx is incomplete and consists of the upper surface of the soft palate.

LYMPHATICS. There is an extensive submucosal lymphatic capillary plexus. Tumor cells spread along three different lymph node pathways: the jugular chain, the spinal accessory chain, and the retropharyngeal pathway (Fig. 26.2-16).[146] The

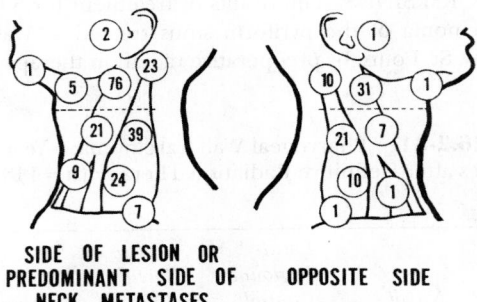

SIDE OF LESION OR PREDOMINANT SIDE OF NECK METASTASES   OPPOSITE SIDE

FIGURE 26.2-16.   Distribution of metastases to lymph node areas in epithelial tumors of the nasopharynx. The circled numbers indicate the number of times the particular lymph node was involved. Note the high incidence of involvement of the lymph nodes of the spinal accessory chain. Total cases = 99. No lymph nodes were involved in 10 patients (10%); lymph nodes were involved in 89 patients (89%). There was unilateral involvement in 38 patients (39%) and bilateral involvement in 51 patients (51%). (From ref. 146, with permission. Copyright 1965, American Roentgen Ray Society.)

lateral retropharyngeal nodes lie in the retropharyngeal space and medial to the carotid artery. Directly behind the nodes are the lateral masses for C-1 and C-2. Marked nodal enlargement, such as that which occurs in lymphoma, may distort the posterior tonsillar pillar, shifting it medially and anteriorly. Otherwise, diagnosis depends on contrast-enhanced CT or MRI. Inconstant lymphatic vessels are described as draining directly to the midjugular nodes and to the spinal accessory nodes.[3]

Pathology

Most histologic varieties of malignant tumor have been reported to arise from the nasopharynx and its immediate supporting structures. Carcinomas compose approximately 85% and lymphomas approximately 10% of the malignant lesions. The World Health Organization (WHO) has classified nasopharyngeal carcinomas as follows: WHO-1, squamous cell carcinoma; WHO-2, nonkeratinizing carcinoma; and WHO-3, undifferentiated carcinoma. Lymphoepithelioma is included in the WHO-3 category.[147] A miscellaneous group of malignant tumors includes melanoma, plasmacytoma,[148] juvenile angiofibroma,[149] carcinosarcoma, sarcomas, nonchromaffin paragangliomas, and minor salivary gland tumors.

Patterns of Spread

PRIMARY. Inferior extension along the lateral pharyngeal walls and tonsillar pillars is recognized in almost one-third of patients. Extension into the posterior nasal cavity is frequent but usually limited to less than 1 cm. Invasion of the posterior ethmoids, the maxillary antrum, and the orbit occurs fairly often and is important to recognize because it dictates a modification of treatment techniques. Invasion into or through the base of the skull is recognized radiographically or clinically in at least 25% of patients before treatment. The sphenoid sinus frequently is invaded. Tumor may erode through the foramen ovale, the foramen lacerum, and the foramen spinosum. Tumor eventually reaches the cavernous sinus and has access to cranial nerves II to VI (Fig. 26.2-17).

The lateral muscular wall of the nasopharynx is incomplete superiorly. The defect, termed the *sinus of Morgagni*, is traversed by the cartilaginous portion of the eustachian tube and the levator palatine muscle, providing access for cancer of the nasopharynx to the lateral pharyngeal space and base of the skull.

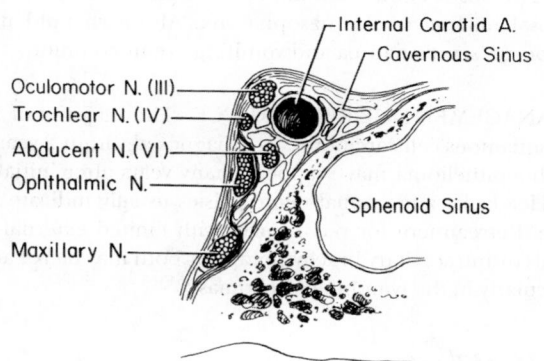

FIGURE 26.2-17. Coronal section of the cavernous sinus. (From ref. 147, with permission.)

LYMPHATICS. There is an 80% to 90% incidence of metastatic neck node disease on presentation; approximately 50% of patients have bilateral lymph node metastases (see Fig. 26.2-16). Low-grade squamous cell carcinomas produce fewer metastases (73%) than high-grade carcinomas (92%). Metastases to submental and occipital nodes may appear when there is blockage of the common lymphatic pathways either by massive neck disease or by an untimely neck dissection.

Clinical Picture

The most common presenting complaint is a painless upper neck mass or masses, which may be quite large when first discovered. Nasal obstruction, epistaxis, and otitis media are caused by local tumor effect. Sore throat occurs in approximately 15% of patients and is related to spread into the oropharyngeal wall. Facial pain may be referred from any of the three divisions of the trigeminal nerve, usually the mandibular division. Occipital or temporal headache frequently is seen. Pain in the scalp over the left mastoid area is related to involvement of a high jugular lymph node that has become fixed to the skull and spine. Pain in lifting the head and extending the neck is related to posterior infiltration of the prevertebral muscles. Proptosis occurs with posterior orbital invasion and usually displaces the eyeball anteriorly. Trismus is related to the invasion of the pterygoid region.

Neurologic symptoms and signs occur in approximately 25% of patients. Involvement of cranial nerves II to VI indicates intracranial extension into the cavernous sinus. Cranial nerves IX to XII and the sympathetic chain are involved in the lateral pharyngeal space.

Examination of the nasopharynx shows a lesion on the lateral wall or roof; the nasopharyngeal surface of the soft palate is rarely involved. In early lesions, the findings may be subtle with only slight fullness in the fossa of Rosenmüller or a small submucosal bulge in the roof. Lymphomas tend to remain submucosal until quite large.

Fiberoptic examination may show tumor growing into the posterior and superior nasal cavity. Tumor may be seen infiltrating submucosally along the posterior tonsillar pillars but infrequently grows very far down the posterior pharyngeal wall. The posterior tonsillar pillars may bulge into the oropharynx if an enlarged node develops in the lateral pharyngeal space. The cranial nerves should be carefully evaluated; cranial nerve VI is the one most commonly involved. The eyes should be evaluated for proptosis. Ear examination may show findings of otitis media or, rarely, gross tumor.

AJCC Staging

The AJCC staging system for primary tumors of the nasopharynx is as follows[16]:

Primary Tumor (T)

T1   Tumor confined to the nasopharynx
T2   Tumor extends to soft tissues
T2a Tumor extends to the oropharynx and/or nasal cavity without parapharyngeal extension [Parapharyngeal extension denotes posterolateral infiltration of tumor beyond the pharyngobasilar fascia]

T2b   Any tumor with parapharyngeal extension [Parapharyngeal extension denotes posterolateral infiltration of tumor beyond the pharyngobasilar fascia]
T3   Tumor involves bony structures and/or paranasal sinuses
T4   Tumor with intracranial extension and/or involvement of cranial nerves, infratemporal fossa, hypopharynx, orbit, or masticator space

Regional Lymph Nodes (N)

NX   Regional lymph nodes cannot be assessed
N0   No regional lymph node metastasis
N1   Unilateral metastasis in lymph node(s), 6 cm or less in greatest dimension, above the supraclavicular fossa [Midline nodes are considered ipsilateral nodes]
N2   Bilateral metastasis in lymph node(s), 6 cm or less in greatest dimension, above the supraclavicular fossa
N3a   Metastasis in a lymph node(s) greater than 6 cm
N3b   Extension to the supraclavicular fossa

Stage Grouping

0	Tis	N0	M0
I	T1	N0	M0
IIA	T2a	N0	M0
IIB	T1	N1	M0
	T2a	N1	M0
	T2b	N0–N1	M0
III	T1	N2	M0
	T2a–T2b	N2	M0
	T3	N0–N2	M0
IVA	T4	N0–N2	M0
IVB	Any T	N3	M0
IVC	Any T	Any N	M1

Treatment

SELECTION OF TREATMENT MODALITY. The treatment of almost all malignancies of the nasopharynx is by radiation therapy because complete surgical resection is usually not feasible. Neck dissection is used less often in the management of neck disease because of the relatively high success rate with radiation therapy alone, particularly for lymphoepithelioma. Neck dissection should be added for large masses, persistence, or recurrence after irradiation. A small adenocarcinoma or sarcoma may be excised. Juvenile angiofibromas are preferably excised because of the young age of the patient, although the tumors are quite successfully cured by radiation therapy when complete resection is unlikely or dangerous.[149] Although the benefit of adjuvant chemotherapy for nasopharyngeal carcinomas is questioned by some investigators, most patients with advanced disease should be evaluated for concomitant chemotherapy.[150–153]

IRRADIATION TECHNIQUE. The anatomic radiation treatment planning is the same for squamous cell carcinoma, transitional cell carcinoma, and lymphoepithelioma. If the tumor is thought to be limited to the nasopharynx or to have minimal soft tissue extension, the following areas are included in the treatment volume: (1) nasopharynx proper, (2) posterior 2 cm of the nasal cavity, (3) posterior ethmoid sinuses, (4) entire sphenoid sinus and basioccipital bone, (5) cavernous sinus, (6) base of the skull (7 to 8 cm width encompassing the foramen ovale,

carotid canal, and foramen spinosum laterally), (7) pterygoid fossae, (8) posterior one-third of maxillary sinus, (9) oropharyngeal wall to the level of the mid-tonsillar fossa, (10) retropharyngeal nodes, and (11) neck nodes on both sides.

Extension to the base of the skull or involvement of cranial nerves II to VI requires the superior border be raised to include the entire pituitary, the base of the brain in the suprasellar area, the adjacent middle cranial fossa, and the posterior portion of the anterior cranial fossa. Patients with anterior invasion into the orbit, ethmoids, or maxillary sinus require an individualized plan to produce a satisfactory dose distribution. The use of three-dimensional CT-based treatment planning allows for the use of more conformal fields. IMRT is useful to reduce the dose to parotid glands and the temporal lobes to reduce long-term morbidity. Patients may be treated once daily at 2 Gy/fraction to doses of 66 Gy for T1 or T2 cancers or to 70 Gy for T3 or T4 lesions. The authors currently treat patients to 74.4 to 76.8 Gy at 1.2 Gy/fraction twice daily. Patients treated with IMRT receive 72 Gy in 42 fractions using the M. D. Anderson Hospital concomitant boost technique.

Neck Nodes. A comprehensive *en bloc* plan must be developed to irradiate the neck to the level of the clavicles. The retropharyngeal nodes are included in the treatment of the primary lesion. The upper neck nodes are included in the primary fields to the level of the thyroid notch. In the case of a clinically negative neck, the posterior margin is placed 1 to 2 cm behind the posterior border of the sternocleidomastoid to encompass the high spinal accessory nodes and upper internal jugular nodes. The portals are extended anteriorly into the submental area only if there is disease in the submandibular triangle or if the patient had a neck dissection before irradiation. The lower neck is treated through an anterior portal with a shield over the larynx.

Acute Sequelae. The large volume of mucosa irradiated produces significant side effects during treatment. The addition of adjuvant chemotherapy increases the acute toxicity. Sore throat begins at the end of the second week of therapy and persists for 1 to 2 months after the completion of treatment. Dryness is always present and may be severe. Loss of taste and appetite is often quite profound, but both return 1 to 6 months after completion of treatment. The auditory tube is in the high-dose area, and obstruction may occur with secondary otitis media and hearing loss. Polyethylene tubes inserted through the eardrums to drain the middle ears can correct this condition. The obstruction often improves or clears completely after mucosal healing of the nasopharynx. Although mild nausea may occur, severe nausea and vomiting are uncommon.

MANAGEMENT OF RECURRENCE. The majority of recurrent squamous cell carcinomas are diagnosed within 2 years, but lymphoepithelioma may reappear many years after initial therapy. Headache and cranial nerve palsies usually indicate recurrence. Retreatment for recurrences with limited external-beam portals or intracavitary brachytherapy or both may be rewarding, particularly in the lymphoepitheliomas.[154,155]

Results of Treatment

Lee and coworkers[156] reported the following 10-year outcomes in a series of 5037 patients treated with radiation therapy at the

Queen Elizabeth Hospital, Hong Kong, between 1976 and 1985: local control, 61%; regional control, 64%; distant metastasis–free survival, 59%; and survival, 42%. Chua et al.[157] evaluated 290 patients and found that primary tumor volume of more than 60 cc was associated with a lower likelihood of local control after radiation therapy. Teo and colleagues[158] evaluated a series of 903 patients treated at the Prince of Wales Hospital, Hong Kong, and observed that local control was adversely affected by advanced patient age, skull-base invasion, and cranial nerve involvement. Prognostic factors associated with an increased rate of distant metastases and poor survival were male sex, skull-base and cranial nerve(s) involvement, advanced neck stage, nodal fixation, and bilateral positive neck nodes.[158]

Follow-Up

Follow-up includes careful observation and laboratory testing for possible endocrine hypofunction of the thyroid and pituitary. Dental care must be closely monitored because of the severe xerostomia.

Detection of a local-regional recurrence is important, because salvage is occasionally possible, especially if the recurrence is a marginal miss or the initial doses were low.

Complications of Treatment

The irradiation of part of the brain including the hypothalamus, frontal and temporal lobes, and pituitary to doses between 60 Gy and 75 Gy has only rarely been associated with brain necrosis. Primary or secondary hypopituitarism (from a hypothalamic lesion) has been reported. Hypothyroidism may result from either a direct effect on the thyroid gland or an indirect effect on the pituitary. Delayed bone age and growth failure may be seen in young patients. A transient CNS syndrome may appear 2 to 3 months after irradiation and may require several months to resolve. General weakness and extreme fatigue may be symptoms of low serum cortisol levels. Radiation myelitis of the cervical cord or brainstem is the most severe CNS complication. IMRT may be used to reduce the dose to the CNS, particularly the temporal lobes.

Trismus occurs to varying degrees because of fibrosis of the pterygoid muscles; this is more likely in those treated with two opposing portals for the entire course. Palsy of cranial nerves IX to XII may occur several years after treatment and is related to nerve entrapment in the lateral pharyngeal space. Eye complications (e.g., retrobulbar optic neuritis) may develop owing to irradiation of the optic nerve. Irradiation of the posterior eyeball to high doses may produce a radiation retinopathy with decreased vision or even total loss of vision.

NASAL VESTIBULE, NASAL CAVITY, AND PARANASAL SINUSES

Tumors of the nasal vestibule are considered separately from nasal cavity tumors because they are essentially skin cancers and have a different natural history.[159] Primary tumors arising from the nasal cavity and paranasal sinuses are considered together because the lesions are frequently advanced when first seen and it is not always possible to determine the site of origin with certainty. Primary lesions of the lower half of the maxillary sinuses and limited lesions of the nasal cavity can be identified as such.

Cancer of the nasal cavity or paranasal sinuses is a relatively rare problem with a yearly risk factor estimated at approximately one case for every 100,000 people. These cancers occur more often in men (2 to 1) and usually appear after the age of 40 except for tumors of minor salivary gland origin and esthesioneuroblastomas, which may even appear before the age of 20.[160] Nasal cavity and ethmoid sinus adenocarcinomas have been linked to occupations associated with wood dust: those in the furniture industry, sawmill work, and carpentry. Other occupations with dust-filled work environments such as shoe making, baking, and flour milling also have been implicated as a cause of adenocarcinomas.[161–164] Thorotrast, containing the radioactive metal thorium, is a known etiologic agent in maxillary sinus carcinomas. Thorotrast was used in past years as a contrast medium for radiographic study of the maxillary sinuses. The Thorotrast was retained in the sinus and was responsible for tumor induction.

Primary carcinomas of the sphenoid sinuses are said to be rare. They mimic nasopharyngeal carcinoma and most often are diagnosed after they penetrate the nasopharynx, at which time they are thought to be advanced nasopharyngeal cancer.

Frontal sinus neoplasms are rare.

Anatomy

The nasal vestibule is the entrance to the nasal cavity. It is lined by skin in which there are numerous hair follicles and sebaceous glands. The vestibule is a three-sided, pear-shaped cavity approximately 1.5 cm in diameter that ends posteriorly at the limen nasi. The alar cartilages form the anterolateral wall. The medial wall is the mobile columella, formed by the medial wing of the alar cartilage and the anterior portion of the cartilaginous septum. The floor is the superior surface of the hard palate (maxilla).

The nasal cavity begins at the limen nasi and ends at the posterior nares, where it communicates directly with the nasopharynx. Each lateral wall is composed of thin bony folds that project into the nasal cavity. These are the inferior, medial, and superior nasal turbinates. The nasolacrimal duct enters the nasal cavity beneath the inferior turbinate. The frontal sinus and ethmoid bullae connect to the nasal cavity with openings that lie under the middle turbinate. The sphenoid sinus communicates with the nasal cavity by an opening on the anterior wall of the sphenoid sinus. The olfactory nerves enter the nasal cavity through the cribriform plate and distribute nerve fibers over the upper one-third of the septum and superior nasal turbinate. Approximately 20 branches of the olfactory nerve penetrate the cribriform plate, and these perforations provide an avenue of tumor spread to the floor of the anterior cranial fossa. The epithelium is nonciliated columnar. The lower half of the nasal cavity is the respiratory portion, and the epithelium is ciliated columnar. There are numerous collections of lymphoid tissue and mucous glands beneath the epithelium.

The maxillary sinuses are single pyramidal cavities with average measurements of approximately 3.7 cm in height by 2.5 cm in transverse diameter by 3 cm anteroposteriorly, and a volume of approximately 15 cc in adults. The medial wall is the lateral wall of the nasal cavity and has one or two openings communicating with the middle meatus under the medial turbinate. The inferior wall, or floor, is the hard palate. The roots of the teeth may penetrate into the cavity. The posterolateral wall is related to the zygomatic process and the pterygomaxillary space. The superior wall is the orbital floor.

The frontal sinuses are two irregular, asymmetrical air cavities separated by a thin bony septum. They connect to the middle meatus of the nasal cavity by the frontonasal duct. Frontal sinus cells may extend far laterally in the orbital process of the frontal bone. They are separated from the anterior ethmoid cells by thin bony walls. The posterior wall separating the frontal sinus from the anterior cranial fossa is relatively thick in most patients.

The ethmoid sinuses consist of a number of air cells lying between the medial walls of the orbits and the lateral wall of the nasal cavity. The lateral wall is the lamina papyracea, a very thin, porous bone easily penetrated by tumor. Medially, the ethmoid air cells bulge into the lateral wall of the nasal cavity and from the superior and medial turbinates. The ethmoid cells communicate with the nasal cavity in the middle meatus. These bony walls are thin and easily traversed by tumor. The ethmoid air cells extend far anteriorly, and for this reason ethmoid lesions may present as a subcutaneous mass at the inner canthus. The lacrimal bone covers the anterior cells laterally. The midline perpendicular plate of the ethmoid separates the right and left ethmoid cells anatomically. There is no anatomic barrier between the anterior, middle, and posterior ethmoids.

The sphenoid sinus is a midline structure in the body of the sphenoid bone. The pituitary lies above, the cavernous sinuses laterally, the nasal cavity and ethmoid sinuses in front, and the nasopharynx beneath. The clivus and brainstem lie posteriorly. The pneumatization is variable and can extend into all portions of the sphenoid bone. The right and left sinuses are partially separated by a septum, but are considered as one in treatment planning because the septum is incomplete and easily penetrated. The sphenoid sinus connects anteriorly with the nasal cavity in the sphenoethmoidal recess.

LYMPHATICS

Nasal Vestibule. The lymphatic trunks run to the submaxillary nodes. There is a small risk for involvement of an intercalated facial node just behind the commissure of the lip along the course of the facial neurovascular bundle. In addition, preauricular nodes occasionally are involved, especially when tumor invades the lip or skin of the ala nasi.

Nasal Cavity and Paranasal Sinuses. The lymphatics of the nasal cavity are separated into the olfactory group and the respiratory group. According to Rouviere,[3] they do not communicate with each other. There is a connection between the lymphatic network of the olfactory region and the subarachnoid spaces, which allows some absorption of cerebrospinal fluid (CSF) into the lymphatic system. The lymphatics of the olfactory region of the nasal cavity run posteriorly to terminate in lymph nodes alongside the jugular vein at the base of the skull in the lateral pharyngeal space. The lymphatics of the respiratory nasal cavity also run posteriorly to terminate a bit lower, either in the lateral retropharyngeal node or the subdigastric node. The capillary lymphatic plexus of the nasal mucosa is probably not very profuse, judged by the relatively low incidence of metastatic nodes even with advanced disease.

The mucosa of the paranasal sinuses has either no capillary lymphatics or a very sparse number of capillary lymphatics.

Metastases from carcinomas of the paranasal sinuses are uncommon, even though lesions frequently are quite advanced. It is unlikely for a paranasal sinus tumor to present with cervical lymphadenopathy and an asymptomatic primary lesion confined to a sinus.

Pathology

BENIGN TUMORS. Many so-called benign tumors destroy bone and soft tissues and, if uncorrected, cause death. The management of some of these problems is not unlike cancer treatment. Inflammatory polyps, giant cell reparative granulomas, benign odontogenic tumors, and necrotizing sialometaplasia are some of the benign lesions appearing in this area.[165]

MALIGNANT TUMORS

Nasal Vestibule. Almost all malignant tumors arising in the nasal vestibule are squamous cell carcinomas; basal cell carcinomas and adnexal carcinomas are also reported.

Nasal Cavity and Paranasal Sinuses. Squamous cell carcinoma or one of its variants is the most common neoplasm. Minor salivary gland tumors account for 10% to 15% of neoplasms in this region. Lymphoma and melanoma account for approximately 5% and 1% of cases, respectively. Esthesioneuroblastoma or olfactory neuroblastoma is a malignant neurogenic tumor that originates from the olfactory mucosa. It occurs at all ages, with cases commonly seen in the second and third decades. A wide range of soft tissue and bone sarcomas is reported for the nasal cavity and paranasal sinus region, including chondrosarcoma, osteosarcoma, and Ewing's sarcoma.

Inverting papilloma of the nasal cavity is a confusing condition often called benign, but for practical reasons it is best classified as malignant because it may have a rather aggressive clinical picture that requires cancer-type management and may be associated with a carcinoma. It is better approached as a "grade one-half" neoplasm than as a benign polyp; it may be lethal if uncontrolled. The histologic picture is that of a papilloma growing into the stroma rather than growing outward. The lesion occurs predominantly in men 40 to 70 years of age. Squamous cell or transitional cell carcinoma is reported in association with inverting papillomas in 5% to 15% of cases and represents conversion of the papilloma to a more malignant tumor.[166]

Midline lethal granuloma is a natural killer nasal T-cell lymphoma that is a progressively destructive condition involving the nose, paranasal sinuses, and hard palate, and produces secondary erosion of contiguous structures. Unchecked, the disease is fatal, usually after an extended illness. Death results from extension to the CNS, hemorrhage, sepsis, or inanition. Treatment is usually radiation therapy. Chemotherapy is used in combination if the patient is medically able to tolerate combined modality therapy.

Patterns of Spread

NASAL VESTIBULE

Primary. Lesions of the nasal vestibule invade the alar and septal cartilages and may extend to the skin surface of the nose. The upper lip is frequently invaded. Posterior growth into the nasal cavity is frequent. Early cancers originating on the columella and anterior septum are often superficial lesions that ulcerate and produce a crust or scab and often present with perforation of the membranous and cartilaginous septum.

Lymphatic. Lymph node spread is usually to a solitary ipsilateral submaxillary node, but may be bilateral. The facial, preauricular, and submental nodes are at small risk. Mendenhall and coworkers[159] reported only 4 of 60 patients (7%) with clinically positive lymph nodes at diagnosis, but 7 patients (12%) later developed positive lymph nodes.

NASAL CAVITY AND PARANASAL SINUSES

Nasal Cavity. The routes of spread for lesions of the nasal cavity are essentially the same for various histologies, with the exception of esthesioneuroblastoma and minor salivary gland tumors. The latter have a greater propensity for perineural spread, although squamous cell carcinoma and esthesioneuroblastoma also may follow nerve pathways.

Lesions arising in the olfactory region invade the ethmoids and the orbit, spread through the sieve-like cribriform plate to the anterior cranial fossa, and spread between bone and dura. Eventually they penetrate dura and invade the frontal lobes. These lesions also tend to destroy the septum and may invade through nasal bone to the skin. Lesions arising on the lateral wall of the nasal cavity invade the maxillary sinus, ethmoids, and orbit.

Esthesioneuroblastomas may show submucosal spread and may grow along olfactory nerves and penetrate through an intact dura to the frontal lobe.

The nasopharynx and sphenoid sinus are secondarily invaded in advanced lesions. Tumor may follow the numerous nasal nerves posteriorly and then superiorly toward the sphenopalatine ganglion near the base of the skull or along the maxillary branch of the trigeminal nerve.

Maxillary Sinus. All walls of the sinus may be penetrated by tumor; the pattern of spread and bone destruction is dependent on site of origin within the sinus. Lesions arising in the anterolateral infrastructure tend to invade through the lateral inferior wall or grow through dental sockets. Cancer presents in the oral cavity when tumor erodes through the maxillary gingiva or into the gingivobuccal sulcus, at first appearing as a submucosal mass, causing elevation of the mucosa, loosening of the teeth, or improper seating of a denture. Ulceration follows, with the development of an oral-antral fistula. Lesions arising on the medial infrastructure readily extend through the thin, porous medial wall into the nasal cavity.

Posterior infrastructure lesions erode through the posterolateral wall and into the infratemporal fossa. Tumor escaping posteriorly has immediate access to the base of the skull and may preclude an operative attempt. Extension of lesions to the orbit occurs either directly through the roof of the maxillary sinus, by a circuitous route through the ethmoids and lamina papyracea, or by way of the infratemporal fossa and then through the infraorbital fissure.

Tumors arising in the suprastructure of the antrum have two general patterns of development. One group develops laterally, invades the malar bone, and produces a mass just below the lateral floor of the orbit that may eventually ulcerate through to the skin. The orbit is invaded laterally and the eye is displaced inward and upward. The temporal fossa is often involved, as is the zygomatic bone in very advanced lesions. The suprastruc-

tural cancers that develop medially invade the nasal cavity, ethmoid and frontal sinuses, lacrimal apparatus, and medial inferior orbit. It is often impossible to determine whether the origin is maxillary antrum, nasal cavity, or ethmoid.

Ethmoid Sinuses. Lesions of the ethmoid sinuses have many options for local spread because of their location and the thin, porous bony walls, none of which offers much resistance to tumor penetration. The lamina papyracea is the lateral wall for the middle and posterior ethmoid air cells, and invasion through it into the medial orbit is common. The anterior ethmoid cells are covered laterally by the small, thin lacrimal bone and the frontal process of the maxilla. Thus, the ethmoid air cells extend anteriorly within a centimeter of the inner canthus. The medial surfaces of the ethmoid labyrinth are the middle and superior nasal conchae, which are formed by thin, convoluted bone; spread into the nasal cavity is common. The more advanced lesions invade the maxillary antrum, nasopharynx, sphenoid sinus, and anterior cranial fossa.

Sphenoid Sinus. There is little information regarding spread patterns for tumors arising in the sphenoid sinus. It is probable that some of the advanced nasopharyngeal lesions are, in reality, primary sphenoid sinus lesions. The fact that a disproportionate number of advanced nasopharyngeal lesions have no neck metastases is suggestive of their origin in the sphenoid sinus, a site with sparse, if any, capillary lymphatics. The sphenoid sinus is closely related to the cranial nerves in the cavernous sinus: III, IV, and VI, and the ophthalmic and maxillary branches of the trigeminal nerve (see Fig. 26.2-17). Cranial nerve palsies and headache are frequently the first clinical evidence of a sphenoid sinus tumor. Diagnosis is usually made, however, when tumor eventually breaks through into the nasopharynx or nasal cavity where it can be seen and biopsy performed.

Inverting Papilloma. A report of 223 cases of inverting papillomas showed that the lateral nasal wall was the most commonly involved site (68%), with ethmoid and maxillary sinus involvement also being common (57%), as was involvement of the septum (28%). However, ethmoid and maxillary sinus involvement without tumor of the lateral nasal wall occurred in 4%. Intracranial extension was usually associated with a carcinoma. Tumor occurred bilaterally when there was spread through the nasal septum; multicentric sites of origin were observed.[167] There are two reports in the literature of cervical metastases from benign-appearing inverted papillomas; the metastases had the microscopic appearance of inverting papillomas.[168,169]

Lymphatic. The incidence of lymphatic metastases at diagnosis is 10% to 15% for nasal cavity and ethmoid sinus tumors and probably lower for antral and sphenoid tumors. The risk of lymphatic metastases is related to extension of tumor outside the sinus to areas with capillary lymphatics. Maxillary sinus tumors that invade the oral cavity and involve the buccal mucosa, maxillary gingiva, or hard palate may spread to the submandibular and jugulodigastric nodes. Lesions that invade the nasal cavity or nasopharynx spread posteriorly to the parapharyngeal nodes and then to the jugulodigastric area. Minor salivary gland tumors, melanoma, and sarcomas have an unknown rate of lymph node metastasis. The risk of cervical node involvement for esthesioneuroblastoma is approximately 20%.[160]

Clinical Picture

NASAL VESTIBULE. Lesions of the nasal vestibule present with symptoms of a slow-growing mass with attendant crusting, and occasional minor bleeding. Pain, if it occurs, is usually modest, even with destruction of cartilage or involvement of the lip. Septal perforation may occur.

NASAL CAVITY AND PARANASAL SINUSES

Nasal Cavity. The earliest symptoms of nasal cavity neoplasms are a low-grade chronic infection with discharge, obstruction, and minor, intermittent bleeding. The symptoms mimic those associated with nasal polyps; because many of the patients with nasal neoplasms have a previous history of nasal operations for polyps, cancer is often missed in an early stage. The patient often complains of "sinus trouble" and intermittent anterior headache. Subsequent symptoms depend on pattern of growth. Lesions arising in the olfactory region may cause unilateral or bilateral nasal expansion of the bridge of the nose, and a submucosal mass may appear near the inner canthus and eventually ulcerate. Obstruction of the nasolacrimal system may be a presenting complaint, with the patient treated by incision and drainage for dacryocystitis. Extension through the cribriform plate or into the ethmoid sinuses is accompanied by frontal headache. Aberration of smell is rare. Invasion of the medial orbit produces proptosis and diplopia; a mass may be palpated in the orbit. Indirect examination of the nasopharynx may show early submucosal invasion through the posterior nares.

Maxillary Sinus. Maxillary sinus cancers develop silently when they are confined to the sinus and produce symptoms after extension through the walls. If the tumor invades toward the oral cavity, the presenting symptoms relate to pain associated with the upper teeth; there may be a loosening and eventually loss of teeth. Tumor may penetrate into the gingivobuccal sulcus or upper gum and eventually progress to an oral-antral fistula. If the patient wears upper dentures, the first symptom is an ill-fitting denture. Palpation and observation of the face may show a mass. Early invasion of the floor of the orbit may be detected by feeling both orbits simultaneously with the tips of the index fingers inserted between the bony rim and eyeball. Posterior invasion of the orbit produces proptosis, diplopia, and edema of the conjunctiva. Invasion of the infraorbital nerve or its branches in the floor of the orbit may cause paresthesia of the skin of the lower eyelid, side of the nose, and anterior premaxillary skin. Nasal obstruction and bleeding are common complaints, along with "sinus pain" or "fullness" over the involved antrum. Trismus and headache are associated with invasion posteriorly into the pterygopalatine fossa, pterygoid muscles, infratemporal fossa, and base of the skull.

Cancers developing in the medial suprastructure of the antrum present with nasal symptoms of discharge or bleeding, mild infraorbital pain, infected lacrimal sac, and displacement of the eye upward and laterally with proptosis, diplopia, and conjunctival edema.

Cancer developing in the lateral suprastructure produces a mass below the lateral canthus with associated pain. The eye may be deviated medially and upward when orbital invasion occurs. There is edema of the conjunctiva, narrowing of the palpebral opening, diplopia, and proptosis. Tumor may extend to the temporal fossa, producing a diffuse fullness.

Ethmoid Sinuses. Mild to moderate sinus ache or pain referred to the frontal-nasal area is an early symptom of ethmoid sinus lesions. A painless mass may present near the inner canthus; the mass may become infected and be misinterpreted as a boil or dacryocystitis. Diplopia develops with invasion of the medial orbit. Proptosis is often present, and a mass may be felt by digital palpation of the orbit. Nasal discharge, epistaxis, and obstruction are frequent presenting complaints. Paresthesia may occur over the distribution of sensory nerves.

Early invasion of the nasal cavity may produce only submucosal bulging into the superior or medial meatus, which is easily confused with allergic rhinitis, polyps, or inflammatory changes. Invasion into the nasopharynx is usually submucosal and appears on the roof and lateral wall. Advanced lesions may obstruct the eustachian canal.

AJCC Staging

The AJCC staging system for tumors of the nasal vestibule, nasal cavity, and paranasal sinuses is as follows[16]:

Nasal Vestibule

The staging system for skin cancer is used.

Maxillary Sinus

TX   Primary tumor cannot be assessed

T0   No evidence of primary tumor

Tis   Carcinoma *in situ*

T1   Tumor limited to the maxillary sinus mucosa with no erosion or destruction of bone

T2   Tumor causing bone erosion or destruction including extension into the hard palate and/or middle nasal meatus, except extension to posterior wall of maxillary sinus and pterygoid plates

T3   Tumor invades any of the following: bone of the posterior wall of maxillary sinus, subcutaneous tissues, floor of medial wall of orbit, pterygoid fossa, ethmoid sinuses

T4a   Tumor invades anterior orbital contents, skin of cheek, pterygoid plates, infratemporal fossa, cribriform plate, sphenoid or frontal sinuses

T4b   Tumor invades any of the following: orbital apex, dura, brain, middle cranial fossa, cranial nerves other than maxillary division of trigeminal nerve (V2), nasopharynx, or clivus

Nasal Cavity and Ethmoid Sinus

TX   Primary tumor cannot be assessed

T0   No evidence of primary tumor

Tis   Carcinoma *in situ*

T1   Tumor restricted to any one subsite, with or without bony invasion

T2   Tumor invading two subsites in a single region or extending to involve an adjacent region within the nasoethmoidal complex, with or without bony invasion

T3   Tumor extends to invade the medial wall or floor of the orbit, maxillary sinus, palate, or cribriform plate

T4a   Tumor invades any of the following: anterior orbital contents, skin of nose or cheek, minimal extension to anterior cranial fossa, pterygoid plates, sphenoid or frontal sinuses

T4b Tumor invades any of the following: orbital apex, dura, brain, middle cranial fossa, cranial nerves other than V2, nasopharynx, or clivus

Treatment

NASAL VESTIBULE

Selection of Treatment Modality. Both surgery and radiation therapy produce a high degree of success.[159] Radiation therapy is usually the preferred treatment because of the deformity produced by excision. Excision is preferred for very small lesions, the removal of which will not produce cosmetic deformity or require reconstruction; few lesions fit this description. Another subset of patients best treated surgically are those with invasion of the premaxilla. Radiation therapy is selected for the remainder.

Surgical Treatment. Excision of lesions in the nasal vestibule usually involves removal of cartilage as well as skin. Depending on the site of the lesion, either the columella, the septum, or the alar cartilages will have to be removed, with a resulting cosmetic deformity that is difficult to reconstruct. If the alar cartilage has been sacrificed, either a composite graft consisting of skin and cartilage from the ear or a nasolabial flap can be used to repair the defect. If the entire external nose is resected, a prosthesis is used.

Irradiation Technique. External-beam radiation therapy, brachytherapy, or a combination of both may be used. There are two basic external-beam treatment plans: opposed lateral portals and single anterior portal. When the tumor volume can be encompassed by lateral portals, there is an advantage in avoiding unnecessary exit irradiation to the nasal cavity, nasopharynx, and CNS. This technique confines irradiation to the anterior nasal area, but has the disadvantage of full skin reaction because a wax bolus nose block is necessary to ensure homogeneous irradiation. The portals may be angled posteriorly to ensure sufficient posterior coverage; wedges are added to compensate for the angle.

The single anterior portal technique uses a combination of photons and electrons. A wax bolus ensures a homogeneous dose. The advantages of this technique are that the portal may be shaped, shielding the eyes is easier, and the skin of the tip of the nose and sometimes the bridge of the nose need not be covered by wax, which allows some of the skin to receive a lesser dose of radiation. The dose ranges from 66 to 70 Gy at 2 Gy/fraction, once daily in a continuous course.

Interstitial brachytherapy of the nasal vestibule and nasal cavity is highly individualized and uses afterloaded ^{192}Ir needles. The implant is usually composed of two, three, or four planes of sources inserted perpendicularly through the skin surface of the external nose with crossing needles placed in the dorsum of the nose, floor of the nasal cavity, and upper lip. The dose varies depending on the size of the lesion.[159]

NASAL CAVITY

Selection of Treatment Modality. The histology, extent, and location of the malignant tumor in the nasal cavity are all considered when treatment decisions are made.

Inverting papilloma is treated initially by surgical excision. Depending on the procedure, the local recurrence rate may be fairly high, and subsequent excisions required. When the lesion begins to act aggressively with rapid recurrences and invasion of the sinuses, orbit, and anterior cranial fossa, it should be considered a low-grade cancer and treated appropriately by more radical removal. Irradiation is recommended for lesions that are incompletely resected, for patients with multiple recurrences, and for those in which carcinoma is found in the specimen.[166]

Squamous cell carcinoma and adenocarcinoma of the nasal cavity can be treated with surgery, irradiation, or both. Most analyses of nasal cavity carcinomas are included with paranasal sinus cancer series. Because of selection bias, it is difficult to compare the results of various therapies. Regional and distant metastases are relatively uncommon, and therefore local control is tantamount to cure.

Either surgery or radiation therapy is used for discrete early lesions. Operative management may be indicated for early lesions, in which good surgical margins can be expected without cosmetic or functional loss. Excision is also the treatment of choice for melanomas and sarcomas. Combined surgery and adjuvant radiosurgery are preferred at the authors' institution because local control is probably better than after single-modality treatment, and a lower dose can be used compared with definitive irradiation, thus reducing the risk of damage to the visual apparatus.[170] Definitive radiation therapy is used for incompletely resectable tumors.

Surgical Treatment. Lateral rhinotomy provides the best access for resection of lesions of the nasal cavity. Generally, reconstruction is not necessary unless the entire cartilaginous septum has been removed, in which case there will be a saddle deformity of the nose. The lateral wall of the nose may be removed by this approach for resection of inverting papilloma and other localized neoplasms. More advanced lesions require removal of involved sinuses and orbit. A craniofacial procedure may be required.

Irradiation Technique. The external-beam irradiation technique emphasizes an anterior portal with one or two lateral portals. Contiguous structures such as the maxillary sinus, ethmoid sinus, medial orbit, nasopharynx, base of the skull, and sphenoid sinus are generally included in the initial treatment volume as required. The treatment volume is reduced after 50 Gy to include the original gross disease with a margin. IMRT may be used if feasible.

Advanced lesions may require inclusion of an entire orbit. In these cases, loss of vision usually occurs, but an operation would require visual loss in any case. Treatment planning should protect the opposite eye and optic nerve.

Combined Treatment Policies. If combined treatment is planned, the authors prefer to perform the operation first to avoid obscuring the extent of tumor. Irradiation is started 4 to 6 weeks afterward. The dose is usually 60 Gy in 6 weeks to 65 Gy in 7 weeks for clear margins. Patients with positive margins or gross residual tumor after operation receive 74.4 Gy in 62 twice-daily fractions.

Management of Recurrence. Once the patient has had an operation or irradiation, it is difficult to determine the extent of recurrent disease because of changes caused by the previous therapy. The most common situation for salvage is a radiation or surgical therapy failure that can be treated successfully by a craniofacial resection. Tumor extension to the sphenopalatine fossa with definite destruction of a pterygoid plate is a relative contraindication to a craniofacial procedure. Cranial nerve involvement, posterior invasion near the optic chiasm, and sphenoid sinus or cavernous sinus invasion are contraindications to resection. MRI can distinguish between exudate and gross tumor in a sinus. The anterior wall of the sphenoid sinus may be removed, but the sinus itself cannot be completely resected. Postoperative irradiation should be considered whether or not margins are positive.

MAXILLARY SINUS

Selection of Treatment Modality. Surgical resection gives the best results. Early infrastructure lesions may be excised and cured by surgery alone, but for most other cases, irradiation is given postoperatively even if margins are negative. Extension of cancer to the base of the skull, nasopharynx, or sphenoid sinus contraindicates surgical excision. The pterygoid process below the foramen rotundum may be removed along with the attached pterygoid muscles, but destruction of the sphenoid bone above this point is a contraindication to operation. Procedures to resect portions of the base of the skull are described for special clinical situations.

Surgical Treatment. Surgery for carcinoma of the maxillary sinus depends on which walls are involved. If the floor of the orbit is free of disease, then the eye and the orbital rim may be left undisturbed. If, however, there is involvement through the floor of the orbit, then a maxillectomy with resection of the orbital floor with or without an orbital exenteration must be performed. If the posterior wall or the pterygoid plates are involved, they too must be included in the resection. A split-thickness skin graft is used to line the cavity, and a dental prosthesis is then used to fill the resulting deformity in the palate. The prosthesis is constructed before surgery so it can be placed at the time of operation and act as a stent. The permanent prosthesis is constructed approximately 6 months after the operation.

Irradiation Technique. Irradiation treatment planning includes the entire maxilla, the adjacent nasal cavity, ethmoid sinus, nasopharynx, and pterygopalatine fossa. All or part of the orbit is included in patients with extension into or near the orbital fossa; failure to include the orbital contents is one of the most common causes of treatment failure. Definition of the target volume is aided by the use of treatment planning CT, at times combined with image-fusion MRI. The prescribed dose is 65 to 70 Gy for irradiation alone. Altered fractionation should be considered. The dose for preoperative irradiation varies from 50 to 60 Gy, and the dose for postoperative irradiation varies from 60 to 70 Gy.

ETHMOID SINUS

Selection of Treatment Modality. Ethmoid sinus lesions are usually extensive when first diagnosed. Radiation therapy alone produces better results than surgery alone and is the preferred single treatment.[171] If resection is feasible with acceptable functional and cosmetic results, then the operation is carried out, followed by postoperative radiation therapy even if the margins are clear.

Surgical Treatment. Localized lesions require resection of the ethmoids and the ipsilateral maxilla and orbit. Extensive lesions are removed by a craniofacial procedure.

Irradiation Technique. Radiation treatment is entirely by external beam, emphasizing treatment through an anterior field combined with one or two lateral fields. This field arrangement, weighted 2:1 or 3:1 in favor of the anterior field, provides adequate treatment of the tumor volume while avoiding excessive irradiation of the contralateral eye and optic nerve. Wedges are added to achieve a satisfactory dose distribution. Electrons should not be used for the anterior portal. IMRT should be considered if a more conformal dose distribution can be achieved with this technique.

Management of Recurrence. Recurrent disease is heralded by recurrent pain and cranial nerve palsies. Localized recurrence after surgery only may be managed by radiation therapy alone or craniofacial resection and postoperative radiation therapy. Patients with radiation therapy failures may be suitable for maxillectomy or craniofacial resection.

SPHENOID SINUS. The treatment of sphenoid sinus lesions is with radiation therapy, and the technique is similar to that used for advanced carcinoma of the nasopharynx.

Results of Treatment

NASAL VESTIBULE. Goepfert and coworkers[172] reviewed the M. D. Anderson Hospital experience of 26 patients with squamous cell carcinoma of the nasal vestibule. The absolute 5-year survival was 78%. Ten patients were treated initially by surgery; one developed a local recurrence and successfully underwent salvage treatment by radiation. Sixteen patients were treated by radiation therapy; three developed local recurrence, and two successfully underwent a salvage operation.

Mendenhall et al.[159] reviewed results for 56 patients treated by irradiation at the University of Florida for squamous cell carcinoma of the nasal vestibule (Table 26.2-34). Four additional patients with unfavorable T4 cancers were treated with high-dose preoperative radiation therapy and resection. All four patients were cured; three of four experienced significant complications.

NASAL CAVITY AND ETHMOID SINUS

Inverting Papilloma. Weissler and coworkers[167] reported on 233 cases of inverting papilloma seen over a 35-year period. One hundred thirty-four patients had at least 1 year of follow-up. The risk of recurrence was 71% in patients who had an intranasal procedure and 56% in those who had a Caldwell-Luc procedure. Patients having a lateral rhinotomy had the lowest incidence of recurrence (29%). Reports from more modern

TABLE 26.2-34. Five-Year Outcomes of Squamous Cell Carcinoma of the Nasal Vestibule after Definitive Radiation Therapy at the University of Florida (56 Patients)

T Stage	No. of Patients	Local Control (%)	Cause-Specific Survival (%)
T1 or T2	35	94	86
T4	21	71	86
Overall	56	85	91

(Data from ref. 159.)

TABLE 26.2-35. Five-Year Outcomes for Malignancies of the Nasal Cavity and Paranasal Sinuses Treated at the University of Florida (78 Patients)

Disease Extent	No. of Patients	Local Control (%)	Cause-Specific Survival (%)	Survival (%)
Limited to site of origin	22	86	91	82
Extension to adjacent site	21	65	56	52
Destruction of skull base or pterygoid plates, or intracranial extension	35	34	34	29

(Data from ref. 170.)

series show an even lower incidence of recurrence when a lateral rhinotomy approach is used.[173]

Weissler and coworkers[167] also reported on six patients who received radiation therapy for benign inverting papilloma and nine who received radiation therapy for inverting papilloma associated with malignant disease. Twelve of the 15 patients had a complete response to radiation therapy and were free of disease for long periods of follow-up. Gomez et al.[174] reported on 10 patients with advanced or recurrent inverting papillomas who were treated with definitive radiation therapy. Local recurrence developed in four patients at 1.5, 6.5, 12.0, and 13.0 years after treatment. Six patients remained continuously disease free at 7.0, 8.5, 8.5, 9.0, 9.0, and 20.5 years after radiation therapy.

Carcinoma. Cheesman and coworkers[175] selected craniofacial resection for 54 patients with a variety of malignant tumors of the nasal cavity and paranasal sinuses. The majority were recurrent after surgery, radiation therapy, or chemotherapy. The operative mortality was 5%. Seven of 25 patients (28%) were free of disease with a minimum of 3 years of follow-up.

Katz et al.[170] reviewed results for 78 patients treated at the University of Florida for malignancies of the nasal cavity (48 patients), ethmoid sinus (24 patients), sphenoid sinus (5 patients), and frontal sinus (1 patient). Forty-seven patients

were treated with radiation therapy alone, 25 with surgery and postoperative irradiation, 2 with preoperative radiation therapy and surgery, and 4 with chemotherapy in combination with irradiation with or without surgery. Although patients who were treated with surgery and postoperative radiation therapy had improved local control at 5 years compared with those receiving definitive irradiation (79% vs. 49%, $P = .05$), multivariate analysis of local control revealed that only primary stage significantly influenced this end point. The 5-year outcomes are summarized in Table 26.2-35. Of the 67 patients who presented with a clinically negative neck, 39 patients received no elective neck irradiation and 33 patients (85%) remained regionally controlled. Elective neck irradiation was used in 28 patients, most of whom had advanced disease, and the neck remained disease free in 25 patients (89%).

Esthesioneuroblastoma. Elkon and coworkers[176] reviewed the literature on esthesioneuroblastoma and compiled the results of 78 cases (Table 26.2-36). They concluded that either radiation therapy or surgery was sufficient treatment for early-stage disease, but combined treatment might be advantageous for late-stage presentations. The 5-year absolute survival rate was 75% for stage A, 60% for stage B, and 41% for stage C.

Monroe and coworkers[160] reported on 22 patients treated with curative intent at the University of Florida and observed the following 5-year outcomes: local control, 59%; cause-specific survival, 54%; and survival, 48%. The 5-year cause-specific survival rate was lower after definitive radiation therapy (17%) compared with craniofacial resection and postoperative irradiation (56%). Cervical metastases occurred in 6 of 22 patients (27%). Recurrence in the neck was observed in four of nine patients with N0 disease initially who did not receive elective neck irradiation compared with 0 of 11 patients who were electively treated ($P = .02$).

MAXILLARY SINUS. Jesse[177] reviewed results for 63 patients with squamous cell carcinoma of the maxillary antrum who were treated for cure and had a 3-year survival rate of 44%. Three-year survival after surgery alone for selected lesions was 9 of 20 patients. Patients selected for combined treatment had either preoperative or postoperative irradiation; the results were similar for both techniques with an overall local recurrence rate of 38%. Patients with infrastructural lesions and superolateral lesions had a 3-year survival rate of 13 of 19 (68%), whereas

TABLE 26.2-36. Esthesioneuroblastoma: Results of Treatment to Primary Tumor by Modality and Stage for 78 Patients with Follow-Up of 6 Months to 32 Years (Number Controlled/Number Treated)

Modality	Stage A—Confined to Nasal Cavity		Stage B—Confined to Nasal Cavity and Paranasal Sinuses		Stage C—Beyond Nasal Cavity and Paranasal Sinuses	
	Initial Treatment	For Recurrent Disease at Primary Site	Initial Treatment	For Recurrent Disease at Primary Site	Initial Treatment	For Recurrent Disease at Primary Site
Radiation therapy alone	3/5	5/5	6/7	3/4	1/5	1/1
Surgery alone	5/9	2/2	3/6	—	1/1	0/0
Radiation therapy and surgery	9/10	0/0	15/20	0/1	7/15	0/0
Ultimate local control	24/24 (100%)	—	27/33 (82%)	—	10/21 (48%)	—

(Modified from ref. 176.)

those with supermedial or superoposterior lesions had a survival rate of 29%. An update of the M. D. Anderson Hospital experience included 85 patients and revealed no significant improvements in survival.[178]

Bataini and Ennuyer[179] reported the Curie Foundation results for 31 patients with carcinoma of the maxillary antrum treated by megavoltage radiation therapy between 1959 and 1965. Only three patients had limited primary disease; 30% had clinically positive lymph nodes. The 5-year survival rate was 32%. Waldron and coworkers[180] reported on 110 patients treated with curative intent at the Princess Margaret Hospital with definitive radiation therapy (83 patients) or surgery and adjuvant irradiation (27 patients). The 5-year rates of local control and cause-specific survival were 42% and 43%, respectively. Sixty-three patients developed a local recurrence and 25 of 63 underwent salvage surgery with a subsequent 5-year cause-specific survival of 31%.

Complications of Treatment

SURGERY. Complications of maxillectomy include failure of the split-thickness skin graft to heal, trismus, CSF leak, and hemorrhage. Complications of ethmoid sinus surgery include hemorrhage, meningitis, CSF leak, cellulitis and pansinusitis, brain abscess, and stroke. Complications of the craniofacial procedure include meningitis, subdural abscess, CSF leak, diplopia, and hemorrhage.

RADIATION THERAPY. Eye complications are the most frequent and significant complications of radiation therapy.[181-183] When only a portion of the ipsilateral eye is irradiated (medial one-third), it is possible to preserve vision in the majority of patients. When there is extensive disease in the orbit, however, the entire eye is irradiated to a high dose with almost certain loss of vision; however, these same patients would require orbital exenteration if treated by surgery. Katz et al.[170] reported ipsilateral blindness in 21 of 78 patients (27%); the complication was anticipated in most patients. Four patients (5%) developed unanticipated bilateral blindness; all were treated with definitive irradiation. The risk for bilateral blindness can be reduced by use of CT and MRI scans for improved treatment planning and knowledge of the tolerance of the optic nerve.

A few patients will experience a transient CNS syndrome that includes vertigo, headaches, decreased cerebration, and lethargy. This syndrome usually appears 2 to 3 months after completion of treatment, but may occur as late as 12 to 15 months. The early-appearing CNS syndromes usually last 1 to 2 months; the late-appearing syndromes last 6 to 12 months before slowly resolving. Aseptic meningitis, chronic sinusitis, or serous otitis media can occur. High-dose irradiation of the nasal cavity can cause narrowing and synechiae of the nasal cavity. Douching with saltwater and daily self-dilations with petrolatum-coated cotton swabs will reduce the problem. Septal perforations occur when tumor has destroyed part of the septum; these do not usually require treatment. Destruction of the nasal bone and septum by tumor may result in cosmetic deformity. Maxillary necrosis may develop, particularly if teeth are extracted.

CHEMODECTOMAS (GLOMUS BODY TUMORS)

Chemodectomas are an uncommon group of neoplasms that may originate anywhere glomus bodies are found. The lesions

are rare before the age of 20, there is a female predominance in some series, and the lesions occur in multiple sites in 10% to 20% of cases, especially in members of families with a history of this tumor. Carotid body tumors are associated with conditions producing chronic hypoxia, such as high-altitude habitation.

Anatomy

The normal glomus bodies in the head and neck vary from 0.1 to 0.5 mm in diameter. Tumors arising in glomus bodies (i.e., chemodectomas or nonchromaffin paragangliomas) arise most often from the carotid and temporal bone glomus bodies, with rare reports of tumors arising in the orbit, nasopharynx, larynx, nasal cavity, paranasal sinuses, tongue, and jaw. The temporal bone glomus bodies are not found consistently in any location, but vary from person to person. At least one-half of the glomus bodies are found in the general region of the jugular fossa and are located in the adventitia of the superior bulb of the internal jugular vein. The remaining are distributed along the course of the nerve of Jacobson (a branch of cranial nerve X). Approximately 20% of all temporal bone glomus bodies lie in the tympanic canaliculus and approximately 10% in relation to the cochlear promontory. A few glomus bodies are located in the descending part of the facial canal. The carotid bodies are located in relation to the bifurcation of the common carotid. Orbit bodies are in relation to the ciliary nerve, and vagal bodies are adjacent to the ganglion nodosum of the vagus nerve.

Pathology

Chemodectomas are histologically benign tumors resembling the parent tissue and consist of nests of epithelioid cells within stroma-containing, thin-walled blood vessels and nonmyelinated nerve fibers. The tumor mass is well circumscribed, but a true capsule is not seen. The criterion of malignancy is based on the clinical progress of the disease rather than the histologic picture. Chemodectomas without cellular atypia may metastasize to regional nodes or to distant organ sites.

Patterns of Spread

These lesions generally grow slowly; it is usual to have a history of symptoms for a few years and occasionally for 20 years or longer.

CAROTID BODY TUMORS. Carotid body tumors are usually located at the bifurcation of the common carotid and, as they expand, tend to displace and encircle the internal and external carotid vessels. The tumor begins in the adventitia of the artery and initially derives its blood supply from the vasa vasorum. An accessory blood supply may come from branches of the vertebral artery and ascending cervical artery. The tumor is usually closely adherent to the wall of the carotid adjacent to the vascular pedicle, and there may be thinning of the arterial wall owing to pressure by the mass. Large masses extend toward the cervical spine, base of the skull, angle of the mandible, and lateral pharyngeal space and its contents.

TEMPORAL BONE TUMORS. Glomus tympanicum lesions tend to be small when diagnosed because they produce symptoms early in their course. Tumor may involve the ossicles, tympanic membrane, mastoid, external auditory canal, semicircular canal, and the facial Jacobson's and Arnold's nerves.

Glomus jugulare tumors invade the base of the skull, petrous apex, jugular vein, middle ear, and middle and posterior cranial fossae. Cranial nerves V to XII may be involved.

LYMPHATIC METASTASES. Lymphatic metastases occur in approximately 5% of carotid body tumors but are very rare for temporal bone tumors. An upper neck mass may be an inferior extension of a jugular fossa or vagal tumor rather than a lymph node metastasis.

DISTANT METASTASES. Distant metastases have been rarely reported for temporal bone tumors; carotid body tumors have a low risk for distant metastases, probably in the range of 5% or less.

Clinical Picture

CAROTID BODY TUMORS. The most common presenting symptom of carotid body tumors is an asymptomatic, slow-growing mass in the upper neck near the bifurcation of the carotid. Large masses may encroach on the parapharyngeal space and produce dysphagia, pain, and cranial nerve palsies. A carotid sinus syndrome may occur because of the pressure of the mass.

On examination, the mass usually is found to lie deep to the sternocleidomastoid muscle and to be tethered to surrounding structures. Fixation occurs only in large tumors extending to the spine and base of the skull. A submucosal bulge may be seen in the tonsillar area. A bruit may be heard.

TEMPORAL BONE TUMORS. Because glomus bodies are distributed throughout the temporal bone, the initial symptoms and signs depend on the site of origin. Tumor arising in or near the middle ear presents with an insidious conductive hearing loss, pulsatile tinnitus, vertigo, and headache. Patients with lesions developing in or around the jugular fossa develop headache, often pulsatile in nature, referred to the orbit or temple. Cranial nerves V to XII and the sympathetic nerves become affected. Lesions developing in the facial canal present with facial nerve symptoms. Otorrhea and hemorrhage may occur when tumor breaks through into the external auditory canal.

A characteristic blue-red mass may be seen bulging in the tympanic membrane. A mass may be appreciated in the upper neck between the mandible and mastoid. Paralysis of cranial nerves V to XII and sympathetic nerves may occur.

Differential Diagnosis

CAROTID BODY TUMORS. The differential diagnosis for carotid body tumors includes enlarged lymph nodes, aneurysm of the carotid artery, branchial cleft cyst, benign tumors (e.g., lipoma), and direct extension of a lateral pharyngeal wall or pyriform sinus cancer into the soft tissues of the neck.

CT or MRI scan with contrast or both provide the diagnosis. A biopsy usually produces serious hemorrhage and is not recommended. Angiography is usually unnecessary unless resection is anticipated.

TEMPORAL BONE TUMORS. The differential diagnosis for temporal bone tumors includes the presentation of an internal carotid artery in the middle ear either as an aberrant vessel or as an aneurysm, and these patients also present with hearing loss, pulsatile tinnitus, and a pulsatile mass behind the eardrum. A high jugular bulb may present as a vascular mass in the middle ear and mimic a glomus tumor. Other diagnoses to be considered include the following: polyp of ear canal, malignant tumor of the nasopharynx with extension to the temporal bone, acoustic neuroma, carcinoma of the middle ear, metastatic carcinoma (especially breast cancer), cholesteatoma, histiocytosis, chronic serous otitis, and mastoiditis.

Staging

There is no accepted staging scheme for chemodectomas. Patients are considered to have an early lesion when there is little or no bone destruction and to have an advanced lesion when there is extensive bone destruction or cranial nerve deficits.

Treatment

SELECTION OF TREATMENT MODALITY. Although chemodectomas have a low potential for metastatic spread and a slow growth pattern, they can cause major disability and eventually death if unchecked. It may be appropriate to recommend no treatment in selected cases, but the great majority should be treated.

Temporal Bone Tumors. Surgical excision is satisfactory for small temporal bone lesions that can be removed without risk of operative death or damage to normal structures. Stereotactic radiosurgery is an option for early lesions, although long-term results are limited.

Early lesions of the tympanic cavity are managed successfully by excision without loss of hearing or vestibular function. The remainder of the lesions are managed best by irradiation, with a very high success rate and minimal morbidity with current techniques. Partial removal of the tumor before irradiation does not improve the results and only increases the overall morbidity. Local control after radiation therapy is defined as stable disease or partial regression with no evidence of growth after long-term follow-up.

Carotid Body Tumors. Small lesions (1 to 5 cm) of the carotid body may be successfully removed with little risk to the patient. However, if replacement of the carotid vessels is anticipated or if a large lesion is fixed or unresectable because of size, radiation therapy is the preferred initial treatment. These lesions are identical histologically to temporal bone chemodectomas, and the response to radiation is similar. It is preferable to use radiation therapy rather than risk the possibility of a stroke or other operative calamity. A radiation dose of 45 Gy at 1.8 Gy/fraction once daily does not exclude the possibility of surgical excision.

SURGICAL TREATMENT
Temporal Bone Tumors. Small glomus tympanicum lesions are approached through the eardrum or mastoid area and are removed. Hearing loss may occur from the operation, but if there is conductive hearing loss from the tumor, it may be correctable.

For the glomus jugulare tumors, surgery is reserved for radiation treatment failure, in which case a radical mastoidectomy or a subtotal temporal bone resection would be required. Some surgeons advocate a base of skull approach.

Carotid Body Tumors. When an adequate workup indicates that the most likely diagnosis is a carotid body tumor, hypertension, if present, should be treated. A standard neck incision is made in a skin crease at the level of the carotid bulb, and the carotid sheath and its contents are identified. The tumor mass is usually lying at the crotch of the internal and external carotid arteries, often displacing these vessels. Marked drops in blood pressure and bradycardia can be avoided by injecting the bulb area with lidocaine. Troublesome bleeding may be avoided by using the bipolar electrode before excising the mass. The mass is then removed, with the carotid arteries preserved.

IRRADIATION TECHNIQUE. The current treatment plan is 45 Gy in 5 weeks, 1.8 Gy/fraction, to the tumor volume. The dose is well below the tolerance of all normal tissues included, even if the brainstem and cord must be included for a large lesion. Patients are treated with CT-based treatment planning and one of the following techniques: wedge pair, stereotactic radiation therapy, or IMRT.

Acute sequelae of treatment should be almost nil at 1.8 Gy/fraction. The patient will have temporary hair loss in the entrance and exit areas beginning approximately the third week. Mild nausea may occur. Late sequelae are few. The hair should regrow over a period of 2 to 4 months but may show a slightly different texture or color. The patient may develop an otitis media, especially if the middle ear is involved with tumor.

MANAGEMENT OF RECURRENCE. Patients have follow-up with annual CT or MRI scans. The tumor usually stabilizes or partially regresses after successful irradiation. Tumor growth after complete resection or irradiation is defined as a recurrence.

Documented recurrence after operation usually is treated by irradiation. The complication rate in this group is higher than for those treated initially by irradiation. Recurrence after irradiation should be treated by operation if feasible; if operation is not possible, reirradiation may be considered. The potential for a complication would be significant, but, in the face of advancing neoplasm, the risk probably would be acceptable.

Results of Treatment

TEMPORAL BONE TUMORS. O'Leary et al.[184] reported on 64 patients treated surgically with a mean follow-up of 4.9 years; the local control rate was 95%. Woods and coworkers[185] observed a local control rate of 89% in 71 patients treated surgically who were followed from 1 to 22 years.

Local control for 53 patients with 55 temporal bone chemodectomas treated with definitive radiation therapy at the University of Florida was 92% at 15 years.[186] Powell et al.[187] reported a local control rate of 90% after radiation therapy for 46 patients who had a median follow-up of 9 years.

CAROTID BODY TUMORS. Biller et al.[188] reported on 18 patients treated surgically who were followed from 1 to 16 years; the local control rate was 89%. Green and coworkers[189] reported a local control rate of 89% after surgery in 18 patients who had a mean follow-up of 8 years.

Verniers et al.[190] reported on 22 patients treated with radiation therapy alone or radiation therapy combined with a subtotal resection and followed for an average of 10 years. Local control was achieved in all. Hinerman et al.[186] reported on 18 patients treated with definitive radiation therapy and having an average follow-up of 9 years. Local control was obtained in 96%.

Complications of Treatment

SURGERY. Fatalities have been reported from biopsy and resection. The major risks during operation are hemorrhage and injury to the cranial nerves. Other complications include hemiparesis, spinal fluid leak, and hearing loss.

IRRADIATION. There have been isolated reports of brain necrosis after radiation treatment. These cases were associated with high doses, high daily fractions, or repeat courses of irradiation. This complication should not occur at a dose of 45 Gy or less given at 1.8 Gy/d, 5 days a week. Other complications include cholesteatoma and sequestrum of the mastoid and otitis media. Detectable damage to the hearing mechanism and vestibular apparatus is very unlikely after 40 to 45 Gy to the normal temporal bone. Cranial nerves may regain function, especially if the deficit is of recent onset. Cranial nerve palsy due to irradiation should not occur at 45 Gy.

MAJOR SALIVARY GLANDS

Tumors of the major salivary glands account for 3% to 4% of all head and neck neoplasms. The average age of patients with malignant neoplasms is approximately 55 years; and of those with benign tumors, approximately 40 years. Approximately one-fourth of parotid tumors and one-half of submandibular tumors are malignant.

Anatomy

The parotid gland is a relatively simple structure that is formed by the muscles, bones, vessels, and nerves that come in contact with the gland. The major bulk of the parotid gland is superficial, extending superiorly to the zygomatic arch and anterior aspect of the external auditory canal. The anterior border is variable, but does not extend beyond the opening of the parotid duct into the oral cavity opposite the second molar. Inferiorly, the gland extends between the mastoid and the angle of the mandible. The gland lies in front of and below the external auditory canal. A deep lobe extends into the parapharyngeal area, where it is in relationship to the lateral process of C-1, the styloid process, and the contents of the parapharyngeal space.

The parotid gland is encompassed by fascia that is sufficient to contain most parotid infections in addition to benign and low-grade malignant tumors. However, the fascia between the parotid gland and the conchal and tragal cartilages is thin; this is a weak spot that tumor quickly traverses. The fascia separating the deep lobe from the parapharyngeal space (stylomandibular fascial membrane) may be sufficiently thin to allow tumor or infection easy access to the parapharyngeal space and pharynx.

The sensory nerve supply to the parotid area and part of the pinna is from the greater auricular nerve (C-2 to C-3). This nerve is severed in removal of the parotid gland with permanent loss of sensation. The facial nerve (VII) penetrates the parotid gland almost immediately on leaving the stylomastoid canal and forms an extensive anastomotic network within the gland and gives off branches to the muscles of expression.

The parotid gland is richly supplied from several arteries that freely anastomose and create arteriovenous bleeding during parotidectomy. The external carotid, internal maxillary and superficial temporal arteries, and posterior facial vein lie deep to cranial nerve VII.

The superficial preauricular nodes lie outside the fascia of the parotid gland and immediately in front of the tragus. They drain the skin of the anterior ear, temple, and upper face, including the eye and nose. They are involved most frequently by metastatic skin cancer and lymphoma, but not usually from parotid neoplasms. The preauricular nodes then empty into the superficial cervical nodes along the external jugular vein, or they may communicate with the jugular chain of nodes.

There are two groups of nodes within the fascia of the parotid gland. Within the substance of the parotid gland are numerous lymph follicles and four to ten small lymph nodes scattered along the posterior facial and external jugular veins. Thus, they may lie deep to cranial nerve VII. Outside the gland but within the fascia are subparotid nodes that lie in front of the tragus and between the inferior aspect of the tail of the parotid and the anterior border of the sternocleidomastoid muscle. When enlarged, the subparotid nodes are difficult to distinguish from a mass in the tail of the parotid gland.

Pathology

BENIGN TUMORS

Benign Mixed Tumors. Benign mixed tumors, also called pleomorphic adenomas, are slow-growing neoplasms surrounded by an imperfect pseudocapsule traversed by fingers of tumor. Enucleation or removal of a narrow cuff of normal tissue usually results in recurrence. The age of appearance is as low as the early 20s and the mean age of occurrence is 40.

Papillary Cystadenoma Lymphomatosum. Also called Warthin's tumor, a papillary cystadenoma lymphomatosum is encased by a thin but complete capsule. It occurs predominantly in older men, is bilateral in approximately 10% of cases, and may be multiple on one or both sides.

Benign Lymphoepithelial Lesions. Benign lymphoepithelial lesions (Godwin's tumors) account for approximately 5% of benign lesions. The tumor may be bilateral and is more common in women.

Oncocytoma. Oncocytoma is a benign, slow-growing tumor found mostly in the older age group. The encapsulated tumor has a dark appearance similar to melanoma.

Basal Cell Adenoma. The basal cell adenoma is an uncommon benign lesion, usually appearing in older people. It is cured by simple excision. Basal cell adenoma must be distinguished from basal cell carcinoma of the skin metastatic to parotid lymph nodes.

MALIGNANT TUMORS

Low-Grade Malignancy

ACINIC CELL TUMOR. Acinic cell tumors typically are indolent low-grade neoplasms appearing in all age groups and are most common in women. Metastases occur in a small percentage of cases and cannot be predicted by the histologic picture.

MUCOEPIDERMOID CARCINOMA, LOW-GRADE. Most mucoepidermoid carcinomas are indolent lesions readily cured by adequate excision. They may appear in any age group and grow slowly. There is little or no capsule. They are usually well circumscribed, but they may widely infiltrate the normal gland or become fixed to skin.

High-Grade Malignancy

MUCOEPIDERMOID CARCINOMA, HIGH-GRADE. High-grade mucoepidermoid carcinomas behave aggressively, widely infiltrating the salivary gland and producing lymph node and distant metastases. They may be difficult to distinguish from high-grade epidermoid carcinoma.

ADENOCARCINOMA, POORLY DIFFERENTIATED CARCINOMA, ANAPLASTIC CARCINOMA, SQUAMOUS CELL CARCINOMA. Adenocarcinoma, poorly differentiated carcinoma, anaplastic carcinoma, and squamous cell carcinoma tend to appear late in life and have an aggressive behavior. True squamous cell carcinoma arising from the salivary gland occurs rarely. Almost all of the so-called squamous cell carcinomas of the parotid are metastatic from skin cancer, especially from the temple area.[191]

MALIGNANT MIXED TUMOR. A small percentage of benign mixed tumors may develop into frank malignancy.

ADENOID CYSTIC CARCINOMA. Adenoid cystic carcinoma is uncommon in the major salivary glands. It varies in growth rate from slow to fast. Metastases to regional lymph nodes and distant sites occur, perineural involvement is characteristic, and recurrences may appear many years after initial treatment.[192]

LYMPHOEPITHELIOMA (MALIGNANT LYMPHOEPITHELIAL LESION, "ESKIMOMA"). Lymphoepithelioma occurs rarely in the parotid and submandibular gland. The histologic picture is that of lymphoepithelioma with varying degrees of nonmalignant lymphoid stroma.

Patterns of Spread

BENIGN MIXED TUMORS. Benign mixed tumors of the parotid gland grow by expansion and local infiltration. Most tumors begin in the superficial lobe. Because of their slow growth, they rarely cause VII nerve palsy, although the nerve may be stretched by large masses. When incompletely excised, multiple tumor nodules develop within the tumor bed. Skin invasion may occur in recurrent lesions; bone invasion does not occur, but a mass may cause pressure defects of adjacent bone.

MALIGNANT TUMORS. Malignant neoplasms infiltrate the parotid gland, invade the VII nerve and the auriculotemporal nerve, and spread along nerve sheaths. Tumor may invade the adjacent skin, muscles, and bone. Deep lobe lesions invade the parapharyngeal space, infratemporal fossa, and base of the skull, and compromise additional cranial nerves.

Malignant tumors of the submandibular gland invade the gland, fix the tumor to the adjacent mandible, and invade the mylohyoid muscle and eventually the tongue, hypoglossal nerve, and oral cavity or oropharynx. Skin invasion occurs in advanced cases.

Sublingual gland neoplasms usually present as a submucosal mass in the floor of the mouth. The advanced lesions show an ulcerated mass in the floor of the mouth with extension to the tongue, mandible, and submental soft tissues.

LYMPHATIC SPREAD. Lymph node metastases may occur from all of the malignant neoplasms. Twenty percent to 25% of patients with malignant tumors have clinically positive or occult metastases in lymph nodes at the time of diagnosis. Low-grade mucoepidermoid carcinoma and acinic cell adenocarcinoma have a low rate of lymph node metastasis. There is little difference in the rate of lymph node metastasis among the various high-grade lesions. The risk for lymph node metastasis increases with recurrent disease and increased size of the primary lesion.

Clinical Picture

PAROTID GLAND. The great majority of patients with either benign or malignant parotid tumors present with a mass that is easily appreciated. Mild, intermittent pain is occasionally present, but does not distinguish between benign and malignant tumors. Facial nerve palsy is an infrequent presenting complaint and indicates malignancy. Tumors of the deep lobe may produce dysphagia. The mobility of the mass depends on its size and location. Fixation or reduced mobility may occur in both benign and malignant neoplasms and does not distinguish between the two. Tumors presenting in the deep lobe may cause bulging of the palate and tonsillar area. Advanced malignant lesions may rarely affect cranial nerves IX to XII and the sympathetic chain if the parapharyngeal space is invaded. The mandibular branch of cranial nerve V may be involved when tumor tracks along the auriculotemporal nerve to the base of the skull; pain is an associated finding.

SUBMANDIBULAR GLAND. Both benign and malignant neoplasms present as a mass usually associated with mild pain. Nerve palsy is rarely present. The skin may be infiltrated in advanced lesions. The tumor mass usually is partially fixed to the mandible unless quite small. Loss of mobility occurs with both benign and malignant lesions.

SUBLINGUAL GLAND. Sublingual gland lesions are clinically similar to squamous cell carcinomas of the floor of the mouth. They produce a mass, submucosal at first, that may be felt by the tongue. There is mild discomfort, if any, in the early stages.

Differential Diagnosis

PAROTID GLAND. Gallia and Johnson[193] reviewed findings for 140 patients who eventually underwent parotidectomy for diagnosis. Only 11% had malignant masses; the remainder had benign neoplasms (62%) or nonneoplastic conditions (27%). Conditions that may be confused with a parotid tumor include the following: (1) metastatic cancer, lymphoma, or leukemia involving parotid area lymph nodes; (2) fatty replacement, tail of parotid; (3) chronic parotitis; (4) Boeck's sarcoid; (5) stone in duct; (6) cysts (branchial cleft, dermoid); (7) hypertrophy associated with diabetes; (8) hypertrophy of masseter muscle, unilateral or bilateral; (9) neoplasms of the mandible; (10) prominent transverse process of C-1 (atlas); (11) penetrating foreign bodies; (12) hemangioma or lymphangioma; and (13) lipoma.

SUBMANDIBULAR GLAND. The differential diagnosis of a submandibular mass centers around inflammatory disease, squamous cell carcinoma metastatic to a lymph node, and a primary neoplasm of the submandibular gland.

Gallia and Johnson[193] reviewed findings for 110 submandibular lesions in patients who underwent biopsy. Ninety-three lesions (85%) were nonneoplastic, usually inflamed glands, and nine lesions (8%) were benign tumors. Eight patients (7%) had malignant lesions, of which three lesions were lymphoma, three were metastatic carcinoma, and two were primary submandibular gland carcinoma.

Biopsy Technique

PAROTID GLAND. The biopsy and definitive surgical treatment are often the same for parotid masses. Biopsy of lesions lying in the superficial lobe is best accomplished by performing a superficial parotidectomy. For lesions involving both the superficial and deep lobes or just the deep lobe, "biopsy" is performed by total parotidectomy. Incisional and excisional biopsy may contaminate the tumor bed, increasing the risk of tumor recurrence and facial nerve damage as well as increasing the extent of the definitive surgical procedure by necessitating wide removal of the biopsy site.

There are advocates of FNA for diagnosis. It is essential that the pathologist be familiar with this method. A negative FNA finding does not necessarily mean that there is no tumor, so that surgical decisions often rely heavily on clinical and radiographic findings. FNA can be used in the inoperable or recurrent lesions when radiation therapy is planned as the initial treatment.

SUBMANDIBULAR GLAND. FNA is helpful when results are positive for tumor but may delay diagnosis when findings are falsely negative. When needle biopsy results are negative but history, physical examination, and radiographic studies suggest neoplasm, and a careful search of the head and neck area fails to reveal a primary mucosal lesion, the submandibular triangle is dissected as the biopsy procedure. Incisional or excisional biopsy increases the risk of tumor recurrence, even when followed by appropriate treatment, and increases the surgical morbidity by requiring excision of the biopsy site.

AJCC Staging

The AJCC staging system for tumors of the major salivary glands is as follows[16]:

Primary Tumor (T)

TX   Primary tumor cannot be assessed

T0   No evidence of primary tumor

T1   Tumor 2 cm or less in greatest dimension without extraparenchymal extension[a]

T2   Tumor more than 2 cm but not more than 4 cm in greatest dimension without extraparenchymal extension[a]

T3   Tumor more than 4 cm and/or tumor having extraparenchymal extension[a]

T4a Tumor invades skin, mandible, ear canal, and/or facial nerve

T4b Tumor invades skull base and/or pterygoid plates and/or encases carotid artery

*a*Extraparenchymal extension is clinical or macroscopic evidence of invasion of soft tissues. Microscopic evidence alone does not constitute extraparenchymal extension for classification purposes.

Treatment

SELECTION OF TREATMENT MODALITY

Parotid Gland. The initial management of resectable superficial lobe parotid masses is *en bloc* superficial lobectomy. The tumor usually can be dissected free of the facial nerve. If the tumor involves the deep portion of the gland, the nerve is retracted and the deep portion excised (i.e., total parotidectomy). Skin, bone, and muscle may also be resected as needed.

Low-grade malignant neoplasms are usually managed by operation only. Radiation therapy is given postoperatively for nearly all high-grade lesions. Radiation therapy is advised for low-grade malignant lesions that are recurrent and those with positive margins or narrow margins on the facial nerve. Tumor spill at the time of operation is a controversial indication for postoperative irradiation. Postoperative radiation therapy is advised for selected benign mixed tumors when there is microscopic residual disease after operation, and for nearly all patients operated on for recurrent disease. Radiation therapy alone is unlikely to control gross disease, and if possible, resection of any gross residual benign mixed tumor should be performed before radiation therapy. Inoperable malignancies are treated by radiation therapy with occasional success.

Chemotherapy has been reserved for patients with incurable disease and those in prospective clinical trials.

Submandibular Gland. If frozen-section diagnosis shows a malignant submandibular gland lesion and there is no involvement of nerves, mandible, or soft tissues, submandibular triangle dissection is performed and postoperative irradiation is given to the submandibular bed and ipsilateral neck. If there is perineural invasion, bone invasion, a clinically positive node, or extension to contiguous soft tissues, then the resection is enlarged to encompass the necessary areas. This may include the mandible, mylohyoid muscle, digastric muscle, adjacent floor of the mouth or tongue, and involved nerves. Postoperative radiation therapy is added in nearly all cases.

SURGICAL TREATMENT

Superficial Parotidectomy. The parotid gland is a unilobular gland and is artificially divided into superficial and deep portions by the VII nerve. A superficial mass in the parotid gland is best approached by a superficial parotidectomy and frozen-section diagnosis because this affords the best method of diagnosis and often is the definitive treatment. The facial nerve is not sacrificed unless it is grossly involved with disease.

The incision is made in the preauricular crease and then curves under the ear lobe posteriorly and then into the neck. The facial nerve must be identified in all superficial and total parotidectomies. Once this is accomplished, the dissection is carried out between the mass and the facial nerve. A margin of at least 1 cm around the mass is necessary if a benign tumor is suspected, and a larger margin if the mass is malignant. The adequacy of treatment is determined by frozen sections.

Total Parotidectomy. Total parotidectomy is recommended for tumors that arise in the superficial lobe and extend into the deep lobe. A superficial parotidectomy is generally performed; then the nerve is dissected free from the underlying deep lobe and the deep lobe and tumor are removed. Occasionally, the mandible must be divided to gain access to the retromandibular portion of the deep lobe of the parotid gland. A partial mandibulectomy is required when the mandible is invaded by tumor. When pain is present, the auriculotemporal nerve should be explored to the base of the skull.

The paraparotid nodes are removed with the primary lesion. If the nodes are positive, a neck dissection is added. Neck dissection is always included for clinically positive nodes. Elective neck dissection is not done for low-grade lesions.

A radical parotidectomy implies removal of the entire parotid, the facial nerve, and other involved tissues such as skin, bone, or muscle. If the branch of the facial nerve or the entire nerve must be sacrificed, an immediate autologous nerve graft may be done. Postoperative radiation therapy is delayed for 6 weeks, and the chance of successful function is reported to be good.[194]

RADIATION THERAPY.
Radiation therapy plays its major role as an adjunct to surgery and is usually given postoperatively, although preoperative treatment is advised in special situations. Postoperative irradiation is indicated for nearly all high-grade lesions, for low-grade neoplasms with close or positive margins, for tumors of the deep lobe, for perineural invasion, for recurrent tumors, and for multiple regional node metastases. According to Spiro and coworkers,[195] tumor spill at the time of operation may not be a single prognostic factor for recurrence.

The minimum treatment volume for parotid lesions includes the parotid bed and upper neck nodes. Perineural involvement indicates enlargement of the portals to cover the nerve pathways. The entire ipsilateral neck is included for high-grade lesions or for clinically positive nodes in the neck dissection specimen. The tumor dose to the primary area is 60 to 65 Gy over 6 to 7 weeks if there is no gross residual disease. Higher doses using altered fractionation are used for patients with microscopically positive margins or gross disease.

Submandibular space external-beam portals are tailored to the extent of disease found in the surgical dissection. The entire ipsilateral neck is included. The postoperative dose is 65 to 70 Gy because the rate of recurrence, even with combined treatment, is substantial.

Results of Treatment

PAROTID GLAND

Benign Mixed Tumors. For benign mixed tumors, enucleation or excision with a narrow rim of normal tissue results eventually in a local recurrence rate of approximately 20% after 10 to 15 years of follow-up.

Rafla-Demetrious[196] reported only a 2.7% recurrence rate when enucleation or excision was followed by postoperative radiation therapy. Superficial parotidectomy (or excision for selected small lesion) results in a recurrence rate of approximately 5%. Spiro[197] reported a 7% recurrence rate, with a minimum of 10 years of follow-up, for 1342 benign parotid tumors treated by surgery.

The surgical success rate for recurrent lesions depends on the number of previous operations and the size and extent of recurrence. It may be necessary to sacrifice one or several branches of the seventh nerve and to repair the defect with a nerve graft. Postoperative irradiation of 60 to 65 Gy is added in selected cases in which there are close margins or microscopic residual disease, or in cases in which a subsequent recurrence would be almost impossible to manage surgically or would result in loss of the facial nerve.

Death because of benign mixed tumors is unlikely.

Malignant Tumors. The surgical results for low-grade malignant lesions are quite good, and radiation therapy is not often required. The local recurrence rate for operation alone is 50% to 60% for high-grade tumors.[195,198]

Garden and coworkers[199] reported on 166 patients treated with surgery and postoperative radiation therapy for parotid malignancies at the M. D. Anderson Hospital between 1965 and 1989. Forty patients (24%) developed a recurrent disease that was local in 9% and regional in 6%. Histologic type did not significantly influence the likelihood of local control (*P* = .36). Twenty-five patients (15%) developed distant metastases with disease control above the clavicles. The 10- and 15-year survival rates were 60% and 52%, respectively.

The 5-year absolute survival rates by histologic type for patients treated with surgery and postoperative radiation therapy added on a selective basis at the M. D. Anderson Hospital were as follows: acinic cell carcinoma (n = 12), 92%; low-grade mucoepidermoid carcinoma (n = 28), 76%; adenocarcinoma (n = 12), 66%; malignant mixed carcinoma (n = 27), 50%; adenoid cystic carcinoma (n = 10), 50%; squamous cell carcinoma (n = 6), 50%; high-grade mucoepidermoid carcinoma (n = 13), 46%; and undifferentiated carcinoma (n = 12), 33%.[200]

Theriault and Fitzpatrick[201] reviewed results for 271 patients with parotid cancer seen at the Princess Margaret Hospital between 1958 and 1980. The minimum follow-up was 5 years and the median follow-up was 10 years. Thirty-five patients had only radiation therapy, 67 had surgery alone, and 169 had surgery plus postoperative radiation therapy, 45 to 55 Gy in 20 fractions. Relapse-free survival and cause-specific survival rates are compared for different treatment modalities in Table 26.2-37. Local-regional control at 10 years was obtained in 12% by radiation therapy, in 22% by surgery, and in 71% by surgery plus radiation therapy. Significant prognostic factors for survival were tumor stage, regional metastases, age (young better than old), histologic type, and facial nerve involvement.

CHEMOTHERAPY RESULTS. The development of effective chemotherapy for patients with salivary gland carcinomas has been limited by the heterogeneity of this disease, the relative efficacy of surgery and radiation therapy, and the lack of effective chemotherapeutic agents.

SUBMANDIBULAR GLAND. Byers and coworkers[202] reported the results of treatment for 22 malignant tumors of the submandibular gland with no prior therapy. Treatment was resection followed selectively by postoperative irradiation. The local control rate was 64% and the survival rate was 50%.

Spiro[197] reported the results of surgery for 129 malignant submandibular gland carcinomas seen between 1939 and 1973. All patients had a minimum of 10 years of follow-up. Adenoid cystic

TABLE 26.2-37. Parotid Carcinoma: Survival in 269 Patients Treated at Princess Margaret Hospital, 1958–1980 (5-Year Minimum Follow-Up)

	Relapse-Free		Cause-Specific	
	5-Y (%)	10-Y (%)	5-Y (%)	10-Y (%)
Surgery plus radiation therapy	69	63	78	72
Surgery	30	23	63	48
Radiation therapy	9	9	23	18

(Data from ref. 201.)

carcinoma occurred in 35%, mucoepidermoid carcinoma in 29%, and malignant mixed tumor in 19%. Cervical lymph nodes were malignant in 28%. The local-regional control rate was 40% and the cause-specific cure rate was 31% at 5 years and 22% at 10 years.

Benign tumors of the submandibular gland were resected in 106 patients; only 2 developed a local recurrence.[197]

Complications of Treatment

SURGERY. Temporary facial nerve palsy may occur due to manipulation of the nerve during operation, and function gradually returns over a few months' time. Persistent weakness of the lower lip may occur, even though the remainder of the nerve recovers. Tarsorrhaphy may be required to protect the eye until function returns. Spontaneous return of facial movement has been reported to occur after surgical division of the VII nerve. Facial nerve palsy may be repaired by a nerve graft. If grafting is not possible, a nerve crossover technique may be used that connects the ipsilateral hypoglossal nerve to branches of the seventh nerve. Gustatory sweating (Frey's syndrome) occurs in approximately 10% of patients after parotidectomy. This problem rarely requires treatment. Persistent salivary fistula is rare.

RADIATION THERAPY. Xerostomia is avoided by techniques that spare the contralateral salivary tissues. There may be trismus to fibrosis of the masseter and pterygoid muscles and the temporomandibular joint. It should be possible to exclude the temporomandibular joint from high doses in most situations.

Otitis media may occur if the ear is irradiated. Localized hair loss may occur with some techniques. Osteoradionecrosis may rarely occur with high doses.

MINOR SALIVARY GLANDS

Tumors of minor salivary gland origin are uncommon, accounting for 2% to 3% of all malignant neoplasms of the upper aerodigestive tract. They may appear at any age, but are uncommon before age 20 and rare under age 10. They tend to occur most often in the hard palate, nasal cavity, and paranasal sinuses, areas infrequently involved by squamous cell carcinomas. Thus, the site of origin is related more to the density of the minor salivary glands in a particular tissue than to an environmental factor.

Anatomy

Minor salivary glands are ubiquitous in mucosa of the upper aerodigestive tract with the exception of the gingivae and the anterior portion of the hard palate, which are free of minor salivary glands. They are distributed on the undersurface of the anterior and lateral oral tongue and the base of the tongue. Aberrant salivary tissue sometimes is seen in lymph nodes, the body of the mandible just behind the third molar teeth, the vestigial remnant of the nasopalatine canal in the anterior maxilla, the middle ear, the lower neck, the sternoclavicular joint, the thyroglossal duct, and other sites.

Pathology

Approximately one-half of minor salivary gland tumors are malignant. The histologic varieties of malignant tumors include adenoid cystic carcinoma, mucoepidermoid carcinoma, adenocarcinoma, malignant mixed, acinic cell, and oncocytic carcinomas. Approximately two-thirds are adenoid cystic. The mucoepidermoid carcinoma and adenocarcinomas arise predominantly in the oral cavity.

The benign tumors are benign mixed (pleomorphic adenoma) in the great majority of cases, with a few cases of intraductal papillomas, papillary cystadenomas, basal cell adenomas, and benign oncocytomas.[203]

Patterns of Spread

Tongue lesions usually originate from the tongue. There are no minor salivary glands in the anterior half of the hard palate, so tumors arise on the posterolateral hard palate and all of the soft palate. The site of origin for floor of mouth salivary gland tumors is moot—either the sublingual gland or a minor salivary gland. The nasopharynx is an uncommon site of origin.

These tumors grow by local infiltration with eventual invasion of muscle, bone, and cartilage. Perineural spread is a common feature, particularly for adenoid cystic carcinoma. Tumor may track both centrally and peripherally along nerves, but the central spread is the more common event because most lesions arise near the terminations of the nerves. Extension along nerves eventually may traverse the base of the skull and surface intracranially, although this spread pattern may not become manifest for several years after the original treatment. Tumor growth along a nerve may be characterized by skipped areas, so that a normal nerve segment is no assurance of free margins. Adenoid cystic carcinoma may grow along the haversian systems of bone without showing bone destruction.[204]

The risk of positive lymph nodes is related to the site of origin and the histologic type. Lymph node metastases are most likely from sites with a dense capillary lymphatic network, similar to the pattern for squamous carcinoma. Adenoid cystic carcinoma, low-grade mucoepidermoid carcinoma, and acinic cell carcinoma are at low risk to spread to lymph nodes; approximately 20% of adenoid cystic carcinomas spread to lymph nodes, but this low incidence may be related partly to their frequent site of origin in the hard palate and paranasal sinuses, areas that infrequently produce lymph node metastases. The high-grade tumors (high-grade mucoepidermoid carcinoma, adenocarcinoma, and malignant mixed tumor) have a 30% incidence of lymph node involvement on admission, and eventually 51% show lymph node metastases.

Clinical Picture

The clinical picture obviously depends on the site of origin. The signs and symptoms differ somewhat from those of squamous cell carcinoma arising in the same area. Many of the lesions are indolent, and the history may go back many months or even years; approximately 25% of patients give a history of a mass being present over 10 years. Because lesions develop under the epithelium, the initial lesion is a submucosal mass that is often painless until ulceration develops. Perineural involvement is expressed as pain or paresthesias. Otherwise, the clinical picture resembles that for squamous cell carcinomas for a given size and site. Lymph node metastases occur at predictable sites. The clinically positive nodes are usually small and mobile, but neck dissection on such a patient may show numerous small, clinically undetectable positive nodes.

The same staging systems applied to squamous cell carcinomas may be used.

Treatment

SELECTION OF TREATMENT MODALITY. Benign mixed-grade tumors are managed by operation. Postoperative irradiation sometimes is advised in cases in which margins are close or positive.

The low-grade carcinomas are treated initially by an operation when feasible, but irradiation is sometimes used as the primary treatment for inaccessible lesions or in cases in which the functional loss would be considerable. Postoperative irradiation is added for close margins or for those lesions that have recurred more than once. If the patient presents after excisional biopsy of a small lesion, irradiation is an alternative to reexcision, particularly if the procedure would produce significant cosmetic or functional loss.

The treatment of high-grade lesions varies immensely, depending on the site of origin, stage of disease, and willingness of the patient to accept a major cosmetic or functional change subsequent to an operation. Because the philosophy at the University of Florida is to accept radiation therapy as a curative therapy, the authors essentially approach most lesions as they would a squamous cell carcinoma of similar stage and similar anatomic site.[205]

When combined treatment is indicated, the operation should precede radiation therapy to facilitate healing and to gain knowledge of tumor extent for radiation treatment planning.

SURGICAL TREATMENT. Benign tumors are removed by wide local excision that includes a cuff of normal tissue. Small low-grade lesions with a long history of slow growth may be treated with a wide local excision including a shell of normal tissue. Large low-grade lesions and high-grade lesions require a more radical resection. When perineural invasion is present, it is not possible, of course, to remove all the nerves potentially involved, but the nerves that are involved should be sacrificed wherever it is reasonable to do so. As an alternative, postoperative irradiation may be used to cover the perineural routes of spread. Because unsuccessfully treated patients often live many years before they eventually die of the disease, careful planning must go into reconstruction and rehabilitation.

IRRADIATION TECHNIQUE. The irradiation techniques and doses are similar to those for squamous cell carcinomas of the same anatomic site and similar tumor size, with the exception that nerve pathways must be covered for adenoid cystic

TABLE 26.2-38. Incidence of Recurrence of Pleomorphic Adenoma of Minor Salivary Glands in the Royal Marsden Series Distributed According to the Method of Treatment

Method of Treatment	No. of Patients	No. with Recurrence	Length of Follow-Up
Radiation alone	11	0	5 for 5+ y
Preoperative radiation and surgery	14	2	9 for 5+ y
Surgery and postoperative radiation	18	0	14 for 5+ y
			9 for 10+ y
Surgery alone	1	0	5 y
Total	44	2	29 for 5+ y

(From ref. 196, with permission.)

carcinomas. Subclinical perineural spread for adenoid cystic carcinomas must be considered to be present even though not seen on the biopsy specimen or surgical sections. Recurrences frequently are manifested in and about the base of the skull at the termination of the cranial nerves.

The regression rate of adenoid cystic carcinoma during treatment is similar to that of squamous cell carcinoma. Successfully treated adenocarcinomas or low-grade mucoepidermoid carcinomas may require several weeks or months to disappear after completion of treatment. The regional lymphatics are irradiated electively, depending on the site of origin and grade of the lesion.

Results of Treatment

Spiro and coworkers[206] reported the Memorial Sloan-Kettering results for 434 malignant minor salivary gland tumors, of which 90% were treated surgically. The cause-specific 5-, 10-, and 15-year cure rates were 44%, 32%, and 21%, respectively; 51% died of the original cancer. Patients with adenoid cystic carcinoma had the poorest prognosis, with approximately 20% surviving without recurrence. Those with adenocarcinoma had an intermediate outlook, with approximately 35% surviving without recurrence. Mucoepidermoid carcinomas had the best control rate, with approximately 70% long-term cures. Bardwil and coworkers[207] reported a similar series from M. D. Anderson Hospital with shorter follow-up (3 to 20 years) in which surgery was the sole treatment in 88% of cases. Local control rate was reported to be 75%, but 47% of patients died of their original cancer, a percentage similar to that in the Memorial Sloan-Kettering series.

Parsons and coworkers[205] reported on 95 patients treated at the University of Florida for minor salivary gland carcinomas between 1964 and 1992. The 20-year actuarial local control rate was 57% with no significant difference according to histologic type or primary site. The 12-year probability of distant metastases was 40%. Absolute survival rates were as follows: 5 years, 65%; 10 years, 41%; and 15 years, 34%.

Benign mixed tumors of minor salivary gland origin have a good prognosis. Enucleation, however, is followed by recurrence, and a cuff of normal tissue is required. Spiro[197] reported on 81 benign tumors. Sixty occurred on the palate and 13 on the lip or cheek. With a minimum follow-up of 10 years, the local recurrence rate was 6%.

Rafla-Demetrious[196] reported the Royal Marsden Hospital experience of 44 cases of benign mixed tumor (Table 26.2-38). Eleven patients were treated by radiation therapy alone, and none of the tumors regrew, although not all had complete regression. Local recurrence of benign mixed tumor may appear after many, many years, and an occasional patient may eventually die of uncontrolled disease.

REFERENCES

1. Jemal A, Murray T, Samuels A, et al. Cancer statistics, 2003. *CA Cancer J Clin* 2003;53:5.
2. Erkal HS, Mendenhall WM, Amdur RJ, et al. Synchronous and metachronous squamous cell carcinomas of the head and neck mucosal sites. *J Clin Oncol* 2001;19:1358.
3. Rouviere H. *Anatomy of the human lymphatic system.* Ann Arbor, MI: Edwards Brothers, 1938, Tobias MJ, translator.
4. Nathu RM, Mendenhall NP, Almasri NM, et al. Non-Hodgkin's lymphoma of the head and neck: a 30-year experience at the University of Florida. *Head Neck* 1999;21:247.
5. Ward JR, Feigenberg SJ, Mendenhall NP, et al. Radiation therapy for angiosarcoma. *Head Neck* 2003;25:873.
6. Maddox WA, Urist MM. Histopathological prognostic factors of certain primary oral cavity cancers. *Oncology (Huntingt)* 1990;4:39.
7. Mendenhall WM, Mancuso AA, Parsons JT, et al. Diagnostic evaluation of squamous cell carcinoma metastatic to cervical lymph nodes from an unknown head and neck primary site. *Head Neck* 1998;20:739.
8. Mendenhall WM, Mancuso AA, Amdur RJ, et al. Squamous cell carcinoma metastatic to the neck from an unknown head and neck primary site. *Am J Otolaryngol* 2001;22:261.
9. Erkal HS, Mendenhall WM, Amdur RJ, et al. Squamous cell carcinomas metastatic to cervical lymph nodes from an unknown head-and-neck mucosal site treated with radiation therapy alone or in combination with neck dissection. *Int J Radiat Oncol Biol Phys* 2001;50:55.
10. Lindberg RD. Distribution of cervical lymph node metastases from squamous cell carcinoma of the upper respiratory and digestive tracts. *Cancer* 1972;29:1446.
11. O'Sullivan B, Warde P, Grice B, et al. The benefits and pitfalls of ipsilateral radiotherapy in carcinoma of the tonsillar region. *Int J Radiat Oncol Biol Phys* 2001;51:332.
12. Fisch U. *Lymphography of the cervical lymphatic system.* Philadelphia: WB Saunders, 1968, Tobias MJ, translator.
13. McLaughlin MP, Mendenhall WM, Mancuso AA, et al. Retropharyngeal adenopathy as a predictor of outcome in squamous cell carcinoma of the head and neck. *Head Neck* 1995;17:190.
14. Al-Othman MOF, Morris CG, Hinerman RW, et al. Distant metastases after definitive radiotherapy for squamous cell carcinoma of the head and neck. *Head Neck* 2003;25:629.
15. Merino OR, Lindberg RD, Fletcher GH. An analysis of distant metastases from squamous cell carcinoma of the upper respiratory and digestive tracts. *Cancer* 1977;40:145.
16. American Joint Committee on Cancer. *AJCC cancer staging manual,* 6th ed. New York: Springer, 2002.
17. Mendenhall WM, Parsons JT, Million RR, et al. A favorable subset of AJCC stage IV squamous cell carcinoma of the head and neck. *Int J Radiat Oncol Biol Phys* 1984;10:1841.
18. Fu KK, Pajak TF, Trotti A, et al. A Radiation Therapy Oncology Group (RTOG) phase III randomized study to compare hyperfractionation and two variants of accelerated fractionation to standard fractionation radiotherapy for head and neck squamous cell carcinomas: first report of RTOG 9003. *Int J Radiat Oncol Biol Phys* 2000;48:7.
19. Chao CKS, Ozyigit G, Tran BN, et al. Patterns of failure in patients receiving definitive and postoperative IMRT for head-and-neck cancer. *Int J Radiat Oncol Biol Phys* 2003;55:312.
20. Mendenhall WM, Villaret DB, Amdur RJ, et al. Planned neck dissection after definitive radiotherapy for squamous cell carcinoma of the head and neck. *Head Neck* 2002;24:1012.
21. Mendenhall WM, Million RR. Elective neck irradiation for squamous cell carcinoma of the head and neck: analysis of time-dose factors and causes of failure. *Int J Radiat Oncol Biol Phys* 1986;12:741.
22. Mendenhall WM, Million RR, Cassisi NJ. Elective neck irradiation in squamous-cell carcinoma of the head and neck. *Head Neck Surg* 1980;3:15.
23. Mendenhall WM, Parsons JT, Stringer SP, et al. Squamous cell carcinoma of the head and neck treated with irradiation: management of the neck. *Semin Radiat Oncol* 1992;2:163.
24. Barkley HT Jr, Fletcher GH, Jesse RH, et al. Management of cervical lymph node metastases in squamous cell carcinoma of the tonsillar fossa, base of tongue, supraglottic larynx, and hypopharynx. *Am J Surg* 1972;124:462.
25. Byers RM. Modified neck dissection: a study of 967 cases from 1970 to 1980. *Am J Surg* 1985;150:414.
26. Mendenhall WM, Amdur RJ, Hinerman RW, et al. Postoperative radiation therapy for squamous cell carcinoma of the head and neck. *Am J Otolaryngol* 2003;24:41.
27. McGuirt WF, McCabe BF. Significance of node biopsy before definitive treatment of cervical metastatic carcinoma. *Laryngoscope* 1978;88:594.
28. Ellis ER, Mendenhall WM, Rao PV, et al. Incisional or excisional neck-node biopsy before definitive radiotherapy, alone or followed by neck dissection. *Head Neck* 1991;13:177.
29. Million RR, Cassisi NJ. General principles for treatment of cancers in the head and neck: selection of treatment for the primary site and for the neck. In: Million RR, Cassisi NJ, eds. *Management of head and neck cancer: a multidisciplinary approach,* 1st ed. Philadelphia: JB Lippincott Company, 1984:43.
30. Schantz SP, Harrison LB, Forastiere AA. Tumors of the nasal cavity and paranasal sinuses, nasopharynx, oral cavity, and oropharynx. In: DeVita VT, Hellman S, Rosenberg SA, eds.

Cancer: principles and practice of oncology, 6th ed. Philadelphia: Lippincott Williams & Wilkins, 2001:797.

31. Munro AJ. Chemotherapy for head and neck cancer. In: Souhami RL, Tannock I, Hohenberger P, et al, eds. *Oxford textbook of oncology,* 2nd ed. New York: Oxford University Press Inc., 2002:1345.

32. Khuri FR, Shin DM, Glisson BS, et al. Treatment of patients with recurrent or metastatic squamous cell carcinoma of the head and neck: current status and future directions. *Semin Oncol* 2000;27:25.

33. Pivot X, Cals L, Cupissol D, et al. Phase II trial of a paclitaxel-carboplatin combination in recurrent squamous cell carcinoma of the head and neck. *Oncology* 2001;60:66.

34. Glisson BS, Murphy BA, Frenette G, et al. Phase II trial of docetaxel and cisplatin combination chemotherapy in patients with squamous cell carcinoma of the head and neck. *J Clin Oncol* 2002;20:1593.

35. Johnson NW. General principles. Epidemiology of premalignant and malignant lesions. In: Souhami RL, Tannock I, Hohenberger P, et al., eds. *Oxford textbook of oncology,* 2nd ed. New York: Oxford University Press Inc., 2002:1247.

36. Papadimitrakopoulou VA. Chemoprevention of head and neck cancer: an update. *Curr Opin Oncol* 2002;14:318.

37. Papadimitrakopoulou VA, Hong WK. Biomolecular markers as intermediate end points in chemoprevention trials of upper aerodigestive tract cancer. *Int J Cancer* 2000;88:852.

38. Wang Z, Qiu W, Mendenhall WM. Influence of radiation therapy on reconstructive flaps after radical resection of head and neck cancer. *Int J Oral Maxillofac Surg* 2003;32:35.

39. Huang DT, Johnson CR, Schmidt-Ullrich R, et al. Postoperative radiotherapy in head and neck carcinoma with extracapsular lymph node extension and/or positive resection margins: a comparative study. *Int J Radiat Oncol Biol Phys* 1992;23:737.

40. Lundahl RE, Foote RL, Bonner JA, et al. Combined neck dissection and postoperative radiation therapy in the management of the high-risk neck: a matched-pair analysis. *Int J Radiat Oncol Biol Phys* 1998;40:529.

41. Department of Veterans Affairs Laryngeal Cancer Study Group. Induction chemotherapy plus radiation compared with surgery plus radiation in patients with advanced laryngeal cancer. *N Engl J Med* 1991;324:1685.

42. Lefebvre J-L, Chevalier D, Luboinski B, et al. Larynx preservation in pyriform sinus cancer: preliminary results of a European Organization for Research and Treatment of Cancer phase III trial. EORTC Head and Neck Cancer Cooperative Group. *J Natl Cancer Inst* 1996;88:890.

43. Pignon JP, Bourhis J, Domenge C, et al. Chemotherapy added to locoregional treatment for head and neck squamous-cell carcinoma: three meta-analyses of updated individual data. *Lancet* 2000;355:949.

44. Pameijer FA, Mancuso AA, Mendenhall WM, et al. Can pretreatment computed tomography predict local control in T3 squamous cell carcinoma of the glottic larynx treated with definitive radiotherapy? *Int J Radiat Oncol Biol Phys* 1997;37:1011.

45. Mancuso AA, Mukherji SK, Schmalfuss I, et al. Preradiotherapy computed tomography as a predictor of local control in supraglottic carcinoma. *J Clin Oncol* 1999;17:631.

46. Nathu RM, Mancuso AA, Zhu TC, et al. The impact of primary tumor volume on local control for oropharyngeal squamous cell carcinoma treated with radiotherapy. *Head Neck* 2000;22:1.

47. Mukherji SK, O'Brien SM, Gerstle RJ, et al. The ability of tumor volume to predict local control in surgically treated squamous cell carcinoma of the supraglottic larynx. *Head Neck* 2000;22:282.

48. Calais G, Alfonsi M, Bardet E, et al. Randomized trial of radiation therapy versus concomitant chemotherapy and radiation therapy for advanced-stage oropharynx carcinoma. *J Natl Cancer Inst* 1999;91:2081.

49. Adelstein DJ, Lavertu P, Saxton JP, et al. Mature results of a phase III randomized trial comparing concurrent chemoradiotherapy with radiation therapy alone in patients with stage III and IV squamous cell carcinoma of the head and neck. *Cancer* 2000;88:876.

50. Adelstein DJ, Li Y, Adams GL, et al. An Intergroup phase III comparison of standard radiation therapy and two schedules of concurrent chemoradiotherapy in patients with unresectable squamous cell head and neck cancer. *J Clin Oncol* 2003;21:92.

51. Forastiere AA, Berkey B, Maor M, et al. Phase III trial to preserve the larynx: induction chemotherapy and radiotherapy versus concomitant chemoradiotherapy versus radiotherapy alone, Intergroup Trial R91-11. *Proc Am Soc Clin Oncol* 2001;20:2a(abst).

52. Brizel DM, Albers ME, Fisher SR, et al. Hyperfractionated irradiation with or without concurrent chemotherapy for locally advanced head and neck cancer. *N Engl J Med* 1998;338:1798.

53. Jeremic B, Shibamoto Y, Milicic B, et al. Hyperfractionated radiation therapy with or without concurrent low-dose daily cisplatin in locally advanced squamous cell carcinoma of the head and neck: a prospective randomized trial. *J Clin Oncol* 2000;18:1458.

54. Olmi P, Crispino S, Fallai C, et al. Locoregionally advanced carcinoma of the oropharynx: conventional radiotherapy vs. accelerated hyperfractionated radiotherapy vs. concomitant radiotherapy and chemotherapy—a multicenter randomized trial. *Int J Radiat Oncol Biol Phys* 2003;55:78.

55. Staar S, Rudat V, Stuetzer H, et al. Intensified hyperfractionated accelerated radiotherapy limits the additional benefit of simultaneous chemotherapy—results of a multicentric randomized German trial in advanced head-and-neck cancer. *Int J Radiat Oncol Biol Phys* 2001;50:1161.

56. Steiner W, Ambrosch P, Hess CF, et al. Organ preservation by transoral laser microsurgery in piriform sinus carcinoma. *Otolaryngol Head Neck Surg* 2001;124:58.

57. Laccourreye O, Veivers D, Hans S, et al. Chemotherapy alone with curative intent in patients with invasive squamous cell carcinoma of the pharyngolarynx classified as T1-T4 N0M0 complete clinical responders. *Cancer* 2001;92:1504.

58. Mendenhall WM, Riggs CE, Amdur RJ, et al. Altered fractionation and/or adjuvant chemotherapy in definitive irradiation of squamous cell carcinoma of the head and neck. *Laryngoscope* 2003;113:546.

59. Mendenhall WM, Amdur RJ, Stringer SP, et al. Stratification of stage IV squamous cell carcinoma of the oropharynx [Letter]. *Head Neck* 2000;22:626.

60. Kies MS, Haraf DJ, Rosen F, et al. Concomitant infusional paclitaxel and fluorouracil, oral hydroxyurea, and hyperfractionated radiation for locally advanced squamous head and neck cancer. *J Clin Oncol* 2001;19:1961.

61. Robbins KT, Kumar P, Wong FS, et al. Targeted chemoradiation for advanced head and neck cancer: analysis of 213 patients. *Head Neck* 2000;22:687.

62. Regine WF, Valentino J, Arnold SM, et al. High-dose intra-arterial cisplatin boost with hyperfractionated radiation therapy for advanced squamous cell carcinoma of the head and neck. *J Clin Oncol* 2001;19:3333.

63. Suntharalingam M, Haas ML, Van Echo DA, et al. Predictors of response and survival after concurrent chemotherapy and radiation for locally advanced squamous cell carcinomas of the head and neck. *Cancer* 2001;91:548.

64. Parsons JT, Mendenhall WM, Stringer SP, et al. Twice-a-day radiotherapy for squamous cell carcinoma of the head and neck: the University of Florida experience. *Head Neck* 1993;15:87.

65. Siemann DW, Mendenhall WM. Role of carbogen in the treatment of head and neck cancer. *Cancer Control* 1999;6:606.

66. Kaanders JH, Pop LA, Marres HA, et al. ARCON: experience in 215 patients with advanced head-and-neck cancer. *Int J Radiat Oncol Biol Phys* 2002;52:769.

67. Siemann DW, Warrington KH, Horsman MR. Targeting tumor blood vessels: an adjuvant strategy for radiation therapy. *Radiother Oncol* 2000;57:5.

68. Licitra L, Grandi C, Guzzo M, et al. Primary chemotherapy in resectable oral cavity squamous cell cancer: a randomized controlled trial. *J Clin Oncol* 2003;21:327.

69. Fitzpatrick PJ. Cancer of the lip. *J Otolaryngol* 1984;13:32.

70. Byers RM, O'Brien J, Waxler J. The therapeutic and prognostic implications of nerve invasion in cancer of the lower lip. *Int J Radiat Oncol Biol Phys* 1978;4:215.

71. MacKay EN, Sellers AH. A statistical review of carcinoma of the lip. *Can Med Assoc J* 1964;90:670.

72. Hendricks JL, Mendelson BC, Woods JE. Invasive carcinoma of the lower lip. *Surg Clin North Am* 1977;57:837.

73. Mohs FE, Snow SN. Microscopically controlled surgical treatment for squamous cell carcinoma of the lower lip. *Surg Gynecol Obstet* 1985;160:37.

74. Fletcher GH. Elective irradiation of subclinical disease in cancers of the head and neck. *Cancer* 1972;29:1450.

75. Ange DW, Lindberg RD, Guillamondegui OM. Management of squamous cell carcinoma of the oral tongue and floor of mouth after excisional biopsy. *Radiology* 1974;116:143.

76. Chu A, Fletcher GH. Incidence and causes of failures to control by irradiation the primary lesions in squamous cell carcinomas of the anterior two-thirds of the tongue and floor of the mouth. *Am J Roentgenol Radium Ther Nucl Med* 1973;117:501.

77. Fu KK, Lichter A, Galante M. Carcinoma of the floor of the mouth: an analysis of treatment results and the sites and causes of failures. *Int J Radiat Oncol Biol Phys* 1976;1:829.

78. Mendenhall WM, Van Cise WS, Bova FJ, et al. Analysis of time-dose factors in squamous cell carcinoma of the oral tongue and floor of mouth treated with radiation therapy alone. *Int J Radiat Oncol Biol Phys* 1981;7:1005.

79. Marcus RB Jr, Million RR, Mitchell TP. A preloaded, custom-designed implantation device for stage T1-T2 carcinoma of the floor of mouth. *Int J Radiat Oncol Biol Phys* 1980;6:111.

80. Tapley N. *Clinical applications of the electron beam.* New York: John Wiley & Sons, 1976.

81. Rodgers LW Jr, Stringer SP, Mendenhall WM, et al. Management of squamous cell carcinoma of the floor of mouth. *Head Neck* 1993;15:16.

82. Sessions DG, Spector GJ, Lenox J, et al. Analysis of treatment results for floor-of-mouth cancer. *Laryngoscope* 2000;110:1764.

83. Pernot M, Hoffstetter S, Peiffert D, et al. Epidermoid carcinomas of the floor of the mouth treated by exclusive irradiation: statistical study of a series of 207 cases. *Radiother Oncol* 1995;35:177.

84. Wang CC, Biggs PJ. Technical and radiotherapeutic considerations of intra-oral cone electron beam radiation therapy for head and neck cancer. *Semin Radiat Oncol* 1992;2:171.

85. Byers RM, Weber RS, Andrews T, et al. Frequency and therapeutic implications of "skip matastases" in the neck from squamous carcinoma of the oral tongue. *Head Neck* 1997;19:14.

86. Mendenhall WM, Parsons JT, Stringer SP, et al. T2 oral tongue carcinoma treated with radiotherapy: analysis of local control and complications. *Radiother Oncol* 1989;16:275.

87. Wendt CD, Peters LJ, Delclos L, et al. Primary radiotherapy in the treatment of stage I and II oral tongue cancers: importance of the proportion of therapy delivered with interstitial therapy. *Int J Radiat Oncol Biol Phys* 1990;18:1287.

88. Fein DA, Mendenhall WM, Parsons JT, et al. Carcinoma of the oral tongue: a comparison of results and complications of treatment with radiotherapy and/or surgery. *Head Neck* 1994;16:358.

89. Sessions DG, Spector GJ, Lenox J, et al. Analysis of treatment results for oral tongue cancer. *Laryngoscope* 2002;112:616.

90. Pernot M, Malissard L, Hoffstetter S, et al. The study of tumoral, radiobiological, and general health factors that influence results and complications in a series of 448 oral tongue carcinomas treated exclusively by irradiation. *Int J Radiat Oncol Biol Phys* 1994;29:673.

91. Nair MK, Sankaranarayanan R, Padmanabhan TK. Evaluation of the role of radiotherapy in the management of carcinoma of the buccal mucosa. *Cancer* 1988;61:1326.

92. Diaz EM Jr, Holsinger FC, Zuniga ER, et al. Squamous cell carcinoma of the buccal mucosa: one institution's experience with 119 previously untreated patients. *Head Neck* 2003;25:267.

93. Ash CL. Oral cancer: a 25 year study. *Am J Roentgenol Radium Ther Nucl Med* 1962;87:417.

94. Small IA, Waldron CA. Ameloblastomas of the jaws. *Oral Surg Oral Med Oral Pathol* 1955;8:281.

95. Sinclair NA. Cysts and ameloblastomas: a relationship. *Aust Dent J* 1977;22:27.

96. Pandya NJ, Stuteville OH. Treatment of ameloblastoma. *Plast Reconstr Surg* 1972;50:242.

97. Byers RM, Anderson B, Schwarz EA, et al. Treatment of squamous cell carcinoma of the retromolar trigone. *Am J Clin Oncol* 1984;7:647.

98. McIvor J. The radiological features of ameloblastoma. *Clin Radiol* 1974;25:237.

99. Sehdev MK, Huvos AG, Strong EW, et al. Proceedings: ameloblastoma of maxilla and mandible. *Cancer* 1974;33:324.

100. Rankow RM, Hickey MJ. Adamantinoma of the mandible: analysis of surgical treatment. *Surgery* 1954;36:713.

101. Overholt SM, Eicher SA, Wolf P, et al. Prognostic factors affecting outcome in lower gingival carcinoma. *Laryngoscope* 1996;106:1335.

102. Huang CJ, Chao KSC, Tsai J, et al. Cancer of retromolar trigone long-term radiation therapy outcome. *Head Neck* 2001;23:758.

103. Shibuya H, Horiuchi J-I, Suzuki S, Amagasa M, Mashima K. Oral carcinoma of the upper jaw: results of radiation treatment. *Acta Radiol Oncol* 1984;23:331.

104. Lindberg RD, Barkley HT Jr, Jesse RH, et al. Evolution of the clinically negative neck in patients with squamous cell carcinoma of the faucial arch. *Am J Roentgenol Radium Ther Nucl Med* 1971;111:60.

105. Steiner W, Fierek O, Ambrosch P, et al. Transoral laser microsurgery for squamous cell carcinoma of the base of the tongue. *Arch Otolaryngol Head Neck Surg* 2003;129:36.

106. Parsons JT, Mendenhall WM, Stringer SP, et al. Squamous cell carcinoma of the oropharynx: surgery, radiation or both. *Cancer* 2002;94:2967.

107. Al-Othman MOF, Amdur RJ, Morris CG, et al. Does feeding tube placement predict for long-term swallowing disability after radiotherapy for head and neck cancer? *Head Neck* 2003;25:741.

108. Mendenhall WM, Amdur RJ, Stringer SP, et al. Radiation therapy for squamous cell carcinoma of the tonsillar region: a preferred alternative to surgery? *J Clin Oncol* 2000;18:2219.

109. Ratzer ER, Schweitzer RJ, Frazell EL. Epidermoid carcinoma of the palate. *Am J Surg* 1970;119:294.

110. Erkal HS, Serin M, Amdur RJ et al. Squamous cell carcinomas of the soft palate treated with radiation therapy alone or followed by planned neck dissection. *Int J Radiat Oncol Biol Phys* 2001;50:359.

111. Wynder EL. The epidemiology of cancers of the upper alimentary and upper respiratory tracts. *Laryngoscope* 1978;88:50.

112. Vincent RG, Marchetta F. The relationship of the use of tobacco and alcohol to cancer of the oral cavity, pharynx or larynx. *Am J Surg* 1963;106:501.

113. Pillsbury HRC, Kirchner JA. Clinical vs histopathologic staging in laryngeal cancer. *Arch Otolaryngol* 1979;105:157.

114. Mendenhall WM, Amdur RJ, Morris CG, et al. T1–T2 N0 squamous cell carcinoma of the glottic larynx treated with radiation therapy. *J Clin Oncol* 2001;19:4029.

115. Olsen KD, DeSanto LW, Pearson BW. Positive delphian lymph node: clinical significance in laryngeal cancer. *Laryngoscope* 1987;97:1033.

116. Lederman M. Place de la radiotherapie dans le traitment du cancer du larynx (The place of radiotherapy in the treatment of cancer of the larynx). *Ann Radiol* (Paris) 1961;4:443.

117. Garcia-Serra A, Hinerman RW, Amdur RJ, et al. Radiotherapy for carcinoma in situ of the true vocal cords. *Head Neck* 2002;24:390.

118. Burns HP, van Nostrand AW, Bryce DP. Verrucous carcinoma of the larynx: management by radiotherapy and surgery. *Ann Otol Rhinol Laryngol* 1976;85:538.

119. Mendenhall WM, Parsons JT, Stringer SP, et al. Stage T3 squamous cell carcinoma of the glottic larynx: a comparison of laryngectomy and irradiation. *Int J Radiat Oncol Biol Phys* 1992;23:725.

120. Mendenhall WM, Parsons JT, Mancuso AA, et al. Definitive radiotherapy for T3 squamous cell carcinoma of the glottic larynx. *J Clin Oncol* 1997;15:2394.

121. Mendenhall WM, Million RR, Sharkey DE, et al. Stage T3 squamous cell carcinoma of the glottic larynx treated with surgery and/or radiation therapy. *Int J Radiat Oncol Biol Phys* 1984;10:357.

122. Mendenhall WM, Amdur RJ, Mancuso AA, et al. T3–T4 squamous cell carcinoma of the larynx treated with radiation therapy. *J Hong Kong Coll Radiol* 2001;4:27.

123. Weinstein GS, El-Sawy MM, Ruiz C, et al. Laryngeal preservation with supracricoid partial laryngectomy results in improved quality of life when compared with total laryngectomy. *Laryngoscope* 2001;111:191.

124. Mendenhall WM, Morris CG, Stringer SP, et al. Voice rehabilitation after total laryngectomy and postoperative radiation therapy. *J Clin Oncol* 2002;20:2500.

125. Gluckman JL, Hamaker RC, Schuller DE, et al. Surgical salvage for stomal recurrence: a multi-institutional experience. *Laryngoscope* 1987;97:1025.

126. Mendenhall WM, Parsons JT, Mancuso AA, et al. Radiotherapy for squamous cell carcinoma of the supraglottic larynx: an alternative to surgery. *Head Neck* 1996;18:24.

127. Hinerman RW, Mendenhall WM, Amdur RJ, et al. Carcinoma of the supraglottic larynx: treatment results with radiotherapy alone or with planned neck dissection. *Head Neck* 2002;24:456.

128. Mendenhall WM, Morris CG, Amdur RJ, et al. Parameters that predict local control after definitive radiotherapy for squamous cell carcinoma of the head and neck. *Head Neck* 2003;25:535.

129. Somerset JD, Mendenhall WM, Amdur RJ, et al. Planned postradiotherapy bilateral neck dissection for head and neck cancer. *Am J Otolaryngol* 2001;22:383.

130. Thomas JV, Olsen KD, Neel HB 3rd, et al. Early glottic carcinoma treated with open laryngeal procedures. *Arch Otolaryngol Head Neck Surg* 1994;120:264.

131. Som ML. Cordal cancer with extension to vocal process. *Laryngoscope* 1975;85:1298.

132. Foote RL, Olsen KD, Buskirk SJ, et al. Laryngectomy alone for T3 glottic cancer. *Head Neck* 1994;16:406.

133. Harwood AR, Beale FA, Cummings BJ, et al. T3 glottic cancer: an analysis of dose-time-volume factors. *Int J Radiat Oncol Biol Phys* 1980;6:675.

134. Neel HB 3rd, Devine KD, DeSanto LW. Laryngofissure and cordectomy for early cordal carcinoma: outcome in 182 patients. *Otolaryngol Head Neck Surg* 1980;88:79.

135. Ballantyne AJ. Principles of surgical management of cancer of the pharyngeal walls. *Cancer* 1967;20:663.

136. Kirchner JA. Pyriform sinus cancer: a clinical and laboratory study. *Ann Otol Rhinol Laryngol* 1975;84:793.

137. Ogura JH, Biller HF, Wette R. Elective neck dissection for pharyngeal and laryngeal cancers: an evaluation. *Ann Otol Rhinol Laryngol* 1971;80:646.

138. Amdur RJ, Mendenhall WM, Stringer SP, et al. Organ preservation with radiotherapy for T1-T2 carcinoma of the pyriform sinus. *Head Neck* 2001;23:353.

139. Pameijer FA, Mancuso AA, Mendenhall WM, et al. Evaluation of pretreatment computed tomography as a predictor of local control in T1/T2 pyriform sinus carcinoma treated with definitive radiotherapy. *Head Neck* 1998;20:159.

140. Hull MC, Morris CG, Tannehill SP, et al. Definitive radiotherapy alone or combined with a planned neck dissection for squamous cell carcinoma of the pharyngeal wall. *Cancer* 2003;98(10):2224.

141. Marks JE, Freeman RB, Lee F, et al. Pharyngeal wall cancer; an analysis of treatment results complications and patterns of failure. *Int J Radiat Oncol Biol Phys* 1978;4:587.

142. Meoz-Mendez RT, Fletcher GH, Guillamondegui O. Analysis of the results of radiation in the treatment of squamous cell carcinomas of the pharyngeal walls. *Int J Radiat Oncol Biol Phys* 1978;4:579.

143. Marks JE, Kurnick B, Powers WE, et al. Carcinoma of the pyriform sinus: an analysis of treatment results and patterns of failure. *Cancer* 1978;41:1008.

144. El-Badawi SA, Goepfert H, Fletcher GH. Squamous cell carcinoma of the pyriform sinus. *Laryngoscope* 1982;92:357.

145. Ho JHC. An epidemiologic and clinical study of nasopharyngeal carcinoma. *Int J Radiat Oncol Biol Phys* 1978;4:183.

146. Fletcher GH, Million RR. Malignant tumors of the nasopharynx. *Am J Roentgenol Radium Ther Nucl Med* 1965;93:44.

147. Mendenhall WM, Million RR, Mancuso AA, et al. Nasopharynx. In: Million RR, Cassisi NJ, eds. *Management of head and neck cancer: a multidisciplinary approach*, 2nd ed. Philadelphia: JB Lippincott Company, 1994:599.

148. Mendenhall WM, Mendenhall CM, Mendenhall NP. Solitary plasmacytoma of bone and soft tissues. *Am J Otolaryngol* 2003;24(6):395.

149. Mendenhall WM, Werning JW, Hinerman RW, et al. Juvenile nasopharyngeal angiofibroma. *J Hong Kong Coll Radiol* 2003;6:15.

150. Al-Sarraf M, LeBlanc M, Shanker Giri PG, et al. Chemoradiotherapy versus radiotherapy in patients with advanced nasopharyngeal cancer: phase III randomized intergroup study 0099. *J Clin Oncol* 1998;16:1310.

151. Chan AT, Teo PM, Ngan RK, et al. Concurrent chemotherapy-radiotherapy compared with radiotherapy alone in locoregionally advanced nasopharyngeal carcinoma: progression-free survival analysis of a phase III randomized trial. *J Clin Oncol* 2002;20:2038.

152. Chi KH, Chang YC, Guo WY, et al. A phase III study of adjuvant chemotherapy in advanced nasopharyngeal carcinoma patients. *Int J Radiat Oncol Biol Phys* 2002;52:1238.

153. Chow E, Payne D, O'Sullivan B, et al. Radiotherapy alone in patients with advanced nasopharyngeal cancer: comparison with an intergroup study. Is combined modality treatment really necessary? *Radiother Oncol* 2002;63:269.

154. Teo PM, Kwan WH, Chan AT, et al. How successful is high-dose (60 Gy or more) reirradiation using mainly external beams in salvaging local failures of nasopharyngeal carcinoma? *Int J Radiat Oncol Biol Phys* 1998;40:897.

155. Leung TW, Tung SY, Sze WW, et al. Salvage radiation therapy for locally recurrent nasopharyngeal carcinoma. *Int J Radiat Oncol Biol Phys* 2000;48:1331.

156. Lee AWM, Poon YF, Foo W, et al. Retrospective analysis of 5037 patients with nasopharyngeal carcinoma treated during 1976-1985: overall survival and patterns of failure. *Int J Radiat Oncol Biol Phys* 1992;23:261.

157. Chua DTT, Sham JST, Kwong DLW, et al. Volumetric analysis of tumor extent in nasopharyngeal carcinoma and correlation with treatment outcome. *Int J Radiat Oncol Biol Phys* 1997;39:711.

158. Teo P, Yu P, Lee WY, et al. Significant prognosticators after primary radiotherapy in 903 nondisseminated nasopharyngeal carcinoma evaluated by computer tomography. *Int J Radiat Oncol Biol Phys* 1996;36:291.

159. Mendenhall WM, Stringer SP, Cassisi NJ, et al. Squamous cell carcinoma of the nasal vestibule. *Head Neck* 1999;21:385.

160. Monroe AT, Hinerman RW, Amdur RJ, et al. Radiation therapy for esthesioneuroblastoma: rationale for elective neck irradiation. *Head Neck* 2003;25:529.

161. Acheson ED, Cowdell RH, Hadfield E, et al. Nasal cancer in woodworkers in the furniture industry. *Br Med J* 1968;2:587.

162. Acheson ED, Cowdell RH, Jolles B. Nasal cancer in the Northamptonshire boot and shoe industry. *Br Med J* 1970;1:385.

163. Acheson ED, Hadfield EH, Macbeth RG. Carcinoma of the nasal cavity and accessory sinuses in woodworkers. *Lancet* 1967;1:311.

164. Ironside P, Matthews J. Adenocarcinoma of the nose and paranasal sinuses in woodworkers in the state of Victoria, Australia. *Cancer* 1975;36:1115.

165. Maisel RH, Johnston WH, Anderson HA, et al. Necrotizing sialometaplasia involving the nasal cavity. *Laryngoscope* 1977;87:429.

166. Mendenhall WM, Million RR, Cassisi NJ, et al. Biologically aggressive papillomas of the nasal cavity: the role of radiation therapy. *Laryngoscope* 1985;95:344.

167. Weissler MC, Montgomery WM, Turner PA, et al. Inverted papilloma. *Ann Otol Rhinol Laryngol* 1986;95:215.

168. Schoub L, Timme AH, Uys CJ. A well-differentiated inverted papilloma of the nasal space associated with lymph node metastases. *S Afr Med J* 1973;47:1663.

169. Fechner RE, Sessions RB. Inverted papilloma of the lacrimal sac, paranasal sinus, and cervical region. *Cancer* 1977;40:2303.

170. Katz TS, Mendenhall WM, Morris CG, et al. Malignant tumors of the nasal cavity and paranasal sinuses. *Head Neck* 2002;24:821.

171. Ellingwood KE, Million RR. Cancer of the nasal cavity and ethmoid/sphenoid sinuses. *Cancer* 1979;43:1517.

172. Goepfert H, Guillamondegui OM, Jesse RH, et al. Squamous cell carcinoma of nasal vestibule. *Arch Otolaryngol* 1974;100:8.
173. Myers EN, Schramm VL Jr, Barnes EL Jr. Management of inverted papilloma of the nose and paranasal sinuses. *Laryngoscope* 1981;91:2071.
174. Gomez JA, Mendenhall WM, Tannehill SP, et al. Radiation therapy in inverted papillomas of the nasal cavity and paranasal sinuses. *Am J Otolaryngol* 2000;21:174.
175. Cheesman AD, Lund VJ, Howard DJ. Craniofacial resection for tumors of the nasal cavity and paranasal sinuses. *Head Neck Surg* 1986;8:429.
176. Elkon D, Hightower SI, Lim ML, et al. Esthesioneuroblastoma. *Cancer* 1979;44:1087.
177. Jesse RH. Preoperative versus postoperative radiation in the treatment of squamous cell carcinoma of the paranasal sinuses. *Am J Surg* 1965;110:552.
178. Stern SJ, Goepfert H, Clayman G, et al. Squamous cell carcinoma of the maxillary sinus. *Arch Otolaryngol Head Neck Surg* 1993;119:964.
179. Bataini JP, Ennuyer A. Advanced carcinoma of the maxillary antrum treated by cobalt teletherapy and electron beam irradiation. *Br J Radiol* 1971;44:590.
180. Waldron JN, O'Sullivan B, Gullane P, et al. Carcinoma of the maxillary antrum: a retrospective analysis of 110 cases. *Radiother Oncol* 2000;57:167.
181. Parsons JT, Bova FJ, Fitzgerald CR, et al. Radiation optic neuropathy after megavoltage external-beam irradiation: analysis of time-dose factors. *Int J Radiat Oncol Biol Phys* 1994;30:755.
182. Parsons JT, Bova FJ, Fitzgerald CR, et al. Radiation retinopathy after external-beam irradiation: analysis of time-dose factors. *Int J Radiat Oncol Biol Phys* 1994;30:765.
183. Parsons JT, Bova FJ, Fitzgerald CR, et al. Severe dry-eye syndrome following external beam irradiation. *Int J Radiat Oncol Biol Phys* 1994;30:775.
184. O'Leary MJ, Shelton C, Giddings NA, et al. Glomus tympanicum tumors: a clinical perspective. *Laryngoscope* 1991;101:1038.
185. Woods CI, Strasnick B, Jackson CG. Surgery for glomus tumors: the Otology Group experience. *Laryngoscope* 1993;103:65.
186. Hinerman RW, Mendenhall WM, Amdur RJ, et al. Definitive radiotherapy in the management of chemodectomas arising in the temporal bone, carotid body, and glomus vagale. *Head Neck* 2001;23:363.
187. Powell S, Peters N, Harmer C. Chemodectoma of the head and neck: results of treatment in 84 patients. *Int J Radiat Oncol Biol Phys* 1992;22:919.
188. Biller HF, Lawson W, Som P, et al. Glomus vagale tumors. *Ann Otol Rhinol Laryngol* 1989;98:21.
189. Green JD Jr, Brackmann DE, Nguyen CD, et al. Surgical management of previously untreated glomus jugulare tumors. *Laryngoscope* 1994;104:917.
190. Verniers DA, Keus RB, Schouwenburg PF, et al. Radiation therapy, an important mode of treatment for head and neck chemodectomas. *Eur J Cancer* 1992;28A:1028.
191. DelCharco JO, Mendenhall WM, Parsons JT, et al. Carcinoma of the skin metastatic to the parotid area lymph nodes. *Head Neck* 1998;20:369.
192. Mendenhall WM, Morris CG, Amdur RJ, et al. Radiotherapy alone or combined with surgery for adenoid cystic carcinoma of the head and neck. *Head Neck* 2004;26(2):154.
193. Gallia LJ, Johnson JT. Incidence of neoplastic versus inflammatory disease in major salivary gland masses diagnosed by surgery. *Laryngoscope* 1981;91:512.
194. Gullane PJ, Havas TJ. Facial nerve grafts: effects of postoperative irradiation. *J Otolaryngol* 1987;16:112.
195. Spiro RH, Huvos AG, Strong EW. Cancer of the parotid gland: a clinicopathologic study of 288 primary cases. *Am J Surg* 1975;130:452.
196. Rafla-Demetrious S. *Mucous and salivary gland tumors*. Springfield, IL: Charles C. Thomas, 1970:118.
197. Spiro RH. Salivary neoplasms: overview of a 35-year experience with 2,807 patients. *Head Neck Surg* 1986;8:177.
198. Woods JE, Chong GC, Beahrs OH. Experience with 1360 primary parotid tumors. *Am J Surg* 1975;130:460.
199. Garden AS, El-Naggar AK, Morrison WH, et al. Postoperative radiotherapy for malignant tumors of the parotid gland. *Int J Radiat Oncol Biol Phys* 1997;37:79.
200. Guillamondegui O, Byers RM, Luna MA. Aggressive surgery in treatment for parotid cancer. The role of adjunctive postoperative radiotherapy. *AJR Am J Roentgenol* 1975; 123:49.
201. Theriault C, Fitzpatrick PJ. Malignant parotid tumors: prognostic factors and optimum treatment. *Am J Clin Oncol* 1986;9:510.
202. Byers RM, Jesse RH, Guillamondegui OM, et al. Malignant tumors of the submaxillary gland. *Am J Surg* 1973;126:458.
203. Thawley SE, Ward SP, Ogura JH. Basal cell adenoma of the salivary glands. *Laryngoscope* 1974;84:1756.
204. Ranger D, Thackray AC, Lucas RB. Mucous gland tumors. *Br J Cancer* 1956;10:1.
205. Parsons JT, Mendenhall WM, Stringer SP, et al. Management of minor salivary gland carcinomas. *Int J Radiat Oncol Biol Phys* 1996;35:443.
206. Spiro RH, Koss LG, Haidu SI, et al. Tumors of minor salivary origin: a clinicopathologic study of 492 cases. *Cancer* 1973;31:117.
207. Bardwil JM, Reynolds CT, Ibanez ML, et al. Report of one hundred tumors of the minor salivary glands. *Am J Surg* 1966;112:493.
208. American Joint Committee on Cancer. *Manual for staging of cancer*, 2nd ed. Philadelphia: JB Lippincott Company, 1983:27.
209. Mendenhall WM, Parsons JT, Mancuso AA, et al. Head and neck: management of the neck. In: Perez CA, Brady LW, eds. *Principles and practice of radiation oncology*, 2nd ed. Philadelphia: JB Lippincott Company, 1992:790.
210. Ojiri H, Mendenhall WM, Stringer SP, et al. Post-RT CT results as a predictive model for the necessity of planned post-RT neck dissection in patients with cervical metastatic disease from squamous cell carcinoma. *Int J Radiat Oncol Biol Phys* 2002;52:420.
211. Nisi KW, Foote RL, Bonner JA, et al. Adjuvant radiotherapy for squamous cell carcinoma of the tongue base: improved local-regional disease control compared with surgery alone. *Int J Radiat Oncol Biol Phys* 1998;41:371.
212. Machtay M, Perch S, Markiewicz D, et al. Combined surgery and postoperative radiotherapy for carcinoma of the base of tongue: analysis of treatment outcome and prognostic value of margin status. *Head Neck* 1997;19:494.
213. Kraus DH, Vastola AP, Huvos AG, et al. Surgical management of squamous cell carcinoma of the base of the tongue. *Am J Surg* 1993;166:384.
214. Thawley SE, Simpson JR, Marks JE, et al. Preoperative irradiation and surgery for carcinoma of the base of the tongue. *Ann Otol Rhinol Laryngol* 1983;92:485.
215. Harrison LB, Lee HJ, Pfister DG, et al. Long term results of primary radiotherapy with/without neck dissection for squamous cell cancer of the base of tongue. *Head Neck* 1998;20:668.
216. Lusinchi A, Eskandari J, Son Y, et al. External irradiation plus curietherapy boost in 108 base of tongue carcinomas. *Int J Radiat Oncol Biol Phys* 1989;17:1191.
217. Crook J, Mazeron JJ, Marinello G, et al. Combined external irradiation and interstitial implantation for T1 and T2 epidermoid carcinomas of base of tongue: the Creteil experience (1971–1981). *Int J Radiat Oncol Biol Phys* 1988;15:105.
218. Spanos WJ Jr, Shukovsky LJ, Fletcher GH. Time, dose, and tumor volume relationships in irradiation of squamous cell carcinomas of the base of the tongue. *Cancer* 1976;37:2591.
219. Mak AC, Morrison WH, Garden AS, et al. Base-of-tongue carcinoma: treatment results using concomitant boost radiotherapy. *Int J Radiat Oncol Biol Phys* 1995;33:289.
220. Jaulerry C, Rodriguez J, Brunin F, et al. Results of radiation therapy in carcinoma of the base of the tongue: the Curie Institute experience with about 166 cases. *Cancer* 1991;67:1532.
221. Mendenhall WM, Stringer SP, Amdur RJ, et al. Is radiation therapy a preferred alternative to surgery for squamous cell carcinoma of the base of tongue? *J Clin Oncol* 2000;18:35.
222. Dupont JB, Guillamondegui OM, Jesse RH. Surgical treatment of advanced carcinomas of the base of the tongue. *Am J Surg* 1978;136:501.
223. Puthawala AA, Syed AMN, Eads DL, et al. Limited external beam and interstitial ^{192}iridium irradiation in the treatment of carcinoma of the base of the tongue: a ten year experience. *Int J Radiat Oncol Biol Phys* 1988;14:839.
224. Weber RS, Gidley P, Morrison WH, et al. Treatment selection for carcinoma of the base of the tongue. *Am J Surg* 1990;160:415.
225. Perez CA, Patel MM, Chao KSC, et al. Carcinoma of the tonsillar fossa: prognostic factors and long-term therapy outcome. *Int J Radiat Oncol Biol Phys* 1998;42:1077.
226. Foote RL, Schild SE, Thompson WM, et al. Tonsil cancer. Patterns of failure after surgery alone and surgery combined with postoperative radiation therapy. *Cancer* 1994; 73:2638.
227. Hicks WL, Kuriakose MA, Loree TR, et al. Surgery versus radiation therapy as single-modality treatment of tonsillar fossa carcinoma: the Roswell Park Cancer Institute experience (1971–1991). *Laryngoscope* 1998;108:1014.
228. Puthawala AA, Syed AM, Eads DL, et al. Limited external irradiation and interstitial ^{192}iridium implant in the treatment of squamous cell carcinoma of the tonsillar region. *Int J Radiat Oncol Biol Phys* 1985;11:1595.
229. Pernot M, Malissard L, Hoffstetter S, et al. Influence of tumoral, radiobiological, and general factors on local control and survival of a series of 361 tumors of the velotonsillar area treated by exclusive irradiation (external beam irradiation + brachytherapy or brachytherapy alone). *Int J Radiat Oncol Biol Phys* 1994;30:1051.
230. Bataini JP, Asselain B, Jaulerry C, et al. A multivariate primary tumour control analysis in 465 patients treated by radical radiotherapy for cancer of the tonsillar region: clinical and treatment parameters as prognostic factors. *Radiother Oncol* 1989;14:265.
231. Wong CS, Ang KK, Fletcher GH, et al. Definitive radiotherapy for squamous cell carcinoma of the tonsillar fossa. *Int J Radiat Oncol Biol Phys* 1989;16:657.
232. Amornmarn R, Prempree T, Jaiwatana J, et al. Radiation management of carcinoma of the tonsillar region. *Cancer* 1984;54:1293.
233. Mizono GS, Diaz RF, Fu KK, et al. Carcinoma of the tonsillar region. *Laryngoscope* 1986;96:240.
234. Gwozdz JT, Morrison WH, Garden AS, et al. Concomitant boost radiotherapy for squamous carcinoma of the tonsillar fossa. *Int J Radiat Oncol Biol Phys* 1997;39:127.
235. Gluckman JL, Black RJ, Crissman JD. Cancer of the oropharynx. *Otolaryngol Clin North Am* 1985;18:451.
236. Givens CD Jr, Johns ME, Cantrell RW. Carcinoma of the tonsil. Analysis of 162 cases. *Arch Otolaryngol* 1981;107:730.
237. Rabuzzi DD, Mickler AS, Clutter DJ, et al. Treatment results of combined high-dose preoperative radiotherapy and surgery for oropharyngeal cancer. *Laryngoscope* 1982;92: 989.
238. Schuller DE, McGuirt WF, Krause CJ, et al. Symposium: adjuvant cancer therapy of head and neck tumors. Increased survival with surgery alone vs. combined therapy. *Laryngoscope* 1979;89:582.
239. Garrett PG, Beale FA, Cummings BJ, et al. Carcinoma of the tonsil: the effect of dose-time-volume factors on local control. *Int J Radiat Oncol Biol Phys* 1985;11:703.
240. Lusinchi A, Wibault P, Marandas P, et al. Exclusive radiation therapy: the treatment of early tonsillar tumors. *Int J Radiat Oncol Biol Phys* 1989;17:273.
241. Jesse RH. The evaluation of treatment of patients with extensive squamous cancer of the vocal cords. *Laryngoscope* 1975;85:1424.
242. Ogura JH, Sessions DG, Spector GJ. Analysis of surgical therapy for epidermoid carcinoma of the laryngeal glottis. *Laryngoscope* 1975;85:1522.
243. Skolnik EM, Yee KF, Wheatley MA, et al. Carcinoma of the laryngeal glottis: therapy and end results. *Laryngoscope* 1975;85:1453.
244. Vermund H. Role of radiotherapy in cancer of the larynx as related to the TNM system of staging. A review. *Cancer* 1970;25:485.
245. Stewart JG, Jackson AW. The steepness of the dose response curve both for tumor cure and normal tissue injury. *Laryngoscope* 1975;85:1107.
246. Harwood AR, Beale FA, Cummings BJ, et al. T4N0M0 glottic cancer: an analysis of dose-time-volume factors. *Int J Radiat Oncol Biol Phys* 1981;7:1507.
247. Davis RK, Kelly SM, Hayes J. Endoscopic CO_2 laser excisional biopsy of early supraglottic cancer. *Laryngoscope* 1991;101:680.

248. Steiner W. Results of curative laser microsurgery of laryngeal carcinomas. *Am J Otolaryngol* 1993;14:116.

249. Zeitels SM, Koufman JA, Davis RK, et al. Endoscopic treatment of supraglottic and hypopharynx cancer. *Laryngoscope* 1994;104:71.

250. Csanády M, Iván L, Czigner J. Endoscopic CO$_2$ laser therapy of selected cases of supraglottic marginal tumors. *Eur Arch Otorhinolaryngol* 1999;256:392.

251. Rudert HH, Werner JA, Höft S. Transoral carbon dioxide laser resection of supraglottic carcinoma. *Ann Otol Rhinol Laryngol* 1999;108:819.

252. Fletcher GH, Hamberger AD. Causes of failure in irradiation of squamous-cell carcinoma of the supraglottic larynx. *Radiology* 1974;111:697.

253. Ghossein NA, Bataini JP, Ennuyer A, et al. Local control and site of failure in radically irradiated supraglottic laryngeal cancer. *Radiology* 1974;112:187.

254. Wang CC, Montgomery WM. Deciding on optimal management of supraglottic carcinoma. *Oncology* 1991;5:41.

255. Nakfoor BM, Spiro IJ, Wang CC, et al. Results of accelerated radiotherapy for supraglottic carcinoma: a Massachusetts General Hospital and Massachusetts Eye and Ear Infirmary experience. *Head Neck* 1998;20:379.

256. Sykes AJ, Slevin NJ, Gupta NK, et al. 331 cases of clinically node-negative supraglottic carcinoma of the larynx: a study of a modest size fixed field radiotherapy approach. *Int J Radiat Oncol Biol Phys* 2000;46:1109.

257. Ogura JH, Sessions DG, Spector GJ. Conservation surgery for epidermoid carcinoma of the supraglottic larynx. *Laryngoscope* 1975;85:1808.

258. Bocca E. Sixteenth Daniel C. Baker Jr, memorial lecture. Surgical management of supra-glottic cancer and its lymph node metastases in a conservative perspective. *Ann Otol Rhinol Laryngol* 1991;100:261.

259. Lee NK, Goepfert H, Wendt CD. Supraglottic laryngectomy for intermediate-stage cancer: UT MD Anderson Cancer Center experience with combined therapy. *Laryngoscope* 1990;100:831.

260. DeSanto LW. Early supraglottic cancer. *Ann Otol Rhinol Laryngol* 1990;99:593.

261. Steiniger JR, Parnes SM, Gardner GM. Morbidity of combined therapy for the treatment of supraglottic carcinoma: supraglottic laryngectomy and radiotherapy. *Ann Otol Rhinol Laryngol* 1997;106:151.

262. Spriano G, Antognoni P, Piantanida R, et al. Conservative management of T1-T2N0 supraglottic cancer: a retrospective study. *Am J Otolaryngol* 1997;18:299.

263. Burstein FD, Calcaterra TC. Supraglottic laryngectomy: series report and analysis of results. *Laryngoscope* 1985;95:833.

264. Isaacs JH Jr, Slattery WH 3rd, Mendenhall WM, et al. Supraglottic laryngectomy. *Am J Otolaryngol* 1998;19:118.

265. Lutz CK, Johnson JT, Wagner RL, et al. Supraglottic carcinoma: patterns of recurrence. *Ann Otol Rhinol Laryngol* 1990;99:12.

266. Gall AM, Sessions DG, Ogura JH. Complications following surgery for cancer of the larynx and hypopharynx. *Cancer* 1977;39:624.

267. Weber PC, Johnson JT, Myers EN. Impact of bilateral neck dissection on recovery following supraglottic laryngectomy. *Arch Otolaryngol Head Neck Surg* 1993;119:61.

268. Beckhardt RN, Murray JG, Ford CN, et al. Factors influencing functional outcome in supraglottic laryngectomy. *Head Neck* 1994;16:232.

SECTION **3**

MICHAEL A. CRARY
GISELLE D. CARNABY (MANN)

Rehabilitation after Treatment for Head and Neck Cancer

During the last two decades, head and neck cancer management strategies have focused on an increase in organ preservation approaches, conservative laryngopharyngeal surgery, and advances in reconstructive surgery. As a result of these conservative approaches, patients and practitioners anticipated enhanced posttreatment functions within head and neck organ systems. Despite this evolution in cancer treatment, communication (speech and voice) and swallowing limitations remain prevalent among posttreatment head and neck cancer patients. In fact, posttreatment functional limitations may result from any treatment for head and neck cancer. Moreover, combined modality treatments compound the risks for functional deficits after treatment. After treatment for head and neck cancer, a wide range of functional limitations in speech, voice, and swallowing may occur. This dispersion of potential deficits extends beyond the scope of any single professional. Consequently, patients benefit most from a multidisciplinary rehabilitation effort from the time of diagnosis.

This chapter reviews speech, voice, and swallowing deficits that occur secondary to various treatments for head and neck cancer. First, general consequences of various treatments are described, followed by specific details of speech, voice, and swallowing deficits. Evaluation strategies are then described for speech, voice, and swallowing deficits in head and neck cancer patients, as well as specific rehabilitation strategies for these functional limitations. Throughout this chapter, the multidisciplinary nature of the deficits encountered by head and neck cancer patients is emphasized and various roles of the multidisciplinary cancer management team are described.

GENERAL FUNCTIONAL CONSEQUENCES OF TREATMENT FOR HEAD AND NECK CANCER

Surgery, radiation therapy, and chemotherapy, either in isolation or in combination, remain the primary treatment avenues for head and neck cancer. Each treatment option has its own impact on head and neck functions, and this impact is enhanced in combination. Understanding the general consequences of these treatment modalities will facilitate a better comprehension of the impact of each modality on speech, voice, and swallowing functions.

SURGERY

Resection of structures involved in speech, voice, and swallowing functions is likely to result in some degree of functional deficit. The type and extent of surgery and the nature of any reconstruction have a direct impact on postsurgical functional limitations. Some deficits are limited to the immediate postoperative time period, whereas others are long lasting. Specific surgical changes that may impact communication and swallowing functions are swelling, reduced mobility, and sensory loss. Moreover, if head/neck anatomy is significantly revised, this alteration may be additive to these general impact factors.

RADIATION THERAPY

Similar to surgery, procedural variations in the application of radiation therapy may differentially impact posttreatment function. Although the degree of functional deficits may change depending on the extent and type of radiation therapy used, side effects are common and directly influence communication and swallowing functions. Effects of radiation therapy change over time and may involve mucosal tissue and muscle function. Radiation therapy side effects include severe pain, reduced salivary flow, edema, restricted movement, nausea and vomiting, reduced appetite, reduced senses of taste and smell, and dental problems.

CHEMOTHERAPY

Like radiation therapy, chemotherapy can be applied in combination with other modalities simultaneously, before or after the cotherapy. Side effects of chemotherapy are often significant for the patient with head/neck cancer and can directly impair communication and swallowing functions. Chemotherapy side effects include fatigue, nausea and vomiting, loss of appetite, reduced senses of taste and smell, gastrointestinal irregularities, oral dryness, and sores in the mouth.

SPEECH, VOICE, AND SWALLOWING DEFICITS AFTER TREATMENT FOR HEAD AND NECK CANCER

In the prior section general functional consequences of the primary treatment options for head and neck cancer were introduced. As a result of these posttreatment changes, patients treated for head and neck cancer may experience a variety of speech, voice, and swallowing problems. A basic understanding of these problems and the factors that may determine their presence or characteristics can assist clinicians in developing effective assessment and rehabilitation strategies. This section begins with a basic overview of speech, voice, and swallowing functions. Subsequently, the impact of surgical and radiation interventions on these head and neck functions are reviewed.

Speech and Voice Deficits

Patients may encounter a variety of speech or voice deficits after treatment for head/neck cancer. Speech production is largely a function of movement of the lips, tongue, and jaw. Restricted movement or tissue loss in these structures has a negative impact on a patient's ability to articulate sound patterns. When palatal or velopharyngeal structures are altered, patients may experience increased nasal resonance during speech resulting from excessive nasal airflow. In severe cases, excessive nasal airflow can result in nearly unintelligible speech production. Voice deviations result from alterations in laryngeal function. They may range from a mild hoarseness to complete aphonia depending on the degree of disruption to laryngeal anatomy or physiology.

Swallowing Deficits (Dysphagia)

Swallowing function requires adequate anatomy and physiology of structures in the oral cavity, pharynx, and esophagus. Oral swallowing functions include the ability to ingest material into the mouth, masticate, and manipulate this material toward delivery of a bolus to the pharynx. The pharynx guides and safely transports swallowed material through the pharyngoesophageal (PE) segment and into the proximal esophagus. Esophageal motor action directs this material through the lower esophageal sphincter and into the stomach. Varying types and degrees of dysphagia result from disruption to these structures or functions, either by surgical resection (with or without reconstruction) or changes induced by radiation therapy.

SURGICAL IMPACT ON SPEECH, VOICE, AND SWALLOWING FUNCTIONS

Removal, rearrangement, or reconstruction of head/neck structures may contribute to varying degrees of speech, voice, or swallowing difficulties. A general, historic perception is that patients will develop more severe speech, voice, or swallowing problems if they experience greater than 50% tissue removal or large composite resections compared to patients with less involved resections.[1,2] More recently, however, investigators have challenged this rule,[3] as reconstruction techniques offer the potential for improved postsurgical anatomy and movement. Given the range of surgical approaches available, the cancer management team should evaluate each patient before and after surgery to identify any speech, voice, or swallowing impairment. Generally, the more tissue removed or relocated, the higher the probability of postoperative functional deficits. Table 26.3-1 summarizes the impact of surgery on speech, voice, and swallowing functions.

As the postsurgical time period increases, so does the likelihood of movement restrictions contributing to functional limitations. For example, data specific to swallowing function suggest that performance at 3 postsurgical months is similar to that at 12 months. This observation suggests that the first 3 months after surgery is a critical period for rehabilitation efforts.[4,5]

The cancer management team should consider the location of surgical intervention as to its potential to disrupt speech, voice, or swallowing functions. For example, limitations in speech and swallowing functions are common after partial and total glossectomy procedures. After lingual resections, speech and swallowing functional outcomes are directly related to the reconstruction technique used.[6] Restrictions in mobility of the residual tongue result in the loss of linguopalatal contact and precise lingual movement for speech articulation.[7] These same limitations impair a patient's ability to form, control, and transport an oral bolus during swallowing attempts. Poorer speech and swallowing function can result from significant reduction of the tongue stump or reconstruction of a flat, depressed tongue shape.[8]

Frequently, extensive composite resections require removal or alteration of nasal and palatal structures. These surgical changes may result in reduced velopharyngeal closure. This inability to separate the nasal and oral cavities during speech limits a patient's ability to create oral pressure for the production of sounds such as *t*, *d*, *k*, and *g* and to distinguish nasal from nonnasal sounds. Communication between the oral and nasal cavities also has an impact on a patient's ability to clear a bolus from the oropharynx and can result in food or liquid entering the nasopharynx during swallowing attempts (e.g., nasopharyngeal reflux). Composite resections of integrated oral and pharyngeal structures likewise have a multifactorial effect on speech and swallowing functions subserved by these structures.

Laryngeal resection may range from small, localized excisions to total removal of laryngeal structures. If the resection is limited to a single vocal cord or involves the hemilarynx only, the impact on voice and swallowing will be minimized. In general, postsurgical voice characteristics include lowered fundamental frequency (pitch), reduced intensity (loudness), and increased air escape (breathiness).[9] Postsurgical swallowing deficits may include subglottic aspiration of food or liquid secondary to reduced glottal closure. Combined surgical procedures (e.g., extended hemilaryngectomy with neck dissection and flap) result in greater anatomic revision and further restrictions to mobility. These procedures have an enhanced negative effect on voice and swallow functions.

TABLE 26.3-1. Common Speech, Voice, and Swallowing Disorders Resulting from Various Surgeries in the Treatment of Head and Neck Cancer

Resection	Physiologic Effect	Speech Defect	Swallowing
Partial glossectomy	Removes <50%—anterior tissue removal ↑ difficulties	Minor articulation errors	Difficulty holding and preparing a bolus for swallowing
Total glossectomy	Removal >50% of tongue; flap technique influences result	Vowels only preserved; consonant production incomplete; ↓ speech intelligibility; free flaps show better speech outcomes	Difficulty moving materials out of the oral cavity; reduced tongue driving force; may show reduced pharyngeal clearance
Tonsil/base of tongue	Reduced anterior tongue range	Minor speech defects	Reduced tongue driving force; difficulty moving materials through the oropharynx
Palatal resection	Removal of >50% of soft palate; incomplete velar seal	Increased nasalance, reduced word intelligibility; may benefit from prosthetic device to fill defect and increase contacts for speech	Velar leak results in retrograde movement of materials into the nasopharynx
Anterior/lateral floor of mouth	Reduced anterior tongue range; unable to lateralize tongue; reduced ability to elevate hyoid/larynx; reduced opening of upper esophageal sphincter	Articulation deficits; reduced speech intelligibility	Reduced control of oral bolus; reduced tongue driving force; difficulty moving material through the oropharynx; delayed triggering of pharyngeal swallow; reduced clearance of bolus from pharynx
Partial pharyngeal resection	Reduced pharyngeal wall contraction; reduced elevation of hyoid/larynx	Voice and speech preserved; ↓ secretion management; impairment of vocal clarity	Difficulty clearing materials from the pharynx; delayed triggering of pharyngeal swallow
Hemilaryngectomy	Unilateral resection; partial airway closure	Voice and speech preserved; ↓ secretion management may impair vocal clarity	Unilateral pharyngeal weakness; reduced airway protection
Supraglottic laryngectomy	Incomplete posterior tongue movement; restricted arytenoids motion; partial airway closure	No speech problems—mild loss of voice quality (breathiness)	Delay in bolus propulsion; difficulty with elevation of structures for swallow; reduced airway protection
Total laryngectomy	Removal of vibratory source; alternative source surgically developed	Loss of voice; articulation preserved; alaryngeal speech aid/TEP required	Issues with reduced negative pressure, bolus transit; anatomic or physiologic stenosis of PE segment possible

↑, increase; ↓, decrease; PE, pharyngoesophageal; TEP, tracheoesophageal puncture.

Total laryngectomy is the extreme example of laryngeal surgery. This procedure results in significant functional changes for the patient. A primary alteration is the separation of the airway and the swallowing tract. Redirection of airflow to a surgically created stoma in the anterior neck results in loss of natural voice and reduction in the senses of taste and smell. Swallowing function is further altered by the surgical creation of a "neopharynx" after removal of laryngeal structures. Between 10% and 58% of total laryngectomees report some difficulty with swallowing function.[10] These difficulties have been associated with loss of pharyngeal driving force or increased resistance to bolus flow through the PE segment from either anatomic or physiologic stenosis. Larger resections with more complicated reconstructions increase the risk of significant functional limitations after surgery.

TRACHEOSTOMY ISSUES

The primary roles of tracheostomy in the treatment of head and neck cancer after surgical interventions are to maintain an open airway and provide access for pulmonary toilet during the recovery period. On some occasions, a tracheostomy tube can be placed during or after radiation treatment to alleviate respiratory distress resulting from edema of the airway. Whatever the initial purpose of tracheostomy tube placement, the physiologic impact is considerable on speech and swallowing functions. Placement of a tracheostomy tube reduces airflow and air pressures within the upper aerodigestive tract that support speech and swallowing functions.[11] Reduction or elimination of expiratory airflow reduces cough effectiveness and disturbs the normal apneic interval during swallowing.[12] Furthermore, studies of chronic upper airway bypass have demonstrated a negative impact on laryngopharyngeal reflexes.[13] The alteration in airflow, air pressure, and protective reflexes subsequent to tracheostomy tube placement has been implicated in the development of dysphagia and voice problems after decannulation in these patients.[14]

Placement of a tracheostomy tube has been associated with increased risk of aspiration resulting from disruption to normal swallow biomechanics. This procedure may tether the larynx, reducing laryngeal excursion during swallowing.[15] A more pronounced tethering effect may result from large-diameter or inflated-cuff tracheostomy tubes. Reduction in laryngeal excursion contributes to incomplete clearance of materials from the pharynx during swallowing. Subsequently, post-swallow residue can be aspirated. Also, use of a high-pressure cuffed tracheostomy tube may increase pressure in the upper esophagus or impinge on the esophagus, causing backflow and aspiration of contents into the airway.[16] Patients continue to aspirate around the cuff because of incomplete sealing or leaks after movement or subsequent to large-volume swallows.[17] For these reasons, clinicians should exercise caution when initiating oral feeding in patients with a tracheostomy tube with an inflated cuff.

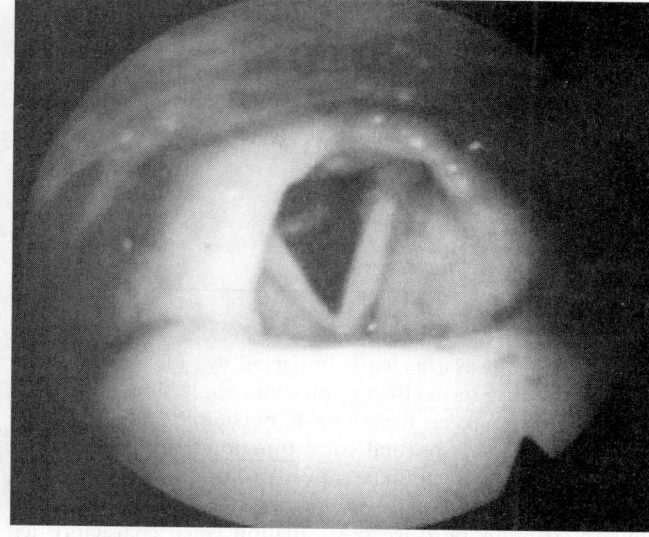

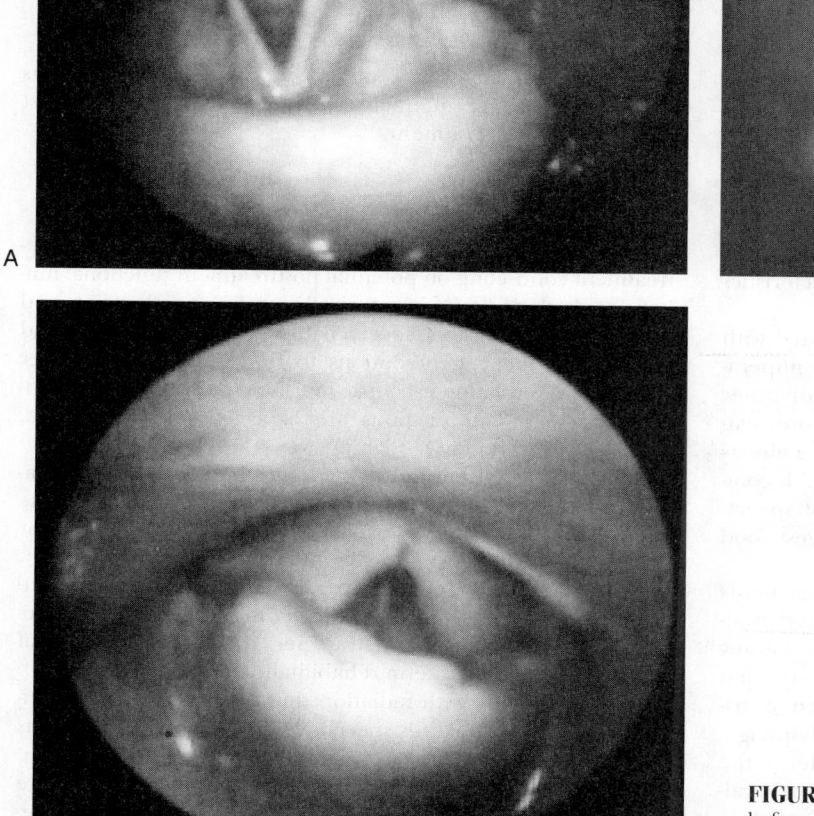

FIGURE 26.3-1. **A:** Endoscopic image of larynx and pharynx before initiation of radiation therapy. **B:** Same patient at conclusion of radiation therapy (6 weeks). **C:** Same patient at 6-month follow-up examination.

Clinicians must be aware of factors that can predict and facilitate decannulation outcome to improve clinical decision making. Premature or inappropriate decannulation of a tracheostomy tube can result in ongoing voice and swallowing difficulties, including possible aspiration of swallowed materials and extended hospitalization. Team members should consider each patient's mental status, respiratory capacity, presence of upper airway obstruction, secretion volume, effectiveness of cough, and feeding readiness to facilitate successful tracheostomy tube removal.

RADIATION THERAPY IMPACT ON SPEECH, VOICE, AND SWALLOWING FUNCTIONS

Radiation therapy contributes to a variety of mucosal and muscle tissue changes, which can complicate existing speech, voice, or swallowing difficulties and create new problems. Frequent side effects of radiation therapy that may have a negative impact on speech, voice, or swallowing functions include mucositis, xerosto-

mia, and edema. These complications occur to some degree in nearly every patient receiving radiation therapy in the treatment of head and neck cancer. As a result of these complications, patients may experience pain, dryness, and limited mobility of structures required for successful speech, voice, or swallowing functions. Difficulties that persist after completion of radiation therapy may be linked to fibrosis or atrophy in muscles or peripheral nerve deficits, or both. Each contributes to reduced mobility within head and neck structures. In addition, thickened secretions in the oropharynx, hypopharynx, or larynx alter speech and voice clarity and contribute to reduced swallow efficiency. Consequently, reduced swallowing efficiency results in prolonged mealtimes, post-swallow residue requiring multiple swallows to clear, and difficulty controlling the direction of a swallowed bolus, leading to potential risks of tracheal aspiration. Figure 26.3-1 depicts changes to the larynx and pharynx viewed endoscopically over a 6-month period subsequent to radiation therapy. Table 26.3-2 summarizes some of the more salient oropharyngeal swallowing problems encountered by patients treated with radiation therapy for head and neck cancer.

TABLE 26.3-2.   Salient Oropharyngeal Swallowing Problems Associated with Radiation Therapy for Head/Neck Cancer

Bolus control deficits (63%)
Small amounts per bolus
Multiple swallow attempts per bolus
Increased mealtimes
Reduced frequency of swallowing
Dry mouth (92%)
Pain (58%)
Altered taste (75%)

Speech functions are clearly impacted by radiation therapy; however, the long-term effect is questionable.[18] Moreover, long-term impact on voice functions is debatable. Some studies describe a return to normal vocal functions within 3 months after treatment,[19] but others report prolonged alterations in vocal fold movement parameters and voice characteristics.[20,21] Similarly, patients perceive postradiation voice characteristics as deviant for up to 2 years after treatment.[22]

Oral health is a major concern in the patient treated with radiation therapy. A pretreatment dental consult is imperative and may result in extraction of diseased teeth or other corrective/preventive action. Even with appropriate pretreatment care, remaining teeth frequently suffer from the effects of radiation therapy. Poor dentition or other oral health complications may also have an impact on the clarity of speech production and a patient's ability to successfully ingest food by mouth.

After radiation therapy, speech and voice impairments may not be severe or long lasting. However, impaired swallowing ability is a serious consequence of radiation therapy in head and neck cancer, as it can further complicate what may, in some patients, be an already compromised nutritional state. Consequently, the specific pattern of dysphagia and the tissue or muscle changes, or both, that underlie the overt symptoms should be identified during the clinical evaluation and become the focus of intervention for the rehabilitation team.

EVALUATION OF SPEECH, VOICE, AND SWALLOWING AFTER HEAD AND NECK CANCER TREATMENT

In preceding sections of this chapter, the general and specific consequences of head and neck cancer treatments on speech, voice, and swallowing functions have been described. In this section, the basic components of the clinical and instrumental evaluation of these functional impairments are outlined, beginning with a brief introduction of the cancer rehabilitation team and proceeding to a discussion of the importance of pretreatment counseling. Subsequently, the basic components of the clinical interview, physical examination, and instrumental examinations that are appropriate for evaluation of speech, voice, or swallowing functions are described. The section concludes with a discussion of the importance of assessing impact factors, those factors that can influence outcome of treatment, and a brief commentary on the timing of the initial and follow-up evaluations.

CANCER REHABILITATION TEAM

Patients with head and neck cancer may encounter a wide range of posttreatment functional limitations. To address this range of limitations effectively, a diverse team of medical and allied health specialists must interact effectively from the time of disease identification. Often, these team members function independently within a consult system driven by the oncologist or surgeon providing primary cancer care to the patient. However, most effective cancer teams use a formal review board or meeting in which all major team members participate and have input into the plan of care. This formal sharing of information facilitates enhanced care to the patient, as team members are interactively engaged from the earliest phases of cancer treatment.

PRETREATMENT EVALUATION AND COUNSELING

Beyond the cancer treatment plan, patients benefit from pretreatment counseling on potential posttreatment functional limitations. As these limitations typically involve speech, voice, and swallowing functions, the speech pathologist on the team should discuss with the patient options to function maximally after treatment. Pretreatment counseling should be provided whenever posttreatment functions are expected to be impaired, regardless of treatment modality.

Patients treated surgically experience immediate postoperative changes for which they should be well prepared. These changes could involve nonoral feeding sources and altered or even nonverbal modes of communication. Consequently, patients should be counseled regarding the extent and duration of postsurgical limitations, including a discussion of specific options for short-term strategies to adjust for functional limitations and longer-term rehabilitation plans.

Patients treated with radiation therapy should also be educated on the potential for speech, voice, or swallowing deficits that occur during or subsequent to the course of treatment. Counseling should include discussion of the potentially acute side effects of radiation therapy that may cause speech, voice, or swallowing difficulties. The counseling clinician should identify to the patient methods to limit the functional impact of these treatment side effects, in addition to rehabilitation efforts that can be used to combat more long-lasting functional limitations.

Pretreatment counseling is a delicate undertaking for the patient and the speech pathologist. The patient has recently learned of the cancer diagnosis and treatment plan and likely does not prioritize or understand posttreatment functional limitations at this time.[23,24] The paradox to this situation is that pretreatment counseling is important to help the patient adjust to posttreatment conditions, some of which may be immediate and severe. Therefore, the speech pathologist must be sensitive to the patient's situation and identify educational approaches to maximize retention of information from counseling. Family members should be included in pretreatment counseling. The speech pathologist may provide the patient and family with simple written material to take away from counseling, along with the opportunity to pose questions later that might arise from this written material. If appropriate, the speech pathologist can demonstrate to patients any devices that will be required for speaking, swallowing, or breathing after treatment. Patients scheduled for a total laryngectomy should be informed about the multiple communication options available to them after surgery and, when appropriate, an artificial larynx should be provided to the patient for pre-surgery practice. Furthermore, all patients should be provided with information on local support mechanisms that will be of assistance to them after treatment. The most prevalent coping strategy among patients with head and neck cancer is to seek social support mechanisms.[25] Finally, patients may benefit from a social visit with a cancer survivor who has experienced the type of treatment that the patient is about to enter. This individual can provide important information on functional limitations, rehabilitation efforts, and support mechanisms from a personal, empathic perspective.

EVALUATION OF SPEECH, VOICE, AND SWALLOWING FUNCTIONS

A comprehensive evaluation of speech, voice, and swallowing functions is essential to focus any rehabilitative effort. This evaluation should incorporate a detailed description of the patient's symptoms; a physical examination of speech, voice, and swallow mechanism; and instrumental examinations as indicated to verify, grade, and document anatomic and physiologic contributors to functional deficits. Finally, the evaluation should consider what might be termed *impact factors*. Impact factors may directly or indirectly affect speech, voice, or swallowing functions or the outcome of rehabilitative efforts.

PATIENT SYMPTOMS: CLINICAL INTERVIEW. Patients' perceptions of functional deficits are helpful in focusing subsequent aspects of the evaluation. For example, patients tend to be adept at localizing dysphagia symptoms and in perceiving changes in swallowing function.[26] In addition to a list of patient symptoms, this component of evaluation is helpful in identifying patient strategies for coping with perceived limitations and consequences of those functional limitations. If swallowing is impaired, many patients attempt a variety of compensatory activities and, if unsuccessful, avoid problematic foods or liquids. When this latter pattern is identified, nutritional issues become more important in the assessment. Likewise, patients with speech or voice limitations may self-impose restrictions on communicative interactions that result in negative social or even employment consequences. In fact, at least one report identified speech articulation function as the primary reason for dropout from a longitudinal study.[27]

Physical Examination

The physical examination of speech, voice, and swallowing functions includes components that are common to all patients, as well as components that are specific to the respective functional deficits. Common components include assessment of altered anatomy that might have an impact on speech, voice, or swallowing functions; assessment of movement limitations related to anatomic or physiologic changes; and assessment of mucosal integrity and associated problems (dryness, pain, sores, altered secretions). For patients who retain some ability to speak, evaluation should include an omnibus measure of speech intelligibility in addition to a more detailed description of specific sounds that are misartic-

ulated. Evaluation of perceived hypernasality should consider reduced oral resonance from limited mouth opening or anatomic alterations and increased nasal resonance from a compromised velopharyngeal mechanism. Voice characteristics should be examined in reference to clarity (quality) of vocal tone and ability to control pitch and loudness changes. Perceptions of breathiness during phonation should be noted in reference to the potential for reduced glottal closure.

Evaluation of swallowing performance may overlap with that for speech and voice abilities, as the three share a common anatomy and physiology. For example, patients with oral changes contributing to speech deficits may also demonstrate limitations in oral aspects of chewing and swallowing. Patients with severe dysphonia characterized by breathiness may have limitations in airway protection during swallowing. Patients with swallowing complaints should be observed during swallowing attempts. As a precaution, clinicians must use comprehensive information from the patient and the physical examination in deciding whether it is safe to ask a given patient to swallow and, if so, which material should be used for swallowing attempts. If the clinician is concerned about safety of the swallow (relating to potential for aspiration into the airway), initial swallow attempts should be completed under instrumental guidance (endoscopy or fluoroscopy).

INSTRUMENTAL EXAMINATIONS. Various instrumental options are available for more objective analysis of speech, voice, and swallowing abilities. Although many of these are important for detailed evaluations, especially in research activities, daily clinical practice may not require their inclusion. For example, a variety of acoustic and aerodynamic techniques are available for detailed description of speech and voice deviations. Although these measures provide increased objectivity, they have not yet been shown to be essential in the clinical management of these functional deficits in patients with head and neck cancer. Conversely, imaging techniques are essential to evaluate movement capabilities of structures in the upper aerodigestive tract that relate to speech, voice, and swallowing functions. Two primary imaging techniques are useful in assessing movement capabilities of these mechanisms: fluoroscopy and transnasal endoscopy.

Both imaging techniques are helpful in evaluating movement of the velar, pharyngeal, and laryngeal components of the upper aerodigestive tract that are essential to speech, voice, and swallowing functions. Although used to evaluate the same functions, each technique has its own strengths and limitations. Fluoroscopic inspection provides valuable information on movement characteristics during speaking or swallowing attempts. This information is often essential in directing appropriate rehabilitation efforts. Endoscopic evaluation of these same structures also provides related but slightly different information to that obtained by fluoroscopic evaluation. Endoscopic imaging is superior to the fluoroscopic technique in the inspection of anatomic (including mucosal) changes and in the evaluation of pooled secretions. The fluoroscopic technique is superior to the endoscopic technique in providing a more comprehensive perspective (mouth to stomach) of the swallowing mechanism.

Videostroboscopy is an extension of the endoscopic technique. This technique evaluates vocal fold mucosal integrity. In simple terms, stroboscopy permits inspection of the flexibility of vocal fold mucosa. Movement of the vocal fold mucosa is observed as a "mucosal wave" or apparent movement of tissue from the medial to the lateral vocal fold. Inspection of the mucosal wave identifies a variety of vocal fold vibratory characteristics associated with normal or impaired phonation. These characteristics assist in explanation of dysphonia and help to direct the rehabilitative effort.

Assessing Impact Factors

Impact factors are those patient characteristics that directly or indirectly contribute to impaired speech, voice, or swallowing functions. Impact factors prominent among head and neck cancer patients are pain, xerostomia, taste and smell, nutritional status, and psychological status.

Many patients experience cancer-related pain. If pain is experienced within the speech/swallowing tract, functional limitations may result from reduced range or frequency of movement, or both. From this perspective, patients should be asked to comment on the presence of pain within the speech/swallowing mechanism and to rate the severity of any reported pain.

Xerostomia is commonly cited as a side effect of radiation therapy. However, oral dryness secondary to reduced salivary flow may not have a direct impact on motor aspects of swallowing in patients with head and neck cancer. Rather, xerostomia may affect sensory processes in the oral cavity that change patient perception of comfort during eating.[28] From either perspective, xerostomia should be assessed during the clinical evaluation along with the patient's perception of the impact of this condition.

The senses of taste and smell are cardinal factors in the enjoyment of eating. Impairment of these senses may contribute to impaired appetite and resultant reduction of food and liquid intake. Although standard protocols exist for the systematic evaluation of taste and smell functions, patient reporting is often sufficient to document the presence of these sensory deficits and their impact on oral intake of food and liquid.

Malnutrition in cancer patients is multifactorial and contributes to altered quality of life, reduced survival, and treatment-related morbidity. Between 30% and 50% of patients with head and neck cancer experience a degree of malnutrition at some point before, during, or after treatment.[29–31] Reasons for malnutrition include dysphagia and odynophagia, dysgeusia, reduced appetite, poor absorption/utilization of nutrients, and increased caloric needs. Nutritional status can be evaluated by a variety of techniques, including body mass index, anthropomorphic measures, analysis of dietary journals, and blood serum levels. The nutritional specialist on the rehabilitation team plays a key role in identifying nutritional deficits and suggesting directions for improving nutritional status.

Psychological status is an additional factor that may have an impact on the outcome of treatment and rehabilitation. Cancer patients often must cope with pain, fatigue, disfigurement, communication limitations, and altered ability to ingest food and liquid. These conditions are chronic in many cases and may contribute to distress and depression. These latter factors may have a negative impact on treatment outcome and on patient participation in the rehabilitation process. Psychological consultation is helpful in identifying these factors and suggesting directions for minimizing their impact on treatment outcome and rehabilitation efforts.

Timing of the Evaluation

The timing of posttreatment evaluation depends on the type of treatment and the individual patient's condition. Many practitioners prefer to use a baseline evaluation to help focus the posttreatment rehabilitation effort and identify findings that may be predictive of treatment outcome. Surgical patients may be seen in the hospital for assessment of speech/swallowing abilities. Typically, these early assessments are directed at identifying temporary strategies for effective communication and safe swallowing. Long-term rehabilitation efforts are not usually the focus of these early evaluations, as the patient's condition is expected to improve from the immediate postoperative state.

Patients who receive radiation therapy should be evaluated for acute side effects and subsequently followed for the emergence of late-occurring difficulties. Acute toxicity side effects may not develop. If they are experienced, however, they may resolve subsequent to completion of radiation therapy. In addition, late effects of radiation therapies are being noted more frequently.[32] Consequently, patients should participate in long-term follow-up to identify any speech, voice, or swallowing deficits that may emerge at a future point.

Cancer rehabilitation reflects a multidisciplinary effort. The rehabilitative effort begins with a comprehensive evaluation of functional abilities and limitations. Timing of this evaluation may be patient dependent, but a pretreatment or baseline evaluation may help to focus the team and the patient on potential posttreatment deficits and rehabilitation directions. The next section describes rehabilitation strategies for the head and neck patient after treatment. It begins with a review of general considerations for speech, voice, and swallow rehabilitation and progresses to a more detailed description of specific examples of rehabilitation for these functions.

REHABILITATION OF POSTTREATMENT FUNCTIONAL LIMITATIONS

GENERAL CONSIDERATIONS FOR SPEECH, VOICE, AND SWALLOW REHABILITATION

Patients who have been treated for head and neck cancer present challenges to rehabilitation efforts resulting from cancer and its treatment. Clinicians must consider the impact of altered anatomy, mucosal changes, and muscle changes in developing a treatment plan toward a specified functional outcome. Furthermore, clinicians must address the underlying causes of functional limitations to facilitate improved performance. Although the speech pathologist leads the rehabilitation effort for speech, voice, and swallowing functions, this professional must work with other members of the cancer rehabilitation team to remediate, minimize, or compensate for anatomic, mucosal, or muscle changes to maximize the potential for functional improvement.

SPECIFIC THERAPY APPROACHES FOR SPEECH, VOICE, AND SWALLOWING FUNCTIONAL LIMITATIONS

Rehabilitation of Underlying Factors Contributing to Speech, Voice, or Swallowing Difficulties

Changes to mucosal or muscle tissue may have a direct impact on speech, voice, or swallowing functions. Alterations in muco-

TABLE 26.3-3. Common Interventions Used in the Treatment of Mucosal or Muscle Changes Secondary to Radiation Therapy

Mucosal Changes	Muscle Changes
Salivary supplements	Cold stimulation
Water	Stretching to increase movement range
Analgesics	Exercises to strengthen muscle groups
Ice chips	
Mouthwash	
Gels	
Prescription medications	
Mechanical cleansing	

sal or muscle tissue are prevalent after radiation therapy either with or without surgery. In some cases, the rehabilitation team must address these "underlying factors" as part of the rehabilitation process. Table 26.3-3 summarizes some of the more common interventions used in the treatment of mucosal or muscle changes secondary to radiation therapy.

Xerostomia is a common sequela of radiation therapy. Oral dryness can be reduced with a variety of simple strategies. So-called synthetic saliva can be obtained in many forms, including mouthwash, sprays, gels, and even chewing gum. Applications such as mouthwash and chewing gum are easily merged into a patient's daily routine. Patients also often report use of a water bottle or spray bottle with water to provide moisture in the mouth. Furthermore, prescription medications can also be used in an attempt to increase salivary flow; however, they often require extended use and may be cost prohibitive to patients. Ultimately, patients often experiment with a variety of methods to combat xerostomia. Clinicians can help in this process by providing a wide range of options and information.

Pain in the oral cavity or pharynx may contribute to reduced movement during speech or swallowing. Few strategies have been proven successful to combat this problem; however, a review of evidence in this area[33] suggests that the strongest support exists for using ice chips during the course of radiation therapy. Another strategy that has some evidence-based support is mechanical cleansing with saline. Analgesic gels and over-the-counter liquid medications are also used. In severe cases, prescription medications may be required to control pain.

Changes in muscle tissue often result in reduced range of movement in structures supporting speech and swallowing functions. Stretching muscle groups is a general strategy to increase range of movement in cases of scarring or fibrosis. Repetitive stretching has been shown to improve movement, especially in the jaw.[34] To facilitate this approach, commercial and improvised devices are available. Patients may also engage in exercises that facilitate volitional stretching of muscle groups and increased range and frequency of movement. Consultation with the physical therapist on the rehabilitation team is beneficial in many cases.

Treatment of underlying factors is intended to provide the patient with the best possible mechanism to minimize functional limitations. In some instances, treating the underlying deficits is sufficient to restore adequate function to the patient. In other situations, treating the underlying deficits is only the first step in the rehabilitation process. Speech, voice, and swallowing deficits often require intensive and focused rehabilita-

tion with contributions from many professionals on the cancer rehabilitation team.

Rehabilitation Strategies for Oral Deficits

Structural changes within the oral cavity contribute to reduced movement of remaining structures and limit contact among structures required for swallowing and speech articulation functions. Speech articulation abilities and oral transport of materials during swallow attempts are impaired when the residual or reconstructed tongue makes poor contact with the hard palate. If the soft palate is compromised, speech resonance characteristics become hypernasal when excessive air escapes through the velopharynx. In this latter condition, liquid or food materials may reflux into the nasal cavity during swallowing attempts. Remediation of these deficits is best approached by a combination of the speech pathologist and the maxillofacial prosthodontist. This team can design and fabricate maxillary shaping devices, palatal lifts, obturators, or other intraoral prostheses that contribute to improved speech and swallow function.

A maxillary shaping prosthesis can function to fill a defect in the hard palate or to reduce the distance from the hard palate to the residual or reconstructed tongue, or both. In the latter instance, the prosthetic device can be thickened and shaped to facilitate maximal contact between the palate and tongue. Increased linguopalatal contact results in improved speech articulation and improved oral bolus transport during swallow attempts. Prosthetic rehabilitation of the hard palate is reported to be highly successful in improving speech and swallow functions.[35]

Oral-nasal separation is facilitated by either a palatal lift or obturator. A palatal lift helps elevate the existing soft palate into a raised position. A palatal obturator fills a gap created by tissue removal. These prosthetic devices function to improve anatomic separation of the oral and nasal cavities. This separation improves speech performance by reducing hypernasality during speech. In addition, swallow performance is improved by eliminating nasal reflux of food and liquid materials and perhaps by increasing pharyngeal pressures during swallow attempts.

Beyond prosthetic management, speech functions may also require behavioral therapy. Behavioral therapy strategies for speech articulation typically focus on increasing range and speed of motion of compromised structures. If appropriate contact cannot be realized between structures needed to produce specific speech sounds, the speech pathologist can instruct the patient in strategies to produce sounds that are similar in character. This compensatory strategy cannot render error-free speech patterns, but it can serve to enhance overall intelligibility of spoken communication.

Fortunately, many behavioral options are available to patients to combat swallowing deficits related to alterations in oral functions. Changes in head posture, use of feeding devices, and/or altered diet consistencies all may contribute to improved swallowing function. For instance, patients with limited tongue movement can facilitate oral bolus transport by raising the chin to allow gravity to transport materials to the posterior oral cavity or into the pharynx, where they can be swallowed. Effective use of this technique is predicated on adequate airway protection and functioning of the PE segment

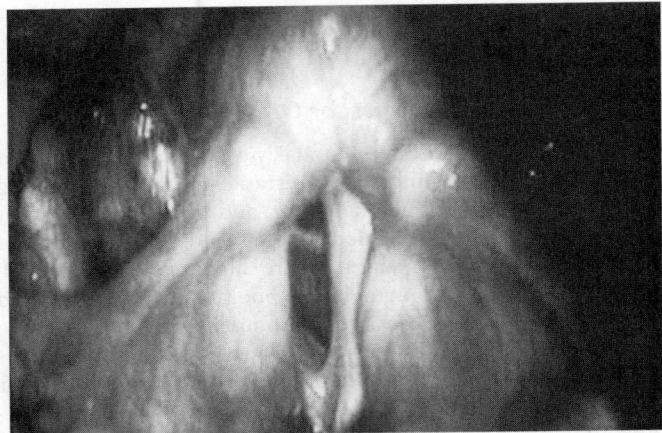
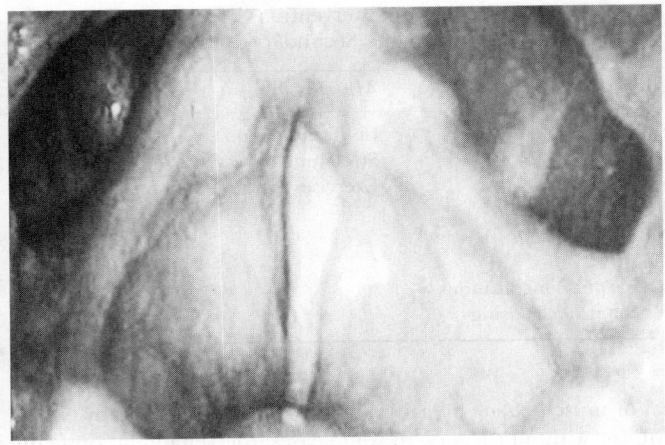

A
B

FIGURE 26.3-2. **A:** Adducted larynx after right laser cordectomy. **B:** Same larynx after medialization of right true vocal fold remnant via thyroplasty.

during swallow attempts. Also, the patient who relies on this technique may have to tolerate a liquid diet or very soft, liquefied foods, as heavier foods are not likely to move efficiently through the oral mechanism via gravity only. Feeding devices are available[36] that allow patients to place more solid foods in the posterior oral cavity. Often called *glossectomy spoons*, these devices are used to place soft food in the posterior mouth in those patients who have reduced tongue mass or restricted lingual movement. Other options available to patients include using syringes or soft catheters to place food in the posterior oral cavity or pharynx or even in the proximal esophagus.

Rehabilitation Strategies for Laryngopharyngeal Deficits

Changes to the larynx or pharynx as a result of cancer treatment have a direct impact on voice and swallow functions. When laryngeal closure is compromised, either from movement or structural deviations, patients experience reduced vocal volume, breathy voice quality, and reduced ability to protect the airway during swallowing attempts. If laryngeal deficits are accompanied by limitations in pharyngeal musculature, swallowing deficits are magnified.

Reduced glottal closure can be improved surgically or, in the case of milder deviations, with behavioral therapy. Surgical medialization to improve glottal closure typically involves thyroplastic medialization of a lateralized vocal fold or injection of biomaterials into the submucosal vocal fold. The determining factors in selection of the specific technique may be the degree of glottal closure, the patient's overall health status, and the surgeon's experience with the respective techniques. Figure 26.3-2 depicts glottal incompetence resulting from a right laser cordectomy and subsequent improved closure secondary to thyroplasty. This patient experienced improved voice abilities and reduced aspiration of liquids.

Behavioral therapy techniques are commonly used when reduced glottal closure limits airway protection during swallowing attempts. To improve swallow efficiency and reduce or eliminate aspiration, patients can use a variety of simple maneuvers. These techniques include the chin-down position, the supraglottic swallow, and the super supraglottic swallow. The chin-down

position may be helpful when a patient demonstrates a delay in initiating the pharyngeal component of the swallow. This head position narrows the oropharyngeal opening and causes the patient to swallow upward over the tongue base. The supraglottic and super supraglottic swallow maneuvers focus on closing the airway before swallow onset and coughing gently post-swallow to clear any residue in the larynx immediately after the swallow. The difference between the two maneuvers is the amount of effort used by the patient during the swallow attempt.

Side lying is another technique to facilitate improved airway protection. This position is intended to reduce the influence of gravity on bolus movement, allowing the patient increased time to adjust the swallow and protect the airway. If clinicians identify pharyngeal asymmetry during the swallowing evaluation, they should recommend that the stronger side be lower during swallow attempts.

Patients may improve airway protection by improving coordination of the swallow or reducing the amount of post-swallow residue, or both, with three additional swallow maneuvers. First, the effortful or hard swallow results in increased lingual pressure during swallowing, which may help move a bolus through the swallowing tract more efficiently.[37] Second, the Mendelsohn maneuver requires patients to maintain the most superior and contracted swallow position for a few seconds. This technique may improve swallow coordination,[38,39] resulting in less potential for aspiration or residue. Finally, a simple head turn maneuver may help patients with hemipharyngeal asymmetries by redirecting the bolus to the more intact side and by reducing the pressure within the PE segment on the contralateral side. A brief summary of each of these swallow maneuvers is provided in Table 26.3-4.

Rehabilitation Strategies for the Laryngectomized Patient

Clinicians can recommend an artificial speaking device in most cases immediately after total laryngectomy. Artificial speaking devices simulate sound and function as either a primary or auxiliary speech system. Such devices are relatively inexpensive and easy to operate. Two primary alternatives are available: pneumatic and electronic. Pneumatic devices consist of a dia-

TABLE 26.3-4. Summary of Behavioral Swallowing Maneuvers Commonly Used in Dysphagia Therapy

Technique	How Done	Intended to...	Physiology	Outcomes
Side lying	Lie down with stronger side lower	Slow down bolus; provides time to adjust and protect airway	Emphasizes pharyngeal contraction	Less aspiration
Chin up	Elevate chin	Propel bolus to back of mouth	Widens oropharynx; increases PES pressure	Better oral transport
Chin down	Lower chin	Improve airway protection	Narrows oropharynx	Reduced aspiration
Head turn	Turn head to right or left	Reduce post-swallow residue and aspiration	Redirect bolus to stronger side of pharynx; lowers PES pressure	Increased amount swallowed; less residue and lower risk of aspiration
Supraglottic swallow	Hold breath...swallow...gentle cough...	Reduce aspiration by increasing glottal closure	Horizontal glottal closure; increased movement of swallowing structures	Reduced aspiration; increased laryngeal elevation
Super supraglottic swallow	Hold breath...bear down...swallow...gentle cough...	Reduce aspiration by increasing glottal closure	Horizontal and A-P glottal closure; increased movement of swallowing structures	Reduced aspiration; increased laryngeal elevation
Mendelsohn maneuver	Squeeze swallow at apex	Improve swallowing coordination	Increased and prolonged hyolaryngeal elevation	Improved swallowing coordination; less post-swallow residue; less aspiration
Effortful swallow	Swallow harder	Increase lingual force on bolus	Increased tongue-palate pressures; increased duration of swallow; increased tongue base movement	Less residue

A-P, anterior-posterior; PES, pharyngoesophageal segment.

phragm, a reed that generates the sound, and a tube that directs the sound into the mouth for shaping into speech. Battery-operated devices (electrolarynxes) include either intraoral or neck type. Intraoral devices may be superior immediately after surgery, when edema may make neck placement difficult, if not impossible.

Laryngectomized patients may benefit from yet another rehabilitation option, esophageal speech. Esophageal speech requires the patient to inject or inhale air into the esophagus and expel the air through the surgically created (PE) segment. Esophageal speech is an inexpensive and noninvasive rehabilitation method. Although this method of speech production can be introduced early (1 to 2 weeks postoperatively) in the recovery period, reported success rates in learning esophageal voice vary between 26% and 71%.[40] Still, debate surrounds the efficacy and utility of this method of voice rehabilitation.[41,42] Some authors have suggested that lower pitch levels resulting from this technique function as a detractor to this method, especially in women. Others have implicated reduced intensity and duration of voicing as problematic.[43] As with other forms of alaryngeal speech restoration, issues such as age, gender, cognitive function, treatment modality, functionality of the PE segment, and the rehabilitation program offered may all have an impact on success rates.

In recent years, clinicians have considered the tracheoesophageal puncture (TEP) technique as the "state of the art" in voice restoration after total laryngectomy. Rather than injecting or trapping air into the esophagus for speech, TEP involves the surgical creation of a permanent puncture through the tracheoesophageal wall that shunts pulmonary air into the esophagus. In this way, vibration of the PE segment is achieved for voicing and is limited only by the expiratory capacity of the patient. The tracheoesophageal shunt is fitted with a one-way valve, which prevents aspiration from the esophagus into the trachea.

TEP valves are available in various resistance and profile types to match an individual's physiologic requirements. An outer housing or tracheostoma valve can also be fitted that contains a soft diaphragm covering the stoma to allow normal respiration and to divert air through the valve for hands-free operation during speech. This external valve system is popular, as it can be worn under normal clothing and eliminates the need for manual occlusion of the stoma when speaking. TEP valves are designed to last for at least 3 to 6 months; however, continued wear without cleaning can result in decreased vocal clarity over time, and regular cleaning is recommended.

TEP can be performed as either a primary or secondary surgical procedure. Primary TEP is performed at the time of the laryngectomy. During surgery, a catheter is placed into a newly created fistula that penetrates the posterior wall of the trachea entering the esophageal lumen. The catheter functions to maintain the fistula in the postsurgical period. Approximately 10 days after surgery, the catheter is removed and the voice prosthesis is placed into the fistula. If radiation treatment is planned, the patient is advised that speech may worsen because of edema and mucositis resulting from the radiation treatment. In addition, the voice prosthesis may malfunction secondary to accumulation of secretions resulting from alterations in saliva consistency and abnormal swallowing that may occur in this period. In secondary TEP, a fistula is created and the prosthesis is inserted anywhere from 1 to 3 months after surgery. Before the initial fitting of the speaking valve, the patient must be provided with alternate means of communication.

Controversy surrounds the value of primary versus secondary TEP. Proponents of secondary placement claim that waiting 1 to 3 months after laryngectomy facilitates better control of factors such as stoma size, patency of the PE segment, migration of the puncture site after radiation treatment, and motivation.[44] Those surgeons and speech pathologists who support the primary puncture technique, however, cite the technical simplicity, effectiveness, low morbidity, and cost effectiveness of a one-stage procedure. In addition, practitioners claim that patients benefit psychologically by being able to speak sooner after the primary operation.[45] Nevertheless, success rates do not currently reflect major differences between the two methods.[46]

Studies reviewing predictors of esophageal and TEP voicing have identified tonicity of the PE segment as one of the most important factors for "good" voicing.[47] With this in mind, surgeons who frequently perform a pharyngeal constrictor myotomy, unilateral pharyngeal plexus neurectomy, or a combined procedure at the time of primary surgery[48] advocate the pharyngeal plexus neurectomy as the procedure of choice, suggesting that it preserves residual resting tone in the PE segment, allowing higher speaking frequency compared to other methods. To assess the tone in the PE segment, clinicians complete an air insufflation test. Commonly referred to as the *Taub test,* this examination requires a transnasal catheter to be inserted approximately 25 cm into the esophagus. The catheter is filled with air, and the patient is asked to inhale, occlude the stoma, and attempt a sustained vowel. The length and quality of sound produced determine success. The procedure can be repeated and the placement of the catheter adjusted to assess tonicity at various points along the PE segment.

Further assessment of the tonicity of the PE segment can be achieved using a lidocaine block of the pharyngeal plexus. If the PE segment appears hypertonic and highly resistant to air flow, chemodenervation via botulinum toxin injection should be considered before surgical options. When speech produced under insufflation testing is faint, however, hypotonicity may be suspected. In these instances, techniques such as external pressure or neck band placement can be used to increase the vibratory source and enhance sound production.

Finally, manometry is another method available to examine PE segment function. Manometric evaluation has been advocated as an easy and reliable technique by which to measure opening pressures (15 to 20 mm Hg) that correlate with good esophageal voicing.[49]

The development of low resistance and self-retaining valves has reduced the impact of manual dexterity and visual acuity in prosthetic voice restoration.[50,51] Many surgeons and speech pathologists believe that the indwelling prosthesis has advantages over traditional prostheses in patient acceptability, speaking effort, compliance, and maintenance.[52] However, significant differences in speech intelligibility have not been consistently demonstrated between traditional versus indwelling speaking valves.

Ultimately, TEP, like other forms of voice restoration, is not suited for every postlaryngectomy patient. Consequently, each patient must be carefully evaluated for candidacy. TEP success appears to be heavily influenced by candidacy choice and the procedure used to train patients in the use and maintenance of the prosthesis. In addition, factors such as stoma construction, placement and angle of the TEP, age, pulmonary status, cognitive function, and desire for communication have been noted to affect success of this technique.[53]

Initial success rates for TEP procedures have been reported to range between 73% and 95%.[54] Interestingly, reports have identified declining success rates over time.[55] This declining success rate may result from many patient-related factors, including population aging, inadequate prosthetic care or maintenance, and dislodgment of the prosthesis.

Regardless of the method of alaryngeal speech chosen, a successfully restored voice minimizes social, mental, and vitality limitations.[56] Recent literature has emphasized the training and use of multiple communication methods for the laryngectomized patient. Just as laryngeal speakers have access to vocal and nonvocal means of communication, so too should the laryngectomy speaker be offered more than one communication mode. With alterations in surgically created systems, multiple speech alternatives can facilitate flexibility and support the maintenance of health-related quality of life.

CONCLUSION

This chapter has provided an overview of common disruptions to speech, voice, and swallow functions that may result from treatment for head and neck cancer. Just as the problems encountered by patients are rarely singular, neither are the treatments. The cancer rehabilitation team must be multidisciplinary to afford patients the best opportunities for rehabilitation after cancer treatment. Successful rehabilitation and resultant enhanced health-related quality of life are a direct outcome of coordinated and timely multidisciplinary team efforts.

REFERENCES

1. Hsiao HT, Leu YS, Lin CC. Tongue reconstruction with free radial forearm flap after hemiglossectomy: a functional assessment. *J Reconstr Microsurg* 2003;19:137.
2. Wheeler RL, Logemann JA, Rosen MS. Maxillary reshaping prostheses: effectiveness in improving speech and swallowing of post surgical oral cancer patients. *J Prosthet Dent* 1980;43:313.
3. Seikaly H, Rieger J, Wolfaardt J, et al. Functional outcomes after primary oropharyngeal cancer resection and reconstruction with the radial forearm free flap. *Laryngoscope* 2003;113:897.
4. Pauloski BR, Logemann JA, Rademaker AW, et al. Speech and swallowing function after oral and oropharyngeal resections: one-year follow-up. *Head Neck* 1994;16:313.
5. Zuydam AC, Rogers SN, Brown JS, et al. Swallowing rehabilitation after oro-pharyngeal resection for squamous cell carcinoma. *Br J Oral Maxillofac Surg* 2000;38:513.
6. Su WF, Chen SG, Sheng H. Speech and swallowing function after reconstruction with a radial forearm free flap or a pectoralis major flap for tongue cancer. *J Formos Med Assoc* 2002;101:472.
7. Furia CL, Kowalski LP, Latorre MR, et al. Speech intelligibility after glossectomy and speech rehabilitation. *Arch Otolaryngol Head Neck Surg* 2001;127:877.
8. Kimata YSM, Hishinuma S, Ebihara S, et al. Analysis of the relations between the shape of the reconstructed tongue and postoperative functions after subtotal or total glossectomy. *Laryngoscope* 2003;113:905.
9. Leeper HA, Heeneman H, Reynolds C. Vocal function following vertical hemilaryngectomy: a preliminary investigation. *J Otolaryngol* 1990;19:62.
10. McConnel FM MM, Logemann JA. Examination of swallowing after total laryngectomy using manofluorography. *Head Neck Surg* 1986;9:3.
11. Dettelbach MA, Gross RD, Mahlmann J, et al. Effect of the Passy-Muir valve on aspiration in patients with tracheostomy. *Head Neck* 1995;17:297.
12. Shaker R, Milbrath M, Ren J, et al. Deglutitive aspiration in patients with tracheostomy: effect of tracheostomy on the duration of vocal cord closure. *Gastroenterology* 1995;108:1357.
13. Sasaki CT, Suzuki M, Horiuchi M, et al. The effect of tracheostomy on the laryngeal closure reflex. *Laryngoscope* 1977;87:1428.
14. Chadda K LB, Benaissa L, Annane D, et al. Physiological effects of decannulation in tracheostomized patients. *Intensive Care Med* 2002;28:1761.
15. Martin F. Dysphagia due to tracheotomy. *Med Klin(Munich)* 1999;94:43.
16. Leverment JN, Pearson FG, Rae S. A manometric study of the upper esophagus in the dog following cuffed-tube tracheostomy. *Br J Anaesth* 1976;48:83.
17. Pinkus NB. The dangers of oral feeding in the presence of cuffed tracheostomy tubes. *Med J Aust* 1973;1:1238.
18. Pauloski BR, Rademaker AW, Logemann JA, et al. Speech and swallowing in irradiated and nonirradiated postsurgical oral cancer patients. *Otolaryngol Head Neck Surg* 1998; 118:616.
19. Harrison LB, Solomon B, Miller S, et al. Prospective computer-assisted voice analysis for patients with early stage glottic cancer: a preliminary report of the functional result of laryngeal irradiation. *Int J Radiat Oncol Biol Phys* 1990;19:123.

20. Fung K, Yoo J, Leeper HA, et al. Vocal function following radiation for non-laryngeal versus laryngeal tumors of the head and neck. *Laryngoscope* 2001;111:1920.

21. Hocevar-Boltezar I, Zargi M, Honocodeevar-Boltezar I. Voice quality after radiation therapy for early glottic cancer. *Arch Otolaryngol Head Neck Surg* 2000;126:1097.

22. Dagli AS, Mahieu HF, Festen JM. Quantitative analysis of voice quality in early glottic laryngeal carcinomas treated with radiotherapy. *Eur Arch Otorhinolaryngol* 1997;254:78.

23. List MA, Stracks J, Colangelo L, et al. How do head and neck cancer patients prioritize treatment outcomes before initiating treatment? *J Clin Oncol* 2000;18:877.

24. Zeine L, Larson M. Pre- and post-operative counseling for laryngectomees and their spouses: an update. *J Commun Disord* 1999;32:51.

25. List MA, Lee RJ, Stracks J, et al. An exploration of the pretreatment coping strategies of patients with carcinoma of the head and neck. *Cancer* 2002;95:98.

26. Pauloski BR, Rademaker AW, Logemann JA, et al. Swallow function and perception of dysphagia in patients with head and neck cancer. *Head Neck* 2002;24:555.

27. Colangelo LA, Logemann JA, Rademaker AW, et al. Relating speech and swallow function to dropout in a longitudinal study of head and neck cancer. *Otolaryngol Head Neck Surg* 1999;121:713.

28. Logemann JA, Smith CH, Pauloski BR, et al. Effects of xerostomia on perception and performance of swallow function. *Head Neck* 2001;23:317.

29. Bokhorst-de van dS, van Leeuwen PA, Kuik DJ, et al. The impact of nutritional status on the prognoses of patients with advanced head and neck cancer. *Cancer* 1999;86:519.

30. Lees J. Incidence of weight loss in head and neck cancer patients on commencing radiotherapy treatment at a regional oncology centre. *Eur J Cancer Care (Engl)* 1999;8:133.

31. Johnston CA, Keane TJ, Prudo SM. Weight loss in patients receiving radical radiation therapy for head and neck cancer: a prospective study. *JPEN J Parenter Enteral Nutr* 1982;6:399.

32. Zackrisson PMC, Strander H, Wennerberg J, et al. A systematic overview of radiation therapy effects in head and neck cancer. *Acta Oncol* 2003;42:443.

33. Symonds RP. Treatment induced mucositis: an old problem with new remedies. *Br J Cancer* 1998;77:1689.

34. Lubit EC. An appliance for jaw dilation in prolonged posttraumatic and post surgical trismus and fibrosis. *J Oral Surg* 1980;38:541.

35. Bernhart BJ, Huryn JM, Disa J, et al. Hard palate resection, microvascular reconstruction, and prosthetic restoration: a 14-year retrospective analysis. *Head Neck* 2003;25:671.

36. Fleming S. Treatment of mechanical swallowing disorders. In: Groher ME, ed. *Dysphagia: diagnosis and management*, 3rd ed. Boston: Butterworth-Heinemann, 1997:265.

37. Hind JA, Nicosia MA, Roecker EB, et al. Comparison of effortful and noneffortful swallows in healthy middle-aged and older adults. *Arch Phys Med Rehabil* 2001;82:1661.

38. Lazarus C, Logemann JA, Gibbons P. Effects of maneuvers on swallowing function in a dysphagic oral cancer patient. *Head Neck* 1993;15:419.

39. Crary MA. A direct intervention program for chronic neurogenic dysphagia secondary to brainstem stroke. *Dysphagia* 1995;10:6.

40. Koike M, Kobayashi N, Hirose H, et al. Speech rehabilitation after total laryngectomy. *Acta Otolaryngol Suppl* 2002:107.

41. Mjones AB, Olofsson J, Danbolt C, et al. Oesophageal speech after laryngectomy: a study of possible influencing factors. *Clin Otolaryngol* 1991;16:442.

42. Frowen J, Perry A. Reasons for success or failure in surgical voice restoration after total laryngectomy: an Australian study. *J Laryngol Otol* 2001;115:393.

43. Smithwick L, Davis P, Dancer J, et al. Female laryngectomees' satisfaction with communication methods and speech-language pathology services. *Percept Mot Skills* 2002;94:204.

44. Kao W MR, Kimmel CA, Getch C, et al. The outcome of techniques of primary and secondary tracheoesophageal puncture. *Arch Otolaryngol Head Neck Surg* 1994;120:301.

45. Yoshida GY, Hamaker R, Singer M, et al. Primary voice restoration at laryngectomy. *Laryngoscope* 1989;99:1093.

46. Karlen RG, Maisel RH. Does primary tracheoesophageal puncture reduce complications after laryngectomy and improve patient communication? *Am J Otolaryngol* 2001;22:324.

47. Ramachandran KAP, Hurren A , March RL, et al. Botulinum toxin injection for failed tracheoesophageal voice in laryngectomees: the Sunderland experience. *J Laryngol Otol* 2003;117:544.

48. Singer MI, Hamaker RC, Blom ED, et al. Applications of the voice prosthesis during laryngectomy. *Ann Otol Rhinol Laryngol* 1989;98:921.

49. Baugh RF, Lewin JS, Baker S. Preoperative assessment of tracheoesophageal speech. *Laryngoscope* 1987;97:461.

50. Hotz MA, Baumann A, Schaller I, et al. Success and predictability of Provox prosthesis voice rehabilitation. *Arch Otolaryngol Head Neck Surg* 2002;128:687.

51. Manni JJ, van den Hoogen FJ, Oudes M. Experiences with the Groningen voice prosthesis after laryngectomy. *HNO* 1994;42:358.

52. Chung RP, Patel P, Ter Keurs M, et al. In vitro and in vivo comparison of the low-resistance Groningen and the Provox tracheoesophageal voice prostheses. *Rev Laryngol Otol Rhinol (Bord)* 1998;119:301.

53. Fagan JJ, Lentin R, Oyarzabal MF, et al. Tracheoesophageal speech in a developing world community. *Arch Otolaryngol Head Neck Surg* 2002;128:50.

54. Izdebski K, Reed CG, Ross JC, et al. Problems with tracheoesophageal fistula voice restoration in totally laryngectomized patients. A review of 95 cases. *Arch Otolaryngol Head Neck Surg* 1994;120:840.

55. Quer M, Burgues-Vila J, Garcia-Crespillo P. Primary tracheoesophageal puncture vs esophageal speech. *Arch Otolaryngol Head Neck Surg* 1992;118:188.

56. Schuster M LJ, Kummer P, Hoppe U, et al. Quality of life in laryngectomees after prosthetic voice restoration. *Folia Phoniatr Logop* 2003;55:211.

CHAPTER **27**

Cancer of the Lung

SECTION **1**

YOSHITAKA SEKIDO
KWUN M. FONG
JOHN D. MINNA

Molecular Biology of Lung Cancer

A number of genetic and epigenetic molecular lesions are necessary to transform normal bronchial epithelium to overt lung cancer. These various molecular lesions ultimately result in the abrogation of key cellular regulatory and growth control pathways. Of the three major classes of human "cancer" genes, the protooncogenes and tumor suppressor genes (TSGs) are involved in lung carcinogenesis, whereas evidence for DNA repair gene dysfunction is not yet conclusive. Many of the protooncogene and TSG changes are common to both major lung cancer subtypes, small cell lung cancer (SCLC) and non-SCLC (NSCLC). Although some subtypes may be more prone to certain mutations (Table 27.1-1), these differing mutations can, nonetheless, ultimately result in the abrogation of common, critical pathways. After the formation of an overt cancer, these and other cancer hallmark changes may influence the processes of invasion, metastases, and resistance against cancer therapy. In "translating" these laboratory discoveries into the clinic, it is important to identify the nature and frequency of these various changes, test whether they have clinically important associations (e.g., with smoking, histologic type, stage, survival, response to therapy), and determine whether they have clinical use for early diagnosis, monitoring prevention and treatment efforts, or as targets for the development of new treatment.

GENETIC AND EPIGENETIC ALTERATIONS IN LUNG CANCERS

GENOMIC INSTABILITY AND DNA REPAIR GENES

Lung cancer cells display chromosomal instability—that is, numeric abnormalities (aneuploidy) of chromosomes, as well as structural cytogenetic abnormalities.[1] The latter include nonreciprocal translocations and deletions, representing changes in TSGs, whereas double minutes and homogeneously staining regions indicate gene amplification. Although the specific genes associated with the chromosomal changes are being rapidly identified, the underlying mechanisms for this chromosomal instability are not yet known. Alterations in microsatellite polymorphic repeat sequences are another type of instability, found in 35% of SCLCs and 22% of NSCLCs.[2] However, the DNA repair genes affected in lung cancer that give these changes are still unknown. Regardless of the underlying mechanism, the possibility of exploiting the microsatellite alteration phenotype for the early diagnosis of lung cancer in body fluids and sputum is being explored. 8-Hydroxyguanine is an oxidatively damaged mutagenic base that causes G:C→T:A transversions in DNA, which are frequently found in lung cancer. *8-Oxo guanine glycosylase (OGG1)* encodes a DNA glycosylase that specifically excises 8-hydroxyguanine from DNA. Thus, it is of great interest that individuals with low OGG activity have a greatly increased risk of developing lung cancer,[3] whereas lung adenoma/carcinoma spontaneously develops in *Ogg1* knockout mice, with 8-oxyguanine accumulated in their genome.[4]

ABERRANT DNA METHYLATION

Abnormal DNA hypermethylation at cytosine residues within the CpG islands, clustered around the 5' ends of many genes, is an

TABLE 27.1-1.   Most Frequently Acquired Molecular Abnormalities in Lung Cancer

Abnormalities	Small Cell Lung Cancer	Non–Small Cell Lung Cancer
Microsatellite instabilities	~35%	~22%
Autocrine loops	GRP/GRP receptor	TGF-α/EGFR; heregulin/HER2/neu
	SCF/KIT	HGF/MET
RAS point mutation	<1%	15–20%
MYC family overexpression	15–30%	5–10%
p53 inactivation	~90%	~50%
RB inactivation	~90%	15–30%
p16^{INK4A} inactivation	0–10%	30–70%
FHIT inactivation	~75%	50–75%
RASSF1A inactivation	~90%	~40%
SEMA3B inactivation	~90%	~75%
Frequent allelic loss	3p, 4p, 4q, 5q, 8p, 10q, 13q, 17p, 22q	3p, 6q, 8p, 9p, 13p, 17p, 19q
Telomerase activity	~100%	80–85%
BCL2 expression	75–95%	10–35%

EGFR, epidermal growth factor receptor; FHIT, fragile histidine triad; GRP, gastrin-releasing peptide; HGF, hepatocyte growth factor; RB, retinoblastoma protein; SCF, stem cell factor; TGF-α, transforming growth factor-α.

alternative mechanism to gene mutation for down-regulating TSG expression. *p16^{INK4A}* and *RASSF1A* are examples of the TSG targets that are frequently epigenetically silenced in lung cancer. Other genes have also been found to undergo somatically acquired aberrant promoter methylation in lung cancer, including death-associated protein kinase, E-cadherin (*CDH1*), glutathione S-transferase (*GSTP1*), H-cadherin (*CDH13*), O^6-methylguanine-DNA-methyltransferase, retinoic acid receptor beta-2 (RAR-β), and tissue inhibitor of metalloproteinase 3.[5] Furthermore, the discovery of approximately 200 CpG islands differentially methylated in lung adenocarcinoma cells suggests that there are yet other unidentified target genes for epigenetic inactivation.[6] Methylated DNA sequences can be detected in the body fluids (serum, bronchoscopic specimens, and sputum) of patients whose tumors demonstrate the same aberrantly hypermethylated genes, probably by the shedding of tumor DNA. Thus, aberrantly methylated DNA sequences that can be sensitively detected among a background of normal DNA represent an attractive strategy for early molecular detection. Histone deacetylation is another epigenetic mechanism for down-regulation of gene expression. Thus, it may be possible to reverse methylation pharmacologically with agents such as 5-aza-cytidine (decitabine) and 5-aza-2'-deoxycytidine. Clinical trials with demethylating agents with or without histone deacetylase inhibitors are under way.

Loss of imprinting (associated with hypomethylation of the promoter region) of the insulin-like growth factor-2 gene and the *H19* gene is found in lung cancer, leading to reexpression of the genes. Additionally, in cigarette smokers, messenger RNA up-regulation of the active *H19* allele was observed in airway epithelium, suggesting that monoallelic up-regulation is an early response to smoking and may progress to loss of imprinting of the paternal *H19* gene as smoking exposure drives the cell to malignant transformation.[7]

PROTOONCOGENES AND GROWTH STIMULATION

Many growth factor/receptor systems are expressed by either the lung tumor or adjacent normal cells, thus providing autocrine or paracrine growth stimulatory loops (Fig. 27.1-1). These are excellent new therapeutic targets. Overexpression of epidermal growth factor receptor (EGFR) is observed in approximately 70% of NSCLCs and may be a prognostic factor for poor survival. Coexpression of EGFRs and their ligands, especially transforming growth factor-α, by lung cancer cells indicates the presence of an autocrine (self-stimulatory) growth factor loop. Gefitinib (ZD1839, Iressa) is a specific inhibitor of EGFR–tyrosine kinase that demonstrates antitumor activity in xenograft models of human lung cancer and has clinical activity in patients with NSCLC.[8] Monoclonal antibodies against the extracellular domain of EGFR, such as C225, are another way of therapeutically targeting this key pathway. In 2004, two reports identified somatically acquired mutations in the EGFR in patients whose lung cancers responded to gefitinib.[8a,8b] These mutations (both deletions and point mutations) occurred in the kinase domain and caused the receptor to have prolonged activation after stimulation with EGF and also made the receptor very sensitive to gefitinib. The mutations occurred more frequently in tumors from nonsmokers, adenocarcinomas, women, and in Asian populations, explaining the increased clinical response to gefitinib seen in these subpopulations. It will be of great importance to see whether other lung cancers with increased expression of EGFR but without mutation also show clinical benefit from treatment with this class of drugs or a related therapeutic attack on this signaling pathway.

ERBB2 (HER2/neu) is highly expressed in more than one-third of NSCLCs, especially adenocarcinomas, although gene amplification as seen in breast cancer is not usually the underlying mechanism in lung cancer. A metaanalysis suggested that overexpression of ERBB2 is a factor of poor prognosis for survival in NSCLC.[9] Trastuzumab (Herceptin), a recombinant humanized monoclonal antibody that recognizes HER2 and thus blocks its activity, is being tested for efficacy in NSCLC as a single agent or in combination with chemotherapy.[10]

KIT and its ligand, stem cell factor, are both preferentially expressed in many SCLCs. Activation of this putative autocrine loop may provide a growth advantage or mediate chemoattraction. The stem cell factor/KIT signal transduction pathway has been shown to be associated with Lck, an src-related tyrosine kinase. Potential inhibitors of the KIT kinase, including imatinib (STI 571, Gleevec), inhibit cell proliferation and induce cell death in several SCLC lines. However, a phase II trial of imatinib did not show any objective response for 19 patients with SCLC, although only four were positive for KIT immunostaining.[11] MET and its ligand, hepatocyte growth factor, are involved in fetal lung development. Coexpression of this putative loop is observed in most NSCLCs, and high hepatocyte growth factor levels were associated with a poor outcome in resectable NSCLC patients.

Besides protooncogene products, other growth stimulatory loops are found in lung cancer. The best known is that governed by gastrin-releasing peptide and other bombesin-like peptides together with their receptors, which participate in lung development and repair, as well as promoting SCLC growth via an autocrine loop. Immunohistochemical studies showed that gastrin-releasing peptide is expressed in 20% to 60% of SCLC but less frequently in NSCLCs. Although this loop is a possible therapeu-

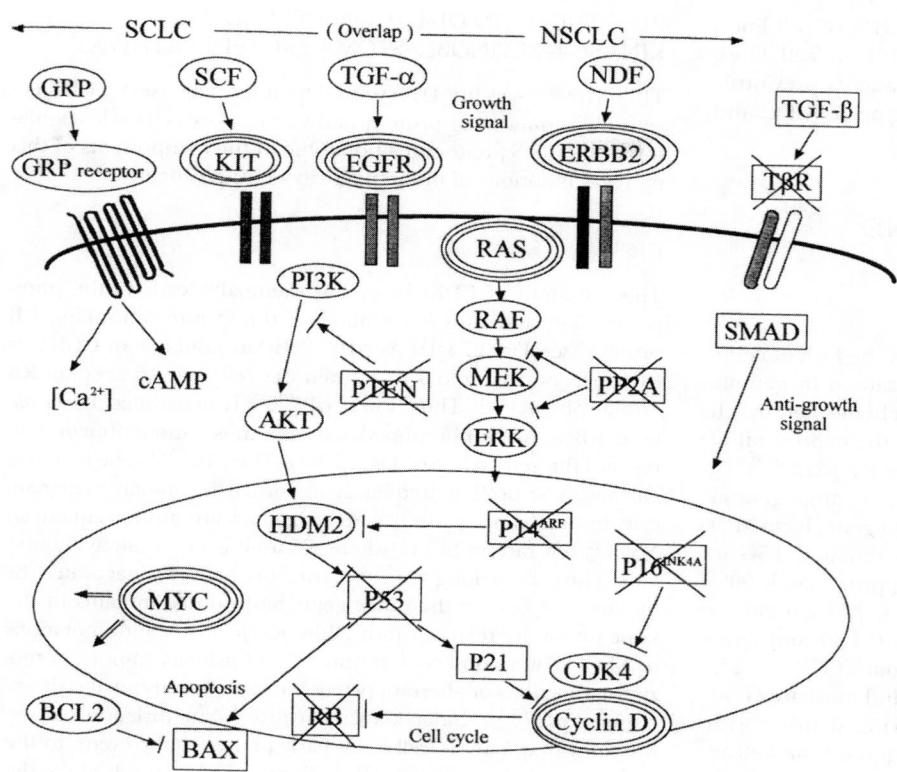

FIGURE 27.1-1. Common growth stimulatory and inhibitory cascades involved in lung cancer cells. A single circle denotes growth stimulatory molecules, and multiple circles indicate activation caused by some tumor-acquired abnormality. A box denotes growth inhibitory molecules, whereas their inactivation is indicated by a cross within the box, again acquired, for example, by mutation in the tumor. Double arrows indicate transcriptional activation of target genes that regulate cell growth. cAMP, cyclic adenosine monophosphate; CDK4, cyclin-dependent kinase-4; EGFR, epidermal growth factor receptor; ERK, extracellular regulated kinase; GRP, gastrin-releasing peptide; NSCLC, non-small cell lung cancer; PI3K, phosphoinositide 3 kinase; RB, retinoblastoma protein; SCF, stem cell factor; SCLC, small cell lung cancer; TGF-α, transforming growth factor-α.

tic target, a phase I clinical trial of the anti–gastrin-releasing peptide monoclonal antibody 2A11 did not result in an objective antitumor response in patients with lung cancer.[12]

Other signaling pathways likely to be relevant for lung carcinogenesis include sonic hedgehog (Shh), which mediates epithelial-mesenchymal interactions in lung development by signaling to adjacent lung mesenchyme. Extensive activation of the hedgehog pathway has been demonstrated within the airway epithelium during repair of acute airway injury as well as in a subset of SCLC.[13]

As downstream effectors are needed to transduce incoming growth factor/receptor signals to the nucleus, it is not surprising that cytoplasmic signal transduction cascades are also implicated in carcinogenesis. For instance, the receptor tyrosine kinases initially signal the guanosine triphosphate–binding RAS protein. The *RAS* gene family (*KRAS*, *HRAS*, and *NRAS*) can be activated by point mutations at codons 12, 13, or 61, and one member of this family is mutated in approximately 20% to 30% of NSCLCs (particularly adenocarcinomas), but hardly ever in SCLCs. *KRAS* accounts for 90% of the *RAS* mutations in lung adenocarcinomas, with approximately 85% of the *KRAS* mutations affecting codon 12. Moreover, transgenic mice with oncogenic *K-ras* alleles that are activated by spontaneous recombination events in the whole animal are highly predisposed to early-onset lung cancer.[14] Further, the remaining wild-type *RAS* allele may play a key role in controlling tumorigenesis as a potential tumor suppressor, as mice susceptible to the chemical induction of lung tumors frequently lose wild-type *Kras2* during lung tumor progression.[15] Characteristically, approximately 70% of *KRAS* mutations are G→T transversions, with the substitution of the normal glycine by either cysteine or valine. Similar G→T transversions also affect the *P53* gene in lung cancer and represent the type of DNA damage expected from bulky DNA adducts caused by the polycyclic hydrocarbons and nitrosamines in tobacco smoke. Further evidence for a causative role for tobacco smoke is the correlation of *KRAS* mutations with cigarette consumption. A metaanalysis of 881 NSCLC patients, 217 of whom had tumor *KRAS* mutations, suggested poor prognosis associated with mutant *KRAS*.[16] However, a prospective study showed that neither chemosensitivity nor survival correlated with *KRAS* mutation in advanced lung adenocarcinomas.[17] Therapeutically, farnesyltransferase and geranylgeranyltransferase inhibitors that interfere with *RAS* function were developed to inhibit the growth of tumor cells with *RAS* mutations. However, an early phase II study of the farnesyltransferase inhibitor R115777 showed no objective responses in patients with NSCLC.[18]

A direct downstream effector of RAS is the *RAF1* protooncogene product. However, mutations in the *RAF1* gene have not been detected in human lung cancers. Its role is complex, as growth arrest of SCLC by activated RAF1 suggests that it has a TSG-like function, and one copy of *RAF1* is frequently lost in lung cancer.[19] *BRAF*, another member of the *RAF* family, was shown to be mutated in malignant melanomas and colon cancers and is the subject of clinical trials with RAF kinase inhibitors. However, *BRAF* was very rarely mutated in lung cancer.

Ultimately, signal transduction cascades result in the activation of nuclear protooncogene products, such as those encoded by the *myc* family genes (*MYC*, *MYCN*, and *MYCL*). MYC, when heterodimerized with a protein called MAX, functions as a transcription factor, necessary for normal cell-cycle progression, differentiation, and programmed cell death. *MYC* is frequently activated via gene amplification or transcriptional dysregulation in SCLC and NSCLC. *MYCL* was originally isolated from an SCLC cell line, and abnormalities of *MYCL* or *MYCN* generally occur in SCLC. One member of the *MYC* family is amplified in 18% of SCLC tumors and 31% of cell lines, compared to 8% of NSCLC tumors and 20% of cell lines. Amplification appeared more frequent in patients previously treated with chemotherapy, the "variant" subtype of SCLC, and its presence correlates with adverse survival.

TUMOR SUPPRESSOR GENES AND GROWTH SUPPRESSION

P53 PATHWAY

p53 (or TP53) maintains genomic integrity in the face of cellular stress from DNA damage (for example, caused by gamma and ultraviolet irradiation, carcinogens, and chemotherapy). It functions as a transcription factor to activate the expression of genes that control cell-cycle checkpoints (e.g., *p21WAF1/CIP1*), apoptosis (*BAX*), DNA repair (*GADD45*), and angiogenesis (thrombospondin); (see Fig. 27.1-1). The *p53* gene, located at chromosome 17p13, is the most frequently mutated TSG in human malignancies, and mutations affect approximately 90% of SCLCs and 50% of NSCLCs. In NSCLCs, *p53* alterations occurred more frequently in squamous cell (51%) and large cell (54%) carcinomas than adenocarcinomas (39%).[20] *p53* mutations correlate with cigarette smoking, and most are G→T transversions. Other evidence linking smoking damage with *p53* mutations is the finding that a major cigarette smoke carcinogen, benzo[a]pyrene, selectively forms adducts at *p53* mutational hot spots.[21] Missense mutations prolong the half-life of the p53 protein, leading to increased levels detectable by immunohistochemistry. Whether the occurrence of *p53* mutations (detected by either immunohistochemistry or molecular analysis) in a patient's tumor affect survival is controversial.[22] The Li-Fraumeni syndrome of inherited susceptibility to cancer due to an inherited germline mutation of *p53* may also lead to increased susceptibility to lung cancer in adults in these pedigrees. This increased risk is modified by tobacco smoking, as carriers who smoked had a 3.16-fold higher risk for lung cancer than those who did not smoke.[23] Several promising gene therapy clinical trials have been reported in which lung cancers are treated by intratumoral injection (endobronchially or by computed tomography–guided needle injection), introducing a wild-type *p53* gene using retroviral or adenoviral vectors. Future therapeutic gains may come from combining gene and conventional therapies. For example, a phase II study of intratumoral injection of adenoviral transduced *p53* in combination with radiation therapy demonstrated evidence of tumor regression at the primary injected tumor.[24]

Other components of the p53 pathway may be abnormal in lung tumors that are wild type for *p53*. One upstream component is the kinase encoded by the ataxia-telangiectasia gene that phosphorylates p53. However, mutations have not yet been found in lung cancer. Other upstream regulators of p53 are the *HDM2* oncogene product and *p14ARF* TSG product. Abnormal overexpression of HDM2 is found in lung cancers and can abrogate p53 function by complexing with p53, facilitating its degradation by the ubiquitin pathway. p14ARF controls cell growth by abrogating HDM2 inhibition of p53 activity, with loss of expression of p14ARF also seen in lung cancer. Thus, HDM2 overexpression and p14ARF inactivation may be mutually exclusive events in human lung cancers.[25]

P16INK4A–CYCLIN D1–CYCLIN-DEPENDENT KINASE-4–RETINOBLASTOMA PROTEIN PATHWAY

The p16INK4A–cyclin D1–cyclin-dependent kinase-4 (CDK4)–retinoblastoma (RB) protein pathway is a key cell-cycle regulator at the G1/S phase transition. One of the components of this pathway is abnormal in the majority of lung cancers.

P16INK4A

The activation of CDKs by cyclins eventually leads to the phosphorylation and thus inactivation of the growth-controlling RB protein (see Fig. 27.1-1). As p16INK4A is an inhibitor of CDK4 or CDK6, its normal role is to restrain the cell cycle by keeping RB unphosphorylated. Thus, when p16INK4A is inactivated by mutation, RB remains phosphorylated and thus cannot function to restrain the cell cycle (see Fig. 27.1-1). The *p16INK4A* gene locus on chromosome 9p21 is frequently abnormal in human malignancies. In lung cancer, *p16INK4A* abnormalities are more frequent in NSCLC but rare in SCLC, where *RB* itself is nearly always abnormal. Thus, most lung cancers have this pathway inactivated by mutation of one or the other gene, and double mutants in the same tumor are relatively rare. Although *p16INK4A* point mutations in NSCLCs were observed in only 14% of primary tumors, homozygous deletions or aberrant promoter methylation can also downregulate *p16INK4A*.[2] Indeed, aberrant *p16INK4A* methylation may be the most frequent, as well as an early preneoplastic event, in the pathogenesis of squamous cell carcinomas.[26] As a result of the different mechanisms, p16INK4A is absent in approximately 40% of primary NSCLCs and thus the most common component of the p16INK4A–cyclin D1–CDK4–RB pathway inactivated in NSCLC. A further complexity is that p16INK4A and p14ARF are derived by alternative reading of the same DNA locus. Thus, changes at the *p16INK4A* locus may not only abrogate p16INK4A function but also disrupt the other major p53 pathway through p14ARF by means of the ability of p14ARF to stabilize p53. Thus, changes at this one p16INK4A/p14ARF site can affect the RB and the p53 TSG pathways.

CYCLINS AND CYCLIN-DEPENDENT KINASES

As cyclin D1/CDK4 complex inhibits RB activity by phosphorylation, cyclin D1 or CDK4 overexpression is another way of disrupting this p16INK4A–cyclin D1–CDK4–RB pathway. Immunohistochemically, cyclin D1 is overexpressed in 12% to 47% of primary NSCLCs and, in some reports, associated with a poor prognosis. How this overexpression occurs in lung cancer is currently unknown. Another cell-cycle regulator at the G1/S transition, cyclin E, is overexpressed in NSCLCs and also appears to be an unfavorable prognostic factor.

RETINOBLASTOMA PROTEIN

The RB gene (*RB*) located at chromosomal region 13q14 encodes a growth-suppressive nuclear phosphoprotein. When in its active (hypophosphorylated) form, RB binds and inactivates proteins such as transcription factor E2F-1, which is essential for G1/S transition of the cell cycle (see Fig. 27.1-1). Mutations of one *RB* allele together with loss of the other wild-type *RB* allele are frequent in SCLC. The RB protein is absent or structurally abnormal in more than 90% of SCLCs and 15% to 30% of NSCLCs. The infrequency of *RB* abnormalities in

NSCLC is not surprising, given that the p16^INK4A–cyclin D1–CDK4–RB pathway is otherwise already impaired from abnormalities in the other components. In effect, lung cancers can be characterized as having either *RB* mutation (mostly SCLC) or *p16^INK4A* inactivation (mostly NSCLC). Gene therapy to replace RB is difficult because of the large size of the *RB* coding region and the need for systemic delivery. As a susceptibility factor, patients with retinoblastoma or their relatives who carry a mutant *RB* in the germline have an excess risk of developing SCLC if they survive into adult life. Mutations of two other *RB*-related genes, *p107* and *RB2/p130*, have also occasionally been implicated in lung cancer.

OTHER PUTATIVE TUMOR SUPPRESSOR GENE SITES, INCLUDING THOSE AT CHROMOSOME REGION 3P

Besides the *p53*, *p16^INK4A*, and *RB* loci, cytogenetic and allelotyping studies show nonrandom, hemiallelic loss at many other chromosome regions in lung cancer. Such tumor-specific, somatically acquired loss of heterozygosity (LOH) is a traditional feature of TSG inactivation, suggesting the existence of underlying TSGs at multiple chromosomal regions. Genome-wide techniques searching for LOH in lung cancers indicated that there are 22 different regions with LOH in more than 60% of the tumors and noted significant differences in the regions involved between SCLC and NSCLC.[27] The exact genes involved at these many different sites are the subject of current investigation.

Multiple distinct chromosome 3p regions of allele loss have been identified, including 3p25-26, 3p21.3-22, 3p14, and 3p12, indicating the presence of multiple 3p TSGs. Chromosome 3p allele loss stands out as a very frequent event in lung cancer pathogenesis, occurring in more than 90% of SCLCs and more than 80% of NSCLCs. It is also an early event and often is detected in bronchial dysplasias or even in histologically normal epithelium.

In addition, the 3p21.3 site appears to have four or five TSGs all located together in one small region. The 3p21.3 TSGs include *RASSF1A*, *FUS1*, *SEMA3B*, and *BLU*. *RASSF1A* is one of several candidate TSGs at 3p21.3, being epigenetically inactivated in more than 90% of SCLCs and 40% to 50% of NSCLCs, although another alternative splicing form, *RASSF1C*, is expressed in most cases.[28,29] Replacement of *RASSF1A* leads to lung tumor suppression *in vitro* and *in vivo*. *SEMA3B*, located at the 3p21.3, has also been shown to be inactivated by promoter methylation, and its replacement leads to apoptosis in lung cancer.[30] The *FUS1* gene located immediately next to *RASSF1A* loses expression of its protein by a novel mechanism being investigated. Of clinical importance, *FUS1* gene therapy delivered systemically by liposomes can cure mice with widely metastatic NSCLC xenografts. Because of this, it has entered clinical trials in patients also delivered systemically by liposomes.

The fragile histidine triad (*FHIT*) gene is found at 3p14.2, and FHIT protein is absent in many lung cancers, including the squamous cell type (87%) and adenocarcinoma (57%). The loss of FHIT protein is strongly associated with smoking and occurs in some preneoplastic lesions. Functionally, transfection of wild-type *FHIT* into lung cancer cells induces apoptosis and suppresses tumorigenicity.[31] In addition, the *DUTT1/ROBO1* gene located at 3p12-13 is also a candidate TSG, and mice created with germline abnormalities at this locus show inadequate lung development and bronchial hyperplasia.[32] Lung cancer cells have resistance to retinoids, which is due to dysfunction of RAR-β that is located in chromosome region 3p24. Loss of expression of RAR-β protein is detected in approximately 50% of lung cancers due to the promoter hypermethylation. The loss of RAR-β function in lung cancer preneoplasia may explain why retinoids failed in multiple clinical trials to prevent lung cancer development.

PTEN located at 10q23 is mutated in only a subset of lung cancer. It encodes a phosphatase whose expression is down-regulated in 10% to 25% of NSCLCs. *TSLC1* located at 11q23 is another candidate TSG, which can be inactivated by concordant promoter hypermethylation and LOH in NSCLC.[33] *MYO18B* located at 22q12 has also been found to undergo deletion, somatic mutations, and hypermethylation in lung cancer; however, its function is unknown.[34]

OTHER BIOLOGIC ABNORMALITIES FOR LUNG CANCER DEVELOPMENT

CELLULAR IMMORTALITY RESULTING FROM INCREASED TELOMERASE ACTIVITY

During normal cell division, telomere shortening leads to cell senescence and thus governs normal cell "mortality." Telomeres are maintained in normal stem cells by the enzyme telomerase. However, abnormal expression of telomerase contributes to human cell immortalization and cancer pathogenesis. Telomerase is a ribonucleocomplex, and ectopic expression in tumors of its catalytic subunit, human telomerase reverse transcriptase (hTERT), appears critical for the cellular immortalization. For instance, immortalization of primary human airway epithelial cells can be achieved through the successive introduction of the simian virus 40 early region and hTERT.[35] Immortalized cells were then responsive to malignant transformation by a *ras* oncogene. Approximately 100% of SCLCs and 80% to 85% of NSCLCs were demonstrated to express high levels of telomerase activity. High telomerase activity was associated with increased cell proliferation rates and advanced stage in NSCLCs, whereas expression of hTERT messenger RNA was associated with poor survival of patients with stage I NSCLC.[36] Telomerase activity or expression of its RNA component, or both, are also deregulated in carcinoma *in situ* lesions, indicating the temporal role for telomerase activation during lung preneoplasia. Thus, telomerase activity or expression can be used as a potential biomarker to detect premalignant as well as tumor cells. For these reasons, there is much interest in developing antitelomerase drugs as new therapeutics.

FAILURE OF APOPTOSIS RESULTING FROM MULTIPLE GENETIC CHANGES

Unlike normal cells, tumors have acquired the ability to escape from programmed cell death (apoptosis), which occurs with DNA damage. The loss of a normal apoptosis program can make lung cancer cells resistant to chemotherapy and radiation therapy. Multiple molecules of the apoptotic signaling pathways are abnormal in lung cancer cells, the most prominent being p53. Another is the antiapoptotic gene, *BCL2*, which is abnormally overexpressed in SCLC (75% to 95%) and some NSCLCs (25% to 35% of squamous cell carcinoma and approximately 10% of adenocarcinoma). Because of the potent role that BCL2 plays in suppressing apoptosis and thus in inhibiting responses to chemotherapy and radiotherapy, considerable effort is being made to develop antisense BCL2 therapeutics, which are entering clinical trials. Also, extracellular matrix proteins may protect SCLC against chemotherapy-induced apoptosis via β1 integrin–stimulated tyrosine kinase activation.[37] In addition, Fas (CD95) and its ligand (FasL), which play key roles in the initiation of one apoptotic pathway, were also implicated in lung cancer. Lung cancers express Fas ligand but not the receptor. However, as T cells express Fas, a model that may help explain the resistance of lung cancer cells from immune surveillance implicates the clonal deletion (by Fas apoptosis) of immune T cells that would otherwise be directed against lung cancer antigens.

METASTASIS AND ANGIOGENESIS ARISE FROM GENETIC AND EPIGENETIC CHANGES IN LUNG CANCER

Many potential factors influencing metastasis from primary lung cancers have been studied, including cell adhesion molecules. For instance, reduced E-cadherin expression, which can occur by promoter hypermethylation, was associated with tumor dedifferentiation, increased lymph node metastasis, and poor survival in NSCLC patients. Reduced α_3 integrin expression correlated with a poor prognosis of patients with lung adenocarcinoma. Specific CD44 isoforms may also be associated with lung cancer metastasis. Matrix metalloproteinases that induced stromal degradation are also involved in lung cancer invasion: Gelatinase A expression was observed in approximately 50% of SCLCs and 65% of NSCLCs, and stromelysin-3 overexpression was detected in stromal elements of primary NSCLCs. Several clinical trials of matrix metalloproteinase inhibitors to mimic their natural counterparts are being tested in the treatment of lung cancer.

Highly metastatic NSCLC variants show up-regulation in various proinflammatory cytokines and angiogenic chemotactic chemokines.[38] Furthermore, metastatic lesions from four organs (lung, liver, kidney, and bone), which were induced by intravenous injection of SCLC cells in mice, had different gene expression profiles, depending on the organ to which they had spread.[39]

Tumor angiogenesis is necessary for a tumor mass to grow beyond a few millimeters in size and is regulated by the balance of inducers and inhibitors that are released by tumor cells and host cells. Vascular endothelial growth factor, basic fibroblast growth factor, and angiogenic CXC chemokines, such as interleukin-8, have all been implicated in lung cancer. Overall, it is thought that lung cancers produce factors that stimulate angiogenesis and stop producing others that would inhibit this process. Thus, tumor angiogenesis has become a major new therapeutic target for lung cancer. Clinical trials in lung cancer with humanized recombinant anti–vascular endothelial growth factor monoclonal antibody combined with chemotherapy in NSCLC have shown great promise. In some cases, the responses have been so dramatic that major bleeding occurred in necrotic tumors, especially squamous cell cancers.

CARCINOGENS IN TOBACCO SMOKE AND GENETIC SUSCEPTIBILITY TO LUNG CANCER (GENETIC EPIDEMIOLOGY)

The major cause of lung cancer comes from smoking, and tobacco smoke contains many substances, including carcinogens, cocar-cinogens, and tumor promoters. Among them, 20 carcinogens convincingly cause lung tumors in laboratory animals or humans and are likely to be involved in lung cancer induction.[40] Of the three major classes of carcinogens in tobacco smoke [polycyclic aromatic hydrocarbons (such as benzo[a]pyrene), nitrosamines, and aromatic amines], much interest focuses on the nitrosamines, especially 4-(methylnitrosamino)-1-(3-pyridyl)-1-butanone (NNK), because they induce tumors of the lung, mainly adenomas and adenocarcinomas, independent of the route of administration in mice. The carcinogenic effects of tobacco smoke in the lung involve the induction of carcinogen-activating and inactivating enzymes, as well as covalent DNA adduct formation, which may cause DNA misreplication and mutation. DNA adducts have been identified in the bronchial tissue of patients with lung cancer, and adduct levels correlate with the amount of tobacco smoke exposure. In former smokers, age at smoking initiation was inversely associated with DNA adduct levels,[41] mandating efforts to prevent the onset of smoking in children and young people. In addition, for reasons that are not yet clear, it appears that women are more susceptible to development of lung cancer from cigarette smoking than men.

The finding that lung cancer does not develop in every heavy smoker has led to the concept of interindividual variation and the hypothesis that individuals may exhibit genetic polymorphisms in carcinogen metabolizing, DNA repair, and other homeostatic pathways that determine individual lung cancer risk. It is likely that such genetic factors only modify the risk from smoking ("gene-environment" interaction). Among genes for carcinogen-metabolizing enzymes, polymorphisms in the cytochrome P-450 genes *CYP1A1*, *CYP2D6*, and *CYP2E1* and in mu-class glutathione S-transferase (*GSTM1*) have received the most attention. Although studies have suggested that there may be a modest association of *GSTM1* null polymorphism with lung cancer, studying single candidate genes may not be adequate to predict lung cancer risk, due to the complexity of carcinogen metabolism, gene-gene and gene-environment interactions, and the relatively small effect of an individual gene. In addition, it also appears that persons may inherit different susceptibility to smoking behaviors, for example, through polymorphisms in one of the dopamine receptors. Researchers have much optimism that molecular epidemiology will help identify individuals at highest risk of developing lung cancer. Such information, in addition to the smoking history, will be of great value in new lung cancer screening trials (e.g., with spiral computed tomography scans) and in chemoprevention trials to identify persons at highest risk of developing lung cancer.

MOLECULAR CHANGES IN PRENEOPLASIA

Before lung cancer is clinically recognizable, a series of morphologically distinct changes (hyperplasia, metaplasia, dysplasia, and carcinoma *in situ*) can be observed in the bronchial epithelium of smokers. It is believed that dysplasia and carcinoma *in situ* represent true preneoplastic (precancerous) changes. These sequential changes found with squamous cell cancers arising from central bronchi have long been recognized, whereas other changes in peripheral bronchioles and alveoli (adeno- and large cell cancers), such as adenomatous and alveolar hyperplasia, are more recently described.

It is now clear that preneoplastic cells contain several genetic abnormalities identical to some of the abnormalities

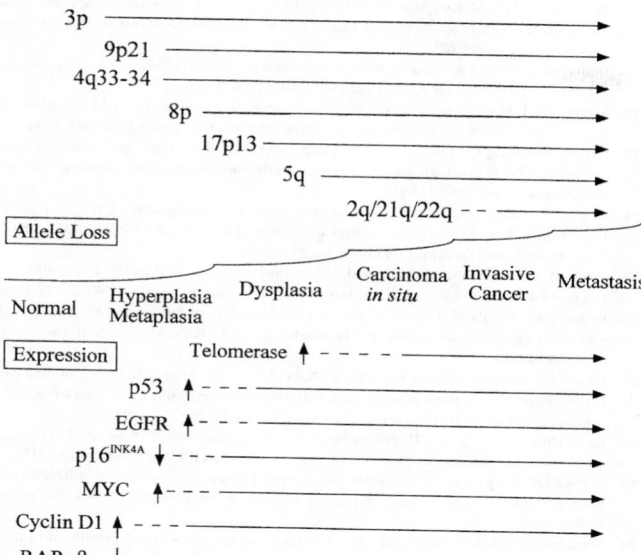

FIGURE 27.1-2. Timing of genetic changes found in preneoplastic lesions in respiratory epithelium, best studied to date in squamous cell lung carcinoma. Note that not every change is necessary and that the sequence may not always be the same. EGFR, epidermal growth factor receptor; RAR-β, retinoic acid receptor beta.

found in overt lung cancer cells. For squamous cell cancers, immunohistochemical analysis has confirmed abnormal expression of protooncogenes (cyclin D1) and TSGs (p53) in these lesions.[42] Allelotyping of precisely microdissected, preneoplastic foci of cells shows that 3p allele loss is currently the earliest known change, suggesting that one or more 3p TSGs may act as "gatekeeper" for lung cancer pathogenesis.[43] This is followed by 9p, 8p, and 17p allele loss (and *p53* mutation; Fig. 27.1-2). Even histologically normal bronchial epithelium has been shown to have genetic losses. Similarly, atypical alveolar hyperplasia, the potential precursor lesion of adenocarcinomas, also harbors *KRAS* mutations and allele losses of 3p, 9p, and 17p.[44] Other genetic alterations, such as inactivation of *LKB1*, whose germline mutations cause Peutz-Jeghers syndrome, have also been implicated in the development of adenocarcinoma. These observations are also consistent with the multistep model of carcinogenesis and a "field cancerization" process, whereby the whole tissue region is repeatedly exposed to carcinogenic damage (tobacco smoke) and is at risk for development of multiple, separate foci of neoplasia.[45]

Although all types of lung cancers have associated molecular abnormalities in their normal and preneoplastic lung epithelium, SCLC patients in particular appear to have multiple genetic alterations occurring in their histologically normal-appearing respiratory epithelium. Molecular changes have been found not only in the lungs of patients with lung cancer but also in the lungs of current and former smokers without lung cancer. These molecular alterations are thus important targets for use in the early detection of lung cancer and for use as surrogate biomarkers in following the efficacy of lung cancer chemoprevention. In this regard, it appears that the smoking-damaged respiratory epithelium has thousands of clonal patches, each containing clones of cells with 3p and other allele loss abnormalities.[46] The challenge is to identify not only

the prevalence and temporal sequence of molecular lesions in lung preneoplasia but to determine which are rate limiting and indispensable and thus represent potential candidates for intermediate biomarker monitoring and therapeutic efforts.

GLOBAL GENE EXPRESSION PROFILING

Analysis of gene expression patterns through microarrays reveals that patterns of gene expression correspond to the four major morphologic classes of lung cancer.[47,48] Adenocarcinomas were further subclassified, indicating that microarray studies may help refine the clinical and histologic classification of tumors and may possibly predict their behavior and response to therapy.[49] In combination with laser capture microdissection, microarray expression analyses of NSCLCs revealed tobacco smoking– and prognosis-related molecular profiles[50] and identified genes for prediction of lymph node metastasis and sensitivity to anticancer drugs.[51] SCLC cell lines, xenografts, and primary tumors analyzed with expression profiling were also grouped into distinct gene expression clusters that need to be characterized clinically.[52] Using matrix-assisted laser desorption/ionization mass spectrometry, proteomic patterns were obtained directly from small amounts of frozen-tissue sections of NSCLC, which grouped patients into histologic types and predicted prognosis.[53] These RNA and protein approaches have great potential for altering the bioclassification of lung tumors in the future, aiding in early detection and in helping predict what would be optimal chemotherapy regimens.

MOLECULAR TOOLS IN THE LUNG CANCER CLINIC

Our understanding of the molecular genetic changes in lung cancer pathogenesis is advancing rapidly, particularly from genomic, proteomic, and transgenic animal models. Some abnormalities are common to other human cancers, whereas others appear more specific for lung cancer, perhaps because of unique types, dosage, and tissue deposition of carcinogen exposure. Where their biochemical function is known, the proteins rendered abnormal appear to fall into several growth regulatory pathways. Thus, the "wiring" diagram of the lung cancer cell is becoming clear. A substantial effort has been made to "translate" this current scientific knowledge of these abnormalities from the bench to the bedside. These approaches fall into four general categories:

1. Identification of persons at highest risk of developing lung cancer to enable chemoprevention and intensified smoking cessation efforts. In this regard, with improved methods of molecular identification of true precancerous lesions, our paradigm will become "treatment" of precancerous lesions rather than "chemoprevention." Because this treatment would occur in individuals without clinically evident cancer, we need to make sure the treatments have high therapeutic and benefit-risk ratios.
2. Early detection tools to identify primary and recurrent disease. Again, such "early detection" of invasive but clinically occult disease would require careful analysis of risk-benefit ratios. Because lung cancer eventually develops in only one of ten cigarette smokers, the identification of persons with a genetic susceptibility to lung

cancer should allow targeting and intensification of smoking cessation, early detection, and chemoprevention efforts. In this regard, the encouraging new information on spiral computed tomography scanning for the early detection of lung cancer should be greatly targeted and enhanced by combining radiologic screening with identification of genetic epidemiology markers and acquired respiratory genetic alterations to identify the most at-risk individuals.

3. Identification of prognostic biomarkers that would also include markers to predict the response to various therapies, particularly the targeted biologic therapy but also conventional chemo- and radiotherapy.

4. Designing new cancer-specific therapies based on knowledge of genetic abnormalities. The latter includes replacing mutant TSGs, drugs targeted against activated protooncogenes, interfering with autocrine or paracrine loops, and inhibiting angiogenesis, metastasis, and apoptotic pathways in cancer cells. Although these new therapies may be effective by themselves, it is more reasonable to assume that they would complement, rather than replace, existing therapies.

REFERENCES

1. Balsara BR, Testa JR. Chromosomal imbalances in human lung cancer. *Oncogene* 2002;21:6877.
2. Sekido Y, Fong KM, Minna JD. Molecular genetics of lung cancer. *Annu Rev Med* 2003;54:73.
3. Paz-Elizur T, Krupsky M, Blumenstein S, et al. DNA repair activity for oxidative damage and risk of lung cancer. *J Natl Cancer Inst* 2003;95:1312.
4. Sakumi K, Tominaga Y, Furuichi M, et al. *Ogg1* knockout-associated lung tumorigenesis and its suppression by *Mth1* gene disruption. *Cancer Res* 2003;63:902.
5. Toyooka S, Toyooka KO, Maruyama R, et al. DNA methylation profiles of lung tumors. *Mol Cancer Ther* 2001;1:61.
6. Shiraishi M, Sekiguchi A, Terry MJ, et al. A comprehensive catalog of CpG islands methylated in human lung adenocarcinomas for the identification of tumor suppressor genes. *Oncogene* 2002;21:3804.
7. Kaplan R, Luettich K, Heguy A, et al. Monoallelic up-regulation of the imprinted H19 gene in airway epithelium of phenotypically normal cigarette smokers. *Cancer Res* 2003;63:1475.
8. Fukuoka M, Yano S, Giaccone G, et al. Multi-institutional randomized phase II trial of gefitinib for previously treated patients with advanced non-small-cell lung cancer. *J Clin Oncol* 2003;21:2237.
8a. Lynch TJ, Bell DW, Sordella R, et al. Activating mutations in the epidermal growth factor receptor underlying responsiveness of non-small-cell lung cancer to gefitinib. *N Engl J Med* 2004;350:2129.
8b. Paez JG, Jänne PA, Lee JC, et al. EGFR mutations in lung cancer: correlation with clinical response to gefitinib therapy. *Science* 2004;304.
9. Meert AP, Martin B, Paesmans M, et al. The role of HER-2/neu expression on the survival of patients with lung cancer: a systematic review of the literature. *Br J Cancer* 2003;89:959.
10. Langer CJ, Stephenson P, Thor A, et al. Trastuzumab in the treatment of advanced non-small-cell lung cancer: is there a role? Focus on Eastern Cooperative Oncology Group study 2598. *J Clin Oncol* 2004;22:1180.
11. Soria JC, Johnson BE, Chevalier TL. Imatinib in small cell lung cancer. *Lung Cancer* 2003;41:S49.
12. Chaudhry A, Carrasquillo JA, Avis IL, et al. Phase I and imaging trial of a monoclonal antibody directed against gastrin-releasing peptide in patients with lung cancer. *Clin Cancer Res* 1999;5:3385.
13. Watkins DN, Berman DM, Burkholder SG, et al. Hedgehog signalling within airway epithelial progenitors and in small-cell lung cancer. *Nature* 2003;422:313.
14. Johnson L, Mercer K, Greenbaum D, et al. Somatic activation of the *K-ras* oncogene causes early onset lung cancer in mice. *Nature* 2001;410:1111.
15. Zhang Z, Wang Y, Vikis HG, et al. Wildtype Kras2 can inhibit lung carcinogenesis in mice. *Nat Genet* 2001;29:25.
16. Huncharek M, Muscat J, Geschwind JF. K-ras oncogene mutation as a prognostic marker in non-small cell lung cancer: a combined analysis of 881 cases. *Carcinogenesis* 1999;20:1507.
17. Rodenhuis S, Boerrigter L, Top B, et al. Mutational activation of the K-ras oncogene and the effect of chemotherapy in advanced adenocarcinoma of the lung: a prospective study. *J Clin Oncol* 1997;15:285.
18. Adjei AA, Mauer A, Bruzek L, et al. Phase II study of the farnesyl transferase inhibitor R115777 in patients with advanced non-small-cell lung cancer. *J Clin Oncol* 2003;21:1760.
19. Ravi RK, Weber E, McMahon M, et al. Activated Raf-1 causes growth arrest in human small cell lung cancer cells. *J Clin Invest* 1998;101:153.
20. Tammemagi MC, McLaughlin JR, Bull SB. Meta-analyses of p53 tumor suppressor gene alterations and clinicopathological features in resected lung cancers. *Cancer Epidemiol Biomarkers Prev* 1999;8:625.
21. Denissenko MF, Pao A, Tang M, et al. Preferential formation of benzo[a]pyrene adducts at lung cancer mutational hotspots in P53. *Science* 1996;274:430.
22. Mitsudomi T, Hamajima N, Ogawa M, et al. Prognostic significance of p53 alterations in patients with non-small cell lung cancer: a meta-analysis. *Clin Cancer Res* 2000;6:4055.
23. Hwang SJ, Cheng LS, Lozano G, et al. Lung cancer risk in germline p53 mutation carriers: association between an inherited cancer predisposition, cigarette smoking, and cancer risk. *Hum Genet* 2003;113:238.
24. Swisher SG, Roth JA, Komaki R, et al. Induction of p53-regulated genes and tumor regression in lung cancer patients after intratumoral delivery of adenoviral p53 (INGN 201) and radiation therapy. *Clin Cancer Res* 2003;9:93.
25. Eymin B, Gazzeri S, Brambilla C, et al. Mdm2 overexpression and p14^ARF inactivation are two mutually exclusive events in primary human lung tumors. *Oncogene* 2002;21:2750.
26. Belinsky SA, Nikula KJ, Palmisano WA, et al. Aberrant methylation of *p16^INKa* is an early event in lung cancer and a potential biomarker for early diagnosis. *Proc Natl Acad Sci U S A* 1998;95:11891.
27. Girard L, Zöchbauer-Müller S, Virmani AK, et al. Genome-wide allelotyping of lung cancer identifies new regions of allelic loss, differences between small cell lung cancer and non-small cell lung cancer, and loci clustering. *Cancer Res* 2000;60:4894.
28. Dammann R, Li C, Yoon JH, et al. Epigenetic inactivation of a RAS association domain family protein from the lung tumour suppressor locus 3p21.3. *Nat Genet* 2000;25:315.
29. Burbee DG, Forgacs E, Zochbauer-Muller S, et al: Epigenetic inactivation of RASSF1A in lung and breast cancers and malignant phenotype suppression. *J Natl Cancer Inst* 2001;93:691.
30. Tomizawa Y, Sekido Y, Kondo M, et al. Inhibition of lung cancer cell growth and induction of apoptosis after reexpression of 3p21.3 candidate tumor suppressor gene SEMA3B. *Proc Natl Acad Sci U S A* 2001;98:13954.
31. Roz L, Gramegna M, Ishii H, et al. Restoration of fragile histidine triad (*FHIT*) expression induces apoptosis and suppresses tumorigenicity in lung and cervical cancer cell lines. *Proc Natl Acad Sci U S A* 2002;99:3615.
32. Xian J, Clark KJ, Fordham R, et al. Inadequate lung development and bronchial hyperplasia in mice with a targeted deletion in the *Dutt1/Robo1* gene. *Proc Natl Acad Sci U S A* 2001;98:15062.
33. Kuramochi M, Fukuhara H, Nobukuni T, et al. TSLC1 is a tumor-suppressor gene in human non-small-cell lung cancer. *Nat Genet* 2001;27:427.
34. Nishioka M, Kohno T, Tani M, et al. MYO18B, a candidate tumor suppressor gene at chromosome 22q12.1, deleted, mutated, and methylated in human lung cancer. *Proc Natl Acad Sci U S A* 2002;99:12269.
35. Lundberg AS, Randell SH, Stewart SA, et al. Immortalization and transformation of primary human airway epithelial cells by gene transfer. *Oncogene* 2002;21:4577.
36. Wang L, Soria JC, Kemp BL, et al. hTERT expression is a prognostic factor of survival in patients with stage I non-small cell lung cancer. *Clin Cancer Res* 2002;8:2883.
37. Sethi T, Rintoul RC, Moore SM, et al. Extracellular matrix proteins protect small cell lung cancer cells against apoptosis: a mechanism for small cell lung cancer growth and drug resistance in vivo. *Nat Med* 1999;5:662.
38. Kozaki K, Koshikawa K, Tatematsu Y, et al. Multi-faceted analyses of a highly metastatic human lung cancer cell line NCI-H460-LNM35 suggest mimicry of inflammatory cells in metastasis. *Oncogene* 2001;20:4228.
39. Kakiuchi S, Daigo Y, Tsunoda T, et al. Genome-wide analysis of organ-preferential metastasis of human small cell lung cancer in mice. *Mol Cancer Res* 2003;1:485.
40. Hecht SS. Tobacco smoke carcinogens and lung cancer. *J Natl Cancer Inst* 1999;91:1194.
41. Wiencke JK, Thurston SW, Kelsey KT, et al. Early age at smoking initiation and tobacco carcinogen DNA damage in the lung. *J Natl Cancer Inst* 1999;91:614.
42. Lonardo F, Rusch V, Langenfeld J, et al. Overexpression of cyclins D1 and E is frequent in bronchial preneoplasia and precedes squamous cell carcinoma development. *Cancer Res* 1999;59:2470.
43. Wistuba II, Behrens C, Virmani AK, et al. High resolution chromosome 3p allelotyping of human lung cancer and preneoplastic/preinvasive bronchial epithelium reveals multiple, discontinuous sites of 3p allele loss and three regions of frequent breakpoints. *Cancer Res* 2000;60:1949.
44. Westra WH. Early glandular neoplasia of the lung. *Respir Res* 2000;1:163.
45. Braakhuis BJM, Tabor MP, Kummer JA, et al. A genetic explanation of Slaughter's concept of field cancerization: evidence and clinical implications. *Cancer Res* 2003;63:1727.
46. Park IW, Wistuba, II, Maitra A, et al. Multiple clonal abnormalities in the bronchial epithelium of patients with lung cancer. *J Natl Cancer Inst* 1999;91:1863.
47. Garber ME, Troyanskaya OG, Schluens K, et al. Diversity of gene expression in adenocarcinoma of the lung. *Proc Natl Acad Sci U S A* 2001;98:13784.
48. Bhattacharjee A, Richards WG, Staunton J, et al. Classification of human lung carcinomas by mRNA expression profiling reveals distinct adenocarcinoma subclasses. *Proc Natl Acad Sci U S A* 2001;98:13790.
49. Beer DG, Kardia SLR, Huang CC, et al. Gene-expression profiles predict survival of patients with lung adenocarcinoma. *Nat Med* 2002;8:816.
50. Miura K, Bowman ED, Simon R, et al. Laser capture microdissection and microarray expression analysis of lung adenocarcinoma reveals tobacco smoking- and prognosis-related molecular profiles. *Cancer Res* 2002;62:3244.
51. Kikuchi T, Daigo Y, Katagiri T, et al. Expression profiles of non-small cell lung cancers on cDNA microarrays: identification of genes for prediction of lymph-node metastasis and sensitivity to anti-cancer drugs. *Oncogene* 2003;22:2192.
52. Pedersen N, Mortensen S, Sorensen SB, et al. Transcriptional gene expression profiling of small cell lung cancer cells. *Cancer Res* 2003;63:1943.
53. Yanagisawa K, Shyr Y, Xu BJ, et al. Proteomic patterns of tumour subsets in non-small-cell lung cancer. *Lancet* 2003;362:433.

DAVID S. SCHRUMP
NASSER K. ALTORKI
CLAUDIA L. HENSCHKE
DARRYL CARTER
ANDREW T. TURRISI
MARTIN E. GUTIERREZ

SECTION 2

Non–Small Cell Lung Cancer

TABLE 27.2-1. Major Mutagens, Carcinogens, and Related Substances in Tobacco Smoke

Substance	Effect	Model
PARTICULATE PHASE		
Neutral fraction	C	Rodents
Benzo[a]pyrene	C	
Dibenz[a]anthracene	C	
Basic fraction	C	
Nicotine		
Tobacco-specific nitrosamines	C	Rodents
Acidic fraction	C + TP	
Cathecol		
Unidentified	TP	
Residue	C	
Nickel	C	
Cadmium	C	
^{210}Po	C	
GASEOUS PHASE	C + M	
Hydrazine	C	Mice
Vinyl chloride	M	Ames

C, carcinogenic; M, mutagenic; ^{210}Po, polonium 210; TP, toxic product.

INCIDENCE

Lung cancer ranks among the most commonly occurring malignancies and currently is the leading cause of cancer-related deaths worldwide.[1] In the United States, lung cancer is the most common cause of cancer-related deaths in men as well as in women, with an incidence approximating 70 per 100,000 individuals.[2] In the year 2003, an estimated 171,900 Americans were diagnosed with lung cancer, and approximately 157,200 succumbed to this disease. Claiming 187,000 lives annually, lung cancer currently accounts for one-third of all cancer-related deaths in the European Union.[3] Whereas accumulated risks for lung cancer are highest in North America and Europe,[4] this disease is rapidly emerging as a major cause of mortality in Asia as well. For instance, in Japan, lung cancer is responsible for approximately 55,000 cancer-related deaths per year.[5] In China, the mortality rate from lung cancer in males now approximates 33 per 100,000, and death rates are expected to substantially increase over the next several decades.[6]

The global rise in lung cancer incidence, together with the fact that the overall 5-year survival of patients with this disease is less than 15%, underscore the magnitude of the lung cancer epidemic. The current chapter focuses on recent developments regarding the diagnosis, treatment, and prevention of non–small cell lung cancer (NSCLC).

ETIOLOGY

SMOKING

The vast majority of NSCLCs are caused by cigarette smoking. In the United States approximately 80% of lung cancer deaths in men and women are directly attributable to tobacco abuse. The incidence of lung cancer throughout the world reflects the prevalence of cigarette smoking, and evolving patterns of lung cancer appear attributable to the use of filters, tar content, and variations in tobacco blends implemented to produce a more palatable nicotine delivery system.[7] Cigarette smoke contains over 300 chemicals, 40 of which are known to be potent carcinogens (Table 27.2-1). Of particular significance, nitrosamine 4-(methylnitrosamino)-1-(3-pyridil)-1-butanone (NNK), and polycyclic aromatic hydrocarbons (PAHs) such as benzo[a]pyrene induce pulmonary carcinomas in rodents that exhibit histologic and molecular genetic profiles virtually identical to those of human lung cancers.[8] For instance, NNK induces mutations involving the K-ras proto-oncogene, and up-regulates DNA methyltransferase activity in type II pneumocytes—events that correlate with progression to adenocarcinoma in murine lung cancer models.[8,9] Mutations involving K-ras have been observed in 40% of human pulmonary adenocarcinomas and correlate with tobacco exposure[10]; aberrant DNA methylation is a hallmark of human lung cancers.[11] PAHs in tobacco smoke form DNA adducts, the extent of which correlates with tobacco exposure in target tissues.[12] In addition, PAHs induce mutations within the p53 tumor suppressor gene, which regulates cell-cycle progression, DNA repair, and apoptosis. Mutations involving p53 have been observed in 50% to 70% of all lung cancers. Mutations induced by PAHs typically are manifested as G→T transversions involving the nontranscribed strand, which indicates preferential repair of the transcribed DNA. G→T transversions involving p53 in lung cancers are observed more frequently in smokers.[13]

Since 1965, the prevalence of smoking in the United States has declined by nearly 50%.[7] In 2000, the prevalence of smoking among United States adults was 23% overall, and varied considerably among ethnic groups. Prevalence was highest in Native Americans (40%), intermediate for whites and African Americans (24%), and lowest among Hispanic Americans (18%) and Asian Americans (15%). Whereas smoking prevalence was equal in Native American males and females, in other ethnic groups smoking was much more prevalent in males.[7] As in the United States, prevalence of smoking in males has generally declined in the European Union; smoking trends in women vary among the constituent countries.[14] In Asia, smoking is far more prevalent in males.[6]

The vast majority of cigarettes consumed in industrialized nations contain filters. This has reduced particle size in inhaled smoke, facilitating deposition of carcinogens deeper in the lungs. In addition, newer tobacco blends contain higher amounts of nitrates, which on burning form nitrosamines such as NNK. Although it was initially believed that the low tar and nicotine content in modern cigarettes would diminish carcinogen exposure, smokers of low-yield cigarettes often compensate by engaging in more vigorous puffing and inhalation.[15] These data may account, in part, for the emergence of adenocarcinomas as the dominant histologic type in lung cancer during recent years. Furthermore, the Cancer Prevention Study II trial, involving more than 940,000 individuals 30 years of age or older who were either current or former smokers or never smoked, demonstrated that lung cancer risk was higher in males and females smoking high-tar (more than 22 mg) nonfilter brands, than in those smoking medium-tar (15 to 21 mg) cigarettes.[16] Of interest, lung cancer risk for smokers of low-tar or very low tar cigarettes was comparable to risk for smokers of medium-tar blends. Menthol does not appear to increase lung cancer risk.[17]

Tobacco-associated lung cancer risk is not restricted to cigarettes. Cigars contain more tobacco per unit and generate more carbon monoxide than cigarettes. Cigars tend to have increased nitrate content, which results in the formation of nitrogen oxides, nitrosamines, and ammonia. Indeed, cigar smoke is as carcinogenic as, if not more carcinogenic than, cigarette smoke.[12]

The risk of lung cancer is related to duration as well as intensity of smoking. Using data from two large case-control studies in Britain, Peto et al.[18] observed that persistent smoking was associated with a 16-fold increase in cumulative lung cancer risk, and that this risk doubled if smoking commenced before age 15. Data from the Cancer Prevention Study II trial indicate that smoking one pack of cigarettes per day for 30 years increases risk of lung cancer–specific mortality 20- to 60-fold in men and 14- to 20-fold in women compared to risk in those who never smoked. The risk nearly doubles if consumption persists for 40 years.[19]

Doll and Peto[20] established a model for lung cancer risk in which duration was more significant than intensity of smoking in individuals with comparable pack-year tobacco exposure. In this model, the relationship between the number of cigarettes smoked per day and lung cancer risk was relatively linear; however, duration of smoking was associated with an exponential increase in lung cancer risk. For instance, a threefold increase in cigarettes smoked per day increased lung cancer risk threefold, whereas a threefold increase in duration of smoking was associated with a 100-fold increase in lung cancer risk.

Lung cancer risk in smokers can be significantly diminished in a time-dependent manner after smoking cessation. For instance, analysis of a large cohort of U.S. veterans revealed that the relative risk of lung cancer in former smokers compared to those who never smoked was 16 for the first 5 years of abstinence, 8 for the next 5 years, and gradually declined to 2 over the next 30 years.[19,21] These data indicate that lung cancer risk can be substantially reduced after smoking cessation, yet never reaches baseline—a fact that may account for the observation that nearly 50% of lung cancers in the U.S. currently arise in former smokers.[22,23]

Whereas the link between tobacco and lung cancer risk is well established for people who actively smoke, the relationship between environmental tobacco smoke (ETS) exposure (passive smoking) and lung cancer risk in nonsmokers appears somewhat more controversial.[19] Individuals exposed to ETS inhale tobacco carcinogens at levels significantly lower than the levels inhaled by active smokers. Nevertheless, case-control as well as cohort studies indicate that ETS contributes to 25% of all lung cancers in nonsmokers (approximately 3000 cases per year in the United States).[24] The risk of lung cancer is proportional to the level of ETS exposure. Overall, available data indicate that nonsmokers have a significantly increased risk of lung cancer if their spouses smoke[12,25]; female nonsmokers exposed to ETS experience a 25% increased risk, whereas male nonsmokers have nearly a 35% increase in lung cancer risk if their spouses smoke. ETS exposure in the workplace may increase lung cancer risk in nonsmokers by 20%. Nonsmokers exposed to ETS excrete tobacco-specific carcinogens in the urine at levels 1% to 5% of those detected in active smokers.[12,26] The levels of urinary tobacco–specific carcinogens are consistent with relative risks of lung cancer in ETS-exposed nonsmokers and active smokers.

Tobacco abuse has global economic, social, and medical ramifications. Whereas lung cancer trends in males in the United States and the European Union have plateaued or decreased, lung cancer incidence in women continues to increase.[3,27] Overall, the trends in lung cancer incidence and mortality reflect tobacco consumption in these countries. Presently, China is the largest producer and consumer of tobacco products. An estimated 67% of males and 4% of females over 15 years of age are smokers. The total of 320 million Chinese smokers constitutes approximately one-third of all smokers worldwide.[6] In China, the average daily consumption of cigarettes rose from one in 1950 to ten in 1990—a rate that was similar to that seen in the United States between 1910 and 1950. In addition, the prevalence of passive smoking in China exceeds 50%; much of this exposure occurs in the home among women and children.[6] As a result of current tobacco exposure, the incidence of lung cancer in China will increase dramatically over the next several decades, with predicted death rates attributable to tobacco approaching 3 million by the year 2050.

Incontrovertible evidence linking cigarette smoking with lung cancer, and the devastating social and economic impact of tobacco abuse have prompted many countries to initiate programs to decrease tobacco addiction. These efforts have included legislation to increase taxes on cigarettes and to ban tobacco advertisements as well as smoking in public places. In addition, educational programs have been implemented in schools to limit the number of adolescents who start smoking, because data indicate that if individuals do not initiate smoking as adolescents, they are unlikely to smoke thereafter. In addition, smoking cessation clinics have been established to decrease the number of individuals who continue to smoke despite knowing the risks of such behavior. Such tobacco control efforts may favorably impact smoking prevalence and lung cancer mortality. For instance, Jemal et al.[28] observed that lung cancer death rates in the United States correlate strongly and inversely with state tobacco control efforts; furthermore, tobacco control indices significantly correlate in a positive manner with cessation of smoking between the ages of 30 and 39.

Despite tobacco control efforts in the United States and other industrialized nations, global tobacco consumption and lung cancer mortality rates continue to rise. To address this issue, the American Society of Clinical Oncology published a policy statement advocating a variety of measures that should be taken immediately to curb global tobacco use.[29] These include (1) increasing efforts to limit tobacco use, particularly in young individuals; (2) substantially raising cigarette taxes and using future cigarette tax increases as a primary means to enhance state revenues; (3) ensuring that tobacco settlement funds be used solely for research related to the treatment and prevention of tobacco related illnesses; (4) mandating full disclosure of all ingredients in tobacco products; (5) restructuring third-party payments to compensate for tobacco cessation programs; (6) further limiting ETS exposure by extension of current cigarette bans in public places; and (7) curtailing government-sponsored promotion of tobacco and tobacco-related products.

GENETIC PREDISPOSITION

Whereas the vast majority of lung cancers are attributable to cigarette smoking, fewer than 20% of smokers develop this disease. Although these observations suggest a genetic predisposition to lung cancer, to date, the genes conferring susceptibility to this disease remain elusive. Braun et al.[30] conducted a large twin cohort study and observed no genetic factors to be predictive of lung cancer. However, several recent studies indicate an increased risk of lung cancer among first-degree relatives of probands with this disease. Hemminki et al.[31] observed a threefold increase in lung cancer risk among siblings of patients with lung cancer. Etzel et al.[32] observed a significant familial aggregation of lung cancer among patients with late-onset but not early-onset (before 50 years of age) lung cancer. A rare autosomal dominant, genetic trait may confer susceptibility in individuals with limited tobacco exposure who develop lung cancer at an early age. Hwang et al.[33] observed a threefold increase in lung cancer risk in patients with Li-Fraumeni syndrome who smoke compared to smokers without p53 germline mutations.

A number of studies have focused on polymorphisms affecting expression, function, or both, of enzymes regulating metabolism of tobacco carcinogens, DNA repair, or inflammation. Dialyna et al.[34] examined polymorphisms involving CYP1A1, GSTM1, and GSTT1 in Greek lung cancer patients and observed that the GSTT1 null genotype was more common in those with adenocarcinomas and correlated with advanced age at diagnosis. Le Marchand et al.[35] noted a slight but significant association between an exon 7 CYP1A1 polymorphism and lung cancer risk in the United States and observed significant interactions for smoking status and gender; the effect of the polymorphism was more pronounced in female smokers and those who had never smoked. Kiyohara et al.[36] observed that the GSTM1 null genotype was associated with a slightly increased overall risk of lung cancer in Japanese patients [odds ratio (OR), 1.37; 95% confidence interval (CI), 0.90 to 2.09]; of interest, the GSTM1 null genotype and high ETS exposure (more than 40 pack-years by husbands) was associated with markedly higher risk (OR, 2.27; 95% CI, 1.13 to 4.5) compared to GSTM1 null genotype and low ETS exposure. In an additional study, Nazar-Stewart et al.[37] noted that the GSTM1 null genotype was associated with a modestly increased lung cancer risk overall, which was more pronounced for squamous cell cancer and adenocarcinoma. The risk associated with GSTM1 null genotype was increased twofold to sixfold in heavy smokers. Miller et al.[38] reported that the GSTP1GG polymorphism nearly doubled the lung cancer risk associated with pack-year tobacco exposure; at 26 pack-years, the GSTP1GG polymorphism was associated with an OR of 13 (95% CI, 6.5 to 25.0) compared with 6 for the more common GSTP1AA genotype. In contrast, Ariyoshi et al.[39] observed that the CYP2AG*4 polymorphism that results in the complete loss of CYP2A6 expression was associated with reduced lung cancer risk.

A number of carcinogens in tobacco smoke are potential mutagens, and several studies indicate that polymorphisms involving genes that regulate DNA repair may be associated with increased risk of lung cancer. In a case-control study involving 2300 patients, Zhou et al.[40] examined polymorphisms within the XRCC1 (x-ray cross-complementing group 1) and ERCC2 (excision repair cross-complementing group 2) genes in relation to smoking and lung cancer. These authors had previously reported an association between ASP312ASN and LYS751GLN polymorphisms and lung cancer risk. In the new study, the authors examined the ARG339GLN polymorphism, and observed that the OR was 1.3, which decreased with increasing pack-year tobacco exposure. The ORs were 5.0 in nonsmokers and 0.3 in heavy smokers when extreme genotype combinations of the three variant alleles were compared with the wild-type genotype, indicating that tobacco exposure can modulate the direction and magnitude of cancer risk associated with XRCC1 and ERCC2 polymorphisms. Wang et al.[41] observed that a polymorphism of XRCC3, producing a variant T allele genotype was significantly associated with lung cancer risk in African Americans and Mexican Americans (OR, 5.2; 95% CI, 1.6 to 17.0). A joint effect of the variant T allele and heavy smoking was observed (OR, 37.3), which suggests that the association of XRCC3 polymorphism with lung cancer risk is heavily dependent on tobacco exposure.

Studies have suggested that inflammation and reactive oxygen species contribute to the pathogenesis of lung cancer.[42] Campa et al.[43] examined polymorphisms involving the cyclooxygenase-2 (COX-2), interleukin-6, and interleukin-8 genes and observed that patients exhibiting the C allele of a polymorphism involving the 3' untranslated region of COX-2 had a significantly increased risk of lung cancer (OR, 4.28 and 2.12 for homozygotes and heterozygotes, respectively). A polymorphism involving the interleukin-6 gene coincided with risk of squamous cell carcinoma, whereas a polymorphism involving the interleukin-8 gene was associated with diminished lung cancer risk. Kantarci et al.[44] observed that the −463 (G→4A) homozygote polymorphism involving the myeloperoxidase gene correlated inversely with lung cancer risk.

OCCUPATIONAL AND ENVIRONMENTAL EXPOSURE

A variety of occupational and environmental exposures have been implicated as potential risk factors for the development of lung cancer. These include exposure to asbestos and silica fibers, organic compounds such as chloral methyl ether and PAHs, diesel fumes and air pollution, metals such as chromium and nickel, arsenic, and ionizing radiation. Assessment of risk related to individual occupational and environmental factors poses considerable challenges, due to imprecise methodologies for quantifying prolonged low-level exposure, the lag time between exposure and the development of cancer, and exposure to other factors such as smoking that confound the analysis.[19,45] In general, cigarette smoking potentiates the effects of many occupational and environmental carcinogens. A full discussion of these risk factors is beyond the scope of this presentation; however, several pertinent exposures are briefly discussed. Occupational and environmental factors associated with lung cancer have been extensively reviewed in several articles.[19,45-47]

Asbestos exposure, which is a major risk factor for the development of malignant pleural mesothelioma, has been associated with increased risk of lung cancer. In several studies dating back to the 1950s, a sevenfold to tenfold increase in lung cancer risk was observed in individuals exposed to asbestos dust in textile mills in the United Kingdom or to insulation in North America.[48,49] All of the common types of commercial asbestos have been associated with lung cancer, with an apparent dose-response relationship; asbestos and cigarette smoking exhibit multiplicative effects.[50] Lung cancers typically develop 30 to 35 years after asbestos exposure—a latency period comparable to that observed for malignant pleural mesothelioma. Although use of asbestos in shipyards and building construction throughout the industrialized world has declined in recent years, asbestos exposure will continue to be a relevant occupational risk factor for lung cancer for the next several decades.

Analysis of the risk of lung cancer after residential asbestos exposure, either from living with an individual working with asbestos or residing near asbestos mines, has produced variable results. In studies in South Africa and China, a small increase in lung cancer risk was noted after residential asbestos exposure; however, these risks have not been observed in studies performed in Europe and North America.[46]

A variety of metals, including nickel, cobalt, cadmium, and chromium, have been implicated as potential pulmonary carcinogens.[46,47] Exposure to these metals typically occurs among foundry workers and welders, with lung cancer risk appearing to be increased in individuals with high levels of exposure. The mechanisms by which these metals induce lung cancer appear complex, and the effects of these agents may be potentiated by cigarette smoke.[51] For instance, nickel and cobalt induce oxidative stress in cultured cells and up-regulate expression of hypoxia-inducible factor and downstream hypoxia-related genes through reactive oxygen species–independent mechanisms.[52] Furthermore, nickel enhances benzo[a]pyrene-diol-epoxide mutagenesis in cultured human cells via inhibition of nucleotide excision repair.[53] Of interest, lung cancer patients exhibit diminished DNA repair capacity compared with healthy individuals.[54] Because benzo[a]pyrene-diol-epoxide is the active metabolite of benzo[a]pyrene (a major carcinogen in tobacco smoke), these observations may explain, in part, the mechanisms by which nickel and tobacco smoke exhibit multiplicative effects with regard to lung cancer risk.[55] Collectively, these data highlight the complexity of the relationships between occupational and environmental factors, smoking, and genetic predisposition in lung cancer risk.

Ionizing radiation induces DNA damage, and exposure to high-energy-transfer agents such as neutrons, plutonium, or radon as well as low-energy-transfer sources such as x-rays and gamma rays increases lung cancer risk. The latency period between radiation exposure and cancer development depends on the source and duration of exposure.

Radon is an inert gas that results from the radioactive decay of uranium. Radon exposure is believed to contribute to 15,000 to 20,000 lung cancer cases per year in the United States. The α-particles emitted by radon induce DNA damage in respiratory epithelial cells and can mediate inactivation of the p16 tumor suppressor gene via methylation mechanisms.[56] Methylation of p16 is a very early and critical molecular event in the pathogenesis of NSCLC.[57]

A number of epidemiologic studies have clearly demonstrated markedly increased lung cancer risk in uranium miners, with radon exposure and cigarette smoking exhibiting synergistic effects. Of particular concern is radon exposure in household dwellings. Even though residential radon levels are 50- to 100-fold less than the lowest levels in uranium mines, indoor radon exposure has been associated with increased lung cancer risk. Because of the number of people exposed and the potential duration of this exposure, household radon appears to be a significant environmental risk factor for lung cancer.[58]

The effects of low-energy-transfer radiation appear variable. Patients with tuberculosis or ankylosing spondylitis who received

numerous radiation treatments over prolonged periods have exhibited minimal increases in lung cancer risk; in contrast, increased lung cancer risk has been noted in lymphoma or breast cancer patients receiving high doses of external-beam radiation to axillary, supraclavicular, or mediastinal lymph nodes.[59,60] The latency period for these radiation-induced lung cancers is typically 5 to 10 years.

In light of the fact that the average male adult inhales over 10,000 L of air per day, the potential role of air pollution in terms of lung cancer risk is a major public health issue. Numerous studies have been performed to define the risk of lung cancer associated with exposure to specific pollutants in environmental air, such as metals from smelting and refining industries as well as PAHs and particulate carcinogens resulting from combustion of fossil fuels.[19,45,46] Additional studies have focused on the association of indoor pollutants and lung cancer risk. Although these studies have been difficult to control for all potential confounding variables, available data suggest that 1% to 2% of lung cancers are directly attributable to air pollution.

In a well-designed, prospective cohort study involving over 8000 males from six U.S. cities, Dockerty et al.[61] observed a positive correlation between air pollution and lung cancer risk (adjusted mortality rate ratio, 1.26). In an additional study, Pope et al.[62] observed that sulfate content in air correlated with moderately increased lung cancer risk in the United States. Blot and Fraumeni[63] observed an increased lung cancer risk in people living in U.S. counties with lead, copper, or zinc smelting and refining industries. Increased lung cancer risk was also observed in studies by Xu et al.[64] and Brown et al.[65] involving individuals working in, or residing near, nonferrous smelters.

Epidemiologic data suggest that lung cancer risk is associated with urbanization and that vehicle density may be an excellent predictor of cancer mortality. Bofetta et al.[66] observed a positive exposure-response relationship for diesel exhaust and lung cancer in Swedish males. In a retrospective cohort study of 55,395 U.S. railroad workers adjusted for tobacco exposure, Larkin et al.[67] noted an increased risk of lung cancer (relative risk, 1.4; 95% CI, 1.01 to 2.05) after exposure to diesel exhaust. In an additional case-reference study adjusted for tobacco smoking, Gustavsson et al.[68] observed that diesel fume exposure was associated with a relative risk of 1.63 (95% CI, 1.14 to 2.33). These data, together with the findings of studies by Risom et al.[69] and Belinsky et al.[70] demonstrating that inhaled diesel exhaust mediates oxidative DNA damage as well as methylation of p16 in respiratory epithelial cells, provide compelling evidence for the potential carcinogenic effects of environmental air pollution.

In addition to external air pollution, indoor air contaminants have been associated with increased risk of lung cancer, particularly in developing countries. In addition to ETS and radon exposure, the use of coal for cooking and heating has been linked to lung cancer in several studies in China, and this exposure may account, in part, for the geographic variation of lung cancer in that country.[71,72] Exposure to coal burning in preadult years has been previously associated with increased lung cancer risk in the United States[73]; however, this exposure presently is no longer common in this country.

DIET

Observations in the 1970s that lung cancer patients had low levels of vitamin A prompted intense interest in the potential role of diet in modulating lung cancer risk. Subsequent studies suggested that, by inhibiting DNA damage, antioxidant micronutrients might reduce lung cancer risk. As with the occupational and environmental risk factors previously addressed in Occupational and Environmental Exposure, the potential impact of dietary factors in reducing lung cancer risk is difficult to assess due to the overwhelming carcinogenic effects of tobacco smoke.[19,74] Of particular interest in this regard are the effects of consumption of fruits and vegetables, as well as of micronutrients such as retinols, carotenoids, vitamin C, and folate.

Data regarding fruit and vegetable consumption and lung cancer risk are somewhat contradictory. A protective effect of fruit consumption has been suggested in some but not all studies.[19] On the other hand, the majority of studies performed to date indicate that increased vegetable consumption diminishes lung cancer risk. Although carrots and tomatoes appear to have a protective effect, the specific vegetables that reduce lung cancer risk have not been fully defined.

Overall, the data pertaining to the impact of vitamins and micronutrients and lung cancer risk are inconclusive. Presently, studies have not clearly established an association between dietary retinol intake or circulating retinol levels and reduced lung cancer risk. In contrast, despite several negative reports, numerous studies suggest that dietary intake of total carotenoids, and specifically β-carotene, as well as circulating levels of these carotenoids have a protective effect regarding lung cancer. Similarly, most studies suggest that vitamin C intake and serum ascorbic acid concentrations may be associated with diminished lung cancer risk.[19,74]

Johanning et al.[75] reported that squamous cell lung cancers exhibit decreased DNA methylation as well as reduced folate and vitamin B_{12} concentrations relative to matched normal tissues. Shen et al.[76] observed that dietary folate intake was significantly lower in lung cancer patients than in matched healthy controls ($P<.001$) and that dietary intake above the control median value was associated with a 40% reduction in lung cancer risk. The inverse correlation between dietary folate intake and lung cancer risk appeared most pronounced in patients who drank alcohol, smoked more, did not take supplemental folate, and had a family history of lung cancer. Using host cell reactivation assays that measure nucleotide excision repair in peripheral blood leukocytes, Wei et al.[77] observed that individuals with low dietary folate intake had markedly diminished DNA repair capacity. Interestingly, Bosken et al.[54] reported that lung cancer patients have reduced DNA repair capacity compared to healthy individuals. Collectively, observations that low folate levels enhance DNA damage, together with the fact that lung cancer patients exhibit reduced folate levels and diminished DNA repair capacity, provide a compelling rationale for the evaluation of folate supplements as a means to prevent lung cancer.

PATHOLOGY

The designation *non–small cell carcinoma of the lung* refers to a group of commonly observed pulmonary neoplasms that are typically associated with cigarette smoking and share the common property of not being responsive to small cell carcinoma treatment protocols (Table 27.2-2). Through the 1960s, the predominant type of non–small cell carcinoma was squamous cell carcinoma. Although the overall incidence of lung cancer has dramatically increased over the past 30 years, the relative incidence of

TABLE 27.2-2. World Health Organization Histologic Classification of Epithelial Tumors of the Lung

---

PREINVASIVE LESIONS
Squamous dysplasia/carcinoma *in situ*
Atypical adenomatous hyperplasia
Diffuse idiopathic pulmonary neuroendocrine cell hyperplasia
INVASIVE MALIGNANT LESIONS
Squamous cell carcinoma
Variants
    Papillary
    Clear cell
    Small cell
    Basaloid
Small cell carcinoma
Variant
    Combined small cell carcinoma
Adenocarcinoma
Acinar
Papillary
Bronchioloalveolar carcinoma
    Nonmucinous (Clara cell/type II pneumocyte) type
    Mucinous (goblet cell) type
    Mixed mucinous and nonmucinous (Clara cell/type II pneumocyte
      and goblet cell) type, or indeterminate cell type
Solid adenocarcinoma with mucin formation
Adenocarcinoma with mixed subtypes
    Variants
      Well-differentiated fetal adenocarcinoma
      Mucinous ("colloid") adenocarcinoma
      Mucinous cystadenocarcinoma
      Signet-ring adenocarcinoma
      Clear cell adenocarcinoma
Large cell carcinoma
Variants
    Large cell neuroendocrine carcinoma
    Combined large cell neuroendocrine carcinoma
    Basaloid carcinoma
    Lymphoepithelioma-like carcinoma
    Clear cell carcinoma
    Large cell carcinoma with rhabdoid phenotype
Adenosquamous carcinoma
Carcinomas with pleomorphic, sarcomatoid, or sarcomatous elements
Carcinomas with spindle or giant cells
    Pleomorphic carcinoma
    Spindle cell carcinoma
    Giant cell carcinoma
Carcinosarcoma
Pulmonary blastoma
Carcinoid tumors
Typical carcinoid
Atypical carcinoid
Carcinomas of salivary gland type
Mucoepidermoid carcinoma
Adenoid cystic carcinoma
Others
Unclassified

[From Travis WD, Colby TD, Corrin B. *Histologic Typing of Lung and Pleural Tumors—The World Health Organization (WHO) Classification of Lung Cancer 1999* (rev. 10 October 1998). Geneva: World Health Organization, 1999, with permission.]

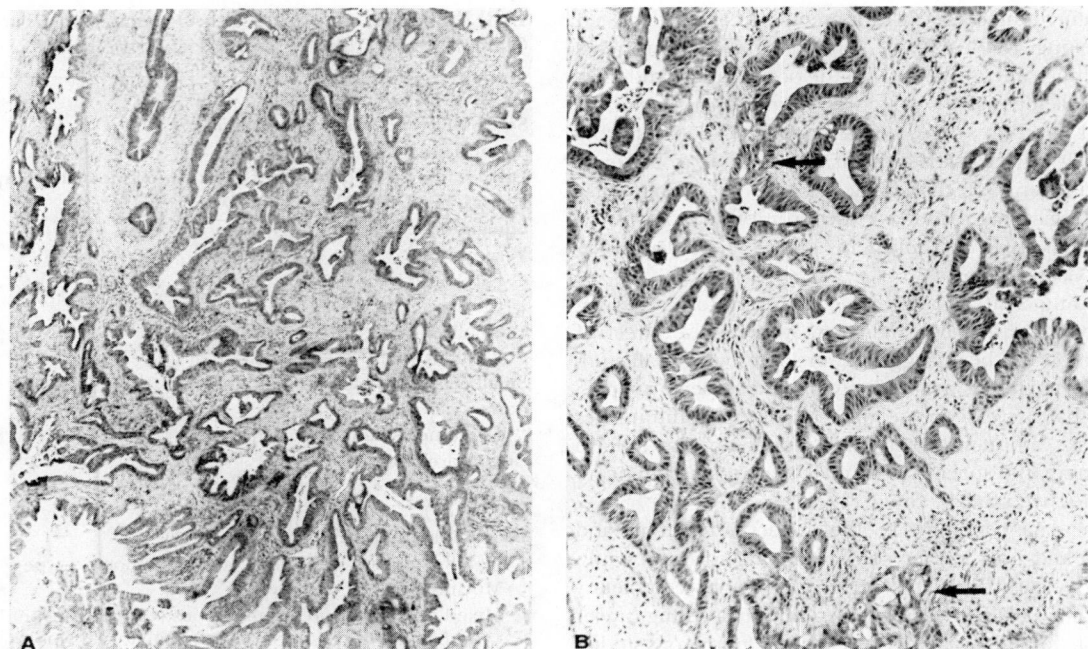

FIGURE 27.2-1. Well-differentiated adenocarcinoma. Well-formed glands with a focal cribriform arrangement (*arrows*) are surrounded by a cellular stroma. **A:** Low-power magnification. **B:** High-power magnification.

squamous cell carcinoma has decreased, and adenocarcinoma has become the dominant cell type—a phenomenon that has been temporally associated with the changes in tobacco blends and the use of filters in cigarettes.[78]

ADENOCARCINOMA

Adenocarcinomas are most often located in the periphery of the lung radiographically and in the smaller airways histologically. Therefore, they are not readily amenable to detection by sputum cytology or other types of cytology, at least in their early stages; however, they may become apparent in the relatively translucent pulmonary periphery on computed tomography (CT) scan in the earliest stages and then on chest radiograph. The 1999 World Health Organization histologic typing of lung cancers recognizes 14 subtypes of adenocarcinoma of the lung, but only a few types account for the great majority of cases (Fig. 27.2-1).

The precursor lesion for pulmonary adenocarcinoma is considered to be atypical alveolar hyperplasia (AAH).[79] Typically found incidentally in pulmonary specimens removed because of the presence of other, more advanced, neoplasms, AAH frequently measures less than 5 mm in diameter and is composed of atypical type II pneumocytes proliferating on an alveolar wall that is either normal in thickness or altered by inactive fibrous scarring. AAH and small nonmucinous bronchoalveolar carcinoma (BAC) fall on a histologic spectrum, and these neoplasms are difficult to differentiate by cytologic, histologic, and genetic techniques. Lesions 5 mm in diameter or less are usually made up of relatively small cells with limited nuclear atypia in comparison to larger lesions, which exhibit progressively more abnormal cells. The rate of progression from AAH to cancer is considered to be quite low, in the range of 1% to 5% over a period of years.

BRONCHOALVEOLAR CARCINOMA

BAC is found in mucinous and nonmucinous variants. The mucinous type is characterized by the growth of malignant mucus-containing goblet cells on the surface of alveolar walls. As such, it is often characterized by pools of mucus and may be associated with the colloid variant of adenocarcinoma in which mucus is predominant over tumor cells. Mucinous BAC has a tendency to be multifocal and fatal (Fig. 27.2-2).

Nonmucinous BAC is comprised of type II pneumocytes or Clara cells exhibiting nuclear anaplasia and pleomorphism greater than that of AAH, but less than that of other types of adenocarcinoma. The malignant cells spread over the alveolar walls in a monolayer, which presents a barrier to gas exchange in the affected alveolar sac and leads to right-to-left intrapulmonary shunt.

Early-stage peripheral adenocarcinomas have been studied intensely and reported as having a good prognosis. Noguchi et al.[80] reported five different subtypes, A to E. In type A, BAC proliferates on the alveolar surface of essentially normal alveolar walls, and in type B, alveolar walls are scarred with well-established collagen free of fibroblasts[81]; elastotic fibers may also be prominent and are considered evidence of parenchymal collapse. Types A and B are associated with a 100% survival rate and are considered noninvasive or carcinoma *in situ* and therefore incapable of metastasizing because they have not invaded the stroma or angiolymphatic vessels of the lung. However, their lepidic growth pattern may allow spread within the airways. Thus defined, BAC is an uncommon type of adenocarcinoma of the lung.

A BAC pattern is often seen at the periphery of invasive types of adenocarcinoma in a *mixed subtype*. When invasive carcinoma is present, the term *BAC* should not be used. Invasive subtypes include acinar (gland forming), papillary, and solid. Noguchi et al.[80] recognized these mixed carcinomas as type C, with the dis-

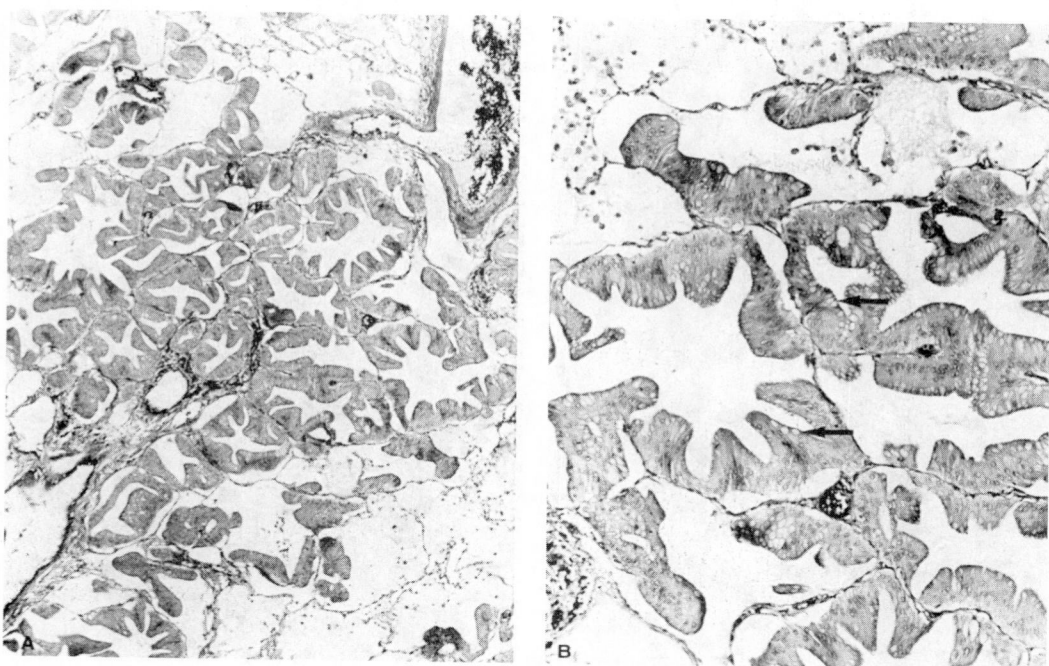

FIGURE 27.2-2. Bronchoalveolar carcinoma. Columnar cells with minimal nuclear atypia are arranged along intact alveolar septa. The lepidic growth pattern is associated with no stromal reaction. Mucin vacuoles are present in the apical cytoplasm (*arrows*). **A:** Low-power magnification. **B:** High-power magnification.

criminating feature of a desmoplastic stroma in which there is proliferation of fibroblasts leading to an actively enlarging fibrous stroma, considered evidence of stromal invasion. Five-year mortality rates for patients with Noguchi type C adenocarcinomas approximate 20%, which indicates a capacity of these neoplasms to invade angiolymphatic spaces and to metastasize to lymph nodes and other sites. Types D and E adenocarcinomas have progressively higher mortality rates due to higher nuclear and histologic grades in an invasive stroma.

Fetal adenocarcinomas are rare tumors that resemble the developing lung in the pseudoglandular period characterized by dichotomous branching of bronchi. Histologically, they are characterized by columnar cells with subnuclear vacuoles rich in glycogen.[82]

Categorization of three other subtypes of primary pulmonary adenocarcinomas stresses the ever-present differential diagnosis of primary from metastatic adenocarcinoma. Mucinous adenocarcinoma with goblet cells mimics colon cancer,[83] signet-ring carcinoma with single cells and small groups exhibiting anaplastic nuclei and eccentric intracellular vacuoles of mucus resembles gastric carcinoma,[83,84] and clear cell carcinoma with a centrally placed nucleus in a clear cytoplasm may be mistaken for renal cell carcinoma.[84] Distinctions are often made on clinical grounds, with recognition of a prior or concurrent carcinoma in another organ, and may be aided by the use of immunohistochemical staining.[85] In particular, the antibody to thyroid transcription factor-1 is useful as a marker of origin in the lung (or thyroid), whereas CK-20 antigen is characteristic of adenocarcinomas of the gastrointestinal tract (especially colon), and gross cystic disease fluid protein-15 is observed in breast cancers.[86]

Other adenocarcinomas are composed of a solid type of large cell carcinoma in which mucin production can only be demonstrated with the aid of histochemical stains. The differ-

ential diagnosis in these lesions is between adenocarcinoma and large cell cancer of the lung or other organs.

LARGE CELL CARCINOMA

Large cell carcinomas are composed of large cells without cytoplasmic differentiation and account for approximately 15% of all lung cancers. With more extensive sampling and electron-microscopical examination, many undifferentiated large cell carcinomas can be classified more appropriately as poorly differentiated adenocarcinomas or, rarely, squamous cell carcinomas (Fig. 27.2-3).

Although the World Health Organization classification recognizes basaloid, lymphoepithelioma-like, and clear cell types, these differ little clinically.[87,88] The prognosis of large cell undifferentiated carcinoma is similar to that of adenocarcinoma, and, in most clinical trials, the two histologic types are grouped together. Large cell carcinoma may show a partial neuroendocrine phenotype recognized from carcinoid histologic features, immunostaining for chromogranin A or synaptophysin, or the ultrastructural demonstration of dense core granules. When accompanied by necrosis, high mitotic rate, and tumor necrosis, these carcinomas are associated with a poor prognosis.

SQUAMOUS CELL CARCINOMA

Squamous cell carcinoma may present clinically in the periphery of the lung as a small subpleural nodule with the gross appearance and overall prognosis of a peripheral adenocarcinoma (Fig. 27.2-4). However, squamous cell carcinoma typically arises in proximal segmental bronchi via progression through stages of dysplasia. In its earliest form (carcinoma *in situ*), malignant squamous cells spread over the bronchial surface, often involving submucosal glands, without invasion through the basement mem-

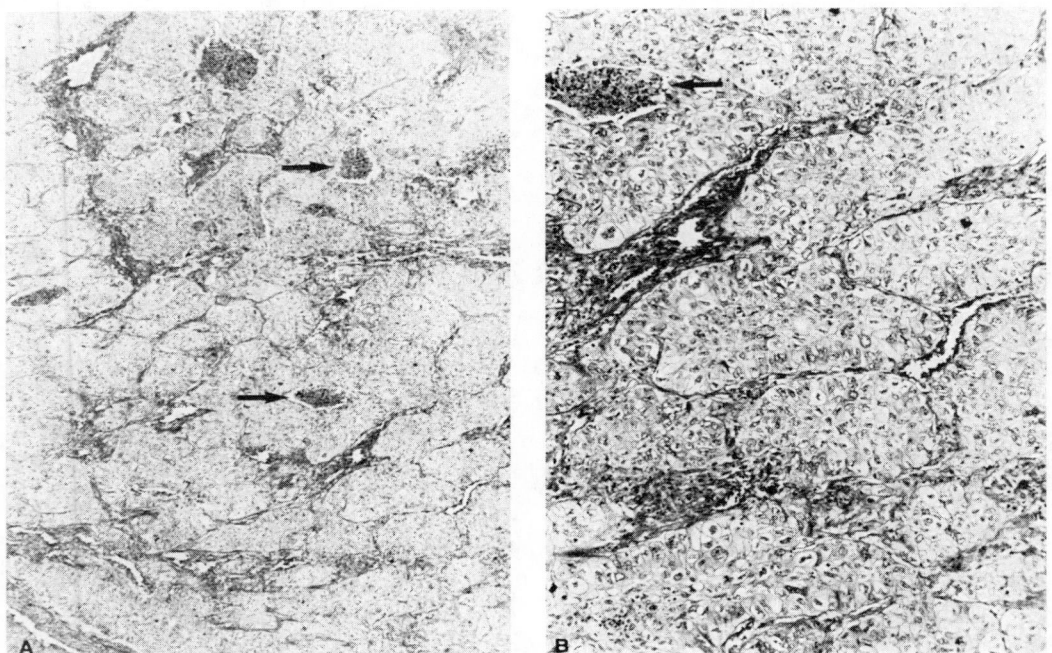

FIGURE 27.2-3.   Large cell undifferentiated carcinoma. Sheets of highly atypical cells with focal necrosis (*arrows*) are present. There is no evidence of keratinization of gland formation. **A:** Low-power magnification. **B:** High-power magnification.

brane. Because there is exfoliation of the malignant cells from the bronchial surface, squamous cell carcinoma can be detected by cytologic examination at its earliest stage, occasionally before it is evident on chest radiograph, due to its origin in the electron-dense bronchi, which render it radiographically occult. Localiza-

tion may be problematic before therapy. With further growth, squamous cell carcinoma invades the basement membrane and extends into the parenchyma and bronchial lumen, producing obstruction with resultant atelectasis or pneumonia. Histologically, squamous cell carcinoma is composed of sheets of epithelial

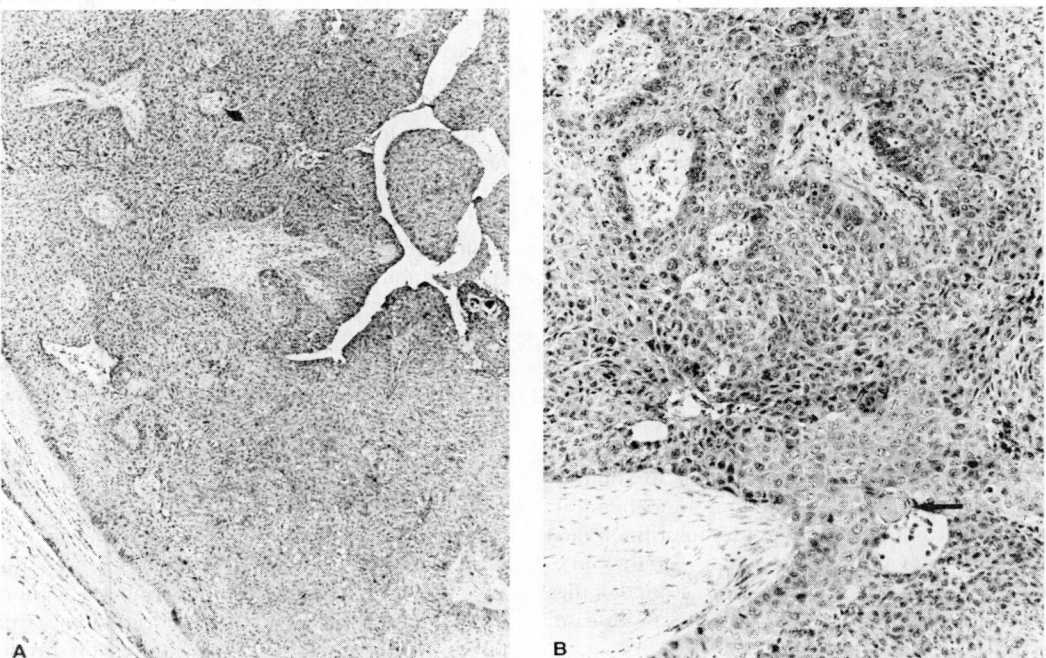

FIGURE 27.2-4.   Moderately differentiated squamous cell carcinoma. Sheets of tumor cells with variable amounts of cytoplasm and moderate nuclear atypia are present. Focal keratinization is evident (*arrow*). **A:** Low-power magnification. **B:** High-power magnification.

cells with individual cell keratinization, intercellular bridges, or pearl formation.[89] Squamous cell carcinoma tends to be slow growing, and it is estimated that the progression from *in situ* carcinoma to a clinically apparent tumor takes 3 to 4 years.

ADENOSQUAMOUS CARCINOMA

As the name implies, adenosquamous carcinomas have histologic areas differentiated as both squamous cell carcinoma and adenocarcinoma. They are predominantly found in the periphery of the lung and have clinical behavior more like that of adenocarcinoma. Studies suggest that they are a cytogenetically distinct entity.[90]

PLEOMORPHIC CARCINOMAS

The pleomorphic group of tumors includes carcinomas with giant and usually multinucleated cells; carcinomas with a spindle cell, pseudosarcomatous configuration; and those with both carcinoma and sarcoma morphologic features, including the rare pulmonary blastoma.[91,92] All are aggressive malignancies and are usually found at high stage, but survival is stage dependent.

CARCINOMAS OF SALIVARY GLAND TYPE

Carcinomas of the salivary gland type include mucoepidermoid carcinomas (low and high grade), recognized by their characteristic intermediate or transitional cells; adenoid-cystic carcinomas, which share the aggressiveness of their salivary gland counterparts; and low-grade, acinic cell carcinomas.[93,94] All are predominantly found in large bronchi and are thought to arise from submucosal gland epithelia.

CARCINOID

Carcinoids manifest a prominent neuroendocrine phenotype in morphologic, immunohistochemical, and ultrastructural features. Histologically they are characterized by organoid, ribbon or festoon pseudorosette, and sometimes spindle patterns of cuboidal cells with small and hyperchromatic nuclei. Typical carcinoids are usually found in large bronchi and feature an organoid pattern. Peripheral carcinoids are often spindle cell tumors. Both are low-grade neoplasms with a low incidence of metastases. Carcinoids with necrosis, mitotic figures, or progressive nuclear anaplasia are classified as atypical and have a higher rate of metastases.[95] The very mitotically active, necrotic, and anaplastic carcinoids are classified as large cell neuroendocrine carcinomas and have a very poor prognosis.[96]

MOLECULAR MARKERS OF PROGNOSIS

During the past 10 years, considerable insight has been achieved regarding the molecular basis of lung cancer.[11] As a result, numerous studies have been performed to ascertain if specific mutational events have unique prognostic significance. In particular, these translational efforts have focused on common aberrations regarding expression of genes regulating cell-cycle progression, apoptosis, invasion, and metastasis. For instance, well-designed studies suggest that overexpression of epidermal growth factor receptor (EGFR), particularly in conjunction with erbB2 correlates with diminished survival in lung cancer patients after curative resec-

tions.[97,98] Additional studies suggest that increased expression of mitogen-activated protein kinase as well as K-ras and p53 mutations correlate with adverse outcome in lung cancer patients.[99–102] Loss of FHIT (fragile histidine triad) expression as well as overexpression of COX-2 have also been reported to correlate with poor prognosis in lung cancer patients.[103,104] Unfortunately, none of these markers is sufficiently robust for use in the clinical management of lung cancer patients at this time.

Given the molecular heterogeneity of lung cancers, it is not surprising that no single biomarker has emerged that uniformly correlates with prognosis in lung cancer patients. On the other hand, combinations of markers, identified either by standard immunohistochemical techniques or by more novel complementary DNA arrays, and proteomic profiling may prove quite useful for the diagnosis and treatment of lung cancer. In one study, Miura et al.[105] used laser capture microdissection and complementary DNA microarrays to identify 45 genes that distinguished lung cancers in smokers from those in nonsmokers. Additional analysis revealed 27 genes that were differentially expressed in long-term survivors compared to nonsurvivors after potentially curative lung cancer resections. A number of these pertinent genes regulate the mitotic spindle checkpoint and are involved in maintaining genomic stability. Volm et al.[106] evaluated expression of 21 gene products in lung cancer specimens from 216 patients. Using hierarchical clustering techniques, these investigators observed that expression of FOS, JUN, erbB1, cyclin A, and proliferating cell nuclear antigen were decreased in tumors from long-term survivors. Using complementary DNA array techniques, Beer et al.[107] identified a cluster of genes (some of which were not previously associated with prognosis) that predicted survival in patients with early-stage pulmonary adenocarcinomas. Similar studies performed by Wigle et al.[108] have confirmed that gene expression profiles may prove extremely useful for determining prognosis of lung cancer patients. Additional studies have indicated that methylation profiles may also coincide with tumor histologic type, stage, and prognosis in lung cancer patients.[109,110]

Several studies indicate that proteomic techniques may be extremely valuable for discriminating tumor histologic type and stage of lung cancers. Chen et al.[111] used quantitative two-dimensional gel electrophoresis to evaluate protein expression in 107 lung cancer specimens and observed that aberrant expression of 11 proteins associated with the glycolysis pathway correlated with poor survival; in particular, elevated levels of phosphoglycerate kinase-1 in sera correlated with poor outcome. Using proteomic techniques, Yanagisawa et al.[112] observed a pattern of 15 distinct mass spectroscopic peaks in lung cancer cells that distinguished between patients with good outcome and those with poor survival (median survival, 33 months vs. 6 months, respectively; $P < .001$). Collectively, these data indicate that gene expression profiling and tissue proteomics may prove highly useful for ascertaining the histologic type, stage, and prognosis of lung cancers.

MODES OF METASTASIS

After a variable period of growing within lung parenchyma or within the bronchial wall, the primary tumor invades the vascular and lymphatic channels, thereby metastasizing to regional lymph nodes and distant sites. In most instances, regional lymph node metastases precede systemic dissemination. The regional lym-

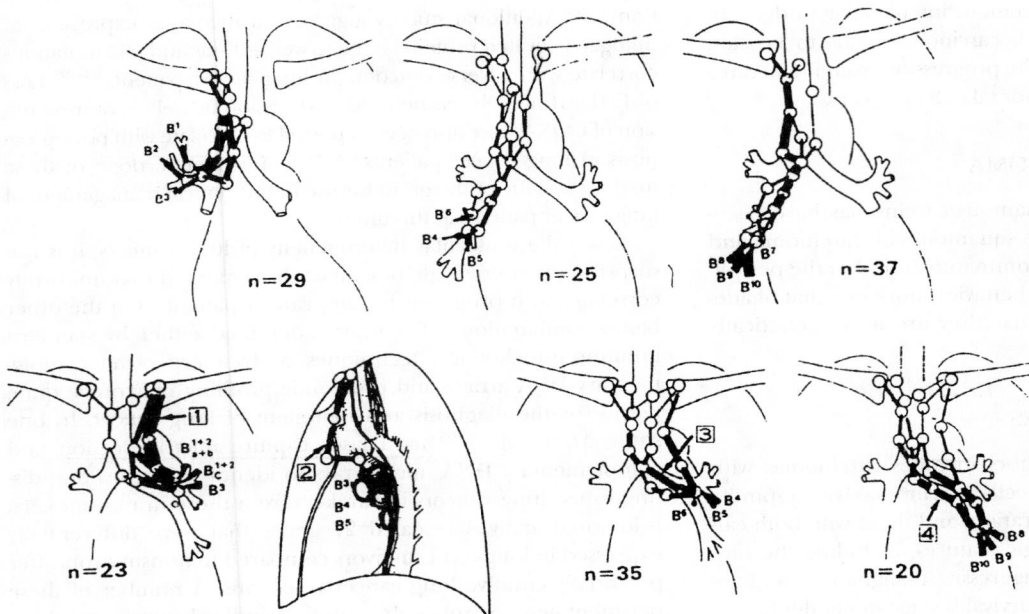

FIGURE 27.2-5. The regional lymphatic drainage of the lung as described by Noel. Most of the lymphatic drainage ultimately reaches the right superior mediastinum and right supraclavicular regions. (From ref. 358, with permission.)

phatic drainage of the lung is outlined in Figure 27.2-5. In lung tissue, lymphatic drainage parallels the bronchoarterial system, with lymph nodes situated adjacent to the segmental or lobar bronchi. Lower lobe lymphatics drain to the posterior mediastinum and the subcarinal lymph nodes. Right upper lobe lymphatics drain toward the superior mediastinum, whereas the left upper lobe lymphatics typically course lateral to the aorta and subclavian artery in the anterior mediastinum, as well as along the left main bronchus to the superior mediastinum. Ultimately, all of these lymphatic channels drain into the right lymphatic or left thoracic ducts, which empty into the subclavian veins. Although skip metastases can occur, antegrade lymphatic metastases most commonly exhibit sequential involvement of bronchopulmonary (N1), mediastinal (N2 and N3), and supraclavicular (N3) lymph nodes. Retrograde lymphatic spread to the pleural surface can occur, particularly with peripheral tumors.

By direct extension, the primary tumor can invade contiguous structures, such as the mediastinal pleura, great vessels, heart, esophagus, diaphragm, or chest wall. Once vascular or lymphatic invasion occurs, metastatic dissemination to distant sites is common. Although bone, liver, adrenals, and brain are the most common sites of distant disease, lung cancer can metastasize to virtually every organ of the body. Metastases within the lung result from a variety of mechanisms, including endobronchial embolization and retrograde lymphatic and hematogenous dissemination.

CLINICAL MANIFESTATIONS

The signs and symptoms manifested by patients suffering from lung cancer depend on the histologic features of the tumor and the extent of locoregional invasion, as well as the location, size, and number of distant metastases (Table 27.2-3). Many patients present with an asymptomatic lesion discovered incidentally on chest radiograph.

Tumors arising in the larger airways may cause persistent cough, wheezing, or hemoptysis. Typically, patients with hemoptysis experience blood-streaked sputum; massive bleeding is

rarely seen at presentation. Continued growth of endobronchial tumors frequently results in atelectasis with or without pneumonia and abscess. If pleural surfaces are involved, either by the primary tumor or associated infection, pleuritic pain may develop with or without detectable pleural effusion. The loss of lung

TABLE 27.2-3. Common Signs and Symptoms of Lung Cancer

SYMPTOMS SECONDARY TO CENTRAL OR ENDOBRONCHIAL GROWTH OF THE PRIMARY TUMOR
Cough
Hemoptysis
Wheeze and stridor
Dyspnea from obstruction
Pneumonitis from obstruction (fever, productive cough)
SYMPTOMS SECONDARY TO PERIPHERAL GROWTH OF THE PRIMARY TUMOR
Pain from pleural or chest wall involvement
Cough
Dyspnea on a restrictive basis
Lung abscess syndrome from tumor cavitation
SYMPTOMS RELATED TO REGIONAL SPREAD OF THE TUMOR IN THE THORAX BY CONTIGUITY OR BY METASTASIS TO REGIONAL LYMPH NODES
Tracheal obstruction
Esophageal compression with dysphagia
Recurrent laryngeal nerve paralysis with hoarseness
Phrenic nerve paralysis with hemidiaphragm elevation and dyspnea
Sympathetic nerve paralysis with Horner's syndrome
Eighth cervical and first thoracic nerves with ulnar pain and Pancoast's syndrome
Superior vena cava syndrome from vascular obstruction
Pericardial and cardiac extension with resultant tamponade, arrhythmia, or cardiac failure
Lymphatic obstruction with pleural effusion
Lymphangitic spread through lungs with hypoxemia and dyspnea

(From Cohen MH. Signs and symptoms of bronchogenic carcinoma. In: Straus MJ, ed. *Lung cancer: clinical diagnosis and treatment.* New York: Grune & Stratton, 1977:85, with permission.)

function usually is associated with dyspnea, the severity of which depends on the amount of lung involved and the patient's underlying pulmonary reserve.

Depending on its location, the primary tumor can invade the chest wall, producing either stabbing or burning radicular pain and pleural effusion. With apical tumors, classic Pancoast's syndrome (lower brachial plexopathy, Horner's syndrome, and shoulder pain) may arise due to invasion of a lower brachial plexus (T-1 and C-8 nerve routes), stellate ganglion, and chest wall. Invasion or encasement of the structures within the mediastinum may cause superior vena cava (SVC) syndrome, recurrent nerve or phrenic nerve palsy, esophageal dysphagia, or pericardial effusion. Recurrent nerve palsy resulting in hoarseness and cricopharyngeal dysphagia is often observed with advanced left upper lobe tumors. Nodal involvement associated with lower lobe tumors or their direct extension within the posterior mediastinum may produce partial or complete obstruction of the esophagus that results in dysphagia with or without tracheoesophageal fistula. In addition to specific symptoms directly related to the tumor or associated lymphadenopathy, vague chest discomfort frequently occurs in patients suffering from lung cancer. This pain is usually of visceral origin and appears unrelated to direct invasion of local structures.

Nearly all patients with advanced, inoperable NSCLC exhibit symptoms referable to their disease at the time of initial presentation. Fatigue and decreased activity are reported by more than 80% of individuals, and most also experience cough, dyspnea, decreased appetite, and weight loss. The frequency and multitude of symptoms in most patients and the severity of these complaints mandates prompt treatment of the underlying malignancy and management of each symptom while definitive therapy is under way.

The presenting complaints of a patient with metastatic disease are largely determined by the specific sites involved. For example, patients with bone metastases present with pain and limitation of function. In contrast, pericardial effusions of malignant or cancer-associated but nonmalignant origin either may be asymptomatic or may produce dyspnea, cough, and chest discomfort, symptoms identical to those produced by pulmonary tumors with pleural metastases. Most adrenal and hepatic metastases are initially asymptomatic; however, in advanced disease, these metastases can cause considerable pain, either from capsular expansion or invasion into adjacent organs. Adrenal insufficiency due to bilateral metastases may occur on rare occasions.

The anorexia-cachexia syndrome, as well as generalized weakness and fatigue, are the most common systemic manifestations of NSCLC. In addition, a variety of paraneoplastic syndromes may be associated with lung cancer. Many of these conditions are not specific to lung cancer but have been documented to occur frequently in individuals with this disease (Table 27.2-4). Hypertrophic pulmonary osteoarthropathy occurs frequently in NSCLC patients and is manifested as bone and joint pain. Clubbing of the digits is observed. Serum alkaline phosphatase level is often elevated, whereas hepatic enzyme levels are normal. Plain radiographs of affected bones demonstrate periosteal inflammation and elevation, and radionuclide bone scans reveal intense, symmetric radiolabel uptake in the distal ends of long bones. Symptoms associated with hypertrophic pulmonary osteoarthropathy may respond dramatically to either aspirin or nonsteroid antiinflammatory

TABLE 27.2-4. Paraneoplastic Syndromes in Patients with Lung Cancer

ENDOCRINE
Hypercalcemia (ectopic parathyroid hormone)
Cushing's syndrome
Syndrome of inappropriate antidiuretic hormone
Carcinoid syndrome
Gynecomastia
Hypercalcitonemia
Elevated growth hormone
Elevated prolactin, follicle-stimulating hormone, luteinizing hormone
Hypoglycemia
Hyperthyroidism
NEUROLOGIC
Encephalopathy
Subacute cerebellar degeneration
Progressive multifocal leukoencephalopathy
Peripheral neuropathy
Polymyositis
Autonomic neuropathy
Eaton-Lambert syndrome
Optic neuritis
SKELETAL
Clubbing
Pulmonary hypertrophic osteoarthropathy
HEMATOLOGIC
Anemia
Leukemoid reactions
Thrombocytosis
Thrombocytopenia
Eosinophilia
Pure red cell aplasia
Leukoerythroblastosis
Disseminated intravascular coagulation
CUTANEOUS
Hyperkeratosis
Dermatomyositis
Acanthosis nigricans
Hyperpigmentation
Erythema gyratum repens
Hypertrichosis lanuginosa acquista
OTHER
Nephrotic syndrome
Hypouricemia
Secretion of vasoactive intestinal peptide with diarrhea
Hyperamylasemia
Anorexia or cachexia

(Adapted from Maddaus M, Ginsberg RJ. Diagnosis and staging. In: Pearson FG, Deslauriers J, Ginsberg R, eds. *Thoracic surgery*. New York: Churchill Livingstone, 1995:671, with permission.)

agents and typically resolve after definitive treatment of the primary lesion. Digital clubbing may also resolve with curative therapy.

STAGING AND DIAGNOSIS

In 1985, the American Joint Committee on Cancer, the International Union Against Cancer, and the Japanese Cancer Committee established a worldwide tumor-node-metastasis (TNM) staging system, which was rapidly adopted and extensively used in the

TABLE 27.2-5. Tumor, Node, Metastasis (TNM) Staging System for Lung Cancer

PRIMARY TUMOR

TX	Positive malignant cell; no lesion seen
T1	<3-cm diameter
T2	>3-cm diameter
	Distal atelectasis
T3	Extension to parietal pleura, chest wall diaphragm, or pericardium
	<2 cm from carina or total atelectasis
T4	Invasion of mediastinal organs
	Malignant pleural effusion

REGIONAL LYMPH NODE INVOLVEMENT

N0	No nodal involvement
N1	Ipsilateral bronchopulmonary or hilar nodes
N2	Ipsilateral or subcarinal mediastinal nodes
	Ipsilateral supraclavicular nodes
N3	Contralateral mediastinal hilar or supraclavicular nodes

METASTATIC INVOLVEMENT

M0	No metastases
M1	Metastases present

Stage	*TNM*	*5-Y Survival Rate (%)*
REVISED STAGING SYSTEM		
IA	T1, N0, M0	>70
IB	T2, N0, M0	60
IIA	T1, N1, M0	50
IIB	T2, N1, M0	30
	T3, N0–N1, M0	40
IIIA	T1–T3, N2, M0	10–30
IIIB	Any T4, any N3, M0	<10
IV	Any M1	<5

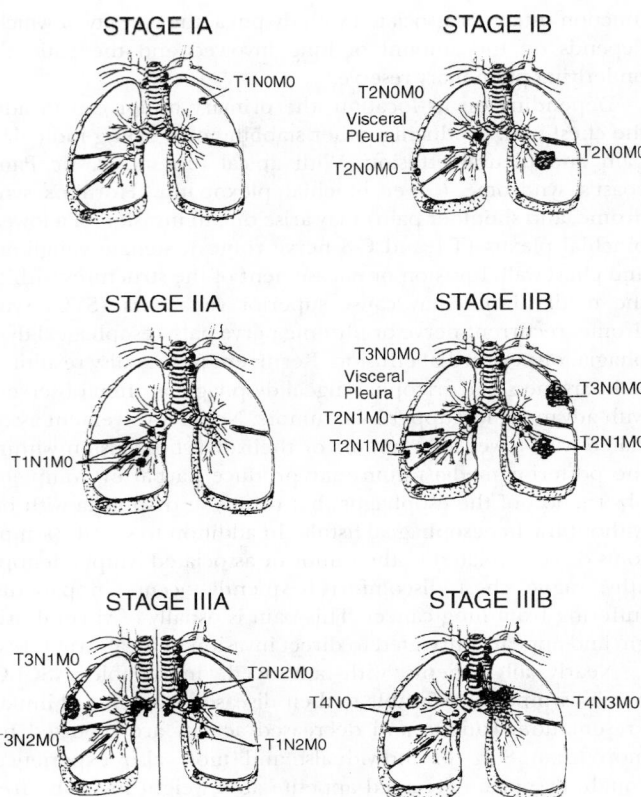

FIGURE 27.2-6. New International Staging System. Categories of stage IA, IB, IIA, IIB, IIIA, and IIIB disease. (From Mountain CF. A new international staging system for lung cancer. *Chest* 1986;89[Suppl]:225, with permission.)

management of lung cancer. A revised staging system was accepted by the American Joint Committee on Cancer and the International Union Against Cancer in 1997 (Table 27.2-5; Fig. 27.2-6). In the current staging system, the primary tumor is subdivided into four categories (T1 to T4) depending on size, site, and local involvement. Lymph node involvement has been subdivided into bronchopulmonary (N1), ipsilateral mediastinal (N2), and contralateral or supraclavicular disease (N3). Metastases are absent (M0) or present (M1). Using the TNM system, four stages of lung cancer have been identified that are associated with significant differences in 5-year survival depending on the stage of disease at diagnosis (Fig. 27.2-7). The TNM system includes clinical as well as pathologic criteria. When clinical parameters alone are used, a significant percentage of tumors are under-staged, compared to the stage ultimately identified by pathologic analysis. Although the 1997 staging system lacks uniformity regarding definition and prognosis within certain subtypes of locally advanced disease (T3 vs. T4 and N2 vs. N3), it is a functional system that should be used for the management of all lung cancer patients.

In patients suspected of harboring lung cancer, accurate tissue diagnosis and staging are critical determinants of therapy and overall prognosis. Because of this, the evaluation of any patient suspected of having lung cancer should proceed in an expedient, cost-efficient manner (Fig. 27.2-8). A detailed history taking and physical examination remain the most important steps in initially assessing a patient with possible lung cancer. Smoking history, occupational and environmental exposure, and family history

should be documented. Review of systems should focus on new symptoms, including persistent or recurrent respiratory infections, cough, hemoptysis, or pain, as well as symptoms referable to recurrent nerve palsy or SVC obstruction. In addition, review of systems should ascertain symptoms referable to metastatic disease, including focal neurologic deficits, bone pain, weight loss, or paraneoplastic syndromes. Physical examination should focus on the presence of supraclavicular or cervical lymphadenopathy, signs of partial or complete airway obstruction and pneumonia or pleural effusion, as well as organomegaly or pain indicative of metastatic disease. Extremity examination should rule out the presence of hypertrophic pulmonary osteoarthropathy, as well as deep venous thrombosis, which may be a manifestation of cancer-associated hypercoagulopathy. Neurologic examination should rule out cognitive as well as focal motor deficits.

Once the physical examination has been completed, posteroanterior and lateral chest radiographs as well as CT scans of the chest and upper abdomen should be obtained. Typically, patients with symptoms or signs of pulmonary disease (i.e., volume loss, wheezing, chest wall pain) manifest abnormalities on routine chest radiographs. In general, plain chest radiographs can reveal peripheral nodules and volume loss suggestive of bronchial obstruction, as well as hilar and mediastinal lymphadenopathy, pleural effusions, and bony destruction. Whereas routine chest radiographs generally rule out a large peripheral lung cancer or central obstructing lesion, a normal chest radiograph does not exclude a primary lung cancer. For instance, Sone et al.[113]

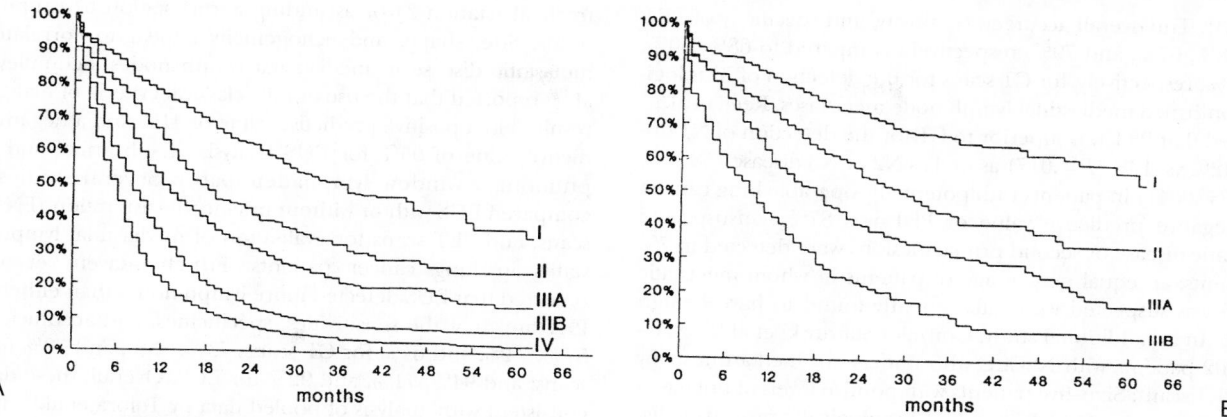

FIGURE 27.2-7. Actuarial survival curves according to different stages (1986 staging). **A:** Survival after clinical staging. **B:** Survival after final pathologic staging. Note that early-stage cancers are under-staged by clinical staging, which results in a poorer survival rate than after pathologic staging. However, the higher the stage, the less likely that clinical staging under-stages the disease. (From Mountain CF. A new international staging system for lung cancer. *Chest* 1986;89[Suppl]:225, with permission.)

reported that conventional chest radiographs failed to reveal 77% of CT-detected, histologically proven lung cancers, including 79% (33 of 42) of tumors smaller than 2.0 cm. Seventy-four percent of these tumors were located in well-penetrated regions of the lung, and 71% of these were missed on chest radiograph. Twenty-six percent of tumors were adjacent to, or obscured by, hilar structures, and none of these tumors was detected by chest radiograph. Ninety-three percent of tumors smaller than 2 cm were adenocarcinomas, and 79% of these were not detected by chest radiograph. Bepler et al.[114] noted that, compared to conventional chest radiographs, CT scans have a threefold higher overall detection rate, with a fivefold increase in detection of resectable lung cancers. Hence, CT scans of the chest are the standard of care for any patient suspected of having a primary lung cancer. In general, conventional CT scans have a sensitivity of 60% and specificity of approximately 80% to 90% for the detection of lung cancer. The diagnostic accuracy of CT scans, particularly for small peripheral lesions, can be further improved through the use of super high-resolution scanning techniques. Finkelstein et al.[115] reported that modern, super high-resolution CT scans have a sensitivity and specificity of approximately 83% and 100%, respectively, for the detection of malignant endoluminal or obstructive lesions involving the airway.

Once an abnormality is detected on CT scan that is suspicious for cancer, additional studies should be obtained to determine the extent and malignancy status of the lesion. Of particular importance in this regard is ascertaining if the lesion is a primary NSCLC or a small cell lung cancer, management of which is comprehensively discussed in Chapter 27.3. The size and location of the primary lesion and possible metastases determine which additional imaging studies and biopsy methods are most appropriate for establishing tissue diagnosis and confirming the stage of the disease (see Fig. 27.2-8).

Although important for the preliminary assessment of mediastinal lymphadenopathy, CT scans cannot be used to assess mediastinal lymph node metastases reliably. In general, by CT criteria, a "normal" mediastinal lymph node must be smaller than 1 cm in transverse diameter. The presence of any lymph node larger than this suggests malignant lymphadenopathy. On the other hand, enlarged lymph nodes are not always

malignant, particularly in the context of tumors associated with volume loss or postobstructive pneumonitis. Similarly, lymph nodes smaller than 1 cm may contain foci of malignant cells, the frequency of which is as high as 15% in certain series. Because of this, the size of mediastinal lymph nodes does not necessarily rule in or rule out metastatic disease.

In the United States and Europe, whole body [18F]fluorodeoxyglucose positron emission tomography (FDG-PET) is currently being used for evaluation of patients with known or suspected malignant disease.[116] Although FDG-PET cannot be used routinely to identify intracranial metastases, these imaging studies appear particularly useful for the detection of mediastinal lymph node metastases as well as visceral and bony metastases in lung cancer patients due to the avid uptake of the fluorodeoxyglucose radiolabel by most common histologic types of lung cancer. Luketich et al.[117] compared PET scans with standard CT scans for staging the mediastinum in lung cancer patients who subsequently underwent mediastinal lymph node dissection

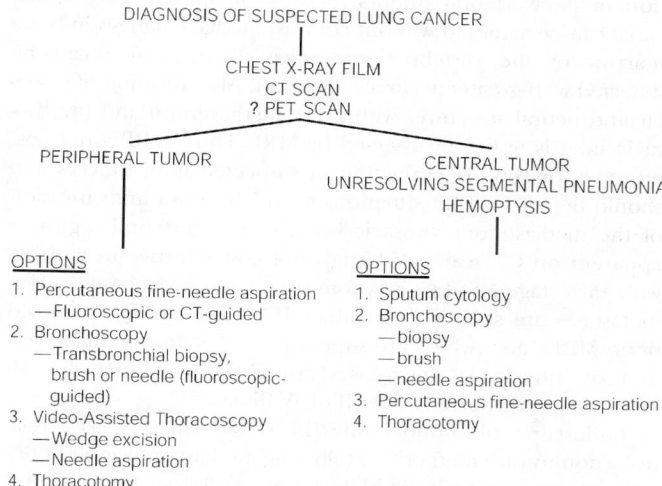

FIGURE 27.2-8. Schema to indicate the diagnostic procedures depending on the presenting lesion. CT, computed tomography; PET, positron emission tomography.

(MLND). The overall accuracy, sensitivity, and specificity of PET were 78%, 67%, and 79%, respectively, compared to 68%, 50%, and 71%, respectively, for CT scans for the detection of histologically confirmed mediastinal lymph node metastases. Reed et al.[118] reported that PET was superior to CT for the detection of N1 disease (42% vs. 13%; $P = .017$) as well as N2 or N3 disease (58% vs. 32%; $P = .0041$) in patients with potentially operable lung cancer. The negative predictive value of PET was 87%. Unsuspected metastatic disease or second primary lesions were detected in 7% of patients; an equal percentage of patients in whom metastatic disease was suspected were subsequently found to have benign disease. In an additional study, Gonzalez-Stawinski et al.[119] evaluated 202 patients with NSCLC who underwent mediastinoscopy after PET scans. Sixty-five patients with positive levels of uptake in the mediastinum on PET scan had histologically proven malignant disease in corresponding nodal stations. Of 137 patients with "negative" levels of mediastinal uptake, 16 were subsequently found to have N2 or N3 malignant disease at mediastinoscopy. The sensitivity, specificity, positive predictive value, negative predictive value, and accuracy for PET were 64%, 77%, 45%, 88%, and 74%, respectively. Granulomatous inflammation, silicosis, and sinus histiocytosis contributed to false-positive PET images of mediastinal lymph nodes in lung cancer patients. Data indicate that integration of PET and CT scans can enhance the accuracy of these individual modalities for the detection of lung cancer.[120]

FDG-PET scanning appears superior to either CT imaging or bone scans for identification of occult metastatic disease at presentation. Additional studies suggest that PET scans may be superior to CT scans for assessing response to radiation or chemoradiation therapy in lung cancer patients.[121,122] Although PET scans may be useful for differentiating benign from malignant solitary pulmonary nodules, granulomatous inflammation can result in false-positive results, and BACs may be metabolically inactive, which results in a false-negative scan. Hence, PET cannot be used to determine definitively the cause of a mass lesion or associated lymphadenopathy; tissue diagnosis remains the standard of care.

Standard magnetic resonance imaging (MRI) investigation of pulmonary lesions does not appear to improve diagnosis in most lung cancer cases. However, MRI is particularly useful for evaluation of paravertebral tumors, because imaging of the spinal canal can be achieved without contrast media. Changes in bone marrow of the vertebrae suggestive of carcinoma can be detected with greater accuracy with MRI. Also, invasion of vascular and neural structures within the mediastinum and the thoracic inlet is optimally assessed by MRI. Thus, MRI is not cost effective for routine evaluation of suspected lung cancers and should be reserved for situations in which local tumor invasion of the mediastinum, thoracic inlet, or paravertebral region is apparent on CT scans. Although not cost effective in patients with early-stage NSCLC, in whom occult central nervous system metastases are seen in fewer than 15%, gadolinium-enhanced brain MRI scans (which are superior to CT scans for the detection of intracranial metastases) should be obtained for all patients with suspected stage III or IV disease.[123]

Endoscopic ultrasonography (EUS) has emerged as a relatively noninvasive method of evaluating mediastinal lymph nodes in lung cancer patients.[124] EUS can detect lesions larger than 3 mm in the paratracheal region (stations 2 and 4 bilaterally) aortopulmonary window (station 5), subcarinal region (station 7), and paraesophageal region (station 8) but cannot assess pre-

tracheal (station 3) or ascending aorta (station 6) lymph node status. Size, shape, and echogenicity appear to correlate with metastatic disease in mediastinal lymph nodes. Schmulewitz et al.[125] reported that the use of four classical criteria of malignancy resulted in a positive predictive value of 41% and a negative predictive value of 95% for EUS analysis of subcarinal and aortopulmonary window lymphadenopathy. Several studies have compared EUS with or without fine-needle aspiration (FNA), CT scans, and PET scans for evaluation of mediastinal lymph node status in lung cancer patients. Fritscher-Ravens et al.[124,126] reported that EUS detected more lymph nodes than either CT or PET and that the sensitivities, specificities, and accuracies were 57%, 74%, and 67% for CT scans; 73%, 83%, and 79% for PET scans; and 94%, 71%, and 92% for EUS. Overall, these data are consistent with analysis of pooled data by Toloza et al.[127] indicating sensitivities and specificities of 57% and 47% for CT scans, 84% and 89% for PET imaging, and 78% and 71% for EUS. As was also noted by other investigators, Fritscher-Ravens et al.[124,126] observed that PET imaging could be improved when combined with CT, which resulted in a sensitivity of 81%, specificity of 94%, and accuracy of 88%. The specificity of EUS increased to 100% when combined with FNA.

METHODS TO ESTABLISH TISSUE DIAGNOSIS

SPUTUM CYTOLOGY

Cytologic analysis of exfoliated cells in sputum is a rapid, relatively inexpensive means to establish a tissue diagnosis in an individual with an apparent pulmonary carcinoma. Sputum can be either spontaneously collected or induced with hypertonic saline. Pooling of three daily specimens increases the diagnostic yield. Sputum samples are considered representative if alveolar macrophages as well as bronchial epithelial cells are present. Overall, the sensitivity of sputum cytology is 65% (range, 22% to 98%) in the setting of established cancers. The diagnostic yield of sputum cytology is enhanced for centrally located lesions, squamous cell carcinomas, and large tumors, particularly if multiple sputum samples are examined.[128]

A variety of molecular techniques have been evaluated as a means to increase the diagnostic yield of sputum cytology. These include nuclear image analysis, immunohistochemical evaluation of p53 and heterogeneous nuclear riboprotein A2/B1 expression, and analysis of K-ras and p53 mutations, loss of heterozygosity, aberrant promoter methylation, and DNA adduct levels in genomic DNA. Additional studies have focused on the evaluation of gene expression profiles in tumor cells.[129] Overall, the feasibility and efficacy of use of these newer methodologies in the context of sputum cytology for established carcinomas have not been fully investigated. Furthermore, the usefulness of these techniques for the detection of occult pulmonary malignancies has not been established.

PERCUTANEOUS FINE-NEEDLE ASPIRATION

FNA is an excellent method for obtaining tissue samples for cytologic and histologic confirmation of malignancy. This can be performed using fluoroscopically guided or CT-guided techniques. The positive yield in experienced hands exceeds 95%.

However, indeterminate biopsy results must be interpreted with caution. FNA cannot rule out malignancy unless a true-positive benign diagnosis (i.e., hamartoma or infectious process) can be definitively established. Abnormalities involving bone, liver, and adrenal glands suggestive of metastatic disease on staging studies can be readily confirmed by FNA using ultrasonographically guided or CT-guided techniques. Frequently, biopsy of one of these sites simultaneously establishes tissue diagnosis and stage of the disease.

BRONCHOSCOPY

Fiberoptic bronchoscopy (FOB) can be performed with or without sedation, and with minimal morbidity and exceptional safety. FOB enables visualization of the tracheobronchial tree to the second or third segmental divisions. Cytologic or histologic specimens can be obtained from identified lesions. In general, the diagnostic yield of FOB with cytologic brushings or biopsy of visible lesions exceeds 90%. Even when no visible lesion is identified, the bronchus draining the area of suspicion can be lavaged and effluent obtained for cytologic analysis. With FOB and fluoroscopy, peripheral lesions identified by high-resolution CT scans can be reached by cytologic brushes, needle, or biopsy forceps.

In addition to establishing tissue diagnosis, FOB may be used to evaluate mediastinal lymph nodes. Transbronchoscopic needle aspiration through the airway wall as popularized by Wang can confirm the presence of malignancy in enlarged mediastinal lymph nodes without the necessity of mediastinoscopy, thoracoscopy, or EUS and FNA.

MEDIASTINOSCOPY, MEDIASTINOTOMY, AND ENDOSCOPIC ULTRASONOGRAPHY PLUS FINE-NEEDLE ASPIRATION

Mediastinoscopy was developed by Carlens more than 50 years ago to facilitate staging of superior mediastinal lymph nodes (N2 or N3) in patients with lung cancer. It remains the most accurate technique to assess superior mediastinal lymph nodes, which are frequently involved in this disease. The procedure is safe and effective in experienced hands. In two large trials the mortality rate was 0% and the major morbidity rate was less than 1%. Patients suspected of having locally advanced disease on the basis of direct tumor extension to the mediastinum, enlarged lymph nodes on CT scan, or mediastinal uptake on PET scan, should undergo mediastinoscopy for definitive staging of their disease.

Standard mediastinoscopy is useful for biopsying lymph nodes in the upper and lower paratracheal regions, precarinal sites, and subcarinal lymph node stations. Lymph nodes within the aortopulmonary window and along the ascending aorta (stations 5 and 6) that are not accessible by standard mediastinoscopy techniques can be evaluated by extended mediastinoscopy, anterior mediastinotomy (Chamberlain procedure), or video-assisted thoracoscopic techniques. Data suggest that EUS plus FNA may also be a reliable method for evaluation of station 5 lymph nodes.[124] Because this is often the first level of mediastinal nodes involved in left upper lobe cancers, many practitioners defer such examinations when cervical mediastinoscopy fails to demonstrate metastatic disease in the superior mediastinum unless these lymph nodes appear involved on imaging studies. Patients without superior mediastinal lymph node involvement may have a relatively good prognosis after resection, even when anterior mediastinal lymph nodes (stations 5 or 6) are microscopically involved.

The routine use of mediastinoscopy before surgical intervention for lung cancer remains controversial. With mediastinoscopy, inoperable superior (N3) mediastinal disease can be identified and unnecessary thoracotomies thereby avoided. Some investigators argue that mediastinoscopy is not necessary for the management of peripheral nodules smaller than 3 cm in diameter (T1) with no abnormalities detected on chest radiograph or chest CT scan, because the likelihood of occult metastatic disease in N2 lymph nodes in these circumstances is 10% to 15%.[130] Currently, it is reasonable to forego mediastinoscopy in patients with clinical stage I disease who have no evidence of mediastinal uptake on FDG-PET scan given the negative predictive value of this imaging modality. However, any patient entering prospective trials for treatment of early lung cancer should undergo mediastinoscopy (or other invasive procedure) for definitive staging of their tumor. Furthermore, patients with more locally advanced disease (clinical stage II or III) should undergo mediastinoscopy to rule out inoperable N3 disease and identify those individuals with N2 disease who might be considered for induction therapy before surgery.

THORACENTESIS

Thoracentesis of a pleural effusion associated with presumed lung cancer can identify inoperable pleural disease (T4). Typically, a bloody pleural effusion is malignant; however, unless malignant cells are identified, a bloody pleural effusion should be considered traumatic. In general, thoracentesis can yield a diagnosis of cancer in 70% of malignant effusions. If the initial thoracentesis result is negative, additional percutaneous thoracenteses may improve the diagnostic yield; otherwise, thoracoscopy can be used to simultaneously drain the pleural fluid for cytologic examination and obtain pleural as well as lymph node tissue for diagnosis.

THORACOSCOPY

Video-assisted thoracoscopy has been used in the diagnosis, staging, and resection of lung cancer with increasing frequency. Peripheral nodules can be identified and excised using video-assisted, minimally invasive techniques, and mediastinal lymph nodes can be sampled for histologic examination. This technique is also extremely valuable for evaluation and palliation of suspected pleural disease, particularly when thoracentesis has been nondiagnostic. Currently, thoracoscopy is ideal for assessment of mediastinal nodes not accessible by standard mediastinoscopy or EUS-FNA techniques and for evaluation of suspected T4 lesions.

THORACOTOMY

More than 95% of tumors can and should be accurately diagnosed and staged before thoracotomy. Nevertheless, in a small minority of individuals, the diagnosis of lung cancer is only made at thoracotomy. In general, these are cases in which there is a large inflammatory component associated with a small focus of cancer that obscures diagnosis. During thoracotomy the diagnosis often can be obtained via multiple FNAs with immediate cytologic analysis or incisional (or preferably excisional) biopsy with frozen-section examination. Additional intraoperative biopsies of hilar and mediastinal lymph nodes should be performed, with resection of the primary lesion and complete MLND undertaken if indicated on the basis of intra-operative staging. Not infrequently, unsuspected involvement of adjacent structures is recognized only at the time of surgery.

LUNG CANCER SCREENING

Given the data that survival of lung cancer patients is contingent on disease stage at the time of detection and that most patients present with advanced incurable disease, it would seem that early detection might result in more favorable outcomes for these individuals. To date, however, there are no prospective randomized trials demonstrating that screening has a survival impact in patients destined to develop lung cancer.

The interest in mass screening for lung cancer dates back to the 1950s. At that time resection was, and to date remains, the treatment of choice, especially in patients with stage I disease. Numerous population-based as well as randomized, controlled trials were conducted from the 1960s through the 1980s, all of which used plain chest radiography (CXR) with or without sputum cytology for cancer detection.[131–141] Overall, these trials demonstrated no benefit from either screening modality alone or in combination regarding reduction of lung cancer–specific mortality. These data are the basis for the recommendations of the National Cancer Institute (NCI) and the American Cancer Society that screening should not be offered routinely to patients at high risk for lung cancer and that people with signs and symptoms of this disease should consult their physicians. Recently, low-dose CT (LDCT) has become available as a screening tool, once again prompting interest in mass screening for lung cancer and reigniting old controversies regarding this disease.[141–144]

PLAIN RADIOGRAPHY SCREENING TRIALS

Between 1952 and 1972, at least five nonrandomized trials were conducted in Europe and the United States to evaluate CXR, with or without sputum cytology, as a screening modality for lung cancer.[131,132] The most notable of these studies was the North London Lung Cancer Study in which 55,034 patients were nonrandomly assigned to receive a plain CXR every 6 months for 3 years (screened group) or a single CXR at the beginning and end of the 3-year period (control group).[132] After 3 years, there were more cases of lung cancer in the screened group than in the control group (132 vs. 96). In addition, more of the cancers in the screened group were resected (44% vs. 29%). Nonetheless, after 5 years of screening and a median follow-up of 3 years, no difference in lung cancer–specific mortality was noted between the two groups.

RANDOMIZED TRIALS

In the 1970s, the NCI reexamined the question of mass screening for lung cancer through the establishment and funding of the Co-operative Early Lung Cancer Group. This group in turn initiated randomized trials at the Johns Hopkins Hospital, the Memorial Sloan-Kettering Cancer Center (MSKCC), and the

Mayo Clinic Foundation.[134,135,137] The trials at Johns Hopkins Hospital and MSKCC assessed the incremental benefit of sputum cytology as a screening tool in individuals undergoing radiographic screening. At each center, nearly 10,000 men older than 45 years of age who smoked at least one pack of cigarettes daily were randomly assigned to receive an annual CXR alone or an annual CXR and sputum cytology every 4 months. After 5 years of screening and 5 years of follow-up, there was no difference between the two groups in the number of detected cancers, resectability rates, or lung cancer–specific deaths. The authors concluded that the addition of routine sputum cytology to a program of periodic radiographic examination did not decrease lung cancer mortality.[137,139]

The Mayo Lung Project (MLP) examined the combined impact of CXR and sputum cytology compared to usual care.[136] Males older than 45 years of age who were current smokers (at least one pack per day) were randomly assigned after baseline screening either to receive annual CXR with sputum cytology every 4 months or to receive advice to follow the Mayo Clinic recommendations concerning annual CXR and sputum cytology (no reminders were sent). After a median follow-up of 3 years (range, 1.0 to 5.5 years), there were more cancers in the screened group than in the unscreened group (206 cases vs. 160 cases). In addition, the screened group had significantly more stage I and II tumors (48% vs. 32%). The 5-year survival rate was also higher for the cases in the screened group (33% vs. 15%). Of interest, there was no difference between the two groups in the number of cases with advanced disease (123 vs. 119) or lung cancer–specific deaths (122 vs. 115).[137] Another analysis done 15 years later[138] confirmed no significant difference in disease-specific mortality (the primary requisite of successful screening) between the two groups.

A fourth trial was conducted in Czechoslovakia in which 6364 men were randomly assigned to receive annual CXR and sputum cytology for 3 years or an initial screening with CXR and sputum cytology, both of which were repeated at the end of the 3-year period.[140,141] After the initial 3-year period, both groups were screened annually for an additional 3 years. The results were essentially the same as those for the MLP, with more cancers and more earlier-stage tumors detected in the screened group. Nonetheless, disease-specific mortality was unchanged by the more intensive screening regimen.

PERSPECTIVE

Despite the consistency of the results from all four randomized trials, the recommendation against screening remains controversial. An important observation put forward by the International Union Against Cancer in 1984 was that none of the studies, including the MLP, incorporated a completely unscreened control group.[145] In the Johns Hopkins Hospital and MSKCC studies, an annual CXR was performed in the control as well as in the screened groups, and in the Czech study the control group was screened in 4 of the 6 years of the study period. In the MLP trial, individuals in the control group were given the standard Mayo advice of annual CXR and sputum cytology, and 50% of them followed surveillance recommendations. The absence of a genuine control arm almost certainly confounded these studies, which potentially missed a modest yet clinically important effect of screening, such as a 10% to 20% reduction in lung cancer mortality.[146,147] A number of other potentially important design flaws have been reviewed, including the short duration of screening, which may have precluded realization of its full impact, as well as the use of average mortality across all study years as the outcome measure—a likely insensitive indicator of successful screening, because disease-specific mortality changes over time as screening continues.[148]

LOW-DOSE COMPUTED TOMOGRAPHY

Since its introduction into clinical practice in the early 1980s, CT has proven to be more sensitive than CXR for the detection of pulmonary nodules. Technologic advances in the early 1990s significantly reduced the radiation dose and enabled scanning of the entire chest within a single breath-hold. These advances contributed to a resurgence of interest in screening for lung cancer. Projects were initiated by the National Cancer Center in Tokyo, Japan,[142] and the Early Lung Cancer Action Project (ELCAP) in New York.[143] In Japan, chest LDCT was added to an existing lung cancer screening program using CXR.[142] A report summarized the Tokyo experience for a total of 1611 individuals. The majority (88%) were men who were either current or former smokers (86%) between 40 and 79 years of age.[149] All participants also underwent simultaneous CXR and sputum cytologic analysis. At the initial screen, a positive test result was noted in 11.5%, 3.4%, and 0.8% using LDCT, CXR, and sputum cytology, respectively. Fourteen lung cancers (0.87%) were detected among all 1611 participants at baseline, ten of which (72%) were stage I disease with a mean tumor diameter of 19.8 mm. At repeat screening, LDCT gave a positive result in 9.1% of patients versus 2.6% and 0.7% for CXR and sputum cytology, respectively. Twenty-two additional cancers were detected (0.28%), 82% of which were stage IA with a mean tumor diameter of 14.6 mm. Of the 36 cancers detected, 70% were discovered on CT alone. Five-year survival was 76% for those patients whose cancers were detected at baseline and 64% for those whose cancers were detected on the repeat screen. ELCAP conducted a prospective study at Weill Medical College of Cornell University, recruiting 1000 asymptomatic individuals at risk for lung cancer for baseline and annual repeat screening. At enrollment, participants had a median age of 67 years and a median 47-pack-year smoking history.[143] All had simultaneous CXR and CT scans. At baseline, 233 individuals (23%) had an abnormality detected by CT scans. Lung cancer was diagnosed in 27 patients (2.7%), 23 (85%) of whom had stage IA disease. Only 7 (25%) of the 27 malignancies were seen on CXR. Two additional cases were diagnosed as a result of symptoms before the first annual repeat screening. These findings show that CT screening led to a high proportion of screening-related diagnoses (27 of 29), a result that was different from the experience for screening by CXR.[148] On the annual repeat screen, 2.5% of individuals had a positive finding on CT.[148] Nine cancers were detected (0.6%), of which seven were stage IA.

The largest study reported to date was conducted by Sone et al.[144] in Japan. Using a mobile CT unit, these investigators performed baseline screening on 5483 individuals (aged 40 to 74 years) in the general population, an important distinction from the aforementioned studies, which only evaluated high-risk individuals. Abnormal scans were noted in 5% of individuals, and the malignancy rate was 0.48%. On annual repeat, 3.8% of participants had an abnormal scan, and the malig-

nancy rate was 0.41%. Of the 60 detected cancers, 55 (88%) were stage IA.

LDCT screening trials have now been conducted by various centers in the United States and Europe. Results of these studies are consistent with data reported by ELCAP and Japanese investigators.[150–153] All studies have shown that LDCT is superior to traditional CXR for lung cancer detection. Although the rate of false-positive findings at baseline (prevalence) screening was relatively high, the rate has been generally lower on the repeat (incidence) scans. These studies have also confirmed the influence of age and smoking history on the rate of malignancy, with the lowest rate reported in patients over 40 years of age without a smoking history (0.4%) and the highest rate among 60-year-old current or former smokers. Finally, the majority of lung cancers detected in these LDCT screening programs were stage IA. Collectively, these data warrant further studies to define more precisely the cohorts at risk, refine the screening and subsequent diagnostic algorithms, and establish the most appropriate design to assess the eventual impact of LDCT screening on lung cancer–specific mortality. Criticism of LDCT screening pertains to its unproven impact on lung cancer mortality, its cost effectiveness, and the potential harm to a patient faced with what eventually proves to be a false-positive finding. A detailed rebuttal of these concerns is beyond the scope of this chapter; however, a point of particular concern is the impact of CT screening on lung cancer–specific mortality. The concern is based mainly on the concept of overdiagnosis, one of several biases believed to be inherent in mass screening programs.

OVERDIAGNOSIS

Overdiagnosis is defined as the detection of tumors—usually in the context of screening programs—that despite histologic evidence of malignancy represent biologically indolent diseases that would not manifest during the individual's natural life span. Although this concept may seem almost heretical to practicing lung cancer clinicians, it is an acknowledged bias of any mass screening program. Much of the evidence for overdiagnosis in lung cancer is based on the finding of more cases of lung cancer in the screened cohort of the MLP than in the control cohort (206 vs. 160). Because the lung cancer–specific mortality was essentially similar in both cohorts (3.2 of 1000 vs. 3.0 of 1000), it is possible that the 46 additional cancers detected in the screened cohort were due to overdiagnosis, that is, represented pseudodisease that had no apparent ill effect.[154,155] The same reasoning was proposed by the extended follow-up of the MLP, because on reanalysis, disease-specific mortality remained nearly the same (4.4 of 1000 vs. 3.9 of 1000) despite an excess of cases of early-stage disease in the screened cohort.[138] On the other hand, the evidence against overdiagnosis on CXR screening in the MLP is compelling. When left unresected, screen-detected stage I lung cancer had a virulently malignant course, with fewer than 10% of patients remaining alive at 5 years.[156] A more detailed analysis of the growth rate of lung cancers in the MLP and MSKCC projects provides compelling evidence supporting the aggressive nature of these lesions.[157] Nearly all screen-detected stage I cancers found on CXR were not seen on prior chest radiographs. With a median size of 2 cm at diagnosis, the growth rate of these lesions is well within the growth rate typical of aggressive malignancies. However, one cannot dismiss altogether the probability of overdiagnosis within the context of CT screening. There is strong evidence that some categories of malignancy identified only on CT, such as the nonsolid or ground-glass opacities, may have no tendency toward nodal metastases and 100% curability with resection.[156] Although these lesions may represent truly indolent, overdiagnosed neoplasms, ground-glass opacities can have a solid component harboring invasive adenocarcinoma. To date, the natural history of ground-glass opacity has not been clearly defined.

CURRENT LUNG CANCER SCREENING TRIALS

Prostate, Lung, Colorectal, Ovarian Cancer Screening Trial

The Prostate, Lung, Colorectal, Ovarian Cancer screening trial is a complex, multicenter trial sponsored by the NCI with a target accrual of 150,000 people aged 55 to 74 years. Individuals are randomly assigned to undergo annual CXR for 2 to 3 years or routine medical care (no screening). Participants will be followed for 13 years. Accrual began in 1994 and was completed in 2001. The trial has an 89% power to detect a 10% reduction in lung cancer–specific mortality. Final analysis is expected around 2014.

National Lung Screening Trial

The National Lung Screening Trial is sponsored by the NCI's Division of Cancer Prevention. Participants will be men and women 55 to 74 years of age who have smoked at least 30 pack-years. A total of 15,300 subjects will be randomly assigned to receive either LDCT or CXR with annual screening for 3 years and a 5-year follow-up period. The study is powered to detect a 50% reduction in lung cancer mortality by LDCT. The similarity of this design to that of the MLP leaves it subject to the same concerns previously discussed in Perspective.

New York Early Lung Cancer Action Project

The baseline results of the ELCAP[148] sparked considerable interest in screening for lung cancer and led to augmentation of the original 2-institution ELCAP conducted in New York City to another study, the NY-ELCAP, involving 12 institutions throughout New York State. A baseline and a single annual repeat screening were performed in more than 6000 high-risk individuals using the same indications for screening and design as in the original ELCAP. The design distinguishes between the diagnostic and intervention components of screening and addresses each component separately using a "diagnostic-prognostic" design.[158,159] The focus of the study is the assessment of the merits of a particular regimen of CT screening for lung cancer in terms of its diagnostic yield.

International Early Lung Cancer Action Project

The goal of the international ELCAP is to perform 30,000 baseline and repeat screenings at institutions throughout the world with the goal of addressing the issue of overdiagnosis and curative effectiveness of early intervention in a LDCT-screened population. It was started in 2001 and left each institution free to set its own indications for screening, provided that a standardized protocol was used for screening. This study will permit pooling of data to estimate the extent of overdiagnosis by comparing the curability of resected and unresected early-stage disease.

CHEMOPREVENTION

In light of the fact that lung cancers arise from the stochastic accumulation of genetic events that activate protooncogenes and silence tumor suppressors,[11] it is conceivable that compounds that ameliorate these effects might prove efficacious for lung cancer prevention. Considerable efforts have been under way to investigate a variety of agents for the prevention of lung cancer in high-risk patients. Overall, despite encouraging preclinical data, the results of large chemoprevention trials evaluating primary prevention (in healthy high-risk smokers), secondary prevention (in those with premalignant lesions), and tertiary prevention (in previously treated individuals with second primary tumors) have been discouraging.[160] At least seven well-designed phase II and phase III trials have failed to demonstrate efficacy of retinoids, including retinal, retinal palmitate, isotretinoin, and β-carotene, for primary, secondary, or tertiary prevention of lung cancer. Interestingly, β-carotene appears to increase lung cancer risk in current as well as former smokers, apparently via formation of oxidative metabolites that induce P-450 enzymes and decrease the levels of retinoic acid receptor beta and retinoid X receptor. Additional studies have shown no decrease in lung cancer risk in patients receiving vitamin E (α-tocopherol) or selenium supplements.[160]

Data have implicated erbB1 and erbB2, ras, COX-2, and protein kinase C in modulating growth and metastasis of lung cancer cells. For this reason, inhibitors of these pathways are attractive agents for evaluation in lung cancer prevention trials.[161,162] Furthermore, given the relevance of epigenetic mechanisms of gene expression in lung cancer cells, it is conceivable that DNA demethylating agents and histone deacetylase inhibitors may also prove beneficial for lung cancer prevention.[163] In general these newer compounds, which target critical signal transduction pathways and alter global chromatin structure, appear more potent than retinoids, and clinical trials evaluating a number of these agents either are currently under way or will be initiated in the near future.

OVERVIEW OF INVASIVE LUNG CANCER MANAGEMENT: TREATMENT MODALITIES

Historically, surgery has provided the best chance of cure for resectable NSCLC. Whenever surgery is not an option in patients with potentially resectable cancers who are unable to tolerate resection, radiotherapy has been used for local control of the primary tumor and regional lymphatic metastases. As a single modality, chemotherapy is rarely curative in lung cancer patients; however, complete responses and prolonged survivals occasionally have been seen in patients with advanced locoregional as well as metastatic disease. During the past 20 years, combined modality therapies have been extensively evaluated as a means to enhance survival in patients with resectable as well as unresectable disease.

SURGERY

In general, surgery is the best treatment modality for patients whose lung cancers are limited to the hemithorax and can be

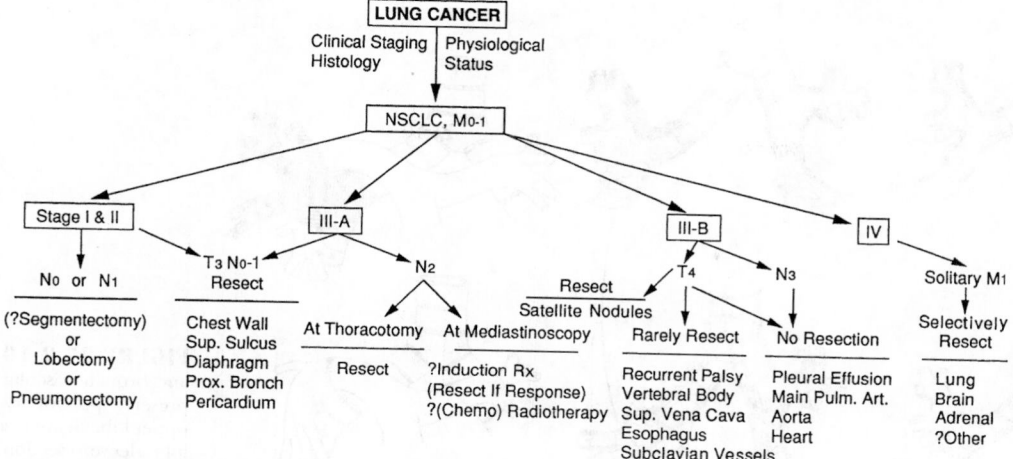

FIGURE 27.2-9.   Schema for operability at the various stages of non–small cell lung cancer (NSCLC). See text for details. Chemo, chemotherapy; Prox. Bronch, proximal bronchus; Pulm. Art., pulmonary artery; Rx, therapy; Sup., superior.

totally encompassed by excision (Fig. 27.2-9). In stage I and stage II disease, when the tumor has not extended beyond the bronchopulmonary lymph nodes, complete (R0) resections are almost always feasible. Currently, controversy arises regarding the management of N2 disease. Ipsilateral N2 mediastinal lymph node involvement, despite being potentially resectable, typically portends limited survival after resection alone. Because of this, pathologic staging of the mediastinum is critical for determining treatment and prognosis for individuals with locally advanced lung cancer. Patients in whom N2 disease is identified preoperatively have a much poorer prognosis than individuals with occult N2 disease discovered only at the time of thoracotomy (less than 10% vs. 30% 5-year survival rates, respectively).

Stage IIIB disease by virtue of incontrovertible evidence of contralateral (N3) lymph node metastases or invasion of vital structures such as carina, heart, or great vessels (T4) or the presence of a malignant pleural effusion (T4) typically is inoperable. Similarly, lung cancer that has metastasized to distant organs (stage IV disease) is generally incurable by surgery. Occasionally individuals with solitary brain or adrenal gland metastases may achieve long-term survival after resection of the primary and metastatic lesions.

Patient Selection

The preoperative evaluation of patients considered for surgical treatment of lung cancer includes clinical staging of the disease to determine resectability and assessment of the cardiopulmonary reserve of the patient to determine whether the intended pulmonary resection can be performed with acceptable perioperative risk. Studies best suited to assess cardiopulmonary reserve include spirometry with diffusion capacity, arterial blood gas concentrations, quantitative ventilation-perfusion scans, and oxygen consumption studies, as well as echocardiography, cardiac radionuclide scans, and cardiac MRI. Traditionally, patients have been deemed suitable candidates for pulmonary resection if the expected postoperative forced expiratory volume in 1 second (FEV_1) and diffusing

capacity of the lung for carbon monoxide (DLCO) equal or exceed 40% of the predicted value and the patient does not suffer from hypercapnia or pulmonary hypertension. More recent data[164] suggest that individuals in whom preoperative FEV_1 and DLCO values exceed 60% of the predicted values are at low risk for adverse effects from pulmonary resection including pneumonectomy and need no additional pulmonary studies. In contrast, patients with preoperative FEV_1 and DLCO values of less than 60% should undergo quantitative ventilation-perfusion scans to predict the impact of the intended resection on overall pulmonary reserve. Patients in whom postoperative predicted FEV_1 or DLCO values, or both, are less than 40% or individuals with pCO_2 of more than 45% should undergo exercise testing (oxygen consumption studies) using cycle ergometry with increasing workloads to further assess perioperative risk. In general, patients with expected postoperative FEV_1 and DLCO values of less than 40% of predicted values but with a maximal oxygen consumption (MVO_2) of more than 15 mL/kg can undergo pulmonary resection including pneumonectomy with acceptable risk. Patients with expected postoperative FEV_1 and DLCO values of less than 40% predicted and an MVO_2 of less than 15 mL/kg have increased risk of perioperative pulmonary complications and death, and should be considered for nonsurgical, palliative therapy. However, some individuals with small peripheral lesions and MVO_2 of less than 15 mL/kg may be candidates for limited resection, although such interventions should be individualized and patients should be informed regarding the increased risk of these procedures.

Surgical Procedures

Whereas pneumonectomy was initially considered the operation of choice for managing all lung cancers, lobectomy is currently the standard of care, provided it will result in complete *en bloc* resection of the tumor mass.[165] Recently, there has been a resurgence of interest in smaller resection for early-stage carcinomas. Jensik et al.[166] reported that survival as well as morbidity and mortality of segmentectomy for T1 to 2/N0 peripheral

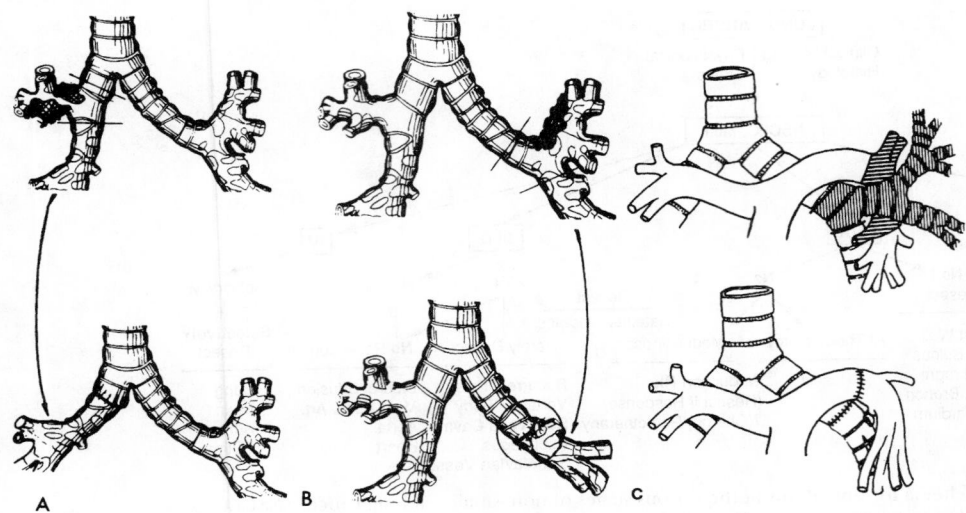

FIGURE 27.2-10. Bronchoplastic and bronchovascular sleeve resections to preserve pulmonary function. **A:** Right upper lobe sleeve resection. **B:** Left upper lobe sleeve resection. **C:** Left upper lobe bronchovascular sleeve resection.

lung cancers were equivalent to lobectomy. However, more recent data suggest that locoregional recurrence may be increased and survival decreased when less than a lobectomy is performed for early-stage adenocarcinomas. For proximally situated tumors (T3) for which pneumonectomy traditionally would be required for total excision, parenchyma-preserving operations using bronchoplastic or angioplastic techniques [e.g., sleeve lobectomy (SL)] (Fig. 27.2-10) yield survival results equivalent to those for pneumonectomy, and should be performed whenever possible.

The most common complications after lung cancer surgery are not related to technical failures of the operation but rather are due to cardiopulmonary problems, particularly supraventricular arrhythmias and respiratory failure. Because of improved surgical and anesthetic techniques and perioperative care, the postoperative mortality rates for surgical resection in lung cancer patients have decreased remarkably during the past 50 years. Currently, pneumonectomy can typically be performed with a mortality rate of less than 6%, lobectomy with a mortality rate of less than 3%, and smaller resections with a mortality rate of 1% or less.

RADIOTHERAPY

Radiotherapy is perhaps the most versatile treatment for NSCLC of any stage because it does not require fitness for surgery or the ability to tolerate chemotherapy. Regardless of comorbidities or age, radiotherapy can be used safely by modifying dose, volume of treatment, fractionation of total dose, and how and if it is integrated with other modalities. In unresectable disease, it remains the primary modality in conjunction with chemotherapy for the cure of tumor. In the postoperative setting, its role as an adjuvant treatment to improve local control continues to be postulated. Radiotherapy palliates advanced and metastatic lung cancer.

The vast bulk of radiotherapy for NSCLC is delivered via external-beam radiotherapy, most commonly with a linear accelerator. Newer techniques, such as three-dimensional conformal radiotherapy (3D-CRT) and intensity-modulated radiotherapy (IMRT), improve delivery of external-beam radiotherapy by more accurately defining targets to treat and protect and thereby causing fewer side effects. This permits delivery of higher doses of radi-

ation to the tumor target and increased sparing of normal tissues. Brachytherapy is another treatment modality that is used with both curative and palliative intent. Alterations in dose fractionation, such as hyperfractionation, are attempts to take advantage of the biologic behavior of tumors and normal tissue to optimize repair of radiation damage and limit tumor repopulation.

The maximum tolerated dose of radiotherapy to the thorax has yet to be established. Standard therapy for unresectable disease in North America and Europe has consisted of 60 to 65 Gy over approximately 6 weeks, commonly treating the gross tumor and regional lymph nodes. When patients receiving 65 Gy were carefully evaluated for local tumor control, only 15% were found to be free of disease after treatment.[167] Radiation resistance to the moderate dose levels (60 to 65 Gy) typically used represents a major factor contributing to the high incidence of local failure. Higher doses appear to be required for improved local control.[168] A phase I to II protocol[169] of hyperfractionated radiotherapy established that a dose of 69.2 Gy can be safely delivered using a twice-daily scheme of 1.2 Gy/fraction, which is intended to lower late effects. Currently, dose-escalation protocols using accepted once-daily treatment investigated the upper limits of dose that can be tolerated. Doses as high as 102.9 Gy for small tumors and 81 Gy for large tumors have been delivered safely.[170–172] The issue of dose escalation needs to be considered in the context of volume of irradiation and integration with chemotherapy, which has become a standard part of therapy in many stages.

External-Beam Radiotherapy

External-beam radiotherapy produced by high-energy photon beams generated by a linear accelerator is the workhorse of radiotherapy departments throughout the world. Radiation oncologists balance the toxicity to the lung, spinal cord, esophagus, and other thoracic structures against the need to deliver effective doses to control locoregional tumor. Beam delivery and weighting as well as energy, number of beams, and beam direction all require treatment planning. Currently, this sophistication requires treatment-planning systems that allow for precise definition of tumor and target volumes and definition of structures to be protected. What constitutes the target (surely the observed tumor and any regional nodes clearly harboring cancer) is being rethought in light of the fact that the former total nodal method required a very large volume and that volume may preclude dose escalation to levels that may control tumors of any size. With volume reduction targets, higher doses can be achieved, but clinical studies have yet to demonstrate the appropriate volume of treatment, given dose escalation and integration of chemotherapy. New imaging modalities, such as FDG-PET scanning, have been used to help to define tumor volumes.[173] The treatment field should be verified on the treatment machine before the initiation of radiotherapy. Treatment fields should also be checked weekly so that adjustments can be made.

Acute side effects occurring during the course of radiotherapy are organ specific. These side effects depend on what organs and how much of the organs is included in what proportion of the treatment dose and are related to the fractionation scheme, total dose, and use of sequential or concomitant chemotherapy or radiosensitizers. They typically manifest in the second to third week of treatment. A significant concern of combined therapy is the increased toxicity, which may outweigh the benefit from using both modalities.

Delayed acute radiation toxicity typically occurs within 1 to 3 months after completing treatment but has been known to occur as late as 6 months after completion of therapy. Organs at risk include normal lung, esophagus, spinal cord, and heart. Radiation factors include fraction size, overall treatment time, radiation dose, and volume of normal organ treated, all of which contribute to acute and delayed toxicity for conventional fractionation with radiotherapy. Similarly, the use of concurrent chemotherapy, as well as novel fractionation regimens, can lower the threshold for delayed tissue reactions.[174]

PULMONARY TOXICITY. Animal models have demonstrated increased vascular permeability after thoracic irradiation.[175] Alveolar surfactant levels also increase after thoracic irradiation and, owing to increased vascular permeability, surfactant is detectable in the serum.[176] This endothelial injury may lead to an inflammatory response, causing the clinical syndrome of radiation pneumonitis. Elevated serum levels of transforming growth factor-α, a growth factor known to stimulate connective tissue formation, have been demonstrated in patients developing lung toxicity.[177]

Radiation-induced clinical pneumonitis is a diagnosis of exclusion and consists of a syndrome of cough, dyspnea, fever, and an abnormal chest radiograph. It is the most commonly observed delayed acute reaction, usually occurring between 1 and 3 months after completion of radiotherapy. Patients with pneumonitis typically present with shortness of breath on exertion, tachypnea, tachycardia, fever, and nonproductive cough. CXR often shows an infiltrate within the irradiated volume[178]; however, with the use of conformal ports, the shape of the infiltrate may be less easy to discern. Chest CT scanning is often helpful in showing characteristic changes that do not conform to known anatomic planes. Often one can see pneumonitis that forms a "straight line" on CT—a finding that is not commonly seen with either infection or inflammatory states of the lung. These symptoms mimic a respiratory infection, which must be ruled out before starting treatment with steroids. Lymphangitic spread of tumor must be considered in the differential diagnosis as well. Although the effects of radiation

pneumonitis are sometimes self-limiting, it is a potentially life-threatening process. The use of corticosteroids (prednisone) at a starting dosage of 1 mg/kg/d, followed by a carefully controlled slow taper, usually resolves most clinical symptoms of pneumonitis. Corticosteroids, however, appear to reduce the ability of alveolar macrophages to release tumor necrosis factor in response to infectious agents, which can lead to recurrent respiratory tract infections in patients treated chronically with these drugs.[179]

Enhancement of radiation injury by chemotherapy in terms of acute and late effects appears to be increased with concurrent treatment, with a tendency for damage to decline as the interval between drug and radiation is increased.[180,181] Roach et al.[182] retrospectively analyzed radiotherapy parameters in 24 combined modality Radiation Therapy Oncology Group (RTOG) trials completed before 1994, involving more than 1911 patients with both small cell lung cancer and NSCLC, to determine potential risk factors for radiation pneumonitis when radiation is combined with chemotherapy. Multiple fractionation schemes, total doses, and fraction sizes, along with several chemotherapeutic regimens, were used. The overall incidence of pneumonitis was 7.8%. Factors associated with a higher risk included fraction size higher than 2.67 Gy and total dose. Twice-daily radiation, however, appeared to reduce the risk expected if the same total daily dose were given as a single fraction. Based on this analysis, radiotherapy at a high dose per fraction combined with chemotherapy should be avoided. Confounding these findings is the relatively constant large treatment portals used in that era. Safety and efficacy of conformal, small-volume, stereotactic radiotherapy for lung cancer is now being explored.

Late radiation injury may be related more to the dose per fraction and total dose. The degree of late pulmonary toxicity and fibrosis is directly proportional to the volume of normal lung irradiated and the total dose delivered, as well as the fraction size. It is not clear whether chemotherapy actually modifies the latency period for the development of late pulmonary reactions or increases the incidence. For patients presenting with reduced pulmonary function, however, and for patients who develop severe clinical pneumonitis, a distortion of the pulmonary architecture by fibrosis can have a major impact on the quality of life and functional status. Most of these findings antedate use of reduced volume and conformal techniques, and it is accepted that volume is a critical factor contributing to frequency and intensity of radiation-related pneumonitis. Similarly, concurrent chemotherapy is more frequently employed, and certain drugs are clearly difficult to use with thoracic radiotherapy, namely, bleomycin, doxorubicin, and busulfan. Probably detrimental are all alkylators, but especially the nitrosoureas, and mitomycin C. Of the newer drugs, the taxanes and gemcitabine are potential pulmonary toxins alone. Platinum and carboplatinum are well suited for use with thoracic radiotherapy.

ESOPHAGEAL TOXICITY. Because the esophagus has a central location adjacent to mediastinal lymph nodes, it is exposed to high-dose radiation during the treatment of NSCLCs, especially when elective nodal irradiation is used. Radiation may induce acute esophagitis during the course of therapy. Histologic changes occur during the first week of treatment,[183] although clinical symptoms typically begin during the second through fourth weeks of treatment. Esophagitis presents with mild to severe swallowing difficulty requiring diet modification, topical anesthesia (viscous lidocaine), and nonnarcotic or narcotic analgesics, depending on severity. It is caused by an inflammatory response of the esophageal mucosa.[183] Some have considered acute esophageal toxicity dose limiting; however, the transient discomfort almost always resolves. Stricture is unacceptable, but most patients can be coaxed through esophagitis with liquids and narcotics without requiring hospitalization or developing stricture. If the patient can be supported and there are no long-term effects, it does not measure up to a dose-limiting standard. Stricture may be related to total dose, volume, fraction size, and chemotherapy agents used and how they are sequenced.

Chemotherapy and radiosensitizers appear to accelerate the onset and severity of esophageal symptoms. It is rare to see grade 3 or worse esophagitis with radiation alone, yet this is common in patients treated with combined modality (chemotherapy and radiation) regimens. In a randomized prospective Intergroup trial, the rate of grade 3 or worse esophagitis increased from 1.3% to 65.0% with the addition of concurrent cisplatin and etoposide to 50.4-Gy thoracic radiation.[184] When radiotherapy is used concurrently with carboplatin and paclitaxel, the rate of grade 3 or 4 esophageal toxicity has been reported to be approximately 25%.[183] Agents such as 5-fluorouracil, doxorubicin, cisplatin, and mitomycin intensify radiation-induced esophageal toxicity.[185–187] Acute esophagitis generally resolves shortly after the completion of radiotherapy, with few patients progressing to chronic esophagitis. The patient with chronic esophagitis may benefit from serial dilatation to prevent or relieve stricture formation. The factors of length of esophagus, total dose, and chemotherapeutic agent weigh heavily. Strictures occur only infrequently with cisplatin and etoposide combinations, even when higher doses of thoracic radiotherapy are used.

Hyperfractionated treatment increases acute esophageal toxicity. When 60 Gy given via accelerated hyperfractionation was compared to the same dose delivered via standard fractionation, the rate of grade 3 or worse acute esophageal toxicity increased from 9% to 35% ($P = .0017$).[188]

NEUROTOXICITY. A transient myelopathic syndrome (Lhermitte's syndrome) occurs rarely during the first 6 to 12 months after therapy and is manifested by dysesthesias and paresthesias affecting the upper extremities and shoulder girdles on flexion of the neck.[189] It is related to the total radiation dose, dose per fraction, and length of spinal cord irradiated. Lhermitte's syndrome is self-limiting and does not appear to be related to the development of late radiation myelitis.[190]

The spinal cord can tolerate conventionally fractionated radiotherapy doses in the range of 45 to 50 Gy. In some cases, depending on the volume of spinal cord treated and the dose per fraction, the tolerance has been reported to be as high as 60 to 70 Gy. In selected cases in which the tumor is paraspinal, it may be appropriate to treat a small portion of the cord to this dose with the patient's understanding of the potential toxicity.[191] There has been a concern that altered fractionation might lead to increased myelitis. Jeremic et al.[192] have reported no cases of radiation myelitis in 158 patients who lived at least 1 year after receiving hyperfractionated radiotherapy in fraction sizes of 1.2 Gy/d to a total dose of 50.4 Gy. Once it develops, radiation-induced transverse myelitis is irreversible.

CARDIAC TOXICITY. Cardiac toxicity has been reported after radiation therapy for Hodgkin's disease and breast cancer but is not a common late effect in lung cancer patients. Drawing an analogy between lung cancer and either breast cancer or Hodgkin's disease does not hold up. Some worry that the survival has been too poor and too short to assess the frequency of the problem. Old techniques limited cardiac silhouette doses to 40 to 45 Gy, a dose low enough to rarely cause problems in the diseases with longer survival. Radiation injury to the heart is usually manifested as pericarditis, although other complications such as myocardial ischemia and chronic pericardial effusions can occur. Because the tolerance for the entire heart is approximately 40 Gy and up to one-third of the heart can tolerate approximately 60 Gy,[193] the former standard dose delivered, one cannot have confidence about the tolerable doses to produce 5% toxicity. It is not clear that lung cancer patients have been reported to be harmed by cardiac toxicity, but the analogy to other diseases has guided protocols. Three-dimensional techniques (discussed later in Three-Dimensional Conformal Radiotherapy) allow the entire heart and the pericardium, chambers, and valves to be identified and doses recorded. The coronary arteries and their orifices cannot be detected at this time, but 3D-CRT allows increased dose to tumor and a cataloging of dose to all of the normal structures subtended by beams.

Three-Dimensional Conformal Radiotherapy

The technique of 3D-CRT allows for increasing dose to tumor targets and better restriction of dose away from normal structures to improve the local outcome of radiotherapy in NSCLC.[194,195] The major aim of this method is accurate definition of the target and delivery of dose to it. Three-dimensional technology and more sophisticated IMRT assure target dose but also record partial organ doses to tissues through which beams pass. Analytic tools are evolving that provide relative risks depending on dose and volume treated. This ability provides a potential for increasing the tumor dose to levels beyond those feasible with conventional radiotherapy, with a concomitant decrease in the probability of normal tissue complication. Single-institution and cooperative group studies of dose escalation to evaluate the efficacy of this strategy have been conducted.[170,171] The concept of V20, the volume of total lung that receives 20 Gy, has been introduced as a potential benchmark for comparing plans and assessing the relative risk for toxicity in the form of pneumonitis, grade 3 or 4 pneumonitis, and death from pneumonitis. The V20 concept has been embraced by some groups as established, but in fact more data are needed to determine the risk for higher cumulative doses. On the other hand, as more numerous and smaller beams are used to come at a variety of angles cross-firing at tumor targets, the total or integral lung doses, albeit small, may increase. Determination of the risk (especially long term) of the integral dose requires more data from long-term survivors regarding toxicity as well as induction of second tumors.

3D-CRT requires a CT data set for treatment planning. 3D-CRT provides tools such as beam's eye view, dose-volume histograms, and digitally reconstructed radiographs in addition to normal tissue and target rendering. A clinical tumor volume is defined in the axial plane of the CT images. A margin is subsequently added to the clinical tumor volume to generate the planning target volume. This margin compensates for tumor motion during treatment caused by breathing, patient movement, and setup error. The treatment beams are subsequently constructed using the beam's eye view technique. Because time also implies that there is motion, this has been called the fourth dimension. Compensating for motion with enlarging margin has been and continues to be used, but research is now probing other means such as automated breath-holding, gating, and tracking as means to assure target dose but minimize normal tissue exposure.

The use of 3D-CRT also allows investigators to predict more accurately the toxicity of a given course of radiotherapy. The normal tissue complication probability is an estimate of clinical toxicity based on the dose delivered to the volume of normal lung. It has been shown to correlate with incidence of radiation pneumonitis. Other institutions use either the mean lung dose or the dose that a given volume of lung receives as a determinant of lung toxicity. For example, in the RTOG dose-escalation protocol, the volume of lung receiving 20 Gy (V20) is used as a guide to what dose to deliver.[170] The frequency of grade 3 or 4 pneumonitis rises as a function of percentage of normal lung treated, but fatal pneumonitis is really only seen after 30% of normal lung is included.

Intensity-Modulated Radiotherapy

IMRT represents a new approach to radiotherapy in which the beam penetrance and target dose coverage change dynamically, with wafer-thin multileaf collimators either exposing target or protecting defined regions to give more radiotherapy to areas with tumor and less to areas of normal tissue.[196] Although the technology is widely available and used, its role in treatment of thoracic malignancies is not established and requires further evaluation.

Gated Radiotherapy

Motion of the tumor defeats attempts to use IMRT. Because of physiologic dynamic motions (heart beat, respiratory expansion and contraction, coughing, swallowing), the standard solution opened fields to accommodate the motion. This technique unnecessarily exposes normal lung, risks toxicity, and restricts dose escalation. It is impossible to use IMRT on moving targets. Lung tumors have been shown to move substantially during quiet breathing, which causes inaccuracies in treatment delivery.[197,198] Underdosage of the clinical tumor volume may result if the tumor target moves outside the treatment volume during the administration of radiotherapy. To compensate for this motion, a large margin is generally used, which consequently increases the amount of normal lung tissue in the high-dose volume and limits the amount of radiation that can be delivered.

To overcome this, techniques have been developed to "freeze-frame" the tumor during radiotherapy. Two techniques have been used to reduce the effect of respiratory motion. The first confines the radiation delivery to a specified phase in the breathing cycle by beaming the linear accelerator on during some phases of the respiratory cycle and off during others as the patient breathes freely. Breathing is monitored with devices that trigger radiation delivery during specific phases of the patient's respiratory cycle when the target is relatively frozen in

motion.[199] Gated treatments have been evaluated[199,200] and offer the advantage of allowing patients to breathe spontaneously during their radiation therapy. In the second approach, breathing is controlled either voluntarily by the patient[200] or by an occlusion valve.[201] This technique is less cumbersome electronically but requires more patient cooperation.

Stereotactic Radiotherapy

Stereotactic radiotherapy and stereotactic radiosurgery have been shown to be effective in treating brain metastases. Stereotactic radiotherapy is a technique in which a high dose of radiation is delivered to a small lesion, which minimizes dose to surrounding structures. This technique has been applied to lung tumors and has provided good local control.[202] Pilot studies have examined the role of body frame and single-fraction radiotherapy as well as fractionated techniques using multiple, very large doses (22 Gy/fraction for two or three fractions) or hypofractionated doses given over the course of 4 to 7 weeks.[203–211] The concept of targeting lung lesions without nodes but accommodating for respiratory motion requires further investigation. No clear data establish an optimal dose, and despite the nearly one dozen preliminary papers, toxicity end points and rates have not been established. The potential for this therapy includes treatment of very early lesions defined by screening studies, if the toxicity profile is not prohibitive. Furthermore, substituting these treatments for surgery requires information from controlled studies with longer follow-up. The clearly eligible patient subset is patients with medically inoperable lung cancer who do not have surgical options.

Neutron Therapy

Radiotherapy with fast neutrons has been examined as a potential modality to improve the results of therapy for NSCLC. The biologic properties of neutrons differ from those of conventional photons, with the former possessing the advantage of high linear energy transfer. This high linear energy transfer results in a number of effects, including greater relative biologic effectiveness, reduced oxygen enhancement ratio, less sublethal and potentially lethal damage repair, and less cell-cycle specificity than photons.[212]

A randomized trial involving 200 patients compared modern neutron therapy to a dose of 20.4 neutron Gy with 66 Gy of standard photons[213]; no difference in overall survival was noted in the two groups. Grade 3 or worse radiation pneumonitis occurred in 24% and 11% of the patients in the neutron and photon groups, respectively. Therefore, the role of neutron therapy for NSCLC remains unproven at this time, and the toxicity profile seems worse. The potential application of three-dimensional techniques and intensity modulation may be revisited at centers at which neutron-beam therapy is available. Restricted volumes may allow for higher doses, which may lead to improved tumor control and lower toxicity.

Brachytherapy

INTRAOPERATIVE INTERSTITIAL BRACHYTHERAPY AND RADIOTHERAPY. Intraoperative interstitial brachytherapy has been applied in the curative and palliative treatment of NSCLC. Implantation of radioactive sources offers an advantage over external irradiation because of the limited penetrability from source to prescription point, which results in rapid dose fall-off and sparing of surrounding normal tissues.

Indications for implantation include unresectable or incompletely resected tumors found at thoracotomy; hilar tumors adherent to major vasculature with no clearance for safe dissection; attachment of tumors to mediastinal structures, such as the trachea, pericardium, or esophagus; extensive tumor involvement of the chest wall, spine, or paravertebral tissue for which a complete resection is not possible; and recurrent or metastatic endobronchial lesions.[214]

For curative techniques, the selection of radioactive sources depends on the tumor location and the amount of gross disease remaining after surgery. In circumstances in which more than 1 cm of tumor is left behind, a permanent volume implant is usually required. The area to be implanted is determined, and its dimensions are measured. A nomogram is applied to determine the number of radioactive sources [iodine 125 (^{125}I) or palladium 103 (^{103}Pd)] needed and the proper spacing of the needles, which in turn are based on the strength of the sources and the average dimension of the tumor volume. Hollow needles are inserted into the tumor, and radioactive sources are permanently implanted. For close and positive margins or in the presence of a minimal plaque of residual gross disease, either a permanent planar or temporary interstitial implant may be used. For situations requiring permanent placement of radioactive sources, ^{125}I seeds encapsulated in Vicryl or ^{103}Pd seeds can either be directly sutured onto the area at risk or sewn into a premeasured Dexon or Vicryl mesh, which in turn is sutured onto the target area. A similar technique using ^{125}I embedded in a Gelfoam plaque has been described.[215] Both techniques allow implantation of radioactive seeds in areas near vital structures that cannot be directly sutured.[216]

Temporary implants containing iridium 192 (^{192}Ir) or ^{125}I provide either a low or a high dose-rate method of delivering radiation using afterloading catheters. Temporary implants have been advocated for tumors invading the chest wall, superior sulcus, mediastinum, and paravertebral regions when a complete resection is not certain. In general, the catheters are spaced 1 cm apart, with a 1-cm margin around the defined target, and exit out the chest wall. The catheters are then loaded with radioactive sources (^{125}I or ^{192}Ir) 4 or 5 days after surgery to allow for proper wound healing.

INTRALUMINAL BRACHYTHERAPY. Intraluminal brachytherapy or endobronchial brachytherapy (EBB) is generally used as a palliative treatment for obstructive recurrent tumors causing such symptoms as dyspnea and hemoptysis. This treatment directly introduces a high-activity ^{192}Ir source directly into the lumen of the tracheal or bronchial airway. Flexible bronchoscopic guidance is used to localize the tumor and to position a catheter beyond the site of disease. Patients are generally treated under a combination of monitored intravenous sedation and the application of local anesthesia to the larynx and trachea. The radioactive ^{192}Ir source is then introduced into the catheter and positioned. Treatment lasts only a couple of minutes because of the high activity of the source. High dose-rate intraluminal brachytherapy has largely replaced both direct interstitial implantation of ^{125}I seeds into endobronchial tumors and low dose-rate endobronchial irradiation.[217]

Side effects after intraluminal brachytherapy include massive hemoptysis, fistula formation, chronic mucosal sloughing, and airway edema.[218] Langendijk et al.[219] examined risk factors for massive hemoptysis. The highest complication rate occurred in patients receiving EBB for recurrent tumor (43%) or combination external-beam therapy and EBB (25%). They also found that patients receiving a single fraction of 15 Gy prescribed to 1 cm had a 50% rate of massive hemoptysis, whereas patients receiving 7.5 Gy two times or 10 Gy in a single fraction had an 11% rate. Hennequin et al.[220] theorized that most massive hemoptysis is from disease progression and not treatment toxicity. They reported a 7% risk of massive hemoptysis and concluded that all but one case had evidence of tumor progression. They also reported an 8.7% rate of radiation bronchitis. The risk factors for toxicity in their series included palliative intent of treatment and the length of bronchus treated.

Intraoperative Radiotherapy

Experience with the use of intraoperative radiotherapy for NSCLC is limited. This modality does not appear to show a significant benefit over external-beam irradiation alone or in combination with chemotherapy. The technique involves the modification of a linear accelerator through the attachment of an intraoperative cone for electron-beam treatment.[221] Both the optimal dose and threshold tolerance of mediastinal structures are unknown; however, one fraction is generally delivered intraoperatively at a dose of 10 to 20 Gy. The published results are conflicting. With no reported phase III trials, this modality must be considered experimental.

CHEMOTHERAPY

Overall, only 15% of all patients who present with NSCLC are cured. This dismal outcome is not due to the failure of surgery and radiation therapy to eradicate local regional disease but is the result of micrometastases present at the time of diagnosis. Therefore, to enhance the outcome of patients with lung cancer, systemic therapies must be developed that not only improve the cure rate for locoregional disease but also prolong survival in a significant manner for those individuals who present with metastatic disease.

Platinum-based combinations have become the standard of care for treating NSCLC. In 1988, Rapp et al.[222] reported that cisplatin-based chemotherapy improved survival of patients with metastatic lung cancer. Additional trials have confirmed these findings (Table 27.2-6) prompting widespread use of chemotherapy for palliation in patients with metastatic lung cancer. Cisplatin- or carboplatin-based doublets (often using docetaxel, gemcitabine, irinotecan, paclitaxel, or vinorelbine) are now standard for patients with stage IV and "wet" (pleural effusion) stage IIIB disease. There does not appear to be any advantage for the use of more than two drugs or the use of maintenance chemotherapy (see later in Stage IV Disease).

In addition to improving survival for patients with stage IV disease, chemotherapy may improve outcome for patients with locoregional disease. When used either in sequence or concurrently with radiation, platinum-based therapy prolongs median survival and increases the fraction of patients with stage III disease who are long-term survivors. Whereas some of this benefit may be due to improved local control, eradication of

TABLE 27.2-6. Results of Chemotherapy for Advanced Lung Cancer

Study	Regimen	No. of Patients	RR (%)	Survival Median (Mo)	Survival 1-Y (%)
Le Chevalier et al.[465]	Cisplatin and vinorelbine	206	30	9.3	35
	Cisplatin and vindesine	206	19	7.4	27
	Vinorelbine	206	14	7.2	30
Bonomi et al.[468]	Cisplatin and VP-16	150	12	7.7	32
	Cisplatin and paclitaxel, 135 mg 24 h	150	26.5	9.6	37
	Cisplatin and paclitaxel, 250 mg 24 h	150	32.1	10.0	39
Kelly et al.[488]	Carboplatin and paclitaxel	208	25	8	38
	Cisplatin and vinorelbine	202	25	8	36
Schiller et al.[572]	Cisplatin and paclitaxel, 135 mg 24 h	303	21.3	7.8	3.5
	Cisplatin and gemcitabine	301	21	8.1	4.5
	Cisplatin and docetaxel	304	17.3	7.4	3.6
Scagliotti et al.[512]	Cisplatin and gemcitabine	205	30	9.8	37
	Carboplatin and paclitaxel	201	32	9.9	43
	Cisplatin and vinorelbine	201	30	9.5	37

RR, response rate.

micrometastatic disease appears to be the principal mechanism by which chemotherapy improves survival of patients with locally advanced lung cancer.

Before 2003 there was little evidence to support the routine use of adjuvant chemotherapy after potentially curative resections in lung cancer patients. The International Adjuvant Lung Trial (IALT) and Cancer and Leukemia Group B (CALGB) studies suggest that adjuvant platinum-based chemotherapy used after surgical resection may improve survival of patients undergoing resection of stage I, II, or IIIA NSCLC.[223]

Neoadjuvant chemotherapy in which a specified number of chemotherapy cycles is administered before definitive local therapy with surgery or radiotherapy appears to be beneficial for locally advanced NSCLC. The simultaneous use of chemotherapy and radiotherapy (concomitant chemoradiotherapy) has also been intensively investigated. In theory, adjuvant and induction chemotherapy are administered to improve control of occult metastatic disease. Decreasing the size (down-staging) of the locoregional tumor burden may also be observed after induction therapy. The delay of radiotherapy to allow for administration of induction chemotherapy has been of theoretic concern, because this could lead to the proliferation of clonogenic tumor cells in an unresponsive tumor. Concomitant chemoradiotherapy may also result in systemic antitumor activity. However, this will be realized only if systemically active doses and schedules of the drugs are administered. In clinical practice, the latter has been challenging, because radiation-related toxicities (i.e., esophagitis and radiation pneumonitis) are usually increased in the presence of chemotherapy. Therefore, the primary goal of concomitant chemoradiotherapy may be to enhance the antitumor activity of radiation and increase locoregional control (radiation sensitization or enhancement).

Induction chemotherapy followed by radiotherapy prolongs the median survival time in patients with unresectable stage III disease compared with patients receiving radiotherapy alone.[224,225] Trials by Furuse et al.[226] and the RTOG[227] conclusively support the use of concurrent chemotherapy and radiation compared to sequential chemotherapy when treating locally advanced disease.

However, the toxicity of concurrent chemoradiotherapy is substantial, and for patients with an impaired performance status, sequential chemotherapy and radiation is preferred.

Chemotherapy has an emerging role in stage IIIA (N2) disease. The use of induction chemotherapy in the surgical setting (stage IIIA),[228,229] alone or in conjunction with radiotherapy,[230] results in a 5-year survival of 20% to 30% compared with 5% to 10% for surgery alone for clinical N2 disease. Intergroup data indicated a significant increase in progression-free survival in patients treated with chemoradiotherapy followed by surgery, but the anticipated improvement in survival of 10% was not evident.[231]

SPECIFICS OF LUNG CANCER MANAGEMENT

LOCALIZED "RESECTABLE" (STAGES I, II, AND IIIA) DISEASE

When disease is localized to the lung or includes only regional lymphatics, treatment typically involves surgery or radiation or both. Despite apparent eradication of local disease, patients most frequently succumb to distant metastases, which suggests that occult micrometastases were present at the time of initial treatment. In light of this, combined modality treatments presently are being evaluated in patients with resectable disease in an attempt to prolong survival by eliminating micrometastatic foci at the time of initial therapy.

Primary Surgery

Stage I and II lung cancer denotes disease limited to the hemithorax, with tumor extension no farther than the adjacent resectable structures peripherally (T3) or hilar nodes proximally (N1). In these cases, whenever possible, surgical excision is the treatment of choice.

In most instances, lobectomy is the procedure required. When the primary tumor or lymph node involvement extends to the proximal bronchus or proximal pulmonary artery (T3) or crosses the major fissure so that a complete resection is only possible by pneumonectomy, this more extensive procedure should be performed. When resectable adjacent structures (chest wall, diaphragm) are involved, an *en bloc* resection encompassing all sites of disease is necessary.

The role of mediastinal lymphadenectomy as part of the surgical procedure remains controversial. Whereas complete ipsilateral or bilateral mediastinal lymphadenopathy may improve accuracy of staging,[232] some investigators also feel that aggressive lymph node dissections improve survival. Keller et al.[233] randomly assigned 373 lung cancer patients to receive pulmonary resection with either systematic sampling (SS) or complete ipsilateral MLND. Although the percentages of patients with N1 and N2 disease were comparable in the two arms, more patients were found to have multilevel N2 disease in the MLND group. Patients who underwent MLND had statistically longer survivals compared to those evaluated by SS (64 vs. 25 months, respectively); the survival advantage in the MLND group was restricted to individuals with right-sided cancers (possibly due to the lack of complete resection of L2 and L4 lymph node stations in the MLND group). In another randomized trial involving 471 evaluable patients, Wu et al.[234] noted statistically significant improvement in survival of patients with stage I, II, and IIIA NSCLC after pulmonary resection with MLND compared to those undergoing lung resection with mediastinal lymph node sampling. In light of the fact that, in experienced hands, MLND does not significantly increase operative time or morbidity, it is reasonable to consider complete ipsilateral MLND dissection as standard of care in all lung cancer resections until unequivocal data indicate appropriate alternatives. A small randomized trial comparing mediastinal lymphadenectomy to mediastinoscopy plus intraoperative lymph node sampling showed no difference in survival, locoregional recurrence, or accuracy of the two staging procedures as applied to stage I or II lung cancer.[235] A larger phase III trial is under way in North America to address this issue.

In peripheral T1N0 tumors, the role of lesser resection (segmentectomy, wedge excision, or precision cautery dissection) has yet to be fully defined. A randomized trial conducted by the Lung Cancer Study Group (LCSG)[236] demonstrated that after long-term follow-up, the locoregional recurrence rate was threefold higher with limited resection than with lobectomy (15% vs. 5%), although morbidity, mortality, and pulmonary function were equal in both arms. A marginally significant long-term survival benefit was noted for lobectomy. In a retrospective review, Warren et al.[237] observed that locoregional recurrence was higher after segmentectomy than after lobectomy. However, this difference was primarily seen in stage II carcinomas; no survival difference was observed for T1N0 carcinomas resected by lobectomy or segmentectomy. To date, many of the studies comparing lobectomy to lesser resection for early-stage lung cancers have not been prospective randomized trials. Therefore, patients selected for segmentectomy or wedge resections tended to have more impaired pulmonary reserve and to exhibit other significant comorbidities. For this reason, overall survivals in these studies are difficult to assess because patients receiving limited resections suffered relatively more non–cancer-related deaths. Kodama et al.[238] compared segmentectomy to lobectomy for treatment of T1N0 carcinomas in patients with adequate pulmonary reserve for lobectomy. Overall 5-year survival, recurrence rates, and lung cancer–related deaths were comparable in the

two treatment arms; of note, however, the average tumor diameter was significantly larger in the lobectomy group than in the segmentectomy group (2.29 vs. 1.67 cm). Koike et al.[239] compared the results of limited resection in 74 patients with lobectomy in 159 patients for treatment of T1 (smaller than 2 cm) peripheral lung cancers. All patients had adequate pulmonary reserve for lobectomy. No significant differences were noted in 3-year or 5-year survival rates for these individuals.

Available data indicate that within the T1 category, increasing tumor size is associated with diminished survival after resection.[240] Watanabe et al.[241] observed mediastinal lymph node involvement in 11% of patients undergoing resection of clinical T1N0M0 lung cancers smaller than 2 cm in diameter; the majority of the lymph node metastases were associated with adenocarcinomas. Konaka et al.[242] retrospectively reviewed data for 171 consecutively treated patients undergoing resection of peripheral clinical T1N0M0 carcinomas smaller than 2 cm in diameter. Lymph node metastases were noted in 18% of patients (6% N1, 12% N2) and were more frequently associated with tumors 1.5 to 2.0 cm than with those less than 1.5 cm in diameter. No lymph node metastases were noted in patients with tumors smaller than 1 cm in diameter. In another retrospective series, Miller et al.[243] reviewed the Mayo Clinic experience pertaining to surgical treatment of 100 patients with lung carcinomas 1 cm or less in diameter. Seventy-five patients underwent lobectomy or bilobectomy, whereas 25 individuals had segmentectomy or wedge resections. Tumor diameters ranged from 3 to 10 mm. Seven patients had lymph node metastases. Lung cancer–specific 5-year survival was 85.4%; patients undergoing lobectomy had improved survival and fewer recurrences than those undergoing limited resections.

In summary, current data do not clearly support the routine use of limited resection for peripheral stage I lung cancers in patients who are candidates for lobectomy. Nevertheless, anatomic segmentectomy may be reasonable for individuals with peripheral tumors smaller than 3 cm that exhibit no endobronchial extension or intrapulmonary metastases and do not involve N1 or N2 lymph node stations on the basis of intraoperative staging. The role of limited resection for very small (less than 1 cm) tumors, such as those detected by CT screening methods, needs to be evaluated in well-designed, prospective studies.

Although the vast majority of lobectomies are performed via thoracotomy, a number of surgeons have advocated video-assisted lobectomy whenever feasible for resection of lung cancer.[244] Proponents of video-assisted thoracic surgery (VATS) claim that the pulmonary resections and MLNDs performed by VATS are comparable to those performed during thoracotomy. VATS lobectomy is performed with lung isolation and the placement of several 2-cm port sites as well as a 5- to 8-cm "utility" incision, through which instruments are placed for hilar dissection. Typically, cancers not amenable to VATS resection include tumors larger than 5 cm in diameter, T3 lesions, and those with extensive lymph node involvement. Several investigators no longer exclude patients with lymph node metastases or individuals who have received induction therapy.

VATS lung resections are less invasive than those performed by thoracotomy and typically enable patients to return to normal activity sooner than patients undergoing comparable lung resection by thoracotomy. In general, hospital stay is decreased, postoperative pain is diminished, and chest tubes are removed sooner in patients undergoing VATS procedures than in those undergoing thoracotomy. However, no apparent late differences in pain or morbidity have been noted in patients undergoing VATS procedures compared to those undergoing thoracotomy. For this reason, the adequacy of VATS resection for lung cancer has not been clearly established.[245] McKenna et al.[246] reported a 4-year survival rate of 70% for patients with stage I lung cancer undergoing VATS resection. Walker et al.[247] reported 5-year survival rates of 78% for stage I, 51% for stage II, and 29% for stage III carcinomas—results that are comparable with those for open procedures. Sugi et al.[248] prospectively randomly assigned 100 patients with stage IA lung cancer to undergo VATS lobectomy or conventional resection. MLNDs were performed in all patients. The average size of the tumors in both groups was 2 cm. Overall 5-year survival in the VATS and open lobectomy groups was 90% and 85%, respectively.

Although in experienced hands, VATS lobectomy appears comparable to conventional lobectomy for treatment of early-stage disease, the role of VATS in more advanced lung cancer has yet to be determined. Overall, the prognosis of the patient depends on the extent of the pulmonary resection and MLND, and the surgical technique should be that which the surgeon is most competent to perform.

After resection for stage I and II lung cancer, the 5-year survival rate without recurrence exceeds 50% in stage I disease and 35% in stage II disease. In completely resected T1N0 tumors, 5-year survival rates exceed 70% and in some series surpass 80%.[240,249]

T3N0 Tumors

Lung cancers invading the chest wall, diaphragm, or mediastinum are designated T3 tumors. In general, the deeper the invasion, the worse the prognosis. In all instances, it is recommended that these tumors be resected *en bloc* within all involved structures. Prognosis is related to completeness of resection, depth of invasion, and lymph node status.

Involvement of the chest wall occurs relatively frequently in patients with peripheral carcinomas. Because of the inability to precisely define the extent of chest wall invasion at the time of surgery and the low morbidity of chest wall resections in experienced hands, *en bloc* removal of ribs and intervening musculature is standard of care for local control of these tumors. Inoue et al.[250] reported 5-year survival rates of 35%, 29%, and 27% for patients undergoing resection of lung cancers exhibiting parietal pleural, subpleural, and intercostal muscle invasion, respectively. Magdeleinat et al.[251] reported results pertaining to chest wall resections in 201 lung cancer patients. Complete resections were achieved in 83% of individuals. Five-year survival rates were 25% for patients with T3N0 tumors. Completeness of resection, depth of invasion, and nodal status impacted survival in these individuals. In an additional study, Roviaro et al.[252] observed a remarkable 78% 5-year survival rate in 23 patients with stage IIB (T3N0) disease compared to a 7% survival rate for patients with stage IIIA disease, which attests to the impact of mediastinal lymph node metastases in patients with lung cancers invading the chest wall. Chapelier et al.[253] reported their experience with 100 lung cancers invading the chest wall. Five-year survival rates were 22%, 9%, and 0% for patients with T3N0, T3N1, and T3N2 tumors, respectively. Histologic differentiation and depth of chest wall invasion were the main factors influencing long-term survival.

Tumors invading the diaphragm frequently spread along the diaphragmatic pleura; because of this, most patients present with a malignant pleural effusion (T4) indicating incurable disease. In rare instances, however, tumors with direct focal diaphragmatic invasion may be amenable to lobectomy with *en bloc* resection and reconstruction of the diaphragm. Yokoi et al.[254] identified 63 patients with lung cancers invading the diaphragm out of 16,771 individuals undergoing lung cancer resections in Japan. Complete resections were achieved in 55 patients, 26 of whom had T3N0 disease. Overall survival of patients undergoing complete resections was 23%. Survival of patients with T3N0 and with T3N1 to 2 tumors was 28% and 18%, respectively. Depth of diaphragm invasion impacted survival; patients with either parietal pleural or subpleural invasion had a 33% 5-year survival rate, compared to 14% for individuals with deep muscle or peritoneal invasion. Rocco et al.[255] reported an actuarial 5-year survival rate of 27% for patients with T3N0 tumors invading the diaphragm. The extent of diaphragmatic involvement, evidenced by the need for prosthetic reconstruction, correlated adversely with survival.

Invasion of the mediastinal pleura, pericardium, or mediastinal fat may occasionally be seen in lung cancer patients. In many instances, *en bloc* resection of the involved mediastinal tissue can accomplish a complete resection; however, the results of surgery for these lesions are not well known, because most tumors with mediastinal invasion also involve major vascular structures (T4) as well as mediastinal lymph nodes. Because of this, it is important to determine resectability preoperatively using CT and MRI scans to delineate invasion of vascular structures, and mediastinoscopy to rule out N2 or N3 disease. Burt et al.[256] reported their experience with 225 lung cancers invading the mediastinum at MSKCC. Only 22% of tumors could be completely resected, 34% were incompletely resected, and 44% were totally unresectable. Among patients with completely resected T3N0 disease involving the mediastinum, a 30% 5-year survival rate may be seen.

Tumors within 2 cm of the carina are also designated T3. Although these neoplasms can be resected by pneumonectomy, parenchyma-preserving operations using bronchoplastic or angioplastic techniques are preferable alternatives. Studies indicate that SL yields survival rates and quality of life comparable to if not better than those obtained by standard pneumonectomy. Fadel et al.[257] evaluated 139 patients undergoing SL with or without angioplasty for NSCLC. The overall operative mortality was 3%, and overall 5-year survival rate was 52%. Multivariate analysis revealed that nodal status (N0 or N1 vs. N2) and microscopic invasion of the bronchial stump were independent determinants of long-term survival. In another large series, Chunwei et al.[258] evaluated the results of SL in 78 patients with NSCLC. Twenty-one individuals required resection and reconstruction of the pulmonary artery. Five-year survival rate was 63% for patients with stage II disease; no individual with N2 disease survived 5 years. Patients requiring bronchovascular reconstruction did significantly worse than those having bronchoplasty alone. Multivariate analysis revealed nodal status to be the most important determinant of long-term survival in patients undergoing complete resections. Deslauriers et al.[259] compared the results for 184 sleeve lobectomies with those for 1046 standard pneumonectomies performed at a single institution. The operative mortality was 1.6% for SL and 5.3% for pneumonectomy. Five-year survival was 52% for SL and 33% for pneumonectomy. The survival rates for patients with stage I or II disease who were treated using SL were significantly better than those for similarly staged individuals undergoing pneumonectomies. Local recurrence was comparable in the two groups. These data, together with those reported by De Leyn et al.[260] and Ferguson and colleagues,[261] confirm that SL is associated with a lower perioperative mortality, affords comparable if not improved overall survival rates, and enables better exercise tolerance and quality of life than pneumonectomy for centrally located tumors.

Stage IIIA Disease

T3N1 DISEASE. Stage IIIA disease includes T3N1 tumors. As with any other T status, once lymph nodes are involved, the prognosis is much worse; thus, these tumors are categorized as IIIA rather than IIB. Historically, fewer than 20% of patients with T3 lesions associated with N1 metastases survive 5 years, and few if any survive 5 years when mediastinal nodes are involved.[262]

T1 TO 3N2 DISEASE. The existence of N2 disease remains the most controversial area for primary surgical management of lung cancer. Although such tumors are potentially resectable, once ipsilateral mediastinal or subcarinal lymph nodes (or both) are involved by tumor, the ultimate prognosis is much worse. When disease is diagnosed preoperatively either by noninvasive or invasive staging techniques, fewer than 10% of all patients treated with primary surgery survive 5 years, despite adjuvant therapy. Adverse prognostic factors include multiple levels of N2 disease, multiple lymph nodes from one station involved with tumor, adenocarcinoma, and extranodal extension of disease. More than 75% of patients with N2 disease present with disease extending beyond one lymph node station.

"Minimal" N2 Disease. Single-station lymph node involvement with microscopic foci of disease not apparent on clinical staging constitutes most of the subset of minimal N2 disease. This stage of disease is usually discovered at the time of thoracotomy or at pretreatment mediastinoscopy. Five-year survival rates after surgical resection are 10% to 20% and are higher when a complete resection is performed. After incomplete (R1 or R2) resections, few if any patients survive beyond 3 years. Patients found to have involvement of multiple lymph node stations at final pathologic staging also fare poorly.

"Bulky" N2 Disease. Patients with tumors with mediastinal involvement beyond that described as minimal N2 disease constitute the large segment of patients presenting with stage IIIA disease. This more advanced, bulky, or multistation N2 disease usually can be identified preoperatively and is termed clinical N2 disease. It is considered by most surgeons to be inoperable, since few individuals are cured by resection alone.[263-265] Because of this, induction chemotherapy and chemoradiotherapy have been evaluated in these patients. For most of these patients, chemoradiotherapy is considered the standard treatment for local control.

Combined Modality Approaches (Including Surgery)

SITES OF FAILURE. Recognition of prognostic and surgical factors that predict for specific anatomic failure patterns can allow selection of patients for local, systemic, or combined

therapy. After surgical resection, patients with pathologic stage T1 to 2N0 tumors who have negative resection margins have survival rates in excess of 50%. For these individuals, isolated mediastinal or primary site recurrences are unusual, and there is no rationale for the routine use of postoperative radiation therapy (PORT). Patients with T1N1 tumors have an isolated local failure rate of 12%. The rate of isolated distant failure for T1N1 patients is 33%, which indicates a need for effective chemotherapy to prevent systemic and central nervous system recurrences. For T2N1 disease, the isolated local failure rate is 14% and the distant failure rate is 36%, which again demonstrates the need for effective adjuvant systemic therapy.[266] In view of the fact that isolated N1 metastases are rare in these large surgical series, it is reasonable to consider adjuvant local therapy in patients with documented N1 disease when the mediastinal nodes were neither sampled nor dissected, because occult N2 disease may be present.

Survival decreases for patients with N2 disease discovered intraoperatively. When no adjuvant therapy is used, thoracic recurrence is seen in approximately 20% of patients, even if the resection margins are negative, and distant metastases become even more common, which suggests that both failure patterns need to be addressed if survival is to be improved.[267] Second primary lung cancers occur in all surviving patients at a rate of approximately 1% each year.[268,269]

ADJUVANT RADIOTHERAPY

Stage I Disease. The results for selected patients managed with surgery alone (T1 to 2N0) are reasonably good, and in general these patients do not benefit from adjuvant radiotherapy. Randomized trials of PORT including N0 patients have found no benefit from the addition of adjuvant treatment,[270-272] and it is not recommended. In fact, some trials have shown a survival disadvantage in patients receiving PORT, presumably from the toxicity of the radiation. The Medical Research Council performed a metaanalysis of nine trials involving 2128 patients who underwent complete resection and were randomly assigned to either no treatment or PORT.[273] Doses of PORT varied from 30 to 60 Gy, and most of the trials used cobalt 60 radiotherapy. Patients with stage I disease were included in many of the trials. A significantly increased hazard ratio for mortality was observed for patients with stage I disease receiving PORT.

Stage II and Stage III Disease. The role of adjuvant radiotherapy for stage II (N1) NSCLC is controversial, but it has been recommended in the past because the incidence of local failure with surgery alone is high. A locoregional intrathoracic failure rate of 31% was observed by the Ludwig Lung Cancer Study Group (LCSG) for patients with completely resected stage II disease.[274] The Medical Research Council metaanalysis reported a trend toward decreased survival in patients with stage II disease receiving PORT.

The LCSG investigated the efficacy of postoperative mediastinal irradiation in completely resected stage II and III squamous cell carcinoma of the lung. This trial randomly assigned 210 patients to receive 50 Gy in 25 fractions after surgery or observation alone. The rate of locoregional failure (as first site of failure) was reduced from 41% to 3% with radiotherapy for all node-positive patients. Despite enhancing locoregional control, radiotherapy did not improve survival for stage II patients because more than two-thirds of first failures were distant.[267] The LCSG failed to separate patients with N1 and N2 disease but rather analyzed them as a single group.[267] A trend toward improved survival was observed in N2 patients receiving radiotherapy.

The Medical Research Council of the United Kingdom also completed a randomized adjuvant trial in which 308 patients with stage II and III disease were treated with either 40 Gy of radiation or no further therapy. Although a trend toward improved survival with radiotherapy was seen in the T2N2 subgroup, no overall survival benefit was observed.[275] The metaanalysis performed by the Medical Research Council confirmed these results. The council reported higher local recurrences in 276 patients in the surgery-only arms of the trials. There were fewer local recurrences in patients receiving PORT. In addition, there was a trend toward improved survival in patients with stage III and N2 disease in this arm, although it did not reach significance.[273] PORT has also been advocated for resected NSCLC invading pleura or chest wall without nodal metastases (T3N0). This issue has never been properly examined in a prospective fashion, although the LCSG attempted to address this question in a study that was closed due to poor patient accrual.[256,276] The survival rate approaches 50% for patients with chest wall tumors undergoing *en bloc* complete resection (R0), and there appears to be little gained with additional local treatment.[277] Therefore, the role of PORT remains controversial. It has not been shown to produce a benefit in early-stage disease. It has been shown to improve local control in patients with mediastinal nodal disease but has no proven survival benefit. There is likely a subgroup of patients, such as those with micrometastatic disease, who will have an improved survival with PORT; however, this patient population has yet to be identified.

Positive Margins (R1, R2 Resections). The presence of microscopic disease after curative surgery for early-stage disease at the bronchial resection margin, chest wall, or vascular margin may adversely affect the prognosis of patients. Yet, despite data that suggest that adjuvant radiotherapy reduces local recurrence, the retrospective literature regarding the efficacy of radiotherapy to improve local control is conflicting.[278–280]

ADJUVANT CHEMOTHERAPY WITH OR WITHOUT RADIOTHERAPY. Adjuvant chemotherapy improves outcome for patients with breast cancer, colorectal cancer, and gastric cancer. Until recently there was very little evidence that adjuvant chemotherapy was beneficial in patients with completely resected NSCLC. In the 1980s, a number of important studies were performed by the LCSG. The LCSG published two large randomized trials using the cyclophosphamide plus doxorubicin and cisplatin (CAP) regimen. The first trial included patients with completely resected stage II or III adenocarcinoma or large cell carcinoma.[281] Patients were randomly assigned to receive either CAP chemotherapy or immunotherapy with intrapleural bacille Calmette-Guérin and levamisole administered for 18 months. In 141 randomly assigned patients, there was a significant 6-month delay in median time to recurrence and a 15% survival advantage at 1 year favoring chemotherapy. The survival of the control immunotherapy group was similar to that of earlier patients treated with surgery alone, and the authors attributed the improved survival in the chemotherapy arm to the effects of chemotherapy.

Another LCSG study involved patients with incompletely resected disease who were randomly assigned to receive PORT alone or radiotherapy and six cycles of CAP.[282] Incomplete resection was defined as postoperative residual microscopic or macroscopic disease, or disease in the highest resected paratracheal lymph node. Data for 164 patients were analyzed. The chemotherapy group had a significantly longer time to progression ($P = .066$); median survival was only marginally improved with chemotherapy, and there was no 5-year survival benefit.

Studies involving patients with less advanced disease have also been published. The LCSG compared four cycles of CAP to no further therapy in 269 patients with stage I disease. No benefit was identified for chemotherapy, but only 53% of assigned patients completed chemotherapy.[283] A study testing a lower-dose, six-cycle CAP regimen in T1 to 3N0 disease showed a benefit in time to recurrence and survival; however, an imbalance in the randomization process resulted in the assignment of more patients with advanced disease to the observation arm.[284]

Efforts to develop effective adjuvant therapies have included chemotherapy and radiation strategies. Radiation offers the potential to improve local control, which remains a problem for patients with stage III lung cancer. Concurrent chemoradiotherapy is superior to sequential therapy in nonsurgical treatment of stage III disease.[226,285,286] This finding was the major rationale for examining the potential role of adjuvant concurrent chemoradiotherapy after resection of lung cancer.

Keller et al.[287] randomly assigned patients with stage II and IIIA disease to receive either radiation alone (50.4 Gy) or radiation (50.4 Gy) given concurrently with four cycles of cisplatin and etoposide. There was no difference in overall survival between the two groups. The median survival was 39 months for the radiation-alone arm versus 38 months for the chemotherapy plus radiotherapy arm. A major concern with the Keller et al. study is that the radiation and chemotherapy were administered concurrently. Although superior for bulk disease, it is not clear that concurrent chemotherapy and radiation therapy is optimal for treating minimal residual disease in the adjuvant setting. Furthermore, toxicity is more pronounced with concurrent chemotherapy and radiation therapy regimens. For this reason, concurrent chemoradiation in the adjuvant setting cannot be recommended for patients undergoing complete resection. It may be considered for patients with positive margins or residual disease after surgery.

Much of the uncertainty regarding adjuvant chemotherapy has been the result of studies that were not large enough to demonstrate small, yet potentially meaningful, differences in outcome. The Non–Small Cell Lung Cancer Collaborative Group performed a metaanalysis examining survival in 9387 patients (7151 deaths) in 52 randomized clinical trials.[288] Included in this metaanalysis were data from 14 randomized trials pertaining to 4357 patients receiving surgical resection alone or surgery plus adjuvant chemotherapy. Cisplatin-based chemotherapy regimens appeared to improve survival in patients undergoing resection by 5%. Whereas the benefit was not statistically significant, this observation prompted additional studies to address the issue of adjuvant chemotherapy in patients with resected lung cancer.

In 2003, several trials were reported that provide important insight into the role of adjuvant chemotherapy. The Adjuvant Lung Project Italy trial enrolled more than 1200 patients who were randomly assigned to receive surgery with or without three cycles of adjuvant mitomycin, vindesine, and cisplatin.[289] At 5 years, the group that received adjuvant chemotherapy had a nonsignificant (2% to 3%) improvement in overall survival. However, the trial was limited by the fact that compliance with chemotherapy was poor, with only 69% of patients receiving the full three cycles of chemotherapy. Furthermore, given the size of the Adjuvant Lung Project Italy trial, it is not possible to exclude a small but clinically important survival benefit for adjuvant chemotherapy.

In the IALT study, patients with completely resected stage I, II, or IIIA lung cancer were randomly assigned to observation or to three or four cycles of cisplatin-based chemotherapy.[223] A unique feature of the trial was that each participating facility chose one of the following chemotherapy regimens: cisplatin plus vindesine, cisplatin plus etoposide, cisplatin plus vinorelbine, or cisplatin with vinblastine. Radiation treatment was also left to the discretion of each institution, but a consistent standard had to be maintained. Patients were enrolled at 148 centers in 33 countries, with 36% of individuals having pathologic stage I disease, 25% having stage II disease, and 39% having stage III disease. Although the initial accrual target was 3300 patients, the trial was closed after 1867 patients had been enrolled, because a planned interim analysis detected a significant impact of therapy on survival (the primary end point). The hazard ratio for death in patients receiving adjuvant chemotherapy was 0.86 (95% CI, 0.76 to 0.98). The median overall survival improved from 44 months to 50 months. This translated into a 4% improvement in overall survival at 5 years (44.5% vs. 40.4%; $P < .03$). Approximately 1% of individuals receiving chemotherapy died as a result of this intervention.[223]

Results of the IALT study show a clear, albeit small, survival benefit to adjuvant platinum-based chemotherapy. Subset analysis revealed no trend for benefit based on either stage of disease or chemotherapy regimen. The IALT trial was the first well-designed study with patient accrual sufficient to demonstrate a benefit in the expected range for adjuvant cisplatin-based therapy. The modest degree of efficacy demonstrated by this study is plausible and confirms the results of the 1995 metaanalysis.[288]

UFT is an oral antimetabolite comprised of a fixed ratio of uracil and tegafur. This compound has been studied extensively in Japan as adjuvant treatment after complete surgical resection. Kato et al.[290] reported the results of an adjuvant trial that randomly assigned 979 patients with stage I disease to observation alone or 2 years of UFT (250 mg/m^2/d). At a median of 70 months of follow-up, adjuvant UFT therapy was associated with a small (3%) but statistically significant improvement in 5-year survival. Subgroup analysis suggested that the magnitude of benefit was substantial for patients with T2N0 carcinomas (84.9% vs. 73.5%) but not for patients with T1N0 tumors.

Additional data regarding the potential benefit of adjuvant therapy will be available when several additional studies mature. CALGB announced in early 2004 that an adjuvant trial comparing carboplatin and paclitaxel treatment to observation alone after resection of T2N0 disease was closed early after an interim analysis by the data safety monitoring committee detected a survival advantage in the treatment arm.[290a,290b] The National Cancer Institute of Canada has also conducted a trial of adjuvant cisplatin and vinorelbine versus observation alone in stage I and stage II (except T3N0) lung cancer patients undergoing complete resection. A significant treatment effect was noted in the patients receiving adjuvant chemotherapy.[290b]

The findings of the IALT study[223] as well as the data of Kato et al.[290] suggest that adjuvant chemotherapy should be considered for patients with resected lung cancer. Clearly every patient should not be treated. It is reasonable to restrict treatment to patients with a good performance status and adequate end-organ function. Age alone should not be a criteria for treatment, because presently there are no data to suggest that older patients do not benefit from adjuvant chemotherapy.

Significant questions remain regarding systemic treatment for resectable lung cancer. Should treatment be given preoperatively or postoperatively? How many cycles of treatment are optimal? Is cisplatin superior, or can carboplatin-based regimens be used? How should novel agents be incorporated into the treatment algorithm? These questions will be the focus of future studies.

PREOPERATIVE RADIOTHERAPY. After publication of the initial investigations on the use of preoperative irradiation as a component of treatment of NSCLC, many studies using this induction approach were undertaken in the hope of improving both local control and survival of patients with marginally resectable disease.[291–293] Acceptance of preoperative irradiation was based on improved resectability as well as complete responses in surgical specimens after such therapy. Reports of survival of patients with superior sulcus tumors after combined preoperative radiotherapy (when no previous survivals had occurred) bolstered enthusiasm for an approach of preoperative radiotherapy alone. Subsequently, several randomized trials were initiated to answer this question with larger cohorts of patients. The first such major randomized trial was performed by the U.S. Veterans Administration. After a minimum follow-up of 4 years in surviving patients, no increase in survival was noted in the pretreatment group. The overall survival rate was 12.5% in the pretreatment arm, compared with 21.0% in the surgery-alone arm, although this was not statistically significant.[293] In 1975, the NCI published results of two separate but integrated multi-institutional randomized trials addressing the use of preoperative radiotherapy followed by surgery in both operable and inoperable NSCLC without evidence of preoperative radiotherapy advantage.[294]

It is clear from both the nonrandomized and randomized data that preoperative irradiation alone does not improve long-term survival in the population studied, and has no established role as a single-induction modality for the management of marginally resectable or unresectable stage IIIA or IIIB disease. Because of this, most current trials are investigating the use of preoperative concomitant chemoradiotherapy or chemotherapy alone.

INDUCTION (NEOADJUVANT) CHEMOTHERAPY
Early-Stage Disease. Induction (neoadjuvant) chemotherapy before resection has several theoretic advantages, including enhancing local control, reducing tumor volume, treating micrometastatic disease, and being better tolerated than postoperative chemotherapy. The role of induction chemotherapy in early-stage (IB to IIIA) NSCLC has been evaluated by the Bimo-

dality Lung Oncology Team trial. In this phase II study, 94 patients with stage IB, II, and selected IIIA NSCLC received two courses of paclitaxel (225 mg/m^2 in a 3-hour infusion) and carboplatin [area under the curve (AUC) = 6] administered every 21 days, followed by surgery. Patients with completely resected tumors received three additional courses of paclitaxel-carboplatin therapy. Ninety-two patients completed preoperative chemotherapy, with major responses observed in 59% of the enrolled individuals. Of the 92 patients potentially eligible for surgery, 80 (93%) underwent exploration, and 70 (82%) underwent complete resection. The 1-year survival was estimated at 85%.[295] This trial demonstrated that induction chemotherapy could be administered with acceptable toxicity in patients with early-stage lung cancer who were potentially curable with surgery alone. In a phase III study, the French Thoracic Cooperative Group randomly assigned 355 patients to receive two courses of mitomycin C, ifosfamide, and cisplatin followed by surgery and two postoperative chemotherapy cycles in responding patients, or surgery alone.[296] In both arms, patients with pT3 or pN2 disease received thoracic radiotherapy. Overall response to induction chemotherapy was 64%. The median survival was 37 months for the combined modality arm and 26 months for the surgical arm. Survival differences between arms increased from 3.8% at 1 year to 8.6% at 4 years. Interestingly, the survival benefit was observed only in patients with stage I or II disease. Based on these studies, a randomized Intergroup trial (S9900) comparing three cycles of induction paclitaxel-carboplatin plus surgery to surgery alone in early-stage NSCLC is under way.

Stage IIIA Nonbulky or Resectable Disease. Interpretation of numerous phase II studies of neoadjuvant chemotherapy for stage IIIA patients is very difficult due to differences in the chemotherapeutic regimens, mediastinal staging procedures, and radiation therapy used in these trials. Overall, the results of these phase II trials indicate an average response rate of 60%, with 55% of individuals undergoing thoracotomy and 49% of patients having complete resections. Median survival has been reported to be 16 months, with a 5-year survival rate of 30% in chemoresponsive patients and 50% in patients exhibiting pathologic complete response. Neoadjuvant chemotherapy-radiotherapy results in higher rates of downstaging of the primary tumor. In a phase III trial, Rosell et al.[229] randomly assigned 60 patients with stage IIIA NSCLC to receive induction chemotherapy (three courses of cisplatin 50 mg/m^2/cycle, mitomycin C, and ifosfamide) followed by resection and postoperative radiation therapy (50 Gy), or to resection plus postoperative radiation therapy. A threefold survival advantage was seen in patients receiving induction chemotherapy (median survival, 26 vs. 8 months). Long-term results of this study continued to support a survival difference (median survival, 22 months for chemotherapy plus surgery vs. 10 months for surgery alone).[297] In an additional phase III trial, Roth et al.[298] randomly assigned 60 patients with stage IIIA lung cancer to surgery alone or to induction chemotherapy (three cycles of cyclophosphamide, etoposide, and cisplatin) plus surgery. Although not included in the formal protocol, radiotherapy was administered to over one-half of patients in both groups. Induction chemotherapy was associated with a sixfold increase in median survival (64 vs. 11 months) and significantly better 3-year survival (56% vs. 15%). In a subsequent report, 32% of patients who underwent neoadjuvant chemotherapy versus 16% of those who had surgery alone remained alive with a median follow-up of 82 months.[299] The median survival in

the perioperative chemotherapy arm (21 months), although less than initially reported, was consistent with that observed by Rosell et al.[297] In the trial conducted by the French Thoracic Cooperative Group discussed previously in Induction (Neoadjuvant) Chemotherapy: Early-Stage Disease, no improvement in survival was seen in patients with N2 disease who received chemotherapy.[296] A second French study revealed that preoperative chemotherapy was associated with a better prognosis for patients with bulky N2 disease: 5-year survival rates were 18% and 5% for patients treated with and without preoperative chemotherapy, respectively (*P* <.001). However, a similar advantage could not be demonstrated for those with minimal N2 disease.[300] Based on the contradictory results and limitations of phase II and III clinical trials, the benefit of induction chemotherapy in patients with resectable stage IIIA (N2) disease remains uncertain, and additional studies are warranted to further address this issue.

INDUCTION CHEMOTHERAPY WITH RADIOTHERAPY. Cisplatin-based combination chemotherapy has been used before and concurrently with radiotherapy in an effort to improve results. Faber et al.[301] conducted two consecutive trials in patients with clinically evident N2 NSCLC. The first combined 5-fluorouracil, cisplatin, and 40 Gy of chest radiotherapy; the second added etoposide to the regimen. The complete resection rate was 68% in the first trial, and 76% in the second study. Median survivals were 21 months and 34 months, respectively. The difference in survival was not significant. Four treatment-related deaths occurred in the two trials. The LCSG combined 5-fluorouracil, cisplatin, and 30 Gy of chest radiotherapy.[302] Overall, 42% of patients underwent a complete surgical resection, and a median survival of 11 months was observed. These results were similar to those of an earlier trial conducted by the LCSG using the CAP regimen with 30 Gy of chest radiotherapy; a 33% resection rate and 11-month median survival were seen in patients with stage III disease.[303] CALGB tested the combination of 5-fluorouracil, vinblastine, and cisplatin plus 30 Gy of irradiation in 32 patients with stage IIIA disease.[304] The complete resection rate was 62%, and three treatment-related deaths occurred. The Southwest Oncology Group (SWOG) combined 45 Gy of radiotherapy with etoposide and cisplatin and documented a 65% complete resection rate.[305]

More recently, a significant effort has been put forth in phase I and II trials to optimize the locoregional therapy in a select group of patients with marginally resectable stage IIIA and IIIB disease. The goals of induction therapy are to convert marginally resectable or unresectable disease, improve locoregional control, and eliminate distant micrometastases.

SEQUENTIAL CHEMOTHERAPY AND RADIOTHERAPY. Two phase II trials reported results with induction chemotherapy followed by preoperative radiotherapy and surgery for stage III NSCLC. Skarin et al.[306] treated 41 patients with pathologically determined marginally resectable stage IIIA NSCLC. Included within this group were patients with T3N0 disease and patients with N2 mediastinal metastases. Forty-one patients received two cycles of CAP chemotherapy followed by 30 Gy of radiation. A complete resection was accomplished in 36 of 41 patients (88%). The median survival was 32 months, and the 3-year survival rate was 30%. Systemic treatment failed in 18 of 36 patients (50%), and local treatment failed in four patients. Sherman et al.[307] treated 21 patients with vinblastine and cisplatin followed by 30 Gy of radiation to the mediastinum. The radiographically determined response rate, resection rate, and median survival were similar to those reported by Skarin et al.[306]

CONCURRENT CHEMOTHERAPY AND RADIOTHERAPY. Several phase II trials have tested the feasibility of combining a variety of induction chemotherapy regimens concurrently with radiotherapy before surgery to maximize induction results through a trimodal strategy. A North American Intergroup has completed a phase III trial evaluating the role of surgery in conjunction with standard chemoradiotherapy for the treatment of stage IIIA and selected stage IIIB NSCLC. The preliminary results demonstrate a benefit in disease-free survival but no benefit in overall survival from surgery in this setting.[231]

Phase II trials cannot establish optimal treatment because of the heterogeneity of both the patients entered and the treatments delivered,[308] and the lack of statistical power due to small sample size. Different chemotherapeutic regimens were used, mostly cisplatin-based. Significant variability among the different trials can be seen in the sequencing of the chemotherapy in relation to the radiation, radiation total dose, dose per fraction, continuous-course versus split-course strategy, timing of surgery, inclusion by some studies of T3N0 versus clinically evident N2 disease, inclusion of stage IIIB disease, staging methods, performance criteria, and toxicity of individual regimens. Although a number of phase II trials have reported promising results, wide variation exists in terms of initial response rates (range, 50% to 90%), complete resection rates (range, 28% to 88%), pathologic complete response rates (range, 9% to 21%), median survival rates (range, 13 to 32 months), and 2-year survival rates (range, 20% to 40%).

Several trials have evaluated altered fractionation schemes (especially hyperfractionation) combined with concurrent chemotherapy using a variety of drugs and dosage regimens to enhance the response rates and optimize resection rates and local control.[309–311] Overall, these trials suggest that a bimodal or trimodal approach combining neoadjuvant chemotherapy with or without radiotherapy followed by surgery provides a potentially superior method of enhancing resectability and improving locoregional control and survival compared to radiotherapy alone followed by surgery. Some series also demonstrated a doubling of both local control and survival rates over those reported with preoperative radiotherapy with or without chemotherapy. The use of altered fractionation also appears to result in higher response rates and local control rates than the use of standard-fraction irradiation combined with chemotherapy and has seemingly acceptable toxicity.

A major issue concerning the use of induction regimens in patients with potentially resectable NSCLC pertains to perioperative morbidity and mortality. Roberts et al.[312] reported that induction chemotherapy significantly increased life-threatening perioperative complications in patients undergoing potentially curative operations. Martin et al.[313] reported significantly increased risk of mortality in patients undergoing right pneumonectomy after preoperative chemotherapy with or without radiation therapy. On the other hand, Siegenthaler et al.[314] observed no increase in perioperative morbidity or mortality in 76 patients undergoing resection for NSCLC after induction therapy compared to 259 individuals treated with surgery alone at M. D. Anderson Cancer Center. Ohta et al.[315] reported that induction chemoradiation therapy did not affect perioperative

morbidity or mortality in lung cancer patients undergoing sleeve resection. Collectively, these data indicate that induction therapy regimens (particularly those with radiation therapy) may increase perioperative morbidity and that appropriate patient selection, as well as diligent intraoperative and postoperative management, may diminish this risk.

The role of induction therapies followed by surgery in treatment of resectable lung cancer remains to be defined, particularly for individuals who experience pathologic complete response or a significant down-staging of disease.[316–318] In N2 disease, it appears to improve long-term survival, although the role of surgery vis-à-vis radiotherapy as the primary control mechanism is unclear, particularly in light of the data of Taylor et al.[319] demonstrating that local control and survival rates in patients with stage IIIA NSCLC treated with concurrent chemoradiation were comparable to those observed in patients receiving induction chemotherapy followed by surgery. Whether induction therapies have an impact on earlier-stage (non-T1N0) disease has yet to be defined; once again, it is hoped that current phase III trials will resolve this question.

SUPERIOR SULCUS TUMORS. Tumors arising in the apex of the lung that invade the first rib and are associated with involvement of the brachial plexus and stellate ganglion produce Pancoast's syndrome. These tumors require aggressive multidisciplinary intervention. Failure to achieve local control of these neoplasms results in debilitating pain, loss of arm function, and high-level spinal cord compression. During the past decade, treatment of these neoplasms has evolved considerably so that even tumors with vertebral body or subclavian vessel invasion, as well as those with clinically evident N2 disease, should be considered for resection.[320,321] Presently, optimal standard of care consists of induction chemotherapy with concurrent radiation therapy, aggressive surgical resection, including resection of all involved structures, or induction chemotherapy, surgery, and PORT.

Pfannschmidt et al.[322] reported results of treatment of 56 lung cancers invading the superior sulcus. Fifteen patients underwent preoperative radiation therapy, 10 patients had preoperative and postoperative radiation therapy, 22 had resection and PORT, and 9 individuals had surgery without radiation therapy. Five-year survival rates for patients with completely resected N0 or N1 disease was 34%. Complete resection and mediastinal lymph nodes status correlated with prolonged survival. No significant differences regarding radiation therapy regimens were observed in this study. Komaki et al.[323] retrospectively reviewed data for a series of 143 patients with superior sulcus tumors resected at M. D. Anderson Cancer Center. The overall predictors of 5-year survival included weight loss, tumor extension into the supraclavicular fossa or vertebral body, stage of the disease, and surgical treatment. Patients with IIB tumors had a 47% 5-year survival rate compared to 15% for individuals with stage IIIA or IIIB disease. PORT appeared to improve survival in patients undergoing complete resection. In an additional study at M. D. Anderson Cancer Center, Gandhi et al.[324] reported a 2-year actuarial survival rate of 54% in patients undergoing resection of superior sulcus tumors invading the vertebral body. Local recurrence rate was 9% in individuals with negative surgical margins and 100% in individuals with residual disease at the margins of resection. Alifano et al.[325] reported a 47% 5-year survival rate for 67 patients undergoing resection of T3N0 superior sulcus tumors and observed that completeness of resection and absence of associated illnesses—but not histologic type, tumor size, or lymph node status—were predictors of survival in these patients. Bilsky et al.[326] observed that completeness of resection, regardless of the extent of involvement of the spine, correlated with survival in patients with superior sulcus tumors with spinal or brachial plexus involvement.

Data indicate that cisplatin-based therapy with concurrent radiation improves local control and possibly prolongs survival in patients with superior sulcus carcinomas. Wright et al.[326a] reported their experience with 35 patients treated with either induction radiotherapy or induction chemotherapy plus radiotherapy and surgery at the Massachusetts General Hospital. All of these patients had N0 status at final pathology. A pathologic complete or near-complete response was observed in 35% of patients receiving radiation therapy alone, compared to 87% of individuals receiving induction chemotherapy plus radiotherapy. Four-year survival rates were 49% in the radiation therapy arm and 84% in the chemotherapy plus radiotherapy arm. Rusch et al.[327] reported results of Intergroup trial 0160 evaluating induction chemotherapy plus radiotherapy and surgical resection in 111 patients with mediastinoscopy-negative T3 to 4N0 to 1 NSCLC involving the superior sulcus. Induction therapy consisted of two cycles of cisplatin-etoposide chemotherapy with concurrent radiotherapy (45 Gy). Of 95 patients who were eligible, 83 individuals underwent surgery, of whom 76 had complete resections. Fifty-four patients (65%) had a pathologic complete response or minimal microscopic disease after induction therapy. Two-year survival rate was 70% for all individuals who underwent complete resection. Collectively, these data indicate that aggressive multimodality therapy is feasible in patients with superior sulcus carcinomas, and individuals with invasion of adjacent structures can achieve significant palliation and survival benefit after complete resection.

EXTERNAL-BEAM RADIOTHERAPY AS DEFINITIVE THERAPY.

Selection Criteria. The selection of patients for definitive management with radiotherapy depends on several factors, the most important of which are extent of disease, performance status, and pulmonary function. Accurate staging is required to identify and exclude patients with distant metastasis from undergoing radical treatment. In addition to distant metastases, malignant pleural and pericardial effusions are contraindications for definitive radiotherapy. In some circumstances, however, a small pleural effusion not seen on chest radiograph is discovered on staging CT scanning, which renders the decision to proceed with definitive management less clear. Patients with this finding in the setting of no other significant clinical, laboratory, or radiographic findings that suggest distant spread should be considered for curative treatment.[328]

No specific criteria exist to define the extent of tumor bulk considered unsuitable for treatment with curative intent using conventional treatment planning. In general, however, an intrathoracic tumor size of 8 cm or larger is considered relatively prohibitive for high-dose treatment (55 to 70 Gy) due to excessive pulmonary toxicity. Patients with such large tumors without evidence of extrathoracic spread should be considered for induction chemotherapy to attempt tumor shrinkage and

reduce the volume of lung that must be targeted. Large tumors or bulky nodal disease may potentially receive high-dose radiotherapy with 3D-CRT. This approach has the potential to maximize delivery of the prescribed high dose to the target volume and minimize the dose to surrounding normal tissues. This issue is being investigated in ongoing phase I dose-escalation trials.[170–172] It may be that large tumors cannot be safely treated to a high dose, and the bulk of target size (tumor plus involved nodes) may make treatment for cure an unrealistic goal.

Many patients considered for definitive radiotherapy have compromised lung function from smoking and resultant chronic obstructive pulmonary disease. Physiologic changes in pulmonary function after radiotherapy depend on several factors, including pulmonary reserve before radiotherapy, the anatomic region of lung treated, total dose, dose per fraction, prior chemotherapy or the desire to incorporate chemotherapy concurrently with radiotherapy, and the presence of more than a 10% shift of the ventilation or perfusion to the contralateral lung from tumor or nodal disease causing central bronchial or major pulmonary vessel obstruction.[329] Some investigators have found that the postradiation decrease in pulmonary function as determined by pulmonary function tests and single photon emission CT imaging studies correlates with the amount of lung receiving 30 Gy.[330]

For patients with clinical stage I and II NSCLC that otherwise is technically resectable but in whom surgery is prohibited because of severe medical contraindications, as well as for patients who refuse surgery or have clinically evident but minimal N2 disease, primary radiotherapy alone offers a reasonable alternative approach and potential for locoregional control and cure.[331–336] Although surgery has resulted in the highest reported survival rates for those with stage I and II disease, no modern randomized studies have compared surgery to radiation in a comparable group of patients. The observed differences in results between surgery and radiation are due in part to selection bias, because in many instances patients referred for radiation treatment have worse performance status, have less rigorously staged disease, and have poor pulmonary function combined with other comorbidities.[334] In addition, most surgical series report results after pathologic staging. Surgical series reveal that in 25% to 50% of patients with clinically defined stage I disease, disease is up-staged at surgery. The rate of occult N1 or N2 disease is as high as 56% if the patient has a positive result on preoperative bronchoscopy.[337] Therefore, it is important to evaluate cause-specific survival as an end point in these studies, because many patients die of intercurrent disease. In addition, many historical series reporting results with radiation therapy alone used inferior equipment and treatment planning by today's standards and delivered inadequate doses.

More modern series have examined the issues of dose and dose escalation in relation to tumor size, local control, and survival for stage I and II disease. The evidence suggests that radical radiotherapy is an effective treatment primarily for tumors smaller than 3 cm (T1) when treated to doses of 65 Gy or higher. This treatment has a greater probability of complete response, local control, and disease-free survival, with rates almost comparable to those in some surgical series.[338] Complete response and local control of larger tumors, however, appear less likely with standard radiation fractionation schedules and doses, despite availability of modern equipment and CT-based planning.

The need to treat the mediastinum in patients with no evidence of nodal spread has been challenged. The inclusion of large volumes of lung within a radiation port to prevent regional failure, especially for peripheral T1 and T2 tumors, must be balanced against the potential for increased toxicity. Treatment of the local tumor volume alone appears justified when the patient's outcome is not subject to negative impact if the regional lymph nodes are not included. The evidence appears to support the use of smaller target volumes to deliver higher doses without compromise of the regional outcome.[333] The regional failure rate is typically less than 10% in reported series in which elective nodal areas were not treated.[333,335,339] In one series,[340] most patients did receive elective nodal irradiation but still had a treatment failure rate approaching 10%, which suggests that a typical elective dose of 40 Gy is not enough to control occult disease. Selection for this approach would be improved by pretreatment invasive mediastinal staging.

Medically Inoperable Lung Cancer. Two of the earliest studies demonstrating the curability of medically inoperable lung cancer with radiation alone were reported by Hilton[341] and Smart.[342] Thirty-eight patients with stage I or II NSCLC were treated with curative intent. Doses of 50 to 55 Gy were prescribed for squamous cell cancers, delivered to the primary site only, and doses of 40 to 45 Gy were prescribed for undifferentiated cancers, delivered to the primary site and mediastinum. Despite inadequate doses, frequent treatment breaks to allow recovery for acute reactions, orthovoltage equipment, unsatisfactory staging, and a mix of tumor histologic types, the 2-year and 5-year survival rates were 47% and 17%, respectively.[341,342]

In 1963, Morrison et al.[343] reported the results of the only randomized trial comparing surgery with radiation for stage I and II NSCLC. Although the outcome for surgery was superior to that for radiotherapy alone, the trial was severely flawed. In this study of patients randomly assigned to radiation alone, patient numbers were small, the patients received radiation doses in the range of 45 Gy, and the study included tumors with small cell histology (approximately 30%). Additionally, almost 30% of patients undergoing surgery received adjuvant PORT.[343]

Series investigating radiotherapy alone often suffer from selection bias. Many of the medical contraindications that prohibit surgery, such as older age, poor performance status, severe intercurrent medical illness, and poor pulmonary function, are known to be significant prognostic factors for survival.[344,345] Patients referred for radiotherapy are more likely to be elderly and to be at greater risk for death from intercurrent diseases. Patients receiving radiotherapy alone generally have also undergone less extensive staging (clinical vs. pathologic) than those in surgical series reporting pathologic versus clinical outcome. Some patients discovered on mediastinoscopy to harbor N2 disease may be excluded or separated from outcome analyses in surgical series.[344] Sandler et al.[334] demonstrated the importance of rigorous clinical staging in selecting true stage I NSCLC for primary radiotherapy. In their series of 77 patients with clinical stage I NSCLC treated with primary radiotherapy, treatment in only 2 of 12 patients who underwent "excellent" staging evaluation failed locoregionally at 3 years; in contrast, locoregional failure occurred in 22 of 24 (87%) with "good" staging and 30 of 41 (79%) with staging categorized as "other." With the advent of noninvasive assessment of nodal regions through CT and PET, some of this discrepancy might diminish.[344,345]

Tumor size is a prognostic factor in almost every retrospective series reported. For example, Krol et al.[333] found that patients with tumors smaller than 4 cm had a 35% overall survival at 3 years and those with tumors larger than 4 cm had a 13% 3-year survival. There has also been some evidence that higher radiation doses (more than 65 Gy) lead to improved survival.[335,338] Jeremic et al.[339] and Morita et al.[336] have treated patients with some of the highest doses seen in the literature, 69.6 Gy and 65 Gy, respectively, and report favorable overall survival. These two factors (tumor size and dose) are interrelated, because a very large tumor, technically T2, is often difficult to treat to high doses because of the danger of pulmonary toxicity. Squamous cell histologic type has been shown to be a positive prognostic factor, as has younger age.[334,340] The results from many modern series appear in Table 27.2-7. Patients with smaller tumors that can be treated to higher doses appear to be the best candidates for primary radiotherapy. Treatment of elective nodal regions prophylactically is probably not needed. The best radiotherapy results are still inferior to the results of most surgical series, although there are many confounding factors to account for a portion

TABLE 27.2-7.   Results for Patients Treated with Radiation Therapy Alone for Early-Stage Non–Small Cell Lung Cancer

Study	No. of Patients	Dose (Gy)	Overall Survival, 3-Y (%)	Overall Survival, 5-Y (%)	Cause-Specific Survival, 3-Y (%)	Cause-Specific Survival, 5-Y (%)	Local Control, 5-Y (%)
Dosoretz et al.[338]	152	60–69	40[a]	10	—	—	—
Jeremic et al.[339]	49	69.6[b]	46	30	—	—	55
Krol et al.[333]	108	60–65	31	15	42	31	~25
Kaskowitz et al.[340]	53	63	19	6	33	13	0
Morita et al.[346]	149	65	34	22	—	—	—
Slotman et al.[379]	31	48 (4-Gy fractions)	42	8	76	—	—
Graham et al.[573]	103	60	35[b]	14	—	—	—
Sandler et al.[334]	77	60	17	—	22	—	44
Sibley et al.[335]	141	55–70	24	13	—	—	—
Zhang et al.[574]	44	55–70	55[c]	32[c]	—	—	—

[a]2-Year.
[b]Hyperfractionated.
[c]Crude survival.

of this difference. It is hoped that with improved staging and dose delivery, the results with primary radiotherapy will improve.

"UNRESECTABLE" STAGE IIIA AND IIIB NON–SMALL CELL LUNG CANCER

Whether stage IIIA or IIIB disease is considered unresectable depends, to a large degree, on the experience and attitudes of the physician treating the patient. What one surgeon considers unresectable, another with an aggressive surgical attitude may deem completely resectable. Nevertheless, when stage IIIA disease is extremely bulky and enlarged lymph nodes surround vital structures in the mediastinum, it is unlikely that any primary surgical approach will be beneficial. In centers with more aggressive attitudes, patients with these "unresectable" tumors have been evaluated for combined modality protocols that include surgery.

Patients with unresectable stage IIIA or IIIB NSCLC have traditionally been treated with radiotherapy alone. Because all known macroscopic disease is confined to the chest, therapy is given with "curative" intent. However, only 5% to 10% of such patients survive beyond 5 years, primarily due to progression of disease outside the radiation field (occurring in up to 70% of patients), which reflects the presence of systemic micrometastases at the time of initial therapy.[346] In a large proportion of patients, disease also progresses within the irradiated field, which indicates the failure of radiotherapy alone to eliminate all macroscopic tumor. Consequently, efforts to increase cure rates have focused simultaneously on increasing both locoregional and systemic control of disease. In practice, induction chemotherapy or concomitant chemoradiotherapy (or both) have been evaluated to achieve these goals.

Aggressive Surgery

Primary surgery has limited value in patients with stage IIIA NSCLC exhibiting biopsy-proven bulky, multilevel, or extracapsular N2 disease. Because of this, induction therapies combined with surgery or radiotherapy have been intensively investigated in these patients. When these individuals are treated, imaging results must be correlated with invasive staging, because findings on CT and PET scans do not accurately reflect treatment response.[347]

Stage IIIB NSCLC encompasses a heterogeneous group of neoplasms exhibiting invasion of the carina, great vessels, or vertebral bodies (T4), as well as tumors associated with a malignant pleural effusion (T4) and tumors exhibiting ipsilateral supraclavicular or contralateral mediastinal lymph node metastases (N3). In general, tumors in patients with IIIB disease are inoperable. Because of this, combined modality regimens using chemotherapy and radiation are most appropriate for patients with good performance status. Nevertheless, in highly selected patients, T4 tumors can be completely resected, with long-term survival achieved in some of these individuals who receive combined modality treatment.[348,349]

Although primary lung cancer invading the carina is generally considered unresectable, pneumonectomy with tracheal sleeve resection and direct reanastomosis of the trachea to the contralateral main-stem bronchus can be performed. In some patients, "extended" SL (resection of the carina) can be used to preserve pulmonary function. Five-year survival rates for highly selected patients undergoing carinal resection approach 40% in some series.[350] Survival is contingent on complete resection and nodal status. Mitchell et al.[351] observed 5-year survival rates of 51%, 32%, and 12% for patients with carinal tumors with N0, N1, and N2 disease, respectively. Anastomotic dehiscence with bronchial fistula formation and postoperative pulmonary insufficiency are the most common postoperative problems in these individuals. Given the present survival rates, only highly selected patients without N2 disease should undergo carinal resection. For this reason, before resection of such a tumor, mediastinoscopy should be considered mandatory.

Involvement of the SVC has been treated occasionally by *en bloc* resection and graft replacement. Several reviews indicate the feasibility of concomitant pulmonary resection with SVC resection and reconstruction, with patient survival contingent on completeness of resection and nodal status. Preoperative differentiation of SVC invasion by the tumor (T4) or by involved mediastinal lymph nodes (N2) can be difficult. Invasive staging of the mediastinum is mandatory in these individuals, because patients with N2 disease typically do not benefit from SVC resection and reconstruction.[352,353]

Complete excision of a primary tumor exhibiting mediastinal organ invasion is usually not possible, and incomplete resections do not afford survival or palliation benefit.[354] In the series at MSKCC, there were no 5-year survivors among 19 patients with aorta involvement and three patients with atrial invasion, but one patient of seven (14%) with esophageal invasion lived beyond 5 years.[256] Despite these results, a tumor with limited invasion of the atrial wall can occasionally be completely resected with the hope of an occasional cure.

En bloc resection of the lung with part of the involved aorta, esophagus, or vertebral body, not uncommon in the treatment of superior sulcus tumors, may result in long-term survival for selected patients. PORT may be of benefit in these situations to augment local control. An analysis by Japanese investigators suggested that long-term survival is limited to patients with minimal atrial or aortic adventitial involvement in tumors invading great vessels.[355]

Five percent to 10% of patients with lung cancer present with a nonmalignant pleural effusion due to atelectasis, obstructive pneumonitis, lymphatic or venous obstruction, or pulmonary embolus. Even if nonmalignant, an effusion evident on a prior chest radiograph has a poor prognosis. Investigators at the Mayo Clinic demonstrated that even cytologically negative pleural effusions evident on chest radiographs were predictive of unresectability in 95% of patients. However, they concluded that in patients with cytologically negative pleural effusions, unresectability must be documented. On the other hand, Naruke et al.[356] reported a 40% 5-year survival rate in 112 patients with nonmalignant effusions—a survival rate identical to that observed for 1298 patients without effusions.

Even in patients with malignant pleural effusions, occasional 5-year survivals have been documented when all disease has been eradicated.[356,357] In general, however, cytologically proven malignant pleural effusions indicate disease incurable via surgical approaches, and the tumors are usually treated with primary chemotherapy.

The role of surgery in preoperatively identified N3 disease previously considered totally inoperable has been examined in phase II trials. Hata et al.[358] investigated the use of two-field lymphadenectomy, including total mediastinal exenteration and supraclavicular node dissection. The exact role of postoperative therapies combined with this procedure was not discussed. The long-term results of such treatment are unknown. In addition, induction therapies (particularly chemoradiation) have been investigated by SWOG and other intergroups.[359,360] Overall, the data indicate that, after very intensive induction therapies, some patients survive long term; however, it does not appear that surgery improves survival in these individuals. In fact, in many phase II trials, no attempt was made to remove the involved N3 lymph nodes. Surgery was directed toward removal of the primary tumor and N2 nodes.

Adjuvant and Neoadjuvant Therapies

After complete resection in patients proven to have T4 or N3 disease, radiotherapy has been usually recommended as adjuvant treatment because of the high incidence of locoregional failure after aggressive surgery for these advanced tumors. Because of the paucity of patients reported to have undergone this treatment, the exact role of adjuvant radiotherapy cannot be assessed. It is for this subset of tumors that neoadjuvant therapies have been investigated in many phase II trials. It does appear that clinically staged T4 tumors (especially T4N0 disease) do reasonably well after this combined modality approach.[348,361,362] In one such study,[362] patients with clinically evident T4 tumors, including SVC syndrome, tracheal involvement, and posterior mediastinal invasion, were treated with mitomycin, vinblastine, and cisplatin (MVP) chemotherapy followed by surgery. Sixty-three percent of patients underwent a complete resection, and overall survival at 4 years was 19.5%. Despite these encouraging results, most T4 and N3 tumors cannot be resected completely. In such instances, these tumors should be treated by combined modality regimens, using radiotherapy to achieve local control.

RADIOTHERAPY. Although it seems clear that contemporary thoracic radiotherapy may offer a modest survival advantage to patients with disease limited to the thorax, the poor results from earlier studies led the RTOG to investigate methods of improving outcome with radiation alone, initially by concentrating on dose intensification with conventional fractionation and more recently by using altered fractionation. In addition, RTOG investigators have attempted to identify appropriate selection criteria and prognostic factors for the various approaches and to apply innovative treatment planning and technology.

Standard External-Beam Radiotherapy. The earliest trial by the RTOG for unresectable NSCLC attempted to establish the optimal schedule of standard fractionated radiation alone. Protocol 73-01 was limited to 379 patients with either medically inoperable stage I or II disease or unresectable stage III NSCLC of various histologic types. Patients in this trial were randomly assigned to one of four dose-escalating arms, including 40-Gy split-course or 40-Gy, 50-Gy, or 60-Gy continuous-course thoracic radiation delivered in 4, 5, or 6 weeks with a daily fraction size of 2 Gy. Analysis of patterns of failure and survival showed a higher complete response rate (24%) and 3-year survival rate (15%) with 60-Gy continuous-course radiotherapy than with lower doses of continuous- and split-course radiation treatment (40 to 50 Gy). The failure rate

within the irradiated volume was 53% to 58% for 40 Gy, 49% for 50 Gy, and 35% for 60 Gy. This improvement in local control was still apparent nearly 5 years later. The median time to any failure increased from 8 to 19 months as dose was increased from 40 to 60 Gy. Overall, patients who achieved a complete tumor response also experienced increased survival, compared with partial responders or patients with stable disease. The 3-year survival rate in complete responders was 23%, compared with 10% in partial responders and 15% in patients with stable disease.[363]

By escalating the total dose from 40 to 60 Gy, this trial established a dose-response relation between local control and short-term survival. Despite the preliminary local control and survival advantages in patients experiencing a complete response and in patients receiving a dose of 60 Gy, the overall median survival for patients receiving 40 Gy was 9.6 months, compared with 10.1 months for patients receiving 50 to 60 Gy. In addition, the 5-year survival rate for all patients in this trial was approximately 6%, with no significant differences among the four arms.

Three-Dimensional Conformal Radiotherapy. In a dose-escalation protocol using 3D-CRT at the University of Michigan, patients were treated at doses that ranged from 69.3 to 102.9 Gy. The researchers reported a single case of acute grade 3 pneumonitis and five cases of acute grade 2 pneumonitis.[171] Patients with advanced disease have now been receiving neoadjuvant chemotherapy in addition to radiotherapy. The median survival in patients with stage III or recurrent disease was 16 months, and 2-year overall survival was 36%.

Graham et al.[170,364] reported the results of 3D-CRT for NSCLC at Washington University. They treated tumors to a dose of 60 to 74 Gy. Elective nodal irradiation was given to all except those patients with poor pulmonary function. These investigators reported a 2-year survival rate of 53% with this technique. Investigators at the University of Chicago reported a 2-year local control rate of 23% and a survival rate of 37% in patients treated with doses ranging from 60 to 70 Gy.[365] The MSKCC reported 2-year local control, disease-free survival, and overall survival rates of 36%, 11%, and 22%, respectively, in a group of patients with advanced-stage disease treated with 3D-CRT.[172]

Elective Nodal Irradiation. Standard radiotherapy typically involves a dose of 40 Gy to the entire mediastinum, supraclavicular fossa, and ipsilateral hilum, even if there is no evidence of disease in these areas (e.g., T4N0 tumors). It has been shown that this elective treatment can add significantly to the morbidity of the radiation therapy.[366,367] Many centers have made the decision to eliminate elective nodal irradiation in an effort to increase the dose to the tumor. When RTOG trial results were reviewed to estimate the clinical impact of omitting nodal irradiation, it was found that when the ipsilateral hilum and mediastinum were incorrectly treated, there was an increased risk of progression.[368] The MSKCC reported an elective nodal failure rate of 8% and a local failure rate of 65%,[369] which suggests that, until regions of known disease can be better controlled, there is probably no need to treat the entire mediastinum and supraclavicular region electively when T4N0 tumors are being treated. Invasive staging or PET scanning may improve decision making.

ALTERED FRACTIONATION RADIOTHERAPY. Altered fractionation implies any deviation from the standard fractionation of 1.8 to 2.0 Gy delivered once daily, 5 days weekly for 6 to 7 weeks. Several forms of altered fractionation, such as continuous hyperfractionation accelerated radiotherapy (CHART), and variations of these regimens have been investigated.[441] The basic goal of altered fractionation strategies is to deliver higher total doses of radiation to improve the local outcome without increasing late normal tissue toxicity. Altered fractionation schemes exploit the significant differences in the capacity of late-responding and early-responding tissues to repair radiation cellular damage.

Hyperfractionation. Hyperfractionated radiotherapy uses more than 1 fraction/d, delivered in fraction sizes that are smaller than those used with standard fractionation (1.1 to 1.5 Gy/fraction vs. 1.8 to 2.0 Gy/fraction). Thus, hyperfractionation uses multiple small fractions per day to deliver a higher total daily dose and final total dose to improve tumor cell kill without increasing late toxicity and accepts increased but resolvable acute toxicity.[370]

The RTOG initiated a phase I and II trial to evaluate radiotherapy with 1.2-Gy twice-daily fractionation for locally advanced unresectable disease. Eight hundred eighty-four patients were randomly selected to receive doses of 60.0, 64.8, and 69.6 Gy, in 1.2-Gy fractions twice daily with a minimum of a 4-hour interfraction interval. After reasonable time had elapsed to evaluate both acute and late effects, which were considered tolerable, patients were further assigned to either 74.4 or 79.2 Gy of radiotherapy, with closure of the two lowest-dose arms. In a favorable subgroup of patients, the 69.6-Gy dose results appeared significantly better ($P = .002$) than results with standard fractionation in comparable patients from an earlier RTOG study and the other arms of the trial.[331] No increased toxicity was seen in the higher-dose arms to account for the decreased survival compared to that in the 69.6-Gy arm.

Based on these results, the RTOG began a phase III trial comparing radiotherapy of 69.6 Gy given via hyperfractionation and 60 Gy given via standard fractionation in thirty 2-Gy fractions. The third arm of the trial replicated the study arm of CALGB protocol 8433: induction chemotherapy with cisplatin and vinblastine followed by 60 Gy of radiation. The 5-year survivals for standard radiotherapy, hyperfractionated radiotherapy, and induction chemotherapy plus radiation were 4%, 5%, and 8%, respectively. The survival in the chemotherapy-plus-radiotherapy arm was significantly higher.[371] As yet, there is no clear survival advantage that can be demonstrated for hyperfractionation compared to standard radiotherapy. However, many trials continue to use this hyperfractionation regimen of 69.6 Gy. Further studies are needed to find the maximum tolerable dose of radiation with either hyperfractionation or standard fractionation and compare it to results for 60 Gy of radiation.

Accelerated Radiotherapy. RTOG trial 8407 examined the role of an accelerated concomitant boost of radiotherapy. Patients received 45 Gy over 5 weeks to the primary tumor and mediastinal lymph nodes. Two to three times a week, a concomitant boost of 1.8 Gy would be delivered only to the primary tumor and involved lymph nodes. A dose of 25.2 Gy via concomitant boost (to a total of 70.2 Gy) was found to be tolerable.[372] Two-year survival was 21% for the patients receiving the higher-dose radiotherapy. Another RTOG phase II trial (8312) demonstrated a 2-year survival rate of 25% and a 3-year survival rate of 18%.[364]

Continuous Radiotherapy. CHART uses many radiobiologic principles in an effort to improve the therapeutic ratio. CHART delivers 54 Gy in three daily doses of 1.5 Gy over 12 continuous days, including weekends. With CHART, treatment is given every day to counteract rapidly proliferating cells. Hyperfractionation with many smaller doses of radiation may reduce long-term toxicity. Accelerating the treatment time from 6 to 2 weeks also may counteract tumor repopulation.

CHART was first examined in a small prospective phase II trial.[373] Some degree of esophageal toxicity was present in all patients. Ten percent of patients developed acute radiation pneumonitis. Two-year survival was 34%.

A phase III randomized study was performed in 13 centers in the United Kingdom. Patients were assigned to receive either standard radiation to 60 Gy in 30 daily doses of 2 Gy over 6 weeks or to CHART. Approximately one-half the patients had stage III disease; the remainder had early-stage disease or disease of unknown stage. No other therapeutic modality was used. Two-year survival was significantly increased from 20% to 29% in the CHART arm. In addition, local control significantly improved from 15% to 23%.[374] Severe esophageal toxicity also increased from 3% to 19%, and acute radiation pneumonitis was 19% in the conventional group and 10% in the CHART arm. However, late pulmonary toxicity and fibrosis requiring treatment at 2 years was present in 16% of living patients who received CHART compared to 4% who received conventional radiotherapy. The physical and psychological symptoms caused by this aggressive regimen have been shown to be tolerable.[375]

The use of CHART has been limited by the need to reorganize radiation departments to accommodate the demanding radiation treatment schedule. In addition, patients are hospitalized during the entire course of radiation therapy, which may significantly increase the cost of treatment. Therefore, trials have been conducted using CHART without treatment on weekends.[376]

An Eastern Cooperative Oncology Group (ECOG) trial examined the feasibility of hyperfractionated accelerated radiotherapy.[377] Twenty-eight patients received 57.6 Gy over 15 days (12 treatment days) in 1.6-Gy fractions delivered three times daily, 4 hours apart. The need to wait 6 hours between fractions was avoided by not treating consecutively those fields containing spinal cord. The investigators found that this regimen was tolerable, with the main toxicities being esophagitis and moist desquamation of the skin. Median survival of 13 months was similar to that for combined modality approaches.

A North Central Cancer Treatment Group trial compared standard radiotherapy (60 Gy in 30 daily fractions of 2 Gy over 6 weeks) to an accelerated hyperfractionated approach (60 Gy in 40 fractions of 1.5 Gy twice daily over 4 weeks). A third arm received the accelerated hyperfractionated regimen with concomitant cisplatin and etoposide. Results for the two radiation-alone arms were not significantly different, although there was a trend toward improved local control and overall survival when the two hyperfractionation arms were combined.[378]

Hypofractionated Radiotherapy. The reality for most physicians treating unresectable NSCLC is that, in many patients, favorable parameters are not present. In these patients with unresectable stage III tumors, the results with either radiotherapy alone or combined modality treatment are poor, and the chance for cure is low. Studies have examined the use of hypofractionated radiotherapy for unresectable stage III disease and compared the results to those for standard fractionation to 60

Gy in RTOG trials. Depending on one's philosophy, the use of hypofractionated radiotherapy may simply be a palliative treatment or it may be a curative approach with low expectation, based on known results for radiotherapy alone. One study revealed that patients with stage III disease treated with 40-Gy split-course irradiation had longer survival times and lower local relapse rates but higher distant failure rates than those receiving 24 to 32 Gy. Survival rates for patients with stage IIIA disease treated with 40 Gy at 1, 2, and 5 years were 47%, 22%, and 7%, respectively. In patients with stage IIIB disease, the radiation scheme did not correlate with survival and relapse rates. Survival rates at 1, 2, and 5 years were 30%, 9%, and 2%, respectively. The hypofractionated schemes were extremely well tolerated, and no severe complications were observed.[379] Although the data for both schedules of treatment appear comparable, split-course irradiation cannot be routinely recommended based on the available literature on treatment of locally advanced NSCLC.

RADIOSENSITIZERS. Schaake-Koning et al.[380] demonstrated a survival advantage when cisplatin given weekly or daily was added to thoracic radiotherapy. Three-year overall survival improved from 2% to 16% with the addition of daily cisplatin. The benefit was due to increased local control with cisplatin. It is not clear whether cisplatin actually enhances the effect of radiation or whether it is independently cytotoxic, with its effectiveness more dependent on dosing and dose level. Other studies have shown no benefit from the addition of concomitant chemotherapy to thoracic radiation.[381–383]

A CALGB-ECOG study examined induction chemotherapy with cisplatin and vinblastine followed by 60 Gy radiotherapy with or without radiosensitization with carboplatin, 100 mg/m².[384] This study differs from those described heretofore because it used cytotoxic chemotherapy for induction in both arms and therefore was solely testing the value of radiosensitization. There was no difference in overall survival, failure-free survival, or response between the two arms. There was a higher local control rate in the carboplatin arm, but this did not have an impact on survival.

RADIATION PROTECTORS. The radioprotectant amifostine is a sulfhydryl compound, the metabolites of which scavenge free radicals that are generated in tissues exposed to radiation.[385] A phase II clinical trial using amifostine with sequential chemotherapy and standard radiation (60 Gy) demonstrated no episodes of grade 3 or worse esophagitis or pneumonitis.[386] Komaki et al.[387] reported that amifostine diminished esophagitis, pneumonitis, and neutropenia in patients receiving concurrent chemotherapy and radiation therapy for inoperable lung cancer. In both of these studies, there was no evidence of tumor protection. Amifostine might allow for the use of higher doses of chemotherapy and radiation with acceptable toxicity.

Prophylactic Cranial Irradiation for Locally Advanced Disease

The hypothesis that prophylactic cranial irradiation (PCI) can improve survival is based on the assumption that isolated brain failures occur commonly and lead to death and that these can be effectively prevented by tolerable doses of radiation. PCI has been shown on metaanalysis to improve survival in patients with

small cell lung cancer.[388] However, isolated brain failures are not common in NSCLC, and it is not possible to predict which patients are at risk. Consequently, it is unlikely that survival would be improved to a detectable degree if effective prophylaxis were delivered to the entire population of patients with resected disease. Of 1532 patients treated surgically in prospective trials of the LCSG, only 6.8% (104 of 1532) had first recurrences in the brain. However, 71% of the patients in this series had T1 to 2N0 tumors. Patients with locally advanced disease treated with thoracic irradiation on the RTOG protocols had an initial brain failure rate of 7% for squamous histology, 19% for adenocarcinoma, and 13% for large cell carcinoma. Even for adenocarcinoma, the brain is a less common site of initial failure than bone (24%) or opposite lung (21%).[389,390]

Four randomized trials of PCI added to chest irradiation (with or without chemotherapy) have been reported for patients with locally advanced NSCLC and have not demonstrated improved survival, although treatment did reduce the rate of development of brain metastasis.[391–394] Thus, until systemic treatment and local therapy are sufficient to render the brain the main site of clinical failure, PCI cannot be recommended for patients with any stage of NSCLC, and its use remains investigational.

The use of PCI after combined modality therapy that includes surgery has not been sufficiently investigated. However, one study involved 75 patients who had stage IIIA or IIIB NSCLC treated by induction therapy and who were treated with PCI (30 Gy over 3 weeks). In this phase II trial, PCI was started after the end of the final chemotherapy cycle and before surgery. In those patients who had partial or complete responses to the induction chemotherapy, there were no relapses in the brain as the first site of recurrence. Further study is warranted, because the brain is the most common site of first relapse in most induction therapy reports.[394]

Combined Modality Treatments Including Radiotherapy

SEQUENTIAL CHEMOTHERAPY AND RADIOTHERAPY (INDUCTION OR NEOADJUVANT CHEMOTHERAPY). The use of induction chemotherapy is based on several theoretic considerations.[395–398] It has been suggested that the early use of chemotherapy lowers the systemic tumor burden and prevents the growth of microscopic systemic disease, and that bulky locoregional macroscopic disease is decreased and addressed more easily by subsequent surgery, radiotherapy, or both.

Several large randomized studies of induction chemotherapy in unresectable NSCLC have been published. Generally, studies using more intensive chemotherapeutic regimens and larger study cohorts have favored the use of chemotherapy. Metaanalyses of chemotherapy in this setting also suggest a significant therapeutic benefit but are compromised by the limitations of this technique, which reflect the poor design or execution of many of the randomized trials.[288,399]

When the role of chemotherapy for unresectable stage III disease is assessed, it is beneficial to concentrate on specific well-designed and well-conducted trials. In 1984, CALGB initiated a randomized study comparing standard radiotherapy to two cycles of induction chemotherapy with cisplatin plus vinblastine followed by radiotherapy.[400,401] Eligible patients had stage III unresectable NSCLC; eligibility was restricted to those with only 5% weight loss before study entry and a performance status of 0 or 1. Patients with supraclavicular lymph node involvement or cytologically positive pleural effusion were also excluded. Thus, eligible patients were selected to be in a generally favorable state of health and to be treated with curative intent. This study was closed after an interim analysis, with only 155 eligible patients entered, when a survival difference became apparent. The median survival time favored chemotherapy (14 vs. 10 months; *P* = .0066). Thus, the addition of 1 month of chemotherapy to radiation resulted in a 4-month prolongation of life. More interestingly, the chemotherapy also resulted in a doubling of the number of long-term survivors. On both study arms, few patients were noted to have recurrences after 2 years of follow-up. Seventeen percent of patients were alive at 5 years' follow-up on the chemotherapy arm, compared with 7% of patients receiving standard radiotherapy alone.

A confirmatory Intergroup study was subsequently organized.[225,402] In this trial, the two study arms of the CALGB trial were repeated; a third arm was added to test the hypothesis that use of intensified radiotherapy as a single modality might also result in increased survival rates. Eligibility criteria were identical to those spelled out in the CALGB study. This study largely confirmed the results of the CALGB study: Median survival times for radiotherapy alone, hyperfractionated radiotherapy, and induction chemotherapy were 11, 12, and 14 months, respectively. This difference again favored the addition of chemotherapy to radiotherapy. The use of hyperfractionated radiotherapy alone resulted in no significant benefit. Long-term survival data from this study suggest that 3-year survival rates are similar for induction chemotherapy and hyperfractionated radiotherapy (and superior to those for standard fractionation radiotherapy).

Given the systemic activity of chemotherapy, it might be expected that the increased survival rate observed with induction chemotherapy would be due to increased systemic control. However, not all studies have included an analysis of the pattern of failure. A European study tested three cycles of induction chemotherapy with vindesine, lomustine, cisplatin, and cyclophosphamide in patients with squamous cell and large cell lung carcinoma and showed a small survival benefit favoring chemotherapy. Increased systemic control due to chemotherapy was also shown in the Intergroup trial, whereas there was no effect on intrathoracic control.[167,403,404]

These results have been confirmed by at least two metaanalyses. The first one analyzed 14 randomized trials involving 1887 patients with stage IIIA or IIIB disease. When cisplatin-based chemotherapy regimens were considered (ten randomized trials), chemoradiotherapy was associated with a 24% and 30% reduction in mortality at 1 and 2 years, respectively, but no significant survival benefit beyond 2 years.[405] The second metaanalysis included 22 trials encompassing 3033 patients and compared radical radiation therapy with chemoradiotherapy; 11 of the chemotherapy regimens were cisplatin based. Cisplatin-based combined therapy was associated with an absolute survival benefit at 2 and 5 years of 3% and 2%, respectively.[288]

In summary, induction chemotherapy has been shown in large randomized studies to increase survival rates of patients with unresectable stage III NSCLC. This appears to be due to increased systemic disease control and is therefore compatible with the observations of activity for chemotherapy in patients with stage IV disease and the theoretic models supporting induction chemotherapy. For this reason, induction chemotherapy is a current standard therapy for these patients.

CONCOMITANT CHEMORADIOTHERAPY. The simultaneous use of chemotherapy and radiotherapy has also been widely investigated. This approach is based on considerations similar to those for sequential chemoradiotherapy in that chemotherapy may cover systemic disease, whereas radiotherapy can treat locoregional disease. The concomitant approach provides the additional theoretic benefit of increasing locoregional control through a direct interaction of the two modalities, which is not the case when the two modalities are administered in sequence.[395,406] Clinically, the administration of intensive concomitant chemoradiotherapy is complicated by increased toxicities. These include esophagitis, a risk of radiation pneumonitis, and increased myelosuppression because the thoracic bone marrow is exposed to the radiation. As a result, the chemotherapy frequently has been administered using single-agent regimens at suboptimal doses, or the radiotherapy schedule has been interrupted to allow for recovery of normal tissues. It is known that prolongation of a course of radiotherapy decreases its single-modality efficacy.

Results of several single-drug chemoradiotherapeutic trials have been published. In particular, cisplatin as a single agent has been tested in several randomized trials. A study of weekly cisplatin (15 mg/m²/wk) plus radiotherapy to 50.4 Gy found no survival benefit.[381] Similarly, studies of radiotherapy with low daily doses of cisplatin[382] or cisplatin given every 3 weeks[383] showed no survival benefit. Only one study showed improved local control and survival for daily cisplatin added to radiotherapy; however, the patients on the control arm received protracted radiotherapy.[380] Thus, concomitant chemoradiotherapy using single-agent cisplatin or other drugs has largely failed to improve the survival rates of patients with locoregionally advanced NSCLC, although it may provide a locoregional sensitization effect. This appears to be due to the lack of systemic activity of low-dose single-agent therapy; thus, the predominant mode of failure in these patients (distant disease) is inadequately addressed.

Results of several studies testing combination chemotherapy with concomitant radiotherapy or using hyperfractionated radiotherapy have also been published.[395,407–413] These studies largely have been performed in the phase I and II settings. Results uniformly indicate increased toxicity. However, some studies have also suggested therapeutic benefit and have found encouraging survival data.

The SWOG has published results of two phase II trials using cisplatin and etoposide with concurrent radiotherapy. In the first trial,[230] concomitant chemoradiotherapy to 45 Gy was administered in the preoperative setting. The response rate for this regimen before surgery was 59%, and 71% of patients were able to undergo resection. The 3-year survival rate was 26%. This study formed the basis for the current large Intergroup trial evaluating concomitant chemoradiotherapy plus chemoradiotherapy boost versus resection in patients with marginally resectable stage IIIA NSCLC. A second study, SWOG trial 9019,[414,415] evaluated this chemoradiotherapy regimen in patients with unresectable disease (T4N0 to 1, T4N2, or T4N3 stage IIIB NSCLC). Induction therapy was two cycles of cisplatin plus etoposide concurrent with once-daily thoracic radiotherapy (45 Gy). In the absence of

TABLE 27.2-8. A Randomized Phase III Study of Concurrent versus Sequential Radiotherapy with Mitomycin, Vindesine, and Cisplatin (Platinum) (MVP) in Stage III Non–Small Cell Lung Cancer

Treatment Arm	No. of Patients	Response Rate (%)	Survival Median (mo)	2-Y (%)	3-Y (%)	P Value
Concurrent	156	84	16.5	37	27	.0473
Sequential	158	66.4	13.3	25.6	12.5	

progressive disease, radiotherapy was completed to 61 Gy, with two additional cycles of cisplatin plus etoposide. At a median follow-up of 52 months, the overall median survival was 15 months. Three- and 5-year survivals were 17% and 15%, respectively. The SWOG has evaluated a similar regimen of carboplatin, etoposide, and concurrent radiotherapy in patients with poor prognostic features.[416] Pilot data in this group of patients indicated similar median and 2-year survival times, which indicates the feasibility of chemoradiotherapy for a suboptimal patient population.

Definitive testing of combination chemotherapy with concurrent radiotherapy in the phase III setting has been limited. Of three randomized trials comparing concurrent with sequential chemotherapy with radiotherapy, two have demonstrated a statistically significant benefit for concurrent therapy. A three-arm study investigated the combination of carboplatin and etoposide at two dosage levels added to hyperfractionated radiotherapy (1.2 Gy twice daily; total dose, 64.8 Gy).[410] Administration of carboplatin (100 mg/m^2) on days 1 and 2 and etoposide (100 mg/m^2) on days 1 to 3 of each week of radiotherapy resulted in a significant increase in median survival compared to hyperfractionated radiotherapy alone (median survival, 8 vs. 18 months). A similar comparison of twice-daily radiotherapy to 69.6 Gy with and without daily intravenous carboplatin (50 mg) and etoposide (50 mg) showed a significant increase in median survival time (22 vs. 14 months) and 4-year survival rates (23% vs. 9%).[411] These studies support the addition of chemotherapy to radiotherapy but do not clarify whether twice-daily radiotherapy is superior to single daily fractions. Intensified radiotherapy schedules are mainly supported by the British CHART study.[374] A similar study has been reported by Japanese investigators. Furuse et al.[226,285] compared the administration of the MVP regimen as induction chemotherapy to its administration with concurrent radiotherapy. Median survival times were 16 months versus 13 months in favor of the concurrent administration of chemoradiotherapy. A pattern-of-failure analysis indicated a higher relapse in the brain for patients treated with concurrent chemoradiotherapy, with the possibility of higher intrathoracic control (Table 27.2-8). In a French trial,[286] 212 patients were randomly assigned to receive induction chemotherapy with cisplatin plus vinorelbine followed by thoracic radiotherapy (66 Gy) or to receive concurrent treatment (the same dose of thoracic radiotherapy started on day 1 with concurrent cisplatin plus etoposide followed by two additional cycles of chemotherapy with cisplatin plus vinorelbine). Concurrent therapy was associated with a nonsignificant trend toward improved median survival (15.0 vs. 13.8 months), and 2-year survival (35% vs. 23%).

Because both induction chemotherapy and concomitant chemoradiotherapy prolong survival, it can be asked which of the two approaches is superior. Based on previous pilot studies, 611 patients with stage III NSCLC were randomly chosen to receive induction chemotherapy with cisplatin plus vinblastine (standard) followed by thoracic radiation to a total dose of 60 Gy delivered in daily fractions; concurrent cisplatin plus vinblastine with radiation to a total dose of 60 Gy delivered in daily fractions; or cisplatin with orally administered etoposide and concomitant hyperfractionated radiotherapy to a total dose of 69.6 Gy delivered in twice-daily fractions.[417,418] Although nonhematologic toxicity was higher on the concurrent arms, median survival was significantly better in the concurrent standard radiotherapy arm (17.0 months vs. 14.6 and 15.2 months in the sequential and twice-daily radiotherapy arms; P = .046 for the comparison with sequential therapy), as was 4-year survival (21% vs. 12% and 17%, respectively).[227]

INDUCTION AND CONCOMITANT CHEMORADIATION. An alternative strategy to a direct comparison of induction versus concomitant combined modality therapy is the administration of both. This strategy is supported by the suggestion that induction chemotherapy and concomitant chemoradiotherapy may exert their favorable influences on survival by different mechanisms. In particular, induction chemotherapy appears to improve systemic disease control, whereas concomitant chemoradiotherapy leads to higher locoregional control. This hypothesis has been evaluated in several studies. CALGB compared administration of cisplatin and vinblastine followed by radiotherapy with administration of the same induction chemotherapeutic regimen followed by radiotherapy with weekly doses of concomitant carboplatin.[384] This study showed a median survival time of 13 months on both arms but suggested increased locoregional control for patients receiving carboplatin. This study adds to the evidence that single-agent radiation sensitization with a platinum agent is of clinical benefit.

More recently, similar investigations have focused on the integration of novel chemotherapeutic single agents into chemoradiation treatment. Preclinical and early clinical data suggest that taxanes, gemcitabine, vinorelbine, and topoisomerase I inhibitors act as radiation enhancers.[419-433] Additional trials have evaluated the administration of paclitaxel with or without carboplatin on a weekly schedule with concurrent chest radiotherapy. Phase II trials indicate high response and promising 1- and 2-year survival rates with this approach. Pilot studies using paclitaxel are summarized in Table 27.2-9. A three-arm randomized phase II study by CALGB (study

TABLE 27.2-9. Selected Phase II Trials of Weekly Paclitaxel-Based Chemotherapy with Concurrent Radiotherapy in Patients with Stage III Unresectable Non–Small Cell Lung Cancer

Author	No. of Patients	Concurrent Chemotherapy	Radiotherapy	Relative Risk (%)	Survival 1-Y (%)	Survival 2-Y (%)
Choy et al.[423]	29	Paclitaxel	60 Gy[a]	86	73	NA
Choy et al.[424]	39	Paclitaxel and carboplatin	66 Gy[a]	75.7	56.3	38.3
Choy et al.[425]	43	Paclitaxel and carboplatin	69.6 Gy[b]	78.6	63	NA
Belani et al.[426]	38	Paclitaxel and carboplatin	60–65 Gy[a]	NA	63	54

NA, not available.
[a]Once-daily radiation.
[b]Twice-daily radiation.

9431)[434] evaluated new drugs in combination with cisplatin in unresectable stage III NSCLC. One hundred seventy-five eligible patients received four cycles of cisplatin at 80 mg/m² on days 1, 22, 43, and 64 along with one of the following: gemcitabine, 1250 mg/m² on days 1, 8, 22, and 29 and 600 mg/m² on days 43, 50, 64, and 71 (arm 1); paclitaxel 225 mg/m² for 3 hours on days 1 and 22 and 135 mg/m² on days 43 and 64 (arm 2); or vinorelbine 25 mg/m² on days 1, 8, 15, 22, and 29 and 15 mg/m² on days 43, 50, 64, and 71 (arm 3). Radiotherapy was initiated on day 43 at 2 Gy/d (total dose, 66 Gy). Median survival for all patients was 17 months, with no clearly superior arm in this phase II trial. The observed survival rates exceeded those of previous CALGB trials and may be attributable to the use of concomitant chemoradiotherapy. An additional trial evaluating three novel agents (gemcitabine, paclitaxel, or vinorelbine in combination with cisplatin) in the induction and concomitant setting is under way. The radiation dose in this trial is 66 Gy.[431]

To evaluate further the role of induction chemotherapy within the context of concomitant chemoradiotherapy, the CALGB is conducting a randomized trial in which concomitant chemoradiotherapy with carboplatin, paclitaxel, and concurrent radiotherapy is compared with two cycles of induction chemotherapy using carboplatin and paclitaxel followed by the same concomitant chemoradiotherapeutic regimen. This trial will evaluate whether induction chemotherapy is of benefit in patients receiving concomitant chemoradiotherapy.

Additional trials are expanding on observations with accelerated radiotherapy. The aforementioned British trial has indicated that administration of accelerated radiotherapy is superior to standard radiotherapy as a single-treatment modality.[374,413] Because accelerated radiotherapy has an impact on locoregional control only, its administration after induction chemotherapy is being evaluated in a randomized ECOG trial.[435]

A second randomized multi-institutional phase II trial compared two different schedules of paclitaxel-based induction chemotherapy and concurrent chemoradiotherapy with sequential paclitaxel-based chemotherapy followed by radiotherapy in patients with stage III NSCLC.[436] Two hundred seventy-six patients were randomly assigned to arm 1 (sequential), which received two cycles of paclitaxel (200 mg/m²) plus carboplatin (AUC = 6) followed by daily thoracic irradiation (to 63.0 Gy); arm 2 (induction/concurrent), which received induction chemotherapy (two cycles) followed by

weekly paclitaxel (45 mg/m²) and carboplatin (AUC = 2) with thoracic irradiation for 7 weeks; or arm 3 (concurrent/consolidation), which received concurrent chemotherapy and radiation followed by two cycles of paclitaxel (200 mg/m²) plus carboplatin (AUC = 6). Arm 3 (concurrent/consolidation) appeared to have the best therapeutic outcome; at a median follow-up of 26 months, the median survival in this arm was 16.1 months.

When these studies of combined modality therapy for unresectable NSCLC are reviewed, it is clear that induction chemotherapy using new agents, followed by concomitant chemoradiotherapy, has led to a significant increase in survival rates. The existing data indicate that patients can be treated with induction chemotherapy or concomitant chemoradiotherapy outside of a clinical trial (as a standard therapy); however, the impact of these strategies on survival is small, and participation in clinical trials is strongly encouraged.

STAGE IV DISEASE

General Principles

Of the nearly 169,000 Americans who will develop NSCLC in any given year, 55% will present with stage IIIB or IV disease that is not amenable to curative treatment. More than half of the remaining 45% of individuals treated with curative intent will experience relapse and eventually succumb to their disease. With the exception of the rare patient with oligometastases, patients with stage IV NSCLC typically die from their disease, with an overall median survival time of 8 to 16 months. The fraction of patients who are alive 1 year after diagnosis has increased slightly over the past decade; presently approximately one-third of patients with stage IIIB or IV disease are alive at 1 year, and 10% to 21% of these individuals are alive 2 years after diagnosis. Although these data reflect improvements in the care of patients with advanced lung cancer, treatment remains palliative, with the goal of compassionate and effective end-of-life care.

Prolongation of Survival by Chemotherapy

In the 1970s and 1980s, combination chemotherapy (usually cisplatin based) was shown to reproducibly achieve objective responses in 20% to 30% of lung cancer patients.[437,438] Despite

TABLE 27.2-10. Selected Randomized Trials of Chemotherapy versus Best Supportive Care in Advanced Non–Small Cell Lung Cancer

Study	Chemotherapy	No. of Patients BSC/Chemo	Median Survival (wk) BSC/Chemo	P Value
Rapp et al.[222]	CAP/VP	50/43/44[a]	17/25/33[a]	.05/.01[b]
Cartei et al.[575]	CCM	50/52	17/37	.0001
Woods et al.[576]	VP	91/97	17/27	.33
Cellerino et al.[577]	CEP/MEC	57/58	21/34	.135
Kaasa et al.[578]	VP	43/44	17/22	.28
ELVIS[447]	VNR	81/80	21/28	.03
Cullen et al.[456]	MIC	176/175	21/29	.03
Stephens et al.[579]	Platinum based	364/361	24.5/33.1	.0016

BSC, best supportive care; CAP/VP, cyclophosphamide (Cytoxan), doxorubicin (Adriamycin), cisplatin (platinum)/vinblastine, cisplatin; CCM, cisplatin, cyclophosphamide/mitomycin; CEP/MEC, cyclophosphamide, etoposide + platinum/mitomycin, etoposide + cisplatin; Chemo, chemotherapy; ELVIS, Elderly Lung Cancer Vinorelbine Italian Study Group; MIC, mitomycin, ifosfamide, cisplatin; VNR, vinorelbine; VP, vindesine/platinum.
[a]BSC/chemo/chemo.
[b]CAP vs. BSC/VP vs. BSC.

the fact that cytotoxic regimens appear to have activity in stage IV NSCLC, overall median survival of patients receiving chemotherapy was only 6 to 8 months, with few patients surviving longer than 1 year. Because of this, the value of chemotherapy in the routine management of patients with stage IV NSCLC was unclear.[439–444] Indeed, some investigators hypothesized that the survival benefits derived from chemotherapy were not sufficient to justify the toxicities and costs. At least 12 randomized studies, involving over 2000 patients, were initiated to compare combination chemotherapy with best supportive care (BSC) in patients with advanced NSCLC (Table 27.2-10). Seven of these trials showed a statistically significant survival benefit in favor of chemotherapy. The Canadian study remains the most frequently cited study in this category.[222] In this trial, 150 patients with advanced NSCLC were randomly assigned to receive cisplatin plus vindesine, the CAP regimen, or BSC. The median survival times were significantly longer in the cisplatin plus vindesine and CAP groups than in the BSC arm (33 and 25 weeks, respectively); survival prolongation was achieved with acceptable costs.[445] In a subsequent Big Lung Trial, Stephens et al.[446] randomly assigned 725 patients to receive either short-term cisplatin-based chemotherapy (three cycles) or BSC and confirmed that chemotherapy improved median survival by 8 weeks. The Elderly Lung Cancer Vinorelbine Italian Study Group[447] randomly assigned 161 elderly patients (older than 70 years) to receive BSC with or without single-agent therapy with vinorelbine (30 mg/m^2 on days 1 and 8 of every 21-day cycle for up to six cycles) and observed a statistically significant

prolongation in median survival with a possible improvement in overall quality of life in the vinorelbine-treated group (P = .03). Anderson et al.[448] randomly assigned 300 patients to receive BSC with or without single-agent chemotherapy with gemcitabine (1000 mg/m^2 on days 1, 8, and 15 of each 28-day cycle); the chemotherapy-arm patients scored better than control patients on the quality-of-life scale and reported fewer lung cancer–related symptoms.

Because these trials were limited due to insufficient numbers of patients or suboptimal chemotherapy regimens, metaanalyses were performed, the results of which are summarized in Table 27.2-11.[288,405,449–451] Overall, these metaanalyses indicate that chemotherapy is associated with a cost-efficient reduction in the OR for death in the first 6 months and a modest but statistically significant prolongation in median survival time. As a result, many physicians consider the use of chemotherapy to be standard for most patients with advanced NSCLC.[437,439,452,453]

Quality of Life

With the limited survival benefit for patients with stage IV NSCLC, quality of life has been considered a relevant end point for chemotherapeutic trials involving these individuals. Validated questionnaires have been developed to accurately assess quality of life. Early randomized trials suggested that chemotherapy can improve quality of life. For instance, in a Canadian study, patients receiving chemotherapy had a lower incidence of disease-related complications, leading to

TABLE 27.2-11. Metaanalysis of Best Supportive Care versus Chemotherapy

Study	No. of Studies	Results	Conclusion
Souquet et al.[449]	7	Reduced mortality at 3 and 6 mo.	CT to be offered
Grilli et al.[450]	6	6-Wk gain in survival (24% reduction in probability of death).	CT for selected patients
Marino et al.[451]	8	Median survival, 3.9 vs. 6.7 mo (20% more at 6 mo).	CT to be offered
NSCLC Collaborative Group[288]	11 (8 cisplatin-based)	Median survival, 6 vs. 8 mo; 1-y survival: 16% vs. 26%. Data best for cisplatin-based therapy.	CT improves survival

CT, chemotherapy; NSCLC, non–small cell lung cancer.

fewer hospital admissions.[445,454,455] Typically, disease-related symptoms improved after chemotherapy, sometimes even in the absence of a measurable tumor response.[456–458] Quality-of-life scores improved with chemotherapy, whereas they declined over the first 6 weeks with BSC. Improved survival and quality of life were also demonstrated with single-agent chemotherapy in a population of patients older than age 70 years.[447]

A number of large analyses have been performed to validate prognostic factors in patients with stage IV NSCLC disease receiving chemotherapy. The SWOG analyzed their database of 2531 patients with advanced NSCLC using Cox modeling, recursive partitioning, and amalgamation techniques,[459] and reported that good performance status, female gender, age of 70 years or older, low tumor burden, normal lactate dehydrogenase and serum calcium levels, and a hemoglobin level of more than 11 g/dL were associated with favorable response to chemotherapy. The use of cisplatin was an additional, favorable predictor of survival. A European group conducted a similar analysis of 1052 patients and observed that lower tumor burden, good performance status, older age, and female gender were associated with a more favorable response to therapy.[460]

Therapeutic Options for Patients with Advanced Disease

Patients with newly diagnosed stage IV NSCLC should be informed of the therapeutic options that will provide the best palliation. In many circumstances, the best initial treatment is a local modality. For example, brain metastases, spinal cord compression, and impending fractures of weight-bearing bones are usually treated with radiation or surgery before systemic therapy commences. Patients who present with postobstructive pneumonia are often treated initially by radiotherapy with the addition of either an endobronchial stent or EBB; after some resolution of the pneumonia, systemic therapy can be considered.

Based on available data from randomized trials, optimal chemotherapy regimens for advanced NSCLC include cisplatin and vinorelbine, cisplatin and gemcitabine, or, alternatively, cisplatin or carboplatin and paclitaxel. Performance status is the single best factor for identifying those individuals who can tolerate and are most likely to benefit from chemotherapy. Patients with an ECOG performance status of 0 or 1 are the best candidates for chemotherapy and can achieve both prolongation of survival and improvement in quality of life. Patients with an ECOG performance status of 2 typically experience symptom relief, but as a group do not obtain substantial survival benefit. Individuals with an ECOG performance status of 3 or 4 do not benefit from chemotherapy; because of this, BSC is the preferred means of palliation. Age does not predict adverse outcome; thus patients who are elderly with a good performance status should be offered systemic treatment.

First-Line Chemotherapy

Randomized studies during the 1980s established the value of chemotherapy compared to BSC. The combination of cisplatin with etoposide or vinblastine emerged as a standard in the United States, whereas in Europe, cisplatin plus vindesine was most frequently administered. In the 1990s, reproducible single-agent activity was demonstrated for paclitaxel, docetaxel, vinorelbine, gemcitabine, and irinotecan. Evaluation of these newer agents frequently has included a comparison of the drugs administered with cisplatin versus cisplatin alone. Currently, platinum-based combination chemotherapy regimens are preferred for the treatment of NSCLC. Etoposide, vindesine, and vinblastine have traditionally been considered as first-generation agents when combined with cisplatin. The second generation of regimens includes platinum combinations with vinorelbine, docetaxel, paclitaxel, and gemcitabine, and nonplatinum regimens (i.e., gemcitabine plus vinorelbine or paclitaxel). Current regimens (particularly those that are carboplatin based) appear less toxic; however, the overall outcome of patients treated with these newer drug combinations is only marginally better than that reported for patients treated with older regimens.

Standard of Care: Platinum-Based Doublets

Between 1981 and 1991, more than 1900 patients participated in three different randomized trials evaluating a wide range of cisplatin-based chemotherapy regimens. ECOG trial EST 1581[461] evaluated cyclophosphamide, doxorubicin, methotrexate, and procarbazine (CAMP); MVP; etoposide and cisplatin; and vindesine and cisplatin. ECOG trial EST 1583[462] compared MVP; vinblastine and cisplatin; MVP alternating with CAMP; carboplatin followed by the MVP regimen at the time of progression; and iproplatin followed by MVP at the time of progression. A SWOG trial[463] randomly assigned patients to receive cisplatin plus etoposide with or without methylglyoxal bisguanylhydrazone; cisplatin and vinblastine; cisplatin and vinblastine alternating with vinblastine and mitomycin; or fluorouracil, vincristine, mitomycin/cyclophosphamide, doxorubicin, and cisplatin. The response rates ranged between 6% and 31%, and median survival times were 24.5 to 31.0 months. Median survival durations were not significantly different among the studies. No particular cisplatin-based combination emerged as a superior regimen for advanced NSCLC.

In 1985, 108 patients with stage III NSCLC were randomly assigned to receive cisplatin (120 mg/m^2) with either vindesine (3 mg/m^2) or vinblastine (6 mg/m^2). No significant differences were observed in response rate (33% vs. 41%) or median survival (18.4 vs. 16.2 months). The two regimens demonstrated comparable response and survival data, but patients on the vinblastine arm had an increased incidence of neutropenia.[464] In 1993, Le Chevalier et al. were the first to use a second-generation agent along with platinum,[465] reporting that cisplatin plus vinorelbine was superior to cisplatin plus vindesine. The median survival time for patients receiving cisplatin and vinorelbine was significantly longer than that noted for patients treated with cisplatin and vindesine (40 vs. 30 weeks, respectively). This study also demonstrated that cisplatin was required in the doublet, because cisplatin plus vinorelbine was superior to vinorelbine alone. Further analysis revealed that this chemotherapy regimen had acceptable efficacy and cost effectiveness compared to other common medical interventions.[454] In a more recent, randomized trial, cisplatin plus vinorelbine (P-NVB) was compared with vinorelbine plus ifosfamide plus cisplatin (NIP). The overall response rate was 34.6% for P-NVB and 35.7% for NIP. Median survival time and 1-year survival rate were 10.0 months and 38.4% for P-NVB and 8.2 months and 33.7% for NIP, respectively. The SWOG randomly assigned 432 chemotherapy-naive patients to receive cisplatin and vinorelbine or single-agent cisplatin. The median progression-free and overall survival times were modestly yet significantly better in patients receiving combined therapy than in those treated with cisplatin alone (4 vs. 2 months, and 8 vs. 6 months, respectively).[466]

The cisplatin-etoposide combination was initially developed as an effective regimen for patients with small cell lung cancer and remains standard of care for this disease. The efficacy of cisplatin-etoposide for NSCLC has also been documented. In a phase II study of 94 patients with advanced NSCLC, the response rate was 38% and median survival was 7.5 months.[467] In a phase III trial, the ECOG randomly assigned patients to one of three regimens: cisplatin plus etoposide; paclitaxel, cisplatin, and granulocyte colony-stimulating factor; or paclitaxel plus cisplatin. Significant differences were observed between the cisplatin-etoposide and paclitaxel-cisplatin groups (response rate, 12% vs. 26.31%, respectively). These data suggested that paclitaxel regimens may be associated with superior survival compared to the ECOG standard of cisplatin plus etoposide.[468]

Gemcitabine has been evaluated in randomized phase II and III trials.[469–472] A European trial compared cisplatin and gemcitabine with cisplatin and etoposide, and suggested a favorable impact on median survival.[470] Another randomized trial demonstrated, that compared to cisplatin alone, gemcitabine plus cisplatin improved median survival by 2 months but was associated with an increase in hematologic toxicities.[469] In a phase III trial comparing gemcitabine alone with gemcitabine plus carboplatin in 332 patients with advanced NSCLC, Sederholm[473] observed overall response rates of 30% in the combination arm and 12% in the gemcitabine arm; the median survival in the combination arm (9 months) was superior to that in the arm receiving gemcitabine alone.

Two randomized phase III trials failed to demonstrate any difference in efficacy between gemcitabine plus cisplatin and the combination of mitomycin, ifosfamide, and cisplatin or between gemcitabine plus carboplatin and the combination of either mitomycin, ifosfamide, and cisplatin or mitomycin, vinblastine, and cisplatin in treatment of stage IIIB or stage IV disease.[474,475] A multicenter, randomized phase II study established the use of gemcitabine as safe and feasible when the agent is combined with carboplatin or cisplatin. Median survival durations were identical for gemcitabine with either cisplatin or carboplatin (10.4 vs. 10.8 months).[476] A phase II study evaluated the response rate and toxicity of a regimen of gemcitabine (1000 mg/m^2 over 30 minutes on days 1 and 8) plus oxaliplatin (65 mg/m^2 over 120 minutes on days 1 and 8) every 21 days for six cycles in 32 patients with poor-prognosis NSCLC. The response rate was 19%, and the median overall survival was 27 weeks; toxicity was acceptable.[477] In an additional phase II study using a different oxaliplatin schedule (130 mg/m^2 on day 1, every 21 days), Crino et al.[478] observed a response rate of 20%. In clinical trial 08975 of the European Organization for Research and Treatment of Cancer (EORTC), 480 chemotherapy-naive patients with advanced lung cancer were randomly assigned to receive one of three different chemotherapy regimens: paclitaxel and cisplatin; gemcitabine and cisplatin; or paclitaxel and gemcitabine. Median survival times were 8.1 months, 8.9 months, and 6.7 months, respectively, for these regimens.[479]

Numerous studies have indicated that paclitaxel has single-agent activity against NSCLC (Table 27.2-12).[480–482] A European trial demonstrated that cisplatin plus paclitaxel resulted in a median survival of 10 months—a response similar to that for cisplatin and teniposide—and was better tolerated.[483] In the mid-1990s, several groups reported successful phase II trials using carboplatin combined with a 3-hour infusion of paclitaxel. The most optimistic of these trials was by Langer et al.,[484] who administered carboplatin (AUC = 7.5) and paclitaxel (175 mg/m^2 over 1 hour) to chemotherapy-naive patients with advanced NSCLC at three weekly intervals for six cycles. They noted a response rate in excess of 50%, and median survival of 48.5 weeks. Additional phase II trials confirmed that the carbo-

TABLE 27.2-12. Single-Agent Activity of New Chemotherapeutic Agents for Non–Small Cell Lung Cancer

Agent	No. of Studies[a]	No. of Patients	Total CR + PR	Median Survival[b]	No. of Studies[c]	1-Y Survival (%)	No. of Studies[d]
Paclitaxel[e]	10	317	84 (26%)	37 (24–56)	6	41	7
Docetaxel[f]	8	300	77 (26%)	41 (27–48)	5	52	3
Vinorelbine	6	621	126 (20%)	33 (29–40)	6	24	3
Gemcitabine[g]	9	572	122 (21%)	41 (31–49)	5	39	2
Irinotecan	4	138	37 (27%)	35 (27–42)	2	NR	NR
Topotecan	5	119	15 (13%)	38 (33–40)	4	35	2

CR, complete response; NR, not reported; PR, partial response.
[a]Number of studies reporting results.
[b]Average median survival in weeks (range).
[c]Number of studies with median survival data.
[d]Number of studies with 1-year survival data.
[e]Includes both short (1- to 3-hour) and long (24-hour) infusion schedules. There were no differences in response or survival based on infusion duration.
[f]Includes doses of 60–100 mg/m^2. The response rates were 23% at 60 mg/m^2 and 29% at 100 mg/m^2. Survival data were similar.
[g]Includes doses of 800 mg/m^2 given on days 1, 8, and 15 of a 28-day cycle. At doses >1000 mg/m^2, there were no obvious dose responses.
(Adapted from ref. 437.)

TABLE 27.2-13. Comparison of Various Combination Chemotherapy Regimens

Study	Regimen	Response Rate (%)	Median Survival (mo)	1-Y Survival (%)	P Value
OLD VS. NEW COMBINATION CHEMOTHERAPY REGIMENS					
Le Chevalier et al.[465]	Vinorelbine	14	7.2	35	—
	Cisplatin + vindesine	19	7.4	35	.04
	Cisplatin + vinorelbine	30	9.3	40	.01
Bonomi et al.[468]	Cisplatin + etoposide	12.5	7.6	32	—
	Cisplatin + paclitaxel	25	9.5	37	NA
	Cisplatin + paclitaxel + G-CSF	28	10.1	40	—
Giaccone et al.[483]	Cisplatin + teniposide	28	9.9	41	—
	Cisplatin + paclitaxel	41	9.7	43	NS
Belani et al.[487]	Cisplatin + etoposide	14	9.9	37	—
	Carboplatin + paclitaxel	22	9.5	32	NS
Crino et al.[485]	Mitomycin, ifosfamide, cisplatin	28	8.8	—	
	Cisplatin + gemcitabine	40	8.1	—	NS
Cardenal et al.[470]	Cisplatin + etoposide	22	7.2	25	—
	Cisplatin + gemcitabine	41	8.7	32	.18
NEW VS. NEW COMBINATION CHEMOTHERAPY REGIMENS					
Kelly et al.[488]	Cisplatin + vinorelbine	27	8.0	36	—
	Carboplatin + paclitaxel	27	8.0	33	NS

G-CSF, granulocyte colony-stimulating factor; NA, not available; NS, not significant.

platin-paclitaxel combination could be given with acceptable toxicity. Other randomized trials have confirmed the activity of regimens of cisplatin or carboplatin plus paclitaxel, and the favorable toxicity profile of the latter combination (Table 27.2-13).[483,485–489] The first phase III cooperative group trial to compare two second-generation regimens was performed by SWOG. This trial compared vinorelbine plus cisplatin to paclitaxel plus carboplatin and found that these regimens resulted in comparable response rates and median survival times (approximately 8 months).[490] ECOG conducted a randomized study comparing two different doses of 24-hour infusion of paclitaxel (135 mg/m² or 250 mg/m² with granulocyte colony-stimulating factor support) plus cisplatin with cisplatin plus etoposide in chemotherapy-naive patients with stage IIIB or IV NSCLC. When data for the two paclitaxel-cisplatin arms were analyzed together, a higher response rate as well as a significantly longer median survival time were seen with the cisplatin-paclitaxel combination than with the etoposide-cisplatin regimen (9.9 vs. 7.6 months, respectively). The higher paclitaxel dose did not improve the response rate.[491,492] CALGB conducted a phase III randomized trial in which 584 patients with stage IIIB (malignant effusion) or IV NSCLC were randomly assigned to receive carboplatin (AUC = 6) and paclitaxel (225 mg/m² over 3 hours) or paclitaxel alone every 3 weeks for up to 6 cycles. The response rates and median survival were significantly improved in the carboplatin-paclitaxel arm.[493] The ease of administration of carboplatin combined with 3-hour paclitaxel infusion established this as a treatment standard for many oncologists in the United States.

Docetaxel has been shown to have activity as second-line therapy in patients with cisplatin-refractory disease.[494,495] Although response rates of 42% and median survival of 16 months have been observed for docetaxel plus vinorelbine, this combination has been associated with significant neutropenia.[496] A docetaxel-platinum combination was evaluated in

the TAX 326 trial[497] in which 1218 patients with advanced NSCLC were randomly assigned to receive docetaxel (75 mg/m²) with either carboplatin (AUC = 6) or cisplatin (75 mg/m²) every 3 weeks; or vinorelbine (25 mg/m²/wk) with cisplatin (100 mg/m²) every 4 weeks. Although the response rates were higher in the docetaxel-cisplatin arm (31.6% vs. 24.5%; P = .029), the median survival and 2-year survival rate in the docetaxel-cisplatin and vinorelbine-cisplatin arms were not significantly different (11.3 vs. 10.1 months and 21% vs. 14%, respectively); docetaxel plus carboplatin was not significantly better than either vinorelbine plus cisplatin or docetaxel plus cisplatin for any end point. Patients treated with either of the docetaxel-containing regimens reported improved quality of life, whereas the quality of life for those treated with cisplatin and vinorelbine generally decreased.[497,498] Based on this study, the U.S. Food and Drug Administration approved docetaxel in combination with cisplatin for first-line use in patients with advanced NSCLC in December 2002.

Kubota et al.[499] evaluated the combinations of cisplatin (80 mg/m²) plus docetaxel (60 mg/m²) or vindesine (3 mg/m² on days 1, 8, and 15). The docetaxel-cisplatin regimen was significantly better than the vindesine-cisplatin therapy (response rate, 37% vs. 21%, and median survival 11.3 vs. 9.6 months, respectively).[499] Sequential docetaxel–nonplatinum drug combinations have also been explored. In a phase II trial evaluating gemcitabine (1000 mg/m²) and vinorelbine (25 mg/m²) given intravenously on days 1 and 8 every 3 weeks for three cycles followed by docetaxel (60 mg/m²) administered intravenously at 3-week intervals for three cycles in 44 patients with advanced NSCLC, Hosoe et al.[500] observed a response rate of 47.7%, a median survival of 15.7 months, and a 1-year survival rate of 59%. Grade 3 pneumonitis was seen in 4.5% of patients on gemcitabine cycles. Based on these data, a phase III trial comparing this nonplatinum triplet with a standard platinum doublet combination (carboplatin plus paclitaxel) has been proposed.

Encouraging data also exist for irinotecan.[501–504] In phase II trials, irinotecan-cisplatin regimens produced response rates of 35%, with a median survival of 6 to 8 months and 1-year survival from 40% to 60% in chemotherapy-naive patients with advanced NSCLC.[505–507] In a phase III trial of irinotecan with and without cisplatin versus cisplatin plus vindesine in previously untreated patients with advanced NSCLC, survival among patients with stage IV disease was significantly better in the group given irinotecan plus cisplatin than in the groups receiving irinotecan alone or vindesine plus cisplatin (median survival, 50 weeks vs. 46.0 and 45.6 weeks, respectively).[508] Multiple phase I and II studies have combined irinotecan with taxanes, either alone or in combination with carboplatin, and have found similar response and survival rates.

The current standard of care for patients with advanced NSCLC is chemotherapy with a platinum-based doublet. At least four randomized clinical trials have compared cisplatin with carboplatin doublets in the treatment of advanced NSCLC. Only one out of the four trials has shown a modest but significant improvement in median survival.[509] The EORTC 07861 protocol compared cisplatin plus etoposide with carboplatin plus etoposide. The response rates favored the cisplatin-etoposide arm, but the difference did not reach statistical significance, and median survival was similar in both arms.[510] Rosell et al.[509] randomly assigned 618 patients to paclitaxel plus cisplatin or paclitaxel plus carboplatin and observed that the response rates were similar in both arms. The median survival was modestly but significantly better in the cisplatin-paclitaxel group (9.8 vs. 8.2 months). The ECOG 1594 trial demonstrated similar outcomes in patients treated with carboplatin plus paclitaxel, cisplatin plus docetaxel, cisplatin plus gemcitabine, or cisplatin plus paclitaxel,[511] and in a European trial, Scagliotti et al.[512] observed similar activities for cisplatin plus gemcitabine, carboplatin plus paclitaxel, and cisplatin plus vinorelbine. Collectively, these randomized trials indicate that none of these regimens is superior to the others.

Non–platinum-based regimens using gemcitabine combinations such as paclitaxel plus gemcitabine, vinorelbine plus gemcitabine, and docetaxel plus gemcitabine have been evaluated in several phase II clinical trials. Rodriguez et al.[513] evaluated the combination of paclitaxel (135 mg/m^2 given intravenously over 3 hours) on day 1, cisplatin (120 mg/m^2 given intravenously in 6 hours) on day 1, and gemcitabine (800 mg/m^2 given intravenously over 30 minutes) on days 1 and 8, every 4 weeks. The response rate, median survival time, and 1-year survival rate were 74%, 16 months, and 51%, respectively. In a phase II study, Douillard et al.[514] evaluated paclitaxel plus gemcitabine as first-line treatment for metastatic NSCLC and observed a response rate of 36%, a median survival of 12 months, and a 1-year survival rate of 48%. Because the survival reports were similar in these phase II trials, the contribution of cisplatin to the paclitaxel plus gemcitabine combination is unclear. Douillard et al.[514] evaluated the efficacy and toxicity of a non–platinum-based regimen (paclitaxel, 200 mg/m^2 on day 1, plus gemcitabine, 1000 mg/m^2 on days 1 and 8 every 3 weeks) versus a platinum-based regimen (paclitaxel, 200 mg/m^2 on day 1 plus carboplatin on day 1). The objective response rates and median survival

times for the paclitaxel-gemcitabine and paclitaxel-carboplatin arms were comparable (28% and 9.8 months vs. 35% and 10.4 months, respectively). The EORTC 08975 study[479] randomly assigned 480 patients to three arms: two cisplatin-based and one non–cisplatin-based paclitaxel and gemcitabine regimens. Response rates ranged from 27.7% to 36.6%, and median survivals ranged from 6.7 to 8.9 months, with no statistically significant differences in any of the clinical end points among arms. Overall, phase III trial data indicate no statistically significant survival advantage for platinum-containing doublets compared to gemcitabine in conjunction with docetaxel, paclitaxel, or vinorelbine.[515–519]

Elderly Patients and Chemotherapy Treatment

Randomized trials have demonstrated that elderly patients receiving chemotherapy do not have worse outcomes than younger patients.[492,520,521] Furthermore, randomized trials restricted to elderly patients have shown that single-agent vinorelbine is superior to BSC,[447] but there are conflicting data regarding whether doublet chemotherapy regimens are superior to single-agent therapy in those individuals. Frasci et al.[522] reported that, compared to vinorelbine alone, gemcitabine-vinorelbine therapy prolonged median survival time and 1-year survival rates (29 vs. 18 weeks, and 30% vs. 13%, respectively).[522,523] Contrasting results were observed in the Multicenter Italian Lung Cancer in the Elderly Study involving 698 patients older than 70 years of age who were randomly assigned to receive gemcitabine alone (1200 mg/m^2 days 1 and 8 every 3 weeks), vinorelbine alone (30 mg/m^2 on days 1 and 8, every 3 weeks), or gemcitabine (1000 mg/m^2) plus vinorelbine (25 mg/m^2), both administered on days 1 and 8, every 3 weeks. The response rate, time to progression, and median survival in the groups receiving cisplatin were not significantly better than those observed for patients treated with single-agent chemotherapy.[524]

Second-Line Chemotherapy

In a landmark study, Shepherd et al.[525] demonstrated that second-line chemotherapy can improve outcome in patients who have received cisplatin therapy. Individuals receiving docetaxel had better median and 1-year survivals compared to those given BSC (7.5 vs. 4.6 months, and 37% vs. 11%, respectively). For patients receiving second-line treatment, weekly docetaxel may provide similar efficacy with a better toxicity profile.[526] The Shepherd et al. study established docetaxel as the standard regimen against which other regimens will be compared. Presently, there is no evidence that combination therapy using standard agents is beneficial in second-line treatment. Nevertheless, because the overall outcome of second-line therapy is so poor, a great deal of effort has focused on improving the efficacy of this salvage therapy. Pemetrexed, a multitargeted antifolate approved for the treatment of malignant pleural mesothelioma, appears to have similar efficacy to docetaxel but with less myelosuppression.[527] As first-line chemotherapy, pemetrexed combinations mediate response rates of 30% to 40% and median survivals of 8.9 to 10.9 months.[528–531] Phase II studies support the efficacy of pemetrexed in combination with cisplatin, carboplatin, or oxaliplatin in patients with advanced NSCLC. Efforts to combine novel, biologically targeted agents with docetaxel as second-line treatment are ongoing. Among the most promising agents for second-line therapy are antisense oligonucleotides, COX-2 inhibitors, and antiangiogenic compounds. It remains to be seen if these novel combinations will be superior to docetaxel alone.

Optimal Duration of Chemotherapy

The goal of chemotherapy is to maximize survival benefit and palliate symptoms. It is intuitive that the duration of chemotherapy should be short to minimize potential toxicity. Socinski et al.[532] attempted to address the issue of optimal duration of chemotherapy in a study of 230 patients with advanced NSCLC. Individuals were randomly assigned to four courses of paclitaxel plus carboplatin followed by salvage therapy with single-agent paclitaxel at the time of progression, or to continuous treatment with both agents until radiographically determined progression. Overall response rates as well as median and 1-year survival rates were similar, but the incidence of treatment-related grade 2 or higher neurotoxicity increased from 20% to 43% between the fourth and eighth cycles of continuous treatment. Four cycles of carboplatin-paclitaxel chemotherapy was as effective as continuous treatment until progression. Data suggest that, although response correlates with improved survival, stable disease remains an end point beneficial to patients.[533] Currently there is no evidence that maintenance chemotherapy prolongs the survival of patients exhibiting stabilization of disease after four or six cycles of chemotherapy. For this reason, it is recommended that chemotherapy be given for two cycles, at which point response should be assessed with appropriate imaging. Patients who show a clear response and those who have stable disease should receive two additional cycles before response is again evaluated. A maximum of six cycles should be administered, after which the standard of care would be to follow patients carefully and allow a treatment break.

Novel Agents for Non–Small Cell Lung Cancer

Because lung cancer is the leading cause of cancer-related deaths throughout the world, there is a major public health reason to improve outcome for patients with this disease. Substituting one active drug for another in a platinum-based doublet or using more than four cycles of therapy has not improved outcome. Triplet regimens appear no better than doublet regimens for NSCLC. Hence, if outcome is to be improved, drugs must be developed that have novel mechanisms of action and toxicity profiles that differ from those of traditional chemotherapy agents.

GEFITINIB AND ERLOTINIB. EGFR is expressed in 40% to 80% of lung cancers, which makes this an attractive target for molecular intervention in this disease. Gefitinib and erlotinib were the first two agents to target the tyrosine kinase of the EGFR. Both of these agents have activity in NSCLC. Phase I trials of gefitinib showed that this oral agent was well tolerated, with rash and diarrhea as the major side effects. In the phase I series, impressive activity was seen in patients with NSCLC. This led to phase II trials in patients who had previously been treated with chemotherapy. In the Iressa Dose Evaluation in Advanced Lung 1 (IDEAL-1) trial conducted in Japan and Europe,[534] a response rate of 18% was observed among patients who were mostly receiving second-line chemotherapy. In the IDEAL-2 study conducted in the United States, gefitinib was administered to patients who had received prior cisplatin and docetaxel therapy (hence, therapy was mostly third line). The response rate was 11% in this trial. In both of these trials, gefitinib was well tolerated; once again, rash and diarrhea were the principal side effects. The speed of response was remarkable: The median time to response was 8 days. In a report of 100 patients with an advanced chemotherapy-refractory BAC subtype of NSCLC receiving gefitinib on a compassionate-use basis, partial responses were noted in 6 of 94 evaluable individuals; minor responses or stabilization of disease was noted in 19 patients.[535,536] The ability of gefitinib to provide meaningful benefit to patients with lung cancer who had received prior first-line therapy with a platinum-based regimen and second-line therapy with docetaxel led to Food and Drug Administration approval for this setting. Enthusiasm for gefitinib has been somewhat tempered by the development of interstitial pneumonitis in 0.3% to 1.0% of patients receiving this drug.[536,537] Although this condition often responds to steroids, this risk is an important consideration when treating lung cancer patients, who often exhibit significantly compromised pulmonary function.

Erlotinib is an EGFR tyrosine kinase inhibitor that has activity in NSCLC. In a phase II study of patients with previously treated lung cancer, erlotinib produced a response rate of 13%.[538] The toxicity profile is very similar to that of gefitinib, with rash and diarrhea being the most common side effects.

Although preclinical data suggested that inhibition of EGFR activity potentiates the effects of cytotoxic chemotherapy agents, combining either gefitinib or erlotinib with standard chemotherapy regimens has not been successful. More than 3500 patients have been entered onto randomized trials of chemotherapy combined with either erlotinib or gefitinib. Unfortunately none of the four studies have shown a benefit to combining an EGFR tyrosine kinase inhibitor with standard chemotherapy.[539] This is an issue that may be addressed again once it is better known who responds to these novel agents or once agents are available that yield response in a larger number of individuals.

ANTI–EPIDERMAL GROWTH FACTOR RECEPTOR MONOCLONAL ANTIBODIES. Cetuximab (IMC-C225, Erbitux), a human-mouse chimeric monoclonal antibody,[540] and ABX-EGF, a fully humanized monoclonal antibody, bind specifically to human EGFR. Phase III studies comparing carboplatin plus paclitaxel with and without cetuximab as well as phase II trials of ABX-EGF in NSCLC are under way.

The nonreceptor tyrosine kinase protein kinase C pathway has been targeted with small molecules such as Bryostatin and ISIS 3525 (protein kinase C–α messenger RNA inhibitor). A phase II clinical trial of Bryostatin in combination with paclitaxel is in progress. Based on the results of the phase II trial of the combination of ISIS 3525 plus paclitaxel and ISIS 3525 plus cisplatin and gemcitabine in which response rates ranged from 37% to 48% and the median survival was 15.9 months,[541,542] two phase III trials have been initiated to evaluate the combinations of carboplatin and paclitaxel plus ISIS 3525, and cisplatin and gemcitabine plus ISIS 3525 as first-line treatment for advanced NSCLC.

A variety of strategies have been used to target the ras pathway, including the use of farnesyl transferase inhibitors, antisense molecules (ISIS 2503), peptide vaccines, and raf kinase inhibitors (BAY 43-9006 and antisense ISIS 5132). Some of the early results with the use of farnesyl transferase inhibitors (tipifarnib) and antisense molecules (ISIS 5132) have been disappointing.[543–545] Additional novel agents such as bexarotene, flavopiridol, and Prinomastat targeting retinoic acid signal transduction, cyclin-dependent kinases, and matrix metalloproteinases, respectively, have also yielded disappointing results in phase II clinical trials.[546–548] Phase I and II clinical trials of single-agent therapy or combinations of cyclic guanosine monophosphate inhibitors (exisulind), histone deacetylase inhibitors (SAHA, FR901228), Akt inhibitors, proteasome inhibitors (bortezimib), and antiangiogenesis agents such as anti–vascular endothelial growth factor monoclonal antibodies (bevacizumab) and vascular endothelial growth factor receptor tyrosine kinase inhibitors (SU5416, SU6668, ZD6474), COX-2 inhibitors, and inhibitors of methionine aminopeptidase (TNP-470) are under way. A major issue regarding molecularly targeted therapy in future clinical trials is how best to integrate these novel molecules into the multidisciplinary treatment of NSCLC.

Local Therapies and Palliation

SOLITARY METASTASES

Metastasis (M1) to Lung. Differentiating between a second primary lung cancer and a metastasis in synchronous lung lesions or among local recurrence, a new primary lung cancer, and a pulmonary metastasis from a previously resected lung cancer can be difficult. A second or recurrent lung lesion is considered a metastasis if the histology is identical to that of the primary tumor and the lesion occurs in the opposite lung or a noncontiguous area of the ipsilateral lung.

Deslauriers et al.[549] reported that the presence of satellite nodules discovered at surgery clearly separated from the primary tumor but with identical histologic characteristics is a poor prognostic factor. In patients with satellite nodules from all stages of lung cancer, 5-year survival was 21.6%, compared to 44% if no nodules were present. The mechanism of tumor dissemination in the lung is not well known, but metastases may develop as a result of airborne or hematogenous spread from a primary bronchogenic carcinoma. The present TNM staging system fails to classify these synchronous lung lesions specifically.

Metastasis (M1) to Brain. Brain metastases constitute more than 25% of all observed recurrences in patients with resected NSCLC and are seen with greater frequency at autopsy.[550] In a review by the LCSG, the brain was the sole site of first recurrence in only 6.4% of patients with completely resected NSCLC but accounted for approximately 20% of all recurrences.[551] Nearly one-half of patients with brain metastases have solitary lesions on CT scan. When these lesions are symptomatic, the median survival without therapy is limited to 1 month. Corticosteroids and whole brain irradiation can offer effective palliation of symptoms but only modestly increase survival up to 6 months.[552]

A synchronous or metachronous solitary brain metastasis can be treated, whenever possible, by resection, with 5-year survival rates of 10% to 20%. Excision of a brain metastasis followed by radiation therapy appears superior to whole brain radiotherapy alone in prolonging median survival (9.2 vs. 3.4 months), preventing local recurrence, and providing a better quality of life.[553] Data suggest that stereotactic radiotherapy may yield results comparable to those of surgery and whole brain radiotherapy.[554,555]

Metastasis (M1) to the Adrenal Gland. Adrenal metastases from bronchogenic carcinoma are found in approximately one-third of patients at autopsy. Routine preoperative upper abdominal CT scanning reveals an adrenal mass in approximately 10% of patients.[556] In selected patients, excision of the primary lung tumor and of an isolated adrenal metastasis may improve survival.[557–560] The ultimate role of such an approach in the context of multimodality therapy has yet to be defined.

Metastasis (M1) to Liver, Bone, or Skin. No reports of long-term survival after combined surgical excision of a primary lung cancer and a synchronous solitary liver, bone, or skin metastasis have been published. It is rare that these lesions are truly solitary metastatic foci. However, patients with solitary metachronous sites fare reasonably well after complete surgical excision.[561]

PALLIATION. In view of the poor survival rate of patients with locally advanced NSCLC and patients with metastatic disease, effective palliation is an important objective. Carroll et al.[562] followed 134 patients with inoperable disease and observed that 64% needed immediate local palliation. One-half of individuals with no thoracic symptoms at presentation required subsequent local treatment. Thus, a watch-and-wait policy is appropriate for only a minority of patients, and it is critical that they be followed carefully to prevent the development of serious local complications that may be less easily palliated. In particular, it is important to intervene before SVC obstruction, lobar collapse, or obstructive pneumonia develops. The latter two conditions produce a radiographic picture in which tumor and other processes are not easily distinguishable, and large radiation fields may be necessary for effective control.

Numerous trials have demonstrated the palliative benefit of radiotherapy in patients with inoperable NSCLC.[562–565] Various regimens produce a high rate of palliation that often is sustained for a significant proportion of the patient's survival. Randomized trials suggest that certain symptoms, such as hemoptysis and pain, are more effectively palliated, whereas dyspnea and poor performance status appear to be more refractory to treatment. Investigators in Italy used radiotherapy of either 5.5 or 8.8 Gy once a week for a total dose of 44 Gy and reported that 80% of 45 patients experienced an average improvement of 20 points in the Karnofsky performance score.[348,566]

An RTOG trial showed that even regimens with larger fraction sizes had a low incidence (8%) of severe complications. An early Medical Research Council trial showed no difference in survival or toxicity between a regimen of 17 Gy given in two fractions 1 week apart and a more conventional palliative fractionation (30 Gy in ten fractions or 27 Gy in six fractions).[563] A follow-up study, however, demonstrated an increase in median survival from 7 months to 9 months when a regimen of 17 Gy in 2 fractions was compared to a regimen of 36 to 39 Gy in 12 to 13 fractions.[567] However, palliation was quicker and more durable in the hypofractionated arm.

A variety of surgical interventions may be required to palliate symptoms in patients with advanced NSCLC: bronchoscopic ablation of tumor to relieve endobronchial obstruction or hemoptysis, pleurodesis or placement of stents to relieve symptomatic malignant pleural effusions, or pericardial fenestration for malignant pericardial effusions. On rare occasions, resection of primary tumors and lung parenchyma may be required to control septic complications or massive hemoptysis, or to palliate unstable vertebral body involvement.

Bronchoscopic removal of endobronchial tumor is an efficient way of relieving endobronchial obstruction. Simple mechanical débridement with the use of the bronchoscope is often sufficient. Coagulative techniques such as use of a carbon dioxide, argon, or neodymium:yttrium aluminum garnet laser, electrocautery, and cryotherapy have been used in conjunction with mechanical débridement.[568–570] There has been increased interest in the use of photodynamic therapy for relieving endobronchial obstructions.[571] Massive hemorrhage is infrequently seen because of the judicious use of coagulative techniques. Frequently, endobronchial stents are used for long-term palliation. Malignant pleural and pericardial effusions frequently observed in patients with advanced NSCLC can be effectively palliated with a variety of techniques as outlined in Chapter 51.5.

REFERENCES

1. Peto R, Chen ZM, Boreham J. Tobacco—the growing epidemic. *Nat Med* 1999;5:15.
2. Jemal A, Tiwari RC, Murray T, et al. Cancer statistics, 2004. *CA Cancer J Clin* 2004;54:8.
3. Bray F, Tyczynski JE, Parkin DM. Going up or coming down? The changing phases of the lung cancer epidemic from 1967 to 1999 in the 15 European Union countries. *Eur J Cancer* 2004;40:96.
4. Ezzati M, Lopez AD. Measuring the accumulated hazards of smoking: global and regional estimates for 2000. *Tob Control* 2003;12:79.
5. Ando M, Wakai K, Seki N, et al. Attributable and absolute risk of lung cancer death by smoking status: findings from the Japan Collaborative Cohort Study. *Int J Cancer* 2003;105:249.
6. Zhang H, Cai B. The impact of tobacco on lung health in China. *Respirology* 2003;8:17.
7. Giovino GA. Epidemiology of tobacco use in the United States. *Oncogene* 2002;21:7326.
8. Malkinson AM. Primary lung tumors in mice: an experimentally manipulable model of human adenocarcinoma. *Cancer Res* 1992;52:2670s.
9. Belinsky SA, Nikula KJ, Baylin SB, Issa JP. Increased cytosine DNA-methyltransferase activity is target-cell-specific and an early event in lung cancer. *Proc Natl Acad Sci U S A* 1996;93:4045.
10. Slebos RJ, Hruban RH, Dalesio O, et al. Relationship between K-ras oncogene activation and smoking in adenocarcinoma of the human lung. *J Natl Cancer Inst* 1991;83:1024.
11. Sekido Y, Fong KM, Minna JD. Molecular genetics of lung cancer. *Annu Rev Med* 2003;54:73.
12. Vineis P, Alavanja M, Buffler P, et al. Tobacco and cancer: recent epidemiological evidence. *J Natl Cancer Inst* 2004;96:99.
13. Hainaut P, Pfeifer GP. Patterns of p53 G→T transversions in lung cancers reflect the primary mutagenic signature of DNA-damage by tobacco smoke. *Carcinogenesis* 2001;22:367.
14. Quinn MJ. Cancer trends in the United States—a view from Europe. *J Natl Cancer Inst* 2003;95:1258.
15. Djordjevic MV, Stellman SD, Zang E. Doses of nicotine and lung carcinogens delivered to cigarette smokers. *J Natl Cancer Inst* 2000;92:106.
16. Harris JE, Thun MJ, Mondul AM, Calle EE. Cigarette tar yields in relation to mortality from lung cancer in the cancer prevention study II prospective cohort, 1982–8. *BMJ* 2004;328:72.
17. Brooks DR, Palmer JR, Strom BL, Rosenberg L. Menthol cigarettes and risk of lung cancer. *Am J Epidemiol* 2003;158:609.
18. Peto R, Darby S, Deo H, et al. Smoking, smoking cessation, and lung cancer in the UK since 1950: combination of national statistics with two case-control studies. *BMJ* 2000;321:323.
19. Alberg AJ, Samet JM. Epidemiology of lung cancer. *Chest* 2003;123:21S4.
20. Doll R, Peto R. Cigarette smoking and bronchial carcinoma: dose and time relationships among regular smokers and lifelong non-smokers. *J Epidemiol Community Health* 1978;32:303.
21. Hrubec Z, McLaughlin JK. Former cigarette smoking and mortality among US veterans: a 26-year follow-up, 1954–1980. In: Burns DM, Garfinkel L, Samet J, eds. *Changes in cigarette-related disease risks and their implication for prevention and control.* Bethesda, MD: US Government Printing Office, 1997:501.
22. Tong L, Spitz MR, Fueger JJ, Amos CA. Lung carcinoma in former smokers. *Cancer* 1996;78:1004.
23. Fellows JL, Trosclair A. Annual smoking-attributable mortality, years of potential life lost and economic cost—United States 1995–1999. *MMWR Morb Mortal Wkly Rep* 2002;51:300.
24. US Environmental Protection Agency. *Respiratory health effects of passive smoking: lung cancer and other disorders.* Washington: US Government Printing Office;1992; EPA No. 600/006F.
25. International Agency for Research on Cancer. *IARC Monographs on the evaluation of carcinogenic risks to humans, Vol 83. Tobacco smoking and involuntary smoking.* Lyons, France: IARC Press, 2003.
26. Hecht SS. Human urinary carcinogen metabolites: biomarkers for investigating tobacco and cancer. *Carcinogenesis* 2002;23:907.
27. Patel JD, Bach PB, Kris MG. Lung cancer in US women: a contemporary epidemic. *JAMA* 2004;291:1763.
28. Jemal A, Cokkinides VE, Shafey O, Thun MJ. Lung cancer trends in young adults: an early indicator of progress in tobacco control (United States). *Cancer Causes Control* 2003;14:579.
29. American Society of Clinical Oncology policy statement update: tobacco control—reducing cancer incidence and saving lives. *J Clin Oncol* 2003;21:2777.
30. Braun MM, Caporaso NE, Page WF, Hoover RN. Genetic component of lung cancer: cohort study of twins. *Lancet* 1994;344:440.
31. Hemminki K, Li X, Czene K. Familial risk of cancer: data for clinical counseling and cancer genetics. *Int J Cancer* 2004;108:109.
32. Etzel CJ, Amos CI, Spitz MR. Risk for smoking-related cancer among relatives of lung cancer patients. *Cancer Res* 2003;63:8531.
33. Hwang SJ, Cheng LS, Lozano G, et al. Lung cancer risk in germline p53 mutation carriers: association between an inherited cancer predisposition, cigarette smoking, and cancer risk. *Hum Genet* 2003;113:238.
34. Dialyna IA, Miyakis S, Georgatou N, Spandidos DA. Genetic polymorphisms of CYP1A1, GSTM1 and GSTT1 genes and lung cancer risk. *Oncol Rep* 2003;10:1829.
35. Le Marchand L, Guo C, Benhamou S, et al. Pooled analysis of the CYP1A1 exon 7 polymorphism and lung cancer (United States). *Cancer Causes Control* 2003;14:339.
36. Kiyohara C, Wakai K, Mikami H, et al. Risk modification by CYP1A1 and GSTM1 polymorphisms in the association of environmental tobacco smoke and lung cancer: a case-control study in Japanese nonsmoking women. *Int J Cancer* 2003;107:139.
37. Nazar-Stewart V, Vaughan TL, Stapleton P, et al. A population-based study of glutathione S-transferase M1, T1 and P1 genotypes and risk for lung cancer. *Lung Cancer* 2003;40:247.
38. Miller DP, Neuberg D, de Vivo I, et al. Smoking and the risk of lung cancer: susceptibility with GSTP1 polymorphisms. *Epidemiology* 2003;14:545.
39. Ariyoshi N, Miyamoto M, Umetsu Y, et al. Genetic polymorphism of CYP2A6 gene and tobacco-induced lung cancer risk in male smokers. *Cancer Epidemiol Biomarkers Prev* 2002;11:890.
40. Zhou W, Liu G, Miller DP, et al. Polymorphisms in the DNA repair genes XRCC1 and ERCC2, smoking, and lung cancer risk. *Cancer Epidemiol Biomarkers Prev* 2003;12:359.
41. Wang Y, Liang D, Spitz MR, et al. XRCC3 genetic polymorphism, smoking, and lung carcinoma risk in minority populations. *Cancer* 2003;98:1701.
42. Ballaz S, Mulshine JL. The potential contributions of chronic inflammation to lung carcinogenesis. *Clin Lung Cancer* 2003;5:46.
43. Campa D, Zienolddiny S, Maggini V, et al. Association of a common polymorphism in the cyclooxygenase 2 gene with risk of non-small cell lung cancer. *Carcinogenesis* 2003;25:229.
44. Kantarci OH, Lesnick TG, Yang P, et al. Myeloperoxidase-463 (G→A) polymorphism associated with lower risk of lung cancer. *Mayo Clin Proc* 2002;77:17.
45. Whitrow MJ, Smith BJ, Pilotto LS, Pisaniello D, Nitschke M. Environmental exposure to carcinogens causing lung cancer: epidemiological evidence from the medical literature. *Respirology* 2003;8:513.
46. Boffetta P, Nyberg F. Contribution of environmental factors to cancer risk. *Br Med Bull* 2003;68:71.
47. Gottschall EB. Occupational and environmental thoracic malignancies. *J Thorac Imaging* 2002;17:189.
48. Selikoff IJ, Hammond EC, Seidman H. Mortality experience of insulation workers in the United States and Canada, 1943–1976. *Ann N Y Acad Sci* 1979;330:91.
49. Doll R. Mortality from lung cancer in asbestos workers. *Br J Ind Med* 1955;12:81.
50. Hammond EC, Selikoff IJ, Seidman H. Asbestos exposure, cigarette smoking and death rates. *Ann N Y Acad Sci* 1979;330:473.
51. Jarup L. Hazards of heavy metal contamination. *Br Med Bull* 2003;68:167.
52. Salnikow K, Su W, Blagosklonny MV, Costa M. Carcinogenic metals induce hypoxia-inducible factor-stimulated transcription by reactive oxygen species-independent mechanism. *Cancer Res* 2000;60:3375.
53. Hu W, Feng Z, Tang MS. Nickel (II) enhances benzo[a]pyrene diol epoxide-induced mutagenesis through inhibition of nucleotide excision repair in human cells: a possible mechanism for nickel (II)-induced carcinogenesis. *Carcinogenesis* 2004;25:455.
54. Bosken CH, Wei Q, Amos CI, Spitz MR. An analysis of DNA repair as a determinant of survival in patients with non-small-cell lung cancer. *J Natl Cancer Inst* 2002;94:1091.
55. Andersen A, Berge SR, Engeland A, Norseth T. Exposure to nickel compounds and smoking in relation to incidence of lung and nasal cancer among nickel refinery workers. *Occup Environ Med* 1996;53:708.
56. Belinsky SA, Klinge DM, Liechty KC, et al. Plutonium targets the p16 gene for inactivation by promoter hypermethylation in human lung adenocarcinoma. *Carcinogenesis* 2004;25:1063.

57. Schrump DS, Nguyen DM. Targets for molecular intervention in multistep pulmonary carcinogenesis. *World J Surg* 2001;25:174.

58. US Department of Health and Human Services. *The health consequences of involuntary smoking: a report of the Surgeon General.* Washington, DC: US Government Printing Office; 1986; USDHHSA Publication No. DCD 87.

59. Deutsch M, Land SR, Begovic M, et al. The incidence of lung carcinoma after surgery for breast carcinoma with and without postoperative radiotherapy. Results of National Surgical Adjuvant Breast and Bowel Project (NSABP) clinical trials B-04 and B-06. *Cancer* 2003;98:1362.

60. Matesich SM, Shapiro CL. Second cancers after breast cancer treatment. *Semin Oncol* 2003;30:740.

61. Dockery DW, Pope CA III, Xu X, et al. An association between air pollution and mortality in six U.S. cities. *N Engl J Med* 1993;329:1753.

62. Pope CA III, Thun MJ, Namboodiri MM, et al. Particulate air pollution as a predictor of mortality in a prospective study of U.S. adults. *Am J Respir Crit Care Med* 1995;151:669.

63. Blot WJ, Fraumeni JF Jr. Arsenical air pollution and lung cancer. *Lancet* 1975;2:142.

64. Xu ZY, Blot WJ, Xiao HP, et al. Smoking, air pollution, and the high rates of lung cancer in Shenyang, China. *J Natl Cancer Inst* 1989;81:1800.

65. Brown LM, Pottern LM, Blot WJ. Lung cancer in relation to environmental pollutants emitted from industrial sources. *Environ Res* 1984;34:250.

66. Boffetta P, Dosemeci M, Gridley G, et al. Occupational exposure to diesel engine emissions and risk of cancer in Swedish men and women. *Cancer Causes Control* 2001;12:365.

67. Larkin EK, Smith TJ, Stayner L, et al. Diesel exhaust exposure and lung cancer: adjustment for the effect of smoking in a retrospective cohort study. *Am J Ind Med* 2000;38:399.

68. Gustavsson P, Jakobsson R, Nyberg F, et al. Occupational exposure and lung cancer risk: a population-based case-referent study in Sweden. *Am J Epidemiol* 2000;152:32.

69. Risom L, Dybdahl M, Bornholdt J, et al. Oxidative DNA damage and defence gene expression in the mouse lung after short-term exposure to diesel exhaust particles by inhalation. *Carcinogenesis* 2003;24:1847.

70. Belinsky SA, Snow SS, Nikula KJ, et al. Aberrant CpG island methylation of the p16(INK4a) and estrogen receptor genes in rat lung tumors induced by particulate carcinogens. *Carcinogenesis* 2002;23:335.

71. Chen BH, Hong CJ, Pandey MR, Smith KR. Indoor air pollution in developing countries. *World Health Stat Q* 1990;43:127.

72. Mumford JL, He XZ, Chapman RS, et al. Lung cancer and indoor air pollution in Xuan Wei, China. *Science* 1987;235:217.

73. Wu AH, Henderson BE, Pike MC, Yu MC. Smoking and other risk factors for lung cancer in women. *J Natl Cancer Inst* 1985;74:747.

74. Key TJ, Allen NE, Spencer EA, Travis RC. The effect of diet on risk of cancer. *Lancet* 2002;360:861.

75. Johanning GL, Heimburger DC, Piyathilake CJ. DNA methylation and diet in cancer. *J Nutr* 2002;132:3814S.

76. Shen H, Wei Q, Pillow PC, et al. Dietary folate intake and lung cancer risk in former smokers: a case-control analysis. *Cancer Epidemiol Biomarkers Prev* 2003;12:980.

77. Wei Q, Shen H, Wang LE, et al. Association between low dietary folate intake and suboptimal cellular DNA repair capacity. *Cancer Epidemiol Biomarkers Prev* 2003;12:963.

78. Valaitis J, Warren S, Gambel D. Increasing incidence of adenocarcinoma of the lung. *Cancer* 1981;47:1042.

79. Nakanishi K. Alveolar epithelial hyperplasia and adenocarcinoma of the lung. *Arch Pathol Lab Med* 1990;114:363.

80. Noguchi M, Morikawa A, Kawasaki M, et al. Small adenocarcinoma of the lung. Histologic characteristics and prognosis. *Cancer* 1995;75:2844.

81. Madri JA, Carter D. Scar cancers of the lung: origin and significance. *Hum Pathol* 1984;15:625.

82. Priest JR, McDermott MB, Bhatia S, et al. Pleuropulmonary blastoma: a clinicopathologic study of 50 cases. *Cancer* 1997;80:147.

83. Kish JRJ, et al. Primary mucinous adenocarcinoma of the lung with signet-ring cells: a histochemical comparison with signet-ring cell carcinomas of other sites. *Hum Pathol* 1989;21:459.

84. Katzenstein AL, Prioleau PG, Askin FB. The histologic spectrum and significance of clear-cell change in lung carcinoma. *Cancer* 1980;45:943.

85. Hammar SP. Metastatic adenocarcinoma of unknown primary origin. *Hum Pathol* 1998;29:1393.

86. Folpe AL, Gown AM, Lamps LW, et al. Thyroid transcription factor-1: immunohistochemical evaluation in pulmonary neuroendocrine tumors. *Mod Pathol* 1999;12:5.

87. Chan JK, Hui PK, Tsang WY, et al. Primary lymphoepithelioma-like carcinoma of the lung. A clinicopathologic study of 11 cases. *Cancer* 1995;76:413.

88. Moro D, Brichon PY, Brambilla E, et al. Basaloid bronchial carcinoma. A histologic group with a poor prognosis. *Cancer* 1994;73:2734.

89. Carter D. Squamous cell carcinoma of the lung: an update. *Semin Diagn Pathol* 1985;2:226.

90. Takamori S, Noguchi M, Morinaga S, et al. Clinical pathologic characteristics of adenosquamous carcinoma of the lung. *Cancer* 1991;67:649.

91. Ginsberg SS, Buzaid AC, Stern H, Carter, D. Giant cell carcinoma of the lung. *Cancer* 1992;70:606.

92. Fishback NF, Travis WD, Moran CA, et al. Pleomorphic (spindle/giant cell) carcinoma of the lung. A clinicopathologic correlation of 78 cases. *Cancer* 1994;73:2936.

93. Yousem SA, Hochholzer L. Mucoepidermoid tumors of the lung. *Cancer* 1987;60:1346.

94. Moran CA, Suster S, Koss MN. Primary adenoid cystic carcinoma of the lung. A clinicopathologic and immunohistochemical study of 16 cases. *Cancer* 1994;73:1390.

95. Arrigoni MG, Wollner LB, Bernatz PE. Atypical carcinoid tumors of the lung. *J Thorac Cardiovasc Surg* 1972;64:413.

96. Travis WD, Rush W, Flieder DB, et al. Survival analysis of 200 pulmonary neuroendocrine tumors with clarification of criteria for atypical carcinoid and its separation from typical carcinoid. *Am J Surg Pathol* 1998;22:934.

97. Selvaggi G, Novello S, Torri V, et al. Epidermal growth factor receptor overexpression correlates with a poor prognosis in completely resected non-small-cell lung cancer. *Ann Oncol* 2004;15:28.

98. Onn A, Correa AM, Gilcrease M, et al. Synchronous overexpression of epidermal growth factor receptor and HER2-neu protein is a predictor of poor outcome in patients with stage I non-small-cell lung cancer. *Clin Cancer Res* 2004;10:136.

99. Blackhall FH, Pintilie M, Michael M, et al. Expression and prognostic significance of kit, protein kinase B, and mitogen-activated protein kinase in patients with small cell lung cancer. *Clin Cancer Res* 2003;9:2241.

100. Kim DH, Kim JS, Park JH, et al. Relationship of Ras association domain family 1 methylation and K-ras mutation in primary non-small cell lung cancer. *Cancer Res* 2003;63:6206.

101. Huncharek M, Muscat J, Geschwind JF. K-ras oncogene mutation as a prognostic marker in non-small cell lung cancer: a combined analysis of 881 cases. *Carcinogenesis* 1999;20:1507.

102. Ahrendt SA, Hu Y, Buta M. p53 mutations and survival in stage I non-small-cell lung cancer: results of a prospective study. *J Natl Cancer Inst* 2003;95:961.

103. Toledo G, Sola JJ, Lozano MD, Soria E, Pardo J. Loss of FHIT protein expression is related to high proliferation, low apoptosis and worse prognosis in non-small-cell lung cancer. *Mod Pathol* 2004;17:440.

104. Brattstrom D, Wester K, Bergqvist M, et al. HER-2, EGFR, COX-2 expression status correlated to microvessel density and survival in resected non-small cell lung cancer. *Acta Oncol* 2004;43:80.

105. Miura K, Bowman ED, Simon R, et al. Laser capture microdissection and microarray expression analysis of lung adenocarcinoma reveals tobacco smoking- and prognosis-related molecular profiles. *Cancer Res* 2002;62:3244.

106. Volm M, Koomagi R, Mattern J, Efferth T. Expression profile of genes in non-small cell lung carcinomas from long-term surviving patients. *Clin Cancer Res* 2002;8:1843.

107. Beer DG, Kardia SL, Huang CC, et al. Gene-expression profiles predict survival of patients with lung adenocarcinoma. *Nat Med* 2002;8:816.

108. Wigle DA, Jurisica I, Radulovich N, et al. Molecular profiling of non-small cell lung cancer and correlation with disease-free survival. *Cancer Res* 2002;62:3005.

109. Fruhwald MC. DNA methylation patterns in cancer: novel prognostic indicators? *Am J Pharmacogenomics* 2003;3:245.

110. Toyooka S, Toyooka KO, Maruyama R, et al. DNA methylation profiles of lung tumors. *Mol Cancer Ther* 2001;1:61.

111. Chen G, Gharib TG, Wang H, et al. Protein profiles associated with survival in lung adenocarcinoma. *Proc Natl Acad Sci U S A* 2003;100:13537.

112. Yanagisawa K, Shyr Y, Xu BJ, et al. Proteomic patterns of tumour subsets in non-small-cell lung cancer. *Lancet* 2003;362:433.

113. Sone S, Li F, Yang ZG, et al. Characteristics of small lung cancers invisible on conventional chest radiography and detected by population based screening using spiral CT. *Br J Radiol* 2000;73:137.

114. Bepler G, Goodridge CD, Djulbegovic B, Clark RA, Tockman M. A systematic review and lessons learned from early lung cancer detection trials using low-dose computed tomography of the chest. *Cancer Control* 2003;10:306.

115. Finkelstein SE, Summers RM, Nguyen DM, et al. Virtual bronchoscopy for evaluation of malignant tumors of the thorax. *J Thorac Cardiovasc Surg* 2002;123:967.

116. Vansteenkiste JF. PET scan in the staging of non-small cell lung cancer. *Lung Cancer* 2003;42[Suppl 1]:S27.

117. Luketich JD, Friedman DM, Meltzer CC, et al. The role of positron emission tomography in evaluating mediastinal lymph node metastases in non-small-cell lung cancer. *Clin Lung Cancer* 2001;2:229.

118. Reed CE, Harpole DH, Posther KE, et al. Results of the American College of Surgeons Oncology Group Z0050 trial: the utility of positron emission tomography in staging potentially operable non-small cell lung cancer. *J Thorac Cardiovasc Surg* 2003;126:1943.

119. Gonzalez-Stawinski GV, Lemaire A, Merchant F, et al. A comparative analysis of positron emission tomography and mediastinoscopy in staging non-small cell lung cancer. *J Thorac Cardiovasc Surg* 2003;126:1900.

120. Lardinois D, Weder W, Hany TF, et al. Staging of non-small-cell lung cancer with integrated positron-emission tomography and computed tomography. *N Engl J Med* 2003;348:2500.

121. Mac Manus MP, Hicks RJ, et al. Positron emission tomography is superior to computed tomography scanning for response-assessment after radical radiotherapy or chemoradiotherapy in patients with non-small-cell lung cancer. *J Clin Oncol* 2003;21:1285.

122. Weber WA, Petersen V, Schmidt B, et al. Positron emission tomography in non-small-cell lung cancer: prediction of response to chemotherapy by quantitative assessment of glucose use. *J Clin Oncol* 2003;21:2651.

123. Hochstenbag MM, Twijnstra A, Hofman P, Wouters EF, ten Velde GP. MR-imaging of the brain of neurologic asymptomatic patients with large cell or adenocarcinoma of the lung. Does it influence prognosis and treatment? *Lung Cancer* 2003;42:189.

124. Fritscher-Ravens A, Bohuslavizki KH, Brandt L, et al. Mediastinal lymph node involvement in potentially resectable lung cancer: comparison of CT, positron emission tomography, and endoscopic ultrasonography with and without fine-needle aspiration. *Chest* 2003;123:442.

125. Schmulewitz N, Wildi SM, Varadarajulu S, et al. Accuracy of EUS criteria and primary tumor site for identification of mediastinal lymph node metastasis from non-small-cell lung cancer. *Gastrointest Endosc* 2004;59:205.

126. Fritscher-Ravens A, Davidson BL, Hauber HP, et al. Endoscopic ultrasound, positron emission tomography, and computerized tomography for lung cancer. *Am J Respir Crit Care Med* 2003;168:1293.

127. Toloza EM, Harpole L, Detterbeck F, McCrory DC. Invasive staging of non-small cell lung cancer: a review of the current evidence. *Chest* 2003;123:157S.

128. Petty TL. Sputum cytology for the detection of early lung cancer. *Curr Opin Pulm Med* 2003;9:309.

129. Thunnissen FB. Sputum examination for early detection of lung cancer. *J Clin Pathol* 2003;56:805.

130. Choi YS, Shim YM, Kim J, Kim K. Mediastinoscopy in patients with clinical stage I non-small cell lung cancer. *Ann Thorac Surg* 2003;75:364.

131. Bretz G. Earlier diagnosis and survival in lung cancer. *BMJ* 1969;4,260.

132. Bretz G. The value of lung cancer detection by six-monthly chest radiographs. *Thorax* 1968;23:414.

133. Flehinger BJ, Kimmel M, Melamed MR. Natural history of adenocarcinoma-large cell carcinoma of the lung: conclusions from screening programs in New York and Baltimore. *J Natl Cancer Inst* 1988;80:337.

134. Frost JK, Ball WC Jr, Levin ML, et al. Early lung cancer detection: results of the initial (prevalence) radiologic and cytologic screening in the Johns Hopkins study. *Am Rev Respir Dis* 1984;130:549.

135. Flehinger BJ, Melamed MR, Zaman MB, et al. Early lung cancer detection: results of the initial (prevalence) radiologic and cytologic screening in the Memorial Sloan-Kettering study. *Am Rev Respir Dis* 1984;130:555.

136. Fontana RS. Meta-analysis of computed tomography for staging non-small cell lung cancer. *Am Rev Respir Dis* 1990;141:1093.

137. Fontana RS, Sanderson DR, Woolner LB, et al. Lung cancer screening: the Mayo program. *J Occup Med* 1986;28:746.

138. Marcus PM, Bergstralh EJ, Fagerstrom RM, et al. Lung cancer mortality in the Mayo Lung Project: impact of extended follow-up. *J Natl Cancer Inst* 2000;92:1308.

139. Melamed MR, Flehinger BJ, Zaman MB, et al. Screening for early lung cancer: results of the Memorial-Sloan Kettering study in New York. *Chest* 1984;86:44.

140. Kubik AK, Parkin DM, Zatloukal P. Czech study on lung cancer screening: post-trial follow-up of lung cancer deaths up to year 15 since enrollment. *Cancer* 2000;89:2363.

141. Kubik A, Polak J. Lung cancer detection. Results of a randomized prospective study in Czechoslovakia. *Cancer* 1986;57:2427.

142. Kaneko M, Eguchi K, Ohmatsu H, et al. Peripheral lung cancer: screening and detection with low-dose spiral CT versus radiography. *Radiology* 1996;201:798.

143. Henschke CI, McCauley DI, Yankelevitz DF, et al. Early lung cancer action project: overall design and findings from baseline screening. *Lancet* 1999;354:99.

144. Sone S, Takashima S, Li F, et al. Mass screening for lung cancer with mobile spiral computed tomography scanner. *Lancet* 1998;351:1242.

145. Prorok PC, Chamberlain J, Day NE, Hakama M, Miller AB. UICC workshop on the evaluation of screening programmes for cancer. *Int J Cancer* 1984;34:1.

146. Fontana RS, Sanderson DR, Woolner LB, et al. Screening for lung cancer. A critique of the Mayo Lung Project. *Cancer* 1991;67:1155.

147. Strauss GM, Gleason RE, Sugarbaker DJ. Screening for lung cancer. Another look; a different view. *Chest* 1997;111:754.

148. Henschke CI, Yankelevitz DF, Kostis WJ. CT screening for lung cancer. *Semin Ultrasound CT MR* 2003;24:23.

149. Sobue T, Moriyama N, Kaneko M, et al. Screening for lung cancer with low-dose helical computed tomography: anti-lung cancer association project. *J Clin Oncol* 2002;20:911.

150. Diederich S, Wormanns D, Semik M, et al. Screening for early lung cancer with low-dose spiral CT: prevalence in 817 asymptomatic smokers. *Radiology* 2002;222:773.

151. Nawa T, Nakagawa T, Kusano S, et al. Lung cancer screening using low-dose spiral CT: results of baseline and 1-year follow-up studies. *Chest* 2002;122:15.

152. Swensen SJ, Jett JR, Hartman TE, et al. Lung cancer screening with CT: Mayo Clinic experience. *Radiology* 2003;226:756.

153. Pastorino U, Bellomi M, Landoni C, et al. Early lung-cancer detection with spiral CT and positron emission tomography in heavy smokers: 2-year results. *Lancet* 2003;362:593.

154. Eddy DM. Screening for lung cancer. *Ann Intern Med* 1989;111:232.

155. Marcus PM. Lung cancer screening: an update. *J Clin Oncol* 2001;19:83S.

156. Flehinger BJ, Kimmel M, Melamed MR. The effect of surgical treatment on survival from early lung cancer. Implications for screening. *Chest* 1992;101:1013.

157. Yankelevitz DF, Kostis WJ, Henschke CI, et al. Overdiagnosis in chest radiographic screening for lung carcinoma: frequency. *Cancer* 2003;97:1271.

158. Henschke CI, Yankelevitz DF, Smith JP, Miettinen OS. Screening for lung cancer: the early lung cancer action approach. *Lung Cancer* 2002;35:143.

159. Henschke CI, Wisnivesky JP, Yankelevitz DF, Miettinen OS. Small stage I cancers of the lung: genuineness and curability. *Lung Cancer* 2003;39:327.

160. Winterhalder RC, Hirsch FR, Kotantoulas GK, Franklin WA, Bunn PA Jr. Chemoprevention of lung cancer—from biology to clinical reality. *Ann Oncol* 2004;15:185.

161. Khuri FR. Primary and secondary prevention of non-small-cell lung cancer: the SPORE trials of lung cancer prevention. *Clin Lung Cancer* 2003;5[Suppl 1]:S36.

162. Harris RE, Beebe-Donk J, Schuller HM. Chemoprevention of lung cancer by non-steroidal anti-inflammatory drugs among cigarette smokers. *Oncol Rep* 2002;9.

163. Kopelovich L, Crowell JA, Fay JR. The epigenome as a target for cancer chemoprevention. *J Natl Cancer Inst* 2003;95:1747.

164. Datta D, Lahiri B. Preoperative evaluation of patients undergoing lung resection surgery. *Chest* 2003;123:2096.

165. Churchill ED, Sweet RH, Sutter L, et al. The surgical management of carcinoma of the lung: the study of cases treated at the Massachusetts General Hospital from 1930–50. *J Thorac Cardiovasc Surg* 1950;20:349.

166. Jensik RJ, Faber LP, Milloy FJ, Monson DO. Segmental resection for lung cancer. A fifteen-year experience. *J Thorac Cardiovasc Surg* 1973;66:563.

167. Le Chevalier T, Arriagada R, Quoix E, et al. Radiotherapy alone versus combined chemotherapy and radiotherapy in nonresectable non-small-cell lung cancer: first analysis of a randomized trial in 353 patients. *J Natl Cancer Inst* 1991;83:417.

168. Emami B. Three-dimensional conformal radiation therapy in bronchogenic carcinoma. *Semin Radiat Oncol* 1996;6:92.

169. Cox JD, Azarnia N, Byhardt RW, et al. A randomized phase I/II trial of hyperfractionated radiation therapy with total doses of 60.0 Gy to 79.2 Gy: possible survival benefit with greater than or equal to 69.6 Gy in favorable patients with Radiation Therapy Oncology Group stage III non-small-cell lung carcinoma: report of Radiation Therapy Oncology Group 83-11. *J Clin Oncol* 1990;8:1543.

170. Graham MV. Predicting radiation response. *Int J Radiat Oncol Biol Phys* 1997;39:561.

171. Hayman JA, Martel MK, Ten Haken RK, et al. Dose escalation in non-small cell lung cancer (NSCLC) using conformal 3-dimensional radiation therapy (C3DRT): update of a phase I trial. *Proc Am Soc Clin Oncol* 1999;18:(abst).

172. Rosenzweig KE, Hanley J, Mychalczak B, et al. Final report of the 70.2 Gy and 75.6 Gy dose levels of a phase I dose escalation study using three dimensional conformal radiotherapy in the treatment of inoperable lung cancer. *Int J Radiat Oncol Biol Phys* 1998;42:(abst).

173. Munley MT, Marks LB, Scarfone C, et al. Multimodality nuclear medicine imaging in three-dimensional radiation treatment planning for lung cancer: challenges and prospects. *Lung Cancer* 1999;23:105.

174. Dische S, Saunders MI. Continuous, hyperfractionated, accelerated radiotherapy (CHART): an interim report upon late morbidity. *Radiother Oncol* 1989;16:65.

175. Evans ML, Graham MM, Mahler PA, Rasey JS. Changes in vascular permeability following thorax irradiation in the rat. *Radiat Res* 1986;107:262.

176. Rubin P, McDonald S, Maasilta P, et al. Serum markers for prediction of pulmonary radiation syndromes. Part I: surfactant apoprotein. *Int J Radiat Oncol Biol Phys* 1989;17:553.

177. Anscher MS, Murase T, Prescott DM, et al. Changes in plasma TGF beta levels during pulmonary radiotherapy as a predictor of the risk of developing radiation pneumonitis. *Int J Radiat Oncol Biol Phys* 1994;30:671.

178. Marks LB. The pulmonary effects of thoracic irradiation. *Oncology (Huntingt)* 1994;8:89.

179. Martinet N, Vaillant P, Charles T, Lambert J, Martinet Y. Dexamethasone modulation of tumour necrosis factor-alpha (cachectin) release by activated normal human alveolar macrophages. *Eur Respir J* 1992;5:67.

180. Steel GG. The search for therapeutic gain in the combination of radiotherapy and chemotherapy. *Radiother Oncol* 1988;11:31.

181. Von der Masse H, Overgaard JJ, Vaeth M. Effect of cancer chemotherapeutic drugs on radiation-induced lung damage in mice. *Radiother Oncol* 1986;5:245.

182. Roach M III, Gandara DR, Yuo HS, et al. Radiation pneumonitis following combined modality therapy for lung cancer: analysis of prognostic factors. *J Clin Oncol* 1995;13:2606.

183. Choy H, LaPorte K, Knill-Selby E, Mohr P, Shyr Y. Esophagitis in combined modality therapy for locally advanced non-small cell lung cancer. *Semin Radiat Oncol* 1999;9:90.

184. Keller SM, Adak S, Wagner H, et al. Prospective randomized trial of postoperative adjuvant therapy in patients with completely resected stages II and IIIa non-small cell lung cancer: an intergroup trial (E3590). *Proc Am Soc Clin Oncol* 1999;18:465a(abst).

185. Sadeghi A, Payne D, Rubinstein L, Lad T. Combined modality treatment for resected advanced non-small cell lung cancer: local control and local recurrence. *Int J Radiat Oncol Biol Phys* 1988;15:89.

186. Eagan RT, Lee RE, Frytak S, et al. Thoracic radiation therapy and adriamycin/cisplatin-containing chemotherapy for locally advanced non-small cell lung cancer. *Cancer Clin Trials* 1981;4:381.

187. Umsawasdi T, Valdivieso M, Barkley HT Jr, et al. Esophageal complications from combined chemoradiotherapy (cyclophosphamide + Adriamycin + cisplatin + XRT) in the treatment of non-small cell lung cancer. *Int J Radiat Oncol Biol Phys* 1985;11:511.

188. Ball D, Bishop J, Smith J, et al. A phase III study of accelerated radiotherapy with and without carboplatin in non-small cell lung cancer: an interim toxicity analysis of the first 100 patients. *Int J Radiat Oncol Biol Phys* 1995;31:267.

189. van Houtte P, Danhier S, Mornex F. Toxicity of combined radiation and chemotherapy in non-small cell lung cancer. *Lung Cancer* 1994;10 [Suppl 1]: S271.

190. Sheline GE, Wara WM, Smith V. Therapeutic irradiation and brain injury. *Int J Radiat Oncol Biol Phys* 1980;6:1215.

191. McCunniff AJ, Liang MJ. Radiation tolerance of the cervical spinal cord. *Int J Radiat Oncol Biol Phys* 1989;16:675.

192. Jeremic B, Shibamoto Y, Milicic B, Acimovic L, Milisavljevic S. Absence of thoracic radiation myelitis after hyperfractionated radiation therapy with and without concurrent chemotherapy for stage III non-small-cell lung cancer. *Int J Radiat Oncol Biol Phys* 1998;40:343.

193. Emami B, Lyman J, Brown A, et al. Tolerance of normal tissue to therapeutic irradiation. *Int J Radiat Oncol Biol Phys* 1991;21:109.

194. Armstrong J, Raben A, Zelefsky M, et al. Promising survival with three-dimensional conformal radiation therapy for non-small cell lung cancer. *Radiother Oncol* 1997;44:17.

195. Robertson JM, Ten Haken RK, Hazuka MB, et al. Dose escalation for non-small cell lung cancer using conformal radiation therapy. *Int J Radiat Oncol Biol Phys* 1997;37:1079.

196. Derycke S, De Gersem WR, Van Duyse BB, De Neve WC. Conformal radiotherapy of stage III non-small cell lung cancer: a class solution involving non-coplanar intensity-modulated beams. *Int J Radiat Oncol Biol Phys* 1998;41:771.

197. Ekberg L, Holmberg O, Wittgren L, Bjelkengren G, Landberg T. What margins should be added to the clinical target volume in radiotherapy treatment planning for lung cancer? *Radiother Oncol* 1998;48:71.

198. Ross CS, Hussey DH, Pennington EC, Stanford W, Doornbos JF. Analysis of movement of intrathoracic neoplasms using ultrafast computerized tomography. *Int J Radiat Oncol Biol Phys* 1990;18:671.

199. Kubo HD, Hill BC. Respiration gated radiotherapy treatment: a technical study. *Phys Med Biol* 1996;41:83.

200. Hanley J, Debois MM, Mah D, et al. Deep inspiration breath-hold technique for lung tumors: the potential value of target immobilization and reduced lung density in dose escalation. *Int J Radiat Oncol Biol Phys* 1999;45:603.
201. Wong JW, Sharpe MB, Jaffray DA, et al. The use of active breathing control (ABC) to reduce margin for breathing motion. *Int J Radiat Oncol Biol Phys* 1999;44:911.
202. Uematsu M, Shioda A, Tahara K, et al. Focal, high dose, and fractionated modified stereotactic radiation therapy for lung carcinoma patients: a preliminary experience. *Cancer* 1998;82:1062.
203. Timmerman R, Papiez L, McGarry R, et al. Extracranial stereotactic radioablation: results of a phase I study in medically inoperable stage I non-small cell lung cancer. *Chest* 2003;124:1946.
204. Nagata Y, Negoro Y, Aoki T, et al. Clinical outcomes of 3D conformal hypofractionated single high-dose radiotherapy for one or two lung tumors using a stereotactic body frame. *Int J Radiat Oncol Biol Phys* 2002;52:1041.
205. Onishi H. Stereotactic three dimensional (3-D) conformal multiple dynamic arc radiotherapy for stage II non-small cell lung cancer using a linear accelerator unified with self-moving CT scanner and patient's self-breath and beam control technique. *Proc Am Soc Clin Oncol* 2003;22.
206. Onishi H, Nagata Y, Shirato H, et al. Stereotactic hypofractionated high-dose irradiation for patients with stage I non-small cell lung carcinoma: clinical outcomes in 241 cases of a Japanese multi-institutional study. *Int J Radiat Oncol Biol Phys* 2003;27.
207. Harada T, Shirato H, Ogura S, et al. Real-time tumor tracking radiation therapy (RTRT) for stage I non-small cell lung cancers (NSCLCa). *Proc Am Soc Clin Oncol* 2003;22.
208. Niibe Y, Karasawa M, Shibuya M, et al. Prospective study of three-dimensional radiation therapy (3D-CRT) using middle fraction size for small-sized lung tumor in elderly patients. *Proc Am Soc Clin Oncol* 2003;22.
209. Hof H, Herfarth K, Munter M, et al. Stereotactic single-dose radiotherapy of stage I non-small cell lung cancer (NSCLC). *Int J Radiat Oncology Biol Phys* 2003;56:335.
210. Whyte RI, Crownover R, Murphy MJ, et al. Stereotactic radiosurgery for lung tumors: preliminary report of a phase I trial. *Ann Thorac Surg* 2003;75:1097.
211. Fukumoto S, Shirato H, Shimzu S, et al. Small-volume image-guided radiotherapy using hypofractionated, coplanar, and noncoplanar multiple fields for patients with inoperable stage I non-small cell lung carcinomas. *Cancer* 200;95:1546.
212. Budach V. The role of fast neutrons in radiooncology: a critical reappraisal. *Strahlenther Onkol* 1991;176:677.
213. Koh WJ, Krall JM, Peters LJ, et al. Neutron vs. photon radiation therapy for inoperable regional non-small cell lung cancer: results of a multicenter randomized trial. *Int J Radiat Oncol Biol Phys* 1993;27:499.
214. Nori D. Intraoperative brachytherapy in non-small cell lung cancer. *Semin Surg Oncol* 1993;9:99.
215. Marchese M, Nori D, Anderson L, et al. A versatile permanent planar implant technique utilizing I-125 seed embedded in Gelfoam. *Int J Radiat Oncol Biol Phys* 1981;194:747.
216. Nori D. Role of intraoperative brachytherapy in non-small cell lung cancer. In: Nori D, ed. *Proceedings of the international conference on thoracic oncology.* New York: Booth Memorial Medical Center, 1991:143.
217. Raben A, Mychalczak B. Brachytherapy for non-small cell lung cancer and selected neoplasms of the chest. *Chest* 1997;112:276S.
218. Mehta M, Shahabi S, Jarjour N, Steinmetz M, Kubsad S. Effect of endobronchial radiation therapy on malignant bronchial obstruction. *Chest* 1990;97:662.
219. Langendijk JA, Tjwa MK, de Jong JM, ten Velde GP, Wouters EF. Massive haemoptysis after radiotherapy in inoperable non-small cell lung carcinoma: is endobronchial brachytherapy really a risk factor? *Radiother Oncol* 1998;49:175.
220. Hennequin C, Tredaniel J, Chevret S, et al. Predictive factors for late toxicity after endobronchial brachytherapy: a multivariate analysis. *Int J Radiat Oncol Biol Phys* 1998;42:21.
221. Abe M, Takahashi M, Yabumoto E, et al. Clinical experiences with intraoperative radiotherapy of locally advanced cancers. *Cancer* 1980;45:40.
222. Rapp E, Pater JL, Wilan A, et al. Chemotherapy can prolong survival in patients with advanced non-small-cell lung cancer—report of a Canadian multicenter randomized trial. *J Clin Oncol* 1988;6:633.
223. Arriagada R, Bergman B, Dunant A, et al. Cisplatin-based adjuvant chemotherapy in patients with completely resected non-small-cell lung cancer. *N Engl J Med* 2004;350:351.
224. Schaake-Koning C, van den Bogaert W, Dalesio O, et al. Effects of concomitant cisplatin and radiotherapy on inoperable non-small cell lung cancer. *N Engl J Med* 1992;326:524.
225. Sause WT, Scott C, Taylor S, et al. Radiation tHerapy Oncology Group (RTOG) 88-08 and Eastern Cooperative Oncology Group (ECOG) 4588: preliminary results of a phase III trial in regionally advanced, unresectable non-small-cell lung cancer. *J Natl Cancer Inst* 1995;87:198.
226. Furuse K, Fukuoka M, Kawahara M, et al. Phase III study of concurrent versus sequential thoracic radiotherapy in combination with mitomycin, vindesine, and cisplatin in unresectable stage III non-small-cell lung cancer. *J Clin Oncol* 1999;17:2692.
227. Curran W, Scott C, Langer C, et al. Long-term benefit is observed in a phase III comparison of sequential vs concurrent chemo-radiation for patients with unresected stage III non-small cell lung cancer: RTOG 9410. *Proc Am Soc Clin Oncol* 2003;22 (abst).
228. Roth JA, Fossella F, Komaki R, et al. A randomized trial comparing perioperative chemotherapy and surgery with surgery alone in resectable stage III non-small cell lung cancer. *J Natl Cancer Inst* 1994;86:673.
229. Rosell R, Gomez-Codina J, Camps C, et al. A randomized trial comparing preoperative chemotherapy plus surgery with surgery alone in patients with non-small cell lung cancer. *N Engl J Med* 1994;330:153.
230. Albain KS, Rusch VW, Crowley JJ, et al. Concurrent cisplatin/etoposide plus chest radiotherapy followed by surgery for stages IIIA (N2) and IIIB non-small-cell lung cancer: mature results of Southwest Oncology Group phase II study 8805. *J Clin Oncol* 1995;13:1880.
231. Turrisi AT, Scott CB, Rusch VR, et al. Randomized trial of chemoradiotherapy to 61 Gy [no S] versus chemoradiotherapy to 45 Gy followed by surgery [S] using cisplatin etoposide in stage IIIa non-small cell lung cancer (NSCLC): intergroup trial 0139, RTOG (9309). *Int J Radiat Oncol Biol Phys* 2003;57:S125.
232. Gajra A, Newman N, Gamble GP, Kohman LJ, Graziano SL. Effect of number of lymph nodes sampled on outcome in patients with stage I non-small-cell lung cancer. *J Clin Oncol* 2003;21:1029.
233. Keller SM, Adak S, Wagner H, Johnson DH. Mediastinal lymph node dissection improves survival in patients with stages II and IIIa non-small cell lung cancer. Eastern Cooperative Oncology Group. *Ann Thorac Surg* 2000;70:358.
234. Wu Y, Huang ZF, Wang SY, Yang XN, Ou W. A randomized trial of systematic nodal dissection in resectable non-small cell lung cancer. *Lung Cancer* 2002;36:1.
235. Izbicki JR, Thetter O, Habekost M, et al. Radical systematic mediastinal lymphadenectomy in non-small cell lung cancer—a randomized controlled trial. *Br J Surg* 1994;81:229.
236. Ginsberg RJ, Rubinstein LV. Randomized trial of lobectomy versus limited resection for T1 N0 non-small cell lung cancer. Lung cancer study group. *Ann Thorac Surg* 1995;60:615.
237. Warren WH, Faber LP. Segmentectomy versus lobectomy in patients with stage I pulmonary carcinoma. Five-year survival and patterns of intrathoracic recurrence. *J Thorac Cardiovasc Surg* 1994;107:1087.
238. Kodama K, Doi O, Higashiyama M, Yokouchi H. Intentional limited resection for selected patients with T1 N0 M0 non-small-cell lung cancer: a single-institution study. *J Thorac Cardiovasc Surg* 1997;114:347.
239. Koike T, Yamato Y, Yoshiya K, Shimoyama T, Suzuki R. Intentional limited pulmonary resection for peripheral T1 N0 M0 small-sized lung cancer. *J Thorac Cardiovasc Surg* 2003;125:924.
240. Gajra A, Newman N, Gamble GP, et al. Impact of tumor size on survival in stage IA non-small cell lung cancer: a case for subdividing stage IA disease. *Lung Cancer* 2003;42:51.
241. Watanabe S, Oda M, Tsunezuka Y, et al. Peripheral small-sized (2 cm or less) non-small cell lung cancer with mediastinal lymph node metastasis; clinicopathologic features and patterns of nodal spread. *Eur J Cardiothorac Surg* 2002;22:995.
242. Konaka C, Ikeda N, Hiyoshi T, et al. Peripheral non-small cell lung cancers 2.0 cm or less in diameter: proposed criteria for limited pulmonary resection based upon clinicopathological presentation. *Lung Cancer* 1998;21:185.
243. Miller DL, Rowland CM, Deschamps C, et al. Surgical treatment of non-small cell lung cancer 1 cm or less in diameter. *Ann Thorac Surg* 2002;73:1545.
244. Endo C, Sagawa M, Sakurada A, et al. Surgical treatment of stage I non-small cell lung carcinoma. *Ann Thorac Cardiovasc Surg* 2003;9:283.
245. Chang MY, Sugarbaker DJ. Surgery for early stage non-small cell lung cancer. *Semin Surg Oncol* 2003;21:74.
246. McKenna RJ Jr, Wolf RK, Brenner M, Fischel RJ, Wurnig P. Is lobectomy by video-assisted thoracic surgery an adequate cancer operation? *Ann Thorac Surg* 1998;66:1903.
247. Walker WS, Codispoti M, Soon SY, et al. Long-term outcomes following VATS lobectomy for non-small cell bronchogenic carcinoma. *Eur J Cardiothorac Surg* 2003;23:397.
248. Sugi K, Kaneda Y, Esato K. Video-assisted thoracoscopic lobectomy achieves a satisfactory long-term prognosis in patients with clinical stage IA lung cancer. *World J Surg* 2000;24:27.
249. Nonaka M, Kadokura M, Yamamoto S, et al. Tumor dimension and prognosis in surgically treated lung cancer: for intentional limited resection. *Am J Clin Oncol* 2003;26:499.
250. Inoue K, Sagawa M, Sato M, et al. Prognosis of T3 patients with resected non-small cell lung cancer according to the invaded organs *Kyobu Geka* 1998;51:907.
251. Magdeleinat P, Alifano M, Benbrahem C, et al. Surgical treatment of lung cancer invading the chest wall: results and prognostic factors. *Ann Thorac Surg* 2001;71:1094.
252. Roviaro G, Varoli F, Grignani F, et al. Non-small cell lung cancer with chest wall invasion: evolution of surgical treatment and prognosis in the last 3 decades. *Chest* 2003;123:1341.
253. Chapelier A, Fadel E, Macchiarini P, et al. Factors affecting long-term survival after en-bloc resection of lung cancer invading the chest wall. *Eur J Cardiothorac Surg* 2000;18:513.
254. Yokoi K, Tsuchiya R, Mori T, et al. Results of surgical treatment of lung cancer involving the diaphragm. *J Thorac Cardiovasc Surg* 2000;120:799.
255. Rocco G, Rendina EA, Meroni A, et al. Prognostic factors after surgical treatment of lung cancer invading the diaphragm. *Ann Thorac Surg* 1999;68:2065.
256. Burt ME, Pomerantz AH, Bains MS, et al. Results of surgical treatment of stage III lung cancer invading the mediastinum. *Surg Clin North Am* 1987;67:987.
257. Fadel E, Yildizeli B, Chapelier AR, et al. Sleeve lobectomy for bronchogenic cancers: factors affecting survival. *Ann Thorac Surg* 2002;74:851.
258. Chunwei F, Weiji W, Xinguan Z, et al. Evaluations of bronchoplasty and pulmonary artery reconstruction for bronchogenic carcinoma. *Eur J Cardiothorac Surg* 2003;23:209.
259. Deslauriers J, Gregoire J, Jacques LF, et al. Sleeve lobectomy versus pneumonectomy for lung cancer: a comparative analysis of survival and sites or recurrences. *Ann Thorac Surg* 2004;77:1152.
260. De Leyn P, Rots W, Deneffe G, et al. Sleeve lobectomy for non-small cell lung cancer. *Acta Chir Belg* 2003;103:570.
261. Ferguson MK, Lehman AG. Sleeve lobectomy or pneumonectomy: optimal management strategy using decision analysis techniques. *Ann Thorac Surg* 2003;76:1782.
262. Downey RJ, Martini N, Rusch VW, et al. Extent of chest wall invasion and survival in patients with lung cancer. *Ann Thorac Surg* 1999;68:188.
263. Martini N, Flehinger BJ, Zaman MB, Beattie EJ Jr. Results of resection in non-oat cell carcinoma of the lung with mediastinal lymph node metastases. *Ann Surg* 1983;198:386.
264. Martini N, Flehinger BJ. The role of surgery in N2 lung cancer. *Surg Clin North Am* 1987;67:1037.
265. Shields TW. The significance of ipsilateral mediastinal lymph node metastasis (N2 disease) in non-small cell carcinoma of the lung. *J Thorac Cardiovasc Surg* 1990;99:48.
266. Martini N, Flehinger BJ, Nagasaki F, Hart B. Prognostic significance of N1 disease in carcinoma of the lung. *J Thorac Cardiovasc Surg* 1983;86:646.
267. Effects of postoperative mediastinal radiation on completely resected stage II and stage III epidermoid cancer of the lung. The Lung Cancer Study Group. *N Engl J Med* 1986;315:1377.
268. Feld R, Rubinstein L, Weisenburger T, et al. Site of recurrence in resected stage I non-small cell lung cancer: a guide for future studies. *J Clin Oncol* 1984;2:1352.

269. Pairolero PC, Williams DE, Bergstralh EJ, et al. Postsurgical stage I bronchogenic carcinoma: morbid implications of recurrent disease. *Ann Thorac Surg* 1984;38:331.

270. Bangma P. Post-operative radiotherapy. In: Deeley T, ed. *Carcinoma of the bronchus: modern radiotherapy.* New York: Appleton-Century-Crofts, 1972:163.

271. Paterson R, Russell MH. Clinical trials in malignant disease. IV-Lung cancer. value of post-operative radiotherapy. *Clin Radiol* 1962;13:141.

272. van Houtte P, Rocmans P, Smets P, et al. Postoperative radiation therapy in lung caner: a controlled trial after resection of curative design. *Int J Radiat Oncol Biol Phys* 1980;6:983.

273. Postoperative radiotherapy in non-small-cell lung cancer: systematic review and meta-analysis of individual patient data from nine randomized controlled trials. PORT Meta-analysis Trialists Group. *Lancet* 1998;352:257.

274. Patterns of failure in patients with resected stage I and II non-small-cell carcinoma of the lung. The Ludwig Lung Cancer Study Group. *Ann Surg* 1987;205:67.

275. Stephens RJ, Girling DJ, Bleehen NM, et al. The role of post-operative radiotherapy in non-small-cell lung cancer: a multicentre randomized trial in patients with pathologically staged T1–2, N1–2, M0 disease. Medical Research Council Lung Cancer Working Party. *Br J Cancer* 1996;74:632.

276. Allen MS, Mathisen DJ, Grillo HC, et al. Bronchogenic carcinoma with chest wall invasion. *Ann Thorac Surg* 1991;51:948.

277. McCaughan BC. Primary lung cancer invading the chest wall. *Chest Surg Clin N Am* 1994;4:17.

278. Gebitekin C, Gupta NK, Satur CM, et al. Fate of patients with residual tumour at the bronchial resection margin. *Eur J Cardiothorac Surg* 1994;8:339.

279. Law MR, Henk JM, Lennox SC, Hodson ME. Value of radiotherapy for tumour on the bronchial stump after resection for bronchial carcinoma. *Thorax* 1982;37:496.

280. Kaiser LR, Fleshner P, Keller S, et al. The significance of extramucosal residual tumor at the bronchial resection margin. *Ann Thorac Surg* 1989;47:265.

281. Holmes EC. Surgical adjuvant therapy of non-small cell lung cancer. *Chest* 1986;89:295S.

282. Lad T, Rubinstein L, Sadeghi A. The Lung Cancer Study Group: the benefits of adjuvant treatment for resected locally advanced non-small cell lung cancer. *J Clin Oncol* 1988;6:9.

283. Feld R, Rubinstein L, Thomas PA. Adjuvant chemotherapy with cyclophosphamide, doxorubicin, and cisplatin in patients with completely resected stage I non-small-cell lung cancer. The Lung Cancer Study Group. *J Natl Cancer Inst* 1993;85:299.

284. Niiranen A, Niitamokorhonen S, Kouri M, et al. Adjuvant chemotherapy after radical surgery for non-small–cell lung cancer—a randomized study. *J Clin Oncol* 1992;10:1927.

285. Furuse K, Kubota K, Kawahara M, et al. Phase II study of concurrent radiotherapy and chemotherapy for unresectable stage III non-small-cell lung cancer. Southern Osaka Lung Cancer Study Group. *J Clin Oncol* 1995;13:869.

286. Pierre F, Maurice P, Gilles R, et al. A randomized phase III trial of sequential chemo-radiotherapy versus concurrent chemo-radiotherapy in locally advanced non-small cell lung cancer: RTOG 9410. *Proc Am Soc Clin Oncol* 2001;20:(abst).

287. Keller SM, Adak S, Wagner H, et al. A randomized trial of postoperative adjuvant therapy in patients with completely resected stage II or IIIA non-small-cell lung cancer. Eastern Cooperative Oncology Group. *N Engl J Med* 2000;343:1217.

288. Chemotherapy in non-small cell lung cancer: a meta-analysis using updated data on individual patients from 52 randomized clinical trials. Non-small Cell Lung Cancer Collaborative Group. *BMJ* 1995;311:899.

289. Scagliotti GV, Fossati R, Torri V, et al. Randomized study of adjuvant chemotherapy for completely resected stage I, II, or IIIA non-small-cell lung cancer. *J Natl Cancer Inst* 2003;95:1453.

290. Kato H, Ichinose Y, Ohta M, et al. A randomized trial of adjuvant chemotherapy with uracil-tegafur for adenocarcinoma of the lung. *N Engl J Med* 2004;350:1713.

290a. Strauss GM, Herndon J, Maddaus MA, et al. Randomized clinical trial of adjuvant chemotherapy with paclitaxel and carboplatin following resection in stage IB non-small cell lung cancer (NSCLC): Report of Cancer and Leukemia Group B (CALGB) Protocol 9633. *Proc Am Soc Clin Oncol* 2004;(abst 7019).

290b. Winton TL, Livingston R, Johnson D, et al. A prospective randomised trial of adjuvant vinorelbine (VIN) and cisplatin (CIS) in completely resected stage 1B and II non small cell lung cancer (NSCLC) Intergroup JBR.10. *Proc Am Soc Clin Oncol* 2004;(abst 7018).

291. Bromley LL, Szur L. Combined radiotherapy and resection for carcinoma of the bronchus. *Lancet* 1995;5:937.

292. Bloedorn FG, Cowley RA, Cuccia CA, et al. Preoperative irradiation in bronchogenic carcinoma. *Am J Roentgenol Radiat Ther Nucl Med* 1964;92:77.

293. Shields TW, Higgins GA Jr, Lawton R, Heilbrunn A, Keehn RJ. Preoperative x-ray therapy as an adjuvant in the treatment of bronchogenic carcinoma. *J Thorac Cardiovasc Surg* 1970;59:49.

294. Warram J. Preoperative irradiation of cancer of the lung: final report of a therapeutic trial. A collaborative study. *Cancer* 1975;36:914.

295. Pisters KM, Ginsberg RJ, Giroux DJ, et al. Induction chemotherapy before surgery for early-stage lung cancer: a novel approach. Bimodality Lung Oncology Team. *J Thorac Cardiovasc Surg* 2000;119:429.

296. Depierre A, Milleron B, Moro-Sibilot D, et al. Preoperative chemotherapy followed by surgery compared with primary surgery in resectable stage I (except T1N0), II, and IIIa non-small-cell lung cancer. *J Clin Oncol* 2002;20:247.

297. Rosell R, Gomez-Codina J, Camps C, et al. Preresectional chemotherapy in stage IIIA non-small-cell lung cancer: a 7-year assessment of a randomized controlled trial. *Lung Cancer* 1999;26:7.

298. Roth JA, Fossella F, Komaki R, et al. A randomized trial comparing perioperative chemotherapy and surgery with surgery alone in resectable stage IIIa non-small-cell lung cancer. *J Natl Cancer Inst* 1994;86:673.

299. Roth JA, Atkinson EN, Fossella F, et al. Long-term follow-up of patients enrolled in a randomized trial comparing perioperative chemotherapy and surgery with surgery alone in resectable stage IIIA non-small-cell lung cancer. *Lung Cancer* 1998;21:1.

300. Andre F, Grunenwald D, Pignon JP, et al. Survival of patients with resected N2 non-small-cell lung cancer: evidence for a subclassification and implications. *J Clin Oncol* 2000;18:2981.

301. Faber LP, Kittle CF, Warren WH, et al. Preoperative chemotherapy and radiation for stage III non-small cell lung cancer. *Ann Thorac Surg* 1989;47:669.

302. Weiden P, Piantadosi S. Preoperative chemotherapy in stage III non-small cell lung cancer (NSCLC): a phase II study of the Lung Cancer Study Group (LCSG). *Proc Am Soc Clin Oncol* 1988;7:197.

303. Eagan RT, Ruud C, Lee RE, Pairolero PC, Gail MH. Pilot study of induction therapy with cyclophosamide, doxorubicin, and cisplatin (CAP) and chest irradiation prior to thoracotomy in initially inoperable stage III M0 non-small-cell lung cancer. *Cancer Treat Rep* 1987;71:895.

304. Strauss G, Sherman L, Mathisen D, et al. Concurrent chemotherapy (CT) and radiotherapy (RT) followed by surgery (S) in marginally resectable stage IIIA non-small cell carcinoma of the lung (NSCLC): a cancer and leukemia group B study. *Proc Am Soc Clin Oncol* 1988;7:203.

305. Albain K, Rusch V, Crowley J, et al. Concurrent cisplatin (DDP) VP-16 and chest, irradiation (RT) followed by surgery for stages IIIa and IIIb non-small cell lung cancer (NSCLC): a Southwest Oncology Group (SWOG) study 8805. *Proc Am Soc Clin Oncol* 1991;10:244.

306. Skarin A, Jochelson M, Sheldon T, et al. Neoadjuvant chemotherapy in marginally resectable stage III M0 non-small-cell lung cancer: long-term follow-up in 41 patients. *J Surg Oncol* 1989;40:266.

307. Sherman D, Strauss G, Schwartz J, et al. Combined modality therapy for regionally advanced stage III non-small cell carcinoma of the lung (NSCLC) employing neo-adjuvant chemotherapy. *Proc Am Soc Clin Oncol* 1978;6:167.

308. Albain KS. Induction therapy followed by definitive local control for stage III non-small-cell lung cancer. A review, with a focus on recent trimodality trials. *Chest* 1993;103:43S.

309. Choi NC, Carey RW, Daly W, et al. Potential impact on survival of improved tumor downstaging and resection rate by preoperative twice-daily radiation and concurrent chemotherapy in stage IIIA non-small-cell lung cancer. *J Clin Oncol* 1997;15:712.

310. Grunenwald D, Le Chavalier T, Arriagada R, et al. Surgical resection of stage IIIb non-small cell lung cancer after concomitant induction chemotherapy: preliminary results of a pilot study. *Proc Am Soc Clin Oncol* 1995;14:(abst).

311. Eberhardt W, Wilke H, Stamatis G, et al. Preoperative chemotherapy followed by concurrent chemoradiation therapy based on hyperfractionated accelerated radiotherapy and definitive surgery in locally advanced non-small-cell lung cancer: mature results of a phase II trial. *J Clin Oncol* 1998;16:622.

312. Roberts JR, Eustis C, DeVore R, et al. Induction chemotherapy increases perioperative complications in patients undergoing resection for non-small cell lung cancer. *Ann Thorac Surg* 2001;72:885.

313. Martin J, Ginsberg RJ, Abolhoda A, et al. Morbidity and mortality after neoadjuvant therapy for lung cancer: the risks of right pneumonectomy. *Ann Thorac Surg* 2001;72:1149.

314. Siegenthaler MP, Pisters KM, Merriman KW, et al. Preoperative chemotherapy for lung cancer does not increase surgical morbidity. *Ann Thorac Surg* 2001;71:1105.

315. Ohta M, Sawabata N, Maeda H, Matsuda H. Efficacy and safety of tracheobronchoplasty after induction therapy for locally advanced lung cancer. *J Thorac Cardiovasc Surg* 2003;125:96.

316. Sawabata N, Keller SM, Matsumura A, et al. The impact of residual multi-level N2 disease after induction therapy for non-small cell lung cancer. *Lung Cancer* 2003;42:69.

317. Betticher DC, Hsu Schmitz SF, Totsch M, et al. Mediastinal lymph node clearance after docetaxel-cisplatin neoadjuvant chemotherapy is prognostic of survival in patients with stage IIIA pN2 non-small-cell lung cancer: a multicenter phase II trial. *J Clin Oncol* 2003;21:1752.

318. Trodella L, Granone P, Valente S, et al. Neoadjuvant concurrent radiochemotherapy in locally advanced (IIIA-IIIB) non-small-cell lung cancer: long-term results according to downstaging. *Ann Oncol* 2004;15:389.

319. Taylor NA, Liao ZX, Cox JD, et al. Equivalent outcome of patients with clinical stage IIIA non-small-cell lung cancer treated with concurrent chemoradiation compared with induction chemotherapy followed by surgical resection. *Int J Radiat Oncol Biol Phys* 2004;58:204.

320. Dartevelle P, Macchiarini P. Surgical management of superior sulcus tumors. *Oncologist* 1999;4:398.

321. Wright CD, Mathisen DJ. Superior sulcus tumors. *Curr Treat Options Oncol* 2001;2:43.

322. Pfannschmidt J, Kugler C, Muley T, Hoffmann H, Dienemann H. Non-small-cell superior sulcus tumor: results of en bloc resection in fifty-six patients—non-small-cell Pancoast. *Thorac Cardiovasc Surg* 2003;51:332.

323. Komaki R, Roth JA, Walsh GL, et al. Outcome predictors for 143 patients with superior sulcus tumors treated by multidisciplinary approach at the University of Texas M. D. Anderson Cancer Center. *Int J Radiat Oncol Biol Phys* 2000;48:347.

324. Gandhi S, Walsh GL, Komaki R, et al. A multidisciplinary surgical approach to superior sulcus tumors with vertebral invasion. *Ann Thorac Surg* 1999;68:1778.

325. Alifano M, D'Aiuto M, Magdeleinat P, et al. Surgical treatment of superior sulcus tumors: results and prognostic factors. *Chest* 2003;124:996.

326. Bilsky MH, Vitaz TW, Boland PJ, et al. Surgical treatment of superior sulcus tumors with spinal and brachial plexus involvement. *J Neurosurg* 2002;97:301.

326a. Wright CD, Menard MT, Wain JC, et al. Induction chemoradiation compared with induction radiation for lung cancer involving the superior sulcus. *Ann Thorac Surg* 2002;73:1541.

327. Rusch VW, Giroux DJ, Kraut MJ, et al. Induction chemoradiation and surgical resection for non-small cell lung carcinomas of the superior sulcus: initial results of Southwest Oncology Group Trial 9416 (Intergroup Trial 0160). *J Thorac Cardiovasc Surg* 2001;121:472.

328. Bleehen NM, Ball D, Belani CP, et al. Combined radiation and chemotherapy for unresectable non-small cell lung carcinoma. *Lung Cancer* 1994;10[Suppl 1]:S19.

329. Choi NC, Kanarek DJ, Grillo HC. Effect of postoperative radiotherapy on changes in pulmonary function in patients with stage II and IIIA lung carcinoma. *Int J Radiat Oncol Biol Phys* 1990;18:95.

330. Marks LB, Munley MT, Bentel GC, et al. Physical and biological predictors of changes in whole-lung function following thoracic irradiation. *Int J Radiat Oncol Biol Phys* 1997;39:563.

331. Cox JD, Azarnia N, Byhardt RW, et al. A randomized phase I/II trial of hyperfractionated radiation therapy with total doses of 60.0 Gy to 79.2 Gy: possible survival benefit

with greater than or equal to 69.6 Gy in favorable patients with Radiation Therapy Oncology Group stage III non-small-cell lung carcinoma: report of Radiation Therapy Oncology Group 83-11. *J Clin Oncol* 1990;8:1543.
332. Haffty BG, Goldberg NB, Gerstley J, Fischer DB, Peschel RE. Results of radical radiation therapy in clinical stage I, technically operable non-small cell lung cancer. *Int J Radiat Oncol Biol Phys* 1988;15:69.
333. Krol AD, Aussems P, Noordijk EM, Hermans J, Leer JW. Local irradiation alone for peripheral stage I lung cancer: could we omit the elective regional nodal irradiation? *Int J Radiat Oncol Biol Phys* 1996;34:297.
334. Sandler HM, Curran WJ Jr, Turrisi AT III. The influence of tumor size and pre-treatment staging on outcome following radiation therapy alone for stage I non-small cell lung cancer. *Int J Radiat Oncol Biol Phys* 1990;19:9.
335. Sibley GS, Jamieson TA, Marks LB, Anscher MS, Prosnitz LR. Radiotherapy alone for medically inoperable stage I non-small-cell lung cancer: the Duke experience. *Int J Radiat Oncol Biol Phys* 1998;40:149.
336. Morita K, Fuwa N, Suzuki Y, et al. Radical radiotherapy for medically inoperable non-small cell lung cancer in clinical stage I: a retrospective analysis of 149 patients. *Radiother Oncol* 1997;42:31.
337. Sawyer TE, Bonner JA, Gould PM, et al. Predictors of subclinical nodal involvement in clinical stages I and II non-small cell lung cancer: implications in the inoperable and three-dimensional dose-escalation settings. *Int J Radiat Oncol Biol Phys* 1999;43:965.
338. Dosoretz DE, Galmarini D, Rubenstein JH, et al. Local control in medically inoperable lung cancer: an analysis of its importance in outcome and factors determining the probability of tumor eradication. *Int J Radiat Oncol Biol Phys* 1993;27:507.
339. Jeremic B, Shibamoto Y, Acimovic L, Milisavljevic S. Hyperfractionated radiotherapy alone for clinical stage I non-small cell lung cancer. *Int J Radiat Oncol Biol Phys* 1997;38:521.
340. Kaskowitz L, Graham MV, Emami B, Halverson KJ, Rush C. Radiation therapy alone for stage I non-small cell lung cancer. *Int J Radiat Oncol Biol Phys* 1993;27:517.
341. Hilton G. The present position relating to cancer of the lung. Results with radiotherapy alone. *Thorax* 1960;15:17.
342. Smart J. Can lung cancer be cured by irradiation alone? *JAMA* 1966;195:134.
343. Morrison R, Deeley TJ, Cleland W. The treatment of carcinoma of the bronchus: a clinical trial to compare surgery and super-voltage radiotherapy. *Lancet* 1963;1:683.
344. Armstrong JG, Minsky BD. Radiation therapy for medically inoperable stage I and II non-small cell lung cancer. *Cancer Treat Rev* 1989;16:247.
345. Vansteenkiste JF, Stroobants SG, De Leyn PR, et al. Lymph node staging in non-small-cell lung cancer with FDG-PET scan: a prospective study on 690 lymph node stations from 68 patients. *J Clin Oncol* 1998;16:2142.
346. Arriagada R, Le Chevalier T, Rekacewicz E, et al. Cisplatin-based chemoradiotherapy (CT) in patients with locally advanced non-small cell lung cancer (NSCLC): late analysis of a French randomized trial. *Proc Am Soc Clin Oncol* 1997;16:446a.
347. Port JL, Kent MS, Korst RJ, et al. Positron emission tomography scanning poorly predicts response to preoperative chemotherapy in non-small cell lung cancer. *Ann Thorac Surg* 2004;77:254.
348. Rusch VW, Albain KS, Crowley JJ, et al. Neoadjuvant therapy: a novel and effective treatment for stage IIIb non-small cell lung cancer. Southwest Oncology Group. *Ann Thorac Surg* 1994;58:290.
349. Macchiarini P, Chapelier AR, Monnet I, et al. Extended operations after induction therapy for stage IIIb (T4) non-small cell lung cancer. *Ann Thorac Surg* 1994;57:966.
350. Mitchell JD. Carinal resection and reconstruction. *Chest Surg Clin N Am* 2003;13:315.
351. Mitchell JD, Mathisen DJ, Wright CD, et al. Resection for bronchogenic carcinoma involving the carina: long-term results and effect of nodal status on outcome. *J Thorac Cardiovasc Surg* 2001;121:465.
352. Fukuse T, Wada H, Hitomi S. Extended operation for non-small cell lung cancer invading great vessels and left atrium. *Eur J Cardiothorac Surg* 1997;11:664.
353. Spaggiari L, Regnard JF, Magdeleinat P, et al. Extended resections for bronchogenic carcinoma invading the superior vena cava system. *Ann Thorac Surg* 2000;69:233.
354. Doddoli C, Role G, Thomas P, et al. Is lung cancer surgery justified in patients with direct mediastinal invasion? *Eur J Cardiothorac Surg* 2001;20:339.
355. Tsuchiya R, Asamura H, Kondo H, Goya T, Naruke T. Extended resection of the left atrium, great vessel, or both for lung cancer. *Ann Thorac Surg* 1994;57:960.
356. Naruke T, Goya T, Tsuchiya R, Suemasu K. Prognosis and survival in resected lung carcinoma based on the new international staging system. *J Thorac Cardiovasc Surg* 1988;96:440.
357. Reyes L, Parvez Z, Regal AM, Takita H. Neoadjuvant chemotherapy and operations in the treatment of lung cancer with pleural effusion. *J Thorac Cardiovasc Surg* 1991;101:946.
358. Hata E, Miyamoto H, Kohiyama R, et al. Resection of N2/N3 mediastinal disease. In: Motta G, ed. *Lung cancer frontiers in science and treatment.* Genoa: Grafica LP, 1994:431.
359. Stamatis G, Eberhardt W, Stuben G, et al. Preoperative chemoradiotherapy and surgery for selected non-small cell lung cancer IIIB subgroups: long-term results. *Ann Thorac Surg* 1999;68:1144.
360. Albain KS. Induction chemotherapy with/without radiation followed by surgery in stage III non-small-cell lung cancer. *Oncology (Huntingt)* 1997;11:51.
361. Choi NC, Carey RW, Myojin JD, et al. Preoperative chemo-radiotherapy (CT-RT) using concurrent boost radiation (RT) and resection for good responders in stage IIIb (T4 or N3) non-small cell lung cancer (NSCLC): a feasibility study. *Lung Cancer* 1997;18[Suppl 1]:76(abst).
362. Rendina EA, Venuta F, De Giacomo T, et al. Induction chemotherapy for T4 centrally located non-small cell lung cancer. *J Thorac Cardiovasc Surg* 1999;117:225.
363. Perez CA, Bauer M, Edelstein S, Gillespie BW, Birch R. Impact of tumor control on survival in carcinoma of the lung treated with irradiation. *Int J Radiat Oncol Biol Phys* 1986;12:539.
364. Graham PH, Gebski VJ, Langlands AO. Radical radiotherapy for early non-small cell lung cancer. *Int J Radiat Oncol Biol Phys* 1995;31:261.
365. Sibley GS, Mundt AJ, Shapiro C, et al. The treatment of stage III non-small cell lung cancer using high dose conformal radiotherapy. *Int J Radiat Oncol Biol Phys* 1995;33:1001.
366. Armstrong J, McGibney C. The impact of three-dimensional radiation on the treatment of non-small cell lung cancer. *Radiother Oncol* 2000;56:157.
367. Pu AT, Harrison AS, Robertson JM. The toxicity of elective nodal irradiation in the definitive treatment of non-small cell carcinoma. *Int J Radiat Oncol Biol Phys* 1997;39 (abst).
368. Emami B. Three-dimensional conformal radiation therapy in bronchogenic carcinoma. *Semin Radiat Oncol* 1996;6:92.
369. Rosenzweig KE, Sim SE, Mychalczak B. Elective nodal irradiation in the treatment of non-small cell lung cancer with three-dimensional conformal radiation therapy. *Int J Radiat Oncol Biol Phys* 1999;45:23.
370. Byhardt R. The evolution of Radiation Therapy Oncology Group (RTOG) protocols for non-small cell lung cancer. *Int J Radiat Oncol Biol Phys* 1995;32:1513.
371. Sause W, Kolesar P, Taylor S, et al. Five-year results: phase III trial of regionally advanced unresectable non-small cell lung cancer. *Proc Am Soc Clin Oncol* 1998;7(abst).
372. Byhardt RW, Pajak TF, Emami B, et al. A phase I/II study to evaluate accelerated fractionation via concomitant boost for squamous, adeno, and large cell carcinoma of the lung: report of Radiation Therapy Oncology Group 8407. *Int J Radiat Oncol Biol Phys* 1993;26:459.
373. Saunders MI, Dische S. Continuous, hyperfractionated, accelerated radiotherapy (CHART) in non-small cell carcinoma of the bronchus. *Int J Radiat Oncol Biol Phys* 1990;19:1211.
374. Saunders M, Dische S, Barrett A, et al. Continuous hyperfractionated accelerated radiotherapy (CHART) versus conventional radiotherapy in non-small-cell lung cancer: a randomized multicentre trial. CHART Steering Committee. *Lancet* 1997;350:161.
375. Bailey AJ, Parmar MK, Stephens RJ. Patient-reported short-term and long-term physical and psychologic symptoms: results of the continuous hyperfractionated accelerated [correction of accelerated] radiotherapy (CHART) randomized trial in non-small-cell lung cancer. CHART Steering Committee. *J Clin Oncol* 1998;16:3082.
376. Saunders MI, Rojas A, Lyn BE, et al. Experience with dose escalation using CHARTWEL (continuous hyperfractionated accelerated radiotherapy weekend less) in non-small-cell lung cancer. *Br J Cancer* 1998;78:1323.
377. Mehta MP, Tannehill SP, Adak S. Phase II trial of hyperfractionated accelerated radiation therapy for nonresectable non-small-cell lung cancer: results of Eastern Cooperative Oncology Group 4593. *J Clin Oncol* 1998;16:3518.
378. Bonner JA, McGinnis WL, Stella PJ, et al. The possible advantage of hyperfractionated thoracic radiotherapy in the treatment of locally advanced non-small cell lung carcinoma: results of a North Central Cancer Treatment Group Phase III Study. *Cancer* 1998;82:1037.
379. Slotman BJ, Njo KH, de Jonge A, Meijer OW, Karim AB. Hypofractionated radiation therapy in unresectable stage III non-small cell lung cancer. *Cancer* 1993;72:1885.
380. Schaake-Koning C, van den BW, Dalesio O, et al. Effects of concomitant cisplatin and radiotherapy on inoperable non-small-cell lung cancer. *N Engl J Med* 1992;326:524.
381. Soresi E, Clerici M, Grilli R, et al. A randomized clinical trial comparing radiation therapy v radiation therapy plus cis-dichlorodiammine platinum (II) in the treatment of locally advanced non-small cell lung cancer. *Semin Oncol* 1988;15:20.
382. Trovo MG, Minatel E, Franchin G, et al. Radiotherapy versus radiotherapy enhanced by cisplatin in stage III non-small cell lung cancer. *Int J Radiat Oncol Biol Phys* 1992;24:11.
383. Blanke C, Ansari R, Mantravadi R, et al. Phase III trial of thoracic irradiation with or without cisplatin for locally advanced unresectable non-small-cell lung cancer: a Hoosier Oncology Group protocol. *J Clin Oncol* 1995;13:1425.
384. Clamon G, Herndon J, Cooper R, et al. Radiosensitization with carboplatin for patients with unresectable stage III non-small-cell lung cancer: a phase III trial of the Cancer and Leukemia Group B and the Eastern Cooperative Oncology Group. *J Clin Oncol* 1999;17:4.
385. Smoluk GD, Fahey RC, Calabro-Jones PM, et al. Radioprotection of cells in culture by WR-2721 and derivatives: form of the drug responsible for protection. *Cancer Res* 1988;48:3641.
386. Tannehill SP, Mehta MP, Larson M, et al. Effect of amifostine on toxicities associated with sequential chemotherapy and radiation therapy for unresectable non-small-cell lung cancer: results of a phase II trial. *J Clin Oncol* 1997;15:2850.
387. Komaki R, Lee JS, Milas L, et al. Effects of amifostine on acute toxicity from concurrent chemotherapy and radiotherapy for inoperable non-small-cell lung cancer: report of a randomized comparative trial. *Int J Radiat Oncol Biol Phys* 2004;58:1369.
388. Auperin A, Arriagada R, Pignon JP, et al. Prophylactic cranial irradiation for patients with small-cell lung cancer in complete remission. Prophylactic Cranial Irradiation Overview Collaborative Group. *N Engl J Med* 1999;341:476.
389. Kris MG, Gralla RJ, Wertheim MS, et al. Trial of the combination of mitomycin, vindesine, and cisplatin in patients with advanced non-small cell lung cancer. *Cancer Treat Rep* 1986;70:1091.
390. Perez CA, Pajak TF, Rubin P, et al. Long-term observations of the patterns of failure in patients with unresectable non-oat cell carcinoma of the lung treated with definitive radiotherapy. Report by the Radiation Therapy Oncology Group. *Cancer* 1987;59:1874.
391. Cox JD, Stanley K, Petrovich Z, Paig C, Yesner R. Cranial irradiation in cancer of the lung of all cell types. *JAMA* 1981;245:469.
392. Umsawasdi T, Valdivieso M, Chen TT, et al. Role of elective brain irradiation during combined chemoradiotherapy for limited disease non-small cell lung cancer. *J Neurooncol* 1984;2:253.
393. Mira J, Miller T, Crowley J. Chest irradiation (RT) versus chest RT + chemotherapy +/ prophylactic brain RT in localized non-small cell lung cancer: a Southwest Oncology Group randomized study. *Int J Radiat Oncol Biol Phys* 1990;19:45.
394. Stuschke M, Eberhardt W, Pottgen C, et al. Prophylactic cranial irradiation in locally advanced non-small-cell lung cancer after multimodality treatment: long-term follow-up and investigations of late neuropsychologic effects. *J Clin Oncol* 1999;17:2700.
395. Gordon GS, Vokes EE. Chemoradiation for locally advanced, unresectable NSCLC. New standard of care, emerging strategies. *Oncology (Huntingt)* 1999;13:1075.
396. Lilenbaum RC, Langenberg P, Dickersin K. Single agent versus combination chemotherapy in patients with advanced non-small cell lung carcinoma: a meta-analysis of response, toxicity, and survival. *Cancer* 1998;82:116.

397. Vokes EE, Weichselbaum RR. Concomitant chemoradiotherapy: rationale and clinical experience in patients with solid tumors. *J Clin Oncol* 1990;8:911.
398. Vokes EE, Green MR. Clinical studies in non-small cell lung cancer: the CALGB experience. *Cancer Invest* 1998;16:72.
399. Pritchard RS, Anthony SP. Chemotherapy plus radiotherapy compared with radiotherapy alone in the treatment of locally advanced, unresectable, non-small-cell lung cancer—a meta-analysis. *Ann Intern Med* 1996;125:723.
400. Dillman RO, Seagren SL, Propert KJ, et al. A randomized trial of induction chemotherapy plus high-dose radiation versus radiation alone in stage III non-small-cell lung cancer. *N Engl J Med* 1990;323:940.
401. Dillman RO, Herndon J, Seagren SL, Eaton WL Jr, Green MR. Improved survival in stage III non-small-cell lung cancer: seven-year follow-up of cancer and leukemia group B (CALGB) 8433 trial. *J Natl Cancer Inst* 1996;88:1210.
402. Komaki R, Scott CB, Sause WT, et al. Induction cisplatin/vinblastine and irradiation vs. irradiation in unresectable squamous cell lung cancer: failure patterns by cell type in RTOG 88-08/ECOG 4588. Radiation Therapy Oncology Group. Eastern Cooperative Oncology Group. *Int J Radiat Oncol Biol Phys* 1997;39:537.
403. Le Chevalier T, Arriagada R, Tarayre M, et al. Significant effect of adjuvant chemotherapy on survival in locally advanced non-small-cell lung carcinoma. *J Natl Cancer Inst* 1992;84:58.
404. Tredaniel J, Hennequin C, Zalcman G, et al. Prolonged survival after high-dose rate endobronchial radiation for malignant airway obstruction. *Chest* 1994;105:767.
405. Marino P, Preatoni A, Cantoni A. Randomized trials of radiotherapy alone versus combined chemotherapy and radiotherapy in stages IIIa and IIIb non-small cell lung cancer. A meta-analysis. *Cancer* 1995;76:593.
406. Vokes EE, Vijayakumar S, Bitran JD, Hoffman PC, Golomb HM. Role of systemic therapy in advanced non-small-cell lung cancer. *Am J Med* 1990;89:777.
407. Mirimanoff RO. Concurrent chemotherapy (CT) and radiotherapy (RT) in locally advanced non-small cell lung cancer (NSCLC): a review. *Lung Cancer* 1994;11[Suppl 3]:S79.
408. Shaw EG, McGinnis WL, Jett JR, et al. Pilot study of accelerated hyperfractionated thoracic radiation therapy plus concomitant etoposide and cisplatin chemotherapy in patients with unresectable stage III non-small-cell carcinoma of the lung. *J Natl Cancer Inst* 1993;85:321.
409. Langer CJ, Curran WJ Jr, Keller SM, et al. Report of phase II trial of concurrent chemoradiotherapy with radical thoracic irradiation (60 Gy), infusional fluorouracil, bolus cisplatin and etoposide for clinical stage IIIB and bulky IIIA non-small cell lung cancer. *Int J Radiat Oncol Biol Phys* 1993;26:469.
410. Jeremic B, Shibamoto Y, Acimovic L, Djuric L. Randomized trial of hyperfractionated radiation therapy with or without concurrent chemotherapy for stage III non-small-cell lung cancer. *J Clin Oncol* 1995;13:452.
411. Jeremic B, Shibamoto Y, Acimovic L, Milisavljevic S. Hyperfractionated radiation therapy with or without concurrent low-dose daily carboplatin/etoposide for stage III non-small-cell lung cancer: a randomized study. *J Clin Oncol* 1996;14:1065.
412. Jeremic B, Shibamoto Y, Milicic B, et al. A phase II study of concurrent accelerated hyperfractionated, radiotherapy and carboplatin/oral etoposide for elderly patients with stage III non-small cell lung cancer. *Int J Radiat Oncol Biol Phys* 1999;44:343.
413. Bailey AJ, Parmar MK, Stephens RJ. Patient-reported short-term and long-term physical and psychologic symptoms: results of the continuous hyperfractionated accelerated [correction of accelerated] radiotherapy (CHART) randomized trial in non-small-cell lung cancer. CHART Steering Committee. *J Clin Oncol* 1998;16:3082.
414. Albain KS, Crowley JJ, Turrisi AT III, et al. Concurrent cisplatin, etoposide, and chest radiotherapy in pathologic stage IIIB non-small-cell lung cancer: a Southwest Oncology Group phase II study, SWOG 9019. *J Clin Oncol* 2002;20:3454.
415. Albain KS, Crowley JJ, Turrisi AT et al. Concurrent cisplatin/etoposide plus radiotherapy for pathologic stage IIIB non-small cell lung cancer: a Southwest Oncology Group phase II study (S9019). *Proc Am Soc Clin Oncol* 1997;16:446a (abst).
416. Lau DH, Crowley JJ, Gandara DR, et al. Southwest Oncology Group phase II trial of concurrent carboplatin, etoposide, and radiation for poor-risk stage III non-small-cell lung cancer. *J Clin Oncol* 1998;16:3078.
417. Lee JS, Scott C, Komaki R, et al. Concurrent chemoradiation therapy with oral etoposide and cisplatin for locally advanced inoperable non-small-cell lung cancer: radiation therapy oncology group protocol 91-06. *J Clin Oncol* 1996;14:1055.
418. Komaki R, Scott C, Ettinger D, et al. Randomized study of chemotherapy/radiation therapy combinations for favorable patients with locally advanced inoperable non-small cell lung cancer: Radiation Therapy Oncology Group (RTOG) 92-04. *Int J Radiat Oncol Biol Phys* 1997;38:149.
419. Vokes EE, Gregor A, Turrisi AT. Gemcitabine and radiation therapy for non-small cell lung cancer. *Semin Oncol* 1998;25:66.
420. Masters GA, Haraf DJ, Hoffman PC, et al. Phase I study of vinorelbine, cisplatin, and concomitant thoracic radiation in the treatment of advanced chest malignancies. *J Clin Oncol* 1998;16:2157.
421. Mauer AM, Masters GA, Haraf DJ, et al. Phase I study of docetaxel with concomitant thoracic radiation therapy. *J Clin Oncol* 1998;16:159.
422. Choy H, Akerley W, DeVore R. Paclitaxel, carboplatin and radiation therapy for non-small-cell lung cancer. *Oncology (Huntingt)* 1998;12:80.
423. Choy H, Akerley W, Safran H, et al. Phase II trial of weekly paclitaxel and concurrent radiation therapy for locally advanced non-small cell lung cancer. *Proc Am Soc Clin Oncol* 1996;15:371(abst).
424. Choy H, Akerley W, Safran H, et al. Multiinstitutional phase II trial of paclitaxel, carboplatin, and concurrent radiation therapy for locally advanced non-small-cell lung cancer. *J Clin Oncol* 1998;16:3316.
425. Choy H, DeVorse RD, Hande KR, et al. Phase II study of paclitaxel, carboplatin, and hyperfractionated radiation therapy for locally advanced inoperable non-small cell lung cancer: a Vanderbilt Cancer Center Affiliate Network (VCCAN) trial. *Proc Am Soc Clin Oncol* 1998;17:467(abst).
426. Belani CP, Aisner J, Day R, et al. Weekly paclitaxel and carboplatin with simultaneous thoracic radiotherapy for locally advanced non-small cell lung cancer: three year follow-up. *Proc Am Soc Clin Oncol* 1997;16:448a (abst).
427. Wagner H, Antonia S, Shaw G, et al. Induction chemotherapy with carboplatin and paclitaxel followed by hyperfractionated accelerated radiation for patients with unresectable stage IIIA and IIIB non-small cell lung cancer. *Proc Am Soc Clin Oncol* 1998;17:469a (abst).
428. Lau DH, Ryu JK, Gandara DR, et al. Twice-weekly paclitaxel and radiation for stage III non-small cell lung cancer. *Semin Oncol* 1997;24:S12.
429. Hudes R, Langer C, Movasas B, et al. Induction paclitaxel and carboplatin followed by concurrent chemoradiotherapy in unresectable, locally advanced non-small cell lung carcinoma: report of FCCC 94001. *Proc Am Soc Clin Oncol* 1997;16:448a(abst).
430. Greco FA, Stroup SL, Gray JR, Hainsworth JD. Paclitaxel in combination chemotherapy with radiotherapy in patients with unresectable stage III non-small-cell lung cancer. *J Clin Oncol* 1996;14:1642.
431. Vokes EE, Leopold KA, Herndon JE II, et al. A randomized phase II study of gemcitabine or paclitaxel or vinorelbine with cisplatin as induction chemotherapy (Ind CT) and concomitant chemoradiotherapy (XRT) for unresectable stage II non-small cell lung cancer (NSCLC) (CALGB Study 9431). *Proc Am Soc Clin Oncol* 1999;18:459a(abst).
432. Saka H, Shimokata K, Yoshida S, et al. Irinotecan (CPT-11) and concurrent radiotherapy in locally advanced non-small cell lung cancer (NSCLC): a phase II study of the Japan Clinical Oncology Group (JCOG 9504). *Proc Am Soc Clin Oncol* 1997;16:447a(abst).
433. Niell HB, Kumar P, Miller AA, Griffin JP. Induction paclitaxel and cisplatin followed by concomitant chemoradiation therapy in stage III non-small cell lung cancer. *Cancer Ther* 1999;2:67.
434. Vokes EE, Herndon JE, Crawford J, et al. Randomized phase II study of cisplatin with gemcitabine or paclitaxel or vinorelbine as induction chemotherapy followed by concomitant chemoradiotherapy for stage IIIB non-small-cell lung cancer: cancer and leukemia group B study 9431. *J Clin Oncol* 2002;20:4191.
435. Mehta MP, Tannehill SP, Adak S, et al. Phase II trial of hyperfractionated accelerated radiation therapy for nonresectable non-small-cell lung cancer: results of Eastern Cooperative Oncology Group 4593. *J Clin Oncol* 1998;16:3518.
436. Choy H, Curran WJ Jr, Scott CB. Preliminary report of locally advanced multimodality protocol (LAMP): ACR 427: a randomized phase II study of three chemo-radiation regimens with paclitaxel, carboplatin, and thoracic radiation (TRT) for patients with locally advanced non-small cell lung cancer (LA-NSCLC). *Proc Am Soc Clin Oncol* 2002 (abst).
437. Bunn PA Jr, Kelly K. New chemotherapeutic agents prolong survival and improve quality of life in non-small cell lung cancer: a review of the literature and future directions. *Clin Cancer Res* 1998;4:1087.
438. Shepherd FA. Treatment of advanced non-small cell lung cancer. *Semin Oncol* 1994;21:7.
439. Clinical practice guidelines for the treatment of unresectable non-small-cell lung cancer. Adopted on May 16, 1997 by the American Society of Clinical Oncology. *J Clin Oncol* 1997;15:2996.
440. Bonomi PD, Finkelstein DM, Ruckdeschel JC, et al. Combination chemotherapy versus single agents followed by combination chemotherapy in stage IV non-small-cell lung cancer: a study of the Eastern Cooperative Oncology Group. *J Clin Oncol* 1989;7:1602.
441. Masters GA, Vokes EE. Should non-small cell carcinoma of the lung be treated with chemotherapy? Pro: chemotherapy is for non-small cell lung cancer. *Am J Respir Crit Care Med* 1995;151:1285.
442. Johnson DH. Chemotherapy for metastatic non-small-cell lung cancer—can that dog hunt? *J Natl Cancer Inst* 1993;85:766.
443. Slevin ML, Stubbs L, Plant HJ, et al. Attitudes to chemotherapy: comparing views of patients with cancer with those of doctors, nurses, and general public. *BMJ* 1990;300:1458.
444. Douglas IS, White SR. Should non-small cell carcinoma of the lung be treated with chemotherapy? Con: therapeutic empiricism—the case against chemotherapy in non-small cell lung cancer. *Am J Respir Crit Care Med* 1995;151:1288.
445. Jaakkimainen L, Goodwin P, Pater J, et al. Counting the costs of chemotherapy in a National Cancer Institute randomized trial in non-small cell lung cancer. *J Clin Oncol* 1990;8:1301.
446. Stephens R, Fairclimb D, Gower N, et al. The Big Lung Trial (BLT): determining the value of cisplatin-based chemotherapy for all patients with NSCLC. *Proc Am Soc Clin Oncol* 2002;38.
447. Effects of vinorelbine on quality of life and survival of elderly patients with advanced non-small-cell lung cancer. The Elderly Lung Cancer Vinorelbine Italian Study Group. *J Natl Cancer Inst* 1999;91:66.
448. Anderson H, Hopwood P, Stephens RJ, et al. Gemcitabine plus best supportive care (BSC) vs BSC in inoperable non-small cell lung cancer—a randomized trial with quality of life as the primary outcome. UK NSCLC Gemcitabine Group. Non-small cell lung cancer. *Br J Cancer* 2000;83:447.
449. Souquet PJ, Chauvin F, Boissel JP, et al. Polychemotherapy in advanced non small cell lung cancer: a meta-analysis. *Lancet* 1993;342:19.
450. Grilli R, Oxman AD, Julian JA. Chemotherapy for advanced non-small-cell lung cancer: how much benefit is enough? *J Clin Oncol* 1993;11:1866.
451. Marino P, Pampallona S, Preatoni A, Cantoni A, Invernizzi F. Chemotherapy vs supportive care in advanced non-small-cell lung cancer. Results of a meta-analysis of the literature. *Chest* 1994;106:861.
452. Johnson DH. Treatment strategies for metastatic non small-cell lung cancer. *Clin Lung Cancer* 1999;1:34.
453. Vokes EE, Bitran JD. Non-small-cell lung cancer. Toward the next plateau. *Chest* 1994;106:659.
454. Smith TJ, Hillner BE, Neighbors DM, McSorley PA, Le Chevalier T. Economic evaluation of a randomized clinical trial comparing vinorelbine, vinorelbine plus cisplatin, and vindesine plus cisplatin for non-small-cell lung cancer. *J Clin Oncol* 1995;13:2166.
455. Goodwin PJ, Shepherd FA. Economic issues in lung cancer: a review. *J Clin Oncol* 1998;16:3900.

456. Cullen MH, Billingham LJ, Woodroffe CM, et al. Mitomycin, ifosfamide, and cisplatin in unresectable non-small-cell lung cancer: effects on survival and quality of life. *J Clin Oncol* 1999;17:3188.
457. Ellis PA, Smith IE, Hardy JR, et al. Symptom relief with MVP (mitomycin C, vinblastine and cisplatin) chemotherapy in advanced non-small-cell lung cancer. *Br J Cancer* 1995;71:366.
458. Tummarello D, Graziano F, Isidori P, Cellerino R. Symptomatic, stage IV, non-small-cell lung cancer (NSCLC): response, toxicity, performance status change and symptom relief in patients treated with cisplatin, vinblastine and mitomycin-C. *Cancer Chemother Pharmacol* 1995;35:249.
459. Albain KS, Crowley JJ, LeBlanc M, Livingston RB. Survival determinants in extensive-stage non-small-cell lung cancer: the Southwest Oncology Group experience. *J Clin Oncol* 1991;9:1618.
460. Paesmans M, Sculier JP, Libert P, et al. Response to chemotherapy has predictive value for further survival of patients with advanced non-small cell lung cancer: 10 years experience of the European Lung Cancer Working Party. *Eur J Cancer* 1997;33:2326.
461. Ruckdeschel JC, Finkelstein DM, Ettinger DS, et al. A randomized trial of the four most active regimens for metastatic non-small-cell lung cancer. *J Clin Oncol* 1986;4:14.
462. Bonomi PD, Finkelstein DM, Ruckdeschel JC, et al. Combination chemotherapy versus single agents followed by combination chemotherapy in stage IV non-small-cell lung cancer: a study of the Eastern Cooperative Oncology Group. *J Clin Oncol* 1989;7:1602.
463. Weick JK, Crowley J, Natale RB, et al. A randomized trial of five cisplatin-containing treatments in patients with metastatic non-small-cell lung cancer: a Southwest Oncology Group study. *J Clin Oncol* 1991;9:1157.
464. Kris MG, Gralla RJ, Kalman LA, et al. Randomized trial comparing vindesine plus cisplatin with vinblastine plus cisplatin in patients with non-small cell lung cancer with an analysis of methods of response assessment. *Cancer Treat Rep* 1985;69:387.
465. Le Chevalier T, Brisgand D, Douillard J, et al. Randomized study of vinorelbine and cisplatin versus vindesine and cisplatin versus vinorelbine alone in advanced non-small-cell lung cancer: results of a European multicenter trial including 612 patients. *J Clin Oncol* 1994;12:360.
466. Wozniak AJ, Crowley JJ, Balcerzak SP, et al. Randomized trial comparing cisplatin with cisplatin plus vinorelbine in the treatment of advanced non-small-cell lung cancer: a Southwest Oncology Group study. *J Clin Oncol* 1998;16:2459.
467. Capon DJ, Seeburg P, McGrath JP, et al. Activation of K-ras 2 gene in human colon and lung carcinomas by 2 different point mutations. *Nature* 1983;304:507.
468. Bonomi P, Kim K, Chang A, et al. Phase III trial comparing etoposide (E), cisplatin (C), versus Taxol (T) with cisplatin-G-CSF (G), versus Taxol-cisplatin in advanced non-small cell lung cancer. An Eastern Cooperative Oncology Group (ECOG) trial. *Proc Am Soc Clin Oncol* 1996;15:382a (abst).
469. Sandler A, Nemunaitis J, Deehnam C, et al. Phase III study of cisplatin (C) with or without gemcitabine (G) in patients with advanced non-small cell lung cancer (NSCLC). *Proc Am Soc Clin Oncol* 1998;17:454a(abst).
470. Cardenal F, Lopez-Cabrerizo MP, Anton A, et al. Randomized phase III study of gemcitabine-cisplatin versus etoposide-cisplatin in the treatment of locally advanced or metastatic non-small-cell lung cancer. *J Clin Oncol* 1999;17:12.
471. Perng RP, Chen YM, Ming-Liu J, et al. Gemcitabine versus the combination of cisplatin and etoposide in patients with inoperable non-small-cell lung cancer in a phase II randomized study. *J Clin Oncol* 1997;15:2097.
472. Manegold CH, Stahel R, Mattson K, et al. Randomized phase II study of gemcitabine (GEM) monotherapy versus cisplatin plus etoposide (C/E) in patients (pts) with locally advanced or metastatic non-small cell lung cancer (NSCLC). *Proc Am Soc Clin Oncol* 1997;16:1651.
473. Sederholm C. Gemcitabine versus gemcitabine/carboplatin in advanced non-small cell lung cancer: preliminary findings in a phase III trial of the Swedish Lung Cancer Study Group. *Semin Oncol* 2002;29:50.
474. Crino L, Scagliotti GV, Ricci S, et al. Gemcitabine and cisplatin versus mitomycin, ifosfamide, and cisplatin in advanced non-small-cell lung cancer: a randomized phase III study of the Italian Lung Cancer Project. *J Clin Oncol* 1999;17:3522.
475. Danson S, Middleton MR, O'Byrne KJ, et al. Phase III trial of gemcitabine and carboplatin versus mitomycin, ifosfamide, and cisplatin or mitomycin, vinblastine, and cisplatin in patients with advanced non-small cell lung carcinoma. *Cancer* 2003;98:542.
476. Mazzanti P, Massacesi C, Rocchi MB, et al. Randomized, multicenter, phase II study of gemcitabine plus cisplatin versus gemcitabine plus carboplatin in patients with advanced non-small cell lung cancer. *Lung Cancer* 2003;41:81.
477. Franciosi V, Barbieri R, Aitini E, et al. Gemcitabine and oxaliplatin: a safe and active regimen in poor prognosis advanced non-small cell lung cancer patients. *Lung Cancer* 2003; 41:101.
478. Crino L, De Marinis F, et al. Gemcitabine-oxaliplatin (GEMOX) chemotherapy as first-line treatment in advanced non-small cell lung cancer (NSCLC): preliminary results of a multicenter phase II study. *Proc Am Soc Clin Oncol* 2003;22.
479. Smit EF, van Meerbeeck JP, Lianes P, et al. Three-arm randomized study of two cisplatin-based regimens and paclitaxel plus gemcitabine in advanced non-small-cell lung cancer: a phase III trial of the European Organization for Research and Treatment of Cancer Lung Cancer Group—EORTC 08975. *J Clin Oncol* 2003;21:3909.
480. Murphy WK, Fossella FV, Winn RJ, et al. Phase II study of Taxol in patients with untreated advanced non-small cell lung cancer. *J Natl Cancer Inst* 1993;85:384.
481. Chang AY, Kim K, Glick J, et al. Phase II study of Taxol, merbarone, and piroxantrone in stage IV non-small-cell lung cancer: the Eastern Cooperative Oncology Group Results. *J Natl Cancer Inst* 1993;85:388.
482. Hainsworth JD, Thompson DS, Greco FA. Paclitaxel by 1-hour infusion: an active drug in metastatic non-small-cell lung cancer. *J Clin Oncol* 1995;13:1609.
483. Giaccone G, Splinter TA, Debruyne C, et al. Randomized study of paclitaxel-cisplatin versus cisplatin-teniposide in patients with advanced non-small-cell lung cancer. The European Organization for Research and Treatment of Cancer Lung Cancer Cooperative Group. *J Clin Oncol* 1998;16:2133.
484. Langer CJ, McAleer CA, Bonjo CA, et al. Paclitaxel by 1-h infusion in combination with carboplatin in advanced non-small cell lung carcinoma (NSCLC). *Eur J Cancer* 2000; 36:183.
485. Crino L, Mosconi AM, Scagliotti GV, et al. Gemcitabine as second-line treatment for relapsing or refractory advanced non-small cell lung cancer: a phase II trial. *Semin Oncol* 1998;25:23.
486. Gatzemeier U, von Pawel J, Gottfried M, et al. Phase III comparative study of high-dose cisplatin (HD-CIS) versus a combination of paclitaxel (TAX) and cisplatin (CIS) in patients with advanced non-small cell lung cancer (NSCLC). *Proc Am Soc Clin Oncol* 1998;17:454a (abst).
487. Belani C, Natale R, Lee J, et al. Randomized phase III trial comparing cisplatin/etoposide versus carboplatin/paclitaxel in advanced and metastatic non-small cell lung cancer (NSCLC). *Proc Am Soc Clin Oncol* 1998;455a(abst).
488. Kelly K, Crowley J, Bunn P, et al. A randomized phase III trial of paclitaxel plus carboplatin (PC) versus vinorelbine plus cisplatin (VC) in untreated advanced non-small cell lung cancer (NSCLC): a Southwest Oncology Group (SWOG) trial. *Proc Am Soc Clin Oncol* 1999;18a(abst).
489. Kosmidis P, Mylonakis N, Skarlos D, et al. A multicenter randomized trial of paclitaxel (175 mg/m^2) plus carboplatin (6 AUC) versus paclitaxel (225 mg/m^2) plus carboplatin (6 AUC) in advanced non-small cell lung cancer (NSCLC). *Proc Am Soc Clin Oncol* 1999;18a(abst).
490. Kelly K, Crowley J, Bunn PA Jr, et al. Randomized phase III trial of paclitaxel plus carboplatin versus vinorelbine plus cisplatin in the treatment of patients with advanced non–small-cell lung cancer: a Southwest Oncology Group trial. *J Clin Oncol* 2001;19:3210.
491. Bonomi P, Kim K, Fairclough D, et al. Comparison of survival and quality of life in advanced non-small-cell lung cancer patients treated with two dose levels of paclitaxel combined with cisplatin versus etoposide with cisplatin: results of an Eastern Cooperative Oncology Group trial. *J Clin Oncol* 2000;18:623.
492. Langer CJ, Manola J, Bernardo P, et al. Cisplatin-based therapy for elderly patients with advanced non-small-cell lung cancer: implications of Eastern Cooperative Oncology Group 5592, a randomized trial. *J Natl Cancer Inst* 2002;94:173.
493. Rogerio C, Lilenbaum R, List M, et al. Single-agent (SA) versus combination chemotherapy (CC) in advanced non-small cell lung cancer (NSCLC): a CALGB randomized trial of efficacy, quality of life (QOL), and cost-effectiveness. *Proc Am Soc Clin Oncol* 2002.
494. Fossella FV, DeVore R, Kerr R, et al. Phase II trial of docetaxel 100 mg/m^2 or 75 mg/m^2 vs vinorelbine/ifosfamide for non-small cell lung cancer (NSCLC) previously treated with platinum-based chemotherapy (PBC). *Proc Am Soc Clin Oncol* 1999;18(abst).
495. Shepherd F, Ramlau R, Mattson K, et al. Randomized study of Taxotere (TAX) versus best supportive care (BSC) in non-small cell lung cancer (NSCLC) patients previously treated with platinum-based chemotherapy. *Proc Am Soc Clin Oncol* 1999;18:463a(abst).
496. Sanchez JM, Balana C, Font A, et al. Phase II non-randomized study of three different sequences of docetaxel and vinorelbine in patients with advanced non-small cell lung cancer. *Lung Cancer* 2002;38:309.
497. Fossella F, Pereira JR, von Pawel J, et al. Randomized, multinational, phase III study of docetaxel plus platinum combinations versus vinorelbine plus cisplatin for advanced non-small-cell lung cancer: the TAX 326 study group. *J Clin Oncol* 2003;21:3016.
498. Gralla R, von Pawel J, Pluzanska A, et al. Prospective analysis of quality of life (QOL) in a randomized multinational phase II study comparing docetaxel (D) plus either cisplatin (C) or carboplatin (Cb) with vinorelbine plus cisplatin (VC) in patients with advanced non-small cell lung cancer (NSCLC). *Proc Am Soc Clin Oncol* 2002.
499. Kubota K, Watanabe K, Kunitoh H, et al. Phase III randomized trial of docetaxel plus cisplatin versus vindesine plus cisplatin in patients with stage IV non-small-cell lung cancer: the Japanese Taxotere Lung Cancer Study Group. *J Clin Oncol* 2004;22:254.
500. Hosoe S, Komuta K, Shibata K, et al. Gemcitabine and vinorelbine followed by docetaxel in patients with advanced non-small-cell lung cancer: a multi-institutional phase II trial of nonplatinum sequential triplet combination chemotherapy (JMTO LC00-02). *Br J Cancer* 2003;88:342.
501. Iaffaioli RV, Tortoriello A, Facchini G, et al. Phase I-II study of gemcitabine and carboplatin in stage IIIB–IV non-small-cell lung cancer. *J Clin Oncol* 1999;17:921.
502. DeVore RF, Johnson DH, Crawford J, et al. Phase II study of irinotecan plus cisplatin in patients with advanced non-small-cell lung cancer. *J Clin Oncol* 1999;17:2710.
503. Fukuoka M, Niitani H, Suzuki A, et al. A phase II study of CPT-11, a new derivative of camptothecin, for previously untreated non-small-cell lung cancer. *J Clin Oncol* 1992;10:16.
504. Oshita F, Noda K, Nishiwaki Y, et al. Phase II study of irinotecan and etoposide in patients with metastatic non-small-cell lung cancer. *J Clin Oncol* 1997;15:304.
505. Socinski MA, Sandler AB, Israel VK, et al. Phase II trial of irinotecan, paclitaxel and carboplatin in patients with previously untreated stage IIIB/IV non-small cell lung carcinoma. *Cancer* 2002;95:1520.
506. Cardenal F, Domine M, Massuti B, et al. Three-week schedule of irinotecan and cisplatin in advanced non-small cell lung cancer: a multicentre phase II study. *Lung Cancer* 2003;39:201.
507. Langer CJ. Treatment of non-small-cell lung cancer in North America: the emerging role of irinotecan. *Oncology (Huntingt)* 2001;15:19.
508. Negoro S, Masuda N, Takada Y, et al. Randomized phase III trial of irinotecan combined with cisplatin for advanced non-small-cell lung cancer. *Br J Cancer* 2003;88:335.
509. Rosell R, Gatzemeier U, Betticher DC, et al. Phase III randomized trial comparing paclitaxel/carboplatin with paclitaxel/cisplatin in patients with advanced non-small-cell lung cancer: a cooperative multinational trial. *Ann Oncol* 2002;13:1539.

510. Klastersky J, Sculier JP, Lacroix H, et al. A randomized study comparing cisplatin or carboplatin with etoposide in patients with advanced non-small-cell lung cancer: European Organization for Research and Treatment of Cancer Protocol 07861. *J Clin Oncol* 1990;8:1556.

511. Schiller JH, Harrington D, Belani CP, et al. Comparison of four chemotherapy regimens for advanced non-small-cell lung cancer. *N Engl J Med* 2002;346:92.

512. Scagliotti GV, De Marinis F, Rinaldi M, et al. Phase III randomized trial comparing three platinum-based doublets in advanced non-small-cell lung cancer. *J Clin Oncol* 2002;20:4285.

513. Rodriguez J, Cortes J, Calvo E, et al. Paclitaxel, cisplatin, and gemcitabine combination chemotherapy within a multidisciplinary therapeutic approach in metastatic non-small cell lung carcinoma. *Cancer* 2000;89:2622.

514. Douillard JY, Lerouge D, Monnier A, et al. Combined paclitaxel and gemcitabine as first-line treatment in metastatic non-small cell lung cancer: a multicentre phase II study. *Br J Cancer* 2001;84:1179.

515. Popa IE, Smith FP, Rizvi NA. A phase II trial of gemcitabine and docetaxel in patients with chemotherapy-naive, advanced non-small cell lung carcinoma. *Proc Am Soc Clin Oncol* 2002.

516. Georgoulias V, Papadakis E, Alexopoulos A, et al. Platinum-based and non-platinum-based chemotherapy in advanced non-small-cell lung cancer: a randomized multicentre trial. *Lancet* 2001;357:1478.

517. Alberola V, Camps C, Provencio M, et al. Cisplatin plus gemcitabine versus a cisplatin-based triplet versus nonplatinum sequential doublets in advanced non-small-cell lung cancer: a Spanish Lung Cancer Group phase III randomized trial. *J Clin Oncol* 2003;21:3207.

518. Gridelli C, Gallo C, Shepherd FA, et al. Gemcitabine plus vinorelbine compared with cisplatin plus vinorelbine or cisplatin plus gemcitabine for advanced non-small-cell lung cancer: a phase III trial of the Italian GEMVIN Investigators and the National Cancer Institute of Canada Clinical Trials Group. *J Clin Oncol* 2003;21:3025.

519. van Meerbeeck J, Smit E, Lianes P. An EORTC randomized phase III trial of three chemotherapy regimens in advanced non-small cell lung cancer. *Proc Am Soc Clin Oncol* 2004;20(abst).

520. Sandler AB, Nemunaitis J, Denham C. Phase III trial of gemcitabine plus cisplatin versus cisplatin alone in patients with locally advanced or metastatic non-small-cell lung cancer. *J Clin Oncol* 2000;18:122.

521. Wozniak AJ, Crowley JJ, Balcerzak SP, et al. Randomized trial comparing cisplatin with cisplatin plus vinorelbine in the treatment of advanced non-small-cell lung cancer: a Southwest Oncology Group study. *J Clin Oncol* 1998;16:2459.

522. Frasci G, Lorusso V, Panza N, et al. Gemcitabine plus vinorelbine versus vinorelbine alone in elderly patients with advanced non-small-cell lung cancer. *J Clin Oncol* 2000;18:2529.

523. Fosella FV, Cea B. Phase III study (TAX 326) of docetaxel-cisplatin (DC) and docetaxel-carboplatin (DCb) versus vinorelbine-cisplatin (VC) for the first-line treatment of advanced/metastatic non-small cell lung cancer (NSCLC): analyses in elderly patients. *Proc Am Soc Clin Oncol* 2003;22:629(abst).

524. Gridelli C, Perrone F, Gallo C, et al. Chemotherapy for elderly patients with advanced non-small-cell lung cancer: the Multicenter Italian Lung Cancer in the Elderly Study (MILES) phase III randomized trial. *J Natl Cancer Inst* 2003;95:362.

525. Shepherd FA, Dancey J, Ramlau R, et al. Prospective randomized trial of docetaxel versus best supportive care in patients with non-small-cell lung cancer previously treated with platinum-based chemotherapy. *J Clin Oncol* 2000;18:2095.

526. Lilenbaum RC, Schwartz MA, Seigel L, et al. Phase II trial of weekly docetaxel in second-line therapy for non-small cell lung carcinoma. *Cancer* 2001;92:2158.

527. Hanna N, Shepherd FA, Rosell R, et al. A phase III study of pemetrexed vs docetaxel in patients with recurrent non-small cell lung cancer who were previously treated with chemotherapy. *Proc Am Assoc Cancer Res* 2003;22(abst).

528. Manegold C, Gatzemeier U, von Pawel J, et al. Front-line treatment of advanced non-small-cell lung cancer with MTA (LY231514, pemetrexed disodium, ALIMTA) and cisplatin: a multicenter phase II trial. *Ann Oncol* 2000;11:435.

529. Shepherd FA, Dancey J, Arnold A, et al. Phase II study of pemetrexed disodium, a multi-targeted antifolate, and cisplatin as first-line therapy in patients with advanced non-small cell lung carcinoma: a study of the National Cancer Institute of Canada Clinical Trials Group. *Cancer* 2001;92:595.

530. Zinner R, Obasaju CK, Fosella FV, et al. Alimta plus carboplatin in patients with advanced non-small cell lung cancer: a phase II trial. *Proc Am Soc Clin Oncol* 2003;22(abst).

531. Scagliotti G, Kortsik C, Calstellano D, et al. Phase II randomized study of pemetrexed + carboplatin or oxaliplatin, as first-line chemotherapy in patients with locally advanced or metastatic non-small cell lung cancer. *Proc Am Soc Clin Oncol* 2003;22(abst).

532. Socinski MA, Schell MJ, Peterman A, et al. Phase III trial comparing a defined duration of therapy versus continuous therapy followed by second-line therapy in advanced-stage IIIB/IV non-small-cell lung cancer. *J Clin Oncol* 2002;20:1335.

533. Kelly K. The benefits of achieving stable disease in advanced lung cancer. *Oncology (Huntingt)* 2003;17:957.

534. Fukuoka M, Yano S, Giaccone G, et al. Multi-institutional randomized phase II trial of gefitinib for previously treated patients with advanced non-small-cell lung cancer. *J Clin Oncol* 2003;21:2237.

535. Janne P, Ostler PA, Lucca J, et al. ZD 1839 (Iressa) shows antitumor activity in patients with recurrence non-small cell lung cancer treated on a compassionate use protocol. *Proc Am Soc Clin Oncol* 2002;21(abst).

536. Miller V, Patel J, Shah N, et al. The epidermal growth factor receptor tyrosine kinase inhibitor erlotinib shows promising activity in patients with bronchoalveolar cell carcinoma (BAC): preliminary results of a phase II trial. *Proc Am Soc Clin Oncol* 2003;22:619a(abst).

537. Kinoshita A, Fukuda M, Kanda T, et al. Pulmonary damage during gefitinib monotherapy in patients with non-small cell lung cancer. *Proc Am Soc Clin Oncol* 2003;22(abst).

538. Perez-Soler R, Chachoua A, Huberman M, et al. A phase II trial of the epidermal growth factor tyrosine kinase inhibitor OSI-774 following platinum-based chemotherapy in patients with advanced, EGFR-expressing, non-small cell lung cancer. *Proc Am Soc Clin Oncol* 2003;20(abst).

539. Herbst RS, Schiller J, Miller V, et al. Subset analyses of INTACT results for gefitinib (ZD 1839) when combined with platinum-based chemotherapy (CT) for advanced non-small cell lung cancer (NSCLC). *Proc Am Soc Clin Oncol* 2003;22(abst).

540. Kim E, Maurer AM, Fosella F, et al. A phase II study of Erbitux (IMC-C225), an epidermal growth factor receptor (EGFR) blocking antibody, in combination with docetaxel in chemotherapy refractory/resistant patients with advanced non-small cell lung cancer (NSCLC). *Proc Am Soc Clin Oncol* 2002;21(abst).

541. Yuen A, Halsey J, Fisher G, et al. Phase I/II trial of ISIS 3521, an antisense inhibitor of PKC-alpha, with carboplatin and paclitaxel in non-small cell lung cancer. *Proc Am Soc Clin Oncol* 2001;20(abst).

542. Ritch P, Belt R, George S, et al. Phase I/II trial of ISIS 3521/LY90003. An antisense inhibitor of PKC-alpha with cisplatin and gemcitabine in advanced non-small cell lung cancer. *Proc Am Soc Clin Oncol* 2002;21(abst).

543. Dang T, Johnson DH, Kelly K, et al. Multicenter phase II trial of an antisense inhibitor of H-ras (ISIS 2503) in advanced non-small cell lung cancer. *Proc Am Soc Clin Oncol* 2001;10(abst).

544. Wojtowicz J, Hamilton MJ, Bernstein S, et al. Clinical trial of mutant ras peptide vaccination along with IL-2 or GM-CSF. *Proc Am Soc Clin Oncol* 2000;19(abst).

545. Adjei AA, Mauer A, Bruzek L, et al. Phase II study of the farnesyl transferase inhibitor R115777 in patients with advanced non-small-cell lung cancer. *J Clin Oncol* 2003;21:1760.

546. DeGrendele H. Current data with bexarotene (Targretin) in non-small-cell lung cancer. *Clin Lung Cancer* 2003;4:210.

547. Shapiro GI, Supko JG, Patterson A, et al. A phase II trial of the cyclin-dependent kinase inhibitor flavopiridol in patients with previously untreated stage IV non-small cell lung cancer. *Clin Cancer Res* 2001;7:1590.

548. Sridhar SS, Shepherd FA. Targeting angiogenesis: a review of angiogenesis inhibitors in the treatment of lung cancer. *Lung Cancer* 2003;42[Suppl 1]:S81.

549. Deslauriers J, Brisson J, Cartier R, et al. Carcinoma of the lung: evaluation of satellite nodules as a factor influencing prognosis after resection. *J Thorac Cardiovasc Surg* 1989;97:504.

550. Magilligan DJ Jr, Duvernoy C, Malik G, et al. Surgical approach to lung cancer with solitary cerebral metastasis: twenty-five years' experience. *Ann Thorac Surg* 1986;42:360.

551. Figlin RA, Piantadosi S, Feld R. Intracranial recurrence of carcinoma after complete surgical resection of stage I, II, and III non-small cell lung cancer. *N Engl J Med* 1988;318:1300.

552. Martini N. Rationale for surgical treatment of brain metastasis in non-small cell lung cancer. *Ann Thorac Surg* 1986;42:357.

553. Patchell RA, Tibbs PA, Walsh JW, et al. A randomized trial of surgery in the treatment of single metastases to the brain. *N Engl J Med* 1990;322:494.

554. Harpole D, Arnos A, Alexander E, et al. Stage of the primary is important when treating isolated brain metastases from lung cancer. *Proc Am Soc Clin Oncol* 1996;15:382.

555. Petrovich Z, Yu C, Giannotta SL, O'Day S, Apuzzo ML. Survival and pattern of failure in brain metastasis treated with stereotactic gamma knife radiosurgery. *J Neurosurg* 2002;97:499.

556. Allard P, Yankaskas BC, Fletcher RH, Parker LA, Halvorsen RA Jr. Sensitivity and specificity of computed tomography for the detection of adrenal metastatic lesions among 91 autopsied lung cancer patients. *Cancer* 1990;66:457.

557. Twomey P, Montgomery C, Clark O. Successful treatment of adrenal metastases from large-cell carcinoma of the lung. *JAMA* 1982;248:581.

558. Raviv G, Klein E, Yellin A, Schneebaum S, Ben Ari G. Surgical treatment of solitary adrenal metastases from lung carcinoma. *J Surg Oncol* 1990;43:123.

559. Reyes L, Parvez Z, Nemoto T, Regal AM, Takita H. Adrenalectomy for adrenal metastasis from lung carcinoma. *J Surg Oncol* 1990;44:32.

560. Porte H, Siat J, Guibert B, et al. Resection of adrenal metastases from non-small cell lung cancer: a multicenter study. *Ann Thorac Surg* 2001;71:981.

561. Schuchert MJ, Luketich JD. Solitary sites of metastatic disease in non-small cell lung cancer. *Curr Treat Options Oncol* 2003;4:65.

562. Carroll M, Morgan SA, Yarnold JR, Hill JM, Wright NM. Prospective evaluation of a watch policy in patients with inoperable non-small cell lung cancer. *Eur J Cancer Clin Oncol* 1986;22:1353.

563. Inoperable non-small-cell lung cancer (NSCLC): a Medical Research Council randomized trial of palliative radiotherapy with two fractions or ten fractions. Report to the Medical Research Council by its Lung Cancer Working Party. *Br J Cancer* 1991;63:265.

564. Teo P, Tai TH, Choy D, Tsui KH. A randomized study on palliative radiation therapy for inoperable non small cell carcinoma of the lung. *Int J Radiat Oncol Biol Phys* 1988;14:867.

565. Simpson JR, Francis ME, Perez-Tamayo R, Marks RD, Rao DV. Palliative radiotherapy for inoperable carcinoma of the lung: final report of a RTOG multi-institutional trial. *Int J Radiat Oncol Biol Phys* 1985;11:751.

566. Bindi M, Tucci E, Pepi F, Bellezza A, Pirtoli L. Changes in performance status in patients with pulmonary carcinoma treated with mono-fractionation radiotherapy once a week. *G Ital Oncol* 1990;10:89.

567. Macbeth FR, Bolger JJ, Hopwood P, et al. Randomized trial of palliative two-fraction versus more intensive 13-fraction radiotherapy for patients with inoperable non-small cell lung cancer and good performance status. Medical Research Council Lung Cancer Working Party. *Clin Oncol (R Coll Radiol)* 1996;8:167.

568. Shin JH, Kim SW, Shim TS, et al. Malignant tracheobronchial strictures: palliation with covered retrievable expandable nitinol stent. *J Vasc Interv Radiol* 2003;14:1525.

569. Stockton PA, Ledson MJ, Hind CR, Walshaw MJ. Bronchoscopic insertion of Gianturco stents for the palliation of malignant lung disease: 10 year experience. *Lung Cancer* 2003;42:113.

570. Morris CD, Budde JM, Godette KD, Kerwin TL, Miller JI Jr. Palliative management of malignant airway obstruction. *Ann Thorac Surg* 2002;74:1928.

571. Lee P, Kupeli E, Mehta AC. Therapeutic bronchoscopy in lung cancer. Laser therapy, electrocautery, brachytherapy, stents, and photodynamic therapy. *Clin Chest Med* 2002;23:241.

572. Schiller JH, Harrington D, Sandler A, et al. A randomized phase III trial of four chemotherapy regimens in advanced non-small cell lung cancer. *Proc Am Soc Clin Oncol* 2000;1a (abst).

573. Graham PH, Gebski VJ, Langlands AO. Radical radiotherapy for early non-small cell lung cancer. *Int J Radiat Oncol Biol Phys* 1995;31:261.

574. Zhang HX, Yin WB, Zhang LJ, et al. Curative radiotherapy of early operable non-small cell lung cancer. *Radiother Oncol* 1989;14:89.

575. Cartei G, Cartei F, Cantone A, et al. Cisplatin-cyclophosphamide-mitomycin combination chemotherapy with supportive care versus supportive care alone for treatment of metastatic non-small cell lung cancer. *J Natl Cancer Inst* 1993;85:794.

576. Woods RL, Williams CJ, Levi J, et al. A randomized trial of cisplatin and vindesine versus supportive care only in advanced non-small cell lung cancer. *Br J Cancer* 1990;61:608.

577. Cellerino R, Tummarello D, Guidi F, et al. A randomized trial of alternating chemotherapy versus best supportive care in advanced non-small cell lung cancer. *J Clin Oncol* 1991;9:1453.

578. Kaasa S, Lund E, Thorud E, Hatlevoll R, Host H. Symptomatic treatment versus combination chemotherapy for patients with extensive non-small cell lung cancer. *Cancer* 1991;67:2443.

579. Stephens R, Fairclimb D, Gower N, et al. The Big Lung Trial (BLT): determining the value of cisplatin-based chemotherapy for all patients with NSCLC. Preliminary results in the supportive care setting. *Proc Am Soc Clin Oncol* 2002;21:1161 (abst).

JOHN R. MURREN
ANDREW T. TURRISI
HARVEY I. PASS

SECTION 3

Small Cell Lung Cancer

EPIDEMIOLOGY AND ETIOLOGY

Small cell lung cancer (SCLC) is the histologic diagnosis in approximately 15% of the more than 173,700 patients diagnosed with lung cancer annually in the United States.[1] Across the world, the proportion of lung cancers that are of the small cell histology tends to be between 10% and 20% in men and 10% to 30% in women.[2] The predominant risk factor for lung cancer is tobacco exposure, which is the cause of up to 90% of cases diagnosed.[3] Among the major histologic subtypes of lung cancer, the association between the extent of tobacco exposure and risk is particularly strong for squamous cell cancer and SCLC.[4,5] Thus, the incidence of SCLC has paralleled trends in cigarette smoking after a 20- to 50-year lag period. In the twentieth century, manufactured cigarettes first became popular among men and then among women, and successive generations began smoking at progressively earlier ages. Per capita consumption in the United States increased from approximately 54 cigarettes per adult in 1900 to a peak of 4345 cigarettes per adult in 1963.[6] Between 1965 and 1995, the number of adult males who were active smokers declined from 52% to 27%. For women, smoking prevalence declined from 28% to 23% in this time period. Unfortunately, smoking prevalence for the adult population has changed little over the last several years, and currently it remains at 23%.[7] Furthermore, there have been increasing trends in tobacco smoking among adolescents, particularly girls.[6,8] This highlights the importance of antitobacco programs, which, when implemented, are effective in reducing tobacco use among adolescents.[9]

Exposure to other environmental respiratory carcinogens, such as asbestos, benzene, coal tar, and other industrial chemicals, may interact with tobacco smoke to increase risk.[10–13] Underlying lung disease and diet have also been implicated.[11,14,15] The risk associated with household exposure to radon gas remains controversial.[11] Pedigree studies and specific metabolic phenotypes have identified familial clusters and populations at increased risk for lung cancer, which is not surprising because several nonrandom genetic defects are associated with this disease.[16–18] Germline

mutations of genes such as p53 are not likely to contribute to susceptibility to lung cancer. Rather, genetic polymorphisms in genes involved in the activation and metabolism of the procarcinogens in tobacco smoke probably contribute to risk.[19]

The trends in smoking prevalence have important implications for the current and future population demographics of SCLC. Over the next few decades, the incidence of lung cancer should continue to decline in the United States, and as the birth cohorts most heavily exposed to tobacco age, the median age at diagnosis for SCLC will also grow older. Among males, the incidence rates peaked in 1984 and have been declining at a rate of approximately 1.4% per year, with the largest declines noted in the incidence of small cell and squamous cell cancers.[6] Among women, the peak incidence appeared to be in 1994. However, if the increase in popularity of cigarette smoking among adolescents does not change, the declining incidence of lung cancer can be predicted to reverse. Furthermore, there may be gender and racial differences regarding susceptibility to tobacco smoke carcinogens, although this remains controversial.[20–22] These factors, along with the changing demographics of the smoking population worldwide, will define the patient population in which SCLC develops in future generations.

PATHOLOGY

A diagnosis of SCLC is based primarily on light microscopy. In 1981, the World Health Organization proposed a histologic classification that gained wide acceptance.[23] In this classification, SCLC was divided into three subtypes that consist of oat cell, intermediate cell type, and combined oat cell (SCLC combined with squamous carcinoma or adenocarcinoma). It soon became clear that the morphologic features used to distinguish oat cell from the intermediate cell histology were imprecise and that, even when strict criteria were used, pure SCLC, whether it was classified as oat cell or intermediate cell, behaved identically. Consequently, the International Association for the Study of Lung Cancer (IASLC) proposed a revised classification in 1988 that recognized pure small cell cancer and two less common variants: mixed small cell/large cell carcinoma and combined small cell carcinoma.[24] This classification schema is what is typically used today.

SCLC is composed of neoplastic cells that are typically arranged in clusters, sheets, or trabeculae separated by a delicate fibrovascular stroma. The tumor typically arises in the central airways and initially infiltrates the submucosa, gradually obstructing the lumen by extrinsic or endobronchial spread. The cells are generally 1.5 to 2.5 times the diameter of a small resting lymphocyte.[25] They have scant cytoplasm and a finely granular nuclear chromatin. Nucleoli are absent or inconspicuous. Mitotic rates are high, and necrosis of individual tumor cells within cell clusters is common. Crush artifact, resulting in smearing of nuclear chromatin, and hematoxyphilic encrustation of vessel walls are common.[24,26] More than 90% of untreated SCLC falls into this category.

In the mixed small cell/large cell variant, there is a subset of cells that resemble large cell carcinoma. These cells may be larger than, or equivalent in size to, the small cell component. These cells are distinguished by the presence of prominent, frequent nucleoli and a nuclear chromatin pattern that is more coarsely granular or open. Variable amounts of cytoplasm are present. The other subtype recognized in the IASLC classification is combined SCLC. In this tumor, small cell carcinoma typically coexists with squamous carcinoma, although adenocarcinoma or one of the less common non–small cell histologies may be present.[24]

In most series, the frequency of the small cell/large cell variant is between 3% and 6%, and for combined SCLC it is 1% to 3%.[24,27–29] Less concordance is found among pathologists on the diagnosis of the mixed-cell variant than there is for pure SCLC.[27,28] Furthermore, the ability to identify a mixed population is influenced by the size of the biopsied material, with examination of a lymph node more likely than a typical bronchial biopsy to result in identification of a mixed-cellular population. It remains unclear whether the presence of a mixed-cell or a combined histology confers a different prognosis or response to treatment than pure small cell carcinoma. For the mixed small cell subtype, there are series that have identified survival that is inferior,[30,31] superior,[28] or comparable[27,32] to pure SCLC. Little information is available regarding the outcome of patients with combined SCLC. A review of 429 patients treated at Vanderbilt University for SCLC identified 9 (2%) with combined small cell and non–small cell histologies.[29] Two of these patients were long-term survivors, and both of them underwent surgical resection in addition to chemotherapy. Thus, surgery may play a role in the management of combined SCLC, and the presence of non–small cell elements, although uncommon, must be considered in patients who might potentially benefit from resection of residual non-SCLC when the initial diagnosis is based on the limited material available by needle or bronchoscopic sampling.

Although the diagnosis of small cell carcinoma rests primarily on morphologic assessment, immunocytochemistry plays a role, and electron microscopy is of occasional value in difficult cases. Virtually all SCLC are immunoreactive for keratin and epithelial membrane antigen, so that if a tumor does not stain for these markers other diagnoses should be considered.[33] One or more markers of neuroendocrine differentiation, such as chromogranin, neuron-specific enolase, Leu-7, and synaptophysin, can be detected in approximately 75% of SCLC.[26,33] The presence of these markers, however, is not mandatory for the diagnosis and does not distinguish small cell from non-SCLC, because 10% to 20% of non-SCLC exhibit neuroendocrine differentiation. By electron microscopy, the cells are closely apposed, with a high nuclear-cytoplasmic ratio. Chromatin is finely clumped but uniformly dispersed within the nucleus. Few organelles and only occasional, uniformly small, dense core granules are located in the cytoplasm. The presence of large granules should raise the diagnosis of a carcinoid tumor.[26]

The major differential diagnostic considerations for a small cell carcinoma are non-SCLC, other small round cell tumors, reserve cell hyperplasia, and a lymphocytic proliferation. Small cell carcinoma composed of larger tumor cells may be difficult to differentiate from a poorly differentiated non-SCLC, particularly if neuroendocrine features are present. Reserve cells are progenitors for bronchial epithelial cells and proliferate in response to chronic irritation of the airways. Features that distinguish reserve cells from small cell carcinoma include retention of cell boundaries within a cell cluster, a lack of the extreme nuclear molding found in small cell carcinoma, and an absence of granularity of the chromatin.[26]

CLINICAL PRESENTATION

In general, the clinical presentation of SCLC is similar to the other histologies of bronchogenic carcinoma. Few patients are asymptomatic at diagnosis. In screening studies only 4% to 12% of the lung cancers detected as a solitary pulmonary nodule are small cell carcinoma.[34,35] The initial complaints usually reflect the local presence of a tumor. Cough is the most common symptom. Recent acceleration of cough or accompanying hemoptysis increases the likelihood that an underlying cancer is present. Dyspnea and chest pain are reported in 30% to 40% of patients at diagnosis.[36] Because SCLC typically develops in the central airways, hemoptysis, postobstructive pneumonitis, wheezing, or hoarseness due to vocal chord paralysis may be present. Superior vena caval obstruction is present at diagnosis in 10% of patients with SCLC.[37] Chest imaging typically shows hilar and mediastinal invasion and regional adenopathy. One-third of patients have some degree of atelectasis present.[36] A peripheral location or chest-wall involvement by the tumor is uncommon. For example, no more than 2% of SCLC present as a superior sulcus tumor.[38,39]

Most patients with SCLC have clinically detectable metastases at diagnosis (Table 27.3-1). Bone involvement is usually characterized by osteolytic lesions, often in the absence of bone pain, or elevations in the serum calcium or alkaline phosphatase.[40–42] However, marked osteoblastic activity is present in a minority of patients. Hepatic and adrenal lesions are typically asymptomatic. Elevation of the serum lactate dehydrogenase (LDH), alkaline phosphatase, or hepatic transaminases is present in the majority of patients in whom liver metastases are identified. In contrast, radiographically confirmed brain metastases are symptomatic in more than 90% of cases. Endovascular metastases (tumor emboli) or lymphangitic spread can be among the underlying causes of dyspnea. Constitutional symptoms, including weight loss, anorexia, and fatigue, are common and correlate with the presence of extensive-stage disease.

The spectrum of paraneoplasia associated with SCLC differs to some degree from the syndromes observed with non-SCLC. Small cell carcinoma is the histology in only 5% of patients with lung cancer diagnosed with hypertrophic pulmonary osteoarthropathy. Humorally mediated hypercalcemia is very rare. On the other hand, the vast majority of lung cancer patients in whom the syndrome of inappropriate antidiuretic hormone (SIADH), Cushing's syndrome, or neurologic paraneoplasia develops have SCLC. SCLC accounts for approximately 75% of the tumors associated with SIADH. Although serum concentrations of antidiuretic hormone are elevated in the majority of those with SCLC, only approximately 10% of patients fulfill the criteria of SIADH, and

TABLE 27.3-1. Sites of Involvement of Small Cell Lung Cancer at Diagnosis and Autopsy

	Clinical Data		Autopsy Data		
Site	All Patients	Single Site	LD at Presentation	ED at Presentation	All Patients
Liver	21–36	6–7	60	73	69
Bone	27–41	9–13	45[a]	56[a]	54
Bone marrow	15–30	2–4	35	NA	NA
Adrenals	5–31	8–11	32	35	65
Brain	10–14	4–6	32	37–65	28–65
Retroperitoneal lymph nodes	3–12	NA	28	29	52
Mediastinal lymph nodes	66–80	80	73	83	87
Supraclavicular lymph nodes	17	5	NA	NA	42
Contralateral lung	1–12	1–4	14	8	27
Pleural effusion	16–20	2–7	28	30	NA
Subcutaneous tissues	5	NA	NA	NA	19 (and other soft tissues)
Pancreas	NA	NA	10–14	17	51

ED, extensive stage; LD, limited stage; NA, not available.

[a]Bone and bone marrow.

[Modified from Agiris A, Murren JR. Staging and prognostic factors in small cell lung cancer. In: Pass HI, Carbone DP, Johnson DH, et al., eds. *Lung cancer: principles and practice*, 3rd ed. Philadelphia: Lippincott Williams & Wilkins, 2004(*in press*).]

symptoms are present in no more than 5%. In some cases, ectopic production of atrial natriuretic factor contributes to the disorder in sodium homeostasis. Similarly, increased serum levels of adrenocorticotropic hormone can be detected in up to 50% of patients with lung cancer, but Cushing's syndrome develops in only 5% of patients with SCLC. In approximately one-half of these cases, it is present at diagnosis. Some of the cutaneous manifestations of Cushing's syndrome may not be prominent, perhaps because of the rapid growth and clinical course of SCLC. A few studies have demonstrated that a low serum sodium is an adverse prognostic factor,[43,44] and patients with Cushing's syndrome have a very limited survival.[45,46]

Neurologic paraneoplastic syndromes include sensory, sensorimotor, and autoimmune neuropathies and encephalomyelitis. These syndromes are thought to occur through autoimmune mechanisms, and antinuclear antibodies that bind to SCLC and to neuronal tissues have been identified.[47] Symptoms may precede the diagnosis by many months and are often the presenting complaint.[48] They may also be the initial sign of relapse from remission. In contrast to the endocrine syndromes, for which successful treatment of the tumor effectively controls the symptoms, the severity of the neurologic symptoms is unrelated to tumor bulk and often does not improve despite successful antineoplastic therapy. Subacute peripheral neuropathy may be the most frequent neurologic syndrome. The Lambert-Eaton syndrome is characterized by proximal muscle weakness that improves with continued use, hyporeflexia, and dysautonomia. Characteristic electromyographic findings confirm the diagnosis. The cause is related to autoantibody impairment of acetylcholine from the cholinergic nerve terminals.[49] Rare neurologic entities include cerebellar ataxia, retinal degeneration, intestinal dysmotility, limbic encephalomyelitis, and necrotizing myelopathy.

STAGING EVALUATION AND PROGNOSTIC FACTORS

The goal of staging is to establish the prognosis, to identify patients with disease confined to the chest who are appropriate

for combined modality therapy, and to assess whether an individual patient will be at increased risk of mortality if treated with an aggressive chemotherapy program. Surgery plays a minor role in the management of this disease, and fewer than 10% of patients are candidates for thoracotomy. As a result, a simple two-stage system, introduced by the Veterans' Administration Lung Study Group (VALSG) when radiotherapy was the major therapeutic option, is still generally used.[50] In the VALSG system, limited stage is defined as disease confined to one hemithorax that can be encompassed in a tolerable radiation field. These patients are currently treated with a combined modality approach. All other patients are considered to have extensive-stage disease. At presentation, 60% to 70% of patients with SCLC have extensive disease, and 30% to 40% limited-stage disease.

In the VALSG staging system, the appropriate classification of selected sites remains controversial. These sites include an ipsilateral pleural effusion, supraclavicular lymphadenopathy (ipsilateral or contralateral), or contralateral mediastinal lymphadenopathy. Several large series have failed to identify a difference in survival between patients with an isolated ipsilateral pleural effusion and other patients with limited SCLC,[51–54] and some groups have included patients with ipsilateral pleural effusions within their definition of limited-stage disease.[55–58] However, only 2% to 7% of all patients with otherwise limited SCLC have an isolated pleural effusion,[53,59] so that small differences in outcome associated with this clinical factor might be missed. Analyses of two large cooperative group databases, which included *in toto* more than 4000 patients, showed that the survival of individuals with an isolated effusion was similar to that of patients with one site of extensive disease.[56,59] In one of these analyses, an isolated effusion conferred a poorer survival compared to other patients classified as having limited disease, which was of borderline significance ($P = .051$).[56] In clinical practice, it is assumed that an effusion is malignant, unless the fluid is a transudate, nonhemorrhagic, and cytologically negative on repeated examinations. Patients with a malignant effusion are appropriate to exclude from combined modality treatment because hemithoracic radiotherapy to encompass the entirety of the pleura makes little sense and has few, if any, advocates. The tolerable dose for an entire lung that is already compromised from smoking is not evidence based or predicted by pulmonary function testing. Moreover, the dose to eradicate small cell carcinoma likely exceeds this tolerability.

Although most randomized trials evaluating the role of combined modality therapy in limited-stage SCLC have excluded patients with an ipsilateral pleural effusion, they have usually included those with ipsilateral, and sometimes contralateral, supraclavicular lymph node metastases. The presence of supraclavicular lymphadenopathy is commonly associated with extensive disease but, when encountered in patients with otherwise limited disease (5% of cases), carries a trend toward poorer survival.[59,60] Contralateral mediastinal involvement is also usually classified as limited-stage disease. However, two randomized studies that evaluated the use of a more aggressive, twice-a-day (b.i.d.) radiation regimen excluded patients with contralateral hilar disease[61,62] to reduce the normal lung volume irradiated and the risk for toxicity. Patients with limited-stage disease who present with superior vena cava syndrome have a similar prognosis to other patients with limited-stage disease[54] and have been included in randomized studies investigating the role of combined modality therapy.[63,64]

Several series have identified an especially favorable outcome for patients with limited disease who undergo surgical resection and have an absence of mediastinal metastases. Survival in this select group is between 50% and 60%.[65,66] Retrospective analysis of the University of Toronto database demonstrated that these patients with "very limited"–stage disease, which was defined as patients without evidence of mediastinal metastases by computed tomography (CT) scan or mediastinoscopy, treated with chemotherapy and radiation, had a more favorable prognosis than other patients with limited-stage disease.[58] In this group, the median survival was almost 16 months, and the projected survival at 5 years was 18%. The 5-year survival for patients with mediastinal involvement was 6%, and for the 49 patients with supraclavicular adenopathy, pleural effusion, or pneumonic consolidation or atelectasis it was only 2%. Among the patients with extensive disease, a number of studies have shown that the number of metastatic sites is an important parameter.[51,54,56,59]

As a result of these inconsistencies, the IASLC has suggested that the tumor, node, metastasis (TNM) staging system be used. In the IASLC system, patients with disease confined to the thorax, including those with ipsilateral and contralateral regional nodal metastases (N2 to N3) and patients with an ipsilateral pleural effusion, regardless of whether it is cytologically positive or negative, are classified as having limited disease. The IASLC panel also recommended that extensive disease be limited to patients with distant metastasis and defined stage IVA as a metastasis to a single extrathoracic organ and stage IVB as dissemination to more than one organ. Micke et al.[67] compared the prognostic utility of the two systems in a retrospective analysis of 109 consecutive patients treated between 1989 and 1999. The number of patients with limited disease was 29 (27%) according to the VALSG system and 52 (48%) in the IASLC system. The IASLC criteria had greater discriminatory power in predicting survival.

TNM staging is especially important for early-stage patients being considered for surgical resection. However, because many current studies in limited disease are testing more intensive schedules of radiation, it is probable that patients with supraclavicular and contralateral hilar lymphadenopathy will continue to be excluded from these studies based on the potential for excessive toxicity.

CLINICAL AND SEROLOGIC PROGNOSTIC FACTORS

Besides disease extent based on VALSG stage, multivariate analyses suggest that performance status is the most reproducible prognostic factor. Performance status reflects the underlying extent of the disease and partially dictates tolerance for the intensity of treatment. Although patients with a poorer performance status are at a higher risk for treatment-related complications, they may still benefit from a combined modality approach.[68] Several other clinical parameters have been proposed. Male gender was an adverse prognostic factor in some, but not all, studies.[44,51,53,56,59,69–71] Older age has been an independent adverse prognostic factor in patients with SCLC in some series[44,56,59,72,73] but not in others.[74–77] Older age has been associated with decreased performance status and comorbidities[77] and often results in compromised chemotherapy dose intensity,[74,77] which may partially explain its prognostic implications. Certain metastatic sites, such as liver,[53,70,79] brain,[51,70] bone marrow,[80] and bone,[51] as well as the total number of metastatic sites involved,[51,56,59,70,81] have been found to be of prognostic significance for patients with extensive-stage disease. The development of Cushing's syndrome as a paraneoplastic manifestation in SCLC has been correlated with a poor response to therapy and short survival.[45] Continued use of tobacco during the administration of combined modality therapy was identified as an adverse prognostic factor in a group of 186 patients with limited disease.[82] Antitumor immunity plays an important role in determining the prognosis in cancer. Although immune response is not generally thought to be as important a determinant in SCLC as some other malignancies, a retrospective analysis of 56 SCLC specimens surgically removed before any therapy demonstrated that a high number of tumor-infiltrating lymphocytes and CD8 cells had a significantly better survival than those with lower numbers of T cells,[83] and two small studies correlated a low CD4-CD8 ratio in peripheral blood with shorter survival.[84,85]

Multiple series have reported that an abnormal LDH is found in 33% to 57% of all patients with SCLC and up to 85% of patients with extensive-stage disease and that it is a strong predictor of poor outcome.[53,56,70] Other serum markers shed from tumor that have been proposed to have prognostic significance include neuron-specific enolase,[70,76] chromogranin, and precursors of gastrin-releasing peptide.[86–88] Serum markers shed from epithelial neoplasms, such as carcinoembryonic antigen,[72,81] cytokeratin fragment CYFRA 21-1,[86] and syndecan-1[89] have demonstrated prognostic significance in some models.

Tumor Cell–Associated Factors

Molecular hallmarks of SCLC that have been identified include inactivation of Rb, mutation of p53, and the overexpression of bcl-2 and of c-myc. A number of investigators are attempting to correlate the expression of these biomarkers with clinical outcomes. The results to date are conflicting and reflect the use of different methodologies in small populations. Biomarkers used to assess angiogenesis include tumor microvessel density and the expression of proangiogenic proteins in tumor or serum. Microvascular count was associated with a shorter disease-free and overall survival in one study of 75 patients with limited-stage SCLC[90] but was not a prognostic factor in another study of equal size.[83] Serum levels of vascular endothelial growth factor (VEGF) have been correlated with the extent of disease and inferior response to chemotherapy. Serum and tumor levels of

VEGF have been associated with poorer survival in some,[90,91] but not all, studies.[92] The high prevalence of VEGF expression in tumor cells supports the further investigation of this protein as a therapeutic target. Analysis of tumor blocks of 93 patients demonstrated that high topoisomerase IIb expression was associated with a lower rate of response to the chemotherapy and that high levels of expression of topoisomerase IIa, Ki67, and bcl-2 were predictive of worse survival.[93] Resistance in SCLC may also be mediated by the overexpression of membrane drug efflux proteins such as P-glycoprotein and the multidrug resistance–associated protein (MRP-1).[94] Technetium 99–methoxy-isobutylisonitrile (sestamibi) is a substrate for P-glycoprotein and MRP-1 and may be a method for assessing the activity of tumor-associated drug transporters.[95]

ASSESSMENT OF RISK

In many respects, treatment for SCLC is as demanding as a thoracotomy and pulmonary resection. In some large cooperative group trials, treatment-related mortality has exceeded 10%. Accordingly, a careful assessment of a patient's ability to undergo aggressive therapy, particularly if concurrent chemotherapy and radiation are planned, is warranted. Several retrospective analyses have attempted to identify patients at increased risk for treatment-related mortality. An analysis of 382 patients treated in a single institution identified age greater than 50 years, Karnofsky performance status of 50 or less, treatment with a regimen containing three drugs or more, and a prior septic episode during chemotherapy as risk factors for septic complications.[96] In this study, older patients with a poor performance status had a 22-fold greater risk of septic death than individuals without those risk factors. In another study involving 610 patients, each one of the 71 fatalities that occurred during the first cycle of VP-16–based chemotherapy was matched to the next patient enrolled on the trial.[97] Patients dying early were more likely to have a poor performance status, clinical hepatomegaly, a low serum albumin, and elevations of the blood urea nitrogen and serum alkaline phosphatase. The Copenhagen Lung Cancer Group compared 937 patients treated on its two most recent studies to 819 patients treated on early clinical studies.[98] The mortality during the first cycle of chemotherapy in the recent studies was threefold higher (12.6% vs. 4.2%) than in the earlier trials. An algorithm was developed that defined patients at high risk if they had a poor performance status [Eastern Cooperative Oncology Group (ECOG) 3 or 4] or if they were 65 years old or older and had a serum LDH that was more than twice the upper normal level. Based on this algorithm, 21% of the 937 patients would be considered at high risk. In this high-risk group, the median survival time was 133 days, and the 2-year survival was 4.5%. Mortality during the first chemotherapy cycle was 33%. Of note, more than half of these early deaths occurred in older patients with an elevated LDH who had a preserved performance status.

STAGING PROCEDURES

Autopsy and clinical studies have shown that SCLC commonly disseminates to soft tissue and multiple viscera (see Table 27.3-1). Outside of the context of a clinical trial, it is reasonable to discontinue the staging survey once disease beyond the chest has been identified. Exceptions include the presence of additional symptomatic areas that may require prompt therapy, such as symptoms

and signs suggestive of metastases to a weight-bearing bone or to the neuraxis. Algorithms have been proposed that use each diagnostic modality in a stepwise fashion to reduce the costs of the staging workup.[57,99]

History; clinical examination, including neurologic examination; a complete blood count; a biochemical panel, including electrolytes, liver function tests, and LDH determination; and a chest x-ray film comprise the first line of pretreatment evaluation in SCLC. Selected biochemical parameters, in particular the serum LDH, have been shown to be predictive of the extent of disease.[53,56,100–102] Symptoms and abnormalities detected in these tests often direct subsequent testing. CT scanning of the chest delineates the extent of the primary tumor and detects mediastinal lymphadenopathy. A pericardial effusion is infrequently seen at presentation, but thickening of the pericardium detected on CT scan of the chest is a common finding of unknown significance.[103] A CT is necessary for purposes of planning the radiation portal field for evaluation of the few who are candidates for surgical resection and response assessment. However, its capability to assess tumor response is limited in areas of atelectasis and radiation-induced fibrosis where the presence of active tumor cannot be ascertained. The role of positron emission tomography (PET) scanning in distinguishing residual tumor versus benign radiographic abnormalities needs to be further investigated.

CT scanning detects intraabdominal lesions in approximately 35% of patients with SCLC at presentation.[104] By the use of chest and abdominal CT, locally advanced or distant disease is diagnosed in 94% to 96% of patients.[105] CT has an accuracy of 85% in detecting liver metastases in SCLC overall,[104] and that increases in patients with abnormalities in liver function tests. Involvement of the adrenal glands by metastatic tumor is almost always clinically silent. Clinical studies have implicated the adrenals as the only metastatic site in SCLC in 8% to 11% of patients at diagnosis; however, the majority of these cases were not biopsy proven. In autopsy series, adrenal metastases are seen in 35% to 65% of patients with SCLC. The accuracy of noninvasive imaging in differentiating between adenomas and adrenal metastases in patients with lung cancer has been suboptimal, although newer magnetic resonance imaging (MRI) techniques, such as chemical shift imaging, may improve the accuracy of MRI in differentiating adenomas from metastatic deposits.[106]

Brain metastases are found in 10% of SCLC patients at the time of diagnosis.[107] The cumulative risk for brain metastases increases with survival. Multiple lesions are usually found at autopsy in patients with central nervous system (CNS) involvement. Leptomeningeal involvement is extremely rare at presentation but may develop antemortem in 2% to 13% of patients. The majority of these patients have simultaneous brain metastases.[108] Although the yield of brain CT in patients with neurologic abnormalities is very high (42% to 88%), it is only 3% to 8% in asymptomatic patients with SCLC.[109] If asymptomatic brain metastases are present, chemotherapy may be adequate treatment,[109,110] and the early detection and treatment of asymptomatic brain metastases with radiation therapy have not been shown to significantly improve patient outcome.[109] As a result, there is not a compelling rationale to routinely image the brain of patients with known metastatic disease. If brain metastases are the single site of distant disease, the prognosis may not be significantly altered because the median survival compared to patients with limited disease has been comparable in some series,[111] although not in others.[108] A CT or MRI of the brain assesses patients considered for prophylactic cranial irradiation (PCI), because demonstrable metastases alter intent, dose, and fractionation.

Up to 40% of patients with SCLC have a positive radionuclide bone scan at diagnosis; in fewer than 10% of cases, this is the only site of metastatic disease.[40,112] Bone involvement by bone scan is frequently detected in asymptomatic patients with SCLC and correlates with an elevated alkaline phosphatase and bone marrow positivity. Further diagnostic evaluation with a plain radiograph, and in some cases with a bone CT scan or MRI, may be required to investigate areas of equivocal findings that could be due to osteoarthritis or trauma. In assessing response, repeat bone scanning is helpful but not sufficiently reliable.[112] In some cases, patients demonstrate a more intense uptake of metastatic lesions on bone scan that reflects bone regeneration and is a sign of response to therapy.

The bone marrow is involved in 15% to 30% of patients with SCLC at presentation but is uncommonly the only site of metastatic disease.[40,53,113] As a result, performing routine bone marrow examinations rarely modifies staging. The yield of bone marrow biopsy can be increased by immunostaining with anti-SCLC monoclonal antibodies, which is positive in 15% to 66% of histologically negative bone marrow, respectively.[114,115] However, the clinical significance of bone marrow involvement demonstrated by these methods has not yet been determined. A leukoerythroblastic picture on the peripheral blood, which is present in 8% to 19% of all cases at presentation, is highly specific for extensive bone marrow infiltration by SCLC.[42,113,116] Severe thrombocytopenia, with a platelet count of less than 50 × 10^9/L, and an elevated LDH are also suggestive of bone marrow metastases.[42,102,116] Bone marrow involvement usually coincides with bone and liver metastases, but not with CNS involvement.[116] At least half of the patients with a positive bone marrow have bone metastases detected by bone scan.[40,117] In patients with a normal bone scan, normal LDH, and no evidence of thrombocytopenia or peripheral blood leukoerythroblastosis, the yield of bone marrow biopsy is extremely low,[117] and it can be omitted.

MRI allows for the noninvasive evaluation of large volumes of bone marrow and is a sensitive method for detecting bone marrow involvement by SCLC. Bone marrow positivity by MRI has been reported in 30% to 60% of patients with SCLC and identifies marrow involvement missed in the initial biopsy in 3% to 19% of patients.[118,119] Circulating malignant cells detected can be found in the peripheral blood of 27% of SCLC patients.[120] The significance of this finding needs to be investigated.

Studies of PET in SCLC have been predominantly retrospective and of small sample size;[121,122,126] no randomized studies or even large prospective studies have yet been conducted. Nevertheless, preliminary data show that SCLC tumors demonstrate avid uptake of [18F]fluorodeoxyglucose (FDG) and that a staging evaluation with PET complements conventional staging. PET scan was superior in some cases in detecting bone metastases, which is consistent with the preliminary observations in other malignant diseases.[123,124] The intensity of metabolic activity as determined by the standard uptake value has been identified as a prognostic factor for non-SCLC[125] and may have a similar utility in SCLC.[122]

Technetium-labeled monoclonal antibody imaging has been evaluated as a staging method in SCLC,[127] as has indium-labeled pentetreotide.[128] Although the capacity to image the entire body in a single scan makes these approaches attractive, they are not commonly used because of limited sensitivity.

TREATMENT

Early efforts at the management of SCLC with surgery were characterized by incomplete staging before and during thoracotomy. Nevertheless, in the 1960s, some studies reported 5-year or longer survival in more than 10% of the patients. These results, however, were overshadowed by two studies in the 1970s that provided philosophic justification for not using a surgical approach in this disease. The British Medical Research Council published a 144-patient trial (Table 27.3-2) that demonstrated the modest superiority of radiotherapy as primary treatment for "operable" SCLC.[129] Shortly thereafter, an American study[130] compared the survival of 146 "operable" but nonresected patients with 41 resected patients and found no differences.

The inadequate results with surgery or radiation alone, even in carefully selected patients, highlighted the need for systemic treatment in SCLC, and the primary role of chemotherapy in the management of this disease is now well established. In a study conducted more than 30 years ago testing various alkylating agents, cyclophosphamide was shown to double survival compared with supportive care in patients with extensive disease, and shortly thereafter a combination of cyclophosphamide with radiation was shown to improve survival compared to radiation alone in patients with limited disease.[131,132] An extensive evaluation of the drugs then available demonstrated that anthracyclines and vinca alkaloids, along with certain alkylating drugs, produced single-agent response rates of up to 50%. The antimetabolites appeared to be less active with the response rates reported of 20% to 30%. In the 1980s, the epipodophyllotoxins (VP-16 and VM-26) and the platinum analogues were introduced, and their activity ranged from 40% to 60% in previously untreated patients. During the past decade, two new classes of chemotherapeutic agents, the taxanes and the camptothecins, have entered clinical practice and are establishing a role in the management of this disease.

DEFINITIONS OF ACTIVE CHEMOTHERAPY AND STRATEGIES FOR EVALUATING NEW AGENTS

As agents such as cyclophosphamide and doxorubicin became established in the management of SCLC, it became clear in the

TABLE 27.3-2. Survival in Patients with Operable Small Cell Lung Cancer Randomized to Surgery or Radiotherapy

Group	Patients	Mean Survival (Mo)	Survival Rate		
			1 Y	2 Y	5 Y
Surgery	71	6.5	21	4	1^a
Radiotherapy	73	10^b	22	10	4

^{a}One patient unable to receive surgery; given irradiation.
^{b}Significant survival difference (*P* = .04) in favor of radiotherapy. (Modified from ref. 129.)

evaluation of new drugs that exposure to prior chemotherapy and response to this therapy were at least as important as other known prognostic factors in predicting response to the new agent. For example, the epipodophyllotoxins produce response rates of 40% to 90% in untreated patients,[133,134] but in relapsed patients the response rates to VP-16 and VM-26 were 5% to 12% and 20%, respectively.[135,136] Based on retrospective analysis of the activity of effective chemotherapy drugs in different populations, response rates of 10% or greater in patients with refractory disease, 20% or greater in patients in "sensitive relapse" (typically defined as response to initial therapy and a treatment-free interval of more than 3 months before disease progression), and 30% or greater in patients with previously untreated extensive disease have been proposed as the appropriate targets to declare a new chemotherapy drug active.[137,138] Because of the biologic aggressiveness of SCLC, the patient population that should be selected to test new drugs remains controversial. Clinical trials that enroll patients with refractory disease, for example, pose the least risk that outcome might be compromised if the new agent turns out to be inactive. However, substantially more patients would need to be evaluated to establish a response rate of 10% or greater than would be necessary to establish a response rate of 30% or greater in previously untreated patients. This means that a much larger number of patients would be exposed to the toxicity of a new drug before it was rejected. Thus, the initial testing of new drugs in patients with sensitive relapse has been proposed as a reasonable compromise,[139] although evaluation in previously untreated patients may be reasonable for new drugs of particular promise.[137]

COMBINATION CHEMOTHERAPY

A number of chemotherapy drugs fulfill the criteria for activity outlined in the previous section. Several of these drugs, such as nitrogen mustard, methotrexate, altretamine, and carmustine (BCNU), are seldom used today. During the past decade, five drugs, or analogues of these five drugs, have been used in the management of SCLC (Table 27.3-3). Current treatment recommendations are based on the experience with these agents.

Several additional chemotherapy drugs introduced in the past decade have established a role in the management of non-SCLC. With the exception of topoisomerase I poisons, adoption of the newer agents in SCLC has been limited. Most of the experience with these drugs has been in patients previously treated with chemotherapy. As a result, the newer agents are typically used alone as palliation for patients who have received prior chemotherapy. However, if the results reported from a Japanese study that demonstrated superior activity for the combination of irinotecan and cisplatin compared to etoposide and cisplatin (EP) is confirmed, this newer agent will be more widely used as initial therapy. Furthermore, some of the newer agents, such as gemcitabine and vinorelbine (Navelbine), are better tolerated in the elderly than is cisplatin and are being evaluated as initial therapy for older and more debilitated patients.

After the activity of cyclophosphamide was established in SCLC, multidrug combinations were developed and tested (Table 27.3-4). Randomized trials of these early combinations demonstrated superior activity to single-agent cyclophosphamide. The combination of cyclophosphamide, doxorubicin,

TABLE 27.3-3. Active Agents in Small Cell Lung Cancer

Drug	Dose (mg/m²)[a]	No Prior Chemotherapy		Prior Chemotherapy	
		Patient (n)	% Response	Patient (n)	% Response
Cyclophosphamide	1000	112	22	—	—
Ifosfamide	5000–8000	103	54	14	43
Doxorubicin	60	8	12	14	29
Epirubicin	100–120	182	48	—	—
Carboplatin	250–450	52	63	54	13
Cisplatin	50–120	—	—	118	14
Vincristine	1.5[b]	10	40	9	44
Vindesine	3–4[b]	—	—	50	24
Vinorelbine	30[b]	17	24	49	14
VP-16	100–300[c]	66	82	91	5
Teniposide	60–100[c]	109	52	80	22
Paclitaxel	250	75	45	24	29
Docetaxel	75–100	12	8	28	25
Irinotecan	100[b]	—	—	59	24
	350	—	—	32	16
Topotecan	1.5–2.0[c]	48	39	362	17
Gemcitabine	1000–1250[b]	31	48	64	19

Note: Response rates are weighted averages obtained from selected published trials that administered the chemotherapy drug intravenously in doses and schedules currently used. The duration of drug infusion was variable. Response rates should be regarded as approximate because patient populations were heterogeneous.
[a]Cycles repeated every 3 to 4 weeks unless otherwise specified.
[b]Treatment was given weekly or biweekly.
[c]Treatment was given daily or every other day for 3 to 5 days, repeated every 3 to 4 weeks.
(Modified from Agiris A, Murren JR. Advances in chemotherapy for small cell lung cancer. *Cancer J* 2001;7:228.)

TABLE 27.3-4. Commonly Used Chemotherapy Regimens

Regimen	Dose (mg/m^2)	Schedule
CDE		
Cyclophosphamide	1000	d 1
Doxorubicin	40	d 1
VP-16	120	d 1–3
CAV		
Cyclophosphamide	1000	d 1
Doxorubicin	45	d 1
Vincristine	1.4	d 1
EP		
VP-16	100	d 1–3
Cisplatin	80	d 1
VIP		
VP-16	75	d 1–4
Ifosfamide	1.2	d 1–4
Cisplatin	20	d 1–4
ICE		
Ifosfamide	5000[a]	d 1
Carboplatin	400	d 1
VP-16	100	d 1–3
CP		
Carboplatin	AUC = 7[b]	d 1
Paclitaxel	175	d 1
IRINOP		
Irinotecan	60	d 1, d 8, d 15[c]
Cisplatin	60	d 1

Note: Cycles are repeated every 3 to 4 weeks. Intravenous route of administration is used, although the oral formulation of VP-16 has been substituted for the intravenous formulation, assuming that it has a bioavailability of 0.50. Mesna is also required in regimens that include ifosfamide.

[a] Administered as a 24-hour continuous infusion.
[b] Area under the curve (AUC) dosing according to the formula of Calvert or Chatulet.
[c] Day 15 dose omitted in some regimens.

and dacarbazine produced a higher response rate and survival when compared with an equally toxic dose of single-agent cyclophosphamide.[140] Hansen et al.[141] demonstrated that the addition of vincristine to the combination of cyclophosphamide, methotrexate, and CCNU (lomustine) improved survival compared to the three-drug combination, highlighting the usefulness of this relatively nonmyelotoxic agent in combination therapy. Livingston et al.[78] developed the CAV (cyclophosphamide, doxorubicin, vincristine) combination, and this became a standard.

With the identification of VP-16 as an important agent, several modifications of the CAV regimen that included VP-16 were tested. In extensive disease a slight improvement in survival was noted when VP-16 replaced either doxorubicin or vincristine, although greater myelosuppression was evident in the cyclophosphamide, doxorubicin, and etoposide (CDE) arm in the latter trial.[142] Hong et al.[142] compared intensive CV (with the dose of cyclophosphamide increased from 1000 to 2000 mg/m^2) to CAV and to CEV (cyclophosphamide, VP-16, and vincristine) and reported that patients treated with CV had a shorter survival and experienced more myelosuppression than those treated on the other two arms. Substitution of VP-16 for methotrexate in the LCOM regimen (lomustine, cyclophosphamide, vincristine, methotrexate) also improved survival.[143] Administration of the VP-16 beginning on day 3 produced bet-

ter survival but more myelosuppression than beginning the VP-16 on day 14 of the cycle, perhaps because this schedule provided greater dose density, or perhaps because it delivered the VP-16 at a point at which more tumor cells were in cell cycle and therefore more susceptible to the drug.[144]

Five randomized trials have evaluated the addition of VP-16 (CAVE) to the CAV regimen.[145–149] In three studies the doses of CAV were equivalent in each arm.[145–147] Not surprisingly, in these studies the addition of VP-16 resulted in increased hematologic toxicity. Although a better response rate was evident in the arm containing VP-16 in at least some patient subsets in each of these studies, an improvement in response duration (of 3 months) and survival (of 6 weeks, $P = .08$) was seen in only one study.[146] Jett et al.[147] compared CAVE to CAV in 231 patients with limited disease. Despite a reduction of the dose of cyclophosphamide by 33%, there was still greater myelosuppression in the CAVE arm. A small improvement occurred in median and 2-year survival with CAVE, which was not statistically significant. Two randomized studies intensified components of this regimen: In one the cyclophosphamide was increased from 1000 to 1200 mg/m^2, and the dose of doxorubicin increased from 40 to 75 mg/m^2 in the CAV arm compared to the CAVE arm.[149] The regimens produced equivalent myelotoxicity, response rates, and survival. These results were comparable to the outcomes with less intensive CAV regimens in extensive disease.

The EP regimen was tested in SCLC because this combination produced synergistic activity in preclinical systems and was established as an active regimen in other diseases. Evan et al.[150,151] reported response rates of 55% in patients previously treated with CAV and 86% in newly diagnosed patients. Einhorn et al.[152] reported that two cycles of consolidation with EP added to the treatment of patients with limited disease who were responding to six cycles of CAV produced a longer survival than that of patients randomized to CAV only. Three randomized trials have compared EP to cyclophosphamide, vincristine, and an anthracycline.[153–155] Less myelosuppression occurred with EP, and, if given with radiation, patients experienced less esophagitis and interstitial pneumonitis. Furthermore, the largest trial included limited- and extensive-stage disease and showed that EP overall produced a better median (14.5 vs. 8.0 months) and 5-year (10% vs. 3%) survival with comparable toxicities and impact on quality-of-life parameters.[155] Three metaanalyses support the superiority of platinum-containing chemotherapy for SCLC.[156–158] As a result, EP is now the standard regimen for limited-stage disease. Because none of the randomized studies detected a difference in survival among patients with extensive-stage disease, a nonplatinum regimen is an acceptable alternative for patients with extensive-stage SCLC.

Carboplatin can be substituted for cisplatin with no apparent loss of activity and improved tolerance.[159,160] In combination with VP-16, Bishop et al.[161] reported a response rate of 77% and 58% for limited and extensive disease, respectively. Moreover, randomized trials of multiagent regimens in which the two platinum analogues were compared suggested that they were at least equivalent. The Hellenic Cooperative Oncology Group randomized 147 patients to receive VP-16, 100 mg/m^2 days 1 to 3, and cisplatin, 100 mg/m^2, or carboplatin, 300 mg/m^2, along with concurrent radiation.[159] Response and survival were similar in the two arms, although the toxicity, particularly nausea, vomiting, nephrotoxicity, and neurotoxicity, were significantly lower in the patients who received carboplatin. Myelosuppression was also less in the carboplatin arm, but this was not statistically significant. However, this was designed as a phase II study and was not powered to prove equivalence. In a larger randomized trial, induction with teniposide, vincristine, and either carboplatin or cisplatin produced equivalent activity and toxicity.[160] The survival was also similar for the two treatment arms, but relative differences between the two platinum drugs may not be apparent because six other drugs were included in the regimen.

Based on the activity of paclitaxel in relapsed and newly diagnosed disease, combinations of a platinum drug, etoposide, and paclitaxel have been developed. Two studies compared EP to EP plus paclitaxel. Despite the addition of granulocyte colony-stimulating factor (G-CSF), the addition of the third drug increased the toxicity without improving the survival.[162,163] Notably, these studies reported a treatment-related mortality in the three-drug arm of 6.4%[163] and 13%.[162] One of these trials was terminated after the accrual of 132 patients because of the excessive toxicity,[162] and the other trial was limited to patients with extensive disease.[164] In contrast, a German study that evaluated carboplatin and etoposide with or without paclitaxel demonstrated a significantly better median survival (12.7 vs. 11.7 months) and 3-year (17% vs. 9%) survival for the group treated with the three-drug regimen.[165] The survival advantage was confined to patients with limited disease. The dose of the etoposide was 20% higher in the two-drug arm. Transfusions and treatment delays were more common in this group.

Ifosfamide produces less myelosuppression than cyclophosphamide and has significant single-agent activity. The three-drug regimen of VP-16, ifosfamide, and cisplatin (VIP), which was tested in refractory germ cell tumors initially, has also been evaluated in SCLC. In this population, which is older and has more comorbid illness than patients with germ cell tumors, a 20% reduction in dose intensity was necessary to avoid excessive myelosuppression.[166] In randomized trials comparing VIP to EP, one study, which included patients with limited and extensive disease, found no difference in survival between the two treatment groups, and the other, which was larger and enrolled only patients with extensive disease, identified a significant, although small, difference in median survival (9 vs. 7.3 months) and 2-year survival rates (13% vs. 5%).[167] In both studies myelosuppression was more severe in the arm treated with ifosfamide. Carboplatin has been substituted for cisplatin in this regimen (ICE), and in single-arm studies impressive response rates and cumulative myelosuppression have been reported.[168,169] A large trial comparing ICE plus a midcycle dose of vincristine to other standard therapy demonstrated improvement in the median and the 1-year survival rates.[170] The majority of patients in the control arm were treated with cyclophosphamide, doxorubicin, and etoposide, and the results may reflect the superiority of a platinum-containing regimen.

Several studies are in progress evaluating camptothecin (topotecan or irinotecan)-based regimens in SCLC. In combination with platinum agents, response rates are between 17% and 29% in previously treated patients and 75% to 84% in newly diagnosed patients.[171,172] Noda et al.[173] compared cisplatin and irinotecan to EP as initial treatment in extensive disease. The study was terminated after 154 of the planned 230 patients were enrolled because median (12.8 vs. 9.4 months) and 2-year (19.5% vs. 5.2%) survival were significantly better in the group treated with cisplatin and irinotecan. Myelosuppression was the most common severe toxicity in both groups and was more frequently observed with EP. Significant diarrhea occurred only in the irinotecan group and was observed in 16% of the patients. Additional studies comparing these two-drug regimens are being conducted. Combinations of camptothecins with agents other than a platinum drug are also being evaluated, and many of the studies have reported significant activity, albeit with substantial associated myelosuppression.

DURATION OF CHEMOTHERAPY

Through the 1970s, sensitive tumors were often treated with chemotherapy for periods as long as 2 years. This meant that most patients with SCLC continued chemotherapy until disease progression or death. In 1984, Feld et al.[174] reported a large study demonstrating that six cycles of CAV and thoracic irradiation produced survival comparable to the results of a previous treatment program that included 12 months of maintenance therapy. Subsequently, a large number of randomized studies examined whether maintenance chemotherapy prolonged survival.[175–184]

Three studies that randomized patients in complete remission after induction therapy to maintenance treatment or observation identified improved survival with the prolonged treatment program in certain patient subsets.[175,176,179] The Cancer and Leukemia Group B (CALGB) randomized 258 patients to one of four chemotherapy regimens, and 57 patients in complete remission underwent a second randomization to maintenance therapy or observation. Among the 46 patients with limited disease who proceeded to the second randomization, the median survival was improved with maintenance chemotherapy (16.8 vs. 6.8 months).[175] However, the induction regimens used in this study might be considered inferior to currently used treatments. In a second study, patients treated with six cycles of CAV and in complete remission were randomized to six additional cycles of the same chemotherapy or observation.[176] For the patients with extensive disease, the median survival was improved by approximately 4 months with maintenance treatment. An additional trial, organized by the ECOG, randomized patients to CAV alternating with another three-drug combination or CAV alone.[179] After six to eight cycles of induction, patients in complete remission underwent a second randomization to maintenance treatment or observation. Patients assigned to CAV and maintenance therapy had a longer progression-free survival and overall survival (P = .09) than patients who received only CAV with no maintenance. In contrast, for the patients who received the six-drug regimen, those who were given no maintenance survived longer than the patients who received maintenance treatment. These studies suggest that there may be a subset of patients, perhaps those with particularly chemotherapy-sensitive disease, who derive a benefit from a maintenance program if they are treated with a CAV induction regimen. In unselected patients, however, clinical trials that have evaluated treatment programs that extend beyond six cycles of chemotherapy have not demonstrated an advantage in survival and may be associated with inferior quality of life.

The Medical Research Council randomized 265 patients who had responded to six cycles of induction chemotherapy to an additional six cycles of maintenance or observation.[178] Overall, there was no difference in survival between patients treated with 6 or 12 cycles of chemotherapy, although for patients in complete remission at the time of randomization a subset analysis suggested that maintenance provides a survival benefit. Three other large studies that randomized patients responding to 5 or 6 cycles of induction to a total of 12 cycles of chemotherapy or observation found no difference in outcome.[180,181,183] Another study that randomized patients with limited disease from the start of chemotherapy to a total of 6 cycles or 12 cycles identified inferior survival in the arm treated with the longer course of therapy.[177]

A second Medical Research Council trial randomized a total of 458 patients to treatment with VP-16, cyclophosphamide, methotrexate, and vincristine (ECMV) for three cycles; ECMV for six cycles; or VP-16 and ifosfamide for six cycles.[185,186] The median survival for patients treated for only three cycles was approximately 1 month shorter than for those who received one of the regimens given for six cycles. Although this difference was not statistically significant, the study was not sufficiently powered to exclude a small advantage with longer treatment programs.[186] Among the more symptomatic patients, palliation of symptoms was slightly better for those treated with the ifosfamide and VP-16 combination, but the differences between the three arms were small.[185]

Other studies have evaluated whether four cycles of chemotherapy are adequate.[182,184,187] Spiro et al.[187] designed a study that included a double randomization at diagnosis. Patients received four or eight cycles of CEV and on relapse were given additional chemotherapy or supportive care. Of the four treatment arms, patients who received four cycles of chemotherapy and only supportive care at relapse had a significantly inferior median survival of 30 weeks. Thus, in this study, four cycles of treatment were adequate, provided that chemotherapy was offered to patients appropriate for additional therapy at relapse. Two additional studies evaluated four cycles of induction with longer treatment programs.[182,184] A European trial randomized patients who responded to four cycles of EP to CAV for up to ten additional cycles or to observation.[182] No survival differences were identified, but the study had limited power based on a small sample size that included limited and extensive disease. The ECOG enrolled 402 eligible patients with extensive-stage disease onto a trial that delivered four cycles of EP followed by a randomization of patients with at least stable disease to four additional cycles of topotecan or to observation.[184] Although maintenance therapy increased the time before documentation of disease progression, there was no difference in quality-of-life measurement or overall survival. Despite a predicted favorable distribution into the cerebrospinal fluid, topotecan maintenance did not reduce the incidence of CNS metastases.

In summary, four to six cycles of induction chemotherapy appear to be optimal in the management of limited and extensive SCLC. Maintenance chemotherapy beyond induction is of unproven value but may play a role in selected patients, depending on the sensitivity of their disease to chemotherapy and the induction regimen they received. Treatment at relapse should be considered if clinically appropriate.

APPROACH TO PATIENTS WITH LIMITED DISEASE

An overview of the management of patients with limited disease is shown in Figure 27.3-1. An occasional patient has stage I

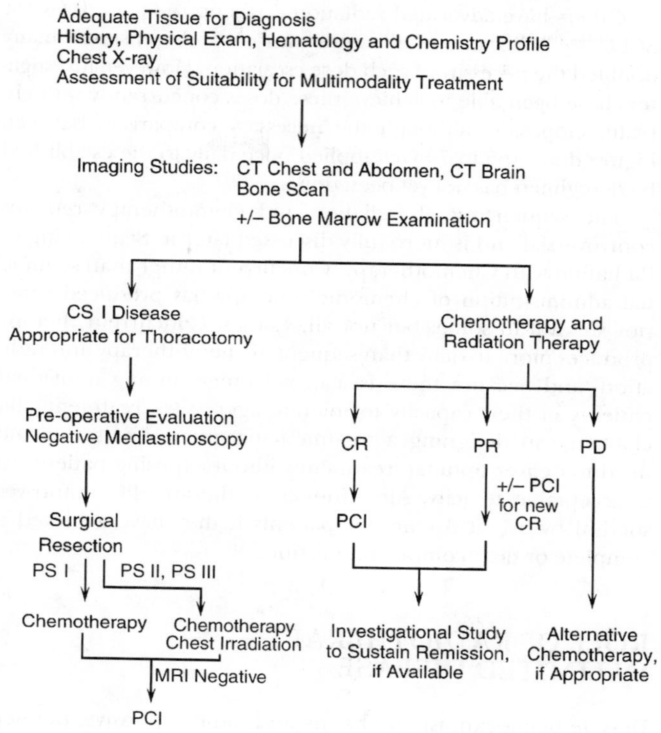

FIGURE 27.3-1. Algorithm outlining management of patients with limited disease. CR, complete response; CS I, clinical stage I; CT, computed tomography; MRI, magnetic resonance imaging; PCI, prophylactic cranial irradiation; PD, progressive disease; PR, partial response; PS, pathologic stage.

disease by noninvasive staging; if this patient is a candidate for thoracotomy, a mediastinoscopy should be considered to ensure that mediastinal nodal metastases are not present before thoracotomy is attempted. Adjuvant chemotherapy is indicated in patients who are resected. Other patients with limited disease should be carefully evaluated to determine their capacity to undergo combined modality therapy. Most patients who are not candidates for a clinical protocol should receive four to six cycles of chemotherapy and radiation to the chest. In limited disease, the CAV regimen produces an overall response rate of 80% to 90%, a complete remission rate of 50% to 60%, a median survival time of only 12 to 16 months, and a 3-year disease-free survival of 10% to 15%. The VP-16 and cisplatin regimen is more effective than CAV and is associated with less toxicity if given with concurrent radiation.[155]

The best results in limited SCLC occur with the combination of cisplatin/etoposide and thoracic radiotherapy optimally administered with 150 cGy b.i.d. to a total dose of 4500 cGy in 3 weeks.[61] At least 4 (and preferably 6) hours elapse between treatments. Targeting and beam shaping limit exposures to normal tissues throughout the entire 3-week period. In the initial study, portals delivered radiotherapy anteriorly and posteriorly each day, switching to a posterior obliqued field to limit direct spinal cord dose to approximately 3600 Gy. Today, these fields would be planned to deliver the dose to a defined target with three-dimensional treatment planning, which allows concentration of the dose to the targeted areas and lower graded doses to adjacent normal structures.

Others have advocated radiation doses up to 60 to 70 Gy for SCLC.[188,189] Because this tumor was so radiosensitive, many doubted the necessity of such dose escalation. However, investigators have been able to achieve these doses concurrently with cisplatin etoposide, although the necessary comparison between higher doses (55 to 70 Gy) applied once daily to the established b.i.d. regimen has not yet been done.

The sequencing of radiation and chemotherapy remains controversial and is more fully discussed later in Sequencing of Radiation with Chemotherapy. Concurrent rather than sequential administration of chemoradiotherapy has produced superior survival in some, but not all, studies. Concurrent therapy produces more toxicity than sequential chemotherapy and radiation, and because there is a broad range among individual patients in their capacity to tolerate aggressive treatment, the challenge in designing a treatment program is to satisfy the need to deliver optimal treatment without exposing patients to unacceptable toxicity. After induction therapy, PCI improves survival by 5% at 3 years for patients if they have achieved a complete or near complete remission.[190]

ROLE OF RADIOTHERAPY IN LIMITED DISEASE

Despite being exquisitely chemo- and radioresponsive, neither modality alone controls all aspects of disease. The CALGB trial of the late 1980s demonstrated that 90% of patients treated with chemotherapy alone failed locally.[63] The Pignon and Arriagada metaanalysis provided more data to mandate thoracic radiotherapy, but the sequence of modalities, dose, volume of target, and fractionation issues were not clarified by this overview of studies that used cyclophosphamide- or doxorubicin-based regimens.[191] As a result, the integration of chemotherapy and radiation therapy continues to be debated.

SEQUENCING OF RADIATION WITH CHEMOTHERAPY

Concurrent therapy is defined as combined modality treatment in which chemotherapy and radiation therapy are administered throughout the same time period. Sequential therapy is defined as the administration of chemotherapy and radiotherapy separately in time, with one modality begun only after completion of the other, often associated with a delay for the second modality to allow the patient an adequate recovery from the initial treatment modality. Several randomized studies reported borderline or significantly improved survival using combined modality treatment. Two of these studies used concurrent radiotherapy,[63,192] one alternating radiotherapy,[193] and two studies sequential radiation.[194,195] The magnitude of survival benefit was modest, ranging from 1 to 4 months in improvement in median survival and increases in the 2-year survival from 7% to 17%. The two studies with the longest follow-up[192,195] demonstrated less advantage beyond 5 years for patients given radiotherapy, partially because of second primary lung cancers. Of the studies not demonstrating improved survival without chest irradiation, two used sequential radiation therapy and one a concurrent regimen in which only a single drug was given simultaneously with irradiation. The negative trial conducted exclusively in patients in complete remission from chemotherapy was initiated because of earlier uncontrolled data suggesting marked improvement in disease-free survival when radiation was given to complete responders at the completion of drug administration. The randomized trial showed a lack of survival benefit from "consolidation" treatment when irradiation was given after chemotherapy has been completed. Combined modality therapy also increased the complete response rate in most of the trials and significantly reduced chest recurrence rates.

A 1992 metaanalysis evaluated randomized trials in which more than 2100 patients with limited-stage SCLC were randomized to receive either chemotherapy alone or in combination with chest irradiation.[68] Patients given combined modality therapy had a 14% reduction in death rate and an absolute 5.4% improvement in 3-year survival compared with those receiving chemotherapy alone. Both differences were highly significant in this metaanalysis. This study reinforces the results of individual studies that demonstrated modest but statistically significant improvement in survival after combined modality treatment. A second and independent metaanalysis reached similar conclusions.[196]

Whether the variations in the temporal relationships of the radiation therapy and chemotherapy components of combined modality treatment influence the antitumor effects is by no means resolved. Concurrent and alternating combined modality programs that do not incorporate planned delays in chemotherapy for radiotherapy administration may possess superior efficacy. Among the randomized trials, three of four concurrent or alternating programs yielded improved survival, whereas one of three sequential programs produced only marginally significant improvement favoring radiation. However, indirect comparisons from the metaanalysis do not document significant survival advantages for any of the three methods of combining chemotherapy with irradiation.[68] Unfortunately, the trials that were included in the metaanalyses all used cyclophosphamide- and doxorubicin-based chemotherapy, combinations that are incompatible with thoracic radiotherapy. No study used today's standard: cisplatin and etoposide with concurrent radiotherapy.

The dose of thoracic irradiation needed to control locoregional SCLC was thought initially to be lower when chemotherapy was given with irradiation.[197] Because improved drug treatment yielded better control of distant metastases, however, a high frequency of local failures with lower dose schedules, such as 3000 cGy in 2 weeks, became apparent.[198] Retrospective data in patients given combined modality therapy suggested that doses higher than 5000 cGy were needed for optimal prevention of locoregional failure,[199] and one randomized trial demonstrated superior local tumor control with 3750 cGy compared with 2500 cGy.[200] Many authorities recommend higher doses in the range of 5000 to 6000 cGy or more[201–203] for optimal local control. The proof of a better therapy is ultimately in improved survival without long-term consequences. Improved local control may point to the value of a method; however, systemic and local control needs to be adequate to produce improved survival.

Randomized trials have yielded conflicting results on whether concurrent irradiation is best given early or late in the chemotherapy program. Although the CALGB study reported by Perry et al.[63] found better results with delayed irradiation, the immediate concurrent arm had markedly attenuated subsequent dose intensity of chemotherapy. Perhaps because of the use of cyclophosphamide and etoposide causing marked myelosuppression, investigators were reluctant to push onward with full doses of chemotherapy. Moreover, these results really show that, using 1980s staging and treatment techniques, all treatment arms produced unacceptable survival by today's benchmarks, and therefore it is not at all clear that the intended focus of timing has any relevance to today's treatment. The National Cancer Institute Canada trial came to the opposite conclusion.[64] This trial used full doses with etoposide (EP)/cisplatin, randomizing the radiotherapy to be concurrent with cycle 2 or cycle 6. The radiotherapy delivered 4000 cGy in 3 weeks and added an additional week for recovery in the early treatment. Indirect comparisons from the metaanalysis could not resolve this issue.[68] The Japanese Clinical Oncology Group randomized patients to concurrent cycle 1 EP with sequential therapy after four cycles, with b.i.d. radiotherapy delivering 4500 cGy in 3 weeks.[204] Unfortunately, the trial was underpowered, but it points toward early concurrent therapy being superior to sequential therapy. This trial verifies that only four cycles of EP and 4500 cGy delivered in an accelerated fraction scheme produce credible response, survival, and local control.

Although minimizing the toxicities of the combined modality approach without compromising therapeutic efficacy is worthy of further research, the addition of chest irradiation has increased myelosuppressive, pulmonary, and esophageal complications of treatment, particularly with concurrent cyclophosphamide-based regimens.[192,205,206] One study analyzed the frequency of radiation pneumonitis in lung cancer patients treated with chemotherapy and chest irradiation.[207] Almost 80% of the patients in this series had SCLC. In a multivariate analysis the only factors that significantly correlated with the increased frequency of radiation-related pulmonary injury were individual fraction sizes of more than 2.50 Gy/d, b.i.d. fractionation as opposed to once-a-day fractions, and the total cumulative dose. Somewhat surprisingly, there were no significant differences among concurrent, alternating, and sequential combined modality treatments. Several trials reported high rates of esophagitis (with occasional strictures) and weight loss in patients given combined modality therapy.[192,206]

Not all concurrent combined modality programs report excessive pulmonary toxicity,[63] suggesting that the selection of drugs combined with irradiation is influential in inducing some of these complications. Platinum and etoposide may be an especially suitable regimen for concurrent treatment in small cell carcinoma of the lung. After two successive trials of sequential combined modality treatment in limited-stage patients produced 4-year survival figures of approximately 10% in the Southwest Oncology Group, a subsequent trial in which a platinum-etoposide combination was given concurrently with chest irradiation beginning on the first day of therapy resulted in 30% 4-year survival, and severe pulmonary toxicity was seen only in one patient.[208]

ALTERED FRACTIONATION RADIATION

Delivering chest irradiation in multiple daily fractions was theorized on experimental grounds to reduce long-term pulmonary toxicity while still maintaining antitumor efficacy. In fact, using even smaller doses per fraction has a theoretic basis because small cells are exponentially killed with very low doses and very low dose rates.[209] SCLC would appear to be an ideal neoplasm for b.i.d. treatment in that it has a high growth fraction, short cell-cycle time, and small to absent shoulder on the *in vitro* cell survival curve. Pilot studies in the late 1980s combining etoposide and platinum plus b.i.d. chest irradiation were promising, with median survivals greater than 2 years and

in most series low rates of associated pneumonitis.[210–212] An intergroup study randomized 417 patients with limited-stage SCLC to a program that included EP for four cycles and radiation therapy beginning on day 1 of the first cycle.[61] The cumulative dose was 4500 rads in both arms, with one arm receiving the radiation in 180-cGy fractions daily and the other arm receiving 150-cGy fractions on a b.i.d. basis. Although the fractionation might be the obvious variable, the duration of therapy (total time) varied between the arms as well (3 vs. 5 weeks). Of importance, higher doses using conventional fractions lengthen time of treatment, and longer treatment times may exert selective pressure on the emergence of resistant clones. The target volume included the primary tumor plus bilateral mediastinal nodes and the ipsilateral hilum but included the supraclavicular nodes only when involved. Local failure was reduced from 52% with the daily schedule to 36% with the b.i.d. schedule ($P = .06$). Of interest, patients who failed in local and in distant sites had a frequency of 23% with daily treatment, versus only 6% with the b.i.d. approach ($P = .01$). More importantly, although statistically significant differences in survival were not seen at 24 months,[211] the curves deviated so that at 5 years the survival was only 16% with once-a-day treatment, as opposed to 26% with the b.i.d. schedule ($P = .04$).[61] All patients who achieved less than complete response were scored as local failures, but those treated with the accelerated scheme achieving only a partial response survived, as well as those with a complete response, implying that the local failure rate was overcalled by imaging on that arm. Overall long-term morbidities were not significantly different between the two arms, although there was a higher frequency of grade 3 esophagitis with b.i.d. treatment.

A North Central Cancer Treatment Group trial attempted to reduce morbidity of twice-daily radiation by inserting a 2.5-week pause between two equally balanced 2400-cGy split courses.[62] After three cycles of induction chemotherapy, fit and responding patients were randomized to receive either 4800 cGy delivered in a twice-daily regimen as split courses of 2400 cGy or 5400 cGy in a once-daily regimen in 6 weeks. Chemotherapy was delivered every 28 days for two additional cycles. Thus, the 4800-cGy dose was delivered in 5.5 weeks, longer than standard time, *not* an accelerated regimen.[213] The 20% 5-year survival percentage was notably less than the benchmark 26% from the intergroup trial when 4500 cGy was delivered in 3 weeks.

Combined modality therapy is the standard treatment. It requires close coordination between medical and radiation oncologists. Selection for combined modality treatment requires patients with an excellent performance status. Because not all patients are sufficiently fit for combined modality treatment, single modality therapy may be appropriate for those who are debilitated or have serious comorbidities. Because single modality therapy is suboptimal, reassessment after initial chemotherapy or radiotherapy may allow for sequencing of the other modality if the patient's condition sufficiently improves to warrant this. A substantial clinical challenge continues to be inadequate control of local and systemic disease, in addition to failure in sanctuary sites. In the last 15 years, gains have been realized, with better integration of radiotherapy with CT-aided targeting and beam delivery and fewer cycles of chemotherapy, each of which contributes to lower morbidity. The enthusiasm for newer drugs, marketed with great promise, has had a disappointing lesser impact, and to date none of the newer drugs can stake a claim to a role in initial management in treatment of limited disease.

PROPHYLACTIC CRANIAL IRRADIATION

Brain metastases are detected in fewer than 10% of SCLC patients at the time of presentation and are subsequently diagnosed during life in another 20% to 25%, with an increasing likelihood of development seen with lengthening survival.[214,215] In the absence of radiation therapy to the CNS, actuarial analysis reveals a probability of brain metastases ranging from 50% to 80% in terms of those patients who survive 2 years.[214,216] At postmortem examination, they are found in up to 65% of patients.[217] Because these metastases are sometimes the sole site of clinical relapse from complete remission and are frequently clinically disabling, PCI has been recommended by many,[218] but not all,[219] over the past 10 to 15 years to curtail their development. The rationale is essentially an extrapolation from original strategies used in acute lymphocytic leukemia of childhood.

A large number of early prospective randomized trials assessed the benefit of PCI given at or within a few months of diagnosis in patients who were initially free of CNS involvement.[175,220–224] When these trials were considered together, doses of PCI ranging from 2000 to 4000 cGy reduced the frequency of clinically detectable brain metastases from 24% to 6%. In most of these trials, a significant reduction of intracranial tumor spread was observed. However, no significant impact of PCI on survival was seen in any of those studies. Retrospective analyses suggested that virtually all benefit in preventing intracranial metastases with PCI was confined to patients who achieved a complete remission to their initial treatment.[216] In actuarial analysis, partial responders or nonresponders have similar risks of recurrence in the brain regardless of whether or not PCI was administered. This is not surprising because persisting systemic cancer could readily metastasize to the CNS after completion of PCI.

More recently, in a metaanalysis of almost 1000 patients in seven trials between 1977 and 1995, patients were evaluated with and without PCI[190] after initially obtaining a complete response. The primary end point was overall survival, and the analysis was based on intent to treat. PCI doses ranged from 24 to 40 Gy in most patients, although the metaanalysis did include one series of 25 patients who received only 8 Gy in one fraction. The metaanalysis suggested that a significant gain in survival was seen with PCI in patients who achieved complete remission, with 3-year survival figures increasing from 15% to almost 21%. PCI significantly decreased the probability of brain metastases and increased the likelihood of disease-free survival. Going to higher doses appeared to have no obvious impact on survival, although it seemed to have an increasing effect of eliminating brain metastases. A trend was also seen toward a decreased risk of brain metastases when PCI was administered earlier. The metaanalysis was not able to assess the impact of PCI on cognitive function, because most of the studies included did not include neurocognitive assessments, at baseline or beyond 2 years. Two studies[225,226] that assessed baseline neuropsychological function before treatment demonstrated that many patients appear to have abnormalities of cognitive function as initial manifestations of their cancer, even when brain metastases were not detected and before any treatment.

Another factor that produces considerable controversy about recommending PCI to patients who achieve a complete response is the significant risk of toxicity associated with it. Because the 5-year survival appears to have improved, it is evident that some patients have neurologic and intellectual impairment as well as abnormalities on CT scan that may be related to PCI.[227–229] In one study, CT scan and CNS abnormalities were significantly more frequent in patients who had received PCI or therapeutic brain irradiation than in those who had not.[230] These findings were especially disturbing because complete responders are at greater risk for possible complications. Many deficits on neuropsychological testing have been unsuspected on casual examination, but a few patients have obvious major impairments. CT scan abnormalities continue to worsen for several years after treatment has ended, although the abnormalities may eventually stabilize.[231] Neurologic abnormalities were most prominent in one series of patients who were given PCI concurrently with high-dose chemotherapy or in individual radiation fractions of 400 cGy.[228] Some authorities suggest that PCI should be administered only in standard fractions of 200 cGy after completion of chemotherapy.[232] Two ongoing studies, one predominantly in Europe and the other in North America, address whether a higher dose 3600 cGy provides better control than a lower, commonly used dose of 2500 cGy. These studies are powered to demonstrate a reduction in relapse because the required number of entrants to prove a survival difference was prohibitive. Neurocognitive tests are suggested but not mandated. In one study, a third accelerated treatment arm uses 150-cGy fractions b.i.d. in 12 treatment days to deliver 3600 cGy.

The neuropsychological and imaging abnormalities may or may not be due to PCI. Chemotherapy, possible paraneoplastic syndromes, and the effects of chronic cigarette and alcohol abuse are some of the factors that may be important contributors. In one study that evaluated cognitive function in patients before and after chemoradiation but before any PCI, deficits were discovered in verbal memory, frontal lobe function, and motor coordination within both groups of patients.[226] Administration of methotrexate, procarbazine, and lomustine has decreased over the last 15 years; these particular agents have been incriminated in neuropsychological dysfunction.

One of the studies included in the metaanalysis had almost 300 patients who were randomized to receive PCI after having achieved a complete remission to initial treatment.[224] Twenty percent of these patients had extensive-stage disease, virtually all of whom are ultimately expected to relapse and die. The mean time between the initiation of treatment and the randomization was 5 months. The actuarial likelihood of isolated brain metastasis as the first site of treatment failure was 19% in patients given PCI and 45% in those who did not receive PCI. Corresponding figures for total brain metastases were 40% and 67%, respectively; both differences were highly significant. However, in this one study overall survival was not significantly improved. The important observation was that there were no obvious differences in the neuropsychological function between the two groups, but only 33 patients underwent a complete reassessment at 18 months. Inasmuch as neuropsychological abnormalities possibly due to PCI progress over time, these data are insufficient to exclude radiation-associated cognitive damage, but they are nonetheless relevant.

It is important to understand that PCI as opposed to therapeutic irradiation should not require a dose that approaches tissue tolerance. Higher doses may be more successful at eliminating brain metastases, but there appears to be prophylactic benefit with relatively modest doses of 2400 cGy in 300-cGy fractions, to 2500 cGy in 250-cGy fractions. Because of concern about larger doses per fraction on brain function, 200-cGy fractions to 3000 cGy have been adopted as a standard. If PCI is administered at a time when no chemotherapeutic agents are being administered, radiation-induced permeability alterations that allow more chemotherapeutic agent into brain parenchyma should be obviated. The authors' guidelines for PCI, after thorough discussion with the patient of potential risks and benefits, are (1) PCI is typically recommended 2 weeks after completion of all chemotherapy to complete and very good partial responders after induction therapy, and (2) radiotherapy fractions of 200 to 300 cGy are given over 2 to 3 weeks to a total dose of 2400 to 3000 cGy.

ROLE OF SURGERY IN LIMITED DISEASE

Surgery is reserved for selected patients. In contrast to the majority of patients with limited disease, careful TNM staging is important in those patients being considered for surgical resection. Higgins et al.[34] reported that SCLC was present in only 1% of the solitary pulmonary nodules resected and that the 5-year survival rate was 36% for 11 patients who would now be classified as having stage I disease. The Veterans Administration Surgical Oncology Group conducted a series of four trials that included 148 patients, 132 of whom survived a potentially curative resection and were randomized to receive either adjuvant chemotherapy or observation.[233] A 23% overall 5-year survival was recorded, with survival patterns that were more favorable in less advanced stages: T1 to 2N0, 28% to 60%; T1 to 2N1, 9% to 31%; and T3 or N2, 3.6%. Although survival was marginally better with the addition of postoperative chemotherapy, it was clear that the small group of patients with localized disease after sophisticated surgical staging techniques could enjoy much better survival with surgical resection alone than was previously appreciated.

Several factors have strengthened the rationale for incorporating surgical therapy into the total "package" of treatment for selected SCLC patients.[234] Despite the high response rate to present chemotherapy regimens, the rate of relapse in the thorax can approach 75% in the absence of properly administered radiotherapy. A gradual shift toward identification of more localized potentially resectable subgroups of limited-disease patients with clinical staging occurred, encouraged by the use of invasive procedures, including Wang needle biopsy, mediastinotomy, and mediastinoscopy, and the recognition that the new international staging system for lung cancer[235] can provide a common language for discussing these issues.

One of the chief theoretic justifications for adding surgery to the treatment regimen for SCLC is the possibility of influencing relapse in the tumor bed or the mediastinum. In patients who have had surgery at diagnosis, local recurrences are infrequent,[236,237] possibly because patients with stage I or II disease are overrepresented in this group. Patients who have been pretreated with chemotherapy more often had clinical stage IIIA disease, and their local relapse rate is higher, in the range of 18% to 28%.[238,239] These local relapse rates still appear considerably less than in patients given chemotherapy

with or without radiation therapy with no surgical intervention. Patients given initial chemotherapy who have a negative biopsy of the primary tumor site at the time of surgery and therefore do not have resection performed have a high frequency of local recurrence.[240] No cancer is present in the resected specimen in 10% to 20% of cases resected for CT,[27,241,242] and this particular patient subset enjoys a better prognosis.

Only a modest quantity of data exist on how often surgical resection at the diagnosis of SCLC is possible. Prospective studies of the feasibility of initial thoracotomy by their nature cannot include patients discovered only at thoracotomy to have small cell carcinoma. A review of the literature[243] suggests that as many as 16% of patients with SCLC are operative candidates, but this is likely to be an unrealistically high estimate because those patients who are evaluated by a thoracic surgeon constitute a highly selected group.

A marked increase in mortality does not seem to occur in patients who have operative removal of small cell carcinoma. In the few studies that describe operative risks after chemotherapy and radiotherapy, the mortality varies between 0% and 10%,[238–240,244–246] with many studies reporting no operative mortality or increased morbidity compared to expected outcomes in patients undergoing pulmonary resection for other indications. The extent of resection—pneumonectomy or lobectomy—has generally been dictated by the intraoperative findings rather than the original extent of the tumor in patients given preoperative chemotherapy.

SURGERY FOLLOWED BY CHEMOTHERAPY

The exceedingly poor long-term survival rates with surgery of SCLC were obtained in patients with clinical stages I through III; these patients for the most part underwent only minimal staging procedures by current standards. Only when results are categorized by tumor stages can the potential curative effects of surgery alone be demonstrated. One report, for example, documents 5-year survival of 35% in stage I and 23% in stage II patients.[246] The only randomized trials of surgery compared to surgery with postoperative chemotherapy were begun approximately 20 years ago and used inferior drug regimens by today's standards.[247–250] Nonetheless, they did in the aggregate reveal a survival advantage from chemotherapy (Table 27.3-5). Suffice it to say that thoracic oncologists should never recommend surgery as sole treatment for SCLC.[251]

Statements regarding the efficacy of combined modality approaches for SCLC that include surgical resection can be evaluated only when stratified by the temporal relationships among the different modalities. A number of programs of initial surgery followed by adjunctive chemotherapy after surgery have been reported; patients with multiple stages of tumor are included.[66,236,245,252–257] In general, modern combination che-

TABLE 27.3-5. Pooled Results from Randomized Surgical Adjuvant Studies in Small Cell Lung Cancer

Adjuvant Therapy	Patients (n)	2-Y Survival Rate (%)
Chemotherapy	92	26
Placebo	61	8

(Data from refs. 247–250.)

motherapy programs, usually including CAV or etoposide, have been used. Survival experience is quite heterogeneous, ranging from a 5-year survival of 9% in earlier to as high as 83% in more recent studies.

Nodal status and primary tumor or T status have significant effects on the survival of patients who have undergone resection. The significance of mediastinoscopy for SCLC is unclear, however, due to the small number of surgical cases. In a review,[258] 4 of 37 patients with SCLC (10.8%) were found to have mediastinal lymph node metastasis. A thoracotomy was performed in 33 patients, and 6 additional patients (18.2%) were found to have N2 disease after examination of the surgical specimens. In the identification of all mediastinal metastases, mediastinoscopy was 40.0% sensitive, 100% specific, and 83.8% accurate. When the superior mediastinal, paratracheal, pretracheal, tracheobronchial, and subcarinal lymph nodes were defined as approachable nodes, mediastinoscopy was 66.7% sensitive, 100% specific, and 94.6% accurate in the evaluation of these restricted nodes. In view of these data, mediastinoscopy should be performed in all patients who are being considered for resection of known SCLC.

Nodal status and primary tumor or T status were addressed directly in a few studies. Angeletti et al.[237] and Shepherd et al.[236] reported increased survival of node-negative compared to N1 and N2 patients after surgical resection and postoperative chemotherapy, whereas Macchiarini et al.[253] found a decrease in 5-year survival with increasing T category in surgically resected patients without nodal metastases. Retrospective reviews published by Rea et al.[256] and Lucchi et al.[257] have reinforced the importance of surgical staging in evaluating the outcomes for surgery and SCLC. Rea reported that 51 stage I/II SCLC patients resected and given chemotherapy after resection had 5-year survival rates of 52.2% (stage I) and 30% (stage II). In the review by Lucchi et al.,[257] stage I or II resected SCLC patients who underwent postoperative chemotherapy had 5-year survival rates of 47% and 14.8%, respectively. Stage III patients from this series who underwent surgery followed by adjuvant therapy had a 5-year survival of 14.4%. In general, 5-year survival is rare in patients given postoperative chemotherapy after mediastinal node disease has been documented at initial surgical resection,[245,246] although this observation is not universal.[236]

The largest experience as a cooperative group trial examining the role of surgery followed by adjuvant therapy in SCLC was conducted by the International Society of Chemotherapy Lung Cancer Study Group.[66] Four-year survival rates for completely resected, pathologically staged SCLC patients with N0 (n = 69), N1 (n = 58), and N2 (n = 36) who received postoperative therapy were 60%, 36%, and 33%, respectively. Based on these studies, most authorities believe that any survival benefits of initial surgical resection will likely be confined to patients with pathologic stages (p-stage) I and II, and conventional wisdom currently holds that surgical resection at diagnosis in patients with N2 disease is considered experimental.

Further studies from Japan have investigated the role of induction therapy and surgery for SCLC. A retrospective study of 91 patients who had undergone pulmonary resection for SCLC revealed a 5-year overall probability of survival of 37.1%. The 5-year survival rate was 100% for p-stage 0, 56.1% for p-stage IA, 30.0% for p-stage IB, 57.1% for p-stage IIA, and 42.9% for p-stage IIB. In the p-stage IA to IIB patients who underwent a complete resection, the 5-year survival rate of those treated by operation with chemotherapy was better than that of patients treated by operation alone, and the 5-year survival rate of the patients who had four or more courses of chemotherapy was 80%.[259] Kobayashi et al.[260] reported a cohort of 59 patients with clinical stage I through III resectable SCLC who underwent surgery. Postoperative adjuvant chemotherapy was based on an *in vitro* sensitivity. The 5-year survival rates for p-stage I, p-stage II, and p-stage III were 55%, 33%, and 23%, respectively.[260]

Because most available data on outcome of patients who receive surgery and postoperative chemotherapy is uncontrolled, one can only observe that the survival of such patients is clearly better than the survival of patients with limited disease who receive chemotherapy alone and better than the reported outcome of all but a few series of patients, most of them recent, given chemotherapy and chest irradiation. An extremely important point concerning initial surgical resection that remains unresolved is whether the superior outcome of patients with more localized (i.e., stages I and II) disease who undergo complete resection before initiation of chemotherapy is attributable to the resection itself or to an inherently better prognosis in patients with a tumor burden small enough to permit resection.

A controlled trial to address this question cannot be done because of the impossibility of randomizing patients whose small cell carcinoma is diagnosed only at the time of thoracotomy to undergo or not undergo surgical extirpation of their cancers, and therefore institutional data on patients with similar tumor burden after clinical staging who do and do not proceed to thoracotomy may be relevant. In Denmark, survival of "clinically operable" patients is similar whether or not an operation with the intent of completely resecting the tumor is performed,[261] although both these groups live much longer than other limited-stage patients. At the University of Toronto, a similar analysis, evaluating only patients without evidence of mediastinal metastases on chest radiograph or mediastinoscopy, produced similar conclusions.[58] At present, one can only conclude that early-stage patients may benefit from surgical resection. Certainly, if a resectable SCLC is documented for the first time at thoracotomy, we recommend the surgeon proceed with the operation if mediastinal node metastases are absent. In patients with a proven pathologic diagnosis, thoracotomy for tumor resection in clinical stage I disease should be considered only after complete staging procedures, including mediastinoscopy or mediastinotomy, reveal no evidence of tumor spread.

The whole question of the SCLC presenting as a solitary pulmonary nodule is somewhat controversial at this time. In a retrospective review of 408 small cell carcinoma patients, Quoix et al.[262] found that those with solitary pulmonary nodules have a median survival of 24 months. A number of factors could explain the improved prognosis, not the least of which is simply very early diagnosis (lead-time bias). Another possibility is that the solitary nodule may represent a fundamentally different category of SCLC or not be small lung cancer at all. Warren[263] reevaluated 50 cases of surgically resected SCLC. Thirty-four were pathologically confirmed to be SCLC, and stage I cases had a surprisingly low 9% 2-year survival. Twelve cases, however, were reclassified as well-differentiated neuroendocrine carcinoma, and 2-year survival of these stage I patients was 75%. The significance of these findings is presently unclear.

CHEMOTHERAPY FOLLOWED BY SURGERY

Surgical resection in SCLC might theoretically be more effective if performed after initial chemotherapy rather than at the time

TABLE 27.3-6.　Survival Data with Chemotherapy Followed by Surgical Resection

Study	Patients (n)	Stage	Response Rate (%)	Resected Patients (n)	Median Survival	% Survival (Y)
Prager et al.[265]	40	Limited	85	8 (20%)	NR	50 (1–2)
Holoye et al.[264]	26[a]	Limited	100	17 (65%)	R: 61 mo U: 16 mo	65 (5)
Baker et al.[244]	37	Limited	73	20 (54%)	R: 26 mo U: 12 mo	65 (2–3)
Johnson et al.[240]	24[a]	Limited	100	17 (53%)	R: 20 mo U: 18 mo	NR
Williams et al.[239]	38	Limited	84	21 (55%)	R: 33 mo U: 10 mo	48 (3–5)
Shepherd et al.[267]	72	I, II, IIIA	80	33 (46%)	R: 21 mo U: 12 mo	36 (5)
Lad et al.[268]	70	Limited	66	56 (83%)	R: 12 mo U: 12 mo	20 (2)
Fujimori et al.[269]	22	I, II, IIIA	96	21 (96%)	R: 62 mo	73 (3) I, II 43 (3) IIIA

NR, not reported; R, resected; U, unresectable.
[a]Patients deemed surgical candidates only after response to chemotherapy.

of diagnosis. Chemotherapy could be given in an immediate attempt to eradicate occult distant metastatic disease, the major cause of treatment failure. Only patients who respond to the chemotherapy, that is, those most likely to benefit, would undergo thoracotomy. Comprehensive initial preoperative staging procedures could be avoided, or at least be less rigorous, because chemotherapy would be the first treatment. Finally, after response to chemotherapy a larger fraction of patients might be surgical candidates.

Since 1984, there has been a steady increase in the fraction of cases reported to be resectable after chemotherapy response. Moreover, there is more uniformity in presurgical staging procedures, including mediastinoscopy, used to identify patients who might benefit from postchemotherapy surgery. As shown in Table 27.3-6,[238–240,244,264,265] resection rates in some series can exceed 50%, with estimated 5-year survivals in resected patients of 35% to 65%. Factors that prevent thoracotomy include poor response to chemotherapy, poor pulmonary function or other medical problems, and patient refusal.[239] The selection criteria for potential surgical candidates often exclude those with such adverse prognostic factors as supraclavicular adenopathy, superior vena cava syndrome, bulky mediastinal involvement, and pleural effusions.

The approach of chemotherapy followed by surgery has led to higher survival rates compared to chemotherapy (often with chest irradiation) in patients with stage I disease, with median survival not yet reached in patients from Toronto.[236] Stage II and III patients had median survivals of 69 and 52 weeks, respectively, and significant differences in survival were noted in all resected patients compared to 19 eligible patients who did not receive surgery after the chemotherapy. The median survival of stage II and III patients was no different, however, than in otherwise eligible patients not receiving thoracotomy (51 weeks). The best results, not surprisingly, are found in patients with no malignant cells in the surgical specimen.[239] Some,[266] but not all,[236] authors report absence of long-term survival in patients with initial mediastinal node involvement who undergo postchemotherapy resection.

Whether surgery is best performed before or after chemotherapy in patients with known SCLC who are considered oper-

able at diagnosis is not known. Survival of patients with surgery followed by chemotherapy and with chemotherapy followed by surgery was quite similar in Toronto.[267] The more fundamental question, whether postchemotherapy surgery improves survival, also cannot be regarded as settled, although in one institution survival of limited-stage patients who were considered eligible or ineligible for eventual surgical resection should they respond to chemotherapy was similar.[239] A Lung Cancer Study Group trial in which 217 patients who responded to chemotherapy (66% of those beginning chemotherapy) were randomized to undergo or not undergo thoracotomy for attempted surgical resection has matured. This study did not reveal survival differences, and the median survival and 2-year survival were 12 months and 20%, respectively, for both arms.[268] The results of this study, however, are difficult to interpret because only 42% of the registered patients were randomized, 10% did not receive protocol-specified therapy, and the response rate of 65% was low compared to modern response rates with SCLC regimens. This point is emphasized when one considers a more recent pilot study from Japan. Treatment in this study consisted of induction chemotherapy with cisplatin, doxorubicin, vincristine, and etoposide followed by surgical resection. In the 28 patients reported, the response rate was 96% and the resection rate was 95%. The 3-year survival rates were 73% for stage I and II disease and 43% for stage IIIA disease.[269] The majority of patients in the Lung Cancer Study Group study were stage III (N2 or T3, or both) tumors, and, notwithstanding the above data from Japan, the role of surgery in N2 disease is of debate not only in SCLC but in non-SCLC.

Newer phase II–type studies of induction therapy and surgery for SCLC have been reported from Poland and Germany. In the Polish study,[270] 75 patients, stage I through IIIA, were exposed to VP-16–based cytoreductive chemotherapy, and after three courses of treatment, 46 patients underwent thoracotomy, of whom 35 had resection. The complete response rate was 16%, and 4 weeks after surgery, chemotherapy was resumed. Three patients experienced local relapse (3 of 33), among them the single patient with incomplete resection, and local and distant failure developed in two other patients (2 of

33). The median survival in all 35 resected patients was 18 months, and the median survival in the cN0 + N1 subsets was 25.09 months, whereas in cN2 disease, it was 13.75 months.

Eberhardt et al.[271] described the original German experience with multimodality therapy of SCLC in 1999. After mediastinoscopy, 46 consecutive patients (stage IB, 6; IIA, 2; IIB/IIIA, 22; IIIB, 16) received four cycles of EP and surgery (IB/IIA) or three cycles of EP followed by one cycle of concurrent chemoradiation, including hyperfractionated radiation therapy and surgery (IIB/IIIA). Forty-three patients showed an objective response. Twenty-three patients were completely resected (R0). An update of this trial[272] reveals an actuarial 5- and 10-year survival of 39% and 35% for all the patients in the trial. In 22 patients who had initial disease involvement in the mediastinum, the 5- and 10-year survival rates are 44% and 41%, and local and locoregional tumor control is 100%. Patients with relapse events beyond 4 years were associated with second malignancies with other aerodigestive cancers or prostate cancer. Based on these data, the German group is considering a phase II trial with patients randomized to operation or small volume radiation boost after induction chemoradiation therapy. At present, the West Japan Lung Cancer Group is performing a prospective randomized trial of trimodality therapy in limited-disease SCLC, and another multicenter randomized trial in Germany is using sequential instead of concurrent chemoradiotherapy and surgery for SCLC.[272]

APPROACH TO PATIENTS WITH EXTENSIVE DISEASE

For more than 90% of patients, extensive SCLC is a fatal disease within 2 years of diagnosis. Nevertheless, compared with supportive care, chemotherapy offers substantial benefit by improving the quality and the quantity of survival within this limited window. Treatment with current chemotherapy produces an overall response rate of 60% to 80%, and the median survival time is 7 to 12 months. Once distant metastases have been identified during staging, further radiographic staging studies are necessary only if dictated by a clinical protocol or as necessary to evaluate a symptomatic complaint (Fig. 27.3-2). Combination chemotherapy is superior to any single agent tested thus far, including oral VP-16.[273,274] Treatment should be administered for a total of four to six cycles. Because many of these patients have poor functional status and other adverse prognostic factors, less aggressive chemotherapy programs are acceptable and may provide comparable palliation with less toxicity. Because relapse invariably occurs, enrollment on an investigational study evaluating new targets designed to impair tumor growth is warranted if available. When disease progression does occur, additional chemotherapy should be offered to most patients with a good functional status.

ROLE OF CHEST IRRADIATION IN EXTENSIVE DISEASE

Retrospective reviews of the literature demonstrate that the addition of chest irradiation plus chemotherapy for patients who have extensive-stage SCLC may reduce the frequency of progressive disease in the thorax, but the overall response rates, median survival, and 2-year disease-free survival figures remain unchanged.[203,275] Because patients with extensive dis-

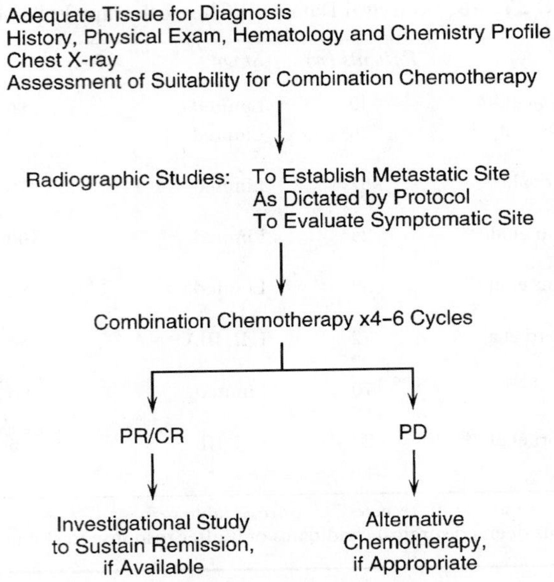

FIGURE 27.3-2. Algorithm outlining management of patients with extensive disease. CR, complete response; PD, progressive disease; PR, partial response.

ease generally achieve complete response rates of only 20% to 25% with current chemotherapy regimens and frequently relapse in distant metastatic sites, it is logical that an additional localized form of treatment would have minimal impact on survival. Successive large studies by the Southwest Oncology Group also confirm that, although thoracic radiotherapy can substantially reduce the frequency of initial relapse at the primary tumor site, it has no apparent effect on survival.[276,277]

Several clinical trials have randomized patients with extensive disease to chemotherapy alone or in combination with irradiation to the chest disease as well as to some or all sites of overt distant metastases.[198,277–279] With one exception,[278] no worthwhile advantages in survival have been seen with the addition of radiotherapy for patients with extensive disease. At present, except as part of a clinical trial, there is no indication for chest irradiation in extensive SCLC other than symptomatic palliation.

ROLE OF CHEMOTHERAPY AND RADIATION THERAPY TO THE NEURAXIS

For overt metastatic lesions within the CNS, doses of 300 rads daily to doses of 3000 to 3600 Gy typically are used. Overt intracranial metastases appear to be more difficult to sterilize than intrathoracic disease.[280] If there are only one or two clinically documented intracranial lesions, a boost to 5000 cGy can be considered if the patient has excellent performance status. Based on experience in other clinical settings, stereotactic treatment can also be used.

Chemotherapy is also a therapeutic option for brain metastases, perhaps because the blood–brain barrier is disrupted in the setting of macroscopic metastatic disease. Small series of patients in whom brain metastases were present at diagnosis have been treated with standard chemotherapy regimens without radiation, and the majority have demonstrated clinical and radiographic improvement.[110] Chemotherapy has also been used at the time of relapse, and response rates of 33% to 43% have been reported.[110,281,282] In previously treated patients, the response to chemotherapy in the brain appears to be comparable to the response rates in other organs, and it is not dissimilar from the activity of irradiation, which in one series produced a partial response rate of 50%; the median survival was 4.7 months in a series of 22 patients.[283] Thus, although brain irradiation remains the standard for patients who have not been previously irradiated, chemotherapy is a reasonable option for those in whom recurrent disease develops after prior brain radiation, particularly if active systemic disease is also present.

STRATEGIES TO OPTIMIZE CHEMOTHERAPY RESPONSE

A number of strategies have been investigated in an attempt to improve treatment outcome using the currently available drugs. These approaches include increasing the number of active agents used in the treatment program, often by the use of cyclic alternation between two combination regimens, increasing the dose intensity, frequently with the support of hematopoietic growth factors or blood progenitor cells, and weekly chemotherapy regimens, which increase the dose intensity by shortening the interval between treatment rather than increasing the dose. A confounding limitation in all of these studies is the use of body surface area to determine the drug dose. The correlation between body surface area and pharmacokinetic parameters is poor, which can result in a four- to tenfold variation in systemic exposure. Analysis of 23 patients treated with doxorubicin, ifosfamide, and etoposide demonstrated a significant correlation between systemic exposure to etoposide measured on the first cycle and survival.[284]

These strategies are invariably associated with substantial morbidity because most patients with SCLC are older, have comorbid conditions and a poor functional status, and are at risk for postobstructive pneumonia. As a result, support with prophylactic oral antibiotics may play a role in the management of this disease even though this approach is not commonly used for patients with solid tumors treated with chemotherapy that induces modest myelosuppression. A European study comparing broad-spectrum oral antibiotics versus placebo for patients treated with CDE demonstrated a 50% reduction in the incidence of febrile neutropenia along with a significant reduction in the incidence of infectious deaths (0% vs. 6%).[285] Although the use of prophylactic antibiotics cannot be recommended routinely, they can be considered in patients at increased risk due to host factors, extent of disease, or treatment with an intensified chemotherapy program.

ALTERNATING CYCLIC COMBINATION CHEMOTHERAPY

The recognition of clonal heterogeneity within a tumor and the inability to develop treatment regimens that included more than four drugs due to overlapping toxicity led to an interest in alternating chemotherapy combinations. The somatic mutation model developed by Goldie and Coldman provided a theoretic underpinning to this approach, because this model predicted that the best probability of cure was achieved by the earliest possible introduction and most rapid alternation of all active agents.[286,287] If two equally effective non–cross-resistant regimens were available, the model predicted that alternating between regimens every other cycle would be more effective than alternating after every three cycles or giving one regimen continuously for five cycles before switching to the second regimen.[287]

A large number of clinical trials have been conducted attempting to evaluate alternating multidrug combinations, particularly in extensive disease.[153,179,276,288–290] The EP regimen was initially tested in patients who had progressed after cyclophosphamide-based chemotherapy, suggesting that these drug combinations were non–cross resistant.[291] The National Cancer Institute of Canada conducted a study in which 289 patients were randomized to CAV or CAV alternating with EP.[288] Chemotherapy was given for a total of six cycles. The response rate (65% vs. 47%), progression-free survival, and median survival time (9.6 vs. 8.0 months) favored the patients who had received alternating therapy. The results could be explained by the inclusion of a more active regimen (EP) within the alternating arm, an advantage due to greater drug diversity with five effective drugs rather than three, or as support of the Goldie and Coldman concept. Roth et al.[153] subsequently evaluated 437 patients with extensive disease in a randomized trial comparing EP for four cycles, CAV for six cycles, or CAV alternating with EP for a total of six cycles. Although a slight improvement occurred in progression-free survival ($P = .052$) with the alternating regimen, there was no significant difference in response rate or overall survival between the treatment arms. Nonresponders to CAV crossed over to EP were twice as likely to respond to second-line therapy as nonresponders to EP that crossed over to CAV, although these differences were not statistically significant (28% vs. 14% for induction responders who relapsed and 15% vs. 8% for patients with primary resistance, respectively). An assumption of the Goldie and Coldman hypothesis is that the alternating regimens are non–cross resistant, which is not the case with the CAV and EP combinations, as demonstrated by the modest activity when nonresponding patients are crossed over from one of these regimens to the other. The European Organization for Research and Treatment of Cancer developed a regimen consisting of vincristine, ifosfamide, mesna, and carboplatin (VIMP) and randomized patients with extensive disease to CDE or CDE alternating with VIMP.[289] The study was closed after 143 patients had been registered and demonstrated no significant differences in survival. Although it did not reach its planned accrual, it still had sufficient power to have detected an increase in median survival time of 2 months with alternating therapy, had it existed. These studies, therefore, do not support the superiority of an alternating chemotherapy combination in patients with extensive disease.

Alternating non–cross-resistant chemotherapy has also been investigated in patients with limited disease.[154,292–295] The National Cancer Institute of Canada randomized 300 patients with limited disease to either CAV for three cycles followed by EP for three cycles or CAV alternating with EP for a total of six cycles.[293] No differences were noted in response rates, time to treatment failure, or survival. A Japanese study compared CAV to EP to alternating CAV/EP.[154] Patients with limited disease received four cycles of chemotherapy followed by thoracic irradiation. Patients with extensive disease who responded to chemotherapy continued treatment for 1 year. A total of 288 patients were enrolled. No differences in survival based on treatment were noted in the patients with extensive disease. Patients with limited disease had improved survival, even after adjusting for other prognostic factors with the alternating regimen compared with CAV ($P = .058$) or EP ($P = .032$). In contrast, Urban et al.[295] reported inferior survival with an alternating seven-drug regimen compared to a four-drug regimen, although the seven-drug combination was less intensive based on the magnitude of myelosuppression. These results suggest that an equally intensive alternating regimen is a reasonable alternative for patients with limited disease, despite the fact that the survival advantage noted in the Japanese trial has not been confirmed by another study.

Additional studies have evaluated alternating chemotherapy introduced after achieving a response to an induction regimen.[292,296,297] For example, Wolf et al.[292] randomized 321 patients, 135 of who had limited disease, to treatment with ifosfamide and VP-16 (IE) to response plateau followed by CAV, or IE alternating with CAV. A total of six cycles of chemotherapy were delivered in each arm. No difference in outcome was noted based on treatment arm in either limited or extensive disease. Other studies have compared alternating regimens that were designed based on the suggestion of *in vitro* synergy[298] or have compared an alternating multidrug combination to a different standard regimen.[299] For example, a German multicenter trial demonstrated that an alternating eight-drug regimen was slightly superior to CAV.[299] In sum, these studies can be viewed as suggesting a modest advantage for regimens that introduce greater diversity of active drugs into treatment rather than a test of the Goldie-Coldman hypothesis.

DOSE INTENSIFICATION

In experimental models, numerous chemotherapy drugs display log-linear or near linear dose-response curves.[300,301] Increasing the dose of chemotherapy delivered has been demonstrated to improve survival in a number of clinical settings.[302–304] In SCLC, several approaches to increase dose intensity have been evalu-

ated. These include dose intensification without or with hematopoietic growth factor support, dose intensification with marrow or peripheral blood stem cell support, and compression of the time in which chemotherapy is delivered using a weekly schedule.

Hryniuk and Bush[305] developed a methodology that expresses dose intensity as the drug dose administered per meter squared per week. Limitations of this method include the assumption that all drugs and schedules of administration are therapeutically equivalent. Nevertheless, this method has been used to demonstrate a positive correlation between dose intensity and treatment outcome in advanced breast cancer and ovarian cancer.[305,306] In SCLC, however, an analysis of 60 clinical trials using this methodology found limited and conflicting correlations between dose intensity, response rates, and median survival.[307]

Several randomized trials have attempted to determine whether a modest increase in dose intensity improves survival in this disease.[308–314] In a small trial comparing different doses of a regimen consisting of cyclophosphamide (500 vs. 1000 mg/m^2), lomustine (50 vs. 100 mg/m^2), and methotrexate (50 vs. 100 mg/m^2), survival was inferior in the lower-dose arm.[308] Preliminary findings of a cooperative group study in which the dose of cyclophosphamide was increased from 700 to 1500 mg/m^2 in a regimen that also included lomustine and methotrexate also demonstrated improved survival in the patients treated with the more intensive regimen.[309] These early studies confirm that the use of lower than standard doses of drugs can compromise survival in a chemotherapy-sensitive disease.

More recently, several investigators evaluated whether increasing the dose of drugs beyond the dose used in current regimens improves survival. Most of these studies were conducted in patients with extensive disease[312,313,315–317] (Table 27.3-7). A trial comparing dose-intensified to standard-dose CAV[312] and a study comparing high-dose to standard-dose EP[313] identified increased toxicity without improvement in survival. Neither of these studies used a hematopoietic growth factor in the intensified arm. Standard doses of cyclophosphamide, 4'-epidoxorubicin, etoposide,

TABLE 27.3-7. Randomized Trials Evaluating Dose Intensity in Small Cell Lung Cancer

Study	Regimen	Patients (n)	Disease Stage	Dose Intensity Variable	Relative Dose Intensity[a]	Toxicity: High vs. Standard	2-Y Survival: High vs. Standard
Johnson et al.[312]	CAV	247	Extensive	Dose C, A	1.27 Cycles 1–3	Increased myelotoxicity, increased nausea	NSD
Figueredo et al.[310]	CAV	103	Extensive	Dose C, A	1.17 Cycles 1–4	Increased myelotoxicity, increased stomatitis	NSD
Arriagada et al.[311]	CAPE	105	Limited	Dose C, P	1.11 Cycle 1	NSD	43% vs. 26%
Le Chevalier et al.[314]	CAPE	295	Limited	Dose C	1.33 Cycle 1	NSD	NSD
Ihde et al.[313]	EP	90	Extensive	Dose E, P	1.46 Cycles 1–2	Increased myelotoxicity, increased weight loss	NSD
Pujol et al.[317]	EpCPE	125	Extensive	Dose	0.9 Total	Increased myelotoxicity	8.9 vs. 11.0 mo[b]
Steward et al.[319]	ICaE-V	300	60% Limited	Interval	1.26 Total	NSD	33% vs. 18%
Lorigan et al.[320]	ICaE	318	88% Limited	Interval	1.82 Total	Less neutropenic infections	NSD
Thatcher et al.[321]	CDE	403	77% Limited	Interval	1.34 Total	Increased transfusions	13% vs. 8%
Ardizzoni et al.[322]	CDE	244	57% Limited	Dose, interval	1.70 Total	Increased myelotoxicity, increased stomatitis	NSD

A, doxorubicin; C, cyclophosphamide; Ca, carboplatin; D, doxorubicin; E, etoposide; Ep, 4'-epidoxorubicin; I, ifosfamide; NSD, no significant difference; P, cisplatin; V, vincristine.
[a]Relative dose intensity delivered in the high-dose arm, compared with control arm over specified number of cycles.
[b]Median survival time.

and cisplatin given for six cycles were compared to an intensified schedule in which three of the four drugs were given at a 50% higher dose for four cycles.[317] This study demonstrated a shorter response duration and survival in the dose-intensified arm. Although the planned cumulative doses of chemotherapy were equivalent for three of the drugs, the intensified arm actually received a lower total dose because of toxicity. The Danish group reported a study in which patients were treated with a five-drug regimen that contained carboplatin without or with the addition of cisplatin.[318] Survival was better for patients with limited disease treated with the intensified platinum regimen. However, it is not certain that the activity of these platinum analogues is identical, and therefore this study may not have been a true assessment of increased dose. Furthermore, radiotherapy was not included as part of the planned treatment for patients with limited disease, making the results of trial difficult to extrapolate to current management programs.

The only study that has suggested that the administration of higher drug doses within a standard regimen was beneficial was conducted in patients with limited disease. This French study randomized 105 patients with limited disease to a higher dose of cisplatin (100 vs. 80 mg/m^2) and cyclophosphamide (1200 vs. 1000 mg/m^2) in a regimen that also included doxorubicin and VP-16.[311] The increased doses of chemotherapy were only given on the first cycle. At 2 years, the progression-free (28% vs. 8%) and the overall survival (43% vs. 26%) were improved in the higher-dose arm. A subsequent trial evaluated whether further escalation of the cyclophosphamide during cycle 1 from 1200 mg/m^2 to 2000 mg/m^2 provided further benefit.[314] No further improvement occurred in survival with this additional increase in cyclophosphamide dose during the first cycle. These studies indicate that a modest intensification of the dose of the commonly used agents does not improve outcome for patients with SCLC and may even compromise survival by producing excessive toxicity. However, the French data are compatible with earlier trials that suggest a minimum threshold dose is necessary to maximize survival. Beyond this threshold, whether we face a plateau with current drugs or further improvement is feasible by using growth factor and stem cell support to substantially increase dose remains a reasonable setting for further investigation.

DOSE INTENSIFICATION BY INTERVAL COMPRESSION

A number of studies have evaluated whether shortening the interval between chemotherapy cycles improves survival. In patients with extensive disease, delivering CAVE on days 1 and 8 of the first few courses of chemotherapy did not appear promising.[315] A multicenter study randomized 300 patients to six cycles of vincristine, ifosfamide, carboplatin, and VP-16 (ICE-V) delivered every 4 weeks or every 3 weeks.[319] Most of the patients included in the study had limited disease. In the group receiving chemotherapy every 3 weeks, the delivered dose intensity was increased by 26% over the entire treatment program compared with the group treated every 4 weeks. The median survival (443 vs. 351 days) and the 2-year survival rate (33% vs. 18%) were better in the intensified arm ($P = .0014$), even after adjustment in a multivariate analysis. In a subsequent study, ICE given every 4 weeks was compared to ICE given every 2 weeks with support of G-CSF and autologous blood collected before the cycle and reinfused 24 hours after

the chemotherapy.[320] Most patients had limited-stage disease. Although the median delivered dose intensity was increased by 82% without significant increased toxicity, no survival benefit was identified.

Two studies have evaluated the importance of cycle duration for the CDE regimen. The first multicenter study randomized 403 patients, 77% of whom had limited disease, to cyclophosphamide, doxorubicin, and VP-16 delivered on an every-3-week schedule or on an every-2-week schedule. Patients treated every 2 weeks received G-CSF support.[321] The delivered dose intensity was 34% greater on the every-2-week schedule, and the complete remission rate and the overall survival were better in this group. Improved survival was observed in patients with limited- and those with extensive-stage disease treated on the every-2-week schedule. In contrast, a study comparing standard CDE given every 3 weeks to increased doses of the drugs given every 2 weeks with G-CSF support demonstrated no differences in survival between the groups despite an increase in the delivered dose intensity of 70% in the experimental arm.[322] The former study enrolled a larger number of patients and had a higher percentage of patients with limited disease. In addition, the dose of chemotherapy was similar in the two arms, and the only parameter evaluated was a reduction in interval between cycles. Overall, these studies fail to demonstrate that compression of the treatment cycle, even if this can be accomplished without a significant increase in toxicity, is an effective means to improve survival. These data mirror the conclusions that can be drawn from the weekly chemotherapy programs.

WEEKLY DOSE-INTENSIVE CHEMOTHERAPY REGIMENS

Some groups have developed weekly regimens that use six or seven drugs.[323–325] Three weekly programs have been tested in randomized multi-institutional settings.[325–327] A multidrug combination developed by Sculier et al.,[325] which included seven drugs, was compared to standard treatment consisting of CAV. Overall, there was no difference in median survival (49 vs. 43 weeks) or in 2-year survival rates (8.5% vs. 7.9%) between the treatment arms. A second randomized trial evaluated a regimen consisting of EP alternating on a weekly basis with ifosfamide plus doxorubicin. This was compared to a standard chemotherapy regimen consisting of alternating 3-week cycles of CAV and EP.[326] Included in this study were 438 patients, the majority of whom had limited disease. No differences in either median or 2-year survival rates were evident. In both of these randomized studies, myelosuppression was a dominant side effect, and the actual dose intensity delivered was a lower percentage of the planned dose in the weekly treatment arms. However, treatment-related mortality was low and no worse with weekly treatment than with standard therapy.

A more intensive weekly program that included cisplatin, vincristine, doxorubicin, and VP-16 (CODE) delivered higher doses of chemotherapy by infusing myelosuppressive and relatively nonmyelosuppressive drugs on alternate weeks and by using an aggressive supportive regimen consisting of corticosteroids, gastroprotective agents, and prophylactic antibiotics. The Japan Clinical Oncology Group compared CODE plus G-CSF to a standard regimen consisting of alternate 3-week cycles of CAV and EP[327]; 220 patients with extensive disease were enrolled in this study. The overall response rate and the complete remission rate (15%) were similar in the two treatment arms. The median survival time (11.6 vs. 10.9 months) and 2-year survival rates (11.7% vs. 8.5%) were also comparable. The incidence of neutropenic fever was significantly higher, and there were four toxic deaths in the weekly treatment arm. In North America, a randomized intergroup study compared CODE to alternating CAV and EP over 18 weeks.[328] A total of 219 patients with extensive disease with a good performance status were enrolled. Although the response rate was improved (87% vs. 70%) with the weekly program, the response duration and median survival were equivalent between the two treatment arms. Moreover, febrile neutropenia was more common in the patients treated with CODE, and there were more toxic deaths (8.2% vs. 1.0%) compared with the standard treatment arm. In aggregate, these studies demonstrate that weekly chemotherapy programs offer no advantage to standard treatment given every 3 weeks, and, if given at the maximum tolerated dose, weekly chemotherapy is significantly more toxic than standard therapy.

HEMATOPOIETIC GROWTH FACTORS

G-CSF and granulocyte-macrophage colony-stimulating factor (GM-CSF) are members of a group of glycoproteins that stimulate the production and maturation of hematopoietic progenitor cells and regulate the function of mature blood cells.[329] Two randomized, placebo-controlled trials demonstrated that the use of G-CSF as an adjuvant to CAE chemotherapy significantly reduced the duration of neutropenia, incidence of febrile neutropenia, and the use of hospital resources.[330,331] A decision analysis based on the results of one of these trials concluded that the routine use of G-CSF led to a net decrease in the total cost per treatment cycle based on billed charges but was associated with an increased cost based on actual provider costs or payments by the U.S. Medicare system.[332] Moreover, this analysis was extrapolated from the rate of hospitalization due to febrile neutropenia during the first cycle of chemotherapy, which in this study was 55% in the placebo arm and 26% in the group treated with G-CSF. Another decision analysis suggested that, from an economic perspective, a rate of hospitalization of 40% or greater was necessary to justify the routine inclusion of G-CSF into a chemotherapy regimen.[333] These conclusions are consistent with the guidelines of the American Society of Clinical Oncology, which recommended primary prophylaxis (G-CSF administration concomitant with the first chemotherapy cycle) only when the expected incidence of febrile neutropenia exceeded 40%.[334] The incidence of febrile neutropenia after conventional chemotherapy for SCLC is approximately 18%.[335] The differences in the reported rates of febrile neutropenia between studies were related to the chemotherapy regimen used and also to the diligence with which fever was sought and with how febrile neutropenia was defined. Two analyses that compared the use of G-CSF as secondary prophylaxis (G-CSF administered with all subsequent courses of chemotherapy if febrile neutropenia occurred on the previous cycle) suggested that this approach was more costly than a strategy of reducing the dose of the chemotherapy by 25%.[335,336]

Maintaining the dose of chemotherapy with growth factor support, rather than reducing or delaying the dose because of hematologic toxicity, would be appropriate if this translated into improved treatment efficacy. The results of studies designed to determine whether hematopoietic growth factors can increase the delivered dose intensity have been mixed.[317,319,321,322,337,338] A trial randomized patients to treatment with ICE-V every 3 weeks or every 4 weeks.[319] In a second randomization, patients were given GM-CSF or placebo after each chemotherapy cycle. Survival was improved for patients treated every 3 weeks, but the addition of GM-CSF did not reduce the incidence or the duration of febrile neutropenia, and there was no difference in survival between the patients who received GM-CSF or placebo. In a subsequent study, ICE given every 4 weeks was compared to ICE given every 2 weeks. In the dose-dense arm, support of G-CSF and autologous blood collected before the cycle and reinfused 24 hours after the chemotherapy prevented excessive toxicity.[320]

With the use of G-CSF, treatment-intensified doses of CDE are feasible every 2 weeks. Two randomized trials comparing ACE given every 2 weeks with G-CSF or every 3 weeks without the growth factor demonstrated conflicting results regarding an impact on survival.[321,322] In both studies, the intensified group required more transfusions of red cells and platelets. The incidence of febrile neutropenia was not increased in the patients receiving the greater dose intensity, but in one study there was a second randomization that evaluated the addition of prophylactic oral antibiotics that confounded the supportive benefit attributable to the G-CSF.[322] Symptom scales were measured in one study, and dose intensification did not compromise the overall quality of life.[321]

Two studies evaluated G-CSF as an adjunct to weekly chemotherapy programs.[337,338] In one trial G-CSF did not increase the delivered dose intensity,[337] whereas in the other study dose intensity and survival were improved in the arm that included G-CSF support.[338] A subsequent trial, however, compared this latter regimen with G-CSF support to a standard chemotherapy regimen that was given every 3 weeks and found no survival advantage with the intensified program.[327] An attempt to use G-CSF to increase the dose of three myelotoxic drugs in a four-drug regimen by 50% was not feasible and resulted in increased marrow toxicity, a reduction in cumulative drug dose received, and inferior survival.[317] Inclusion of GM-CSF in a combined modality program that consisted of EP plus concurrent radiation in patients with limited disease demonstrated that, although the neutrophil nadirs were higher in the arm receiving GM-CSF, these patients developed more episodes of febrile neutropenia requiring intravenous antibiotics and hospitalization.[339] Serious thrombocytopenia and blood transfusions were also increased in the group receiving GM-CSF.

These data suggest that the inclusion of a hematopoietic growth factor within a chemotherapy regimen may permit a modest escalation in the dose intensity of some regimens, but not others. Whether this dose intensification is clinically meaningful is a separate issue, and broad generalizations are difficult. Another issue that has not been resolved is whether patients who are at higher risk of toxicity due to age or other adverse prognostic factors, and patients in whom febrile neutropenia has developed on a previous treatment cycle, are better managed by reducing the dose of standard chemotherapy regimens or by adding a myeloid growth factor so that standard regimens can be given at full dose. Thus, dose, treatment interval, drug diversity, and patient selection are all parameters that define clinical outcome. The current data do not support the routine use of hematopoietic growth factors to escalate or maintain dose intensity for the regimens listed in Table 27.3-4.

However, it is possible that special populations who are at increased risk of infectious complications, such as the elderly and immunoincompetent, profit from the use of growth factor support. Similarly, there may be populations who benefit from maximizing the dose intensity of a specific chemotherapy regimen, such as patients with limited disease treated with CDE.

MARROW AND PERIPHERAL BLOOD STEM CELL TRANSPLANTATION

Dose intensification with high-dose chemotherapy, supported by stem cells collected from the peripheral blood or bone marrow, has provided a survival advantage to select groups of patients with hematologic malignancies. In contrast, reviews of the efficacy of high-dose therapy in adult solid tumors have concluded that no role for this approach has been established, even in the diseases most sensitive to chemotherapy and radiation. However, the efficacy of high-dose therapy in SCLC has been evaluated in a relatively limited number of patients when compared to other diseases, such as breast cancer. Many of the earliest studies in SCLC enrolled patients with relapsed or chemotherapy-resistant disease. Although response rates were higher than would be anticipated with additional standard doses of chemotherapy, response duration was brief (ranging from 2 to 8 months) and the median survival was often less than 4 months.[340–342] Subsequent studies evaluated high-dose therapy as an early component of treatment in newly diagnosed patients. With this strategy, patients received little or no induction chemotherapy before the high-dose regimen. It was hoped that by avoiding exposure to multiple cycles of conventional chemotherapy the risk of developing drug resistance in the tumor could be reduced. Response durations and survival, however, were comparable to those achieved with standard chemotherapy.[343]

A more commonly applied approach has been to use high-dose therapy as late intensification after standard treatment.[344,345] Theoretic support for this strategy is provided by the mathematical model proposed by Norton and Simon, which predicts that, as the tumor volume is reduced, relative resistance to chemotherapy develops. These studies differ in the number of cycles and type of regimen used for induction, the extent of tumor response required before high-dose consolidation, the composition of the high-dose regimen, and whether radiation or surgery, or both, was included as part of the treatment program.

The only reported phase III trial administered five cycles of induction therapy and then randomized patients who achieved a good response to consolidation with cyclophosphamide, BCNU, and etoposide with bone marrow support, or one additional cycle of conventional doses of these same drugs.[346] A total of 101 patients were registered and 45 were randomized, which included 13 patients who initially had extensive disease. The complete remission rate and the median relapse-free survival ($P = .002$) were superior in the high-dose arm. Although the median survival time was improved (68 vs. 55 weeks), this was not statistically significant ($P = .13$), and long-term survival was achieved in only 2 of the 23 patients treated with the high-dose regimen. A criticism of this study has been that thoracic irradiation was not included as part of the treatment plan, and in most patients the site of initial relapse was confined to the chest. Accordingly, many groups that have continued to investigate consolidative high-dose therapy have used a multimodality

program. For example, the Southwest Oncology Group treated 58 patients with limited disease with induction chemotherapy and radiation followed by consolidation with high-dose cyclophosphamide and autologous marrow support.[347] Only 21 patients received the consolidation, but 9 achieved long-term disease-free remissions, and the median survival of the patients receiving consolidation was 27 months.

At the Dana-Farber Cancer Institute, patients responding to conventional chemotherapy have been treated with high doses of BCNU, cyclophosphamide, and cisplatin along with stem cell or marrow support followed by thoracic irradiation and PCI. The initial report described 19 patients, and this has been updated to include 36 patients.[343] With the period of observation after completion of the high-dose therapy ranging from 21 months to 9 years, 52% of these patients with limited disease have remained in remission. The majority of patients (81%) were in complete remission or near complete remission at the time they received high-dose consolidation, and compared with patients transplanted in a partial remission, maximal cytoreduction with induction therapy appears to have been an important prognostic factor for long-term survival. Despite treatment with 50 to 60 Gy radiation to the chest, approximately half of the relapses occurred at the primary site.

Fetscher et al.[345] have described a program whereby patients received two to four cycles of induction chemotherapy followed by dose-intensive VP-16, ifosfamide, carboplatin, and epirubicin along with peripheral blood stem cell support. Additional locoregional therapy consisted of surgical resection or thoracic irradiation. Complete responders received PCI. Over a 6-year period, 100 patients (67 with extensive disease and 33 with limited disease) were treated with this approach. Only 19 of the 33 patients with limited disease proceeded to high-dose therapy. Excluding the favorable subset of patient with early-stage disease who underwent complete surgical resection, 5-year survival was 33%.[345] Leyvraz et al.[348] have shown that multiple cycles of high-dose therapy can be given within a cooperative group. In this study, treatment consisted of mobilization with epirubicin, collection of stem cells, and then three cycles of dose-intensified ICE given at 4-week intervals. Compared with standard doses of ICE, a two to threefold escalation of each chemotherapy drug was feasible. The median duration of severe leukopenia was 4 days, and there was no evidence of cumulative toxicity with the multiple cycles of high-dose treatment. This program is now being compared to standard therapy in patients with a favorable prognosis in a randomized trial.

In sum, high-dose consolidative therapy has been evaluated in a selected population that is younger and healthier than the general population of patients with SCLC. Even in this more favorable subset, it is not clear whether survival is better than would have been expected with conventional treatment. Treatment-related complications have been reduced with the substitution of peripheral blood stems cells for bone marrow and with improvements in supportive care, but even the most recent series report treatment-related mortality that exceeds the 2% to 5% mortality currently expected with high-dose therapy in other settings. This may be the result of more comorbid illness, even in the best subset of patients with SCLC, or it may simply be due to the small numbers of patients included in the reported series. Among the technical issues that need to be clarified is whether tumor cell contamination of the harvested stem cell product is a significant cause of treatment failure. Tumor cell contamination of leukapheresis products may be as high as 80%.[349] Several randomized studies are evaluating the role of high-dose consolidation in SCLC and should help define whether this approach, as currently practiced, is of value in this disease.

MANAGEMENT OF SMALL CELL LUNG CANCER IN THE ELDERLY AND INFIRM

At diagnosis, 25% to 40% of patients with SCLC are 70 years old or older.[350–352] Compared to younger patients, the elderly have a poorer performance status and more comorbidity.[350,351] Physiologic changes in body composition, a relative hypoalbuminemia or anemia, and a reduction in glomerular filtration rate contribute to altered pharmacokinetics and enhanced risk of drug toxicity that lead to more frequent complications from intensive treatment.[96,98] Cognitive and nutritional deficiencies may exist. As a result, many physicians treat elderly patients less aggressively.[77] For example, one retrospective review management for 20 of 123 (16%) elderly patients consisted only of radiation therapy and another 23 patients (19%) received only supportive care.[350] Another review of the management of 312 patients diagnosed between 1985 and 1991 showed that in the management of the elderly population, 23% of the patients received only supportive care and in the subset of patients with limited disease only 43% received chemotherapy as well as radiation.[351] In contrast, in patients between the ages of 60 and 69 fewer than 10% received supportive care and 65% with limited disease received combined modality therapy.

When chemotherapy is given to elderly patients, it is usually administered at attenuated doses and often for fewer cycles.[78,350,351] In one study the median nadir white blood cell count was 2800/μL and the nadir platelet count was 198,000/μL.[350] Patients who are treated with chemotherapy derive a survival benefit despite attenuation of the dose and duration of treatment, and in some series the response and survival for the elderly have been comparable to that of younger patients.[74,350,351]

Very few elderly patients have been included in clinical trials, and those who have been enrolled are among a minority with less comorbidity and better functional status.[351] As a result, extrapolation of the published data for standard therapies to the general population of elderly patients may be inaccurate. In a population-based study, increasing age was associated with a poorer functional status and increased comorbidities. As a result, age was associated with less intensive treatment, but it was not an independent variable affecting survival.[77] Consequently, several chemotherapy programs have been developed for the elderly and for patients unfit for participation in standard therapy protocols that aim to optimize palliation with acceptable risks. One approach has been to use monotherapy with the epipodophyllotoxins. VP-16 can be given orally, making it particularly attractive in the palliative setting.[353] The Medical Research Council designed a trial comparing oral VP-16, 50 mg b.i.d. for 10 days, to standard combination chemotherapy consisting of VP-16 and vincristine or CAV.[273] In each arm, chemotherapy was repeated every 3 weeks for a total of four cycles. The median age enrolled on this study was 67 years, and 38% of the patients had a performance status equal to 3 to 4. The study was prematurely stopped after an interim analysis that showed inferior survival in

the patients treated with VP-16 monotherapy. Hematologic toxicity was also worse with oral VP-16, and 17 deaths occurred during the first month of treatment in this arm compared to 10 deaths on the control group. A second British trial comparing oral VP-16 given at 100 mg b.i.d. for 5 days to VP-16 and cisplatin alternating with CAV in poor-prognosis patients was also stopped early because of inferior progression-free and overall survival in the VP-16 monotherapy arm.[274] Moreover, palliation of symptoms and quality of life were better with combination chemotherapy. Based on the results of these two trials, monotherapy with oral VP-16 cannot be recommended as adequate treatment for patients with SCLC. Monotherapy with carboplatin has been compared to CAV in a randomized phase II study.[354] Myelosuppression and complications requiring hospitalization were lower with the single agent, but equivalent survival was not assessed by this trial design.

An alternative approach for providing palliative chemotherapy explored in Britain was the delivery of chemotherapy as needed to palliate symptoms, rather than at fixed 3- or 4-week treatment intervals. A total of 300 patients were randomized to receive CEV every 3 weeks for a total of eight cycles or to an "as needed" treatment program.[355] In this arm patients were evaluated at 3-week intervals after the first treatment cycle and were re-treated only if they were symptomatic or had evidence of tumor growth while not receiving treatment. Patients randomized to receive chemotherapy as needed had a median interval between cycles of 42 days and received only 50% as much total chemotherapy as the patients treated on the fixed schedule. Although the median survival times were equivalent, better symptomatic control was achieved with the fixed-interval treatment.

Another investigation of less intensive therapy compared the VP-16, ECMV regimen to EV.[356] Three cycles were planned for each arm because a prior study comparing three and six cycles of ECMV showed equivalent survival.[186] A total of 310 patients with extensive disease or limited disease and poor performance status were registered. The response rates and survival were comparable between the two arms.[356] Twice as many early fatalities (death during the first treatment cycle) occurred in patients who received the four-drug ECMV regimen (37 vs. 18). Nevertheless, ECMV produced better palliation of symptoms than did EV. Another study compared a regimen of EP alternating with CAV every 3 weeks at standard doses to EP alternating with CAV every 10 to 11 days at 50% of the standard dose.[357] Response and survival were comparable with both schedules, and toxicity was not reduced with the more frequent administration of lower doses.

Elderly patients with limited disease and a good functional status should be treated with combined modality therapy. In a study of 75 elderly patients with reasonably good performance status and limited disease, two cycles of carboplatin and prolonged oral VP-16 were given with concurrent hyperfractionated radiation and a median survival of 15 months, and a 5-year survival of 13% was observed.[358] In 55 patients with limited disease unfit for standard treatment, Murray et al.[352] administered one cycle of CAV followed by one cycle of VP-16 and cisplatin along with 20 to 30 Gy concurrent thoracic irradiation. The complete remission rate was 51%, and 28% of the patients were alive and disease free at 2 years. Yuen et al.[75] retrospectively analyzed the intergroup 0096 study and observed similar response rate and survival for patients older than 70 years compared to younger patients, albeit at the cost of a greater myelotoxicity. These data indicate that curative therapy can be delivered to this population.

Patients with extensive disease tend to be more frail than those with limited-stage disease, and the treatment delivered must be done with even greater caution. Carboplatin-based regimens are often used and, if given in standard dose, may be associated with unacceptable mortality.[359] The Vancouver group developed a four-drug regimen consisting of attenuated doses of cisplatin, doxorubicin, vincristine, and VP-16 (PAVE) administered for four cycles to patients older than 65 years and with a performance status of 3.[360] Concurrent thoracic irradiation was given to patients with limited disease and selected patients with extensive disease. The delivered total dose was 80% of the intended dose. Survival at 2 years was 38% and 18% for patients with limited and extensive disease, respectively. Hospitalization was necessary for 42% of patients receiving combined modality treatment and for 15% of the patients treated with chemotherapy alone. Just one septic death occurred. Comparison of single-institution phase II trials to the outcomes observed in controlled cooperative group studies is difficult. Nevertheless, it highlights the challenge of delivering a maximally effective treatment regimen with manageable toxicity to elderly and high-risk patients and may be a setting in which primary supportive therapies, such as hematopoietic growth factor and prophylactic oral antibiotics, may be indicated.

BIOLOGIC RESPONSE MODIFIERS AND OTHER TREATMENTS

Although cytotoxic therapy is very effective in reducing the disease burden in SCLC, it is rarely curative. The immune response to SCLC appears to be modest. Efforts to augment the immune response have included treatment with nonspecific immunomodulators, therapy with interferons and interleukin-2, and active immunization with anti-idiotypic antibodies. Studies that have evaluated bacillus Calmette-Guérin (BCG), the methanol-extracted residue of BCG, or thymosin fraction V, a soluble product of calf thymus thought to reconstitute immune function, have failed to demonstrate a beneficial effect on response rate, response duration, or survival.[361,362]

The expression of major histocompatibility complex antigens is reduced in SCLC and thus may play a role in this tumor's ability to escape immune surveillance.[363,364] Interferon has been shown to increase the expression of major histocompatibility antigens on SCLC cells *in vitro* and *in vivo*.[365] Small studies in newly diagnosed patients treated with either interferon-α or interferon-γ, however, showed a total absence of activity. Because immune augmentation may be most effective in patients with low disease burden, larger studies have evaluated interferons as maintenance treatment in patients responding to chemotherapy. Mattson et al.[366] conducted a study in which patients responding to induction chemotherapy were randomized to a maintenance chemotherapy, natural interferon-α, or observation. Although there were no differences overall, a subset analysis showed improved survival for patients with limited disease who received interferon. Another study that administered interferon-α along with the induction chemotherapy and as maintenance reported a higher complete response rate and improved median survival.[367] Due to poor accrual, however, the study was stopped prematurely, and only 77 patients were evaluable. Two other randomized trials, one in which interferon-α was included as part of the induction and maintenance regimen and a sec-

ond, cooperative group trial in which interferon-α maintenance was evaluated in patients with limited disease who had responded to induction chemotherapy[368,369] showed no survival advantage. Interferon-γ maintenance therapy in patients with complete or near complete remissions has also been evaluated in two randomized trials.[370,371] Although the dose and schedule selected from one trial were confirmed to be biologically active as demonstrated by a significant increase in the expression of HLA-DR and Fc receptors on monocytes,[372] neither study demonstrated an impact on survival. In addition to the typical influenza-like side effects and myelosuppression, a few of the studies in lung cancer have suggested that the interferons may enhance radiation-induced lung injury, and at least one case of fatal pneumonitis occurred.[371]

High-dose interleukin-2 has also been evaluated in a group of patients with extensive disease who experienced less than a complete remission to induction chemotherapy.[373] The overall response rate was 21%, but the toxicity was severe, and treatment was discontinued in 11 of 24 patients because of life-threatening side effects. These studies indicate that at the present time treatment with cytokine therapy has not established a role in the management of this disease.

SCLC displays a variety of markers of neuroendocrine differentiation that could serve as targets for biologic agents. Neural cell adhesion molecule is one such target to which an immunotoxin, consisting of a murine monoclonal antibody linked to a modified ricin molecule, has been developed. In a dose-escalation trial, 1 of 21 patients had a partial response that lasted 3 months.[374] Because this antibody proved too toxic, a chimeric humanized antibody bound to maytansinoid toxin is being tested. In an alternate strategy, a monoclonal antibody directed against gastrin-releasing peptide was developed with the intent of interrupting this autocrine growth loop. One of 12 evaluable patients had a complete remission that lasted 6 months.[375] The patients treated with these two biologic agents all had disease resistant to chemotherapy. The activity noted is encouraging for further clinical development.

The increasing knowledge of the signal transduction pathways that determine cellular survival has provided multiple new targets for the development of anticancer therapies. Evaluation of many of these agents in SCLC has lagged behind the testing in non-SCLC, but prototypic studies in SCLC include the assessment of G3139, a bcl-2 antisense oligonucleotide, by Rudin et al.[376] The c-kit protooncogene encodes a transmembrane tyrosine kinase growth factor receptor that belongs to the platelet-derived growth factor receptor family. It can be detected in roughly half of SCLC tumors by immunochemistry and expression has been implicated as a poor prognostic factor. However, in one study no activating mutations in the c-kit exon 11 were found in 22 samples positive by immunohistochemistry, suggesting that imatinib might not play a significant therapeutic role for SCLC.[377] In fact, a small study reported disappointing activity.[378]

The variable region of an antibody mirrors its antigen. Therefore, a second antibody raised against this variable region structurally mimics the original antigen. Infusion of this second anti-idiotypic antibody often induces a more effective immune response than does infusion of the antigen of interest. Thus, a limitation of monoclonal antibody therapy, the development of a host immune response to the infused mouse protein (human antimouse antibody, or HAMA, reaction) can be exploited by infusing a mouse anti-idiotypic antibody to augment immunity to antigens preferentially expressed on tumor cells. An anti-idiotypic antibody, BEC2, which resembles a ganglioside expressed on SCLC cells, has been tested in 15 patients who had responded to conventional chemotherapy.[379] Side effects of the vaccination were modest and consisted primarily of skin reactions to the BCG adjuvant. Comparison to a historic matched control group suggested that progression-free and overall survival were substantially improved. Preliminary results of a randomized phase III trial evaluating this vaccine as a means to sustain remission in patients with limited disease that had responded to combined modality therapy, failed to show improvement in progression-free survival.[380] Anti-idiotypic antibodies are being developed that resemble other poorly immunogenetic antigens expressed by SCLC cells. Because the expression of any one of these antigens is variable, a polypeptide vaccine containing multiple immunogenetic antigens will probably be needed to effectively target every SCLC cell.

A potential role of the coagulation system in the propagation of cancer has been recognized for many years. Thrombin is generated *in situ* and may function as a growth factor for the tumor.[381] Initial studies evaluating whether the addition of warfarin to the chemotherapy regimen improved survival yielded mixed results. In a randomized trial involving a total of 50 patients, the addition of warfarin significantly improved progression-free and overall survival.[382] In a larger cooperative group study, patients receiving warfarin (Coumadin) with chemotherapy had a higher response rate ($P = .012$) and a 6-week improvement in median progression-free and overall survival, although the difference for the latter two end points was not statistically significant.[383] The addition of 1 g/d aspirin, a dose sufficient to inhibit platelet aggregation, failed to demonstrate a benefit.[384] A subsequent trial by the same group of investigators demonstrated that the subcutaneous administration of unfractionated heparin at therapeutic doses given during the first 5 weeks of chemotherapy resulted in a higher complete remission rate and improved survival.[381] More recently, several drugs designed to inhibit matrix metalloproteinases, a family

of nearly 30 enzymes capable of remodeling extracellular matrix and basement membrane that may play a role in the process of metastasis, have been tested in patients after initial chemotherapy. Studies to date have demonstrated toxicity without improved survival.[385,386]

TREATMENT AT RELAPSE

The majority of patients with SCLC relapse within a year of initial therapy, and many are candidates for second-line treatment[153,154,387–392] (Table 27.3-8). Factors that predict the likelihood of response to subsequent chemotherapy include the interval between completion of induction and relapse, the extent of tumor regression achieved with the induction regimen, and the composition of the induction program.[393] For example, the activity of teniposide in previously treated patients was 53% if the chemotherapy-free interval was greater than 2.6 months, compared with 12% if the treatment-free interval was shorter.[394] As a consequence, "sensitive relapse" is often, and somewhat arbitrarily, defined as a chemotherapy-free interval of 3 months or greater. In patients in sensitive relapse, response rates to second-line therapy often exceed 50%, and any chemotherapy regimen active in SCLC appears to be effective, including the drug regimen that was initially used for induction.[139,395–397] The likelihood of a secondary response appears to be better in patients who have not previously been treated with a platinum agent.[398]

For patients who relapse early, the regimen used for second-line and the induction regimen may be important in determining the likelihood of a secondary response.[291] For example, in patients treated with CAV as the induction regimen, second-line treatment EP produces a response rate of approximately 35%.[387,388] Only approximately half as many patients (15%) who experience early relapse after EP induction respond to CAV as a second-line therapy.[389] In some of the randomized trials that have compared CAV to EP, patients not responding to

TABLE 27.3-8. Activity of Combination Chemotherapy Regimens at Relapse

Study	Evaluable Patients (n)	Previous Chemotherapy (n)	Chemotherapy	Response (%)	Response Duration (Wk)	Median Survival (Wk)
Evans et al.[387]	34	CAV (23)	EP	44	NR	17
Lopez et al.[388]	30	CAV (23)	EP	27	20	16
Roth et al.[153] and Fukuoka et al.[154]	66	CAV	EP	20	NR	NR
Roth et al.[153] and Fukuoka et al.[154]	26	EP	CAV	8	NR	NR
Shepherd et al.[389]	13	EP	CAV	15	24	15
Ardizzoni et al.[400]	108	P or J (48)	PT	28	12 (s) 19 (r)	24 (s) 26 (r)
Smit et al.[390]	22	CDE (13)[a]	JV	36	NR	18
Postmus et al.[391]	25	CDE	VIMP	60	NR	19
Groen et al.[401]	34	CDE (33)	JT	73.5	21	31
Monnet et al.[392]	20	CIV	APE	45	NR	NR
	10	APE	CIV	0	—	—
Postmus et al.[391]	43	JV (22) IMJ (21)	CDE	51	NR	22

APE, doxorubicin, cisplatin, VP-16; CAV, cyclophosphamide, doxorubicin, vincristine; CDE, cyclophosphamide, doxorubicin, VP-16; CIV, carboplatin, ifosfamide, vincristine; EP, VP-16, cisplatin; IMJ, ifosfamide, mesna, carboplatin; J, carboplatin; JT, carboplatin, paclitaxel; JV, carboplatin, vincristine; NR, not reported; P, cisplatin; PT, cisplatin, topotecan; r, resistant; s, sensitive relapse; VIMP, vincristine, ifosfamide, mesna, cisplatin.
[a]Treated with specified regimen.

initial therapy (primarily refractory) and crossed over the alternative regimen were more likely to respond to EP than to CAV, although, in this more resistant group of patients, the response rates to second-line treatment overall were lower and were 15% to 23% for EP and approximately 8% for CAV.[153,154]

Drugs that have been reported to be active as second-line agents include carboplatin, topotecan, and paclitaxel, although the reported response rates have been variable, reflecting the small, heterogeneous populations tested. Topotecan has been most thoroughly evaluated and produces a response of 18% in patients in sensitive relapse, and in resistant patients it is less than 10%.[399,400] Results of combination therapy that includes these drugs have been variable. Ardizzoni et al.[171] reported a response rate of 29% for patients in sensitive relapse and 24% for those with resistant disease treated with cisplatin and topotecan. The activity in patients with resistant disease may have reflected the exclusion of prior cisplatin treatment in this group. Overall, 17% of patients experienced febrile neutropenia, and the treatment-related mortality was 5%. The combination of carboplatin and paclitaxel was evaluated in two studies and was reported to be 25% and 74%.[401,402] The survival from the start of second-line therapy is rarely more than 4 to 6 months and does not appear to be better with the use of combination therapy. These studies indicate that, for patients with a reasonable performance status, second-line therapy is appropriate. If a combination regimen is used, it is best reserved for patients who are not resistant to cisplatin. Symptomatic sites of disease can frequently be managed with radiation.

SURGICAL MANAGEMENT OF PERSISTENT OR RECURRENT LOCAL DISEASE

Histologically mixed disease is a not uncommon occurrence when SCLC is resected after chemotherapy. Non–small cell lung and mixed small and non–small cell elements occur in 5% to 35% of specimens.[239,244,264,403] Whether these pathologic findings may be attributable to selection by chemotherapy of non–small cell elements present in the original tumor, histologic changes

induced by chemotherapy, the presence of a second lung cancer, or incorrect initial diagnosis is not resolved. Nevertheless, surgery may prove therapeutically efficacious if the only residual cancer is non–small cell in type. Because of this frequency of mixed histologies at the time of resection after chemotherapy, the Toronto group reported a retrospective analysis of salvage surgery in limited SCLC.[267] Twenty-eight selected patients underwent thoracotomy after lack of response to induction chemotherapy or relapse after initial response. A surprising resection rate of 82% was possible, and 10 patients (36%) had mixed elements histologically. Projected 5-year survival is 23%. The authors believe it is important to verify these findings in other patients who are prospectively identified by specific selection criteria before such an approach is recommended.

TREATMENT OUTCOME AND LONG-TERM SURVIVAL

Although current therapy has a significant impact on the natural history of this disease, the number of patients cured remains frustratingly small (Table 27.3-9). Patients are at greatest risk of dying during the first 24 months after diagnosis; this risk declines between years 2 and 3 and is further reduced beyond the third year. In the Surveillance, Epidemiology, and End Results program database, overall survival at 2, 3, and 5 years was 11.6%, 7.1%, and 4.6%, respectively.[404] In an analysis of 2196 patients treated on clinical trials in Britain, the hazard fell by a factor of 10 after 3 years but was still approximately seven times that of the general population.[405] Excessive mortality in long-term survivors is due to late relapse with SCLC and to the development of second primary tumors. Late relapse occurs in approximately 10% of patients who are free of disease at 5 years.[406] Second primary tumors pose an even greater risk than relapse in long-term survivors. Overall, the relative risk of a second primary tumor in patients who survive beyond 2 years is increased by 3.5-fold.[407] Most of these second primary tumors are non-SCLC or other malignancies of the upper aerodigestive

TABLE 27.3-9. Effect of Treatment on Survival in Small Cell Lung Cancer According to Extent of Disease

Therapy	Median Survival (Mo)		2- to 3-Y Survival Rate (%)	
	Limited Disease[a]	Extensive Disease	Limited Disease	Extensive Disease
Supportive care	3	1.5	—	—
Surgery	5–6[a]	—	4–5[a]	—
	11[b]		30–35[b]	
Thoracic radiotherapy	10[a]	—	10[a]	—
	3–9		2–7	
Single-agent chemotherapy	6	4	—	—
Combination chemotherapy	10–14	7–11	5–15	1–3
Combination chemotherapy with chest irradiation	15–26	7–11	10–40	1–2

[a]Operable patients in prechemotherapy era.
[b]Selected, carefully evaluated, pathologically staged patients.
(Modified from Morstyn G, Ihde DC, Lichter AS, et al. Small cell lung cancer 1973–1983: early progress and recent obstacles. *Int J Radiat Oncol Biol Phys* 1984;10:51; and ref. 61, with permission.)

tract, indicating that field cancerization due to tobacco exposure has occurred.[407,408] The risk of a second primary tumor increases significantly over time, and continued smoking after the initial diagnosis of SCLC, radiation to the chest, and treatment with alkylating agents magnifies this risk.[407] For example, the risk of a second lung cancer in patients who continue to smoke was approximately fourfold more than those who stopped before the diagnosis of SCLC and twofold greater in patients who received chest irradiation compared to nonirradiated patients. The cumulative risk of a second lung cancer was 32% at 12 years and continued to increase beyond that time point. Consequently, patients successfully treated for SCLC constitute an extraordinarily high-risk group and deserve close medical follow-up. This population would be appropriate for studies evaluating new screening technologies, such as spiral CT scanning, and are candidates for chemoprevention trials.

Long-term survivors are also at increased risk for non–cancer-related morbidity. In a French study of patients surviving beyond 30 months, treatment-related sequelae included neurologic impairment in 13% of the patients, pulmonary fibrosis in 18%, and cardiac disorders in 10%.[409] Return to work was possible in 40% of these patients and was not influenced by the presence of late treatment-related complications. In a Danish analysis of patients surviving 5 years or more, there was a sixfold increased risk of death from nonneoplastic causes, particularly cardiovascular and pulmonary diseases.[410]

Very few patients with extensive disease attain long-term survival. At 2 years after diagnosis, no more than 5% of these patients remain alive, and the survival rate at 5 years is only 1%.[80,404] Although the impact of combination chemotherapy on survival is unambiguous, it is not clear whether any of the agents, treatment schedules, or supportive measures introduced since 1980 have improved survival for patients with extensive disease compared to the therapies available in the 1970s. Analysis of 21 phase III trials conducted in North America between 1972 and 1990 showed an improvement in median survival time from 7.0 months to 8.9 months when studies initiated in the first decade were compared to studies begun in the second.[411] In contrast, an analysis of 1111 consecutive patients treated on clinical trials in Scandinavia between 1973 and 1992 demonstrated no improvement in survival over those two decades.[412] In this series, severe myelosuppression and febrile neutropenia were significantly more common in patients treated between 1981 and 1992, suggesting that more intensive therapies in a relatively unselective population increase toxicity without improving survival. Progress in the management of limited-stage disease is clearer; an analysis of North American randomized trials conducted between 1972 and 1992 demonstrated a doubling of long-term survivors over this time period.[413] Although stage migration may be a contributing factor, this increased survival probably reflects improved treatment as a result of the use of platinum-based rather than cyclophosphamide-based chemotherapy in combined modality programs.

EXTRAPULMONARY SMALL CELL CARCINOMA

Extrapulmonary small cell anaplastic carcinoma is a clinicopathologic entity distinct from SCLC. It is estimated that approximately 1000 cases are diagnosed in the United States annually.[414] On routine histopathologic examination, pulmonary and extrapulmo-

nary small cell carcinomas are indistinguishable. Mixed tumors, which include a variety of cell types, may occur more frequently and deletions of chromosome 3p may be less common with extrapulmonary tumors.[415] Primary small cell carcinomas have been identified in virtually every organ site.[416] The most common sites include the esophagus and other gastrointestinal organs, the head and neck region, the cervix, and the bladder. A sex predilection appears to be present based on the primary site; most of the small cell carcinomas of the head and neck region, esophagus, and bladder are found in males. With the exception of primary tumors arising in the cervix, in which a younger age group is affected, the majority of patients are middle-aged or older.

A history of tobacco use is common, particularly in tumors that occur in the head and neck region and the esophagus, but there is not as strong an association with smoking as there is with pulmonary small cell carcinoma. Paraneoplastic syndromes due to the ectopic production of adrenocorticotropic and antidiuretic hormones also occur with extrapulmonary small cell cancer, and in at least one case report humorally mediated hypercalcemia was identified.[417]

By definition, patients with extrapulmonary small cell cancers must have a normal CT scan of the chest and preferably a normal bronchoscopic examination. Merkel-cell carcinoma is a distinct entity that is primarily found in the skin and can be distinguished by certain immunocytochemical characteristics. Extrapulmonary small cell carcinomas can disseminate widely, and the recommended staging studies are similar for pulmonary small cell carcinoma.[416] A two-stage system is generally used. Limited disease is defined as tumor confined to the organ of origin and the locoregional nodes that are encompassable within a radiation portal. Tumors that have spread beyond one radiation portal are defined as extensive. In contrast to SCLC, most patients in whom a primary site is identified have limited disease at the time of diagnosis. In a series of 71 patients from the Mayo Clinic, 76% of the tumors were localized at diagnosis.[418] In this series, the only sites that presented 50% or more of the time with extensive disease were primary tumors of the gastrointestinal tract and tumors of unknown primary site.

In many respects, the natural history and response to treatment for small cell carcinoma are similar for pulmonary and extrapulmonary sites. Patients with extensive disease are candidates for treatment with combination chemotherapy. In several reports in the literature, a proportion of patients with limited disease managed with local therapies alone, particularly surgical resection, achieve a long-term progression-free survival.[414,416,418] Success of local therapy appears to vary depending on the primary site of the small cell carcinoma. Although some patients with small volume disease confined to the organ of origin can be cured with surgery alone, the risk of relapse remains high even in this most favorable subset, and in most patients adjuvant chemotherapy should be strongly considered. For patients with locoregional disease, the combination of chemotherapy and radiation is a reasonable alternative to surgery. Overall, the prognosis for extrapulmonary small cell carcinoma is poor. In the Mayo Clinic series, 3- and 5-year survival rates were 38% and 13%, respectively.[418]

REFERENCES

1. Jemal A, Tiwari RC, Murray T, et al. Cancer statistics, 2004. *CA Cancer J Clin* 2004;54:8.
2. Parkin DM, Sankaranarayanan R. Overview on small cell lung cancer in the world: industrialized countries, third world, Eastern Europe. *Anticancer Res* 1994;14:277.

3. Shopland DR, Eyre HJ, Pechacek TF. Smoking-attributable cancer mortality in 1991: is lung cancer now the leading cause of death among smokers in the United States? *J Natl Cancer Inst* 1991;83:1142.

4. Lubin JH, Blot WJ. Assessment of lung cancer risk factors by histologic category. *J Natl Cancer Inst* 1984;73:383.

5. Morabia A, Wynder EL. Cigarette smoking and lung cancer cell types. *Cancer* 1991;68:2074.

6. Wingo PA, Ries LA, Giovino GA, et al. Annual report to the nation on the status of cancer, 1973–1996, with a special section on lung cancer and tobacco smoking. *J Natl Cancer Inst* 1999;91:675.

7. Prevalence of current cigarette smoking among adults and changes in prevalence of current and some day smoking—United States, 1996–2001. *MMWR Morb Mortal Wkly Rep* 2003;52:303.

8. Barrueco M, Cordovilla R, Hernandez Mezquita MA, et al. Sex differences in experimentation and tobacco consumption by children, adolescents and young adults. *Arch Bronconeumol* 1998;34:199.

9. Chen X, Li G, Unger JB, et al. Secular trends in adolescent never smoking from 1990 to 1999 in California: an age-period-cohort analysis. *Am J Public Health* 2003;93:2099.

10. Saracci R. The interactions of tobacco smoking and other agents in cancer etiology. *Epidemiol Rev* 1987;9:175.

11. Ernster VL. Female lung cancer. *Annu Rev Public Health* 1996;17:97.

12. Hayes RB, Yin SN, Dosemeci M, et al. Mortality among benzene-exposed workers in China. *Environ Health Perspect* 1996;[104 Suppl 6]:1349.

13. Steenland K, Loomis D, Shy C, et al. Review of occupational lung carcinogens. *Am J Ind Med* 1996;29:474.

14. Alavanja MC, Brownson RC, Boice JD Jr, et al. Preexisting lung disease and lung cancer among nonsmoking women. *Am J Epidemiol* 1992;136:623.

15. Mayne ST, Buenconsejo J, Janerich DT. Previous lung disease and risk of lung cancer among men and women nonsmokers. *Am J Epidemiol* 1999;149:13.

16. Brownson RC, Alavanja MC, Caporaso N, et al. Family history of cancer and risk of lung cancer in lifetime non-smokers and long-term ex-smokers. *Int J Epidemiol* 1997;26:256.

17. Sellers TA, Bailey-Wilson JE, Elston RC, et al. Evidence for mendelian inheritance in the pathogenesis of lung cancer [see comments]. *J Natl Cancer Inst* 1990;82:1272.

18. Mayne ST, Buenconsejo J, Janerich DT. Familial cancer history and lung cancer risk in United States nonsmoking men and women. *Cancer Epidemiol Biomarkers Prev* 1999;8:1065.

19. Bennett WP, Hussain SP, Vahakangas KH, et al. Molecular epidemiology of human cancer risk: gene-environment interactions and p53 mutation spectrum in human lung cancer. *J Pathol* 1999;187:8.

20. Zang EA, Wynder EL. Differences in lung cancer risk between men and women: examination of the evidence [see comments]. *J Natl Cancer Inst* 1996;88:183.

21. Ramalingam S, Pawlish K, Gadgeel S, et al. Lung cancer in young patients: analysis of a Surveillance, Epidemiology, and End Results database. *J Clin Oncol* 1998;16:651.

22. Jemal A, Travis WD, Tarone RE, et al. Lung cancer rates convergence in young men and women in the United States: analysis by birth cohort and histologic type. *Int J Cancer* 2003;105:101.

23. World Health Organization. *Histologic typing of lung tumors*, 2nd ed. Geneva: World Health Organization, 1981.

24. Hirsch FR, Matthews MJ, Aisner S, et al. Histopathologic classification of small cell lung cancer. Changing concepts and terminology. *Cancer* 1988;62:973.

25. Carter D, Eggleston JC. Tumors of the lower respiratory tract. In: *Atlas of tumor pathology, second series, fascicle* 17. Washington, DC: Armed Forces Institute of Pathology, 1980.

26. Travis WD, Linder J, Mackay B. Classification, histology, cytology, and electron microscopy. In: Pass HI, Mitchell JB, Johnson DH, et al. eds. *Lung cancer: principles and practice*. Philadelphia: Lippincott–Raven, 1996.

27. Aisner SC, Finkelstein DM, Ettinger DS, et al. The clinical significance of variant-morphology small-cell carcinoma of the lung. *J Clin Oncol* 1990;8:402.

28. Fraire AE, Johnson EH, Yesner R, et al. Prognostic significance of histopathologic subtype and stage in small cell lung cancer. *Hum Pathol* 1992;23:520.

29. Mangum MD, Greco FA, Hainsworth JD, et al. Combined small-cell and non-small-cell lung cancer. *J Clin Oncol* 1989;7:607.

30. Radice PA, Matthews MJ, Ihde DC, et al. The clinical behavior of "mixed" small cell/large cell bronchogenic carcinoma compared to "pure" small cell subtypes. *Cancer* 1982;50:2894.

31. Fushimi H, Kukui M, Morino H, et al. Detection of large cell component in small cell lung carcinoma by combined cytologic and histologic examinations and its clinical implication. *Cancer* 1992;70:599.

32. Bepler G, Neumann K, Holle R, et al. Clinical relevance of histologic subtyping in small cell lung cancer. *Cancer* 1989;64:74.

33. Guinee DG Jr, Fishback NF, Koss MN, et al. The spectrum of immunohistochemical staining of small-cell lung carcinoma in specimens from transbronchial and open-lung biopsies. *Am J Clin Pathol* 1994;102:406.

34. Higgins GA, Shields TW, Keehn RJ. The solitary pulmonary nodule. Ten-year follow-up of Veterans Administration-Armed Forces Cooperative Study. *Arch Surg* 1975;110:570.

35. Muhm JR, Miller WE, Fontana RS, et al. Lung cancer detected during a screening program using four-month chest radiographs. *Radiology* 1983;148:609.

36. Chute CG, Greenberg ER, Baron J, et al. Presenting conditions of 1539 population-based lung cancer patients by cell type and stage in New Hampshire and Vermont. *Cancer* 1985;56:2107.

37. Sculier JP, Evans WK, Feld R, et al. Superior vena caval obstruction syndrome in small cell lung cancer. *Cancer* 1986;57:847.

38. Paulson DL. Carcinomas in the superior pulmonary sulcus. *J Thorac Cardiovasc Surg* 1975;70:1095.

39. Johnson DH, Hainsworth JD, Greco FA. Pancoast's syndrome and small cell lung cancer. *Chest* 1982;82:602.

40. Levitan N, Byrne RE, Bromer RH, et al. The value of the bone scan and bone marrow biopsy staging small cell lung cancer. *Cancer* 1985;56:652.

41. Michel F, Soler M, Imhof E, et al. Initial staging of non-small cell lung cancer: value of routine radioisotope bone scanning. *Thorax* 1991;46:469.

42. Tritz DB, Doll DC, Ringenberg QS, et al. Bone marrow involvement in small cell lung cancer. Clinical significance and correlation with routine laboratory variables. *Cancer* 1989;63:763.

43. Souhami RL, Bradbury I, Geddes DM, et al. Prognostic significance of laboratory parameters measured at diagnosis in small cell carcinoma of the lung. *Cancer Res* 1985;45:2878.

44. Osterlind K, Andersen PK. Prognostic factors in small cell lung cancer: multivariate model based on 778 patients treated with chemotherapy with or without irradiation. *Cancer Res* 1986;46:4189.

45. Shepherd FA, Laskey J, Evans WK, et al. Cushing's syndrome associated with ectopic corticotropin production and small-cell lung cancer. *J Clin Oncol* 1992;10:21.

46. Dimopoulos MA, Fernandez JF, Samaan NA, et al Paraneoplastic Cushing's syndrome as an adverse prognostic factor in patients who die early with small cell lung cancer. *Cancer* 1992;69:66.

47. Dalmau J, Furneaux HM, Gralla RJ, et al. Detection of the anti-Hu antibody in the serum of patients with small cell lung cancer—a quantitative Western blot analysis. *Ann Neurol* 1990;27:544.

48. Patel AM, Jett JR. Clinical presentation and staging of lung cancer. In: Aisner J, Arriagada R, Green MR, et al. eds. *Comprehensive textbook of thoracic oncology*. Baltimore: Williams & Wilkins, 1996:293.

49. O'Neill JH, Murray NM, Newsom-Davis J. The Lambert-Eaton myasthenic syndrome. A review of 50 cases. *Brain* 1988;111:577.

50. Zelen M. Keynote address on biostatistics and data retrieval, part 3. *Cancer Chemother Rep* 1973;4:31.

51. Sagman U, Maki E, Evans WK, et al. Small-cell carcinoma of the lung: derivation of a prognostic staging system. *J Clin Oncol* 1991;9:1639.

52. Livingston RB, McCracken JD, Trauth CJ, et al. Isolated pleural effusion in small cell lung carcinoma: favorable prognosis. A review of the Southwest Oncology Group experience. *Chest* 1982;81:208.

53. Dearing MP, Steinberg SM, Phelps R, et al. Outcome of patients with small-cell lung cancer: effect of changes in staging procedures and imaging technology on prognostic factors over 14 years. *J Clin Oncol* 1990;8:1042.

54. Maestu I, Pastor M, Gomez-Codina J, et al. Pretreatment prognostic factors for survival in small-cell lung cancer: a new prognostic index and validation of three known prognostic indices on 341 patients. *Ann Oncol* 1997;8:547.

55. Stahel RA, Ginsberg RJ, Haddad K, et al. Staging and prognostic factors in small cell lung cancer: a consensus report. *Lung Cancer* 1989;5:119.

56. Albain KS, Crowley JJ, LeBlanc M, et al. Determinants of improved outcome in small-cell lung cancer: an analysis of the 2,580-patient Southwest Oncology Group data base. *J Clin Oncol* 1990;8:1563.

57. Chauvin F, Trillet V, Court-Fortune I, et al. Pretreatment staging evaluation in small cell lung carcinoma. A new approach to medical decision making. *Chest* 1992;102:497.

58. Shepherd FA, Ginsberg RJ, Haddad R, et al. Importance of clinical staging in limited small-cell lung cancer: a valuable system to separate prognostic subgroups. The University of Toronto Lung Oncology Group. *J Clin Oncol* 1993;11:1592.

59. Spiegelman D, Maurer LH, Ware JH, et al. Prognostic factors in small-cell carcinoma of the lung: an analysis of 1,521 patients. *J Clin Oncol* 1989;7:344.

60. Urban T, Chastang C, Vaylet F, et al. Prognostic significance of supraclavicular lymph nodes in small cell lung cancer: a study from four consecutive clinical trials, including 1,370 patients. "Petites Cellules" Group. *Chest* 1998;114:1538.

61. Turrisi AT 3rd, Kim K, Blum R, et al. Twice-daily compared with once-daily thoracic radiotherapy in limited small-cell lung cancer treated concurrently with cisplatin and etoposide. *N Engl J Med* 1999;340:265.

62. Bonner JA, Sloan JA, Shanahan TG, et al. Phase III comparison of twice-daily split-course irradiation versus once-daily irradiation for patients with limited stage small-cell lung carcinoma. *J Clin Oncol* 1999;17:2681.

63. Perry MC, Eaton WL, Propert KJ, et al. Chemotherapy with or without radiation therapy in limited small-cell carcinoma of the lung. *N Engl J Med* 1987;316:912.

64. Murray N, Coy P, Pater JL, et al. Importance of timing for thoracic irradiation in the combined modality treatment of limited-stage small-cell lung cancer. The National Cancer Institute of Canada Clinical Trials Group. *J Clin Oncol* 1993;11:336.

65. Kreisman H, Wolkove N, Quoix E. Small cell lung cancer presenting as a solitary pulmonary nodule. *Chest* 1992;101:225.

66. Karrer K, Ulsperger E. Surgery for cure followed by chemotherapy in small cell carcinoma of the lung. For the ISC-Lung Cancer Study Group. *Acta Oncol* 1995;34:899.

67. Micke P, Faldum A, Metz T, et al. Staging small cell lung cancer: Veterans Administration Lung Study Group versus International Association for the Study of Lung Cancer—what limits limited disease? *Lung Cancer* 2002;37:271.

68. Pignon JP, Arriagada R, Ihde DC, et al. A meta-analysis of thoracic radiotherapy for small-cell lung cancer [see comments]. *N Engl J Med* 1992;327:1618.

69. Wolf M, Holle R, Hans K, et al. Analysis of prognostic factors in 766 patients with small cell lung cancer (SCLC): the role of sex as a predictor for survival. *Br J Cancer* 1991;63:986.

70. Bremnes RM, Sundstrom S, Aasebo U, et al. The value of prognostic factors in small cell lung cancer: results from a randomized multicenter study with minimum 5 year follow-up. *Lung Cancer* 2003;39:303.

71. Rawson NS, Peto J. An overview of prognostic factors in small cell lung cancer. A report from the Subcommittee for the Management of Lung Cancer of the United Kingdom Coordinating Committee on Cancer Research. *Br J Cancer* 1990;61:597.

72. Gronowitz JS, Bergstrom R, Nou E, et al. Clinical and serologic markers of stage and prognosis in small cell lung cancer. A multivariate analysis. *Cancer* 1990;66:722.

73. Allan SG, Stewart ME, Love S, et al. Prognosis at presentation of small cell carcinoma of the lung. *Eur J Cancer* 1990;26:703.
74. Siu LL, Shepherd FA, Murray N, et al. Influence of age on the treatment of limited-stage small-cell lung cancer. *J Clin Oncol* 1996;14:821.
75. Yuen AR, Zou G, Turrisi AT, et al. Similar outcome of elderly patients in intergroup trial 0096: Cisplatin, etoposide, and thoracic radiotherapy administered once or twice daily in limited stage small cell lung carcinoma. *Cancer* 2000;89:1953.
76. Jorgensen LG, Osterlind K, Genolla J, et al. Serum neuron-specific enolase (S-NSE) and the prognosis in small-cell lung cancer (SCLC): a combined multivariable analysis on data from nine centres [published erratum appears in Br J Cancer 1996;74:2043]. *Br J Cancer* 1996;74:463.
77. Ludbrook JJ, Truong PT, MacNeil MV, et al. Do age and comorbidity impact treatment allocation and outcomes in limited stage small-cell lung cancer? A community-based population analysis. *Int J Radiat Oncol Biol Phys* 2003;55:1321.
78. Livingson RB, Moore TN, Heilbrun L, et al. Small-cell carcinoma of the lung: combined chemotherapy and radiaiton. A Southwest Oncology Group Study. *Ann Intern Med* 1978;88:194.
79. Christodoulou C, Pavlidis N, Samantas E, et al. Prognostic factors in Greek patients with small cell lung cancer (SCLC). A Hellenic Cooperative Oncology Group study. *Anticancer Res* 2002;22:3749.
80. Lassen U, Osterlind K, Hansen M, et al. Long-term survival in small-cell lung cancer: posttreatment characteristics in patients surviving 5 to 18+ years—an analysis of 1,714 consecutive patients. *J Clin Oncol* 1995;13:1215.
81. Kawahara M, Fukuoka M, Saijo N, et al. Prognostic factors and prognostic staging system for small cell lung cancer. *Jpn J Clin Oncol* 1997;27:158.
82. Videtic GM, Stitt LW, Dar AR, et al. Continued cigarette smoking by patients receiving concurrent chemoradiotherapy for limited-stage small-cell lung cancer is associated with decreased survival. *J Clin Oncol* 2003;21:1544.
83. Eerola AK, Soini Y, Paakko P. A high number of tumor-infiltrating lymphocytes are associated with a small tumor size, low tumor stage, and a favorable prognosis in operated small cell lung carcinoma. *Clin Cancer Res* 2000;6:1875.
84. Studnicka M, Wirnsberger R, Neumann M, et al. Peripheral blood lymphocyte subsets and survival in small-cell lung cancer. *Chest* 1994;105:1673.
85. Nakamura H, Saji H, Ogata A, et al. Immunologic parameters as significant prognostic factors in lung cancer. *Lung Cancer* 2002;37:161.
86. Pujol JL, Quantin X, Jacot W, et al. Neuroendocrine and cytokeratin serum markers as prognostic determinants of small cell lung cancer. *Lung Cancer* 2003;39:131.
87. Drivsholm L, Paloheimo LI, Osterlind K. Chromogranin A, a significant prognostic factor in small cell lung cancer. *Br J Cancer* 1999;81:667.
88. Shingyoji M, Takiguchi Y, Watanabe R, et al. Detection of tumor specific gene expression in bone marrow and peripheral blood from patients with small cell lung carcinoma. *Cancer* 2003;97:1057.
89. Anttonen A, Leppa S, Ruotsalainen T, et al. Pretreatment serum syndecan-1 levels and outcome in small cell lung cancer patients treated with platinum-based chemotherapy. *Lung Cancer* 2003;41:171.
90. Fontanini G, Faviana P, Lucchi M, et al. A high vascular count and overexpression of vascular endothelial growth factor are associated with unfavorable prognosis in operated small cell lung carcinoma. *Br J Cancer* 2002;86:558.
91. Lucchi M, Mussi A, Fontanini G, et al. Small cell lung carcinoma (SCLC): the angiogenic phenomenon. *Eur J Cardiothorac Surg* 2002;21:1105.
92. Dowell J, Amirkhan R, Lai W, et al. Survival in small cell lung cancer (SCLC) is independent of vascular endothelial growth factor (VEGF) and cyclooxygenase (COX2) expression. *Proc Am Soc Clin Oncol* 2003;22:632.
93. Dingemans AM, Witlox MA, Stallaert RA, et al. Expression of DNA topoisomerase IIalpha and topoisomerase IIbeta genes predicts survival and response to chemotherapy in patients with small cell lung cancer. *Clin Cancer Res* 1999;5:2048.
94. Hsia TC, Lin CC, Wang JJ, et al. Relationship between chemotherapy response of small cell lung cancer and P-glycoprotein or multidrug resistance-related protein expression. *Lung* 2002;180:173.
95. Kao A, Shiun SC, Hsu NY, et al. Technetium-99m methoxyisobutylisonitrile chest imaging for small-cell lung cancer. Relationship to chemotherapy response (six courses of combination of cisplatin and etoposide) and p-glycoprotein or multidrug resistance related protein expression. *Ann Oncol* 2001;12:1561.
96. Radford JA, Ryder WDJ, Dodwell D, et al. Predicting septic complications from chemotherapy: an analysis of 382 patients treated for small cell lung cancer without dose reduction after major sepsis. *Eur J Cancer* 1993;29A:81.
97. Morittu L, Earl HM, Souhami RL, et al. Patients at risk of chemotherapy-associated toxicity in small cell lung cancer. *Br J Cancer* 1989;59:801.
98. Lassen UN, Osterlind K, Hirsch FR, et al. Early death during chemotherapy in patients with small-cell lung cancer: derivation of a prognostic index for toxic death and progression. *Br J Cancer* 1999;79:515.
99. Richardson GE, Venzon DJ, Edison M, et al. Application of an algorithm for staging small-cell lung cancer can save one third of the initial evaluation costs. *Arch Intern Med* 1993;153:329.
100. Byhardt RW, Hartz A, Libnoch JA, et al. Prognostic influence of TNM staging and LDH levels in small cell carcinoma of the lung (SCCL). *Int J Radiat Oncol Biol Phys* 1986;12:771.
101. Sagman U, Feld R, Evans WK, et al. The prognostic significance of pretreatment serum lactate dehydrogenase in patients with small-cell lung cancer. *J Clin Oncol* 1991;9:954.
102. Stokkel MP, van Eck-Smit BL, Zwinderman AH, et al. Pretreatment serum lactate dehydrogenase as additional staging parameter in patients with small-cell lung carcinoma. *J Cancer Res Clin Oncol* 1998;124:215.
103. Whitley NO, Fuks JZ, McCrea ES, et al. Computed tomography of the chest in small cell lung cancer: potential new prognostic signs. *AJR Am J Roentgenol* 1984;142:885.
104. Ihde DC, Dunnick NR, Johnston-Early A, et al. Abdominal computed tomography in small cell lung cancer: assessment of extent of disease and response to therapy. *Cancer* 1982;49:1485.
105. Norlund JD, Byhardt RW, Foley WD, et al. Computed tomography in the staging of small cell lung cancer: implications for combined modality therapy. *Int J Radiat Oncol Biol Phys* 1985;11:1081.
106. Schwartz LH, Ginsberg MS, Burt ME, et al. MRI as an alternative to CT-guided biopsy of adrenal masses in patients with lung cancer. *Ann Thorac Surg* 1998;65:193.
107. Giannone L, Johnson DH, Hande KR, et al. Favorable prognosis of brain metastases in small cell lung cancer. *Ann Intern Med* 1987;106:386.
108. van Oosterhout AG, van de Pol M, ten Velde GP, et al. Neurologic disorders in 203 consecutive patients with small cell lung cancer. Results of a longitudinal study. *Cancer* 1996;77:1434.
109. Hardy J, Smith I, Cherryman G, et al. The value of computed tomographic (CT) scan surveillance in the detection and management of brain metastases in patients with small cell lung cancer. *Br J Cancer* 1990;62:684.
110. Kristensen CA, Kristjansen PE, Hansen HH. Systemic chemotherapy of brain metastases from small-cell lung cancer: a review. *J Clin Oncol* 1992;10:1498.
111. Kochhar R, Frytak S, Shaw EG. Survival of patients with extensive small-cell lung cancer who have only brain metastases at initial diagnosis. *Am J Clin Oncol* 1997;20:125.
112. Levenson RM Jr, Sauerbrunn BJ, Ihde DC, et al. Small cell lung cancer: radionuclide bone scans for assessment of tumor extent and response. *AJR Am J Roentgenol* 1981;137:31.
113. Bezwoda WR, Lewis D, Livini N. Bone marrow involvement in anaplastic small cell lung cancer. Diagnosis, hematologic features, and prognostic implications. *Cancer* 1986;58:1762.
114. Trillet-Lenoir VN, Arpin D, Brune J. Bone marrow metastases detection in small cell lung cancer. A review. *Anticancer Res* 1994;14:2795.
115. Canon JL, Humblet Y, Lebacq-Verheyden AM, et al. Immunodetection of small cell lung cancer metastases in bone marrow using three monoclonal antibodies. *Eur J Cancer Clin Oncol* 1988;24:147.
116. Campling B, Quirt I, DeBoer G, et al. Is bone marrow examination in small-cell lung cancer really necessary? *Ann Intern Med* 1986;105:508.
117. Hamrick RMD, Murgo AJ. Lactate dehydrogenase values and bone scans as predictors of bone marrow involvement in small-cell lung cancer. *Arch Intern Med* 1987;147:1070.
118. Seto T, Imamura F, Kuriyama K, et al. Effect on prognosis of bone marrow infiltration detected by magnetic resonance imaging in small cell lung cancer. *Eur J Cancer* 1997;33:2333.
119. Layer G, Steudel A, Schuller H, et al. Magnetic resonance imaging to detect bone marrow metastases in the initial staging of small cell lung carcinoma and breast carcinoma. *Cancer* 1999;85:1004.
120. Peck K, Sher YP, Shih JY, et al. Detection and quantitation of circulating cancer cells in the peripheral blood of lung cancer patients. *Cancer Res* 1998;58:2761.
121. Chin R Jr, McCain TW, Miller AA, et al. Whole body FDG-PET for the evaluation and staging of small cell lung cancer: a preliminary study. *Lung Cancer* 2002;37:1.
122. Pandit N, Gonen M, Krug L, et al. Prognostic value of [(18)F]FDG-PET imaging in small cell lung cancer. *Eur J Nucl Med Mol Imaging* 2003;30:78.
123. Schirrmeister H, Guhlmann A, Elsner K, et al. Sensitivity in detecting osseous lesions depends on anatomic localization: planar bone scintigraphy versus 18F PET. *J Nucl Med* 1999;40:1623.
124. Bury T, Barreto A, Daenen F, et al. Fluorine-18 deoxyglucose positron emission tomography for the detection of bone metastases in patients with non-small cell lung cancer. *Eur J Nucl Med* 1998;25:1244.
125. Vansteenkiste JF, Stroobants SG, Dupont PJ, et al. Prognostic importance of the standardized uptake value on (18)F-fluoro-2-deoxy-glucose-positron emission tomography scan in non-small-cell lung cancer: an analysis of 125 cases. Leuven Lung Cancer Group. *J Clin Oncol* 1999;17:3201.
126. Kamel EM, Zwahlen D, Wyss MT, et al. Whole-body (18)F-FDG PET improves the management of patients with small cell lung cancer. *J Nucl Med* 2003;44:1911.
127. Balaban EP, Walker BS, Cox JV, et al. Detection and staging of small cell lung carcinoma with a technetium-labeled monoclonal antibody. A comparison with standard staging methods. *Clin Nucl Med* 1992;17:439.
128. Reisinger I, Bohuslavitzki KH, Brenner W, et al. Somatostatin receptor scintigraphy in small-cell lung cancer: results of a multicenter study [see comments]. *J Nucl Med* 1998;39:224.
129. Fox W, Scadding JG. Medical Research Council comparative trial of surgery and radiotherapy for primary treatment of small-celled or oat-celled carcinoma of bronchus. Ten-year follow-up. *Lancet* 1973;2:63.
130. Mountain CF. Clinical biology of small cell lung carcinoma: relationship to surgical therapy. *Semin Oncol* 1978;5:272.
131. Green RA, Humphrey E, Close H. Alkylating agents in bronchogenic carcinoma. *Am J Med* 1969;46:516.
132. Radiotherapy alone or with chemotherapy in the treatment of small-cell carcinoma of the lung: the results at 36 months. 2nd report to the Medical Research Council on the 2nd small-cell study. *Br J Cancer* 1979;40:1.
133. Bork E, Ersboll J, Dombernowsky P, et al. Teniposide and etoposide in previously untreated small cell lung cancer: a randomized study. *J Clin Oncol* 1991;9:1627.
134. Clark PI, Slevin ML, Joel SP, et al. A randomized trial of two etoposide schedules in small-cell lung cancer: the influence of pharmacokinetics on efficacy and toxicity. *J Clin Oncol* 1994;12:1427.
135. Wolff SN, Birch R, Sarma P, et al. Randomized dose-response evaluation of etoposide in small cell carcinoma of the lung: a Southeastern Cancer Study Group Trial. *Cancer Treat Rep* 1986;70:583.
136. Hansen HH, Dombernowsky P, Hansen M, et al. Teniposide in the treatment of small cell lung cancer: a review. *Semin Oncol* 1992;19:65.
137. Ettinger DS, Finkelstein DM, Ritch PS, et al. Study of either ifosfamide or teniposide compared to a standard chemotherapy for extensive disease small cell lung cancer: an Eastern Cooperative Oncology Group randomized study (E1588). *Lung Cancer* 2002;37:311.
138. Moore TD, Korn EL. Phase II trial design considerations for small-cell lung cancer. *J Natl Cancer Inst* 1992;84:150.

139. Giaccone G, Ferrati P, Donadio M, et al. Reinduction chemotherapy in small cell lung cancer. *Eur J Cancer Clin Oncol* 1987;23:1697.
140. Lowenbraun S, Bartolucci A, Smalley RV, et al. The superiority of combination chemotherapy over single agent chemotherapy in small cell lung carcinoma. *Cancer* 1979;44:406.
141. Hansen HH, Dombernowsky P, Hansen M, et al. Chemotherapy of advanced small-cell anaplastic carcinoma. Superiority of a four-drug combination to a three-drug combination. *Ann Intern Med* 1978;89:177.
142. Hong WK, Nicaise C, Lawson R, et al. Etoposide combined with cyclophosphamide plus vincristine compared with doxorubicin plus cyclophosphamide plus vincristine and with high-dose cyclophosphamide plus vincristine in the treatment of small-cell carcinoma of the lung: a randomized trial of the Bristol Lung Cancer Study Group. *J Clin Oncol* 1989;7:450.
143. Hirsch FR, Hansen HH, Hansen M, et al. The superiority of combination chemotherapy including etoposide based on in vivo cell cycle analysis in the treatment of extensive small-cell lung cancer: a randomized trial of 288 consecutive patients. *J Clin Oncol* 1987;5:585.
144. Vindelov LL, Hansen HH, Gersel A, et al. Treatment of small-cell carcinoma of the lung monitored by sequential flow cytometric DNA analysis. *Cancer Res* 1982;42:2499.
145. Jackson DV Jr, Zekan PJ, Caldwell RD, et al. VP-16-213 in combination chemotherapy with chest irradiation for small-cell lung cancer: a randomized trial of the Piedmont Oncology Association. *J Clin Oncol* 1984;2:1343.
146. Jackson DV Jr, Case LD, Zekan PJ, et al. Improvement of long-term survival in extensive small-cell lung cancer. *J Clin Oncol* 1988;6:1161.
147. Jett JR, Everson L, Therneau TM, et al. Treatment of limited-stage small-cell lung cancer with cyclophosphamide, doxorubicin, and vincristine with or without etoposide: a randomized trial of the North Central Cancer Treatment Group. *J Clin Oncol* 1990;8:33.
148. Messeih AA, Schweitzer JM, Lipton A, et al. Addition of etoposide to cyclophosphamide, doxorubicin, and vincristine for remission induction and survival in patients with small cell lung cancer. *Cancer Treat Rep* 1987;71:61.
149. Lowenbraun S, Birch R, Buchanan R, et al. Combination chemotherapy in small cell lung carcinoma. A randomized study of two intensive regimens. *Cancer* 1984;54:2344.
150. Evans WK, Osoba D, Feld R, et al. Etoposide (VP-16) and cisplatin: an effective treatment for relapse in small-cell lung cancer. *J Clin Oncol* 1985;3:65.
151. Evans WK, Shepherd FA, Feld R, et al. VP-16 and cisplatin as first-line therapy for small-cell lung cancer. *J Clin Oncol* 1985;3:1471.
152. Einhorn LH, Crawford J, Birch R, et al. Cisplatin plus etoposide consolidation following cyclophosphamide, doxorubicin, and vincristine in limited small-cell lung cancer. *J Clin Oncol* 1988;6:451.
153. Roth BJ, Johnson DH, Einhorn LH, et al. Randomized study of cyclophosphamide, doxorubicin, and vincristine versus etoposide and cisplatin versus alternation of these two regimens in extensive small-cell lung cancer: a phase III trial of the Southeastern Cancer Study Group. *J Clin Oncol* 1992;10:282.
154. Fukuoka M, Furuse K, Saijo N, et al. Randomized trial of cyclophosphamide, doxorubicin, and vincristine versus cisplatin and etoposide versus alternation of these regimens in small-cell lung cancer. *J Natl Cancer Inst* 1991;83:855.
155. Sundstrom S, Bremnes RM, Kaasa S, et al. Cisplatin and etoposide regimen is superior to cyclophosphamide, epirubicin, and vincristine regimen in small-cell lung cancer: results from a randomized phase III trial with 5 years follow-up. *J Clin Oncol* 2002;20:4665.
156. Chute JP, Venzon DJ, Hankins L, et al. Outcome of patients with small-cell lung cancer during 20 years of clinical research at the US National Cancer Institute. *Mayo Clin Proc* 1997;72:901.
157. Mascaux C, Paesmans M, Berghmans T, et al. A systematic review of the role of etoposide and cisplatin in the chemotherapy of small cell lung cancer with methodology assessment and meta-analysis. *Lung Cancer* 2000;30:23.
158. Pujol JL, Carestia L, Daures JP. Is there a case for cisplatin in the treatment of small-cell lung cancer? A meta-analysis of randomized trials of a cisplatin-containing regimen versus a regimen without this alkylating agent. *Br J Cancer* 2000;83:8.
159. Skarlos DV, Samantas E, Kosmidis P, et al. Randomized comparison of etoposide-cisplatin vs. etoposide-carboplatin and irradiation in small-cell lung cancer. A Hellenic Co-operative Oncology Group study. *Ann Oncol* 1994;5:601.
160. Lassen U, Kristjansen PE, Osterlind K, et al. Superiority of cisplatin or carboplatin in combination with teniposide and vincristine in the induction chemotherapy of small-cell lung cancer. A randomized trial with 5 years follow up. *Ann Oncol* 1996;7:365.
161. Bishop JF, Raghavan D, Stuart-Harris R, et al. Carboplatin (CBDCA, JM-8) and VP-16-213 in previously untreated patients with small-cell lung cancer. *J Clin Oncol* 1987;5:1574
162. Mavroudis D, Papadakis E, Veslemes M, et al. A multicenter randomized clinical trial comparing paclitaxel-cisplatin-etoposide versus cisplatin-etoposide as first-line treatment in patients with small-cell lung cancer. *Ann Oncol* 2001;12:463.
163. Niell H, Herndon J, Miller A, et al. Randomized phase III intergroup trial (CALGB 9732) of etoposide (VP-16) and cisplatin (DDP) with or without paclitaxel (TAX) and G-CSF in patients with extensive stage small cell lung cancer (ED-SCLC). *Proc Am Soc Clin Oncol* 2002;21:293a.
164. Neill HB, Miller AA, Clamon GH, et al. A phase II study evaluating the efficacy of carboplatin, etoposide, and paclitaxel with granulocyte colony-stimulating factor in patients with stage IIIB and IV non-small cell lung cancer and extensive small cell lung cancer. *Semin Oncol* 1997;24:S12-130.
165. Reck M, von Pawel J, Macha HN, et al. Randomized phase III trial of paclitaxel, etoposide, and carboplatin versus carboplatin, etoposide, and vincristine in patients with small-cell lung cancer. *J Natl Cancer Inst* 2003;95:1118.
166. Loehrer PJ Sr, Rynard S, Ansari R, et al. Etoposide, ifosfamide, and cisplatin in extensive small cell lung cancer. *Cancer* 1992;69:669.
167. Loehrer PJ Sr, Ansari R, Gonin R, et al. Cisplatin plus etoposide with and without ifosfamide in extensive small-cell lung cancer: a Hoosier Oncology Group study. *J Clin Oncol* 1995;13:2594.
168. Thatcher N, Lind M, Stout R, et al. Carboplatin, ifosfamide and etoposide with mid-course vincristine and thoracic radiotherapy for 'limited' stage small cell carcinoma of the bronchus. *Br J Cancer* 1989;60:98.
169. Wolff AC, Ettinger DS, Neuberg D, et al. Phase II study of ifosfamide, carboplatin, and oral etoposide chemotherapy for extensive-disease small-cell lung cancer: an Eastern Cooperative Oncology Group pilot study. *J Clin Oncol* 1995;13:1615.
170. Thatcher N, Quian W, Girling D. Ifosfamide, carboplatin and etoposide with mid-cycle vincristine (ICE-V) versus standard chemotherapy (C) in patients with small cell lung cancer (SCLC) and good performance status (PS): results of an MRC randomized trial (LU21). *Proc Am Soc Clin Oncol* 2003;22:619.
171. Ardizzoni A, Manegold C, Debruyne C, et al. European Organization for Research and Treatment of Cancer (EORTC) 08957 phase II study of topotecan in combination with cisplatin as second-line treatment of refractory and sensitive small cell lung cancer. *Clin Cancer Res* 2003;9:143.
172. Kudoh S, Fujiwara Y, Takada Y, et al. Phase II study of irinotecan combined with cisplatin in patients with previously untreated small-cell lung cancer. West Japan Lung Cancer Group. *J Clin Oncol* 1998;16:1068.
173. Noda K, Nishiwaki Y, Kawahara M, et al. Irinotecan plus cisplatin compared with etoposide plus cisplatin for extensive small-cell lung cancer. *N Engl J Med* 2002;346:85.
174. Feld R, Evans WK, DeBoer G, et al. Combined modality induction therapy without maintenance chemotherapy for small cell carcinoma of the lung. *J Clin Oncol* 1984;2:294.
175. Maurer LH, Tulloh M, Weiss RB, et al. A randomized combined modality trial in small cell carcinoma of the lung: comparison of combination chemotherapy-radiation therapy versus cyclophosphamide-radiation therapy effects of maintenance chemotherapy and prophylactive whole brain irradiation. *Cancer* 1980;45:30.
176. Cullen M, Morgan D, Gregory W, et al. Maintenance chemotherapy for anaplastic small cell carcinoma of the bronchus: a randomized, controlled trial. *Cancer Chemother Pharmacol* 1986;17:157.
177. Byrne MJ, van Hazel G, Trotter J, et al. Maintenance chemotherapy in limited small cell lung cancer: a randomized controlled clinical trial. *Br J Cancer* 1989;60:413.
178. Controlled trial of twelve versus six courses of chemotherapy in the treatment of small-cell lung cancer. Report to the Medical Research Council by its Lung Cancer Working Party. *Br J Cancer* 1989;59:584.
179. Ettinger DS, Finkelstein DM, Abeloff MD, et al. A randomized comparison of standard chemotherapy versus alternating chemotherapy and maintenance versus no maintenance therapy for extensive-stage small-cell lung cancer: a phase III study of the Eastern Cooperative Oncology Group. *J Clin Oncol* 1990;8:230.
180. Lebeau B, Chastang C, Allard P, et al. Six vs. twelve cycles for complete responders to chemotherapy in small cell lung cancer: definitive results of a randomized clinical trial. The "Petites Cellules" Group. *Eur Respir J* 1992;5:286.
181. Giaccone G, Dalesio O, McVie GJ, et al. Maintenance chemotherapy in small-cell lung cancer: long-term results of a randomized trial. European Organization for Research and Treatment of Cancer Lung Cancer Cooperative Group. *J Clin Oncol* 1993;11:1230.
182. Beith JM, Clarke SJ, Woods RL, et al. Long-term follow-up of a randomized trial of combined chemoradiotherapy induction treatment, with and without maintenance chemotherapy in patients with small cell carcinoma of the lung. *Eur J Cancer* 1996;32A:438.
183. Sculier JP, Paesmans M, Bureau G, et al. Randomized trial comparing induction chemotherapy versus induction chemotherapy followed by maintenance chemotherapy in small-cell lung cancer. European Lung Cancer Working Party. *J Clin Oncol* 1996;14:2337.
184. Schiller JH, Adak S, Cella D, et al. Topotecan versus observation after cisplatin plus etoposide in extensive-stage small-cell lung cancer: E7593—a phase III trial of the Eastern Cooperative Oncology Group. *J Clin Oncol* 2001;19:2114.
185. Bleehen NM, Girling DJ, Machin D, et al. A randomized trial of three or six courses of etoposide cyclophosphamide methotrexate and vincristine or six courses of etoposide and ifosfamide in small cell lung cancer (SCLC). II: Quality of life. Medical Research Council Lung Cancer Working Party. *Br J Cancer* 1993;68:1157.
186. Bleehen NM, Girling DJ, Machin D, et al. A randomized trial of three or six courses of etoposide cyclophosphamide methotrexate and vincristine or six courses of etoposide and ifosfamide in small cell lung cancer (SCLC). I: Survival and prognostic factors. Medical Research Council Lung Cancer Working Party. *Br J Cancer* 1993;68:1150.
187. Spiro SG, Souhami RL, Geddes DM, et al. Duration of chemotherapy in small cell lung cancer: a Cancer Research Campaign trial. *Br J Cancer* 1989;59:578.
188. Ajaikumar BS, Barkley HT Jr. The role of radiation therapy in the treatment of small cell undifferentiated bronchogenic cancer. *Int J Radiat Oncol Biol Phys* 1979;5:977.
189. Roof KS, Fidias P, Lynch TJ, et al. Radiation dose escalation in limited-stage small-cell lung cancer. *Int J Radiat Oncol Biol Phys* 2003;57:701.
190. Auperin A, Arriagada R, Pignon JP, et al. Prophylactic cranial irradiation for patients with small-cell lung cancer in complete remission. Prophylactic Cranial Irradiation Overview Collaborative Group [see comments]. *N Engl J Med* 1999;341:476.
191. Pignon JP, Arriagada R. Role of thoracic radiotherapy in limited-stage small-cell lung cancer: quantitative review based on the literature versus meta-analysis based on individual data [letter; comment]. *J Clin Oncol* 1992;10:1819.
192. Bunn PA Jr, Lichter AS, Makuch RW, et al. Chemotherapy alone or chemotherapy with chest radiation therapy in limited stage small cell lung cancer. A prospective, randomized trial. *Ann Intern Med* 1987;106:655.
193. Perez CA, Einhorn L, Oldham RK, et al. Randomized trial of radiotherapy to the thorax in limited small-cell carcinoma of the lung treated with multiagent chemotherapy and elective brain irradiation: a preliminary report. *J Clin Oncol* 1984;2:1200.
194. Fox RM, Woods RL, Tattersall MH, et al. A randomized study of adjuvant immunotherapy with levamisole and Corynebacterium parvum in operable non-small cell lung cancer. *Int J Radiat Oncol Biol Phys* 1980;6:1043.
195. Rosenthal S, Tattersa MHN, Fox RM, et al. Adjuvant thoracic radiotherapy in small cell lung cancer: ten-year follow-up of a randomized study. *Lung Cancer* 1991;7:235.
196. Warde P, Payne D. Does thoracic irradiation improve survival and local control in limited-stage small-cell carcinoma of the lung? A meta-analysis [see comments]. *J Clin Oncol* 1992;10:890.

197. Cox JD, Byhardt R, Komaki R, et al. Interaction of thoracic irradiation and chemotherapy on local control and survival in small cell carcinoma of the lung. *Cancer Treat Rep* 1979;63:1251.
198. Williams C, Alexander M, Glatstein EJ, et al. Role of radiation therapy in combination with chemotherapy in extensive oat cell cancer of the lung: a randomized study. *Cancer Treat Rep* 1977;61:1427.
199. Choi NC, Carey RW. Importance of radiation dose in achieving improved loco-regional tumor control in limited stage small-cell lung carcinoma: an update. *Int J Radiat Oncol Biol Phys* 1989;17:307.
200. Coy P, Hodson I, Payne DG, et al. The effect of dose of thoracic irradiation on recurrence in patients with limited stage small cell lung cancer. Initial results of a Canadian Multicenter Randomized Trial. *Int J Radiat Oncol Biol Phys* 1988;14:219.
201. Arriagada R, Kramar A, Le Chevalier T, et al. Competing events determining relapse-free survival in limited small-cell lung carcinoma. The French Cancer Centers' Lung Group. *J Clin Oncol* 1992;10:447.
202. Papac RJ, Son Y, Bien R, et al. Improved local control of thoracic disease in small cell lung cancer with higher dose thoracic irradiation and cyclic chemotherapy [published erratum appears in Int J Radiat Oncol Biol Phys 1988;14:213]. *Int J Radiat Oncol Biol Phys* 1987;13:993.
203. Lichter AS, Bunn PA Jr, Ihde DC, et al. The role of radiation therapy in the treatment of small cell lung cancer. *Cancer* 1985;55:2163.
204. Takada M, Fukuoka M, Kawahara M, et al. Phase III study of concurrent versus sequential thoracic radiotherapy in combination with cisplatin and etoposide for limited-stage small-cell lung cancer: results of the Japan Clinical Oncology Group Study 9104. *J Clin Oncol* 2002;20:3054.
205. Brooks BJ Jr, Seifter EJ, Walsh TE, et al. Pulmonary toxicity with combined modality therapy for limited stage small-cell lung cancer. *J Clin Oncol* 1986;4:200.
206. Osterlind K, Hansen HH, Hansen HS, et al. Chemotherapy versus chemotherapy plus irradiation in limited small cell lung cancer. Results of a controlled trial with 5 years follow-up. *Br J Cancer* 1986;54:7.
207. Roach M 3rd, Gandara DR, Yuo HS, et al. Radiation pneumonitis following combined modality therapy for lung cancer: analysis of prognostic factors [see comments]. *J Clin Oncol* 1995;13:2606.
208. McCracken JD, Janaki LM, Crowley JJ, et al. Concurrent chemotherapy/radiotherapy for limited small-cell lung carcinoma: a Southwest Oncology Group Study. *J Clin Oncol* 1990;8:892.
209. Carney DN, Mitchell JB, Kinsella TJ. In vitro radiation and chemotherapy sensitivity of established cell lines of human small cell lung cancer and its large cell morphological variants. *Cancer Res* 1983;43:2806.
210. Turrisi AT 3rd, Glover DJ. Thoracic radiotherapy variables: influence on local control in small cell lung cancer limited disease. *Int J Radiat Oncol Biol Phys* 1990;19:1473.
211. Turrisi AT 3rd, Glover DJ, Mason BA. A preliminary report: concurrent twice-daily radiotherapy plus platinum-etoposide chemotherapy for limited small cell lung cancer. *Int J Radiat Oncol Biol Phys* 1988;15:183.
212. Ihde DC, Grayson J, Woods E, et al. Twice daily chest irradiation an adjuvant to etoposide/cisplatin therapy of limited stage small cell lung cancer. In: Salmon S, ed. *Adjuvant therapy of cancer,* 6th ed. Philadelphia: WB Saunders, 1990.
213. Schild S, Brindle J, Geyer S, et al. Long term results of a phase III trial comparing once a day radiotherapy (QD RT) or twice a day radiotherapy (BID RT) in limited stage small cell lung cancer. *Proc Am Soc Clin Oncol* 2003;22:631.
214. Komaki R, Cox JD, Whitson W. Risk of brain metastasis from small cell carcinoma of the lung related to length of survival and prophylactic irradiation. *Cancer Treat Rep* 1981;65:811.
215. Nugent JL, Bunn PA Jr, Matthews MJ, et al. CNS metastases in small cell bronchogenic carcinoma: increasing frequency and changing pattern with lengthening survival. *Cancer* 1979;44:1885.
216. Rosen ST, Makuch RW, Lichter AS, et al. Role of prophylactic cranial irradiation in prevention of central nervous system metastases in small cell lung cancer. Potential benefit restricted to patients with complete response. *Am J Med* 1983;74:615.
217. Hirsch FR, Paulson OB, Hansen HH, et al. Intracranial metastases in small cell carcinoma of the lung: correlation of clinical and autopsy findings. *Cancer* 1982;50:2433.
218. Glantz MJ, Choy H, Yee L. Prophylactic cranial irradiation in small cell lung cancer: rationale, results, and recommendations. *Semin Oncol* 1997;24:477.
219. Einhorn L. The case against prophylactic cranial irradiation in limited small cell lung cancer. *Semin Radiat Oncol* 1995;5:57.
220. Hansen HH, Dombernowsky P, Hirsch FR, et al. Prophylactic irradiation in bronchogenic small cell anaplastic carcinoma. A comparative trial of localized versus extensive radiotherapy including prophylactic brain irradiation in patients receiving combination chemotherapy. *Cancer* 1980;46:279.
221. Cox JD, Petrovich Z, Paig C, et al. Prophylactic cranial irradiation in patients with inoperable carcinoma of the lung: preliminary report of a cooperative trial. *Cancer* 1978;42:1135.
222. Seydel HG, Creech R, Pagano M, et al. Prophylactic versus no brain irradiation in regional small cell lung carcinoma. *Am J Clin Oncol* 1985;8:218.
223. Kristjansen PE, Hansen HH. Prophylactic cranial irradiation in small cell lung cancer—an update. *Lung Cancer* 1995;[12 Suppl 3]:S23.
224. Arriagada R, Le Chevalier T, Borie F, et al. Prophylactic cranial irradiation for patients with small-cell lung cancer in complete remission. *J Natl Cancer Inst* 1995;87:183.
225. Gregor A, Cull A, Stephens RJ, et al. Prophylactic cranial irradiation is indicated following complete response to induction therapy in small cell lung cancer: results of a multicentre randomized trial. United Kingdom Coordinating Committee for Cancer Research (UKCCCR) and the European Organization for Research and Treatment of Cancer (EORTC) [see comments]. *Eur J Cancer* 1997;33:1752.
226. Meyers CA, Byrne KS, Komaki R. Cognitive deficits in patients with small cell lung cancer before and after chemotherapy. *Lung Cancer* 1995;12:231.
227. Fleck JF, Einhorn LH, Lauer RC, et al. Is prophylactic cranial irradiation indicated in small-cell lung cancer? *J Clin Oncol* 1990;8:209.
228. Johnson BE, Becker B, Goff WB 2nd, et al. Neurologic, neuropsychologic, and computed cranial tomography scan abnormalities in 2- to 10-year survivors of small-cell lung cancer. *J Clin Oncol* 1985;3:1659.
229. Laukkanen E, Klonoff H, Allan B, et al. The role of prophylactic brain irradiation in limited stage small cell lung cancer: clinical, neuropsychologic, and CT sequelae. *Int J Radiat Oncol Biol Phys* 1988;14:1109.
230. Lee JS, Umsawasdi T, Lee YY, et al. Neurotoxicity in long-term survivors of small cell lung cancer. *Int J Radiat Oncol Biol Phys* 1986;12:313.
231. Johnson BE, Patronas N, Hayes W, et al. Neurologic, computed cranial tomographic, and magnetic resonance imaging abnormalities in patients with small-cell lung cancer: further follow-up of 6- to 13-year survivors. *J Clin Oncol* 1990;8:48.
232. Turrisi AT. Brain irradiation and systemic chemotherapy for small-cell lung cancer: dangerous liaisons? [see comments]. *J Clin Oncol* 1990;8:196.
233. Shields TW, Higgins GA Jr, Matthews MJ, et al Surgical resection in the management of small cell carcinoma of the lung. *J Thorac Cardiovasc Surg* 1982;84:481.
234. Meyer JA. Indications for surgical treatment in small cell carcinoma of the lung. *Surg Clin North Am* 1987;67:1103.
235. Mountain CF. Revisions in the International System for Staging Lung Cancer. *Chest* 1997;111:1710.
236. Shepherd FA, Evans WK, Feld R, et al. Adjuvant chemotherapy followed by surgical resection for small cell carcinoma of the lung. *J Clin Oncol* 1988;6:832.
237. Angeletti CA, Macchiarini P, Mussi A, et al. Influence of T and N stages on long-term survival in resectable small cell lung cancer. *Eur J Surg Oncol* 1989;15:337.
238. Shepherd FA, Ginsberg RJ, Patterson GA, et al. A prospective study of adjuvant surgical resection after chemotherapy for limited small cell lung cancer. A University of Toronto Lung Oncology Group study. *J Thorac Cardiovasc Surg* 1989;97:177.
239. Williams CJ, McMillan I, Lea R, et al. Surgery after initial chemotherapy for localized small-cell carcinoma of the lung. *J Clin Oncol* 1987;5:1579.
240. Johnson DH, Einhorn LH, Mandelbaum I, et al. Postchemotherapy resection of residual tumor in limited stage small cell lung cancer. *Chest* 1987;92:241.
241. Gazdar AF, Linnoila RI. The pathology of lung cancer—changing concepts and newer diagnostic techniques. *Semin Oncol* 1988;15:215.
242. Carney DN, Gazdar AF, Bepler G, et al. Establishment and identification of small cell lung cancer cell lines having classic and variant features. *Cancer Res* 1985;45:2913.
243. Sridhar KS, Hussein AM, Thurer RJ. Evolving role of surgical treatment in limited-disease small cell lung carcinoma. *J Surg Oncol* 1989;40:155.
244. Baker RR, Ettinger DS, Ruckdeschel JD, et al. The role of surgery in the management of selected patients with small-cell carcinoma of the lung. *J Clin Oncol* 1987;5:697.
245. Hara N, Ohta M, Ichinose Y, et al. Influence of surgical resection before and after chemotherapy on survival in small cell lung cancer. *J Surg Oncol* 1991;47:53.
246. Prasad US, Naylor AR, Walker WS, et al. Long term survival after pulmonary resection for small cell carcinoma of the lung [see comments]. *Thorax* 1989;44:784.
247. Higgins GA, Shields TW. Experience of the Veterans Administration Surgical Adjuvant Group. In: Muggia FM, Rozencweig M, eds. *Lung cancer: progress in therapeutic research.* New York: Raven, 1979:433.
248. Karrer K, Pridun N, Denck H. Chemotherapy as an adjuvant to surgery in lung cancer. *Cancer Chemother Pharmacol* 1978;1:145.
249. Shields TW, Humphrey EW, Eastridge CE, et al. Adjuvant cancer chemotherapy after resection of carcinoma of the lung. *Cancer* 1977;40:2057.
250. Wingfield HV. Combined surgery and chemotherapy for carcinoma of the bronchus. *Lancet* 1970;1:470.
251. Karrer K, Shields TW, Denck H, et al. The importance of surgical and multimodality treatment for small cell bronchial carcinoma [see comments]. *J Thorac Cardiovasc Surg* 1989;97:168.
252. Friess GG, McCracken JD, Troxell ML, et al. Effect of initial resection of small-cell carcinoma of the lung: a review of Southwest Oncology Group Study 7628. *J Clin Oncol* 1985;3:964.
253. Macchiarini P, Hardin M, Basolo F, et al. Surgery plus adjuvant chemotherapy for T1-3N0M0 small-cell lung cancer. Rationale for current approach [see comments]. *Am J Clin Oncol* 1991;14:218.
254. Hayata Y, Funatsu H, Suemasu K, et al. Surgical indications in small cell carcinoma of the lung. *Jpn J Clin Oncol* 1978;8:93.
255. Osterlind K, Hansen M, Hansen HH, et al. Influence of surgical resection prior to chemotherapy on the long-term results in small cell lung cancer. A study of 150 operable patients. *Eur J Cancer Clin Oncol* 1986;22:589.
256. Rea F, Callegaro D, Favaretto A, et al. Long term results of surgery and chemotherapy in small cell lung cancer. *Eur J Cardiothorac Surg* 1998;14:398.
257. Lucchi M, Mussi A, Chella A, et al. Surgery in the management of small cell lung cancer. *Eur J Cardiothorac Surg* 1997;12:689.
258. Inoue M, Nakagawa K, Fujiwara K, et al. Results of preoperative mediastinoscopy for small cell lung cancer. *Ann Thorac Surg* 2000;70:1620.
259. Inoue M, Miyoshi S, Yasumitsu T, et al. Surgical results for small cell lung cancer based on the new TNM staging system. Thoracic Surgery Study Group of Osaka University, Osaka, Japan. *Ann Thorac Surg* 2000;70:1615.
260. Kobayashi S, Okada S, Hasumi T, et al. Combined modality therapy including surgery for stage III small-cell lung cancer on the basis of the sensitivity assay in vitro. *Surg Today* 2000;30:127.
261. Osterlind K, Hansen M, Hansen HH, et al. Treatment policy of surgery in small cell carcinoma of the lung: retrospective analysis of a series of 874 consecutive patients. *Thorax* 1985;40:272.
262. Quoix E, Fraser R, Wolkove N, et al. Small cell lung cancer presenting as a solitary pulmonary nodule. *Cancer* 1990;66:577.
263. Warren WH, Memoli VA, Jordan AG, et al. Reevaluation of pulmonary neoplasms resected as small cell carcinomas. Significance of distinguishing between well-differentiated and small cell neuroendocrine carcinomas. *Cancer* 1990;65:1003.

264. Holoye PY, Shirinian M. Adjuvant surgery in the multimodality treatment of small-cell lung cancer. *Am J Clin Oncol* 1991;14:251.
265. Prager RL, Foster JM, Hainsworth JD, et al. The feasibility of adjuvant surgery in limited-stage small cell carcinoma: a prospective evaluation. *Ann Thorac Surg* 1984;38:622.
266. Meyer JA, Gullo JJ, Ikins PM, et al. Adverse prognostic effect of N2 disease in treated small cell carcinoma of the lung. *J Thorac Cardiovasc Surg* 1984;88:495.
267. Shepherd FA, Ginsberg R, Patterson GA, et al. Is there ever a role for salvage operations in limited small-cell lung cancer? [see comments]. *J Thorac Cardiovasc Surg* 1991;101:196.
268. Lad T, Piantadosi S, Thomas P, et al. A prospective randomized trial to determine the benefit of surgical resection of residual disease following response of small cell lung cancer to combination chemotherapy. *Chest* 1994;106[6 Suppl]:320S.
269. Fujimori K, Yokoyama A, Kurita Y, et al. A pilot phase 2 study of surgical treatment after induction chemotherapy for resectable stage I to IIIA small cell lung cancer. *Chest* 1997;111:1089.
270. Lewinski T, Zulawski M, Turski C, et al. Small cell lung cancer I–III A: cytoreductive chemotherapy followed by resection with continuation of chemotherapy. *Eur J Cardiothorac Surg* 2001;20:391.
271. Eberhardt W, Stamatis G, Stuschke M, et al. Prognostically orientated multimodality treatment including surgery for selected patients of small-cell lung cancer patients stages IB to IIIB: long-term results of a phase II trial. *Br J Cancer* 1999;81:1206.
272. Eberhardt W, Korfee S. New approaches for small-cell lung cancer: local treatments. *Cancer Control* 2003;10:289.
273. Girling DJ. Comparison of oral etoposide and standard intravenous multidrug chemotherapy for small-cell lung cancer: a stopped multicentre randomized trial. Medical Research Council Lung Cancer Working Party. *Lancet* 1996;348:563.
274. Souhami RL, Spiro SG, Rudd RM, et al. Five-day oral etoposide treatment for advanced small-cell lung cancer: randomized comparison with intravenous chemotherapy. *J Natl Cancer Inst* 1997;89:577.
275. Seifter EJ, Ihde DC. Therapy of small cell lung cancer: a perspective on two decades of clinical research. *Semin Oncol* 1988;15:278.
276. Livingston RB, Mira JG, Chen TT, et al. Combined modality treatment of extensive small cell lung cancer: a Southwest Oncology Group study. *J Clin Oncol* 1984;2:585.
277. Livingston RB, Schulman S, Mira JG, et al. Combined alkylators and multiple-site irradiation for extensive small cell lung cancer: a Southwest Oncology Group Study. *Cancer Treat Rep* 1986;70:1395.
278. Jeremic B, Shibamoto Y, Nikolic N, et al. Role of radiation therapy in the combined-modality treatment of patients with extensive disease small-cell lung cancer: a randomized study. *J Clin Oncol* 1999;17:2092.
279. Wilson HE, Stanley K, Vincent RG, et al. Comparison of chemotherapy alone versus chemotherapy and radiotherapy for extensive small cell carcinoma of the lung. *J Surg Oncol* 1983;23:181.
280. Carmichael J, Crane JM, Bunn PA, et al. Results of therapeutic cranial irradiation in small cell lung cancer. *Int J Radiat Oncol Biol Phys* 1988;14:455.
281. Groen HJ, Smit EF, Haaxma-Reiche H, et al. Carboplatin as second line treatment for recurrent or progressive brain metastases from small cell lung cancer. *Eur J Cancer* 1993;12:1696.
282. Postmus PE, Smit EF, Haaxma-Reiche H, et al. Teniposide for brain metastases of small-cell lung cancer: a phase II study. European Organization for Research and Treatment of Cancer Lung Cancer Cooperative Group. *J Clin Oncol* 1995;13:660.
283. Postmus PE, Haaxma-Reiche H, Gregor A, et al. Brain-only metastases of small cell lung cancer; efficacy of whole brain radiotherapy. An EORTC phase II study. *Radiother Oncol* 1998;46:29.
284. Freyer G, Ligneau B, Tranchand B, et al. The prognostic value of etoposide area under the curve (AUC) at first chemotherapy cycle in small cell lung cancer patients: a multicenter study of the groupe Lyon-Saint-Etienne d'Oncologie Thoracique (GLOT). *Lung Cancer* 2001;31:247.
285. Tjan-Heijnen VC, Postmus PE, Ardizzoni A, et al. Reduction of chemotherapy-induced febrile leucopenia by prophylactic use of ciprofloxacin and roxithromycin in small-cell lung cancer patients: an EORTC double-blind placebo-controlled phase III study. *Ann Oncol* 2001;12:1359.
286. Goldie JH, Coldman AJ. A mathematical model for relating the drug sensitivity of tumors to their spontaneous mutation rate. *Cancer Treat Rep* 1979;63:1727.
287. Goldie JH, Coldman AJ, Gudauskas GA. Rationale for the use of alternating non-cross-resistant chemotherapy. *Cancer Treat Rep* 1982;66:439.
288. Evans WK, Feld R, Murray N, et al. Superiority of alternating non-cross-resistant chemotherapy in extensive small cell lung cancer. A multicenter, randomized clinical trial by the National Cancer Institute of Canada [published erratum appears in *Ann Intern Med* 1988;108:496]. *Ann Intern Med* 1987;107:451.
289. Postmus PE, Scagliotti G, Groen HJ, et al. Standard versus alternating non-cross-resistant chemotherapy in extensive small cell lung cancer: an EORTC Phase III trial. *Eur J Cancer* 1996;32A:1498.
290. Osterlind K, Sorenson S, Hansen HH, et al. Continuous versus alternating combination chemotherapy for advanced small cell carcinoma of the lung. *Cancer Res* 1983;43:6085.
291. Andersen M, Kristjansen PE, Hansen HH. Second-line chemotherapy in small cell lung cancer. *Cancer Treat Rev* 1990;17:427.
292. Wolf M, Pritsch M, Drings P, et al. Cyclic-alternating versus response-oriented chemotherapy in small-cell lung cancer: a German multicenter randomized trial of 321 patients. *J Clin Oncol* 1991;9:614.
293. Feld R, Evans WK, Coy P, et al. Canadian multicenter randomized trial comparing sequential and alternating administration of two non-cross-resistant chemotherapy combinations in patients with limited small-cell carcinoma of the lung. *J Clin Oncol* 1987;5:1401.
294. Goodman GE, Crowley JJ, Blasko JC, et al. Treatment of limited small-cell lung cancer with etoposide and cisplatin alternating with vincristine, doxorubicin, and cyclophosphamide versus concurrent etoposide, vincristine, doxorubicin, and cyclophosphamide and chest radiotherapy: a Southwest Oncology Group Study. *J Clin Oncol* 1990;8:39.
295. Urban T, Baleyte T, Chastang CL, et al. Standard combination versus alternating chemotherapy in small cell lung cancer: a randomized clinical trial including 394 patients. 'Petites Cellules' Group. *Lung Cancer* 1999;25:105.
296. Aisner J, Whitacre M, Van Echo DA, et al. Combination chemotherapy for small cell carcinoma of the lung: continuous versus alternating non-cross-resistant combinations. *Cancer Treat Rep* 1982;66:221.
297. Ettinger DS, Lagakos S. Phase III study of CCNU, cyclophosphamide, adriamycin, vincristine, and VP-16 in small-cell carcinoma of the lung. *Cancer* 1982;49:1544.
298. Osterlind K, Hansen M, Hirsch FR, et al. Combination chemotherapy of limited-stage small-cell lung cancer. A controlled trial on 221 patients comparing two alternating regimens. *Ann Oncol* 1991;2:41.
299. Havemann K, Wolf M, Holle R, et al. Alternating versus sequential chemotherapy in small cell lung cancer. A randomized German multicenter trial. *Cancer* 1987;59:1072.
300. Teicher BA. Preclinical models for high-dose therapy. In: Armitage JO, Antman KH, eds. *High-dose chemotherapy: pharmacology, hematopoietins, stem cells.* Baltimore: Williams & Wilkins, 1992:14.
301. Schabel FM Jr, Griswold DP Jr, Corbett TH, et al. Increasing the therapeutic response rates to anticancer drugs by applying the basic principles of pharmacology. *Cancer* 1984;54:1160.
302. Linch DC, Winfield D, Goldstone AH, et al. Dose intensification with autologous bone-marrow transplantation in relapsed and resistant Hodgkin's disease: results of a BNLI randomized trial. *Lancet* 1993;341:1051.
303. Attal M, Harousseau JL, Stoppa AM, et al. A prospective, randomized trial of autologous bone marrow transplantation and chemotherapy in multiple myeloma. *N Engl J Med* 1996;335:91.
304. Shipp MA, Abeloff MD, Antman KH, et al. International consensus conference on high-dose therapy with hematopoietic stem cell transplantation in aggressive non-Hodgkin's lymphomas: report of the jury. *J Clin Oncol* 1999;17:423.
305. Hryniuk W, Bush H. The importance of dose intensity in chemotherapy of metastatic breast cancer. *J Clin Oncol* 1984;2:1281.
306. Levin L, Hryniuk W. The application of dose intensity to problems in chemotherapy of ovarian and endometrial cancer. *Semin Oncol* 1987;14:12.
307. Klasa RJ, Murray N, Coldman AJ. Dose-intensity meta-analysis of chemotherapy regimens in small-cell carcinoma of the lung. *J Clin Oncol* 1991;9:499.
308. Cohen MH, Creaven PJ, Fossieck BE Jr, et al. Intensive chemotherapy of small cell bronchogenic carcinoma. *Cancer Treat Rep* 1977;61:349.
309. Mehta C, Vogl SE, Farber S, et al. High-dose cyclophosphamide (c) in the induction (ind) chemotherapy (ct) of small cell lung cancer (sclc)—minor improvements in the rate of remission and survival. *Proc Am Assoc Cancer Res* 1982;23:165(abst).
310. Figueredo AT, Hryniuk WM, Strautmanis I, et al. Co-trimoxazole prophylaxis during high-dose chemotherapy of small-cell lung cancer. *J Clin Oncol* 1985;3:54.
311. Arriagada R, Le Chevalier T, Pignon JP, et al. Initial chemotherapeutic doses and survival in patients with limited small-cell lung cancer. *N Engl J Med* 1993;329:1848.
312. Johnson DH, Einhorn LH, Birch R, et al. A randomized comparison of high-dose versus conventional-dose cyclophosphamide, doxorubicin, and vincristine for extensive-stage small-cell lung cancer: a phase III trial of the Southeastern Cancer Study Group. *J Clin Oncol* 1987;5:1731.
313. Ihde DC, Mulshine JL, Kramer BS, et al. Prospective randomized comparison of high-dose and standard-dose etoposide and cisplatin chemotherapy in patients with extensive-stage small-cell lung cancer. *J Clin Oncol* 1994;12:2022.
314. Le Chevalier T, Riviere A, Pignon JP, et al. Is there an optimal dose for frontline chemotherapy in limited small cell lung cancer? *Proc Am Soc Clin Oncol* 2002;21:294a.
315. Brower M, Ihde DC, Johnston-Early A, et al. Treatment of extensive stage small cell bronchogenic carcinoma. Effects of variation in intensity of induction chemotherapy. *Am J Med* 1983;75:993.
316. Gridelli C, Perrone F, D'Aprile M, et al. Phase II study of intensive CEV (carboplatin, epirubicin and VP-16) plus G-CSF (granulocyte-colony stimulating factor) in extensive small cell lung cancer [Letter]. *Eur J Cancer* 1995;31A:2424.
317. Pujol JL, Douillard JY, Riviere A, et al. Dose-intensity of a four-drug chemotherapy regimen with or without recombinant human granulocyte-macrophage colony-stimulating factor in extensive-stage small-cell lung cancer: a multicenter randomized phase III study. *J Clin Oncol* 1997;15:2082.
318. Hirsch FR, Osterlind K, Jeppesen N, et al. Superiority of high-dose platinum (cisplatin and carboplatin) compared to carboplatin alone in combination chemotherapy for small-cell lung carcinoma: a prospective randomized trial of 280 consecutive patients. *Ann Oncol* 2001;12:647.
319. Steward WP, von Pawel J, Gatzemeier U, et al. Effects of granulocyte-macrophage colony-stimulating factor and dose intensification of V-ICE chemotherapy in small-cell lung cancer: a prospective randomized study of 300 patients. *J Clin Oncol* 1998;16:642.
320. Lorigan P, Woll P, O'Brien M, et al. Randomized phase 3 trial of dose dense ICE chemotherapy versus standard ICE in good prognosis small cell lung cancer (SCLC). *Proc Am Soc Clin Oncol* 2003;22:619.
321. Thatcher N, Girling DJ, Hopwood P, et al. Improving survival without reducing quality of life in small-cell lung cancer patients by increasing the dose-intensity of chemotherapy with granulocyte colony-stimulating factor support: results of a British Medical Research Council multicenter randomized trial. Medical Research Council Lung Cancer Working Party. *J Clin Oncol* 2000;18:395.
322. Ardizzoni A, Tjan-Heijnen VC, Postmus PE, et al. Standard versus intensified chemotherapy with granulocyte colony-stimulating factor support in small-cell lung cancer: a prospective European Organization for Research and Treatment of Cancer-Lung Cancer Group phase III trial-08923. *J Clin Oncol* 2002;20:3947.
323. Taylor CW, Crowley J, Williamson SK, et al. Treatment of small-cell lung cancer with an alternating chemotherapy regimen given at weekly intervals: a Southwest Oncology Group pilot study. *J Clin Oncol* 1990;8:1811.

324. Alba E, Breton JJ, Alonso L, et al. Alternating chemotherapy for small-cell lung cancer. A twelve-week schedule of six drugs. *Ann Oncol* 1992;3:31.

325. Sculier JP, Paesmans M, Bureau G, et al. Multiple-drug weekly chemotherapy versus standard combination regimen in small-cell lung cancer: a phase III randomized study conducted by the European Lung Cancer Working Party. *J Clin Oncol* 1993;11:1858.

326. Souhami RL, Rudd R, Ruiz de Elvira MC, et al. Randomized trial comparing weekly versus 3-week chemotherapy in small-cell lung cancer: a Cancer Research Campaign trial. *J Clin Oncol* 1994;12:1806.

327. Furuse K, Fukuoka M, Nishiwaki Y, et al. Phase III study of intensive weekly chemotherapy with recombinant human granulocyte colony-stimulating factor versus standard chemotherapy in extensive-disease small-cell lung cancer. The Japan Clinical Oncology Group. *J Clin Oncol* 1998;16:2126.

328. Murray N, Livingston R, Shepherd F, et al. Randomized study of CODE versus alternating CAV/EP for extensive-stage small-cell lung cancer: an intergroup study of the National Cancer Institute of Canada Clinical Trials Group and the Southwest Oncology Group. *J Clin Oncol* 1997;17:2300.

329. Clark SC, Kamen R. The hematopoietic colony-stimulating factors. *Science* 1987;236:1229.

330. Crawford J, Ozer H, Stoller R, et al. Reduction by granulocyte colony-stimulating factor of fever and neutropenia induced by chemotherapy in patients with small-cell lung cancer. *N Engl J Med* 1991;325:164.

331. Trillet-Lenoir V, Green J, Manegold C, et al. Recombinant granulocyte colony stimulating factor reduces the infectious complications of cytotoxic chemotherapy. *Eur J Cancer* 1993;29A:319.

332. Glaspy JA, Bleecker G, Crawford J, et al. The impact of therapy with filgrastim (recombinant granulocyte colony-stimulating factor) on the health care costs associated with cancer chemotherapy. *Eur J Cancer* 1993;29A:S23.

333. Lyman GH, Lyman CG, Sanderson RA, et al. Decision analysis of hematopoietic growth factor use in patients receiving cancer chemotherapy. *J Natl Cancer Inst* 1993;85:488.

334. Ozer H, Armitage JO, Bennett CL, et al. 2000 update of recommendations for the use of hematopoietic colony-stimulating factors: evidence-based, clinical practice guidelines. American Society of Clinical Oncology Growth Factors Expert Panel. *J Clin Oncol* 2000;18:3558.

335. Nichols CR, Fox EP, Roth BJ, et al. Incidence of neutropenic fever in patients treated with standard-dose combination chemotherapy for small-cell lung cancer and the cost impact of treatment with granulocyte colony-stimulating factor. *J Clin Oncol* 1994;12:1245.

336. Chouaid C, Bassinet L, Fuhrman C, et al. Routine use of granulocyte colony-stimulating factor is not cost-effective and does not increase patient comfort in the treatment of small-cell lung cancer: an analysis using a Markov model. *J Clin Oncol* 1998;16:2700.

337. Miles DW, Fogarty O, Ash CM, et al. Received dose-intensity: a randomized trial of weekly chemotherapy with and without granulocyte colony-stimulating factor in small-cell lung cancer. *J Clin Oncol* 1994;12:77.

338. Fukuoka M, Masuda N, Negoro S, et al. CODE chemotherapy with and without granulocyte colony-stimulating factor in small-cell lung cancer. *Br J Cancer* 1997;75:306.

339. Bunn PA Jr, Crowley J, Kelly K, et al. Chemoradiotherapy with or without granulocyte-macrophage colony-stimulating factor in the treatment of limited-stage small-cell lung cancer: a prospective phase III randomized study of the Southwest Oncology Group [published erratum appears in *J Clin Oncol* 1995;13:2860]. *J Clin Oncol* 1995;13:1632.

340. Stahel RA, Takvorian RW, Skarin AT, et al. Autologous bone marrow transplantation following high-dose chemotherapy with cyclophosphamide, BCNU and VP-16 in small cell carcinoma of the lung and a review of current literature. *Eur J Cancer Clin Oncol* 1984;20:1233.

341. Eder JP, Antman K, Elias A, et al. Cyclophosphamide and thiotepa with autologous bone marrow transplantation in patients with solid tumors. *J Natl Cancer Inst* 1988;80:1221.

342. Lazarus HM, Spitzer TR, Creger RJ. Phase I trial of high-dose etoposide, high-dose cisplatin, and reinfusion of autologous bone marrow for lung cancer. *Am J Clin Oncol* 1990;13:107.

343. Elias A. Hematopoietic stem cell transplantation for small cell lung cancer. *Chest* 1999;116[3 Suppl]:531S.

344. Elias AD, Ayash L, Frei Ed, et al. Intensive combined modality therapy for limited-stage small-cell lung cancer. *J Natl Cancer Inst* 1993;85:559.

345. Fetscher S, Brugger W, Engelhardt R, et al. Standard- and high-dose etoposide, ifosfamide, carboplatin, and epirubicin in 100 patients with small-cell lung cancer: a mature follow-up report. *Ann Oncol* 1999;10:561.

346. Humblet Y, Symann M, Bosly A, et al. Late intensification chemotherapy with autologous bone marrow transplantation in selected small-cell carcinoma of the lung: a randomized study. *J Clin Oncol* 1987;5:1864.

347. Goodman GE, Crowley J, Livingston RB, et al. Treatment of limited small-cell lung cancer with concurrent etoposide/cisplatin and radiotherapy followed by intensification with high-dose cyclophosphamide: a Southwest Oncology Group study. *J Clin Oncol* 1991;9:453.

348. Leyvraz S, Perey L, Rosti G, et al. Multiple courses of high-dose ifosfamide, carboplatin, and etoposide with peripheral-blood progenitor cells and filgrastim for small-cell lung cancer: a feasibility study by the European Group for Blood and Marrow Transplantation. *J Clin Oncol* 1999;17:3531.

349. Perey L, Benhattar J, Peters R, et al. High tumour contamination of leukaphereses in patients with small cell carcinoma of the lung: a comparison of immunocytochemistry and RT-PCR. *Br J Cancer* 2001;85:1713.

350. Shepherd FA, Amdemichael E, Evans WK, et al. Treatment of small cell lung cancer in the elderly. *J Am Geriatr Soc* 1994;42:64.

351. Dajczman E, Fu LY, Small D, et al. Treatment of small cell lung carcinoma in the elderly. *Cancer* 1996;77:2032.

352. Murray N, Grafton C, Shah A, et al. Abbreviated treatment for elderly, infirm, or non-compliant patients with limited-stage small-cell lung cancer. *J Clin Oncol* 1998;16:3323.

353. Johnson DH, Greco FA, Strupp J, et al. Prolonged administration of oral etoposide in patients with relapsed or refractory small-cell lung cancer: a phase II trial. *J Clin Oncol* 1990;8:1613.

354. White S, Lorigan P, Middleton M, et al. Randomized phase II study of cyclophosphamide, doxorubicin, and vincristine compared with single-agent carboplatin in patients with poor prognosis small cell lung cancer. *Cancer* 2001;92:601.

355. Earl HM, Rudd RM, Spiro SG, et al. A randomized trial of planned versus as required chemotherapy in small cell lung cancer: a Cancer Research Campaign trial. *Br J Cancer* 1991;64:566.

356. Randomized trial of four-drug vs less intensive two-drug chemotherapy in the palliative treatment of patients with small-cell lung cancer (SCLC) and poor prognosis. Medical Research Council Lung Cancer Working Party [published erratum appears in *Br J Cancer* 1996;74:997]. *Br J Cancer* 1996;73:406.

357. James LE, Gower NH, Rudd RM, et al. A randomized trial of low-dose/high-frequency chemotherapy as palliative treatment of poor-prognosis small-cell lung cancer: a Cancer Research Campaign trial. *Br J Cancer* 1996;73:1563.

358. Jeremic B, Shibamoto Y, Acimovic L, et al. Carboplatin, etoposide, and accelerated hyperfractionated radiotherapy for elderly patients with limited small cell lung carcinoma: a phase II study. *Cancer* 1998;82:836.

359. Larive S, Bombaron P, Riou R, et al. Carboplatin-etoposide combination in small cell lung cancer patients older than 70 years: a phase II trial. *Lung Cancer* 2002;35:1.

360. Westeel V, Murray N, Gelmon K, et al. New combination of the old drugs for elderly patients with small-cell lung cancer: a phase II study of the PAVE regimen. *J Clin Oncol* 1998;16:1940.

361. McCracken JD, Chen T, White J, et al. Combination chemotherapy, radiotherapy, and BCG immunotherapy in limited small-cell carcinoma of the lung: a Southwest Oncology Group study. *Cancer* 1982;49:2252.

362. Scher HI, Shank B, Chapman R, et al. Randomized trial of combined modality therapy with and without thymosin fraction V in the treatment of small cell lung cancer. *Cancer Res* 1988;48:1663.

363. Tanio Y, Watanabe M, Osaki T, et al. High sensitivity to peripheral blood lymphocytes and low HLA-class I antigen expression of small cell lung cancer cell lines with diverse chemo-radiosensitivity. *Jpn J Cancer Res* 1992;83:736.

364. Yazawa T, Kamma H, Fujiwara M, et al. Lack of class II transactivator causes severe deficiency of HLA-DR expression in small cell lung cancer. *J Pathol* 1999;187:191.

365. Ball ED, Sorenson GD, Pettengill OS. Expression of myeloid and major histocompatibility antigens in small cell carcinoma of the lung cell lines by cytofluorography: modulation by gamma interferon. *Cancer Res* 1986;46:2335.

366. Mattson K, Niiranen A, Pyrhonen S, et al. Natural interferon alfa as maintenance therapy for small cell lung cancer. *Eur J Cancer* 1992;1387.

367. Prior C, Oroszy S, Oberaigner W, et al. Adjunctive interferon-alpha-2c in stage IIIB/IV small-cell lung cancer: a phase III trial [published erratum appears in *Eur Respir J* 1997;10:963]. *Eur Respir J* 1997;10:392.

368. Ruotsalainen TM, Halme M, Tamminen K, et al. Concomitant chemotherapy and IFN-alpha for small cell lung cancer: a randomized multicenter phase III study. *J Interferon Cytokine Res* 1999;19:253.

369. Kelly K, Crowley JJ, Bunn PA Jr, et al. Role of recombinant interferon alfa-2a maintenance in patients with limited-stage small-cell lung cancer responding to concurrent chemoradiation: a Southwest Oncology Group study. *J Clin Oncol* 1995;13:2924.

370. Jett JR, Maksymiuk AW, Su JQ, et al. Phase III trial of recombinant interferon gamma in complete responders with small-cell lung cancer. *J Clin Oncol* 1994;12:2321.

371. van Zandwijk N, Groen HJ, Postmus PE, et al. Role of recombinant interferon-gamma maintenance in responding patients with small cell lung cancer. A randomized phase III study of the EORTC Lung Cancer Cooperative Group. *Eur J Cancer* 1997;33:1759.

372. Pujol JL, Gibney DJ, Su JQ, et al. Immune response induced in small-cell lung cancer by maintenance therapy with interferon gamma. *J Natl Cancer Inst* 1993;85:1844.

373. Clamon G, Herndon J, Perry MC, et al. Interleukin-2 activity in patients with extensive small-cell lung cancer: a phase II trial of Cancer and Leukemia Group B. *J Natl Cancer Inst* 1993;85:316.

374. Lynch TJ Jr, Lambert JM, Coral F, et al. Immunotoxin therapy of small-cell lung cancer: a phase I study of N901-blocked ricin. *J Clin Oncol* 1997;15:723.

375. Kelley MJ, Linnoila RI, Avis IL, et al. Antitumor activity of a monoclonal antibody directed against gastrin-releasing peptide in patients with small cell lung cancer. *Chest* 1997;112:256.

376. Rudin CM, Otterson GA, Mauer AM, et al. A pilot trial of G3139, a bcl-2 antisense oligonucleotide, and paclitaxel in patients with chemorefractory small-cell lung cancer. *Ann Oncol* 2002;13:539.

377. Burger H, den Bakker MA, Stoter G, et al. Lack of c-kit exon 11 activating mutations in c-KIT/CD117-positive SCLC tumour specimens. *Eur J Cancer* 2003;39:793.

378. Johnson BE, Fischer T, Fischer B, et al. Phase II study of imatinib in patients with small cell lung cancer. *Clin Cancer Res* 2003;9:5880.

379. Grant SC, Kris MG, Houghton AN, et al. Long survival of patients with small cell lung cancer after adjuvant treatment with the anti-idiotypic antibody BEC2 plus Bacillus Calmette-Guerin. *Clin Cancer Res* 1999;5:1319.

380. Giaccone G, Debruyne C, Felip E, et al. Phase III study of BEC2/BCG vaccination in limited disease small cell lung cancer (LD-SLSC) patients, following response to chemotherapy and thoracic irradiation (EORTC 08971, the SILVA study). *Proc Am Soc Clin Oncol* 2004;23:7020(abst).

381. Lebeau B, Chastang C, Brechot JM, et al. Subcutaneous heparin treatment increases survival in small cell lung cancer. "Petites Cellules" Group. *Cancer* 1994;74:38.

382. Zacharski LR, Henderson WG, Rickles FR, et al. Effect of warfarin on survival in small cell carcinoma of the lung. Veterans Administration Study No. 75. *JAMA* 1981;245:831.

383. Chahinian AP, Propert KJ, Ware JH, et al. A randomized trial of anticoagulation with war-

farin and of alternating chemotherapy in extensive small-cell lung cancer by the Cancer and Leukemia Group B. *J Clin Oncol* 1989;7:993.

384. Lebeau B, Chastang C, Muir JF, et al. No effect of an antiaggregant treatment with aspirin in small cell lung cancer treated with CCAVP16 chemotherapy. Results from a randomized clinical trial of 303 patients. The "Petites Cellules" Group. *Cancer* 1993;71:1741.

385. Shepherd FA, Giaccone G, Seymour L, et al. Prospective, randomized, double-blind, placebo-controlled trial of marimastat after response to first-line chemotherapy in patients with small-cell lung cancer: a trial of the National Cancer Institute of Canada-Clinical Trials Group and the European Organization for Research and Treatment of Cancer. *J Clin Oncol* 2002;20:4434.

386. Rigas J, Denham C, Rinaldi D, et al. Randomized placebo-controlled trials of the matrix metalloproteinase inhibitor (MMPI), BAY12-9566 as adjuvant therapy for patients with small cell and non-small cell lung cancer. *Proc Am Soc Clin Oncol* 2003;22:628.

387. Evans WK, Feld R, Osoba D, et al. VP-16 alone and in combination with cisplatin in previously treated patients with small cell lung cancer. *Cancer* 1984;53:1461.

388. Lopez JA, Mann J, Grapski RT, et al. Etoposide and cisplatin salvage chemotherapy for small cell lung cancer. *Cancer Treat Rep* 1985;69:369.

389. Shepherd FA, Evans WK, MacCormick R, et al. Cyclophosphamide, doxorubicin, and vincristine in etoposide- and cisplatin-resistant small cell lung cancer. *Cancer Treat Rep* 1987;71:941.

390. Smit EF, Berendsen HH, de Vries EG, et al. A phase II study of carboplatin and vincristine in previously treated patients with small-cell lung cancer. *Cancer Chemother Pharmacol* 1989;25:202.

391. Postmus PE, Smit EF, Kirkpatrick A, et al. Testing the possible non-cross resistance of two equipotent combination chemotherapy regimens against small-cell lung cancer: a phase II study of the EORTC Lung Cancer Cooperative Group. *Eur J Cancer* 1993;2:204.

392. Monnet I, Chariot P, Quoix E, et al. Extensive small-cell lung cancer. A randomized comparison of two chemotherapy programs with early crossover in instances of failure. Association pour le Traitement des Tumeurs Intra-Thoraciques (ATTIT). *Ann Oncol* 1992;3:813.

393. Ebi N, Kubota K, Nishiwaki Y, et al. Second-line chemotherapy for relapsed small cell lung cancer. *Jpn J Clin Oncol* 1997;27:166.

394. Giaccone G, Donadio M, Bonardi G, et al. Teniposide in the treatment of small-cell lung cancer: the influence of prior chemotherapy. *J Clin Oncol* 1988;6:1264.

395. Batist G, Ihde DC, Zabell A, et al. Small-cell carcinoma of lung: reinduction therapy after late relapse. *Ann Intern Med* 1983;98:472.

396. Postmus PE, Berendsen HH, van Zandwijk N, et al. Retreatment with the induction regimen in small cell lung cancer relapsing after an initial response to short term chemotherapy. *Eur J Cancer Clin Oncol* 1987;23:1409.

397. Vincent M, Evans B, Smith I. First-line chemotherapy rechallenge after relapse in small cell lung cancer. *Cancer Chemother Pharmacol* 1988;21:45.

398. Albain KS, Crowley JJ, Hutchins L, et al. Predictors of survival following relapse or progression of small cell lung cancer. Southwest Oncology Group Study 8605 report and analysis of recurrent disease data base. *Cancer* 1993;72:1184.

399. Eckardt J, Depierre A, Ardizzoni A, et al. Pooled analysis of topotecan in the second-line treatment of patients with sensitive small cell lung cancer. *Proc Am Soc Clin Oncol* 1997;16:A1624.

400. Ardizzoni A, Hansen H, Dombernowsky P, et al. Topotecan, a new active drug in the second-line treatment of small-cell lung cancer: a phase II study in patients with refractory and sensitive disease. The European Organization for Research and Treatment of Cancer Early Clinical Studies Group and New Drug Development Office, and the Lung Cancer Cooperative Group. *J Clin Oncol* 1997;15:2090.

401. Groen HJ, Fokkema E, Biesma B, et al. Paclitaxel and carboplatin in the treatment of small-cell lung cancer patients resistant to cyclophosphamide, doxorubicin, and etoposide: a non-cross-resistant schedule. *J Clin Oncol* 1999;17:927.

402. Kakolyris S, Mavroudis D, Tsavaris N, et al. Paclitaxel in combination with carboplatin as salvage treatment in refractory small-cell lung cancer (SCLC): a multicenter phase II study. *Ann Oncol* 2001;12:193.

403. Shepherd FA, Ginsberg RJ, Feld R, et al. Surgical treatment for limited small-cell lung cancer. The University of Toronto Lung Oncology Group experience. *J Thorac Cardiovasc Surg* 1991;101:385.

404. Merrill RM, Henson DE, Barnes M. Conditional survival among patients with carcinoma of the lung [see comments]. *Chest* 1999;116:697.

405. Stephens RJ, Bailey AJ, Machin D. Long-term survival in small cell lung cancer: the case for a standard definition. Medical Research Council Lung Cancer Working Party. *Lung Cancer* 1996;15:297.

406. Sekine I, Nishiwaki Y, Kakinuma R, et al. Late recurrence of small-cell lung cancer: treatment and outcome. *Oncology* 1996;53:318.

407. Tucker MA, Murray N, Shaw EG, et al. Second primary cancers related to smoking and treatment of small-cell lung cancer. Lung Cancer Working Cadre [see comments]. *J Natl Cancer Inst* 1997;89:1782.

408. Kawahara M, Ushijima S, Kamimori T, et al. Second primary tumours in more than 2-year disease-free survivors of small-cell lung cancer in Japan: the role of smoking cessation. *Br J Cancer* 1998;78:409.

409. Jacoulet P, Depierre A, Moro D, et al. Long-term survivors of small-cell lung cancer (SCLC): a French multicenter study. Groupe d'Oncologie de Langue Francaise. *Ann Oncol* 1997;8:1009.

410. Osterlind K, Hansen HH, Hansen M, et al. Long-term disease-free survival in small-cell carcinoma of the lung: a study of clinical determinants. *J Clin Oncol* 1986;4:1307.

411. Chute JP, Chen T, Feigal E, et al. Twenty years of phase III trials for patients with extensive-stage small-cell lung cancer: perceptible progress. *J Clin Oncol* 1999;17:1794.

412. Lassen UN, Hirsch FR, Osterlind K, et al. Outcome of combination chemotherapy in extensive stage small-cell lung cancer: any treatment related progress? *Lung Cancer* 1998;20:151.

413. Janne PA, Freidlin B, Saxman S, et al. Twenty-five years of clinical research for patients with limited-stage small cell lung carcinoma in North America. *Cancer* 2002;95:1528.

414. Remick SC, Hafez GR, Carbone PP. Extrapulmonary small-cell carcinoma. A review of the literature with emphasis on therapy and outcome. *Medicine (Baltimore)* 1987;66:457.

415. Johnson BE, Whang-Peng J, Naylor SL, et al. Retention of chromosome 3 in extrapulmonary small cell cancer shown by molecular and cytogenetic studies. *J Natl Cancer Inst* 1989;81:1223.

416. Remick SC, Ruckdeschel JC. Extrapulmonary and pulmonary small-cell carcinoma: tumor biology, therapy, and outcome. *Med Pediatr Oncol* 1992;20:89.

417. Hobbs RD, Stewart AF, Ravin ND, et al. Hypercalcemia in small cell carcinoma of the pancreas. *Cancer* 1984;53:1552.

418. Galanis E, Frytak S, Lloyd RV. Extrapulmonary small cell carcinoma. *Cancer* 1997;79:1729.

Robert B. Cameron
Patrick J. Loehrer, Sr.
Charles R. Thomas, Jr.

CHAPTER **28**

Neoplasms of the Mediastinum

Tumors involving the mediastinum may be primary or secondary in nature. Primary neoplasms can originate from any mediastinal organ or tissue but most commonly arise from thymic, neurogenic, lymphatic, germinal, and mesenchymal tissues. All primary mediastinal neoplasms, except those of thymic origin, also occur elsewhere in the body and are discussed in other chapters. Secondary (metastatic) mediastinal tumors are more common than primary neoplasms and most frequently represent lymphatic involvement from primary tumors of the lung or infradiaphragmatic organs, such as pancreatic, gastroesophageal, and testicular cancer. This chapter provides an overview of primary mediastinal neoplasms. Specific tumors are covered in detail, including thymic, primary mediastinal germ cell, mesenchymal, cardiac, and neurogenic tumors. Esophageal cancer and lymphomas are covered in Chapters 29.1 and 41, respectively.

ANATOMY

The mediastinum occupies the central portion of the thoracic cavity. It is bounded by the pleural cavities laterally, by the thoracic inlet superiorly, by the diaphragm inferiorly, by the sternum anteriorly, and by the chest wall posteriorly. The mediastinum can be divided into three clinically relevant compartments: anterior, middle, and posterior (Fig. 28-1). The anterior mediastinum lies posterior to the sternum and anterior to the pericardium and great vessels, extends from the thoracic inlet to the diaphragm, and contains the thymus gland, lymph nodes, and, rarely, ectopic thyroid and parathyroid glands. The middle mediastinum is defined as the space occupied by the heart, pericardium, proximal great vessels, and central airways, including phrenic nerves and lymph nodes. The posterior mediastinum is bounded by the heart and great vessels anteriorly, the thoracic inlet superiorly, the diaphragm inferiorly, and the chest wall of the back posteriorly and includes the paravertebral gutters, esophagus, descending aorta, sympathetic chains and vagus nerves, azygos vein, thoracic duct, and lymph nodes. Although other anatomic mediastinal divisions have been proposed, these other schemes have limited clinical use.

INCIDENCE AND PATHOLOGY

Mediastinal neoplasms are uncommon tumors that can occur at any age but are most often seen in the third through the fifth decades of life.[1,2] Table 28-1 reviews the classification and distribution of mediastinal masses. The incidence of primary mediastinal tumors was documented in a review of 1900 patients (Table 28-2).[1] In addition, 439 patients (18% of all mediastinal masses) were found to have cystic lesions. Thymic neoplasms predominate in the anterior mediastinum, followed in frequency by lymphomas, germ cell tumors, and carcinoma. Bronchial, enteric, and pericardial cysts are the most common masses in the middle mediastinum, followed by lymphomas, mesenchymal tumors, and carcinoma.[3] In the posterior mediastinum, neurogenic tumors and esophageal cancers are most common, followed by enteric cysts, mesenchymal tumors, and endocrine neoplasms.[1]

The incidence of mediastinal tumors in each anatomic compartment also varies with age. In adults, 54% of mediastinal neoplasms occur in the anterior, 20% in the middle, and 26% in the posterior mediastinum.[1] In pediatric populations, 43%, 18%, and 40% of neoplasms occur in the anterior, middle, and posterior mediastinum, respectively.[2] A higher incidence of thymic tumors and lymphomas in adults and neurogenic tumors in children account for these differences. Azarow et al.[2] compared mediastinal masses in 195 adult and 62 pediatric patients (Table 28-3). Cysts were not included but accounted for 16% to 18% of adult and 24% of pediatric mediastinal masses.[2] Therefore, age as well as location establishes the probable diagnosis.[1,2,4]

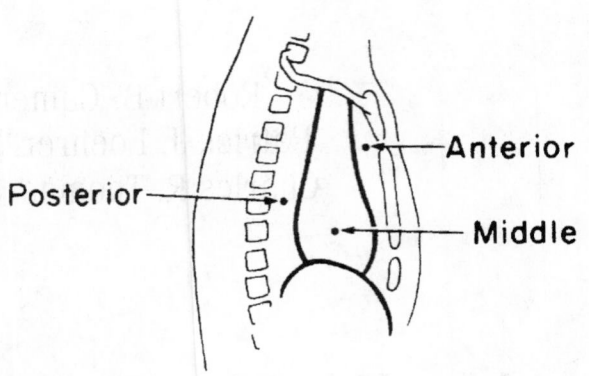

FIGURE 28-1. Mediastinal compartments. (Adapted from Fraser RS, Pare JAP, Fraser RF, et al. *Synopsis of diseases of the chest*, 2nd ed. Philadelphia: WB Saunders, 1994:73.)

pathologic techniques, the majority of patients no longer require open surgical biopsy before planning definitive therapy.

SYMPTOMS AND SIGNS

Approximately 40% of mediastinal masses are asymptomatic and discovered incidentally on a routine chest radiograph.[1] The remaining 60% of cases have symptoms related to either compression/direct invasion of surrounding mediastinal structures or to paraneoplastic syndromes. Asymptomatic patients are more likely to have benign lesions, whereas symptomatic patients more often harbor malignancies.[1] Davis et al.[5] found that 85% of patients with a malignancy were symptomatic, but only 46% of patients with benign neoplasms had identifiable complaints. The most commonly described symptoms are chest pain, cough, and dyspnea.[1] Superior vena cava syndrome, Horner's syndrome, hoarseness, and neurologic deficits more commonly occur with malignancies.[5] Systemic syndromes associated with mediastinal neoplasms are shown in Tables 28-4 and 28-5.

DIAGNOSTIC CONSIDERATIONS

A meticulous history and physical examination, along with a variety of imaging, serologic, and invasive tests, often can confirm the suspected diagnosis. With improved imaging, biopsy, and

RADIOGRAPHIC IMAGING STUDIES

Radiographic imaging studies initially localize mediastinal neoplasms. The posteroanterior and lateral chest radiographs

TABLE 28-1. Classification of Mediastinal Tumors

NEUROGENIC (POSTERIOR)	**THYMIC (ANTERIOR)**
Arising from peripheral nerves	Thymoma
Neurofibroma	Carcinoid
Neurilemoma (schwannoma)	Thymolipoma
Neurosarcoma	Thymic carcinoma
Arising from sympathetic ganglion	**ANEURYSMS (MIDDLE AND POSTERIOR)**
Ganglioneuroblastoma	Ascending aortic
Ganglioneuroma	Transverse arch
Neuroblastoma	Descending aortic
Arising from paraganglionic tissue	Great vessels
Pheochromocytoma	**MESENCHYMAL TUMORS (ALL THREE COMPARTMENTS)**
Chemodectoma (paraganglioma)	Fibroma, fibrosarcoma
GERM CELL (ANTERIOR—PRIMARY; MIDDLE AND POSTERIOR—METASTATIC)	Lipoma, liposarcoma
Seminoma	Myxoma
Nonseminomatous	Mesothelioma
Pure embryonal cell	Leiomyoma, leiomyosarcoma
Mixed embryonal cell	Rhabdomyosarcoma
With seminomatous elements	Xanthogranuloma
With trophoblastic elements	Mesenchymoma
With teratoid elements	Hemangioma
With endodermal sinus elements	Hemangioendothelioma
Teratoma, benign	Hemangiopericytoma
HERNIAS (ALL THREE COMPARTMENTS)	Lymphangioma
Hiatal	Lymphangiopericytoma
Morgagni	Lymphangiomyoma
CYSTS (ALL THREE COMPARTMENTS)	**LYMPHADENOPATHY (ALL THREE COMPARTMENTS)**
Pericardial	Inflammatory
Bronchogenic	Granulomatous
Enteric	Sarcoid
Thymic	**LYMPHOMA (ANTERIOR, MIDDLE, AND RARELY POSTERIOR)**
Thoracic duct	Hodgkin's disease
Meningoceles	Histiocytic lymphoma
	Undifferentiated
	ENDOCRINE (ANTERIOR AND MIDDLE)
	Thyroid
	Parathyroid

TABLE 28-2. Relative Frequency of Primary Mediastinal Tumors

Tumor	Incidence (%)
Neurogenic	25.3
Thymoma	23.3
Lymphoma	15.3
Germ cell neoplasm	12.2
Endocrine tumor	7.8
Mesenchymal tumor	7.3
Primary carcinoma	5.7
Other	2.9

(Adapted from ref. 1, with permission.)

define the location, size, density, and calcification of a mass, which helps focus the initial diagnostic testing; however, an intravenous contrast-enhanced computed tomography (CT) scan is by far the best imaging modality to accurately assess the nature (cystic vs. solid) of the lesion, detect fat and calcium, determine the relationship to surrounding structures, and, in some instances, predict invasiveness of some tumors.[6–8]

Magnetic resonance imaging (MRI) is used less frequently than CT.[9,10] Its advantages include multiplanar imaging and absence of ionizing radiation.[6] MRI scans are superior to CT in defining vascular involvement and in distinguishing recurrent tumor from radiation fibrosis.[9,10] However, patient claustrophobia, time, and expense limit the use of MRI scanning. Other imaging modalities that may be useful include transthoracic sonography, transesophageal echocardiography, and ultrasonography.[11–13]

Although the use of positron emission tomography (PET) is well established for the assessment of mediastinal lymph nodes in lung cancer and lymphoma, the use of PET in the evaluation of primary mediastinal neoplasms has not been fully defined. Some evidence exists that PET may help clarify the nature of mediastinal masses and detect the presence of neoplasm in residual mediastinal tissue after therapy.[14]

SEROLOGY AND CHEMISTRY

Some mediastinal neoplasms release tumor markers into the serum that can be measured to confirm a diagnosis, evaluate response to therapy, and monitor for tumor recurrence. α-Fetoprotein (AFP), human chorionic gonadotropin-β (β-HCG), and

TABLE 28-3. Relative Frequency of Primary Mediastinal Tumors in Adults and Children

Tumor	Incidence (%) Adults	Children
Thymic	31	28
Neurogenic	15	47
Lymphoma	26	9
Germ cell	15	9
Vascular	1	6
Miscellaneous	13	2

(Adapted from ref. 2, with permission.)

TABLE 28-4. Systemic Syndromes Associated with Mediastinal Neoplasms

Tumor	Syndrome
Thymoma	Acute pericarditis, Addison's disease, agranulocytosis, alopecia areata, Cushing's syndrome, hemolytic anemia, hypogammaglobulinemia, limbic encephalopathy, myasthenia gravis, myocarditis, nephrotic syndrome, panhypopituitarism, pernicious anemia, polymyositis, pure red cell aplasia, rheumatoid arthritis, sarcoidosis, scleroderma, sensorimotor radiculopathy, stiff-person syndrome, thyroiditis, ulcerative colitis
Hodgkin's disease	Alcohol-induced pain, Pel-Ebstein fever
Neurofibroma	von Recklinghausen's disease, osteoarthritis
Thymic carcinoid	Multiple endocrine neoplasia
Neuroblastoma	Opsomyoclonus, erythrocyte abnormalities
Neurilemoma	Peptic ulcer

lactate dehydrogenase are elaborated by some germ cell tumors and should be obtained in male patients with anterior mediastinal masses. Also, adrenocorticotropic hormone, thyroid hormone, and parathormone may help differentiate certain mediastinal tumors (see Table 28-5).

INVASIVE DIAGNOSTIC TESTS

An accurate histologic diagnosis is essential for appropriate treatment of mediastinal masses. Previously, most patients required surgical biopsies; however, improvements in cytopathologic techniques have greatly improved the ability to determine pathologic diagnoses with very small tissue samples.[15,16] CT-guided percutaneous needle biopsy, using either fine-needle aspiration techniques and cytologic assessment or larger-core needle biopsy and histologic evaluation, now are standard in the initial evaluation of most mediastinal masses.[15] Although fine-needle specimens are usually adequate to distinguish carcinomatous lesions, core biopsies are recommended for most other mediastinal neoplasms, especially lymphoma and thymoma.[15] Most recent series report diagnostic yields for

TABLE 28-5. Systemic Manifestations of Hormone Production by Mediastinal Neoplasms

Symptoms	Hormone	Tumor
Hypertension	Catecholamines	Pheochromocytoma, chemodectoma, neuroblastoma, ganglioneuroma
Hypercalcemia	Parathyroid hormone	Parathyroid adenoma
Thyrotoxicosis	Thyroxine	Thyroid
Cushing's syndrome	ACTH	Carcinoid tumor
Gynecomastia	HCG	Germ cell tumor
Hypoglycemia	? Insulin	Mesenchymal tumors
Diarrhea	VIP	Ganglioneuroma, neuroblastoma, neurofibroma

ACTH, adrenocorticotropic hormone; HCG, human chorionic gonadotropin; VIP, vasoactive intestinal polypeptide.

percutaneous needle biopsy in excess of 90%.[15,16] Complications include simple pneumothorax (25%), pneumothorax requiring chest tube placement (5%), and hemoptysis (7% to 15%).[15] In some circumstances, fine-needle aspiration of posterior and middle mediastinal tumors can be performed endoscopically using transesophageal ultrasonography.[13]

Surgical procedures occasionally are still required in the diagnosis of mediastinal tumors. Mediastinoscopy is a relatively simple procedure with a diagnostic accuracy of more than 90% for biopsies of the upper middle, anterior, and posterior mediastinum.[16,17] Anterior parasternal mediastinotomy (Chamberlain procedure) yields a diagnosis in 95% of anterior mediastinal masses and, if necessary, can be accomplished under local anesthesia.[18] Thoracoscopy is minimally invasive and provides a diagnostic accuracy of nearly 100% in most areas of the mediastinum.[17] Currently, thoracotomy is almost never necessary as a solely diagnostic procedure.

THYMIC NEOPLASMS

The thymus is an incompletely understood lymphatic organ functioning in T-lymphocyte maturation. It is composed of thymocytes/lymphocytes and an epithelial stroma. Although lymphomas, carcinoid tumors, and germ cell tumors all may arise within the thymus, only thymomas, thymic carcinomas, and thymolipomas arise from true thymic elements.

THYMIC ANATOMY AND PHYSIOLOGY

The thymus develops from a paired epithelial anlage in the ventral portion of the third pharyngeal pouch and is closely associated with the developing parathyroid glands.[19] The thymic epithelial stromal cells are likely derived from ectodermal and endodermal components.[20] During weeks 7 and 8 of development, the thymus elongates and descends caudally and ventromedially into the anterior mediastinum. Lymphoid cells arrive from the liver and bone marrow during week 9 and are separated from the perivascular spaces by a flat layer of epithelial cells that create the blood–thymus barrier. Maturation and differentiation occur in this antigen-free environment. By week 12, a separate cortex and medulla become evident. By the fourth fetal month, lymphocytes circulate to peripheral lymphoid tissue.[20]

Six subtypes of epithelial cells have been identified in mature thymus.[20] Four exist primarily in the cortical region and two in the medullary region. Type 6 cells form Hassall's corpuscles that are characteristic of thymus. These cells have an ectodermal origin and are displaced into the thymic medulla, where they hypertrophy and form tonofilaments, finally appearing as concentric cells without nuclei.[19,20]

At maturity, the thymus gland is an irregular, lobulated organ. It attains its greatest relative weight at birth, but its absolute weight increases to 30 to 40 g by puberty. During adulthood, it slowly involutes and is replaced by adipose tissue.[20] Ectopic thymic tissue has been found to be widely distributed throughout the mediastinum and neck, particularly the aortopulmonary window and retrocarinal area, and often is indistinguishable from mediastinal fat.[21,22] This ectopic tissue is the likely explanation for thymomas outside the anterior mediastinum and possibly for the failure of limited thymectomy to improve myasthenia gravis (MG) in some cases.[21–23]

THYMOMA

Thymic neoplasms, mostly thymomas, constitute 30% of anterior mediastinal masses in adults[1,2,24] but only 15% of anterior mediastinal masses in children.[4] A review of Surveillance, Epidemiology, and End Results program (SEER) data suggests that thymomas occur in 15 of every 100,000 person-years, are more common in males and Pacific Islanders, and increase in frequency into the eighth decade of life.[25] Nearly one-half of thymomas are asymptomatic and discovered only on routine radiographs. In symptomatic patients, 40% have MG (diplopia, ptosis, dysphagia, fatigue, etc.), whereas others complain of chest pain and symptoms of hemorrhage or compression of mediastinal structures.[26]

Pathology and Classification

Ninety percent of thymomas occur in the anterior mediastinum, and the remainder arise in the neck or other areas of the mediastinum.[21,22] Grossly, they are lobulated, firm, tan-pink to gray tumors that may contain cystic spaces, calcification, or hemorrhage. They may be encapsulated, adherent to surrounding structures, or frankly invasive. Microscopically, thymomas arise from thymic epithelial cells, although thymocytes/lymphocytes may predominate histologically. True thymomas contain cytologically bland cells and should be distinguished from thymic carcinomas, which have malignant cytologic characteristics. Confusion exists because of previous "benign" or "malignant" designations. Currently, the terms *noninvasive* and *invasive* are preferred. Noninvasive thymomas have an intact capsule, are movable, and are easily resected, although they can be adherent to adjacent organs. In contrast, invasive thymomas involve surrounding structures and can be difficult to remove without *en bloc* resection of adjacent structures, despite their cytologic benign appearance. Metastatic disease can occur and is most commonly seen as pleural implants and pulmonary nodules. Metastases to extrathoracic sites are rare.[26]

Originally, in 1976, Rosai and Levine[27] proposed that thymomas be divided into three types, depending on the predominant architecture of the tumor: lymphocytic, epithelial, or mixed (lymphoepithelial); however, there has been little direct correlation between this classification system and prognosis. In 1985, Marino and Muller-Hermelink[28] proposed a histologic classification system determined by the thymic site of origin; that is, tumors arising from epithelial cells of the cortex are termed cortical *thymomas*, corresponding to traditional epithelial thymomas. Those arising from spindle cells of the medullary areas are called *medullary thymomas*, corresponding to traditional spindle cell thymomas. *Mixed thymomas* have features of both. The Muller-Hermelink classification was later further divided into medullary, mixed, predominantly cortical, and cortical thymomas and well-differentiated and high-grade thymic carcinomas.[29] Medullary and mixed thymomas were considered benign with no risk of recurrence, even with capsular invasion. Predominantly cortical and cortical thymomas exhibited intermediate invasiveness and a low but definite risk of late relapse, regardless of their invasiveness. Well-differentiated thymic carcinomas were always invasive, with a high risk of relapse and death.[30] Controversy regarding the pathology of thymic neoplasms[31,32] led the World Health Organization Committee on the Classification of Thymic Tumors to adopt a new classification system for thymic neoplasms based on prognosti-

TABLE 28-6. World Health Organization Staging System for Thymic Epithelial Tumors

Tumor Type	Cells	Clinicopathologic Classification	Histologic Terminology
A	Spindle or oval	Benign thymoma	Medullary
B	Epithelioid or dendritic	Category I malignant thymoma	Cortical; organoid
B1			Lymphocyte-rich; predominately cortical
B2			Cortical
B3			Well-differentiated thymic carcinoma
AB		Benign thymoma	Mixed
C		Category II malignant thymoma	Nonorganotypic; thymic carcinoma, epidermoid keratinizing and nonkeratinizing carcinoma, lymphoepithelioma-like carcinoma, sarcomatoid carcinoma, clear-cell carcinoma, basaloid carcinoma, mucoepidermoid carcinoma, undifferentiated carcinoma

cally significant cytologic similarities between normal thymic epithelial cells and neoplastic cells (Table 28-6).[33]

In 1981, Masaoka et al.[34] developed a staging system based on the previous work of Bergh et al. The four stages are shown in Table 28-7. The Masaoka stage II classification assesses microscopic invasion (occult in 28%) and gross tumor adherence determined at surgery.[30] Staging was found to correlate with prognosis, with 5-year survival rates of 96% for stage I, 86% for stage II, 69% for stage III, and 50% for stage IV.[34] The Groupe d'Etudes des Tumeurs Thymiques (GETT) is another surgically oriented staging system that demonstrates 90% concordance with the Masaoka system.[35] Of interest, the expression of genes c-JUN and AL050002 were found using microarray technology and real-time reverse transcriptase-polymerase chain reaction to correlate with Masaoka stage and prognosis; in addition, AL050002 expression was found to correlate with the World Health Organization tumor classification system.[36]

Associated Systemic Syndromes

A wide variety of systemic disorders occur in 71% of thymomas, with autoimmune diseases (systemic lupus erythematosus, polymyositis, myocarditis, Sjögren's syndrome, ulcerative colitis, Hashimoto's thyroiditis, rheumatoid arthritis, sarcoidosis, and scleroderma) and endocrine disorders (hyperthyroidism, hyperparathyroidism, Addison's disease, and panhypopituitarism) being the most common.[36] Symptoms of these associated disorders often lead to the original discovery of the mediastinal tumor.

Blood disorders, such as red cell aplasia, hypogammaglobulinemia, T-cell deficiency syndrome, erythrocytosis, pancytopenia, megakaryocytopenia, T-cell lymphocytosis, and pernicious anemia, also have been noted. Other than myasthenia, neuromuscular syndromes include myotonic dystrophy, myositis, and Eaton-Lambert syndrome. Miscellaneous diseases include hypertrophic osteoarthropathy, nephrotic syndrome, minimal-change nephropathy, pemphigus, and chronic mucocutaneous candidiasis. A second malignancy, such as Kaposi's sarcoma, chemodectoma, multiple myeloma, acute leukemia, non-Hodgkin's lymphoma, sarcomas, and various carcinomas (e.g., lung, colon), develops in nearly 15% of patients with thymoma.[36]

MYASTHENIA GRAVIS. MG is the most common associated autoimmune disorder, occurring in 30% to 50% of patients with thymomas. Younger women and older men usually are affected, with a female-male ratio of 2:1. Myasthenia is a disorder of neuromuscular transmission. Symptoms begin insidiously and result from the production of antibodies to the postsynaptic nicotinic acetylcholine receptor at the myoneural junction. Ocular symptoms are the most frequent initial complaint, eventually progressing to generalized weakness in 80%. The role of the thymus in myasthenia remains unclear, but autosensitization of T lymphocytes to acetylcholine receptor proteins or an unknown action of thymic hormones remains a likely possibility.[37]

Pathologic changes in the thymus are noted in 70% of patients with MG. Lymphoid hyperplasia, characterized by the proliferation of germinal centers, is most commonly seen. Thymomas are identified in only approximately 15% of patients with myasthenia.[37]

The treatment of MG involves the use of anticholinesterase-mimetic agents [i.e., pyridostigmine bromide (Mestinon)]. In severe cases, plasmapheresis may be required to remove high antibody titers. Thymectomy has become an increasingly accepted procedure in the treatment of MG, although the indications, timing, and surgical approach remain controversial.[23] Some improvement in myasthenic symptoms almost always occurs after thymectomy, but complete remission rates vary from 7% to 63%.[23] Patients with MG and thymomas or thymic carcinomas do not respond as well to thymectomy as do those without thymomas. Age older than 55 and a duration of symptoms of less than 1 year also were found to be associated with a poor outcome.[38] Overall survival for myasthenia patients is lower for those with thymomas as well, but no differences were noted based on the extent of invasion present.[39]

RED CELL APLASIA. Pure red cell aplasia is considered an autoimmune disorder and is found in 5% of patients with thymomas.[40] Of patients with red cell aplasia, 30% to 50% have

TABLE 28-7. Thymoma Staging System of Masaoka

Stage	Description
I	Macroscopically completely encapsulated and microscopically no capsular invasion
II	Macroscopic invasion into surrounding fatty tissue or mediastinal pleura
	Microscopic invasion into capsule
III	Macroscopic invasion into neighboring organs (pericardium, great vessels, lung)
IVa	Pleural or pericardial dissemination
IVb	Lymphogenous or hematogenous metastasis

(From ref. 34, with permission.)

associated thymomas. Ninety-six percent of the patients affected are older than 40 years of age. Examination of the bone marrow reveals an absence of erythroid precursors and, in 30%, an associated decrease in platelet and leukocyte numbers. Thymectomy has produced remission in 38% of patients. Octreotide and prednisone were effective in one patient with recurrent disease.[41] The pathologic basis of these responses is poorly understood.

HYPOGAMMAGLOBULINEMIA. Hypogammaglobulinemia is seen in 5% to 10% of patients with thymoma, and 10% of those with hypogammaglobulinemia have been shown to have thymoma. Defects in cellular and humoral immunity have been described, and many patients also have red cell hypoplasia. Thymectomy has not proved beneficial in this disorder.

Treatment

Thymomas are slow-growing neoplasms that should be considered potentially malignant. Surgery, radiation, and chemotherapy all may play a role in their management.

SURGERY. Complete surgical resection is the mainstay of therapy for thymomas and is the most important predictor of long-term survival.[42,43] Although median sternotomy with a vertical or submammary incision is most commonly used, bilateral anterolateral thoracotomies with transverse sternotomy, or "clamshell procedure," is preferred with advanced or laterally displaced tumors. Video-assisted thoracoscopy also has been reported, but long-term results remain unproven.[44] Because of concern about tumor seeding, biopsy procedures are not routinely performed. During surgery, a careful assessment of areas of possible invasion and adherence should be made by the surgeon, who is the best judge of tumor invasiveness. Extended total thymectomy, including all tissue anterior to the pericardium from the diaphragm to the neck and laterally from phrenic nerve to phrenic nerve, is recommended in all cases. Complete surgical resection is associated with an 82% overall 7-year survival rate, whereas survival with incomplete resection is 71% and with biopsy is only 26%.[42] Survival after complete tumor resection has been similar in patients with noninvasive and invasive thymomas in several studies.[34,45] Patients with MG and thymoma were studied by Crucitti et al.,[46] who reported a 78% 10-year survival rate and a 3% recurrence rate with 4.8% (1.7% since 1980) operative mortality after extended thymectomy. Aggressive resection, including lung, phrenic nerve, pericardium, pleural implants, and pulmonary metastases, is occasionally helpful.[34,42,44]

The role of debulking or subtotal resection in stage III and IV disease remains controversial. Several studies have documented 5-year survival rates from 60% to 75% after subtotal resection and 24% to 40% after biopsy alone.[34,42,43,45] More recent studies, however, suggest no survival advantage to debulking followed by radiation when compared to radiation alone.[47] The use of surgery in recurrent disease remains to be defined. Maggi et al.[42] reported a 71% 5-year survival rate in 12 surgery patients and a 41% survival rate in 11 patients treated with radiation and chemotherapy alone. Prolonged tumor-free survival also was reported by Kirschner[48] in 23 patients. Urgesi et al.,[49] however, noted a 74% 5-year survival rate in 11 patients undergoing surgery and radiation, compared with 65% in 10 patients treated with radiation alone (not statistically different).

RADIATION THERAPY. Thymomas are radiosensitive tumors and, consequently, radiation has been used to treat all tumor stages as well as recurrent disease.[42,43,45] In stage I thymomas, adjuvant radiotherapy has been administered but has not improved on the excellent results with surgery alone (more than 80% 10-year survival rate).[42,43,45] In stage II and III invasive disease, adjuvant radiation can decrease recurrence rates after complete surgical resection from 28% to 5%.[47,50] In addition, Pollack et al.[51] reported an increase in 5-year disease-free survival for stage II to IVa from 18% to 62% with the addition of adjuvant radiation. Others have documented similar results.[45] Stage II patients with cortical tumors[52,53] and microscopic invasion of pleura or pericardium are most likely to benefit from postoperative radiation.[54] Preoperative radiotherapy for extensive tumors has been reported in limited studies that suggest a decreased tumor burden and potential for tumor seeding at the time of surgery.[42,43]

Radiation therapy has proved beneficial in the treatment of extensive disease.[43,47,51,54] Radiotherapy after incomplete surgical resection produces local control rates of 35% to 74% and 5-year survival rates ranging from 50% to 70% for stage III and 20% to 50% for stage IVa tumors.[43,47,49] In addition, Ciernik et al.[47] and others[49] have reported similar survival rates (87% 5-year and 70% 7-year) in patients treated with radiation alone compared with partial surgical resection and adjuvant radiation in small numbers of stage III and IV patients and patients with intrathoracic recurrences. Large variations in the amount of tumor treated and radiation delivered, however, make interpretation of these results difficult.[43,47,51,55]

Radiation therapy is delivered in doses ranging from 30 to 60 Gy in 1.8- or 2.0-cGy fractions over 3 to 6 weeks.[42,45,51,56] No improvement in local control has been shown with doses exceeding 60 Gy[47]; however, completely resected and microscopic residual disease can be well controlled with only 40 to 45 Gy.[43,47] Treatment portals have included single anterior field, unequally weighted (2:1 or 3:2) opposed anterior-posterior fields, wedge-pair, and multifield arrangements.[47,57] The gross tumor volume is defined by visible tumor or surgical clips seen on a treatment-planning CT scan. Areas of possible microscopic disease and a small border to account for daily variability and respiratory motion are added to define the clinical and planning target volumes. Gating techniques to minimize respiratory variation and intensity-modulated radiation therapy are new techniques that can minimize the dose heterogeneity, increase total dose and fraction size, and minimize toxicity.[58–60] Prophylactic supraclavicular and hemithorax fields have been used but are not warranted because of increased risks of pulmonary fibrosis, pericarditis, and myelitis.[43,47,48,61]

CHEMOTHERAPY. Chemotherapy has been used with increasing frequency in the treatment of invasive thymomas. Single-agent and combination therapy have both demonstrated activity in the adjuvant and neoadjuvant settings. Doxorubicin, cisplatin, ifosfamide, corticosteroids, and cyclophosphamide all have been used as single-agent therapy.[62] The most active agents are cisplatin, ifosfamide, and corticosteroids; however, only cisplatin and ifosfamide have undergone phase II testing.[24,63] Cisplatin, at doses of 100 mg/m^2, has produced complete responses lasting up to 30 months, but lower doses (50 mg/m^2) have associated response rates of only 11%.[62] Ifosfamide (with mesna) at a single dose of 7.5 g/m^2 or as a continuous infusion of 1.5 g/m^2/d for 5 days every 3 weeks has resulted in 50% complete and 57% overall response rates. Duration of complete remission ranged from 6 to 66 months.[63] Varying regimens of corticosteroids have shown effectiveness in the treatment of all histologic subtypes of thymoma (with and without myasthenia), with a 77% overall response rate in limited numbers of patients.[62,64] Corticosteroids also have been effective for patients who are unsuccessful with chemotherapy[62]; however, the actual impact may only be on the lymphocytic and not the malignant epithelial component of the tumor.

Combination chemotherapy regimens have shown higher response rates and have been used in adjuvant and in neoadjuvant settings in the treatment of advanced invasive, metastatic, and recurrent thymoma. Cisplatin-containing regimens appear to be the most active. Fornasiero et al.[65] reported a 43% complete and 91.8% overall response rate with a median survival of 15 months in 37 previously untreated patients with stage III or IV invasive thymoma treated with monthly (median, 5 months) cisplatin, 50 mg/m^2 on day 1; doxorubicin, 40 mg/m^2 on day 1; vincristine, 0.6 mg/m^2 on day 3; and cyclophosphamide, 700 mg/m^2 on day 4. Loehrer et al.[66] documented 10% complete and 50% overall response rates with a median survival of 37.7 months in 29 patients with metastatic or locally progressive recurrent thymoma treated with cisplatin, 50 mg/m^2; doxorubicin, 50 mg/m^2; and cyclophosphamide, 500 mg/m^2, given every 3 weeks for a maximum of eight cycles after radiotherapy. Park et al.[67] retrospectively described 35% complete and 64% overall response rates with a median survival of 67 months in responding and 17 months in nonresponding patients in 17 patients with invasive stage II and IV thymoma initially treated after relapse with cyclophosphamide, doxorubicin, and cisplatin, with or without prednisone. The European Organization for Research and Treatment of Cancer noted 31% complete and 56% overall response rates with a median survival of 4.3 years in a small study of 16 patients with advanced thymoma treated with cisplatin and etoposide.[68] The addition of ifosfamide to cisplatin and etoposide had a lower than anticipated response rate (approximately 32%) in patients with thymoma and thymic carcinoma.[69]

COMBINED MODALITY APPROACHES. The use of neoadjuvant chemotherapy as part of a multimodality approach to stage III and IV thymoma was reviewed by Tomiak and Evans.[62] Six combined reports document 31% complete and 89% overall response rates in 61 total patients treated with a variety of neoadjuvant chemotherapy regimens (80% cisplatin based). Twenty-two patients (36%) underwent surgery, with 11 (18%) achieving a complete resection (all treated with cisplatin). Nineteen patients were treated with radiotherapy, but only five patients had disease-free survivals exceeding 5 years.[62] Rea et al.[70] reported 43% complete and 100% overall response rates with median and 3-year survival rates of 66 months and 70%, respectively, in 16 stage III and IVa patients treated initially with cisplatin, doxorubicin, vincristine, and cyclophosphamide, followed by surgery. At surgery, 69% were completely resected and the other 31% received postoperative radiation. Macchiarini et al.[71] reported similar findings. Twenty-five percent complete and 92% overall response rates with a remarkable 83% 7-year disease-free survival rate were reported in 12 patients at the M. D. Anderson Cancer Center who received cisplatin, doxorubicin, cyclophosphamide, and prednisone

induction chemotherapy followed by surgical resection (80% complete) and adjuvant radiotherapy for locally advanced (unresectable) thymoma.[72] The degree of chemotherapy-induced tumor necrosis correlated with Ki-67 expression.

A multi-institutional prospective trial demonstrated a 22% complete and 70% overall response rate with a median survival of 93 months and a Kaplan-Meier 5-year failure-free survival rate of 54.3% in 23 patients with stage III (22 of 23) unresectable thymoma (GETT stage IIIA/IIIB), stage IV (1 of 23) thymoma, and thymic carcinoma (2 of 23) treated with two to four cycles of cisplatin, doxorubicin, and cyclophosphamide chemotherapy and sequential radiation therapy (54 Gy).[73,74] Just more than 25% had MG. Although these results compare favorably to those obtained with neoadjuvant therapy followed by surgical resection and radiation, further confirmation is needed.

Results of Treatment

Five- and 10-year survival rates for stage I, III, and IV tumors are reported to be 89% to 95% and 78% to 90%, 70% to 80% and 21% to 80%, and 50% to 60% and 30% to 40%,[34,75] respectively. Disease-free survival rates of 74%, 71%, 50%, and 29% also have been reported for stage I, II, III, and IV disease, respectively.[42] Although Maggi et al.[42] reported a 10% overall recurrence rate in 241 patients, fewer than 5% of noninvasive thymomas and 20% of invasive thymomas were noted to recur. A large multi-institutional experience was reported from Japan involving 1093 thymomas with documented 5-year survival rates of 100%, 98.4%, 88.7%, 70.6%, and 52.8% for Masaoka stages I, II, III, IVa, and IVb, respectively.[76] Although MG was once considered an adverse prognostic factor, this is no longer the case because of improvements in perioperative care. Currently, myasthenia actually may lead to improved survival as a result of earlier detection of thymomas.[77]

THYMIC CARCINOMA

Thymic carcinoma is a rare aggressive thymic neoplasm that has a poor prognosis. Like thymoma, it is an epithelial tumor, but cytologically it exhibits malignant features. Extensive local invasion and distant metastases are common. Suster and Rosai[78] reported on 60 patients ranging in age from 10 to 76 years and with a slight male predominance. Nearly 70% of patients had symptoms of cough, chest pain, or superior vena cava syndrome. Myasthenia and other thymoma-associated syndromes are rare.

The histologic classification of thymic carcinoma was proposed by Levine and Rosai[79] and revised by Suster and Rosai.[78] The tumors are classified broadly as low or high grade. Low-grade tumors include squamous cell carcinoma, mucoepidermoid carcinoma, and basaloid carcinoma. High-grade neoplasms include lymphoepithelioma-like carcinoma and small cell, undifferentiated, sarcomatoid, and clear-cell carcinomas.[78,80–82] The classification of thymic carcinoma has prognostic significance, with low-grade tumors following a favorable clinical course (median survival rates of 25.4 months to more than 6.6 years) because of a low incidence of local recurrence and metastasis and high-grade malignancies exhibiting an aggressive clinical course (median survival of only 11.3 to 15.0 months).[78,80] Although the Masaoka thymoma staging system[78,80] and a proposed tumor-node-metastasis classification system[83] have been used in staging thymic carcinoma, their use is unproven. The histologic grade remains the best prognostic indicator.

The optimal treatment of thymic carcinoma remains undefined, but currently a multimodality approach, including surgical resection, postoperative radiation, and chemotherapy, is recommended. Initial surgical resection followed by radiation has been used in most studies.[69,78,80,81,83] Complete resection should be attempted but usually is not possible.[80,84] One analysis noted a 9.5-month median survival after resection and postoperative electron-beam radiation therapy,[69] with a trend toward improved survival in other studies.[78,80,81] Chemotherapy with cisplatin-based regimens similar to those used with thymomas has produced variable responses in small numbers of patients.[78,80,81] Combinations of doxorubicin, cyclophosphamide, and vincristine also have generated partial responses, as has the combination of 5-fluorouracil and leucovorin. Use of neoadjuvant chemotherapy has been reported in a small number of patients.[85]

The prognosis of thymic carcinoma is poor because of early metastatic involvement of pleura; lung; mediastinal, cervical, and axillary lymph nodes; bone; and liver.[78] The overall survival rate at 5 years is approximately 35%.[78,80] A reported Japanese experience noted an 88.2%, 51.7%, and 37.6% 5-year survival in patients with stages I/II, III, and IV, respectively.[76] Improved survival has been correlated with encapsulated tumors, lobular growth pattern, low mitotic activity, early-stage tumors, low histologic grade, and complete surgical resection.[78,84]

THYMIC CARCINOID

Thymic carcinoid tumors are rare, with fewer than 125 reported cases.[86-89] They occur predominantly in males[87] and originate from normal thymic Kulchitsky cells, which are part of the amine precursor uptake and decarboxylation group. Most have the ability to manufacture peptides, amines, kinins, and prostaglandins. They are aggressive tumors that invade locally and commonly metastasize to regional lymph nodes. Metastases occur in 70% of patients within 8 years of initial diagnosis.[89]

The gross appearance of thymic carcinoids is similar to that of thymomas, but they rarely are encapsulated. Microscopically, the tumors exhibit a ribbon-like growth pattern with rosette formation in a fibrovascular stroma. The cells are small, round, or oval with eosinophilic cytoplasm and uniformly round nuclei.[87] Immunohistochemical studies reveal argyrophilic cells that stain with cytokeratin and neuronal-specific enolase. Electron microscopy reveals the presence of secretory granules.[88] Thymic carcinoids, like other foregut carcinoids, are associated with Cushing's syndrome, multiple endocrine neoplasia, and, rarely, the carcinoid syndrome.[87-90]

The diagnosis of thymic carcinoid often requires open surgical biopsy. Complete surgical resection is recommended, although recurrence is common.[87-89] The effectiveness of adjuvant therapy is unproven, but most reports advocate adjuvant radiotherapy for incompletely resected tumors.[87-89] Chemotherapy rarely has been used in cases of metastatic or recurrent disease.[87-89]

Although a 5-year survival rate of 60% has been reported with complete surgical resection,[88] local recurrences are common and distant metastases occur in approximately 30% of patients.[87] The long-term prognosis is generally poor.

THYMOLIPOMA

Thymolipomas are rare benign neoplasms composed of mature adipose and thymic tissue, and they account for 1% to 5% of thymic neoplasms.[91] These tumors are also known as *lipothymomas, mediastinal lipomas with thymic remnants,* and *thymolipomatous hamartomas.*[91,92] In a review of 27 patients, Rosado-de-Christenson et al.[92] noted an equal gender distribution and a mean age of 27 years. Approximately 50% of patients presented with symptoms of vague chest pain, dyspnea, and tachypnea. Others have reported, in adults only, an association with MG, red cell aplasia, hypogammaglobulinemia, lichen planus, and Graves' disease.[91,93]

Thymolipomas are soft, lobulated, encapsulated tumors that originate in the anterior mediastinum. They often attain a large size before becoming symptomatic. They frequently conform to the shape of the cardiac and mediastinal structures and are found in the anterior inferior mediastinum "draped along the diaphragm" and connected to the thymus by a small pedicle.[92] Microscopically, the tumors are composed of thymic tissue, often with calcified Hassall's corpuscles, and more than 50% adipose tissue.[92] Histologically, thymolipomas do not appear malignant, and malignant transformation does not occur. Treatment involves complete resection. Long-term follow-up is not available, but recurrences have not been reported.

GERM CELL TUMORS

The vast majority of germ cell tumors arise within gonadal tissue, but the mediastinum is the most common site for the development of extragonadal germ cell tumors. They are most commonly seen in the anterior mediastinum and account for 10% to 15% of all primary mediastinal tumors.[1] These tumors have generated considerable interest because of their uncertain histogenesis.

ETIOLOGY

Extragonadal germ cell tumors are found along the body's midline from the cranium (pineal gland) to the presacral area. This line corresponds to the embryologic urogenital ridge. It is presumed that these tumors arise from malignant transformation of germ cells that have abnormally migrated during embryonic development.[94] Mediastinal germ cell neoplasms account for only 2% to 5% of all germinal tumors, but they constitute 50% to 70% of all extragonadal tumors.[94]

CLASSIFICATION

Mediastinal germ cell tumors are broadly classified as benign or malignant. Benign tumors include mature teratomas and mature teratomas with an immature component of less than 50%. Malignant germ cell tumors are divided into seminomas (dysgerminomas) and nonseminomatous tumors. Nonseminomatous tumors include embryonal carcinomas, choriocarcinomas, yolk sac tumors, and immature teratomas.[95] Seminomas may exist in a pure form, but any elevation of AFP indicates the presence of an element of a nonseminomatous tumor. In addition, mediastinal germ cell tumors have a propensity to develop a component of non–germ cell malignancy (e.g., rhabdomyosarcoma, adenocarcinoma, permeative neuroectodermal tumor), which can become the predominant histology.

INCIDENCE AND CLINICAL PRESENTATION

In adults, benign germ cell tumors have no gender predilection, but 90% of malignant germ cell tumors occur in men. In the pediatric population, benign and malignant extragonadal germ cell tumors occur with equal gender distribution. Mediastinal germ cell tumors are most commonly diagnosed in the third decade of life, but patients as old as 60 years of age have been reported. The incidence of these neoplasms is equal in all races. Many patients with benign tumors, including 50% of teratomas, are asymptomatic; however, 90% to 100% of patients with malignant tumors have symptoms of chest pain, dyspnea, cough, fever, or other findings related to compression or invasion of surrounding mediastinal structures.[96,97]

DIAGNOSIS

Mediastinal germ cell tumors are most often detected on the basis of standard chest radiographs. More than 95% of the chest films are abnormal, with almost all masses noted in the anterior mediastinum. Three percent to 8% of tumors arise within the posterior mediastinum.[97] Chest CT scans demonstrate the extent of disease, relationship to surrounding structures, and presence of cystic areas and calcification within the tumor. Abdominal imaging should be performed to assess for possible liver metastases. Although careful examination of the testes, including a testicular ultrasound, should always be performed, an isolated tumor mass in the anterior mediastinum without retroperitoneal involvement is not consistent with a primary testicular tumor. It is not necessary to perform blind orchiectomy or testicular biopsy in patients with normal physical examinations and unremarkable ultrasound findings.[94] Mediastinal sonography imaging patterns have been suggested as a means to improve the diagnostic accuracy of mediastinal teratomas.[98]

Determination of serum tumor markers is important in the diagnosis and follow-up of mediastinal germ cell tumors. Immunoassays for β-HCG and AFP should be obtained in all patients who possess mediastinal masses that are suspicious for germ cell tumors. Elevations of β-HCG and AFP confirm a malignant component to the tumor. AFP, β-HCG, or both are elevated in 80% to 85% of nonseminomatous germ cell tumors, with AFP being detected in 60% to 80% of these tumors and β-HCG in 30% to 50%.[96] Patients with benign teratomas have normal markers, and patients with pure seminoma may have low levels of β-HCG, but AFP is not detected.

TERATOMAS

Benign teratomas are the most common mediastinal germ cell tumor, accounting for 70% of the mediastinal germ cell tumors in children and 60% of those in adults. They can be seen in any age group but most commonly occur in adults from 20 to 40 years of age; there is no gender predilection.

Teratomas may be solid or cystic in appearance and are often referred to as *dermoid cysts* if unilocular. Teratomas contain elements from all three germ cell layers, with a predominance of the ectodermal component in most tumors, including skin, hair, sweat glands, sebaceous glands, and teeth. Mesoderm is represented by fat, smooth muscle, bone, and cartilage. Respiratory and intestinal epithelium are often seen as the endodermal component. The majority of mediastinal teratomas are composed of mature ectodermal, mesodermal, and endodermal elements and exhibit a benign course. Immature teratomas phenotypically may appear as a malignancy derived from these ectodermal, mesodermal, and endodermal elements. These latter tumors behave aggressively and generally are not responsive to systemic therapy.

Treatment of "benign" mediastinal teratoma includes complete surgical resection, which results in excellent long-term cure rates. Radiotherapy and chemotherapy play no role in the management of this tumor. The tumor may be adherent to surrounding structures, necessitating resection of pericardium, pleura, or lung. Complete resection of teratomas should be the goal of treatment. Resection of mature teratomas has been shown to result in prolonged survival with little chance of recurrence.[95] Immature teratomas are potentially malignant tumors; their prognosis is influenced by the anatomic site of the tumor, patient age, and the fraction of the tumor that is immature.[95] In patients younger than 15 years, immature teratomas behave similarly to their mature counterparts. In older patients, they may behave as highly malignant tumors. Currently, a trial of cisplatin-based combination chemotherapy (up to four cycles of cisplatin, etoposide, and bleomycin or vinblastine, ifosfamide, and cisplatin, if responding) is frequently administered before attempted surgical resection.[95]

SEMINOMA

Primary pure mediastinal seminoma accounts for approximately 35% of malignant mediastinal germ cell tumors; it is principally seen in men aged 20 to 40 years.[99] Seminomas grow slowly and metastasize later than their nonseminomatous counterparts, and they may have reached a large size by the time of diagnosis. Symptoms are usually related to compression or even invasion of surrounding mediastinal structures. Twenty percent to 30% of mediastinal seminomas are asymptomatic when discovered,[99] but metastases are present in 60% to 70% of patients. Pulmonary and other intrathoracic metastases are most commonly seen. Extrathoracic metastases usually involve bone.[99]

The treatment of mediastinal seminoma has evolved since the early 1970s. Definitive conclusions regarding treatment are difficult, because several potentially curative treatment modalities exist. Seminomas are extremely radiosensitive tumors, and for many years, high-dose mediastinal radiation has been used as initial therapy, resulting in long-term survival rates of 60% to 80%.[100] A review of recommendations for radiation therapy treatment in extragonadal seminoma was reported by Hainsworth and Greco.[99] Thirty-five to 40 Gy is the most commonly used radiation dose. Doses as low as 20 Gy have been reported to be curative, but most reports note a significant local recurrence rate with doses of less than 45 Gy.[99] Radiation portals should include a shaped mediastinal field and both supraclavicular areas.[99]

Mediastinal seminoma often presents as bulky, extensive, and locally invasive disease, requiring large radiotherapy portals. These portals result in excessive irradiation of surrounding normal lung, heart, and other mediastinal structures. Additionally, for 20% to 40% of patients in whom local control is achieved, treatment can be expected to fail at distant sites.[99]

Chemotherapy was previously used only in advanced gonadal seminoma, but encouraging results and the above-mentioned problems with radiotherapy have led to broadened indications;

chemotherapy is now being used as initial therapy in many patients with bulky tumors. Pure mediastinal seminoma falls into the intermediate-risk category of the new International Staging System for Germ Cell Tumors. Even patients with visceral metastases fall into this intermediate category and, as such, have a prognosis with cisplatin-based combination chemotherapy exceeding 75% for 5-year survival. Standard systemic therapy consists of cisplatin-based combination chemotherapy. Lemarie et al.[96] reported that 12 of 13 patients treated experienced complete remission, with two recurrences after treatment. Bokemeyer et al.[101] reported an international analysis of 51 patients with mediastinal seminoma. In this study, patients were treated with chemotherapy (38 = 74.5%), chemotherapy and radiation (10 = 19.6%), or radiation alone (3 = 5.9%). Chemotherapy was primarily cisplatin based (45/48 = 94%) but included carboplatin (3 = 6%), which had an inferior objective response rate (80% vs. 93%). The progression-free survival and overall survival were 77% and 88%, respectively, but patients with extrathoracic metastases (6 = 11.8%) had a worse prognosis. A collective review of 52 patients was undertaken by Hainsworth and Greco.[99] Fourteen patients had received prior radiation therapy, but all underwent chemotherapy with cisplatin and various combinations of cyclophosphamide, vinblastine, bleomycin, or etoposide. Complete responses to treatment were noted in 85% of patients, and 83% were long-term disease-free survivors.[99] Although radiotherapy is less toxic, chemotherapy appears to be superior, and therefore, cisplatin-based combination chemotherapy currently is recommended either with or without supradiaphragmatic radiation.

The management of patients with residual radiographic abnormalities after chemotherapy is controversial. Studies have shown that the residual mass is a dense scirrhous reaction in 85% to 90% of patients, and the presence of viable seminoma is rare. Others have shown a 25% incidence of residual viable seminoma in these patients treated with chemotherapy followed by resection of residual masses larger than 3 cm.[102] Close observation without surgery is recommended for residual masses after chemotherapy unless the mass enlarges.[102,103] Evaluation with PET scans has not proved helpful, and empiric radiation therapy is not recommended.[99,104]

Despite a report of 76.9% long-term survival using primary surgical resection followed by adjuvant therapy,[105] most authors believe that surgery does not play a role in the definitive treatment of seminoma.[100] In addition, surgical debulking of large tumors has not been shown to be of benefit in improving local control or survival.[99]

All patients with mediastinal seminoma should be treated with curative intent. Isolated mediastinal seminoma with minimal disease and without evidence of metastatic disease is most often managed with radiotherapy alone, with an excellent prognosis and long-term survival. Locally advanced and bulky disease should be treated initially with cisplatin-based combination chemotherapy, usually four cycles of cisplatin and etoposide, with radiotherapy, and followed by salvage chemotherapy (vinblastine, ifosfamide, and cisplatin) in the event of recurrence.[106] Patients with distant metastases should undergo cisplatin-based combination chemotherapy as initial treatment.

NONSEMINOMATOUS GERM CELL TUMORS

Nonseminomatous germ cell tumors include choriocarcinoma, embryonal carcinoma, teratoma, and endodermal sinus (yolk sac) tumors. They may occur in pure form, but in approximately one-third of cases, multiple cell types are present. Other malignant components, including adenocarcinomas, squamous cell carcinomas, and sarcomas, may be present or even represent the predominant tissue type, as usually occurs in immature teratomas.

Nearly 85% of nonseminomatous germ cell tumors occur in men, with a mean age of 29 years. Karyotypic analyses have been performed on a number of these patients, and the 47XXY pattern of Klinefelter's syndrome has been found in up to 20% of patients.[107] Mediastinal nonseminomatous germ cell tumors are most commonly found in the anterior mediastinum and appear grossly as lobulated masses with a thin capsule. They are frequently invasive at the time of diagnosis, with almost 90% of patients exhibiting symptoms. They appear on CT scans as large inhomogeneous masses containing areas of hemorrhage and necrosis. Elevated levels of β-HCG are seen in 30% to 50% of patients, and AFP is detected in 60% to 80%.

Nonseminomatous germ cell tumors carry a poorer prognosis than either pure extragonadal seminoma or their gonadal nonseminomatous counterparts, and all patients with primary mediastinal nonseminomatous germ cell tumors fall into the poor-risk category of the International Germ Cell Consensus Classification.[108] Eighty-five percent to 95% of patients have obvious distant metastases at the time of diagnosis. Common metastatic sites include lung, pleura, lymph nodes, liver, and, less commonly, bone.[99]

A number of non–germ cell malignant processes have been found in association with nonseminomatous germ cell tumors. One of the most interesting is that found in association with acute megakaryocytic leukemia. Other hematologic malignancies, such as acute myeloid leukemia, acute nonlymphocytic leukemia, erythroleukemia, myelodysplastic syndrome, malignant histiocytosis, and thrombocytosis, have all been reported. These malignancies may antedate the discovery of the germ cell tumor or occur synchronously. Solid tumors, such as embryonal rhabdomyosarcoma, small cell undifferentiated carcinoma, neuroblastoma, and adenocarcinoma have been described and occur more frequently in primary mediastinal tumors compared to gonadal germ cell neoplasms.[94]

The diagnosis of nonseminomatous germ cell tumors can often be made without tissue biopsy.[100] In many centers, the presence of an anterior mediastinal mass in a young male with elevated serum tumor markers (AFP and β-HCG) is adequate to initiate treatment. If a tissue diagnosis is deemed necessary, fine-needle–guided aspiration with cytologic staining for tumor markers can be used for confirmation. An anterior mediastinotomy provides the best exposure for open biopsy if necessary.[100]

Treatment of nonseminomatous germ cell tumors incorporates cisplatin-based chemotherapy, which has markedly improved the prognosis in these patients. In the past, long-term survival after treatment of nonseminomatous germ cell tumors was very rare; today, however, overall complete remission rates of 40% to 50% are obtained in most series.[95,96,99,101] Treatment is initiated with cisplatin-containing combination chemotherapy, which often includes etoposide and bleomycin. Treatment should be administered every 3 weeks for four courses; patients should then be restaged with serum tumor markers and CT scans of the chest and abdomen.[99] In a collective review of 158 patients undergoing a variety of combination chemotherapeutic regimens for the initial treatment of nonseminomatous germ cell tumors, complete responses were noted in 54% of patients, and 42% were long-term disease-free survivors.[99] In an international review of 287 patients, responses were noted in 178 of 278 patients who received chemotherapy (64%) and the progression-free and overall survival were 44% and 45%, respectively.[101]

Patients with negative tumor markers and no radiographic evidence of residual disease after initial chemotherapy require no further treatment. Persistent elevation of serum tumor markers, particularly if they begin to rise again, usually requires salvage chemotherapy.[99] Patients with normal serum tumor markers but radiographic evidence of residual masses after induction chemotherapy should undergo surgical resection 4 to 6 weeks after completion of chemotherapy.[99,100] Complete resection should be attempted, because debulking procedures provide no benefit. Patients found to have residual viable germ cell tumor undergo two additional cycles of chemotherapy. Patients with immature teratoma or non–germ cell malignancies can simply be observed after complete resection. Nichols[94] reports complete remissions in 18 of 31 patients using this regimen, and other series report complete remission rates of 50% to 70%, with long-term survival rates approximating 50%.[108] Equivalent results are obtained in all histologic subtypes.

The treatment of recurrent disease is difficult, because patients with relapsing mediastinal nonseminomatous germ cell tumors do extraordinarily poorly with salvage therapy, such as vinblastine, ifosfamide, and cisplatin[109]; optimal therapy has not been determined. Standard salvage chemotherapy has not proved beneficial, with only 9 of 79 patients (11%) becoming disease free in one study[101] and few patients ever achieving durable remissions. High-dose chemotherapy with stem cell rescue is effective in only a few selected patients.[110] Occasionally, surgical resection of residual disease despite persistently elevated tumor markers can be beneficial.[111]

MESENCHYMAL TUMORS

Mediastinal mesenchymal tumors, or soft tissue tumors, originate from the connective tissue elements of the mediastinum. Smooth and striated muscle, lymphatic tissue, fat, and vascular tissue all give rise to a variety of neoplasms, which may be benign or malignant. Most of these tumors also occur in other parts of the body and are discussed in detail in Chapter 35.1.

Mesenchymal tumors account for approximately 6% of primary mediastinal neoplasms.[1] They are less common in the mediastinum than in other locations. Approximately 55% are malignant, and there is no gender predilection. In general, treatment of malignant mesenchymal tumors involves combination therapy, including surgical resection, radiation therapy, and chemotherapy. Benign tumors should be excised completely, after which little chance of recurrence remains.

Lipomas are the most common mesenchymal tumor of the mediastinum, representing 2% of all mediastinal neoplasms.[1] Benign lipomas are most often located in the anterior mediastinum. They may grow to large size without symptoms. Treatment is complete resection, and although local recurrence is possible, it is unusual. Malignant liposarcoma is more commonly found in the posterior mediastinum.

Fibromas are encapsulated asymptomatic tumors that may grow to a very large size. Fibrosarcomas often are symptomatic malignancies associated with hypoglycemia. Fibromas

are cured with complete surgical excision, but fibrosarcomas are usually unresectable and respond poorly to radiation and chemotherapy.[10] Leiomyomas, leiomyosarcomas, rhabdomyomas, rhabdomyosarcomas, synovial cell sarcomas, mesotheliomas, and xanthogranulomas also occasionally occur in the mediastinum.[1,112]

Vascular tumors of the mediastinum include hemangiomas, hemangioendotheliomas, and benign and malignant hemangiopericytomas.[1,112] Ten percent to 30% of all vascular tumors are malignant. Mediastinal hemangiomas represent 0.5% of all mediastinal neoplasms but are the most common vascular tumor. They may be cavernous or capillary and are often associated with hemangiomas in other areas of the body.[113] Sixty percent occur in the anterior mediastinum, and 25% occur posteriorly. Diagnosis is best accomplished by CT scan or MRI, in which phleboliths may be seen in 30% of these tumors. Angiography is important in identifying and embolizing major feeding vessels before surgery.[113] Total excision is considered the treatment of choice; however, large, incompletely resected hemangiomas usually do not recur.

Lymphangiomas, also known as *cystic hygromas*, often extend into the anterior mediastinum from the cervical area. Seventeen percent are located exclusively in the mediastinum. They tend to enlarge as patients grow, particularly during puberty. Treatment involves surgical resection, but this is often difficult because of adherence to surrounding structures. Response to radiation is variable. Other lymphatic soft tissue tumors include lymphangiosarcoma and lymphangiopericytoma.

NEUROGENIC TUMORS

Thoracic neurogenic tumors occur most commonly in the posterior mediastinum but occasionally are found in the anterior mediastinum and elsewhere. They compose between 19% and 39% of all mediastinal tumors[114] and 75% of posterior mediastinal tumors. They originate from peripheral nerves (nerves of the brachial plexus and intercostal nerves), autonomic sympathetic ganglia, and, rarely, from the vagus nerve. Neurogenic tumors in the anterior mediastinum originate in chemoreceptor paragangliomas.

Whereas neurogenic tumors in infants and children are frequently malignant and often present with metastatic disease, in adults the majority of these tumors are benign. They occur without gender predilection at any age but are more likely in young adults. Often asymptomatic, they are solitary (except in neurofibromatosis) and found on a routine chest x-ray. Benign tumors can attain a considerable size. They frequently arise in the paravertebral sulcus from the posterior roots of the spinal nerves at the zone of transition between the central and peripheral myelin. They also may arise on the posterior portion of the spinal nerve root in the spinal canal and grow through the intervertebral foramen into the paravertebral area, giving rise to the appearance of a dumbbell- or hourglass-shaped tumor. These tumors must be recognized to plan an appropriate operation in conjunction with a neurosurgeon. Depending on their size and location, lesions may cause spinal cord compression, pain, paresthesias, Horner's syndrome, and muscle atrophy. Superior vena cava syndrome, dyspnea, cough, and bony erosions, which wrongly suggest a malignant process, also have been described.

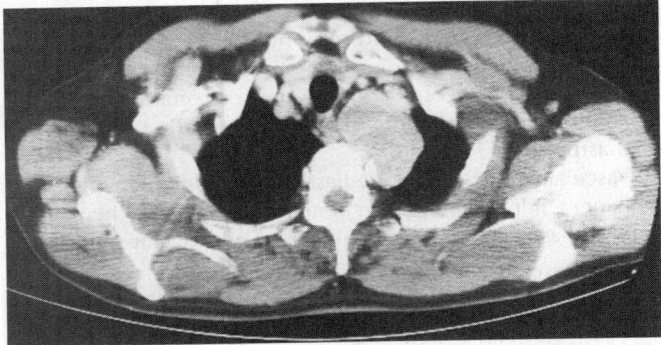

FIGURE 28-2. Schwannoma in the paravertebral area in the apex of the left chest.

NEURILEMOMA (SCHWANNOMA)

Neurilemoma (schwannoma) is the most common tumor in the paravertebral sulcus. Arising from the intercostal nerve sheath, the tumor is encapsulated, white or yellowish pink in color, with calcifications and cystic degeneration. Histologically, it is composed of uniform, slender, biphasic fusiform cells with elongated, twisted nuclei that have a tendency to align in a regimented or palisaded appearance.[115] The tumor may contain large blood vessels and may be a source of considerable blood loss during surgical removal. Schwannoma can be further differentiated into melanotic, adenomatous, or psammomatous tumors (Fig. 28-2).[115]

NEUROFIBROMA

Neurofibromas are most often benign and asymptomatic. However, they can have an intradural as well as an extradural component and may cause symptoms of cord compression. They are not encapsulated and may have a plexiform appearance. Microscopically, neurofibromas have a heterogeneous cell population, but Schwann cell differentiation is not always present. Neurogenic tumors can be differentiated from leiomyomas, meningiomas, and fibrous histiocytomas by the immunohistochemical identification of S-100 protein. Solitary neurofibromas are cured by surgical excision.

Neurofibromas can occur as multiple lesions in von Recklinghausen's disease. Neurofibromatosis is inherited as an autosomal dominant trait affecting both genders equally; however, approximately one-half of the cases are sporadic.[116] The clinical features vary and include hyperpigmented café au lait skin spots, skin and subcutaneous multiple neurofibromas (hamartomas), scoliosis, bowing of long bones, disorders of sexual development, and multiple neurogenic tumors and malignancies, such as malignant schwannomas.[117] Mediastinal neurofibromas may be multiple and appear as long plexiform masses. Histologically, they consist of large nerve fibers mixed with connective tissue stroma containing Schwann cells and fibroblasts. Surgical intervention is justified for lesions located in the spinal canal that cause spinal cord or nerve root compression. The prognosis generally is poor.[118]

MALIGNANT SCHWANNOMA

Malignant schwannomas are the malignant counterparts of neurilemomas and neurofibromas. Ultrastructural studies, however, cannot always document Schwann cells in these tumors derived from nerve sheaths, and therefore the terms *malignant nerve sheath tumor, neurogenic sarcoma,* and *neurofibrosarcoma* are sometimes used.[118] Malignant nerve sheath tumors commonly are large. They are painful and may cause superior vena cava obstruction, Horner's syndrome, dyspnea, dysphagia, hoarseness, and invasion of the lung, bones, and aorta, depending on their location and size.

The diagnostic criteria for malignant nerve sheath tumors are controversial.[116] Origin from a major nerve, presence of Schwann cells and S-100 protein, the diagnosis of neurofibromatosis, and nuclear palisading are important features. Histologic findings include hypercellularity, pleomorphic dense nuclei, multiple and abnormal mitoses, and invasion of the surrounding structures. The malignant nerve sheath tumors are usually large (often larger than 5 cm in diameter), partially encapsulated, soft, and gray, with hemorrhage and necrosis. Histologically, they are composed of spindle cells with comma-shaped, irregular nuclei. Neural and perineural invasion, mature cartilage, bone, striated muscle, squamous differentiation, and mucin-secreting glands also may be seen.[119,120]

Clinically, these tumors are aggressive, locally invasive, and highly metastatic. They often recur after resection, leading to a 75% 5-year survival rate. Patients with neurofibromatosis and a malignant nerve sheath tumor have a 15% to 30% 5-year survival rate. Combination chemotherapy is recommended in stage III and IV disease (Fig. 28-3).

TUMORS OF SYMPATHETIC GANGLIA

Mediastinal ganglioneuromas are found in the posterior mediastinum along the sympathetic chain in children older than 4 years and in adults in the third and fourth decades of life. Occasionally, a neuroblastoma may mature into a benign ganglioneuroma.[121] The tumor usually is asymptomatic but sometimes presents with Horner's syndrome and, rarely, with diarrhea caused by production of vasoactive intestinal polypeptide. Ganglioneuromas have a smooth contour and contain areas of stippled calcification. They may resemble other benign neurogenic tumors, causing rib erosions.[122] Microscopically, spindle cell proliferation is seen that appears identical to that in a neurofibroma, except that ganglioneuromas exhibit the presence of large ganglion cells. Ganglioneuromas are benign tumors, although regional lymph nodes may contain islands of tumor cells attributed to matured neuroblasts.[116] They require complete excision.

NEUROBLASTOMAS

Although neuroblastomas usually originate in the adrenal glands and along nerve plexuses, they can be found in any location where embryonic neuroblasts from the neural crest migrate. In the chest, they occur along the sympathetic trunk in the paravertebral sulcus. This tumor is the most common malignancy of early childhood, occurring most commonly in the first 2 years of life. Patients with mediastinal neuroblastomas usually are symptomatic and frequently have metastatic disease.[123] Symptoms are related to local compression (Horner's syndrome and heterochromia of the iris) or to systemic release of vasoactive peptides, such as catecholamines, vanil-

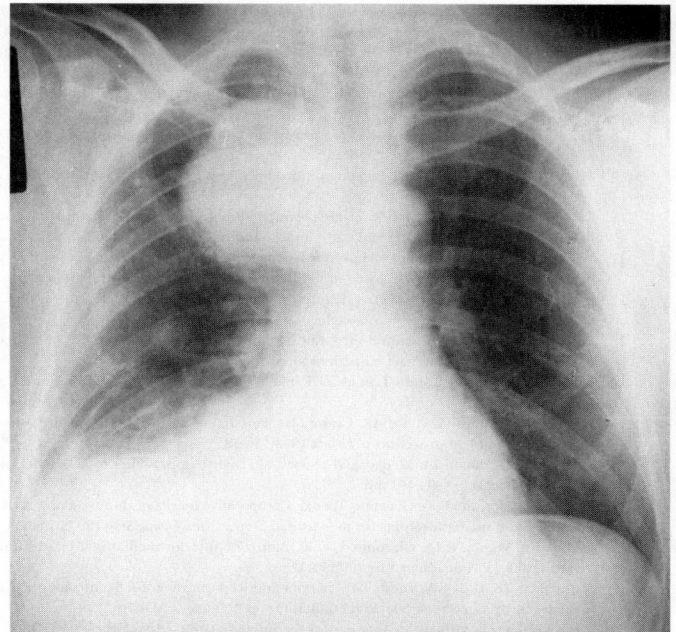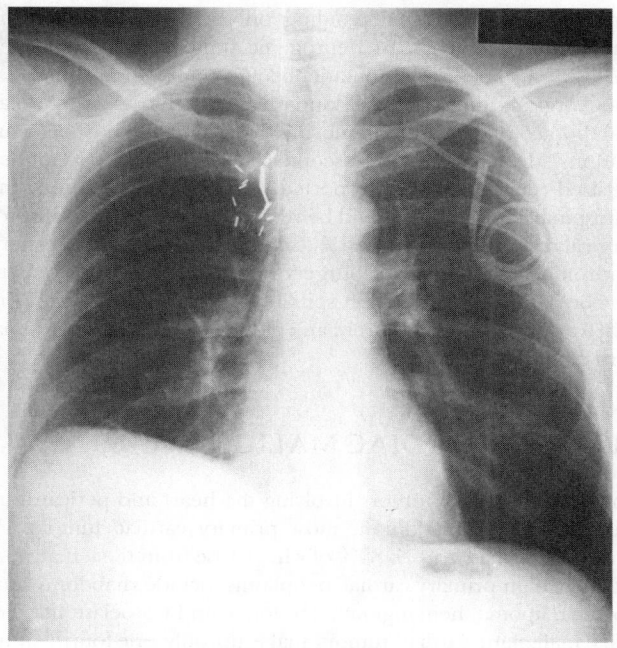

FIGURE 28-3. **A:** Malignant neurofibroma, initially considered to be nonresectable, in a 34-year-old man. **B:** The tumor was resected after a combination of chemotherapy and radiation therapy.

lylmandelic acid, homovanillic acid, and 3-methoxy-4-hydroxyphenylglycol. Encephalopathy, myasthenia, and Cushing's syndrome may be present.[124] Radiographically, a mass is seen in the posterior mediastinum, with stippled calcifications, skeletal erosion, and occasional extension into the spinal canal.

Pathology reveals lobulated gray or red tumors with hemorrhagic areas. Microscopically, small cells with scant cytoplasm and polygonal nuclei exhibit various degrees of differentiation. Intracytoplasmic neurofilaments and neurosecretory granules and extracellular material seen on electron microscopy distinguish neuroblastoma from other childhood tumors, such as lymphoma, Ewing's sarcoma, and rhabdomyosarcoma.

Neuroblastomas are highly aggressive tumors. Survival depends on the age of the patient, the stage of disease, the location of the tumor, and histologic differentiation. The prognosis is better in patients younger than 1 year of age and in those with limited, well-differentiated tumors. Neuroblastomas may regress spontaneously or undergo maturation into ganglioneuromas. Ganglioneuroblastomas have a better prognosis than neuroblastomas.[125] The staging system for neuroblastoma is shown in Table 28-8. Treatment for stage I and II disease is surgical resection; adjuvant postoperative radiotherapy is recommended only for stage II tumors. For stage III and IV, a combination of chemotherapy and radiation is advised.

GRANULAR CELL TUMOR

Granular cell tumors (granular cell myoblastomas) are considered benign. They are found in the posterior mediastinum and are derived from Schwann cells. They are soft, gray, and poorly circumscribed tumors consisting of uniform polygonal cells either in nests or strands with eosinophilic granular cytoplasm and a stroma of fibrous connective tissue.[126] Resection is always curative.

DIAGNOSIS

Although posterior mediastinal neoplasms are predominately neurogenic, other tumors also must be considered in the differential diagnosis. Goiters, esophageal leiomyomas, solitary fibrous tumors, and bronchial/esophageal duplication cysts all have been reported. Once identified, the nature of these lesions, their relationship to other structures, and the presence of distant metastases can be determined by CT scans. MRI scans can define vascular involvement and provide multiplanar views that are valuable in assessing tumor extension into paravertebral foramina. An iodine 131 nuclear scan may be helpful if a goiter is suspected.

Histologic diagnosis is not necessary before surgery. However, if surgical resection is not contemplated, a definitive diagnosis is required for further treatment planning. This diagnosis generally requires a generous biopsy obtained by an open surgical procedure or a CT-guided core-needle biopsy.

MANAGEMENT

If no contraindication is present, resection of all neurogenic tumors is advised. Neurogenic tumors grow and can cause life-

TABLE 28-8. Staging System for Neuroblastoma

Stage	Description
I	Tumor is limited to site of origin.
II	Tumor extends beyond site of origin or, when limited to site of origin, has metastatic regional lymph nodes present on same side.
III	Tumor extends to contralateral side.
IV	Metastases are present beyond regional lymph nodes.

threatening symptoms, depending on their size and location. Therefore, observation of neurogenic tumors may be justified only with a stable, asymptomatic, benign tumor in an otherwise poor surgical candidate. The standard approach uses a posterolateral thoracotomy incision, removing the tumor with normal tissue margins. More recently, thorascopic resection of small- to moderate-sized tumors has been reported.[127] In dumbbell tumors, the intraspinal component should be removed first. The mortality for surgical resection is less than 1%. Complications include Horner's syndrome and chylothorax. Surgery with spinal canal involvement may be complicated by direct spinal cord trauma, ischemia from spinal artery injury, and, rarely, an epidural hematoma with spinal cord compression.

PRIMARY CARDIAC MALIGNANCIES

The vast majority of tumors involving the heart and pericardium are metastatic. In addition, most primary cardiac tumors are benign myxomas, 75% to 80% of which arise from the left atrium. Other benign primary cardiac neoplasms include rhabdomyoma, fibroma, lipoma, hemangioma, teratoma, and fibroelastoma. Primary malignant cardiac tumors make up only one-fourth of all primary cardiac neoplasms and most commonly originate from the atria.[128] Many are sarcomas,[129] including angiosarcoma,[130] rhabdomyosarcoma, leiomyosarcoma,[131] fibrosarcoma,[132] lymphoma, malignant fibrous histiocytoma,[133] and mesothelioma of the pericardium.[134] Pheochromocytomas also occur.

A high index of suspicion is imperative in establishing a diagnosis, because presenting symptoms often mimic other nonneoplastic cardiac diseases, such as right heart failure and even tamponade requiring drainage. Whole body gallium scans,[135] echocardiography, CT, and MRI all may serve to localize a primary cardiac neoplasm. With the advent of electrocardiographic gating, MRI has taken the forefront in imaging of cardiac lesions.[136] Although complete surgical resection is required for cure, negative margins usually are not possible,[137]and up to 80% of primary cardiac malignancies present with systemic metastases.[138]

Adjuvant chemotherapy and external-beam radiotherapy can be administered, but a report from the Institut Gustave Roussy does not support the routine use of adjuvant chemotherapy for primary cardiac sarcomas.[133] Neoadjuvant (induction) chemotherapy has been reported with a response and subsequent surgical resection.[139]

New surgical techniques, including orthotopic and autotransplantation, may be beneficial in highly selected patients.[140] With the advent of "gating" technology and sophisticated treatment planning, more accurate targeting with electron-beam radiation therapy may be possible, similar to stereotactic radiosurgery of the brain. Currently, long-term survival is rare.

REFERENCES

1. Davis RD, Oldham HN, Sabiston DC. Primary cysts and neoplasms of the mediastinum: recent changes in clinical presentation, methods of diagnosis, management, and results. *Ann Thorac Surg* 1987;44:229.
2. Azarow KS, Pearl RH, Zurcher R, Edwards FH, Cohen AJ. Primary mediastinal masses: a comparison of adult and pediatric populations. *J Thorac Cardiovasc Surg* 1993;106:67.
3. Strollo DC, Rosado-de-Christenson ML, Jett JR. Primary mediastinal tumors. Part II. Tumors of the middle and posterior mediastinum. *Chest* 1997;112:1344.
4. Simpson I, Campbell PE. Mediastinal masses in childhood: a review from a pediatric pathologist's point of view. *Prog Pediatr Surg* 1991;27:93.
5. Davis RD, Oldham HN, Sabiston DC. The mediastinum. In: Sabiston DC, Spencer FC, eds. *Surgery of the chest*, 5th ed. Philadelphia: WB Saunders, 1989.
6. Weisbrod GL, Herman SJ. Mediastinal masses: diagnosis with non-invasive techniques. *Semin Thorac Cardiovasc Surg* 1992;4:3.
7. Naidich DP. Helical computed tomography of the thorax: clinical applications. *Radiol Clin North Am* 1994;32:759.
8. Tomiyama H, Muller NL, Ellis SJ, et al. Invasive and noninvasive thymoma: distinctive CT features. *J Comput Assist Tomogr* 2001;25:388.
9. Mayo JR. Magnetic resonance imaging of the chest: where we stand. *Radiol Clin North Am* 1994;32:795.
10. Rinadi TP, Batocchi AP, Evoli A, et al. Thymic lesions and myasthenia gravis: diagnosis based on mediastinal imaging and pathological findings. *Acta Radiol* 2002;43:380.
11. Wernecke K, Vassallo P, Potter R, Lukener HG, Peters PE. Mediastinal tumors: sensitivity of detection with sonography compared with CT and radiography. *Radiology* 1990;175:137.
12. Faletra F, Ravini M, Moreo A, et al. Transesophageal echocardiography in the evaluation of mediastinal masses. *J Am Soc Echocardiogr* 1992;5:178.
13. Larsen SS, Krasnik M, Vilmann P, et al. Endoscopic ultrasound guided biopsy of mediastinal lesions has a major impact on patient management. *Thorax* 2002;57:98.
14. Kubota K, Yamada S, Kondo T, et al. PET imaging of primary mediastinal tumours. *Br J Cancer* 1996;73:882.
15. Morrissey B, Adams H, Gibbs AR, Crane MD. Percutaneous needle biopsy of the mediastinum: review of 94 procedures. *Thorax* 1993;48:632.
16. Bressler EL, Kirkham JA. Mediastinal masses: alternative approaches to CT-guided needle biopsy. *Radiology* 1994;191:391.
17. Rendina EA, Venuta F, DeGiacomo T, et al. Comparative merits of thoracoscopy, mediastinoscopy, and mediastinotomy for mediastinal biopsy. *Ann Thorac Surg* 1994;57:992.
18. Redina EA, Venuta F, De Giacomo T, et al. Biopsy of anterior mediastinal masses under local anesthesia. *Ann Thorac Surg* 2002;74:1720.
19. Skandalakis JE, Gray SW, Todd NW. Pharynx and its derivatives. In: Skandalakis JE, Gray SW, eds. *Embryology for surgeons*, 2nd ed. Baltimore: Williams & Wilkins, 1994.
20. VonGaudecker B. Functional histology of the human thymus. *Anat Embryol* 1991;183:1.
21. Jaretski A, Wolff M. "Maximal" thymectomy for myasthenia gravis: surgical anatomy and operative technique. *J Thorac Cardiovasc Surg* 1988;96:711.
22. Fukai I, Funato Y, Mizuno T, Hasimoto T, Masaoka A. Distribution of thymic tissue in the mediastinal adipose tissue. *J Thorac Cardiovasc Surg* 1991;101:1099.
23. Blossom GB, Ernstoff RM, Howells GA, Bendick PJ, Glover JL. Thymectomy for myasthenia gravis. *Arch Surg* 1993;128:855.
24. Thomas CR Jr, Wright CD, Loehrer PJ Sr. Thymoma: state of the art. *J Clin Oncol* 1999;17:2280.
25. Engels EA, Pfeiffer RM. Malignant thymoma in the United States: demographic patterns in incidence and associations with subsequent malignancies. *Int J Cancer* 2003;105:546.
26. Patterson GA. Thymomas. *Semin Thorac Cardiovasc Surg* 1992;4:39.
27. Rosai J, Levine GD. Tumors of the thymus. In: *Atlas of tumor pathology*. Series 2, Fascicle 13. Washington, DC, Armed Forces Institute of Pathology, 1976;34:55.
28. Marino M, Muller-Hermelink HK. Thymoma and thymic carcinoma: relation of thymoma epithelial cells to the cortical and medullary differentiation of thymus. *Virchows Arch A Pathol Anat Histopathol* 1985;407:119.
29. Kirchner T, Muller-Hermelink H. New approaches to the diagnosis of thymic epithelial tumors. *Prog Surg Pathol* 1989;10:167.
30. Quintanilla-Martinez L, Wilkins EW, Choi N, et al. Thymoma: histologic subclassification is an important prognostic factor. *Cancer* 1994;74:606.
31. Shimosato Y. Controversies surrounding the subclassification of thymoma. *Cancer* 1994;74:542.
32. Suster S, Moran CA. Primary thymic epithelial neoplasms: current concepts and controversies. In: Fechner RE, Rosen PP, eds. *Anatomic pathology*, vol 2. Chicago: ASCP Press, 1997:1.
33. Marx A, Muller-Hermelink HK. From basic immunobiology to the upcoming WHO-classification of tumors of the thymus. *Pathol Res Pract* 1999;195:515.
34. Masaoka A, Monden Y, Nakahara K, Tanioka T. Follow-up study of thymomas with special reference to their clinical stages. *Cancer* 1981;48:2485.
35. Gamondes JP, Balawi A, Greenland T, et al. Seventeen years of surgical treatment of thymoma: factors influencing survival. *Eur J Cardiothorac Surg* 1991;5:124.
36. Sasaki H, Ide N, Fukai I, et al. Gene expression analysis of human thymoma correlates with tumor stage. *Int J Cancer* 2002;101:342.
37. Berrih-Akin S, Morel E, Raimond F, et al. The role of the thymus in myasthenia gravis: immunohistological and immunological studies in 115 cases. *Ann N Y Acad Sci* 1987;505:51.
38. Lopez-Cano M, Ponseti-Bosch JM, Espin-Basany E, Sanchez-Garcia JL, Armengol-Carrasco M. Clinical and pathologic predictors of outcome in thymoma-associated myasthenia gravis. *Ann Thorac Surg* 2003;76:1643.
39. Palmisani MT, Evoli A, Batocchi AP, Provenzano C, Torali P. Myasthenia gravis associated with thymoma: clinical characteristics and long term outcome. *Eur Neurol* 1993;34:78.
40. Masaoka A, Hashimoto T, Shibata K, Yamakowa Y, Nakamae K. Thymomas associated with pure red cell aplasia: histology and follow-up studies. *Cancer* 1989;64:1872.
41. Palmieri G, Lastoria S, Cala O, et al. Successful treatment of a patient with a thymoma and pure red cell aplasia with octreotide and prednisone. *N Engl J Med* 1997;336:263.
42. Maggi G, Casadio C, Cavallo A, et al. Thymoma: results of 241 operated cases. *Ann Thorac Surg* 1991;51:152.
43. Cowen D, Mornex RF, Bachelot T, et al. Thymoma: results of a multicentric retrospective series of 149 non-metastatic irradiated patients and review of the literature. *Radiother Oncol* 1995;34:9.
44. Kaiser LR. Thymoma: the use of minimally invasive resection techniques. *Chest Surg Clin N Am* 1994;4:185.
45. Nakahara K, Ohno K, Hashimoto J, et al. Thymoma: results of complete resection and adjuvant postoperative irradiation in 141 consecutive patients. *J Thorac Cardiovasc Surg* 1988;95:1041.

46. Crucitti F, Daghetto GB, Bellantone R, et al. Effects of surgical treatment in thymoma with myasthenia gravies: our experience in 103 patients. *J Surg Oncol* 1992;50:43.

47. Ciernik IF, Meier U, Lutolf UM. Prognostic factors and outcome of incompletely resected invasive thymoma following radiation therapy. *J Clin Oncol* 1994;12:1484.

48. Kirschner PA. Reoperation for thymoma: report of 23 cases. *Ann Thorac Surg* 1990;49:550.

49. Urgesi A, Monetti U, Rossi G, et al. Aggressive treatment of intrathoracic recurrences of thymoma. *Radiother Oncol* 1992;24:221.

50. Koh WJ, Loehrer PJ Sr, Thomas CR Jr. Thymoma: the role of radiation and chemotherapy. In: Wood DE, Thomas CR Jr, eds. Mediastinal tumors: update 1995. Medical radiology-diagnostic imaging and radiation oncology volume. Heidelberg, Germany: Springer-Verlag, 1995:19.

51. Pollack A, Komaki R, Cox JD, et al. Thymoma: treatment and prognosis. *Int J Radiat Oncol Biol Phys* 1992;23:1037.

52. Quintanilla-Martinez L, Wilkins EW Jr, Ferry JA, et al. Thymoma: morphologic subclassification correlates with invasiveness and immunohistologic features. A study of 122 cases. *Hum Pathol* 1993;24:958.

53. Harris N. Classification of thymic epithelial neoplasms. In: Marx A, Muller-Hermelink HK, eds. *Epithelial tumors of the thymus. Pathology, biology, treatment.* New York: Plenum Publishing, 1997:1.

54. Haniuda M, Miyazawa M, Yoshida K, et al. Is postoperative radiotherapy for thymoma effective? *Ann Surg* 1996;224:219.

55. Mornex F, Resbeut M, Richard P, et al. Radiotherapy and chemotherapy for invasive thymomas: a multicentric retrospective review of 90 cases. *Int J Radiat Oncol Biol Phys* 1995;32:651.

56. Latz D, Schraube P, Oppitz U, et al. Invasive thymoma: treatment with postoperative radiation therapy. *Radiology* 1997;204:859.

57. Graham MV, Emami B. Mediastinum and trachea. In: Perez CA, Brady LW, eds. *Principles and practice of radiation oncology,* 3rd ed. Philadelphia: Lippincott–Raven Publishers, 1997:1221.

58. Roach M III, Vijayakumar S. The role of three-dimensional conformal radiotherapy in the treatment of mediastinal tumors. In: Wood DE, Thomas CR Jr, eds. *Mediastinal tumors: update 1995. Medical radiology-diagnostic imaging and radiation oncology volume.* Heidelberg, Germany: Springer-Verlag, 1995:117.

59. Marks LB. The impact of organ structure on radiation response. *Int J Radiat Oncol Biol Phys* 1996;34:1165.

60. Thomas CR Jr, Williams TE, Turrisi AT III. Lung toxicity in the treatment of lung cancer: thoughts at the end of the millennium. In: Meyer J, Karger T, eds. *Radiation injury: prevention and treatment. Frontiers of radiation therapy and oncology.* Basel, Switzerland: Karger Medical and Scientific Publishers, 1999.

61. Bogart J, Sagerman RH. High-dose hemithorax irradiation in a patient with recurrent thymoma: a study of pulmonary and cardiac radiation tolerance. *Am J Clin Oncol* 1999;22:441.

62. Tomiak EM, Evans WK. The role of chemotherapy in invasive thymoma: a review of the literature and considerations for future clinical trials. *Crit Rev Oncol Hematol* 1993;15:113.

63. Harper P, Highly M, Rankin E, et al. The treatment of malignant thymoma with single agent ifosfamide. *Br J Cancer* 1991;63[Suppl 13]:7.

64. Kirkove C, Berghmans J, Noel H, Van de Merckt J. Dramatic response of recurrent invasive thymoma to high dose corticosteroids. *Clin Oncol* 1992;4:64.

65. Fornasiero A, Danilele O, Ghiotto C, et al. Chemotherapy for invasive thymoma: a 13 year experience. *Cancer* 1991;68:30.

66. Loehrer PJ, Kim KM, Aisner SC, et al. Cisplatin plus doxorubicin plus cyclophosphamide in metastatic or recurrent thymoma: final results of an intergroup trial. *J Clin Oncol* 1994;12:1164.

67. Park HS, Shin DM, Lee JS, et al. Thymoma: a retrospective study of 87 cases. *Cancer* 1994;73:2491.

68. Giaccone G, Ardizzoni A, Kirkpatrick A, et al. Cisplatin and etoposide combination chemotherapy for locally advanced or metastatic thymoma: a phase II study of the European organization for research and treatment of lung cancer cooperative group. *J Clin Oncol* 1996;14:814.

69. Loehrer PJ, Jiroutek M, Aisner S, et al. Phase II trial of etoposide (V), ifosfamide (I), plus cis-platin (P) in patients with advanced thymoma (T) or thymic carcinoma (TC): preliminary results from a ECOG coordinated intergroup trial. *Proc Am Soc Clin Oncol* 1998;17:30(abst 118).

70. Rea F, Sartori F, Lay M, et al. Chemotherapy and operation for invasive thymoma. *J Cardiovasc Surg* 1993;106:543.

71. Macchiarini P, Chella A, Ducci F, et al. Neoadjuvant chemotherapy, surgery and postoperative radiation therapy for invasive thymoma. *Cancer* 1991;68:706.

72. Shin DM, Walsh GL, Komaki R, et al. A multidisciplinary approach to therapy for unresectable malignant thymoma. *Ann Intern Med* 1998;129:100.

73. Loehrer PJ Sr, Chen M, Kim KM, et al. Cisplatin, doxorubicin, and cyclophosphamide plus thoracic radiation therapy for limited-stage unresectable thymoma: an intergroup trial. *J Clin Oncol* 1997;15:3093.

74. Bernatz PE, Harrison EG, Clagget OT. Thymomas: a clinicopathologic study. *J Thorac Cardiovasc Surg* 1961;42:424.

75. Muller-Hermelink HK, Marx A, Gender K, Kirchner T. The pathological basis of thymoma-associated myasthenia gravis. *Ann N Y Acad Sci* 1993;681:56.

76. Kondo K, Monden Y. Therapy for thymic epithelial tumors: a clinical study of 1,320 patients from Japan. *Ann Thorac Surg* 2003;76:878.

77. Nieto IP, Robledo JP, Pajuelo MC, et al. Prognostic factors for myasthenia gravis treated by thymectomy: review of 61 cases. *Ann Thorac Surg* 1999;67:1568.

78. Suster S, Rosai J. Thymic carcinoma: a clinicopathologic study of 60 cases. *Cancer* 1991;67:1025.

79. Levine GD, Rosai J. Thymic hyperplasia and neoplasia: a review of current concepts. *Hum Pathol* 1978;9:495.

80. Hsu CP, Chan CY, Chen CL, et al. Thymic carcinoma: ten years' experience in twenty patients. *J Thorac Cardiovasc Surg* 1994;107:615.

81. Weide LG, Ulbright TM, Loehrer PJ, Williams SD. Thymic carcinoma: a distinct clinical entity responsive to chemotherapy. *Cancer* 1993;71:1219.

82. Suster S, Moran CA. Spindle cell thymic carcinoma: clinicopathologic and immunohistochemical study of a distinctive variant of primary thymic epithelial neoplasm. *Am J Surg Pathol* 1999;23:681.

83. Shimizu J, Hayashi Y, Monita K, et al. Primary thymic carcinoma: a clinicopathological and immunohistochemical study. *J Surg Oncol* 1994;56:159.

84. Liu H, Hsu W, Chen Y, et al. Primary thymic carcinoma. *Ann Thorac Surg* 2002;73:1076.

85. Yano T, Hara N, Ichinose Y, et al. Treatment and prognosis of primary thymic carcinoma. *J Surg Oncol* 1993;52:255.

86. Rosai J, Higa E. Mediastinal endocrine neoplasm of probable thymic origin related to carcinoid tumors. *Cancer* 1972;29:1061.

87. Wang DY, Chang DB, Kuo SH, et al. Carcinoid tumors of the thymus. *Thorax* 1994;49:33.

88. Vietri F, Illuminati R, Guglielmi R, et al. Carcinoid tumor of the thymus gland. *Eur J Surg* 1994;160:645.

89. Asbun HJ, Calabria RP, Calmes S, Lang AG, Bloch JH. Thymic carcinoid. *Am Surg* 1991;57:442.

90. Zeiger MA, Swartz SE, Macgillivary DC, Linnoila I, Shakir M. Thymic carcinoid in association with MEN syndromes. *Am Surg* 1992;58:430.

91. McManus KG, Allen MS, Trastek VF, et al. Lipothymoma with red cell aplasia, hypogammaglobulinemia and lichen planus. *Ann Thorac Surg* 1994;58:1534.

92. Rosado-de-Christenson ML, Pugatch RD, Moran CA, Galobardes J. Thymolipoma: analysis of 27 cases. *Radiology* 1994;193:121.

93. Litano Y, Yokomari K, Ohkura M, et al. Giant thymolipoma in a child. *J Pediatr Surg* 1993;28:1622.

94. Nichols CR, Fox EP. Extra-gonadal and pediatric germ cell tumors. *Hematol Oncol Clin North Am* 1991;5:1189.

95. Dulmet EM, Macchiarini P, Suc B, Verley J. Germ cell tumors of the mediastinum: a 30 year experience. *Cancer* 1993;72:1994.

96. Lemarie E, Assouline PS, Diot P, et al. Primary mediastinal germ cell tumors: results of a French retrospective study. *Chest* 1992;102:1477.

97. Luna M, Valenzuela-Tamaritz J. Germ cell tumors of the mediastinum: postmortem findings. *Am J Clin Pathol* 1976;65:450.

98. Wu T, Wang H, Chang Y, et al. Mature mediastinal teratoma: sonographic imaging patterns and pathologic correlation. *J Ultrasound Med* 2002;21:759.

99. Hainsworth JD, Greco FA. Extragonadal germ cell tumors and unrecognized germ cell tumors. *Semin Oncol* 1992;19:119.

100. Ginsberg RJ. Mediastinal germ cell tumors: the role of surgery. *Semin Thorac Cardiovasc Surg* 1992;4:51.

101. Bokemeyer C, Nichols CR, Draz J, et al. Extragonadal germ cell tumors of the mediastinum and retroperitoneum: results from an international analysis. *J Clin Oncol* 2002;20:1864.

102. Schultz S, Einhorn L, Conces D, et al. Management of residual mass in patients with advanced seminoma: Indiana University experience. *J Clin Oncol* 1989;7:1497.

103. Horwich A, Paluchowska B, Norman A, et al. Residual mass following chemotherapy of seminoma. *Ann Oncol* 1997;8:37.

104. Ganjoo KN, Chan RJ, Sharma M, Einhorn LH. Positron emission tomography scans in the evaluation of postchemotherapy residual masses in patients with seminoma. *J Clin Oncol* 1999;17:3457.

105. Takeda S, Miyoshi A, Ohta M, et al. Primary germ cell tumors in the mediastinum: a 50-year experience at a single Japanese institution. *Cancer* 2003;97:367.

106. Miller KD, Loehrer PJ, Gonin R, et al. Salvage chemotherapy with vinblastine, ifosfamide, and cisplatin in recurrent seminoma. *J Clin Oncol* 1997;15:1427.

107. Luna M, Valenzuela-Tamaritz J. Germ cell tumors of the mediastinum: postmortem findings. *Am J Clin Pathol* 1976;65:450.

108. International Germ Cell Collaborative Group. International germ cell consensus classification: a prognostic factor–based staging system for metastatic germ cell cancers. *J Clin Oncol* 1997;15:594.

109. Loehrer PJ, Gonin R, Nichols CR, et al. Vinblastine plus ifosfamide plus cisplatin as initial salvage therapy in recurrent germ cell tumor. *J Clin Oncol* 1998;16:2500.

110. Broun ER, Nichols CR, Einhorn LH, Tricot GJK. Salvage therapy with high dose chemotherapy and autologous bone marrow support in the treatment of primary non-seminomatous mediastinal germ cell tumors. *Cancer* 1991;68:1513.

111. Hartmann JT, Einhorn L, Nichols CR, et al. Second-line chemotherapy in patients with relapsed extragonadal nonseminomatous germ cell tumors: results of an international multicenter analysis. *J Clin Oncol* 2001;19:1641.

112. Mack TM. Sarcomas and other malignancies of soft tissue, retroperitoneum, peritoneum, pleura, heart, mediastinum, and spleen. *Cancer* 1995;75:211.

113. Worthy SA, Gholkar A, Walls TJ, Todd NV. Case report: multiple thoracic hemangiomas: a rare cause of spinal cord compression. *Br J Radiol* 1995;68:770.

114. Davidson KG, Walbaum PR, McCormack RJM. Intrathoracic neural tumors. *Thorax* 1978;33:359.

115. Wick MR, Sterenberg SS. *Diagnostic surgical pathology.* New York: Raven Press, 1994:1141.

116. Enzinger FM, Weiss SW. *Soft tissue tumors.* St. Louis: Mosby, 1983.

117. Brasfield RD, Das Gupta TK. Von Recklinghausen's disease: a clinical pathologic study. *Ann Surg* 1972;175:1986.

118. Akwari OE, Payne WS, Onforio BM, et al. Dumbbell neurogenic tumors of the mediastinum. *Mayo Clin Proc* 1978;53:353.

119. Woodruff JM. Peripheral nerve tumors showing glandular differentiation. *Cancer* 1976;37:2399.

120. MacKay B, Osborne BM. The contribution of electron microscopy to the diagnoses of tumors. *Pathobiology annual,* vol 8. New York: Raven Press, 1978:359.

121. Adam A, Hochholzer L. Ganglioneuroblastoma of the posterior mediastinum: a clinico-pathologic review of 80 cases. *Cancer* 1981;47:373.

122. Bar-Ziv J, Nogrady MB. Mediastinal neuroblastoma and ganglioneuroma: the differentiation between primary and secondary involvement on the chest roentgenogram. *AJR Am J Roentgenol* 1975;125:380.

123. Robinson MG, McCorquodale MM. Trisomy 18 and neurogenic neoplasia. *J Pediatr* 1981;99:428.

124. Evans AE, D'Angio GJ, Koop CE. Diagnosis and treatment of neuroblastoma. *Pediatr Clin North Am* 1976;23:161.

125. Fortner J, Nicastri A, Murphy ML. Neuroblastoma: natural history and results of treating 133 cases. *Ann Surg* 1968;167:132.

126. Rosenbloom PM, Barrows GH, Kmetz DR, et al. Granular cell myoblastoma arising from the thoracic sympathetic nerve chain. *J Pediatr Surg* 1975;10:819.

127. Liu HP, Yim APC, Wan J, et al. Thorascopic removal of intrathoracic neurogenic tumors: a combined Chinese experience. *Ann Surg* 2000;232:187.

128. Chen HZ, Jiang L, Rong WH, et al. Tumours of the heart. An analysis of 79 cases. *Chin Med J* 1992;105:153.

129. Raaf HN, Raaf JH. Sarcomas related to the heart and vasculature. *Semin Surg Oncol* 1994;10:374.

130. Stein M, Deitling F, Cantor A, et al. Primary cardiac angiosarcoma: a case report and review of therapeutic options. *Med Pediatr Oncol* 1994;23:149.

131. Han P, Drachtman RA, Amenta P, Ettinger LJ. Successful treatment of a primary cardiac leiomyosarcoma with ifosfamide and etoposide. *J Pediatr Hematol Oncol* 1996;18:314.

132. Jyothirmayi R, Jacob R, Nair K, Rajan B. Primary fibrosarcoma of the right ventricle—a case report. *Acta Oncol* 1995;34:972.

133. Llombart-Cussac A, Pivot X, Contesso G, et al. Adjuvant chemotherapy for primary cardiac sarcomas: the IGR experience. *Br J Cancer* 1998;78:1624.

134. Thomason R, Schlegel W, Lucca M, et al. Primary malignant mesothelioma of the pericardium: case report and literature review. *Tex Heart Inst J* 1994;21:170.

135. Teramoto N, Hayashi K, Miyatani K, et al. Malignant fibrous histiocytoma of the right ventricle of the heart. *Pathol Int* 1995;45:315.

136. Gilkeson RC, Chiles C. MR evaluation of cardiac and pericardial malignancy. *Magn Reson Imaging Clin N Am* 2003;11:173.

137. Hermann MA, Shankerman RA, Edwards WD, et al. Primary cardiac angiosarcoma: a clinicopathologic study of six cases. *J Thorac Cardiovasc Surg* 1992;103:655.

138. Thomas CR Jr, Johnson GW Jr, Stoddard MF, et al. Primary malignant cardiac tumors: update 1992. *Med Pediatr Oncol* 1992;20:519.

139. Baat P, Karwande SV, Kushner JP, et al. Successful treatment of a cardiac angiosarcoma with combined modality therapy. *J Heart Lung Transplant* 1994;13:923.

140. Michler RE, Goldstein DJ. Treatment of cardiac tumors by orthotopic cardiac transplantation. *Semin Oncol* 1997;24:534.

CHAPTER **29**

Cancers of the Gastrointestinal Tract

MITCHELL C. POSNER
ARLENE A. FORASTIERE
BRUCE D. MINSKY

SECTION **1**

Cancer of the Esophagus

Esophageal cancer is unique among the gastrointestinal tract malignancies because it embodies two distinct histopathologic types, squamous cell carcinoma and adenocarcinoma. Which type of cancer occurs in a given patient or predominates in a given geographic area depends on many variables, including individual lifestyle, socioeconomic pressures, and environmental factors. The United States, along with many other Western countries, has witnessed in recent decades a profound increase in incidence rates of adenocarcinoma, whereas squamous cell carcinoma continues to predominate worldwide. Although it would seem appropriate to individualize treatment of these tumors, often they are managed as a single entity. Unfortunately, present-day therapeutic interventions have had little impact on survival, as evidenced by the equivalence of incidence and mortality rates. A more thorough understanding of the initiating events, the molecular biologic basis, and treatment successes and failures will hopefully spawn a new era of therapy effectively targeting both adenocarcinoma and squamous cell carcinoma of the esophagus.

EPIDEMIOLOGY

The epidemiology of esophageal cancer is defined by its substantial variability as a function of histologic type, geographic area, gender, race, and ethnic background.[1] Because of the recent increase in incidence rates of adenocarcinoma, especially in the Western hemisphere, epidemiologic studies are now distinguishing between histologic types when reporting results, whereas in the past, incidence rates of esophageal cancer only reflected squamous cell carcinoma. This still remains true in high-incidence areas where published rates are not obtained from population-based tumor registries. These high-incidence areas include Turkey, northern Iran, southern republics of the former Soviet Union, and northern China, where incidence rates exceed 100 per 100,000 person-years. Incidence rates of squamous cell carcinoma may vary 200-fold between different populations in the same geographic area due to unique cultural practices. The highest incidence rates for males (more than 15 per 100,000 person-years) reported from population-based tumor registries were in Calvados, France; Hong Kong; and Miyagi, Japan; and the highest rates for females (more than 5 per 100,000 person-years) were in Bombay, India; Shanghai, China; and Scotland.[2]

Esophageal cancer is relatively uncommon in the United States and the lifetime risk of being diagnosed with the disease is less than 1%.[3] It was estimated that 13,900 new cases would be identified in 2003 with 13,000 individuals expected to die of the disease, which emphasizes its virulence.[4] Incidence, mortality, and survival patterns in the United States vary greatly depending on race, gender, and histologic type. Age-adjusted incidence rates are highest among African American men and the predominant histologic type is squamous cell carcinoma (Fig. 29.1-1). The incidence rates for African American men peaked in the early 1980s and since then have shown a marked decline to the current rate of approximately 12 per 100,000 person-years.[3] Incidence rates among white men continue to increase and now exceed 6 per 100,000 person-years and reflect the marked increase in the incidence of adenocarcinoma of the esophagus of more than 400% in the past two decades.[1] Although the incidence of adenocarci-

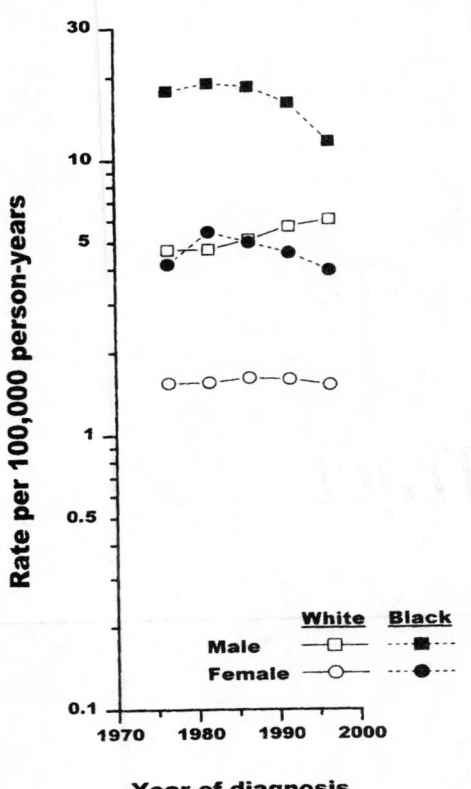

FIGURE 29.1-1. Trends in age-adjusted incidence rates for esophageal cancer in the United States by race.

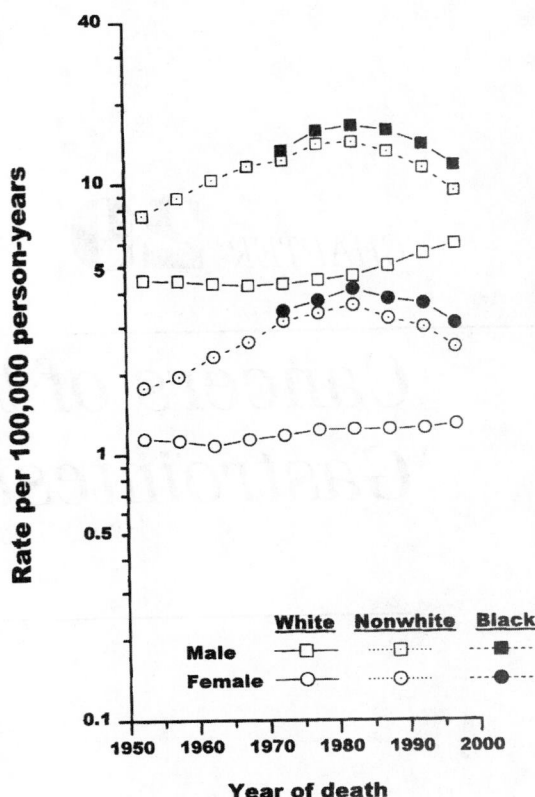

FIGURE 29.1-2. Trends in esophageal cancer mortality rates in the United States by race and gender.

noma in white females is lower than that in white men, rates of adenocarcinoma have increased in women by more than 300% over the past 20 years. Similar trends have been noted in Western European countries. This trend of increased incidence of adenocarcinoma of the esophagus has paralleled the upward trend in rates of both gastroesophageal reflux disease and obesity.

Mortality rates for esophageal cancer also are race dependent (Fig. 29.1-2). A steady decline in esophageal cancer mortality has been noted since the mid-1980s in the nonwhite United States population, whereas over the same period, a marked increase in mortality was noted among white men and women.[1] The mortality rates among African Americans exceed those for all other populations combined. Although survival rates for all esophageal cancer patients are uniformly dismal, regardless of race or gender, 5-year relative survival rates have significantly improved since the 1970s based on Surveillance, Epidemiology, and End Results (SEER) population-based tumor registry reporting.[3] African Americans have poorer 5-year survival rates than white Americans, and men fare poorly compared to women. There is no survival difference related to cell type (squamous cell carcinoma vs. adenocarcinoma).

ETIOLOGIC FACTORS AND PREDISPOSING CONDITIONS

Squamous cell carcinoma and adenocarcinoma of the esophagus share some risk factors, whereas other risk factors are specific to one histologic type or the other.

TOBACCO AND ALCOHOL USE

Tobacco and alcohol use are considered the major contributing factors in the development of esophageal cancer worldwide. It is estimated that up to 90% of the risk of squamous cell carcinoma of the esophagus in Western Europe and North America can be attributed to tobacco and alcohol use.[5] Population-based studies demonstrate that tobacco and alcohol use are independent risk factors and their effects are multiplicative, as evidenced by the association of the highest risk of developing esophageal cancer with heavy use of both agents. Approximately 65% and 57% of squamous cell carcinomas of the esophagus have been attributed to smoking tobacco for longer than 6 months in white and African American men, respectively, in the United States.[6] There appears to be a dose-response effect related to the duration and intensity of smoking and, importantly, there is an impressive (up to 50%) reduction in risk of developing squamous cell carcinoma of the esophagus for those who quit smoking and an inverse relationship between risk and the length of time since cessation of tobacco use.[7] Cigarette smoking is also a risk factor in the development of adenocarcinoma of the esophagus, leading to a twofold increase in risk for heavy smokers (more than one pack per day).[7,8] Although the effect is less for adenocarcinoma than for squamous cell carcinoma, quitting smoking does not appear to decrease the risk of adenocarcinoma, which remains elevated for decades after smoking cessation.[7,8] This suggests that tobacco carcinogens may affect carcinogenesis early on in esophageal adenocarcinoma and has, therefore, not been impacted by the decline in prevalence of smoking in the United States. Although tobacco smoke contains known or putative carcinogens such as nitrosamines, 2-naphthylamine, benzo[a]pyrene, and benzene, causative agents and their mechanisms of action for esophageal cancer have not been elucidated.

The consumption of alcoholic beverages is a major contributing factor in the increased risk of esophageal squamous cell carcinoma in Western countries. In the United States, approximately 80% of squamous cell carcinoma of the esophagus in men can be attributed to drinking more than one alcoholic beverage per day.[6] A dose-response relationship exists between the amount of alcohol ingested and the risk of developing squamous cell carcinoma, and the benefit of cessation of drinking alcohol varies in specific geographic areas.[9,10] The type of alcoholic beverage has also been implicated as a risk factor, although in most studies the most commonly consumed beverage in a specific geographical region is the one most frequently associated with increased risk.[1] Although specific carcinogens may be present in a variety of alcoholic beverages, in all likelihood it is alcohol itself, either as a mechanical irritant, promoter of dietary deficiency, or contributor to susceptibility to other carcinogens, that leads to carcinogenesis. If there is an association between alcohol consumption and the risk of adenocarcinoma of the esophagus, the risk is significantly lower than that for squamous cell carcinoma, and a large population-based case-control study in the United States revealed no relationship between alcohol intake and risk of esophageal adenocarcinoma.[8]

DIET AND NUTRITION

For both squamous cell carcinoma and adenocarcinoma of the esophagus, case-control studies provide evidence of a protective effect of fruits and vegetables, especially those eaten raw.[7,11] These food groups contain a number of micronutrients and dietary components such as vitamins A, C, and E, selenium, carotenoids, and fiber that may prevent carcinogenesis. For example, vitamin C has been shown to block the endogenous formation of N-nitrosocompounds, which have been implicated as a risk factor for development of esophageal cancer.[12] Deficiencies of the aforementioned nutrients and dietary components have been associated with increased risk of esophageal squamous cell carcinoma in some parts of the world. Consumption of hot beverages has been suggested as a risk factor for esophageal cancer in South America.[13]

SOCIOECONOMIC STATUS

Low socioeconomic status as defined by income, education, or occupation is associated with increased risk for esophageal squamous cell carcinoma and, to a lesser degree, for adenocarcinoma.[8,14] In the United States it is estimated that 39% and 69% of squamous cell carcinomas of the esophagus in white men and African American men, respectively, are related to low annual income.[6] A number of occupational and industrial hazards, including exposure to perchlorethylene (dry cleaners, metal polishers), combustion products and fossil fuels (chimney sweeps, printers, gas station attendants, asphalt and metal workers), silica and metal dust, and asbestos, as well as viral exposure via meat packing and slaughtering, have been suggested as possible risk factors for squamous cell carcinoma but not adenocarcinoma of the esophagus.[2]

OBESITY

The prevalence of obesity in the United States markedly increased from 12.8% in the early 1960s to almost 23% between 1988 and 1994.[15] This upward trend parallels that seen for incidence rates of esophageal adenocarcinoma. Increased body mass index is a risk factor for adenocarcinoma of the esophagus, and individuals with the highest body mass index have up to a sevenfold greater risk of esophageal cancer than those with a low body mass index.[7,16–18] The mechanism by which obesity contributes to an increased risk of esophageal adenocarcinoma is uncertain, although the linkage between obesity and gastroesophageal reflux disease is presumed to be a chief, but not the sole, factor. Because of the influence of nutritional and socioeconomic factors, the risk of squamous cell carcinoma of the esophagus increases with decreasing body mass index.

GASTROESOPHAGEAL REFLUX DISEASE

Gastroesophageal reflux disease has been implicated as one of the strongest risk factors for the development of adenocarcinoma of the esophagus.[19,20] Chronic reflux is associated with Barrett's esophagus, the premalignant precursor of esophageal adenocarcinoma. Population-based case-control studies examining the relationship between symptomatic reflux and risk of adenocarcinoma of the esophagus have demonstrated that increased frequency, severity, and chronicity of reflux symptoms are associated with a 2-fold to 16-fold increased risk of adenocarcinoma of the esophagus.[19,20] In a study in Sweden, this association was noted regardless of the presence of Barrett's esophagus.[19] Trends in incidence rates of gastroesophageal reflux disease over the past three decades parallel the time trends of increasing incidence of adenocarcinoma in the United States.

HELICOBACTER PYLORI INFECTION

Infection with *Helicobacter pylori* and particularly with cagA+ strains is inversely associated with the risk of adenocarcinoma of the esophagus.[21] The mechanism of action is unclear, although *H pylori* infection can result in chronic atrophic gastritis leading to decreased acid production, which negates the effects of chronic reflux, including the potential for development of Barrett's esophagus. *H pylori* infection has no association with the risk of squamous cell carcinoma of the esophagus.

BARRETT'S ESOPHAGUS

Barrett's esophagus is defined by the presence of intestinal metaplasia (mucin-producing goblet cells) in columnar cell–lined epithelium that replaces the normal squamous epithelium of the distal esophagus.[22–24] Although other types of mucosa (gastric fundic or junctional type) have been identified in Barrett's esophagus, specialized intestinal metaplasia confirmed by histologic examination of biopsy specimens is required for the diagnosis of Barrett's esophagus and is the prerequisite preneoplastic process associated with the development of adenocarcinoma. A diagnosis of Barrett's esophagus confers a 40- to 125-fold higher risk of progressing to esophageal carcinoma compared with the risk in the general population and is the single most important risk factor for developing adenocarcinoma.[25,26] The absolute risk that any single patient with Barrett's esophagus will develop adenocarcinoma in a year is approximately 1 in 200 (absolute risk, 0.5% per patient-year).[26–29] The definition of Barrett's esophagus used to include only those patients with columnar cell–lined epithelium of more than 3 cm; however, intestinal metaplasia is well documented within columnar epithelium less than 3 cm in length, and patients with short segment Barrett's esophagus are at risk of developing dysplasia and subsequently adenocarcinoma, not unlike their counterparts with long segment Barrett's esophagus.[30]

Barrett's esophagus is an acquired condition secondary to chronic tissue injury caused by gastroesophageal reflux disease. The frequency of Barrett's esophagus in the general population undergoing endoscopy is less than 1%,[31] whereas for those with long-term reflux symptoms, Barrett's esophagus of some length is identified in 5% to 15%.[32] The strategy of surveillance endoscopy for patients with long-standing symptomatic gastroesophageal reflux disease, especially those at high risk for Barrett's esophagus (middle-aged to elderly white males) and subsequent adenocarcinoma, seems logical. However, the utility of screening in such individuals is unproven and unlikely to have a significant impact on reducing death from cancer, because 40% of patients with adenocarcinoma of the esophagus have no history of reflux[19] and fewer than 5% of patients undergoing resection for adenocarcinoma were documented to have Barrett's esophagus before seeking medical attention for their symptomatic cancer.[33] Both medical and surgical antireflux therapies are effective at reducing or eliminating the symptoms of gastroesophageal reflux, but no clear-cut evidence exists that either therapy reduces the risk of esophageal adenocarcinoma. A randomized Veterans Affairs Cooperative Study of medical and surgical antireflux treatment in patients with severe gastroesophageal reflux disease demonstrated superior control of reflux symptoms in the surgical treatment group but no difference between medical and surgical therapy groups in the incidence of esophageal cancer.[28] Overall survival was significantly decreased in the surgical treatment group as a result of an unexpected excess of deaths from heart disease.

Practice guidelines published by the American College of Gastroenterology recommend surveillance endoscopy for patients with the diagnosis of Barrett's esophagus, and the grade of dysplasia should determine the endoscopy interval.[24] The driving force behind this recommendation is the findings from noncontrolled studies suggesting that adenocarcinomas identified by surveillance methods are detected at an earlier stage and are associated with a more favorable outcome after esophagectomy.[34–36] In addition, Barrett's esophagus can be identified in 80% to 100% of resected specimens from patients undergoing esophagectomy for esophageal carcinoma.[37,38] However, the efficacy of screening endoscopy is unclear, and there are no convincing data demonstrating that surveillance prevents cancer or improves life expectancy. Numerous studies are available examining the incidence of adenocarcinoma in patients with Barrett's esophagus undergoing surveillance.[27,39,40] For example, Macdonald et al.[40] followed 143 patients with Barrett's esophagus for an average of 4.4 years with surveillance endoscopy and identified only one patient with asymptomatic esophageal adenocarcinoma. Similar findings were reported by O'Connor et al.,[27] who followed 136 patients for a mean of 4.2 years in an endoscopic surveillance program during which 2 patients developed adenocarcinoma for an incidence of 1 in 285 patient-years. These studies suggest that routine surveillance of patients with Barrett's esophagus is unlikely to alter the

natural history of this disease due to the low incidence of adenocarcinoma and the morbidity and mortality associated with the recommended treatment, esophageal resection. Although some authors suggest that surgical antireflux therapy causes regression of metaplastic epithelium or interrupts progression from Barrett's esophagus to low-grade and high-grade dysplasia,[41–43] convincing evidence is lacking to support this contention. Furthermore, although aggressive antireflux therapy would halt continued irritation of the mucosa at risk before malignant transformation, it may have no effect on the molecular genetic events responsible for stimulation and control of cellular proliferation activated early in the malignant process.

Progression from intestinal metaplasia to dysplasia in Barrett's esophagus signifies an unequivocal neoplastic change in the epithelium characterized by cytologic or architectural abnormalities that are associated with the potential for malignant degeneration. The severity of these cytologic changes dictates classification of dysplasia as being low grade or high grade. The experience of the pathologist is crucial in correctly diagnosing high-grade dysplasia, which is the most important predictor for esophageal adenocarcinoma.[44] Although, among experienced pathologists, the differentiation of high-grade dysplasia from either low-grade dysplasia, indefinite dysplasia, or absence of dysplasia is straightforward (85% interobserver agreement), the diagnosis of low-grade dysplasia as differentiated from either indefinite dysplasia or findings negative for dysplasia is less reproducible (50% to 75% interobserver agreement).[45,46] Any degree of dysplasia warrants endoscopic surveillance, the frequency of which is dictated by the degree of dysplasia. Annual endoscopy is recommended for those patients with low-grade dysplasia and more frequent screening is recommended for those patients with high-grade dysplasia. The controversy regarding the management of patients with high-grade dysplasia is fully discussed in Treatment, later in this chapter.

The proposed stepwise carcinogenic sequence in which specialized intestinal metaplasia proceeds to low-grade dysplasia, high-grade dysplasia, and frank carcinoma suggests a potential opportunity for chemoprevention to disrupt the succession to cancer. This approach is attractive because there is no convincing evidence to suggest that control of acid reflux, either medically or surgically, prevents the development of intestinal metaplasia or reverses or eradicates Barrett's esophagus or dysplasia once it has been diagnosed. Buttar et al.,[47] recognizing that carcinogenesis in Barrett's esophagus is associated with increased expression of cyclooxygenase-2 (COX-2), examined the effect of COX-2 inhibitors on the development of Barrett's esophagus and adenocarcinoma in a preclinical model. Both selective and nonselective COX-2 inhibitors were effective in inhibiting Barrett's esophagus–related adenocarcinoma. This study provides a platform for exploring the potential for COX-2 inhibitors and other agents as potential chemopreventive agents in patients at risk of developing adenocarcinoma.

TYLOSIS

Tylosis (focal nonepidermolytic palmoplantar keratoderma) is a rare disease inherited in an autosomal dominant manner that is characterized by hyperkeratosis of the palms and soles and esophageal papillomas. Patients with this condition exhibit abnormal maturation of squamous cells and inflammation within the esophagus and are at extremely high risk of developing esophageal cancer.[48,49] The tylosis esophageal cancer (TOC) gene has been mapped to 17q25 by linkage analysis of pedigrees associated with high risk of esophageal cancer development.[50] In addition to being mutated in tylosis, the TOC gene is frequently deleted in sporadic human esophageal cancers.[51,52] Iwaya et al.[52] used 20 microsatellite markers focusing on the TOC locus to investigate loss of heterozygosity (LOH) in 58 sporadic esophageal squamous cell carcinomas. LOH was observed in 37 of 52 informative cases (71%), of which 80% (33 of 37) involved the TOC locus. Envoplakin, encoding a protein component of desmosomes that is expressed in esophageal keratinocytes, has been mapped to the TOC region[52]; however, no tylosis-specific mutations involving this gene have been observed.[53] Further studies are required to define the tumor suppressor gene(s) mapping to 17q25 that are inactivated in tylosis-associated as well as sporadic esophageal carcinomas.

PLUMMER-VINSON/PATERSON-KELLY SYNDROME

Plummer-Vinson/Paterson-Kelly syndrome is characterized by iron-deficiency anemia, glossitis, cheilitis, brittle fingernails, splenomegaly, and esophageal webs. Approximately 10% of individuals with Plummer-Vinson/Paterson-Kelly syndrome develop hypopharyngeal or esophageal epidermoid carcinomas.[54] The mechanisms by which these tumors arise have not been fully defined, although nutritional deficiencies as well as chronic mucosal irritation from retained food particles at the level of the webs may contribute to the pathogenesis of these neoplasms.[55]

CAUSTIC INJURY

Squamous cell carcinomas may arise in lye strictures, often developing 40 to 50 years after caustic injury.[56] The majority of these cancers are located in the middle third of the esophagus. The pathogenesis of these neoplasms may be similar to that implicated in esophageal cancers arising in patients with Plummer-Vinson/Paterson-Kelly syndrome. These cancers are often diagnosed late due to the fact that chronic dysphagia and pain caused by the lye strictures obscure symptoms of esophageal cancer.

ACHALASIA

Achalasia is an idiopathic esophageal motility disorder characterized by increased basal pressure in the lower esophageal sphincter, incomplete relaxation of this sphincter after deglutition, and aperistalsis of the body of the esophagus. A 16- to 30-fold increase in esophageal cancer risk has been noted in achalasia patients.[57,58] In a retrospective analysis, Aggestrup et al.[59] observed the development of esophageal carcinomas in 10 of 147 patients undergoing esophagomyotomy for achalasia. These neoplasms typically are squamous cell carcinomas, believed to result from prolonged irritation from retained foods at the air–fluid interface in the mid-esophagus, and arise an average of 17 years after onset of achalasia symptoms. The insidious nature of carcinomas arising in the context of chronic dysphagia and pain attributable to megaesophagus contributes to their late diagnosis in achalasia patients.[60]

HUMAN PAPILLOMAVIRUS INFECTION

Several studies suggest that human papillomavirus (HPV) infection may contribute to the pathogenesis of esophageal squamous cell cancers in high-incidence areas in Asia and South Africa.[61] This oncogenic virus, which has been associated with cervical and oropharyngeal cancers,[62,63] encodes two proteins (E6 and E7) that sequester the Rb and p53 tumor suppressor gene products. Using polymerase chain reaction techniques, de Villiers et al.[64] detected HPV DNA sequences in 17% of esophageal squamous cell cancers from China. In an additional study using similar techniques, Lavergne and de Villiers[65] identified a broad spectrum of HPV in approximately one-third of esophageal cancer specimens obtained from patients living in high-incidence areas in China and South Africa. Shibagaki et al.[66] detected HPV sequences in 15 of 72 (21%) esophageal cancer specimens obtained from Japanese patients. In contrast, HPV sequences have not been observed in cancers arising in low-incidence areas. Poljack et al.[67] observed no evidence of HPV in 121 formalin-fixed, paraffin-embedded esophageal cancer specimens obtained from patients in Slovenia. Similarly, Rugge et al.[68] detected no HPV in 18 carcinomas arising in Italian patients. Turner et al.[69] observed no evidence of HPV in 51 formalin-fixed, paraffin-embedded esophageal cancer specimens obtained from patients in North America. In a large population-based control study, Lagergren et al.[70] compared 121 patients with esophageal squamous cell cancers and 173 adenocarcinoma patients with 302 population-based controls in Sweden. These authors observed no association between HPV infection and risk of esophageal cancer in this low-incidence area. Collectively, these data suggest that HPV may contribute to the pathogenesis of esophageal squamous cancers in high-incidence regions; however, this oncogenic virus appears to have little, if any, role in the pathogenesis of esophageal malignancies arising in low-incidence areas.

PRIOR AERODIGESTIVE TRACT MALIGNANCY

Carcinomas of the aerodigestive tract arise as a consequence of multistep processes in cancerization fields. Patients with upper aerodigestive tract cancers develop second primary cancers at a rate of approximately 4% per year.[71] Nearly 10% of secondary neoplasms arising in patients with prior histories of oropharyngeal carcinoma arise in the esophagus.[71] Levi et al.[72] observed that approximately 10% of second primary cancers in patients with prior histories of lung carcinoma arose in the esophagus. The increased risk of second primary tobacco-related carcinomas[73] warrants close surveillance of patients with histories of aerodigestive tract malignancy.

Interestingly, p53 mutational analysis of multiple primary cancers of the aerodigestive tract in 17 patients demonstrated complete discordance of p53 genotype between separate primary tumors from the same patient, which suggests that p53 is not functioning as a tumor susceptibility gene in this setting.[74]

APPLIED ANATOMY AND HISTOLOGY

ANATOMY

The esophagus bridges three anatomic compartments: the neck, thorax, and abdomen (Fig. 29.1-3). The esophagus extends from the cricopharyngeus muscle at the level of the cricoid cartilage to the gastroesophageal junction.[75] The borders of the cervical esophagus are the cricopharyngeus to the thoracic inlet (approximately 18 cm from the incisors). The remainder of the esophagus is commonly divided into thirds,

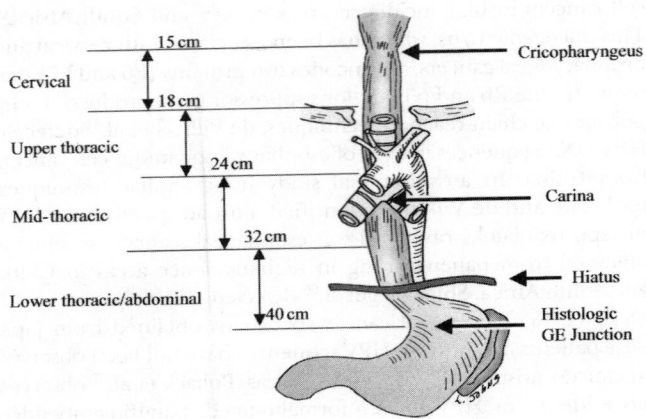

FIGURE 29.1-3.   Anatomy of the esophagus with landmarks and recorded distance from the incisors used to divide the esophagus into topographic compartments. GE, gastroesophageal.

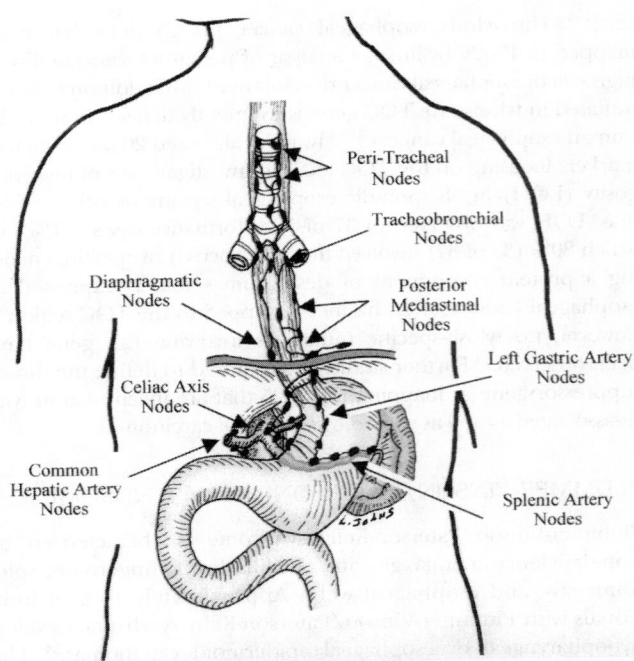

FIGURE 29.1-4.   Lymphatic drainage of the esophagus with anatomically defined lymph node basins.

with the upper third extending from the thoracic inlet to the carina (approximately 24 cm from the incisors), the middle third extending from the carina to the inferior pulmonary veins (32 cm from the incisors), and the distal esophagus traversing the remaining distance into the abdomen to the gastroesophageal junction (40 cm from the incisors). Squamous cell carcinoma of the esophagus is the predominant histology in the cervical esophagus and upper and middle thirds of the thoracic esophagus, whereas adenocarcinoma predominates in the distal esophagus.

Knowledge of the lymphatic drainage of the esophagus is critical to understanding how the numerous surgical approaches for esophageal cancer have evolved and explains why some surgeons recommend a specific procedure based on tumor location in the esophagus (Fig. 29.1-4). Tumors of the cervical and upper third of the thoracic esophagus drain to cervical and superior mediastinal lymph nodes. Tumors of the middle third of the esophagus drain both cephalad and caudad with lymph nodes at risk in the paratracheal, hilar, subcarinal, periesophageal, and pericardial nodal basins. Lesions in the distal esophagus primarily drain to lymph nodes in the lower mediastinum and celiac axis region. Due to the extensive lymphatic network and rich mucosal and submucosal lymphatics within the wall of the esophagus, skip metastases for upper third lesions have been noted in celiac axis nodal basins, and likewise, cervical lymph node metastases have been noted in as many as 30% of patients with distal esophageal lesions. This forms the basis for some surgeons' recommendation of a more thorough oncologic procedure, a combined transthoracic and abdominal approach for lesions of the mid- and distal esophagus,[76,77] and for others' recommendation of a three-field (cervical, mediastinal, and abdominal) lymphadenectomy for all tumors of the mid- through distal esophagus.[78,79] However, lymphatic spread correlates with pathologic T category of the primary esophageal tumor, and lymph node metastases are initially limited in an overwhelming majority of patients to regional lymph nodes. Lymph node involvement in lymphatic basins distant from the primary tumor are rarely identified unless metastases to regional lymph nodes have already occurred.[80] These data challenge the validity of extensive lymphadenectomy and also suggest the potential value of sentinel lymph node sampling to direct surgical dissection.[81]

HISTOLOGY

The overwhelming majority of esophageal malignancies may be classified as either squamous cell carcinomas or adenocarcinomas. Squamous cell carcinomas account for approximately 40% of esophageal malignancies diagnosed in the United States and the vast majority of cancers arising in high-incidence areas throughout the world.[82] Approximately 60% of these neoplasms are located in the middle third of the esophagus, whereas 30% and 10% arise in the distal third and proximal third of the intrathoracic esophagus, respectively.[83,84] Typically, these tumors are associated with contiguous or noncontiguous carcinoma *in situ* as well as widespread submucosal lymphatic dissemination.[85,86]

Adenocarcinomas frequently arise in the context of Barrett's esophagus; because of this, these tumors tend to be localized in the distal third of the esophagus and may be fungating or stenotic in appearance.[87,88] The vast majority of the tumors are associated with intestinal metaplasia or dysplasia.[89] No significant survival differences have been noted in adenocarcinoma patients compared with individuals with similarly staged squamous cell cancers.[90,91]

Several rare cancers of the esophagus have been described, including squamous cell carcinoma with sarcomatous features, as well as adenoid cystic and mucoepidermoid carcinomas.[92–96] These neoplasms are indistinguishable clinically and prognostically from the more common types of esophageal carcinoma.

Small cell carcinomas account for approximately 1% of esophageal malignancies and arise from argyrophilic cells in the basal layer of the squamous epithelium.[97,98] These neoplasms are usually located in the middle or lower third of the esophagus and may be associated with ectopic production of a variety of hormones, including parathormone, secretin, granulocyte colony-stimulation factor, and gastrin-releasing peptide; individuals with these cancers often present with systemic disease.[99,100] Although small cell carcinomas frequently respond to radiation therapy and chemotherapy, patients with these neoplasms typically succumb to widespread distant metastases.[101–103]

Leiomyosarcoma is the most common mesenchymal tumor affecting the esophagus, accounting for fewer than 1% of all esophageal malignancies.[92,104] These neoplasms usually arise as lower third tumors and typically present as bulky masses with significant hemorrhage and necrosis.[105,106] Malignant lymphoma and Hodgkin's disease rarely involve the esophagus; esophageal involvement typically is secondary to extension from other sites, although primary malignant lymphoma of the esophagus has occasionally been observed.[107,108] Patients with acquired immunodeficiency syndrome may exhibit Kaposi's sarcoma involving the esophagus.[109,110] Malignant melanoma involving the esophagus is exceedingly rare and presents as a bulky polypoid intraesophageal tumor of varying color depending on melanin production.[92,111] The prognosis is extremely poor for these patients even with aggressive therapy.

MOLECULAR BIOLOGY

The appearance of the hallmarks of tumorigenesis and acquisition of the malignant phenotype with all of its biologic perturbations require, as described by Hanahan and Weinberg,[112] obtainment of certain capabilities by the cell, including growth signal autonomy, ability to ignore antigrowth signals, evasion of apoptosis, unlimited replicative ability, angiogenesis, and invasion and metastatic potential. The molecular alterations and mechanisms underlying these acquired characteristics in many human tumors, including esophageal cancer, have become evident as the understanding of molecular biology has exponentially increased in recent years (Table 29.1-1). Many of the genetic alterations resulting in unchecked growth and proliferation and avoidance of programmed cell death exert their effect by modifying the cell cycle. Evidence for specific molecular events linked to the carcinogenic process has been found for both squamous cell carcinoma and adenocarcinoma of the esophagus.[113]

In the cell cycle during transition from the G_1 phase to the S phase, a crucial decision point (restriction point) is reached in which cells either complete the cell cycle and go on to divide or withdraw from the cycle.[114] Many of the mutations that lead to gain of function (oncogenes) or loss of function (tumor suppressor genes) exert their effects at this critical juncture. Control of the restriction point is mediated by retinoblastoma (Rb) protein via complex interactions with cyclins and cyclin-dependent kinases (CDKs). Active nonphosphorylated Rb protein blocks passage through the restriction point to the S phase, whereas phosphorylation inactivates Rb protein, negating its blocking function and facilitating completion of the cell cycle.[115] Cyclins are a group of specialized proteins that bind to and activate CDK molecules, which leads to phosphorylation of target proteins regulating the cell cycle. Cyclin D1 binds with CDK-4 during G_1 and these complexes phosphorylate Rb, inactivating its suppressor effect and promoting cells' entry into the S phase. Both cyclin D1 and cyclin E have been detected in biopsy specimens from patients with either premalignant conditions or cancer of the esophagus.[116,117] Overexpression of cyclin D1 has been identified in approximately 30% of patients with Barrett's esophagus[118] or esophageal squamous dysplasia[119] and in up to 70% of patients with squamous cell carcinoma of the esophagus.[120] In multiple studies, cyclin D1 overexpression is a predictor of poor outcome as measured by correlation of cyclin D1 overexpression with regional and distant metastases, advanced tumor grade and stage, poor response to chemotherapy, and decreased overall survival.[119,121] Cyclin E overexpression was identified in patients with

TABLE 29.1-1.   Molecular Genetic Events Linked to the Acquired Malignant Phenotype in Esophageal Cancer

Gene/Protein Product	Alteration	Mechanism	Acquired Functional Capability
Cyclin D1/E	Gene amplification	Promotes entry into S phase	Growth self-sufficiency
Rb (retinoblastoma)	Mutation, LOH	Tumor suppressor—blocks passage to S phase	Growth self-sufficiency
EGF/EGFR	Gene amplification	Growth factor/growth factor receptor	Growth self-sufficiency
TGF-α	Gene amplification	Growth factor	Growth self-sufficiency
erbB2	Gene amplification	Growth factor receptor	Growth self-sufficiency
p53	Mutation, LOH	Tumor suppressor—causes G_1 arrest of DNA-damaged cells	Resistance to antigrowth signals
p16	Mutation, LOH, promoter hyper-methylation	Tumor suppressor—inhibits CD/CDK complex	Resistance to antigrowth signals
p15	Mutation, LOH, promoter hyper-methylation	Tumor suppressor—inhibits CD/CDK copies	Resistance to antigrowth signals
COX-2	Overexpression	Inhibition of apoptotic pathways	Avoidance of apoptosis
FAS/FAS ligand	Underexpression, overexpression	Death receptor/death receptor ligand	Inhibition of apoptosis (cancer cell)
			Promotion of apoptosis (lymphocyte)
			Inhibition of immune surveillance
Telomerase	Up-regulation	Maintenance of telomere length	Unlimited DNA replication
VEGF/VEGFR	Overexpression	Endothelial cell growth factor/receptor	Sustained angiogenesis
E-cadherin	Down-regulation	Cellular adhesion	Invasion and metastasis

CD/CDK, cyclin D1/cyclin-dependent kinase; COX-2, cyclooxygenase-2; EGF, epidermal growth factor; EGFR, epidermal growth factor receptor; LOH, loss of heterozygosity; TGF-α, transforming growth factor-α; VEGF, vascular endothelial growth factor; VEGFR, vascular endothelial growth factor receptor.

Barrett's esophagus with dysplasia and adenocarcinoma and in patients with squamous cell carcinoma of the esophagus.[117,122]

Although mutations of the Rb gene in Barrett's esophagus, adenocarcinoma, and squamous cell carcinoma have not been documented, suggestive evidence exists implicating altered Rb function in the carcinogenic process. Allelic loss of 13q where the locus of the Rb gene resides can render the Rb gene to be nonfunctional. LOH has been noted in up to 50% of patients with Barrett's adenocarcinoma and squamous cell carcinoma.[120,123] Loss of immunostaining for Rb protein has been noted in Barrett's esophagus with dysplasia, adenocarcinoma, and squamous cell carcinoma of the esophagus.[124,125] Growth factors and their receptors can activate proliferative pathways by inducing cyclin expression. Exogenous growth factors or endogenous growth ligands can bind to growth factor receptors, leading to uncontrolled cell division. Tyrosine kinase growth factor receptors and their ligands, epidermal growth factor (EGF), and transforming growth factor-α have been incriminated in the carcinogenic process of both squamous cell carcinoma and adenocarcinoma.[126,127] Increased expression of transforming growth factor-α and the EGF receptor have been detected in Barrett's esophagus, esophageal adenocarcinoma, and squamous cell carcinoma of the esophagus.[126–130] EGF overexpression has been detected in Barrett's adenocarcinoma and esophageal squamous cell carcinoma.[127] EGF receptor overexpression may predict a poor response to chemoradiotherapy and be associated with poor outcome.[131,132] Itakura et al. reported that EGF receptor immunoreactivity was associated with decreased survival in patients with squamous cell carcinoma.[131] Kitagawa et al.[133] and Shimada et al.[134] noted that EGF receptor overexpression was associated with regional and distant recurrence and diminished overall survival in patients undergoing esophagectomy for squamous cell carcinoma.

Like other oncogenes, mutated erbB2 is associated with unchecked proliferative activity.[135] Some investigators have detected erbB2 overexpression in Barrett's esophagus, high-grade dysplasia, and adenocarcinoma,[136,137] whereas others have found no evidence for increased expression in biopsy samples from patients with Barrett's esophagus, either with or without dysplasia.[138] The same conflicting results have been seen for squamous cell carcinoma of the esophagus.[139,140]

Antigrowth signals disrupt the cell cycle at the restriction point by causing cells to become quiescent or initiating growth arrest and differentiation. The majority of these events are a consequence of the effects of antigrowth signals on the Rb pathway. The p53 gene product prevents cells with DNA damage from replicating by causing arrest in the G_1 phase and allowing repair mechanisms to act before entry into the S phase.[141] The p53 can exert its effects in varied ways. One mechanism to regulate cell-cycle progression involves inhibiting the function of the cyclin and CDK complex, which effectively blocks inactivation of the Rb protein by phosphorylation. If the tumor suppressor function of p53 is lost, Rb phosphorylation occurs, inactivating that tumor suppressor and allowing cell-cycle progression through the restriction point and replication of damaged DNA.[113] Multiple mechanisms exist to inactivate tumor suppressor genes and render their protein products functionless, including mutation, LOH, and promoter hypermethylation preventing gene transcription.

Detection of mutated p53 protein by immunohistochemistry has been demonstrated with increasing frequency during histologic progression from Barrett's esophagus (5%) through dysplasia (65% to 75%) to frank adenocarcinoma (up to 90%).[142–145] Loss of allele 17p, the site of the p53 gene locus, has been detected in 50% to 90% of Barrett's adenocarcinoma.[146,147] Identification of both mutant p53 protein and LOH of 17p in Barrett's specialized intestinal metaplasia suggests that p53 inactivation occurs early in the carcinogenic process. Both mutant p53 protein detected by immunohistochemistry and specific p53 gene mutations detected by genomic sequencing have been identified in 40% to 75% of patients with squamous cell carcinoma of the esophagus.[148–151] Point mutations in p53 predominately occur in exons 5 to 8, that segment of the genome responsible for DNA binding. The presence of a p53 point mutation detected by direct sequencing of p53 exons 5 to 8 significantly correlated with response to induction chemoradiotherapy and predicted survival after esophagectomy in patients with either squamous cell carcinoma or adenocarcinoma of the esophagus.[152]

Both p16 and p15, members of the INK4 protein family, are tumor suppressor gene products that inhibit cyclin D1–CDK complexes, preventing Rb protein phosphorylation and maintaining its ability to exert control over the cell cycle at the restriction point.[153] Inactivation of these tumor suppressor genes by any mechanism would result in inactivation of the Rb protein by phosphorylation and subsequently unchecked cellular proliferation. LOH of 9p21, the locus for both p16 and p15, has been demonstrated with high frequency in both dysplastic Barrett's epithelium and Barrett's adenocarcinoma (90% and more than 80% of cases, respectively).[154,155] Although point mutations of p15 and p16 have been infrequently identified or have been nonexistent in Barrett's esophagus and Barrett's-associated adenocarcinoma,[154] promoter hypermethylation, which prevents tumor suppressor function by blocking transcription, has been documented and correlates with the degree of dysplasia in Barrett's esophagus. It is present in up to 75% of specimens with high-grade dysplasia and is found in almost 50% of patients with adenocarcinoma of the esophagus.[123,156] These data provide supportive evidence for the role of p16 as a tumor suppressor gene in cancer progression in Barrett's esophagus. Point mutations of p16 in invasive squamous cell carcinoma have been found, but conflicting results have been reported regarding its frequency.[157–159] Altered expression of p16 protein documented by immunohistochemistry has been noted in half of sampled patients with squamous cell carcinoma of the esophagus and appears to correlate with overexpression of cyclin D1 and poor outcome.[160] Promoter hypermethylation silencing of p16 tumor suppressor function has been noted in up to 50% of squamous cell carcinomas of the esophagus.[161,162] As with adenocarcinoma, conflicting results have been reported regarding the frequency of genetic alterations of p15 in squamous cell carcinoma.[161,163]

Avoidance of apoptosis is another characteristic the cancer cell acquires through gene-altering events. As mentioned earlier, p53 protein prevents DNA damaged cells from progressing through the cell cycle until that DNA damage is repaired. Another mechanism by which p53 protein exerts its tumor suppressor effects is by activating proapoptotic pathways in the presence of severe DNA damage.[113] Tumor cells may avoid programmed cell death by increased synthesis of enzymes such as COX-2, which inhibits apoptotic pathways. COX-2 overexpression has been demonstrated in premalignant and malignant epithelium in both squamous cell carcinoma and adenocarcinoma of the esophagus.[164–167] The second mechanism that allows tumor cells to avoid apoptosis is alteration of the expression of death receptors. FAS is expressed by normal cells and when bound by the FAS ligand activates proapoptotic pathways.[168] Reduced expression of FAS would inhibit apoptosis of tumor cells, whereas overexpression of FAS ligand by tumor cells would activate apoptotic mechanisms in lymphocytes responsible for immune surveillance.[169] FAS ligand overexpression has been detected in both adenocarcinoma and squamous cell carcinoma of the esophagus as well as in premalignant squamous epithelium.[162,170] Contradictory results regarding reduced expression of the FAS receptor have been reported in Barrett's esophagus and Barrett's esophagus–associated adenocarcinoma[124,171,172]; however, decreased expression of the FAS receptor has been demonstrated in dysplastic squamous cell epithelium and invasive squamous cell carcinoma.[173,174] In addition, FAS receptor expression in squamous cell carcinoma of the esophagus has been correlated with prognostic variables associated with improved outcome and is an independent predictor for disease-free survival.[173]

Maintenance of telomere length allows DNA replication to be sustained indefinitely. After normal DNA replication, telomeres are shortened, which halts cell division. Tumor cells abrogate this ability to limit DNA replication by activation of telomerase, which stabilizes telomere length.[175] Aberrant expression of telomerase has been observed in the vast majority of esophageal cancers examined to date. Koyanagi et al.[176] detected telomerase expression in 100% of 57 esophageal squamous cell carcinomas. Morales et al.[177] observed increased telomerase expression in 100% of adenocarcinomas and Barrett's esophagus cases with high-grade dysplasia. High telomerase expression was associated with increasing degrees of dysplasia, up to and including invasive carcinoma, a finding confirmed by Lord et al.[178]

The acquired capability of angiogenesis facilitates tumor growth, invasion, and metastases formation. Vascular endothelial growth factor expression has been detected in epithelial and endothelial cells in Barrett's esophagus with dysplasia and invasive carcinoma.[179] Vascular endothelial growth factor receptors are also up-regulated in Barrett's esophagus.[180] Loss of cell-cell adhesion can lead to both invasion and metastases. Alterations in expression of E-cadherin, a cell-cell adhesion molecule, or its associated catenins disrupt cell-cell interactions, which results in the potential for tumor progression.[181] Reduced expression of E-cadherin has been correlated with progression from Barrett's esophagus to dysplasia and finally to adenocarcinoma.[182]

NATURAL HISTORY AND PATTERNS OF FAILURE

Natural history data and patterns of failure after specific treatment modalities provide insight into the biologic tendencies of esophageal carcinoma and suggest potential therapeutic avenues to explore. At presentation, the overwhelming majority of patients have locally or regionally advanced or disseminated cancer, irrespective of histologic type.[4,183] The lack of a serosal envelope and the rich submucosal lymphatic network of the esophagus provide a favorable milieu for extensive local infiltration by tumor and lymph node involvement. If distant disease is not clinically evident at the time that patients are initially diagnosed with esophageal carcinoma, evidence suggests that occult micrometastases are invariably present, and recurrence patterns confirm that distant failure is a significant and universally fatal component of relapse.[184–188] Bone marrow samples obtained during rib resec-

tions performed as part of curative esophagectomy and evaluated by immunohistochemical and quantitative polymerase chain reaction techniques revealed disseminated tumor cells in up to 90% of patients sampled.[189,190] The clinical relevance of these findings is unclear, but they suggest the need to focus not only on local-regional therapeutic modalities but on systemic interventions. The lung, liver, and bone are the most common sites of distant disease with depth of tumor invasion and lymph node involvement predictive of tumor dissemination.[75,184,185]

Median survival after esophagectomy for patients with localized disease is 15 to 18 months with a 5-year overall survival rate of 20% to 25%. Patterns of failure after esophagectomy suggest that both location of tumor and histologic type may influence the distribution of recurrence. In patients with cancers of the upper and middle thirds of the esophagus, which are predominately squamous cell carcinomas, local-regional recurrence predominates over distant recurrence, whereas in patients with lesions of the lower third, where adenocarcinomas are more frequently located, distant recurrence is more common.[184,185] Although one of the rationales for a three-field lymph node dissection for esophageal cancer is evidence of metastases in up to 30% of cervical lymph nodes, only a very small percentage of patients (fewer than 5%) develop clinically evident recurrence at cervical sites.[80]

The addition of chemotherapy, radiotherapy, or chemoradiotherapy to surgery may alter patterns of failure, although reported results are not consistent. Preoperative radiotherapy and preoperative chemoradiotherapy may reduce the rate of local-regional recurrence but has no obvious effect on the rate of distant metastases.[188,191,192] In two prospective randomized trials of preoperative chemotherapy plus surgery versus surgery alone, one study showed a slight but non–statistically significant decrease in distant relapse with chemotherapy,[185] whereas the other demonstrated equivalent distant recurrence rates in both the preoperative chemotherapy and surgery-alone arms.[187] Treatment failure patterns after definitive chemoradiotherapy without surgical resection reveal that concurrent administration of chemotherapy and radiotherapy provides better local control than radiotherapy alone but that distant recurrence was not significantly affected and was the major contributor to death.[193] Although the addition of surgery further reduces local failure from 45% to 32%,[194] it does not diminish systemic recurrence and, in fact, may enhance it by allowing patients to manifest distant disease because they do not succumb to local-regional failure. These patterns of relapse suggest that any further improvement in overall outcome for patients with esophageal cancer will be achieved through advances in systemic therapy.

CLINICAL PRESENTATION

The symptoms most commonly associated with esophageal cancer are dysphagia and weight loss. Unfortunately, in most instances dysphagia signifies locally advanced disease or distant metastases or both. At presentation, patients usually describe progressive dysphagia, with difficulty initially in swallowing solids, then liquids, and, in the most extreme circumstances, their own saliva. Taking into account that cure is an unlikely end result with even the most aggressive forms of treatment, palliation of this single symptom impacts most on the patient's quality of life. Other symptoms and patient demographic characteristics are closely aligned with the underlying histology. Patients with squamous cell carcinoma of the esophagus more often are of African American heritage and a low socioeconomic class, and have a history of tobacco or alcohol abuse or both. Substantial weight loss accompanying dysphagia is seen in approximately 90% of patients with squamous cell carcinoma. Patients with adenocarcinoma of the esophagus tend to be white males from middle to upper socioeconomic classes who are overweight, have a history of symptomatic gastroesophageal reflux, and have been treated with antireflux therapy.

Approximately 20% of patients experience odynophagia (painful swallowing). Additional presenting symptoms may include dull retrosternal pain resulting from invasion of mediastinal structures, bone pain secondary to bone metastases, and cough or hoarseness secondary to paratracheal nodal or recurrent laryngeal nerve involvement. These types of symptoms suggest unresectable locally advanced disease or metastases. Unusual presentations are pneumonia secondary to tracheoesophageal fistula or exsanguinating hemorrhage due to aortic invasion.

DIAGNOSTIC STUDIES AND PRETREATMENT STAGING

Patients who present with symptoms suggestive or pathognomic of cancer of the esophagus should undergo upper endoscopy to determine whether a mass is present, and biopsy to establish a tissue diagnosis. Analysis of specimens from biopsies combined with cytologic brushings has a diagnostic accuracy that approaches 100%.[195,196] Targeted biopsy can be enhanced by the use of chromoendoscopy techniques, which use dyes such as indigo carmine, Lugol's solution, methylene blue, and toluidine blue to highlight topographic features and epithelial changes and lead to improved diagnostic accuracy.[197,198] A focused history taking should elicit information on predisposing factors for esophageal cancer, including tobacco use, alcohol use, symptomatic reflux, diagnosis of Barrett's esophagus, and history of head and neck malignancy. Prior surgery on the stomach or colon should be documented because it may influence the choice of reconstructive conduit to restore alimentary continuity at the time of esophagectomy. Findings on physical examination that would prompt further diagnostic testing or tissue sampling include hoarseness due to recurrent laryngeal nerve involvement, cervical or supraclavicular lymphadenopathy, pleural effusion, and new onset of bone pain.

Routine chest radiography should be performed, but liquid oral contrast examination of the esophagus and stomach is no longer mandatory and, in many instances, is unnecessary in the era of flexible endoscopy. Esophagogastroscopy allows precise evaluation of the extent of esophageal and gastric involvement and can precisely measure the distance of the tumor from the incisors to appropriately categorize the tumor's location. Upper endoscopy also allows identification of "skip" lesions or second primaries as well as indicating the presence and extent of Barrett's esophagus. In addition, dilation of a stenotic lesion visualized at endoscopy may provide relief, albeit temporarily, from dysphagia. In the event the strictured area cannot be successfully dilated at endoscopy, a barium swallow test can provide information regarding extent of disease. Bronchoscopy should be reserved for those patients with tumors of the mid-

and upper esophagus to rule out invasion of the membranous trachea and possible tracheoesophageal fistula. In the absence of symptoms, bone scans should not be part of the routine workup because their yield is extremely low.

On completion of the initial diagnostic workup and after a tissue diagnosis of esophageal cancer, pretreatment staging procedures are essential to accurately determine the depth of esophageal wall penetration, the status of regional lymph node basins, and the presence or absence of distant metastases so that patients can be guided to the appropriate treatment options and provided with prognostic information. All patients should undergo a computed tomography (CT) scan of the chest, abdomen, and pelvis as the initial evaluation for extent of disease. CT scans are highly accurate (approaching 100%) in detecting liver or lung metastases and suggesting peritoneal carcinomatosis (ascites, omental infiltration, peritoneal tumor studding, etc.).[199–201] Accuracy for detecting aortic involvement or tracheobronchial invasion exceeds 90%.[200,202,203] Because of this, initial staging by CT renders further, more costly staging studies unnecessary and avoids consideration of patients with obvious metastatic disease for resection. CT is inaccurate in determining T stage, because it cannot define individual layers of the esophageal wall and will miss small T1 and T2 tumors. CT assessment of regional or distant lymph nodes is hindered by relatively low sensitivity (50% to 70%) due to its reliance on size criteria (larger than 1 cm) alone.[199,200,202,204–206] Because lymph node involvement is frequently seen in small or normal-size lymph nodes, the false-negative rate is high, and despite a reasonable specificity of 85%, accuracy in determining lymph node involvement is limited (approximately 60%).

Endoscopic ultrasonography (EUS) and EUS-guided fine-needle aspiration (FNA) are now considered to be invaluable tools for accurate pretreatment staging of esophageal cancer. The accuracy of EUS in determining both T and N stage is a function of its ability to clearly delineate the multiple layers of the esophageal wall[207,208] and its reliance on multiple criteria, including shape, border pattern, echogenicity, and size, to determine lymph node involvement.[209,210] Numerous studies have demonstrated that EUS is superior to CT in both T and N staging of esophageal cancer.[211,212] In these studies the overall accuracy for T staging is approximately 85% and for N staging is approximately 75%.[213] The accuracy of determining lymph node involvement has been increased with the use of linear-array EUS with a channel that allows passage of a needle to perform tissue aspiration for cytology. Studies of EUS FNA report an overall accuracy of 85% to 100% with sensitivity and specificity of more than 90%.[206,214,215] EUS is as accurate as CT in identifying aortic invasion[216,217] and can detect distant metastases to lung, liver, and peritoneum (ascites, omental implantation, etc.) but with less accuracy than CT.[211] EUS is highly operator dependent with regard to procurement of adequate images and correct interpretation. EUS is also limited in its ability to define relatively superficial lesions as either T1 or T2.[213,218,219] Making this distinction is critical because it may allow the use of minimal resection techniques for T1 lesions and avoidance of potentially toxic preoperative chemoradiotherapy for both T1 and T2 tumors. To address this issue, miniprobe high-frequency (20-MHz) sonographic catheters that can be passed through the working channel of the standard endoscope are now being used and provide improved accuracy.[220,221] In the past, presence of a malignant obstruction was considered a relative contraindication to the use of EUS because it required dilation to pass the instrument and increased the risk of perforation. A new generation of endoscopes that are thin caliber and can be passed over a guidewire can traverse almost all obstructing lesions, allowing EUS assessment for proper staging.[222] The accuracy of EUS in assessing response to induction chemoradiotherapy is severely limited, and its use frequently leads to overstaging because the fibrotic changes induced by treatment mimic residual tumor.[223,224]

Although it is a relatively recent addition to the armamentarium of staging procedures for esophageal cancer, [18F]fluorodeoxyglucose (FDG) positron emission tomography (PET) is being widely used, both appropriately and inappropriately, in the management of esophageal cancer. The accuracy of FDG-PET in assessing regional lymph nodes falls somewhere between the low and high accuracy of CT and EUS, respectively, and therefore its value in this respect is uncertain.[225,226] However, numerous studies confirm that, in the detection of distant metastases, FDG-PET is superior to CT, with a sensitivity, specificity, and accuracy all in the range of 80% to 90%.[226,227] This translates into the detection of unsuspected metastatic disease (up-staging) in approximately 15% of patients and refutation of suspected disease (down-staging) in 10%, which leads to alteration of the intended treatment plan in at least 20% of patients. FDG-PET appears to have some value in evaluating response to chemotherapy and radiotherapy. Weber et al.[228] demonstrated that decreased FDG uptake significantly correlated with pathologically confirmed response in patients treated with induction chemotherapy before esophagectomy for esophageal adenocarcinoma. Brücher et al.,[229] from the same institution, Technische Universität München, showed a similar result of decreased FDG uptake in responders compared to nonresponders in patients with squamous cell carcinoma of the esophagus treated with preoperative chemoradiotherapy. Downey et al.[230] examined the use of FDG-PET in a series of patients with predominately adenocarcinoma of the esophagus and found that PET did not identify disease progression or unresectable disease after induction therapy but that a greater decrease in the standardized uptake value was associated with a nonsignificant improvement in disease-free and overall survival. It remains uncertain whether the use of FDG-PET in assessing response alters the treatment approach; however, its utility in detecting additional distant disease not previously identified by other imaging modalities confirms a role for PET that is complimentary to that of other staging procedures for carcinoma of the esophagus, although it should not supplant them.

Minimally invasive surgical techniques (laparoscopy, thoracoscopy, or both) are being used for staging of both local-regional and distant disease. Performing laparoscopy as the initial procedure at the time of planned esophagectomy adds little in the way of time and cost to the procedure and allows detection of unsuspected distant metastases, which spares the morbidity of laparotomy in 10% to 15% of cases.[231,232] Luketich et al.,[233] in a study comparing staging laparoscopy and thoracoscopy with CT and EUS in 53 patients with esophageal cancer, demonstrated either up-staging or down-staging in 32% when the combined laparoscopic and thoracoscopic technique was used. The same group from the University of Pittsburgh, using minimally invasive staging techniques to assess the utility of FDG-PET scans, noted that minimally invasive techniques were superior, showing greater sensitivity than FDG-PET.[234] Krasna et al.[235] reported improved accuracy in evaluating local invasion, lymph node metastases, and distant metastases with thoracoscopic and laparoscopic staging. Although these studies suggest improved pretreatment staging with the minimally invasive surgical approaches, such approaches have not been embraced as standard staging procedures by most surgeons due to the morbidity, length of hospital stay, and cost associated with what is considered an additional procedure.

Finally, a study comparing the health care costs and efficacy of staging procedures including CT scan, EUS FNA, PET, and thoracoscopy-laparoscopy reported that CT plus EUS FNA was the least expensive and offered the most quality-adjusted life-years on average than all the other strategies. PET plus EUS FNA was somewhat more effective but also more expensive.[236]

PATHOLOGIC STAGING

The guidelines established by the American Joint Committee on Cancer for staging of esophageal cancer are outlined in Tables 29.1-2 and 29.1-3.[75] The primary tumor (T) stage is based on depth of tumor invasion into and through the wall of the esophagus. The nodal (N) stage is determined by the presence of involved regional lymph nodes. The designation of a lymph node as regional is based on its relationship to the location of the primary tumor. For primary tumors located in the distal esophagus, celiac lymph node involvement is considered distant metastasis and designated as M1A. For tumors located in the upper thoracic esophagus metastases to cervical lymph nodes also carry the designation M1A. Any other lymph nodes involved by tumor are classified with other distant sites of involvement as M1B. It has been recommended that lymph node status be based on examination of at least 6 lymph nodes in the resected specimen; however, one analysis noted an improvement in sensitivity to over 90% when 12 or

TABLE 29.1-2. Tumor (T), Node (N), Metastasis (M) Staging System for Esophageal Cancer

PRIMARY TUMOR (T)	
TX	Primary tumor cannot be assessed
T0	No evidence of primary tumor
Tis	Carcinoma *in situ*
T1	Tumor invades lumina propria or submucosa
T2	Tumor invades muscularis propria
T3	Tumor invades adventitia
T4	Tumor invades adjacent structures
REGIONAL LYMPH NODES (N)	
NX	Regional lymph nodes cannot be assessed
N0	No regional lymph node metastasis
N1	Regional lymph node metastasis
DISTANT METASTASIS (M)	
MX	Distant metastasis cannot be assessed
M0	No distant metastasis
M1	Distant metastasis
Tumors of the lower thoracic esophagus	
M1a	Metastasis in celiac lymph nodes
M1b	Other distant metastasis
Tumors of the mid-thoracic esophagus	
M1a	Not applicable
M1b	Nonregional lymph nodes and/or other distant metastasis
Tumors of the upper thoracic esophagus	
M1a	Metastasis in cervical lymph nodes
M1b	Other distant metastasis

TABLE 29.1-3. Classification of Stage Groupings for Esophageal Cancer

Stage Groupings	TNM Classifications		
0	Tis	N0	M0
I	T1	N0	M0
IIA	T2	N0	M0
	T3	N0	M0
IIB	T1	N1	M0
	T2	N1	M0
III	T3	N1	M0
	T4	Any N	M0
IV	Any T	Any N	M1
IVA	Any T	Any N	M1a
IVB	Any T	Any N	M1b

more lymph nodes were examined as is recommended for colorectal carcinoma.[237]

Successive pathologically determined stage groups are predictive of length of survival.[75,183] It has been suggested that extensive nodal disease may be associated with better survival than visceral metastases, and it does appear that survival with stage IVA disease more closely mimics that with stage III disease than that with stage IVB disease.

TREATMENT

Optimal treatment of esophageal cancer in every major stage grouping (premalignant or intramucosal lesions, localized resectable tumors, and unresectable metastatic disease) remains elusive and a work in progress that continues to engender substantial controversy. The paucity of appropriately designed studies to scientifically determine the most effective therapeutic strategy for any given clinical situation fuels the ongoing debate and undermines the potential for achieving consensus. Although there is no disagreement that esophageal resection prevents progression from high-grade dysplasia to invasive carcinoma and is curative for T1 lesions limited to the mucosa, the morbidity and mortality associated with esophagectomy has created enthusiasm for alternative approaches such as mucosal ablation and endoscopic resection. Surgery has always been considered the most effective way of ensuring both local-regional control and long-term survival for patients with tumors invading into or beyond the submucosa with or without lymph node involvement. Some investigators suggest that extending the limits of resection will further improve outcome. However, surgery alone or any other single modality fails in the vast majority of patients, which has led many oncologists to embrace combined modality therapy and some to question the necessity for surgical intervention. Despite the lack of convincing evidence to support its use, chemoradiotherapy with or without resection is the most common therapeutic regimen offered to patients with esophageal carcinoma in the United States.[183] A full understanding of these issues and others regarding the treatment of carcinoma of the esophagus requires careful scrutiny of the available literature with an attempt to separate bias from fact in developing a rational therapeutic approach for patients regardless of the stage of their disease.

TREATMENT OF PREMALIGNANT AND T1 DISEASE (LOCALIZED TO THE MUCOSA ONLY)

Pathologic confirmation of high-grade dysplasia in Barrett's esophagus is the most powerful predictor of subsequent invasive adenocarcinoma and therefore warrants instituting a therapeutic plan. The rationale for esophagectomy is that resection completely eradicates the mucosa at risk, which prevents progression to invasive carcinoma. This approach is further supported by numerous surgical series reporting that, for patients with high-grade dysplasia who undergo esophagectomy, previously unidentified invasive cancer is present in up to 40% of resected specimens.[34,238–240] Those who assert that esophagectomy is not indicated would argue that the vast majority of patients with high-grade dysplasia do not go on to develop invasive carcinoma in their lifetimes, and that management of such patients using endoscopic methods ranging from surveillance to mucosal ablative and resection techniques allows identification of patients with an early invasive lesion that is readily amenable to cure or elimination of the mucosa at risk, preventing progression. Patients with superficial invasive tumors confined to the mucosa have little or no risk of lymph node metastases and are considered candidates for potentially less morbidity-producing resection methods.

Surveillance

The management of high-grade dysplasia with endoscopic surveillance is based on the assumptions that the majority of patients will not progress to invasive carcinoma during their lifetimes, that a prolonged interval exists between the time of diagnosis of high-grade dysplasia and development of adenocarcinoma, and that cancers detected by surveillance are at an earlier stage and are therefore highly curable.[241] Studies demonstrating that patients with Barrett's esophagus–associated adenocarcinomas detected by surveillance have an earlier stage of disease and have better survival than those whose cancers are detected at initial endoscopy provide supportive evidence for this approach.[34–36] Critics counter this argument with results from numerous surgical series that report identification of invasive adenocarcinoma in up to 45% of esophagectomy specimens from patients referred with a diagnosis of high-grade dysplasia.[238–240] Proponents of surveillance management argue that these patients were not entered into an endoscopic surveillance program with strict biopsy criteria developed with the intent of providing early detection of malignant degeneration. Proposed guidelines for surveillance includes serial endoscopy at 3- to 6-month intervals with multiple four-quadrant biopsies at 1- to 2-cm intervals.[24] Schnell et al. entered 75 patients with high-grade dysplasia into organized surveillance programs similar to that described and identified invasive cancer in 16% over a mean follow-up period of 7.3 years.[242] In 11 of the 12 patients, adenocarcinoma was detected at an early stage and was considered cured with subsequent resection or ablation. Of note, patients whose cancer was detected during the first year of protocol management were excluded from analysis. The downside of endoscopic vigilance is that in a certain percentage of patients invasive cancer goes undetected and the patients will not be candidates for potentially curative treatment.[243–245] This must be weighed against the morbidity and mortality of esophagectomy, which are especially poignant in those patients who undergo the risks of surgery and are found not to have invasive carcinoma. It is important to note that the extent of high-grade dysplasia does not predict the presence of occult adenocarcinoma identified at esophagectomy and therefore cannot necessarily be applied to a subjective quantification of disease.[246] In a final analysis, the patient must be well informed about the issues related to both surveillance and alternative measures and must make a decision based on individual needs and expectations.

Ablative Methods

The mechanism of action of all mucosal ablative techniques, including photodynamic therapy (PDT), laser ablation, and argon plasma coagulation, is destruction of the mucosal layer. The premise for managing high-grade dysplasia with endoscopic ablative therapy is that mucosal injury in an acid-controlled environment eliminates the premalignant mucosa and resurfaces the esophageal lining with regenerated squamous epithelium.[241]

PDT involves administration of an inactive photosensitizing agent that when exposed to light of the proper wavelength results in oxygen radical production and tissue destruction. The largest experience with this technique has been reported by Overholt et al.[247] In their study, 80% of patients had eradication of high-grade dysplasia with PDT combined with acid-suppressive therapy over a mean follow-up period of 50 months. Eight percent of patients developed carcinomas, half of which were subsquamous adenocarcinomas detected during extended follow-up. PDT was also used in nine patients with "early-stage cancer," and treatment was declared to have failed in almost 60% of these patients. Early interim results of a phase III randomized study comparing PDT plus omeprazole with omeprazole alone demonstrated improved eradication of high-grade dysplasia in the PDT arm (80% vs. 40%) at a 6-month follow-up.[248] With further follow-up a marked reduction in the number of cancers was noted in the PDT-treated group (17% vs. 39%); however, the results emphasize the risk of development of invasive cancer in a relatively short follow-up interval of only 12 months. These results highlight the limitations of PDT, and because tissue is not obtained to properly stage disease, at the present time this modality should only be offered to patients with severe comorbid disease who are not candidates for other more definitive therapy. Complications of PDT include stricture formation and photosensitivity. Limited experience with thermal ablation for high-grade dysplasia has been reported. Small series of either laser ablation[249,250] or argon plasma coagulation[251,252] of high-grade dysplasia suggest that high-grade dysplasia can be eradicated; however, the follow-up period in these studies was short and invasive carcinoma has subsequently been documented. The major risk of thermal ablation is esophageal perforation.

Endoscopic Mucosal Resection

Endoscopic mucosal resection (EMR) is a relatively recent addition to the endoscopic therapeutic options available for patients with either high-grade dysplasia or superficial esophageal cancers. EMR technique involves the submucosal injection of fluid to lift and separate the lesion from the underlying muscular layer, which allows full resection and tissue retrieval for appropriate histologic examination.[253] Ell et al.[254] prospec-

tively examined the utility of EMR in 64 patients, 3 of whom had high-grade dysplasia and the remainder of whom had early esophageal carcinoma. Eradication of disease was achieved in all patients with high-grade dysplasia; of the 35 patients with favorable lesions (2 cm or less, well or moderately differentiated, and limited to the mucosa) 34 were in complete remission at a mean follow-up of 12 months. The complete remission rate in patients with less favorable lesions was 59%, which emphasizes the need to adhere to strict criteria to optimize disease eradication. These results and similar findings in smaller series examining EMR[255,256] confirm that use of this technique is feasible for treatment of high-grade dysplasia and carcinoma limited to the mucosa and provides an alternative to esophagectomy, especially in those patients considered high risk for surgical intervention.

Minimally Invasive Esophagectomy

There is little debate that esophageal resection is the most definitive intervention for eliminating high-grade dysplasia and is extremely effective treatment for carcinoma limited to the mucosa. However, the substantial morbidity and potential for mortality associated with esophagectomy, even in the most experienced hands, has resulted in considerable controversy regarding its acceptance as optimal therapy in this setting. In an attempt to reduce morbidity and mortality while achieving an equivalent oncologic outcome, minimally invasive techniques for esophageal resection have been designed and are being investigated. A variety of minimally invasive approaches have been used for esophagectomy, including laparoscopic, thoracoscopic, combined laparoscopic and thoracoscopic, and hand-assisted techniques (Table 29.1-4).[257–260] These techniques have been described and are similar in conduct to open procedures of transthoracic and transhiatal esophagectomy detailed in Surgical Resection, later in this chapter, except for the nuances of the minimally invasive approach (Figs. 29.1-5 and 29.1-6). These procedures have been applied to the treatment of all stages of potentially resectable esophageal cancer but would seem to be most applicable in the management of premalignant and early-stage disease. The largest experience with minimally invasive esophagectomy has been reported by Luketich et al.[258] in a study of 77 patients with premalignant disease or esophageal cancer, the majority of whom underwent a combined laparoscopic and thoracoscopic procedure. Fourteen patients had either high-grade dysplasia or stage I carcinoma of the esophagus. Median operative time was 7.5 hours, median length of hospital stay was 7 days, and a 30-day perioperative mortality was zero. Median follow-up was 20 months, and a 3-year survival of 90% was achieved in patients with either high-grade dysplasia or stage I disease. The outcome appears to be similar to that seen with open esophagectomy and the conduct of the operation from an oncologic standpoint (margin status and lymph

TABLE 29.1-4. Minimally Invasive Approaches to Resection of Esophageal Cancer

Endoscopic mucosal resection
Combined thoracoscopic/laparoscopic esophagectomy
Laparoscopic transhiatal esophagectomy
Thoracoscopically assisted esophagectomy
Hand-assisted laparoscopic transhiatal esophagectomy

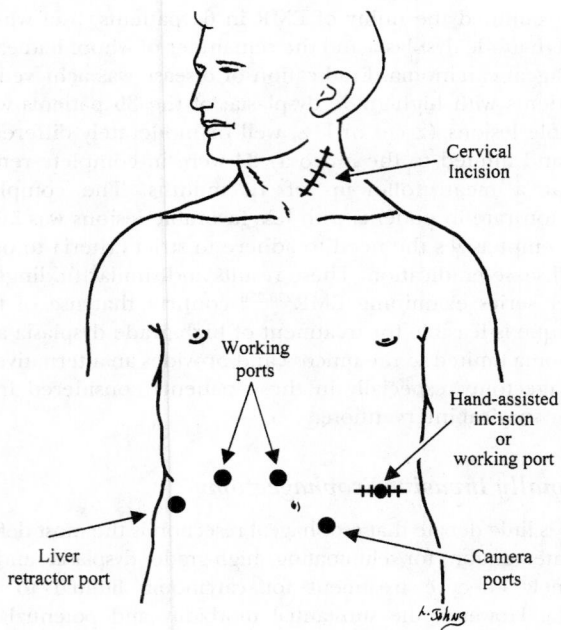

FIGURE 29.1-5. Abdominal port sites and incisions used for minimally invasive esophagectomy. If a thoracoscopic approach is not used to dissect and mobilize the thoracic esophagus, a 6-cm incision is used instead of the left-sided abdominal working port to perform a hand-assisted transhiatal esophagectomy.

node retrieval) seems adequate. These results are promising, but whether they are durable or reproducible must be determined through further study. Initial experience with the hand-assisted laparoscopic esophagectomy technique has been reported. By providing tactile feedback to the surgeon, this approach closely mimics open esophagectomy and may be more widely applicable in the surgical community.[259] Whether the theoretical advantages of decreased postoperative pain, reduced length of hospital stay, and cost effectiveness of minimally invasive esophagectomy translate into actual benefits and outcome equivalent to that of more conventional resection techniques remain unproven and must be determined through controlled comparative studies.[261,262]

TREATMENT OF LOCALIZED DISEASE

Surgery has traditionally been the treatment of choice for patients with localized, resectable carcinoma of the esophagus

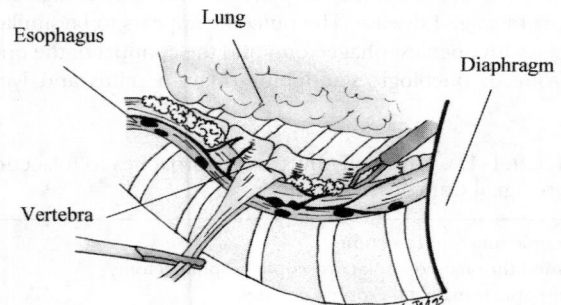

FIGURE 29.1-6. Thoracoscopic view and dissection of intrathoracic esophagus.

and continues to be a component of a more comprehensive approach to esophageal cancer in a substantial number of patients. Failure of surgery alone to significantly alter the natural history of esophageal cancer has resulted in considerable enthusiasm for combined modality therapy. The shift toward multimodal treatment, although theoretically sound, is not convincingly supported by data from phase III clinical trials comparing preoperative therapeutic regimens (radiation, chemotherapy, or chemoradiotherapy) to surgery alone. Similarly, although it is appropriate to question the role of surgery in a multimodal approach to treatment of esophageal cancer, no data are currently available from studies designed to examine the necessity of surgery, and therefore the wisdom of eliminating resection from the treatment algorithm is questionable. The treatment options available to patients with localized disease are detailed and supportive data, when available, are presented.

Surgical Resection

Many controversies exist regarding the surgical treatment of esophageal cancer, including the optimal surgical approach, the extent of local resection and lymph node retrieval, selection of a reconstructive conduit, and location of the anastomosis. Decisions regarding surgical technique are routinely based from personal bias, comfort level of the surgeon, and a subjective view of tumor biology, because solid evidence from scientifically designed trials is marginal and, in most instances, nonexistent. However, there is a growing body of evidence which suggests that outcome after esophagectomy is directly related to both surgeon and hospital volume. Numerous studies that used health services–linked databases have demonstrated a statistically significant association between performance of surgery in hospitals designated as high-volume esophagectomy institutions and lower complication and mortality rates.[263–266] Although this link has been shown for other complex surgical procedures, the association between volume and outcome for esophageal resection appears to be one of the strongest.[267]

TRANSHIATAL ESOPHAGECTOMY. The transhiatal route for esophageal resection has gained favor, especially among surgeons in the United States, concurrent with the rising incidence of adenocarcinoma of the distal esophagus, which is readily approachable and effectively dissected through the diaphragmatic hiatus (Table 29.1-5). The technique is as follows.[268,269] It is prudent to initially perform laparoscopic exploration to rule out disseminated disease and, if it is confirmed, to abort the intended resection before exposing the patient to the risks of laparotomy. Through a midline incision, the stomach is mobilized by dividing all vascular attachments while preserving the right gastroepiploic and right gastric vessels on whose pedicle the reconstructive conduit will be based. The duodenum is fully mobilized via a Kocher maneuver and a pyloric drainage procedure is performed, which has been demonstrated in prospective randomized trials to reduce gastric stasis and minimize pulmonary complications such as aspiration.[270,271] Cautery division of the diaphragmatic crus allows wide access to the mediastinum and dissection under direct vision of the middle and lower third of the esophagus. A left cervical incision provides exposure to the cervical esophagus, and circumferential dissection of the cervical esophagus is carried down to below the thoracic inlet to the upper thoracic esophagus, with care to avoid injury to the recurrent laryngeal nerve. The remain-

TABLE 29.1-5. Conventional Approaches to Esophageal Resection for Cancer

TRANSHIATAL
Laparotomy and cervical approach
Peritumoral or two-field lymph node dissection
En bloc resection feasible for distal esophageal tumors
Cervical anastomosis

TRANSTHORACIC

Ivor Lewis
Right thoracotomy and laparotomy
Peritumoral or two-field lymph node dissection
En bloc resection feasible for mid-/distal thoracic tumors

McKeown or "three hole"
Right thoracotomy, laparotomy, cervical approach
Peritumoral, two-field or three-field lymph node dissection
En bloc resection feasible for mid-/distal thoracic tumors
Cervical anastomosis

Left thoracotomy
Left thoracotomy with or without cervical approach
Peritumoral lymph nodes dissection
Intrathoracic or cervical anastomosis

Left thoracoabdominal
Left thoracoabdominal approach
Peritumoral or two-field lymph node dissection
Intrathoracic anastomosis

---

der of the dissection at the level of and superior to the carina is completed by blunt dissection through the esophageal hiatus. The cervical esophagus is then divided, the stomach and attached intrathoracic esophagus are delivered through the abdominal wound, and a gastric tube, which will serve as the reconstructive conduit, is fashioned using multiple applications of a linear stapling device. The gastric tube is then transposed through the posterior mediastinum to the cervical wound, where a cervical esophagogastric anastomosis is performed. The stomach is considered by most surgeons as the replacement conduit of choice for the resected esophagus. A segment of colon, usually based on the ascending branch of the inferior mesenteric artery, is an effective esophageal substitute if for any reason the stomach is deemed unsuitable for reconstruction or the surgeon prefers. Although the original intent of this approach was not to perform a methodical lymph node dissection, a standard two-field lymphadenectomy (abdominal and lower mediastinal) can readily be achieved, and for that matter, if the surgeon is so inclined, a radical *en bloc* resection can be performed as described by Bumm et al.[272]

The stated advantages attributed to the transhiatal approach to esophagectomy include avoidance of a thoracotomy incision, which thereby minimizes pain and subsequent postoperative pulmonary complications; elimination of the lethal complications of mediastinitis associated with an intrathoracic anastomotic leak; and a shorter duration of operation, which results in decreased morbidity and mortality.[269] Limitations and disadvantages of transhiatal esophagectomy include poor visualization of upper and mid-thoracic esophageal tumors, increased anastomotic leak rate with subsequent stricture formation, possibility of chylothorax, and possibility of recurrent laryngeal nerve injury. The largest experience with transhiatal esophagectomy was reported by Orringer et al.[273] and included 800 patients with esophageal cancer, 69% of whom had adenocarcinoma and 28% of whom had squamous cell carcinoma. Tumors were located in the lower third of the esophagus in 74.5%, in the middle third in 22%, and in the upper third in 4.5%. In-hospital mortality was 4.5%. The most common complications were anastomotic leak (13%) and recurrent laryngeal nerve palsy (7%). Leak of a cervical esophageal gastric anastomosis was handled simply in the vast majority of patients with opening of the cervical wound, followed by local wound care. Hoarseness from recurrent laryngeal nerve injury resolved spontaneously in 99% of cases. Overall 5-year survival was 23%, and stage-specific 5-year survival was 59% for stage I, 22% for stage II, 29% for stage IIB, and 10% for stage III. These results reflect those reported from other surgical series of transhiatal esophagectomy (Table 29.1-6).[273–278]

TRANSTHORACIC ESOPHAGECTOMY. Transthoracic esophagectomy has been the most common surgical approach used to resect carcinomas of the esophagus and is the standard procedure against which all other techniques are measured (see Table 29.1-5). Although a left thoracotomy provides adequate exposure to tumors of the distal esophagus, a right thoracotomy affords access to upper, mid-, and distal esophageal lesions and is the preferred route for transthoracic exposure. A right thoracotomy combined with an upper midline laparotomy (Ivor Lewis esophagectomy) is the technique most commonly used for esophageal resection and is briefly described here.[269] The abdominal portion of the procedure duplicates that of the transhiatal approach detailed earlier in Transhiatal Esophagectomy and includes mobilization of the stomach and distal esophagus, upper abdominal lymphadenectomy, pyloromyotomy, and placement of a feeding jejunostomy before abdominal wound closure and repositioning for the thoracic component of the procedure. A muscle-sparing right lateral thoracotomy is performed through the fifth or sixth intercostal space. The azygos vein is divided, the mediastinal pleura incised, the intrathoracic esophagus mobilized, and a mediastinal lymph node dissection performed. After

TABLE 29.1-6. Results of Transhiatal Esophagectomy for Esophageal Cancer

Study	Year	Patients (n)	Histologic Type	Perioperative Mortality (%)	5-Y Survival (%)
Gelfand et al.[274]	1992	160	A	0.9	21
Gertsch et al.[276]	1993	100	A/S	3	23
Vigneswaran et al.[275]	1993	131	A/S	2.3	21
Dudhat and Shinde[278]	1998	80	S	7.5	37
Orringer et al.[273]	1999	800	A/S	4.5	23
Bolton and Teng[277]	2002	124	A/S	1.6	27.3

A, adenocarcinoma; S, squamous cell carcinoma.

TABLE 29.1-7. Results of Transthoracic Esophagectomy for Esophageal Cancer

Study	Year	Patients (n)	Histologic Type	Perioperative Mortality (%)	5-Y Survival (%)
Wang et al.[284]	1992	368	S	6.5	7.6
Lieberman et al.[285]	1995	258	A/S	5	27
Adam et al.[283]	1996	597	A/S	6.9	16.3
Sharpe and Moghissi[281]	1996	562	A/S	9	18
Bossett et al.[286]	1997	139	S	3.6	26
Ellis[282]	1999	455	A/S	3.3	24.7

A, adenocarcinoma; S, squamous cell carcinoma.

division of the proximal esophagus in the chest ensuring an adequate margin, the gastroesophageal junction and stomach are pulled into the thoracic cavity. The stomach is then divided with a linear stapler, the specimen is removed and an esophagogastric anastomosis performed. An alternative approach has been described in which the right thoracotomy is the initial stage of the procedure followed by repositioning of the patient supine for an abdominal and left cervical incision to achieve a cervical esophagogastric anastomosis.[279,280]

The transthoracic approach provides direct visualization and exposure of the intrathoracic esophagus facilitating a wider dissection to achieve a more adequate radial margin around the primary tumor and more thorough lymph node dissection, which theoretically results in a more sound cancer operation. In patients with significant comorbid conditions, the combined effects of an abdominal and thoracic incision may compromise cardiorespiratory function. An intrathoracic anastomotic leak can lead to mediastinitis, sepsis, and death. In addition, esophagitis in the nonresected thoracic esophagus may occur secondary to bile reflux. The three-incision (cervical, thoracic, and abdominal) modification of the procedure effectively eliminates the potential for complications associated with an intrathoracic esophagogastric anastomosis.

Numerous authors have reported results of transthoracic esophagectomy; however, most, if not all, of these reports include patients who were resected via other surgical approaches and underwent a more extended lymphadenectomy (Table 29.1-7).[281–286] Suffice it to say that both overall and stage-specific 5-year survival rates were similar to those seen with transhiatal esophagectomy. The cleanest data may be derived from prospective randomized trials exploring the role of induction therapy before esophagectomy in which there is a surgery-alone control arm. In only one of those trials, that conducted by Bossett et al.,[286] was a transthoracic approach the only surgical procedure allowed. In that trial, 139 patients were randomly assigned to the surgery-alone group. Median survival time was 18.6 months and 5-year survival rate was 26%.

TRANSHIATAL VERSUS TRANSTHORACIC ESOPHAGECTOMY. The controversy regarding the optimal surgical approach for esophageal cancer remains unresolved. Proponents of transthoracic esophagectomy claim superior oncologic outcome secondary to wider tumor clearance and more thorough lymphadenectomy. Supporters of transhiatal esophagectomy argue that a cervicoabdominal approach minimizes postoperative morbidity and mortality and is oncologically equivalent to the transthoracic approach.

Two large metaanalyses have compared transhiatal esophagectomy to transthoracic esophagectomy based on collective reviews of numerous individual studies.[287,288] Both reports include studies that compared transhiatal to transthoracic esophagectomy, studies of transhiatal esophagectomy only, and studies of transthoracic esophagectomy only. The vast majority of these studies were retrospective and were not standardized with regard to techniques used, use of additional therapy, and results reporting. The collective review by Rindani et al.[287] encompassed 5483 patients from 44 series published between 1986 and 1996. Perioperative mortality was significantly higher in the transthoracic esophagectomy group than in the transhiatal group (9.5% vs. 6.3%), whereas overall perioperative complications were not significantly different in the two groups. Patients who underwent transhiatal esophagectomy had a higher incidence of anastomotic leak, anastomotic stricture, and recurrent laryngeal nerve injury. Overall 5-year survival was similar for the two groups: 24% for the transhiatal esophagectomy group and 26% for the transthoracic esophagectomy group. Hulscher et al.[288] performed a collective review of 50 studies performed between 1990 and 1999 yielding 7527 patients for comparison of the transthoracic versus the transhiatal route. Postoperative mortality was significantly greater in the transthoracic group than in transhiatal group (9.2% vs. 5.7%). Transthoracic esophagectomy was associated with a significantly higher risk of pulmonary complications (18.7% vs. 12.7%), whereas patients treated with transhiatal esophagectomy had a higher anastomotic leak rate (13.6% vs. 7.2%). Five-year survival was not significantly different, with 23% 5-year survival for transthoracic esophagectomy and 21.7% 5-year survival with transhiatal esophagectomy. A prospective database based on the Veterans Administration National Surgical Quality Improvement Program was used to analyze perioperative outcome in 945 patients, 562 who underwent transthoracic esophagectomy and 383 who underwent resection through a transhiatal approach.[289] There was no difference in overall mortality (10% for transthoracic approach vs. 9.9% for transhiatal approach) or morbidity (47% for transthoracic vs. 49% for transhiatal).

Four phase III trials have prospectively examined the outcomes for patients randomly assigned to undergo either transhiatal or transthoracic esophagectomy.[290–293] No definitive conclusions can be drawn from three of these trials due to the extremely small sample size. The trial in the Netherlands, however, deserves special attention. Hulscher et al.[293] randomly assigned 220 patients with mid- or distal esophageal carcinoma to undergo either transhiatal esophagectomy or transthoracic esophagectomy. The transthoracic group underwent a systematic mediastinal and upper abdominal lymph node dissection. Although the number of lymph nodes retrieved was significantly higher in

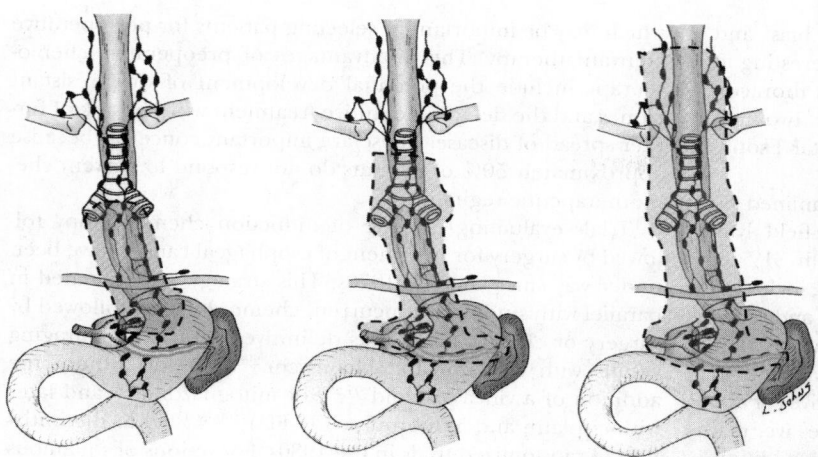

FIGURE 29.1-7. Standard, two-field, and three-field lymphadenectomy.

the transthoracic group (31 vs. 16; *P* <.001), there was no difference in the radicality of the two procedures with equivalent R0, R1, and R2 resections. Postoperative pulmonary complications, ventilatory time, intensive care unit stay, and hospital stay were significantly higher in those patients assigned to the transthoracic group. Despite the higher perioperative morbidity, there was no statistically significant increase in in-hospital mortality (4% vs. 2% for transthoracic vs. transhiatal esophagectomy, respectively; *P* <.5). At a median follow-up of 4.7 years, there were no significant differences between the transhiatal and transthoracic esophagectomy groups with respect to median disease-free interval (1.4 vs. 1.7 years, respectively) and median overall survival time (1.8 vs. 2.0 years, respectively). Likewise, no significant differences were noted in local-regional recurrence, distant recurrence, and combined local-regional and distant recurrence for patients randomly allocated to the transthoracic or transhiatal esophagectomy arm. The investigators point out that a trend toward improved disease-free survival (39% vs. 27%) and overall survival (39% vs. 29%) at 5 years favored the transthoracic approach group.

From the data presented, one could reasonably conclude that either the transhiatal or transthoracic procedure can be performed with acceptable morbidity and mortality in experienced hands and that, with either technique, the outcome is remarkably similar—that is, poor.

EXTENDED ESOPHAGECTOMY. In an attempt to improve on the dismal results reflected in high local recurrence rates and poor overall survival with standard transhiatal and transthoracic esophagectomy techniques, some surgeons have advocated and examined extending the limits of resection to accomplish a more effective primary tumor excision and lymph node dissection. Two concepts guide the intent of these more extended resections: *en bloc* resection of the primary tumor with its adjacent surrounding tissue, and systematic lymph node dissection encompassing either two (mediastinal and abdominal) or three (cervical, mediastinal, and abdominal) lymph node basins (Fig. 29.1-7). Although some investigators have focused and reported separately on *en bloc* esophagectomy and extended lymphadenectomy, most of the techniques described encompass both components of this "radical" approach. *En bloc* esophagectomy involves resection of mid- and lower esophageal tumors with an envelope of adjacent tissue that includes the mediastinal pleura laterally, the pericardium anteriorly, and the azygos vein and tho-

racic duct posterolaterally with the surrounding periesophageal tissue and lymph nodes. For tumors traversing the esophageal hiatus, a cuff of diaphragm is resected. In addition to a thorough mediastinal lymph node dissection extending from the tracheal bifurcation to the esophageal hiatus, an upper abdominal lymph node dissection incorporating lymph nodes along the portal vein, common hepatic artery, celiac trunk, left gastric artery, and splenic artery is included to achieve a two-field lymph node dissection.[294] A three-field lymph node dissection extends the lymphadenectomy to the superior mediastinum including nodes along the course of the right and left recurrent laryngeal nerves and, through a separate collar incision in the neck, completes the dissection with removal of the lower cervical nodes including the deep external and lateral cervical lymph node basins.[78,79]

Most of the series examining the utility of extended esophagectomy are retrospective and involve a single institution. Hagen et al.[76] reported on 100 consecutively treated patients who had undergone an *en bloc* esophagectomy with two-field lymphadenectomy; none of the patients received additional preoperative or postoperative chemotherapy or radiotherapy. The perioperative mortality was 6%, with the most common complications being pneumonia (19%), subphrenic abscess (13%), respiratory failure (9%), anastomotic leak (10%), and empyema (7%). Local recurrence was detected in only one patient and overall actuarial 5-year survival was 52%. Patients with stage III lesions had a 25% actuarial 5-year survival. Altorki et al.[77] reviewed the results for 128 patients who underwent esophagectomy at a single institution; 61% received an *en bloc* esophagectomy and the remainder underwent a standard esophageal resection. Approximately 40% of those undergoing the more extended resection had a three-field lymphadenectomy; the others had a systematic two-field lymphadenectomy. The in-hospital mortality for the *en bloc* resection group was 5.1%, similar to that for those undergoing a standard resection. The most common postoperative complications in the extended resection group were respiratory events (24%) and anastomotic leak (12.8%), but no significant differences were noted in comparison to the standard resection group. Four-year survival for the *en bloc* group was 41.5% overall and 34.5% for stage III patients, with both of these survival figures markedly better than those for the standard resection group. However, both of the studies described here are single-institution, retrospective analyses for which the results, at least in part if not completely, can be attributed to selection bias and enhanced staging leading to stage migration. It is interesting to note that similar results have been achieved without thoracotomy using a transhiatal approach with systematic two-field lymphadenectomy as described earlier in Transhiatal Esophagectomy.[272]

A group at Cornell University also separately examined 80 patients who underwent esophagectomy with three-field lymphadenectomy.[79] Overall 30-day mortality was 5% with 31% of patients developing major postoperative complications, including need for reintubation (16%), anastomotic leak (11%), and recurrent laryngeal nerve injury (9%). Overall 5-year survival was 51%. Cervical lymph node metastases were identified in 36% of patients, and the 5-year survival rate for those with positive cervical lymph nodes was 25%. These results, although impressive, may also reflect both selection bias and stage migration. In addition, the expertise required to perform these technically demanding procedures effectively limits their application to only specialized centers and a fraction of the patients who might benefit from these procedures if an actual advantage were proven.

Results from phase III trials would potentially clarify the role of extended esophagectomy. As described in detail earlier in Transhiatal versus Transthoracic Esophagectomy, Hulscher et al.[288] performed a prospective randomized study of extended transthoracic resection versus transhiatal resection involving 220 patients with adenocarcinoma of the esophagus. Those patients who underwent an extended transthoracic resection had *en bloc* resection of the ipsilateral pleura, thoracic duct, azygos vein, and adjacent periesophageal tissue with a methodical two-field lymph node dissection. The study was performed in two academic medical centers with extensive expertise in esophageal resection. No significant difference was noted in local-regional recurrence, median disease-free survival, and median overall survival. There were trends toward improved disease-free and overall survival at 5 years in favor of the extended resection group. A small study by Nishihira et al.[295] of 62 patients randomly assigned to either three-field or two-field lymphadenectomy showed an improved, but not statistically significant, survival advantage for extended lymphadenectomy (66.2% vs. 48%; *P* = .19). Patients in this study were randomly assigned to receive either chemoradiotherapy or chemotherapy alone after surgery, which confounds the interpretation of the results.

The body of evidence confirms that extended resections improve staging and may enhance local-regional control; however, these procedures should still be considered investigational pending the availability of reliable data supporting their worth.

Adjuvant Therapy

PREOPERATIVE CHEMOTHERAPY. Nearly three-fourths of patients newly diagnosed with esophageal cancer present with locally advanced (stage IIB or III) disease. The poor survival rate achieved with surgery alone has provided the impetus for the evaluation of preoperative (induction) chemotherapy in patients with resectable esophageal cancer.

The potential benefits of induction chemotherapy include down-staging of the disease to facilitate surgical resection, improvement in local control, and eradication of micrometastatic disease. Esophagectomy after induction therapy enables comprehensive pathologic assessment of treatment response,

which may be important in selecting patients for postoperative adjuvant therapy. The disadvantages of preoperative chemotherapy include the potential development of drug-resistant clones and the delay in definitive treatment with the risk of further spread of disease. These are important concerns, because approximately 50% of patients do not respond to current chemotherapeutic regimens.

Trials evaluating the use of induction chemotherapy followed by surgery for treatment of esophageal cancer have been under way since the late 1970s. This strategy was evaluated in parallel with studies of concurrent chemoradiation followed by surgery or chemoradiation as definitive therapy. Encouraging results with cisplatin and bleomycin,[296] with or without the addition of a vinca alkaloid[297,298] or mitoguazone,[299] and later with cisplatin and 5-fluorouracil (5-FU),[300–304] led to the initiation of randomized trials in the 1980s. For lesions of squamous histology, the response rate to two or three cycles of cisplatin (100 mg/m^2 day 1) and 5-FU (1000 mg/m^2/d for 96 or 120 hours) every 3 weeks ranged between 42% and 66%, with a 0% to 10% pathologically confirmed complete response rate; curative resection rates were between 40% and 80%, and median survival was from 18 to 28 months.[300–304] Lesions were staged with a barium esophagogram and CT scan initially and then again before surgery to assess response to induction therapy.

Six randomized trials evaluating the use of preoperative chemotherapy in esophageal cancer patients are summarized in Table 29.1-8.[186,187,305–308] Four of the trials enrolled only patients with squamous cell carcinoma,[305–308] whereas half to two-thirds of patients enrolled in the two more recent and largest trials (U.S. Intergroup and Medical Research Council) had adenocarcinoma of the esophagus, gastroesophageal junction, or cardia.[186,187]

No improvement in survival was noted in three small trials enrolling under 100 patients each, reported by Nygaard et al.,[305] Roth et al.,[307] and Schlag.[308] The first randomized trial in the United States was conducted by Roth and colleagues[307] at M. D. Anderson Cancer Center. They enrolled a total of 39 patients, who were randomly assigned equally to preoperative cisplatin, bleomycin, and vindesine therapy for three courses or to immediate surgery. Six months of postoperative adjuvant cisplatin and vindesine was planned for patients in the preoperative chemotherapy arm. A 47% major response rate, including one pathologically confirmed complete response, was documented. Although resectability rates were similar in the two groups, a higher percentage of patients receiving preoperative chemotherapy had negative surgical margins, and those who responded to chemotherapy had significantly longer survival than those who did not respond (median of 20 vs. 6.2 months; *P* = .008). However, differences in overall survival at 3 years (25% vs. 5%) were not significant.

A multicenter trial in Germany reported by Schlag[308] compared cisplatin and 5-FU (three cycles) followed by surgery with surgery alone. The trial was stopped early after enrolling 46 patients because of a substantial increase in operative morbidity and mortality in the chemotherapy group. A 41% major response rate was observed, including pathologically confirmed complete response in two patients. There was no difference in median survival in the overall comparison; however, those who responded to preoperative chemotherapy survived longer than those who did not respond (13 vs. 5 months).

Kok and colleagues[306] reported a survival advantage for preoperative chemotherapy in a preliminary communication. This

TABLE 29.1-8. Randomized Trials of Preoperative Chemotherapy

Series	Treatment	Patients (n)	Histologic Type	Survival Median	2-Y (%)	3-Y (%)
Nygaard et al.[305]	Preop cisplat/bleo	50	S			3
	Surgery	41				9
Roth et al.[307]	Preoperative cisplat/VDS/bleo and adjuvant cisplat/VDS	19	S	9 mo		25
	Surgery	20		9 mo		5
Schlag[308]	Preop cisplat/5-FU	34	S	10 mo		
	Surgery	41		10 mo		
Kok et al.[306]	Preop cisplat/etoposide	86	S	18.5 mo		
	Surgery	85		11 mo		
Kelsen et al. (Intergroup 0013)[186]	Preop cisplat/5-FU and adjuvant cisplat/5-FU	213	S/A	15 mo	35	26
	Surgery	227		16 mo	37	23
MRCOCWG[187]	Preop cisplat/5-FU	400	S/A	16.8 mo	43	32
	Surgery	402		13.3 mo	34	25

A, adenocarcinoma; bleo, bleomycin; cisplat, cisplatin; 5-FU, 5-fluorouracil; MRCOCWG, Medical Research Council Oesophageal Cancer Working Group; Preop, preoperative; S, squamous cell carcinoma; VDS, vindesine.

study, enrolling 171 patients with squamous cell carcinoma, differed from other trials by requiring response assessment after two courses of preoperative chemotherapy. Patients showing no response underwent immediate surgery, whereas patients showing a response received two more courses of chemotherapy before surgery. The regimen consisted of cisplatin (80 mg/m^2 day 1) and etoposide (100 mg/m^2 intravenously on days 1 to 2 and 200 mg/m^2 orally on days 3 to 5). In a preliminary communication, at a median follow-up for surviving patients of 15 months, the median survival of the preoperative chemotherapy group was significantly longer than for those randomly assigned to immediate surgery (18.5 vs. 11.0 months; P = .002). These data raise the question of possible benefit from more intensive therapy and the potential relevance of identifying patients with chemosensitive tumors. However, a final report has never been published.

The small numbers of patients enrolled in these trials and the lack of prospective randomized controlled data for patients with adenocarcinoma of the esophagus led the U.S. Intergroup to mount a large, definitive trial, INT 0113. A total of 467 patients with resectable esophageal cancer were randomly assigned to one of two treatment groups: (1) three cycles of cisplatin and 5-FU followed by surgery and then, for those patients whose resection was curative (R0), two additional cycles of cisplatin and 5-FU as adjuvant treatment; or (2) immediate surgery.[186] In contrast to other trials, barium esophagogram was the only test required to assess clinical response to preoperative chemotherapy. Thus, it is not surprising that only a 19% response rate was reported. Survival and pattern of failure were the major study end points. No differences were observed between the surgery control group and the preoperative cisplatin and 5-FU group in terms of curative resection rate (59% vs. 62%), treatment mortality (6% vs. 7%), overall median survival (16.1 vs. 14.9 months), or 3-year survival (26% vs. 23%). Furthermore, the median survival of patients who had a curative resection was the same in both treatment groups (27.4 vs. 25.0 months). The pattern of failure was also similar for the two treatment groups (local recurrence 31% vs. 32%, and distant recurrence 50% vs. 41% in the surgery-alone group compared to those receiving

induction chemotherapy followed by surgery, respectively). Tumor histologic type did not influence response to treatment. Although no improvement in survival was demonstrated, the trial importantly provides a contemporary surgical experience in the treatment of esophageal squamous carcinoma and adenocarcinoma. Important outcomes in this trial include the postoperative death rate well below 10%, the lack of difference in survival for lesions of different histologic types, and the fact that an R0 curative resection (regardless of treatment) conferred a median survival time of over 2 years.

In contrast to the results of the 467-patient U.S. Intergroup trial, the Medical Research Council Oesophageal Cancer Working Group demonstrated a statistically significant 9% improvement in 2-year survival rate (43% vs. 34%) with preoperative cisplatin and 5-FU.[187] A total of 802 patients, 31% with squamous lesions and 69% with adenocarcinoma or lesions of undifferentiated histologic type, were enrolled. Patients were randomly assigned either to receive two courses of cisplatin (80 mg/m^2) and 5-FU (1000 mg/m^2/d, continuous infusion for 4 days) 3 weeks apart followed by surgery or to undergo immediate surgery. The curative resection (R0) rate (60% vs. 54%) and the percentage of randomly assigned patients undergoing surgery (92% vs. 97%) were similar for the two treatment groups. Patients receiving preoperative chemotherapy had improved median survival (16.8 months vs. 13.3 months) and 2-year survival rate (43% vs. 34%). Overall survival was significantly improved with preoperative chemotherapy (P = .004; hazard ratio, 0.79; 95% confidence interval, 0.67 to 0.93). The estimated reduction in risk of death was 21%. The postoperative mortality rate was 10% in both treatment groups.

There is no clear explanation for the discrepancy in survival outcome for the experimental treatment groups in these two trials, whereas survival of the surgery control groups was essentially the same. The Medical Research Council study had the advantage of a larger sample size and greater power to observe a small difference. One proposed explanation is that a greater proportion of patients who received chemotherapy underwent surgery in the Medical Research Council study, 92% compared to 80% in the Intergroup trial, and a microscopically complete resection (R0) was performed in similar proportions.

As a consequence of these outcomes, preoperative cisplatin and 5-FU is now the standard of care for resectable esophageal cancer (squamous cell carcinoma and gastroesophageal junction adenocarcinoma) in the United Kingdom, whereas this approach remains investigational in the United States. In North America, the focus has shifted to the evaluation of preoperative concurrent chemoradiation strategies that may have a greater likelihood of achieving histologic complete response and improving long-term survival.

PREOPERATIVE RADIATION THERAPY. The rationale for adjuvant radiation therapy is based on the patterns of failure after potentially curative surgery in patients with clinically resectable disease. Unfortunately, few surgical series report these data. The incidence of local failure in the surgical control arms of the randomized trials of preoperative radiation therapy reported by Mei et al.[309] and Gignoux et al.[310] was 12% and 67%, respectively. The local failure rate in the surgical control arm of the randomized trial of postoperative radiation therapy conducted by Teniere et al.[311] was 35% for patients with negative local-regional lymph nodes and 38% for patients with positive local-regional lymph nodes. The surgical control arm of INT 0113 provides a modern, more relevant baseline for the results of surgery alone. As discussed earlier in Preoperative Chemotherapy, there was a 31% local failure rates in patients undergoing an R0 resection and a total local failure rate (including the additional 30% of patients with persistent disease) of 61%. Although the majority of patients with esophageal cancer die of distant metastasis, the incidence of local failure after surgery alone is high enough to examine the use of adjuvant radiation therapy.

Six randomized trials of preoperative radiation therapy for patients with clinically resectable disease are summarized in Table 29.1-9.[305,309,310,312–314] The series reported by Launois et al.,[312] Gignoux et al.,[310] and Nygaard et al.[305] are limited to patients with squamous cell carcinoma. Patients with both squamous cell carcinoma and adenocarcinoma are included in the series by Arnott et al.[313] The histologic type was not indicated in the series reported by Huang et al.[314] and Mei et al.[309]

Overall, preoperative radiation therapy did not increase the resectability rate, and only two series reported local failure rates. Although Mei and colleagues[309] reported no difference in local failure, Gignoux et al.[310] observed a significantly lower local failure rate in patients who received preoperative radiation therapy than in those treated with surgery alone (46% vs. 67%, respectively).

Two trials have reported an improvement in survival. The series of Nygaard and associates was a four-arm trial in which patients were randomly assigned to receive chemotherapy (two cycles of cisplatin and bleomycin), radiation therapy, chemoradiation, or surgery alone.[305] Patients who received preoperative radiation therapy (with or without chemotherapy) had a significant improvement in overall 3-year survival (18% vs. 5%; P = .009). The 48 patients who received preoperative radiation therapy without chemotherapy had a 20% 3-year survival rate; however, this did not reach statistical significance. Therefore, this was not a pure radiation study, and the benefit may have been due, in part, to the chemotherapy. A similar improvement in survival was reported by Huang et al. (46% vs. 25%); however, a statistical analysis was not performed.[314] Furthermore, a metaanalysis from the Oesphageal Cancer Collaborative Group also showed no clear evidence of a survival advantage with preoperative radiation therapy.[191]

The randomized preoperative radiation therapy trials discussed earlier used suboptimal design. Conventional doses of radiation therapy were not used, and some used a split-course radiation therapy regimen. Furthermore, none allowed an adequate interval between the completion of radiation therapy and surgery. In general, a 4- to 7-week interval is recommended. Consequently, radiation-related morbidity cannot be appropriately assessed in these trials.

The only study that allows analysis of the effect of radiation fractionation is a randomized trial performed in France involving patients with squamous cell carcinomas who received chemoradiation using continuous-course versus split-course radiation.[315] The 95 patients who received a continuous-course regimen had a significantly higher local control rate (57% vs. 29%) and 2-year event-free survival rate (33% vs. 23%), and a borderline significantly higher 2-year survival rate (37% vs. 23%). Because it is less effective than continuous-course therapy, split-course radiation therapy is not recommended.

In summary, because only two of the six series have reported local failure rates, it is difficult to draw firm conclusions regarding the influence of preoperative radiation therapy on local control. Two series reported an improvement in survival; in one, half of the patients received chemotherapy, and in the other, a

TABLE 29.1-9.   Randomized Trials of Preoperative Radiation Therapy for Esophageal Cancer

Series	Type	Patients (n)	Total Dose (cGy)	Fraction Size (cGy)	Resectable (%) Surgery	Resectable (%) Radiation Therapy	Local Failure (%) Surgery	Local Failure (%) Radiation Therapy	5-Y Survival (%) Surgery	5-Y Survival (%) Radiation Therapy
Arnott et al.[313]	SCC + adeno-carcinoma	176	2000	200	NR	NR	NR	NR	17	9
Gignoux et al.[310]	SCC	229	3300	330	58	47	67	46[a]	8	10
Nygaard et al.[305]	SCC	186	3500[b]	175	NR	NR	NR	NR	5	18 (3-y)[a]
Launois et al.[312]	SCC	109	4000	NR	70	76	NR	NR	10	10
Huang et al.[314]	NR	160	4000	200	90	92	NR	NR	25	46[c]
Mei et al.[309]	NR	206	4000	NR	85	93	12	13	30	35

NR, information not reported in the manuscript; SCC, squamous cell carcinoma.
[a]P = .009.
[b]With or without chemotherapy.
[c]Statistical analysis was not performed.

statistical analysis was not performed. Four of the six series reported no advantage in overall survival. Nonrandomized trials performed by Yadava et al.[316] and Sugimachi and associates[317] also reported no survival benefit. Based on the available, albeit limited, data from randomized trials, preoperative radiation therapy does not appear to significantly decrease local failure rate or improve survival in esophageal cancer patients.

PREOPERATIVE CHEMORADIOTHERAPY. The survival outcome after single-modality treatment (radiation therapy or surgery) for the primary management of esophageal cancer is poor. Furthermore, the absence of survival improvement when radiotherapy is added either preoperatively or postoperatively has focused research efforts on the integration of chemotherapy before surgery in conjunction with radiotherapy. The rationale for trimodal therapy, chemoradiotherapy followed by surgery, is based on the pattern of both local and distant failure associated with surgery alone or chemoradiotherapy without surgery, which are the two treatment options established as standards of care based on data from randomized controlled trials. The results for patients randomly assigned to the surgery control arm of the INT 0113 trial revealed a high rate of failure in controlling local disease. Ninety-two of 227 patients (41%) either had a noncurative resection or did not have surgery performed, and the local recurrence rate among those who did undergo curative resection was 31% (39 or 129).[186] Similarly, the two Intergroup trials (R85-01 and INT 0123) evaluating nonsurgical treatment (concurrent cisplatin and 5-FU, and radiotherapy) showed unacceptably high rates of local failure. Persistent or recurrent local-regional disease at 1 year was documented in 44% of patients treated in the R85-01 trial[318] and 53% of patients in the INT 0123 trial.[319] Both trials combined chemotherapy and standard fractionation radiotherapy (1.8 to 2.0 Gy/fraction). The total radiation dose ranged from 50 Gy (R85-01) to 64.8 Gy (INT 0123); however, increasing the radiation dose from 50 to 64.8 Gy, as tested in INT 0123, did not improve local-regional control.

Trials of preoperative chemotherapy followed by surgery have had limited success in improving local control as discussed in Preoperative Chemotherapy, earlier in this chapter. Notably, the curative resection rates for the experimental treatment groups (two or three cycles of cisplatin and 5-FU followed by surgery) were 62% and 60%, respectively, for the U.S. INT 0113 trial[186] and the Medical Research Council trial.[187] Among the proportion of patients undergoing a curative resection, neither study showed an effect of preoperative chemotherapy in suppressing distant metastases or reducing local-regional failure compared to results for the patients in the surgery-alone treatment group.

Most of the agents active against esophageal cancer (i.e., 5-FU, cisplatin, mitomycin C, paclitaxel) are known to enhance radiosensitivity in cancer cells. Conceivably, chemotherapy in conjunction with radiotherapy may prevent dissemination of tumor cells during surgery and thus decrease the rate of distant metastases in patients receiving potentially curative resections. Treatment with chemoradiation followed by esophagectomy has the potential (1) to down-stage the disease, (2) to remove microscopic persistent disease after chemoradiation, (3) to increase the rate of complete resection with negative circumferential margins, and (4) to have an adjuvant affect against micrometastatic disease.

Nonrandomized Trials. This discussion focuses on journal-reported series limited to patients with clinically resectable squamous cancer of the esophagus or adenocarcinoma of the esophagus, gastroesophageal junction, or cardia. Most of the trials have used 5-FU and cisplatin–based chemotherapy (Table 29.1-10),[192,320-337] although more recent trials incorporate paclitaxel or irinotecan in two- or three-drug combination regimens (Table 29.1-11).[338-346]

The results of selected phase II series in which patients have undergone preoperative combined modality therapy followed by a planned operation are summarized in Table 29.1-10.[192,320-337] Leichman and colleagues at Wayne State University[347] were the first to report use of a combination of cisplatin and infusional 5-FU and concurrent radiotherapy (30 Gy) followed by surgery for the treatment of patients with squamous cell carcinoma of the esophagus. In a series of 21 patients receiving this preoperative regimen, 5 (24%) had no residual tumor in the resection specimen. All five were surviving at 2 years, which suggests an association between attaining pathologically confirmed complete response status and potential cure. This pilot trial was expanded into a Southwest Oncology Group trial (8037) for patients with squamous cell carcinoma. Of 113 patients enrolled in this trial, only 71 underwent an operation.[320] The pathologically confirmed complete response rate was 16%, and the operative mortality was 11%. Although the median survival for all patients was 12 months and the 2-year survival rate was 28%, the median survival of those showing a pathologically confirmed complete response was 32 months.

Since these initial reports, results of more than 50 phase II single-institution or multicenter trials have been published.[348] The vast majority used cisplatin (75 to 100 mg/m²) and 5-FU (1000 mg/m²/d continuous infusion for 4 or 5 days) with concurrent radiotherapy followed by surgery in 4 to 8 weeks. In most series, the pathologically determined complete response rate (based on total number treated) was approximately 25%. Intensive combined modality regimens using hyperfractionated radiotherapy were evaluated by Forastiere et al.[322,323] as well as Raoul et al.[333] and Adelstein et al.[330] Some of these regimens achieved higher pathologically determined complete response rates and survival rates, usually with corresponding increases in acute toxicity. However, no clear advantage to altered fractionation schedules has been shown.

The total dose of radiotherapy with concurrent chemotherapy varied from 30 Gy in earlier series up to 60 Gy, followed by surgery. Pathologically determined complete response rates are uniformly in the 15% to 20% range with lower doses of radiation,[320,324,335,336] whereas total doses exceeding 50 Gy are associated with increased toxicity and perioperative complications.[334] Doses of 44 to 50 Gy using standard fractionation and concurrent therapy with cisplatin plus 5-FU generally result in pathologically determined complete response rates of 25% to 40%[192,322-325,328-330,333,337] and acceptable toxicity with postoperative mortality rates well below 10%.

More conventional doses of chemotherapy and radiotherapy have been advocated by Stahl et al.,[327] Jones et al.,[329] Forastiere et al.,[328] and Bates et al.[325] In addition, these investigators have sought to determine whether preoperative endoscopy with biopsy can accurately assess response to treatment, and whether achievement of pathologically confirmed complete response after chemoradiation improves overall survival. Bates et al.[325] reported a 65% 3-year survival rate in patients who achieved a pathologically confirmed complete response, compared with a 25% survival rate in those who did not. Forastiere

TABLE 29.1-10. Results of Preoperative Combined Modality Therapy for Esophageal Cancer: Selected Nonrandomized Trials

Series	Patients (n)	Histology	Chemotherapy	RT (Gy)	Resection (%)	Pathologic CR (%)[a]	Survival	Operative Mortality (%)
Poplin et al., 1987[320]	113	S	CF	30	49	16	12 mo (median), 28% (2-y)	11
Naunheim et al., 1992[321]	47	S/A	CF	30–36	72	17	23 mo (median), 40% (3-y)	5
Forastiere et al., 1990, 1993[322,323]	43	S/A	CFV	38–45	91	23	29 mo (median), 46% (3-y), 34% (5-y)	2
Hoff et al., 1993[324]	68	S/A	CFLE	30	75	18	24 mo (median), 51% (2-y)	2
Bates et al., 1996[325]	39	S/A	CF	45	90	46	22 mo (median), 40% (3-y)	9
Malhaire et al., 1996[326]	56	S	CF	37	79	38	37 mo (median), 55% (3-y), 30% (5-y)	11
Stahl et al., 1996[327]	72	S/A	CFLE	40	67	22	17 mo (median), 33% (3-y)	15
Forastiere et al., 1997[328]	50	S/A	CF	44	90	38	31 mo (median), 58% (2-y)	0
Jones et al., 1997[329]	66	S/A	CF	45	82	33	19 mo (median), 32% (3-y)	7
Adelstein et al., 1997[330]	72	S/A	CF	45	88	27	44% (4-y)	18
Posner et al., 1998, 2001[331,332]	44	S/A	CFIfn	40–45	82	24	28 mo (median), 52% (2-y), 32% (5-y)	8
Raoul et al., 1998[333]	32	S	CFL	45	81	56	52% (3-y)	10
Keller et al., 1998[334]	46	A	FM	60	72	17	17 mo (median), 27% (2-y)	17
Bedenne et al., 1998[335]	96	S	CF	30	82	20	17 mo (median), 40% (2-y), 25% (5-y)	9
Laterza et al., 1999[336]	111	S	CF	30	78	15	14 mo (median), 32% (2-y)	10
Heath et al., 2000[337]	42	S/A	CF	44	93	26	NR (median), 62% (2-y)	0
Kleinberg et al., 2003[192]	92	S/A	CF	44	93	33	35 mo (median), 57% (2-y), 40% (5-y)	0

A, adenocarcinoma; C, cisplatin; CR, complete response; E, etoposide; F, 5-fluorouracil; Ifn, interferon; L, leucovorin; M, mitomycin; NR, not reached; RT, radiation therapy; S, squamous cell carcinoma; V, vinblastine.
[a]Percent of patients enrolled.

and colleagues[328] reported 2-year survival rates of 78% for those with a pathologically confirmed complete response compared with 46% for those showing residual tumor in the resected esophagus (P = .006). In trials with long-term follow-up,[192,322] investigators observed 5-year survival rates of 60% to 67% and 27% to 32% for those with pathologically confirmed complete response and those with residual disease after induction therapy, respectively.[192,322] These data from nonrandom-

TABLE 29.1-11. Early Results of Recent Phase I and II Trials of Preoperative Chemoradiation

Series	Patients (n)	Histologic Type	Preoperative Treatment	Outcome
Khushalani et al.[338]	38	S/A	Ph I Oxali F + RT 50.4 Gy	pCR 38% (13 patients selected for resection)
Safran et al.[339]	41	S/A	Ph II C Pac + RT 39.6 Gy	pCR 29%, 2-y survival 42%
Adelstein et al.[340]	40	S/A	Ph II C Pac + RT 45 Gy (b.i.d.)[a]	pCR 23%, 3-y survival 30%
Wright et al.[341]	40	S/A	Ph I–II C F Pac + RT 58.5 Gy (b.i.d.)[a]	pCR 35%, 2-y survival 61%
Meluch et al.[342]	130	S/A	Ph II Carbo F Pac + RT 45 Gy	pCR 36%, 3-y survival 41%
Bains et al.[343]	41	S/A	Ph II C Pac × 2 then C Pac (96 h) + RT 50.4 Gy	pCR 22%
Swisher et al.[344]	38	S/A	Ph II C F Pac × 2 then C F + RT 45 Gy	pCR 21%, 3-y survival 63%, 5-y survival 39%
Ajani et al.[345]	43	S/A	Ph II C Irin then F Pac + RT	pCR 28%
Ilson et al.[346]	19	S/A	Ph I C Irin then C Irin + RT 50.4 Gy	pCR 27% (15 patients selected for resection)

A, adenocarcinoma; C, cisplatin; Carbo, carboplatin; F, 5-fluorouracil; Irin, irinotecan; Oxali, oxaliplatin; Pac, paclitaxel; pCR, pathologically confirmed complete response; Ph, phase; S, squamous cell carcinoma; RT, radiation therapy.
[a]Regimen not recommended due to toxicity.

ized trials suggest that, with preoperative chemoradiotherapy, patients who are down-staged to pathologically negative status have a survival advantage. In addition, the fact that long-term survival was observed in approximately 30% of patients with residual tumor in the resected specimen suggests that surgery is an important component of the multimodal regimens.

At present, no methods short of surgical resection can accurately determine which patients will be found to have no residual tumor in the resected esophageal specimen after chemoradiotherapy. Bates and colleagues[325] noted a 41% false-negative rate with preoperative endoscopy and biopsy. Jones and colleagues[349] reported that CT had a sensitivity of 65%, a specificity of 33%, a positive predictive value of 58%, and a negative predictive value of 41% in evaluating pathologically determined response after preoperative combined modality therapy in esophageal cancer patients. Many studies show that EUS performed after chemoradiotherapy is also a poor predictor of complete response due to the inability to distinguish postirradiation fibrosis and inflammation from residual tumor. Reported staging accuracy is below 50%.[350-352] The value of FDG-PET for staging after chemoradiation needs to be further studied. Several studies of esophageal cancer patients show that an early decrease in FDG uptake after chemotherapy can predict clinical response.[228,230,353] Flamen and colleagues[353] evaluated the predictive value of PET after chemoradiotherapy in patients receiving preoperative treatment. The sensitivity and positive predictive value of PET for identifying a pathologically determined complete response were 67% and 50%, respectively. Both false-positive PET findings (residual FDG activity in an area of intense inflammatory activity on histopathologic analysis) and false-negative findings occurred at the primary tumor site.

Several investigators have reported documentation of downstaging by performing comprehensive pretreatment staging.[337,354] In a prospective trial of preoperative cisplatin plus protracted infusion 5-FU and radiation (44 Gy), investigators at Johns Hopkins and Yale Cancer Centers staged lesions in 42 patients using spiral CT scans of the chest, abdomen, and pelvis, EUS, and laparoscopy including biopsy of suspicious regional and celiac nodes.[337] Pretreatment staging demonstrated 26% of lesions to be stage IIA and 74% to be stages IIB, III, and IVA. Postresection pathologic staging showed that 69% of patients had down-staging of disease, including 26% to pathologically determined complete response status and 7% to stage I disease; 12% had no change and 19% had up-staging of disease (progression). Patients achieving pathologically determined complete response included those with pretreatment stage IIA, IIB, and III disease. The 2-year survival rate for those showing pathologically determined complete response was 91% compared with 51% for patients with a complete resection but residual tumor in the specimen. All of the patients with up-staged lesions died of their disease within 2 years of completing treatment. A Cox proportional hazards survival analysis of pathologically determined stages 0 (pathologically confirmed complete remission) to IV showed that the relative risk of death was similar for stages 0 or I disease and significantly increased for disease of stages II, III, and IV. Thus, this analysis supports the importance of down-staging to pathologically confirmed complete response or minimal residual disease.

Few studies have reported long-term follow-up to determine actual survival rates at 5 years. Those available are indicated in Table 29.1-10, and rates range from 25% reported by Bedenne et al.[335] for a series of 96 patients with squamous cell esoph-

ageal cancer to 40% reported by Kleinberg and colleagues[192] in a 10-year update of trials of involving predominantly esophageal adenocarcinoma patients conducted at Johns Hopkins and Yale.

Taken together, these uncontrolled trial data (see Table 29.1-10) accumulated over nearly two decades suggest approximately a 10% improvement in survival compared with historical surgery controls. However, substantially greater improvement in survival seems to be afforded patients who are down-staged to pathologically confirmed complete response or minimal residual disease (stage I).

Pattern of failure after chemoradiotherapy and resection is influenced by histologic type, with a greater likelihood of local recurrence for patients with squamous cell carcinoma of the esophagus and predominantly distant recurrence for those with adenocarcinoma of the distal esophagus, gastroesophageal junction, and cardia. In a literature review of trials of preoperative chemoradiotherapy published between 1980 and 2000, Geh and colleagues[348] found that the overall risk of relapse was 46% but that the majority of relapses, 80%, were at distant sites; local-regional recurrence alone constituted only 9% of treatment failures. These cumulative data correspond with individual reports from major centers in the United States[192,325,330,332] and suggest that trimodal therapy leads to better local-regional control than does surgery alone or chemoradiotherapy without surgery.

The preliminary results of phase I and II trials of preoperative chemoradiotherapy integrating oxaliplatin, paclitaxel, and irinotecan into combination chemotherapy regimens are listed in Table 29.1-11. In two phase I trials,[338,346] surgery was performed only on selected patients; otherwise, pathologically determined complete response rates are based on the total number of patients initiating treatment and range from 21% to 36%.[339-345] These pathologically determined complete response rates appear similar to those for previous cisplatin and 5-FU plus radiotherapy preoperative regimens, as do survival rates. Adelstein and colleagues[340] found less mucosal toxicity associated with a regimen of cisplatin and paclitaxel plus radiotherapy than with the cisplatin and 5-FU plus radiotherapy regimen they used earlier.[330] However, the incidence of grade 3 or 4 neutropenia, fever, and unplanned hospitalizations was significantly higher with the paclitaxel regimen, without any improvement in either pathologically determined complete response rate or survival estimates. Wright and colleagues[341] reported unacceptable toxicity with a regimen of cisplatin, 5-FU, and paclitaxel plus concurrent hyperfractionated radiotherapy (total dose, 58.5 Gy); follow-up time was insufficient to obtain meaningful survival data. Meluch and colleagues[342] reported mature trial results for a combination of carboplatin, 5-FU, and paclitaxel plus concurrent radiotherapy evaluated through the Minnie Pearl Cancer Research Network. Among a total of 123 patients, the pathologically determined complete response rate was 38%, and after a median follow-up of 45 months, the 3-year survival rate was 41%. Grade 3 or 4 leukopenia (73% of patients), esophagitis (43%), and hospitalization (57%) suggest that this regimen, as well, added toxicity without providing incremental improvement in survival.

Swisher et al.,[344] Ajani et al.,[345] and Ilson et al.[346] have published pilot experiences in administration of induction chemotherapy before chemoradiotherapy and then surgery as a strategy to increase pathologically determined complete response rate and reduce distant recurrence. In the study by Swisher and colleagues,

Adjuvant Chemotherapy

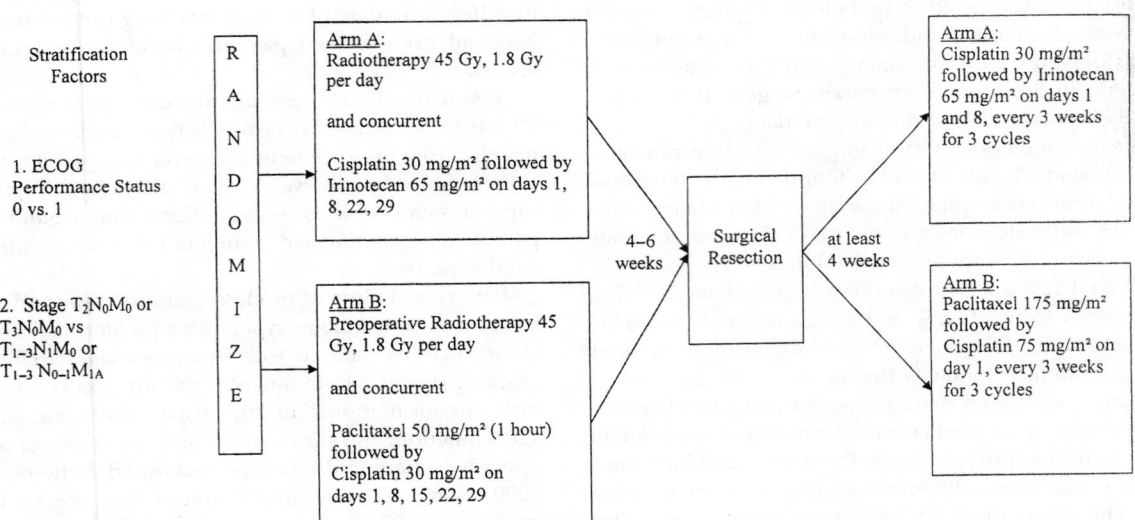

FIGURE 29.1-8. Schema of Eastern Cooperative Oncology Group (ECOG) trial E1201, a randomized phase II study of operable adenocarcinoma of the esophagus to measure response rate and toxicity of preoperative combined modality paclitaxel and cisplatin plus radiation therapy or irinotecan and cisplatin plus radiation therapy followed by postoperative chemotherapy.

two cycles of an intensive regimen of cisplatin, 5-FU, and paclitaxel with growth factor support was followed by cisplatin and infusional 5-FU with concurrent radiotherapy (total, 45 Gy), then surgery.[344] The pathologically determined complete response rate was 21%, and after a median follow-up of 58 months, 3- and 5-year survival estimates were 63% and 39%, respectively. Ilson et al.[346] and Ajani et al.[345] tested induction regimens of irinotecan and cisplatin. Ilson et al. continued irinotecan and cisplatin with concurrent radiotherapy followed by surgery.[346] They noted improvement in dysphagia during the induction chemotherapy phase and less esophagitis than with 5-FU–containing regimens. Ajani et al. followed induction chemotherapy with a regimen of paclitaxel and 5-FU with concurrent radiotherapy and then surgery.[345] Pathologically determined complete response rates in the two trials were 28% and 27%, respectively.

In summary, these newer regimens need to be further studied. Some appear more toxic than cisplatin and 5-FU plus radiotherapy, and the pathologically determined complete response rates and survival estimates show no obvious gain, but longer follow-up is needed. Interpretation of survival rates from these studies must be done cautiously given the likelihood of stage migration due to the incorporation of EUS and PET into routine staging evaluation.

The Eastern Cooperative Oncology Group is currently testing two of these combinations in a randomized phase II trial (E1201) limited to patients with resectable adenocarcinoma of the distal esophagus, gastroesophageal junction and cardia (Fig. 29.1-8). The two preoperative treatments being tested are (1) paclitaxel (50 mg/m^2, 1-hour infusion) followed by cisplatin (30 mg/m^2) on days 1, 8, 15, 22, 29, and concurrent radiotherapy (45 Gy); and (2) cisplatin (30 mg/m^2) followed by irinotecan (65 mg/m^2) on days 1, 8, 22, 29, and concurrent radiotherapy (45 Gy). Patients in each arm then proceed to esophagectomy followed by three cycles of adjuvant paclitaxel and cisplatin (arm 1) or cisplatin and irinotecan (arm 2). Stag-

ing with esophageal EUS is an eligibility requirement. This multicenter trial in a larger and more homogeneous patient population will provide better estimates of efficacy and associated toxicity for these two regimens.

Randomized Trials. Three randomized trials compared preoperative combined modality therapy with surgery alone in patients with clinically resectable disease (Table 29.1-12).[188,286,355,356] The series of Le Prise et al.[357] is not included because patients received sequential rather than concurrent chemotherapy and radiotherapy. The three trials combined cisplatin and 5-FU[355,356] or single-agent cisplatin[286] with concurrent radiotherapy.

The Bosset et al.[286] trial was limited to patients with stage I or II squamous cell carcinoma based on a previously defined CT staging system, whereas the Urba et al.[188] and Walsh et al. trials[355,356] were designed for locally advanced, resectable adenocarcinoma only (Walsh et al.) or adenocarcinoma and squamous cell cancers (Urba et al.). A significant difference in the median and 3-year survival rates was observed only in the Walsh et al. trial. It is noteworthy that the pathologically determined complete response rate was consistent for all studies, 25% to 28%, as was the 3-year survival rate for patients in each of the investigational treatment groups, 30% to 34%.

Urba and associates at the University of Michigan[188] randomly assigned 100 patients (75 with adenocarcinoma, 25 with squamous cell carcinoma) to receive (1) preoperative cisplatin (20 mg/m^2 on days 1 to 5 and 17 to 21), vinblastine (1 mg/m^2 on days 1 to 4 and 17 to 20), 5-FU (300 mg/m^2/24 h on days 1 to 21), and concurrent radiotherapy (1.5 Gy twice a day to 45 Gy), followed on day 42 by a transhiatal esophagectomy; or (2) immediate surgery. Survival analysis after a median follow-up of 8.2 years for surviving patients revealed a nonsignificant improvement favoring preoperative combined modality therapy (3-year survival, 30% vs. 16%; *P* = .15). A significant decrease in local-regional recurrence as a component of first failure was observed

TABLE 29.1-12. Preoperative Combined Modality Therapy for Esophageal Cancer: Randomized Trials

Series	Patients (n)	Histologic Type	Treatment	R0 Resection (%)	pCR (%)	Survival Median	Survival 3-Y (%)	Local Failure (%)
Urba et al.[188]	100	75% A, 25% S	Preop CFV + RT	90	28	1.46 y	30	19[a]
			Surgery	90	0	1.48 y	16	39
Walsh et al.[355,356]	113	A	Preop CF + RT	NR	25	16 mo[a]	32[a]	—
			Surgery	NR	0	11 mo	6	—
Bosset et al.[286]	282	S	Preop C + RT	81	26	19 mo	34	—
			Surgery	69	0	19 mo	36	—

A, adenocarcinoma; C, cisplatin; F, 5-fluorouracil; NR, not reported; pCR, pathologically confirmed complete response; Preop, preoperative; RT, radiation therapy; S, squamous cell carcinoma; V, vinblastine.
[a]Difference statistically significant.

(19% recurrence rate for the combined treatment group vs. 42% for the group undergoing immediate surgery; $P = .02$). However, there was no difference in the rates of distant metastases, 60% and 65%, respectively. In a multivariant analysis, tumors more than 5 cm in size, squamous cell histologic type, and age older than 70 years were independently associated with shorter survival. Although overall survival rates were not significantly different, there was a 31% lower risk of death, after adjustment for other prognostic factors, for patients randomly assigned to receive trimodal therapy, which suggests a possible benefit and the need for a trial adequately powered to detect a smaller survival difference. Consistent with phase II trial data, patients achieving a pathologically confirmed complete response had better survival outcome, with a median survival time of 50 months and 3-year survival rate of 64%, compared to those with residual disease in the resected specimen, who had a median survival time of 12 months and a 3-year survival rate of 19%.

In a series in Dublin, Walsh and colleagues[355] reported a significant survival advantage for patients receiving preoperative combined modality therapy. A total of 113 patients with adenocarcinoma of the esophagus, gastroesophageal junction, and cardia were randomly assigned to receive (1) two cycles (weeks 1 and 6) of 5-FU (15 mg/kg/24 h on days 1 to 5), cisplatin (75 mg/m² on day 7), plus concurrent radiotherapy (2.67 cGy/d to 40 Gy) followed by esophagectomy; or (2) immediate surgery alone. Combined modality therapy was well tolerated. The incidence of acute toxicity of grade 3 or higher was 15%. The operative mortality was 9% in the multimodality treatment arm compared with 4% in the surgery control arm. After a median follow-up of surviving patients of 18 months, a significant improvement in both median survival time (16 vs. 11 months; $P = .01$) and 3-year survival rate (32% vs. 6%; $P = .01$) was observed in patients receiving preoperative therapy compared with those treated with surgery alone. A major criticism of this trial was the low 3-year survival rate (6%) in the surgical control arm. This probably reflects a patient population with more advanced disease than in those enrolled in the other two trials. CT staging was not required. Over 80% of patients had lymph node metastases.[356]

A third randomized trial of preoperative combined modality therapy was reported by Bosset and colleagues[286] of the European Organization for Research and Treatment of Cancer (EORTC). A total of 282 patients with clinically resectable (early stage I and II) squamous cell carcinoma were randomly assigned to undergo either preoperative combined modality therapy or surgery alone. The preoperative regimen consisted of five daily fractions of 3.7 Gy each followed by a 2-week rest and another 3.7 Gy for 5 days. Chemotherapy was limited to cisplatin, 80 mg/m², 0 to 2 days before starting each 5 days of radiotherapy. After a median follow-up of 55 months, patients who received preoperative combined modality therapy had a significantly better 3-year disease-free survival rate (40% vs. 28%) and local disease-free survival (relative risk, 0.6), yet had no improvement in median survival time (19 months) or overall 3-year survival (36%) compared with patients treated with surgery alone. However, this combined modality therapy regimen was unconventional in design; not only was the radiation split course and delivered with unusually high doses per fraction, but the doses of chemotherapy would not be considered adequate for systemic therapy.

Although two of the three randomized trials demonstrated a survival advantage for combined modality therapy, they are limited by small numbers of patients. To help clarify the benefit of this approach, the Intergroup developed a randomized trial of preoperative combined modality therapy (Cancer and Leukemia Group B C9781), in which patients were randomly assigned to receive (1) immediate surgery or (2) two cycles of cisplatin, 5-FU, and concurrent radiotherapy (total dose, 50.4 Gy) followed by surgery. Unfortunately, this trial, activated in July 1998, was terminated early due to failure to enroll enough patients.

In summary, the efficacy of preoperative combined modality treatment for patients with resectable esophageal cancer remains controversial. The accumulated experience from phase II and phase III trials indicates the following concerning chemoradiotherapy using cisplatin and infusional 5-FU–based therapy followed by esophagectomy:

1. In approximately two-thirds of patients disease is down-staged.
2. A survival advantage exists for patients experiencing down-staging to pathologically confirmed complete response or minimal residual disease status.
3. Surgery appears to be an important component of treatment to eliminate persistent disease after chemoradiotherapy. Twenty percent to 30% of this group will be long-term survivors.
4. Local-regional control is improved, whereas distant failure is frequent and is the major cause of death.

In the absence of a much larger controlled trial than either the Urba et al. or Walsh et al. studies, preoperative chemoradiotherapy, by strict criteria, has not been designated as "standard of care." However, the benefits outlined and the improved survival of patients in the studies by Urba et al. and Walsh et al. have led both academic centers and community practices to adopt this combined modality approach for locally advanced (stage IIB, III) disease, particularly distal esophageal and gastroesophageal junction adenocarcinoma. Due to the substantial toxicity associated with this therapy, it should be used cautiously and priority should be given to enrolling patients in clinical trials.

POSTOPERATIVE CHEMOTHERAPY. Widespread dissemination of disease is the primary cause of death of patients with esophageal cancer. Because of this, considerable effort is under way to identify novel chemotherapeutic agents and to intensify exposure to agents with documented activity against this disease. Administering chemotherapy after surgery to patients who have already received chemotherapy or chemoradiation preoperatively has not been easily achieved in phase II[299,300,337] and phase III trials.[186,307] This is exemplified by the INT 0113 trial, in which only 38% of patients who were candidates for adjuvant cisplatin and 5-FU therapy received the two planned courses.[186]

The use of adjuvant chemotherapy in patients who have had surgery alone as their primary curative treatment is more feasible from the standpoint of patient tolerance, but it remains unclear whether therapy with current agents confers a survival advantage. In Japan, surgery includes removal of the primary lesion plus extended dissection of lymph nodes in the mediastinum, neck, and abdomen. The Japanese Oncology Group has evaluated postoperative chemotherapy in a series of randomized trials.[358–361] One study of patients who had undergone resection compared observation with two courses of adjuvant cisplatin and vindesine.[360] A total of 205 patients who underwent complete resection were randomly assigned to treatment groups after stratification for regional node involvement. Median follow-up was 59 months, and the 5-year survival rate was 45% in the control arm and 48% in the adjuvant treatment arm, which indicated no survival benefit from this chemotherapy regimen.

A second trial of adjuvant chemotherapy had the same study design as that previously described, except that the chemotherapy was cisplatin and 5-FU administered for two courses after curative resection.[359,361] A total of 242 patients were randomly assigned to the various study arms with stratification for N0/N1 status. At a median follow-up of 40.4 months, no differences were observed in the 5-year survival estimates (51% for controls and 61% for chemotherapy patients; $P = .3$). However, the estimated 5-year disease-free survival rate was improved with chemotherapy (58% for the chemotherapy group vs. 46% for the observation group; $P = .05$). When data were analyzed according to lymph node status, the disease-free survival rates for node-negative patients were 77% in the surgery-alone group versus 82% in the adjuvant treatment group ($P = .3$), and rates for node-positive patients were 35% in the surgery-alone group versus 53% in the adjuvant treatment group ($P = .06$). These data suggest that adjuvant chemotherapy may benefit patients with regional node involvement. The trend for improvement in disease-free survival for this subgroup is intriguing. Further evaluation of adjuvant chemotherapy in both histologic types of esophageal cancer seems warranted.

The Eastern Cooperative Oncology Group completed a phase II trial (E8296) evaluating adjuvant therapy consisting of cisplatin (75 mg/m^2) and paclitaxel (175 mg/m^2 over 3 hours)

every 3 weeks for four courses in patients with completely resected, node-positive adenocarcinoma of the esophagus, gastroesophageal junction, or cardia.[362] Eligible patients had surgically staged T2N1M0 or T3 to 4 N0 to 1 M0 margin-negative disease. A total of 55 eligible patients were analyzed, of whom 49 (89%) had lymph node involvement. The paclitaxel-cisplatin regimen was reasonably well tolerated, with leukopenia being the most common toxicity (grade 3 or 4 reported in 56% of patients), and 46 patients (84%) were able to complete all four cycles of chemotherapy. After a median follow-up for surviving patients of 2.9 years (minimum follow-up of 2 years), the actual 2-year survival rate was 60%. This compares favorably with results for contemporary historical controls.[186]

In summary, the available data for postoperative adjuvant chemotherapy suggests a possible prolongation of survival for patients who have had a potentially curative (R0) resection and have lymph node–positive (N1) disease. There are no data to indicate or suggest that administration of postoperative adjuvant chemotherapy will prolong survival for patients who have undergone a curative resection and have negative nodes (N0). Patients who have positive margins of resection should be considered for postoperative radiation. Those who have had R0 resections but have regional nodal metastases (stages IIB and III) should be enrolled in clinical trials evaluating adjuvant therapies.

POSTOPERATIVE RADIATION THERAPY. Several reports of nonrandomized trials have suggested that postoperative radiation therapy may be effective after esophagectomy. Yamamoto and associates reported a 94% 2-year local control rate in node-positive patients.[363] For patients who underwent a three-field dissection, Hosokawa and associates added intraoperative radiation followed by 45 Gy postoperatively. The 5-year survival rate was 34%.[364] Among patients who received the highest dose of intraoperative radiation (25 Gy), 22% developed fatal tracheal ulceration. No treatment-related deaths were seen with doses lower than 20 Gy.

Two randomized trials were limited to patients treated in the adjuvant setting (Table 29.1-13). Teniere and colleagues[311] reported the results for 221 patients with squamous cell carcinoma randomly assigned to receive either surgery alone or postoperative radiation therapy (45 to 55 Gy at 1.8 Gy/fraction). At a minimum follow-up of 3 years, postoperative radiation therapy was found to have no significant impact on survival. In the series of Fok et al.,[365] patients with both squamous cell carcinomas and adenocarcinomas receiving either curative or palliative resections were evaluated; although the total dose of radiation therapy was conventional, the dose per fraction (3.5 Gy) was unconventional. No significant decrease in local failure or distant failure, or improvement in the median survival time was achieved with the addition of postoperative radiation therapy.

POSTOPERATIVE CHEMORADIOTHERAPY. The only randomized trial of postoperative chemoradiation is the Intergroup trial INT 0116 (see Table 29.1-13).[366] Although the goal of this trial was to examine the role of postoperative adjuvant chemoradiation in gastric cancer, 20% of patients had adenocarcinoma of the gastroesophageal junction. Eligible patients included those with stage IB, II, IIIA, IIIB, or IV nonmetastatic adenocarcinoma of the stomach or gastroesophageal junction. After an *en bloc* resection with negative margins, patients were randomly assigned

TABLE 29.1-13. Postoperative Radiation Therapy for Esophageal Cancer: Randomized Trials

Series	Patients (n)	Median Survival Time	Survival Rate (%)	Local Failure (%) LN+	LN−	Overall	Distant Failure (%)
Teniere et al.[311]							
Radiation	119		19	30	10[a]		
Surgery	102		19	38	35		
Fok et al.[365]							
Radiation	30	15 mo				10	40
Surgery	30	21 mo				13	30
MacDonald et al.[366]							
Chemoradiation	281	36 mo	50 (3-y)[a]			19	33
Surgery	275	27 mo	41 (3-y)			29	18

LN+, lymph node positive; LN−, lymph node negative.
Note: The MacDonald et al. trial (Intergroup 0116) primarily included patients with stage IB to IIIB gastric cancer. However, 20% of patients enrolled in the trial had adenocarcinoma of the gastroesophageal junction.
[a]Statistically significant.

to receive either observation alone or postoperative chemoradiation consisting of four monthly cycles of bolus 5-FU and leucovorin plus 45 Gy concurrent radiation with cycle 2. A total of 603 patients were registered. Pretreatment characteristics were similar in both arms, and most patients had locally advanced disease. Approximately two-thirds had T3 or T4 tumors and approximately 85% had positive local-regional nodes.

Patients randomly assigned to receive postoperative combined modality therapy had a significant decrease in local failure as the first site of failure (19% vs. 29%) and an increase in median survival (36 months vs. 27 months), 3-year relapse-free survival (48% vs. 31%), and overall survival (50% vs. 41%; *P* = .005). The most common acute toxicities were hematologic and gastrointestinal, and the incidence of grade 4 toxicity was higher with combined modality therapy (41% vs. 32%). Although 17% of patients could not complete all therapy as planned, there was only one treatment-related death.

Individual grade 3+ toxicities included 54% hematological, 33% gastrointestinal, 6% infection, and 4% neurological toxicities. To minimize radiation-related toxicity, careful pretreatment review of the simulation films was performed. This frequently resulted in the recommendation to the treating radiation oncologist to modify the design or volume (or both) of the radiation fields. Based on the positive results of the INT 0116 trial, the standard of care for patients with T3 or node-positive gastric cancer after a complete resection with negative margins is postoperative chemoradiation. Because 20% had adenocarcinoma of the gastroesophageal junction, those patients should also receive this treatment if they have not received preoperative therapy.

In summary, the role of postoperative chemoradiation is controversial. Because the INT 0116 trial revealed a survival advantage with postoperative chemoradiation and patients with adenocarcinoma of the gastroesophageal junction were entered in that trial, it is reasonable to offer postoperative chemoradiation to patients with stages T3 or N1–2 disease.

The other role for postoperative radiation therapy is in cases of positive surgical margins. Based on the positive survival results from chemoradiation trials such as Radiation Therapy Oncology Group (RTOG) 85-01, patients selected for treated with postoperative radiation should receive systemic chemotherapy with radiation.[318,367]

Definitive Chemoradiotherapy

Although definitive chemoradiation is a treatment option for patients with localized resectable esophageal carcinoma, especially those with cervical esophageal squamous cell carcinoma or those not considered ideal resection candidates, this therapeutic approach is discussed in detail in Combined Modality Therapy under Treatment of Locally Advanced Disease, later in this chapter.

TREATMENT OF LOCALLY ADVANCED DISEASE

Radiation Therapy

There is considerable controversy as to the ideal therapeutic approach for esophageal cancer. The 1992–1994 Patterns of Care study examined 400 patients treated at 61 academic and nonacademic radiation oncology practices to determine practice patterns in the United States.[368] During that period, treatment approaches included primary chemoradiation, 54%; radiation alone, 20%; preoperative chemoradiation, 13%; postoperative combined modality therapy, 8%; postoperative radiation, 4%; and preoperative radiation, 1%. In a more recent Patterns of Care analysis from 1996 to 1999, 414 patients who received radiation therapy as part of definitive or adjuvant management at 59 institutions were surveyed.[369] Compared with the 1992–1994 survey, more patients underwent EUS staging (18% vs. 2%; *P*<.0001) and more patients received preoperative chemoradiation (27% vs. 10%; *P* = .007); preoperative chemoradiation was used more frequently in the subset of patients with adenocarcinoma (46% vs. 19%; *P*=.0002), and the use of paclitaxel-based chemotherapy increased (22% vs. 0.2%; *P* = .001). Brachytherapy was used in 6% of patients. In a similar patterns of care study of 767 patients treated in Japan from 1998 to 2001, 220 (28%) received preoperative or postoperative radiation or both, with or without chemotherapy.[370] Various oncology groups have published treatment guidelines; however, there is still no consensus at the present time.[371–373]

The effect of histologic type (adenocarcinoma vs. squamous cell carcinoma) is unclear. At present the data are conflicting, with some series reporting different results by histologic type but other series reporting no difference. Fortunately, the National Cancer Institute Intergroup randomized trials stratify patients by lesion histologic type. Until these data are available, the impact of histologic type cannot be adequately assessed, and it is reasonable to treat both types of lesions in a similar fashion.

PRIMARY NONSURGICAL THERAPY. Primary therapy for esophageal cancer is either surgical or nonsurgical. Although the overall results of these approaches are similar, the patient population selected for treatment with each modality is usually different. For several reasons, this results in a selection bias against nonsurgical therapy. First, patients with unfavorable prognostic features are more commonly selected for treatment with nonsurgical therapy. These features include medical contraindications and primary unresectable or metastatic disease. Second, surgical series report results based on pathologically determined stage, whereas nonsurgical series report results based on clinically determined stage. Pathologic staging has the advantage of excluding some patients with metastatic disease not identified during clinical staging. Third, because some patients treated without surgery are approached in a palliative rather than a curative fashion, the intensity of chemotherapy and the doses and techniques of radiation therapy can be suboptimal.

The difficulty of accurately staging esophageal cancer preoperatively is discussed in Diagnostic Studies and Pretreatment Staging, earlier in this chapter. Not only are CT and EUS used, but the efficacy of FDG-PET must be emphasized. Studies have examined the effectiveness of PET in the staging of esophageal cancer. After standard staging for esophageal cancer (including CT and endoscopy), undetected metastatic disease was identified by PET in 15% of patients in the series by Flamen et al.[353] and in 20% of patients in the series by Downey and associates.[230] Although PET is investigational, its use is highly encouraged for all patients who are selected for a nonoperative approach.

Radiation Therapy Alone. Many series have reported results of external-beam radiation therapy alone. Most include patients with unfavorable features such as clinical T4 disease and multiple positive lymph nodes. For example, in the series of De-Ren, 184 of the 678 patients had stage IV disease.[374] Overall, the 5-year survival rate for patients treated with conventional doses of radiation therapy alone is 0% to 10%.[374–376] The use of radiation therapy as a potentially curative modality requires doses of at least 50 Gy at 1.8 to 2.0 Gy/fraction. Shi and colleagues reported a 33% 5-year survival rate with the use of late-course accelerated fractionation to a total dose of 68.4 Gy.[377] However, in the radiation-therapy-alone arm of the RTOG 85-01 trial in which patients received 64 Gy at 2 Gy/d with modern techniques, all patients were dead of their disease by 3 years.[318,367]

There is limited experience in the use of radiation therapy alone for patients with superficial[378] or clinically determined T1 disease.[379] The trial by Sykes et al. was limited to 101 patients (90% with squamous cell carcinoma) with tumors smaller than 5 cm who received 45 to 52.5 Gy in 15 to 16 fractions. The 5-year survival was 20%.[380]

Collectively, these data indicate that radiation therapy alone should be reserved for palliation or for patients who are medically unable to receive chemotherapy. As is discussed in the following section, the results of chemoradiation are more favorable, and it remains the standard of care.

Combined Modality Therapy (Definitive Chemoradiation)
CONVENTIONAL APPROACHES. There are many single-arm, non-randomized trials of chemoradiation alone and they have included patients with disease at a variety of stages.[381–385] Few series examine patients with T1 or T2 disease.[378,383,386] In the series reported by Coia and associates, patients received 5-FU and mitomycin C concurrently with 60 Gy of radiation therapy.[383] When results for clinical stage I and II disease are combined, the local failure rate was 25%, the 5-year actuarial local relapse-free survival was 70%, and the 5-year actuarial survival was 30%.

Six randomized trials compared radiation therapy alone with chemoradiation (Table 29.1-14).[193,305,318,387–391] Of these six trials, five used suboptimal doses of radiation and three used inadequate doses of systemic chemotherapy. For example, in the series of Araujo and colleagues,[392] patients received only one cycle of 5-FU, mitomycin C, and bleomycin. The EORTC trial used subcutaneous methotrexate.[387] In the Scandinavian trial reported by Nygaard and associates, patients received low doses of chemotherapy (cisplatin, 20 mg/m², and bleomycin, 10 mg/m², for a maximum of two cycles).[305] An analysis of pooled data from these trials reported a significant local control and survival benefit at 1 year for chemoradiation compared with radiation therapy alone.[372] Chemoradiation was associated with a significant increase in adverse effects, including life-threatening toxicities.

In the ECOG EST-1282 trial,[390] patients who received combined modality therapy had a significantly increased median survival compared with those receiving radiation alone (15 months vs. 9 months; $P = .04$) but experienced no improvement in 5-year survival (9% vs. 7%). However, this was not a pure nonsurgical trial because approximately 50% of patients in each arm underwent surgery after receiving 40 Gy of radiation. Furthermore, this decision was dependent on the individual investigator's preference. The operative mortality was 17%. Finally, the Pretoria trial reported by Slabber et al., which was limited to a total of 70 patients with T3 squamous cell cancers, used a low-dose (40 Gy) split-course radiation schedule.[389]

The only trial that was designed to deliver adequate doses of systemic chemotherapy with concurrent radiation therapy was the RTOG 85-01 trial reported by Herskovic et al. (Fig. 29.1-9).[193,318,388] This Intergroup trial primarily included patients with squamous cell carcinoma. Patients received four cycles of 5-FU (1000 mg/m²/24 h × 4 days) and cisplatin (75 mg/m² on day 1). Radiation therapy (50 Gy at 2 Gy/d) was given concurrently with day 1 of chemotherapy. Curiously, cycles 3 and 4 of chemotherapy were delivered every 3 weeks (weeks 8 and 11) rather than every 4 weeks (weeks 9 and 13). This intensification may explain, in part, why only 50% of the patients finished all four cycles of the chemotherapy. The control arm was given radiation therapy alone, albeit at a higher dose (64 Gy) than the chemoradiation arm.

Patients who received chemoradiation had a significant improvement in median survival (14 months vs. 9 months) and 5-year survival (27% vs. 0%; $P < .0001$).[388] There was a clear plateau in the survival curve. Minimum follow-up was 5 years, and the 8-year survival was 22%.[193] Histologic type did not significantly influence the results: 21% of patients with squamous cell carcinomas (n = 107) were alive at 5 years compared with 13% of patients with adenocarcinoma (n = 23) (P was not significant). Although African Americans had larger primary tumors and all were squamous cell cancers, there was no difference in their survival compared with whites.[393] The incidence of local failure as the first site of failure (defined as local persistence or recurrence) was also decreased in the combined modality arm (47% vs. 65%). The protocol was closed early due to the posi-

TABLE 29.1-14. Randomized Trials of Radiation Therapy versus Combined Modality Therapy for Esophageal Cancer

Series	Patients (n)	Overall Survival (%)	Median Survival Failure (Mo)	Local (%)
Herskovic et al. (Radiation Therapy Oncology Group)[193,318,388]				
Radiation alone	62	0% 5-y[a]	9	68[b]
Combined modality therapy	61	27% 5-y	14	47[c]
		22% 8-y		
Combined modality therapy	69	NR	17	52
Araujo et al. (National Cancer Institute Brazil)[391]				
Radiation alone	31	6% 5-y		84
Combined modality therapy	28	16%		61
Roussel et al. (European Organization for Research and Treatment of Cancer)[387]				
Radiation alone	69	6% 3-y		
Combined modality therapy	75	12%		
Nygaard et al. (Scandinavia)[305]				
Radiation alone	51	6% 3-y		
Combined modality therapy	46	0%		
Slabber et al.[d] (Pretoria)[389]				
Radiation alone	36		5	
Combined modality therapy	34		6	
Smith et al.[e] (Eastern Cooperative Oncology Group EST-1282)[390]				
Radiation alone	60	7% 5-y	9[c]	
Combined modality therapy	59	9%	15	

NR, information not reported in the manuscript.
[a]Nonrandomized group treated following early closure of the randomization.
[b]Radiation Therapy Oncology Group reported local failure as local persistance + local recurrence.
[c]Statistically significant difference.
[d]Limited to patients with squamous cell cancer with T3 disease.
[e]Approximately 50% in each arm underwent surgery.

tive results; however, after this early closure, an additional 69 eligible patients were treated with the same chemoradiation regimen. In this nonrandomized combined modality group, the 5-year survival was 14% and local failure was 52%.

Chemoradiation not only improves the results compared with radiation alone but also is associated with a higher incidence of toxicity. In the 1997 report of the RTOG 85-01 trial, patients who received chemoradiation had a higher incidence of acute grade 3 toxicity (44% vs. 25%) and acute grade 4 toxicity (20% vs. 3%) compared with those who received radiation therapy alone. Including the one treatment-related death (2%), the incidence of total acute grade 3+ toxicity was 66%.[388] The 1999 report examined late toxicity. The incidence of late grade 3+ toxicity was similar in the combined modality arm and in the radiation-alone arm (29% vs. 23%).[193] However, grade 4+ toxicity remained higher in the combined modality arm (10% vs. 2%). Interestingly, the nonrandomized chemoradiation group experienced a similar incidence of late grade 3+ toxicity (28%) but a lower incidence of grade 4 toxicity (4%), and there were no treatment-related deaths.

Based on the positive results from the RTOG 85-01 trial, the conventional nonsurgical treatment for esophageal carcinoma is chemoradiation. Notwithstanding, the local failure rate in the RTOG 85-01 chemoradiation arm was 45%, and there is room for improvement. Therefore, new approaches such as intensification of chemoradiation and escalation of the radiation dose have been developed in an attempt to help improve these results.

COMPARISON OF DEFINITIVE CHEMORADIATION AND SURGERY. Although there are a number of trials comparing preoperative chemoradiation with surgery alone, there is no trial that directly compares the two standard treatments for nonmetastatic esophageal cancer: nonoperative chemoradiation and surgery alone. It is an important issue for the practicing oncologist and for the establishment of standards of care. The positive results of RTOG 85-01, demonstrating a 27% 5-year survival rate for patients treated with definitive chemoradiation compared with no 5-year survival after treatment with radiotherapy alone, is a major advance. This treatment option has influenced the selection of patients for nonsurgical management because it provides an alternative for restoring swallowing function in patients with locally advanced disease for whom resection would likely be palliative.

For patients with earlier-stage disease that appears resectable, definitive chemoradiation may also be appropriate treatment;

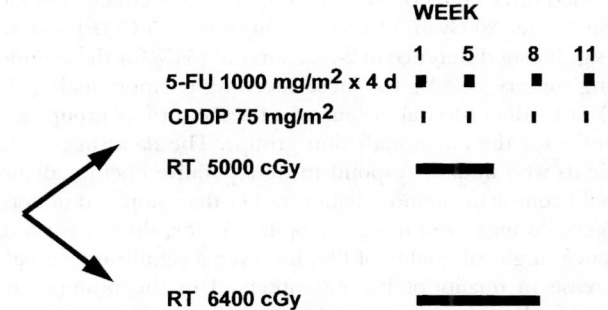

FIGURE 29.1-9. Phase III Intergroup trial Radiation Therapy Oncology Group 85-10 for patients with squamous cell and adenocarcinoma of the esophagus selected for a nonoperative approach. 5-FU, 5-fluorouracil; CDDP, cisplatin; RT, radiation therapy.

however, prospective trials comparing this approach with surgery, stratified by stage, have yet to be performed. Nonetheless, contemporary series suggest that the nonsurgical approach offers a survival rate that is the same or better than that achievable with surgery alone. For example, the median survival time and 5-year survival rate were 14 months and 27%, respectively, in the chemoradiation arm of RTOG 85-01 and 20 months and 20%, respectively, in INT 0122.[394] In comparison, the median survival in the surgical control arm of the Dutch trial reported by Kok et al.[306] was 11 months, and the median survival time and 5-year survival rate in the surgical control arm of INT 0113 were 16 months and 20%, respectively. Likewise, the local failure rates were similar. The incidence of local failure (local recurrence plus local persistence of disease) as the first site of failure was 45% in RTOG 85-01 and 39% in INT 0122. Although local failure as the first site of failure was 31% in INT 0113, this analysis was limited to patients who underwent a complete resection with negative margins (R0 resection). Because an additional 30% of patients had residual local disease, if one were to score these patients also as having locally persistent disease (as was done in the RTOG 85-01 analysis), the comparable local failure rate with surgery alone would be 30% + 31% = 61%. The treatment-related mortality rates were also similar (2% in RTOG 85-01, 9% in INT 0122, and 6% in INT 0113).

In summary, the local failure, survival, and treatment-related mortality rates for nonsurgical and surgical therapies are similar. Although the results are comparable, it is clear that both the nonsurgical and surgical approaches have limited success.

NECESSITY FOR SURGERY AFTER CHEMORADIATION. Two trials examine whether surgery is necessary after chemoradiation. The Federation Francaise de Cancerologie Digestive (FFCD) trial addresses the issue of whether patients who respond midway through chemoradiation should continue with the treatment or undergo surgery.[395,396] The German Oesophageal Cancer Study Group examined the question of whether chemoradiation followed by surgery is equivalent to nonoperative chemoradiation.[397]

In the FFCD 9102 trial, all 445 patients with clinically resectable T3 to 4 N0 to 1 M0 squamous cell carcinoma or adenocarcinoma of the esophagus received chemoradiation; however, the randomization was limited to patients who responded to initial chemoradiation. Patients initially received two cycles of 5-FU and cisplatin plus concurrent radiation (either 46 Gy at 2 Gy/d or a split-course regimen of 15 Gy in weeks 1 and 3).[395] The 259 patients who had at least a partial response were then randomly assigned to receive surgery or additional chemoradiation, which included three cycles of 5-FU and cisplatin, plus concurrent radiation (either 20 Gy at 2 Gy/d or split-course 15 Gy). There was no significant difference in 2-year survival (34% for those undergoing surgery vs. 40% for those receiving chemoradiation; $P = .56$) or median survival (18 months for the surgery group vs. 19 months for the chemoradiation group). The data suggest that patients who initially respond to nonoperative chemoradiation should complete chemoradiation rather than stop and undergo surgery. As measured using the Spitzer index, there was no difference in global quality of life; however, a significantly greater decrease in quality of life was observed in the postoperative period in the surgery arm (7.52 vs. 8.45; $P<.01$).[396]

The German Oesophageal Cancer Study Group compared preoperative chemoradiation followed by surgery with chemoradiation alone.[397] In this trial, 177 patients with uT3–4N0–

1M0 squamous cell cancers of the esophagus were randomly assigned to receive preoperative therapy (three cycles of 5-FU, leucovorin, etoposide, and cisplatin, followed by concurrent etoposide and cisplatin, plus 40 Gy of radiation) followed by surgery or chemoradiation alone (the same chemotherapy regimen, but the radiation dose was increased to 60 Gy). Despite an improvement in local control for those who were randomly assigned to receive preoperative therapy followed by surgery compared with those receiving chemoradiation alone (81% vs. 64%), there was no significant difference in 3-year survival (28% vs. 20%). Although the difference in the radiation dose in the two arms makes the interpretation of the data difficult, there does not appear to be a benefit to surgery after nonoperative chemoradiation.

TUMOR MARKERS AND PREDICTORS OF RESPONSE TO CHEMORADIATION. It would be helpful to predict which tumors have a higher likelihood of responding to radiation or chemoradiation. In 38 patients with squamous cell carcinoma who received chemoradiation with or without surgery, tumors without p53 expression and tumors with weak Bcl-X_L expression showed a higher response to chemotherapy (56% and 53%, respectively) than tumors positive for p53 or with strong Bcl-X_L expression (30% and 32%, respectively; P not significant).[398] After preoperative chemoradiation, patients with p53-negative tumors had a significantly better mean survival than those with p53-positive tumors (31 months vs. 11 months; $P = .0378$). No prognostic impact was seen for the expression of apoptosis-regulating genes. By multivariate analysis, Pomp et al. found that overexpression of p53 resulted in a decrease in survival in 69 patients with squamous cell carcinoma or adenocarcinoma treated with radiation alone.[399] In one study, there was a correlation between decreasing levels of four phospholipids and increasing T stage and grade.[400]

Kishi and associates reported that, of 77 patients treated with chemoradiation for squamous cell cancer, those with p53- and metallothionein-positive tumors had a poor response to treatment, whereas strong expression of CDC25B was associated with a good response.[401] In 73 patients with T2 to 4 M0 esophageal cancer treated with 60 Gy of radiation plus 5-FU and cisplatin, Hironaka et al. examined pretreatment biopsy specimens for a variety of markers, including p53, Ki-67, EGF receptor, cyclin D1, vascular endothelial growth factor, microvessel density (MVD), thymidylate synthase, dihydropyrimidine dehydrogenase, and glutathione S-transferase.[402] By multivariate analysis MVD, T stage, and performance status were independent prognostic variables ($P = .002$, .02, and .02, respectively). Patients with high-MVD tumors had a better 3-year survival rate than those with low-MVD tumors (61% vs. 33%; $P = .02$). Morita et al. found that patients with lymphocyte infiltration around the tumor had a 5-year survival rate of 46% to 76% compared with 28% ($P<.05$) in patients whose tumors did not have lymphocytic infiltration.[403] With the further discovery and understanding of various tumor suppressor genes, these data may be used to help select patients for chemoradiation.

INTENSIFICATION OF CHEMORADIATION. The phase II Intergroup trial 0122 [ECOG PE289/RTOG 90-12] was designed to intensify treatment in the RTOG 85-01 combined modality arm.[394] The development of the neoadjuvant chemotherapy approach used in INT 0122 was based, in part, on the results of a randomized trial of preoperative radiation therapy (55 Gy) versus preoperative chemotherapy (5-FU, cisplatin, and vindesine) conducted at Memorial Sloan-Kettering Cancer Center. This trial revealed that the resectability (65% vs. 58%), objective response (64% vs. 55%), and local failure rates (15% vs. 6%) with either preoperative radiation therapy or preoperative chemotherapy, respectively, were similar.[404] Both the chemotherapy and radiation therapy in INT 0122 were intensified as follows: (1) the 5-FU continuous infusion (1000 mg/m^2/24 hours) was increased from 4 days to 5 days, (2) the total number of cycles of chemotherapy was increased from four to five cycles, (3) three cycles of full-dose neoadjuvant 5-FU and cisplatin were delivered before the start of chemoradiation, and (4) the radiation dose was increased from 50 Gy to 64.8 Gy. The study was limited to 45 patients with squamous cell carcinoma and 38 were eligible.

For the 38 eligible patients, the primary tumor response rate was as follows: 47% complete response, 8% partial response, and 3% stable disease.[404] The first site of clinical treatment failure was local in 39% and distant in 24%. In the total patient group, there were six deaths during treatment, four of which were treatment related (9% of 45 patients). The median survival time was 20 months and the 5-year actuarial survival rate was 20%. Therefore, this intensive neoadjuvant approach did not appear to offer a benefit compared with conventional doses and techniques of chemoradiation. Similar toxicities were reported by Ishikura et al. for 139 patients with squamous cell cancers treated with 5-FU, cisplatin, and 60 Gy of radiation.[405] However, the higher radiation dose (64.8 Gy) in INT 0122 was tolerated and was compared with 50.4 Gy of radiation in the Intergroup trial INT 0123 (Fig. 29.1-10). This trial is discussed in External-Beam Therapy, later in this chapter.

A limited number of phase I and II trials have tested the use of neoadjuvant chemotherapy before radiation therapy or chemoradiation. Valerdi et al. reported the results for 40 patients with clinical stage II and III squamous cell cancers who received two cycles of neoadjuvant cisplatin, vindesine, and bleomycin (days 1 and 29) followed by 60 Gy of radiation.[384] In contrast with the INT 0122 trial, no chemotherapy was delivered with the radiation therapy. The pathologically determined complete response rate was 53%. After a median follow-up of 78 months, the local failure rate was 62%, the median survival time was 11 months, and the 5-year actuarial survival rate was 15%. These results are similar to those obtained for the RTOG 85-01 combined modality arm with the exception of the higher treatment-related death rate of 5%.

Using a five-drug neoadjuvant regimen, Roca and colleagues treated 55 patients (54 with squamous cell cancer) with bolus cisplatin, 5-FU, leucovorin, bleomycin, and mitomycin C for 15 days followed by 60 Gy of radiation plus concurrent chemotherapy with 5-FU, leucovorin, and cisplatin.[406] No maintenance chemotherapy was delivered. Patients with lesions at all anatomic sites within the esophagus were eligible and 53% had clinical stage III disease. Although the treatment-related mortality was only 4% and the 3-year survival was 35%, local failure as a component of failure was 42%, which was similar to the 45% rate reported in the RTOG 85-01 chemoradiation arm.

More recent trials using newer regimens for neoadjuvant chemotherapy such as paclitaxel and cisplatin[343] or CPT-11 and cisplatin[346] before the start of chemoradiation have reported more favorable results. Bains and associates reported that, of 38 patients who presented with dysphagia, 92% had relief after the completion of two cycles (weeks 1 and 4) of neoadjuvant paclitaxel (175 mg/m^2, 3-hour infusion) and cisplatin (75-mg/m^2 bolus).[343] Similar results have been reported by Ilson et al. for 19 patients who received two cycles of neoadjuvant CPT-11 (65 mg/m^2) plus cisplatin (30 mg/m^2) weeks 1, 2, 4, and 5 before the start of chemoradiation.[346] Treatment was well tolerated with no grade 3+ nonhematologic toxicity, and only 5% of patients required a feeding tube. Of the 16 patients who presented with dysphagia, 81% had dysphagia relief after the completion of neoadjuvant chemotherapy.

Another potential advantage of neoadjuvant chemotherapy is the early identification of those patients who may or may not respond to the chemotherapeutic regimen being delivered. Ott et al. performed FDG-PET in 35 patients with adenocarcinoma of the gastroesophageal junction or stomach 2 weeks after the start of cisplatin, 5-FU, and leucovorin neoadjuvant chemotherapy, which was followed by surgery; results of the FDG-PET scan were able to predict which patients showed a response to the full course of chemotherapy, as judged from the surgical specimens.[407] Although this study was investigational, if the nonresponders can be identified early, changing the chemotherapeutic regimen may be helpful.

In summary, although the early trials primarily using neoadjuvant regimens based on 5-FU and cisplatin did not suggest a benefit, more recent trials using paclitaxel- and CPT-11–based regimens reveal more favorable response rates and improvement of dysphagia.

INTENSIFICATION OF THE RADIATION DOSE. Another approach to the dose intensification of chemoradiation is increasing the radiation dose above 50.4 Gy. There are two methods by which to increase the radiation dose to the esophagus: brachytherapy and external-beam radiation therapy.

BRACHYTHERAPY. Intraluminal brachytherapy allows the escalation of the dose to the primary tumor while protecting the surrounding dose-limiting structures such as the lung, heart, and spinal cord.[408] A radioactive source is placed intraluminally via bronchoscopy or a nasogastric tube. Brachytherapy has been used both as primary therapy (usually as a palliative modality)[409–413] and as boost after external-beam radiation therapy or combined modality therapy.[409,414–417] It can be delivered by high dose rate or low dose rate.[418] Although there are technical and radiobiologic

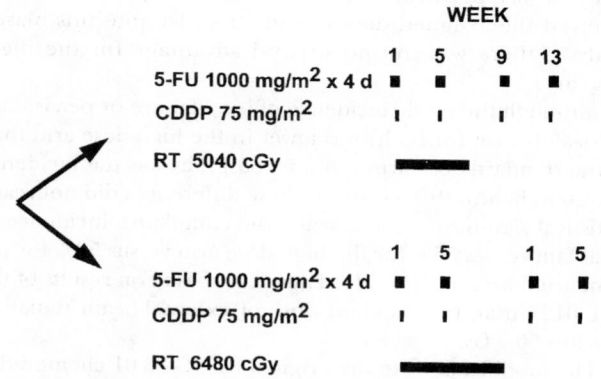

FIGURE 29.1-10.   Phase III Intergroup trial 0123 (Radiation Therapy Oncology Group 94-05) for patients with squamous cell or adenocarcinoma of the esophagus. 5-FU, 5-fluorouracil; CDDP, cisplatin; RT, radiation therapy.

differences between the two dose rates, there are no clear therapeutic advantages for either.

Series that combine brachytherapy with external-beam radiation therapy or chemoradiation report results similar to those for conventional chemoradiation. Calais et al. reported a local failure rate of 43% and a 5-year actuarial survival of 18%.[414] Even for a more favorable subset of patients with clinical T1 to 2 disease, Yorozu et al. reported a local failure rate of 44% and a 5-year survival of 26%.[419]

In the RTOG 92-07 trial, 75 patients with squamous cell cancers (92%) or adenocarcinomas (8%) of the thoracic esophagus received the RTOG 85-01 combined modality regimen (5-FU, cisplatin, 50 Gy of radiation) followed by a boost during cycle 3 of chemotherapy with either low dose-rate or high dose-rate intraluminal brachytherapy.[420] The choice of the dose rate was at the discretion of the investigator. Due to low accrual the low dose-rate option was discontinued and the analysis was limited to patients who received the high dose-rate treatment. High dose-rate brachytherapy was delivered in weekly fractions of 5 Gy during weeks 8, 9, and 10. After the development of several fistulas, the fraction delivered at week 10 was discontinued.

Although the complete response rate was 73%, at a median follow-up of only 11 months, rate of local failure as the first site of failure was 27%. Rates of acute toxicity were 58% for grade 3, 26% for grade 4, and 8% for grade 5 (treatment-related death). The cumulative incidence of fistula was 18% per year and the crude incidence was 14%. Of the six treatment-related fistulas, three were fatal. Given the significant toxicity, this treatment approach should be used with caution.

The American Brachytherapy Society has developed guidelines for esophageal brachytherapy.[421] Its recommendations include the following. For patients treated in the curative setting brachytherapy should be limited to tumors 10 cm or less with no evidence of distant metastasis. Contraindications include tracheal or bronchial involvement, cervical esophagus location, or stenosis that cannot be bypassed. The applicator should have an external diameter of 6 to 10 cm. If combined modality therapy is used (defined as 5-FU–based chemotherapy plus 45 to 50 Gy of radiation) the recommended doses of brachytherapy are 10 Gy in two weekly fractions of 5 Gy each for high dose rate and 20 Gy in a single fraction at 4 to 10 Gy/h for low dose rate. The doses should be prescribed to 1 cm from the source. Finally, brachytherapy should be delivered after the completion of external-beam radiation therapy and not concurrently with chemotherapy.

In patients treated in the curative setting, the addition of brachytherapy does not appear to improve the results compared with those for radiation therapy or combined modality therapy alone. Therefore, although it seems reasonable to assume that adding intraluminal brachytherapy to radiation or combined modality therapy would provide an additional benefit, whether such a benefit exists remains unclear.

EXTERNAL-BEAM THERAPY. There are a limited number of phase II trials examining patient tolerance for external-beam radiation doses of 60 Gy or more when delivered concurrently with chemotherapy. In a separate toxicity analysis performed by Coia and associates, the results for 90 patients with clinical stage I to IV squamous cell carcinomas and adenocarcinomas of the esophagus were reported.[383] The incidence of grade 3 toxicity was 22% and of grade 4 toxicity was 6%. There were no treatment-related deaths.

Calais et al. reported the results for 53 patients with clinically unresectable disease who received 5-FU, cisplatin, and mitomycin C plus 65 Gy of radiation.[422] The full dose of radiation could be delivered in 96% of patients. The incidence of World Health Organization grade 3+ toxicity was 30% and the overall 2-year survival rate was 42%. It should be noted that the chemotherapy in this trial was not delivered at doses adequate to treat systemic disease.

Because almost all patients in both the INT 0122 trial and the Calais trials (96% and 94%, respectively) who started radiation therapy were able to complete the full dose (64.8 to 65.0 Gy), this higher dose of radiation was used in the experimental arm of the Intergroup esophageal trial INT 0123 (RTOG 94-05). The INT 0123 trial[423] was the follow-up to RTOG 85-01. In this trial, patients with either squamous cell carcinoma or adenocarcinoma who were selected for nonsurgical treatment were randomly assigned to receive a slightly modified RTOG 85-01 combined modality regimen with 50.4 Gy of radiation versus the same chemotherapy with 64.8 Gy of radiation (see Fig. 29.1-10).

The modifications to the original RTOG 85-01 chemoradiation arm includes (1) using 1.8-Gy fractions to 50.4 Gy rather than 2-Gy fractions to 50 Gy; (2) treating with 5-cm proximal and distal margins for 50.4 Gy rather than treating the whole esophagus for the first 30 Gy followed by a cone down with 5 cm margins to 50 Gy; (3) cycle 3 of 5-FU and cisplatin did not begin until 4 weeks after the completion of radiation therapy rather than 3 weeks after; and (4) cycles 3 and 4 of chemotherapy were delivered every 4 weeks rather than every 3 weeks.

INT 0123 was closed to accrual in 1999 when an interim analysis revealed that it was unlikely that the high-dose arm would achieve superior survival compared with the standard-dose arm. For the 218 eligible patients, there was no significant difference in median survival time (13.0 months vs. 18.1 months) or 2-year survival rate (31% vs. 40%) between the high-dose and standard-dose arms.[423] Although 11 treatment-related deaths occurred in the high-dose arm compared with 2 in the standard-dose arm, 7 of the 11 deaths occurred in patients who had received 50.4 Gy or less.

To help determine if this unexplained increase in treatment-related deaths in the high-dose arm was the factor responsible for the inferior survival rate, a separate survival analysis was performed that included only patients who received the assigned dose of radiation. Despite this biased analysis, there was still no survival advantage for the high-dose arm.

Although the crude incidence of local failure or persistence of local disease (or both) was lower in the high-dose arm than in the standard-dose arm (50% vs. 55%), as was the incidence of distant failure (9% vs. 16%), these differences did not reach statistical significance. At 2 years, the cumulative incidence of local failure was 56% for the high-dose arm versus 52% for the standard-dose arm ($P = .71$). Therefore, based on results of the INT 0123 trial, the standard dose of external-beam radiation remains 50.4 Gy.

The modifications to the original RTOG 85-01 chemoradiation arm outlined earlier did not adversely affect the local control or survival rate in the control arm of INT 0123. Therefore, the radiation doses and field design used in the control arm of INT 0123 should be used.

TABLE 29.1-15.   Results of Primary High-Dose Accelerated Fractionation/Hyperfractionation Combined Modality Therapy: Selected Series

Series	No.	Histologic Type	Treatment	Local Control	Survival	Grade 3+ Toxicity
Girinsky et al.[424]	88	—	65 Gy (2 Gy b.i.d.) ± 5-FU/CDDP before radiation	48% 3-y	12% 3-y	13%
Jeremic et al.[425]	28	Squamous	54 Gy (1.5 Gy b.i.d.) 5-FU/CDDP × 4	71%	29% 5-y	50%
Wang et al.[426] (randomized)	101	Squamous	66 Gy (1.5 Gy b.i.d.) vs.	56% 3-y	38% 3-y	61% esophagitis
			68.4 Gy total, 41.4 Gy (1.8 Gy/d), then 27 Gy (1.5 Gy b.i.d.)	57% 3-y	41% 3-y	10% esophagitis

CDDP, cisplatin; 5-FU, 5-fluorouracil.

Radiation can be intensified not only by increasing the total dose but also by using accelerated fractionation or hyperfractionation. Selected series using the latter approach for radiotherapy given as primary treatment (without surgery) are listed in Table 29.1-15.[424–426] Wang et al. randomly assigned 101 patients with squamous cell cancer to receive either continuous accelerated hyperfractionated radiation (66 Gy) or late-course accelerated hyperfractionated radiation (68.4 Gy).[426] Compared with patients who received late-course accelerated hyperfractionated radiation, those treated with continuous accelerated hyperfractionated radiation had a significantly higher incidence of grade 3+ esophagitis (61% vs. 10%; $P < .001$); however, no benefit was seen in local control or survival. Although these approaches are reasonable, most series report an increase in acute toxicity without any clear therapeutic benefit. These regimens remain investigational.

NEW COMBINED MODALITY REGIMENS. Because 75% to 80% of patients die of metastatic disease, advances in systemic therapies are necessary for further improvement of results. The most widely used chemotherapeutic regimen to be combined with radiation for the treatment of esophageal cancer is 5-FU and cisplatin. There are new chemotherapeutic agents both in current practice and in development for esophageal cancer. Most are being developed for use in preoperative regimens and are combined with radiation doses of 45 to 50.4 Gy. These include both cytotoxic and targeted small molecules. Chemoradiation regimens using paclitaxel[343,427,428] and docetaxel[429] have shown encouraging results. The RTOG randomized phase II trial E-0113 compares paclitaxel plus cisplatin, with or without 5-FU (Fig. 29.1-11). The ECF (epirubicin, cisplatin, and 5-FU) regimen has been combined with postoperative radiation,[430] and will be given to the experimental arm of the Intergroup postoperative adjuvant trial for gastric and gastroesophageal junction cancers (CALGB 80101). Other agents such as irinotecan,[346,431,432] herceptin,[433] oxaliplatin,[338] and celecoxib[434] are being used as the foundations for new regimens. Whether these investigational approaches offer improved results compared to conventional chemoradiation regimens based on 5-FU and cisplatin is not known. The development of the ideal regimens and schedules remains an active area of clinical investigation.

PALLIATION OF ESOPHAGEAL CANCER WITH RADIATION THERAPY

Palliation of Dysphagia and Bleeding. Dysphagia is a common problem in patients with esophageal cancer. Not only is it the most frequently presenting symptom, but it can remain a problem up to the time of the patient's death. Many of the series examining dysphagia are retrospective, and most do not use objective criteria to define and assess dysphagia. Some do not report the number of patients presenting with dysphagia or the percentage who receive palliative treatment until the time of death. Furthermore, few series carefully examine other variables that may influence the results, such as histologic type, stage, and location of the primary tumor.

There are a number of options for palliation such as stents, feeding tubes, chemotherapy, and external-beam radiation therapy or brachytherapy (or both). The selection of the technique is variable and is commonly based on physician preference. The SORTIE (Stent Or Radiation Therapy Intervention for Esophageal cancer) trial is randomly assigning patients to receive a stent or radiation therapy in a dose of 20 Gy. The preliminary results for the first 32 patients suggest that stents offer more immediate relief; however, radiation results in more durable palliation.[435] Final results are pending.

Patients for whom stents fail are commonly treated with radiation. Li and colleagues report that the presence of a metal stent increases the radiation dose 5% to 10% at a 0.5-cm depth in the esophageal wall.[436] Therefore, the radiation dose should be decreased by 5% to 10% when a metal stent is in the radiation field. Nishimura and colleagues reported a high grade 3+ complication rate in 47 patients who underwent stent placement before or during radiation treatment and recommend that stent placement be delayed until radiation therapy has failed.[437]

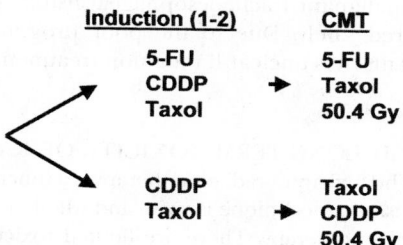

Induction (1-2)		**CMT**
5-FU CDDP Taxol	→	5-FU Taxol 50.4 Gy
CDDP Taxol	→	Taxol CDDP 50.4 Gy

FIGURE 29.1-11.   RTOG randomized phase II trial E-0113 comparing paclitaxel (Taxol) plus cisplatin (CDDP), with or without 5-fluorouracil (5-FU). CMT, combined modality therapy.

TABLE 29.1-16.   Palliation of Dysphagia with Radiation Therapy with or without Chemotherapy

| Series | Total No. Patients | Palliation of Dysphagia[a] | |
		At the End of Treatment (%)	Duration
Radiation therapy alone			
Wara et al.[438]	103	89	6-mo average
Petrovich et al.[439]	133	87	34% ≥ 6 mo
			18% ≥ 3 mo
			35% ≤ 3 mo
Roussel et al.[387]	69	70	—
Caspers et al.[441]	127	71	54% until death
Whittington et al.[440]	25	—	5% at 9 mo
Combined modality therapy			
Coia et al.[445]	102	88	67–100% until death
Seitz et al.[381]	35	100[b]	—
Whittington et al.[440]	26	—	87% 3-y actuarial
Algan et al.[442]	8	100	—
Gill et al.[443]	71	60	—
Urba and Turrisi[444]	27	—	59% until death
Izquierdo et al.[382]	25	64	Median, 5 mo

[a]See text for definition and number of patients presenting with dysphagia.
[b]Patients had dilation or neodymium Yttrium aluminum garnet laser treatment at the start of therapy.

As seen in Table 29.1-16, a limited number of series have examined the palliative benefits of either radiation alone[387,438–441] or combined modality therapy.[381,382,440,442–445] Overall, external-beam radiation therapy alone provides palliation of dysphagia in 70% to 80% of patients.

The most comprehensive and carefully performed analysis of swallowing function in patients receiving chemoradiation is by Coia et al.[445] Using a swallowing score modified from O'Rourke et al.,[446] they analyzed 102 patients treated with three 5-FU–based combined modality regimens. Before the start of therapy, 95% of patients had some degree of dysphagia. Within 2 weeks after the start of treatment, 45% had improvement in dysphagia, and by the completion of the 6-week therapy, 83% had improvement. Overall, 88% experienced an improvement in dysphagia. The median time to maximum improvement was 4 weeks (range, 1 to 21 weeks), and all but two patients could swallow at least soft or solid foods at the time of maximum symptomatic improvement.

Variables such as intent of treatment, tumor histologic type, and tumor location were examined. Of the 25 patients treated with a curative intent who survived more than 1 year, all were able to eat soft or solid foods after treatment. The rate of benign stricture (defined as a stricture in the absence of recurrent disease) was 12%. Even among patients treated in the noncurative setting, 91% had an initial improvement in swallowing and 67% had palliation until the time of death. Histologic type and stage had no impact on the rate of palliation. However, patients with lesions in the distal third of the esophagus had a significantly greater improvement in dysphagia than those with tumors in the upper two-thirds of the esophagus (95% vs. 79%; $P<.05$).

Intraluminal brachytherapy is also an effective, albeit more limited, method of palliation. It achieves palliation of dysphagia in 35% to 80% of patients and results in a median survival of approximately 5 months.[409–412] A major limitation of brachyther-apy is the effective treatment distance. The primary isotope is iridium 192, which is usually prescribed to treat to a distance of 1 cm from the source. Therefore, any portion of the tumor that is more than 1 cm from the source will receive a suboptimal radiation dose. This limitation has been confirmed by pathologic analysis of surgical specimens.[447] There is a selection bias against benefits from brachytherapy because it is commonly used either for patients for whom external-beam radiation therapy has failed or for patients who are medically unable to travel for daily outpatient treatment. Even when account is taken of this selection bias, given its limited effective range, it is usually not as successful as external-beam radiation therapy in treating the entire tumor volume. However, in the randomized trial reported by Sur et al., there was no significant difference in local control or survival with high dose-rate brachytherapy and with external-beam radiation therapy.[410]

In summary, external-beam radiation therapy, either alone or in combination with chemotherapy, provides palliation of dysphagia in approximately 80% of patients, with half experiencing palliation until the time of death. If a patient requires rapid palliation (within a few days), alternative approaches such as laser treatment or stent placement are recommended. Although external-beam radiation with or without chemotherapy takes at least 2 weeks to produce palliation, once palliation is achieved it is more durable than that provided by the other palliative modalities because external-beam radiation treats the problem (the gross tumor mass), not just the symptom. If external-beam radiation is not possible, then intraluminal brachytherapy should be considered, because it is an effective modality for decreasing symptoms such as dysphagia and bleeding.

Treatment in the Setting of a Tracheoesophageal Fistula. The presence of a malignant tracheoesophageal fistula is an unfavorable prognostic feature. Although the survival of such patients is poor, occasionally they may survive for a prolonged period. Historically, radiation therapy was believed to be contraindicated in these patients for fear of exacerbating the fistula as the tumor responded. More recently there have been reports to the contrary. In a Mayo Clinic series, ten patients with malignant tracheoesophageal fistulas received 30- to 66-Gy external-beam radiation, and the median survival time was 5 months.[448] Most importantly, none of the patients experienced an enlarging or more debilitating fistula after radiation. In one case report, a patient who developed a fistula while receiving external-beam radiation continued to receive treatment to a total dose of 56.5 Gy, and the fistula healed 2 months after the completion of radiation treatment.[449]

Although the experience is very limited, the data suggest that radiation treatment does not necessarily increase the severity of a malignant tracheoesophageal fistula and it may be administered safely. Due to the poor prognosis of this group of patients, it is unclear if radiation treatment improves outcome.

ACUTE AND LONG-TERM TOXICITY OF RADIATION THERAPY.   The toxicity of radiation therapy is a function of what the total dose is, what technique is used, and whether the patient has received chemotherapy. There are limited toxicity data for patients who received conventional doses of radiation therapy. Essentially all patients experience lethargy and esophagitis commencing 2 to 3 weeks after the start of radiation therapy; these symptoms usually resolve 1 to 2 weeks after the completion of therapy.

The most carefully documented acute toxicity data for patients receiving radiation therapy alone (without chemotherapy) are from the control arm of RTOG 85-01 in which patients received radiation therapy alone to a dose of 64 Gy.[318,388] The incidence of acute grade 3 toxicity was 25% and the incidence of acute grade 4 toxicity was 3%. There were no treatment-related deaths. The incidence of long-term grade 3+ toxicity was 23% and of long-term grade 4+ toxicity was 2%.[193]

As can surgery, radiation therapy can produce esophageal strictures. The total incidence of stricture (benign plus malignant) in patients receiving radiation therapy alone or radiation combined with chemotherapy is 20% to 40% in modern series and up to 60% in historical series.[450] It should be noted that almost half of these strictures are malignant because they are associated with local recurrence. Furthermore, the incidence of stricture is lower in series in which careful radiation techniques were used. For example, Coia et al. examined a subset of 25 patients who experienced local control and survived at least 1 year. The incidence of benign stricture was 12%.[445]

One series examined the functional results in patients who developed benign or malignant strictures.[446] Eighty patients received 45 to 56 Gy and 53% received some form of chemotherapy. Of the 24 patients (30%) who developed a benign stricture, 71% were able to tolerate a full or soft diet and required dilation, with a median interval between dilations of 5 months. Therefore, even in the subset of patients who develop a benign stricture, dilation is effective in the majority of patients. In contrast, in the 28% of patients who developed a malignant stricture, dilation was unsuccessful and esophageal intubation was required.

The high incidence of fistula reported in the RTOG 92-07 trial of chemoradiation plus intraluminal brachytherapy (18% actuarial, 14% crude) has not been seen in series using radiation therapy or chemoradiation without intraluminal brachytherapy. The incidence of other long-term grade 3+ toxicities such as pneumonitis or pericarditis is 5%. If appropriate radiation doses and techniques are used, spinal cord myelitis should not occur.

The effect of radiation on pulmonary function was examined by Gergel and associates.[451] Patients received 39.6 Gy with anterior-posterior fields followed by radiation with oblique fields to a total dose of 50.4 Gy, plus concurrent chemotherapy with oxaliplatin and 5-FU. Results of pulmonary function tests administered before and a median of 16 days after radiation revealed significant declines in diffusing capacity for carbon monoxide and total lung capacity.

The issue of treatment-related deaths in patients receiving chemoradiation is complex. Although the incidence was only 2% in RTOG 85-01, subsequent trials have reported a higher treatment-related mortality rate (i.e., 9% in INT 0122 and 8% in RTOG 92-07). These mortality rates are lower than the 10% to 15% incidence reported in the historical surgical series, although only slightly higher than the 6% reported in the surgical control arm of INT 0113.[186] It is interesting to note that, as the mortality rate with surgery has decreased, there has been a corresponding increase in the treatment-related mortality rate reported in the nonoperative trials. As discussed earlier in Primary Nonsurgical Therapy, this may be related, in part, to bias in selecting patients to be treated with the nonoperative approach. Only a randomized trial of surgical versus nonsurgical therapy can address this issue.

RADIATION FIELD DESIGN AND TREATMENT TECHNIQUES. Just as expert surgical skills are required for a successful esophagectomy, radiation field design for esophageal cancer requires careful techniques.[452] There are a number of sensitive organs that, depending on the location of the primary tumor, may be in the radiation field. These include but are not limited to skin, spinal cord, lung, heart, intestine, stomach, kidney, and liver. Minimizing the dose to these structures while delivering an adequate dose to the primary tumor and local-regional lymph nodes requires patient immobilization and CT-based treatment planning for organ identification, lung correction, and development of dose-volume histograms.

Although CT can identify adjacent organs and structures, it may be limited in defining the extent of the primary tumor. To assess the consistency of target volume delineation, Tai and colleagues sent sample cases with CT scans to 48 radiation oncologists throughout Canada and asked them to fill out questionnaires regarding treatment techniques as well as to outline the boost target volumes.[453] There was substantial inconsistency in defining the planning target volume, both in the transverse and longitudinal dimensions. Therefore, in addition to a CT scan, it is helpful to obtain results of a barium swallow test at the time of radiation therapy simulation. The integration of other imaging modalities such as EUS, PET, and magnetic resonance imaging into radiation treatment planning is under active investigation.

In a separate study reported by Tai et al., 12 Canadian radiation oncologists drew cervical esophagus target volumes based on the RTOG 94-05 protocol design both before and after a one-on-one training session.[454] Pretraining and posttraining survey revealed less variability in the longitudinal positions of the target volumes after training, which illustrates the importance of specialized training.

Nutting and colleagues compared two-phase conformal radiotherapy with intensity-modulated radiotherapy (IMRT) in five patients who received 55 Gy of radiation plus concurrent chemotherapy.[428] Treatment plans using both techniques were carried out and were compared using dose-volume histograms and normal tissue complication probabilities. The IMRT using nine equispaced fields provided no improvement over conformal radiation because the larger number of fields in the IMRT plan distributed a low dose over the entire lung. In contrast, IMRT using four fields equal to the conformal fields offered an improvement in lung sparing.

From a radiation treatment–planning viewpoint, tumors at or above the carina are treated as a cervical primary and the supraclavicular nodes are included in the radiation field. Tumors below the carina but not extending to the gastroesophageal junction are considered mid-esophageal, and the radiation field does not include the supraclavicular or celiac nodes. Tumors that involve the gastroesophageal junction are considered distal and the celiac nodes are included. This simplistic but practical definition is helpful in designing radiation therapy fields.

The standard radiation dose for patients selected for curative nonoperative chemoradiation is 50.4 Gy at 1.8 Gy/fraction. The radiation field should include the primary tumor with 5-cm superior and inferior margins and 2-cm lateral margins. The primary local-regional lymph nodes should receive the

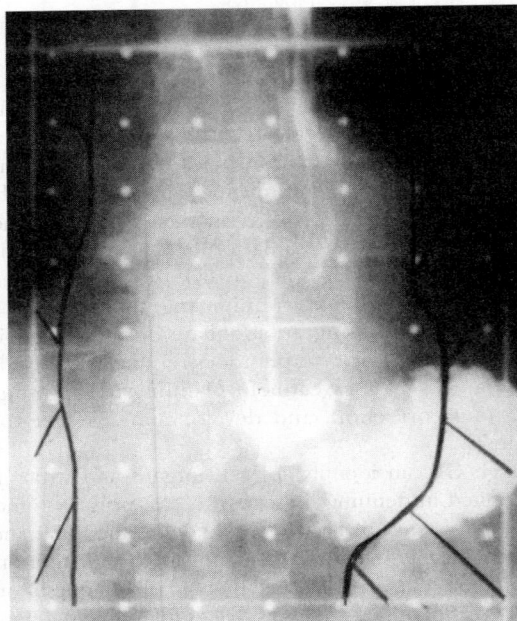
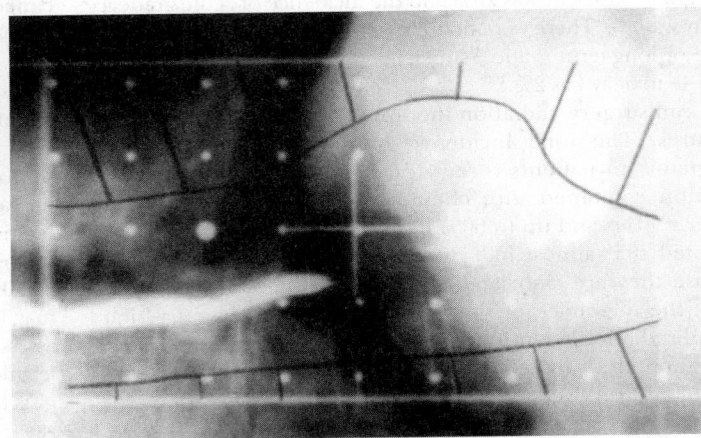

FIGURE 29.1-12.   An example of a four-field technique for the treatment of a distal esophageal cancer.

same dose. An example of a four-field technique for distal esophageal cancer is seen in Figure 29.1-12.

For cervical esophageal tumors, patients are placed supine. Various field designs are possible, and the choice depends on the geometry of the primary tumor in relation to the spinal cord. Field designs include a three-field plan (two anterior oblique fields and a posterior field) or, more commonly, anteroposterior-posteroanterior to 39.6 to 41.4 cGy followed by a left or right opposed oblique pair with photons plus an electron boost to the contralateral supraclavicular area, both to a total dose of 50.4 Gy. For mid-esophageal tumors, patients are placed prone to help exclude the spinal cord from the radiation field and a four-field design is used (anteroposterior, posteroanterior, and opposed lateral fields). For distal tumors, patients are treated supine using the same four-field technique. Care should be taken to exclude as much of the normal stomach as possible, especially if the patient is receiving radiation preoperatively. CT-based three-dimensional treatment planning should be performed, and all fields should be treated each day. Dose-volume histograms help guide the radiation oncologist in choosing a radiation plan that minimizes the loss of normal organ function.

In the palliative setting there are a variety of radiation treatment regimens. Because the goal is rapid palliation of symptoms, the most common approach is to treat anteroposteriorly and posteroanteriorly, including the primary tumor with 2-cm margins, in ten 3-Gy fractions to a total dose of 30 Gy.

The most critical normal structures that lie in proximity to the esophagus are the spinal cord, heart, lungs, and kidneys. When radiation is combined with chemotherapy, the radiation fractionation should be 1.8 Gy/d. The spinal cord dose should not exceed 45 Gy. All fields should be treated each day. Doses to the heart, lungs, and kidneys depend to a large extent on the volume of these organs in the treatment field. Dose-volume histograms are the most effective way to modify treatment techniques to decrease the acute and long-term radiation-related toxicity. In the rare situations when whole heart irradiation is needed, the dose should be limited to 25 to 30 Gy. In the thorax, radiation fields frequently include substantial volumes of lung, especially with oblique or lateral fields. Decreased pulmonary function occurs after irradiation, particularly if large volumes of lung are exposed to doses greater than 20 Gy. There is progressive decreased ventilatory and diffusing capacity as a result of endothelial degeneration and interstitial fibrosis. Fields that include such substantial volumes of lung should be limited to 20 Gy. Except for the spinal cord, it is acceptable for small volumes of normal tissue in immediate proximity to the esophagus to receive doses as high as 60 Gy. However, because the standard total dose of radiation is 50.4 Gy, this degree of inhomogeneity should be uncommon. Fortunately, even with tumors as distal as the gastroesophageal junction, there is a limited amount of liver and kidney in the treatment fields.

Endoluminal Palliation Techniques

A substantial number of patients with esophageal cancer present with locally advanced or metastatic disease that is not amenable to any treatment with curative intent, and therefore palliation of symptoms is the primary, and in many instances the only, goal of treatment. Symptoms of locally advanced or progressive tumor invasion that require immediate intervention are dysphagia (present in the vast majority of patients) and tracheoesophageal fistula. In the setting of either unresectable or disseminated disease, surgical approaches to palliation have been relegated to a historical footnote with the advances in endoscopic technology that achieve comparable or superior efficacy with less morbidity and mortality than the more invasive surgical techniques of resection and bypass.[455] These endoscopic techniques include dilation, stent placement, and ablation, mainly in the form of PDT or neodymium:yttrium aluminum garnet (Nd:YAG) laser treatment.

Esophageal dilation can be effective in relieving dysphagia in up to 90% of patients.[456] However, the effect is transient (lasting 4 weeks or less) so that repeated dilations are required, and the procedure is associated with a 5% to 10% rate of complications, including perforation.[457] Because the duration of dysphagia relief is limited, dilation is most commonly performed to allow for proper placement of a self-expanding stent device.

Fixed-diameter plastic endoluminal prostheses, associated with significant morbidity and mortality and a low rate of dysphagia relief,[458] have largely been abandoned as a stenting tool in favor of self-expandable metal stents. These stents are relatively easy to insert under fluoroscopic and endoscopic guidance with a technical success rate of approximately 95% and an efficacy of 85% to 100% in relieving dysphagia.[455,459,460] The duration of response is 5 to 6 months and complications occur in 10% to 15% of patients, the most common being stent migration and tumor ingrowth.[460] Placement of stents with barbs can reduce stent migration, whereas the use of stents coated with silicone or polyurethane may prevent or delay tumor ingrowth and subsequent esophageal obstruction.[461] Tumor ingrowth may be addressed by insertion of another stent or by tumor ablation. Placement of stents through proximally located tumors, especially those near the cricopharyngeus, is often not well tolerated by patients. In addition, stents placed across the gastroesophageal junction have a greater tendency to migrate and may result in symptomatic acid reflux. Coated stents have been used with good success (more than 90%) for the treatment of tracheoesophageal fistula.[462] Finally, stents have been successfully deployed after chemoradiotherapy to improve dysphagia, although exsanguinating hemorrhage has been reported with their use in patients with aortic invasion.[463]

Nd:YAG laser therapy delivers high-energy beams through an endoscopically introduced fiber to vaporize tumor tissue and create an esophageal lumen. Nd:YAG laser treatment is effective in relieving dysphagia in 70% to 90% of patients, with a duration of response of 1 to 3 months.[464–467] Tumors of the mid-esophagus are most amenable to laser therapy, although tumors in other locations can be treated. Complications occur in 2% to 4% of patients and include perforation and bleeding.[467] Multiple treatments may be required to achieve satisfactory relief of dysphagia.

PDT, as described earlier in Ablative Methods, uses a photosensitizing agent that is introduced intravenously, is absorbed by tumor tissue, and, when activated with light of a certain wavelength, leads to tumor necrosis. Relief of dysphagia has been reported in 60% to 90% of patients, with a duration of response of 1 to 3 months.[468,469] Complications occur in 10% to 25% of patients and include chest pain, pleural effusion, tracheoesophageal fistula, and sun sensitivity. A multicenter randomized trial compared PDT to Nd:YAG laser therapy in 218 esophageal cancer patients with dysphagia.[470] Objective tumor response was significantly greater in those patients in the PDT arm; however, no differences were noted in dysphagia relief between the two treatment groups. Photosensitivity was noted in 19% of patients treated with PDT, and there was a significantly higher risk of perforation in the Nd:YAG group than in the PDT group (7% vs. 1%).

Other forms of ablative therapy, including argon plasma coagulation and electrocautery, produce tumor necrosis with efficacy rates similar to those of the ablative methods mentioned earlier.[455,471–473] Electrocautery is associated with higher perforation rates because it requires dilation, whereas argon plasma coagulation is most appropriate for smaller, vascular lesions.

All of the aforementioned methods are effective in relieving dysphagia for varying periods of time, and frequently more than one method is required to achieve effective palliation of symptoms during the patient's lifetime. Therefore, the endoluminal techniques described are considered complimentary methods for palliation in the patient with esophageal cancer, and all options should be considered and potentially used to relieve debilitating symptoms.

TREATMENT OF METASTATIC DISEASE

Major centers in the United States report 5-year survival rates of 15% to 20% for esophageal cancer patients undergoing resection.[474,475] Although radical esophagectomy may save some patients with locally advanced carcinoma, the vast majority of individuals succumb to their disease, which suggests that most patients have occult metastases at presentation. Studies of patterns of recurrence and data from autopsy series confirm the potential for tumor spread to all organs.[87,476–479] These data have provided the rationale for using systemic therapy in conjunction with surgery, radiation, or both in patients with apparently localized disease or as the primary treatment for patients with clinically evident disseminated disease.

Standard criteria for evaluating treatment response require that serial measurement of disease be possible. For the esophageal cancer patient with metastatic disease to distant organ sites or lymph nodes, treatment response can be reliably assessed using spiral CT or magnetic resonance imaging. Serial tumor measurement for response assessment in patients with disease limited to the esophagus is less reliable. Endoscopy with brushings and biopsy may be performed to confirm a clinically determined complete response; however, biopsy is subject to sampling error, and biopsy findings are not a reliable indicator of complete histologic resolution of disease. Whole body FDG-PET performed before and during or after chemotherapy may be a valuable noninvasive method of predicting tumor response and a favorable treatment outcome. Several studies have shown that a reduction in tumor FDG uptake (median decrease in standardized uptake value) correlates with response and longer survival.[228–230] A variety of single agents and combination regimens have been evaluated in patients with recurrent or metastatic carcinoma of the esophagus. These patients often have a high tumor burden and poor performance status with little prospect for prolongation of survival. Phase II clinical trials in this population have identified drugs with activity that have been integrated into combined modality regimens for the treatment of earlier-stage disease.

Until the mid-1990s, the accumulated experience with chemotherapy was almost entirely in patients with squamous cell tumors. With the well-documented rising incidence of adenocarcinoma of the distal esophagus, gastroesophageal junction, and cardia in the United States and Western industrialized countries, patients with this histologic type now make up well over half of referrals for chemotherapy. Most trials of new agents and combined modality regimens now include patients with both tumor types.

Single-Agent Chemotherapy

Studies of single-agent chemotherapy for esophageal cancer are summarized in Table 29.1-17.[480–509] Response data for many

TABLE 29.1-17.   Trials of Single Agents with Activity against Carcinoma of the Esophagus

Drug	Dosage	Patients (n)	Histologic Type	% CR + PR	Reference(s)
Bleomycin	15–30 mg/m^2, 10–20 mg/m^2/d IV or IM	80	S	15	480–484
5-Fluorouracil	300 mg/m^2 CIVI × 6 wk	13[a]	S	85	485
	500 mg/m^2 IV daily × 5	26	S	16	486
Mitomycin	20 mg/m^2 IV every 4–5 wk	31	S	35	487,488
Doxorubicin	40–60 mg/m^2 IV every 3 wk	33	S	18	486,489
Methotrexate	200 mg/m^2 every 10 d	44[a]	S	48	490
Cisplatin	50–120 mg/m^2 IV every 3–4 wk	131	S	21	487,490–494
	120 mg/m^2 IV d 1 & 15	15[a]	S	73	495
Vindesine	3–4 mg/m^2 IV every 2 wk	83	S	26	496–498
Mitoguazone	400–700 mg/m^2 IV weekly	64	S	23	499–501
Vinorelbine	20–25 mg/m^2 IV weekly	30	S	20	502
	30 mg/m^2 every 2 wk	16	S	25	509
Docetaxel	75 mg/m^2 every 3 wk	22	A	18	505
Gemcitabine	1250 mg/m^2 d 1, 8, 15 every 4 wk	21	S/A	0	506
Topotecan	1.5 mg/m^2/24 h d 1, 8, 15 every 6 wk	45	S/A	2	507
	1.5 mg/m^2 every day × 5 every 3 wk	17	S	0	508
Paclitaxel	250 mg/m^2/24 h IV every 3 wk	51	S/A	32	503
	140 mg/m^2 over 96 h every 3 wk	14	S/A	0	504

A, adenocarcinoma; CR, complete response; PR, partial response; S, squamous cell carcinoma.
[a]Neoadjuvant.

of the older drugs have come from broad phase I and II trials conducted in the early 1970s, which included small numbers of esophageal cancer patients. Bleomycin, 5-FU, mitomycin, and cisplatin have been most frequently used because of their single-agent activity and additive or synergistic effects with radiation. Because of the potential for pulmonary toxicity, bleomycin is no longer included in combination regimens, having been replaced by 5-FU. Similarly, mitomycin is less often used because of its toxicity profile, which includes hemolytic-uremic syndrome and cumulative myelosuppression.

Seven trials examined the use of cisplatin for single-agent therapy in esophageal cancer patients,[487,490–495] six of which used dosages ranging from 50 to 120 mg/m^2 every 3 to 4 weeks. The cumulative response rate in patients with metastatic or recurrent disease was 21%.[487,490–495] Administration of the drug as a single-bolus dose once every 3 weeks and in a divided dose over 5 days every 3 weeks appeared to be equally efficacious. Using a more dose-intense schedule of cisplatin (120 mg/m^2 on day 1 and 15), Miller et al.[495] observed a 73% response rate in 15 patients before surgery.

A randomized phase II trial of cisplatin alone and cisplatin in combination with 5-FU in 92 patients with metastatic squamous cell carcinoma of the esophagus was reported by the EORTC.[494] A 19% response rate was observed in 45 patients receiving single-agent cisplatin (100 mg/m^2 every 3 weeks). The response rate in the combination therapy arm was 35%. No studies of single-agent cisplatin have been performed in patients with adenocarcinoma of the esophagus.

Vinorelbine is a semisynthetic vinca alkaloid that has less neurotoxicity than vincristine and vinblastine. Phase II trials in metastatic squamous cell cancer of the esophagus report response rates of 20% to 25% using weekly or biweekly dosing schedules.[502,509] In a subsequent trial, Conroy and colleagues evaluated the doublet of vinorelbine and cisplatin.[510] A total of 71 patients with metastatic squamous cell cancer were treated and a 34%

response rate was observed. Use of vinorelbine has not been evaluated in patients with adenocarcinoma of the esophagus.

The taxane paclitaxel was the first entirely new compound to be tested in both adenocarcinoma and squamous cell carcinoma of the esophagus. Paclitaxel promotes the stabilization of microtubules and is a cycle-specific agent affecting cells in the G_2/M phase. Paclitaxel also enhances radiation effects and may be both concentration and schedule dependent.[511] Two trials of single-agent paclitaxel have been reported. One used the maximum tolerable dose of 250 mg/m^2, derived from initial phase I trials using a 24-hour infusion schedule.[503] The overall response rate was 32% (34% in 33 patients with adenocarcinoma, and 28% in 18 patients with squamous cell carcinoma). All patients had good performance status, were chemotherapy naive, and had distant metastases. The second trial tested a regimen of 140 mg/m^2 infused over 96 hours in patients previously treated using a shorter infusion schedule of paclitaxel containing combination chemotherapy.[504] No responses were observed.

There is one small trial of docetaxel (75 mg/m^2 every 3 weeks) in patients with metastatic adenocarcinoma.[505] An 18% response rate was observed in chemotherapy-naive patients, whereas no responses were seen among previously treated patients.

Drugs that have been adequately tested in squamous cell cancer of the esophagus and have response rates of less than 5% are the methotrexate analog dichloromethotrexate[512] and trimetrexate,[513,514] and etoposide,[515,516] ifosamide,[517,518] and carboplatin.[519–522] Carboplatin has been studied in both adenocarcinoma and squamous cell carcinoma using a fixed dose schedule of 300 to 400 mg/m^2 in individuals with normal renal function. In contrast to the activity observed in phase II evaluations of cisplatin, responses to carboplatin were observed in only 3 of 59 chemotherapy-naive patients. Therefore, substitution of carboplatin for cisplatin is not recommended when

TABLE 29.1-18.   Selected Combination Chemotherapy Regimens for Recurrent and Metastatic Carcinoma of the Esophagus

Regimen	Evaluable Patients (n)	Histologic Type	% CR + PR	Reference(s)
Cisplatin + bleomycin	17	S	17	296
Cisplatin + bleomycin + vindesine	51	S	31	297,523
Cisplatin + bleomycin + methotrexate	40	S	30	524,525
Cisplatin + mitoguazone + vindesine	20	S	40	526
Cisplatin + mitoguazone + vinblastine	36	S	11	527
Cisplatin + 5-FU	82	S	35	494
Carboplatin + vinblastine	16	S	0	528
Cisplatin + vinorelbine	71	S	34	510
13-*cis* retinoic acid + interferon-α_{2a}	15	S/A	0	531
5-FU + interferon-α_{2a}	57	S/A	26	529,533
Cisplatin + 5-FU + interferon-α_{2a}	66	S/A	53 (62% S, 32% A)	530,534
Cisplatin + etoposide	65	S	48	532
Cisplatin + etoposide + 5-FU + leucovorin	69	S	34	535
Paclitaxel (24 h) + cisplatin every 3 wk	32	S/A	44 (25% S, 46% A)	538
Paclitaxel (3 h) + cisplatin every 2 wk	51	S/A	43	536
Paclitaxel (3 h) + cisplatin every wk × 6	24	A	50	537
Paclitaxel (3 h) + cisplatin + 5-FU every 4 wk	60	S/A	48 (56% S, 46% A)	540
Irinotecan + cisplatin every wk × 4, every 6 wk	35	S/A	57 (66% S, 52% A)	541
Irinotecan + cisplatin every wk × 4, every 6 wk	25	A	51	542
Docetaxel + irinotecan every wk × 3, every 4 wk	24	S/A	13	544
Docetaxel + irinotecan every 3 wk	46	A	26	543
Mitomycin + cisplatin + 5-FU	285	A/G	46% A, 38% G	545
Vs.				
Epirubicin + cisplatin + 5-FU	289	A/G	44% A, 36% G	

A, adenocarcinoma of esophagus, gastroesophageal junction, cardia; 5-FU, 5-fluorouracil; G, gastric cancer; S, squamous cell carcinoma.

treating patients with either adenocarcinomas or squamous cell carcinomas of the esophagus. Topotecan and gemcitabine have been separately evaluated in both histologic tumor types and have been shown to be inactive.[506–508]

Combined-Agent Chemotherapy

Older trials (before the mid-1990s) and those in Europe were almost exclusively limited to patients with squamous cell carcinoma. Because esophageal cancer is a relatively uncommon malignancy, many studies include a heterogeneous population of treatment-naive patients with locally advanced intrathoracic disease as well as patients with recurrent or metastatic disease. Not only is there variation in the patient population, but more recent trials usually limit eligibility to patients with no prior chemotherapy and performance status of 0 or 1. Thus, in the absence of comparative trials, newer regimens may appear more effective.

The results for platinum-based combination chemotherapy regimens are detailed in Table 29.1-18.[296,297,361,510,523–532] Most series consist of small numbers of patients, and therefore the 95% confidence intervals are large and nearly all responses are partial. On average, duration of response ranges from 3 to 6 months.

Trials conducted in the 1980s testing three-drug regimens such as cisplatin, bleomycin, and vindesine[297,523] and cisplatin and mitoguazone combined with vindesine[526] or vinblastine[527] yielded response rates of 30% to 40% in patients with squamous cell carcinoma. Toxicity was primarily moderate myelosuppression. Bleomycin and mitoguazone were subsequently replaced by 5-FU to reduce toxicity and to take advantage of its synergistic activity with cisplatin.

The two-drug combination of cisplatin (100 mg/m^2 on day 1) and 5-FU (1000 mg/m^2/d continuous infusion for 96 to 120 hours) has been the standard regimen for two decades to treat patients with either squamous cell carcinoma or adenocarcinoma. A 35% response rate was observed in patients with metastatic, recurrent, or locally advanced incurable squamous cell cancer of the esophagus.[494] Higher response rates (in the 40% to 60% range) were reported in trials administering two or three cycles of cisplatin and 5-FU as induction therapy before surgery. The difference in response rates may be related to better performance status, better nutrition, and smaller-volume disease in the surgical candidates. Attempts to substitute carboplatin for cisplatin have been unsuccessful; in a phase II trial of carboplatin and vinblastine,[528] investigators at Memorial Sloan-Kettering Cancer Center observed no responses in 16 patients even though 11 had previously untreated inoperable cancers and 15 had Karnofsky performance scores of 70 or higher.

Four trials using interferon-α_{2a} as a biomodulator of 5-FU suggested possible benefit.[529,530,533,534] Preclinical data indicated synergistic cytolytic activity when interferon was combined with 5-FU, possibly due to interferon-mediated stimulation of thymidine phosphorylase, which increases the conversion of 5-FU to its active metabolite, fluorodeoxyuridylate. Ilson and colleagues[530] treated 26 incurable esophageal cancer patients with interferon-α_{2a} (3 million U subcutaneously daily), cisplatin (100 mg/m^2 on day 1), and continuous-infusion 5-FU (750 mg/m^2/d for 5 days) recycled every 28 days. The complete plus partial response rate was 50%, and the duration of response ranged from 11 to 74 weeks. Treatment responses were observed in 8 of 11 patients with squamous cell carcinoma (73%; 95% confidence interval, 47% to 99%) and 5 of 15 patients with adenocarcinoma (33%;

95% confidence interval, 9% to 57%). Similar results were reported by Bazarbashi and colleagues: 61% response rate for squamous cell cancer and 29% for adenocarcinoma.[534]

Despite the lack of single-agent activity for etoposide, the Rotterdam Oesophageal Tumour Study Group[532] reported a 48% response rate in patients with unresectable or metastatic squamous cell carcinoma given combination chemotherapy including this drug. This experience in the use of cisplatin (80 mg/m² on day 1) and etoposide (100 mg/m² intravenously on days 1 and 2 and 200 mg/m² orally on days 3 to 5 every 4 weeks) served as the basis for a phase III evaluation of this regimen in the preoperative setting.[306] A subsequent trial adding infusional 5-FU and leucovorin to cisplatin plus etoposide showed similar activity (34% complete plus partial responses) but more mucosal toxicity.[535]

Combination regimens including paclitaxel have been evaluated in esophageal cancer patients. In three phase II trials of paclitaxel and cisplatin, response rates ranged from 43% to 50%; activity was comparable in both histologic tumor types.[536–538] In a study evaluating paclitaxel (24-hour infusion) in doses of 200 to 250 mg/m² with growth factor support combined with cisplatin (75 mg/m²), toxicity (primarily myelosuppression) was severe, leading to one or more hospitalizations in 50% of patients and five treatment-related deaths.[538] This particular regimen cannot be recommended. Others have evaluated alternative dosing schedules.[536,537] An evaluation of escalating doses of paclitaxel (100 to 200 mg/m²) in 3-hour infusions combined with a fixed dose of cisplatin (60 mg/m²) administered every 2 weeks demonstrated a 43% response rate in 51 patients.[536] Doses of paclitaxel above 180 mg/m² caused dose-limiting neurotoxicity.[539] A second trial evaluated a weekly regimen of cisplatin (70 mg/m²) and 3-hour paclitaxel infusion.[537] The maximum tolerable dose of paclitaxel was 100 mg/m²/wk, and the response rate was 50%. The antitumor activity reported for these three regimens was comparable, but toxicity varied considerably.

The three-drug combination of paclitaxel, 175 mg/m² (3-hour infusion), combined with cisplatin (20 mg/m²/d × 5) and 5-FU (1000 mg/m²/d continuous infusion × 120 hours) was evaluated in 60 patients at four centers.[540] A 48% response rate was reported (56% in patients with squamous cell cancer and 46% in patients with adenocarcinoma); significantly more complete responses were observed in patients with squamous cell carcinoma. Toxicity resulted in unplanned hospitalizations for 48% of patients, primarily for severe stomatitis, fever, and neutropenia. The addition of paclitaxel to the established cisplatin and 5-FU regimen did not raise the response rate sufficiently to warrant further evaluation in a larger comparative trial.

It is clear that the optimal dose and schedule of paclitaxel in combination with other active drugs remains to be determined. In general, shorter infusion schedules of paclitaxel result in less myelotoxicity but more neurotoxicity when combined with cisplatin.

Other regimens of interest include those containing irinotecan. First reported was the doublet of irinotecan and cisplatin administered in low dose on a weekly schedule.[541,542] *In vitro* studies demonstrated sequence-dependent synergy for cisplatin followed by irinotecan, which prevents removal of cisplatin-induced DNA interstrand cross-links. Two trials yielded encouraging results with a regimen of cisplatin (30 mg/m²) followed by irinotecan (65 mg/m²) administered weekly for 4 weeks, repeated every 6 weeks.[541,542] Ilson and colleagues[541] observed a 57% response rate in 35 patients [12 of 23 patients with adenocarcinoma (52%) and 8 of 12 patients with squamous cell cancer (66%)]; median duration of response was 4.2 months.[541] Dysphagia and global quality of life were improved in the majority of patients. Ajani and colleagues[542] observed a 51% response rate using the same regimen in 25 patients with adenocarcinoma, but recommended reduction of the irinotecan dose to 50 mg/m² in previously treated patients. These investigators also noted that 66% of the third or fourth weekly doses were delayed or canceled due to toxicity. In both studies toxicity consisted of myelosuppression, diarrhea, and fatigue. Diarrhea was ameliorated with prophylactic use of antidiarrheal agents, dose reduction, or both.

Docetaxel and irinotecan are another doublet tested on a schedule of once every 3 weeks (at 40 mg/m² and 100 mg/m², respectively)[543] and on a low-dose weekly schedule for 3 out of 4 weeks (at 25 mg/m² and 55 mg/m², respectively).[544] The weekly schedule appears less active than the every-3-weeks dosing schedule (13% response rate in 24 patients with adenocarcinoma or squamous cell cancers contrasted with 26% response rate in 46 patients with adenocarcinoma of the esophagus, gastroesophageal junction, or cardia).

Investigators in the United Kingdom have developed the three-drug regimen ECF as the reference regimen for treatment of upper gastrointestinal tract adenocarcinomas. A randomized trial comparing ECF to mitomycin, cisplatin, and 5-FU (MCF) enrolled 580 patients, of whom 40 had squamous cell carcinoma of the esophagus and the remainder had adenocarcinoma (125, esophagus; 125, gastroesophageal junction; 243, stomach).[545] There was no difference in response rate or survival time with ECF and MCF. However, there was a significantly higher response rate among patients with gastroesophageal junction cancers than among those with distal gastric cancers (48% vs. 37%; *P* = .041). This is consistent with the concept that the biology and natural history of gastroesophageal junction and cardia cancers is different from those of gastric cancers.

Two small phase II trials at the University of Glasgow substituted either capecitabine[546] or raletrexed[547] for 5-FU in the ECF regimen and reported response rates of 24% to 29% in a mix of patients with advanced gastric and distal esophageal and gastroesophageal junction cancers. Further evaluation of the combination with capecitabine was planned.

In summary, recent trials of combination regimens that include paclitaxel or irinotecan appear to have higher response rates than previous regimens; however, duration of response remains brief. In addition, the toxicities recorded in many of these phase II single-institution experiences have been excessive.

Additional patient trials using the most promising regimens are needed. No specific paclitaxel-based regimen has yet emerged as more efficacious and less toxic than cisplatin and 5-FU. The combination of irinotecan and cisplatin may have the most favorable response and toxicity profile and is undergoing further evaluation with schedule modification (day 1 and 8 dosing every 21 days) in patients with metastatic disease and in combination with radiotherapy as preoperative neoadjuvant treatment. Regimens that exclude cisplatin appear less efficacious. Comparative trials are needed to determine if any of the newer regimens is indeed more active or has a better toxicity profile than cisplatin and 5-FU. No data have as yet emerged regarding the incorporation of molecularly targeted therapeutic agents such as inhibitors of angiogenesis or of the EGF receptor and its downstream pathway intermediates.

STAGE-DIRECTED TREATMENT RECOMMENDATIONS

Although, in many clinical situations, level I evidence is lacking to support ironclad recommendations regarding the most effective treatment of patients grouped by stage, reasonable trial-generated information exists to suggest appropriate therapeutic interventions for patients catalogued under broad staging categories.

Resection remains the standard by which all other treatment options must be measured for patients with high-grade dysplasia in the setting of Barrett's esophagus or T1 disease limited to the mucosa with the caveat that esophagectomy-associated mortality must be extremely low. With more experience and longer follow-up data, ablative methods or the more attractive therapeutic option, EMR, may become universally accepted as treatment alternatives considered comparable to surgery. Intensive long-term endoscopic surveillance for patients with Barrett's esophagus–associated high-grade dysplasia is necessary to limit both cancer- and treatment-related mortality.

Esophagectomy is an appropriate method for treating patients with stage I, II, III, and select IVA disease. Alternatively, definitive chemoradiation is a therapeutic option for patients with stage II and III disease and the majority of those with stage IVA lesions, especially those who are not considered surgical candidates or who have squamous cell carcinoma at or above the carina. The high rate of persistent or recurrent local-regional disease after definitive chemoradiation suggests that additional local therapy in the form of surgery may be necessary and beneficial. This potential benefit may only be realized if perioperative mortality is minimized. Although preoperative chemoradiotherapy has not been definitively proven to be more effective than surgery alone, it remains an attractive approach that has been embraced by oncologists for patients with resectable stage IIB, III, and selected IVA esophageal cancers and should continue to be examined in well-designed clinical trials. Postoperative chemoradiotherapy should be reserved for patients with resected adenocarcinoma of the gastroesophageal junction. Preoperative chemotherapy is an accepted standard of care in the United Kingdom but is still considered investigational in the United States. All patients with unresectable or stage IV disease are ideally suited for clinical trials exploring novel therapeutic agents and approaches.

REFERENCES

1. Brown LM, Devesa SS. Epidemiologic trends in esophageal and gastric cancer in the United States. *Surg Oncol Clin N Am* 2002;11:235.
2. Brown LM, Devesa SS, Fraumeni JF. Epidemiology of esophageal cancer. In: Posner M, Vokes EE, Weichselbaum RR, eds. *Cancer of the upper gastrointestinal tract.* Hamilton, Ontario, Canada: BC Decker, 2002:1.
3. Ries LAG EM, Kososy CL, et al. *Cancer statistics review SEER 1973–1998,* 2001.
4. Jemal A, Murray T, Samuels A, et al. Cancer statistics, 2003. *CA Cancer J Clin* 2003;53:5.
5. Schottenfeld D. Epidemiology of cancer of the esophagus. *Semin Oncol* 1984;11:92.
6. Brown LM, Hoover R, Silverman D, et al. Excess incidence of squamous cell esophageal cancer among US Black men: role of social class and other risk factors. *Am J Epidemiol* 2001;153:114.
7. Kabat GC, Ng SK, Wynder EL. Tobacco, alcohol intake, and diet in relation to adenocarcinoma of the esophagus and gastric cardia. *Cancer Causes Control* 1993;4:123.
8. Gammon MD, Schoenberg JB, Ahsan H, et al. Tobacco, alcohol, and socioeconomic status and adenocarcinomas of the esophagus and gastric cardia. *J Natl Cancer Inst* 1997;89:1277.
9. Castellsague X, Munoz N, De Stefani E, et al. Independent and joint effects of tobacco smoking and alcohol drinking on the risk of esophageal cancer in men and women. *Int J Cancer* 1999;82:657.
10. Castellsague X, Munoz N, De Stefani E, et al. Smoking and drinking cessation and risk of esophageal cancer (Spain). *Cancer Causes Control* 2000;11:813.
11. Yu MC, Garabrant DH, Peters JM, et al. Tobacco, alcohol, diet, occupation, and carcinoma of the esophagus. *Cancer Res* 1988;48:3843.
12. Munoz N, Day NE. *Esophageal cancer.* In: Schottenfeld D, Fraumeni JF, eds. *Cancer epidemiology and prevention,* 2nd ed. New York: Oxford University Press, 1996:681.
13. Castellsague X, Munoz N, De Stefani E, et al. Influence of mate drinking, hot beverages and diet on esophageal cancer risk in South America. *Int J Cancer* 2000;88:658.
14. Gorey K, Vena JE. Cancer differentials among US blacks and whites: quantitative estimates of socioeconomic-related risks. *J Natl Med Assoc* 1994;86:209.
15. National Center for Health Statistics. *Health, United States 2000, with adolescent health chart book.* Hyattsville, MD: NCHS, 2000.
16. Vaughan TL, Davis S, Kristal A, et al. Obesity, alcohol, and tobacco as risk factors for cancers of the esophagus and gastric cardia: adenocarcinoma versus squamous cell carcinoma. *Cancer Epidemiol Biomarkers Prev* 1995;4:85.
17. Brown LM, Swanson CA, Gridley G, et al. Adenocarcinoma of the esophagus: role of obesity and diet. *J Natl Cancer Inst* 1995;87:104.
18. Chow WH, Blot WJ, Vaughan TL, et al. Body mass index and risk of adenocarcinomas of the esophagus and gastric cardia. *J Natl Cancer Inst* 1998;90:150.
19. Lagergren J, Bergstrom R, Lindgren A, et al. Symptomatic gastroesophageal reflux as a risk factor for esophageal adenocarcinoma. *New Engl J Med* 1999;340:825.
20. Chow WH, Finkle WD, McLaughlin JK, et al. The relation of gastroesophageal reflux disease and its treatment to adenocarcinomas of the esophagus and gastric cardia. *JAMA* 1995;274:474.
21. Chow WH, Blaser MJ, Blot WJ, et al. An inverse relation between cagA+ strains of *Helicobacter pylori* infection and risk of esophageal and gastric cardia adenocarcinoma. *Cancer Res* 1998;58:588.
22. Cameron AJ. Management of Barrett's esophagus. *Mayo Clin Proc* 1998;73:457.
23. Spechler SJ. Clinical practice. Barrett's esophagus. *N Engl J Med* 2002;346:836.
24. Sampliner RE. Updated guidelines for the diagnosis, surveillance, and therapy of Barrett's esophagus. *Am J Gastroenterol* 2002;97:1888.
25. Cameron AJ, Ott BJ, Payne WS, The incidence of adenocarcinoma in columnar-lined (Barrett's) esophagus. *N Engl J Med* 1985;313:857.
26. Drewitz DJ, Sampliner RE, Garewal HS. The incidence of adenocarcinoma in Barrett's esophagus: a prospective study of 170 patients followed 4.8 years. *Am J Gastroenterol* 1997;92:212.
27. O'Connor JB, Falk GW, Richter JE. The incidence of adenocarcinoma and dysplasia in Barrett's esophagus: report on the Cleveland Clinic Barrett's Esophagus Registry. *Am J Gastroenterol* 1999;94:2037.
28. Spechler SJ, Lee E, Ahnen D, et al. Long-term outcome of medical and surgical therapies for gastroesophageal reflux disease: follow-up of a randomized controlled trial. *JAMA* 2001;285:2331.
29. Shaheen NJ, Crosby MA, Bozymski EM, et al. Is there publication bias in the reporting of cancer risk in Barrett's esophagus? *Gastroenterology* 2000;119:333.
30. Rudolph RE, Vaughan TL, Storer BE, et al. Effect of segment length on risk for neoplastic progression in patients with Barrett esophagus. *Ann Intern Med* 2000;132:612.
31. Cameron AJ, Zinsmeister AR, Ballard DJ, et al. Prevalence of columnar-lined (Barrett's) esophagus. Comparison of population-based clinical and autopsy findings. *Gastroenterology* 1990;99:918.
32. Csendes A, Smok G, Burdiles P, et al. Prevalence of Barrett's esophagus by endoscopy and histologic studies: a prospective evaluation of 306 control subjects and 376 patients with symptoms of gastroesophageal reflux. *Dis Esophagus* 2000;13:5.
33. Dulai GS, Guha S, Kahn KL, et al. Preoperative prevalence of Barrett's esophagus in esophageal adenocarcinoma: a systematic review. *Gastroenterology* 2002;122:26.
34. Peters JH, Clark GW, Ireland AP, et al. Outcome of adenocarcinoma arising in Barrett's esophagus in endoscopically surveyed and nonsurveyed patients. *J Thorac Cardiovasc Surg* 1994;108:813.
35. Ferguson MK, Durkin A. Long-term survival after esophagectomy for Barrett's adenocarcinoma in endoscopically surveyed and nonsurveyed patients. *J Gastrointest Surg* 2002;6:29.
36. Corley DA, Levin TR, Habel LA, et al. Surveillance and survival in Barrett's adenocarcinomas: a population-based study. *Gastroenterology* 2002;122:633.
37. Hamilton SR, Smith RR, Cameron JL. Prevalence and characteristics of Barrett esophagus in patients with adenocarcinoma of the esophagus or esophagogastric junction. *Hum Pathol* 1988;19:942.
38. Theisen J, Stein HJ, Dittler HJ, et al. Preoperative chemotherapy unmasks underlying Barrett's mucosa in patients with adenocarcinoma of the distal esophagus. *Surg Endosc* 2002;16:671.
39. van der Burgh A, Dees J, Hop WC, et al. Oesophageal cancer is an uncommon cause of death in patients with Barrett's oesophagus. *Gut* 1996;39:5.
40. Macdonald CE, Wicks AC, Playford RJ. Final results from 10 year cohort of patients undergoing surveillance for Barrett's oesophagus: observational study. *BMJ* 2000;321:1252.
41. DeMeester SR, DeMeester TR. Columnar mucosa and intestinal metaplasia of the esophagus: fifty years of controversy. *Ann Surg* 2000;231:303.
42. Gurski RR, Peters JH, Hagen JA, et al. Barrett's esophagus can and does regress after antireflux surgery: a study of prevalence and predictive features. *J Am Coll Surg* 2003;196:706.

43. Katz D, Rothstein R, Schned A, et al. The development of dysplasia and adenocarcinoma during endoscopic surveillance of Barrett's esophagus. *Am J Gastroenterol* 1998;93:536.
44. Haggitt RC. Barrett's esophagus, dysplasia, and adenocarcinoma. *Hum Pathol* 1994;25:982.
45. Skacel M, Petras RE, Gramlich TL, et al. The diagnosis of low-grade dysplasia in Barrett's esophagus and its implications for disease progression. *Am J Gastroenterol* 2000;95:3383.
46. Montgomery E, Bronner MP, Goldblum JR, et al. Reproducibility of the diagnosis of dysplasia in Barrett esophagus: a reaffirmation. *Hum Pathol* 2001;32:368.
47. Buttar NS, Wang KK, Leontovich O, et al. Chemoprevention of esophageal adenocarcinoma by COX-2 inhibitors in an animal model of Barrett's esophagus. *Gastroenterology* 2002;122:1101.
48. Ashworth MT, Nash JR, Ellis A, et al. Abnormalities of differentiation and maturation in the oesophageal squamous epithelium of patients with tylosis: morphological features. *Histopathology* 1991;19:303.
49. Risk JM, Mills HS, Garde J, et al. The tylosis esophageal cancer (TOC) locus: more than just a familial cancer gene. *Dis Esophagus* 1999;12:173.
50. Risk JM, Field EA, Field JK, et al. Tylosis oesophageal cancer mapped. *Nat Genet* 1994;8:319.
51. von Brevern M, Hollstein MC, Risk JM, et al. Loss of heterozygosity in sporadic oesophageal tumors in the tylosis oesophageal cancer (TOC) gene region of chromosome 17q. *Oncogene* 1998;17:2101.
52. Iwaya T, Maesawa C, Ogasawara S, et al. Tylosis esophageal cancer locus on chromosome 17q25.1 is commonly deleted in sporadic human esophageal cancer. *Gastroenterology* 1998;114:1206.
53. Risk JM. Envoplakin, a possible candidate gene for focal NEPPK/esophageal cancer (TOC): the integration of genetic and physical maps of the TOC region on 17q25. *Genomics* 1999; 59:234.
54. Shamma'A MH, Benedict EB. Esophageal webs; a report of 58 cases and an attempt at classification. *N Engl J Med* 1958;259:378.
55. Ribeiro U Jr, Posner MC, Safatle-Ribeiro AV, et al. Risk factors for squamous cell carcinoma of the oesophagus. *Br J Surg* 1996;83:1174.
56. Csikos M, Horvath O, Petri A, et al. Late malignant transformation of chronic corrosive oesophageal strictures. *Langenbecks Arch Chir* 1985;365:231.
57. Sandler RS, Nyren O, Ekbom A, et al. The risk of esophageal cancer in patients with achalasia. A population-based study. *JAMA* 1995;274:1359.
58. Meijssen MA, Tilanus HW, van Blankenstein M, et al. Achalasia complicated by oesophageal squamous cell carcinoma: a prospective study in 195 patients. *Gut* 1992;33:155.
59. Aggestrup S, Holm JC, Sorensen HR. Does achalasia predispose to cancer of the esophagus? *Chest* 1992;102:1013.
60. Loviscek LF, Cenoz MC, Badaloni AE, et al. Early cancer in achalasia. *Dis Esophagus* 1998;11:239.
61. Sur M, Cooper K. The role of the human papilloma virus in esophageal cancer. *Pathology* 1998;30:348.
62. Stoler MH. Human papillomaviruses and cervical neoplasia: a model for carcinogenesis. *Int J Gynecol Cancer* 2000;19:16.
63. Mineta H, Ogino T, Amano HM, et al. Human papilloma virus (HPV) type 16 and 18 detected in head and neck squamous cell carcinoma. *Anticancer Res* 1998;18:4765.
64. de Villiers EM, Lavergne D, Chang F, et al. An interlaboratory study to determine the presence of human papillomavirus DNA in esophageal carcinoma from China. *Int J Cancer* 1999;81:225.
65. Lavergne D, de Villiers EM. Papillomavirus in esophageal papillomas and carcinomas. *Int J Cancer* 1999;80:681.
66. Shibagaki I, Tanaka H, Shimada Y, et al. p53 mutation, murine double minute 2 amplification, and human papillomavirus infection are frequently involved but not associated with each other in esophageal squamous cell carcinoma. *Clin Cancer Res* 1995;1:769.
67. Poljak M, Cerar A, Seme K. Human papillomavirus infection in esophageal carcinomas: a study of 121 lesions using multiple broad-spectrum polymerase chain reactions and literature review. *Hum Pathol* 1998;29:266.
68. Rugge M, Bovo D, Busatto G, et al. p53 alterations but no human papillomavirus infection in preinvasive and advanced squamous cancer in Italy. *Cancer Epidemiol Biomarkers Prev* 1997;6:171.
69. Turner JR, Shen LH, Crum CP, et al. Low prevalence of human papillomavirus infection in esophageal squamous cell carcinomas from North America: analysis by a highly sensitive and specific polymerase chain reaction-based approach. *Hum Pathol* 1997; 28:174.
70. Lagergren J, Wang Z, Bergstrom R, et al. Human papillomavirus infection and esophageal cancer: a nationwide seroepidemiologic case-control study in Sweden. *J Natl Cancer Inst* 1999;91:156.
71. Leon X, Quer M, Diez S, et al. Second neoplasm in patients with head and neck cancer. *Head Neck* 1999;21:204.
72. Levi F, Randimbison L, Te VC, et al. Second primary cancers in patients with lung carcinoma. *Cancer* 1999;86:186.
73. Narayana A, Vaughan AT, Fisher SG, et al. Second primary tumors in laryngeal cancer: results of long-term follow-up. *Int J Radiat Oncol Biol Phys* 1998;42:557.
74. Ribeiro U, Safatle-Ribeiro AV, Posner MC, et al. Comparative p53 mutational analysis of multiple primary cancers of the upper aerodigestive tract. *Surgery* 1996;120:45.
75. American Joint Commission on Cancer. *AJCC Cancer Staging Manual*, 6th ed. New York: Springer Verlag, 2002:91.
76. Hagen JA, DeMeester SR, Peters JH, et al. Curative resection for esophageal adenocarcinoma. Analysis of 100 en bloc esophagectomies. *Ann Surg* 2001;234:520.
77. Altorki NK, Girardi L, Skinner DB. En bloc esophagectomy improves survival for stage III esophageal cancer. *J Thorac Cardiovasc Surg* 1997;114:948.
78. Akiyama H, Tsurumaru M, Udagawa H, et al. Radical lymph node dissection for cancer of the thoracic esophagus. *Ann Surg* 1994;220:364.
79. Altorki N, Kent M, Ferrara C, et al. Three-field lymph node dissection for squamous cell and adenocarcinoma of the esophagus. *Ann Surg* 2002;236:177.
80. Feith M, Stein HJ, Siewert JR. Pattern of lymphatic spread of Barrett's cancer. *World J Surg* 2003;27:1052.
81. Kitagawa Y, Fujii H, Mukai M, et al. Intraoperative lymphatic mapping and sentinel lymph node sampling in esophageal and gastric cancer. *Surg Oncol Clin N Am* 2002;11:293.
82. Blot WJ. *Epidemiology and genesis of esophageal cancer in thoracic oncology.* In: Ruckdeschel RJ, Weisenburger JC, eds. Philadelphia: WB Saunders, 1995.
83. Sons HU. Esophageal cancer: autopsy findings in 171 cases. *Arch Pathol Lab Med* 1984; 108:983.
84. Anderson LL, Lad TE. Autopsy findings in squamous-cell carcinoma of the esophagus. *Cancer* 1982;50:1587.
85. Mandard A, Tourneux, J, Gignoux, M, et al. In situ carcinoma of the esophagus. Macroscopic study with particular reference to the Lugol test. *Endoscopy* 1980;12:51.
86. Mandard AM, Marnay J, Gignoux M, et al. Cancer of the esophagus and associated lesions: detailed pathologic study of 100 esophagectomy specimens. *Hum Pathol* 1984;15:660.
87. Begin LR. The pathobiology of esophageal cancer in thoracic oncology. In: Roth JA, Ruckdeschel JC, Weisenburger TH, eds. Philadelphia: WB Saunders, 1995:288.
88. Steiger Z, Wilson RF, Leichman L, et al. Primary adenocarcinoma of the esophagus. *J Surg Oncol* 1987;36:68.
89. Haggitt RC, Tryzelaar J, Ellis FH, et al. Adenocarcinoma complicating columnar epithelium-lined (Barrett's) esophagus. *Am J Clin Pathol* 1978;70:1.
90. Altorki NK, Skinner DB. Occult cervical nodal metastasis in esophageal cancer: preliminary results of three-field lymphadenectomy. *J Thorac Cardiovasc Surg* 1997;113:540.
91. Lerut T, De Leyn P, Coosemans W, et al. Surgical strategies in esophageal carcinoma with emphasis on radical lymphadenectomy. *Ann Surg* 1992;216:583.
92. Caldwell CB, Bains MS, Burt M. Unusual malignant neoplasms of the esophagus. Oat cell carcinoma, melanoma, and sarcoma. *J Thorac Cardiovasc Surg* 1991;101:100.
93. Osamura RY, Shimamura K, Hata J, et al. Polypoid carcinoma of the esophagus. A unifying term for "carcinosarcoma" and "pseudosarcoma." *Am J Surg Pathol* 1978;2:201.
94. Matsusaka T, Watanabe H, Enjoji M. Pseudosarcoma and carcinosarcoma of the esophagus. *Cancer* 1976;37:1546.
95. Sweeney EC, Cooney T. Adenoid cystic carcinoma of the esophagus: a light and electron microscopic study. *Cancer* 1980;45:1516.
96. Burt M. *Unusual malignancies. Esophageal surgery.* In: Pearson F, Deslauriers J, Ginsberg RJ, et al., eds. New York: Churchill Livingstone, 1995.
97. Reyes CV, Chejfec G, Jao W, et al. Neuroendocrine carcinomas of the esophagus. *Ultrastruct Pathol* 1980;1:367.
98. Tateishi R, Taniguchi H, Wada A, et al. Argyrophil cells and melanocytes in esophageal mucosa. *Arch Pathol* 1974;98:87.
99. Nagashima R, Mabe K, Takahashi T. Esophageal small cell carcinoma with ectopic production of parathyroid hormone-related protein (PTHrp), secretin, and granulocyte colony-stimulating factor (G-CSF). *Dig Dis Sci* 1999;44:1312.
100. Suzuki H, Takayanagi S, Otake T, et al. Primary small cell carcinoma of the esophagus with achalasia in a patient in whom pro-gastrin-releasing peptide and neuron-specific enolase levels reflected the clinical course during chemotherapy. *J Gastroenterol* 1999;34:378.
101. Medgyesy CD, Wolff RA, Putnam JB Jr, et al. Small cell carcinoma of the esophagus: the University of Texas MD Anderson Cancer Center experience and literature review. *Cancer* 2000;88:262.
102. Maier A, Woltsche M, Fell B, et al. Local and systemic treatment in small cell carcinoma of the esophagus. *Oncol Rep* 2000;7:187.
103. Kimura H, Konishi K, Maeda K, et al. Highly aggressive behavior and poor prognosis of small-cell carcinoma in the alimentary tract: flow-cytometric analysis and immunohistochemical staining for the p53 protein and proliferating cell nuclear antigen. *Dig Surg* 1999;16:152.
104. Adad SJ, Etchebehere RM, Hayashi EM, et al. Leiomyosarcoma of the esophagus in a patient with chagasic megaesophagus: case report and literature review. *Am J Trop Med Hyg* 1999;60:879.
105. Levine MS, Buck JL, Pantongrag-Brown L, et al. Leiomyosarcoma of the esophagus: radiographic findings in 10 patients. *AJR Am J Roentgenol* 1996;167:27.
106. Rocco G, Trastek VF, Deschamps C, et al. Leiomyosarcoma of the esophagus: results of surgical treatment. *Ann Thorac Surg* 1998;66:894.
107. Herrmann R, Panahon AM, Barcos MP, et al. Gastrointestinal involvement in non-Hodgkin's lymphoma. *Cancer* 1980;46:215.
108. Agha FP, Schnitzer B. Esophageal involvement in lymphoma. *Am J Gastroenterol* 1985;80:412.
109. Haller JO, Cohen HL. Gastrointestinal manifestations of AIDS in children. *AJR Am J Roentgenol* 1994;162:387.
110. Lim SG, Lipman MC, Squire S, et al. Audit of endoscopic surveillance biopsy specimens in HIV positive patients with gastrointestinal symptoms. *Gut* 1993;34:1429.
111. Chalkiadakis G, Wihlm JM, Morand G, et al. Primary malignant melanoma of the esophagus. *Ann Thorac Surg* 1985;39:472.
112. Hanahan D, Weinberg RA. The hallmarks of cancer. *Cell* 2000;100:57.
113. Souza RF. Molecular and biologic basis of upper gastrointestinal malignancy—esophageal carcinoma. *Surg Oncol Clin N Am* 2002;11:257.
114. Pardee AB. A restriction point for control of normal animal cell proliferation. *Proc Natl Acad Sci U S A* 1974;71:1286.
115. Weinberg RA. The retinoblastoma protein and cell cycle control. *Cell* 1995;81:323.
116. Arber N, Gammon MD, Hibshoosh H, et al. Overexpression of cyclin D1 occurs in both squamous carcinomas and adenocarcinomas of the esophagus and in adenocarcinomas of the stomach. *Hum Pathol* 1999;30:1087.
117. Sarbia M, Stahl M, Fink U, et al. Prognostic significance of cyclin D1 in esophageal squamous cell carcinoma patients treated with surgery alone or combined therapy modalities. *Int J Cancer* 1999;84:86.

118. Arber N, Lightdale C, Rotterdam H, et al. Increased expression of the cyclin D1 gene in Barrett's esophagus. *Cancer Epidemiol Biomarkers Prev* 1996;5:457.
119. Shamma A, Doki Y, Shiozaki H, et al. Cyclin D1 overexpression in esophageal dysplasia: a possible biomarker for carcinogenesis of esophageal squamous cell carcinoma. *Int J Oncol* 2000;16:261.
120. Roncalli M, Bosari S, Marchetti A, et al. Cell cycle-related gene abnormalities and product expression in esophageal carcinoma. *Lab Invest* 1998;78:1049.
121. Sarbia M, Bektas N, Muller W, et al. Expression of cyclin E in dysplasia, carcinoma, and nonmalignant lesions of Barrett esophagus. *Cancer* 1999;86:2597.
122. Matsumoto M, Furihata M, Ishikawa T, et al. Comparison of deregulated expression of cyclin D1 and cyclin E with that of cyclin-dependent kinase 4 (CDK4) and CDK2 in human oesophageal squamous cell carcinoma. *Br J Cancer* 1999;80:256.
123. Boynton RF, Huang Y, Blount PL, et al. Frequent loss of heterozygosity at the retinoblastoma locus in human esophageal cancers. *Cancer Res* 1991;51:5766.
124. Coppola D, Schreiber RH, Mora L, et al. Significance of Fas and retinoblastoma protein expression during the progression of Barrett's metaplasia to adenocarcinoma. *Ann Surg Oncol* 1999;6:298.
125. Ikeguchi M, Oka S, Gomyo Y, et al. Clinical significance of retinoblastoma protein (pRB) expression in esophageal squamous cell carcinoma. *J Surg Oncol* 2000;73:104.
126. Jankowski J, McMenemin R, Hopwood D, et al. Abnormal expression of growth regulatory factors in Barrett's oesophagus. *Clin Sci (Lond)* 1991;81:663.
127. Yoshida K, Kuniyasu H, Yasui W, et al. Expression of growth factors and their receptors in human esophageal carcinomas: regulation of expression by epidermal growth factor and transforming growth factor alpha. *J Cancer Res Clin Oncol* 1993;119:401.
128. Jankowski J, Hopwood D, Wormsley KG. Flow-cytometric analysis of growth-regulatory peptides and their receptors in Barrett's oesophagus and oesophageal adenocarcinoma. *Scand J Gastroenterol* 1992;27:147.
129. Brito MJ, Filipe MI, Linehan J, et al. Association of transforming growth factor alpha (TGFA) and its precursors with malignant change in Barrett's epithelium: biological and clinical variables. *Int J Cancer* 1995;60:27.
130. Yacoub L, Goldman H, Odze RD. Transforming growth factor-alpha, epidermal growth factor receptor, and MiB-1 expression in Barrett's-associated neoplasia: correlation with prognosis. *Mod Pathol* 1997;10:105.
131. Itakura Y, Sasano H, Shiga C, et al. Epidermal growth factor receptor overexpression in esophageal carcinoma. An immunohistochemical study correlated with clinicopathologic findings and DNA amplification. *Cancer* 1994;74:795.
132. Hickey K, Grehan D, Reid IM, et al. Expression of epidermal growth factor receptor and proliferating cell nuclear antigen predicts response of esophageal squamous cell carcinoma to chemoradiotherapy. *Cancer* 1994;74:1693.
133. Kitagawa Y, Ueda M, Ando N, et al. Further evidence for prognostic significance of epidermal growth factor receptor gene amplification in patients with esophageal squamous cell carcinoma. *Clin Cancer Res* 1996;2:909.
134. Shimada Y, Imamura M, Watanabe G, et al. Prognostic factors of oesophageal squamous cell carcinoma from the perspective of molecular biology. *Br J Cancer* 1999;80:1281.
135. Alroy I, Yarden Y. The ErbB signaling network in embryogenesis and oncogenesis: signal diversification through combinatorial ligand-receptor interactions. *FEBS Lett* 1997;410:83.
136. Jankowski J, Coghill G, Hopwood D, et al. Oncogenes and onco-suppressor gene in adenocarcinoma of the oesophagus. *Gut* 1992;33:1033.
137. Kim R, Clarke MR, Melhem MF, et al. Expression of p53, PCNA, and C-erbB-2 in Barrett's metaplasia and adenocarcinoma. *Dig Dis Sci* 1997;42:2453.
138. Flejou JF, Paraf F, Muzeau F, et al. Expression of c-erbB-2 oncogene product in Barrett's adenocarcinoma: pathological and prognostic correlations. *J Clin Pathol* 1994;47:23.
139. Shiga K, Shiga C, Sasano H, et al. Expression of c-erbB-2 in human esophageal carcinoma cells: overexpression correlated with gene amplification or with GATA-3 transcription factor expression. *Anticancer Res* 1993;13:1293.
140. Suwanagool P, Parichatikanond P, Maeda S. Expression of c-erbB-2 oncoprotein in primary human tumors: an immunohistochemistry study. *Asian Pac J Allergy Immunol* 1993;11:119.
141. Giaccia AJ, Kastan MB. The complexity of p53 modulation: emerging patterns from divergent signals. *Genes Dev* 1998;12:2973.
142. Hamelin R, Flejou JF, Muzeau F, et al. TP53 gene mutations and p53 protein immunoreactivity in malignant and premalignant Barrett's esophagus. *Gastroenterology* 1994;107:1012.
143. Ramel S, Reid BJ, Sanchez CA, et al. Evaluation of p53 protein expression in Barrett's esophagus by two-parameter flow cytometry. *Gastroenterology* 1992;102:1220.
144. Younes M, Lebovitz RM, Lechago LV, et al. p53 protein accumulation in Barrett's metaplasia, dysplasia, and carcinoma: a follow-up study. *Gastroenterology* 1993;105:1637.
145. Casson AG, Mukhopadhyay T, Cleary KR, et al. p53 gene mutations in Barrett's epithelium and esophageal cancer. *Cancer Res* 1991;51:4495.
146. Blount PL, Ramel S, Raskind WH, et al. 17p allelic deletions and p53 protein overexpression in Barrett's adenocarcinoma. *Cancer Res* 1991;51:5482.
147. Meltzer SJ, Yin J, Huang Y, et al. Reduction to homozygosity involving p53 in esophageal cancers demonstrated by the polymerase chain reaction. *Proc Natl Acad Sci U S A* 1991;88:4976.
148. Gaur D, Arora S, Mathur M, et al. High prevalence of p53 gene alterations and protein overexpression in human esophageal cancer: correlation with dietary risk factors in India. *Clin Cancer Res* 1997;3:2129.
149. Kato H, Yoshikawa M, Miyazaki T, et al. Expression of p53 protein related to smoking and alcoholic beverage drinking habits in patients with esophageal cancers. *Cancer Lett* 2001;167:65.
150. Lam KY, Tsao SW, Zhang D, et al. Prevalence and predictive value of p53 mutation in patients with oesophageal squamous cell carcinomas: a prospective clinico-pathological study and survival analysis of 70 patients. *Int J Cancer* 1997;74:212.
151. Taniere P, Martel-Planche G, Saurin JC, et al. TP53 mutations, amplification of P63 and expression of cell cycle proteins in squamous cell carcinoma of the oesophagus from a low incidence area in Western Europe. *Br J Cancer* 2001;85:721.
152. Ribeiro U Jr, Finkelstein SD, Safatle-Ribeiro AV, et al. p53 sequence analysis predicts treatment response and outcome of patients with esophageal carcinoma. *Cancer* 1998;83:7.
153. Malumbres M, Pellicer A. RAS pathways to cell cycle control and cell transformation. *Front Biosci* 1998;3:d887.
154. Barrett MT, Sanchez CA, Galipeau PC, et al. Allelic loss of 9p21 and mutation of the CDKN2/p16 gene develop as early lesions during neoplastic progression in Barrett's esophagus. *Oncogene* 1996;13:1867.
155. Wong DJ, Barrett MT, Stoger R, et al. p16INK4a promoter is hypermethylated at a high frequency in esophageal adenocarcinomas. *Cancer Res* 1997;57:2619.
156. Klump B, Hsieh CJ, Holzmann K, et al. Hypermethylation of the CDKN2/p16 promoter during neoplastic progression in Barrett's esophagus. *Gastroenterology* 1998;115:1381.
157. Zhou X, Tarmin L, Yin J, et al. The MTS1 gene is frequently mutated in primary human esophageal tumors. *Oncogene* 1994;9:3737.
158. Esteve A, Martel-Planche G, Sylla BS, et al. Low frequency of p16/CDKN2 gene mutations in esophageal carcinomas. *Int J Cancer* 1996;66:301.
159. Mori T, Miura K, Aoki T, et al. Frequent somatic mutation of the MTS1/CDK4I (multiple tumor suppressor/cyclin-dependent kinase 4 inhibitor) gene in esophageal squamous cell carcinoma. *Cancer Res* 1994;54:3396.
160. Takeuchi H, Ozawa S, Ando N, et al. Altered p16/MTS1/CDKN2 and cyclin D1/PRAD-1 gene expression is associated with the prognosis of squamous cell carcinoma of the esophagus. *Clin Cancer Res* 1997;3:2229.
161. Xing EP, Nie Y, Wang LD, et al. Aberrant methylation of p16INK4a and deletion of p15INK4b are frequent events in human esophageal cancer in Linxian, China. *Carcinogenesis* 1999;20:77.
162. Maesawa C, Tamura G, Nishizuka S, et al. Inactivation of the CDKN2 gene by homozygous deletion and de novo methylation is associated with advanced stage esophageal squamous cell carcinoma. *Cancer Res* 1996;56:3875.
163. Suzuki H, Zhou X, Yin J, et al. Intragenic mutations of CDKN2B and CDKN2A in primary human esophageal cancers. *Hum Mol Genet* 1995;4:1883.
164. Shirvani VN, Ouatu-Lascar R, Kaur BS, et al. Cyclooxygenase 2 expression in Barrett's esophagus and adenocarcinoma: ex vivo induction by bile salts and acid exposure. *Gastroenterology* 2000;118:487.
165. Wilson KT, Fu S, Ramanujam KS, et al. Increased expression of inducible nitric oxide synthase and cyclooxygenase-2 in Barrett's esophagus and associated adenocarcinomas. *Cancer Res* 1998;58:2929.
166. Zimmermann KC, Sarbia M, Weber AA, et al. Cyclooxygenase-2 expression in human esophageal carcinoma. *Cancer Res* 1999;59:198.
167. Shamma A, Yamamoto H, Doki Y, et al. Up-regulation of cyclooxygenase-2 in squamous carcinogenesis of the esophagus. *Clin Cancer Res* 2000;6:1229.
168. Suda T, Takahashi T, Golstein P, et al. Molecular cloning and expression of the Fas ligand, a novel member of the tumor necrosis factor family. *Cell* 1993;75:1169.
169. Strand S, Hofmann WJ, Hug H, et al. Lymphocyte apoptosis induced by CD95 (APO-1/Fas) ligand-expressing tumor cells—a mechanism of immune evasion? *Nat Med* 1996;2:1361.
170. Younes M, Schwartz MR, Ertan A, et al. Fas ligand expression in esophageal carcinomas and their lymph node metastases. *Cancer* 2000;88:524.
171. Hughes SJ, Nambu Y, Soldes OS, et al. Fas/APO-1 (CD95) is not translocated to the cell membrane in esophageal adenocarcinoma. *Cancer Res* 1997;57:5571.
172. Younes M, Lechago J, Ertan A, et al. Decreased expression of Fas (CD95/APO1) associated with goblet cell metaplasia in Barrett's esophagus. *Hum Pathol* 2000;31:434.
173. Shibakita M, Tachibana M, Dhar DK, et al. Prognostic significance of Fas and Fas ligand expressions in human esophageal cancer. *Clin Cancer Res* 1999;5:2464.
174. Gratas C, Tohma Y, Barnas C, et al. Up-regulation of Fas (APO-1/CD95) ligand and down-regulation of Fas expression in human esophageal cancer. *Cancer Res* 1998;58:2057.
175. Morales CP, Souza RF, Spechler SJ. Hallmarks of cancer progression in Barrett's oesophagus. *Lancet* 2002;360:1587.
176. Koyanagi K, Ozawa S, Ando N, et al. Clinical significance of telomerase activity in the non-cancerous epithelial region of oesophageal squamous cell carcinoma. *Br J Surg* 1999;86:674.
177. Morales CP, Lee EL, Shay JW. In situ hybridization for the detection of telomerase RNA in the progression from Barrett's esophagus to esophageal adenocarcinoma. *Cancer* 1998;83:652.
178. Lord RV, Salonga D, Danenberg KD, et al. Telomerase reverse transcriptase expression is increased early in the Barrett's metaplasia, dysplasia, adenocarcinoma sequence. *J Gastrointest Surg* 2000;4:135.
179. Couvelard A, Paraf F, Gratio V, et al. Angiogenesis in the neoplastic sequence of Barrett's oesophagus. Correlation with VEGF expression. *J Pathol* 2000;192:14.
180. Auvinen MI, Sihvo EI, Ruohtula T, et al. Incipient angiogenesis in Barrett's epithelium and lymphangiogenesis in Barrett's adenocarcinoma. *J Clin Oncol* 2002;20:2971.
181. Christofori G, Semb H. The role of the cell-adhesion molecule E-cadherin as a tumour-suppressor gene. *Trends Biochem Sci* 1999;24:73.
182. Swami S, Kumble S, Triadafilopoulos G. E-cadherin expression in gastroesophageal reflux disease, Barrett's esophagus, and esophageal adenocarcinoma: an immunohistochemical and immunoblot study. *Am J Gastroenterol* 1995;90:1808.
183. Daly JM, Karnell LH, Menck HR. National cancer database report on esophageal carcinoma. *Cancer* 1996;78:1820.
184. Mariette C, Balon JM, Piessen G, et al. Pattern of recurrence following complete resection of esophageal carcinoma and factors predictive of recurrent disease. *Cancer* 2003;97:1616.
185. Katayama A, Mafune K, Tanaka Y, et al. Autopsy findings in patients after curative esophagectomy for esophageal carcinoma. *J Am Coll Surg* 2003;196:866.
186. Kelsen DP, Ginsberg R, Pajak TF, et al. Chemotherapy followed by surgery compared with surgery alone for localized esophageal cancer. *N Engl J Med* 1998;339:1979.
187. Group MRCOCW. Surgical resection with or without preoperative chemotherapy in oesophageal cancer: a randomised controlled trial. *Lancet* 2002;359:1727.

188. Urba SG, Orringer MB, Turrisi A, et al. Randomized trial of preoperative chemoradiation versus surgery alone in patients with locoregional esophageal carcinoma. *J Clin Oncol* 2001;19:305.
189. O'Sullivan GC, Sheehan D, Clarke A, et al. Micrometastases in esophagogastric cancer: high detection rate in resected rib segments. *Gastroenterology* 1999;116:543.
190. Bonavina L, Soligo D, Quirici N, et al. Bone marrow-disseminated tumor cells in patients with carcinoma of the esophagus or cardia. *Surgery* 2001;129:15.
191. Arnott SJ, Duncan W, Gignoux M, et al. Preoperative radiotherapy in esophageal carcinoma: a meta-analysis using individual patient data (Oesophageal Cancer Collaborative Group). *Int J Radiat Oncol Biol Phys* 1998;41:579.
192. Kleinberg L, Knisely JP, Heitmiller R, et al. Mature survival results with preoperative cisplatin, protracted infusion 5-fluorouracil, and 44-Gy radiotherapy for esophageal cancer. *Int J Radiat Oncol Biol Phys* 2003;328.
193. Cooper JS, Guo MD, Herskovic A, et al. Chemoradiotherapy of locally advanced esophageal cancer. Long-term follow-up of a prospective randomized trial (RTOG 85-01). *JAMA* 1999;281:1623.
194. Denham JW, Steigler A, Kilmurray J, et al. Relapse patterns after chemo-radiation for carcinoma of the oesophagus. *Clin Oncol (R Coll Radiol)* 2003;15:98.
195. Cusso X, Mones-Xiol J, Vilardell F. Endoscopic cytology of cancer of the esophagus and cardia: a long-term evaluation. *Gastrointest Endosc* 1989;35:321.
196. Zargar SA, Khuroo MS, Jan GM, et al. Prospective comparison of the value of brushings before and after biopsy in the endoscopic diagnosis of gastroesophageal malignancy. *Acta Cytol* 1991;35:549.
197. Jung M, Kiesslich R. Chromoendoscopy and intravital staining techniques. *Baillieres Best Pract Res Clin Gastroenterol* 1999;13:11.
198. Acosta MM, Boyce HW Jr. Chromoendoscopy—where is it useful? *J Clin Gastroenterol* 1998;27:13.
199. Lea JW, Prager RL, Bender HW Jr. The questionable role of computed tomography in preoperative staging of esophageal cancer. *Ann Thorac Surg* 1984;38:479.
200. Quint LE, Glazer GM, Orringer MB. Esophageal imaging by MR and CT: study of normal anatomy and neoplasms. *Radiology* 1985;156:727.
201. Watt I, Stewart I, Anderson D, et al. Laparoscopy, ultrasound and computed tomography in cancer of the oesophagus and gastric cardia: a prospective comparison for detecting intra-abdominal metastases. *Br J Surg* 1989;76:1036.
202. Becker CD, Barbier P, Porcellini B. CT evaluation of patients undergoing transhiatal esophagectomy for cancer. *J Comput Assist Tomogr* 1986;10:607.
203. Vilgrain V, Mompoint D, Palazzo L, et al. Staging of esophageal carcinoma: comparison of results with endoscopic sonography and CT. *AJR Am J Roentgenol* 1990;155:277.
204. Picus D, Balfe DM, Koehler RE, et al. Computed tomography in the staging of esophageal carcinoma. *Radiology* 1983;146:433.
205. Yoon YC, Lee KS, Shim YM, et al. Metastasis to regional lymph nodes in patients with esophageal squamous cell carcinoma: CT versus FDG PET for presurgical detection prospective study. *Radiology* 2003;227:764.
206. Romagnuolo J, Scott J, Hawes RH, et al. Helical CT versus EUS with fine needle aspiration for celiac nodal assessment in patients with esophageal cancer. *Gastrointest Endosc* 2002;55:648.
207. Aibe T, Fuji T, Okita K, et al. A fundamental study of normal layer structure of the gastrointestinal wall visualized by endoscopic ultrasonography. *Scand J Gastroenterol Suppl* 1986;123:6.
208. Tio TL, den Hartog Jager FC, Tytgat GN. The role of endoscopic ultrasonography in assessing local resectability of oesophagogastric malignancies. Accuracy, pitfalls, and predictability. *Scand J Gastroenterol Suppl* 1986;123:78.
209. Aibe T, Ito T, Yoshida T, et al. Endoscopic ultrasonography of lymph nodes surrounding the upper GI tract. *Scand J Gastroenterol Suppl* 1986;123:164.
210. Catalano MF, Sivak MV Jr, Rice T, et al. Endosonographic features predictive of lymph node metastasis. *Gastrointest Endosc* 1994;40:442.
211. Botet JF, Lightdale CJ, Zauber AG, et al. Preoperative staging of gastric cancer: comparison of endoscopic US and dynamic CT. *Radiology* 1991;181:426.
212. Tio TL, Cohen P, Coene PP, et al. Endosonography and computed tomography of esophageal carcinoma. Preoperative classification compared to the new (1987) TNM system. *Gastroenterology* 1989;96:1478.
213. Rosch T, Endosonographic staging of esophageal cancer: a review of literature results. *Gastrointest Endosc Clin N Am* 1995;5:537.
214. Vazquez-Sequeiros E, Norton ID, Clain JE, et al. Impact of EUS-guided fine-needle aspiration on lymph node staging in patients with esophageal carcinoma. *Gastrointest Endosc* 2001;53:751.
215. O'Toole D, Palazzo L, Arotcarena R, et al. Assessment of complications of EUS-guided fine-needle aspiration. *Gastrointest Endosc* 2001;53:470.
216. Chak A, Canto M, Gerdes H, et al. Prognosis of esophageal cancers preoperatively staged to be locally invasive (T4) by endoscopic ultrasound (EUS): a multicenter retrospective cohort study. *Gastrointest Endosc* 1995;42:501.
217. Fockens P, Kisman K, Merkus MP, et al. The prognosis of esophageal carcinoma staged irresectable (T4) by endosonography. *J Am Coll Surg* 1998;186:17.
218. Souquet JC, Napoleon B, Pujol B, et al. Endoscopic ultrasonography in the preoperative staging of esophageal cancer. *Endoscopy* 1994;26:764.
219. Yoshikane H, Tsukamoto Y, Niwa Y, et al. Superficial esophageal carcinoma: evaluation by endoscopic ultrasonography. *Am J Gastroenterol* 1994;89:702.
220. McLoughlin RF, Cooperberg PL, Mathieson JR, et al. High resolution endoluminal ultrasonography in the staging of esophageal carcinoma. *J Ultrasound Med* 1995;14:725.
221. Wu LF, Wang BZ, Feng JL, et al. Preoperative TN staging of esophageal cancer: comparison of miniprobe ultrasonography, spiral CT and MRI. *World J Gastroenterol* 2003;9:219.
222. Mallery S, Van Dam J. Increased rate of complete EUS staging of patients with esophageal cancer using the nonoptical, wire-guided echoendoscope. *Gastrointest Endosc* 1999;50:53.
223. Willis J, Cooper GS, Isenberg G, et al. Correlation of EUS measurement with pathologic assessment of neoadjuvant therapy response in esophageal carcinoma. *Gastrointest Endosc* 2002;55:655.
224. Saltzman JR. Section III: endoscopic and other staging techniques. *Semin Thorac Cardiovasc Surg* 2003;15:180.
225. Flamen P, van Cutsem E, Lerut T, et al. The utility of positron emission tomography with 18F-fluorodeoxyglucose (FDG-PET) to predict the pathologic response and survival of esophageal cancer after preoperative chemoradiation therapy (CRT). *Proc ASCO* 2001;20:127a.
226. Luketich JD, Schauer PR, Meltzer CC, et al. Role of positron emission tomography in staging esophageal cancer. *Ann Thorac Surg* 1997;64:765.
227. Kole AC, Plukker JT, Nieweg OE, et al. Positron emission tomography for staging of oesophageal and gastroesophageal malignancy. *Br J Cancer* 1998;78:521.
228. Weber WA, Ott K, Becker K, et al. Prediction of response to preoperative chemotherapy in adenocarcinomas of the esophagogastric junction by metabolic imaging. *J Clin Oncol* 2001;19:3058.
229. Brücher BL, Weber W, Bauer M, et al. Neoadjuvant therapy of esophageal squamous cell carcinoma: response evaluation by positron emission tomography. *Ann Surg* 2001;233:300.
230. Downey RJ, Akhurst T, Ilson D, et al. Whole body 18FDG-PET and the response of esophageal cancer to induction therapy: results of a prospective trial. *J Clin Oncol* 2003;21:428.
231. Dagnini G, Caldironi MW, Marin G, et al. Laparoscopy in abdominal staging of esophageal carcinoma. Report of 369 cases. *Gastrointest Endosc* 1986;32:400.
232. Mortensen MB, Scheel-Hincke JD, Madsen MR, et al. Combined endoscopic ultrasonography and laparoscopic ultrasonography in the pretherapeutic assessment of resectability in patients with upper gastrointestinal malignancies. *Scand J Gastroenterol* 1996;31:1115.
233. Luketich JD, Meehan M, Nguyen NT, et al. Minimally invasive surgical staging for esophageal cancer. *Surg Endosc* 2000;4:700.
234. Meltzer CC, Luketich JD, Friedman D, et al. Whole-body FDG positron emission tomographic imaging for staging esophageal cancer comparison with computed tomography. *Clin Nucl Med* 2000;25:882.
235. Krasna MJ, Jiao X, Mao YS, et al. Thoracoscopy/laparoscopy in the staging of esophageal cancer: Maryland experience. *Surg Laparosc Endosc Percutan Tech* 2002;12:213.
236. Wallace MB, Nietert PJ, Earle C, et al. An analysis of multiple staging management strategies for carcinoma of the esophagus: computed tomography, endoscopic ultrasound, positron emission tomography, and thoracoscopy/laparoscopy. *Ann Thorac Surg* 2002;74:1026.
237. Dutkowski P, Hommel G, Bottger T, et al. How many lymph nodes are needed for an accurate pN classification in esophageal cancer? Evidence for a new threshold value. *Hepatogastroenterology* 2002;49:176.
238. Heitmiller RF, Redmond M, Hamilton SR. Barrett's esophagus with high-grade dysplasia. An indication for prophylactic esophagectomy. *Ann Surg* 1996;224:66.
239. Falk GW, Rice TW, Goldblum JR, et al. Jumbo biopsy forceps protocol still misses unsuspected cancer in Barrett's esophagus with high-grade dysplasia. *Gastrointest Endosc* 1999;49:170.
240. Nigro JJ, Hagen JA, DeMeester TR, et al. Occult esophageal adenocarcinoma: extent of disease and implications for effective therapy. *Ann Surg* 1999;230:433.
241. Pacifico RJ, Wang KK. Nonsurgical management of Barrett's esophagus with high-grade dysplasia. *Surg Oncol Clin N Am* 2002;11:321.
242. Schnell TG, Sontag SJ, Chejfec G, et al. Long-term nonsurgical management of Barrett's esophagus with high-grade dysplasia. *Gastroenterology* 2001;120:1607.
243. Romagnoli R, Collard JM, Gutschow C, et al. Outcomes of dysplasia arising in Barrett's esophagus: a dynamic view. *J Am Coll Surg* 2003;197:365.
244. Levine DS, Haggitt RC, Blount PL, et al. An endoscopic biopsy protocol can differentiate high-grade dysplasia from early adenocarcinoma in Barrett's esophagus. *Gastroenterology* 1993;105:40.
245. Cameron AJ. Barrett's esophagus: does the incidence of adenocarcinoma matter? *Am J Gastroenterol* 1997;92:193.
246. Dar MS, Goldblum JR, Rice TW, et al. Can extent of high grade dysplasia in Barrett's oesophagus predict the presence of adenocarcinoma at oesophagectomy? *Gut* 2003;52:486.
247. Overholt BF, Panjehpour M, Halberg DL. Photodynamic therapy for Barrett's esophagus with dysplasia and/or early stage carcinoma: long-term results. *Gastrointest Endosc* 2003;58:183.
248. Overholt B HR, Branner MP, et al. A multicenter, partially blinded, randomized study of the efficacy of photodynamic therapy (PDT) using portimer sodium (POR) for the ablation of high grade dysplasia (HGD) in Barrett's esophagus (BE): results of 6-month follow-up. *Gastroenterology* 2001;120:[Suppl 1]:A-79.
249. Gossner L, May A, Stolte M, et al. KTP laser destruction of dysplasia and early cancer in columnar-lined Barrett's esophagus. *Gastrointest Endosc* 1999;49:8.
250. Sharma P, Jaffe PE, Bhattacharyya A, et al. Laser and multipolar electrocoagulation ablation of early Barrett's adenocarcinoma: long-term follow-up. *Gastrointest Endosc* 1999;49:442.
251. Morris CD, Byrne JP, Armstrong GR, et al. Prevention of the neoplastic progression of Barrett's oesophagus by endoscopic argon beam plasma ablation. *Br J Surg* 2001;88:1357.
252. Van Laethem JL, Jagodzinski R, Peny MO, et al. Argon plasma coagulation in the treatment of Barrett's high-grade dysplasia and in situ adenocarcinoma. *Endoscopy* 2001;33:257.
253. Dye C, Waxman I. Interventional endoscopy in the diagnosis and staging of upper gastrointestinal malignancy. *Surg Oncol Clin N Am* 2002;11:305.
254. Ell C, May A, Gossner L, et al. Endoscopic mucosal resection of early cancer and high-grade dysplasia in Barrett's esophagus. *Gastroenterology* 2000;118:670.
255. Nijhawan PK, Wang KK. Endoscopic mucosal resection for lesions with endoscopic features suggestive of malignancy and high-grade dysplasia within Barrett's esophagus. *Gastrointest Endosc* 2000;52:328.
256. Yoshida M, Hanashi T, Momma K, et al. Endoscopic mucosal resection for radical treatment of esophageal cancer. *Gan To Kagaku Ryoho* 1995;22:847.
257. Swanstrom LL, Hansen P. Laparoscopic total esophagectomy. *Arch Surg* 1997;132:943.
258. Luketich JD, Schauer PR, Christie NA, et al. Minimally invasive esophagectomy. *Ann Thorac Surg* 2000;70:906.

259. Posner MC, Alverdy J. Hand-assisted laparoscopic surgery for cancer. *Cancer J* 2002;8:144.

260. Osugi H, Takemura M, Higashino M, et al. Video-assisted thoracoscopic esophagectomy and radical lymph node dissection for esophageal cancer. A series of 75 cases. *Surg Endosc* 2002;16:1588.

261. Law S, Wong J. Use of minimally invasive oesophagectomy for cancer of the oesophagus. *Lancet Oncol* 2002;3:215.

262. Wu PC, Posner MC. The role of surgery in the management of oesophageal cancer. *Lancet Oncol* 2003;4:481.

263. Swisher SG, Deford L, Merriman KW, et al. Effect of operative volume on morbidity, mortality, and hospital use after esophagectomy for cancer. *J Thorac Cardiovasc Surg* 2000;119:1126.

264. Begg CB, Cramer LD, Hoskins WJ, et al. Impact of hospital volume on operative mortality for major cancer surgery. *JAMA* 1998;280:1747.

265. Birkmeyer JD, Siewers AE, Finlayson EV, et al. Hospital volume and surgical mortality in the United States. *N Engl J Med* 2002;346:1128.

266. Dimick JB, Pronovost PJ, Cowan JA, et al. Surgical volume and quality of care for esophageal resection: do high-volume hospitals have fewer complications? *Ann Thorac Surg* 2003;75:337.

267. Halm EA, Lee C, Chassin MR. Is volume related to outcome in health care? A systematic review and methodologic critique of the literature. *Ann Intern Med* 2002;137:511.

268. Posner MC. Techniques of esophageal resection, in cancer of the upper gastrointestinal tract. In: Posner MC, Vokes EE, Weichselbaum RR, eds. Hamilton, Ontario, Canada: BC Decker, 2002:1.

269. Park JO, Posner MC. Standard surgical approaches in the management of esophageal cancer. *Surg Oncol Clin N Am* 2002;11:351.

270. Fok M, Cheng SW, Wong J. Pyloroplasty versus no drainage in gastric replacement of the esophagus. *Am J Surg* 1991;162:447.

271. Urschel JD, Blewett CJ, Young JE, et al. Pyloric drainage (pyloroplasty) or no drainage in gastric reconstruction after esophagectomy: a meta-analysis of randomized controlled trials. *Dig Surg* 2002;19:160.

272. Bumm R, Feussner H, Bartels H, et al. Radical transhiatal esophagectomy with two-field lymphadenectomy and endodissection for distal esophageal adenocarcinoma. *World J Surg* 1997;21:822.

273. Orringer MB, Marshall B, Iannettoni MD. Transhiatal esophagectomy: clinical experience and refinements. *Ann Surg* 1999;230:392.

274. Gelfand GA, Finley RJ, Nelems B, et al. Transhiatal esophagectomy for carcinoma of the esophagus and cardia. Experience with 160 cases. *Arch Surg* 1992;127:1164.

275. Vigneswaran WT, Trastek VF, Pairolero PC, et al. Transhiatal esophagectomy for carcinoma of the esophagus. *Ann Thorac Surg* 1993;56:838.

276. Gertsch P, Vauthey JN, Lustenberger AA, et al. Long-term results of transhiatal esophagectomy for esophageal carcinoma. A multivariate analysis of prognostic factors. *Cancer* 1993;72:2312.

277. Bolton JS, Teng S. Transthoracic or transhiatal esophagectomy for cancer of the esophagus—does it matter? *Surg Oncol Clin N Am* 2002;11:365.

278. Dudhat SB, Shinde SR. Transhiatal esophagectomy for squamous cell carcinoma of the esophagus. *Dis Esophagus* 1998;11:226.

279. McKeown KC. Total three-stage oesophagectomy for cancer of the oesophagus. *Br J Surg* 1976;63:259.

280. Linden PA, Sugarbaker DJ. Section V: techniques of esophageal resection. *Semin Thorac Cardiovasc Surg* 2003;15:197.

281. Sharpe DA, Moghissi K. Resectional surgery in carcinoma of the oesophagus and cardia: what influences long-term survival? *Eur J Cardiothorac Surg* 1996;10:359.

282. Ellis FH Jr. Standard resection for cancer of the esophagus and cardia. *Surg Oncol Clin N Am* 1999;8:279.

283. Adam DJ, Craig SR, Sang CT, et al. Oesophagogastrectomy for carcinoma in patients under 50 years of age. *J R Coll Surg Edinb* 1996;41:371.

284. Wang LS, Huang MH, Huang BS, et al. Gastric substitution for resectable carcinoma of the esophagus: an analysis of 368 cases. *Ann Thorac Surg* 1992;53:289.

285. Lieberman MD, Shriver CD, Bleckner S, et al. Carcinoma of the esophagus. Prognostic significance of histologic type. *J Thorac Cardiovasc Surg* 1995;109:130.

286. Bosset JF, Gignoux M, Triboulet JP, et al. Chemoradiotherapy followed by surgery compared with surgery alone in squamous cell cancer of the esophagus. *N Engl J Med* 1997;337:161.

287. Rindani R, Martin CJ, Cox MR. Transhiatal versus Ivor-Lewis oesophagectomy: is there a difference? *Aust N Z J Surg* 1999;69:187.

288. Hulscher JB, Tijssen JG, Obertop H, et al. Transthoracic versus transhiatal resection for carcinoma of the esophagus: a meta-analysis. *Ann Thorac Surg* 2001;72:306.

289. Rentz J, Bull D, Harpole D, et al. Transthoracic versus transhiatal esophagectomy: a prospective study of 945 patients. *J Thorac Cardiovasc Surg* 2003;125:1114.

290. Goldminc M, Maddern G, Le Prise E, et al. Oesophagectomy by a transhiatal approach or thoracotomy: a prospective randomized trial. *Br J Surg* 1993;80:367.

291. Jacobi CA, Zieren HU, Muller JM, et al. Surgical therapy of esophageal carcinoma: the influence of surgical approach and esophageal resection on cardiopulmonary function. *Eur J Cardiothorac Surg* 1997;11:32.

292. Chu KM, Law SY, Fok M, et al. A prospective randomized comparison of transhiatal and transthoracic resection for lower-third esophageal carcinoma. *Am J Surg* 1997;174:320.

293. Hulscher JB, van Sandick JW, de Boer AG, et al. Extended transthoracic resection compared with limited transhiatal resection for adenocarcinoma of the esophagus. *N Engl J Med* 2002;347:1662.

294. Skinner DB. En bloc resection for neoplasms of the esophagus and cardia. *J Thorac Cardiovasc Surg* 1983;85:59.

295. Nishihira T, Hirayama K, Mori S. A prospective randomized trial of extended cervical and superior mediastinal lymphadenectomy for carcinoma of the thoracic esophagus. *Am J Surg* 1998;175:47.

296. Coonley CJ, Bains M, Hilaris B, et al. Cisplatin and bleomycin in the treatment of esophageal carcinoma. A final report. *Cancer* 1984;54:2351.

297. Kelsen D, Hilaris B, Coonley C, et al. Cisplatin, vindesine, and bleomycin chemotherapy of local-regional and advanced esophageal carcinoma. *Am J Med* 1983;75:645.

298. Schlag P, Herrmann R, Raeth V, et al. Preoperative chemotherapy in esophageal cancer. A phase II study. *Acta Oncol* 1988;27:811.

299. Forastiere AA, Gennis M, Orringer MB, et al. Cisplatin, vinblastine, and mitoguazone chemotherapy for epidermoid and adenocarcinoma of the esophagus. *J Clin Oncol* 1987;5:1143.

300. Carey RW, Hilgenberg AD, Wilkins EW Jr, et al. Long-term follow-up of neoadjuvant chemotherapy with 5-fluorouracil and cisplatin with surgical resection and possible postoperative radiotherapy and/or chemotherapy in squamous cell carcinoma of the esophagus. *Cancer Invest* 1993;11:99.

301. Kies MS, Rosen ST, Tsang TK, et al. Cisplatin and 5-fluorouracil in the primary management of squamous esophageal cancer. *Cancer* 1987;60:2156.

302. Ajani JA, Ryan B, Rich TA, et al. Prolonged chemotherapy for localized squamous carcinoma of the oesophagus. *Eur J Cancer* 1992;28A:880.

303. Vignoud J, Visset J, Paineau J, et al. Preoperative chemotherapy in squamous cell carcinoma of the esophagus: clinical and pathological analysis, 48 cases. *Ann Oncol* 1990;1:45.

304. Wright CD, Mathisen DJ, Wain JC, et al. Evolution of treatment strategies for adenocarcinoma of the esophagus and gastroesophageal junction. *Ann Thorac Surg* 1994;58:1574.

305. Nygaard K, Hagen S, Hansen HS, et al. Pre-operative radiotherapy prolongs survival in operable esophageal carcinoma: a randomized, multicenter study of pre-operative radiotherapy and chemotherapy. The second Scandinavian trial in esophageal cancer. *World J Surg* 1992;16:1104.

306. Kok TC, Lanschot JV, Siersema PD, et al. Neoadjuvant chemotherapy in operable esophageal squamous cell cancer: final report of a phase III multicenter randomized trial. *Proc ASCO* 1997;16:277.

307. Roth JA, Pass HI, Flanagan MM, et al. Randomized clinical trial of preoperative and postoperative adjuvant chemotherapy with cisplatin, vindesine, and bleomycin for carcinoma of the esophagus. *J Thorac Cardiovasc Surg* 1988;96:242.

308. Schlag PM. Randomized trial of preoperative chemotherapy for squamous cell cancer of the esophagus. The Chirurgische Arbeitsgemeinschaft Fuer Onkologie der Deutschen Gesellschaft Fuer Chirurgie Study Group. *Arch Surg* 1992;127:1446.

309. Mei W, Xian-Zhi G, Weibo Y, et al. Randomized clinical trial on the combination of preoperative irradiation and surgery in the treatment of esophageal carcinoma: report on 206 patients. *Int J Radiat Oncol Biol Phys* 1989;16:325.

310. Gignoux M, Roussel A, Paillot B, et al. The value of preoperative radiotherapy in esophageal cancer: results of a study of the E.O.R.T.C. *World J Surg* 1987;11:426.

311. Teniere P, Hay J-M, Fingerhut A, et al. Postoperative radiation therapy does not increase survival after curative resection for squamous cell carcinoma of the middle and lower esophagus as shown by a multicenter controlled trial. *Surg Gynecol Obstet* 1991;173:123.

312. Launois B, Delarue D, Campion JP, et al. Preoperative radiotherapy for carcinoma of the esophagus. *Surg Gynecol Obstet* 1981;153:690.

313. Arnott SJ, Duncan W, Kerr GR, et al. Low dose preoperative radiotherapy for carcinoma of the oesophagus: results of a randomized clinical trial. *Radiother Oncol* 1993;24:108.

314. Huang GJ, Gu XZ, Wang LJ, et al. Combined preoperative irradiation and surgery for esophageal carcinoma. In: Delarue NC, ed. *International trends in general thoracic surgery.* St. Louis: CV Mosby, 1988:315.

315. Jacob JH, Seitz JF, Langlois C, et al. Definitive concurrent chemo-radiation therapy (CRT) in squamous cell carcinoma of the esophagus (SCCE): preliminary results of a French randomized trial comparing standard vs. split course irradiation (FNCLCC-FFCD 9305). *Proc ASCO* 1999;18:270a.

316. Yadava OP, Hodge AJ, Matz LR, et al. Esophageal malignancies: is preoperative radiotherapy the way to go? *Ann Thorac Surg* 1991;51:189.

317. Sugimachi K, Matsufuji H, Kai H, et al. Preoperative irradiation for carcinoma of the esophagus. *Surg Gynecol Obstet* 1986;162:174.

318. Herskovic A, Martz K, Al-Sarraf M, et al. Combined chemotherapy and radiotherapy compared with radiotherapy alone in patients with cancer of the esophagus. *N Engl J Med* 1992;326:1593.

319. Minsky B, Pajak T, Ginsberg R, et al. INT 0123 (Radiation Therapy Oncology Group 94-05) phase III trial of combined-modality therapy for esophageal cancer: high-dose versus standard-dose radiation therapy. *J Clin Oncol* 2002;20:1167.

320. Poplin E, Fleming T, Leichman L, et al. Combined therapies for squamous-cell carcinoma of the esophagus, a Southwest Oncology Group Study (SWOG-8037). *J Clin Oncol* 1987;5:622.

321. Naunheim KS, Petruska P, Roy TS, et al. Preoperative chemotherapy and radiotherapy for esophageal carcinoma. *J Thorac Cardiovasc Surg* 1992;103:887.

322. Forastiere A, Orringer MB, Perez-Tamayo C, et al. Preoperative chemoradiation followed by transhiatal esophagectomy for carcinoma of the esophagus: final report. *J Clin Oncol* 1993;11:1118.

323. Forastiere A, Orringer MB, Perez-Tamayo C, et al. Concurrent chemotherapy and radiation therapy followed by transhiatal esophagectomy for local-regional cancer of the esophagus. *J Clin Oncol* 1990;8:119.

324. Hoff SJ, Stewart JL, Murray MJ, et al. Preliminary results with neoadjuvant therapy and resection for esophageal carcinoma. *Ann Thorac Surg* 1993;56:282.

325. Bates BA, Detterbeck FC, Bernard SA, et al. Concurrent radiation therapy and chemotherapy followed by esophagectomy for localized esophageal carcinoma. *J Clin Oncol* 1996;14:156.

326. Malhaire JP, Labat JP, Lozach P, et al. Preoperative concomitant radiochemotherapy in squamous cell carcinoma of the esophagus: results of a study of 56 patients. *Int J Radiat Oncol Biol Phys* 1996;34:429.

327. Stahl M, Wilke H, Fink U, et al. Combined preoperative chemotherapy and radiotherapy in patients with locally advanced esophageal cancer: interim analysis of a phase II trial. *J Clin Oncol* 1996;14:829.

328. Forastiere AA, Heitmiller RF, Lee DJ, et al. Intensive chemoradiation followed by esophagectomy for squamous cell and adenocarcinoma of the esophagus. *Cancer J Sci Am* 1997;3:144.

329. Jones DR, Detterbeck FC, Egan TM, et al. Induction chemoradiotherapy followed by esophagectomy in patients with carcinoma of the esophagus. *Ann Thorac Surg* 1997;64:185.

330. Adelstein DJ, Rice TW, Becker M, et al. Use of concurrent chemotherapy, accelerated fractionation radiation, and surgery for patients with esophageal cancer. *Cancer* 1997;80:1011.

331. Posner MC, Gooding WE, Landreneau RJ, et al. Preoperative chemoradiotherapy for carcinoma of the esophagus and gastroesophageal junction. *Cancer J Sci Am* 1998;4:237.

332. Posner MC, Gooding WE, Lew JI, et al. Complete 5-year follow-up of a prospective phase II trial of preoperative chemoradiotherapy for esophageal cancer. *Surgery* 2001;130:620.

333. Raoul JL, Le Prise E, Meunier B, et al. Neoadjuvant chemotherapy and hyperfractionated radiotherapy with concurrent low-dose chemotherapy for squamous cell esophageal carcinoma. *Int J Radiat Oncol Biol Phys* 1998;42:29.

334. Keller SM, Ryan L, Coia LR, et al. High dose chemoradiotherapy followed by esophagectomy for adenocarcinoma of the esophagus and gastroesophageal junction. Results of a phase II study of the Eastern Cooperative Oncology Group. *Cancer* 1998;83:1908.

335. Bedenne L, Seitz JF, Milan C, et al. Cisplatin, 5-FU and preoperative radiotherapy in esophageal epidermoid cancer. Multicenter phase II FFCD 8804 study. *Gastroenterol Clin Biol* 1998;22:273.

336. Laterza E, de'Manzoni G, Tedesco P, et al. Induction chemo-radiotherapy for squamous cell carcinoma of the thoracic esophagus: long-term results of a phase II study. *Ann Surg Oncol* 1999;6:777.

337. Heath EI, Burtness BA, Heitmiller RF, et al. Phase II evaluation of preoperative chemoradiation and postoperative adjuvant chemotherapy for squamous cell and adenocarcinoma of the esophagus. *J Clin Oncol* 2000;18:868.

338. Khushalani KI, Leichman CG, Proulx G, et al. Oxaliplatin in combination with protracted-infusion fluorouracil and radiation: report of a clinical trial for patients with esophageal cancer. *J Clin Oncol* 2002;20:2844.

339. Safran H, Gaissert H, Akerman P, et al. Paclitaxel, cisplatin, and concurrent radiation for esophageal cancer. *Cancer Invest* 2001;19:1.

340. Adelstein DJ, Rice TW, Rybicki LA, et al. Does paclitaxel improve the chemoradiotherapy of locoregionally advanced esophageal cancer? A nonrandomized comparison with fluorouracil-based therapy. *J Clin Oncol* 2000;18:2032.

341. Wright CD, Wain JC, Lynch TJ, et al. Induction therapy for esophageal cancer with paclitaxel and hyperfractionated radiotherapy: a phase I and II study. *J Thorac Cardiovasc Surg* 1997;114:811.

342. Meluch AA, Greco FA, Gray JR, et al. Preoperative therapy with concurrent paclitaxel/carboplatin/infusional 5-FU and radiation therapy in locoregional esophageal cancer: final results of a Minnie Pearl Cancer Research Network phase II trial. *Cancer J* 2003;9:251.

343. Bains MS, Stojadinovic A, Minsky B, et al. A phase II trial of preoperative combined-modality therapy for localized esophageal carcinoma: initial results. *J Thorac Cardiovasc Surg* 2002;124:270.

344. Swisher SG, Ajani JA, Komaki R, et al. Long term outcome of a phase II trial evaluating chemotherapy, chemoradiotherapy, and surgery for locoregionally advanced esophageal cancer. *Int J Radiat Oncol Biol Phys* 2003;57:120.

345. Ajani JA, Faust J, Yao J, et al. Irinotecan/cisplatin followed by 5-FU/paclitaxel/radiotherapy and surgery in esophageal cancer. *Oncology (Huntingt)* 2003;17:[Suppl 8]:20.

346. Ilson DH, Bains M, Kelsen DP, et al. Phase I trial of escalating-dose irinotecan given weekly with cisplatin and concurrent radiotherapy in locally advanced esophageal cancer. *J Clin Oncol* 2003;21:2926.

347. Leichman L, Steiger Z, Seydel HG, et al. Preoperative chemotherapy and radiation therapy for patients with cancer of the esophagus: a potentially curative approach. *J Clin Oncol* 1984;2:75.

348. Geh JI, Crellin AM, Glynne-Jones R. Preoperative (neoadjuvant) chemoradiotherapy in oesophageal cancer. *Br J Surg* 2001;88:338.

349. Jones DR, Parker LA, Detterbeck FC, et al. Inadequacy of computed tomography in assessing patients with esophageal carcinoma after induction chemoradiotherapy. *Cancer* 1999;85:1026.

350. Zuccaro G Jr, Rice TW, Goldblum J, et al. Endoscopic ultrasound cannot determine suitability for esophagectomy after aggressive chemoradiotherapy for esophageal cancer. *Am J Gastroenterol* 1999;94:906.

351. Laterza E, de Manzoni G, Guglielmi A, et al. Endoscopic ultrasonography in the staging of esophageal carcinoma after preoperative radiotherapy and chemotherapy. *Ann Thorac Surg* 1999;67:1466.

352. Beseth BD, Bedford R, Isacoff WH, et al. Endoscopic ultrasound does not accurately assess pathologic stage of esophageal cancer after neoadjuvant chemoradiotherapy. *Am Surg* 2000;66:827.

353. Flamen P, Van Cutsem E, Lerut A, et al. Positron emission tomography for assessment of the response to induction radiochemotherapy in locally advanced oesophageal cancer. *Ann Oncol* 2002;13:361.

354. Jiao X, Sonett J, Gamliel Z, et al. Trimodality treatment versus surgery alone for esophageal cancer. A stratified analysis with minimally invasive pretreatment staging. *J Cardiovasc Surg (Torino)* 2002;43:531.

355. Walsh TN, Noonan N, Hollywood D, et al. A comparison of multimodal therapy and surgery for esophageal adenocarcinoma. *N Engl J Med* 1996;335:462.

356. Walsh TN, Grennell M, Mansoor S, et al. Neoadjuvant treatment of advanced stage esophageal adenocarcinoma increases survival. *Dis Esophagus* 2002;15:121.

357. Le Prise E, Etienne PL, Meunier B, et al. A randomized study of chemotherapy, radiation therapy, and surgery versus surgery for localized squamous cell carcinoma of the esophagus. *Cancer* 1994;73:1779.

358. Group J. A comparison of chemotherapy and radiotherapy as adjuvant treatment to surgery for esophageal carcinoma. *Chest* 1993;104:203.

359. Iizuka AT, Isono KK, Watanabe H, et al. A randomized trial comparing surgery to surgery plus postoperative chemotherapy for localized squamous carcinoma of the thoracic esophagus: the Japan Clinical Oncology Study Group (JCOG) study. *Proc Am Soc Clin Oncol* 1998;17:282a.

360. Ando N, Iizuka T, Kakegawa T, et al. A randomized trial of surgery with and without chemotherapy for localized squamous carcinoma of the thoracic esophagus: the Japan Clinical Oncology Group Study. *J Thorac Cardiovasc Surg* 1997;114:205.

361. Iizuka T, Surgical adjuvant treatment of esophageal carcinoma: a Japanese Esophageal Oncology Group Experience. *Semin Oncol* 1994;21:462.

362. Armanios MY, Xu R, Forastiere A, et al. Phase II adjuvant chemotherapy for resected adenocarcinoma of the esophagus, gastro-esophageal (GE) junction and cardia (8296): a trial of the Eastern Cooperative Oncology Group. *Proc Am Soc Clin Oncol* 2003;22:296(abst).

363. Yamamoto M, Yamashita T, Matsubara T, et al. Reevaluation of postoperative radiotherapy for thoracic esophageal carcinoma. *Int J Radiat Oncol Biol Phys* 1997;37:75.

364. Hosokawa M, Shirato H, Ohara K, et al. Intraoperative radiation therapy to the upper mediastinum and nerve-sparing three-field lymphadenectomy followed by external beam radiotherapy for patients with thoracic esophageal carcinoma. *Cancer* 1999;86:6.

365. Fok M, Sham JST, Choy D, et al. Postoperative radiotherapy for carcinoma of the esophagus: a prospective, randomized controlled trial. *Surgery* 1993;113:138.

366. MacDonald JS, Smalley SR, Benedetti J, et al. Chemoradiotherapy after surgery compared with surgery alone for adenocarcinoma of the stomach or gastroesophageal junction. *N Engl J Med* 2001;345:725.

367. Al-Sarraf M, Martz K, Herskovic A, et al. Superiority of chemo-radiotherapy (CT-RT) vs radiotherapy (RT) in patients with esophageal cancer. Final report of an Intergroup randomized and confirmed study. *Proc ASCO* 1996;15:206.

368. Coia LR, Minsky BD, Berkey BA, et al. Outcome of patients receiving radiation for cancer of the esophagus: results of the 1992–1994 patterns of care study. *J Clin Oncol* 2000;18:455.

369. Suntharalingam M, Moughhan J, Coia LR, et al. The national practice for patients receiving radiation therapy for carcinoma of the esophagus: results of the 1996–1999 Patterns of Care Study. *Int J Radiat Oncol Biol Phys* 2003;56:981.

370. Gomi K, Oguchi M, Hirokawa Y, et al. Process and preliminary outcome of a patterns of care study of esophageal cancer in Japan: patients treated with surgery and radiotherapy. *Int J Radiat Oncol Biol Phys* 2003;56:813.

371. Coia LR, Minsky BD, John MJ, et al. Patterns of care study decision tree and management guidelines for esophageal cancer. *Radiat Med* 1998;16:321.

372. Wong RKS, Malthaner RA, Zuraw L, et al. Combined modality radiotherapy and chemotherapy in nonsurgical management of localized carcinoma of the esophagus: a practice guideline. *Int J Radiat Oncol Biol Phys* 2003;55:930.

373. Members NCCNP. Esophageal cancer—clinical practice guidelines in oncology. *J Natl Comp Cancer* 2003;1:14.

374. De-Ren S. Ten-year follow-up of esophageal cancer treated by radical radiation therapy: analysis of 869 patients. *Int J Radiat Oncol Biol Phys* 1989;16:329.

375. Newaishy GA, Read GA, Duncan W, et al. Results of radical radiotherapy of squamous cell carcinoma of the esophagus. *Clin Radiol* 1982;33:347.

376. Okawa T, Kita M, Tanaka M, et al. Results of radiotherapy for inoperable locally advanced esophageal cancer. *Int J Radiat Oncol Biol Phys* 1989;17:49.

377. Shi X, Yao W, Liu T. Late course accelerated fractionation in radiotherapy of esophageal carcinoma. *Radiother Oncol* 1999;51:21.

378. Seki K, Karasawa K, Kohno M, et al. The treatment result of definitive radiotherapy for superficial esophageal cancer. *Int J Radiat Oncol Biol Phys* 2001;51:264.

379. Nemoto K, Zhao HJ, Goto T, et al. Radiation therapy for limited-stage small-cell esophageal cancer. *Am J Clin Oncol* 2002;25:404.

380. Sykes AJ, Burt PA, Slevin NJ, et al. Radical radiotherapy for carcinoma of the oesophagus: an effective alternative to surgery. *Radiother Oncol* 1998;48:15.

381. Seitz JF, Giovannini M, Padaut-Cesana J, et al. Inoperable nonmetastatic squamous cell carcinoma of the esophagus managed by concomitant chemotherapy (5-fluorouracil and cisplatin) and radiation therapy. *Cancer* 1990;66:214.

382. Izquierdo MA, Marcuello E, Gomez de Segura G, et al. Unresectable nonmetastatic squamous cell carcinoma of the esophagus managed by sequential chemotherapy (cisplatin and bleomycin) and radiation therapy. *Cancer* 1993;71:287.

383. Coia LR, Engstrom PF, Paul AR, et al. Long-term results of infusional 5-FU, mitomycin-C, and radiation as primary management of esophageal cancer. *Int J Radiat Oncol Biol Phys* 1991;20:29.

384. Valerdi JJ, Tejedor M, Illarramendi JJ, et al. Neoadjuvant chemotherapy and radiotherapy in locally advanced esophagus carcinoma: long term results. *Int J Radiat Oncol Biol Phys* 1994;27:843.

385. Poplin EA, Jacobson J, Herskovic A, et al. Evaluation of multimodality treatment of locoregional esophageal carcinoma by Southwest Oncology Group 9060. *Cancer* 1996;78:1851.

386. Nemoto K, Yamada S, Hareyama M, et al. Radiation therapy for superficial esophageal cancer: a comparison of radiotherapy methods. *Int J Radiat Oncol Biol Phys* 2001;50:639.

387. Roussel A, Jacob JH, Jung GM, et al. Controlled clinical trial for the treatment of patients with inoperable esophageal carcinoma: a study of the EORTC Gastrointestinal Tract Cancer Cooperative Group, in recent results in cancer research. In: Schlag P, Hohenberger P, Metzger U, eds. Berlin: Springer-Verlag, 1988:21.

388. Al-Sarraf M, Martz K, Herskovic A, et al. Progress report of combined chemoradiotherapy versus radiotherapy alone in patients with esophageal cancer: an intergroup study. *J Clin Oncol* 1997;15:277.

389. Slabber CF, Nel JS, Schoeman L, et al. A randomized study of radiotherapy alone versus radiotherapy plus 5-fluorouracil and platinum in patients with inoperable, locally advanced squamous cell cancer of the esophagus. *Am J Clin Oncol* 1998;21:462.

390. Smith TJ, Ryan LM, Douglass HO, et al. Combined chemoradiotherapy vs. radiotherapy alone for early stage squamous cell carcinoma of the esophagus: a study of the Eastern Cooperative Oncology Group. *Int J Radiat Oncol Biol Phys* 1998;42:269.

391. Araujo CM, Souhami L, Gil RA, et al. A randomized trial comparing radiation therapy versus concomitant radiation therapy and chemotherapy in carcinoma of the thoracic esophagus. *Cancer* 1991;67:2258.
392. Araujo CMM, Souhami L, Gil RA, et al. A randomized trial comparing radiation therapy versus concomitant radiation therapy and chemotherapy in carcinoma of the thoracic esophagus. *Cancer* 1991;67:2258.
393. Streeter OE, Martz KL, Gaspar LE, et al. Does race influence survival for esophageal cancer patients treated on the radiation and chemotherapy arm of RTOG # 85-01? *Int J Radiat Oncol Biol Phys* 1999;44:1047.
394. Minsky BD, Neuberg D, Kelsen DP, et al. Final report of intergroup trial 0122 (ECOG PE-289, RTOG 90-12): phase II trial of neoadjuvant chemotherapy plus concurrent chemotherapy and high-dose radiation for squamous cell carcinoma of the esophagus. *Int J Radiat Oncol Biol Phys* 1999;43:517.
395. Bedenne L, Michel P, Bouche O, et al. Randomized phase III trial in locally advanced esophageal cancer: radiochemotherapy followed by surgery versus radiochemotherapy alone (FFCD 9102). *Proc ASCO* 2002;21:130a.
396. Bonnetain F, Bedenne L, Michel P, et al. Definitive results of a comparative longitudinal quality of life study using the Spitzer index in the randomized multicentric phase III trial FFCD 9102 (surgery vs. radiochemotherapy in patients with locally advanced esophageal cancer). *Proc ASCO* 2003;22:250.
397. Stahl M, Wilke H, Walz MK, et al. Randomized phase III trial in locally advanced squamous cell carcinoma (SCC) of the esophagus: chemoradiation with and without surgery. *Proc ASCO* 2003;22:250.
398. Sarbia M, Stahl M, Fink U, et al. Expression of apoptosis-regulating proteins and outcome of esophageal cancer patients treated by combined therapy modalities. *Clin Cancer Res* 1998;4:2991.
399. Pomp J, Davelaar J, Blom J, et al. Radiotherapy for oesophagus carcinoma: the impact of p53 on treatment outcome. *Radiother Oncol* 1998;46:179.
400. Merchant TE, Minsky BD, Lauwers GY, et al. Esophageal cancer phospholipids correlated with histopathologic findings: a 31P NMR study. *NMR Biomed* 1999;12:184.
401. Kishi K, Doki Y, Miyata H, et al. Prediction of the response to chemoradiation and prognosis in oesophageal squamous cancer. *Br J Surg* 2002;89:597.
402. Hironaka S, Hasebe T, Kamijo T, et al. Biopsy specimen microvessel density is a useful prognostic marker in patients with T2-4M0 esophageal cancer treated with chemoradiotherapy. *Clin Cancer Res* 2002;8:124.
403. Morita M, Kuwano H, Araki K, et al. Prognostic significance of lymphocytic infiltration following preoperative chemoradiotherapy and hyperthermia for esophageal cancer. *Int J Radiat Oncol Biol Phys* 2001;49:1259.
404. Kelsen DP, Minsky B, Smith M, et al. Preoperative therapy for esophageal cancer: a randomized comparison of chemotherapy versus radiation therapy. *J Clin Oncol* 1990:1352.
405. Ishikura S, Nihei K, Ohtsu A, et al. Long-term toxicity after definitive chemoradiotherapy for squamous cell carcinoma of the thoracic esophagus. *J Clin Oncol* 2003;21:2697.
406. Roca E, Pennella E, Sardi M, et al. Combined intensive chemoradiotherapy for organ preservation in patients with resectable and non-resectable oesophageal cancer. *Eur J Cancer* 1996;32A:429.
407. Ott K, Fink U, Becker K, et al. Prediction of response to preoperative chemotherapy in gastric carcinoma by metabolic imaging: results of a prospective trial. *J Clin Oncol* 2003;21:4604.
408. Armstrong JG, High dose rate remote afterloading brachytherapy for lung and esophageal cancer. *Semin Radiat Oncol* 1993;4:270.
409. Moni J, Armstrong JG, Minsky BD, et al. High dose rate intraluminal brachytherapy for carcinoma of the esophagus. *Dis Esophagus* 1996;9:123.
410. Sur RK, Singh DP, Sharma SC. Radiation therapy of esophageal cancer: role of high dose rate brachytherapy. *Int J Radiat Oncol Biol Phys* 1992;22:1043.
411. Jager J, Langendijk H, Pannebakker M, et al. A single session of intraluminal brachytherapy in palliation of esophageal cancer. *Radiother Oncol* 1995;37:237.
412. Sur RK, Donde B, Levin VC, et al. Fractionated high dose rate intraluminal brachytherapy in palliation of advanced esophageal cancer. *Int J Radiat Oncol Biol Phys* 1998;40:447.
413. Maingon P, d'Hombres A, Truc G, et al. High dose rate brachytherapy for superficial cancer of the esophagus. *Int J Radiat Oncol Biol Phys* 2000;46:71.
414. Calais G, Dorval E, Louisot P, et al. Radiotherapy with high dose rate brachytherapy boost and concomitant chemotherapy for stages IIB and III esophageal carcinoma: results of a pilot study. *Int J Radiat Oncol Biol Phys* 1997;38:769.
415. Akagi Y, Hirokawa Y, Kagemoto M, et al. Optimum fractionation for high-dose-rate endoesophageal brachytherapy following external irradiation of early stage esophageal cancer. *Int J Radiat Oncol Biol Phys* 1999;43:525.
416. Schraube P, Fritz P, Wannenmacher MF. Combined endoluminal and external irradiation of inoperable oesophageal carcinoma. *Radiother Oncol* 1997;44:45.
417. Okawa T, Dokiya T, Nishio M, et al. Multi-institutional randomized trial of external radiotherapy with and without intraluminal brachytherapy for esophageal cancer in Japan. *Int J Radiat Oncol Biol Phys* 1999;45:623.
418. Caspers RJL, Zwinderman AH, Griffioen G, et al. Combined external beam and low dose rate intraluminal radiotherapy in oesophageal cancer. *Radiother Oncol* 1993;27:7.
419. Yorozu A, Dokiya T, Oki Y, et al. Curative radiotherapy with high-dose-rate brachytherapy boost for localized esophageal carcinoma: dose-effect relationship of brachytherapy with the balloon type applicator system. *Radiother Oncol* 1999;51:133.
420. Gaspar LE, Qian C, Kocha WI, et al. A phase I/II study of external beam radiation, brachytherapy and concurrent chemotherapy in localized cancer of the esophagus (RTOG 92-07): preliminary toxicity report. *Int J Radiat Oncol Biol Phys* 1997;37:593.
421. Gaspar LE, Nag S, Herskovic A, et al. American Brachytherapy Society (ABS) consensus guidelines for brachytherapy of esophageal cancer. *Int J Radiat Oncol Biol Phys* 1997;38:127.
422. Calais G, Jadaud E, Chapet S, et al. High dose radiotherapy (RT) and concomitant chemotherapy for nonresectable esophageal cancer. Results of a phase II study. *Proc ASCO* 1994;13:197.
423. Minsky BD, Pajak T, Ginsberg RJ, et al. INT 0123 (RTOG 94-05) phase III trial of combined modality therapy for esophageal cancer: high dose (64.8 Gy) vs. standard dose (50.4 Gy) radiation therapy. *J Clin Oncol* 2002;20:1167.
424. Girinsky T, Auperin A, Marsiglia H, et al. Accelerated fractionation in esophageal cancers: a multivariate analysis on 88 patients. *Int J Radiat Oncol Biol Phys* 1997;38:1013.
425. Jeremic B, Shibamoto Y, Acimovic L, et al. Accelerated hyperfractionated radiation therapy and concurrent 5-fluorouracil/cisplatin chemotherapy for locoregional squamous cell carcinoma of the thoracic esophagus: a phase II study. *Int J Radiat Oncol Biol Phys* 1998;40:1061.
426. Wang Y, Shi XH, He SQ, et al. Comparison between continuous accelerated hyperfractionated and late-course accelerated hyperfractionated radiotherapy for esophageal carcinoma. *Int J Radiat Oncol Biol Phys* 2002;54:131.
427. Goldberg M, Lampert C, Colarusso P, et al. Survival following intensive preoperative combined modality therapy with paclitaxel, cisplatin, 5-fluorouracil, and radiation in resectable esophageal carcinoma: a phase I report. *Proc ASCO* 2002;21:154a.
428. Nutting CM, Bedford JL, Cosgrove VP, et al. A comparison of conformal and intensity-modulated techniques for oesophageal radiotherapy. *Radiother Oncol* 2001;61:157.
429. Font A, Garcia-Alfonso P, Arellano A, et al. Preoperative combined multimodal therapy with docetaxel plus 5-fluorouracil and concurrent hyperfractionated radiotherapy for locally advanced esophageal cancer. *Proc ASCO* 2002;21:128b.
430. Fuchs C, Fitzgerald T, Mamon H, et al. Postoperative adjuvant chemoradiation for gastric or gastroesophageal adenocarcinoma using epirubicin, cisplatin, and infusional (CI) 5-FU (ECF) before and after CI 5-FU and radiotherapy (RT): a multicenter study. *Proc ASCO* 2003;22:257.
431. Ilson DH, Minsky B, Kelsen D. Irinotecan cisplatin and radiation in esophageal cancer. *Oncology* 2002;16s:11.
432. D'Adamo DR, Bains M, Minsky B, et al. A phase I trial of paclitaxel, cisplatin, irinotecan, and concurrent radiation therapy in locally advanced esophageal cancer. *Proc ASCO* 2003;22:349.
433. Safran H, DiPetrillo T, Nadeem A, et al. Neoadjuvant Herceptin, paclitaxel, cisplatin, and radiation for adenocarcinoma of esophagus: a phase I study. *Proc ASCO* 2002;21:141a.
434. Enzinger PC, Mamon H, Bueno R, et al. Phase II cisplatin, irinotecan, celecoxib and concurrent radiation therapy followed by surgery for locally advanced esophageal cancer. *Proc ASCO* 2003;22:361.
435. Turrisi AT, Hawes RH, Redmond C, et al. Palliation with stent (S) or radiation therapy (RT) 20 Gy in 5 fractions intervention for esophageal (SORTIE) cancer dysphagia: a multicenter trial for T-4, N-any, M +/− squamous or adenocarcinoma of the esophagus. A randomized trial relief from dysphagia and quality of life (QOL) analysis. *Proc ASCO* 2002;21:138a.
436. Li XA, Chibani O, Greenwald B, et al. Radiotherapy dose perturbation of metallic esophageal stents. *Int J Radiat Oncol Biol Phys* 2002;54:1276.
437. Nishimura Y, Nagata K, Katano S, et al. Severe complications in advanced esophageal cancer treated with radiotherapy after intubation of esophageal stents: a questionnaire survey of the Japanese Society for Esophageal Diseases. *Int J Radiat Oncol Biol Phys* 2003;56:1327.
438. Wara WM, Mauch PM, Thomas AN, et al. Palliation for carcinoma of the esophagus. *Radiology* 1976;121:717.
439. Petrovich Z, Langholz B, Formenti S, et al. Management of carcinoma of the esophagus: the role of radiotherapy. *Am J Clin Oncol* 1991;14:80.
440. Whittington R, Coia LR, Haller DG, et al. Adenocarcinoma of the esophagus and esophago-gastric junction: the effects of single and combined modalities on the survival and patterns of failure following treatment. *Int J Radiat Oncol Biol Phys* 1990;19:593.
441. Caspers RJL, Welvaart K, Verkes RJ, et al. The effect of radiotherapy on dysphagia and survival in patients with esophageal cancer. *Radiother Oncol* 1988;12:15.
442. Algan O, Coia LR, Keller SM, et al. Management of adenocarcinoma of the esophagus with chemoradiation alone or chemoradiation followed by esophagectomy: results of sequential nonrandomized phase II studies. *Int J Radiat Oncol Biol Phys* 1995;32:753.
443. Gill PG, Denham JW, Jamieson GG, et al. Patterns of treatment failure and prognostic factors associated with the treatment of esophageal carcinoma with chemotherapy and radiotherapy either as sole treatment of followed by surgery. *J Clin Oncol* 1992;10:1037.
444. Urba SG, Turrisi AT. Split-course accelerated radiation therapy combined with carboplatin and 5-fluorouracil for palliation of metastatic or unresectable carcinoma of the esophagus. *Cancer* 1995;75:435.
445. Coia LR, Soffen EM, Schultheiss TE, et al. Swallowing function in patients with esophageal cancer treated with concurrent radiation and chemotherapy. *Cancer* 1993;71:281.
446. O'Rourke IC, Tiver K, Bull C, et al. Swallowing performance after radiation therapy for carcinoma of the esophagus. *Cancer* 1988;61:2022.
447. Sur M, Sur R, Cooper K, et al. Morphologic alterations in esophageal squamous cell carcinoma after preoperative high dose rate intraluminal brachytherapy. *Cancer* 1996;77:2200.
448. Gschossmann JM, Bonner JA, Foote RL, et al. Malignant tracheoesophageal fistula in patients with esophageal cancer. *Cancer* 1993;72:1513.
449. Arlington A, Bohorquez J. Irradiation of carcinoma of the esophagus containing a tracheoesophageal fistula. *Cancer* 1993;71:3808.
450. Minsky BD. Radiation therapy in the treatment of esophagus cancer. *Chest Surg Clin N Am* 1994;4:285.
451. Gergel TJ, Leichman LL, Nava HR, et al. Effect of concurrent radiation therapy and chemotherapy on pulmonary function in patients with esophageal cancer: dose-volume histogram analysis. *Cancer J* 2002;8:451.
452. Phillips TL, Minsky BD, Dicker A. Cancer of the esophagus. In: Leibel S, Phillips TL, eds. *Textbook of radiation oncology*. Philadelphia: WB Saunders, 1998:601.
453. Tai P, van Dyk J, Yu E, et al. Variability of target volume delineation in cervical esophageal cancer. *Int J Radiat Oncol Biol Phys* 1998;42:277.
454. Tai P, van Dyk J, Battista J, et al. Improving the consistency in cervical esophageal target volume definition by special training. *Int J Radiat Oncol Biol Phys* 2002;53:766.
455. Nash CL, Gerdes H. Methods of palliation of esophageal and gastric cancer. *Surg Oncol Clin N Am* 2002;11:459.

456. Moses FM, Peura DA, Wong RK, et al. Palliative dilation of esophageal carcinoma. *Gastrointest Endosc* 1985;31:61.

457. Lundell L, Leth R, Lind T, et al. Palliative endoscopic dilatation in carcinoma of the esophagus and esophagogastric junction. *Acta Chir Scand* 1989;155:179.

458. Siersema PD, Dees J, van Blankenstein M. Palliation of malignant dysphagia from oesophageal cancer. Rotterdam Oesophageal Tumor Study Group. *Scand J Gastroenterol Suppl* 1998;225:75.

459. Kubba AK, Krasner N. An update in the palliative management of malignant dysphagia. *Eur J Surg Oncol* 2000;26:116.

460. Segalin A, Bonavina L, Carazzone A, et al. Improving results of esophageal stenting: a study on 160 consecutive unselected patients. *Endoscopy* 1997;29:701.

461. Vakil N, Morris AI, Marcon N, et al. A prospective, randomized, controlled trial of covered expandable metal stents in the palliation of malignant esophageal obstruction at the gastroesophageal junction. *Am J Gastroenterol* 2001;96:1791.

462. Raijman I, Siddique I, Ajani J, et al. Palliation of malignant dysphagia and fistulae with coated expandable metal stents: experience with 101 patients. *Gastrointest Endosc* 1998;48:172.

463. Sumiyoshi T, Gotoda T, Muro K, et al. Morbidity and mortality after self-expandable metallic stent placement in patients with progressive or recurrent esophageal cancer after chemoradiotherapy. *Gastrointest Endosc* 2003;57:882.

464. Mitty RD, Cave DR, Birkett DH. One-stage retrograde approach to Nd:YAG laser palliation of esophageal carcinoma. *Endoscopy* 1996;28:350.

465. Maciel J, Barbosa J, Leal AS. Nd-YAG laser as a palliative treatment for malignant dysphagia. *Eur J Surg Oncol* 1996;22:69.

466. Barr H, Krasner N. Prospective quality-of-life analysis after palliative photoablation for the treatment of malignant dysphagia. *Cancer* 1991;68:1660.

467. Naveau S, Chiesa A, Poynard T, et al. Endoscopic Nd-YAG laser therapy as palliative treatment for esophageal and cardial cancer. Parameters affecting long-term outcome. *Dig Dis Sci* 1990;35:294.

468. Adler DG, Baron TH. Endoscopic palliation of malignant dysphagia. *Mayo Clin Proc* 2001;76:731.

469. Heier SK, Rothman KA, Heier LM, et al. Photodynamic therapy for obstructing esophageal cancer: light dosimetry and randomized comparison with Nd:YAG laser therapy. *Gastroenterology* 1995;109:63.

470. Lightdale CJ, Heier SK, Marcon NE, et al. Photodynamic therapy with porfimer sodium versus thermal ablation therapy with Nd:YAG laser for palliation of esophageal cancer: a multicenter randomized trial. *Gastrointest Endosc* 1995;42:507.

471. Jensen DM, Machicado G, Randall G, et al. Comparison of low-power YAG laser and BICAP tumor probe for palliation of esophageal cancer strictures. *Gastroenterology* 1988;94:1263.

472. Johnston JH, Fleischer D, Petrini J, et al. Palliative bipolar electrocoagulation therapy of obstructing esophageal cancer. *Gastrointest Endosc* 1987;33:349.

473. Heindorff H, Wojdemann M, Bisgaard T, et al. Endoscopic palliation of inoperable cancer of the oesophagus or cardia by argon electrocoagulation. *Scand J Gastroenterol* 1998;33:21.

474. Roth JA, Putnam JB Jr. Surgery for cancer of the esophagus. *Semin Oncol* 1994;21:453.

475. Salazar JD, Doty JR, Lin JW, et al. Does cell type influence post-esophagectomy survival in patients with esophageal cancer? *Dis Esophagus* 1998;11:168.

476. Mantravadi RV, Lad T, Briele H, et al. Carcinoma of the esophagus: sites of failure. *Int J Radiat Oncol Biol Phys* 1982;8:1897.

477. Mandard AM, Chasle J, Marnay J, et al. Autopsy findings in 111 cases of esophageal cancer. *Cancer* 1981;48:329.

478. Attah EB, Hajdu SI. Benign and malignant tumors of the esophagus at autopsy. *J Thorac Cardiovasc Surg* 1968;55:396.

479. Aisner JA, Forastiere A, RA. Patterns of recurrence for cancer of the lung and esophagus. *Cancer Treat Symp* 1983;2:87(abst).

480. Yagoda A, Mukherji B, Young C, et al. Bleomycin, an antitumor antibiotic. Clinical experience in 274 patients. *Ann Intern Med* 1972;77:861.

481. Stephens FO. Bleomycin—a new approach in cancer chemotherapy. *Med J Aust* 1973;1:1277.

482. Ravry M, Moertel CG, Schutt AJ, et al. Treatment of advanced squamous cell carcinoma of the gastrointestinal tract with bleomycin (NSC-125066). *Cancer Chemother Rep* 1973;57:493.

483. Tancini G, Bajetta E, Bonadonna G. Bleomycin alone and in combination with methotrexate in the treatment of carcinoma of the esophagus (author's transl). *Tumori* 1974;60:65.

484. Kolaric K, Maricic Z, Dujmovic I, et al. Therapy of advanced esophageal cancer with bleomycin, irradiation and combination of bleomycin with irradiation. *Tumori* 1976;62:255.

485. Lokich JJ, Shea M, Chaffey J. Sequential infusional 5-fluorouracil followed by concomitant radiation for tumors of the esophagus and gastroesophageal junction. *Cancer* 1987;60:275.

486. Ezdinli EZ, Gelber R, Desai DV, et al. Chemotherapy of advanced esophageal carcinoma: Eastern Cooperative Oncology Group experience. *Cancer* 1980;46:2149.

487. Engstrom PF, Lavin PT, Klaassen DJ. Phase II evaluation of mitomycin and cisplatin in advanced esophageal carcinoma. *Cancer Treat Rep* 1983;67:713.

488. Whitington R, Clos H. Clinical experience with mitomycin C. *Cancer Chemother Rep* 1970;54:195.

489. Kolaric K, Maricic Z, Roth A, et al. Combination of bleomycin and adriamycin with and without radiation on the treatment of inoperable esophageal cancer. A randomized study. *Cancer* 1980;45:2265.

490. Advani SH, Saikia TK, Swaroop S, et al. Anterior chemotherapy in esophageal cancer. *Cancer* 1985;56:1502.

491. Davis S, Shanmugathasa M, Kessler W. cis-Dichlorodiammineplatinum(II) in the treatment of esophageal carcinoma. *Cancer Treat Rep* 1980;64:709.

492. Ravry M, Moore M. Phase II pilot study of cisplatinum (II) in advanced squamous cell esophageal cancer. *Proc Am Soc Clin Oncol* 1980;21:353.

493. Panettiere FJ, Leichman LP, Tilchen EJ, et al. Chemotherapy for advanced epidermoid carcinoma of the esophagus with single-agent cisplatin: final report on a Southwest Oncology Group study. *Cancer Treat Rep* 1984;68:1023.

494. Bleiberg H, Conroy T, Paillot B, et al. Randomised phase II study of cisplatin and 5-fluorouracil (5-FU) versus cisplatin alone in advanced squamous cell oesophageal cancer. *Eur J Cancer* 1997;33:1216.

495. Miller JI, McIntyre B, Hatcher CR Jr. Combined treatment approach in surgical management of carcinoma of the esophagus: a preliminary report. *Ann Thorac Surg* 1985;40:289.

496. Kelsen DP, Bains M, Cvitkovic E, et al. Vindesine in the treatment of esophageal carcinoma: a phase II study. *Cancer Treat Rep* 1979;63:2019.

497. Bedikian AY, Valdivieso M, Bodey GP, et al. Phase II evaluation of vindesine in the treatment of colorectal and esophageal tumors. *Cancer Chemother Pharmacol* 1979;2:263.

498. Bezwoda WR, Derman DP, Weaving A, et al. Treatment of esophageal cancer with vindesine: an open trial. *Cancer Treat Rep* 1984;68:783.

499. Kelsen D, Chapman R, Bains M, et al. Phase II study of methyl-GAG in the treatment of esophageal carcinoma. *Cancer Treat Rep* 1982;66:1427.

500. Ravry MJ, Omura GA, Hill GJ, et al. Phase II evaluation of mitoguazone in cancers of the esophagus, stomach, and pancreas: a Southeastern Cancer Study Group Trial. *Cancer Treat Rep* 1986;70:533.

501. Falkson G. Methyl-GAG (NSC-32946) in the treatment of esophagus cancer. *Cancer Chemother Rep* 1971;55:209.

502. Conroy T, Etienne PL, Adenis A, et al. Phase II trial of vinorelbine in metastatic squamous cell esophageal carcinoma. European Organization for Research and Treatment of Cancer Gastrointestinal Treat Cancer Cooperative Group. *J Clin Oncol* 1996;14:164.

503. Ajani JA, Ilson DH, Daugherty K, et al. Activity of Taxol in patients with squamous cell carcinoma and adenocarcinoma of the esophagus. *J Natl Cancer Inst* 1994;86:1086.

504. Anderson SE, O'Reilly EM, Kelsen DP, et al. Phase II trial of 96-hour paclitaxel in previously treated patients with advanced esophageal cancer. *Cancer Invest* 2003;21:512.

505. Heath EI, Urba S, Marshall J, et al. Phase II trial of docetaxel chemotherapy in patients with incurable adenocarcinoma of the esophagus. *Invest New Drugs* 2002;20:95.

506. Sandler AB, Kindler HL, Einhorn LH, et al. Phase II trial of gemcitabine in patients with previously untreated metastatic cancer of the esophagus or gastroesophageal junction. *Ann Oncol* 2000;11:1161.

507. Macdonald JS, Jacobson JL, Ketchel SJ, et al. A phase II trial of topotecan in esophageal carcinoma: a Southwest Oncology Group study (SWOG 9339). *Invest New Drugs* 2000;18:199.

508. Asbury RF, Lipsitz S, Graham D, et al. Treatment of squamous cell esophageal cancer with topotecan: an Eastern Cooperative Oncology Group Study (E2293). *Am J Clin Oncol* 2000;23:45.

509. Bidoli P, Stani SC, De Candis D, et al. Single-agent chemotherapy with vinorelbine for pretreated or metastatic squamous cell carcinoma of the esophagus. *Tumori* 2001;87:299.

510. Conroy T, Etienne PL, Adenis A, et al. Vinorelbine and cisplatin in metastatic squamous cell carcinoma of the oesophagus: response, toxicity, quality of life and survival. *Ann Oncol* 2002;13:721.

511. Milas L, Hunter NR, Mason KA, et al. Enhancement of tumor radio response of a murine mammary carcinoma by paclitaxel. *Cancer Res* 1994;54:3506.

512. Bajorin D, Kelsen D, Heelan R. Phase II trial of dichloromethotrexate in epidermoid carcinoma of the esophagus. *Cancer Treat Rep* 1986;70:1246.

513. Alberts AS, Falkson G, Badata M, et al. Trimetrexate in advanced carcinoma of the esophagus. *Invest New Drugs* 1988;6:319.

514. Brown T, Fleming T, Tangen C, et al. A phase II trial of trimetrexate in the treatment of esophageal cancer. A Southwest Oncology Group Trial. *Proc Am Soc Clin Oncol* 1992;11:A479(abst).

515. Coonley C, Bains M, Kelsen DP. VP-16-213 in the treatment of esophageal cancer: a phase II trial. *Cancer Treat Rep* 1983;67:397.

516. Radice PA, Bunn PA Jr, Ihde DC. Therapeutic trials with VP-16-213 and VM-26: active agents in small cell lung cancer, non-Hodgkin's lymphomas, and other malignancies. *Cancer Treat Rep* 1979;63:1231.

517. Nanus DM, Kelsen DP, Lipperman R, et al. Phase II trial of ifosfamide in epidermoid carcinoma of the esophagus: unexpectant severe toxicity. *Invest New Drugs* 1988;6:239.

518. Kok TC, van der Gaast A, Splinter TA, et al. Ifosfamide in advanced adenocarcinoma of the oesophagus or oesophageal-gastric junction area. Rotterdam Esophageal Tumor Study Group. *Eur J Cancer* 1991;27:1112.

519. Mannell A, Winters Z. Carboplatin in the treatment of oesophageal cancer. *S Afr Med J* 1989;76:213.

520. Queisser W, Preusser P, Mross KB, et al. Phase II evaluation of carboplatin in advanced esophageal carcinoma. A trial of the Phase I/II Study Group of the Association for Medical Oncology of the German Cancer Society. *Onkologie* 1990;13:190.

521. Sternberg C, Kelsen D, Dukeman M, et al. Carboplatin: a new platinum analog in the treatment of epidermoid carcinoma of the esophagus. *Cancer Treat Rep* 1985;69:1305.

522. Steel A, Cullen MH, Robertson PW, et al. A phase II study of carboplatin in adenocarcinoma of the oesophagus. *Br J Cancer* 1988;58:500.

523. Dinwoodie WR, Bartolucci AA, Lyman GH, et al. Phase II evaluation of cisplatin, bleomycin, and vindesine in advanced squamous cell carcinoma of the esophagus: a Southeastern Cancer Study Group Trial. *Cancer Treat Rep* 1986;70:267.

524. De Besi P, Salvagno L, Endrizzi L, et al. Cisplatin, bleomycin and methotrexate in the treatment of advanced oesophageal cancer. *Eur J Cancer Clin Oncol* 1984;20:743.

525. Vogl SE, Greenwald E, Kaplan BH. Effective chemotherapy for esophageal cancer with methotrexate, bleomycin, and cis-diamminedichloroplatinum II. *Cancer* 1981;48:2555.

526. Kelsen DP, Fein R, Coonley C, et al. Cisplatin, vindesine, and mitoguazone in the treatment of esophageal cancer. *Cancer Treat Rep* 1986;70:255.

527. Chapman R, Fleming TR, Van Damme J, et al. Cisplatin, vinblastine, and mitoguazone in squamous cell carcinoma of the esophagus: a Southwest Oncology Group Study. *Cancer Treat Rep* 1987;71:1185.

528. Lovett D, Kelsen D, Eisenberger M, et al. A phase II trial of carboplatin and vinblastine in the treatment of advanced squamous cell carcinoma of the esophagus. *Cancer* 1991;67:354.

529. Wadler S, Fell S, Haynes H, et al. Treatment of carcinoma of the esophagus with 5-fluorouracil and recombinant alfa-2a-interferon. *Cancer* 1993;71:1726.

530. Ilson DH, Sirott M, Saltz L, et al. A phase II trial of interferon alpha-2A, 5-fluorouracil, and cisplatin in patients with advanced esophageal carcinoma. *Cancer* 1995;75:2197.

531. Enzinger PC, Ilson DH, Saltz LB, et al. Phase II clinical trial of 13-cis-retinoic acid and interferon-alpha-2a in patients with advanced esophageal carcinoma. *Cancer* 1999;85:1213.

532. Kok TC, Van der Gaast A, Dees J, et al. Cisplatin and etoposide in oesophageal cancer: a phase II study. Rotterdam Oesophageal Tumour Study Group. *Br J Cancer* 1996;74:980.

533. Kelsen D, Lovett D, Wong J, et al. Interferon alfa-2a and fluorouracil in the treatment of patients with advanced esophageal cancer. *J Clin Oncol* 1992;10:269.

534. Bazarbashi S, Rahal M, Raja MA, et al. A pilot trial of combination cisplatin, 5-fluorouracil and interferon-alpha in the treatment of advanced esophageal carcinoma. *Chemotherapy* 2002;48:211.

535. Polee MB, Kok TC, Siersema PD, et al. Phase II study of the combination cisplatin, etoposide, 5-fluorouracil and folinic acid in patients with advanced squamous cell carcinoma of the esophagus. *Anticancer Drugs* 2001;12:513.

536. Polee MB, Eskens FA, van der Burg ME, et al. Phase II study of biweekly administration of paclitaxel and cisplatin in patients with advanced oesophageal cancer. *Br J Cancer* 2002; 86:669.

537. Polee MB, Verweij J, Siersema PD, et al. Phase I study of a weekly schedule of a fixed dose of cisplatin and escalating doses of paclitaxel in patients with advanced oesophageal cancer. *Eur J Cancer* 2002;38:1495.

538. Ilson DH, Forastiere A, Arquette M, et al. A phase II trial of paclitaxel and cisplatin in patients with advanced carcinoma of the esophagus. *Cancer J* 2000;6:316.

539. van der Gaast A, Kok TC, Kerkhofs L, et al. Phase I study of a biweekly schedule of a fixed dose of cisplatin with increasing doses of paclitaxel in patients with advanced oesophageal cancer. *Br J Cancer* 1999;80:1052.

540. Ilson DH, Ajani J, Bhalla K, et al. Phase II trial of paclitaxel, fluorouracil, and cisplatin in patients with advanced carcinoma of the esophagus. *J Clin Oncol* 1998;16:1826.

541. Ilson DH, Saltz L, Enzinger P, et al. Phase II trial of weekly irinotecan plus cisplatin in advanced esophageal cancer. *J Clin Oncol* 1999;17:3270.

542. Ajani JA, Baker J, Pisters PW, et al. CPT-11 plus cisplatin in patients with advanced, untreated gastric or gastroesophageal junction carcinoma: results of a phase II study. *Cancer* 2002;94:641.

543. Jatoi A, Tirona MT, Cha SS, et al. A phase II trial of docetaxel and CPT-11 in patients with metastatic adenocarcinoma of the esophagus, gastroesophageal junction, and gastric cardia. *Int J Gastrointest Cancer* 2002;32:115.

544. Lordick F, von Schilling C, Bernhard H, et al. Phase II trial of irinotecan plus docetaxel in cisplatin-pretreated relapsed or refractory oesophageal cancer. *Br J Cancer* 2003;89: 630.

545. Ross P, Nicolson M, Cunningham D, et al. Prospective randomized trial comparing mitomycin, cisplatin, and protracted venous-infusion fluorouracil (PVI 5-FU) with epirubicin, cisplatin, and PVI 5-FU in advanced esophagogastric cancer. *J Clin Oncol* 2002; 20:1996.

546. Evans TR, Pentheroudakis G, Paul J, et al. A phase I and pharmacokinetic study of capecitabine in combination with epirubicin and cisplatin in patients with inoperable oesophago-gastric adenocarcinoma. *Ann Oncol* 2002;13:1469.

547. Mackay HJ, McInnes A, Paul J, et al. A phase II study of epirubicin, cisplatin and raltitrexed combination chemotherapy (ECT) in patients with advanced oesophageal and gastric adenocarcinoma. *Ann Oncol* 2001;12:1407.

PETER W. T. PISTERS
DAVID P. KELSEN
STEVEN M. POWELL
JOEL E. TEPPER

SECTION 2

Cancer of the Stomach

Adenocarcinoma of the stomach was the leading cause of cancer-related death worldwide through most of the twentieth century. It now ranks second only to lung cancer, and an estimated 875,000 new cases are diagnosed annually worldwide.[1] In many parts of the world, however, the incidence of gastric cancer has gradually decreased, principally because of changes in diet, food preparation, and other environmental factors. The declining incidence has been dramatic in the United States, where this disease ranks seventh as a cause of cancer-related deaths. It is estimated that 22,700 new cases are diagnosed annually in the United States, with approximately 11,800 deaths per year.[2]

The prognosis for this disease remains poor, except in a few countries. The explanations for these poor results are multifactorial. The lack of defined risk factors and specific symptoms and the relatively low incidence have contributed to the late stage at diagnosis seen in most Western countries. In Japan, where gastric cancer is endemic, more patients are diagnosed at an early stage, which is reflected by higher overall survival rates.

Although the incidence of gastric cancer has decreased dramatically over the past century, the decline has been limited to cancers below the esophagogastric junction. The number of newly diagnosed cases of proximal gastric and esophagogastric junction adenocarcinomas has increased markedly since the mid-1980s.[3,4] These tumors are thought to be biologically more aggressive than distal tumors and more complex to treat.

The only proven, potentially curative treatment for gastric cancer is surgical resection of all gross and microscopic disease. Even after what is believed to be a "curative" gastrectomy,

disease recurs in regional or distant sites, or both, in the majority of patients. Efforts to improve these poor results have focused on developing effective pre- and postoperative systemic and regional adjuvant therapies. This chapter details the current concepts regarding the origins, diagnosis, and treatment of this worldwide health problem.

EPIDEMIOLOGY AND ETIOLOGY

The incidence and mortality for gastric cancer vary widely in different regions of the world. The highest incidences of stomach cancer can be found in Japan, South America, and Eastern Europe, with incidence rates as high as 30 to 85 cases per 100,000 population.[5] In contrast, low-incidence areas such as the United States, Israel, and Kuwait have incidence rates of only 4 to 8 cases per 100,000 women.[5] Mortality figures approximate incidence figures in many high-incidence countries. However, in Japan, there has been a decline in mortality, perhaps as a result of mass screening.[6]

Immigrants gradually acquire the incidence rates of the country to which they move, strongly suggesting that environmental factors are of primary importance in etiology.[7,8] In one study, Japanese migrating to lower-risk areas had a risk of stomach cancer that was intermediate between that of the Western population and that of the Japanese population in Japan.[9] The risk of stomach cancer was also high in second-generation offspring who continued to consume a Japanese-style diet but was low in those who adopted a Western-style diet.[10] A study of Polish migrants living in the United States for 10 years found that the incidence of gastric cancer decreased and became intermediate between the usual incidences in the countries of origin and adoption.[11] These studies suggest that environmental exposure in early life is essential in determining risk but that other environmental or cultural factors continue to influence the predisposition to cancer.

In the United States, gastric cancer is now the seventh most common cause of cancer-related death,[2] although a century ago it was the most common cause. Incidence rates increase and survival decreases with increasing age of the population. Substantial racial variations are found in incidence and death rates. The highest death rates are among African American men (approximately 15 cases per 100,000 population annually), followed by white men (approximately half that incidence), African American women (slightly less than in white men), and white women (approximately half the rate of white men).

U.S. survival statistics have shown continued improvement in survival rates over the past two decades, although the reason for this improvement is not clear. Surveillance, Epidemiology, and End Results (SEER) cancer statistics showed a 15.4% 5-year overall survival rate in 1973, compared with 21.8% by 1997. Survival rates are best in the groups with the lowest incidence of gastric cancer.

One of the most striking epidemiologic observations has been the increasing incidence of adenocarcinomas involving the proximal stomach and distal esophagus.[12–15] These tumors are thought to have different etiologic factors; for example, gastric body lesions are associated with low acid production and *Helicobacter pylori* infection (see later), whereas cardia lesions are not associated with either. Cardia lesions also have a higher male-female ratio and are more common in whites than in African Americans. In 1991, Blot et al.,[12] reviewing the National Cancer Institute's (SEER) database, reported that during the period 1976 to 1987, a shift to proximal gastric lesions was noted. The annual rate of increase for proximal gastric lesions was 4.3% for white men, 4.1% for white women, 3.6% for African American men, and 5.6% for African American women, and these increases were occurring at the same time as decreases in the incidence of tumors of the gastric body and antrum. These annual rates of increase are greater than those of lung cancer or melanoma. By 1984 to 1987, cancers of the cardia made up 47% of all gastric cancers in white men. European investigators have reported similar data.[15] This trend is worrisome because proximal gastric cancers are thought to have a poorer prognosis, stage for stage, compared with distal cancers.[16–18]

For the endemic forms of gastric cancer, primarily the intestinal type, Correa[19] has postulated a progression from normal tissue to chronic atrophic gastritis, to intestinal metaplasia, and then to dysplasia.[7] He has also suggested that this progression is associated with varying risk factors, with *H pylori* and high salt intake associated with chronic atrophic gastritis and high nitrate intake leading to intestinal metaplasia.

The etiology of gastric cancer is likely multifactorial. A list of factors associated with increased risk of gastric adenocarcinoma is outlined in Table 29.2-1. The following paragraphs address specific areas of interest in the literature addressing the etiology of gastric cancer.

The etiologic basis for the rising incidence of proximal gastric and gastroesophageal junction cancers is being aggressively pursued. The increasing prevalence of obesity in the United States may be one contributing factor. Elevated body mass index[20,21] and high caloric consumption[22] have been associated with adenocarcinoma of the distal esophagus and gastric cardia. Gastroesophageal reflux disease may be another risk factor, although one also associated with obesity. A population-based, case-control study performed in Sweden found that for persons with recurrent symptoms of reflux, as compared to those without such symptoms, the odds ratio (OR) was 7.7 [95% confidence interval (CI), 5.3 to 11.4] for esophageal adenocarcinoma and 2.0 (95%

TABLE 29.2-1. Factors Associated with Increased Risk of Developing Stomach Cancer

ACQUIRED FACTORS
Nutritional
   High salt consumption
   High nitrate consumption
   Low dietary vitamin A and C
   Poor food preparation (smoked, salt cured)
   Lack of refrigeration
   Poor drinking water (well water)
Occupational
   Rubber workers
   Coal workers
Cigarette smoking
Helicobacter pylori infection
Epstein-Barr virus
Radiation exposure
Prior gastric surgery for benign gastric ulcer disease
GENETIC FACTORS
Type A blood
Pernicious anemia
Family history
Hereditary nonpolyposis colon cancer
Li-Fraumeni syndrome
PRECURSOR LESIONS
Adenomatous gastric polyps
Chronic atrophic gastritis
Dysplasia
Intestinal metaplasia
Menetrier's disease

CI, 1.4 to 2.9) for developing adenocarcinoma of the gastric cardia.[21] Other studies have found tobacco use to be associated with tumors at these sites.[23] Gammon et al.[24] observed an OR of 2.4 (95% CI, 1.7 to 3.4) for the development of gastric cancer in cigarette smokers. Conversely, the use of aspirin and nonsteroidal and inflammatory drugs has been associated with a lower risk of esophageal and cardia cancers,[25] implicating inflammation in the etiology of gastric cancer.

In 1965, Lauren[26] described two histologic types of gastric adenocarcinoma, intestinal and diffuse, which provided a model to understand better the etiology and epidemiology of the disease. The intestinal variant arises from precancerous lesions such as gastric atrophy or intestinal metaplasia within the stomach, occurs more commonly in men than in women, is more frequent in older people, and represents the dominant histologic type in regions where stomach cancer is endemic, suggesting a predominantly environmental etiology. The diffuse form does not typically arise from recognizable precancerous lesions. It is more common in low-incidence regions, occurs slightly more frequently in women and in younger patients, and has a higher association with familial occurrence (blood type A), suggesting a genetic etiology.[27] Changes in the incidence of gastric cancer over time appear to reflect primarily a change in the incidence of the intestinal form.[367]

Gastric adenocarcinomas of the body and antrum of the stomach have a strong association with *H pylori* infection. This is a common infection in many parts of the world and was associated with a doubled risk of such cancers in a metaanalysis of multiple studies.[28,29] The precise mechanism by which *H pylori* infection increases gastric cancer incidence is unclear, but it appears to increase the incidence of chronic atrophic gastritis, which produces a low-acidity environment, and the incidence of metaplasia and dysplasia.[30–32] However, because *H pylori* infection is present in more than 50% of the population in many parts of the world, it is clearly not a sufficient event for the development of gastric cancer. Reports suggest that gastric cancer develops in 5% of *H pylori*–positive persons over 10 years.[33] Multiple factors have been suggested that may interact with *H pylori* in producing gastric cancer, including tobacco use, age at infection, gender, and diet (e.g., low intake of ascorbic acid, carotene, and vitamin E). The precise type of *H pylori* infection may also be a factor. A number of studies have suggested that *cag*A strains, which are associated with cytotoxin expression, produce more gastric inflammation and have a strong association with gastric cancer.[34–36]

A number of other factors have been studied for their relationship with gastric cancer formation. Relatively little information is available to support a strong relationship between gastric cancer and alcohol use, although there may be a weak association between alcohol and tumors of the gastric cardia.[24,37] A moderate association between tobacco use and gastric cancer formation appears to be present (overall risk, 1.5 to 2.5),[38–40] with a long time interval after smoking cessation necessary before a decrease in risk is seen.

Evidence is fairly strong that eating fruits and vegetables (especially when raw) has a protective effect against gastric cancer, and there is a suggestion that eating foods high in antioxidants, including vitamins C and E, carotenoids, and flavonoids, may be beneficial. Green tea, which contains large amounts of phenols, could also be protective, but results have been inconsistent.[41–44]

The data on nitrates found in preserved foods and gastric cancer are mixed. Nitrates can be converted to nitrites and then to N-nitroso compounds, which produce gastric cancer in laboratory animals.[43,45] Some studies have shown a strong association between high intake of nitrates and gastric cancer, and other studies have shown no association.

Radiation exposure, especially at a young age, has been shown to produce a high risk of gastric cancer.[46] Gastric ulcer disease is also associated with an increased risk of gastric cancer, whereas duodenal ulcer disease is associated with a modest risk reduction.[32]

ANATOMIC CONSIDERATIONS

The stomach begins at the gastroesophageal junction and ends at the pylorus (Fig. 29.2-1). Above it lie the diaphragm and left lobe of the liver; before it is the abdominal wall; and below it are the transverse colon, mesocolon, and greater omentum. Behind and to the sides are the spleen, pancreas, left adrenal gland, left kidney, and splenic flexure of the colon. Cancers arising from the proximal greater curvature may directly involve the splenic hilum and tail of the pancreas, whereas more distal tumors may invade the transverse colon. Proximal cancers may extend into the diaphragm, spleen, or left lateral segment of the liver.

The blood supply to the stomach is extensive and is based on vessels arising from the celiac axis (see Fig. 29.2-1). The right gastric artery, arising from the hepatic artery, and the left gastric artery, arising from the celiac axis directly, course along the lesser curvature. Along the greater curvature are

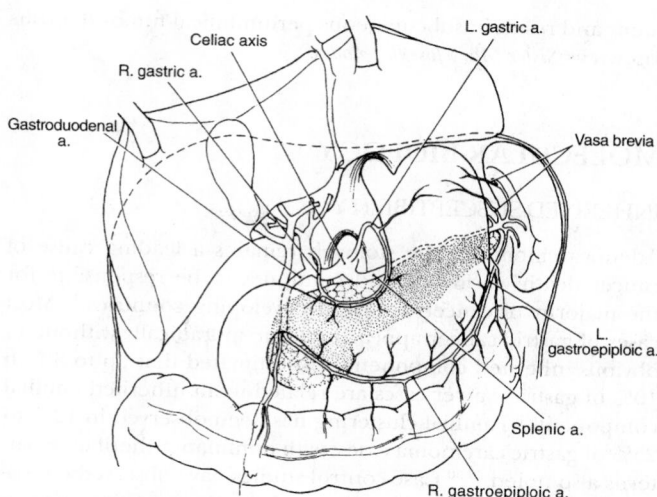

FIGURE 29.2-1. Blood supply to the stomach and anatomic relationships of the stomach with other adjacent organs likely to be involved by direct extension of a T4 gastric tumor.

the right gastroepiploic artery, which originates from the gastroduodenal artery at the inferior border of the proximal duodenum, and the left gastroepiploic artery, branching from the splenic artery laterally. The short gastric arteries (vasa brevia) arise directly from the splenic artery and make a relatively small contribution to the blood supply to the proximal portion of the stomach. The preservation of any of these vessels in the course of a subtotal gastrectomy for carcinoma is not necessary (and is not possible if the operation is performed correctly), and the most proximal few centimeters of remaining stomach are well supplied by collateral flow from the lower segmental esophageal arcade. The rich submucosal blood supply of the stomach is an important factor in its ability to heal rapidly and produce a low incidence of anastomotic disruption.

The venous supply of the stomach tends to parallel the arterial supply. The venous efflux ultimately passes the portal venous system and is reflected in the fact that the liver is a primary site for distant metastatic spread.

The lymphatic drainage of the stomach is extensive, and distinct anatomic groups of perigastric lymph nodes have been defined according to their relationship to the stomach and its blood supply. The six perigastric lymph node groups are the subpyloric and gastroepiploic nodes along the greater curvature and the suprapyloric and the lesser curvature lymph nodes along the lesser curvature and, proximally, the right and left pericardial nodes. The second echelon (extraperigastric) nodes include the common hepatic, left gastric, splenic hilum, and splenic artery lymphatics, which drain into the celiac and periaortic lymphatics. Proximally are the lower esophageal lymph nodes; extensive spread of gastric cancer along the intrathoracic lymph channels may be manifested clinically by a metastatic lymph node in the left supraclavicular fossa (Virchow's node) or left axilla (Irish's node). As the submucosal lymphatic supply of the stomach becomes extensively involved with tumor, other routes of lymphatic drainage may be recruited. Tumor spread to the lymphatics in the hepatoduodenal ligament can extend along the falciform ligament and result in subcutaneous periumbilical tumor deposits known as *Sister Mary Joseph's nodes.*

MOLECULAR BIOLOGY

INHERITED SUSCEPTIBILITY

Adenocarcinoma of the stomach remains a leading cause of cancer death worldwide and continues to be responsible for the majority of cancer deaths in developing countries.[47] Most cases of gastric cancer appear to occur sporadically without an obvious inherited component. It is estimated that up to 8% to 10% of gastric cancer cases are related to an inherited familial component.[48] Familial clustering has been observed in 12% to 25% of gastric carcinoma cases, with dominant inheritance patterns also noted.[49,50] Case-control studies have observed consistent, up to threefold, increases in risk for gastric cancer among relatives of patients with gastric cancer.[51,52] A population-based control study found increased risk for gastric cancer when first-degree relatives were affected (OR = 1.7 with a parent, OR = 2.6 with a sibling), with the risk increasing (OR up to 8.5) if more than one first-degree relative was affected.[53] Interestingly, a higher risk was noted in individuals with an affected mother versus an affected father. Studies of monozygotic twins have even shown a slight trend toward increased concordance of gastric cancers compared to dizygotic twins.[54,55]

Large families with an obvious autosomal dominant, highly penetrant inherited predisposition for the development of gastric cancer are rare. However, a large Maori kindred manifesting early-onset diffuse gastric cancers was able to be investigated for linkage analysis, and this disease was found to be linked to the *E-cadherin/CDH1* locus on 16q and associated with mutations in this gene.[56] Subsequently, several kindreds from a variety of ethnic backgrounds manifesting a diffuse, poorly differentiated gastric cancer predisposition trait have been shown to harbor germline *E-cadherin* alterations that co-segregate with these cancers at a relatively high (67% to 83%) penetrant rate.[56–60] Thus, E-cadherin mutation testing should be considered in the appropriate clinical setting.

Hereditary nonpolyposis colon cancer is a now well-characterized inherited predisposition trait that can involve gastric cancer development.[61] Germline genetic abnormalities of mismatch repair genes underlying this disease entity have been unveiled and include potential tumor development in a variety of tissue types.[62] Gastric carcinomas that occur in this setting were predominantly diagnosed at a mean age of 56 years, of the intestinal type, and without *H pylori* infection detected, and most exhibited microsatellite instability in a Finnish hereditary nonpolyposis colon cancer registry study.[63] Gastric carcinoma in an extended Li-Fraumeni kindred with an underlying *p53* germline alteration has even been reported.[64] Gastric cancers have also been noted to occur in patients with gastrointestinal polyposis disease entities such as familial adenomatous polyposis and Peutz-Jeghers.[65] Interestingly, an increased risk of gastric cancer associated with familial adenomatous polyposis (patients with germline *APC* mutations) has been reported in high-risk regions such as Asia,[66] whereas no increased risk was exhibited in other populations.[67] Overall, gastric carcinoma is rare in these settings, and the exact contribution of the polyposis and underlying germline alterations of *APC* and *LKB1/*

STK11 to gastric adenocarcinoma development in these cases is unclear. Finally, rare kindreds exhibiting site-specific gastric cancer predilection have been reported, occasionally associated with other inherited abnormalities.[68,69]

HOST AND ENVIRONMENTAL OBSERVATIONS

H pylori infection appears to lead to a five- to sixfold increase in risk of gastric malignancy, adenocarcinoma, and primary non-Hodgkin's lymphoma.[70–72] Yet, gastric cancer does not develop in most of those infected with this microorganism. The relative importance of bacterial virulence factors, environmental factors, and host factors (i.e., age of acquisition, immune responses, acid secretion changes) involved in the clinical outcome of this infection are currently pressing issues. Several allelic variants of polymorphisms in proinflammatory cytokines such as interleukin-1β, a potent inhibitor of acid secretion, have been associated with gastric cancers, suggesting that the host response may be an important determinant in the clinical outcome of infection.[73]

A population association study demonstrated the more frequent occurrence (54%) of the HLA DQB1*0301 allele in white patients with gastric cancer than in a control noncancerous group (27%).[74] If confirmed not to represent ethnic heterogeneity, this association may imply that this locus itself directly influences susceptibility to gastric cancer development or is a marker in linkage disequilibrium with a nearby cancer-predisposing locus. In another study, the frequency of allele DQB1*0401 was significantly higher in those infected with *H pylori* who developed atrophic gastritis than those who were infected and did not develop atrophic gastritis or those not infected.[75] The potential role of the HLA locus in gastric tumorigenesis has implications for the importance of a potential escape mechanism from immune surveillance as a causative factor for this disease. The fact that gastric cancer does not develop in most people with these alleles illustrates the complexity of this multifactorial disease.

In the 1950s, the blood group A phenotype was reported to be associated with gastric cancers.[27,76,77] Of interest, *H pylori* was shown to adhere to the Lewis[b] blood group antigen, indicating a potentially important host factor that might facilitate this chronic infection and subsequent risk of gastric cancer.[78] Additionally, small variant alleles of a mucin gene, *Muc1*, were found to be associated with gastric cancer patients compared to a blood donor control population.[79] Confirmatory studies demonstrating the relevance of these findings are still awaited. In fact, one study found no correlation between blood group phenotype including A and Lewis[b] and the occurrence of gastric cancer.[80]

Evidence of Epstein-Barr virus infection has been noted in several gastric carcinomas, although its significance is unclear. Although dietary irritants (i.e., salts or preservatives) and potential carcinogens (i.e., nitrates) have been suggested as etiologic factors of gastric cancer, as have several protective factors (i.e., ascorbic acid, fruits, vegetables, α-tocopherol, onions, and gastric acidity),[81] no specific agent has been definitively indicted or proved beneficial. Molecular studies may help discern the true influential factors.

MOLECULAR ALTERATIONS

Most cases of stomach cancer are sporadic in nature. Multiple gastric tumor classification systems have been formulated in efforts to identify various subgroups with different biologic behavior and prognostic indicators. It is anticipated that molecular markers will facilitate the classification of the various subgroups of gastric carcinomas.

Cytogenetic studies have been unrevealing in identifying consistent, overt chromosomal aberrations in gastric cancers. However, loss of heterozygosity studies and comparative genomic hybridization analyses have identified several DNA loci with significant allelic loss; these loci may harbor a tumor suppressor gene important in gastric tumorigenesis.[368–370] The exact targets of loss or gain in most of these chromosomal regions, including 4, 5q, 9p, 18q, and 20q, remain to be clarified.

Microsatellite Instability

Microsatellite instability and associated alterations of the *transforming growth factor (TGF)-β II receptor, IGFRII, BAX, E2F-4, hMSH3,* and *hMSH6* genes are found in a subset of gastric carcinomas.[82–86] Although the majority of gastric cancers exhibit significant aneuploidy, microsatellite instability has been found in 13% to 44% of sporadic gastric carcinomas.[87] In one study, abnormal loss of expression of either hMLH1 or hMSH2 protein was demonstrated in all gastric cancer cases exhibiting a high rate of microsatellite instability (MSI-H).[88] In another study, altered expression of hMLH1 was associated with abnormal methylation of the promoter region of *hMLH1* in MSI-H cases, suggesting a silencing role of hypermethylation.[89,90] The degree of genome-wide instability varies in gastric cancers, with the high degree of microsatellite instability (e.g., greater than 33% abnormal loci in MSI-H cases) occurring in only 16% of gastric cancers, usually of the subcardinal intestinal or mixed type, and associated with less frequent lymph node or vessel invasion, prominent lymphoid infiltration, and better prognosis.[91]

Specific Somatic Changes

Multiple somatic alterations have been described in gastric carcinomas at the molecular level. The significance of these changes in gastric tumorigenesis remains to be established in most instances. Once fully characterized, critical molecular alterations that are prevalent in these cancers are anticipated to provide new avenues to combat this lethal disease.

The *p53* gene is consistently altered in a majority of gastric cancers.[92] Many studies have used immunohistochemical analysis of tumors in an effort to detect excessive expression of p53 as an indirect means to identify mutations of this gene, but this finding does not appear to have consistent prognostic value in patients with gastric cancers.[93,94]

A target of amplification on 17q in gastric cancers was identified using a combination of comparative genomic hybridization and oligonucleotide microarray studies.[95] DARP32 and a novel isoform t-DARP were both discovered to be overexpressed in the majority of gastric carcinomas.[96] Additional studies should define its role in gastric tumorigenesis.

No inactivating somatic mutations of *p16^{INK4}* were detected in more than 70 cases of gastric carcinoma screened by polymerase chain reaction–single-stranded conformational polymorphism analysis.[97] On the other hand, *p16^{INK4}* somatic mutations were noted along with loss of heterozygosity of 9p in several esophageal adenocarcinomas, which are related to gastroesophageal junctional cancers.[98,99] Other cases of these cancers were observed to have loss of p16 expression associated with abnormal hypermethylation of the *p16^{INK4}* promoter, suggesting that this epigenetic gene expression silencing may play a role in esophageal tumorigenesis.[100] In a study of p16's promoter region in gastric cancers, a significant number (41%) exhibited CpG island methylation.[101] Many cases with hypermethylation of promoter regions displayed the MSI-H phenotype and multiple sites of methylation, including the *hMLH1* promoter region.[102]

Many sporadic diffuse gastric cancers display altered E-cadherin. E-cadherin is a transmembrane, calcium ion–dependent adhesion molecule important in epithelial cell homotypic interactions and, when decreased in expression, is associated with tumor invasiveness.[103] In one study, reduced E-cadherin expression, as determined by immunohistochemical analysis, was noted in 92% of gastric carcinomas and observed to be significantly associated with undifferentiated, diffuse-type cancers.[104] Genetic abnormalities of the *E-cadherin* gene (located on chromosome 16q22.1) and transcripts have been demonstrated in half of diffuse gastric cancers on reverse transcriptase–polymerase chain reaction analysis.[105] A significant proportion of sporadic diffuse gastric carcinomas, including specifically the diffuse component of mixed-type tumors, contain somatic *E-cadherin* gene mutations.[106,107] Additionally, promoter hypermethylation of *E-cadherin* is associated with decreased expression of this gene.[108] Furthermore, a study found that α-catenin, which binds to the intracellular domain of E-cadherin and links it to actin-based cytoskeletal elements, had reduced immunohistochemical expression in 70% of gastric carcinomas and that its expression correlated with infiltrative growth and poor differentiation.[109]

Evidence of a tumor suppressor locus on chromosome 3p has accumulated from a variety of studies and includes allelic loss at 3p in primary gastric tumors (46%) and homozygous deletion of 3p in a gastric cancer cell line (KATO III).[110] The *FHIT* gene was isolated from the common fragile site region (FRA3B) at 3p14.2 and found to have abnormal transcripts with deleted exons in five of nine gastric cancers.[111] Furthermore, loss of FHIT protein expression was demonstrated immunohistochemically in the majority of gastric carcinomas in one study.[112] Also, a somatic missense mutation was identified in exon 6 of the *FHIT* gene during a coding region analysis of 40 gastric carcinomas.[113] Additional studies are needed to identify the critically altered targets on chromosome 3p and clarify the role that *FHIT* plays in gastric tumorigenesis. The role that the fragile site FRA3B plays in gastric cancer development remains to be determined.

Loss of the trefoil peptide TFF1 has been described in approximately 50% of gastric carcinomas.[114] Mice with homozygous deletion of *Tff1* by homologous recombination all developed antral dysplasia, and 30% were reported to have multifocal gastric carcinoma.[115] Tff1, originally called *pS2,* resides on chromosome 21q and was first identified as an estrogen-inducible gene in a breast cancer cell line.

Alterations of other gene products, including those involved in cell-cycle regulation, growth factor signaling, telomerase activity, angiogenesis, and extracellular matrix structure, have been described. Loss of p27, a cell-cycle regulator, have been observed to correlate with advanced stage in gastric cancer.[116] Amplification and overexpression of the *c-met* gene, which encodes a tyrosine kinase receptor for the hepatocyte growth factor, have been reported in gastric carcinomas,[117] and the epidermal growth factor and its receptor are expressed in approximately one-fourth of gastric cancers. Alterations of fibroblast growth factor receptors, including *K-sam* mutations, have been observed in a number of gastric tumors.[118,119] Telomerase activity has frequently been detected by a polymerase chain reaction–based assay in late-stage gastric tumors and observed to be associated with a poor prognosis. Amplification of *c-erbB-2* has been demonstrated in a small subset (approximately 10%) of gastric cancers and overexpression observed to be associated with a poor prognosis.[120] The expression of angiogenesis factors such as vascular endothelial growth factor has been observed in a subset of gastric cancers, indicating the potential role of angiogenesis inhibitor therapy. Membrane-type matrix metalloproteinase is preferentially expressed in some gastric cancer cells with colocalization and activation of the zymogen proMMP-2.[121] Increased plasminogen activation has been reported as well in several gastric tumors. Specific alterations such as these need true prevalence determination and further characterization in gastric cancer before genetic tests can be designed for clinical use.

High-throughput assays such as microarrays that comprehensively determine gene expression or DNA copy number patterns are just beginning to be explored. Potential biomarkers such as phospholipase A_2 or profiles of expression identified with these analyses may provide some prognostic as well as diagnostic information about gastric cancer.[122–124] Comprehensive serial analysis of gene expression has also identified novel genetic alterations, including overexpression of calcium-binding proteins.[96]

PATHOLOGY AND TUMOR BIOLOGY

Approximately 95% of all malignant gastric neoplasms are adenocarcinomas, and in general, the term *gastric cancer* refers to adenocarcinoma of the stomach. Other malignant tumors are very rare and include squamous cell carcinoma, adenoacanthoma, carcinoid tumors, and leiomyosarcoma.[125] Although no normal lymphoid tissue is found in the gastric mucosa, the stomach is the most common site for lymphomas of the gastrointestinal tract. The increased awareness of association between mucosa-associated lymphoid tissue lymphomas and *H pylori* may explain, in part, the rise in incidence.[126] The differentiation between adenocarcinoma and lymphoma can sometimes be difficult but is essential because staging, treatment, and prognosis are different for each disease.[127]

HISTOPATHOLOGY

Several staging schemas have been proposed based on the morphologic features of gastric tumors. The Borrmann classification divides gastric cancer into five types depending on macroscopic appearance. Type I represents polypoid or fungating cancers, type II encompasses ulcerating lesions surrounded by elevated borders, type III represents ulcerated lesions infiltrating the gastric wall, type IV are diffusely infiltrating tumors, and type V are unclassifiable cancers.[128] The gross morphologic appearance of gastric cancer and the degree of histologic differentiation are not independent prognostic variables.[129,130] Ming[130] has proposed a histomorphologic staging system that divides gastric cancer into either a prognostically favorable expansive type or a poor-prognosis infiltrating type. Based on an analysis of 171 gastric cancers, the expansive-type tumors were uniformly polypoid or superficial on gross appearance, whereas the infiltrative tumors were almost always diffuse. Grossly ulcerated lesions were equally divided between the expanding or infiltrative forms. Broder's classification of gastric cancer grades tumors histologically from 1 (well differentiated) to 4 (anaplastic). Bearzi and Ranaldi[131] have correlated the degree of histologic differentiation with the gross appearance of 41 primary gastric cancers seen on endoscopy. Ninety percent of protruding or superficial cancers were well differentiated (Broder's grade 1), whereas almost one-half of all ulcerated tumors were poorly differentiated or diffusely infiltrating (Broder's grades 3 and 4).

The most widely used classification of gastric cancer is by Lauren.[26] It divides gastric cancers into either intestinal or diffuse forms. This classification scheme, based on tumor histology, effectively characterizes two varieties of gastric adenocarcinomas that manifest distinctively different pathology, epidemiology, and etiologies. The intestinal variety represents a differentiated cancer with a tendency to form glands. In contrast, the diffuse form exhibits very little cell cohesion and has a predilection for extensive submucosal spread and early metastases. Although the diffuse-type cancers are generally associated with a worse outcome than the intestinal type, this finding is not independent of tumor, node, metastasis (TNM) stage.

PATTERNS OF SPREAD

Carcinomas of the stomach can spread by local extension to involve adjacent structures and can develop lymphatic metastases, peritoneal metastases, and distant metastases. These extensions can occur by the local invasive properties of the tumor, lymphatic spread, or hematogenous dissemination. The initial growth of the tumor occurs by penetration into the gastric wall, extension through the wall, and involvement of an increasing percentage of the stomach. The two modes of local extension that can have a major therapeutic impact are tumor penetration through the gastric serosa, where the risk of tumor invasion of adjacent structures or peritoneal spread is increased, and involvement of lymphatics. Zinninger[132] has evaluated the spread in the gastric wall and has found a wide variation in its extent. Tumor spread is often through the intramural lymphatics or in the subserosal layers. Local extension can also occur into the esophagus or the duodenum. Duodenal extension is principally through the muscular layer by direct infiltration and through the subserosal lymphatics, but is not generally of great extent. Extension into the esophagus occurs primarily through the submucosal lymphatics.

Local extension does not occur solely by radial intramural spread but also by deep invasion through the wall to involve adjacent structures. Extension can occur through the gastric serosa to involve omentum, spleen, adrenal gland, diaphragm, liver, pancreas, or colon. Data from several large older series indicated that 60% to 90% of patients had primary tumors penetrating the serosa or invading adjacent organs and that at least 50% had lymphatic metastases.[133,134] Of the 1577 primary gastric cancer cases admitted to Memorial Sloan-Kettering Cancer Center between July 1, 1985, and June 30, 1998, 60% of the 1221 resected cases had evidence of serosal penetration, and 68% had positive nodes. Lymph node metastases were found in 18% of pT1 lesions after R0 resection in 941 patients. This rate increased significantly to 60% in pT2 lesions. The highest inci-

TABLE 29.2-2. Pattern of Nodal Metastases from Gastric Cancer

	Upper Third (%)	Middle Third (%)	Lower Third (%)
Paracardia	22	9	4
Lesser or greater curvature	25	36	37
Right gastric artery/suprapyloric	2	3	12
Infrapyloric	3	15	49
Left gastric artery	19	22	23
Common hepatic artery	7	11	25
Celiac axis	13	8	13
Splenic artery/hilum	11	3	2
Hepatoduodenal ligament	1	2	8
Others	0–5	0–5	0–5

(Modified from ref. 335, with permission.)

dence of lymphatic metastasis was seen in tumors diffusely involving the entire stomach. Tumors located at the gastroesophageal junction also had a high incidence relative to other sites. The pattern of nodal metastases also varies depending on the location of the primary site (Table 29.2-2), with the left gastric artery nodes being consistently at increased risk for nodal metastases, regardless of tumor location.

Gastric cancer recurs in multiple sites, locoregionally and systemically (Table 29.2-3). The literature reveals disagreements over failure patterns (see Table 29.2-3); these disagreements are likely related to the patient cohorts accepted for evaluation, the time at which failure was determined, and the method of determination of failure patterns. In two older autopsy series, the rate of locoregional failure [defined as tumor in perigastric tissues (e.g., in the retroperitoneal "gastric bed," perigastric lymph nodes, gastric remnant)] after potentially curative resection was 40% to 80%.[135,136] Many patients had multiple sites of local failure. Shiu and coworkers[133] found a 23% local recurrence rate in 169 patients treated for carcinoma of the body of the stomach.

Gunderson and Sosin[137] reanalyzed the reoperation series performed by Wangensteen at the University of Minnesota, where patients had a second-look laparotomy after resection of the primary tumor. This type of analysis is valuable because it can demonstrate the early (and perhaps most treatable) modes of failure, rather than simply showing diffuse metastatic disease at autopsy. Sixty-nine percent of patients had evidence of a locoregional recurrence, and 42% had peritoneal seeding. Most of the local failures were located in the gastric bed (81%),

although recurrences also occurred in the anastomosis or stump (39%) or in the regional lymph nodes (63%). A trial from the British Stomach Cancer Group found the incidence of local failure in patients treated with surgery alone to be 37 of 69 (54%).[138] A series evaluating local failure patterns reported by Landry et al.[139] showed a total locoregional failure rate of 38%, with most of the local recurrences in the gastric bed, the anastomosis, or the gastric stump. The incidence of local failure increased when the primary disease extended through the gastric wall or when lymph nodes were involved at the initial surgery. Liver metastases occurred in 30% of patients and peritoneal seeding in 23%. Extraabdominal failure was relatively rare and occurred in 13% of patients.

Some newer series suggest a higher incidence of peritoneal seeding as a failure pattern. Wisbeck et al.[371] evaluated autopsy and clinical records of 85 patients who died of gastric cancer. Sixteen patients had a resection with curative intent; 15 of these developed a locoregional recurrence, 8 developed peritoneal seeding, and 7 developed lung metastases. Of the entire cohort, 40 of 85 (47%) developed peritoneal seeding. Ajani et al.[140] treated 25 patients with preoperative chemotherapy. At the time of surgery, eight had peritoneal carcinomatosis, and it developed subsequently in an additional five patients. Because imaging studies were not done routinely postoperatively, they could not accurately determine the risk of locoregional failure. These data suggest that increased attention to methods of controlling local and regional disease as well as systemic disease is needed to improve long-term results.

CLINICAL PRESENTATION AND PRETREATMENT EVALUATION

SIGNS AND SYMPTOMS

Because of the vague, nonspecific symptoms that characterize gastric cancer, most patients are diagnosed with advanced-stage disease. Patients may have a combination of signs and symptoms such as weight loss, anorexia, fatigue, or epigastric discomfort, none of which unequivocally indicates gastric cancer.

Weight loss is a common symptom, and its clinical significance should not be underestimated. Dewys and colleagues[141] found that, in 179 patients with advanced, nonmeasurable gastric cancer, more than 80% had a greater than 10% decrease in body weight before diagnosis. Furthermore, patients with weight loss had a significantly shorter survival than did those without weight loss.

TABLE 29.2-3. Recurrence Patterns after Primary Surgery for Gastric Cancer

Author (Y)	Analysis	Local-Regional	Peritoneal	Distant
Landry et al.[139] (1990)	130 pts—clinical	38% (49/130)	—	—
Gunderson and Sosin[137] (1982)	105 pts—surgery	69% (74/105)	42% (44/105)	—
Wisbeck[371] (1986)	145 pts—autopsy	94% (15/16)	50% (8/16)	44% liver, 13% lung
Roviello et al.[336] (2003)	441 pts—first site of failure	22%—lymph node, 11%; gastric bed/adjacent organs, 8%; gastric stump, 3%	17%	17%
Allum et al.[337] (1989)	145 pts—clinical	27%	—	22%

pts, patients.

In some patients, symptoms may suggest the presence of a lesion at a specific location. A history of dysphagia may indicate the presence of a tumor in the cardia with extension through the gastroesophageal junction. Early satiety is an infrequent symptom of gastric cancer but is indicative of a diffusely infiltrative tumor that has resulted in loss of distensibility of the gastric wall. Persistent vomiting is consistent with an antral carcinoma obstructing the pylorus. Significant gastrointestinal bleeding is uncommon with gastric cancer; however, hematemesis does occur in approximately 10% to 15% of patients. Ascites, jaundice, or a palpable mass indicates extensive and incurable disease. Signs and symptoms at presentation are often related to spread of disease. Because the transverse colon is held in proximity to the stomach by the gastrocolic ligament, the transverse colon is a potential site of malignant fistulization and obstruction from a gastric primary tumor. Diffuse peritoneal spread of disease frequently produces other sites of intestinal obstruction. A large ovarian mass (Krukenberg's tumor) or a large peritoneal implant in the pelvis (Blumer's shelf), which can produce symptoms of rectal obstruction, may be felt on pelvic or rectal examination. Nodular metastases in the subcutaneous tissue around the umbilicus or in peripheral lymph nodes represent areas in which a tissue diagnosis can be established with minimal morbidity.

SCREENING

Mass screening programs for gastric cancer have been most successful in high-risk areas, especially in Japan.[142] A variety of screening tests have been studied in Japanese patients, with a sensitivity and specificity of approximately 90%.[6] Screening typically includes the use of double-contrast barium radiographs or upper endoscopy.[6]

The yield in screened populations has been substantial; in some Japanese studies, up to 60% of patients actively participating in routine mass screening programs have the disease and up to 60% of newly diagnosed patients have early gastric cancer (EGC).[142] The latter is clinically important because, as discussed in Stage I Disease (Early Gastric Cancer), later in this chapter, EGC has a very high cure rate with surgical treatment. However, the fact that gastric cancer remains the number one cause of death in Japan indicates the limitations of a mass screening program when the entire population at risk is not effectively screened. Studies have verified that a low serum pepsinogen I/II ratio can be used to better select patients at increased risk for atrophic gastritis and gastric cancer.[143]

PRETREATMENT STAGING

Tumor Markers

The carcinoembryonic antigen (CEA) level is elevated in approximately one-third of patients with primary gastric cancer.[144] The sensitivity of CEA as a marker of gastric cancer is low, but when the CEA level is elevated, it generally correlates with stage. Combining CEA with other markers, such as the sialylated Lewis antigens CA19-9 or CA50, can increase sensitivity, compared with CEA alone.[145–147]

A large study of patients with gastric cancer evaluated the prognostic significance of serum levels of CEA (n = 237), α-fetoprotein (n = 164), human chorionic gonadotropin-β (β-HCG; n = 165), CA19-9 (n = 64), and CA125 (n = 104), as well

as tissue staining for C-erb B-2 (n = 160) and β-HCG (n = 160). In a multivariate analysis, only a serum β-HCG level of 4 IU/L or greater (hazard ratio, 1.7; 95% CI, 2.8 to 1.1) and a CA125 level of 350 U/mL or greater (hazard ratio, 2.2; 95% CI, 4.2 to 1.2) had prognostic significance. Elevated serum β-HCG and CA125 levels in gastric cancer before chemotherapy may reflect not just tumor burden but also aggressive biology; however, the utility of these markers in staging must be compared to that of other known preoperative markers of stage, such as on T- and N-stage endoscopic ultrasonography (EUS).[148]

Endoscopy

Endoscopy is generally considered to be the best method to diagnose gastric cancer. Endoscopy directly visualizes the gastric mucosa and allows biopsy of tissue for a histologic diagnosis.

EUS is presently available in many centers, and, although mainly used to further stage previously diagnosed tumors, it may be helpful in identifying early diffuse-type gastric carcinoma lesions that might otherwise be overlooked. EUS has the added capability to evaluate the deeper layers of the gastric wall to help define the T stage of the tumor and provide information on the morphologic status of surrounding lymph nodes. EUS has an accuracy of up to 90% for T staging of gastric tumors and 75% for N staging; these rates are higher than those for preoperative computed tomography (CT) scans.[149,150]

Computed Tomography

Once gastric cancer is suspected, CT of the abdomen and pelvis is an important part of the staging evaluation. Patients with Siewert type I or II tumors (see Siewert classification later in Classification of Esophagogastric Junction Cancers) should also undergo a chest CT.

CT is useful for noninvasive assessment of perigastric lymphadenopathy, peritoneal disease, and intraabdominal visceral (primary liver) metastatic disease and for estimation of the degree of tumor penetration through the gastric wall. With modern multiphase, multidetector spiral CT imaging, there is increased accuracy in the assessment of extragastric disease and mural penetration (particularly for T2 and greater tumors).[151,152] The accuracy of CT assessment of tumor location and T stage can be enhanced over that of conventional helical CT by use of water as an oral contrast agent—so called helical hydro-CT.[153,154]

Positron Emission Tomography

Whole body 2-[^{18}F]fluoro-2-deoxyglucose (FDG)–positron emission tomography (PET) is being applied increasingly in the evaluation of gastrointestinal malignancies. A relative paucity of data is available on the role of PET in the staging of gastric cancer. A few pilot studies of PET imaging for gastric cancer (all stages)[155] and the use of PET in the detection of recurrent disease have been reported.[156] The absence of meaningful data on PET for staging gastric cancer contrasts with esophageal cancer, for which PET has an increasingly well-defined role in pretreatment staging.

Important differences in tumor biology may limit the role for PET in gastric cancer. For example, the glucose transporter-1, an important transporter of FDG into tumor cells, is rarely present in common subtypes of gastric carcinoma, including signet-ring cell carcinoma and mucinous adenocarcinoma (2.0% and 6.3%, respectively).[157] This may contribute to false-negative FDG-PET imaging.[156] Interestingly, the presence of glucose transporter-1 and FDG-avid gastric cancers is associated with decreased overall survival.[156,157]

Laparoscopy

Staging laparoscopy has become an accepted part of the pretreatment staging evaluation of patients who are believed to have localized gastric cancer after initial helical CT assessment. The rationale for laparoscopic staging is based on the fact that sensitivity of CT for detection of extragastric disease declines with the size of metastases. Indeed, current CT techniques cannot consistently identify low-volume macroscopic metastases that are 5 mm or less in size. Laparoscopy allows for direct inspection of the peritoneal and visceral surfaces for detection of CT-occult small-volume metastases. Staging laparoscopy also allows for assessment of peritoneal cytology and intraperitoneal evaluation with adjunctive diagnostic techniques such as laparoscopic ultrasound (LUS). Patients who are found to have occult metastatic disease at laparoscopy are considered incurable, and the use of laparoscopy allows them to avoid laparotomy.

The rate of detection of CT-occult M1 disease by laparoscopy is dependent on the quality of CT scanning and interpretation. Studies from the 1990s (during which time there was inconsistent use of the more sensitive helical CT technique) demonstrated that CT-occult disease could be identified in 13% to 37% of patients.[158–160] It is likely that the yield of laparoscopy may be somewhat lower than this with more widespread use of higher-quality helical CT preliminary staging. Nonetheless, even high-quality helical CT is insufficiently sensitive for detection of low-volume extragastric disease, and, thus, laparoscopy, CT, and EUS are complementary staging studies.

A number of unresolved issues remain regarding the timing and extent of laparoscopy that should be performed for optimal staging. Laparoscopy can be performed as a separate staging procedure before definitive treatment planning or immediately before planned laparotomy for gastrectomy. When performed as a separate procedure, laparoscopy has the disadvantage of the additional risks and expense of a second general anesthetic. However, separate procedure laparoscopy allows the additional staging information acquired at laparoscopy to be reviewed and discussed with the patient and multidisciplinary treatment group before definitive treatment planning. This is important in some settings because laparoscopic staging findings that may alter therapeutic options and prognosis (e.g., peritoneal cytology) are not always available on a real-time basis during laparoscopy. Consequently, the timing of laparoscopy varies in different centers depending on factors such as the availability of intraoperative cytology assessment and the use of preoperative treatment approaches.

The extent of laparoscopic evaluation is another unresolved staging issue. LUS and "extended laparoscopy" are techniques that may increase the diagnostic yield of laparoscopy. LUS involves examination of the stomach, perigastric region, and peritoneal cavity using a laparoscopic ultrasound probe, whereas extended laparoscopy involves a more detailed laparoscopic examination of the perigastric region that includes laparoscopic examination of the lesser sac and retrogastric space (i.e., more than simple inspection of the stomach and peritoneal cavity). Preliminary results reveal conflicting data on the added benefit

of LUS and extended laparoscopy.[161–163] Further studies are required to evaluate the cost-benefit relationship of these advanced laparoscopic techniques to better define whether LUS and extended laparoscopy have a routine or selective role in patients undergoing conventional laparoscopic staging.

STAGING, CLASSIFICATION, AND PROGNOSIS

The uniform and accurate staging of gastric cancer is essential to predict prognosis and assess outcome meaningfully. For patients

TABLE 29.2-4. American Joint Committee on Cancer Staging of Gastric Cancer, 2002

Definition of TNM			
PRIMARY TUMOR (T)			
TX	Primary tumor cannot be assessed		
T0	No evidence of primary tumor		
Tis	Carcinoma *in situ*: intraepithelial tumor without invasion of the lamina propria		
T1	Tumor invades lamina propria or submucosa		
T2	Tumor invades muscularis propria or subserosa		
T2a	Tumor invades muscularis propria		
T2b	Tumor invades subserosa		
T3	Tumor penetrates serosa (visceral peritoneum) without invasion of adjacent structures		
T4	Tumor invades adjacent structures		
REGIONAL LYMPH NODES (N)			
NX	Regional lymph node(s) cannot be assessed		
N0	No regional lymph node metastasis		
N1	Metastasis in 1–6 regional lymph nodes		
N2	Metastasis in 7–15 regional lymph nodes		
N3	Metastases in more than 15 regional lymph nodes		
DISTANT METASTASIS (M)			
MX	Presence of distant metastasis cannot be assessed		
M0	No distant metastasis		
M1	Distant metastasis		
STAGE GROUPING			
O	Tis	N0	M0
IA	T1	N0	M0
IB	T1	N1	M0
	T2a/b	N0	M0
II	T1	N2	M0
	T2	N1	M0
	T3	N0	M0
IIIA	T2a/b	N2	M0
	T3	N1	M0
	T4	N0	M0
IIIB	T3	N2	M0
IV	T4	N1–3	M0
	T1–3	N3	M0
	Any T	Any N	M1

TNM, tumor, node, metastasis.
(From ref. 199, with permission.)

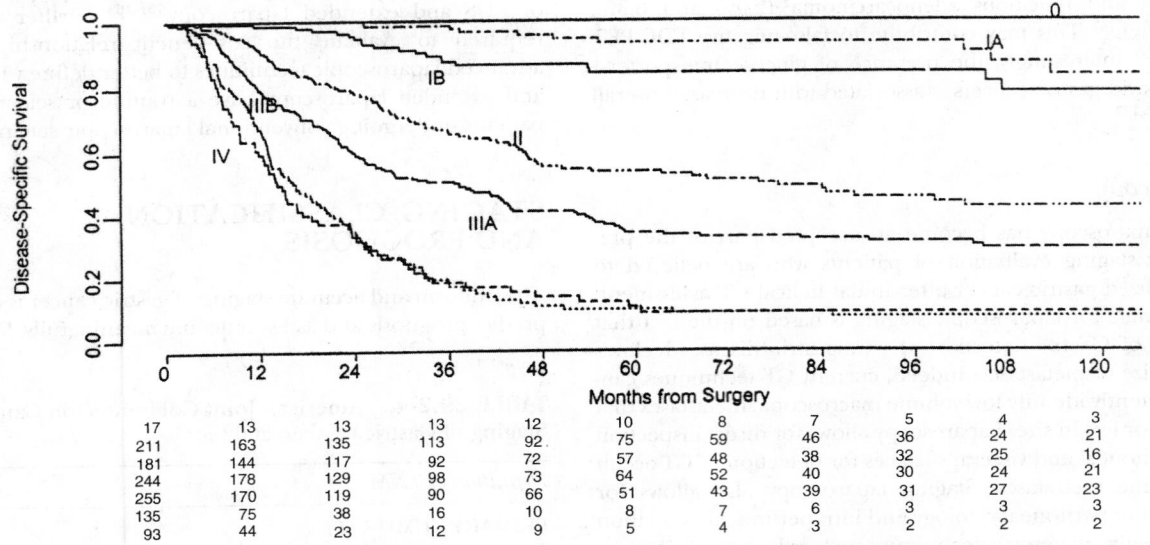

FIGURE 29.2-2.   Disease-specific survival by American Joint Committee on Cancer stage grouping. Numbers beneath x-axis indicate patients at risk. (From ref. 183, with permission.)

with surgically treated gastric adenocarcinoma, pathologic staging [American Joint Committee on Cancer/International Union Against Cancer (AJCC/UICC), or Japanese system] and classification of the completeness of resection (R) should be done. In addition, although not formal components of AJCC stage grouping, the histopathologic grade and type and, when available, the peritoneal lavage cytology status should be recorded. The latter is important because the presence of free peritoneal cancer cells has been shown by a number of investigators to carry a prognosis comparable to that of visceral metastatic disease.[164–166]

AMERICAN JOINT COMMITTEE ON CANCER/ INTERNATIONAL UNION AGAINST CANCER TUMOR, NODE, METASTASIS STAGING

The AJCC/UICC TNM staging system for gastric cancer is outlined in Table 29.2-4.[167] The AJCC/UICC stage-stratified sur-

vival rates of a cohort of 1039 patients treated by complete (R0) surgical resection at a single Western center are shown in Figure 29.2-2.

In the AJCC/UICC staging system, tumor (T) stage is determined by depth of tumor invasion into the gastric wall and extension into adjacent structures (Fig. 29.2-3). The relationship between T stage and survival is well defined (Fig. 29.2-4; Table 29.2-5).

Nodal stage (N) is based on the number of involved lymph nodes—a criterion that may predict outcome more accurately than the location of involved lymph nodes.[168,169] Tumors with 1 to 6 involved nodes are classified as pN1, 7 to 15 involved nodes as pN2, and more than 15 involved nodes as pN3. The use of numeric thresholds for nodal classification has become increasingly more accepted, although the extent of lymphadenectomy and rigor of pathologic assessment may affect results.[170] The threshold approach is based on observa-

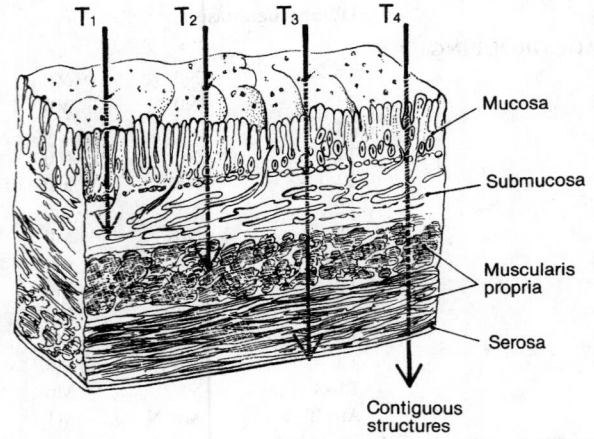

FIGURE 29.2-3.   Definition of American Joint Committee on Cancer/International Union Against Cancer T stage based on depth of penetration of the gastric wall.

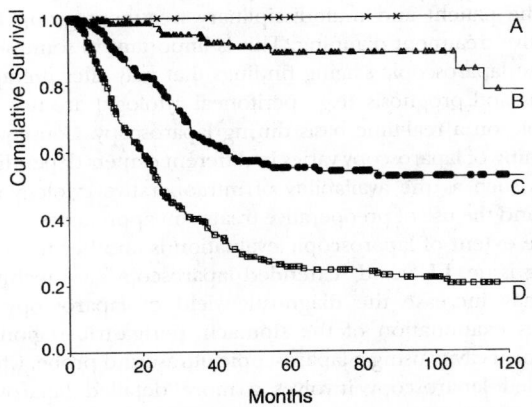

FIGURE 29.2-4.   Kaplan-Meier curves of disease-specific survival according to American Joint Committee on Cancer T stage. **A:** Tis (tumor *in situ;* n = 16). **B:** T1 (n = 168). **C:** T2 (n = 265). **D:** T3 (n = 464). T4 (not shown) (n = 28).

TABLE 29.2-5. Survival after Curative Resection for Gastric Cancer by TNM Stage

		5-Y Survival (%)					
		T1		T2		T3	T4
Study	Number of Patients	M	SM	PM	SS	SE	SI/SEI
Noguchi et al.[338] (Japan)	3143	94	87	75	51	23 (S2)	5
Maruyama et al.[335] (Japan)	3176	95	87	82	65	34 (S2)	14
Boku et al.[339] (Japan)	238	—	—	90	—	42 (S2)	29
Baba et al.[340] (Japan)	142	—	—	55	—	34	32
Hermanek[182] (Germany)	977	84	75	73	40	24	25
Shiu et al.[341] (United States)	246	—	—		56	32	—
Bozzetti et al.[342] (Italy)	361	82	69	38		—	—
MSKCC[169] (United States)	944		91		56	26	—

M, mucosa; MSKCC, Memorial Sloan-Kettering Cancer Center; PM, muscularis propria; S2, serosal invasion; SE, cancer cells exposed to the peritoneal cavity; SEI, the coexistence of SE and SI; SI, cancer cells infiltrating neighboring tissue; SM, submucosa; SS, subserosa, TNM, tumor, node, metastasis.

tions that survival decreases as the number of metastatic lymph nodes increases[169,171] and that there are decreases in survival at four or more involved[172,173] and again at seven or more involved lymph nodes.[168,174] Given the reliance on numeric thresholds for nodal staging, it is extremely important that surgeons and pathologists work together to ensure that adequate numbers of lymph nodes are retrieved and examined. Indeed, reports document poor compliance with AJCC staging primarily because the numbers of lymph nodes removed or examined, or both, were insufficient (15 or less).[175,176]

Ratio-based lymph node classification is an alternative to the threshold-based system currently used for AJCC/UICC staging. This alternative approach may minimize the confounding effects of regional variations in the extent of lymphadenectomy and in pathologic evaluation of the lymphadenectomy specimen on lymph node staging and thereby reduce the impact of stage migration. Several reports have evaluated ratio-based lymph node staging.[167,170,177,178] Bando et al.[177] evaluated the ratio of metastatic to uninvolved lymph nodes (RML) in a group of 650 patients who underwent R0 gastrectomy with D2 lymph node dissection. The anatomic location, number of positive lymph nodes (as used in the current AJCC/UICC system), and RML were analyzed for staging accuracy and relationship to patient survival. RML was found to be an independent prognostic factor for survival and reduced the frequency of stage migration from 15% (when numeric thresholds were used for staging) to 7%. These findings were confirmed in a separate analysis of 1019 patients treated by R0 gastrectomy at Kansai Medical University in Japan.[178] On the basis of these reports, ratio-based lymph node staging should be considered for future versions of gastric cancer staging systems.

JAPANESE STAGING SYSTEM

The most recent Japanese Classification for Gastric Carcinoma was published in 1998.[179] The Japanese classification and staging system are more detailed than the AJCC/UICC staging system and place more emphasis on the distinction between clinical, surgical, pathologic, and "final" staging (prefixes "c," "s," "p," and "f," respectively). For example, a surgically treated and staged patient with locally advanced, nonmetastatic gastric cancer might be staged as pT3, pN2, sH0, sM0, f stage IIIB (where

H0 denotes no hepatic metastases and the "f" prefix denotes final clinicopathologic stage). The Japanese classification system also includes a classification system for EGC [Fig. 29.2-5; see Stage I Disease (Early Gastric Cancer), later in this chapter].

Similar to the AJCC/UICC staging system, primary tumor (T) stage in the Japanese system is based on the depth of invasion and extension to adjacent structures, as outlined in Table 29.2-6. However, the assignment of lymph node (N) stage involves much more rigorous pathologic assessment than is required for AJCC/UICC staging. The Japanese system extensively classifies 18 lymph node regions into four N categories depending on their relationship to the primary tumor and anatomic location.[179] Most perigastric lymph nodes (nodal stations 1 to 6) are considered group 1. Lymph nodes situated along the proximal left gastric artery (station 7), common hepatic artery (8), celiac axis (9), splenic artery (11), and proper hepatic artery (12) are defined as group 2. Paraaortic lymph nodes (16) are defined as group 3. The presence or absence of pathologically positive lymph nodes in each lymph node group is reflected in the assigned N stage.

Subtypes of Type 0

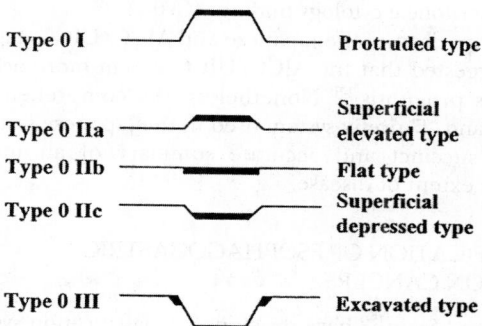

FIGURE 29.2-5. Japanese classification system for early gastric cancer. *Notes*: In the combined superficial types, the type occupying the largest area should be described first, followed by the next type, for example, IIc + III. Type 0 I and type 0 IIa are distinguished as follows: Type 0 I: The lesion has a thickness of more than twice that of the normal mucosa. Type 0 IIa: The lesion has a thickness up to twice that of the normal mucosa. (From ref. 179, with permission.)

TABLE 29.2-6. Japanese Gastric Cancer Association Staging System for Gastric Cancer

TUMOR STAGE (T)

T1	Tumor invasion of mucosa and/or muscularis mucosa (M) or submucosa (SM)
T2	Tumor invasion of muscularis propria (MP) or subserosa (SS)
T3	Tumor penetration of serosa (SE)
T4	Tumor invasion of adjacent structures (SI)
TX	Unknown

NODAL STAGE (N)

N0	No evidence of lymph node metastasis
N1	Metastasis to group 1 lymph nodes but no metastasis to groups 2 to 3 lymph nodes
N2	Metastasis to group 2 lymph nodes but no metastasis to group 3 lymph nodes
N3	Metastasis to group 3 lymph nodes
NX	Unknown

HEPATIC METASTASIS STAGE (H)

H0	No liver metastasis
H1	Liver metastasis
HX	Unknown

PERITONEAL METASTASIS STAGE (P)

P0	No peritoneal metastasis
P1	Peritoneal metastasis
PX	Unknown

PERITONEAL CYTOLOGY STAGE (CY)

CY0	Benign/indeterminate cells on peritoneal cytology
CY1	Cancer cells on peritoneal cytology
CYX	Peritoneal cytology was not performed

OTHER DISTANT METASTASIS (M)

M0	No other distant metastases (although peritoneal, liver, or cytologic metastases may be present)
M1	Distant metastases other than the peritoneal, liver, or cytologic metastases
MX	Unknown

STAGE GROUPING

	N0	N1	N2	N3
T1				
T2	IA	IB	II	
T3	IB	II	IIIA	
T4	II	IIIA	IIIB	IV
H1, P1, CY1, M1	IIIA	IIIB		

Note: Cytology believed to be "suspicious for malignancy" should be classified as CY0.
(From ref. 179, with permission.)

The Japanese staging system also includes elements not included in the AJCC/UICC system (see Table 29.2-6). These are macroscopic description of the tumor (EGC subtype or Borrmann type for more advanced tumors), extent of peritoneal metastases (classified as P0-1), extent of hepatic metastases (H0-1), and peritoneal cytology findings (CY0-1).[179]

A comparison of the Japanese and AJCC/UICC staging systems suggested that the AJCC/UICC system more accurately estimates prognosis.[170] Nonetheless, the comprehensive "c," "s," "p," and "f" prefix system used in the Japanese system provides a succinct and accurate summary of an individual patient's extent of disease.

CLASSIFICATION OF ESOPHAGOGASTRIC JUNCTION CANCERS

Siewert and Stein[180] have developed a classification system for adenocarcinoma of the esophagogastric junction. Now commonly referred to as the *Siewert classification*, this system recognizes three distinct clinical entities that arise within 5 cm of the junction of the tubular esophagus and the stomach:

Type 1—adenocarcinoma of the distal esophagus, which usually arises from an area with specialized intestinal metaplasia of the esophagus (i.e., Barrett's esophagus) and may infiltrate the esophagogastric junction from above

Type II—adenocarcinoma of the cardia, which arises from the epithelium of the cardia or from short segments with intestinal metaplasia at the esophagogastric junction

Type III—adenocarcinoma of the subcardial stomach, which may infiltrate the esophagogastric junction or distal esophagus from below

The assignment of tumors to one of these subtypes is based on morphology and the anatomic location of the epicenter of the tumor. Classification can be performed based on the results of contrast radiography, endoscopy, CT, and operative findings. The Siewert classification system has been endorsed by the International Society for Diseases of the Esophagus and the International Gastric Cancer Association.

The Siewert classification has important therapeutic implications.[181] The lymphatic drainage routes differ for type 1 versus type II and III lesions. As shown on lymphographic studies, the lymphatic pathways from the lower esophagus pass cephalad (into the mediastinum) and caudad (toward the celiac axis). In contrast, the lymphatic drainage from the cardia and subcardial regions is toward the celiac axis, splenic hilus, and paraaortic nodes. Thus, the Siewert classification provides a practical means

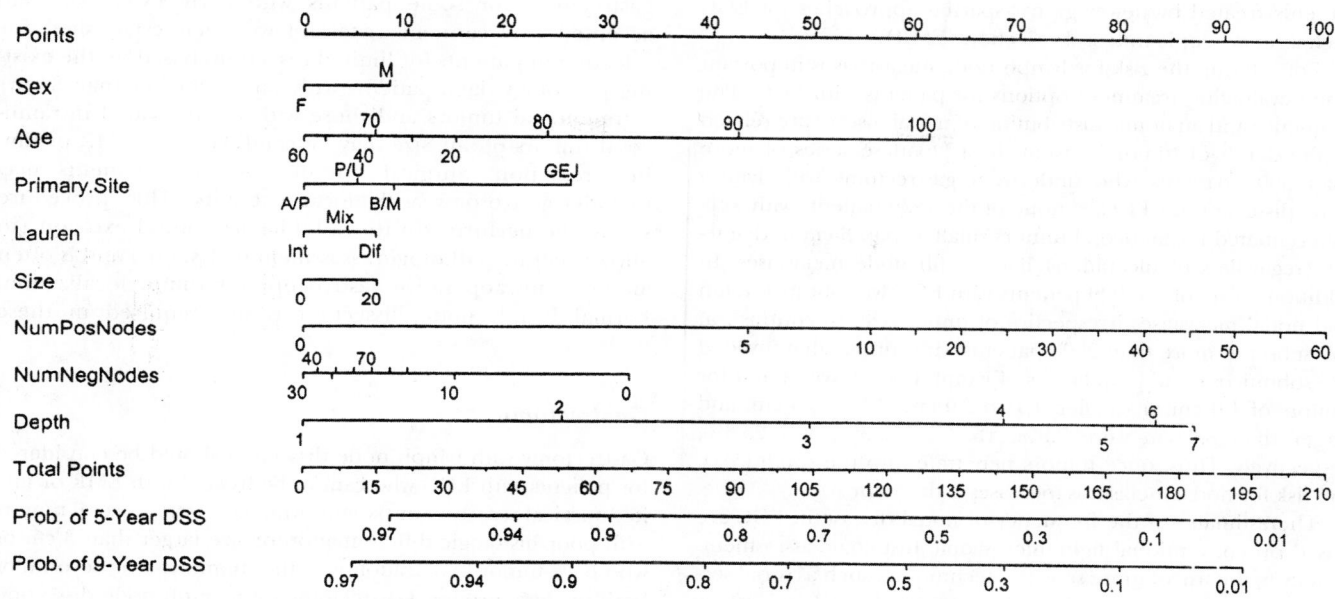

FIGURE 29.2-6. Nomogram for disease-specific survival (DSS). Instructions for physician: Locate the patient's sex on the **Sex** axis. Draw a line straight upward to the **Points** axis to determine how many points toward gastric cancer–specific death the patient received for his or her sex. Sum the points achieved for each predictor, and locate this sum on the **Total Points** axis. Draw a line straight down to the disease-specific survival axes to find the patient's probability of surviving gastric cancer, assuming he or she does not die of another cause first. A/P, antrum or pyloric; B/M, body or middle one-third, Dif, diffuse; GEJ, gastroesophageal junction; int, intestinal; mix, mixed; NumPosNodes, number of positive nodes; NumNegNodes, number of negative nodes; Prob.; probability; P/U, proximal or upper one-third. (From ref. 183, with permission.)

for choosing among surgical options. For type I tumors, esophagectomy is required, whereas type II and III tumors can be treated by transabdominal extended gastrectomy (resection of the stomach and distal intraabdominal esophagus).[181]

R CLASSIFICATION

The R classification system indicates the amount of residual disease left after tumor resection.[182] R0 indicates no gross or microscopic residual disease; R1 indicates microscopic residual disease, and R2 signifies gross residual disease. The R classification has implications for individual patient care and clinical research. Surgeons should wait for the final pathology results before completing their operative summaries so that patient records include the R classification for the gastrectomy. Results of clinical trials that include surgery should include information on R status.

Readers should be aware of the dual use of the "R" terminology in the gastric cancer literature. Before 1995, the Japanese staging and treatment descriptive vernacular included an "R level," which described the extent of lymphadenectomy according to the highest echelon of lymph nodes included in the lymphadenectomy. The latter is now classified by "D" (for dissection) level. Care should be exercised in current use of the R classification, restricting such use to describe the completeness of resection (R0-2).

PREDICTING INDIVIDUAL PATIENT PROGNOSIS

Kattan et al.[183] have developed a nomogram for estimating 5-year disease-specific survival using established prognostic factors derived from a population of 1039 gastric cancer patients

treated by R0 surgical resection at a single institution (Fig. 29.2-6). Clinicopathologic factors incorporated in the nomogram include patient age and gender, primary tumor site, Lauren classification, tumor size and depth, and the numbers of positive and negative lymph nodes. For patients with surgically treated gastric carcinoma, the nomogram estimates the probability of individual (i.e., personal) survival unencumbered by specific knowledge of prognostic factors, relative risk, or the risk group in which he/she may belong. This tool may be useful for individual patient counseling, follow-up scheduling, and clinical trial eligibility assessment and is available for personal hand-held computer devices at http://www.nomograms.org.

TREATMENT OF LOCALIZED DISEASE

STAGE I DISEASE (EARLY GASTRIC CANCER)

Classification of Early Gastric Cancer and Risk for Nodal Metastases

The Japanese Research Society for Gastric Cancer has classified EGC based on endoscopic criteria first established by the Japanese Endoscopy Society for the description of T1 tumors. The current classification system is used for *in situ* and invasive tumors and categorizes tumors based on endoscopic findings as follows: protruded, type 0 I; superficial elevated, type 0 IIa; flat, type 0 IIb; superficial depressed, type 0 IIc; and excavated, type 0 III.[179] The English-language version of the Japanese EGC classification contains excellent color photos of these subtypes.[179] This classification system is important in describing patients treated by newer gastric-sparing approaches for EGC such as endoscopic mucosal resection (EMR).

Considering the risk for lymph node metastasis is important when evaluating treatment options for patients with EGC. The frequency and anatomic distribution of nodal disease are related to the depth of tumor invasion. In a Japanese series of more than 5000 patients who underwent gastrectomy with lymph node dissection for EGC,[184] none of the 1230 patients with well-differentiated intramucosal tumors smaller than 3 cm in diameter (regardless of ulceration) had lymph node metastases. In addition, none of the 929 patients with EGC without ulceration had nodal metastases irrespective of tumor size. In contrast, in the subset of more than 2000 patients with tumors that invaded the submucosa, the frequencies of lymph node involvement for tumors of 1.0 cm or smaller, 1.1 to 2.0 cm, 2.1 to 3.0 cm, and larger than 3.0 cm were 7.9%, 13.3%, 15.55%, and 23.3%, respectively. Thus, once tumors penetrate into the submucosa, the risk for nodal metastasis increases with tumor size.

The estimates of the frequency of nodal disease in EGC are based on conventional light-microscopic histologic assessment. However, the use of more sensitive techniques, such as serial sectioning of individual lymph nodes, immunohistochemistry, or reverse transcriptase–polymerase chain reaction, may increase the frequency of detection of occult micrometastatic disease.[185] The clinical significance of micrometastases is unknown. Treatment options for patients with EGC include EMR, limited surgical resection, and gastrectomy.

Endoscopic Mucosal Resection

A subset of patients with EGC can undergo an R0 resection (see R Classification, earlier in this chapter) without lymphadenectomy or gastrectomy. The Japanese have popularized EMR for EGC. This approach involves the submucosal injection of fluid to elevate the lesion and facilitate complete mucosal resection under endoscopic guidance. Most centers reporting significant experience with EMR are in Japan (Table 29.2-7) owing primarily to the relative preponderance of EGC in Japan and the technical proficiency of many endoscopists in academic centers there. In Western countries, there is less experience with EMR.

Only patients with tumors that have extremely low metastatic potential should be offered EMR.[186,187] These are generally well-differentiated, superficial type IIa or IIc lesions smaller than 3 cm in diameter and located in an easily manipulated area. Tumors invading the submucosa are at increased risk for metastasizing to lymph nodes and are not usually considered candidates for EMR.

As illustrated in Table 29.2-7, complete resection of selected EGCs can be accomplished in a majority of cases (73.4%). Emerging variations of EMR techniques include the cap suction and cut versus a ligating device. Most EMRs use the saline lift technique. EMR-related complication rates including bleeding and perforation have been extremely low in most studies. As outcome studies accumulate demonstrating favorable survival, EMR is emerging as the definitive management of selected EGCs and is not just reserved for patients in whom gastrectomy cannot be considered.

Limited Surgical Resection

Given the low rate of nodal involvement for patients with EGC, limited resection may be a reasonable alternative to gastrectomy for some patients with early EGC. No well-accepted pretreatment criteria have been established for selection of patients for limited resection. Based on the existing pathology data, patients with small (smaller than 3 cm) intramucosal tumors and those with nonulcerated intramucosal tumors of any size may be candidates for EMR or limited resection. Surgical options for these patients may include gastrotomy with local excision. This procedure should be performed with full-thickness mural excision (to allow accurate pathologic assessment of T status) and is often aided by intraoperative gastroscopy for tumor localization. Formal lymph node dissection is not required in these patients.

Gastrectomy

Gastrectomy with lymph node dissection should be considered for patients with EGC who cannot be treated with EMR or limited surgical resection or patients who have intramucosal tumors with poor histologic differentiation or size larger than 3 cm or who have tumor penetration into the submucosa or beyond, or both of these groups. Gastrectomy with lymph node dissection allows for adequate pathologic staging and local therapy for these higher-risk patients.

No consensus has been reached on the extent of lymphadenectomy that should be performed as part of gastrectomy for EGC. Dissection of level I lymph nodes is a reasonable minimum standard at this time. The roles for nodal "sampling" without formal node dissection (D0 dissection) and sentinel lymph node (SLN) biopsy in the treatment of EGC remain undefined at this time (see Sentinel Lymph Node Biopsy, later in the chapter).

STAGE II AND STAGE III DISEASE

Surgery

Surgical resection is the cornerstone of treatment for patients with localized gastric cancer; indeed, surgical resection can be curative in most patients with EGC. However, for stage II and III disease, surgery is necessary but often not sufficient for cure. The general therapeutic goal is to achieve a micro- and macroscopically complete resection (R0). A complete discussion of all the technical details of gastric resection and reconstruction is beyond the scope of this chapter. However, specific surgical issues believed to be of oncologic significance are addressed in the following sections, including the extent of gastrectomy, extent of lymph node dissection, and role of partial pancreatectomy and splenectomy. Additional technical details and description of the operative procedures for gastric cancer can be found in surgical atlases.[188,189]

EXTENT OF RESECTION FOR MID AND DISTAL GASTRIC CANCERS. The extent of gastrectomy required for satisfactory primary tumor treatment depends mostly on the gross and microscopic status of surgical margins. For most clinical situations, a 5-cm grossly negative margin around the tumor and microscopically negative surgical margins (R0) are the treatment goals. When gastrectomy is performed with curative intent, frozen-section assessment of proximal and distal resec-

TABLE 29.2-7. Selected Clinical Series of Endoscopic Mucosal Resection for Patients with Early Gastric Cancer

Study	n	Indications	Method (%)					% Resection		Resectability (%)		Complications	
			2CS	ICS	EMRC	EMRL	Injection	En Bloc	Piecemeal	Complete	Incomplete	Bleeding	Perforation
Takekoshi et al.[343]	308	S	308	—	—	—	No	266	42	74.0	26.0	—	—
Tani et al.[344]	86	S	—	—	86	—	HSE	53	33	97.7	2.3	10	3
Chonan et al.[345]	123	S	46	31	46	—	Saline	—	—	69.9	30.1	0-3	0-1-2
Fujisaki et al.[346]	187	S	—	—	—	187	HSE	—	—	61.5	38.5	—	—
Misaka et al.[347]	115	El ≤30 mm Dep ≤20 mm	115	—	—	—	HSE	—	—	47.0	53.0	—	—
Honmyo et al.[348]	62	S	62	—	—	—	Saline	44	18	69.4	30.6	—	—
Tada et al.[349]	599	S	599	—	—	—	Saline	—	—	70.3	29.7	—	—
Abe and Ihto[350]	60	S	25	35	—	—	Saline	—	—	61.7	38.3	—	—
Hiki[351]	48	S	48	—	—	—	Saline	—	—	70.8	29.2	—	—
O-izumi et al.[352]	256	Dep ≤20 mm UI– ≤10 mm UI+	256	—	—	—	No	—	—	90.6	9.4	3	1
Atsumi et al.[353]	113	S + CIS	113	—	—	—	Saline	—	—	62.8	37.2	—	—
Takahashi et al.[354]	140	S + CIS	140	—	—	—	Saline	85	55	77.1	22.9	9	2
Kojima et al.[355]	185	S + CIS	185	—	—	—	Saline	99	86	78.9	21.1	9	2
Ono et al.[356]	479	S + diam ≤30 mm	479[a]	—	—	—	Unknown	—	—	69.0	31.0	—	25
Sakai et al.[357]	341	S	341	—	—	—	Unknown	341	0	84.5	14.4	—	—
Total	3102	—	2532 (81.6)	66 (2.1)	132 (4.3)	187 (6.0)	—	888 (28.6)	234 (7.5)	2278 (73.4)	820 (26.4)	34 (1.1)	36 (1.2)

CIS, contraindication for surgery; ICS, 1-channel scope; 2CS, 2-channel scope; Dep, depressed; diam, diameter; El, elevated; n, number of cases; EMRC, cap-fitted endoscopic mucosal resection; EMRL, ligating device endoscopic mucosal resection; HSE, hypertonic saline epinephrine; S, standard.
[a]Needle-knife technique was used in an unspecified small minority of the cases in this series.
(Modified from ref. 355.)

tion margins should be used intraoperatively to improve the likelihood that an R0 resection has been performed.

Three relatively small, prospective randomized controlled trials (RCTs) have compared total gastrectomy to partial (subtotal) gastrectomy for distal gastric cancer.[190–192] Overall morbidity, mortality, and oncologic outcome were comparable in each of these RCTs. As a result, when the general oncologic goal of an R0 resection can be achieved by a gastric-preserving approach, partial gastrectomy is preferred over total gastrectomy. This is particularly relevant for distal gastric cancers, for which a gastric-preserving R0 approach may minimize the risks of specific sequelae of total gastrectomy, such as early satiety, weight loss, and the need for vitamin B_{12} supplementation.

EXTENT OF RESECTION FOR PROXIMAL GASTRIC CANCER. Many choices are available for surgical management of adenocarcinomas arising at the esophagogastric junction or in the proximal stomach (Siewert types II and III). Many abdominal surgeons have advocated transabdominal approaches with resection of the lower esophagus and proximal stomach or total gastrectomy. Surgeons trained in thoracic surgery have frequently advocated a combined abdominal and thoracic procedure (often termed *esophagogastrectomy*), with an intrathoracic or cervical anastomosis between the proximal esophagus and the distal stomach, or a procedure termed *transhiatal* (or blunt) *esophagectomy* (THE), which involves resection of the esophagus and gastroesophageal junction, with mediastinal dissection performed in a blunt fashion through the esophageal hiatus of the diaphragm. When THE is performed for adenocarcinoma of the esophagogastric junction, gastrointestinal continuity is restored by low cervical anastomosis of the stomach (usually advanced through the esophageal bed in the mediastinum) to the low cervical esophagus. Selection among the options has been dependent primarily on individual surgeon training and experience.

The optimal surgical procedure for patients with localized tumors of the esophagogastric junction and proximal stomach is a matter of considerable debate. A Dutch RCT compared transthoracic esophagogastrectomy (TTEG, with abdominal and thoracic incisions) to THE in 220 patients with adenocarcinoma of the esophagus and esophagogastric junction.[193] Although this trial was designed for patients with esophageal cancer, 40 (18%) of the patients had adenocarcinomas of the esophagogastric junction (Siewert type II), and the operations evaluated are among those considered for patients with Siewert type II or III cancers. Perioperative morbidity was higher after THE, but there was no significant difference in in-hospital mortality compared to TTEG. Although median overall, disease-free, and quality-adjusted survival did not differ significantly between the groups, there was a trend toward improved overall survival at 5 years with TTEG. These results are believed to be equivocal,[194] and there is currently no consensus on the optimal surgical approach for patients with Siewert type II tumors. Until longer follow-up of the Dutch trial is available or additional RCTs are performed, or both, the surgical approach to these patients will continue to be individualized—determined by a constellation of factors, including surgeon factors (training and experience), patient factors (age, comorbidity, and performance status), and tumor factors (pretreatment T and N stage).

EXTENT OF LYMPHADENECTOMY. The dialogue surrounding lymphadenectomy involves at least two important issues:

(1) staging—removal and histopathologic analysis of an "adequate" number of lymph nodes, and (2) therapy—are some forms of lymphadenectomy therapeutic for patients with gastric cancer? These issues are too complex to review in detail here but have been addressed in many reviews.[195–197]

Single-institution reports suggest that the number of pathologically positive lymph nodes is of prognostic significance[174,198] and that removal and pathologic analysis of at least 15 lymph nodes are required for adequate pathologic staging.[169] Indeed, the current AJCC staging system (6th edition) accounts for these issues and therefore requires analysis of 16 or more lymph nodes to assign a pathologic N stage.[199] The multidisciplinary clinical correlates of this are obvious: (1) Surgeons must perform an adequate lymphadenectomy, and (2) pathologists must retrieve and examine at least 16 lymph nodes to provide optimal pathologic staging.

The possible therapeutic benefit of extended lymph node dissection has been the focus of four RCTs, which are summarized in Table 29.2-8.[190,200–202] These trials were performed because retrospective[203,204] and prospective nonrandomized[205] evidence suggested that extended lymph node dissection may be associated with improved long-term survival. The RCTs tested the hypothesis that removal of additional pathologically positive lymph nodes (not generally removed as part of a standard lymph node dissection) improves survival. The larger RCTs attempted to follow what are referred to as the *Japanese rules* for lymph node classification and dissection[206] that govern the extent of nodal dissection required based on anatomic location of the primary tumor. Using these Japanese definitions, the RCTs compared limited lymphadenectomy of the perigastric lymph nodes (D1 dissection) to *en bloc* removal of second-echelon lymph nodes (D2 dissection). At least two of the trials[190,200] are underpowered for their primary end point—overall survival. The most recent trials from the Medical Research Council (MRC) of the United Kingdom[201] and the Dutch Gastric Cancer Group[202] have received the most attention and discussion.

The MRC trial registered 737 patients with gastric adenocarcinoma; 337 (46%) patients were ineligible by staging laparotomy because of advanced disease, and 400 (54%) were randomized at the time of laparotomy to undergo D1 or D2 lymph node dissections. Postoperative morbidity was significantly greater (46% vs. 28%; $P < .001$), and in-hospital mortality was significantly higher in the D2 group than in the D1 group (13% vs. 6%, $P < .04$; 95% CI for D2, 4% to 11%).[207] The excess morbidity and mortality seen in the D2 group was thought to be related to the routine use of distal (left) pancreatectomy and splenectomy. Partial pancreatectomy and splenectomy were performed to maximize clearance of lymph nodes at the splenic hilum—primarily for patients with proximal tumors; however, many surgeons now believe that adequate lymph node dissection can be performed with pancreas- and spleen-preserving techniques. Long-term follow-up analysis of patients in the MRC trial demonstrated comparable 5-year overall survival rates of 35% and 33% in the D1 and D2 dissection groups, respectively (difference, –2%; 95% CI, –12% to 8%). Survival based on death from gastric cancer as the event was also similar in the D1 and D2 groups (hazard ratio = 1.05; 95% CI, 0.79 to 1.39), as was recurrence-free survival (hazard ratio = 1.03; 95% CI, 0.82 to 1.29).[201] The authors concluded that classic Japanese-style D2 lymphadenectomy (with partial pancreatectomy and splenectomy) offered no survival advantage over D1 lymphadenectomy.

TABLE 29.2-8.   Prospective Randomized Trials Comparing D1 versus D2–3 Resection for Potentially Curable Gastric Carcinoma

	Extent of Lymphadenectomy		
	D1	D2	P Value
GROOTE SCHUUR HOSPITAL, CAPE TOWN[200]			
Number of patients	22	21	—
Length of operation (h)	1.7 ± 0.6	2.33 ± 0.7	<.005
Transfusions (units/group)	4	25	<.05
Postoperative stay (d)	9.3 ± 4.7	13.9 ± 9.7	<.05
5-Y survival (log rank test)	0.69	0.67	NS
PRINCE OF WALES HOSPITAL, HONG KONG[190]			
Number of patients	25	29	—
Length of operation (h)	140	260	<.05
Operative blood loss (mL)	300	600	<.05
Postoperative stay	8	16	<.05
Median survival (d)	1511	922	<.05
MEDICAL RESEARCH COUNCIL TRIAL, UNITED KINGDOM[201,207]			
Number of patients	200	200	—
Operative mortality (%)	6.5	13	<.04
Postoperative complications (%)	28	46	<.001
5-Y survival (%)	35	33	NS
DUTCH GASTRIC CANCER TRIAL, THE NETHERLANDS[202]			
Number of patients	380	331	—
Operative mortality rate (%)	4	10	.004
Postoperative complications (%)	25	43	<.001
Postoperative stay (d)	18	25	<.001
5-Y survival (%)	42	47	NS

NS, not stated.

The Dutch Gastric Cancer Group conducted a larger RCT with optimal surgical quality control comparing D1 to D2 lymph node dissection for patients with gastric adenocarcinoma; 996 patients were registered, and 711 (71%) were randomized to D1 dissection (n = 380) or D2 dissection (n = 331). To maximize surgical quality control, all operations were monitored.[208] Initially, this oversight was done by a Japanese surgeon who trained a group of Dutch surgeons; they, in turn, acted as supervisors during surgery at 80 participating centers. Notwithstanding the extraordinary efforts to ensure quality control of the two types of lymph node dissection, noncompliance (not removing all lymph node stations) and contamination (removing more than was indicated) occurred, blurring the distinction between the two operations and confounding the interpretation of the oncologic end points.[209] The postoperative morbidity was higher in the D2 group (43% vs. 25%, *P* <.001), and the mortality was also significantly higher in the D2 group (10% vs. 4%, *P* = .004). Patients treated with D2 dissection also required a longer hospitalization.[210] As in the MRC trial, partial pancreatectomy and splenectomy were performed *en passant* in the D2 group. Five-year survival rates were similar in the two groups: 45% for the D1 group and 47% for the D2 group (95% CI for the difference, –9.6% to 5.6%). The subset of patients who had R0 resections, excluding those who died postoperatively, had cumulative risks of relapse at 5 years of 43% with D1 dissection and 37% with D2 dissection (95% CI for the difference, –2.4% to 14.4%). The Dutch investigators concluded that there was no role for the routine use of D2 lymph node dissection in patients with gastric cancer.

Interpretation of the existing level 1 evidence is encumbered by a number of issues that have been discussed in detail elsewhere.[196,197] The primary concerns relate to whether (1) the increased operative mortality associated with protocol-mandated partial pancreatectomy and splenectomy for patients with proximal tumors undergoing D2 dissection prevented identification of a potential therapeutic impact of extended lymph node dissection, and (2) the phenomena of noncompliance and contamination led to homogenization of the operative procedures to such an extent that the fundamental hypothesis was not tested. Owing to these interpretation issues, the question of a possible therapeutic benefit of D2 dissection remains unsettled, and additional RCTs are under way in Italy and Taiwan.

Many Japanese gastric surgeons have considered the caveats associated with the MRC and Dutch trials and believe that, notwithstanding inherent patient selection and stage migration biases,[196,209] the existing retrospective data provide sufficient proof of a clinical benefit of D2 dissection. On this basis, D2 dissection has been adopted as the standard of care for patients with localized, higher-risk gastric cancer in many centers in Japan and some specialized centers in the West.[211] In Japan, the Japan Clinical Oncology Group (JCOG) has investigated an even more aggressive surgical approach in an RCT evaluating paraaortic lymphadenectomy in the management of completely resected (R0) T2 to T4 gastric cancer. Between July 1995 and April 2001, 523 patients from 25 institutions were registered. Patients were randomized intraoperatively to undergo D2 lymphadenectomy alone or D2 lymphadenectomy plus paraaortic lymph node dissection (D3). The primary end point is overall survival; only preliminary morbidity and mortality results have been reported.[372] The patients treated with D3 dissection had longer operation times, greater blood loss, and a higher frequency of blood transfusion than did the group that underwent D2 dissection. However, the groups had no significant differences in postoperative complications, and only two patients (0.8%, one in each group) died of postoperative complications. These findings demonstrate that the addition of paraaortic lymph node dissection to D2 dissection in Japanese patients does not significantly increase the rate of postoperative morbidity or mortality. Preliminary analysis of overall survival is scheduled for late 2004.

PARTIAL PANCREATECTOMY AND SPLENECTOMY: RESECT OR PRESERVE? Partial (left, distal) pancreatectomy and splenectomy have been performed as part of D2 lymph node dissection to remove the lymph nodes along the splenic artery (station 11) and at the splenic hilum (station 12)—primarily for patients with tumors located in the proximal and mid stomach. Indeed, partial pancreatectomy and splenectomy were required for patients with proximal tumors in the D2 arm of the Dutch and MRC RCTs but were required only for direct tumor extension in the D1 arm. A summary of the association between splenectomy and operative morbidity, early surgical mortality, and long-term survival are provided in Table 29.2-9. Splenectomy is associated with an increased risk for surgical complications and postoperative death. In addition, a multivariate analysis suggested that splenectomy is associated with inferior long-term survival. The frequent performance of splenectomy (e.g., 30% of patients in the D2 arm vs. 3% in the D1 arms of the Dutch trial) with its associated adverse effects on short- and long-term mortality confounds the interpretation of the Dutch and MRC RCTs. Thus, the hypothesis that spleen- and pancreas-preserving D2 lymph node dissection improves survival remains unproven.

Increasingly, experienced gastric surgeons have acknowledged the adverse effects of splenectomy. The evolving consensus is that splenectomy should be performed only in cases with intraoperative evidence of direct tumor extension into the spleen or when the primary tumor is located in the proximal stomach along the greater curvature. Partial pancreatectomy should be performed only in cases of direct tumor extension to the pancreas.

Reports have described pancreas- and spleen-preserving forms of D2 dissection.[212–214] This organ-preserving modification of classic D2 dissection allows for dissection of some sta-

TABLE 29.2-9. Impact of Splenectomy Observed in Randomized Clinical Trials of Extended Lymph Node Dissection

End Point	Dutch Trial	MRC Trial	Comment
Operative morbidity	Yes	Yes	Independent risk factor
Operative mortality	Yes	Yes	Independent risk factor
Survival	Yes	No	HR = 1.36; P = .07

HR, hazard ratio; MRC, Medical Research Council.

tion 11 and 12 lymph nodes without the potential adverse effects of pancreatectomy or splenectomy, or both. In a small single-institution RCT reported from Chile, Csendes et al.[215] randomized 187 patients with localized proximal gastric adenocarcinoma to treatment by total gastrectomy with D2 lymph node dissection plus splenectomy or total gastrectomy with D2 lymphadenectomy alone. Operative mortality was similar in the two groups (splenectomy group, 3%; control group, 4%). However, septic complication rates were higher in the splenectomy arm than in the control arm (P <.04). No difference was seen in 5-year overall survival rates, although it is not clear that the trial was designed with survival as the primary end point.

The JCOG is conducting a multiinstitutional RCT (JCOG 0110-MF) comparing D2 dissection with and without splenectomy for patients with proximal gastric cancer.[216] The hypothesis to be tested is that the 5-year overall survival of patients treated by D2 dissection without splenectomy is 5% less than that of patients treated by D2 dissection with splenectomy. With a planned accrual of 500 patients, this design will provide a 70% power to reject the null hypothesis when 5-year overall survival is 3% greater after splenic preservation compared with splenectomy.[216] The results of this trial will elucidate the short- and long-term effects of splenectomy for patients with proximal gastric cancers.

INDIVIDUALIZED ASSESSMENTS OF LYMPH NODE INVOLVEMENT. Attention has focused on methods of individual assessment of risk of lymphatic spread. These techniques offer the possibility of tailoring surgical therapy for an individual patient based on clinicopathologic risk assessment of the primary tumor or pre- or intraoperative identification of SLNs or primary draining lymph nodes, or both. In the future, it is hoped that molecular determinants of lymph node metastasis will supplant these approaches. At present, at least three approaches to individual nodal risk assessment have been evaluated: computer modeling, preoperative endoscopic injection, and SLN biopsy.

Preoperative Computer Modeling of Individual Patient Nodal Involvement. Maruyama and colleagues have developed a computer program to estimate the probability of spread to specific nodal regions for an individual patient using his or her pretreatment clinicopathologic data. As initially developed, the program incorporated data on tumor size, depth of infiltration, location, grade, type, and macroscopic appearance of primary tumors from 2000 patients with surgically resected gastric cancers treated at the National Cancer Center of Tokyo.[217] The data set used for matching individual patient data is continuously updated and now includes more than 8000 patients. The Maruyama computer model has been validated in non-Japanese patients in studies done in Germany[218] and Italy.[219] In the United States, Hundahl et al.[220] retrospectively applied this computer model to evaluate the surgical treatment of patients entered into the Intergroup trial of adjuvant fluorouracil (FU)-based chemoradiation. The Maruyama program was used to estimate the likelihood of disease in undissected regional node stations, defining the sum of these estimates as the Maruyama index of unresected disease. Of the participating patients, 54% underwent D0 lymphadenectomy. The median index was 70 (range, 0 to 429). In contrast to D level, the Maruyama index proved to be an independent prognostic factor of survival, even with adjustment for the potentially linked variables of T stage and number of positive nodes.

Preoperative Endoscopic Peritumoral Injection. The hypothesis that peritumoral injection of compounds designed to optimize lymph node dissection improves lymph node clearance was addressed in a small RCT evaluating preoperative endoscopic vital staining with CH40 before D2 dissection. The frequency of positive lymph nodes in patients injected with CH40 before D2 dissection was greater than that observed in patients treated by D2 dissection alone.[221] This approach optimized the yield of lymph node dissection, presumably by directing surgeons to include specific lymph nodes in the dissection that would have otherwise been left *in situ* or by directing pathologists to examine specific areas of the lymphadenectomy specimens, or both. Further prospective studies of this approach are required to confirm the feasibility of this technique and assess its impact on intraoperative decision making regarding the extent of lymphadenectomy.

Sentinel Lymph Node Biopsy. The goal of SLN biopsy is to identify the node or nodes believed to be the first peritumoral lymph nodes in the orderly spread of gastric adenocarcinoma from the primary site to the regional lymph nodes. Sampling of this lymph node may allow for prediction of the nodal status of the entire lymph node basin—possibly obviating node dissection and its attendant morbidity in patients found to have a negative SLN. Pilot studies have evaluated the feasibility, sensitivity, and specificity of SLN biopsy for patients with gastric cancer.[222–226] These pilot studies demonstrated that SLN identification is feasible in approximately 95% of patients. However, most patients with gastric cancer have multiple "sentinel" nodes, with mean numbers of SLNs per patient ranging from 2.6 to 6.3. It is likely that the numbers of identified SLNs depend on a number of factors, including anatomic location of the primary tumor, pathologic stage, and the node identification technique used. Most pilot studies of SLN biopsy have involved subsequent D2 lymph node dissection, thereby allowing assessment of the false-negative rate of SLN biopsy. The aggregate experience to date suggests that, among patients with pathologically involved lymph nodes, SLN results in false-negative assessment of pathologic nodal status in 11% to 60% of patients. Thus, the preliminary data available suggest that SLN biopsy cannot reliably replace lymph node dissection as a means of accurately staging regional nodal basins. Until further data are available, SLN biopsy should remain an investigational approach.

VOLUME RELATIONSHIPS FOR GASTRECTOMY. Studies have established a clear relationship between institutional gastrectomy volume and perioperative mortality. The analysis of a national database by Birkmeyer et al.[227] of 31,854 patients who underwent gastrectomy between 1994 and 1999 demonstrated an inverse relationship between institutional gastrectomy volume and operative mortality. The OR for gastrectomy-related death was lowest among patients treated at the hospitals in the highest gastrectomy volume quintile (OR, 0.72; 95% CI, 0.63 to 0.83). A separate analysis evaluating surrogate end points for morbidity demonstrated that gastrectomy at high-volume centers was associated with the shortest duration of hospital stay and the lowest readmission rates.[228]

Similar findings were noted by Hannan et al.[229] in an analysis of the New York State Department of Health's administrative database. Their analysis of 3711 patients who underwent

gastrectomy between 1994 and 1997 included adjustments for covariates such as age, demographic variables, organ metastasis, socioeconomic status, and comorbidities. Patients who had gastrectomy at hospitals in the highest-volume quartile had an absolute risk-adjusted mortality rate that was 7.1% lower (*P* <.0001) than those treated at hospitals in the lowest-volume quartile even though the overall mortality for gastrectomy was only 6.2%. These studies demonstrate that the risk-adjusted mortality for gastectomy is significantly lower when gastrectomy is performed by high-volume providers.

It is likely that the variations in gastrectomy-related mortality relate in part to surgeon training[230] and experience with the procedure. Data on gastrectomy volume obtained from general surgeons undergoing recertification after a minimum of 7 years in practice demonstrate that the mean number of gastric resections performed by recertifying general surgeons in the United States is only 1.4 per year.[231] Thus, given the data supporting a relationship between hospital and provider volumes and the morbidity and mortality of gastric resection, there are reasons to consider regionalization of the surgical treatment of gastric cancers.

OUTCOME IN JAPAN VERSUS WESTERN COUNTRIES. Stage-stratified survival rates for gastric adenocarcinoma are higher in Japan than in most Western countries. The reasons for this are complex, are incompletely understood, and cannot be fully addressed within the context of a chapter covering all aspects of gastric cancers.

Important differences in the epidemiology of gastric cancer may contribute to observed differences in outcome in Japan versus Western countries. First, the better-prognosis intestinal-type (Lauren classification[26]) tumors are seen more commonly in Japan, whereas the diffuse-type cancers that are associated with a poorer prognosis are more frequent in Western series. These regional differences in the frequencies of intestinal and diffuse cancers are believed to be related to the higher incidence of *H pylori* infection and atrophic gastritis in Japanese populations. Second, poorer-prognosis proximal gastric cancers are less frequent in Japanese than in Western populations.[232,233] Indeed, the increase in proximal gastric cancers observed in the West[12] has not been observed in Japanese populations.[234] These important differences in tumor location and Lauren subtype may contribute to observed differences in stage-specific outcome between Japan and Western countries.

Regional differences in the diagnostic criteria for EGC also may contribute to regional differences in observed outcome. In Japan, gastric carcinoma is diagnosed based on its structural and cytologic features without consideration of invasion of the lamina propria. In contrast, Western pathologists consider invasion of the lamina propria to be an essential element of the diagnosis of carcinoma.[235,236] As a consequence, unequivocally neoplastic noninvasive lesions are classified as carcinoma in Japan but as dysplasia by Western pathologists.[235] To overcome these differences, the Padvova,[237] Vienna,[238] and revised Vienna[239] classifications have been proposed. However, until there is worldwide consensus and implementation of uniform diagnostic criteria for EGC, comparative assessments of the outcome of patients with EGC treated in Japan and Western countries should acknowledge the selection bias associated with different diagnostic criteria.

Stage migration is a well-documented factor contributing to the stage-specific differences in outcome between Japanese and

Western patients.[196] Stage migration arises because there is widespread use of extensive D2 or D3 lymphadenectomy combined with rigorous pathologic assessment of the lymphadenectomy specimen in Japan. In contrast, these techniques are infrequently used in Western countries. More accurate stage assignment of Japanese patients leads to secondary stage migration—improvement in stage-specific survival without improvement in overall survival. The frequency and impact of stage migration were quantified by the Dutch Gastric Cancer Group in their RCT comparing D1 and D2 lymph node dissection.[202,240] Stage migration occurred in 30% of patients in the D2 group, and the stage-specific decreases in survival rates attributable to stage migration were 3% for AJCC/UICC stage I disease, 8% for stage II, 6% for stage III, and 12% for stage IIIB, with the more accurately staged D2 group having higher survival rates.[240]

In addition to regional differences in epidemiology, diagnostic criteria for early-stage cancers, and stage migration, other factors may contribute to the observed differences in stage-stratified survival. Such factors may include genetic, environmental, and biologic differences between Japanese and Western patients and tumors. These factors have been less well studied but were addressed in a comprehensive review by Davis and Sano.[241]

Combined-Modality Treatment

RATIONALE FOR ADJUVANT THERAPY. The prognosis for patients with gastric cancer is, to a large extent, dependent on the stage of disease at the time of diagnosis. In the future, other factors may become equally or more important as information becomes available from molecular analyses of tumor tissue (e.g., gene expression arrays). Such analyses may allow physicians to identify patients with apparent early-stage disease who will not be cured by surgery alone and, conversely, patients with stage IIIA or IIIB cancer who will not have residual disease after surgery and in whom additional therapy is not needed. At present, as a group, patients with early-stage gastric cancers [for example, Tis (tumor *in situ*), T1N0M0, or shallow penetrating T2N0M0 tumors] have a good to excellent prognosis, and cure rates can exceed 80% with surgery alone. Unfortunately, these patients make up a minority of Western patients, who are usually symptomatic at the time of diagnosis. The majority of patients with operable stage II, IIIA, or IIIB disease have at least a 60% chance of tumor recurrence and death within 5 years of diagnosis. This group thus might benefit from adjuvant therapy.

The preoperative identification of patients with lower-risk disease (for whom surgery alone may be adequate) and those with higher-risk disease (for whom adjuvant therapy may be beneficial) remains difficult. Preoperative staging techniques, including laparoscopy, EUS, and, to a lesser extent, PET, have been able to identify patients with stage IV (incurable) disease more accurately. However, these techniques still have a relatively low sensitivity for separating patients with early-stage disease from those with tumors that are more advanced locally and regionally.

Because the risk of recurrence with surgery alone is high, the use of adjuvant systemic therapy and, in the postoperative setting, additional regional treatment with radiation have been extensively explored. Two different strategies have been tested: postoperative (adjuvant) chemotherapy or chemoradiation therapy or preoperative (also known as *neoadjuvant* or *primary*) chemotherapy. More recently, some clinical trials have begun

exploring preoperative chemoradiation. The rationale for neoadjuvant therapy is that systemic treatment with its attendant risks is best given when a patient is most fit to tolerate treatment (i.e., before surgery), that tumor regression with neoadjuvant therapy may improve the likelihood of an R0 resection, and that the early introduction of systemic therapy allows simultaneous treatment of regional and distant disease. In contrast, the rationale for postoperative therapy is that higher-risk patients will have already been identified by more accurate pathologic staging and lower-risk patients will be spared the risks for toxicity associated with preoperative treatment based on less accurate pretreatment staging. In addition, because surgery is the most effective therapeutic modality, with initial surgical resection one would not be taking the risk of giving potentially ineffective therapy while delaying effective treatment.

POSTOPERATIVE ADJUVANT CHEMOTHERAPY. Table 29.2-10 summarizes the results of a number of prospective randomized trials testing the hypothesis that postoperative systemic therapy increases cure rates for patients with resected stage II to IIIB gastric cancers. Earlier studies from the 1960s, 1970s, and 1980s were discussed in detail in previous editions of this text and in other reviews and are not covered in detail here. In essence, the majority of trials using older systemic regimens for adjuvant therapy failed to demonstrate a consistent reduction in the risk of recurrence. However, these studies included nitrosourea-containing and mitomycin-containing regimens, which are in general no longer being studied.

Anthracycline-Containing Regimens. Results with several doxorubicin-containing adjuvant regimens have been reported (see Table 29.2-10). Coombes et al.[242] studied 315 patients (281 of whom were evaluable) who had curatively resected gastric cancer and who were randomized to receive postoperative FU, doxorubicin (Adriamycin), and mitomycin (FAM), or no postoperative therapy. Chemotherapy could be started as late as 6 weeks after surgery. No significant differences were reported in the 3- or 5-year disease-free survival or overall survival rates (FAM, 45.7%; control, 35.4%). In a second RCT of postoperative FAM, the Southwest Oncology Group also failed to note an improvement in survival for the FAM group.[243]

Krook et al.[244] studied a different doxorubicin-containing combination in the adjuvant setting. After curative resection, 125 evaluable patients were randomized to receive observation alone or three cycles of FU (for 5 days) plus doxorubicin (on day 1). No differences were noted in overall survival between the two groups (median survival in observation group, 31 months; treatment group, 36 months). The 5-year overall survival rates were almost identical (33% vs. 32%).

The FU, doxorubicin, and methotrexate (FAMTX) regimen has been extensively studied in patients with advanced metastatic disease, and in randomized trials it was superior to regimens such as FAM.[244] A small randomized trial from the Netherlands compared neoadjuvant FAMTX plus surgery (27 patients) to surgery alone (29 patents). Patients receiving FAMTX chemotherapy had no significant advantages. The authors concluded that more active regimens than FAMTX will be required for future randomized trials.[245]

In another small study, Neri et al.[246] compared a postoperative regimen of epirubicin, FU, and leucovorin (55 patients) to

TABLE 29.2-10. Intravenous Postoperative Adjuvant Therapy for Gastric Cancer: Selected Phase III Trials

Study	Regimen	No. of Patients	Median Survival	5-Y Survival Rate (%)	P Value
Carrato et al.[358]	Control	75	2.6 y	NS	—
	Mitomycin C-UFT	69	2.3 y	NS	NS
Nakajima et al.[359]	Control	285	>5 y	83	—
	Mitomycin C–FU-UFT	288	>5 y	86	.17
Allum et al.[337]	Control	130	15 mo	18	—
	Mitomycin C–FU	141	16 mo	28	.98
	Mitomycin C–FU-CMFV	140	16 mo	10	—
Nakajima et al.[360]	Control	79	>5 y	51	—
	Mitomycin C–FU–Ara-C	81	>5 y	68	.09
	Mitomycin C–UFT–Ara-C	83	>5 y	63	—
Coombes et al.[242]	Control	130	15 mo	18	—
	FAM	133	36 mo	46	.17
Estape et al.[361]	Control	66	NS	26	.025
	Mitomycin	68	NS	41	—
Tsavaris et al.[247]	Control	42	NS	81	NS
	FU-epirubicin-mitomycin	42	NS	64	—
Italian GITSG[362]	Control	69	NS	~50	.9
	MACCNU-FU	75	NS	~50	—
	MACCNU-FU-levamisole	69	NS	~50	—
Neri et al.[246]	Control	55	13.9 mo	13	.01
	FU-leucovorin-epirubicin	48	20.4 mo	25	—
Hallissey et al.[270]	Control	145	14.7	20	.14
	RT, 4500 cGy	153	12.9	12	—
	FAM	138	17.3	19	—
EORTC Lise et al.[363]	Control	159	NS	~43	.3
	FAM	155	NS	~43	—
Macdonald et al.[243]	Control	100	NS	31	.45
	FAM	93	NS	33	—
Krook et al.[244]	Control	64	36 mo	33	.88
	FA	61	34 mo	32	.88
FFCD Ducreux et al.[248]	Control	133	46 mo	48 (4 y)	—
	Cisplatin-FU	127	44 mo	40	.25

Ara-C, arabinosylcytosine (cytarabine); CCNU, chloroethylcyclohexylnotrisourea; CMFV, cyclophosphamide, methotrexate, fluorouracil, vincristine; EORTC, European Organization for Research and Treatment of Cancer; FAM, fluorouracil, doxorubicin (Adriamycin), and mitomycin; FU, fluorouracil; GITSG, Gastrointestinal Tumor Study Group; NS, not stated; RT, radiation therapy; UFT, uracil and tegafur.

surgery only (48 patients) for stage III disease. The median survival for patients receiving adjuvant chemotherapy (20.4 months) was superior to that for patients undergoing surgery only (13.6 months; *P* = .01). Although these results are encouraging, they are at odds with the study by Krook et al.[244] in a similar number of patients. Use of this regimen should be considered investigational.

Tsavaris et al.[247] performed a small randomized trial (84 patients) in which epirubicin was substituted for doxorubicin to create the FU, epirubicin, and mitomycin adjuvant regimen. Recurrence or death occurred in 64% of patients receiving adjuvant therapy versus 81% of the control group; this difference was not statistically significant.

Cisplatin-Containing Regimens. Prospective randomized studies in patients with stage IV disease have not consistently demonstrated a significant improvement in survival for patients receiving cisplatin-containing regimens when compared to other chemotherapy combinations or single agents. However, response rates have in general been higher when cisplatin has been included. Therefore, there has been substantial interest in the use of cisplatin-containing regimens in the adjuvant setting.

Ducreux et al.[248] reported in abstract form the use of postoperative cisplatin and FU in patients undergoing gastric resection with curative intent. The planned accrual, to allow identification of a difference of 15% in 5-year survival, was 400 patients. However, only 278 patients (260 evaluable patients) were studied, and the trial was stopped due to insufficient accrual. The 3-year overall survival rate was 54.5% for surgery alone and 55.6% for surgery plus chemotherapy.[247]

Metaanalysis of Adjuvant Chemotherapy Trials. Many adjuvant therapy studies reported to date involved relatively small numbers of patients and therefore could identify only large differences in outcome. Several metaanalyses have been performed using pooled data to evaluate the magnitude of benefit from postoperative adjuvant chemotherapy.

Earle and Maroun[249] performed a metaanalysis involving 12 trials from Western countries. In this analysis, the crude ratio for death for patients receiving adjuvant therapy was 0.81 (0.67 to 0.98), with a relative risk of death of 0.94 (0.88 to 1.01). The authors concluded that there was only a small survival benefit from postoperative chemotherapy in the 12 trials analyzed.

Hermans et al.[250] reviewed 11 trials reported since 1980 involving postoperative chemotherapy versus observation alone after potentially curative resection in 2096 patients. The OR for death was 0.88 (95% CI, 0.78 to 1.08), which was not statistically significant compared to observation alone. Hermans et al.[251] later updated their data in a brief report that included two additional trials. The later analysis suggested a slight benefit from postoperative adjuvant chemotherapy.

Janunger et al.[252] reported a metaanalysis of studies published through 2001. They identified 21 randomized studies published in the English-language literature with a surgery-only control group and an experimental arm that included postoperative chemotherapy. Importantly, data on individual patients were not used. For the 3962 patients, the overall OR of death was 0.84 (95% CI, 0.74 to 0.96) in the postoperative-chemotherapy group, indicating a modest but statistically significant survival benefit with adjuvant chemotherapy. However, in a separate analysis of Western trials versus Asian trials, the benefit appeared to be confined to the Asian studies only. The reasons for this are unclear.[252] In a similar metaanalysis of 20 studies, Mari et al.[253] also noted a modest advantage from adjuvant chemotherapy.

In summary, clinical studies to date have not yet shown compelling evidence that postoperative chemotherapy using any of the currently available regimens should be considered a standard of care in patients who have undergone potentially curative resections for gastric cancer (the role of chemoradiation is discussed in Adjuvant Chemoradiation Therapy, later in this chapter). Of note, the reported metaanalyses involved trials with relatively small numbers of patients and did not use individual patient data. Furthermore, stratification for known prognostic indicators was not usually done in the trials.

PREOPERATIVE CHEMOTHERAPY. Locally advanced gastric cancers usually are defined as potentially resectable T3 or T4 tumors without radiologically or laparoscopically definable distant metastases. The use of preoperative (neoadjuvant) chemotherapy before attempted resection in patients with high-risk nonmetastatic disease should be studied for several reasons. For these patients with locally advanced gastric cancers, performing a potentially curative resection (R0) frequently is difficult, and the risk of distant failure, even with R0 resection, is high. However, because pretreatment assessment of lymph node involvement is difficult with the preoperative staging techniques currently available, T2 lesions, particularly those with suspicious lymph nodes, are also frequently included in preoperative treatment protocols.

Assessing Response to Preoperative Treatment. Assessing response to neoadjuvant therapy in patients with localized tumors is difficult. The accuracy of repeat endoscopy after neoadjuvant chemotherapy has been poor.[254] Serial CT studies after neoadjuvant chemotherapy also have a low overall sensitivity and accuracy in assessing response.[255] Kelsen et al.[254] investigated the use of EUS and CT in predicting pathologic stage in patients undergoing neoadjuvant chemotherapy. Preoperative EUS stage before and after neoadjuvant chemotherapy was compared to the pathologic stage in the context of a clinical trial of preoperative FAMTX. Postchemotherapy EUS was found to be inaccurate in distinguishing T2 from T3 tumors and in assessing lymph node status.[254]

PET is another technique for predicting response to neoadjuvant therapy. A decrease in FDG uptake has been proposed as an early marker of tumor regression in patients receiving systemic chemotherapy.[256] Although preliminary studies with FDG-PET in gastric cancer have now been reported, definitive large-scale trials correlating survival outcome with changes in PET findings are still awaited. Consequently, there is currently no available accurate means of assessing response to preoperative treatment. Thus, clinical trials of preoperative treatment suggesting treatment-related down-staging using preoperative primary tumor reassessment should be interpreted with caution, as there are no reliable means to accurately assess response before surgery.

Results of Preoperative Treatment. Although assessing the degree of tumor regression remains difficult, phase II studies of neoadjuvant chemotherapy have demonstrated that preoperative treatment can be given with acceptable toxicity and with no apparent increase in operative morbidity or mortality. Many pilot and phase II trials of neoadjuvant chemotherapy have been reported, in either final or abstract form, during the past 5 years. Results from selected trials are shown in Table 29.2-11. Almost all of these trials have involved the use of systemic chemotherapeutic regimens that have demonstrated moderate response rates in patients with measurable metastatic gastric cancer.

Lowy et al.[257] summarized the long-term results of cisplatin-based neoadjuvant chemotherapy in three sequential M. D. Anderson neoadjuvant therapy trials with a total of 83 patients. Seventy-three percent of patients underwent R0 resections, and 4% had pathologic complete responses. Despite the inherent difficulty in assessing response (discussed in Assessing Response to Preoperative Treatment, earlier in this chapter), response to chemotherapy as assessed clinically was an independent predictor of survival in this study.

Crookes et al.[258] reported the long-term results of a phase II study using preoperative cisplatin plus FU followed by postoperative intraperitoneal floxuridine (FUDR) and cisplatin in 59 patients. A 71% R0 resection rate was noted, the operative mortality was 5%, and the median overall survival was estimated to exceed 4 years. Because these patients did not undergo pretreatment laparoscopy or EUS, however, the trial may have included patients with early-stage tumors.

Kelsen et al.[254] performed two trials of preoperative chemotherapy followed by postoperative intraperitoneal treatment. The first study used the FAMTX regimen preoperatively and gave FU and cisplatin postoperatively.[254] Fifty-six evaluable patients were identified by EUS as having locally advanced disease; most had stage IIIA or IIIB tumors. The major side effect of FAMTX was myelosuppression, which led to at least one hospitalization for neutropenic fever in 60% of patients. The operability rate was 89%, and the resectability rate was 81%; 34 of the 56 patients (61%) underwent potentially curative resections, and 10 (18%) underwent palliative resections. With a median follow-up of 28 months, the median overall survival duration for all patients was 15.3 months. In a follow-up study, the same group of investigators treated 35 patients with preoperative cisplatin and FU for two cycles followed by postoperative intraperitoneal FUDR plus leucovorin.[259] All patients underwent pretreatment laparoscopy and EUS, and all had T3 or lymph node–positive tumors. The toxicity of preoperative chemotherapy was tolerable, without any increase in operative morbidity or mortality. The R0 resection rate was 82%, and the estimated median duration of overall survival was 22.5 months.

Fink et al.[260] treated a group of 49 patients with preoperative cisplatin, FU, and leucovorin (PLF). The R0 resection rate

TABLE 29.2-11. Neoadjuvant Therapy for Locally Advanced Gastric Cancer: Selected Phase II and Phase III Trials

Study	Regimen	No. of Patients	Operable	Resectable	Median Survival	2-Y Survival Rate (%)
PHASE II TRIALS						
Wilke et al.[364]	EAP	34	19 (56%)	10 (29%)	18 mo	26
Ajani et al.[140]	EAP	48	41 (85%)	37 (77%)	16 mo	42
Ajani et al.[365]	EFP	25	12 (48%)	18 (72%)	15 mo	44
Crookes et al.[258]	Cisplatin-FU-LV/IP FUdR-Cisplatin	59	(95%)	(71%)	>4 y	64
Siewert et al.[205]	Cisplatin-FU-LV	41	(88%)	(73%)	NS	56[a]
Kelsen et al.[254]	FAMTX-IP FP	56	50 (89%)	34 (61%)	15 mo	40
Alexander[341]	FU/LV IFN	22	20 (90%)	18 (82%)	18 mo	52
PHASE III TRIALS						
Kang et al.[261]	Cisplatin-etoposide-FU	53	(89%)	(71%)	33 mo	55
	Control	54	(89%)	(61%)	32 mo	55
Alum and Weeden[262]	ECF	250	NS	(79%)	NS	48
	Control	253	NS	(69%)	NS	40

EAP, etoposide, doxorubicin (Adriamycin), and cisplatin; ECF, epirubicin, cisplatin-fluorouracil; EFP, etoposide, fluorouracil, cisplatin; FAMTX, fluorouracil, doxorubicin (Adriamycin), and methotrexate; FU, fluorouracil; FUdR, 5-fluorodeoxyuridine; IFN, interferon; IP, intraperitoneal; LV, leucovorin; NS, not stated.
[a]Median follow-up, 18 months.

was 76%; the median duration of overall survival for all patients was 36 months, and at a median follow-up of 28 months, the median survival for the patients who underwent R0 resection had not been reached.[260]

Several phase III studies of neoadjuvant chemotherapy have now been reported in preliminary form. Kang et al.[261] reported the preliminary results of a small randomized trial of neoadjuvant cisplatin, etoposide, and FU plus surgery (53 patients) versus surgery alone (54 patients). No significant difference was noted in operability rate (89% vs. 100%), resection rate (71% vs. 61%), or median overall survival (33 vs. 32 months).

The MRC Clinical Trials Unit reported the preliminary results of a randomized trial in patients with gastric and lower esophageal cancers comparing perioperative chemotherapy with the epirubicin, cisplatin-FU (ECF) regimen to surgery alone (the MAGIC trial).[262] In this study, 503 patients (89% with gastric or gastroesophageal junction cancers) were randomly assigned to receive three preoperative and three postoperative cycles of ECF given at 3-week intervals. The surgery-only and perioperative chemotherapy groups appeared to be similar in age, gender ratio, and performance status; but early-stage tumors were more frequent in the latter group. In the preliminary report (in abstract form), 88% of patients were able to complete preoperative chemotherapy, but only 55% began postoperative treatment.[262] Forty percent completed all six planned cycles. Potentially curative resections were performed in 79% of perioperative chemotherapy patients, compared to 69% of surgery-only patients (P = .02). No difference was found in operative morbidity or mortality (6% for chemotherapy vs. 7% for surgery-alone patients). At the time of abstract presentation, an improved disease-free survival rate was noted, but the overall survival rate was not significantly different. The final results of the MAGIC trial are pending.

In summary, approaches involving preoperative chemotherapy with or without postoperative chemotherapy are now under way in the United States and in Europe. To date, the data indicate no increase in operative morbidity or mortality with neoadjuvant chemotherapy. Because evaluating the effect on the primary tumor is difficult, the extent of down-staging with neoadjuvant therapy can only be estimated. The perioperative chemotherapy approach used in the MAGIC trial, although promising, requires confirmation in definitive randomized phase III trials before firm conclusions regarding its value can be reached.

INTRAPERITONEAL CHEMOTHERAPY. The rationale for the use of intraperitoneal chemotherapy after resection of primary gastric cancer is the high risk of peritoneal metastasis as an initial component of treatment failure. Autopsy series and second-look laparotomy series have reported that up to 50% of gastric cancer patients who undergo potentially curative resections have clinically evident peritoneal carcinomatosis as a site (sometimes the only site) of failure.

Intraperitoneal therapy thus is a rational experimental technique to maximize the effectiveness of currently available antineoplastic agents by using intraperitoneal treatment as a portion of the adjuvant therapy for gastric cancer.

As a summary of these data, intraperitoneal chemotherapy with or without hyperthermia (CHIP), given with curative intent, is a rational experimental strategy to pursue until such time as more effective systemic agents are developed. However, the amount of clinical trials data is very limited. Future studies will require cooperative group or international trials to accrue adequate numbers of patients in a timely fashion.

IMMUNOCHEMOTHERAPY. Japanese and Korean investigators have performed a number of trials studying the use of immunochemotherapy as adjuvant treatment after curative resection of gastric cancer. Many of these trials involve using a protein-bound polysaccharide (PSK) alone or combined with chemotherapy after gastrectomy. PSK is a polysaccharide extracted from *Coriolis versicolor*, whose mechanism of action is not fully understood. The control arm in most of these studies, however, also received chemotherapy. Nakazato et al.[263] reported the results of a study involving patients who were randomly assigned to receive mitomycin plus FU (given by mouth) or the same chemotherapy plus PSK. The experimental arm received treatment with PSK for 36 months after surgery. As part of the eligibility process, patients had to have a positive purified protein derivative of tuberculin (PPD) test. Both groups received ten cycles of chemotherapy. With a minimum follow-up of 5 years, a significant survival advantage was seen for the PSK group; 70.7% of the PSK group versus 59.4% of the standard treatment group were alive and disease free at 5 years. Ochiai et al.[264] compared chemotherapy versus chemoimmunotherapy after resection. The immunotherapy used was a *Nocardia rubra* cell wall skeleton extract. No surgery-only control group was established; both groups received mitomycin, FU, and cytosine arabinoside chemotherapy. In this study, therapy was started perioperatively: Patients received mitomycin during surgery and on day 1 and then began weekly mitomycin, FU, and cytosine arabinoside. The chemotherapy group had 90 patients, and the chemotherapy immunotherapy group had 97 patients. No difference in survival for patients who had curative resections was seen. A subgroup of 71 patients did not undergo a curative resection and were analyzed separately. A survival advantage for those receiving immunochemotherapy was seen.

In other trials, Korean investigators have studied the use of chemotherapy plus immunostimulants after potentially curative resection. In one trial, chemotherapy with mitomycin, FU, and cytosine arabinoside plus OK432 (a *Streptococcus pyogenes* preparation) was given to 74 patients, whereas a control group of 64 patients underwent surgery alone.[265] Of the group receiving postoperative treatment, 44.6% were alive at 5 years, compared to 23.4% of those randomized to surgery only. In a follow-up three-arm trial, patients were randomized to receive immunotherapy with OK432 plus chemotherapy with mitomycin and FU. A second group received chemotherapy alone, whereas the third arm was a control arm of observation after surgery. At 5 years, 45.3% of the immunochemotherapy group were alive, compared to 29.8% of the chemotherapy group and 24.4% of the surgery group. Kim et al.[266] performed a similar trial using FAM chemotherapy with or without OK432. Fifty patients received chemotherapy alone, and 49 patients received chemotherapy plus OK432. These authors reported a significant improvement in survival for chemotherapy plus immunotherapy versus chemotherapy alone (62% vs. 52%, $P = .04$).

In summary, data from Japanese and Korean investigators suggest that immunotherapy may improve outcome for patients undergoing potentially curative resection. The number of patients in any given trial is small, and it is unclear how these trials should be translated to Western patient populations. Large-scale confirmatory trials are necessary before immunochemotherapy is accepted as a standard of care.

RANITIDINE AND TAMOXIFEN. Preliminary data had suggested that ranitidine or cimetidine might be useful in preventing recurrence of resected gastric cancer. Primrose et al.[267] performed a double-blind placebo-controlled trial of ranitidine, 150 mg twice daily, versus placebo taken for up to

5 years. No other adjuvant therapy was allowed. Patients with resectable gross disease, including those with stage IV tumors, were allowed entrance into this trial. The study, as is the case with other adjuvant trials, has only a small number of patients (41 in one arm and 46 in the other). No difference was seen in overall outcome, although a trend to benefit in stage IV patients was noted. In a second trial with a similar design using cimetidine, a similar lack of benefit was noted. Thus, to date, therapy using histamine-2 blockers has not shown benefit in preventing recurrence in patients with resected gastric tumors.

Using a hormonal approach, Harrison et al.[268] treated 100 patients in a randomized trial with tamoxifen as a single agent. This study allowed entrance of patients who had residual gross disease; thus, the study was not evaluating truly adjuvant chemotherapy. Slightly more than one-half (55.8%) of tumors were estrogen receptor positive. Tamoxifen had no effect on survival outcome; in fact, the control group did slightly better than the treated group.

ADJUVANT RADIATION THERAPY. Interest has been shown in the use of adjuvant radiation therapy in the treatment of gastric cancer owing to the substantial incidence of local and regional failure after primary surgical resection (discussed in Patterns of Spread, earlier in this chapter). Relatively few studies have evaluated radiation therapy alone (with no concomitant chemotherapy) as an adjuvant to surgical resection of gastric cancer. A study from China randomized 370 patients with tumors of the gastric cardia to receive surgery alone or with preoperative radiation therapy to a dose of 40 Gy in 20 fractions. Adjuvant radiation therapy improved the 5-year overall survival (20% vs. 13% with surgery alone, $P = .009$), local control (61% vs. 48%), and regional nodal control rates (61% vs. 45%).[269] A British Stomach Cancer Group study randomized patients to receive postoperative radiation therapy; postoperative chemotherapy with 5-FU, doxorubicin, and mitomycin C; or surgery alone. At 5 years follow-up, there were no significant survival differences between any of the three arms, but the local recurrence rate was lowered in the radiation therapy arm (10% vs. 27% with surgery alone, $P < .01$).[270]

Other adjuvant radiation approaches have been tried in an effort to increase the total radiation dose that can be delivered safely (Table 29.2-12). One such approach is intraoperative electron-beam radiation therapy, pioneered by Abe and Taka-

TABLE 29.2-12. Gastric Cancer: Surgery Alone versus Surgery and Intraoperative Radiation Therapy (IORT), Japan

	5-Y Survival			
	Surgery		Surgery + IORT	
Stage	No. of Patients	%	No. of Patients	%
I	43	93	20	88.1
II	11	54.5	18	77.6
III	38	36.8	19	44.6
IV (no distant metastases)	18	0	27	19.5

(Modified from ref. 271, with permission.)

hashi in Japan.[271,272] With this approach, patients receive a single dose of high-energy electrons delivered to the tumor bed at the time of gastrectomy. Because most of the radiosensitive normal structures can be retracted out of the radiation field, the risk of significant bowel complications is reduced. In a nonrandomized trial, Abe and Takahashi demonstrated an improved 5-year overall survival rate (20%) in patients with locally advanced disease (usually because of posterior infiltration) who were treated with intraoperative radiation therapy compared to surgery alone. In contrast, a small randomized trial using a similar approach at the U.S. National Cancer Institute[273] did not demonstrate a significant survival advantage, although it did show improved local control, compared with surgery alone. A number of phase II trials have been performed that demonstrate the feasibility of this approach in a large number of centers, but these trials do not allow any conclusions regarding efficacy[271,274–276] (see Table 29.2-12).

ADJUVANT CHEMORADIATION THERAPY. Most studies that have evaluated radiation therapy as an adjuvant have also used concomitant 5-FU chemotherapy. Some of the earliest data come from the Mayo Clinic, where studies were performed in the 1960s on the use of radiation therapy and 5-FU for a variety of gastrointestinal malignancies. Although these studies were for patients with locally advanced tumors, they laid the groundwork for subsequent adjuvant therapy studies. Childs et al.[277] reported a study of patients with locally advanced gastric cancer who were randomized to receive radiation therapy alone to a dose of approximately 40 Gy or radiation therapy combined with 5-FU (15-mg/kg/d bolus for 3 days) as a radiation sensitizer. A significant improvement was seen in survival with the combination of 5-FU and radiation compared with radiation alone. Because the dose of 5-FU was extremely low, most physicians have interpreted these data as indicating that 5-FU serves as a radiation sensitizer. This is consistent with data obtained for cancers at other gastrointestinal sites, for which 5-FU combined with radiation therapy has improved survival.

Dent et al.[278] treated 142 gastric cancer patients with surgery alone or surgery followed by 20 Gy radiation given in eight fractions over 10 days plus 5-FU (12.5 mg/kg/d) for 4 days immediately before radiation. A second chemoradiation cycle was given starting on day 28. Some patients had no gross residual disease but may have had incomplete resection. No survival difference was seen between the surgery-alone and chemoradiation groups.[279] Moertel et al.[279] reported the results of a small randomized trial of postoperative radiation therapy (3750 cGy in 24 fractions) plus 5-FU (15 mg/kg/d for 3 days) versus surgery alone for poor-prognosis gastric cancer patients, including those with serous carcinoma, metastases to regional lymph nodes, invasion of adjacent structures, or tumors originating in the gastric cardia. Eighty percent of patients had nodal disease, and approximately 25% had invasion of adjacent structures. The chemoradiation group had a 5-year overall survival rate of 20% versus a 4% 5-year overall survival rate in the surgery-only controls. Local-regional recurrence was decreased from 54% in the surgery-alone arm to 39% in the combined-modality arm. The survival results in this study are similar to those reported in a nonrandomized series by Slot et al.[280] in which 57 patients with poor prognostic factors received postoperative radiation therapy to a dose of 30 to 50 Gy combined with 5-FU. The 5-year overall survival rate was 26%, with 16 patients having a local-regional recurrence as their first site of relapse.

The major change in adjuvant therapy for gastric cancer in the past 5 years comes from the results of the gastrointestinal Intergroup trial, which tested the value of postoperative adjuvant radiation therapy and chemotherapy for patients with T2 to T4 or N1, or both, M0 gastric cancer after surgery with no evidence of residual disease. Patients had to have adequate nutritional intake (1500 kcal) at the time of study entry. The treatment scheme used two cycles of 5-FU and leucovorin followed by concurrent chemoradiation therapy with 45 Gy radiation given using fields that encompassed the entire gastric bed. A total of 550 patients were entered in the study; 84% had node-positive tumors, and 69% had T3 or T4 disease. Toxicity was acceptable, although major radiation therapy quality control issues had to be addressed as the study progressed. This study demonstrated a major advantage in overall survival, disease-free survival, and local-regional control with the use of adjuvant chemoradiation therapy, with much of the advantage attributable to improved local and regional control (Fig. 29.2-7; Table 29.2-13).[281]

The Intergroup study has been criticized for not having good surgical quality control; only a minimal number of nodes were found in many surgical specimens, and D2 dissections (defined as more than 10 nodes recovered by the pathologist) were performed in only 10% of patients. However, commentators often overlook the fact that the Intergroup protocol was a study of postoperative chemoradiation for patients with completely resected high-risk gastric cancer; gastrectomy and lymph node dissection were not part of the protocol treatment, and patients were evaluated for protocol eligibility only after recovery from gastrectomy. As such, the "surgical results" of the Intergroup trial are best viewed as a reflection of the standard practices of American surgeons and pathologists. It is likely that future combined-modality protocols that include gastrectomy and lymph node dissection with standardized pathologic evaluation of the gastrectomy and node dissection specimens will result in different rates of R0 resection, D2 dissection, and lymph node retrieval. The chemoradiation group in the Inter-

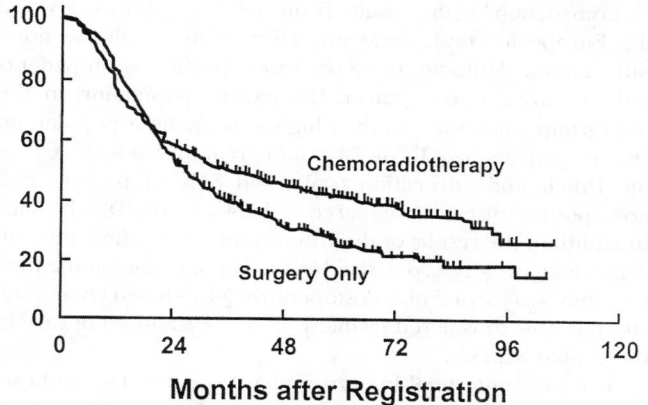

FIGURE 29.2-7.   Intergroup trial. Overall survival in the gastrointestinal Intergroup study of surgery alone versus surgery plus postoperative chemoradiation therapy, according to assigned treatment arm. The median survival duration was 27 months in the surgery-alone group and 36 months in the surgery plus chemoradiotherapy group. The hazard ratio for death in the surgery-alone group was 1.35 (95% confidence interval, 10.9 to 1.66, *P* = .005). (From ref. 281, with permission.)

TABLE 29.2-13. Outcomes from Gastrointestinal Intergroup Trial of Adjuvant Chemoradiation Therapy for Surgically Resected Gastric Cancer

	Surgery Alone	Surgery + Postoperative Chemoradiation
Local recurrence (n)	51	21
Regional recurrence (n)	126	76
Distant recurrence (n)	32	36
3-y DFS ($P = .001$)	32%	49%
3-y survival ($P = .03$)	41%	52%

DFS, disease-free survival.

group study had long-term survival results similar to those in the Dutch Gastric Cancer Group and MRC lymph node dissection trials,[201,202] in which surgery alone was the standard treatment. Comparison of the Intergroup results with those of the Dutch and MRC trials has led some to speculate that the chemoradiation was offsetting the adverse effects of suboptimal surgical therapy.[282] This school of thought is supported by the pattern of relapse in the Intergroup study: First relapse occurred locally in 29% of patients in the surgery-alone arm versus 19% in the postoperative chemoradiation arm; distant recurrences were the first site of relapse in 18% of patients in the surgery-alone arm versus 33% in the postoperative chemoradiation arm. A statistical assessment of the differences in these relapse rates was not performed because the protocol required documentation of a single site of first relapse and it was thought that statistical assessment of the differences in these relapse rates would be biased by incomplete recording of sites of treatment failure. Nevertheless, these data suggest that the primary effect of postoperative chemoradiation in the Intergroup study was a reduction in local and regional recurrence rates without apparent differences in distant relapse rates. Hence, comparable local control might be achievable with optimal surgery that includes D2 lymph node dissection, and it is possible that the extent and quality of surgery have an impact on the value of adjuvant treatment.

Comparison of the results from the Intergroup study and the European lymph node dissection trials should be done with caution. Although these trials were performed in patients with localized gastric cancer, the patient population in the Intergroup study was clearly a higher-risk patient population; 69% of patients had T3 or T4 tumors (compared with 26% in the Dutch node dissection trial), and 84% of patients had node-positive disease (compared with 54% in the Dutch trial). In addition, the results of the Intergroup study reflect the outcomes with surgery as practiced in the United States at the time the study was carried out. Postoperative 5-FU–based chemoradiation is now considered by many to be the standard of care in the United States.

The gastrointestinal Intergroup has launched a second randomized prospective trial [Cancer and Leukemia Group B (CALGB) 80101] in patients with completely resected high-risk gastric cancer comparing two chemotherapy regimens given before and after 5-FU–based chemoradiation. Based on randomized data demonstrating the superiority of the ECF regimen in patients with metastatic esophagogastric cancer,[283] CALGB 80101 is testing the use of one cycle of postoperative

ECF (epirubicin, 50 mg/m²; cisplatin, 60 mg/m²; and continuous-infusion 5-FU, 200 mg/m²/d for 21 days) followed by radiation therapy with concurrent continuous-infusion 5-FU (200 mg/m²/d) and two additional cycles of ECF. This will be compared to one cycle of postoperative 5-FU and leucovorin followed by concurrent continuous-infusion 5-FU (200 mg/m²/d) and two additional cycles of 5-FU and leucovorin. The planned accrual is 824 patients to detect a 25% improvement in overall survival in the ECF plus chemoradiation arm versus the 5-FU–leucovorin plus chemoradiation arm.

TREATMENT OF ADVANCED DISEASE (STAGE IV)

CHEMOTHERAPY

Among the palliative treatments for advanced gastric cancer, systemic therapy has probably been studied the most. Many studies of single cytotoxic agents have been reported, and chemotherapeutic agents with activity have been combined in a variety of regimens in an attempt to increase response rates and survival, as well as quality of life. Although some newer combinations studied in randomized trials have been reported to induce higher response rates than single agents, the effects on medium- and long-term survival are more questionable. Targeted agents that act through mechanisms other than cytotoxicity are under development.

Single-Agent Chemotherapy

The objective response rates reported using single agents in patients with advanced gastric cancer are shown in Table 29.2-14. Many of these are older agents, and the data regarding them are summarized in the previous edition of this text as well as in many reviews.[284]

FU has been extensively studied as a single agent in metastatic gastric cancer. The reported overall objective response rate of 21% is probably an overestimate, however. In the past, the most widely used schedules for administering FU as a single agent were daily intravenous injections for 5 days, repeated every 4 to 5 weeks, or weekly intravenous injections. More recently, combination regimens giving FU as a continuous intravenous infusion for several days to several weeks have been reported. The response rates to infusional therapy given alone or with leucovorin appear to be similar. The toxicity profile of infusional FU is different from that of bolus FU. The major side effects of infusional FU are mucositis, diarrhea, myelosuppression, and an erythroderma of the palms and soles. This erythroderma syndrome (hand-foot syndrome) is also a prominent toxic effect of some oral forms of fluorinated pyrimidines.

The antitumor antibiotics mitomycin C and doxorubicin were extensively used for metastatic gastric cancer in the past. Reported response rates of up to 30% for mitomycin C (again, probably an overestimate) and a lower response rate of 17% for doxorubicin date from older studies. The anthracycline analogue epirubicin has more recently been used widely in place of doxorubicin as part of the ECF regimen, described in more detail in Cisplatin-Based Chemotherapy, later in this chapter.

Among the most widely used single agents undergoing study in the 1970s and 1980s was the platinum analogue cisplatin. As a

TABLE 29.2-14. Response Rates to Single-Agent Chemotherapy in Patients with Stage IV Gastric Adenocarcinoma

Drug	No. of Patients	Response Rate (%)
ANTIMETABOLITES		
Fluorouracil	416	21
Methotrexate	28	11
Trimetrexate glucuronate	26	19
Trizinate	26	15
Gemcitabine hydrochloride	15	0
ORAL ANTIMETABOLITES		
UFT	188	28
S1	51	49
Capecitabine	31	19
Hydroxyurea (oral)	31	19
Camofur (oral)	31	27
Tegafur (oral)	19	19
ANTIBIOTICS		
Mitomycin C	211	30
Doxorubicin hydrochloride	141	17
Epirubicin hydrochloride	80	19
HEAVY METALS		
Cisplatin	139	30
Carboplatin	41	17
TAXANES		
Paclitaxel	98	17
Docetaxel	123	21
CAMPTOTHECANS		
Irinotecan hydrochloride	66	23
Topotecan hydrochloride	33	6

UFT, uracil and tegafur.

single agent, it was reported to induce major objective regressions in 19% of patients with metastatic gastric cancer, including patients who had received prior chemotherapy. Controversy exists as to whether carboplatin is as active as cisplatin in gastric cancer. Recently, attention has focused on oxaliplatin. Oxaliplatin is now being studied in combination with a variety of other agents, primarily fluorinated pyrimidines such as FU, and with irinotecan. This platinum analogue plays an important role in the treatment of colorectal cancer and is now undergoing study in gastric and gastroesophageal junction adenocarcinomas.

Two new classes of compounds have been reported to have activity in upper gastrointestinal tract adenocarcinomas. The taxanes paclitaxel and docetaxel have both undergone phase II trials. Several different dosing schedules for paclitaxel have been studied (e.g., 1-hour weekly infusions and 3-hour and 24-hour infusions given every 3 weeks). Approximately 20% of patients treated with paclitaxel have had major objective regressions, primarily partial remissions.[285–290] The response rate has generally been lower in patients who received prior chemotherapy. No obvious advantage to any particular schedule has been identified, and no trial comparing schedules has been performed. The overall response rate with docetaxel has been slightly higher (approximately 20% to 25%) than with paclitaxel, and most studies have used a once-every-3-weeks dosing schedule. The median duration of response with docetaxel and paclitaxel is approximately 4 to 6 months. No direct comparison between the two taxanes in gastric cancer has yet been reported.

Irinotecan, a camptothecin, represents the second new class of agents with reported activity in gastric cancer. When it has

been used as a single agent, responses have been seen in previously treated and previously untreated patients, with acceptable toxicity.

Combination Chemotherapy

Numerous attempts have been made to develop more effective therapies for metastatic gastric cancer by combining drugs with known single-agent activity. In addition to the many phase II trials reported in the past, several larger, randomized phase III studies have been completed more recently. With few exceptions, results from multicenter phase III trials have shown lower response rates for combination regimens than have phase II studies of the same drug regimens (30% to 50%).[291–298] Only phase III trials allow a definitive evaluation of the ability of combination regimens to prolong survival.

FAM and FAMTX

The FAM combination was widely used for metastatic gastric cancer in the 1980s[299,300] but is rarely used in current clinical practice. Phase III trials failed to demonstrate a significant improvement in survival with FAM, and the response rates in those trails were substantially lower than the rates reported in the initial studies of FAM.

Biochemical modulation of FU by methotrexate and leucovorin led to the development of the FAMTX regimen. Phase II studies in patients with metastatic gastric cancer indicated high response rates to FAMTX, and phase III studies comparing FAMTX with etoposide, doxorubicin, and cisplatin (EAP) showed FAMTX to be better tolerated. These led to a European Organization for Research and Treatment of Cancer study comparing FAMTX and the older FAM regimen.[301] The response rate with FAMTX was superior to that with FAM. The 2-year overall survival rate for patients receiving FAMTX was 9%, compared with 0% for those receiving FAM; this was not better than the rate expected with the best supportive care. Subsequently, FAMTX was found to be inferior to cisplatin-containing combinations, and it is not widely used currently.

Cisplatin-Based Chemotherapy

Although many phase II studies of cisplatin-containing regimens have been performed, only a few RCTs have been reported. Several recent trials have compared cisplatin-based combinations to non–cisplatin-based combinations, allowing a fuller evaluation of these regimens.

The *in vitro* synergy between cisplatin and FU, the activity of cisplatin as a single agent in gastric cancer, and the potential advantage of cisplatin over older drugs such as mitomycin C led to the development of cisplatin-FU regimens. Response rates to many of these regimens are in the 30% to 50% range.[302] For example, the cumulative overall response rate for FU, doxorubicin, and cisplatin (FAP) is approximately 35%. As is the case for other combinations, only 3% to 5% of patients achieve complete clinical remissions.[294,303] Cunningham et al.[304] substituted epirubicin for doxorubicin in the ECF combination (epirubicin, cisplatin, and FU). In phase II trials of ECF, the overall response rate ranged from 37% to 71%.

These preliminary results led Waters et al.[305] to perform a comparison of ECF to FAMTX. In a randomized MRC study,[306]

126 patients received ECF and 130 patients received FAMTX. The overall response rate for ECF was significantly higher than that for FAMTX (46% vs. 21%). Median survival was also longer for ECF (8.7 vs. 6.1 months). In an update by Waters et al., the 2-year overall survival rate was 14% for patients receiving ECF versus 5% for those receiving FAMTX.

Ross et al.[306] performed a two-arm randomized trial comparing ECF (289 patients; reference arm) to mitomycin, cisplatin, and protracted infusional FU (MCF; 285 patients). The trial allowed entrance of patients who had esophageal or gastric cancers, and the overwhelming majority of patients had adenocarcinoma. Patients with locally advanced disease were also allowed to take part; only a small percentage of these patients subsequently underwent operation. No significant difference was seen in response (42% for ECF vs. 44% for MCF), median survival (9.4 months vs. 8.7 months), or 1- and 2-year overall survival rates. The analysis included a quality-of-life assessment in which ECF was generally superior to MCF. The authors concluded that ECF should continue to be one of the reference treatments for advanced esophagogastric cancer.

Other trials, primarily phase II studies, have been performed that included epirubicin.[307,308] In general, they have shown response rates similar to those reported for other cisplatin-containing combinations.

Cisplatin-Etoposide Variants

Because etoposide and cisplatin may be synergistic, these drugs have been combined in the treatment of many tumors. Several phase II studies in patients with metastatic gastric cancer demonstrated that the combination is well tolerated.[309,310] Preusser et al.[311] then added doxorubicin to create the EAP regimen. Phase II trials of EAP reported high response rates. In subsequent phase III studies, although response rates of approximately 50% were reported, toxicity was high, with treatment-related mortality ranging between 10% and 14%. In a randomized comparison of EAP to FAMTX, Kelsen et al.[312] showed similar response rates for the two regimens but significantly less toxicity with FAMTX.

Wilke et al.[313] developed etoposide, leucovorin, and 5-FU (ELF). Because of the toxicity of EAP, particularly in older patients, phase II study data indicated a substantial response rate, approximately 50%, and a median duration of response of 9 to 10 months. ELF was subsequently studied in phase III trials (see the next section, Cisplatin-Fluorouracil).

Cisplatin-Fluorouracil

The combination of cisplatin and FU has also been extensively studied in gastric cancer. Phase II studies have indicated substantial activity with acceptable toxicity. This regimen has been considered by some U.S. investigators to be a reference regimen and typically consists of 75 to 100 mg/m^2 cisplatin and 750 to 1000 mg/m^2 FU given as a 4- or 5-day infusion.

Two phase III randomized studies compared cisplatin-FU to other regimens. Vanhoefer et al.[314] compared ELF, cisplatin-FU, and FAMTX in 399 patients with advanced gastric cancer. No significant differences were seen in response rates among the patients with measurable disease (9% for ELF, 20% for cisplatin-FU, and 12% for FAMTX). Also, no differences were found in median survival, which ranged from 6.7 to 7.2 months. Ohtsu et al.[315] compared cisplatin-FU to FU alone and to uracil and tegafur (UFT) plus mitomycin C in 280 Japanese patients with unresectable advanced gastric cancer. The UFT-mitomycin arm was inferior and was closed after an interim analysis. The overall response rate was higher for cisplatin-FU (34%) than for FU alone (11%) or for UFT-mitomycin (9%), as was the progression-free-survival rate. However, there was no difference in overall survival. Both groups of investigators concluded that there was no clear advantage to the cisplatin-FU regimen over other treatments.

Docetaxel-Containing Therapy

Phase II trial results for taxane-containing, irinotecan-containing, and oxaliplatin-containing regimens are being reported, but there are no reports of completed phase III trials involving these regimens. Interim results of one randomized study comparing a docetaxel, cisplatin, and FU regimen to a cisplatin and FU regimen have been reported in abstract form. In this study, Ajani et al.[290] compared 75 mg/m^2 docetaxel plus 75 mg/m^2 cisplatin on day 1 plus 750 mg/m^2/d FU by continuous intravenous infusion over 5 days every 3 weeks with 100 mg/m^2 cisplatin followed by a 5-day infusion of 1000 mg/m^2 FU every 4 weeks. The primary end point was time to progression, with secondary end points being overall survival and response rate. At the time of the interim analysis, 111 patients receiving the three-drug regimen and 112 receiving the two-drug regimen had been analyzed. A significantly higher time to tumor progression was reported for the docetaxel, cisplatin, and FU arm. The response and survival rates also appear to be higher in this arm. However, the final results of this study have not yet been reported.

Another area of investigation is the use of irinotecan-containing regimens. Preliminary results of a randomized phase II trial comparing cisplatin and irinotecan to irinotecan, FU, and leucovorin have been reported. Both of these combinations were found in earlier studies to have substantial response rates. In this study, the two arms (approximately 70 patients in each) were well balanced for major prognostic variables. Toxicity was slightly greater in the cisplatin-irinotecan arm, and the overall response rate was higher and median survival longer for patients receiving irinotecan, FU, and leucovorin. Therefore, the three-drug arm was chosen for a definitive phase III trial comparing it to cisplatin-FU. This study has completed the accrual, and no data are available at this time.

In addition to new classes of cytotoxic agents, there is also interest in the use of oral fluorinated pyrimidines. These are FU prodrugs that offer the ease of oral administration and mimic the benefits of long-term infusional therapy. Different mechanisms of action offer another advantage. Three fluorinated pyrimidines have been studied in gastric cancer as single agents: UFT, S1, and capecitabine. In most studies, the overall response rate for all three drugs is approximately 20% to 30%, similar to the rate reported in the past for FU. Whether the oral fluoropyrimidines are equivalent to infusional FU in gastric cancer is not yet clear.

Targeted Therapy

The demonstration in other tumor types of the effectiveness of anticancer agents with a mechanism of action different from that of cytotoxic chemotherapy, particularly when used in combination with cytotoxic agents, has spurred interest in their evaluation in gastric cancer. Herceptin, cetuximab, and signal transduction inhibitors such as erlotinib (Tarceva) and gefitinib (Irressa) are now being studied in gastric cancer, so far with negative results. No data are currently available for several agents that have demonstrated substantial activity in other gastrointestinal malignancies, such as bevacizuimab (Avastin), an antibody to the vascular endothelial growth factor ligand (see Chapter 29.8). Studies combining bevacizuimab with cytotoxic chemotherapy in gastric cancer are in the advanced planning stage.

Predicting Response

The development of techniques that will allow physicians to prospectively choose chemotherapeutic agents that are most likely to work in an individual patient is a high priority. This is particularly important because currently available cytotoxic chemotherapy for gastric cancer has only modest to moderate effectiveness, with objective regressions in 25% to 40% of all patients treated, and toxicities can be substantial. *In vitro* assays of live tumor cells have not proved to have adequate sensitivity; however, several studies have suggested that molecular analysis of tumor tissue might provide a more accurate predictor of outcome. The hypothesis is that levels of expression of molecular targets or of molecules associated with the mechanism of action of an individual agent are associated with response or resistance.

Preliminary studies of several new techniques for molecular analysis have been performed in gastric cancer. These studies were generally retrospective evaluations of prospectively accrued data and tissue. For example, the majority of correlative studies have involved collecting tissue before therapy, treating a group of patients with the same treatment (e.g., cisplatin-FU chemotherapy), and then correlating the molecular analysis findings with clinical outcome. In some cases, tissue has been collected at the time of definitive surgery after initial chemotherapy; these studies are more difficult to evaluate because the correlative analysis is performed after treatment.

The molecular analysis approaches used to date include evaluation of single genes or small numbers of genes by immunohistochemistry or by the use of reverse transcriptase–polymerase chain reaction. Gene expression profiling involving hundreds or thousands of genes has also been studied. These techniques are being explored extensively for cancers in general, but data on their use in gastric cancer are limited. Most of the data currently available involve small groups of patients treated with preoperative chemotherapy in whom molecular analysis of pretreatment biopsy specimens and posttreatment surgically resected tissue is performed. In older trials from the University of Southern California, Metzer et al.[316] and Lenz et al.[317] reported on an analysis of a subgroup of patients who received neoadjuvant cisplatin-FU chemotherapy, followed by resection and intraperitoneal floxuridine. Response and survival were correlated with molecular markers assessed by reverse transcriptase–polymerase chain reaction for several genes of interest, primarily thymidilate synthase (TS) and ERCC1 (excision repair cross complementing gene), a putative marker of cisplatin sensitivity. Patients with low levels of relative expression of these two genes had a significantly longer median survival and higher long-term survival rate than did patients with high levels of expression.

Several other groups have investigated the use of similar molecular markers. Boku et al.[339] used immunohistochemistry to measure TS, p53, vascular endothelial growth factor, and glutathione transferase expression in 39 patients with unresectable gastric cancer treated with cisplatin-FU chemotherapy. Patients with a lower level of expression of TS (as indicated by a negative immunohistochemical stain) had a higher response rate and longer survival than did patients with higher expression (positive stains). Similarly, patients whose samples were negative for p53, BCL-2, and glutathione S-transferase had improved clinical outcome. Conversely, patients with higher expression of vascular endothelial growth factor had a higher response rate. In a multivariate analysis, a combination of favorable molecular phenotypes had a greater impact on survival than did performance status or other clinical parameters.

Resistance to chemotherapy has been reported by many investigators to be associated with mutations of the p53 oncogene. Several studies of this association have been performed in gastric cancer. Cascinu et al.[318] performed immunohistochemical analysis of pretreatment endoscopic biopsies from 30 patients with locally advanced but not metastatic gastric cancer. Assessing response to treatment in such patients can be difficult, but 10 of 12 responding patients had p53-negative tumors, whereas patients overall had high levels of p53 expression. On the other hand, neither Ikeguchi et al.[319] nor Yeh et al.[320] found a relationship between p53 status and intraperitoneal chemotherapy response. A definitive study in which adequate numbers of patients with advanced gastric cancer receive the same chemotherapy irrespective of their molecular marker profile and are followed prospectively has not yet been performed.

Histopathologic Assessment of Response

The use of preoperative systemic therapy has led to an interest in evaluating histologic changes as a surrogate marker of efficacy. Histologic assessment of response typically includes identification of residual cancer cells and determination of the extent of fibrosis.[321] In one study, a tumor regression scale of grades 1 to 5 was used, with 1 denoting a complete pathologic regression and 5 meaning no evidence of chemotherapy effect.

Regression was defined by the replacement of cancer with fibrous tissue and scattered inflammatory cells. Percent histologic response was determined, ranging from no evidence of treatment effect (0%) to a complete response with no viable tumor identified (100%). Complete or near complete responses were associated with improved long-term survival rates.[322,323]

The use of immunohistochemistry in assessing treatment response has also been evaluated. In one study, p53, Ki-67, and epidermal growth factor receptor expression were the most reliable tissue markers of response.[324] Initial evaluations of the induction of apoptosis by chemotherapy in gastric cancer have used the TUNEL assay.[325,326] Satomi et al. correlated traditional assessment of histologic response and TUNEL assay findings.[326] However, the use of histology as a surrogate for therapeutic effect is still an experimental approach.

FDG–Positron Emission Tomography and Treatment Response

Another potential role for FDG-PET is the evaluation of treatment response. A growing body of evidence suggests that FDG-

PET can be used to identify response to therapy early in treatment. This approach has been studied in several tumors, including non-Hodgkin's lymphoma,[17,18] breast cancer,[20] and tumors of the gastroesophageal junction.[327] In these studies, PET was used to assess response to chemotherapy or to chemoradiation, and results were correlated with histology, traditional imaging modalities, and survival.

Weber et al. studied 40 patients with cancers of the esophagus and gastroesophageal junction treated with preoperative cisplatin-FU chemotherapy.[327] They compared FDG-PET findings for the primary tumor at day 14 with histologic response to chemotherapy in the resected specimen. Histologic responders had a significantly greater drop in standard uptake value (SUV; 54%) than did nonresponders. The optimal cutpoint for differentiating between responders and nonresponders in this small series was estimated to be an SUV decline of 39%. Using this value as a predictor of histologic response, a sensitivity of 93% and specificity of 95% were seen for PET. Histologic regression was achieved in 53% of patients with a metabolic response and in only 5% of those without a metabolic response.

This group presented similar results in a subsequent study for advanced gastric cancer in which a 35% SUV decline cutpoint for responders versus nonresponders was used.[373] The positive and negative predictive values for FDG-PET for histologic response were 77% and 86%, respectively. The 2-year overall survival rates of PET responders versus PET nonresponders were 89% and 26% ($P = .0005$). The authors concluded that a significant decrease in FDG-PET SUV identified at day 14 is associated with histologic response and with survival.

A similar approach has been used to evaluate the effects of chemoradiation for esophageal and gastroesophageal junction tumors. Downey et al.[328] have reported that a significant drop in FDG-PET SUV after preoperative chemoradiation treatment can distinguish responders from nonresponders, as determined by histology, and can predict for an improved survival rate.

Chemotherapy versus Best Supportive Care

During the late 1980s and early 1990s, there was considerable debate over whether chemotherapy for patients with advanced gastric cancer had any advantages over best supportive care. This issue is important, not only in helping patients with advanced disease choose the best options for care but also in its implications for adjuvant therapy in patients with localized, high-risk, potentially curable tumors.

Four randomized trials have been reported in which patients with metastatic gastric cancer were assigned to receive either chemotherapy and best supportive care or best supportive care alone. In all of these trials, the chemotherapy could be initiated at the time of symptomatic or objective progression at the discretion of the treating physician. Although these studies included relatively small numbers of patients (indicating the difficulty of performing such studies) and studies had to be stopped early if a benefit was seen in the chemotherapy-receiving arm, the data were fairly consistent. Patients randomized to receive best supportive care alone, even when allowed to receive chemotherapy at a later date, had a median survival of 3 to 5 months, whereas patients randomized to receive immediate chemotherapy had a median survival of 9 to 11 months.

TABLE 29.2-15. Chemotherapy for Advanced Gastric Cancer: Treatment versus Best Supportive Care (BSC)

Regimen	No. of Patients	Median Survival (Mo)	Survival Rate (%) 1 Y	Survival Rate (%) 2 Y
FAMTX	30	10	40	6
BSC	10	3	10	0
FEMTX	17	12	—	—
BSC	19	3	—	—
EtopLF	10	10	—	—
BSC	8	4	—	—
ELF	52	10.2	34.6	9.6
BSC	51	5	7.8	0

A, doxorubicin (Adriamycin); E, epirubicin; Etop, etoposide; F, fluorouracil; L, leucovorin; MTX, methotrexate.
(Modified from ref. 366, with permission.)

The 1-year overall survival rates were 35% to 40% for patients receiving chemotherapy versus approximately 10% for those receiving only best supportive care (Table 29.2-15). The 2-year overall survival rates were 6% to 10% for patients receiving chemotherapy versus 0% for the other patients. These data indicate that systemic chemotherapy has a real although modest effect on survival in patients with advanced gastric cancer. Furthermore, the results support the use of systemic cytotoxic chemotherapy as part of multimodality therapy in patients with less advanced but high-risk cancers. None of the regimens used in the best supportive care trials included cisplatin, paclitaxel, docetaxel, or irinotecan.

SURGERY FOR PALLIATION

Because the survival for patients with advanced gastric cancer is so poor, any proposed operation should have a good chance of providing sustained symptomatic relief while minimizing the attendant morbidity and need for prolonged hospitalization. Ekbom and Gleysteen[329] have reviewed the results of palliative resection versus intestinal bypass (gastrojejunostomy) in 75 patients with advanced gastric cancer. The most frequent symptoms for which patients underwent operation included pain, hemorrhage, nausea, dysphasia, or obstruction. Operative mortality was 25% for gastrojejunostomy, 20% for palliative partial or subtotal gastrectomy, and 27% for total or proximal palliative gastrectomy. The most common and often fatal complication was anastomotic leak. After gastrojejunostomy, 80% of patients had relief of symptoms for a mean of 5.9 months, compared with palliative resection, which provided relief of symptoms in 88% of patients for a mean of 14.6 months. Although the duration of palliation was significantly longer after resection ($P < .01$), the selection criteria for resection versus bypass were not controlled, and some bias against performing a palliative resection in high-risk patients with more advanced disease may have occurred.

Meijer et al.[330] also have reported a retrospective analysis of 51 patients undergoing either palliative intestinal bypass or resection. In 20 of 26 patients (77%) undergoing resection, palliation was considered moderate to good, with a mean survival of 9.5 months. After gastroenterostomy, some palliation was noted in 8 of 25 patients (32%), and survival was 4.2

months. Butler et al.[331] have presented the results of total gastrectomy for palliation in 27 patients with advanced gastric cancer. Operative mortality was only 4%, whereas morbidity occurred in 48% of patients. Median survival was 15 months, with a survival rate of 38% at 2 years. This substantial survival rate at 2 years reflects the fact that, although all patients were symptomatic before surgery, only one-half had stage IV disease. Patients with linitis plastica present a very difficult therapeutic challenge. Resection may provide palliation of symptoms; however, survival after total gastrectomy is exceedingly poor, ranging from 3 months to 1 year.[332]

Bozzetti et al.[333] have reviewed the outcomes of 246 patients with advanced gastric cancer who underwent simple exploratory laparotomy alone, gastrointestinal bypass, or palliative resection at the National Cancer Institute of Milan. When survival was compared in patients with similar type and extent of disease, a consistent trend was seen for improved median survival with palliative resection in patients with local spread (4.4 vs. 8.0 months) and distant spread of disease (3 vs. 8 months). Boddie et al.[334] have reported similar results in 45 patients undergoing palliative resection at the M. D. Anderson Cancer Center for advanced gastric cancer. Operative mortality for resection was 22%. In 21 patients who had undergone a palliative bypass procedure, survival was significantly shorter than for those undergoing resection ($P<.01$).

In select patients with symptomatic advanced gastric cancer, resection of the primary disease appears to provide symptomatic relief with acceptable morbidity and mortality, even in the presence of macroscopic residual disease. The criteria for deciding which patients may benefit from palliative operation have not been established, and the data available represent retrospective analyses of patients selected for operation. The choice of procedure in these studies may have been influenced by differences in opinion regarding the value of palliative surgery in patients with such a grave prognosis.

RADIATION FOR PALLIATION

To date, no studies have evaluated the use of radiation therapy in patients with locally recurrent or metastatic carcinoma of the stomach. Its use is likely to be limited to palliation of symptoms—such as bleeding or controlling pain secondary to local tumor infiltration. Although minimal data are available, radiation therapy seems to be fairly effective (from anecdotal experience) in controlling bleeding, as is true in other sites. This can often be accomplished at relatively low radiation doses. Pain from local tumor invasion can also be palliated, although the doses required are higher (45 Gy). On rare occasions, a case may arise of a patient with a focal local recurrence without metastases who would be amenable to relatively high-dose radiation therapy to try to prolong survival or in whom radiation therapy would be given as an adjuvant to surgical resection. At present, however, no data support such an approach.

REFERENCES

1. International Agency for Research on Cancer (IARC), 2000.
2. Jemal A, Tiwari RC, Murray T, et al. Cancer statistics, 2004. *CA Cancer J Clin* 2004;54:8.
3. Boring CC, Squires TS, Tong T. Cancer statistics, 1991. *CA Cancer J Clin* 1991;41:19.
4. Salvon-Harman JC, Cady B, Nikulasson S, et al. Shifting proportions of gastric adenocarcinomas. *Arch Surg* 1994;129:381.
5. Parkin DM. Studies of cancer in migrant populations: methods and interpretation. *Rev Epidemiol Sante Publique* 1992;40:410.
6. Murakami R, Tsukuma H, Ubukata T, et al. Estimation of validity of mass screening program for gastric cancer in Osaka, Japan. *Cancer* 1990;65:1255.
7. Correa P, Cuello C, Duque E. Carcinoma and intestinal metaplasia of the stomach in Colombian migrants. *J Natl Cancer Inst* 1970;44:297.
8. Stadtlander CT, Waterbor JW. Molecular epidemiology, pathogenesis and prevention of gastric cancer. *Carcinogenesis* 1999;20:2195.
9. Kamineni A, Williams MA, Schwartz SM, et al. The incidence of gastric carcinoma in Asian migrants to the United States and their descendants. *Cancer Causes Control* 1999;10:77.
10. Haenszel W, Segi M, Lee RK. Stomach cancer among Japanese in Hawaii. *J Natl Cancer Inst* 1972;49:969.
11. Staszewski J. Migrant studies in alimentary tract cancer. *Recent Results Cancer Res* 1972;39:85.
12. Blot WJ, Devesa SS, Kneller RW, et al. Rising incidence of adenocarcinoma of the esophagus and gastric cardia. *JAMA* 1991;265:1287.
13. Cady B, Rossi RL, Silverman ML, et al. Gastric adenocarcinoma. A disease in transition. *Arch Surg* 1989;124:303.
14. Powell J, McConkey CC. Increasing incidence of adenocarcinoma of the gastric cardia and adjacent sites. *Br J Cancer* 1990;62:440.
15. Powell J, McConkey CC. Increasing incidence of adenocarcinoma and gastric cardia. *Eur J Cancer Prev* 1990;1:265.
16. Harrison LE, Karpeh MS, Brennan MF. Proximal gastric cancers resected via a transabdominal-only approach. Results and comparisons to distal adenocarcinoma of the stomach. *Ann Surg* 1997;225:678.
17. Maehara Y, Moriguchi S, Kakeji Y, et al. Prognostic factors in adenocarcinoma in the upper one-third of the stomach. *Surg Gynecol Obstet* 1991;173:223.
18. Ohno S, Tomisaki S, Oiwa H, et al. Clinicopathologic characteristics and outcome of adenocarcinoma of the human gastric cardia in comparison with carcinoma of other regions of the stomach. *J Am Coll Surg* 1995;180:577.
19. Correa P. Human gastric carcinogenesis: a multistep and multifactorial process—First American Cancer Society award lecture on cancer epidemiology and prevention. *Cancer Res* 1992;52:6735.
20. Chow WH, Blot WJ, Vaughan TL, et al. Body mass index and risk of adenocarcinomas of the esophagus and gastric cardia. *J Natl Cancer Inst* 1998;90:150.
21. Lagergren J, Bergstrom R, Lindgren A, et al. Symptomatic gastroesophageal reflux as a risk factor for esophageal adenocarcinoma. *N Engl J Med* 1999;340:825.
22. Zhang ZF, Kurtz RC. Adenocarcinomas of the esophagus and gastric cardia: the role of diet. *Nutr Cancer* 1997;27:298.
23. Zhang ZF, Kurtz RC, Sun M, et al. Adenocarcinomas of the esophagus and gastric cardia: medical conditions, tobacco, alcohol, and socioeconomic factors. *Cancer Epidemiol Biomarkers Prev* 1996;5:761.
24. Gammon MD, Schoenberg JB, Ahsan H, et al. Tobacco, alcohol, and socioeconomic status and adenocarcinomas of the esophagus and gastric cardia. *J Natl Cancer Inst* 1997;89:1277.
25. Farrow DC, Vaughan TL, Hansten PD, et al. Use of aspirin and other nonsteroidal anti-inflammatory drugs and risk of esophageal and gastric cancer. *Cancer Epidemiol Biomarkers Prev* 1998;7:97.
26. Lauren P. The two histological main types of gastric carcinoma: diffuse and so-called intestinal-type carcinoma. *Acta Pathol Microbiol Scand* 1965;64:31.
27. Aird I, Bentall H, Roberts JAF. A relationship between cancer of the stomach and the ABO blood group. *Br Med J* 1953;1:799.
28. Huang JQ, Sridhar S, Hunt RH. Meta-analysis of the relationship between *Helicobacter pylori* seropositivity and gastric cancer. *Gastroenterology* 1998;114:1169.
29. Eslick GD, Lim LL, Byles JE, et al. Association of *Helicobacter pylori* infection with gastric carcinoma: a meta-analysis. *Am J Gastroenterol* 1999;94:2373.
30. Brown L. *Helicobacter pylori*: epidemiology and routes of transmission. *Epidemiol Rev* 2000;22:283.
31. Zhang ZF, Kurtz RC. *Helicobacter pylori* infection on the risk of stomach cancer and chronic atropic gastritis. *Cancer Detect Prev* 1999;23:357.
32. Terry MB, Gaudet MM, Gammon MD. The epidemiology of gastric cancer. *Semin Radiat Oncol* 2002;12:111.
33. Uemura N, Okamoto S, Yamamoto S, et al. *Helicobacter pylori* infection and the development of gastric cancer. *N Engl J Med* 2001;345:784.
34. Enroth H, Kraaz W. *Helicobacter pylori* strain types and risk of gastric cancer. *Cancer Epidemiol Biomarkers Prev* 2000;9:981.
35. Parsonnet J. Risk for gastric cancer in people with CagA positive or CagA negative Helicobacter pylori infection. *Gut* 1997;40:297.
36. Queiroz D, Mendes E, Rocha G. cagA-positive Helicobacter pylori and risk for developing gastric carcinoma in Brazil. *Int J Cancer* 1998;78:135.
37. Zaridze D, Borisova E, Maximovitch D, et al. Alcohol consumption, smoking and risk of gastric cancer: case-control study from Moscow, Russia. *Cancer Causes Control* 2000;11:363.
38. Hansson LE, Baron JA, Nyren O, et al. Tobacco, alcohol and the risk of gastric cancer: a population-based case-control study in Sweden. *Int J Cancer* 1994;57:26.
39. De Stephani E, Boffetta P, Carzoglio J, et al. Tobacco smoking and alcohol drinking as risk factors for stomach cancer: a case-control study in Uruguay. *Cancer Causes Control* 1998;9:321.
40. Chow WH, Swanson C, Lissowska J, et al. Risk of stomach cancer in relation to consumption of cigarettes, alcohol, tea, and coffee in Warsaw, Poland. *Int J Cancer* 1999;81:871.
41. Ji BT, Chow WH, Yang G. The influence of cigarette smoking, alcohol, and green tea consumption on the risk of carcinoma of the cardia and distal stomach in Shanghai, China. *Cancer* 1996;77:2449.
42. Tsubono Y, Nishino Y, Komatsu S, et al. Green tea and risk of gastric cancer in Japan. *N Engl J Med* 2001;344:632.

43. *Food, nutrition, and the prevention of cancer: a global perspective.* Washington, DC: American Institute for Cancer Research, 1997.
44. Nomura AM. *Stomach cancer in cancer epidemiology and prevention.* New York: Oxford University Press, 1996.
45. Kono S, Hirohata T. Nutrition and stomach cancer. *Cancer Causes Control* 1996;7:41.
46. Kai M, Luebeck EG, Moolgavkar S. Analysis of the incidence of solid cancer among atomic bomb survivors using a two-stage model of carcinogenesis. *Radiat Res* 1997;148:348.
47. Boyle P. Global burden of cancer. *Lancet* 1997;349[Suppl 2]:SII23.
48. La Vecchia C, Negri E, Franceschi S, et al. Family history and the risk of stomach and colorectal cancer. *Cancer* 1992;70:50.
49. Goldgar DE, Easton DF, Cannon-Albright LA, et al. Systematic population-based assessment of cancer risk in first-degree relatives of cancer probands. *J Natl Cancer Inst* 1994;86:1600.
50. Jones E. Familial gastric cancer. *N Z Med J* 1964;63:287.
51. Zanghieri G, Di Gregorio C, Sacchetti C, et al. Familial occurrence of gastric cancer in the 2-year experience of a population-based registry. *Cancer* 1990;66:2047.
52. Mecklin JP, Nordling S, Saario I. Carcinoma of the stomach and its heredity in young patients. *Scand J Gastroenterol* 1988;23:307.
53. Palli D, Galli M, Caporaso NE, et al. Family history and risk of stomach cancer in Italy. *Cancer Epidemiol Biomarkers Prev* 1994;3:15.
54. Gorer P. Genetic interpretation of studies on cancer in twins. *Ann Eugen* 1938;8:219.
55. Lee FI. Carcinoma of the gastric antrum in identical twins. *Postgrad Med J* 1971;47:622.
56. Guilford P, Hopkins J, Harraway J, et al. E-cadherin germline mutations in familial gastric cancer. *Nature* 1998;392:402.
57. Gayther SA, Gorringe KL, Ramus SJ, et al. Identification of germ-line E-cadherin mutations in gastric cancer families of European origin. *Cancer Res* 1998;58:4086.
58. Yoon KA, Ku JL, Yang HK, et al. Germline mutations of E-cadherin gene in Korean familial gastric cancer patients. *J Hum Genet* 1999;44:177.
59. Shinmura K, Kohno T, Takahashi M, et al. Familial gastric cancer: clinicopathological characteristics, RER phenotype and germline p53 and E-cadherin mutations. *Carcinogenesis* 1999;20:1127.
60. Pharoah PD, Caldas C. Incidence of gastric cancer and breast cancer in CDH1 (E-cadherin) mutation carriers from hereditary diffuse gastric cancer families. *Gastroenterology* 2001;121:1348.
61. Lynch HT, Smyrk TC, Watson P, et al. Genetics, natural history, tumor spectrum, and pathology of hereditary nonpolyposis colorectal cancer: an updated review. *Gastroenterology* 1993;104:1535.
62. Kinzler KW, Vogelstein B. Lessons from hereditary colorectal cancer. *Cell* 1996;87:159.
63. Aarnio M, Salovaara R, Aaltonen LA, et al. Features of gastric cancer in hereditary nonpolyposis colorectal cancer syndrome. *Int J Cancer* 1997;74:551.
64. Varley JM, McGown G, Thorncroft M, et al. An extended Li-Fraumeni kindred with gastric carcinoma and a codon 175 mutation in TP53. *J Med Genet* 1995;32:942.
65. Lindor NM, Greene MH. The concise handbook of family cancer syndromes. Mayo Familial Cancer Program. *J Natl Cancer Inst* 1998;90:1039.
66. Utsunomiya J. The concept of hereditary colorectal cancer and the implications of its study. *Clin Colorectal Cancer* 1990;3.
67. Offerhaus GJ, Giardiello FM, Krush AJ, et al. The risk of upper gastrointestinal cancer in familial adenomatous polyposis. *Gastroenterology* 1992;102:1980.
68. Maimon S, Zinninger M. Familial gastric cancer. *Gastroenterology* 1953;25:139.
69. Wolf C, Isaacson E. An analysis of 5 stomach cancer families in the state of Utah. *Cancer* 1961;14:1005.
70. Parsonnet J, Friedman GD, Vandersteen DP, et al. Helicobacter pylori infection and the risk of gastric carcinoma. *N Engl J Med* 1991;325:1127.
71. Parsonnet J, Hansen S, Rodriguez L, et al. Helicobacter pylori infection and gastric lymphoma. *N Engl J Med* 1994;330:1267.
72. Blaser MJ, Chyou PH, Nomura A. Age at establishment of Helicobacter pylori infection and gastric carcinoma, gastric ulcer, and duodenal ulcer risk. *Cancer Res* 1995;55:562.
73. El Omar EM, Rabkin CS, Gammon MD, et al. Increased risk of noncardiac gastric cancer associated with proinflammatory cytokine gene polymorphisms. *Gastroenterology* 2003; 124:1193.
74. Lee JE, Lowy AM, Thompson WA, et al. Association of gastric adenocarcinoma with the HLA class II gene DQB10301. *Gastroenterology* 1996;111:426.
75. Sakai T, Aoyama N, Satonaka K, et al. HLA-DQB1 locus and the development of atrophic gastritis with Helicobacter pylori infection. *J Gastroenterol* 1999;34[Suppl 11]:24.
76. Billington BP. Gastric cancer relationships between blood groups, site, and epidemiology. *Lancet* 1956;2:859.
77. Buckwalter JA, Wholwend CB, Colter DC. The association of the ABO blood groups to gastric carcinoma. *Surg Gynecol Obstet* 1957;104:176.
78. Boren T, Falk P, Roth KA, et al. Attachment of Helicobacter pylori to human gastric epithelium mediated by blood group antigens. *Science* 1993;262:1892.
79. Carvalho F, Seruca R, David L, et al. MUC1 gene polymorphism and gastric cancer—an epidemiological study. *Glycoconj J* 1997;14:107.
80. Umlauft F, Keeffe EB, Offner F, et al. Helicobacter pylori infection and blood group antigens: lack of clinical association. *Am J Gastroenterol* 1996;91:2135.
81. Fuchs CS, Mayer RJ. Gastric carcinoma. *N Engl J Med* 1995;333:32.
82. Kim SJ, Bang YJ, Park JG, et al. Genetic changes in the transforming growth factor beta (TGF-beta) type II receptor gene in human gastric cancer cells: correlation with sensitivity to growth inhibition by TGF-beta. *Proc Natl Acad Sci U S A* 1994;91:8772.
83. Yamamoto H, Sawai H, Perucho M. Frameshift somatic mutations in gastrointestinal cancer of the microsatellite mutator phenotype. *Cancer Res* 1997;57:4420.
84. Yin J, Kong D, Wang S, et al. Mutation of hMSH3 and hMSH6 mismatch repair genes in genetically unstable human colorectal and gastric carcinomas. *Hum Mutat* 1997;10:474.
85. Souza RF, Appel R, Yin J, et al. Microsatellite instability in the insulin-like growth factor II receptor gene in gastrointestinal tumours. *Nat Genet* 1996;14:255.
86. Souza RF, Yin J, Smolinski KN, et al. Frequent mutation of the E2F-4 cell cycle gene in primary human gastrointestinal tumors. *Cancer Res* 1997;57:2350.
87. Seruca R, Santos NR, David L, et al. Sporadic gastric carcinomas with microsatellite instability display a particular clinicopathologic profile. *Int J Cancer* 1995;64:32.
88. Halling KC, Moskaluk CA, Thibodeau SN, et al. Origin of microsatellite instability in gastric cancer. *Am J Pathol* 1999;155:205.
89. Leung SY, Yuen ST, Chung LP, et al. hMLH1 promoter methylation and lack of hMLH1 expression in sporadic gastric carcinomas with high-frequency microsatellite instability. *Cancer Res* 1999;59:159.
90. Fleisher AS, Esteller M, Wang S, et al. Hypermethylation of the hMLH1 gene promoter in human gastric cancers with microsatellite instability. *Cancer Res* 1999;59:1090.
91. dos Santos NR, Seruca R, Constancia M, et al. Microsatellite instability at multiple loci in gastric carcinoma: clinicopathologic implications and prognosis. *Gastroenterology* 1996;110:38.
92. Hollstein M, Shomer B, Greenblatt M, et al. Somatic point mutations in the p53 gene of human tumors and cell lines: updated compilation. *Nucleic Acids Res* 1996;24:141.
93. Gabbert HE, Muller W, Schneiders A, et al. The relationship of p53 expression to the prognosis of 418 patients with gastric carcinoma. *Cancer* 1995;76:720.
94. Hurlimann J, Saraga EP. Expression of p53 protein in gastric carcinomas. Association with histologic type and prognosis. *Am J Surg Pathol* 1994;18:1247.
95. Varis A, Wolf M, Monni O, et al. Targets of gene amplification and overexpression at 17q in gastric cancer. *Cancer Res* 2002;62:2625.
96. El Rifai W, Moskaluk CA, Abdrabbo MK, et al. Gastric cancers overexpress S100A calcium-binding proteins. *Cancer Res* 2002;62:6823.
97. Igaki H, Sasaki H, Tachimori Y, et al. Mutation frequency of the p16/CDKN2 gene in primary cancers in the upper digestive tract. *Cancer Res* 1995;55:3421.
98. Wong DJ, Barrett MT, Stoger R, et al. p16INK4a promoter is hypermethylated at a high frequency in esophageal adenocarcinomas. *Cancer Res* 1997;57:2619.
99. Klump B, Hsieh CJ, Holzmann K, et al. Hypermethylation of the CDKN2/p16 promoter during neoplastic progression in Barrett's esophagus. *Gastroenterology* 1998;115:1381.
100. Barrett MT, Sanchez CA, Galipeau PC, et al. Allelic loss of 9p21 and mutation of the CDKN2/p16 gene develop as early lesions during neoplastic progression in Barrett's esophagus. *Oncogene* 1996;13:1867.
101. Suzuki H, Itoh F, Toyota M, et al. Distinct methylation pattern and microsatellite instability in sporadic gastric cancer. *Int J Cancer* 1999;83:309.
102. Toyota M, Ahuja N, Suzuki H, et al. Aberrant methylation in gastric cancer associated with the CpG island methylator phenotype. *Cancer Res* 1999;59:5438.
103. Birchmeier W, Behrens J. Cadherin expression in carcinomas: role in the formation of cell junctions and the prevention of invasiveness. *Biochem Biophys Acta* 1994;1198:11.
104. Mayer B, Johnson JP, Leitl F, et al. E-cadherin expression in primary and metastatic gastric cancer: down-regulation correlates with cellular dedifferentiation and glandular disintegration. *Cancer Res* 1993;53:1690.
105. Becker KF, Atkinson MJ, Reich U, et al. E-cadherin gene mutations provide clues to diffuse type gastric carcinomas. *Cancer Res* 1994;54:3845.
106. Machado JC, Soares P, Carneiro F, et al. E-cadherin gene mutations provide a genetic basis for the phenotypic divergence of mixed gastric carcinomas. *Lab Invest* 1999;79:459.
107. Ascano JJ, Moskaluk CA, Harper JC, et al. Inactivation of the E-cadherin gene in sporadic diffuse-type gastric cancer. *Mod Pathol* 2001;14:942.
108. Grady WM, Willis J, Guilford PJ, et al. Methylation of the CDH1 promoter as the second genetic hit in hereditary diffuse gastric cancer. *Nat Genet* 2000;26:16.
109. Matsui S. Immunohistochemical evaluation of alpha-catenin expression in human gastric cancer. *Virchows Arch* 1997;424:375.
110. Kastury K, Baffa R, Druck T, et al. Potential gastrointestinal tumor suppressor locus at the 3p14.2 FRA3B site identified by homozygous deletions in tumor cell lines. *Cancer Res* 1996;56:978.
111. Ohta M, Inoue H, Cotticelli MG, et al. The FHIT gene, spanning the chromosome 3p14.2 fragile site and renal carcinoma-associated t(3;8) breakpoint, is abnormal in digestive tract cancers. *Cell* 1996;84:587.
112. Baffa R, Veronese ML, Santoro R, et al. Loss of FHIT expression in gastric carcinoma. *Cancer Res* 1998;58:4708.
113. Gemma A, Hagiwara K, Ke Y, et al. FHIT mutations in human primary gastric cancer. *Cancer Res* 1997;57:1435.
114. Hibi K, Robinson CR, Wu L, et al. Molecular detection of genetic alterations in the serum of colorectal cancer patients. *Cancer Res* 1998;58:1405.
115. Lefebvre O, Chenard MP, Masson R, et al. Gastric mucosa abnormalities and tumorigenesis in mice lacking the pS2 trefoil protein. *Science* 1996;274:259.
116. Chetty R. p27 protein and cancers of the gastrointestinal tract and liver: an overview. *J Clin Gastroenterol* 2003;37:23.
117. Kuniyasu H, Yasui W, Kitadai Y, et al. Frequent amplification of the c-met gene in scirrhous type stomach cancer. *Biochem Biophys Res Commun* 1992;189:227.
118. Jang JH, Shin KH, Park JG. Mutations in fibroblast growth factor receptor 2 and fibroblast growth factor receptor 3 genes associated with human gastric and colorectal cancers. *Cancer Res* 2001;61:3541.
119. Tahara E, Semba S, Tahara H. Molecular biological observations in gastric cancer. *Semin Oncol* 1996; 23:307.
120. Mizutani T, Onda M, Tokunaga A, et al. Relationship of C-erbB-2 protein expression and gene amplification to invasion and metastasis in human gastric cancer. *Cancer* 1993;72:2083.
121. Powell SM. Stomach cancer. In: Kinzler KW, ed. *The genetics of human cancer.* New York: McGraw-Hill Companies, Inc., 1998:647.
122. Guan XY, Fang Y, Sham J, et al. Recurrent chromosome alterations in hepatocellular carcinoma detected by comparative genomic hybridization. *Genes Chromosomes Cancer* 2001;30:110.
123. Leung SY, Chen X, Chu KM, et al. Phospholipase A_2 group IIA expression in gastric adenocarcinoma is associated with prolonged survival and less frequent metastasis. *Proc Natl Acad Sci U S A* 2002;99:16203.

124. Hippo Y, Taniguchi H, Tsutsumi S, et al. Global gene expression analysis of gastric cancer by oligonucleotide microarrays. *Cancer Res* 2002;62:233.
125. Lewin JK, Appelman HD. Carcinoma of the stomach. In: Rosai JSL, ed. *Tumors of the esophagus and stomach.* Washington, DC: Armed Forces Institute of Pathology, 1995:245.
126. Isaacson PG. Gastric MALT lymphoma: from concept to cure. *Ann Oncol* 1999;10:637.
127. Haber DA, Mayer RJ. Primary gastrointestinal lymphoma. *Semin Oncol* 1988;15:154.
128. The general rules for the gastric cancer study in surgery. *Jpn J Surg* 1973;3:61.
129. Kitamura K, Beppu R, Anai H, et al. Clinicopathologic study of patients with Borrmann type IV gastric carcinoma. *J Surg Oncol* 1995;58:112.
130. Ming SC. Gastric carcinoma. A pathobiological classification. *Cancer* 1977;39:2475.
131. Bearzi I, Ranaldi R. Early gastric cancer: a morphologic study of 41 cases. *Tumori* 1982;68:223.
132. Zinninger M. Extension of gastric cancer in the intramural lymphatics and its relation to gastrectomy. *Am Surg* 1954;20:920.
133. Shiu MH, Papacristou DN, Kosloff C, Eliopoulos G. Selection of operative procedure for adenocarcinoma of the midstomach. Twenty years' experience with implications for future treatment strategy. *Ann Surg* 1980;192(6):730.
134. Papachristou DN, Shiu MH. Management by en bloc multiple organ resection of carcinoma of the stomach invading adjacent organs. *Surg Gynecol Obstet* 1981;152:483.
135. McNeer G, Bowden L, Booner RJ, et al. Elective total gastrectomy for cancer of the stomach: end results. *Ann Surg* 1974;180:252.
136. Wisbeck WM, Becher EM, Russell AH. Adenocarcinoma of the stomach: autopsy observations with therapeutic implications for the radiation oncologist. *Radiother Oncol* 1986;7:13.
137. Gunderson LL, Sosin H. Adenocarcinoma of the stomach: areas of failure in a re-operation series (second or symptomatic look) clinicopathologic correlation and implications for adjuvant therapy. *Int J Radiat Oncol Biol Phys* 1982;8:1.
138. Allum WH, Hallissey MT, Ward LC, et al. A controlled, prospective, randomised trial of adjuvant chemotherapy or radiotherapy in resectable gastric cancer: interim report. British Stomach Cancer Group. *Br J Cancer* 1989;60:739.
139. Landry J, Tepper JE, Wood WC, et al. Patterns of failure following curative resection of gastric carcinoma. *Int J Radiat Oncol Biol Phys* 1990;19:1357.
140. Ajani JA, Ota DM, Jessup JM, et al. Resectable gastric carcinoma. An evaluation of preoperative and postoperative chemotherapy. *Cancer* 1991;68:1501.
141. Dewys WD, Begg C, Lavin PT, et al. Prognostic effect of weight loss prior to chemotherapy in cancer patients. Eastern Cooperative Oncology Group. *Am J Med* 1980;69:491.
142. Kaneko E, Nakamura T, Umeda N, et al. Outcome of gastric carcinoma detected by gastric mass survey in Japan. *Gut* 1977;18:626.
143. Yoshihara M, Sumii K, Haruma K, et al. Correlation of ratio of serum pepsinogen I and II with prevalence of gastric cancer and adenoma in Japanese subjects. *Am J Gastroenterol* 1998;93:1090.
144. Nakane Y, Okamura S, Akehira K, et al. Correlation of preoperative carcinoembryonic antigen levels and prognosis of gastric cancer patients. *Cancer* 1994;73:2703.
145. Ikeda Y, Oomori H, Koyanagi N, et al. Prognostic value of combination assays for CEA and CA 19-9 in gastric cancer. *Oncology* 1995;52:483.
146. Kodera Y, Yamamura Y, Torii A, et al. The prognostic value of preoperative serum levels of CEA and CA19-9 in patients with gastric cancer. *Am J Gastroenterol* 1996;91:49.
147. Pectasides D, Mylonakis A, Kostopoulou M, et al. CEA, CA 19-9, and CA-50 in monitoring gastric carcinoma. *Am J Clin Oncol* 1997;20:348.
148. Botet JF, Lightdale CJ, Zauber AG, et al. Preoperative staging of gastric cancer: comparison of endoscopic US and dynamic CT. *Radiology* 1991;181:426.
149. Dittler HJ, Siewert JR. Role of endoscopic ultrasonography in gastric carcinoma. *Endoscopy* 1993;25:162.
150. Matsumoto Y, Yanai H, Tokiyama H, et al. Endoscopic ultrasonography for diagnosis of submucosal invasion in early gastric cancer. *J Gastroenterol* 2000;35:326.
151. Cho JS, Kim JK, Rho SM, et al. Preoperative assessment of gastric carcinoma: value of two-phase dynamic CT with mechanical iv. injection of contrast material. *AJR Am J Roentgenol* 1994;163:69.
152. Fukuya T, Honda H, Kaneko K, et al. Efficacy of helical CT in T-staging of gastric cancer. *J Comput Assist Tomogr* 1997;21:73.
153. Dux M, Richter GM, Hansmann J, et al. Helical hydro-CT for diagnosis and staging of gastric carcinoma. *J Comput Assist Tomogr* 1999;23:913.
154. D'Elia F, Zingarelli A, Palli D, et al. Hydro-dynamic CT preoperative staging of gastric cancer: correlation with pathological findings. A prospective study of 107 cases. *Eur Radiol* 2000;10:1877.
155. Yeung HW, Macapinlac H, Karpeh M, et al. Accuracy of FDG-PET in Gastric Cancer. Preliminary Experience. *Clin Positron Imaging* 1998;1:213.
156. De Potter T, Flamen P, Van Cutsem E, et al. Whole-body PET with FDG for the diagnosis of recurrent gastric cancer. *Eur J Nucl Med Mol Imaging* 2002;29:525.
157. Kawamura T, Kusakabe T, Sugino T, et al. Expression of glucose transporter-1 in human gastric carcinoma: association with tumor aggressiveness, metastasis, and patient survival. *Cancer* 2001;92:634.
158. Asencio F, Aguilo J, Salvador JL, et al. Video-laparoscopic staging of gastric cancer. A prospective multicenter comparison with noninvasive techniques. *Surg Endosc* 1997;11:1153.
159. Burke EC, Karpeh MS, Conlon KC, et al. Laparoscopy in the management of gastric adenocarcinoma. *Ann Surg* 1997;225:262.
160. Lowy AM, Mansfield PF, Leach SD. Laparoscopic staging for gastric cancer. *Surgery* 1996;119:611.
161. Smith A, John TG, Garden OJ, et al. Role of laparoscopic ultrasonography in the management of patients with oesophagogastric cancer. *Br J Surg* 1999;86:1083.
162. Lavonius MI, Gullichsen R, Salo S, et al. Staging of gastric cancer: a study with spiral computed tomography, ultrasonography, laparoscopy, and laparoscopic ultrasonography. *Surg Laparosc Endosc Percutan Tech* 2002;12:77.
163. Hulscher JB, Nieveen van Dijkum EJ, de Wit LT, et al. Laparoscopy and laparoscopic ultrasonography in staging carcinoma of the gastric cardia. *Eur J Surg* 2000;166:862.
164. Nekarda H, Gess C, Stark M, et al. Immunocytochemically detected free peritoneal tumour cells (FPTC) are a strong prognostic factor in gastric carcinoma. *Br J Cancer* 1999;79:611.
165. Ribeiro U Jr, Gama-Rodrigues JJ, Safatle-Ribeiro AV, et al. Prognostic significance of intraperitoneal free cancer cells obtained by laparoscopic peritoneal lavage in patients with gastric cancer. *J Gastrointest Surg* 1998;2:244.
166. Burke EC, Karpeh MS Jr, Conlon KC, et al. Peritoneal lavage cytology in gastric cancer: an independent predictor of outcome. *Ann Surg Oncol* 1998;5:411.
167. Nitti D, Marchet A, Olivieri M, et al. Ratio between metastatic and examined lymph nodes is an independent prognostic factor after D2 resection for gastric cancer: analysis of a large European monoinstitutional experience. *Ann Surg Oncol* 2003;10:1077.
168. Roder JD, Bottcher K, Busch R, et al. Classification of regional lymph node metastasis from gastric carcinoma. German Gastric Cancer Study Group. *Cancer* 1998;82:621.
169. Karpeh MS, Leon L, Brennan MF. Lymph node staging in gastric cancer: is location more important than number? An analysis of 1,038 patients. *Ann Surg* 2000;232:362.
170. Ichikura T, Tomimatsu S, Uefuji K, et al. Evaluation of the New American Joint Committee on Cancer/International Union against cancer classification of lymph node metastasis from gastric carcinoma in comparison with the Japanese classification. *Cancer* 1999;86:553.
171. Ichikura T, Ogawa T, Chochi K, et al. Minimum number of lymph nodes that should be examined for the International Union Against Cancer/American Joint Committee on Cancer TNM classification of gastric carcinoma. *World J Surg* 2003;27:330.
172. de Manzoni G, Verlato G, Guglielmi A, et al. Prognostic significance of lymph node dissection in gastric cancer. *Br J Surg* 1996;83:1604.
173. Jatzko GR, Lisborg PH, Denk H, et al. A 10-year experience with Japanese-type radical lymph node dissection for gastric cancer outside of Japan. *Cancer* 1995;76:1302.
174. Adachi Y, Kamakura T, Mori M, et al. Prognostic significance of the number of positive lymph nodes in gastric carcinoma. *Br J Surg* 1994;81:414.
175. Hundahl SA, Phillips JL, Menck HR. The National Cancer Data Base Report on poor survival of U.S. gastric carcinoma patients treated with gastrectomy, 5th ed. American Joint Committee on Cancer staging, proximal disease, and the "different disease" hypothesis. *Cancer* 2000;88:921.
176. Mullaney PJ, Wadley MS, Hyde C, et al. Appraisal of compliance with the UICC/AJCC staging system in the staging of gastric cancer. Union International Contra la Cancrum/American Joint Committee on Cancer. *Br J Surg* 2002;89:1405.
177. Bando E, Yonemura Y, Taniguchi K, et al. Outcome of ratio of lymph node metastasis in gastric carcinoma. *Ann Surg Oncol* 2002;9:775.
178. Inoue K, Nakane Y, Iiyama H, et al. The superiority of ratio-based lymph node staging in gastric carcinoma. *Ann Surg Oncol* 2002;9:27.
179. Japanese Gastric Cancer Association. Japanese classification of gastric carcinoma, 2nd English ed. *Gastric Cancer* 1998;1:10.
180. Siewert JR, Stein HJ. Classification of adenocarcinoma of the oesophagogastric junction. *Br J Surg* 1998;85:1457.
181. Rudiger SJ, Feith M, Werner M, et al. Adenocarcinoma of the esophagogastric junction: results of surgical therapy based on anatomical/topographic classification in 1,002 consecutive patients. *Ann Surg* 2000;232:353.
182. Hermanek P. Prognostic factors in stomach cancer surgery. *Eur J Surg Oncol* 1986;12:241.
183. Kattan MW, Karpeh MS, Mazumdar M, et al. Postoperative nomogram for disease-specific survival after an r0 resection for gastric carcinoma. *J Clin Oncol* 2003;21:3647.
184. Gotoda T, Yanagisawa A, Sasako M, et al. Incidence of lymph node metastasis from early gastric cancer: estimation with a large number of cases at two large centers. *Gastric Cancer* 2000;3:219.
185. Matsumoto M, Natsugoe S, Ishigami S, et al. Lymph node micrometastasis and lymphatic mapping determined by reverse transcriptase-polymerase chain reaction in pN0 gastric carcinoma. *Surgery* 2002;131:630.
186. Miyata M, Yokoyama Y, Okoyama N, et al. What are the appropriate indications for endoscopic mucosal resection for early gastric cancer? Analysis of 256 endoscopically resected lesions. *Endoscopy* 2000;32:773.
187. Yamao T, Shirao K, Ono H, et al. Risk factors for lymph node metastasis from intramucosal gastric carcinoma. *Cancer* 1996;77:602.
188. Cady B. Subtotal gastric resection. In: Daly JM, Cady B, Low D, eds. *Atlas of surgical oncology.* St. Louis: Mosby-Year Book, Inc., 1993:221.
189. Lawrence JW. Total gastrectomy. In: Daly JM, Cady B, Low D, eds. *Atlas of surgical oncology.* St. Louis: Mosby-Year Book, Inc., 1993:241.
190. Robertson CS, Chung SC, Woods SD, et al. A prospective randomized trial comparing R1 subtotal gastrectomy with R3 total gastrectomy for antral cancer. *Ann Surg* 1994;220:176.
191. Gouzi JL, Huguier M, Fagniez PL, et al. Total versus subtotal gastrectomy for adenocarcinoma of the gastric antrum. A French prospective controlled study. *Ann Surg* 1989;209:162.
192. Bozzetti F, Marubini E, Bonfanti G, et al. Subtotal versus total gastrectomy for gastric cancer: five-year survival rates in a multicenter randomized Italian trial. Italian Gastrointestinal Tumor Study Group. *Ann Surg* 1999;230:170.
193. Hulscher JBF, van Sandick JW, de Boer AGEM, et al. Extended transthoracic resection compared with limited transhiatal resection for adenocarcinoma of the esophagus. *N Engl J Med* 2002;347:1662.
194. Kitajima M, Kitagawa Y. Surgical treatment of esophageal cancer—the advent of the era of individualization. *N Engl J Med* 2002;347:1705. World Wide Web URL: http://content.nejm.org/cgi/content/full/347/21/1705, 2004.
195. Hundahl SA. Gastric cancer nodal metastases: biologic significance and therapeutic considerations. *Surg Oncol Clin N Am* 1996;5:129.
196. Hundahl SA. Staging, stage migration, and patterns of spread in gastric cancer. *Semin Radiat Oncol* 2002;12:141.
197. Kodera Y, Schwarz RE, Nakao A. Extended lymph node dissection in gastric carcinoma: where do we stand after the Dutch and British randomized trials? *J Am Coll Surg* 2002;195:855.
198. Kodera Y, Yamamura Y, Shimizu Y, et al. The number of metastatic lymph nodes: a promising prognostic determinant for gastric carcinoma in the latest edition of the TNM classification. *J Am Coll Surg* 1998;187:597.

199. Stomach. In: Greene F, Page D, Fleming ID, et al., eds. *AJCC cancer staging manual.* New York: Springer-Verlag, 2002:99.
200. Dent DM, Madden MV, Price SK. Randomized comparison of R1 and R2 gastrectomy for gastric carcinoma. *Br J Surg* 1988;75:110.
201. Cuschieri A, Weeden S, Fielding J, et al. Patient survival after D1 and D2 resections for gastric cancer: long-term results of the MRC randomized surgical trial. Surgical Co-operative Group. *Br J Cancer* 1999;79:1522.
202. Bonenkamp JJ, Hermans J, Sasako M, et al. Extended lymph-node dissection for gastric cancer. Dutch Gastric Cancer Group. *N Engl J Med* 1999;340:908.
203. Kodama Y, Sugimachi K, Soejima K, et al. Evaluation of extensive lymph node dissection for carcinoma of the stomach. *World J Surg* 1981;5:241.
204. Otsuji E, Toma A, Kobayashi S, et al. Long-term benefit of extended lymphadenectomy with gastrectomy in distally located early gastric carcinoma. *Am J Surg* 2000;180:127.
205. Siewert JR, Bottcher K, Roder JD, et al. Prognostic relevance of systematic lymph node dissection in gastric carcinoma. German Gastric Carcinoma Study Group. *Br J Surg* 1993;80:1015.
206. Kajitani T. The general rules for the gastric cancer study in surgery and pathology. Part I. Clinical classification. *Jpn J Surg* 1981;11:127.
207. Cuschieri A, Fayers P, Craven J, et al. Postoperative morbidity and mortality after D1 and D2 resections for gastric cancer: preliminary results of the MRC randomised controlled surgical trial. The Surgical Cooperative Group. *Lancet* 1996;347:995.
208. Bonenkamp JJ, Hermans J, Sasako M, et al. Quality control of lymph node dissection in the Dutch randomized trial of D1 and D2 lymph node dissection for gastric cancer. *Gastric Cancer* 1998;1:152.
209. Bunt TM, Bonenkamp HJ, Arends JW, et al. Factors influencing noncompliance and contamination in a randomized trial of "Western" (r1) versus "Japanese" (r2) type surgery in gastric cancer. *Cancer* 1994;73:1544.
210. Bonenkamp JJ, Songun I, Sasako M, et al. Randomised comparison of morbidity after D1 and D2 dissection for gastric cancer in 996 Dutch patients. *Lancet* 1995;345:745.
211. Brennan MF. Lymph-node dissection for gastric cancer. *N Engl J Med* 1999;340:956.
212. Furukawa H, Hiratsuka M, Ishikawa O, et al. Total gastrectomy with dissection of lymph nodes along the splenic artery: a pancreas-preserving method. *Ann Surg Oncol* 2000;7:669.
213. Doglietto GB, Pacelli F, Caprino P, et al. Pancreas-preserving total gastrectomy for gastric cancer. *Arch Surg* 2000;135:89.
214. Schwarz RE .Spleen-preserving splenic hilar lymphadenectomy at the time of gastrectomy for cancer: technical feasibility and early results. *J Surg Oncol* 2002;79:73.
215. Csendes A, Burdiles P, Rojas J, et al. A prospective randomized study comparing D2 total gastrectomy versus D2 total gastrectomy plus splenectomy in 187 patients with gastric carcinoma. *Surgery* 2002;131:401.
216. Sano T, Yamamoto S, Sasako M. Randomized controlled trial to evaluate splenectomy in total gastrectomy for proximal gastric carcinoma: Japan clinical oncology group study JCOG 0110-MF. *Jpn J Clin Oncol* 2002;32:363.
217. Kampschoer GH, Maruyama K, van de Velde CJ, et al. Computer analysis in making preoperative decisions: a rational approach to lymph node dissection in gastric cancer patients. *Br J Surg* 1989;76:905.
218. Bollschweiler E, Boettcher K, Hoelscher AH, et al. Preoperative assessment of lymph node metastases in patients with gastric cancer: evaluation of the Maruyama computer program. *Br J Surg* 1992;79:156.
219. Guadagni S, de Manzoni G, Catarci M, et al. Evaluation of the Maruyama computer program accuracy for preoperative estimation of lymph node metastases from gastric cancer. *World J Surg* 2000;24:1550.
220. Hundahl SA, MacDonald JS, Benedetti J, et al. Surgical treatment variation in a prospective, randomized trial of chemoradiotherapy in gastric cancer: the effect of undertreatment. *Ann Surg Oncol* 2002;9:278.
221. Catarci M, Guadagni S, Zaraca F, et al. Prospective randomized evaluation of preoperative endoscopic vital staining using CH-40 for lymph node dissection in gastric cancer. *Ann Surg Oncol* 1998;5:580.
222. Aikou T, Higashi H, Natsugoe S, et al. Can sentinel node navigation surgery reduce the extent of lymph node dissection in gastric cancer? *Ann Surg Oncol* 2001;8:90S.
223. Kitagawa Y, Fujii H, Mukai M, et al. Radio-guided sentinel node detection for gastric cancer. *Br J Surg* 2002;89:604.
224. Ichikura T, Morita D, Uchida T, et al. Sentinel node concept in gastric carcinoma. *World J Surg* 2002;26:318.
225. Miwa K, Kinami S, Taniguchi K, et al. Mapping sentinel nodes in patients with early-stage gastric carcinoma. *Br J Surg* 2003;90:178.
226. Hayashi H, Ochiai T, Mori M, et al. Sentinel lymph node mapping for gastric cancer using a dual procedure with dye- and gamma probe-guided techniques. *J Am Coll Surg* 2003;196:68.
227. Birkmeyer JD, Siewers AE, Finlayson EV, et al. Hospital volume and surgical mortality in the United States. *N Engl J Med* 2002;346:1128.
228. Goodney PP, Stukel TA, Lucas FL, et al. Hospital volume, length of stay, and readmission rates in high-risk surgery. *Ann Surg* 2003;238:161.
229. Hannan EL, Radzyner M, Rubin D, et al. The influence of hospital and surgeon volume on in-hospital mortality for colectomy, gastrectomy, and lung lobectomy in patients with cancer. *Surgery* 2002;131:6.
230. Callahan MA, Christos PJ, Gold HT, et al. Influence of surgical subspecialty training on in-hospital mortality for gastrectomy and colectomy patients. *Ann Surg* 2003;238:629.
231. Ritchie WP Jr, Rhodes RS, Biester TW. Work loads and practice patterns of general surgeons in the United States, 1995–1997: a report from the American Board of Surgery. *Ann Surg* 1999;230:533.
232. Noguchi Y, Yoshikawa T, Tsuburaya A, et al. Is gastric carcinoma different between Japan and the United States? *Cancer* 2000;89:2237.
233. Gill S, Shah A, Le N, et al. Asian ethnicity-related differences in gastric cancer presentation and outcome among patients treated at a Canadian cancer center. *J Clin Oncol* 2003;21:2070.
234. Kodera Y, Yamamura Y, Shimizu Y, et al. Adenocarcinoma of the gastroesophageal junction in Japan: relevance of Siewert's classification applied to 177 cases resected at a single institution. *J Am Coll Surg* 1999;189:594.
235. Schlemper RJ, Itabashi M, Kato Y, et al. Differences in diagnostic criteria for gastric carcinoma between Japanese and western pathologists. *Lancet* 1997;349:1725.
236. Lauwers GY, Shimizu M, Correa P, et al. Evaluation of gastric biopsies for neoplasia: differences between Japanese and Western pathologists. *Am J Surg Pathol* 1999;23:511.
237. Rugge M, Correa P, Dixon MF, et al. Gastric dysplasia: the Padova international classification. *Am J Surg Pathol* 2000;24:167.
238. Schlemper RJ, Riddell RH, Kato Y, et al. The Vienna classification of gastrointestinal epithelial neoplasia. *Gut* 2000;47:251.
239. Schlemper RJ, Kato Y, Stolte M. Diagnostic criteria for gastrointestinal carcinomas in Japan and Western countries: proposal for a new classification system of gastrointestinal epithelial neoplasia. *J Gastroenterol Hepatol* 2000;15[Suppl]:G49.
240. Bunt AM, Hermans J, Smit VT, et al. Surgical/pathologic-stage migration confounds comparisons of gastric cancer survival rates between Japan and Western countries. *J Clin Oncol* 1995;13:19.
241. Davis PA, Sano T. The difference in gastric cancer between Japan, USA and Europe: what are the facts? What are the suggestions? *Crit Rev Oncol Hematol* 2001;40:77.
242. Coombes RC, Schein PS, Chilvers CE, et al. A randomized trial comparing adjuvant fluorouracil, doxorubicin, and mitomycin with no treatment in operable gastric cancer. International Collaborative Cancer Group. *J Clin Oncol* 1990;8:1362.
243. MacDonald JS, Fleming TR, Peterson RF, et al. Adjuvant chemotherapy with 5-FU, adriamycin, and mitomycin-C (FAM) versus surgery alone for patients with locally advanced gastric adenocarcinoma: a Southwest Oncology Group study. *Ann Surg Oncol* 1995;2:488.
244. Krook JE, O'Connell MJ, Wieand HS, et al. A prospective, randomized evaluation of intensive-course 5-fluorouracil plus doxorubicin as surgical adjuvant chemotherapy for resected gastric cancer. *Cancer* 1991;67:2454.
245. Songun I, Keizer HJ, Klementschitsch P, et al. Chemotherapy for operable gastric cancer: results of the Dutch randomised FAMTX trial. The Dutch Gastric Cancer Group (DGCG). *Eur J Cancer* 1999;35:558.
246. Neri B, de LV, Romano S, et al. Adjuvant chemotherapy after gastric resection in node-positive cancer patients: a multicentre randomised study. *Br J Cancer* 1996;73:549.
247. Tsavaris N, Tentas K, Kosmidis P, et al. A randomized trial comparing adjuvant fluorouracil, epirubicin, and mitomycin with no treatment in operable gastric cancer. *Chemotherapy* 1996;42:220.
248. Ducreux MP, Nordlinger B, Ychou M, et al. Resected gastric adenocarcinoma: randomized trial of adjuvant chemotherapy with 5-FU-Cisplatin (FUP). Final results of the FFCD 8801 trial. *Proc Am Soc Clin Oncol* 2000;19:241a.
249. Earle CC, Maroun JA. Adjuvant chemotherapy after curative resection for gastric cancer in non-Asian patients: revisiting a meta-analysis of randomised trials. *Eur J Cancer* 1999;35:1059.
250. Hermans J, Bonenkamp HJ, Boon MC, et al. Adjuvant therapy after curative resection for gastric cancer: meta-analysis of randomized trials. *J Clin Oncol* 1993;11:1441.
251. Hermans J, Bonenkamp HJ, Nakajima T, et al. Meta-analyses need time, collaboration, and funding. *J Clin Oncol* 1994;12:878.
252. Janunger KG, Hafstrom L, Glimelius B. Chemotherapy in gastric cancer: a review and updated meta-analysis. *Eur J Surg* 2002;168:597.
253. Mari E, Floriani I, Tinazzi A, et al. Efficacy of adjuvant chemotherapy after curative resection for gastric cancer: a meta-analysis of published randomised trials. A study of the GISCAD (Gruppo Italiano per lo Studio dei Carcinomi dell'Apparato Digerente). *Ann Oncol* 2000;11:837.
254. Kelsen D, Karpeh M, Schwartz G, et al. Neoadjuvant therapy of high-risk gastric cancer: a phase II trial of preoperative FAMTX and postoperative intraperitoneal fluorouracil-cisplatin plus intravenous fluorouracil. *J Clin Oncol* 1996;14:1818.
255. Ng CS, Husband JE, MacVicar AD, et al. Correlation of CT with histopathological findings in patients with gastric and gastro-oesophageal carcinomas following neoadjuvant chemotherapy. *Clin Radiol* 1998;53:422.
256. Ichiya Y, Kuwabara Y, Sasaki M, et al. A clinical evaluation of FDG-PET to assess the response in radiation therapy for bronchogenic carcinoma. *Ann Nucl Med* 1996;10:193.
257. Lowy AM, Mansfield PF, Leach SD, et al. Response to neoadjuvant chemotherapy best predicts survival after curative resection of gastric cancer. *Ann Surg* 1999;229:303.
258. Crookes P, Leichman CG, Leichman L, et al. Systemic chemotherapy for gastric carcinoma followed by postoperative intraperitoneal therapy: a final report. *Cancer* 1997;79:1767.
259. Brenner B, Shah M, Karpeh M, et al. Cisplatin-fluorouracil followed by postoperative intraperitoneal A phase II trial of neoadjuvant floxuridine-leucovorin in patients with locally advanced gastric cancer. *Ann Surg* 2004 (*in press*).
260. Fink U, Ott K, Dittler H. Neoadjuvant cisplatin leucovorin and fluorouracil (PLF) in adequately staged patients with locally advanced gastric carcinoma. *Proc Am Soc Clin Oncol* 1999;272a.
261. Kang Y, Choi D, Im Y. A phase III randomized comparison of neoadjuvant chemotherapy followed by surgery versus surgery for locally advanced stomach cancer. *Proc Am Soc Clin Oncol* 1996;15:215.
262. Allum WH, Weeden S. Perioperative chemotherapy and operable gastric and lower esophageal cancer: a randomized, controlled trial (the MAGIC trial ISRCNT93793971). *Proc Am Soc Clin Oncol* 2003;22.
263. Nakazato H, Koike A, Saji S, et al. Efficacy of immunochemotherapy as adjuvant treatment after curative resection of gastric cancer. Study Group of Immunochemotherapy with PSK for gastric cancer. *Lancet* 1994;343:1122.
264. Ochiai T, Sato H, Sato H, et al. Randomly controlled study of chemotherapy versus chemoimmunotherapy in postoperative gastric cancer patients. *Cancer Res* 1983;43:3001.
265. Kim JP, Kwon OJ, Oh ST, et al. Results of surgery on 6589 gastric cancer patients and immunochemosurgery as the best treatment of advanced gastric cancer. *Ann Surg* 1992; 216:269.

266. Kim SY, Park HC, Yoon C, et al. OK-432 and 5-fluorouracil, doxorubicin, and mitomycin C (FAM-P) versus FAM chemotherapy in patients with curatively resected gastric carcinoma: a randomized Phase III trial. *Cancer* 1998;83:2054.

267. Primrose JN, Miller GV, Preston SR, et al. A prospective randomised controlled study of the use of ranitidine in patients with gastric cancer. Yorkshire GI Tumour Group. *Gut* 1998;42:17.

268. Harrison JD, Morris DL, Ellis IO, et al. The effect of tamoxifen and estrogen receptor status on survival in gastric carcinoma. *Cancer* 1989;64:1007.

269. Zhang ZX, Gu XZ, Yin WB, et al. Randomized clinical trial on the combination of preoperative irradiation and surgery in the treatment of adenocarcinoma of gastric cardia (AGC)—report on 370 patients. *Int J Radiat Oncol Biol Phys* 1998;42:929.

270. Hallissey MT, Dunn JA, Ward LC, et al. The second British Stomach Cancer Group trial of adjuvant radiotherapy or chemotherapy in resectable gastric cancer: five-year follow-up. *Lancet* 1994;343:1309.

271. Abe M, Takahashi M. Intraoperative radiotherapy: the Japanese experience. *Int J Radiat Oncol Biol Phys* 1981;7:863.

272. Abe M, Takahashi M, Ono K, et al. Japan gastric trials in intraoperative radiation therapy. *Int J Radiat Oncol Biol Phys* 1988;15:1431.

273. Sindelar W, Chen P, Tepper J, et al. Intraoperative radiotherapy in retroperitoneal sarcomas: final results of a prospective, randomized, clinical trial. *Arch Surg* 1993;128:402.

274. Sindelar WF, Kinsella TJ, Tepper JE, et al. Randomized trial of intraoperative radiotherapy in carcinoma of the stomach. *Am J Surg* 1993;165:178.

275. Ogata T, Araki K, Matsuura K, et al. A 10-year experience of intraoperative radiotherapy for gastric carcinoma and a new surgical method of creating a wider irradiation field for cases of total gastrectomy patients. *Int J Radiat Oncol Biol Phys* 1995;32:341.

276. Calvo FA, Aristu JJ, Azinovic I, et al. Intraoperative and external radiotherapy in resected gastric cancer: updated report of a phase II trial. *Int J Radiat Oncol Biol Phys* 1992;24:729.

277. Childs DS Jr, Moertel CG, Holbrook MA, et al. Treatment of unresectable adenocarcinomas of the stomach with a combination of 5-fluorouracil and radiation. *Am J Roentgenol Radium Ther Nucl Med* 1968;102:541.

278. Dent DM, Werner ID, Novis B, et al. Prospective randomized trial of combined oncological therapy for gastric carcinoma. *Cancer* 1979;44:385.

279. Moertel CG, O'Fallon JR, Holbrook MA, et al. Combined 5-fluorouracil and radiation therapy as a surgical adjuvant for poor prognosis gastric carcinoma. *J Clin Oncol* 1984;2:1249.

280. Slot A, Meerwaldt JH, van Putten WL, et al. Adjuvant postoperative radiotherapy for gastric carcinoma with poor prognostic signs. *Radiother Oncol* 1989;16:269.

281. MacDonald JS, Smalley S, Benedetti J, et al. Chemoradiotherapy after surgery compared with surgery alone for adenocarcinoma of the stomach or gastroesophageal junction. *N Engl J Med* 2001;345:725.

282. van de Velde CJ, Peeters KC. The gastric cancer treatment controversy. *J Clin Oncol* 2003;21:2234.

283. Webb A, Scarffe JH, Harper P, et al. Randomized trial comparing epirubicin, cisplatin, and fluorouracil versus fluorouracil, doxorubicin, and methotrexate in advanced esophagogastric cancer. *J Clin Oncol* 1997;15:261.

284. Kelsen DP, Minsky BD. Gastric cancer: clinical management. In: Kelsen DP, Daly JM, Kern SE, et al., eds. *Gastrointestinal oncology: principles and practice*. Philadelphia: Lippincott Williams & Wilkins, 2001:383.

285. Ohtsu A, Boku N, Tamura F, et al. An early phase II study of a 3-hour infusion of paclitaxel for advanced gastric cancer. *Am J Clin Oncol* 1998;21:416.

286. Cascinu S, Graziano F, Cardarelli N, et al. Phase II study of paclitaxel in pretreated advanced gastric cancer. *Anticancer Drugs* 1998;9:307.

287. Ajani JA, Ilson DH, Kelsen DP. Paclitaxel in the treatment of patients with upper gastrointestinal carcinomas. *Semin Oncol* 1996;23:55.

288. Sulkes A, Smyth J, Sessa C, et al. Docetaxel (Taxotere) in advanced gastric cancer: results of a phase II clinical trial. EORTC Early Clinical Trials Group. *Br J Cancer* 1994;70:380.

289. Einzig AI, Neuberg D, Remick SC, et al. Phase II trial of docetaxel (Taxotere) in patients with adenocarcinoma of the upper gastrointestinal tract previously untreated with cytotoxic chemotherapy: the Eastern Cooperative Oncology Group (ECOG) results of protocol E1293. *Med Oncol* 1996;13:87.

290. Ajani JA, Fairweather J, Pisters PW, et al. Phase III study of CPT-11 plus cisplatin in patients with advanced gastric and GE junction carcinomas. *Proc Am Soc Clin Oncol* 1999;18:241a.

291. Douglass HO Jr, Lavin PT, Goudsmit A, et al. An Eastern Cooperative Oncology Group evaluation of combinations of methyl-CCNU, mitomycin C, Adriamycin, and 5-fluorouracil in advanced measurable gastric cancer (EST 2277). *J Clin Oncol* 1984;2:1372.

292. Levi JA, Fox RM, Tattersall MH, et al. Analysis of a prospectively randomized comparison of doxorubicin versus 5-fluorouracil, doxorubicin, and BCNU in advanced gastric cancer: implications for future studies. *J Clin Oncol* 1986;4:1348.

293. Lacave AJ, Clavel M, Planting A, et al. cis-Platinum as second-line chemotherapy in advanced gastric adenocarcinoma. A phase II study of the EORTC Gastrointestinal Tract Cancer Cooperative Group. *Eur J Cancer Clin Oncol* 1985;21:1321.

294. Epelbaum R, Haim N, Stein M, et al. Treatment of advanced gastric cancer with DDP (cisplatin), adriamycin, and 5-fluorouracil (DAF). *Oncology* 1987;44:201.

295. Schnitzler G, Queisser W, Heim ME, et al. Phase III study of 5-FU and carmustine versus 5-FU, carmustine, and doxorubicin in advanced gastric cancer. *Cancer Treat Rep* 1986;70:477.

296. Lopez M, Di Lauro L, Papaldo P, et al. Treatment of advanced measurable gastric carcinoma with 5-fluorouracil, adriamycin, and BCNU. *Oncology* 1986;43:288.

297. Janieson G, Gill P. A prospective trial of 5-FU and BCNU in the treatment of advanced gastric cancer. *Aust N Z J Surg* 1985;5:16.

298. Levi JA, Dalley DN, Aroney RS. Improved combination chemotherapy in advanced gastric cancer. *Br Med J* 1979;2:1471.

299. MacDonald JS, Schein PS, Woolley PV, et al. 5-Fluorouracil, doxorubicin, and mitomycin (FAM) combination chemotherapy for advanced gastric cancer. *Ann Intern Med* 1980;93:533.

300. Loggie BW, Fleming RA, McQuellon RP, et al. Cytoreductive surgery with intraperitoneal hyperthermic chemotherapy for disseminated peritoneal cancer of gastrointestinal origin. *Am Surg* 2000;66:561.

301. Wils JA, Klein HO, Wagener DJ, et al. Sequential high-dose methotrexate and fluorouracil combined with doxorubicin—a step ahead in the treatment of advanced gastric cancer: a trial of the European Organization for Research and Treatment of Cancer Gastrointestinal Tract Cooperative Group. *J Clin Oncol* 1991;9:827.

302. Los G, Smals OA, van Vugt MJ, et al. A rationale for carboplatin treatment and abdominal hyperthermia in cancers restricted to the peritoneal cavity. *Cancer Res* 1992;52:1252.

303. Gastrointestinal Tumor Study Group. Triazinate and platinum efficacy in combination with 5-fluorouracil and doxorubicin: results of a three-arm randomized trial in metastatic gastric cancer. *J Natl Cancer Inst* 1988;80:1011.

304. Cunningham D, Cahn A, Menzies-Gow N. Cisplatin, epirubicin and 5-flourouracil (CEF) has significant activity in advanced gastric cancer. *Proc Am Soc Clin Oncol* 1990;9:123.

305. Waters JS, Norman A, Scarffe JH, et al. Long-term survival after epirubicin, cisplatin and fluorouracil for gastric cancer: results of a randomized trial. *Br J Cancer* 1999;80:269.

306. Ross P, Nicolson M, Valle J, et al. Prospective randomized trial comparing mitomycin, cisplatin, and protracted venous-infusion fluorouracil (PVI 5-FU) with epirubicin, cisplatin, and PVI 5-FU in advanced esophagogastric cancer. *J Clin Oncol* 2002;20:1996.

307. Barone C, Cassano A, Astone A, et al. Association of epirubicin, etoposide and cisplatin in gastric cancer. A phase II study. *Oncology* 1991;48:353.

308. Icli F, Celik I, Aykan F, et al. A randomized Phase III trial of etoposide, epirubicin, and cisplatin versus 5-fluorouracil, epirubicin, and cisplatin in the treatment of patients with advanced gastric carcinoma. Turkish Oncology Group. *Cancer* 1998;83:2475.

309. Kelsen DP, Buckner J, Magill G, et al. Phase II trial of cisplatin and etoposide in adenocarcinomas of the upper gastrointestinal tract. *Cancer Treat Rep* 1987;71:329.

310. Elliott TE, Moertel CG, Wieand HS, et al. A phase II study of the combination of etoposide and cisplatin in the therapy of advanced gastric cancer. *Cancer* 1990;65:1491.

311. Preusser P, Achterrath W, Wilke H, et al. Chemotherapy of gastric cancer. *Cancer Treat Rev* 1988;15:257.

312. Kelsen D, Atiq OT, Saltz L, et al. FAMTX (fluorouracil, methotrexate, Adriamycin) is as effective and less toxic than EAP (etoposide, Adriamycin, cisplatin): a random assignment trial in gastric cancer. *Proc Am Soc Clin Oncol* 1991;10:137.

313. Wilke H, Preusser P, Fink U, et al. High dose folinic acid/etoposide/5-fluorouracil in advanced gastric cancer—a phase II study in elderly patients or patients with cardiac risk. *Invest New Drugs* 1990;8:65.

314. Vanhoefer U, Rougier P, Wilke H, et al. Final results of a randomized phase III trial of sequential high-dose methotrexate, fluorouracil, and doxorubicin versus etoposide, leucovorin, and fluorouracil versus infusional fluorouracil and cisplatin in advanced gastric cancer: a trial of the European Organization for Research and Treatment of Cancer Gastrointestinal Tract Cancer Cooperative Group. *J Clin Oncol* 2000;18:2648.

315. Ohtsu A, Shimada Y, Shirao K, et al. Randomized phase III trial of fluorouracil alone versus fluorouracil plus cisplatin versus uracil and tegafur plus mitomycin in patients with unresectable, advanced gastric cancer: The Japan Clinical Oncology Group Study (JCOG9205). *J Clin Oncol* 2003;21:54.

316. Metzger R, Leichman CG, Danenberg KD, et al. ERCC1 mRNA levels complement thymidylate synthase mRNA levels in predicting response and survival for gastric cancer patients receiving combination cisplatin and fluorouracil chemotherapy. *J Clin Oncol* 1998;16:309.

317. Lenz HJ, Leichman CG, Danenberg KD, et al. Thymidylate synthase mRNA level in adenocarcinoma of the stomach: a predictor for primary tumor response and overall survival. *J Clin Oncol* 1996;14(1):176.

318. Cascinu S, Graziano F, Del Ferro E, et al. Expression of p53 protein and resistance to preoperative chemotherapy in locally advanced gastric carcinoma. *Cancer* 1998;83:1917.

319. Ikeguchi M, Saito H, Katano K, et al. Relationship between the long-term effects of intraperitoneal chemotherapy and the expression of p53 and p21 in patients with gastric carcinoma at stage IIIa and stage IIIb. *Int Surg* 1997;82:170.

320. Yeh KH, Shun CT, Chen CL, et al. High expression of thymidylate synthase is associated with the drug resistance of gastric carcinoma to high dose 5-fluorouracil-based systemic chemotherapy. *Cancer* 1998;82:1626.

321. Mandard AM, Dalibard F, Mandard JC, et al. Pathologic assessment of tumor regression after preoperative chemoradiotherapy of esophageal carcinoma. Clinicopathologic correlations. *Cancer* 1994;73:2680.

322. Weisburger JH, Marquardt H, Mower HF, et al. Inhibition of carcinogenesis: vitamin C and the prevention of gastric cancer. *Prev Med* 1980;9:352.

323. Dorgan JF, Schatzkin A. Antioxidant micronutrients in cancer prevention. *Hematol Oncol Clin North Am* 1991;5:43.

324. Forman D. Are nitrates a significant risk factor in human cancer? *Cancer Surv* 1989;8:443.

325. Burstein M, Monge E, Leon-Barua R, et al. Low peptic ulcer and high gastric cancer prevalence in a developing country with a high prevalence of infection by Helicobacter pylori. *J Clin Gastroenterol* 1991;13:154.

326. Satomi D, Takiguchi N, Koda K, et al. Apoptosis and apoptosis-associated gene products related to the response to neoadjuvant chemotherapy for gastric cancer. *Int J Oncol* 2002;20(6):1167.

327. Weber WA, Ott K, Becker K, et al. Prediction of response to preoperative chemotherapy in adenocarcinomas of the esophagogastric junction by metabolic imaging. *J Clin Oncol* 2001;19(12):3058.

328. Downey RJ, Akhurst T, Ilson D, et al. Whole body 18FDG-PET and the response of esophageal cancer to induction therapy: results of a prospective trial. *J Clin Oncol* 2003;21:428.

329. Ekbom GA, Gleysteen JJ. Gastric malignancy: resection for palliation. *Surgery* 1980;88:476.

330. Meijer S, De Bakker OJ, Hoitsma HF. Palliative resection in gastric cancer. *J Surg Oncol* 1983;23:77.

331. Butler JA, Dubrow TJ, Trezona T, et al. Total gastrectomy in the treatment of advanced gastric cancer. *Am J Surg* 1989;158:602.

332. Aranha GV, Georgen R. Gastric linitis plastica is not a surgical disease. *Surgery* 1989;106:758.

333. Bozzetti F, Bonfanti G, Audisio RA, et al. Prognosis of patients after palliative surgical procedures for carcinoma of the stomach. *Surg Gynecol Obstet* 1987;164:151.

334. Boddie AW Jr, McMurtrey MJ, Giacco GG, et al. Palliative total gastrectomy and esophagogastrectomy. A reevaluation. *Cancer* 1983;51:1195.

335. Maruyama K, Gunven P, Okabayashi K, et al. Lymph node metastases of gastric cancer. General pattern in 1931 patients. *Ann Surg* 1989;210:596.

336. Roviello F, Marrelli D, de Manzoni G, et al. Prospective study of peritoneal recurrence after curative surgery for gastric cancer. *Br J Surg* 2003;90:1113.

337. Allum WH, Hallissey MT, Kelly KA. Adjuvant chemotherapy in operable gastric cancer. Five-year follow-up of first British Stomach Cancer Group trial. *Lancet* 1989;1:571.

338. Noguchi Y, Imada T, Matsumoto A, et al. Radical surgery for gastric cancer. A review of the Japanese experience. *Cancer* 1989;64:2053.

339. Boku N, Chin K, Hosokawa K, et al. Biological markers as a predictor for response and prognosis of unresectable gastric cancer patients treated with 5-fluorouracil and cis-platinum. *Clin Cancer Res* 1998;4(6):1469.

340. Baba H, Korenaga D, Okamura T, et al. Prognostic factors in gastric cancer with serosal invasion. Univariate and multivariate analyses. *Arch Surg* 1989;124:1061.

341. Alexander HR, Grem JL, Pass HI, et al. Neoadjuvant chemotherapy for locally advanced gastric adenocarcinoma. *Oncology (Huntingt)* 1993;7(5):37.

342. Bozzetti F, Bonfanti G, Morabito A, et al. A multifactorial approach for the prognosis of patients with carcinoma of the stomach after curative resection. *Surg Gynecol Obstet* 1986;162:229.

343. Takekoshi T, Baba Y, Ota H, et al. Endoscopic resection of early gastric carcinoma: results of a retrospective analysis of 308 cases. *Endoscopy* 1994;26:352

344. Tani M, Inoue H, Kando F, et al. Endoscopic mucosal resection for early gastric cancer—usefulness of planning fractionated resection. *Prog Digest Endosc* 1995;47:64.

345. Chonan A, Mochizuki F, Ando M, et al. Endoscopic mucosal resection (EMR) of early gastric cancer—usefulness of aspiration EMR using a capfitted scope. *Digest Endosc* 1998;10:31.

346. Fujisaki J, Ikegami M, Oota Y, et al. Endoscopic mucosal resection for early gastric cancers: its follow-up and management for problematic cases. *Prog Digest Endosc* 1997;50:70.

347. Misaka R, Kawaguchi M, Saitoh T. A study of the efficiency of endoscopic mucosal resection and the additional treatment as the total planning treatment for early gastric cancer. *Prog Digest Endosc* 1997;50:79.

348. Honmyo U, Misumi A, Murakami A, et al. A clinicopathological study on surgically resected stomachs in patients with preceding endoscopic mucosal resection for early gastric cancer. *Digest Endosc* 1996;8:192.

349. Tada M, Matsumoto Y, Murakami A, et al. Problems and their solutions in curative endoscopic resection of early gastric carcinomas. *Digest Endosc* 1993;5:1169.

350. Abe T, Ihto M. Endoscopic mucosal resection for the early gastric cancer. *Prog Digest Endosc* 1995;17:146.

351. Hiki Y. Surgical treatment for gastric cancer from the surgical perspective. *Gastrointest Endosc* 1991;33:2285.

352. O-izumi H, Matsuda T, Fukase K, et al. Endoscopic resection for early gastric cancer. The actual procedure and clinical evaluation. *Stomach Intestine* 1991;26:289.

353. Atsumi M, Kodama T, Uehira H, et al. Surveillance after endoscopic resection and early diagnosis of local recurrence. *Stomach Intestine* 1993;28:1433.

354. Takahashi H, Kojima T, Parra A, et al. Clinical evaluation of endoscopic therapy for early gastric cancer. *Endoscopy* 1997;29.

355. Kojima T, Parra-Blanco A, Takahashi H, et al. Outcome of endoscopic mucosal resection for early gastric cancer: review of the Japanese literature. *Gastrointest Endosc* 1998;48:550.

356. Ono H, Kondo H, Gotoda T, et al. Endoscopic mucosal resection for treatment of early gastric cancer. *Gut* 2001;48:225.

357. Sakai T, Takekoshi T, Kaku S. Endoscopic resection (ER) 3—double snare method. In: Nakamura K, ed. *Practical gastroenterology*. Tokyo: Bunkodo, 1998:62.

358. Carrato A, Diaz-Rubio E, Medrano J. Phase III trial of surgery versus adjuvant chemotherapy with mitomycin C and tegafur plus uracil, starting within the first week after surgery, for gastric adenocarcinoma. *Proc Am Soc Clin Oncol* 1995;14:198.

359. Nakajima T, Nashimoto A, Kitamura M, et al. Adjuvant mitomycin and fluorouracil followed by oral uracil plus tegafur in serosa-negative gastric cancer: a randomised trial. Gastric Cancer Surgical Study Group. *Lancet* 1999;354:273.

360. Nakajima T, Takahashi T, Takagi K, et al. Comparison of 5-fluorouracil with ftorafur in adjuvant chemotherapies with combined inductive and maintenance therapies for gastric cancer. *J Clin Oncol* 1984;2:1366.

361. Estape J, Grau JJ, Lcobendas F, et al. Mitomycin C as an adjuvant treatment to resected gastric cancer. A 10-year follow-up. *Ann Surg* 1991;213:219.

362. Adjuvant treatments following curative resection for gastric cancer. The Italian Gastrointestinal Tumor Study Group. *Br J Surg* 1988;75:1100.

363. Lise M, Nitti D, Marchet A, et al. Prognostic factors in resectable gastric cancer: results of EORTC study no. 40813 on FAM adjuvant chemotherapy. *Ann Surg Oncol* 1995;2:495.

364. Wilke H, Preusser P, Fink U, et al. Preoperative chemotherapy in locally advanced and nonresectable gastric cancer: a phase II study with etoposide, doxorubicin, and cisplatin. *J Clin Oncol* 1989;7:1318.

365. Ajani JA, Roth JA, Putnam JB, et al. Feasibility of five courses of pre-operative chemotherapy in patients with resectable adenocarcinoma of the oesophagus or gastrooesophageal junction. *Eur J Cancer* 1995;31A:665.

366. Wils J. The treatment of advanced gastric cancer. *Semin Oncol* 1996;23:397.

367. Fortner JG, Lauwers GY, Thaler HT, et al. Nativity, complications, and pathology are determinants of surgical results for gastric cancer. *Cancer* 1994;73:8.

368. El Rifai W, Harper JC, Cummings OW, et al. Consistent genetic alterations in xenografts of proximal stomach and gastro-esophageal junction adenocarcinomas. *Cancer Res* 1998;58:34.

369. Yustein AS, Harper JC, Petroni GR, et al. Allelotype of gastric adenocarcinoma. *Cancer Res* 1999;59:1437.

370. Schneider BG, Pulitzer DR, Brown RD, et al. Allelic imbalance in gastric cancer: an affected site on chromosome arm 3p. *Genes Chromosomes Cancer* 1995;13:263.

371. Wisbeck WM, Becher EM, Russell AH. Adenocarcinoma of the stomach: autopsy observations with therapeutic implications for the radiation oncologist. *Radiother Oncol* 1986;7:13.

372. Sano T, Sasako M, Nashimoto A, et al. Gastric cancer surgery: results of morbidity and mortality of a prospective randomized controlled trial (JCOG 9501) comparing D2 and extended para-aortic lymphadenectomy. *J Clin Oncol* 2004 (*in press*).

373. Ott K, Fink U, Becker K, et al. Prediction of response to preoperative chemotherapy in gastric carcinoma by metabolic imaging: results of a prospective trial. *J Clin Oncol* 2003;21:4603.

CHARLES J. YEO
THERESA PLUTH YEO
RALPH H. HRUBAN
SCOTT E. KERN
CHRISTINE A. IACOBUZIO-DONOHUE
ANIRBAN MAITRA
MICHAEL GOGGINS
MARCIA I. CANTO
WELLS MESSERSMITH
ROSS A. ABRAMS
DANIEL A. LAHERU
MANUEL HIDALGO
ELIZABETH M. JAFFEE

SECTION 3

Cancer of the Pancreas

EPIDEMIOLOGY AND RISK FACTORS

EPIDEMIOLOGY

Pancreatic cancer (PC) is the fifth leading cause of cancer death in the United States, with 28,000 to 30,300 newly diagnosed cases (ductal adenocarcinoma being the most common form) per year.[1] Approximately an equal number of deaths occur annually from PC.[1] The incidence rate for PC is approximately nine new cases per 100,000 people, with the peak incidence in the seventh and eighth decades of life and an average age of 60 to 65 years at diagnosis.[1] The incidence rate is slightly higher in men than in women (relative risk, 1.35) and 30% to 40% higher in African American men.

Survival in patients with untreated PC is poor. For all stages combined, the 1-year survival rate is 19% and the 5-year survival rate is 4%.[1] The majority (80%) of PCs are metastatic at the time of diagnosis. Surgical resection (when margin negative, node negative) offers the best possibility for cure, with 5-year survival approaching 40% when performed at specialized major medical institutions.[2,3]

In the United States, incidence rates of PC increased threefold between 1920 and 1978, an increase that has also been observed in other developed countries.[3,4] Rates for men and for women have modestly declined since 1978 and appear to have stabilized at the current rates. A portion of the increased incidence may have been attributable to more accurate disease diagnosis and less disease misclassification. Additionally, improved surveillance may account for a small portion of the increased incidence.

A positive relationship exists between certain environmental exposures and cases of PC, including personal cigarette smoking, environmental tobacco smoke (ETS), and chemical exposures.[3,4] Cigarette smoking in the United States and in other countries increased greatly in the first half of the twentieth century. In fact, 40% of adult Americans were smokers in 1965. Increased cigarette smoking likely accounts for a large portion of the increased incidence of PC. By 1990, the prevalence of smoking among Americans had decreased to 25%, with modest declines again noted in 1999.[3] Because of the long latency period before diagnosis, it remains to be seen if this will translate into lower PC incidence rates in the future.

ETIOLOGIC (RISK) FACTORS

Tobacco Smoke Exposure

Tobacco smoke exposure plays a significant role in the development of PC. It has been estimated that tobacco smoking contributes to the development of 20% to 30% of PCs.[4] The strongest associations between cigarette smoking and PC have been observed when the pack-years smoked were within the previous 10 years.[3] Smoking cessation can reduce this risk. Indeed, Mulder et al.[5] have estimated that moderate reduction in smoking in Europe could save almost 68,000 lives that would otherwise be lost to PC by the year 2020.

Environmental Tobacco Smoke

ETS contains the same toxins, irritants, and carcinogens, such as carbon monoxide, nicotine, cyanide, ammonia, benzene, nitrosamines, vinyl chloride, arsenic, and hydrocarbons, as do cigarettes. Thirty-seven percent of American adult nonsmokers report that they either live with a smoker or are exposed to ETS at work.[6] A Department of Health and Human Services' Centers for Disease Control and Prevention study estimated that nearly 9 out of 10 nonsmoking Americans are exposed to ETS, as measured by the level of cotinine in their blood.[6]

Demographic and Host Risk Factors

A number of demographic risk factors have been associated with the development of PC worldwide and are summarized in Table 29.3-1. Included are older age (most PCs occur between the ages of 60 and 80), African American race, low socioeconomic status, and Ashkenazi Jewish heritage (related to germline mutations).[4]

Diabetes Mellitus

Host etiologic factors associated with an increased risk of PC include a history of diabetes mellitus (DM), chronic cirrhosis, pancreatitis, a high-fat/cholesterol diet, and prior cholecystectomy.[3,4] The association between DM, pancreatitis, and the

TABLE 29.3-1. Factors Associated with Increased Risk of Pancreatic Cancer

Advancing age
African American males
Low socioeconomic status
Native female Hawaiians
Ashkenazi Jewish heritage
Cigarette smoking
Six genetic syndromes (see Table 29.3-2)
Diabetes mellitus
Chronic pancreatitis
Cirrhosis
Obesity
Increased height
Low level of physical activity
High-fat and cholesterol diet
Occupational exposure to carcinogens (PCBs, DDT, NNK, benzidine)

DDT, dichlorodiphenyl trichloroethane; PCBs, polychlorinated biphenyls.

development of PC is complex because PC, by destroying the pancreatic parenchyma, can itself cause DM and pancreatitis.

Metaanalysis of 20 epidemiologic studies on the association between DM and PC confirms that the pooled relative risk of PC in persons with DM for 5 years is double (relative risk, 2.0; confidence interval, 1.3 to 2.2) the risk of persons without DM.[3] The analysis further suggested that impaired glucose tolerance, insulin resistance, and hyperinsulinemia are involved in the etiology of PC.

Obesity and Physical Activity

High body mass index (a measure of obesity), increased height, and a low level of physical activity all increased the risk of PC, as demonstrated in a cohort study of 160,000 health professionals.[7] Moderate physical activity resulted in decreased PC rates, and merely walking or hiking 1.5 hours or more per week was associated with a 50% reduction in PC. Likewise, body mass index had no effect if the participant was a moderate exerciser. For cigarette smoking, the strongest associations with PC were observed when the pack-years smoked were within the previous 15 years. These findings clearly suggest that weight loss and exercise may reduce the risk of developing PC independent of smoking cessation.

Occupational Factors

A metaanalysis of 20 population studies of occupational exposures and PC from journal publications during the period 1969 to 1998 was performed.[8] Exposure to chlorinated hydrocarbon solvents, nickel and nickel compounds, chromium compounds, polycyclic aromatic hydrocarbons, organochlorine insecticides, silica dust, and aliphatic solvents conveyed elevated risk ratios. Overall, the occupational etiologic fraction for PC was estimated at 12%, but it increased to 29% when the chlorinated hydrocarbon solvents were considered in a subpopulation.

Elevated serum levels of organochloride compounds (dichlorodiphenyltrichlorethane, dichlorodiphenyldichloroethylene, and polychlorinated biphenyls), are also associated with the development of PC.[9] Approximately 90% of PC patients have an acquired K-ras oncogene mutation. In a case-control study, PC patients with K-ras mutations had significantly higher levels of dichlorodiphenyltrichlorethane, dichlorodiphenyldichloroethylene, and three polychlorinated biphenyl compounds compared to PC patients without the K-ras mutation and to those in the control group. These compounds are postulated to enhance the actions of K-ras rather than cause the mutation, suggesting a gene-environment interaction or effect modification. It may also be that these compounds interact with premalignant ductal precursor lesions and accelerate their malignant progression.

Other Possible Factors

Factors that have been repeatedly studied, with no consistent association with the development of PC, include moderate alcohol intake, nonhereditary and acute pancreatitis, and coffee drinking.

GENETIC PREDISPOSITIONS

PC is characterized by inherited and acquired genetic mutations.[10] Genetic predisposition plays a small but significant role in PC risk. Activation of the oncogene K-ras plus inactivation of

tumor suppressor genes (p53, DPC4, p16, and BRCA2) are associated with the development of PC. Nearly 90% of all cases of PC have p16 mutations, 75% have p53 mutations, and 55% have DPC4 mutations. Fewer than 4% of PC cases appear to involve dysfunction of the various DNA mismatch repair genes [microsatellite instability (MIN)].

It is estimated that 10% to 20% of PCs are hereditary or have a familial link. Multiple lines of evidence support this. Cohort studies have shown an increased risk of developing PC among individuals who report a family history of PC. Tersmette et al.[11] have shown that this risk increases with the number of affected members in the family. Risk was estimated by comparing new observed cases of PC to expected cases based on the United States population-based Surveillance, Epidemiology, and End Results program data. An 18-fold increased risk of PC was found in familial PC kindreds compared to sporadic groups. When three or more family members were affected with PC, there was a 57-fold increased risk. When stratified according to age, the risk of PC was largely confined to relatives older than 60 years of age.

Segregation analyses suggest that aggregation of PC in families has a genetic rather than an environmental basis.[12] Nongenetic transmission models were rejected ($P < .0001$) in the segregation analysis of 287 families, ascertained through an index case diagnosed with PC. The most parsimonious model included autosomal dominant inheritance of a rare allele (still to be identified), estimated to be carried by approximately 0.5% of the population.[12]

INHERITED SYNDROMES

Although accounting for less than 20% of the familial aggregation of PC, several genetic syndromes (caused by germline mutations) associated with an increased risk of PC have been identified.[3,10] These are summarized in Table 29.3-2 and include

1. Familial breast cancer with germline mutations in the *BRCA2* gene. Carriers of germline BRCA2 mutations have a 3.5- to 10.0-fold increased risk of developing PC, and 17% (1 in 6) of patients with PC and a strong family history of PC (at least 3 family members with PC) have been shown to have germline *BRCA2* mutations. This makes BRCA2 mutation the most common germline mutation in patients with hereditary PC.
2. Familial atypical multiple mole melanoma syndrome with germline mutations in the *p16* gene. Carriers of *p16* germline mutations have a 12- to 20-fold increased risk of developing PC, as well as an increased risk of melanoma.

TABLE 29.3-2.   Genetic Syndromes and Gene Alterations Associated with Familial Pancreatic Cancer

Syndrome	Gene Alteration (Chromosomal Locus)
Hereditary pancreatitis	*PRSSI* (7q35)
Hereditary nonpolyposis colorectal cancer (Lynch II variant)	hMSH2, hMLH1, others
Hereditary breast and ovarian cancer	BRCA2 (13q12q13)
Familial atypical multiple mole melanoma (FAMMM) syndrome	p16 (9p21)
Peutz-Jeghers syndrome	STK11/LKB1 (19p13)
Ataxia-telangiectasia	ATM (11q22-23)

TABLE 29.3-3. Solid Exocrine Neoplasms of the Pancreas

Neoplasm	Age (Y)	Direction of Differentiation	Most Common Genetic Alterations	Overall 5-Y Survival Rates (%)
Ductal adenocarcinoma	Most, 60–80	Infiltrating glands with an intense desmoplastic reaction	Activating mutations in *K-ras*, inactivation of DPC4, p16, p53	4
Acinar cell carcinoma	Mean, 58	Pancreatic exocrine enzymes, including trypsin, chymo-trypsin, and lipase	One-fourth have APC/β-cate-nin mutations	6
Pancreatoblastoma	Mean age, 2.5 in children, 40 in adults	Multiple, including acinar; distinctive squamoid nests	LOH on 11p	55

APC, advanced pancreatic cancer; LOH, loss of heterozygosity.

3. The Peutz-Jeghers syndrome (PJS), characterized by muco-cutaneous melanocytic macules and hamartomatous polyps of the gastrointestinal (GI) tract. Patients with the PJS have a greater than 100-fold increased risk of developing PC.
4. The hereditary nonpolyposis colorectal cancer syndrome, characterized by germline mutations in one of the DNA mismatch repair genes (*hMSH1, hMSH2*, etc.).
5. Hereditary pancreatitis with germline mutations in the *PRSS1* (cationic trypsinogen) gene. Patients develop severe pancreatitis at a young age (often children and adolescents) and have a 50-fold excess risk of developing PC.
6. Ataxia-telangiectasia, a rare autosomal recessive inherited disorder, characterized by cerebellar ataxia, oculocutaneous telangiectasias, and cellular and humoral immune deficiencies. The gene, ATM, is also associated with an increased risk of leukemia, lymphoma, and cancers of the breast, ovaries, biliary tract, stomach, and, occasionally, the pancreas.

A seventh syndrome, that of PC, pancreatic insufficiency, and DM, has been described in a family (called *Family X*), and the phenotype has been linked to chromosome 4q32-34.[3]

DATA FROM THE NATIONAL FAMILIAL PANCREAS TUMOR REGISTRY

The above genetic syndromes do not explain the vast majority of cases in which there is a familial aggregation of PC. The National Familial Pancreas Tumor Registry has therefore been established at Johns Hopkins, with the hope of identifying the causes for the aggregation of PC in families. To date, more than 1200 families have enrolled in this registry. Early analyses of the kindreds enrolled in the National Familial Pancreas Tumor Registry have shown that the risk of cancer is 18-fold greater in first-degree relatives of familial PC cases (at least 2 first-degree relatives with PC in the family) than it is in first-degree relatives of sporadic PC cases (families in which there has been only 1 member with PC).[11] In addition, the increased risk of PC in familial PC kindreds extends to second-degree relatives, as a significantly increased rate of PC was identified in second-degree relatives of familial cases compared with sporadic pancreatic cases (3.7% vs. 0.6%; *P*<.0001).

PATHOLOGY

Although we tend to think of "PC" as a single entity, in fact, an array of biologically and clinically distinct neoplasms can arise in the pancreas. Neoplasms of the pancreas can be broadly grouped into those with predominantly exocrine differentiation and those with endocrine differentiation. Exocrine neoplasms of the pancreas can be further subdivided into cystic and solid tumors. The vast majority of malignancies of the pancreas are solid infiltrating ductal adenocarcinomas, and the term *PC* is therefore often used synonymously with infiltrating ductal adenocarcinoma.

SOLID NEOPLASMS OF THE EXOCRINE PANCREAS

The most common solid neoplasms of the exocrine pancreas are the infiltrating ductal adenocarcinoma and variants of ductal adenocarcinoma, acinar cell carcinoma, and pancreatoblastoma (Table 29.3-3). *Infiltrating ductal adenocarcinomas* are malignant epithelial neoplasms that show glandular or ductal differentiation.[13] Most arise in patients between the ages of 60 and 80 years, and men outnumber women (male-female ratio, 1.35:1.0). The majority of ductal adenocarcinomas arise in the head of the gland, but they can also arise in the body or in the tail or even diffusely involve multiple parts of the pancreas. Grossly, infiltrating ductal adenocarcinomas form firm, poorly defined white-yellow masses. These carcinomas often extend beyond the grossly identifiable tumor, and invasion into large vessels and adjacent organs is common.

Three features characterize infiltrating ductal adenocarcinomas at the light microscopic level.[13] First, by definition, the neoplastic cells show evidence of glandular/ductal differentiation. The second feature that characterizes ductal adenocarcinomas is that they induce an intense nonneoplastic desmoplastic stromal reaction. This desmoplastic stroma contains myofibroblasts, lymphocytes, extracellular collagen, and trapped nonneoplastic pancreatic tissue, including trapped islets of Langerhans. An infiltrative growth pattern is the third feature that characterizes infiltrating ductal adenocarcinoma. This infiltrative growth is manifested in the haphazard arrangement of the neoplastic glands; in extension of the carcinoma beyond the pancreas into adjacent structures, including large vessels, the duodenum, the stomach, the adrenals, and the peritoneum; and by perineural and lymphovascular invasion (Fig. 29.3-1). Growth along nerves is one route by which infiltrating ductal adenocarcinomas extend out of the gland and into the retroperitoneum, and lymphovascular invasion is associated with lymph node and more distant metastases.

A growing body of evidence suggests that histologically well-defined noninvasive epithelial proliferations begin in the

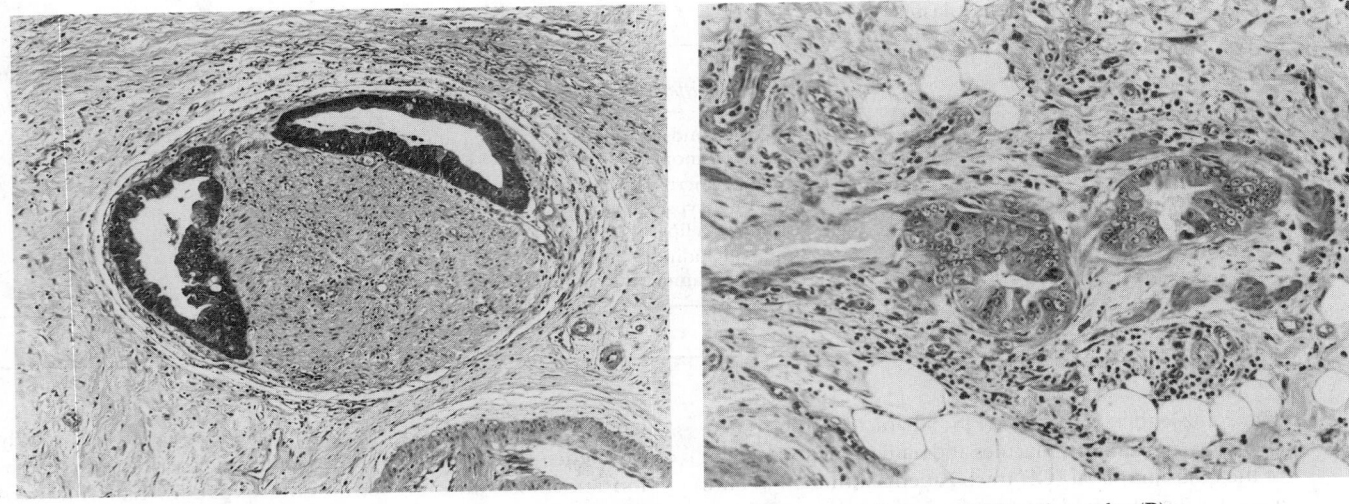

FIGURE 29.3-1.   Infiltrating ductal adenocarcinoma of the pancreas. Perineural **(A)** and vascular **(B)** invasion are common.

smaller pancreatic ducts (Fig. 29.3-2A) and progress to invasive ductal adenocarcinoma. These lesions, called *pancreatic intraepithelial neoplasia* (PanIN), often accompany infiltrating ductal adenocarcinomas, and PanINs harbor many of the same molec-

ular genetic alterations as are found in infiltrating ductal adenocarcinomas.[14] PanINs are important to recognize because they can mimic an infiltrating carcinoma microscopically and because they are reasonable targets for chemoprevention and

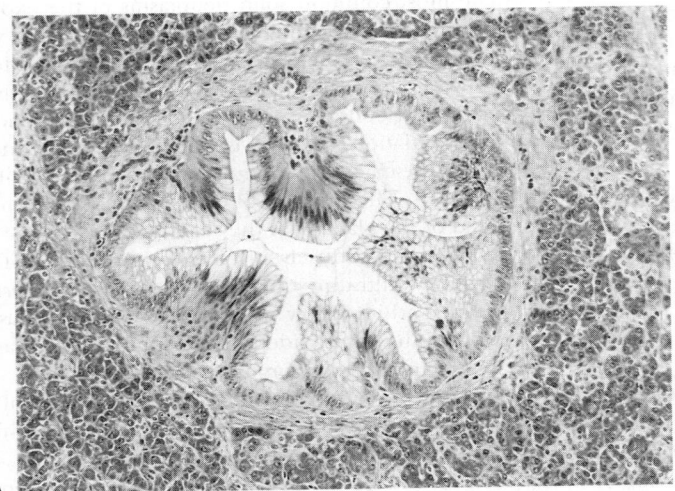

FIGURE 29.3-2.   **A:** Pancreatic intraepithelial neoplasia (PanIN). These lesions in the small pancreatic ducts can progress to an infiltrating ductal adenocarcinoma. **B:** Histologic-genetic progression model of infiltrating pancreatic ductal adenocarcinoma from PanIN. (From Wilentz RE, Iacobuzio-Donahue CA, Argani P, et al. Loss of expression of Dpc4 in pancreatic intraepithelial neoplasia: evidence that DPC4 inactivation occurs late in neoplastic progression. *Cancer Res* 2000;60:2002, with permission.)

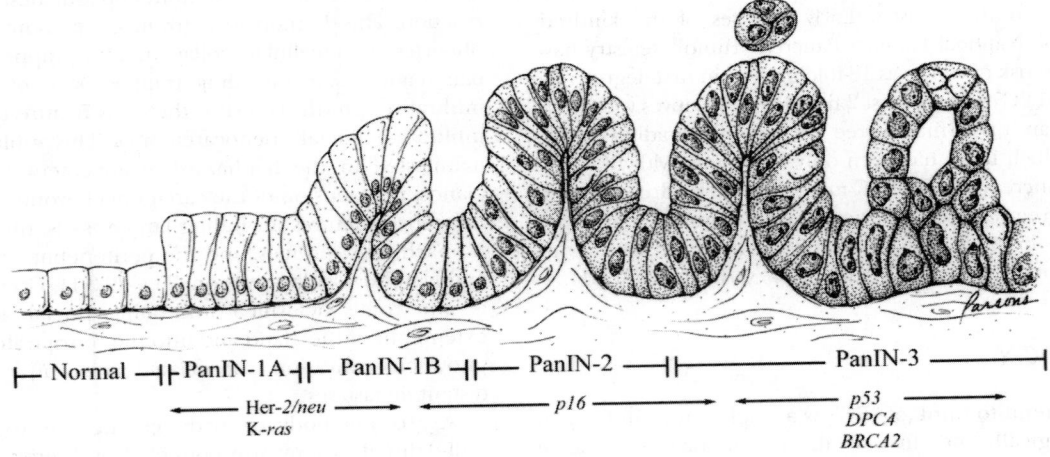

screening for early pancreatic neoplasia. Figure 29.3-2*B* depicts the postulated progression model from PanIN to invasive ductal adenocarcinoma.

Immunohistochemically, most infiltrating ductal adenocarcinomas express cytokeratins 7 and 19, carcinoembryonic antigen, epithelial membrane antigen, CA 19-9, and the mucins (MUC1, MUC3, MUC4, and MUC5).[13] Fifty-five percent of ductal adenocarcinomas show a complete loss of DPC4 protein expression.

Infiltrating ductal adenocarcinomas are fully malignant neoplasms. The overall 5-year survival rate is less than 4%, but 5-year survival approaches 20% for all patients who undergo surgical resection.

Several variants of infiltrating adenocarcinoma exist. These include *signet-ring cell, medullary, adenosquamous, colloid ductal* (mucinous noncystic), and *anaplastic carcinomas*, as well as the *undifferentiated carcinoma with osteoclast-like giant cells*.[13] Of importance, signet-ring cell carcinomas have to be distinguished from metastases from a gastric or breast primary, and medullary carcinomas of the pancreas are associated with specific genetic alterations (inactivation of one of the DNA mismatch repair genes).

Acinar cell carcinomas are malignant epithelial neoplasms that show evidence of exocrine enzyme production.[15,16] Most acinar cell carcinomas arise in adults (mean age, 58 years), although cases have been reported in children. The male-female ratio is 3.6:1.0. Most patients present nonspecifically with signs and symptoms related to a large pancreatic mass, but 15% present with the syndrome of metastatic fat necrosis (subcutaneous fat necrosis, peripheral eosinophilia, and polyarthralgias) caused by the release of lipase into the circulation. Grossly acinar cell carcinomas are usually softer than most ductal adenocarcinomas, and by light microscopy they grow in sheets and at least focally form acinar structures. Acini are composed of pyramidal cells with basal nuclei and granular cytoplasm, oriented around small lumina. Immunohistochemical labeling is often needed to establish a diagnosis. In most cases the neoplastic cells label with antibodies to trypsin, chymotrypsin, and/or lipase. At the ultrastructural level the presence of zymogen granules can be used to confirm acinar differentiation. Acinar cell carcinomas are fully malignant neoplasms.

Pancreatoblastomas are malignant epithelial neoplasms that show several directions of differentiation.[13,17,18] At a minimum, acinar differentiation and distinctive squamous nests are present. In addition, many pancreatoblastomas show endocrine, ductal, and even mesenchymal differentiation. Most pancreatoblastomas arise in children, but up to a third may arise in adults. At the genetic level, pancreatoblastomas frequently show loss of heterozygosity (LOH) on the short arm of chromosome 11 near the WT-2 locus, a finding that links them with other embryonal neoplasms such as hepatoblastomas.[18] Pancreatoblastomas are malignant neoplasms. A third of the patients have metastases at diagnosis. The outcome for children is slightly better than for adults.

CYSTIC NEOPLASMS OF THE EXOCRINE PANCREAS

The most common cystic neoplasms of the pancreas include mucinous cystic neoplasms, intraductal papillary mucinous neoplasms (IPMNs), serous cystic neoplasms, and solid and pseudopapillary neoplasms (Table 29.3-4). A review of the diagnostic features of cystic neoplasms of the pancreas can be found on the Web (http://pathology2.jhu.edu/pancreascyst/index.cfm).

Mucinous cystic neoplasms are much more common in women (90%) than in men.[19] These distinctive neoplasms arise in the tail of the gland more frequently than in the head of the gland. Grossly, mucinous cystic neoplasms are composed of large cysts that contain thick tenacious mucin.[13,19] The cysts are separated by thick septae and do not communicate with the larger pancreatic ducts. These cysts are lined by a columnar mucin-producing epithelium, and the stroma surrounding the cysts has a histologic appearance similar to ovarian stroma. The epithelium can show varying degrees of cytologic and architectural atypia, and one-third of mucinous cystic neoplasms are associated with an invasive carcinoma, usually an invasive ductal adenocarcinoma. Based on the degree of cytologic and architectural atypia and the presence or absence of an invasive carcinoma, mucinous cystic neoplasms have been categorized into mucinous cystadenoma (no atypia, no invasion), borderline mucinous cystic neoplasm (moderate atypia, no invasion), mucinous cystic neoplasm with *in situ* carcinoma (marked atypia, no invasion), and mucinous cystadenocarcinoma (an associated invasive carcinoma).[13] The critical prognosticator for patients with a mucinous cystic neoplasm is the presence or absence of an invasive

TABLE 29.3-4. Cystic Neoplasms of the Exocrine Pancreas

Neoplasm	Gender	Involvement of Larger Ducts	Cyst Contents	Cyst Lining	Stroma	Immunolabeling
Mucinous cystic neoplasm	90% female	No	Mucoid	Columnar mucinous epithelium	Distinctive ovarian type	Cytokeratin, MUC2, CEA, stroma labels for inhibin and progesterone receptors
Intraductal papillary mucinous neoplasm	60% male	Yes	Mucoid	Columnar mucinous epithelium	Collagenous	Cytokeratin, MUC2, CEA
Serous cystic neoplasm	70% female	No	Clear, watery	Low cuboidal glycogen-rich	Collagenous	Cytokeratin
Solid pseudopapillary neoplasm	90% female	No	Hemorrhagic necrotic	Discohesive uniform cells	Collagenous	CD10, nuclear β-catenin

CEA, carcinoembryonic antigen; MUC, mucin.

carcinoma. Patients with completely resected mucinous neoplasms without an associated invasive carcinoma are cured.[19] By contrast, the 5-year survival rate for patients with a completely resected invasive mucinous cystadenocarcinoma is approximately 50%.

IPMNs also produce mucin, but in contrast to mucinous cystic neoplasms, IPMNs involve the larger pancreatic ducts and lack a distinctive stroma.[13,20] Because these neoplasms involve the larger pancreatic ducts, mucin can often be seen on endoscopy oozing from a patulous ampulla of Vater. Grossly, IPMNs reveal villous projections into a dilated pancreatic duct that contains thick mucin. By light microscopy IPMNs are composed of papillae lined by tall columnar mucin-producing epithelium. One-third of IPMNs have an associated invasive carcinoma, and this invasive carcinoma often shows abundant extracellular mucin production (colloid carcinoma). The 5-year survival rate for patients with resected invasive carcinomas arising in association with IPMNs is approximately 40%.

Serous cystic neoplasms are almost always benign.[13,21] The average age is 65 years, and the male-female ratio is 3:7. Serous cystic neoplasms have a characteristic gross appearance. They are well demarcated and on cross section are composed of multiple (at times innumerable) small cysts, often with a central stellate scar. By light microscopy the cysts are lined by low cuboidal cells with uniform centrally placed nuclei and clear cytoplasm. Special stains will demonstrate that the cytoplasmic clearing is caused by abundant amounts of glycogen.

Solid pseudopapillary neoplasms are distinctive neoplasms of uncertain histogenesis that almost always arise in young women (90% female; average age, 26 years).[13,22] They are well demarcated and grossly are composed of solid areas admixed with cystic areas with hemorrhage and necrosis. By light microscopy the solid areas are composed of sheets of relatively uniform cells and delicate blood vessels. The nuclei are uniform, and the cells appear somewhat discohesive. In some areas the neoplastic cells appear to "drop out," forming pseudopapillae around small blood vessels. Immunohistochemically, the neoplastic cells label for CD 10 and α_1-antitrypsin and show an abnormal nuclear labeling for β-catenin. The abnormal nuclear labeling for β-catenin is a manifestation of genetic mutations in the β-catenin gene. Surgical resection is the treatment of choice for these neoplasms, and, if completely resected, most patients are cured of their disease.

MOLECULAR GENETICS

Four categories of mutated genes play a role in the pancreatic tumorigenesis: oncogenes, tumor suppressor genes, genome-maintenance genes, and tissue-maintenance genes (summarized in Table 29.3-5). Some of these mutations are germline;

TABLE 29.3-5. Genetic Profile of Pancreatic Carcinoma[a]

Gene	Gene Locations	Frequency in Cancers (%)	Timing during Tumorigenesis[b]	Mutation Origin
ONCOGENES				
KRAS2	12p	95	Early-mid	Som.
BRAF	7q	4	—	Som.
AKT2	19q	10–20	—	Som.
MYB	6q	10	—	Som.
EBY genome		<1	—	
TUMOR SUPPRESSORS/GENOME-MAINTENANCE GENES				
P16/RB1	9p/13q	>90	Mid-late	Som.>germ.
TP53	17p	50–75	Late	Som.
MADH4	18q	55	Late	Som.
BRCA2	13q	7	Late	Germ.>som.
FANCC/FANCG	9q/9p	3	—	Germ. or som.
MKK4	17p	4	—	Som.
LKB1/STK11	19p	4	—	Som.>germ.
ACVR1B	12q	2	—	Som.
TGFBR1	9q	1	—	Som.[c]
MS1⁻/TGFBR2	3p	1	—	Som.[c]
MS1⁺/TGFBR2	3p	4	—	Som.>germ.[d]
ACVR2	2q	4	—	Som.>germ.[d]
BAX	19q	4	—	Som.>germ.[d]
MLH1	3p	4	—	Som.>germ.[d]
FBXW7/cyclin E deregulation	4q	6	—	Som.[e]
TISSUE-MAINTENANCE GENES				
PRSS1	7q	<1	Prior	Germ.

Germ., (prevalence of) germline mutation; som., (prevalence of) somatic mutation or methylation.
[a]References are given in the text.
[b]Stage of appearance of the genetic changes during the intraductal precursor phase of the neoplasm, where known. For BRCA2, most mutations are inherited, but the loss of the second allele is reported only in a single advanced pancreatic intraepithelial neoplasm.
[c]Single examples of homozygous deletion of the TGFBRI gene and TGFBR2 gene have been identified in MS1⁻ pancreatic cancer.
[d]In MS1⁺ tumors, the mismatch repair defect is usually somatic in origin; the TGFBR2, ACVR2, and BAX alterations are somatic.
[e]A single example of homozygous mutation of the FBXW7 gene is reported in a series having a 6% prevalence of cyclin E overexpression. Cyclin E amplification is reported to date only in cell lines.

that is, they are transmitted within a family. Others that are mutated during life, termed *somatic mutations*, contribute to tumorigenesis within a tissue but are not passed to offspring. Telomere abnormalities and signs of chromosome instability are the most common alterations. Four genes are mutated in most cases (the *KRAS2*, *p16*, *p53*, and *MADH4* genes). Other genetic abnormalities are seen at a much lower frequency: *BRCA2*, *FANCC*, *FANCG*, *FBXW7*, *BAX*, *RB1*, the transforming growth factor-β (TGF-β) receptors *TGFBR1* and *TGFBR2*, the activin receptors *ACBR1B* and *ACVR2*, *MKK4*, *STK11*, *p300*, sites of gene amplification, various deletion patterns, the mitochondrial genome, the DNA mismatch-repair genes, cationic trypsinogen, and the Epstein-Barr virus genome, among others.

The analysis of these genes has had direct clinical impact. For example, many cases occur on an inherited basis, and these patients and their families may benefit from genetic counseling. A routine distinction must be made between conventional ductal adenocarcinoma and a histologically and genetically distinct variant having a medullary growth pattern.[23] The analysis of the genetic alterations in preinvasive pancreatic neoplasia has indicated that most carcinomas arise by a process of progressive intraductal tumorigenesis (see Fig. 29.3-2*B*).

COMMON GENETIC CHANGES

Telomere shortening is the earliest and most prevalent genetic change identified in the precursor lesions.[24] Telomere erosion is thought to predispose to chromosome fusion (translocations) and their missegregation during mitosis. Later during tumorigenesis, telomerase is reactivated,[25] moderating the telomere erosive process while permitting continued chromosomal instability.

The KRAS2 gene mediates signals from growth factor receptors and other signaling inputs. The mutations convert the normal K-ras protein (a protooncogene) to an oncogene, causing the protein to become overactive in transmitting the growth factor–initiated signals. The gene is mutated in more than 90% of conventional pancreatic ductal carcinomas.[26] The first genetic change in the ducts is probably not (or not always) a KRAS2 mutation, for the prevalence of this mutation rises in the more advanced lesions (see Table 29.3-5).[27]

The Smad pathway mediates signals initiated on the binding of the extracellular proteins TGF and activin to their receptors. These signals are transmitted to the nucleus by the SMAD family of related genes that includes MADH4 (*SMAD4*, *DPC4*). SMAD protein complexes bind specific recognition sites on DNA and cause the transcription of certain genes. Mutations in the DPC4 gene are found in 55% of pancreatic carcinomas, and these include homozygous deletions and intragenic mutations combined with LOH.[28]

The p16/Rb1 pathway is a key control of the cell division cycle. The retinoblastoma protein (Rb1) is a transcriptional regulator and regulates the entry of cells into S phase. A complex of cyclin D and a cyclin-dependent kinase (Cdk4 and Cdk6) phosphorylates and thereby regulates Rb1. The p16 protein is a Cdk inhibitor that binds Cdk4 and Cdk6. Virtually all pancreatic carcinomas suffer a loss of p16 function, through homozygous deletions, mutation/LOH, or promoter methylation associated with a lack of gene expression.[29] In addition, inherited mutations of the *p16* gene cause familial melanoma/PC, the familial atypical multiple mole melanoma.[30]

The p53 protein binds to specific sites of DNA and activates the transcription of certain genes. The *p53* gene has point mutations that inhibit its ability to bind DNA in 50% to 75% of PCs.

Most human carcinomas have chromosomal instability, which produces changes in chromosomal copy numbers or aneuploidy. Most PCs have complex karyotypes, including deletions of whole chromosomes and subchromosomal regions. Chromosomal instability is the process that causes most of the tumor deletions (LOH). Some tumors, however, do not have significant gross or numeric chromosomal changes and have a different form of genetic instability; they have defects in DNA mismatch repair, producing high mutation rates at sites of simple repetitive sequences termed *microsatellites*.[31] MIN occurs in a small percentage of PCs.[23,32] The pattern of genetic damage in these tumors differs considerably from that in tumors with chromosomal instability.

LOW-FREQUENCY GENETIC CHANGES

The causative genes of Fanconi's anemia play a role in human tumorigenesis. The *BRCA2* gene represents Fanconi complementation group D1 and is thought to aid DNA strand repair. Because of this function, it is perhaps best to categorize *BRCA2* as a genome-maintenance gene rather than a standard tumor suppressor. Of "sporadic" PCs, 7% to 10% (more in instances of familial aggregation) harbor an inactivating intragenic inherited mutation of one copy of the *BRCA2* gene, accompanied by LOH.[33] The *FANCC* and *FANCG* genes have somatic or germline mutations in some PC patients, again with loss of the wild-type allele in the cancer.[34] The known hypersensitivity of Fanconi's cells to interstrand DNA–cross-linking agents, such as cisplatin and mitomycin C (MMC), has suggested that PCs with Fanconi's pathway genetic defects would be especially susceptible to treatment with such agents.

The mitochrondrial genome may be mutated in a majority of PCs. These mutations most likely represent genetic drift and perhaps do not directly contribute to the process of tumorigenesis.[35] Such mutations, however, could potentially serve as a diagnostic target because of the large number of copies of the mitochondrial genome in human carcinoma cells.

The *MKK4* gene participates in a stress-related protein kinase pathway. It is stimulated by various influences, including chemotherapy, and its downstream effects, including apoptosis and cellular differentiation. The *MKK4* gene has homozygous deletions or mutation/LOH in approximately 4% of PC cases.[36]

Germline mutations of the *STK11* (*LKB1*) gene, a serine-threonine kinase, are responsible for the PJS. PJS was anecdotally associated with PC decades ago. A follow-up study examined lifetime risk, finding PC to develop in nearly a third of PJS patients. Sporadic PCs, independent of PJS, also lose the STK11 gene by homozygous deletion or by somatic mutation/LOH in approximately 4% of cases.[37]

Gene amplification occurs occasionally in PC. Amplified regions include the *AKT2* gene within an amplicon on chromosome 19q and the *MYB* gene on 6q, involving approximately 10% to 20% of cases studied.[38] Approximately 6% of PCs overexpress the oncogene, *CCNE1* (cyclin E). Two mechanisms have been demonstrated: cyclin E gene amplification and the genetic inactivation of the *FBXW7* (AGO) gene, which normally serves to degrade cyclin E during the normal phases of the cell division cycle.[39]

The patterns of chromosomal deletion in PC are complex. In one study, an average of 40% of all chromosomal arms in each cancer had a deletion. For most lost regions, no particular tumor suppressor genes are known to be targeted by the deletions. Conversely, in some regions known to harbor tumor suppressor genes, the known mutated genes do not justify the high observed prevalence rates of LOH. Individual homozygous deletions are found at some additional genetic locations, again without a definitive target gene for these events.

Defects in DNA mismatch repair (MIN) are seen in some PCs.[23,39] These cancers typically have a medullary histologic phenotype and mutations of the type II TGF-β (*TGFBR2*) and activin (*ACVR2*) receptor genes. They can also have mutations of the proapoptotic *BAX* gene and of the growth factor pathway mediator *BRAF* gene (analogous, presumably, to mutations of the *KRAS2* gene). The MIN tumors do not have the propensity for large chromosomal alterations and gross aneuploidy.[40] In a study of four cases of PCs having MIN, all lacked expression of the Mlh1 protein.[23] Not all medullary phenotype cancers have MIN. Yet, medullary pancreatic carcinomas as a whole have a number of clinical and genetic differences compared to those with conventional histologic appearance; the tumors have pushing rather than infiltrative borders, the *KRAS2* gene often is wild-type, and the patient frequently has a family history of malignancy.[23,32]

Inherited mutations of the cationic trypsinogen (*PRSS1*) gene permit the premature activation of the proenzyme within the pancreas, causing a familial recurrent form of acute pancreatitis. Some affected kindreds have a cumulative risk of PC that approaches 40% by the time the affected individuals reach 60 years of age.[41] This cancer diathesis falls in a unique category of cancer susceptibility in that the predisposition emanates from genetic alterations of a gene tissue-maintenance gene, one that is neither an oncogene, tumor suppressor gene, nor a genome-maintenance gene.

GENE EXPRESSION PROFILING AND BEYOND

Studies using global gene expression methodologies have provided a unique opportunity to better understand this lethal tumor and to have a potential impact on patient care. These methods include serial analysis of gene expression, complementary DNA microarrays, oligonucleotide arrays, and proteomics.

Gene and protein expression profiling using each of these technologies has advanced our understanding of pancreatic ductal adenocarcinoma in three important ways. First, in excess of 200 genes have been identified that are highly expressed in pancreatic duct adenocarcinomas but not in normal pancreatic ductal epithelium. Each of these highly expressed genes offer new opportunities for development of diagnostic tests or therapeutic targets. Second, many genes relating to the clinicopathologic features of infiltrating ductal adenocarcinomas have been identified, providing new insights into the biology of this PC. Third, gene expression studies have revealed novel features related to the process of tissue invasion by PCs. In this regard, new possibilities for drug delivery focused on tumor-stromal interactions have been identified. Each of these advances is discussed in more detail below.

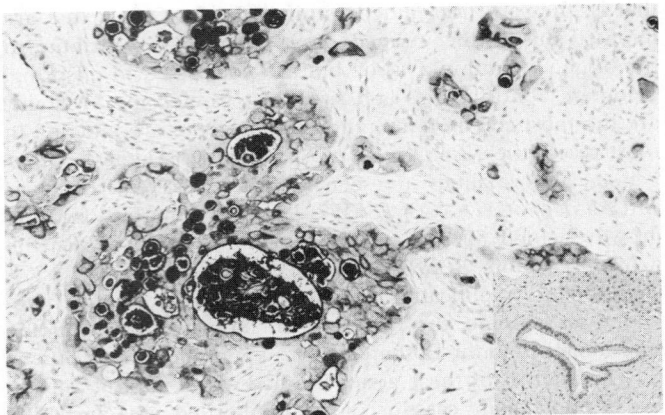

FIGURE 29.3-3.   Immunohistochemical staining of mesothelin protein in infiltrating pancreatic ductal adenocarcinoma. Intense protein labeling is seen within the neoplastic epithelium in a membranous distribution. Luminal secretions also strongly label for mesothelin protein. In contrast, normal ductal epithelium is negative (*inset*). (See Color Fig. 29.3-3 in the CD-ROM.)

NOVEL MARKERS OF PANCREATIC DUCTAL ADENOCARCINOMA

Perhaps the most urgent need in the battle against PC is the identification of specific tumor markers for the interpretation of difficult biopsies and for early diagnosis (Fig. 29.3-3). Overexpressed genes now recognized as potentially important in PC are depicted in Table 29.3-6.[42–47] These potential tumor markers represent a variety of protein functions, including cell adhesion, cell motility, cytoskeletal assembly, proteolysis, or matrix remodeling. Some have now been validated as specific markers of pancreatic carcinoma, whereas others are in the process of being confirmed.

NEW INSIGHTS INTO THE BIOLOGY OF PANCREATIC DUCTAL ADENOCARCINOMA

Gene expression profiling has also provided novel insight into the complex biology of PC.[48,49] Recent evidence provided through global gene expression profiling has revealed that certain cellular processes play a more prominent role in PCs than were previously recognized. For example, genes whose protein products are involved in cell membrane junctions and cell/matrix interactions have consistently been identified as upregulated in PCs by several investigators. This observation could correspond to altered cellular attachments and cell surface architecture, resulting in aberrant cell-cell interactions that are a reproducible characteristic of cancer cells. Several ion-homeostasis–dependent proteins, especially those specific for the calcium ion (Ca²⁺), such as S100A4, S100A10, or Trop-2, have been identified as overexpressed in PC. The consistent expression of these genes in PCs may indicate key homeostatic mechanisms necessary for cancer cell survival, and interference with their expression may promote cancer cell death. Finally, several genes whose protein products may contribute to chemoradioresistance in PCs have also been identified, such as ataxia-telangiectasia group D–associated protein (ATDC), topoisomerase II alpha, and transglutaminase II. ATDC protein has been shown to be induced by ionizing radiation and to

TABLE 29.3-6.   Examples of Novel Markers of Pancreatic Ductal Adenocarcinoma Identified by Gene Expression Profiling

Name	Normal Cellular Function	Expression in Pancreatic Cancer	Potential Use
Claudin 4	Component of epithelial tight junctions	Overexpressed in neoplastic epithelium; membranous distribution	Radioimaging, immunotherapy
Fascin	Cytoskeletal protein, cellular motility	Overexpressed in neoplastic epithelium; cytoplasmic distribution	Diagnostic marker
HIP/PAP	?	Normal acinar cells; released during acute/chronic pancreatitis	Screening marker
Hsp47	Collagen-specific chaperone	Desmoplastic stromal cells	Diagnostic marker/radioimaging
Mesothelin	GP1-anchored protein, ?adhesion	Overexpressed in neoplastic epithelium; membranous distribution	Diagnostic marker immunotherapy screening
Muc4	Apomucin, epithelial protection	Overexpressed in neoplastic epithelium; membranous distribution	Diagnostic marker/immunotherapy
PSCA	GP1-anchor protein, ?adhesion	Overexpressed in neoplastic epithelium; membranous distribution	Diagnostic marker immunotherapy screening
S100A4	S100 calcium-binding protein	Overexpressed in neoplastic epithelium; cytoplasmic distribution	Diagnostic marker

HIP/PAP, hepatocarcinoma-intestine-pancreas/pancreatitis-associated protein I.

suppress the radiosensitivity of ataxia-telangiectasia fibroblast cell lines, whereas expressed genes such as topoisomerase II alpha or transglutaminase II may relate to the chemotherapeutic resistance often observed for PCs. Thus, global gene expression technologies can provide important insights into pancreatic carcinomas, many of which may affect how future therapies are designed and administered.

NEW INSIGHTS INTO THE INVASIVE PROCESS IN PANCREATIC DUCTAL ADENOCARCINOMA

Gene expression profiling of PC has also provided new insights into the process of tumor invasion. Specifically, gene expression studies of PC tissues have been used to identify expression patterns associated with the exuberant desmoplastic response.[50] These genes were found to be expressed in surgically resected PC tissues, but not in normal pancreas tissue or in cultured PC cell lines, thus reflecting the cellular components of the host stromal response seen in the presence of infiltrating carcinoma. Investigations into the cellular localization of these genes using *in situ* hybridization have identified a specific "architecture" for their expression in invasive pancreatic carcinomas. Gene expression within invasive PCs can be segregated into distinct and reproducible compartments: the neoplastic epithelium, angioendothelium, juxtatumoral stroma (those stromal cells immediately adjacent to the invasive neoplastic epithelium), or the panstromal compartment (all stromal tissue within the host response), indicating that a highly organized and structured process of tumor invasion exists in the pancreas. The finding of genes expressed by the neoplastic epithelium in invasive carcinomas, but not in cancer cell lines derived from invasive carcinomas, also highlights the importance of gene expression related to a neoplastic cell's interactions with its environment.

SCREENING AND EARLY DETECTION

APPROACHES TO CLINICAL SCREENING

Most pancreatic ductal adenocarcinomas (approximately 85%) are diagnosed at a late, incurable stage. Because complete resection of small cancers may improve the outcome of this deadly disease, there is great interest in improving the early detection of PC. The optimal approach for early detection of PC is still under study. Ideally, one would like to identify lesions that have a high chance of cure after surgical resection, such as a high-grade benign PanIN 3 lesion, a benign IPMN, or less than 1 cm pancreatic ductal adenocarcinoma using a noninvasive imaging test or a biomarker.[51]

Currently, imaging modalities for screening and early detection include computed tomography (CT) scan, magnetic resonance imaging (MRI)/magnetic resonance (MR) cholangiopancreatography, and endoscopic ultrasonography (EUS). With the development of multidetector techniques, CT angiography, and three-dimensional reconstruction, CT imaging continues to improve.[52] For early detection, EUS may be the imaging modality of choice because it detects smaller pancreatic lesions than those detected with thin-section dual-phase spiral CT.[53] The accuracy of diagnosis of PC in patients with pancreatic masses who are suspected of having cancer is close to 100% for EUS and approaches 92% for dual-phase CT. Furthermore, EUS can readily discriminate between solid and cystic lesions (unlike CT) and, when combined with fine-needle aspiration (FNA), provides a cytologic diagnosis of minute lesions as small as 2 to 5 mm that are not visualized by CT, ultrasound, or MRI. FNA performed during an EUS procedure can help to establish a diagnosis of malignancy, although the diagnostic yield from cytology in this setting is variable. Endoscopic retrograde cholangiopancreatography (ERCP) is less likely to detect small tumors, and it is a relatively more invasive test for screening due to the risk of developing pancreatitis (5% to 10%).

Serum CA 19-9, the only widely used tumor marker, is valuable for following the therapeutic response of patients with PC who have an elevated serum CA 19-9 level.[54] CA 19-9 is of limited value as a screening marker, however, as approximately 10% to 15% of individuals do not secrete CA 19-9 because of their Lewis antigen status. In addition, CA 19-9 levels may be within the normal range while the cancer is still at a small and asymptomatic stage, and CA 19-9 can be elevated in benign biliary or pancreatic conditions. Similar problems with diagnostic accuracy have been observed for other investigational markers. Attempts have been made to combine markers to improve the diagnostic performance of CA 19-9 by combining it with other markers.

One current approach to screen high-risk individuals uses EUS of the pancreas, multidetector CT with three-dimensional reconstruction, and serum CA 19-9 measurements as the initial screening tests. ERCP, EUS-FNA, and other investigations can be performed if abnormalities are found on EUS or CT, or both. In an ongoing clinical trial at Johns Hopkins using this approach in patients with PJS and at-risk relatives from familial PC kindreds, six pancreatic masses were found by EUS (four also detected by CT) in 37 individuals screened. One invasive PC, one IPMN, two cystic neoplasms, and two nonneoplastic masses (chronic pancreatitis) were detected, corresponding to a diagnostic yield of 10.5% for pancreatic neoplasms.[55] The one patient with an invasive adenocarcinoma was resected and is still alive and disease free 5 years after surgery. Overall, these data suggest that it may be worthwhile to screen for pancreatic neoplasia in high-risk populations. However, there is not yet enough information to determine the clinical use and cost effectiveness of such a screening approach, the risks involved, and the appropriate screening intervals and optimal type of surgery (partial vs. total pancreatectomy). Brentnall et al.[56] at the University of Washington in Seattle reported their experience with screening three high-risk families with unique phenotypic features (including DM and chronic pancreatitis). Of 14 patients from three families surveyed primarily by EUS, 7 were found to have EUS and ERCP abnormalities suggestive of unique pancreatic duct lesions (saccular or grape-like deformities) and chronic pancreatitis. Pathologic analysis of total pancreatectomy resection specimens revealed diffuse, often high-grade pancreatic duct lesions (PanIN). However, total pancreatectomy is associated with a significant morbidity and obligate insulin-dependent diabetes and at present probably should only be considered for patients with a very high lifetime risk of PC, such as those with hereditary pancreatitis and a confirmed PRSS1 mutation.

DEVELOPING BIOMARKERS FOR EARLY DETECTION

Better markers of PC are needed for early diagnosis of symptomatic individuals whose initial workup fails to yield a diagnosis and as a screening test to permit the early detection of PC in asymptomatic individuals at high risk of developing the disease. Although a serum test would have wide application, the inability to find an accurate diagnostic serum test for PC and the need to identify small pancreatic lesions have led to interest in using pancreatic juice as a specimen for searching for novel markers of PC. The potential high concentration of DNA and proteins makes pancreatic juice a potentially optimal specimen to use when screening high-risk patients for PC, analogous to sputum for lung cancer or nipple aspirates for breast cancer. Pancreatic juice can be collected during routine upper GI endoscopy after secretin stimulation without the need for ERCP. Often when PC is suspected, imaging tests fail to identify a pancreatic mass. Molecular markers could facilitate early diagnosis by aiding in the interpretation of inconclusive cytology specimens obtained by sampling the pancreatic duct or from fine-needle aspirates obtained during EUS.

Biomarkers can be divided into three biochemical targets: DNA, RNA, and proteins. DNA-based techniques aim to detect cancer-specific DNA alterations. The diagnostic potential of DNA- and RNA-based markers has improved with the use of quantitative polymerase chain reaction. Markers that have prom-

ise are the detection of DNA methylation changes and mitochondrial mutations that arise during PC development. DNA methylation abnormalities may be particularly suitable for use in early detection strategies. Numerous aberrant methylation events occur during carcinogenesis (e.g., methylation of *hMLH1* and *p16*), and they can be detected in secondary sources using the very sensitive methylation-specific polymerase chain reaction technique. Pancreatic carcinomas harbor aberrant methylation of a number of cancer-related genes (*SPARC*, *ppENK*, *p16*, *TSLC1*, and others).[57] Efforts to use DNA methylation as a diagnostic tool in the pancreas are complicated by tissue-specific differences in normal methylation patterns. Many genes that are aberrantly methylated in PCs, whereas not normally methylated in the pancreas, are often methylated in normal duodenum. Therefore, quantification of DNA methylation changes in pancreatic juice obtained directly from the pancreatic duct may be needed if these markers are to be diagnostically useful in the differential diagnosis of pancreatic lesions in the clinical setting. Mitochondrial mutations are commonly found in cancers of multiple types and may be amenable to assay in the clinical setting. Mutations occur throughout the mitochondrial genome in pancreatic and other cancers, and thus sophisticated assays are needed to reliably identify such mutations.

As with detection of PC DNA, detection of PC messenger RNA is more appropriate for the analysis of pancreatic juice or fine-needle aspirates. The main RNA-based marker investigated to date has been hTERT. Approximately 90% of cancers express the telomerase hTERT subunit, and approximately 90% of patients with PC have detectable telomerase activity in their pancreatic juice.[58] The detection of telomerase enzymatic activity or the

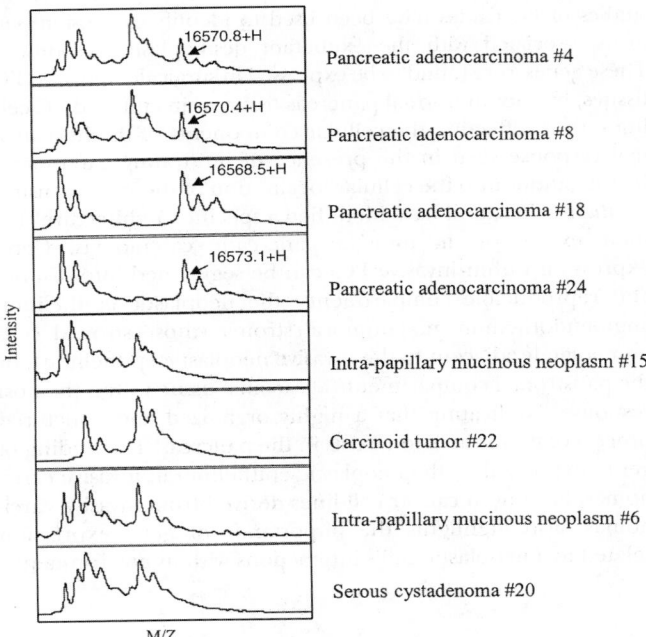

FIGURE 29.3-4. Representative spectrum examples of SELDI (surface-enhanced laser desorption ionization mass spectrometry) analysis of pancreatic juice samples bound to IMAC-3 copper protein chip array. A peak at approximately 16,570 d (*arrow*) was present in the four pancreatic juice samples from patients with pancreatic adenocarcinoma (PC4, PC8, PC18, PC24) but absent in four patients with other pancreatic diseases (bottom 4 spectra). (From ref. 4, with permission.)

hTERT subunit may be helpful in differentiating PC from benign pancreatic disease. Because telomerase is expressed in inflammatory cells, however, it may not be sufficiently specific for use as a cancer screening marker. Many genes have been identified as overexpressed at the RNA level in PCs compared to normal pancreas.[48] Gene-chip profiling or other RNA-based methodologies may be promising approaches for the early detection of PC.

Protein-based markers ultimately may have the most application for PC diagnostics. The ultimate goal of such a marker would be a "prostate-specific antigen test" for PC. One approach toward the identification of protein markers involves the large-scale analysis of proteins in biologic fluids or cells, termed *proteomics*. One such proteomics technique is SELDI (surface-enhanced laser desorption ionization mass spectrometry), which analyzes protein profiles of samples applied to protein chips.[59] SELDI profiling of pancreatic juice led to the identification of markedly elevated hepatocarcinoma-intestine-pancreas/pancreatitis-associated protein I (HIP/PAP) levels in pancreas juice samples from patients with PC compared to patients with other pancreatic diseases (Fig. 29.3-4). Serum profiling using SELDI and other mass spectrometry approaches is being explored as a diagnostic tool in a variety of cancers.

CLINICOPATHOLOGIC STAGING

Staging of pancreatic exocrine cancers depends on the size and extent of the primary tumor, as well as the status of regional lymph node involvement and metastasis to distant sites.[60] The newest version of the American Joint Committee on Cancer (AJCC) *Cancer Staging Manual*, published in 2002, updated and revised the PC staging system (Table 29.3-7). Because only a minority of patients with PC undergo surgical resection, this system applies to clinical and to pathologic staging.

ANATOMY

The pancreas is a coarsely lobulated yellowish gland that lies somewhat obliquely in the retroperitoneum, extending from the duodenal C loop and running cephalad to the splenic hilum (Fig. 29.3-5). The gland is divided into somewhat arbitrary sections: the head (with a small, posterior uncinate process), neck, body, and tail. Tumors of the pancreatic head arise to the right of the superior mesenteric vein–portal vein confluence and include tumors of uncinate origin. Tumors of the pancreatic body arise between the superior mesenteric vein–portal vein confluence and the left lateral aspect of the aorta. Tumors of the pancreatic tail are located lateral to the aorta, extending out to the splenic hilum.

STAGING

Unfortunately, only a minority of patients with PC are able to undergo surgical resection of the pancreas and adjacent structures, and therefore a single TNM (tumor, node, metastasis) classification system is best applied to the clinical and the pathologic staging. The newest edition of the AJCC *Cancer Staging Manual* has

TABLE 29.3-7. American Joint Committee on Cancer Cancer Staging: Exocrine Pancreas

PRIMARY TUMOR (T)

TX	Primary tumor cannot be assessed
T0	No evidence of primary tumor
Tis	Carcinoma *in situ* (also PanIN 3)
T1	Tumor limited to pancreas, 2 cm or less in greatest dimension
T2	Tumor limited to pancreas, more than 2 cm in greatest dimension
T3	Tumor extends beyond the pancreas but without involvement of the celiac axis or the superior mesenteric artery
T4	Tumor involves the celiac axis or the superior mesenteric artery (unresectable primary tumor)

REGIONAL LYMPH NODES (N)

NX	Regional lymph nodes cannot be assessed
N0	No regional lymph node metastasis
N1	Regional lymph node metastasis

DISTANT METASTASIS (M)

MX	Distant metastasis cannot be assessed
M0	No distant metastasis
M1	Distant metastasis

STAGE GROUPING

Stage 0	Tis	N0	M0
Stage IA	T1	N0	M0
Stage IB	T2	N0	M0
Stage IIA	T3	N0	M0
Stage IIB	T1	N1	M0
	T2	N1	M0
	T3	N1	M0
Stage III	T4	Any N	M0
Stage IV	Any T	Any N	M1

PanIN, pancreatic intraepithelial neoplasia.
(From ref. 60, with permission.)

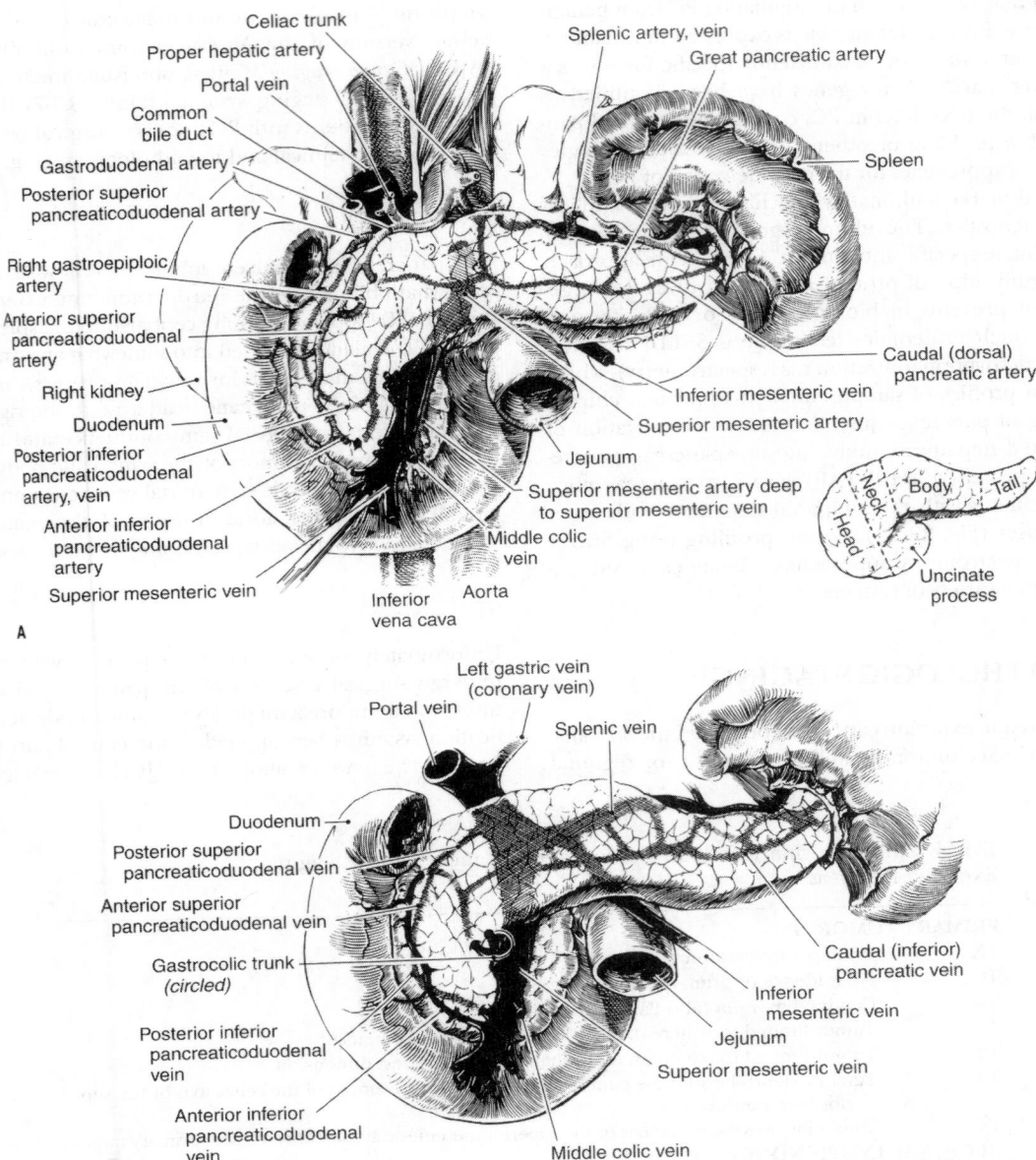

FIGURE 29.3-5. **A:** Gross anatomy and vascular anatomy of the pancreas. The pancreas is divided into five major regions: the head, neck, uncinate process, body, and tail (*inset*). The arterial blood supply to the pancreas consists of the gastroduodenal artery and a branch of the celiac trunk, which divides into the posterior and anterior superior pancreaticoduodenal arteries. These two vessels form an arcade and communicate with the anterior and posterior inferior pancreaticoduodenal arteries, which are branches of the proximal superior mesenteric artery. The body and tail of the pancreas are supplied by branches from the splenic artery. **B:** The venous drainage of the pancreas parallels the arterial supply, with an anterior and posterior venous arcade around the head of the pancreas, draining into the superior mesenteric vein below and the portal vein above. The body and tail of the pancreas drain to the inferior pancreatic vein and to the branches of the splenic vein. (From Bastidas JA, Niederhuber JE. Pancreas. In: Abeloff MD, et al., eds. *Clinical oncology.* New York: Churchill Livingstone, 1995:1374, with permission.)

made two changes, altering the key classification to a more clinically relevant system (see Table 29.3-7). First, because pancreatic tumors are judged unresectable when they encase or encircle large arterial structures such as branches of the celiac axis or superior mesenteric artery, T1, T2, and T3 lesions all fulfill criteria for local resectability, whereas T4 lesions that involve the branches of the celiac axis or the superior mesenteric artery are considered

unresectable. The second major change involves stage grouping III. In the current edition, stage III is used to classify patients with unresectable, locally advanced PC, with major visceral arterial involvement. Stage III no longer is used to denote the presence of lymph node metastasis.

Although the extent of resection is not part of the TNM staging system, the extent of resection is quite important for pancreatic adenocarcinoma. Patients with complete resection, including grossly and microscopically negative margins of resection, are considered to have R0 disease. Patients with grossly negative but positive microscopic margins of resection are considered to have R1 disease. Patients with grossly and microscopically positive margins of resection are considered to have R2 disease.

CLINICAL PRESENTATION AND EVALUATION

CLINICAL PRESENTATION

The majority of patients with PC present clinically with the development of jaundice. This occurs as a result of a right-sided neoplasm obstructing the intrapancreatic portion of the common bile duct. Seen with the jaundice are accompanying signs and symptoms, such as abdominal pain, dark urine, light stools, weight loss, pruritus, weakness, and anorexia.[3]

In a minority of patients, PC presents without jaundice. In patients with left-sided tumors, a gnawing epigastric or back pain may be present. New-onset DM may be the first clinical feature in approximately 10% of all patients. Occasionally, acute pancreatitis may be the first manifestation of a PC, related to partial obstruction of the pancreatic duct, which causes pancreatic inflammation. It is important to consider the diagnosis of a pancreatic tumor in elderly patients presenting with pancreatitis, particularly when there is no obvious cause for the pancreatitis such as gallstones or alcohol abuse.[3]

Additional symptoms found in a small percentage of patients may include nausea or vomiting, or both, related to mechanical gastroduodenal obstruction. Mechanical obstruction of the proximal duodenum can be related to right-sided neoplasms, or an obstruction at the ligament of Treitz can be seen with cancers of the midbody of the pancreas.

The most common physical finding at initial presentation is jaundice. Often, patients with deep jaundice may exhibit cutaneous signs of scratching, related to pruritus. Hepatomegaly, temporal wasting, and a palpable gallbladder may also be present. In patients with disseminated advanced PC, findings may include palpable hepatic metastases, left supraclavicular adenopathy (Virchow's node), periumbilical lymphadenopathy (Sister Mary Joseph's nodes), or the unusual finding of drop metastases in the pelvis encircling the perirectal region (Blumer's shelf).[3]

Laboratory studies in patients with cancer of the right side of the pancreas often reveal elevated serum bilirubin, alkaline phosphatase, and γ-glutamyl transpeptidase, with mild elevations of the hepatic aminotransferases. A normochromic anemia and mild hypoalbuminemia may reflect the chronic nature of the neoplastic process and its nutritional sequelae. Hepatitis serologies are often assessed, and they are typically negative. Although uncommon, patients with ductal adenocarcinoma of the pancreas may have hyperamylasemia or hyperlipasemia, findings more commonly seen in patients with IPMN. A prolongation of the prothrombin time may be seen in deeply jaundiced patients due to malabsorption of fat-soluble vitamins.[3]

DIAGNOSTIC IMAGING

At the current time, diagnostic and staging imaging for PC best uses multidetector CT acquisition with three-dimensional

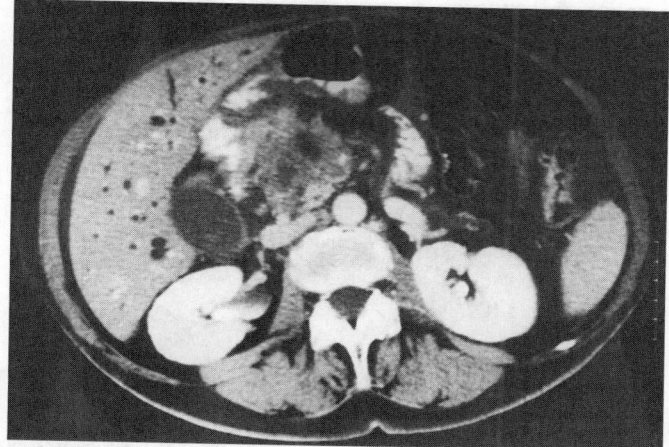

FIGURE 29.3-6. Late arterial phase of a spiral computed tomographic scan, using contrast as the oral agent. The kidneys and aorta are contrast enhanced, as is the inferior vena cava. Dilated bile ducts are seen in the liver, and the gallbladder is distended. A large (5 cm) hypodense mass is seen in the head of the pancreas, and the superior mesenteric vein (SMV) is not seen. Additional caudal images confirmed occlusion of the SMV, with numerous mesenteric venous collaterals. This tumor was deemed unresectable based on the advanced local disease. (From ref. 4, with permission.)

reconstruction.[61] This technology was introduced in the late 1990s and has supplanted spiral or helical CT as the preferred noninvasive imaging modality for the diagnosis and staging of PC. Multidetector CT incorporates dual-phase imaging in the arterial and the venous phases of enhancement. Water is used as the oral contrast agent of choice. Nonionic contrast medium is administered via a peripheral intravenous catheter at a rate of 3 mL/sec, and slices through the pancreas are obtained every 1.25 mm, with all images being acquired during one 20-second breath hold. For visualizing the study on film, 3- to 5-mm slices are printed. However, the 1.25-mm acquired slices are reviewed at a three-dimensional work station using a standard software platform, allowing for three-dimensional viewing of the data sets to improve detection, staging, and surgical planning. Using this technology, adenocarcinoma of the pancreas typically appears as a low-density (hypodense) mass within the pancreas, generally best seen on the venous phase of enhancement (Figs. 29.3-6 to 29.3-8). Right-sided pancreatic tumors typically obstruct the common bile duct or the pancreatic duct, or both, resulting in intrahepatic and extrahepatic bile ductal dilatation and pancreatic ductal dilatation in the body and tail of the gland. Left-sided pancreatic tumors may obstruct the pancreatic duct toward the splenic side of the gland and may obstruct the splenic vein, creating splenic vein thrombosis and the sequelae of perigastric varices. Tumor involvement of the major peripancreatic vascular structures can be seen as circumferential hypodense tissues surrounding the branches of the celiac axis, the superior mesenteric artery or vein, or the splenic artery or vein. CT scanning also has the ability to detect hepatic metastases or peripancreatic lymph node enlargement, although a pathologic diagnosis cannot be obtained from imaging alone.

Advances in MRI, including high-resolution imaging, fast imaging, volume acquisitions, functional imaging, and MR cholangiopancreatography, have led to an improved ability of MRI to

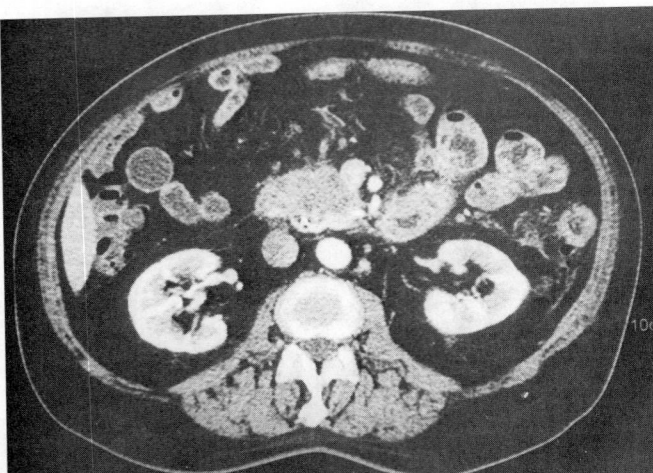

FIGURE 29.3-7. Arterial phase of a multidetector computed tomography scan, using water as the oral agent. The kidneys and aorta are contrast enhanced. A 3-cm hypodense tumor mass is seen in the pancreatic uncinate process, anterior to the aorta and inferior vena cava. The tumor abuts the right lateral aspect of the superior mesenteric vein. The superior mesenteric artery is contrast enhanced, patent, and not approached by tumor. This tumor was resected via pancreaticoduodenectomy, with negative resection margins. (From ref. 4, with permission.)

diagnose and stage PC.[62,63] Arterial and venous patency can be evaluated using appropriate phase studies. Because the majority of PCs have significant desmoplasia with sparse vascularity, most tumors appear with low signal intensity on T1-weighted fat-suppressed images and diminished enhancement on dynamic contrast-enhanced images (Fig. 29.3-9). Although some controversy exists, current, modern multidetector CT acquisition and MRI appear comparable for tumor detection and staging. No advantage appears to be gained by obtaining CT as well as MR studies in patients with suspected, apparently resectable, PC.

ERCP has lost favor as a routine imaging test for patients being evaluated for PC. Although ERCP does allow direct imaging of the pancreatic duct, and its sensitivity for the diagnosis of PC remains high, the use of endoscopic pancreatography for diagnosis is rarely necessary. Of course, the finding of a long irregular stricture in an otherwise normal pancreatic duct, without a past history of pancreatitis, is highly suspicious for PC (Fig. 29.3-10). However, with the current technologic advances in CT scanning and MRI, the routine practice of diagnostic ERCP is unsupported.

EUS has gained popularity and is now increasingly available for pancreatic imaging.[64] Numerous studies have evaluated EUS in distinguishing benign from malignant pancreatic masses (Fig. 29.3-11). In general, EUS performed by a well-trained observer has generally been shown to be more sensitive and specific than either CT or MR in the assessment of pancreatic masses. However, EUS is time intensive and invasive. EUS can be combined with FNA to acquire cellular material for cytologic analysis. EUS-FNA appears to be most efficacious in acquiring a tissue diagnosis of PC when such a diagnosis is required before surgical treatment. Of note, unless protocol-based neoadjuvant chemotherapy or chemoradiation therapy is planned, in most patients with a resectable tumor seen by imaging, such a tissue diagnosis is not necessary. Thus, although EUS-FNA is able to yield a tissue diagnosis of PC in many patients, it must be stressed that patients with resectable lesions suspicious for PC do not require such a tissue diagnosis before surgical resection.

Although CT or MRI remains the mainstay of imaging of patients with suspected PC, the newer technique of positron emission tomography (PET) provides additional imaging opportunities. PET uses the increased metabolism of glucose by PC cells as the basis of imaging. PET scanning for PC uses fluorine 18 (a positron-emitting tracer) as a glucose-like substrate *in vivo*.[65] Fluorine 18 is labeled to fluorodeoxyglucose (FDG), which is rapidly taken up by tumor cells and imaged. FDG-PET has been reported to be highly sensitive and specific

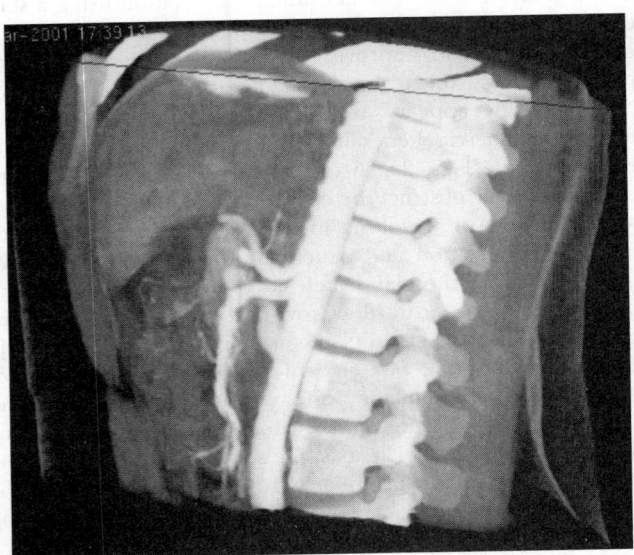

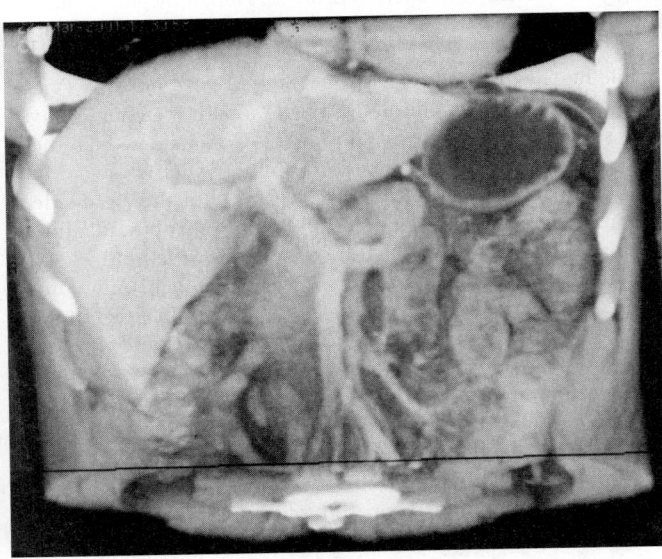

FIGURE 29.3-8. Multidetector computed tomographic images from a patient with a small cancer in the head of the pancreas. **A:** Sagittal three-dimensional (3D) reconstruction, showing normal aorta, celiac axis, and superior mesenteric artery. **B:** Coronal 3D reconstruction showing normal liver, gastric fundus, and portal vein, as well as intact superior mesenteric artery and vein. (From ref. 4, with permission.)

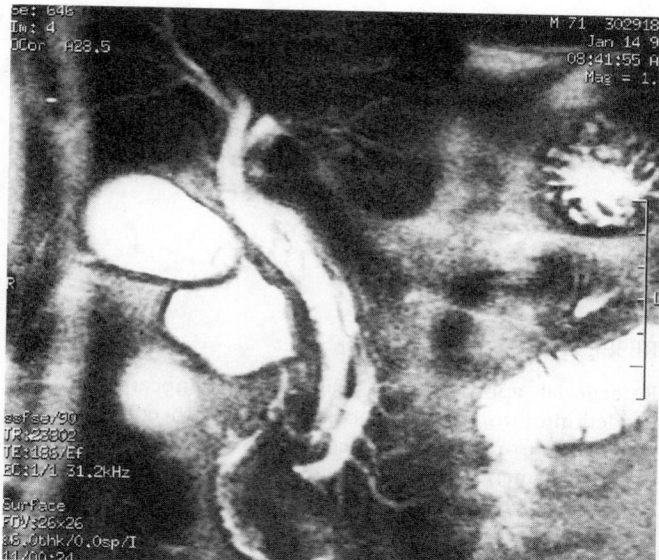

FIGURE 23.3-9. Single-shot, spin-echo magnetic resonance cholangiopancreatogram in a patient with obstructive jaundice. The common bile duct and the pancreatic duct are both dilated, and a hypointense area of tumor is apparent in the periampullary region. (From Yeo CJ, Cameron JL. Pancreatic cancer. *Curr Probl Surg* 1999;36:57, with permission.)

for PC in recent small series. Importantly, FDG localizes not only at tumor sites but at sites of inflammation and infection. Future information about FDG-PET will clarify its role in predicting prognosis and tumor dissemination and in distinguishing between benign and malignant tumors.

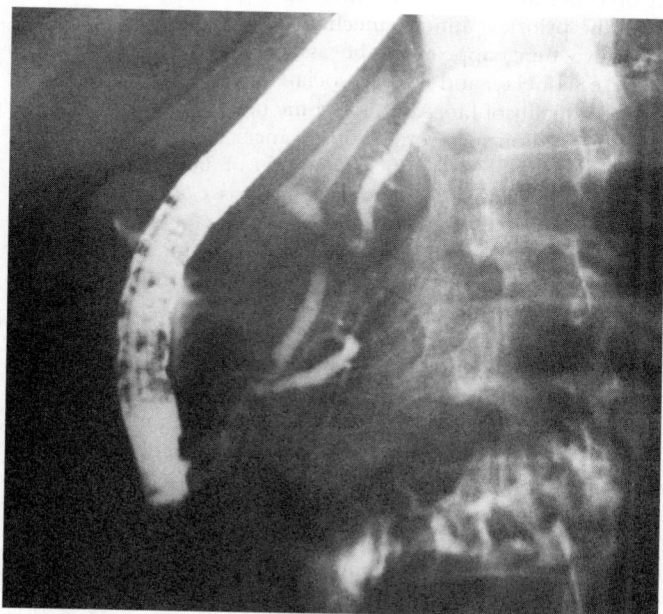

FIGURE 29.3-10. Endoscopic retrograde cholangiopancreatography in a patient with obstructive jaundice, revealing a classic "double-duct" sign. No evidence of tumor is seen at the gems (knee) of the common bile duct and pancreatic duct. (From Yeo CJ, Cameron JL. Pancreatic cancer. *Curr Probl Surg* 1999;36:57, with permission.)

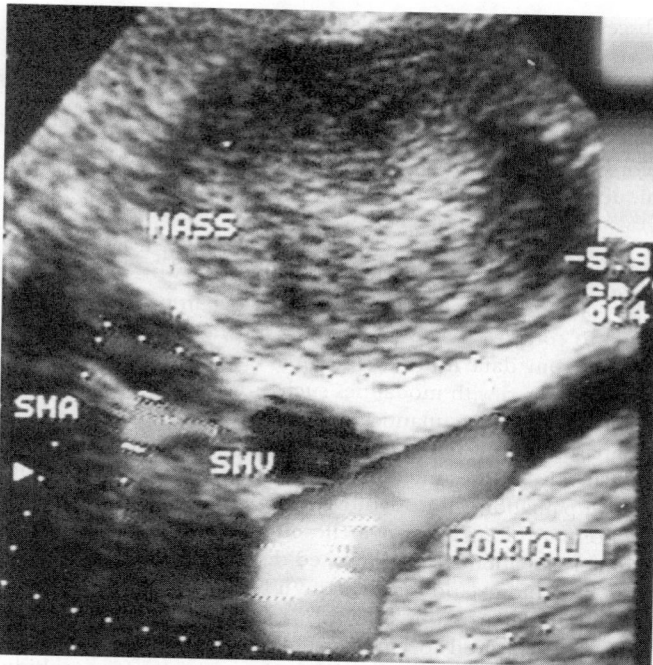

FIGURE 29.3-11. Endoscopic ultrasonography image using linear array echoendoscope, revealing a mass in the head of the pancreas with no vascular invasion of the superior mesenteric artery (SMA), superior mesenteric vein (SMV), or portal vein (portal). (From Yeo CJ, Cameron JL. Pancreatic cancer. *Curr Probl Surg* 1999;36:57, with permission.)

HISTOPATHOLOGIC DIAGNOSIS

It has been the authors' practice at the Johns Hopkins Medical Institutions not to perform routine pancreatic biopsy either preoperatively or intraoperatively in patients who present with obstructive jaundice from a mass in the head of the pancreas. The authors believe that such a biopsy is not indicated in the setting of a good-risk patient who is an operative candidate harboring a clinically resectable pancreatic mass. This is because a positive biopsy result would lead to the recommendation for exploration and resection, and a negative biopsy would also lead to the recommendation for exploration and resection, because we could not be certain there was not an underlying neoplastic lesion requiring resection. As noted in Neoadjuvant Strategies, there is a role for pancreatic biopsy (or biopsy of distant metastases in liver or subcutaneous lymph nodes) in poor-risk patients in whom a major pancreatic resection is not possible or indicated, as they may be candidates for palliative chemoradiation therapy or chemotherapy alone. Additionally, some form of tissue diagnosis to document adenocarcinoma is mandatory in patients who are to undergo preoperative neoadjuvant protocols. Furthermore, biopsy may be considered in patients whose clinical presentation and imaging studies are not suggestive of pancreatic carcinoma but rather of more uncommon entities such as pancreatic lymphoma. In this situation, the diagnosis of lymphoma would preclude surgical exploration and allow treatment via multiple-drug chemotherapy.

In situations in which a pancreatic biopsy is necessary, options include either a percutaneous or an endoscopic approach. Although percutaneous biopsy is generally safe, serious complications, such as hemorrhage, pancreatitis, fistula, abscess, and death, have been reported. Additionally, there have been reports of tumor seeding along the subcutaneous tract of the needle and concerns regarding tumor dissemination by the act of capsular disruption of the neoplasm. In general, it is has been the authors' practice, when a pancreatic biopsy is needed, to proceed with the apparently safer technique of EUS combined with FNA.[3]

LAPAROSCOPY

The role of diagnostic/staging laparoscopy in patients with PC remains controversial. The rationale for the use of laparoscopy comes from data indicating that between 20% and 40% of patients staged with modalities such as CT, MR, or EUS will be determined to have unanticipated peritoneal or liver metastases at laparotomy. Of note, part of the rationale for using laparoscopy involves a presumed but unproven equivalence of nonoperative palliation with operative palliation in patients with PC. Proponents of laparoscopy believe it can identify a substantial number of patients with advanced disease who will not benefit from laparotomy and recommend it be applied to all patients.

Routine laparoscopy only makes sense if the percentage of patients discovered to have disseminated or unresectable disease remains high (20% to 40%) in the era of modern multidetector CT or MRI. In addition, it is important that patients who undergo laparoscopy to be spared laparotomy can be optimally palliated nonoperatively. Diagnostic/staging laparoscopy can unquestionably be performed with minimal morbidity and mortality on an outpatient basis. Any suspicious lesions are biopsed under direct vision with frozen-section analysis. Of note, there are varying degrees of expertise in the application of laparoscopy, with some highly experienced groups performing a more extensive laparoscopic evaluation.[3,66,67]

At the current time the authors' practice uses staging laparoscopy on a selected basis in patients with suspected adenocarcinoma of the body and tail of the pancreas. In such cases, up to 50% of patients can be expected to have peritoneal metastases not seen by modern imaging studies. In contrast, patients presenting with obstructive jaundice secondary to tumors in the head of the pancreas typically have less than a 20% incidence of unexpected intraperitoneal metastases after modern staging studies. Patients with left-sided tumors do not typically have either biliary or gastric outlet obstruction, and therefore they do not require routine palliation of biliary or gastric obstruction. Thus, in the group of patients with left-sided tumors, laparoscopy can spare the patient an unnecessary laparotomy, because there is little role for operative palliation. However, in patients with right-sided tumors who present with obstructive jaundice, vague symptoms of gastric outlet obstruction, and tumor-related abdominal and back pain, the opportunity to proceed, even if unresectable, to biliary-enteric bypass, gastrojejunostomy, and alcohol celiac nerve block for optimal operative palliation makes it unnecessary to proceed to preoperative laparoscopy.[3]

A report by Barreiro et al.[68] underscores this practice of selective laparoscopy based on primary tumor site. In this retrospective review of 188 patients with pancreatic or periampullary cancer, all patients underwent high-quality CT and laparotomy over a 3-year period. The overall resectability rate for all right-sided cancers was 67%, compared to only 18% for left-sided tumors. After patients undergoing operative pallia-

tion were excluded, a nontherapeutic laparotomy could have been avoided by the use of diagnostic laparoscopy in only 2% of patients with right-sided tumors. In contrast, for patients with left-sided tumors, 53% of patients would have benefited from laparoscopy, and 35% of all patients with left-sided tumors could have avoided an unnecessary laparotomy.

TREATMENT OF POTENTIALLY RESECTABLE DISEASE

RESECTIONAL APPROACHES

Resectional approaches to pancreatic adenocarcinoma are divided into two types of procedures. First, procedures that are performed to resect right-sided tumors typically involve some form of pancreaticoduodenectomy. Second, procedures to resect left-sided tumors involve distal or caudal pancreatectomy.

Pancreaticoduodenectomy for Tumors of the Head, Neck, or Uncinate Process

The first successful resection of the duodenum and portion of the pancreas for an ampullary tumor was reported in 1912 by Kausch, a German surgeon from Berlin. More than 20 years later, Allen O. Whipple and his associates in New York City reported three cases of pancreaticoduodenal resection, again for ampullary cancer. Although the early reports describe pancreaticoduodenal resections that spared the pylorus and retained the entire stomach, in the 1950s and 1960s, pancreaticoduodenectomy was most commonly performed in combination with a distal gastrectomy (Fig. 29.3-12A). In the 1970s, the concept of pylorus preservation during pancreaticoduodenectomy was repopularized (Fig. 29.3-12B). Pylorus preservation is favored because it preserves the entire gastric reservoir, maintains the pyloric sphincter mechanism, somewhat shortens the operative time, appears to be associated with no consistent adverse sequelae, and is not associated with a long-term decrement in quality of life. Although some have cautioned that pylorus preservation may compromise cancer therapy, this has not been supported by a significant number of data.[3,69,70] In 80% to 90% of the authors' patients, the pylorus can be successfully preserved. The two most common causes for sacrificing the pylorus and performing a distal gastrectomy include (1) intraoperative findings of tumor involvement of the first portion of the duodenum, pylorus, or distal stomach or (2) ischemia of the duodenal cuff after resection, related to devascularization.[3]

OPERATIVE TECHNIQUE. In those patients who are being explored for potential pancreaticoduodenectomy, the initial portion of the operative procedure is designed to assess for resectability.[3] Tumor involvement is searched for within the liver, on the parietal and visceral peritoneal surfaces, at the level of the celiac axis lymph nodes, and throughout the abdomen. By elevating the duodenum and head of the pancreas out of the retroperitoneum (Kocher maneuver), retroperitoneal involvement can be assessed and the superior mesenteric vein and its branches and the palpable superior mesenteric artery pulse can be identified. The porta hepatis is also carefully assessed by mobilizing the gallbladder out of the gallbladder fossa and following the cystic duct down to its junction with the

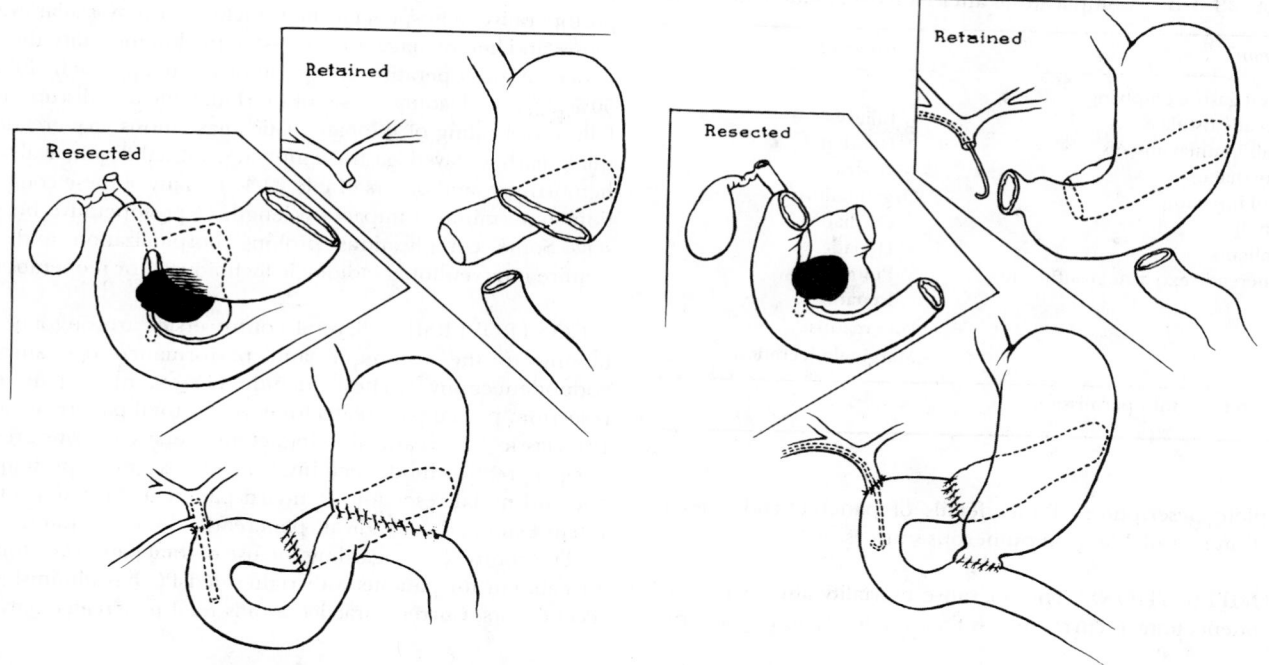

FIGURE 29.3-12. **A:** Classic pancreaticoduodenectomy, to include distal gastrectomy. *Top left:* The structures resected include the distal stomach; entire duodenum and proximal jejunum; head, neck, and uncinate process of the pancreas with tumor (black); gallbladder; and distal extrahepatic biliary tree. *Top right:* The structures retained include the proximal stomach, body and tail of the pancreas, proximal biliary tree, and jejunum distal to the ligament of Treitz. *Bottom:* Reconstruction is shown as a proximal end-to-end pancreaticojejunostomy, hepaticojejunostomy decompressed via a T tube, and a distal gastrojejunostomy. **B:** Pylorus-preserving pancreaticoduodenectomy. *Top left:* The structures resected include the duodenum (except for the initial 1 to 2 cm beyond the pylorus and proximal jejunum); head, neck, and uncinate process of the pancreas, with tumor (black); gallbladder; and distal extrahepatic biliary tree. *Top right:* The structures retained include the entire stomach, pylorus and proximal 1 to 2 cm of duodenum, body and tail of the pancreas, proximal biliary tree, and jejunum distal to the ligament of Treitz. *Bottom:* The reconstruction is shown as a proximal end-to-end pancreaticojejunostomy, hepaticojejunostomy decompressed via a percutaneous transhepatic catheter, and a distal duodenojejunostomy. (From Yeo CJ, Cameron JL. The pancreas. In: Hardy JD, ed. *Hardy's textbook of surgery*, 2nd ed. Philadelphia: JB Lippincott Co, 1988:717, with permission.)

common hepatic duct. In those cases that prove resectable, the intraoperative assessment will determine that the tumor is localized only to the area of the head, neck, or uncinate process of the pancreas, with no tumor involvement outside of the resection zone.

Several maneuvers can speed the performance of a pancreaticoduodenectomy and improve the safety of the operation. Early division of the extrahepatic biliary tree allows caudal retraction of the distal common bile duct, opening the plane to visualize the anterior portion of the portal vein in an inferior direction. The division of the proximal GI tract is typically performed approximately 2 cm distal to the pylorus, and distally the jejunum 10 to 20 cm beyond the ligament of Treitz is divided. The superior mesenteric vein is identified in the plane between the transverse mesocolon and the uncinate process, running anterior to the third portion of the duodenum, frequently surrounded by adipose tissue and receiving tributaries from the uncinate process and the transverse mesocolon. The proximal jejunum and distal duodenum can be delivered dorsal to the superior mesenteric vessels from the patient's left to the right side, allowing easier dissection of the uncinate process off the right lateral aspect of the superior mesenteric vein.

Further steps in pancreaticoduodenal resection involve the division of the pancreatic neck overlying the superior mesenteric vein–portal vein confluence and the final cautious dissection of the head and uncinate process from the right lateral aspects of the superior mesenteric vein, portal vein, and superior mesenteric artery.

Multiple options exist for the reconstruction of the pancreas, bile duct, and GI tract.[3] Most commonly the reconstructive technique involves an anastomosis of the pancreas first, followed by the bile duct and the duodenum or stomach (see Fig. 29.3-12). The pancreatic-enteric anastomosis is typically performed as a pancreaticojejunostomy, in either an end-to-end or end-to-side fashion. Controversy continues regarding the importance of duct to mucosal sutures, the use of pancreatic ductal stenting, and the optimal configuration of the pancreaticojejunostomy. An alternative for pancreatic-enteric reconstruction involves the use of a pancreaticogastrostomy.[71] The biliary-enteric anastomosis is typically performed in end-to-side fashion, approximately 10 cm downstream on the jejunal limb from the pancreaticojejunal anastomosis. The third anastomosis is the duodenojejunostomy, performed 10 to 15 cm downstream from the biliary-enteric anastomosis. A more

TABLE 29.3-8. Complications after Pancreaticoduodenectomy

Common	Uncommon
Delayed gastric emptying	Fistula
Pancreatic fistula	Biliary
Intraabdominal abscess	Duodenal
Hemorrhage	Gastric
Wound infection	Organ failure
Metabolic	Cardiac
Diabetes	Hepatic
Pancreatic exocrine insufficiency	Pulmonary
	Renal
	Pancreatitis
	Marginal ulceration

(From ref. 75, with permission.)

complete description of the details of pancreaticoduodenal resection is available from numerous sources.[72,73]

COMPLICATIONS. The operative mortality after pancreaticoduodenectomy is currently less than 2% to 3% in major surgical centers with significant experience. The leading causes of postoperative in-hospital mortality include cardiovascular events, sepsis, and hemorrhage. In contrast to the low mortality, the incidence of postoperative complications can approach 40% to 50%.[74–76] The leading causes of morbidity include disruption or failure of healing of the pancreatic anastomosis (pancreatic fistula), early delayed gastric emptying, intraabdominal abscess, hemorrhage, and others (Table 29.3-8). Many of these complications have minimal impact on length of postoperative hospital stay. Some complications prolong hospitalization and may require interventional radiologic techniques[76] or reoperation.

CONTROVERSIES. Several controversies are ongoing pertaining to the technique and performance of pancreaticoduodenectomy.[77] These include (1) extent of pancreatic resection: partial pancreatectomy versus total pancreatectomy, (2) classic pancreaticoduodenectomy versus pylorus-preserving pancreaticoduodenectomy, and (3) extent of peripancreatic and nodal resection: standard pancreaticoduodenectomy versus extended (or radical) pancreaticoduodenectomy.

The controversy regarding the use of total pancreatectomy as a treatment for patients with right-sided PC has diminished in recent years. Current practice avoids total pancreatectomy and

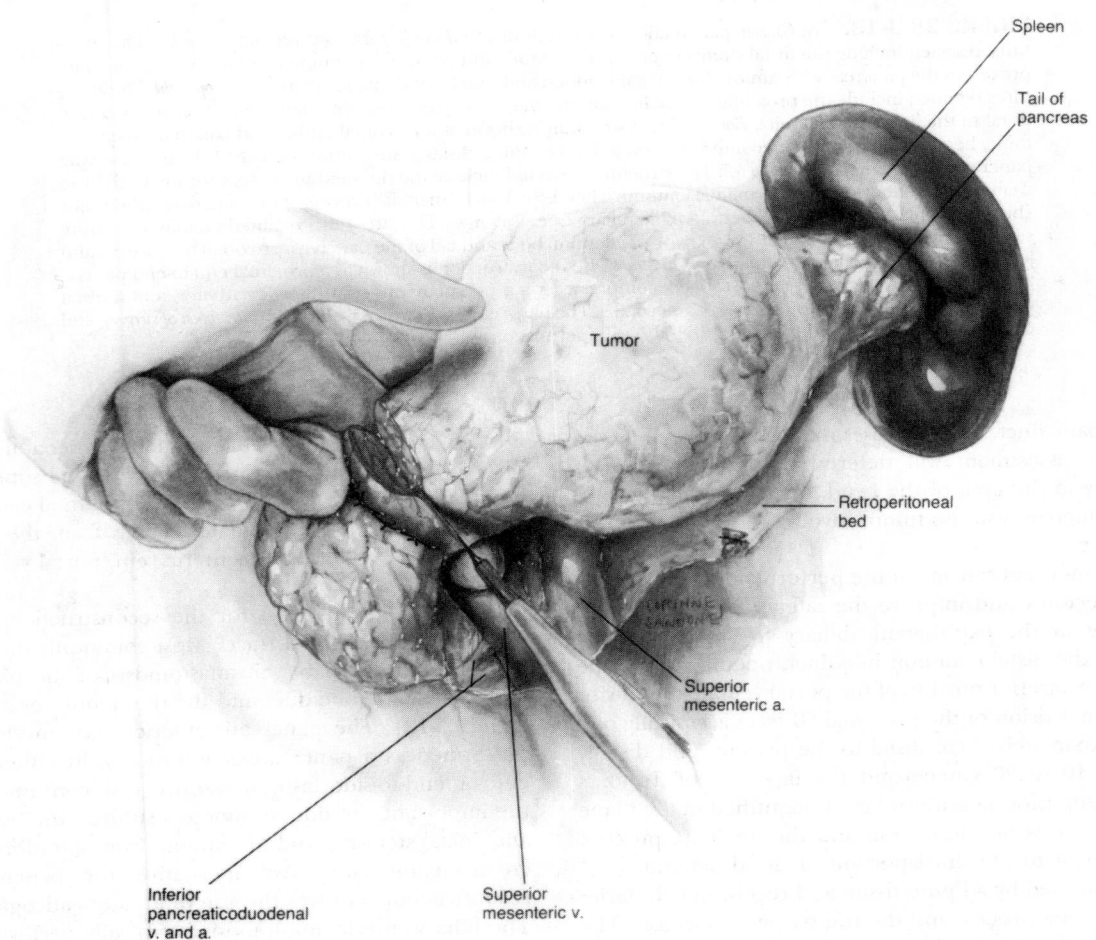

FIGURE 29.3-13. Illustration near the completion of a distal pancreatectomy and splenectomy for a large tumor in the body of the pancreas. The spleen and tail of the pancreas have been mobilized out of the retroperitoneum. The pancreatic parenchyma is being divided using the electrocautery. (From Cameron JL. *Atlas of surgery.* Vol 1. Toronto: BC Decker, 1990:435, Image H, with permission.)

favors the performance of a partial resection. By avoiding total pancreatectomy, one avoids the obligate requirements for exogenous pancreatic enzyme supplements, avoids the inevitable development of insulin-dependent DM, reduces the potential for increased intraoperative blood loss, and avoids splenectomy and the loss of splenic function. Total pancreatectomy is currently reserved for cases in which the pancreatic adenocarcinoma extends from the right side of the gland to the left or in rare cases in which the pancreatic remnant is too soft, friable, or inflamed to allow a safe pancreatic-enteric anastomosis.

Because pylorus-preserving pancreaticoduodenectomy does not appear to be associated with a consistent increased rate of adverse sequelae and has equivalent survival and quality of life as compared to classic resection, most groups are now favoring pylorus-preserving resections in patients with pancreatic adenocarcinoma. Additional reasons to support pylorus preservation include maintenance of pyloric sphincter function, maintenance of the entire gastric reservoir, and more normal physiology as regards gastric acid secretion and hormone release.

Several retrospective reports and a few prospective trials have suggested that extended (radical) pancreaticoduodenectomy may improve survival in patients with pancreatic adenocarcinoma.[78,79] However, a prospective randomized trial at Johns Hopkins failed to reveal a survival advantage for one type of extended resection.[69] In this trial, 294 patients with periampullary adenocarcinoma were analyzed, having been allocated to standard pylorus-preserving pancreaticoduodenectomy or radical pancreaticoduodenectomy (which included distal gastrectomy and retroperitoneal lymphadenectomy). Although the mortality between the two groups was similar (2% to 4%), significantly more complications occurred in the radical group (29% standard vs. 43% radical; *P* <.01). Patients with pancreatic adenocarcinoma (n = 163) had no differences in either median, 1-year, 3-year, or 5-year actuarial survival when comparing between the standard and radical groups (median survival, 20 to 21 months; 2-year survival, 75%; 3-year survival, 37%; 5-year survival, 17%). From this, the largest prospective, randomized clinical trial of standard versus radical resection, no survival benefit appears to be derived from the addition of distal gastrectomy and retroperitoneal lymphadenectomy over a pylorus-preserving pancreaticoduodenectomy.

Distal Pancreatectomy for Tumors of the Body and Tail

A minority of patients with pancreatic adenocarcinoma have tumors arising in the left side of the pancreas. Such tumors do not obstruct the intrapancreatic portion of the bile duct, do not present with early jaundice, and typically grow to a larger size before diagnosis. Left-sided tumors are associated with a much higher incidence of metastatic disease, and the likelihood that curative resection will be possible is therefore lower for such left-sided tumors. However, if the tumor is discovered when it is localized, not encasing in the celiac axis or the superior mesenteric or portal venous systems, resection remains a surgical option. Importantly, involvement of either the splenic artery or the splenic vein, or both, does not alone render the patient unresectable, as the entirety of these vessels can be resected *en bloc* with the tumor. In addition to routine imaging studies including either multidetector three-dimensional CT or modern MR, there appears to be an important role for staging laparoscopy in patients with left-sided tumors.[3]

At exploration the entire abdomen is evaluated for metastatic disease. The lesser omentum is opened to allow assessment of the celiac axis and periaortic region. Similarly, the greater omentum is divided through the gastrocolic ligament, allowing the entirety of the pancreatic body and tail to be assessed. Furthermore, the ligament of Treitz is carefully evaluated because tumors in the body of the pancreas may invade the fourth portion of the duodenum at this site.

Localized tumors without extensive vascular or retroperitoneal involvement are appropriate for surgical resection. Splenic preservation is typically not indicated when the resection is being performed for pancreatic adenocarcinoma. Therefore, the spleen is mobilized out of the retroperitoneum, often with early ligation of the splenic artery. The short gastric vessels along the gastric greater curvature require division, as do the vessels within the splenocolic ligament. Mobilization of the spleen from the retroperitoneum facilitates dissection of the tail of the pancreas and elevation of the tumor toward the midline (Fig. 29.3-13).

The resectability rates for adenocarcinoma of the left side of the pancreas in the era before routine staging laparoscopy were approximately 10%. The use of staging laparoscopy, in addition to modern CT and MR, has improved the resectability rates. A comparison between the results for right-sided pancreatic resection (pancreaticoduodenectomy) and left-sided pancreatic resection (distal pancreatectomy) is shown in Table 29.3-9. In general, at the time of resection, left-sided tumors are larger, have a lesser degree of lymph node involvement, and are associated with a somewhat poorer outcome.[3,80,81]

PALLIATIVE SURGERY

Palliative surgery for pancreatic adenocarcinoma is appropriate in patients discovered to have unresectable disease at the time of planned resection or in good-risk patients whose tumor-related symptoms are poorly alleviated by nonoperative means. Pallia-

TABLE 29.3-9. Right-Sided versus Left-Sided Pancreatic Resection: Johns Hopkins Experience (1984–1999)

	Right-Sided (Pancreaticoduodenectomy; n = 564)	Left-Sided (Distal Pancreatectomy; n = 52)	P Value
Tumor diameter	3.1 cm	4.7 cm	<.001
Positive resection margins	30%	20%	NS
Positive lymph node status (N1)	73%	59%	.03
Postoperative mortality	2.3%	1.9%	NS
Overall complications	31%	25%	NS
Median length of postoperative hospital stay	11 d	7 d	NS
Survival			
1 y	64%	50%	NS
5 y	17%	15%	NS
Median	18 mo	12 mo	NS

NS, not significant.
(From ref. 2, with permission.)

tive surgery is most appropriate for patients with right-sided tumors and is designed to relieve biliary obstruction, avoid or treat duodenal obstruction, palliate tumor-associated pain, and improve quality of life.[3]

The surgical procedures for palliation of obstructive jaundice all include some form of an internal biliary bypass. The three most common techniques used include hepatico- or choledochojejunostomy, choledochoduodenostomy, or cholecystojejunostomy. The preferred technique is hepatico- or choledochojejunostomy, with the gallbladder being removed before mobilization of the biliary tree. Although choledochoduodenostomy provides effective relief of obstructive jaundice in a number of benign conditions, it has generally been avoided in patients with PC due to concerns regarding the proximity of the biliary-enteric anastomosis to the tumor, with the possibility of recurrent jaundice. Although cholecystojejunostomy has been advocated by some surgeons (because it can be performed quickly and can be done laparoscopically) and does not require dissection of the extrahepatic biliary tree, data do not support its use because of recurrent jaundice. A number of retrospective reviews have compared the short- and long-term results after hepatico(choledocho)jejunostomy and cholecystojejunostomy for palliation of obstructive jaundice. In a classic review,[82] although operative mortality and long-term sur-

vival were similar, the incidence of recurrent jaundice was zero after hepatico(choledocho)jejunostomy, compared to 8% in patients undergoing cholecystojejunostomy. Furthermore, a metaanalysis[83] found that cholecystojejunostomy carried only an 89% success rate for alleviating jaundice, compared to a 97% success rate with hepatico(choledocho)jejunostomy.[3]

At the time of diagnosis of right-sided PC, up to one-third of patients have some symptoms of nausea, early satiety, and/or vomiting. Over the years, information has accrued regarding the natural history of duodenal obstruction associated with PC. In a review of more than 8000 surgically managed patients, 13% who did not undergo gastrojejunostomy at their initial operation required gastrojejunostomy before their death, and an additional 20% of patients died with symptoms of duodenal obstruction.[82] In addition, an analysis of more than 1600 cases found that 17% of patients who underwent biliary bypass alone developed duodenal obstruction at a mean of 8.6 months after operation and required subsequent gastric bypass.[83] To date, only one prospective randomized trial has evaluated the role of prophylactic gastrojejunostomy in patients found at laparotomy to have unresectable right-sided PC.[84] In this study, 87 patients without evidence of preoperative duodenal obstruction or intraoperative tumor encroachment around the duodenal C loop were randomized to

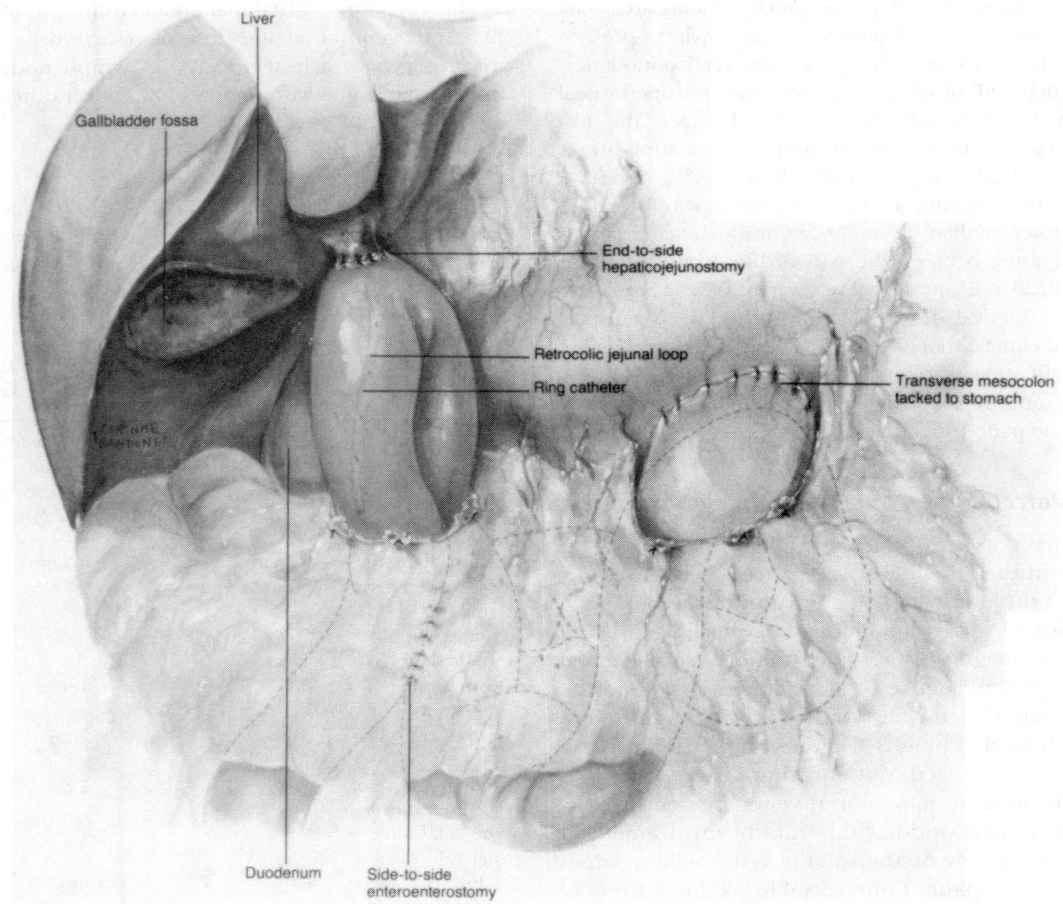

FIGURE 29.3-14.   Anatomy after one method of a completed double-bypass procedure. *Right:* Retrocolic gastrojejunostomy, performed to the dependent portion of the gastric greater curvature. *Left:* End-to-side hepaticojejunostomy to a retrocolic jejunal loop, with a downstream side-to-side enteroenterostomy. The gallbladder has been removed. (From Cameron JL. *Atlas of surgery.* Vol 1. Toronto: BC Decker, 1990:427, Image V, with permission.)

receive either a prophylactic retrocolic gastrojejunostomy or no such procedure. Although the postoperative mortality, morbidity, postoperative length of hospital stay, and mean survival were similar, 8 of 43 patients (19%) without gastrojejunostomy developed late gastric outlet obstruction requiring intervention, whereas no patient in the prophylactic gastrojejunostomy group required repeat intervention (*P*<.01). Based on these data and the results of previous retrospective analyses, the authors typically performed retrocolic gastrojejunostomy in patients found at laparotomy to have unresectable right-sided pancreatic adenocarcinoma.[3] The gastrojejunostomy is usually performed as an isoperistaltic loop procedure, using the jejunum 20 to 30 cm beyond the ligament of Treitz, and placing the horizontal gastrotomy posterior, in the most dependent portion of the gastric greater curvature (Fig. 29.3-14). Using this technique the incidence of gastric-emptying problems appears to be low, and hospital discharge is not delayed.[84] Importantly, vagotomy is not performed for the palliation of PC, as it may further contribute to delayed gastric emptying. Instead, proton pump inhibitors are given to reduce gastric acid secretion, designed to prevent marginal ulceration.[3]

The abdominal and back pain associated with an unresected pancreatic adenocarcinoma can be unremitting, narcotic requiring, and a major debilitating symptom for the patient. At the time of palliative surgery, this symptom can be addressed by intraoperative chemical (alcohol) block. Only one prospective, randomized placebo-controlled trial of intraoperative alcohol block has been reported. In this study from Johns Hopkins, the alcohol block (chemical splanchnicectomy) was performed by injection of either 20 mL 50% alcohol or a saline placebo of either side of the aorta at the level of the celiac axis.[85] Data analyses indicated that mean pain scores (as recorded on a visual analog scale) were significantly lower in the patients who received the alcohol block, as compared to the patients who were given the saline placebo. These data support the routine performance of intraoperative alcohol block in patients undergoing operative palliation for unresectable pancreatic adenocarcinoma.

The most recently published Johns Hopkins experience with surgical palliation of unresectable pancreatic adenocarcinoma is summarized in Table 29.3-10. Over a 6-year period, 256 patients underwent such operative palliation.[86] In this group, 68% of the patients were unresectable due to liver or peritoneal metastases, and 32% were unresectable due to local vascular invasion. The most common operative procedures were alcohol block (75%), biliary plus gastric bypass (51%), and gastric bypass alone (19%). Some patients had prior operative procedures for biliary bypass, whereas some individuals had prior nonoperative biliary decompression (via endoprosthesis or percutaneous drain) that was left intact. The postoperative in-hospital mortality was 3.1%, the complication rate was 22%, and the length of postoperative hospital stay was 10 days. The median survival was 6.5 months, with 1- and 2-year survivals of 25% and 9%, respectively.

POSTOPERATIVE ADJUVANT THERAPY

Despite insights into the overall understanding of PC at the molecular level, improved imaging techniques to identify disease at an earlier stage, and improved surgical techniques, the 5-year survival is still approximately 15% to 20% for resectable disease and 3% for all stages combined.[3,80] The role of adjuvant

TABLE 29.3-10. Johns Hopkins Experience with Surgical Palliation (n = 256 patients)

Age	64 y
Gender	57% male
Presenting symptoms	
Abdominal pain	64%
Jaundice	57%
Procedures	
Chemical splanchnicectomy	75%
Biliary and gastric bypass	51%
Gastric bypass	19%
Operative time	3.9 h
Transfusions (mean)	0
Operative mortality	3.1%
Overall morbidity	22%
Postoperative length of stay	10 d
Median survival	6.5 mo
1-y survival	25%
2-y survival	9%

(From Sohn TA, Lillemoe KD, Cameron JL, et al. Surgical palliation of unresectable periampullary adenocarcinoma in the 1990s. *J Am Coll Surg* 1999;188:658, with permission.)

therapy for patients with resected disease is underscored by the pattern of disease relapse after surgical resection. Several retrospective analyses have demonstrated that, in addition to the development of distant metastases, local-regional recurrence occurs in greater than 50% of patients who have undergone potentially curative resection. The combined use of chemotherapy with regionally directed radiation has long been proposed as a method to control local-regional disease as well as to treat microscopic metastatic disease.

The current standard of 5-fluorouracil (5-FU)–based combined modality chemoradiotherapy is based on *in vitro* data, animal studies, and a series of human studies, the most notable being those from the Gastrointestinal Tumor Study Group (GITSG). This study, using split-course irradiation in modest doses with concurrent bolus (5-FU) followed by maintenance 5-FU, demonstrated a survival advantage for the therapy in comparison to surgery alone.[87] Although criticized for slow and limited accrual, the GITSG study was the first to document that adjuvant therapy after surgical resection for pancreatic surgery prolonged survival. Additional studies by the GITSG demonstrated the benefit of combined chemoradiotherapy versus chemotherapy alone or radiation therapy alone for patients with resectable disease.[88]

A number of groups have further developed this approach (Table 29.3-11).[89–100] The Johns Hopkins Hospital published results of a single-institution prospective but nonrandomized trial that was designed to evaluate survival benefit in patients with PC after surgical resection.[88] This report, involving 174 patients, demonstrated that patients receiving GITSG-style chemoradiotherapy with maintenance 5-FU truncated at 6 months (rather than 2 years), or a more intensive regimen (involving higher doses of irradiation as well as hepatic irradiation administered without interruption and with continuous-infusion 5-FU chemotherapy augmented with leukovorin), did better than patients receiving no postsurgical therapy. The median survival for the more standard regimen was 21 months, with 1- and 2-year survivals at 80% and 44%. For the intensive regi-

TABLE 29.3-11. Adjuvant Studies in Pancreatic Cancer

Adjuvant Study	No. of Patients	EBRT Dose (Gy)	Chemotherapy	Median Survival (Mo)	1-Y Survival (%)	2-Y Survival (%)	5-Y Survival (%)
GITSG, 1985[87]	22 surgery alone	None	None	11	49	15	NR
	21 to chemorad	40 split course	5-FU bolus	20 (P = .01)	63	42	NR
GITSG, 1987[88]	30	40 split course	5-FU bolus	18	67	46	NR
Whittington et al., 1991[241]	33 surgery alone	None	None	15	70 (est)	30 (est)	8 (3 y)
	10 rad alone	45–63	None	15	72 (est)	40 (est)	5 (3 y)
	28 chemorad	45–63	5-FU bolus and MMC	16	75 (est)	55 (est)	34 (3 y)
Foo et al., 1993[242]	29	35.1–60.0	5-FU bolus	22.8	NR	48	12
Spitz et al., 1997[97]	19	50.4	5-FU CI	22	70 (est)	42 (est)	40 (est)
Yeo et al., 1997[89]	53 surgery alone	None	None	13.5	54	30	NR
	99 "standard"	40–45 split course	5-FU bolus	21 (P = .002)	80	44	NR
	21 "intensive"	50.4–57.6 split course With liver 23.4–27.0	5-FU CI + leuko-vorin	17.5 (P = .252)	70	22	NR
Demeure et al., 1998[243]	30 surgery alone	None	None	16.9	90 (est)	20 (est)	0
(Stage I: 29 patients)	31 chemorad	50.4–54.0	5-FU bolus or CI	24.2 (P < .05)	100 (est)	50 (est)	50 (est)
Pendurthi and Hoff-man, 1998[234]	23	50.4	5-FU bolus or CI	25			
Abrams et al., 1999[90]	23	50.4–57.6, with liver 23.4–27.0	5-FU CI	15.9	62 (est)	25 (est)	NR
EORTC, 1999[244]	54 surgery alone	None	None	12.6	40 (est)	23	10
	60 chemorad	40	5-FU bolus	17.1 (P = .099)	65 (est)	37	20
Paulino et al., 1999[98]	30 chemorad	30.6–64.8	5-FU bolus or CI	26 (P = .004)	84	52	NR
	8 rad alone	30.6–64.8	None	5.5	0	0	0
Mehta et al., 2000[92]	52	54	5-FU CI	32	80	62	39
Nukui et al., 2000[93]	16	45–54	5-FU bolus or CI	18.5	92 (est)	84	Not reached
	17	45–54	5-FU CI with cis-platin and IFN-α	Not reached	80 (est)	50 (est)	25 (est)
Chakravarthy et al., 2000[99]	29	50 split course	5-FU CI with MMC and DPM	16	84	60	NR
Sohn et al., 2000[80]	119 surgery alone	None	None	11	48	22 (est)	9
(Retrospective study)	333 adjuvant tx	40–50	5-FU/± MMC, DPM	19 (P < .0001)	71	38 (est)	20
ESPAC1, 2001[245]	200 surgery alone	None	None	16.1	NA	NA	NR
	103 chemorad	40 split course	None	15.5	NA	NA	NR
	166 chemo alone	None	5-FU bolus	19.7	60 (est)	39 (est)	16 (est)
	72 chemorad with addi-tional chemo	40 split course	5-FU bolus	NA	NA	NA	NR
Picozzi et al., 2003[94]	53	45–50	5-FU CI with cis-platin and IFN-α	46	88	53	49
Van Laethem et al., 2003[246]	22	40 split course	Gemcitabine	15	50 (est)	15 (est)	NR

chemorad, chemoradiotherapy; CI, continuous infusion; DPM, dipyridamole; EBRT, external-beam radiation therapy; EORTC, European Organization for Research and Treatment of Cancer; est, estimated; 5-FU, 5-fluorouracil; GITSG, Gastrointestinal Tumor Study Group; IFN, interferon; MMC, mitomycin C; NA, not available; NR, not reported; rad, radiotherapy; tx, therapy.

men, the median survival was 17.5 months, with 1- and 2-year survivals at 70% and 22%. For the control arm, the median survival was 13.5 months, with survival at 1 and 2 years at 54% and 30%. This approach has been further refined by Sohn et al.[80] and Abrams et al.[90] The critical prognostic factors appear to be the status of resection margins, lymph node involvement (especially having more than 3 lymph nodes involved), tumor size greater than 3 cm, and the presence of a poorly differentiated component within the tumor. Using these factors, patients can be segregated into high-risk and low-risk groups, with median survival after standard adjuvant therapy being 30.5 months for low-risk patients and 14 months for high-risk patients.

In an effort to enhance the activity of chemotherapy in PC, other agents have been examined in combination with 5-FU. MMC is an antitumor antibiotic with activity in several GI cancers including PC. The University of California at Los Angeles group has published their experience using MMC (10 mg/m² IV every 6 weeks) and 5-FU (200 mg/m²/d administered via continuous infusion), in combination with leukovorin (30 mg/m² weekly) and dipyridamole (75 mg PO daily), in 38 patients with locally advanced pancreatic carcinoma.[91] Of these, there were 14 partial responders with one complete response. The median survival for all patients was 15.5 months, which is an improvement over historic data for local-regional advanced disease. This regimen has subsequently been applied to resected PC in combination with radiotherapy. The Johns Hopkins group has presented data on 39 patients with PC after surgical resection, treated with combined radiotherapy (50 Gy in 25 fractions with a planned 2-week break after 25 Gy) and chemotherapy consisting of 5-FU, 400 mg/m² days 1 to 3; MMC, 10 mg/m² day 1; leukovorin, 20 mg/m² days 1 to 3; and dipyridamole, 75 mg PO q.i.d. days 0 to 4 administered on weeks 1 and 4. One month after combined chemoradiotherapy, patients received four additional cycles (4 months) of the same chemotherapy alone. At 12.6 months median follow-up, median survival was 16 months.[90]

The Virginia Mason Medical Center published their experience with 33 patients with resected pancreatic adenocarcinoma who received combined radiotherapy (external beam at a dose of 45 to 54 Gy in standard fractions days 1 to 35) and chemotherapy (5-FU, 200 mg/m²/d as continuous infusion; weekly cisplatin, 30 mg/m² IV bolus; and interferon-α, 3 million units subcutaneously every other day) during radiation or GITSG-type chemotherapy with radiation therapy.[93] After combined modality chemoradiotherapy, chemotherapy alone was administered (5-FU, 200 mg/m²/d as continuous infusion) in two 6-week courses during weeks 9 to 14 and 17 to 22. Of note, 13 of 17 patients randomized to the interferon-based chemoradiotherapy had positive lymph nodes compared to only 7 of 16 patients randomized to the GITSG-based chemoradiotherapy. Significant grade III/IV GI toxicities occurred, including vomiting, mucositis, diarrhea, and GI bleeding in the interferon-based chemotherapy group, requiring hospitalization in 35% of patients. However, the majority of patients were still able to receive more than 80% of the planned therapy. The median overall survival and 2-year actuarial survival rates were 18.5 months and 54% for patients receiving the GITSG-based chemoradiotherapy. In contrast, the median survival and 2-year survivals were greater than 24 months and 84% for the interferon-based chemoradiotherapy. The Virginia Mason group has presented a follow-up study of 53 patients with resected pancreas cancer treated with similar interferon-based chemoradiotherapy. Toxicities including anorexia, dehydration, diarrhea, mucositis, nausea, and vomiting necessitated hospitalization in 23 of 53 patients. However, the clinical efficacy remains very encouraging, with a median survival of 46 months and a 2-year survival of 53%.[94] The American College of Surgeons Oncology Group is coordinating a multiinstitutional phase II study of this interferon-based chemoradiation regimen in patients with pancreatic adenocarcinoma who have undergone resection.

In July 2002, the Radiation Therapy Oncology Group closed R97-04. This phase III study of 518 PC patients randomized patients between two arms: (1) 5-FU continuous infusion (250 mg/m²/d for 3 weeks), followed by 5-FU continuous infusion (250 mg/m²/d) during radiation therapy (50.4 Gy in 1.8-Gy fractions), followed by two cycles 5-FU continuous infusion; and (2) gemcitabine, 1000 mg/m² weekly × 3, followed by 5-FU continuous infusion during radiation therapy, followed by three cycles gemcitabine alone. The experimental question being asked was whether gemcitabine before and after 5-FU–based chemoradiotherapy would be more efficacious than continuous-infusion 5-FU before and after the same 5-FU–based chemoradiotherapy. In 1997, when this study was designed, there was inadequate knowledge regarding how to safely administer gemcitabine concurrently with irradiation to allow for concurrent gemcitabine and radiotherapy. This study was the first North American cooperative group trial since the GITSG trial. Although the survival results for this trial will not be known until late 2004, a number of important observations have already been made. These include the fact that neither arm was associated with unacceptable acute toxicity during the trial; that accrual was quite rapid (12 to 14 patients per month), reflecting the support of the Eastern Cooperative Oncology Group (ECOG) and the Southwest Oncology Group; and the willingness of patients and their physicians to participate in adjuvant trials for PC.[3]

Despite a growing body of literature supporting the benefit of adjuvant combined modality therapy after potentially definitive resection in patients with high risk for recurrence, adjuvant chemoradiation has not been universally accepted as standard of care. One of the criticisms has been that none of these studies included an observation-only arm. Two studies have questioned the benefits of adjuvant chemoradiation.

A European Organization for Research and Treatment of Cancer (EORTC) trial randomized 218 patients with pancreatic and nonpancreatic periampullary adenocarcinoma 2 to 8 weeks after potentially curative resection to either observation alone or to combined radiotherapy (40 Gy using a three- or four-field technique in 2-Gy fractions with a 2-week break at midtreatment) and chemotherapy (5-FU administered as a continuous infusion, 25 mg/kg/d during the first week of each 2-week radiation therapy module only).[95] No postradiation chemotherapy was administered. Median progression-free survival was 16 months in the observation arm versus 17.4 months in the treatment arm (P = .643). Median survival was 19 months in the observation group versus 24.5 months in the treatment group but was not statistically significant (P = .737). For the subgroup of patients with pancreatic adenocarcinoma (n = 114), the median survival was 12.6 months in the observation group versus 17.1 months in the treatment arm but was not statistically significant (P = .099). Of note, 21 of 104 patients randomized to the treatment arm were not treated. In addition, although the original dose of 5-FU was already modest, 35 patients in the treatment arm received only 3 days of 5-FU during the second module of radiotherapy, secondary to grade I/II toxicities. Therefore, this study could be reinterpreted as an underpowered, possibly positive study.

The European Study Group for Pancreatic Cancer randomized 541 patients with pancreatic adenocarcinoma in a four-arm trial, based on a two-by-two factorial design: (1) observation, (2) concomitant chemoradiotherapy alone (20 Gy in 10 fractions over 2 weeks with 500 mg/m^2 5-FU IV bolus during the first 3 days of radiation therapy; the module is repeated after a planned 2-week break) followed by no additional chemotherapy, (3) chemotherapy alone (leukovorin, 20 mg/m^2 bolus, followed by 5-FU, 425 mg/m^2 administered for 5 consecutive days repeated every 28 days for 6 cycles), and (4) chemoradiotherapy followed by chemotherapy.[96] No significant difference was found in survival between patients assigned to chemoradiotherapy (median survival, 15.5 months) versus observation (median survival, 16.1 months; $P = .24$). The survival data were similar in the subset (n = 285 patients) randomized through the two-by-two design. In contrast, there was a survival advantage for those patients treated with chemotherapy alone (median survival, 19.7 months) versus the observation arm (median survival, 14 months; $P = .0005$). For the same subset randomized through the original two-by-two design, survival demonstrated a trend toward improved survival for chemotherapy alone (median survival, 17.4 months) versus observation alone (15.9 months) but was not statistically significant ($P = .19$). Multivariate analysis for known prognostic factors, including margin status, lymph node involvement, tumor grade, and size, did not alter the effect for chemoradiotherapy treatment. The study authors concluded that there was no survival benefit for adjuvant chemoradiotherapy and that a potential benefit existed for adjuvant chemotherapy alone after surgical resection.

Although this European Study Group for Pancreatic Cancer trial was a randomized study consisting of more than 500 patients, its conclusions should be carefully measured.[3] To encourage maximal patient recruitment, the study was modified in that 68 patients were assigned separately and randomized to either chemoradiotherapy or observation. In addition, 188 patients were subsequently assigned separately and randomized to either chemotherapy alone or observation. In a sense, three randomizations were possible for inclusion into the same study. Also, patients in the additional two randomizations could have potentially received "background chemotherapy or chemotherapy" that was not specifically defined. The background treatment was not known in 82 eligible patients. Of note, these patients were still assigned into an arm of the study despite lack of definitive knowledge of prior therapy. Finally, 25 of the eligible 541 patients refused to accept their randomization, and an additional 25 patients withdrew secondary to treatment toxicities.

NEOADJUVANT STRATEGIES

Neoadjuvant therapy is a potentially attractive alternative to current postoperative adjuvant chemoradiation for several reasons:

1. Radiation is more effective on well-oxygenated cells that have not been devascularized by surgery.
2. Contamination and subsequent seeding of the peritoneum with tumor cells secondary to surgery could theoretically be reduced.
3. Patients with metastatic disease on restaging after neoadjuvant therapy would not need to undergo definitive resection and might benefit from palliative intervention.
4. The risk of delaying adjuvant therapy would be eliminated because it would be delivered in the neoadjuvant setting.

A number of groups have further developed this approach (Table 29.3-12).[91,97,101–107]

The M. D. Anderson Cancer Center (MDACC) published their experience of 132 patients with localized resectable pancreatic adenocarcinoma treated preoperatively with radiation therapy (45.0 to 50.4 Gy in standard 1.8-Gy fractions or consisting of 30 Gy rapid fractionation in 3 Gy/fraction) combined with chemotherapy (5-FU continuous infusion, 300 mg/m^2/d, or gemcitabine, 400 mg/m^2/wk, or paclitaxel, 60 mg/m^2/wk) followed by surgical resection.[101] No surgical delays occurred in the neoadjuvant group, but delays were noted in 6 of 25 patients who underwent surgical resection first. At a median follow-up of 19 months, no significant differences in survival were noted between treatment groups, with overall median survivals of 21 months.

The Fox Chase Cancer Center published their experience of 53 patients with localized resectable PC who were treated preoperatively with radiation therapy (50.4 Gy in 180-cGy fractions) and chemotherapy (MMC, 10 mg/m^2 day 2, with 5-FU, 1000 mg/m^2/d continuous infusion days 2 to 5 and 29 to 32).[102] Forty-one patients subsequently underwent exploratory laparotomy at the conclusion of preoperative chemoradiation. From this group of patients, 17 were not resectable (including 11 patients with hepatic or peritoneal metastases and 6 patients with local extension that precluded resection). Twenty-four patients eventually underwent potentially curative resection. Significant treatment-related hematologic and nonhematologic toxicities were identified, including one patient with treatment-related toxicities that precluded reexploration. Median survival for the entire group was 9.7 months and 15.7 months for the group that underwent surgical resection.

The Fox Chase group has since published a follow-up study of 30 patients with localized resectable PC of whom 26 received preoperative radiation therapy (50.4 Gy) with 5-FU continuous infusion.[103] Fourteen patients who received preoperative therapy subsequently underwent resection. Median survival was 34 months for the resected group, compared to 8 months in the group that could not be resected.

The MDACC have also used neoadjuvant paclitaxel, 60 mg/m^2 over 3 hours weekly with 30 Gy radiation therapy rapid fractionation.[104] Of note, if patients could undergo surgical resection, they could also have received intraoperative radiation therapy. Grade III hematologic and nonhematologic toxicities were identified in 16 patients. No delays in surgery were attributable to preoperative therapy. Twenty of 25 patients who underwent exploratory laparotomy underwent surgical resection; there were no histologic complete responders. With a median follow-up of 45 months, 3-year survival for these patients after potentially curative resection was 28%, with an overall median survival of 19 months.

Although the distinction between resectable and locally advanced unresectable disease has been clarified by the AJCC sixth edition staging (locally advanced unresectable = T4, stage III), the distinction between potentially resectable versus unresectable disease can be challenging and can have important implications from a therapeutic and from a reporting perspective. Currently, ECOG is planning to open a prospective randomized trial, allocating patients to intensified gemcitabine-based or gemcitabine/5-FU/platinum–based chemoradiotherapy in a neoadjuvant setting. This trial makes an important distinction between clearly unresectable disease and potentially resectable disease, especially around the issues of partial versus complete encasement of the superior mesenteric artery and

TABLE 29.3-12. Neoadjuvant Studies in Patients with Resectable Pancreatic Cancer

Study	Evaluable Patients	% Resected	EBRT (Gy)	Chemotherapy	Median Survival (All Patients in Mo)	Median Survival (Resected Patients in Mo)	1-Y Survival (%)	2-Y Survival (%)	5-Y Survival (%)
Evans et al., 1992[232]	28	17 (61%)	50.4 + IORT	5-FU CI	NA	NA	NA	NA	NA
Hoffman et al., 1995[233]	34	11 (32%)	50.4	5-FU bolus and MMC	NA	45	70 (est)	60 (est)	40 (est)
Staley et al., 1996[105]	39	39 (100%)	30 or 50.4 and IORT	5-FU CI	19	19	75 (est)	35 (est)	NA
Spitz et al., 1997[97]	91	52 (57%)	30 or 50.4	5-FU CI	20.2	19.2	76 (est)	38 (est)	28 (est)
Pendurthi and Hoffman, 1998[234]	70	25 (36%)	50.4	5-FU bolus and MMC	NA	20	75 (est)	40 (est)	8 (est)
Hoffman et al., 1998[102]	53	24 (45%)	50.4	5-FU bolus and MMC	9.7	15.7	72	27	8
Pisters et al., 1998[235]	35	20 (74%)	30 + IORT	5-FU CI	7	25	84	56 (est)	NA
Todd et al., 1998[91]	38	4 (10%)	None	5-FU CI/MMC/ DPM	15.5	41	100	75	NA
White et al., 2001[106]	53 resectable	28 (53%)	45	5-FU CI and MMC/CDDP	Not reached	Not reached	100	52 (est)	38 (est)
	58 advanced	11 (19%)	45	5-FU CI and MMC/CDDP	Not reached	Not reached	65 (est)	16 (est)	0
Breslin et al., 2001[101]	132	132 (100%)	30.0–50.4 and/or IORT	5-FU CI or Gem or paclitaxel (Taxol)	21	21	78 (est)	50 (est)	23
Moutardier et al., 2002[107]	19	15 (79%)	30 or 45	5-FU bolus and CDDP	20	30	NA	52	NA
Arnoletti et al., 2002[103]	26	14 (54%)	50.4	5-FU and/or MMC or Gem	NA	34	75 (est)	68	45
Pisters et al., 2002[104]	35	20 (57%)	30 and IORT	Paclitaxel	12	19	75 (est)	35 (est)	10 (est)
Magnin et al., 2003[236]	32	19 (59%)	30 or 45	5-FU CI + CDDP	16	30	82 (est)	59	NA

CDDP, cisplatin; CI, continuous infusion; DPM, dipyridamole; EBRT, external-beam radiation therapy; IFN, interferon; IORT, intraop radiation therapy; 5-FU, 5-fluorouracil; Gem, gemcitabine; MMC, mitomycin-C; NA, not available.

the length of superior mesenteric vein involved by tumor at initial presentation.

To date, the current data demonstrate that, although neoadjuvant chemoradiotherapy can be administered safely, there is no clear survival advantage to this strategy compared to postoperative therapy. In the realm of marginally resectable patients, it remains to be seen whether there is a meaningful cohort of patients for whom this approach may represent an important therapeutic advantage based on "down-staging" and subsequent improved surgical outcomes.

TREATMENT OF LOCALLY ADVANCED DISEASE

Locally advanced PC is most commonly defined as patients with AJCC sixth edition T4 lesions, in which the primary tumor involves branches of the celiac axis or the superior mesenteric artery. Such involvement connotes an unresectable primary tumor and represents stage III disease. Such patients may require nonoperative palliation of disease-related processes such

as obstructive jaundice, gastroduodenal obstruction, or abdominal pain. In some settings operative palliation can additionally be used. Focused anticancer treatment for such locally advanced pancreatic adenocarcinoma can involve chemoradiation approaches, chemotherapy alone, or locally directed therapy.

NONOPERATIVE PALLIATION

The nonoperative palliative management of patients with PC can be applied to those with unresectable locally advanced disease, less frequently to patients with distant metastases, or to patients with acute or chronic debilitating diseases that make anesthesia and surgery prohibitive.[3] The one exception to these indications favoring nonoperative management are those patients with symptomatic upper GI obstruction (from tumors that obstruct at the duodenal C loop or at the ligament of Treitz) in whom nonoperative palliation is not reliable and gastrojejunostomy may be the best method of palliation. In patients who are to be managed nonoperatively, a tissue diagnosis can be obtained via biopsy of distant metastases or of local tumor. Jaundice is present in the majority of the patients with pancreatic adenocarcinoma. If untreated, obstructive jaundice can result in progressive liver dysfunction, hepatic failure, and early death.[3] Furthermore, the pruritus associated with obstructive jaundice can be quite debilitating and rarely responds to medications. Fortunately, biliary decompression can now be achieved either by endoscopic or by percutaneous transhepatic techniques in nearly all patients who are not candidates for surgical intervention.

The technique of endoscopic biliary stent insertion for palliation of malignant obstructive jaundice is associated with a technical success rate exceeding 90% in the hands of skilled endoscopists performing such endoscopic stenting on a regular basis. Once biliary cannulation has been accomplished, a guidewire is typically manipulated above the malignant stricture, and a No. 7 to 10 French plastic endoprosthesis is secured in position, being pushed over the guidewire. After stent placement, serial liver function tests are obtained to confirm a decline in the serum bilirubin. Early complications after endoprosthesis placement include cholangitis, pancreatitis, bleeding, and bile duct or duodenal perforation. Late complications include stent occlusion, cholecystitis, and stent migration. Metallic expandable endoprostheses have been developed by a number of manufacturers and have been modified to allow endoscopic placement. Once fully deployed, these metallic endoprostheses become embedded in the wall of the bile duct and should be considered permanent, although they can be removed at surgery. Such metallic endoprostheses greatly reduce the problem of stent migration; however, tumor ingrowth remains a problem, causing late stent occlusion.[3]

Percutaneous transhepatic biliary drainage is now used only if endoscopic biliary endoprosthesis placement cannot be performed. For this technique, diagnostic cholangiography first defines the site of bile duct obstruction and serves as a road map for the advancement of a percutaneous transhepatic biliary catheter through the biliary obstruction, with the catheter being advanced into the duodenum. In most cases biliary drainage with an internal-external catheter serves as the initial management, with subsequent management involving either maintenance of such an internal-external catheter or percutaneous placement of a totally indwelling endoprosthesis. Complications of percutaneous transhepatic catheter drainage include stent occlusion, hemobilia related to the transhepatic route, bile peritonitis, bile pleural effusion, cholangitis, pancreatitis, and acute cholecystitis. The available data support the use of the endoscopic method as the primary approach for nonoperative palliation of jaundice in patients with locally advanced PC.[3]

The pain associated with locally advanced PC can be an incapacitating symptom of the disease. Unfortunately, for many patients, such pain is poorly controlled, and it can remain a significant problem up until their demise.[3] In general, this pain is not relieved by endoscopic or percutaneous biliary decompression. Analgesic therapy is guided by the Three-Step Analgesic Ladder of the World Health Organization.[108] Tumor-associated pain is best treated with long-acting oral analgesics in appropriate doses, with dose escalations as appropriate. In patients who cannot take oral medications, topical analgesics worn as continuous-release patches can be highly effective. Poorly controlled pain is often the result of inadequate analgesic dosing and may require the expertise of pain management specialists. Several nonoperative treatment

modalities, such as percutaneous or endoscopic celiac nerve block or external-beam radiation therapy (EBRT) directed at the primary tumor and celiac plexus, can be considered for management of pain intractable to appropriate oral or topical pain medications. In the authors' experience most patients can be well managed without resorting to such invasive therapies.

OPERATIVE PALLIATION

At times, patients undergo exploration for a presumed resectable pancreatic adenocarcinoma, only to find that they are in fact unresectable due to unanticipated locally advanced disease. At the time of laparotomy, these patients are candidates to undergo palliative procedures such as biliary-enteric bypass, gastrojejunostomy, and chemical (alcohol) nerve block, as discussed previously in Treatment of Potentially Resectable Disease: Palliative Surgery.

CHEMORADIATION APPROACHES

Although EBRT alone can improve symptoms associated with locally advanced disease, the high local failure rate and synergy observed when EBRT is combined with chemotherapy have led to trials using both modalities. Chemoradiation approaches have shown improved survival compared to either modality alone, but the improvements are modest and local control remains a significant challenge. No randomized comparisons have been made of radiation or chemotherapy, or both, versus supportive care (aside from subset analyses in trials for metastatic disease).

Several prospective randomized trials have shown a benefit with chemoradiation compared to either radiation or chemotherapy alone in the management of locally advanced disease (Table 29.3-13). The first trial was published in 1969 and included patients with different types of GI cancers, 64 of whom had locally unresectable PC randomized to either 5-FU or placebo, combined with 35 to 40 Gy radiation.[109] Median survival in the combined modality arm was significantly higher than in the radiation therapy–only arm (10.4 vs. 6.3 months). The GITSG randomized 194 locally advanced PC patients to receive split-course EBRT, either alone (60 Gy) or combined (either 40 or 60 Gy) with 5-FU, 500 mg/m^2 on the first 3 days of each 20 Gy radiation.[110] The EBRT-alone arm was discontinued after an interim analysis showed improved median time to progression and overall survival in the combined modality arms. No significant differences were seen between the high- and low-dose EBRT in the chemoradiation arms, although there were trends favoring the higher-dose arm in time to progression and survival. A second GITSG study compared SMF (streptozotocin, mitomycin, and 5-FU) chemotherapy alone versus SMF combined with EBRT (54 Gy) and showed a significant improvement in median survival (9.7 vs. 7.4 months) for the chemoradiation arm.[111] In contradistinction to the GITSG studies, a randomized ECOG study of 91 patients comparing 5-FU, 600 mg/m^2 weekly with or without EBRT (40 Gy, which has been criticized as an insufficient dose), did not find a significant benefit to combined modality therapy over chemotherapy alone.[111] Thus, three randomized studies have demonstrated a modest survival benefit for combined modality therapy over chemotherapy or EBRT alone, and one ECOG study with a possibly suboptimal dose of EBRT (40 Gy) did not show a benefit over 5-FU alone.

TABLE 29.3-13.   Selected Randomized Trials in Locally Advanced Pancreatic Cancer

Reference	Radiation (Gy)	Chemotherapy	No. of Patients	Median Survival (Mo)	1-Y Survival (%)
CHEMORADIATION VS. RADIATION ALONE					
Moertel et al., 1969[109]	35–40	5-FU	32	10.4[a]	25[a,b]
	35–40	Placebo	32	6.3	6[b]
GITSG, 1981[237]	60	5-FU	111	11.4	44[a]
	40	5-FU	117	8.4	39[a]
	60	—	25	5.3	14
CHEMORADIATION VS. CHEMOTHERAPY ALONE					
ECOG, 1985[238]	40	5-FU	47	8.3	28[b]
	—	5-FU	44	8.2	31[b]
GITSG, 1988[239]	54	5-FU and SMF	22	9.7[a]	41[a]
	—	SMF	21	7.4	19
CHEMORADIATION WITH DIFFERENT CHEMOTHERAPY REGIMENS					
SWOG, 1980[240]	60	mCCNU and 5-FU	33	8.8	40[b]
	60	mCCNU and 5-FU and testo-lactone	29	6.9	27[b]
GITSG, 1985[87]	60	5-FU	73	8.5	33[b]
	40	Doxorubicin	70	7.6	26[b]
Earle et al., 1994[115]	50–60	5-FU	44	7.8	34[b]
	50–60	Hycanthone	43	7.8	26[b]

ECOG, Eastern Cooperative Oncology Group; 5-FU, 5-fluorouracil; GITSG, Gastrointestinal Study Group; Gy, Gray; mCCNU, methyl lomustine; SMF, streptozotocin, mitomycin, 5-FU; SWOG, Southwest Oncology Group.
[a]$P < .05$.
[b]Calculated from survival curve.
[Adapted from Earle CC, Agboola O, Maroun J, et al. The treatment of locally advanced pancreatic cancer: a practice guideline. *Can J Gastroenterol* 2003;17(3):161.]

Several trials have examined the use of different chemotherapy agents with radiation therapy in the locally advanced setting. The first was a Southwest Oncology Group study published in 1980 randomizing 69 patients to mCCNU (methyl lomustine) and 5-FU with or without testolactone, combined with 60 Gy radiation.[113] No significant difference was found in overall survival, and myelosuppression (87%) and GI toxicity (23%) were common. A GITSG study randomized 143 patients to EBRT with either weekly 5-FU or doxorubicin.[114] Median survival was similar in both arms (approximately 8 months), but the doxorubicin arm had more frequent severe toxicity. Finally, a randomized phase II study of 87 patients compared the radiation sensitizer hycanthone to 5-FU, both given with 60 Gy of split-course radiation, and found no difference in survival.[115] Thus, three trials failed to demonstrate a survival advantage of different chemotherapy regimens given with radiation therapy compared to 5-FU, which tended to have less toxicity.

CHEMORADIATION USING GEMCITABINE

Considerable interest has been shown in combining EBRT with gemcitabine due to its clinical benefit in the metastatic setting and potent radiosensitizing properties. Studies combining radiotherapy with gemcitabine have proceeded cautiously because of this synergy. Early trials were designed to determine the maximal tolerated dose of gemcitabine when delivered weekly and integrated with radiation therapy consisting of 50.4 Gy in standard 1.8-Gy fractions.[116] A margin of 3 cm around the gross target volume was required for the initial field of 39.6 Gy. The margin was subsequently reduced to 2 cm for the final 10.8-Gy boost. The starting dose of gemcitabine was 300 mg/m^2. Hematologic and GI toxicities were identified as dose limiting at 700 mg/m^2. Blackstock et al.,[117] in a phase I study, examined gemcitabine (starting at 20 mg/m^2) twice weekly in combination with radiation therapy (total dose 50.4 Gy in 1.8-Gy fractions) in 19 patients with locally advanced pancreatic adenocarcinoma. Thrombocytopenia, neutropenia, and nausea/vomiting were dose-limiting toxicities. Of the 15 patients assessable for response, three partial responses were identified. A dosage of 40 mg/m^2 twice weekly in combination with radiotherapy to a total dose of 50.4 Gy was subsequently examined by the Cancer and Leukemia Group B (CALGB) in a phase II study of 38 patients with locally advanced PC.[118] After chemoradiotherapy, patients without disease progression received gemcitabine alone, 1000 mg/m^2 weekly × 3 every 4 weeks for five additional cycles. Grade III/IV hematologic toxicity was significant and identified in 60% of patients. In addition, grade III/IV GI toxicity was identified in 42% of patients. With a median follow-up of 10 months, median survival was 7.9 months.

The MDACC has since published a corollary phase I study of 18 patients with locally advanced disease using rapid fractionation external-beam radiation.[119] Patients received dose-escalation gemcitabine from 350 mg/m^2 to 500 mg/m^2 weekly × 7 with concurrent rapid fractionation 3000-cGy EBRT during the first 2 weeks of therapy. Hematologic and nonhematologic toxicities were significant in all three patient cohorts; there were eight responses (four minor and four partial). One of two patients who were subsequently explored had a resection. The recommended phase II testing dose of gemcitabine was 350 mg/m^2.

These dose-finding studies suggest that the maximal tolerated dose of gemcitabine when combined with radiation therapy is dependent on the radiation therapy field size. Planned confirmatory studies will follow up on these observations.

The University of Michigan has described an alternative approach using standard doses of gemcitabine at 1000 mg/m^2 weekly × 3 every 4 weeks and administering radiation therapy as dose escalation, beginning at 24 Gy (1.6-Gy fractions in 15 fractions) in 34 patients with locally advanced disease.[120] The majority of patients received chemotherapy after combined modality treatment, at the discretion of the treating physician. Three-fourths of the patients received at least 85% of the planned gemcitabine. Two of six assessable patients experienced dose-limiting toxicity at the final planned radiation dose of 42 Gy in 2.8-Gy fractions. Late GI toxicities developed in an additional two patients at this dose level. Six patients were documented to have a partial response, with a complete radiographic response in two patients. In addition, four patients with documented stable disease at time of study entry experienced objective responses (2 partial and 2 complete responses). Resection was performed in one of three surgically explored patients. With median follow-up of 22 months, median survival for the entire group was 11.6 months. The recommended phase II radiation dose was 36 Gy in 2.4-Gy fractions.

Other chemotherapy agents have been added to gemcitabine combined with radiation therapy. ECOG published a phase I study of seven patients with locally advanced disease using 5-FU/gemcitabine combined with radiation therapy to a maximum dose of 59.4 Gy in 1.8-Gy fractions.[121] 5-FU (200 mg/m^2/d as continuous infusion throughout radiation therapy) was administered with weekly gemcitabine dose escalation beginning at 100 mg/m^2. Because of dose-limiting toxicities seen in two of the first three patients, the study was amended to lower the initial dose of gemcitabine to 50 mg/m^2. However, dose-limiting toxicities were subsequently seen in three of four patients at the 50-mg/m^2 dose. Three of the five dose-limiting toxicities occurred at radiation doses less than 36 Gy. The study was subsequently closed.

Gemcitabine has also been combined with cisplatin and radiation in published phase I trials, following up on promising preclinical synergistic data. A study based at the Mayo Clinic gave twice-weekly gemcitabine and cisplatin for 3 weeks during radiation (50.4 Gy in 28 fractions).[122] Dose-limiting toxicities consisted of grade 4 nausea and vomiting, and the recommended phase II dose was gemcitabine, 300 mg/m^2, and cisplatin, 10 mg/m^2. Another trial used strictly time-scheduled gemcitabine (days 2, 5, 26, and 33 because a weekly regimen was too toxic) and cisplatin (days 1 to 5 and 29 to 33) combined with radiation, with a recommended phase II dose of 20 mg/m^2 for cisplatin and 300 mg/m^2 for gemcitabine.[123] The response to chemoradiation allowed 10 of 30 initially unresectable patients to undergo surgery, with an R0 resection in nine cases and a complete response in two cases.

Given the current published data, would 5-FU or gemcitabine be better suited to be used concurrently with radiation therapy for either resected or locally advanced disease? The MDACC retrospectively examined their database of 114 patients with locally advanced disease treated with combination radiation therapy (rapid fractionation 30 Gy in 10 fractions) with either 5-FU continuous infusion, 200 to 300 mg/m^2 (61 patients), or gemcitabine, 250 to 500 mg/m^2 weekly × 7 (53 patients).[124] A significantly higher incidence of severe acute toxicity (defined as toxicity requiring a hospital stay of more than 5 days, mucosal ulceration with bleeding, more than 3 dose deletions of gemcitabine, or discontinuation of 5-FU, or toxicity resulting in surgical intervention or death) developed in patients receiving gemcitabine compared with those receiving 5-FU (23% vs. 2%, P <.0001). Five of 53 patients treated with gemcitabine/radiation therapy subsequently underwent surgical resection compared to 1 of 61 patients treated with 5-FU/radiation therapy. However, with short median follow-up, median survival was similar (11 months vs. 9 months, P = .19).

CHEMOTHERAPEUTIC APPROACHES ALONE, WITHOUT RADIATION

Because the benefit of chemoradiation is relatively modest, and the aforementioned randomized ECOG study showed no benefit to radiation added to 5-FU alone,[112] some oncologists recommend chemotherapy alone for locally advanced disease. Gemcitabine is the most commonly used agent, extrapolating from the metastatic disease setting. This is based on the randomized trial by Burris et al.,[125] in which 26% of the study subjects had locally advanced disease. Gemcitabine ameliorated symptoms and modestly improved survival compared to 5-FU, but the results for patients with locally advanced disease were not reported separately. An ECOG phase III trial (E4201) comparing gemcitabine (600 mg/m^2 weekly)/radiation (50.4 Gy in 28 fractions) followed by weekly gemcitabine (1000 mg/m^2 weekly, 3 of 4 weeks) versus gemcitabine opened in April 2003 and is examining this issue.

LOCALLY DIRECTED THERAPY

Brachytherapy and intraoperative radiotherapy (IORT) have been used in the setting of locally advanced disease. Both modalities are aimed at improving local-regional tumor control. Given the propensity of this disease to disseminate into the liver, adjacent peritoneum, and systemically, what can be achieved overall for patients by the addition of either of these modalities to external-beam irradiation and chemotherapy is not completely clear.

Mohiuddin et al.[126] reported on 81 patients with localized unresectable carcinoma of the pancreas managed using intraoperative iodine 125 (^{125}I) implants, external-beam irradiation, and perioperative systemic chemotherapy. The radioactive iodine implant was designed to deliver a minimum peripheral dose up to 1200 cGy over 1 year. Patients were also treated with 50 to 55 Gy external-beam irradiation and systemic chemotherapy consisting of 5-FU, mitomycin, and occasionally CCNU. Implants were performed at laparotomy. The mortality was 5%, and a 34% acute morbidity rate occurred, with cholangitis, upper GI bleeding, and gastric outlet obstruction being the most common. In addition, there was a 32% late morbidity rate, with GI bleeding, cholangitis, and radiation enteritis being the most common late developments. Local control was obtained in 39 of 53 (74%) evaluable patients. Of 14 patients undergoing reexploration more than 6 months after implantation, 86% showed extensive fibrosis and had negative biopsies from the region of the tumor. In eight patients undergoing autopsy, five (63%) were without evidence of local or regional tumor. Nevertheless, 52 of these 81 patients (64%) failed, with intraabdominal disease, primarily hepatic and peritoneal. With a minimum follow-up of 2 years at the time of publication, the median survival for the total group was 12 months, the 2-year survival was 21%, and the 5-year survival was 7%. Despite satisfactory local control in several patients, many centers would not be willing to accept this level of therapeutic intensity in a group of patients for whom the management paradigm is not curative.

Nori et al.[127] have reported on a series of 15 patients undergoing similar management but using palladium 103 instead of [125]I. The implant was designed to provide a matched peripheral dose of 1100 cGy. Patients also received external-beam irradiation of 4500 cGy over 4.5 weeks and chemotherapy with 5-FU and MMC. Median survival was 10 months. The authors concluded that palladium 103 is an alternative to ^{125}I for interstitial brachytherapy for unresectable patients and that symptom relief appeared to occur somewhat faster. The study did not show any improvement in the median survival as compared to [125]I. Finally, a note of caution was raised by Raben et al.[128] on the use of palladium brachytherapy for locally unresectable carcinoma of the pancreas. In their series of 11 patients, they found an unacceptably high complication rate, including gastric outlet obstruction, duodenal perforation, and sepsis. They did not find an improvement in median survival over other modalities and did not recommend this approach for further study.

The use of IORT using single-fraction electron-beam treatment has also been extensively studied. In experienced hands, IORT can be given with acceptable morbidity. However, there are occasional reports of unacceptably high complication rates. Generally, intraoperative radiation therapy has been given in combination with EBRT in the range of 45.0 to 50.4 Gy with 5-FU alone or 5-FU–based combination chemotherapy. The Radiation Therapy Oncology Group reported on 51 patients with unresected nonmetastatic PC treated with IORT and EBRT/5-FU, and found a major postoperative complication rate of 12%.[129] Two patients had major morbidity leading to death. Zerbi et al.[130] have suggested that the use of intraoperative radiation therapy as an adjuvant to resection decreases the risk of local recurrence. As reviewed by Willett and Warshaw,[131] the dose of intraoperative radiation therapy is generally in the range of 10 to 20 Gy, with some investigators prescribing to the 90% line and others prescribing to the 100% line.

In addition to local radiation delivery, a variety of other techniques and agents are under development for the treatment of locally advanced PC. One example is intratumoral injection via endoscopic ultrasound of ONYX-015, an engineered adenovirus that selectively replicates in tumor cells. A phase I/II trial of this agent combined with gemcitabine in 21 patients showed that the technique was feasible, and two partial responses were seen.[132] Another novel biologic agent in development is TNFerade, a replication-deficient adenovector carrying a transgene encoding for human tumor necrosis factor-α regulated by a radiation-inducible promoter.[133] Weekly intratumoral injections have been given in combination with chemoradiation (50.4 Gy along with continuous-infusion 5-FU, 200 mg/m² daily). In a phase I trial, 2 of 17 patients converted from unresectable to resectable, and 1 of these had a pathologic complete response.

TREATMENT RECOMMENDATIONS FOR LOCALLY ADVANCED DISEASE

The optimal treatment for locally advanced PC remains controversial. No randomized trials have compared either chemoradi-

ation strategies versus best supportive care or chemotherapy alone (aside from the GITSG trial in which 5-FU and radiation were added to SMF chemotherapy), and the survival benefit from combined modality therapy for locally advanced disease has been modest in various trials. Nonetheless, most practitioners in the United States use radiation therapy (typically, 54 Gy in 1.8-Gy fractions) with simultaneous chemotherapy, the standard being 5-FU. Although several chemotherapy regimens have been compared to 5-FU in randomized trials, none have proven more efficacious, and they are typically more toxic. Various ways of giving 5-FU have been used in these trials, but most practitioners choose either continuous-infusion 200 mg/m²/d during radiation therapy or a 500-mg/m² bolus given on the first 3 days and last 3 days of radiation. Studies are under way that will examine the role of gemcitabine (alone and combined with radiation) for locally advanced disease. In addition, given the limited success of current treatments, several novel approaches are being actively explored, with the aim of allowing patients who present with unresectable disease to undergo curative surgery.

TREATMENT OF METASTATIC AND RECURRENT DISEASE

The standard treatment of patients with advanced metastatic or recurrent pancreatic adenocarcinoma and adequate performance status, or both, is systemic chemotherapy. The natural history of PC with a high intrinsic tendency to early spread to lymph nodes and other organs, as well as the relative inefficacy of existing treatments for localized or locally advanced disease, implies that the vast majority of patients will eventually be considered candidates for systemic treatments.

Several general considerations can be made regarding the role of chemotherapy in patients with PC. First, PC is intrinsically highly resistant to the majority of existing anticancer agents. The outcome of patients treated with currently available drugs is poor, and treatment should be considered palliative. Second, patients with advanced PC are frequently symptomatic and debilitated, with a poor performance status and symptoms such as pain, nausea and vomiting, fatigue, anorexia, weakness, and weight loss that compromise the ability to administer full and rigorous chemotherapy treatments. Third, patients with PC often have elevated bilirubin and alkaline phosphatase as well as alterations in other liver function parameters, which further limit the administration of drugs that are cleared by the liver. Finally, the assessment of objective response to chemotherapy is difficult, because PC patients frequently lack bidimensional measurable disease. This last factor has resulted in a large variation in response rate in phase II studies published in the literature and complicates the evaluation of new drugs in this disease. More recently, the less biased parameters of time to tumor progression, progression-free survival or overall survival, and quality-of-life end points are frequently used for this purpose.

HISTORICAL PERSPECTIVE

The role of chemotherapy in PC has been evaluated in clinical studies that compare the quality of life and survival of patients with PC who received chemotherapy against patients who were treated with supportive care alone. Glimelius et al.[134] randomized 90 patients with advanced pancreatic or biliary tract cancer to chemotherapy with either 5-FU/leucovorin and etoposide or 5-FU/leucovorin alone versus best supportive care. Patients treated with chemotherapy had better improvement in quality of life as determined by the EORTC Quality of Life Questionare-C30 scale (36% improvement in the chemotherapy group vs. 10% in the best supportive group, $P = .01$) and survival (median survival, 6.0 vs. 2.5 months; $P < .01$). A second small randomized trial that compared treatment with 5-FU/adriamycin and MMC with supportive care reported a median survival of 8.5 months in patients treated with chemotherapy and 3.75 months in patients who received best supportive care alone ($P = .002$).[135] Furthermore, in a Japanese study patients with advanced pancreatic and biliary tract cancer were randomized to either treatment with FAM (5-FU, adriamycin, and MMC) or supportive care. Patients treated with FAM had longer time to tumor progression but not overall survival.[136] Altogether these studies indicate that systemic chemotherapy has a palliative role in patients with advanced PC.

5-FU had been considered the most active chemotherapeutic agent in the treatment of patients with advanced PC for many years. Response rates ranged from 0 to 20% in phase II studies in which responses were assessed using modern CT, whereas responses were as high as 28% in studies in which rigorous assessment of tumor response was not applied. Median survival of patients treated with 5-FU ranged from 4 to 5 months in most of these studies. No clear evidence has been shown that the varied administration schedules (bolus vs. infusion regimens) and dose-regimens of 5-FU result in a better outcome. In addition, modulation of 5-FU with other agents, such as leucovorin, methotrexate, interferon-α, or N-(phosphonacetyl)-L-aspartate (PALA) did not result in increased response rate in phase II studies. Because of its single-agent activity, 5-FU was also an important component of multichemotherapy regimens. A number of combination chemotherapy regimens were developed and tested from the 1970s to 1990s, such as combinations of 5-FU with adriamycin and MMC (FAM); cyclophosphamide, methotrexate, vincristine, and MMC (Mallison regimen); epirubicin, cisplatin, carboplatin, caffeine, and high-dose cytarabine (CAG); and streptozotocin. The detailed summary of these studies, which have historic interest, is beyond the scope of this chapter and can be found in previous editions of this textbook.[137] In general, these combination phase II studies showed higher response rates than 5-FU single-agent regimens, with responses as high as 37% to 43% observed in phase II studies with the FAM and SMF regimens. These promising results, however, were not confirmed in randomized phase III studies, in which the survival of patients treated with 5-FU alone was not statistically different from that of patients treated with more aggressive and toxic chemotherapy regimens. In summary, past studies indicated that single-agent 5-FU was the most active agent in PC and that alternate schedules and doses, modulation strategies, and multichemotherapy treatments were not superior to 5-FU alone.

SINGLE-AGENT CHEMOTHERAPY

During the last decade, a large number of chemotherapeutic agents have been tested in phase II and phase III studies in patients with advanced PC. Table 29.3-14 summarizes the most salient features of selected phase II studies with these drugs, and a discussion of the most relevant agents is provided in the following paragraphs.

GEMCITABINE

Gemcitabine (2',2'-difluorodeoxycytidine, dFdC, Gemzar; Eli Lilly, Indianapolis, IN) is a nucleoside analog that showed antitumor activity in various preclinical models of cancer, including PC.[138,139] On the basis of its favorable toxicity profile in phase I studies, gemcitabine was evaluated in phase II studies in patients with PC. Table 29.3-15 summarizes single-agent gemcitabine phase II and III studies, comparing gemcitabine with other chemotherapy agents in PC. Studies comparing gemcitabine with novel drugs are discussed in Combination Chemotherapy Regimen, later in this chapter. In a multicenter phase II study in which gemcitabine was given at a dose of 800 mg/m² as a 30-minute intravenous injection weekly for 3 consecutive weeks followed by 1 week of rest, 5 of 44 patients (11%) had an objective response.[161] In a similar study that enrolled 34 patients, 2 (6.3%) had an objective response, and the median survival was 6.3 months.[162] An important observation in these initial studies was that despite a very modest objective response rate, patients improved in other clinically relevant parameters, such as weight loss, pain, requirements of analgesia, and performance status. This finding prompted the evaluation of the drug in two subsequent studies incorporating a new clinical end point called *clinical benefit response* (CBR). CBR was defined as a composite measurement in two primary parameters, Karnofsky performance status and pain, and a secondary parameter, weight gain. Patients needed to be stable in pain and analgesic consumption before study entry. They were classified as having a positive response if they had an improvement that lasted more than 4 weeks in any of the parameters, without simultaneous deterioration in any other parameter. The first study evaluated the activity of gemcitabine in 74 patients with 5-FU–refractory PC.[163] Sixty-three patients completed a prestudy pain stabilization phase and were treated with 1000 mg/m² gemcitabine administered weekly for 7 consecutive weeks followed by 1-week rest and then weekly for 3 consecutive weeks every 4 weeks. Seventeen of 63 patients (27%) attained a CBR. The median duration of CBR was 14 weeks, and the median survival for patients treated with gemcitabine was 3.85 months.

A second randomized phase III clinical trial compared the CBR, time to progression, and survival of patients with advanced metastatic adenocarcinoma of the pancreas who had not received prior systemic therapy.[164] One hundred twenty-six patients with advanced symptomatic PC completed a lead-in period to characterize and stabilize pain and then were randomized to receive either gemcitabine at the same dose and schedule described above (63 patients) or to 5-FU, 600 mg/m² once a week (63 patients). More than 70% of the patients had stage IV disease and a Karnofsky performance status of 50% to 70%. A positive CBR was experienced by 23.8% of gemcitabine-treated patients compared with 4.8% of 5-FU–treated patients ($P = .0022$). The median survival durations were 5.65 and 4.41 months for gemcitabine-treated and 5-FU–treated patients, respectively ($P = .0025$). The survival rate at 12 months was 18% for gemcitabine patients and 2% for 5-FU patients. The response rate was 5.4% for gemcitabine and 0% for 5-FU, supporting the notion that the response rate is a poor marker of clinical benefit

TABLE 29.3-14. Selected Single-Agent Chemotherapy Studies in Patients with Advanced Pancreatic Cancer

Class	Agent	No. of Patients	Patient Characteristics	RR	Median Survival (Mo)	1-Y Survival	Reference
Antimicrotubule	Docetaxel	43	First line	15	7	NR	Rougier et al., 2000[140]
	Docetaxel	33	First line	6	9	36.4	Androulakis et al., 1999[141]
	Docetaxel	21	First line	4.7	5.9	NR	Lenzi et al., 2002[142]
	Docetaxel	21	First line	0	3.9	NR	Okeda et al., 1999[143]
	Paclitaxel	18	Second line	5.5	NR	NR	Oettle et al., 2000[144]
	DHA-paclitaxel	42	First line	3.3	7.6	NR	Jacobs et al., 2003[145]
Platinum	Oxaliplatin	18	NR	0	2.6	NR	Rougier et al., 2000[146]
Topoisomerase I inhibitors	Irinotecan	34	First line	9	5.2	NR	Wagener et al., 1995[147]
	Rubitecan	19	First and second line	28.6	5.25	16.7	Konstadoulakis et al., 2001[148]
	Exatecan	39	First and second line	5	5.5	27	D'Adamo et al., 2001[149]
Fluoropyrimidines	Capecitabine	42	First line	7.3	6	NR	Cartwright et al., 2002[150]
	UFT	14	NR	0	3.75	NR	Mani et al., 1998[151]
	S-1	31	First line	22.6	15.3	NR	Hayashi et al., 2003[152]
	5-FU–eniluracil	116	First and second line	8 (first line), 2 (second line)	3.6 (first line), 3.4 (second line)	16 (first line), 10 (second line)	Rothenberg et al., 2002[153]
Antifolate	Pemetrexed	42	First line	5.7	6.5	28	Miller et al., 2000[154]
	Raltitrexed	42	NR	5	NR	NR	Pazdur et al., 1996[155]
	Raltitrexed[a]	19	Second line	0	4.3	—	Ulrich-Pur et al., 2003[156]
	ZD9331[b]	30	First line	3	5	NR	Smith and Gallagher, 2003[157]
Nucleoside analog	Troxacitabine	55	First line	0	NR	NR	Lapointe et al., 2002[158]
Antiandrogen	Flutamide	14	Second line	0	4.7	—	Sharma et al., 1997[159]
	Flutamide[c]	24	First line	NR	8	NR	Greenway, 1998[160]

DHA, decosahexanoic acid; NR, not reported; RR, response rates; UFT, uracil/ftorafur.
[a]Randomized versus raltitrexed + irinotecan.
[b]Randomized comparison to gemcitabine.
[c]Randomized comparison to placebo. Statistically significant better survival for flutamide group versus placebo group (4 months, $P = .01$).

in patients with PC. Because of the CBR advantage observed in these studies, gemcitabine was made available through an investigational new drug program before regulatory approval. This program enrolled 3023 patients, 80% of whom had stage IV disease. A retrospective analysis of these patients indicated that 18.4% had improvement in symptoms. The response rate in 982 evaluable patients was 12%, and median progression-free survival and overall survival were 2.7 and 4.8 months in 2012 and 2380 evaluable patients, respectively.[165,166] Based on these studies, gemcitabine was approved for the treatment of patients with advanced PC in the United States and many other countries and is currently considered the standard agent for the treatment of this disease, as well as the accepted control with which to compare new drugs and interventions.

Other studies have explored alternative schedules for administering gemcitabine. Based on the mechanism of action of the drug, it was postulated that a prolonged administration schedule would result in a more sustained intracellular accumulation of the active metabolite dFdCTP.[167] Phase I studies of gemcitabine using a fixed-dose-rate administration in patients with solid tumors showed that the maximum tolerated dose was 1500 mg/m² administered as 10 mg/m²/min.[168] This promising approach was subsequently tested in a randomized phase II study in patients with chemotherapy-naive PC.[169] Ninety patients were randomized to receive gemcitabine at a dose of 2200 mg/m² as a 30-minute infusion or 1500 mg/m² at a fixed dose rate of 10 mg/m²/min. The drug was given weekly for 3 consecutive weeks every 4 weeks in both arms of the study.

TABLE 29.3-15. Studies of Single-Agent Gemcitabine in Pancreatic Cancer

Authors	Phase	Dose/Schedule	No. of Patients	Patient Characteristics	RR (%)	CBR (%)	Median Survival (Mo)	1-Y Survival (%)
Casper et al., 1994[161]	II	Gemcitabine, 800 mg/m² days 1, 8, 15 q4wk	44	First line	11	NR	5.6	23
Carmichael et al., 1996[162]	II	Gemcitabine, 800 mg/m² days 1, 8, 15 q4wk	34	First line, 58% stage IV	6	NR	3.3	NR
Rothenberg et al., 1996[163]	II	Gemcitabine, 1000 mg/m² weekly × 7; 1 wk rest; days 1, 8, 15 q4wk	63	5-FU refractory	10.5	27	3.8	4
Burris et al., 1997[164]	III	Gemcitabine, 1000 mg/m² weekly × 7; 1 wk rest; days 1, 8, 15 q4wk	63	First line, >70% stage IV	5.4	23.8 ($P =$ .0022)	5.6 ($P =$ .0025)	18
		5-FU, 600 mg/m² weekly	63		0	4.8	4.4	2
Storniolo et al., 1999[165]	TIND	Gemcitabine, 1000 mg/m² weekly × 7; 1 wk rest; days 1, 8, 15 q4wk	3023	First and second line	12.1	17.2	5.7	15

CBR, clinical benefit response; 5-FU, 5-fluorouracil; NR, not reported; RR, response rate; TIND, treatment investigational new drug.

Patients treated with the fixed-dose-rate regimen experienced more toxicities, with 49% and 37% occurrence of neutropenia and thrombocytopenia versus 28% and 10%, respectively, in patients treated in the conventional schedule. Patients on the fixed-dose-rate had a higher response rate (11.6% vs. 4.1%), median survival (8 vs. 5 months), and 1-year survival (23.8% vs. 7.3%) than patients treated on the conventional schedule. Consistent with prior observations, the fixed-dose-rate infusion resulted in higher intracellular levels of dFdCTP in peripheral blood mononuclear cells. This strategy is now being tested in randomized phase III studies.

COMBINATION CHEMOTHERAPY REGIMENS

The superiority of single-agent gemcitabine versus 5-FU in patients with advanced PC led to the acceptance of this drug as the standard of care for these patients and introduced an agent with which to combine other existing and new drugs. Since the approval of gemcitabine, a large number of phase I/II and, more recently, phase III clinical trials have tested the safety and tolerability of gemcitabine in combination with other drugs and compared the efficacy of the combination regimens with single-agent gemcitabine. In general, the rationale to develop these regimens has been based on clinical and pharmacologic criteria, with the goal to combine drugs with demonstrated single-agent activity, not overlapping toxicity, and different mechanisms of action. Most of the studies have used the conventional 30-minute infusion regimen of gemcitabine, whereas more recent studies have also incorporated the fixed-dose-rate infusion regimens. The next section describes the main features of some of these regimens.

Gemcitabine-Fluoropyrimidine Combinations

The combination of gemcitabine and 5-FU has been extensively studied in multiple clinical trials, the most relevant of which are summarized in Table 29.3-16. The fluoropyrimidine studied has varied substantially and has included single-agent 5-FU (given as bolus, 24- and 48-hour infusion, and protracted continuous infusion), modulated 5-FU, and oral fluoropyrimidines such as capecitabine and uracil/ftorafur. The combination of gemcitabine and 5-fluoropyrimidines has been, in general, very well tolerated and has permitted the administration of both agents at full dose in most clinical trials. In noncomparative studies, the combination regimens have been associated with a modest increase in response rate, median survival, and 1-year survival, although a substantial variability is seen among trials. Of interest, the majority of studies that assessed CBR have reported a high rate of symptom improvements in these trials, with responses in the 40% to 50% range.

Three studies have compared the toxicity and efficacy of gemcitabine combined with fluoropyrimidines versus gemcitabine alone. Di Constanzo et al.[181] compared a combination of gemcitabine plus continuous-infusion 5-FU with gemcitabine alone in 92 patients with advanced PC in a randomized phase II design. Patients treated with the combined treatment arm experienced more frequent thrombocytopenia and mucositis. No differences in outcome were observed in this trial, which reported 8% and 11% response rates in the single and combined arm, respectively, and an identical 6-month median survival. A similar randomized phase II study compared the combination of gemcitabine plus the oral fluoropyrimidine capecitabine with gemcitabine alone,[188] with no differences in any outcome parameter being observed. Berlin et al.[182] reported a randomized phase III study conducted by the ECOG, in which patients with locally advanced or advanced PC were treated with either gemcitabine alone or the combination of gemcitabine plus weekly bolus 5-FU. Patients treated with the combination arm had a significantly longer progression-free survival (3.4 months) than patients treated with single-agent gemcitabine (2.2 months). No differences were observed with regard to response rate and overall survival. In summary, although the combination of gemcitabine with a fluoropyrimidine is well tolerated, there is no evidence of meaningful improvement in any relevant parameter of outcome, and therefore the combination cannot be recommended for routine use.

TABLE 29.3-16. Gemcitabine-Fluoropyrimidine Combinations in Advanced Pancreatic Cancer

Author	Gemcitabine Dose/Schedule	Fluoropyrimidine Dose/Schedule	Phase	No. of Patients	Response Rate (%)	CBR (%)	Median Survival (Mo)	1-Y Survival (%)
Cascinu et al., 1999[170]	1000 mg/m² d 1, 8, 15 q4wk	5-FU, 600 mg/m² bolus d 1, 8, 15 q4wk	II	54	3.7	51	7	22
Hidalgo et al., 1999[171]	900 mg/m² d 1, 8, 15 q4wk	5-FU, 200 mg/m²/d continuous infusion	I/II	26	19	45	10.3	39.5
Berlin et al., 2000[172]	1000 mg/m² d 1, 8, 15 q4wk	5-FU, 600 mg/m² bolus d 1, 8, 15 q4wk	II	36	14	NR	4.4	8.6
Cascinu et al., 2000[173]	1500 mg/m² at 10 mg/m²/min d 1, 8 q3wk	5-FU, 600 mg/m² bolus d 1, 8 q3wk	II	34	17	17	5.7	
Oettle et al., 2000[174]	1000 mg/m² d 1, 8, 15 q4wk	Leucovorin, 200 mg/m² 2-h infusion, and 5-FU, 750 mg/m² 24-h infusion d 1, 8, 15 q5wk	II	38	5	NR	9.3	32
Matano et al., 2000[175]	1000 mg/m² d 1, 8, 15 q4wk	5-FU, 500 mg/m² continuous infusion d 1–5	II	11	9	64	NR	NR
Feliu et al., 2000[176]	1000 mg/m² d 1, 8, 15 q4wk	6S-stereoisomer of leucovorin (6SLV), 250 mg/m² 2-h infusion on d 1; oral 6SLV, 7.5 mg/12 h on d 2–14; and oral UFT, 390 mg/m²/d (in 2 doses) on d 1–14	II	42	16	47	7	21
Kurtz et al., 2000[177]	1000 mg/m² d 1, 8, 15 q4wk	5-FU, 200 mg/m²/d continuous infusion d 1, 8, 15 q4wk	II	29	10	39	4	NR
Rauch et al., 2001[178]	1000 mg/m² d 1, 8, 15 q4wk	5-FU, 200 mg/m²/d continuous infusion	II	25	20	65	7	NR
Louvet et al., 2001[179]	1000–1500 mg/m² on d 3 q2wk	Leucovorin, 400 mg/m² over 2 h, followed by 5-FU, 400 mg/m² bolus and 2–3 g/m² infused over 46 h q2wk	II	62	26	49	9	32
Marantz et al., 2001[180]	1000 mg/m² d 1, 8, 15 q4wk	Leucovorin, 20 mg/m²; 5-FU, 600 mg/m² bolus d 1, 8, 15 q4wk	II	29	21	NR	8.4	36
Di Constanzo et al., 2001[181]	Arm A: 1000 mg/m² weekly × 7; 1 wk rest; d 1, 8, 15 q4wk	Arm A: None	II	48	8	NR	6	NR
	Arm B: 1000 mg/m² weekly × 7; 1 wk rest; d 1, 8, 15 q4wk	Arm B: 5-FU, 200 mg/m²/d continuous infusion 6 wk on 2 wk off		44	11	NR	6	NR
Berlin et al., 2002[182]	Arm A: 1000 mg/m² d 1, 8, 15 q4wk	Arm A: None	III	163	5.6	NR	5.4	NR
	Arm B: 1000 mg/m² d 1, 8, 15 q4wk	Arm B: 5-FU, 600 mg/m² bolus d 1, 8, 15 q4wk		164	6.9		6.7 (P = .9)	
Feliu et al., 2002[183]	1200 mg/m² at 10 mg/m²/min d 1, 8, 15 q4wk	Oral UFT, 400 mg/m²/d (in 2–3 doses/d) for 3 consecutive wk q4wk	II	43	33	64	11	32
Barone et al., 2003[184]	1000–1200 mg/m² d 1, 8, 15 q4wk	5-FU, 2000–2250 mg/m² 24-h infusion d 1, 8, 15 q4wk	I/II	21	9.5	50	11	33
Murad et al., 2003[185]	1000 mg/m² d 1, 8, 15 q4wk	5-FU, 500 mg/m² bolus days 1, 8, 15 q4wk	II	26	29	41	9	30
Correale et al., 2003[186]	1000 mg/m² d 1, 8 q3wk	Leucovorin, 100 mg/m², by 5-FU, 400 mg/m² bolus d 1–3 q2wk	II	42	31	NR	13.1	NR
Hess et al., 2003[187]	1000 mg/m² 2 wk on 1 wk off	Capecitabine, 500–800 mg/m² b.i.d. continuously for 2 wk q3wk	I/II	36	15	NR	6.3	33
Scheithauer et al., 2003[188]	Arm A: 2200 mg/m² every other wk	Arm A: None	II	42	14	33	8.2	37
	Arm B: 2200 mg/m² every other wk	Arm B: Capecitabine, 1250 mg/m² b.i.d. 1 wk on 1 wk off		41	17	48.4	9.5	31.8

CBR, clinical benefit response; 5-FU, 5-fluorouracil; NR, not reported; UFT, uracil/ftorafur.

Gemcitabine-Cisplatin Combinations

Studies testing the combination of gemcitabine with cisplatin are summarized in Table 29.3-17. The rationale for this combination is based on preclinical studies demonstrating synergistic activity between the two drugs, likely due to a decreased ability of the cell to repair DNA damage induced by cisplatin in the presence of gemcitabine. In addition, cisplatin has modest single-agent activity in PC, with a 21% objective response rate and a 5-month median survival in phase II studies.[195] Furthermore, the toxicity profile of cisplatin (with nausea and vomiting and nephro-, neuro-, and ototoxicity) does not overlap with the preferential hematologic toxic effects of gemcitabine. The combination studies have used a weekly administration schedule of the two drugs and have demonstrated a reasonable tolerability profile. As occurred in the combination studies with fluoropyrimidines, the response rates and median survivals of patients treated with gemcitabine in combination with cisplatin have been higher than those reported with gemcitabine alone and have ranged from response rates of 9% to 31%, with median survival figures ranging from 5.0 to 9.6 months. In a randomized phase II study conducted by Colucci et al.,[192] the combination of gemcitabine and cisplatin resulted in a higher response rate (26.4% vs. 11.0%) and time to tumor progression (5 vs. 2 months) but no significant differences in median or 1-year survival. The combination arm resulted in higher hematologic toxicity. The preliminary results from a phase III randomized clinical trial have also been presented.[194] The trial enrolled a total of 198 patients with advanced or locally advanced PC. The combined gemcitabine-cisplatin regimen resulted in a statistically significant prolongation of time to tumor progression from 2.5 to 6.4 months, with no significant improvement in the objective response rate or overall survival.

Gemcitabine-Oxaliplatin Combinations

The combination of gemcitabine with oxaliplatin has been reported in two published phase II studies. The GERCOR (Oncology Multidisciplinary Research Group) cooperative group assessed the efficacy and toxicity of a biweekly regimen of oxaliplatin, 100 mg/m², and gemcitabine, 1000 mg/m² administered as a 10-mg/m² fixed-dose-rate infusion in patients with advanced or locally advanced PC.[196] Sixty-four patients were treated, and 30% of them achieved an objective response. Symptom improvement was noticed in 40% of the patients. The median survival and 1-year survival were 5.3 months and 36%, respectively. Overall, the treatment was very well tolerated, with fewer than 15% of the patients having grade 3 to 4 toxicity. The second study was conducted by the North Central Cancer Treatment Group cooperative and enrolled 47 patients in a regimen of oxaliplatin, 100 mg/m² on day 1, and gemcitabine, 1000 mg/m² on days 1 and 8, with cycles repeated every 3 weeks, a regimen based on a prior phase I study conducted by the same group.[197,198] The overall response rate was 10.9%, and the median survival was 6.2 months. In a preliminary report of a phase III study, the combination of gemcitabine-oxaliplatin using the GERCOR regimen described above resulted in an increase in progression-free survival from 4 to 6 months.[199] The study, however, included two variables: the addition of oxaliplatin and the use of a fixed-dose-rate infusion rather than the conventional 30-minute infusion, making it difficult to determine which one is responsible for the apparent improvement. Based on these data, ECOG 6201 is comparing standard gemcitabine, with fixed-dose-rate infusion gemcitabine, with the gemcitabine-oxaliplatin combination as developed by the GERCOR group. This study will provide definitive data with regard to the relative merits of adding oxaliplatin to gemcitabine, as well as the dosing schedule of gemcitabine.

TABLE 29.3-17. Gemcitabine-Cisplatin Combinations in Advanced Pancreatic Cancer

Author	Gemcitabine Dose/Schedule	Cisplatin Dose/Schedule	Phase	No. of Patients	Response Rate (%)	CBR (%)	Median Survival (Mo)	1-Y Survival (%)
Brodowicz et al., 2000[189]	1000 mg/m² d 1, 8, 15 q4wk	35 mg/m² d 1, 8, 15 q4wk	II	16	31	NR	9.6	NR
Heinemann et al., 2000[190]	1000 mg/m² d 1, 8, 15 q4wk	50 mg/m² d 1 and 15 q4wk	II	41	11.4	NR	8.2	27
Philip et al., 2001[191]	1000 mg/m² d 1, 8, 15 q4wk	50 mg/m² d 1 and 15 q4wk	II	42	26	NR	7.1	19
Colucci et al., 2002[192]	Arm A: 1000 mg/m² weekly × 7; 1 wk rest; d 1, 8, 15 q4wk	Arm A: None	II	44	9.2	49	5	11
	Arm B: 1000 mg/m² weekly × 7; 1 wk rest; d 1, 8, 15 q4wk	Arm B: 25 mg/m² weekly × 7; 1 wk rest; d 1, 8, 15 q4wk		53	26.4 (P = .02)	53	7.5	11.3
Cascinu et al., 2003[193]	1000 mg/m² d 1, 8 q3wk	25 mg/m² d 1, 8 q3wk	II	45	9	24	5.6	NR
Heinemann et al., 2003[194]	Arm A: 1000 mg/m² d 1, 8, 15 q4wk	Arm A: None	III	100	8	NR	6	NR
	Arm B: 1000 mg/m² d 1 and 15 q4wk	Arm B: 50 mg/m² d 1 and 15 q4wk		98	10.2	NR	7.6 (P = .1)	NR

CBR, clinical benefit response; NR, not reported.

Gemcitabine-Docetaxel Combination

The combination of gemcitabine and docetaxel was developed based on early reports suggesting that docetaxel was very active as a single agent in patients with PC.[140] Cascinu et al.[200] from the GIS-CAD (Italian Group for the Study of Digestive Tract Cancer) reported a phase I/II study of docetaxel, 70 to 80 mg/m^2 on day 8, and gemcitabine, 1000 mg/m^2 on days 1 and 8 every 21 days. The maximum tolerated dose of the regimen was 70 mg/m^2 docetaxel, with higher doses resulting in dose-limiting hematologic toxicity. Eighteen patients were treated in the phase II portion of the study, with only one partial response (5.5%) and a median survival of 5.4 months, which resulted in early termination of the study. Jacobs[201] conducted a phase II study of docetaxel, 75 mg/m^2 on day 1, and standard gemcitabine, 1000 mg/m^2 on days 1, 8, and 15 every 28 days. The regimen had to be modified to a weekly docetaxel schedule of 40 mg/m^2 on days 1 and 8, with gemcitabine, 1000 mg/m^2, administered the same days every 21 days, because grade 2 to 3 hematologic toxicity developed in 13 of the first 18 patients. Overall, seven patients achieved a partial response, for a median time to progression of 5.25 months. The combination of gemcitabine-docetaxel (gemcitabine, 800 mg/m^2 on days 1 and 8, and docetaxel, 85 mg/m^2 every 3 weeks) has been compared to cisplatin-docetaxel (cisplatin, 75 mg/m^2 on day 1, and docetaxel, 75 mg/m^2 on day 1 every 21 days) in a randomized phase II study conducted by the EORTC.[202] Preliminary data from this study indicate that the regimens are equally effective, with a response rate of 16% and a median survival of 7.6 and 7.1 months, respectively. The combination of docetaxel-gemcitabine is currently one of the experimental arms of CALGB 89904, a phase III randomized clinical trial in which patients with advanced PC are randomized to treatment with fixed-dose-rate gemcitabine (10 mg/m^2/min × 150 minutes on days 1, 8, and 15 every 28 days), gemcitabine-cisplatin (gemcitabine, 1000 mg/m^2 on days 1, 8, and 15, and cisplatin, 50 mg/m^2 on days 1 and 15), gemcitabine-docetaxel (gemcitabine, 1000 mg/m^2 on days 1 and 8, and docetaxel, 40 mg/m^2 on days 1 and 8 every 21 days), or gemcitabine-irinotecan (gemcitabine, 1000 mg/m^2 on days 1 and 8, and irinotecan, 100 mg/m^2 on days 1 and 8).

Gemcitabine-Topoisomerase I Inhibitor Combination Studies

The topoisomerase inhibitor most widely studied in PC is irinotecan. In a phase I study of gemcitabine combined with irinotecan, the maximum tolerated dose of the drugs was 1000 mg/m^2 gemcitabine and 100 mg/m^2 irinotecan on days 1 and 8 every 21 days.[202] A subsequent phase II study with this regimen showed a 20% objective response rate in 45 patients treated, and 30% of the patients had a greater than 50% reduction in CA 19-9 levels.[203] Median and 1-year survival were 5.7 months and 27%, respectively. These results are very similar to those obtained by Stathopoulos et al.[204] using a different regimen in which patients received gemcitabine, 1000 mg/m^2 on days 1 and 8, and irinotecan, 300 mg/m^2 on day 8, with cycles repeated every 21 days.[204] A total of 60 patients were treated, reporting an objective response rate of 24.7%, median survival of 7 months, and 1-year survival of 22.5%. Despite these encouraging results, a phase III randomized trial that compared gemcitabine with gemcitabine plus irinotecan using the day 1 and 8 schedule mentioned above in a total of 360 patients with locally advanced or advanced PC failed to demonstrate a survival

benefit for the combination.[205] Patients treated with the combination had a higher response rate of 16.1% versus 4.4% ($P = .001$) but similar time to tumor progression (3.5 to 3.0 months; $P = .352$) and survival (6.3 vs. 6.6 months; $P = .789$). Toxicity was similar in the two groups, with patients treated with the combination arm having a higher occurrence of diarrhea (19% vs. 2%) and the groups having similar quality-of-life scores. As mentioned earlier, CALGB 89904 is currently testing the gemcitabine-irinotecan combination in a phase III study. Phase II and III studies of other topoisomerase inhibitors such as exatecan and rubitecan are also being conducted, but results are not available.

Gemcitabine-Antifolate Combinations

The two antifolates that have been studied in combination regimens in PC are raltitrexed and pemetrexed. The combination of raltitrexed (3 mg/m^2 as a 15-minute infusion on day 1 and gemcitabine, 1000 mg/m^2 on days 1 and 8 every 21 days) was tested in 25 patients with advanced or locally advanced PC.[206] Three partial remissions (12%) occurred, and the median survival of the entire cohort was 6.1 months. Pemetrexed is synergistic with gemcitabine *in vitro*, and in a phase I study the combination was well tolerated.[207] A subsequent phase II study combining gemcitabine, 1250 mg/m^2 on days 1 and 8, with pemetrexed, 500 mg/m^2 on day 8 with folic acid and vitamin B$_{12}$ supplementation, enrolled 42 patients.[208] The response rate was 15%, median survival was 6.5 months, and 1-year survival was 29%. Based on these results, a multicenter phase III study targeting a sample size of 520 patients has been completed.[209,210]

Other Combination Chemotherapy Regimens in Pancreatic Cancer

The anthracycline epirubicin has single-agent activity in patients with PC, which, in a randomized trial, was similar to a 5-FU–based combination.[211] Several phase II studies have explored the activity of epirubicin in combination with gemcitabine. Neri et al.[212] administered epirubicin, 20 mg/m^2 on days 1, 8, and 15, with gemcitabine, 1000 mg/m^2 on days 1, 8, and 15, every 4 weeks to 44 patients with locally advanced or metastatic pancreatic adenocarcinoma, or both. The overall response rate was 25%, and the median survival was 10.9 months. A total of 12 of 27 (44.4%) eligible patients attained a CBR. Other gemcitabine-based combinations that have been tested in phase II studies included gemcitabine-celecoxib and gemcitabine-flutamide.[167,213]

Few studies have evaluated three or more drug combination regimens in PC. Reni et al.[214] published a phase II study of gemcitabine, 600 mg/m^2 on days 1 and 8; cisplatin, 40 mg/m^2 on day 1; epirubicin, 40 mg/m^2 on day 1; and continuous-infusion 5-FU, 200 mg/m^2 on days 1 to 28. A total of 49 patients were treated in the study, with a response rate of 58%, median survival of 10 months, and 1-year survival of 39%. Twenty-eight percent and 51% of the cycles were complicated by grade 3 and 4 thrombocytopenia and neutropenia, respectively. Several other triple- and quadruple-drug combinations have also been reported.

NEW DRUGS IN PANCREATIC CANCER

During the last few years, an increasing number of new drugs, many of them targeted to specific alterations in malignant cells, have been tested in PC, as well as in other tumors. The rationale

TABLE 29.3-18.   Studies with Novel Drugs in Advanced Pancreatic Cancer

Novel Agent	Author	Gemcitabine Dose/Schedule	Novel Drug Dose/Schedule	Phase	No. of Patients	Response Rate (%)	Median Survival (Mo)	1-Y Survival (%)
MMPI	Rosemurgy et al., 1999[226]	—	Marimastat, 5–75 mg PO b.i.d., 10–25 mg PO/d	I	64	NR	5.3	21
MMPI	Evans et al., 2001[217]	—	Marimastat, 10–100 mg PO b.i.d.[a]	II	130	—	3.8	—
MMPI	Bramhall et al., 2001[218]	Arm A: 1000 mg/m² weekly × 7; 1 wk rest; d 1, 8, 15 q4wk Arm B, C, D: —	Arm A: —	III	103	26	5.6	19
			Arm B: marimastat, 5 mg b.i.d.		104	3	3.7	14
			Arm C: marimastat, 10 mg b.i.d.		105	3	3.5	14
			Arm D: marimastat, 25 mg b.i.d.		102	3	4.2	20
MMPI	Bramhall et al., 2002[219]	1000 mg/m² weekly × 7; 1 wk rest; d 1, 8, 15 q4wk	Arm A: marimastat, 10 mg b.i.d.	III	120	11	5.5	NR
			Arm B: placebo		119	16	5.5	NR
MMPI	Moore et al., 2003[220]	Arm A: 1000 mg/m² weekly × 7; 1 wk rest; d 1, 8, 15 q4wk	Arm B: BAY12-9566, 800 mg PO b.i.d.	III	139	6	6.59	25
					138	0.9	3.74 (P<.001)	10
Angiogenesis inhibitor	Kindler et al., 2003[221]	1000 mg/m² d 1, 8, 15 q4wk	Bevacizumab, 10 mg/kg IV, days 1 and 15	II	30	27	Not reached	53[b]
FTI	Cohen et al., 2003[223]	—	Tipifarnib, 300 mg PO b.i.d.	II	20	0	4.8	NR
FTI	Van Cutsem et al., 2002[224]	1000 mg/m² weekly × 7; 1 wk rest; d 1, 8, 15 q4wk	Arm A: tipifarnib, 200 mg PO b.i.d. Arm B: placebo	III	688	NR	6.4 6.1	27 24
FTI	Lersch et al., 2001[225]	Arm A: 1000 mg/m² weekly × 7; 1 wk rest; d 1, 8, 15 q4wk	Arm B: lonafarnib, 200 mg PO b.i.d.	II	30	3	4.4	NR
					33	6	3.3	
EGFR	Safran and Schwartz, 2001[227]	1000 mg/m² weekly × 7; 1 wk rest; d 1, 8, 15 q4wk	Trastuzumab, 2 mg/kg/wk[c]	II	23	24	7.5	24
	Abbruzzese et al., 2001[228]	1000 mg/m² weekly × 7; 1 wk rest; d 1, 8, 15 q4wk	Cetuximab, 250 mg/kg/wk[d]	II	41	12.5	6.7	33

EGFR, epidermal growth factor receptor; FTI, farnesyltransferase inhibitor; MMPI, matrix metalloproteinase inhibitor; NR, not reported.
[a]Ninety percent of the patients received 25-mg dose.
[b]Actuarial estimated.
[c]Loading dose of 4 mg/kg/wk.
[d]Loading dose of 400 mg/kg/wk.

to develop these drugs in PC comes from better understanding of the biologic basis of the disease that has made possible the identification and validation of some of these targets in PC. In addition, the poor prognosis of patients with this disease, and the evidence from clinical trials discussed above that conventional chemotherapy may have reached a plateau with regard to improving outcome, has also motivated an aggressive evaluation of new drugs in PC.[215] Table 29.3-18 summarizes the key features of selected studies conducted with novel drugs in PC.

Matrix Metalloproteinase Inhibitors

The matrix metalloproteinase (MMP) inhibitors are a group of closely related proteases, which are dysregulated in the majority of human neoplasms including PC. The increased activity of these enzymes has been related to tumor growth, progression, invasion, generation of blood vessels, and metastasis. Several inhibitors of the MMPs have been developed as anticancer agents, and two of them, marimastat and BAY12-9566, have been more extensively studied in PC.[216]

Marimastat is a hydroxamate peptidomimetic broad-spectrum inhibitor of the MMP family, including MMP 1, 2, and 9. In phase I studies in PC, dosages from 10 to 25 mg orally twice a day were well tolerated. In a large phase II study that enrolled 113 patients, 90% of whom were treated with 25 mg once a day, a 30% decline or stabilization in the tumor marker CA 19-9 was reported, with a median survival of 3.8 months.[217] Arthralgias, the most common toxicity encountered with marimastat, developed in 29% of the patients. The efficacy and toxicity of marimastat at dosages of 5, 10, and 25 mg twice a day were compared to those of gemcitabine in a phase III study. Patients treated with gemcitabine had a longer progression-free survival of 3.8 months versus 1.9 to 2.0 months for the marimastat-treated group ($P = .001$).[218] Overall survival was also better for gemcitabine and significantly worse for patients treated with marimastat at doses of 5 and 10 mg, whereas no statistically significant differences were observed in overall survival with the 25-mg twice-a-day dose. A subset analysis in this study showed that the benefit of gemcitabine was restricted to patients with advanced disease and that those with locally advanced tumors benefited from marimastat, supporting the hypothesis that these drugs may be more active in situations of early disease. Finally, the combination of gemcitabine with marimastat was tested against gemcitabine alone in a randomized phase III study, with no improvement in any parameter of outcome in the combined-treatment group.[219]

The second MMP inhibitor extensively studied in PC is BAY12-9566, a peptidomimetic inhibitor specific for the MMPs 2 and 9. The drug was compared in a phase III study to single-agent gemcitabine.[220] Of a planned sample of 350 patients, 270 were enrolled, after an interim analysis demonstrated that patients treated with gemcitabine had a significantly better time to tumor progression (3.5 vs. 1.6 months; $P <.001$) and overall survival (6.59 vs. 3.74; $P <.001$). Quality-of-life analysis also favored gemcitabine. In summary, these studies suggest that current MMP inhibitors do not have relevant antitumor activity in patients with advanced PC. Whether or not these drugs or newer-generation analogs will be effective in earlier stages of PC remains to be determined.

Angiogenesis Inhibitors

The angiogenesis inhibitor that appears most promising in PC is bevacizumab, a recombinant, humanized monoclonal antibody against the vascular endothelial growth factor, which is a growth factor that has been implicated in PC progression in several preclinical studies. Bevacizumab has been studied in combination with gemcitabine in a phase II study in patients with PC.[221] Patients with advanced or locally advanced PC received gemcitabine, 1000 mg/m^2 on days 1, 8, and 15 every 28 days, and bevacizumab, 10 mg/kg intravenously on days 1 and 15. Results on the first 26 evaluable patients have been reported, with a response rate of 27%, median time to tumor progression of 6 months, and estimated 1-year survival of 53%. Correlative studies suggest that patients with higher baseline levels of vascular endothelial growth factor tend to have poorer outcomes.

Inhibitors of the Ras Oncogene

Mutations in the oncogene Ras are the most frequent genetic abnormality in PC. Because Ras must be farnesylated to be active (a posttranslational modification mediated by the enzyme farnesyltransferase), inhibitors of this enzyme have been developed as potential Ras inhibitors.[222] Two of these farnesyltransferase inhibitors, tipifarnib and lonafarnib, have been studied in disease-oriented studies in PC. Tipifarnib was tested in a single-agent phase II study in patients with advanced PC, administered at a dosage of 300 mg orally twice a day.[223] Twenty patients were treated, with no objective responses and a median survival of less than 5 months. Correlative studies conducted in peripheral blood mononuclear cells demonstrated partial inhibition of the target farnesyltransferase enzyme. In parallel to this study, a randomized phase III study compared the combination of tipifarnib plus gemcitabine versus gemcitabine plus placebo in patients with advanced PC[224]; 688 patients were treated, without demonstrating any improvement in out-

come in those given tipifarnib plus gemcitabine. Lonafarnib was evaluated in a randomized phase II study in comparison to gemcitabine.[225] The 3-month progression-free survival rate for patients treated with lonafarnib was 23%, compared to 31% for gemcitabine, and the median overall survivals were 3.3 months and 4.4 months, respectively. Two partial responses occurred in patients treated with lonafarnib, and one partial response was observed in the gemcitabine-treated group.

Inhibitors of the Epidermal Growth Factor Receptor Family of Receptors

Pharmacologically, the inhibitors of the epidermal growth factor receptors (EGFR) belong to two broad classes of drugs: monoclonal antibodies against the extracellular domain of the receptor and small-molecule inhibitors of the intracellular TK domain. The studies conducted in PC have mainly tested the combination of these drugs with gemcitabine.

Several studies have evaluated monoclonal antibodies. Safran and Schwartz[227] reported a phase II study of trastuzumab, a monoclonal antibody that targets the Her-2 receptor, in combination with gemcitabine in patients with PC. Up to 21% of PCs are Her-2 positive, and preclinical studies have shown that inhibition of Her-2 signaling with trastuzumab is associated with antitumor effects in PC models. Patients with Her-2–positive pancreatic adenocarcinoma received gemcitabine, 1000 mg/m^2 weekly for 7 consecutive weeks followed by 1 week of rest and then weekly for 3 weeks every 4 weeks, and trastuzumab, 2 mg/kg/wk after an initial loading dose of 4 mg/kg. Data on 23 patients have been reported thus far. Five patients had a partial response (response rate 24%), and the median survival and 1-year survival were 7.5 months and 24%, respectively. Nine of 18 evaluable patients (50%) have had greater than 50% reduction in CA 19-9. Abbruzzese et al.[228] conducted a phase II study of gemcitabine and cetuximab, a monoclonal antibody against the EGFR in EGFR-positive PC patients. Forty-one patients were treated in the study. The overall response rate was 12.5%, with a median survival of 6.7 months and 1-year survival of 33%.

The second clinically relevant classes of agents that inhibit the EGFR are small-molecule inhibitors of the receptor TK. Several of these agents are currently in clinical development. Two of these compounds, EKB-569 and erlotinib, have been specifically developed for PC. EKB-569, an irreversible inhibitor of the EGFR and of the Her-2 receptor, has completed a phase I study in combination with gemcitabine. Furthermore, a randomized phase III study of gemcitabine plus erlotinib or placebo has completed enrollment.

TREATMENT RECOMMENDATIONS

The standard treatment for patients with advanced PC remains single-agent gemcitabine. This strategy is also appropriate for patients with locally advanced disease, although these individuals are commonly managed with combined modality approaches. Either a conventional 30-minute or fixed-dose-rate gemcitabine infusion is appropriate, based on existing data. Combinations of gemcitabine with other agents, such as cisplatin, irinotecan, oxaliplatin, and fluoropyrimidines, have not resulted in improvement in survival or quality of life in studies available thus far. Such combinations should not be considered standard of care at the present time, although this could change as the results of randomized studies become available. Because the main effect of chemotherapy in PC is symptom palliation, this should be the primary criterion to guide chemotherapy treatments. More recently, the serum marker CA 19-9 has been used as a predictor of clinical and radiologic response. Finally, considering the poor outcome of patients treated with conventional treatments, enrollment in clinical trials testing new treatment strategies should be encouraged.

IMMUNOTHERAPY

Immunotherapy has the potential to provide non–cross-resistant mechanisms of antitumor activity that can be integrated with surgery, radiation, and chemotherapy. A major advantage of immune-based therapies is their ability to specifically target the transformed tumor cell relative to the normal cell of origin. As a result, minimal and less severe nonspecific toxicities are expected when compared with other PC treatment modalities. Immunotherapy is extensively discussed elsewhere in this text.

ANTIGEN-BASED VACCINES

A few candidate pancreatic antigens recognized by B and T cells have already been identified and fall into several categories, including reactivated embryonic genes (carcinoembryonic antigen), mutated oncogenes/suppressor genes (*k-ras* and *p53*), altered mucins (MUC1), and overexpressed tissue-specific genes (*HER-2/neu* and *Gastrin-17*). Viral vector, protein, and peptide vaccines using some of these antigens have been tested in phase I and II clinical trials. Although T-cell responses have been observed, they have not yet been correlated with clinical regressions.[229,230]

Mutated *k-ras* vaccines have been the most extensively studied peptide/protein–based vaccine approach in patients with pancreatic adenocarcinoma. In the largest study, patients with either resected or advanced pancreatic adenocarcinoma were intradermally administered a 17 amino acid peptide containing either the specific *k-ras* codon 12 mutation (resected disease) or a mixture of four *k-ras* peptides containing the four most common mutations (advanced disease). Human granulocyte-macrophage colony-stimulating factor (GM-CSF; 40 g) was administered intradermally 15 minutes before peptide vaccination. Patients were vaccinated weekly for 4 weeks and were given booster injections at weeks 6 and 20. Peptide vaccination was well tolerated in all 48 patients. Of the 48 vaccinated patients, 43 were evaluable for induction of immune response. A positive delayed-typed hypersensitivity (DTH; measured as less than 5 mm induration 48 hours after vaccination) was observed in 21 of 43 evaluable patients. In addition, the peptide vaccine elicited a positive mutated *k-ras*–specific proliferative T-cell response in the peripheral blood of 17 of 43 evaluable patients. Mean survival of patients after resection was 25.6 months. In the group with advanced disease, stable disease was seen in 11 of 34 evaluable patients. An immune response (defined as either a positive DTH or a proliferative T-cell response) was observed in 20 of the 34 treated patients, including all 11 patients demonstrating stable disease. The median survival in the group that demonstrated an immune response was 148 days, versus 61 days in the group that did not demonstrate an immune response ($P = .0002$).

WHOLE TUMOR CELL VACCINES

Whole tumor cell vaccine approaches involve the use of autologous or allogeneic tumor cells to stimulate an immune response. However, studies aimed at dissecting antitumor immune responses have confirmed that most tumors are not naturally immunogenic. A preclinical model suggests that the failure of the immune system to reject spontaneously arising tumors is unrelated to the absence of sufficiently immunogenic tumor antigens. Instead, the problem is derived from the immune system's inability to respond appropriately to these antigens.[230] These findings have led to the concept that a tumor cell can become more immunogenic if engineered to secrete immune activating cytokines.

The results of a phase I study testing irradiated allogeneic pancreatic tumor cell lines transfected with GM-CSF as adjuvant treatment administered in sequence with adjuvant chemoradiation in patients with resected pancreatic adenocarcinoma have been reported.[231] Fourteen patients with stage 2 or 3 disease received an initial vaccination 8 weeks after pancreaticoduodenectomy. This was a dose-escalation study in which three patients each received 1×10^7, 5×10^7, and 1×10^8, and five patients received 5×10^8 vaccine cells. Study patients were jointly enrolled in an adjuvant chemoradiation protocol for 6 months. After the completion of adjuvant chemoradiation, patients were reassessed, and those who were still in remission were treated with three additional vaccinations given 1 month apart at the same original dose that they received for the first vaccination. Few toxicities were observed. Systemic GM-CSF levels were measured to assess the longevity of vaccine cells at the immunizing site. Serum GM-CSF levels could be detected for up to 96 hours after vaccination. Postvaccination DTH responses to autologous tumor cells were observed in one of three patients receiving 1×10^8 and in two of four patients receiving 5×10^8 vaccine cells. Follow-up studies are ongoing.

REFERENCES

1. American Cancer Society. *Facts and figures.* Atlanta, GA: American Cancer Society, 2002.
2. Sohn TA, Yeo CJ, Cameron JL, et al. Resected adenocarcinoma of the pancreas—616 patients: results, outcomes, and prognostic indicators. *J Gastrointest Surg* 2000;4:567.
3. Yeo TP, Hruban RH, Leach SD, et al. Pancreatic cancer. *Curr Probl Cancer* 2002;26:176.
4. Lowenfels AB, Maisonneuve P. Environmental factors and risk of pancreatic cancer. *Pancreatology* 2003;3:1.
5. Mulder I, van Genugten MLL, Hoogenveen R, de Hollander AE, Bueno-de-Mesquita HB. The impact of smoking on future pancreatic cancer: a computer simulation. *Ann Oncol* 1999;10:S74.
6. Centers for Disease Control and Prevention. National Center for Environmental Health Publication No. 01-0164, March 2001. World Wide Web URL: http://www.cdc.gov/nceh/dls/report/, 2001.
7. Michaud DS, Giovannucci E, Willett WC, et al. Physical activity, obesity, height, and the risk of pancreatic cancer. *JAMA* 2001;286:921.
8. Ojajarvi I, Partanen T, Ahlbom A, et al. Occupational exposures and pancreatic cancer: a meta-analysis. *Occup Environ Med* 2000;57:316.
9. Hoppin J, Tolbert P, Holly E, et al. Pancreatic cancer and serum organochlorine levels. *Cancer Epidemiol Biomarkers Prev* 2000;9:199.
10. Hruban RH, Petersen GM, Ha PK, Kern SE. Genetics of pancreatic cancer: from genes to families. *Surg Oncol Clin N Am* 1998;7:1.
11. Tersmette AC, Petersen GM, Offerhaus GJA, et al. Increased risk of incident pancreatic cancer among first-degree relatives of patients with familial pancreatic cancer. *Clin Cancer Res* 2001;7:738.
12. Klein AP, Petersen GM, Beaty TH, Bailey-Wilson JE, Hruban RH. Statistical evidence for a novel major gene involved in pancreatic cancer. *Genet Epidemiol* 2002;23:133.
13. Solcia E, Capella C, Klöppel G. *Atlas of tumor pathology: tumors of the pancreas,* 3rd ed. Washington, DC: Armed Forces Institute of Pathology, 1997.
14. Hruban RH, Adsay NV, Albores-Saavedra J, et al. Pancreatic Intraepithelial Neoplasia (PanIN): a new nomenclature and classification system for pancreatic duct lesions. *Am J Surg Pathol* 2001;25:579.

15. Klimstra DS, Heffess CS, Oertel JE, Rosai J. Acinar cell carcinoma of the pancreas. A clinicopathologic study of 28 cases. *Am J Surg Pathol* 1992;16:815.
16. Abraham SC, Wu TT, Hruban RH, et al. Genetic and immunohistochemical analysis of pancreatic acinar cell carcinoma: frequent allelic loss on chromosome 11p and alterations in the APC/beta catenin pathway. *Am J Pathol* 2002;160:953.
17. Klimstra DS, Wenig BM, Adair CF, Heffess CS. Pancreatoblastoma. A clinicopathologic study and review of the literature. *Am J Surg Pathol* 1995;19:1371.
18. Abraham SC, Wu TT, Klimstra DS, Finn L, Hruban RH. Distinctive molecular genetic alterations in sporadic and familial adenomatous polyposis-associated pancreatoblastomas: frequent alterations in the AIIX/B-catenin pathway and chromosome 11p. *Am J Pathol* 2001;159:1619.
19. Wilentz RE, Albores-Saavedra J, Zahurak M, et al. Pathologic examination accurately predicts prognosis in mucinous cystic neoplasms of the pancreas. *Am J Surg Pathol* 1991; 23:1320.
20. Adsay NV, Longnecker DS, Klimstra DS. Pancreatic tumors with cystic dilatation of the ducts: intraductal papillary mucinous neoplasms and intraductal oncocytic papillary neoplasms. *Semin Diagn Pathol* 2000;17:16.
21. Compton CC. Serous cystic tumors of the pancreas. *Semin Diagn Pathol* 2999:17:43.
22. Abraham SC, Klimstra DS, Wilentz RE, et al. Solid-pseudopapillary tumors of the pancreas almost always harbor mutations in the beta-catenin gene. *Am J Pathol* 2002;160: 1361.
23. Wilentz RE, Goggins M, Redston M, et al. Genetic, immunohistochemical, and clinical features of medullary carcinomas of the pancreas: a newly described and characterized entity. *Am J Pathol* 2000;156:1641.
24. van Heek NT, Meeker AK, Kern SE, et al. Telomere shortening is nearly universal in pancreatic intraepithelial neoplasia. *Am J Pathol* 2002;161:1541.
25. Hiyama E, Kodama T, Shinbara K, et al. Telomerase activity is detected in pancreatic cancer but not in benign tumors. *Cancer Res* 1997;57:326.
26. Almoguera C, Shibata D, Forrester K, et al. Most human carcinomas of the exocrine pancreas contain mutant c-K-ras genes. *Cell* 1988;53:549.
27. Caldas C, Hahn SA, Hruban RH, et al. Detection of K-ras mutations in the stool of patients with pancreatic adenocarcinoma and pancreatic ductal hyperplasia, *Cancer Res* 1994;54:3568.
28. Hahn SA, Schutte M, Hoque AT, et al. DPC4, a candidate tumor-suppressor gene at 18q21.1. *Science* 1996;271:350.
29. Schutte M, Hruban RH, Geradts J, et al. Abrogation of the Rb/p16 tumor-suppressive pathway in virtually all pancreatic carcinomas. *Cancer Res* 1997;57:3126.
30. Goldstein AM, Fraser MC, Struewing JP, et al. Increased risk of pancreatic cancer in melanoma-prone kindreds with p16INK4 mutations. *N Engl J Med* 1995;333:970.
31. Ionov Y, Peinado MA, Malkhosyan S, Shibata D, Perucho M. Ubiquitous somatic mutations in simple repeated sequences reveal a new mechanism for colonic carcinogenesis. *Nature* 1993;363:558.
32. Yamamoto H, Itoh F, Nakamura H, et al. Genetic and clinical features of human pancreatic ductal adenocarcinomas with widespread microsatellite instability, *Cancer Res* 2001;61:3139.
33. Goggins M, Schutte M, Lu J, et al. Germline BRCA2 gene mutations in patients with apparently sporadic pancreatic carcinomas. *Cancer Res* 1996;56:5360.
34. van der Heijden MS, Yeo CJ, Hruban RH, Kern SE. Fanconi anemia gene mutations in young-onset pancreatic cancer. *Cancer Res* 2003;63:2585.
35. Jones JB, Song JJ, Hempen PM, et al. Detection of mitochondrial DNA mutations in pancreatic cancer offers a "mass"-ive advantage over detection of nuclear DNA mutations. *Cancer Res* 2001;61:1299.
36. Teng DH-F, Perry III WL, Hogan JK, et al. Human mitogen-activated protein kinase 4 as a candidate tumor suppressor. *Cancer Res* 1997;57:4177.
37. Su GH, Hruban RH, Bova GS, et al. Germline and somatic mutations of the STK11/LKB1 Peutz-Jeghers gene in pancreatic and biliary cancers. *Am J Pathol* 1999;154:1835.
38. Batra SK, Metzgar RS, Hollingsworth MA. Molecular cloning and sequence analysis of the human ribosomal protein S16. *J Biol Chem* 1991;266:6830.
39. Calhoun E, Jones J, Ashfaq R, et al. BRAF and FBXW7 (CDC4, FBW7, AGO, SEL10) mutations in distinct subsets of pancreatic cancer: potential therapeutic targets. *Am J Pathol* 2003;163:1255.
40. Lengauer C, Kinzler KW, Vogelstein B. Genetic instability in colorectal cancers. *Nature* 1997;386:623.
41. Lowenfels AB, Maisonneuve P, DiMagno EP, et al. Hereditary pancreatitis and the risk of pancreatic cancer. International Hereditary Pancreatitis Study Group. *J Natl Cancer Inst* 1997;89:442.
42. Ryu B, Jones J, Blades NJ, et al. Relationships and differentially expressed genes among pancreatic cancers examined by large-scale serial analysis of gene expression. *Cancer Res* 2002;62:819.
43. Argani P, Iacobuzio-Donahue C, Ryu B, et al. Mesothelin is overexpressed in the vast majority of ductal adenocarcinomas of the pancreas: identification of a new pancreatic cancer marker by serial analysis of gene expression (SAGE). *Clin Cancer Res* 2001;7:3862.
44. Argani P, Rosty C, Reiter RE, et al. Discovery of new markers of cancer through serial analysis of gene expression: prostate stem cell antigen is overexpressed in pancreatic adenocarcinoma. *Cancer Res* 2001;61:4320.
45. Maitra A, Iacobuzio-Donahue C, Rahman A, et al. Immunohistochemical validation of a novel epithelial and a novel stromal marker of pancreatic ductal adenocarcinoma identified by global expression microarrays: sea urchin fascin homolog and heat shock protein 47. *Am J Clin Pathol* 2002;118:52.
46. Rosty C, Christa L, Kuzdzal S, et al. Identification of hepatocarcinoma-intestine-pancreas/pancreatitis- associated protein I as a biomarker for pancreatic ductal adenocarcinoma by protein biochip technology. *Cancer Res* 2002;62:1868.
47. Conejo JR, Kleeff J, Koliopanos A, et al. Syndecan-1 expression is up-regulated in pancreatic but not in other gastrointestinal cancers. *Int J Cancer* 2000;88:12.
48. Iacobuzio-Donahue CA, Maitra A, Shen-Ong GL, et al. Discovery of novel tumor markers of pancreatic cancer using global gene expression technology. *Am J Pathol* 2002;160:1239.
49. Iacobuzio-Donahue CA, Maitra A, Olsen M, et al. Exploration of global gene expression patterns in pancreatic adenocarcinoma using cDNA microarrays. *Am J Pathol* 2003;162: 1151.
50. Iacobuzio-Donahue CA, Ryu B, Hruban RH, et al. Exploring the host desmoplastic response to pancreatic carcinoma: gene expression of stromal and neoplastic cells at the site of primary invasion. *Am J Pathol* 2002;160:91.
51. Sohn TA, Yeo CJ, Cameron JL, et al. Intraductal papillary mucinous neoplasms of the pancreas: an increasingly recognized clinicopathologic entity. *Ann Surg* 2001;234:313.
52. Fishman EK, Horton KM, Urban BA. Multidetector CT angiography in the evaluation of pancreatic carcinoma: preliminary observations. *J Comput Assist Tomogr* 2000;24:849.
53. Legmann P, Vignaux O, Dousset B, et al. Pancreatic tumors: comparison of dual-phase helical CT and endoscopic sonography. *AJR Am J Roentgenol* 1998;170:1315.
54. Abrams RA, Grochow LB, Chakravarthy A, et al. Intensified adjuvant therapy for pancreatic and periampullary adenocarcinoma: survival results and observations regarding patterns of failure, radiotherapy dose and CA19-9 levels. *Int J Radiat Oncol Biol Phys* 1999;44:1039.
55. Canto MI, Jagannath S, Griffin C, et al. Screening for pancreatic neoplasia in high-risk individuals. *J Gastroenterol Hepatol (in press).*
56. Brentnall TA, Bronner MP, Byrd DR, Haggitt RC, Kimmey MB. Early diagnosis and treatment of pancreatic dysplasia in patients with a family history of pancreatic cancer. *Ann Intern Med* 1999;131:247.
57. Sato N, Fukushima N, Maitra A, et al. Discovery of novel targets for aberrant methylation in pancreatic carcinoma using high-throughput microarrays. *Cancer Res* 2003;63:3735.
58. Iwao T, Hiyama E, Yokoyama T, et al. Telomerase activity for the preoperative diagnosis of pancreatic cancer. *J Natl Cancer Inst* 1997;89:1621.
59. Rosty C, Christa L, Kuzdzal S, et al. Identification of hepatocarcinoma-intestine-pancreas/pancreatitis-associated protein I as a biomarker for pancreatic ductal adenocarcinoma by protein biochip technology. *Cancer Res* 2002;62:1868.
60. Exocrine pancreas. In: *AJCC cancer staging manual*, 6th ed. New York: Springer, 2002:157.
61. Horton KM. Multidetector CT and three-dimensional imaging of the pancreas: state of the art. *J Gastrointest Surg* 2002;6:126.
62. Bluemke DA, Fishman EK. CT and MR evaluation of pancreatic cancer. *Surg Oncol Clin N Am* 1998;7:103.
63. Reinhold C. Magnetic resonance imaging of the pancreas in 2001. *J Gastrointest Surg* 2002;6:133.
64. Wiersema MJ. Endoscopic ultrasonography. *J Gastrointest Surg* 2002;6:129.
65. Alazraki N. Imaging of pancreatic cancer using fluorine-18 fluorodeoxyglucose positron emission tomography. *J Gastrointest Surg* 2002:6:136.
66. Conlon KC, Dougherty E, Klimstra DS, et al. The value of minimal access surgery in the staging of patients with potentially resectable peripancreatic malignancy. *Ann Surg* 1996;223:134.
67. Fernandez-del Castillo C, Warshaw AL. Laparoscopic staging and peritoneal cytology. *Surg Oncol Clin N Am* 1998;7:135.
68. Barreiro CJ, Lillemoe KD, Koniaris LG, et al. Diagnostic laparoscopic for periampullary and pancreatic cancer: what is the true benefit? *J Gastrointest Surg* 2002:6:75.
69. Yeo CJ, Cameron JL, Lillemoe KD, et al. Pancreaticoduodenectomy with or without distal gastrectomy and extended retroperitoneal lymphadenectomy for periampullary adenocarcinoma—part 2: randomized controlled trial evaluating survival, morbidity and mortality. *Ann Surg* 2002;236:355.
70. Nguyen TC, Sohn TA, Cameron JL, et al. Standard versus radical pancreaticoduodenectomy for periampullary adenocarcinoma: a prospective randomized trial evaluating quality of life in pancreaticoduodenectomy survivors. *J Gastrointest Surg* 2003;7:1.
71. Yeo CJ, Cameron JL, Maher MM, et al. A prospective randomized trial of pancreaticogastrostomy versus pancreaticojejunostomy after pancreaticoduodenectomy. *Ann Surg* 1995;222:580.
72. Yeo CJ, Cameron JL, Sohn TA, et al. Pancreaticoduodenectomy with or without extended retroperitoneal lymphadenectomy for periampullary adenocarcinoma: comparison of morbidity and mortality and short-term outcome. *Ann Surg* 1999;229:613.
73. Yeo CJ. The Whipple procedure in the 1990s. *Adv Surg* 1999;32:271.
74. Yeo CJ, Cameron JL, Sohn TA, et al. Six hundred fifty consecutive pancreaticoduodenectomies in the 1990s; pathology, complications, outcomes. *Ann Surg* 1997;226:248.
75. Yeo CJ. Management of complications following pancreaticoduodenectomy. *Surg Clin North Am* 1995;75:913.
76. Sohn TA, Yeo CJ, Cameron JL, et al. Pancreaticoduodenectomy: role of interventional radiologists in managing patients and complications. *J Gastrointest Surg* 2003;7:209.
77. Yeo CJ, Cameron JL. Pancreatic cancer: current controversies. In: Schein M, Wise L, eds. *Clinical controversies in surgery.* Basel, Switzerland: Karger Landes,1998:70.
78. Satake K, Nishiwaki H, Yokomatsu H, et al. Surgical curability and prognosis for standard versus extended resections for T1 carcinoma of the pancreas. *Surg Gynecol Obstet* 1992;175:259.
79. Pedrazzoli S, DiCarlo V, Dionigi R, et al. Standard versus extended lymphadenectomy associated with pancreaticoduodenectomy in the surgical treatment of adenocarcinoma of the head of the pancreas. A multicenter, prospective, randomized study. *Ann Surg* 1998;228:508.
80. Sohn TA, Yeo CJ, Cameron JL, et al. Resected adenocarcinoma of the pancreas—616 patients: results, outcomes and prognostic indicators. *J Gastrointest Surg* 2000;4:567.
81. Wade TP, Virgo KS, Johnson FE. Distal pancreatectomy for cancer: results in US Department of Veterans Affairs Hospitals, 1987–1991. *Pancreas* 1995;11:341.
82. Sarr MG, Cameron JL. Surgical management of unresectable carcinoma of the pancreas. *Surgery* 1983;91:123.

83. Watanapa P, Williamson RCN. Surgical palliation for pancreatic cancer: developments during the past two decades. *Br J Surg* 1992;79:8.

84. Lillemoe KD, Cameron JL, Hardacre JM, et al. Is prophylactic gastrojejunostomy indicated for unresectable periampullary cancer? A prospective randomized trial. *Ann Surg* 1999;230:322.

85. Lillemoe KD, Cameron JL, Kaufman HS, et al. Chemical splanchnicectomy in patients with unresectable pancreatic cancer: a prospective randomized trial. *Ann Surg* 1993;217:447.

86. Sohn TA, Lillemoe KD, Cameron JL, et al. Surgical palliation of unresectable periampullary adenocarcinoma in the 1990s. *J Am Coll Surg* 1999;188:658.

87. Kalser MH, Ellenberg SS. Pancreatic cancer: adjuvant combined radiation and chemotherapy following curative resection. *Arch Surg* 1985;120:899.

88. Gastrointestinal Tumor Study Group. Further evidence of effective adjuvant combined radiation and chemotherapy following curative resection of pancreatic cancer. *Cancer* 1987;59:2006.

89. Yeo CJ, Abrams RA, Grochow LB, et al. Pancreaticoduodenectomy for pancreatic adenocarcinoma: postoperative adjuvant chemoradiation improves survival. *Ann Surg* 1997;225:621.

90. Abrams RA, Grochow LB, Chakravarthy A, et al. Intensified adjuvant therapy for pancreatic and periampullary adenocarcinoma: survival results and observations regarding patterns of failure, radiotherapy dose and CA19-9 levels. *Int J Radiat Oncol Biol Phys* 1999;44:1039.

91. Todd KE, Gloor B, Lane JS, et al. Resection of locally advanced pancreatic cancer after downstaging with continuous infusion 5-fluorouracil, mitomycin-C, leucovorin and dipyridamole. *J Gastrointest Surg* 1998;2:159.

92. Mehta VK, Fisher GA, Ford JM, et al. Adjuvant radiotherapy and concomitant 5-fluorouracil by protracted venous infusion for resected pancreatic cancer. *Int J Radiat Oncol Biol Phys* 2000;48:1483.

93. Nukui Y, Picozzi VJ, Traverso LW. Interferon based adjuvant chemoradiation therapy improves survival after pancreaticoduodenectomy for pancreatic adenocarcinoma. *Am J Surg* 2000;179:367.

94. Picozzi VJ, Kozarek RE, Jacobs AD, et al. Adjuvant therapy for resected pancreas cancer (PC) using alpha-interferon (IFN)-based chemoradiation: completion of a phase II trial. *Proc Am Soc Clin Oncol* 2003;22:265(abst).

95. Klinkenbijl JH, Jeekel J, Sahmoud T, et al. Adjuvant radiotherapy and 5-fluorouracil after curative resection of cancer of the pancreas and periampullary region. *Ann Surg* 1999;230:776.

96. Neoptolemos JP, Dunn JA, Stocken DD, et al. Adjuvant chemoradiotherapy and chemotherapy in resectable pancreatic cancer: a randomized controlled trial. *Lancet* 2001;358:1576.

97. Spitz FR, Abbruzzese JL, Lee JE, et al. Preoperative and postoperative chemoradiation strategies in patients treated with pancreaticoduodenectomy for adenocarcinoma of the pancreas. *J Clin Oncol* 1997;15:928.

98. Paulino AC. Resected pancreatic cancer treated with adjuvant radiotherapy with or without 5-fluorouracil: treatment results and patterns of failure. *Am J Clin Oncol* 1999;22:489.

99. Chakravarthy A, Abrams RA, Yeo CJ. Intensified adjuvant combined modality therapy for resected periampullary adenocarcinoma: acceptable toxicity and suggestion of improved 1 year survival. *Int J Radiat Oncol Biol Phys* 2000;48:1089.

100. Van-Laethem JL, Demols A, Gay F, et al. Postoperative adjuvant gemcitabine and concurrent radiation after curative resection of pancreatic head carcinoma: a phase II study. *Int J Radiat Oncol Biol Phys* 2003;56:974.

101. Breslin TM, Hess KR, Harbison DB, et al. Neoadjuvant chemoradiotherapy for adenocarcinoma of the pancreas: treatment variables and survival duration. *Ann Surg Oncol* 2001;8:123.

102. Hoffman JP, Lipsitz S, Pisansky T, et al. Phase II trial of preoperative radiation therapy and chemotherapy for patients with localized, resectable adenocarcinoma of the pancreas: an Eastern Cooperative Oncology Group study. *J Clin Oncol* 1998;16:317.

103. Arnoletti JP, Hoffman JP, Ross EA, et al. Pre-operative chemoradiation in the management of adenocarcinoma of the body of the pancreas. *Am Surg* 2002;68:330.

104. Pisters PWT, Wolff RA, Janjan NA, et al. Preoperative paclitaxel and concurrent rapid fractionation radiation for resection pancreatic adenocarcinoma: toxicities, histologic response rates and event-free outcome. *J Clin Oncol* 2002;20:2537.

105. Staley CA, Lee JE, Cleary KR, et al. Preoperative chemoradiation, pancreaticoduodenectomy, and intraoperative radiation therapy for adenocarcinoma of the pancreatic head. *Am J Surg* 1996;171:118.

106. White RR, Hurwitz HI, Morse MA, et al. Neoadjuvant chemoradiation for localized adenocarcinoma of the pancreas. *Ann Surg Oncol* 2001;8:758.

107. Moutardier V, Giovanni M, Lelong B, et al. A phase II single institutional experience with pre-operative radiochemotherapy in pancreatic adenocarcinoma. *Eur J Surg Oncol* 2002;28:531.

108. Levy MH. Pharmacology treatment of cancer pain. *N Engl J Med* 1996;335:1124.

109. Moertel CG, Childs DS Jr, Reitemeier RJ, et al. Combined 5-fluorouracil and supervoltage radiation therapy of locally unresectable gastrointestinal cancer. *Lancet* 1969;2:865.

110. Moertel CG, Frytak S, Hahn RG, et al. Therapy of locally unresectable pancreatic carcinoma: a randomized comparison of high dose (6000 rads) radiation alone, moderate dose radiation (4000 rads + 5-fluorouracil), and high dose radiation + 5-fluorouracil. The Gastrointestinal Tumor Study Group. *Cancer* 1981;48:1705.

111. Gastrointestinal Tumor Study Group. Treatment of locally unresectable carcinoma of the pancreas: comparison of combined-modality therapy (chemotherapy plus radiotherapy) to chemotherapy alone. *J Natl Cancer Inst* 1988;80:751.

112. Klaassen DJ, MacIntyre JM, Catton GE, et al. Treatment of locally unresectable cancer of the stomach and pancreas: a randomized comparison of 5-fluorouracil alone with radiation plus concurrent and maintenance 5-fluorouracil—an Eastern Cooperative Oncology Group Study. *J Clin Oncol* 1985;3:373.

113. McCracken JD, Ray P, Heilbrun LK, et al. 5-Fluorouracil, methyl-CCNU, and radiotherapy with or without testolactone for localized adenocarcinoma of the exocrine pancreas. A Southwest Oncology Group Study. *Cancer* 1980;46:1518.

114. Gastrointestinal Tumor Study Group. Radiation therapy combined with adriamycin or 5-fluorouracil for the treatment of locally unresectable pancreatic carcinoma. *Cancer* 1985;56:2563.

115. Earle JD, Foley JF, Wieand HS, et al. Evaluation of external-beam radiation therapy plus 5-fluorouracil (5-FU) versus external-beam radiation therapy plus hycanthone (HYC) in confined, unresectable pancreatic cancer. *Int J Radiat Oncol Biol Phys* 1994;28:207.

116. McGinn CJ, Zalupski MM. Radiation therapy with once-weekly gemcitabine in pancreatic cancer: current status of clinical trials. *Int J Radiat Oncol Biol Phys* 2003;56:[Suppl]10.

117. Blackstock AW, Bernard SA, Richards F, et al. Phase I trial of twice-weekly gemcitabine and concurrent radiation in patients with advanced pancreatic cancer. *J Clin Oncol* 1999;17:2208.

118. Blackstock AW, Tempero MA, Niedwiecki D, et al. Phase II chemoradiation trial using gemcitabine in patients with locoregional adenocarcinoma of the pancreas. *Proc Am Soc Clin Oncol* 2001;20:158a(abst).

119. Wolff RA, Evans DB, Gravel DM, et al. Phase I trial of gemcitabine combined with radiation for the treatment of locally advanced pancreatic adenocarcinoma. *Clin Cancer Res* 2001;2246:2246.

120. McGinn CJ, Zalupski MM, Shureiqi I, et al. Phase I trial of radiation dose escalation with concurrent weekly full-dose gemcitabine in patients with advanced pancreatic cancer. *J Clin Oncol* 2001;19:4202.

121. Talamonti MS, Catalano PJ, Vaughn DJ, et al. Eastern Cooperative Oncology Group phase I trial of protracted venous infusion fluorouracil plus weekly gemcitabine with concurrent radiation therapy in patients with locally advanced pancreas cancer: a regimen with unexpected early toxicity. *J Clin Oncol* 2000;18:3384.

122. Martenson JA, Vigliotti APG, Pitot HC, et al. A phase I study of radiation therapy and twice-weekly gemcitabine and cisplatin in patients with locally advanced pancreatic cancer. *Int J Radiat Oncol Biol Phys* 2003;55:1305.

123. Brunner TB, Grabenbauer GG, Klein P, et al. Phase I trial of strictly time-scheduled gemcitabine and cisplatin with concurrent radiotherapy in patients with locally advanced pancreatic cancer. *Int J Radiat Oncol Biol Phys* 2003;55:144.

124. Crane CH, Abbruzzese JL, Evans DB, et al. Is the therapeutic index better with gemcitabine based chemoradiation than with 5-fluorouracil based chemoradiation in locally advanced pancreatic cancer? *Int J Radiat Oncol Biol Phys* 2002;52:1293.

125. Burris HA 3rd, Moore MJ, Andersen J, et al. Improvements in survival and clinical benefit with gemcitabine as first-line therapy for patients with advanced pancreas cancer: a randomized trial. *J Clin Oncol* 1997;15:2403.

126. Mohiuddin M, Rosato F, Barbot D, et al. Long-term results of combined modality treatment with I-125 implantation for carcinoma of the pancreas. *Int J Radiat Oncol Biol Phys* 1992;23:305.

127. Nori D, Merimsky O, Osian AD, et al. Palladium-103: a new radioactive source in the treatment of unresectable carcinoma of the pancreas: a phase I-II study. *J Surg Oncol* 1996;61:300.

128. Raben A, Mychalczak B, Brennan MF, et al. Feasibility study of the treatment of primary unresectable carcinoma of the pancreas with 103PD brachytherapy. *Int J Radiat Oncol Biol Phys* 1996;35:351.

129. Tepper JE, Noyes D, Krall JM, et al. Intraoperative radiation therapy of pancreas carcinoma: a report of RTOG-8505. Radiation Therapy Oncology Group. *Int J Radiat Oncol Biol Phys* 1991;21:1145.

130. Zerbi A, Fossati V, Parolini D, et al. Intraoperative radiation therapy adjuvant to resection in the treatment of pancreatic cancer. *Cancer* 1994;73:2930.

131. Willett CG, Warshaw AL. Intraoperative electron beam irradiation in pancreatic cancer. *Front Biosci* 1998;3:e207.

132. Hecht JR, Bedford R, Abbruzzese JL, et al. A phase I/II trial of intratumoral endoscopic ultrasound injection of ONYX-015 with intravenous gemcitabine in unresectable pancreatic carcinoma. *Clin Cancer Res* 2003;9:555.

133. Hanna N, Chung T, Hecht R, et al. TNFerade in pancreatic cancer: results of a run-in phase of a major randomized study in patients with locally advanced pancreatic cancer. *Proc Am Soc Clin Oncol* 2003;22:271(abst).

134. Glimelius B, et al. Chemotherapy improves survival and quality of life in advanced pancreatic and biliary cancer. *Ann Oncol* 1996;7:593.

135. Palmer KR, et al. Chemotherapy prolongs survival in inoperable pancreatic carcinoma. *Br J Surg* 1994;81:882.

136. Takada T, et al. Prospective randomized trial comparing 1/2 FAM (5-fluorouracil (5-FU) + adriamycin + mitomycin C) versus palliative therapy for the treatment of unresectable pancreatic and biliary tract carcinomas (the 2nd trial in non-resectable patients). Japanese Study Group of Surgical Adjuvant Therapy for Carcinomas of the Pancreas and Biliary Tract. *Gan To Kagaku Ryoho* 1996;23:707.

137. Evans DB AJ, Willet CG. Cancer of the pancreas. In: DeVita VT Jr, Rosenberg SA, eds. *Cancer: principles and practice of oncology.* Philadelphia: Lippincott Williams & Wilkins, 2001:1126.

138. Shewach DS, Lawrence TS. Gemcitabine and radiosensitization in human tumor cells. *Invest New Drugs* 1996;14:257.

139. Von Hoff DD. Activity of gemcitabine in a human tumor cloning assay as a basis for clinical trials with gemcitabine. San Antonio Drug Development Team. *Invest New Drugs* 1996;14:265.

140. Rougier P, et al. A phase II study: docetaxel as first-line chemotherapy for advanced pancreatic adenocarcinoma. *Eur J Cancer* 2000;36:1016.

141. Androulakis N, et al. Treatment of pancreatic cancer with docetaxel and granulocyte colony-stimulating factor: a multicenter phase II study. *J Clin Oncol* 1999;17:1779.

142. Lenzi R, et al. Phase II study of docetaxel in patients with pancreatic cancer previously untreated with cytotoxic chemotherapy. *Cancer Invest* 2002;20:464.

143. Okada S, et al. Phase II study of docetaxel in patients with metastatic pancreatic cancer: a Japanese cooperative study. Cooperative Group of Docetaxel for Pancreatic Cancer in Japan. *Br J Cancer* 1999;80:438.

144. Oettle H, et al. Paclitaxel as weekly second-line therapy in patients with advanced pancreatic carcinoma. *Anticancer Drugs* 2000;11:635.

145. Jacobs A, Planting A, Ferry D, et al. Efficacy of DHA-paclitaxel (TXP) in pancreatic cancer. *Proc Am Soc Clin Oncol* 2003;22:272.

146. Rougier P, DM, Ould Kaci M, et al. Randomized phase II study of Oxaliplatin alone (OXA), 5-Fluorouracil (5FU) alone, and the two drugs combined (OXA-FU) in advanced or metastatic pancreatic adenocarcinoma (APC). *Proc Am Soc Clin Oncol* 2000.

147. Wagener DJ, et al. Phase II trial of CPT-11 in patients with advanced pancreatic cancer, an EORTC early clinical trials group study. *Ann Oncol* 1995;6:129.

148. Konstadoulakis MM, et al. A phase II study of 9-nitrocamptothecin in patients with advanced pancreatic adenocarcinoma. *Cancer Chemother Pharmacol* 2001;48:417.

149. D'Adamo D, Hammond L, Donehower R, et al. Final results of a phase II study of DX-8951f (Exatecan Mesylate, DX) in advanced pancreatic cancer. *Proc Am Soc Clin Oncol* 2001;20:134a.

150. Cartwright TH, et al. Phase II study of oral capecitabine in patients with advanced or metastatic pancreatic cancer. *J Clin Oncol* 2002;20:160.

151. Mani S, et al. Phase II trial of uracil/tegafur (UFT) plus leucovorin in patients with advanced pancreatic carcinoma: a University of Chicago phase II consortium study. *Ann Oncol* 1998;9:1035.

152. Hayashi K, Imoizumi T, Kuramochi H, Uchida K, Takasaki K. High response rates in patients with pancreatic cancer using the oral fluoropyrimidine S-1. *Oncol Rep* 2002;9:1355.

153. Rothenberg ML, et al. Phase II trial of 5-fluorouracil plus eniluracil in patients with advanced pancreatic cancer: a Southwest Oncology Group study. *Ann Oncol* 2002;13:1576.

154. Miller KD, et al. Phase II study of the multitargeted antifolate LY231514 (ALIMTA, MTA, pemetrexed disodium) in patients with advanced pancreatic cancer. *Ann Oncol* 2000;11:101.

155. Pazdur R, et al. Phase II trial of ZD1694 (Tomudex) in patients with advanced pancreatic cancer. *Invest New Drugs* 1996;13:355.

156. Ulrich-Pur H, et al. Irinotecan plus raltitrexed vs raltitrexed alone in patients with gemcitabine-pretreated advanced pancreatic adenocarcinoma. *Br J Cancer* 2003;88:1180.

157. Smith D, Gallagher N. A phase II/III study comparing intravenous ZD9331 with gemcitabine in patients with pancreatic cancer. *Eur J Cancer* 2003;39:1377.

158. Lapointe R, Letourneau R, Steward W, et al. Phase 2 study of troxacitabine in chemotherapy naive patients with advanced cancer of the pancreas. *Proc Am Soc Clin Oncol* 2002;565.

159. Sharma JJ, et al. Phase II study of flutamide as second line chemotherapy in patients with advanced pancreatic cancer. *Invest New Drugs* 1997;15:361.

160. Greenway BA. Effect of flutamide on survival in patients with pancreatic cancer: results of a prospective, randomized, double blind, placebo controlled trial. *BMJ* 1998;316:1935.

161. Casper ES, et al. Phase II trial of gemcitabine (2,2'-difluorodeoxycytidine) in patients with adenocarcinoma of the pancreas. *Invest New Drugs* 1994;12:29.

162. Carmichael J, et al. Phase II study of gemcitabine in patients with advanced pancreatic cancer. *Br J Cancer* 1996;73:101.

163. Rothenberg ML, et al. A phase II trial of gemcitabine in patients with 5-FU-refractory pancreas cancer. *Ann Oncol* 1996;7:347.

164. Burris HA 3rd, et al. Improvements in survival and clinical benefit with gemcitabine as first-line therapy for patients with advanced pancreas cancer: a randomized trial. *J Clin Oncol* 1997;15:2403.

165. Storniolo AM, et al. An investigational new drug treatment program for patients with gemcitabine: results for over 3000 patients with pancreatic carcinoma. *Cancer* 1999;85:1261.

166. Haller DG. Chemotherapy for advanced pancreatic cancer. *Int J Radiat Oncol Biol Phys* 2003;56:[Suppl 4]16.

167. Hochster HS. Newer approaches to gemcitabine-based therapy of pancreatic cancer: fixed-dose-rate infusion and novel agents. *Int J Radiat Oncol Biol Phys* 2003;56[Suppl 4]:24.

168. Brand R, Capadano M, Tempero M. A phase I trial of weekly gemcitabine administered as a prolonged infusion in patients with pancreatic cancer and other solid tumors. *Invest New Drugs* 1997;15:331.

169. Tempero M, et al. Randomized phase II comparison of dose-intense gemcitabine: thirty-minute infusion and fixed dose rate infusion in patients with pancreatic adenocarcinoma. *J Clin Oncol* 2003;21:3402.

170. Cascinu S, et al. A combination of gemcitabine and 5-fluorouracil in advanced pancreatic cancer, a report from the Italian Group for the Study of Digestive Tract Cancer (GISCAD). *Br J Cancer* 1999;80:1595.

171. Hidalgo M, et al. Phase I-II study of gemcitabine and fluorouracil as a continuous infusion in patients with pancreatic cancer. *J Clin Oncol* 1999;17:585.

172. Berlin JD, et al. A phase II study of gemcitabine and 5-fluorouracil in metastatic pancreatic cancer: an Eastern Cooperative Oncology Group Study (E3296). *Oncology* 2000;58:215.

173. Cascinu S, et al. A combination of a fixed dose rate infusion of gemcitabine associated to a bolus 5-fluorouracil in advanced pancreatic cancer, a report from the Italian Group for the Study of Digestive Tract Cancer (GISCAD). *Ann Oncol* 2000;11:1309.

174. Oettle H, et al. A phase II trial of gemcitabine in combination with 5-fluorouracil (24-hour) and folinic acid in patients with chemonaive advanced pancreatic cancer. *Ann Oncol* 2000;11:1267.

175. Matano E, et al. Gemcitabine combined with continuous infusion 5-fluorouracil in advanced and symptomatic pancreatic cancer: a clinical benefit-oriented phase II study. *Br J Cancer* 2000;82:1772.

176. Feliu J, et al. Phase II trial of gemcitabine and UFT modulated by leucovorin in patients with advanced pancreatic carcinoma. The ONCOPAZ Cooperative Group. *Cancer* 2000;89:1706.

177. Kurtz JE, et al. Gemcitabine and protracted 5-FU for advanced pancreatic cancer. A phase II study. *Hepatogastroenterology* 2000;47:1450.

178. Rauch DP, et al. Activity of gemcitabine and continuous infusion fluorouracil in advanced pancreatic cancer. *Oncology* 2001;60:43.

179. Louvet C, et al. Phase II trial of bimonthly leucovorin, 5-fluorouracil and gemcitabine for advanced pancreatic adenocarcinoma (FOLFUGEM). *Ann Oncol* 2001;12:675.

180. Marantz A, et al. Phase II study of gemcitabine, 5-fluorouracil, and leucovorin in patients with pancreatic cancer. *Semin Oncol* 2001;28[Suppl 10]:44.

181. Di Costanzo F, SA, Carlini P, et al. Gemcitabine (GEM) alone or in combination with 5-FU continuous infusion (CI) in the treatment of advanced pancreatic cancer (APC): a GOIRC randomized phase II trial. *Proc Am Soc Clin Oncol* 2001:20.

182. Berlin JD, et al. Phase III study of gemcitabine in combination with fluorouracil versus gemcitabine alone in patients with advanced pancreatic carcinoma: Eastern Cooperative Oncology Group Trial E2297. *J Clin Oncol* 2002;20:3270.

183. Feliu J, et al. Phase II study of a fixed dose-rate infusion of gemcitabine associated with uracil/tegafur in advanced carcinoma of the pancreas. *Ann Oncol* 2002;13:1756.

184. Barone C, et al. Weekly gemcitabine and 24-hour infusional 5-fluorouracil in advanced pancreatic cancer: a phase I-II study. *Oncology* 2003;64:139.

185. Murad AM, et al. Phase II trial of the use of gemcitabine and 5-fluorouracil in the treatment of advanced pancreatic and biliary tract cancer. *Am J Clin Oncol* 2003;26:151.

186. Correale P, et al. A novel biweekly pancreatic cancer treatment schedule with gemcitabine, 5-fluorouracil and folinic acid. *Br J Cancer* 2003;89:239.

187. Hess V, et al. Combining capecitabine and gemcitabine in patients with advanced pancreatic carcinoma: a phase I/II trial. *J Clin Oncol* 2003;21:66.

188. Scheithauer W, et al. Biweekly high-dose gemcitabine alone or in combination with capecitabine in patients with metastatic pancreatic adenocarcinoma: a randomized phase II trial. *Ann Oncol* 2003;14:97.

189. Brodowicz T, et al. Phase II study of gemcitabine in combination with cisplatin in patients with locally advanced and/or metastatic pancreatic cancer. *Anticancer Drugs* 2000;11:623.

190. Heinemann V, et al. Gemcitabine and cisplatin in the treatment of advanced or metastatic pancreatic cancer. *Ann Oncol* 2000;11:1399.

191. Philip PA, et al. Phase II study of gemcitabine and cisplatin in the treatment of patients with advanced pancreatic carcinoma. *Cancer* 2001;92:569.

192. Colucci G, et al. Gemcitabine alone or with cisplatin for the treatment of patients with locally advanced and/or metastatic pancreatic carcinoma: a prospective, randomized phase III study of the Gruppo Oncologia dell'Italia Meridionale. *Cancer* 2002;94:902.

193. Cascinu S, et al. Weekly gemcitabine and cisplatin chemotherapy: a well-tolerated but ineffective chemotherapeutic regimen in advanced pancreatic cancer patients. A report from the Italian Group for the Study of Digestive Tract Cancer (GISCAD). *Ann Oncol* 2003;14:205.

194. Heinemann V, QD, Gieseler F, et al. A phase III trial comparing gemcitabine plus cisplatin vs. gemcitabine alone in advanced pancreatic carcinoma. *Proc Am Soc Clin Oncol* 2003.

195. Wils JA, et al. Activity of cisplatin in adenocarcinoma of the pancreas. *Eur J Cancer* 1993;29A:203.

196. Louvet C, et al. Gemcitabine combined with oxaliplatin in advanced pancreatic adenocarcinoma: final results of a GERCOR multicenter phase II study. *J Clin Oncol* 2002;20:1512.

197. Alberts SR, et al. Gemcitabine and oxaliplatin for patients with advanced or metastatic pancreatic cancer: a North Central Cancer Treatment Group (NCCTG) phase I study. *Ann Oncol* 2002;13:553.

198. Alberts SR, et al. Gemcitabine and oxaliplatin for metastatic pancreatic adenocarcinoma: a North Central Cancer Treatment Group phase II study. *Ann Oncol* 2003;14:580.

199. Louvet C, LR, Hammel P, et al. Gemcitabine versus GEMOX (gemcitabine + oxaliplatin) in non resectable pancreatic adenocarcinoma: interim results of the GERCOR /GISCAD Intergroup Phase III. *Proc Am Soc Clin Oncol* 2003.

200. Cascinu S, et al. A phase I-II study of gemcitabine and docetaxel in advanced pancreatic cancer: a report from the Italian Group for the Study of Digestive Tract Cancer (GISCAD). *Ann Oncol* 1999;10:1377.

201. Jacobs AD. Gemcitabine-based therapy in pancreas cancer: gemcitabine-docetaxel and other novel combinations. *Cancer* 2002;95[Suppl 4]:923.

202. Rocha Lima CM, et al. Irinotecan and gemcitabine in patients with solid tumors: phase I trial. *Oncology (Huntingt)* 2002;16[Suppl 5]:19.

203. Rocha Lima CM, et al. Irinotecan plus gemcitabine induces both radiographic and CA 19-9 tumor marker responses in patients with previously untreated advanced pancreatic cancer. *J Clin Oncol* 2002;20:1182.

204. Stathopoulos GP, et al. Treatment of pancreatic cancer with a combination of irinotecan (CPT-11) and gemcitabine: a multicenter phase II study by the Greek Cooperative Group for Pancreatic Cancer. *Ann Oncol* 2003;14:388.

205. Rocha Lima CMS, RR, Jeffery M, et al. A randomized phase 3 study comparing efficacy and safety of gemcitabine (GEM) and irinotecan (I), to GEM alone in patients (pts) with locally advanced or metastatic pancreatic cancer who have not received prior systemic therapy. *Proc Am Soc Clin Oncol* 2003.

206. Kralidis E, et al. Activity of raltitrexed and gemcitabine in advanced pancreatic cancer. *Ann Oncol* 2003;14:574.

207. Adjei AA. Preclinical and clinical studies with combinations of pemetrexed and gemcitabine. *Semin Oncol* 2002;29[Suppl 18]:30.

208. Kindler HL, DW, Hochster H, et al. Clinical outcome in patients (pts) with advanced pancreatic cancer treated with pemetrexed/gemcitabine. *Proc Am Soc Clin Oncol* 2003.

209. Kindler HL. The pemetrexed/gemcitabine combination in pancreatic cancer. *Cancer* 2002;95[Suppl 4]:928.

210. Kindler HL. Pemetrexed in pancreatic cancer. *Semin Oncol* 2002;29:[Suppl 18]49.

211. Topham C, et al. Randomized trial of epirubicin alone versus 5-fluorouracil, epirubicin and mitomycin C in locally advanced and metastatic carcinoma of the pancreas. *Br J Cancer* 1991;64:179.

212. Neri B, et al. Weekly gemcitabine plus epirubicin as effective chemotherapy for advanced pancreatic cancer: a multicenter phase II study. *Br J Cancer* 2002;87:497.

213. Corrie P, et al. Phase II study to evaluate combining gemcitabine with flutamide in advanced pancreatic cancer patients. *Br J Cancer* 2002;87:716.

214. Reni M, et al. Definitive results of a phase II trial of cisplatin, epirubicin, continuous-infusion fluorouracil, and gemcitabine in stage IV pancreatic adenocarcinoma. *J Clin Oncol* 2001;19:2679.

215. Von Hoff DD, Bearss D. New drugs for patients with pancreatic cancer. *Curr Opin Oncol* 2002;14:621.

216. Hidalgo M, Eckhardt SG. Development of matrix metalloproteinase inhibitors in cancer therapy. *J Natl Cancer Inst* 2001;93:178.

217. Evans JD, et al. A phase II trial of marimastat in advanced pancreatic cancer. *Br J Cancer* 2001;85:1865.

218. Bramhall SR, et al. Marimastat as first-line therapy for patients with unresectable pancreatic cancer: a randomized trial. *J Clin Oncol* 2001;19:3447.

219. Bramhall SR, et al. A double-blind placebo-controlled, randomised study comparing gemcitabine and marimastat with gemcitabine and placebo as first line therapy in patients with advanced pancreatic cancer. *Br J Cancer* 2002;87:161.

220. Moore MJ, et al. Comparison of gemcitabine versus the matrix metalloproteinase inhibitor BAY 12-9566 in patients with advanced or metastatic adenocarcinoma of the pancreas: a Phase III Trial of the National Cancer Institute of Canada Clinical Trials Group. *J Clin Oncol* 2003;21:3296.

221. Kindler HL, AR, Lester E, et al. Bevacizumab (B) plus gemcitabine (G) in patients (pts) with advanced pancreatic cancer (PC). *Proc Am Soc Clin Oncol* 2003.

222. Adjei AA. Blocking oncogenic Ras signaling for cancer therapy. *J Natl Cancer Inst* 2001;93:1062.

223. Cohen SJ, et al. Phase II and pharmacodynamic study of the farnesyltransferase inhibitor R115777 as initial therapy in patients with metastatic pancreatic adenocarcinoma. *J Clin Oncol* 2003;21:1301.

224. Van Cutsem E, Karasek P, Oettle H, et al. Phase III trial comparing gemcitabine + R115777 (Zarnestra) versus gemcitabine + placebo in advanced pancreatic cancer (PC). *Proc Am Soc Clin Oncol* 2002;517a.

225. Lersch C, VCE, Amado R, et al. Randomized phase II study of SCH 66336 and gemcitabine in the treatment of metastatic adenocarcinoma of the pancreas. *Proc Am Soc Clin Oncol* 2001.

226. Rosemurgy A, et al. Marimastat in patients with advanced pancreatic cancer: a dose-finding study. *Am J Clin Oncol* 1999;22:247.

227. Safran H, RR, Schwartz J, Herceptin and gemcitabine for metastatic pancreatic cancer. *Eur J Cancer* 2001;37[Suppl 6]:S310.

228. Abbruzzese JL, RA, Xiong Q, et al. Phase II study of anti-epidermal growth factor receptor (EGFR) antibody Cetuximab (IMC-C225) in combination with gemcitabine in patients with advanced pancreatic cancer. *Proc Am Soc Clin Oncol* 2001.

229. Greten TF, Jaffee EM. Cancer vaccines. *J Clin Oncol* 1999;17:1047.

230. Wolf AM, Wolf D, Steurer M, et al. Increase of regulatory T cells in the peripheral blood of cancer patients. *Clin Cancer Res* 2003;9:606.

231. Jaffee EM, Hruban RH, Biedrzycki B, et al. Novel allogeneic granulocyte-macrophage colony-stimulating factor-secreting tumor vaccine for pancreatic cancer: a phase I trial of safety and immune activation. *J Clin Oncol* 2001;19:145.

232. Evans DB, Rich TA, Byrd DR, et al. Pre-opeartive chemoradiation and pancreaticoduodenectomy for adenocarcinoma of the pancreas. *Arch Surg* 1992;127:1335.

233. Hoffman JP, Weese JL, Solin LJ, et al. A pilot study of pre-operative chemoradiation for patients with localized adenocarcinoma of the pancreas. *Am J Surg* 1995;169:71.

234. Pendurthi TK, Hoffman JP. Pre-operative versus postoperative chemoradiation for patients with resected pancreatic adenocarcinoma. *Am Surg* 1998;64:686.

235. Pisters PW, Abbruzzese JL, Janjan NA, et al. Rapid fractionation pre-operative chemoradiation, pancreaticoduodenectomy, and intraoperative radiation therapy for resectable pancreatic adenocarcinoma. *J Clin Oncol* 1998;16:3843.

236. Magnin V, Moutardier V, Giovannini MH, et al. Neoadjuvant pre-operative chemoradiation in patients with pancreatic cancer. *Int J Radiat Oncol Biol Phys* 2003;55:1300.

237. Moertel CG, Frytak S, Hahn RG, et al. Therapy of locally unresectable pancreatic carcinoma: a randomized comparison of high dose (6000 rads) radiation alone, moderate dose radiation (4000 rads + 5-fluorouracil), and high dose radiation + 5-fluorouracil. The Gastrointestinal Tumor Study Group. *Cancer* 1981;48:1705.

238. Klaassen DJ, MacIntyre JM, Catton GE, et al. Treatment of locally unresectable cancer of the stomach and pancreas: a randomized comparison of 5-fluorouracil alone with radiation plus concurrent and maintenance 5-fluorouracil—an Eastern Cooperative Oncology Group Study. *J Clin Oncol* 1985;3:373.

239. Gastrointestinal Tumor Study Group. Treatment of locally unresectable carcinoma of the pancreas: comparison of combined-modality therapy (chemotherapy plus radiotherapy) to chemotherapy alone. *J Natl Cancer Inst* 1988;80:751.

240. McCracken JD, Ray P, Heilbrun LK, et al. 5-Fluorouracil, methyl-CCNU, and radiotherapy with or without testolactone for localized adenocarcinoma of the exocrine pancreas. A Southwest Oncology Group Study. *Cancer* 1980;46:1518.

241. Whittington R, Bryer MP, Haller DG, et al. Adjuvant therapy of resected adenocarcinoma of the pancreas. *Int J Radiat Oncol Biol Phys* 1991;21:1137.

242. Foo ML, Gunderson LL, Nagorney DM, et al. Patterns of failure in grossly resected pancreatic ductal adenocarcinoma treated with adjuvant irradiation ± 5 fluorouracil. *Int J Radiat Oncol Biol Phys* 1993;26:483.

243. Demeure MJ. Doffek KM, Komorowski RA, et al. Molecular metastases in stage I pancreatic cancer: improved survival with adjuvant chemoradiation. *Surgery* 1998;124:663.

244. Klinkenbijl JH, Jeekel J, Sahmoud T, et al. Adjuvant radiotherapy and 5-fluorouracil after curative resection of cancer of the pancreas and periampullary region. *Ann Surg* 1999;230:776.

245. Neoptolemos JP, Dunn JA, Stocken DD, et al. Adjuvant chemoradiotherapy and chemotherapy in resectable pancreatic cancer: a randomized controlled trial. *Lancet* 2001;358:1576.

246. Van Laethem JL, Demols A, Gay F, et al. Postoperative adjuvant gemcitabine and concurrent radiation after curative resection of pancreatic head carcinoma: a phase II study. *Int J Radiat Oncol Biol Phys* 2003;56:974.

DAVID L. BARTLETT
BRIAN I. CARR
J. WALLIS MARSH

SECTION 4

Cancer of the Liver

Primary tumors of the liver represent one of the most common malignancies worldwide. The annual international incidence of the disease is some 1 million cases, with a male to female ratio of approximately 4:1. In the United States, approximately 15,400 new tumors of the liver and biliary passages are diagnosed each year, with 12,300 deaths estimated annually.[1] Approximately one-half of these tumors are of the gallbladder, a third are tumors of the intrahepatic and extrahepatic biliary ducts, and the remainder are primary hepatocellular carcinomas (HCCs), accounting for 4000 to 6000 cases per year in the United States.[2,3]

The death rates in males in low-incidence countries such as the United States are 1.9 per 100,000 per year, in intermediate-incidence areas such as Austria and South Africa they range from 5.1 to 20.0, and in high-incidence areas such as Asia (China and Korea) they are as high as 23.1 to 150 per 100,000 per year. The incidence of HCC in the United States is currently thought to be around 3 per 100,000 persons, with significant gender, ethnic, and geographic variations.[4] The highest rate was in Hawaii at 4.5 and the lowest was in Utah at 1.0 patients per 100,000 population. These numbers for the United States are rapidly increasing and may be a gross underestimate.[4–8] There are thought to be around 4 million chronic hepatitis C virus (HCV) carriers alone in the United States. Approximately 10% of them, or 400,000, are likely to develop cirrhosis. Of these, it is estimated that around 5%, or 20,000, may develop HCC. Add to this the two other common predisposing factors—hepatitis B virus (HBV) infection and chronic alcohol consumption—and 60,000 new HCC cases annually seem possible. There appears to be evidence for increasing incidence of HCV-based HCC (Fig. 29.4-1). Because most HCC patients have a multiyear history of hepatitis B, hepatitis C, or alcohol abuse and cirrhosis, possibly the death certificates record the chronic liver failure, rather than HCC, as a cause of death. Since the last edition of this text, better imaging studies have become available to further define intrahepatic spread of hepatic malignancies, liver transplantation has been increasingly applied and its role better defined, and new treatment methods such as yttrium 90 (^{90}Y) microspheres have become available. The twin problems of major derangements in hepatic physiology associated with many neoplasms of the biliary tree, and the associated high incidence of recurrence of most of these tumors, will require new basic information about hepatobiliary biology and the tumors arising from them to allow significant progress. It is likely that future advances in the management of these malignancies will be dependent in part on immunization strategies for HBV and HBC, as well as develop-

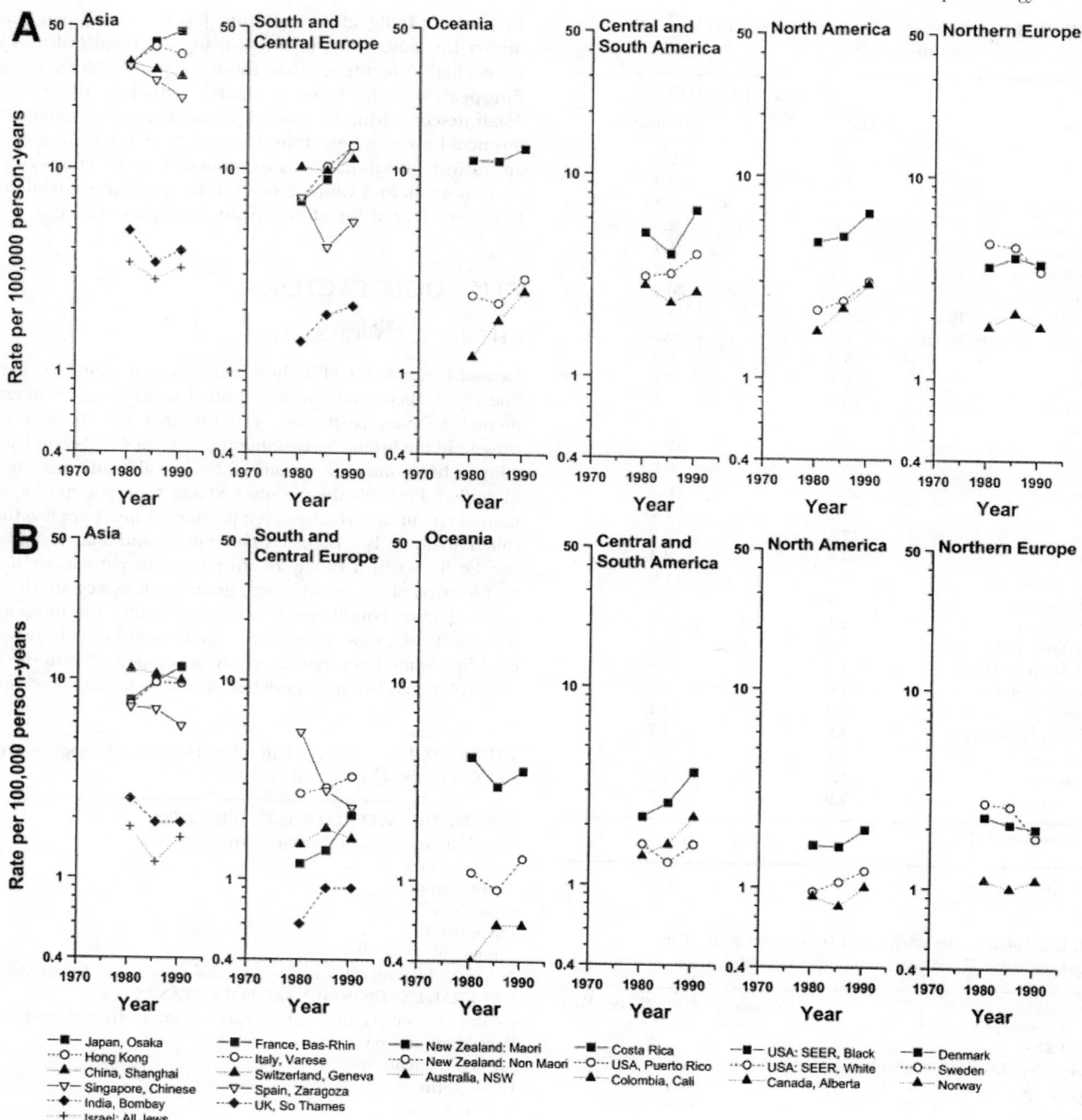

FIGURE 29.4-1. **A:** Age-adjusted primary liver cancer incidence trends: 1978–1982 to 1988–1992 (males). **B:** Age-adjusted primary liver cancer incidence trends: 1978–1982 to 1988–1992 (females). (From ref. 292, with permission.)

ment of means to decrease cirrhosis of any origin and provide earlier diagnosis by surveillance screening of patients at risk of HCC development who have known predisposing diseases.

EPIDEMIOLOGY

There are two general types of epidemiologic study of HCC: those of country-based incidence rates (Table 29.4-1) and those of rates among migrants (Table 29.4-2).[9] Table 29.4-1

shows a sampling of incidence rates in various countries in South America, Asia, Africa, and Europe. Hyperendemic hot spots occur in areas of China and sub-Saharan Africa. In Asia and Africa, high incidence rates have been associated both with high endemic hepatitis B carrier rates and with mycotoxin contamination of foodstuffs, stored grains, drinking water, and soil. Ethnic factors appear also to be important, because incidence rates can vary in the same population according to ethnic origins. Examples of variations in a given population are found in studies such as those performed in Los Angeles and

TABLE 29.4-1. Age-Adjusted Incidence Rates for Hepatocellular Carcinoma

	Persons per 100,000 per Year	
Country	Male	Female
Argentina	6.0	2.5
Peru	4.0	2.9
Brazil, Recife	9.2	8.3
Brazil, São Paulo	3.8	2.6
Colombia	2.8	1.4
Costa Rica	5.1	2.2
Mozambique	112.9	30.8
South Africa, Cape: Black	26.3	8.4
South Africa, Cape: White	1.2	0.6
Senegal	25.6	9.0
Nigeria	15.4	3.2
Swaziland	10.5	3.0
Algeria	1.5	1.4
Gambia	33.1	12.6
Burma	25.5	8.8
Philippines	19.9	6.2
Japan	7.2	2.2
Korea	13.8	3.2
Thailand	6.8	2.3
China, Shanghai	34.4	11.6
India, Bombay	4.9	2.5
India, Madras	2.1	0.7
Israel, born in Europe	3.4	4.7
Israel, born in Africa	7.4	1.5
United Kingdom	1.6	0.8
France	6.9	1.2
Germany, Hamburg	4.5	1.7
Italy, Varese	7.1	2.7
Norway	1.8	1.1
Spain, Navarra	7.9	4.7

(Data from ref. 179.)

TABLE 29.4-2. Age-Adjusted Incidence Rates for Hepatocellular Carcinoma among Male Migrants

Population	Persons per 100,000 per Year
CHINESE	
People's Republic of China, Shanghai	31.7
Hong Kong	34.4
Singapore	32.2
San Francisco	18.1
Los Angeles	12.0
Hawaii	7.8
JEWS	
Born in Israel	1.5
Born in Europe and USA	3.1
Born in Asia and Africa	3.6
JAPANESE	
Osaka	5.5
Miyagi	2.5
UNITED STATES	
Hawaii	5.7
San Francisco	3.0
Los Angeles	2.7

(Data from ref. 9.)

Israel (see Table 29.4-2). Ethnic Japanese in Japan have a higher incidence than Japanese living in Hawaii, who in turn have a higher incidence than those living in California. Jews of European descent, when compared with Jews of African or Asian descent living in Israel, do have a lower incidence.[9] Differences have also been found according to ethnic origin when an individual population is examined. Los Angelinos of Japanese, Korean, and Chinese descent have a higher incidence of hepatoma than those of European or Hispanic descent.

ETIOLOGIC FACTORS

CHEMICAL CARCINOGENS

Causative agents for HCC have been studied along two general lines. First, agents have been identified as carcinogenic in experimental animals, particularly rodents, that are thought to be present in the human environment (Table 29.4-3). Second, association of hepatoma with various other clinical conditions has been identified. Probably the best-studied and most potent ubiquitous natural chemical carcinogen is a product of the *Aspergillus* fungus called aflatoxin B_1. *Aspergillus flavus* mold and aflatoxin product can be found in a variety of stored grains, particularly in hot, humid parts of the world, where grains such as rice are stored in unrefrigerated conditions. In the months after the monsoon in Southeast Asia, most village-based grains can be seen to be covered by a white layer that can easily be scraped off with the nails. This substance is highly enriched in aflatoxin and is consumed

TABLE 29.4-3. Rodent Chemical Hepatocarcinogens Known to Exist in the Human Environment

SYNTHETIC MATERIALS AND MEDICINES
Sex hormones (e.g., androgens, estrogen)
Vinyl chloride
Aurothioglucose
Oxazepam
Phenobarbital
Thiouracil
Industrial dyes and colorants (e.g., *p*-aminoazobenzene, *O*-aminotoluene)
GENERAL ENVIRONMENTAL POLLUTANTS
N-nitrosodimethylamine (e.g., nitrite- and nitrate-treated foods)
Polychlorinated biphenyls
Carbon tetrachloride
Chloroform
Vinyl chloride
Dichlorodiphenyltrichloroethane (DDT), aldrin, dieldrin, heptachlor (pesticides)
Bis-(2-choroethyl) ether (soil fumigant, insecticide)
Diallate (herbicide)
Dioxane (solvent)
Hydrazine (rocket fuel)
Trichloroethylene (dry-cleaning solvent)
NATURAL PRODUCTS
Aflatoxins
Sterigmatocystins (*Aspergillus versicolor*)
Luteoskyrin, cyclochlorotine (rice toxins)
Pyrrolizidine alkaloids (*Senecio* plants, bush tea)
Cycasin (cycad plants)
Safrole (sassafras oil)
Tannic acid, tannins
Griseofulvin

TABLE 29.4-4.   Global Epidemiology of Hepatocellular Carcinoma and Hepatitis C Virus

Area/Country	Overall Anti-HCV Positivity Rate in HCC Patients (%)	Anti-HCV According to HB$_s$Ag Status		Anti-HCV in Controls without HCC (%)
		Positive	Negative	
Central Japan	73.5 (61/83)	10/29 (35%)	51/54 (94%)	0.9–1.2
Northern Italy	65 (86/132)	22/41 (54%)	64/91 (70%)	Not determined
Sicily, Italy	76 (152/200)	18/31 (58%)	134/169 (79%)	Not determined
Barcelona, Spain	75 (72/96)	5/9 (55.5%)	67/87 (77%)	7.3
Miami, USA	52.5 (31/59)	11/18 (61.1%)	20/41 (48.8%)	0.5
South Africa	28.9 (110/380)	47/184 (25.5%)	63/196 (32.1%)	0.7
Taiwan	33.3 (22/26)	7/42 (16.7%)	15/24 (62.5%)	0.95

HB$_s$Ag, hepatitis B surface antigen; HCC, hepatocellular carcinoma; HCV, hepatitis C virus.
(Data from ref. 17.)

with the grain by most of the village over the following months. Data on aflatoxin contamination of foodstuffs correlate well with incidence rates in Africa and to some extent in China. In hyperendemic areas of China, even farm animals such as ducks have HCC.

The most potent hepatocarcinogens appear to be natural products that occur in the environment that are synthesized by plants, fungi, and bacteria. In large areas of the world people ingest *Senecio* plants and bush trees containing pyrrolizidine alkaloids as well as tannic acid, safrole, and, in the Pacific, the cycad plants. These are suspected carcinogens. Although some human medical compounds are hepatocarcinogens for rodents (see Table 29.4-3), there is little evidence that they play an important role in human hepatocarcinogenesis except for sex hormones. A considerable literature exists on the hepatocarcinogenicity of anabolic steroids as well as the induction of benign adenomas by estrogens.[10] Although estrogens are capable of causing HCC in rodents, an epidemiologic association in humans has never clearly been shown. In an industrial society, a large number of environmental pollutants, particularly pesticides and insecticides, are known rodent carcinogens.

HEPATITIS AND HEPATOCELLULAR CANCER

Both case-control studies and cohort studies have shown a strong association between chronic HBV carriage rates and increased incidence of HCC (Tables 29.4-4 and 29.4-5).[11] Among Taiwan-

ese male postal carriers who tested positive for hepatitis B surface antigen (HB$_s$Ag) and were followed by Beasley and colleagues,[11] an annual incidence of HCC of 495 per 100,000 was found. This represented a 98-fold greater risk than observed in HB$_s$Ag-negative individuals. The incidence of primary HCC in Alaskan natives is markedly increased, again related to a high prevalence of HBV infection. A bimodal distribution with tumors occurring in the age range of both 15 to 25 and 40 to 65 was noted.[12,13] Based on this information, a similar prospective study was carried out in surviving family members of the identified HCC patients [24 members screened biannually for α-fetoprotein (AFP) and HBV]. A single 19-year-old man was identified with elevated AFP levels who subsequently underwent apparent hepatic resection with curative intent. Interestingly, the pathologic findings in this patient population demonstrate chronic portal inflammation in the noninvolved liver.[13,14] In 17 specimens examined, 14 had chronic portal inflammation and only 3 had advanced cirrhosis. This suggests that induction of HCC may simply involve rounds of hepatic destruction with subsequent proliferation and not necessarily frank cirrhosis.

By evaluating apparently asymptomatic HB$_s$Ag-positive blood donors at American Red Cross centers,[15] a minimum relative risk of 12.7 was noted for liver cancer compared to HB$_s$Ag-negative individuals. In men aged 30 to 35 years, three deaths due to hepatoma were noted, which equates to a 248-fold greater risk for such individuals compared with the general population. HB$_s$Ag-

TABLE 29.4-5.   Role of Hepatitis B in Hepatocellular Carcinoma (Case-Control Studies)

Study Population	No. of Patients		HB$_s$Ag Positive		Relative Risk (95% CI)	Attributable Risk (%)
	HCC	Controls	HCC (%)	Controls (%)		
HIGH-RISK AREAS						
Senegal	165	328	61.2	11.3	12.4 (7.7–19.3)	56.3
South Africa	289	213	61.6	11.3	12.6 (7.7–20.1)	56.7
Hong Kong	107	107	82.0	22.0	21.3 (10.1–45.9)	78.5
People's Republic of China	50	50	86.0	22.0	17.0 (4.3–99.4)	77.9
Philippines	104	84	70.0	18.0	10.83 (5.3–20.9)	63.9
INTERMEDIATE-RISK AREA						
Greece	194	451	45.9	7.3	10.7 (6.8–16.6)	41.6
LOW-RISK AREA						
United States	86	161	17.9	0.0	(10.0–100)	—

CI, confidence interval; HB$_s$Ag, hepatitis B surface antigen; HCC, hepatocellular carcinoma.
(Data modified from ref. 180.)

positive individuals who are at greatest risk are those who are male, who have a family history of the disease, whose age is over 45, and who have cirrhosis.[16]

Although up to a 200-fold excess incidence of HCC was found in Taiwan, the association of chronic HBV infection in different populations of Southeast Asia who have HCC is somewhat varied.[11] An apparent increase with time of HCC in Japan is associated with a stable incidence of chronic hepatitis B (see Fig. 29.4-1).[17] This increase in Japanese HCC incidence rates is currently thought to be from previously undiagnosed hepatitis C.[17,18] The relative roles of HBV and HCV is currently under examination. Several animal models that develop HCC are available for the study of HBV, including the woodchuck, the Peking duck, and the ground squirrel, which are infected with HBV-like viruses (hepadnaviruses). A large-scale World Health Organization–sponsored intervention study is currently under way in Asia involving HBV vaccination of the newborn. Ten percent to 15% of those populations have chronic hepatitis B, most of which is thought to be transmitted at birth through the vaginal canal. It will take another 40 years to prove whether this step reduces the indigenous incidence of HCC.

The role of hepatitis in HCC appears complicated (Table 29.4-6). There appear to be clinical differences between HCC patients with HBV infection in various geographic areas and between HCC patients with HBV infection and those with HCV infection.[17,18] HCC in African blacks is not associated with severe cirrhosis but is poorly differentiated and very aggressive compared with HCC in U.S. patients. Despite uniform HBV carrier rates among the South African Bantu, there is a ninefold difference in HCC incidence between Mozambicans living along the coast and those living inland. These differences are attributed to the additional exposure to dietary aflatoxin B_1 and other carcinogenic mycotoxins.[19] The role of HBV and HCV as direct carcinogens is unclear, because the HCV genome is not integrated into the human host, and the HBV genome is integrated in a seemingly random fashion. Specific human genes with which HBV sequences are regularly associated have not been identified. Furthermore, it is not clear whether most HBV carriers first progress to acquire HCC. Thus, Koch's postulates are not yet fulfilled for HBV (or HCV) and subsequent HCC development. At best, an association can be claimed at this point. It is thought that rounds of hepatic destruction after replicative repair lead to the accumulation of mutations associated with cancer development. The precise timing of HCV infection from blood transfusions has allowed a comparison of latent periods for HCC development after HCV infection (transfusions) and after HBV infection (often at birth). The average age for HBV-associated HCC is around 52 years, compared with 62 years for HCV association. The typical interval between HCV-contaminated transfusion and subsequent HCC is only approximately 30 years (compared with 40 to 50 years for HCC after HBV transmission). HCV-based HCC thus evolves much faster. The state of the liver also differs in that patients with HCV-associated HCC tend to have more frequent and more advanced cirrhosis. However, in HBV-associated HCC, only half the patients have cirrhosis; the remainder have chronic active hepatitis.

OTHER ETIOLOGIC CONDITIONS

The 60% to 80% rate of association of HCC with underlying cirrhosis has long been recognized. More typically the association occurs with macronodular cirrhosis in Southeast Asia, but an association is also seen with micronodular cirrhosis in Europe

TABLE 29.4-6.   Conditions Associated with Hepatocellular Carcinoma

Condition	Risk
CIRRHOSIS	
Hepatitis B virus infection	High
Hepatitis C virus infection	High
Alcohol use	High
Autoimmune chronic active hepatitis	High
Cryptogenic cirrhosis	Moderate
Primary biliary cirrhosis	Low
METABOLIC DISEASES	
Genetic hemochromatosis	High
Hereditary tyrosinemia	High
α_1-Antitrypsin deficiency	Moderate
Ataxia telangiectasia	Moderate
Types 1 and 3 glycogen-storage disease	Moderate
Galactosemia	Moderate
Citrullinemia	Moderate
Hereditary hemorrhagic telangiectasia	Moderate
Porphyria cutanea tarda	Moderate
Wilson's disease	Low
Orotic aciduria	Moderate
Alagille's syndrome (congenital cholestatic syndrome)	Moderate
ENVIRONMENTAL AGENTS	
Thorotrast	Moderate
Androgenic steroids	Moderate
Cigarette smoking	ND
Aflatoxin	ND
Pyrrolizidine alkaloids	ND
Cycasin	ND
N-Nitrosylated compounds	ND

ND, not determined in humans.

and the United States.[20] It is still not clear whether cirrhosis itself is a predisposing factor to the development of HCC or whether the underlying causes of the cirrhosis are actually the carcinogenic factors. However, approximately 20% of North American patients with HCC do not have underlying cirrhosis, and probably no more than 70% have associated hepatitis B. Several underlying conditions have been found to be associated with an increased risk for the development of HCC (see Table 29.4-6). These include hepatitis-associated cirrhosis and alcohol-associated cirrhosis, autoimmune chronic active hepatitis, cryptogenic cirrhosis, and other virus-associated cirrhosis. A less common association is with primary biliary cirrhosis, which is more typically associated with subsequent development of cholangiocarcinoma. Several metabolic diseases are also associated with an increased risk for the development of HCC. These include hemochromatosis (iron accumulation), Wilson's disease (copper accumulation), α_1-antitrypsin deficiency, tyrosinemia, porphyria cutanea tarda, glycogen-storage disease types 1 and 3, citrullinemia, and orotic aciduria. Approximately 50% of patients in the authors' experience have some form of underlying and preexisting hepatitis, 28% have a history of chronic alcohol consumption without hepatitis, and 80% have some form of cirrhosis (Table 29.4-7). The etiology of HCC in those 20% of patients who have no cirrhosis is currently unclear, nor is the natural history of their HCC well defined. In children, congenital cholestatic syndrome (Alagille's syndrome) is associated with a familial type of HCC.

TABLE 29.4-7. Etiologic Factors in Hepatocellular Carcinoma Patients, University of Pittsburgh, Liver Cancer Center (1989 to 2001) (n = 547)

Factor	No. of Patients	%
HEPATITIS	279	51
HCV	117	21
HBV	68	12
HBV and HCV	44	8
Hepatitis status unknown	50	10
CIRRHOSIS	441	81
NO CIRRHOSIS	106	19
CIRRHOSIS, HEPATITIS NEGATIVE (EXCLUDES UNKNOWNS)	131	24
Alcohol, chronic consumption	287	52
Alcohol, hepatitis negative	153	28
Alcohol and HCV	67	12
Alcohol and HBV	35	6
Alcohol and HCV and HBV	32	7

HBV, hepatitis B virus; HCV, hepatitis C virus.

PATHOLOGY

Tumors of the liver can be classified as either benign or malignant (Table 29.4-8) and by the tissue of origin (mesenchymal tumors or the more common epithelial neoplasms).[21] Malignant epithelial neoplasms constitute 85% to 95% of all tumors of the liver. Six percent to 12% are benign and again are largely of epithelial origin. Mixed HCC and cholangiocarcinoma can also be found, typically in 2% of the authors' patient population in Pittsburgh. One percent to 3% are malignant mesenchymal tumors.[21] Approximately half of the hepatobiliary tumors in the United States arise in the gallbladder or in the extrahepatic biliary tree. Other distinctions made clinically and reflected in the staging system include the size of the tumor, with those smaller than 2 cm often representing tumors with the very best prognosis.[22] Tumors having a well-defined

TABLE 29.4-8. Hepatic Neoplasms

BENIGN TUMORS

Hepatocellular hyperplasia: macroregenerative nodule, nodular hyperplasia, mixed hamartoma
Hepatocellular adenoma: typical, associated with anabolic steroids
Hepatic cysts: simple, polycystic
Bile duct adenoma
Benign mesenchymal tumors and tumor-like conditions: mesenchymal hamartoma, hemangioma, infantile hemangioendothelioma, lymphangiomatosis, lipoma, leiomyoma, fibroma, inflammatory pseudotumor, myxoma
Tumor of heterotopic tissue and uncertain origin: adrenal rest tumor, pheochromocytoma, pancreatic rest, carcinoid, neuroendocrine infantile sinusoidal tumor, teratoma, yolk sac tumor, malignant trophoblastic tumor, hepatic malignant mixed tumor

PRIMARY MALIGNANT EPITHELIAL TUMORS

Hepatocellular carcinoma variants: childhood, fibrolamellar, combined, spindle cell, clear cell, giant cell, carcinosarcoma, sclerosing hepatoblastoma
Cholangiocarcinoma and cholangiocellular carcinoma
Hepatic cystadenocarcinoma, squamous cell carcinoma

PRIMARY MALIGNANT MESENCHYMAL TUMORS

Angiosarcoma, hemangioendothelioma, leiomyosarcoma, malignant schwannoma, fibrosarcoma, malignant fibrous, histiocytoma, lymphoma, osteosarcoma, rhabdomyosarcoma, mesenchymal sarcoma

rim on computed tomography (CT) scan or on subsequent pathologic examination have a better prognosis. Tumors arising in patients from the West may even be less aggressive than those arising in individuals from Asian countries. Rare inflammatory pseudomasses and pseudotumors associated with either infarction or inflammation can be recognized and need to be distinguished from true tumors arising in the liver. Many other tumors have a propensity to metastasize to the liver or to the adjacent biliary tree. Metastases appear to obtain access to the systemic circulation, usually by hematogenous spread through either the portal vein or the hepatic artery.[23] The lymphatics of the liver course between lobules and drain primarily through vessels surrounding the portal veins directly into the liver hilum and cisterna chyli. The remaining 20% of the liver is drained by vessels ascending along the vena cava.[22] Grossly, metastatic tumors are often peripheral and multiple and cause umbilication of the surface of the liver, whereas primary liver tumors are more often central and can be solitary, but are usually hypervascular on the arterial phase of a helical CT scan.

A characteristic of HCC is invasion of the portal vein and to a lesser extent the hepatic vein. Such invasion is unquestionably the most important negative prognostic factor for resection and for liver transplantation, after positive margins and lymph nodes. It is typically seen on dynamic CT as an obstruction of portal flow with venous expansion, which thus distinguishes malignant from benign thrombosis. Malignant thrombi are often hypervascular on the arterial phase of the CT, whereas bland thrombi are not hypervascular.

The tumors most frequently metastasizing to the liver during their natural course include melanoma (especially uveal melanoma with the clinical picture of one affected eye and an enlarged liver), gallbladder carcinoma, and colon, pancreatic, and breast carcinomas. By absolute number, the most frequent tumors of nonhepatic origin in the liver include lung cancer, colon cancer, pancreatic cancer, breast cancer, and gastric carcinoma, in decreasing order of frequency.[21]

Specialized immunohistochemical staining can be used to distinguish primary tumors of the liver from metastatic deposits. Specifically, positive staining for AFP, polyclonal but not monoclonal carcinoembryonic antigen, and loss of reticulin staining are very useful. More specialized pathologic staining techniques, including flow-cytometric DNA analysis, are also useful in the evaluation of HCC.[24-27] Seventy-eight percent of HCCs are aneuploid and 22% are diploid. Elevated AFP level has been shown to be significantly associated with aneuploid tumors, but appears to provide no information regarding survival. This is different from what is observed with other gastrointestinal tumors, including gastric and esophageal cancers, in which clinical outcome is more clearly related to this DNA pattern. The rapidity of proliferation of cells within the HCC can be detected by *in vitro* incorporation of 5'-bromodeoxyuridine, and by the cell-cycle stains proliferating cell nuclear antigen and Ki-67, which can be used to obtain additional prognostic information. Those individuals with low DNA synthetic capacity had higher rates of 2-year survival after surgery and a lower incidence of intrahepatic metastases than those with high DNA synthetic capacity. This is similar to the findings for patients with breast cancer.

CLINICAL FEATURES

Common symptoms in patients affected with HCC include abdominal pain, weight loss, weakness, fullness and anorexia,

TABLE 29.4-9. Clinical Presentation of Hepatocellular Carcinoma, University of Pittsburgh, Liver Cancer Center (1989 to 2001) (n = 547)

Symptom	No. of Patients	%
No symptom	129	24
One symptom	254	46
Two symptoms	109	20
Three or more symptoms	55	10
Abdominal pain	219	40
Other (workup of anemia, various diseases)	64	12
Routine physical examination findings, elevated results on liver function tests	129	24
Weight loss	112	20
Appetite loss	59	11
Weakness and malaise	83	15
Jaundice	30	5
Routine screening of known cirrhosis	92	17
Routine screening of known hepatitis	71	13
Cirrhosis symptoms (ankle swelling, abdominal bloating, increased girth, pruritus, encephalopathy, gastrointestinal bleeding)	98	18
Diarrhea	7	1
Tumor rupture	1	
PATIENT CHARACTERISTICS		
Mean age (y)	56 ± 13	
Male/female ratio	105:1	
Ethnicity		
White		72
Middle Eastern		10
Asian		13
African American		5
TUMOR CHARACTERISTICS		
Number of hepatic tumors		
1		20
2		25
3 or more		65
Portal vein invasion		75
Lobar distribution		
Unilobar		25
Bilobar		75

abdominal swelling, jaundice, and vomiting (Table 29.4-9). Common physical signs include hepatomegaly, hepatic bruit, ascites, splenomegaly, jaundice, wasting, and fever.[28] Some differences are observed in presenting signs and symptoms between high- and low-incidence areas. The most common symptom is abdominal pain, particularly in high-risk areas. It is usually present in South African blacks, whereas only a minority (40% to 50%) of Chinese and Japanese patients present with abdominal pain. An abdominal mass or swelling may be noticed by patients and is often associated with pain. Abdominal swelling may occur as a consequence of ascites due to the underlying chronic liver disease or may be due to a rapidly expanding tumor. Occasionally, central necrosis or acute hemorrhage into the peritoneal cavity leads to death. It occurs in 10% to 20% of Asians and approximately 6% of blacks but is rare among Europeans. Hemoperitoneum from bleeding HCC is also a well-recognized complication of needle biopsy of highly vascular hepatomas. Weakness and malaise occur in approximately 70% of Asians, although only 30% of African blacks and Europeans present with this symptom. Similarly, weight loss occurs in most Asians and Europeans but in fewer than 5% of Japanese. This may be due to the fact that Japa-

nese hepatoma is typically diagnosed at an earlier stage, due to a rigorous surveillance program.

Unexplained weight loss in a patient known to have cirrhosis should suggest a diagnosis of HCC. Anorexia and abdominal fullness occur in approximately 60% of Chinese patients but only in 30% of European and African patients. All of these symptoms apply to large (more than 2 cm) HCCs. In countries where there is an active surveillance program such as Japan, HCC tends to be identified at an earlier stage, when symptoms may be few or attributable only to the underlying disease. Jaundice is infrequent and, when present, is usually due to underlying liver disease. However, only 10% of patients presenting with jaundice have jaundice attributable to the HCC. This may be due to obstruction of the main intrahepatic ducts, obstruction of the common hepatic duct at the porta hepatis, infiltration into the biliary radicals, or, extremely rarely, blood in the biliary tree. Hematemesis may occur due to esophageal varices from the underlying chronic liver disease with portal hypertension. Bone pain is seen in 3% to 12% of patients, but necropsies show pathologic bone metastases in approximately 20% of patients. Respiratory symptoms may occur on presentation but are rare. They are usually due to elevated hemidiaphragm consequent to hepatomegaly or pain from rib metastases. Pleural effusions may occur, but symptomatic lung metastases are rare. A summary of common presentations in the authors' experience is presented in Table 29.4-9. Interestingly, 25% of the authors' patients, mostly with advanced-stage HCC, had no symptoms at all.

PHYSICAL SIGNS

Hepatomegaly is the most frequent physical sign, occurring in 50% to 90% of patients. The size of the liver may be massive, particularly in endemic areas. Abdominal bruits arising from the HCC, presumably from the associated vascularity, have a variable incidence, ranging from 6% to 25%. Ascites occurs in 30% to 60% of patients. It is usually due to the underlying liver disease, although occasionally may be caused by hemoperitoneum. It is important to tap the ascites of any HCC patient and send it for cytologic examination, because positive cytological results have a major adverse impact on prognosis. Splenomegaly occurs commonly, mainly due to the associated portal hypertension from the underlying liver disease. Acute splenomegaly may be due to portal vein occlusion by the tumor. Weight loss and muscle wasting are common, particularly with rapidly growing or large tumors. Fever is found in 10% to 50% of patients with HCC. The cause is not clear, although tumor necrosis has been invoked as an explanation. The signs of chronic liver disease may often be present, including jaundice, dilated abdominal veins, palmar erythema, gynecomastia, testicular atrophy, and peripheral edema. Budd-Chiari syndrome has been reported in several series due to HCC invasion of the hepatic veins. This causes tense ascites and a large, tender liver. Virchow-Trosier nodes occur in the supraclavicular region but are rarely observed. Cutaneous metastases have also been reported as red-blue nodules.

PARANEOPLASTIC SYNDROMES

A variety of paraneoplastic syndromes have been described. Most of these are biochemical abnormalities without associated clinical consequences. The most important ones include hypoglycemia (also caused by end-stage liver failure), erythrocytosis, hypercalcemia, hypercholesterolemia, dysfibrinogenemia, carcinoid syndrome, increased thyroxin-binding globulin levels, sexual changes (gynecomastia, testicular atrophy, and precocious puberty), and porphyria cutanea tarda. Hypoglycemia occurs in two settings. Relatively mild hypoglycemia occurs in rapidly growing HCC among the Chinese as part of a terminal illness. In the other setting, the HCC is more slowly growing, but the hypoglycemia may be profound. Its pathogenesis is unclear. Erythrocytosis occurs in 3% to 12% of patients. Hypercholesterolemia may occur in 10% to 40% of patients. This has been shown to be due to an absence of normal feedback control in hepatoma cells and is due to a deletion in β-hydroxyβ-methylglutaryl-coenzyme A reductase.

STAGING

Multiple clinical staging systems for hepatic tumors have been described. The most widely used is the American Joint Committee on Cancer TNM system (Table 29.4-10). However, the new Cancer of the Liver Italian Program system is also now in wide use (Table 29.4-11).[29] Other staging systems have been proposed, and a consensus is needed.[30,31] Stage I, solitary tumors of less than 2 cm diameter without vascular invasion clearly have the best prognosis. Adverse prognostic features include multiple tumors, vascular invasion, and lymph node spread. Vascular invasion in particular has profound effects on prognosis. Vascular invasion may be macroscopic or microscopic. In general, large tumors invariably have microscopic invasion, which cannot be appreciated until after resection. As a consequence, full staging can usually be done only after surgical extirpation of the tumor. Stage III disease contains a mixture of lymph node–positive and lymph node–negative tumors. Stage III tumors with positive lymph node disease have a poor prognosis, and few such patients survive 1 year. The prognosis of stage IV disease is poor after either resection or transplantation, and there are few 1-year survivors. A working staging system based entirely on clinical features that incorporates the contribution of the underlying liver disease was originally developed by Okuda et al. as shown in Table 29.4-12.[28] Adverse prognostic signs include tumor size (more than 50% of liver), ascites (with positive or negative cytologic findings), hypoalbuminemia (less than 3 g/dL), and hyperbilirubinemia (more than 3 mg/dL). Patients with Okuda stage III (advanced) disease—namely, those with three or more positive features—have a dire prognosis because curative resection is usually impossible, and the condition of the liver typically precludes chemotherapy. The current TNM–American Joint Committee on Cancer–International Union Against Cancer staging system still has some limitations and has been revised. Stage should be reported using this system to allow comparison of treatment results across institutions.

CLINICAL EVALUATION

HISTORY AND PHYSICAL EXAMINATION

The history is important in evaluating putative predisposing factors, including a history of hepatitis or jaundice, blood transfusion, or use of intravenous drugs. It should include any family history of HCC or hepatitis and detailed social history, including job descriptions to identify industrial exposure to possible car-

TABLE 29.4-10. American Joint Committee on Cancer Staging System

PRIMARY TUMOR (T)

TX	Primary tumor cannot be assessed
T0	No evidence of primary tumor
T1	Solitary tumor without vascular invasion
T2	Solitary tumor with vascular invasion, or Multiple tumors ≤5 cm
T3	Multiple tumors >5 cm or Tumor involving a major branch of the portal or hepatic vein(s)
T4	Tumor(s) with direct invasion of adjacent organs other than the gallbladder or with perforation of visceral peritoneum

REGIONAL LYMPH NODES (N)

NX	Regional lymph nodes cannot be assessed
N0	No regional lymph node metastasis
N1	Regional lymph node metastasis

DISTANT METASTASIS (M)

MX	Distant metastasis cannot be assessed
M0	No distant metastasis
M1	Distant metastasis

STAGE GROUPING

I	T1	N0	M0
II	T2	N0	M0
IIIA	T3	N0	M0
IIIB	T4	N0	M0
IIIC	Any T	N1	M0
IV	Any T	Any N	M1

(From ref. 22, with permission.)

TABLE 29.4-11. Cancer of the Liver Italian Program Staging System

	Points		
Variables	0	1	2
i. Morphology and Hepatic replacement (%)	Single <50	Multiple <50	— >50
ii. Child-Pugh score	A	B	C
iii. α-Fetoprotein level (ng/mL)	<400	≥400	—
iv. Portal vein thrombosis	No	Yes	—
Score = Sum of points for the four variables.			

Note. This staging system was developed using classic techniques of analysis of variance. It was developed using only patients with cirrhosis, and uses Child-Pugh score rather than its individual components.

TABLE 29.4-12. Okuda Staging System

Parameter	Value	Points
Tumor size	>50%	1
	<50%	0
Ascites	Present	1
	Absent	0
Serum albumin level	>3 g/dL	0
	<3 g/dL	1
Serum bilirubin level	>3 mg/dL	1
	<3 mg/dL	0
Stage 1	0 points	
Stage 2	1–2 points	
Stage 3	3–4 points	

Note. This was the first staging system, developed in 1984. (Data from ref. 28.)

cinogenic drugs as well as sex hormones. Physical examination is important and should include examination for signs and symptoms of underlying liver disease such as jaundice, ascites, peripheral edema, spider nevi, palmar erythema, and weight loss. Evaluation of the abdomen for hepatic size, presence of masses, hepatic nodularity and tenderness, and presence of splenomegaly should be carried out. Assessment of overall performance status is essential for management decisions.

SEROLOGIC ASSAYS

The first serologic assay for detection and clinical follow-up of patients with HCC was measurement of AFP. AFP was found in the serum of animals bearing transplantable hepatomas and was later detected in humans.[32] Improvements in this assay, including the development of radioimmunoassays for AFP,[33] allowed sequential studies in high-risk patients and patients being treated with either surgical resection or chemotherapy.[34–36] Although AFP level is elevated in approximately 70% of individuals in Asian countries bearing hepatomas, it is only increased in approximately 50% of patients in the United States and Europe.[37] Although AFP elevations can be detected early in the course of the disease, most clinical studies suggest that ultrasonography is an even more sensitive screening modality. Still, increased AFP level is the standard against which other assays must be judged. The other most widely used assay is that for des-γ-carboxy prothrombin (DCP) protein induced by vitamin K abnormality (PIVKA-2). The level of this protein is increased in as many as 80% of patients with HCC but may also be elevated in patients with vitamin K deficiency.[37–42] It may even have prognostic use.[43] The elevations of both AFP and PIVKA-2 observed in chronic hepatitis and cirrhosis sometimes make it difficult to interpret these assays. Although many other assays have been developed, none has greater aggregate sensitivity and specificity.[40–42,44–50]

In a patient presenting with either a new hepatic mass or other indications of recent hepatic decompensation, measurement of levels of carcinoembryonic antigen, vitamin B_{12}, AFP, ferritin, and PIVKA-2 as well as standard liver function tests should be performed. Prothrombin time, partial thromboplastin time, and albumin level, which reflect hepatic synthetic function, as well as traditional liver function tests (levels of transaminases, lactate dehydrogenase, and alkaline phosphatase) should be performed. Platelet count and white blood cell count decreases may reflect portal hypertension and associated hypersplenism. Serologic testing for hepatitis A, B, C, and D viruses should be performed. If HBV serologic test results are positive, quantitative measurements of HBV DNA or RNA should be obtained.

RADIOLOGY

An ultrasonographic examination of the liver is an excellent screening tool. To assess the local extent of tumor and accurately determine its size and spread, a good-quality CT scan, with and without intravenous contrast (to include the arterial phase) or with coincident administration of contrast material delivered into the superior mesenteric artery (CT portography), should be performed. Magnetic resonance imaging (MRI) can also provide detailed information. Ethiodol (Lipiodol) is an ethiodized oil emulsion retained by liver tumors that can be delivered by hepatic artery injection (5 to 15 mL) for CT imaging 1 week later.[51,52] For small tumors, Lipiodol injection is very helpful

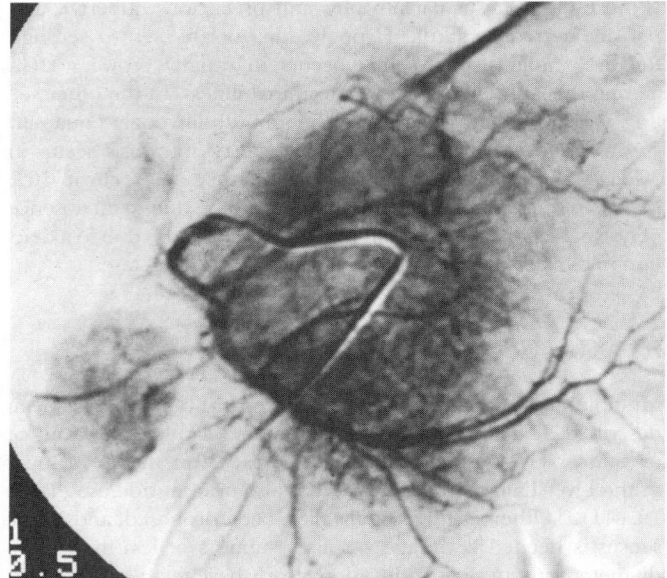

FIGURE 29.4-2. Hypervascularity of a primary hepatocellular carcinoma as shown by arteriography. Notice the straightening of vessels within the tumor and early venous filling.

before biopsy because the histologic presence of Lipiodol constitutes proof that the needle biopsy specimen is really the mass under suspicion. Celiac arteriography with selective lobar or superselective studies is occasionally useful to delineate the relationship of the tumor to vessels and to distinguish it from the rare hypovascular pseudotumor (Fig. 29.4-2). Hepatic tumors are usually hypervascular; show tortuosity of the vessels, vascular pooling, and hepatic staining; and often demonstrate rapid entry of contrast into the associated hepatic veins. Arterial portal shunting in the presence of portal hypertension can also be observed.

In prospective studies ultrasonographic screening has been shown to be more sensitive than repetitive AFP testing, especially for small tumors in high-risk patients, and fewer than 50% of the authors' HCC patients have elevated AFP levels.[53] Using transducers of 3.5 or 5.0 MHz, both diagnosis and biopsy of suspicious lesions can be carried out. Ultrasonography is widely used in the diagnosis of HCC, particularly in surveillance programs for patients with chronic liver disease who are at risk for the development of HCC. The instrumentation is inexpensive and widely available. Ultrasonography is particularly useful for the diagnosis of portal venous thrombosis. Ultrasonography is also helpful in distinguishing HCC from metastatic tumors, because HCC has a typical ring sign when smaller than 2 cm. When patients have only persistent elevation of liver enzyme levels, it is probably useful to obtain a blind-needle biopsy specimen to establish the nature of the underlying disease.[51] Blind-needle biopsy, however, is successful in fewer than 40% of instances in establishing a diagnosis of HCC unless massive replacement of the liver is noted. For patients with suspected malignancy with a normal CT scan, laparoscopy with laparoscopic ultrasonography may be helpful to direct the biopsy.

Questions that need to be addressed with imaging studies are what are the location and number of masses in the liver, whether there is evidence of extrahepatic tumor spread, and whether the vessels are patent or not. CT scan appears to display tumor extent better than sonography, but both imaging modalities can miss lesions smaller than 1 to 2 cm, especially in the presence of a nodular, cirrhotic liver.[52,54,55] Angioportography, in which contrast material is directly infused into the mesenteric vessels, has been demonstrated in a number of studies to detect very small lesions and to be superior to conventional dynamic CT.[54–56] Direct comparisons of individual imaging modalities have sometimes been limited by the lack of a gold standard to define the number and size of lesions identified. However, the standard is continuously changing with CT improvements, such as the multihead scanner.[57–63] Studies done at the University of Pittsburgh using resected livers from individuals undergoing liver transplantation indicated that lesions were detectable by sonography in 81% and by CT in 94% of instances. Although vascular invasion was demonstrated after histologic examination in 53% of cases, it was only detectable by CT in 31% and by sonography in 17%. It is particularly difficult in patients with underlying cirrhosis to make the fine distinctions necessary regarding number of lesions and vascular invasion that are critical for operative decision making. CT scanning can also identify details, such as the characteristic central scarring of fibrolamellar tumors.[64] CT portography has a high sensitivity, but drawbacks include the detection of small abnormalities that represent flow voids or benign lesions. False-negatives have also been identified, especially in instances in which there is fatty infiltration of the liver. Triple-phase helical CT (Fig. 29.4-3) appears to be a current standard, especially with a fast bolus of contrast injection to detect small vascular HCCs.

MRIs, especially T2-weighted studies, are particularly good at detecting intrahepatic lesions. Some difficulty in distinguishing hemangiomas that have a very high T2 signal can be obviated because a less intense signal is observed with hepatomas.[65,66] One of the major problems with such techniques is the requirement for long data acquisition time and poor anatomic definition because of a low signal-to-noise ratio. The use of paramagnetic contrast agents such as gadolinium and the use of T1-weighted sequences appear to provide somewhat better contrast. The T2-weighted spin-echo sequences appear to be the most efficient to detect tumor. The use of magnetic resonance angiography in HCC has also been reported. A prospective study comparing triphasic helical CT scan to magnetic resonance angiography revealed a greater sensitivity

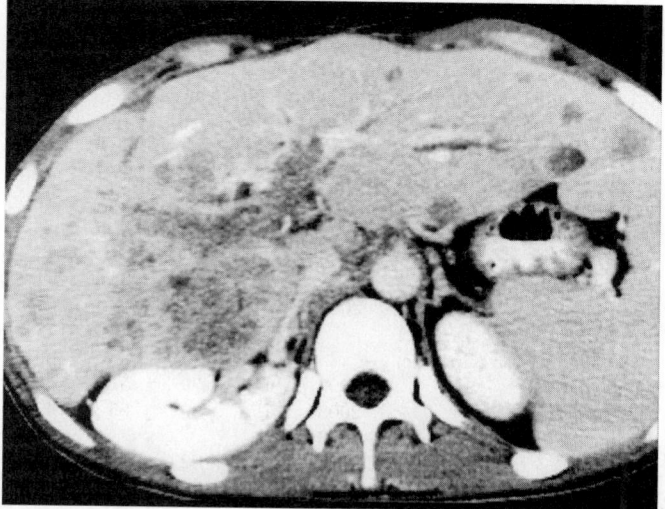

FIGURE 29.4-3. Portal venous phase of triphasic computed tomography scan demonstrating advanced hepatocellular cancer involving the main portal vein.

for magnetic resonance angiography (76% vs. 61%) as determined from examination of the explanted liver after transplantation.[67]

Technetium 99m sulfur colloid is used for hepatic scintigraphy. This is based on the uptake of the colloid by the hepatic reticuloendothelial system. Scintigraphy reveals photopenic areas in HCC images. A variation of this is single photon emission CT using a rotating gamma camera. This modality gives more precise spatial orientation and clearer images.

The role of [18F]fluorodeoxyglucose positron emission tomography (FDG-PET) scans in the evaluation of HCC has been carefully studied. In one retrospective study, FDG-PET imaging was only successful in detecting 64% of lesions. Nevertheless, it had a clinically significant impact in 28% of cases above and beyond standard imaging, including the detection of unsuspected metastatic disease.[68] A prospective comparison of triphasic CT, gadolinium-enhanced MRI, ultrasonography, and FDG-PET was reported and verified by examination of explanted liver specimens after transplant. This study revealed similar results for CT, MRI, and ultrasonography, whereas none of the lesions was detected by FDG-PET imaging.[69]

PATHOLOGIC DIAGNOSIS

Histologic proof of the presence of HCC is mandatory for clinical trials. In the authors' practice, this requires a core liver biopsy of the mass under ultrasonographic or CT guidance. Obtaining a pathologic diagnosis has its hazards in patients with HCC. Not only are results of bleeding studies often abnormal due to thrombocytopenia and decreases in levels of liver-dependent clotting factors, but these tumors tend to be hypervascular. Spillage of tumor has also been suggested as a problem after percutaneous biopsy. Only two such instances, however, were found in the last 600 biopsies performed at the University of Pittsburgh. Fine-needle aspirates can provide sufficient material for diagnosis of cancer,[70] but core biopsy specimens are most preferred because of the tissue architecture given by this technique, which usually allows the distinguishing of HCC from adenocarcinoma. In addition, laparoscopic approaches can also be used. For patients suspected of having portal vein involvement, a core biopsy of the portal vein may be performed safely.[70–72] A portal vein biopsy specimen demonstrating cancer is now regarded as an exclusion criterion for hepatic transplantation for HCC. Patients with a high clinical suspicion of HCC who are deemed appropriate surgical candidates may be taken to surgery without a preoperative biopsy.

SCREENING OF HIGH-RISK POPULATIONS

Many discrete patient populations are susceptible to hepatoma. Because of the availability of sensitive serum markers and the high prevalence of disease, it is possible that certain populations could be screened on a regular basis. A workshop on screening for HCC[16] was held to determine which patient populations might benefit. Prospective studies in high-risk populations have generally concluded that ultrasonography is more sensitive than AFP elevations.[73–76] A study conducted in Italian patients with cirrhosis identified a yearly incidence of 3% but no appreciable increase in the rate of detection of potentially curable tumors with aggressive screening.[75] Although high-risk patients continue to be screened, it is likely that major changes in longevity of patients with these

TABLE 29.4-13. Treatment Options for
Hepatocellular Carcinoma

SURGERY
Partial hepatectomy
Liver transplantation
LOCAL ABLATIVE THERAPIES
Cryosurgery
Microwave ablation
Ethanol injection
Acetic acid injection
Radiofrequency ablation
**REGIONAL THERAPIES: HEPATIC ARTERY TRANSCATHETER
 TREATMENTS**
Transarterial chemotherapy
Transarterial embolization
Transarterial chemoembolization
Transarterial radiotherapy
  Yttrium 90 microspheres
  Iodine 131 Lipiodol
CONFORMAL EXTERNAL-BEAM RADIATION THERAPY
SYSTEMIC THERAPIES
Chemotherapy
Immunotherapy
Hormonal therapy + growth control
SUPPORTIVE CARE

---

disorders will come not through screening but through prevention strategies, including universal vaccination against HBV.[77]

CLINICAL MANAGEMENT

The clinical management choices for hepatocellular cancer can be complex, because of the numerous options that exist for treatment and the underlying liver disease that affects the majority of HCC patients (Table 29.4-13).[78] The natural history of HCC is variable, and prolonged survival without treatment has been reported.[79] Patients presenting with advanced tumors (vascular invasion, symptoms, extrahepatic spread) have a median survival of approximately 5 months with no treatment. Treatment results reported in the literature are difficult to interpret, because survival as an end point may reflect more the underlying liver disease than progression of HCC. Treatment strategies may be more dependent on the underlying liver disease than on the stage of the tumor. A focused multidisciplinary team, including a hepatologist, interventional radiologist, surgical oncologist, transplant surgeon, and medical oncologist, is important for the comprehensive management of HCC patients.

STAGE I AND II HEPATOCELLULAR CARCINOMA

Early-stage tumors can be managed successfully using a variety of techniques, including surgical resection, local ablation (radiofrequency ablation), and local injection therapies (ethanol injection).[80,81] Because the majority of patients with HCC suffer from a field defect in the liver, they are at risk for multiple primary tumors throughout the liver in their lifetime. As discussed earlier in Etiologic Factors, the majority of patients have significant underlying liver disease and may not tolerate major loss of hepatic parenchyma. Also, because of the underlying liver disease, patients may be eligible for liver transplantation in the future.

Therefore, the most important principle to follow in early-stage HCC is to use treatment that allows for maximal sparing of the hepatic parenchyma. Avoiding major open surgery may also improve the results of subsequent transplant surgery if required.

Surgical Excision

Open surgical excision is a reliable method for treating stage I HCC[82] (Table 29.4-14). The goal is to obtain a 1-cm margin of normal tissue around the tumor. Beyond that requirement, the type of excision does not impact in any way on cancer treatment outcome. The excision of surface tumors is best accomplished as a nonanatomic wedge excision, in which the tumor is simply excised with a 1-cm margin and no more. The hepatic parenchyma can be divided using a variety of techniques, with the goal to minimize blood loss and maintain adequate exposure to ensure that accurate margins are obtained. This can be performed safely for tumors up to 5 cm in diameter with minimal blood loss. Deep tumors within the hepatic parenchyma and

TABLE 29.4-14. Survival after Liver Resection for
Hepatocellular Carcinoma Reported by Large Series

Study	Year	n	Survival (%) 1-Y	3-Y	5-Y
Kanematsu et al.[181]	1990	107	83	51	26
Yamanaka et al.[182]	1990	295	76	44	31
Liver Cancer Study Group of Japan[183]	1990	2174	67	40	29
Ringe et al.[184]	1991	131	68	42	36
Sasaki et al.[185]	1992	186	—	—	44
Nagasue et al.[186]	1993	229	80	51	26
Takenaka et al.[187]	1994	229	89	76	76
Lai et al.[188]	1995	343	60	33	24
Vauthey et al.[189]	1995	106	—	—	41
Kawasaki et al.[190]	1995	112	92	79	—
Llovet et al.[191]	1999	77	85	—	51
Yamamoto et al.[192]	1999	294	—	71	—
Arii et al.[193,a]	2000				
T1 <2 cm		1318	96	—	72
T1 2–5 cm		2722	95	—	58
T2 <2 cm		502	92	—	55
T2 2–5 cm		1548	95	—	58
Wayne et al.[194]	2002	249	83	—	41
Yeh et al.[195]	2002	218	63	42	32
Ziparo et al.[196]	2002	81	75	62	51
Belghiti et al.[197]	2002	328	81	57	37
Kanematsu et al.[198]	2002	303	84	67	51
Grazi et al.[199]	2003				
Cirrhotic		308	86	64	42
Noncirrhotic		135	84	68	51
Lang et al.[200]	2003				
Major resection (cirrhotic)		84	90[b]	78[b]	73
Minor resection (cirrhotic)		134	85[b]	76[b]	60
Cha et al.[201]	2003	164	79	51	40
De Carlis et al.[202]	2003	154	90[b]	65[b]	47
Chen et al.[203]	2003				
<3 cm		145	82	59	42
>3 cm		340	56	39	31

[a]Nationwide survey in Japan.
[b]Estimated from manuscript based on survival curves.

tumors larger than 5 cm must be managed by an anatomic resection, in which the most distal portal triad to the region involved by the tumor is controlled and the segment or segments are resected. Centrally located tumors may require a lobectomy, and large tumors may require an extended hepatectomy. The risk of major hepatectomy is high (5% to 10% mortality) due to the underlying liver disease and the potential for liver failure but is acceptable in selected cases.[83] Preoperative portal vein occlusion can sometimes be performed to cause atrophy of the HCC-involved lobe and compensatory hypertrophy of the noninvolved liver.[84] This allows for a safer resection. Intraoperative ultrasonography is useful for planning the surgical approach for HCC.[85] The ultrasonography can image the proximity of major vascular structures that may be encountered during the dissection. For deep tumors, the ultrasonography may identify the portal pedicle supplying the segment involved with HCC, and early control of this triad can be obtained. Intraoperative ultrasonography is also helpful for screening the rest of the liver for small tumors.

The use of inflow occlusion (Pringle maneuver) in liver resection in patients with cirrhosis has been studied. Concern exists regarding whether ischemic injury to the liver will lead to liver failure or result in worsening cirrhosis. Numerous studies, including a randomized trial, have demonstrated no ill effects to inflow occlusion. In fact, the most significant predictor of postoperative mortality is blood loss, and the Pringle maneuver decreases blood loss and leads to an improvement in perioperative morbidity.[86–88]

The morbidity and mortality of a simple wedge excision should be minimal, but even slight manipulation of a cirrhotic liver may lead to liver failure and other complications, such as respiratory failure (adult respiratory distress syndrome, pneumonia), cardiovascular compromise, ascites, and infection. Cirrhotic patients are fragile with respect to the tolerance of any major surgery. Any significant postoperative complications may lead to liver failure (Table 29.4-15).

The Child-Pugh classification of liver failure is still the most reliable prognosticator for tolerance of hepatic surgery (Table 29.4-16). Only patients with disease classified as Child's A should be considered for surgical resection. Patients with Child's B and C disease with stage I HCC tumors should be referred for transplant if appropriate. Patients with ascites or a recent history of variceal bleeding should be treated with transplantation. A variety of hepatic functional tests have been described for quantitative assessment of hepatic reserve, but these techniques have not been adopted in routine practices. The most validated is the indocyanine green clearance test. Indocyanine green is delivered systemi-

TABLE 29.4-15. Hepatic Resection Operative Morbidity and Mortality in Cirrhotic Patients

Study	Year	n	% Mortality
Tsuzuki et al.[204]	1990	119	13
Nagasue et al.[186]	1993	177	12
Yeh et al.[195]	2002	218	8.8
Wei et al.[83]	2002	155	8.4[a]
Ziparo et al.[196]	2002	88	8.7
Belghiti et al.[197]	2002	328	6.4
Kanematsu et al.[198]	2002	303	1.6
Grazi et al.[199]	2003	308	5

[a]Extended hepatectomy only.

TABLE 29.4-16. Child-Pugh Classification of Cirrhosis

Parameter	Points		
	1	2	3
Bilirubin level (mg/dL)	1–1.9	2–2.9	>2.9
Prolongation of pro-thrombin time (s)	1–3	4–6	>6
Albumin level (g/dL)	>3.5	2.8–3.4	<2.8
Ascites	None	Mild	Moderate/severe
Encephalopathy	None	Grade 1 or 2	Grade 3 or 4

Note: Grade A, 5–6 points; Grade B, 7–9 points; Grade C, 10–15 points.

cally and the hepatic retention is measured at 15 minutes. When the retention rate is less than 10%, all resections are possible. If it is 10% to 20%, a bisegmentectomy is well tolerated; if 20% to 29%, a single segment can be excised safely; if 30% or higher, then the risk of liver failure with any form of resection is high. In one study, the operative mortality was reduced to 1% when these criteria were used.[89]

Even Child's A cirrhotic patients or noncirrhotic patients may be better served with a less invasive option than open excision. Although open surgical excision is the most reliable, the patient may be better served with a laparoscopic approach to resection, laparoscopic radiofrequency ablation, percutaneous radiofrequency ablation, or percutaneous ethanol injection. Minimizing the risk of the procedure may improve the outcome and allow for all options in the future. No adequate comparisons of these different techniques have been undertaken to determine their relative success. In general, the choice of treatment is based on physician and patient preference.

Laparoscopic Resection

Laparoscopic surgical resection is a minimally invasive technique for resecting liver tumors.[90–92] The abdomen can be insufflated with carbon dioxide or lifted with specialized retractors.[93] Visualization is accomplished with a camera, and instruments are placed through the abdominal wall for hepatic parenchymal dissection. A laparoscopic approach to resection of small surface liver tumors is safe and feasible with widely available laparoscopic instruments. Larger lobectomies and segmentectomies are not commonly performed using a minimally invasive approach. The risk of bleeding and air embolus, and the number of required instrument ports have prevented this from becoming a common procedure to date. Nevertheless, many centers have reported major laparoscopic hepatectomies with the proposed advantage of less morbidity and quicker recovery.[94] Laparoscopic surgical resection has the advantage over local ablative techniques of allowing assessment of margins pathologically but has the same risk of bleeding, hepatic failure, and ascites as open excision. Laparoscopic surgery for cancer has the theoretic downside of spreading tumor cells at the time of laparoscopy. In general, surgeons have been reluctant to adopt laparoscopic approaches for cancer resection until randomized studies fail to demonstrate a negative impact on tumor recurrence compared to open surgery. Trials of more common procedures for cancer such as colectomies have not demonstrated a negative impact of the laparoscopic technique to date.[95] This experience may transfer to other procedures such as liver resection as long as the same oncologic principles of resection are used with the laparoscopic approach as are used with the open approach.

Local Ablation Strategies

Radiofrequency ablation is a technique that uses heat to thermally ablate tumors.[96,97] A thin probe (18 gauge) is inserted into the middle of the tumor, then needle electrodes are deployed to adjustable distances. An alternating electrical current (400 to 500 kHz) is delivered through the electrodes. The current causes agitation of the particles of the surrounding tissues, generating frictional heat. The heat leads to a reliable sphere of necrosis. The size of the sphere depends on the length of deployment of the electrodes. Currently, the maximum size of the probe arrays allows for a 7-cm zone of necrosis. This would be adequate for a 5-cm tumor. The heat reliably kills cells within the zone of necrosis. The lack of uniform success is due to the difficulty of positioning the probe accurately in three dimensions using ultrasonographic or CT guidance. Also, large blood vessels may act as heat sinks, preventing adequate cytodestruction of cells adjacent to these structures.[98] Finally, treatment of tumors close to the main portal pedicles can lead to bile duct injury and obstruction. This limits the location of tumors that are optimally suited for this technique. In series examining the results of treatment of HCC with radiofrequency ablation, the data suggest a uniformly excellent response, with a local recurrence rate (at the site of ablation) of between 5% and 20%.[97,99–103] The treatment can be performed percutaneously with CT or ultrasonographic guidance, or at the time of laparoscopy with ultrasonographic guidance. The disadvantage of the laparoscopic approach is the requirement for general anesthesia, but some have suggested better results with this approach.[104] Use of the percutaneous approach may also be limited by the presence of structures at risk for injury around the tumor, such as the diaphragm, colon, or gallbladder. These structures can be retracted free in a laparoscopic approach. In general, radiofrequency ablation is reliable as a single treatment. A single ablation can take up to 20 minutes for a 7-cm ablation. The procedure is well tolerated and can be performed on an outpatient basis. It can be repeated numerous times and frequently, especially if performed percutaneously. This technique is best suited overall to small tumors (less than 3 cm) deep within the hepatic parenchyma and away from the hepatic hilum. Complete preservation of hepatic parenchyma is possible with reliable tumor killing. A theoretical risk of needle tract tumor seeding exists.[105] The tract can be thermally ablated while retracting the needle, which decreases this risk.

Local Injection Therapy

Numerous agents have been used for local injection into tumors, but the most commonly used agent has been ethanol. Ethanol injection into HCC is the most widely used therapy worldwide. The relatively soft HCC within the hard background cirrhotic liver allows injection of large volumes of ethanol into the tumor without diffusion into the hepatic parenchyma or leakage out of the liver. Ethanol causes a direct destruction of cancer cells, but it is in no way selective for cancer and will destroy normal cells in the vicinity. The key to success is the accuracy of the injection. This technique is associated with a 15% risk of recurrence at the site of treatment. It has the advantage of being minimally invasive, because a very small needle can be used for injection, and it is quite inexpensive. The disadvantage

is that a response usually requires multiple injections (average of three). The maximum size of tumor that can be reliably treated is 3 cm, even with multiple injections. For this reason, radiofrequency ablation is preferable to most clinicians. Nevertheless, the cost of radiofrequency ablation may be prohibitive in many places. Acetic acid is another agent with established success as a local injection for HCC. A randomized trial suggested that local recurrence is lower with acetic acid than with ethanol.

Transplantation

A viable option for stage I and II tumors in the setting of cirrhosis is transplantation. The expected morbidity and mortality for transplantation for non–cancer-related liver disease has improved with appropriate patient selection and established expertise of liver transplant programs. With this acceptable morbidity and mortality, the major considerations regarding liver transplantation become the long-term outcome in terms of cancer recurrence. The National Institutes of Health Consensus Conference on liver transplantation in 1983 concluded that primary hepatic malignancy confined to the liver but not amenable to resection may be an indication for transplantation, although it was noted that the results indicated a strong likelihood of recurrence of the malignancy. As predicted, recurrence proved to be the rule rather than the exception, and results were dismal (Table 29.4-17). As survival data gradually accumulated, transplantation in advanced HCC cases was abandoned. However, no consensus existed among transplant surgeons and physicians as to the acceptable limits of HCC for which transplant could be beneficial, which left each program free to perform transplantation for any patient it deemed deserving.

Transplant centers realized over time that earlier tumors in the setting of severe cirrhosis could be treated successfully with transplantation. Originally proposed by Bismuth et al.[106] and then later studied prospectively by Mazzaferro et al.,[107] liver transplantation for patients with a single lesion of 5 cm or smaller or multifocal disease limited to three or fewer nodules, each 3 cm or smaller, resulted in excellent tumor-free survival (70% or higher at 5 years) (Table 29.4-18). These guidelines have become widely accepted, both in the United States and Europe, and were incor-

TABLE 29.4-17. Overall Survival after Liver Transplantation for Nonselected Patients with Hepatocellular Carcinoma

Study	Year	No. HCC Patients	Survival (%) 3-Y	Survival (%) 5-Y
O'Grady et al.[205]	1988	50	38	30
Olthoff et al.[206]	1990	16	NA	31
Iwatsuki et al.[207]	1991	105	39	36
Penn (registry)[208]	1991	365	30	18
Ringe et al.[209]	1991	61	NA	15
Bismuth et al.[106]	1993	60	47	NA
Tan et al.[210]	1995	15 (<8 cm)	63	NA
Klintmalm[211] (registry)	1998	422	50	44
Otto et al.[212]	1998	50	48	NA
Pichlmayr et al.[213]	1998	135	32	27
Hemming et al.[214]	2001	112	63	57
All liver transplantations in USA[215] (all indications)	2000	—	79	74

HCC, hepatocellular carcinoma; NA, not available.

TABLE 29.4-18. Results of Liver Transplantation for Early Hepatocellular Carcinoma

Study	Year	No. HCC Patients	Tumor (Size and Number)	Neoadjuvant Therapy	Survival (%)
Bigourdan et al.[216]	2003	17	1 ≤5 cm; 3 ≤3 cm	TACE	71 (5 y)
Yao et al.[109]	2001	46	1 ≤5 cm; 3 ≤3 cm	TACE/ETOH	72 (5 y)
Tamura et al.[217]	2001	56	<5 cm	±TACE	71 (5 y)
Regalia et al.[111]	2001	122	1 ≤5 cm; 3 ≤3 cm	TACE	80 (5 y)
Jonas et al.[218]	2001	120	1 ≤5 cm; 3 ≤3 cm	None	71 (5 y)
Harnois et al.[219]	1999	27	n ≤3, ≤5 cm	TACE	84 (2 y)
Llovet et al.[220]	1998	58	<5 cm	None	74 (5 y)
Figueras et al.[221]	1997	38	<5 cm	TACE	79 (5 y)
Mazzaferro et al.[107]	1996	48	1 ≤5 cm; 3 ≤3 cm	TACE	75 (4 y)
Venook et al.[222]	1995	13	n ≤3, ≤5 cm	TACE	77 (3.3 y)
Romani et al.[223]	1994	27	<5 cm	TACE/ETOH	71 (3 y)

ETOH, ethanol; HCC, hepatocellular carcinoma; n, number; TACE, transcatheter arterial chemoembolization.

porated into the United Network for Organ Sharing (UNOS) policy, even though the Mazzaferro et al. study was based on a limited number of patients and there were no data concerning the fate of those who did not meet these criteria who did not receive a transplant. Subsequent studies in Pittsburgh,[108] the University of California at San Francisco,[109,110] and Milan[111] have shown that acceptable tumor-free survival can be obtained for many patients not meeting these strict criteria who do not receive liver transplants under current UNOS guidelines.

As of 2001, the indications for transplantation for hepatocellular cancer included the following: (1) the patient is not a liver resection candidate; (2) the tumor(s) is smaller than or equal to 5 cm in diameter; (3) there is no macrovascular involvement; and (4) there is no identifiable extrahepatic spread of tumor to surrounding lymph nodes, lungs, abdominal organs, or bone. Reports on the results of transplantations complying with these restrictions demonstrated 5-year survival rates in the range of 70% to 75%.[112] Even with acceptance of the fact that preoperative imaging is far from perfect, 5-year tumor-free survival rates above 70% can be expected with adherence to the current guidelines. In an evaluation of living donor transplantations for HCC in which the only exclusion criteria were extrahepatic metastasis and vascular invasion detected during the preoperative evaluation, Kaihara et al. reported 1- and 3-year survival rates of 73% and 55%, respectively.[113] These results have to be considered quite remarkable given that 54% of their patients had pathologically determined TNM stage IVA disease and 45% were outside the Milan-UNOS criteria at the time of transplantation.

These strict criteria led to better results for those undergoing transplantation, but priority scoring for transplantation led to cancer patients waiting too long for their transplants. Tumors would often become too advanced during the patient's time on the waiting list for a donated liver. Survival statistics may be skewed due to selection of candidates who did not progress during their wait on the transplant list. A variety of nonresection therapies were used as a bridge to transplantation, including radiofrequency ablation, ethanol injection, and transarterial embolization procedures. At a minimum, it seems clear that these pretransplantation treatment regimens allow patients to remain on the transplant waiting list longer and thereby give them greater opportunities to undergo transplantation.[114] What remains unclear, however, is whether this translates into prolonged survival after transplantation.[115,116] Furthermore, it is not known whether patients who have had their tumors treated preoperatively follow the recurrence pattern predicted by their tumor status at the time of transplantation (i.e., after local ablative therapy) or if they follow the course indicated by tumor parameters present before such treatment.

The UNOS point system for priority scoring of liver transplant recipients now includes additional points for patients with HCC. This allows patients with early-stage disease to receive a priority score that leads to rapid transplantation. Now, even patients who are resection candidates can be treated with transplantation. The controversy over appropriate management of these patients will remain until more data on the long-term results for transplantation of patients with early-stage disease are reported. To date, it is known that survival for early-stage disease treated with surgery is 50% to 75%, whereas with transplantation it is reportedly higher than 70%. Longer-term intention-to-treat studies will be necessary to define the better treatment.

The success of living related donor liver transplantation programs has also led to patients' receiving transplantation earlier for HCC. In cases of living related donations, the UNOS guidelines are often exceeded, with a lower potential for long-term survival accepted in this setting in which there is no competition for the organ. Gondolesi et al. reported 2-year survival of 60% after living donor liver transplantation in 36 HCC patients, of whom 53% exceeded UNOS priority criteria.[117]

Adjuvant Therapy

The role of adjuvant chemotherapy for patients with HCC after resection or transplantation remains undefined. Both adjuvant and neoadjuvant approaches have been studied. Two randomized controlled trials and seven nonrandomized trials have evaluated preoperative transarterial chemotherapy. No clear advantage in disease-free or overall survival was found in these studies.[118] Postoperative transarterial chemotherapy has been examined in four randomized controlled trials and three nonrandomized controlled trials. A metaanalysis of these trials revealed a significant improvement in disease-free and overall survival.[118] The regimens consisted of Lipiodol and chemotherapy agents, including doxorubicin, mitomycin C, and cisplatin. An analysis of postoperative adjuvant systemic chemotherapy trials demonstrates no disease-free or overall survival advantage. Neoadjuvant approaches such as chemoembolization have been successful as a bridge to transplantation and have decreased tumor burden in resection candidates to improve resectability. Numerous studies of adjuvant therapy after resection and liver transplantation have been performed, but the results are not definitive.[119–122]

STAGE III AND IV HEPATOCELLULAR CARCINOMA

Fewer surgical options exist for stage III tumors involving major vascular structures. In patients without cirrhosis, a major hepatectomy is feasible and provides the best chance of long-term survival, although prognosis is poor. Patients with Child's A cirrhosis may undergo resection, but a lobectomy is associated with significant morbidity and mortality, and long-term prognosis is poor. Nevertheless, a small percentage of patients will achieve long-term survival, which justifies an attempt at resection when feasible. Preoperative portal vein occlusion to induce compensatory hypertrophy preoperatively may improve the results or help define which patients will tolerate a major hepatectomy. Because of the advanced nature of these tumors, even successful resection is met with rapid recurrence. These patients are not considered candidates for transplantation, because of the high tumor recurrence rates, unless their tumors can be down-staged with adjuvant therapy. Although the therapy is unproven, these patients are ideal for neoadjuvant treatment approaches such as embolization. Decreasing the size of the primary tumor allows for less surgery, and the delay in surgery allows for extrahepatic disease to manifest on imaging studies so that unnecessary surgery on the primary tumor can be avoided. Successful regional therapy strategies may make the patient eligible for transplantation. The prognosis is poor for stage IV tumors, and no surgical treatment is recommended. Care must be taken to differentiate multifocal disease from intrahepatic metastases, because the latter has a much worse prognosis. Molecular genotyping may be the best way to make this differentiation.

Systemic Chemotherapy

A large number of controlled and uncontrolled clinical studies have been performed for most of the major classes of cancer chemotherapy, given intravenously as a single agent or in combination. The reader is referred to reviews and some of the larger studies (Table 29.4-19).[123–126] Although there were initial encouraging reports of single-agent doxorubicin therapy in Uganda, subsequent studies have failed to confirm the early enthusiastic reports for this or any other single agent. The consensus is that no single agent or combination of agents given systemically reproducibly leads to greater than 25% response rates or has any effect on survival. Drugs that appear clearly to have no reproducible response when given systemically as single agents include 5-fluorouridine, doxorubicin, cisplatin, VP-16, and neocarzinostatin. No combination of these drugs has been associated with survival beyond that of untreated controls. There appears to be little justification for treating patients with single or combination drugs in a systemic fashion outside a cancer clinical trial, probably in phase II trials of new agents.

Regional Chemotherapy

Although the results of systemic chemotherapy for either regional or metastatic HCC are dismal, a large number of encouraging reports have appeared concerning a variety of regional chemotherapies for HCC confined to the liver (Table 29.4-20). Much of the experience has come from Europe and Asia, where the large number of cases has allowed systematic studies to be performed. Despite the fact that increased hepatic extraction of chemotherapy has

TABLE 29.4-19. Selected Studies of Chemotherapy for Hepatocellular Carcinoma

Investigation	Drug	Partial Response Rate (%)
SYSTEMIC CHEMOTHERAPY		
Sciarrino et al., 1985[224]	Doxorubicin	0
Chlebowski et al., 1984[225]	Doxorubicin	11
Ihde et al., 1977[226]	Doxorubicin	15
Falkson et al., 1984[227]	Doxorubicin, 5-FU, methyl-CCNU	19
Falkson et al., 1984[228]	Neocarzinostatin	8
Ravry et al., 1984[229]	Doxorubicin, bleomycin	16
Cavalli et al., 1981[230]	VP-16 (etoposide)	13
Melia et al., 1983[231]	VP-16	18
Melia et al., 1981[232]	Cisplatin	1
Ravry et al., 1986[233]	Cisplatin	0
Falkson et al., 1987[234]	Cisplatin	17
Falkson et al., 1987[234]	Mitoxantrone	8
Colleoni et al., 1993[235]	Mitoxantrone	23
Chao et al., 1998[236]	Paclitaxel	0
Patt et al., 2003[237]	5-FU + IFN	18
Patt et al., 2000[238]	5-FU + IFN + cisplatin + doxorubicin	20
Okada et al., 1999[239]	Cisplatin, mitoxantrone + 5-FU	33
Reviews[123–125,162,240,241]		
INTRAHEPATIC ARTERIAL CHEMOTHERAPY		
Onohara et al., 1988[242]	Cisplatin	55
Kajanti et al., 1986[243]	Cisplatin	40
Nagasue et al., 1987[244]	Epirubicin	15
Carr et al., 1996[136]	Cisplatin dose escalation	50

5-FU, 5-fluorouracil; IFN, interferon; methyl-CCNU, methyl-chloroethylcyclohexylnitrosourea.

been shown for very few drugs, some drugs such as cisplatin, doxorubicin, mitomycin C, and possibly neocarzinostatin have been found to produce substantial objective responses when administered regionally. In contrast to the Western experience for metastatic colon cancer to the liver, few data are available regarding continuous hepatic arterial infusion for HCC, although pilot studies are suggestive.[127,128] Almost all studies have been done using bolus administration. Because almost none of the reports have stratified responses or survival based on TNM staging, it is difficult to know long-term prognosis in relation to tumor extent. Many but not all of the studies on regional intrahepatic arterial chemotherapy also use an embolizing agent such as Lipiodol, gelatin (Gelfoam), starch (Spherex), microspheres, or polyvinyl alcohol (Ivalon).[129–132] The last is rarely used now, due to increased hepatotoxicity. Two new products have now come to market using microspheres of defined size ranges. They are Embosphere (BioSphere) and Contour SE (Boston Scientific). The optimal diameter of the particles for transcatheter arterial chemoembolization (TACE) has yet to be defined. Consistently higher objective response rates are reported for arterial administration of drugs together with some form of hepatic artery occlusion than for any form of systemic chemotherapy to date. The widespread use of some form of embolization (TACE) in addition to chemotherapy has added to its toxicities. These include the almost universal presence of high fever (more than 95%), abdominal pain (more than 60%), and anorexia (more than 60%). In addition, more than 20% of patients have increased ascites or transient elevation of transaminases. Cystic artery spasm and cholecystitis are also not uncommon. However,

TABLE 29.4-20. Intrahepatic Artery Chemotherapy with or without Embolization for Hepatocellular Carcinoma

Investigation	Agents	No. of Patients	Response Rate (%)
Sasaki et al., 1987[245]	Platinum + gelatin sponge	20	65
Kasugai et al., 1989[246]	Platinum + ethiodized oil	25	38
Ohnishi et al., 1984[247]	MMC + microcapsules	20	32
Lin et al., 1988[248]	5-FU + polyvinyl alcohol (Ivalon)	21	32
Fujimoto et al., 1985[249]	5-FU/MMC + starch	19	68
Audisio et al., 1990[250]	MMC + microcapsules	30	43
Kobayashi et al., 1986[251]	Doxorubicin + ethiodized oil	33	42
Kanematsu et al., 1989[252]	Doxorubicin + ethiodized oil	70	47
Shibata et al., 1989[253]	Platinum + ethiodized oil	71	47
Konno et al., 1983[254]	SMANCS + ethiodized oil	44	90
Pelletier et al., 1990[255]	Doxorubicin + gelatin sponge	42	17
Carr, 1991[256]	Doxorubicin/cisplatin	25	50
Venook et al., 1990[257]	Doxorubicin/cisplatin/MMC + gelatin sponge	50	24
Ohnishi et al., 1987[258]	MMC + microcapsules	32	28
Ohnishi et al., 1987[258]	MMC + gelatin sponge + microcapsules	34	57
Beppu et al., 1991[259]	Cisplatin + ethiodized oil + aclarubicin microspheres	62	50
Groupe d'Etude et de Traitement du Carcinome Hepatocellulaire, 1995[260]	Cisplatin + ethiodized oil	43	16
	vs. no therapy	38	0
Chang et al., 1994[271]	Cisplatin + Gelfoam + ethiodized oil	22	68[a]
	vs. Gelfoam + ethiodized oil	24	67[a]
Stuart et al., 1993[137]	Doxorubicin, ethiodized oil + Gelfoam	47	43
Bruix et al., 1994[261]	Gelfoam, no chemotherapy	50	81
Carr et al., 1997[130]	Doxorubicin, cisplatin + Spherex	35	63
Carr et al., 1993[129]	Doxorubicin, cisplatin + ethiodized oil	37	57
	vs. doxorubicin + cisplatin	34	47
Carr et al., 2002[262]	Cisplatin	155	58
Ngan et al., 1993[263]	Cisplatin, ethiodized oil, Gelfoam	232	41
Yamamoto et al., 1993[265]	Interleukin-2		
Kawai et al., 1994[264]	Epirubicin + Gelfoam vs. doxorubicin + Gelfoam	192	a
Yoshimi et al., 1992[266]	Resection	66	a
	vs. TAE	29	a
Epstein et al., 1991[31]	Cisplatin + hepatic irradiation	21	48
Rougier et al., 1993[267]	Doxorubicin + Gelfoam	232	41

5-FU, 5-fluorouracil; MMC, mitomycin C; SMANCS, styrene maleic acid conjugates of neocarzinostatin and mitomycin C; TAE, transcatheter arterial embolization.
[a]Similar survival.

higher responses have also been found, and this regimen has also been used as therapy and neoadjuvant therapy in children.[133–135]

Several studies have examined response rates and survival for mixtures of both chemotherapy and transhepatic arterial embolization or occlusion. Results have been conflicting. Several studies have compared intrahepatic arterial chemotherapy, usually with addition of Lipiodol and Gelfoam embolization, to no treatment, to embolization (with or without chemotherapy), or to other chemotherapy (Tables 29.4-21 and 29.4-22). All of these studies used either doxorubicin or cisplatin at rather low doses compared with what is used systemically. None of the studies found response rates higher than 50%. As a consequence, few of these studies showed any survival advantage. Nonrandomized studies reported higher responses to platinum or showed greater survival, but only when compared with historical controls.[136] One study reported promising survival figures suggesting decreased postresection recurrences.[121] The hepatic toxicities associated with embolization have been ameliorated by the use of degradable starch microspheres, with 50% to 60% response rates.[130,131] Similar results were achieved in a randomized study of doxorubicin and cisplatin with or without Lipiodol or with doxorubicin and Gelfoam.[126,137]

Because there is no standard chemotherapy drug for HCC, combinations are used differently by different groups and often at suboptimal dosages. The best strategy now is to take one step backward and find the optimum intraarterial dosages for each of what are probably the two current best drugs, cisplatin and doxorubicin, and then to combine a single drug at optimal dosing with an arterial occluding agent. Once regimens that reliably and consistently induce greater than 50% partial responses are available, effects on survival should be detectable. In addition, different studies report noncomparable patients. Tumor stage has been rarely given, so that different studies report responses of patients with differing tumor burdens and degrees of cirrhosis. Reports have questioned the value of any chemotherapy added to embolization due to lack of apparent survival advantages.[138,139] A high percentage of HCC patients die of their cirrhosis and not of their tumor. A reasonable target now should be to improve patient survival and quality of life,[140] with or without higher tumor response rates. In addition, it is not clear that the formal CT response criteria for oncologic partial responses are adequate for HCC. It appears that a loss of vascularity on CT without size change is also a reasonable index of loss of viability and thus tumor response to TACE.[141]

TABLE 29.4-21. Selected Randomized Clinical Trials of Transhepatic Artery Chemoembolization versus Other Chemotherapy for Hepatocellular Carcinoma

Study	Year	Agents 1	Agents 2	Effects on Survival
Kawai et al.[268]	1992	Doxorubicin + embo	Embo	None
Kawai et al.[269]	1997	Epirubicin + embo	Doxorubicin + embo	None
Watanabe et al.[270]	1994	Epirubicin + embo	Doxorubicin + embo	None
Chang et al.[271]	1994	Cisplatin + embo	Embo	None
Hatanaka et al.[272]	1995	Cisplatin, doxorubicin + embo	Same + Lipiodol	None
Uchino et al.[273]	1993	Cisplatin, doxorubicin + oral FU	Same + tamoxifen	None
Madden et al.[274]	1993	Cisplatin + ADMOS	5-epi-doxorubicin	None
Chung et al.[275]	2000	Cisplatin + interferon	Cisplatin	None
Lin et al.[276]	1988	Embo	Embo + IV FU	None
Yoshikawa et al.[277]	1994	Epirubicin + Lipiodol	Epirubicin	None
Kajanti et al.[278]	1992	Epirubicin + FU	IV Epirubicin + FU	None
Tzoracoleftherakis et al.[279]	1999	Doxorubicin	IV doxorubicin	None
Bhattacharya et al.[280]	1995	Epirubicin + Lipiodol	Iodine 131 Lipiodol	None

ADMOS, Adriamycin (doxorubicin)/mitomycin C oil suspension; Embo, chemoembolization; FU, 5-fluorouracil.

Two randomized controlled trials have shown a survival advantage for TACE, mainly in a selected subset of patients (see Table 29.4-22).[138,139] However, these trials provide the first evidence of survival benefit for TACE, or indeed for any medical treatment for surgically unresectable HCC.

Newer Therapies

Various new therapies have been introduced and evaluated (Table 29.4-23). The effects of systemic interferon therapy have generally been poor.[142–145] The combination of chemotherapy and interferon has had only marginal effect. However, there are indications that interferon may be useful in reducing recurrence rates after more definitive treatment.[122] Similarly, tamoxifen has been attractive because of its low toxicity, and its use appears to be rational because of the high male to female gender bias in HCC epidemiology. However, results have been entirely mixed, and on the whole there appears to be little support for its use from the evidence of randomized control trials.[146–149] Studies have shown no objective responses to tamoxifen or to the antiandrogen keto-conazole. Results of a European Organization for Research and Treatment of Cancer trial of the antiandrogen nilutamide (Anandron) and the luteinizing hormone–releasing hormone agonist goserelin (Zoladex) were disappointing. So far, conflicting results have been found for octreotide (Sandostatin), with minor or low response rates from thalidomide, megestrol, and vitamin K. These agents are attractive because of minimal toxicities, but responses so far are disappointing. Epidermal growth factor receptor anti-

bodies are currently in the process of clinical evaluation as are various antiangiogenic therapies, and no results can yet be reported on response rates or survival. Similarly, gene therapy strategies are attractive because of the feasibility of local-regional application, but thus far no positive results have been reported. New ways of mixing or exploring old therapies are also being evaluated.[150] These include continuous chemotherapy infusion intravenously and continuous infusion of drugs into the hepatic artery,[127,128] the combination of radiation and chemotherapy,[151] and more particularly the use of adjuvant therapies after resection and after liver transplantation.[120–122,151]

Several forms of radiation have been used in the treatment of HCC, including external-beam radiation and conformal external-beam radiation.[152–157] There are suggestions of a dose-response relationship, but radiation hepatitis remains a significant problem.[155] Several studies have used iodine 131 as a radiolabel either attached to antiferritin antibodies or attached to Lipiodol, but there was no enhancement of survival when compared to that of controls.[119,151,158] More recently, treatment with the pure β-emitter ^{90}Y attached to either glass or resin microspheres has been assessed in HCC in phase II trials. There appear to be encouraging survival effects with minimal toxicities.[159–163] However, randomized control trials have yet to be performed.

Studies that are currently prepared or under way include research investigating the addition of degradable starch micro-

TABLE 29.4-22. Randomized Clinical Trials of Transhepatic Arterial Chemoembolization Chemotherapy versus No Treatment

Study	Year	Agents	Effects on Survival
Pelletier et al.[281]	1990	Doxorubicin + Gelfoam	None
Trinchet[260]	1995	Cisplatin + Gelfoam	None
Bruix et al.[282]	1998	Coils + Gelfoam	None
Pelletier et al.[283]	1998	Cisplatin + Lipiodol	None
Lo et al.[138]	2002	Cisplatin + Lipiodol	Yes
Llovet et al.[139]	2002	Doxorubicin + Lipiodol	Yes
Reviews[123,240,284]	—	—	—

TABLE 29.4-23. Various Medical Treatments (Nonchemotherapeutic) for Hepatocellular Carcinoma

Tamoxifen[146–149]
Luteinizing hormone–releasing hormone agonists[285]
Interferon[142–145]
Octreotide (Sandostatin)[286,287]
Megestrol[288,289]
Vitamin K[164–167]
Thalidomide[290]
Epidermal growth factor receptor antibody
Interleukin-2[265]
Iodine 131 Lipiodol[119,151]
Iodine 131 ferritin[158]
Yttrium 90 microspheres[159–161,163,291]
Antiangiogenesis strategies

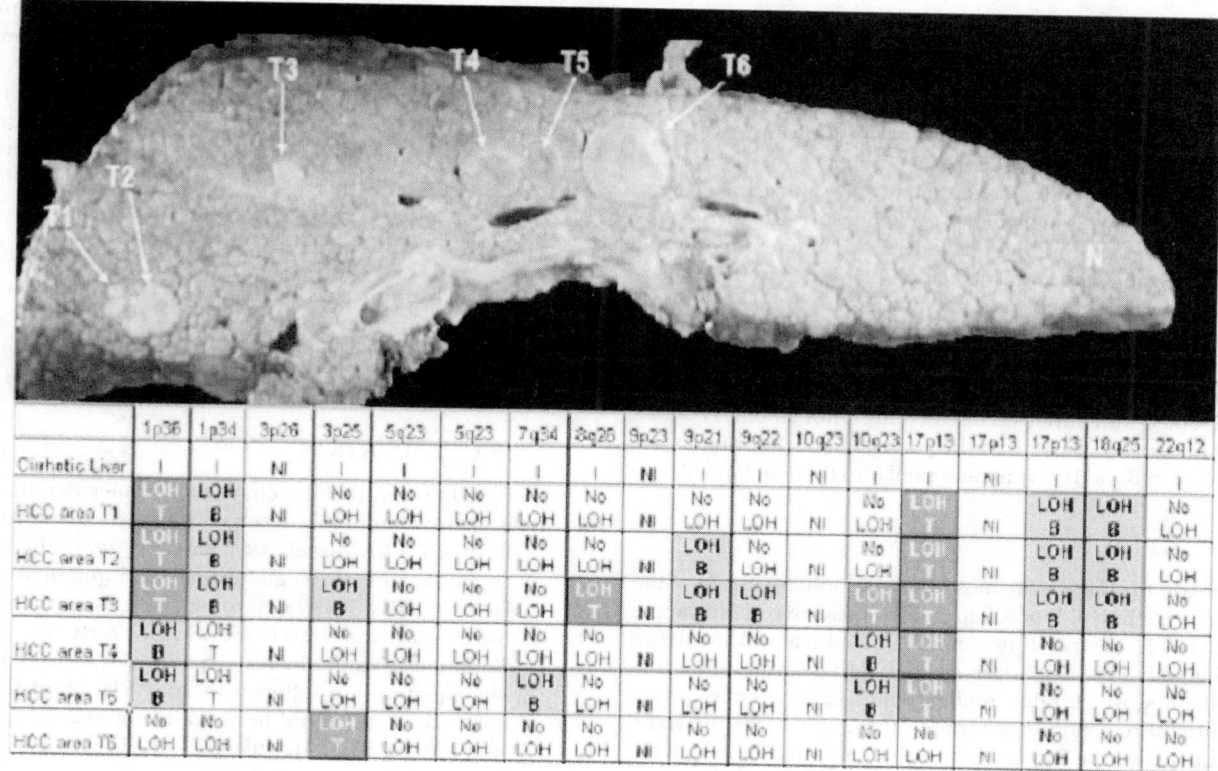

FIGURE 29.4-4. Shown are the genotyping results for the six tumor nodules (T1 to T6) detected in this cirrhotic liver. The blue and red shading are used to indicate opposite alleles. This diagram illustrates that lesions T1, T2, and T3 are intrahepatic metastases and separate from the other lesions; similarly, lesions T4 and T5 are distinct from the other lesions but not from each other (i.e., intrahepatic metastases); T6 is a completely separate and distinct nodule from all other lesions. HCC, hepatocellular carcinoma; LOH, loss of heterozygosity; T, top; B, bottom. (Courtesy of Syd Finkelstein, MD.) (See Color Fig. 29.4-4 in the CD-ROM.)

spheres (Spherex) as embolization agents to reduce the toxicities of embolization. Phase I studies of antiangiogenic drugs and the evaluation of immunosuppressant drugs such as rapamycin that also have growth-inhibitory or antihepatotrophic actions are under way. The use of genetically engineered cells that overexpress either lymphokines or growth-inhibitory factors is currently also under investigation.

Vitamin K has been assessed in clinical trials at high dosage for its HCC-inhibitory actions.[164–167] This idea is based on the characteristic biochemical defect in HCC of elevated plasma levels of immature prothrombin (DCP or PIVKA-2), due to a defect in the activity of prothrombin carboxylase, which is a vitamin K–dependent enzyme. Addition of vitamin K to HCC cell lines *in vitro* results in a correction of this defect and growth inhibition.[166,167] Even massive vitamin K doses appear to be free of any human toxicity. This approach appears to be encouraging, especially because several long-term survivors are now accumulating in these studies.

The contribution of serum biomarkers such as serum proteomics will likely identify patient subsets who can benefit most from TACE or other therapies. Better predictors of the biology of HCC will allow for more selective application of different therapies and better prognostication. The best example of this is in transplantation, in which competition for organs exists, and patients die awaiting transplantation for benign disease. It would be advantageous to be able to predict which patients will experience treatment failure with systemic disease within months of transplantation. Marsh et al. described 103 cases in which micro-

dissection genotyping techniques were used to establish the degree of malignancy for each nodule by (1) assessing the accumulated mutational load through loss of heterozygosity at ten different loci, and (2) calculating the fractional allelic loss rate.[168] By comparing the genotyping of multiple lesions in the liver, one can define whether these are multiple primary tumors or intrahepatic metastases, which have a much worse prognosis[169] (Fig. 29.4-4). It has been found that, among multiple *de novo* tumors, 94.4% are bilobar, whereas multiple intrahepatic metastases are bilobar 62.9% of the time (*P* <.02). The measure of allelic loss of heterozygosity combined with tumor number, tumor size, vascular invasion, lobar distribution, and patient gender provided a highly discriminatory model for predicting cancer recurrence after liver transplantation. The use of previously developed artificial neural network models in combination with the genotyping results could predict those who survived for 5 years in 88% of cases. This result needs to be further validated in prospective studies but provides the potential for better measurements of outcome using molecular characteristics.

TREATMENT OF OTHER PRIMARY LIVER TUMORS

FIBROLAMELLAR HEPATOCELLULAR CARCINOMA

Fibrolamellar HCC (FL-HCC) is a rare histologic variant of HCC and differs in several respects from the normal-variant

HCC. FL-HCC occurs in a much younger age group (peak incidence in the third decade), is uncommonly associated with cirrhosis, and affects males and females equally. Additionally, a much higher percentage of patients with FL-HCC than of those with normal-variant HCC present with positive lymph nodes.

Whether the diagnosis of FL-HCC portends a more favorable outcome after surgical treatment remains controversial.[170–173] As is true for essentially all malignant liver lesions, resection remains the first-line therapy. For those patients in whom the tumor is felt to be unresectable, liver transplantation provides a valuable alternative. Pinna described 13 patients with FL-HCC who underwent transplantation between 1968 and 1995, and reported 1-, 3-, and 5-year patient survival rates of approximately 90%, 75%, and 38%, respectively.[174] Given that most patients undergoing transplantation presented with advanced disease, this is not an unacceptable survival rate, particularly given the young age of the patients. El-Gazzaz et al. reported survival rates similar to those of Pinna.[175]

HEPATOBLASTOMA

Hepatoblastoma (HB) is the most common primary cancer of the liver occurring in childhood. The annual incidence of HB ranges from 0.5 to 1.5 cases per 1 million children, with a peak incidence occurring within the first 2 years of life.[176] HB is highly sensitive to chemotherapy, which often renders unresectable tumors resectable. Surgical resection is considered first-line therapy; however, most patients whose tumors cannot be converted to resectable lesions but who do not have distant metastases can be rescued with liver transplantation. Survival rates for these children after liver transplantation are excellent, with 1-, 3-, and 5-year survival reported at 92%, 92%, and 83%, respectively.[177]

EPITHELIOID HEMANGIOENDOTHELIOMA

Epithelioid hemangioendothelioma (EHE) is a very rare tumor of vascular origin that can originate in the liver. It occurs predominantly in females. The tumor is often confused with other more aggressive cancers, particularly cholangiocarcinoma, angiosarcoma, and HCC. The clinical course of EHE is quite variable. In the review by Makhlouf et al., 137 cases were described, and survival ranged from 4 months to 28 years.[178] Of interest, one patient who received no treatment survived for 27 years without evidence of metastasis. Surgical resection is considered to be the treatment of choice; however, this particular cancer is often multifocal, which makes liver transplantation the only surgical option. The presence of metastatic disease does not seem to influence survival and should not be considered an absolute contraindication to either surgical resection or transplantation.

SUMMARY: PRACTICAL GUIDE TO THE MANAGEMENT OF PATIENTS WITH HEPATOCELLULAR CARCINOMA

PRESENTATION

The most common modes of patient presentation:

1. A patient with a known history of hepatitis, jaundice, or cirrhosis, with an abnormality on the twice-yearly screen by liver ultrasonography or CT scan, or rising AFP or DCP (PIVKA-2) level

2. A patient with an abnormal result on a liver function test done for other reasons or as part of a routine medical examination

3. A patient undergoing radiologic workup for liver transplantation for cirrhosis in whom a tumor is detected

4. A patient with symptoms of HCC including tumor rupture (hemoperitoneum), cachexia, abdominal pain, or fever

HISTORY AND PHYSICAL EXAMINATION

1. Clinical jaundice, asthenia, itching (scratches), tremors, or disorientation

2. Hepatomegaly, splenomegaly, ascites, peripheral edema, skin signs of liver failure, or palpable lymph nodes

CLINICAL EVALUATION

1. Blood tests: full blood count (splenomegaly), liver function tests, ammonia levels, electrolyte levels, AFP and DCP or PIVKA-2 levels, Ca^{2+} and Mg^{2+} levels; hepatitis B, C, and D virus serologic testing (and quantitative HBV DNA or HCV RNA, if serologic test for either is positive); neurotensin level (specific for FL-HCC).

2. Triphasic dynamic helical (spiral) CT scan of liver (if inadequate, then follow with an MRI); chest CT scan; bone scan; upper and lower gastrointestinal endoscopy (for varices, bleeding, ulcers); and brain scan (only if symptoms suggest)

3. Biopsy: core-needle biopsy (unless curative surgery is planned)

THERAPY

1. HCC smaller than 2 cm: radiofrequency ablation, percutaneous ethanol injection, or resection (Fig. 29.4-5)

2. HCC larger than 2 cm, no vascular invasion: liver resection, radiofrequency ablation, or liver transplantation

3. Multiple unilobar tumors or tumor with vascular invasion: aggressive intrahepatic arterial chemoembolization followed by liver transplantation

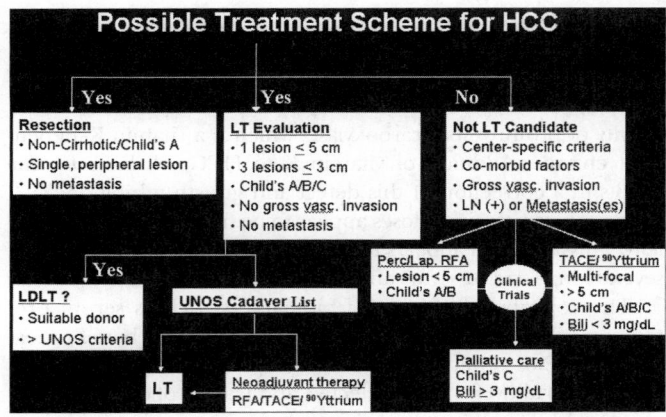

FIGURE 29.4-5. Algorithm for management of hepatocellular cancer (HCC). Bili, bilirubin level; LDLT, living donor liver transplantation; LN, lymph nodes; LT, liver transplantation; Perc/Lap, percutaneous/laparoscopic; RFA, radiofrequency ablation; TACE, transarterial chemoembolization; UNOS, United Network for Organ Sharing.

4. Bilobar disease: aggressive intrahepatic artery chemoembolization, with liver transplantation for those patients whose tumors have shown at least a formal partial response and who do not have major portal vein thrombosis
5. Extrahepatic HCC: results of phase I and II studies should be applied in this setting

REFERENCES

1. Parker SL, Tong T, Bolden S, Wingo PA. Cancer statistics. *CA Cancer J Clin* 1996;46:5.
2. Simonetti RG, Camma C, Fiorello F, et al. Hepatocellular carcinoma. A worldwide problem and the major risk factors. *Dig Dis Sci* 1991;36:962.
3. Di Bisceglie AM, Rustgi VK, Hoofnagle JH, Dusheiko GM, Lotze MT. NIH conference. Hepatocellular carcinoma. *Ann Intern Med* 1988;108:390.
4. El-Serag HB, Davila JA, Petersen NJ, McGlynn KA. The continuing increase in the incidence of hepatocellular carcinoma in the United States: an update. *Ann Intern Med* 2003;139:817.
5. El-Serag HB, Mason AC. Rising incidence of hepatocellular carcinoma in the United States. *N Engl J Med* 1999;340:745.
6. El-Serag HB, Mason AC, Key C. Trends in survival of patients with hepatocellular carcinoma between 1977 and 1996 in the United States. *Hepatology* 2001;33:62.
7. El-Serag HB. Hepatocellular carcinoma: an epidemiologic view. *J Clin Gastroenterol* 2002;35[Suppl 2]:S72:35.
8. Davila JA, Petersena NJ, Nelson HA, El-Serag HB. Geographic variation within the United States in the incidence of hepatocellular carcinoma. *J Clin Epidemiol* 2003;56:487.
9. Steinitz R, Parkin DM, Young JL, Bieber CA, Katz L. Cancer incidence in Jewish migrants to Israel, 1961–1981. *IARC Sci Publ* 1989;1.
10. Henderson BE, Preston-Martin S, Edmondson HA, Peters RL, Pike MC. Hepatocellular carcinoma and oral contraceptives. *Br J Cancer* 1983;48:437.
11. Beasley RP, Hwang LY, Lin CC, Chien CS. Hepatocellular carcinoma and hepatitis B virus. A prospective study of 22,707 men in Taiwan. *Lancet* 1981;2:1129.
12. Heyward WL, Lanier AP, Bender TR, et al. Primary hepatocellular carcinoma in Alaskan natives, 1969–1979. *Int J Cancer* 1981;28:47.
13. Heyward WL, Lanier AP, Bender TR, et al. Early detection of primary hepatocellular carcinoma by screening for alpha-fetoprotein in high-risk families. A case-report. *Lancet* 1983;2:1161.
14. Popper H, Thung SN, McMahon BJ, et al. Evolution of hepatocellular carcinoma associated with chronic hepatitis B virus infection in Alaskan Eskimos. *Arch Pathol Lab Med* 1988;112:498.
15. Dodd RY, Nath N. Increased risk for lethal forms of liver disease among HBsAg-positive blood donors in the United States. *J Virol Methods* 1987;17:81.
16. McMahon BJ, London T. Workshop on screening for hepatocellular carcinoma. *J Natl Cancer Inst* 1991;83:916.
17. Okuda K. Hepatocellular carcinomas associated with hepatitis B and C virus infections: are they any different? *Hepatology* 1995;22:1883.
18. Shiratori Y, Shiina S, Imamura M, et al. Characteristic difference of hepatocellular carcinoma between hepatitis B- and C- viral infection in Japan. *Hepatology* 1995;22:1027.
19. Lutwick LI. Relation between aflatoxin, hepatitis-B virus, and hepatocellular carcinoma. *Lancet* 1979;1:755.
20. Tiribelli C, Melato M, Croce LS, et al. Prevalence of hepatocellular carcinoma and relation to cirrhosis: comparison of two different cities of the world—Trieste, Italy, and Chiba, Japan. *Hepatology* 1989;10:998.
21. Craig JR, Peter RL, Edwardson HA. *Tumors of the liver and intrahepatic bile ducts.* Washington, DC: Armed Forces Institute of Pathology, 1989.
22. Greene FL. *AJCC cancer staging manual,* 6th ed. New York: Springer-Verlag, 2002.
23. Katyal S, Oliver JH III, Peterson MS, et al. Extrahepatic metastases of hepatocellular carcinoma. *Radiology* 2000;216:698.
24. Nalesnik MA, Lee RG, Carr BI. Transforming growth factor alpha (TGFalpha) in hepatocellular carcinomas and adjacent hepatic parenchyma. *Hum Pathol* 1998;29:228.
25. Minervini MI, Demetris AJ, Lee RG, et al. Utilization of hepatocyte-specific antibody in the immunocytochemical evaluation of liver tumors. *Mod Pathol* 1997;10:686.
26. Chen MF, Hwang TL, Tsao KC, Sun CF, Chen TJ. Flow cytometric DNA analysis of hepatocellular carcinoma: preliminary report. *Surgery* 1991;109:455.
27. Tarao K, Shimizu A, Harada M, et al. In vitro uptake of bromodeoxyuridine by human hepatocellular carcinoma and its relation to histopathologic findings and biologic behavior. *Cancer* 1991;68:1789.
28. Okuda K, Obata H, Nakajima Y, et al. Prognosis of primary hepatocellular carcinoma. *Hepatology* 1984;4:3S.
29. CLIP investigators. A new prognostic system for HCC: a retrospective study of 435 patients. *Hepatology* 1998;28:751.
30. Llovet JM, Bru C, Bruix J. Prognosis of hepatocellular carcinoma: the BCLC staging classification. *Semin Liver Dis* 1999;19:329.
31. Epstein B, Ettinger D, Leichner PK, Order SE. Multimodality cisplatin treatment in non-resectable alpha-fetoprotein-positive hepatoma. *Cancer* 1991;67:896.
32. Abelev GI, Perova SD, Khramkova NI, Postnikova ZA, Irlin IS. Production of embryonal alpha-globulin by transplantable mouse hepatomas. *Transplantation* 1963;1:174.
33. Waldmann TA, McIntire KR. The use of radioimmunoassay for alpha-fetoprotein in the diagnosis of malignancy. *Cancer* 1974;34:1510.
34. McIntire KR, Vogel CL, Primack A, Waldmann TA, Kyalwazi SK. Effect of surgical and chemotherapeutic treatment on alpha-fetoprotein levels in patients with hepatocellular carcinoma. *Cancer* 1976;37:677.
35. Buamah PK, Cornell C, James OF, Skillen AW, Harris AL. Serial serum AFP heterogeneity changes in patients with hepatocellular carcinoma during chemotherapy. *Cancer Chemother Pharmacol* 1986;17:182.
36. Matsumoto Y, Suzuki T, Asada I, et al. Clinical classification of hepatoma in Japan according to serial changes in serum alpha-fetoprotein levels. *Cancer* 1982;49:354.
37. Piper M, Carr BI, Virji MA. Alpha-fetoprotein (AFP) and des-gamma-carboxy-prothrombin (DCP) in hepatocellular carcinoma (HCC) and chronic liver diseases. *Hepatology* 1992;16:538.
38. Sakon M, Monden M, Gotoh M, et al. The effects of vitamin K on the generation of des-gamma-carboxy prothrombin (PIVKA-II) in patients with hepatocellular carcinoma. *Am J Gastroenterol* 1991;86:339.
39. Nakao A, Virji A, Iwaki Y, et al. Abnormal prothrombin (DES-gamma-carboxy prothrombin) in hepatocellular carcinoma. *Hepatogastroenterology* 1991;38:450.
40. Melia WM, Johnson PJ, Carter S, Munro-Neville A, Williams R. Plasma carcinoembryonic antigen in the diagnosis and management of patients with hepatocellular carcinoma. *Cancer* 1981;48:1004.
41. Paradinas FJ, Melia WM, Wilkinson ML, et al. High serum vitamin B12 binding capacity as a marker of the fibrolamellar variant of hepatocellular carcinoma. *BMJ* 1982;285:840.
42. Collier NA, Weinbren K, Bloom SR, et al. Neurotensin secretion by fibrolamellar carcinoma of the liver. *Lancet* 1984;1:538.
43. Nagaoka S, Yatsuhashi H, Hamada H, et al. The des-gamma-carboxy prothrombin index is a new prognostic indicator for hepatocellular carcinoma. *Cancer* 1993;98:2671.
44. Sawabu N, Nakagen M, Ozaki K, et al. Clinical evaluation of specific gamma-GTP isoenzyme in patients with hepatocellular carcinoma. *Cancer* 1983;51:327.
45. Melia WM, Bullock S, Johnson PJ, Williams R. Serum ferritin in hepatocellular carcinoma. A comparison with alpha-fetoprotein. *Cancer* 1983;51:2112.
46. Kew MC, Fisher JW. Serum erythropoietin concentrations in patients with hepatocellular carcinoma. *Cancer* 1986;58:2485.
47. Derynck R, Goeddel DV, Ullrich A, et al. Synthesis of messenger RNAs for transforming growth factors alpha and beta and the epidermal growth factor receptor by human tumors. *Cancer Res* 1987;47:707.
48. Ito N, Kawata S, Tamura S, et al. Elevated levels of transforming growth factor beta messenger RNA and its polypeptide in human hepatocellular carcinoma. *Cancer Res* 1991;51:4080.
49. Grieco A, De Stefano V, Cassano A, et al. Hepatocarcinoma in cirrhosis. Is antithrombin III a neoplastic marker? *Dig Dis Sci* 1991;36:990.
50. Haglund C, Lindgren J, Roberts PJ, Nordling S. Difference in tissue expression of tumour markers CA 19-9 and CA 50 in hepatocellular carcinoma and cholangiocarcinoma. *Br J Cancer* 1991;63:386.
51. Brady PG, Peebles M, Goldschmid S. Role of laparoscopy in the evaluation of patients with suspected hepatic or peritoneal malignancy. *Gastrointest Endosc* 1991;37:27.
52. Merine D, Takayasu K, Wakao F. Detection of hepatocellular carcinoma: comparison of CT during arterial portography with CT after intraarterial injection of iodized oil. *Radiology* 1990;175:707.
53. Sheu JC, Sung JL, Chen DS, et al. Early detection of hepatocellular carcinoma by real-time ultrasonography. A prospective study. *Cancer* 1985;56:660.
54. Hosoki T, Chatani M, Mori S. Dynamic computed tomography of hepatocellular carcinoma. *AJR Am J Roentgenol* 1982;139:1099.
55. Heiken JP, Weyman PJ, Lee JK, et al. Detection of focal hepatic masses: prospective evaluation with CT, delayed CT, CT during arterial portography, and MR imaging. *Radiology* 1989;171:47.
56. Nelson RC, Chezmar JL, Sugarbaker PH, Bernardino ME. Hepatic tumors: comparison of CT during arterial portography, delayed CT, and MR imaging for preoperative evaluation. *Radiology* 1989;172:27.
57. Brancatelli G, Federle MP, Grazioli L, Carr BI. Hepatocellular carcinoma in noncirrhotic liver: CT, clinical, and pathologic findings in 39 U.S. residents. *Radiology* 2002;222:89.
58. Kanematsu M, Oliver JH III, Carr B, Baron RL. Hepatocellular carcinoma: the role of helical biphasic contrast-enhanced CT versus CT during arterial portography. *Radiology* 1997;205:75.
59. Baron RL, Oliver JH III, Dodd GD III, et al. Hepatocellular carcinoma: evaluation with biphasic, contrast-enhanced, helical CT. *Radiology* 1996;199:505.
60. Kim T, Murakami T, Hori M, et al. Small hypervascular hepatocellular carcinoma revealed by double arterial phase CT performed with single breath-hold scanning and automatic bolus tracking. *AJR Am J Roentgenol* 2002;178:899.
61. Kawata S, Murakami T, Kim T, et al. Multidetector CT: diagnostic impact of slice thickness on detection of hypervascular hepatocellular carcinoma. *AJR Am J Roentgenol* 2002;179:61.
62. Murakami T, Kim T, Kawata S, et al. Evaluation of optimal timing of arterial phase imaging for the detection of hypervascular hepatocellular carcinoma by using triple arterial phase imaging with multidetector-row helical computed tomography. *Invest Radiol* 2003;38:497.
63. Murakami T, Kim T, Hori M, Federle MP. Double arterial phase multi-detector row helical CT for detection of hypervascular hepatocellular carcinoma. *Radiology* 2003;229:931.
64. Soyer P, Roche A, Levesque M, Legmann P. CT of fibrolamellar hepatocellular carcinoma. *J Comput Assist Tomogr* 1991;15:533.
65. Ohtomo K, Itai Y, Furui S, et al. Hepatic tumors: differentiation by transverse relaxation time (T2) of magnetic resonance imaging. *Radiology* 1985;155:421.
66. Itai Y, Ohtomo K, Furui S, et al. MR imaging of hepatocellular carcinoma. *J Comput Assist Tomogr* 1986;10:963.
67. Burrel M, Llovet JM, Ayuso C, et al. MRI angiography is superior to helical CT for detection of HCC prior to liver transplantation: an explant correlation. *Hepatology* 2003;38:1034.
68. Wudel LJ Jr, Delbeke D, Morris D, et al. The role of [18F]fluorodeoxyglucose positron emission tomography imaging in the evaluation of hepatocellular carcinoma. *Am Surg* 2003;69:117.

69. Teefey SA, Hildeboldt CC, Dehdashti F, et al. Detection of primary hepatic malignancy in liver transplant candidates: prospective comparison of CT, MR imaging, US, and PET. *Radiology* 2003;226:533.

70. Dusenbery D, Ferris JV, Thaete FL, Carr BI. Percutaneous ultrasound-guided needle biopsy of hepatic mass lesions using a cytohistologic approach. Comparison of two needle types. *Am J Clin Pathol* 1995;104:583.

71. Dodd GD III, Carr BI. Percutaneous biopsy of portal vein thrombus: a new staging technique for hepatocellular carcinoma. *AJR Am J Roentgenol* 1993;161:229.

72. Dusenbery D, Dodd GD III, Carr BI. Percutaneous fine-needle aspiration of portal vein thrombi as a staging technique for hepatocellular carcinoma. Cytologic findings of 46 patients. *Cancer* 1995;75:2057.

73. Cottone M, Turri M, Caltagirone M, et al. Early detection of hepatocellular carcinoma associated with cirrhosis by ultrasound and alfa-fetoprotein: a prospective study. *Hepatogastroenterology* 1988;35:101.

74. Kanematsu T, Sonoda T, Takenaka K, et al. The value of ultrasound in the diagnosis and treatment of small hepatocellular carcinoma. *Br J Surg* 1985;72:23.

75. Colombo M, de Franchis R, Del Ninno E, et al. Hepatocellular carcinoma in Italian patients with cirrhosis. *N Engl J Med* 1991;325:675.

76. Colombo M, Mannucci PM, Brettler DB, et al. Hepatocellular carcinoma in hemophilia. *Am J Hematol* 1991;37:243.

77. Hoofnagle JH. Toward universal vaccination against hepatitis B virus. *N Engl J Med* 1989;321:1333.

78. Bilimoria MM, Lauwers GY, Doherty DA, et al. Underlying liver disease, not tumor factors, predicts long-term survival after resection of hepatocellular carcinoma. *Arch Surg* 2001;136:528.

79. Llovet JM, Bustamante J, Castells A, et al. Natural history of untreated nonsurgical hepatocellular carcinoma: rationale for the design and evaluation of therapeutic trials. *Hepatology* 1999;29:62.

80. Poon RT, Fan ST, Tsang FH, Wong J. Locoregional therapies for hepatocellular carcinoma: a critical review from the surgeon's perspective. *Ann Surg* 2002;235:466.

81. Varela M, Sala M, Llovet JM, Bruix J. Treatment of hepatocellular carcinoma: is there an optimal strategy? *Cancer Treat Rev* 2003;29:99.

82. Donckier V, Van Laethem JL, Van Gansbeke D, et al. New considerations for an overall approach to treat hepatocellular carcinoma in cirrhotic patients. *J Surg Oncol* 2003;84:36.

83. Wei AC, Tung-Ping PR, Fan ST, Wong J. Risk factors for perioperative morbidity and mortality after extended hepatectomy for hepatocellular carcinoma. *Br J Surg* 2003;90:33.

84. Makuuchi M, Imamura H, Sugawara Y, Takayama T. Progress in surgical treatment of hepatocellular carcinoma. *Oncology* 2002;62[Suppl 1]:74.

85. Torzilli G, Makuuchi M. Intraoperative ultrasonography in liver cancer. *Surg Oncol Clin N Am* 2003;12:91.

86. Makuuchi M, Imamura H, Sugawara Y, Takayama T. Progress in surgical treatment of hepatocellular carcinoma. *Oncology* 2002;62[Suppl 1]:74.

87. Belghiti J, Noun R, Malafosse R, et al. Continuous versus intermittent portal triad clamping for liver resection: a controlled study. *Ann Surg* 1999;229:369.

88. Man K, Fan ST, Ng IO, et al. Prospective evaluation of Pringle maneuver in hepatectomy for liver tumors by a randomized study. *Ann Surg* 1997;226:704.

89. Miyagawa S, Makuuchi M, Kawasaki S, Kakazu T. Criteria for safe hepatic resection. *Am J Surg* 1995;169:589.

90. Laurent A, Cherqui D, Lesurtel M, et al. Laparoscopic liver resection for subcapsular hepatocellular carcinoma complicating chronic liver disease. *Arch Surg* 2003;138:763.

91. Gigot JF, Glineur D, Santiago AJ, et al. Laparoscopic liver resection for malignant liver tumors: preliminary results of a multicenter European study. *Ann Surg* 2002;236:90.

92. Cherqui D, Husson E, Hammoud R, et al. Laparoscopic liver resections: a feasibility study in 30 patients, *Ann Surg* 2000;232:753.

93. Itamoto T, Katayama K, Miura Y, et al. Gasless laparoscopic hepatic resection for cirrhotic patients with solid liver tumors. *Surg Laparosc Endosc Percutan Tech* 2002;12:325.

94. Kurokawa T, Inagaki H, Sakamoto J, Nonami T. Hand-assisted laparoscopic anatomical left lobectomy using hemihepatic vascular control technique. *Surg Endosc* 2002;16:1637.

95. Weeks JC, Nelson H, Gelber S, Sargent D, Schroeder G. Short-term quality-of-life outcomes following laparoscopic-assisted colectomy vs open colectomy for colon cancer: a randomized trial. *JAMA* 2002;287:321.

96. Livraghi T, Meloni F. Treatment of hepatocellular carcinoma by percutaneous interventional methods. *Hepatogastroenterology* 2002;49:62.

97. Bleicher RJ, Allegra DP, Nora DT, et al. Radiofrequency ablation in 447 complex unresectable liver tumors: lessons learned. *Ann Surg Oncol* 2003;10:52.

98. Lu DS, Raman SS, Limanond P, et al. Influence of large peritumoral vessels on outcome of radiofrequency ablation of liver tumors. *J Vasc Interv Radiol* 2003;14:1267.

99. Harrison LE, Koneru B, Baramipour P, et al. Locoregional recurrences are frequent after radiofrequency ablation for hepatocellular carcinoma. *J Am Coll Surg* 2003;197:759.

100. Kitamoto M, Imagawa M, Yamada H, et al. Radiofrequency ablation in the treatment of small hepatocellular carcinomas: comparison of the radiofrequency effect with and without chemoembolization. *AJR Am J Roentgenol* 2003;181:997.

101. Giovannini M, Moutardier V, Danisi C, et al. Treatment of hepatocellular carcinoma using percutaneous radiofrequency thermoablation: results and outcomes in 56 patients. *J Gastrointest Surg* 2003;7:791.

102. Guglielmi A, Ruzzenente A, Battocchia A, et al. Radiofrequency ablation of hepatocellular carcinoma in cirrhotic patients. *Hepatogastroenterology* 2003;50:480.

103. Scaife CL, Curley SA. Complication, local recurrence, and survival rates after radiofrequency ablation for hepatic malignancies. *Surg Oncol Clin N Am* 2003;12:243.

104. Kuvshinoff BW, Ota DM. Radiofrequency ablation of liver tumors: influence of technique and tumor size. *Surgery* 2002;132:605.

105. Llovet JM, Vilana R, Bru C, et al. Increased risk of tumor seeding after percutaneous radiofrequency ablation for single hepatocellular carcinoma. *Hepatology* 2001;33:1124.

106. Bismuth H, Chiche L, Adam R, et al. Liver resection versus transplantation for hepatocellular carcinoma in cirrhotic patients. *Ann Surg* 1993;218:145.

107. Mazzaferro V, Regalia E, Doci R, et al. Liver transplantation for the treatment of small hepatocellular carcinomas in patients with cirrhosis. *N Engl J Med* 1996;334:693.

108. Marsh JW, Dvorchik I. Liver organ allocation for hepatocellular carcinoma: are we sure? *Liver Transpl* 2003;9:693.

109. Yao FY, Ferrell L, Bass NM, et al. Liver transplantation for hepatocellular carcinoma: expansion of the tumor size limits does not adversely impact survival. *Hepatology* 2001;33:1394.

110. Yao FY, Ferrell L, Bass NM, et al. Liver transplantation for hepatocellular carcinoma: comparison of the proposed UCSF criteria with the Milan criteria and the Pittsburgh modified TNM criteria. *Liver Transpl* 2002;8:765.

111. Regalia E, Coppa J, Pulvirenti A, et al. Liver transplantation for small hepatocellular carcinoma in cirrhosis: analysis of our experience. *Transplant Proc* 2001;33:1442.

112. Steinmuller T, Jonas S, Neuhaus P. Review article: liver transplantation for hepatocellular carcinoma. *Aliment Pharmacol Ther* 2003;17[Suppl 2]:138.

113. Kaihara S, Kiuchi T, Ueda M, et al. Living-donor liver transplantation for hepatocellular carcinoma. *Transplantation* 2003;75[3 Suppl]:S37.

114. Graziadei IW, Sandmueller H, Waldenberger P, et al. Chemoembolization followed by liver transplantation for hepatocellular carcinoma impedes tumor progression while on the waiting list and leads to excellent outcome. *Liver Transpl* 2003;9:557.

115. Oldhafer KJ, Chavan A, Fruhauf NR, et al. Arterial chemoembolization before liver transplantation in patients with hepatocellular carcinoma: marked tumor necrosis, but no survival benefit? *J Hepatol* 1998;29:953.

116. Majno PE, Adam R, Bismuth H, et al. Influence of preoperative transarterial lipiodol chemoembolization on resection and transplantation for hepatocellular carcinoma in patients with cirrhosis. *Ann Surg* 1997;226:688.

117. Gondolesi GE, Roayaie S, Munoz L, et al. Adult living donor liver transplantation for patients with hepatocellular carcinoma: extending UNOS priority criteria. *Ann Surg* 2004;239:142.

118. Curran RD, Billiar TR, Stuehr DJ, et al. Multiple cytokines are required to induce hepatocyte nitric oxide production and inhibit total protein synthesis. *Ann Surg* 1990;212:462.

119. Lau WY, Leung TW, Ho SK, et al. Adjuvant intra-arterial iodine-131-labelled lipiodol for resectable hepatocellular carcinoma: a prospective randomized trial. *Lancet* 1999;353:797.

120. Muto Y, Moriwaki H, Ninomiya M, et al. Prevention of second primary tumors by an acyclic retinoid, polyprenoic acid, in patients with hepatocellular carcinoma. Hepatoma Prevention Study Group. *N Engl J Med* 1996;334:1561.

121. Wu CC, Ho YZ, Ho WL, et al. Preoperative transcatheter arterial chemoembolization for resectable large hepatocellular carcinoma: a reappraisal. *Br J Surg* 1995;82:122.

122. Shiratori Y, Shiina S, Teratani T, et al. Interferon therapy after tumor ablation improves prognosis in patients with hepatocellular carcinoma associated with hepatitis C virus. *Ann Intern Med* 2003;138:299.

123. Martin RC, Jarnagin WR. Randomized clinical trials in hepatocellular carcinoma and biliary cancer. *Surg Oncol Clin N Am* 2002;11:193.

124. Simonetti RG, Liberati A, Angiolini C, Pagliaro L. Treatment of hepatocellular carcinoma: a systematic review of randomized controlled trials. *Ann Oncol* 1997;8:117.

125. Mathurin P, Rixe O, Carbonell N, et al. Review article: Overview of medical treatments in unresectable hepatocellular carcinoma—an impossible meta-analysis? *Aliment Pharmacol Ther* 1998;12:111.

126. Lee YT. Systemic and regional treatment of primary carcinoma of the liver. *Cancer Treat Rev* 1977;4:195.

127. Murata K, Shiraki K, Kawakita T, et al. Low-dose chemotherapy of cisplatin and 5-fluorouracil or doxorubicin via implanted fusion port for unresectable hepatocellular carcinoma. *Anticancer Res* 2003;23:1719.

128. Ando E, Tanaka M, Yamashita F, et al. Hepatic arterial infusion chemotherapy for advanced hepatocellular carcinoma with portal vein tumor thrombosis: analysis of 48 cases. *Cancer* 2002;95:588.

129. Carr BI, Zajko A, Bron K. Prospective randomized study of intrahepatic artery chemotherapy with cisplatin and doxorubicin, with or without Lipiodol in the treatment of advanced-stage hepatocellular carcinoma. *Am Soc Clin Oncol* 1993;668:12.

130. Carr BI, Zajko A, Bron K, et al. Phase II study of Spherex (degradable starch microspheres) injected into the hepatic artery in conjunction with doxorubicin and cisplatin in the treatment of advanced-stage hepatocellular carcinoma: interim analysis. *Semin Oncol* 1997;24:S6.

131. Furuse J, Ishii H, Satake M, et al. Pilot study of transcatheter arterial chemoembolization with degradable starch microspheres in patients with hepatocellular carcinoma. *Am J Clin Oncol* 2003;26:159.

132. Alexander HR Jr, Allegra CJ, Lawrence TS. Metastatic cancer to the liver. In: DeVita VT Jr, Hellman S, Rosenberg SA, eds. *Cancer: principles and practice of oncology*. Philadelphia: Lippincott Williams & Wilkins, 2001.

133. Reyes JD, Carr B, Dvorchik I, et al. Liver transplantation and chemotherapy for hepatoblastoma and hepatocellular cancer in childhood and adolescence. *J Pediatr* 2000;136:795.

134. Gerber DA, Arcement C, Carr B, et al. Use of intrahepatic chemotherapy to treat advanced pediatric hepatic malignancies. *J Pediatr Gastroenterol Nutr* 2000;30:137.

135. Arcement CM, Towbin RB, Meza MP, et al. Intrahepatic chemoembolization in unresectable pediatric liver malignancies. *Pediatr Radiol* 2000;30:779.

136. Carr BI. Escalating cisplatin doses by hepatic artery infusion (HAI) for advanced-stage hepatocellular carcinoma (HCC). 367. 6th International Conference on Anti-Cancer Treatment, 1996.

137. Stuart K, Stokes K, Jenkins R, Trey C, Clouse M. Treatment of hepatocellular carcinoma using doxorubicin/ethiodized oil/gelatin powder chemoembolization. *Cancer* 1993;72:3202.

138. Lo CM, Ngan H, Tso WK, et al. Randomized controlled trial of transarterial lipiodol chemoembolization for unresectable hepatocellular carcinoma. *Hepatology* 2002;35:1164.

139. Llovet JM, Real MI, Montana X, et al. Arterial embolization or chemoembolization versus symptomatic treatment in patients with unresectable hepatocellular carcinoma: a randomized controlled trial. *Lancet* 2002;359:1734.

140. Steel J, Baum A, Carr B. Quality of life in patients diagnosed with primary hepatocellular carcinoma: hepatic arterial infusion of Cisplatin versus 90-Yttrium microspheres (Therasphere). *Psychooncology* 2004;13:73.
141. Ebied OM, Federle MP, Carr BI, et al. Evaluation of responses to chemoembolization in patients with unresectable hepatocellular carcinoma. *Cancer* 2003;97:1042.
142. Lai CL, Wu PC, Lok AS, et al. Recombinant alpha 2 interferon is superior to doxorubicin for inoperable hepatocellular carcinoma: a prospective randomized trial. *Br J Cancer* 1989;60:928.
143. Llovet JM, Sala M, Castells L, et al. Randomized controlled trial of interferon treatment for advanced hepatocellular carcinoma. *Hepatology* 2000;31:54.
144. Lai CL, Lau JY, Wu PC, et al. Recombinant interferon-alpha in inoperable hepatocellular carcinoma: a randomized controlled trial. *Hepatology* 1993;17:389.
145. Falkson G, Lipsitz S, Borden E, Simson I, Haller D. Hepatocellular carcinoma. An ECOG randomized phase II study of beta-interferon and menogaril. *Am J Clin Oncol* 1995;18:287.
146. Farinati F, De Maria N, Fornasiero A, et al. Prospective controlled trial with antiestrogen drug tamoxifen in patients with unresectable hepatocellular carcinoma. *Dig Dis Sci* 1992;37:659.
147. Martinez Cerezo FJ, Tomas A, Donoso L, et al. Controlled trial of tamoxifen in patients with advanced hepatocellular carcinoma. *J Hepatol* 1994;20:702.
148. Liu CL, Fan ST, Ng IO, et al. Treatment of advanced hepatocellular carcinoma with tamoxifen and the correlation with expression of hormone receptors: a prospective randomized study *Am J Gastroenterol* 2000;95:218.
149. Tamoxifen in treatment of hepatocellular carcinoma: a randomized controlled trial. CLIP Group. *Lancet* 1998;352:17.
150. Yuen MF, Ooi CG, Hui CK, et al. A pilot study of transcatheter arterial interferon embolization for patients with hepatocellular carcinoma. *Cancer* 2003;97:2776.
151. Brans B, Van Laere K, Gemmel F, et al. Combining iodine-131 Lipiodol therapy with low-dose cisplatin as a radiosensitizer: preliminary results in hepatocellular carcinoma. *Eur J Nucl Med Mol Imaging* 2002;29:928.
152. Abrams RA, Pajak TF, Haulk TL, Flam M, Asbell SO. Survival results among patients with alpha-fetoprotein-positive, unresectable hepatocellular carcinoma: analysis of three sequential treatments of the RTOG and Johns Hopkins Oncology Center. *Cancer J Sci Am* 1998;4:178.
153. Lawrence TS, Dworzanin TM, Walker-Andrews SC, et al. Treatment of cancers involving the liver and porta hepatis with external beam irradiation and intraarterial hepatic fluorodeoxyuridine. *Int J Radiat Oncol Biol Phys* 1991;20:555.
154. Seong J, Park HC, Han KH, Chon CY. Clinical results and prognostic factors in radiotherapy for unresectable hepatocellular carcinoma: a retrospective study of 158 patients. *Int J Radiat Oncol Biol Phys* 2003;55:329.
155. Park HC, Seong J, Han KH, et al. Dose-response relationship in local radiotherapy for hepatocellular carcinoma. *Int J Radiat Oncol Biol Phys* 2002;54:150.
156. Robertson JM, Lawrence TS, Dworzanin LM, et al. Treatment of primary hepatobiliary cancers with conformal radiation therapy and regional chemotherapy. *J Clin Oncol* 1993;11:1286.
157. Leung WT, Lau WY, Ho S, et al. Selective internal radiation therapy with intra-arterial iodine-131-Lipiodol in inoperable hepatocellular carcinoma. *J Nucl Med* 1994;35:1313.
158. Order S, Pajak T, Leibel S, et al. A randomized prospective trial comparing full dose chemotherapy to 131I antiferritin: an RTOG study. *Int J Radiat Oncol Biol Phys* 1991;20:953.
159. Carr BI, Amesur N, Zajko A, et al. Safety and efficacy of hepatic artery microspheres in unresectable hepatocellular carcinoma (HCC). *Proc Am Soc Clin Oncol* 2003;22(abst 1046).
160. Lau WY, Ho S, Leung TW, et al. Selective internal radiation therapy for nonresectable hepatocellular carcinoma with intraarterial infusion of 90yttrium microspheres. *Int J Radiat Oncol Biol Phys* 1998;40:583.
161. Carr B. Hepatic arterial 90-Yttrium glass microspheres (Therasphere) for unresectable hepatocellular carcinoma: interim safety and survival data on 65 patients. *Liver Transpl* 2004;10:S107.
162. Leung TW, Johnson PJ. Systemic therapy for hepatocellular carcinoma. *Semin Oncol* 2001; 28:514.
163. Dancey JE, Shepherd FA, Paul K, et al. Treatment of nonresectable hepatocellular carcinoma with intrahepatic 90Y-microspheres. *J Nucl Med* 2000;41:1673.
164. Carr BI. A phase I/phase II study of high-dose vitamin K in patients with advanced, inoperable hepatocellular carcinoma. Proc AASLD. *Hepatology* 1994;20:727.
165. Zamibone A, Biasi L, Graffeo M, et al. Phase II study of high-dose vitamin K1 in hepatocellular carcinoma. *Proc Am Soc Clin Oncol* 1998;17:307A.
166. Carr BI, Wang Z, Kar S. K vitamins, PTP antagonism, and cell growth arrest. *J Cell Physiol* 2002;193:263.
167. Carr BI. Complete suppression of DCP/PIVKA 2 levels by vitamin K1 administration to patients with hepatocellular carcinoma. *Hepatology* 1993;18:500.
168. Marsh JW, Finkelstein SD, Demetris AJ, et al. Genotyping of hepatocellular carcinoma in liver transplant recipients adds predictive power for determining recurrence-free survival. *Liver Transpl* 2003;9:664.
169. Finkelstein SD, Marsh W, Demetris AJ, et al. Microdissection-based allelotyping discriminates de novo tumor from intrahepatic spread in hepatocellular carcinoma. *Hepatology* 2003;37:871.
170. Ringe B, Wittekind C, Weimann A, Tusch G, Pichlmayr R. Results of hepatic resection and transplantation for fibrolamellar carcinoma. *Surg Gynecol Obstet* 1992;175:299.
171. Soreide O, Czerniak A, Bradpiece H, Bloom S, Blumgart L. Characteristics of fibrolamellar hepatocellular carcinoma. A study of nine cases and a review of the literature. *Am J Surg* 1986;151:518.
172. Ruffin MT. Fibrolamellar hepatoma. *Am J Gastroenterol* 1990;85:577.
173. Vauthey JN, Klimstra D, Franceschi D, et al. Factors affecting long-term outcome after hepatic resection for hepatocellular carcinoma. *Am J Surg* 1995;169:28.
174. Pinna AD, Iwatsuki S, Lee RG, et al. Treatment of fibrolamellar hepatoma with subtotal hepatectomy or transplantation. *Hepatology* 1997;26:877.
175. El Gazzaz G, Wong W, El Hadary MK, et al. Outcome of liver resection and transplantation for fibrolamellar hepatocellular carcinoma. *Transpl Int* 2000;13[Suppl 1]:S406.
176. Al Qabandi W, Jenkinson HC, Buckels JA, et al. Orthotopic liver transplantation for unresectable hepatoblastoma: a single center's experience. *J Pediatr Surg* 1999;34:1261.
177. Reyes JD, Carr B, Dvorchik I, et al. Liver transplantation and chemotherapy for hepatoblastoma and hepatocellular cancer in childhood and adolescence. *J Pediatr* 2000;136:795.
178. Makhlouf HR, Ishak KG, Goodman ZD. Epithelioid hemangioendothelioma of the liver: a clinicopathologic study of 137 cases. *Cancer* 1999;85:562.
179. Parkin DM, Muir C, Whelan SL, et al. *Cancer incidence in five continents.* Lyon, France: IARC Scientific Publications, 1987.
180. Bosch X, Munoz N. Epidemiology of hepatocellular carcinoma. In: Okuda K, Ishak KG, eds. *Neoplasms of the liver.* New York: Springer-Verlag, 1987:3.
181. Kanematsu T, Shirabe K, Sugimachi K. Surgical strategy for primary hepatocellular carcinoma associated with cirrhosis. *Semin Surg Oncol* 1990;6:36.
182. Yamanaka N, Okamoto E, Toyosaka A, et al. Prognostic factors after hepatectomy for hepatocellular carcinomas. A univariate and multivariate analysis. *Cancer* 1990;65:1104.
183. Liver Cancer Study Group Japan. Primary liver cancer in Japan. Clinicopathologic features and results of surgical treatment. *Ann Surg* 1990;211:277.
184. Ringe B, Pichlmayr R, Wittekind C, Tusch G. Surgical treatment of hepatocellular carcinoma: experience with liver resection and transplantation in 198 patients. *World J Surg* 1991;15:270.
185. Sasaki Y, Imaoka S, Masutani S, et al. Influence of coexisting cirrhosis on long-term prognosis after surgery in patients with hepatocellular carcinoma. *Surgery* 1992;112:515.
186. Nagasue N, Kohno H, Chang YC, et al. Liver resection for hepatocellular carcinoma. Results of 229 consecutive patients during 11 years. *Ann Surg* 1993;217:375.
187. Takenaka K, Shimada M, Higashi H, et al. Liver resection for hepatocellular carcinoma in the elderly. *Arch Surg* 1994;129:846.
188. Lai EC, Fan ST, Lo CM, et al. Hepatic resection for hepatocellular carcinoma. An audit of 343 patients. *Ann Surg* 1995;221:291.
189. Vauthey JN, Klimstra D, Franceschi D, et al. Factors affecting long-term outcome after hepatic resection for hepatocellular carcinoma. *Am J Surg* 1995;169:28.
190. Kawasaki S, Makuuchi M, Miyagawa S, et al. Results of hepatic resection for hepatocellular carcinoma *World J Surg* 1995;19:31.
191. Llovet JM, Fuster J, Bruix J. Intention-to-treat analysis of surgical treatment for early hepatocellular carcinoma: resection versus transplantation. *Hepatology* 1999;30:1434.
192. Yamamoto J, Iwatsuki S, Kosuge T, et al. Should hepatomas be treated with hepatic resection or transplantation? *Cancer* 1999;86:1151.
193. Arii S, Yamaoka Y, Futagawa S, et al. Results of surgical and nonsurgical treatment for small-sized hepatocellular carcinomas: a retrospective and nationwide survey in Japan. The liver cancer study group of Japan. *Hepatology* 2000;32:1224.
194. Wayne JD, Lauwers GY, Ikai I, et al. Preoperative predictors of survival after resection of small hepatocellular carcinomas. *Ann Surg* 2002;235:722.
195. Yeh CN, Chen MF, Lee WC, Jeng LB. Prognostic factors of hepatic resection for hepatocellular carcinoma with cirrhosis: univariate and multivariate analysis. *J Surg Oncol* 2002;81:195.
196. Ziparo V, Balducci G, Lucandri G, et al. Indications and results of resection for hepatocellular carcinoma. *Eur J Surg Oncol* 2002;28:723.
197. Belghiti J, Regimbeau JM, Durand F, et al. Resection of hepatocellular carcinoma: a European experience on 328 cases. *Hepatogastroenterology* 2002;49:41.
198. Kanematsu T, Furui J, Yanaga K, et al. A 16-year experience in performing hepatic resection in 303 patients with hepatocellular carcinoma: 1985–2000. *Surgery* 2002;131[1 Suppl]:S153.
199. Grazi GL, Cescon M, Ravaioli M, et al. Liver resection for hepatocellular carcinoma in cirrhotics and noncirrhotics. Evaluation of clinicopathologic features and comparison of risk factors for long-term survival and tumour recurrence in a single centre. *Aliment Pharmacol Ther* 2003;17[Suppl 2]:119.
200. Lang BH, Poon RT, Fan ST, Wong J. Perioperative and long-term outcome of major hepatic resection for small solitary hepatocellular carcinoma in patients with cirrhosis. *Arch Surg* 2003;138:1207.
201. Cha CH, Ruo L, Fong Y, et al. Resection of hepatocellular carcinoma in patients otherwise eligible for transplantation. *Ann Surg* 2003;238:315.
202. De Carlis L, Giacomoni A, Pirotta V, et al. Surgical treatment of hepatocellular cancer in the era of hepatic transplantation. *J Am Coll Surg* 2003;196:887.
203. Chen JY, Chau GY, Lui WY, et al. Clinicopathologic features and factors related to survival of patients with small hepatocellular carcinoma after hepatic resection. *World J Surg* 2003;27:294.
204. Tsuzuki T, Sugioka A, Ueda M, et al. Hepatic resection for hepatocellular carcinoma. *Surgery* 1990;107:511.
205. O'Grady JG, Polson RJ, Rolles K, Calne RY, Williams R. Liver transplantation for malignant disease. Results in 93 consecutive patients. *Ann Surg* 1988;207:373.
206. Olthoff KM, Millis JM, Rosove MH, et al. Is liver transplantation justified for the treatment of hepatic malignancies? *Arch Surg* 1990;125:1261.
207. Iwatsuki S, Starzl TE, Sheahan DG, et al. Hepatic resection versus transplantation for hepatocellular carcinoma. *Ann Surg* 1991;214:221.
208. Penn I. Hepatic transplantation for primary and metastatic cancers of the liver. *Surgery* 1991;110:726.
209. Ringe B, Pichlmayr R, Wittekind C, Tusch G. Surgical treatment of hepatocellular carcinoma: experience with liver resection and transplantation in 198 patients. *World J Surg* 1991;15:270.
210. Tan KC, Rela M, Ryder SD, et al. Experience of orthotopic liver transplantation and hepatic resection for hepatocellular carcinoma of less than 8 cm in patients with cirrhosis. *Br J Surg* 1995;82:253.
211. Klintmalm GB. Liver transplantation for hepatocellular carcinoma: a registry report of the impact of tumor characteristics on outcome. *Ann Surg* 1998;228:479.
212. Otto G, Heuschen U, Hofmann WJ, et al. Survival and recurrence after liver transplantation versus liver resection for hepatocellular carcinoma: a retrospective analysis. *Ann Surg* 1998;227:424.

213. Pichlmayr R, Weimann A, Oldhafer KJ, et al. Appraisal of transplantation for malignant tumours of the liver with special reference to early stage hepatocellular carcinoma. *Eur J Surg Oncol* 1998;24:60.
214. Hemming AW, Cattral MS, Reed AI, et al. Liver transplantation for hepatocellular carcinoma. *Ann Surg* 2001;233:652.
215. HHS/HRSA/OSP/DOT and UNOS. 2000 Annual Report of the U.S. Scientific Registry of Transplant Recipients and the Organ Procurement and Transplantation Network: Transplant Data: 1989–1998. 2004. Rockville, MD and Richmond, VA, 2-16-2001.
216. Bigourdan JM, Jaeck D, Meyer N, et al. Small hepatocellular carcinoma in Child A cirrhotic patients: hepatic resection versus transplantation. *Liver Transpl* 2003;9:513.
217. Tamura S, Kato T, Berho M, et al. Impact of histological grade of hepatocellular carcinoma on the outcome of liver transplantation. *Arch Surg* 2001;136:25.
218. Jonas S, Bechstein WO, Steinmuller T, et al. Vascular invasion and histopathologic grading determine outcome after liver transplantation for hepatocellular carcinoma in cirrhosis. *Hepatology* 2001;33:1080.
219. Harnois DM, Steers J, Andrews JC, et al. Preoperative hepatic artery chemoembolization followed by orthotopic liver transplantation for hepatocellular carcinoma. *Liver Transpl Surg* 1999;5:192.
220. Llovet JM, Bruix J, Fuster J, et al. Liver transplantation for small hepatocellular carcinoma: the tumor-node-metastasis classification does not have prognostic power. *Hepatology* 1998;27:1572.
221. Figueras J, Jaurrieta E, Valls C, et al. Survival after liver transplantation in cirrhotic patients with and without hepatocellular carcinoma: a comparative study. *Hepatology* 1997;25:1485.
222. Venook AP, Ferrell LD, Roberts JP, et al. Liver transplantation for hepatocellular carcinoma: results with preoperative chemoembolization. *Liver Transpl Surg* 1995;1:242.
223. Romani F, Belli LS, Rondinara GF, et al. The role of transplantation in small hepatocellular carcinoma complicating cirrhosis of the liver. *J Am Coll Surg* 1994;178:379.
224. Sciarrino E, Simonetti RG, Le Moli S, Pagliaro L. Adriamycin treatment for hepatocellular carcinoma. Experience with 109 patients. *Cancer* 1985;56:2751.
225. Chlebowski RT, Brzechwa-Adjukiewicz A, Cowden A, et al. Doxorubicin (75 mg/m^2) for hepatocellular carcinoma: clinical and pharmacokinetic results. *Cancer Treat Rep* 1984;68:487.
226. Ihde DC, Kane RC, Cohen MH, McIntire KR, Minna JD. Adriamycin therapy in American patients with hepatocellular carcinoma. *Cancer Treat Rep* 1977;61:1385.
227. Falkson G, MacIntyre JM, Moertel CG, Johnson LA, Scherman RC. Primary liver cancer. An Eastern Cooperative Oncology Group Trial. *Cancer* 1984;54:970.
228. Falkson G, MacIntyre JM, Schutt AJ, et al. Neocarzinostatin versus m-AMSA or doxorubicin in hepatocellular carcinoma. *J Clin Oncol* 1984;2:581.
229. Ravry MJ, Omura GA, Bartolucci AA. Phase II evaluation of doxorubicin plus bleomycin in hepatocellular carcinoma: a Southeastern Cancer Study Group trial. *Cancer Treat Rep* 1984;68:1517.
230. Cavalli F, Rozencweig M, Renard J, Goldhirsch A, Hansen HH. Phase II study of oral VP-16-213 in hepatocellular carcinoma. *Eur J Cancer Clin Oncol* 1981;17:1079.
231. Melia WM, Johnson PJ, Williams R. Induction of remission in hepatocellular carcinoma. *Cancer* 1983;51:206.
232. Melia WM, Westaby D, Williams R. Diamminedichloride platinum (cis-platinum) in the treatment of hepatocellular carcinoma. *Clin Oncol* 1981;7:275.
233. Ravry MJ, Omura GA, Bartolucci AA, et al. Phase II evaluation of cisplatin in advanced hepatocellular carcinoma and cholangiocarcinoma: a Southeastern Cancer Study Group trial. *Cancer Treat Rep* 1986;70:311.
234. Falkson G, Ryan LM, Johnson LA, et al. A random phase II study of mitoxantrone and cisplatin in patients with hepatocellular carcinoma. An ECOG study. *Cancer* 1987;60:2141.
235. Colleoni M, Buzzoni R, Bajetta E, et al. A phase II study of mitoxantrone combined with beta-interferon in unresectable hepatocellular carcinoma. *Cancer* 1993;72:3196.
236. Chao Y, Chan WK, Birkhofer MJ, et al. Phase II and pharmacokinetic study of paclitaxel therapy for unresectable hepatocellular carcinoma patients. *Br J Cancer* 1998;78:34.
237. Patt YZ, Hassan MM, Lozano RD, et al. Phase II trial of systemic continuous fluorouracil and subcutaneous recombinant interferon alfa-2b for treatment of hepatocellular carcinoma. *J Clin Oncol* 2003;21:421.
238. Patt YZ, Hassan MM, Lozano RD, et al. Durable clinical response of refractory hepatocellular carcinoma to orally administered thalidomide. *Am J Clin Oncol* 2000;23:319.
239. Okada S, Ueno H, Okusaka T, et al. Phase II trial of cisplatin, mitoxantrone and continuous infusion 5-fluorouracil for hepatocellular carcinoma. *Proc Am Soc Clin Oncol* 1999;18:248a (abst 952).
240. Llovet JM, Bruix J. Systematic review of randomized trials for unresectable hepatocellular carcinoma: chemoembolization improves survival. *Hepatology* 2003;37:429.
241. Koda M, Murawaki Y, Mitsuda A, et al. Combination therapy with transcatheter arterial chemoembolization and percutaneous ethanol injection compared with percutaneous ethanol injection alone for patients with small hepatocellular carcinoma: a randomized control study. *Cancer* 2001;92:1516.
242. Onohara S, Kobayashi H, Itoh Y, Shinohara S. Intra-arterial cis-platinum infusion with sodium thiosulfate protection and angiotensin II induced hypertension for treatment of hepatocellular carcinoma. *Acta Radiol* 1988;29:197.
243. Kajanti M, Rissanen P, Virkkunen P, Franssila K, Mantyla M. Regional intra-arterial infusion of cisplatin in primary hepatocellular carcinoma. A phase II study. *Cancer* 1986;58:2386.
244. Nagasue N, Yukaya, H, Okamura J. Intra-arterial administration of epirubicin in the treatment of non-resectable hepatocellular carcinoma. *Cancer Chemother Pharmacol* 1987;19:183.
245. Sasaki Y, Imaoka S, Kasugai H, et al. A new approach to chemoembolization therapy for hepatoma using ethiodized oil, cisplatin, and gelatin sponge. *Cancer* 1987;60:1194.
246. Kasugai H, Kojima J, Tatsuta M, et al. Treatment of hepatocellular carcinoma by transcatheter arterial embolization combined with intraarterial infusion of a mixture of cisplatin and ethiodized oil. *Gastroenterology* 1989;97:965.
247. Ohnishi K, Tsuchiya S, Nakayama T, et al. Arterial chemoembolization of hepatocellular carcinoma with mitomycin C microcapsules. *Radiology* 1984;152:51.
248. Lin DY, Liaw YF, Lee TY, Lai CM. Hepatic arterial embolization in patients with unresectable hepatocellular carcinoma—a randomized controlled trial. *Gastroenterology* 1988;94:453.
249. Fujimoto S, Miyazaki M, Endoh F, et al. Biodegradable mitomycin C microspheres given intra-arterially for inoperable hepatic cancer. With particular reference to a comparison with continuous infusion of mitomycin C and 5-fluorouracil. *Cancer* 1985;56:2404.
250. Audisio RA, Doci R, Mazzaferro V, et al. Hepatic arterial embolization with microencapsulated mitomycin C for unresectable hepatocellular carcinoma in cirrhosis. *Cancer* 1990;66:22.
251. Kobayashi H, Hidaka H, Kajiya Y, et al. Treatment of hepatocellular carcinoma by transarterial injection of anticancer agents in iodized oil suspension or of radioactive iodized oil solution. *Acta Radiol Diagn* 1986;27:139.
252. Kanematsu T, Furuta T, Takenaka K, et al. A 5-year experience of lipiodolization: selective regional chemotherapy for 200 patients with hepatocellular carcinoma. *Hepatology* 1989;10:98.
253. Shibata J, Fujiyama S, Sato T, et al. Hepatic arterial injection chemotherapy with cisplatin suspended in an oily lymphographic agent for hepatocellular carcinoma. *Cancer* 1989;64:1586.
254. Konno T, Maeda H, Iwai K, et al. Effect of arterial administration of high-molecular-weight anticancer agent SMANCS with lipid lymphographic agent on hepatoma: a preliminary report. *Eur J Cancer Clin Oncol* 1983;19:1053.
255. Pelletier G, Roche A, Ink O, et al. A randomized trial of hepatic arterial chemoembolization in patients with unresectable hepatocellular carcinoma. *J Hepatol* 1990;11:181.
256. Carr BI. Aggressive treatment for advanced hepatocellular carcinoma (HCC): high response rates and prolonged survival. *Hepatology* 1991;14:243.
257. Venook AP, Stagg RJ, Lewis BJ, et al. Chemoembolization for hepatocellular carcinoma. *J Clin Oncol* 1990;8:1108.
258. Ohnishi K, Sugita S, Nomura F, Iida S, Tanabe Y. Arterial chemoembolization with mitomycin C microcapsules followed by transcatheter hepatic artery embolization for hepatocellular carcinoma. *Am J Gastroenterol* 1987;82:876.
259. Beppu T, Ohara C, Yamaguchi Y, et al. A new approach to chemoembolization for unresectable hepatocellular carcinoma using aclarubicin microspheres in combination with cisplatin suspended in iodized oil. *Cancer* 1991;68:2555.
260. Groupe d'Etude et de Traitement du Carcinome Hepatocellulaire. A comparison of lipiodol chemoembolization and conservative treatment for unresectable hepatocellular carcinoma. *N Engl J Med* 1995;332:1256.
261. Bruix J, Castells A, Montana X, et al. Phase II study of transarterial embolization in European patients with hepatocellular carcinoma: need for controlled trials. *Hepatology* 1994;20:643.
262. Carr BI. Hepatic artery chemoembolization for advanced stage HCC: experience of 650 patients. *Hepatogastroenterology* 2002;49:79.
263. Ngan H, Lai CL, Fan ST, et al. Treatment of inoperable hepatocellular carcinoma by transcatheter arterial chemoembolization using an emulsion of cisplatin in iodized oil and gelfoam. *Clin Radiol* 1993;47:315.
264. Kawai S, Tani M, Okamura J, et al. Prospective and randomized clinical trial for the treatment of hepatocellular carcinoma—a comparison between L-TAE with farmorubicin and L-TAE with adriamycin: preliminary results (second cooperative study). Cooperative study group for liver cancer treatment of Japan. *Cancer Chemother Pharmacol* 1994;33[Suppl]:S97.
265. Yamamoto M, Iizuka H, Fujii H, Matsuda M, Miura K. Hepatic arterial infusion of interleukin-2 in advanced hepatocellular carcinoma. *Acta Oncol* 1993;32:43.
266. Yoshimi F, Nagao T, Inoue S, et al. Comparison of hepatectomy and transcatheter arterial chemoembolization for the treatment of hepatocellular carcinoma: necessity for prospective randomized trial. *Hepatology* 1992;16:702.
267. Rougier P, Roche A, Pelletier G, et al. Efficacy of chemoembolization for hepatocellular carcinomas: experience from the Gustave Roussy Institute and the Bicetre Hospital. *J Surg Oncol* 1993;3[Suppl]:94.
268. Kawai S, Okamura J, Ogawa M, et al. Prospective and randomized clinical trial for the treatment of hepatocellular carcinoma—a comparison of lipiodol-transcatheter arterial embolization with and without adriamycin (first cooperative study). The cooperative study group for liver cancer treatment of Japan. *Cancer Chemother Pharmacol* 1992;31[Suppl]:S1.
269. Kawai S, Tani M, Okamura J, et al. Prospective and randomized trial of lipiodol-transcatheter arterial chemoembolization for treatment of hepatocellular carcinoma: a comparison of epirubicin and doxorubicin (second cooperative study). The cooperative study group for liver cancer treatment of Japan. *Semin Oncol* 1997;24:S6.
270. Watanabe S, Nishioka M, Ohta Y, et al. Prospective and randomized controlled study of chemoembolization therapy in patients with advanced hepatocellular carcinoma. *Cancer Chemother Pharmacol* 1994;33[Suppl]:S93.
271. Chang JM, Tzeng WS, Pan HB, Yang CF, Lai KH. Transcatheter arterial embolization with or without cisplatin treatment of hepatocellular carcinoma. A randomized controlled study. *Cancer* 1994;74:2449.
272. Hatanaka Y, Yamashita Y, Takahashi M, et al. Unresectable hepatocellular carcinoma: analysis of prognostic factors in transcatheter management. *Radiology* 1995;195:747.
273. Uchino J, Une Y, Sato Y, et al. Chemohormonal therapy of unresectable hepatocellular carcinoma. *Am J Clin Oncol* 1993;16:206.
274. Madden MV, Krige JE, Bailey S, et al. Randomized trial of targeted chemotherapy with lipiodol and 5-epidoxorubicin compared with symptomatic treatment for hepatoma. *Gut* 1993;34:1598.
275. Chung YH, Song IH, Song BD, et al. Combined therapy consisting of intra-arterial cisplatin infusion and systemic interferon-alpha for hepatocellular carcinoma patients with major portal vein thrombosis or distant metastases. *Cancer* 2000;88:1986.
276. Lin DY, Liaw YF, Lee TY, Lai CM. Hepatic arterial embolization in patients with unresectable hepatocellular carcinoma—a randomized controlled trial. *Gastroenterology* 1988;94:453.
277. Yoshikawa M, Saisho H, Ebara M, et al. A randomized trial of intrahepatic arterial infusion of 4'-epidoxorubicin with Lipiodol versus 4'-epidoxorubicin alone in the treatment of hepatocellular carcinoma. *Cancer Chemother Pharmacol* 1994;33[Suppl]:S149.

278. Kajanti M, Pyrhonen S, Mantyla M, Rissanen P. Intra-arterial and intravenous use of 4' epidoxorubicin combined with 5-fluorouracil in primary hepatocellular carcinoma. A randomized comparison. *Am J Clin Oncol* 1992;15:37.

279. Tzoracoleftherakis EE, Spiliotis JD, Kyriakopoulou T, Kakkos SK. Intra-arterial versus systemic chemotherapy for non-operable hepatocellular carcinoma. *Hepatogastroenterology* 1999;46:1122.

280. Bhattacharya S, Novell JR, Dusheiko GM, et al. Epirubicin-Lipiodol chemotherapy versus 131iodine-Lipiodol radiotherapy in the treatment of unresectable hepatocellular carcinoma. *Cancer* 1995;76:2202.

281. Pelletier G, Roche A, Ink O, et al. A randomized trial of hepatic arterial chemoembolization in patients with unresectable hepatocellular carcinoma. *J Hepatol* 1990;11:181.

282. Bruix J, Llovet JM, Castells A, et al. Transarterial embolization versus symptomatic treatment in patients with advanced hepatocellular carcinoma: results of a randomized, controlled trial in a single institution. *Hepatology* 1998;27:1578.

283. Pelletier G, Ducreux M, Gay F, et al. Treatment of unresectable hepatocellular carcinoma with lipiodol chemoembolization: a multicenter randomized trial. Groupe CHC. *J Hepatol* 1998;29:129.

284. Camma C, Schepis F, Orlando A, et al. Transarterial chemoembolization for unresectable hepatocellular carcinoma: meta-analysis of randomized controlled trials. *Radiology* 2002;224:47.

285. Grimaldi C, Bleiberg H, Gay F, et al. Evaluation of antiandrogen therapy in unresectable hepatocellular carcinoma: results of a European Organization for Research and Treatment of Cancer multicentric double-blind trial. *J Clin Oncol* 1998;16:411.

286. Rabe C, Pilz T, Allgaier HP, et al. Clinical outcome of a cohort of 63 patients with hepatocellular carcinoma treated with octreotide. *Z Gastroenterol* 2002;40:395.

287. Dimitroulopoulos D, Xinopoulos D, Tsamakidis K, et al. The role of Sandostatin LAR in treating patients with advanced hepatocellular cancer. *Hepatogastroenterology* 2002;49:1245.

288. Villa E, Ferretti I, Grottola A, et al. Hormonal therapy with megestrol in inoperable hepatocellular carcinoma characterized by variant oestrogen receptors. *Br J Cancer* 2001;84:881.

289. Chao Y, Chan WK, Wang SS, et al. Phase II study of megestrol acetate in the treatment of hepatocellular carcinoma. *J Gastroenterol Hepatol* 1997;12:277.

290. Patt YZ, Hassan MM, Lozano RD, et al. Durable clinical response of refractory hepatocellular carcinoma to orally administered thalidomide. *Am J Clin Oncol* 2000;23:319.

291. Salem R, Thurston KG, Carr BI, Goin JE, Geschwind JF. Yttrium-90 microspheres: radiation therapy for unresectable liver cancer. *J Vasc Interv Radiol* 2002;13:S223.

292. McGlynn KA, Tsao L, Hsing AW, Devessa SS, Fraumeni JF. International trends and patterns of primary liver cancer. *Int J Cancer* 2001;94:290.

SECTION 5

DAVID L. BARTLETT
RAMESH K. RAMANATHAN
MELVIN DEUTSCH

Cancer of the Biliary Tree

The biliary tract or the biliary drainage system includes the intrahepatic and extrahepatic bile ducts and the gallbladder. The terminology of biliary tract cancers has varied, and semantic confusion still exists (Fig. 29.5-1). The term *cholangiocarcinoma* refers to all tumors arising from bile duct epithelium. Cholangiocarcinomas are differentiated by the anatomic site of origin: intrahepatic, hilar, and distal. Intrahepatic cholangiocarcinomas present as liver masses. Hilar cholangiocarcinomas involve the confluens of the left and right duct and usually both intrahepatic and extrahepatic ducts. They are also known as Klatskin's tumors.[1] Distal cholangiocarcinomas involve the common or proper hepatic duct or both without extension to the confluens of the right and left ducts. Distal cholangiocarcinomas usually involve the intrapancreatic portion of the bile duct. Because of their distinctly different epidemiology, etiology, and treatment, tumors of the gallbladder are considered separate entities.[2]

What is common among all biliary tract cancers is general rarity, difficulty in diagnosis, and overall poor prognosis. This leads to a paucity of data from which to define the natural history and optimal treatment regimens. Overall, these are highly lethal cancers, with reported 1- and 2-year survival rates after diagnosis of 25% and 13% respectively, with few reported long-term survivors.[3] There are grounds for optimism, however, because studies have shown improved survival in patients with cholangiocarcinomas over the last decade.[4,5] The management of patients with biliary tract cancer is complex because of the obstruction of bile drainage and the subsequent risk of cholangitis and liver failure. A dedicated, multidisciplinary team that includes a surgeon, gastroenterologist, interventional radiologist, pathologist, medical oncologist, and radiation oncologist is required for the effective management of these patients.

CHOLANGIOCARCINOMAS

EPIDEMIOLOGY

Cholangiocarcinomas are uncommon cancers in the United States. There are an estimated 7000 new cases of gallbladder cancer and cholangiocarcinoma diagnosed annually in the United States, with approximately 3500 deaths in the same period.[6] Cholangiocarcinomas are less common than gallbladder cancers and probably account for 2000 to 3000 cases per year.[7] The incidence and mortality from cholangiocarcinomas has been on the rise in the United States and other countries.[8] The incidence of cholangiocarcinoma increases with age, and the majority of patients are older than 65 years. The peak incidence is in the eighth decade of life, and cholangiocarcinomas are slightly more common in men.[9,10] Hilar cholangiocarcinomas are the most common (67%), followed by distal cholangiocarcinomas (27%), then intrahepatic cholangiocarcinomas (6%).[11] Patients with a defined cause, such as primary sclerosing cholangitis (PSC) or choledochal cysts, tend to develop cholangiocarcinoma at a younger age.[7]

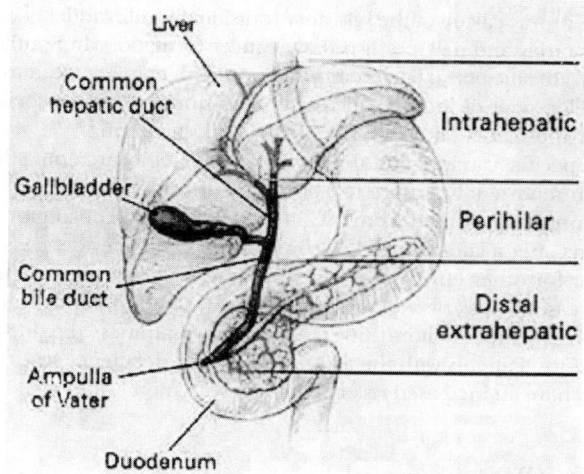

FIGURE 29.5-1. Terminology for biliary tract cancers based on anatomic site of involvement. (Adapted from ref. 2, with permission.)

ETIOLOGY

In most patients, cholangiocarcinomas are sporadic, and no precipitating factor can be identified. In a minority of patients, a number of risk factors can be identified. These predisposing factors all cause chronic inflammation of the bile duct.[12] PSC and choledochal cysts are the most common known predisposing factors found in the United States.[13] Unlike in gallbladder cancer, cholelithiasis has minimal impact as a risk factor for cholangiocarcinomas.

PSC is an autoimmune condition strongly associated with ulcerative colitis. In early stages, PSC results in inflammation of the bile ducts. Subsequent chronic disease can lead to multifocal strictures of the biliary system.[14] In patients with PSC, the risk of developing a biliary malignancy is approximately 160 times that in the general population, with 10% to 13% of such patients developing a hepatobiliary cancer.[15,16] In patients with PSC, cholangiocarcinoma occurs at a young age, and approximately one-third of cancers are diagnosed within 1 year of diagnosis of PSC. Patients have a poor prognosis, because they often have multifocal cancer, and underlying liver dysfunction complicates surgery or specific cancer therapy.[17]

Choledochal cyst is a rare condition manifest by congenital cystic dilatation(s) of the bile ducts. Bile stasis in the cysts leads to chronic inflammation of the duct and a greatly increased risk of cholangiocarcinoma. Ten percent to 20% of patients with choledochal cysts will develop cholangiocarcinoma if left untreated or managed with surgical drainage alone.[18,19] Early excision of the choledochal cyst may reduce the risk of cholangiocarcinoma. Caroli's disease is a rare variant of choledochal cysts that results in intrahepatic ductal dilatation. It is also a risk factor for developing cholangiocarcinoma.[20]

Liver fluke infestation is estimated to afflict 17 million people worldwide, mostly in Southeast Asia and China. These parasites lead to chronic inflammation of the bile duct. The incidence of cholangiocarcinoma in these countries ranks among the highest in the world (87 per 100,000).[21] The liver flukes responsible for cholangiocarcinomas are *Opisthorchis viverrini* and *Clonorchis sinensis*.[22] In patients with liver fluke infestation, early detection of bile duct malignancy is difficult. The prognosis if cancer develops appears similar to that reported in patients without liver fluke infestation.

Chronic calculi of the bile duct (outside the gallbladder) occurs very rarely and may predispose to cancer formation. In Southeast Asia, chronic portal bacteremia and portal phlebitis can lead to the development of intrahepatic pigmented stones. This is associated with approximately a 10% risk of cholangiocarcinoma.[23,24]

Specific carcinogens that lead to cholangiocarcinoma have been reported. Exposure to Thorotrast (thorium dioxide), a radiocontrast agent used from 1930 to 1960, leads to cholangiocarcinoma after a latent period of 16 to 45 years.[25] The evidence is less clear for other environmental exposures. Cigarette smoking may increase the risk of cholangiocarcinoma.[26] Other potential carcinogens include radionuclides, radon, nitrosamines, dioxin, and asbestos. Patients with the acquired immune deficiency syndrome may have an increased risk of cholangiocarcinoma.[27]

ANATOMY

The liver is divided into eight segments based on the blood supply and venous drainage of the liver. Bile ducts are included along with the hepatic artery and portal vein in the portal triad, which is directed to each segment of the liver. The main left hepatic duct exits the liver at the base of the umbilical fissure, and the main right hepatic duct exits the liver between segments V and VI. The caudate lobe drains directly into the left main hepatic duct via numerous small branches. The confluens of the right and left hepatic ducts occurs in the hilum of the liver. The cystic duct may enter the common duct near the confluens of the right and left ducts, or distally near the duodenum. It may also enter the right hepatic duct. This aspect of biliary anatomy is quite variable. The distal bile duct travels posteriorly within the head of the pancreas and then joins the pancreatic duct in a common channel leading to the ampulla of Vater. The type of surgery required for cholangiocarcinoma varies greatly depending on the location and extent of the tumor.

The porta hepatis consists of (from right to left) the bile duct, the portal vein, and the hepatic artery. At the hilum of the liver, the portal vein is posterior; the right hepatic artery generally passes between the common bile duct and the portal vein; and the cystic artery generally passes anterior to the bile duct. The proximity of the portal vein and hepatic artery to the bile duct leads to early vessel involvement or occlusion from cholangiocarcinoma, which affects the surgical resection options. Care must also be taken to map out the blood supply to the liver, because arterial anomalies are common, and this can lead to inadvertent injury of the arterial system during dissection within the porta hepatis.

The lymph node drainage of the bile ducts involves the periportal lymph nodes first, then the peripancreatic, celiac, and interaortocaval lymph nodes.[28] Lymph nodes in the porta hepatis may be difficult to remove because of attached venous branches from the portal vein or fixation of tumor-involved lymph nodes to the bile duct, portal vein, hepatic artery, or the head of the pancreas.

PATHOLOGY

More than 90% of cholangiocarcinomas are adenocarcinomas.[29] Other types, which account for fewer than 5% each, are squamous cell carcinomas, sarcomas, small cell cancer, and lymphomas. Local invasion within the porta hepatis is common, as is metastatic or direct involvement of the liver and peritoneal carcinomatosis.[30] Cholangiocarcinomas may be divided into sclerosing, nodular (mass forming), and papillary types, with the sclerosing type most frequently seen.[11] The sclerosing type causes an intense desmoplastic reaction and is seen as diffuse thickening of the ducts without a defined mass. This form is the most difficult to treat. The nodular type tends to result in a mass lesion and usually arises within the liver. The papillary type is rare. It is a low-grade adenocarcinoma that is represented by a polypoid mass filling the lumen of the bile duct, with minimal invasion and no desmoplastic reaction. It is associated with a favorable outcome.[31]

The reporting of cholangiocarcinoma should include the type and location of the tumor. The type often corresponds with the location. Intrahepatic forms are more likely to be nodular and mass forming, whereas hilar and extrahepatic cholangiocarcinomas are more likely to be sclerosing. Nevertheless, examples exist of sclerosing intrahepatic tumors and vice versa.

Histologically, cholangiocarcinomas are mucin-producing adenocarcinomas consisting of acinar and solid structures.[32]

The sclerosing type, which is the most common, is characterized by extensive fibrosis. Single tumor cells may be found within extensive fibrous stroma. The papillary form appears histologically as papillary fronds extending into the lumen of the ducts. These may produce extracellular mucin. The nodular type demonstrates histologic heterogeneity at advanced stages. At early stages it appears similar to the sclerosing type, with abundant fibrous stroma and a tubular pattern. Satellites are common, representing spread distally down bile duct branches or invasion of small portal vein branches and metastases. Intrahepatic mass-forming nodular-type cholangiocarcinomas are easily misinterpreted as metastatic cancers from other gastrointestinal primary tumors. Search for another primary tumor will be unproductive. Cytokeratin 20 staining may differentiate these tumors, because cytokeratin 20 staining is common and diffuse in colorectal cancers but focal and rare in cholangiocarcinoma.[33]

The molecular biology of cholangiocarcinomas is not well understood. It is likely that the sequence of progression from normal mucosa to adenomatous hyperplasia, dysplasia, carcinoma *in situ*, and then invasive cancer takes place similarly to the pathogenesis of other cancers and that this progression is characterized by a number of genomic mutations.[34] As in other cancers, the tumor suppressor genes p53 and K-ras are mutated in the majority of biliary tract cancers.[35–38] Mutations of Her-2/neu and c-met have also been reported.[39] Autocrine growth loops have been identified involving HGF/met and interleukin-6/gp130.[40] Alterations in the glycosylation of mucins (MUC proteins) and sialosyl Tn antigen may be important in the pathogenesis of cholangiocarcinomas as well.[41]

The TNM system devised by the American Joint Committee on Cancer (*AJCC cancer staging manual*, 6th edition) should be used for staging cholangiocarcinoma.[42] The staging for intrahepatic bile duct tumors is similar to that for primary hepatocellular cancer (Table 29.5-1). The TNM system for hilar and distal cholangiocarcinomas is shown in Table 29.5-2. It has been suggested that the TNM system is not helpful in defining surgical resectability and therefore may not adequately predict outcome.[43]

TABLE 29.5-1. *American Joint Committee on Cancer Staging of Intrahepatic Cholangiocarcinoma (Same as for All Forms of Intrahepatic Primary Tumors)*

T1	Solitary tumor without vascular invasion		
T2	Solitary tumor with vascular invasion or multiple tumors none >5 cm		
T3	Multiple tumors >5 cm or tumor involving a major branch of the portal or hepatic veins		
T4	Tumor(s) with direct invasion of adjacent organs other than the gallbladder or with perforation of visceral peritoneum		
N1	Nodal metastases to the hepatoduodenal ligament		
M1	Any distant metastases		
Stage I	T1	N0	M0
Stage II	T2	N0	M0
Stage IIIA	T3	N0	M0
Stage IIIB	T4	N0	M0
Stage IIIC	Any T	N1	M0
Stage IV	Any T	Any N	M1

(From ref. 175, with permission.)

TABLE 29.5-2. American Joint Committee on Cancer Staging for Extrahepatic Cholangiocarcinoma

T1	Tumor confined to the bile duct		
T2	Tumor invades beyond the wall of the bile duct		
T3	Tumor invades the liver, gallbladder, pancreas, and/or unilateral branches of the portal vein (right or left) or hepatic artery (right or left)		
T4	Tumor invades any of the following: main portal vein or its branches bilaterally, common hepatic artery, or other adjacent structures, such as the colon, stomach, duodenum, or abdominal wall		
N1	Regional lymph node metastasis		
M1	Distant metastasis		
Stage IA	T1	N0	M0
Stage IB	T2	N0	M0
Stage IIA	T3	N0	M0
Stage IIB	T1–T3	N1	M0
Stage III	T4	Any N	M0
Stage IV	Any T	Any N	M1

(From ref. 175, with permission.)

CLINICAL PRESENTATION

Early-stage tumors remain asymptomatic. In most patients a diagnostic workup is initiated when there are signs and symptoms of obstruction of the biliary system. Painless jaundice is most commonly a result of malignant obstruction. Pancreatic cancer is the most likely, followed by cholangiocarcinoma, then other parenchymal liver tumors. Painless jaundice is the most common complaint of patients with cholangiocarcinoma, seen in 70% to 90% of patients, followed by pruritus (66%), abdominal pain, weight loss (30% to 50%), and fever (approximately 20%).[11,44,45] These symptoms, especially jaundice, tend to occur early with distal and hilar cholangiocarcinomas but late with intrahepatic cholangiocarcinomas.[46] It is important to realize that obstruction of the right or left bile duct alone usually does not lead to jaundice or an elevated bilirubin level. Levels of other hepatic enzymes, such as alkaline phosphatase and γ-glutamyltransferase, are markedly elevated due to cellular damage related to the obstruction, but the other lobe of the liver compensates for the loss of bile drainage by producing enough bile to maintain a normal serum bilirubin level. Over time the obstructed lobe may become atrophic, especially when the portal vein has also been blocked by the tumor. It is only when the unilateral tumor becomes large enough to cause pain or anorexia and weight loss that a diagnostic workup is initiated. The unilateral tumor may also extend down the bile ducts to involve the confluens of the right and left ducts, at which time the patient may become jaundiced.

On physical examination, a palpable liver may be noted in patients with intrahepatic cholangiocarcinoma. A palpable gallbladder, also called Courvoisier's sign, due to obstruction of the cystic duct (or common bile duct distal to the cystic duct), may be found. Obstruction of the bile duct and biliary stasis may lead to bacterial colonization and cholangitis. Patients with cholangitis present in a dramatic fashion, with high fever, pain, nausea, vomiting, and rigors. They are bacteremic with typical biliary tract flora (*Escherichia coli, Klebsiella, Proteus, Pseudomonas aeruginosa, Serratia, Streptococcus,* and *Enterobacter*). In general, although bile is a rich medium for bacterial growth, it is sterile, and therefore obstruction should not lead directly to cholangitis. Once a free communication is made between the gastrointestinal tract and the biliary system (as with a stent), the bile becomes contaminated, and cholangitis is a more frequent problem. Patients with biliary stones are more likely to have contaminated bile and may present earlier with cholangitis in the face of biliary obstruction.

DIAGNOSTIC EVALUATION

Laboratory Tests

Liver function tests generally reveal elevated markers of cholestasis—elevated bilirubin, alkaline phosphatase, and γ-glutamyltransferase levels. Serum aminotransferase levels may be normal or mildly elevated in the early stages. Serum tumor marker levels may aid in diagnosis. Serum carcinoembryonic antigen (CEA) and carbohydrate antigen 19-9 (CA 19-9) levels are most commonly elevated in cholangiocarcinoma. CEA levels may be elevated but have a low predictive value for cholangiocarcinoma. CEA is therefore not helpful for diagnosis.[46a] Most patients with cholangiocarcinomas have elevated CA 19-9 levels. CA 19-9 levels above 100 U/mL were found to be 89% sensitive and 86% specific for the diagnosis of bile duct carcinoma in patients with PSC.[47] Other studies have demonstrated a lower predictive value of CA 19-9 for cholangiocarcinoma in patients with PSC.[47a,52] Benign biliary tract disease may result in elevated CA 19-9 levels, and the optimal cutoff value for suspicion of cancer is not clear. High values (more than 180 U/mL) tend to be more specific at the expense of sensitivity.[46a] CA 19-9 and CEA levels have also been measured in bile specimens and may be elevated in the presence of cancer.[47b] A combined index of CA 19-9 and CEA has been proposed, with studies showing mixed results in predicting cancer.[47a] The presence of cholangitis or hepatolithiasis or both can cause elevations of tumor marker levels, and these tests should be repeated after symptoms have resolved. Also, CA 19-9 is a carbohydrate cell surface antigen related to the Lewis blood group antigens. Patients with negative Lewis blood group antigen (representing 10% of the population) cannot synthesize CA 19-9 and cannot manifest an elevation in this marker.[48] Additional potential markers for cholangiocarcinoma include CA 242, CA 72-4, CA 50, CA 125, and serum MUC5AC. These have all been evaluated with mixed results.[49–52]

Radiologic Evaluation

When a patient presents with jaundice, or when the laboratory examination is consistent with biliary obstruction (elevated alkaline phosphatase and γ-glutamyltransferase levels), workup should begin with ultrasonography to rule out biliary stones as the cause. If the cause is not cholelithiasis, then a computed tomography (CT) scan of the abdomen may be obtained. A helical CT scan with dynamic contrast and 5-mm cuts through the liver and head of the pancreas is preferred. The CT scan characteristically demonstrates thickening of the bile duct and dilated ducts proximal to the abnormality.[53] Attention should be given to associated portal vein patency and any evidence of liver atrophy. Also, attention should be given to lymphadenopathy in the periportal, celiac, and interaortocaval regions, and any mass in the head of the pancreas or liver.

The next test should be some form of cholangiography. The appearance and location of the bile duct stricture can be helpful. Smooth, tapering strictures of the distal bile duct are more consistent with benign scarring, whereas irregular strictures at the confluens are more consistent with hilar cholangiocarcinoma. Typically, endoscopic retrograde cholangiopancreatography (ERCP) is performed, in which not only can the duct be completely imaged, but the obstruction can be stented and brushes of the duct can be obtained for pathologic evaluation. Hilar cholangiocarcinoma should be studied with a percutaneous transhepatic approach [percutaneous transhepatic cholangiography (PTC)]. This is more invasive than ERCP but allows better visualization of the proximal bile ducts, which often define resectability.

Frequently, complete obstruction of the bile duct does not allow for complete imaging using either a transhepatic or endoscopic approach. A better test, therefore, may be magnetic resonance cholangiography (Fig. 29.5-2). Heavily T2-weighted magnetic resonance imaging (MRI) of the liver and pancreas with projection images of the bile duct and pancreatic duct can provide images of the entire biliary tract. This is obviously less invasive for the patient and may provide better information than ERCP or PTC. In addition, associated masses and malignant thickening can be defined with the biliary obstruction. Hyperintense regions on T2-weighted MRI may be consistent with cholangiocarcinoma. If available and cost effective, this test could replace CT scans and other forms of cholangiography.

Although biliary obstruction can be defined anatomically with ultrasonography, CT, ERCP, PTC, or magnetic resonance cholan-

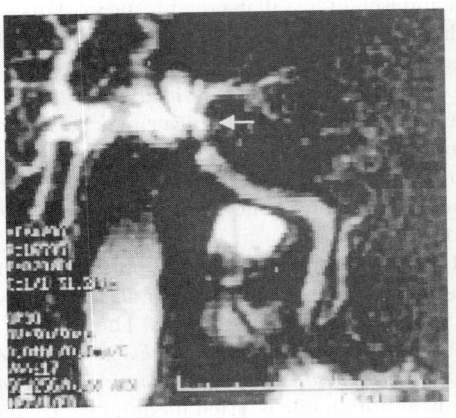
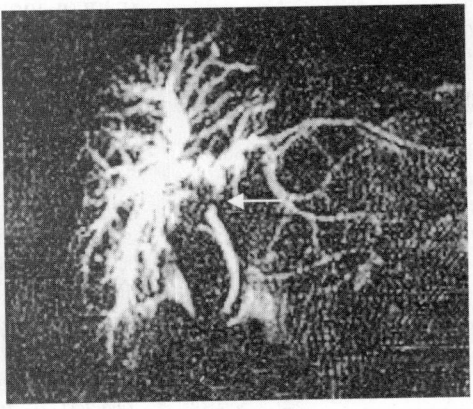

FIGURE 29.5-2. Magnetic resonance cholangiopancreatography (MRCP) for cholangiocarcinoma. **A:** MRCP image for a patient with resectable hilar cholangiocarcinoma. Arrow marks the clear definition of the proximal right and left main hepatic ducts. **B:** MRCP for a patient with hilar cholangiocarcinoma. The arrow marks the hilum. There is no clear delineation of the main right or left hepatic ducts. This patient underwent exploratory surgery and was found to have disease that was unresectable for cure. (**A** adapted from ref. 240, with permission.)

A,B

giopancreatography (MRCP), the differentiation of benign from malignant causes of obstruction can be difficult. The CA 19-9 level can be helpful, as discussed in Laboratory Tests earlier in this chapter. Endoscopic ultrasonography may be useful for distal common bile duct cancers for defining a mass or abnormal thickening, which can direct biopsies.[54] Positron emission tomography (PET) has been described as helpful in differentiating malignant from benign strictures of the bile duct; however, as with pancreatic cancer, the density of metabolically active cells in the setting of intense fibrosis is not always amenable to successful PET imaging.[55] The presence of inflammation from benign causes of biliary obstruction can provide falsely intense PET images. Intrahepatic cholangiocarcinomas are usually PET positive.

Choledochoscopy

Direct visualization of the duct with directed biopsies is the ideal technique for workup of cholangiocarcinoma.[56] Techniques performed at the time of both ERCP and PTC have been developed and described. As the technology improves and becomes more widely available, more reports will define the accuracy of this technique. A visual assessment of proximal ducts at the time of PTC may be helpful to define resectability. Often, however, the tumor infiltrates the wall of the bile duct and cannot be seen involving the epithelium. Visual inspection may underestimate the true margin.

Biopsy and Cytologic Analysis

Cells can be obtained for cytologic analysis using a variety of means. Bile can be collected for cytologic examinations, brushings of the bile duct can be obtained at the time of ERCP or PTC, and CT-guided percutaneous aspiration can be performed. A positive cytologic finding eases the decision making for management and allows for more focused discussion with the patient regarding therapy and prognosis. The tumors are often hypocellular and difficult to diagnose by biopsy. A review of eight reports in the literature from 1980 to 1997 summarized 223 cytologic examinations in patients with bile duct tumors.[57] The sensitivity for diagnosing cancer was 62%. This is unsatisfactory and leads to a resection to treat or rule out cancer regardless of the biopsy results. The future possibility of neoadjuvant therapy may bring more importance to the preoperative pathologic assessment of cholangiocarcinoma. Fine-needle aspiration directed by endoscopic ultrasonography has been reported to have an accuracy of 91%, a sensitivity of 89%, and a specificity of 100% in the diagnosis of patients with strictures at the hilum.[54] Newer techniques, such as mutational analysis of shed cells, may improve the sensitivity and usefulness of cytologic analysis.

Summary of Diagnostic Evaluation

Intrahepatic cholangiocarcinomas present with pain, weight loss, and nausea and vomiting. Laboratory examination usually reveals subtle abnormalities in liver enzyme levels with a normal bilirubin level. A high level of α-fetoprotein directs the workup toward hepatocellular cancer, whereas a high CA 19-9 level directs it toward cholangiocarcinoma or metastatic pancreatic cancer. The typical intrahepatic cholangiocarcinoma presents as a dominant mass with multiple satellite tumors. Findings from fine-needle aspiration are accurate at making the diagnosis of adenocarcinoma and

differentiating from hepatocellular carcinoma, but it may be impossible to use histologic criteria to differentiate intrahepatic cholangiocarcinoma from metastatic carcinoma from other gastrointestinal primary tumors. Lack of cytokeratin 20 staining on immunohistochemistry may be the best method for differentiation as described earlier in Pathology. If the staining is not helpful, then upper and lower endoscopy (in addition to the CT scan) should be performed to rule out another gastrointestinal primary tumor. If no primary is identified, the diagnosis of exclusion should be intrahepatic cholangiocarcinoma.

The diagnostic evaluation for obstructive jaundice requires the interpretation of tests within the context of the clinical picture, which often leads to surgical treatment without a definitive diagnosis. Once the biopsy result is positive, or the suspicion is high for cholangiocarcinoma, the determination of resectability must be made. This involves careful assessment of the performance status and comorbidities of the patient, and the patient's ability to tolerate major surgery. Also, the extent of involvement of the bile ducts must be assessed. It is helpful to know the extent of surgery required to resect the tumor. If the intrapancreatic duct is involved, then a pancreaticoduodenectomy is required. If the tumor extends along the bile ducts into a lobe of the liver, then a hepatic lobectomy is necessary.

Often the most difficult assessment is evaluation the status of the proximal bile ducts for determining resectability and planning which lobe of the liver (if any) needs to be resected. Cholangiograms are important for this determination. As long as either the main right or left hepatic duct appears normal, the tumor is potentially resectable for cure. Further assessment of the opposite lobe can be made at the time of surgery. The success of nonsurgical palliation allows the avoidance of major surgery in patients whose tumors are clearly unresectable for cure. The accuracy of this diagnostic assessment is quite important. If the main portal vein is invaded, or the portal vein supplying the lobe of the liver that is planned to be left behind is occluded, then the tumor is unresectable. A common limit to surgical resection is involvement of the proximal bile ducts in both lobes of the liver. Cholangiogram assessment of these ducts is essential as discussed in Radiologic Evaluation, earlier in the chapter, and they are perhaps most expeditiously examined using MRCP.

SURGERY FOR CHOLANGIOCARCINOMA

Preoperative Stenting of the Bile Duct

The usefulness of preoperative stenting for obstructive jaundice in the setting of resectable tumors is controversial. The major advantage is the rapid palliation of symptoms, and the potential utility of transhepatic stents as postoperative stents.[58] The disadvantage is the subsequent bacterial colonization of bile that leads to cholangitis and that may increase the risk of infectious complications at the time of surgery.[59] The stent itself may lead to a dense fibrous reaction that can be difficult to differentiate from the tumor. The common use of MRCP as a diagnostic modality and the ability to move rapidly to surgical resection could alleviate the need for more invasive cholangiography and stenting.

Intrahepatic Cholangiocarcinoma

The long-term results and natural history of surgery for intrahepatic cholangiocarcinomas is difficult to define due to its

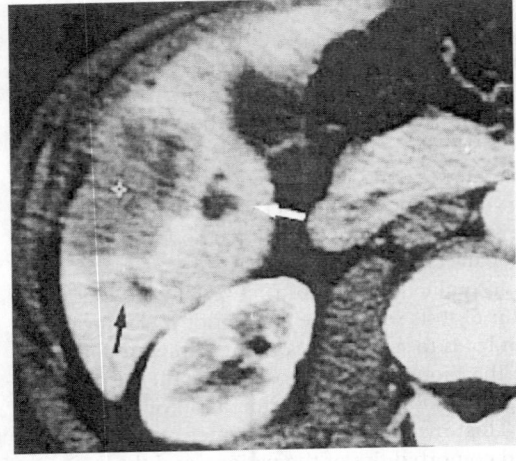
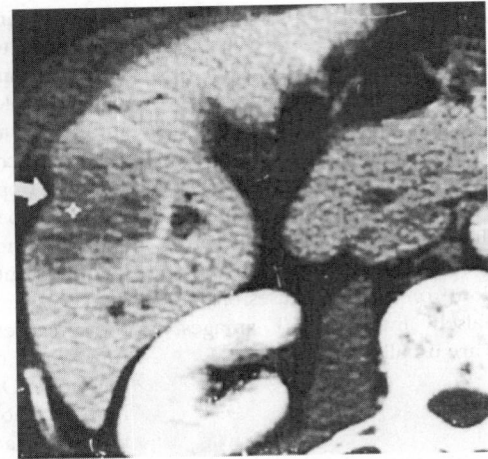

A,B

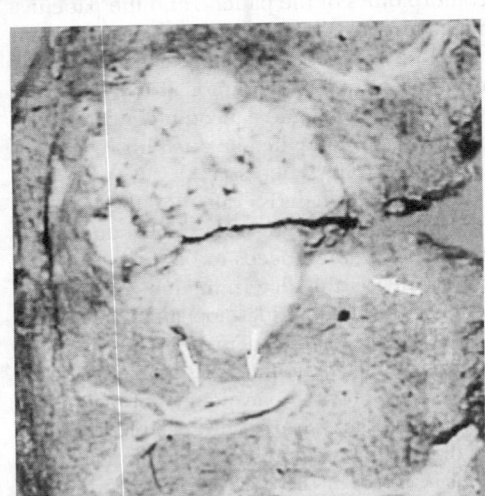
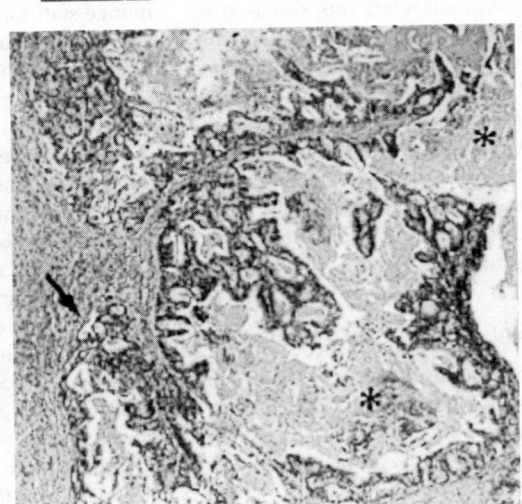

C,D

FIGURE 29.5-3. Intrahepatic cholangiocarcinoma. **A:** Arterial phase computed tomography (CT) scan demonstrating classic ring enhancement, central necrosis (*star*), satellitosis (*white arrow*), and dilated, thickened peripheral biliary ducts (*black arrow*). **B:** Portal venous phase CT scan demonstrating loss of enhancement, central necrosis (*star*) and dimpling of the surface of the liver (*arrow*). **C:** Gross pathologic photograph of specimen demonstrating satellitosis and diffuse fibrous thickening of the peripheral bile ducts (*arrows*). **D:** Low-power microscopy with hematoxylin and eosin staining of same specimen demonstrating extensive necrosis (*star*) and invasion into the hepatic parenchyma (*arrow*). (From ref. 53, with permission.)

rarity, and therefore the indications for resectability are not well described. Consequently, resectability is determined based on anatomic considerations. Intrahepatic metastases tend to occur as multiple satellites, and although their presence affects prognosis, it should not define resectability (Fig. 29.5-3). For resection, the satellites should be confined to a lobe or segment. In this setting, cells may not have contaminated the contralateral lobe, and curative resection is still possible. The goal of resection is to remove all liver parenchyma at risk for intrahepatic metastases based on the proximal extent of the tumor. Usually this requires a lobectomy. If both lobes of the liver are involved with metastases, then curative resection is unlikely, and other forms of therapy should be considered. Extrahepatic spread portends a poor prognosis and in general should be considered a contraindication to resection.

Small series in the literature describe the outcome after surgical resection for intrahepatic cholangiocarcinoma (Table 29.5-3). The resectability rate ranges from 32% to 90%. The mortality of resection is slightly higher than in series of hepatic resection for other indications but is generally less than 10%. The median survival after resection for intrahepatic cholangiocarcinoma ranges from 15 to 59 months. Five-year survival rates range from 13% to 42%. Prognostic factors include margin status, satellite metastases, nodal metastases, vascular invasion (hepatic vein or portal vein), and tumor size. Although they

are rare, intrahepatic intraductal papillary tumors have an excellent prognosis if completely resected.[60]

Hilar Cholangiocarcinoma

The surgical management of hilar cholangiocarcinoma is complex, usually requiring an *en bloc* resection of at least one lobe of the liver and the extrahepatic bile duct, and a complete peripor-

TABLE 29.5-3. Patient Outcome after Surgical Resection for Intrahepatic Cholangiocarcinoma

Study	Year	n	Median Survival (Mo)	5-Y Survival (%)
Pichlmayr et al.[176]	1995	32	20	13
Berdah et al.[177]	1996	31	15	35
Lieser et al.[178]	1998	61	—	22
Chu et al.[179]	1999	48	16	22
Valverde et al.[180]	1999	30	28	—
Shimada et al.[181]	2001	49	26	28
Weber et al.[182]	2001	33	37	—
Ebata et al.[183]	2003	160	—	28
Ohtsuka et al.[184]	2003	50	26	23
Uenishi et al.[185]	2003	54	—	17

tal lymphadenectomy. The intraoperative assessment of extent of disease can be difficult, because of the chronic inflammation that is associated with chronic biliary obstruction and the presence of a stent. Based on preoperative assessment of the proximal bile ducts, a plan should be in place regarding the extent of resection. This usually involves hepatic lobectomy in cases in which the duct is abnormal past the first sectoral or segmental branches of the main right or left hepatic duct, respectively. The contralateral preserved bile duct should be transected at the level of the first segmental branch. This maximizes the chance of obtaining a negative margin while maintaining adequate drainage of the lobe. It is sometimes possible to extend the resection into the segmental branches, then re-create a main drainage channel by suturing the individual segmental or sectoral ducts together. Intraoperative decisions can be aided by pathologic examination of the transected duct margins. In the case of tumor involving the left main hepatic duct, careful assessment of the caudate lobe branches need to be made. Several early branches of the left hepatic duct drain the caudate lobe and can be involved early with tumor. Consideration of routine caudate lobectomy should be made in these cases.[61] Studies demonstrate that 46% of hilar cholangiocarcinomas microscopically involve the caudate lobe.[62]

The entire extrahepatic bile duct should be resected down to the level of the duodenum. A frozen section of the distal bile duct should be obtained for determination of margins. A pancreaticoduodenectomy may be required if the only residual disease is the distal intrapancreatic portion of the bile duct. This is rare for hilar cholangiocarcinoma. Lymphadenectomy should include all soft tissue in the porta hepatis, excluding the portal vein and hepatic artery. Assessment of the common hepatic artery nodes, the celiac artery nodes, the peripancreatic nodes, and the interaortocaval lymph nodes should be made. Under some circumstances, dissection of these regions may be indicated.

Many single-institution studies (mostly retrospective) exist describing the results of surgical resection for hilar cholangiocarcinoma (Table 29.5-4). Approximately one-third of patients presenting with the suspected diagnosis of cholangiocarcinoma had resectable disease.[13] Operative mortality averaged approximately

8%, which indicates the high-risk population that this tumor affects and the complexity of the procedure.[63] Twenty percent to 25% of patients survived 5 years after surgical resection. Recurrences occurred most commonly at the bed of resection, followed by retroperitoneal lymph nodes. Distant metastases occurs in one-third of cases. The most common site was the lung or mediastinum, followed by liver, then peritoneum. Comparisons of outcome over time suggest improved outcome in more recent series as a result of routine inclusion of liver resection. Prognostic factors for survival include microscopic margin status, lymph node status, tumor size, tumor grade, preoperative serum albumin level, and postoperative sepsis.[58,64]

Distal Cholangiocarcinoma

Extrahepatic cholangiocarcinoma not involving the confluens of the right and left main hepatic ducts involves the common hepatic duct and commonly involves the intrapancreatic portion of the duct. This usually requires a pancreaticoduodenectomy with resection of the extrahepatic bile duct to the level of the confluens for complete clearance of disease. Rarely, the tumor may be confined to a small region of the duct, and an extrahepatic bile duct resection can be performed without a pancreaticoduodenectomy. Intraoperative assessment with the help of the pathologist must dictate the extent of resection. In any case, the resection should again include a complete clearance of the periportal lymph nodes—all tissue in the porta hepatis excluding the portal vein and hepatic artery. For extensive involvement of the bile duct without distant spread, consideration can be made for *en bloc* combined hepatic and pancreatic resections. The morbidity of such extensive surgery is high, and the overall prognosis is poor with extensive disease, so careful consideration is required before embarking on such extensive surgery.[61]

The incidence of distal common bile duct tumors compared to hilar cholangiocarcinomas is low, but the resectability rate is higher. A pancreaticoduodenectomy has a reasonable chance of providing a margin-negative resection for tumors of the distal bile duct. They less frequently involve the portal vein and are not limited by liver involvement, as is seen with hilar cholangiocarcinomas. The risk of pancreaticoduodenectomy and distal bile duct resection is high, with morbidity rates between 40% and 60% and mortality rates between 2% and 10%. Probably because of the higher rate of resectability with negative margins, the outcome is improved, although still poor. Median survival is expected to be between 20 and 33 months, and expected 5-year survival rate is between 14% and 50% (Table 29.5-5).

TABLE 29.5-4. Patient Outcome after Surgical Resection for Hilar Cholangiocarcinoma

Study	Year	n	Median Survival (Mo)	5-Y Survival (%)
Sugiura et al.[186]	1994	83	—	20
Nakeeb et al.[187]	1996	109	19	11
Klempnauer et al.[64]	1997	151	24	28
Miyazaki et al.[188]	1998	76	—	26
Nagino et al.[189]	1998	138	—	—
Neuhaus et al.[190]	1999	95[a]	—	22
Gazzaniga et al.[191]	2000	74	17	11
Launois et al.[192]	2000	82[b]	22	10
Lee et al.[193]	2000	111[c]	37	22
Nimura et al.[61]	2000	142	25	21
Jarnagin et al.[194]	2001	80	—	—
Kawarada et al.[195]	2002	87	15	26

[a]Includes 15 patients treated with liver transplantation.
[b]Perioperative deaths excluded.
[c]Only examines those treated with liver resection, and median follow-up only 16 months.

TABLE 29.5-5. Patient Outcome after Surgical Resection for Distal Cholangiocarcinoma

Author	Year	n	Median Survival (Mo)	5-Y Survival (%)
Nagorney et al.[196]	1993	22	24	50
Fong et al.[197]	1996	45	33	27
Wade et al.[198]	1997	34	22[a]	14
Yeo et al.[199]	1997	65	20	16[b]
Sasaki et al.[28]	2001	59	—	34
Yoshida et al.[200]	2002	26	20	37

[a]Mean survival.
[b]Three-year survival.

Transplantation for Cholangiocarcinoma

Transplantation as a primary treatment modality for hilar and intrahepatic cholangiocarcinoma is a viable treatment option.[65] Organ availability has been the most limiting factor in the use of this modality, but the success of living related donor transplantation may rejuvenate the use of transplantation for hilar and intrahepatic cholangiocarcinoma. Complete hepatectomy provides the best chance of a complete resection for these tumors. Nevertheless, the historic results of liver transplantation for cholangiocarcinoma have been dismal. Meyer et al. reported the results of liver transplantation for cholangiocarcinoma in 207 patients listed in the Cincinnati Transplant Tumor Registry.[66] Fifty-one percent of the patients undergoing transplantation suffered recurrence. The median time from transplantation to recurrence was 9.7 months, and the median time between recurrence and death was 2 months.

In 1993, physicians at the Mayo Clinic developed a protocol using external-beam radiation therapy and bolus 5-fluorouracil (5-FU), followed by brachytherapy, protracted intravenous infusion of 5-FU, and liver transplantation for highly selected patients with early-stage cholangiocarcinoma.[67] Twenty-eight patients underwent exploratory surgery, at which time 11 were excluded due to metastatic disease. Seventeen patients proceeded to liver transplantation; seven patients had no identifiable tumor in the explanted specimen. Of the ten patients with identifiable tumor, two died of non–cancer-related causes. Of the remaining patients, two developed recurrent disease, one at 40 months and another at 54 months after transplantation. The median duration of follow-up was 41.8 months (range, 2.8 to 105.5). The 5-year actuarial survival rate for those undergoing transplantation was 87%.

Other small series have demonstrated 3-year survival rates from 0% to 53%.[68] Studies suggest expected 3-year survival of 30% to 40%. Extrahepatic nodal disease or metastases are a contraindication to transplantation. The 1-year mortality rate for transplantation in major centers is around 20%.[69]

Follow-Up after Resection

No clear guidelines exist for surveillance and follow-up after surgery. A physical examination with routine laboratory tests every 3 to 4 months for the first 3 years after surgery and then at longer intervals of 6 months until year 5 is reasonable. The role of CA 19-9 level in surveillance is not clear, but persistently rising levels often precede radiologic evidence of recurrence by a number of months. The role of CT scans for surveillance has not been evaluated in clinical trials, but due to the high risk of recurrence, radiologic evaluation with CT scans of the abdomen every 6 months for 2 to 3 years after surgery may be useful detect recurrent disease.

The pattern of failure after curative resection includes peritoneal spread, hepatic metastases, local extrahepatic recurrence, and distant metastases (most commonly to lung). As with pancreatic, gallbladder, and hepatocellular cancers, cholangiocarcinomas have a propensity to seed and can recur in needle biopsy tracts, abdominal wall incision wounds, and the peritoneal cavity. Surgery is generally not indicated for recurrent cholangiocarcinoma. Close surveillance and early diagnosis of recurrences may allow for eligibility for clinical trials, which may someday improve the outcome for this disease.

NEOADJUVANT THERAPY

The use of preoperative chemotherapy and radiation in treatment of cholangiocarcinoma remains investigational. Neoadjuvant therapy may be an option for patients with marginally resectable cancers; however, down-staging of a categorically unresectable cancer to an operable state rarely, if ever, occurs.[70,71]

ADJUVANT RADIOTHERAPY

In general, postoperative adjuvant radiotherapy is radiotherapy administered after resection with curative intent or at least a gross total resection, in which there is a substantial risk of local recurrence. Naturally, the administered radiotherapy must be able to decrease significantly the incidence of local recurrence. Clinicians often debate the amount of local recurrence risk and the clinical consequences of local recurrence (in terms of morbidity and mortality) that warrants postoperative radiotherapy. Also, the magnitude of benefit in terms of a decrease in local recurrence rates, improvement in disease-free and overall survival rates, and the associated morbidity of treatment must be considered before administering adjuvant radiotherapy. Ideally, adjuvant postoperative radiotherapy should produce a statistically significant decrease in the local-regional recurrence rate, increase the disease-free and overall survival rates, and have minimum morbidity.

For most solid tumors in adults in which adjuvant postoperative radiotherapy is used for minimal residual tumor, the usual administered doses are in the range of 5000 to 6000 cGy at 180 to 200 cGy/d. For those tumors such as breast cancer and rectal cancer for which adjuvant systemic chemotherapy has been demonstrated to provide a significant disease-free survival benefit, the administered radiotherapy dose may be closer to the 5000-cGy level. For those malignancies such as upper respiratory tract cancers in which the benefits of chemotherapy are less evident, postoperative radiotherapy to 6000 cGy or more is commonly used.

The irradiated volume after surgery should include the operative bed and regional nodal sites likely to be involved. After cholangiocarcinoma surgery, the irradiated volume includes multiple organs intolerant of high-dose radiation, such as the spinal cord, right kidney, liver, stomach, duodenum, and small bowel. This limits the volume that can be safely irradiated to a high dose. Increasing the volume irradiated necessarily leads to inclusion of more normal tissues, and increasing the doses administered increases the incidence and severity of both acute and chronic sequelae.

Extrahepatic cholangiocarcinomas have a high incidence of local-regional recurrence after resection in addition to metastases involving the liver and other distant sites.[72,73] Whereas postoperative radiotherapy is not likely to impact the incidence of metastases to the liver, peritoneum, and other distant sites, it is administered with the expectation that the local recurrence rate will decrease. Because of the rarity of cholangiocarcinoma cases with resection for cure, there are no large prospective randomized studies evaluating adjuvant radiotherapy in this setting. Data on the use of adjuvant radiotherapy for biliary tract cancer are derived mainly from retrospective reviews with small numbers of nonrandomized patients.

Postoperative adjuvant radiotherapy for biliary tract cancer can be administered either by external-beam radiotherapy, brachytherapy, intraoperative radiotherapy (IORT), or a combination of radiotherapy modalities. External-beam radiotherapy is the most commonly used radiotherapy modality for biliary tract cancer.

Advantages of external-beam radiotherapy include the widespread availability of this modality, its noninvasive nature, and the ability to deliver a homogeneous high dose to a large volume. Most commonly, radiotherapy is administered in a continuous course over 5 to 6 weeks. Most retrospective reviews of radiotherapy for biliary cancer have used external-beam radiotherapy to a dose of at least 4000 to 5000 cGy at 180 cGy/d to a large volume. Some patients have been treated with additional external-beam radiotherapy to a smaller volume to a total dose of 6000 cGy or more, or additional radiotherapy has been administered by intraluminal brachytherapy or IORT. The relative ease of placing a catheter by which brachytherapy can be administered into the involved portion of the biliary tract makes brachytherapy an attractive modality for treating a localized portion (boost volume) of the biliary tract cancer to a high dose. Similarly, IORT, where available, has occasionally been used to administer a single large dose to the operative bed or the intact tumor at the time of surgery.

Brachytherapy in which catheters are placed within the biliary duct has been used to administer a "boost" after external-beam radiotherapy or even as the only form of radiotherapy for biliary tract tumors. The usual dose delivered is 2000 to 3000 cGy at 1 cm from the sources over several days or, when the high-dose afterloading method is used, 500 cGy daily for 3 days. Brachytherapy has the advantage of providing a high dose to a localized, relatively small volume over several days. However, the disadvantage is that the fall-off in dose is rather rapid. Thus, although a high dose is administered to the tissue immediately adjacent to the radioactive sources, there is very little dose more than 2 cm away. Also, brachytherapy requires the insertion of a catheter into the biliary tract, which increases the risk of cholangitis and hemorrhage.

IORT, in which a single dose of radiation is administered using an electron beam at the time of surgery, usually immediately after resection and before closure of the abdominal cavity, offers the theoretical advantage of being able to deliver a high dose of radiation, usually more than 2000 cGy, to the operative bed while at the same time sensitive structures such as the stomach and small intestine are displaced away from the beam. However, IORT is a logistical problem unless a linear accelerator with high-energy electron-beam capabilities is situated within, or very close to, the operating room. This latter difficulty, and also the lack of any randomized studies demonstrating benefit of IORT for cholangiocarcinomas, have precluded its widespread use.

At the University of Pittsburgh, split-course radiotherapy has frequently been used to treat bile duct and pancreatic cancers, either after resection or for advanced unresectable lesions.[74,75] For postresection cases with likely minimal residual tumor, 2500 cGy in ten fractions is administered, and then after a 3- to 4-week interruption, a second course of 2500 cGy in ten fractions is administered if there has been no evidence of tumor progression. Radiobiologically, the total dose of 5000 cGy in 20 fractions with the interruption is equivalent to a dose of approximately 5200 cGy in 26 fractions administered continuously at 200 cGy/d or 5580 cGy in 31 fractions at 180 cGy/d. The main advantage of split-course radiotherapy is that the treatment course is administered in fewer overall sessions and those patients with progressive tumors during the interruption are spared further unnecessary treatments. Also, the therapy appears to be well tolerated. One theoretical disadvantage is the possibility of tumor repopulation during the interruption and a possible increase in late sequelae with the higher daily doses. In the experience at the University of Pittsburgh with relatively short follow-up due to the high mortality of bile duct and pancreatic cancer, there seemed to be no increase in acute or late sequelae from the split-course regimen and no difference in survival between those patients treated with split-course radiotherapy and those receiving continuous radiotherapy.

Kim et al. reported on a series of 84 patients with hilar and distal cholangiocarcinoma treated between 1982 and 1994 with surgery and postoperative radiotherapy.[76] Seventy-two patients had a gross total resection. Margins of resection were negative in 47 and positive in 25. Twelve patients had gross residual tumor. Seventy-one patients were treated with a split-course regimen consisting of 2000 cGy in ten fractions followed by a 2-week rest and then an additional 2000 cGy in ten fractions using relatively large (10 cm × 10 cm) anterior-posterior fields with blocks. This regimen is equivalent to 3800 cGy in 19 fractions or 3960 cGy in 22 fractions. Bolus 5-FU was given for the first 3 days of each course. Thirteen patients with more advanced disease were treated with 4000 to 4500 cGy in a continuous course. The 5-year survival rates were 36%, 35%, and 0% for patients with complete surgical resection, resection with microscopic residual tumor, and resection with gross residual disease, respectively, and the median survival times for these same groups were 25, 24, and 13 months, respectively. The observation that the 5-year survival rates and median survival times were equivalent for patients with microscopic residual cancers and for those with negative margins, all of whom received radiotherapy, suggests that postoperative adjuvant radiotherapy may have improved the outcome for patients with microscopic residual tumor.

Todoroki et al. reported on a 23-year experience with 63 patients who underwent resection of locally advanced cholangiocarcinoma involving the main hepatic duct.[77] Forty-seven patients had microscopic residual tumor and 28 were treated with adjuvant radiotherapy. Seventeen of the 28 were treated by both IORT and postoperative external-beam radiotherapy. No details were presented concerning the external-beam radiotherapy. Six patients underwent resection and IORT and five underwent resection and postoperative external-beam radiotherapy. The 5-year survival rate after treatment with IORT and postoperative external-beam radiotherapy after resection was 39.2% compared to 16.7% for IORT alone and 0% for external-beam radiotherapy alone. The 5-year survival rate for patients treated with IORT and external-beam radiotherapy after resection was statistically significantly improved compared to that for patients undergoing resection alone (39.2% vs. 13.5%). IORT was administered using high-energy electron beams to a dose of 2750 or 3500 cGy. The investigators did report an increase in complication rate with the higher dose and with larger electron-beam fields of 8 cm in diameter. They subsequently reduced the single dose of IORT to 2000 cGy and the electron energy beam to 8 MeV instead of 16 or 18 MeV. The field diameter was also reduced to less than 6 cm. Subsequently, there were no severe complications related to the IORT.

Todoroki et al., in a review of results for patients with middle and lower third cholangiocarcinoma, reported a trend toward improved 5-year survival rate in 8 patients who received radiotherapy after resection with microscopic residual disease compared with 17 patients who underwent resection alone (8% vs. 0%; P = .137).[78] Radiotherapy was associated with significantly prolonged median survival in six patients who had a resection with gross residual disease compared with those who had inoperable cancers. The median dose of external-beam radiotherapy was 4720 cGy at 180 to 200 cGy/d. IORT was administered to three patients, and two patients had intraluminal brachytherapy after external-beam radiotherapy.

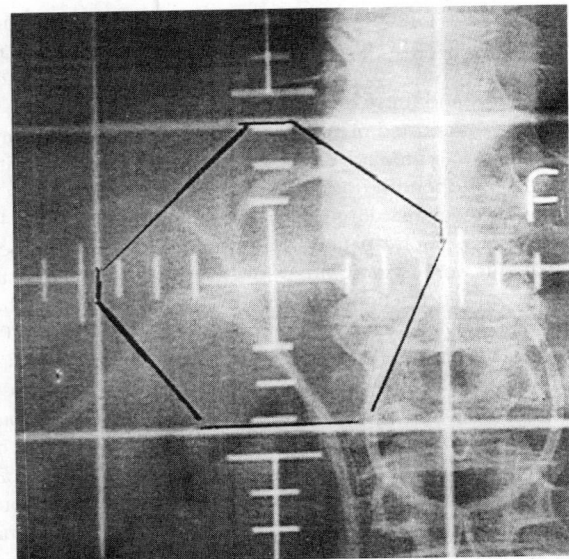
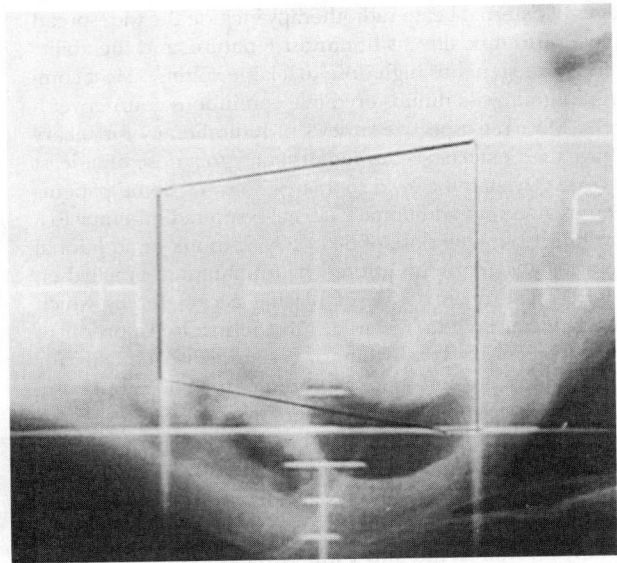

FIGURE 29.5-4. Treatment volumes for a 65-year-old patient with advanced cancer of the common hepatic duct. The patient received 2500 cGy in ten fractions. This course was repeated after a 4-week interval, and then an additional 1000 cGy in five fractions was administered after a second 4-week interval. The patient died 11 months later with metastases to the liver and lung but with local control.

Kurosaki et al. reported a 20-year experience using IORT after resection in 35 patients with cholangiocarcinoma.[79] All were treated with electron-beam radiation in the 5- to 19-MeV energy range. The IORT dose was 1500 to 3000 cGy, but four of the five patients who received 3000 cGy were in the early death group. Sixteen patients also received external-beam radiotherapy, 880 to 5400 cGy. In 11 patients without lymph node involvement and negative margins, the addition of external-beam radiotherapy did not influence survival. However, for 24 patients with lymph node involvement, there was a significant difference in survival between those who received IORT and external-beam radiotherapy and those who received IORT alone. The benefit of adding external-beam radiotherapy to IORT was also observed in patients who underwent a "noncurative" resection with involved margins.

At the University of Pittsburgh, the volumes used for split-course irradiation for cholangiocarcinoma (Fig. 29.5-4) are smaller than what others have recommended.[80–82] The use of split-course irradiation to a relatively smaller volume has not resulted in a decrease in therapeutic outcome. However, the number of patients treated is still relatively small, and patients were nonrandomly allocated to either split-course or continuous irradiation.[74]

In summary, adjuvant radiotherapy is recommended for all patients who have had a resection with curative intent for cholangiocarcinoma, especially if the tumor has invaded into or through the muscularis layer, the margins of resection are involved, or regional lymph nodes are involved. A minimum of 5000 cGy at 180 to 200 cGy/d should be given, with additional external-beam radiotherapy administered to a more limited volume to a total dose of at least 6000 cGy. Split-course radiotherapy as described earlier should be considered as an alternative way of administering the external-beam radiotherapy. IORT at the time of the resection makes sense theoretically and certainly should be considered in those institutions that have the capability. Additional radiotherapy using brachytherapy should also be considered for those patients for whom it is feasible. Newer methods of conformal treatment planning including intensity-modulated radiotherapy allow for the administration of high doses of external-beam radiotherapy, usually more than 6000 cGy, to a volume such as is shown in Figure 29.5-4 and yet avoid an intolerable dose to adjacent normal structures. Improved therapeutic results await the introduction of more effective chemotherapy regimens that would improve on the results of radiation alone in the adjuvant and even the advanced disease setting.

ADJUVANT CHEMOTHERAPY

Complete surgical resection offers the best chance of long-term disease-free survival and a possible cure. However most patients, except those with the most favorable characteristics, will have local or regional recurrence. Due to the lack of randomized studies, there are few data on which to base treatment recommendations for adjuvant therapy, and clearly more studies are warranted. Only one randomized study has been published evaluating the effect of chemotherapy after surgery (Table 29.5-6). Takeda et al. conducted a randomized study of chemotherapy consisting of mitomycin C and 5-FU compared to observation alone in patients with resected pancreaticobiliary cancers. A total of 508 patients were entered after surgery. Sites of disease were pancreas (n = 173), bile duct (n = 139), gallbladder (n = 140), and ampulla of Vater (n = 56). There were no apparent differences in 5-year disease-free survival or overall survival for patients with pancreatic, bile duct, or ampulla of Vater carcinomas. However, patients with gallbladder cancer had a significantly better 5-year survival with chemotherapy. Nevertheless, when an intent-to-treat analysis was applied, the survival differences were no longer apparent.[83]

ADJUVANT CHEMORADIOTHERAPY

Retrospective analysis and small phase II studies of chemoradiotherapy have suggested superior outcomes for patients receiving adjuvant therapy. The results of some phase II studies or retro-

TABLE 29.5-6. Randomized Studies of Adjuvant Therapy for Gallbladder Cancer and Cholangiocarcinoma

Study	No. of Patients		Therapy	Survival		Comments
	Periampullary			Median (Mo)	5-Y	
Klinkenbijl et al.,[201] 1999	49		Observation vs.	40.1	36%	Study also included pancreatic cancer
	44		RT 40 Gy[a] + 5-FU	39.5	38%	

Study	No. of Patients			Therapy	5-Y Survival			Comments
	Bile Duct	Gallbladder	Ampullary		Bile Duct	Gallbladder	Ampullary	
Takada et al.,[83] 2002	60	43	24	Observation vs.	34.3%	14%	34.3%	Survival differences significant only for gallbladder cancer
	58	69	24	MMC + 5-FU[b]	28%	26%	28.3%	

5-FU, 5-fluorouracil; MMC, mitomycin C; RT, radiotherapy.
[a]RT 2 Gy × 5 fractions/wk for 2 wk then repeated for 2 wk after a 2-wk delay to total of 40 Gy; 5-FU 25 mg/kg/d during RT.
[b]5-FU 310 mg/m^2 × 5 d (wk 1 and wk 3) followed by oral 5-FU (100 mg/m^2 from wk 5 until recurrence); MMC 6 mg/m^2 IV on day 1.

spective analysis have shown encouraging outcomes.[4,11,83a–83i] In one of the larger studies, 91 patients with extrahepatic cholangiocarcinoma underwent radiation therapy after surgery to a total of 40 Gy. Concurrent chemotherapy with 5-FU was administered in 71 patients. The overall 5-year survival was 31%. In this study, on multivariate analysis, only nodal status was a predictor for survival, and adjuvant therapy had no effect.[76] It should be kept in mind that patients who are offered adjuvant therapy tend not to have significant comorbidities, tend to have an uneventful postoperative course and a good performance status allowing initiation of adjuvant therapy, and may have an improved outcome with or without adjuvant therapy.

No large randomized studies have been conducted evaluating the role of adjuvant chemoradiotherapy for patients undergoing resection of cholangiocarcinomas. One randomized study by Klinkenbijl et al. evaluated the effectiveness of adjuvant chemoradiotherapy for periampullary tumors (see Table 29.5-6). In this study, periampullary tumors were stratified separately from pancreatic cancers. After surgery, patients were randomly assigned to observation or chemoradiation with 5-FU. There were a total of 93 patients with periampullary tumors in this study; however, no differences in outcome were seen with adjuvant therapy.[201]

Due to the small numbers of patients in clinical trials, possible selection bias, and lack of randomized data showing a benefit, routine adjuvant therapy for all patients is not recommended. The authors' practice is to administer adjuvant radiotherapy with concurrent 5-FU or 5-FU plus leucovorin (LV) to patients with high-risk characteristics such as regional lymph node involvement or positive postoperative surgical margins.

ADVANCED DISEASE

Palliative Procedures

The goal of palliation for bile duct tumors is drainage of the biliary system to avoid jaundice. In many cases, patients die of liver failure as a direct result of inadequate biliary drainage. The hepatocytes would otherwise function normally. In most cases it is unnecessary to drain both sides of the liver. However, this is dependent on the level of baseline hepatic dysfunction and any atrophy caused by long-term biliary obstruction or concomitant portal vein obstruction. Drainage of the bile ducts

can be performed using ERCP-placed stents, PTC-placed stents, or surgical bypass techniques.[84]

Hilar cholangiocarcinomas are best palliated using PTC-placed stents. An attempt should be made to drain the most functional lobe of the liver with a stent that traverses the malignant obstruction and allows for internal drainage. The catheter will exit the skin but can remain capped. This allows for irrigation and easy access for cholangiography and stent changes as needed. The downside is that the exposed catheter can be a factor in diminishing the quality of life.

Operative drainage procedures for hilar cholangiocarcinomas can be technically challenging but quite effective. The best long-term palliation is performed by creating a bypass to intraparenchymal bile ducts, using a defunctionalized limb of jejunum. The segment III bile duct can be accessed through the liver parenchyma anteriorly; the surgeon must stay well away from the hilar region, which is at risk for cancer progression.[85] The right lobe can be drained through a bypass to the anterior sectoral bile duct. Either bypass should be sufficient to avoid jaundice and maintain liver function. The obvious downside of operative drainage is the morbidity and recovery from surgery when overall life expectancy is limited. The best time for operative drainage is at the time of exploration for presumed resectable tumors. The "cost" of surgery has already been paid, and the additional morbidity of the bypass is acceptable. The advantage of surgical bypass is the avoidance of long-term catheter presence within the bile duct, which leads to accumulation of sludge and intermittent cholangitis. Cholangitis is a significant cause of morbidity and mortality in patients with cholangiocarcinoma.

Distal bile duct tumors can be successfully palliated with an ERCP-placed stent, which allows for completely internal drainage. Silastic stents need to be replaced every 3 months for best results and to minimize cholangitis.[86] This requires repeated endoscopic procedures. Surgical bypass to the common bile duct is easier than with hilar cholangiocarcinoma, and as successful, but still requires the morbidity and recovery of a laparotomy and bowel anastomosis. Again, this is best considered at the time of exploration for presumed resectable disease. Laparoscopic bypass of distal bile duct obstruction can be performed.[87] This is usually accomplished using a cholecystojejunostomy. This will be unsuccessful if the common bile duct at the level of the cystic duct is involved with tumor. This is often the case with unresectable cholangiocarcinoma.

Metal expandable stents can be placed via PTC or ERCP to open malignant strictures of the bile duct. Physician preference often dictates whether metal or Silastic stents are used. The advantage of the metal stents is that they maintain biliary drainage longer than the Silastic stents and therefore are associated with less cholangitis.[86] They do not require changing every 3 months. The disadvantage is that they cannot be removed, and they will eventually become obstructed due to advancement of the tumor. It can be difficult or impossible to pass a new stent through an obstructed metal stent. In general, it is recommended that replaceable Silastic stents be used for those with a life expectancy of less than 6 months, and metal stents be used for those with a longer life expectancy.[86]

Radiotherapy

Most of the discussion already presented concerning adjuvant radiotherapy for cholangiocarcinoma also applies to advanced cholangiocarcinoma that is unresectable or that has been resected leaving gross residual tumor. However, with gross residual disease, the radiation doses necessary for control are higher than those used in the clinical setting in which only microscopic disease is being irradiated. Thus, using external-beam radiotherapy alone, total doses should be at least 6500 cGy at 180 to 200 cGy/d. When possible, IORT or brachytherapy should be administered as a boost dose. Data regarding radiotherapy in advanced-stage cholangiocarcinoma, either unresectable or resected with gross residual tumor, indicate that radiotherapy does provide a benefit in terms of overall survival. Morganti et al. reported on a small series of 20 patients with unresectable tumor or gross residual tumor after resection, all treated with external-beam radiotherapy, 3960 to 5040 cGy, with 12 patients also receiving brachytherapy, 3000 to 5000 cGy administered at 1 cm from the sources. Two patients who had external-beam radiotherapy and brachytherapy for unresected tumors were 5-year survivors.[82]

Shin et al. reported on 31 patients with inoperable carcinoma of the extrahepatic bile ducts treated with external-beam radiotherapy alone (17 patients) or external-beam radiotherapy and high dose-rate brachytherapy (14 patients).[81] The administered external-beam radiotherapy dose was 3600 to 5500 cGy (median, 5040 cGy). Brachytherapy was administered in single doses of 500 cGy/d for 3 days using an afterloading technique. There was no statistically significant difference in local recurrence, but prolongation of the median time to tumor recurrence increased with the use of external-beam radiotherapy and brachytherapy (9 months vs. 5 months; $P = .06$). The 2-year survival for patients treated with a combination of external-beam therapy and brachytherapy was 21% versus 0% for those treated with external-beam radiotherapy alone ($P = .015$), but the external-beam radiotherapy doses were higher in the group receiving brachytherapy. Also, it must be noted that this is a retrospective review of patients nonrandomly assigned to either treatment.

A small series of 24 patients with advanced bile duct tumor reported by Aldin and Mohiuddin were treated with external-beam radiotherapy or brachytherapy or both.[88] The external-beam radiotherapy doses ranged from 2700 to 6000 cGy and the brachytherapy dose was 2500 cGy at 1 cm. Nineteen patients also received chemotherapy. The 2-year survival rates

and median survival intervals improved as the total dose of administered radiotherapy increased.

Flickinger et al. of the University of Pittsburgh reported on 63 patients who received radiotherapy for primary cancers of the extrahepatic biliary duct (55 patients) and gallbladder (8 patients).[74] Three patients received brachytherapy alone, 2800 to 5500 cGy, and 60 patients received external-beam radiotherapy, 540 to 6160 cGy, of whom 9 also received additional intraluminal brachytherapy, 1400 to 4500 cGy. There were only two long-term survivors at 50 months, and both had liver transplantation followed by radiotherapy. The total dose of administered radiotherapy did not have an impact on length of survival.

Crane et al. reported on 52 patients with localized but unresectable biliary tract cancer treated with external-beam radiotherapy.[89] Three patients also had brachytherapy and one patient had treatment with IORT. Total administered doses ranged from 3000 cGy to 8500 cGy. The median time to local progression was not influenced by the total radiation dose administered.

Buskirk et al. reported on 34 patients with subtotal resected or unresectable carcinoma of the extrahepatic bile ducts.[90] All received external-beam radiotherapy to a minimum of 4500 cGy with or without 5-FU. Seventeen patients received additional external-beam radiotherapy, 500 to 1500 cGy, and ten other patients received brachytherapy and an additional seven other patients received additional radiotherapy with IORT. Local control and length of survival seemed to be better in those patients who had external-beam radiotherapy plus brachytherapy or IORT.

At the University of Pittsburgh, split-course radiotherapy is occasionally used for advanced bile duct tumors, and in such cases, in addition to the two courses of 2500 cGy in ten fractions, a third course of 1000 cGy in four or five fractions is administered 3 to 4 weeks after the second course—again, if there has been no evidence of tumor progression in the interim. Radiobiologically, the three courses of radiotherapy are equivalent to a continuous course of 180 cGy daily for 35 treatments (6300 cGy) or 200 cGy daily for 30 treatments (6000 cGy). This regimen has been well tolerated.

Chemotherapy

Due to the rarity of these tumors, almost all clinical trials have broadened eligibility to include all tumors arising from the biliary tract. Because of the small numbers of patients with biliary tract cancers in clinical trials, it is not possible to know whether there are differences in response to chemotherapy for tumors in different anatomic sites of the biliary tract, such as gallbladder carcinomas and cholangiocarcinomas.

Based on review of published studies of chemotherapy, there is no consensus as to the best agent or regimen for unresectable or metastatic cholangiocarcinoma. Due to the rarity of the disease, randomized studies have not been conducted. In addition, a significant number of patients present with biliary obstruction and elevated levels on liver function tests, which severely curtails the ability to administer chemotherapy.

As with most gastrointestinal malignancies, 5-FU as a single agent or in combination is the most evaluated drug for gallbladder and bile duct malignancies and appears to have some activity (Table 29.5-7). Single-agent studies using other agents such as cisplatin, mitomycin, and amsacrine have been disappointing.[203,204] Despite the wide range of activity reported with 5-FU, in most studies the time to progression is a few months,

TABLE 29.5-7. Chemotherapy Trials for Advanced Biliary Tree Carcinomas

Study	No. of Patients			Therapy	Response Rate (%)	Median Survival (Mo)
	Gallbladder	Bile Duct	Total			
Falkson et al.,[202] 1984	18	12	30	Oral 5-FU	10	5.2–6.5
	16	10	36	Oral 5-FU + STZ	7.7	3.0–3.5
	19	12	31	Oral 5-FU + MeCCNU	9.7	2.0–2.5
Bukowski et al.,[203] 1983	12	11	23	m-AMSA (amsacrine)	8.7	2.0–2.8
Ravry et al.,[204] 1986	—	9	9	CDDP	0	—
Taal et al.,[173] 1993	13	16	39	MMC	10	4.5
Whittington et al.,[205] 1995	—	9	9	CI 5-FU + RT	—	11.9
Harvey et al.,[206] 1984	—	14	14	FAM	31	11.5
Takada et al.,[207] 1998	10	4	14	FAM	14.3	4.1–5.2
Kajanti et al.,[208] 1994	6	11	17	Epirubicin + MTX + 5-FU	0	9.0
Sanz-Altamira et al.,[209] 1998	4	10	14	5-FU + LV + carboplatin	21	5.0
Choi et al.,[210] 2000	9	19	28	5-FU + LV	32	6.0
Patt et al.,[211] 1996	10	25	35	CI 5-FU + IFN	34	12.0
Patt et al.,[212] 2001	19	22	41	CI 5-FU + IFN + Dox + CDDP	21.1	14.0
Chen et al.,[213] 1998	6	13	19	CI 5-FU + LV	33	7.0
Chen et al.,[214] 2001	3	22	25	CI 5-FU + LV + MMC	26	6.0
Mani et al.,[215] 1999	0	13	13	UFT + LV	0	7.0
Jones et al.,[216] 1996	4	11	15	Paclitaxel	0	—
Pazdur et al.,[217] 1999	0	17	17	Docetaxel	0	—
Papakostas et al.,[218] 2001	16	10	26	Docetaxel	20	8.0
Kubicka et al.,[219] 2001	—	23	23	Gemcitabine	30	9.3
Penz et al.,[91] 2001	10	22	32	Gemcitabine	22	11.5
Gebbia et al.,[220] 2001	12	6	18	Gemcitabine	22	4.5
	10	12	22	Gemcitabine/5-FU/LV	36	6.0
Kuhn et al.,[221] 2002	26	17	43	Gemcitabine/docetaxel	9.3	11.0
Eng et al.,[222] 2003	9	6	15	Gemcitabine	0	5.0
Fiebiger et al.,[223] 2002	14	6	20	Lanreotide	5	4.5

CDDP, cisplatin; CI, continuous infusion; Dox, doxorubicin; FAM, 5-fluorouracil, Adriamycin (doxorubicin), mitomycin; 5-FU, 5-fluorouracil; IFN, interferon-α; LV, leucovorin; MeCCNU, methyl-chloroethylcyclohexylnitrosourea; MMC, mitomycin; MTX, methotrexate; RT, radiation therapy; STZ, streptozocin; UFT, uracil and tegafur.

and median survival of patients is in the range of 6 months. For locally advanced biliary tract cancers, concurrent chemotherapy and radiation is commonly used, although use of this approach is supported by a study involving only nine patients. In this study, continuous infusion of 5-FU with radiation therapy was found to be well tolerated.[205]

The addition of LV to 5-FU generally results in a higher response rate in other tumors, and this combination has been evaluated in treatment of cholangiocarcinoma. One study reported a response rate of 32% in 28 patients with cholangiocarcinoma; however, the median survival was only 6 months.[210] A weekly regimen of high-dose 5-FU with LV was reported to have a 33% response rate with a median patient survival of 7 months.[90a] However, the same high-dose 5-FU plus LV regimen with the addition of mitomycin proved intolerable with severe toxicity.[214]

Continuous-infusion 5-FU, compared to bolus 5-FU, is more active and better tolerated, especially in colorectal cancer. Oral formulations of 5-FU mimic a continuous infusion schedule, and have the advantage of easy administration. A number of oral pro–5-FU drugs such as capecitabine, uracil-tegafur, and eniluracil are now available and are being evaluated in a number of tumor types. Mani et al. evaluated uracil-tegafur in combination with LV in 13 patients with cholangiocarcinoma, but no responses were reported. The median survival was 7 months.[215] In the United States only capecitabine has gained regulatory approval and is commercially available. Preliminary results with capecitabine and

another oral 5-FU drug termed S1 indicate possible activity in patients with hepatobiliary cancers.[90b]

Combination chemotherapy with 5-FU has been reported to increase response rates but at the expense of increased toxicity. Median survival rates in some of these studies appear to be promising; however, the apparent benefit may be due to patient selection. In one study, Patt et al. treated 35 patients with biliary tree cancers with continuous-infusion 5-FU and subcutaneous interferon-α$_{2b}$. The response rate was 34%, with a median survival of 12 months.[211] The same investigators added cisplatin and doxorubicin to a modified 5-FU and interferon-α schedule (PIAF regimen). Forty-one patients were treated, and overall response rate was 21%. The median survival was 14 months; however, most patients experienced significant toxicity.[212] Other investigators have evaluated 5-FU with or without LV with carboplatin, cisplatin, doxorubicin, or epirubicin with similar results.[206–209]

Over the last decade, newer chemotherapeutic agents have been evaluated without much success. The taxanes, both docetaxel and paclitaxel, have been evaluated in biliary tract cancers and appear to have minimal activity.[216–218] Gemcitabine has proven activity in pancreatic cancer, which has led to a number of studies of its use in biliary tract cancers, with mixed results. Kubicka et al. treated 23 patients with cholangiocarcinomas with gemcitabine; the response rate was 30%, with median survival of 9.5 months.[219] In a study of gemcitabine given every 2 weeks, Penz et al. found this regimen to be active, with a response rate of 22%

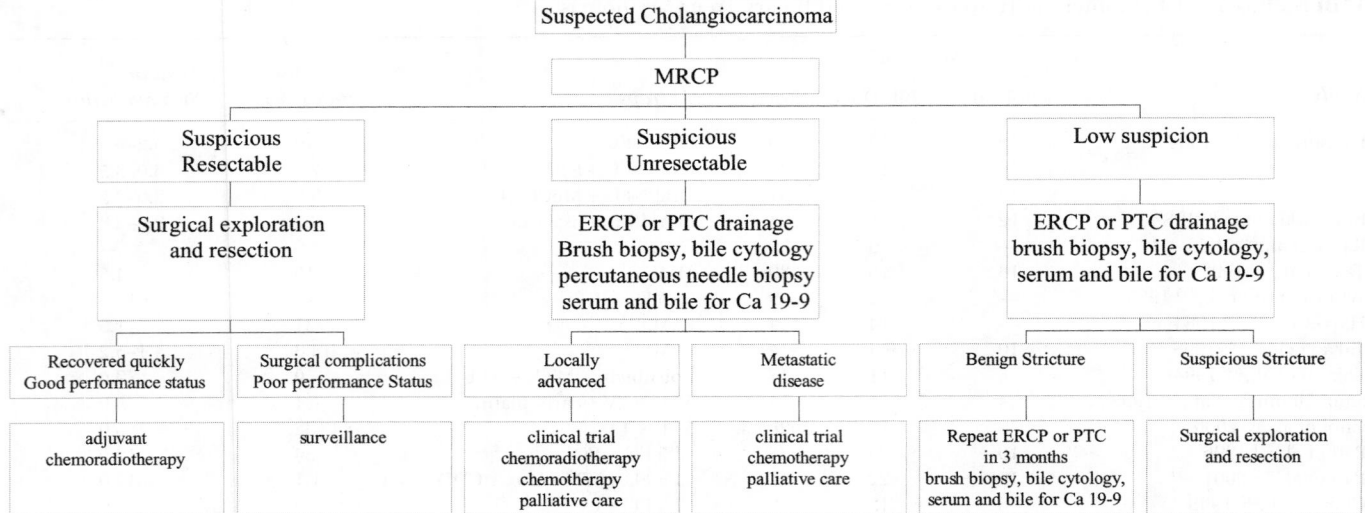

FIGURE 29.5-5. Algorithm for management of suspected cholangiocarcinoma. Ca 19-9, carbohydrate antigen 19-9; ERCP, endoscopic retrograde cholangiopancreatography; MRCP, magnetic resonance cholangiopancreatography; PTC, percutaneous transhepatic cholangiography.

and median survival of 11.5 months.[91] A preliminary report by Gebbia et al. documented a response rate of 22% and median survival of 4.5 months with single-agent gemcitabine, and a response rate of 36% and median survival of 6.0 months in 22 patients treated with the combination of gemcitabine plus 5-FU and LV.[220] In contrast, Eng et al. evaluated a fixed dose rate of gemcitabine (1500 mg/m^2 over 150 minutes) in 14 patients with biliary tract cancers. No objective responses were documented, and the median survival was only 5 months.[222] Gemcitabine combinations continue to be evaluated, and in one study, the combination of docetaxel and gemcitabine resulted in a response rate of 9.3% and a median survival of 11.0 months.[221] Preliminary results for the use of gemcitabine with either cisplatin or irinotecan in biliary tree cancers have also been reported.[91a,91b]

A number of new combinations and novel drugs are undergoing evaluation in biliary tract cancers. One such agent is the somatostatin analog lanreotide, which was found to be inactive.[223] Other agents and modalities investigated are a rebeccamycin analog (NSC 655649), liposomal doxorubicin, and whole body hyperthermia with chemotherapy. In particular, a rebeccamycin analog, which is a novel antitumor antibiotic with both topoisomerase I and II activity as well as DNA-intercalating properties, appears to have promising activity, with reported median survival of 10 months at interim analysis of a phase II study.[91a,91c–91g]

Although hepatic arterial infusion therapy is widely used for primary hepatocellular cancers, its role in cholangiocarcinomas remains investigational, with few reported studies.[91h,91i] The blood supply to the biliary tract is primarily from the hepatic artery, and hepatic arterial infusion is a logical approach. Tanaka et al. reported on a series of 11 patients with intrahepatic cholangiocarcinomas who received chemotherapy with 5-FU through an implanted hepatic arterial pump. Responses were noted, with a median survival of 26 months.[91j] Mezawa et al. evaluated use of a carboplatin-coated percutaneous transhepatic biliary catheter in five patients with cholangiocarcinomas and noted activity.[91k] Photodynamic therapy is a new approach used to treat endoluminal lesions of the lung and esophagus. Tumors of the biliary tract frequently encroach on the lumen of the bile ducts, and photody-

namic therapy is being evaluated in cholangiocarcinoma, with preliminary evidence of activity in some patients.[91l–91n]

SUMMARY OF TREATMENT RECOMMENDATIONS

An algorithm for treatment of cholangiocarcinoma is shown in Figure 29.5-5. When possible, the first line of therapy is surgical resection with the goal of achieving negative microscopic margins. Adjuvant chemoradiotherapy is considered in patients with a good performance status. In patients with locally advanced disease, concurrent 5-FU given by continuous infusion or bolus infusion with LV and radiation therapy can be used for palliation, especially if there is pain. There is no proven benefit for combination chemotherapy in patients with advanced surgically unresectable biliary tract cancers. The authors' practice is to enroll patients with biliary tract cancers into clinical trials whenever possible. Due to lack of standardized therapy, phase I studies involving previously untreated or treated patients would be appropriate. Chemotherapy should only be offered to patients with a good performance status, because those who have significant cancer-related symptoms have a short life expectancy and are unlikely to benefit from therapy. In patients with evidence of metastatic disease a trial of 5-FU plus LV, continuous-infusion 5-FU, capecitabine, or gemcitabine could be tried. There is no proven benefit for second-line therapy, and in this setting, enrollment in phase I studies or best supportive care would be appropriate.

TUMORS OF THE GALLBLADDER

Histologically, gallbladder cancer resembles other biliary neoplasms and therefore is appropriate to be considered together in the same chapter. However, its epidemiology, clinical presentation, staging, and surgical treatment are distinct from those of cholangiocarcinoma, and therefore gallbladder cancer is considered separately in this chapter. Chemotherapy and radiation therapy trials often combine patients with gallbladder cancers and cholangiocarcinomas, so there may be some overlap in the description of these treatments. Gallbladder cancer tends to be an aggressive tumor that spreads early and leads to rapid death. DeStoll described the gross appearance and invasive nature of gallbladder cancer in 1788 based on his study of two autopsy cases.[92] The clinical pessimism surrounding gallbladder cancer is due to its late presentation and lack of effective therapy. Gallbladder cancer spreads early by lymphatic metastasis, hematogenous metastasis, and direct invasion into the liver, and as with cholangiocarcinoma has a uniquely high propensity to seed the peritoneal surfaces after tumor spillage and cause tumor implants in biopsy tracts, abdominal wounds, and the peritoneal cavity. Classically, the 5-year survival in most large series is less than 5%, and the median survival is less than 6 months.[92a,92b] It is important for the oncology clinician to understand the natural history, biology, staging, and surgical treatment of this tumor, so that appropriate decisions are made at the time of initial diagnosis. Given the high chance of these lesions' being found incidentally at the time of cholecystectomy, the general surgeon must be familiar with the appropriate management in that setting. Inappropriate procedures may allow spread of this tumor throughout the abdominal cavity, to laparoscopic port sites, or to biopsy needle tracts, which renders the disease untreatable. On the other hand, it is important to understand the limitations of surgical resection so that operations with unreasonably high morbidity but minimal chance of success are avoided.

EPIDEMIOLOGY

The incidence of gallbladder cancer varies by geographic region and racial-ethnic group. Gallbladder cancer is up to 25 times more common in some geographic regions than in others.[92c] The highest incidences are reported in Chileans, Bolivians, Central Europeans, Israelis, American Indians, and Americans of Mexican origin.[93] Gallbladder cancer is the main cause of death from cancer among women in Chile.[94] Japanese men have been reported to have the highest mortality rate from gallbladder carcinoma.[95] The lowest rates are seen in the people of Spain and India, black Rhodesians, and black Americans. Within the United States and the United Kingdom, urban areas show higher incidences than rural regions.[96,97] It has been suggested that lower socioeconomic status may lead to delayed access to cholecystectomy, which may increase gallbladder cancer rates.[98]

In the United States, women are two to six times more likely to develop gallbladder cancer than men. As with cholangiocarcinoma, the incidence steadily increases with age, reaching its maximum in the seventh decade of life.[99] Nevertheless, reports exist of a 21-year-old Chilean girl[94] and an 11-year-old American Indian girl[100] with the diagnosis of gallbladder cancer. Trends in gallbladder cancer mortality show a variable pattern. Germany and the Netherlands have relatively high mortality rates from gallbladder cancer and have shown declines in most age groups. Sweden, France, and Bulgaria show steady upward trends.[97] Gallbladder cancer incidence in the United States, Britain, and Canada has stabilized or declined, coincident with the rise in the number of laparoscopic cholecystectomies.

In the United States, gallbladder cancer is the most common biliary tract malignancy and the fifth most common gastrointestinal malignancy. Estimates of the Surveillance, Epidemiology, and End Results (SEER) program revealed an incidence of 1.2 cases per 100,000 population per year in the United States.[101] Based on SEER data and data from the National Cancer Database, there are approximately 2800 deaths per year secondary to gallbladder cancer in the United States.[101,102]

ETIOLOGY

The etiology of gallbladder cancer is similar to that of cholangiocarcinoma, in that some form of chronic inflammation leads to malignant transformation. In the case of the gallbladder, the overwhelming inciting factor for chronic inflammation is gallstones. Seventy-five percent to 98% of all patients with carcinoma of the gallbladder have cholelithiasis.[103] The epidemiology of gallbladder cancer is closely linked to the epidemiology of gallbladder stones.[104] Calcification of the gallbladder (porcelain gallbladder) is associated with gallbladder cancer in 10% to 25% of cases.[105] Calcification is the end stage of a long-standing inflammatory process and is therefore associated with an increased risk of gallbladder cancer.

Case-control studies have identified a history of biliary problems, older age, and female sex as risk factors for the development of gallbladder cancer.[106,107] The presence of an anomalous pancreaticobiliary duct junction is a risk factor for gallbladder cancer independent of the presence of gallstones.[108] This may establish a chronic inflammatory state of the gallbladder. Typhoid carriers may also suffer chronic inflammation of the gallbladder and have a sixfold higher risk of gallbladder cancer.[109] Other rare associations with gallbladder cancer include inflammatory bowel disease[110] and polyposis coli.[111] Reports of familial clusters of gallbladder cancer exist in the literature,[112] but any inherited predisposition has not been found in large series of gallbladder cancer.[113]

Although gallstones and chronic inflammation of the gallbladder are involved in the pathogenesis of this tumor, the incidence of gallbladder cancer in a population of patients with gallstones is only 0.3% to 3.0%. Chronic inflammation seems to act as a promoter for some other carcinogenic exposure. Experimentally, Kowalewski and Todd[114] showed that carcinoma of the gallbladder was induced in 68% of hamsters who had cholesterol pellets inserted into the gallbladder and were given the carcinogen dimethylnitrosamine versus only 6% of controls fed the carcinogen alone. Exposure to methyldopa,[115] oral contraceptives,[116] and isoniazid,[117] and occupational exposure in the rubber industry[118] have been implicated in carcinogenesis of gallbladder cancer, but none of these associations have been proven.

ANATOMIC CONSIDERATIONS

Certain anatomic considerations are important in the management of gallbladder cancer. The location of the primary tumor within the gallbladder and the proximity of the portal vein, hepatic artery, and bile duct are all important factors in the surgical management of this tumor. The gallbladder is attached to segments IVb and V of the liver, and these segments are involved early in tumors of the fundus and body of the gallbladder. Tumors of the infundibulum or cystic duct readily obstruct the common bile duct and may involve the portal vein. As with cholangiocarcinoma, the tumor may be unresectable early in its course.

The lymphatic drainage of the gallbladder has been carefully mapped using a blue dye technique.[119] The lymph descends around the bile duct and involves cystic and pericholedochal nodes first. From there connections are made to nodes posterior to the pancreas, portal vein, and common hepatic artery. Finally, the flow reaches the interaortocaval,

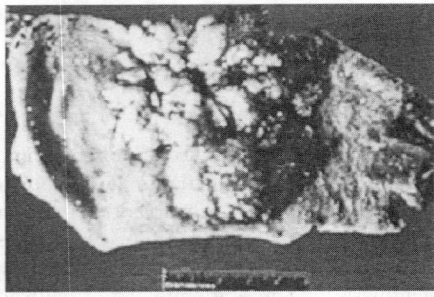
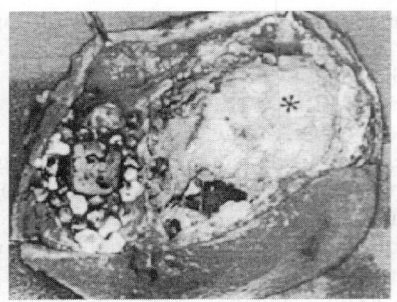
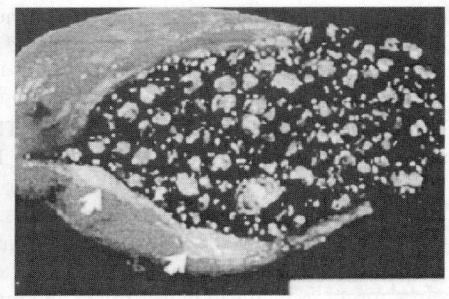

A–C

FIGURE 29.5-6.   Photographs of the typical forms of gallbladder cancer. **A:** Cauliflower-like intraluminal growth of a papillary adenocarcinoma. **B:** Moderately well differentiated adenocarcinoma (*asterisk*) in an opened gallbladder specimen with associated gallstones. **C:** Poorly differentiated adenocarcinoma with diffuse mural thickening of the gallbladder (*arrows*) and associated gallstones. (From ref. 241, with permission.)

celiac, and superior mesenteric artery lymph nodes. Importantly, the dye never ascended toward the hepatic hilum, whereas it stained node-bearing adipose tissue posterior to the head of the pancreas and portal vein as an early event. Some connections are made directly from the pericholedochal nodes to interaortocaval nodes, which explains the difficulty in controlling this disease with a regional lymph node dissection.

PATHOLOGY

Gallbladder cancers demonstrate progression from dysplasia to carcinoma *in situ* to invasive carcinoma.[120] Severe dysplasia and carcinoma *in situ* are identified in surrounding gallbladder epithelium in more than 90% of gallbladder cancer cases.[121] The time of progression of precursor lesions to invasive carcinoma is 5 to 15 years.[120,122] Adenomas are present in up to 1.1% of cholecystectomy specimens.[123] The precancerous nature of adenomas of the gallbladder is controversial. Benign adenomas do not have the same association with cholecystitis as do invasive carcinomas; therefore, it is unlikely that the majority of carcinomas arise in adenomas. Nevertheless, 19% of invasive carcinomas are found to have adenomatous components.[124] Papillary cancers may represent malignant degeneration of papillary adenomas.

Sixty percent of tumors originate in the fundus of the gallbladder, 30% in the body, and 10% in the neck.[120] Tumors that arise in the neck and Hartmann's pouch may infiltrate the cystic and common bile duct, making it clinically and radiographically indistinguishable from hilar cholangiocarcinomas. Gallbladder cancer can be categorized into infiltrative, nodular, and papillary forms[125] (Fig. 29.5-6). This directly parallels the forms of cholangiocarcinoma discussed in Cholangiocarcinomas: Pathology earlier in this chapter. As with cholangiocarcinoma, the most common form is the infiltrative form, and the papillary forms have the best prognosis.

The infiltrative tumors cause thickening and induration of the gallbladder wall, sometimes extending to involve the entire gallbladder. These tumors spread in a subserosal plane, which is the same plane used by the surgeon for routine cholecystectomy. If the tumor is unrecognized at the time of cholecystectomy, this plane will be violated and tumor cells will seed the peritoneal cavity. As the infiltrative tumor becomes more advanced, it invades the liver and can result in a thick wall of tumor encasing the gallbladder. Nodular or mass-forming gallbladder cancers can show early invasion through the gallbladder wall into the liver or neighboring structures. Despite this

invasiveness, they may be easier to control surgically than the infiltrative form in which the margins are less defined. Papillary carcinomas exhibit a polypoid or cauliflower-like appearance and fill the lumen of the gallbladder with only minimal invasion of the gallbladder wall. Papillary carcinomas have a much better prognosis than the other types.

The most common histologic type of gallbladder carcinoma is adenocarcinoma. However, unlike with cholangiocarcinomas, the gallbladder can be involved with a number of different histologic types. The histologic types of gallbladder cancer and their incidences as recorded by the SEER program of the National Cancer Institute are listed in Table 29.5-8. Primary malignant mesenchymal tumors of the gallbladder have been described, including embryonal rhabdomyosarcoma, leiomyosarcoma, malignant fibrous histiocytoma, angiosarcoma, and Kaposi's sarcoma. Other primary rare tumors of the gallbladder that have been described in the literature include carcinosarcoma, carcinoid, lymphoma, and melanoma. In addition, the gallbladder can be involved with metastatic cancers from numerous sites. Many tumors exhibit more than one histologic pattern. The only histologic type with clear prognostic significance is the papillary adenocarcinoma, which has a markedly improved survival compared to all other histologic types.[101] There is also evidence to suggest that oat cell carcinomas[9] and adenosquamous tumors[95] have a poorer survival rate.

Gallbladder cancer has a remarkable propensity to seed and grow in the peritoneal cavity, as well as along needle biopsy sites and in laparoscopic port sites. It can also spread early by direct extension into the liver and other adjacent organs. The gallbladder has a thin wall, a narrow lamina propria, and only a single

TABLE 29.5-8.   Relative Incidence of Gallbladder Cancer by Histologic Type, as Reported by Carriaga and Henson

Histologic Type	Relative Incidence (%)
Adenocarcinoma	80
Papillary adenocarcinoma	6
Mucinous and mucin-producing adenocarcinoma	5
Squamous cell carcinoma	2
Sarcoma	0.2
Other and unspecified	7

(Data from ref. 101.)

muscle layer. Tumor invades into the liver at a thickness at which in other organs it would be encountering a second muscle layer. Once it penetrates the thin muscle layer, it has access to major lymphatic and vascular channels. Gallbladder cancer therefore tends to have early lymphatic and hematogenous spread. At autopsy, gallbladder cancer patients have a 91% to 94% incidence of lymphatic metastasis, 65% to 82% incidence of hematogenous metastasis, and 60% incidence of peritoneal spread.[126,127] Hematogenous metastasis tends to be from invasion into small veins extending directly from the gallbladder into the portal venous system, leading to hepatic metastases in segments IV and V of the liver.[128] The incidence of regional invasion and metastasis at the time of diagnosis and treatment is summarized in Table 29.5-9. There is a high propensity for intraabdominal recurrence after resection with distant metastasis occurring late in the course. The only common extraabdominal site of metastasis is the lung. It is rare, however, to have metastasis to the lung in the absence of advanced local-regional disease.

Multiple staging systems have been described for gallbladder cancer taking into account pathologic and clinical characteristics with prognostic significance. The different staging systems create confusion when one attempts to compare the treatment results of different series in the literature. It is essential to standardize the staging system for the purpose of reporting and comparing treatment results. The main staging systems referred to in the literature include the modified Nevin system,[129,130] the Japanese Biliary Surgical Society system,[131] and the AJCC TNM staging system (Table 29.5-10). It is the stage according to the latter system that should be reported uniformly for standardization.

The TNM system includes tumors invading the mucosa or muscle layer in stage I. It is important to realize that tumors can arise in Rokitansky-Aschoff sinuses and be considered stage I in a subserosal position. Tumors with invasion into the perimuscular connective tissue are considered stage II, and those with liver invasion are stage III. In addition, tumors with nodal metastasis to the hepatoduodenal ligament are included in stage III. In contrast, stage IV includes tumors with distant metastasis. It should be noted that, although grade does not factor into staging, it does have prognostic significance. Gallbladder cancers undergo histopathologic grading from G1 (well differentiated) to G4 (undifferentiated). High-grade tumors have a worse prognosis.[9] The majority of patients present with grade 3, poorly differentiated tumors.

K-ras and p53 mutations are common in gallbladder cancer.[93,132] Mutant p53 is found in 92% of invasive carcinomas, 86%

TABLE 29.5-9. Incidence of Regional Invasion and Metastasis at the Time of Diagnosis and Treatment Based on a Literature Review by Boerma[128]

Pathologic Finding	Relative Incidence (%)
Confined to gallbladder wall	10
Liver invasion	59
Common bile duct infiltration	35
Lymphatic invasion and regional lymphatic metastases	45
Gallbladder vein infiltration	39
Portal vein or hepatic artery invasion	15
Adjacent organ invasion (excluding liver)	40
Perineural invasion	42
Liver metastasis	34
Distant metastasis (excluding liver)	20

TABLE 29.5-10. American Joint Committee on Cancer Staging System for Gallbladder Cancer

T1	Tumor with invasion into muscularis layer		
T2	Tumor with transmural invasion of gallbladder wall		
T3	Tumor perforates the serosa (visceral peritoneum) and/or directly invades the liver and/or one other adjacent organ or structure, such as the stomach, duodenum, colon, pancreas, omentum, or extrahepatic bile ducts		
T4	Tumor invades main portal vein or hepatic artery or invades multiple extrahepatic organs or structures		
N1	Regional lymph node metastasis		
Stage IA	T1	N0	M0
Stage IB	T2	N0	M0
Stage IIA	T3	N0	M0
Stage IIB	T1–T3	N1	M0
Stage III	T4	Any N	M0
Stage IV	Any T	Any N	M1

(From ref. 175, with permission.)

of carcinomas *in situ*, and 28% of dysplastic epithelia.[133,134] K-ras mutations are identified in 39% of gallbladder carcinomas.[135] Overexpression of the c-erbB2 gene[136] and decreased expression of the nm23 gene product[137] also may play an important role in the development of gallbladder cancer. A few studies have demonstrated that CDKN2 (also known as *MTS1* or *p19^{ink4}*) may play a role in gallbladder carcinogenesis.[138] Another candidate suppressor gene implicated in the development of gallbladder cancer is fragile histidine triad (FHIT) gene.[139]

CLINICAL PRESENTATION

The clinical presentation of gallbladder cancer is identical to the symptoms of biliary colic or chronic cholecystitis. This leads to a low index of suspicion for cancer in most cases and results in the incidental finding of gallbladder cancer at the time of surgery for cholecystitis or on pathologic review of the resected gallbladder. Patients older than 70 years with a history of recent weight loss and persistent right upper quadrant pain should be suspected of having gallbladder cancer. Careful history taking may reveal patients with gallbladder cancer to have a more continuous, diffuse abdominal pain than the crampy right upper quadrant pain associated with biliary colic. Jaundice and anorexia are a sign of advanced disease.[140] The presence of a right upper quadrant mass in association with gallbladder cancer reflects unresectability in 92% of patients. Clinical jaundice represented unresectability in 18 of 18 patients in one study.[141]

DIAGNOSTIC EVALUATION

Laboratory Tests

As with cholangiocarcinoma, CA 19-9 is the best serum marker for gallbladder cancer. A level above 20 U/mL has 79% sensitivity and 79% specificity for the diagnosis of gallbladder cancer.[142] This can be used to aid in the diagnosis in suspicious clinical situations, but it is not cost effective as a general screen for all patients undergoing cholecystectomy. A CEA level higher than 4 ng/mL is 93% specific for the diagnosis of gallbladder cancer compared to controls undergoing cholecystectomy or upper abdominal surgery for benign conditions, but it is only 50% sen-

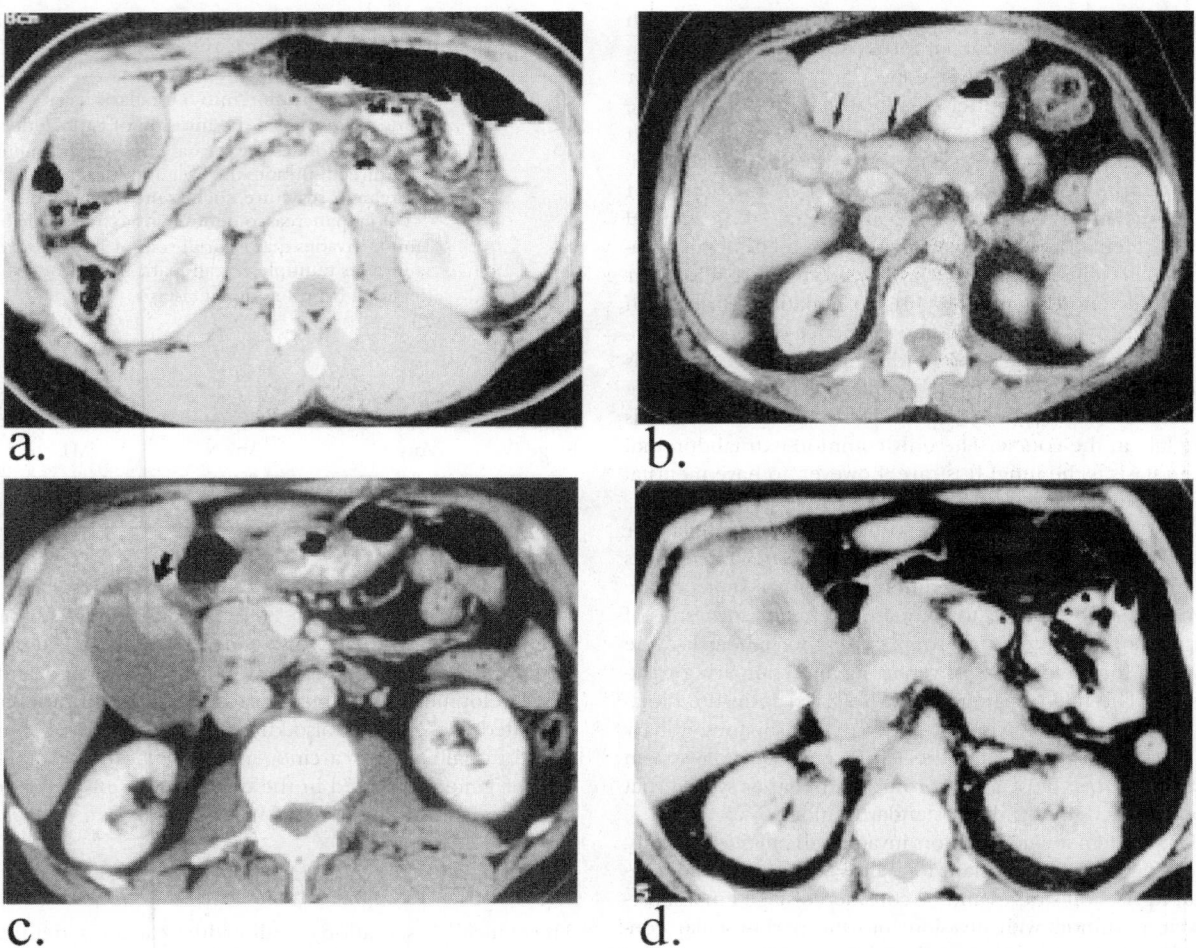

FIGURE 29.5-7.   Classic contrast-enhanced computed tomography findings of gallbladder cancer. **a:** Focal mass in the gallbladder fundus representing adenocarcinoma in a 35-year-old woman. **b:** Advanced diffusely infiltrative gallbladder cancer with hepatic invasion and periportal lymphadenopathy (*arrows*). **c:** Sessile, soft tissue mass in gallbladder representing a moderately well differentiated adenocarcinoma in a 55-year-old man. **d:** Diffusely thickened gallbladder with a mass extending into the adjacent liver parenchyma and a peripancreatic lymph node (*arrow*) representing poorly differentiated adenocarcinoma in a 67-year-old man. (From ref. 241, with permission.)

sitive for detecting cancer.[142] Increased alkaline phosphatase and bilirubin levels are found in cases of advanced gallbladder cancer. A trend toward anemia and leukocytosis has also been identified as an indicator of advanced disease.[141]

Radiologic Evaluation

The most common initial radiologic evaluation for symptoms of right upper quadrant pain is an ultrasonographic examination. Ultrasonography typically demonstrates gallstones and gallbladder wall thickening, which is nonspecific for gallbladder cancer. A comparison of ultrasonographic features of early malignancy and benign gallbladder disease revealed some findings that were important in the differentiation. Discontinuous gallbladder mucosa, echogenic mucosa, and submucosal echolucency were significantly more common in gallbladder cancer than in benign gallbladder disease. A polypoid mass was present in 27% and a gallbladder-replacing or invasive mass was present in 50% of patients with gallbladder cancer examined.[143]

CT scanning reveals a mass partially obliterating the gallbladder lumen in 42% of cases, a polypoidal mass in 26%, and diffuse wall thickening in 6% of cases[144] (Fig. 29.5-7). However, only 38% of pathologically positive nodes are identified preoperatively by CT scan.[145] Endoscopic ultrasonography may be helpful as an adjunct to other imaging modalities for the evaluation of periportal and peripancreatic adenopathy. Unfortunately, large inflammatory lymph nodes are difficult to differentiate from metastatic tumor without pathologic confirmation. Endoscopic ultrasonography–directed needle biopsy may be useful if the information would prevent a laparotomy. The use of MRI for the diagnostic workup of gallbladder cancer can be helpful.[146] MRCP may provide more detailed information than can be provided by ultrasonography or CT.[147]

Biopsy and Cytologic Analysis

Once a mass suspicious for gallbladder cancer has been identified, whether a biopsy should be performed before definitive exploration and resection is controversial. It is clear that cholecystectomy as a diagnostic biopsy before definitive resection is unacceptable, and all emphasis should be placed on being prepared for definitive resection at the time of initial exploration. Diagnosis by cytologic examination of bile is one way to avoid violating the tumor and seeding cells in the peritoneal cavity or abdominal wound. The diagnostic accuracy of combined ERCP and bile cytologic analysis is 50% for gallbladder cancers.[148] The sensitivity of bile cytologic analysis alone for the diagnosis of gallbladder cancer has been reported between 50% and 73%.[149,150] For any patient suspected of having gallbladder cancer who undergoes ERCP or PTC, bile should be collected for cytologic examination.

Percutaneous fine-needle aspiration or core-needle biopsy should be performed on masses that are not considered for surgical resection. The accuracy of percutaneous fine-needle aspiration has been reported to be 88% for gallbladder cancers. The false-positive rate is negligible.[150] Percutaneous core-needle biopsy has a higher chance of resulting in needle tract seeding than fine-needle aspiration and should be kept in reserve for cases in which fine-needle aspiration is unsuccessful. In cases in which a diagnosis of gallbladder cancer would result in referral to another institution for definitive surgical management, bile cytologic analysis or percutaneous fine-needle aspiration cytologic analysis would be preferable to any form of operative or laparoscopic biopsy.

SURGERY FOR GALLBLADDER CANCER

Prophylactic Cholecystectomy

The incidence of gallbladder cancer is low compared to the incidence of gallstones in the population, so prophylactic cholecystectomy for asymptomatic cholelithiasis to prevent the development of carcinoma is not indicated. Nevertheless, any abnormality in the gallbladder wall consistent with an early cancer needs to be taken seriously and consideration given to further workup. Only early diagnosis and treatment of gallbladder cancer is currently able to alter its natural history. A calcified or porcelain gallbladder is an indication for cholecystectomy in the asymptomatic patient, because up to 25% of cases are associated with gallbladder cancer.[105] It may be in these high-risk situations that serum CA 19-9 evaluation and bile cytologic analysis can be helpful in making a preoperative diagnosis of cancer. Laparoscopic cholecystectomy is usually not reasonable in this setting, because of the risk for incidental cancer and inadvertent seeding of the peritoneal cavity.

Benign Polyps

Benign tumors of the gallbladder are common and can be detected on ultrasonography. They can be classified into epithelial tumors (adenoma), mesenchymal tumors (fibroma, lipoma, hemangioma), and pseudotumors (cholesterol polyps, inflammatory polyps, and adenomyoma). The majority of polyps are cholesterol polyps.[151] Four percent to 7% of patients with polypoid lesions of the gallbladder are found to have gallbladder cancer.[151,152] Malignant lesions are significantly more likely to be found in patients older than 50 years and are more likely to be present as a solitary lesion larger than 1 cm in diameter. Based on these findings, the indication for cholecystectomy for asymptomatic benign polyps includes the presence of any solitary polyp larger than 1 cm in diameter in a patient older than 50 years of age. For lesions that do not fit these characteristics, it is reasonable to obtain follow-up scans every 6 to 12 months, and any suspicious findings (focal thickening of the gallbladder wall) should be an indication for further workup as described in Tumors of the Gallbladder: Diagnostic Evaluation, earlier in this chapter.

Extended (Radical) Cholecystectomy

A rational approach to surgery for gallbladder carcinoma was described by Glenn and Hays in 1954 and included wedge resection of the gallbladder bed and regional lymphadenectomy of the hepatoduodenal ligament.[153] Figure 29.5-8 is a diagrammatic representation of the extent of dissection in an extended or radical cholecystectomy. Definitive resection for gallbladder cancer depends on the stage and location of the tumor as well as whether or not the procedure is a re-resection after a previous simple cholecystectomy. T1 (stage IA) tumors can be treated with simple cholecystectomy. Any suspicious nodes should be removed for a frozen-section pathologic diagnosis. Stage IB, II, and selected stage III (T4N0) tumors should be treated with *en bloc* resection of the gallbladder, segments IVb and V of the liver, and regional lymph node dissection. Stage IV tumors should be treated with appropriate palliation when indicated. Because of the high incidence of local-regional recurrence, strict operative principles should be maintained for liver resection and lymph node dissection. Recommendations for liver resection for gallbladder cancer have ranged from a limited wedge excision of 2 cm of liver around the gallbladder bed to routine extended right hepatic lobectomy. The goal is to achieve a negative margin on the tumor, encompassing cells that have directly infiltrated the liver. Sometimes after prior cholecystectomy or biliary procedures it can be difficult to differentiate scar and tumor in the porta hepatis. The best management in these cases may be an extended right hepatectomy and extrahepatic bile duct resection. The complication rate for extended resection can be as high as 50%, with a mortality rate of

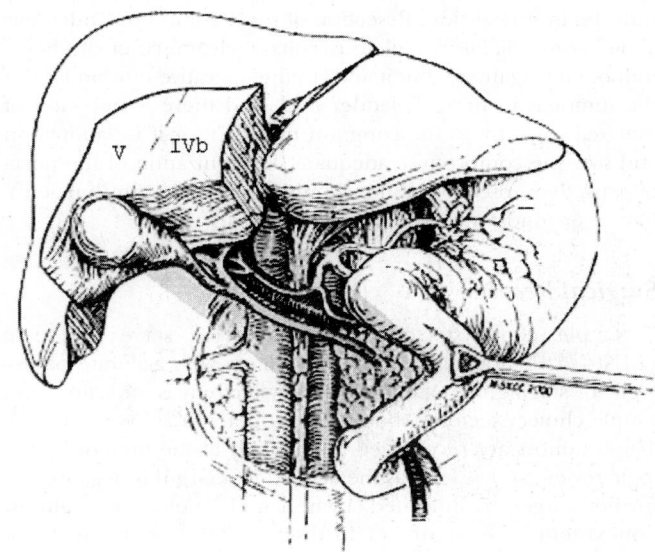

FIGURE 29.5-8. Schematic representing surgical treatment for gallbladder carcinoma. An extended cholecystectomy includes the gallbladder *en bloc* with segments IVb and V of the liver. Lymph nodes should be dissected completely from the shaded region. (From ref. 242, with permission.)

TABLE 29.5-11. Actuarial Survival Results Reported in Retrospective Reviews after Resection of T1 Gallbladder Cancers

Study	Year	n	Procedure	Survival (%)	
				3-Y	5-Y
Ouchi et al.[224]	1987	14	Not specified	78	71.4
Yamaguchi et al.[95]	1988	11	Not specified	100	—
Donohue et al.[129]	1990	6	83% simple cholecystectomy	100	100
Gall et al.[225]	1991	7	Simple cholecystectomy	86	86
Ogura et al.[166,a]	1991	366	Not specified	87	78
Shirai et al.[157]	1992	39	Simple cholecystectomy	100	100
Yamaguchi et al.[227]	1992	6	Simple cholecystectomy	100	100
Shirai et al.[226]	1992	56	Simple cholecystectomy	100	100
		38	Extended cholecystectomy	100	100
Matsumoto et al.[154]	1992	4	Extended cholecystectomy	100	100
Oertli et al.[140]	1993	6	Simple cholecystectomy	100	100
de Aretxabala et al.[158]	1997	32	69% simple cholecystectomy	94	94
Todoroki et al.[228]	1999	13	Simple cholecystectomy	100	100
Wakai et al.[229]	2002	12	Simple cholecystectomy	—	90
Toyonaga et al.[230]	2003	23	Simple cholecystectomy	100	100

[a]Multi-institutional survey.

5%. The potential gain of the procedure must justify the risk. Good patient and tumor selection are essential in these cases.

Recommendations for lymph node dissection for gallbladder cancer have ranged from excision of the cystic duct node alone to *en bloc* pancreaticoduodenectomy to clear the pancreaticoduodenal lymph nodes.[154] In general, a full Kocher maneuver should be performed, and lymphatic tissue should be dissected behind the duodenum and pancreas and swept superiorly. Any interaortocaval nodes or superior mesenteric nodes should be included in the specimen if possible. Also the soft tissue anterior to the duodenum and pancreas should be swept superiorly. The portal vein and hepatic artery should be skeletonized and all tissue swept superiorly. Skeletonization should be continued as far into the liver hilum as possible, ideally maintaining continuity with the liver resection. Resection of the common bile duct may allow more reliable complete lymphatic clearance of the hepatoduodenal ligament, but it adds to the operative morbidity.[155] If the tumor is in the gallbladder neck and there is suspicion of mucosal spread into the common bile duct, or if inflammation and scarring compromise adequate skeletonization of the porta hepatis, then resection of the common bile duct with Roux-en-Y hepaticojejunostomy should be performed.

Surgical Results

A simple cholecystectomy is curative for stage I disease (T1N0)[156–158] (Table 29.5-11). For tumors with accurate pathologic T1 staging, no extended cholecystectomy is indicated, and simple cholecystectomy should result in a 100% 5-year survival. These tumors are recognized incidentally at the time of pathologic review, and as long as the cystic duct margin is negative, no further surgery is indicated. Lymph node metastasis is almost nonexistent in the setting of T1 disease.[159] If there is any doubt as to whether the pathologic staging is accurate, a more extensive re-resection is justified.

Patients with stage II disease (T2N0) are best treated with an extended cholecystectomy. As discussed in Tumors of the Gallblad-

der: Pathology, earlier in this chapter, ideally the cancer is recognized and diagnosed before disrupting the subserosal plane during simple cholecystectomy. Unfortunately, because most of these cases are initially addressed laparoscopically, intraoperative diagnosis is uncommon for T2 disease. It is in these patients that radical re-resection leads to the best chance of long-term cure. When an extended cholecystectomy is performed for T2 disease the 5-year survival has been reported to be as high as 100%[154] but probably falls in the range of 70% to 90%[157,158,160] (Table 29.5-12). Simple cholecystectomy alone is associated with a 5-year survival rate of 20% to 40.5%.[157,158] Lymph node metastases are seen in 46% of patients with T2 primary tumors, which provides another reason in favor of radical re-resection after simple cholecystectomy.[159]

For patients with stage IIB disease (T3N1), an extended cholecystectomy is the recommended treatment approach. This may include *en bloc* resection of the common bile duct for grossly positive periportal lymph nodes to improve periportal lymph node clearance. Patients with metastases to N1 nodes (cystic duct or periportal lymph nodes) can be cured, which thus further justifies re-resection for all tumors with transmural invasion. Five-year survival ranges from 45% to 63% for patients with metastatic disease to N1 nodes.[131,155,161] Three-year survival has ranged from 38% to 80% in various trials[129,154,160] (Table 29.5-13). Simple cholecystectomy or a lesser operation would not be expected to result in long-term survival.

Stage III gallbladder cancer represents an advanced malignancy that is generally beyond surgical treatment. However, patients with T4N0 disease representing a mass-forming gallbladder cancer may achieve long-term survival after an extended resection.[155] Patients with nodal metastases beyond the hepatoduodenal ligament have a poor prognosis, and in general the authors would advocate palliative care. Some investigators have reported anecdotal cases of long-term cures in patients with distant nodal disease (formerly N2 disease),[154,161] but most have reported a poor outcome that does not justify the morbidity of the extended resection.

In series of extended cholecystectomies the operative morbidity ranges from 5% to 46% and the mortality from 0% to

TABLE 29.5-12. Actuarial Survival Results Reported in Retrospective Reviews after Resection of T2 Gallbladder Cancers

Study	Year	n	Procedure	Survival (%)	
				3-Y	5-Y
Yamaguchi et al.[95]	1988	73	Not specified	40.1	—
Donohue et al.[129]	1990	12	67% extended cholecystectomy	58	22
Ogura et al.[166,a]	1991	499	Not specified	53	37
Gall et al.[225]	1991	7	86% simple cholecystectomy	86	86
Shirai et al.[226]	1992	35	Simple cholecystectomy	57	40.5
		10	Extended cholecystectomy	90	90
Yamaguchi et al.[156]	1992	25	Simple cholecystectomy	36	36
Matsumoto et al.[154]	1992	9	Extended cholecystectomy	100	100
Oertli et al.[140]	1993	17	Simple cholecystectomy	29	24
Cubertafond et al.[231,a]	1994	52	88% simple cholecystectomy	20	—
Bartlett et al.[232]	1996	8	Extended cholecystectomy	100	88
Paquet[233]	1998	5	Extended cholecystectomy	100	80
Todoroki et al.[228]	1999	19	Extended cholecystectomy	—	78
Wakai et al.[229]	2002	7	Extended cholecystectomy	100	100
Toyonaga et al.[230]	2003	43	Extended cholecystectomy	68	54
Muratore et al.[234]	2003	11	Extended cholecystectomy	—	64

[a]Multi-institutional survey.

21%.[129,162–165] The reported morbidity and mortality rate of major liver resections has decreased, even in the aged population, so with careful patient selection extended cholecystectomy should be safe.[162] In a multiple-institution review of 1686 gallbladder cancer resections in Japan, the authors reported a 12.8% morbidity for a simple cholecystectomy, 21.9% for extended cholecystectomy, and 48.3% for hepatic lobectomy.[166] The mortality rates were 2.9%, 2.3%, and 18%, respectively. They reported 150 hepatopancreaticoduodenectomies for gallbladder cancer with a 54% morbidity and a 15.3% mortality rate. The risk of resection for each patient and for each type of resection needs to be weighed against the patient's chance of benefiting from the procedure based on the tumor stage.

ADJUVANT THERAPY

As with cholangiocarcinoma, reports on adjuvant radiotherapy after resection for gallbladder cancer are difficult to interpret. They involve small numbers of patients nonrandomly allocated to various combinations of resection (complete and incomplete), external-beam radiotherapy, brachytherapy, and IORT. Kresl et al. reported the Mayo Clinic experience from 1985 to 1997 in which 21 consecutively treated gallbladder carcinoma patients all underwent surgery and then external-beam radiotherapy to a median dose of 5400 cGy in fractions of 180 to 200 cGy/d.[167] One patient also was treated with 1500 cGy IORT after external-beam radiotherapy. For patients with gross residual tumor, microscopic residual tumor, and no residual disease, the median survival times were 0.6, 1.4, and 15.1 years, respectively ($P = .02$). Two-year local control rates were 0%, 80%, and 88% for patients with gross residual tumor, microscopic residual tumor, and no residual tumor, respectively ($P < .01$). For six patients who received more than 5400 cGy, the 3-year local control rate was 100% versus 65% for 15 patients who received less than 5400 cGy. All patients also received 5-FU with or without LV. It is interesting that the local control rate with a relatively high dose of external-beam radiotherapy seemed to be equivalent for patients with microscopic residual tumor and for those with no residual tumor after resection. There was also a suggestion that increasing the external-beam radiotherapy dose above 5400 cGy led to an improved local control rate. It should be noted that the 64% 5-year survival of the 12 patients with no residual tumor after resection but with postoperative radiotherapy seemed to be better than historical results from the same institution using surgery alone in patients undergoing a complete resection.

In the report by Flickinger et al., eight patients with primary carcinoma of the gallbladder treated with radiotherapy had a much worse survival than those with cholangiocarcinoma.[74] The

TABLE 29.5-13. Actuarial Survival Results Reported in Retrospective Reviews after Extended Resection of T3 and T4 Gallbladder Cancers

Author	Year	n	T Stage	Survival (%)	
				3-Y	5-Y
Matsumoto et al.[154]	1992	8	T3	38	—
Onoyama et al.[131]	1995	12	T3	44	44
Bartlett et al.[232]	1996	8	T3	63	63
Ouchi et al.[224]	1987	12	T3, T4	17	—
Nakamura et al.[235]	1989	13	T3, T4	16	16
Donohue et al.[129]	1990	17	T3, T4	50	29
Gall et al.[225]	1991	8	T3, T4	50	—
Shirai et al.[226]	1992	20	T3, T4	—	45
Ogura et al.[166]	1991	453	T4	18	8
Todoroki et al.[236]	1991	27	T4	7	—
Nimura et al.[237]	1991	14	T4	10	—
Matsumoto et al.[154]	1992	27	T4	25	—
Onoyama et al.[131]	1995	14	T4	8	8
Bartlett et al.[232]	1996	7	T4	25	25
Schauer et al.[238]	2001	25	T3, T4	20	0
Kondo et al.[239]	2002	68	T3, T4	44	33
Behari et al.[163]	2003	29	T3, T4	35	28
Toyonaga et al.[230]	2003	7	T3, T4	14	0

eight patients with primary gallbladder carcinoma were all dead within 1 year. Similarly, Buskirk et al. reported on four patients with gallbladder carcinoma, who were all dead by 10 months.[90]

For external-beam radiotherapy, the volume to be irradiated should include the gallbladder fossa and adjacent liver as determined from the preoperative CT scans plus the regional nodal areas. The radiation dose administered, either in the adjuvant setting or for unresectable residual disease, must be relatively high. Using conformal three-dimensional treatment planning, doses of external-beam radiotherapy alone should be at least 6000 cGy in 30 to 35 treatments. Lower doses of external-beam radiotherapy may be administered if supplemented by a boost with IORT or brachytherapy or both. As with bile duct carcinomas, split-course radiotherapy as described earlier in Adjuvant Radiotherapy in the section on cholangiocarcinoma has been used at the University of Pittsburgh and appears to be well tolerated.

Adjuvant chemotherapy for gallbladder cancer has been discussed earlier in Adjuvant Chemotherapy in the section on cholangiocarcinoma, because the two are often combined in studies. In general, gallbladder cancer does not respond well to currently available systemic chemotherapy. Nevertheless, because of the poor prognosis in patients with regionally confined disease, combinations of adjuvant chemotherapy (5-FU, mitomycin C) and radiation therapy have been studied.[168] Chao and Greager reported on 15 patients who received some form of chemotherapy or radiation therapy or both after resection for gallbladder cancer, and there was no significant improvement in survival compared to 7 patients who did not receive adjuvant therapy.[169] Oswalt and Cruz reported a median survival of 20 weeks for patients treated with adjuvant chemotherapy compared to 8 weeks for patients treated with surgery alone.[170] Morrow et al. reported a median survival of 4.5 months for patients receiving adjuvant chemotherapy or radiation therapy or both versus 3 months for patients treated with surgery alone.[171] All of these trials compared patients receiving treatment to control patients in a nonrandomized fashion. It may be that the patients with better performance status received adjuvant therapy, and therefore it is difficult to say whether the treatment had an effect on survival.

ADVANCED DISEASE

The median survival time for patients presenting with unresectable disease is 2 to 4 months, with a 1-year survival rate of less than 5%.[140,172] This aggressive disease course needs to be considered when deciding on palliative management. The goals of palliation should be relief of pain, jaundice, and bowel obstruction and prolongation of life. These goals should be accomplished as simply as possible given the aggressive nature of this disease. Resection of gross disease probably provides the best palliation and a chance for cure in some instances but is usually not possible. Palliation of biliary obstruction is performed identically to that in cholangiocarcinoma as discussed in Cholangiocarcinomas: Advanced Disease, earlier in this chapter. Percutaneous stents are effective and should be used, because the expected survival does not usually warrant a surgical bypass.

Chemotherapy has been used for palliation of unresectable disease. A European Organization for Research and Treatment of Cancer cooperative study examined the use of bolus mitomycin C in advanced gallbladder and biliary tract carcinoma, but no significant activity was identified.[173] Others have examined the use of 5-FU, doxorubicin (Adriamycin), and nitrosoureas alone and in combination for gallbladder cancer, with some reports of minimal responses.[127] Regional therapy has been examined using intraarterial mitomycin C for gallbladder cancer. A 48% overall response rate and a prolongation of median survival from 5 months to 14 months compared to that of historical controls was reported.[174]

Radiation therapy has also been examined in palliation for gallbladder cancer. The results of Houry et al.[168] suggest that radiotherapy may increase survival after no resection or palliative resection of gallbladder carcinoma. The benefit is

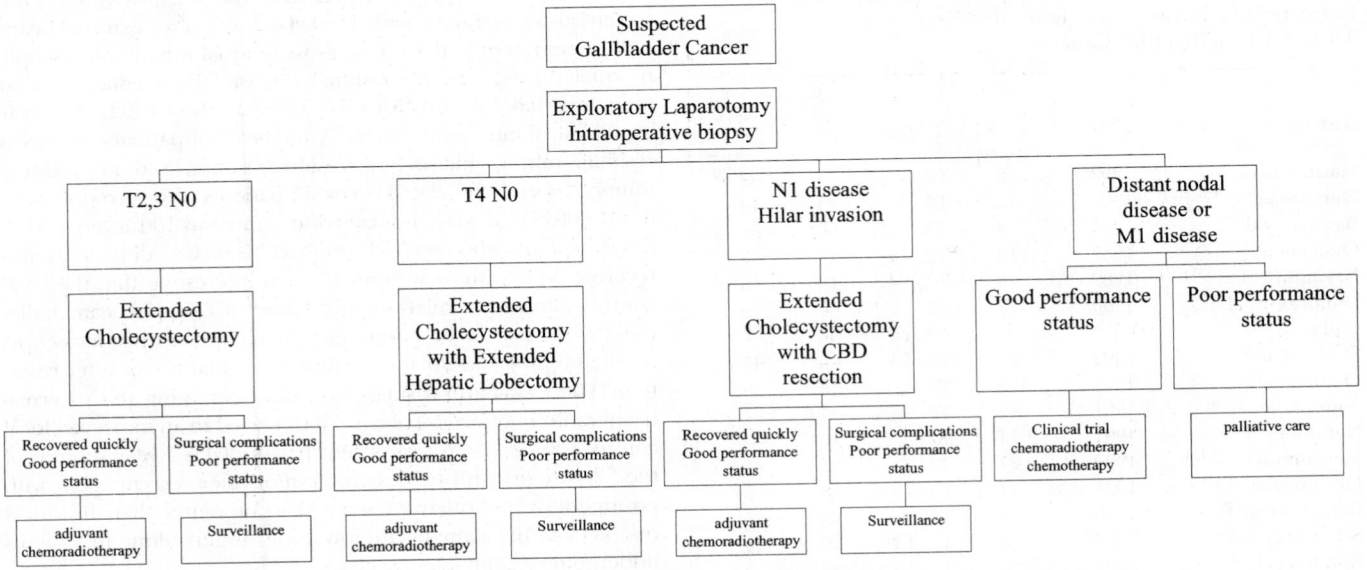

FIGURE 29.5-9. Algorithm for management of gallbladder carcinoma identified on preoperative imaging. T1 tumors should not be recognized preoperatively except for papillary tumors, which can be managed with simple cholecystectomy. CBD, common bile duct.

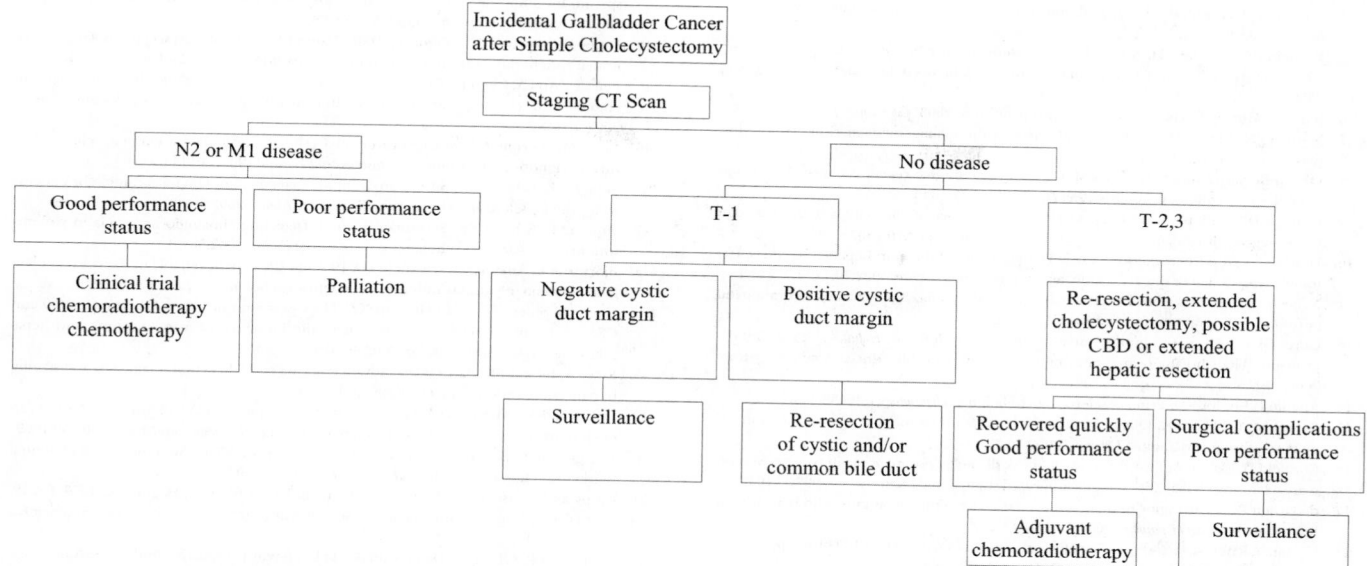

FIGURE 29.5-10. Algorithm for management of gallbladder cancer found as an incidental finding on pathologic examination of a cholecystectomy specimen. CBD, common bile duct; CT, computed tomography.

minimal, with a median survival of only 6 to 8 months. Radiotherapy does appear to be well tolerated and, although of unproven benefit, may improve symptoms and prolong survival in selected patients.

SUMMARY OF TREATMENT RECOMMENDATIONS

Gallbladder cancer is an aggressive disease with a dismal prognosis. It should not, however, be approached with a fatalistic attitude, because appropriate workup and extended resection can result in a cure. The areas that can be improved are more careful preoperative imaging for patients undergoing cholecystectomy for symptoms of cholecystitis and appropriate workup of all suspicious lesions. The authors believe that providing definitive surgical treatment as the initial procedure allows the best chance for cure. Workup may include measurement of CA 19-9 level, ERCP with bile cytologic examination, and fine-needle aspiration cytologic analysis. In addition, appropriate intraoperative decision making is essential, and palpable suspicious thickenings of the gallbladder wall should be diagnosed with careful examination of a biopsy specimen. A diagnosis of cancer should be treated with definitive *en bloc* liver resection and lymph node dissection without interruption of the subserosal gallbladder resection plane, which often includes tumor. Advanced tumors recognized on preoperative radiologic imaging or at the time of laparotomy can be treated with aggressive surgical resection, which can result in long-term survival. This approach needs to be individualized based on the patient's concomitant health and extent of disease. Resection of hematogenous metastasis is not justified, nor is resection of distant nodal disease. Many reports of long-term survival after resection of locally advanced T4 lesions and N1 metastasis justify an aggressive surgical resection in selected patients. This may include a bile duct resection and extended hepatic lobectomy. Patients with a good performance status should be con-

sidered for adjuvant chemotherapy. Patients with advanced disease should be considered for clinical trials. An algorithm for management is shown in Figures 29.5-9 and 29.5-10.

NEW ADVANCES FOR TREATMENT OF BILIARY TRACT CANCERS

It is unlikely that significant improvements in the survival of patients with biliary tract cancers will be seen with currently available chemotherapeutic agents, and new approaches are needed. Understanding the molecular biology of the biliary tract cancers will be crucial in developing targeted agents. Her-2/neu and C-kit are overexpresssed in breast cancer and gastrointestinal stromal tumors, respectively, and can be therapeutically targeted; however, in cancers of the biliary tract, the overexpression of these proteins appear to be low. Aberrant signaling of epidermal growth factor receptors is important in the development and progression of cancer, and a number of agents targeting this pathway are in clinical trials. In biliary tree cancers, the prevalence of epidermal growth factor receptor expression and its role in tumorigenesis needs to be elucidated, and epidermal growth factor receptor inhibitors need to be evaluated in clinical trials. Similarly, antiangiogenic drugs and agents inhibiting the vascular endothelial growth factor receptor need to be evaluated in well-designed clinical trials with relevant translational studies.

REFERENCES

1. Klatskin G. Adenocarcinoma of the hepatic duct at its bifurcation within the porta hepatis. An unusual tumor with distinctive clinical and pathological features. *Am J Med* 1965;38:241.
2. de Groen PC, Gores GJ, LaRusso NF, Gunderson LL, Nagorney DM. Biliary tract cancers. *N Engl J Med* 1999;341:1368.
3. Patel T. Worldwide trends in mortality from biliary tract malignancies. *BMC Cancer* 2002;2:10.

4. Nakeeb A, Tran KQ, Black MJ, et al. Improved survival in resected biliary malignancies. *Surgery* 2002;132:555.

5. Weimann A, Varnholt H, Schlitt HJ, et al. Retrospective analysis of prognostic factors after liver resection and transplantation for cholangiocellular carcinoma. *Br J Surg* 2000;87:1182.

6. Jemal A, Murray T, Samuels A, et al. Cancer statistics, 2003. *CA Cancer J Clin* 2003;53:5.

7. Vauthey JN, Blumgart LH. Recent advances in the management of cholangiocarcinomas. *Semin Liver Dis* 1994;14:109.

8. Okuda K, Nakanuma Y, Miyazaki M. Cholangiocarcinoma: recent progress. Part 1: epidemiology and etiology. *J Gastroenterol Hepatol* 2002;17:1049.

9. Henson DE, Albores-Saavedra J, Corle D. Carcinoma of the gallbladder. Histologic types, stage of disease, grade, and survival rates. *Cancer* 1992;70:1493.

10. Henson DE, Albores-Saavedra J, Corle D. Carcinoma of the extrahepatic bile ducts. Histologic types, stage of disease, grade, and survival rates. *Cancer* 1992;70:1498.

11. Nakeeb A, Pitt HA, Sohn TA, et al. Cholangiocarcinoma. A spectrum of intrahepatic, perihilar, and distal tumors. *Ann Surg* 1996;224:463.

12. Gores GJ. Cholangiocarcinoma: current concepts and insights. *Hepatology* 2003;37:961.

13. Jarnagin WR. Cholangiocarcinoma of the extrahepatic bile ducts. *Semin Surg Oncol* 2000;19:156.

14. Angulo P, Lindor KD. Primary sclerosing cholangitis. *Hepatology* 1999;30:325.

15. Bergquist A, Ekbom A, Olsson R, et al. Hepatic and extrahepatic malignancies in primary sclerosing cholangitis. *J Hepatol* 2002;36:321.

16. Kornfeld D, Ekbom A, Ihre T. Survival and risk of cholangiocarcinoma in patients with primary sclerosing cholangitis. A population-based study. *Scand J Gastroenterol* 1997;32:1042.

17. de Groen PC. Cholangiocarcinoma in primary sclerosing cholangitis: who is at risk and how do we screen? *Hepatology* 2000;31:247.

18. Chapman RW. Risk factors for biliary tract carcinogenesis. *Ann Oncol* 1999;10[Suppl 4]:308.

19. O'Neill JA Jr. Choledochal cyst. *Curr Probl Surg* 1992;29:361.

20. Taylor AC, Palmer KR. Caroli's disease. *Eur J Gastroenterol Hepatol* 1998;10:105.

21. Watanapa P, Watanapa WB. Liver fluke-associated cholangiocarcinoma. *Br J Surg* 2002;89:962.

22. International Agency for Research on Cancer. Infection with liver flukes (Opisthorchis viverrini, Opisthorchis felineus and Clonorchis sinensis). *IARC Monogr Eval Carcinog Risks Hum* 1994;61:121.

23. Chen MF, Jan YY, Wang CS, et al. A reappraisal of cholangiocarcinoma in patient with hepatolithiasis. *Cancer* 1993;71:2461.

24. Kim MH, Sekijima J, Lee SP. Primary intrahepatic stones. *Am J Gastroenterol* 1995;90:540.

25. Lipshutz GS, Brennan TV, Warren RS. Thorotrast-induced liver neoplasia: a collective review. *J Am Coll Surg* 2002;195:713.

26. Mitacek EJ, Brunnemann KD, Hoffmann D, et al. Volatile nitrosamines and tobacco-specific nitrosamines in the smoke of Thai cigarettes: a risk factor for lung cancer and a suspected risk factor for liver cancer in Thailand. *Carcinogenesis* 1999;20:133.

27. Hocqueloux L, Gervais A. Cholangiocarcinoma and AIDS-related sclerosing cholangitis. *Ann Intern Med* 2000;132:1006.

28. Sasaki R, Takahashi M, Funato O, et al. Prognostic significance of lymph node involvement in middle and distal bile duct cancer. *Surgery* 2001;129:677.

29. Lim JH. Cholangiocarcinoma: morphologic classification according to growth pattern and imaging findings. *AJR Am J Roentgenol* 2003;181:819.

30. Burke EC, Jarnagin WR, Hochwald SN, et al. Cholangiocarcinoma: patterns of spread, the importance of hepatic resection for curative operation, and a presurgical clinical staging system. *Ann Surg* 1998;228:385.

31. Martin RC, Klimstra DS, Schwartz L, et al. Hepatic intraductal oncocytic papillary carcinoma. *Cancer* 2002;95:2180.

32. Weinbren K, Mutum SS. Pathological aspects of cholangiocarcinoma. *J Pathol* 1983;139:217.

33. Rullier A, Le Bail B, Fawaz R, et al. Cytokeratin 7 and 20 expression in cholangiocarcinomas varies along the biliary tract but still differs from that in colorectal carcinoma metastasis. *Am J Surg Pathol* 2000;24:870.

34. Okuda K, Nakanuma Y, Miyazaki M. Cholangiocarcinoma: recent progress. Part 2: molecular pathology and treatment. *J Gastroenterol Hepatol* 2002;17:1056.

35. Laurent-Puig P, Legoix P, Bluteau O, et al. Genetic alterations associated with hepatocellular carcinomas define distinct pathways of hepatocarcinogenesis. *Gastroenterology* 2001;120:1763.

36. Stern MC, Umbach DM, Yu MC, et al. Hepatitis B, aflatoxin B(1), and p53 codon 249 mutation in hepatocellular carcinomas from Guangxi, People's Republic of China, and a meta-analysis of existing studies. *Cancer Epidemiol Biomarkers Prev* 2001;10:617.

37. Masuhara S, Kasuya K, Aoki T, et al. Relation between K-ras codon 12 mutation and p53 protein overexpression in gallbladder cancer and biliary ductal epithelia in patients with pancreaticobiliary maljunction. *J Hepatobiliary Pancreat Surg* 2000;7:198.

38. Ahrendt SA, Rashid A, Chow JT, et al. p53 overexpression and K-ras gene mutations in primary sclerosing cholangitis-associated biliary tract cancer. *J Hepatobiliary Pancreat Surg* 2000;7:426.

39. Aishima SI, Taguchi KI, Sugimachi K, et al. c-erbB-2 and c-Met expression relates to cholangiocarcinogenesis and progression of intrahepatic cholangiocarcinoma. *Histopathology* 2002;40:269.

40. Sugawara H, Yasoshima M, Katayanagi K, et al. Relationship between interleukin-6 and proliferation and differentiation in cholangiocarcinoma. *Histopathology* 1998;33:145.

41. Amaya S, Sasaki M, Watanabe Y, et al. Expression of MUC1 and MUC2 and carbohydrate antigen Tn change during malignant transformation of biliary papillomatosis. *Histopathology* 2001;38:550.

42. AJCC (American Joint Committee on Cancer). Extrahepatic bile duct tumor. In: Green FL, ed. *Cancer staging manual*, 6th ed. New York: Springer-Verlag, 2002.

43. Burke EC, Jarnagin WR, Hochwald SN, et al. Hilar cholangiocarcinoma: patterns of spread, the importance of hepatic resection for curative operation, and a presurgical clinical staging system. *Ann Surg* 1998;228:385.

44. Farley DR, Weaver AL, Nagorney DM. "Natural history" of unresected cholangiocarcinoma: patient outcome after noncurative intervention. *Mayo Clin Proc* 1995;70:425.

45. Lee CC, Wu CY, Chen JT, Chen GH. Comparing combined hepatocellular-cholangiocarcinoma and cholangiocarcinoma: a clinicopathological study. *Hepatogastroenterology* 2002;49:1487.

46. Chen MF. Peripheral cholangiocarcinoma (cholangiocellular carcinoma): clinical features, diagnosis and treatment. *J Gastroenterol Hepatol* 1999;14:1144.

46a. Siqueira E, Schoen RE, Silverman W, et al. Detecting cholangiocarcinoma in patients with primary sclerosing cholangitis. *Gastrointest Endosc* 2002;56:40.

47. Siqueira E, Schoen RE, Silverman W, et al. Detecting cholangiocarcinoma in patients with primary sclerosing cholangitis. *Gastrointest Endosc* 2002;56:40.

47a. Bjornsson E, Kilander A, Olsson R. CA 19-9 and CEA are unreliable markers for cholangiocarcinoma in patients with primary sclerosing cholangitis. *Liver* 1999;19:501.

47b. Chen CY, Shiesh SC, Tsao HC, Lin XZ. The assessment of biliary CA 125, CA 19-9 and CEA in diagnosing cholangiocarcinoma—the influence of sampling time and hepatolithiasis. *Hepatogastroenterology* 2002;49:616.

48. Riker A, Libutti SK, Bartlett DL. Advances in the early detection, diagnosis, and staging of pancreatic cancer. *Surg Oncol* 1997;6:157.

49. Ozkan H, Kaya M, Cengiz A. Comparison of tumor marker CA 242 with CA 19-9 and carcinoembryonic antigen (CEA) in pancreatic cancer. *Hepatogastroenterology* 2003;50:1669.

50. Wongkham S, Sheehan JK, Boonla C, et al. Serum MUC5AC mucin as a potential marker for cholangiocarcinoma. *Cancer Lett* 2003;195:93.

51. Carpelan-Holmstrom M, Louhimo J, Stenman UH, Alfthan H, Haglund C. CEA, CA 19-9 and CA 72-4 improve the diagnostic accuracy in gastrointestinal cancers. *Anticancer Res* 2002;22:2311.

52. Hultcrantz R, Olsson R, Danielsson A, et al. A 3-year prospective study on serum tumor markers used for detecting cholangiocarcinoma in patients with primary sclerosing cholangitis. *J Hepatol* 1999;30:669.

53. Han JK, Choi BI, Kim AY, et al. Cholangiocarcinoma: pictorial essay of CT and cholangiographic findings. *Radiographics* 2002;22:173.

54. Fritscher-Ravens A, Broering DC, Knoefel WT, et al. EUS-guided fine-needle aspiration of suspected hilar cholangiocarcinoma in potentially operable patients with negative brush cytology. *Am J Gastroenterol* 2004;99:45.

55. Anderson CD, Rice MH, Pinson CW, et al. Fluorodeoxyglucose PET imaging in the evaluation of gallbladder carcinoma and cholangiocarcinoma. *J Gastrointest Surg* 2004;8:90.

56. Siddique I, Galati J, Ankoma-Sey V, et al. The role of choledochoscopy in the diagnosis and management of biliary tract diseases. *Gastrointest Endosc* 1999;50:67.

57. Soreide O, Sondenaa K. Fine needle biopsy and aspiration cytology. In: Blumgart L, Fong Y, eds. *Surgery of the liver and biliary tract.* United Kingdom: W.B. Saunders, 2001:419.

58. Lillemoe KD, Cameron JL. Surgery for hilar cholangiocarcinoma: the Johns Hopkins approach. *J Hepatobiliary Pancreat Surg* 2000;7:115.

59. Hochwald SN, Burke EC, Jarnagin WR, Fong Y, Blumgart LH. Association of preoperative biliary stenting with increased postoperative infectious complications in proximal cholangiocarcinoma. *Arch Surg* 1999;134:261.

60. Nakanuma Y, Sasaki M, Ishikawa A, et al. Biliary papillary neoplasm of the liver. *Histol Histopathol* 2002;17:851.

61. Nimura Y, Kamiya J, Kondo S, et al. Aggressive preoperative management and extended surgery for hilar cholangiocarcinoma: Nagoya experience. *J Hepatobiliary Pancreat Surg* 2000;7:155.

62. Tabata M, Kawarada Y, Yokoi H, Higashiguchi T, Isaji S. Surgical treatment for hilar cholangiocarcinoma. *J Hepatobiliary Pancreat Surg* 2000;7:148.

63. Nagino M, Kamiya J, Uesaka K, et al. Complications of hepatectomy for hilar cholangiocarcinoma. *World J Surg* 2001;25:1277.

64. Klempnauer J, Ridder GJ, von Wasielewski R, et al. Resectional surgery of hilar cholangiocarcinoma: a multivariate analysis of prognostic factors. *J Clin Oncol* 1997;15:947.

65. Pascher A, Jonas S, Neuhaus P. Intrahepatic cholangiocarcinoma: indication for transplantation. *J Hepatobiliary Pancreat Surg* 2003;10:282.

66. Meyer CG, Penn I, James L. Liver transplantation for cholangiocarcinoma: results in 207 patients. *Transplantation* 2000;69:1633.

67. Hassoun Z, Gores GJ, Rosen CB. Preliminary experience with liver transplantation in selected patients with unresectable hilar cholangiocarcinoma. *Surg Oncol Clin N Am* 2002;11:909.

68. Shimoda M, Farmer DG, Colquhoun SD, et al. Liver transplantation for cholangiocellular carcinoma: analysis of a single-center experience and review of the literature. *Liver Transpl Surg* 2001;7:1023.

69. Edwards EB, Roberts JP, McBride MA, Schulak JA, Hunsicker LG. The effect of the volume of procedures at transplantation centers on mortality after liver transplantation. *N Engl J Med* 1999;341:2049.

70. McMasters KM, Tuttle TM, Leach SD, et al. Neoadjuvant chemoradiation for extrahepatic cholangiocarcinoma. *Am J Surg* 1997;174:605.

71. Sudan D, DeRoover A, Chinnakotla S, et al. Radiochemotherapy and transplantation allow long-term survival for nonresectable hilar cholangiocarcinoma. *Am J Transplant* 2002;2:774.

72. Mittal B, Deutsch M, Iwatsuki S. Primary cancers of extrahepatic biliary passages. *Int J Radiat Oncol Biol Phys* 1985;11:849.

73. Kopelson G, Galdabini J, Warshaw AL, Gunderson LL. Patterns of failure after curative surgery for extra-hepatic biliary tract carcinoma: implications for adjuvant therapy. *Int J Radiat Oncol Biol Phys* 1981;7:413.

74. Flickinger JC, Epstein AH, Iwatsuki S, Carr BI, Starzl TE. Radiation therapy for primary carcinoma of the extrahepatic biliary system. An analysis of 63 cases. *Cancer* 1991;68:289.

75. Flickinger JC, Jawalekar K, Deutsch M, Webster J. Split course radiation therapy for adenocarcinoma of the pancreas. *Int J Radiat Oncol Biol Phys* 1988;15:359.

76. Kim S, Kim SW, Bang YJ, Heo DS, Ha SW. Role of postoperative radiotherapy in the management of extrahepatic bile duct cancer. *Int J Radiat Oncol Biol Phys* 2002;54:414.
77. Todoroki T, Ohara K, Kawamoto T, et al. Benefits of adjuvant radiotherapy after radical resection of locally advanced main hepatic duct carcinoma. *Int J Radiat Oncol Biol Phys* 2000;46:581.
78. Todoroki T, Kawamoto T, Koike N, et al. Treatment strategy for patients with middle and lower third bile duct cancer. *Br J Surg* 2001;88:364.
79. Kurosaki H, Karasawa K, Kaizu T, et al. Intraoperative radiotherapy for resectable extrahepatic bile duct cancer. *Int J Radiat Oncol Biol Phys* 1999;45:635.
80. Hayes JK Jr, Sapozink MD, Miller FJ. Definitive radiation therapy in bile duct carcinoma. *Int J Radiat Oncol Biol Phys* 1988;15:735.
81. Shin HS, Seong J, Kim WC, et al. Combination of external beam irradiation and high-dose-rate intraluminal brachytherapy for inoperable carcinoma of the extrahepatic bile ducts. *Int J Radiat Oncol Biol Phys* 2003;57:105.
82. Morganti AG, Trodella L, Valentini V, et al. Combined modality treatment in unresectable extrahepatic biliary carcinoma. *Int J Radiat Oncol Biol Phys* 2000;46:913.
83. Takada T, Amano H, Yasuda H, et al. Is postoperative adjuvant chemotherapy useful for gallbladder carcinoma? A phase III multicenter prospective randomized controlled trial in patients with resected pancreaticobiliary carcinoma. *Cancer* 2002;95:1685.
83a. Urego M, Flickinger JC, Carr BI. Radiotherapy and multimodality management of cholangiocarcinoma. *Int J Radiat Oncol Biol Phys* 1999;44:121.
83b. Figueras J, Llado L, Valls C, et al. Changing strategies in diagnosis and management of hilar cholangiocarcinoma. *Liver Transpl* 2000;6:786.
83c. Kraybill WG, Lee H, Picus J, et al. Multidisciplinary treatment of biliary tract cancers. *J Surg Oncol* 1994;55:239.
83d. Minsky BD, Kemeny N, Armstrong JG, Reichman B, Botet J. Extrahepatic biliary system cancer: an update of a combined modality approach. *Am J Clin Oncol* 1991;14:433.
83e. Robertson JM, Lawrence TS, Dworzanin LM, et al. Treatment of primary hepatobiliary cancers with conformal radiation therapy and regional chemotherapy. *J Clin Oncol* 1993;11:1286.
83f. Mehta VK, Fisher GA, Ford JM, et al. Adjuvant chemoradiotherapy for "unfavorable" carcinoma of the ampulla of Vater: preliminary report. *Arch Surg* 2001;136:65.
83g. Koyama K, Tanaka J, Sato Y, et al. Experience in twenty patients with carcinoma of hilar bile duct treated by resection, targeting chemotherapy and intracavitary irradiation. *Surg Gynecol Obstet* 1993;176:239.
83h. Kawarada Y, Yamagiwa K, Das BC. Analysis of the relationships between clinicopathologic factors and survival time in intrahepatic cholangiocarcinoma. *Am J Surg* 2002;183:679.
83i. Serafini FM, Sachs D, Bloomston M, et al. Location, not staging, of cholangiocarcinoma determines the role for adjuvant chemoradiation therapy. *Am Surg* 2001;67:839.
84. Abraham NS, Barkun JS, Barkun AN. Palliation of malignant biliary obstruction: a prospective trial examining impact on quality of life. *Gastrointest Endosc* 2002;56:835.
85. Jarnagin WR, Burke E, Powers C, Fong Y, Blumgart LH. Intrahepatic biliary enteric bypass provides effective palliation in selected patients with malignant obstruction at the hepatic duct confluence. *Am J Surg* 1998;175:453.
86. Prat F, Chapat O, Ducot B, et al. A randomized trial of endoscopic drainage methods for inoperable malignant strictures of the common bile duct. *Gastrointest Endosc* 1998;47:1.
87. Burdiles P, Rossi RL. Laparoscopy in pancreatic and hepatobiliary cancer. *Surg Oncol Clin N Am* 2001;10:531.
88. Alden ME, Mohiuddin M. The impact of radiation dose in combined external beam and intraluminal Ir-192 brachytherapy for bile duct cancer. *Int J Radiat Oncol Biol Phys* 1994;28:945.
89. Crane CH, Macdonald KO, Vauthey JN, et al. Limitations of conventional doses of chemoradiation for unresectable biliary cancer. *Int J Radiat Oncol Biol Phys* 2002;53:969.
90. Buskirk SJ, Gunderson LL, Schild SE, et al. Analysis of failure after curative irradiation of extrahepatic bile duct carcinoma. *Ann Surg* 1992;215:125.
90a. Chen JS, Jan YY, Lin YC, et al. Weekly 24 h infusion of high-dose 5-fluorouracil and leucovorin in patients with biliary tract carcinomas. *Anticancer Drugs* 1998;9:393.
90b. Lozano R, Patt Y, Hassan M, et al. Oral Capecitabine (Xeloda) for the treatment of hepatobiliary cancers (hepatocellular carcinoma, cholangiocarcinoma, and gallbladder cancer). *Proc Am Soc Clin Oncol* 2000;1025(abst).
91. Penz M, Kornek GV, Raderer M, et al. Phase II trial of two-weekly gemcitabine in patients with advanced biliary tract cancer. *Ann Oncol* 2001;12:183.
91a. Carraro S Servienti PJ, Bruno MF, et al. Gemcitabine and cisplatin in locally advanced or metastatic gallbladder and bile duct adenocarcinomas. *Proc Am Soc Clin Oncol* 2001;21:A2333.
91b. Stieler JM, Roll L, Arnig M, et al. Gemcitabine and irinotecan—a pilot study for patients with non-resectable cancer of the bile duct system. *Proc Am Soc Clin Oncol* 2003;22:1233.
91c Dowlati A, Hoppel CL, Ingalls ST, et al. Phase I clinical and pharmacokinetic study of rebeccamycin analog NSC 655649 given daily for five consecutive days. *J Clin Oncol* 2001;19:2309.
91d. Dowlati A, Posey J, Ramanathan RK, et al. Multicenter phase II and pharmacokinetic study of rebeccamycin analogue (RA) in advanced biliary cancer. *Proc Am Soc Clin Oncol* 2003;22:1070.
91e. Hegewisch-Becker S, Corovic A, Jaeger E, et al. Whole body hyperthermia (WBH, 41.8 C) combined with carboplatin and etoposide in advanced biliary tract cancer. *Proc Am Soc Clin Oncol* 2003;22:1247.
91f. Miller RL, Bowen KE, Chun HG, et al. A phase II study of liposomal doxorubicin (LD, Doxil) in patients with advanced hepatocellular carcinoma (HCC) or cholangiocarcinoma. *Proc Am Soc Clin Oncol* 2002;21:2324.
91g. Doval DC, Sekhon JS, Fuloria J, et al. Gemcitabine and cisplatin in chemotherapy-naive, unresectable gallbladder cancer: a large multicenter, phase II study. *Proc Am Soc Clin Oncol* 2001;20:622.
91h. Smith GW, Bukowski RM, Hewlett JS, Groppe CW. Hepatic artery infusion of 5-fluorouracil and mitomycin C in cholangiocarcinoma and gallbladder carcinoma. *Cancer* 1984;54:1513.
91i. Robertson JM, McGinn CJ, Walker S, et al. A phase I trial of hepatic arterial bromodeoxyuridine and conformal radiation therapy for patients with primary hepatobiliary cancers or colorectal liver metastases. *Int J Radiat Oncol Biol Phys* 1997;39:1087.
91j. Tanaka N, Yamakado K, Nakatsuka A, et al. Arterial chemoinfusion therapy through an implanted port system for patients with unresectable intrahepatic cholangiocarcinoma—initial experience. *Eur J Radiol* 2002;41:42.
91k. Mezawa S, Homma H, Sato T, et al. A study of carboplatin-coated tube for the unresectable cholangiocarcinoma. *Hepatology* 2000;32:916.
91l. Zoepf T, Jakobs R, Rosenbaum A, et al. Photodynamic therapy with 5-aminolevulinic acid is not effective in bile duct cancer. *Gastrointest Endosc* 2001;54:763.
91m. Ortner M. Photodynamic therapy for cholangiocarcinoma. *J Hepatobiliary Pancreat Surg* 2001;8:137.
91n. Rumalla A, Baron TH, Wang KK, et al. Endoscopic application of photodynamic therapy for cholangiocarcinoma. *Gastrointest Endosc* 2001;53:500.
92. DeStoll M. Rationis Mendendi. Nosocomio practico vendobonensi. Edited by Lugduni B. Hongkoop, Haak et Socios et A. et J., 1788.
92a. Perpetuo MO, Valdivieso M, Heilbrun LK, et al. Natural history study of gallbladder cancer: a review of 36 years experience at M.D. Anderson hospital and tumor institute. *Cancer* 1978;42:330.
92b. Piehler JM, Crichlow RW. Primary carcinoma of the gallbladder. *Surg Gyn Obstet* 1978;147:929.
92c. Diehl AK. Epidemiology of gallbladder cancer: a synthesis of recent data. *J Natl Cancer Inst* 1980;65:1209.
93. Lazcano-Ponce EC, Miquel JF, Munoz N, et al. Epidemiology and molecular pathology of gallbladder cancer. *CA Cancer J Clin* 2001;51:349.
94. de Aretxabala X, Roa I, Araya JC, et al. Gallbladder cancer in patients less than 40 years old. *Br J Surg* 1994;81:111.
95. Yamaguchi K, Enjoji M. Carcinoma of the gallbladder: a clinicopathology of 103 patients and a newly proposed staging. *Cancer* 1988;62:1425.
96. Diehl AK. Epidemiology of gallbladder cancer: a synthesis of recent data. *J Natl Cancer Inst* 1980;65:1209.
97. Zatonski W, LaVecchia C, Levi F, Negri E, Lucchini F. Descriptive epidemiology of gallbladder cancer in Europe. *J Cancer Res Clin Oncol* 1993;119:165.
98. Serra I, Calvo A, Bez S, Yamamoto M. Risk factors for gallbladder cancer. An international collaborative case-control study. *Cancer* 1996;78:1515.
99. Nakayama F. Recent progress in the diagnosis and treatment of carcinoma of the gallbladder—introduction. *World J Surg* 1991;15:313.
100. Rudolph R, Cohen JJ. Cancer of the gallbladder in an 11-year-old Navajo girl. *J Pediatr Surg* 1972;7:66.
101. Carriaga MT, Henson DE. Liver, gallbladder, extrahepatic bile ducts and pancreas. *Cancer* 1995;75[Suppl 1]:171.
102. Donohue JH, Stewart AK, Menck HR. The National Cancer Data Base report on carcinoma of the gallbladder, 1989–1995. *Cancer* 1998;83:2618.
103. Wanebo HJ, Vezeridis MP. Treatment of gallbladder cancer. [Review]. *Cancer Treat Res* 1994;69:97.
104. Zatonski W, La Vecchia C, Levi F, Negri E, Lucchini F. Descriptive epidemiology of gallbladder cancer in Europe. *J Cancer Res Clin Oncol* 1993;119:165.
105. Berk RN, Armbuster TG, Saltzstein SL. Carcinoma in the porcelain gallbladder. *Radiology* 1973;106:29.
106. Ghadirian P, Simard A, Baillargeon J. A population-based case-control study of cancer of the bile ducts and gallbladder in Quebec, Canada. *Rev Epidemiol Sante Publique* 1993;41:107.
107. Kodama M, Kodama T. Epidemiological peculiarities of cancers of the gall-bladder and larynx that distinguish them from other human neoplasias. *Anticancer Res* 1994;14:2205.
108. Chijiiwa K, Tanaka M, Nakayama F. Adenocarcinoma of the gallbladder associated with anomalous pancreaticobiliary ductal junction. *Am Surg* 1993;59:430.
109. Welton JC, Marr JS, Friedman SM. Association between hepatobiliary cancer and typhoid carrier state. *Lancet* 1979;1:791.
110. Joffe N, Antolioli DA. Primary carcinoma of the gallbladder associated with chronic inflammatory bowel disease. *Clin Radiol* 1981;32:319.
111. Wilson SA, Princenthal RA, Law B, Leopold GR. Gallbladder carcinoma in association with *polyposis coli*. *Br J Radiol* 1987;60:771.
112. Trajber HJ, Szego T, Junior H, et al. Adenocarcinoma of the gallbladder in two siblings. *Cancer* 1982;50:1200.
113. Fernandez E, La Vecchia C, D'Avanzo B, Negri E, Franceschi S. Family history and the risk of liver, gallbladder, and pancreatic cancer. *Cancer Epidemiol Biomarkers Prev* 1994;3:209.
114. Kowalewski K, Todd EF. Carcinoma of the gallbladder induced in hamsters by insertion of cholesterol pellets and feeding dimethylnitrosamine. *Proc Soc Exp Biol Med* 1971;136:482.
115. Broden G, Bengtsson L. Biliary carcinoma associated with methyldopa therapy. *Acta Chir Scand* 1980;500:7.
116. Ellis EF, Gordon PR, Gottlieb LS. Oral contraceptives and cholangiocarcinoma. *Lancet* 1978;1:207.
117. Lowenfels AB, Norman J. Isoniazid and bile duct cancer. *JAMA* 1978;240:434.
118. Mancuso TF, Brennan MJ. Epidemiological considerations of cancer of the gallbladder, bile ducts and salivary glands in the rubber industry. *J Occup Med* 1970;12:333.
119. Shirai Y, Yoshida K, Tsukada K, Ohtani T, Muto T. Identification of the regional lymphatic system of the gallbladder by vital staining. *Br J Surg* 1992;79:659.
120. Albores-Saavedra J, Henson DE. *Atlas of tumor pathology, second series fascicle 22: tumors of the gallbladder and extrahepatic bile ducts.* Bethesda: Armed Forces Institute of Pathology, 1986.
121. Black WC. The morphogenesis of gall bladder carcinoma. In: Fenoglio CM, Wolff M, eds. *Progress in surgical pathology.* New York: Masson Publishing Inc., 1984:207.

122. Roa I, Araya JC, Villaseca M, et al. Preneoplastic lesions and gallbladder cancer: an estimate of the period required for progression. *Gastroenterology* 1996;111:232.

123. Aldridge MC, Bismuth H. Gallbladder cancer: the polyp-cancer sequence. *Br J Surg* 1990;77:363.

124. Kozuka S, Tsubone M, Yasui A, Hachisuka K. Relation of adenoma to carcinoma in the gallbladder. *Cancer* 1982;50:2226.

125. Sumiyoshi K, Nagai E, Chijiiwa K, Nakayama F. Pathology of carcinoma of the gallbladder. *World J Surg* 1991;15:315.

126. Kimura W, Nagai H, Kuroda A, Morioka Y. Clinicopathologic study of asymptomatic gallbladder carcinoma found at autopsy. *Cancer* 1989;64:98.

127. Perpetuo MO, Valdivieso M, Heilbrun LK, et al. Natural history study of gallbladder cancer: a review of 36 years experience at M.D. Anderson hospital and tumor institute. *Cancer* 1978;42:330.

128. Boerma EJ. Towards an oncological resection of gall bladder cancer. [Review]. *Eur J Surg Oncol* 1994;20:537.

129. Donohue JH, Nagorney DM, Grant CS, et al. Carcinoma of the gallbladder: does radical resection improve outcome? *Arch Surg* 1990;125:237.

130. Nevin JE, Moran TJ, Kay S, King R. Carcinoma of the gallbladder: staging, treatment, and prognosis. *Cancer* 1976;37:141.

131. Onoyama H, Yamamoto M, Tseng A, Ajiki T, Saitoh Y. Extended cholecystectomy for carcinoma of the gallbladder. *World J Surg* 1995;19:758.

132. Itoi T, Watanabe H, Ajioka Y, et al. APC, K-ras codon 12 mutations and p53 gene expression in carcinoma and adenoma of the gall-bladder suggest two genetic pathways in gallbladder carcinogenesis. *Pathol Int* 1996;46:333.

133. Wee A, Teh M, Raju GC. Clinical importance of p53 protein in gall bladder carcinoma and its precursor lesions. *J Clin Pathol* 1994;47:453.

134. Wistuba II, Sugio K, Hung J, et al. Allele-specific mutations involved in the pathogenesis of endemic gallbladder carcinoma in Chile. *Cancer Res* 1995;55:2511.

135. Imai M, Hoshi T, Ogawa K. K-ras codon 12 mutations in biliary tract tumors detected by polymerase chain reaction denaturing gradient gel electrophoresis. *Cancer* 1994;73:2727.

136. Chow NH, Huang SM, Chan SH, et al. Significance of c-erbB-2 expression in normal and neoplastic epithelium of biliary tract. *Anticancer Res* 1995;15:1055.

137. Fujii K, Yasui W, Shimamoto F, et al. Immunohistochemical analysis of nm23 gene product in human gallbladder carcinomas. *Virchows Arch* 1995;426:355.

138. Wistuba II, Albores-Saavedra J. Genetic abnormalities involved in the pathogenesis of gallbladder carcinoma. *J Hepatobiliary Pancreat Surg* 1999;6:237.

139. Koda M, Yashima K, Kawaguchi K, et al. Expression of Fhit, Mlh1, and P53 protein in human gallbladder carcinoma. *Cancer Lett* 2003;199:131.

140. Oertli D, Herzog U, Tondelli P. Primary carcinoma of the gallbladder: operative experience during a 16 year period. *Eur J Surg* 1993;159:415.

141. Thorbjarnarson B, Glenn G. Carcinoma of the gallbladder. *Cancer* 1959;12:1009.

142. Strom BL, Maislin G, West SL, et al. Serum CEA and CA 19-9: potential future diagnostic or screening tests for gallbladder cancer? *Int J Cancer* 1990;45:821.

143. Wibbenmeyer LA, Sharafuddin MJ, Wolverson MK, et al. Sonographic diagnosis of unsuspected gallbladder cancer: imaging findings in comparison with benign gallbladder conditions. *AJR Am J Roentgenol* 1995;165:1169.

144. Kumar A, Aggarwal S. Carcinoma of the gallbladder: CT findings in 50 cases. *Abdom Imaging* 1994;19:304.

145. Ohtani T, Shirai Y, Tsukada K, Hatakeyama K, Muto T. Carcinoma of the gallbladder: CT evaluation of lymphatic spread. *Radiology* 1993;189:875.

146. Wilbur AC, Gyi B, Renigers SA. High-field MRI of primary gallbladder carcinoma. *Gastrointest Radiol* 1988;13:142.

147. Schwartz LH, Coakley FV, Sun Y, et al. Neoplastic pancreaticobiliary duct obstruction: evaluation with breath-hold MR cholangiopancreatography. *AJR Am J Roentgenol* 1998;170:1491.

148. Harada H, Saski T, Yamamoto N. Assessment of endoscopic aspiration cytology and endoscopic retrograde cholangio-pancreatography in patients with cancer of the hepatobiliary tract. *Gastroenterol Jpn* 1977;12:59.

149. Mohandas KM, Swaroop VS, Gullar SU, et al. Diagnosis of malignant obstructive jaundice by bile cytology: results improved by dilating the bile duct strictures [see comments]. *Gastrointest Endosc* 1994;40:150.

150. Akosa AB, Barker F, Desa L, Benjamin I, Krausz T. Cytologic diagnosis in the management of gallbladder carcinoma. *Acta Cytol* 1995;39:494.

151. Shinkai H, Kimura W, Muto T. Surgical indications for small polypoid lesions of the gallbladder. *Am J Surg* 1998;175:114.

152. Yang HL, Sun YG, Wang Z. Polypoid lesions of the gallbladder: diagnosis and indications for surgery. *Br J Surg* 1992;79:227.

153. Glenn F, Hayes DM. The scope of radical surgery in the treatment of malignant tumors of the extrahepatic biliary tract. *Surg Gynecol Obstet* 1954;99:529.

154. Matsumoto Y, Fujii H, Aoyama H, et al. Surgical treatment of primary carcinoma of the gallbladder based on the histologic analysis of 48 surgical specimens. *Am J Surg* 1992;163:239.

155. Bartlett DL, Fong Y, Brennan MF, Fortner JG, Blumgart LH. Long-term results after resection for gallbladder cancer—implications for staging and management. *Ann Surg* 1996;224:639.

156. Yamaguchi K, Tsuneyoshi M. Subclinical gallbladder carcinoma. *Am J Surg* 1992;163:382.

157. Shirai Y, Yoshida K, Tsukada K, Muto T. Inapparent carcinoma of the gallbladder. An appraisal of a radical second operation after simple cholecystectomy. *Ann Surg* 1992;215:326.

158. de Aretxabala XA, Roa IS, Burgos LA, Araya JC, Villaseca MA, Silva JA. Curative resection in potentially resectable tumours of the gallbladder. *Eur J Surg* 1997;163:419.

159. Tsukada K, Kurosaki I, Uchida K, et al. Lymph node spread from carcinoma of the gallbladder. *Cancer* 1997;80:661.

160. Chijiiwa K, Tanaka M. Carcinoma of the gallbladder: an appraisal of surgical resection. *Surgery* 1994;115:751.

161. Shirai Y, Yoshida K, Tsukada K, Muto T, Watanabe H. Radical surgery for gallbladder carcinoma. Long-term results. *Ann Surg* 1992;216:565.

162. Onoyama H, Ajiki T, Takada M, Urakawa T, Saitoh Y. Does radical resection improve the survival in patients with carcinoma of the gallbladder who are 75 years old and older? *World J Surg* 2002;26:1315.

163. Behari A, Sikora SS, Wagholikar GD, et al. Long-term survival after extended resections in patients with gallbladder cancer. *J Am Coll Surg* 2003;196:82.

164. Nakamura S, Sakaguchi S, Suzuki S, Muro H. Aggressive surgery for carcinoma of the gallbladder. *Surgery* 1989;106:467.

165. Ouchi K, Suzuki M, Tominaga T, Saijo S, Matsuno S. Survival after surgery for cancer of the gallbladder. *Br J Surg* 1994;81:1655.

166. Ogura Y, Mizumoto R, Isaji S, et al. Radical operations for carcinoma of the gallbladder: present status in Japan. *World J Surg* 1991;15:337.

167. Kresl JJ, Schild SE, Henning GT, et al. Adjuvant external beam radiation therapy with concurrent chemotherapy in the management of gallbladder carcinoma. *Int J Radiat Oncol Biol Phys* 2002;52:167.

168. Houry S, Schlienger M, Huguier M, et al. Gallbladder carcinoma: role of radiation therapy. *Br J Surg* 1989;76:448.

169. Chao TC, Greager JA. Primary carcinoma of the gallbladder. *J Surg Oncol* 1991;46:215.

170. Oswalt C, Cruz AB. Effectiveness of chemotherapy in addition to surgery in treating carcinoma of the gallbladder. *Rev Surg* 1977;34:436.

171. Morrow CE, Sutherland DE, Florack G. Primary gallbladder carcinoma: significance of subserosal lesions and results of aggressive surgical treatment and adjuvant chemotherapy. *Surgery* 1983;94:709.

172. Wanebo HJ, Castle WN, Fechner RE. Is carcinoma of the gallbladder a curable lesion? *Ann Surg* 1982;195:624.

173. Taal BG, Audisio RA, Bleiberg H, et al. Phase II trial of mitomycin C (MMC) in advanced gallbladder and biliary tree carcinoma. An EORTC gastrointestinal tract cancer cooperative group study. *Ann Oncol* 1993;4:607.

174. Makela JT, Kairaluoma MI. Superselective intra-arterial chemotherapy with mitomycin for gallbladder cancer. *Br J Surg* 1993;80:912.

175. Green FL. *AJCC cancer staging manual*, 6th edition. New York: Springer-Verlag, 2002.

176. Pichlmayr R, Lamesch P, Weimann A, Tusch G, Ringe B. Surgical treatment of cholangiocellular carcinoma. *World J Surg* 1995;19:83.

177. Berdah SV, Delpero JR, Garcia S, Hardwigsen J, Le Treut YP. A Western surgical experience of peripheral cholangiocarcinoma. *Br J Surg* 1996;83:1517.

178. Lieser MJ, Barry MK, Rowland C, Ilstrup DM, Nagorney DM. Surgical management of intrahepatic cholangiocarcinoma: a 31-year experience. *J Hepatobiliary Pancreat Surg* 1998;5:41.

179. Chu KM, Fan ST. Intrahepatic cholangiocarcinoma in Hong Kong. *J Hepatobiliary Pancreat Surg* 1999;6:149.

180. Valverde A, Bonhomme N, Farges O, et al. Resection of intrahepatic cholangiocarcinoma: a Western experience. *J Hepatobiliary Pancreat Surg* 1999;6:122.

181. Shimada M, Yamashita Y, Aishima S, et al. Value of lymph node dissection during resection of intrahepatic cholangiocarcinoma. *Br J Surg* 2001;88:1463.

182. Weber SM, Jarnagin WR, Klimstra D, et al. Intrahepatic cholangiocarcinoma: resectability, recurrence pattern, and outcomes. *J Am Coll Surg* 2001;193:384.

183. Ebata T, Nagino M, Kamiya J, et al. Hepatectomy with portal vein resection for hilar cholangiocarcinoma: audit of 52 consecutive cases. *Ann Surg* 2003;238:720.

184. Ohtsuka M, Ito H, Kimura F, et al. Extended hepatic resection and outcomes in intrahepatic cholangiocarcinoma. *J Hepatobiliary Pancreat Surg* 2003;10:259.

185. Uenishi T, Hirohashi K, Kubo S, et al. Clinicopathologic features in patients with long-term survival following resection for intrahepatic cholangiocarcinoma. *Hepatogastroenterology* 2003;50:1069.

186. Sugiura Y, Nakamura S, Iida S, et al. Extensive resection of the bile ducts combined with liver resection for cancer of the main hepatic duct junction: a cooperative study of the Keio Bile Duct Cancer Study Group. *Surgery* 1994;115:445.

187. Nakeeb A, Pitt HA, Sohn TA, et al. Cholangiocarcinoma. A spectrum of intrahepatic, perihilar, and distal tumors. *Ann Surg* 1996;224:463.

188. Miyazaki M, Ito H, Nakagawa K, et al. Aggressive surgical approaches to hilar cholangiocarcinoma: hepatic or local resection? *Surgery* 1998;123:131.

189. Nagino M, Nimura Y, Kamiya J, et al. Segmental liver resections for hilar cholangiocarcinoma. *Hepatogastroenterology* 1998;45:7.

190. Neuhaus P, Jonas S, Bechstein WO, et al. Extended resections for hilar cholangiocarcinoma. *Ann Surg* 1999;230:808.

191. Gazzaniga GM, Filauro M, Bagarolo C, Mori L. Surgery for hilar cholangiocarcinoma: an Italian experience. *J Hepatobiliary Pancreat Surg* 2000;7:122.

192. Launois B, Reding R, Lebeau G, Buard JL. Surgery for hilar cholangiocarcinoma: French experience in a collective survey of 552 extrahepatic bile duct cancers. *J Hepatobiliary Pancreat Surg* 2000;7:128.

193. Lee SG, Lee YJ, Park KM, Hwang S, Min PC. One hundred and eleven liver resections for hilar bile duct cancer. *J Hepatobiliary Pancreat Surg* 2000;7:135.

194. Jarnagin WR, Fong Y, DeMatteo RP, et al. Staging, resectability, and outcome in 225 patients with hilar cholangiocarcinoma. *Ann Surg* 2001;234:507.

195. Kawarada Y, Das BC, Naganuma T, Tabata M, Taoka H. Surgical treatment of hilar bile duct carcinoma: experience with 25 consecutive hepatectomies. *J Gastrointest Surg* 2002;6:617.

196. Nagorney DM, Donohue JH, Farnell MB, Schleck CD, Ilstrup DM. Outcomes after curative resections of cholangiocarcinoma. *Arch Surg* 1993;128:871.

197. Fong Y, Blumgart LH, Lin E, Fortner JG, Brennan MF. Outcome of treatment for distal bile duct cancer. *Br J Surg* 1996;83:1712.

198. Wade TP, Prasad CN, Virgo KS, Johnson FE. Experience with distal bile duct cancers in U.S. Veterans Affairs hospitals: 1987–1991. *J Surg Oncol* 1997;64:242.

199. Yeo CJ, Cameron JL, Sohn TA, et al. Six hundred fifty consecutive pancreaticoduodenectomies in the 1990s: pathology, complications, and outcomes. *Ann Surg* 1997;226:248.

200. Yoshida T, Matsumoto T, Sasaki A, et al. Prognostic factors after pancreatoduodenectomy with extended lymphadenectomy for distal bile duct cancer. *Arch Surg* 2002;137:69.

201. Klinkenbijl JH, Jeekel J, Sahmoud T, et al. Adjuvant radiotherapy and 5-fluorouracil after curative resection of cancer of the pancreas and periampullary region: phase III trial of the EORTC gastrointestinal tract cancer cooperative group. *Ann Surg* 1999;230:776.

202. Falkson G, MacIntyre JM, Moertel CG. Eastern Cooperative Oncology Group experience with chemotherapy for inoperable gallbladder and bile duct cancer. *Cancer* 1984;54:965.

203. Bukowski RM, Leichman LP, Rivkin SE. Phase II trial of m-AMSA in gallbladder and cholangiocarcinoma: a Southwest Oncology Group Study. *Eur J Cancer Clin Oncol* 1983;19:721.

204. Ravry MJ, Omura GA, Bartolucci AA, et al. Phase II evaluation of cisplatin in advanced hepatocellular carcinoma and cholangiocarcinoma: a Southeastern Cancer Study Group Trial. *Cancer Treat Rep* 1986;70:311.

205. Whittington R, Neuberg D, Tester WJ, Benson AB, III, Haller DG. Protracted intravenous fluorouracil infusion with radiation therapy in the management of localized pancreaticobiliary carcinoma: a phase I Eastern Cooperative Oncology Group Trial. *J Clin Oncol* 1995;13:227.

206. Harvey JH, Smith FP, Schein PS. 5-Fluorouracil, mitomycin, and doxorubicin (FAM) in carcinoma of the biliary tract. *J Clin Oncol* 1984;2:1245.

207. Takada T, Nimura Y, Katoh H, et al. Prospective randomized trial of 5-fluorouracil, doxorubicin, and mitomycin C for non-resectable pancreatic and biliary carcinoma: multicenter randomized trial. *Hepatogastroenterology* 1998;45:2020.

208. Kajanti M, Pyrhonen S. Epirubicin-sequential methotrexate-5-fluorouracil-leucovorin treatment in advanced cancer of the extrahepatic biliary system. A phase II study. *Am J Clin Oncol* 1994;17:223.

209. Sanz-Altamira PM, Ferrante K, Jenkins RL, et al. A phase II trial of 5-fluorouracil, leucovorin, and carboplatin in patients with unresectable biliary tree carcinoma. *Cancer* 1998;82:2321.

210. Choi CW, Choi IK, Seo JH, et al. Effects of 5-fluorouracil and leucovorin in the treatment of pancreatic-biliary tract adenocarcinomas. *Am J Clin Oncol* 2000;23:425.

211. Patt YZ, Jones DV Jr, Hoque A, et al. Phase II trial of intravenous fluorouracil and subcutaneous interferon alfa-2b for biliary tract cancer. *J Clin Oncol* 1996;14:2311.

212. Patt YZ, Hassan MM, Lozano RD, et al. Phase II trial of cisplatin, interferon alpha-2b, doxorubicin, and 5-fluorouracil for biliary tract cancer. *Clin Cancer Res* 2001;7:3375.

213. Chen H, Hardacre JM, Uzra A, Cameron JL, Choti MA. Isolated liver metastases from neuroendocrine tumors: does resection prolong survival? *J Am Coll Surg* 1998;187:88.

214. Chen JS, Lin YC, Jan YY, Liau CT. Mitomycin C with weekly 24-h infusion of high-dose 5-fluorouracil and leucovorin in patients with biliary tract and periampullar carcinomas. *Anticancer Drugs* 2001;12:339.

215. Mani S, Sciortino D, Samuels B, et al. Phase II trial of uracil/tegafur (UFT) plus leucovorin in patients with advanced biliary carcinoma. *Invest New Drugs* 1999;17:97.

216. Jones DV Jr, Lozano R, Hoque A, Markowitz A, Patt YZ. Phase II study of paclitaxel therapy for unresectable biliary tree carcinomas. *J Clin Oncol* 1996;14:2306.

217. Pazdur R, Royce ME, Rodriguez GI, et al. Phase II trial of docetaxel for cholangiocarcinoma. *Am J Clin Oncol* 1999;22:78.

218. Papakostas P, Kouroussis C, Androulakis N, et al. First-line chemotherapy with docetaxel for unresectable or metastatic carcinoma of the biliary tract. A multicentre phase II study. *Eur J Cancer* 2001;37:1833.

219. Kubicka S, Rudolph KL, Tietze MK, Lorenz M, Manns M. Phase II study of systemic gemcitabine chemotherapy for advanced unresectable hepatobiliary carcinomas. *Hepatogastroenterology* 2001;48:783.

220. Gebbia V, Giuliani F, Maiello E, et al. Treatment of inoperable and/or metastatic biliary tree carcinomas with single-agent gemcitabine or in combination with levofolinic acid and infusional fluorouracil: results of a multicenter phase II study. *J Clin Oncol* 2001;19:4089.

221. Kuhn R, Hribaschek A, Eichelmann K, et al. Outpatient therapy with gemcitabine and docetaxel for gallbladder, biliary, and cholangio-carcinomas. *Invest New Drugs* 2002;20:351.

222. Eng C, Ramanathan RK, Remick S, et al. Phase II trial of fixed dose rate gemcitabine in patients with advanced biliary tree carcinoma. *Am J Clin Oncol* 2003 (*in press*).

223. Fiebiger WC, Scheithauer W, Traub T, et al. Absence of therapeutic efficacy of the somatostatin analogue lanreotide in advanced primary hepatic cholangiocellular cancer and adenocarcinoma of the gallbladder despite in vivo somatostatin-receptor expression. *Scand J Gastroenterol* 2002;37:222.

224. Ouchi K, Owada Y, Matsuno S, Sato T. Prognostic factors in the surgical treatment of gallbladder carcinoma. *Surgery* 1987;101:731.

225. Gall FP, Kockerling F, Scheele J, Schneider C, Hohenberger W. Radical operations for carcinoma of the gallbladder: present status in Germany. *World J Surg* 1991;15:328.

226. Shirai Y, Yoshida K, Tsukada K, Muto T. Inapparent carcinoma of the gallbladder. An appraisal of a radical second operation after simple cholecystectomy. *Ann Surg* 1992;216:565.

227. Yamaguchi A, Tsukioka Y, Fushida S, et al. Intraperitoneal hyperthermic treatment for peritoneal dissemination of colorectal cancers. *Dis Colon Rectum* 1992;35:964.

228. Todoroki T, Kawamoto T, Takahashi H, et al. Treatment of gallbladder cancer by radical resection. *Br J Surg* 1999;86:622.

229. Wakai T, Shirai Y, Hatakeyama K. Radical second resection provides survival benefit for patients with T2 gallbladder carcinoma first discovered after laparoscopic cholecystectomy. *World J Surg* 2002;26:867.

230. Toyonaga T, Chijiiwa K, Nakano K, et al. Completion radical surgery after cholecystectomy for accidentally undiagnosed gallbladder carcinoma. *World J Surg* 2003;27:266.

231. Cubertafond P, Gainant A, Cucchiaro G. Surgical treatment of 724 carcinomas of the gallbladder. Results of the French Surgical Association Survey. *Ann Surg* 1994;219:275.

232. Bartlett D, Fong Y, Blumgart LH. Complete resection of the caudate lobe of the liver: technique and results. *Br J Surg* 1996;83:1076.

233. Paquet KJ. Appraisal of surgical resection of gallbladder carcinoma with special reference to hepatic resection. *J Hep Bil Panc Surg* 1998;5:200.

234. Muratore A, Amisano M, Vigano L, Massucco P, Capussotti L. Gallbladder cancer invading the perimuscular connective tissue: results of reresection after prior non-curative operation. *J Surg Oncol* 2003;83:212.

235. Nakamura S, Sakaguchi S, Suzuki S, Muro H. Aggressive surgery for carcinoma of the gallbladder. *Surgery* 1989;106:467.

236. Todoroki T, Iwasaki Y, Orii K, et al. Resection combined with intraoperative radiation therapy (IORT) for stage IV (TNM) gallbladder carcinoma. *World J Surg* 1991;15:357.

237. Nimura Y, Hayakawa N, Kamiya J, et al. Hepatopancreatoduodenectomy for advanced carcinoma of the biliary tract. *Hepato-gastroenterol* 1991;38:170.

238. Schauer RJ, Meyer G, Baretton G, Schildberg FW, Rau HG. Prognostic factors and long-term results after surgery for gallbladder carcinoma: a retrospective study of 127 patients. *Langenbecks Arch Surg* 2001;386:110.

239. Kondo S, Nimura Y, Hayakawa N, et al. Extensive surgery for carcinoma of the gallbladder. *Br J Surg* 2002;89:179.

240. Manfredi R, Masselli G, Maresca G, et al. MR imaging and MRCP of hilar cholangiocarcinoma. *Abdom Imaging* 2003;28:319.

241. Levy AD, Murakata LA, Rohrmann CA Jr. Gallbladder carcinoma: radiologic-pathologic correlation. *Radiographics* 2001;21:295.

242. Bartlett DL, Fong Y. Gallbladder cancer. In: Blumgart LH, Fong Y, Jarnagin WR, eds. *American Cancer Society atlas of clinical oncology: hepatobiliary cancer*. London: B.C. Decker, Inc., 2001:213.

SECTION **6**

HERBERT J. ZEH III

Cancer of the Small Intestine

Cancer arising in the small intestine presents significant diagnostic and therapeutic challenges to the cancer clinician because (1) it is not a single pathologic entity but rather a diverse group of histologically benign and malignant tumors; (2) it is relatively rare, making collection, collation, and analysis of epidemiologic data, as well as treatment outcomes, difficult; and (3) it usually presents with vague or nonspecific symptoms, making early diagnosis difficult. A majority of the information we have about these tumors is derived from retrospective review of large cancer databases (that have limited clinical details) or from single-institutional series. As a result our knowledge about this diverse collection of tumors is often incongruously merged, leading to an incomplete picture of the natural history of each subtype. This chapter starts by reviewing those features shared by all cancers arising in the small intestine, including epidemiology, pathogenetic mechanisms, clinical presentation, and diagnostic workup. Next, the four most common subtypes, adenocarcinoma, carcinoid, lymphoma, and sarcoma/gastrointestinal stromal tumor (GIST), which account for greater than 98% of malignancies arising in the small intestine, are reviewed individually.

TABLE 29.6-1.   Large Population-Based Studies of Small Intestinal Cancer[a]

Author/Database	No. of Cases	Histology	% of Total	Cases in Millions
Ross et al.[3] (1972–1985)	1190	Adenocarcinoma	37	—
		Carcinoid	42	—
		Lymphoma	12	—
		Sarcoma	7.5	—
Weiss and Yang[4] (1973–1982)	1832	Adenocarcinoma	40	3.9
		Carcinoid	29	1.9
		Lymphoma	17	1.2
		Sarcoma	12	1.6
Gabos et al.[5] (1975–1989)	1244	Adenocarcinoma	41	—
		Carcinoid	26	—
		Lymphoma	19	—
		Sarcoma	11	—
DiSario et al.[2] (1966–1990)	328	Adenocarcinoma	24	—
		Carcinoid	41	—
		Lymphoma	19	—
		Sarcoma	11	—
Chow et al.[8] (1973–1990)	1718	Adenocarcinoma	36	3.7
		Carcinoid	35	3.8
		Lymphoma	9	1.3
		Sarcoma	13	1.1
Severson et al.[6] (1973–1991)	3292	Adenocarcinoma	NA	6.5
		Carcinoid	NA	6.5
		Lymphoma	NA	—
		Sarcoma	NA	—
Howdle et al.[7] (1998–2000)	395	Adenocarcinoma	44	—
		Carcinoid	20	—
		Lymphoma	27	—
		Sarcoma	9	—

NA, not available.

[a]Distribution of most common histologic subtypes is consistent, with adenocarcinoma and carcinoid tumors being most common.

INCIDENCE

Cancer arising in the small intestine is extremely rare. In 2004, there are expected to be 5200 new cases, accounting for just 0.3% of all new expected cancer cases in the United States. It accounts for approximately 2% of all gastrointestinal (GI) cancers, with a much lower incidence than cancer of the colon and rectum (135,000), stomach (25,000), and pancreas (35,000). Mortality from small bowel tumors is dependent on the histologic subtype, with overall survival for all types approximately 50%. The incidence of malignant tumors arising in the small intestine has been estimated to be between 5.9 and 9.9 per million people in the United States and 5.1 per million people in the United Kingdom.

The incidence of benign small bowel tumors is difficult to ascertain from the large retrospective reviews, as they are inherently biased toward the reporting of symptomatic tumors. In one large study of 9721 consecutive autopsies, 112 neoplasms of the small bowel were discovered, 72 of which were benign lesions. This suggests that the prevalence of asymptomatic tumors is much higher than predicted by the overall incidence reported by these large reviews.[1] More than 40 different histologically distinct tumors have been described to arise in the small intestine; however, greater than 95% of the time that malignancy is discovered it is either adenocarcinoma, carcinoid, leiomyoma/leiomyosarcoma (GIST), or lymphomas. Most of the information that we have regarding the incidence of individual histologic sub-

types of cancers arising in the small intestine is derived from a handful of reviews of large cancer databases or large single-institutional retrospective case series[2–8] (Table 29.6-1).[9–16] These studies demonstrate a consistent demographic distribution of these tumor types: adenocarcinoma (24% to 44%), carcinoid (20% to 42%), sarcoma/GIST (7% to 9%), and lymphoma (12% to 27%). Unique demographic features of each of these common cancers arising in the small intestine are discussed in further detail later in the text.

PATHOGENETIC MECHANISMS IN SMALL INTESTINAL CARCINOGENESIS

The small bowel constitutes approximately 75% of the entire length of the GI tract and 90% of its absorptive surface. Despite this, small bowel malignancies account for only approximately 1% to 2% of all GI malignancies. The incidence of cancers arising in the small intestine is approximately 40- to 60-fold less than that of colon tumors. Several theories have been forwarded in the literature as to the reason why the small bowel seems to be relatively protected from development of cancer. They are as follows: (1) The contents of the small bowel are liquid and therefore have a much faster transit time, resulting in less time for exposure to potential carcinogens; (2) the pH in the small bowel tends to be neutral to alkaline, making it less susceptible to acidic conditions under which most carcinogens act; (3) the bacterial content of the small bowel is less anaerobic, which predisposes to less degradation of bowel salts, which some believe are carcinogenic in the colon; (4) the small bowel has high receptors for uptake of folate, and this results in high folate levels that some believe are protective against carcinogenesis; (5) the small bowel has high levels of benzopyrene hydroxylase, which leads to breakdown of benzopyrene, a potential carcinogen that is used as a food additive in a variety of over-the-counter foods; (6) the small bowel has a high level of lymphoid tissue and especially of immunoglobulin A, which may be immunoprotective against the development of cancer; and (7) the small bowel contains fewer stem cells, which may be the target of carcinogens, and therefore less predisposed to development of cancers. Given the rare occurrence and diverse histologic makeup of cancers arising in the small intestine, none of these theories has received sufficient study to be accepted as medical fact; however, they provide substrate for future research into these cancers and may provide insight into cancers arising in other parts of the GI tract.

GENETIC AND ENVIRONMENTAL FACTORS THAT PREDISPOSE TO MALIGNANCY ARISING IN THE SMALL INTESTINE

Several environmental, as well as genetic, syndromes have been clearly documented to predispose to an increased risk of developing malignancy in the small intestine (Table 29.6-2).

1. Familial adenomatous polyposis (FAP). Patients with FAP have multiple adenomas in the colon and, if left untreated, run a relative risk of 100% of developing colon cancer. Many investigators have documented that these patients are also at risk for development of adenomas and adenocarcinomas of the small intestine. In fact, periampullary adenocarcinoma is the leading cause of death in patients with FAP who have undergone total colonic resection. Most of these tumors are clustered in the periampullary duodenum, but they may occur anywhere in the small intestine. The lifetime relative risk of developing small bowel adenocarcinoma in patients with FAP has been rated to be as high as 330.

2. Hereditary nonpolyposis colorectal cancer. Patients with hereditary nonpolyposis colorectal cancer also have an increased risk for small bowel cancer.[17] Lifetime risk is

estimated to be approximately 1%, which is significantly higher than that of the general population.[18,19]

3. Other primary cancers. Several reviews of large databases of patients with cancers arising from the small intestine have noted increased rates of other malignancies.[18] The relative risk of developing small bowel malignancy has been shown to be elevated in patients with prior colon and rectal, prostate, lung, and breast cancers.[11,18,20] Ripley and Weinerman,[21] in a review of the tumor registry of two Canadian provinces, identified a greater than eightfold increased risk of having a second primary malignancy in patients with small bowel adenocarcinoma. A majority of the patients (73%) with second malignancies had their small bowel primary diagnosed after the other cancer.

4. Crohn's disease. Adenocarcinoma of the small bowel occurs with a higher frequency in patients with Crohn's disease.[18,22] These tumors tend to occur in younger individuals, with an average age of 48.2 compared to the average age overall of 65, and usually in those patients with long-standing Crohn's disease of greater than 10 years.[23] Unlike sporadic adenocarcinomas, which most often arise in the duodenum, Crohn's disease–associated tumors are most commonly found in the ileum.[24–26]

5. Celiac disease. The association between development of small bowel malignancy and celiac disease has been examined in a large survey of all small bowel malignancies in the United Kingdom.[7,11,18] In this clinical pathologic study, approximately 395 cases of small bowel cancer were reported, of which 107 were lymphomas, 175 were adenocarcinomas, and 79 were carcinoid tumors. Thirteen percent of the adenocarcinomas and 39% of the lymphomas were found to be associated with celiac disease. The adenocarcinomas appeared to be histologically similar to other adenocarcinomas arising spontaneously. Adenocarcinomas associated with celiac disease occur more often in the jejunum. Lymphomas arising in the setting of celiac disease are referred to as *enteropathy-associated T-cell lymphoma* (EATL). These lymphomas are primarily found in the jejunum and are T cell in origin. The use of a gluten-free diet appears to decrease the risk of malignancy.

6. Peutz-Jeghers. Peutz-Jeghers disease is a rare autosomal dominant disease that is characterized by multiple hamartomatous-like polyps of the small bowel and focal melanin deposits with pigmentation of the skin and mucous membranes. Peutz-Jeghers syndrome polyps are not true polyps, as they tend to have a core of smooth muscle arising from the muscular mucosa extending into the polyp. These polyps in and of themselves can present problems with obstruction, bleeding, and small bowel intussusception. The relative risk of developing small bowel cancer in patients with Peutz-Jeghers is approximately 18-fold greater than that of the general population.[27] This is believed to be secondary to a germline defect in the LKB1 tumor suppressor gene found in these patients. Whether or not these malignancies arise from atypical transformation of the hamartomatous polyps has not been clearly defined.

7. Several other diseases have been linked to increased risk of benign and malignant neoplasm of the small intes-

TABLE 29.6-2. Genetic and Environmental Conditions That Predispose to Cancer of the Small Intestine

Condition	Histology
Familial adenomatous polyposis	Adenocarcinoma
Hereditary nonpolyposis colon cancer	Adenocarcinoma
Crohn's disease	Adenocarcinoma
Peutz-Jeghers	Adenocarcinoma, hamartomas
Gardner's syndrome	Adenocarcinoma, desmoid
Celiac disease	Adenocarcinoma, lymphoma
Neurofibromatosis	Paraganglioma
Acquired immunodeficiency syndrome	Lymphoma
History of other primary[a]	Adenocarcinoma, carcinoid

[a]See ref. 18.

tine, including neurofibromatosis (paragangliomas), acquired immunodeficiency syndrome (lymphomas), Gardner's syndrome (desmoid tumors), and cystic fibrosis (adenocarcinoma).

PRESENTATION AND DIAGNOSIS OF CANCERS ARISING IN THE SMALL INTESTINE

No specific signs or symptoms indicate the presence of malignancy in the small intestine. The typical presentation for these cancers is often vague and nonspecific. However, a few generalizations can be made after review of the large case series in the literature:

1. It appears that malignant lesions are symptomatic earlier in their natural history and for a shorter period of time before diagnosis, as opposed to benign lesions, which are more frequently discovered incidentally.[28]
2. Approximately one-half of all small bowel tumors present as an acute event; 77% of the time this is either an obstruction or a perforation.[7,18]
3. The most frequently presenting signs and symptoms are nonspecific and include abdominal pain, nausea and vomiting (obstruction), weight loss, and GI bleed.[7,9,10,15,18]

The small numbers of each histologic subtype reported in each of these case series make it difficult to draw generalizations about specific signs and symptoms for each of the more common histologic subtypes. It does appears that adenocarcinomas are more frequently associated with pain and obstruction when compared to those of sarcomas or carcinoids. Sarcomas (GIST) are more frequently associated with acute GI hemorrhage than the other common subtypes, and lymphomas appear to be associated with a higher rate of presentation with intestinal perforation (Table 29.6-3).

Early diagnosis of small bowel tumors is hampered by this lack of early and specific clinical symptoms. Several authors have retrospectively reviewed the diagnostic workup of small bowel tumors and found significant delays in the time from presentation to definitive diagnosis.[28–30] Ciresi and Scholten[28] examined a series of 49 patients with primary small bowel intestinal tumors from 1981 to 1993. They found that the average delay in diagnosis from the time of symptoms was approximately 30.2 weeks. Only 31% of the patients in this series had a definitive diagnosis before surgical resection. The average number of diagnostic

tests performed on these patients was 2.5 before the diagnosis. Similarly, Maglinte et al.[30,31] examined a series of 77 patients and found a delay from time of symptoms to time of diagnosis of 7.8 months. In this series of 77 patients, 14 had the appropriate study but it was misread (3 were read as benign when there was really a malignancy, and 11 were read out as normal but were clearly abnormal), and 26 of these patients had no test or the wrong test ordered. The relative delay attributed to each of these scenarios was as follows: (1) the patient failed to report symptoms (less than 2-month delay), (2) the physician did not order the appropriate diagnostic test (8.2-month delay), and (3) the appropriate test was ordered but was misread (12-month delay).

These two studies highlight the difficulty in diagnosing small bowel tumors. The reason for this is that the standard workup for vague abdominal pain, nausea and vomiting, or weight loss usually includes esophagogastroduodenoscopy, colonoscopy, plain abdominal films, and abdominal ultrasound. These radiologic techniques are relatively insensitive except for very advanced tumors of the small bowel. Therefore, the clinician must have a high degree of suspicion for patients who present repetitively with vague or nonspecific symptoms and use advanced diagnostic imaging to assist in the diagnosis. The two best-described radiologic evaluations for the diagnosis of tumors arising in the small bowel are double-contrast barium study (enteroclysis) and computed tomography (CT).

SMALL BOWEL ENTEROCLYSIS STUDY

Barium contrast studies are often one of the first studies ordered by the clinician in the primary fruition for evaluation of vague abdominal pain and weight loss that are common in cancers arising in the small intestine. It has been estimated that the sensitivity of a simple small bowel follow-through with barium is quite low: Only approximately 50% of the time is it able to indirectly diagnose the problem, and only 30% to 40% of the time does it reveal direct evidence of the cancer. In contrast, the addition of double contrast in the form of a formal enteroclysis study results in significant improvement in sensitivity and specificity, with a sensitivity of 95% for detecting either direct or indirect evidence of a cancer and 90% sensitivity for directly diagnosing the tumor, often with accurate histologic predictions.[32]

Several authors have reviewed the radiographic findings of enteroclysis study of the four major histologic subtypes of cancers arising in the small bowel.[33–37]

1. Adenocarcinoma on enteroclysis study often presents as an annular lesion with a very short segment of bowel being affected. Overhanging edges or an apple-core appearance with mucosal alterations are often present. The radiographic appearances of simple polypoid adenomas can be contrasted from the adenocarcinoma by the findings of thickening of the local small bowel and the presence of luminal obstruction or dilation (Table 29.6-4).
2. Similarly, carcinoid tumors have classic features found on enteroclysis studies. They are found in the ileum tenfold more commonly. They present as smooth mucosal elevations, often with evidence of intussusception mass displacement. If they are larger than 2 cm, there is sometimes evidence of mass displacement of surrounding bowel loops.

TABLE 29.6-3. Presenting Signs and Symptoms of Cancer Arising in the Small Bowel in Several Larger Series[7,9,10,15,18]

Sign/ Symptom	Adenocarcinoma	Carcinoid	Sarcoma (GIST)	Lymphoma
Abdominal pain	38–46	34	25	39–55
Obstruction	45–77	22–49	15	22
Perforation	2	0–2	0–2	15
GI bleed	12–26	0–2	30	4
Weight loss	21	25	0–5	52

GIST, gastrointestinal stromal tumor.

TABLE 29.6-4. Radiographic Appearance of Cancer Arising in the Small Intestine

Tumor	Enteroclysis	Computed Tomography
Adenocarcinoma	Annular stricture, apple core, short segment, mucosal irregularity	Eccentric thickening of bowel wall, annular narrowing
Carcinoid	Ileal location, smooth mucosal elevation, mass displacement of surrounding bowel loops	Ill-defined, homogeneous mass, stellate soft tissue stranding (desmoplastic response) calcifications
Sarcoma/GIST	Submucosal: Punched-out filling defect Intramural: Smooth blank filling defect "Dumbbell": Combination	Submucosal: Homogeneous mass, hypervascular mass Intramural: Homogeneous mass, hypervascular mass, central necrosis
Lymphoma	Focal aneurysmal dilatation followed by narrowing, broad-based mucosal ulceration	Filling defect, target lesion, long bowel thickening, cavitary lesions with aneurysmal thickening

GIST, gastrointestinal stromal tumor.

3. The radiographic appearances of sarcoma/GIST on enteroclysis study have been well characterized into four different growth patterns. These include the submucosal pattern, which often presents as a punched-out or filling defect on enteroclysis study, and the intramural or subserosal, which often results in the appearance of a blank space or mass effect on the small bowel wall. Another pattern is the dumbbell-type growth pattern of the GIST tumor that results in a combination of mucosal filling defect and mass effect on the local small bowel.

4. Lymphoma on enteroclysis study reveals narrowing of the lumen, usually nonobstructing. When it represents the only feature of lymphoma, it may be indistinguishable from adenocarcinoma, except that it is mostly located distally. Discrete broad-based ulceration or a large cavitating lesion, secondary to central necrosis of a large, rapidly dividing mass, is characteristic. The cavitating mass may erode adjacent ileal loops and may result in fistula formation. Focal aneurysmal dilatation, featuring an aperistaltic, ballooned, thick-walled segment filled with amorphous barium collection, is another characteristic feature of lymphoma.

COMPUTED TOMOGRAPHY

Similar to the enteroclysis study, a significant amount of literature has been accumulated on the characteristic radiologic findings of each of the histologic subtypes of cancers arising in the small bowel found on CT.[35,38] In a small retrospective series, Dudiak et al.[39] found that the radiologic findings on CT scan allow for specific diagnosis in 60% of adenocarcinomas, 58% of lymphomas, and 33% of carcinoids (see Table 29.6-4).

Adenocarcinoma

CT findings of an adenocarcinoma of the small bowel usually manifest as annular narrowing with abrupt concentric or irregular "overhanging edges." Eccentric thickening of the small bowel wall is usually present as well as potential narrowing of the lumen and dilation of the proximal small bowel. In addition to helping in diagnosing the presence of an adenocarcinoma arising in the small bowel, the CT scan can be used to stage these patients. This method has been examined by Buckley et al.[40] and found to be quite reproducible. The classic findings include mesenteric stranding or fat stranding in and around the root of the mesentery as well as overt lymph nodes. This group has noted that the large, aggressive ulcerated adenocarcinoma can often be mistaken for a lymphoma. However, in the adenocarcinoma the lymph nodes are usually less bulky and a shorter segment of the small bowel is generally involved.

Lymphoma

The findings of primary small bowel lymphoma on CT scan include the absence of lymphadenopathy in other places in the body, including the superficial lymph node basins, the hilar and mediastinal lymph node basins, and the retroperitoneal area. Primary small bowel lymphoma usually presents as a nodular filling defect, larger and more varied in shape than just simple lymphoid hyperplasia. Often a discrete polyp can form the lead point as an intussusception that can be identified as a target lesion on the CT scan. These are usually longer segments of the small bowel that are involved, as opposed to the adenocarcinoma, and classic findings of aneurysmal dilatation of the small bowel with intermittent obstruction are present. Aneurysmal dilatation of the small bowel lumen is not usually found in adenocarcinomas. With aggressive large cell lymphomas, there can often be findings of cavitary masses that appear arising from the mesentery. Low-grade lymphomas, including EATL, that are associated with celiac disease, often present as just segment nodular wall thickening, a nonspecific finding that is frequently difficult to distinguish from other forms of lymphoid hyperplasia or ischemia or other insults to the small intestine.

Carcinoid

On CT, carcinoid tumors appear as ill-defined, homogeneous masses with displaced small bowel loops. Often a stellate pattern of soft tissue stranding the "desmoplastic reaction" is present, with some calcifications that can be found in the mesentery. This is quite characteristic of these tumors and leads to correct diagnosis when these findings are present.

Gastrointestinal Stromal Tumor

CT findings associated with GISTs include a submucosal mass that is usually very well circumscribed, is either extrinsic or exocentric, and often, depending on the size, displaces adjacent bowel loops. Classically, these are hypervascular lesions that enhance greatly and are very homogeneous in nature. However, sometimes the larger lesions are associated with necrotic centers. This finding of central liquefactive necrosis in the center of a large GIST-like tumor has been correlated with a higher finding on final pathology of a malignant GIST.

OTHER DIAGNOSTIC TECHNIQUES

Endoscopy of the duodenum, push enteroscopy, and extended colonoscopy all play a role in the diagnostic workup of cancers that arise in the small bowel. These studies allow direct visualization of the tumor and biopsy to confirm the diagnosis, making them the gold standard for specificity. However, each of them is severely limited in its ability to completely examine the entire surface area of the small intestine, making them quite insensitive. Newer endoscopic techniques, such as wireless capsule endoscopy, that allow for direct visualization of the entire surface area of the small intestine hold great promise in the early evaluation of patients with early small bowel pathology. Wireless capsule endoscopy has already been demonstrated to have higher sensitivity and specificity than barium small bowel follow-through studies in detecting causes of obscure GI bleeding.[41]

The octreotide scan is another useful scan in diagnosing carcinoid tumors carcinoids that arise in the small bowel. It is based on binding of the radioactive somatostatin analog to the receptor on carcinoid cells. It appears that octreotide scanning is particularly good in identifying extraabdominal metastasis.[42]

ADENOCARCINOMA ARISING IN THE SMALL INTESTINE

Adenocarcinoma is the most common histologic subtype of cancer arising in the small intestine. It accounts for between 37% and 40% of all neoplasms, arising in the small intestine in large case series and cancer database reviews.[4–6,8,11,18,43] The overall incidence of adenocarcinoma arising in the small intestines is estimated to be approximately 14 per 100 million population. Review by Severson et al.[6] of the Surveillance, Epidemiology, and End Results program (SEER) database has revealed an increase in the rate of adenocarcinoma among black males rising from 8.2 per 1 million to 16 cases per 1 million in the years 1987 through 1999 versus 1973 to 1977. A similar increase was noted among white males, from 6.2 to 8.5. Peak incidence is in the sixth and seventh decades of life, with the average age of onset 65 years of age. Adenocarcinoma arising in the small intestine most commonly occurs in the duodenum (50%), followed by the jejunum (17% to 23%) and the ileum (13% to 15%). Interestingly, there also appears to be a slight predisposition to development of adenocarcinoma of the small bowel in a Meckel's diverticulum, with an overrepresentation of cases in Meckel's diverticula reported. The majority of these patients present with advanced disease, with American Joint Committee on Cancer stage 3 or greater. In a review of the National Cancer Database by Howe et al.,[44] the overall 5-year disease-free survival rate was 30.5%, with 60.2% at 1 year, 44.2% at 2 years, and 37% at 3 years. Mean survival was 19.7 months. These survival rates were also somewhat dependent on the primary tumor site, with duodenal cancer of 5-year survival

being 28.2%, jejunal cancer 37.6%, and ileal cancer 37.8%. In addition, patients older than 75 had a worse prognosis, 5-year survival of 22% versus 33.9%. Similarly, those patients with poorly differentiated tumors had worse outcome versus those with moderate to low to well-differentiated tumors.[44]

GENETICS OF ADENOCARCINOMA ARISING IN THE SMALL INTESTINE

The histologic progression of invasive colorectal cancer has been well studied and appears to develop through one of several distinct genetic mutational pathways. The first is the classic adenoma to carcinoma pathway as elucidated by Voglestien and colleagues. In this pathway early lesions show mutations in the cyclooxygenase and APC genes followed later by K-ras, SMAD4, and p53. In the second pathway tumors arise in the setting of germline mutations in the DNA mismatch repair genes, the so-called replication error or RER phenotype. Inability to correct random mutations ultimately leads to many of the mutational changes described in the classic adenoma to carcinoma pathway. Adenocarcinoma arising in the small intestine shares many morphologic characteristics and risk factors with colorectal carcinoma. Both tumors arise from preexisting polyps. Both are associated with increased risk in patients with FAP, hereditary nonpolyposis colorectal cancer, and inflammatory bowel disease. These similarities suggest that these two diseases may share similar genetic pathways. This would be an interesting finding because the much lower incidence of small bowel tumors, despite 40- to 60-fold greater surface area, may suggest that there is some intrinsic protection in the small bowel to development of cancer. Multiple authors have examined genetic alterations in adenocarcinomas arising in the small bowel. These are summarized in Table 29.6-5.

Blaker et al.[45] examined 17 cases of sporadic adenocarcinoma arising in the jejunum. In this study they found that only 3 of 17 patients had mutations in the APC gene, which was similar to that of spontaneously arising colorectal cancer; 2 of 17 were found to have evidence of microsatellite instability; and 80% of them were found to have loss of the 18q21 through q22, an upstream gene from the SMAD4 gene, which is also frequently lost in colorectal cancer.[45]

Wheeler et al.[46] examined 21 cases of sporadic adenocarcinoma arising in the small intestines for mismatch repair genes. They found that 1 of 21 (5%) of the tumors were RER positive. Similarly, they found no evidence of any significant mutations in the mutational cluster region of the APC gene. The majority of these (greater than 30%) were also found to have mutations in the β-catenin, E-cadherin, and p53 genes.[46]

Arai et al.[47] examined 15 cases of jejunal adenocarcinoma and found that the mutational rate of K-ras and the p53 and APC were similar to or lower than those of colorectal cancer. This suggests that there is a distinct genetic pathway that does not follow the well-defined polyp-to-adenocarcinoma sequence found in colon cancer.[47]

In the largest study to date, Planck et al.[47a] examined 89 small bowel adenocarcinomas arising in the small intestine.[46] They found that 15 of 89 of these were positive for microsatellite instability. This microsatellite instability was traced to mutations in the mismatch repair gene mutation in the majority of these cases. Interestingly, the majority of the microsatellite instability found in the adenocarcinomas arising in

TABLE 29.6-5. Genetic Abnormalities Found in Adenocarcinomas Arising in the Small Intestine[a]

Study	No. of Tumors Examined	Mutations in p53	Mutations in K-ras	Mutations in APC	Mutations in RER
Blaker et al.[45]	17	—	—	3/17	2/17
Arai et al.[47]	15	4/15	—	3/15	NA
Wheeler et al.[46]	21	5/21	—	0/21	1/21
Planck et al.[47a]	89	—	—	—	16/89
Nishyama et al.[b]	35	14/35	2/35	—	—
Scarpa et al.[c]	12	8/12	5/12	6/10	3/12
Expected colon cancer	—	40–80%	40–80%	40–60%	15–20%

NA, not available.

[a]It does not appear that adenocarcinoma of the small bowel is associated with significant rates of mutations in the APC gene similar to colorectal cancer.
[b]Nishiyama K, Yao T, Yonemasu H, et al. Overexpression of p53 protein and point mutation of K-ras genes in primary carcinoma of the small intestine. *Oncol Rep* 2002;9:293.
[c]Scarpa A, Zamboni G, Achille A, et al. ras-Family gene mutations in neoplasia of the ampulla of Vater. *Int J Cancer* 1994;59:39.

the small bowel were not found to be the cause of mutations of the MLH-1 gene, as is found in the majority of colorectal carcinomas.

ADENOMAS AND ADENOCARCINOMAS ARISING IN THE SETTING OF FAMILIAL ADENOMATOUS POLYPOSIS

Approximately 90% of patients with FAP develop duodenal involvement with polyps. These polyps are of malignant potential, and 2% to 5% of all patients with FAP develop adenocarcinoma of the duodenum at some time during their lifetime.[6,48] In fact, the leading cause of death among patients with FAP who have had proctocolectomy is adenocarcinoma of the duodenum. In a large series of 952 families with FAP, the lifetime risk of developing duodenal cancer by the age of 70 years was 4%.[48,49] Although the association between these duodenal polyps in the setting of FAP and the development of adenocarcinoma is well defined, the natural history of these polyps is unknown.[50–52] In a study over a 4-year period, only 32% increased in number and 11 increased in histologic grade. A similar study of longer than 11 years with 98 patients showed a 73% progression rate of untreated duodenal ampullary adenomas in patients with FAP.[53,54]

Perhaps the best-known staging system for these polyps has been proposed by Spigelman et al.[55,56] It is based on the number, size, histologic type, and degree of dysplasia in the polyps (Table 29.6-6). Based on these staging criteria, the polyps can be categorized into either major or minor ampullary polyposis. This staging system has been prospectively examined by several authors.[57,58] Patients with major ampullary polyposis (stage III/IV) have been found to have a rate of progression to cancer approximately fourfold higher than those with minor ampullary adenomas. Current recommendations based on these criteria are that patients with stage I or II disease can be evaluated with endoscopy every 3 to 4 years, whereas those with stage III or IV disease should have endoscopy and annual biopsy. Findings on screening endoscopy that should lead to definitive treatment include enlarging lesion greater than 1 cm, severe dysplasia, villous histology, or frank adenocarcinoma. Similarly, bleeding or symptomatic ulceration should warrant intervention.

Isolated resection, either surgical or through endoscopy of duodenal polyps in the setting of FAP, has been reported by

several groups but has been found to be almost universally followed by progression of the disease.[6,48,50,53] Surgical prophylactic pyloric-preserving pancreaticoduodenectomy or pancreas-preserving duodenectomy for severe polyposis has been advocated. Several groups have shown this to be safe and effective in preventing the development of duodenal cancer in these patients.[52,59,60]

PROGNOSTIC CLINICOPATHOLOGIC CORRELATES

In a review of institutional series at the Cleveland Clinic, Abrahams et al.[61] examined in detail 37 cases of adenocarcinoma arising in the small bowel. These excluded periampullary lesions. In this series of 37 patients, there were 22 segmental resections, 10 pancreaticoduodenectomies, and 1 polypectomy, with 4 undergoing palliative bypass or an unknown treatment. The 5-year survival for this small cohort of patients was 52% at 5 years and 47% at 10 years, with a mean follow-up of 50 months. Prognostic factors on univariate analysis were shown to be positive surgical margins, extramural venous spread, the presence of lymph node metastasis, or poor tumor differentiation. In another review, an institutional series by Veyrieres et

TABLE 29.6-6. Spigelman Staging System of Duodenal Polyps in the Setting of Familial Adenomatous Polyposis[a]

	Points		
Characteristic	1	2	3
Number of polyps	1–4	5–20	>20
Size of polyps	1–4 mm	5–10 mm	>10 mm
Histology	Tubulo	Tubulovillous	Villous
Dysplasia	Mild	Moderate	Severe

Stage	Points
0	0
1	1–4
2	5–6
3	7–8
4	9–12

[a]It is recommended that patients with stage III/IV undergo yearly endoscopic screening.

al.[62] examined 100 cases of adenocarcinoma arising in the small bowel. The overall 5-year survival was 63% in localized disease and 52% in those in which there was lymph node involvement. In this case series, only tumor differentiation was found to be significantly associated with improved 5- and 10-year survival rate, and the site of the tumor, including duodenum, jejunum, and ileum, did not seem to be affected; further, the size of the tumor of 5 cm or greater did not significantly predict survival.

TREATMENT OF LOCALIZED DISEASE

Surgery is the mainstay of treatment of adenocarcinoma arising in the small bowel. Complete surgical resection with negative margins remains the single best curative regimen. For those tumors arising in the duodenum, there are a variety of surgical options, including segmental duodenal resection, pancreaticoduodenectomy, or pancreas-preserving duodenal resection. For duodenal tumors, it appears that segmental resection leads to overall less survival.[63–65] Sohn et al.[64] reported improved overall survival in patients undergoing pancreaticoduodenectomy versus segmental resection (only a 14% disease-free survival rate was reported in patients undergoing segmental resection). Similarly, Rose et al.[65] from Memorial Sloan-Kettering reported a 60% 5-year survival rate with a combination of a pancreas-preserving and pancreas-resecting technique.

The rare nature of adenocarcinomas arising in the small bowel has led to a paucity of information in the literature as to the benefits of adjuvant chemotherapy and radiation therapy. In the National Cancer Database series reviewed by Howe et al.,[44] only approximately 8.2% of the patients with localized disease received radiotherapy and 15.6% of those with regional involvement received radiation therapy. Similarly, chemotherapy was given to 14.2% of those with local disease, 35% with regional disease, and 36% with distant metastasis. In this retrospective review with very little clinical information and large selection bodies, there appeared to be overall better survival for those patients treated with combination treatment. Most chemotherapy regimens that have been examined consist of 5-fluorouracil (5-FU) alone in combination with a variety of other agents, including doxorubicin, cisplatin, mitomycin C, and cyclophosphamide. One study by the Royal Marsden Hospital showed that protracted venous infusion of 5-FU has activity in primary adenocarcinoma of the small bowel.[66] Several other isolated studies have reported response rates with 5-FU and methotrexate.

CARCINOID TUMORS ARISING IN THE SMALL INTESTINE

The traditional classification of carcinoid tumors is according to the embryonal site of origin, which includes foregut (lung, thymus, stomach, pancreas, and proximal duodenum), midgut (distal duodenal to proximal colon), and hindgut carcinoids (distal colon and rectum). Midgut carcinoids are usually referred to as *classic* carcinoids. They are thought to arise from the neuroendocrine cells of Kulchitsky in the intestinal tract. Midgut carcinoids have an early propensity of local-regional spread but generally follow an indolent course,

with many patients with metastatic disease surviving longer than 5 years.

DEMOGRAPHICS OF CARCINOIDS ARISING IN THE SMALL INTESTINE

Modlin et al.[67] have performed a comprehensive review of all carcinoid tumors in the United States: 10,878 carcinoid tumors were identified in the SEER database from 1973 to 1999 and an additional 2837 carcinoid tumors that were registered previously by the two earlier National Cancer Institute programs. In this large database the most frequent site for occurrence of carcinoid tumors was the GI tract (67.5%). Within the GI tract, a majority of the carcinoid tumors occurred in the small intestine (41.8%) or the rectum (27.4%), with the stomach accounting for 8.7%. The age-, race-, and gender-adjusted incidence rates for small intestinal carcinoids were 0.88 for white men and 0.63 for white women and 0.82 for African American men and 0.52 per 100,000 population for African American women. The average age at diagnosis for patients with small intestinal carcinoids was 65.4 years, which was within 2 months of the average age of diagnosis for patients with noncarcinoid tumors of the same site (65.3 years). Within the small intestine, the majority of the carcinoid tumors were identified in the ileum, followed by the duodenum and then the jejunum. In contrast to adenocarcinomas, which occur most frequently in the duodenum, there was a significantly higher incidence of tumors arising in Meckel's diverticulum than would be expected. Approximately 22.4% of carcinoid tumors were associated with other noncarcinoid neoplasms. This was specifically true for carcinoids arising in the small intestine, where 29% of these were associated with other noncarcinoid neoplasms. The meaning of this is unknown; however, some have hypothesized that the pericarcinoid milieu may promote the development of other noncarcinoid cancers. Carcinoid tumors have a high propensity for early local-regional spread and metastatic dissemination. In this large database, 58.3% of the patients were found to have local-regional or metastatic spread at the time of presentation.

CLINICOPATHOLOGIC CORRELATE OF PROGNOSIS

For carcinoid tumors arising in the small bowel, it appears that size of the primary and depth of invasion are the best predictors of risk for local-regional and distant spread of the tumor.[42,68–70] Soga[70] has examined the clinical behavior of 1102 cases of jejunoileal carcinoids (largest review in the literature of carcinoids arising in the small intestine). In this large series, the risk of local-regional or distant spread was directly related to the tumor size and the depth of invasion (Tables 29.6-7 and 29.6-8). The three cutoff points were with (1) tumors of less than 6 mm (15.8%), (2) tumors of 6 to 10 mm in size (31.5%), and (3) tumors of 11 to 20 mm (73.6%). In addition, those lesions with transmural invasion were found to have metastasis 68.4% of the time, as opposed to those with just submucosal invasion (30.8%). Overall 5-year survival for all patients was approximately 73.3%. It was significantly better for those patients who presented without metastasis, with a 5-year survival of 90.9% as opposed to 68.2% for patients presenting with the presence of metastasis. Others have noted even higher rates of lymph node metastases in jejunoileal carcinoids. Makri-

TABLE 29.6-7. Risk of Metastases from Carcinoid Tumors Arising in the Small Intestine[a]

Size of Primary Tumor (mm)	Risk of Metastases (%)
<6	15
6–10	31
>10	73

[a]Risk of local-regional or distant metastases in a single large review of 1102 carcinoids arising in the small intestine. Even small carcinoids less than 6 mm are associated with a significant rate of metastases. (From ref. 70, with permission.)

dis et al.,[68] in a small series of patients undergoing surgery for symptomatic carcinoid, observed a very high incidence of lymph node metastases: (1) less than 0.5 cm (69%), (2) 0.5 to 1.0 cm (94%), and (3) greater than 1.0 to 2.0 cm or larger (100%). Shebani et al.[69] found that jejunal carcinoids greater than 2 cm in size and with greater depth of invasion were statistically associated with a higher rate of lymph node or distant metastasis.

TREATMENT OF LOCALIZED DISEASE

Segmental resection of the tumor with accompanying draining lymph nodes is the treatment of choice for primary carcinoids arising in the small bowel. As noted above even very small carcinoids (less than 0.5 cm) arising in the small intestine are associated with a substantial risk of nodal metastases. Therefore, even incidentally discovered, small tumors should be resected with their nodal basins. Five-year survival after resection of localized disease has been reported to range between 50% and 85%.[68–73] Given the slow indolent course of most carcinoids, several authors have advocated resection of the primary tumor with the metastatic lymph nodes, irrespective of the presence of widespread metastatic disease. In a small retrospective series, Soreide et al.[74] found better survival for patients with midgut lesions subjected to primary resection of the tumor and mesenteric lymph nodes versus those who did not undergo the

TABLE 29.6-8. Pathologic Correlates of Malignant Potential of Gastrointestinal Stromal Tumors Arising in the Small Intestine[a]

Tumor size	Probably benign	<2 cm
	Uncertain potential	>2 but <5 cm
	Probably malignant	<5 cm
Mitotic activity	Probably benign	<5 mitoses per 50 hpf
	Probably malignant	<5 mitoses per 50 hpf
KIT-activating mutations	Exon 11 mutations correlated more often with malignant behavior	
	Exon 9 mutations highly correlated with malignant behavior	

hpf, high-power field.
[a]Pathologic correlates of malignant potential in gastrointestinal stromal tumors (GIST) from the small intestine. GIST arising in the small intestine are more aggressive, being associated with development of metastatic disease at a smaller size than gastric GIST. Mutational analysis of the c-KIT gene reveals several mutations that appear to confer worse prognosis.

debulking, with a median survival of 139 versus 69 months. In this series, even patients with hepatic metastasis showed improvement, and median survival was 216 months versus 48 months without treatment. The decision to perform palliative resection in a patient with disseminated carcinoid arising in the small bowel should carefully balance the risks and benefits of the procedure, including the premorbid condition of the patient and other comorbid medical conditions, as well as the severity of the symptoms.

CARCINOID SYNDROME

The carcinoid syndrome is a constellation of symptoms, including flushing, diarrhea, and wheezing, that is caused by release into the systemic circulation of tumor-derived substances and their metabolites. These substances include serotonin, bradykinin, prostaglandin, and catecholamines. The liver and lung usually metabolize some of these substances, preventing their release into the systemic circulation. Therefore, it is generally believed that the development of carcinoid syndrome requires the presence of pulmonary or hepatic metastasis before it develops. Only 10% to 17% of patients with small bowel carcinoids present with carcinoid syndrome; however, symptoms develop in approximately 60% to 70% of them during some point of their disease. The symptoms of the carcinoid syndrome are often provoked by eating, alcohol, or stress. The etiology of the carcinoid syndrome and the flushing and diarrhea that occur with it is controversial, and no clear direct etiologic origin of any of the symptoms has been correlated directly to an individual substance. The most effective tool for relieving symptoms of carcinoid syndrome is the use of the long-acting somatostatin analog octreotide. This has been found in multiple series to improve, and even prevent, flushes as well as diarrhea.[75–77]

TREATMENT OF ADVANCED DISEASE

The goal of treatment of metastatic carcinoid tumor remains twofold: Improve survival and control symptoms through cytoreduction. Cytoreductive treatments for metastatic carcinoid include (1) surgery, (2) hepatic arterial embolization with or without regional delivery of chemotherapy, and (3) systemic chemotherapy.

Surgery/Local Ablative Therapy

The most common site of metastasis from the carcinoid syndromes after the original lymph nodes is the liver. A majority of these patients present with bilobar disseminated liver metastasis; however, in several anecdotal and small case series, those patients with a small number of metastases who underwent surgical excision of these enjoyed prolonged disease-free survival.[78–80] A retrospective review of all patients at the Mayo Clinic undergoing hepatic metastasectomy for neuroendocrine tumors between 1977 and 1998 was published by Sarmiento and Que.[80] This included 120 patients with hepatic metastasis from carcinoid tumors that had arisen in the ileum. Major hepatectomy was performed in 54% of the patients, and the postoperative complication rate was 14%, with a mortality of 1.2%. Surgical debulking of the tumor controlled symptoms of carcinoid syndrome in 104 of 108 patients. The recurrence rate was 59% at 5 years for carcinoid syndrome and 84% at 5 years for tumor. Overall survival was 61% and 35% at 5 and 10 years compared to historic 5-year survival of 36%. This retrospective series suggests that cytoreduction through hepatic metastasectomy may prolong survival and control symptoms in a carefully selected group of patients.

Orthotopic liver transplantation has been reported in a series of patients with metastatic carcinoid.[81–83] In a series of 31 patients undergoing orthotopic liver transplantation for metastatic neuroendocrine tumors (15 carcinoid patients), Le Treut et al.[81] reported an overall 5-year survival of 73% and a disease-free survival of 47%. Lehnert et al.[83a] reported 47% and 24% overall survival and recurrence-free survival from 103 patients. Other cytoreductive techniques for treatment of carcinoid tumors have been reported as well. These include local ablative techniques such as radiofrequency ablation. Preliminary reports on radiofrequency ablation by Berber et al.[84] demonstrate that it is safe, and in a small series of seven patients, no postoperative complications were reported and several patients were able to reduce their dose of octreotide, corresponding to a decrease in overall symptoms.

Chemoembolization Therapy

In a retrospective review of all patients treated with hepatic arterial chemoembolization at the M. D. Anderson Institute from the year 1992 to December 2000, 81 patients with carcinoid tumor underwent hepatic chemoembolization.[84] Fifty patients underwent strictly straightforward embolization, and 31 underwent a combination of intraarterial chemotherapy and embolization. Sixty-nine patients could be evaluated for response. In these, 67% were found to have a partial response, greater than a 50% reduction of their tumors. Minimal response occurred in 6 (8.7%) patients and stable disease in 11 (16%). Only six patients, or 8.7%, had progressive disease during the median follow-up period. The mean duration of the response in the 42 patients who had a partial response was 17 months. Sixty-two percent of the patients had reduction in their tumor-related symptoms. The probability of progression and increased survival in this series was estimated to be 75%, 35%, and 11% at 1, 2, and 3 years, respectively. The median overall survival was 31 months. The probability of survival at 1 year was 93%, 60% at 2 years, and 24% at 5 years. This series shows the effectiveness as well as the relative safety of this technique and demonstrates that it should be considered for all patients with unresectable hepatic metastases from carcinoid tumors who can tolerate it.

Chemotherapy

A variety of chemotherapeutic agents have been examined, alone or in combination, for the treatment of metastatic carcinoid.[85] The two most successful regimens have included streptozotocin combined with cyclophosphamide or 5-FU, showing response rates for the 5-FU combination of 44% and 37% for cyclophosphamide regimens to biochemical response rates. Other groups have examined the use of, or addition of, doxorubicin to the 5-FU, cyclophosphamide, streptozotocin regimen and found that they could increase the biochemical response rates.[86] However, in general these response rates were limited. The use of a combination of chemotherapy with interferon-α has also been examined and found to increase the biochemical as well as the tumor response rates when compared to the chemotherapy regimens used alone. Some groups have examined the efficacy of interferon-α and found that it could synergize with current chemotherapies.[87] It was reported by Saltz et al.,[88] in 1993, that octreotide can prevent the progression of metastatic carcinoid tumors. In a series of 34 patients treated with octreotide, 50% have stable disease that lasted a median of 5 months.

LYMPHOMA ARISING IN THE SMALL INTESTINE

Lymphoma accounts for the third most common neoplasm arising in the small intestine, accounting for approximately 15% to 20% of all malignant small bowel tumors. Extranodal lymphoma or lymphoma arising within the solid organs occurs in up to 40% of all cases of lymphoma. Primary malignant lymphoma that occurs extranodally was first recognized by Virkow in 1863; however, it was Dawson et al. who first established the criteria for primary GI lymphoma: (1) absence of palpable lymphadenopathy; (2) normal peripheral blood smear and bone marrow biopsy; (3) absence of mediastinal lymphadenopathy on chest x-ray; (4) disease grossly confined to the affected small bowel segment as confirmed by diagnostic imaging, endoscopy, or laparotomy; (5) regional lymphadenopathy only; and (6) absence of hepatic or splenic tumor involvement except via direct extension from the primary bowel involvement. The GI tract is the most frequently involved extranodal site, accounting for up to half of all extranodal disease.

The stomach is the most common primary site for GI involvement with lymphoma, accounting for as high as 50% or 60% of all extranodal lymphomas, followed by the small intestine, colon, and other organs, including the pancreas and the liver. On a recent review from the University of Rochester over a 3-year period, 48% of all GI lymphomas were gastric, 26% small intestinal, and 12% colonic. The incidence of intestinal lymphoma has been reported to be increasing in the United States, doubling from 1985 to 1990. This has been attributed to an upsurge in the lymphoma among immunocompromised patients, as well as immigration from the Middle East and Near East.

STAGING

Tumor spread is the most important factor in the prognosis of intestinal lymphoma. A variety of staging systems exists for primary intestinal neoplasms that are all based on the classic Ann Arbor staging system. The two modifications to the Ann Arbor system for specific primary intestinal lymphomas include the Blackledge staging system and the Musshoff and Schmidt-Volmer modification. In this last staging system, stage I is a lymphoma limited to a single site. Stage II is intestinal lymphomas that are confined below the diaphragm and separated into two subgroups with regional (stage II 1E and distant stage II 2E) lymph node involvement. Stage III is when organs on both sides of the diaphragm are involved, and stage IV is widespread dissemination including the liver and the spleen. All of these systems, the Ann Arbor and the Musshoff and Blackledge modifications, have similar common aspects, including stage I for limited local disease, stage II for regional involvement, and stages III and IV for an advanced disease stage. More recently, a TNM (tumor, node, metastasis)-like staging system for primary

TABLE 29.6-9. Most Common Lymphomas Arising in the Small Intestine (Revised European-American Lymphoma Classification)

Histology	Percent of Small Bowel Lymphomas
Diffuse large B-cell lymphoma	55
MALT lymphoma	20
Peripheral T-cell/EATL	15
Burkitt's lymphoma	5

EATL, enteropathy-associated T-cell lymphoma; MALT, mucosal-associated lymphoid tissue lymphoma.

GI lymphomas has been proposed by the European Gastrointestinal Lymphoma Study Group. This classification system is believed to be well suited for the unique aspects of primary GI lymphomas in terms of being able to predict the response to therapy, as well as the clinical staging of the disease.

SUBTYPES OF LYMPHOMA ARISING IN THE SMALL INTESTINE

Numerous classification schemes exist for non-Hodgkin's lymphomas. These include the Kiel-Rappaport, Lukes-Collins, Revised European-American Lymphoma (REAL), Working Formulation, and World Health Organization classifications. Under the most recent of these classification schemes (World Health Organization classification, as well as the REAL classification), lymphomas arising in the GI tract generally fall into one of four categories (Table 29.6-9): (1) diffuse large B-cell lymphoma, (2) mucosal-associated lymphoid tissue (MALT)–associated lymphomas, (3) peripheral T-cell lymphoma, and (4) Burkitt's lymphomas.

Diffuse Large B-Cell Lymphoma

Diffuse large B-cell lymphoma is the most common non-Hodgkin's lymphoma occurring in the GI tract, developing most often in the ileocecal region. Other names for the large diffuse B-cell lymphoma include the large cell immunoblastic, large-cleaved follicular center cell, centroblastic D immunoblastic cell, and diffuse mixed lymphocytic and histiocytic cells. Morphologically, these tumors are composed of diffuse large B cells with large nuclei that are twice the size of a normal lymphocyte. These tumor cells are CD19, positive CD20, positive CD22, positive CD79a. They tend to have a high percentage of BCL2 gene that is rearranged in approximately 30% of them. Immunodeficiency virus, as well as general immunodepressed states, have been found to be risk factors for the development of this lymphoma.

These tumors commonly occur in adult males, with a median age of 54 to 61 years. They usually present as focal or segmental lesions in the distal small intestine. Treatment of localized disease consists primarily of surgical resection followed by adjuvant radiation or chemotherapy.[89–91] Overall 5-year survival has been reported to be between 50% and 70% for tumors treated with multimodality therapy.

Mucosal-Associated Lymphoid Tissue Lymphoma

In the REAL classification, MALT is known as the marginal zone B-cell lymphoma. These lymphomas are characterized by cellular heterogeneity, including marginal zone cells similar to those of Peyer's patch and mesenteric nodal tissue. Reactive follicles are usually present, with the neoplastic marginal zone occupying the marginal zone or intrafollicular region. These tumor cells express immunoglobulin M greater than immunoglobulin G or immunoglobulin A. They express B-cell–associated antigens, including CD19, CD20, CD22, and CD79a. They are usually CD5 negative, CD10 negative, CD23 negative, and CD43 variable. Unlike the large diffuse B cells, they are not associated with BCL2 or BCL1 rearrangements. Clinically, these tumors are associated with histories of chronic inflammation, including autoimmune disorders such as Sjögren's syndrome or Hashimoto's thyroiditis and *Helicobacter* gastritis. The majority of the patients present with localized stage I or II extranodal disease involving the small intestine. Studies suggest that proliferation in some early MALT-like–type tumors may be antigen driven, as from the *Helicobacter pylori* bacteria. Treatment is multimodality, including surgical resection and adjuvant chemoradiation therapy. Survival from small MALT arising in the small intestine has been reported to be better than MALT arising in the stomach.[92]

Burkitt's Lymphoma

Burkitt's lymphoma has also been described arising in the GI tract, accounting for fewer than 5% of all small intestinal lymphomas. Burkitt's lymphoma cells are monomorphic medium-sized cells with round nuclei and abundant basophilic cytoplasm. The tumor has an extremely high rate of proliferation, giving it a starry-eyed pattern that is usually present, imparted by the numerous benign macrophages that have ingested apoptotic tumor cells. Burkitt's lymphoma is most common in children and accounts for approximately one-third of all non-African pediatric lymphomas. The GI tract is the third most common site for involvement of endemic Burkitt's lymphoma. The majority of cases of non-African and nonendemic types present in the abdomen, most often in the distal ileum and cecum. In the National Cancer Institute series of sporadic Burkitt's lymphoma, one-fourth of the patients presented with a mass in the right lower quadrant mimicking an appendicitis. Burkitt's lymphoma is a rapidly growing tumor with short doubling time. Treatment consists primarily of chemotherapy, usually vincristine, cyclophosphamide, doxorubicin, and methotrexate.

T-Cell Lymphomas of the Small Intestine

This tumor was originally termed *malignant histiocytosis of the intestine* but has since been shown to be conclusively T-cell lymphoma arising in the small intestine. It accounts for approximately 15% of all lymphomas arising in the small intestine. Tumor cells contain a variable mixture of small, medium, and large cells and a high content of intraepithelial T cells in the adjacent mucosa. The tumor cells are CD3 positive, CD7 positive, CD8 positive, CD4 negative, and CD103 positive. These tumors are often found to have T-cell receptor beta changes clonally rearranged. EATL was first defined by O'Farrelly in 1986.[93] This is a lymphoma that has been found to arise in the setting of malabsorption and steatorrhea and to be closely associated with celiac disease. The exact risk of EATL and celiac disease is difficult to discern given the significant amount of subclinical celiac disease. However, it has been estimated to arise in approximately 5% to 10% of all patients with celiac disease. It is believed that the relative risk of developing a lymphoma in the setting of celiac disease is 25- to 100-fold higher than in normal patients.[94] In one study non-Hodgkin's lymphoma was the most common cause of death in celiac patients. In a large series of 30 EATL lymphomas from Ireland, there appeared to be an equal number of men and women. The majority of the patients had the lymphoma diagnosed concurrently with diagnosis of the celiac disease. Fully one-third of the patients presented with a surgical emergency, perforation, or obstruction as their mode of presentation. Of these 30 patients with lymphomas associated with celiac disease, 24 were found to be of EATL type arising in the jejunum or the proximal ileum. Treatment consisted of surgery and chemotherapy. The 5-year survivor rate was quite poor, approximately 11%.[95] The exact phenotypic type of the cell in EATL lymphoma has been examined, and they appear to fall into one of two distinct cell types, a CD3-positive, CD4-negative, CD8-negative, CD3-positive, CD8-positive, or CD56-positive type. The link between refractory sprue disease that is not responsive to a gluten-free diet and the development of lymphoma is controversial at this point.[95] Several authors have suggested that development of a lymphoma may be simply a monoclonal outgrowth of reactive T cells. However, others have pointed to the polyclonal nature of EATL, suggesting that this is, in fact, not a result of simple monoclonal outgrowth and reaction to a gluten diet.

MESENCHYMAL TUMORS ARISING IN THE SMALL INTESTINE

Since the last edition of this text, a paradigm shift has occurred in our understanding and treatment of mesenchymal tumors arising in the small intestine. It is now recognized that a vast majority of the tumors that had been previously identified as leiomyoma and leiomyosarcoma are actually CD117-positive GIST. In fact, GISTs are now thought to be the most common mesenchymal tumors arising from the small intestine. True leiomyomas and leiomyosarcomas are rare in the GI tract, with the exception of the esophagus.

Adding to the excitement over our improved understanding of these common tumors of the GI tract was the discovery of a drug that could successfully treat these sometimes aggressive tumors. STI 571, which is now known by its trade name Gleevec, is a compound that was specifically designed to inhibit the Abl protein tyrosine kinase, which is present in 95% of patients with chronic myelogenous leukemia. This compound can inhibit several families of tyrosine kinases, including c-kit. Clinical trials have found that this compound is very effective in treating GISTs without many of the side effects associated with traditional chemotherapies.

DEMOGRAPHICS OF GASTROINTESTINAL STROMAL TUMORS

It is very difficult to know accurately the true incidence of GIST, as only in the last 5 years have we been able to define these tumors as distinct subtypes. According to a population-based sample, the incidence of all GISTs in the GI tract is estimated as 10 to 20 per million of the population.[96]

The largest review of smooth muscle tumors of the small intestine has been reported by Blanchard et al.[97] They have reviewed the entire world's literature from 1881 to 1996, identifying 1074 patients with leiomyomas and 1686 with the designa-

tion *leiomyosarcomas*. Because the majority of all mesenchymal tumors of the GI tract (except the esophagus) are believed to be GISTs, older data on leiomyomas and leiomyosarcomas arising in the intestinal smooth muscle largely reflect GISTs.[96] The peak incidence was between the ages of 50 and 59, with the youngest age being 7 months and the oldest being 90. In this series, benign GISTs were two to three times more common than malignant GISTs. The frequency of GIST in the small intestine was proportional to the length of that segment, with most commonly being found in the jejunum, followed by the ileum, and lastly by the duodenum. Interestingly, the exception to this was that there was a higher than expected prevalence of tumors that were found to arrive in Meckel's diverticulum, representing 1% to 2% of all the small bowel malignant GISTs reported in this large series. These authors also found that the second portion of the duodenum contained the highest number of GISTs. These tumors tended to be more common intraluminally or intramurally, as opposed to the rest of the small intestine, where they were most commonly extraluminal. In this very large series, approximately one-half of the GISTs were found to be 5 cm or less. Those identified as malignant GISTs were found to be between 5 and 9 cm. The most common signs and symptoms in presentation of these tumors tended to be pain, intussusception, and bleeding for benign GIST, and pain, weight loss, and bleeding for malignant GIST. Diagnosis in this very large series was most commonly made by either barium swallow or CT scan. CT scan was found to be very successful, diagnosing correctly 89.5% of leiomyomas and 98% of leiomyosarcomas in this review. Only one-third of the patients in this study were found to have metastasis. The only significant prognostic variable found to correlate with the ability to metastasize was that tumors greater than 5 cm had a higher instance of metastasis. Survival in this series was reported in 22 of the series reviewed, for a total number of 705 patients. Five-year survival was 27.8%, ranging from 10% to 48%. This survival rate incorporated all tumors and did not stratify or stage them according to benign or malignant characteristics.

HISTOLOGY OF GASTROINTESTINAL STROMAL TUMOR ARISING IN THE SMALL INTESTINE

It has been reported by Miettinen et al.[98,99] that the GISTs arising at different anatomic sites display differences in immunohistochemical staining. In a review of 292 GISTs arising throughout the GI tract, these authors found that the majority of the GISTs arising in the small bowel stained equal positivity for CD34 and smooth muscle actin. However, GISTs arising in the colon and rectum as well as in the stomach were rarely positive for smooth muscle actin and always 100% positive for CD34, as opposed to the small bowel GISTs, which were only positive approximately 50% of the time. Similarly, S100 positivity was rarely found but was most frequently seen in small intestinal GISTs (15% of the time). These tumors were more often found to contain extracellular collagen globules (skeinoid fibers).

CLINICOPATHOLOGIC CORRELATES OF MALIGNANT POTENTIAL

The identification of the C-KIT overexpression mutation that identifies GISTs has allowed a wealth of information to be gathered in the last 5 years regarding the clinicopathologic correlates of this tumor. In addition, the emergence of an effective treatment for malignant GIST in STI 571 has heightened the importance of correctly identifying those GISTs with malignant behavior. The percentage of malignant small intestinal GIST has been estimated to be between 50% and 64%.[100–102] The following have been found to be critical to predicting the metastatic malignant behavior of GISTs.

1. Size and mitotic count. Factors indicating malignant potential for duodenal GIST have been reported to be size greater than 4.5 cm and greater than two mitoses per 50 high-power fields. For jejunoileal GIST, size greater than 5 cm and five or more mitoses per 50 high-power field suggest malignant potential.[101,103] Interestingly, the significance of size and mitotic count on malignant potential in GIST is site dependent. Multiple studies have demonstrated that GIST arising in the small intestine displays a greater biologic aggressiveness than that arising in the stomach and colon.

2. Site. GISTs arising in the small intestine appear to have a more malignant behavior at a smaller size than those found in the stomach or in the colon and rectum. Emory et al.[103a] have reported on a very large series of GI smooth muscle (stromal tumors) from a variety of anatomic sites and found that these differ greatly in prognostic significance. In this series of 1004 GISTs, multivariate analysis revealed that location in the small intestine was significantly associated with worse overall survival than GIST from the colon and stomach.

3. Other clinical histologic correlates of malignant behavior that have been examined include cellularity and nuclear atypia, mucosal invasion, specific genetic mutations,[104] and ulceration, but none of these have been shown to correlate well with prognosis.

The ability to completely discriminate between a benign and malignant GIST tumor remains somewhat difficult, as there are clearly cases in all of the series showing that even those patients with small tumors and no mitotic failures have been observed to die of their disease; therefore, at this point there remain no complete criteria that can be predictive of malignancy and outcome in GI tumors. A GIST workshop was held at the National Institutes of Health, and the recommendations were not to categorize GISTs as benign or malignant but, rather, to categorize them as to their malignant potential.

TREATMENT OF LOCALIZED DISEASE

The principal treatment for primary GISTs arising in the small intestine is complete surgical excision. Great care has to be taken during the operative procedure, as these tumors are somewhat soft, fleshy, and prone to rupture, which has been reported to lead to early and diffuse intraabdominal recurrence. The goal for the surgical margins should be gross margins. It is not believed that negative microscopic margins lead to improved survival, especially when certain tumors that are extremely large, or greater than 15 cm, are resected. In these situations it is likely that there is already diffuse spreading and shedding of tumor cells throughout the abdomen, and gross surgical margins are all that is required. Lymph node metastases are rare, and therefore an extensive lymph node dissection is not recommended.

In a retrospective review of 200 patients with GISTs who underwent primary surgery with complete excision of their tumors at Memorial Sloan-Kettering, disease-specific survival rate was 88% at 1 year, 65% at 3 years, and 54% at 5 years.[103,105] The median survival of those patients who undergo a complete excision was 66 months, as opposed to those who had incomplete resection at 22 months. In this series 86% of 93 patients with primary disease were able to undergo complete resection, justifying the removal of adjacent organs when necessary to achieve complete negative gross margins. Microscopic margin status did not influence outcome in this series.

In a majority of patients, distant or local recurrence develops at some point in their disease course. In fact, only 13 of 132 patients in a series from M. D. Anderson Cancer Center, who underwent complete resection of the primary tumor, were disease free after median follow-up of 68 months.[106] Initial recurrence for GISTs is often widespread intraperitoneal, as well as hepatic, metastasis. One-half of the patients have recurrence in the peritoneum and two-thirds in the liver and the peritoneum. Currently, there are no data to support adjuvant chemotherapy or radiation therapy for the management of completely resected GISTs. Because of the risk of local recurrence after primary resection of GISTs, the efficacy of conventional chemotherapy and radiotherapy in preventing this, and the demonstration of considerable activity of STI 571 and metastatic disease, there has been an increased interest in examining the use of this drug in the adjuvant setting. Several authors have hypothesized that STI 571 may in fact be more beneficial in a setting of minimal disease, especially when one examines the fact that there were few complete responders in the early trials but that a large majority of patients were nonprogressors. The American College of Surgeons Oncology Group is leading a phase II intergroup trial, which is supported by the Cancer Therapy Evaluation Program, that is examining the use of STI 571, 400 mg/d for 1 year, after complete resection of high-risk GISTs. For the purpose of this trial, high risk is to find a tumor size growing within 10 cm, tumor rupture or tumor hemorrhage at the time, or markedly focal tumors. In addition, the American College of Surgeons Group is also opening up a randomized trial looking at patients with tumors greater than 3 cm and a randomized double-blind placebo trial of 400 mg STI 571 versus placebo. The primary end point in this trial is survival, and it is a crossover design, so that patients who experience recurrence can then be crossed over to STI 571.

OTHER MESENCHYMAL LESION TUMORS ARISING IN THE SMALL INTESTINE

Overwhelmingly, the majority of the mesenchymal tumors that arise in the small intestine are GISTs. The other tumors that need to be differentiated from GISTs include inflammatory fibroid polyps, fibromatoses, inflammatory and myofibroblastic tumors, solitary fibrous tumors, schwannomas, simple leiomyomas, and true leiomyomas.

Leiomyomas and Leiomyosarcomas

True leiomyomas and leiomyosarcomas are now believed to be nearly nonexistent in the small intestine. These lesions resemble mature smooth muscle and have low cellularity and few mitoses. They are positive for desmin and actin and are negative for CD117 (c-kit and CD34).

Inflammatory Fibroid Polyps

Inflammatory fibroid polyps are benign lesions infrequently encountered in the small intestine. They are typically submucosal and consist of a mixture of small granulation tissue-like vessels, spindle cells, and inflammatory cells. These lesions can stain positively for CD34; however, they do not stain for CD117 with the exception of very small areas of stroma within these tumors.

Fibromatosis (Desmoid Tumors)

These spindle cell tumors are frequently confused with GISTs. Histologically, they are bland, spindled stellate cells in parallel and evenly arranged around the blood vessels. These lesions can be locally aggressive and confused with GISTs, as it has been reported that some 75% of them in one series stained positive for CD117; however, they tend to have lower mitotic activity, more collagen than a GIST tumor, and less cytologic pleomorphism.

Inflammatory and myofibroblastic tumors, also known as *inflammatory pseudotumors* or *inflammatory fibrosarcomas*, are inflammatory uncommon mesenchymal tumors that are characterized by spindle cells admixed with lymphocytes and plasma cells. These lesions are believed to be benign reactions to infectious processes. Others have been shown to be clonal or oligoclonal rarely; however, they behave in a malignant fashion. Histologically, these tumors can resemble GISTs and can be differentiated from these by the presence of plasma cells. Numerous stains for desmin and actin may be positive, but CD117 and CD34 are negative in these lesions. Sixty percent of these lesions were stained for anaplastic lymphoma kinase.

Schwannomas

Schwannomas of the gut have been recorded to occur in the small intestine, although rarely, and they are more commonly found in the stomach, the colon, or the esophagus. These lesions are characterized by lymph node aggregates around their periphery, with nuclear palisading Verocay bodies and hyalinized vessels similar to schwannomas found elsewhere in the body. They stain strongly for S100 or CD117 negative. These lesions almost always behave as benign lesions.

REFERENCES

1. Alexander JW, Altemeier WA. Association of neoplasms of the small intestine with other neoplastic growths. *Ann Surg* 1967;167:958.
2. DiSario JA, Burt RW, Vargas H, McWhorter WP. Small bowel cancer: epidemiological and clinical characteristics from a population-based registry. *Am J Gastroenterol* 1994;89:699.
3. Ross RK, Hartnett NM, Bernstein L, Henderson BE. Epidemiology of adenocarcinomas of the small intestine: is bile a small bowel carcinogen? *Br J Cancer* 1991;63:143.
4. Weiss NS, Yang CP. Incidence of histologic types of cancer of the small intestine. *J Natl Cancer Inst* 1987;78:653.
5. Gabos S, Berkel J, Band P, et al. Small bowel cancer in western Canada. *Int J Epidemiol* 1993;22:198.
6. Severson RK, Schenk M, Gurney JG, et al. Increasing incidence of adenocarcinomas and carcinoid tumors of the small intestine in adults. *Cancer Epidemiol Biomarkers Prev* 1996;5:81.
7. Howdle PD, Jalal PK, Holmes GK, Houlston RS. Primary small-bowel malignancy in the UK and its association with coeliac disease. *QJM* 2003;96:345.
8. Chow JS, Chen CC, Ahsan H, Neugut AI. A population-based study of the incidence of malignant small bowel tumours: SEER, 1973-1990. *Int J Epidemiol* 1996;25:722.
9. Cunningham JD, Aleali R, Aleali M, et al. Malignant small bowel neoplasms: histopathologic determinants of recurrence and survival. *Ann Surg* 1997;225:300.
10. Ito H, Perez A, Brooks DC, et al. Surgical treatment of small bowel cancer: a 20-year single institution experience. *J Gastrointest Surg* 2003;7:925.
11. Frost DB, Mercado PD, Tyrell JS. Small bowel cancer: a 30-year review. *Ann Surg Oncol* 1994;1:290.
12. Martin RG. Malignant tumors of the small intestine. *Surg Clin North Am* 1986;66:779.
13. Brucher BL, Stein HJ, Roder JD, et al. New aspects of prognostic factors in adenocarcinomas of the small bowel. *Hepatogastroenterology* 2001;48:727.
14. Brucher BL, Roder JD, Fink U, et al. Prognostic factors in resected primary small bowel tumors. *Dig Surg* 1998;15:42.
15. Talamonti MS, Goetz LH, Rao S, Joehl RJ. Primary cancers of the small bowel: analysis of prognostic factors and results of surgical management. *Arch Surg* 2002;137:564.
16. Minardi AJ Jr, Zibari GB, Aultman DF, et al. Small-bowel tumors. *J Am Coll Surg* 1998;186:664.
17. Watson P, Lynch HT. Cancer risk in mismatch repair gene mutation carriers. *Fam Cancer* 2001;1:57.
18. Neugut AI, Jacobson JS, Suh S, et al. The epidemiology of cancer of the small bowel. *Cancer Epidemiol Biomarkers Prev* 1998;7:243.
19. Watson P, Lynch HT. Extracolonic cancer in hereditary nonpolyposis colorectal cancer. *Cancer* 1993;71:677.
20. Neugut AI, Santos J. The association between cancers of the small and large bowel. *Cancer Epidemiol Biomarkers Prev* 1993;2:551.
21. Ripley D, Weinerman BH. Increased incidence of second malignancies associated with small bowel adenocarcinoma. *Can J Gastroenterol* 1997;11:65.
22. Hutchins RR, Bani HA, Kojodjojo P, et al. Adenocarcinoma of the small bowel. *ANZ J Surg* 2001;71:428.
23. Fresko D, Lazarus SS, Dotan J, Reingold M. Early presentation of carcinoma of the small bowel in Crohn's disease ("Crohn's carcinoma"). Case reports and review of the literature. *Gastroenterology* 1982;82:783.
24. Donohue JH. Malignant tumours of the small bowel. *Surg Oncol* 1994;3:61.
25. Lashner BA. Risk factors for small bowel cancer in Crohn's disease. *Dig Dis Sci* 1992;37:1179.
26. Munkholm P, Langholz E, Davidsen M, Binder V. Intestinal cancer risk and mortality in patients with Crohn's disease. *Gastroenterology* 1993;105:1716.
27. Hemminki A. The molecular basis and clinical aspects of Peutz-Jeghers syndrome. *Cell Mol Life Sci* 1999;55:735.
28. Ciresi DL, Scholten DJ. The continuing clinical dilemma of primary tumors of the small intestine. *Am Surg* 1995;61:698.
29. Yang YS, Huang QY, Wang WF, et al. Primary jejunoileal neoplasm: a review of 60 cases. *World J Gastroenterol* 2003;9:862.
30. Maglinte DD, Chernish SM, Bessette J, et al. Factors in the diagnostic delays of small bowel malignancy. *Indiana Med* 1991;84:392.
31. Maglinte DD, O'Connor K, Bessette J, et al. The role of the physician in the late diagnosis of primary malignant tumors of the small intestine. *Am J Gastroenterol* 1991;86:304.
32. Bessette JR, Maglinte DD, Kelvin FM, Chernish SM. Primary malignant tumors in the small bowel: a comparison of the small-bowel enema and conventional follow-through examination. *AJR Am J Roentgenol* 1989;153:741.
33. Gourtsoyiannis N, Mako E. Imaging of primary small intestinal tumours by enteroclysis and CT with pathological correlation. *Eur Radiol* 1997;7:625.
34. Buckley JA, Fishman EK. CT evaluation of small bowel neoplasms: spectrum of disease. *Radiographics* 1998;18:379.
35. Buckley JA, Jones B, Fishman EK. Small bowel cancer. Imaging features and staging. *Radiol Clin North Am* 1997;35:381.
36. Laurent F, Drouillard J, Lecesne R, Bruneton JN. CT of small-bowel neoplasms. *Semin Ultrasound CT MR* 1995;16:102.
37. Maglinte DT, Reyes BL. Small bowel cancer. Radiologic diagnosis. *Radiol Clin North Am* 1997;35:361.
38. Horton KM, Fishman EK. The current status of multidetector row CT and three-dimensional imaging of the small bowel. *Radiol Clin North Am* 2003;41:199.
39. Dudiak KM, Johnson DC, Stephens DH. Primary tumors of the small intestine: CT evaluation. *AJR Am J Roentgenol* 1995;152:995.
40. Buckley JA, Siegelman SS, Jones B, Fishman EK. The accuracy of CT staging of small bowel adenocarcinoma: CT/pathologic correlation. *J Comput Assist Tomogr* 1997;21:986.
41. Costamagna G, Shah SK, Riccioni ME, et al. A prospective trial comparing small bowel radiographs and video capsule endoscopy for suspected small bowel disease. *Gastroenterology* 2002;123:999.
42. Stinner B, Kisker O, Zielke A, Rothmund M. Surgical management for carcinoid tumors of small bowel, appendix, colon, and rectum. *World J Surg* 1996;20:183.
43. North JH, Pack MS. Malignant tumors of the small intestine: a review of 144 cases. *Am Surg* 2000;66:46.
44. Howe JR, Karnell LH, Menck HR, Scott-Conner C. The American College of Surgeons Commission on Cancer and the American Cancer Society. Adenocarcinoma of the small bowel: review of the National Cancer Data Base, 1985-1995. *Cancer* 1999;86:2693.
45. Blaker H, von Herbay A, Penzel R, et al. Genetics of adenocarcinomas of the small intestine: frequent deletions at chromosome 18q and mutations of the SMAD4 gene. *Oncogene* 2002;21:158.
46. Wheeler JM, Warren BF, Mortensen NJ, et al. An insight into the genetic pathway of adenocarcinoma of the small intestine. *Gut* 2002;50:218.
47. Arai M, Shimizu S, Imai Y, et al. Mutations of the Ki-ras, p53 and APC genes in adenocarcinomas of the human small intestine. *Int J Cancer* 1997;70:390.

47a. Planck M, Ericson K, Piotrowska Z, et al. Microsatellite instability and expression of MLH1 and MSH2 in carcinomas of the small intestine. *Cancer* 2003;97:1551.

48. Vasen HF, Bulow S, Myrhoj T, et al. Decision analysis in the management of duodenal adenomatosis in familial adenomatous polyposis. *Gut* 1997;40:716.

49. Bulow S, Alm T, Fausa O, et al. Duodenal adenomatosis in familial adenomatous polyposis. DAF Project Group. *Int J Colorectal Dis* 1995;10:43.

50. Alarcon FJ, Burke CA, Church JM, van Stolk RU. Familial adenomatous polyposis: efficacy of endoscopic and surgical treatment for advanced duodenal adenomas. *Dis Colon Rectum* 1999;42:1533.

51. Burke CA, Beck GJ, Church JM, van Stolk RU. The natural history of untreated duodenal and ampullary adenomas in patients with familial adenomatous polyposis followed in an endoscopic surveillance program. *Gastrointest Endosc* 1999;49:358.

52. Penna C, Bataille N, Balladur P, et al. Surgical treatment of severe duodenal polyposis in familial adenomatous polyposis. *Br J Surg* 1998;85:665.

53. Penna C, Phillips RK, Tiret E, Spigelman AD. Surgical polypectomy of duodenal adenomas in familial adenomatous polyposis: experience of two European centres. *Br J Surg* 1993;80:1027.

54. Heiskanen I, Kellokumpu I, Jarvinen H. Management of duodenal adenomas in 98 patients with familial adenomatous polyposis. *Endoscopy* 1999;31:412.

55. Spigelman AD, Talbot IC, Penna C, et al. Evidence for adenoma-carcinoma sequence in the duodenum of patients with familial adenomatous polyposis. The Leeds Castle Polyposis Group (Upper Gastrointestinal Committee). *J Clin Pathol* 1994;47:709.

56. Nugent KP, Spigelman AD, Williams CB, et al. Follow-up in familial adenomatous polyposis. *Lancet* 1993;341:1225.

57. Kashiwagi H, Kanazawa K, Koizumi M, et al. Development of duodenal cancer in a patient with familial adenomatous polyposis. *J Gastroenterol* 2000;35:856.

58. Kashiwagi H, Spigelman AD, Debinski HS, et al. Surveillance of ampullary adenomas in familial adenomatous polyposis. *Lancet* 1994;344:1582.

59. Ruo L, Coit DG, Brennan MF, Guillem JG. Long-term follow-up of patients with familial adenomatous polyposis undergoing pancreaticoduodenal surgery. *J Gastrointest Surg* 2002;6:671.

60. Kalady MF, Clary BM, Tyler DS, Pappas TN. Pancreas-preserving duodenectomy in the management of duodenal familial adenomatous polyposis. *J Gastrointest Surg* 2002;6:82.

61. Abrahams NA, Halverson A, Fazio VW, et al. Adenocarcinoma of the small bowel: a study of 37 cases with emphasis on histologic prognostic factors. *Dis Colon Rectum* 2002;45:1496.

62. Veyrieres M, Baillet P, Hay JM, et al. Factors influencing long-term survival in 100 cases of small intestine primary adenocarcinoma. *Am J Surg* 1997;173:237.

63. Santoro E, Sacchi M, Scutari F, et al. Primary adenocarcinoma of the duodenum: treatment and survival in 89 patients. *Hepatogastroenterology* 1997;44:1157.

64. Sohn TA, Lillemoe KD, Cameron JL, et al. Adenocarcinoma of the duodenum: factors influencing long-term survival. *J Gastrointest Surg* 1998;2:79.

65. Rose DM, Hochwald SN, Klimstra DS, Brennan MF. Primary duodenal adenocarcinoma: a ten-year experience with 79 patients. *J Am Coll Surg* 1996;183:89.

66. Crawley C, Ross P, Norman A, et al. The Royal Marsden experience of a small bowel adenocarcinoma treated with protracted venous infusion 5-fluorouracil. *Br J Cancer* 1998;78:508.

67. Modlin IM, Lye KD, Kidd M. A 5-decade analysis of 13,715 carcinoid tumors. *Cancer* 2003;97:934.

68. Makridis C, Oberg K, Juhlin C, et al. Surgical treatment of mid-gut carcinoid tumors. *World J Surg* 1990;14:377.

69. Shebani KO, Souba WW, Finkelstein DM, et al. Prognosis and survival in patients with gastrointestinal tract carcinoid tumors. *Ann Surg* 1999;229:815.

70. Soga J. Carcinoids of the small intestine: a statistical evaluation of 1102 cases collected from the literature. *J Exp Clin Cancer Res* 1997;16:353.

71. de Vries H, Verschueren RC, Willemse PH, et al. Diagnostic, surgical and medical aspect of the midgut carcinoids. *Cancer Treat Rev* 2002;28:11.

72. Soreide JA, van Heerden JA, Thompson GB, et al. Gastrointestinal carcinoid tumors: long-term prognosis for surgically treated patients. *World J Surg* 2000;24:1431.

73. Gronbech JE, Soreide O, Bergan A. The role of resective surgery in the treatment of the carcinoid syndrome. *Scand J Gastroenterol* 1992;27:433.

74. Soreide O, Berstad T, Bakka A, et al. Surgical treatment as a principle in patients with advanced abdominal carcinoid tumors. *Surgery* 1992;111:48.

75. Kvols LK, Moertel CG, O'Connell MJ, et al. Treatment of the malignant carcinoid syndrome. Evaluation of a long-acting somatostatin analogue. *N Engl J Med* 1986;315:663.

76. Janson ET, Oberg K. Long-term management of the carcinoid syndrome. Treatment with octreotide alone and in combination with alpha-interferon. *Acta Oncol* 1993;32:225.

77. Oberg K, Norheim I, Theodorsson E. Treatment of malignant midgut carcinoid tumours with a long-acting somatostatin analogue octreotide. *Acta Oncol* 1991;30:503.

78. McEntee GP, Nagorney DM, Kvols LK, et al. Cytoreductive hepatic surgery for neuroendocrine tumors. *Surgery* 1990;108:1091.

79. Sarmiento JM, Heywood G, Rubin J, et al. Surgical treatment of neuroendocrine metastases to the liver: a plea for resection to increase survival. *J Am Coll Surg* 2003;197:29.

80. Sarmiento JM, Que FG. Hepatic surgery for metastases from neuroendocrine tumors. *Surg Oncol Clin N Am* 2003;12:231.

81. Le Treut YP, Delpero JF, Dousset B, et al. Results of liver transplantation in the treatment of metastatic neuroendocrine tumors. A 31-case French multicentric report. *Ann Surg* 1997;225:355.

82. Frilling A, Rogiers X, Malago M, et al. Liver transplantation in patients with liver metastases of neuroendocrine tumors. *Transplant Proc* 1998;30:3298.

83. Routley D, Ramage JK, McPeake J, et al. Orthotopic liver transplantation in the treatment of metastatic neuroendocrine tumors of the liver. *Liver Transpl Surg* 1995;1:118.

83a. Lehnert T. Liver transplantation for metastatic neuroendocrine carcinoma: an analysis of 103 patients. *Transplantation* 1998;66:1307.

84. Berber E, Flesher N, Siperstein AE. Laparoscopic radiofrequency ablation of neuroendocrine liver metastases. *World J Surg* 2002;26:985.

85. Moertel CG, Johnson CM, McKusick MA, et al. The management of patients with advanced carcinoid tumors and islet cell carcinomas. *Ann Intern Med* 1994;120:302.

86. Bukowski RM, Johnson KG, Peterson RF, et al. A phase II trial of combination chemotherapy in patients with metastatic carcinoid tumors. A Southwest Oncology Group Study. *Cancer* 1987;60:2891.

87. Oberg K, Eriksson B, Janson ET. Interferons alone or in combination with chemotherapy or other biologicals in the treatment of neuroendocrine gut and pancreatic tumors. *Digestion* 1994;[55 Suppl 3]:64.

88. Saltz L, Trochanowski B, Buckley M, et al. Octreotide as an antineoplastic agent in the treatment of functional and nonfunctional neuroendocrine tumors. *Cancer* 1993;72:244.

89. Gray GM, Rosenberg SA, Cooper AD, et al. Lymphomas involving the gastrointestinal tract. *Gastroenterology* 1982;82:143.

90. Rawls RA, Vega KJ, Trotman BW. Small bowel lymphoma. *Curr Treat Options Gastroenterol* 2003;6:27.

91. Koniaris LG, Drugas G, Katzman PJ, Salloum R. Management of gastrointestinal lymphoma. *J Am Coll Surg* 2003;197:127.

92. Nakamura S, Matsumoto T, Takeshita M, et al. A clinicopathologic study of primary small intestine lymphoma: prognostic significance of mucosa-associated lymphoid tissue-derived lymphoma. *Cancer* 2000;88:286.

93. O'Farrelly C, Feighery C, O'Briain DS, et al. Humoral response to wheat protein in patients with coeliac disease and enteropathy associated T cell lymphoma. *Br Med J (Clin Res Ed)* 1986;293:908.

94. Green PH, Fleischauer AT, Bhagat G, et al. Risk of malignancy in patients with celiac disease. *Am J Med* 2003;115:191.

95. Egan LJ, Walsh SV, Stevens FM, et al. Celiac-associated lymphoma. A single institution experience of 30 cases in the combination chemotherapy era. *J Clin Gastroenterol* 1995;21:123.

96. Miettinen M, Lasota J. Gastrointestinal stromal tumors (GISTs): definition, occurrence, pathology, differential diagnosis and molecular genetics. *Pol J Pathol* 2003;54:3.

97. Blanchard DK, Budde JM, Hatch GF, III, et al. Tumors of the small intestine. *World J Surg* 2000;24:421.

98. Miettinen M, Lasota J. Gastrointestinal stromal tumors—definition, clinical, histological, immunohistochemical, and molecular genetic features and differential diagnosis. *Virchows Arch* 2001;438:1.

99. Miettinen M, Sobin LH, Sarlomo-Rikala M. Immunohistochemical spectrum of GISTs at different sites and their differential diagnosis with a reference to CD117 (KIT). *Mod Pathol* 2000;13:1134.

100. Brainard JA, Goldblum JR. Stromal tumors of the jejunum and ileum: a clinicopathologic study of 39 cases. *Am J Surg Pathol* 1997;21:407.

101. Goldblum JR, Appelman HD. Stromal tumors of the duodenum. A histologic and immunohistochemical study of 20 cases. *Am J Surg Pathol* 1995;19:71.

102. Tworek JA, Appelman HD, Singleton TP, Greenson JK. Stromal tumors of the jejunum and ileum. *Mod Pathol* 1997;10:200.

103. Miettinen M, El Rifai W, Sobin HL, Lasota J. Evaluation of malignancy and prognosis of gastrointestinal stromal tumors: a review. *Hum Pathol* 2002;133:478.

103a. Emory TS, Sobin LH, Lukes L, Lee DH, O'Leary TJ. Prognosis of gastrointestinal smooth-muscle (stromal) tumors: dependence on anatomic site. *Am J Surg Pathol* 1999;23:82.

104. Hirota S, Nishida T, Isozaki K, et al. Gain-of-function mutation at the extracellular domain of KIT in gastrointestinal stromal tumours. *J Pathol* 2001;193:505.

105. DeMatteo RP, Lewis JJ, Leung D, et al. Two hundred gastrointestinal stromal tumors: recurrence patterns and prognostic factors for survival. *Ann Surg* 2000;231:51.

106. Ng EH, Pollock RE, Munsell MF, et al. Prognostic factors influencing survival in gastrointestinal leiomyosarcomas. Implications for surgical management and staging. *Ann Surg* 1992;215:68.

SECTION **7**   GEORGE D. DEMETRI

Gastrointestinal Stromal Tumors

TABLE 29.7-1. Pathology Terms That Encompass the Spectrum of Gastrointestinal Stromal Tumors

Gastrointestinal stromal tumor
Leiomyoblastoma
Gastrointestinal leiomyosarcoma
Gastrointestinal autonomic nerve tumor
Gastrointestinal pacemaker cell tumor
Plexosarcoma
Gastrointestinal neurofibrosarcoma

The exceptionally rapid development of knowledge regarding the molecular pathobiology of gastrointestinal stromal tumor (GIST) and the translation of that knowledge into a highly effective, molecularly targeted therapy represent an important milestone in solid tumor oncology. Rarely in the history of medicine does the opportunity arise to watch an entire field of investigation evolve so quickly and have such a major effect on the lives of patients who have a life-threatening malignancy. Although abdominal sarcomas have been described for more than two decades, the molecular understanding of the subset of sarcomas known as GISTs has only recently been achieved. From this understanding, a series of worldwide investigations has led to novel and effective ways to approach patients with this disease, with attendant improvements in the recognition, diagnosis, imaging, staging, and treatment of GIST. In this chapter, the highlights of these recent critical advances are summarized, and the relevance to current clinical practice and future basic and applied cancer research is emphasized.

HISTOPATHOLOGIC FEATURES AND HISTOGENESIS

BACKGROUND AND HISTORICAL PERSPECTIVE: DEFINITION OF GASTROINTESTINAL STROMAL TUMOR AS A CLINICOPATHOLOGICALLY UNIQUE FORM OF SARCOMA

Although relatively rare, the sarcomas classified under the term *gastrointestinal stromal tumor* represent the most common mesenchymal malignancy of the gastrointestinal (GI) tract. The incidence of GIST was vastly underrecognized (and therefore underreported in cancer registry databases) before the year 2000, but this neoplasm was estimated to account for approximately 1% to 3% of all malignant GI tumors. Before 1999, the diagnostic criteria for GIST remained controversial and somewhat confusing. The term *GIST* was initially a purely descriptive term developed in 1983 by Mazur and Clark[3] to define intraabdominal tumors that were not carcinomas and also failed to exhibit features of either smooth muscle or nerve cells. However, pathologists recognized that there was not a completely clear differential expression of muscle or nerve antigenic markers when careful immunohistochemical analyses were performed on certain mesenchymal tumors of the gut. There was, in fact, variability of expression of differentiation antigens used as markers for muscle cells (e.g., smooth muscle actin) and nerve cells (such as S-100). Several names were applied to these tumors based on the variable patterns of cell lineage markers described by a variety of pathologists across the world (Table 29.7-1).

GISTs were often previously diagnosed as leiomyomas or leiomyosarcomas because of their histologic resemblance to these smooth muscle neoplasms. Despite this, it had long been recognized that a subset of these tumors that arose in the bowel wall had a number of peculiar histologic features and likely represented a different entity altogether.[1,2] These GI tract "leiomyosarcomas" were also noted to be particularly resistant to standard chemotherapy regimens used to treat leiomyosarcomas elsewhere (with greater success in leiomyosarcomas arising in the uterus or vascular sites). Additional differences between many GISTs and leiomyosarcomas became apparent with the application of modern immunohistochemical techniques in the 1980s. By these assays, a significant subset of these tumors was noted to lack the characteristic muscle antigens that defined leiomyosarcomas located elsewhere in the body. Given these findings, in 1983 Mazur and Clark introduced the generic term *GIST* in an effort to segregate and subclassify these tumors.[3] However, the term *GIST* was still controversial and not fully specific in its definition. Other terms were generated based on the fact that neural crest antigens such as neuron-specific enolase and S-100 could be demonstrated in GIST cells, which led to the terms *plexosarcomas*[4] and *gastrointestinal autonomic nerve tumors.*[5] Additional research in immunohistochemical analysis of GISTs in the early 1990s revealed that a significant proportion of these tumors expressed the CD34 antigen (an antigen that is shared between hematopoietic stem cells as well as vascular and myofibroblastic cells). It was initially hoped that CD34 might prove to be a key differentiating feature between GISTs and other spindle cell tumors of the GI tract, such as schwannomas or leiomyomas. However, this was not the case. CD34 expression characterized only approximately half of GIST cases, and a proportion of smooth muscle and Schwann cell tumors could also express CD34. Therefore, CD34 was neither a sensitive nor a specific marker to distinguish GIST from other mesenchymal neoplasms.[9,10]

Pathologists also proposed that some GIST cells differentiated along smooth muscle lineages, whereas others were neurogenic in origin; still, over a third of them lacked any detectable immunostaining for lineage-specific markers (null phenotype).[6–8] The reproducible diagnostic classification of these spindle cell tumors remained elusive and relied on the purely descriptive use of the term *GIST.*

Before the year 2000, therefore, there were no reproducible, clearly defined, objective criteria to classify GIST, and it is likely that several types of epithelioid and spindle cell tumors were included in the clinical diagnostic category of GIST. Similarly, many true GIST cases were put into different diagnostic frameworks, such as leiomyoblastomas and GI autonomic nerve tumors. This makes the interpretation of published clinical results before the year 2000 difficult, given the likely heterogeneity in the diagnostic term GIST before the recognition of the role of the KIT and platelet-derived growth factor receptor (PDGFR) tyrosine kinase receptors in these diseases.

LINEAGE RELATIONS BETWEEN GASTROINTESTINAL STROMAL TUMOR AND THE MESENCHYMAL PRECURSOR CELLS THAT GIVE RISE TO THE INTERSTITIAL CELLS OF CAJAL

A conceptual advance in thinking about GIST occurred in the late 1990s with the notion that these tumors bore certain histopathologic similarities to a specific cell type inherent in the GI tract, known as the *interstitial cells of Cajal* (ICC).[11] ICCs are the unique "pacemaker cells" that are normally present in the myenteric plexus and act to coordinate gut peristalsis by linking the smooth muscle cells of the bowel wall with the autonomic nervous system. GIST cells and ICCs were noted to have similar ultrastructural features combining neural and myogenic differentiation, and both cell types were documented to express the KIT receptor tyrosine kinase (KIT RTK); therefore, it has been widely accepted that the cells of both GISTs and normal ICCs share a common precursor cell.[12,13] The KIT RTK and its ligand, stem cell factor, are documented to play an essential role in the development and maintenance of normal ICCs as well as of other cells, including melanocytes, erythrocytes, germ cells, and mast cells. KIT expression is noted in the vast majority (more than 95%) of GISTs, but KIT is not expressed by other smooth muscle tumors of the GI tract or other non-GIST stromal tumors (e.g., there is no KIT expression in endometrial stromal tumors).

The origin of the neoplastic cells of GIST remains a matter of active investigation, and the signaling pathways that result in the malignant behavior of GIST are poorly understood. Certain data suggest that GISTs originate from CD34+ stem cells residing within the wall of the gut, which can then differentiate toward the ICC phenotype.[13–15]

RATIONALE LEADING TO A MOLECULAR UNDERSTANDING OF GASTROINTESTINAL STROMAL TUMORS

The molecular understanding of GIST pathogenesis was advanced greatly by a key observation made by Hirota, Kitamura, and colleagues in Japan in 1998.[16] This group was interested in the role played by KIT in ICC and other cell growth and development signaling, and they went on to define the relationship between GIST and certain mutations in the *KIT* protooncogene that conferred uncontrolled activation to the KIT signaling enzyme.[16] Normally, the KIT protein serves as a transmembrane RTK; the CD117 antigen can be detected by immunohistochemical staining as a marker for the presence of the KIT protein. In normal cell signaling, KIT binds its ligand, known also as stem cell factor or *Steel* factor, and this ligand binding brings together two molecules of KIT (the signaling cascade is summarized in Fig. 29.7-1). These two KIT receptors form a homodimer with crossphosphorylation of critical tyrosine residues in the intracellular domains of KIT. These phosphorylation events then activate the signal transduction pathways downstream of KIT. The net physiologic effect of KIT activation is the stimulation of cell proliferation and enhanced cell survival; therefore, uncontrolled activation could theoretically lead to neoplastic growth of cells. The Japanese team provided the critical confirmation of this theory at both the cellular and molecular level.[16] This elegant work was derived from a recognition of the key biologic similarities between GIST and ICC cells.[17–20] *KIT* gene mutations were identified in five of six cases of human GIST studied by this team, and they went on to document that the mutations led to uncontrolled, ligand-independent phosphorylation by the KIT kinase.[16] Genetically engineered cells harboring the mutant, overactive KIT proteins also grew into tumors when injected into nude mice, a proof of concept for the malignant phenotype induced by the aberrant signaling pathways associated with KIT overactivity.[16]

The oncogenic potential of mutant, uncontrollably active KIT in the pathogenesis of GIST in humans was further supported by the identification of a family that exhibited an autosomal dominant inheritance pattern of GIST. Genetic analysis of this kindred revealed that they harbored a germline activating *KIT* mutation, similar to the mutations that were seen in sporadic cases of GIST.[21] Several other families have since been identified with germline *KIT* mutations and an abnormally high incidence of GIST, usually occurring as multiple foci within any affected individual.[22,23] Often, these tumors may not present clinically until the second or third decade of life, and some even present in far advanced age. *KIT* mutations have also been documented in very small (less than 1-cm) GISTs that were detected incidentally and that appear morphologically benign.[24] These findings support the hypothesis that activating mutations in the *KIT* protooncogene represent an early

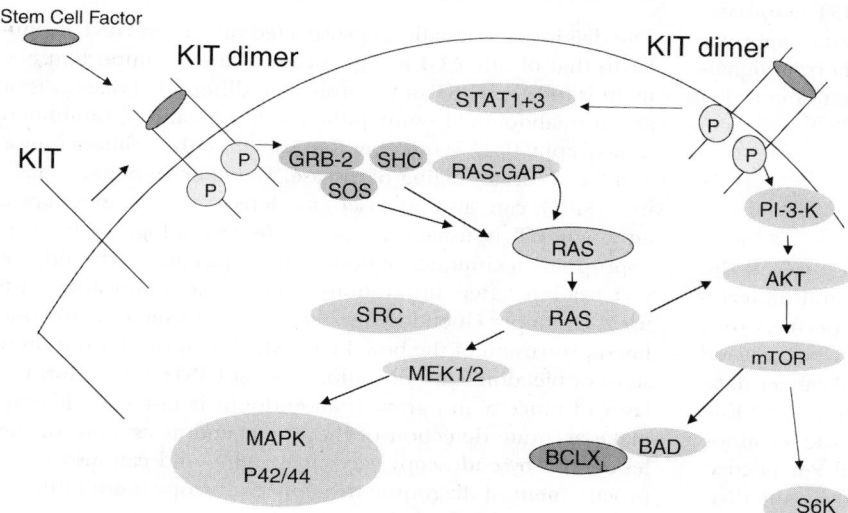

FIGURE 29.7-1. Simplified schema of the molecular cascade involved in KIT-mediated cell signaling. Other steps may be operative as well, and the relative contribution of each of these downstream signaling events to different aspects of aberrant KIT signaling in gastrointestinal stromal tumor remains the subject of active investigation. Each step may be a potential future target for therapeutic development. MAPK, mitogen-activated protein kinase; mTOR, mammalian target of rapamycin; P, phosphorus; PI-3-K, phosphatidylinositol 3 kinase; S6K, S6 kinase. (Modified from A. Fletcher, *unpublished data*, 2004; and ref. 24a.)

event in the mechanisms that ultimately result in GIST oncogenesis. The other key signaling steps that confer a malignant phenotype to GIST cells remain obscure. However, the unique aspects of the signaling cascades in GIST are being actively elucidated, and these appear to differ from KIT signaling in hematologic neoplasia in that the STAT5 pathway is not typically activated in GIST, whereas STAT1 and STAT3 are activated at a high level.[24a]

The literature before the year 2000 was somewhat confusing about whether mutations were relevant to the differentiation between "benign GIST" and "malignant GIST." With the recognition that *KIT* mutations can be found in even the smallest GISTs,[24] there is now consensus that *KIT* genotype alone cannot account for differences between GISTs that may behave in an indolent manner (and that may be functionally "benign") and those that are clearly aggressive and malignant by any functional definition. Additionally, it is clear also that well-differentiated "benign" cell morphology cannot be used to ensure that any individual GIST will pursue a benign clinical course.

With further analyses and use of sophisticated technology, it has become clear that *KIT* mutations can be noted in more than 90% of GIST cells.[25–27] Constitutive activation of the KIT enzymatic function has been reported to characterize every GIST sample analyzed by immunoblotting technique, even in cases in which there are no detectable mutations in the *KIT* gene.[25] The mechanisms by which nonmutated KIT is kept in an uncontrollably phosphorylated state are poorly understood and are the subject of active molecular scrutiny.

Importantly, the vast majority of GIST cells at initial presentation demonstrate only a single site of mutation in the *KIT* gene; complex genetic changes are truly rare. Gain-of-function mutations have been identified most commonly (up to 70% of cases) in exon 11 of *KIT*, which translates into the intracellular juxtamembrane domain of the KIT protein. Mutations in the *KIT* gene locus have also been described (in decreasing order of prevalence) in exon 9 (representing the KIT extracellular domain), exon 13 (kinase domain), and exon 17 (kinase domain).[25–27] It is not yet known with certainty how the structural alterations of these mutations confer constitutive activation onto the KIT protein product, although certain insights have been derived from studies of the activated KIT complex.[27a]

Another key advance in the understanding of GIST has been the recognition that signaling through other uncontrolled kinase activation besides KIT could give rise to GIST neoplastic transformation. Specifically, it is now recognized that approximately 5% of GIST cells show not activation and aberrant signaling of the KIT receptor, but rather mutational activation of a structurally related kinase, PDGFR-α (PDGFRA).[27b,27c]

CLINICAL CONSIDERATIONS

Before the year 2000, the number of new GIST cases in the United States had been grossly underestimated and underreported; experts had proposed that there were perhaps only 300 to 500 new cases per year. However, it is now recognized that many GISTs were not captured in traditional cancer databases such as that of the Surveillance, Epidemiology, and End Results program due to the problems of diagnostic terminology noted earlier in Background and Historical Perspective. Given the significant progress made only recently in the diagnosis and reporting of these tumors and the extremely rapid

rate of accrual to clinical trials in GIST, the estimated incidence of GIST has been revised upward to approximately 5000 new cases per year in the United States alone.[28,28a] It is important to note that not all of these cases will prove to be life-threatening, because many GISTs in cases of limited disease may be small and curable with appropriate surgery as the first-line therapy. A population-based study to define the incidence of GIST using the most up-to-date criteria has reported an incidence of approximately 15 cases per million population.[28b] GIST occurs predominantly in adults at a median age of 58 years but can occur across the age spectrum from infancy to old age. The incidence is slightly higher in men than in women. The majority of GISTs (60% to 70%) have been reported to arise in the stomach, whereas 20% to 30% originate in the small intestine, and fewer than 10% in the esophagus, colon, and rectum. GISTs can also occur in extraintestinal abdominopelvic sites such as the omentum, mesentery, or retroperitoneum.[29–31]

The clinical presentation of patients with GIST can vary tremendously based on the anatomic location of the tumor as well as the tumor size and aggressiveness. For many patients, the detection of GIST may be due to evaluation of nonspecific symptoms or may even be an incidental finding. Symptoms tend to arise only when tumors reach a large size or are in critical anatomic localizations (e.g., constricting gastric outflow). Most symptomatic patients present with tumors that are larger than 5 cm in maximal dimension. Symptoms at presentation may include abdominal pain, an abdominal mass, nausea, vomiting, anorexia, and weight loss. Certain series have reported that up to 40% of patients present with acute hemorrhage into the intestinal tract or peritoneal cavity from tumor rupture, although this certainly is dependent on the size of the tumor. The vast majority of GIST metastases at presentation are intraabdominal, either to the liver, omentum, or peritoneal cavity.[29] Metastatic spread to lymph nodes and to other regions via lymphatics is very rare: Most lesions thought to be nodal metastases simply represent metastatic deposits of tumor nodules in the omentum or peritoneum rather than true lymphatic spread of the disease.

DIAGNOSTIC EVALUATION AND APPROACH TO THE PATIENT

The diagnostic evaluation of suspected or proven GIST is similar to that of other GI malignancies. The most important element is to keep GIST in the suspected differential diagnosis of an intraabdominal nonepithelial malignancy. Computed tomography (CT) is essential for evaluating the primary tumor and for accurate staging of disease. Magnetic resonance imaging (MRI) can also be used to detect hepatic metastases, although CT is usually an adequate technology as long as appropriate techniques of both noncontrast and early and late visualization after intravenous contrast administration are used. On upper GI endoscopy, there may be a smooth, mucosa-lined protrusion of the bowel wall, which may or may not show signs of bleeding and ulceration.[32] Most GISTs arise below the layer of mucosa and grow in an endophytic fashion. This can make accurate detection of the tumor and assessment of the lesion size by endoscopy very challenging and can also make procurement of diagnostic tissue by endoscopy more difficult. Ultrasonographically enhanced endoscopy may prove to have added value in the detection of GIST in the upper GI tract because of this growth pattern.

DIFFERENTIAL DIAGNOSIS OF GASTROINTESTINAL STROMAL TUMOR: DILEMMAS OF DIAGNOSTIC HISTOPATHOLOGY AND CYTOLOGY

GIST was originally described as a monomorphic spindle cell neoplasm. However, it is very clear that this disease can exhibit a wide variety of appearances with characteristics of either an epithelioid (larger, rounder cells) or spindle cell histology. Because the accurate diagnosis of GIST is now critical for appropriate patient management, it is of crucial importance that pathologists consider GIST in the differential diagnosis of tumors arising along the GI tract or in the abdomen and pelvis. The spindle cell pattern of GIST is far more common, occurring in approximately 70% of cases. This subset corresponds to tumors often diagnosed before the year 2000 as GI leiomyosarcomas. The epithelioid, or round cell, pattern represents a majority of the remaining 30% and may have an admixture of spindle cell features. Tumors in the epithelioid subset generally were previously diagnosed as leiomyoblastomas, although some may have been mistaken for poorly differentiated carcinomas. GISTs account for approximately 80% of mesenchymal tumors of the GI tract. There are definitely true smooth muscle neoplasms of the GI tract, including true leiomyomas and leiomyosarcomas, which account for approximately 15% of GI nonepithelial neoplasms; schwannomas account for the remaining 5%. Rarely, other malignancies, such as melanomas of the GI tract, can occur. Therefore, the differential diagnosis is complex and requires expert pathologic review, as well as adequate and appropriately processed and fixed diagnostic tissues.

As noted earlier in Rationale Leading to a Molecular Understanding of Gastrointestinal Stromal Tumors, GISTs characteristically exhibit expression of CD117 by immunohistochemical assays,[28] and the levels of expression can vary from generally diffuse and strong (most common in the spindle cell subtype) to focal and weakly positive in a dot-like pattern (characteristic of the epithelioid subtype).[28] CD34 expression is not specific for GIST, because it can also be noted in desmoid tumors, and approximately 60% to 70% of GIST lesions are positive for CD34.[12,16,28] True leiomyosarcomas express the smooth muscle markers smooth muscle actin and desmin but fail to express CD117. Schwannomas are usually positive for the neural antigen S-100 but are also negative for CD117.[28] Normal mast cells and ICCs in the surrounding stromal tissues serve as ideal positive internal controls, because these normal cells strongly express CD117.

The definitive diagnostic criteria of CD117-negative GIST are not clear at this time. Certainly, expert pathologists can define a rare subset (fewer than 5%) of GISTs that fail to express CD117, and these are most likely to be driven by an alternative kinase such as PDGFRA.[27b] Expert analysis of the *KIT* and *PDGFRA* genotype may be useful to define with certainty the group of rare patients with CD117-negative GISTs in the future.

It is important to recognize that expression of KIT is not limited to GIST cells. Normal ICCs and mast cells express CD117 and are dependent on KIT for normal growth and development. A relatively limited number of other tumors may also express immunohistochemically detectable CD117. These include certain subsets of soft tissue sarcomas, including Ewing's sarcoma and angiosarcoma, as well as other neoplasms such as occasional small cell lung cancers, melanomas, desmoid tumors, seminomas, ovarian carcino-

mas, mastocytomas, neuroblastomas, adenoid cystic carcinomas, and rare subsets of lymphoma and acute myeloid leukemia.[17,18,33,33a] It is most important to recognize that expression of the CD117 antigen does not imply the activation of the KIT target, nor does it necessarily correlate with any *KIT* gene mutation. The same CD117 antigen is expressed by cells harboring normal (wild-type) *KIT* as those that have activating *KIT* mutations. Additionally, expression of KIT protein does not necessarily mean that the protein is involved in the pathogenesis of that specific cancer. In all these regards, GIST was a very special example of a disease in which expression did correlate universally with kinase activation, and this activation was truly pathogenetically crucial to the malignancy. In general, with certain rare exceptions, there is little reason to expect that these other tumors would exhibit clinically important activity from an agent designed to block signaling through the KIT kinase.

PROGNOSTIC FEATURES OF GASTROINTESTINAL STROMAL TUMOR

What is the risk that a patient with primary GIST will develop metastases? The answer to this remains somewhat vague. However, it is clear that even small tumors with benign-appearing cellular morphology can occasionally metastasize. Reports of patient outcomes in studies before 1999 are difficult to interpret, given the problems of diagnostic imprecision in that era. The current consensus among pathologists is to regard all GISTs, including those that seem to have a benign appearance by conventional histopathologic criteria, as having the potential to behave in a malignant fashion (i.e., to metastasize or to infiltrate sufficiently into surrounding tissues that resection for cure is impossible, or both).[28]

A consensus has been reached among expert pathologists with an interest in GIST that the most reliable prognostic factors are the size of the primary tumor and the mitotic index, which measures the proliferative activity of the cells (Fig. 29.7-2). Other factors, such as the specific histologic subtype (epithelioid vs. spindle cell), the degree of cellular pleomorphism, and patient age, may make some contribution to prognosis but are most likely to play a minor role in determining the clinical outcome. Recurrence and survival rates have been reported to correlate with the location of the primary GIST lesion, with small bowel tumors showing a somewhat worse prognosis.

Certain reports before the year 2000 suggested that GISTs showing *KIT* mutations were associated with a less favorable prognosis than cases of GIST with no detectable mutation.[34,35] However, these studies were technically limited, analyzing mutations in

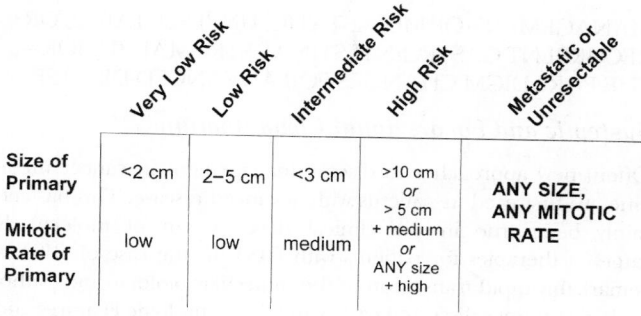

FIGURE 29.7-2. Risk assessment for gastrointestinal tumors. (Adapted from ref. 28.)

exon 11 and finding mutations in only 60% of samples, much lower than the more than 90% rate of mutations seen in a more recent series searching for potential mutations in each of exons 11, 9, 13, and 17.[25] In another study, mutations in exon 11 of *KIT* conferred a somewhat better prognosis for GIST.[36] It remains unclear whether *KIT* genotype is an independent prognostic factor or whether this marker tracks with other clinical features to identify patients with a favorable prognosis more clearly.

DIAGNOSTIC IMAGING OF PATIENTS WITH GASTROINTESTINAL STROMAL TUMORS

One of the most impressive aspects of GIST diagnostic imaging is the use of fluorine ^{18}F-fluorodeoxyglucose (FDG) positron emission tomography (PET) to add complementary information to that obtained by conventional anatomic imaging. Although CT or MRI scanning can assess the size of GIST lesions quite accurately, the functional imaging of GISTs with FDG-PET can give additional information that can assist clinicians in the management of GIST patients. The actual mechanisms responsible for the high-level avidity of GISTs for the FDG tracer used most commonly in PET imaging are not yet known; however, it is likely that there is a direct connection between signaling through the overactive KIT RTK and glucose transport proteins. In this way, one could explain the very rapid changes in PET imaging associated with inhibition of KIT signaling by pharmacologic means.[46,46a] Large GISTs can demonstrate centers with predominately "cystic" or low attenuation characteristics noted on CT or MRI scans. It is clear by FDG-PET scans that the internal mass of large GIST lesions can often be viewed as metabolically quiescent. This is likely due to the endogenous necrosis of very large lesions in their central portions: Even though GIST lesions can be very vascular, the internal portion can nonetheless represent a confluent mass of necrotic material, with the more viable aspects of the GIST pushing out toward the edges of the lesion. In addition, occasionally metastatic GIST lesions in the omentum can be subtle and easy to overlook on CT scans, because small lesions can blend into the folds of the bowel walls and be difficult for even the most experienced radiologist to detect. FDG-PET imaging can detect lesions approximately 1 cm in size without difficulty, because neither the normal bowel nor omentum takes up the FDG tracer with excess avidity.

TREATMENT OPTIONS AND MANAGEMENT DECISIONS IN THE ERA OF MOLECULARLY TARGETED THERAPIES FOR GASTROINTESTINAL STROMAL TUMOR

MANAGEMENT OF METASTATIC, UNRESECTABLE, OR RECURRENT GASTROINTESTINAL STROMAL TUMOR— THE PARADIGM CHANGES FOR ADVANCED DISEASE

Systemic and Locoregional Chemotherapy

Often, new approaches to disease management in cancer medicine are first tried in patients with advanced disease. This has certainly been true in the clinical development of molecularly targeted therapies for patients with GIST. In the case of GIST, a remarkably rapid translation of the molecular biologic and pathobiologic findings discussed earlier in Histopathologic Features and Histogenesis has led to dramatic changes in the management of patients with advanced GIST. Therefore, this chapter first discusses

the management of patients with advanced disease and then moves to the management of patients with early-stage, limited GIST.

In GIST, there was universal opinion that advanced disease represented a pressing unmet medical need before the advent of molecularly targeted therapy. Efforts of medical oncologists to treat GISTs with conventional cytotoxic chemotherapy were essentially universally dismal. The rates of objective antitumor response to a variety of chemotherapy agents for patients with GIST or abdominal leiomyosarcomas were routinely reported as 0% to, at best, less than 5%.[38,46] Other investigators attempted to boost the benefits of chemotherapy by administering the drugs via an intraperitoneal route.[38a] However, because few GISTs remain confined to the peritoneal surfaces, and because the majority of the life-threatening complications of GIST arise from hepatic involvement or other bulky sites of omental disease, this has been viewed as less than optimal. Based on these disappointing results, conventional cytotoxic chemotherapy has generally been regarded as an overall failure in the treatment of GIST.

There are limited data regarding the potential to control metastatic GIST by locoregional techniques such as hepatic artery embolization or chemoembolization. Although a subset of patients with metastatic GIST involving the liver can show antitumor responses and limited progression-free survival after chemoembolization, the benefits are generally measured in months rather than years, and this has not been viewed as a particularly promising strategy for management of most GIST patients.[38b,38c]

The mechanisms of the highly reproducible resistance to chemotherapy exhibited by GIST may be explained, in part, by the demonstration of the increased levels of P-glycoprotein [the product of the multidrug resistance-1 (MDR-1) gene] and the MDR protein that have been reported in GISTs and other intraabdominal sarcomas. In one study evaluating the differences in outcome between GIST and leiomyosarcomas, significantly higher levels of expression of P-glycoprotein (38.4% vs. 13.4%) and MDR protein-1 (35.4% vs. 13.3%) were demonstrated in the GIST cells.[39] It has been postulated that these cellular efflux pumps may prevent chemotherapy from establishing therapeutic concentrations in the target GIST cells.

Radiotherapy rarely plays any role in the management of patients with metastatic GIST. There are remarkably few instances in which radiotherapy has been carefully studied in this disease, most likely because the delivery of therapeutic doses of radiotherapy to the liver or the GI tract usually causes more morbidity than benefit. However, it is possible that targeting radiotherapy with newer techniques such as intensity-modulated radiotherapy or proton beam irradiation might be used for palliation in patients suffering from focal bleeding from a specific site of GIST recurrence. Radiotherapy may also be useful occasionally as a palliative maneuver for pain control in patients with limited although bulky liver metastasis or with a single large metastatic lesion fixed to the wall of the abdomen or pelvis. However, the diffuse pattern of disease recurrence in GIST does not allow radiotherapy to function as an effective therapeutic modality for the majority of patients with advanced disease. Similarly, surgery has traditionally not played a significant role in the management of patients with metastatic GIST, because in most patients liver and peritoneal metastases from GIST are judged unresectable due to multifocal hepatic metastases or multiple sites of intraabdominal metastatic disease.

Clearly, for patients with metastatic or unresectable GIST, the prognosis was dismal before the advent of molecularly targeted therapy. For patients with metastatic or recurrent GIST or GI sarcomas (the majority of which were likely to have been true GISTs), most studies have documented very poor survival rates, with fatal outcomes from disease progression generally occurring within 2 years from the date of first recurrence or metastasis.[29,38,39a]

Development of the First Molecularly Targeted Therapy for Gastrointestinal Stromal Tumor: Imatinib Mesylate [Signal Transduction Inhibitor 571 (STI 571)]

GIST represented a malignancy in which the stage was perfectly set for translational therapeutics. There was agreement among practitioners that no other systemic therapy was useful, and there was a pressing unmet medical need for thousands of patients across the world. There had been rapid and significant advances in understanding the critical molecular abnormalities that characterize the neoplastic cells of GIST. There was also a tremendous stroke of serendipity in that a medication being developed for an entirely different purpose showed dramatic activity in inhibiting the uncontrollably activated KIT RTK, which was critical to the pathobiology of GIST. The rapid evolution of this therapeutic advance came from the coordinated efforts of many investigative teams sharing results across the world, with many patients being the beneficiaries of this rapid diffusion of technology and therapeutic knowledge.

The initial concept for this molecularly targeted approach came from studies of Drs. Brian Druker, Nicholas Lydon, and colleagues,[40] who were screening small molecules with the goal of inhibiting the constitutively active tyrosine kinase enzymatic function of the BCR-ABL oncoprotein, which was known to be critical to the pathogenesis of chronic myeloid leukemia (CML). A team of scientists at Ciba-Geigy (later to become Novartis Pharmaceuticals) had identified a small molecule in the 2-phenylaminopyrimidine class, which could potentially inhibit ABL and the dysregulated BCR-ABL *in vitro*.[40] Additional screening studies by Brian Druker and Elisabeth Buchdunger demonstrated that this agent, named signal transduction inhibitor 571 (STI 571) and later known by the generic name of imatinib mesylate, could also potently inhibit the tyrosine kinase activity of both KIT and PDGFR.[41,42] Studies were subsequently performed in a human mast cell leukemia cell line harboring a *KIT* mutation that was similar to the mutations noted in GIST, and imatinib was shown to inhibit both mutant and wild-type KIT protein.[43] Laboratory experiments testing imatinib in human GIST cell lines with defined activating *KIT* mutations revealed dramatic evidence of anti-GIST activity from this agent. The addition of imatinib to GIST cells in culture rapidly and completely blocked the constitutive activation of KIT, arrested cell proliferation, and induced apoptosis in the tumor cells.[44] By all criteria, therefore, imatinib appeared to be a very promising and scientifically rational approach to the treatment of GIST.

There has now been extraordinary expansion in the worldwide clinical development of imatinib as a molecularly targeted therapy of GIST. These data are summarized in Table 29.7-2. The first clinical experience with this agent in the treatment of GIST began in March 2000 with a 50-year-old woman who had far-advanced, heavily pretreated, and widely metastatic GIST. This patient was treated with imatinib in a single-patient pilot study in Helsinki, Finland. The case history of this patient has been published and documents the rapid response and sustained clinical benefit from imatinib dosing that this patient enjoyed.[45] However, after approximately 3 years, resistance to imatinib developed, and ultimately the patient succumbed to metastatic GIST.

Nonetheless, based on the dramatic and durable benefits in this patient, as well as the striking scientific rationale and strong preclinical data, other studies testing imatinib in GIST were also performed. Taking cues from the clinical development of imatinib in CML patients, a multicenter United States–Finland collaborative study was begun in July 2000 that randomly assigned patients with metastatic GIST to receive one of two dose levels of the drug (either 400 or 600 mg of imatinib administered orally each day continuously as long as the disease was stable or responding to therapy).[46] Nearly concurrently, a dose-finding study was also begun in Europe under the auspices of the European Organization for

TABLE 29.7-2. Summary of Clinical Studies of Imatinib Mesylate in Patients with Metastatic or Unresectable Gastrointestinal Stromal Tumors (GISTs)

Study	n	Imatinib Dosage	Results
Joensuu et al., 2001[45]	1	400 mg daily	Major response, durable for more than 2 y
van Oosterom et al., 2001[46b]	40 (36 GIST)	400 to 1000 mg daily	Partial remissions in 19/36 (53%) GIST patients with additional minor responses in 6/36 (17%)
			Total clinical benefit rate = 70%
			No responses in non-GIST patients
Demetri et al., 2002[46]	147	400 or 600 mg daily	Partial remissions in 97/147 (66%) with additional minor responses and durable stable disease in 25/147 (17%)
			Total clinical benefit rate = 83%, no differences for different doses
Verweij et al., 2003[46c]	51 (27 GIST)	800 mg daily	Complete remissions in 4%, partial remissions in 67%, with additional minor responses and durable stable disease in 18%
			Total clinical benefit rate = 89%
Verweij et al., 2003[49]	946	400 or 800 mg daily	Complete remissions in 5%, partial remissions in 45%, with additional minor responses and durable stable disease in 32%
			Total clinical benefit rate = 82%, no differences for different doses
Benjamin et al., 2003[48]	746	400 or 800 mg daily	Complete remissions in 2%, partial remissions in 46%, with additional minor responses and durable stable disease in 26%
			Total clinical benefit rate = 74%, no differences for different doses

Research and Treatment of Cancer (EORTC) Sarcoma Group to ensure the tolerability of this agent and to gain early experience with this agent in both GIST and other forms of sarcoma.[46b] The maximal tolerated dose of imatinib identified in the EORTC dose-ranging phase I trial was judged to be 800 mg/d (given as 400 mg twice daily); at the higher dose level of 500 mg twice daily, unacceptably severe toxicities, including nausea, vomiting, and severe edema, were noted and were considered dose limiting.[46b]

The United States–Finland trial accrued 147 patients with metastatic GIST between July 2000 and April 2001.[46] The results from each of these trials in the United States and Europe confirmed the exceptional activity of imatinib in controlling metastatic GIST, inducing objective responses in the majority of patients, providing control of symptoms, and undoubtedly prolonging the survival of these patients. The remarkable concordance of results from these wholly independent trials further confirms the impressive activity of this new therapeutic strategy in a disease that was previously resistant to all systemic therapies. The results from both the United States–Finland and the EORTC studies demonstrate that the majority of patients with advanced GIST exhibited objective responses (nearly all partial responses) with imatinib therapy, with an additional subset of patients experiencing durable arrest of disease progression and objectively stable disease. The median time to objective response was more than 3 months, although some patients experienced dramatic disease regressions within a week after starting oral dosing of imatinib. There were no significant differences in response rates or duration of disease control between the 400- and 600-mg daily dose levels of imatinib in the United States–Finland trial, although the study was relatively underpowered to detect any differences.[46] Imatinib was very well tolerated overall in both studies. On the basis of these trials, the U.S. Food and Drug Administration approved the use of imatinib for the treatment of metastatic or unresectable GIST on February 1, 2002. Approval in Europe and the rest of the world followed quickly thereafter.

The EORTC group went on in a subsequent trial to expand its exploration of imatinib in treatment of GIST and other forms of sarcoma. In this trial, the high levels of antitumor activity against GIST were again confirmed, whereas there was no demonstrable benefit for patients with other forms of soft tissue sarcomas.[46c] This work supports the hypothesis that specific molecular targeting of a key pathophysiologic signaling pathway in GIST is critical to the extraordinary activity of imatinib in that disease. Without inhibition of such a target, imatinib treatment does not have obvious anticancer activity in most other solid tumors, although certain exceptions have been documented. In particular, it is relevant to note that the activation of the PDGFR signaling pathway in dermatofibrosarcoma protuberans has been targeted successfully using imatinib as well, with evidence of clinical benefit for dermatofibrosarcoma protuberans patients.[46d,46e,46f]

With reference to the molecular targeting of kinase inhibition in GIST, correlative science studies performed in conjunction with the United States–Finland trial have documented differences in the activity of imatinib based on the genotype of the GIST lesions treated. Specifically, patients whose GIST harbored *KIT* mutations in exon 11 (the most common molecular subtype) had higher rates of objective response and more durable disease control over time with continuous dosing of imatinib than those patients whose disease had exon 9 *KIT* mutations or no detectable *KIT* mutations at all.[46g] Imatinib-sensitive *PDGFRA* mutations can explain responses in certain GIST patients whose disease does not have any *KIT* mutations.[46g] Larger studies are in progress to con-

firm these early results and to examine the prognostic power of these correlations between tumor genotype and the degree of imatinib clinical activity against GIST.

One of the more impressive aspects of this work has been the outstanding tolerability of imatinib overall. It is quite fortunate that blockage by imatinib therapy of the normal physiologic processes that are dependent on the controlled receptor-ligand signaling through normal KIT does not become life-threatening. The adverse effects of imatinib are generally mild (grade 1 or 2 by the National Cancer Institute common toxicity criteria) and include toxicities such as edema (in approximately 74% of patients; especially notable in the loose subcutaneous tissues of the facial periorbital region), diarrhea (45%), myalgia or musculoskeletal pain (40%), skin rashes (30%), and headache (25%). Myelotoxicity was markedly less common in GIST patients than in patients with CML, which suggests that hematologic toxicities result in large part from the underlying marrow dysfunction of CML, rather than from treatment-associated toxicity with imatinib. Nonetheless, GIST patients treated with imatinib can occasionally exhibit severe cytopenias, and they should be monitored carefully.

In general, the most worrisome adverse event observed in the imatinib treatment of patients with advanced GIST was hemorrhages from abdominal or GI sites; this was noted in approximately 5% of GIST patients. It is very likely that these hemorrhagic events were related to bleeding from bulky tumor masses, and this may have been induced by the potent and rapid antitumor effects of imatinib. There were no deaths directly attributable to the study drug.[46]

There appears to be a tachyphylaxis with certain side effects of imatinib therapy. For example, the edema associated with imatinib therapy of GIST often improves with continued dosing over time, although diuretics may be used judiciously and are often effective in managing this side effect. Counseling GIST patients to consume a low-salt diet may also be highly effective in controlling this side effect of treatment. Nausea with imatinib administration is usually mild and self-limited; for most patients, taking the daily dose with food and dividing the dose may be useful. Muscle cramps, frequently reported in the calves, are usually transient and self-limited; many patients have noted that increased fluid intake can help alleviate the frequency or severity of the muscle cramping. In general, imatinib is reasonably well tolerated, and patients have been able to comply with long-term dosing without an excessively negative impact on their functional status.

Another fascinating aspect of this work was the finding that imatinib could rapidly and dramatically affect tumor avidity for FDG on PET scans (Fig. 29.7-3). The down-modulation of tumor avidity for FDG on PET scanning could be detected as early as 24 hours after a single dose of imatinib. These changes could indicate the biologic activity of imatinib far earlier than any detectable changes on CT scanning. The findings of PET scans were also highly reliable, both correlating with beneficial response to imatinib and documenting progressive disease that was resistant to imatinib. These data indicate that functional imaging of GIST with FDG-PET represents a useful diagnostic technique for very early assessment of response to imatinib therapy.[46a,47] FDG-PET should also be a very useful tool for future drug development efforts, because the signal of drug activity can be detected clearly in patients within a very short period of time after drug dosing begins if effective target inhibition occurs.

The optimal dose of imatinib for treatment of advanced GIST remains uncertain. Although there were no documented benefits to the higher dose of 600 mg/d in the United States–

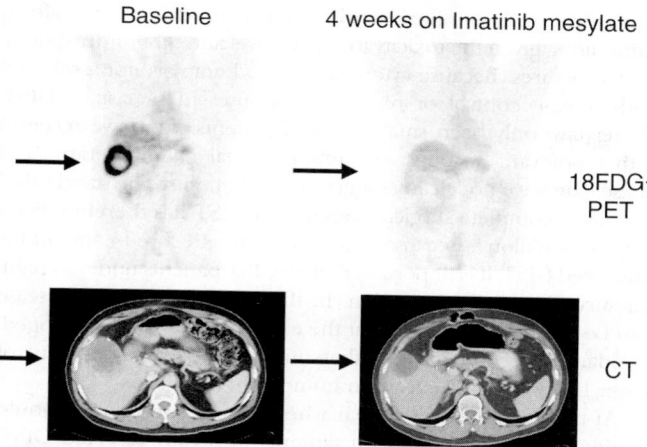

Baseline   4 weeks on Imatinib mesylate

18FDG-PET

CT

FIGURE 29.7-3. Rapid response to imatinib as imaged by ^{18}F-fluoro-deoxyglucose–positron emission tomography (FDG-PET; *top*) and computed tomography (CT) scans (*bottom*). Baseline images (*left*) show large, FDG-avid gastrointestinal stromal tumor metastasis in the right lobe of liver. After 4 weeks of daily imatinib therapy, there is no evidence of FDG avidity remaining in the tumor, although the tumor is still prominent and hypodense on CT imaging. (Images from A. van den Abbeele and G. Demetri, Dana-Farber Cancer Institute.)

Finland trial, there were a few patients who regained disease control when crossed over from the lower dose (400 mg daily) to the higher dose level. Therefore, some marginal benefit might be obtained from modest dose escalation of imatinib in a subset of patients whose disease progresses despite continued dosing at lower therapeutic levels of imatinib.

To explore more definitively whether there is a clinically significant dose response above the lowest recommended daily dose of 400 mg, two very large phase III randomized studies were designed and conducted. One of these studies has been performed by the North American Sarcoma Intergroup with the support of the U.S. National Cancer Institute and the National Cancer Institute of Canada, whereas the other has been conducted by the EORTC in conjunction with the Australasian GI Trials Group and the Italian Sarcoma Group. In both studies, patients with advanced metastatic or unresectable GIST, or both, were randomly assigned to receive imatinib at a dose of either 400 mg or 800 mg daily. Patients were allowed to cross over from the lower dose to the higher dose if there was progression of disease at the lower dose. These studies should be adequately powered to determine whether this large difference in imatinib dosing translates into any benefits in response rates, duration of disease control, or survival for patients with advanced unresectable or metastatic GIST. The most recent updates of these studies have been presented,[48,49] and the studies are closed to accrual, having registered nearly 1700 GIST patients between the two trials.

Although there was no survival difference documented in either trial between patients receiving these two dose levels, there were discordant results in terms of duration of disease control. The North American Sarcoma Intergroup trial demonstrated that the two doses were equivalent in terms of response rates and duration of disease control, as well as overall survival. The EORTC-led study noted a modest but statistically significant benefit in favor of the higher-dose arm in progression-free survival, although no difference was seen in overall survival. In both trials, the higher dose of imatinib was associated with greater incidence of adverse effects and led to a greater number of dose reductions for toxicity. It is unclear why these two large trials have generated discordant data

in terms of progression-free survival, and this remains the subject of active investigation in these ongoing studies.

The optimal duration of imatinib therapy for patients with metastatic GIST remains somewhat uncertain, but most experts consider this as lifelong therapy. Studies in which patients have interrupted imatinib dosing have reported that disease progression often follows shortly after the imatinib is stopped.[49a] This clinical experience supports the hypothesis that continuous exposure to imatinib is necessary to maintain control over a population of GIST cells that may remain quiescent long term as long as aberrant KIT signaling is inhibited. However, if the drug is withdrawn and the uncontrolled KIT activity is allowed to resume, the disease reactivates and progresses. Therefore, for GIST patients who achieve any measure of disease control, continued dosing with imatinib as long as the disease is not progressive appears to be the optimal course of management.

It is critical to emphasize the importance of multidisciplinary management in the care of GIST patients. For optimal management of metastatic disease, medical oncologists, surgeons, radiologists, and nuclear medicine imaging experts must all collaborate closely to determine the best course of action for any given patient. This important message has been emphasized in the Task Force Report on GIST Clinical Practice Guidelines of the National Comprehensive Cancer Network.[59] For example, disease that is initially judged as unresectable may become amenable to surgical excision after a major response induced by imatinib therapy. Most centers recommend surgical resection for such patients, because it is feared that residual GIST may develop secondary mutations that could result in clinical resistance to imatinib and progression of disease.

Resistance to Imatinib

Resistance to imatinib may be primary and manifest as rapid progression of disease despite imatinib dosing, although this appears in far fewer than 20% of patients (see Table 29.7-2). Alternatively, clonal evolution of GIST may be detected clinically, with the emergence of resistant disease after more than a year or two of durable response and disease control. Several mechanisms of resistance to imatinib in GIST have been described,[49a] and these are somewhat similar to the resistance mechanisms that have been demonstrated in CML.[49b] It is unclear what role should ideally be played by other modalities, such as radiofrequency ablation or other locoregional approaches, in managing metastatic GIST once imatinib has achieved the optimal effect or after the appearance of limited resistance to imatinib with oligoclonal progression.[49c] Certainly, it has been described that many GIST lesions may remain controlled while limited clonal progression appears as the first sign of resistance to imatinib.[50] It may be feasible in such patients to resect the resistant clonal growth while maintaining control over the majority of the disease by continuation of imatinib dosing. These strategies will be tested in future trials, as new kinase inhibitors of varying target specificities are used to combat GIST that has become refractory to imatinib.[51]

EXTRAPOLATION OF EMERGING MANAGEMENT PARADIGMS TO EARLY-STAGE GASTROINTESTINAL STROMAL TUMOR

Definitive expert surgery remains the mainstay of treatment for patients with localized, primary GIST. It is important to recognize that surgical resection of GIST should probably be undertaken only if there is a very low risk of functional deficit. If a very large GIST were to be detected, it might be judicious to consider such a lesion unresectable for cure, which could be done without causing unacceptable risk for morbidity; in such a case, preoperative administration of imatinib could be given, with follow-up at close intervals to ensure appropriate response to therapy. In this situation, early assessment of therapeutic response by FDG-PET scanning could be very valuable to confirm that the patient's disease is indeed exhibiting the desired response to imatinib. This should minimize the risk of disease progression, which might put the patient at risk for further growth and invasion into other vital structures. After maximal response (usually occurring within 3 to 6 months), definitive surgery could be performed. A clinical trial is being performed to test more formally the use of preoperative imatinib in patients with resectable or potentially resectable GISTs.

The surgical approach to resection of primary disease must take into account the specific growth and behavior characteristics of GIST. GIST rarely involves the locoregional lymph nodes, and so extensive lymph node exploration or resection is rarely indicated. GIST lesions may exhibit a fragile pseudocapsule, and intraoperative procedures must be optimized to minimize the risk of tumor rupture, which could increase the risk of peritoneal dissemination.[37] The margins of resection from the tumor specimen should be carefully oriented and examined, and biopsy samples from several different areas of the tumor should be evaluated by the surgical pathologist.

The natural history of early-stage, primary GIST has been examined in studies from single-institution referral centers. These are certainly prone to selection bias, and it is clear in this evolving field that many early-stage GIST patients have likely been managed by physicians in multiple specialties (including gastroenterology, general surgery, and others). However, one of the larger series that studied GISTs evaluated 200 patients followed prospectively at the Memorial Sloan-Kettering Cancer Center.[29] Eighty of these patients who had primary disease were managed with complete surgical resection. This group of patients with primary resected GIST demonstrated a 5-year disease-specific survival rate of 54%, which indicates the fact that GIST can recur and ultimately prove to be a life-threatening disease after recurrence. On multivariate analysis, large tumor size (more than 10 cm) was the only predictive factor that impacted negatively on disease-specific survival.[29] In an earlier study of "GI leiomyosarcomas" (of which a sizable proportion were very likely to have been true GISTs), investigators at the M. D. Anderson Cancer Center reported that smaller tumor size (less than 5 cm), complete surgical resection without tumor rupture, and low grade of tumor were significant favorable prognostic factors in their series of 191 patients. The propensity of GIST to recur was confirmed by these data as well, because only 10% of these patients were disease-free with long-term follow-up.[37]

ADJUVANT THERAPY TO IMPROVE OUTCOMES FOR PATIENTS WITH RESECTED EARLY-STAGE GASTROINTESTINAL STROMAL TUMORS

To date, there have only been a limited number of case reports and small series that have investigated the role of adjuvant treatment using conventional modalities such as radiotherapy after surgical resection. As noted earlier in Management of Metastatic, Unresectable, or Recurrent Gastrointestinal Stromal Tumor, radiotherapy does not appear to have an important role in the treatment of GIST, with only minimal activity seen at doses that are safe to administer, given the toxicity to small bowel and other intraabdominal structures. Because cytotoxic chemotherapy is not associated with disease control or objective responses in metastatic GIST, there have only been small series of patients who have received either adjuvant systemic or intraperitoneal chemotherapy, and these data have not clearly suggested any benefits. The standard of care after complete surgical resection of GIST has therefore been observation alone. Because there is now an effective treatment for advanced GIST, it is important that all GIST patients undergo regular surveillance after resection. In this way, any recurrent disease can be detected and treated at the earliest point, with, it is hoped, avoidance of complications that might stem from treatment of large, bulky disease such as intratumoral hemorrhage.

At the present, it is unclear whether imatinib therapy would confer significant benefit on patients with fully resected GIST. Certainly, because imatinib exhibits such impressive activity in the treatment of advanced disease, it is reasonable to hypothesize that this should translate into benefit for the treatment of minimal residual disease after complete surgical resection. However, this requires prospective testing and confirmation. Additionally, because adjuvant therapy is generally time limited, it is possible that the duration of drug exposure may determine the therapeutic impact. Specifically, too short a period of imatinib dosing in the adjuvant postresection setting may not confer optimal benefit to patients. The potential activity of adjuvant imatinib in GIST patients who are at moderate to high risk of recurrence is currently being investigated in a large multicenter phase III trial being conducted under the auspices of the American College of Surgeons Oncology Group in study Z9001; this trial administers imatinib or placebo to patients with fully resected primary GIST for 1 year. It is certainly possible that a longer duration of adjuvant therapy might improve outcomes further, and this is being tested in another trial that will be activated in Europe by the EORTC. Given the potential toxicities and costs of imatinib, as well as the excellent activity of imatinib as therapy for recurrent disease, it is very importance to generate evidence on which to base rational medical practice and critical that these well-designed adjuvant studies of imatinib be completed and analyzed so that patients and physicians can manage this disease with the best knowledge and therapies.

SPECIAL CONSIDERATIONS IN GASTROINTESTINAL STROMAL TUMOR

FAMILIAL SYNDROMES OF GASTROINTESTINAL STROMAL TUMOR

GIST can be associated with rare familial inheritance patterns in which several members of a kindred have the disease.[52–54] In several of these reported families, mutations in *KIT* loci have been reported. Additional characteristics of affected family members include cutaneous lesions such as hyperpigmentation or skin lesions that appear clinically like urticaria pigmentosa. These skin pigmentation abnormalities are no doubt due to the effect of the overactive mutated KIT RTK on melanocyte growth and development. The mechanisms by which such pigmentation disorders remain focal, rather than disseminated, may provide clues as to why GIST lesions may take decades to appear in these rare familial cases.

RELATION OF GASTROINTESTINAL STROMAL TUMOR TO OTHER GENETIC SYNDROMES PREDISPOSING TO NEOPLASMS

Several syndromes that predispose to the development of neoplasms have been described in association with the occurrence of GIST. One of the more widely known of these is the Carney triad, which encompasses GIST (often multifocal) in addition to pulmonary chondromas and extraadrenal paragangliomas.[55] A variant of this syndrome has been described with only GIST and familial paragangliomas.[56] Additionally, a linkage between neurofibromatosis type 1 and an increased incidence of GIST has been widely noted.[57,58] Molecular analysis of GIST lesions arising in patients with neurofibromatosis type 1 has documented that these GISTs are characterized by the wild-type *KIT* gene.[58] It is unclear whether GISTs that arise in the setting of a genetic predisposition syndrome have the same response to imatinib as sporadically occurring GISTs.

NEW CHALLENGES AND ALTERNATIVE APPROACHES

The remarkable developments that have occurred in GIST research and clinical care in the past several years have only further intensified the research in this field. GIST remains a very informative disease for cancer biologists seeking the root causes of neoplastic transformation and maintenance of the malignant phenotype. Similarly, GIST has served as a paradigm for rationally designed translational therapeutics in a solid tumor. In many ways, GIST research is likely to inform many avenues of fundamental discovery research that can be applied to other more common malignancies.

Although imatinib has proven to be a highly effective treatment for patients with metastatic GIST, it is clear that this single agent is not curing the vast majority of patients with advanced disease. Although imatinib-associated control of GIST can be highly durable and last for years, a subset of patients may be either resistant to or intolerant of treatment with this drug. Very few patients with metastatic disease achieve a complete response, and it is important to seek out the mechanisms by which GIST cells go into a state of "hibernation" while still living under the selection pressure of chronic imatinib dosing. Most importantly, it has become clear that acquired resistance to imatinib will occur with increasing frequency over time, even in patients who benefit initially from outstanding clinical responses to this agent. Unusual patterns of recurrence have been seen in some patients, including development of isolated nodules within preexistent tumors[50] and the progression of individual disease sites while the overall tumor burden remains stable and under good control. These findings are consistent with clonal evolution of GIST, with the outgrowth of resistant clones of tumor cells. Multidisciplinary approaches to control of these localized sites of imatinib-resistant disease, such as surgical resection, or other local therapies, such as tumor ablation, may have the best chance of offering some additional benefit to patients while continuing to allow control of the imatinib-sensitive tumor clones elsewhere by continuation of imatinib dosing despite limited progression. Molecular analyses of these resistant clones will provide an important opportunity to determine resistance mechanisms, perhaps even on an individual basis. This is an opportunity to meld structural biology and drug development to

clinical medicine with unparalleled precision. Several clinical trials are already in progress using next-generation agents that target the KIT receptor via different mechanisms or that target alternate pathways thought to be important to the pathobiology of GIST. Many of these trials take advantage of the power of functional imaging with PET scanning to provide early signals of activity, along with correlative molecular analysis of tumor samples to explain clinical phenomena in a scientifically robust manner.

It is also clear that imatinib, as a therapy that targets the fundamental molecular pathophysiology of GIST and CML, does not have an obvious major impact in several other common diseases, such as carcinomas. Studies are ongoing to define whether the PDGFR inhibitory activity of imatinib might prove therapeutically useful in some way. For the moment, imatinib has also proven highly effective in the PDGF-driven malignancies known as dermatofibrosarcoma protuberans and in certain myeloproliferative diseases.

In summary, it is clear that the acquisition of a deeper scientific understanding of GIST has led to the development of powerful new therapeutic tools such as imatinib to disable the malignant potential of GIST cells. It is also clear, however, that new therapies will continue to be needed to improve outcomes for patients with this disease. With improved technology and rational molecular targeting, this translation of science into applied therapeutics should continue to move forward at a very rapid pace, aided by the efforts of collaborating investigators and physicians of multiple specialties around the world.

REFERENCES

1. Golden T, Stout AP. Smooth muscle tumors of the gastrointestinal tract and retroperitoneal tissues. *Gynecol Obstet* 1941;73:784.
2. Stout AP. Bizarre smooth muscle tumors of the stomach. *Cancer* 1962;15:400.
3. Mazur MT, Clark HB. Gastric stromal tumors. Reappraisal of histogenesis. *Am J Surg Pathol* 1983;7:507.
4. Herrera GA, Pinto de Moraes H, Grizzle WE, et al. Malignant small bowel neoplasm of enteric plexus derivation (plexosarcoma). Light and electron microscopic study confirming the origin of the neoplasm. *Dig Dis Sci* 1984;29:275.
5. Walker P, Dvorak AM. Gastrointestinal autonomic nerve (GAN) tumor. Ultrastructural evidence for a newly recognized entity. *Arch Pathol Lab Med* 1986;110:309.
6. Newman PL, Wadden C, Fletcher CD. Gastrointestinal stromal tumours: correlation of immunophenotype with clinicopathological features. *J Pathol* 1991;164:107.
7. Hurlimann J, Gardiol D. Gastrointestinal stromal tumours: an immunohistochemical study of 165 cases. *Histopathology* 1991;19:311.
8. Pike AM, Lloyd RV, Appelman HD. Cell markers in gastrointestinal stromal tumors. *Hum Pathol* 1988;19:830.
9. Miettinen M, Virolainen M, Maarit Sarlomo R. Gastrointestinal stromal tumors—value of CD34 antigen in their identification and separation from true leiomyomas and schwannomas. *Am J Surg Pathol* 1995;19:207.
10. Miettinen M, Monihan JM, Sarlomo-Rikala M, et al. Gastrointestinal stromal tumors/ smooth muscle tumors (GISTs) primary in the omentum and mesentery: clinicopathologic and immunohistochemical study of 26 cases. *Am J Surg Pathol* 1999;23:1109.
11. Perez-Atayde AR, Shamberger RC, Kozakewich HW. Neuroectodermal differentiation of the gastrointestinal tumors in the Carney triad. An ultrastructural and immunohistochemical study. *Am J Surg Pathol* 1993;17:706.
12. Kindblom LG, Remotti HE, Aldenborg F, et al. Gastrointestinal pacemaker cell tumor (GIPACT): gastrointestinal stromal tumors show phenotypic characteristics of the interstitial cells of Cajal. *Am J Pathol* 1998;152:1259.
13. Sircar K, Hewlett BR, Huizinga JD, et al. Interstitial cells of Cajal as precursors of gastrointestinal stromal tumors. *Am J Surg Pathol* 1999;23:377.
14. Sakurai S, Fukasawa T, Chong JM, et al. Embryonic form of smooth muscle myosin heavy chain (SMemb/MHC-B) in gastrointestinal stromal tumor and interstitial cells of Cajal. *Am J Pathol* 1999;154:23.
15. Wang L, Vargas H, French SW. Cellular origin of gastrointestinal stromal tumors: a study of 27 cases. *Arch Pathol Lab Med* 2000;124:1471.
16. Hirota S, Isozaki K, Moriyama Y, et al. Gain-of-function mutations of c-kit in human gastrointestinal stromal tumors. *Science* 1998;279:577.
17. Furitsu T, Tsujimura T, Tono T, et al. Identification of mutations in the coding sequence of the proto-oncogene c-kit in a human mast cell leukemia cell line causing ligand-independent activation of c-kit product. *J Clin Invest* 1993;92:1736.

18. Longley BJ, Tyrrell L, Lu SZ, et al. Somatic c-KIT activating mutation in urticaria pigmentosa and aggressive mastocytosis: establishment of clonality in a human mast cell neoplasm. *Nat Genet* 1996;12:312.
19. Nagata H, Worobec AS, Oh CK, et al. Identification of a point mutation in the catalytic domain of the protooncogene c-kit in peripheral blood mononuclear cells of patients who have mastocytosis with an associated hematologic disorder. *Proc Natl Acad Sci U S A* 1995;92:10560.
20. Tsujimura T, Furitsu T, Morimoto M, et al. Ligand-independent activation of c-kit receptor tyrosine kinase in a murine mastocytoma cell line P-815 generated by a point mutation. *Blood* 1994;83:2619.
21. Nishida T, Hirota S, Taniguchi M, et al. Familial gastrointestinal stromal tumours with germline mutation of the KIT gene. *Nat Genet* 1998;19:323.
22. Maeyama H, Hidaka E, Ota H, et al. Familial gastrointestinal stromal tumor with hyperpigmentation: association with a germline mutation of the c-kit gene. *Gastroenterology* 2001;120:210.
23. Isozaki K, Terris B, Belghiti J, et al. Germline-activating mutation in the kinase domain of KIT gene in familial gastrointestinal stromal tumors. *Am J Pathol* 2000;157:1581.
24. Corless CL, McGreevey L, Haley A, et al. KIT mutations are common in incidental gastrointestinal stromal tumors one centimeter or less in size. *Am J Pathol* 2002;160:1567.
24a. Duensing A, Medeiros F, McConarty B, et al. Mechanisms of oncogenic KIT signal transduction in primary gastrointestinal stromal tumors (GISTs). *Oncogene* 2004;23:3999.
25. Rubin BP, Singer S, Tsao C, et al. KIT activation is a ubiquitous feature of gastrointestinal stromal tumors. *Cancer Res* 2001;61:8118.
26. Lux ML, Rubin BP, Biase TL, et al. KIT extracellular and kinase domain mutations in gastrointestinal stromal tumors. *Am J Pathol* 2000;156:791.
27. Lasota J, Wozniak A, Sarlomo-Rikala M, et al. Mutations in exons 9 and 13 of KIT gene are rare events in gastrointestinal stromal tumors. A study of 200 cases. *Am J Pathol* 2000;157:1091.
27a. Mol CD, Lim KB, Sridhar V, et al. Structure of a c-kit product complex reveals the basis for kinase transactivation. *J Biol Chem* 2003;278:31461.
27b. Heinrich MC, Corless CL, Duensing A, et al. PDGFRA activating mutations in gastrointestinal stromal tumors. *Science* 2003;299:708.
27c. Hirota S, Ohashi A, Nishida T, et al. Gain-of-function mutations of platelet-derived growth factor receptor alpha gene in gastrointestinal stromal tumors. *Gastroenterology* 2003;125:660.
28. Fletcher CD, Berman JJ, Corless C, et al. Diagnosis of gastrointestinal stromal tumors: a consensus approach. *Hum Pathol* 2002;33:459.
28a. Miettinen M, El-Rifai W, Sobin LH, Lasota J. Evaluation of malignancy and prognosis of gastrointestinal stromal tumors: a review. *Hum Pathol* 2002;33:478.
28b. Kindblom LG, Meis-Kindblo J, Bümming P, et al. Incidence, prevalence, phenotype and biologic spectrum of gastrointestinal stromal cell tumors (GIST)—a population-based study of 600 cases. *Ann Oncol* 2002;13[Suppl 5]:157(abst).
29. DeMatteo RP, Lewis JJ, Leung D, et al. Two hundred gastrointestinal stromal tumors: recurrence patterns and prognostic factors for survival. *Ann Surg* 2002;231:51.
30. Miettinen M, Lasota J. Gastrointestinal stromal tumors—definition, clinical, histological, immunohistochemical, and molecular genetic features and differential diagnosis. *Virchows Arch* 2001;438:1.
31. Emory TS, Sobin LH, Lukes L, et al. Prognosis of gastrointestinal smooth-muscle (stromal) tumors: dependence on anatomic site. *Am J Surg Pathol* 1999;23:82.
32. Pidhorecky I, Cheney RT, Kraybill WG, et al. Gastrointestinal stromal tumors: current diagnosis, biologic behavior, and management. *Ann Surg Oncol* 2000;7:705.
33. Coffin CM, Dehner LP, Meis-Kindblom JM. Inflammatory myofibroblastic tumor, inflammatory fibrosarcoma, and related lesions: an historical review with differential diagnostic considerations. *Semin Diagn Pathol* 1998;15:102.
33a. Hornick JL, Fletcher CD. Immunohistochemical staining for KIT (CD117) in soft tissue sarcomas is very limited in distribution. *Am J Clin Pathol* 2002;117:188.
34. Ernst SI, Hubbs AE, Przygodzki RM, et al. KIT mutation portends poor prognosis in gastrointestinal stromal/smooth muscle tumors. *Lab Invest* 1998;78:1633.
35. Taniguchi M, Nishida T, Hirota S, et al. Effect of c-kit mutation on prognosis of gastrointestinal stromal tumors. *Cancer Res* 1999;59:4297.
36. Singer S, Rubin BP, Lux ML, et al. Prognostic value of KIT mutation type, mitotic activity, and histologic subtype in gastrointestinal stromal tumors. *J Clin Oncol* 2002;20:3898.
37. Ng EH, Pollock RE, Munsell MF, et al. Prognostic factors influencing survival in gastrointestinal leiomyosarcomas. Implications for surgical management and staging. *Ann Surg* 1992;215:68.
38. Goss GA, Merriam P, Manola J, et al. Clinical and pathological characteristics of gastrointestinal stromal tumors (GIST). *Proc Am Soc Clin Oncol* 2000;19.
38a. Eilber FC, Rosen G, Forscher C, et al. Recurrent gastrointestinal stromal sarcomas. *Surg Oncol* 2000;9:71
38b. Rajan DK, Soulen MC, Clark TW, et al. Sarcomas metastatic to the liver: response and survival after cisplatin, doxorubicin, mitomycin-C, Ethiodol, and polyvinyl alcohol chemoembolization. *J Vasc Interv Radiol* 2001;12:187.
38c. Mavligit GM, Zukwiski AA, Ellis LM, et al. Gastrointestinal leiomyosarcoma metastatic to the liver. Durable tumor regression by hepatic chemoembolization infusion with cisplatin and vinblastine. *Cancer* 1995;75:2083.
39. Plaat BE, Hollema H, Molenaar WM, et al. Soft tissue leiomyosarcomas and malignant gastrointestinal stromal tumors: differences in clinical outcome and expression of multidrug resistance proteins. *J Clin Oncol* 2000;18:3211.
39a. Mudan SS, Conlon KC, Woodruff J, et al. Salvage surgery in recurrent gastrointestinal sarcoma: prognostic factors to guide patient selection. *Cancer* 1999;88:66.
40. Druker BJ, Tamura S, Buchdunger E, et al. Effects of a selective inhibitor of the Abl tyrosine kinase on the growth of Bcr-Abl positive cells. *Nat Med* 1996;2:561.
41. Buchdunger E, Zimmermann J, Mett H, et al. Inhibition of the Abl protein-tyrosine kinase in vitro and in vivo by a 2-phenylaminopyrimidine derivative. *Cancer Res* 1996;56:100.
42. Buchdunger E, Cioffi CL, Law N, et al. Abl protein-tyrosine kinase inhibitor STI571 inhibits in vitro signal transduction mediated by c-kit and platelet-derived growth factor receptors. *J Pharmacol Exp Ther* 2000;295:139.
43. Heinrich MC, Griffith DJ, Druker BJ, et al. Inhibition of c-kit receptor tyrosine kinase activity by STI 571, a selective tyrosine kinase inhibitor. *Blood* 2000;96:925.
44. Tuveson DA, Willis NA, Jacks T, et al. STI571 inactivation of the gastrointestinal stromal tumor c-KIT oncoprotein: biological and clinical implications. *Oncogene* 2001;20:5054.
45. Joensuu H, Roberts PJ, Sarlomo-Rikala M, et al. Effect of the tyrosine kinase inhibitor STI571 in a patient with a metastatic gastrointestinal stromal tumor. *N Engl J Med* 2001;344:1052.
46. Demetri GD, von Mehren M, Blanke CD, et al. Efficacy and safety of imatinib mesylate in advanced gastrointestinal stromal tumors. *N Engl J Med* 2002;347:472.
46a. Stroobants S, Goeminne J, Seegers M, et al. 18FDG-Positron emission tomography for the early prediction of response in advanced soft tissue sarcoma treated with imatinib mesylate (Glivec). *Eur J Cancer* 2003;39:2012.
46b. van Oosterom AT, Judson I, Verweij J, et al. European Organization for Research and Treatment of Cancer soft tissue and bone sarcoma group. Safety and efficacy of imatinib (STI571) in metastatic gastrointestinal stromal tumours: a phase I study. *Lancet* 2001;358:1421.
46c. Verweij J, van Oosterom A, Blay JY, et al. Imatinib mesylate is an active agent for gastrointestinal stromal tumors but does not yield responses in other soft-tissue sarcomas that are unselected for a molecular target. *Eur J Cancer* 2003;39:2006.
46d. Maki RG, Awan RA, Dixon RH, Jhanwar S, Antonescu CR. Differential sensitivity to imatinib of 2 patients with metastatic sarcoma arising from dermatofibrosarcoma protuberans. *Int J Cancer* 2002;100:623.
46e. Rubin BP, Schuetze SM, Eary JF, et al. Molecular targeting of platelet-derived growth factor B by imatinib mesylate in a patient with metastatic dermatofibrosarcoma protuberans. *J Clin Oncol* 2002;20:3586.
46f. McArthur GA, Demetri GD, Heinrich M, et al. Imatinib target exploration study. Molecular and clinical analysis of response to imatinib for locally advanced dermatofibrosarcoma protuberans. *Proc Am Soc Clin Oncol* 2001;22:(abst 781).
46g. Heinrich MC, Corless CL, Demetri GD, et al. Kinase mutations and imatinib response in patients with metastatic gastrointestinal stromal tumor. *J Clin Oncol* 2003;21:4342.
47. Van den Abbeele A, Badawi RD, Cliché JP, et al. 18F-FDG-PET predicts response to imatinib mesylate (Gleevec) in patients with advanced gastrointestinal stromal tumors (GIST). *Proc Am Soc Clin Oncol* 2002;21:(abst 1610).
48. Benjamin R, Rankin C, Fletcher C, et al. Phase III dose-randomized study of imatinib mesylate (IM) for GIST: Intergroup S0033 early results. *Proc Am Soc Clin Oncol* 2003;22:814(abst 3271).
49. Verweij J, Casali PG, Zalcberg J, et al. Early efficacy comparison of two doses of imatinib for the treatment of advanced gastrointestinal stromal tumors (GIST): interim results of a randomized phase III trial from the EORTC-STBSG, ISG and AGITG *Proc Am Soc Clin Oncol* 2003;22:814(abst 3272).
49a. Blay JY, Berthaud P, Perol D, et al. Continuous vs intermittent imatinib treatment in advanced GIST after one year: a prospective randomized phase III trial of the French Sarcoma Group. *Proc Am Soc Clin Oncol* 2004;(abst 9006).
49b. Shah NP, Sawyers CL. Mechanisms of resistance to STI571 in Philadelphia chromosome-associated leukemias. *Oncogene* 2003;22:7389.
49c. Dileo P, Randhawa R, Vansonnenberg E, et al. Safety and efficacy of percutaneous radiofrequency ablation (RFA) in patients (pts) with metastatic gastrointestinal stromal tumor (GIST) with clonal evolution of lesions refractory to imatinib mesylate (IM). *Proc Am Soc Clin Oncol* 2004;(abst 9024).
50. Shankar S, Desai J, Potter A, et al. Novel patterns of progression following initial response to imatinib in patients with malignant gastrointestinal stromal tumors (GIST). *Proc Am Soc Clin Oncol* 2003;22:230(abst 923).
51. Demetri GD, George S, Heinrich MC, et al. GIST SU11248 Study Group. Clinical activity and tolerability of the multi-targeted tyrosine kinase inhibitor SU11248 in patients (pts) with metastatic gastrointestinal stromal tumor (GIST) refractory to imatinib mesylate. *Proc Am Soc Clin Oncol* 2003;22:814(abst 3273).
52. Nishida T, Hirota S, Taniguchi M, et al. Familial gastrointestinal stromal tumours with germline mutation of the KIT gene. *Nat Genet* 1998;19:323.
53. Isozaki K, Terris B, Belghiti J, et al. Germline-activating mutation in the kinase domain of KIT gene in familial gastrointestinal stromal tumors. *Am J Pathol* 2000;157:1581.
54. Maeyama H, Hidaka E, Ota H, et al. Familial gastrointestinal stromal tumor with hyperpigmentation: association with a germline mutation of the c-kit gene. *Gastroenterology* 2001;120:210.
55. Carney JA. Gastric stromal sarcoma, pulmonary chondroma, and extra-adrenal paraganglioma (Carney triad): natural history, adrenocortical component, and possible familial occurrence. *Mayo Clin Proc* 1999;74:543.
56. Carney JA, Stratakis CA. Familial paraganglioma and gastric stromal sarcoma: a new syndrome distinct from the Carney triad. *Am J Med Genet* 2002;108:132.
57. Zoller ME, Rembeck B, Oden A, et al. Malignant and benign tumors in patients with neurofibromatosis type 1 in a defined Swedish population. *Cancer* 1997;79:2125.
58. Kinoshita K, Hirota S, Isozaki K, et al. Absence of c-kit gene mutations in gastrointestinal stromal tumours from neurofibromatosis type 1 patients. *J Pathol* 2004;202:80.
59. Demetri G, et al. Optimal management of patients with gastrointestinal stromal tumors—task force report of the clinical practice guidelines from the national comprehensive cancer network. *J NCCN* 2004;2[Suppl 1]:S1.

STEVEN K. LIBUTTI
LEONARD B. SALTZ
ANIL K. RUSTGI
JOEL E. TEPPER

SECTION 8

Cancer of the Colon

Significant advances have been made in the study of colorectal cancer over the last few years. A more thorough understanding of the molecular basis for this disease, coupled with the development of new therapeutic approaches, has dramatically altered the way in which patients are managed. New strategies for screening and for the detection of recurrent disease have also impacted the way physicians approach the workup and disease staging of their patients. This chapter and Chapter 29.9 endeavor to provide an up-to-date description of the current state of the science and outline a multidisciplinary approach to the patient with colon or rectal cancer.

EPIDEMIOLOGY

INCIDENCE AND MORTALITY

Globally, nearly 800,000 new colorectal cancer cases are believed to occur each year, which account for approximately 10% of all incident cancers, and mortality from colorectal cancer is estimated at nearly 450,000 per year.[1] In 1998, there were an estimated 131,600 new cases of colorectal cancer and 56,500 deaths in the United States.[2] Thus, colorectal cancer accounts for nearly 11% of cancer mortality in the United States.[2] Prevalence estimates[3–6] reveal that in unscreened individuals aged 50 years or older, there is a 0.5% to 2% chance of harboring an invasive colorectal cancer, a 1% to 1.6% chance of an *in situ* carcinoma, a 7% to 10% chance of a large (1 cm or more) adenoma, and a 25% to 40% chance of an adenoma of any size.

Age impacts colorectal cancer incidence more than any other demographic factor. The incidence of sporadic colorectal cancer increases dramatically above the age of 45 or 50 years for all groups. In almost all countries, age-standardized incidence rates are lower for women than for men; in 1990 colorectal cancer incidence per 100,000 was 19.4 for men and 15.3 for women.[1] In the United States from 1992 to 1995, the age-standardized incidence was 50.5 for men and 37.0 for women when combined for all races.[2] Interestingly, however, the lifetime risk of a colorectal cancer diagnosis in the United States is nearly 6% for men and women, but the lifetime risk of colorectal cancer mortality is higher for women at 2.7% than for men at 2.6%.[2] These disparate characteristics between standardized and lifetime rates may be attributable to the longer life expectancy of women.

Although decreases in age-standardized colorectal cancer incidence and mortality rates are apparent in the United States over the past 10 to 15 years, such trends may be counterbalanced by prolonged longevity. At the current time, there are an estimated 250,000 colorectal cancer–related hospitalizations per year at an associated cost of $5 billion annually[7] and with a significant disparity along ethnic and racial lines.

GEOGRAPHIC VARIATION

Geographic variation in colorectal cancer incidence implies, and to a large extent proves, the critical nature of environmental factors. A 30- to 40-fold difference is seen between the highest and lowest incidence rates. As an illustration, the incidence rate for Alaskan natives exceeds 70 per 100,000,[8] whereas that for residents of Gambia and Algeria is less than 2 per 100,000.[1] Generally speaking, colorectal cancer incidence and mortality rates are greatest in developed Western nations.[1,2,9,10] The reader is referred to detailed statistics on incidence and mortality rates in different countries over time according to gender, ethnicity, and anatomic site compiled by the National Cancer Institute (http://www3.cancer.gov/atlasplus/).

As mentioned, there appears to be a recent decrease in age-standardized colorectal cancer incidence and mortality rates in the United States. From 1985 to 1995, colorectal cancer incidence decreased by approximately 20% and mortality by nearly 23%. Furthermore, 5-year survival improved. These trends are apparent regardless of gender, race, or ethnic group, except for native Americans. Although, at an initial glance, one might invoke alterations in dietary and lifestyle factors or the use of chemopreventive agents, it is clear that enhanced use of colonoscopy with polypectomy represents a significant reason for the improvements in trends in some areas.[11]

EMIGRATION PATTERNS IN POPULATION GROUPS

Seminal studies[12–15] have revealed that migrants from low-incidence areas to high-incidence areas assume the incidence of the host country within one generation. For example, for Chinese immigrating to the United States, higher colorectal cancer rates have been ascribed to greater meat consumption and diminished physical activity in contrast to controls within their original country.[13] These and other studies underscore the importance of environmental exposure in colorectal cancer incidence and provide a platform for attention to dietary and lifestyle modification as preventive measures.

RACE AND ETHNICITY

Although dietary and lifestyle factors are of paramount importance in low-incidence regions of the world, especially Asia and Africa, nonetheless there are certain trends along racial or ethnic lines. For example, an inherited APC gene mutation, I1307K, confers a higher risk of colorectal cancer within certain Ashkenazi Jewish families that is not apparent in other ethnic groups.[16,17] Inherited mutations in the DNA mismatch repair genes may be more common among African Americans.[18] This may account in part for anatomic variation in colon cancers between races in the United States,[19,20] an area that is receiving much attention in epidemiology and biology-based research.

SOCIOECONOMIC FACTORS

Generally, cancer incidence and mortality rates have been higher in economically advantaged countries.[2,21] This may be related to consumption of a high-fat and high-red-meat diet, lack of physical activity with resulting obesity, and variations in mortality causes over a longitudinal period of time. Yet, if dietary and lifestyle factors in lower income groups start to mirror those in higher income groups in the years to come, the differences in colorectal cancer incidence and mortality rates may start to converge.

ANATOMIC SHIFT

Classically, colon cancer was believed to be a disease of the left or distal colon. However, the incidence of right-sided or proximal colon cancer has been increasing in North America[20,22,23] and Europe.[24,25] Similar trends have been observed in Asian countries.[26] This anatomic shift is likely multifactorial: (1) longevity has increased, (2) response to luminal procarcinogens and carcinogens may vary between different sites of the colon and rectum, and (3) genetic factors may preferentially involve defects in mismatch repair genes with resulting microsatellite instability (MSI) in proximal colon cancers, and the chromosomal instability pathway may be predominant in left-sided colon and rectal cancers. These developments in anatomic variation necessarily impact considerably on screening procedures,[27] response to chemoprevention, response to chemotherapy,[28,29] and, ultimately, disease-specific survival.

ETIOLOGY: GENETIC AND ENVIRONMENTAL RISK FACTORS

The etiology of colorectal cancer is complex, involving an interplay of environmental and genetic factors (Table 29.8-1). These factors can conspire to change the normal mucosa to a premalignant adenomatous polyp to a frank colorectal cancer over the course of many years. This section briefly mentions inherited predisposition; the genetic underpinnings of colorectal cancer are elaborated on in Biology of Colorectal Cancer: Clinical and Molecular Genetic Risk Factors, later in this chapter. The key environmental factors are considered.

INHERITED PREDISPOSITION

Family history of colorectal cancer confers an increased lifetime risk of colorectal cancer, but that enhanced risk varies depending on the nature of the family history. Familial factors contribute importantly to the risk of sporadic colorectal cancer, depending on the involvement of first-degree or second-degree relatives, or both, and the age at onset of colorectal cancer. Involvement of at least one first-degree relative with colorectal cancer doubles the risk of colorectal cancer.[30,31] There is further enhancement of the risk if such a relative is affected before the age of 60. Similarly, the likelihood of harboring premalignant adenomas or colorectal cancer is increased in first-degree relatives of persons with colorectal cancer.[32–36] The National Polyp Study[34] reveals compelling data: The relative risk for parents and siblings of patients with adenomas compared to spousal controls was 1.8, which increased to 2.6 if the proband was younger than age 60 years at adenoma detection.

Provocative assessments of population groups suggest a dominantly inherited susceptibility to colorectal adenomas and cancer, which may account for the majority of sporadic colorectal cancer, but dominantly inherited susceptability may have variable inheritance based on the degree of exposure to environmental factor(s).[37,38] What are these susceptibility factors? The answer has yet to emerge. Nonetheless, genetic polymorphisms may be of paramount importance, such as those in glutathione S-transferase,[39] ethylenetetrahydrofolate reductase,[40,41] and N-acetyltransferases, especially N-acetyltransferase-1 and N-acetyltransferase-2.[39,42–44] In fact, genetic polymorphisms may vary among different racial and ethnic groups, which may provide clues into the geographic variation of colorectal cancer as well.[42,45]

ENVIRONMENTAL FACTORS

Seminal studies have underscored the importance of environmental factors as contributors to the pathogenesis of colorectal cancer. One must interpret the results of population-based studies in the context of the methodologies used, lead-time bias, time-lag issues, definition of surrogate and true end points, and the role of susceptibility factors.

Diet

TOTAL CALORIES. Obesity and total caloric intake are independent risk factors for colorectal cancer as revealed by cohort and case-control studies.[46,47] Increased body mass may result in a twofold increase in colorectal cancer risk with a strong association in men with colon but not rectal cancer.

MEAT, FAT, AND PROTEIN. Ingestion of red meat but not white meat is associated with an increased colorectal cancer risk,[21,45–48] and because of this, per capita consumption of red meat is a potent independent risk factor. Whether the total abstinence from red meat leads to a decreased colorectal cancer incidence has not been clarified, because there are studies with opposing results.[49] Fried, barbecued, and processed meats are also associated with colorectal cancer risk, especially risk for rectal cancer, with an odds ratio of 6.[42,50]

Although high protein intake may augment carcinogenesis, definitive proof of this is lacking. Mechanistically, a high-protein diet is associated with accelerated epithelial proliferation.[51]

Fatty components of red meat may be tumor promoters, because fats may be metabolized by luminal bacteria to carcinogens,[45,52] which would cause abnormal colonic epithelial proliferation. There is controversy as to whether the type of fat is important. Some studies suggest that saturated animal fats may confer especially high risk,[21,45] yet other investigations suggest

TABLE 29.8-1. Etiology of Colon Cancer: Environmental Factors

Increased Incidence	*Decreased Incidence*
High-calorie diet	Antioxidant vitamin consumption
High red meat consumption	
Overcooked red meat consumption	Consumption of fresh fruit and vegetables
High saturated fat consumption	Use of nonsteroidal antiinflammatory drugs
Excess alcohol consumption	High-calcium diet
Cigarette smoking	
Sedentary lifestyle	
Obesity	

Note: Coffee or tea consumption has no effect on incidence.

that there is no evidence for increased risk for any specific dietary fat after adjustment for total energy intake.[53]

FIBER. Classically, a high-fiber diet was associated with a low incidence of colorectal cancer in Africa,[54] with numerous studies substantiating this premise.[55,56] Protection was believed to be afforded by wheat bran, fruit, and vegetables.[48] A high-fiber diet was believed to dilute fecal carcinogens, decrease colon transit time, and generate a favorable luminal environment.[45] However, these canonical concepts have been challenged by more recent large, well-controlled studies that showed no inverse relationship between colorectal cancer and fiber intake.[48,57] In a study of nearly 90,000 women aged 34 to 59 years who were followed for 16 years, no protective association was noted between fiber intake and incidence of either adenomatous polyp or colorectal cancer.[57] This result was further corroborated by two large randomized controlled trials that evaluated consumption of high-fiber diets[58,59] for moderate duration and discovered a lack of effect on the number, size, and histologic characteristics of polyps found on colonoscopy. At this point, therefore, the majority of evidence suggests that dietary fiber does not play a role in the risk of developing colorectal cancer.

VEGETABLES AND FRUIT. Vegetable and fruit consumption is generally believed to have a protective effect against colorectal cancer.[21,45] This has been observed for raw, green, and cruciferous vegetables. Whether certain agents such as antioxidant vitamins (E, C, and A), folate, thioethers, terpenes, and plant phenols[60] may be applied in effective chemopreventive strategies requires further investigation, although the data for folate intake are sound.

Calcium also has been historically implicated as having a protective effect. Mechanistically, calcium can be viewed as being able to bind injurious bile acids with reduction of colonic epithelial proliferation.[45,61] This is supported through cell culture models. However, results of population-based studies are not definitive.[21,45]

Lifestyle

Physical inactivity has been associated with colorectal cancer risk,[13,21,45] for colon cancer more than for rectal cancer. A sedentary lifestyle may account for an increased colorectal cancer risk, although the mechanism is unclear.

Most studies have demonstrated a minimally positive effect of alcohol use on risk for colorectal cancer. Associations are strongest between alcohol consumption in men and risk of rectal cancer. Perhaps interference with folate metabolism through acetaldehyde is responsible.[62]

Prolonged cigarette smoking is associated with a higher risk of colorectal cancer.[21,45,63] Cigarette smoking for longer than 20 pack-years was associated with increased large adenoma risk and for longer than 35 pack-years with increased cancer risk.

No reproducible association has been found between the chronic use of either coffee or tea and colorectal cancer risk.[64,65]

Nonsteroidal Antiinflammatory Drugs

Population-based studies strongly support inverse associations between the use of aspirin and other nonsteroidal antiinflammatory drugs (NSAIDs) and the incidences of both colorectal cancer and adenomas.[66–69] In a cohort study,[70] the relative risk of colorectal cancer was 0.49 [95% confidence interval (CI), 0.24 to 1.0] for regular NSAID users compared with nonusers. Duration of NSAID use is important, and right-sided colon cancers may benefit more than left-sided colorectal cancers. Interestingly, the type of NSAID use was not important. As a result of this and other studies, use of NSAIDs and selective cyclooxygenase-2 (COX-2) inhibitors in familial adenomatous polyposis (FAP) and sporadic colorectal cancer has been investigated intensively.

BIOLOGY OF COLORECTAL CANCER: CLINICAL AND MOLECULAR GENETIC RISK FACTORS

Genetic factors play important roles in the initiation, development, and progression of adenomatous polyps and colorectal cancer (Table 29.8-2). The normal colonic epithelium involves an exquisite migration of cells from the proliferating crypt compartment (where stem cells reside) to differentiating surface colonocytes. Cells then are sloughed, and the intestinal epithelium is renewed every 5 to 6 days, which makes it very susceptible to the deleterious effects of chemotherapy and radiation therapy. Insights into the mechanisms that orchestrate cellular processes such as proliferation, differentiation, and apoptosis have been gained from developmental (embry-

TABLE 29.8-2. Familial and Nonfamilial Causes of Colorectal Cancer

SYNDROMES WITH ADENOMATOUS POLYPS
APC gene mutations (1%)
    Familial adenomatous polyposis
    Attenuated APC
    Turcot's syndrome (two-thirds of families)
MMR gene mutations (3%)
    Hereditary nonpolyposis colorectal cancer types I and II
    Muir-Torre syndrome
    Turcot's syndrome (one-third of families)
SYNDROMES WITH HAMARTOMATOUS POLYPS (<1%)
Peutz-Jeghers (*LKB1*)
    Juvenile polyposis (*SMAD4, PTEN*)
    Cowden (*PTEN*)
        Bannayan-Ruvalcaba-Riley syndrome
    Mixed polyposis
OTHER FAMILIAL CAUSES (UP TO 20–25%)
Family history of adenomatous polyps (*MYH*)
Family history of colon cancer
    Risk >3× if two first-degree relatives or one first-degree relative <50 y with colon cancer
    Risk 2× if second-degree relative affected
Familial colon-breast cancer
NONFAMILIAL CAUSES
Personal history of adenomatous polyps
Personal history of colorectal cancer
Inflammatory bowel disease (ulcerative colitis, Crohn's colitis)
Radiation colitis
Ureterosigmoidostomy
Acromegaly
Cronkhite-Canada syndrome

onic and neonatal) studies in the mouse as well as cell culture model systems. Gene overexpression or ablation in the mouse colon through transgenic or knockout approaches has revealed key concepts that are discussed here. The normal colonic epithelium or mucosa is a dynamic system. The progression to an intermediate adenomatous polyp and eventually to frank colorectal cancer, although studied intensively in cell culture and animal models, has natural platforms in inherited disorders. Thus, this subsection covers the inherited forms of human colorectal cancer and uses that as the bridge to an understanding of the pathogenesis of both inherited and sporadic colorectal cancer.

FAMILIAL ADENOMATOUS POLYPOSIS

FAP constitutes 1% of all colorectal cancers. Hallmark features include the development of hundreds to thousands of colonic polyps in patients in their teens to thirties, and if the colon is not surgically removed, 100% of patients progress to colorectal cancer. Extracolonic manifestations include various benign conditions—congenital hypertrophy of the retinal pigment epithelium, mandibular osteomas, supernumerary teeth, epidermal cysts, adrenal cortical adenomas, desmoid tumors (although these tumors may lead to obstruction)—as well as malignant conditions—thyroid tumors, gastric and small intestinal polyps with a 5% to 10% risk of duodenal or ampullary adenocarcinoma or both, and brain tumors.[71] The brain tumors may be of two types, glioblastoma multiforme or medulloblastoma, and the particular association of brain tumors with colonic polyposis is called Turcot's syndrome.[72] The colonic polyps in Turcot's syndrome are fewer and larger than in classic FAP. Patients with an attenuated form of FAP harbor up to 100 colonic polyps and have a predisposition to colorectal cancer when they are in their fifties or sixties.[73]

FAP is an autosomal dominant disorder with nearly 100% penetrance. However, approximately 30% of patients have *de novo* mutations and no apparent family history. Based on karyotypic analysis revealing an interstitial deletion on human chromosome arm 5q and subsequent genetic linkage analysis to 5q21, the gene responsible for FAP was identified as *APC* for *adenomatosis polyposis coli*. FAP patients inherit a mutated copy of the *APC* gene, which predisposes them to early-onset polyposis. During life, FAP patients acquire inactivation of the remaining *APC* gene copy, which accelerates the progression to colorectal cancer. Interesting genotypic-phenotypic associations exist between the location of the *APC* gene mutation and certain clinical manifestations such as congenital hypertrophy of the retinal pigment epithelium, desmoid tumors, and classic FAP versus attenuated FAP.

The *APC* gene comprises 15 exons and encodes a protein of nearly 2850 amino acids (310 kD). Nearly all germline mutations in the *APC* gene lead to a truncated protein, which can be detected through molecular diagnostic assays that can be integrated into genetic counseling and genetic testing of affected patients and at-risk family members.[74–76] The functions of the APC protein and the interrelated pathways and regulatory molecules are dealt with later in Pathogenesis of Sporadic Colorectal Cancer.

HEREDITARY NONPOLYPOSIS COLORECTAL CANCER

Hereditary nonpolyposis colorectal cancer (HNPCC) accounts for approximately 3% of all colorectal cancers. Salient features

TABLE 29.8-3.   Criteria for Diagnosis of Hereditary Nonpolyposis Colorectal Cancer

AMSTERDAM I CRITERIA
At least three relatives with colorectal cancer
One relative should be a first-degree relative of the other two
At least two successive generations should be affected
At least one colorectal cancer case before age 50 y
Familial adenomatous polyposis should be excluded
Tumors should be verified histopathologically

AMSTERDAM II CRITERIA
At least three relatives with HNPCC-associated cancer (colorectal, endometrial, small bowel, ureter, or renal pelvis)
At least two successive generations should be affected
At least one case before age 50 y
Familial adenomatous polyposis should be excluded
Tumors should be verified histopathologically

BETHESDA CRITERIA (FOR IDENTIFICATION OF PATIENTS WITH COLORECTAL TUMOR WHO SHOULD UNDERGO TESTING FOR MICROSATELLITE INSTABILITY)
Cancer in families that meet Amsterdam criteria
Two HNPCC-related cancers, including colorectal or extracolonic
Colorectal cancer and a first-degree relative with colorectal cancer and/or HNPCC-related cancer
Extracolonic cancer and/or colorectal adenoma: one cancer before age 45 y and adenoma before age 40 y
Colorectal cancer or endometrial cancer before age 45 y
Right-sided colorectal cancer before age 45 y with an undifferentiated pattern on histopathologic analysis
Signet-ring–type colorectal cancer before age 45 y
Adenoma before age 40 y

HNPCC, hereditary nonpolyposis colorectal cancer.

include the presence of up to 100 colonic polyps (hence, the term *nonpolyposis*), preferentially, albeit not exclusively, in the right or proximal colon.[77] There is an accelerated rate of progression to colorectal cancer in these diminutive, and at times flat, polyps with mean age of onset of colorectal cancer being 43 years. This is designated HNPCC type I. HNPCC type II is distinguished by extracolonic tumors originating in the stomach, small bowel, bile duct, renal pelvis, ureter, bladder, uterus and ovary, skin, and perhaps the pancreas. The lifetime risk of cancer in HNPCC is 80% for colorectal cancer, approximately 40% for endometrial cancer, and less than 10% for all other cancers.[78] Of note, a variant of HNPCC involves skin tumors and is designated as Muir-Torre syndrome. HNPCC is defined classically by the modified Amsterdam criteria (Table 29.8-3).

HNPCC is an autosomal dominant disorder with approximately 80% penetrance. Genetic and biochemical approaches led to the discovery of the involvement of human DNA mismatch repair genes in HNPCC. Recognized as the human orthologues of mismatch repair genes described in bacteria and yeast, human mismatch repair genes encode enzymes that repair errors during DNA replication, which may occur spontaneously or on exposure to an exogenous agent (e.g., ultraviolet light, chemical carcinogen). Mutation in one of these mismatch repair genes results in MSI, which creates a milieu of somatic mutations of target genes—*TGFβII* receptor, *bax*, and *IGF* type I receptor, among others—in HNPCC-associated tumors.[77] Approximately 60% of germline mutations in HNPCC are found in either the *hMLH1* gene or the *hMSH2* gene, but mutations in other members of this family—*hMSH6, hPMS1, hPMS2*—are rare, which indicates that

TABLE 29.8-4.   Genetic Testing in Inherited Colorectal Cancer

Familial adenomatous polyposis	APC protein truncating testing (preferred)
	If APC mutation found, screen for mutation in family
	Less desirable alternatives: gene sequencing, linkage testing
Hereditary nonpolyposis colorectal cancer	Microsatellite instability (MSI) testing in tumor[a]
	If MSI present, proceed to sequencing of both hMLH1 and hMSH2 genes
	If mutation found, screen for mutation in family
Peutz-Jeghers syndrome, juvenile polyposis, Cowden's disease	Gene mutation analysis

[a]Immunohistochemistry may be an option.

other genes are involved but have yet to be discovered. Genetic testing is not easy for HNPCC as it is for FAP but involves sequencing of both the *hMLH1* and *hMSH2* genes (Table 29.8-4). If a germline mutation is found, then the remaining family members at risk can be genetically screened. MSI testing and hMLH1/hMSH2 immunohistochemistry can be performed on tumor specimens as a possible prelude to genetic testing.

HAMARTOMATOUS POLYPOSIS SYNDROMES

Hamartomatous polyposis syndromes are rare, mostly affecting the pediatric and adolescent population, and represent fewer than 1% of colorectal cancers annually. Peutz-Jeghers syndrome involves large but few colonic and small bowel polyps that can manifest by gastrointestinal bleeding or obstruction and an increased risk of colorectal cancer. The polyps are distinguished by a smooth muscle band in the submucosa. Hallmark clinical features on physical examination include freckles on the hands, around the lips, in the buccal mucosa, and periorbitally. Associated characteristics include sinus, bronchial, and bladder polyps, and 5% to 10% of patients have sex cord tumors. Patients can also develop lung and pancreatic adenocarcinomas. The gene responsible for this syndrome is called *LKB1*, a serine threonine kinase.

Juvenile polyposis has overlapping clinical manifestations with Peutz-Jeghers syndrome, but the polyps tend to be confined to the colon, although cases of gastric and small bowel polyps have been described and there is an increased risk of colorectal cancer. Extracolonic manifestations are not prevalent. This is a polygenic disease involving germline mutations in *PTEN*, *SMAD4*, *BMPR1*, or other genes yet to be identified.

Cowden's disease harbors hamartomatous polyps anywhere in the gastrointestinal tract, and surprisingly, there is no increased risk of colorectal cancer. However, approximately 10% of patients have thyroid tumors and nearly 50% of patients have breast tumors. Germline *PTEN* mutations have been reported.

FAMILIAL COLORECTAL CANCER

It is estimated that 20% to 30% of colorectal cancers are compatible with an inherited predisposition, independent of known syndromes.[79] The identification of other responsible genes will have great clinical impact. Intensive approaches are being pursued through sibling-pair studies and other familial studies. As mentioned earlier in Inherited Predisposition, patients may be predisposed to an increased risk of adenomatous polyps as well in the context of a family history of sporadic adenomatous polyps.

PATHOGENESIS OF SPORADIC COLORECTAL CANCER

Insights gained from inherited colorectal cancer have been applied to sporadic colorectal cancer. Elegant studies have led to the elucidation of colorectal cancer progression as a paradigm for cancer biology and genetics in general. Taking advantage of the knowledge that the transition from normal colonic mucosa to adenomatous polyp to colorectal cancer may take over one decade, investigators have defined two genetic pathways. The first recognizes that because nearly 80% of adenomatous polyps harbor *APC* gene mutations, the APC protein has a gatekeeper function, and dysfunction of this protein leads to chromosomal instability. The APC protein associates with the β-catenin oncoprotein in the cytoplasm and together with glycogen synthase kinase-3β (GSK3β) transphosphorylates β-catenin to target it for degradation (Fig. 29.8-1A). However, in the context of *APC* mutation, β-catenin escapes degradation and is translocated into the nucleus, where it associates with transcriptional factors such as LEF and TCF, which act in concert to activate critical genes such as c-myc, cyclin D1, and peroxisome proliferator–activated receptor δ, among others. Thus, APC is a critical regulator of normal intestinal homeostasis.

As polyps enlarge, they acquire mutations in the *Ras* oncogene in 40% to 50% of cases. Ras-mediated signal pathways are abundant and crucial in cell proliferation, growth, and transformation (see Fig. 29.8-1B).

Frank colorectal cancer formation is associated with mutations in the *p53* and *SMAD4* tumor suppressor genes in approximately 80% of cases. Normally, wild-type p53 is engaged in constraining cell-cycle progression, regulating apoptosis, and responding to genotoxic stress. *SMAD4* is a critical downstream gene of the transforming growth factor-β (TGF-β) signaling pathway. Clearly, other genetic alterations are involved, and biochemical pathways are perturbed. In aggregate, the chromosomal instability pathway accounts for the preponderance of sporadic colorectal cancers, involving the intricate interplay between activation of oncogenes and inactivation of tumor suppressor genes. The accumulation of genetic alterations and the order in which they occur are important in this pathway. Seventy percent to 80% of adenomatous polyps and colorectal cancers harbor COX-2 overexpression, and COX-2 naturally inhibits apoptosis and promotes angiogenesis. COX-2 is a critical target of aspirin and other NSAIDs and has led to studies of the use of selective COX-2 inhibitors.

Likely approximately 15% of sporadic colorectal cancers are formed through an alternative pathway that is often called the MSI pathway. MSI occurs in the tumors, and mutations are acquired in target genes, which leads to aberrant growth and eventual malignant transformation. Thus, the genetic pathways that conspire to promote FAP and HNPCC converge to foster progression in sporadic colorectal cancer.

ANATOMY OF THE COLON

The colon and rectum make up the segment of the digestive system commonly referred to as the *large bowel*. Defined as the portion of intestine from the ileocecal valve to the anus, the

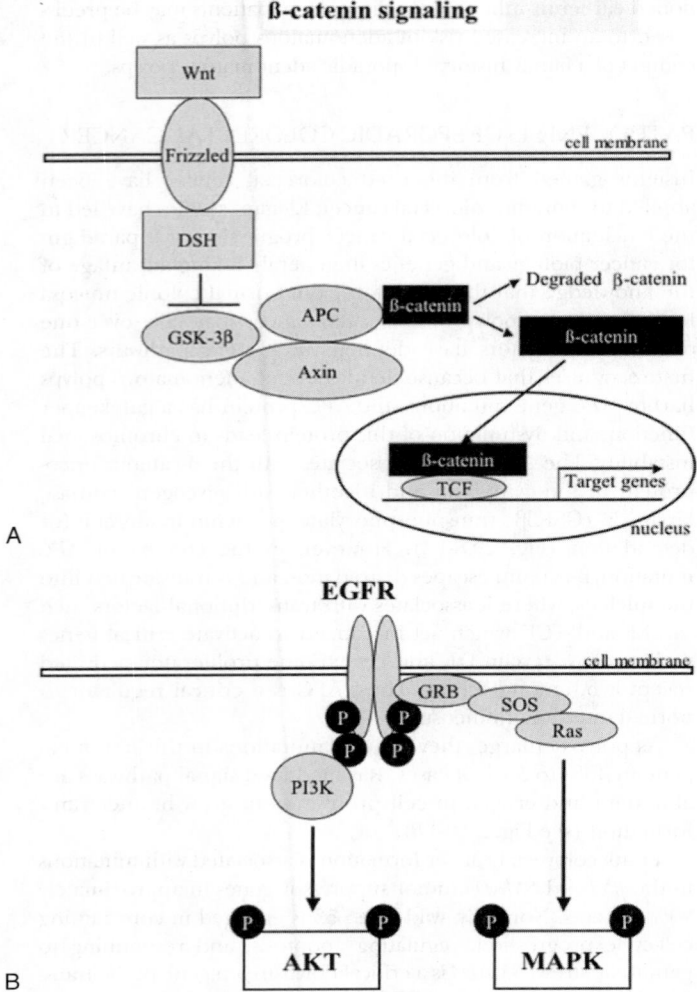

FIGURE 29.8-1. Molecular pathways in sporadic colorectal cancer pathogenesis. **A:** Wnt signaling and APC/β-catenin. **B:** The Ras oncogene and signaling cascades. EGFR, epidermal growth factor receptor; GSK-3β, glycogen synthase kinase-3β; MAPK, mitogen-activated protein kinase; PI3K, phosphatidylinositol 3 kinase; TCF, T-cell factor.

large bowel is approximately 150 cm in length. It is divided into five segments defined by vascular supply and by extraperitoneal or retroperitoneal location. These are (1) the cecum (with appendix) and ascending colon, (2) the transverse colon, (3) the descending colon, (4) the sigmoid colon, and (5) the rectum. The anatomy of the rectum is discussed in detail in Chapter 29.9. The large bowel has a muscular wall and can be distinguished from the small intestine by its increased diameter and the presence of haustra, appendices epiploica, and teniae coli. The teniae consist of condensations of longitudinal muscle fibers starting near the base of the appendix and continuing throughout the abdominal colon to form a continuous longitudinal muscle coat in the upper rectum. Haustra are outpouchings of bowel wall separated by folds that give a classic appearance on radiography or barium enema testing.

The right colon is made up of the cecum (with appendix) and ascending colon. It is anterior to the right kidney and the duodenum. Its vascular supply is from branches of the superior mesenteric artery (SMA). The SMA divides into the middle colic artery and the trunk of the SMA. The middle colic artery immediately forms two to three large arcades in the transverse mesocolon. The SMA ileocolic arterial branches then extend from the SMA. The right colic artery arises as a separate branch from the SMA in 10.7% of cases.[80] The ileocolic artery gives off a right colic artery to the upper ascending colon and forms an anastomosis with branches from the middle colic artery. The ileal branch of the ileocolic artery gives off branches to the distal small bowel and cecum, whereas the colic branch supplies the ascending colon. An anastomosis occurs between the distal SMA and the ileal branch of the ileocolic artery at the junction of the terminal ileum and cecum. The right colon is a retroperitoneal structure.

The transverse colon is supplied by branches of the middle colic artery. It is the first portion of the colon considered to be intraperitoneal, and its length can vary. Its boundaries are defined by the hepatic flexure on the right and the splenic flexure on the left. Both of these points are fixed. The hepatic flexure abuts the gallbladder fossa, whereas the splenic flexure lies anterior to the splenic hilum and the tail of the pancreas. The descending colon is where the colon once again becomes a retroperitoneal structure, and it is defined as the segment of colon from the splenic flexure to the sigmoid colon. The descending colon is the first segment of the left side of the colon and receives its blood supply from the inferior mesenteric artery (IMA). The IMA arises from the aorta and gives off the left colic artery. It also gives off three to four sigmoidal arteries, which supply the intraperitoneal sigmoid colon. The anastomosis between the vessels of the middle colic artery and those of the left colic artery and right colic artery is known as the marginal artery of Drummond. The arcade that effectively connects the left and right circulations is known as the arc of Riolan. The arterial supply to the colon is depicted in Figure 29.8-2.

The venous and lymphatic drainage of the colon parallels the arterial supply and all three vessels course and divide within the colonic mesocolon (Fig. 29.8-3). The mesocolon therefore contains the regional lymph nodes for the segment of colon it supplies and drains. The efferent lymphatic channels pass from the submucosa to the intramuscular and subserosal plexus of the bowel to the first tier of lymph nodes lying adjacent to the large intestine, which are known as *epicolic nodes*.[81] *Paracolic nodes* lie on the marginal vessels along the mesenteric side of the colon and are frequently involved in metastases. *Intermediate nodes* are found along the major arterial branches of the SMA and IMA in the mesocolon. The *principal nodes* are found around the origin of these vessels from the aorta, and they drain into retroperitoneal nodes. The drainage of the superior and inferior mesenteric veins, which drain the ascending, transverse, descending, and sigmoid colon, is to the portal vein. The rectum is drained by rectal tributaries to the vena cava.

The extent of resection of the colon is defined by the vascular supply and by the need to take the regional draining lymph nodes.[82–84] A careful understanding of the colonic anatomy, structure, location, and vascular supply is therefore critical to perform a safe and effective cancer operation. The segmental resections important for removal of lesions in various locations within the colon are described in greater detail later.

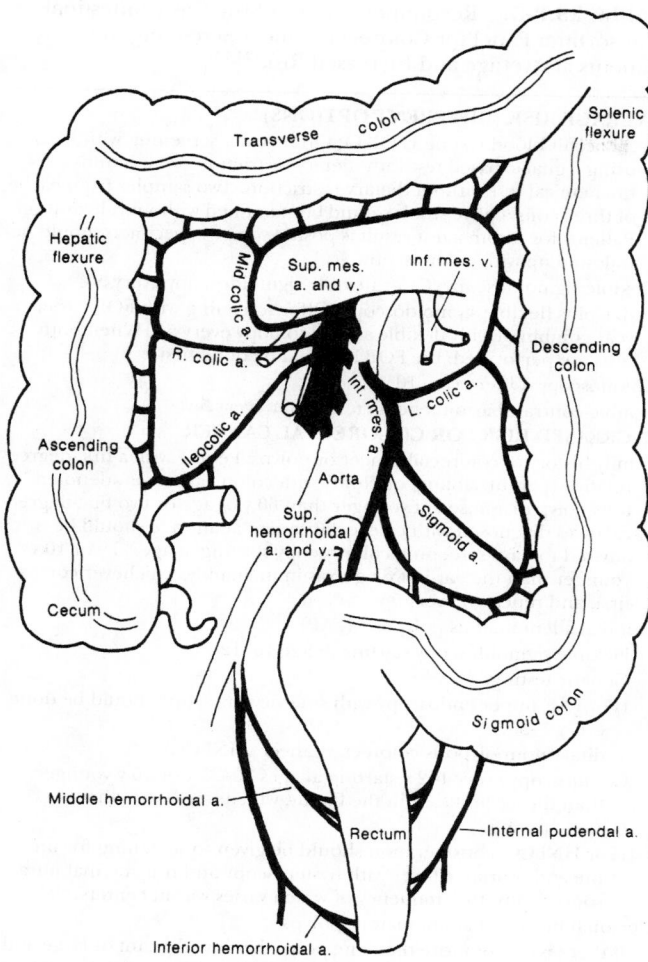

FIGURE 29.8-2. The anatomy of the colon with particular emphasis on the vascular supply.

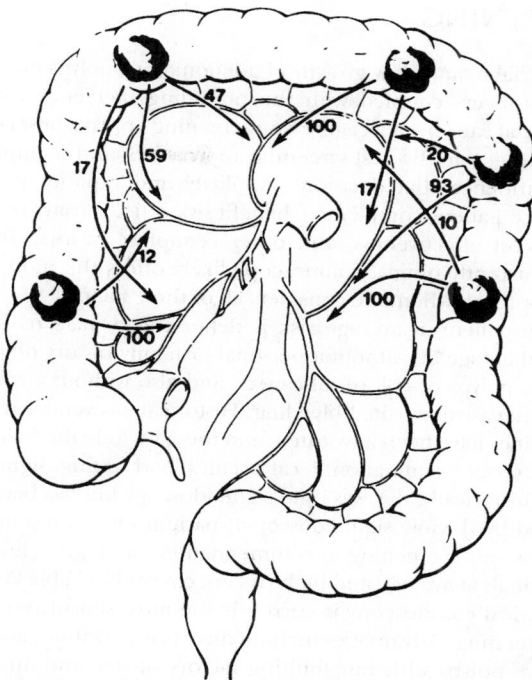

FIGURE 29.8-3. The lymphatic drainage of lesions in various anatomic locations throughout the colon. Numbers represent probability of following that drainage pattern.

DIAGNOSIS

Symptoms associated with colorectal cancer include lower gastrointestinal bleeding, change in bowel habits, abdominal pain, weight loss, change in appetite, and weakness; obstructive symptoms, in particular, are alarming.[85] However, apart from obstructive symptoms, the symptoms do not necessarily correlate with stage of disease or portend a particular diagnosis.[86] Close vigilance is important.

Physical examination may reveal a palpable mass, bright blood through the rectum (usually left-sided colon cancers or rectal cancer) or melena (right-sided colon cancers), or lesser degrees of bleeding (positive result on stool test for occult blood). Adenopathy, hepatomegaly, jaundice, or even pulmonary signs may be present with metastatic disease. Obstruction by colon cancer is usually in the sigmoid or left colon with resulting abdominal distention and constipation, whereas right-sided colon cancers may be more insidious in nature. Complications of colorectal cancer include acute gastrointestinal bleeding, acute obstruction, perforation, and metastasis with impairment of distant organ function.

Laboratory test values may reflect iron-deficiency anemia, electrolyte derangements, and liver function abnormalities.

Level of carcinoembryonic antigen (CEA) may be elevated and is most helpful in postoperative monitoring if the level is reduced to normal as a result of surgery.[87]

Evaluation should include complete history, family history, and physical examination, as well as laboratory tests, colonoscopy, and pan-body computed tomography (CT) scan[88]—the latter if metastatic disease is suspected after the primary diagnosis is made. On completion of the diagnosis and staging (endoscopic ultrasonography should be integrated for staging of rectal cancer), then incorporation of expertise from medical, radiation, and surgical oncologists is required to formulate and implement a treatment plan.

With the advent of molecular biologic techniques, attention has been drawn to stool-based tools and new blood-based tests. Technology now exists to extract genomic DNA or protein from stool and assay for evidence of genetic alterations.[89–93] Large-scale validation studies are in progress. Certainly, in patients with known large adenomatous polyps or colorectal cancer harboring genetic alterations, the same genetic alterations should exist ideally in the stool specimens. One particularly attractive pathway for stool-based diagnostics would be to be able to stratify patients as having high, moderate, or low risk for colorectal cancer, which would influence screening modalities and frequency of screening. In a complementary fashion, functional genomics is being applied to pairwise comparisons of normal colon and colorectal cancers to sample the entire human genome of nearly 30,000 genes to discover those genes, known and novel, that may be up-regulated or down-regulated and possibly linked to detection, prognosis, and therapy. Blood-based tests would certainly be attractive as well for the detection of disease and also for monitoring for recurrence after surgery or surgery with adjuvant therapy.

SCREENING

The variable and slow growth of adenomatous polyps and colorectal cancers coupled with the prevailing incidence rates of colorectal cancer merit aggressive screening approaches. Debate is vigorous as to the best screening approaches, and multiple factors influence that decision: simplicity and rapidity so as to enhance patient compliance, benefit-risk ratio, sensitivity, specificity, cost effectiveness, and other economic factors. To that end, currently optical colonoscopy likely offers the most effective approach when one considers all of these factors.

The patient at average risk is defined as a male or female older than age 50 without a personal or family history of adenomatous polyps or colorectal cancer, and also without any occult or acute gastrointestinal bleeding. Historically, several screening modalities have been advocated, and these include the following: digital rectal examination, fecal occult blood testing, sigmoidoscopy (historically, this was rigid sigmoidoscopy but has been supplanted by flexible sigmoidoscopy), barium enema testing, and colonoscopy. Screening recommendations and guidelines for individuals at average and high risk are covered in Table 29.8-5.

Optical colonoscopy is currently the most sensitive method for screening. Advantages include direct visualization, ability to remove polyps with rate-limiting factors of size and anatomic location, and ability to perform biopsy. Disadvantages involve the preparation required, the invasive nature of the procedure, and potential side effects, including perforation (although this has an incidence of less than 1%).

The digital rectal examination should be part of the general physical examination. Anorectal masses may be palpated. Flexible sigmoidoscopy does not require conscious sedation and hemodynamic monitoring, and typically allows visualization of the rectum, sigmoid colon, and descending colon to the splenic flexure. Flexible sigmoidoscopy should not be considered as a single screening measure but requires coupling with barium enema testing. Barium enema testing permits visualization of the entire colon, but experience is necessary to ensure proper visualization of the rectum. Barium enema testing affords the advantages of ease of preparation, lack of necessity for conscious sedation and hemodynamic monitoring, and ability to visualize polyps and masses. However, small polyps may be missed. Furthermore, if a luminal polyp or mass is identified, then colonoscopy will be necessary for polypectomy or biopsy or both.

New noninvasive technologies are investigational but are receiving attention in clinical studies, and these may provide some initial data demonstrating efficacy. These relate to CT colonography (referred to as "virtual" colonoscopy)[94–101] and even magnetic resonance colonography.[102,103] The findings of one study are consistent with the feasibility of virtual colonoscopy compared to optical colonoscopy,[103] although large-scale population studies are still needed.

STAGING AND PROGNOSIS

Many established factors provide useful prognostication, and many newer indicators appear promising, but only a limited number of criteria have been validated in large prospective trials. In this discussion the focus is primarily on those prognostic and predictive indicators that are best supported by available data and are appropriate for use and consideration in current

TABLE 29.8-5. Recommendations of the Gastrointestinal Consortium Panel for Colorectal Cancer Screening in Patients at Average and Increased Risk[424,425]

AVERAGE RISK (DIFFERENT OPTIONS)

Fecal occult blood testing (FOBT): Offer yearly screening with FOBT using a guaiac-based test with dietary restriction or an immunochemical test without dietary restriction. Two samples from each of three consecutive stools should be examined without rehydration. Patients for whom a test result is positive on any specimen should be followed up with colonoscopy.

Flexible sigmoidoscopy: Offer flexible sigmoidoscopy every 5 y.

FOBT plus flexible sigmoidoscopy: Offer screening with FOBT every year combined with flexible sigmoidoscopy every 5 y. When both tests are performed, the FOBT should be done first.

Colonoscopy: Offer every 10 y.

Double-contrast barium enema test: Offer every 5 y.

INCREASED RISK FOR COLORECTAL CANCER

Family history of colorectal cancer or polyps: People with a first-degree relative (parent, sibling, or child) with colon cancer or adenomatous polyp diagnosed at younger than 60 y of age or two first-degree relatives diagnosed with colorectal cancer at any age should be advised to have screening colonoscopy starting at age 40 y or 10 y younger than the earliest diagnosis in the family, whichever comes first, and repeated every 5 y.

Familial adenomatous polyposis (FAP)

    Flexible sigmoidoscopy starting at age 10–12 y.

    Genetic testing.

    (For FAP, upper endoscopy with side-viewing scope should be done every 1–3 y.)

Hereditary nonpolyposis colorectal cancer (HNPCC)

    Colonoscopy every 1–2 y starting at ages 20–25 y or 10 y younger than the earliest case in the family, whichever comes first.

    Genetic testing.

    (For HNPCC, consideration should be given to screening for uterine and ovarian cancer with hysteroscopy and transvaginal ultrasonography, the frequency of which varies within centers.)

Personal history of adenomatous polyps

    If there is one or more than one polyp that is malignant or large and sessile, or colonoscopy is incomplete, then follow-up colonoscopy in the short term.

    If three or more polyps, follow-up colonoscopy in 3 y.

    If one or two polyps (<1 cm), follow-up colonoscopy in 5 y (or longer).

Personal history of colorectal cancer

    If colonoscopy is incomplete at time of diagnosis of colorectal cancer due to obstruction, then repeat colonoscopy 6 mo after surgical resection.

    If colonoscopy is complete at time of diagnosis of colorectal cancer, then repeat colonoscopy in 3 y; if results are normal, then repeat every 5 y.

Inflammatory bowel disease (ulcerative colitis, Crohn's colitis): Surveillance colonoscopy is recommended.

---

practice. The reader should remain aware of the potential for rapid changes and advances in this area, however.

STAGING

Although many factors have been identified that impact recurrence and survival, none exceeds stage in terms of prognostic significance.[104] Staging of colorectal cancer should be done using the current TNM classification of the American Joint Committee on Cancer (AJCC) and International Union Against Cancer (UICC).[105] Other systems should be regarded as of historical significance only and must be comprehended solely for the purposes of understanding the studies that were performed and reported in the past using these older classifications.

Dukes' Classification and Its Modifications

In the 1930s Cuthbert Dukes, a Scottish pathologist working predominantly on a classification scheme for rectal cancer, developed the classification system that bears his name. This system, which has been widely applied to colon and rectal cancers alike, focuses on information obtained from pathologic examination of the surgical specimen. Tumors were classified as A, B, or C, with stage A indicating tumor restricted to, but not through, the bowel wall; stage B indicating penetration through the bowel wall; and stage C indicating spread to local and regional lymph nodes. Dukes subsequently modified his staging system, first dividing stage C into C1 (local lymph nodes involved) and C2 (lymph nodes at the point of ligature involved) and later adding a fourth stage (subsequently known as stage D) for distant metastasis.

Several investigators made modifications to the Dukes' classifications. In 1949, Kirklin et al. divided Dukes' stage A into a more restricted stage A (mucosal and submucosal involvement only) and a new B1, for disease that involved (but did not fully penetrate) the muscularis propria. The old stage B became B2.

Astler and Coller in 1954 addressed the issue of depth of tumor penetration in patients with positive lymph nodes, breaking stage C into stages C1 (node positive with primary tumor confined to the bowel wall) and C2 (node positive with tumor penetrating the full thickness of bowel wall). Gunderson and Sosin further modified the Astler-Coller system, subdividing tumors based on the presence of microscopic (B2m or C2m) and gross (B2m + g, and C2m + g) penetration through the bowel wall as well as creating stages B3 and C3 for tumors locally invasive into other structures.

Problems not adequately addressed by the Dukes' system or its modifications include lack of determination of adequacy of nodal sampling and lack of consideration of the extent of lymph node involvement. In an analysis of 844 node-positive patients reported by the National Surgical Adjuvant Breast and Bowel Program (NSABP),[106] the two most important prognostic factors were found to be depth of tumor penetration and the number of positive nodes, with patients with one to four positive nodes having a significantly better prognosis than those with greater numbers of involved nodes. The number of positive nodes appeared to be the single most important prognostic factor.

Another potential weakness of the original and modified Dukes' classifications (and most other staging schemes) was the lack of consideration of tumor grade and other pathologic features. Jass attempted to address this issue by assessing a number of histopathologic factors in a Cox regression model.[107] Lymphocytic infiltration was the only histologic variable to be accepted within the model. Number of affected lymph nodes and the depth of penetration of the primary through the bowel wall were also significant predictors. However, the criteria used by Jass for colorectal cancer have been found to be less than optimal in routine practice and are not readily reproducible.[108]

TNM (Tumor, Node, Metastasis) Classification

The current joint AJCC-UICC staging system for colorectal cancer is now the only classification system that should be used.[109] The TNM system classifies colorectal tumors on the basis of the

TABLE 29.8-6. TNM Classification of Colorectal Cancer

Stage	T	N	M
0	Tis	N0	M0
I	T1	N0	M0
	T2	N0	M0
IIA	T3	N0	M0
IIB	T4	N0	M0
IIIA	T1–T2	N1	M0
IIIB	T3–T4	N1	M0
IIIC	Any T	N2	M0
IV	Any T	Any N	M1

(Adapted from Greene FL, et al., eds. *AJCC cancer staging manual*, 6th ed. New York: Springer-Verlag, 2002.)

invasiveness (not size) of the primary tumor (T stage), the number (not size or location) of local and regional lymph nodes containing metastatic cancer (N stage), and the presence or absence of distant metastatic disease (M stage)[105] (Table 29.8-6).

T STAGE. *In situ* adenocarcinoma (Tis) includes cancers confined to the glandular basement membrane or lamina propria. The terms *high-grade dysplasia* and *severe dysplasia* are synonymous with *in situ* carcinoma and are also classified as Tis. T1 tumors invade into but not through the submucosa. T2 tumors invade into but not through the muscularis propria, and T3 tumors invade through the muscularis propria into the subserosa or into nonperitonealized pericolic or perirectal tissue. T4 tumors invade other named organs or structures (T4a) or perforate the visceral peritoneum (T4b). Tumors invading other colorectal segments by way of the serosa (i.e., carcinoma of the cecum invading the sigmoid) are classified as T4a. A tumor that is adherent to other structures or organs macroscopically is classified clinically as T4a; however, if the microscopic examination of the adhesions is negative, then the pathologic classification is pT3. The V and L substaging should be used to identify the presence or absence of vascular or lymphatic invasion. The "p" prefix denotes pathologic (rather than clinical) assessment and the "y" prefix is attached to those tumors that are being reported after neoadjuvant (presurgical) treatment. For example, the pathologic T stage of a tumor showing only penetration into the submucosa after preoperative therapy would be ypT1. Recurrent tumors are reported with an "r" prefix (rpT3).

N STAGE. Because of the prognostic significance associated with increased numbers of lymph nodes inspected (discussed later), the current TNM classification scheme calls for at least 7 to 14 lymph nodes to be analyzed, and both the number of nodes that are positive for tumor and the total number of nodes inspected should be reported. A pN0 designation may be made even if fewer than the recommended number of nodes are present; however, the prognostic significance of this pN0 designation is weaker. N0 denotes that all nodes examined are negative. N1 includes tumors with metastasis in one to three regional lymph nodes. N2 indicates metastasis in four or more regional lymph nodes. Metastatic nodules or foci found in the pericolic, perirectal, or adjacent mesentery without evidence of residual lymph node tissue are regarded as being equivalent to a regional node metastasis and are counted accordingly.

Stage I disease is defined as T1 to T2N0 disease in a patient without distant metastases (M0). Stage II disease is defined as T3 to T4N0M0. The T stage carries prognostic significance for stage II, and therefore T3N0 is classified as stage IIA and T4N0 is classified as stage IIB.

Node positivity in the absence of M1 disease defines stage III colorectal cancer. The prognostic significance of tumor invasiveness (T stage) has now been reincorporated into the assessment of risk in patients with stage III disease. In an exhaustive review of over 50,000 patients, Greene et al. demonstrated the prognostic significance of T stage in node-positive patients.[110] Within the N1 category (one to three positive lymph nodes) T stage was found to be highly prognostic, with patients with T1 or T2 disease faring significantly better than those with T3 or T4 tumors. Within the N2 population (four or more positive nodes), the prognosis was worse than for either subgroup of N1 patients, with T stage no longer carrying prognostic significance. Thus, T stage is prognostic for patients with N0 and N1 disease but not for those with N2 disease. The current TNM staging system takes these findings into account and now stratifies stage III disease into IIIA (T1 to T2N1), IIIB (T3 to T4N1), and IIIC (any T, N2). Stages IIIA, IIIB, and IIIC are highly prognostic for survival.

M STAGE. Patients are designated as having M0 disease if no evidence of distant metastases is present. Identification of distant metastases denotes a classification of M1. Involvement of the external iliac, common iliac, paraaortic, supraclavicular, or other nonregional lymph nodes is classified as distant metastatic (M1) disease.

RESIDUAL TUMOR (R STAGE) AT MARGINS OF RESECTION. Tumors that are completely resected with histologically negative margins are classified as R0. Tumors with a complete gross resection but with microscopically positive margins are classified as R1, with the positive margin indicating that at least microscopic tumor remains in the patient. Patients having incomplete resections with grossly positive margins are classified as having had an R2 resection. The R0, R1, and R2 designations carry strong prognostic implications.

Identification of the proximal and distal margins of resection is relatively straightforward, and definitions of these margins are well understood. A more complex and often misunderstood (as well as underreported) margin of resection is the circumferential radial margin, or CRM. All three margins (proximal, distal, and CRM) should be specifically commented on in the pathology report, as all three have prognostic significance.

The CRM is, by definition, a surgically dissected surface. It is defined as the cut retroperitoneal or perineal soft tissue margin closest to the deepest penetration of tumor. It is considered positive if tumor is present microscopically (R1) or macroscopically (R2) on a *cut* radial or lateral aspect of the surgical specimen. For the ascending colon, descending colon, and upper rectum, which are incompletely encased by peritoneum, the CRM is created by dissection of the retroperitoneal aspect of the bowel. In the case of the lower rectum, which is not encased by peritoneum, the CRM is created by sharp dissection of the mesorectum.

Simple penetration of a tumor into pericolonic or perirectal fat does not necessarily constitute a positive CRM, but rather is simply a description of a T3 primary. Tumor involvement of a peritonealized surface of the bowel and no involvement of a surgically cut surface does not constitute a positive CRM, but rather constitutes a T4b primary. If, however, the cut surface at the deepest penetration of the tumor is positive, then the CRM is positive and the resection is staged R1 (microscopic) or R2 (macroscopic). A positive CRM is highly predictive of local recurrence and should prompt consideration of adjuvant treatment.

HISTOLOGIC GRADE

Although histologic grade has been shown to have prognostic significance, there is significant subjectivity involved in scoring of this variable, and no one set of criteria for determination of grade is universally accepted.[104] The majority of staging systems divide tumors into grade 1 (well differentiated), grade 2 (moderately differentiated), grade 3 (poorly differentiated), and grade 4 (undifferentiated). Many studies collapse this into low grade (well to moderately differentiated) and high grade (poorly differentiated or undifferentiated). Greene et al. demonstrated that grade determined according to this two-tiered split has important prognostic significance.[110]

COLLEGE OF AMERICAN PATHOLOGISTS CONSENSUS STATEMENT

The College of American Pathologists (CAP) has published an expert panel consensus statement outlining its interpretation of the validity and usefulness of a large number of putatively prognostic and predictive factors in colorectal carcinoma.[109] Variables were categorized as belonging to categories I through IV. Category I is defined as those factors proven to be of prognostic import based on evidence from multiple statistically robust, published trials and generally used in patient management. Category IIA includes factors intensively studied biologically or clinically or both and repeatedly shown to have prognostic value for outcome or predictive value for therapy that is of sufficient import to warrant inclusion in the pathology report but that remain to be validated in statistically robust studies. Category IIB includes factors shown to be promising in multiple studies but for which sufficient data are lacking for inclusion in category I or IIA. Category III includes factors felt to be not yet sufficiently studied to determine their prognostic value, and category IV includes those factors that have been adequately studied and have convincingly shown no prognostic significance. A number of these factors are discussed in further detail later.

The T, N, and M categories of the current AJCC-UICC staging system were all classified as category I factors. Other category I inclusions were blood or lymphatic vessel invasion and residual tumor after surgery with curative intent (the R category). Although not assessed pathologically, an elevation of the preoperative CEA level was also felt to merit category I inclusion. Factors in category IIA included tumor grade, radial margin status (for resection of specimens with nonperitonealized surfaces), and residual tumor in the resection specimen after neoadjuvant therapy. Factors in category IIB (many of which are discussed in further detail later) included histologic type, histologic features associated with MSI (i.e., host lymphoid response to tumor and medullary or mucinous histologic type), high degree of MSI (MSI-H), loss of heterozygosity

(LOH) of 18q (DCC gene loss), and tumor border configuration (infiltrating vs. pushing border). Factors grouped in category III included the following: DNA content, all other molecular markers except LOH of 18q/DCC and MSI-H, perineural invasion, microvessel density, tumor cell–associated proteins or carbohydrates, peritumoral fibrosis, peritumoral inflammatory response, focal neuroendocrine differentiation, nuclear organizing regions, and proliferation. Those factors included in category IV (proven to be of no significance) include tumor size and gross tumor configuration.

TOTAL NUMBER OF LYMPH NODES

It has been well established that an adequate number of lymph nodes must be sampled before a patient can be considered node negative. Metastases in lymph nodes may frequently be less than 5 mm in diameter, which makes them easy to overlook. Careful pathologic technique has been demonstrated to be crucial to adequate nodal interpretation. Failure adequately to dissect and display the mesentery leads to underreporting and under-staging.[111,112] It should be noted that reporting of an insufficient number of lymph nodes could be due to a suboptimal nodal dissection at operation, a less than thorough search for nodes by the pathologist, or some combination of the two.

Wong et al. analyzed the pathologic features of 196 colorectal cases and concluded that at least 14 nodes should be evaluated in each specimen in order to provide adequately reliable staging.[112] A much larger analysis was reported on outcome versus nodal sampling in the patients who participated in Intergroup trial INT 0089, a large four-arm trial of different fluorouracil-based adjuvant chemotherapies in colon cancer patients. Multivariate analyses were performed on the node-positive group (2768 patients) and node-negative group (648 patients) separately. The median number of lymph nodes reported for the assessable patients in this trial was 11 (range, 1 to 87). Survival (overall, cancer specific, and disease free) was found to decrease with increasing number of involved lymph nodes (P = .0001 for all three survival end points). However, after the number of involved nodes was controlled for, survival was found to increase with the total number of nodes (positive plus negative) reported (P = .0001 for overall survival, cancer-specific survival, and disease-free survival). Even in patients who were node negative, overall survival (P = .0005) and cancer-specific survival (P = .007) increased significantly as the number of reported lymph nodes increased.

In a different secondary analysis of Intergroup INT 0089, a mathematical model was created to estimate the probability of a true node-negative result on the basis of the number of lymph nodes examined in a subset of patients who had at least ten lymph nodes reported in their resection specimen.[113] A total of 1585 patients with stage III or high-risk stage II colon cancer were evaluated. This model concluded that, when 18 nodes are examined, there is a less than 25% probability of true node negativity in T1 and T2 tumors. However, examination of fewer than ten lymph nodes was needed in T3 and T4 tumors to achieve the same probability. The overall conclusions of this analysis were that disease is under-staged in a very significant proportion of patients and that such under-staging could have important implications for decisions regarding adjuvant therapy and for overall prognosis.

Tepper et al. analyzed data from 1664 patients with T3, T4, or node-positive rectal cancer treated in national Intergroup trial INT 0114.[114] The number of nodes reported was significantly associated with time to relapse and survival among patients who were node negative. For the first through fourth quartiles, the 5-year relapse rates were 0.37, 0.34, 0.26, and 0.19 (P = .003), and the 5-year survival rates were 0.68, 0.73, 0.72, and 0.82 (P = .02). No significant differences were found in this analysis by quartiles among patients who were node positive. The authors suggested that the differences noted were likely to be related primarily to erroneously declaring a patient node negative on the basis of insufficient analysis. These authors concluded that approximately 14 nodes need to be studied to define nodal status accurately.

The CAP consensus statement suggests that a minimum of 12 to 15 lymph nodes should be examined to determine node negativity.[109] Availability of fewer nodes should therefore be regarded as a relative high-risk factor in terms of prognosis and should be factored into decisions regarding adjuvant therapy.

MICROSCOPIC NODAL METASTASES

The advent of improved pathologic techniques and sensitive methods such as immunohistochemistry or polymerase chain reaction (PCR) may have an impact on the number of positive lymph nodes detected[115] and may have important prognostic significance.[116] However, the prognostic value of these positive lymph nodes, which otherwise would not be detected, remains controversial. Jeffers et al. used immunocytochemical staining for cytokeratin AE1:AE3 to evaluate lymph nodes from 77 patients who were found to have negative lymph nodes by routine examination.[117] Nineteen patients (25%) were found to have immunohistochemical evidence of micrometastases; however, there was no difference in survival between patients with microscopically positive and negative nodes. Of course, the limited size of this analysis precludes detection of subtle differences in outcome. Although intuitively the presence of micrometastases detected by either immunohistochemical or reverse transcriptase-PCR (RT-PCR) techniques would seem to carry the prognostic risk associated with nodal positivity, to date such findings are not universally accepted as having prognostic significance, and for staging purposes nodes that harbor individual tumor cells or micrometastases are classified as being negative for tumor.[109,118] It is currently recommended that nodes with tumor foci of 0.2 to 2.0 mm be classified as positive, with an accompanying addendum stating that the biologic and prognostic significance of this finding is unknown.[109,118] If micrometastases are reported, the methodology by which they are detected should be specified, because it is likely that differences in reliability and reproducibility of different techniques will emerge. Although the actual TNM staging is not altered by the presence of micrometastases, many clinicians choose to regard the presence of such a finding as a poor prognostic variable in their consideration of adjuvant treatment.

SENTINEL NODE ANALYSIS

Sentinel node analysis is an approach that has received attention in the management of cutaneous melanoma and breast cancer.[119,120] This technique has been proposed as a means of increasing the yield and the diagnostic information for colon cancer.[121–123]

The technique for sentinel node mapping and biopsy for colon cancer has been described by Saha and colleagues.[124]

Briefly, a dye is injected subserosally around the tumor without injecting the lumen. The first to fourth blue nodes identified are considered the sentinel nodes and are submitted as such for multilevel microsections and analysis. A standard cancer operation is then performed. Unlike sentinel node approaches for melanoma and breast cancer, in which the goal is to potentially limit the extent of an unnecessary formal dissection of a node basin, the goal of the sentinel node technique in colon cancer is to focus the pathologic analysis on fewer nodes so that a more extensive study can be performed. The same extent of node dissection is performed regardless of the use of the sentinel node procedure. However, given the large number of nodes resected, focusing the pathologist on a few "high-risk" nodes may be time and cost effective.

The initial studies of sentinel node biopsy demonstrated that it was technically feasible and, in some cases, resulted in the up-staging of disease.[121,123,125] However, not all subsequent studies have shown equivalent results. False-negative rates as high as 60% have been reported, and some studies have failed to demonstrate any change in the stage determination of the lesion.[126,127]

The technique of sentinel node biopsy for melanoma was first described by Morton et al. of the John Wayne Cancer Institute,[119] and a multicenter phase II trial of sentinel node biopsy for colon cancer was performed at that institution.[128] The study was based on the observation that 30% of patients with TNM stage I or II colorectal cancer developed systemic disease. The investigators hypothesized that by using sentinel node biopsy to identify the first group of draining lymph nodes and performing an RT-PCR–based analysis of those nodes, they could effectively up-stage early-stage lesions to account for this high degree of systemic disease. This study was conducted as a multicenter study, and 40 patients with primary colorectal cancer underwent a dye-directed lymphatic mapping at the time of their colon resection. Each dye-stained "sentinel node" was tagged, and then the tumor and regional nodes were resected using a standard *en bloc* colon resection. All lymph nodes were examined with conventional hematoxylin and eosin (H&E) staining, and in addition each sentinel node was sectioned for cytokeratin immunohistochemical staining and for RT-PCR analysis. The RT-PCR markers that were studied included human choriogonadotropin-β, hepatocyte growth factor receptor, and a universal melanoma-associated antigen. The investigators also, whenever possible, performed an additional RT-PCR analysis on the primary tumor tissue for comparison.

The authors found that 1 to 3 sentinel nodes could be identified in each patient with an average of 15 nodes removed for each colorectal specimen. When the sentinel nodes were found to be negative on histopathologic examination, no non-sentinel nodes were found to have evidence of tumor. Among the 40 patients in the study, H&E staining of sentinel nodes identified tumor in 10 patients (25%), and cytokeratin immunohistochemistry of sentinel nodes identified occult micrometastasis in 4 patients (10%) whose sentinel nodes were negative by H&E. Of the remaining 26 patients without evidence of sentinel node involvement by H&E or immunohistochemistry, 12 (46%) had positive RT-PCR results. The authors found that the number of markers expressed in each sentinel node correlated with the T stage of the primary tumor. They concluded that the identification and focused examination of the sentinel node is a novel method of gauging colorectal cancer spread and that

RT-PCR and cytokeratin immunohistochemistry identified occult micrometastasis in 53% of patients whose sentinel nodes were negative by conventional staging techniques. The sentinel node was the only positive node in 7 of the 40 cases.

One of the problems with evaluating studies of sentinel node biopsy for colorectal cancer is the fact that different techniques for both the performance of the procedure and analysis of the nodes are used at different centers. Some surgeons prefer to perform an *in vivo* mapping in which dye is injected around the lesion and the node is dissected just before resection of the specimen, whereas others prefer to use an *ex vivo* method in which the dye injection and node harvest is performed after the resection has been completed. Furthermore, the analysis of the nodes varies from H&E and immunohistochemical analysis of sections to H&E, immunohistochemical analysis, and RT-PCR techniques. Furthermore, the markers that are examined by both immunohistochemical and RT-PCR techniques vary.

Based on the available data, two conclusions can be reached. First, from a technical standpoint, sentinel node dissection at the time of a colon resection can be performed and the sentinel node accurately identified. Second, the usefulness of this technique has not yet been established.

BLOOD OR LYMPHATIC VESSEL INVASION

Although there have been conflicting reports in the literature, the CAP consensus statement gave blood and lymphatic vessel invasion category I status, which indicates that the preponderance of evidence strongly supports the reliability of these findings as indicators of poorer prognosis.[109] Unfortunately, considerable heterogeneity exists in the methodology for examining for and reporting vessel involvement. The finding of vessel involvement increases with the number of sections examined, and differentiation of postcapillary venules from lymphatics is often not possible. These aspects can make interpretation of some older data on this topic potentially problematic. Current recommendations are that, for each of at least three blocks of tumor (optimally five or more), a single section be examined using H&E stain to look for tumor invasion of vessels. Vessels not definitively interpreted as venules or lymphatics should be reported as angiolymphatic vessels.

HISTOLOGIC TYPE

Several histologic types of colorectal cancer carry specific independent prognostic significance. In signet-ring carcinomas, more than 50% of cells demonstrate the signet-ring morphology in which intracellular mucin accumulation displaces the nucleus and cytoplasm toward the cellular periphery. This histologic type carries an adverse prognosis.[129,130]

The prognostic significance of the finding of mucinous carcinoma (more than 50% mucinous) remains controversial. Although some reports list mucinous type as an adverse histologic feature, this has not been consistently demonstrated. Most findings of adverse prognosis with mucinous histologic type are based on univariate analyses. The one finding in a multivariate analysis of a poor prognostic outcome with mucinous tumors was based on a study of tumors presenting with obstruction, a presentation that is in itself high risk. Some reports have lumped mucinous and signet-cell tumors together and found this to be a negative prognostic factor; however, this may simply reflect the negative impact of the signet-cell tumors, and its meaning regarding the risk of a mucinous histologic type is unclear.

Small cell (extrapulmonary oat cell) tumors are high-grade neuroendocrine tumors with clearly adverse prognostic features. The prognostic significance of focal neuroendocrine differentiation is unclear, however (CAP category III). Most data indicate that extensive neuroendocrine differentiation is associated with a poorer prognosis.[131]

Medullary carcinoma is a subtype characterized by an absence of glands and distinctive growth pattern that previously would have been classified as undifferentiated. It is typically infiltrated with lymphocytes. This histologic subtype is tightly associated with high MSI (MSI-H), and carries a more favorable prognosis.[132] Histologic types other than signet-ring, small cell, and medullary carcinomas are routinely designated in the pathology report; however, the majority of these other histologic types carry no established independent prognostic significance.

MICROSATELLITE INSTABILITY

As discussed earlier in Pathogenesis of Sporadic Colorectal Cancer, there are two distinct mutational pathways that can give rise to colorectal cancer: the MSI pathway and the chromosomal instability pathway. Microsatellites are sections of DNA in which a short sequence of nucleotides (most commonly a dinucleotide) is repeated multiple times.[133] MSI is a situation in which a microsatellite has gained or lost repeat units and so has undergone a change in length, which results in frameshift mutations or base-pair substitutions or both. Approximately 15% of colorectal cancers display these mutations. This form of genetic destabilization is typically associated with defective DNA mismatch-repair function. Studies of HNPCC tumor specimens demonstrated mutations in mismatch repair genes such as MLH1 and MSH2. These genes encode proteins that repair nucleotide mismatches. The phenotype of tumors with this defect is termed the *high-frequency MSI phenotype* (MSI-H).

The majority of colorectal cancer patients (approximately 85%) have cancers characteristic of the chromosomal instability pathway, typically with genetic alterations involving LOH, chromosomal amplifications, and chromosomal translocations. These are known as the microsatellite-stable (MSS) tumors. MSI-H tumors have a number of different features relative to low-MSI (MSI-L) or MSS colorectal tumors.[134,135] MSI-L and MSS tumors tend to behave and present similarly.[27] MSI-H tumors are more frequently right-sided, high grade, and mucinous type.[27,136] They are characteristically associated with increased peritumoral lymphocytic infiltration and are characteristically diploid, whereas MSS tumors are more likely to be aneuploid.[137,138] Patients with MSI-H colorectal cancer are more likely to have a larger primary at the time of diagnosis but are more likely to be node negative. Patients with MSI-H colorectal cancer have a better long-term prognosis than stage-matched patients with cancers exhibiting MSS.[139]

Watanabe et al. evaluated MSI status as well as allelic loss from 18q, 17b, and 8p, as well as cellular levels of p53 and p21$^{\text{WAF1/CIP1}}$ proteins as potential prognostic markers.[140] Tumors were analyzed from 460 patients with stage III and high-risk stage II disease who had been treated with fluorouracil-based

adjuvant therapy. Sixty-two of 298 tumors evaluated for MSI status (21%) were found to be MSI-H. Of the MSI-H tumors, 38 (61%) had a mutation of the gene for the type II receptor of TGF-β1. In this analysis, MSI-H was a favorable prognostic indicator for 5-year disease-free survival (P=.02) and showed a trend toward being a favorable independent prognostic indicator for overall survival but did not reach statistical significance (P=.20). However, the 5-year survival among patients with MSI-H tumors was 74% in the presence of a mutated gene for the type II receptor of TGF-β1 and 46% in patients whose tumors lacked this mutation (relative risk, 2.90; 95% CI, 1.14 to 7.34; P=.04). MSI-H cells are relatively resistant to 5-fluorouracil (5-FU) *in vitro*.[141] All of the patients in the analysis of Watanabe et al. received 5-FU–based chemotherapy. The TGF-β1 pathway inhibits tumor proliferation by causing a late G_1 cell-cycle arrest. Therefore, a mutated, and presumably nonfunctional, TGF-β1 gene could favor increased proliferation, which would be anticipated to confer increased susceptibility to cytotoxic chemotherapy.

Ribic et al. investigated the usefulness of MSI status as a predictor of benefit from fluorouracil-based adjuvant chemotherapy in 570 patients with stage II and III disease from five randomized trials in which a no-treatment control arm was used.[142] Tumors exhibiting MSI-H were found in 95 patients (16.7%), MSI-L tumors in 60 patients (10.5%), and MSS tumors in 415 patients (72.8%). In the 287 patients who did not receive adjuvant chemotherapy, those with tumors exhibiting MSI-H had superior 5-year survival compared to patients with MSI-L or MSS tumors (hazard ratio, 0.31; P=.004). In the population of patients who received adjuvant chemotherapy, there was no difference in survival between the patients with MSI-H tumors and those with non–MSI-H tumors (P=.8).

In the patients with MSI-L or MSS tumors, chemotherapy resulted in improved survival compared to no chemotherapy (hazard ratio, 0.72; P=.04). However, chemotherapy did not improve survival in the patients with MSI-H tumors (Table 29.8-7).

Chemotherapy was associated with improved outcome in patients with both stage II and stage III disease with MSS or MSI-L, with a hazard ratio of 0.67 (95% CI, 0.39 to 1.15) in patients with stage II disease and 0.69 (95% CI, 0.47 to 1.01) in patients with stage III cancer. In contrast, in patients with MSI-H tumors, treatment did not improve survival and in fact was associated

TABLE 29.8-7. Microsatellite Instability Status versus Outcome with 5-Fluorouracil–Based Adjuvant Chemotherapy

	No. of Patients	5-Y Disease-Free Survival (%)	P Value
ALL PATIENTS			
Adjuvant chemotherapy	285	70	
No adjuvant chemotherapy	287	62	.06
PATIENTS WITH MSI-L/MSS			
Adjuvant chemotherapy	230	70	
No adjuvant chemotherapy	245	59	.01
PATIENTS WITH MSI-H			
Adjuvant chemotherapy	53	69	
No adjuvant chemotherapy	42	83	.11

MSI-H, high level of microsatellite instability; MSI-L, low level of microsatellite instability; MSS, microsatellite stable.
(From ref. 142, with permission.)

with a trend toward worse outcome for both stage II cancer (hazard ratio for death, 3.28; 95% CI, 0.86 to 12.48) and stage III cancer (hazard ratio, 1.42; 95% CI, 0.36 to 5.56).

These findings, if corroborated, would potentially provide a powerful predictive tool that could be used for the selection of patients for treatment and for the selection of different treatments for patients with MSI-H tumors versus those with non–MSI-H tumors. The authors of these trials appropriately caution, however, that these findings, although intriguing, require confirmation before being applied in routine practice.

ALLELIC LOSS OF 18Q (DCC GENE LOSS)

Allelic loss (LOH) involving chromosome arm 18q occurs in half or more of all colorectal cancers. Allelic loss of 18q typically involves the DCC (deleted in colon cancer) gene; however other genes in this region, such as *SMAD2* and *SMAD4*, may also be relevant to colorectal cancer development. DCC expression is greatly reduced or absent in many colorectal carcinomas, and loss of DCC is associated with metastasis and an adverse prognosis.[143] The specific product of the DCC gene has been shown to be the netrin-1 receptor. In the nonpathologic state this receptor guides the migration of neuronal axons. DCC induces apoptosis in the absence of netrin-1 binding. DCC is cleaved by caspase, and mutation of the site at which caspase 3 cleaves DCC suppresses the proapoptotic effect of DCC completely. Binding of netrin-1 to DCC blocks apoptosis.[144] Loss of DCC as a result of allelic loss in 18q could therefore be anticipated to impair apoptosis, which results in greater resistance to chemotherapy. This hypothesized mechanism of action of 18q LOH is attractive; however, it should be emphasized that it is not at all clear to what extent DCC is the active moiety in the setting of 18q allelic loss.

Watanabe et al. evaluated allelic loss from chromosome arm 18q as a potential prognostic indicator in archived specimens of tumors from patients who were treated in one of two national Intergroup adjuvant trials (INT 0035 or INT 0089).[140] MSI status was also evaluated, as were 17p, 8p, and cellular levels of p53 and p21^{WAF1/C1P1} proteins. Tumors were analyzed from 460 patients with stage III and high-risk stage II disease who had been treated with fluorouracil-based adjuvant therapy. Allelic loss of 18q was present in 155 of 319 cancers (49%). Allelic loss in 18q was highly prognostically significant in this analysis (Table 29.8-8). In patients with stage III tumors with allelic loss of 18q, 5-year overall survival was 50%, whereas in those with tumors with retained 18q alleles, 5-year survival was 69% (*P* = .005). Other markers evaluated in this analysis were not shown to be prognostically significant.

TABLE 29.8-8. Loss of Heterozygosity (Allelic Loss) at 18q (DDC Gene) and Prognosis in Patients with Stage III Colon Cancer

Allelic Status of 18q	No. of Patients	5-Y Survival (%)	P Value
No loss	112	69	.005
Loss	109	50	.005

(From ref. 140, with permission.)

In another series of 118 patients with stage II and III colon cancer, 18q allelic loss was again shown to be an adverse indicator of prognosis. This was particularly true of the patients with stage II disease, in whom the 5-year disease-free survival rate in those with tumors showing 18q allelic loss was only 54%. Patients with stage II disease whose tumor had no 18q allelic loss demonstrated an excellent clinical outcome, with a 5-year disease-free survival rate of 96%. In a multivariate analysis, 18q allelic loss was a significant independent poor prognostic factor for both disease-free and overall survival.[145]

HOST LYMPHOID RESPONSE

Lymphocytic infiltration has been identified as a favorable prognostic indicator. Whether this is a truly independent predictor of outcome is not clear, however, because this finding is tightly associated with MSI-H, a favorable prognostic factor.

TUMOR BORDER CONFIGURATION

The configuration of the tumor border (infiltrating vs. pushing border) has been shown to have independent prognostic significance. An infiltrating border, characterized by an irregular, infiltrating pattern at the tumor edge (also known as *focal dedifferentiation* or *tumor budding*) has been shown in multivariate analyses to portend a poorer prognosis than tumors with smooth, pushing borders.

CARCINOEMBRYONIC ANTIGEN

An elevated preoperative level of CEA is a poor prognostic factor for cancer recurrence. Although there is variability in the available data regarding the level that denotes a prognostic cutoff, a preoperative CEA level above 5 ng/mL is considered a category I poor prognostic indicator by the CAP consensus panel.[109] Patients in whom elevated CEA levels fail to normalize after a potentially curative operation are at particularly high risk. Several authors have presented evidence indicating that CEA is an independent prognostic factor. In a report of 572 patients who underwent curative resection for node-negative colon cancer,[146] the preoperative CEA level and the stage of disease predicted survival by both univariate and multivariate analysis. Given the prognostic significance of the preoperative CEA level, it is reasonable to recommend that all patients undergoing operation for colorectal cancer have serum CEA level measured before operation.

No other serum markers have been demonstrated to be reliably prognostic or predictive in colorectal cancer. Carbohydrate antigen 19-9 (CA 19-9), a factor that has become widely used in pancreatic cancer, has no role at this time in the routine management of colorectal cancer.

OBSTRUCTION AND PERFORATION

Carcinoma of the colon that is complicated by obstruction or perforation has been recognized as having a poorer prognosis. Data obtained from 1021 patients with Dukes' stage B and C colorectal cancer who were entered into randomized clinical trials of the NSABP showed that the presence of bowel obstruction strongly influenced the outcome. The effect of bowel obstruction was more pronounced when the obstruction was located in the right colon. The larger-sized tumor needed to block the ascending colon completely might allow a longer time for these tumors to grow and spread compared with tumors located in the descending colon.

A review of the Massachusetts General Hospital records compared patients presenting with obstruction or perforation with a control group undergoing curative resection. The actuarial 5-year survival rate in patients presenting with obstruction was 31%, in contrast to 59% in historical controls. For patients with localized perforation, the 5-year actuarial survival rate was 44%. The Gastrointestinal Tumor Study Group (GITSG) multivariate analysis concluded that obstruction was an important indicator of prognosis, independent of Dukes' stage. Bowel perforation was a poor prognostic factor only for disease-free survival.

CATEGORY III FACTORS

Multiple factors, although of investigational interest, are at this time not appropriate for routine clinical use and have so been designated as category III (defined as not sufficiently studied to prove their prognostic value) by the CAP consensus panel. These include DNA content, or ploidy, and proliferation indices. Also included in category III are all molecular markers other than MSI and 18q deletions, such as thymidylate synthase (TS), dihydropyrimidine dehydrogenase (DPD), and p53 mutational status. Perineural invasion, microvessel density, tumor cell–associated proteins or carbohydrates, peritumoral fibrosis, peritumoral inflammatory response, and focal neuroendocrine differentiation are also category III factors. The area of molecular prognostic markers is one of particular activity, however, and it is anticipated that clinical trials that are now ongoing will shed light on these important areas.

PERINEURAL INVASION

The ability of colorectal cancers to invade perineural spaces as far as 10 cm from the primary tumor has long been described. Early reports suggested an increased disease recurrence rate and worse 5-year survival in patients with perineural invasion. Multivariate analyses have failed to show the prognostic significance of this finding. The CAP consensus panel classified perineural invasion as a category III factor (insufficient evidence to determine prognostic significance).

TUMOR SIZE AND CONFIGURATION

Studies have consistently shown that both the size and configuration of the primary tumor in colorectal cancer does not carry prognostic significance (CAP category IV). In a review of data for 391 patients, the mean diameter of Dukes' stage B2 tumors was actually greater than the mean diameter of stage C2 tumors ($P < .001$) and D tumors ($P < .05$). The size of the primary tumor showed no relationship to 5-year adjusted survival. These results were confirmed by the NSABP experience.[106] Tumor configuration is described as exophytic (fungating), endophytic (ulcerative), diffusely infiltrative (linitis plastica), or annular. The vast majority of studies have failed to show any of these configurations to have consistent independent prognostic significance. Linitis plastica has been related to a poor prognosis; however, this may be due to the signet-cell and other high-grade features of the tumors that are typically associated with this morphology.

HEMORRHAGE OR RECTAL BLEEDING

It has been speculated that tumors presenting with bleeding might be found earlier and therefore might be associated with a better prognosis. This has not been confirmed by data. In the GITSG multivariate analysis, the presence of melena or rectal bleeding showed a trend as a prognostic factor for prolonged survival but failed to reach statistical significance ($P = .08$). One large study found bleeding to be a favorable prognostic indicator on univariate analysis; however, this finding disappeared on multivariate analysis. Bleeding at presentation does not appear to carry any significance.

PRIMARY TUMOR LOCATION

Large retrospective reviews of data from the NSABP suggested that right-sided colon cancers carry a worse prognosis than left-sided ones. However, poorer prognosis for patients with disease in the left colon has also been reported. Several investigators report no difference based on the location of the primary tumor. The large GITSG colon cancer experience showed that tumor location (left, right, and rectosigmoid or sigmoid) was of low prognostic value.

ONCOGENES AND MOLECULAR MARKERS

Oncogenes and molecular markers are discussed extensively in Chapter 3. At present none of the markers under investigation has achieved adequate validity to permit routine clinical use. However, the study of molecular markers continues to progress and continues to advanced understanding of the development and treatment of colorectal cancer.

TS continues to be a major area of investigation. Data are conflicting on its prognostic significance; however, preliminary studies suggest that high TS levels may be predictive for resistance to 5-FU–based therapies.[149]

The *p53* gene located on chromosome arm 17p is a well-known tumor suppressor gene. Abnormal *p53* appears to be a late phenomenon in colorectal carcinogenesis. This mutation may allow the growing tumor with multiple genetic alterations to evade cell-cycle arrest and apoptosis. In a retrospective review of data for 141 patients with resected stage II and stage III colon carcinoma, a *p53* mutation was found to increase the risk of death by 2.82 times in patients with stage II disease and by 2.39 times in patients with stage III colon carcinoma. The Southwest Oncology Group (SWOG) assessed the prognostic value of p53 in 66 patients with stage II and 163 patients with stage III colon cancer. Expression of *p53* was found in 63% of cancers and was associated with favorable survival in stage III but not stage II disease. Seven-year survival with stage III disease was 56% with *p53* expression versus 43% with no *p53* expression ($P = .012$).[150] Overall, the data are conflicting on the usefulness of p53 as a prognostic variable, and it does not have a use at this time in standard practice.

GENETIC POLYMORPHISMS

Extensive preliminary work is indicating that genetic polymorphisms can potentially have important predictive implications in terms of both efficacy and toxicity of chemotherapy. For example, the UGT1A1 polymorphism has been correlated with irinotecan (CPT-11) toxicity, and TS and XRCC1 polymorphisms may predict efficacy for oxaliplatin-fluorouracil combinations. These approaches require considerable more validation before they can be considered for standard management, however.[151]

BODY MASS INDEX

Obesity is known to be a risk factor for the development of colon cancer. The influence of body mass index (BMI) on long-term outcomes and treatment-related toxicity was investigated in a group of colon cancer patients. A cohort study was conducted within a large randomized trial of 3759 men and women with high-risk stage II or stage III colon cancer (INT 0089). Obese women with colon carcinoma had significantly worse overall mortality, with a hazard ratio of 1.34 (95% CI, 1.07 to 1.67). BMI was not, however, related to long-term outcomes in men in this cohort. In both men and women, obese patients had significantly lower rates of grade 3 and 4 leucopenia and lower rates of any grade 3 or greater toxicity in comparison with those patients in normal weight categories.

DIABETES MELLITUS

The same population of patients was studied to determine the influence of diabetes mellitus on outcome.[147] At 5 years, patients with diabetes mellitus, compared with patients without diabetes mellitus, experienced a significantly worse disease-free survival (48% vs. 59%; P <.0001). Overall survival was also worse for diabetic patients (57% vs. 66%; P <.0001 and recurrence-free survival was also worse (56% vs. 64%; P = .012). Median survival for diabetic patients was 6.0 years, whereas for nondiabetic patients it was 11.3 years.

BLOOD TRANSFUSION

Considerable controversy has surrounded the question of an association between perioperative blood transfusions and the recurrence rate of colorectal cancer. Some investigators have reported worse disease-free survival in patients who require transfusions. By multivariate analysis in a large prospective study, however, no negative influence of transfusion on survival could be detected, and it does not appear that the need for perioperative blood transfusions carries negative prognostic value. A retrospective analysis evaluating 1051 patients treated with curative surgery for stage II or III colorectal adenocarcinoma at the Mayo Clinic demonstrated that the use of blood components probably had no impact on disease recurrence, and the documented adverse impact of transfusions is more likely due to other variables or to the underlying illness necessitating the transfusion.[148]

APPROACHES TO SURGICAL RESECTION OF COLON CANCER

The management of colon cancer is best understood as a multimodality approach tailored to the stage of disease. However, there are certain basic tenets of surgical management for the resection of the primary lesion that can be applied across various pathologic stages. Therefore, so that a clear description of these techniques can be provided, they are first described based on the type of surgical resection. These procedures are then referred to throughout the discussion of stage-specific treatment.

COLONOSCOPIC RESECTION OF POLYPS

Many lesions of the colon are first detected during endoscopic procedures. These lesions can range from small hyperplastic polyps to large fungating invasive carcinomas. The appearance of these lesions often indicates their relative potential for malignancy. However, the only definitive way to make a diagnosis is through a pathologic examination of the tissue. Therefore, the goal of a colonoscopic biopsy or resection is, whenever feasible, to remove the lesion in its entirety and preserve tissue architecture to achieve both a therapeutic resection and an accurate pathologic diagnosis. Various techniques can be used for the removal of lesions in the colon depending on their size and location. Biopsy forceps and snares are the two instruments most commonly used during a colonoscopy. These devices are fashioned from flexible coated wires that can conform to the shape of the colonoscope and can also conduct bipolar electrical current to achieve coagulation and hemostasis.

Small polypoid lesions that are found during the course of a colonoscopic examination can often be removed in their entirety along with a small amount of normal mucosa using a biopsy forceps. Small amounts of bleeding can be controlled with bipolar electric cording. This is important, because bipolar cautery avoids deep tissue injury that may put the patient at risk for colonic perforation or bleeding. Bleeding and perforation, although uncommon, are seen at an increased frequency during a therapeutic as opposed to a diagnostic colonoscopy.[152,153] Small polyps of up to 5 to 8 mm can be removed very easily with these techniques. Larger, well-pedunculated polyps can often be removed using a snare and electrocautery technique. The snare is placed over the polypoid lesion and cinched down at the base of the polyp. Once it is tightened, an electrical current is applied and the polyp is resected. These polypoid lesions are often too large to be retrieved through the working port of the colonoscope and therefore are held in place with a snare just beyond the tip of the colonoscope where they can be kept in view and are then withdrawn from the patient along with the scope. It is important when sending these specimens to the pathology laboratory to properly orient the polyp so as to indicate the base where the resection took place as well as the other positions of the lesion. This allows the pathologist to provide important information regarding the margin status for the resection. Carcinomas *in situ* as well as stage I invasive carcinomas found in a well-pedunculated polyp can be treated with colonoscopic resection as described earlier, and no further surgical management is necessary as long as the margin of the invasive carcinoma can clearly be seen to be away from the electrocautery artifact at the base of the polyp.[152,153] If this distinction cannot be clearly made, further therapy is required. For this reason, it is often helpful to mark the site of the polyp resection with an agent that will leave a "tattoo" at the point of resection.

For larger lesions with a broad base or sessile lesions, a biopsy is best performed to make a diagnosis rather than resection using the colonoscope. The risk of perforation or inadequate resection margins is greatly increased for broad-based and sessile lesions. Multiple biopsy specimens should be taken to determine whether or not the lesion harbors an invasive cancer, and further resection decisions should be based on the pathologic findings. If such a lesion is left behind, it is of critical importance to note the position of the lesion so that it can be more easily found if a subsequent procedure is required. In addition to a determination of the depth of insertion of the scope, other landmarks should be used to more precisely pinpoint the lesion's location. Landmarks such as haustra, the appendiceal orifice or ileocecal valve in the cecum, or positions within the sigmoid loop can be especially helpful given the inaccuracies of a length measurement using a flexible instrument. In rare cases fluoroscopy can be used to precisely pinpoint the tip of the scope in relationship to its position within the colon.[154,155]

For lesions that cannot be resected through the scope or are found to be invasive carcinomas that are sessile or broad based, a variety of surgical resections can be used depending on the position of the lesion and its T stage. It is important to keep in mind, however, that the formal staging of the lesion does not occur until after the resection is completed, and therefore if one suspects that an invasive carcinoma is present, one should perform a definitive oncologic resection.

For large polyps that are benign on biopsy but are too large to resect through the scope, a simple segmental resection can be performed at the time of an abdominal exploration. Typically, the polyp is located based on the preoperative colonoscopy reports and by careful palpation of the entire colon from the cecum to the peritoneal reflection. Once the lesion is palpated, a small colotomy can be performed opposite the base of the lesion to confirm that the lesion is indeed the polyp that had been noted preoperatively. A resection encompassing 5 cm on either side of the polyp can then be easily accomplished without the need to isolate major vessels, with removal of just the portion of mesentery supplying that segment of colon. A primary anastomosis can be performed using the surgeon's technique of choice. Comparisons of hand-sewn versus stapled anastomoses have been extensively discussed elsewhere.[156]

BOWEL PREPARATION

An important part of the preoperative regimen for a colon resection is the proper cleansing of the bowel to reduce the risk of postoperative complications as well as to allow for easier visualization during the procedure. A variety of regimens have been described and there are many that have demonstrated efficacy.[157,158] Although there are several choices in the literature, the basic components of bowel preparation are a mechanical cleansing of the bowel using a cathartic or volume-displacing agent and appropriate antibiotics administered both intraluminally and intravenously.[159,160]

ANATOMIC RESECTION

For stage I, II, or III invasive carcinomas of the colon, the surgical approach is dictated by the lesion's size and location in the colon.[82,161,162] The location determines what region of bowel is

removed, and the extent of its resection is dictated by its vascular and lymphatic supply.

Resection of the Right Colon

Lesions in the cecum and ascending colon are managed with a right hemicolectomy (Fig. 29.8-4*A* and *B*). The right colon is mobilized from the retroperitoneum by incising its retroperitoneal attachments with care taken to avoid injury to the ureter, inferior vena cava, duodenum, and gonadal vessels. The colon is mobilized from the ileum to the transverse colon with care taken at the hepatic flexure not to injure the gallbladder or duodenum. The ileocolic, right colic, and right branches of the middle colic vessels are then ligated and divided. A proximal ligation to allow for the removal of colonic mesentery along with lymph nodes is performed for staging purposes. Once the vascular supply is divided and the intervening mesenteric tissue is ligated and divided as well, attention can be addressed to the resection of the colonic tissue.

There are a variety of techniques for dividing the colon. This can be done between clamps using a scalpel or using a variety of stapling devices. One method is to use a linear gastrointestinal anastigmatic stapler (GIA stapler). After making a small hole just below the colonic wall through the mesentery at the point chosen for resection, the stapler can be positioned across the colon and fired to divide the tissue. This procedure is then repeated across the ileum just proximal to the ileocecal valve. Once the colon is divided, all remaining mesenteric tissue is carefully ligated and divided, and the colonic specimen can be removed. Although a no-touch technique has been advocated in the past, studies have demonstrated that this has no influence on recurrence or seeding of distant disease.[163] Once the right colon is removed, intestinal continuity can be reestablished by creating an anastomosis between the terminal ileum and the remaining transverse colon using either a hand-sewn or stapled technique.[156]

Resection of the Transverse Colon

For lesions located in the transverse colon, a variety of approaches can be undertaken. Those lesions that are proximal and near the hepatic flexure can be resected with an extended right hemicolectomy. This extension should encompass up to and including the middle colic vessel. The advantages of such a resection over a true transverse colectomy are that the anastomosis performed to restore intestinal continuity involves an anastomosis between the ileum and the remaining colon. Due to the improved blood supply delivered by the small bowel mesentery, there is a decreased risk of an anastomotic leak in an ileocolic compared to a colocolic anastomosis.[156] Likewise, a lesion in the distal transverse colon can be resected with an extended left hemicolectomy, which is described in more detail later in Resection of the Descending Colon. For those lesions that are in the midportion of the transverse colon, however, a transverse colectomy can be performed. This procedure requires a mobilization of the right colon to allow this tissue to be brought over for an anastomosis after the resection.

The omentum is divided from the greater curvature of the stomach up to and including its attachments at the splenic hilum. The omentum can often be a source of micrometastatic

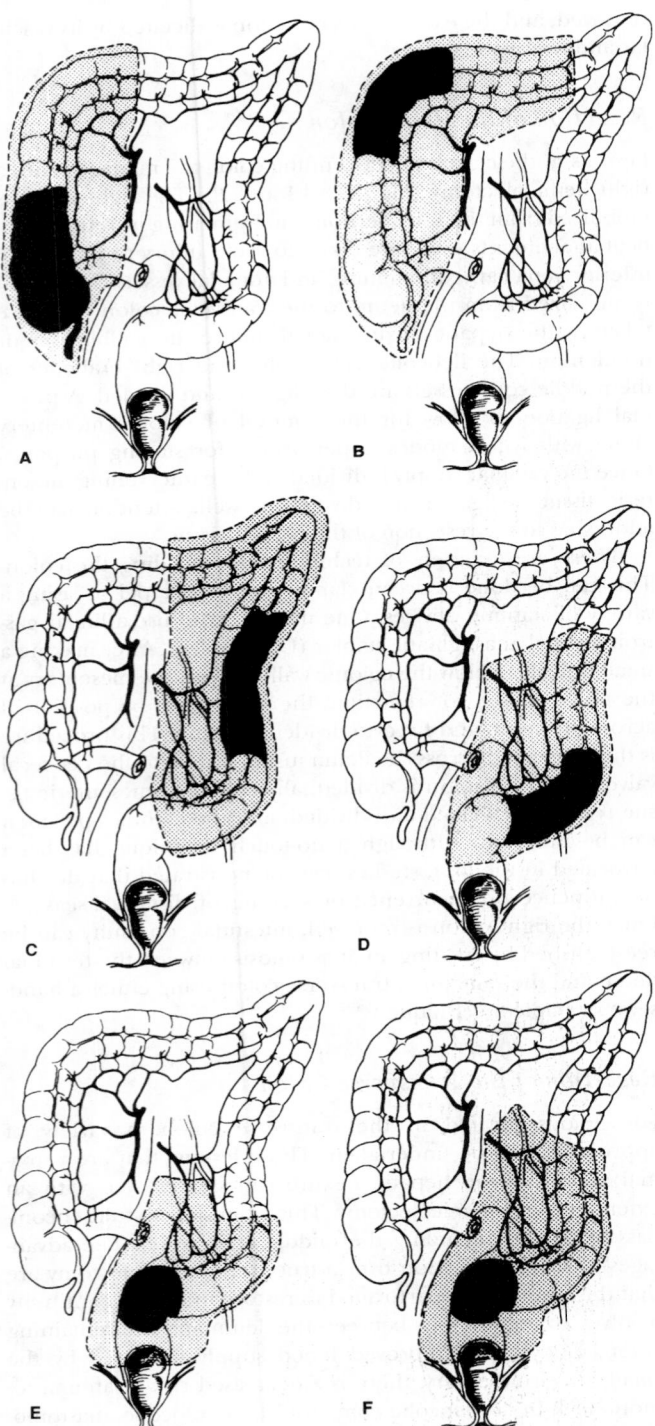

FIGURE 29.8-4. **A:** Surgical resection for a cecal or ascending colon cancer. **B:** Surgical resection for a cancer at the hepatic flexure. **C:** Surgical resection for a descending colon cancer. **D:** Preferred surgical procedure for cancer of the middle and proximal sigmoid colon. In poor-risk patients, the inferior mesenteric artery and the left colic artery may be preserved. **E:** Surgical resection for cancer of the rectosigmoid. **F:** A more radical surgical resection for cancer of the rectosigmoid. (Modified from Enker WE. Surgical treatment of large bowel cancer. In: Enker WE. *Cancer of the colon and rectum.* Chicago: Year Book, 1978:73.)

disease, and therefore its resection at the time of transverse colectomy is indicated. After division of the omentum and mobilization of the right and transverse colon up to and including the splenic flexure, the middle colic artery is ligated at its trunk and smaller vessels from the right and left colic artery branches can be ligated and divided as required. A linear stapler can once again be used to divide the colonic tissue and then the mobilized right colon can be anastomosed to the descending colon in an end-to-end fashion using a hand-sewn anastomosis or a side-to-side stapling technique. Depending on the size of the transverse colon, however, it is often safer and easier to resect the right and transverse colon and connect the ileum to the descending colon. This allows enough colonic reserve for water absorption and normal bowel movements.

Resection of the Descending Colon

For lesions in the proximal descending colon, the splenic flexure is mobilized and the left colic artery can be ligated and divided and the portion of colon removed by mobilizing the splenic flexure and dividing the omentum (see Fig. 29.8-4C and D). The transverse colon can be brought over to the region of the sigmoid colon for anastomosis. For lesions involving the sigmoid colon, a sigmoid colectomy can be performed. More extensive left hemicolectomies for sigmoid lesions have not resulted in improved survival.[164]

The sigmoid colon can be resected with margins on either side of the lesion after mobilizing the descending colon and splenic flexure. The descending colon can then be connected to the rectum using either a hand-sewn technique or a stapling device. For lesions in the midportion of the descending colon, a left hemicolectomy can be performed with care taken to ligate the left colic vessel along with some sigmoidal branches and an adequate portion of mesentery taken for staging purposes. The approaches to the resection of lesions below the peritoneal reflection are discussed in Chapter 29.9.

Total Abdominal Colectomy

For patients with ulcerative colitis or familial polyposis syndrome who either have evidence of invasive carcinoma or are at significant risk for the development of invasive carcinoma, a total abdominal colectomy may be required. This can be performed by mobilization of the right colon, mobilization of the transverse colon along the omentum with the omentum taken as part of the resection, mobilization of the hepatic and splenic flexures, and complete mobilization of the descending colon down to the peritoneal reflection. Ligation of the ileocolic, right colic, middle colic, left colic, and sigmoid branches allows for removal of the colon down to the peritoneal reflection. For patients with ulcerative colitis and familial polyposis syndromes without evidence of carcinoma below the peritoneal reflection, the operation can be terminated at this point with an ileorectal anastomosis and careful surveillance of the remaining rectum via proctoscopy. However, to remove all tissue at risk for further lesions, a total proctocolectomy is often advocated.[165–167] Although this procedure can be performed as an abdominal perineal resection with a permanent end ileostomy, most surgeons now advocate one of many continent pull-through procedures to preserve fecal continence in a patient population that is often very young. Such procedures provide very good control of continence and a relatively normal lifestyle.[168–170]

SURGICAL MANAGEMENT OF COMPLICATIONS FROM PRIMARY COLON CANCER

Patients with primary lesions of the colon can present with obstruction, bleeding, and perforation. The surgical management of these patients can be complex, requiring intraoperative decisions tailored to the situation encountered. Blood per rectum can be one of the most frightening experiences for patient and physician alike. Bleeding from a colorectal cancer can occur anywhere from the cecum to the distal rectum. Although bleeding can be temporized with endoscopic fulguration and the patient supported with transfusion, definitive management of the lesion with either surgery or radiation therapy will ultimately be required. Other maneuvers such as angiographic embolization may provide only a temporary solution. Fortunately, life-threatening hemorrhage due to a colon cancer primary is a rare occurrence. More often these lesions lead to a chronic blood loss resulting in anemia.

Colonic obstruction due to a primary tumor is not uncommon. Obstructing colonic lesions present several important issues.[171] First, the acute obstruction must be managed. An exploration with resection of the tumor and primary anastomosis with or without a diversion is ideal. However, given the fact that the operation will be performed on unprepared bowel and that the patient's physical condition may be less than optimal, resection without an anastomosis and an end colostomy should be considered. In some instances the obstructing lesion may present significant technical hurdles for resection in the setting of an acutely dehydrated and ill patient. In these circumstances a decompression maneuver that can be performed rapidly and with minimal morbidity such as a transverse loop colostomy or a colostomy and mucous fistula can be performed to temporize the situation and allow the patient to be prepared and resuscitated adequately for a definitive resection at a second exploration.

In situations in which a lesion is unresectable or in which there is significant spread of tumor throughout the peritoneum or into contiguous organs that cannot be resected, an internal bypass can be considered to relieve the obstructing process. However, a bypass operation should be reserved for only the most extreme circumstances, because complications after these procedures due to repeated obstructions and leakage with abdominal sepsis are not insignificant.

LAPAROSCOPIC COLON RESECTION

Since its introduction into the field of general surgery for gallbladder resection, the use of laparoscopic surgery has found increasing applications.[172] Laparoscopic surgery has become a particularly important addition to the armamentarium of the surgical oncologist. The use of laparoscopy for the staging of the extent of disease for peritoneal malignancies, pancreatic cancer, colon cancer, and gastric cancer is now widely accepted.[173–175] Laparoscopic resection has also found a niche for the removal of adrenal tumors, the spleen, and the distal pancreas.[176,177] The use of laparoscopic approaches for the resection of malignant lesions in the colon, however, has been met with mixed enthusiasm.

Concerns ranging from inadequacy of resection margins, inadequacy of lymph node sampling, and the potential seeding of port sites with malignant cells have been raised.[178,179] Although these concerns are important, there are several potential advantages for laparoscopic approaches to the surgical management of colon cancer. Issues regarding length of incision, patient recovery time, and return to bowel function are often cited as justification for a laparoscopic approach. However, just as important are the technical advantages of surgery using laparoscopic systems. The improved visualization due to magnification provided by video laparoscopy allows one to perform much more intricate and careful dissections in the deep pelvis, which could potentially reduce postoperative morbidity from low anterior resections using a mesorectal excision technique. The ability to carefully trace vessels in the mesentery under magnification could improve the ability to perform high ligations to retrieve a greater number of lymph nodes for sampling.

The technical difficulties faced during laparoscopic resection of the colon relate, in general, to the size of the specimen being removed and the need to perform an anastomosis. Each of these can be overcome through careful placement of incisions for specimen removal as well as a judicious use of stapling devices to perform both intracorporeal and a combination of intracorporeal and extracorporeal anastomotic techniques. A number of studies looking at the relative risks and benefits of the laparoscopic resection of colon cancer have been performed or are ongoing.[180–183] The largest of these studies is a prospective randomized trial being conducted by the Clinical Outcomes of Surgical Therapy (COST) Study Group. This trial is currently under way at multiple institutions examining both the oncologic outcomes with respect to disease-free and overall survival and the impact of laparoscopic versus open surgery on patient recovery, pain management, and time to return of bowel function. Although the initial report on quality of life showed only a modest short-term benefit for laparoscopic resection versus a conventional open procedure,[184] the overall results of the trial with respect to oncologic outcomes have not yet been reported. Therefore, a definitive discourse on the usefulness of laparoscopic surgery for the management of primary colon cancer will have to await the results of this trial. However, several retrospective and prospective nonrandomized studies have been conducted looking at laparoscopic versus open resection for colorectal adenocarcinoma, and one can glean some information from these smaller investigations.

Over a period of 10 years the group at the Colon and Rectal Clinic of Orlando, Florida, performed a prospective nonrandomized study comparing laparoscopic to open resection for colorectal carcinoma. Laparoscopic resection was offered selectively if there was no large mass or invasion into the abdominal wall or adjacent organs, and if the patient did not have multiple prior operations.[180] All laparoscopic resections were performed with curative intent, and 20% of the patients whose procedures were converted to open resection were included in the laparoscopic resection group based on an intention-to-treat model. The study measured oncologic outcomes and compared them with those of a computer-selected case-matched open resection group using the case-matching variables age, gender, site of primary tumor (colon vs. rectum), and TNM stage. The group receiving laparoscopic resection was followed prospectively and the data were updated on a regular basis. Follow-up of these patients consisted of a combination of office visits, telephone calls, and a review of the U.S. Social Security Death Index Database. There were 172 patients in each group, and the groups were well matched for age, TNM stage, prior chemotherapy or radiation therapy, and site of the primary tumor (colon vs. rectum).

Thirty-day mortality was 1.2% in the laparoscopic resection group and 2.4% in the open resection group; however, this difference was not statistically significant. The local recurrence rate in the laparoscopic group was 3.5% compared to a local recurrence rate in the open group of 2.9%. The stage-for-stage overall 5-year survival rates for the two groups were similar, and the authors, although acknowledging drawbacks based on the nonrandomized nature of the study, concluded that there was no significant difference in outcome between use of a laparoscopic approach versus an open approach in the management of primary colon and rectal tumors. There was no formal cost analysis in this study, however, and therefore, although oncologic outcomes were no different between the two groups, it is impossible to determine whether one group was superior to the other with respect to other outcomes.

A case-matched comparison of clinical and financial outcomes after laparoscopic and open colorectal surgery has been performed.[179] The group at the Cleveland Clinic studied patients from a prospective database who had undergone laparoscopic or open colectomy and were matched for age, gender, and disease-related groupings. A group of 150 patients undergoing laparoscopic colectomy was compared to a matched group of patients undergoing open colectomy. No difference was found between the two groups in diagnosis, complications, or 30-day readmission rate. Although operating room costs were significantly higher for laparoscopic colectomy, this was offset by a decrease in the length of hospital stay, with an overall significant reduction in total costs. This was attributed mainly to a lower level of pharmacy, laboratory, and ward nursing expenses.

The ultimate role of laparoscopic resection in the management of colorectal cancer is yet to be determined. It is hoped that ongoing prospective randomized studies will shed some light on the relative risks and benefits as well as the relative costs of these two procedures. The question will remain, however, if the procedures are equivalent in these prospective studies, whether deviating from the accepted gold standard of open resection for the management of colorectal cancer will be warranted.

POLYPS AND STAGE I COLON CANCER

The management of polyps and stage I colon cancer is through surgical resection. Most cancer in polyps is not diagnosed until after the polypectomy is performed. Therefore, for pedunculated lesions, care should be taken to perform the resection at the junction of the stalk and the mucosa. Invasive early stage I cancer found in a polyp managed by polypectomy does not require further resection if the margin at the stalk is free of cancer.[185,186] Sessile lesions on which biopsy is performed and which are shown to harbor an invasive cancer should be managed with a segmental colon resection. Large polypoid lesions may also require a segmental resection.

Because the stage of the lesion is not determined until after the resection, all colon cancer lesions managed with a segmental resection should be approached the same. The type of resection is dictated by the location of the lesion as has been described in Approaches to Surgical Resection of Colon Cancer. After a complete resection of a stage I lesion, no further adjuvant therapy is required. For patients managed in this way, a 5-year survival of over 95% can be expected.[105,185,187] Lesions that recur were most likely improperly classified stage II or III lesions.

STAGE II AND STAGE III COLON CANCER

The primary management of stage II and III colon cancer is surgical resection using the techniques and approaches described earlier in Approaches to Surgical Resection of Colon Cancer. However, there is a significant risk of residual micrometastatic disease in these patients. Therefore, the role of treatment after resection of a primary colon cancer is to eradicate any residual micrometastatic disease that might be present. Put another way, patients with clinical stage I, II, or III colon cancer are at risk for having occult stage IV disease at a volume that is beneath the level of clinical detectability. The role of adjuvant therapy is to eradicate that microscopic metastatic disease. Because current diagnostic techniques are unable to identify those patients with or without micrometastases, patients at sufficient risk of clinical recurrence (sufficient risk of harboring micrometastases) are treated postoperatively while their residual cancer is small enough so that there is a chance of its being completely destroyed by currently available therapies.

Although patients with stage II cancer as a group have a lower risk of harboring micrometastases than patients with stage III cancer, the rationale behind treatment of these two groups is the same, and many of the trials on which current treatment decisions are based involved patients with both stage II and stage III disease. However, there remains significant controversy regarding the routine use of adjuvant chemotherapy in patients with stage II disease. The development of adjuvant chemotherapy for colon cancer is therefore reviewed for these stages together, and then differences in outcomes and recommendations are highlighted.

EARLY TRIALS

The earliest clinical trials of adjuvant chemotherapy in colon cancer were conducted in the 1950s using the limited arsenal of anticancer agents then available. Many of these agents are now known to have no meaningful activity in metastatic colorectal cancer and so would not be studied in the adjuvant setting today. The adjuvant trials of the 1950s through the mid-1980s tended to be small by current standards. Based perhaps on an unrealistically optimistic expectation of what magnitude of benefit might be achieved from the use of available chemotherapies, the size of the trials did not permit evaluation of more modest clinical benefits. A large metaanalysis of controlled randomized trials of adjuvant therapy published through 1986 indicated a nonsignificant trend toward an overall survival benefit, with a mortality odds ratio of 0.83 in favor of therapy (95% CI, 0.70 to 0.98).[188] This sobering analysis suggested that substantially larger trials would be needed to detect the modest advantages that available chemotherapies might afford.

LARGE-SCALE RANDOMIZED TRIALS

In the C-01 trial, the NSABP cooperative group randomly assigned 1166 patients with Dukes' B and C colon cancer to one of three arms: surgery alone, treatment with bacille Calmette-Guérin (BCG), or the MOF chemotherapy regimen of semustine (methyl CCNU), vincristine (Oncovin), and fluorouracil (5-FU).[189] There were no statistically significant differences between the BCG and surgery-only groups; however, the group treated with MOF had a significantly better disease-free and overall survival than the control group ($P = .02$ and $P = .05$, respectively). This trial was the first to demonstrate that postoperative chemotherapy could result in a survival advantage after resection of locally advanced colon cancer.

FLUOROURACIL PLUS LEVAMISOLE

Levamisole is an antihelminthic that is widely used in veterinary medicine to deworm sheep and cattle. Based on the observation of levamisole's *in vitro* enhancement of immune responses in animals undergoing immunization against *Brucella abortus*, levamisole was extensively investigated as an anticancer agent. Although the majority of these trials yielded negative results, encouraging preliminary data led to a trial of levamisole and levamisole plus fluorouracil in patients with resected colon carcinoma.[190] The results from this trial were encouraging for the levamisole/fluorouracil combination, which led to a large-scale confirmatory trial, INT 0035.

In this trial, 1296 patients (929 patients with stage III colon cancer and 318 patients with stage II cancer) were randomly assigned to receive either surgery alone, surgery followed by a 1-year course of 5-FU plus levamisole, or surgery followed by a 1-year course of levamisole alone.[191] Of the node-positive (stage III) patients treated with surgery alone, 44% remained alive and disease free at 5 years, compared with 61% of patients who received fluorouracil and levamisole. Treatment with levamisole alone had no significant effect. At a median of 6.5 years of follow-up, 5-FU plus levamisole reduced the death rate by 33% and the recurrence rate by 40% ($P = .0007$ and $P < .0001$, respectively).[192,193]

The results of adjuvant treatment for the patients with stage II disease on this trial were less encouraging. At a median follow-up of 7 years, disease-free survival was 79% for patients receiving levamisole plus fluorouracil and 71% for patients receiving surgery alone ($P = .10$). The overall survival was 72% in each arm of the study.[193] In 1990, on the basis of the results of INT 0035, the National Cancer Institute issued a consensus statement establishing adjuvant chemotherapy as the standard of care for patients with node-positive resected colon cancer, in the absence of medical or psychiatric contraindications to such treatment.[187]

FLUOROURACIL PLUS LEUCOVORIN

As trials were progressing with 5-FU plus levamisole in the adjuvant setting, leucovorin was achieving some modicum of success as a modulator of fluorouracil in metastatic disease.[281,284,286] This led to evaluation of fluorouracil plus leucovorin in the adjuvant setting. The NSABP C-03 trial randomly assigned 1081 patients with Dukes' B and C cancer to 1 year of treatment with either the MOF regimen (the superior arm of NSABP C-01 trial) or 5-FU plus leucovorin.[194] The overall survival at 3 years was superior for the 5-FU/leucovorin arm (84% vs. 77%; $P = .003$). Three-year disease-free survival also favored the 5-FU/leucovorin arm (73% vs. 64%; $P = .0004$). These results and the toxicity and secondary leukemias seen with MOF eliminated MOF from further consideration in treatment of colorectal cancer. Semustine has since been withdrawn from clinical development.

Another large-scale study that evaluated the usefulness of fluorouracil and leucovorin in stage II and III colon cancer was the International Multicenter Pooled Analysis of Colon Cancer Trials (IMPACT) study. This was a combined analysis of three nearly identical trials using 5-FU at a dose of 370 to 400 mg/m² plus leucovorin 200 mg/m², each given days 1 to 5 every 28 days for six cycles.[195] Results for a total of 1493 eligible patients were reported. The 3-year event-free survival for patients with Dukes' C disease was 44% for those receiving surgery alone versus 62% for patients randomly assigned to postoperative chemotherapy. The initially reported difference in patients with Dukes' B cancer was substantially smaller, with 76% and 79% of those receiving surgery only and chemotherapy, respectively, remaining event free at 3 years. A subsequent update of results for these 1016 patients with Dukes' B2 disease reported that the benefits for treatment on this trial approached but did not reach statistical significance for either event-free or overall survival.[196]

With the usefulness for both levamisole and leucovorin having been demonstrated, several investigators logically evaluated the combination of fluorouracil, leucovorin, and levamisole. The NSABP C-04 study randomly assigned 2151 patients with Dukes' B and C tumors to one of three arms: weekly 5-FU plus high-dose leucovorin, the same 5-FU plus leucovorin schedule plus oral levamisole, or 5-FU plus levamisole. All treatments were planned for 1 year's duration.[197] The 5-year disease-free survival for 5-FU/leucovorin group was 65%, versus 60% for the 5-FU/levamisole group ($P = .04$). The 5-year overall survival showed a trend in favor of the 5-FU/leucovorin group compared with the 5-FU/levamisole group ($P = .07$). There was no additional advantage gained by addition of levamisole to 5-FU/leucovorin.

The North Central Cancer Treatment Group (NCCTG) and the National Cancer Institute of Canada evaluated whether the addition of leucovorin to 5-FU plus levamisole conferred a benefit. In a two-by-two design, this trial also assessed the efficacy of 6 versus 12 months of postoperative treatment. The results of this trial indicate that the addition of leucovorin to 5-FU/levamisole was not beneficial, and 12 months of chemotherapy did not confer any benefit over 6 months of treatment.[198] Other trials discussed later have further investigated and confirmed the relative lack of benefit for combined leucovorin/levamisole biomodulation of 5-FU, and the acceptability of a shorter duration of therapy.

The question of shortening the duration of adjuvant chemotherapy was further addressed in a randomized study that evaluated a treatment arm of only 12 weeks' duration.[199] Seven hundred sixteen patients with resected Dukes' B and C colorectal cancer were randomly assigned to receive 5-FU and leucovorin (Mayo Clinic schedule) for 6 months or protracted venous infusion (PVI) 5-FU at 300 mg/m²/d for 12 weeks. Relapse-free survival was worse in the patients receiving the Mayo Clinic 5-FU regimen for 6 months than in those receiving PVI 5-FU for 12 weeks (68.6% vs. 80% respectively, $P = .023$). Three-year survival for the 5-FU/leucovorin 6-month group was 83.2% versus 87.9% for the 12-week PVI group (difference not significant, $P = .76$). Grade 3 neutropenia, diarrhea, stomatitis, and alopecia were significantly less in the 3-month PVI 5-FU–treated group. The authors concluded that the 12-week treatment resulted in similar survival but with significantly less toxicity. Although the trend in favor of the 12-week arm is encouraging, the size of the trial makes it difficult to make a statement of noninferiority with certainty. This is the only trial published to date that has evaluated a 12-week treatment arm. Although the results are of interest, in the absence of corroboration, this result should be accepted with caution. It would also be difficult to decide to what degree, if any, the 3-month treatment could be extrapolated to other treatment regimens and schedules.

The QUASAR (Quick and Simple and Reliable) Colorectal Cancer Study Group has reported a large trial with a two-by-two design in which patients with resected colorectal cancer were treated with 5-FU at 370 mg/m^2 and were randomly assigned to receive treatment with either levamisole or placebo, and either low-dose (25-mg) or high-dose (175-mg) *l*-leucovorin.[200] (Note that the *l* isomer of leucovorin, which is available in Europe but not in the United States, is comparable to twice the dose of standard racemic leucovorin. Standard leucovorin is a racemic mixture of *d* and *l* isomers; however, only the *l* isomer is biologically active.) This trial also gave the treating physician the option of treating on a daily × 5 schedule every 4 weeks for 6 months or a once-weekly schedule for 30 weeks.[201] The trial showed no differences in survival between the high- and low-dose leucovorin groups (70% and 71% at 3 years; *P* = .16). Survival was actually modestly worse with levamisole than with placebo (69.4% vs. 71.5%), and this difference approached statistical significance at *P* = .06. There was no difference in outcomes for the daily × 5 and weekly treatment schedules. Although this was a nonrandomized comparison (schedule was selected by physician preference), the arms were well balanced in terms of demographic features. The once-weekly regimen was substantially less toxic in terms of stomatitis, diarrhea, and neutropenia.

Intergroup trial INT 0089 randomly assigned patients to one of four treatment arms: 5-FU plus levamisole for 52 weeks, 5-FU plus weekly high-dose leucovorin for 32 weeks (5-FU, 500 mg/m^2 and leucovorin, 500 mg/m^2 weekly for 6 weeks, repeated every 8 weeks for four cycles), 5-FU plus low-dose leucovorin on a daily × 5 (Mayo Clinic) schedule (5-FU, 425 mg/m^2 and leucovorin, 20 mg/m^2 for five consecutive days, repeated every 28 days for six cycles), or the Mayo Clinic schedule of 5-FU/leucovorin plus levamisole. Results are shown in Table 29.8-9. There were no differences in efficacy between the two 5-FU/leucovorin arms. The shorter leucovorin-based regimens were at least comparable in efficacy to the longer regimen of 5-FU/levamisole. The 5-FU/leucovorin/levamisole regimen was not superior to the 5-FU/leucovorin regimen. The authors concluded that levamisole was not required and that either of the 5-FU/leucovorin regimens could be considered as standard for adjuvant treatment of patients with stage III disease.[202]

Exploiting the different mechanisms of action of bolus and infusional 5-FU, a biweekly (every other week) regimen has been developed in which a 2-hour leucovorin administration is followed by a bolus of 5-FU and then a 22-hour infusion of 5-FU, each given for two consecutive days every 14 days. A comparison of this regimen, known as LV5FU2, with the Mayo Clinic bolus 5-FU/leucovorin regimen in treatment of metastatic disease showed a superior response rate and progression-free survival for the LV5FU2 regimen. Overall survival showed a trend toward improvement, but it was not statistically significant.[203] More recently, a comparison of LV5FU2 and the Mayo Clinic 5-FU/leucovorin regimen in treatment of 905 patients

TABLE 29.8-9. Results of Intergroup Trial INT 0089: 5-FU/Leucovorin versus 5-FU/Levamisole versus 5-FU/Leucovorin/Levamisole in Patients with Stage III Colon Cancer

5-FU–Based Treatment Regimen	Treatment Duration (Wk)	5-Y Disease-Free Survival (%)	5-Y Overall Survival (%)
5-FU plus levamisole	52	56	63
5-FU plus low-dose leucovorin (Mayo Clinic schedule)	24	60	66
5-FU/high-dose leucovorin (Roswell Park schedule)	32	59	65
5-FU plus leucovorin (Mayo Clinic schedule) plus levamisole	24	60	67

5-FU, 5-fluorouracil.
(From ref. 202, with permission.)

with stage II and III cancer has been reported.[204] This randomized, two-by-two factorial study compared LVFU2 with the Mayo Clinic 5-FU/leucovorin regimen, each for either 24 or 36 weeks. Disease-free survival was similar for the LVFU2 and Mayo Clinic 5-FU/leucovorin groups, with a hazard ratio of 1.04 (*P* = .74). No significant differences were seen in overall survival (*P* = .18). Total aggregate toxicities were lower for the LVFU2 group (all toxicities, *P* <.001). This study was designed from a statistical perspective to evaluate whether the LV5FU2 regimen was superior in efficacy to the Mayo Clinic 5-FU/leucovorin regimen. In this respect the trial yielded negative results. Although this study was not powered or designed to rule out inferiority of the LV5FU2 schedule, it would appear that this biweekly schedule could reasonably be considered as comparable in efficacy to other 5-FU/leucovorin regimens in the adjuvant setting.

FLUOROURACIL PLUS INTERFERON-α

Based on encouraging preliminary clinical data for the combination of recombinant interferon-α$_{2a}$ (IFN-α) and 5-FU, the NSABP C-05 trial randomly assigned 2176 patients with Dukes' B and C cancer to receive 5-FU/leucovorin with or without IFN-α. At a median follow-up of 4 years, no significant differences in disease-free or overall survival were seen. The IFN-α–containing arm experienced substantially more toxicity. Thus, there is no role for the use of IFN-α in the adjuvant treatment of colon cancer.

ORAL FLUOROPYRIMIDINE THERAPIES

Oral administration of fluorouracil proved to be problematic because of erratic bioavailability. This was likely due in large part to variable effects of DPD, the rate-limiting enzyme in catabolism of fluorouracil, on the first-pass clearance of oral fluorouracil by the liver. Two oral 5-FU prodrugs, capecitabine and uracil/tegafur (UFT), have demonstrated efficacy in metastatic disease that is comparable to that of the Mayo Clinic schedule of parenteral 5-FU plus leucovorin. Both of these agents have now been studied in the adjuvant setting in com-

TABLE 29.8-10. Results of the MOSAIC Trial: Biweekly Infusional 5-Fluorouracil/Leucovorin (LV5FU2) versus LV5FU2 plus Oxaliplatin (FOLFOX 4) in Patients with Stage II and III Colon Cancer

	LV5FU2 (%) (n = 1123)	FOLFOX 4 (%) (n = 1123)	Hazard Ratio (95% CI)
3-Y disease-free survival of patients with stage III disease (60% of total)	66	72	0.76 (0.02–0.92)
3-Y disease-free survival patients with stage II disease (40% of total)	84	87	0.82 (0.57–1.17)
Overall survival	Not available	Not available	—
Grade 3 or 4 neutropenia	5	41	—
Neutropenic fever	0	1	—
Grade 3 or 4 diarrhea	0	1	—
Grade 3 or 4 vomiting	7	11	—
Neuropathy, any grade	0	92	—
Neuropathy, grade 3	0	12	—
Persistent neuropathy, grade 2 or 3, 1 y after treatment	0	5	—

CI, confidence interval.
(From ref. 206, with permission.)

parison to a Mayo Clinic schedule of 5-FU. In 2004, both trials have been reported in abstract form, and both show comparable efficacy to the Mayo Clinic schedule of 5-FU/leucovorin. UFT/leucovorin and capecitabine also show favorable side-effect profiles compared to the Mayo Clinic 5-FU/leucovorin schedule.[204a,204b]

OXALIPLATIN- AND IRINOTECAN-BASED COMBINATION THERAPIES

Clinical trials in the metastatic setting have established that the antitumor activity of combinations of either irinotecan plus 5-FU/leucovorin or oxaliplatin plus 5-FU/leucovorin is superior to that of 5-FU/leucovorin alone. Clinical trials evaluating these combinations in the adjuvant setting have completed accrual.

Oxaliplatin plus biweekly infusional 5-FU/leucovorin was evaluated in the MOSAIC trial.[206] The results of this trial are summarized in Table 29.8-10. A total of 2246 patients with stage II and III disease were randomly assigned to the LV5FU2 regimen, a biweekly infusional and bolus 5-FU/leucovorin regimen, or the FOLFOX 4 regimen, which is LV5FU2 plus oxaliplatin on day 1. The arms were well balanced for prognostic variables. With a median follow-up of 37 months, the 3-year disease-free survival was superior in the FOLFOX 4 arm, with a hazard ratio of 0.77 (P <.01). For the 1347 patients with stage III disease, the hazard ratio was 0.76 (95% CI, 0.62 to 0.92), with an improvement in 3-year disease-free survival from 66% to 72%. The results for the 899 patients with stage II disease were less definitive, with a hazard ratio of 0.82 (95% CI, 0.57 to 1.17). The 3-year disease-free survival for the patients with stage II cancer was 84% in the control arm and 87% in the FOLFOX 4 arm. At the time of this writing, the results for overall survival from this trial have not yet matured.

The toxicity of the FOLFOX 4 regimen was manageable but was greater than that seen in the control arm, with 41% experiencing grade 3 or 4 neutropenia versus 5% in the control arm,

and 11% experiencing grade 3 or 4 diarrhea versus 7% of controls. All-cause mortality (ACM) in the first 60 days was 0.5% in each arm. Peripheral sensory neuropathy, a toxicity not present in the LV5FU2 control arm, was a frequent occurrence on the FOLFOX 4 arm. Grade 2 neuropathy was reported in 32% of the patients, and grade 3 occurred in 12%. In some cases the duration of the neuropathy was substantial. One year after completion of therapy, 4% of patients still experienced grade 2 neuropathy and 1% still had grade 3 neuropathy. The improved disease-free survival in patients with stage III cancer is encouraging. Whether this will translate into an overall survival advantage and whether the long-term neuropathies will be problematic remains to be determined.

Oxaliplatin has also been combined with a weekly bolus 5-FU regimen in an adjuvant trial. The NSABP has studied a regimen of oxaliplatin plus weekly bolus 5-FU/leucovorin, known as FLOX, versus the standard weekly Roswell Park regimen of 5-FU/leucovorin. This study has completed accrual, and efficacy data are expected in late 2004.

Irinotecan has also been incorporated into investigations of combination therapy in the adjuvant setting. The Cancer and Leukemia Group B (CALGB) studied the weekly schedule of irinotecan plus bolus 5-FU and leucovorin (IFL). Early safety analysis of this trial identified an alarming elevation in early mortality for the experimental arm, with 18 deaths within the first 4 months of treatment on the IFL arm versus 6 deaths within the same time period on the control arm ($P =$ .008).[207] At a median follow-up of 2.1 years in each arm, no differences in either disease-free survival or overall survival were seen. Statistic analysis indicated that the futility boundaries for both of these efficacy parameters had been crossed, which indicates that results for this trial will not be positive for either disease-free or overall survival.[208] Irinotecan should therefore not be used with bolus 5-FU in the adjuvant setting.

Trials of biweekly infusional 5-FU/leucovorin with or without irinotecan have reached full accrual. In one trial, a greater than 90% relative dose intensity of all drugs was administered on both arms of the trial with acceptable toxicity.[209] Efficacy results are anticipated to be available in late 2004.

TREATMENT OF PATIENTS WITH STAGE II DISEASE

The optimal management of patients with stage II colon cancer remains undefined. Although the role of adjuvant therapy in stage II colon cancer has not been firmly established, it is interesting to see what recent practice patterns have been. Using the Surveillance, Epidemiology, and End Results program– and Medicare–linked database, Schrag et al. identified 3151 patients aged 65 to 75 years with resected stage II colon cancer and no adverse prognostic features. Using Medicare billing records, they identified those patients who did or did not receive chemotherapy within 3 months of operation.

Their review ascertained that 27% of patients received chemotherapy during the 3-month postoperative period. Younger age, white race, unfavorable tumor grade, and low comorbidity were associated with a greater likelihood of receiving treatment. The 5-year survival was 75% for untreated patients and 78% for patients who received therapy in this nonrandomized comparison. After adjustment for known between-group differences, the hazard ratio for survival associated with adjuvant treatment was 0.91 (95% CI, 0.77 to 1.09). Thus, despite the lack of proven benefit, a substantial percentage of Medicare beneficiaries have received adjuvant chemotherapy for stage II disease.

Because patients with stage II disease as a group have a relatively favorable prognosis, benefits from treatment could only be expected to be shown if either a highly efficacious therapy were used or extremely large trials were done to detect very subtle differences. The IMPACT metaanalysis provides one of the largest samples of patients with stage II disease.[196] A total of 1016 patients with stage II colon cancer were randomly assigned to receive either 5-FU/leucovorin therapy or surgery alone. The surgery-only arm had a long-term overall survival rate of 81%, versus 83% for patients receiving adjuvant 5-FU/leucovorin. This absolute difference of 2% closely approached, but did not reach, statistical significance.

The NSABP reported a pooled analysis of data from the CO-1, CO-2, CO-3, and CO-4 trials. These trials do not lend themselves well to combination in a metaanalysis. Different regimens were used in the arms of the studies that were combined, and not all of the trials contained a surgery-alone arm. The analysis concluded that a statistically significant benefit for treatment was obtained for stage II cancer patients receiving therapy; however, the methodologic flaws in the analysis limit its interpretability.

Several prognostic indicators have been identified that correlate with a higher risk for subsequent treatment failure in patients with stage II cancer. These include obstruction or perforation of the bowel wall[210] as well as other less established risk factors such as elevated preoperative CEA level, poorly differentiated histologic type, a high S-phase fraction, tumors that do not demonstrate high levels of MSI,[140,211] and tumors with an 18q deletion.[212] It appears that stage II cancer patients with one or more of these risk factors have a poorer prognosis and a prognosis closer to that of patients with stage III disease. Whether adjuvant chemotherapy can provide benefits in these patients similar to those it provides in patients with stage III dis-

ease remains a matter of conjecture at this time. In the absence of definitive data, conclusive recommendations cannot be made at this time. In fully informed high-risk patients with stage II disease, it is reasonable to consider adjuvant treatment using stage III treatment regimens.

TREATMENT OPTIONS FOR PATIENTS WITH STAGE III DISEASE

It is not possible at this time to make a specific general treatment recommendation for all patients with stage III colon cancer. After a period of relative stagnation, the treatment of colorectal cancer is very much in flux, and the clinician must continually remain aware of new information that may alter recommendations. Treatments must be individualized to the needs of each patient. The available data, and the limitations of these data, must be understood by the clinician and discussed with the patient in making treatment decisions and recommendations.

It is clear that in the absence of medical or psychiatric contraindications, patients with node-positive colon cancer should receive postoperative chemotherapy. At the very least, a fluorouracil-based regimen would appear to be appropriate, and approximately a half year of therapy would be supported by the majority of trials. The daily × 5 Mayo Clinic schedule and its variants have been shown to be more toxic than other 5-FU/leucovorin schedules, and therefore daily × 5 schedules should not be used.

Whether to add an additional agent, such as oxaliplatin or irinotecan, is a complicated decision. At the time of this writing, the use of FOLFOX 4 has been shown to improve disease-free survival at 3 years over a 5-FU/leucovorin regimen in patients with stage III disease. Whether this will translate into an overall survival advantage remains unclear. If an overall survival advantage is demonstrated, then use of a FOLFOX-type regimen would become the default position for the majority of stage III cases. In the interim, it seems reasonable to offer FOLFOX as an option to patients with stage III cancer, especially those with stage IIIB or IIIC disease. The risk of peripheral neuropathy and the possibility of long-term neuropathy (1% rate of persistent grade 3 neuropathy at 1 year) must be considered in the selection of therapy.

Weekly irinotecan plus bolus 5-FU/leucovorin should not be used in the adjuvant setting, because randomized data have shown increased risk of early death and no long-term benefit. There are, at the time of this writing, no data to either support or refute the use of any of the following therapies in patients with stage III disease: bolus 5-FU plus oxaliplatin, infusional 5-FU plus irinotecan, capecitabine or UFT, either alone or in combination, and irinotecan plus oxaliplatin combinations. Furthermore, there are no data to support the use of either cetuximab or bevacizumab (BEV) in the adjuvant setting, and adjuvant use of these agents outside of a clinical trial cannot be recommended at this time.

INVESTIGATIONAL ADJUVANT APPROACHES

Portal Vein Infusion

Large, established hepatic metastases derive their blood supply primarily from the hepatic artery. However, tumors smaller than 5 mm in diameter obtain substantial portions of their blood supply from both the hepatic and portal circulations.[213,214] Delivery of chemotherapy directly into the portal vein would appear to be a reasonable maneuver in the adjuvant treatment of colorectal cancer, because the liver is the most common extraregional site of metastases. It would appear that cancer cells enter the liver through the portal vein along the same channels used by nutrients traveling from the gut.

Initial dose-finding studies demonstrated that due to the extraction or first-pass clearance of 5-FU by the liver, substantially higher doses of 5-FU can be safely given by intraportal infusion than by intravenous infusion.[215] The NSABP C-02 trial randomly assigned 1158 patients with Dukes' A, B, or C colon cancer to either a 7-day portal vein infusion of 5-FU (600 mg/ m^2/d) or to surgery alone.[216] A modest, albeit statistically significant, advantage in disease-free survival (74% vs. 64% at 4 years) was demonstrated for the group receiving intraportal chemotherapy; however, no difference was seen in the incidence of hepatic recurrences.

Similar findings were reported from a 533-patient trial performed by the Swiss Group for Clinical Cancer Research.[217,218] In this trial intraportal chemotherapy included 10 mg/m^2 mitomycin C by 2-hour infusion followed by a 7-day infusion of 5-FU at a dose of 500 mg/m^2/d. The 5-year disease-free and overall survival rates were modestly improved in the intraportal treatment group compared with the surgery-only group (57% vs. 48% and 66% vs. 55%, respectively).

Subsequently, a large metaanalysis of intraportal chemotherapy trials involving over 4000 patients in ten randomized studies revealed only a 4% improvement in 5-year overall survival for the patients receiving portal infusion. At present intraportal adjuvant chemotherapy should remain limited to clinical investigations.

Intraperitoneal Chemotherapy

The peritoneal cavity is drained by portal lymphatics into the portal vein. Intraperitoneal chemotherapy therefore delivers high concentrations of drug to the portal circulation without the need for portal vein cannulization. In addition, extremely high concentrations of chemotherapeutic drugs can be given directly onto the peritoneal surfaces, which thereby increases local cytotoxicity. The high first-pass hepatic clearances of floxuridine (FUDR) and 5-FU make these drugs good agents for intraperitoneal administration. Pharmacokinetic studies of intraperitoneal 5-FU and FUDR show that intraperitoneal administration of these agents results in intraperitoneal concentrations 200- to 400-fold higher than those achieved systemically.[219,220]

A small single-arm study explored the feasibility of immediately postoperative treatment with intraperitoneal FUDR and leucovorin plus systemic 5-FU and levamisole.[221] Patients received intraperitoneal FUDR plus leucovorin twice daily for three consecutive days every other week for 3 cycles. Levamisole was begun orally with the second intraperitoneal cycle, and systemic 5-FU by bolus injection daily × 5 was begun with the third intraperitoneal cycle. These systemic doses of 5-FU given concurrently with intraperitoneal chemotherapy were escalated in a phase I manner. On day 29 after the initiation of 5-FU therapy, weekly 5-FU and every-other-week levamisole were started and continued to complete 1 year of therapy. This study regimen was well tolerated. At a median follow-up of 24 months, 24 of 28 patients were alive and free of disease.

A randomized trial involving 241 patients with stage II and III disease compared intraperitoneal plus systemic 5-FU/leucovorin with systemic 5-FU/levamisole.[222] At a median follow-up of 4 years, no benefit was seen for the patients with stage II cancer. Among the 196 eligible patients with stage III disease, however, a 43% reduction in mortality was seen. Results of this small trial are encouraging, but further corroboration is required before this regimen is accepted into standard practice.

Edrecolomab

Edrecolomab, a murine monoclonal immunoglobulin G2a antibody directed against the cell surface glycoprotein 17-1A, was shown in nude mice to inhibit growth of human colon cancer xenografts.[223] Other studies showed that this antibody could induce antibody-dependent cellular cytotoxicity. An initial trial in patients with metastatic disease revealed several minor responses with remarkably little toxicity.[224] Postulating potentially greater effectiveness of this immunologically based therapy on microscopic residual disease, investigators pursued development of this agent in the adjuvant setting. A total of 166 patients were randomly assigned to receive edrecolomab at a dosage of 500 mg by 1-hour infusion 2 weeks after surgery and then 100 mg over 1 hour given every 4 weeks for four doses, or to surgery only. This small trial showed a 32% reduction in mortality for the edrecolomab arm at a median follow-up of 7 years. This encouraging preliminary finding, however, was not supported by a larger confirmatory trial in which 2761 patients with stage III colon cancer were randomly assigned to receive 5-FU/leucovorin (Mayo Clinic schedule) plus edrecolomab, 5-FU/leucovorin alone, or edrecolomab alone. At a median follow-up of 26 months, the overall survival of the patients on edrecolomab plus chemotherapy was essentially the same as that of those on chemotherapy alone (75% and 76%, respectively). Disease-free survival was significantly lower on the edrecolomab-alone arm. Edrecolomab has since been withdrawn from clinical development.

Vaccines

Vaccination strategies endeavor to stimulate the patient's immune system to recognize and eradicate the patient's tumor cells. An ideal immunologic target molecule would be a highly antigenic epitope that is always expressed on the tumor and never expressed on normal tissue. Such an ideal target has yet to be identified; however, a number of approaches have been explored.

CEA is a commonly expressed antigen in colorectal carcinomas. Unfortunately, CEA does not appear to be particularly immunogenic. Several approaches have been pursued in an attempt to increase immune recognition of CEA. One approach has been the development of an anti-idiotype monoclonal antibody vaccine that mimics CEA but with greater immunogenicity.[225] Large-scale trials have yet to be performed. Another approach has been to use a canarypox virus that encodes the gene for CEA and for B7.1, a T-cell costimulatory molecule (ALVAC-CEA B7.1). Administration of ALVAC-CEA B7.1 has been shown to induce CEA-specific T-cell response in patients with advanced adenocarcinoma when given alone[226] but not when given concurrently with granulocyte macrophage-colony stimulating factor.[227]

The canarypox (ALVAC) vector has also been explored as a vehicle for p53-specific vaccination.[228] A recombinant canarypox encoding wild-type human p53 was given to 15 patients with advanced colorectal cancer in a phase I-II trial. Vaccine-mediated enhancement of p53-specific T-cell immunity was found in two patients at the highest dose level. Further studies will explore this approach further in adjuvant treatments.

Another group used the ALVAC vector to facilitate antigen presentation of the epithelial cellular adhesion molecule (Ep-CAM/KSA). The Ep-CAM gene was inserted into the ALVAC vector (ALVAC-KSA). Twelve resected colon cancer patients (with stage I, II, or III disease) were treated. Of six patients treated with ALVAC-KSA alone, two developed a weak T-cell response, whereas of the six treated with ALVAC-KSA plus granulocyte macrophage-colony stimulating factor, five developed a marked IFN-γ response.[229]

Thus, a number of promising avenues of investigation are being pursued; however, at this time the use of vaccine therapy for treatment of resected colon cancer remains highly investigational.

Active Specific Immunotherapy

Irradiated cancer cells maintain their immunogenicity; however, they are unable to proliferate. Active specific immunotherapy (ASI) is a maneuver in which patients are immunized with a preparation of their own irradiated tumor cells plus an immunostimulant such as BCG. This technique has been explored for some time now as a potential adjuvant immunotherapy for colorectal cancer. An initial small, randomized trial involving a total of 80 patients with either colon or rectal cancer showed no survival advantage for the immunized patients.[230] In a retrospective subset analysis, some benefit was seen for those patients with colon cancer, which led to further investigation of this approach.

Another trial was conducted in 213 patients with stage II and III colon cancer.[231] Accrual was slow, and the results were reported with a median follow-up of 5.3 years but a range of 0.7 to 9 years. No benefits were seen in the patients with stage III disease ($P = .52$). In a retrospective subset analysis of the patients with stage II cancer, recurrence-free survival was modestly better ($P = .032$); however, overall survival was not improved ($P = .149$). Thus, current data do not support the use of ASI as an adjuvant treatment for stage II or III colon cancer. A larger trial was performed by the Eastern Cooperative Oncology Group (ECOG).[232] A total of 297 patients with stage II cancer and 115 patients with stage III cancer were randomly assigned to receive ASI or observation after surgery. There were no statistically significant differences in clinical outcomes between the treatment arms at a median follow-up of longer than 7 years; however, there were trends in disease-free survival ($P = .078$) and overall survival ($P = .12$) in favor of ASI in the subset of patients who received the intended treatment and had a delayed cutaneous hypersensitivity response to the third vaccination with an induration of 5 mm. In addition, the 5-year survival was 85% for those with indurations larger than 10 mm, compared with 45% for those with indurations smaller than 5 mm, which possibly suggests benefits for those patients who achieved effective immunization or shows that patients who are capable of getting a hypersensitivity reaction have a better prognosis. Overall, trials have failed to show a benefit for the use of ASI in the management of colon cancer, and its use should remain limited to investigational settings.

RADIATION THERAPY FOR COLON CANCER

Patterns of Failure and the Rationale for Radiation Therapy

The role of adjuvant radiation therapy is poorly defined for colon cancer compared to rectal cancer. This is due to differences in the anatomy, natural history, and possibly the biology of colon cancer and rectal cancer. The most common site of failure after potentially curative surgery in colon cancer is abdominal (liver) rather than locoregional. Because most local failures in colon cancer are extrapelvic, local failure usually does not result in the substantial symptomatology seen in rectal cancer. Methods used to detect local failure (surgery, clinical examination, or imaging) and the times of evaluation (total vs. first failure) are important issues in assessing the importance of locoregional failure in this disease.

Although the overall incidence of local failure is relatively low in colon cancer, local failure rate depends on stage, with local failure rates being as high as 35% for selected disease stages[233-236] (Table 29.8-11). Data suggest that, on the basis of anatomic location and selected pathologic features of their tumors, certain patient subsets have a substantial incidence of local failure and may benefit from more aggressive local therapy. Some authors have considered partially retroperitoneal regions such as the ascending colon, hepatic and splenic flexures, and descending colon to be relatively immobile and thus at higher risk of local failure,[236] but others reported a general trend of increased local failure with more distal colon sites. Willett et al.[235] found no consistent effect of anatomic site on local failure rates (with a suggestion of higher local failure in immobile portions of the colon) but reported a local failure rate of 35% in patients with T4 or T3N+ tumors.

Locoregional Radiation Therapy

The most comprehensive series examining the role of locoregional radiation therapy in colon cancer is a retrospective review by Willett et al.[237,238] (Table 29.8-12). After potentially curative surgery for stages T3 to 4N0 to 2M0 colon cancer, 203 patients received postoperative adjuvant radiation therapy. Those eligible included patients with T4M0 tumors regardless of anatomic site, T3N1 to 2M0 tumors in anatomically immobile regions, and selected high-risk T3N0M0 tumors with close margins. Patients received 45 Gy to the primary tumor bed with a 5-cm margin, including the draining lymph nodes, and a boost to 50.4 to 55.0 Gy depending on the volume of small bowel in the high-dose field. Sixty-three patients received concurrent bolus 5-FU at a variety of doses and schedules.

The treated patients were compared to a historical control group of 395 patients who underwent surgery only. There was a significant improvement in local control and disease-free survival for patients with stage T4N0M0 disease (disease-free survival, 80%) and T4N+M0 disease (disease-free survival, 53%) and for patients with stage T3N0 disease with a perforation or fistula. There was a 37% 5-year disease-free survival in patients

TABLE 29.8-11. Patterns of Failure after Potentially Curative Surgery for Colon Cancer (All Stages)

Series	Detection and Definition of Failure	Stage	No.	No. Experiencing Local Failure (%)		No. Experiencing Abdominal Failure (%)		No. Experiencing Distant Failure	
				Only	Component	Only	Component	Only	Component
Gunderson et al.[236]	Reoperation, cumulative failure	All stages	91	22 (0–30)	48 (0–64)	4 (0–9)	21 (0–36)	7 (0–16)	30 (0–38)
		T3–4 and/or N1–2	72	17	49	6	26	7	35
Willett et al.[426]	Clinical, cumulative failure	All stages	533	6 (0–12)	19 (0–49)	11 (2–24)	21 (3–43)	4 (0–10)	13 (0–25)
		T3–4 and/or N1–2	395	8	26	14	25	5	16
Minsky et al.[427]	Clinical, first failure	All stages	284	6 (0–8)	9 (0–25)	8 (0–29)	13 (0–57)	3 (0–11)	6 (0–25)
		T3–4 and/or N1–2	229	4	10	10	15	5	6

who received radiation therapy with residual disease after subtotal resection.[237] Ten-year results[238] confirm the good outcomes, especially in the T4N0 subset. Schild et al.[239] reported good results for locally advanced tumors with no residual disease, with 47% long-term survival for patients with microscopic residual tumor and 23% for patients with gross residual tumor. These results have been obtained with acceptable acute and late toxicities. Other reports of adjuvant locoregional radiation therapy support these results.[240]

Based on the retrospective data from Willett et al., a randomized phase III Intergroup trial (INT 0130) was developed. Patients with T4 or selected T3N1 to 2 colon tumors were randomly assigned to receive 12 cycles of bolus 5-FU plus levamisole with or without locoregional radiation therapy (45.0 to 50.4 Gy in 25 to 28 fractions) beginning with cycle 2 of chemotherapy. The trial was closed early due to poor accrual, with only 222 of the anticipated 400 patients randomly assigned (189 eligible).[241] Although toxicity was acceptable, there was no significant difference in survival between the two arms. Data on the patterns of failure have not been reported.

Although the routine use of adjuvant postoperative locoregional radiation therapy in colon cancer remains investigational, there are at least two clinical situations in which its use is reasonable. These primarily are situations in which therapy is not truly adjuvant in the conventional sense because the risk of local recurrence is very high due to the known presence or extremely high risk of microscopic or gross residual disease. These include cases of close or positive resection margins and cases of resection of T4 colon cancers that are adherent to structures or tissues and

therefore cannot be fully resected. These cancers have local failure rates similar to like-staged rectal cancers, and it is reasonable to treat them with combined modality therapy, including six cycles of 5-FU–based chemotherapy plus concurrent radiation to the tumor bed. Examples of such situations include cecal tumors invading into the abdominal wall or posteriorly, hepatic flexure tumors with duodenal invasion, and sigmoid cancers with invasion into pelvic structures. Treatment in these situations must be individualized, and radiation should be used only for a clearly surgically defined high-risk population.

Whole abdominal radiation therapy has also been explored in an attempt to cure diffuse intraabdominal and liver disease. However, the total radiation dose is severely limited by normal tissue tolerance. A number of phase II adjuvant trials have been performed delivering 20 to 30 Gy to the whole abdomen, often with concurrent 5-FU therapy.[242,243] SWOG 8572 was a phase II adjuvant pilot trial involving 41 patients with T3N1 to 2M0 disease treated with whole abdominal radiation therapy plus continuous-infusion 5-FU and maintenance 5-FU.[242] The data showed encouraging results in patients with more than four positive nodes, with 5-year disease-free and overall survival rates of 55% and 74%, respectively. Currently, whole abdominal radiation therapy remains investigational.

FOLLOW-UP AFTER MANAGEMENT OF COLON CANCER WITH CURATIVE INTENT

Follow-up after definitive management has two primary goals. First, patients with a history of colorectal cancer are at higher

TABLE 29.8-12. Local Adjuvant Radiation Therapy in Colon Cancer

Group	Stage	Locoregional Failure				5-Y Disease-Free Survival	
		No.	Surgery (%)	No.	Surgery + Radiation (%)	Surgery (%)	Surgery + Radiation (%)
Adjuvant therapy	T3N0	163	10	23	9[a]	70	72
	T4N0	83	31	54	7	63	79
	T3N1–2	100	35	55	30	44	47
	T4N1–2	49	53	39	28	37	53
Residual disease	All stages	—	—	30	47	—	37
Perforation or fistula	T4N0	21	48	23	6	43	91

[a]Actuarial component of total failure.
(From Willett, Massachusetts General Hospital.)

risk than the general population for a second colon cancer primary.[244,245] A colonoscopic screening may be of benefit in the early detection of a second primary malignancy or detection of a benign polyp, which can then be resected to potentially prevent the development of an invasive cancer.

Second, surveillance may increase the change of identifying locoregional or distant recurrence that is potentially curable by surgery. It should be noted that it is this detection of potentially curable recurrent or second primary disease that justifies routine postoperative surveillance. To date there are no compelling data indicating that early detection of unresectable asymptomatic metastatic disease is of benefit to the patient. In other words, if recurrent disease is unresectable and therefore incurable, there is no urgency to identify it. There is no compelling evidence that the early initiation of palliative chemotherapy is of benefit in the patient with asymptomatic, incurable disease. What follow-up routine to use and which studies to include in that follow-up has been the subject of much debate in the colon cancer literature.[246-249] Several studies and imaging modalities have been recommended as important components of a follow-up regimen. These have included (1) measurements of CEA level, (2) careful history and physical examination, (3) liver function tests including transaminase and lactic dehydrogenase levels, (4) complete blood count, (5) fecal occult blood test, (6) chest radiograph, (7) CT, (8) pelvic imaging, (9) flexible proctosigmoidoscopy (rectal cancer), and (10) colonoscopy.

Various retrospective reviews and metaanalyses have argued the relative costs and benefits of each of these individual approaches.[250,251] In 1999 the American Society of Clinical Oncology (ASCO) undertook a review of these various strategies by examining outcomes, including overall and disease-free survival, quality of life, toxicity reduction, and cost effectiveness.[252] The study reviewed all literature published on this subject using a MEDLINE search for the 20 years preceding the initiation of the study. Levels of evidence were graded, possible consequences of false-positive and false-negative tests were examined, and an expert panel reviewed the data and made recommendations. Additional outside reviewers examined the final document and made additional recommendations. The panel reviewed each of the aforementioned ten follow-up assessments, evaluated the costs and benefits, and arrived at a selection of those studies that were thought at the time to have the greatest potential yield in detecting new primaries and recurrent disease.

The role of CEA measurement in patients after definitive management of colorectal cancer has been controversial.[87,250,253] ASCO carefully reviewed the usefulness of this measure in an additional panel in 1996.[254] The recommendation for CEA monitoring then, which was confirmed in a surveillance guideline panel review, was that postoperative serum CEA measurements be performed every 2 to 3 months in patients with stage II or III disease for up to 2 years after diagnosis. An elevated CEA level, if confirmed by retesting, warranted further evaluation for metastatic disease.

The further workup after an elevated CEA level typically consists of colonoscopy, chest radiography, and CT scan of the abdomen and pelvis. If results of these studies are negative, the clinician is faced with a dilemma. The question of what to do in the face of a rising serum CEA level in the absence of disease imageable by conventional imaging modalities is one that has been addressed in clinical trials.[255-260] Strategies to image CEA expression might improve the detection capability of standard imaging studies. Several studies were performed using immunoscintigraphy with an antibody directed against CEA or Tag 72, a CEA-like glycoprotein (CEA scan and OncoScint scan, respectively).[261-263] The results of these studies using antibody-directed immunoscintigraphy were variable. To more directly address this clinical dilemma, a prospective study was performed comparing CEA immunoscintigraphy to positron emission tomography (PET) using fluorine F 18 fluorodeoxyglucose (FDG) and blind second-look laparotomy.[257]

In this study, patients with a rising CEA level without disease imageable by CT of the chest, abdomen, and pelvis or by colonoscopy and abdominal ultrasonography were enrolled, along with patients with a single site of otherwise resectable disease. All patients had a CEA scan performed as well as an FDG-PET scan. All patients for whom there was failure to demonstrate evidence of disease outside of the abdominal cavity went on to have an exploratory laparotomy by a surgeon who had no knowledge of the CEA or the FDG-PET scan results. A second surgeon participated in the remainder of the exploration after thoroughly reviewing all studies, including the nuclear medicine scans. Twenty-eight patients were studied in this fashion. The trial demonstrated that FDG-PET scans were far superior to CEA scans in detecting recurrence, and roughly 30% of the patients in the study potentially benefited by having recurrent disease treated at the time of surgery (Fig. 29.8-5).[257]

Based on these findings, it appears that measurement of serum CEA levels after definitive management of a primary colorectal cancer is a reasonable surveillance technique. If the CEA level is elevated on repeat testing, imaging studies should be performed consisting of CT scans and a thorough evaluation of the colon with colonoscopy. If no recurrence or second primary is detected, an FDG-PET scan can be considered. If disease is discovered, it should be managed as indicated. If no disease is detected, then continued surveillance is warranted with repeated measurement of CEA levels and imaging at intervals.[257,264]

The role of the physical examination has also been evaluated.[252] The ASCO panel noted that no formal examination has been performed of the contribution of the physician's history taking and physical examination to improve outcomes for

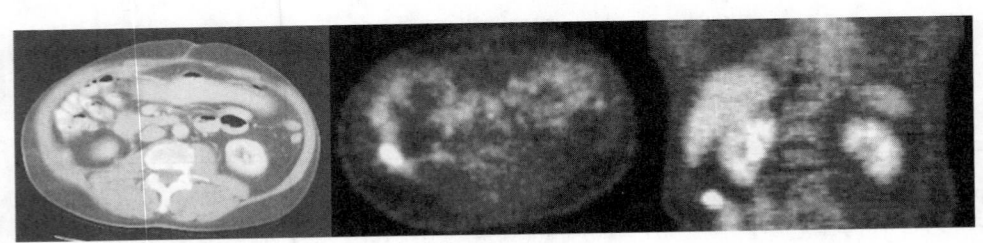

FIGURE 29.8-5. From left to right, the first panel depicts a contrast-enhanced computed tomography scan of a patient with a rising level of carcinoembryonic antigen after a definitive resection of a right colon cancer. The middle and right panels show the same region imaged with fluorine F 18 fluorodeoxyglucose–positron emission tomography.[257]

colorectal cancer. However, data from the larger studies of surveillance showed that 80% of recurrences were found by CEA testing, whereas only 20% were found by routine history taking and physical examination performed at the same time.[265] This has been confirmed by other studies.[266,267] Although no direct effects of history taking or physical examination on detection or outcome in the surveillance period were shown, a physician–patient encounter provides a vital link for other investigations that may influence outcome. Therefore, although their benefit is not in itself substantiated by the data in the literature, it is felt that routine postresection visits should be scheduled every 3 to 6 months for the first 3 years after resection.

The role of liver function tests as a means for detecting colorectal recurrence has also been carefully evaluated. No studies that were reviewed by the ASCO panel demonstrated any benefit for the routine use of liver function test measurements in the postresection surveillance period.[252,268] In fact, studies suggested that other routine blood tests such as CEA level detected recurrence far earlier than abnormal results on liver function tests.[87] Therefore the ASCO consensus panel did not recommend the routine use of liver function tests in the postresection surveillance period.

Routine fecal occult blood testing, routine CT, and routine chest radiography were all thought not to be of benefit in postoperative surveillance. Although the panel was not in uniform agreement with respect to chest radiography, it was thought that all three of these modalities should be reserved for the evaluation of the patient with evidence of recurrence, such as a rising CEA level or positive findings on endoscopy. Each of these modalities in and of itself was not found to be useful.

With respect to colonoscopy and flexible proctosigmoidoscopy, the panel, after reviewing the literature, recommended that all patients undergo colonoscopy to provide preoperative or perioperative documentation of the cancer and to ascertain that the remainder of the colon is free from polyps. Furthermore, the panel agreed that the data were sufficient to recommend colonoscopy every 3 to 5 years to detect new cancers and polyps. However, the panel did not recommend routine annual colonoscopy as follow-up after definitive management of colorectal cancer. Furthermore, the panel concluded that colonoscopy was superior to flexible proctosigmoidoscopy and therefore should be performed as indicated for patients after both colon and rectal cancer surgery. Other studies have also supported the routine use of colonoscopic examination after definitive management of colorectal cancer.[30,33,269–271]

As a follow-up to the ASCO consensus on surveillance, the panel reconvened in 2000 to update their guidelines. The panel affirmed its positive recommendations for the use of serum CEA measurements and colonoscopy in the postoperative surveillance period. Furthermore, it confirmed the importance of physician–patient contact, although acknowledging that no data existed to support physical examination and history taking alone as a means of affecting detection of recurrence. Therefore, in summary, based on the review of the available literature through the ASCO consensus conference and up to the time of the publication of these recommendations, the following are considered reasonable follow-up guidelines after surgical resection of colon and rectal cancer: Patients should have serum CEA level measured every 2 to 3 months for the first 2 years and then every 6 months for up to 5 years if they had stage II or III colorectal cancer managed

definitively. Patients should also have routine colonoscopic examination every 3 to 5 years after the resection.

A metaanalysis and systematic review of randomized trials addressing the impact of close postoperative surveillance on overall survival after definitive management of colorectal cancer was also performed by Renehan and colleagues.[272] A total of five randomized trials that met their inclusion criteria were reviewed, representing 1342 patients. For four of the studies, intensive follow-up consisted of blood tests including serum CEA level, colonoscopy, physical examination, abdominal ultrasonography, and CT scans. In one study, no CEA measurements or CT scans were performed. Follow-up in the intensive arm was every 3 months for 2 years and then every 6 months thereafter up to 5 years, with yearly CT scans and endoscopy. All five studies had a control arm subjected to a less aggressive follow-up regimen, which varied from study to study and ranged from no specific follow-up to periodic laboratory tests and plain radiography or ultrasonography. The investigators found that there was an absolute reduction in mortality of 9% to 13% with use of an aggressive follow-up regimen consisting of serum CEA measurements and CT scans. These two tests, in particular, showed the greatest impact on survival.[272]

Based on the findings of these groups, a rational postoperative surveillance program should include CEA measurements every 3 to 6 months and a yearly CT scan for the first 2 years. Colonoscopy can be performed every 3 to 5 years after the resection. At the time of CEA measurement, a physician encounter should be scheduled in which the patient's symptoms can be discussed and a physical examination performed. If a rising serum CEA level is detected on two consecutive measurements in the absence of imageable disease by CT scan, an FDG-PET scan can be considered. Lesions found on colonoscopy should be managed appropriately either with colonoscopic resection or surgical management. These surveillance guidelines should allow for the early detection of recurrence or second primary lesions and therefore provide the potential to impact patient outcome.

SURGICAL MANAGEMENT OF STAGE IV DISEASE

For a select group of patients with metastatic colorectal cancer, complete surgical resection of stage IV disease may be an option and can provide a long-term survival advantage. This is especially true with respect to metastatic sites in the liver and lung. Numerous regional approaches have also been explored for the treatment of stage IV colon cancer depending on the organ or body cavity involved. Organ-specific infusional therapy, isolated or continuous perfusion therapy, radiofrequency ablation or cryotherapy, surgical debulking, and radiation therapy are all technical approaches that have been used. Many of these regional strategies as well as surgical metastasectomy are discussed in separate chapters and therefore are not specifically addressed here.

MANAGEMENT OF UNRESECTABLE METASTATIC DISEASE

Unresectable metastatic colorectal cancer is generally not curable with current technology. Management centers around palliation and control of symptoms, control of tumor growth, and attempts to lengthen progression-free and overall survival. Given the palliative nature of such treatments, extreme care must be taken to adequately assess each individual's potential for both benefit and harm from chemotherapy. Quality-of-life issues must be frankly and objectively discussed with patients and their caregivers so that informed decisions can be made and expectations can be contained within a realistic framework.

The chemotherapy options available and the developmental work that supports their usefulness are outlined in the following sections. It is of paramount importance to keep in mind that virtually all of the clinical trials involving patients with metastatic disease were restricted by design to patients who were in good overall general medical condition. Entry criteria for most trials require a favorable performance status and acceptable bone marrow, renal, and hepatic function, and often specify evidence of reasonable nutritional intake.

It is not reasonable to extrapolate the results of these trials to patients who do not conform to these entry criteria. The likelihood of benefit in a patient with poor performance status is substantially diminished, and the likelihood of a serious adverse event is greatly increased. Patients with hepatic or renal dysfunction may be particularly prone to additional toxicity if the drug is cleared or metabolized by these organs. Patients with marginal nutritional intake may have their nutritional deficiencies further exacerbated by drugs that produce nausea or anorexia, and patients with partial or complete bowel obstruction or other causes of prolonged gastrointestinal transit time may have increased toxicity from those drugs that undergo an enterohepatic recirculation.

Thus, chemotherapy for patients with incurable metastatic disease should be approached with appropriate caution. Well-motivated patients with good performance status, good bone marrow reserve, and good organ function have a significant potential for substantial benefits from chemotherapy and should be strongly considered for aggressive therapy. Patients with poor performance status and significant comorbidities should be considered either for less aggressive therapies or for supportive care only.

FLUOROURACIL

Virtually the entire history of chemotherapy for colorectal cancer has revolved around 5-FU. Developed by Heidelberger et al. and patented in 1957,[273] it is a source of frustration and humility for investigators working to move beyond it that 45 years later this agent remains at the very core of most chemotherapeutic approaches to colorectal cancer. Following the paradigms of drug development still favored today, 5-FU is a rationally designed, targeted therapy. Heidelberger observed that tumor tissue used a larger amount of uracil than nontumor tissues. He therefore substituted a fluorine atom at the number 5 position of the uracil molecule. Because the effective sizes of fluorine and hydrogen differ by only a minuscule amount (0.15 Å), 5-FU is effectively metabolized by the same enzymatic pathways as uracil.

5-FU must be metabolized before it can exert cytotoxic activity. The details of 5-FU metabolism are covered in Chapter 15.6.

FLUOROURACIL BIOMODULATION

Although 5-FU shows activity in a portion of patients treated, overall response rates are relatively low and cures are virtually nonexistent. Biomodulation is an attempt to exploit the well-

TABLE 29.8-13. Commonly Used 5-Fluorouracil (5-FU) Regimens

Name of Regimen	Reference	Schedule[a]
Mayo Clinic	Poon et al., 1989[280]	LV, 20 mg/m², followed by bolus 5-FU, 425 mg/m², each daily for 5 consecutive days, repeated q28d for first 2 cycles, then q35d thereafter.
Roswell Park	Haller et al., 1998[202]	LV, 500 mg/m² over 2 h; 5-FU, 500 mg/m² by bolus 1-h into LV infusion. Treatments given weekly for 6 consecutive weeks, repeated every 8 wk.
Low-dose weekly LV	Jager et al., 1996[287]	LV, 20 mg/m² over 5–15 min, followed by bolus 5-FU, 500 mg/m²; treatments given weekly for 6 consecutive weeks, repeated every 8 wk.
Protracted venous infusion	Lokich et al., 1989[290]	5-FU, 300 mg/m²/d by continuous infusion.
Arbeitsgemeinschaft Internischiste Onkologie (weekly 24-h infusion)	Kohne et al., 1998[294]	LV, 500 mg/m² over 2 h, followed by 5-FU, 2600 mg/m² over 24 h, repeated weekly.
LV5FU2	de Gramont et al., 1997[296]	LV, 200 mg/m² over 2 h, d 1 and 2, followed by bolus 5-FU, 400 mg/m² d 1 and 2, followed by 5-FU, 600 mg/m² over 22 h, d 1 and 2; cycle repeated every 14 d.
Simplified LV5FU2	Adapted from Andre et al., 1999[352]	LV, 400 mg/m² over 2 h, followed by bolus 5-FU, 400 mg/m², followed by 5-FU, 2400–3000 mg/m² over 46–48 h; cycles repeated every 14 d.

LV, leucovorin.
Note: Dosages listed are recommended starting dosages for patients with good performance status and normal renal, hepatic, and bone marrow function. Individual dosage adjustments may be required.
[a]All agents administered IV.

understood mechanics of 5-FU's interactions with cellular mechanisms to enhance its therapeutic performance. The key to successful biomodulation is selective enhancement of antitumor activity. A maneuver that merely increases the activity of the agent against both malignant and normal tissues is of little benefit. Several of the more prominent biomodulation strategies that have been used are reviewed in the following sections and are summarized in Table 29.8-13.

Leucovorin

The most widely used agent for the biomodulation of 5-FU is the reduced folate leucovorin, also referred to as folinic acid, citrovorum factor, or 5-formyl-tetrahydrofolate. 5-Formyl-tetrahydrofolate is catabolized to 5,10-methylene-tetrathydrofolate, which donates a methyl group to uridylate (deoxyuridine monophosphate, or dUMP) and thereby converts it to thymidylate (deoxythymidine monophosphate, or dTMP), a required building block for DNA synthesis. This process is catalyzed by the enzyme TS through the formation of a ternary complex of dUMP, 5,10-methylene-tetrahydrofolate, and TS.[274] In the presence of 5-FU, fluorodeoxyuridylate (FdUMP), which has greater affinity than dUMP for TS due to the electronegativity of the fluorine atom, preferentially displaces dUMP in this reaction. The covalently linked ternary complex is formed, but the synthesis of thymidylate does not proceed forward, because the methyl group cannot displace the fluorine due to the strength of the fluorine-carbon bond. The stability and durability of the FdUMP–TS–5,10-methylene-tetrahydrofolate ternary complex is increased in the presence of increased quantities of reduced folates such as leucovorin.[274,275] Thus, by potentiating the FdUMP–TS–5,10-methylene-tetrahydrofolate ternary complex, leucovorin potentiates the inhibitory effect of FdUMP on TS and so potentiates the cytotoxic activity of 5-FU.

The laboratory rationale for the biomodulation of 5-FU by leucovorin is so compelling that it is easy to be seduced into the assumption that such an approach must work. Clearly the approach is valid in preclinical systems. The issue of clinical relevance, however, has always been whether or not the therapeutic index of 5-FU can be improved by increasing the antitumor effects without increasing toxicity. Put another way, the issue is whether biomodulation selectively increases the inhibitory effects of 5-FU on malignant over nonmalignant tissue. If so, it is potentially useful; if not, there may be little difference between the biomodulation maneuver and simply increasing the dosage of 5-FU.

Initial uncontrolled pilot trials of 5-FU/leucovorin combinations showed encouraging response rates, although often in the setting of significant toxicity.[276–279] Laboratory data were inconsistent regarding the optimal plasma levels of leucovorin, and multiple treatment schedules were developed using a variety of dosages of both leucovorin and 5-FU. After a large number of uncontrolled phase II explorations, several large randomized trials were conducted.

Poon et al. conducted the trial that, perhaps more than any other, established leucovorin as the biomodulation agent of choice in standard care regimens.[280,281] 5-FU and leucovorin were each given for five consecutive days (Monday through Friday), with treatment cycles repeated at 4 weeks, 8 weeks, and then every 5 weeks thereafter, with either low-dose leucovorin (20 mg/m^2/d) plus 5-FU 425 mg/m^2/d or high-dose leucovorin (200 mg/m^2/d) plus 5-FU 370 mg/m^2/d. The control arm received either 5-FU alone or 5-FU modulated by methotrexate (MTX; which was not found to be effective in this trial). The patients receiving the daily × 5, low-dose leucovorin regimen, which has become widely known as the Mayo Clinic schedule, had the best outcome, with response rates and overall survival superior to those of the control arm both at the *P* <.01 level. On the basis of these data, the Mayo Clinic schedule became both a United States regulatory standard and the most widely used schedule of 5-FU in North America.

There were, however, trials of leucovorin with negative results as well. In a randomized trial involving 181 colorectal patients receiving 5-FU/leucovorin (5-FU 400 mg/m^2/d plus leucovorin 200 mg/m^2/d for 5 days, repeated every 4 weeks) or 5-FU alone (5-FU 13.5 mg/kg/d for 5 days, repeated every 4 weeks), the Italian Oncology Group for Clinical Research reported no statistically significant differences in response rates, time to treatment failure, or overall survival.[282]

Other investigators evaluated the question of whether leucovorin was, in fact, improving the therapeutic index of 5-FU or simply causing higher activity with higher toxicity. Two hun-

dred and ten patients were randomly assigned in a double-blind, placebo-controlled trial to receive 5-FU 375 mg/m^2/d for three consecutive days, followed by weekly treatments starting at 375 mg/m^2 and escalating by prespecified increments until target levels of toxicity were achieved, plus either oral leucovorin or placebo.[283] Again there were no statistically significant differences in response rate, time to tumor progression, or overall survival.

To try to further clarify the contribution of leucovorin, the Advanced Colorectal Cancer Meta-Analysis Project performed a metaanalysis of nine randomized studies that compared 5-FU/leucovorin with 5-FU alone.[284] Leucovorin was found to substantially improve response rate in this analysis (23% vs. 11%; *P* <.0000001), but overall survival did not differ with and without leucovorin (*P* = .57). Of the nine studies included in this metaanalysis, four gave a higher 5-FU dosage in the non–leucovorin-containing arm. The arms of these studies were more likely to show similar levels of both toxicity and activity. The five trials that treated patients with the same dosage of 5-FU in each arm with or without leucovorin tended to show higher activity and higher toxicity for the leucovorin-containing arm. More recently, an update of this metaanalysis has been reported, with longer follow-up and nine additional trials.[285] In an analysis of 2751 patients from 18 trials, a small but statistically significant survival advantage was seen for the leucovorin-containing regimens. The highest benefit (8%) was seen in those trials that used similar 5-FU dosages in each arm.

Other trials have attempted to identify which dosing schedules of 5-FU and leucovorin are optimal. The NCCTG compared the two most widely used leucovorin schedules, the Mayo Clinic low-dose, daily × 5 schedule and the Roswell Park weekly high-dose leucovorin schedule for 6 weeks repeated every 8 weeks.[286] No significant differences in efficacy were seen. The Mayo Clinic regimen produced higher rates of myelosuppression and mucositis, whereas the Roswell Park schedule produced more diarrhea. The Roswell Park schedule in this particular trial was 5-FU 600 mg/m^2 and leucovorin 500 mg/m^2, each given weekly for 6 weeks repeated every 8 weeks. It should be noted that experience has shown the 600 mg/m^2 dose of 5-FU in the original Roswell Park regimen to result in unacceptable toxicity, particularly in terms of diarrhea. The standard dose of 5-FU in the Roswell Park regimen is now considered to be 500 mg/m^2.

A direct comparison of the Roswell Park schedule of weekly 5-FU (500 mg/m^2) with either high-dose (500 mg/m^2) or low-dose (20 mg/m^2) leucovorin showed no significant efficacy differences between the two leucovorin doses. Diarrhea was substantially lessened with the lower dose of leucovorin.[287]

The SWOG performed a randomized phase II trial to assess the activity of several of these biomodulation approaches.[288] The trial was not designed or powered to detect subtle differences, but rather was intended to identify a regimen or regimens that looked most promising on the basis of antitumor activity. A total of 629 chemotherapy-naive patients were randomly assigned to one of six different 5-FU schedules: bolus 5-FU alone, bolus daily × 5-FU/low-dose leucovorin (Mayo Clinic schedule), Roswell Park high-dose weekly leucovorin schedule, 5-FU PVI for 28 days followed by a 1-week rest, 5-FU PVI plus leucovorin, intermittent high-dose weekly 5-FU by 24-hour infusion, and intermittent high-dose weekly infusional 5-FU preceded by 250 mg/m^2 of the now-discontinued investigational agent *N*-phosphonoacetyl-*l*-aspartic acid. None of the biomodulated regimens was superior to single-agent 5-FU bolus in terms of response rate, progression-free survival, or overall survival.

Protracted Venous Infusion

For practical reasons, early trials of 5-FU centered on bolus administration. However, preclinical evidence suggested that increased duration of exposure could improve efficacy.[289] Because the plasma half-life of 5-FU is short (8 to 20 minutes), infusional administration schedules were developed in an attempt to increase efficacy.

The Mid-Atlantic Oncology Program reported a randomized trial of PVI 5-FU at a dosage of 300 mg/m²/d continuously versus 5-FU via bolus administration.[290] There was no difference in survival between the two treatment arms (*P* = .37); however, the PVI treatment was associated with a higher response rate than the bolus regimen (30% vs. 7%, respectively). Improved response rate without survival benefit was also demonstrated in an ECOG trial.[291] A metaanalysis encompassing 1219 patients in six trials comparing PVI 5-FU to bolus 5-FU reported an improved response rate of 22% versus 14% (*P* = .0002) in favor of PVI.[292] Survival time with PVI 5-FU was statistically superior, but this survival advantage was less than 1 month.

High-Dose Intermittent Infusion

In contrast to PVI, in which patients are connected to ambulatory infusion pumps for weeks to months at a time, high-dose intermittent infusion schedules administer 5-FU over 24 to 48 hours, with considerable breaks between treatments. These schedules are far less restrictive for patients than PVI schedules, and discussions of the patient acceptability issues of "infusional" treatment must clarify which sort of infusional schedule is under consideration.

Ardalan et al. reported a small phase II trial of 5-FU 2600 mg/m² given weekly by 24-hour infusion with leucovorin 500 mg/m². Major responses were seen in 10 of 22 patients, including three responses in the 10 patients who had received prior therapy.[293] A larger randomized trial reported by Kohne et al. for the German Arbeitsgemeinschaft Internischiste Onkologie cooperative group confirmed the activity of this regimen, with a major objective response rate of 44% in 91 patients.[294] This trial also found that IFN-α did not add to the activity of this regimen but did add considerable toxicity. A larger phase III confirmatory trial compared the weekly high-dose infusion of 2600 mg/m², either alone or with 500 mg/m² of leucovorin, to the Mayo Clinic bolus daily × 5 schedule of 5-FU. No overall survival differences were seen. The response rates in this confirmatory trial were disappointing at 12% for the bolus regimen versus 10% and 17% for the infusional regimen alone and with leucovorin, respectively (differences not significant). Progression-free survival was increased in the infusion plus leucovorin regimen (*P* = .029), but at the expense of increased incidence of severe diarrhea.[295]

De Gramont et al. developed a regimen with combined bolus and high-dose infusional 5-FU (LV5FU2). Patients received leucovorin 200 mg/m² over 2 hours, followed by a 5-FU bolus of 400 mg/m², followed by 5-FU 600 mg/m² by 22-hour infusion, with all drugs given on days 1 and 2, repeated every 14 days. This LV5FU2 schedule was compared to the daily × 5 Mayo Clinic bolus schedule in a randomized trial.[296] In 433 evaluable patients, the response rate was better for LV5FU2 than for the Mayo Clinic 5-FU schedule (33% vs. 14%; *P* = .0004). The median progression-free survival was modestly but statistically significantly superior for LV5FU2 as well (*P* = .0012). Overall survival for the LV5FU2 group was approximately 5 weeks longer than for the Mayo group. This difference closely approached but did not reach statistical significance (*P* = .067). Patients on the LV5FU2 regimen experienced less overall toxicity than the patients on the Mayo Clinic schedule.

Methotrexate

MTX increases the available intracellular pools of 5'-phospho-ribosyl-1-pyrophosphate (PRPP) as a result of its blocking of purine synthesis. PRPP facilitates the incorporation of 5-FU into RNA by formation of fluorouridine triphosphate RNA building blocks. MTX also increases levels of polyglutamated reduced folates, and this facilitates binding of FdUMP to TS.[274,297] Numerous clinical trials, including a number of randomized trials of MTX modulation of 5-FU, have been performed with conflicting results. A metaanalysis of eight randomized trials comparing MTX/5-FU with 5-FU alone and encompassing 1178 patients found a higher response rate (19% vs. 10%) and a modest 1.6-month survival advantage (odds ratio, 0.87; *P* = .024) for the patients receiving MTX-modulated 5-FU[298]; however, enough negative trial results have been reported to dampen interest in this approach, and MTX modulation is rarely used in colorectal cancer treatments.[281,299]

Trimetrexate

Although MTX and leucovorin were initially thought to have the potential for synergistic "double modulation" of 5-FU, in fact evidence indicates that these two agents compete for the same transport mechanisms for cell entry. They then also compete for intracellular polyglutamation.[300] Trimetrexate (TMTX) is a nonclassical folate that enters the cell by diffusion and does not require polyglutamation for activity.[301] Initial studies did not show single-agent activity in colorectal cancer[302]; however, TMTX was further investigated as a potential biomodulating agent for 5-FU plus leucovorin. It was determined in a phase I trial that 110 mg/m² of TMTX could be safely given 24 hours before each weekly full dose of 5-FU on the Roswell Park regimen (5-FU and leucovorin each at 500 mg/m² weekly for 6 weeks, repeated every 8 weeks).[303] Enthusiasm was raised by a 50% response rate in a multicenter phase II trial of this combination.[304] However, a trial of this combination in patients with 5-FU–refractory cancer did not show appreciable activity.[304a] Furthermore, randomized phase III trials failed to showed benefit to the inclusion of TMTX with 5-FU and leucovorin, and did show that TMTX increased toxicity.[305,306] These results indicate that TMTX does not have a role in the treatment of colorectal cancer.

Interferon-α

Preclinical evidence of enhanced cytotoxicity of 5-FU with addition of IFN-α led to phase I and II development with encouraging initial reports,[307,308] although one phase II study found results for the group receiving the combination to be no better than that for historical controls, with substantial toxicity.[309] Despite the fact that the majority of phase II trials were encouraging, multiple randomized trials of IFN-α plus 5-FU have failed to show a benefit for this approach.[310–313] Two metaanalyses, published together, looked at the results of randomized trials involving 3254 patients. IFN-α was shown to be of no benefit when added to a 5-FU/leucovorin combination compared with 5-FU/leucovorin alone, and 5-FU/IFN-α was shown to be significantly inferior to 5-FU/leucovorin.[314] At this point, the data strongly indicate that IFN-α should not be used in the management of colorectal cancer.

Eniluracil

The rate-limiting step in the degradation of 5-FU is mediated by the enzyme DPD.[315] Eniluracil is a potent, irreversible inhibitor of DPD.[316] In the setting of eniluracil, 5-FU half-life is dramatically prolonged.[317] Because DPD in the liver influences variable first-pass clearance of 5-FU when taken orally, eniluracil permits oral dosing of 5-FU. An ECOG phase II study showed only modest clinical activity,[318] however, and pivotal randomized trials comparing eniluracil-containing regimens against standard 5-FU regimens did not show an advantage for the use of eniluracil. This compound has now been withdrawn from clinical development.

CAPECITABINE

Capecitabine is a 5-FU precursor that is administered orally. It is absorbed intact through the gut and then activated by a series of enzymatic alterations. First, carboxylesterase, predominantly in the liver, metabolizes capecitabine to 5'-deoxy-fluoro-cytidine (5'DFCR). This is then metabolized by cytidine deaminase to 5'-deoxy-5-fluorouridine. 5'-Deoxy-5-fluorouridine is then converted by thymidine phosphorylase into 5-FU. Some data suggest that thymidine phosphorylase levels are higher in tumor than in normal tissue. This could provide a degree of preferential intratumoral activation.[319] Phase II studies demonstrated that capecitabine had substantial activity in colorectal cancer, with an acceptable toxicity profile.[320] Because the addition of leucovorin did not appear to show any benefit, clinical development has gone forward without additional biomodulation. Phase III randomized clinical trials performed both in the United States and Europe have now shown that this orally administered agent is at least as effective as intravenous 5-FU/leucovorin, and the side effect profile of capecitabine is superior to that of the Mayo Clinic schedule of 5-FU.[321,322] The dosage used in these pivotal trials was 1250 mg/m² given twice daily for 14 days followed by a 7-day rest. The major side effects of capecitabine appear to be diarrhea and palmar-plantar erythrodysesthesia, or hand-foot syndrome. This latter toxicity is frequently a dose-limiting side effect, and although the approved starting dosage is 1250 mg/m² twice daily, many clinicians choose to initiate therapy at a lower dosage and escalate if no toxicity is seen. A review of results from two large trials suggests that efficacy was not compromised in those patients who required dosage reductions.[323] Single-agent capecitabine would appear to be a reasonable alternative when 5-FU or biomodulated 5-FU alone is being considered. As is discussed later in Comparisons of Oxaliplatin and Irinotecan-Based Combinations, there is also now considerable interest in combining

capecitabine with other agents, although these combinations are not yet validated in randomized trials. In combination schedules the starting dosage is frequently decreased to 1000 mg/m² twice daily or lower.

URACIL/TEGAFUR PLUS LEUCOVORIN

UFT is a combination of uracil and the fluorouracil prodrug tegafur (ftorafur) in a 4:1 molar ratio. Uracil reversibly and competitively inhibits DPD. Tegafur is a 5-FU prodrug that was previously shown to have antitumor activity in colorectal cancer; however, it produced a neurotoxic metabolite, which limited its clinical usefulness. By inhibiting DPD, uracil allows reliable oral absorption of tegafur and permits small quantities to be used, which greatly reduces the accumulation of metabolites and eliminates the neurotoxicity. DPD inhibition also normalizes the wide range of interpatient DPD activity levels, facilitating dosing estimations and making toxicity more predictable. UFT has been studied most commonly in combination with oral leucovorin on a three-times-daily schedule. Phase II schedules using low-dose leucovorin (5 mg three times daily) with 350 mg/m²/d of UFT divided over three doses daily[324] and high-dose leucovorin (50 mg three times daily)[325] with 300 mg/m² of UFT divided over three doses daily both showed acceptable tolerability, and both showed activity comparable to that which can be achieved with intravenous 5-FU schedules. Two large-scale randomized studies comparing UFT plus oral leucovorin to the parenteral Mayo Clinic schedule of 5-FU/leucovorin were conducted using 300 mg/m²/d of UFT and an intermediate leucovorin dosage of 25 to 30 mg three times daily. Both of these trials showed no significant differences in response rates, time to tumor progression, or overall survival between the oral and parenteral regimens.[326,327] In the United States, the trials did not, however, fulfill the regulatory requirements for noninferiority of UFT/leucovorin, and therefore this compound is not registered in the United States. It is widely used in much of Asia and Europe.

RALTITREXED

Raltitrexed is a nonfluoropyrimidine TS inhibitor that is transported into the tumor reduced folate carriers and then polyglutamated, which results in retained intracellular levels and prolonged inhibition of TS. This allows for once-every-3-weeks dosing. Large-scale trials have demonstrated similar response rates for raltitrexed at 3 mg/m² given once every 3 weeks and standard 5-FU/leucovorin bolus schedules.[328] One trial, however, showed a statistically significantly worse survival for the raltitrexed arm than for the 5-FU/leucovorin arm (9.7 vs. 12.7 months; *P* = .01). An interesting approach to use of this drug is suggested by the observation that low levels of TS predict response to this agent.[329] This could potentially be exploited to favorably select individuals for treatment with raltitrexed. Combination trials with this agent have also been of interest, although randomized data are lacking. The drug is not approved for use in the United States but is available and used in many other parts of the world.

IRINOTECAN

A published review of trials of new agents in treatment of colorectal cancer between 1960 and 1990 found that none of the 72 compounds tested was able to reproducibly exceed the response rate for 5-FU.[330] Given the limitations of accomplishments achievable with biomodulation strategies, new nonfluoropyrimidine agents were clearly needed. The first such agent to show substantial clinical activity in colorectal cancer was irinotecan (CPT-11).

Irinotecan is a semisynthetic derivative of camptothecin, a plant alkaloid extracted from the wood of the Asian tree *Camptotheca acuminate*.[331] Camptothecin was identified as an agent with potential antitumor activity in 1966; however, its poor solubility greatly hampered its initial clinical development. Initial clinical trials in the early 1970s showed antitumor activity but also severe and unpredictable toxicity. Development of camptothecin languished until the mid-1980s, when the identification of camptothecin's mechanism of action led to renewed interest in and renewed efforts to develop soluble derivatives, of which irinotecan (the CPT in CPT-11 is an abbreviation for camptothecin) was one. Irinotecan possesses a bulky dipiperidino side chain linked to the camptothecin molecule via a carboxyl-ester bond. This side chain provides solubility but greatly decreases anticancer activity. Carboxylesterase, a ubiquitous enzyme with primary activity in the liver and gut, cleaves the carboxyl-ester bond to form the more active metabolite, 7-ethyl-10-hydroxycamptothecin (SN-38).[332] SN-38 is as much as 1000-fold more potent in inhibiting topoisomerase I than irinotecan and is thus the predominant active form of the drug. Irinotecan is often considered to be a prodrug for SN-38; however, this concept may be a bit too simplistic, because achieved irinotecan concentrations may be several log units higher than those of SN-38.

Camptothecin, irinotecan, and SN-38 function as inhibitors of topoisomerase I. Topoisomerase I is a nuclear enzyme that aids in DNA uncoiling for replication and transcription. When topoisomerase I binds to DNA, it causes a reversible single-strand break in the DNA, which allows the intact strand to pass through the break to relieve torsional stress on the coiled helix, and then reseals the break. Irinotecan and SN-38 stabilize these single-strand breaks. Although the stabilized breaks do not cause irreversible damage, the collision of replication forks with open single-strand breaks results in double-strand breaks, which leads to lethal DNA fragmentation.

Ironotecan As a Single Agent

A number of different schedules of irinotecan were explored in initial phase I studies, and antitumor activity was seen in a number of patients with colorectal cancer,[333–337] which led to phase II studies of its use in this disease. A phase II trial reported by Shimada et al. found a 22% response rate in a population of previously treated colorectal cancer patients.[338] A subsequent trial reported a 23% response rate and 31% stable disease rate in 43 patients with 5-FU–refractory colorectal cancer.[339]

A combined analysis of data for 304 patients with 5-FU–refractory colorectal cancer from three trials using a 90-minute infusion of irinotecan weekly for 4 weeks followed by a 2-week rest showed a major objective response rate of 13%, with 49% of patients having a minor response or stable disease.[340] Starting dosages ranged from 100 to 150 mg/m²; however, 125 mg/m² was felt to provide the best balance of efficacy and toxicity. Diarrhea and neutropenia were the primary dose-limiting toxicities encountered.

In a phase II trial conducted in France, investigators gave a 350-mg/m² starting dose of irinotecan once every 3 weeks to colorectal cancer patients who were either previously treated with 5-FU or who were chemotherapy naive. An 18% response rate was seen, both in the 48 chemotherapy-naive patients and in the 165 patients who had previously progressed through a 5-FU–based regimen.[341] A U.S. phase II trial of irinotecan in previously untreated colorectal cancer patients reported a 32% response rate using a 125-mg/m² starting dose of irinotecan given weekly for 4 weeks, followed by a 2-week break.[342] Another trial done in the U.S. with this same weekly schedule of irinotecan found a response rate of 26% in 31 previously untreated colorectal cancer patients.[343]

The promising results seen in 5-FU–refractory colorectal cancer in phase II trials were confirmed in randomized phase III trials. Cunningham et al. compared a 350-mg/m² starting dose of irinotecan (300 mg/m² for patients aged 70 years and older) given every 3 weeks to best supportive care in patients with 5-FU–refractory colorectal cancer.[344] This trial showed a 36% 1-year survival for the irinotecan-treated group versus a 14% 1-year survival for the group receiving best supportive care. Quality-of-life parameters for the irinotecan-treated patients, as measured by the EORTC QLQ-C30 questionnaire, were as good as or better than those for patients receiving best supportive care for all major indices.

In a parallel trial, patients with 5-FU–refractory colorectal cancer were randomly assigned to the same schedule of irinotecan as in the previously described trial or to an infusional 5-FU regimen.[345] In this trial as well, the survival of the patients receiving irinotecan was statistically superior, with the 1-year survival for the irinotecan-treated patients being 1.4 times that of the group receiving infusional 5-FU. Quality-of-life data were comparable for the two treatment groups.

Neutropenia and diarrhea were the major toxicities encountered in all of the initial trials of irinotecan, and diarrhea in particular threatened to greatly limit the clinical usefulness of this agent. Two different diarrheal syndromes were identified: early onset and late onset. The early-onset diarrhea, which occurs during or immediately after irinotecan administration, is a cholinergic effect and is readily controlled by the use of atropine.[346] In those patients who experience this symptom (and who do not have a contraindication to atropine administration), 0.5 to 1 mg of atropine gives rapid resolution, and subsequent irinotecan doses can then be given with atropine as a premedication. The late-onset diarrhea is more problematic. A pivotal advance in the development of irinotecan came from Abigerges et al. These investigators identified that aggressive use of intensive loperamide therapy was highly effective in the management of irinotecan-induced late-onset diarrhea.[347] Early and aggressive use of loperamide for management of late-onset diarrhea is now a cornerstone of irinotecan therapy. Although a direct randomized comparison of weekly versus every-3-week administration of single-agent irinotecan showed no substantial differences in terms of efficacy parameters, the once-every-3-weeks schedule was associated with significantly less severe diarrhea.[348]

Irinotecan in First-Line Combination Regimens

The results of first-line trials with single-agent irinotecan did not appear to justify the routine first-line single-agent use of this drug. This finding, and the recognition that 5-FU and irinotecan

TABLE 29.8-14. Commonly Used Irinotecan/5-Fluorouracil (5-FU) Combination Regimens

Name of Regimen	Reference	Schedule[a]
IFL	Saltz et al., 2000[350]	Irinotecan, 125 mg/m^2 over 90 min, followed by LV, 20 mg/m^2 by brief infusion, followed by bolus 5-FU, 500 mg/m^2; all treatments repeated weekly for 4 wk, repeated every 6 wk.
FOLFIRI	Douillard et al., 2000[351]	Irinotecan, 180 mg/m^2 over 2 h; LV, 200 mg/m^2 concurrently with irinotecan (can be given in same line through Y connector), followed by 5-FU bolus, 400 mg/m^2, followed by 5-FU, 600 mg/m^2 infusion over 22 h. Irinotecan given d 1 only. All other agents given d 1 and 2. Cycle repeated every 14 d.
FOLFIRI (simplified)	Andre et al., 1999[352]	Irinotecan, 180 mg/m^2 over 2 h; LV, 400 mg/m^2 concurrently with irinotecan (can be given in same line through Y connector), followed by 5-FU bolus, 400 mg/m^2, followed by 5-FU, 2400–3000 mg/m^2 infusion over 46–48 h. Cycle repeated every 14 d.
FUFIRI	Douillard et al., 2000[351]	Irinotecan, 80 mg/m^2, then LV, 500 mg/m^2, followed by 5-FU, 2300 mg/m^2; all drugs given weekly for 6 wk, repeated every 7 wk.

LV, leucovorin.
Note: Dosages listed are recommended starting dosages for patients with good performance status and normal renal, hepatic, and bone marrow function. Individual dosage adjustments may be required.
[a]All agents administered IV.

appeared to be killing different populations of tumor cells, led to interest in development of combination schedules of irinotecan plus 5-FU. The overlapping toxicity profiles of these agents, with neutropenia and diarrhea figuring prominently in both, constituted the major obstacle in the development of such regimens. Numerous combinations of 5-FU, usually with leucovorin, plus irinotecan, were tested in phase I trials. Saltz et al. reported a phase I trial built on the weekly irinotecan schedule that had been selected for phase I development in North America. A low dose of weekly leucovorin was used to reduce the potential for 5-FU/leucovorin-induced diarrhea. The phase I trial showed that the full single-agent dose of 125 mg/m^2 of irinotecan could be given with 500 mg/m^2 of 5-FU and 20 mg/m^2 of leucovorin, with all drugs given weekly for four consecutive weeks followed by a 2-week break.[349] This and other irinotecan/5-FU/leucovorin regimens are summarized in Table 29.8-14.

This combination of irinotecan, 5-FU, and leucovorin (IFL) was compared to the Mayo Clinic schedule of 5-FU/leucovorin in a multicenter, multinational phase III trial.[350] For regulatory reasons, a single-agent irinotecan arm was included as well. The IFL combination was found to be superior to Mayo Clinic 5-FU/leucovorin in terms of response rate, time to tumor progression, and overall survival. Although it was not the focus of any planned statistical analysis, treatment with irinotecan alone appeared to be comparable in efficacy to treatment with 5-FU/leucovorin. The overall incidence of severe toxicity was similar in all arms of this trial. More serious diarrhea and vomiting were seen with IFL, whereas more neutropenia, neutropenic fever, and stomatitis

were seen with 5-FU/leucovorin. Treatment-related deaths occurred in 1% of patients in each arm of the trial.

In Europe a parallel study investigating the benefit of adding irinotecan to a 5-FU–based schedule was undertaken.[351] Development of irinotecan/5-FU combinations in Europe centered on the use of infusional schedules. Two high-dose intermittent infusional schedules were developed. In France, a biweekly treatment for two consecutive days was explored, whereas German investigators, building on their experience with weekly 24-hour high-dose infusions of 5-FU, combined irinotecan with this schedule. A randomized phase III trial was performed in which a participating center chose which of these two schedules would be used, and then the patients were randomly assigned to that 5-FU/leucovorin schedule plus or minus irinotecan. These combination regimens are outlined in Table 29.8-14. Again, response rate, progression-free survival, and overall survival were superior in the irinotecan-containing arm of the trial. Of note, only the cohort treated with the biweekly schedule demonstrated a statistically superior survival compared with the 5-FU/leucovorin control arm, and the biweekly combination schedule is the only one registered for use in the United States.

More recently, the biweekly schedule of LV5FU2 plus irinotecan has been studied with a simplified LV5FU2 infusion schedule.[352] This schedule, known as FOLFIRI (FOL = folinic acid, F = 5-FU, IRI = irinotecan), was initially studied as a salvage regimen; however, this has now gained widespread acceptance as a first-line treatment option, based on data to be discussed later in Comparisons of Oxaliplatin- and Irinotecan-Based Combinations.

OXALIPLATIN

Oxaliplatin [1,2-diaminocyclohexane (trans-l) oxalatoplatinum] is a third-generation platinum compound of the diaminocyclohexane (DACH) family. Early preclinical testing indicated that DACH platinum compounds had activity in some cancer cell lines and murine models that were resistant to cisplatin. Raymond et al. further characterized the preclinical activity of oxaliplatin using the human tumor cloning assay and demonstrated a broad spectrum of preclinical activity, including activity in colon cancer specimens.[353] Animal studies also demonstrated a toxicity pattern markedly different from that of cisplatin, including a lack of nephrotoxicity.[354]

Oxaliplatin, like other platinum compounds, exerts its cytotoxicity through the formation of platinum-DNA adducts, which cross-link the strands of the DNA double helix, blocking both DNA replication and transcription. The DACH carrier ligand confers additional bulkiness to the platinum adducts, which creates greater disruption of repair mechanisms by steric interference. In contrast to cisplatin-induced adducts, oxaliplatin-induced DNA adducts resist binding of mismatch repair protein complexes and thereby facilitate activation of apoptotic pathways.[355]

Initial single-agent phase I studies established that oxaliplatin could be safely administered and showed evidence of clinical activity.[356,357] No significant nephrotoxicity was seen. Nausea and vomiting, minimal leucopenia, and rare thrombocytopenia were observed. Extra et al.[356] were the first to describe in detail the most notable toxicity encountered with oxaliplatin: neurotoxicity. This neurotoxicity manifested as paresthesias and dysesthesias of the hands, feet, perioral region, and throat. Pharyngolaryngeal dysesthesia, a sensation of choking without overt airway blockage, was described as well. These neurologic toxicities were induced or worsened by exposure to cold. In this early trial the neurotoxic effects were found to be dose dependent, becoming prominent at the 135 mg/m^2 level and escalating in frequency at higher doses. This led to a recommended phase II dose of 130 mg. Initial neurologic symptoms resolved rapidly; however, duration of symptoms increased with additional cycles.

Using a 130-mg/m^2 starting dose over 2 hours every 3 weeks, Diaz-Rubio et al. conducted a phase II trial of single-agent oxaliplatin in chemotherapy-naive colorectal cancer patients.[358] The investigator-reported response rate was 20%; however, an independent radiologic review identified a 12% major objective response rate. Neurotoxicity was common, with 92% of patients experiencing neuropathy and 75% experiencing laryngopharyngeal dysesthesias, but no grade 3 or 4 neurologic events were noted. No nephrotoxicity or ototoxicity was encountered. A second single-agent first-line study of oxaliplatin conducted by the Digestive Group of French Federation of Cancer Centers reported similar results, with a response rate of 24%.[359] Grade 3 neurotoxicity was encountered in 13% of the patients treated. Other toxicities were manageable.

Machover et al. reported two consecutive phase II trials of single-agent oxaliplatin given at 130 mg/m^2 every 3 weeks to previously treated colorectal cancer patients.[360] The response rate for the total of 106 patients was 10%. Neurotoxicity, which was cumulative both in severity and in incidence, was seen to some degree in over 95% of patients in both trials.

Other investigators explored the use of single-agent oxaliplatin using chronomodulation to exploit the potential influence of circadian rhythms on oxaliplatin activity and toxicity. A randomized phase I study indicated that a higher dose of oxaliplatin could be administered with manageable toxicity using a chronomodulated schedule.[361] Patients received either a flat 5-day continuous infusion of oxaliplatin or a chronomodulated infusion. The group on the chronomodulated schedule was able to achieve a 15% higher maximum tolerated dose, with substantially less neurotoxicity and less vomiting. A phase II trial was conducted involving 29 patients with chemotherapy-refractory colorectal cancer using this biomodulated regimen. Starting dosage was 30 mg/m^2/d for 5 days repeated every 3 weeks, with peak administration at 4:00 p.m. (1600 hours), and 5-mg/m^2 dose escalations were introduced over the first three cycles as tolerated. Despite the encouraging results from the previous phase I study, this phase II trial found a response rate of 10%. Seventy-nine percent of patients experienced some degree of neurotoxicity, which reached grade 3 in 12%.

OXALIPLATIN/5-FLUOROURACIL/LEUCOVORIN COMBINATION REGIMENS

Based on a series of phase II trials by Levi et al.[362,363] Giachetti et al. from the same group reported a phase III trial of chronomodulated 5-FU/leucovorin alone or with oxaliplatin.[364] Two hundred patients were randomly assigned to receive a 5-day course every 3 weeks of chronomodulated 5-FU and leucovorin (700 and 300 mg/m^2/d, respectively; peak delivery rate at 0400 hours) with or without oxaliplatin on the first day of each course (125 mg/m^2, as a 6-hour infusion). The group receiving oxaliplatin had a superior response rate (53% vs. 16%; P <.001). Progression-free survival was also superior, just reach-

ing statistical significance (8.7 vs. 7.4 months; P = .048). There were no differences in median overall survival (19.4 and 19.9 months, respectively). Survival outcomes in this trial are somewhat difficult to interpret, because resection of metastatic disease was used extensively in both arms.

Most of the 5-FU/leucovorin/oxaliplatin combination trials have used flat (nonchronomodulated) administration of agents and have centered on variants of the FOLFOX regimen. The term *FOLFOX* [FOL = folinic acid (leucovorin), F = fluorouracil, OX = oxaliplatin] refers to a series of combinations of these agents developed by de Gramont et al. These are biweekly (every-other-week) regimens using 2 days of infusional 5-FU on a 14-day cycle (LV5FU2) as previously described by this group.[296] The FOLFOX 1, 2, and 3 regimens used various alterations in dosing of oxaliplatin, 5-FU, and leucovorin.[365,366] They are of historical interest but were never evaluated in randomized trials. FOLFOX 3 and FOLFOX 4 were reported in a combined series to yield a response rate of 21% in a population of patients whose disease had progressed on the same 5-FU/leucovorin schedule without oxaliplatin.[352] The FOLFOX 4 regimen had a modestly higher response rate and lower toxicity than FOLFOX 3 (which used higher doses of 5-FU and leucovorin), and FOLFOX 4 appeared to be better tolerated. The more commonly used oxaliplatin/5-FU/leucovorin combinations are outlined in Table 29.8-15.

TABLE 29.8-15. Selected Commonly Used Oxaliplatin/5-Fluorouracil (5-FU) Combination Regimens

Name of Regimen	Reference	Schedule[a]
FOLFOX 4	de Gramont et al., 2000[367]	Oxaliplatin, 85 mg/m^2 over 2 h; LV, 200 mg/m^2 concurrently with oxaliplatin (can be given in same line through Y connector), followed by 5-FU bolus, 400 mg/m^2, followed by 5-FU, 600 mg/m^2 infusion over 22 h. Oxaliplatin given d 1 only. All other agents given d 1 and 2. Cycle repeated every 14 d.
FOLFOX 6	Tournigand et al., 2001[371]	Oxaliplatin, 100 mg/m^2 over 2 h; LV, 400 mg/m^2 concurrently with irinotecan (can be given in same line through Y connector), followed by 5-FU bolus, 400 mg/m^2, followed by 5-FU, 2400–3000 mg/m^2 infusion over 46–48 h. Cycle repeated every 14 d.
Modified FOLFOX 6	Widely used in current phase III trials, but not published	Oxaliplatin, 85 mg/m^2 over 2 h; LV, 400 mg/m^2 concurrently with irinotecan (can be given in same line through Y connector), followed by 5-FU bolus, 400 mg/m^2, followed by 5-FU, 2400–3000 mg/m^2 infusion over 46–48 h. Cycle repeated every 14 d.
FUFOX	Grothey et al., 2002[428]	Oxaliplatin, 50 mg/m^2 over 2 h, followed by LV, 500 mg/m^2, followed by 5-FU, 2000 mg/m^2 over 24 h, weekly for 5 wk; repeated every 6 wk.

LV, leucovorin.
Note: Dosages listed are recommended starting dosages for patients with good performance status and normal renal, hepatic, and bone marrow function. Individual dosage adjustments may be required.
[a]All agents administered IV.

A randomized phase III trial was undertaken to evaluate use of the FOLFOX 4 regimen in comparison to the LV5FU2 schedule of 5-FU and leucovorin in patients with previously untreated metastatic colorectal cancer (essentially a trial of LV5FU2 plus or minus oxaliplatin).[367] Four hundred and twenty previously untreated patients with measurable disease were randomly assigned to receive a 2-hour infusion of leucovorin (200 mg/m^2/d) followed by a 5-FU bolus (400 mg/m^2/d) and 22-hour infusion (600 mg/m^2/d) for two consecutive days every 2 weeks, either alone or together with oxaliplatin 85 mg/m^2 as a 2-hour infusion on day 1. Patients treated with FOLFOX 4 had a significantly superior outcome in terms of response rate (51% vs. 22%; P = .001) and progression-free survival (9.0 vs. 6.2 months; P = .0003). The FOLFOX 4 arm had a 1.5-month improvement in median overall survival; however, this did not reach statistical significance (16.2 vs. 14.7 months; P = .12). The number of patients experiencing grade 3 or 4 neutropenia was higher with the FOLFOX 4 than with the LV5FU2 regimen (42% vs. 5% of patients). Grade 3 or 4 diarrhea (12% vs. 5%) was also increased in the FOLFOX 4 arm. Neurotoxicity, virtually absent in the LV5FU2 arm, was frequent in the FOLFOX 4 arm, with 18% of patients experiencing grade 3 neurosensory toxicity. This neurotoxicity did not result in a demonstrable deterioration in quality of life as assessed on this trial.

The FOLFOX 4 regimen has also been evaluated in a multicenter randomized trial as second-line therapy after failure of first-line IFL chemotherapy.[368] Patients were randomly assigned to one of three arms: FOLFOX 4, LV5FU2, or single-agent oxaliplatin. Response rates were 10% for FOLFOX, 0% for LV5FU2, and 1% for oxaliplatin alone (P <.0001 for FOLFOX vs. LV5FU2). Time to tumor progression was also superior for FOLFOX 4 (4.6 months) compared to LV5FU2 (2.7 months) and oxaliplatin alone (1.6 months). These data confirm initial clinical impressions that oxaliplatin/5-FU combinations have activity superior to that of single-agent oxaliplatin, even in 5-FU–refractory disease. FOLFOX 4 has significant activity in IFL-refractory disease; however, single-agent oxaliplatin does not.

Further modifications have been made to the FOLFOX schedule. FOLFOX 5 was designed with an increased dose of oxaliplatin to 100 mg/m^2 every 14 days; however, this regimen was never tested in clinical trials. FOLFOX 6 used this 100-mg/m^2 oxaliplatin dose with a simplified 5-FU/leucovorin schedule.[369] Oxaliplatin 100 mg/m^2 is given over 2 hours, with leucovorin 400 mg/m^2 given concurrently via a T connector. These are then followed by a 400-mg/m^2 bolus of 5-FU and then a 46-hour infusion of 5-FU at 2400 to 3000 mg/m^2. More recently, the FOLFOX 7 regimen has been reported in abstract form, using a 130-mg/m^2 dose of oxaliplatin every 14 days. The simplified leucovorin and 5-FU administration of FOLFOX 6 is maintained, with deletion of the bolus 5-FU. Oxaliplatin is discontinued after 3 months and reintroduced after 12 weeks, or sooner if clinical progression occurs.[370] This regimen appears promising, both for treatment of metastatic disease and for potential use in the adjuvant setting.

COMPARISONS OF OXALIPLATIN- AND IRINOTECAN-BASED COMBINATIONS

With both oxaliplatin- and irinotecan-based regimens showing encouraging activity, the question of which agent to use first was addressed by a number of investigators. Tournigand et al.

TABLE 29.8-16. Comparison of First-Line Use of Irinotecan (FOLFIRI) versus Oxaliplatin (FOLFOX) in Conjunction with the Same Simplified Biweekly Infusional 5-Fluorouracil/Leucovorin Schedule

	FOLFIRI (n = 109 Patients Treated)	FOLFOX 6 (n = 111 Patients Treated)	P Value
Major objective response rate (partial plus complete responses)	56%	54%	.68
Time to tumor progression (on first-line regimen)	8.5 mo	8.1 mo	.65
Time to tumor progression (after first + second-line regimen	14.4 mo	11.5 mo	.65
Overall survival (from initial randomization)	20.4 mo	21.5 mo	.9
2-Y overall survival	41%	45%	—
Grade 3 or 4 neutropenia	25%	44%	—
Neutropenic fever	6%	1%	—
Grade 3 or 4 diarrhea	14%	11%	—
Neuropathy (grade 3)	0%	34%	—
Alopecia (grade 2)	24%	9%	—

(From ref. 371, with permission.)

reported a phase III trial of FOLFOX 6 versus FOLFIRI. This trial used identical simplified LV5FU2 schedules, with the only variable being addition of oxaliplatin or irinotecan. It was planned that all patients would cross over to the other regimen at the time of progression, and the primary end point was time to tumor progression after *both* chemotherapy regimens.[371] Results are shown in Table 29.8-16. Although the study is somewhat underpowered with a total of 226 patients, the results show a striking consistency between regimens, which suggests that use of either FOLFOX 6 or FOLFIRI in first-line treatment is acceptable. As would be anticipated, the oxaliplatin-containing regimen, but not the irinotecan-based one, had a significant degree of neurotoxicity. Diarrhea and alopecia were more problematic in the irinotecan-based regimen. Preliminary results of a somewhat larger trial of 360 patients randomly assigned to receive FOLFOX 4 or the equivalent FOLFIRI schedule using the same LV5FU2 dose and schedule of 5-FU and leucovorin in each arm again showed comparable efficacy data, with differing and predictable toxicity profiles.[372]

The NCCTG-led U.S. Intergroup study N9741, a complex and important trial that underwent many iterations before its completion, initially opened as a four-arm trial comparing the Mayo Clinic 5-FU/leucovorin regimen (control arm) to three different irinotecan/5-FU/leucovorin regimens: weekly bolus IFL as reported by Saltz et al.,[350] a Mayo II schedule of irinotecan on day 1 and bolus 5-FU/low-dose leucovorin on days 2 to 5,[373] and the biweekly infusional schedule of LV5FU2 plus irinotecan as reported by Douillard et al.[351] After accruing a small number of patients, the trial was closed to incorporate three oxaliplatin-containing arms: FOLFOX 4, IROX (a once-every-3-weeks combination of irinotecan and oxaliplatin without 5-FU), and a modified Mayo Clinic schedule of bolus 5-FU plus low-dose leucovorin on days 1 to 5, with oxaliplatin given on day 1. The infusional LV5FU2 plus irinotecan arm was

TABLE 29.8-17.   Results of Intergroup Trial N9741: Irinotecan plus Bolus 5-FU/Leucovorin (IFL), Oxaliplatin plus Infusional 5-FU/Leucovorin (FOLFOX 4), and Irinotecan plus Oxaliplatin (IROX) in First-Line Treatment of Patients with Metastatic Colorectal Cancer

	IFL (n = 264)	FOLFOX 4 (n = 267)	IROX (n = 264)	P Value (IFL vs. FOLFOX)
Major objective response rate (partial plus complete responses)	31%	45%	35%	.03
Time to tumor progression	6.9 mo	8.7 mo	6.5 mo	.001
Overall survival	15.0 mo	19.5 mo	17.4 mo	.0001
Received second-line therapy with active drug not included in first-line regimen	24% (oxaliplatin)	60% (irinotecan)	50% (5-FU)	Not given
Grade 3 or 4 neutropenia	40%	50%	36%	.35
Neutropenic fever	15%	4%	11%	.001
Grade 3 or 4 diarrhea	28%	12%	24%	.001
Grade 3 or 4 nausea	16%	6%	19%	.001
Grade 3 neuropathy	3%	18%	7%	.001
60-d all-cause mortality	4.5%	2.6%	2.7%	Not significant

5-FU, 5-fluorouracil.
(From ref. 375, with permission.)

dropped. This created a six-arm trial. In March 2000, the trial was again halted, based on presentation of evidence that the combination of irinotecan/5-FU/leucovorin, using either bolus or infusional schedules, was superior to 5-FU/leucovorin. The Mayo Clinic control arm of N9741 was now dropped, and weekly bolus IFL became the control arm. At the same time, ongoing real-time monitoring of fatal toxicities identified unacceptably high rates of treatment-related mortality in the oxaliplatin plus Mayo Clinic 5-FU/leucovorin arm and the irinotecan plus 5-FU/leucovorin arm. These schedules were also dropped from the trial, and from further development, which left a three-arm trial of irinotecan plus bolus 5-FU/leucovorin (IFL), oxaliplatin plus infusional LV5FU2, and oxaliplatin plus irinotecan.

The trial was stopped a third time in April 2001, when monitoring of the trial indicated what appeared to be a higher than expected early mortality in the IFL control arm.[207] This observation, however, was based on use of a new metric, the 60-day ACM. This metric records death from *any* cause within 60 days of initial therapy. The 60-day ACM of the IFL arm was initially noted to be 4.5%. Because this was a new metric, however, there were no readily available historical controls; no one had ready access to data to say what the 60-day ACM had been in previous trials, either with IFL or with 5-FU/leucovorin regimens. The 4.5% ACM was therefore compared to the previously reported death rate for the IFL regimen, which was 0.9%. However, the previously reported death rate was the treatment-related death rate, the percentage of deaths judged by the investigators to have been caused by treatment, not all deaths within 60 days of starting therapy. Of further concern to the safety monitoring committee, the experimental arms (FOLFOX 4 and IROX) each showed 60-day ACMs of 1.8% (compared to 4.5% for the IFL control arm). This information was difficult to put into context, however, because the efficacies of the two experimental arms had not yet been established.

In fact, the 60-day ACM on the original phase II trial of IFL (subsequently calculated after N9741 was halted) was 6.7%, and the 60-day ACM for the Mayo Clinic control arm of that trial was found to be 7.3%. Although the 7.3% 60-day ACM appeared subjectively to be unusually high, no historical baseline data on 60-day ACM in 5-FU–based regimens were readily available. To help interpret these data, an analysis was undertaken to determine the 60-day ACM in multiple large-scale randomized trials that had used 5-FU/leucovorin schedules over the prior decade. This analysis confirmed that 60-day ACM regularly was encountered at a rate of 5% to 8% in the treatment of metastatic colorectal cancer.[374] Thus the 60-day ACM for the IFL regimen was actually *lower* in N9741 than in previous trials and was *lower* than that seen consistently with 5-FU/leucovorin regimens alone. In the final analysis of N9741 the 60-day ACMs seen in the IFL, FOLFOX 4, and IROX arms were 4.5%, 2.6%, and 2.7%, respectively, and these differences were not statistically significant.

The differences in efficacy of the regimens in N9741, however, were statistically significant and showed superior outcome for the patients randomly assigned to receive FOLFOX 4, compared to those randomly assigned to receive either IFL or IROX, in terms of response rate, time to tumor progression, and overall survival (Table 29.8-17).[375,376] Toxicity for FOLFOX 4 was also lower for virtually all parameters except, of course, neurotoxicity. The results of the IROX arm did not differ significantly from those of the IFL arm in terms of toxicity, response, or time to tumor progression; however, survival was borderline significantly better in the IROX arm than in the IFL arm (P = .04).

Taken together, where do these trials leave us in terms of first-line use of oxaliplatin- and irinotecan-based regimens? Data from trial N9741 indicate that FOLFOX 4 is superior to IFL in both response rate and time to tumor progression. Overall survival was better in the FOLFOX 4 arm than in the IFL arm as well; however, interpretation of the survival results of N9741 is somewhat complicated, due to imbalances between arms in availability of effective second-line therapy. Second-line irinotecan was available to all patients who had received FOLFOX 4. Oxaliplatin, however, was not commercially available in the United States during the course of N9741. To what degree this imbalance in second-line therapy may have influenced the survival results is unknown. Also, because IFL contains bolus 5-FU whereas FOLFOX 4 contains infusional LV5FU2, it is difficult to isolate the irinotecan versus oxaliplatin component from the 5-FU bolus versus 5-FU infusion component.

Two other trials indicate that the FOLFOX and FOLFIRI regimens have similar safety and efficacy, with differing toxicity profiles.[371,372] Thus, FOLFOX has comparable efficacy to FOLFIRI, whereas FOLFOX has a superior response rate, time to tumor progression, and possibly some degree of survival benefit compared to IFL. Toxicity profiles with irinotecan-based regimens show a higher degree of diarrhea, alopecia, and neutropenia, especially when irinotecan is given with bolus 5-FU. Oxaliplatin-based regimens appear to be relatively well tolerated; however, the neurotoxicity, absent from the irinotecan-based regimens, can be problematic in some patients. It would therefore seem reasonable at this time to favor the use of a high-dose intermittent infusional 5-FU/leucovorin schedule plus either oxaliplatin (i.e., FOLFOX) or irinotecan (i.e., FOLFIRI). Data do not support continued routine use of the bolus IFL schedule, nor are there randomized data to support the routine use of a bolus 5-FU/leucovorin schedule with oxaliplatin. Routine use of IROX is also not supported by the currently available body of data.

Whether to use an irinotecan-based or oxaliplatin-based combination in first-line treatment of patients with good performance status can be considered a matter of patient preference, and discussion of the differing toxicity profiles is appropriate to help individuals decide. It is hoped that in the near future molecular prognostic indicators and pharmacogenomics will provide useful guidance for the individualization of therapies, but such approaches remain investigational at this time.

The only oxaliplatin schedule registered for use in the United States is FOLFOX 4. The LV5FU2 schedule used in this combination is somewhat cumbersome relative to the simplified schedule used in FOLFOX 6. There has not been, and never will be, a randomized trial comparing these two schedules. Most investigators have accepted that the LV5FU2 and simplified LV5FU2 schedules are comparable in efficacy and toxicity, and the simplified schedule has *de facto* replaced the original LV5FU2 in many practices. Investigators in the U.S. cooperative groups have made this assumption as well, and the FOLFOX schedule that is currently being investigated in NCCTG, CALGB, NSABP, and SWOG trials is a modified FOLFOX 6 regimen (see Table 29.8-16) that uses the simplified LV5FU2 doses from FOLFOX 6 with the lower 85 mg/m^2 starting dose of oxaliplatin from FOLFOX 4. This modified FOLFOX 6 schedule appears at this time to be a very reasonable schedule for routine clinical use when the decision is made to use an oxaliplatin/fluorouracil combination.

A regimen of bolus 5-FU, oxaliplatin, and leucovorin has been studied in a phase II trial.[377] The results appear favorable, and a randomized trial comparing this regimen to FOLFOX and to a capecitabine plus oxaliplatin combination has been initiated. However, the use of oxaliplatin with other than infusional 5-FU schedules has not been validated in randomized trials at this time, and therefore cannot be recommended for routine use.

Use of planned sequential administration of FOLFOX and FOLFIRI has also been proposed, both as pretreatment for potentially resectable patients with liver metastases[378] and as adjuvant treatment of earlier-stage disease. Several groups are also exploring the use of "triple therapy" with oxaliplatin, irinotecan, and 5-FU/leucovorin. Phase I and II trials have demonstrated high activity but also substantial toxicity, but no randomized comparisons of this approach are yet available, and it is too soon to say whether or not this approach has a role in either metastatic or earlier-stage disease.[379,380]

A number of investigators have pursued use of an oral fluoropyrimidine, such as capecitabine or UFT, in conjunction with either oxaliplatin or irinotecan. The as yet unanswered question being addressed here is whether chronic oral administration of a fluoropyrimidine will prove to be more acceptable to patients than administration with the ambulatory infusion pumps used in high-dose intermittent 5-FU schedules and whether efficacy will be similar. Phase II data for these combinations are encouraging[381–383]; however, randomized trials, currently ongoing, will be necessary to determine whether these oral fluoropyrimidine-based combinations are acceptable alternatives to parenteral regimens. Until the results of phase III trials are available, these capecitabine- and UFT-based combinations should be regarded as investigational and are not recommended for routine clinical use.

DURATION OF THERAPY

Controversy exists regarding the optimal duration of chemotherapy for palliation of metastatic disease. Traditional practice for many years has been to continue chemotherapy until either unacceptable toxicity, clinical deterioration, or disease progression occurs. Investigators have begun to question the merits of this practice compared to planned discontinuation of chemotherapy after a fixed period of time. Maughan et al. conducted a trial in which 354 patients who were responding or who had stable disease after receiving 12 weeks of either fluorouracil- or raltitrexed-based chemotherapy were randomly assigned either to continue chemotherapy until progression or to stop chemotherapy after the first 12 weeks, followed by a planned restarting on the same chemotherapy at the time of progression.[384] At randomization, 41% of patients had achieved a major objective response and 59% had stable disease. Overall survival was the primary end point of the trial. There was no evidence of a difference in survival between the two groups, with a hazard ratio of 0.87 (P = .23) favoring the intermittent arm. Continuous chemotherapy was noted to delay progression, but the difference was not significant (median of 3.7 months for the intermittent group and 4.9 months for continuous-treatment group; P = .1). Of interest, only 37% of patients on the intermittent treatment arm actually restarted chemotherapy on progression as planned. The use of second-line chemotherapy was comparable in both groups. The authors concluded that the study showed no clear evidence of benefit for continuous therapy versus the intermittent plan. Intermittent therapy showed reduced toxicity, with 17 treatment-related, serious adverse events on the continuous arm compared with 6 on the intermittent treatment arm.

Other investigators specifically addressed the question of whether rechallenge with 5-FU after a planned treatment interruption could produce a response. A pooled analysis was conducted of the data for 613 patients involved in three randomized trials of first-line 5-FU–based therapy.[385] All patients had a planned maximum treatment period of 6 months. Patients with responding or stable disease at the end of that period were observed off treatment with a plan for retreatment at the time of disease progression. Median time to rechallenge was 11.7 months. Seventeen percent of patients had an objective response to rechallenging. Median survival for the group was 14.8 months. These nonrandomized trial data indicate that patients have a significant response rate at time of reinstitution of chemotherapy.

A similar approach was explored in patients receiving second-line irinotecan therapy.[386] A total of 333 patients entered into a trial to receive 24 weeks of irinotecan. Patients remaining on study at the end of that time were to be randomly assigned either to continue treatment or to stop therapy. Of the 333 patients, most came off study due to progression or toxicity before reaching the 24-week mark. Fifty-five patients with responding or stable disease agreed to random assignment. Although the numbers available for comparison were small, there were no differences between the arms in progression-free survival or overall survival, nor were there differences in quality-of-life scores.

Overall there appears to be no compelling evidence that continuation of chemotherapy indefinitely is necessary for optimal control of disease. The option of discontinuation of therapy after a fixed period of time may be a reasonable one to consider in standard practice.

BEVACIZUMAB

BEV is a humanized monoclonal antibody against vascular endothelial growth factor. A randomized phase II trial of two different doses of BEV plus the Roswell Park regimen of 5-FU/leucovorin, or 5-FU/leucovorin alone, has been reported.[387] Response rate, time to tumor progression, and overall survival were superior in the 5-mg/kg (low-dose) BEV arm and the 10-mg/kg (high-dose) BEV arm compared to the 5-FU/leucovorin control arm. Thrombosis was the most significant adverse event and was fatal in one patient. Hypertension, proteinuria, and epistaxis were also seen. Two of 22 patients on the control arm had an unconfirmed response to BEV alone when they were crossed over after progression, but neither of these responses was durable on 4-week follow-up scan. Outcome was best in the 5-mg/kg BEV arm, and this dose was taken forward for phase III studies.

The pivotal phase III trial for BEV has been reported by Hurwitz et al.[388] Four hundred and three patients were randomly assigned to receive standard-dose IFL[350] plus BEV (5 mg/kg every other week) and 412 patients received IFL plus placebo. The addition of BEV resulted in improved response rate (45% vs. 35%; $P < .003$), improved progression-free survival (10.6 vs. 6.2 months; $P < .00001$), and improved overall survival (20.3 vs. 15.6 months; $P = .00003$). Grade 3 hypertension was higher in the BEV arm (11% vs. 2%). Incidences of thromboembolism and proteinuria were the same in the BEV and placebo arms. Six episodes of gastrointestinal perforation were seen on the BEV arm and none on the placebo arm. Although there was significant heterogeneity in the nature of these events, the imbalance is of concern and warrants further attention. Nevertheless, the results of this trial are exciting, both because the 4.7-month survival advantage is the largest seen to date in a randomized trial of therapies for colorectal cancer, and because this trial represents the first randomized phase III validation of the concept of antiangiogenesis in the management of metastatic solid tumors.

It is unclear at this time whether the robust results seen with BEV plus IFL are unique to the particular chemotherapy used or whether other drugs and other regimens would also benefit from combination with IFL. Patients have been accrued to a large randomized trial of FOLFOX 4 plus BEV versus FOLFOX 4 alone versus BEV alone conducted by the ECOG. The BEV alone arm was closed early by the data safety monitoring committee due to inferior outcome. Effi-

cacy and safety reports from this trial are expected in late 2004 or early 2005.

CETUXIMAB

Cetuximab (C225) is a chimeric monoclonal antibody that binds selectively to the epidermal growth factor receptor (EGFR), a 170,000-kD transmembrane glycoprotein that is involved in signaling pathways affecting cellular growth, differentiation, and survival.[389,390] Cetuximab blocks the EGFR binding site, preventing activation of tyrosine kinases on the intracellular portion of the receptor molecule and thereby preventing receptor signaling. Preclinical models indicate that cetuximab has limited single-agent activity but has greater activity in conjunction with cytotoxic chemotherapy. Based on this observation and on a favorable anecdotal experience of a major response in a young patient with irinotecan-refractory disease, a multicenter phase II trial was initiated. This study has been reported in abstract form.[391] Patients were treated with the same dose and schedule of irinotecan that had previously failed, with the addition of cetuximab (400 mg/m^2 loading dose week 1, then weekly 250 mg/m^2 over 1 hour). Prestudy dosage reductions of irinotecan were maintained on entry to this trial. One hundred and twenty patients for whom prior irinotecan therapy had failed, as determined by their treating physicians, were treated. The major objective response rate, as reported by an independent response assessment committee, was 22.5%. Toxicity from irinotecan was moderate, a not unexpected finding because dose modifications had already been made during prestudy treatment. Three percent of patients experienced an allergic, anaphylactoid reaction to cetuximab necessitating cessation of cetuximab therapy. The most common cetuximab-related toxicity was an acne-form skin rash, which was present in 75% of patients, with 12% experiencing a grade 3 rash.

Encouraged by the results of the irinotecan plus cetuximab trial discussed earlier, Saltz et al. initiated a multicenter phase II trial to assess the single-agent activity of cetuximab in patients with irinotecan-refractory colorectal cancer. Five of 57 patients (9%) achieved a partial response on the basis of an independent radiologic review.[392]

Strong confirmatory evidence of the activity of cetuximab was provided in a trial presented by Cunningham et al.[393] These investigators compared cetuximab plus irinotecan versus cetuximab alone in a randomized phase II trial in patients with irinotecan-refractory disease. Three hundred twenty-nine patients were randomly assigned to treatment arms in a 2:1 scheme. The response rates, as reported by independent review, were 22.9% for irinotecan plus cetuximab and 10.8% for irinotecan alone. Time to tumor progression favored the combination as well (4.0 vs. 1.6 months). Survival on the two arms was not significantly different, although this trial was not designed or powered to test this end point.

Cetuximab has been investigated in a preliminary manner in combination with first-line therapy in phase II trials. A small phase II pilot trial of cetuximab in conjunction with weekly bolus IFL demonstrated a 44% response rate.[394] A trial of cetuximab plus irinotecan and weekly infusional 5-FU/LV has also been reported.[395] Twelve of 18 evaluable patients achieved a partial response with predictable and tolerable toxicity. To date, no randomized trials of first-line use of cetuximab plus chemotherapy have been reported. Thus, no data are available on what impact, if any, this drug will have on survival and other efficacy end points in first-line combinations. The CALGB has initiated a large-scale trial of a modified FOLFOX 6 regimen versus the FOLFIRI regimen in a two-by-two randomization with cetuximab treatment to address this question.

OTHER EPIDERMAL GROWTH FACTOR RECEPTOR–TARGETING AGENTS

ABX-EGF, a fully humanized monoclonal antibody that targets the EGFR, has also shown evidence of activity in refractory colorectal cancer. A planned interim analysis of a phase II trial reported a 13% response rate for this agent in 23 patients with chemotherapy-refractory colorectal cancer.[396] Accrual to this trial is ongoing at the time of this writing. Thus far, the limited experiences with the oral EGFR tyrosine kinase inhibitors gefitanib (ZD1839) and erlotanib (OSI-774) have not been encouraging in colorectal cancer.[397,398]

CYCLOOXYGENASE-2 INHIBITORS

COX-2 catalyzes the synthesis of prostaglandins in the inflammatory response process. COX-2 has been frequently shown to be up-regulated in malignant and premalignant tissues. COX-2 expression has been correlated with increased invasiveness, resistance to apoptosis, and increased angiogenesis.[399] Although NSAIDs and selective COX-2 inhibitors clearly can reduce the development of premalignant polyps, evidence that use of either NSAIDs or selective COX-2 inhibitors has a beneficial role in the treatment of colorectal cancer is lacking, and the use of these agents as adjuncts to chemotherapy should be regarded as investigational at this time. Numerous randomized trials are assessing the role of COX-2 inhibitors in combination with chemotherapy in both the adjuvant and metastatic settings. In the absence of any emerging data to the contrary, routine use of COX-2 inhibitors with chemotherapy is not recommended at this time.

OTHER NOVEL AGENTS

The number of agents that are undergoing early evaluation in colorectal cancer is too large to permit a complete discussion of these in this chapter. Several that have entered large-scale phase III trials are briefly mentioned. All of these agents are currently of research interest only and do not have a role in standard treatment of colorectal cancer at this time.

The vascular endothelial growth factor receptor (VEGFR) tyrosine kinase inhibitor PTK787/ZK 22584 is an oral, once-daily, selective angiogenesis inhibitor that targets the VEGFR-1, VEGFR-2, and VEGFR-3 tyrosine kinases.[400] Phase I studies have been completed with this agent plus FOLFIRI.[401] The drug has also been combined with FOLFOX 4 in a phase I study.[402] Large-scale phase III trials are now being initiated with this agent in combination with chemotherapeutic drugs in patients with metastatic colorectal cancer.

Another novel vascular targeting agent that is entering clinical trials in colorectal cancer is ZD6126.[403] This agents binds to tubulin and is thought to induce morphologic changes in tumor endothelial cells, which leads to vessel occlusion and tumor necrosis. A randomized phase III trial of this agent in conjunction with FOLFOX chemotherapy versus FOLFOX alone is also being initiated.

Edotecarin is a noncamptothesian synthetic indolocarbazole topoisomerase I inhibitor that has shown *in vitro* activity against a wide range of tumor cell lines. A phase II study involving patients with colorectal cancer demonstrated three partial responses, four minor responses, and nine cases of stable disease in 24 patients treated with 13 mg/m^2, given as a 2-hour intravenous infusion every 3 weeks.[404] This drug was well tolerated and is now being studied in phase I trials in combination with the standard agents used in chemotherapy of colorectal cancer.

Another agent entering phase III trials in colorectal cancer is tezacitabine, a deoxycytidine nucleoside analog. In a phase II study this agent was given by intravenous infusion on a biweekly schedule. Eleven percent of patients experienced a major response (unconfirmed at the time of report) and an additional six patients (13%) had stability of disease lasting in excess of 6 months. This agent is also entering randomized phase III colorectal trials in conjunction with FOLFOX chemotherapy.

GENE THERAPY

Several aspects of colorectal cancer make the disease a reasonable potential target for gene therapy approaches.[405] Because colorectal cancer may progress within a confined space such as the peritoneal cavity, or within a solitary organ such as the liver, regional administration of a gene vector may be practical. Multiple trials of different gene therapy approaches, including virus-directed enzyme prodrug therapy, immunogenic manipulation, gene correction, and viral therapy, have all been initiated. Major therapeutic benefits from gene therapy in colorectal cancer have yet to be realized, however. These innovative approaches remain extremely interesting and promising but must be regarded as highly investigational at this time.

MOLECULAR PREDICTIVE MARKERS

A decade ago there was little benefit to being able to predict the likelihood of a therapy's working or not, because there was essentially only one therapeutic option to choose: Treatment was limited to 5-FU or some variation on that theme. With the availability now of a number of active agents, the ability to prospectively select a particular drug or drug combination that would have an increased likelihood of efficacy or a decreased likelihood of toxicity would be extremely useful. Such means of rational selection do not yet exist, but evidence suggests that we are rapidly moving closer to such an approach.

One promising avenue of investigation has been the elucidation of markers of resistance to 5-FU based on knowledge of its metabolic pathways. Studies have indicated that high levels of either TS,[149] DPD,[406] or thymidine phosphorylase,[407] as measured in a tumor specimen by RT-PCR, predict for failure to respond to an infusional 5-FU regimen. These observations are intriguing but need to be validated in large-scale prospective trials before being applied to routine practice. There is, at this time, insufficient evidence to support the routine use of these markers in standard practice. Others have investigated genomic analysis as an indicator of response or toxicity. Although these approaches appear promising, they are not yet validated and should not be considered as part of standard care.[151,408]

MANAGEMENT OF SYNCHRONOUS PRIMARY AND METASTATIC DISEASE

Patients who present with potentially resectable metastatic disease, such as those with metastases confined to the liver in a resectable distribution, should undergo resection of both the metastatic and primary tumors. PET scanning should be performed before undertaking such an aggressive surgical approach to assure that other sites of metastatic disease are adequately ruled out.[409,410] Judgment must be exercised in terms of whether to perform both resections at once or to perform staged procedures. Although data to provide guidance are lacking in this area, an approach that is gaining favor in this era of improved drug therapies is to treat with systemic chemotherapy first and then reassess the appropriateness of aggressive surgical intervention. Patients with a favorable response in visible metastases are more likely to have experienced eradication of whatever unidentified micrometastases may have been present and so are more likely to achieve a cure from aggressive surgical intervention. Patients whose disease progresses to the point of unresectability because of the development of additional lesions while on the patient is chemotherapy are not likely to have benefited from initial resection and so are spared the morbidity of what would have been an unsuccessful attempt at curative surgery.

Significant controversy exists regarding the optimal management of patients who present with synchronous unresectable metastatic disease. Historical practice has favored routine palliative resection for these patients; however, more recent data suggest that a reconsideration of this practice is warranted.

In an analysis of linked data from the Surveillance, Epidemiology, and End Results program and Medicare, Temple et al. assessed whether or not surgery was performed within 90 days of diagnosis in patients presenting with synchronous metastatic disease.[411] The records of 5235 patients older than 65 years presenting with stage IV colorectal cancer from 1992 to 1996 were reviewed. Seventy-three percent of these patients with stage IV disease were found to have undergone cancer-directed surgery with 90 days of diagnosis. Among patients older than 80 years, this rate was 68%. Twenty-four percent of all patients undergoing surgery received a colostomy or ileostomy. Of significant concern, 10% of patients undergoing these palliative resections died within 30 days of the operation. This perioperative mortality rose to 15% in patients older than 80 years of age. The vast majority of surgery was performed on the primary tumor. Surgical resection of metastases was rare, occurring in only 4.3% of patients. Overall, the prognosis for the entire cohort was poor, with a 28% mortality at 90 days from diagnosis.

The risk of intestinal complications after chemotherapy for patients with unresected primary colorectal cancer and synchronous metastasis would appear to be low. Tebbutt et al. have summarized the 10-year experience of patients at the Royal Marsden Hospital in London who have been treated with chemotherapy with or without palliative resection of the primary.[412] Eighty-two patients received initial chemotherapy without surgery and 280 patients underwent surgery followed by chemotherapy. The incidences of peritonitis, fistula formation, and intestinal hemorrhage were not significantly different in the resected and unresected patients. Intestinal obstruction occurred in 13% of both groups. Patients undergoing resection did have a lower incidence of requiring three or more blood transfusions (7.5%

vs. 14.6%; $P = .048$), as well as lower rate of palliative abdominal radiotherapy (9.6% vs. 18.3%; $P = .03$).

In a smaller single-institution study, Scoggins et al. retrospectively reviewed a 12-year experience with patients presenting with synchronous metastatic disease.[413] Of 89 patients included in the analysis, 66 underwent initial resection and 23 did not. Of the 23 nonresected patients, 13 received initial chemotherapy, 9 received chemotherapy plus radiation therapy, and 1 received radiation therapy alone. Two of the 23 patients (8.7%) not receiving initial surgery ultimately developed obstruction at the primary site and required diversion. None of the patients experienced tumor-related perforation or hemorrhage.

Current evidence argues against the continued practice of routine noncurative resection for a majority of patients with synchronous metastatic disease. Response rates with initial chemotherapy using the currently available combination regimens discussed in this chapter are substantially higher than those achievable a decade ago. In following the patient's clinical course, the metastatic disease can serve as a clinical indicator of response to systemic chemotherapy. Response in the metastasis is extremely likely to correlate with disease control in the area of the primary as well. Patients felt to be at risk for obstruction within the time period necessary to evaluate the efficacy of first-line chemotherapy should be considered for mechanical stenting using expandable endoscopically placed metal stents.[414]

UNUSUAL COLORECTAL TUMORS

CARCINOID TUMORS

Carcinoid tumors are neuroendocrine tumors characterized by the presence of neurosecretory granules. They are also known as *amine precursor uptake and decarboxylation* (APUD) tumors. Histologically, they are typically characterized by bland, monotonous histologic findings with small nuclei, few nucleoli, and ample cytoplasm. Tumors typically manifest a low-grade histologic type and an indolent clinical course. Approximately half of carcinoid tumors are hormonally nonfunctional in that they produce no clinical evidence of a hormonal syndrome. The hormone typically produced by functional carcinoid tumors is serotonin, and this is best detected by a 24-hour urine collection to measure the breakdown product, 5-hydroxyindolacetic acid. The vast majority of carcinoid tumors are derived from the digestive tract, with a smaller percentage arising in the bronchial pulmonary tree. Rare gonadal carcinoids have also been reported. The majority of gastrointestinal carcinoids originate in the appendix, rectum, and small bowel. True carcinoid of the colon is rare.

Carcinoids of the appendix are relatively common neoplasms with a prevalence of 0.32% among 34,505 patients undergoing routine appendectomy.[415–417] Appendiceal carcinoids smaller than 1 cm in diameter present virtually no risk of distant spread and are adequately managed with simple appendectomy. Carcinoids of the appendix 2 cm or larger in diameter are at significant risk for spread and are appropriately managed with a formal right hemicolectomy to provide adequate resection of the lymph nodes of the right mesocolon, which drain the appendix. Treatment of tumors between 1 and 2 cm is somewhat controversial in terms of whether further surgery is required.

Prognosis of carcinoids of the rectum is similarly differentiated on the basis of size. Carcinoids of the rectum are noted in approximately 1 of every 2500 proctoscopic examinations.[417] Rectal carcinoids are most typically not hormonally functional and usually do not give rise to the carcinoid syndrome. The vast majority are smaller than 1 cm when diagnosed and these small tumors virtually never metastasize. Tumors larger than 2 cm have an extremely high rate of metastasis and again, those of 1 to 2 cm constitutes a variable area in which clinical judgment must be exercised based on the patient's overall medical condition and the extent of surgery required. Endorectal ultrasonography may be useful in identifying regional lymph node metastases, the presence of which would necessitate more radical surgery. Small tumors can be handled by local incision or fulguration. Patients with these small rectal carcinoid tumors do not require hormonal monitoring or routine oncologic evaluation.

HIGH-GRADE NEUROENDOCRINE CARCINOMA

Neuroendocrine carcinomas comprise a spectrum from well-differentiated carcinoid tumors, on one end, to high-grade small cell or oat cell carcinomas, on the other. Extrapulmonary small cell or high-grade neuroendocrine tumors are very uncommon, accounting for fewer than 1000 cases annually. Histologically, small cell cancers arising from different organs are indistinguishable from one another.[418] Because small cell lung cancer is far more common than an extrapulmonary neuroendocrine primary, chest imaging should be performed. As with low-grade neuroendocrine tumors, the rectum is the most common presentation site within the large bowel, and the cecum is the next most common site.

The presentation of high-grade large bowel neuroendocrine tumors is nonspecific and similar to that of adenocarcinomas. Stage IV presentation is most common, with the liver being the most common site of distant spread. Recommendations for management are based on extrapolation from small cell lung cancer paradigms. Systemic chemotherapy, using small cell lung cancer regimens, is the treatment of choice for patients with metastatic disease. Treatment of localized high-grade neuroendocrine carcinoma is controversial. Traditionally a combined modality approach similar to that used in rectal adenocarcinoma has been advocated; however, distant failure is a common occurrence. One reasonable approach is to treat initially with small cell–directed chemotherapy and then consolidate gains in patients with favorable responses using radiation or surgery or both.

LYMPHOMA

Although extranodal presentations of non-Hodgkin's lymphomas are rare, the gastrointestinal tract is the most common site of extranodal involvement. The majority of colorectal lymphomas are non-Hodgkin's type and may present with low-, intermediate-, or high-grade histologies. B-cell diffuse large cell histologic type is most common; however, virtually all B-cell and T-cell types may occur. Approximately 13% to 18% of gastrointestinal tract lymphomas arise in the large bowel[419]; the majority are situated in the cecum or the rectum.[420,421]

Colorectal lymphomas usually present with nonspecific abdominal pain, weight loss, rectal bleeding, mass, or obstruction.[422] The clinical presentation is similar to that of common colorectal carcinoma, and the diagnosis is made on histologic examination of a biopsy specimen. Extensive workup for other sites of disease, including bone marrow biopsy and full body scanning, is necessary both for staging and for acceptance of the diagnosis of the gastrointestinal site as primary.

Owing to the rarity of the disease, data regarding the optimal management of large bowel lymphomas are scarce. Patients with lymphoma of the colon are often treated initially with surgery, although the appropriateness of this practice has not been validated in randomized studies. A combined modality approach, including surgery and chemotherapy, has been advocated by some investigators.[423] The role of radiation therapy also remains unclear, with some investigators favoring its use, especially for treatment of unresectable disease or bulky tumors. Chemotherapy use is based on the appropriate regimens for the particular histologic subtype that is present.

REFERENCES

1. Parkin DM, Pisani P, Ferlay J. Global cancer statistics. *CA Cancer J Clin* 1999;49:33.
2. Landis SH, Murray T, Bolden S, Wingo PA. Cancer statistics 1998. *CA Cancer J Clin* 1998;48:6.
3. Rickert RR, Auerbach O, Garfinkel L, Hammond EC, Frasca JM. Adenomatous lesions of the large bowel: an autopsy survey. *Cancer* 1979;43:1847.
4. DiSario JA, Foutch PG, Mai HD, Pardy K, Manne RK. Prevalence and malignant potential of colorectal polyps in asymptomatic, average-risk men. *Am J Gastroenterol* 1991;86:941.
5. Lieberman DA, Weiss DG, Bond JH, et al. Use of colonoscopy to screen asymptomatic adults for colorectal cancer. Veterans Affairs Cooperative Study Group 380. *N Engl J Med* 2000;343:162.
6. Rex DK, Sledge GW, Harper PA, et al. Colonic adenomas in asymptomatic women with a history of breast cancer. *Am J Gastroenterol* 1993;88:2009.
7. Seifeldin R, Hantsch JJ. The economic burden associated with colon cancer in the United States. *Clin Ther* 1999;21:1370.
8. Brown MO, Lanier AP, Becker TM. Colorectal cancer incidence and survival among Alaska Natives, 1969–1993. *Int J Epidemiol* 1998;27:388.
9. Armstrong B, Doll R. Environmental factors and cancer incidence and mortality in different countries, with special reference to dietary practices. *Int J Cancer* 1975;15:617.
10. Henderson MM. International differences in diet and cancer incidence. *J Natl Cancer Inst Monogr* 1992;599.
11. Nelson RL, Persky V, Turyk M. Determination of factors responsible for the declining incidence of colorectal cancer. *Dis Colon Rectum* 1999;42:741.
12. Staszewski J, Haenszel W. Cancer mortality among the Polish-born in the United States. *J Natl Cancer Inst* 1965;35:291.
13. Whittemore AS, Wu-Williams AH, Lee M, et al. Diet, physical activity, and colorectal cancer among Chinese in North America and China. *J Natl Cancer Inst* 1990;82:915.
14. McMichael AJ, Giles GG. Cancer in migrants to Australia: extending the descriptive epidemiological data. *Cancer Res* 1988;48:751.
15. Kune S, Kune GA, Watson L. The Melbourne colorectal cancer study: incidence findings by age, sex, site, migrants and religion. *Int J Epidemiol* 1986;15:483.
16. Laken SJ, Petersen GM, Gruber SB, et al. Familial colorectal cancer in Ashkenazim due to a hypermutable tract in APC. *Nat Genet* 1997;17:79.
17. Rozen P, Shomrat R, Strul H, et al. Prevalence of the I1307K APC gene variant in Israeli Jews of differing ethnic origin and risk for colorectal cancer. *Gastroenterology* 1999;116:54.
18. Weber TK, Chin HM, Rodriguez-Bigas M, et al. Novel hMLH1 and hMSH2 germline mutations in African Americans with colorectal cancer. *JAMA* 1999;281:2316.
19. Nelson RL, Persky V, Turyk M. Time trends in distal colorectal cancer subsite location related to age and how it affects choice of screening modality. *J Surg Oncol* 1998;69:235.
20. Nelson RL, Dollear T, Freels S, Persky V. The relation of age, race, and gender to the subsite location of colorectal cancer. *Cancer* 1997;80:193.
21. Wilmink AB. Overview of the epidemiology of colorectal cancer. *Dis Colon Rectum* 1997;40:483.
22. Obrand DI, Gordon PH. Continued change in the distribution of colorectal carcinoma. *Br J Surg* 1998;85:246.
23. Fleshner P, Slater G, Aufses AH Jr. Age and sex distribution of patients with colorectal cancer. *Dis Colon Rectum* 1989;32:107.
24. Kemppainen M, Raiha I, Sourander L. A marked increase in the incidence of colorectal cancer over two decades in southwest Finland. *J Clin Epidemiol* 1997;50:147.
25. Thorn M, Bergstrom R, Kressner U, et al. Trends in colorectal cancer incidence in Sweden 1959–93 by gender, localization, time period, and birth cohort. *Cancer Causes Control* 1998;9:145.
26. Ji BT, Devesa SS, Chow WH, Jin F, Gao YT. Colorectal cancer incidence trends by subsite in urban Shanghai, 1972–1994. *Cancer Epidemiol Biomarkers Prev* 1998;7:661.
27. Thibodeau SN, French AJ, Cunningham JM, et al. Microsatellite instability in colorectal cancer: different mutator phenotypes and the principal involvement of hMLH1. *Cancer Res* 1998;58:1713.

28. Fink D, Nebel S, Norris PS, et al. The effect of different chemotherapeutic agents on the enrichment of DNA mismatch repair-deficient tumour cells. *Br J Cancer* 1998;77:703.

29. Karnes WE Jr, Shattuck-Brandt R, Burgart LJ, et al. Reduced COX-2 protein in colorectal cancer with defective mismatch repair. *Cancer Res* 1998;58:5473.

30. Fuchs CS, Giovannucci EL, Colditz GA, et al. A prospective study of family history and the risk of colorectal cancer. *N Engl J Med* 1994;331:1669.

31. Rozen P, Fireman Z, Figer A, et al. Family history of colorectal cancer as a marker of potential malignancy within a screening program. *Cancer* 1987;60:248.

32. Pariente A, Milan C, Lafon J, Faivre J. Colonoscopic screening in first-degree relatives of patients with 'sporadic' colorectal cancer: a case-control study. The Association Nationale des Gastroenterologues des Hopitaux and Registre Bourguignon des Cancers Digestifs (INSERM CRI 9505). *Gastroenterology* 1998;115:7.

33. Guillem JG, Forde KA, Treat MR, et al. Colonoscopic screening for neoplasms in asymptomatic first-degree relatives of colon cancer patients. A controlled, prospective study. *Dis Colon Rectum* 1992;35:523.

34. Winawer SJ, Zauber AG, Gerdes H, et al. Risk of colorectal cancer in the families of patients with adenomatous polyps. National Polyp Study Workgroup. *N Engl J Med* 1996;334:82.

35. Ahsan H, Neugut AI, Garbowski GC, et al. Family history of colorectal adenomatous polyps and increased risk for colorectal cancer. *Ann Intern Med* 1998;128:900.

36. Kerber RA, Slattery ML, Potter JD, Caan BJ, Edwards SL. Risk of colon cancer associated with a family history of cancer or colorectal polyps: the diet, activity, and reproduction in colon cancer study. *Int J Cancer* 1998;78:157.

37. Burt RW, Bishop DT, Cannon LA, et al. Dominant inheritance of adenomatous colonic polyps and colorectal cancer. *N Engl J Med* 1985;312:1540.

38. Ponz de Leon M, Scapoli C, Zanghieri G, et al. Genetic transmission of colorectal cancer: exploratory data analysis from a population based registry. *J Med Genet* 1992;29:531.

39. Harris MJ, Coggan M, Langton L, Wilson SR, Board PG. Polymorphism of the Pi class glutathione S-transferase in normal populations and cancer patients. *Pharmacogenetics* 1998;8:27.

40. Welfare M, Monesola Adeokun A, Bassendine MF, Daly AK. Polymorphisms in GSTP1, GSTM1, and GSTT1 and susceptibility to colorectal cancer. *Cancer Epidemiol Biomarkers Prev* 1999;8:289.

41. Chen J, Giovannucci E, Kelsey K, et al. A methylenetetrahydrofolate reductase polymorphism and the risk of colorectal cancer. *Cancer Res* 1996;56:4862.

42. Chen J, Stampfer MJ, Hough HL, et al. A prospective study of N-acetyltransferase genotype, red meat intake, and risk of colorectal cancer. *Cancer Res* 1998;58:3307.

43. Ma J, Stampfer MJ, Giovannucci E, et al. Methylenetetrahydrofolate reductase polymorphism, dietary interactions, and risk of colorectal cancer. *Cancer Res* 1997;57:1098.

44. Vineis P, McMichael A. Interplay between heterocyclic amines in cooked meat and metabolic phenotype in the etiology of colon cancer. *Cancer Causes Control* 1996;7:479.

45. Potter JD. Colorectal cancer: molecules and populations. *J Natl Cancer Inst* 1999;91:916.

46. Singh PN, Fraser GE. Dietary risk factors for colon cancer in a low-risk population. *Am J Epidemiol* 1998;148:761.

47. Slattery ML, Potter J, Caan B, et al. Energy balance and colon cancer—beyond physical activity. *Cancer Res* 1997;57:75.

48. Willett WC, Stampfer MJ, Colditz GA, Rosner BA, Speizer FE. Relation of meat, fat, and fiber intake to the risk of colon cancer in a prospective study among women. *N Engl J Med* 1990;323:1664.

49. Key TJ, Fraser GE, Thorogood M, et al. Mortality in vegetarians and nonvegetarians: detailed findings from a collaborative analysis of 5 prospective studies. *Am J Clin Nutr* 1999;70:516S.

50. Probst-Hensch NM, Sinha R, Longnecker MP, et al. Meat preparation and colorectal adenomas in a large sigmoidoscopy-based case-control study in California (United States). *Cancer Causes Control* 1997;8:175.

51. Caderni G, Palli D, Lancioni L, et al. Dietary determinants of colorectal proliferation in the normal mucosa of subjects with previous colon adenomas. *Cancer Epidemiol Biomarkers Prev* 1999;8:219.

52. Burnstein MJ. Dietary factors related to colorectal neoplasms. *Surg Clin North Am* 1993;73:13.

53. Howe GR, Aronson KJ, Benito E, et al. The relationship between dietary fat intake and risk of colorectal cancer: evidence from the combined analysis of 13 case-control studies. *Cancer Causes Control* 1997;8:215.

54. Burkitt DP. Epidemiology of cancer of the colon and rectum. 1971. *Dis Colon Rectum* 1993;36:1071.

55. Trock B, Lanza E, Greenwald P. Dietary fiber, vegetables, and colon cancer: critical review and meta-analyses of the epidemiologic evidence. *J Natl Cancer Inst* 1990;82:650.

56. Howe GR, Benito E, Castelleto R, et al. Dietary intake of fiber and decreased risk of cancers of the colon and rectum: evidence from the combined analysis of 13 case-control studies. *J Natl Cancer Inst* 1992;84:1887.

57. Fuchs CS, Giovannucci EL, Colditz GA, et al. Dietary fiber and the risk of colorectal cancer and adenoma in women. *N Engl J Med* 1999;340:169.

58. Schatzkin A, Lanza E, Corle D, et al. Lack of effect of a low-fat, high-fiber diet on the recurrence of colorectal adenomas. Polyp Prevention Trial Study Group. *N Engl J Med* 2000;342:1149.

59. Alberts DS, Martinez ME, Roe DJ, et al. Lack of effect of a high-fiber cereal supplement on the recurrence of colorectal adenomas. Phoenix Colon Cancer Prevention Physicians' Network. *N Engl J Med* 2000;342:1156.

60. Wargovich MJ. New dietary anticarcinogens and prevention of gastrointestinal cancer. *Dis Colon Rectum* 1988;31:72.

61. Bostick RM, Fosdick L, Wood JR, et al. Calcium and colorectal epithelial cell proliferation in sporadic adenoma patients: a randomized, double-blinded, placebo-controlled clinical trial. *J Natl Cancer Inst* 1995;87:1307.

62. Seitz HK, Simanowski UA, Garzon FT, et al. Possible role of acetaldehyde in ethanol-related rectal cocarcinogenesis in the rat. *Gastroenterology* 1990;98:406.

63. Kikendall JW, Bowen PE, Burgess MB, et al. Cigarettes and alcohol as independent risk factors for colonic adenomas. *Gastroenterology* 1989;97:660.

64. Rosenberg L, Werler MM, Palmer JR, et al. The risks of cancers of the colon and rectum in relation to coffee consumption. *Am J Epidemiol* 1989;130:895.

65. Hartman TJ, Tangrea JA, Pietinen P, et al. Tea and coffee consumption and risk of colon and rectal cancer in middle-aged Finnish men. *Nutr Cancer* 1998;31:41.

66. Giovannucci E, Rimm EB, Stampfer MJ, et al. Aspirin use and the risk for colorectal cancer and adenoma in male health professionals. *Ann Intern Med* 1994;121:241.

67. Giovannucci E, Egan KM, Hunter DJ, et al. Aspirin and the risk of colorectal cancer in women. *N Engl J Med* 1995;333:609.

68. Thun MJ, Namboodiri MM, Heath CW Jr. Aspirin use and reduced risk of fatal colon cancer. *N Engl J Med* 1991;325:1593.

69. Rosenberg L, Louik C, Shapiro S. Nonsteroidal antiinflammatory drug use and reduced risk of large bowel carcinoma. *Cancer* 1998;82:2326.

70. Smalley W, Ray WA, Daugherty J, Griffin MR. Use of nonsteroidal anti-inflammatory drugs and incidence of colorectal cancer: a population-based study. *Arch Intern Med* 1999;159:161.

71. Rustgi AK. Hereditary gastrointestinal polyposis and nonpolyposis syndromes. *N Engl J Med* 1994;331:1694.

72. Hamilton SR, Liu B, Parsons RE, et al. The molecular basis of Turcot's syndrome. *N Engl J Med* 1995;332:839.

73. Spirio L, Olschwang S, Groden J, et al. Alleles of the APC gene: an attenuated form of familial polyposis. *Cell* 1993;75:951.

74. Powell SM, Petersen GM, Krush AJ, et al. Molecular diagnosis of familial adenomatous polyposis. *N Engl J Med* 1993;329:1982.

75. Geller G, Botkin JR, Green MJ, et al. Genetic testing for susceptibility to adult-onset cancer. The process and content of informed consent. *JAMA* 1997;277:1467.

76. Giardiello FM. Genetic testing in hereditary colorectal cancer. *JAMA* 1997;278:1278.

77. Chung DC, Rustgi AK. The hereditary nonpolyposis colorectal cancer syndrome: genetics and clinical implications. *Ann Intern Med* 2003;138:560.

78. Marra G, Boland CR. Hereditary nonpolyposis colorectal cancer: the syndrome, the genes, and historical perspectives. *J Natl Cancer Inst* 1995;87:1114.

79. Burt RW. Familial risk and colorectal cancer. *Gastroenterol Clin North Am* 1996;25:793.

80. Garcia-Ruiz A, Milsom JW, Ludwig KA, Marchesa P. Right colonic arterial anatomy. Implications for laparoscopic surgery. *Dis Colon Rectum* 1996;39:906.

81. Chen Y, Liu ZY, Li RX, Guo Z. Structural studies of initial lymphatics adjacent to gastric and colonic malignant neoplasms. *Lymphology* 1999;32:70.

82. Canter RJ, Williams NN. Surgical treatment of colon and rectal cancer. *Hematol Oncol Clin North Am* 2002;16:907.

83. Colquhoun PH, Wexner SD. Surgical management of colon cancer. *Curr Gastroenterol Rep* 2002;4:414.

84. Shatari T, Fujita M, Nozawa K, et al. Vascular anatomy for right colon lymphadenectomy. *Surg Radiol Anat* 2003;25:86.

85. Stein W, Farina A, Gaffney K, et al. Characteristics of colon cancer at time of presentation. *Fam Pract Res J* 1993;13:355.

86. Majumdar SR, Fletcher RH, Evans AT. How does colorectal cancer present? Symptoms, duration, and clues to location. *Am J Gastroenterol* 1999;94:3039.

87. Rocklin MS, Senagore AJ, Talbott TM. Role of carcinoembryonic antigen and liver function tests in the detection of recurrent colorectal carcinoma. *Dis Colon Rectum* 1991;34:794.

88. Stotland BR, Siegelman ES, Morris JB, Kochman ML. Preoperative and postoperative imaging for colorectal cancer. *Hematol Oncol Clin North Am* 1997;11:635.

89. Sidransky D, Tokino T, Hamilton SR, et al. Identification of ras oncogene mutations in the stool of patients with curable colorectal tumors. *Science* 1992;256:102.

90. Smith-Ravin J, England J, Talbot IC, Bodmer W. Detection of c-Ki-ras mutations in fecal samples from sporadic colorectal cancer patients. *Gut* 1995;36:81.

91. Villa E, Dugani A, Rebecchi AM, et al. Identification of subjects at risk for colorectal carcinoma through a test based on K-ras determination in the stool. *Gastroenterology* 1996;110:1346.

92. Eguchi S, Kohara N, Komuta K, Kanematsu T. Mutations of the p53 gene in the stool of patients with resectable colorectal cancer. *Cancer* 1996;77:1707.

93. Nollau P, Moser C, Weinland G, Wagener C. Detection of K-ras mutations in stools of patients with colorectal cancer by mutant-enriched PCR. *Int J Cancer* 1996;66:332.

94. Hara AK, Johnson CD, Reed JE, et al. Detection of colorectal polyps by computed tomographic colography: feasibility of a novel technique. *Gastroenterology* 1996;110:284.

95. Hara AK, Johnson CD, Reed JE, et al. Detection of colorectal polyps with CT colography: initial assessment of sensitivity and specificity. *Radiology* 1997;205:59.

96. Ahlquist DA, Hara AK, Johnson CD. Computed tomographic colography and virtual colonoscopy. *Gastrointest Endosc Clin N Am* 1997;7:439.

97. Dachman AH, Kuniyoshi JK, Boyle CM, et al. CT colonography with three-dimensional problem solving for detection of colonic polyps. *AJR Am J Roentgenol* 1998;171:989.

98. Fenlon HM, Nunes DP, Schroy PC 3rd, et al. A comparison of virtual and conventional colonoscopy for the detection of colorectal polyps. *N Engl J Med* 1999;341:1496.

99. Rex DK, Vining D, Kopecky KK. An initial experience with screening for colon polyps using spiral CT with and without CT colography (virtual colonoscopy). *Gastrointest Endosc* 1999;50:309.

100. Sonnenberg A, Delco F, Bauerfeind P. Is virtual colonoscopy a cost-effective option to screen for colorectal cancer? *Am J Gastroenterol* 1999;94:2268.

101. Johnson CD, Ahlquist DA. Computed tomography colonography (virtual colonoscopy): a new method for colorectal screening. *Gut* 1999;44:301.

102. Morrin MM, LaMont JT. Screening virtual colonoscopy—ready for prime time? *N Engl J Med* 2003;349:2261.

103. Pickhardt PJ, Choi JR, Hwang I, et al. Computed tomographic virtual colonoscopy to screen for colorectal neoplasia in asymptomatic adults. *N Engl J Med* 2003;349:2191.

104. Compton CC. *Surgical pathology of colorectal cancer.* Totowa, NJ: Humana Press, 2002:247.

105. American Joint Committee on Cancer. *Colon and rectum*. Philadelphia: Lippincott–Raven, 2002:113.

106. Wolmark N, Fisher B, Wieand HS. The prognostic value of the modifications of the Dukes' C class of colorectal cancer. An analysis of the NSABP clinical trials. *Ann Surg* 1986;203:115.

107. Jass JR. Lymphocytic infiltration and survival in rectal cancer. *J Clin Pathol* 1986;39:585.

108. Deans G, Heatley M, Anderson N, et al. Jass' classification revisited. *J Am Coll Surg* 1994;179:11.

109. Compton CC, Fielding LP, Burgart LJ, et al. Prognostic factors in colorectal cancer. College of American Pathologists Consensus Statement 1999. *Arch Pathol Lab Med* 2000;124:979.

110. Greene F, Stewart A, Norton H. A new TNM staging strategy for node-positive (stage III) colon cancer: an analysis of 50,042 patients. *Ann Surg* 2002;236:416.

111. Ratto C, Sofo L, Ippoliti M, et al. Accurate lymph-node detection in colorectal specimens resected for cancer is of prognostic significance [Discussion]. *Dis Colon Rectum* 1999;42:143;154.

112. Wong JH, Severino R, Honnebier MB, Tom P, Namiki TS. Number of nodes examined and staging accuracy in colorectal carcinoma. *J Clin Oncol* 1999;17:2896.

113. Joseph NE, Sigurdson ER, Hanlon AL, et al. Accuracy of determining nodal negativity in colorectal cancer on the basis of the number of nodes retrieved on resection. *Ann Surg Oncol* 2003;10:213.

114. Tepper JE, O'Connell MJ, Niedzwicki D, et al. Final report of INT 0114-Aduvant therapy in rectal cancer: analysis by treatment, stage, and gender. *Program/Proc ASCO* 2001;20:123a(abst 489).

115. Liefers GJ, Tollenaar RA, Cleton-Jansen AM. Molecular detection of minimal residual disease in colorectal and breast cancer. *Histopathology* 1999;34:385.

116. Liefers GJ, Cleton-Jansen AM, van de Velde CJ, et al. Micrometastases and survival in stage II colorectal cancer. *N Engl J Med* 1998;339:223.

117. Jeffers MD, O'Dowd GM, Mulcahy H, et al. The prognostic significance of immunohistochemically detected lymph node micrometastases in colorectal carcinoma. *J Pathol* 1994;172:183.

118. Hermanek P, Hutter RV, Sobin LH, Wittekind C. International Union Against Cancer. Classification of isolated tumor cells and micrometastasis. *Cancer* 1999;86:2668.

119. Morton DL, Wen DR, Wong JH, et al. Technical details of intraoperative lymphatic mapping for early stage melanoma. *Arch Surg* 1992;127:392.

120. Canavese G, Gipponi M, Catturich A, et al. Sentinel lymph node mapping in early-stage breast cancer: technical issues and results with vital blue dye mapping and radioguided surgery. *J Surg Oncol* 2000;74:61.

121. Esser S, Reilly WT, Riley LB, Eyvazzadeh C, Arcona S. The role of sentinel lymph node mapping in staging of colon and rectal cancer[discussion]. *Dis Colon Rectum* 2001;44:850.

122. Waters GS, Geisinger KR, Garske DD, Loggie BW, Levine EA. Sentinel lymph node mapping for carcinoma of the colon: a pilot study[discussion]. *Am Surg* 2000;66:943.

123. Paramo JC, Summerall J, Poppiti R, Mesko TW. Validation of sentinel node mapping in patients with colon cancer. *Ann Surg Oncol* 2002;9:550.

124. Saha S, Wiese D, Badin J, et al. Technical details of sentinel lymph node mapping in colorectal cancer and its impact on staging. *Ann Surg Oncol* 2000;7:120.

125. Turner RR, Nora DT, Trocha SD, Bilchik AJ. Colorectal carcinoma nodal staging. Frequency and nature of cytokeratin-positive cells in sentinel and nonsentinel lymph nodes. *Arch Pathol Lab Med* 2003;127:673.

126. Feig BW, Curley S, Lucci A, et al. A caution regarding lymphatic mapping in patients with colon cancer. *Am J Surg* 2001;182:707.

127. Warner EE, Evans SR. The sentinel node biopsy and colon cancer revisited. *Cancer J* 2002;8:435.

128. Bilchik AJ, Saha S, Wiese D, et al. Molecular staging of early colon cancer on the basis of sentinel node analysis: a multicenter phase II trial. *J Clin Oncol* 2001;19:1128.

129. Cusack JC, Giacco GG, Cleary K, et al. Survival factors in 186 patients younger than 40 years old with colorectal adenocarcinoma. *J Am Coll Surg* 1996;183:105.

130. Messerini L, Palomba A, Zampi G. Primary signet-ring cell carcinoma of the colon and rectum. *Dis Colon Rectum* 1995;38:1189.

131. de Bruine AP, Wiggers T, Beek C, et al. Endocrine cells in colorectal adenocarcinomas: incidence, hormone profile and prognostic relevance. *Int J Cancer* 1993;54:765.

132. Jessurun J, Romero-Guadarrama M, Manivel JC. Medullary adenocarcinoma of the colon: clinicopathologic study of 11 cases. *Hum Pathol* 1999;30:843.

133. de la Chapelle A. Microsatellite instability. *N Engl J Med* 2003;349:209.

134. Boland CR, Sato J, Saito K, et al. Genetic instability and chromosomal aberrations in colorectal cancer: a review of the current models. *Cancer Detect Prev* 1998;22:377.

135. Boland CR, Thibodeau SN, Hamilton SR, et al. A National Cancer Institute Workshop on Microsatellite Instability for cancer detection and familial predisposition: development of international criteria for the determination of microsatellite instability in colorectal cancer. *Cancer Res* 1998;58:5248.

136. Thibodeau SN, Bren G, Schaid D. Microsatellite instability in cancer of the proximal colon. *Science* 1993;260:816.

137. Jass J. Diagnosis of hereditary non-polyposis colorectal cancer. *Histopathology* 1998;32:491.

138. Jass JR, Do KA, Simms LA, et al. Morphology of sporadic colorectal cancer with DNA replication errors. *Gut* 1998;42:673.

139. Gryfe R, Kim H, Hsieh ET, et al. Tumor microsatellite instability and clinical outcome in young patients with colorectal cancer. *N Engl J Med* 2000;342:69.

140. Watanabe T, Wu TT, Catalano PJ, et al. Molecular predictors of survival after adjuvant chemotherapy for colon cancer. *N Engl J Med* 2001;344:1196.

141. Carethers JM, Chauhan DP, Fink D, et al. Mismatch repair proficiency and in vitro response to 5-fluorouracil. *Gastroenterology* 1999;117:123.

142. Ribic CM, Sargent DJ, Moore MJ, et al. Tumor microsatellite-instability status as a predictor of benefit from fluorouracil-based adjuvant chemotherapy for colon cancer. *N Engl J Med* 2003;349:247.

143. Fearon E, Cho K, Nigro J, et al. Identification of a chromosome 18q gene that is altered in colorectal cancers. *Science* 1990;247:49.

144. Mehlen P, Rabizadeh S, Snipas S, et al. The DCC gene product induces apoptosis by a mechanism requiring receptor proteolysis. *Nature* 1998;395:801.

145. Lanza G, Matteuzzi M, Gafa R, et al. Chromosome 18q allelic loss and prognosis in stage II and III colon cancer. *Int J Cancer* 1998;79:390.

146. Harrison LE, Guillem JG, Paty P, Cohen AM. Preoperative carcinoembryonic antigen predicts outcomes in node-negative colon cancer patients: a multivariate analysis of 572 patients. *J Am Coll Surg* 1997;185:55.

147. Meyerhardt JA, Catalano PJ, Haller DG, et al. Impact of diabetes mellitus on outcomes in patients with colon cancer. *J Clin Oncol* 2003;21:433.

148. Donohue J, Williams S, Cha S, et al. Perioperative blood transfusions do not affect disease recurrence of patients undergoing curative resection of colorectal carcinoma: a Mayo/North Central Cancer Treatment Group study. *J Clin Oncol* 1995;13:1671.

149. Leichman CG, Lenz H-J, Danenberg K, et al. Quantitation of intratumoral thymidylate synthase expression predicted for disseminated colorectal cancer response and resistance to protracted infusion 5-fluorouracil and weekly leucovorin. *J Clin Oncol* 1997;15:3223.

150. Ahnen DJ, Feigl P, Quan G, et al. Ki-ras mutation and p53 overexpression predict the clinical behavior of colorectal cancer: a Southwest Oncology Group study. *Cancer Res* 1998;58:1149.

151. McLeod HL. Individualized cancer therapy: molecular approaches to the prediction of tumor response. *Expert Rev Anticancer Ther* 2002;2:113.

152. Winawer SJ. Follow-up after polypectomy. *World J Surg* 1991;15:25.

153. Lee MG, Hanchard B. Management of colonic polyps by colonoscopic polypectomy. *West Indian Med J* 1991;40:81.

154. Huang EH, Forde KA. Surgical implications of colonoscopy. *Semin Laparosc Surg* 2003;10:13.

155. Forde KA. Therapeutic colonoscopy. *World J Surg* 1992;16:1048.

156. Libutti SK, Forde KA. Surgical considerations III: bowel anastomosis. In: Cohen A, Weaver S, eds. *Cancer of the colon, rectum and anus*. New York: McGraw-Hill, 1995:445.

157. Guenaga KF, Matos D, Castro AA, Atallah AN, Wille-Jorgensen P. Mechanical bowel preparation for elective colorectal surgery. *Cochrane Database Syst Rev* 2003;CD001544.

158. Makino M, Hisamitsu K, Sugamura K, Kimura O, Kaibara N. Randomized comparison of two preoperative methods for preparation of the colon: oral administration of a solution of polyethylene glycol plus electrolytes and total parenteral nutrition. *Hepatogastroenterology* 1998;45:90.

159. Chen CF, Lin JK, Leu SY, Liang CL. Evaluation of rapid colon preparation with Golytely. *Zhonghua Yi Xue Za Zhi* 1989;44:45.

160. Lewis RT, Goodall RG, Marien B, et al. Is neomycin necessary for bowel preparation in surgery of the colon? Oral neomycin plus erythromycin versus erythromycin-metronidazole. *Can J Surg* 1989;32:265.

161. McGinnis LS. Surgical treatment options for colorectal cancer. *Cancer* 1994;74:2147.

162. Benson AB 3rd, Choti MA, Cohen AM, et al. NCCN practice guidelines for colorectal cancer. *Oncology* 2000;14:203.

163. Garcia-Olmo D, Ontanon J, Garcia-Olmo DC, Vallejo M, Cifuentes J. Experimental evidence does not support use of the "no-touch" isolation technique in colorectal cancer[discussion]. *Dis Colon Rectum* 1999;42:1449.

164. Grinnell RS. Results of ligation of inferior mesenteric artery at the aorta in resections of carcinoma of the descending and sigmoid colon and rectum. *Surg Gynecol Obstet* 1965;120:1031.

165. Ambroze WL Jr, Orangio GR, Lucas G. Surgical options for familial adenomatous polyposis. *Semin Surg Oncol* 1995;11:423.

166. Young CJ, Solomon MJ, Eyers AA, et al. Evolution of the pelvic pouch procedure at one institution: the first 100 cases. *Aust N Z J Surg* 1999;69:438.

167. Regimbeau JM, Panis Y, Pocard M, Hautefeuille P, Valleur P. Handsewn ileal pouch-anal anastomosis on the dentate line after total proctectomy: technique to avoid incomplete mucosectomy and the need for long-term follow-up of the anal transition zone[discussion]. *Dis Colon Rectum* 2001;44:43.

168. Madden MV, Neale KF, Nicholls RJ, et al. Comparison of morbidity and function after colectomy with ileorectal anastomosis or restorative proctocolectomy for familial adenomatous polyposis. *Br J Surg* 1991;78:789.

169. Poppen B, Svenberg T, Bark T, et al. Colectomy-proctomucosectomy with S-pouch: operative procedures, complications, and functional outcome in 69 consecutive patients. *Dis Colon Rectum* 1992;35:40.

170. Fiorentini MT, Locatelli L, Ceccopieri B, et al. Physiology of ileoanal anastomosis with ileal reservoir for ulcerative colitis and adenomatosis coli. *Dis Colon Rectum* 1987;30:267.

171. Hughes ES, McDermott FT, Polglase AL, Nottle P. Total and subtotal colectomy for colonic obstruction. *Dis Colon Rectum* 1985;28:162.

172. Lichten JB, Reid JJ, Zahalsky MP, Friedman RL. Laparoscopic cholecystectomy in the new millennium. *Surg Endosc* 2001;15:867.

173. Mori T, Abe N, Sugiyama M, Atomi Y. Laparoscopic hepatobiliary and pancreatic surgery: an overview. *J Hepatobiliary Pancreat Surg* 2002;9:710.

174. Hartley JE, Monson JR. The role of laparoscopy in the multimodality treatment of colorectal cancer. *Surg Clin North Am* 2002;82:1019.

175. Theodoridis TD, Bontis JN. Laparoscopy and oncology: where do we stand today? *Ann N Y Acad Sci* 2003;997:282.

176. Goletti O, Celona G, Monzani F, et al. Laparoscopic treatment of pancreatic insulinoma. *Surg Endosc* 2003;17:1499.

177. Yoshimura K, Yoshioka T, Miyake O, et al. Comparison of clinical outcomes of laparoscopic and conventional open adrenalectomy. *J Endourol* 1998;12:555.

178. Feliciotti F, Paganini AM, Guerrieri M, et al. Results of laparoscopic vs open resections for colon cancer in patients with a minimum follow-up of 3 years. *Surg Endosc* 2002;16:1158.

179. Delaney CP, Kiran RP, Senagore AJ, Brady K, Fazio VW. Case-matched comparison of clinical and financial outcome after laparoscopic or open colorectal surgery. *Ann Surg* 2003;238:67.

180. Patankar SK, Larach SW, Ferrara A, et al. Prospective comparison of laparoscopic vs. open resections for colorectal adenocarcinoma over a ten-year period. *Dis Colon Rectum* 2003;46:601.
181. Lauter DM, Lau ST, Lanzafame K. Combined laparoscopic-assisted right hemicolectomy and low anterior resection for synchronous colorectal carcinomas. *Surg Endosc* 2003;17:1498.
182. Cobb WS, Lokey JS, Schwab DP, et al. Hand-assisted laparoscopic colectomy: a single-institution experience. *Am Surg* 2003;69:578.
183. Lezoche E, Feliciotti F, Paganini AM, et al. Results of laparoscopic versus open resections for non-early rectal cancer in patients with a minimum follow-up of four years. *Hepatogastroenterology* 2002;49:1185.
184. Weeks JC, Nelson H, Gelber S, Sargent D, Schroeder G. Short-term quality-of-life outcomes following laparoscopic-assisted colectomy vs open colectomy for colon cancer: a randomized trial. *JAMA* 2002;287:321.
185. Nivatvongs S. Surgical management of early colorectal cancer. *World J Surg* 2000;24:1052.
186. Markowitz AJ, Winawer SJ. Management of colorectal polyps. *CA Cancer J Clin* 1997;47:93.
187. NIH consensus conference. Adjuvant therapy for patients with colon and rectal cancer. *JAMA* 1990;264:1444.
188. Buyse M, Zelenicuh-Jacquotte A, Chalmers TC. Adjuvant therapy of colorectal cancer. Why we still don't know. *JAMA* 1988;259:3571.
189. Wolmark N, Fisher B, Rockette H, et al. Postoperative adjuvant chemotherapy or BCG for colon cancer: results from NSABP Protocol C0-1. *J Natl Cancer Inst* 1988;80:30.
190. Laurie JA, Moertel CG, Fleming TR, et al. Surgical adjuvant therapy of large bowel carcinoma: an evaluation of levamisole and the combination of levamisole and fluorouracil. *J Clin Oncol* 1989;7:1447.
191. Moertel C, Fleming T, Macdonald J, et al. Levamisole and fluorouracil for adjuvant therapy of resected colon carcinoma. *N Engl J Med* 1990;322.
192. Moertel CG, Fleming TR, Macdonald J, et al. Fluorouracil plus levamisole as effective adjuvant therapy after resection of stage III colon carcinoma: a final report. *Ann Intern Med* 1995;122:321.
193. Moertel CG, Fleming TR, Macdonald J, et al. Intergroup study of fluorouracil plus levamisole as adjuvant therapy for stage II/Duke's B2 colon cancer. *J Clin Oncol* 1995;13:2936.
194. Wolmark N, Rockette H, Fisher B, et al. The benefit of leucovorin-modulated fluorouracil as postoperative adjuvant therapy for primary colon cancer: results from National Surgical Adjuvant Breast and Bowel Project protocol C-03. *J Clin Oncol* 1993;11:1879.
195. Efficacy of adjuvant fluorouracil and folinic acid in colon cancer. *Lancet* 1995;345:939.
196. Efficacy of adjuvant fluorouracil and folinic acid in B2 colon cancer. *J Clin Oncol* 1999;17:1356.
197. Wolmark N, Rockette H, Mamounas EP, et al. Clinical trial to asses the relative efficacy of fluorouracil and leucovorin, fluorouracil and levamisole, and fluorouracil, leucovorin, and levamisole in patients with Dukes' B and C carcinoma of the colon: results from National Surgical Adjuvant Breast and Bowel Project C-04. *J Clin Oncol* 1999;17:3553.
198. O'Connell MJ, Laurie JA, Kahn M, et al. Prospectively randomized trial of postoperative adjuvant chemotherapy in patients with high-risk colon cancer. *J Clin Oncol* 1998;16:295.
199. Saini A, Norman AR, Cunningham D, et al. Twelve weeks of protracted venous infusion of fluorouracil (5-FU) is as effective as 6 months of bolus 5-FU and folinic acid as adjuvant treatment in colorectal cancer. *Br J Cancer* 2003;88:1859.
200. Comparison of fluorouracil with additional levamisole, higher-dose folinic acid, or both, as adjuvant chemotherapy for colorectal cancer: a randomized trial. QUASAR Collaborative Group. *Lancet* 2000;355:1588.
201. Kerr DJ, Gray R, McConkey C, Barnwell J. Adjuvant chemotherapy with 5-fluorouracil, L-folinic acid and levamisole for patients with colorectal cancer: non-randomized comparison of weekly versus four-weekly schedules—less pain, same gain. QUASAR Colorectal Cancer Study Group. *Ann Oncol* 2000;11:947.
202. Haller D, Catalano P, Macdonald J. Fluorouracil (FU), leucovorin (LV) and levamisole (LEV) adjuvant therapy for colon cancer: five-year final report of INT-0089. *Proc Am Soc Clin Oncol* 1998;17:256a(abst).
203. Andre T, Louvet C, Raymond E, et al. Bimonthly high-dose leucovorin, 5-fluorouracil infusion and oxaliplatin (FOLFOX3) for metastatic colorectal cancer resistant to the same leucovorin and 5-fluorouracil regimen. *Ann Oncol* 1998;9:1251.
204. Andre T, Colin P, Louvet C, et al. Semimonthly versus monthly regimen of fluorouracil and leucovorin administered for 24 or 36 weeks as adjuvant therapy in stage II and III colon cancer: results of a randomized trial. *J Clin Oncol* 2003;21:2896.
204a. Cassidy J, Scheithauer W, McKendrick H. Capecitabine (X) vs bolus 5-FU/leucovorin (LV) as adjuvant therapy for colon cancer (the X-ACT study): efficacy results of a phase III trial. *Proc Am Soc Clin Oncol* 2004;3509(abst).
205. Wolmark N, Wieand S, Lembersky B, et al. A phase III trial comparing oral UFT to FULV in stage II and III carcinoma of the colon: results of NSABP Protocol C-06. *Proc Am Soc Clin Oncol* 2004;3508(abst).
206. Andre T, Boni C, Mouredji-Bardint L, et al. Oxaliplatin, fluorouracil, and leucovorin as adjuvant treatment for colon cancer. *N Engl J Med* 2004;350:2343.
207. Sargent DJ, Niedzwiecki D, O'Connell MJ, Schilsky RL. Recommendation for caution with irinotecan, fluorouracil, and leucovorin for colorectal cancer[author reply]. *N Engl J Med* 2001;345:144.
208. Saltz LB, Niedzwiecki D, Hollis D, et al. Irinotecan plus fluorouracil/leucovorin (IFL) versus fluorouracil/leucovorin alone (FL) in stage III colon cancer (intergroup trial CALGB C89803). *Proc Am Soc Clin Oncol* 2004;3500(abst).
209. Ychou M, Raoul J, Bugat R, et al. LV5FU2+CPT-11 versus LV5FU2 alone in adjuvant colon cancer: interim safety results of the phase III randomized FNCLCC Accord02/FFCD9802 trial. *Proc Am Soc Clin Oncol* 2003;22.
210. Willet CG, Tepper JE, Cohen AM. Obstructive and perforative colonic carcinoma: patterns of failure. *J Clin Oncol* 1985;3:379.
211. Elsaleh H, Iacopetta B. Microsatellite instability is a predictive marker for survival benefit from adjuvant chemotherapy in a population-based series of stage III colorectal carcinoma. *Clin Colorectal Cancer* 2001;1:104.
212. Jen J, Kim H, Piantadosi S, et al. Allelic loss of chromosome 18q and prognosis in colorectal cancer. *N Engl J Med* 1994;331:213.
213. Ackerman N. The blood supply of experimental liver metastases IV. Changes in vascularity with increasing tumor growth. *Surgery* 1974;75:589.
214. Basserman R. Changes of vascular pattern of tumors and surrounding tissue during different phases of metastatic growth. *Cancer Res* 1986;100:256.
215. Almersjo O, Brandberg A, Gustavsson B. Concentration of biologically active 5-fluorouracil in the general circulation during continuous portal infusion in man. *Cancer Lett* 1975;1:113.
216. Wolmark N, Rockette H, Wickerman DL, et al. Adjuvant therapy of Dukes' A, B, and C adenocarcinoma of the colon with portal vein fluorouracil hepatic infusion: preliminary results of National Surgical Adjuvant Breast and Bowel Project Protocol C-02. *J Clin Oncol* 1990;8:1466.
217. Weber W, Laffer U, Metzger U. Adjuvant portal liver infusion with 5-fluorouracil and mitomycin in colorectal cancer. *Anticancer Res* 1993;13:1839.
218. Long term results of single course of adjuvant intraportal chemotherapy for colorectal cancer. *Lancet* 1995;345:349.
219. Speyer JL, Collins JM, Dedrick RL, et al. Phase I and pharmacological studies of 5-fluorouracil administered intraperitoneally. *Cancer Res* 1980;40:567.
220. Speyer JL, Sugarbaker PH, Collins JM, et al. Portal levels and hepatic clearance of 5-fluorouracil after intraportal administration in humans. *Cancer Res* 1981;41:1916.
221. Kelsen DP, Saltz L, Cohen AM, et al. A phase I trial of immediate postoperative intraperitoneal floxuridine and leucovorin plus systemic 5-fluorouracil and levamisole after resection of high risk colon cancer. *Cancer* 1994;74:2224.
222. Scheithauer W, Kornek GV, Marczell A, et al. Combined intravenous and intraperitoneal chemotherapy with fluorouracil + leucovorin vs fluorouracil + levamisole for adjuvant therapy of resected colon carcinoma. *Br J Cancer* 1998;77:1349.
223. Herlyn M, Steplewski Z, Herlyn D, Koprowski H. Colorectal carcinoma-specific antigen: detection by means of monoclonal antibodies. *Proc Natl Acad Sci U S A* 1979;76:1438.
224. Mellstedt H, Frodin JJE, Masuccci G. The therapeutic use of monoclonal antibodies in colorectal carcinoma. *Semin Oncol* 1991;2:462.
225. Foon KA, John WJ, Chakraborty M, et al. Clinical and immune responses in resected colorectal cancer patients treated with anti-idiotype monoclonal antibody vaccine that mimics carcinoembryonic antigen. *J Clin Oncol* 1999;17:2889.
226. Horig H, Lee DS, Conkright W, et al. Phase I clinical trial of a recombinant canarypoxvirus (ALVAC) vaccine expressing human carcinoembryonic antigen and the B7.1 co-stimulatory molecule. *Cancer Immunol Immunother* 2000;49:504.
227. von Mehren M, Arlen P, Gulley J, et al. The influence of granulocyte macrophage colony-stimulating factor and prior chemotherapy on the immunological response to a vaccine (ALVAC-CEA B7.1) in patients with metastatic carcinoma. *Clin Cancer Res* 2001;7:1181.
228. van der Burg SH, Menon AG, Redeker A, et al. Induction of p53-specific immune responses in colorectal cancer patients receiving a recombinant ALVAC-p53 candidate vaccine. *Clin Cancer Res* 2002;8:1019.
229. Ullenhag GJ, Frodin JE, Mosolits S, et al. Immunization of colorectal carcinoma patients with a recombinant canarypox virus expressing the tumor antigen Ep-CAM/KSA (ALVAC-KSA) and granulocyte macrophage colony-stimulating factor induced a tumor-specific cellular immune response. *Clin Cancer Res* 2003;9:2447.
230. Hoover HC, Brandhorst JS, Peters LC, et al. Adjuvant active specific immunotherapy for human colorectal cancer: 6.5-year median follow-up of a phase II prospectively randomized trial. *J Clin Oncol* 1993;11:390.
231. Vermorken JB, Anke ME, van Tinteran H, et al. Active specific immunotherapy for stage II and III human colon cancer: a randomized trial. *Lancet* 1999.
232. Harris JE, Ryan L, Hoover HC Jr, et al. Adjuvant active specific immunotherapy for stage II and III colon cancer with an autologous tumor cell vaccine: Eastern Cooperative Oncology Group Study E5283. *J Clin Oncol* 2000;18:148.
233. Russell AH, Tong D, Dawson LE, Wisbeck W. Adenocarcinoma of the proximal colon. Sites of initial dissemination and patterns of recurrence following surgery alone. *Cancer* 1984;53:360.
234. Russell AH, Tong D, Dawson LE, et al. Adenocarcinoma of the retroperitoneal ascending and descending colon: sites of initial dissemination and clinical patterns of recurrence following surgery alone. *Int J Radiat Oncol Biol Phys* 1983;9:361.
235. Willett C, Tepper JE, Cohen A, et al. Local failure following curative resection of colonic adenocarcinoma. *Int J Radiat Oncol Biol Phys* 1984;10:645.
236. Gunderson LL, Sosin H, Levitt S. Extrapelvic colon—areas of failure in a reoperation series: implications for adjuvant therapy. *Int J Radiat Oncol Biol Phys* 1985;11:731.
237. Willett C, Fung C, Kaufman D, Efird J, Shellito P. Postoperative radiation therapy for high-risk colon carcinoma. *J Clin Oncol* 1993;11:1112.
238. Willett CG, Goldberg S, Shellito PC, et al. Does postoperative irradiation play a role in adjuvant therapy of stage T4 colon cancer? *Cancer J Sci Am* 1999;5:242.
239. Schild SE, Gunderson L, Haddock MG, Wong WW, Nelson H. The treatment of locally advanced colon cancer. *Int J Radiat Oncol Biol Phys* 1997;37:51.
240. Amos EH, Mendenhall WM, McCarty PJ, et al. Postoperative radiotherapy for locally advanced colon cancer. *Ann Surg Oncol* 1996;3:431.
241. Martenson J, Willett C, Sargent J, Donohue RA. Phase III study of adjuvant radiation therapy (RT), 5-fluorouracil (5-FU), and levamisole (LEV) vs 5-FU and LEV in selected patients with resected, high-risk colon cancer: initial results of Int 0130. Proceedings of ASCO 1999;235a.
242. Fabian C, Giri S, Estes N, et al. Adjuvant continuous infusion 5-FU, whole-abdominal radiation, and tumor bed boost in high-risk stage III colon carcinoma: a Southwest Oncology Group pilot study. *Int J Radiat Oncol Biol Phys* 1995;32:457.
243. Ben-Joseph R, Segal R, Russell WL, Oh T. Evaluating the value, accuracy, and operational feasibility of DUE criteria. *Formulary* 1995;30:280.
244. Burt RW. Colon cancer screening. *Gastroenterology* 2000;119:837.
245. Muller AD, Sonnenberg A. Prevention of colorectal cancer by flexible endoscopy and polypectomy. A case-control study of 32,702 veterans. *Ann Intern Med* 1995;123:904.

246. Atkin WS, Morson BC, Cuzick J. Long-term risk of colorectal cancer after excision of rectosigmoid adenomas. *N Engl J Med* 1992;326:658.

247. Burke W, Petersen G, Lynch P, et al. Recommendations for follow-up care of individuals with an inherited predisposition to cancer. I. Hereditary nonpolyposis colon cancer. Cancer Genetics Studies Consortium. *JAMA* 1997;277:915.

248. Graham RA, Wang S, Catalano PJ, Haller DG. Postsurgical surveillance of colon cancer: preliminary cost analysis of physician examination, carcinoembryonic antigen testing, chest x-ray, and colonoscopy. *Ann Surg* 1998;228:59.

249. Mandel JS, Bond JH, Church TR, et al. Reducing mortality from colorectal cancer by screening for fecal occult blood. Minnesota Colon Cancer Control Study. *N Engl J Med* 1993;328:1365.

250. Bruinvels DJ, Stiggelbout AM, Kievit J, et al. Follow-up of patients with colorectal cancer. A meta-analysis. *Ann Surg* 1994;219:174.

251. Bruinvels DJ, Stiggelbout AM, Klaassen MP, et al. Follow-up after colorectal cancer: current practice in The Netherlands. *Eur J Surg* 1995;161:827.

252. Desch CE, Benson AB 3rd, Smith TJ, et al. Recommended colorectal cancer surveillance guidelines by the American Society of Clinical Oncology. *J Clin Oncol* 1999;17:1312.

253. Zeng Z, Cohen AM, Urmacher C. Usefulness of carcinoembryonic antigen monitoring despite normal preoperative values in node-positive colon cancer patients. *Dis Colon Rectum* 1993;36:1063.

254. Clinical practice guidelines for the use of tumor markers in breast and colorectal cancer. Adopted on May 17, 1996 by the American Society of Clinical Oncology. *J Clin Oncol* 1996;14:2843.

255. Ito K, Hibi K, Ando H, et al. Usefulness of analytical CEA doubling time and half-life time for overlooked synchronous metastases in colorectal carcinoma. *Jpn J Clin Oncol* 2002;32:54.

256. Gunderson LL, Sosin H. Areas of failure found at reoperation (second or symptomatic look) following "curative surgery" for adenocarcinoma of the rectum. *Cancer* 1974;34:1278.

257. Libutti SK, Alexander HR Jr, Choyke P, et al. A prospective study of 2-[18F] fluoro-2-deoxy-D-glucose/positron emission tomography scan, 99mTc-labeled arcitumomab (CEA-scan), and blind second-look laparotomy for detecting colon cancer recurrence in patients with increasing carcinoembryonic antigen levels. *Ann Surg Oncol* 2001;8:779.

258. Bruinvels DJ, de Brauw LM, Kievit J, Habbema JD, van de Velde CJ. Attitudes towards detection and management of hepatic metastases of colorectal origin: a second look. *HPB Surg* 1994;8:115.

259. Balz JB, Martin EW, Minton JP. CEA as an early indicator for second-look procedure in colorectal carcinoma. *Rev Surg* 1977;34:1.

260. Martin EW Jr, Minton JP, Carey LC. CEA-directed second-look surgery in the asymptomatic patient after primary resection of colorectal carcinoma. *Ann Surg* 1985;202:310.

261. Beatty JD, Hyams DM, Morton BA, et al. Impact of radiolabeled antibody imaging on management of colon cancer. *Am J Surg* 1989;157:13.

262. Moffat FL Jr, Pinsky CM, Hammershaimb L, et al. Clinical utility of external immunoscintigraphy with the IMMU-4 technetium-99m Fab' antibody fragment in patients undergoing surgery for carcinoma of the colon and rectum: results of a pivotal, phase III trial. The Immunomedics Study Group. *J Clin Oncol* 1996;14:2295.

263. Takenoshita S, Hashizume T, Asao T, et al. Immunoscintigraphy using 99mTc-labeled anti-CEA monoclonal antibody for patients with colorectal cancer. *Anticancer Res* 1995;15:471.

264. Swanson RS. Is an FDG-PET scan the new imaging standard for colon cancer? *Ann Surg Oncol* 2001;8:752.

265. Schoemaker D, Black R, Giles L, Toouli J. Yearly colonoscopy, liver CT, and chest radiography do not influence 5-year survival of colorectal cancer patients. *Gastroenterology* 1998;114:7.

266. Ohlsson B, Breland U, Ekberg H, Graffner H, Tranberg KG. Follow-up after curative surgery for colorectal carcinoma. Randomized comparison with no follow-up. *Dis Colon Rectum* 1995;38:619.

267. Makela J, Laitinen S, Kairaluoma MI. Early results of follow-up after radical resection for colorectal cancer. Preliminary results of a prospective randomized trial. *Surg Oncol* 1992;1:157.

268. Benson AB 3rd, Desch CE, Flynn PJ, et al. 2000 update of American Society of Clinical Oncology colorectal cancer surveillance guidelines. *J Clin Oncol* 2000;18:3586.

269. Fornasarig M, Valentini M, Poletti M, et al. Evaluation of the risk for metachronous colorectal neoplasms following intestinal polypectomy: a clinical, endoscopic and pathological study. *Hepatogastroenterology* 1998;45:1565.

270. Ghahremani GG, Dowlatshahi K. Colorectal carcinomas: diagnostic implications of their changing frequency and anatomic distribution[discussion]. *World J Surg* 1989;13:321.

271. Inadomi JM, Sonnenberg A. The impact of colorectal cancer screening on life expectancy. *Gastrointest Endosc* 2000;51:517.

272. Renehan AG, Egger M, Saunders MP, O'Dwyer ST. Impact on survival of intensive follow up after curative resection for colorectal cancer: systematic review and meta-analysis of randomized trials. *BMJ* 2002;324:813.

273. Heidelberger C, Chaudhuri NK, Danneberg P, et al. Fluorinated pyrimidines: a new class of tumor inhibitory compounds. *Nature* 1957;179:663.

274. Santi DV, McHenry CS, Sommer H. Mechanism of interaction of thymidylate synthetase with 5-fluorodeoxyuridylate. *Biochemistry* 1974;13:471.

275. Lockshin A, Danenberg PV. Biochemical factors affecting the tightness of 5-fluorodeoxyuridylate binding of human thymidylate synthetase. *Biochem Pharmacol* 1981;30:247.

276. Madajewicz, S, Petrelli N, Rustum YM, et al. Phase I-II trial of high dose calcium leucovorin and 5-fluorouracil in advanced colorectal cancer. *Cancer Res* 1984;44:4667.

277. Cunningham J, Bukowski RM, Budd GT, et al. 5-Fluorouracil and folinic acid: a phase I-II trial in gastrointestinal malignancy. *Invest New Drugs* 1984;2:391.

278. Bertrand M, Doroshow J, Multhauf P, et al. High dose continuous infusion folinic acid and bolus 5-fluorouracil in patients with advanced colorectal cancer: a phase II study. *J Clin Oncol* 1986;4:1058.

279. Machover D, Goldschmidt E, Chollet P, et al. Treatment of advanced colorectal and gastric carcinoma with 5-fluorouracil and high dose folinic acid. *J Clin Oncol* 1986;4:685.

280. Poon MA, O'Connell MJ, Moertel CG, et al. Biochemical modulation of fluorouracil: evidence of significant improvement of survival and quality of life in patients with advanced colorectal carcinoma. *J Clin Oncol* 1989;7:1407.

281. Poon M, O'Connell M, Wieand H, et al. Biochemical modulation of fluorouracil with leucovorin: confirmatory evidence of improved therapeutic efficacy in advanced colorectal cancer. *J Clin Oncol* 1991;9:1967.

282. DiCostanzo F, Bartolucci R, Calabresi F, et al. Fluorouracil-alone versus high dose folinic acid and fluorouracil in advanced colorectal cancer: a randomized trial of the Italian Oncology Group for Clinical Research (GOIRC). *Ann Oncol* 1992;3:371.

283. Laufman L, Bukowski RM, Collier MA, et al. A randomized, double-blind trial of fluorouracil plus placebo versus fluorouracil plus oral leucovorin in patients with metastatic colorectal cancer. *J Clin Oncol* 1989;11:1888.

284. Modulation of fluorouracil by leucovorin in patients with advanced colorectal cancer: evidence in terms of response rate. Advanced Colorectal Cancer Meta-Analysis Project. *J Clin Oncol* 1992;10:896.

285. Piedbois P, Michiels S. Survival benefit of 5FU/LV over 5FU bolus in patients with advanced colorectal cancer: an updated meta-analysis based on 2,751 patients. *Proc Am Soc Clin Oncol* 2003;22.

286. Buroker TR, O'Connell MJ, Wieand HS, et al. Randomized comparison of two schedules of fluorouracil and leucovorin in the treatment of advanced colorectal cancer. *J Clin Oncol* 1994;12:14.

287. Jager E, Heike M, Bernhard H, et al. Weekly high-dose leucovorin versus low-dose leucovorin combined with fluorouracil in advanced colorectal cancer: results of a randomized mulitcenter trial. *J Clin Oncol* 1996;14:2274.

288. Leichman CG, Fleming TR, Muggia FM, et al. Phase II study of fluorouracil and its modulation in advanced colorectal cancer: a Southwest Oncology Group study. *J Clin Oncol* 1995;13:1303.

289. Calabro-Jones PM, Byfield JE, Ward JF, Sharp TR. Time-dose relationships for 5-fluorouracil cytotoxicity against human epithelial cancer cells in vitro. *Cancer Res* 1982;42:4413.

290. Lokich JJ, Ahlgren JD, Gullo JJ, Philips JA, Fryer JG. A prospective randomized comparison of continuous infusion fluorouracil with a conventional bolus schedule in metastatic colorectal carcinoma: a Mid-Atlantic Oncology Program Study. *J Clin Oncol* 1989;7:425.

291. O'Dwyer PJ, Ryan LM. Phase III trial of biochemical modulation of 5-fluorouracil by IV or oral leucovorin or by interferon in advanced colorectal cancer: an ECOG/CALGB phase III trial. *Proc Am Soc Clin Oncol* 1996;15:469.

292. Efficacy of intravenous continuous infusion of fluorouracil compared with bolus administration in advanced colorectal cancer. Meta-analysis Group in Cancer. *J Clin Oncol* 1998;16:301.

293. Ardalan B, Chua C, Tian EM, et al. A phase II study of weekly 24-hour infusion with high dose fluorouracil with leucovorin in colorectal carcinoma. *J Clin Oncol* 1991;9:625.

294. Kohne CH, Schoffski P, Wilke H, et al. Effective biomodulation by leucovorin of high-dose infusion fluorouracil given as a weekly 24-hour infusion: results of a randomized trial in patients with advanced colorectal cancer. *J Clin Oncol* 1998;16:418.

295. Kohne CH, Wils J, Lorenz M, et al. Randomized phase III study of high-dose fluorouracil given as a weekly 24-hour infusion with or without leucovorin versus bolus fluorouracil plus leucovorin in advanced colorectal cancer: European Organization of Research and Treatment of Cancer Gastrointestinal Group Study 40952. *J Clin Oncol* 2003.

296. de Gramont A, Bosset JF, Milan C, et al. Randomized trial comparing monthly low-dose leucovorin and fluorouracil bolus with bimonthly high-dose leucovorin and fluorouracil bolus plus continuous infusion for advanced colorectal cancer: a French Intergroup study. *J Clin Oncol* 1997;15:808.

297. Enhancement of 5-fluorodeoxyuridylate binding to thymidylate synthase by dihydropteroylpolyglutamates. *Proc Natl Acad Sci U S A* 1980;77:5663.

298. Meta-analysis of randomized trials testing the biochemical modulation of fluorouracil by methotrexate in metastatic colorectal cancer. *J Clin Oncol* 1994;12:960.

299. Grimelius B. Biochemical modulation of 5-fluorouracil: a randomized comparison of sequential methotrexate, 5-fluorouracil and leucovorin in patients with advanced symptomatic colorectal cancer. *Ann Oncol* 1993;4:235.

300. Romanini A, Li WW, Colofiore JR, Bertino JR. Leucovorin enhances cytotoxicity of trimetrexate/fluorouracil, but not methotrexate/fluorouracil, in CCRF-CEM cells. *J Natl Cancer Inst* 2000;84:1033.

301. Lin JT, Bertino JR. Update on trimetrexate, a folate antagonist with antineoplastic and antiprotozoal properties. *Cancer Invest* 1991;9:159.

302. Ajani JA, Abbruzzese JL, Faintuch JS, et al. A phase II study of trimetrexate therapy for metastatic colorectal carcinoma. *Cancer Invest* 1990;8:619.

303. Conti JA, Kemeny N, Seiter K, et al. Trial of sequential trimetrexate, fluorouracil, and high-dose leucovorin in previously treated patients with gastrointestinal carcinoma. *J Clin Oncol* 1994;12:695.

304. Blanke CD, Kasimis B, Schein P, Capizzi R, Kurman M. Phase II study of trimetrexate, fluorouracil, and leucovorin for advanced colorectal cancer. *J Clin Oncol* 1997;15:915.

304a. Blanke C, Cassidy J, Gerhartz H, James RD, Kasimis B. A phase II trial of trimetrexate (TMTX), 5-fluorouracil (5FU), and leucovorin (LCV) in patients (PTS) with previously treated unresectable or metastatic colorectal cancer (CRC). *Proc Am Soc Oncol* 1999;947(abst).

305. Blanke CD, Shultz J, Cox J, et al. A double-blind placebo-controlled randomized phase III trial of 5-fluorouracil and leucovorin, plus or minus trimetrexate, in previously untreated patients with advanced colorectal cancer. *Ann Oncol* 2002;13:87.

306. Punt CJ, Blanke CD, Zhang J, Hammershaimb L. Integrated analysis of overall survival in two randomized studies comparing 5-fluorouracil/leucovorin with or without trimetrexate in advanced colorectal cancer. *Ann Oncol* 2002;13:92.

307. Wadler S, Wersto R, Weinberg V, et al. Interaction of fluorouracil and interferon in human colon cancer cell lines: cytotoxic and cytokinetic effects. *J Cancer Res* 1990;50:5735.

308. Wadler S, Schwartz EL, Goldman M, et al. Fluorouracil and recombinant alfa-2a-interferon: an active regimen against advanced colorectal carcinoma. *J Clin Oncol* 1989;7:1769.
309. Kelsen D, Sammarco P, Adams L, Murray P. Combination 5-fluorouracil and recombinant alpha interferon in advanced colorectal cancer: activity but significant toxicity. *Proc Am Soc Clin Oncol* 2000;9:109.
310. Hill M, Norman A, Cunningham D, et al. Royal Marsden phase III trial of fluorouracil with or without interferon alfa-2b in advanced colorectal cancer. *J Clin Oncol* 1995;13:1297.
311. Greco FA, Figlin R, York M, et al. Phase II randomized study to compare interferon alfa-2a in combination with fluorouracil versus fluorouracil alone in patients with advanced colorectal cancer. *J Clin Oncol* 1996;2674.
312. Dufour P, Husseini F, Dreyfus B, et al. 5-Fluorouracil versus 5-fluorouracil plus alpha interferon as treatment of metastatic colorectal cancer. A randomized study. *Ann Oncol* 1996;7:575.
313. Phase III randomized study of two fluorouracil combinations with either interferon alfa-2a or leucovorin for advanced colorectal cancer. *J Clin Oncol* 1995;13:921.
314. Thirion P, Piedbois P, Buyse M, et al. Alpha-interferon does not increase the efficacy of 5-fluorouracil in advanced colorectal cancer. *Br J Cancer* 2001;84:611.
315. Diasio RB, Johnson MR. Dihydropyrimidine dehydrogenase: its role in 5-fluorouracil clinical toxicity and tumor resistance. *Clin Cancer Res* 1999;5:2672.
316. Ahmed F, Johnston S, Cassidy J, et al. Eniluracil treatment completely inactivates dihydropyrimidine dehydrogenase in colorectal tumors. *J Clin Oncol* 1999;17:2439.
317. Baccanari DP, Davis ST, Kwick VC, Spector T. 5-Ethynyluracil: effects on the pharmacokinetics and antitumor activity of 5-fluorouracil. *Proc Natl Acad Sci U S A* 1993;90:11064.
318. Marsh JC, Catalano P, Huang J, et al. Eastern Cooperative Oncology Group phase II trial (E4296) of oral 5-fluorouracil and eniluracil as a 28-day regimen in metastatic colorectal cancer. *Clin Colorectal Cancer* 2002;2:43.
319. Schuller J, Cassidy J, Dumont E, et al. Preferential activation of capecitabine in tumor following oral administration to colorectal cancer patients. *Cancer Chemother Pharmacol* 2000;45:291.
320. Van Cutsem E, Findlay M, Osterwalder B, et al. Capecitabine, an oral fluoropyrimidine carbamate with substantial activity in advanced colorectal cancer: results of a randomized phase II study. *J Clin Oncol* 2000;18:1337.
321. Van Cutsem E, Twelves C, Cassidy J, et al. Oral capecitabine compared with intravenous fluorouracil plus leucovorin in patients with metastatic colorectal cancer: results of a large phase III study. *J Clin Oncol* 2001;19:4097.
322. Hoff PM, Ansari R, Batist G, et al. Comparison of oral capecitabine versus intravenous fluorouracil plus leucovorin as first-line treatment in 605 patients with metastatic colorectal cancer: results of a randomized phase III study. *J Clin Oncol* 2001;19:2282.
323. Cassidy J, Twelves C, Van Cutsem E, et al. First-line oral capecitabine therapy in metastatic colorectal cancer: a favorable safety profile compared with intravenous 5-fluorouracil/leucovorin. *Ann Oncol* 2002;13:566.
324. Saltz LB, Leichman CG, Young CW, et al. A fixed-ratio combination of uracil and Ftorafur (UFT) with low dose leucovorin. An active oral regimen for advanced colorectal cancer. *Cancer* 1995;75:782.
325. Pazdur R, Lassere Y, Rhodes V, et al. Phase II trials of uracil and tegafur plus oral leucovorin: an effective oral regimen in the treatment of metastatic colorectal cancer. *J Clin Oncol* 1994;12:2296.
326. Douillard JY, Hoff PM, Skillings JR, et al. Multicenter phase III study of uracil/tegafur and oral leucovorin versus fluorouracil and leucovorin in patients with previously untreated metastatic colorectal cancer. *J Clin Oncol* 2002;20:3605.
327. Carmichael J, Popiela T, Radstone D, et al. Randomized comparative study of tegafur/uracil and oral leucovorin versus parenteral fluorouracil and leucovorin in patients with previously untreated metastatic colorectal cancer. *J Clin Oncol* 2002;20:3617.
328. Cocconi G, Cunningham D, Cutsem E et al. Open, randomized, multicenter trial of raltitrexed versus fluorouracil plus high-dose leucovorin in patients with advanced colorectal cancer. Tomudex Colorectal Cancer Study Group. *J Clin Oncol* 1998;16:2943.
329. Farrugia DC, Ford HE, Cunningham D, et al. Thymidylate synthase expression in advanced colorectal cancer predicts for response to raltitrexed. *Clin Cancer Res* 2003;9:792.
330. Haskell CM, Selch MT. Colon and rectum. In: Haskell CM, ed. *Cancer treatment*. Philadelphia: Saunders, 1990:232.
331. Pizzolato JF, Saltz LB. The camptothecins. *Lancet* 2003;361:2235.
332. Kawato Y, Aonuma M, Hirota Y, Kuga H, Sato K. Intracellular roles of SN-38, a metabolite of the camptothecin derivative CPT-11, in the antitumor effect of CPT-11. *Cancer Res* 1991;51:4187.
333. Negoro S, Fukuoka M, Masuda N, et al. Phase I study of weekly intravenous infusions of CPT-11, a new derivative of camptothecin, in the treatment of advanced non-small-cell lung cancer. *J Natl Cancer Inst* 1991;83:1164.
334. Ohe Y, Sasaki Y, Shinkai T, et al. Phase I study and pharmacokinetics of CPT-11 with 5-day continuous infusion. *J Natl Cancer Inst* 1992;84:972.
335. Rothenberg ML, Kuhn JG, Burris HA 3rd, et al. Phase I and pharmacokinetic trial of weekly CPT-11. *J Clin Oncol* 1993;11:2194.
336. Rowinsky EK., Growchow LB, Ettinger DS, et al. Phase I and pharmacological study of the novel topoisomerase inhibitor 7-ethyl-10-[4-(1-piperidino)-1-piperidino]carbonyloxycamptothecin (CPT-11) administered as a ninety minute infusion every three weeks. *Cancer Res* 1994;54:427.
337. Abigerges D, Chabot GG, Armand JP, et al. Phase I and pharmacologic studies of the camptothecin analogue irinotecan administered every three weeks in cancer patients. *J Clin Oncol* 1995;13:210.
338. Shimada Y, Yoshino M, Wakui A, et al. Phase II study of CPT-11, a new camptothecin derivative, in metastatic colorectal cancer. *J Clin Oncol* 1993;11:909.
339. Rothenberg ML, Ekardt JR, Kuhn JG, et al. Phase II trial of Irinotecan in patients with progressive or rapidly recurrent colorectal cancer. *J Clin Oncol* 1996;14:1128.
340. Von Hoff DD, Rothenberg ML, Pitot HC, et al. Irinotecan therapy for patients with previously treated metastatic colorectal cancer. Overall results of FDA-reviewed pivotal U.S. clinical trials. *Proc Am Soc Clin Oncol* 1997;16:a803.
341. Rougier P, Bugat R, Douillard JY, et al. A phase II study of CPT-11 (irinotecan) in the treatment of advanced colorectal cancer in chemotherapy-naive patients and patients pretreated with 5-FU-based chemotherapy. *J Clin Oncol* 1997;15:251.
342. Conti JA, Kemeny NE, Saltz LB, et al. Irinotecan is an active agent in untreated patients with metastatic colorectal cancer. *J Clin Oncol* 1996;14:709.
343. Pitot HC, Wender MJ, O'Connell M. A phase II trial of CPT-11 (irinotecan) in patients with metastatic colorectal carcinoma: a North Central Cancer Treatment Group (NCCTG) Study. *Proc Am Soc Clin Oncol* 1994;13:a573.
344. Cunningham D, Pyrhonen S, James R, et al. Randomized trial of irinotecan plus supportive care versus supportive care alone after fluorouracil failure for patients with metastatic colorectal cancer. *Lancet* 1998;352:1413.
345. Rougier P, Van Cutsem E, Bajetta E, et al. Randomized trial of irinotecan versus fluorouracil by continuous infusion after fluorouracil failure in patients with metastatic colorectal cancer. *Lancet* 1998;352:1407.
346. Gandia D, Abigerges D, Armand JP, et al. CPT-11 induced cholinergic effects in cancer patients. *J Clin Oncol* 1993;11:196.
347. Abigerges D, Armand JP, Chabot GG, et al. High dose intensity CPT-11 administered as a single dose every 3 weeks: the Institut Gustave Roussy experience. *Proc Am Soc Clin Oncol* 1993;12:133.
348. Fuchs CS, Moore MR, Harker G, et al. Phase III comparison of two irinotecan dosing regimens in second-line therapy of metastatic colorectal cancer. *J Clin Oncol* 2003;21:807.
349. Saltz L, Kanowitz J, Kemeny N, et al. A phase I clinical and pharmacologic trial of irinotecan, 5-fluorouracil, and leucovorin in patients with advanced solid tumors. *J Clin Oncol* 1996;14:2959.
350. Saltz LB, Cox JV, Blanke C, et al. Irinotecan plus fluorouracil and leucovorin for metastatic colorectal cancer. Irinotecan Study Group. *N Engl J Med* 2000;343:905.
351. Douillard JY, Cunningham D, Roth AD, et al. Irinotecan combined with fluorouracil compared with fluorouracil alone as first-line treatment for metastatic colorectal cancer: a multicentre randomized trial. *Lancet* 2000;355:1041.
352. Andre T, Louvet C, Maindrault-Goebel F, et al. CPT-11 (irinotecan) addition to bimonthly, high-dose leucovorin and bolus and continuous-infusion 5-fluorouracil (FOLFIRI) for pretreated metastatic colorectal cancer. GERCOR. *Eur J Cancer* 1999;35:1343.
353. Raymond E, Lawrence R, Izbicka E, Faivre S, Von Hoff DD. Activity of oxaliplatin against human tumor colony-forming units. *Clin Cancer Res* 1998;4:1021.
354. Mathe G, Kidani Y, Segiguchi M, et al. Oxalato-platinum or 1-OHP, a third-generation platinum complex: an experimental and clinical appraisal and preliminary comparison with cis-platinum and carboplatinum. *Biomed Pharmacother* 1989;43:237.
355. Scheeff ED, Briggs JM, Howell SB. Molecular modeling of the intrastrand guanine-guanine DNA adducts produced by cisplatin and oxaliplatin. *Mol Pharmacol* 1999;56:633.
356. Extra JM, Espie M, Calvo F, et al. Phase I study of oxaliplatin in patients with advanced cancer. *Cancer Chemother Pharmacol* 1990;25:299.
357. Raymond E, Chaney SG, Taamma A, Cvitkovic E. Oxaliplatin: a review of preclinical and clinical studies. *Ann Oncol* 1998;9:1053.
358. Diaz-Rubio E, Sastre J, Zaniboni A, et al. Oxaliplatin as single agent in previously untreated colorectal carcinoma patients: a phase II multicentric study. *Ann Oncol* 1998;9:105.
359. Becouarn Y, Ychou M, Ducreux M, et al. Phase II trial of oxaliplatin as first-line chemotherapy in metastatic colorectal cancer patients. Digestive Group of French Federation of Cancer Centers. *J Clin Oncol* 1998;16:2739.
360. Machover D, Diaz-Rubio E, de Gramont A, et al. Two consecutive phase II studies of oxaliplatin (L-OHP) for treatment of patients with advanced colorectal carcinoma who were resistant to previous treatment with fluoropyrimidines. *Ann Oncol* 1996;7:95.
361. Caussanel JP, Levi F, Brienza S, et al. Phase I trial of 5-day continuous venous infusion of oxaliplatin at circadian rhythm-modulated rate compared with constant rate. *J Natl Cancer Inst* 1990;82:1046.
362. Levi F, Zidani R, Misset JL. Randomized multicentre trial of chronotherapy with oxaliplatin, fluorouracil, and folinic acid in metastatic colorectal cancer. International Organization for Cancer Chronotherapy. *Lancet* 1997;350:681.
363. Bertheault-Cvitkovic F, Jami A, Ithzaki M, et al. Biweekly intensified ambulatory chronomodulated chemotherapy with oxaliplatin, fluorouracil, and leucovorin in patients with metastatic colorectal cancer. *J Clin Oncol* 1996;14:2950.
364. Giacchetti S, Perpoint B, Zidani R, et al. Phase III multicenter randomized trial of oxaliplatin added to chronomodulated fluorouracil-leucovorin as first-line treatment of metastatic colorectal cancer. *J Clin Oncol* 2000;18:136.
365. de Gramont A, Vignoud J, Tournigand C, et al. Oxaliplatin with high-dose leucovorin and 5-fluorouracil 48-hour continuous infusion in pretreated metastatic colorectal cancer. *Eur J Cancer* 1997;33:214.
366. Andre T, Bensmaine MA, Louvet C, et al. Multicenter phase II study of bimonthly high-dose leucovorin, fluorouracil infusion, and oxaliplatin for metastatic colorectal cancer resistant to the same leucovorin and fluorouracil regimen. *J Clin Oncol* 1999;17:3560.
367. de Gramont A, Figer A, Seymour M, et al. Leucovorin and fluorouracil with or without oxaliplatin as first-line treatment in advanced colorectal cancer. *J Clin Oncol* 2000;18:2938.
368. Rothenberg ML, Oza AM, Bigelow RH, et al. Superiority of oxaliplatin and fluorouracil-leucovorin compared with either therapy alone in patients with progressive colorectal cancer after irinotecan and fluorouracil-leucovorin: interim results of a phase III trial. *J Clin Oncol* 2003;21:2059.
369. Maindrault-Goebel F, Louvet C, Andre T, et al. Oxaliplatin added to the simplified bimonthly leucovorin and 5-fluorouracil regimen as second-line therapy for metastatic colorectal cancer (FOLFOX6). GERCOR4. *Eur J Cancer* 1999;35:1338.
370. Andre T, Figer A, Cervantes G, et al. FOLFOX7 compared to FOLFOX4. Preliminary results of the randomized optimox study. *Proc Am Soc Clin Oncol* 2003;22.
371. Tournigand C, Louvet C, Quinaux E, et al. FOLFIRI followed by FOLFOX versus FOLFOX followed by FOLFIRI in Metastic Colorectal Cancer (MCRC): final results of a phase III study. *Proc Am Soc Clin Oncol* 2001;20.

372. Colucci G, Maiello E, Gebbia V, et al. Preliminary results of a randomized multicenter trial of the Grupo Oncologico Italia Meridionale (GOIM) comparing FOLFIRI vs FOLFOX in advanced colorectal cancer (ACC) patients. *Proc Am Soc Clin Oncol* 2003;22.

373. Goldberg RM, Kaufmann SH, Atherton P, et al. A phase I study of sequential irinotecan and 5-fluorouracil/leucovorin. *Ann Oncol* 2002;13:1674.

374. Miller L, Emanuel D, Elfring G, Barker K, Saltz L. 60-Day, all-cause mortality with first-line irinotecan/fluorouracil/leucovorin (IFL) or fluorouracil/leucovorin (FL) for metastatic colorectal cancer (MCRC). *Proc Am Soc Clin Oncol* 2002;21.

375. Goldberg R, Morton RF, Sargent DJ, et al. N9741: oxaliplatin (Oxali) or CPT-11 + 5-fluorouracil (5FU)/leucovorin (LV) or oxal + CPT-11 in advanced colorectal cancer (CRC). Updated efficacy and quality of life (QOL) data from an intergroup study. *Proc Am Soc Clin Oncol* 2003;22.

376. Goldberg RM. N9741: a phase III study comparing irinotecan to oxaliplatin-containing regimens in advanced colorectal cancer. *Clin Colorectal Cancer* 2002;2:81.

377. Hochster H, Chachoua A, Speyer J, et al. Oxaliplatin with weekly bolus fluorouracil and low-dose leucovorin as first-line therapy for patients with colorectal cancer. *J Clin Oncol* 2003;21:2703.

378. Artru P, Taieb J, Tournigand C, et al. FOLFOX 7/FOLFIRI (MIROX) regiment as (neo)adjuvant chemotherapy for patients with resectable metastatic colorectal cancer: preliminary results. *Proc Am Soc Clin Oncol* 2002;21.

379. Souglakos J, Mavroudis D, Kakolyris S, et al. Triplet combination with irinotecan plus oxaliplatin plus continuous-infusion fluorouracil and leucovorin as first-line treatment in metastatic colorectal cancer: a multicenter phase II trial. *J Clin Oncol* 2002;20:2651.

380. Falcone A, Masi G, Allegrini G, et al. Biweekly chemotherapy with oxaliplatin, irinotecan, infusional fluorouracil, and leucovorin: a pilot study in patients with metastatic colorectal cancer. *J Clin Oncol* 2002;20:4006.

381. Van Cutsem E, Twelves C, Tabernero J, et al. XELOX: mature results of a multinational, phase II trial of capecitabine plus oxaliplatin, an effective 1st line option for patients (pts) with metastatic colorectal cancer (MCRC). *Proc Am Soc Clin Oncol* 2003;22.

382. Bugat R, Douillard J-Y, Perrier H, et al. France TEGAFIRI, A new combination of UFT/LV and irinotecan as first line treatment in patients (pts) with nonresectable metastatic colorectal cancer (CRC): preliminary results of a multicenter phase II trial. American Society of Clinical Oncology Annual Meeting. 2003;343.

383. Scheithauer W, Kornek GV, Raderer M, et al. Randomized multicenter phase II trial of two different schedules of capecitabine plus oxaliplatin as first-line treatment in advanced colorectal cancer. *J Clin Oncol* 2003;21:1307.

384. Maughan TS, James RD, Kerr DJ, et al. Comparison of intermittent and continuous palliative chemotherapy for advanced colorectal cancer: a multicentre randomized trial. *Lancet* 2003;361:457.

385. Yeoh C, Chau I, Cunningham D, et al. Impact of 5-fluorouracil rechallenge on subsequent response and survival in advanced colorectal cancer: pooled analysis from three consecutive randomized controlled trials. *Clin Colorectal Cancer* 2003;3:102.

386. Lal KR, Norman AR, Ross PJ, et al. A phase II, randomized, multicentre, trial of irinotecan until disease progression (PD) versus up to 8 cycles, in advanced colorectal cancer (CRC) resistant to fluoropyrimidines. American Society of Clinical Oncology Annual Meeting. 2003;254.

387. Kabbinavar F, Hurwitz HI, Fehrenbacher L, et al. Phase II, randomized trial comparing bevacizumab plus fluorouracil (FU)/leucovorin (LV) with FU/LV alone in patients with metastatic colorectal cancer. *J Clin Oncol* 2003;21:60.

388. Hurwitz H, Fehrenbacher L, Novotny W, et al. Bevacizumab plus irinotecan, fluorouracil, and leucovorin for metastatic colorectal cancer. *N Engl J Med* 2004;350:2335.

389. Carpenter G, Cohen S. Epidermal growth factor. *J Biol Chem* 1990;265:7709.

390. Brentjen R, Saltz L. Epidermal growth factor receptor blockade and treatment of solid tumor malignancies. In: DeVita JVT, Hellman S, Rosenberg SA, eds. *Progress in oncology.* Boston: Jones and Bartlett, 2002:113.

391. Saltz L, Rubin M, Hochster H, et al. Cetuximab (IMC-C225) plus irinotecan (CPT-11) is active in CPT-11-refractory colorectal cancer (CRC) that expresses epidermal growth factor receptor (EGFR). *Proc Am Soc Clin Oncol* 2001;20.

392. Saltz L, Meropol NJ, Loehrer PJ, et al. Phase II trial of cetuximab in patients with refractory colorectal cancer that expresses the epidermal growth factor receptor. *J Clin Oncol* 2004;22:1201.

393. Cunningham D, Humblet Y, Siena S, et al. Cetuximab (C225) alone or in combination with irinotecan (CPT-11) in patients with epidermal growth factor receptor (EGFR)-positive, irinotecan-refractory metastatic colorectal cancer (MCRC). American Society of Clinical Oncology Annual Meeting. 2003;252.

394. Rosenberg AH, Loehrer PJ, Needle MN, et al. Erbitux (IMC-C225) plus weekly irinotecan (CPT-11), fluorouracil (5FU) and leucovorin (LV) in colorectal cancer (CRC) that expresses the epidermal growth factor receptor (EGFr). American Society of Clinical Oncology. 2002;135a.

395. Van Laethem JL, Raoul JL, Mitry E, et al. Cetuximab (C225) in combination with biweekly irinotecan (CPT-11), infusional 5-fluorouracil (5-FU) and folinic acid (FA) in patients (pts) with metastatic colorectal cancer (CRC) expressing the epidermal growth factor receptor (EGFR). Preliminary safety and efficacy results. *Proc Am Soc Clin Oncol* 2003;22.

396. Meropol NJ, Berlin J, Hecht JR, et al. CA multicenter study of ABX-EGF monotherapy in patients with metastatic colorectal cancer. *Proc Am Soc Clin Oncol* 2003;256.

397. Dorligschaw O, Kegel T, Jordan K, et al. ZD 1839 (Iressa)-based treatment as last-line therapy in patients with advanced colorectal cancer (ACRC). *Proc Am Soc Clin Oncol* 2003;22.

398. Oza AM, Townsley CA, Siu LL, et al. Phase II study of erlotinib (OSI-774) in patients with metastatic colorectal cancer. *Proc Am Soc Clin Oncol* 2003;22.

399. Blanke CD. Celecoxib with chemotherapy in colorectal cancer. *Oncology (Huntingt)* 2002;16:17.

400. Thomas AL, Morgan B, Drevs J, et al. Vascular endothelial growth factor receptor tyrosine kinase inhibitors: PTK787/ZK 222584. *Semin Oncol* 2003;30:32.

401. Trarbach T, Schleucher N, Riedel U, et al. Phase I study of the oral vascular endothelial growth factor (VEGF) receptor inhibitor PTK787/ZK 222584 (PTK/ZK) in combination with irinotecan/5-fluorouracil/leucovorin in patients with metastatic colorectal cancer. *Proc Am Soc Clin Oncol* 2003;22.

402. Steward WP, Thomas AL, Morgan B, et al. Extended phase I study of the oral vascular endothelial growth factor (VEGF) receptor inhibitor PTK787/ZK 222584 in combination with oxaliplatin/5-fluorouracil (5-FU)/leucovorin as first line treatment for metastatic colorectal cancer. *Proc Am Soc Clin Oncol* 2003;22.

403. Gadgeel SM, LoRusso PM, Wozniak AJ, Wheeler C. A dose-escalation study of the novel vascular-targeting agent, ZD6126, in patients with solid tumors. *Proc Am Soc Clin Oncol* 2002;21.

404. Nahum K, Shiba D, Padavanija P, et al. Phase II efficacy and tolerability study of edotecarin (J-107088) in patients with irinotecan-naïve metastatic colorectal cancer (MCRC). *Proc Am Soc Clin Oncol* 2003;22.

405. Kerr DJ, McArdle CS, Ledermann J, et al. Intrahepatic arterial versus intravenous fluorouracil and folinic acid for colorectal cancer liver metastases: a multicentre randomized trial. *Lancet* 2003;361:3683.

406. Salonga D, Danenberg KD, Johnson M, et al. Colorectal tumors responding to 5-fluorouracil have low gene expression levels of dihydropyrimidine dehydrogenase, thymidylate synthase, and thymidine phosphorylase. *Clin Cancer Res* 2000;6:1322.

407. Metzger R, Danenberg K, Leichman CG, et al. High basal level gene expression of thymidine phosphorylase (platelet-derived endothelial cell growth factor) in colorectal tumors is associated with nonresponse to 5-fluorouracil. *Clin Cancer Res* 1998;4:2371.

408. Iqbal S, Lenz HJ. Targeted therapy and pharmacogenomic programs. *Cancer* 2003;97:2076.

409. Lonneux M, Reffad AM, Detry R, et al. FDG-PET improves the staging and selection of patients with recurrent colorectal cancer. *Eur J Nucl Med Mol Imaging* 2002;29:915.

410. Desai DC, Zervos EE, Arnold MW, et al. Positron emission tomography affects surgical management in recurrent colorectal cancer patients. *Ann Surg Oncol* 2003;10:59.

411. Temple L, Wong WD, Schrag D. Stage IV colorectal cancer: How often do we operate? Insights from the Surveillance, Epidemiology and End Results (SEER)/Medicare Data. *Proc Am Soc Clin Oncol* 2003;22.

412. Tebbutt NC, Norman AR, Cunningham D, et al. Intestinal complications after chemotherapy for patients with unresected primary colorectal cancer and synchronous metastases. *Gut* 2003;52:568.

413. Scoggins CR, Meszoely IM, Blanke CD, Beauchamp RD, Leach SD. Nonoperative management of primary colorectal cancer in patients with stage IV disease. *Ann Surg Oncol* 1999;6:651.

414. Baron TH. Expandable metal stents for the treatment of cancerous obstruction of the gastrointestinal tract. *N Engl J Med* 2001;344:1681.

415. Moertel CG, Weiland LH, Nagorney DM, Dockerty MB. Carcinoid tumor of the appendix: treatment and prognosis. *N Engl J Med* 1987;317:1699.

416. Moertel CG, Dockerty MB, Judd ES. Carcinoid tumors of the vermiform appendix. *Cancer* 1968;21:270.

417. Moertel CG. Karnofsky memorial lecture. An odyssey in the land of small tumors. *J Clin Oncol* 1987;5:1502.

418. Wick M, Weatherby R, Weiland L. Small cell neuroendocrine carcinoma of the colon and rectum: clinical, histologic, and ultrastructural study and immunohistochemical comparison with cloacogenic carcinoma. *Hum Pathol* 1987;18:9.

419. Busch E, Rodriguez-Bigas M, Mamounas E, Barcos M, Petrelli NJ. Primary colorectal non-Hodgkin's lymphoma. *Ann Surg Oncol* 1994;1:222.

420. Shepherd N, Hall P, Coates P, Levison D. Primary malignant lymphoma of the colon and rectum. A histopathological and immunohistochemical analysis of 45 cases with clinicopathological correlations. *Histopathology* 1988;12:235.

421. Cheng P. Unusual tumors of the colon, rectum and anus. In: Raghavan D, Brecher M, Johnson D, et al., eds. In: *Textbook of uncommon cancer.* Chichester: John Wiley & Sons, 1999:439.

422. Fan CW, Changchien CR, Wang JY, et al. Primary colorectal lymphoma. *Dis Colon Rectum* 2000;43:1277.

423. Hwang W, Yao J, Cheng S, Tseng H. Primary colorectal lymphoma in Taiwan. *Cancer* 1992;70:575.

424. Winawer S, Fletcher R, Rex D, et al. Colorectal cancer screening and surveillance: clinical guidelines and rationale—update based on new evidence. *Gastroenterology* 2003;124:544.

425. Rex DK, Johnson DA, Lieberman DA, Burt RW, Sonnenberg A. Colorectal cancer prevention 2000: screening recommendations of the American College of Gastroenterology. American College of Gastroenterology. *Am J Gastroenterol* 2000;95:868.

426. Willett CG, Tepper JE, Cohen AM, Orlow E, Welch CE. Failure patterns following curative resection of colonic carcinoma. *Ann Surg* 1984;200:685.

427. Minsky BD, Mies C, Rich TA, Recht A, Chaffey JT. Potentially curative surgery of colon cancer: patterns of failure and survival. *J Clin Oncol* 1988;6:106.

428. Grothey A, Deschler B, Kroening H, et al. Phase III study of bolus 5-fluorouracil (5-FU)/ folinic acid (FA) (Mayo) vs weekly high-dose 24h 5-FU infusion/FA + oxaliplatin (OXA) (FUFOX) in advanced colorectal cancer (ACRC). *Am Soc Clin Oncol* 2002;129a.

STEVEN K. LIBUTTI
JOEL E. TEPPER
LEONARD B. SALTZ
ANIL K. RUSTGI

SECTION 9

Cancer of the Rectum

Chapter 29.8, Cancer of the Colon, covers information concerning epidemiology, molecular biology, and systemic approaches to the management of colon and rectal cancer. This chapter focuses on issues unique to rectal cancer, with an emphasis on radiation combined modality therapy and sphincter-preserving surgery.

ANATOMY

The anatomy of the rectum can be very confusing, as there are differing definitions of the relevant landmarks. In the upper portion are changes in the musculature of the large bowel and in the relationship to the peritoneal covering, which roughly coincide, and in the lower portion the mucosal changes occur at roughly the same location as the location of the anal sphincter.

The rectum is usually divided into three portions (Fig. 29.9-1). The lower rectum is the area approximately 3 to 6 cm from the anal verge. The midrectum goes from 5 to 6 cm to 8 to 10 cm, and the upper rectum extends approximately from 8 to 10 cm to 12 to 15 cm, from the anal verge, although the retroperitoneal portion of the large bowel often reaches its upper limit at approximately 12 cm from the anal verge. In some patients, especially elderly women, the peritonealized portion of the large bowel can be located much lower than these usual definitions. The determination of the location of the boundary between the rectum and sigmoid colon is important in defining adjuvant therapy, with the rectum usually being operationally defined as that area of the large bowel that is at least partially retroperitoneal.

Externally, the upper extent of the rectum can be identified where the tenia spread to form a longitudinal coat of muscle. The upper third of the rectum is surrounded by peritoneum on its anterior and lateral surfaces but is retroperitoneal posteriorly without any serosal covering. At the rectovesical or rectouterine pouch, the rectum becomes completely extra(retro)peritoneal. The rectum follows the curve of the sacrum in its lower two-thirds. It enters the anal canal at the level of the levator ani. The anorectal ring is at the level of the puborectalis sling portion of the levator muscles.

The location of a rectal tumor is most commonly indicated by the distance between the anal verge, dentate (pectinate or mucocutaneous) line, or anorectal ring and the lower edge of the tumor. These points of reference are all different. Also, these measurements differ depending on the use of a rigid or flexible endoscope. This can be important clinically, as the measurement from a flexible endoscopy can substantially overestimate the distance to the tumor from the anal verge or other landmark. The distance from the anal sphincter musculature is clinically of more importance than the distance from the anal verge, as it has implications for the ability to perform sphincter-sparing surgery. The lack of a peritoneal covering over most of the rectum is a major reason for the higher risk for local failure after primary surgical management than for colon cancer. The mesorectum is

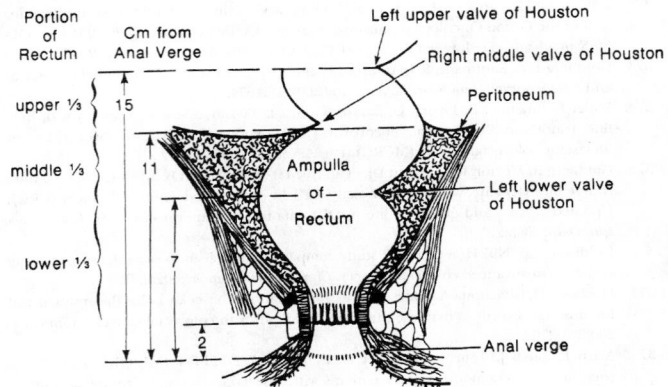

FIGURE 29.9-1. Division of the rectum into upper, middle, and lower thirds.

usually described as the structure defining the extent of a total mesorectal excision (TME), with most of the perirectal fatty tissue and perirectal lymph nodes contained within its boundaries.

LYMPHATIC DRAINAGE

The lymphatic drainage of the upper rectum follows the course of the superior hemorrhoidal artery toward the inferior mesenteric artery. Lymph nodes that are above the midrectum and therefore drain along the superior hemorrhoidal artery are often part of the mesentery that is removed during resections of the intraperitoneal portion of the colon. Lesions that arise in the rectum below approximately 6 cm are in a region of the rectum drained by lymphatics that follow the middle hemorrhoidal artery. Nodes involved from a cancer in this region can include the internal iliac nodes and the nodes of the obturator fossa. These regions deserve particular attention during the resection of lesions in this location. When lesions occur below the dentate line, the lymphatic drainage is via the inguinal nodes, which has major therapeutic implications, especially for the radiation fields. The corollary of this high risk of inguinal node involvement for the very low-lying tumors is that tumors located above the dentate line are at low risk of inguinal node involvement and these nodes, as well as the external iliacs, do not need to be treated.

BOWEL FUNCTION

Fecal continence is maintained through the function of sphincter control and the preservation of the normal muscular anatomy, which creates a neorectal angle or rectal sling. The pelvic floor is composed of the levator ani muscles, which separate the pelvis from the perineum and ischiorectal fossa. The urethra, vagina, and anus pass through the levators.

Preservation of fecal continence during surgery for rectal cancer is therefore dependent on a thorough understanding of the anatomic relationships of the musculature and the sphincter mechanisms. Maintenance of the sphincter apparatus without preservation of the muscular angles will not have the desired result. These anatomic constraints, especially with respect to lateral margins, make the use of adjuvant chemotherapy and radiation therapy critical to a successful surgical outcome. This is true from an oncologic as well as a bowel function perspective.

AUTONOMIC NERVES

The preservation of bladder and sexual function is dependent on the surgeon's understanding of the autonomic nerve supply to the pelvic organs.[1,2] The hypogastric plexus is formed from the sympathetic trunks as they converge over the sacral promontory. These sympathetic nerves are found underneath the pelvic peritoneum along the lateral pelvic sidewalls lateral to the mesorectum. The second, third, and fourth sacral nerve roots give rise to parasympathetic fibers to the pelvic viscera. The parasympathetic fibers proceed laterally as the nervi erigentes to join the sympathetic fibers at the site of the pelvic plexus that is just lateral and somewhat anterior to the tips of the seminal vesicle in men.[1,2] To preserve these structures and therefore sexual and bladder function, a sharp rather than a blunt technique should be used to dissect the region of the mesorectum.[3–6]

STAGING

Standard clinicopathologic staging is the best indicator of prognosis of patients with rectal cancer. For rectal cancer, it is increasingly common to use clinical staging on which to base the decision for neoadjuvant chemoradiation therapy. Therefore, the accuracy of that initial staging is critically important, for management and prognosis. A large number of studies have evaluated other prognostic markers, including pathologic, socioeconomic, molecular, and others, as described more fully in Chapter 29.8. However, even though many of these appear to have prognostic value, none are commonly used to define management. This is related to the large number of tests that could be used, the lack of standardization of these tests, and the lack of knowledge as to how to incorporate them into the patient management scheme. The molecular marker that has engendered the most interest is the deletion of 18q (DCC).[7] These markers have been fully reviewed elsewhere.[8,9]

The staging system, which should be used in the evaluation of patients with rectal cancer, is the American Joint Committee on Cancer/Union Internationale Contre le Cancer tumor, node, metastasis (TNM) staging system, which is fully described in Chapter 29.8 and has been revised to subcategorize patients with stage III (node-positive) tumors. The Dukes' staging system or its multiple modifications were used for many years but provides less information than the TNM system and should not be used. Gradual changes have been made in the TNM system that primarily reflect the stage grouping rather than the system itself. The other systems should be acknowledged for their historic interest and for initially defining many of the high-risk factors for this disease.

Patients now often have a clinical (preoperative) staging, which may define the use of neoadjuvant therapy and a postoperative surgical stage. However, it is important to remember that initial therapy with radiation therapy and chemotherapy can produce substantial down-staging (approximately 15% of patients have a pathologic complete response) and that subsequent therapy should be based on the initial T and N staging determination. Specifically, a good tumor response locally to radiation and chemotherapy does not mean that a patient has any lower risk of having micrometastatic disease and thus does not have a lesser need for adjuvant postoperative chemotherapy. Put another way, in a patient who receives preoperative radiation therapy and chemotherapy, there is no decision point regarding whether or not postoperative chemotherapy should be given on the basis of the surgical pathology result. The plan for postoperative chemotherapy should be carried out even in the setting of a pathologic complete response.

The major change that has occurred in the newest version of the staging system is the acknowledgment that the T stage and the N stage have independent prognostic importance for local control, disease-free survival, and survival.[10,11] Thus, for N0 and N1 patients viewed separately, the extent of the primary tumor in the rectum is of additional prognostic importance. Patients with T1 to T2N1 tumors have a relatively favorable prognosis and an outcome superior to that of other stage III patients. These distinctions may allow us in the future to be more individualized in the adjuvant therapy required.

Although at one level staging is very straightforward, the actualities of proper staging are much more difficult, as it relies on multiple quality control issues, which can mislead the clinician regarding proper therapy. For instance, it has been well demonstrated that, for patients who are pathologically staged as N0, the prognosis is markedly improved for those in whom more than approximately 12 to 14 nodes were identified by the pathologist compared to patients in whom fewer nodes were identified.[12] This could be a surgical issue (fewer nodes were removed) or a pathologist issue (fewer nodes were identified), but it suggests that many patients were inappropriately given a lower stage, which could result in inappropriate therapy. Others have shown that staging accuracy continues to improve as the pathologist recovers more nodes, with accuracy leveling off at approximately 12 to 20 nodes recovered.[13,14] The same issue relates to T-stage determination. If the pathologist does not look carefully for evidence of extension of tumor through the muscularis propria, the patient can be under-staged, resulting in inappropriate treatment. Close or positive circumferential margins are a poor prognosticator, which can only be found if the pathologist assiduously evaluates the radial margins.[15,16]

The standard staging procedure for rectal cancer entails a history, physical examination, complete blood count, liver and renal function studies, and carcinoembryonic antigen (CEA). The routine laboratory studies are quite insensitive to the presence of metastatic disease, but they are usually ordered as a screen of organ function before surgery or chemoradiation therapy. High CEA levels are associated with poorer survival (see Chapter 29.8) and give an indication as to whether follow-up CEA determinations are likely to be useful. A careful rectal examination by an experienced examiner is an essential part of the pretherapy evaluation in determining distance of the tumor from the anal verge or from the dentate line, involvement of the anal sphincter, amount of circumferential involvement, clinical fixation, sphincter tone, and so forth, and has not been replaced by imaging studies or endoscopy. Colonoscopy or barium enema to evaluate the remainder of the large bowel is essential (if the patient is not obstructed) to rule out synchronous tumors or the presence of polyp syndromes.

Imaging studies including computed tomography (CT) or magnetic resonance imaging (MRI) to evaluate the pelvis, abdomen, and liver as well as a chest x-ray to screen for pulmonary metastases are now routine. Much debate has taken place about the relative value of CT versus MRI without a clear resolution. Preference is heavily dependent on the institutional expertise and the equipment available. As the technology continues to change, with fine-cut 16 detector row CT scans, improved MRI contrast agents, and so forth, one technique may become slightly better than another.

Conventional CT lacks sufficient accuracy to be used for preoperative staging of the primary tumor site. For example, in one series using air insufflation of the rectal ampulla and IV contrast, the overall T-stage accuracy was approximately 80%, with 18% overstaging in T2 disease and 21% understaging in T3 tumors.[17] As radiologists have usually defined node positivity on CT based on size (typically 1 cm or greater), the overall accuracy of N staging by CT scan has been less than 80% (nodes involved with rectal cancer are usually not markedly enlarged). The same study demonstrated the expected tradeoff between sensitivity and specificity, but with overall accuracy in a similar range. Endoluminal CT colonography is of increasing interest for screening but at the present time has a minimal role in staging patients with known disease.

MRI suffers from some of the same limitations as CT for evaluating the primary tumor, although endorectal coil MRI allows one to discern the layers of the bowel wall and is similar in accuracy to endorectal ultrasound (EUS) (see later). Thin-section pelvic MRI with a surface coil allows for better visualization of the rectal wall layers, but studies to date still show an overall accuracy for T stage in the range of 80%.[18] Because the presence of nodal disease by MRI is also primarily determined by size, the accuracy is similar to that of CT, although defining node positivity based on irregular border or mixed signal intensity could help improve sensitivity and specificity.[19]

CT, MRI, and positron emission tomography (PET) are all useful for detecting metastatic disease, primarily in the liver. CT has an overall sensitivity of 70% to 85%,[20] which might be improved with multidetector CT, although the data do not yet prove that contention. MRI is superior in characterizing liver lesions and distinguishing cysts and hemangiomas from tumor,[21] especially with the use of enhancement with gadolinium or other agents. PET with [18F]fluorodeoxyglucose has engendered a great deal of interest as a method of better defining patients with metastatic disease, especially in abdominal lymph nodes, where CT and MR are relatively insensitive. However, PET is not standard in the preoperative staging at most institutions, and the incremental gain from routine PET scan appears to be small.[22] PET clearly can be of value in restaging patients with recurrence or suspected recurrence to detect additional metastatic sites before attempted resection of metastatic disease. PET shows promise as the most sensitive study for the detection of metastatic disease, in the liver and elsewhere. A metaanalysis of whole body PET showed a sensitivity of 97% and a specificity of 76% in evaluating for recurrent colorectal cancer,[23] but there is little information on PET as an initial staging study.

In the United States at the present time, contrast CT of the pelvis and the abdomen is the most commonly used imaging study, with MRI or PET being used to clarify abnormalities noted in the liver or abdomen. However, primary use of MRI is acceptable and could become standard with changing technology and availability.

Much interest has been shown in the use of EUS for staging of the primary tumor, and this, at present, is the most effective preoperative staging technique for T and N stage. Endorectal MR provides similar information but is not generally available and will not be discussed further. EUS defines five interface layers of the rectal wall: mucosa, muscularis mucosa, submucosa, muscularis propria, and perirectal fat (as shown in Fig. 29.9-2). Rectal tumors are generally hypoechoic and disrupt the interfaces dependent on the level of tumor extension (Figs. 29.9-3 and 29.9-4). The

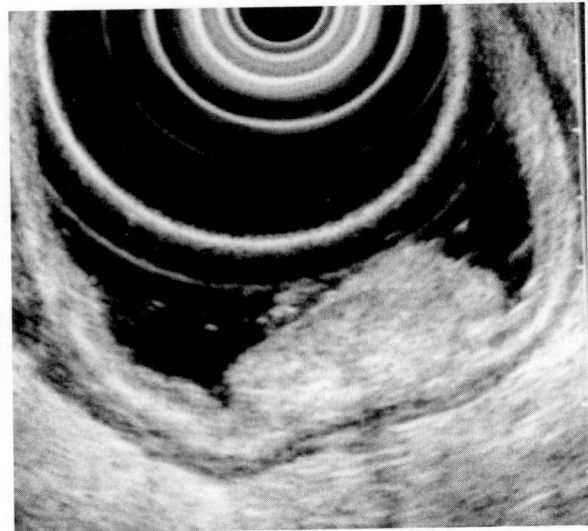

FIGURE 29.9-2. Endorectal ultrasound in a patient with a T1 tumor of the rectum, demonstrating the five layers of the rectal wall. The first layer is hyperechoic and represents the interface between the balloon and the mucosa. The second layer is hypoechoic and is the interface between mucosa and muscularis mucosa. The third layer is hyperechoic and is the submucosa. The fourth layer is hypoechoic and is the muscularis propria. The fifth layer is hyperechoic and is the interface with the perirectal fat. [From Ginsberg GG, Ahmad N. Endoscopic ultrasound for rectal cancer. *VHJOE* 2003;2(2). World Wide Web URL: http://www.vhjoe.org, 2004, with permission.]

accuracy of EUS is heavily dependent on the experience and skill of the operator. The results mentioned below will not be obtained by an inexperienced examiner. However, in experienced hands EUS has an overall accuracy rate for T stage of 75% to 95%, with an overstaging of approximately 10% to 20% in T2 disease, because of an inability to distinguish a desmoplastic response and postbiopsy changes from local tumor invasion and an approximately 10% rate of understaging because of inability to detect microscopic tumor extension.[24–26]

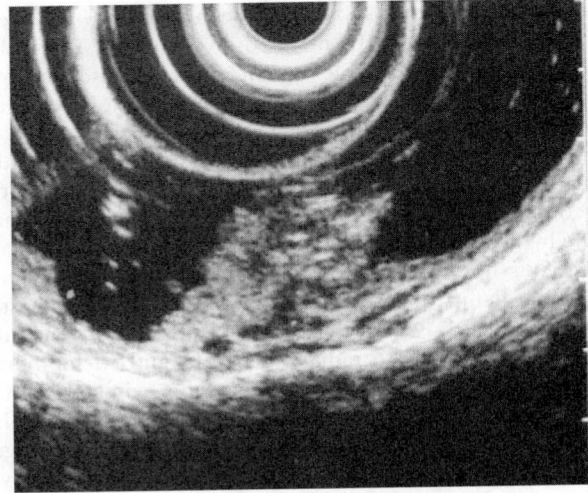

FIGURE 29.9-3. Endorectal ultrasound of a T2 tumor of the rectum; extension into the muscularis propria. [From Ginsberg GG, Ahmad N. Endoscopic ultrasound for rectal cancer. *VHJOE* 2003;2(2). World Wide Web URL: http://www.vhjoe.org, 2004, with permission.]

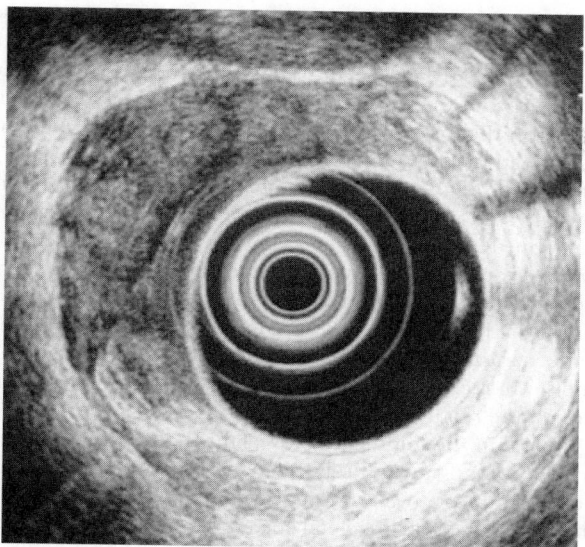

FIGURE 29.9-4. Endorectal ultrasound of a T3 tumor of the rectum; extension through the muscularis propria and into perirectal fat. [From Ginsberg GG, Ahmad N. Endoscopic ultrasound for rectal cancer. *VHJOE* 2003;2(2). World Wide Web URL: http://www.vhjoe.org, 2004, with permission.]

EUS is less accurate in determining N stage than T stage, with an overall accuracy rate of 62% to 83%[24,25] (Fig. 29.9-5). Understaging is due to the fact that many nodal metastases from rectal cancer are small, even micrometastatic, and not easily detected by EUS. In addition, some nodes are located beyond the range of the ultrasound transducer and thus cannot be seen during the procedure. Overstaging is often due to an inflammatory response, perhaps secondary to previous biopsy or manipulation. EUS is not accurate for determining tumor regression after preoperative

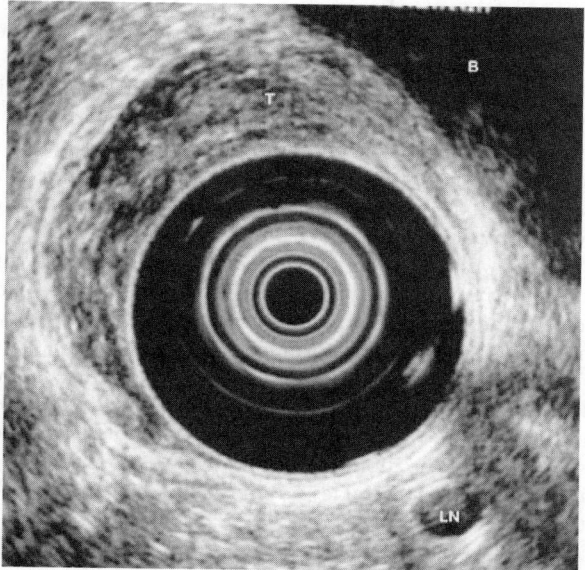

FIGURE 29.9-5. Endorectal ultrasound of a rectal cancer with a positive node in the perirectal fat. B, bladder; LN, lymph node; T, tumor. [From Ginsberg GG, Ahmad N. Endoscopic ultrasound for rectal cancer. *VHJOE* 2003;2(2). World Wide Web URL: http:// www.vhjoe.org, 2004, with permission.]

radiation therapy and chemotherapy, as inflammatory changes and scarring can persist in the rectal wall or in perirectal soft tissue that may not reflect persisting tumor.

SURGERY

The surgical management of primary rectal cancer presents unique problems for the surgeon based, in large part, on the anatomic constraints of the pelvis. Small early-stage lesions of the rectum, which are diagnosed on physical examination or by colonoscopy/proctoscopy, can often be managed with a local resection. Such a local resection can be performed colonoscopically, as described in Chapter 29.8, or lesions can be removed via a transanal excision with the patient positioned in a prone or lithotomy position. Appropriate retractors can provide visualization, and resection should encompass a surrounding margin of normal mucosa[27] and should extend into the perirectal fat.

STAGE I

The treatment of early-stage rectal cancer can be confusing, as many approaches can be used, and patient selection is critical to outcome. In addition, the risk of removal or damage to the anal sphincter is substantial for low-lying tumors and must be taken into consideration, along with the desire not to have a permanent colostomy for early-stage disease. Thus, the options for these patients are primarily those of local therapies without abdominal surgery, abdominal resection of the rectum with anastomosis, and retention of the anal sphincter and abdominal-perineal resection. The last two options are discussed in detail in Stage II and III Rectal Cancer.

For selected T1 and T2 lesions without evidence of nodal disease, transanal excision often provides an adequate resection of the primary tumor mass and can spare the patient the morbidity of a more extensive rectal resection; however, it does not stage the nodal drainage areas and therefore cannot provide as complete staging and management of the tumor as a definitive resection. Tumors considered for local excision must meet a number of criteria to minimize the risk of local-regional failure. Generally, local excision is limited to tumors within 8 to 10 cm of the anal verge, encompass less than 40% of circumference of the bowel wall, are of well-differentiated or moderately well-differentiated histology, and have no pathologic evidence of venous or lymphatic vessel invasion on biopsy. Although it has not been formally proven that these criteria need to be followed, small series have suggested a substantially higher risk of failure after local excision when these criteria have not been met, and most surgeons are reluctant to use local excision for the more extensive T1 or T2 lesions. Even when these criteria have been met, the local recurrence rate can be high after local excision (even when followed by postoperative radiation therapy and chemotherapy), and thus this approach must be used with caution.

Performing a good transanal excision requires substantial surgical expertise, as the surgeon must retain control over the primary tumor and obtain adequate mucosal margins as well as adequate deep resection into perirectal fat. Once removed, the tumor must be well laid out for the pathologist so that all relevant margins can be properly evaluated. For small lesions, there is some experience using preoperative radiation therapy and chemotherapy, but care must be taken to have the site of the primary tumor well marked with a tattoo if this approach is taken, as excellent regression could make identification of the primary site difficult. The staging of such lesions should be performed using EUS to minimize the likelihood of performing a local excision for T3 tumors,[28,29] although there are inaccuracies with this approach.

A posterior proctotomy is useful for large posterior lesions and provides better access to more proximal lesions. This approach is known as a *Kraske's procedure* and is performed by making a posterior longitudinal incision just above the anus to the inferior border of the gluteus maximus. The coccyx is removed, and the underlying levator muscles are divided in a longitudinal fashion in the midline. This approach allows for the mobilization of the rectum and a full-thickness local excision. A transsphincteric excision (Bevan's or York-Mason) involves a similar approach as the posterior proctotomy, except the entire anal sphincter is divided posteriorly in the midline. Most investigators now believe it is appropriate to use adjuvant pelvic radiation therapy with concurrent 5-fluorouracil (5-FU)–based chemotherapy for patients who have had a local excision for T2 tumors and also for selected patients with T1 tumors who have adverse prognostic factors (lymphovascular invasion, close margins, poorly differentiated histology), to decrease the risk of local recurrence.

Another approach that has been used sporadically for patients with early-stage disease is endocavitary radiation therapy. This technique is used for a similar category of patients who are treated with local excision, T1 or T2 tumors less than 3 cm, not poorly differentiated, and with no evidence of nodal involvement. Patients are treated with a special low-energy x-ray machine (50 kVp) that is attached to a rigid endoscopic-type device that can be placed in the rectum directly over the tumor. As the opening of the applicator is 3 cm, it is difficult to treat tumors larger than this, although overlapping fields have been used. Patients typically receive four treatments of 2500 to 3000 cGy each with 2 to 3 weeks between treatments to allow for tumor regression. Although the total dose is extremely high, the minimal penetration of the radiation beam protects the underlying normal tissue. Local control results with this approach have been very good in properly selected patients, but specialized equipment is required and less pathologic information is obtained than after a local excision.

STAGE II AND III RECTAL CANCER

The primary treatment of patients with stage II and III rectal cancer (T3 to T4 and/or N+) is surgical. However, in contrast to the treatment of patients with stage I disease, there is a strong body of information to suggest that combined modality therapy with radiation therapy and chemotherapy should be used in conjunction with surgical resection. This conclusion is based on both patterns of failure data, which demonstrate a substantial incidence of local, regional, and distant disease failure, and the fact that this incidence of tumor recurrence at all sites is decreased with the use of trimodality therapy.

The desire when performing a resection for rectal cancer is to preserve intestinal continuity and the sphincter mechanism whenever possible while still maximizing tumor control. Therefore, careful preoperative screening is crucial in the determination of the location of the lesion and its depth of invasion. Large lesions may respond to preoperative adjuvant chemoradiation and downstage the lesion thereby increasing the likelihood of a successful sphincter-preserving operation. The use of chemotherapy and radiation for this purpose is discussed in greater detail in later sections. As described earlier in Anatomy, it is convenient to think of the rectum as divided into thirds for the purposes of the evaluation and preoperative determination of the surgical approach for resection. The upper third of the rectum is often considered the region of large intestine from the sacral prominence to the peritoneal reflection. These lesions are in almost all cases managed with a low anterior resection in much the same way, as a sigmoid colon cancer (see Chapter 29.8). An adequate 1- to 2-cm distal margin can be achieved for these lesions well above the sphincter mechanism and intestinal continuity restored using either a hand-sewn technique or a circular stapling device inserted through the rectum.[28,30]

Tumors in the middle and lower third of the rectum can be considered as lying entirely below the peritoneal reflection. The resection of these tumors can be challenging due to the confines of the pelvic skeletal structure, and the ability to perform a resection with an adequate distal margin is significantly influenced by the size of the lesion. Nevertheless, tumors of the middle third of the rectum in most cases can be safely resected with a low anterior resection, with restoration of intestinal continuity and preservation of a continent sphincter apparatus.

Lesions in the distal third of the rectum, defined as those within 5 cm of the anal verge, can present the greatest challenge to the surgeon with respect to sphincter preservation. This is often influenced by the extent of lateral invasion of the lesion into the muscles of the sphincter apparatus and how close distally the tumor is to the musculature of the anal canal. The abdominal perineal resection (APR) has historically been considered the standard treatment for patients with rectal cancers located within 6 cm of the anal verge. This procedure requires a transperitoneal as well as a transperineal approach with removal of the entire rectum and sphincter complex. A permanent end-colostomy is created and the perineal wound either closed primarily or left to granulate in after closure of the musculature.

Although an APR is associated with a relatively low rate of local recurrence, it is not without the obvious problems of the need for a permanent colostomy and loss of intestinal continuity and sphincter function. Therefore, intense interest has been focused on developing approaches to the resection of tumors in the distal third of the rectum that would have a high probability of preventing local-regional recurrence and preserve intestinal continuity and sphincter continence.

Tumors within 1 to 2 cm of the dentate line—that is, those that can be removed with at least a 1-cm distal margin—can be resected and intestinal continuity restored with a coloanal anastomosis.[31,32] When performing a very low coloanal anastomosis, it is often prudent to protect the healing suture line with a diverting loop ileostomy, which can be reversed 4 to 6 weeks after the anastomosis has healed. Despite the potential benefits of sphincter preservation, APR is still the most common procedure performed for rectal lesions in the distal and middle third of the rectum.[33]

A review of the published literature demonstrates that between 10% and 67% of procedures for the management of rectal cancers are APR procedures.[31] To increase the number of sphincter-preserving operations performed, several authors cite the use of preoperative chemoradiation as a means to decrease the local recurrence rate.[31,34] They cite statistics that rectal carcinoma responds to preoperative chemoradiation therapy with a 10% to 15% pathologic complete response rate and substantial tumor down-staging. The goal of such an approach would be to reduce the need for APR to an incidence of 10% or less.

When performing a sphincter-preserving operation to preserve the lateral musculature and therefore a functional sphincter complex, the resection by necessity does not have as wide a margin as one performed during an APR. To improve on margin status, intersphincteric resections have been performed.[35] This approach includes a partial sphincteric resection designed to improve margin status without sacrificing sphincter function. In small series, functional results have been comparable to less aggressive sphincter-preserving operations. The impact on oncologic outcome is difficult to interpret and will require larger series.

The choice of a straight coloanal versus a pouch anastomosis is a decision that is based to a large degree on surgeon preference and experience. Some advocate a pouch operation, citing improved anal function as measured by decreased stool frequency and urgency and improved continence.[4] Others have demonstrated that results are equivalent with a straight coloanal anastomosis.[36]

Chemoradiation should be added either preoperatively or postoperatively when performing sphincter-preserving resections for T3 or T4 rectal lesions or for node-positive disease stages II or III. Some evidence has shown that preoperative radiation results in less morbidity than postoperative radiation therapy when a coloanal anastomosis is planned. In a study of 109 patients treated with a low anterior resection and a straight coloanal anastomosis, those receiving preoperative radiation therapy had a lower incidence of adverse effects on anal function than those receiving postoperative radiation.[36] The authors attributed this to sparing of the neorectum from these effects. Relative benefits and outcomes for preoperative chemoradiation versus postoperative chemoradiation are discussed in detail in following sections.

TOTAL MESORECTAL RESECTION

The goal of the resection of rectal tumors is the removal of the tumor with an adequate margin as well as removal of draining lymph nodes and lymphatics to properly stage the tumor and to reduce the risk of recurrence and spread. For lesions in the intraperitoneal colon, the lymphatics and vascular supply are found in the mesentery associated with that region of bowel.

In the rectum, the mesorectum is the structure that contains the blood supply and lymphatics for the upper, middle, and lower rectum. Most involved lymph nodes for rectal cancers are found within the mesorectum, with T1 lesions associated with positive lymph nodes in approximately 57% of cases, T2 lesions with positive lymph nodes in 20% of cases, and T3 and T4 lesions with positive lymph nodes in 65% and 78% of cases.[37]

The anatomy and approach to mesorectal excision are depicted in Figure 29.9-6. This operation involves a sharp dissection occurring in an avascular plane beyond the perirectal fat, which is beyond the region where most of the nodes are located. After a TME the specimen is typically shiny and bilobed, in contrast to the irregular and rough surface after a blunt dissection, where much of the mesorectal fat is left behind. TME attempts not only to clear involved lymph nodes

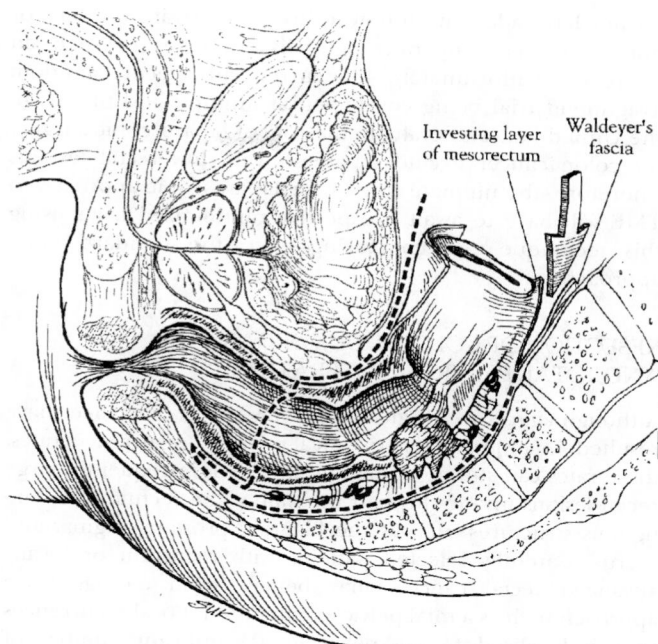

Investing layer of mesorectum

Waldeyer's fascia

FIGURE 29.9-6. Total mesorectal excision.

but also to adequately manage the radial margins of the rectal tumor. These radial margins have been shown to be more important with respect to the risk of local-regional recurrence than the distal mucosal margin.[34,38] Distal mucosal margins of 1 cm or greater are adequate for local control; however, the margin on the mesorectum should extend beyond the distal mucosal margin to ensure a successful surgical outcome.[32,34] A number of studies have demonstrated the benefit of TME, and it is thought by many that this is the procedure of choice for the management of middle- and lower-third rectal cancers.[5,39–41] Although some studies have suggested that an adequate TME might in and of itself be sufficient management for T2 and T3 rectal cancers, the majority of literature still supports the use of adjuvant chemoradiation for stage II and III disease even after a TME.

Large studies of proctectomy with TME have demonstrated a reduction in the overall incidence of local recurrence to less than 10%.[4] The consequences of a TME can be impairment in erectile and bladder function due to disruption of parasympathetic nerves that are located in proximity to the mesorectum. Several authors have stressed the importance of the experience of the surgeon performing the procedure, and some have suggested specific techniques for monitoring modalities that can be used during this procedure to minimize morbidity.[5,6] A careful understanding of the anatomy and adequate visualization during sharp dissection will help in minimizing injury to the parasympathetic nerves and the consequent morbidity.[3,4]

Adequate visualization in the deep pelvis can often be a challenge. This may be a situation in which the visual magnification and ability to enter tight spaces that are unique to the laparoscopic approach may be an advantage. Several groups have demonstrated the feasibility of laparoscopic TME for low rectal cancer as part of a sphincter-preserving operation.[42–44] Some of the larger series, although demonstrating that a TME using laparoscopic techniques can be performed safely, do not have adequate follow-up to demonstrate whether or not there were any oncologic disadvantages to such an approach. Unfortunately, the current prospective random assignment trial being conducted at multiple institutions in the United States to evaluate the role of laparoscopic surgery for colon cancer excludes patients with low rectal lesions. Therefore, the ultimate role of the laparoscopic approach to TME will have to await prospective randomized trials using this technique and comparing it to the standard open approach.

RESECTION OF CONTIGUOUS ORGANS AND TOTAL PELVIC EXENTERATION

Although aggressive surgical approaches to rectal cancer have resulted in improvement in local-regional recurrence rates, these rates can still be as high as 33%. Not infrequently, large rectal lesions invade through the wall of the rectum into contiguous structures such as the bladder, prostate, vagina, and uterus. Carefully selected patients with recurrent or locally advanced rectal cancers may benefit from an aggressive approach such as a total pelvic exenteration. Local recurrences remain localized to the pelvis in a significant number of patients, with autopsy studies demonstrating the incidence of pelvic recurrence to be as high as 50%.[45]

Recurrences in the pelvis can result in significant morbidity, such as tenesmus, pain, bowel obstruction, and fistula. Although some of these can be ameliorated with radiation, these problems are best managed by preventing their occurrence. The impact of total pelvic exenteration on survival has been debated, but the potential benefits on controlling local-regional disease and preventing morbidity keep this technique as one of the tools in the surgeon's armamentarium when approaching large rectal lesions.

COMBINED MODALITY THERAPY (STAGES II AND III)

The use of adjuvant radiation therapy is based on the substantial incidence of local-regional failure with surgical therapy alone[46–52] (Table 29.9-1). The local-regional recurrence rates in these studies are in the range of 25% to 50% for patients with T3 to T4 or N+ disease, or both, and are a dominant pattern of failure, although distant recurrence is also of great importance. Local failure is related not just to the stage of the disease but also the location of the tumor in the rectum (tumors located low in the rectum have a higher incidence of local failure) and the experience and ability of the surgeon. However, the relevance of these older local recurrence data has been brought into question with the advent of the use of TME as described earlier. It is important to realize that the data on local recurrence after primary surgical resection that come from selected series with operations performed by experienced surgeons who have been specially trained in TME may not be relevant to the operations performed by general surgeons who do the operation only occasionally and who are not specially trained.

Although initial studies reported local-regional failure rates of less than 5% after TME without the use of any adjuvant therapy,[39,41,53–55] there was concern that these excellent results could not be replicated in larger population-based studies. A number of European countries or regions have shown that the overall local-regional recurrence risks could be decreased by limiting the surgeons who were authorized to perform rectal surgery to those who were trained and certified in the procedure and by having educational sessions for those who were doing the surgery.[5] This raised the question of what is the true rate of local failure after TME to help define which patients truly require adjuvant therapy.

Undoubtedly the most important piece of information on local recurrence rates with TME are the data from the Dutch TME study,[40] in which patients were randomized to receive either TME alone or a short course of preoperative radiation therapy followed by TME. All patients with rectal cancer were eligible, including those with early-stage disease. Special attempts were made to have good surgical and pathology quality control. The early results (2 years) relating to local tumor recurrence have been reported and are summarized in Table 29.9-2. The study demonstrates that there are subsets of patients in whom TME alone is likely sufficient for obtaining good pelvic control, including individuals with high rectal

TABLE 29.9-1. Local Failure of Rectal Cancer: Surgery Alone (Local Failure Rate/No. of Patients in Cohort)

Analysis	Gunderson and Sosin[49] Reoperation (Crude)	Rich et al.[51] Clinical Exam + Surgery (Crude)	Minsky et al.[107] First Failure; Clinical Exam + Surgery (5-Y Actuarial)	Martling et al.[52] Total Local Recurrence	Mendenhall et al.[46] Total Local Recurrence; 5-Y Follow-Up; Clinical	Pilipshen et al.[48] First Failure; Clinical	Bonadeo et al.[108] Total Local Recurrence; Clinical[a]
T1N0	—	8%/39	11%/11	9%/78	0%/6	0%/5	3%/103
T2N0	—		3%/36		38%/16	14%/128	
T3N0	67%/6	24%/42	23%/60	34%/80	40%/30	30%/111	4%/181
T4N0		53%/15	11%/9			22%/49	
T1–2N+	24%/17	50%/4	14%/11		71%/17		24%/133
T3N+	83%/40	47%/34	25%/31	37%/93	65%/17	49%/89	
T4N+		67%/6	22%/10				
Total	64%/75	30%/142	15%/168	27%/251	46%/90	—	—

[a]Local recurrence highly dependent on site in rectum; 18% overall for tumors 7 cm or less from anal verge.

TABLE 29.9-2. Results of Dutch Total Mesorectal Excision Trial

Technique	Preoperative RT (5 Gy × 5) + TME	TME Alone
NUMBER OF PATIENTS		
Local failure (2 y)	2.4%	8.2%
Local failure (4 y)	3%	10%
LF (DISTANCE FROM ANAL VERGE)		
0–5 cm	5.8%	10%
5–10 cm	1%	10.1%
10–15 cm	1.3%	3.8%
Stage III (4-y estimate)	—	20%

RT, radiation therapy; TME, total mesorectal excision.
Note: Thirty percent of patients had stage 0 or I disease.
(From ref. 40, with permission.)

tumors (some of these may have been sigmoid cancers rather than rectal) and low-stage tumors (T1 to T2, N0). On the other hand, low-lying rectal tumors that are moderately advanced (T3 to T4 and/or N+) had a higher incidence of local-regional failure. Local failure after TME alone was 15% in node-positive patients at 2 years, not corrected for site of the primary, and longer-term follow-up will undoubtedly demonstrate higher local failure rates. In addition, as these results were obtained in a controlled setting, one would likely not obtain similarly good results when surgery is done with less careful quality control. A consistent decrease in local failure rate was achieved by the addition of preoperative radiation therapy, but the absolute magnitude of the effect varied by the tumor characteristics discussed above.

The data are excellent that radiation therapy, especially when combined with chemotherapy, can decrease the local failure rate. This is shown by a Swedish study of preoperative radiation therapy compared to surgery,[56] the Dutch TME trial in the preoperative setting,[40] and multiple studies in the postoperative setting.[57–62] Excellent data are also available to show that local-regional failure is further decreased by the use of concurrent 5-FU–based chemotherapy[57,58,63] (Table 29.9-3). Most studies have demonstrated that local failure

decreases by approximately 50% with the use of adjuvant radiation therapy, with a greater effect when concurrent 5-FU is used with irradiation. This appears to provide a strong justification for the use of adjuvant radiation therapy. What is less clear are the following:

1. Does trimodality therapy with radiation therapy improve survival?
2. Should radiochemotherapy be given preoperatively or postoperatively?
3. Precisely which patients should be irradiated?

DOES ADJUVANT RADIATION THERAPY IMPACT SURVIVAL?

Although multiple randomized trials have addressed the use of adjuvant radiation therapy or chemoradiation therapy, and although they consistently show an improvement in local control with adjuvant radiation therapy, the survival outcome data have been mixed. In the past few years, two metaanalyses have been performed.[64,65] Table 29.9-4 shows the results of a metaanalysis by Camma et al.[65] showing a decreased local recurrence rate, cancer mortality, and overall mortality with the use of preoperative radiation therapy, although without a decrease in distant metastasis rate. The Colorectal Cancer Collaborative Group (Table 29.9-5) study demonstrates no improvement in the likelihood of curative surgery with preoperative therapy or of overall survival with all types of radiation therapy combined. Preoperative radiation therapy, however, was shown to improve local control, disease-free survival, and overall survival compared to surgery alone, although deaths within the first year after surgery were higher after radiation therapy. Local recurrence with preoperative radiation therapy was 46% lower than surgery alone, and cancer deaths were decreased from 50% to 45%. Postoperative radiation therapy was shown to improve local control (although less than preoperative therapy) but did not impact long-term survival. Lending substantial strength to the conclusion that there was a true advantage to radiation therapy is the fact that a dose response was demonstrated for the radiation effect on local control; that is, better control was obtained with higher radiation dose. This observation strengthens the conclusion, as it demonstrates a direct correlation between the amount of

TABLE 29.9-3. Local Control and Survival with and without Radiation Therapy: Preoperative, Postoperative, and ± Chemotherapy[a]

Study/Institution	No. of Patients	Local Failure	Disease-Free Survival	Survival (5-Y)
NSABP-RO-1: surg/surg + RT (postop RT)	184/187	25%/16%	No difference	No difference
NSABP RO-2: surg + chemo/surg + chemo + RT (postop RT)	348/346	13%/8%	—	—
GITSG: surg/surg + RT/surg + chemo + RT (postop RT)	58/50/46	25%/20%/10%	44%/50%/65%	26%/33%/45%
Swedish: surg/surg + RT (preop RT)	—	27%/11%	—	48%/58%
Stockholm II: surg/surg + RT (preop RT)	—	34%/16% (stage II), 37%/21% (stage II)	—	—
MRC: surg/surg + RT (postop RT)	235/234	34%/21%	—	38%/41%

GITSG, Gastrointestinal Tumor Study Group; MRC, Medical Research Council; NSABP, National Surgical Adjuvant Breast and Bowel Project; RT, radiation therapy.
[a]Randomized studies in either all patients or patients with stage II and III disease.

TABLE 29.9-4. Results of Metaanalysis: Preoperative Radiation Therapy versus Surgery Alone

	Camma: Preoperative RT vs. Surgery
Overall 5-y mortality	OR-0.84 (P = .03)
5-y cancer mortality	OR-0.71 (P < .001)
5-y local recurrence	OR-0.49 (P < .001)
5-y distant metastases	OR-0.93 (P = .54)

RT, radiation therapy.
(From ref. 65, with permission.)

therapy and outcome. The data from this analysis are heavily influenced by the results of a single Swedish study showing a long-term survival advantage to the use of preoperative radiation therapy compared to surgery alone.[56] Thus, these data show that improving local control with the use of radiation therapy (and presumably with concurrent chemoradiation therapy) is beneficial and that trimodality therapy, especially when chemoradiation therapy is used preoperatively, can improve survival.

PREOPERATIVE RADIATION THERAPY

The second issue of importance is whether adjuvant therapy should be given preoperatively or postoperatively. Relatively few studies have compared these approaches in a randomized controlled trial. A Swedish study reported in the early 1990s[66,67] evaluated a short course of radiation therapy preoperatively, to a more protracted course and higher total dose delivered postoperatively, and found a decreased local failure with the use of preoperative therapy compared to postoperative therapy (13% vs. 22%). Two trials in the United States have attempted to compare combined chemoradiation therapy delivered preoperatively to the same chemoradiation therapy regimen given postoperatively. However, neither study [NSABP (National Surgical Adjuvant Breast and Bowel Project) or gastrointestinal (GI) intergroup] could accrue a sufficient number of patients to answer the question.[68] The inability to accrue patients to these studies makes it unlikely that such a study will be attempted in the near future in the United States.

In addition to improving survival, another reason for using preoperative chemoradiation therapy is to increase the chance for sphincter preservation for patients with low-lying tumors of the rectum, where an abdominoperineal resection would be conventionally used. The NSABP trial mentioned above was able to obtain worthwhile information regarding this issue.

TABLE 29.9-5. Colorectal Cancer Collaborative Group (2001): Adjuvant Radiation Therapy in Rectal Cancer

	Preoperative RT vs. Surgery	Postoperative RT vs. Surgery
Yearly risk of local recurrence	46% decrease with RT	37% decrease with RT
Death rate	5% less than with surgery	No difference from surgery

RT, radiation therapy.
(From ref. 64.)

When the patient was first seen, the surgeon was asked (for preoperative and for postoperative patients) what operation they thought they would need to perform. In the patients randomized to postoperative radiation therapy (i.e., immediate surgery), the determination in the office corresponded well to the operation actually performed. However, in the patients who received preoperative radiation therapy, sphincter-preserving surgery was performed in 50% of patients, compared to 33% of those who had initial surgery.[69]

Perhaps the most important study addressing the issue of preoperative versus postoperative adjuvant therapy is a German trial of preoperative versus postoperative chemoradiation with radiation therapy given at 180 cGy per fraction and using continuous-infusion 5-FU chemotherapy as a 120-hour infusion, for which preliminary results have been reported in abstract form.[70] This study demonstrates an advantage in sphincter preservation with the use of preoperative therapy. Of the patients thought to need an APR at initial assessment, only 19% had a sphincter-preserving surgery when operation was performed immediately versus 39% after preoperative radiation therapy. A statistically significant decrease also occurred in local failure with preoperative radiation therapy compared to postoperative treatment (7% vs. 11%, P = .02). After a median follow-up of 43 months, there was a small advantage (59% vs. 55%, P = .23) in disease-free survival, which was not statistically significant, but there was a significant decrease in late anastomotic strictures (2.7% vs. 8.5%, P = .001) with preoperative therapy. Acute toxicity was also decreased by the use of preoperative radiation and chemotherapy compared to postoperative therapy. Although final data are required, this provides strong evidence of the superiority of preoperative adjuvant treatment in patients in whom it is determined that adjuvant therapy is needed.

If one is using preoperative RT to try to improve the likelihood of sphincter preservation, the radiation must be given in such a way as to maximize the likelihood of this occurring. Specifically, a "standard" long course of irradiation to a dose of approximately 5000 cGy at 180 to 200 cGy per fraction over 5 to 5.5 weeks (as given in the German trial above) is likely optimal. The short-course therapy with immediate surgery (typically, 500 cGy for 5 fractions given over 1 week) as often used in Europe followed by immediate surgery is not likely to produce enough tumor shrinkage to allow for sphincter preservation in patients with very low-lying tumors. However, there are no data to suggest that the short course is not as effective in producing local control as the longer course of therapy. It is also not as clear as to how to incorporate adjuvant chemotherapy regimens into the short-course therapy given preoperatively.

For theoretical reasons it is believed that radiation therapy delivered preoperatively can decrease the toxicity of therapy. With postoperative radiation therapy the soft tissues of the perineum are at risk for involvement after an APR because of surgical manipulation and therefore need to be irradiated, with its attendant acute skin toxicity. This is not needed with preoperative therapy. With postoperative radiation therapy normal bowel is moved into the pelvis for the anastomosis after a low anterior resection and therefore is irradiated and at risk for late toxicity. In the preoperative setting much of the irradiated bowel is removed with the surgical specimen and therefore is not at risk for producing late bowel injury. It is also likely that there is a higher risk of having small bowel fixed in the pelvis after surgery secondary to adhesions, which could also lead to late toxicity. On the other hand, many studies have demonstrated that acute surgical morbidity and mortality are not substantially increased with the use of preoperative irradiation, although many surgeons routinely perform a temporary diverting colostomy to avoid the problems associated with an anastomotic leak. Except for the German trial mentioned above, which shows decreased acute and late toxicity, data on late toxicity are not available to directly compare the two techniques when used with concurrent chemotherapy and the commonly used dose/fractionation schedules.

As the retrospective metaanalyses have generally shown better tumor control locally and better evidence of a survival advantage secondary to preoperative irradiation, many GI oncologists prefer preoperative radiochemotherapy for the patient who clearly requires adjuvant radiation therapy. The final data from the German randomized trial will be of importance in providing additional information on this issue. A reasonable strategy at present is to use preoperative radiochemotherapy in patients in whom there is little doubt about the advisability of adjuvant therapy (T3N+ or T4 disease) or patients with low-lying tumors in whom an abdominoperineal resection may still be avoided but to use initial surgery for other patient cohorts, with postoperative radiochemotherapy used based on the operative and pathologic findings.

WHICH PATIENTS SHOULD RECEIVE ADJUVANT THERAPY?

For either preoperative or postoperative therapy, one needs to address the issue of precisely which patients need to receive adjuvant radiation therapy and chemotherapy. At the present time these two modalities have been completely linked in U.S. clinical trials, and therefore it is not possible to determine if there are subsets of patients who might benefit from one modality and not the other. In addition, because U.S. trials have all used chemotherapy concurrent with the radiation therapy in addition to postradiation chemotherapy, it is not possible to determine the relative importance of each.

Based on the historic patterns of failure data, which demonstrated high local failure rates with surgery alone for patients with T3 or N+ disease, or both, virtually all U.S. studies have evaluated this entire patient population. However, more detailed analyses have allowed us to define characteristics that help define relatively low-risk and relatively high-risk patient subsets. As mentioned earlier, among the entire group of patients conventionally treated with adjuvant chemoradiation therapy who have been studied in multiple clinical trials, a number of relatively lower-risk categories have been identified. Those include patients with T3N0 or T1 to 2N1 disease,[10,11,71,72] patients with primary tumors located high in the rectum, those with wide circumferential margins on the final pathology specimen,[15,16] those patients with node-negative disease after multiple (greater than 12 to 14) nodes have been evaluated,[12–14,73] and patients in whom TME surgery has been performed by an experienced colorectal oncologic surgeon.[74,75] In the preoperative setting some, but not all, of this information is available at the time a therapeutic decision must be made (including knowledge of the surgeon). In addition, one must consider the known inaccuracy of transrectal ultrasound in staging and the experience of the ultrasonographer.[26,29] However, if most of the above conditions are met, it is possible that routine adjuvant radiation therapy, and perhaps chemotherapy, is not required for the lower-stage tumors. At the present time most patients treated outside clinical trials who have T3 to T4 or N+ disease, or both, should receive adjuvant chemoradiation therapy if there are no extenuating circumstances. However, for patients who meet all of the above-mentioned favorable criteria, not using adjuvant therapy could be considered. Clinical trials need to be performed to help resolve whether some of these patients do not require the use of routine adjuvant radiation therapy.

CONCURRENT CHEMOTHERAPY

Until very recently the use of adjuvant chemotherapy centered on the use of 5-FU chemotherapy, although this drug has existed for almost 50 years and is not very effective for colon or rectal cancer. The initial trials of trimodality therapy in rectal cancer used bolus 5-FU at a dose of 500 mg/m^2/d for 3 days during weeks 1 and 5 of the radiation therapy. This was the approach routinely used until the results of the North Central Cancer Treatment Group study testing the use of long-term continuous-infusion 5-FU during postoperative radiation therapy (bolus 5-FU was used before and after the radiation therapy) were reported.[63] This study demonstrated an advantage to continuous-infusion 5-FU (only during radiation therapy) compared to bolus 5-FU in terms of local control, disease-free survival, and overall survival. Because of this result, and the encouraging results found with more aggressive therapy in colon cancer, it was logical to think that further intensification of chemotherapy would be of value during radiation therapy and when used alone.

Unfortunately, this expectation has not been borne out. Two large U.S. GI intergroup trials have been run testing intensification with either more aggressive 5-FU and leucovorin, additional continuous-infusion 5-FU, or other combinations, with no data demonstrating an advantage.[76,77] Thus, we are left with evidence that continuous-infusion 5-FU during radiation therapy is of value, in improving local control, distant metastases, and survival, but no evidence that anything other than simple 5-FU or 5-FU plus leucovorin should be used during the chemotherapy portion of the therapy. Whether newer agents including cytotoxics with clear efficacy against colon and rectal cancers in the metastatic disease setting such as irinotecan or oxaliplatin, or biologics such as bevacizumab or cetuximab, will be superior to standard 5-FU is unknown at the present time.

In practice, most GI oncologists now use continuous-infusion 5-FU during radiation therapy and weekly 5-FU/leucovorin (Roswell Park Schedule; see Chapter 29.8) as the postradiation chemotherapy. This is used in the preoperative and the postoperative setting, although there is little information to specifically support this precise regimen when much of the therapy is given preoperatively, as the relevant clinical trials have been primarily conducted in the postoperative setting. Based on the promising disease-free survival data seen with the FOLFOX 4 regimen (biweekly oxaliplatin, 5-FU, and leucovorin; see Chapter 29.8) in the adjuvant treatment of colon cancer, use of FOLFOX 4 as postoperative treatment after preoperative infusional 5-FU/radiation is gaining popularity, although specific trials to support this approach have not yet been completed.

Interest has also been shown in the use of oral agents instead of continuous-infusion 5-FU. Capecitabine has generated a great deal of interest as a simpler method of drug delivery. Limited phase I and small phase II studies have been reported confirming feasibility; however, adequately powered large-scale trials to assess the noninferiority of capecitabine versus protracted-infusion 5-FU have not been reported to date. It is noteworthy that capecitabine has yet to be directly compared to an infusional 5-FU regimen, with or without radiation, and therefore the equivalency, or lack thereof, is unknown at this time, and the use of capecitabine plus concurrent radiation for the management of potentially curable rectal cancer should be regarded as investigational pending definitive data.

One must also exert caution in the timing of delivery of oral agents such as capecitabine if one is trying to maximize radiation sensitization, because their kinetics are not identical to that of continuous infusion. Capecitabine should probably be given daily approximately 1 hour before radiation therapy to maximize the interaction between the modalities.

SYNCHRONOUS RECTAL PRIMARY AND METASTASES

The use of pelvic radiotherapy in patients with synchronous presentation of primary and metastatic disease is controversial. Primary combination chemotherapy can provide substantial palliation and can be considered as initial therapy in many rectal cancer patients with metastatic disease.[78] Endoscopically placed expandable metal stents can be considered for palliation or protection from impending obstruction. Control of disease in the pelvis can have important implications for patient quality of life, and therefore combined modality therapy, including radiation, chemotherapy, and, in some cases, palliative surgery, can be appropriate, especially when extrapelvic metastatic disease is small volume and the patient's prognosis is favorable enough that pelvic complications could be anticipated as a long-term problem. Clearly, no firm guidelines can be set in the management of these complex patients, and treatment decisions must be made on an individual basis.

MANAGEMENT OF UNRESECTABLE PRIMARY AND LOCALLY ADVANCED DISEASE (T4)

Although the majority of patients who present with stage II and III disease have primary tumors that are technically easily resectable, a group of patients has T4 tumors with deep local invasion into adjacent structures that makes primary resection for cure difficult, if not impossible. Some T4 tumors invade into the vagina, which is easily resectable, but others invade into pelvic sidewall or sacrum, where a complete surgical resection may be impossible (the coccyx and distal sacrum can be resected if appropriate); others invade into bladder or prostate, where a more extensive surgical resection can be done, but often at the expense of major morbidity or functional loss. Although few randomized trials define optimal therapy in this group of patients, data suggest that it is appropriate to treat these individuals with preoperative radiation therapy combined with chemotherapy, in a manner similar to that described for T3 disease, generally with concurrent 5-FU–based chemotherapy. This often results in a good clinical response that allows for a potentially curative resection to be performed. It is preferable to treat a patient preoperatively to try to avoid leaving residual disease rather than attempting to salvage a patient after a clearly inadequate operation.

The use of adjuvant radiation therapy in this clinical situation also allows for treatment of the lymphatics draining the locally invaded organ, such as the internal or external iliacs, which are not typically resected in an LAR or APR but which may be at substantial risk as secondary involvement from an invaded organ, such as the bladder. Although the definition of "unresectable" at presentation is very subjective, a number of studies have shown that preoperative radiation therapy can convert a substantial number of these patients to having resectable disease with substantial cure rates.[79–82]

Although the use of preoperative radiation therapy with concurrent 5-FU–based chemotherapy, as described above in the adjuvant setting, appears of value in patients with locally advanced disease, there is still a substantial incidence of local failure. Therefore, a number of investigators have explored ways to increase the radiation dose to the highest-risk region to try to improve local tumor control. Three main techniques have been used: supplemental postoperative external-beam radiation boost, intraoperative electron-beam radiation therapy boost, and intraoperative brachytherapy boost.

Relatively few data on the use of postoperative external beam as a boost are available, largely because of concerns of normal tissue tolerance after use of the relatively large fields that would be needed for the boost and the prolonged delay between initial external-beam therapy and the final boost after recovery from surgery. The two intraoperative techniques are philosophically the same, although the technique of radiation delivery is different. After a high dose (5000 cGy) of preoperative chemoradiotherapy and then a 4- to 6-week break, surgical resection is performed, the extent of which depends on the location and extent of tumor. Areas considered at high risk for residual tumor are determined by the surgical findings and by frozen-section pathologic evaluation. For electron-beam intraoperative radiation therapy, a treatment cylinder is placed over the high-risk region, often on a pelvic sidewall or the sacrum, and the cylinder is then aligned to the radiation machine, which is either in the operating room or in the radiation therapy department. The cylinder acts to hold normal tissues outside of the radiation beam and to confine the electron beam. The use of electrons allows the radiation oncologist to adjust the depth of penetration of the beam to conform to the local tumor extent. When using brachytherapy, carriers for the radioactive sources are placed over the high-risk region and then the radiation is given either during the surgery (high-dose rate) or the radioactive sources are inserted approximately 5 days after surgery and left in place for 1 to 2 days (low-dose rate). In all situations the radiation dose is in the range of 1000 to 2000 (most commonly 1500) cGy when used as a boost to conventional therapy. In both approaches care must be taken to be sure that normal tissues such as small bowel are out of the irradiated volume.

Techniques similar to this have been used for a number of years and have shown encouraging results, although formal randomized trials have not been performed. Data suggest fairly good levels of local control and long-term survival if a gross total resection can be accomplished, with poorer results if there is gross residual disease[83–86] (Table 29.9-6). Use of intra-

TABLE 29.9-6. Intraoperative Radiation Therapy for Locally Advanced Rectal Cancer[a]

	Mayo Clinic			*Massachusetts General Hospital*		
	No. of Patients	Local Failure (%)	Overall Survival (5-y) (%)	No. of Patients	Local Failure (%)	Disease-Specific Survival (%)
Complete resection	18[b]	7	69	40	9	63
Partial resection	35	~20	~40	24	37	35
No resection	1	—	0	—	—	—
Total	56	16	46	64	—	—
Recurrent locally advanced tumor	42	40	19	—	—	—

[a]External-beam radiation therapy + resection + intraoperative radiation therapy. No prior radiation therapy.
[b]Two additional patients with no tumor in specimen, both without any tumor recurrence. These are included in the totals.

operative radiation therapy boosts often requires specialized radiation facilities and expertise as well as an experienced team of radiation oncologists, surgical oncologists, urologists, and plastic surgeons. Similar types of intraoperative radiation therapy approaches can produce surprisingly good results (35% 5-year survival) in patients with locally advanced nodal metastases[87] from colon or rectal cancers.

For patients who still cannot have a surgical resection performed, either because of the tumor extent or because of coexisting medical problems, attempts should be made to maximize palliation and perhaps local control. Boost doses of radiation are appropriately delivered to the residual tumor to doses of greater than 6000 cGy if sensitive normal tissues can be removed from the radiation fields. Only a small percentage (5%) of patients with these locally advanced tumors are locally controlled and cured by such an approach, but a substantial percentage will obtain good palliation.[88–90]

RADIATION THERAPY TECHNIQUE

Primarily two dosing schemes for radiation therapy have been used in the treatment of rectal cancer. In the preoperative setting many European centers have favored a rapid short-course treatment of doses of approximately 2500 cGy in five fractions followed by immediate surgery, whereas U.S. centers have generally favored doses of approximately 5040 cGy given at 180 cGy per fraction with a delay of 4 to 8 weeks before surgery. As mentioned earlier in Combined Modality Therapy (Stages II and III), an advantage of the long-course therapy is that it provides time to have tumor regression, which appears to facilitate sphincter preservation, although it is more expensive and time consuming for the patient. In addition, there has been substantial late toxicity from the short-course treatment in earlier series, although this was most evident when the radiation therapy techniques were less sophisticated and simple anteroposterior-posteroanterior fields alone were used, which were, at times, quite large[91]; techniques such as these are not used at present.

Although major late toxicity is relatively uncommon, functional GI disturbances are seen comparatively often. These relate to surgical effects on bowel with lack of a good reservoir function and possible nerve dysfunction, as well as long-term radiation effects on bowel compliance and neural functioning.[67,92] Many patients remain with some rectal urgency and food intolerance (especially to roughage), but symptoms tend to improve over time and most patients can live a relatively normal life related to

their GI tract. Detailed discussions with the patient on the types of foods likely to cause worsening bowel symptoms, attention to the superimposed problems that can occur from other problems such as lactose intolerance, and use of agents such as loperamide can all help the patient deal with bowel problems.

Small bowel–related complications are directly proportional to the volume of small bowel in the radiation field.[93] In patients receiving combined modality therapy, the volume of irradiated small bowel limits the ability to escalate the dose of 5-FU. A number of simple radiotherapeutic techniques are available to decrease radiation-related small bowel toxicity (Table 29.9-7). First, small bowel contrast or CT scanning during treatment planning allows identification of the location of the small bowel to be determined so that fields can be designed to minimize its treatment. Multiple-field techniques (preferably a 3- or 4-field technique) are now standard to minimize normal tissue irradia-

TABLE 29.9-7. Techniques for Minimizing Bowel Toxicity with Pelvic Radiation Therapy; Techniques to Minimize the Acute Toxicity to the Small Bowel from Radiation Therapy

SURGICAL TECHNIQUES FOR POSTOPERATIVE RADIATION THERAPY
Pelvic reconstruction to exclude small bowel from the pelvis
Reperitonealized pelvic floor
Retrovert the uterus
Construct an omental sling
Absorbable mesh
Surgical clips to delineate high-risk areas
RADIATION THERAPY TECHNIQUES
Treatment simulation and planning
Small bowel contrast (especially for postoperative radiation therapy)
Prone position
Multiple-field techniques (3- or 4-field)
Mark perineum after abdominal perineal resection
High energy (≥6 MeV)
Shaped blocks
Computed dosimetry
Limit dose to small bowel to 50.4 Gy
Standard fraction sizes (1.8–2.0 Gy/fraction)
Bladder distention and belly board—providing it does not make the patient uncomfortable, thereby causing movement
During treatment
Treat all fields each day
Low-fiber, low-fat diet
Avoid milk products in lactose-intolerant patients (or use oral lactase supplements)

tion. In one series, the small bowel obstruction rate in patients with rectal cancer who received pelvic radiation therapy was higher with a single-field (21%) as compared with a multiple-field technique (9%). The small bowel obstruction rate increased to 30% when extended-field radiation was used. The use of lateral fields for the boost as well as positioning of the patient in the prone position can further decrease the volume of small bowel in the lateral radiation fields.

The treatment should be designed with the use of computed radiation dosimetry and be delivered by high-energy linear accelerators, which deliver a higher dose to the target volume while relatively sparing surrounding normal structures. The advantage to the combination of a multiple-field technique, high-energy photons, and computed dosimetry produces a homogeneous dose distribution throughout the target volume and minimizes the dose to the small bowel. Although not well studied to date, newer developments in intensity-modulated radiation therapy may allow more conformal radiation dose distributions, which would decrease the irradiation of normal tissues in the pelvis, especially small bowel.

After pelvic surgery, the small bowel commonly fills the pelvis. Adhesions can form, resulting in fixed loops of small bowel in the radiation fields. In this situation, despite treatment of the patient in the prone position, the use of multiple-field techniques may be of limited value. In contrast, when radiation therapy is delivered preoperatively to a patient who has not undergone prior pelvic surgery, the small bowel is usually mobile. When no small bowel fixation is present, treatment in the prone position can exclude much of the small bowel from the posteroanterior field and completely from the lateral fields.

Various physical maneuvers to exclude small bowel from the pelvis have been examined. Gallagher et al.[93] determined the volume, distribution, and mobility of small bowel in the pelvis after a variety of maneuvers. Regardless of the prior surgical history, a significant decrease was seen in the average small bowel volume when the patients were treated in the prone position with abdominal wall compression and bladder distention compared with the supine position and with the use of a four-field technique. Treatment in the prone position without abdominal wall compression was not consistently effective in displacing small bowel and, in some patients (most commonly obese), the volume of small bowel increased.

RADIATION FIELDS

The precise radiation fields that are used should depend on the individual clinical situation, although the principles of the radiation treatment remain the same. The local-regional failures in rectal cancer occur because of residual disease in the soft tissues of the pelvis as well as residual pelvic nodal disease. The nodal disease can be in the internal iliac chain for very low-lying lesions but only involves the external iliac nodes if the anal canal or sphincter is involved or if an organ is involved that drains into the external iliac system. Because the internal iliac nodes are not usually dissected by the surgeon, it is important to treat these for low rectal cancers, but the external iliacs should not be routinely irradiated. The proximal extent of nodal radiation is arbitrary, but the primary drainage of all rectal cancers is along the mesenteric system, which should be treated primarily surgically. Extending radiation fields to cover

paraaortic nodes is not indicated unless there is evidence of disease in these regions.

As many of the local recurrences occur in the soft tissues of the pelvis, the radiation oncologist must be sure to treat the regions where the surgical margins are likely to be least adequate. These include extension to the pelvic sidewall, to the prostate in men and vagina in women, and the presacral space in all patients. The proximal extent of the radiation field should generally extend to the sacral promontory, as that is the level at which there is an attachment of the posterior peritoneum and above which the rectal tumors would become totally intraperitoneal. Above this level there is little risk of pelvic soft tissue invasion for the standard rectal cancer.

The lower extent of the radiation field is more complex. Often the surgeon relies on the radiation oncologist to sterilize the most distal extent of the primary tumor to perform a sphincter-preserving operation, and therefore the distal margins should be at least a couple of centimeters below the primary tumor mass. Although rectal tumors tend to have only a minimal amount of longitudinal spread along the mucosal margin, they can spread further distally in the perirectal fat and in the lymph node regions. This, in fact, is part of the rationale for a TME. Attempts should thus be made to treat to at least the level of the dentate line for most low-lying rectal cancers, although this is likely not necessary for rectal cancers in the proximal third. However, it is also likely the case, although not well proven, that a substantial part of the late toxicity from pelvic radiation therapy is related to dysfunction of the anal sphincter. Thus, it is important to try to minimize the amount of sphincter that is irradiated. Although many textbooks define the lower edge of the radiation field relative to the bones of the pelvis, this is not the proper way to think about irradiating such tumors. The location of bony anatomic landmarks such as the ischial tuberosity has no consistent relationship to the anal sphincter, anal verge, dentate line, or the rectal cancer. The radiation oncologist must identify the location of these structures as best as possible using radiopaque markers and rectal contrast and then determine the balance between adequate distal coverage of the tumor as well as minimizing irradiation of the anal sphincter and the perineum (acute toxicity). For anteroposterior or posteroanterior fields, the lateral borders should extend to treat the pelvic sidewall, a possible region for soft tissue extension. The lateral fields should have a similar superior and inferior margin. The posterior border should include all of the presacral soft tissue so that the posterior extent of the field should cover the anterior border of the sacrum with at least a 1.5-cm margin for patient motion and dosimetric variation. The anterior border of the lateral fields should cover at least the posterior border of the vagina or the prostate, the anterior extent of the primary rectal tumor, and the anterior edge of the sacral promontory. Examples of typical radiation fields are shown in Figure 29.9-7.

IMMOBILIZATION MOLDS AND TISSUE EXPANDERS

A number of investigators have evaluated the effectiveness of custom bowel immobilization molds (belly board), belly drop boards, and other devices to decrease the amount of small bowel irradiated.[94,95] These have generally been partially effective in minimizing bowel irradiation but are dependent on precise location of the device relative to the patient.

areas in the pelvis to better define the tumor volume can be of enormous benefit to the radiation oncologist in limiting the extent of the high-dose region.

DIETARY SUPPLEMENTS AND RADIOPROTECTORS

The benefit of dietary supplements and radioprotectors is controversial. Five randomized trials have examined the efficacy of various compounds to decrease bowel toxicity. These trials have included such compounds as butyric acid to decrease chronic radiation proctitis,[101] sucralfate enemas to decrease acute radiation proctitis,[102] olsalazine to decrease acute enteritis, and mesalazine (5-aminosalicylic acid) to decrease acute radiation enteritis.[103] All of these randomized trials have been negative. In another randomized trial of 73 patients with pelvic malignancies, the addition of 5-aminosalicylic acid increased rather than decreased acute radiation toxicity. The use of an elemental diet has also been studied,[104] which suggested a benefit with decreased GI symptoms, but this has not been aggressively pursued. A lactose-restricted diet has not been effective in decreasing symptoms, and the radioprotector WR-2721 also has not shown benefit in some trials, but there is a suggestion of benefit in others.[105,106] One study suggested that sucralfate may decrease acute and long-term small bowel toxicity in patients receiving pelvic radiation therapy for prostate and bladder cancer.

REFERENCES

1. Havenga K, Enker WE, McDermott K, et al. Male and female sexual and urinary function after total mesorectal excision with autonomic nerve preservation for carcinoma of the rectum. *J Am Coll Surg* 1996;182:495.
2. Havenga K, DeRuiter MC, Enker WE, Welvaart K. Anatomical basis of autonomic nerve-preserving total mesorectal excision for rectal cancer. *Br J Surg* 1996;83:384.
3. Mancini R, Cosimelli M, Filippini A, et al. Nerve-sparing surgery in rectal cancer: feasibility and functional results. *J Exp Clin Cancer Res* 2000;19:35.
4. McNamara DA, Parc R. Methods and results of sphincter-preserving surgery for rectal cancer. *Cancer Control* 2003;10:212.
5. Wibe A, Eriksen MT, Syse A, Myrvold HE, Soreide O. Total mesorectal excision for rectal cancer—what can be achieved by a national audit? *Colorectal Dis* 2003;5:471.
6. Hanna NN, Guillem J, Dosoretz A, et al. Intraoperative parasympathetic nerve stimulation with tumescence monitoring during total mesorectal excision for rectal cancer. *J Am Coll Surg* 2002;195:506.
7. Watanabe T, Wu TT, Catalano PJ, et al. Molecular predictors of survival after adjuvant chemotherapy for colon cancer. *N Engl J Med* 2001;344:1196.
8. Compton CC. *Surgical pathology of colorectal cancer.* Totowa, NJ: Humana Press, 2002:247.
9. Compton CC, Fielding LP, Burgart LJ, et al. Prognostic factors in colorectal cancer. College of American Pathologists Consensus Statement 1999. *Arch Pathol Lab Med* 2000;124:979.
10. Gunderson LL, Sargent D, Tepper J, et al. Impact of TN stage and treatment on survival and relapse in adjuvant rectal cancer pooled analysis. In: *Thirty-ninth annual meeting of the ASCO.* Chicago, IL. 2003:251.
11. Greene FL, Stewart AK, Norton HJ. A new TNM staging strategy for node-positive (stage III) rectal cancer: an analysis of 5,988 patients. In: *Thirty-ninth annual meeting of the ASCO.* Chicago, IL. 2003:251.
12. Tepper JE, O'Connell MJ, Niedzwiecki D, et al. Impact of number of nodes retrieved on outcome in patients with rectal cancer. *J Clin Oncol* 2001;19:157.
13. Goldstein NS, Sanford W, Coffey M, Layfield LJ. Lymph node recovery from colorectal resection specimens removed for adenocarcinoma: trends over time and a recommendation for a minimum number of lymph nodes to be recovered. *Am J Clin Pathol* 1996;106:209.
14. Wong JH, Severino R, Honnebier MB, Tom P, Namiki TS. Number of nodes examined and staging accuracy in colorectal carcinoma. *J Clin Oncol* 1999;17:2896.
15. Quirke P, Durdey P, Dixon M, Williams N. Local recurrence of rectal adenocarcinoma due to inadequate surgical resection: histopathological study of lateral tumour spread and surgical excision. *Lancet* 1986;2:996.
16. Adam I, Mohamdee M, Martin I, et al. Role of circumferential margin involvement in the local recurrence of rectal cancer. *Lancet* 1994;344:707.
17. Chiesura-Corona M, Muzzio PC, Giust G, et al. Rectal cancer: CT local staging with histopathologic correlation. *Abdom Imaging* 2001;26:134.
18. Brown G, Richards CJ, Newcombe RG, et al. Rectal carcinoma: thin-section MR imaging for staging in 28 patients. *Radiology* 1999;211:215.

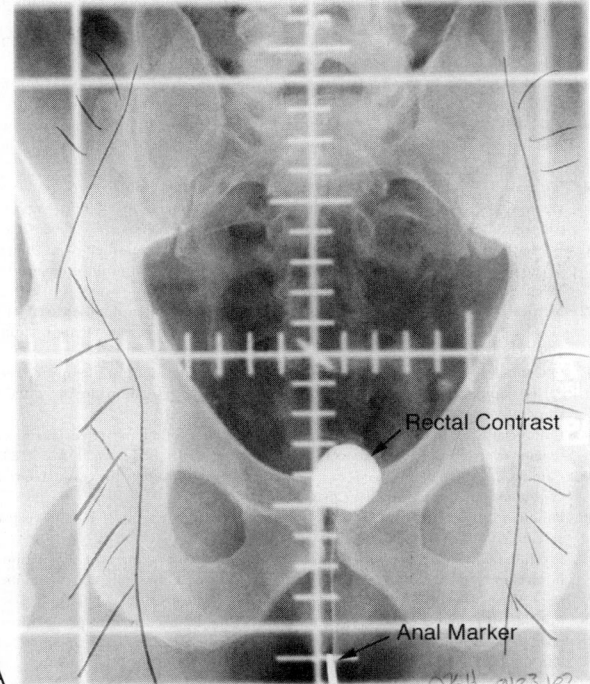

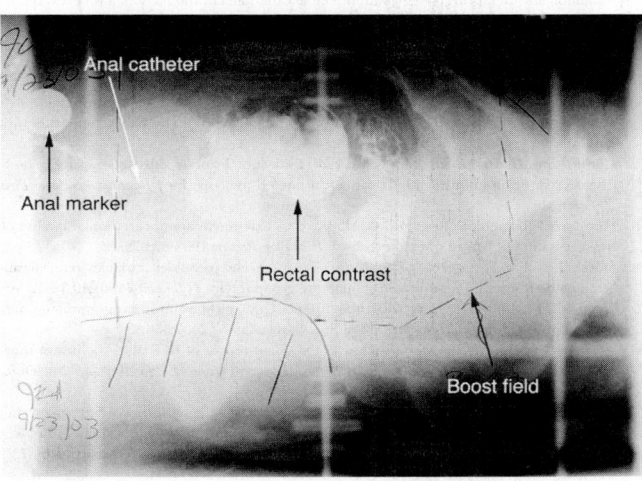

FIGURE 29.9-7. **A,B:** Typical radiation fields for the preoperative treatment of a low-lying rectal cancer. The fields laterally extend to the pelvic sidewall, proximally a short margin above the sacral promontory and distally to the proximal portion of the anal canal, which is marked with a radiopaque marker. On the lateral fields the posterior border is approximately 1.5 cm posterior to the anterior border of the sacrum. The anterior border covers the posterior vaginal wall with margin, the primary tumor, and the sacral promontory.

For patients treated postoperatively, especially after APR, surgical maneuvers to keep small bowel from being fixed in the pelvis can be effective in minimizing bowel irradiation and thus late toxicity. Pelvic tissue expanders have been used by a number of investigators,[96,97] who have reported a significant decrease in small bowel volume in the radiation field and a decrease in acute toxicity. Reperitonealizing the pelvic floor or having a surgical flap inserted into the pelvis can also be of substantial use, and these are the techniques most commonly used at present.[98–100] The placement of surgical clips in high-risk

19. Brown G, Richards CJ, Bourne MW, et al. Morphologic predictors of lymph node status in rectal cancer with use of high-spatial-resolution MR imaging with histopathologic comparison. *Radiology* 2003;227:371.

20. Haider MA, Amitai MM, Rappaport DC, et al. Multi-detector row helical CT in preoperative assessment of small (< or = 1.5 cm) liver metastases: is thinner collimation better? *Radiology* 2002;225:137.

21. Semelka RC, Schlund JF, Molina PL, et al. Malignant liver lesions: comparison of spiral CT arterial portography and MR imaging for diagnostic accuracy, cost, and effect on patient management. *J Magn Reson Imaging* 1996;6:39.

22. Abdel-Nabi H, Doerr RJ, Lamonica DM, et al. Staging of primary colorectal carcinomas with fluorine-18 fluorodeoxyglucose whole-body PET: correlation with histopathologic and CT findings. *Radiology* 1998;206:755.

23. Huebner RH, Park KC, Shepherd JE, et al. A meta-analysis of the literature for whole-body FDG PET detection of recurrent colorectal cancer. *J Nucl Med* 2000;41:1177.

24. Kim NK, Kim MJ, Yun SH, Sohn SK, Min JS. Comparative study of transrectal ultrasonography, pelvic computerized tomography, and magnetic resonance imaging in preoperative staging of rectal cancer. *Dis Colon Rectum* 1999;42:770.

25. Beynon J. An evaluation of the role of rectal endosonography in rectal cancer. *Ann R Coll Surg Engl* 1989;71:131.

26. Garcia-Aguilar J, Pollack J, Lee SH, et al. Accuracy of endorectal ultrasonography in preoperative staging of rectal tumors. *Dis Colon Rectum* 2002;45:10.

27. Canter RJ, Williams NN. Surgical treatment of colon and rectal cancer. *Hematol Oncol Clin North Am* 2002;16:907.

28. Colquhoun PH, Wexner SD. Surgical management of colon cancer. *Curr Gastroenterol Rep* 2002;4:414.

29. Herzog U, von Flue M, Tondelli P, Schuppisser JP. How accurate is endorectal ultrasound in the preoperative staging of rectal cancer? *Dis Colon Rectum* 1996;36:127.

30. Libutti SK, Forde KA. Surgical considerations III: bowel anastomosis. In: Cohen A, Weaver S, eds. *Cancer of the colon, rectum and anus.* New York: McGraw-Hill, 1995:445.

31. Ota DM, Jacobs L, Kuvshinoff B. Rectal cancer: the sphincter-sparing approach. *Surg Clin North Am* 2002;82:983.

32. Moore HG, Riedel E, Minsky BD, et al. Adequacy of 1-cm distal margin after restorative rectal cancer resection with sharp mesorectal excision and preoperative combined-modality therapy. *Ann Surg Oncol* 2003;10:80.

33. Dehni N, McFadden N, McNamara DA, et al. Oncologic results following abdomino-perineal resection for adenocarcinoma of the low rectum. *Dis Colon Rectum* 2003;46:867.

34. Kuvshinoff B, Maghfoor I, Miedema B, et al. Distal margin requirements after preoperative chemoradiotherapy for distal rectal carcinomas: are < or = 1 cm distal margins sufficient? *Ann Surg Oncol* 2001;8:163.

35. Tiret E, Poupardin B, McNamara D, Dehni N, Parc R. Ultralow anterior resection with intersphincteric dissection—what is the limit of safe sphincter preservation? *Colorectal Dis* 2003;5:454.

36. Nathanson DR, Espat NJ, Nash GM, et al. Evaluation of preoperative and postoperative radiotherapy on long-term functional results of straight coloanal anastomosis. *Dis Colon Rectum* 2003;46:888.

37. Sitzler PJ, Seow-Choen F, Ho YH, Leong AP. Lymph node involvement and tumor depth in rectal cancers: an analysis of 805 patients. *Dis Colon Rectum* 1997;40:1472.

38. Willett CG. Sphincter preservation in rectal cancer. *Curr Treat Options Oncol* 2000;1:399.

39. Enker WE, Thaler HT, Cranor ML, Polyak T. Total mesorectal excision in the operative treatment of carcinoma of the rectum. *J Am Coll Surg* 1995;181:335.

40. Kapiteijn E, Marijne CAM, Nagtegaal ID, et al. Preoperative radiotherapy combined with total mesorectal excision for resectable rectal cancer. *N Engl J Med* 2001;345:638.

41. Tocchi A, Mazzoni G, Lepre L, et al. Total mesorectal excision and low rectal anastomosis for the treatment of rectal cancer and prevention of pelvic recurrences. *Arch Surg* 2001;136:216.

42. Zhou ZG, Wang Z, Yu YY, et al. Laparoscopic total mesorectal excision of low rectal cancer with preservation of anal sphincter: a report of 82 cases. *World J Gastroenterol* 2003;9:1477.

43. Tsang WW, Chung CC, Li MK. Prospective evaluation of laparoscopic total mesorectal excision with colonic J-pouch reconstruction for mid and low rectal cancers. *Br J Surg* 2003;90:867.

44. Morino M, Parini U, Giraudo G, et al. Laparoscopic total mesorectal excision: a consecutive series of 100 patients. *Ann Surg* 2003;237:335.

45. Mukherjee A. Total pelvic exenteration for advanced rectal cancer. *S D J Med* 1999;52:153.

46. Mendenhall MW, Million RR, Pfaff WW. Patterns of recurrence in adenocarcinoma of the rectum and rectosigmoid treated with surgery alone: implications in treatment planning with adjuvant radiation therapy. *Int J Radiat Oncol Biol Phys* 1983;9:877.

47. Walz B, Lindstrom E, Butcher H, Baglan R. Natural history of patients after abdominal-perineal resection implications for radiation therapy. *Cancer* 1997;39:2437.

48. Pilipshen S, Heilweil M, Quan S, Sternberg S, Enker W. Patterns of pelvic recurrence following definitive resections of rectal cancer. *Cancer* 1984;53:1354.

49. Gunderson LL, Sosin H. Areas of failure found at reoperation (second or symptomatic look) following "curative surgery" for adenocarcinoma of the rectum. *Cancer* 1974;34:1278.

50. Stockholm Rectal Cancer Study Group. Preoperative short-term radiation therapy in operable rectal carcinoma. *Cancer* 1990;66:49.

51. Rich T, Gunderson L, Lew R, et al. Patterns of recurrence of rectal cancer after potentially curative surgery. *Cancer* 1983;52:1317.

52. Martling A, Holm T, Johansson H, Rutqvist LE, Cedermark B. The Stockholm II trial on preoperative radiotherapy in rectal carcinoma: long-term follow-up of a population-based study. *Cancer* 2001;92:896.

53. Heald RJ. The "Holy Plane" of rectal surgery. *J Royal Soc Med* 1988;81:503.

54. Heald RJ, Moran BJ, Ryall RD, Sexton R, MacFarlane JK. Rectal cancer—the Basingstoke experience of total mesorecal excision, 1978-1997. *Arch Surg* 1998;133:894.

55. Arbman G, Nilsson E, Hallbïik O, Sjïdahl R. Local recurrence following total mesorectal excision for rectal cancer. *Br J Surg* 1996;83:375.

56. Swedish Rectal Cancer Trial. Improved survival with preoperative radiotherapy in resectable rectal cancer. *N Engl J Med* 1997;336:980.

57. Gastrointestinal Tumor Study Group. Prolongation of the disease-free interval in surgically treated rectal carcinoma. *N Engl J Med* 1985;312:1465.

58. Krook JE, Moertel CG, Gunderson L, et al. Effective surgical adjuvant therapy for high-risk rectal carcinoma. *N Engl J Med* 1991;324:709.

59. Fisher B, Wolmark N, Rockette H, et al. Postoperative adjuvant chemotherapy or radiation therapy for rectal cancer: results from NSABP protocol R-01. *J Natl Cancer Inst* 1988;80:21.

60. Wolmark N, Wieand HS, Hayams DM, et al. Randomized trial of postoperative adjuvant chemotherapy with or without radiotherapy for carcinoma of the rectum: National Surgical Adjuvant Breast and Bowel Project protocol R-02. *J Natl Cancer Inst* 2000;92:388.

61. Balslev IB, Pederson M, Teglbjaerg PS, et al. Postoperative radiotherapy in Dukes' B and C carcinoma of the rectum and rectosigmoid: a randomized multicenter study. *Cancer* 1986;58:22.

62. Medical Research Council Rectal Cancer Working Party. Randomised trial of surgery alone versus surgery followed by radiotherapy for mobile cancer of the rectum. *Lancet* 1996;348:1610.

63. O'Connell MJ, Martenson J, Wieand H, et al. Improving adjuvant therapy for rectal cancer by combining protracted-infusion fluorouracil with radiation therapy after curative surgery. *N Engl J Med* 1994;331:502.

64. Colorectal Cancer Collaborative Group. Adjuvant radiotherapy for rectal cancer: a systematic overview of 8507 patients from 22 randomized trials. *Lancet* 2001;358:1291.

65. Camma C, Giunta M, Fiorica F, et al. Preoperative radiotherapy for resectable rectal cancer. A meta-analysis. *JAMA* 2000;284:1008.

66. Pahlman L, Glimelius B. Pre- or postoperative radiotherapy in rectal and rectosigmoid carcinoma. *Ann Surg* 1990;211:187.

67. Frykholm GJ, Glimelius B, Pahlman L. Preoperative or postoperative irradiation in adenocarcinoma of the rectum: final treatment results of a randomized trial and an evaluation of late secondary effects. *Dis Colon Rectum* 1993;36:564.

68. Roh MS, Petrelli N, Wieand L, et al. Phase III randomized trial of preoperative versus postoperative multimodality therapy in patients with carcinoma of the rectum (NSABP R-03). In: ASCO 37th annual meeting, San Francisco, CA, 2001:123(abst 490).

69. Hyams D, Mamunas E, Petrelli N, et al. A clinical trial to evaluate the worth of preoperative multimodality therapy in patients with operable carcinoma of the rectum: a progress report of National Surgical Breast and Bowel Project Protocol R-03. *Dis Colon Rectum* 1997;40:131.

70. Sauer R, Group GRC. Adjuvant versus neoadjuvant combined modality treatment for locally advanced rectal cancer: first results of the German Rectal Cancer Study (CAO/ARO/AIO-94). *Int J Radiat Oncol Biol Phys* 2003;57:S124.

71. Willett CG, Badizadegan K, Ancukiewicz M, Shellito PC. Prognostic factors in stage T3N0 rectal cancer: Do all patients require postoperative pelvic irradiation and chemotherapy? *Dis Colon Rectum* 1999;42:167.

72. Gunderson LL, Sargent DJ, Tepper JE, et al. Impact of T and N substage on survival and disease relapse in adjuvant rectal cancer: a pooled analysis. *Int J Radiat Oncol Biol Phys* 2002;54:386.

73. Hernanz F, Revuelta S, Redondo C, Madrazo C. Colorectal adenocarcinoma: quality of the assessment of lymph node metastases. *Dis Colon Rectum* 1994;37:373.

74. Stocchi L, Nelson H, Sargent D, et al. Impact of surgical and pathologic variables in rectal cancer: a United States community and cooperative group report. *J Clin Oncol* 2001;19:3895.

75. Martling AL, Holm T, Rutqvist LEJ, et al. Effect of a surgical training programme on outcome of rectal cancer in the Country of Stockholm. *Lancet* 2000;356:93.

76. Tepper JE, O'Connell MJ, Niedzwicki D, et al. Final report of INT 0114—adjuvant therapy in rectal cancer: analysis by treatment, stage and gender. *Proc Am Soc Clin Oncol* 2001;123a(abst 489).

77. Smalley S, Benedetti J, Williamson S, et al. Intergroup 0144—phase III trial of 5-FU based chemotherapy regimens plus radiotherapy (XRT) in postoperative adjuvant rectal cancer. Bolus 5-FU vs prolonged venous infusion (PVI) before and after XRT vs bolus-5-FU + leucovorin (LV) + levamisole (LEV) before and after XRT + bolus 5-FU + LV. *ASCO Proceedings* 2003;22:251.

78. Saltz L, Raben D, Minsky BD, et al. Rectal cancer: presentation with metastatic and locally advanced disease. American College of Radiology. ACR appropriateness criteria. *Radiology* 2000;[Suppl 215]:1491.

79. Minsky B, Cohen A, Kemeny N, et al. Pre-operative combined 5-FU, low dose leucovorin, and sequential radiation therapy for unresectable rectal cancer. *Int J Radiat Oncol Biol Phys* 1993;25:821.

80. Dosoretz DE, Gunderson LL, Hedberg S, et al. Preoperative irradiation for unresectable rectal and rectosigmoid carcinomas. *Cancer* 1983;52:814.

81. Emami B, Miller E, Pilepich M, et al. Effect of preoperative irradiation on resectability of colorectal carcinomas. *Int J Radiat Oncol Biol Phys* 1982;8:1295.

82. Marsh R, Chu N, Vauthey J, et al. Preoperative treatment of patients with locally advanced unresectable rectal adenocarcinoma utilizing continuous chronobiologically shaped 5-fluorouracil infusion and radiation therapy. *Cancer* 1996;78:215.

83. Gunderson LL, Nelson H, Martenson JA, et al. Locally advanced primary colorectal cancer: intraoperative electron and external beam irradiation +/- 5-FU. *Int J Radiat Oncol Biol Phys* 1997;37:601.

84. Nakfoor BM, Willett CG, Shellito PC, Kaufman DS, Daly WJ. The impact of 5-fluorouracil and intraoperative electron beam radiation therapy on the outcome of patients with locally advanced primary rectal and rectosigmoid cancer. *Ann Surg* 1998;228:194.

85. Tepper JE, Wood WC, Cohen AM. Treatment of locally advanced rectal cancer with external beam radiation, surgical resection, and intraoperative radiation therapy. *Int J Radiat Oncol Biol Phys* 1989;16:1437.

86. Harrison LB, Minsky BD, Enker WE, et al. High dose rate intraoperative radiation therapy (HDR-IORT) as part of the management strategy for locally advanced primary and recurrent rectal cancer. *Int J Radiat Oncol Biol Phys* 1998;42:325.

87. Haddock MG, Nelson H, Donohue JH, et al. Intraoperative electron radiotherapy as a component of salvage therapy for patients with colorectal cancer and advanced nodal metastases. *Int J Radiat Oncol Biol Phys* 2003;56:966.

88. Wang C, Schulz M. The role of radiation therapy in the management of carcinoma of the sigmoid, rectosigmoid and rectum. *Radiology* 1962;79:1.

89. Overgaard M, Overgaard J. Dose-response relationship for radiation therapy of recurrent, residual, and primarily inoperable colorectal cancer. *Radiother Oncol* 1984;1:217.

90. Brierley JD, Cummings BJ, Wong CS, et al. Adenocarcinoma of the rectum treated by radical external radiation therapy. *Int J Radiat Oncol Biol Phys* 1995;31:255.

91. Frykholm GJ, Isacsson U, Nygard K, et al. Preoperative radiotherapy in rectal carcinoma—aspects of acute adverse effects and radiation technique. *Int J Radiat Oncol Biol Phys* 1996;35:1039.

92. Ooi BS, Tjandra JJ, Green MD. Morbidities of adjuvant chemotherapy and radiotherapy for resectable rectal cancer. *Dis Colon Rectum* 1999;42:403.

93. Gallagher MJ, Brereton HD, Rostock RA, et al. A prospective study of treatment techniques to minimize the volume of pelvic small bowel and reduction of acute and late effects associated with pelvic irradiation. *Int J Radiat Oncol Biol Phys* 1986;12:1565.

94. Shanahan TG, Mehta MP, Bertelrud KL, et al. Minimization of small bowel volume within treatment fields utilizing customized "belly boards." *Int J Radiat Oncol Biol Phys* 1990;19:469.

95. Fu YT, Lam JC, Tze JM. Measurement of irradiated small bowel volume in pelvic irradiation and the effect of a bellyboard. *Clin Oncol (R Coll Radiol)* 1995;7:188.

96. Hoffman JP, Sigurdson ER, Eisenberg BL. Use of saline-filled tissue expanders to protect the small bowel from radiation. *Oncology (Huntingt)* 1998;12:51.

97. Herbert SH, Solin LJ, Hoffman JP, et al. Volumetric analysis of small bowel displacement from radiation portals with the use of a pelvic tissue expander. *Int J Radiat Oncol Biol Phys* 1993;25:885.

98. Thom A, Baumann J, Chandler JJ, Devereux DF. Experience with high-dose radiation therapy and the intestinal sling procedure in patients with rectal carcinoma. *Cancer* 1990;70:581.

99. Lechner P, Cesnik H. Abdominopelvic omentopexy: preparatory procedure for radiotherapy in rectal cancer. *Dis Colon Rectum* 1992;35:1157.

100. Chen JS, ChangChien CR, Wang JY, Fan HA. Pelvic peritoneal reconstruction to prevent radiation enteritis in rectal carcinoma. *Dis Colon Rectum* 1992;35:897.

101. Talley NA, Chen F, King D, Jones M, Talley NJ. Short-chain fatty acids in the treatment of radiation proctitis: a randomized, double-blind, placebo-controlled, cross-over pilot trial. *Dis Colon Rectum* 1997;40:1046.

102. O'Brien PC, Franklin CI, Dear KB, et al. A phase III double-blind randomised study of rectal sucralfate suspension in the prevention of acute radiation proctitis. *Radiother Oncol* 1997;45:117.

103. Resbeut M, Marteau P, Cowen D, et al. A randomized double blind placebo controlled multicenter study of mesalazine for the prevention of acute radiation enteritis. *Radiother Oncol* 1997;44:59.

104. Craighead PS, Young S. Phase II study assessing the feasibility of using elemental supplements to reduce acute enteritis in patients receiving radical pelvic radiotherapy. *Am J Clin Oncol* 1998;21:573.

105. Liu T, Liu Y, He S, Zhang Z, Kligerman MM. Use of radiation with or without WR-2721 in advanced rectal cancer. *Cancer* 1992;69:2820.

106. Athanassiou H, Antonadou D, Coliarakis N, et al. Protective effect of amifostine during fractionated radiotherapy in patients with pelvic carcinomas: results of a randomized trial. *Int J Radiat Oncol Biol Phys* 2003;56:1154.

107. Minsky BD, Mies C, Rich TA, Recht A, Chaffey JT. Potentially curative surgery of colon cancer: patterns of failure and survival. *J Clin Oncol* 1988;6:106.

108. Bonadeo FA, Vaccaro CA, Benati ML, et al. Rectal cancer: local recurrence after surgery without radiotherapy. *Dis Colon Rectum* 2001;44:374.

BERNARD J. CUMMINGS
JAFFER A. AJANI
CAROL J. SWALLOW

SECTION 10

Cancer of the Anal Region

Multimodality treatment intended to preserve anorectal function whenever possible is firmly established as the preferred management for squamous cell cancers of the anal region. Combinations of radiation and chemotherapy, with radical surgery reserved for residual cancer, form the basis of this approach. Recent progress has been made in understanding the epidemiology, etiology, and pathology of anal cancer and in developing more effective treatment schedules.

ANATOMY

The anal region lies at a transition between endoderm and ectoderm and is commonly divided into the anal canal and the perianal skin. The anal canal extends from the rectum to the perianal skin and is 3 to 4 cm long. The superior margin is at the level of the palpable upper border of the anal sphincter and puborectalis muscle of the anorectal ring. The distal margin, the anal verge, is the lowermost level at which the walls of the canal are in contact in their normal resting state. The anus is the distal external opening of the intestinal tract, although the term is sometimes applied to the anal region or to the anal verge. The extent of the perianal skin is not defined but is usually considered to encompass a 5-m radius around the anal verge. The terms *anal margin* and *perianal skin* are now generally regarded as synonymous. However, there are considerable variation and inconsistency in the definition of different parts of the anal region, although a standardized terminology has been proposed.[1]

Four different types of epithelium are found in the region. The perianal skin is similar to hair- and glandular-bearing skin elsewhere and becomes puckered and pigmented near the anal verge. At the verge it blends with the pale mucosa of the distal canal, which is lined by modified squamous epithelium lacking skin appendages. Just below the dentate or pectinate line, the most visible landmark in the canal and formed by the lower end of the anal valves, the squamous epithelium blends with a transitional epithelium that has rectal, urothelial, and squamous features. The purplish-red transitional zone extends proximally for approximately 1 to 2 cm, where it merges with the pink glandular mucosa of the rectum.

The veins of the anal canal communicate with the portal and the systemic venous systems. Venous plexuses in the mucosa and muscles of the anal wall anastomose around the anal verge and distal canal. The distal plexuses communicate with the systemic venous system through the internal pudendal and internal iliac veins. The plexuses of the proximal canal drain principally to the portal system via the inferior mesenteric vein.

The lymphatics of the anal region flow to three lymph node systems. Lymph from the perianal skin and the canal distal to the dentate line drains mainly to the superficial inguinal nodes, with some inconstant communications to the femoral or external iliac nodes. Lymph from about and above the dentate line flows with that from the distal rectum to the internal pudendal, hypogastric, and obturator nodes of the internal iliac system. The drainage of the proximal canal is to the perirectal and superior hemorrhoidal nodes of the inferior mesenteric system. Numerous lymphatic connections exist between the various levels of the anal canal.

The cerebrospinal and autonomic nervous systems contribute to the maintenance of anorectal continence. The striated muscle of the external sphincter is under voluntary control and innervated by the internal rectal nerve, a branch of the pudendal nerve that arises from the second, third, and fourth sacral nerves (S2, S3, S4). Pain, touch, and other sensations from the lining of the anal canal below the dentate line and from the perianal skin are conducted by the internal rectal nerve. Parasympathetic nerves from S2, S3, and S4, and sympathetic fibers from the hypogastric plexus, supply the smooth muscle of the internal sphincter. The upper canal has selective sensitivity for differences in intraluminal pressure, and the autonomic nerves mediate the inhibitor and the facilitator reflexes of the internal sphincter.

PATHOLOGY

The World Health Organization histologic classification of anal tumors has undergone several revisions. The current recommendation, published in 2000,[2] is to use the term *anal intraepithelial neoplasia* (AIN) for precancerous changes in the squamous epithelium of the anal canal and perianal skin (in the skin, such changes are also called *Bowen's disease*). The pathology and molecular biology of AIN have been reviewed in detail.[3] The generic term *anal squamous cell carcinoma* is recommended for the various subtypes described in the previous classification, namely, basaloid (cloacogenic), large cell keratinizing, and large cell nonkeratinizing. This change is based in part on the mixed histopathologic features found in most tumors, the availability for examination in current practice of only small biopsy samples that may not be representative of the whole tumor, and the poor reproducibility of subtype classification among histopathologists. For some years in the clinical literature, many authors grouped the subtypes of squamous cell cancer as "epidermoid" cancer, in recognition of their similar natural histories. The term *epidermoid* does not appear in the current recommended histologic classification. Adenocarcinomas have now also been consolidated into a single grouping. Squamous cell carcinoma with mucinous microcysts and small cell (anaplastic) carcinoma continue to be recognized as subtypes but are rare.

Squamous cell carcinomas of the perianal skin are often of the large cell variant and keratinizing. Verrucous carcinoma or giant malignant condyloma is characterized by local destructive invasion without metastases. Other cancers of the perianal skin, such as basal cell cancer and adenocarcinoma, are similar to those that arise in the skin elsewhere.

EPIDEMIOLOGY

Anal cancers are approximately one-tenth as common as cancers of the rectum. Cancers arise in the canal three to four times more frequently than in the perianal skin. The median age at diagnosis is from 60 to 65 years. Considerable geographic variation is found in the incidence rates and histologic types of anal cancer. For example, in North America and western Europe, squamous cell cancers make up approximately 80% of anal cancers, but in Japan only 20% are squamous, the remainder being mainly adenocarcinomas. Most annual incidence rates lie in the range 0.5 to 1.0 per 100,000 among women and 0.3 to 0.8 per 100,000 among men.[4] Squamous cancers of the anal canal are approximately 1.5 to 4.0 times more common in women, although this difference appears to

have arisen only in the last 50 years[5] and may be declining. Perianal cancers occur with approximately equal frequency in both sexes. Increases in the incidence of anal cancer have been noted in several countries. In the United States, the age-adjusted incidence of squamous anal cancer in white men rose, at an estimated average annual rate of 2.6% per year, from 0.41 per 100,000 in 1973 to 1976 to 0.71 in 1993 to 1996.[6] The corresponding figures for white women were an annual rate of increase of 1.5% per year, from an incidence per 100,000 of 0.78 in 1973 to 1976 to 0.95 in 1993 to 1996. The incidence in black women and men also rose during this period. The incidence of AIN rose even more rapidly, with annual increases in the incidence rates of 4.6% in women and 6.6% in men.[6]

RISK FACTORS AND ETIOLOGY

Evidence has been shown that sexually transmissible agents, such as human papillomavirus (HPV), immunosuppression, and tobacco smoking, are of particular importance. A number of similarities have been noted between squamous cancers of the anal region and of the uterine cervix, vagina, and vulva, the epithelia of which have common features and embryologic origin. It is known that several specific types of HPV are linked to cancers and precursor lesions in the anogenital epithelia and that these HPV types are readily transferred sexually. Many observations first made in squamous cancers of the lower female genital tract have been repeated in anal squamous cancer.[3] HPV type 16 has a particularly high risk of association with anal squamous cancer, as have, to a lesser extent, types 18, 31, 33, 35, and others. These high-risk HPVs (hrHPVs) have been found in approximately 85% of anal squamous cancers in some series, the proportion being partly dependent on the sensitivity of the assay[3,7,8] and subject also to geographic variation.[9] In a series of 386 patients, 86% of whom had invasive cancers, hrHPV were identified in 90% of the anal squamous cancers in women and in 63% of those in men.[7] Squamous cancers arising in the anal canal were hrHPV positive in 92%, compared to 64% in the perianal skin.[7] Because of this discrepancy, it has been suggested that there may be another pathway, not mediated by HPV, by which perianal squamous cancer can develop.[7] The hrHPV E6 and E7 proteins are thought to contribute to the induction of anogenital cancers by interacting with and degrading the function of p53 and pRb, respectively. However, the final progression to invasive anal cancer is not thought to be mediated by HPV oncoproteins. No convincing evidence has been shown that other previously suspect viruses, such as herpes simplex virus, play a role in the etiology of anal squamous cancer.[5]

The identification of a twofold increase in the risk of anal cancer in unmarried men in register-based studies first suggested that sexual behavior might affect the risk of anal cancer. Never-married status among men was assumed to include a relatively high proportion of homosexual men, and more direct studies of this latter group have confirmed their increased risk, presumptively related to anal intercourse. Compared to the overall annual incidence of anal cancer in white men in the United States of approximately 0.7 per 100,000, the estimated incidence in the male homosexual population, before the acquired immunodeficiency syndrome (AIDS) epidemic, ranged from approximately 12 to 37 per 100,000.[10] Recent case-control studies have suggested that a history of multiple sexual partners in homosexual or heterosexual relationships, or of unprotected anal intercourse in men and in women (in the latter, before the age of 30), is predictive of an increased risk of AIN and invasive anal cancer.[5] Such sexual behavior and practices increase the opportunities for transmission of hrHPV.

The ability to prevent or eliminate viral infection is reduced by compromise of cell-mediated immunity. Iatrogenically immunosuppressed organ transplant patients have an increased risk of several types of malignancy, including anogenital squamous cancers.[11] Anal cancer is not at this time an AIDS-defining neoplasm. However, data from the United States AIDS-Cancer registry linkage study do suggest a significant relationship between AIDS and anal squamous cancer.[12] In that study the rate of HPV-associated cancers and precursors was increased in human immunodeficiency virus (HIV)–infected persons for all anogenital sites compared with the general population. The relative risk for anal cancers was 6.8 in women and 37.9 in men. When HIV exposure category was considered, all categories, including male homosexual anal intercourse (the highest anal cancer risk category), injection drug use, transfusion, and heterosexual contact for women, were associated with an increased risk of anal cancer. However, the evidence implicating HIV-induced immunosuppression as a risk factor for anal cancer, independent of sexual practices and behavior, is still considered inconclusive. Although some investigators have identified an incidence of anal squamous cancer in HIV-positive homosexual men approximately double that in those who are HIV negative,[13] others have found little, if any, difference.[5] Whether immunosuppression is iatrogenic or due to HIV infection, those affected have increased rates of anogenital HPV infection, higher progression rates from normal epithelium to AIN and from low to higher-grade AIN, and lower rates of clearance of HPV and regression from abnormal to normal epithelium.[14,15]

In view of the associations between HIV and HPV infections and anal squamous cancers, it has been postulated that the increasing effectiveness of antiretroviral therapy may lead to longer survival of HIV-infected patients and an increased number with anal squamous cancer.[16] Based on observations in renal transplant recipients, the interval between the induction of iatrogenic immunosuppression and the diagnosis of anal cancer is relatively prolonged, averaging 88 months, approximately twice the interval for Kaposi's sarcoma and non-Hodgkin's lymphoma.[11] This prolonged period before the clinical diagnosis of anal cancer may account for the observation that, since the widespread use of highly active antiretroviral therapy (HAART), substantial reductions have occurred in the incidence of Kaposi's sarcoma and lymphoma but, at the time of the review, no significant change in the incidence of other less common malignancies, including anogenital cancers.[17]

Although tobacco smoking is associated with an approximately fivefold increase in risk in several case-control studies,[5,18] it has been suggested that these studies might have been confounded in part by unreported male homosexuality.[5] It has been postulated that an antiestrogenic action of tobacco products may contribute to anogenital squamous carcinogenesis.[19]

Benign anal conditions such as fistulas, fissures, and hemorrhoids do not appear to predispose to cancer, although fissures may facilitate the access of hrHPV to basal epithelial cell layers.[5] The risk of cancer from chronic inflammatory bowel disease appears to be largely discounted by a Danish population-based cohort study of 2723 patients with Crohn's disease and 6334 patients with ulcerative colitis, followed an average of 10 years, which failed to identify any significant increase in the risk of squamous anal cancer.[20]

NATURAL HISTORY

Squamous cell cancers of the anal region, especially the canal, are believed to be preceded by high-grade AIN in most instances.[21] However, it has been estimated that no more than 1% of patients with AIN develop invasive cancer per year,[22] a rate lower than that described for cervical intraepithelial neoplasia.[3] During a 2-year period of observation in a male homosexual group, low-grade AIN was observed to progress to high grade in some patients, particularly those who were HIV positive, but progression to invasive cancer was not detected during the course of the study.[23] The finding of AIN adjacent to invasive cancer is suggestive but not conclusive evidence of progression of AIN.[21] Anal dysplasia frequently recurs after treatment, presumably because of unrecognized wide-field abnormalities and persistence or reinfection with hrHPV.

Squamous cell cancers of the anal canal are characterized by local extension of the primary tumor and lymphatic spread rather than by hematogenous metastases. The primary cancers grow along the length and circumference of the canal and invade the sphincter muscles and perianal connective tissues quite early. At diagnosis, only 12% of tumors were confined to the mucosa and submucosa, and 34% to the sphincter muscles (without regional node metastases) in one series of 137 patients.[24] Cancer extends beyond the canal into the rectum or perianal skin, or both, in approximately half the cases. Deep invasion of the anovaginal septum occurs in approximately 10%, but invasion of the prostate is very uncommon.

Lymphatic spread also occurs early. The regional nodes for the anal canal are now considered to be the perirectal, internal iliac, and inguinal nodes.[25,26] The nodes of the rectosigmoid and sigmoid vascular arcades are regarded as distant metastatic sites. It should be remembered that data on the risk of pelvic nodal involvement are based on surgical series, in which internal iliac nodes were not routinely removed but rectosigmoid and sigmoid nodes were. In surgical series, there were metastatic nodes in the pelvic and inferior mesenteric regions in 26% (279 of 1076 patients in 14 series, range of positive nodes 10% to 40%). In radiation-based and surgical series, inguinal node metastases, not all confirmed by histology, were found at presentation in 22% (320 of 1474 patients, 10 series, range of abnormal nodes 9% to 40%). Based on late relapse rates, inguinal node metastases were present subclinically in a further 10% to 20%.[27–29] Nodal metastases were found with 30% of cancers confined to the sphincter muscles, and with 60% of those that had extended to extrasphincteric tissues or were poorly differentiated.[30] Although some authors found that the rate of lymph node metastases correlated to increasing size of the primary cancer,[30] others observed that, for primary cancers greater than 2 cm in size, increasing size was not a reliable predictor of metastasis to nodes.[24]

Extrapelvic metastases at the time of first presentation are not common and are identified in fewer than 5%.[31] Metastases occur as the sole site of failure in approximately 10% after successful treatment of the primary cancer and regional nodes.

Metastases may occur via the portal or systemic venous systems or via lymphatics. They are found most frequently in the liver, lungs, and extrapelvic lymph nodes and occasionally in bone, skin, brain, and other sites.

Relapse after treatment directed principally to the pelvis, and with only limited systemic therapy, is more common at the site of the primary tumor and regional nodes than outside the pelvis. The risk of local-regional relapse in current practice is up to approximately 30% and extrapelvic failure up to approximately 20%.[24,32,33] The overall 5-year survival rates in population-based registries, generally reflecting treatment practices before current radiation and chemotherapy combinations, are on the order of 55%.[31,34]

Perianal squamous cancers tend to grow locally. They may extend into the anal canal. When there is doubt about the site of origin, it is conventional to classify the cancer as arising in the canal. The most common site of spread is to the ipsilateral inguinal nodes, which are reported to be abnormal in from 5% to 20%. Extrapelvic metastases are uncommon and are usually associated with poorly differentiated cancers, inguinal metastases, or uncontrolled and extensive primary tumors. Overall 5-year cause-specific survival rates usually exceed 80%.

STAGING

The staging system in widest use is the classification endorsed by the American Joint Committee on Cancer[25] and the Union Internationale Contre le Cancer (UICC)[26] (Tables 29.10-1 and 29.10-2). Although this system presents composite TNM (tumor, node, metastasis) stage groups, most reports describe results by T category or N category only.

The size of the primary tumor is established by clinical examination and, less frequently, by imaging such as computed tomography, magnetic resonance imaging, or transanal ultrasound. Direct invasion of adjacent organs (category T4) is uncommon. Vaginal fistulas from primary anal canal cancers are found in fewer than 5% of women, although infiltration of the vaginal mucosa may be found in up to approximately 10%. Invasion of the anovaginal septum without involvement of the vaginal mucosa is generally considered insufficient to categorize a cancer as T4. Invasion of the prostate is rare and is best appreciated by imaging.

Only the inguinal and lower perirectal lymph nodes are accessible to clinical examination. As many as half of all palpable inguinal nodes are enlarged due to reactive hyperplasia,[35] and needle biopsy or simple excision of clinically or radiologically suspicious inguinal nodes for histologic examination is recommended. Most investigators have reported a very low incidence of palpable perirectal node metastases of approximately 1% to 3%,[36] although a few have described rates as high as 30%.[37] In a small series of patients with anal canal primary cancers managed surgically, 44% of the metastatic nodes found in the internal iliac and superior hemorrhoidal chains were less than 0.5 cm in size.[38] Nodes of this size cannot be identified reliably by currently available imaging techniques, although positron emission tomography may eventually prove useful. Although generally technically feasible, abnormal pelvic nodes identified on imaging are not usually subjected to fine-needle biopsy, and the diagnosis of metastasis in these nodes is based on radiologic criteria. The role of sentinel node biopsy for anal cancer has not been defined.[39,40]

TABLE 29.10-1. Anal Canal TNM Classification

PRIMARY TUMOR (T)	
TX	Primary tumor cannot be assessed
T0	No evidence of primary tumor
Tis	Carcinoma *in situ*
T1	Tumor 2 cm or less in greatest dimension
T2	Tumor more than 2 cm but not more than 5 cm in greatest dimension
T3	Tumor more than 5 cm in greatest dimension
T4	Tumor of any size invades adjacent organ(s), for example, vagina, urethra, bladder [involvement of the sphincter muscle(s) *alone* is not classified as T4]
REGIONAL LYMPH NODES (N)	
NX	Regional lymph nodes cannot be assessed
N0	No regional lymph node metastasis
N1	Metastasis in perirectal lymph nodes(s)
N2	Metastasis in unilateral internal iliac and/or unilateral inguinal lymph node(s)
N3	Metastasis in perirectal and inguinal lymph nodes and/or bilateral internal iliac and/or bilateral inguinal lymph nodes
DISTANT METASTASES (M)	
MX	Distant metastasis cannot be assessed
M0	No distant metastasis
M1	Distant metastasis

STAGING GROUPING			
Stage 0	Tis	N0	M0
Stage I	T1	N0	M0
Stage II	T2, T3	N0	M0
Stage IIIA	T1, T2, T3	N1	M0
	T4	N0	M0
Stage IIIB	T4	N1	M0
	Any T	N2, N3	M0
Stage IV	Any T	Any N	M1

TABLE 29.10-2.   Perianal Skin TNM Classification

PRIMARY TUMOR (T)

TX	Primary tumor (T)
T0	No evidence of primary tumor
Tis	Carcinoma *in situ*
T1	Tumor 2 cm or less in greatest dimension
T2	Tumor more than 2 cm but not more than 5 cm in greatest dimension
T3	Tumor more than 5 cm in greatest dimension
T4	Tumor invades deep extradermal structures (i.e., cartilage, skeletal muscle, or bone)

REGIONAL LYMPH NODES (N)

NX	Regional lymph nodes cannot be assessed
N0	No regional lymph node metastasis
N1	Regional lymph node metastasis

DISTANT METASTASIS (M)

MX	Distant metastasis cannot be assessed
M0	No distant metastasis
M1	Distant metastasis

STAGE GROUPING

Stage 0	Tis	N0	M0
Stage I	T1	N0	M0
Stage II	T2, T3	N0	M0
Stage III	T4	N0	M0
	Any T	N1	M0
Stage IV	Any T	Any N	M1

The most common sites of metastases from cancers of the canal are the pelvic or paraaortic nodes, liver, and lungs. These sites can be examined by appropriately directed computed tomography or MR examinations, although a chest film is generally considered an adequate screen for lung metastases. Other investigations, such as skeletal imaging, are indicated only when focal symptoms are present. Imaging studies should be supplemented by full blood count and liver function tests.

For perianal cancers, staging investigations may be restricted to evaluation of the primary cancer and the regional inguinal lymph nodes. Only if the cancer is massive or poorly differentiated, or if inguinal node metastases are confirmed, is more extensive imaging necessary.

PROGNOSTIC FACTORS

Among the many cancer, patient, and treatment factors studied, the anatomic extent of an anal cancer provides the most useful and reproducible prognostic information.[41,42] Extrapelvic metastases carry the worst prognosis.[43] In the absence of distant metastases, the size of the primary tumor is the most useful predictor of local control, preservation of anorectal function, and survival.[32,44] Spread to regional lymph nodes is an adverse factor for survival in most series,[29,32,36,45] and in some series,[45] but not all,[32,46] for control of the primary tumor.

Age and performance status have each been considered prognostic, but case selection affects interpretation of many reports. Women have a better prognosis in some series.[44,45,47] Hemoglobin levels of 10 g/L or less at presentation have been correlated with lower local control and survival rates.[48] Serum markers such as carcinoembryonic antigen and squamous cell carcinoma antigen have not provided consistent results when evaluated as aids to diagnosis or monitoring of response. In HIV-positive patients high viral load, low lymphocyte CD4+ counts, and AIDS have been prognostic of poor local tumor control and survival and, in some series, of impaired tolerance of radiation and chemotherapy.[49,50]

In an extensive review of prognostic factors from the perspective of the pathologist, Fenger[42] surveyed nearly 50 reports on cytogenetic, flow cytometric, immunohistochemical, and other investigations. He considered that these studies, most of which were performed on small groups of patients and without standardization of techniques, offered insights on pathogenesis but did not provide guidance to prognosis of the individual or selection of treatment.

ANAL CANAL SQUAMOUS CANCERS

ANAL INTRAEPITHELIAL NEOPLASIA

The role of screening programs for patients at high risk of AIN has not been established, although it has been argued that screening of men who practice anal intercourse, particularly those who are HIV positive, would be clinically and economically effective.[51] Anoscopy, anal cytology, and high-resolution anal colposcopy each play a role in the assessment of AIN.[3] Although the ideal treatment has not been determined, several local surgical measures are effective in ablating clinically apparent lesions.[3,52] However, high-grade AIN recurs or persists in up to 80% of HIV-positive patients and in fewer than 25% of those who are HIV negative.[3,52] Some authors recommend observation only for wide-field low-grade AIN and even for high-grade AIN when there are no signs of invasive cancer, if the risk of functional damage due to ablative treatment is considered too great.[3] The natural history of areas of AIN adjacent to invasive cancer treated by radiation or radiation and chemotherapy is not known. The presence of specific viral antigens in HPV-related neoplastic conditions such as AIN suggests possible roles in the future for therapeutic and prophylactic vaccines.[53]

TABLE 29.10-3. Selected Results of Radiation Therapy (RT) Alone

| Reference | Radiation | Primary Tumor Control by RT | | | Serious Complications—Colostomy | 5-Y Survival |
		T1	T1, T2	T3, T4		
Newman et al.[47]	50 Gy/20/4 wk	8/9 (≤2 cm)	42/52 (81%) (≤5 cm)	13/20 (65%) (>5 cm or T4)	2/72 (3%)	66%, crude
Martenson and Gunderson[55]	45–50 Gy/ 25–28/5–6 wk plus boost to 55–67 Gy	9/9 (≤2 cm)	17/17 (100%) (≤5 cm)	—	2 temp/17	94%, actuarial
Otim-Oyet et al.[56]	60–65 Gy/ 30–33/6–7 wk (some with boost)	2/2 (≤2 cm)	16/22 (73%) (≤4 cm)	8/17 (47%) (>4 cm)	1/24 (4%)	56%, cause-specific
Deniaud-Alexandre et al.[36]	45 Gy/20/ 4.5 wk plus boost after 5 wk 20 Gy EB or I	21/26 (80%) (≤2 cm)	131/167 (78%) (≤5 cm)	76/138 (55%) (≤5 cm or T4)	17/305 (6%)	67%, actuarial
Papillon et al.[57]	42 Gy/10/ 2.5 wk plus I 20 Gy after 8 wk	NS	29/39 (74%) (≤4 cm)	27/64 (42%) (>4 cm)	6/103 (6%)	60%, crude

EB, external beam; I, interstitial brachytherapy; NS, not stated; temp, temporary.

EARLY-STAGE CANCER (SUPERFICIAL STAGE I)

Local excision can be considered for superficial well- or moderately differentiated squamous cell cancers up to approximately 2 cm in size, because the risk of lymph node metastases from small tumors that have not invaded the sphincter muscles is less than 5%.[24] Although some authors have reported that no patients died of cancer within 5 years of local excision,[24,35] in one series only 12 of 19 patients (63%) survived.[54] Cure rates of up to 100% have been reported for patients with category T1 cancers treated by radiation therapy alone (Table 29.10-3). However, many centers now manage all localized anal cancers by combined radiation and chemotherapy.

The role of local excision alone is controversial for small or microscopic invasive cancers found incidentally in tissues excised for what was thought to be a benign condition. The specimen is often difficult to orient, margins may be uncertain or inadequate, and reexcision may not be practical. Radiation doses on the order of 30 Gy in 3 weeks, combined with chemotherapy, appear to prevent recurrence and carry a low risk of morbidity.[58]

INTERMEDIATE-STAGE CANCER (STAGES I, II, AND III)

Primary Tumor

Combined modality treatment for anal cancer was first described in 1974 by Nigro et al.[59] These investigators observed complete tumor regression in three patients given preoperative radiation, 5-fluorouracil (5-FU), and mitomycin or porfiromycin to reduce the risk of local recurrence commonly associated with abdominoperineal resection. A number of centers subsequently adopted this approach as definitive treatment, reserving radical surgery for the management of residual cancer.

Three randomized trials have established combined modality therapy, using initial radiation therapy, 5-FU, and mitomycin, as well as salvage surgery, as the standard against which other treatments should be compared.[33,45,60] In two of these trials,[33,45] this combination was superior to the same schedule of radiation alone. The third trial[60] demonstrated that combining radiation with 5-FU and mitomycin gave better results than administering 5-FU alone with radiation. Nonrandomized comparisons of this triple-agent radiation-based treatment with radical surgery have shown similar survival rates.[31]

The trials conducted by the United Kingdom Coordinating Committee for Cancer Research (UKCCCR)[33] and the European Organization for Research on Treatment of Cancer (EORTC)[45] both showed statistically significant advantages in the rate of control of the primary cancer and colostomy-free survival rates in patients who received combined modality therapy compared to radiation alone. The UKCCCR trial also showed better cause-specific survival, an end point not described by the EORTC. In neither trial did the improvement in overall survival rates reach statistical significance (Table 29.10-4).

In the UKCCCR trial, 577 patients with all stages of anal squamous cancer (UICC staging system, 1987 edition; same as 2002 edition[26]) were randomized between radiation alone and radiation combined with chemotherapy. In 75%, the primary tumor developed in the anal canal, and in the remainder it arose in the perianal skin. Forty percent had primary tumors larger than 5 cm in size (category T3) or deeply invasive (category T4), 20% had clinically positive nodes, and 2% had known extrapelvic metastases. Chemotherapy consisted of 5-FU (1000 mg/m^2/24 h for 96 hours or 750 mg/m^2/24 h for 120 hours) by continuous peripheral intravenous infusion in the first and final weeks of radiation treatment, plus mitomycin (12 mg/m^2) by bolus intravenous injection on day 1 of the first course of chemotherapy. The radiation dosage was 45 Gy in 20 to 25 fractions in 4 to 5 weeks, by anterior and posterior opposed fields that extended upward from the perineum to

TABLE 29.10-4. Three-Year Results of Randomized Trials of Radiation Alone (RT) versus Radiation, 5-Fluorouracil, and Mitomycin (RTCT) (Percentages)

	UKCCCR (n = 577)			EORTC (n = 103)		
	RT	RTCT	P Value	RT	RTCT	P Value
Local-regional control	39	61	<.0001	55	65	.02
Cause-specific survival	61	72	.02	NS	NS	NS
Overall survival	58	65	.25	65	70	.17

EORTC, European Organization for Research and Treatment of Cancer; NS, not stated; UKCCCR, United Kingdom Coordinating Committee for Cancer Research.

cover the regional nodes to the level of the midsacrum and laterally to encompass the inguinal nodes. Patients were reassessed clinically 6 weeks after treatment. If the primary tumor had not regressed by at least 50%, surgery was recommended. Only 10% of tumors in each study group failed to show at least partial response. All other patients received an additional 15 Gy in six fractions by perineal external-beam irradiation or 25 Gy over 2 to 3 days by temporary iridium 192 implant. Failure in the primary tumor or regional lymph nodes was recorded in 81 of 285 (28%) of those treated by chemoradiation and in 147 of 283 (52%) of those who received radiation alone. The investigators broadened the definition of local-regional failure to include treatment-related morbidity requiring surgery (ten patients in each study group) or inability to close a colostomy opened before treatment (seven patients in each treatment arm). Acute toxicity, particularly hematologic, skin, gastrointestinal, and genitourinary, was increased in the combined modality arm, but late morbidity was comparable in each group. Six deaths (2%) occurred as a result of treatment in the combined modality and two (0.7%) in the irradiation-alone arm.

In the European study, 103 patients with advanced cancers of the anal canal were entered on a trial of similar design.[45] Eighty-five percent had category T3 or T4 tumors (UICC staging system, 1987 edition), and 51% had abnormal nodes. The radiation dose was 45 Gy in 25 fractions over 5 weeks. Chemotherapy consisted of 5-FU (750 mg/m²/24 h by continuous infusion for 120 hours) in the first and fifth week of radiation and a single bolus injection of mitomycin (15 mg/m²) on day 1 of the first course of 5-FU only. Six weeks later, patients in whom a complete regression of the primary tumor had occurred received an additional 15 Gy by interstitial or external-beam radiation. A dose of 20 Gy was given to those who had had partial tumor response. As in the UK trial, the probability of local control and retention of anorectal function was improved by combined modality treatment. One of 51 patients who received chemoradiation died of toxicity. Acute and late toxicity rates were similar. However, the investigators noted that, in this study for which only patients with relatively advanced cancers were eligible, the probability of surviving 3 years or more without relapse, major treatment-related morbidity, or a colostomy was only approximately 30%.

A randomized trial conducted by the Radiation Therapy Oncology Group (RTOG) and Eastern Cooperative Oncology Group showed that it was more effective to give mitomycin and 5-FU with radiation than 5-FU alone.[60] Two hundred and ninety-one patients with squamous cancers of the anal canal of any T or N category (RTOG staging system), and without extrapelvic metastases, were studied. Approximately 40% had cancers larger than 5 cm or invading adjacent organs, and 17% had abnormal nodes. The radiation dosage was 45.0 to 50.4 Gy in 25 to 28 fractions over 5 weeks, by a shrinking field technique that delivered 30.6 Gy in 3.5 weeks to the primary tumor and pelvic and inguinal regional nodes from the perineum to the level of L5 to S1 and higher doses to the lower pelvis. Chemotherapy was given during the first and fifth week of radiation. Each course consisted of 5-FU (1000 mg/m²/24 h by continuous intravenous infusion over 96 hours), with or without mitomycin (10 mg/m² by bolus intravenous injection), on the first day of each course. Patients underwent biopsy of the primary tumor site 6 weeks after treatment. Biopsies were positive in 14% of those who received 5-FU only and in 8% who received both drugs with radiation (P = .14). Patients with positive biopsies from either study group in whom preservation of anal function was considered feasible had the option of receiving an additional 9 Gy in five treatments coupled with a concurrent infusion of 5-FU (1000 mg/m²/24 h for 96 hours) and a single injection of cisplatin (100 mg/m²) on day 2. This treatment resulted in tumor control without colostomy in 7 of 22 patients. At 5 years, the rates of colostomy (11% vs. 22%, P = .02) significantly favored treatment with radiation, 5-FU, and mitomycin.[61] Overall survival rates were similar (67% vs. 65%), but the disease-free survival rate was improved by the combination of radiation with both drugs (67% vs. 50%, P = .006). The rate of hematologic toxicity was increased by mitomycin. Four of 146 (2.7%) patients who received 5-FU and mitomycin experienced fatal toxicity, as did 1 of 145 (0.7%) treated with radiation and 5-FU alone.

Based on tabulation of nonrandomized studies,[62] the combination of radiation, 5-FU, and mitomycin has resulted in 5-year survival rates of approximately 80% for cancers of 2 cm or less in size (T1), 70% for tumors of 2 to 5 cm (T2), 45% to 55% for larger or deeply invasive cancers (T3 or T4), and 65% to 75% overall. The corresponding local control rates (excluding salvage treatment) were approximately 90% to 100% (T1), 65% to 75% (T2), 40% to 55% (T3 or T4), and 60% overall. Up to 5% of patients overall lost anorectal function because of treatment-related morbidity.

Efforts to identify the optimum cytotoxic drug or drug combination schedule and doses continue. The drugs studied most extensively are 5-FU, mitomycin, cisplatin, carboplatin, and bleomycin. Bleomycin is not thought to be of benefit.[34] Over the past decade there has been growing interest in combining 5-FU with cisplatin rather than mitomycin. Cisplatin and 5-FU have proven effective against squamous cell cancer in other sites in the alimentary tract and produce high response rates in metastatic anal cancer; cisplatin may enhance the effects of radiation, whereas mitomycin, as used clinically, does not, and the toxicity of cisplatin is considered by some to be less potentially harmful than that of mitomycin. Selected studies of radiation, 5-FU, and cisplatin are shown in Table 29.10-5.

Several empiric observations suggest that the results of the delivery of chemotherapy concurrently with radiation treatment rather than sequentially may vary with the drugs used. In the case of 5-FU and mitomycin, there is evidence from comparison of nonrandomized series that administration of the drugs

TABLE 29.10-5. Selected Results of Radiation and Concurrent 5-Fluorouracil and Cisplatin

Study	Chemotherapy		Radiation (Dose/ Fractions/Time)	Primary Tumor Complete Response	Survival
	5-FU	Cisplatin			
Gerard et al.[46]	1000 mg/m²/24 h IVI (96 h) D1–4	25 mg/m²IVB D1–4	40 Gy/10/D1–17 plus boost D63–64	76/94 (81%)[a]	84% 5-y actuarial
Martenson et al.[63]	1000 mg/m²/24 h IVI (96 h) D1–4, D43–46	75 mg/m²IVB D1, D43	59.4 Gy/33/D1–59 split at 36 Gy	13/19 (68%)	Maximum follow-up 33 mo
Doci et al.[64]	750 mg/m²/24 h IVI (96 h) D1–4, D22–25 Some plus 3rd cycle	100 mg/m²IVB D1, D22 Some plus 3rd cycle	54 Gy/30/D1–42 some plus boost	32/35 (91%) at 6 mo	Median follow-up 37 mo
Hung et al.[65]	250 mg/m²/24 h IVI (120 h) 5 d/ wk D1–42	4 mg/m²/24 h IVI (120 h) 5 d/wk D1–42	55 Gy/30/D1–42	76/92 (82%)[a]	91% 5-y actuarial

IVB, intravenous bolus injection; IVI, continuous intravenous infusion; NS, not stated.
[a]Local control for at least 12 months; other studies do not report long-term follow-up.

in the week before radiation resulted in outcome inferior to that of concurrent treatment.[66,67] The studies of concurrent 5-FU, cisplatin, and radiation, and of 5-FU and cisplatin as induction chemotherapy before radiation alone[68] or alternating with radiation,[69] all appear to produce high response rates and, at least in those with longer follow-up, enduring tumor control. The importance of controlling the timing of delivery of chemotherapy agents relative to radiation each day is not known. Mainly by analogy with the results of trials already completed in more common cancers, and by general usage, the delivery of 96- to 120-hour infusions of 5-FU, together with bolus injections of cisplatin or mitomycin on the first or second day of the 5-FU infusion, is the schedule used most widely. Continuous infusions of 5-FU and cisplatin throughout a 5- to 7-week course of radiation are feasible.[65,70] The interactions of various combinations of radiation, 5-FU, mitomycin, and cisplatin observed in some laboratory studies continue to lend support to theoretic discussion of the merits and mechanisms of combined modality treatment, but these interactions have not been formally evaluated in the clinic. Randomized trials in progress address directly the value of combining 5-FU and cisplatin with radiation rather than 5-FU and mitomycin (UK) and short versus prolonged infusions of 5-FU (France).

Efforts to improve tumor control rates include increasing the total radiation dose and shortening the overall duration of the radiation schedules. The results of nonrandomized series indicate that, when combined with 5-FU and mitomycin, radiation doses on the order of 30 Gy in 3 weeks eradicate up to about 90% of cancers smaller than approximately 3 cm in size.[62] Higher doses, from 45 Gy in 5 weeks to 54 Gy in 6 weeks, sometimes supplemented by additional radiation after an interval of 6 to 8 weeks, to a total of 60 to 65 Gy over approximately 12 weeks, have controlled from 65% to 75% of primary cancers larger than 4 cm.[62] Improved tumor control was observed in small groups of patients who received continuous-infusion chemotherapy throughout treatment, as the radiation dose was increased from less than 45 Gy in 5 weeks to more than 60 Gy in approximately 6 weeks.[70] Although the patients who had higher radiation doses also received higher total doses of chemotherapy, it was believed that the increase in radiation dose was the more significant factor.

The overall duration of radiation may be prolonged by planned or unplanned interruptions. The acute toxicity of combined modality treatment is greater than that of radiation alone, and short breaks in treatment to allow healing of acute dermatitis and anoproctitis are commonly required.[71] Some authors have recommended longer intervals of up to 8 weeks after the initial course of radiation, to give time for tumor regression before the final boost phase of radiation treatment.[37] The limited data available on the potential doubling time of anal cancers show a median value on the order of 4 days (range, 1 to 30 days; n = 26),[72] similar to that of cervix cancer. The control of cervix cancer, and of many other cancers, by radiation is known to be affected adversely by prolongation of treatment duration. The consensus of studies of anal cancer in which treatment duration has been considered is that improved results are achieved in the subset of patients with the shorter treatment times.[73] However, absolute upper and lower limits for the duration of radiation have not been established.

The tolerance of increased radiation doses and shortened overall treatment times is unpredictable, and careful phase I/II studies are necessary. In preparation for a randomized trial in the UK, patients received 50 Gy in 25 fractions in 5 weeks with a reducing field technique, together with two courses of concurrent 5-FU and mitomycin.[74] Six of 50 patients (12%) needed interruptions of 4 or more treatment days, and 3 patients could not complete the treatment. In an RTOG phase II trial, patients were planned to receive an uninterrupted course of 59.4 Gy in 33 fractions over 6.5 weeks by a reducing field technique, with two courses of concurrent 5-FU and mitomycin. Nine of 18 required a break in treatment of 2 weeks or more.[75,76] These schedules form the basis of current UK and RTOG randomized trials. It is possible that advances in radiation planning and conformal treatment techniques, or the development of pharmacologic agents that protect normal tissues, will reduce the extent of perineal skin reactions and anoproctitis, generally the most difficult side effects for the patient to tolerate.

Severe or moderately severe acute anoproctitis and perineal dermatitis occur in approximately one-third of those who receive concurrent 5-FU–containing chemotherapy and radiation doses of about 30 Gy in 3 weeks, and in approximately one-half to two-thirds of those treated with doses of 54 to 60 Gy in 6

TABLE 29.10-6.   Selected Results of Salvage Surgery

Reference	First Treatment (No.)	Residual Cancer after Surgery (No.)	Surgical Morbidity (%)	Local Relapse after Surgery (%)	Overall Survival (Actuarial)
Ellenhorn et al.[83]	CTRT (38)	NS	26	All (47)	44% median, 47 mo
Pocard et al.[84]	RT (18), CTRT (3)	R0 (20), R1 (1)	24	NS	58%, 3 y
Allal et al.[85]	RT ± C (26)	R0 (21), R1 (1), RX (4)	47	All (42)	45% median, 65 mo
Smith et al.[86]	CTRT (22)	R0 (12), R1-2 (10)	NS	R0 (67)	33% mean, 84 mo
Nilsson et al.[87]	RT (12), CTRT (23)	R0 (32), R1 (3)	66	R0 (44), R1 (100)	52%, 5 y

C, chemotherapy; CTRT, chemoradiation; NS, not stated; R0, no known residual; R1, microscopic residual; R2, gross residual; RT, radiation therapy; RX, residual unknown.

weeks. Most large studies of radiation and concomitant chemotherapy have reported up to approximately 2% mortality, usually as a result of sepsis, not always associated with neutropenia, or of severe anoproctitis, diarrhea, and electrolyte disturbance. Considerable progress has been made by refining radiation techniques to reduce the risk of late complications that require surgery from the 5% to 15% reported in some early series.[62] Side effects of lesser severity, but which affect quality of life adversely, are common and include urgency and frequency of defecation, perineal dermatitis, dyspareunia, and impotence.[77–79] These side effects are managed medically, although with limited success.[77] Prospective studies of quality of life and physiologic studies of anorectal function after combined modality treatment have been infrequent[79,80] but are being incorporated increasingly in randomized and nonrandomized studies. The severity of moderate-grade acute and late toxicity is influenced by radiation technique and dose-time factors.[62]

Although chemoradiation is the preferred initial treatment, some patients have contraindications to chemotherapy or refuse drug therapy. These individuals can be offered radical radiation alone as initial treatment, with reasonable expectations of cure and preservation of function (see Table 29.10-3).[62]

Radical resection of intermediate-stage primary anal canal cancer is reserved for patients who cannot tolerate radiation therapy or chemoradiation or who are incontinent due to irreversible damage of the sphincters or an anovaginal fistula. Patients who have had prior pelvic radiation treatment (most frequently for carcinoma of the cervix) generally cannot be retreated and are managed surgically. Active inflammatory bowel disease affecting the rectum or anal region may be a relative contraindication to pelvic radiation, although most patients in whom inflammatory bowel disease is quiescent tolerate radiation and chemotherapy. The most common indications for radical resection are failure of chemoradiation or radiation and, less frequently, complications of the initial treatment.

Suspected residual cancer should be confirmed by biopsy. Random biopsies from the site of the primary cancer in the absence of clinical features suspicious for cancer were positive in only 2%, and the false-negative rate was approximately 11% (7 of 61).[81] Residual masses after radiation or chemoradiation may take several months to regress fully.[32,82] Frequent examination by an experienced observer is desirable, including, if necessary, examination under anesthesia, to detect recurrence early and forestall progression to technical unresectability. The development of a hard-edged ulcer after previous healing, an enlarging mass, or increasing pain at the primary tumor site should raise suspicion of recurrence.

The results of salvage abdominoperineal resection or composite resection to include adjacent structures vary widely, with survival rates from as low as 0% to better than 50%. Table 29.10-6 summarizes selected features of some of the larger series of salvage surgery. Some authors considered that resection of recurrent disease had a better prognosis than that of cancer that remained clinically residual after chemoradiation, but opinions varied. Strictly, all local recurrences are due to residual cancer. Criteria for attempting surgical salvage were stated infrequently, and factors assessable preoperatively that are prognostic of long-term control have not been established. Decision making in this patient group is complex and should include multidisciplinary consultation. In particular, the need for reconstructive surgery to close defects in irradiated pelvic tissues should be considered. Although no operative or preoperative mortality was reported in the series shown in Table 29.10-6, the morbidity rates were high and likely underestimates, as all were retrospective series. It can be concluded that salvage surgery offers a potential for long-term local control and survival in roughly one-third to one-half of the patients fit for surgery who do not have clearly unresectable cancer or known extrapelvic disease. Palliative surgery can be offered according to the circumstances of individual patients.

Patients who undergo surgery for severe morbidity after radiation-based treatment generally have a good prognosis, reflecting the absence of cancer. However, perineal wound healing may be especially problematic in those who undergo abdominoperineal resection, given the frequent presence of skin breakdown and fistula formation, as well as malnutrition and debility due to pain. Flap reconstruction should be considered to reduce the risk of prolonged delays in healing of the perineal wound. In a few patients, a lesser procedure such as a temporary colostomy may suffice to allow healing of severe proctitis.

Regional Lymph Nodes

Metastases to the regional nodes are controlled by the chemoradiation combinations used for primary anal canal cancer. However, in most studies the 5-year survival rates for patients with regional node metastases are up to 20% lower than in node-negative patients.

Pelvic node metastases are usually diagnosed radiologically, and the response to radiation and chemotherapy can be monitored by imaging. Some authors have recommended surgery after preoperative radiation or radiation and chemotherapy.[37] Because this usually requires abdominoperineal resection rather than pelvic lymphadenectomy,[37] continued radiologic observation is generally preferred. Control rates are usually 80% or better. Even large pelvic node masses may respond completely to radiation and chemotherapy. Incomplete response may be sufficient to allow resection.

Confirmed inguinal node metastases are also controlled by radiation and chemotherapy. When metastases are not fixed to skin or deep structures, the control rate after chemoradiation alone or local excision followed by chemoradiation or radiation is generally 80% or better.[29,32] Formal node dissection is reserved for residual or recurrent metastases after radiation-based treatment. Such patients are at increased risk of significant postoperative wound healing problems or chronic lymphedema.

The rate of late failure in clinically normal inguinal nodes not treated prophylactically ranges from approximately 10% to 25%. Late nodal failures may prove uncontrollable in up to one-half of the patients in whom they occur.[29] Because of the morbidity of node dissection, elective lymphadenectomy of clinically normal inguinal nodes is not recommended.[28] However, elective irradiation of clinically normal inguinal node areas is associated with little morbidity, particularly from the lower doses used in chemoradiation protocols, and reduces the risk of late node failure in the volume irradiated to less than 5%.[62]

ADVANCED CANCER (METASTATIC, STAGE IV)

Extrapelvic metastases have been reported in up to approximately 20% of patients and have assumed increasing significance as control rates for the primary cancer and regional nodes improve. In the patients treated with radiation, 5-FU, and mitomycin in the UKCCCR trial, 27% (21 of 77) of those dying from cancer had metastases only.[33] The overall crude rate of metastases in those treated by chemoradiation was 10% in the UKCCCR trial[33] and 17% in the EORTC trial.[45] The median survival time after diagnosis of extrapelvic metastases is from 8 to 12 months,[43] although longer survival has been recorded when chemotherapy could be combined with potentially curative surgery or radiation.[88]

Squamous anal canal cancer is one of the more sensitive of gastrointestinal tract cancers to currently available chemotherapeutic agents. However, complete and durable responses in metastases or local-regionally recurrent cancer have been elusive. Because of the relative infrequency of anal cancer, most institutional series have included only small numbers of patients. Similarly, relatively few drugs have been studied. The short list includes 5-FU, cisplatin, carboplatin, mitomycin, bleomycin, vincristine, vinblastine,

doxorubicin, and methotrexate. Many more recently developed drugs have not yet been evaluated. Pharmacogenomics may aid in predicting therapeutic efficacy and safety in the future.

The treatment of metastatic anal cancer with single-agent mitomycin or fluoropyrimidines has not been reported since 1985. Cisplatin and carboplatin were noted to produce responses, but attention has shifted to multiple-drug combinations.

The combination studied most extensively, and the most effective, is 5-FU and cisplatin. The usual regimen is a 96- or 120-hour continuous infusion of 5-FU ($1000 \text{ mg/m}^2/24$ h) plus a bolus infusion of cisplatin (100 mg/m^2) on day 1 or 2, repeated at four weekly intervals while tumor response and toxicity permit. Intraarterial cisplatin and floxuridine (5-FUDR) produced responses in liver metastases in two patients.[89] In 17 patients with recurrent or metastatic cancer treated with intravenous 5-FU and cisplatin, 2 achieved complete response and 9 partial responses occurred.[90] A patient with metastatic cancer who received 12 cycles of 5-FU and cisplatin had been free of cancer for more than 3 years at the time of reporting.[91] Responses reported to other cisplatin-based treatment included 5 of 17 to cisplatin, vinblastine, and bleomycin and 2 of 7 to methotrexate, vinblastine, adriamycin, and cisplatin.[92] Other combinations, including mitomycin and 5-FU[93] and bleomycin, vincristine, and high-dose methotrexate,[94] produced few responses. In nonrandomized comparisons, the median survival of patients treated with combinations that did not include cisplatin was similar to that of untreated patients.

Induction or neoadjuvant chemotherapy has been adopted as a strategy by several groups. The principal intent is to reduce the bulk of anal cancer before definitive chemoradiation. The 3-year local recurrence rates after radiation, 5-FU, and mitomycin in the three randomized trials described earlier range from 16% to 45%, reflecting the disparity between the studies but also indicating the need for improvement. By delivering chemotherapy to unirradiated tissues, it is anticipated that drug access will be improved. A secondary benefit of improved local-regional control and the additional courses of chemotherapy may be reduction in the rate of extrapelvic metastases. The results of four pilot studies of induction chemotherapy, three of which used cisplatin and 5-FU[68,95,96] and one carboplatin and 5-FU,[97] are shown in Table 29.10-7. The cumulative major response rate in the 146 patients treated with induction 5-FU and cisplatin is 65% (complete response 15%, partial response 50%). Only 2% showed measurable progression during induction therapy, and only one death from toxicity was reported. After induction chemotherapy and concurrent radiation

TABLE 29.10-7. Selected Results of Induction Chemotherapy

| Reference | No. | Treatment | Courses[a] | Responses after Induction CT[b] | | | | Response after Subsequent RTCT or RT |
				CR	PR	S	Prog	CR
Brunet et al.[68]	22	5-FU, DDP	3	6	13	3	0	20[c]
Peiffert et al.[95]	79	5-FU, DDP	2	8	39	28	1	70
Meropol et al.[96]	45	5-FU, DDP	2	8	21	13	1	36
Svensson et al.[97]	31	5-FU, carbop	3	1	13	14	1	29

Carbop, carboplatin; CR, complete response; CT, chemotherapy; DDP, cisplatin; 5-FU, 5-fluorouracil; Prog, progression; PR, partial response; RT, radiation; RTCT, radiation and concurrent chemotherapy; S, stable.
[a]Planned or most frequent number.
[b]Assessable patients only.
[c]Includes four patients who had surgery.

and chemotherapy or radiation alone, the complete response rate was 86%. The feasibility of this approach in a multi-institutional setting has been established.[96] An intergroup randomized trial (RTOG 98-11) for patients with squamous cancers larger than 2 cm in size is comparing standard therapy with 5-FU, mitomycin, and radiation to two cycles of induction chemotherapy with 5-FU and cisplatin followed by concurrent radiation, 5-FU, and cisplatin.

Adjuvant chemotherapy is also being studied, although, again, the stated intention is to improve local-regional control as much as to reduce extrapelvic metastases. An early nonrandomized study of 5-FU and mitomycin given for up to a year showed no apparent benefit.[98] After an initial phase II study,[99] the UKCCCR is conducting a four-arm randomized trial to evaluate the role of two courses of adjuvant 5-FU and cisplatin, after initial treatment with either radiation, 5-FU and mitomycin, or radiation, 5-FU, and cisplatin.

ADENOCARCINOMAS

Adenocarcinomas comprise approximately 15% of cancers of the anal canal. The majority develop in rectal mucosa that extends below the upper muscular boundary of the canal and are treated similarly to adenocarcinomas that arise in the rectum. The infrequent adenocarcinomas of anal glands or the lining of anal fistulas have usually been managed by abdominoperineal resection.[100] Considerable variation is found between the several small retrospective institutional series.[54,101,102] A small female preponderance is seen, although gender does not appear to be prognostic. No recognized association has been found with hrHPV or immunosuppression. The most useful prognostic factors are T category and N category. Overall 5-year survival rates after all treatments have generally been less than 50%. Although local-regional control is problematic, the risk of distant metastases also appears to be higher than for squamous cell cancers. The merits of surgical adjuvant treatment, using protocols developed for rectal adenocarcinomas or anal squamous cancers, are unproven. Some publications indicate that, at least for smaller adenocarcinomas, up to approximately 4 or 5 cm in size, concomitant treatment with radiation and a 5-FU–based regimen, using protocols similar to those for squamous cancer, offers the prospect of preservation of anorectal function.[101]

SMALL CELL CANCERS

Small cell cancers are rare cancers that should be differentiated by histopathology and immunohistochemistry from poorly differentiated neuroendocrine carcinomas. Small cell anal cancers have a poor prognosis because of early metastasis. Treatment of the primary tumor by radiation-based therapy is intended to preserve anorectal function if possible. Systemic chemotherapy similar to that used for small cell cancers of the lung is sometimes given, but any benefit is unclear.

PERIANAL CANCERS

BOWEN'S DISEASE AND PAGET'S DISEASE

Squamous dysplasia of the perianal skin or Bowen's disease may accompany AIN in the anal canal or the perianal skin.[2] Extra-

mammary Paget's disease often appears as a slowly spreading eczematoid plaque that may extend into the distal canal.[2] Approximately half the cases of anal Paget's disease are associated with a synchronous or metachronous internal malignancy, often a colorectal adenocarcinoma. The remainder are not associated with malignancy elsewhere but have a high local recurrence rate and may become invasive.[2] The preferred treatment for Bowen's disease and Paget's disease (when not associated with an incontinuity adenocarcinoma of the rectum) is wide local excision, with intraoperative microscopic control of margins.[103–105] Local recurrence can often be managed by further local excision. Other less-established treatments for Bowen's disease and noninvasive Paget's disease include topical chemotherapy, topical immune modifiers such as imiquimod, and photodynamic therapy. Radiation therapy, or radiation and chemotherapy, has also been used, but is generally reserved for patients with recurrent or invasive disease in whom adequate excision would entail sacrifice of anorectal function.[106] Although anorectal function can generally be preserved, abdominoperineal resection may be necessary to control extensive or recurrent disease.

INVASIVE CANCERS

The most common histologic type of invasive cancer of the perianal skin is squamous cell carcinoma. These cancers may extend into the distal canal. When the site of origin is uncertain, it is conventional to classify the cancer as arising in the anal canal.

Wide local excision with a 1-cm margin is recommended for perianal cancers, provided anal continence can be preserved.[54] Radiation and radiation combined with chemotherapy are also effective and are the recommended treatment when surgery could impair anal continence. When possible, initial surgical management is preferred to radiation-based treatment of perianal cancers because of the frequent morbidity from long-term changes in the perianal skin after irradiation. In the UKCCCR randomized trial, one in four patients had a cancer that arose in the perianal skin.[33] That trial showed superiority overall for a combination of radiation, 5-FU, and mitomycin, but the investigators did not correlate outcome with the site of origin of the cancers. Nonrandomized studies have demonstrated the effectiveness of radiation alone or radiation and chemotherapy, with local control rates ranging from 60% to 85% in several series.[107] Radical surgery, usually abdominoperineal resection with wide perineal excision and plastic repair, may be required for advanced cancer of tumors recurrent after previous treatment.

The regional nodes for the perianal skin are the inguinal nodes. Perirectal or pelvic node metastases from squamous cancers are very uncommon. The risk of inguinal node metastases is approximately 10%, associated mainly with category T3 or T4 tumors or poorly differentiated cancers. Elective nodal irradiation has been suggested for those categories only. The management of abnormal inguinal nodes is similar to that of anal canal cancer.

The principles of management for the uncommon adenocarcinomas and basal cell cancers of the perianal skin are similar to those for these histologic types elsewhere on the skin. As for squamous cell cancers, every effort is made to preserve anorectal function by preferring initial local excision or radiation therapy to abdominoperineal resection.

SPECIAL CONSIDERATIONS: PATIENTS WITH HUMAN IMMUNODEFICIENCY VIRUS INFECTION/ACQUIRED IMMUNODEFICIENCY SYNDROME

Patients who are HIV positive are at increased risk for development of AIN and of squamous cancers of the anal canal or perianal skin. Local excision is the treatment of first choice for AIN or early stage invasive cancer. Treatment by radiation alone, or combined modality regimens, has been effective in several small groups of HIV-positive patients with more extensive cancer. HIV-infected patients are at increased risk of toxicity, particularly in the perineal skin and anorectal mucosa, when exposed to therapeutic doses of radiation, either alone or combined with chemotherapy. Although the mechanisms for this unpredictable hypersensitivity are not known, the risk of increased toxicity and of lower probability of control of the anal cancer appears to be greater in patients with a lymphocyte CD4+ count less than $200/\mu L$ at the time of starting treatment, or with AIDS.[49,50] The limited data available suggest that HAART does not reliably reduce the severity or incidence of cancer treatment–related toxicity.[22] Complete primary anal cancer remission rates with either radiation or radiation plus chemotherapy on the order of 70% have been described, comparable to or marginally inferior to those in non–HIV-infected patients. It is difficult to obtain reliable data on long-term local control or cancer relapse patterns.[50]

Several reports suggest that it is not necessary to alter standard protocols of radiation or chemotherapy in anticipation of possible toxicity, but modification should be based on the severity of side effects observed in each patient.[49,50] Some patients decline cytotoxic chemotherapy because of their concern that depletion of marrow reserve may impair their ability to tolerate HAART. Radiation alone can be offered to such patients. Radical surgery should be considered for those who cannot tolerate radiation with or without chemotherapy or if such treatment fails.

REFERENCES

1. Wendell-Smith CP. Anorectal nomenclature: fundamental terminology. *Dis Colon Rectum* 2000;43:1349.
2. Fenger D, Frisch M, Marti MC, et al. Tumours of the anal canal. In: Hamilton SR, Aaltonen LA, eds. *Pathology and genetics of tumours of the digestive system.* Lyon: IARC Press, 2000;145.
3. Zbar AP, Fenger C, Efron J, et al. The pathology and molecular biology of anal intraepithelial neoplasia: comparisons with cervical and vulvar intraepithelial carcinoma. *Int J Colorectal Dis* 2002;17:203.
4. International Agency for Research on Cancer. *Cancer incidence in five continents.* Lyon, France, 1997.
5. Frisch M. On the etiology of anal squamous carcinoma. *Dan Med Bull* 2002;49:194.
6. Frisch M, Goodman MT. Human papilloma virus–associated carcinomas in Hawaii and the mainland U.S. *Cancer* 2000;88:1464.
7. Frisch M, Fenger C, van den Brule AJ, et al. Variants of squamous cell carcinoma of the anal canal and perianal skin and their relation to human papilloma virus. *Cancer Res* 1999;59:753.
8. Bjorge T, Engeland A, Luostarinen, et al. Human papilloma virus infection as a risk factor for anal and perianal skin cancer in a prospective study. *Br J Cancer* 2002;87:61.
9. Scholefield JH, Kerr IB, Shepherd NA, et al. Human papillomavirus type 16 DNA in anal cancers from six different countries. *Gut* 1991;32:674.
10. Daling JR, Weiss NS, Klopfenstein LL, et al. Correlates of homosexual behavior and the incidence of anal cancer. *JAMA* 1982;247:1988.
11. Penn I. Cancers of the anogenital region in renal transplant patients. *Cancer* 1986;58:611.
12. Frisch M, Biggar RJ, Engels EA, et al. Association of cancer with AIDS-related immunosuppression in adults. *JAMA* 2001;285:1736.
13. Goedert JJ, Cote TR, Virgo P, et al. Spectrum of AIDS-associated malignant disorders. *Lancet* 1998;351:1833.
14. Critchlow CW, Surawicz CM, Holmes KK, et al. Prospective study of high grade and intraepithelial neoplasia in a cohort of homosexual men: influence of HIV infection, immunosuppression and human papilloma virus infection. *AIDS* 1995;9:1255.
15. Palefsky JM, Holly EA, Ralston ML, et al. High incidence of anal high-grade squamous intraepithelial lesions among HIV-positive and HIV-negative homosexual and bisexual men. *AIDS* 1998;12:495.
16. Palefsky JM. Anal squamous intraepithelial lesions: relation to HIV and human papillomavirus infection. *J Acquir Immune Defic Syndr Hum Retrovirol* 1999;21:542.
17. International Collaboration on HIV and Cancer. Highly active antiretroviral therapy and incidence of cancer in human immunodeficiency virus-infected adults. *JNCI* 2000;92:1823.
18. Daling JR, Sherman KJ, Hislop TG, et al. Cigarette smoking and the risk of anogenital cancer. *Am J Epidemiol* 1992;135:180.
19. Frisch M, Glimelius J, Wohlfahrt J, et al. Tobacco smoking as a risk factor in anal carcinoma: an antiestrogenic mechanism? *J Natl Cancer Inst* 1999;91:708.
20. Frisch M, Johansen C. Anal carcinoma in inflammatory bowel disease. *Br J Cancer* 2000;83:89.
21. Fenger C. Anal neoplasia and its precursors; facts and controversies. *Semin Diag Pathol* 1991;8:190.
22. Klencke BJ, Palefsky JM. Anal cancer: an HIV-associated cancer. *Hematol Oncol Clin North Am* 2003;17:859.
23. Palefsky JM, Holly EA, Hogeboom CJ, et al. Virologic, immunologic, and clinical parameters in the incidence and progression of anal squamous intraepithelial lesions in HIV-positive and HIV-negative homosexual men. *J Acquir Immuno Def Synd Hum Retrovirol* 1998;17:314.
24. Boman BM, Moertel CG, O'Connell M, et al. Carcinoma of the anal canal: a clinical and pathological study of 188 cases. *Cancer* 1984;54:114.
25. Greene FL, Page DL, Fleming D, et al. *AJCC cancer staging manual.* 6th ed. Philadelphia: Lippincott-Raven, 2002.
26. Sobin LH, Wittekind C. *TNM classification of malignant tumours.* 6th ed. New York: Wiley-Liss, 2002.
27. Golden GT, Horsley JS. Surgical management of epidermoid carcinoma of the anus. *Am J Surg* 1976;131:275.
28. Stearns MW, Urmacher C, Sternberg SS, et al. Cancer of the anal canal. *Curr Probl Cancer* 1980;4:1.
29. Gerard JP, Chapet O, Samiei F, et al. Management of inguinal lymph node metastases in patients with carcinoma of the anal canal. Experience in a series of 270 patients treated in Lyon and review of the literature. *Cancer* 2001;92:77.
30. Frost DB, Richards PC, Montague ED, et al. Epidermoid cancer of the anorectum. *Cancer* 1984;53:1285.
31. Myerson RJ, Karnell LH, Menck HR. The national cancer data base report on carcinoma of the anus. *Cancer* 1997;80:805.
32. Cummings BJ, Keane TJ, O'Sullivan B, et al. Epidermoid anal cancer: treatment by radiation and 5-fluorouracil with and without mitomycin C. *Int J Radiat Oncol Biol Phys* 1991;21:1115.
33. UKCCCR Anal Canal Cancer Trial Working Party. Epidermoid anal cancer: results from the UKCCCR randomized trial of radiotherapy alone versus radiotherapy, 5-fluorouracil and mitomycin C. *Lancet* 1996;348:1049.
34. Friberg B, Svensson C, Goldman S, et al. The Swedish National Care Programme for anal carcinoma. Implementation and overall results. *Acta Oncol* 1998;37:25.
35. Pintor MP, Northover JM, Nicholls RJ. Squamous cell carcinoma of the anus at one hospital from 1948 to 1984. *Br J Surg* 1989;76:806.
36. Deniaud-Alexandre E, Touboul E, Tiret E, et al. Results of definitive irradiation in a series of 305 epidermoid carcinoma of the anal canal. *Int J Radiat Oncol Biol Phys* 2003;56:1259.
37. Papillon J. *Rectal and anal cancers: conservative treatment by irradiation—an alternative to radical surgery.* Berlin: Springer-Verlag, 1982.
38. Wade DS, Herrera L, Castillo NB, et al. Metastases to the lymph nodes in epidermoid carcinoma of the anal canal studied by a clearing technique. *Surg Gynecol Obstet* 1989;169:238.
39. Perera D, Pathma-Nathan N, Rabbitt P, et al. Sentinel node biopsy for squamous-cell carcinoma of the anus and anal margin. *Dis Colon Rectum* 2003;46:1027.
40. Cummings BJ. Sentinel node biopsy for squamous cell carcinoma of the anus and anal margin—discussion of Perera D, et al. *Dis Colon Rectum* 2003;46:1030.
41. Cummings BJ. Anal cancer. In: Gospodarowicz MK, Henson DE, Hutter RV, et al., eds. *Prognostic factors in cancer,* 2nd ed. New York: Wiley-Liss, 2001:281.
42. Fenger C. Prognostic factors in anal carcinoma. *Pathology* 2002;34:573.
43. Tanum G, Tveit K, Karlsen KO, et al. Chemotherapy and radiation therapy for anal carcinoma: survival and late morbidity. *Cancer* 1991;67:2462.
44. Goldman S, Auer G, Erhardt K, et al. Prognostic significance of clinical stage, histologic grade, and nuclear DNA content in squamous cell carcinoma of the anus. *Dis Colon Rectum* 1987;30:444.
45. Bartelink H, Roelofsen F, Eschwege F, et al. Concomitant radiotherapy and chemotherapy is superior to radiotherapy alone in the treatment of locally advanced anal cancer: results of a phase III randomized trial of the European Organization for Research and Treatment of Cancer Radiotherapy and Gastrointestinal Cooperative Groups. *J Clin Oncol* 1997;15:2040.
46. Gerard JP, Ayzac L, Hun D, et al. Treatment of anal canal carcinoma with high dose radiation therapy and concomitant fluorouracil-cisplatinum. Long term results in 95 patients. *Radiother Oncol* 1998;46:249.
47. Newman G, Calverley DC, Acker BD, et al. The management of carcinoma of the anal canal by external beam radiotherapy: experience in Vancouver 1971–1988. *Radiother Oncol* 1992;25:196.
48. Constantinou EC, Daly W, Fung CY, et al. Time-dose considerations with treatment of anal cancer. *Int J Radiat Oncol Biol Phys* 1997;39:651.

49. Hoffman R, Welton ML, Klenche B, et al. The significance of pretreatment CD4 count on the outcome and treatment tolerance of HIV-positive patients with anal cancer. *Int J Radiat Oncol Biol Phys* 1999;44:127.

50. Place RJ, Gregorcyk SG, Huber PJ, et al. Outcome analysis of HIV-positive patients with anal squamous cell carcinoma. *Dis Colon Rectum* 2001;44:506.

51. Goldie SJ, Kuntz KM, Weinstein MC, et al. The clinical effectiveness and cost-effectiveness of screening for anal squamous intraepithelial lesions in homosexual and bisexual HIV-positive men. *JAMA* 1999;281:1822.

52. Chang GJ, Berry JM, Jay N, et al. Surgical treatment of high-grade anal squamous intraepithelial lesions: a prospective study. *Dis Colon Rectum* 2002;45:453.

53. Berry JM, Palefsky JM. A review of human papillomavirus vaccines: from basic science to clinical trials. *Front Biosci* 2003;8:S333.

54. Klas JV, Rothenberger DA, Wong WD, et al. Malignant tumors of the anal canal. The spectrum of disease, treatment and outcomes. *Cancer* 1999;85:1686.

55. Martenson JA, Gunderson LL. External radiation therapy without chemotherapy in the management of anal cancer. *Cancer* 1993;71:1736.

56. Otim-Oyet D, Ford H, Fisher C, et al. Radical radiotherapy for carcinoma of the anal canal. *Clin Oncol* 1990;2:84.

57. Papillon J, Mayer M, Montbarbon JF, et al. A new approach to the management of epidermoid carcinoma of the anal canal. *Cancer* 1983;51:1830.

58. Hu K, Minsky BD, Cohen AM, et al. 30 Gy may be an adequate dose in patients with anal cancer treatment with excisional biopsy followed by combined-modality therapy. *J Surg Oncol* 1999;70:71.

59. Nigro ND, Vaitkevicius VK, Considine B. Combined therapy for cancer of the anal canal: a preliminary report. *Dis Colon Rectum* 1974;17:354.

60. Flam M, John M, Pajak TF, et al. The role of mitomycin C in combination with 5-fluorouracil and radiotherapy, and of salvage chemoradiation in the definitive nonsurgical treatment of epidermoid carcinoma of the anal canal: results of a phase III randomized intergroup study. *J Clin Oncol* 1996;14:2527.

61. Flam M. Author update. In: Mayer RJ, ed. *Highlights of clinical gastrointestinal cancer research. Classic papers and current comments.* 1999;3:539.

62. Cummings BJ, Brierley JD. Anal canal. In: Perez CA, Brady LW, Halperin EC, et al., eds. *Principles and practice of radiation oncology,* 4th ed. Philadelphia: Lippincott, Williams and Wilkins 2003:1630.

63. Martenson JA, Lipsitz SR, Wagner H, et al. Initial results of a phase II trial of radiation therapy, 5-fluorouracil and cisplatin for patients with anal cancer. *Int J Radiat Oncol Biol Phys* 1996;35:745.

64. Doci R, Zucali R, La Monica G, et al. Primary chemoradiation therapy with fluorouracil and cisplatin for cancer of the anus: results in 35 consecutive patients. *J Clin Oncol* 1996;14:3121.

65. Hung A, Crane C, Delclos M, et al. Cisplatin-based combined modality therapy for anal carcinoma: a wider therapeutic index. *Cancer* 2003;97:1195.

66. Meeker WR, Sickle-Santanello BJ, Philpott G, et al. Combined chemotherapy, radiation, and surgery for epithelial cancer of the anal canal. *Cancer* 1986;57:525.

67. Miller EJ, Quan SH, Thalar HT. Treatment of squamous cell carcinoma of the anal canal. *Cancer* 1991;67:2038.

68. Brunet R, Becouarn Y, Pigneux J, et al. Cisplatin et fluorouracile en chimiothérapie neo-adjuvante des carcinomas épidermoides du canal anal. *Lyon Chir* 1990;87:77.

69. Roca E, De Simone G, Barugel M, et al. A phase II study of alternating chemoradiotherapy including cisplatin in anal canal carcinoma. *Proc Am Soc Clin Oncol* 1990;9:128(abst).

70. Rich TA, Ajani JA, Morrison WH, et al. Chemoradiation therapy for anal cancer: radiation plus continuous infusion of 5-fluorouracil with or without cisplatin. *Radiother Oncol* 1993;27:209.

71. Cummings BJ. Anal cancer: to split or not to split. *Cancer J Sci Am* 1996;2:194(editorial).

72. Wong CS, Tsang RW, Cummings BJ, et al. Proliferation parameters in epidermoid carcinomas of the anal canal. *Radiother Oncol* 2000;56:349.

73. Graf R, Wust P, Hildebrandt B, et al. Impact of overall treatment time on local control of anal cancer treatment with radiochemotherapy. *Oncology* 2003;65:14.

74. Melcher AA, Sebag-Montefiore D. Concurrent chemoradiotherapy for squamous cell carcinoma of the anus using shrinking field radiotherapy technique without a boost. *Br J Cancer* 2003;88:1352.

75. John M, Pajak T, Flam M, et al. Dose acceleration in chemoradiation for anal cancer: preliminary results of RTOG 9208. *Cancer J Sci Am* 1996;2:205.

76. John M, Pajak T, Krieg R, et al. Dose escalation without split-course chemoradiation for anal cancer: results of a phase II RTOG study. *Proc Am Soc Ther Radiol Oncol. Int J Radiat Oncol Biol Phys* 1997;39[Suppl 2]:203(abst).

77. Cummings BJ. Preservation of structure and function in epidermoid cancer of the anal canal. In: Rosenthal CJ, Rotman M, eds. *Infusion chemotherapy radiotherapy interactions: its biology and significance for organ salvage and prevention of second primary neoplasms.* Amsterdam: Elsevier Science Publishing Co, 1998:167.

78. Allal AS, Sprangers MA, Laurencet F, et al. Assessment of long-term quality of life in patients with anal carcinomas treated by radiotherapy with or without chemotherapy. *Br J Cancer* 1999;80:1588.

79. Vordermark D, Sailer M, Flentje M, et al. Curative intent radiation therapy in anal carcinoma: quality of life and sphincter function. *Radiother Oncol* 1999;52:239.

80. Broens P, Van Limbergen E, Penninckx F, et al. Clinical and manometric effects of combined external beam irradiation and brachytherapy for anal cancer. *Int J Colorect Dis* 1998;13:68.

81. Nigro ND. An evaluation of combined therapy for squamous cell cancer of the anal canal. *Dis Colon Rectum* 1984;27:763.

82. Tanum G, Tveit K, Karlsen KO, et al. Chemoradiotherapy of anal carcinoma: tumour response and acute toxicity. *Oncology* 1993;50:14.

83. Ellenhorn JD, Enker WE, Quan SH. Salvage abdominoperineal resection following combined chemotherapy and radiotherapy for epidermoid carcinoma of the anus. *Ann Surg Oncol* 1994;1:105.

84. Pocard M, Tiret E, Nugent K, et al. Results of salvage abdominoperineal resection for anal canal cancer after radiotherapy. *Dis Colon Rectum* 1998;41:1488.

85. Allal AS, Laurencet FM, Reymond MA, et al. Effectiveness of surgical salvage therapy for patients with locally uncontrolled anal carcinoma after sphincter-conserving surgery. *Cancer* 1999;86:405.

86. Smith AJ, Whelan P, Cummings BJ, et al. Management of persistent or locally recurrent epidermoid cancer of the anal canal with abdominoperineal resection. *Acta Oncol* 2001;40:34.

87. Nilsson PJ, Svensson C, Goldman S, et al. Salvage abdominoperineal resection in anal epidermoid cancer. *Br J Surg* 2002;89:1425.

88. Faivre C, Rougier P, Ducreux M, et al. Carcinoma épidermoide métastatique de l'anus: étude rétrospective de l'éfficacité de l'association de 5-fluoro-uracile en perfusion continue et de cisplatine. *Bull Cancer* 1999;86:861.

89. Ajani JA, Carrasco CH, Jackson DE, et al. Combination of cisplatin plus fluoropyrimidines chemotherapy effective against liver metastases from carcinoma of the anal canal. *Am J Med* 1989;87:221.

90. Mahjoubi M, Sadek H, Francois E, et al. Epidermoid anal canal carcinoma: activity of cisplatin and continuous 5-fluorouracil in metastatic and/or local recurrent disease. *Proc Am Soc Clin Oncol* 1990;9:114(abst 441).

91. Jaiyesimi IA, Pazdur R. Cisplatin and 5-fluorouracil as salvage therapy for recurrent metastatic squamous cell carcinoma of the anal canal. *Am J Clin Oncol* 1993;16:536.

92. Magill GB, Quan S. Salvage chemotherapy of anal epidermoid carcinoma with cisplatin based protocols. *Proc Am Soc Clin Oncol* 1989;8:117(abst).

93. Tanum G. Treatment of relapsing anal carcinoma. *Acta Oncol* 1993;32:33.

94. Wilking N, Petrelli N, Herrera L, et al. A phase II study of combination bleomycin, vincristine, and high-dose methotrexate (BOM) with leukovorin rescue in advanced squamous cell carcinoma of the anal canal. *Cancer Chemother Pharmacol* 1985;15:300.

95. Peiffert D, Giovanni M, Ducreux M, et al. High dose radiation therapy and neoadjuvant plus concomitant chemotherapy with 5fluorouracil and cisplatinum in patients with locally advanced squamous cell anal canal cancer: final results of a phase II study. *Ann Oncol* 2001;12:397.

96. Meropol NJ, Niedzwiecki D, Shank B, et al. Combined modality therapy of poor risk anal carcinoma: a phase II study of the cancer and leukemia group B (CALGB). *Proc Am Soc Clin Oncol* 1999;18:237a(abst).

97. Svensson C, Goldman S, Friberg B, et al. Induction chemotherapy and radiotherapy in loco-regionally advanced epidermoid carcinoma of the anal canal. *Int J Radiat Oncol Biol Phys* 1998;41:863.

98. Michaelson RA, Magill GB, Quan SHQ, et al. Preoperative chemotherapy and radiation therapy in the management of anal epidermoid carcinoma. *Cancer* 1983;51:390.

99. James RD, David C, Neville D, et al. Chemoradiation and maintenance chemotherapy for patients with anal carcinoma: a phase II study of the UK coordinating committee for cancer research (UKCCCR) Anal Cancer Trial Working Party. *Proc Am Soc Clin Oncol* 2000; 19:268a(abst).

100. Tarazi R, Nelson RL. Anal adenocarcinoma: a comprehensive review. *Semin Surg Oncol* 1994;10:235.

101. Belkacemi Y, Berger C, Poortmans P, et al. Management of anal canal adenocarcinoma: a large retrospective study from the Rare Cancer Network. *Int J Radiat Oncol Biol Phys* 2003;56:1274.

102. Papagikos M, Crane CH, Skibber J, et al. Chemoradiation for adenocarcinoma of the anus. *Int J Radiat Oncol Biol Phys* 2003;55:69.

103. Marchesa P, Fazio VW, Oliart S, et al. Perianal Bowen's disease: a clinicopathologic study of 47 patients. *Dis Colon Rectum* 1997;40:1286.

104. Sarmiento JM, Wolff BG, Burgart LJ, et al. Paget's disease of the perianal region—an aggressive disease? *Dis Colon Rectum* 1997;40:1187.

105. McCarter MD, Quan SHQ, Busam K, et al. Long-term outcome of perianal Paget's disease. *Dis Colon Rectum* 2003;46:612.

106. Brown RSD, Lankester KJ, McCormack M, et al. Radiotherapy for perianal Paget's disease. *Clin Oncol* 2002;14:272.

107. Bieri S, Allal AS, Kurtz JM. Sphincter-conserving treatment of carcinomas of the anal margin. *Acta Oncol* 2001;40:29.

CHAPTER **30**

Cancers of the Genitourinary System

SECTION **1**

W. MARSTON LINEHAN
SUSAN E. BATES
JAMES C. YANG

Cancer of the Kidney

Each year in the United States, there are approximately 31,900 cases of kidney and upper urinary tract cancer, resulting in more than 11,900 deaths.[1] These tumors account for approximately 3% of adult malignancies and occur in a male-female ratio of 1.5:1.0. They are more common among urban than rural residents. Although most cases of renal carcinoma occur in persons aged 50 to 70 years, it has been observed in children as young as 6 months of age. Between 1975 and 1995, there was a steady and significant increase in the incidence of renal carcinoma, from 2% to 4% per year, an increase of 43% since 1973.[2-4]

Renal carcinoma was first described by Konig in 1826. As early as 1855, Robin concluded that the renal tubular epithelium was the most probable tissue of origin of the cancer, an observation that was confirmed by Waldeyer in 1867. In 1883, Grawitz, noting that the fatty content of the cancer cells was similar to that of adrenal cells, concluded that the tumors arose from adrenal rests within the kidney and introduced the term *stroma lipomatodes aberrata renis* for these clear cell tumors. The term *hypernephroid tumors* was introduced in 1984 by Birch-Hirschfeld. Since then, the conceptually incorrect term *hypernephroma* has frequently been applied to renal tumors.[5,6]

HISTOLOGIC TYPES OF RENAL CARCINOMA

Kidney cancer is not a single disease; it is made up of a number of different types of cancer that occur in the kidney, including clear cell (75%), type 1 and type 2 papillary (15%), chromophobe (5%), and oncocytoma (5%). These cancers have different histologic types and different clinical courses[7] and are caused by different genetic abnormalities (Fig. 30.1-1).[4,8]

Renal carcinoma occurs in both a sporadic and a hereditary form. There are four main forms of hereditary renal carcinoma. The most studied form of hereditary renal carcinoma is von Hippel-Lindau (VHL). VHL is a hereditary cancer syndrome in which affected individuals are at risk to develop tumors in a number of organs, including the kidney.[4,8] Hereditary papillary renal carcinoma (HPRC) is a hereditary cancer syndrome in which affected individuals are at risk for the development of bilateral, multifocal type 1 papillary renal carcinoma.[9,10] Hereditary leiomyomatosis renal cell carcinoma (HLRCC) is an inherited form of type 2 papillary renal carcinoma,[11] and Birt-Hogg-Dubé (BHD) syndrome is a hereditary form of chromophobe renal carcinoma and oncocytoma.[12] In the hereditary syndromes, the kidney cancer is often bilateral and may occur in a younger age group. An increased incidence of renal carcinoma has also been observed in patients with autosomal dominant polycystic kidney disease and tuberous sclerosis.

ETIOLOGY

A number of environmental, hormonal, cellular, and genetic factors have been studied as possible causal factors in the development of renal carcinoma. In studies of risk of renal adenocarcinoma, cigarette smoking has been found to be a risk factor.[13] A statistically significant dose response has been observed in both sexes for pack-years of cigarette use.[14] It has been estimated that 30% of renal carcinomas in men and 24% in women may be directly related to smoking.[15] Obesity is associated with an increased risk of development of renal carcinoma, particularly in women.[16] Analgesic abuse, which is known to be associated with renal pelvis cancer, is also associated with an increased incidence of kidney cancer. The increased

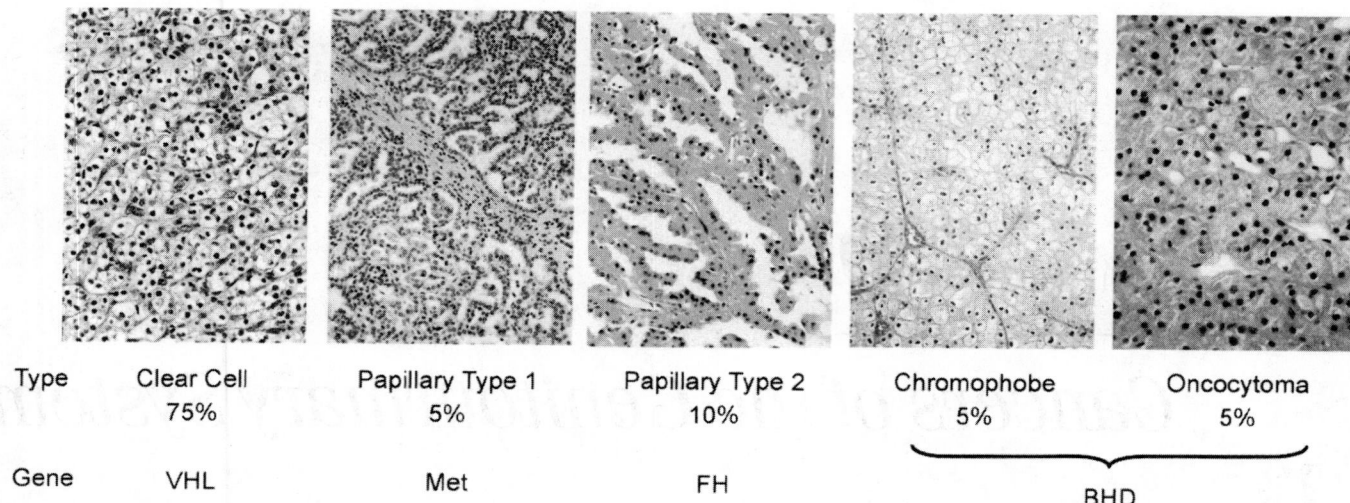

Type	Clear Cell 75%	Papillary Type 1 5%	Papillary Type 2 10%	Chromophobe 5%	Oncocytoma 5%
Gene	VHL	Met	FH	BHD	

FIGURE 30.1-1. Human renal epithelial neopasms. Kidney cancer is not a single disease; it is made up of a number of different types of cancers that occur in the kidney, each with a different histology, a different clinical course, and caused by a different gene.[4,8] BHD, Birt-Hogg-Dubé; FH, fumarate hydratase; VHL, von Hippel-Lindau. (From ref. 8, with permission.) (See Color Fig. 30.1-1 in the CD-ROM.)

risk for the development of renal carcinoma is observed primarily in patients who develop analgesic nephropathy associated with use of phenacetin-containing analgesics.[17–19]

Environmental and occupational factors have also been associated with the development of kidney cancer. Brauch et al. demonstrated an association between the development of renal carcinoma and long-term exposure to high levels of the industrial solvent, trichloroethylene.[20] There is an increased incidence of renal carcinoma among leather tanners, shoe workers, and workers exposed to asbestos.[21] Exposure to cadmium is associated with an increased incidence of kidney cancer, particularly in men who smoke.[22] An association between gasoline exposure and kidney cancer has been observed in animal studies. Although there is an increased incidence of renal carcinoma reported with exposure to petroleum, tar, and pitch products, studies of oil-refinery workers and petroleum products distribution workers do not identify a definite relationship between gasoline exposure and renal cancer. There may be an increased risk of kidney cancer in older workers or in workers exposed to gasoline for prolonged periods of time.[23,24]

There is an increased incidence (100-fold) of renal carcinoma in patients with end-stage renal disease who develop acquired cystic disease of the kidneys.[25] Acquired cystic disease is a recently described phenomenon in which patients on long-term dialysis for renal failure develop renal cysts. Renal carcinoma has been found in association with the papillary hyperplasia observed in the cyst epithelium of these kidneys. The risk of developing kidney cancer has been estimated to be greater than 30 times higher in dialysis patients with cystic changes in their kidney than in the general population.[26] It is estimated that 35% to 47% of patients on long-term dialysis will develop acquired cystic disease, and that approximately 5.8% of the patients with acquired cystic disease will develop renal cancer. Kidney cancer can develop at any time in patients with end-stage renal disease, and it can occur in kidney transplant recipients. Kidney cancer

can occur in patients with end-stage renal disease who are undergoing either hemodialysis or chronic ambulatory dialysis, and it has been reported to occur in patients with end-stage renal disease who are not being dialyzed.[25] Although many of these cancers are clinically insignificant and are found incidentally at autopsy or after bilateral nephrectomy, some will have an aggressive course.[27] Careful surveillance of patients with end-stage renal disease with ultrasonography and computed tomography (CT) is recommended. Family history is also associated with an increased risk of kidney cancer in both men and women.

HEREDITARY FORMS OF KIDNEY CANCER

Like breast cancer, colon cancer, and retinoblastoma, kidney cancer occurs in a sporadic (nonhereditary) as well as a hereditary form. There are at least four forms of hereditary renal carcinoma: VHL, HPRC, HLRCC, and BHD (Table 30.1-1).

TABLE 30.1-1. Genetic Basis of Inherited Forms of Renal Carcinoma

---

VON HIPPEL-LINDAU (VHL)
Histology: clear cell RCC
Gene: VHL
HEREDITARY PAPILLARY RENAL CARCINOMA (HPRC)
Histology: papillary type 1 RCC
Gene: Met
HEREDITARY LEIOMYOMATOSIS RCC (HLRCC)
Histology: papillary type 2 RCC
Gene: fumarate hydratase (FH)
BIRT-HOGG-DUBÉ (BHD)
Histology: chromophobe RCC/oncocytoma
Gene: BHD

RCC, renal cell carcinoma.

TABLE 30.1-2. Clinical Evaluation: von Hippel-Lindau (VHL)

VHL gene germline mutation testing
Magnetic resonance imaging of the brain and spine
Abdominal computed tomography and ultrasound
Ophthalmologic evaluation
Audiometric and ear, nose, throat evaluation
Testicular ultrasound
Metabolic evaluation (catechols)

von Hippel-Lindau: Clear Cell Renal Cell Carcinoma

VHL is a familial cancer syndrome in which affected individuals have a predisposition to develop tumors in a number of organs, including the kidneys, brain, spine, eyes, adrenal glands, pancreas, inner ear, and epididymis.[4,8] Forty percent of VHL patients develop multiple, bilateral tumors or cysts in the kidneys. VHL patients acquire clear cell renal carcinoma[28]; these patients can develop hundreds of small clear cell tumors and cysts in their kidneys. These tumors, which tend to occur early in life, are malignant and can metastasize. VHL patients can also develop pheochromocytoma, pancreatic cysts and islet cell tumors, retinal angiomas, central nervous system hemangioblastomas, inner ear tumors (endolymphatic sac tumors), and epididymal cystadenomas.

VHL GENE. Genetic linkage analysis was used to identify the VHL gene in 1993.[29] Critical to management of VHL patients is the knowledge of who is affected and who is not. Early identification of at-risk individuals is essential for initiation of early intervention for potential prevention of life-threatening complications of the disease, such as metastatic kidney cancer. Identification of the VHL gene has allowed the detection of a germline mutation in nearly 100% of VHL families.[30,31] VHL clinical features can be heterogeneous and manifestations, such as kidney cancer, occult. In some families, VHL can be confused with other hereditary cancer syndromes, such as multiple endocrine neoplasia 2. The availability of germline mutation screening can aid the physician in making the correct diagnosis as well as allowing one to perform presymptomatic screening in at-risk individuals (Table 30.1-2; Fig. 30.1-2).

ROLE OF THE VHL GENE IN CLEAR CELL RENAL CANCER. The VHL gene has been found to be mutated in a high percent of tumors and cell lines from patients with sporadic

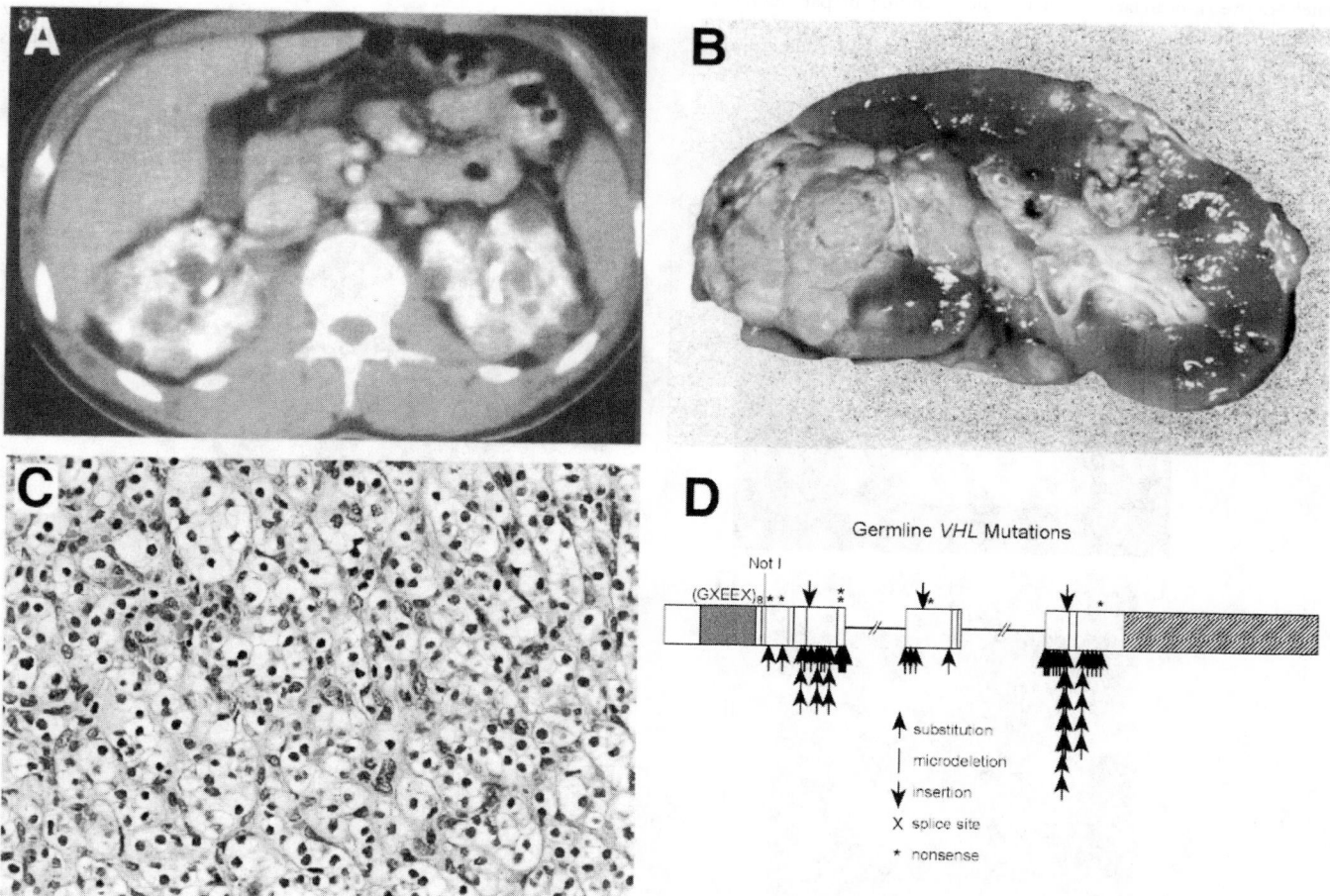

FIGURE 30.1-2. The VHL gene is the gene for the inherited form of clear cell kidney cancer associated with von Hippel-Lindau. Affected individuals in VHL families are at risk for the development of bilateral, multifocal (**A**) clear cell renal carcinoma (**B,C**). The VHL gene is mutated in the germline of affected individuals from VHL kindreds (**D**) and in tumor tissues from patients with sporadic, noninherited clear cell renal carcinoma (data not shown). (From ref. 8, with permission.) (See Color Fig. 30.1-2 in the CD-ROM.)

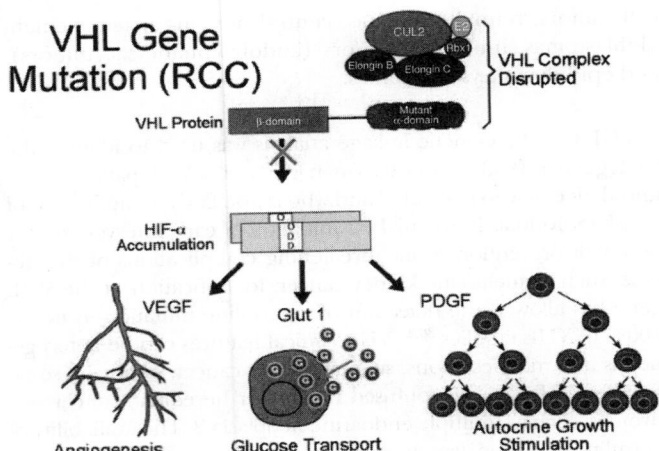

VHL Gene Mutation (RCC)

FIGURE 30.1-3. The von Hippel-Lindau (VHL) kidney cancer tumor suppressor gene product forms a complex that targets the α subunit of the hypoxia-inducible factors (HIF) for ubiquitin-mediated degradation. When the VHL gene is mutated (in clear cell kidney cancer), HIF is not degraded and overaccumulates. This leads to the increased transcription of a number of downstream genes that are thought to be important in the development of kidney cancer, such as vascular endothelial growth factor (VEGF); the glucose transport gene, Glut 1; and growth factors such as platelet-derived growth factor (PDGF). Understanding this pathway has led to the development of a number of molecular therapeutic approaches for clear cell kidney cancer that are currently being evaluated in clinical trials. (Adapted from ref. 8.) (See Color Fig. 30.1-3 in the CD-ROM.)

(nonhereditary) clear cell renal carcinoma.[32,33] VHL gene mutations have not been detected in either tumors from patients with papillary renal carcinoma or from the germline of patients with other hereditary cancers syndromes, such as HPRC (see Hereditary Papillary Renal Carcinoma: Type 1 Papillary Renal Cell Carcinoma, later in this chapter). This has led to the development of a molecular genetic classification of renal carcinoma of papillary versus clear cell (nonpapillary) renal carcinoma, with clear cell renal carcinoma being characterized by inactivation of the VHL gene. The determination that VHL gene mutations can be detected in formalin-fixed tissue from patients with clear cell renal carcinoma[34] provides a potential method for significantly improving clinicians' ability to diagnose this disease, either by analysis of tissue blocks or tissue aspirates from patients suspected of having this disease (Fig. 30.1-3).

Understanding the VHL gene pathway, and how damage to this gene leads to clear cell kidney cancer, has provided the opportunity for the development of disease-specific molecular therapeutic approaches. The VHL protein forms a complex with other proteins and targets the α subunit of the hypoxia-inducible factors (HIF1α and HIF2α) for ubiquitin-mediated degradation. HIF is a transcription factor that regulates production of a number of downstream genes important in cancer, such as vascular endothelial growth factor (VEGF); the glucose transporter, GLUT1; growth factors, such as transforming growth factor-α and platelet-derived growth factor; and erythropoietin. This is normally a hypoxia-mediated process. In normoxia, the VHL

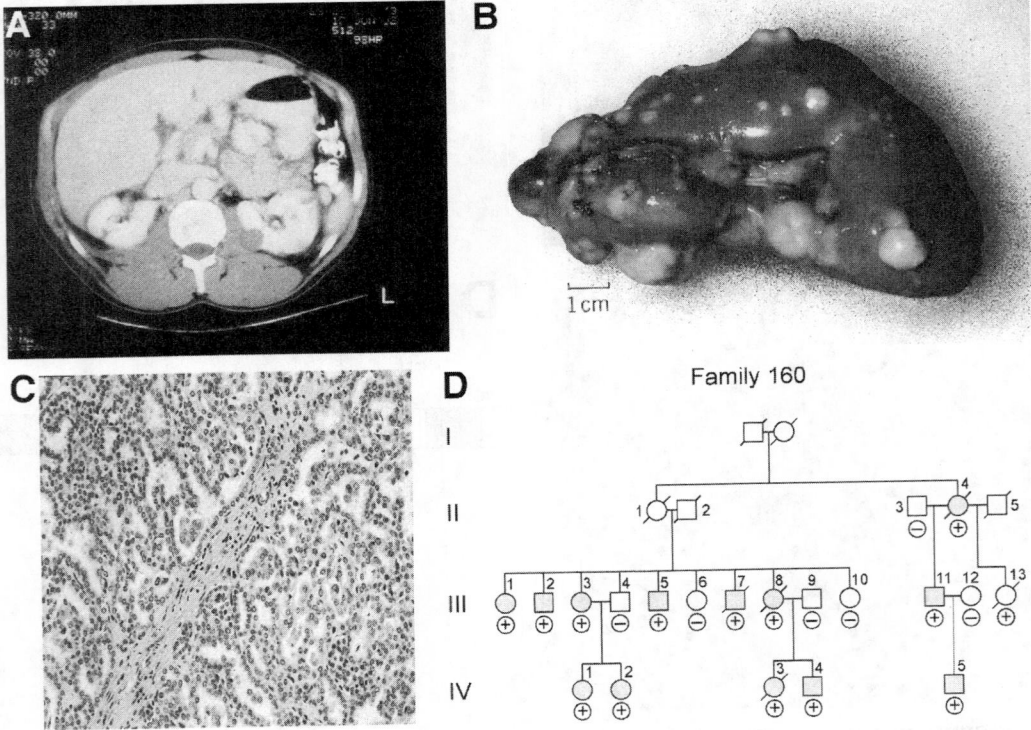

FIGURE 30.1-4. Hereditary papillary renal carcinoma (HPRC) is a hereditary cancer syndrome in which affected individuals are at risk for the development of bilateral (**A**), multifocal (**B**) type 1 papillary renal carcinoma (**C**). HPRC is a hereditary cancer syndrome (**D**) characterized by germline mutation of the c-Met protooncogene. (From ref. 8, with permission.) (See Color Fig. 30.1-4 in the CD-ROM.)

TABLE 30.1-3. Hereditary Papillary Renal Carcinoma

CLINICAL FEATURES
Bilateral, multifocal papillary renal cell carcinoma
Type I papillary renal carcinoma
CLINICAL EVALUATION
c-Met gene germline mutation testing
Abdominal computed tomography and ultrasound

TABLE 30.1-5. Clinical Evaluation: Hereditary Leiomyomatosis Renal Cell Carcinoma

Fumarate hydratase (FH) gene germline mutation testing
Dermatologic evaluation—skin biopsy
Abdominal computed tomography/ultrasound
Pelvic computed tomography/uterine ultrasound

complex targets and degrades HIF. In clear cell kidney cancer, when there is a mutation of the VHL gene, the complex cannot target and degrade HIF. HIF overaccumulates and the result is the increased production of VEGF, transforming growth factor-α, epidermal growth factor receptor, and platelet-derived growth factor. Understanding this pathway has led to the development of a number of targeted molecular therapeutic approaches that involve blocking HIF transcription, the VEGF receptor, or the epidermal growth factor receptor, or all[35] (Fig. 30.1-4).

Hereditary Papillary Renal Carcioma: Type 1 Papillary Renal Cell Carcinoma

HPRC is a form of hereditary renal carcinoma[9,10] in which affected individuals are at risk to develop bilateral, multifocal papillary renal carcinoma. These tumors, which are often detected incidentally, can spread in a fashion similar to sporadic renal carcinoma. Abdominal CT is recommended for evaluation of at-risk individuals, as even large papillary renal tumors are frequently undetectable by renal ultrasound evaluation[36] (Table 30.1-3).

HEREDITARY PAPILLARY RENAL CARCIOMA GENE: MET. Genetic linkage studies in HPRC kindreds localized the HPRC gene and led to the identification of the c-Met protooncogene as the gene responsible for HPRC.[37] Germline mutations in the tyrosine kinase domain of the MET gene have been found in affected individuals in HPRC kindreds.[38]

HEREDITARY PAPILLARY RENAL CARCIOMA GERMLINE TESTING. Germline MET mutation testing is recommended for patients at risk for HPRC. Individuals in HPRC kindreds; those with bilateral, multifocal papillary renal carcinoma; or those with a family history of papillary kidney cancer are considered candidates for germline testing.[38]

Hereditary Leiomyomatosis Renal Cell Carcinoma: Type 2 Papillary Renal Cell Carcinoma

HLRCC is a hereditary cancer syndrome in which affected individuals are at risk for the development of cutaneous and uter-

TABLE 30.1-4. Clinical Features of Hereditary Leiomyomatosis Renal Cell Carcinoma

Cutaneous nodules (leiomyomas)
Uterine leiomyoma (fibroids)
Uterine leiomyosarcoma (rarely)
Renal tumor (type 2 papillary renal cell carcinoma)
  Often solitary
  Aggressive, early to metastasize

ine leiomyoma (uterine fibroids) and type 2 papillary renal carcinoma.[39] The type 2 papillary kidney cancer can be very aggressive and metastasize early. The gene for HLRCC is fumarate hydratase; mutations of this gene are found in the germline of affected individuals in HLRCC kindreds (Tables 30.1-4 and 30.1-5; Fig. 30.1-5).[11,40]

Birt-Hogg-Dubé Syndrome: Chromophobe/Oncocytoma

BHD is a hereditary cancer syndrome in which affected individuals are at risk for the development of benign hair follicle tumors (fibrofolliculoma), pulmonary cysts, and bilateral, multifocal renal tumors[12,41] (Fig. 30.1-6). The renal tumors that occur in BHD syndrome can be chromophobe renal carcinoma (33%), oncocytic neoplasms (50%), clear cell renal carcinoma (10%), or oncocytoma (7%).[42] These tumors are malignant and can metastasize if not detected and treated (Tables 30.1-6 and 30.1-7).

The BHD gene was recently identified, and germline testing is recommended for individuals at risk for BHD. The BHD-associated fibrofolliculomas tend to occur on the face and neck and can be very subtle. A biopsy-positive fibrofolliculoma is considered diagnostic of the disease. The pulmonary cysts in BHD patients are best detected by high-resolution lung CT and have been found in 82% of gene carriers. Twenty-two percent of BHD patients have a history of pneumothorax.[12]

PATHOLOGY

Immunohistologic and ultrastructural analysis have suggested that the proximal renal tubular epithelium is the tissue of origin of most renal tumors. Renal tumors tend to be spherical, but may vary widely in size. The average diameter is approximately 7 cm; however, renal tumors can often grow to fill the entire retroperitoneum. Previously, renal lesions 2 cm or less in diameter were considered to be renal adenomas, whereas lesions 2 cm or more in diameter were considered to be carcinomas. The distinction between benign and malignant tumors is no longer made on the basis of size but on the basis of classic histologic criteria. Although renal carcinoma tends to arise in the cortex of the kidney, it can originate in the interior of the kidney. There is often a pseudocapsule formed around the tumor by compression of surrounding tissue. Hemorrhage and necrosis may be present, and, frequently, large areas of sclerosis and fibrosis are found within the tumor. Calcification and single or multiple fluid-filled cysts may be seen within the tumor. Sporadic renal carcinoma appears in either kidney with equal frequency; it is most often solitary and unilateral.

Renal tumors occur in six main cellular types: clear cell, papillary type 1, papillary type 2, chromophobe, oncocytoma, and collecting duct. Clear cell carcinomas, which make up 75% of kidney

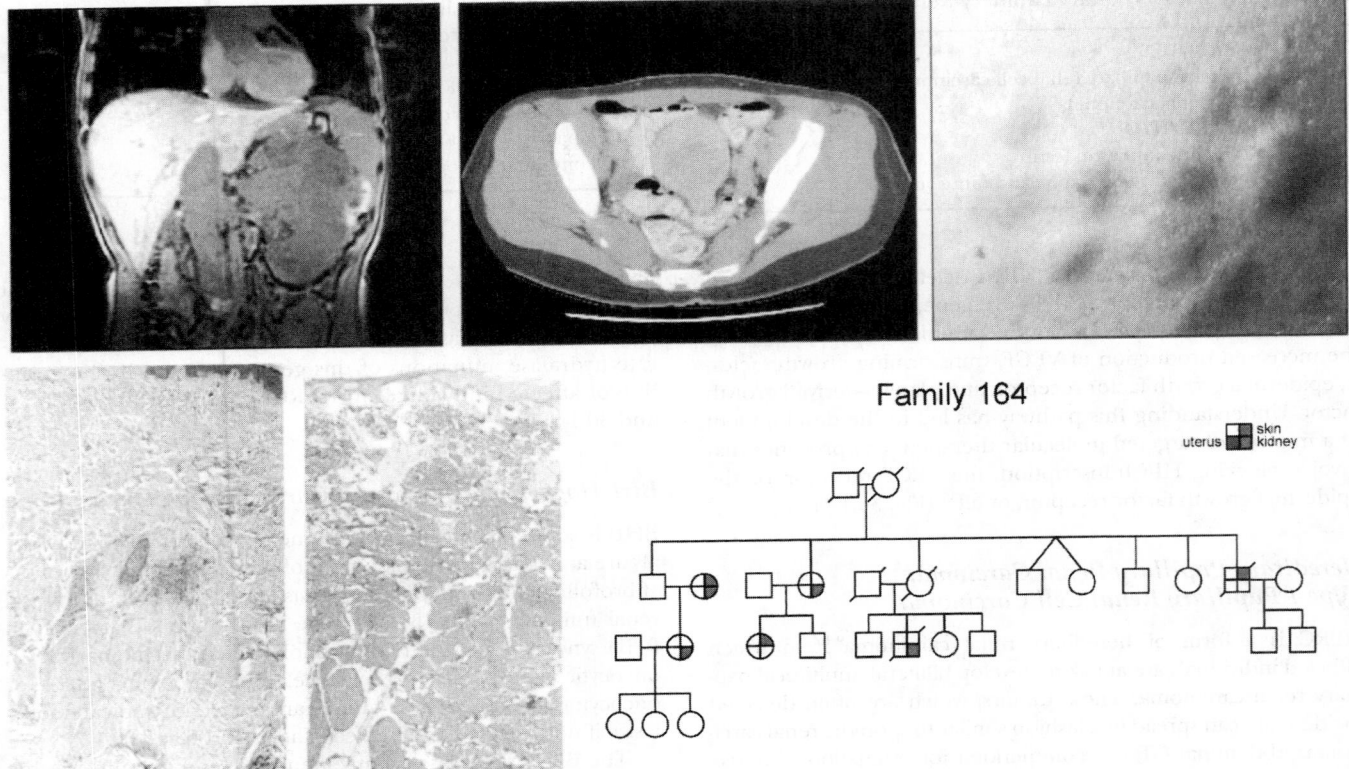

FIGURE 30.1-5.   Hereditary leiomyomatosis renal cell carcinoma (HLRCC) is a hereditary cancer syndrome in which affected individuals are at risk for the development of cutaneous and uterine leiomyoma and type 2 papillary renal carcinoma. HLRCC is characterized by germline mutation of the Krebs cycle enzyme, fumarate hydratase (FH). Germline FH mutation testing is recommended for patients at risk for HLRCC. (From ref. 8, with permission.) (See Color Fig. 30.1-5 in the CD-ROM.)

cancers, contain lightly staining cells with vacuolated cytoplasm containing cholesterol-like substances, neutral lipids, phospholipids, and glycogen. Papillary renal carcinomas make up approximately 15%, with the remainder being chromophobe, collecting duct, and miscellaneous histologic types. Papillary renal carcinoma has been divided into two morphologic subtypes, type 1 and type 2.[43] Collecting duct carcinoma is an unusual variant of renal cell carcinoma that is characterized by a very aggressive clinical course. It is not uncommon for patients with collecting duct carcinoma to present with locally advanced or advanced disease. Chromophobe carcinoma, described by Thoenes et al. in 1985, is characterized by large polygonal cells with pale reticular cytoplasm.[44] Renal oncocytoma, which consists predominantly of eosinophilic cells in a characteristic nested or organoid pattern, is considered to be predominantly a benign lesion. Whether oncocytoma can occur in a malignant form or whether "malignant oncocytoma" is actually a variant of chromophobe renal carcinoma is not completely understood.

The sarcomatoid variant, which can occur with any histologic subtype, represents a localized dedifferentiation of the cancer and is associated with a significantly poorer prognosis than are nonsarcomatous renal carcinomas.[45] A median survival of only 6.6 months in patients with sarcomatoid-type renal carcinoma is in contrast to a 19-month median survival in patients with nonsarcomatous renal carcinoma. Although infrequently used in renal carcinoma, tumor grading may cor-

relate with survival, particularly in patients with nonmetastatic cancer.

CLINICAL PRESENTATION

Renal carcinoma may remain clinically occult for most of its course. The classic presentation of pain, hematuria, and flank mass occurs in a minority of patients and often is indicative of advanced disease. A tumor in the kidney can progress unnoticed to a large size in the retroperitoneum until a metastasis appears. Approximately 30% of patients with renal carcinoma present with metastatic disease, 25% with locally advanced renal carcinoma, and 45% with localized disease.[46] Some 75% of patients with metastatic renal carcinoma have metastases to the lung, 36% to soft tissues, 20% to bone, 18% to liver, 8% to cutaneous sites, and 8% to the central nervous system.[47]

A considerable number of patients with renal carcinoma develop systemic symptoms of this disease (Table 30.1-8). Hypochromic anemia, due to either hematuria or hemolysis, has been observed in 29% to 88% of patients with renal carcinoma. Pyrexia is observed in 20% and cachexia, fatigue, and weight loss in 33%. Secondary amyloidosis is observed in 3% to 5%. Nonmetastatic hepatic dysfunction, initially described by Stauffer in 1961, is a reversible syndrome associated with renal carcinoma that tends to occur in association with fever, fatigue, and weight loss and resolves when the primary tumor is removed. Nonmetastatic hepatic dys-

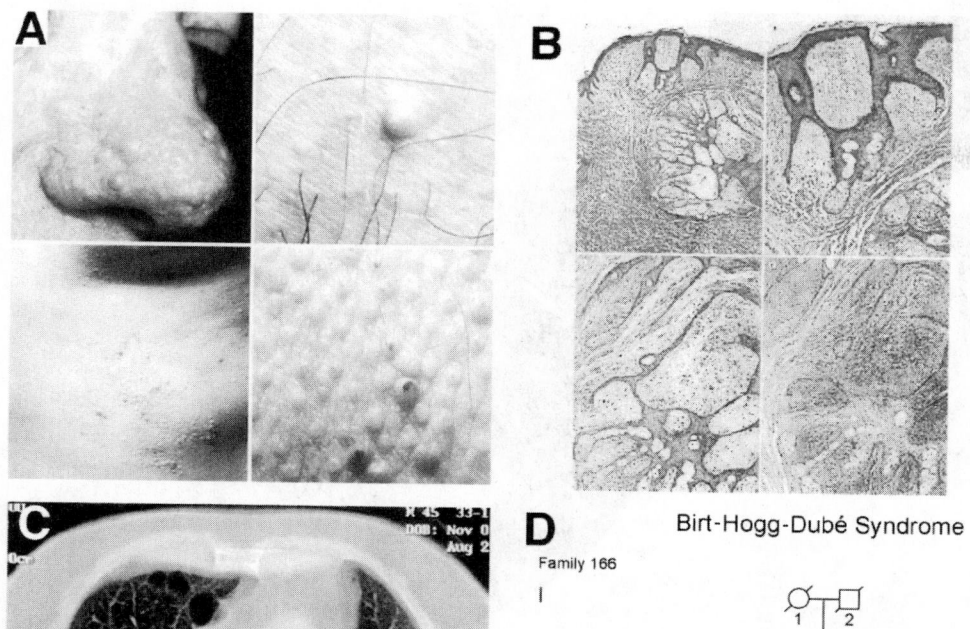

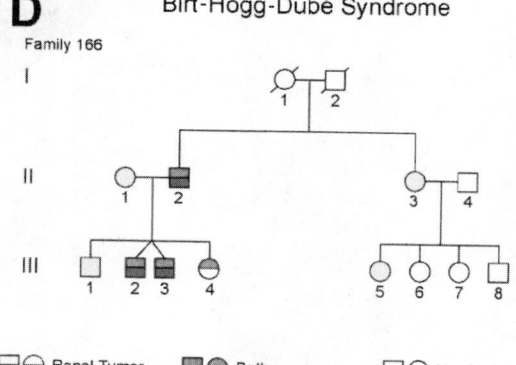

Birt-Hogg-Dubé Syndrome

Family 166

FIGURE 30.1-6. Birt-Hogg-Dubé syndrome is a hereditary kidney cancer syndrome in which affected individuals are at risk for the development of cutaneous (**A**) fibrofolliculoma (**B**), pulmonary cysts (**C**), and pneumothorax and bilateral, multifocal kidney tumors. The kidney tumors in this hereditary cancer syndrome (**D**) are predominantly chromophobe renal carcinoma, hybrid "oncocytic" renal carcinomas and oncocytoma. (From ref. 8, with permission.) (See Color Fig. 30.1-6 in the CD-ROM.)

TABLE 30.1-6.   Clinical Features of Birt-Hogg-Dubé

Cutaneous nodules (hair follicle tumors, fibrofolliculoma) on the face and neck
Pulmonary cysts
Renal tumors
  Chromophobe RCC
  Oncocytic hybrid RCC
  Clear cell RCC
  Oncocytoma

RCC, renal cell carcinoma.

TABLE 30.1-7.   Clinical Evaluation: Birt-Hogg-Dubé (BHD)

BHD gene germline mutation testing
Dermatologic evaluation—skin biopsy
Lung computed tomography
Abdominal computed tomography/ultrasound

TABLE 30.1-8.   Presenting Symptoms, Laboratory Abnormalities, or Abnormalities on Physical Examination and Relationship to Survival in 309 Consecutive Patients Undergoing Nephrectomy for Renal Carcinoma

Presenting Symptom, Abnormal Laboratory Findings, or Abnormalities on Physical Examination	Patients (n = 309)	Patients Surviving 5 Y
Classic triad (gross hematuria, flank mass, pain)	29 (9%)	9/29 (31%)
Hematuria	183 (59%)	74/183 (40%)
Pain	127 (41%)	56/127 (44%)
Abdominal mass	139 (45%)	49/139 (35%)
Fever	21 (7%)	8/21 (38%)
Weight loss	85 (28%)	29/85 (34%)
Anemia	64 (21%)	24/64 (38%)
Erythrocytosis	10 (3%)	4/10 (40%)
Hypercalcemia	11 (3%)	4/11 (36%)
Acute varicocele	7 (2%)	3/7 (43%)
Tumor calcification on x-ray film	39 (13%)	18/39 (46%)
Symptoms of metastases	31 (10%)	1/31 (3%)
Cancer, incidental finding	20 (6%)	13/20 (65%)

(Modified from ref. 186.)

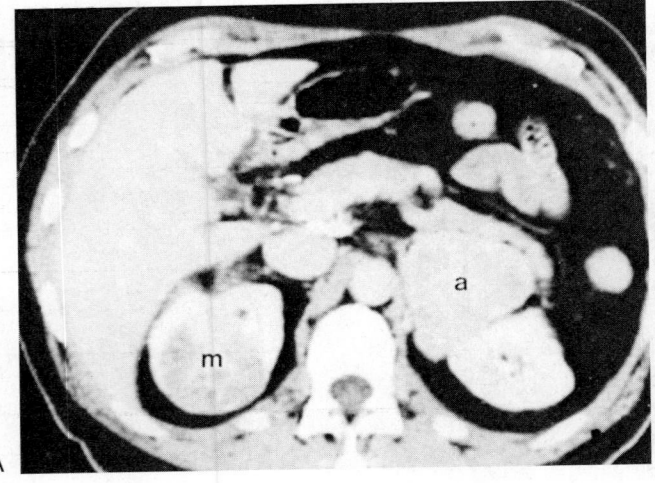

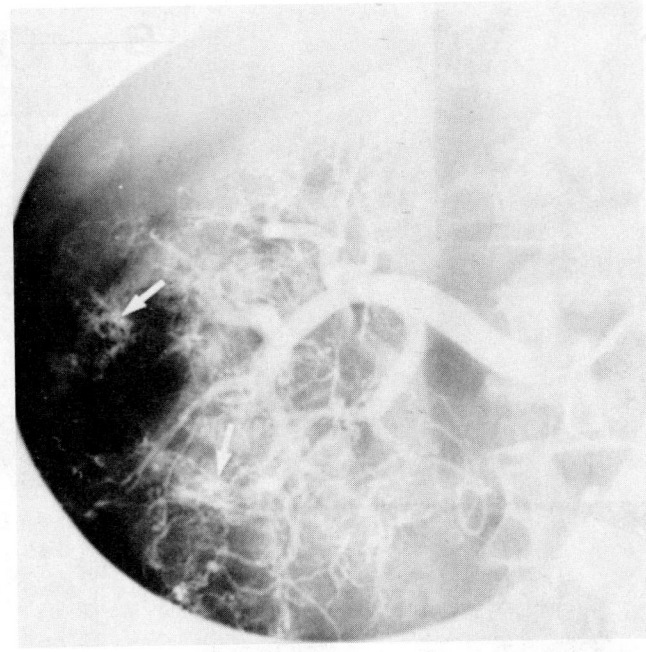

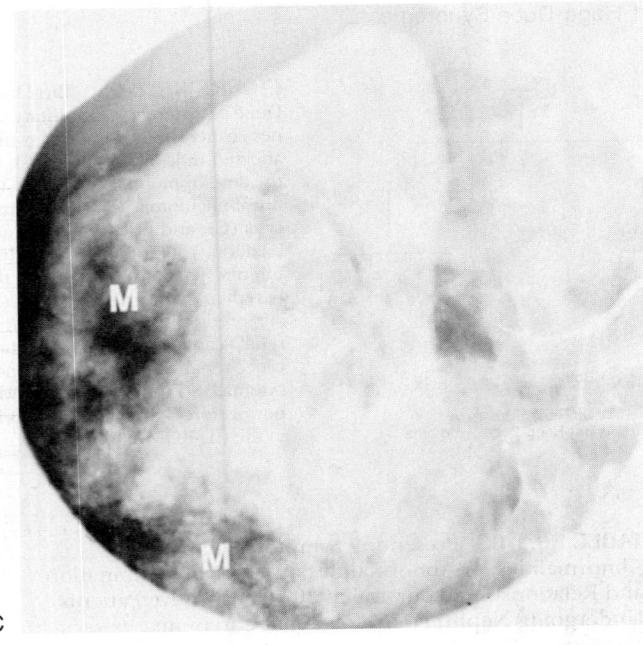

FIGURE 30.1-7. Angiographic appearance of a renal carcinoma. **A:** Computed tomography demonstrates a right renal carcinoma (m) with a large contralateral adrenal metastasis (a). **B:** Early phase of arteriogram demonstrates vascular changes indicative of a malignancy, with puddling and tortuosity (*arrows*). **C:** Late phase of the arteriogram demonstrates that the tumor (M) is relatively avascular despite its early appearance.

function, which is usually associated with poor long-term prognosis, occurs in up to 7% of patients with renal carcinoma.

One to five percent of patients with kidney cancer have polycythemia. Renin levels are often elevated in patients with renal carcinoma but tend to return to normal after the kidney is removed. Whether the tumor itself produces renin or whether it induces renin production by compression of adjacent tissue is unclear. Immunocytochemical studies suggest that renal carcinoma may produce renin, which, however, may be biologically inactive. Plasma fibrinogen levels may be elevated in patients with renal carcinoma and may correlate with tumor stage, disease activity, and response to therapy.

SYTEMICALLY ACTIVE TUMOR-PRODUCED FACTORS

In many patients with renal cell carcinoma, there is evidence of tumor-produced factors that have systemic effects. Pyrexia, cachexia, abnormal liver function, increased alkaline phosphatase levels, hypercalcemia, polycythemia, neuromyopathy, and amyloidosis have all been reported in association with renal cell carcinoma.[48,49]

Humoral hypercalcemia of malignancy, frequently observed in patients with advanced renal cell carcinoma, is thought to be caused by a tumor-produced, systemically active bone-resorbing factor. Kidney cancer produces a factor with parathyroid hormone–like bioactivity. A parathyroid hormone–related protein that has been implicated in malignant hypercalcemia has been cloned from a human lung cancer cell line and is expressed in mammalian cells. Thiede and coworkers demonstrated that human renal carcinoma expresses a parathyroid hormone–like peptide with considerable similarity to parathyroid hormone.[50] Humoral hypercalcemia of malignancy in patients with advanced renal cell carcinoma is associated with a poor prognosis.[51]

RADIOGRAPHIC EVALUATION

Advances in imaging techniques have made the determination of whether a space-occupying renal mass lesion is benign or

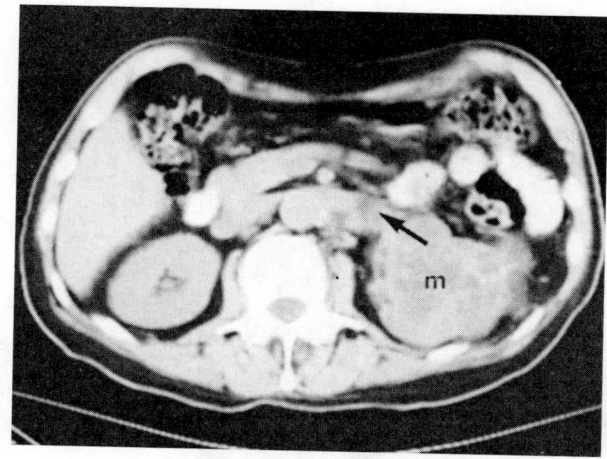
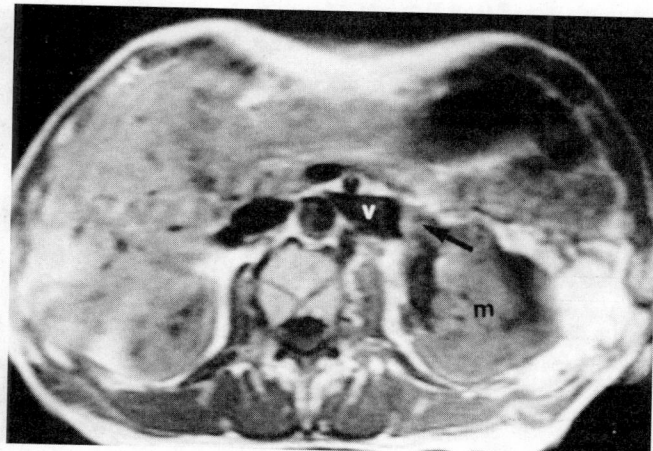

FIGURE 30.1-8. Renal vein invasion by a renal carcinoma as shown by computed tomography (CT) and magnetic resonance imaging. **A:** Nonenhanced CT scan shows large left renal mass with calcification (m) invading the left renal vein (*arrow*). **B:** T1-weighted magnetic resonance image demonstrates tumor (m) and vascular invasion (*arrow*). Flowing blood (v) in the left renal vein is black on this scan.

malignant much more accurate.[52] Diagnostic modalities used to evaluate and stage renal mass lesions have evolved from excretory urography to arteriography, venography, CT, ultrasound, and magnetic resonance imaging (MRI). CT and MRI have evolved to such an extent that excretory urography is currently infrequently used in the initial evaluation of renal mass lesions. Ultrasound examination proves excellent staging and diagnostic information and can provide accurate anatomic detail of extrarenal extension of tumor, adrenal involvement, involvement of lymph nodes, and infiltration of adjacent viscera (Fig. 30.1-7).

Renal arteriography (see Fig. 30.1-7*B* and 30.1-7*C*) is infrequently used in the evaluation of patients with a suspicious renal mass because of advances in MRI imaging. In a renal carcinoma the arteriogram will often show neovascularity, arteriovenous fistulas, pooling of contrast medium, and accentuation of capsular vessels. A renal arteriogram may be useful in evaluating an indeterminate small renal mass lesion or as an aid to the surgeon in defining the vasculature during the surgical removal of a large tumor. Although renal arteriography can be performed with minimal risk, false aneurysms, arterial emboli, hemorrhage, and decreased renal function secondary to contrast agent injection have been encountered. Dual-phase three-dimensional MR angiography is a very useful technique in depicting renal vessels before surgical therapy. This technique is very accurate for the detection of the renal arteries, renal vein involvement, and extension into the inferior vena cava.[53]

CT is the modality of choice for imaging a renal mass (Fig. 30.1-8*A*). With newer techniques using multidetector CT equipment and enhancement technology, it is now possible to obtain thinner cuts (approximately 1 mm) and to compare pre- and postcontrast enhancement of the suspected mass lesion.[52]

Although arteriography and CT are equivalent in depicting renal vein involvement, CT is better for demonstrating local nodal involvement. The use of contrast agent enhancement has greatly increased the sensitivity of CT for abnormal renal mass lesions. Contrast-enhanced CT allows the clinician to detect very small changes in the density of a renal lesion that might indicate the presence of an early neoplastic lesion. Dynamic CT is superior to standard CT arteriography, ultrasonography, and radionuclide scanning and may correctly demonstrate tumor involvement of

the kidney, involvement of the renal fascia, or extension into adjacent organs.

Inferior venacavography may rarely be performed when there is a large renal tumor or when there is uncertainty about tumor involvement of the vena cava. Ultrasound, CT, and MRI (Fig. 30.1-9) can provide information about tumor involvement of the vena cava; however, the inferior venacavagram provides a reliable means of accurately determining the precise extent of vena caval involvement by tumor. This information may be helpful to the surgeon in planning the vascular aspect of the operative procedure. When Horan and coworkers prospectively compared the accuracy of venacavography and MRI, they found that venacavography and MRI offer equal diagnostic accuracy in the identification of venous extension of kidney cancer and that the combination of both tests results in higher diagnostic yield than use of either test alone.[54] MRI is very useful for staging renal carcinoma. MRI can produce a unique three-dimensional picture of the tumor that, in the case of a large tumor, may be an invaluable aid to the surgeon in planning the operative approach. In patients with tumors involving the inferior vena cava, transesophageal echocardiography has been shown to be an accurate diagnostic technique for tumor imaging to document the extent of involvement of the vena cava (see Fig. 30.1-9).

There is no single imaging technique that is best for all patients with renal carcinoma. Depending on the size of the primary tumor and the extent of extrarenal disease, CT, ultrasound, arteriography, venography, and MRI each can provide unique information in an individual case. Because CT, MRI, and ultrasound are outpatient procedures and are less invasive, arteriography is now infrequently used. Multiple imaging modalities are often used to provide the most complete information, particularly when surgical removal of a large tumor is being considered.

STAGING AND PROGNOSIS

Robson Classification

The staging system previously used by most physicians in the United States was the Robson modification of the system of Flocks and Kadesky (Table 30.1-9).[55] In the Robson classification, stage I

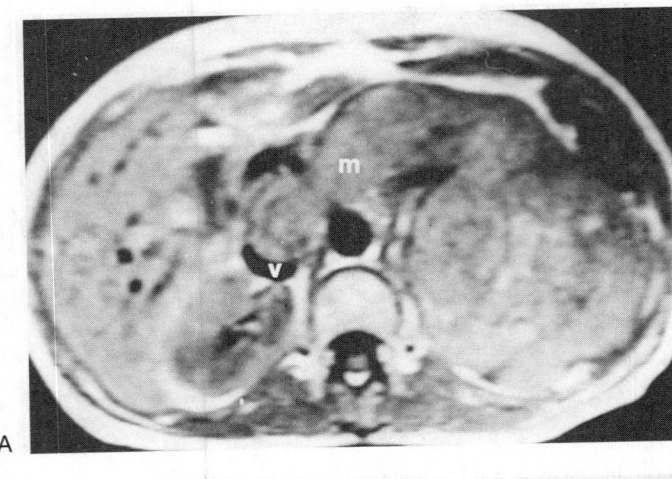

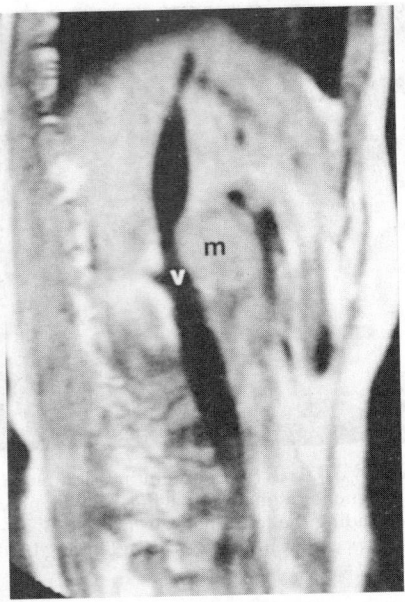

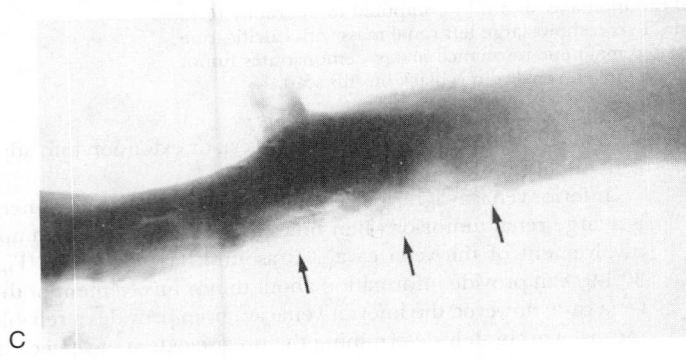

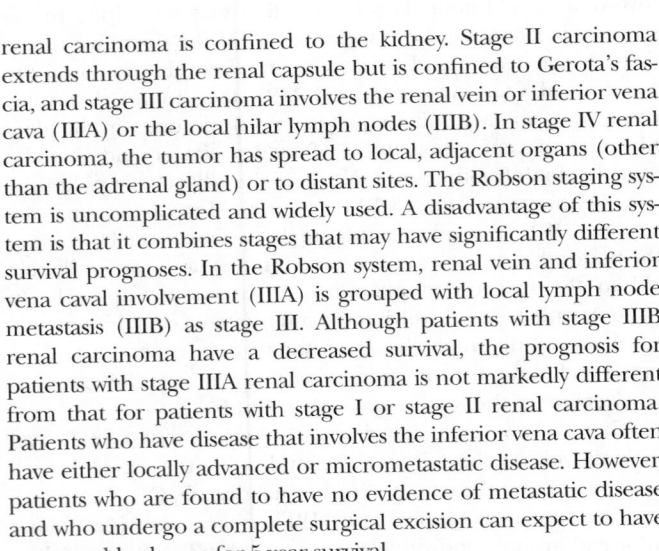

FIGURE 30.1-9.   Invasion of inferior vena cava (IVC) by renal carcinoma demonstrated by magnetic resonance imaging and venography. **A:** Axial T1-weighted image demonstrates a large left renal carcinoma with extension into the left renal vein (m) with protrusion into the IVC (v). **B:** Sagittal T1-weighted image shows the relation of the tumor thrombus (m) to the IVC (v) in the lateral projection. **C:** An anteroposterior image of the interior cavagram demonstrates tumor in the medial aspect of the inferior vena cava.

renal carcinoma is confined to the kidney. Stage II carcinoma extends through the renal capsule but is confined to Gerota's fascia, and stage III carcinoma involves the renal vein or inferior vena cava (IIIA) or the local hilar lymph nodes (IIIB). In stage IV renal carcinoma, the tumor has spread to local, adjacent organs (other than the adrenal gland) or to distant sites. The Robson staging system is uncomplicated and widely used. A disadvantage of this system is that it combines stages that may have significantly different survival prognoses. In the Robson system, renal vein and inferior vena caval involvement (IIIA) is grouped with local lymph node metastasis (IIIB) as stage III. Although patients with stage IIIB renal carcinoma have a decreased survival, the prognosis for patients with stage IIIA renal carcinoma is not markedly different from that for patients with stage I or stage II renal carcinoma. Patients who have disease that involves the inferior vena cava often have either locally advanced or micrometastatic disease. However, patients who are found to have no evidence of metastatic disease and who undergo a complete surgical excision can expect to have a reasonable chance for 5-year survival.

TNM Classification

The TNM (tumor, node, metastasis) classification proves a more accurate method for classifying extent of tumor involvement. In the TNM classification, T1 denotes a tumor that is 7 cm or less in greatest diameter and confined to the kidney. T1 is divided into two categories: T1a refers to a kidney tumor that is 4 cm or less, and T1b is a tumor greater than 4 cm but not more than 7 cm in greatest dimension. T2 denotes a tumor more than 7 cm in greatest dimension, but still confined to the kidney. T3 is a tumor that extends into the major veins or

invades the adrenal gland or perinephric tissues but not beyond Gerota's fascia. T3 is divided into T3a, a tumor that directly invades the adrenal gland or perirenal sinus fat; T3b, a tumor that grossly extends into the renal vein or its segmental branches or vena cava below the diaphragm; and T3c, a tumor that grossly extends into the vena cava above the diaphragm or that invades the wall of the vena cava. T4 denotes a tumor that has extended beyond Gerota's fascia (Table 30.1-10). Unlike the Robson system, the TNM system classifies lymph node involvement (other than a solitary node) as stage IV, leaving tumors with vena cava involvement as stage III. The 2002 TNM classification of renal carcinoma introduced the division of T1 tumors into the a and b groupings based on size and appears to provide improved stratification according to survival.

TABLE 30.1-9.   Comparison of the Two Classification Systems for Staging of Renal Carcinoma

Feature	TNM	Robson
Small tumor, no enlargement of kidney	T1	I (A)
Large tumor, cortex not broken	T2	I (A)
Perinephric or hilar extension	T3a	II (B)
Renal vein involved	T3b	IIIA (C)
Vena cava involved	T3b,c	IIIA (C)
Extension to neighboring organs	T4	IV (D)
Nodal invasion	N+	IIIB (C)
Distant metastases	M+	IV (D)

TNM, tumor, node, metastasis.
(From ref. 56, with permission.)

TABLE 30.1-10. TNM Classification: Kidney

PRIMARY TUMOR (T)

TX	Primary tumor cannot be assessed.
T0	No evidence of primary tumor.
T1	Tumor confined to kidney, <7 cm in greatest diameter.
T1a	Tumor 4 cm or less in greatest dimension, limited to the kidney.
T1b	Tumor >4 cm but not >7 cm in greatest dimension, limited to kidney.
T2	Tumor >7 cm in greatest dimension, limited to the kidney.
T3	Tumor extends into major veins or invades adrenal gland or perinephric tissues but not beyond Gerota's fascia.
T3a	Tumor directly invades adrenal gland or perirenal and/or renal sinus fat but not beyond Gerota's fascia.
T3b	Tumor grossly extends into the renal vein or its segmental (muscle-containing) branches, or vena cava below the diaphragm.
T3c	Tumor grossly extends into vena cava above diaphragm or invades the wall of the vena cava.
T4	Tumor invades beyond Gerota's fascia.

NODAL (N) INVOLVEMENT

The regional lymph nodes are the paraaortic and paracaval nodes. The juxtaregional lymph nodes are the pelvic and mediastinal nodes.

NX	Regional lymph nodes cannot be assessed.
N0	No regional lymph node metastases.
N1	Metastases in a single regional lymph node.
N2	Metastasis in more than one regional lymph node.

DISTANT METASTASIS (M)

MX	Distant metastasis cannot be assessed.
M0	No distant metastasis.
M1	Distant metastasis.

STAGE GROUPING

I	T1	N0	M0
II	T2	N0	M0
III	T3	N0	M0
	T1	N1	M0
	T2	N1	M0
IV	T4	N0	M0
	T4	N1	M0
	Any T	N2	M0
	Any T	Any N	M1

(Data from American Joint Committee on Cancer. *AJCC cancer staging manual*, 6th ed. New York: Springer-Verlag, 2002.)

SURVIVAL

Stage

The 5-year survival initially reported by Robson and coworkers in 1969 was 66% for stage I renal carcinoma, 64% for stage II, 42% for stage III, and only 11% for stage IV.[55] These survival statistics remained essentially the same for a number of years. However, it has since been noted that whereas renal vein involvement does not have a markedly negative effect on prognosis, the 5-year survival for patients with Robson stage IIIB renal cell carcinoma is only 18%. Recent studies have reported better survival for patients with tumors confined to the kidney: 96% 5-year survival for T1 renal carcinoma and an 88% 5-year survival for stage T2 disease (Table 30.1-11). Patients with T3 renal carcinoma had a 64% 5-year survival and those with T4 a 23% 5-year survival.[56-59]

With the expanded use of CT scans or ultrasonography, or both, the rate of incidentally found carcinomas of the kidney has increased. The prognosis for patients whose tumor was diagnosed incidentally is more favorable than that of those who present with

TABLE 30.1-11. Summary of Survival Rates in Renal Carcinoma

Study	Survival (Y)	Survival Rate by TNM Stage (%)			
		I	II	III	IV
Tsui et al., 2000[59]	5	91	74	67	32
Guinan et al., 1997[58]	5	100	69	59	16
Kinouchi et al., 1999[57]	5	96	95	70	24
Javidan et al., 1999[187]	5	95	88	59	20
Average 5-y survival		**96**	**82**	**64**	**23**

TNM, tumor, node, metastasis.
(Modified from ref. 188.)

symptoms, as the former group consists of patients with smaller tumors that usually tend to be confined to the kidney. Patients with metastatic renal carcinoma who present with humoral hypercalcemia of malignancy have a poor prognosis.

Histology

Kidney cancer is not a single disease; rather, it is made up of a number of cancers that occur in the kidney, each with a different histology, a different clinical course, and caused by a different gene. Cheville et al. evaluated outcome in 2385 patients with sporadic kidney cancer who had a nephrectomy between 1970 and 2000.[60] Cancer-specific survival rates at 5 years were 68.9% for clear cell, 87.4% for papillary, and 86.7% for chromophobe renal carcinoma.[60] When papillary renal carcinoma was stratified by type 1 and type 2 papillary renal carcinoma, Mejean et al. found a significantly lower 10-year survival in patients with type 2 papillary renal carcinoma (59%) versus those with type 1 papillary renal carcinoma (80%).[61] Other less frequent types of kidney cancer include collecting duct and medullary renal carcinoma. Collecting duct or Bellini duct carcinoma of the kidney is an uncommon, particularly aggressive form of papillary renal carcinoma. Medullary renal carcinoma is a rare and very aggressive tumor that has been reported in young patients with sickle cell trait. In most of the reported cases, the disease has spread early and has been fatal.[62]

LOCALIZED RENAL CARCINOMA

SURGICAL TREATMENT

Surgery is the only known effective therapy for localized renal carcinoma. The first nephrectomy was performed by Eratus B. Walcott in Milwaukee on June 4, 1861, on a 58-year-old man with a kidney tumor who died 15 days after surgery. Professor Gustave Simon, after completing a number of experimental nephrectomies on dogs, undertook the first deliberate, planned, and successful nephrectomy in Heidelberg on August 2, 1889, in a patient with a persistent ureteral fistula. The first successful nephrectomy in a patient with kidney cancer was performed in 1883 by Grawitz.[63] Since that first nephrectomy, there have been significant advances in surgical techniques involving the introduction of the thoracoabdominal approach to laparoscopic radical nephrectomy and changes in the surgical approach, including the use of partial nephrectomy for small renal tumors.

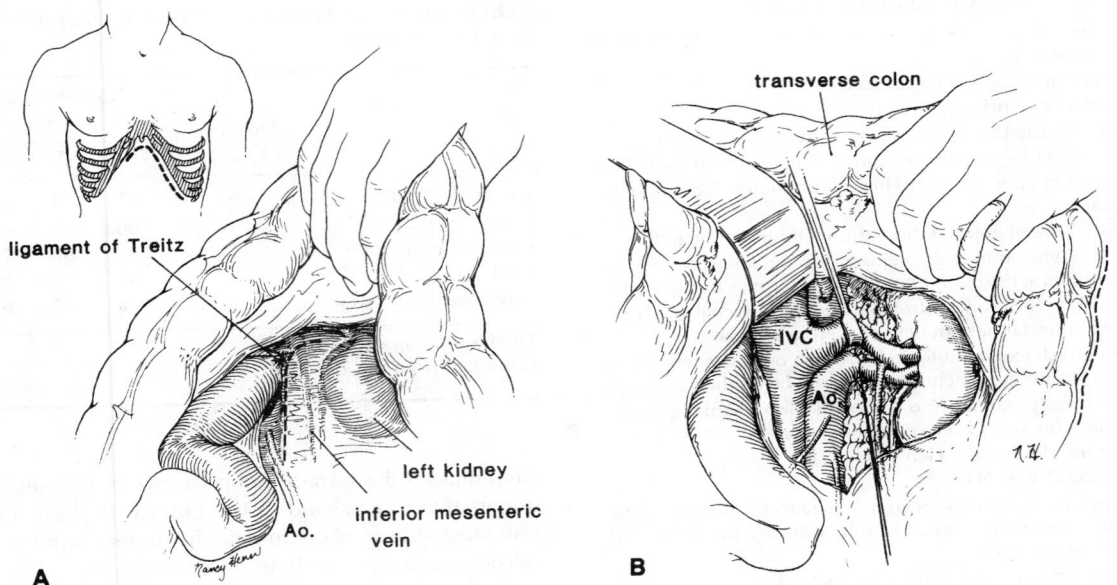

FIGURE 30.1-10.   **A:** Area of dissection for lymph node dissection for radical nephroureterectomy should be from the superior mesenteric artery to the level of the inferior mesenteric artery, with the anatomic structures identified. **B:** The left colon can be reflected from the anterior surface of Gerota's fascia with exposure of the renal artery before ligation and division. The dotted line to the right of the descending colon indicates a line of incision on the left pericolic gutter that should extend superiorly to include division of the splenocolic attachments. IVC, inferior vena cava. (From Paulson DF, Perez CA, Anderson T. Cancer of the kidney and ureter. In: DeVita VT Jr, Hellman S, Rosenberg SA, eds. *Cancer: principles and practice of oncology*, 2nd ed. Philadelphia: JB Lippincott, 1985:898, with permission.)

The standard procedure today for treatment of localized renal carcinoma greater than 4 cm is radical nephrectomy (Fig. 30.1-10). Radical nephrectomy includes complete removal of Gerota's fascia and its contents, including the kidney and the adrenal gland, and provides a better surgical margin than simple removal of the kidney. Many clinicians believe that, in view of the rarity of ipsilateral adrenal metastasis and the potential morbidity associated with adrenalectomy, a macroscopically normal ipsilateral adrenal gland should not be removed with the kidney when the tumor is in the lower pole of the kidney (Fig. 30.1-11).

There are a number of different open surgical approaches to removal of a kidney cancer. Common approaches are the anterior transperitoneal approach, the flank approach, and the thoracoabdominal approach. The choice of surgical approach depends on the location and size of the tumor and the body habitus of the patient. The type of incision is chosen to ensure that the tumor may safely be removed. A flank incision, with or without removal of a portion of the tenth or eleventh rib, is often used for small tumors without venous involvement. A subcostal transabdominal incision may be used when there is a large tumor in the middle or lower aspect of the kidney or when vascular involvement is anticipated and access to the major vessels is essential. A thoracoabdominal incision may be required when there is a large middle or upper pole tumor. In a thoracoabdominal incision, a rib is removed, the thoracic cavity is opened, and the diaphragm is incised. The incision is then carried down transabdominally to allow maximal exposure of the upper abdominal region and the great vessels (see Fig. 30.1-11). If the tumor has grown into the sidewall of the vena cava or if the vena caval involvement is too extensive for a simple partial wall resection, a portion of the vena cava itself may be resected. When the tumor is in the right kidney,

the adjacent vena cava can often be resected safely. If, however, the tumor in the left kidney and the adjacent vena cava is resected, vascular reconstruction of the right renal vein may be needed to establish adequate venous drainage. If the suprahepatic caval extension of a renal tumor thrombus extends up to the right atrium, cardiopulmonary bypass may be required for tumor removal. Regional lymphadenectomy is often performed at the time of radical nephrectomy, although its role in prolonging sur-

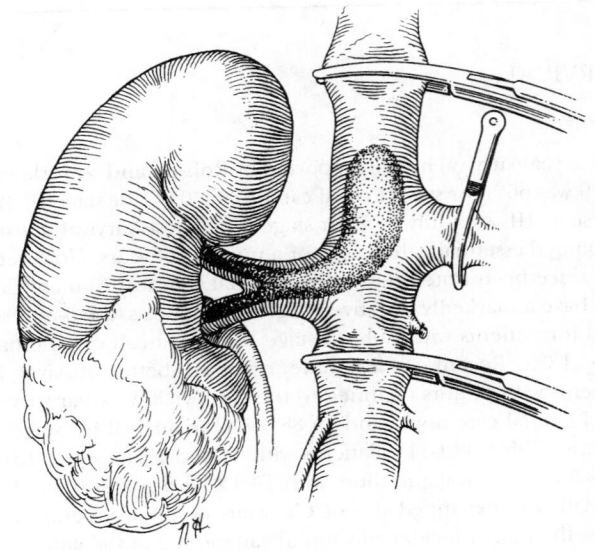

FIGURE 30.1-11.   Surgical removal of a kidney tumor in which there is tumor extension through the renal vein into the inferior vena cava.

vival has not been demonstrated. In a regional lymphadenectomy, ipsilateral nodal tissue from the diaphragm to the bifurcation of the aorta as well as nodal tissue in the interaortocaval region at the hilum of the kidney is removed.

Laparoscopic nephrectomy has quickly become the preferred method for removal of kidney tumors. As advances with this technique are growing, this approach is rapidly becoming the standard of care for management of most renal tumors not amenable to nephron-sparing surgery. The technique is associated with cancer control equivalent to open radical nephrectomy and is associated with decreased hospital stay, more rapid convalescence, decreased postoperative pain, and improved cosmesis.[64] Walther et al. have developed laparoscopic nephrectomy as a means of performing minimally invasive cytoreductive nephrectomy in patients with advanced renal cell carcinoma as preparation for immunologic therapy.[65]

In patients with locally advanced renal cell carcinoma (N+), there is no evidence to date that adjuvant, postsurgical treatment of patients with an agent such as interleukin-2 (IL-2) or interferon-α (IFN-α) increases survival. In patients in whom all visible disease has been resected surgically, most physicians recommend treatment when residual/recurrent disease becomes detectable.

Bilateral Renal Carcinoma, Tumors in Solitary Kidneys, and Renal Tumors Less Than 4 cm

The treatment of patients with either bilateral renal carcinoma or renal carcinoma in a solitary kidney is evolving toward a more minimally invasive approach. Patients with tumor in a solitary kidney may be treated by either partial nephrectomy or nephrectomy followed by dialysis or transplantation, or both, if the tumor is too large for a partial nephrectomy. In selected patients, nephron-sparing surgery may be recommended for patients with sporadic renal cell cancer, particularly those with a small tumor (4 cm or less) or a tumor in a solitary kidney. Nephron-sparing surgery for localized renal tumors has been found to be a safe procedure, providing long-term tumor control and preservation of renal function.[66] Laparoscopic partial nephrectomy provides a minimally invasive alternative for carefully selected patients with renal carcinoma. This technique has been shown to be a viable alternative for selected patients with renal tumors and is associated with excellent tumor control and preservation of renal function.[66,67]

Other approaches for minimally invasive nephron-sparing therapy of renal carcinoma, such as cryotherapy and radiofrequency ablation, are currently under development. These techniques provide promise for the further development of effective forms of therapy with significant decreases in morbidity.[68]

Extracorporeal partial nephrectomy plus autotransplantation is a rarely used technique that allows the surgeon to accurately remove large tumors in the center of a solitary kidney. This *ex vivo* procedure entails radical excision of the kidney and division of the ureter. Under optical magnification, the tumor is carefully dissected from the surrounding renal parenchyma. A small rim of normal tissue is removed along with the tumor to provide a tumor-free margin of resection. After the kidney has been surgically reconstructed, it is autotransplanted back into the iliac space. Vascular anastomosis of the renal artery and vein to the iliac vessels and ureteroureterostomy are performed.[69]

Surgical Management of Patients with Hereditary Forms of Renal Carcinoma

Patients with hereditary forms of renal carcinoma are often challenging to manage. Individuals with VHL, HPRC, or BHD can have widespread renal involvement. Surgical management in these patients involves careful parenchymal-sparing surgery, which is recommended when the renal tumors reach a certain size threshold, generally 3 cm. The use of parenchymal-sparing surgery in these patients is based on a strategy designed to maintain the patient's renal function as long as possible, whereas decreasing the risk for metastasis.[70] Patients who are affected with HLRCC are at risk for the development of an aggressive form of type 2 papillary renal carcinoma that can metastasize early. In these patients, early surgical intervention is recommended.

Management of Small, Incidentally Detected Renal Masses

The experience with expectant management of small renal tumors in VHL, HPRC, and BHD patients has raised the question whether it might be appropriate to conservatively manage small incidentally detected renal masses in the nonhereditary patient population. The report of Volpe et al. suggests that conservative management of patients with renal tumors less than 4 cm may be appropriate for selected patients who are elderly or unsuited for surgery.[71] However, for patients who are surgical candidates, most experienced clinicians recommend surgical therapy. It is currently not possible by preoperative imaging studies to determine which small renal tumors will grow slowly and which will metastasize early. Tumors, such as type 2 papillary renal carcinoma, collecting duct carcinoma, and medullary renal carcinoma, are particularly aggressive and may spread from even a small-sized renal tumor.

METASTATIC RENAL CARCINOMA

CYTOREDUCTIVE NEPHRECTOMY FOR PALLIATION

Adjuvant or palliative nephrectomy is frequently performed in patients with metastatic renal carcinoma, particularly those with pain, hemorrhage, malaise, hypercalcemia, erythrocytosis, or hypertension. Removal of the primary tumor may alleviate some or all of these abnormalities.[51] Although there are isolated reports of regression of metastatic renal carcinoma after removal of the primary tumor, only 4 of 474 patients (0.8%) in nine series who underwent nephrectomy experienced "regression" of metastatic foci.[72]

CYTOREDUCTIVE NEPHRECTOMY IN THE MANAGEMENT OF METASTATIC RENAL CARCINOMA

deKernion and coworkers reported results in 26 patients with metastatic renal carcinoma who underwent palliative nephrectomy and found no increase in survival, compared with survival in the entire group of 79 patients with metastatic renal carcinoma.[73] In the context of metastatic disease, nephrectomy alone has not been shown to be associated with a survival benefit. Nephrectomy is not recommended for the purpose of inducing spontaneous regression; rather, it is performed to control symptoms or to decrease tumor burden in preparation for subsequent therapy.[74]

At the National Cancer Institute Walther et al. developed a strategy of using cytoreductive surgery before systemic immunotherapy in patients with metastatic renal cell carcinoma. This approach—the combination of primary debulking and systemic IL-2—has been associated with durable complete tumor regression in some patients with metastatic renal cell carcinoma.[65,74,75] When the experience with IL-2–based therapies at the National Cancer Institute from 1986 to 1996 was reviewed, among 51 patients treated with the primary kidney in place, no responses were noted in the primary kidney tumor.[76]

Two large randomized trials have been performed to address the role of nephrectomy followed by IFN-α–based immunotherapy compared with IFN-α alone in metastatic renal cell carcinoma. Flanigan et al. found the median survival of 120 patients assigned to surgery followed by IFN to be 11.1 months, compared to 8.1 months in 121 patients assigned to IFN alone (P = .05).[77] Mickisch et al. found time to progression (5 months vs. 3 months) and median duration of survival to be better in patients randomized to surgery plus IFN compared to those randomized to IFN alone.[78] Although there is not data to indicate that nephrectomy alone improves survival, these studies indicate that in well-selected patients with good performance status, nephrectomy plus IFN results in improved outcome among patients with metastatic renal carcinoma than does IFN alone. Nephrectomy in patients with advanced renal cell carcinoma should be considered in the context of a treatment plan including systemic therapy. The recent introduction of laparoscopic nephrectomy in patients with advanced disease[65] provides a potentially less invasive method for cytoreduction as preparation for administration of systemic therapies.

RESECTION OF METASTASES

Of the approximately 30% of patients with renal carcinoma who present with metastases, only 1.5% to 3.5% have a solitary metastasis.[79] Patients with a solitary metastasis synchronous with a primary lesion have decreased survival when compared with patients who develop metastasis after the primary tumor is removed.[80] Surgical resection is appropriate in selected patients with metastatic renal carcinoma. In one study, 59 patients with renal carcinoma who underwent surgical resection for a solitary metastasis had a 45% 3-year survival and a 34% 5-year survival.[79] O'Dea et al. reviewed patients with renal cell cancer and a synchronous or metachronous solitary metastasis.[81] Of the 26 patients who underwent nephrectomy and who later developed metastasis, 23% lived more than 5 years after removal of the metastatic lesions. Three patients were alive 58, 94, and 245 months after resection of the metastatic lesions.[81] In a report in 1999 by van der Poel et al., better survival was found for lung metastases when compared with other sites of metastasis.[80] In this study, 14% were free of disease at 45 months, whereas long-term (more than 5 years) disease-free survival was observed in 7%.[80] Resection of metastases renders few cures but can produce long-term survivors.

SYSTEMIC CHEMOTHERAPY FOR RENAL CELL CARCINOMA

Limited options are available for the systemic therapy of renal cell carcinoma, and no hormonal or chemotherapeutic regimen is accepted as a standard of care. Reviews surveying phase II clinical trials for renal cell carcinoma have appeared at intervals[82–84] without a change in the final conclusion: No systemic chemotherapeutic or hormonal approach has provided a reasonable level of

activity. However, effective therapy may be on the horizon for this most resistant disease in the form of agents aimed at new molecular targets. The discovery of sporadic VHL mutations in clear cell carcinomas led to the identification of increased HIF1α-mediated VEGF activity, and anti-VEGF therapy was shown to be effective in one randomized trial.[85]

What is remarkable is how consistent the results have been with agents developed to date. The development of agents for renal cell cancer has been characterized by an initial, exciting report of activity, followed by later studies that identify the true activity, always much lower, of the agent or combination, a phenomenon that could be described as *response migration*. A comprehensive review by Yagoda et al.[83] encompassed 4542 patients enrolled in 83 clinical trials published from 1983 through 1993. Among 4093 evaluable patients, a 6% response rate was recorded, with 53 complete responses (CRs; 1.3%) and 192 partial responses (PRs; 4.7%). Response rates in excess of 25% were noted in 11 trials; in each case another trial incorporating the same or a comparable treatment regimen reported lower or zero response rates. Thus, randomized studies are needed for confirmation of results obtained in single-agent trials.

Few single agents in the Yagoda review appeared to have activity above the background: 5-fluorouracil (5-FU), the related compound floxuridine, and vinblastine.[83] Fourteen trials with floxuridine yielded response rates ranging from 0% to 43%, with an average rate of 12%. Seven trials had response rates of less than 10%, and four had response rates exceeding 20%. For 5-FU, which has been primarily used in combination with immunotherapy, responses were somewhat fewer, with an overall response rate of 10% for infusional 5-FU alone and 19% for 5-FU in combination with IFN. Similar results were reported for vinblastine, an agent initially thought to have activity in renal cancer, with a 30% response rate reported. In the Yagoda series, seven trials incorporating infusional vinblastine yielded an overall response rate of 7%, and three trials reported no responses.[83] Since 1993, further results with vinblastine have been equally discouraging.[84] For example, in two randomized trials, vinblastine has served as the control arm, producing one PR among 80 patients in one trial and one complete and one PR among 81 patients in another.[86,87] Despite these results, these agents represented the only real choice among standard agents for the treatment of renal cell cancer for many years.

The 83 trials reported in the review by Yagoda et al.[83] included compounds from every class of anticancer agent: taxanes (paclitaxel and docetaxel); vinca alkaloids (vinblastine, vindesine, and vinorelbine); anthracyclines (epirubicin, doxorubicin, and idarubicin); anthracenediones (mitoxantrone, bisantrene); alkylating agents (both nitrosoureas and sulfonylureas, as well as ifosfamide and melphalan); heavy metals (carboplatinum and gallium nitrate); pyrimidines (floxuridine, 5-FU, and gemcitabine); and purines (6-thioguanine, fludarabine, and 2-deoxycoforomycin). Yagoda et al. concluded that the responses could be mediated by an indirect effect on the immune system.[83] Considering that the response rates in these trials are higher than the frequency of spontaneous remissions, and because of the occasional complete remission, one could speculate that the responses involve an effect triggered by the chemotherapy but mediated by the immune system. However, scientific evidence to support this thesis is lacking. Although the majority of patients experiencing a complete remission were noted in trials including cimetidine, vinblastine, 5-FU, and floxuridine, the CR rate ranged between 2% and 4%, which is not very different from the 1.3% CR rate noted in the entire series. These considerations favor a conclusion that little, if any, cytotoxic activity has been exerted in renal cell cancer. It can be concluded that the best recommendation for patients with this disease, after immunotherapy, is participation in clinical trials studying new agents or new approaches.[84]

Hormonal Therapy in Renal Cell Cancer

Hormonal agents have also been used in systemic therapy. Supported by observations in animal models, progestins and androgens have been studied in renal cancer since the 1960s.[82] In the absence of effective chemotherapy, medroxyprogesterone acetate (Megace) was adopted as conventional treatment for renal cell cancer.[82] Although early studies suggested benefit, an overall response rate of 2% more accurately reflects the inactivity of this agent. Except for its value in appetite stimulation, the use of medroxyprogesterone acetate cannot be recommended in the treatment of renal cell cancer today.

Studies with antiestrogens in more recent years have yielded similar results. An overall response rate of 7% (three patients with CR) was identified in four studies treating 146 patients with high-dose tamoxifen (100 mg/m^2/d or more).[83] In 1998, two CRs (3%) were reported in 63 patients receiving 40 mg of oral tamoxifen daily in the control arm of a randomized study.[86] Although one study with high-dose toremifene (300 mg/d), a novel antiestrogen with activity in breast cancer, reported a 17% response rate including one CR, no responses were observed when combined with IFN-α.[87,88] Thus, reported responses to treatment with hormonal therapy most likely mimic the same level of inactivity identified with most single-agent chemotherapeutic trials.

Recent Chemotherapy Trials in Renal Cell Cancer

A limited search for single agents examined in phase II trials in renal cell cancer and reported over the 6-year period through 2003 identified 28 published studies. As shown in Table 30.1-12, the agents are from various pharmaceutical classes and, once again, the refractory nature of renal cell cancer to cytotoxic therapy is observed. Several of the agents studied have antiangiogenic activity (see Antiangiogenic Agents, later in this chapter). One must realize that most studies have not discriminated between his-

TABLE 30.1-12. Phase II Studies in Renal Cell Cancer: 1998–2003

Investigator	Agent	Enter.	Eval.	No. CR	No. PR	RR (%)	TTP	MS	Regimen[a]
Lummen et al., 1998[189]	Titanocene dichloride	14	11	0	0	0	—	11.7	270 mg/m^2 q21d
Vogelzang et al., 1998[190]	Pyrazine diazohydroxide	15	14	0	0	0	—	—	100 mg/m^2/d × 5 q42d
Rigos et al., 1999[191]	Treosulfan	15	10	0	0	0	4	—	10 g/m^2 q28d
Berg et al., 1999[192]	Pyrazoloacridine	12	12	0	0	0	—	—	750 mg/m^2 q21d
Stadler et al., 2000[193]	Flavopiridol	35	34	0	2	6	—	11.2	50 mg/m^2/d CIV × 72 h q14d
Pagliaro et al., 2000[194]	Bryostatin-1	30	30	1	1	7	2.1	13.1	25 µg/m^2 d 1, 8, 15 q28d
Dreicer et al., 2000[195]	Suramin	14	13	0	0	0	—	—	Fixed dose regimen[b]
Small et al., 2000[196]	KW-2189	40	40	0	0	0	3.7	8.2	0.4–0.5 mg/m^2 q35–42d
Berg et al., 2001[197]	Irofulven	13	12	0	0	0	—	—	11 mg/m^2/d × 5 q28d
Kuebler et al., 2001[198]	Pyrazoloacridine	18	13	0	1	6	—	—	750 mg/m^2 q21d
Vogelzang et al., 2001[123]	Ranpirnase	14	14	0	0	0	4	16	480 µg/m^2 q7d
Schroder et al., 2001[199]	Suramin	24	22	0	0	0	—	10	Fixed-dose regimen[b]
Adjei, 2002[200]	Pemetrexed	42	16	0	1	6	—	—	600 mg/m^2 q21d
Skubitz, 2002[201]	Doxil	12	11	0	0	0	—	—	55 mg/m^2 q28d
Vis et al., 2002[202]	Methotrexate-Alb	17	14	0	0	0	—	—	50 mg/m^2 q7d
Wenzel et al., 2002[203]	Capecitabine	26	23	0	2	9	6	13	1250 mg/m^2 PO b.i.d. × 14 d, q21d
Vuky et al., 2002[204]	Arsenic trioxide	14	11	0	0	0	—	—	0.3 mg/kg/d × 5 q28d
Amato et al., 2002[205]	Irofulven	20	19	0	0	0	—	—	11 mg/m^2/d × 5 q28d
Park et al., 2002[206]	Temozolomide	12	12	0	0	0	—	6.8	200 mg/m^2/d PO d 1–5 q28d
Redman et al., 2003[207]	Tetrathiomolybdate	15	13	0	0	0	3	—	40–60 mg PO q.i.d.
Haas et al., 2003[208]	Bryostatin	34	32	0	2	6	3	25	35–40 µg/m^2 q7d × 3 q28d
Madhusudan et al., 2003[209]	Bryostatin	16	13	0	0	0	—	—	25 µg/m^2 q7d × 3 q28d
Motzer et al., 2003[210]	C225 antibody	55	54	0	0	0	1.9	—	400 mg/m^2 × 1, 250 mg/m^2 q7d
Fizazi et al., 2003[211]	Irinotecan	45	34	0	0	0	3[c]	19[c]	350 mg/m^2 q21d
Townsley et al., 2003[212]	Troxacitabine	35	33	0	2	6	3	—	10 mg/m^2 q21d
Whang and Godley, 2003[213]	CCI-779	110	—	—	—	5	6.1	15	25, 75, or 250 mg q7d
Varga et al., 2003[214]	CG250 antibody	36	32	1	0	3	6.3	15	50 mg q7d × 12
Hussain et al., 2003[215]	Rebeccamycin analogue	24	24	0	2	8	—	10	165 mg/m^2 qd × 5, q21d
Davis et al., 2003[216]	PS-341	23	21	0	1	5	—	—	1.5 mg/m^2 twice weekly × 14 d, q21d

CIV, continuous intravenous infusion; CR, complete response; Enter., number of patients entered in study; Eval., number of patients evaluable for response; PR, partial response; RR, response rate; TTP, time to progression in months; MS, median survival in months.
Note: TTP and MS calculated from data provided, assuming 30 days in a month.
[a]Drugs administered as a single intravenous dose unless otherwise noted.
[b]Suramin dose: days 1–5: 1000, 400, 300, 250, 200 mg/m^2; then 275 mg/m^2 on days 11, 15, 19, 22, and then every week.[195,199]
[c]Calculated in a subset of 26 patients who had received prior chemotherapy or immunotherapy.

TABLE 30.1-13.   Randomized Phase III Trials with Interferon and Chemotherapy

Studies		No. of Patients	% Responses	Response Duration (Mo)	Median Survival (Mo)	Survival Benefit for Combination
Kriegmair et al.[226]	Interferon + vinblastine	41	20.5	—	16	No
	Medroxyprogesterone	35	0	—	10	
Pyrhonen et al.[227]	Interferon + vinblastine	79	16.5	3.25	17	Yes
	Vinblastine	81	2.5	2.25	10	
Fossa et al.[228]	Interferon + vinblastine	66	24	6.0	—	No
	Interferon	53	11	8.6	—	
Neidhart et al.[229]	Interferon + vinblastine	83	8	—	—	No
	Interferon	82	12	—	—	
Sagaster et al.[230]	Interferon + coumarin + cimetidine	70	17.1	10	9	No
	Interferon	67	20.8	7.5	8	
Motzer et al.[99]	Interferon + *cis*-retinoic acid	139	11	—	15	No
	Interferon	145	6	—	15	

tologic subtypes, a factor that will become of increasing importance as effective therapies are identified.

An increasing trend to combination chemotherapy regimens can be observed in chemotherapy trials in renal cell cancer. IFN or IL-2 is frequently, but not invariably, included. The combination of gemcitabine and 5-FU warrants mention. In a study reported by Vogelzang at the University of Chicago, seven PRs (17%) were observed among 39 patients receiving gemcitabine at 600 mg/m^2 on days 1, 8, and 15 and continuous-infusion 5-FU at 150 mg/m^2/d for 21 days in 28-day cycles.[89] The response rate initially reported declined in subsequent studies,[90,91] as noted so often for single agents, perhaps owing to the inclusion of patients with advancing disease as experience with the new agent or combination increased. When the University of Chicago experience with gemcitabine and 5-FU was amassed, the overall response rate was 10% among 153 patients treated in five clinical trials.[92] With one complete remission and a median survival of 12.5 months, this was comparable to the 11% response rate, 12 complete remissions, and 13-month median survival observed in 463 patients enrolled in IFN-α–containing trials at the Memorial Sloan-Kettering Cancer Center[93] and suggests that the combination regimen does have a response rate above the background. Although they are better than vinblastine-containing regimens, the results also affirm the need for new therapies.

New agents aimed at new molecular targets continue to be introduced into clinical trials. One agent that has received increasing interest is BAY 43-9006, a Raf-1 kinase inhibitor that induced remissions in renal cancer in the phase I setting and is now under evaluation in a phase II trial.[94] Other agents included are SU-11428, PTK/ZK, and BMS 247550.[95–97] Preliminary results with some of these agents have suggested a level of activity significantly higher than observed with traditional anticancer agents. If significant activity were confirmed in phase II and III clinical trials, such an agent would be readily adopted as standard therapy in this disease that has for so long eluded effective therapy.

Chemotherapy Combined with Interferon in Renal Cell Cancer

IFN-α, one of two immunotherapeutic agents widely used in the treatment of renal cell cancer (as discussed in Biologic Therapy, later in this chapter), has a modest response rate and confers a survival advantage as a single agent. Numerous trials have been conducted combining IFN with cytotoxic chemotherapy in the hope that the immunologic benefit from IFN will improve the response to chemotherapy. However, randomized studies have failed to provide any evidence for combining IFN with chemotherapy (Table 30.1-13). The response migration mentioned earlier for single agents occurred for many of these combinations as well. The most recent example was the combination of IFN-α and *cis*-retinoic acid, when Motzer et al. originally observed a 30% response rate for the combination.[98] Later, a randomized trial comparing IFN-α plus *cis*-retinoic acid with IFN-α alone yielded a 12% response rate for the combination, with no significant survival difference between the two arms.[99] One factor potentially confounding these trials is the inclusion of patients with varying prognoses. Using stratification of patients based on prognostic factors[92,100,101] (Tables 30.1-14 and 30.1-15) may help to eliminate the variation in results long observed in renal carcinoma trials.

TABLE 30.1-14.   Prognostic Factors Identified by Multivariate Analyses

MOTZER ET AL.[100]
Poor performance status
Elevated calcium
Lack of prior nephrectomy
Elevated lactate dehydrogenase
Anemia
STADLER ET AL.[92]
Poor performance status
Elevated calcium
Lack of prior nephrectomy
Elevated alkaline phosphatase
Number of metastatic sites
Low albumin
ATZPODIEN ET AL.[101]
Elevated lactate dehydrogenase
High neutrophil count
Elevated C-reactive protein
Shorter time from diagnosis to metastatic disease
Number of metastatic sites
Presence of bone metastases

TABLE 30.1-15. Median Survival of Patients with Renal Cell Cancer Stratified According to Prognosis at Two Centers

Prognostic Group[a] (No. of Risk Factors)	Memorial Sloan-Kettering Cancer Center (MSKCC) Median Survival (Mo)				University of Chicago Median Survival (Mo)		
	Overall[a] (n = 670)	ChemoRx[b] (n = 274)	Cytokine Rx[b] (n = 396)	Interferon-α[c] (n = 437)	Overall[d] (n = 153)	ChemoRx[d] (n = 112)	Cytokine Rx[e] (n = 41)
All	11	6	13	13	13		
Favorable (0)	20	15	27	30	21	—	—
Intermediate (1–2)	10	7	12	14	12	21	24
Poor (≥3)	4	3	6	5	4	12	12
						4	4

ChemoRx, chemotherapy; Rx, therapy.

Note: Patients were stratified according to the number of risk factors present from the following list: elevated lactate dehydrogenase, anemia, elevated calcium, poor performance status, lack of prior nephrectomy.

[a]Prognostic model developed in 670 patients from MSKCC treated between 1975 and 1996.[100]

[b]Stratification of 670 patients in ref. 100 by cytokine or chemotherapy as first MSKCC therapy.[231]

[c]Stratification of 437 evaluable patients enrolled on interferon-α trials as first systemic therapy at MSKCC between 1982 and 1996.[93]

[d]Application of Motzer prognostic model to 153 patients treated with gemcitabine and 5-fluorouracil in five clinical trials at the University of Chicago between 1997 and 2001.[92]

[e]Patients from gemcitabine/5-fluorouracil trial containing interleukin-2 and interferon-α.[232]

To date, there is no convincing evidence that chemotherapy adds to the effectiveness of single-agent IFN-α.[84] The combination of IFN-α with a cytotoxic agent in patients whose disease progressed after treatment with IL-2 must be considered unproven, and enrollment in clinical trials is the most logical alternative.

SUPPORTIVE CARE IN RENAL CELL CANCER

Although not direct anticancer therapy, progress has been made in supportive care for patients with renal cell cancer, effecting an improvement in quality of life. Bone metastases, which cause significant morbidity due to the lack of effective therapy, occur in roughly one-third of patients with renal cell cancer. Although bisphosphonates were initially shown to be effective in breast cancer and in multiple myeloma, a large placebo-controlled trial extended these results in solid tumors.[102] In a retrospectively analyzed subset of 74 patients with renal cell cancer enrolled in this trial, significant improvement was observed in all skeletal-related events measured.[103] The number of patients experiencing a skeletal-related event was reduced from 74% to 37%, a 50% reduction. The time to development of the first skeletal complication, including first pathologic fracture was delayed, with the median not reached in the treated group. While confirmatory prospective studies are needed, these results suggest that patients with bony metastases due to renal cell cancer will likely benefit from bisphosphonate therapy.

DRUG RESISTANCE IN RENAL CELL CANCER

Intrinsic resistance to chemotherapy has long been a hallmark of renal cancer. Diverse mechanisms of resistance have been studied, although none conclusively demonstrated to be dominant. Molecular prognostic factors that may reflect chemosensitivity or resistance have been examined, but without reliable and effective therapy for renal cell carcinoma their value cannot be determined. As might be expected, in the absence of effective therapy, prognosis will generally relate to the inherent biology of the tumor. Thus, markers of differentiation and indolent biology presently confer a better prognosis because of the limitations of current therapy. Consistently, increased expression of PCNA (proliferating cell nuclear antigen) or MIB-1/Ki-67, both antigens associated with cell prolif-

eration, has been associated with decreased survival.[104–107] Patients with diploid tumors are more likely to have increased disease-free interval.[108] Of interest, response to IFN treatment is also more likely to occur in patients whose tumors manifest a more indolent biology.[109]

P-Glycoprotein and Related ABC Transporters

Overexpression of the 170-kD drug transporter P-glycoprotein (P-gp) and its encoding gene, *MDR-1*, has been most frequently cited as a mechanism of resistance. However, efforts to modulate P-gp by treating patients with antagonists have met with disappointing results to date. Most of the trials attempted modulation of vinblastine. Although the studies, at face value, suggest no role for P-gp in renal carcinoma, it can be argued that this question is not fully resolved.[110] Most of the reversal agents used in the trials were first-generation agents with low potency, selected because they were already in clinical use for other indications. Most of the trials incorporated vinblastine. Although vinblastine is a substrate for P-gp, renal cell cancers may have other mechanisms of resistance to vinblastine that were not addressed by these studies. P-gp inhibition may represent an avenue to increase the intracellular concentration of an agent, but that agent must have intrinsic activity for successful resistance reversal. Recent studies with a third-generation P-gp antagonist, tariquidar, suggest that increased intracellular concentration of a substrate can be achieved in metastatic tumors of patients with renal cell cancer, using nuclear imaging of technetium 99m–labeled sestamibi as a surrogate.[111] Results similar to these were achieved in an earlier study with the P-gp antagonist PSC 833.[112]

Reduced intracellular concentrations of chemotherapy could result from the presence of other ABC transporters on the cell surface.[110] Others, including the family of multidrug resistance–associated proteins (MRP1 through MRP6) that have organic anion transport activity (potentially mediating etoposide, methotrexate, and cisplatin resistance) and an ABC half transporter designated ABCG2 that confers mitoxantrone and camptothecin resistance, extend the spectrum of anticancer agents constrained by reduced drug accumulation. If these transporters are confirmed as being active in renal cell cancer, their inhibition offers a future strategy for increasing drug accumulation in kidney cancer cells. This strategy will become of increasing importance if an effective therapy is identified and then determined to be a substrate for an ABC transporter.

Intracellular Mechanisms

Although drug transporters would directly affect intracellular concentrations of drug, other mechanisms of drug resistance have been identified that confer resistance at the levels of cell survival pathways, drug metabolism, and the drug target. Many of these have been examined as potential molecular markers of prognosis in renal cell cancer, but the findings are preliminary and must be validated.[113] Cell survival in renal carcinoma may be linked to the frequently observed overexpression of the epidermal growth factor receptor and its homologue, ErbB2[114] or to expression of the insulin-like growth factor-1 receptor,[115] or to overexpression of an antiapoptosis protein such as Bcl-2.[107,116,117] Mutation of p53 is not commonly found in renal cell carcinoma.[116,107] Alternatively, increased metabolism of anticancer agents may be promoted by higher levels of enzymes of the cytochrome P-450 family in concert with glutathione and glutathione transferases.[117–119] Decreased levels of topoisomerase II have been observed in renal carcinoma, which could confer resistance to agents that lead to double-strand breaks by trapping topoisomerase II in cleavable complexes.[119] Finally, as potential mediators of drug resistance through survival pathways, altered expression of cellular adhesion molecules, including α-catenin, E-cadherin, and cadherin 6, has been described in renal cancer.[113,120] Thus, multiple mechanisms mediating intracellular resistance can be proposed. The challenge is to determine the importance of such mechanisms and to identify strategies for their circumvention.

Drug Delivery

To some, the generalized resistance supports an argument that drug resistance in renal cell carcinoma is not based primarily on cellular mechanisms. Although investigators have worked principally in other model systems, studies evaluating tumor drug delivery may cast light on the problem of drug resistance in kidney cancer. Factors that influence drug delivery include blood flow, permeability of tumor vasculature, and drug diffusion into the interstitium, which is affected both by properties of the drug and by interstitial pressure within the tumor.[121] Experimental data suggest that interstitial pressure is increased in renal cell cancer[88] and in patients, positron emission tomography scanning has additionally suggested that impaired perfusion is a characteristic finding in renal cancers.[122] Strategies aimed at identifying and reducing these physiologic barriers to drug delivery are under investigation and could have a particular relevance to the very large tumor masses seen in renal cell cancer.

CLINICAL TRIAL DESIGN IN RENAL CELL CANCER

Evaluation of Prognostic Factors

Although patients who have stage IV disease experience a reported median survival of 12 to 24 months, the range of survival times in this group of patients is very broad. A variety of studies have looked at the parameters that predict survival in patients with metastatic renal cancer, and performance status is the most commonly identified predictive parameter. Other factors that have been identified in some studies as predictors of poorer survival of patients with

stage IV disease are shorter interval from diagnosis to detection of metastatic disease, increased number of metastatic sites, multiple organ involvement, recent weight loss, previous chemotherapy, elevated neutrophil count, decreased albumin, elevated alkaline phosphatase, lack of prior nephrectomy, an elevated serum lactate dehydrogenase level, high corrected serum calcium, and low serum hemoglobin (see Table 30.1-14).[92,100,101] Such factors should be considered in evaluating survival in nonrandomized studies. Several prognostic scales have been devised, with the Motzer scale using performance status plus the latter four variables in patients with metastatic disease.[100] As shown in Table 30.1-15, patients can be stratified into risk groups with poor, intermediate, or favorable prognoses, based on the number of adverse risk factors present. This model is quite useful in the interpretation of nonrandomized clinical trial results reporting improvement in stable disease duration, improved survival compared to historical controls, or even responses. In one recent phase II trial, when an overall survival of 16 months was observed, Vogelzang et al. evaluated the number of patients with favorable features and concluded that the patients enrolled had an estimated survival of 15 to 20 months.[123] This allowed the investigators to properly evaluate the outcome of the clinical trial, avoiding the type of cascading repetitive chemotherapy trials so regularly observed in the Yagoda review. Prognostic factor scoring should be routinely included in reports of clinical trials in renal cell cancer. A recent update to the Motzer scale identified three critical variables for prognosis in patients enrolling on clinical trials: performance status, hemoglobin level, and serum calcium.[123b] This scale differentiated a median survival of 22 months in patients with no risk factors from a median survival of 5.4 months in patients with two or three risk factors.

Randomized Discontinuation Design

Randomized trials provide an opportunity to control for differences in varying prognoses among the patients enrolled. In both phase II and III trials, however, it can be difficult to discern the importance of stable disease as a response end point. One clinical trial approach developed to address this problem is the randomized discontinuation design.[124] In this design, patients identified as having stable disease on an experimental therapy are randomized to continue or discontinue the experimental drug. This design was successfully applied to the antiangiogenic agent carboxyaminoimidazole. Reported in abstract form, 9 of 22 patients receiving carboxyaminoimidazole and 13 of 26 patients receiving placebo remained stable for an additional 16 weeks among the first 49 patients with stable disease randomized.[125] The trial enrolled 364 patients before early closure due to lack of efficacy.

Influence of Histologic Subtypes

One question that requires further study is whether the histologic subtype of renal cell cancer influences the response to chemotherapy or cytokine therapy. Although some of the subtypes, such as papillary renal cancer, may have better survival than clear cell renal carcinoma after nephrectomy, this does not extend to survival after therapy for metastatic disease. In a retrospective analysis of 64 patients with non–clear cell renal cancer, only one patient responded to cytokine therapy.[126] The sarcoma-like features of the sarcomatoid variant in renal cancer have led some investigators to treat patients with this dedifferentiated phenotype using regimens developed for sarcoma. Although there are anecdotal reports of response to such therapy, a prospective study was not confirmatory.[127,128] Clinical trials of new agents should stratify patients with different histologies separately.

Conclusion

In conclusion, renal carcinoma is a remarkably refractory solid tumor. More resistant than most other cancers, new phase II agents have failed time and again. The explanation for this drug resistance may lie within the tumor as an entity or within the individual cells. The broad spectrum of drugs to which renal cancers are resistant suggests tumor-based mechanisms, whereas resistance in even the tiniest pulmonary nodule suggests cellular mechanisms. A detailed understanding of drug resistance in renal cell cancer is a major challenge for the future. While novel agents are generating excitement in the field, it is most likely that agents directed against novel targets will be subject to the same mechanisms of resistance that have plagued treatment of this disease for decades.

BIOLOGIC THERAPY

Biologic agents represent the major effective therapies for widespread metastatic renal cell carcinoma. Indeed, their use in treating renal carcinoma has been instrumental in demonstrating the potential for inducing complete and durable regression of human cancer with biotherapy. In the treatment of common metastatic solid tumors, the potential for curative systemic therapy in renal cancer is only exceeded by testicular cancer and matched by melanoma. Yet, this result is only attained by a small proportion of patients with advanced disease, and the factors that predict or produce dramatic, durable responses in such patients have not been elucidated. Nevertheless, the principle that immunotherapy can be curative for some patients has been conclusively established. A new detailed understanding of the molecular events that cause and promote the growth of renal cancer and a better understanding of the immune response to this malignancy should lead to new, targeted therapies using biologic agents.

Spontaneous Tumor Regression

Although spontaneous tumor regression does not represent a bona fide treatment modality, much has been made of this phenomenon in patients with advanced renal cancer, and the mechanism is presumed to be immunologic. The practice of nephrectomy in patients with metastatic disease in the hope of inducing a spontaneous regression has been largely abandoned owing to the rarity of this outcome.[129] In reviews of spontaneous tumor regression, another striking feature is that the majority of regressions are short-lived. In one randomized study of IFN-γ in patients with renal cancer, the placebo-control population demonstrated a singularly high response rate of 6%, but the duration of these regressions were 2 to 13 months with only one ongoing response of 9 months at the time of publication.[130] Other larger reviews show that the true incidence of this phenomenon is probably less than 1% and that the vast majority of documented spontaneous regressions relapse with progressive metastatic disease and require other therapy.[131,132] In addition, the few well-documented cases of durable regressions often occured in patients who had life-threatening infectious or inflammatory events as possible instigators of their regression.[133] These data indicate that spontaneous regression of renal carcinoma is often transient and is not a phenomenon that should be relied on as therapy.

Interferons

Early studies of leukocyte IFN in the treatment of cancer reported sporadic responses in patients with renal cell carcinoma.[134] Subsequently, increased dosages and larger studies were possible using recombinant IFN-α, and this experience was repeated and confirmed. The response rates in the largest studies ranged from 0% to 29% (Table 30.1-16) with few CRs and little long-term survival data.[135,136] In a review of the literature in 1989, Quesada reported an overall response rate of 16% for 654 patients.[137] Factors that seemed to increase the likelihood of responding included good performance status, prior nephrectomy, and metastases confined to the lungs. Nevertheless, these factors could not reliably exclude patients unable to benefit from IFN, and they should serve only as general guidelines. Little data exist on the long-term results from IFN therapy, but, from the very small number of completely responding patients, it is safe to conclude that there are only anecdotal cases of cures of metastatic disease from IFN. Recently, randomized prospective studies have been performed to measure the benefit of IFN-α in patients with advanced renal cancer. A randomized comparison of IFN-α versus medroxyprogesterone acetate in 335 patients demonstrated a significant prolongation of median survival (6 months for medroxyprogesterone acetate and 8.5 months for IFN-α).[138] This modest prolongation of survival was offset by greater symptoms and decreased quality of life in patients on IFN-α. In addition, benefit did not appear durable,

TABLE 30.1-16. Treatment of Metastatic Renal Cell Cancer with Interferon (IFN)

Reference	IFN	Route and Schedule	n	Response Rate (%)	CR (%)
deKernion et al.[233]	IFN-α	6 MU IM q.d.	48	15	2
Quesada et al.[234]	IFN-α	3 MU IM q.d.	50	26	6[a]
Quesada et al.[135]	IFN-α	2 MU IM q.d.	15	0	0
		20 MU IM q.d.	41	29	2
Umeda and Niijima[235]	IFN-α	3–36 MU IM q.d.	153	15	2
	IFN_Lymphoblastoid	5 MU IM 2–7/wk	73	23	1
Muss et al.[236]	IFN-α_2b	2–10 MU SC 3/wk	58	9	2
		30–50 MU IV q.d.	54	6	2

CR, complete response.
[a]Duration of CRs all ≤10 months.

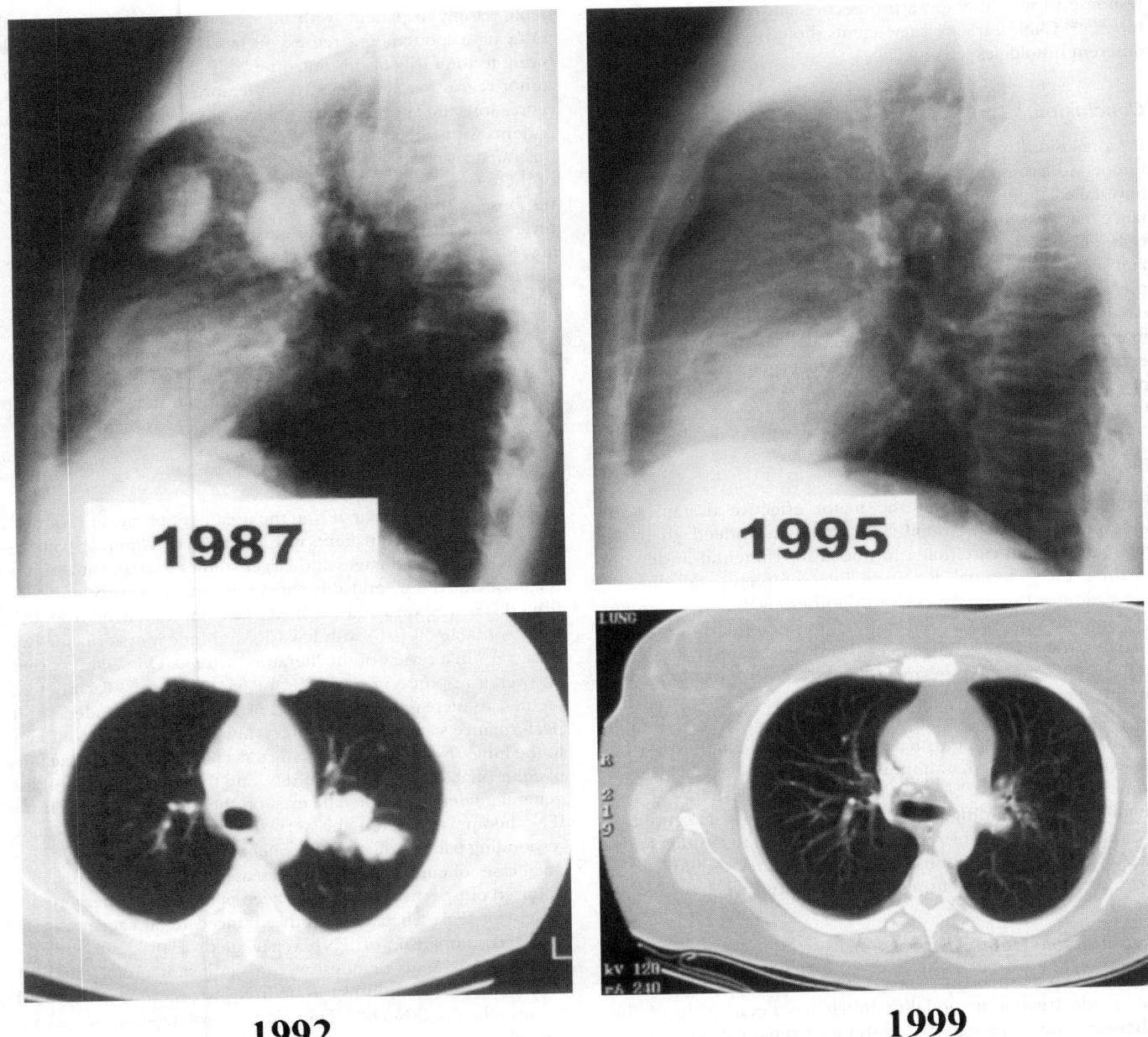

FIGURE 30.1-12.   Radiographs of two patients with long-term complete regressions of pulmonary metastases from renal cancer in response to high-dose therapy with interleukin-2 alone. In most studies, patients with only pulmonary metastases appear to have a slightly higher probability of response.

with estimated progression-free survival at 2 years less than or equal to 5% for both groups.

Many different types and preparations of IFNs have been used in clinical trials. Early trials with "natural" IFN produced from donor leukocytes and subsequent trials with several different subtypes of recombinant IFN-α have not suggested a difference in efficacy between these preparations. Recent trials using IFN-β and IFN-γ have indicated that these agents have either similar or less activity than IFN-α.[139] A randomized comparison of IFN-γ and placebo showed no difference in response rates or survival.[130]

One important consideration in evaluating IFN therapy is that the optimal dose, schedule, and route of IFN administration is not yet known. Although refinement of schedules may have

the potential of increasing response rates somewhat, in view of the small benefit demonstrated to this point, it is unlikely that randomized studies will ever be done to effectively optimize these parameters. In summary, disseminated renal cell cancer shows a small but consistent response rate to IFN (primarily IFN-α), but these benefits must be weighed against the toxicity of chronic therapy and the poor evidence for long-term benefit.

Interleukin-2

After the discovery of interleukin-2 in 1976 and the demonstration of its activities as a T-cell growth factor and activator of T cells and natural killer cells, it was used in clinical trials against a variety of malignancies. From the first trials in 1984, renal cell cancer was identified as a tumor that could respond to IL-2.[140,141] These early trials rapidly escalated the dose of IL-2 to the maximum tolerated dose and then added lymphokine-activated killer (LAK) cells to the therapy based on preclinical results. These trials initially reported response rates of 33% in renal carcinoma, and in a subsequent multicenter experience the response rate was 16%.[142] The remarkable feature of many of these responses is that they appear complete and durable. Median follow-up of more than 10 years is available from those early studies, and review of these patients indicate that 7% to 9% of all patients (nearly one-half of all responding patients) had a CR, and the majority of those completely responding patients have never relapsed.[143–145] This constitutes the most convincing evidence that IL-2 has clinical benefit in the treatment of metastatic renal cell cancer and led to the approval of IL-2 by the U.S. Food and Drug Administration as the only currently approved therapy for this disease in the United States. It should be emphasized that it is the curative potential of these responses and not their frequency, which is of value. Of note is the fact that these studies largely treated clear cell renal cancer and its variants and did not address whether other biologically distinct forms of renal cancer can respond. There is no consistent information documenting responses to IL-2 in patients with pure papillary, chromophobe, medullary, or collecting duct renal cancer. Although some controversy exists as to the response rates of sarcomatoid tumor variants of clear cell tumors, published reports suggest that clear cell tumors with sarcomatoid, granular, or papillary features can all respond to IL-2 treatment[146] (Fig. 30.1-12).

After the initial studies with IL-2, several developments have occurred. The use of LAK cells with IL-2 has been critically examined in randomized studies. Although murine models predicted that the addition of LAK cells to IL-2 would substantially increase therapeutic efficacy, this has not proved to be true in clinical studies. A randomized comparison of high-dose intravenous bolus IL-2 with and without LAK cells showed an insignificant difference in response rate (21% for IL-2 and 31% for IL-2 and LAK cells) with no difference in survival.[147] Other studies have confirmed this,[148] and, currently, there is no evidence to support the use of LAK cells in patients with renal carcinoma.

The initial rapid escalation of IL-2 to its maximum tolerated dose identified 600,000 to 720,000 IU/kg by intravenous bolus given every 8 hours as the maximum tolerated dose. On that schedule, patients tolerated approximately seven to nine consecutive doses before treatment had to be stopped for vascular leak syndrome, hypotension, multiorgan dysfunction, and a variety of other toxicities.[149] These effects rapidly reversed after stopping therapy, but, with hypotension requiring vasopressor support, pulmonary edema, and potential infectious complications, a 2% to 4% treatment-related mortality was initially encountered. Since then, increased experience with IL-2, prophylactic antibiotics when indicated, and patient screening for occult coronary disease have dramatically decreased this mortality rate. A recent report cites 809 consecutive patients who received high-dose bolus IL-2 without a treatment-related morality,[150] a statistic unattainable with most multiagent chemotherapy regimens. Nevertheless, the expense of intensive care unit stay and the precipitous nature of toxicities on high-dose IL-2 led many investigators to try lower-dose regimens. In particular, daily subcutaneous self-administration was adopted as a convenient and inexpensive route. In a scenario replayed many times during the development of IL-2, a multitude of small phase II studies were performed that reported short-term

response rates similar to those seen with high-dose IL-2. An outpatient, daily, self-administered regimen using an initial week (Monday through Friday) of 18 million IU (fixed dose) followed by 5 weeks at one-half that dose was well tolerated and produced a response rate of 23% in 26 evaluable patients.[151] Later, continued experience with a modification of this regimen showed a 20% overall response rate with one ongoing CR in 47 patients,[152] and another group of investigators achieved an 18% response rate with similar regimen.[153] Others reported on the use of continuous infusion IL-2, describing a similar response rate with less toxicity (and less overall IL-2 given for the same time period).[154] A review of the literature (Table 30.1-17) shows response rates to IL-2 monotherapy or IL-2 and LAK cells, delivered on many different schedules and at different doses, ranging from 8% to 35%, and it is clear that smaller nonrandomized studies cannot discern whether one schedule is more effective than another. Nevertheless, lower dose schedules were widely adopted before being critically evaluated. A randomized study addressing this issue has been published.[155] This study randomized patients to receive IL-2 at either 720,000 IU/kg or 72,000 IU/kg every 8 hours by intravenous bolus to maximum tolerance (up to 15 consecutive doses). The lower dose was selected as the maximal dose tolerated without intensive care unit stay and vasopressor support. This two-arm comparison specifically addressed whether the dose of IL-2 was important. Subsequently, a third arm was added to the trial to evaluate the widely used daily, subcutaneous route of administration. This arm delivered 250,000 IU/kg daily for 5 days in the first week and then one-half that dose 5 days a week for the subsequent 5 weeks. Only concurrently randomized patients are compared in this two-stage trial. Although it is clear that the two lower-dose regimens had decreased toxicity, especially for hypotension requiring pressors (36% of courses of high-dose intravenous IL-2 vs. 3% of courses of low-dose intravenous IL-2 vs. none with subcutaneous IL-2), thrombocytopenia, pulmonary distress, and disorientation, it is important to note that there were no deaths or major irreversible toxicities in any of the treatment arms. With a total of 400 patients randomized and a median follow-up of more than 5 years, response rates are as shown in Table 30.1-18. In the two-arm comparison of high- and low-dose intravenous bolus IL-2, the respective response rates are 21% and 13% ($P = .05$). The durations of the responses are notable, as 8 of 11 patients completely responding to high-dose IL-2 remain in CR beyond 4 years, whereas only three of six patients completely responding to low-dose IL-2 were maintaining their responses at 2 years (with a significant difference in the survival of completely responding patients in these two arms). The subset of patients randomized between three treatment arms showed response rates of 21%, 11%, and 10% for high-dose intravenous, low-dose intravenous, and subcutaneous IL-2, respectively, with the decrement in response rates of both low-dose regimens of borderline significance compared to high-dose therapy. As is common for IL-2 studies (in which major benefit is manifested by a small minority of the patients treated), there were no significant differences when overall survival between any arms was assessed. Because the clinical benefit of IL-2 resides in the long-term CRs attained by some patients, this study is most notable for the higher proportion of patients attaining CRs when given high-dose therapy and the greater durability of those same CRs (Figs. 30.1-13 and 30.1-14).

Other studies have addressed the issue of continuous infusion IL-2 versus bolus IL-2. The initial nonrandomized studies using continuous infusion IL-2 reported response rates similar to bolus IL-2 but lesser toxicities. In a subsequent randomized study[156] (in

TABLE 30.1-17. Therapy with Interleukin-2 (IL-2) Alone or with LAK Cells

Study	IL-2 Dose Range[a]	Route and Schedule	n	RR (%)	CR (%)
IL-2 ALONE					
Rosenberg et al.[145]	High	IV bolus q8h	227	19	9
Cytokine Working Group[143,162]	High	IV bolus q8h	71	17	7
Yang et al.[155]	Low	IV bolus q8h	149	13	4
Bukowski et al.[237]	Moderate	IV 3/wk	41	12	2
Gold et al.[157]	High	IV continuous	47	13	6
von der Maase et al.[238]	High	IV continuous	51	16	4
Escudier et al.[239]	Moderate	IV continuous	104	19	4
Negrier et al.[161]	High	IV continuous	138	7	1
Lissoni et al.[240]	Low	SC daily	91	23	2
Buter et al.[152]	Low	SC daily	47	19	4
Tourani et al.[153]	Low	SC 1–2/d	39	18	3
Yang et al.[155]	Low	SC daily	93	10	2
Total			1098	15.4	4.5
IL-2 AND LAK CELLS					
Rosenberg et al.[241]	High	IV bolus q8h	72	35	11
Fisher et al.[142]	High	IV bolus q8h	35	14	6
Weiss et al.[156]	High	IV bolus q8h	46	20	7
Parkinson et al.[242]	High	IV continuous	47	9	4
Negrier et al.[243]	High	IV continuous	51	27	10
Dillman et al.[244,245]	High	IV continuous	46	15	NA
Thompson et al.[246]	High	IV continuous	76	22	8
Weiss et al.[156]	High	IV continuous	48	15	4
Total			421	20.9	8

CR, complete response; LAK, lymphokine-activated killer; NA, not available; RR, response rate.
[a]*High-dose* indicates significant multiorgan toxicity and vasopressors, with intensive care unit support needed in more than one-fourth of treatments. *Moderate-dose* indicates occasional multiorgan toxicity or significant single-organ toxicity with occasional intensive care unit support. *Low-dose* indicates rare or mild multiorgan toxicity and rare intensive care unit support; typically given in the outpatient setting. (Adapted from ref. 247.)

which all patients received LAK cells), patients were assigned to receive either continuous infusion IL-2 at 18.0 to 22.5 million IU/m²/d or 600,000 IU/kg/dose by bolus every 8 hours (the cumulative daily dose by bolus was more than three times the dose by continuous infusion). Both of these doses represented the respective maximally tolerated doses for these regimens, and the few significant differences in toxicities did not favor either regimen. In this study, patients receiving LAK cells and bolus IL-2 had a 20% major

response rate compared to a 15% response rate for patients given LAK cells and continuous infusion IL-2 (the difference was not significant). Fortunately, it has been established that the CRs to high-dose continuous infusion IL-2 can be of long duration. A single institution study of 123 patients (some also receiving LAK cells) with follow-up of 1 to 109 months reported an overall response rate of 19%, with 7% CRs and 78% of those patients sustaining their CRs from 42 to 109+ months[157] (Fig. 30.1-15).

TABLE 30.1-18. A Randomized Study of High- versus Low-Dose Interleukin-2 in Patients with Metastatic Renal Cell Cancer

	High-Dose IV Bolus	Low-Dose IV Bolus	Outpatient SC Daily
TWO-ARM COMPARISON			
No. of patients	155	149	—
Response rate (% PR + CR)	21	13	—
Complete responses (%)	7	4	—
Duration median (range)	100+ mo[a] (19–130+)	30[b] (3–128+)	—
Partial responses (%)	14	9	—
Duration median (range)	14 mo (4–37)	11 mo (4–24)	—
THREE-ARM COMPARISON			
No. of patients	96[c]	92[c]	93
Response rate (% PR + CR)	21	11	10
Complete responses (%)	6	1	2

[a]Eight of 11 CR are ongoing.
[b]Three of six CR are ongoing.
[c]A concurrently randomized subset of the patients analyzed in two-arm comparison.

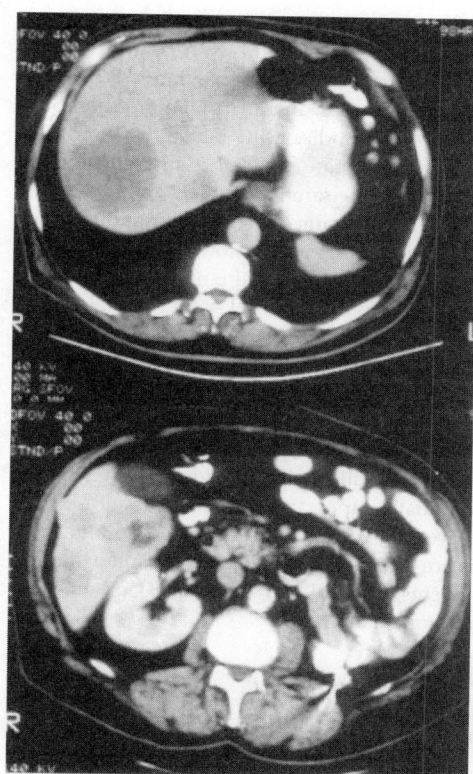
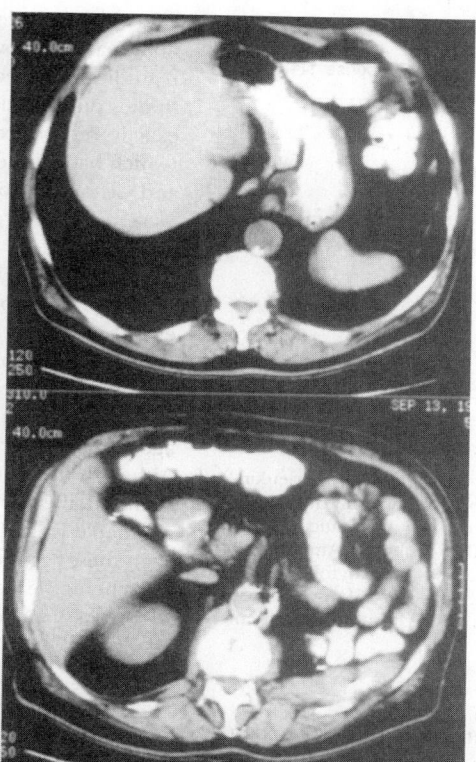

1991   **1999**

FIGURE 30.1-13. Abdominal computed tomography scans of a patient with a durable, ongoing complete response to high-dose interleukin-2 therapy, which included the regression of extensive liver metastases.

A more complex issue is whether any combination of cytokine or chemotherapy added to IL-2 is superior to IL-2 alone. Here again, small, nonrandomized phase II studies have clouded this issue. Numerous small studies combining IL-2 with IFN or chemotherapy (or both) reported improved short-term response rates but generated large, overlapping confidence intervals. The combination of IFN-α and IL-2 is especially appealing because both agents have single-agent activity

against renal carcinoma, and preclinical animal models predict synergistic benefit from combining these agents. Early reports suggested that the response rate for patients with metastatic renal cancer might rise from 18% to 20% with high-dose IL-2 alone, to as much as 31% with high-dose IL-2 plus IFN.[158] However, further accrual and long-term follow-up of the patients in this study did not show sufficient improvement in either response rate or survival (when compared to historical controls

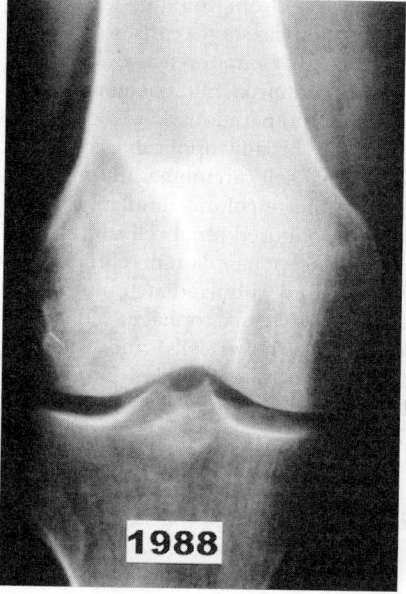
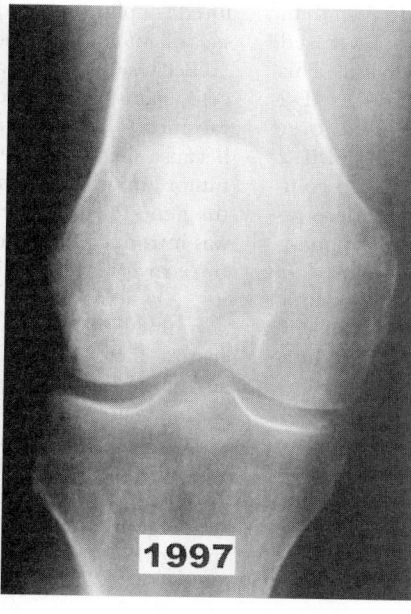

1988   **1997**

FIGURE 30.1-14. Regression and recalcification of a large lytic metastasis of the lateral femoral condyle in a patient with widely metastatic renal cell cancer. This patient also had a durable complete response of all soft tissue metastases with interleukin-2–based immunotherapy.

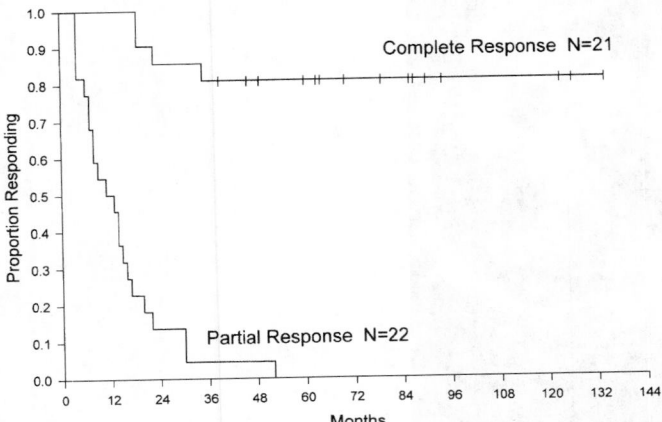

FIGURE 30.1-15. Complete responses to high-dose interleukin-2 (IL-2) in patients with metastatic renal carcinoma are typically durable. An actuarial curve of response duration for patients with metastatic renal cell carcinoma responding to high-dose bolus IL-2 is shown. Among completely responding patients, 81% have not relapsed (median follow-up is 7 years), and no patients have relapsed beyond 3 years. Partial responses can be sustained for years, but, in this study, all partially responding patients eventually relapsed. (Adapted from ref. 185.)

from the same institution) to warrant the additional toxicity seen.[159] Other investigators have been using this combination of cytokines to reduce the dose of IL-2 needed for a response and thus limit toxicity. Most have used outpatient, subcutaneous schedules, as widely described by Atzpodien et al.[160] The initial nonrandomized reports on this regimen emphasized lesser toxicities but similar response rates to high-dose IL-2 monotherapy. Yet, when others have tried the same or similar regimens, their response rates and their toxicity profiles have not been as favorable. Without randomized studies, it is impossible to reconcile these disparate results. Some experience in randomized evaluations of IL-2 and IFN is available. Negrier et al. randomized 425 patients to receive either continuous infusion, high-dose IL-2 alone, subcutaneous IFN-α three times a week, or both agents simultaneously.[161] There was a significantly higher response rate with the combination (18.6%) than with only IL-2 (6.5%) or IFN (7.5%), but this increased response rate did not translate into improved survival. This study demonstrated an unusually low response rate to IL-2 alone, and patients with tumor progression crossed over between therapy arms. Other small randomized studies of IL-2 and IFN have also failed to demonstrate an advantage to combination therapy, but these studies are largely underpowered.[162,163] Preliminary data are available from an ongoing study randomizing patients to either high-dose bolus IL-2 (600,000 IU/kg/dose every 8 hours) or low-dose daily subcutaneous IL-2 with subcutaneous IFN-α added.[164] This study will determine whether the addition of IFN-α to low-dose outpatient IL-2 can compensate for the lower response rates seen when subcutaneous IL-2 was given as monotherapy. After 99 patients were randomized to high-dose bolus and 94 to low-dose IL-2 plus IFN, the response rates for these two groups were 25% and 12%, respectively ($P = .03$). Final results on progression-free and overall survival are still pending.

In a further effort to enhance efficacy by adding other agents, investigators have tried to exploit the reported synergy between 5-FU (which has a low single-agent response rate against renal carcinoma) and IFN by adding this to IL-2 and IFN. Again, early phase II studies reported major increases in response rates,[165] but later studies did not always substantiate this.[166] In fact, an attempt to exactly reproduce the initial studies with 5-FU, IFN, and IL-2 (which had a reported response rate of 49%) resulted in a partial and CR rate of 16%—exactly the same as with IL-2 alone.[167] One issue rarely addressed in evaluating these combinations is the durability of the responses. Long-term follow-up with sufficient patients to evaluate response durations in the minority of patients showing regression is crucial to evaluating IL-2 therapies. Dutcher et al. have raised a possible red flag by reviewing their sequential use of IL-2, IL-2 plus IFN, and IL-2 plus IFN plus 5-FU.[167] Not only did they fail to see an increased response rate as the dose of IL-2 was moderated and other agents added to IL-2, but their percentage of patients attaining durable CRs seemed to decrease. Although their numbers are still small and patients were not randomized, this is a potentially important issue. If durable responses attainable with IL-2 are indeed forfeited by these combinations, then these regimens are indistinguishable from the many ineffective chemotherapy agents with 10% to 15% partial or transient responses and should not be advocated.

Vaccines and Cellular Therapy

There has been an ongoing effort to identify immune cells with reactivity to renal cancer. As described earlier, the use of nonspecific activated killer cells (natural killer or LAK cells) has largely been ineffective, but current efforts have concentrated on T cells and the induction of a T-cell response via vaccination. After the lead of melanoma research, tumor-infiltrating lymphocytes, isolated from renal cancer specimens and cells from mixed lymphocyte-tumor reactions were examined for antitumor reactivity. With some notable exceptions,[168–170] little specific tumor reactivity was seen.[171] Attempts to use tumor-infiltrating lymphocytes clinically have showed some promising early results (usually combined with IL-2 and IFN-α),[172] but a randomized trial of IL-2 with and without CD8-enriched tumor-infiltrating lymphocytes was fraught with technical difficulties and showed no augmentation in response rate or survival with cell transfer.[173] Another small study using cultured lymphocytes (and systemic IL-2) from lymph nodes draining sites of autologous tumor vaccination has shown early promise.[174]

Because of the relative scarcity of tumor-reactive–specific T cells against renal cancer, another approach has been the use of vaccines. Typically, whole tumor preparations have been used because of the failure to identify broadly applicable, common tumor antigens expressed by renal cell carcinoma. In one study, the gene for granulocyte-macrophage colony-stimulating factor was introduced into autologous, cultured renal cell cancer lines by retroviral transduction in a concept based on preclinical studies.[175] Patients were then immunized with irradiated tumor cells secreting large amounts of granulocyte-macrophage colony-stimulating factor (or control nontransduced cells) and evaluated for immune responses and clinical tumor regression. One PR was seen in 16 evaluable patients, and there was evidence of delayed-type hypersensitivity responses generated against tumor as well as an antitumor T-cell response in the responding patient. This approach is limited by the requirement for an autologous, cultured tumor line. Other approaches are investigating the use of tumor lysates and whole tumor cells co-incubated with autologous dendritic cells to vaccinate patients.

TABLE 30.1-19. Phase II Studies of Antiangiogenic Agents in Renal Cell Cancer

Investigator	Agent	Enter.	Eval.	No. CR	No. PR	RR (%)	TTP	MS	Regimen
Eisen et al., 2000[217]	Thalidomide	18	18	0	3	17	—	—	100 mg PO q.d.
Motzer et al., 2001[218]	Thalidomide	26	25	0	0	0	4	—	200–800 mg PO q.d.
Stebbing et al., 2001[219]	Thalidomide	25	22	0	2	9	—	—	600 mg PO q.d.
Daliani et al., 2002[220]	Thalidomide	20	19	0	2	10	4.7	18.1	1200 mg PO q.d.
Minor et al., 2002[221]	Thalidomide	29	24	0	1	4	2.3	3.5	400–1200 mg PO q.d.
Escudier et al., 2002[222]	Thalidomide	40	33	—	2	5	—	10	400–1200 mg PO q.d.
Stadler et al., 1999[223]	TNP-470	33	33	0	1	3	2.8	13.1	60 mg/m²/d IV t.i.w.
Braybrooke et al., 2000[224]	Razoxane	40	38	0	0	0	3	7.3	125 mg b.i.d. PO × 5 d q7d
Batist et al., 2002[225]	Neovastat (AE-941)	22	14	0	2	14	—	16.3	14 patients: 240 mL b.i.d.
Yang et al., 2003[85]	Bevacizumab	39	39	0	4	10	4.8	—	10 mg/kg IV q14d
		37	36	0	0	0	3	—	3 mg/kg IV q14d

CR, complete response; Enter., number of patients entered in study; Eval., number of patients assessable for response; MS, median survival in months; PR, partial response; RR, response rate; TTP, time to progression in months.
Note: TTP and MS calculated from data provided, assuming 30 days in 1 month.

Preliminary data thus far indicate that when vaccines alone are used, only rare responses are seen in patients with metastatic disease, if true objective criteria for response are used.

Another recent approach has used a nonmyeloablative allogeneic peripheral-blood stem-cell transplant, hypothesizing that a graft-versus-tumor response may lead to regression of metastatic renal cancer. With this strategy, tumor regression did not occur until the onset of complete donor chimerism, tapering of immunosuppression and in most cases, the appearance of mild graft-versus-host disease (GVHD), supporting an immunologic mechanism of action related to the allograft.[176] Response rates from different groups vary from 33% to 47%,[177,178] but do include patients who did not respond when given IL-2. It is still not clear whether there is specific recognition of tumor-associated antigens by the matched allograft or whether generalized GVHD is leading to *in situ* production of cytokines that then can treat an intrinsically cytokine-sensitive tumor. Clinical GVHD was highly associated with an improved probability of response. The high frequency of GVHD has also predictably led to substantial treatment-related mortality, ranging from 11% to 33%. As with IL-2 therapy, there are no data to document that this approach produces consistent responses in non–clear cell variants of renal cancer, nor indeed in any other tumor types, but this is still being investigated. Nevertheless, this is an interesting approach that can produce major responses when other modalities have failed, but limiting toxicity and delineating the mechanism of action are important future goals.

Antiangiogenic Agents

The field of angiogenesis and its role as a target for cancer therapy has burgeoned in the last decade. New inhibitors of angiogenesis, such as endostatin and angiostatin,[179] have been discovered, and old compounds, such as thalidomide, have found new life as antiangiogenic agents. Renal cell cancer presents an attractive target for these agents for two reasons. First, it is a tremendously vascular tumor consisting largely of capillaries and blood sinuses surrounded by malignant clear cells. In addition, there appears to be a highly angiogenic environment within clear cell cancers, driven by defects in pVHL and the consequent accumulation of HIFα and the elaboration of VEGF (see Fig. 30.1-3). Thus, the common genetic event that leads to clear cell renal carcinoma involves a deregulation of the VEGF pathway, and, presumably, angiogenesis is a consequence.

Thalidomide, the highly teratogenic sedative thought to have caused deformities via an *in utero* antiangiogenic mechanism, has recently been used in the treatment of metastatic renal cell cancer. In 1998, it was approved by the FDA for treatment of erythema nodosum leprosum. Eisen et al. reported a 17% response rate among 18 patients with renal cell cancer in a trial that enrolled patients with melanoma, renal cell, ovarian, and breast cancer.[217] As shown in Table 30.1-19, other trials have not reproduced that initial response rate, with objective responses ranging from 0% to 10%. Although stable disease was noted in some studies, its use outside clinical trials cannot be recommended. Similarly, endostatin, a 20-kD fragment of collagen XVIII and potent inhibitor of angiogenesis, did not yield the dramatic results anticipated in phase I trials, despite broad preclinical activity observed in mice.[180] No phase II reports in renal cancer have appeared.

More promising are the results with bevacizumab, a humanized monoclonal antibody that neutralizes human VEGF. Preclinical studies suggested that antibody neutralization of VEGF could dramatically inhibit the growth of a number of human tumor xenografts in immunosuppressed mice.[181] This led to a clinical trial conducted in a blinded, placebo-controlled fashion to test whether bevacizumab could affect survival or time to tumor progression in patients with metastatic clear cell renal cancer. One hundred sixteen patients with measurable, metastatic clear cell renal cancer were randomized to placebo, low-dose bevacizumab (3 mg/kg every 2 weeks) or high-dose bevacizumab (10 mg/kg every 2 weeks).[182] There was a highly significant delay in time to tumor progression in patients treated with high-dose bevacizumab (risk ratio for time to tumor progression was 2.55 compared to placebo, $P < .001$) and a minimal delay for those receiving low-dose bevacizumab (Fig. 30.1-16). The cytostatic nature of this drug was emphasized by the low frequency of true tumor regression (seen in only 10% of patients treated with high-dose therapy), a fact that future study designs must consider when choosing study end points. There was no survival benefit demonstrated, but patients were allowed to cross over from placebo to bevacizumab, and maximally tolerated doses of bevacizumab were not used

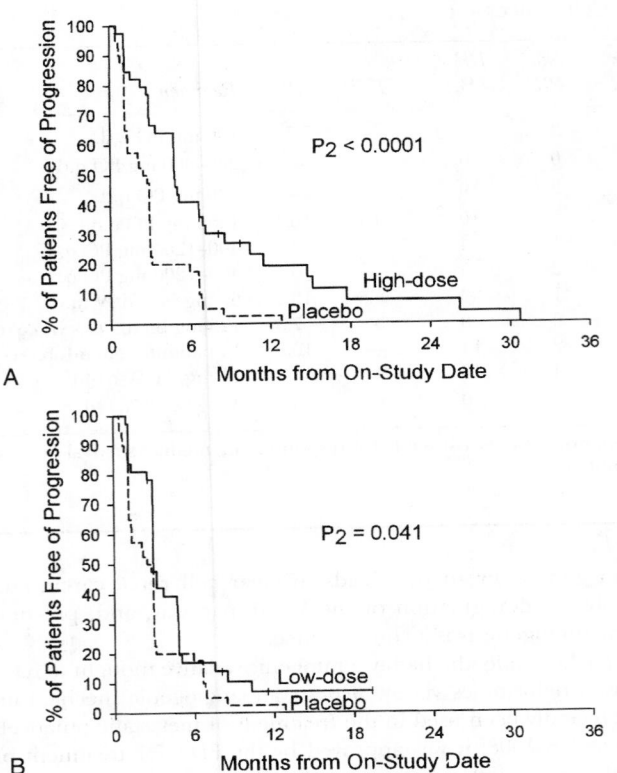

FIGURE 30.1-16. Kaplan-Meier plot of time to progression of patients with metastatic renal cell carcinoma receiving either placebo or one of two doses of bevacizumab (neutralizing antibody to vascular endothelial growth factor). Patients receiving 10 mg/kg/dose every 2 weeks **(A)** showed a highly significant delay in time to tumor progression in this randomized, double-blind trial. A lower dose of 3 mg/kg/dose had minimal benefit **(B)**. (From ref. 85, with permission.)

(indeed toxicity was minimal). This study was the first to demonstrate in a rigorously controlled fashion that an anti-VEGF agent with a putative antiangiogenic mode of action, when given alone, could indeed affect advanced cancer in patients and did so by specifically targeting renal cancer with its prominent angiogenic phenotype. Other early-phase trials of alternative ways to target the VEGF pathway have begun—many using small inhibitory molecules bind to the VEGF tyrosine kinase receptors. Using both receptor blockers and bevacizumab may result in a much more robust blockade of this angiogenic mechanism but may also be limited by shared toxicities, including thromboembolic complications, hypertension, or other sequelae. These trials will require careful design, as investigators have gradually concluded that angiogenesis therapy may block tumor growth rather than induce major clinical responses. Although this is a field with intense activity and interest, it is not yet clear whether a single antiangiogenic agent is sufficient to interrupt the vascular supply of a tumor, producing true patient benefit. It may be that tumors use a variety of angiogenic pathways, and only with carefully combined multi-agent therapy is clinically meaningful tumor arrest or regression seen. Although stable disease and delayed time to progression could be an acceptable outcome in some settings, this outcome is particularly difficult to convincingly prove outside a randomized trial in renal cell carcinoma, because a subset of patients have indolent disease. Reports of phase II trials noting a significant pro-

portion of patients with stable disease should include an analysis of prognostic factors, as described by Motzer et al.[100]

Adjuvant Therapy

Despite the dramatic tumor regressions sometimes attained in patients with metastatic renal cancer who are given biotherapy, frustration remains with the relatively low frequency of these successes. This has led to efforts to apply biotherapies earlier in the course of renal cancer and to the design of adjuvant strategies in the hope that smaller disease volumes might be more responsive. It is important to note that no retrospective analyses have identified lesser tumor burden as a predictor of the probability of responding in the metastatic setting. IFN is one agent that has been tested in a randomized adjuvant study after nephrectomy. Two hundred ninety-four patients with completely resected T3 to T4a or N1, 2, or 3 disease were randomized to observation versus 9 months of subcutaneous lymphoblastoid IFN.[183] With a median follow-up of 4.4 years, patients receiving IFN had similar recurrence rates and significantly worse survival than patients randomized to observation only. In view of these results and the limited response rate to IFN therapy of metastatic disease, there is currently no rationale for recommending adjuvant IFN outside of a protocol setting.

Another recent randomized study tested the administration of one course (two cycles) of high-dose bolus IL-2 versus no therapy in patients who had recently undergone resection of locally advanced or metastatic renal cancer.[184] After enrolling 69 patients, the study was stopped after interim analysis indicated that no significant differences could be demonstrated even if full accrual was attained. This result is not surprising in a study of this size in view of the finding that only a minority of patients with metastatic disease show any tumor regression with IL-2.

Another large, randomized phase III trial of adjuvant therapy has been undertaken to determine whether vaccinating patients with autologous tumor-derived heat-shock proteins (chaperones for tumor antigens and activators of dendritic cells) can reduce the incidence of tumor recurrence in patients with high-risk primary tumors. Again, this intervention has shown little evidence of efficacy in patients with measurable metastatic disease and relies on the adjuvant design of the current trial for its expectations of efficacy. Although there is obvious appeal to testing a chronic, low-toxicity regimen of a cytostatic, antiangiogenic agent such as bevacizumab in patients after resection of a high-risk primary tumor, such trials are not yet under way. In summary, there are no data to support the application of biotherapy in the adjuvant setting, and, in view of the toxicity of some treatments, the lack of a relationship between tumor burden and response rate (in the metastatic setting) and uncertainties regarding the duration of treatment needed, it seems preferable to reserve biotherapies for patients with evaluable disease.

Conclusion

In the last 2 decades, there has been a burgeoning supply of new biologic agents, made available in amounts sufficient for clinical trials by recombinant gene technology. Many of these proteins did not meet the unrealistic expectations generated by preclinical work and entrepreneurial publicity. In the face of these disappointments, several important principles were established by the treatment of renal cell cancer, which should not be overlooked. It has been established that an antiangiogenic strategy, the neutralization of VEGF, can slow the growth rate of advanced cancer in patients. It has also been established that a purely immunologic therapy, IL-2, which has no direct, intrinsic antitumor activity, is able to cause the regression of large, metastatic tumors by stimulating host immune cells. Even more crucial was the demonstration that some of these regressions are potentially curative, with a small but consistent fraction of patients maintaining their CRs to IL-2 beyond 15 years. These long-term responses argue effectively that predicted pitfalls to immunotherapy, such as tumor heterogeneity and antigen loss, immunosuppression by the cancer-bearing state, tumor microenvironment, and a lack of tumor-specific antigens, are not insurmountable problems. To increase the frequency of successful immune attack on renal cell cancer, it is important to understand the mechanisms and cellular elements responsible for these few dramatic responses. Immune effector factors as well as tumor characteristics are likely to be involved in the successful interplay that occurs in responding patients. The treatment of patients with renal cell cancer is likely to contribute to our future understanding of these factors, and this disease remains at the forefront of progress in biologic therapies for cancer.

REFERENCES

1. Jemal A, Murray T, Samuels A, et al. Cancer statistics, 2003. *CA Cancer J Clin* 2003;53:5.
2. Chow W, Devesa S, Warren JL, et al. Rising incidence of renal cell cancer in the United States. *JAMA* 1999;281:1628.
3. Linehan WM, Zbar B, Klausner RD. Renal carcinoma. In: Scriver CR, Beaudet AL, Sly WS, et al., eds. *The metabolic and molecular bases of inherited disease*, 8th ed. New York: McGraw-Hill, 2001:907.
4. Linehan WM, Zbar B, Klausner RD. Renal carcinoma. In: Vogelstein B, Kinzler KW, eds. *The genetic basis of human cancer*, 2nd ed. New York: McGraw-Hill, 2002.
5. Grawitz VP. Die sogenannten lipome der niere. *Beitr Pathol Anat* 1883;93:39.
6. Doderlein A, Birch-Hirschfeld FV. Embryonale drusengeschwulst der nierengegend im kindesalter. *Sex Organe* 1894;3:88.
7. Amin MB, Amin MB, Tamboli P, et al. Prognostic impact of histologic subtyping of adult renal epithelial neoplasms: an experience of 405 cases. *Am J Surg Pathol* 2002;26:281.
8. Linehan WM, Walther MM, Zbar B. The genetic basis of cancer of the kidney. *J Urol* 2003;170:2163.
9. Zbar B, Tory K, Merino M, et al. Hereditary papillary renal cell carcinoma. *J Urol* 1994;151:561.
10. Zbar B, Glenn G, Lubensky IA, et al. Hereditary papillary renal cell carcinoma: clinical studies in 10 families. *J Urol* 1995;153:907.
11. Toro JR, Nickerson ML, Wei MH, et al. Mutations in the fumarate hydratase gene cause hereditary leiomyomatosis and renal cell cancer in families in North America. *Am J Hum Genet* 2003;73:95.
12. Zbar B, Alvord G, Glenn G, et al. Risk of renal and colon neoplasms and spontaneous pneumothorax in the Birt-Hogg-Dube syndrome. *Cancer Epidemiol Biomarkers Prev* 2002;11:393.
13. Mellemgaard A, Engholm G, McLaughlin JK, et al. Risk factors for renal cell carcinoma in Denmark. I. Role of socioeconomic status, tobacco use, beverages, and family history. *Cancer Causes Control* 1994;5:105.
14. Maclure M, Willett W. A case-control study of diet and risk of renal adenocarcinoma. *Epidemiology* 1990;1:430.
15. Yu MC, Mack TM, Hanisch R, et al. Cigarette smoking, obesity, diuretic use, and coffee consumption as risk factors for renal cell carcinoma. *J Natl Cancer Inst* 1986;77:351.
16. Shapiro JA, Williams MA, Weiss NS. Body mass index and risk of renal cell carcinoma. *Epidemiology* 1999;10:188.
17. Tavani A, La Vecchia C. Epidemiology of renal-cell carcinoma. *J Nephrol* 1997;10:93.
18. Vogelzang NJ, Scardino PT, Shipley WU, et al. Epidemiology of renal cell carcinoma. In: Lippincott WW, ed. *Comprehensive textbook of genitourinary oncology*, 2nd ed. 1998.
19. Gago-Dominguez M, Yuan JM, Castelao JE, et al. Regular use of analgesics is a risk factor for renal cell carcinoma. *Br J Cancer* 1999;81:542.
20. Brauch H, Weirich G, Hornauer MA, et al. Trichloroethylene exposure and specific somatic mutations in patients with renal cell carcinoma. *J Natl Cancer Inst* 1999;91:854.
21. Ross RK, Paganini-Hill A, Landolph J, et al. Analgesics, cigarette smoking, and other risk factors for cancer of the renal pelvis and ureter. *Cancer Res* 1989;49:1045.
22. deKernion JB, Smith RB. The kidney and adrenal glands. In: Paulson DF, ed. *Genitourinary surgery*. New York: Churchill Livingstone, 1984:1.
23. Enterline PE, Viren J. Epidemiologic evidence for an association between gasoline and kidney cancer. *Environ Health Perspect* 1985;62:303.
24. McLaughlin JK, Blot WJ, Mehl ES, et al. Petroleum-related employment and renal cell cancer. *J Occup Med* 1985;672.
25. Doublet JD, Peraldi MN, Gattegno B, et al. Renal cell carcinoma of native kidneys: prospective study of 129 renal transplant patients. *J Urol* 1997;158:42.
26. Brennan JF, Stilmant MM, Babayan RK, et al. Acquired renal cystic disease: implications for the urologist. *Br J Urol* 1991;67:342.
27. Grantham JJ, Levin E. Acquired cystic disease: replacing one kidney disease with another. *Kidney Int* 1985;28:99.
28. Walther MM, Lubensky IA, Venzon D, et al. Prevalence of microscopic lesions in grossly normal renal parenchyma from patients with von Hippel-Lindau disease, sporadic renal cell carcinoma and no renal disease: clinical implications. *J Urol* 1995;154:2010.
29. Latif F, Tory K, Gnarra JR, et al. Identification of the von Hippel-Lindau disease tumor suppressor gene. *Science* 1993;260:1317.
30. Chen F, Kishida T, Yao M, et al. Germline mutations in the von Hippel-Lindau disease tumor suppressor gene: correlation with phenotype. *Hum Mutat* 1995;5:66.
31. Stolle CA, Glenn G, Zbar B, et al. Improved detection of germline mutations in the von Hippel-Lindau disease tumor suppressor gene. *Hum Mutat* 1998;12:417.
32. Gnarra JR, Tory K, Weng Y, et al. Mutation of the VHL tumour suppressor gene in renal carcinoma. *Nat Genet* 1994;7:85.
33. Shuin T, Kondo K, Torigoe S, et al. Frequent somatic mutations and loss of heterozygosity of the von Hippel-Lindau tumor suppressor gene in primary human renal cell carcinomas. *Cancer Res* 1994;54:2852.
34. Zhuang Z, Gnarra JR, Zbar B, et al. Detection of the von Hippel-Lindau disease gene mutation by PCR and SSCP in sporadic renal cell carcinoma in paraffin-embedded tissue. *Mod Pathol* 1994;7:86A.
35. Ohh M, Park CW, Ivan M, et al. Ubiquitination of hypoxia-inducible factor requires direct binding to the beta-domain of the von Hippel-Lindau protein. *Nat Cell Biol* 2000;2:423.
36. Choyke PL, Walther MM, Glenn GM, et al. Imaging features of hereditary papillary renal cancers. *J Comput Assist Tomogr* 1997;21:737.
37. Schmidt L, Duh F-M, Chen F, et al. Germline and somatic mutations in the tyrosine kinase domain of the MET proto-oncogene in papillary renal carcinomas. *Nat Genet* 1997;16:68.
38. Schmidt L, Junker K, Weirich G, et al. Two North American families with hereditary papillary renal carcinoma and identical novel mutations in the MET proto-oncogene. *Cancer Res* 1998;58:1719.
39. Launonen V, Vierimaa O, Kiuru M, et al. Inherited susceptibility to uterine leiomyomas and renal cell cancer. *Proc Natl Acad Sci U S A* 2001;98:3387.
40. The Multiple Leiomyoma Consortium. Germline mutations in FH predispose to dominantly inherited uterine fibroids, skin leiomyomata and papillary renal cell cancer. *Nat Genet* 2002;30:1.
41. Toro J, Duray PH, Glenn GM, et al. Birt-Hogg-Dube syndrome: a novel marker of kidney neoplasia. *Arch Dermatol* 1999;135:1195.
42. Pavlovich CP, Hewitt S, Walther MM, et al. Renal tumors in the Birt-Hogg-Dube syndrome. *Am J Surg Pathol* 2002;26:1542.
43. Delahunt B, Eble JN. Papillary renal cell carcinoma: a clinicopathologic and immunohistochemical study of 105 tumors. *Mod Pathol* 1997;10:537.
44. Thoenes W, Storkel S, Rumpelt HJ. Human chromophobe renal cell carcinoma. *Virchows Arch B Cell Pathol Incl Mol Pathol* 1985;48:207.
45. Cangiano T, Liao J, Naitoh J, et al. Sarcomatoid renal cell carcinoma: biologic behavior, prognosis, and response to combined surgical resection and immunotherapy. *J Clin Oncol* 1999;17:523.
46. Golimbu M, Joshi P, Sperber A, et al. Renal cell carcinoma: survival and prognostic factors. *J Urol* 1986;XXVII:291.
47. Maldazys JD, deKernion JB. Prognostic factors in metastatic renal carcinoma. *J Urol* 1986;136:376.
48. Chisholm GD. Nephrogenic ridge tumors and their syndromes. *Ann N Y Acad Sci* 1984;230:403.
49. Evans BK, Fagan C, Arnold T, et al. Paraneoplastic motor neuron disease and renal cell carcinoma: improvement after nephrectomy. *Neurology* 1990;40:960.
50. Thiede MA, Strewler GJ, Nissenson RA, et al. Human renal carcinoma expresses two messages encoding a parathyroid hormone-like peptide: evidence for the alternative splicing of a single-copy gene. *Proc Natl Acad Sci U S A* 1988;85:4605.
51. Walther MM, Patel B, Choyke PL, et al. Hypercalcemia in patients with metastatic renal cell carcinoma: effect of nephrectomy and metabolic evaluation. *J Urol* 1997;158:733.
52. Israel GM, Bosniak MA. Renal imaging for diagnosis and staging of renal cell carcinoma. *Urol Clin North Am* 2003;30:499.
53. Choyke P, Walther MM, Wagner JR, et al. Renal cancer: preoperative evaluation with dual-phase three-dimensional MR angiography. *Radiology* 1997;205:767.
54. Horan JJ, Robertson CN, Choyke PL, et al. The detection of renal carcinoma extension into the renal vein and inferior vena cava: a prospective comparison of venacavography and magnetic resonance imaging. *J Urol* 1989;142:943.
55. Robson CJ, Churchill BM, Anderson W. The results of radical nephrectomy for renal cell carcinoma. *J Urol* 1969;101:297.
56. Javidan J, Stricker HJ, Tamboli P, et al. Prognostic significance of the 1997 TNM classification of renal cell carcinoma. *J Urol* 1999;162:1277.
57. Kinouchi T, Saiki S, Meguro N, et al. Impact of tumor size on the clinical outcomes of patients with Robson State I renal cell carcinoma. *Cancer* 1999;85:689.
58. Guinan P, Stuhldreher D, Frank W, et al. Report of 337 patients with renal cell carcinoma emphasizing 110 with stage IV disease and review of the literature. *J Surg Oncol* 1997;64:295.
59. Tsui KH, Shvarts O, Smith RB, et al. Prognostic indicators for renal cell carcinoma: a multivariate analysis of 643 patients using the revised 1997 TNM staging criteria. *J Urol* 2000;163:1090.
60. Cheville JC, Lohse CM, Zincke H, et al. Comparisons of outcome and prognostic features among histologic subtypes of renal cell carcinoma. *Am J Surg Pathol* 2003;27:612.
61. Mejean A, Hopirtean V, Bazin JP, et al. Prognostic factors for the survival of patients with papillary renal cell carcinoma: meaning of histological typing and multifocality. *J Urol* 2003;170:764.

62. Figenshau RS, Basler JW, Simon JA, et al. Renal medullary carcinoma. *J Urol* 1998; 159:711.
63. Gilbert JB. Diagnosis and treatment of malignant renal tumors. *J Urol* 1937;39:223.
64. Ogan K, Cadeddu JA, Stifelman MD. Laparoscopic radical nephrectomy: oncologic efficacy. *Urol Clin North Am* 2003;30:543.
65. Walther MM, Lyne JC, Libutti SK, et al. Laparoscopic cytoreductive nephrectomy as preparation for administration of systemic interleukin-2 in the treatment of metastatic renal cell carcinoma: a pilot study. *J Urol* 1999;53:496.
66. Gill IS, Matin SF, Desai MM, et al. Comparative analysis of laparoscopic versus open partial nephrectomy for renal tumors in 200 patients. *J Urol* 2003;170:64.
67. Gill IS, Desai MM, Kaouk JH, et al. Laparoscopic partial nephrectomy for renal tumor: duplicating open surgical techniques. *J Urol* 2002;167:469.
68. Gill IS. Minimally invasive nephron-sparing surgery. *Urol Clin North Am* 2003;30:551.
69. Novick AC, Jackson CL, Straffon RA. The role of renal autotransplantation in complex urological reconstruction. *J Urol* 1990;143:452.
70. Herring JC, Enquist EG, Chernoff AC, et al. Parenchymal sparing surgery in patients with hereditary renal cell carcinoma—ten year experience. *J Urol* 2001;165:777.
71. Volpe A, Panzarella T, Rendon RA, et al. The natural history of incidentally detected small renal masses. *Cancer* 2004;100:738.
72. Montie JE, Stewart BH, Straffon RA, et al. The role of adjunctive nephrectomy in patients with metastatic renal cell carcinoma. *J Urol* 1977;117:272.
73. deKernion JB, Ramming KP, Smith RB. The natural history of metastatic renal cell carcinoma: a computer analysis. *J Urol* 1978;120:148.
74. Walther MM, Yang JC, Pass HI, et al. Cytoreductive surgery prior to high dose interleukin-2 based therapy in patients with metastatic renal cell carcinoma. *J Urol* 1997;158:1675.
75. Walther MM, Alexander RB, Weiss GI, et al. Cytoreductive surgery prior to interleukin-2 based therapy in patients with metastatic renal cell carcinoma. *J Urol* 1993;42:250.
76. Wagner JR, Walther MM, Linehan WM, et al. Interleukin-2 based immunotherapy for metastatic renal cell carcinoma with kidney in place. *J Urol* 1999;162:43.
77. Flanigan RC, Salmon SE, Blumenstein BA, et al. Nephrectomy followed by interferon alfa-2b compared with interferon alfa-2b alone for metastatic renal-cell cancer. *N Engl J Med* 2001;345:1655.
78. Mickisch GH, Garin A, Van Poppel H, et al. Radical nephrectomy plus interferon-alfa-based immunotherapy compared with interferon alfa alone in metastatic renal-cell carcinoma: a randomised trial. *Lancet* 2001;358:966.
79. Middleton RG. Surgery for metastatic renal cell carcinoma. *J Urol* 1967;97:973.
80. van der Poel HG, Roukema JA, Horenblas S, et al. Metastasectomy in renal cell carcinoma: a multicenter retrospective analysis. *Eur Urol* 1999;35:197.
81. O'Dea MJ, Zincke H, Utz DC. The treatment of renal cell carcinoma with solitary metastasis. *J Urol* 1978;120:540.
82. Hrushesky WJ, Murphy GP. Current status of the therapy of advanced renal carcinoma. *J Surg Oncol* 1977;9:277.
83. Yagoda A, Abi-Rached B, Petrylak D. Chemotherapy for advanced renal-cell carcinoma: 1983–1993. *Semin Oncol* 1995;22:42.
84. Motzer RJ, Russo P. Systemic therapy for renal cell carcinoma. *J Urol* 2000;163:408.
85. Yang JC, Haworth L, Sherry RM, et al. A randomized trial of Bevacizumab, an anti-vascular endothelial growth factor antibody, for metastatic renal cancer. *N Engl J Med* 2003;349:427.
86. Henriksson R, Nilsson S, Colleen S, et al. Survival in renal cell carcinoma—a randomized evaluation of tamoxifen vs interleukin 2, alpha-interferon (leucocyte) and tamoxifen [see comments]. *Br J Cancer* 1998;77:1311.
87. Gershanovich MM, Moiseyenko VM, Vorobjev AV, et al. High-dose toremifene in advanced renal-cell carcinoma. *Cancer Chemother Pharmacol* 1997;39:547.
88. Rohde D, Wiesner C, Graf D, et al. Interstitial fluid pressure is increased in renal cell carcinoma xenografts. *Urol Res* 2000;28:1.
89. Rini BI, Vogelzang NJ, Dumas MC, et al. Phase II trial of weekly intravenous gemcitabine with continuous infusion fluorouracil in patients with metastatic renal cell cancer. *J Clin Oncol* 2000;18:2419.
90. George CM, Vogelzang NJ, Rini BI, et al. A phase II trial of weekly intravenous gemcitabine and cisplatin with continuous infusion fluorouracil in patients with metastatic renal cell carcinoma. *Ann Oncol* 2002;13:116.
91. Desai AA, Vogelzang NJ, Rini BI, et al. A high rate of venous thromboembolism in a multi-institutional phase II trial of weekly intravenous gemcitabine with continuous infusion fluorouracil and daily thalidomide in patients with metastatic renal cell carcinoma. *Cancer* 2002;95:1629.
92. Stadler WM, Huo D, George C, et al. Prognostic factors for survival with gemcitabine plus 5-fluorouracil based regimens for metastatic renal cancer. *J Urol* 2003;170:1141.
93. Motzer RJ, Bacik J, Murphy BA, et al. Interferon-alfa as a comparative treatment for clinical trials of new therapies against advanced renal cell carcinoma. *J Clin Oncol* 2002;20:289.
94. Strumberg D, Voliotis D, Moeller JG, et al. Results of phase I pharmacokinetic and pharmacodynamic studies of the Raf kinase inhibitor BAY 43-9006 in patients with solid tumors. *Int J Clin Pharmacol Ther* 2002;40:580.
95. Bayes M, Rabasseda X, Prous JR. Gateways to clinical trials. *Methods Find Exp Clin Pharmacol* 2003;25:565.
96. Drevs J. PTK/ZK (Novartis). *IDrugs* 2003;6:787.
97. Abraham J, Agrawal M, Bakke S, et al. Phase I trial and pharmacokinetic study of BMS-247550, an epothilone B analog, administered intravenously on a daily schedule for five days. *J Clin Oncol* 2003;21:1866.
98. Motzer RJ, Schwartz L, Law TM, et al. Interferon alfa-2a and 13-cis-retinoic acid in renal cell carcinoma: antitumor activity in a phase II trial and interactions in vitro. *J Clin Oncol* 1995;13:1950.
99. Motzer RJ, Murphy BA, Bacik J, et al. Phase III trial of interferon alfa-2a with or without 13-cis-retinoic acid for patients with advanced renal cell carcinoma. *J Clin Oncol* 2000;18:2972.
100. Motzer RJ, Mazumdar M, Bacik J, et al. Survival and prognostic stratification of 670 patients with advanced renal cell carcinoma. *J Clin Oncol* 1999;17:2530.
101. Atzpodien J, Royston P, Wandert T, et al. Metastatic renal carcinoma comprehensive prognostic system. *Br J Cancer* 2003;88:348.
102. Rosen LS, Gordon D, Tchekmedyian S, et al. Zoledronic acid versus placebo in the treatment of skeletal metastases in patients with lung cancer and other solid tumors: a phase III, double-blind, randomized trial—the Zoledronic Acid Lung Cancer and Other Solid Tumors Study Group. *J Clin Oncol* 2003;21:3150.
103. Lipton A, Zheng M, Seaman J. Zoledronic acid delays the onset of skeletal-related events and progression of skeletal disease in patients with advanced renal cell carcinoma. *Cancer* 2003;98:962.
104. Visapaa H, Bui M, Huang Y, et al. Correlation of Ki-67 and gelsolin expression to clinical outcome in renal clear cell carcinoma. *J Urol* 2003;61:845.
105. Rioux-Leclercq N, Turlin B, Bansard J, et al. Value of immunohistochemical Ki-67 and p53 determinations as predictive factors of outcome in renal cell carcinoma. *J Urol* 2000;55:501.
106. Morell-Quadreny L, Clar-Blanch F, Fenollosa-Enterna B, et al. Proliferating cell nuclear antigen (PCNA) as a prognostic factor in renal cell carcinoma. *Anticancer Res* 1998;18:677.
107. Sejima T, Miyagawa I. Expression of bcl-2, p53 oncoprotein, and proliferating cell nuclear antigen in renal cell carcinoma. *Eur Urol* 1999;35:242.
108. Di Silverio F, Casale P, Colella D, et al. Independent value of tumor size and DNA ploidy for the prediction of disease progression in patients with organ-confined renal cell carcinoma. *Cancer* 2000;88:835.
109. Papadopoulos I, Rudolph P, Weichert-Jacobsen K, et al. Prognostic indicators for response to therapy and survival in patients with metastatic renal cell cancer treated with interferon alpha-2 beta and vinblastine. *Urology* 1996;48:373.
110. Gottesman MM, Fojo T, Bates SE. Multidrug resistance in cancer: role of ATP-dependent transporters. *Nat Rev Cancer* 2002;2:48.
111. Agrawal M, Abraham J, Balis FM, et al. Increased 99mTc-sestamibi accumulation in normal liver and drug-resistant tumors after the administration of the glycoprotein inhibitor, XR9576. *Clin Cancer Res* 2003;9:650.
112. Chen CC, Meadows B, Regis J, et al. Detection of in vivo P-glycoprotein inhibition by PSC 833 using Tc-99m sestamibi. *Clin Cancer Res* 1997;3:545.
113. Mulders P, Bleumer I, Oosterwijk E. Tumor antigens and markers in renal cell carcinoma. *Urol Clin North Am* 2003;30:455.
114. Stumm G, Eberwein S, Rostock-Wolf S, et al. Concomitant overexpression of the EGFR and erbB-2 genes in renal cell carcinoma (RCC) is correlated with dedifferentiation and metastasis. *Int J Cancer* 1996;69:17.
115. Parker A, Cheville JC, Lohse C, et al. Expression of insulin-like growth factor I receptor and survival in patients with clear cell renal cell carcinoma. *J Urol* 2003;170:420.
116. Vasavada SP, Novick AC, Williams BR. P53, bcl-2, and Bax expression in renal cell carcinoma. *J Urol* 1998;51:1057.
117. Oudard S, Levalois C, Andrieu JM, et al. Expression of genes involved in chemoresistance, proliferation and apoptosis in clinical samples of renal cell carcinoma and correlation with clinical outcome. *Anticancer Res* 2002;22:121.
118. Murray GI, McFadyen MC, Mitchell RT, et al. Cytochrome P450 CYP3A in human renal cell cancer. *Br J Cancer* 1999;79:1836.
119. Volm M, Kastel M, Mattern J, et al. Expression of resistance factors (P-glycoprotein, glutathione S-transferase-pi, and topoisomerase II) and their interrelationship to proto-oncogene products in renal cell carcinomas. *Cancer* 1993;71:3981.
120. Shimazui T, Oosterwijk-Wakka J, Akaza H, et al. Alterations in expression of cadherin-6 and E-cadherin during kidney development and in renal cell carcinoma. *Eur Urol* 2000;38:331.
121. Jain RK. The next frontier of molecular medicine: delivery of therapeutics. *Nat Med* 1998;4:655.
122. Anderson H, Yap JT, Wells P, et al. Measurement of renal tumour and normal tissue perfusion using positron emission tomography in a phase II clinical trial of Razoxane. *Br J Cancer* 2003;89:262.
123. Vogelzang NJ, Aklilu M, Stadler WM, et al. A phase II trial of weekly intravenous ranpirnase (Onconase), a novel ribonuclease in patients with metastatic kidney cancer. *Invest New Drugs* 2001;19:255.
123b. Motzer RJ, Bacik J, Schwartz LH, et al. Prognostic factors for survival in previously treated patients with metastatic renal cell carcinoma. *J Clin Oncol* 2004;22:454.
124. Rosner GL, Stadler W, Ratain MJ. Randomized discontinuation design: application to cytostatic antineoplastic agents. *J Clin Oncol* 2002;20:4478.
125. Stadler WM, Rosner G, Rini B, et al. Successful implementation of the randomized discontinuation trial design (RDTD) with the putative antiangiogenic agent carboxyaminoimidazole (CAI) in renal cell carcinoma (RCC). A Cancer and Leukemia Group B (CALGB) Study. *Proc Am Soc Clin Oncol* 2003;22:193.
126. Motzer RJ, Bacik J, Mariani T, et al. Treatment outcome and survival associated with metastatic renal cell carcinoma of non-clear-cell histology. *J Clin Oncol* 2002;20:2376.
127. Bangalore N, Bhargava P, Hawkins MJ, et al. Sustained response of sarcomatoid renal-cell carcinoma to MAID chemotherapy: case report and review of the literature. *Ann Oncol* 2001;12:271.
128. Escudier B, Droz JP, Rolland F, et al. Doxorubicin and ifosfamide in patients with metastatic sarcomatoid renal cell carcinoma: a phase II study of the Genitourinary Group of the French Federation of Cancer Centers. *J Urol* 2002;168:959.
129. Middleton AWJ. Indications for and results of nephrectomy for metastatic renal cell carcinoma. *Urol Clin North Am* 1980;7:711.
130. Gleave ME, Elhilali M, Fradet Y, et al. Interferon gamma-1b compared to placebo in metastatic renal-cell carcinoma. *N Engl J Med* 1998;338:1265.
131. Bloom HJ. Proceedings: hormone-induced and spontaneous regression of metastatic renal cancer. *Cancer* 1973;32:1066.
132. Snow RM, Schellhammer PF. Spontaneous regression of metastatic renal cell carcinoma. *Urology* 1982;20:177.

133. Marcus SG, Choyke PL, Reiter R, et al. Regression of metastatic renal cell carcinoma after cytoreductive nephrectomy. *J Urol* 1993;150:463.
134. Quesada JR, Swanson DA, Trindade A, et al. Renal cell carcinoma: antitumor effects of leukocyte interferon. *Cancer Res* 1983;43:940.
135. Quesada JR, Rios A, Swanson D, et al. Antitumor activity of recombinant-derived interferon alpha in metastatic renal cell carcinoma. *J Clin Oncol* 1985;3:1522.
136. Moss HB. Interferon therapy for renal cell carcinoma. *Semin Oncol* 1987;14:36.
137. Quesada JR. Role of interferons in the therapy of metastatic renal cell carcinoma. *Urology* 1989;34:80.
138. Medical Research Council Renal Cancer Collaborators. Interferon-α and survival in metastatic renal carcinoma: early results of a randomised controlled trial. *Lancet* 1999;353:14.
139. Small EJ, Weiss GR, Malik UK, et al. The treatment of metastatic renal cell carcinoma patients with recombinant human gamma interferon. *Cancer J Sci Am* 1998;4:162.
140. Rosenberg SA, Lotze MT, Muul LM, et al. A progress report on the treatment of 157 patients with advanced cancer using lymphokine-activated killer cells and interleukin-2 or high-dose interleukin-2 alone. *N Engl J Med* 1987;316:889.
141. Lotze MT, Chang AE, Seipp CA, et al. High-dose recombinant interleukin 2 in the treatment of patients with disseminated cancer: responses, treatment-related morbidity and histologic findings. *JAMA* 1986;256:3117.
142. Fisher RI, Coltman CA, Doroshow JH, et al. Metastatic renal cancer treated with interleukin-2 and lymphokine-activated killer cells. *Ann Intern Med* 1988;108:518.
143. Fisher RI, Rosenberg SA, Sznol M, et al. High-dose aldesleukin in renal cell carcinoma: long-term survival update. *Cancer J Sci Am* 1997;3:S70.
144. Rosenberg SA, Yang JC, Topalian SL, et al. Treatment of 283 consecutive patients with metastatic melanoma or renal cell cancer using high-dose bolus interleukin 2. *JAMA* 1994;271:907.
145. Rosenberg SA, Yang JC, White DE, et al. Durability of complete responses in patients with metastatic cancer treated with high-dose interleukin-2. *Ann Surg* 1998;228:319.
146. Cangiano T, Liao J, Naitoh J, et al. Sarcomatoid renal cell carcinoma: biologic behavior, prognosis, and response to combined surgical resection and immunotherapy. *J Clin Oncol* 1999;17:523.
147. Rosenberg SA, Lotze MT, Yang JC, et al. Prospective randomized trial of high-dose interleukin-2 alone or in conjunction with lymphokine-activated killer cells for the treatment of patients with advanced cancer [published erratum appears in *J Natl Cancer Inst* 1993;85(13):1091]. *J Natl Cancer Inst* 1993;85:622.
148. Law TM, Motzer R, Mazumdar M, et al. Phase III randomized trial of interleukin-2 with or without lymphokine activated killer cells in the treatment of patients with advanced renal cell carcinoma. *Cancer* 1995;76:824.
149. Margolin KA, Rayner AA, Hawkins MJ, et al. Interleukin-2 and lymphokine-activated killer cell therapy of solid tumors: analysis of toxicity and management guidelines. *J Clin Oncol* 1989;7:486.
150. Kammula US, White DE, Rosenberg SA. Trends in the safety of high dose bolus interleukin-2 administration in patients with metastatic cancer. *Cancer* 1998;83:797.
151. Sleijfer DT, Janssen RA, Buter J, et al. Phase II study of subcutaneous interleukin-2 in unselected patients with advanced renal cell cancer on an outpatient basis. *J Clin Oncol* 1992;10:1119.
152. Buter J, Sleijfer DT, Winette TA, et al. A progress report on the outpatient treatment of patients with advanced renal cell carcinoma using subcutaneous recombinant interleukin-2. *Semin Oncol* 1993;20:16.
153. Tourani JM, Lucas V, Mayeur D, et al. Subcutaneous recombinant interleukin-2 (rIL-2) in out-patients with metastatic renal cell carcinoma. Results of a multicenter SCAPP1 trial. *Ann Oncol* 1996;7:525.
154. West WH, Tayer KW, Yannelli JR, et al. Constant-infusion recombinant interleukin-2 plus lymphokine-activated killer cells in metastatic renal cancer. *N Engl J Med* 1987;316:898.
155. Yang JC, Sherry RM, Steinberg SM, et al. Randomized study of high-dose and low-dose interleukin-2 in patients with metastatic renal cancer. *J Clin Oncol* 2003;21:3127.
156. Weiss GR, Margolin KA, Aronson FR, et al. A randomized phase II trial of continuous infusion interleukin-2 or bolus injection interleukin-2 plus lymphokine-activated killer cells for advanced renal cell carcinoma. *J Clin Oncol* 1992;10:275.
157. Gold PJ, Thompson JA, Markowitz DR, et al. Metastatic renal cell carcinoma: long-term survival after therapy with high-dose continuous-infusion interleukin-2 [see comments]. *Cancer J Sci Am* 1997;3:[Suppl 1]S85.
158. Rosenberg SA, Lotze MT, Yang JC, et al. Combination therapy with interleukin-2 and alpha-interferon for the treatment of patients with advanced cancer. *J Clin Oncol* 1989;7:1863.
159. Marincola FM, White DE, Wise AP, et al. Combination therapy with interferon alfa-2a and interleukin-2 for the treatment of metastatic cancer. *J Clin Oncol* 1995;13:1110.
160. Atzpodien J, Hanninen EL, Kirchner H, et al. Multiinstitutional home-therapy trial of recombinant human interleukin-2 and interferon alfa-2 in progressive metastatic renal cell carcinoma. *J Clin Oncol* 1995;13:497.
161. Negrier S, Escudier B, Lasset C, et al. Recombinant human interleukin-2, recombinant human interferon alfa-2a, or both in metastatic renal-cell carcinoma. Groupe Francais d'Immunotherapie [see comments]. *N Engl J Med* 1998;338:1272.
162. Atkins MB, Sparano J, Fisher RI, et al. Randomized phase II trial of high-dose interleukin-2 either alone or in combination with interferon alfa-2b in advanced renal cell carcinoma. *J Clin Oncol* 1993;11:661.
163. Jayson GC, Middleton M, Lee SM, et al. A randomized phase II trial of interleukin 2 and interleukin 2-interferon alpha in advanced renal cancer. *Br J Cancer* 1998;78:366.
164. McDermott D, Flaherty L, Clark J, et al. A randomized phase III trial of high-dose interleukin-2 (HD IL2) versus subcutaneous (SC) IL2/interferon (IFN) in patients with metastatic renal cell carcinoma (RCC). *Proc Am Soc Clin Oncol* 2001:20.
165. Bertolini DR, Nedwin GE, Bringman TS, et al. Stimulation of bone resorption and inhibition of bone formation in vitro by human tumour necrosis factors. *Nature* 1986;319:516.
166. Vindelov LL, Christensen IJ, Nissen NI. Standardization of high-resolution flow cytometry DNA analysis by simultaneous use of chicken and trout red blood cells as internal reference standards. *Cytometry* 1983;3:328.
167. Dutcher JP, Atkins M, Fisher R, et al. Interleukin-2-based therapy for metastatic renal cell cancer: the Cytokine Working Group experience, 1989–1997. *Cancer J Sci Am* 1997;3:[Suppl 1]S73.
168. Gaugler B, Brouwenstijn N, Vantomme V, et al. A new gene coding for an antigen recognized by autologous cytolytic T lymphocytes on a human renal carcinoma. *Immunogenetics* 1996;44:323.
169. Ronsin C, Chung-Scott V, Poullion I, et al. A non-AUG-defined alternative open reading frame of the intestinal carboxyl esterase mRNA generates an epitope recognized by renal cell carcinoma-reactive tumor-infiltrating lymphocytes in situ. *J Immunol* 1999;163:483.
170. Hanada K, Perry-Lalley DM, Ohnmacht GA, et al. Identification of fibroblast growth factor-5 as an overexpressed antigen in multiple human adenocarcinomas. *Cancer Res* 2001;61:5511.
171. Belldegrun A, Muul LM, Rosenberg SA. Interleukin 2 expanded tumor-infiltrating lymphocytes in human renal cell cancer: isolation, characterization, and antitumor activity. *Cancer Res* 1988;48:206.
172. Figlin RA, Pierce WC, Kaboo R, et al. Treatment of metastatic renal cell carcinoma with nephrectomy, interleukin-2 and cytokine-primed or CD8(+) selected tumor infiltrating lymphocytes from primary tumor. *J Urol* 1997;158:740.
173. Figlin RA, Thompson JA, Bukowski RM, et al. Multicenter, randomized, phase III trial of CD8(+) tumor-infiltrating lymphocytes in combination with recombinant interleukin-2 in metastatic renal cell carcinoma [In Process Citation]. *J Clin Oncol* 1999;17:2521.
174. Chang AE, Li Q, Jiang G, et al. Phase II trial of autologous tumor vaccination, anti-CD3-activated vaccine-primed lymphocytes, and interleukin-2 in stage IV renal cell cancer. *J Clin Oncol* 2003;21:884.
175. Simons JW, Jaffee EM, Weber CE, et al. Bioactivity of autologous irradiated renal cell carcinoma vaccines generated by ex vivo granulocyte-macrophage colony-stimulating factor gene transfer. *Cancer Res* 1997;57:1537.
176. Childs R, Chernoff A, Contentin N, et al. Regression of metastatic renal-cell carcinoma after nonmyeloablative allogeneic peripheral-blood stem-cell transplantation. *N Engl J Med* 2000;343:750.
177. Childs R, Srinivasan R. Advances in allogeneic stem cell transplantation: directing graft-versus-leukemia at solid tumors. *Cancer J* 2002;8:2.
178. Rini BI, Zimmerman T, Stadler WM, et al. Allogeneic stem-cell transplantation of renal cell cancer after nonmyeloablative chemotherapy: feasibility, engraftment, and clinical results. *J Clin Oncol* 2002;20:2017.
179. O'Reilly MS, Boehm T, Shing Y, et al. Endostatin: an endogenous inhibitor of angiogenesis and tumor growth. *Cell* 1997;88:277.
180. Herbst RS, Hess KR, Tran HT, et al. Phase I study of recombinant human endostatin in patients with advanced solid tumors. *J Clin Oncol* 2002;20:3792.
181. Kim KJ, Li B, Winer J, et al. Inhibition of vascular endothelial growth factor-induced angiogenesis suppresses tumour growth in vivo. *Nature* 1993;362:841.
182. Yang JC, Haworth L, Sherry RM, et al. A randomized trial of Bevacizumab, an anti-vascular endothelial growth factor antibody, for metastatic renal cancer. *N Engl J Med* 2003;349:427.
183. Trump DL, Elson P, Propert K, et al. Randomized, controlled trial of adjuvant therapy with lymphoblastoid interferon (L-IFN) in resected, high-risk renal cell carcinoma (HR-RCC). *Proc Am Soc Clin Oncol* 1996;15:253.
184. Clark JI, Atkins MB, Urba WJ, et al. Adjuvant high-dose bolus interleukin-2 for patients with high-risk renal cell carcinoma: a cytokine working group randomized trial. *J Clin Oncol* 2003;21:3133.
185. Rosenberg SA, Yang JC, White DE, et al. Durability of complete responses in patients with metastatic cancer treated with high-dose interleukin-2: identification of the antigens mediating response. *Ann Surg* 1998;228:307.
186. Skinner DG, Calvin RB, Vermillion CD, et al. Diagnosis and management of renal cell carcinoma. *Cancer* 1971;28:1165.
187. Javidan J, Stricker HJ, Tamboli P, et al. Prognostic significance of the 1997 TNM classification of renal cell carcinoma. *J Urol* 1999;162:1277.
188. Leibovich BC, Pantuck AJ, Bui MH, et al. Current staging of renal cell carcinoma. *Urol Clin North Am* 2003;30:481.
189. Lummen G, Sperling H, Luboldt H, et al. Phase II trial of titanocene dichloride in advanced renal-cell carcinoma. *Cancer Chemother Pharmacol* 1998;42:415.
190. Vogelzang NJ, Mani S, Schilsky RL, et al. Phase II and pharmacodynamic studies of pyrazine diazohydroxide (NSC 361456) in patients with advanced renal and colorectal cancer. *Clin Cancer Res* 1998;4:929.
191. Rigos D, Wechsel HW, Bichler KH. Treosulfan in the treatment of metastatic renal cell carcinoma. *Anticancer Res* 1999;19:1549.
192. Berg WJ, McCaffrey J, Schwartz LH, et al. A phase II study of Pyrazoloacridine in patients with advanced renal cell carcinoma. *Invest New Drugs* 1998;16:337.
193. Stadler WM, Vogelzang NJ, Amato R, et al. Flavopiridol, a novel cyclin-dependent kinase inhibitor, in metastatic renal cancer: a University of Chicago phase II consortium study. *J Clin Oncol* 2000;18:371.
194. Pagliaro L, Daliani D, Amato R, et al. A phase II trial of bryostatin-1 for patients with metastatic renal cell carcinoma. *Cancer* 2000;89:615.
195. Dreicer R, Smith DC, Williams RD, et al. Phase II trial of suramin in patients with metastatic renal cell carcinoma. *Invest New Drugs* 1999;17:183.
196. Small EJ, Figlin R, Petrylak D, et al. A phase II pilot study of KW-2189 in patients with advanced renal cell carcinoma. *Invest New Drugs* 2000;18:193.
197. Berg WJ, Schwartz L, Yu R, et al. Phase II trial of irofulven (6-hydroxymethylacylfulvene) for patients with advanced renal cell carcinoma. *Invest New Drugs* 2001;19:317.
198. Kuebler JP, King GW, Triozzi P, et al. Phase II study of Pyrazoloacridine in metastatic renal cell carcinoma. *Invest New Drugs* 2001;19:327.
199. Schroder LE, Lew D, Flanigan RC, et al. Phase II evaluation of suramin in advanced renal cell carcinoma. A Southwest Oncology Group study. *Urol Oncol* 2001;6:145.
200. Adjei AA. Pemetrexed in the treatment of selected solid tumors. *Semin Oncol* 2002;29:50.

201. Skubitz KM. Phase II trial of pegylated-liposomal doxorubicin (Doxil) in renal cell cancer. *Invest New Drugs* 2002;20:101.

202. Vis N, van der GA, van Rhijn G, et al. A phase II trial of methotrexate-human serum albumin (MTX-HSA) in patients with metastatic renal cell carcinoma who progressed under immunotherapy. *Cancer Chemother Pharmacol* 2002;49:342.

203. Wenzel C, Locker GJ, Schmidinger M, et al. Capecitabine in the treatment of metastatic renal cell carcinoma failing immunotherapy. *Am J Kidney Dis* 2002;39:48.

204. Vuky J, Yu R, Schwartz L, et al. Phase II trial of arsenic trioxide in patients with metastatic renal cell carcinoma. *Invest New Drugs* 2002;20:327.

205. Amato RJ, Perez C, Pagliaro L. Irofulven, a novel inhibitor of DNA synthesis, in metastatic renal cell cancer. *Invest New Drugs* 2002;20:413.

206. Park DK, Ryan CW, Dolan ME, et al. A phase II trial of oral temozolomide in patients with metastatic renal cell cancer. *Cancer Chemother Pharmacol* 2002;50:160.

207. Redman BG, Esper P, Pan Q, et al. Phase II trial of tetrathiomolybdate in patients with advanced kidney cancer. *Clin Cancer Res* 2003;9:1666.

208. Haas NB, Smith M, Lewis N, et al. Weekly bryostatin-1 in metastatic renal cell carcinoma: a phase II study. *Clin Cancer Res* 2003;9:109.

209. Madhusudan S, Protheroe A, Propper D, et al. A multicentre phase II trial of bryostatin-1 in patients with advanced renal cancer. *Br J Cancer* 2003;89:1418.

210. Motzer RJ, Amato R, Todd M, et al. Phase II trial of antiepidermal growth factor receptor antibody C225 in patients with advanced renal cell carcinoma. *Invest New Drugs* 2003;21:99.

211. Fizazi K, Rolland F, Chevreau C, et al. A phase II study of irinotecan in patients with advanced renal cell carcinoma. *Cancer* 2003;98:61.

212. Townsley CA, Chi K, Ernst DS, et al. Phase II study of troxacitabine (BCH-4556) in patients with advanced and/or metastatic renal cell carcinoma: a trial of the National Cancer Institute of Canada-Clinical Trials Group. *J Clin Oncol* 2003;21:1524.

213. Whang YE, Godley PA. Renal cell carcinoma. *Curr Opin Oncol* 2003;15:213.

214. Varga Z, de Mulder P, Kruit W, et al. A prospective open-label single-arm phase II study of chimeric monoclonal antibody cG250 in advanced renal cell carcinoma patients. *Folia Biol (Praha)* 2003;49:74.

215. Hussain M, Vaishampayan U, Heilbrun LK, et al. A phase II study of Rebeccamycin analog (NSC-655649) in metastatic renal cell cancer. *Invest New Drugs* 2003;21:465.

216. Davis NB, Taber DA, Ansari RH, et al. Phase II trial of PS-341 in patients with renal cell cancer: a University of Chicago phase II consortium study. *J Clin Oncol* 2004;22:115.

217. Eisen T, Boshoff C, Mak I, et al. Continuous low dose thalidomide: a phase II study in advanced melanoma, renal cell, ovarian and breast cancer. *Br J Cancer* 2000;82:812.

218. Motzer RJ, Berg W, Ginsberg M, et al. Phase II trial of thalidomide for patients with advanced renal cell carcinoma. *J Clin Oncol* 2002;20:302.

219. Stebbing J, Benson C, Eisen T, et al. The treatment of advanced renal cell cancer with high-dose oral thalidomide. *Br J Cancer* 2001;85:953.

220. Daliani DD, Papandreou CN, Thall PF, et al. A pilot study of thalidomide in patients with progressive metastatic renal cell carcinoma. *Cancer* 2002;95:758.

221. Minor DR, Monroe D, Damico LA, et al. A phase II study of thalidomide in advanced metastatic renal cell carcinoma. *Invest New Drugs* 2002;20:389.

222. Escudier B, Lassau N, Couanet D, et al. Phase II trial of thalidomide in renal-cell carcinoma. *Ann Oncol* 2002;13:1029.

223. Stadler WM, Kuzel T, Shapiro C, et al. Multi-institutional study of the angiogenesis inhibitor TNP-470 in metastatic renal carcinoma. *J Clin Oncol* 1999;17:2541.

224. Braybrooke JP, O'Byrne KJ, Propper DJ, et al. A phase II study of Razoxane, an antiangiogenic topoisomerase II inhibitor, in renal cell cancer with assessment of potential surrogate markers of angiogenesis. *Clin Cancer Res* 2000;6:4697.

225. Batist G, Patenaude F, Champagne P, et al. Neovastat (AE-941) in refractory renal cell carcinoma patients: report of a phase II trial with two dose levels. *Ann Oncol* 2002;13:1259.

226. Kriegmair M, Oberneder R, Hofstetter A. Interferon alfa and vinblastine versus medroxyprogesterone acetate in the treatment of metastatic renal cell carcinoma. *Urology* 1995;45:758.

227. Pyrhonen S, Salminen E, Ruutu M, et al. Prospective randomized trial of interferon alfa-2a plus vinblastine versus vinblastine alone in patients with advanced renal cell cancer [In Process Citation]. *J Clin Oncol* 1999;17:2859.

228. Fossa SD, Martinelli G, Otto U, et al. Recombinant interferon alfa-2a with or without vinblastine in metastatic renal cell carcinoma: results of a European multi-center phase III study. *Ann Oncol* 1992;3:301.

229. Neidhart JA, Anderson SA, Harris JE, et al. Vinblastine fails to improve response of renal cancer to interferon alfa-n1: high response rate in patients with pulmonary metastases. *J Clin Oncol* 1991;9:832.

230. Sagaster P, Micksche M, Flamm J, et al. Randomised study using IFN-alpha versus IFN-alpha plus coumarin and cimetidine for treatment of advanced renal cell cancer. *Ann Oncol* 1995;6:999.

231. Motzer RJ, Mazumdar M, Bacik J, et al. Effect of cytokine therapy on survival for patients with advanced renal cell carcinoma. *J Clin Oncol* 2000;18:1928.

232. Ryan CW, Vogelzang NJ, Stadler WM. A phase II trial of intravenous gemcitabine and 5-fluorouracil with subcutaneous interleukin-2 and interferon-alpha in patients with metastatic renal cell carcinoma. *Cancer* 2002;94:2602.

233. deKernion JB, Sarna G, Figlin R, et al. The treatment of renal cell carcinoma with human leukocyte alpha-interferon. *J Urol* 1983;130:1063.

234. Quesada JR, Swanson DA, Gutterman JU. Phase II study of interferon alpha in metastatic renal-cell carcinoma: a progress report. *J Clin Oncol* 1985;3:1086.

235. Umeda T, Niijima T. Phase II study of alpha interferon on renal cell carcinoma. Summary of three collaborative trials. *Cancer* 1986;58:1231.

236. Muss HB, Costanzi JJ, Leavitt R, et al. Recombinant alfa interferon in renal cell carcinoma: a randomized trial of two routes of administration. *J Clin Oncol* 1987;5:286.

237. Bukowski RM, Goodman P, Crawford ED, et al. Phase II trial of high-dose intermittent interleukin-2 in metastatic renal cell carcinoma: a Southwest Oncology Group study. *J Natl Cancer Inst* 1990;82:143.

238. Von der M, Geertsen P, Thatcher N, et al. Recombinant interleukin-2 in metastatic renal cell carcinoma—a European multicentre phase II study. *Eur J Cancer* 1991;27:1583.

239. Escudier B, Ravaud A, Fabbro M, et al. High-dose interleukin-2 two days a week for metastatic renal cell carcinoma: a FNCLCC multicenter study. *J Immunother Emphasis Tumor Immunol* 1994;16:306.

240. Lissoni P, Barni S, Tancini G, et al. Clinical response and survival in metastatic renal carcinoma during subcutaneous administration of interleukin-2 alone. *Arch Ital Urol Androl* 1997;69:41.

241. Rosenberg SA, Lotze MT, Yang JC, et al. Experience with the use of high-dose interleukin-2 in the treatment of 652 cancer patients. *Ann Surg* 1989;210:474.

242. Parkinson DR, Fisher RI, Rayner AA, et al. Therapy of renal cell carcinoma with interleukin-2 and lymphokine-activated killer cells: phase II experience with a hybrid bolus and continuous infusion interleukin-2 regimen. *J Clin Oncol* 1990;8:1630.

243. Negrier S, Philip T, Stoter G, et al. Interleukin-2 with or without lymphokine-activated killer cells in metastatic renal cell cancer: a report of the European multi-centre study. *J Clin Oncol* 1989;25:21.

244. Dillman RO, Oldham RK, Tauer KW, et al. Continuous interleukin-2 and lymphokine-activated killer cells for advanced cancer: a national biotherapy study group. *J Clin Oncol* 1991;9:1233.

245. Dillman RO, Church C, Oldham RK, et al. Inpatient continuous-infusion interleukin-2 in 788 patients with cancer. *Cancer* 1993;71:2358.

246. Thompson JA, Shulman KL, Benyunes MC, et al. Prolonged continuous intravenous infusion interleukin-2 and lymphokine-activated killer-cell therapy for metastatic renal cell carcinoma. *J Clin Oncol* 1992;10:960.

247. Yang JC. Interleukin-2: clinical applications. Renal carcinoma. In: Rosenberg S, DeVita V Jr, Hellman S, eds. *Biologic therapy of cancer*, 3rd ed. Philadelphia: Lippincott Williams & Wilkins, 2000.

WILLIAM U. SHIPLEY
DONALD S. KAUFMAN
W. SCOTT McDOUGAL
DOUGLAS M. DAHL
M. DROR MICHAELSON
ANTHONY L. ZIETMAN

SECTION **2**

Cancer of the Bladder, Ureter, and Renal Pelvis

EPIDEMIOLOGY

Bladder cancer is two and one-half times more common in males than in females and more common in whites than in blacks. Approximately 53,000 new cases occur per year in the United States, which is a 20% increase from 20 years ago. The incidence increases with age and peaks in the sixth and seventh decades of life.

Simultaneous or subsequent development of transitional cell carcinomas (TCCs) of the urethra in patients with TCC of the bladder occurs with an incidence of 6% to 16%. Risk factors that make urethral involvement more likely in males and females are recurrent multifocal bladder cancers and bladder neck involvement. In the female, the most predictive risk factor for urethral involvement is the presence of concomitant vaginal extension of the bladder cancer.[1] Carcinoma *in situ* (CIS) involving the bladder neck and trigonal involvement extending to the bladder neck are associated with an increased incidence of urethral involvement.[2]

The incidence of ureteral TCC is 0.7 per 100,000, and renal pelvic TCCs have an incidence of 1 per 100,000.[3] Renal pelvic tumors constitute 5% of all renal tumors, and 90% of them are TCCs. Squamous cell carcinoma and adenocarcinoma constitute the majority of the remainder. Primary upper tract TCCs make up only 5% of all the TCCs of the urinary tract. Patients who have primary TCCs of the upper urinary tract have a 20% to 40% incidence of either synchronous or metachronous bladder cancer. Conversely, patients with bladder cancer have a 1% to 4% incidence of synchronous or metachronous upper tract urothelial tumors.[4,5] If, however, the bladder cancer is grade III, there is associated CIS, or the patient has failed intravesical chemotherapy, some reports suggest a doubling of the incidence of upper tract tumors.[6] Patients with Balkan nephropathy have an increased incidence of upper tract tumors, and these tumors are usually low grade and multiple.[7] In addition there are areas of Taiwan in which TCC of the renal pelvis accounts for 40% of all renal tumors,[8] whereas in other nonendemic areas, upper tract tumors account for only 1% or 2% of renal tumors.[9] Etiologic factors in the Taiwanese endemic region have not been elucidated.

Risk factors for the development of urothelial cancer can be classified into one of three categories: (1) gene abnormalities resulting in perturbations in cell-cycle regulatory processes, (2) chemical exposure, and (3) chronic irritation. Those risk factors involving genetic abnormalities include protooncogene expression, tumor suppressor gene mutation, and abnormalities of specific cell-cycle regulatory proteins, discussed in Molecular Tumor Markers. Protooncogenes implicated in bladder cancer include the Ras p21 proteins.[10] Tumor suppressor genes that have been associated with an altered biology of the disease include p53, p21, p27, and the retinoblastoma gene (pRB).[11] Loss of heterozygosity of chromosome 9 has been implicated in the development of superficial bladder cancer. Abnormalities in specific cell-cycle regulatory proteins, such as CABLES, Ki67, and cyclin D1, have also been implicated in bladder cancer.[12–14]

Epidemiologic evidence in support of chemical exposure as an etiologic factor in bladder cancer has been convincingly documented. Aromatic amines, aniline dyes, nitrites, and nitrates have all been implicated. For those who continue to smoke, tobacco use carries with it a threefold increased risk of developing bladder cancer, and even ex-smokers have a twofold increased risk.[15] Analgesic abuse, particularly phenacetin, is associated with an increased incidence of renal pelvic cancers. Numerous reports have shown strong associations between the development of bladder and upper tract TCCs with industrial contact to chemicals, plastics, coal, tar, and asphalt.[16] Cyclophosphamide administration over the long term, particularly in patients who have upper tract or bladder outlet obstructions, results in an increased incidence of bladder cancer. When drugs such as cyclophosphamide are given, careful attention to hydration and relieving obstruction may be helpful in preventing the development of urothelial cancers. Coffee, tea, and artificial sweeteners have not been shown to act as independent risk factors.

Chronic irritants include catheters, *Schistosoma haematobium,* and irradiation. Chronic irritation due to indwelling catheters associated with chronic infection increases the likelihood of the development of squamous cell carcinoma. *S haematobium* infestation results in an increased incidence of squamous cell cancer and TCC. Pelvic irradiation is also associated with possibly increased incidence of squamous cell cancer.

Studies have suggested that copious water consumption, vitamin intake, and various diets may be beneficial in preventing bladder cancer. None of these actions, however, has shown any clear benefit with respect to prevention.

SCREENING AND EARLY DETECTION

Screening for microhematuria has not been particularly useful in the detection of bladder cancer. If significant microhematuria is detected, specific diagnostic studies are performed. When individuals are screened, 4% to 20% are found to have microhematuria. Of those with microhematuria, only 0.1% to 6.6% have bladder tumors. This translates into a discovery rate of bladder cancer in the population at large varying from 0.005% to 0.2%. None of the patients who had bladder tumors incidentally discovered in these studies had invasive disease. In follow-up, no patient who had grade I, stage Ta tumors discovered through screening progressed at 7 years follow-up. Progressive disease developed only in those with CIS, T1, or high-grade tumors, and that occurred only after 4 years of follow-up.[17,18] Some studies, however, have suggested that routine screening in high-risk populations may increase the early detection rate of high-grade cancers. One might assume that early treatment of these patients would be associated with an increased survival, but this hypothesis has not been substantiated. Screening does not generally improve the detection rate of low-grade tumors because the methodologies used for screening have a large number of false-negatives for low-grade tumors. When urothelial cancer is suspected, noninvasive screening can be performed, including cytology and urinary biomarkers, but the definitive diagnosis can be established only by cystoscopy and biopsy. Cytology is, nevertheless, regarded as the gold standard for noninvasive screening of urine for bladder cancer. It has a sensitivity of 40% to 60% with a specificity in excess of 90%. Nuclear matrix protein (NMP22),[19] fibrin/fibrinogen degradation products,[20] urinary bladder cancer antigen,[21] and basic fetoprotein[22] have all been compared to cytology in bladder cancer screening studies. Other methods used include fluorescence *in situ* hybridization,[23] microsatellite analysis of free DNA,[24] and telomerase reverse transcriptase determination.[25] Unfortunately, all of these tests have a sensitivity that ranges only from 40% to 75% with a specificity of 50% to 90%, thus making it inappropriate to eliminate the need for cystoscopy by the use of these tests.[26] These urinary biomarkers have not been studied yet for sensitivity and specificity in detecting upper tract TCC. Cytology is illustrative of the problems of noninvasive evaluation for tumors in those with unexplained hematuria. Poorly differentiated tumors have a 20% false-negative detection rate, whereas well-differentiated tumors have up to an 80% false-negative detection rate. Most of the other noninvasive screening tests have similar levels of false-positive and false-negative rates but have the benefit of lack of subjectivity by the person reading the test. Thus, all patients with unexplained hematuria require cystoscopic evaluation even if the cytology and urinary biomarkers are negative.

PATHOLOGY

More than 90% of the TCCs throughout the lining of the urinary tract occur in the urinary bladder, and of the remaining 10%, most are in the renal pelvis and fewer than 2% are in the ureter and urethra. Squamous cell carcinomas, defined by the presence of keratinization, account for 5% of bladder tumors. Other even less common bladder tumors include adenocarcinoma and undifferentiated carcinoma variants, such as small cell carcinoma, giant cell carcinoma, and lymphoepitheliomas.[27-29] Tumors of mixed histology consisting of TCC and containing squamous and adenocarcinomatous elements are also identified and are quite common. These are considered variants of TCC, and they do not portend a worse prognosis. Adenocarcinoma may arise in the embryonal remnant of the urachus on or above the bladder dome. Other adenocarcinomas may closely resemble intestinal adenocarcinoma and must be distinguished from direct spread to the bladder from an intestinal primary by careful clinical evaluation. Rarely, these demonstrate a signet-ring cell or clear-cell histology.

The differential diagnosis of TCC usually does not pose a diagnostic difficulty for experienced pathologists, but tumors that are grade I and invasive are occasionally difficult to distinguish from von Brunn's nests.[30] Also, rarely, an invasive TCC may be overdiagnosed when the glandular component of a nephrogenic adenoma is mistaken for TCC with glandular differentiation or a pure adenocarcinoma.[30] When invasion of the lamina propria has occurred, the pathologist must report whether muscularis propria is present in the submitted tissue and whether there is invasion of the muscularis propria. If muscularis propria is not present in the submitted tissue, this should be noted by the pathologist. Identification of invasion of the muscularis propria by tumor may occasionally be difficult, as it may be confused with involvement of the muscularis mucosa, which is in the lamina propria.[31] More than two-thirds of newly diagnosed cases of bladder tumors are exophytic papillary TCCs that are confined to the epithelium (stage Ta) or invade only into the lamina propria (stage T1). These tumors are generally managed endoscopically and, in some cases, by intravesical therapy [see Superficial Bladder Cancer (Ta, Tis, T1), later in this chapter]. Approximately one-half to two-thirds of patients with such tumors have a recurrence or a new TCC in the bladder within 5 years.

Bladder tumors are also classified by their cytologic characteristics as low grade (G1) or high grade (G2, G3).[29] Tumor grade is clinically more significant for noninvasive tumors because nearly all of the invasive neoplasms are high grade at diagnosis. Papillary carcinomas of low grade are considered to be relatively benign tumors that histologically resemble the normal urothelium. They show only very slight pleomorphism or loss of polarity and rarely progress to a higher stage. Primary CIS (stage Tis) that presents without a concurrent exophytic tumor constitutes only 1% to 2% of newly detected cases of bladder cancer, but CIS is found accompanying more than half of bladders presenting with multiple papillary tumors. CIS in this instance is either adjacent to or involving mucosal sites remote from papillary lesions.[32] CIS is believed to be an important precursor of invasive cancer, and if untreated, will develop into muscularis propria–invasive disease within 5 years from the initial diagnosis in more than 50% of patients.

Like bladder tumors, 90% of upper tract tumors are TCCs with similar morphology.[33] Squamous cell carcinomas account for most of the remaining carcinomas, with adenocarcinoma representing at most 1% of upper tract malignancies. The cytologic characteristics for classification of TCC by grade are the same for upper tract TCC and those in the bladder.

MOLECULAR TUMOR MARKERS

As the natural history of superficial urothelial tumors is that of recurrence, an area of controversy is whether tumors that occur at separate sites or at separate times in the urothelial tract are derived from the same clone or are polyclonal in origin. A report by Sidransky et al.[34] demonstrated the clonality of multiple bladder tumors from different sites. Miyao et al.[35] showed concordant genetic alterations in asynchronous tumors from individual patients. These studies suggest that urothelial TCCs appearing at different times and sites can be derived from the same neoplastic clone. Moreover, many studies have reported an increasing frequency of specific genetic abnormalities in bladder tumors of more-advanced stages.[36-38] Many tumor suppressor gene modifications, including those of p53, pRB, p16, p21, thrombospondin-1, glutathione, and factors controlling the expression and function of the epidermal growth factor receptor (EGFR), have been shown in retrospective analyses to influence the outcomes of patients with TCC after various treatments.[39-43] Even in the most intensively studied tumor suppressor gene in advanced TCC, the p53 gene, retrospective analyses give conflicting data on whether a mutation of p53 confers an increased responsiveness or an increased resistance to chemotherapy or radiation.[39,40] Fortunately, this conflict in the predictability of the responsiveness to adjunctive chemotherapy of TCCs with a p53 mutation is now being tested by a prospective phase III trial of postcystectomy methotrexate, vinblastine, doxorubicin, and cisplatin (MVAC) chemotherapy, funded by the National Cancer Institute.[44]

The enthusiasm engendered by the development of novel biologic agents targeted against tumor-specific growth factor pathways or against angiogenesis has been fortified by positive studies in a variety of solid tumors. Two classes of agents that have received great attention are inhibitors of EGFR, including EGFR1 and EGFR2 (or her2/neu), and inhibitors of vascular endothelial growth factor (VEGF) or its receptors. Ample preclinical evidence has shown that (1) many, if not most, bladder tumors express products of the EGFR family, (2) overexpression correlates with an unfavorable outcome, and (3) inhibition of these pathways may have an antitumor effect.[45-50] A number of cooperative groups, including Cancer and Leukemia Group B (CALGB), Radiation Therapy Oncology Group (RTOG), and Southwest Oncology Group (SWOG), are planning to study inhibitors of EGFR1 and her2/neu in the treatment of advanced bladder cancer.

Another avenue for potential selective increase in tumor cytotoxicity relative to normal tissues is the inhibition of angiogenic inducers, which are frequently present in bladder tumors. Several studies have correlated elevated VEGF levels or cyclooxygenase-2 expression with disease recurrence or progression, often as an independent predictor by multivariate analysis.[36,51] This is the basis for combining in prospective clinical trials, anti-VEGF therapy, or various cyclooxygenase-2 inhibitors with other forms of cytotoxic therapy.[52]

The major challenge for clinical and translational investigators is to design appropriate prospective trials that will identify which molecular tumor markers will be prognostic of outcome *and* be predictive of whether a patient will do better treated by surgery, radiation, chemotherapy, molecular targeted therapy, or a combination of these. Only then can molecular tumor markers be incorporated into clinical decision making and allow physicians to make better treatment choices on behalf of their patients.

CANCER OF THE BLADDER

Cancers of the bladder can be grouped into three general categories by their stages at presentation: superficial cancers, muscularis propria–invasive cancers, and metastatic cancers. Each differs in clinical behavior, primary management, and outcome. When treating superficial tumors, the aim is to prevent recurrences and progression to a stage that is life threatening. With muscularis propria–invasive disease, the main issue is to determine which tumors require cystectomy; which can be successfully managed by bladder preservation, using combined modality therapy; and which tumors, by virtue of a high metastatic potential, require an integrated systemic chemotherapeutic approach from the outset. Combination chemotherapy is the standard for treating metastatic disease. Despite reports of complete responses (CRs) in more than 40% of cases, however, the duration of response and overall cure rates remain low. Nonetheless, newer therapies with improved chemotherapeutic regimens, possibly including rationally targeted agents against tumor-specific growth factor pathways, offer the hope that these response rates, long-term control rates, and survival may improve in the future.

CLINICAL PRESENTATION AND STAGING

Bladder cancer is rarely incidentally discovered at autopsy. Indeed, almost all cases are diagnosed premortem. The most common presentation is gross painless hematuria. Unexplained frequency and irritative voiding symptoms should alert one to the possibility of CIS of the bladder or, less commonly, muscularis propria–invasive cancer.

The workup of suspected bladder cancer should include a cytology, a cystoscopy, and an upper tract study. The preference for the upper tract study is spiral computed tomography (CT), as the ureter and the renal pelvis can be particularly well visualized by the use of that technique as well as the relevant lymph nodes and the kidney parenchyma. Careful staging is important, as treatment is dependent on the initial stage of the disease. The clinical stage of the primary tumor is determined by transurethral resection of the bladder tumor (TURBT). This resection should include a sample of the muscularis propria for appropriate diagnosis, particularly if the tumor appears sessile or high grade. Once the specimen has been resected, the base of the resected area should be separately biopsied. Any suspicious areas in the remainder of the bladder should be biopsied, and many advocate additional selected biopsies of the bladder mucosa and a prostatic urethral biopsy as well. Urethral biopsies are clearly indicated in patients with risk factors for urethral involvement as discussed earlier in Epidemiology and in those who have persistent positive cytologies in the absence of a demonstrable bladder lesion. α-Aminolevulinic acid installation and the use of specific wavelengths to visualize the bladder tumor have been recommended to increase the

TABLE 30.2-1. American Joint Committee on Cancer 2002 TNM Bladder Cancer Staging

PRIMARY TUMOR (T)	
Tis	Carcinoma *in situ*
Ta	Noninvasive papillary tumor
T1	Tumor invades the lamina propria, but not beyond
T2	Tumor invades the muscularis propria
pT2a	Tumor invades superficial muscle (inner half)
pT2b	Tumor invades deep muscle (outer half)
T3	Tumor invades perivesical tissue
pT3a	Microscopically
pT3b	Macroscopically (extravesical mass)
T4	Tumor invades any of the following: prostate, uterus, vagina, pelvis or abdominal wall
T4a	Tumor invades prostate, uterus, vagina
T4b	Tumor invades pelvis or abdominal wall
REGIONAL LYMPH NODES (N)	
NX	Regional lymph nodes cannot be assessed
N0	No regional lymph node metastasis
N1	Metastasis in a single lymph node, 2 cm or less in greatest dimension
N2	Metastasis in a single lymph node >2 cm but <5 cm in greatest dimension, or multiple lymph nodes, none >5 cm in greatest dimension
DISTANT METASTASIS (M)	
MX	Distant metastasis cannot be assessed
M0	No distant metastasis
M1	Distant metastasis

(From ref. 53, with permission.)

yield of positive biopsies, but in the authors' experience it is extremely difficult to differentiate inflammatory lesions from urothelial carcinomas using this technique.

The primary bladder cancer is staged according to the depth of invasion into the bladder wall or beyond (Table 30.2-1). The urothelial basement membrane separates superficial bladder cancers into Ta (noninvasive) and T1 (invasive) tumors. The muscularis propria separates superficial disease from deeply (muscularis propria) invasive disease. Stage T2 and higher T-stage tumors invade the muscularis propria, the true muscle of the bladder wall. If the tumor extends through the muscle to involve the full thickness of the bladder and into the serosa, it is classified as T3. If the tumor involves contiguous structures, such as the prostate, the vagina, the uterus, or the pelvic sidewall, the tumor is classified as stage T4.[53] In a TURBT specimen, in contrast to a cystectomy specimen, it is relatively infrequent for the pathologist to be able to make an accurate assessment as to the depth of invasion of the tumor into the muscularis propria, although in some well-oriented pieces of tissue, one can discern that the involvement is only superficial, whereas in other similarly well-oriented specimens one can see that invasion is deep. The fragmentary nature of many TURBT specimens, however, precludes a definitive interpretation of the depth of involvement of the muscularis propria in many instances.[27] Thus, the primary pathologic substages in muscularis propria–invasive tumors of the TNM staging system shown in Table 30.2-1, such as pT2a versus pT2b, cannot be determined from TURBT specimen.[53] CT or magnetic resonance imaging scans (MRIs), even those performed before the TURBT, are not reliable for staging of the pri-

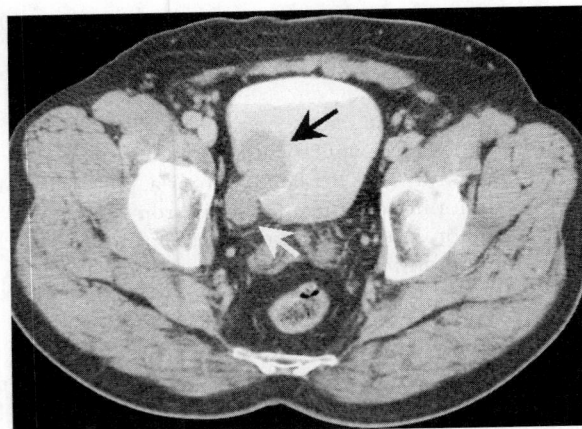

FIGURE 30.2-1. Computed tomography scan of a patient with a muscularis propria–invasive bladder cancer performed before a trans-urethral tumor resection showing unequivocally an extravesical extension of tumor (stage T3). Tumor projecting into the bladder lumen (*black arrow*); portion of the tumor extending into the ureter outside the bladder (*yellow arrow*). (See Color Fig. 30.2-1 in the CD-ROM.)

mary tumor. Neither scan allows for the diagnosis of a Ta/T1 tumor versus a T2/T3 tumor because with neither can the radiologist visualize the depth of invasion of the primary tumor into the bladder wall. These scans, however, are helpful in staging of the primary tumor when they show unequivocal tumor extension outside of the bladder (stage T3; Fig. 30.2-1). CT scans or MRIs after a TURBT also are not reliable for staging of the primary tumor because either surgically induced edema in the resected portion of the bladder wall or postsurgical extravesical inflammatory stranding can be confused with extravesical tumor extension.

Patients who have documented muscularis propria–invasive bladder cancer require an additional set of studies: chest CT, liver function studies, creatinine clearance and electrolytes, and an evaluation of the pelvic and retroperitoneal lymph nodes on CT scan. Bimanual examination is also performed at the time of the TURBT to evaluate for possible extravesical extension of tumor and to determine the degree of mobility of the pelvic contents. An exciting advance in staging bladder cancers involves MRI lymphangiography.[54] With this technology we have found that nodes that appear to be enlarged on CT may be differentiated as to whether or not they are inflammatory or malignant. The sensitivity and specificity of the test is quite high. Having this information preoperatively allows for either neoadjuvant chemotherapy followed by cystectomy or identifies involved lymph nodes in areas not commonly accessed at cystectomy, or both. This is an important new noninvasive technique but will have to be further evaluated in larger studies in patients with invasive bladder cancer if it is to become part of standard practice. If the patient has a history of functional bowel abnormality, a barium study of the segment of bowel to be used for diversion should be performed. It is the authors' practice when using colon in the reconstruction of the urinary tract to obtain a barium enema or colonoscopy, or both, to avoid surprises at the time of surgery. Finally, patients with muscularis propria–invasive bladder cancer must have a prostatic urethral and bulbous urethral biopsy to determine whether or not an orthotopic bladder can be placed or

whether the procedure should encompass the urethra: that is, a cystoprostatourethrectomy in males or a cystourethrectomy and anterior exenteration in females.

TREATMENT

Superficial Bladder Cancer (Ta, Tis, T1)

Seventy percent of patients with bladder cancer have superficial disease at presentation. Approximately 15% to 20% of these patients progress to stage T2 disease or greater over time. Of those who present with Ta or T1 disease, 50% to 70% have a recurrence after initial therapy. Low-grade tumors (grade I or II) and low-stage (Ta) disease tend to have a lower recurrence rate at approximately 50% and a 5% progression rate, whereas high-risk disease (grade III, T1 associated with CIS and multifocal disease) has a 70% recurrence rate and a 30% progression rate to stage T2 or greater disease. Fewer than 5% of patients with superficial bladder cancer develop metastatic disease without developing evidence of muscularis propria invasion (stage T2 disease or greater) of the primary lesion.

Patients who are at significant risk for development of progressive disease or recurrent disease after TURBT are generally considered candidates for adjuvant intravesical drug therapy. For practical purposes this would include those with multifocal CIS, CIS associated with Ta or T1 tumors, any grade III tumor, multifocal tumors, and tumors that rapidly recur after TURBT of the initial bladder tumor. A number of drugs have been used intravesically, including bacillus Calmette-Guérin (BCG), interferon plus BCG, thiotepa, mitomycin C, doxorubicin, and (under study) gemcitabine. Complications generally include frequency, dysuria, and irritative voiding symptoms. Over the long term, bladder contracture may occur with any of these agents. Other complications, which are specific for each drug, are as follows: BCG administration may result in fever, joint pain, granulomatous prostatitis, sinus formation, disseminated tuberculosis, and death; thiotepa may cause myelosuppression; mitomycin C may result in skin desquamation and rash; and doxorubicin may cause gastrointestinal upset and allergic reactions. The proposed benefit of intravesical chemotherapy is to lessen the rate of recurrences and reduce the incidence of progression. Unfortunately, it cannot be clearly stated that any of these drugs accomplishes these goals over the long term. Many studies have demonstrated that over the short term there is a reduction in the recurrence rate of superficial tumors, but in many of these studies the follow-up is less than 2 years.

A number of studies have compared one intravesical chemotherapeutic agent with another. For the most part, BCG in these comparisons has a slight advantage in reducing recurrences.[55] When the follow-up is more than 5 years, however, it appears that reducing the recurrence rate has minimal overall effect when compared to no treatment. Approximately 70% of patients with high-grade disease experience recurrences whether or not they are treated with intravesical therapy. Moreover, there is no well-documented evidence that the use of these agents prevents disease progression, that is, from stage Ta/T1 disease to stage T2 or greater disease. Indeed, approximately one-third of patients who are at high risk for disease progression—those with grade III, T1 disease—progress to stage T2 or greater disease whether or not they are treated with BCG.[56] One-third of patients at 5 years who have disease progression and undergo a cystectomy die of metastatic disease. Thus, approximately 15% of patients with superficial disease are at high risk for disease progression (CIS with associated Ta or T1 disease, rapidly recurrent disease, and/or grade III disease), irrespective of treatment modality, will die of their disease.[57] If definitive therapy (cystectomy) is performed when the disease is found to progress into the muscularis propria (T2 or greater), there is no difference in cure rate when these patients are compared to those who present with T2 or greater disease primarily. These statistics have encouraged some to perform a preemptive cystectomy in those patients at high risk for progression before muscularis propria invasion is documented. Ten-year cancer-specific survivals of 80% are given as justification for this approach, as compared to 50% in patients in whom the cystectomy is performed when the disease progresses to involve the muscularis propria.[58] Unfortunately, this approach subjects approximately two-thirds of these patients to a needless cystectomy.

Muscularis Propria–Invasive Disease

SURGICAL APPROACHES. The standard of care for squamous cell carcinoma, adenocarcinoma, TCC, and spindle cell carcinoma invading the muscularis propria of the bladder is a bilateral pelvic lymph node dissection and a cystoprostatectomy with or without a urethrectomy in the male. In the female an anterior exenteration is performed, which includes the bladder and urethra (the urethra may be spared if uninvolved and an orthotopic bladder reconstruction is to be performed), the ventral vaginal wall, and the uterus. A radical cystectomy may be indicated in non–muscularis propria–invasive bladder cancers when grade III disease is multifocal or associated with CIS, or both, or when bladder tumors rapidly recur, particularly in multifocal areas after intravesical drug therapy. When the prostate stroma is involved with TCC or when there is concomitant CIS of the urethra, a cystoprostatourethrectomy is the treatment of choice. We have described a methodology of performing this procedure *en bloc*, which allows for removal of the entire bladder, prostate, and urethra as a single specimen.[59] If the urethra needs to be removed, the type of urinary reconstruction is limited to an abdominal urinary diversion. In selected circumstances in the male, the neurovascular bundles coursing along the lateral side of the prostate caudally and adjacent to the rectum more cephalad may be preserved, sometimes preserving potency. Partial cystectomies are rarely performed in selected patients, thus preserving bladder function and affording the same cure rate as a radical cystectomy in the properly selected patient. Ideal candidates for partial cystectomy are patients with focal disease located far enough away from the ureteral orifices and bladder neck to allow the surgeon to achieve at least a 2-cm margin around the tumor and a margin sufficient around the ureteral orifices and bladder neck to reconstruct the bladder. Practically, this limits partial cystectomies to those patients who have small tumors located in the dome of the bladder and in whom random bladder biopsies show no evidence of CIS or other bladder tumors.

Survival. The probability of survival from bladder cancer after cystectomy is determined by the pathologic stage of the disease. Survival is markedly influenced by the presence or absence of positive lymph nodes. Some have argued that the

TABLE 30.2-2. Survival after Radical Cystectomy According to Pathologic Stage at 10 Years

Pathologic Stage	Disease-Specific Survival (%)	Overall Survival (%)
pTa, Tis, T1 with high risk of progression	82	—
Organ confined, negative nodes (pT2, pN0)	73	49
Nonorgan confined (pT3–4a or pN1–2)	33	23
Lymph node positive (any T, pN1–2)	28, 34	21

(From refs. 58–61, with permission.)

number of positive nodes impacts survival in that, when resection is performed, there is a potential for cure provided there are fewer than four to eight positive nodes.[55,56] Others are not in complete agreement with this. It is clear, however, that positive perivesical nodes have a less ominous prognosis than involvement of iliac or paraaortic nodes. Pathologic type may also have an impact on outcome, but in most series survival is more dependent on pathologic stage than on the cell type of the cancer. Most large series of survival statistics after treatment include all patients regardless of cell type. These series are generally constituted as to histologic type as follows: TCC, 85% to 90%; combination of TCC and either squamous cell or adenocarcinoma, 6%; pure squamous cell carcinoma, 3%; pure adenocarcinoma, 3%; and small cell and spindle cell carcinoma, 2% (Table 30.2-2).[60,61]

Types of Urinary Diversions. Urinary diversions can be divided into continent and noncontinent. Noncontinent urinary diversions or conduits involve the use of a segment of ileum or colon and less commonly a segment of jejunum. The distal end is brought to the skin, and the ureters are implanted into the proximal end. The patient wears a urinary collection appliance. The advantages of a conduit (ileal or colonic) are its simplicity and the reduced number of immediate and long-term postoperative complications. In most series, the complication rate is approximately 13%; that is, 13% of patients who undergo a cystectomy and urinary diversion of this type will have a significant complication, which impacts on hospital stay or recovery. Generally, the distal ileum is used for the urinary conduit or reservoir, but if the ileum has been irradiated or is otherwise involved, one may select the right colon or a short segment of jejunum. The latter is the least desirable choice, as electrolyte problems may be significant. On occasion during exenterative surgery when an end colostomy is created, a segment of distal bowel is used, thus obviating the need for an intestinal anastomosis.

Continent diversions can be divided into two types: abdominal and orthotopic. Abdominal diversions require a continence valve, whereas an orthotopic neobladder depends on the urethral sphincter for continence. The reservoir is made of bowel that is fashioned into a globular configuration. In the abdominal type of continent diversion, the stoma is brought through the abdominal wall to the skin. The patient must catheterize the pouch every 4 hours. Orthotopic urinary diversions entail the use of bowel brought to the urethra, thus allowing the patient to void by Valsalva (Fig. 30.2-2). Patients must have the ability to

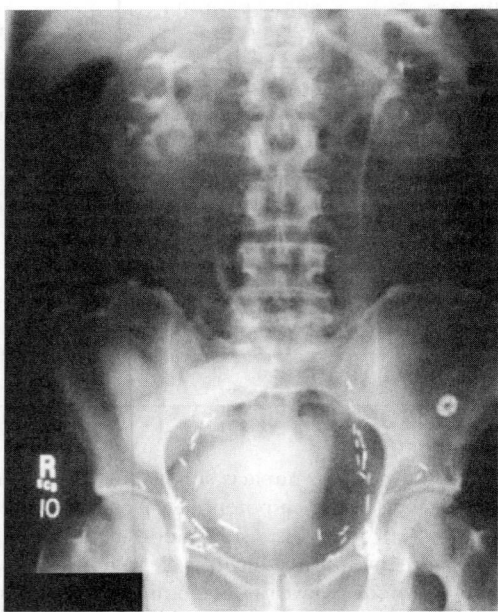

FIGURE 30.2-2. Intravenous urogram of a patient with an orthotopic bladder after radical cystoprostatectomy. The orthotopic bladder was constructed of the right colon and distal ileum.

TABLE 30.2-3. Complications of Cystectomy and Urinary Diversion

---

METABOLIC
Electrolyte abnormalities
Abnormal sensorium/drug metabolism
Infection
Osteomalacia
Growth retardation
Calculi
Short bowel syndrome
Cancer
NEUROMECHANICAL
Atonic segment
Intestinal contractions
Failure of continence mechanism
SURGICAL
Urine leak
Bowel obstruction
Fecal leak
Pyelonephritis
Sepsis
Ureteral intestinal obstruction
Renal failure
Stoma problems
Death
Postoperative complications of any major surgical procedure

---

catheterize themselves, as it is mandatory in the abdominal continent diversion and occasionally necessary in the orthotopic reconstruction. Another type of continent diversion, the ureterosigmoidostomy, is not commonly used due to excessive long-term complications. The advantage of continent diversions is the avoidance of a collection device. The advantage of an orthotopic neobladder over all other types of continent diversions is that it rehabilitates the patient to normal voiding per urethra, often without the need for intermittent catheterization or the need to wear a collection device. Postoperative and long-term complications of continent diversion are increased over the conduit types of diversions. Indeed, in some series postoperative complications range from 13% to 30%. Long-term metabolic complications are also increased.

Complications of Cystectomy and Urinary Diversion. The complications of all types of urinary diversion can be divided into three: metabolic, neuromechanical, and surgical (Table 30.2-3).

METABOLIC COMPLICATIONS. When intestine is interposed in the urinary tract, the potential exists for a number of metabolic complications.[62] These may involve electrolyte abnormalities, altered drug metabolism that may result in altered sensorium, infection, osteomalacia, growth retardation, calculi within the reservoir as well as in the kidney, short bowel syndrome, cancer, and altered bile metabolism.

Perhaps the most significant metabolic complication is an alteration in electrolytes. These abnormalities often have far-reaching consequences. Depending on the segment used, a specific electrolyte abnormality may occur. Thus, when ileum and colon are used, hyperchloremic metabolic acidosis may result. When the jejunum is the segment of choice, a hypochloremic, hyperkalemic metabolic acidosis may occur.

Specific electrolyte abnormalities are more common with certain segments. Thus, hypokalemia is more common when colon is used, hypocalcemia more common when ileum and colon are used, and hypomagnesemia more common when ileum and colon are used.

The most pervasive detrimental effect created by urinary intestinal diversion in all likelihood is due to acidosis. It occurs in general when jejunum, ileum, or colon is interposed in the urinary tract. Acidosis may result in electrolyte abnormalities, osteomalacia, growth retardation, altered sensorium, altered hepatic metabolism, renal calculi, and abnormal drug metabolism. Because jejunum is rarely used, the following discussion relates only to colon and ileum. Moreover, because acidosis is the prime contributor to many metabolic complications, it is of some importance to understand that an acidosis may occur. In general, patients with normal renal function as well as normal hepatic function are less prone to acidosis and its complications.

Treatment for metabolic acidosis is rather straightforward and can be accomplished with bicarbonate, which has the potential to cause gas, or with Bicitra solution, which is sodium citrate and citric acid. Polycitra, which is a combination of potassium citrate, sodium citrate, and citric acid, can also be used. It has the advantage of supplying potassium, which on occasion is deficient. Chlorpromazine and nicotinic acid have been used to block the chloride bicarbonate exchanger and thus lessen the potential for acidosis. They can be used to ameliorate the acidosis in patients who have difficulty taking Polycitra or bicarbonate.

Patients with conduits have a 3% to 4% incidence of renal calculi over the long term. Those with reservoirs have up to a 20% incidence of calculi within the reservoir. The pathogenesis may be a metabolic alteration or infection, or both, whereas reservoir stones are most commonly due to a surgical foreign body or mucus serving as a nidus, or both.

The incidence of bacteriuria is increased in patients with either conduits or pouches. The incidence of sepsis is 13%, with the etiology thought to be transmucosal translocation of bacteria. In addition, the antibacterial activity of the intestinal mucosa appears to be diminished. Thus, the immunoglobulins that are normally secreted by intestinal mucosa are altered. In addition to this, when the bowel is distended, there can be a translocation of bacteria from the lumen into the blood stream.

Because the intestine is interposed in the urinary tract, drugs that are eliminated from the body through the kidney unchanged and have the potential to be reabsorbed by the gut can in fact result in significant alterations in metabolism of that drug. This is particularly true for phenytoin (Dilantin) and for cyclophosphamide. Patients with a urinary diversion, when given systemic chemotherapy, have a higher incidence of complications and are more likely to have their chemotherapy limited when compared to patients without diversion who receive the same drugs and dose.[63]

Removing a segment of bowel from the intestinal tract may result in untoward complications. The loss of the distal ileum may result in B$_{12}$ malabsorption and then manifest itself as anemia and neurologic abnormalities. Bile salt malabsorption may occur and result in diarrhea. Loss of the ileocecal valve may cause diarrhea, with bacterial overgrowth of the ileum and malabsorption of vitamin B$_{12}$ and fat-soluble vitamins A, D, E, and K. Loss of a segment of colon may result in diarrhea and bicarbonate loss.

NEUROMECHANICAL COMPLICATIONS. Neuromechanical complications may be of two types: atonic, resulting in an atonic segment with urinary retention and upper tract deterioration, or hyperperistaltic contractions. The latter is relevant in continent diversions, as this may result in incontinence and a low-capacity reservoir.

SURGICAL COMPLICATIONS. A number of surgical complications occur and can be divided into short-term and long-term complications.[64,65] After any major surgical procedure, a number of complications occur, including thrombophlebitis, pulmonary embolus, wound dehiscence, pneumonia, atelectasis, myocardial infarction, and death. Complications specific to cystectomy and urinary diversion are detailed in Tables 30.2-4 and 30.2-5.

SELECTIVE BLADDER-PRESERVING APPROACHES. The treatment options for muscularis propria–invasive bladder tumors can broadly be divided into those that spare the bladder and those that involve removing it. In the United States, radical cystectomy with pelvic lymph node dissection is the standard method used to treat patients with this tumor, but conservative management with organ preservation is now the standard of care in numerous malignancies, including carcinomas of the breast, the anus, and the head and neck region, where radical surgery can be avoided in the majority of patients. Several reports from North America and Europe have

TABLE 30.2-4. Short-Term Complications after Cystectomy and Urinary Diversion

Complication	Percentage
Acute acidosis requiring therapy	16
Urine leak	3–16
Bowel obstruction	5
Fecal leak	5
Pyelonephritis	5–15
Sepsis	5–15

TABLE 30.2-5. Long-Term Complications after Cystectomy and Urinary Diversion

Complication	Percentage
Ureteral intestinal obstruction	15
Renal deterioration	15
Renal failure	7
Stoma problems	15
Intestinal stricture	10
Bowel obstruction	5

described long-term results using multimodality treatment of muscularis propria–invading bladder cancer, with appropriate safeguards for early cystectomy should this treatment fail. For bladder-conserving therapy to be more widely accepted, this treatment approach must have a high likelihood of eradicating the primary tumor, must preserve good organ function, and must not result in compromised patient survival.

Successful approaches have evolved over the last two decades after the initial reports of the effectiveness of cisplatin against TCC and reports of added efficacy when it is given concurrently with radiation. From 1981 to 1985, the National Bladder Cancer Group first used cisplatin as a radiation sensitizer in 68 patients with muscularis propria–invading bladder cancer that was unsuitable for cystectomy. In a multicenter protocol this approach was shown to be feasible and safe.[66] Furthermore, the long-term survival rate with stage T2 tumors (64%) and stage T3 to T4 tumors (22%) was encouraging. This early result with concurrent cisplatin and pelvic irradiation was validated by the National Cancer Institute–Canada randomized trial of radiation (either definitive or precystectomy) with or without concurrent cisplatin for patients with T3 bladder cancer. The Canadian study showed a significant improvement in pelvic tumor control (67% vs. 47%) in the patients who were assigned cisplatin.[67] Additionally, single-institution studies showed that the combination of a visibly complete TURBT followed by radiation therapy or radiation therapy concurrent with chemotherapy safely improved local control.[68,69] These findings led single institutions and the RTOG to develop the algorithm for bladder preservation of an initial TURBT of as much of the bladder tumor as is safely possible followed by the combination of radiation with concurrent radiosensitizing chemotherapy. One key to the success of such a program is the selection of patients for bladder preservation on the basis of the initial response of each individual patient's tumor to therapy. Thus, bladder conservation is reserved for those patients who have a clinical CR to concurrent chemotherapy and radiation. Prompt cystectomy is recommended for those patients whose tumors respond only incompletely or who subsequently develop an invasive tumor (Fig. 30.2-3). All of the protocols developed at the Massachusetts General Hospital (MGH) or within the RTOG since 1986 explicitly direct discontinuation of the bladder-sparing effort in favor of radical cystectomy at the earliest sign of failure of local control. These protocols require that the patients be medically fit and willing to undergo cystectomy should the initial treatment fail. One-third of the patients entering a potential bladder-preserving protocol with trimodality therapy (initial TURBT followed by concurrent chemotherapy and radiation) will require radical cystectomy.

For almost two decades, the MGH and the RTOG evaluated in phase II and III protocols concurrent radiochemotherapy plus neoadjuvant or adjuvant chemotherapy, and two large centers in

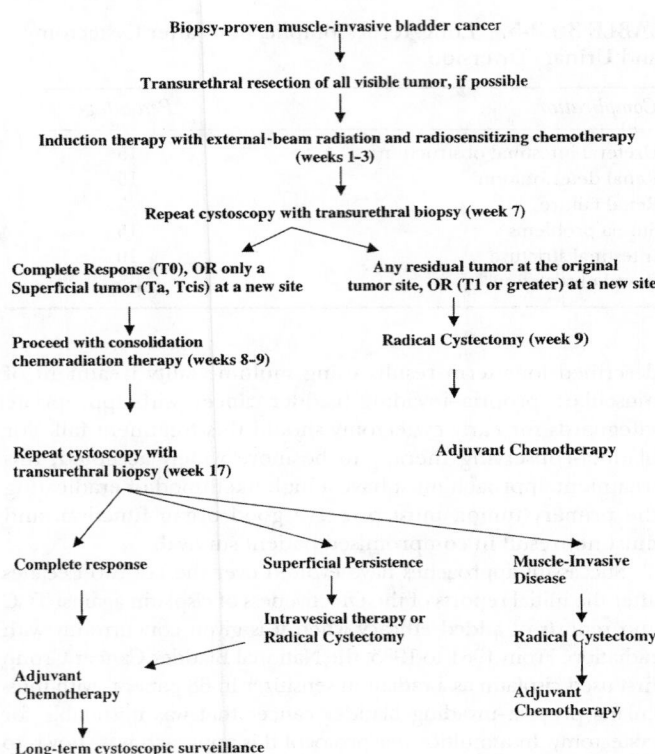

FIGURE 30.2-3. Concurrent schema for trimodality treatment of muscularis propria–invasive bladder cancer with selective bladder preservation. (From Michaelson MD, Zietman AL, Kaufman DS, Shipley WU. Cancer vesical invasion. Papel de las terapias preservadoras de la vejiga y de la quimio terapia neodayuvante. *Urologia Integrada* 2003;8:232, with permission.)

Europe (Erlangen, Germany, and Paris, France) evaluated concurrent radiochemotherapy without neoadjuvant or adjuvant chemotherapy (Table 30.2-6). Radiosensitizing drugs studied in these series, either singly or in various combinations, include cisplatin, carboplatin, paclitaxel, and 5-fluorouracil (5-FU). In addition to these drugs, gemcitabine has been shown to have radiosensitizing properties so intense as to, when used concurrently with bladder radiation, require marked gemcitabine dose reduction to avoid damaging pelvic organs.[70] Preliminary results indicate that in very low gemcitabine doses (33 mg/m^2 twice weekly) treatment is well tolerated and therefore worthy of further study.

Phase II and phase III protocols with concurrent radiochemotherapy are listed in Table 30.2-6 and are described here. The first RTOG study, RTOG 8512, included 42 patients treated with once-daily radiation treatment and concurrent cisplatin, yielding a 5-year survival of 52%.[71] This treatment was well tolerated and resulted in 42% of the patients achieving long-term survival with an intact bladder. RTOG studies 8802 and 8903 used MCV (methotrexate, cisplatin, and vinblastine) chemotherapy as neoadjuvant treatment. In the latter study patients were treated on a phase III trial with or without two cycles of MCV before the combination of cisplatin and once-a-day radiation.[72] No improvement was seen in survival or in local tumor eradication as a result of neoadjuvant therapy.[73] With a median follow-up of 5 years, the overall survival was 48% in patients treated with MCV and 49% in those who received no neoadjuvant treatment. The cystoscopic CR rate was 61% in the MCV arm and 55% in the control arm, not statistically significant. At 5 years, metastases were present in 35% of the patients who received MCV and 42% of those who were given no neoadjuvant chemotherapy. This difference was not statistically significant. The toxicity of the MCV arm was considerable, with only 67% of patients able to complete the planned treatment. This phase III study was not sufficiently powered to settle the question of the place of neoadjuvant chemotherapy in patients undergoing bladder-preserving therapy, but neither the RTOG nor the MGH has revisited the question of the effectiveness of neoadjuvant chemotherapy.

Housset et al.[74] from the University of Paris reported on 120 patients with stage T2 to T4a bladder cancer. The treatment consisted of TURBT followed by cisplatin and 5-FU given concurrently with twice-a-day hypofractionated radiation. The authors reported a 63% overall survival.[74]

The University of Erlangen has updated the largest bladder-sparing study to date, 415 patients treated from 1982 to 2000.[75] This report included 126 patients who received radiation without any chemotherapy and 89 patients who were not clinical stage T2 to T4 but classified as "high-risk T1." The CR rate of all 415 patients was 72%, and local control of the bladder tumor

TABLE 30.2-6. Results of Multimodality Treatment for Muscle-Invading Bladder Cancer

Series	Multimodality Therapy Used	No. of Patients	5-Y Overall Survival (%)	5-Y Survival with Intact Bladder (%)
RTOG 8512 (1993)[71]	External-beam radiation + cisplatin	42	52	42
RTOG 8802 (1996)[72]	TURBT, MCV, external-beam radiation + cisplatin	91	51	44 (4 y)
RTOG 8903 (1998)[73]	TURBT, ± MCV, external-beam radiation + cisplatin	123	49	38
U. Paris (1997)[74]	TURBT, 5-FU, external-beam radiation + cisplatin	120	63	NA
Erlangen (2002)[75]	TURBT, external-beam radiation, cisplatin, carboplatin, or cisplatin and 5-FU	415 (cisplatin, 82; carboplatin, 61; 5-FU/cisplatin, 87)	50	42
MGH (2003)[78]	TURBT, ± MCV, external-beam radiation + cisplatin	190	54	45

5-FU, 5-fluorouracil; MCV, methotrexate, cisplatin, vinblastine; MGH, Massachusetts General Hospital; NA, not available; RTOG, Radiation Therapy Oncology Group; TURBT, transurethral resection of bladder tumor.

after the CR without a muscle-invasive relapse was maintained in 64% of the patients at 10 years. The 10-year disease-specific survival was 42%, and more than 80% of these survivors preserved their bladder. This series, not randomized, included sequential use of radiation with no chemotherapy (126 patients), followed by concurrent cisplatin (145 patients), concurrent carboplatin (95 patients), and concurrent cisplatin with 5-FU (49 patients). The CR rates in these four sequential treatment protocols were 51%, 81%, 64%, and 87%, respectively.[76,77] The 5-year actuarial survival with an intact bladder from these four sequential protocols was 38%, 47%, 41%, and 54%. These results suggest strongly that radiochemotherapy, when given concurrently, is superior to radiation therapy alone; that carboplatin is less radiosensitizing than cisplatin; and that cisplatin plus 5-FU may be superior to cisplatin alone. The authors recognized that this conclusion is compromised by the absence of any randomized trial data from their institution.

From 1994 to 1998, twice-daily radiation therapy was introduced into RTOG protocols with concurrent cisplatin or with cisplatin plus 5-FU as radiosensitizers.[78] From 1999 to 2002, twice-a-day radiation concurrent with cisplatin and paclitaxel as radiosensitizers along with adjuvant cisplatin and gemcitabine was evaluated. The latest North American protocol for bladder-sparing treatment (RTOG 0233) has opened. This is a randomized phase II study comparing two combinations of radiosensitizing chemotherapy (cisplatin plus paclitaxel vs. cisplatin plus 5-FU), each given concurrently with an induction course of twice-daily radiation treatment. This is followed in patients whose tumors initially respond completely by consolidation chemoradiation and in those with incompletely responding tumors by radical cystectomy. All patients then undergo a three-drug adjuvant treatment with cisplatin, gemcitabine, and paclitaxel.[78]

Predictors of Outcome. The update from the MGH includes all 190 patients with muscularis propria–invading bladder cancer clinical stages T2 to T4a on successive, prospective, selective bladder-preserving protocols from 1986 to 1997.[79] Eighty-one patients had been followed for 5 years or more and 28 patients for 10 or more years. The 5- and 20-year overall survival rates are 54% and 36%, respectively. The 5- and 20-year disease-specific survival rates are 63% and 59%. The 5- and 20-year disease-specific survival rates with an intact bladder are 46% and 45%. The disease-specific survival rate stratified by clinical stage is shown in Figure 30.2-4. Clinical stage also significantly influences the CR rate, which is 71% for stage T2 and 57% for stage T3 to T4a. The presence of hydronephrosis, however, significantly reduced the CR rate from 68% to 37% and likely reduces disease-specific survival. As a result of this finding, patients with tumor-associated hydronephrosis are now excluded from our bladder-preserving protocols. The lack of efficacy of neoadjuvant MCV, albeit in one small and poorly powered study, has directed our attention to evaluating the usefulness of adjuvant chemotherapy.

The current schema for trimodality treatment of muscle-invading bladder cancer is provided in Figure 30.2-3. The 5- and 10-year disease-specific survival rate for the 66 patients undergoing cystectomy is 48% and 41%, respectively. This indicates the very important contribution of prompt salvage cystectomy for disease control in the 66 patients who required salvage cystectomy.

Of the 121 patients who were complete responders after induction therapy, 73 developed no further bladder tumors, 32

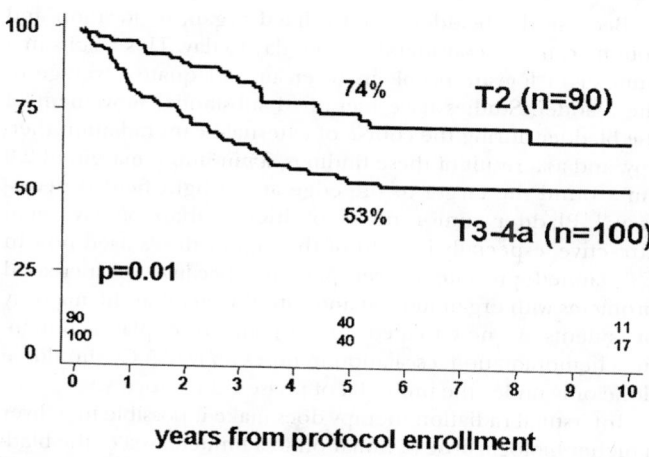

FIGURE 30.2-4. Disease-specific survival with bladder preservation for all 190 patients treated on protocol at the Massachusetts General Hospital from 1986 to 1997. (From ref. 79, with permission.)

subsequently developed a superficial occurrence, and 16 developed an invasive tumor.[80] Twenty-nine patients with superficial recurrence were treated conservatively by TURBT and intravesical chemotherapy, and three underwent immediate cystectomy. However, 7 of the 29 patients required subsequent cystectomy for additional superficial (four patients) or invasive (three patients) recurrence. For these individuals the overall survival was comparable to that of the 73 who had no failure. However, one-third of these patients required a salvage cystectomy.

The pelvic recurrence rate of all 190 patients was 8.4%. This includes 6 of the 41 patients who underwent immediate cystectomy and 6.7% of the remainder, with a median follow-up of 7.3 years.

Radiation Treatment. The most common approach with external-beam irradiation reported from North America and Europe involves the treatment of the whole small pelvis to include the external and internal iliac lymph nodes in the target volume for a total dose of 40 to 45 Gy in 1.8- to 2.0-Gy fractions over 4 to 5 weeks. Subsequently, the target volume is reduced to deliver a final boost dose of 20 to 25 Gy in 15 fractions to the primary bladder tumor. Some protocols call for partial bladder radiation as the boost volume if the location of the tumor in the bladder can be satisfactorily identified by the use of cystoscopic mapping, selected mucosal biopsies, and imaging information from CT or MRI. Plans using conventional fractionation that result in a whole bladder dose of 50 to 55 Gy and a bladder tumor volume dose of 65 Gy in combination with concurrent cisplatin-containing chemotherapy have been widely used. In the United Kingdom, a dose of 50 to 55 Gy at 2.5 to 2.75 Gy per fraction in 4 weeks is common. The available information suggests that the higher dose per fraction may lead to a higher rate of serious late complications. Data from urodynamic and quality-of-life studies indicate that lower dose per fraction irradiation given once or twice a day concurrent with chemotherapy results in excellent long-term bladder function. Twice-a-day fractionation schedules when given as radiation alone have not been shown to be more effective in long-term local tumor control than that achieved with once-per-day schedules.

Because the bladder is not a fixed organ, its location and volume can vary considerably from day to day. This results in a number of logistic problems to ensure adequate coverage of the bladder. Studies have identified substantial movement of the bladder during the course of external-beam radiation therapy, and as a result of these findings, a minimum margin of 2.0 cm around the target to the edge at the light field is necessary.[81] Bladder tumor doses of higher than 65 Gy seem attractive, especially in light of the higher doses used now in CT-planned prostate cancer patients. Because of increased problems with organ motion and with the fact that the majority of patients are now treated with concurrent cisplatin-containing chemoradiation, escalation in doses above 65 Gy should be done only under the umbrella of phase I-II protocols.

Interstitial radiation therapy does make it possible to deliver a higher biologic dose of radiation to a limited area of the bladder within a short period. This approach has been reported from institutions in the Netherlands, Belgium, and France. It is reserved for patients with solitary bladder tumors and as part of combined modality therapy with transurethral resection and external-beam radiation therapy as well as interstitial radiation therapy. External-beam doses of 30 Gy are used in combination with an implant tumor dose of 40 Gy. These groups report that for patients with solitary clinical stage T2 to T3a tumors less than 5 cm in diameter local control rates at 5 years range from 72% to 84% with disease-specific survivals of approximately 80%.[82]

Comparison of Treatment Outcomes of Contemporary Cystectomy Series with Contemporary Selective Bladder-Preserving Series. Comparing the results of selective bladder-preserving approaches with those of radical cystectomy series is confounded by the discordance between clinical (TURBT) staging and pathologic (cystectomy) staging. Clinical staging is more likely to understage the extent of disease with regard to penetration into the muscularis propria or beyond than is pathologic staging.[83] Thus, if any favorable outcome bias exists it is in favor of the pathologically reported radical cystectomy series. Also, most cystectomy series do not report by "intention to treat" and exclude reporting those patients in whom a cystectomy is found to be inappropriate due to advanced disease. In addition, many patients in cystectomy series do not have preoperative proof of a muscle-invading tumor and include 25% to 40% of patients who have tumors of less than pathologic stage T2, in contrast to bladder preservation reports, in which nearly all patients are stage T2 or greater. The University of Southern California reported on 633 patients with pathologic stage T2 to T4a undergoing contemporary radical cystectomy, with an overall survival rate at 5 years of 48% and at 10 years of 32%.[84] Similarly, the report from Memorial Sloan-Kettering Cancer Center contemporary radical cystectomy series reported a 5-year overall survival rate of 36% in patients with tumors of pathologic stage T2 to T4.[85] Also, in a national phase III protocol by SWOG, Eastern Cooperative Oncology Group (ECOG), and CALGB for patients with clinical stage T2 to T4a bladder tumors, in whom the intention to treat was randomly assigned and reported, the 5- and 10-year overall survival rates for all 307 eligible patients were 50% and 34%, respectively.[86] These overall survival rates from contemporary cystectomy series are comparable to those reported from single-institution and cooperative group results using contemporary selective bladder-preserving approaches with trimodality therapy (Table 30.2-7).

Concerns often expressed by urologists are that trimodality therapy is complex, hard to administer, and costly. Although it is correct that trimodality therapy requires close cooperation of urologic, medical, and radiation oncologists, multimodality cancer clinics are now becoming commonplace in North America and provide an ideal setting for ensuring the best treatment.

Bladder Preservation Treatments with Less than Trimodality Therapy. It has been argued that trimodality therapy might represent excessive treatment for many patients with invasive bladder cancer and that comparable results could be obtained by TURBT, either alone or with chemotherapy. Herr[87] reported the outcome of 432 patients initially evaluated by repeat TURBT for muscle-invasive bladder tumors. In that series, 99 patients (23% of the original 432 patients) initially treated conservatively without immediate cystectomy had a 34% rate of progression to a recurrent muscle-invading tumor at 20 years. In series combining TURBT and MVAC chemotherapy, only 50% of those found to have a clinical CR proved to be tumor free at cystectomy.[88] By comparison one of the clearest examples of the improved success of trimodality treatment was reported in the study from the University of Paris.[89] TURBT

TABLE 30.2-7. Muscle-Invasive Bladder Cancer: Survival Outcomes in Contemporary Series

Series	Stages	No. of Patients	Overall Survival (%)	
			5 Y	10 Y
CYSTECTOMY				
U. So. Calif. (2001)[84]	pT2-pT4a	633	48	32
Memorial Sloan-Kettering (2001)[85]	pT2-pT4a	181	36	27
SWOG/ECOG/CALGB[a,b] (2003)[86]	cT2-cT4a	307	50	34
SELECTIVE BLADDER PRESERVATION				
U. Erlangen[a] (2002)[75]	cT2-cT4a	326	45	29
MGH[a] (2003)[78]	cT2-cT4a	190	54	36
RTOG[a] (1998)[73]	cT2-cT4a	123	49	—

CALGB, Cancer and Leukemia Group B; ECOG, Eastern Cooperative Oncology Group; MGH, Massachusetts General Hospital; RTOG, Radiation Therapy Oncology Group; SWOG, Southwest Oncology Group.
[a]These series include all patients by their intention to treat.
[b]Fifty percent of patients were randomly assigned to receive three cycles of neoadjuvant MVAC (methotrexate, vinblastine, doxorubicin, cisplatin).

followed by concurrent cisplatin, 5-FU, and accelerated radiation was used by this group initially as a precystectomy regimen.[89] In the first 18 patients, all of whom demonstrated no residual tumor on cystoscopic evaluation and rebiopsy (a CR) but who all underwent a cystectomy, none had any tumor in the cystectomy specimen (100% had a pathologic CR). Comparing approaches by TURBT plus MVAC chemotherapy alone with trimodality therapy, the 5-year survival rates are comparable (50%), but the preserved bladder rate for all patients studied ranged from 20% to 33% when radiation therapy was not used and from 41% to 45% when radiation therapy was used.[89] Thus, trimodality therapy increases the probability of surviving with an intact bladder by 30% to 40% compared to the results reported with TURBT and chemotherapy alone.

Selective bladder sparing by trimodality therapy should be one of the approaches considered in the treatment of patients with muscle-invading bladder cancer. Although it is not suggested that it will replace radical cystectomy, sufficient data now exist from many national and international prospective studies to demonstrate that it represents a valid alternative. This contribution to the quality of life of patients so treated represents a unique opportunity for urologic surgeons, radiation oncologists, and medical oncologists to work hand in hand. It must be understood, however, that lifelong bladder surveillance is essential because only prompt salvage cystectomy can prevent the focus of a new or a recurrent bladder cancer from disseminating.

EVOLVING STANDARDS FOR SYSTEMIC CHEMOTHERAPY

Neoadjuvant Chemotherapy. Abundant evidence indicates that muscularis propria–invasive transitional cell cancer of the bladder is associated with occult metastases, with the likelihood that micrometastases are present, in many cases, at the time of initial discovery of the bladder tumor. Although down-staging of the primary tumor has been demonstrated, randomized studies using single-agent neoadjuvant chemotherapy have failed to demonstrate a survival benefit or a reduction in the development of distant metastases.

Despite more than two decades of clinical experience and investigation with neoadjuvant chemotherapy, followed either by radiochemotherapy as part of bladder sparing or radical cystectomy, there is still uncertainty as to whether treatment, timed in this way, affects survival. In fact, some hopeful results emerged from early phase I-II trials of single-agent chemotherapy, but several phase II studies done subsequently, using multiagent chemotherapy, several randomized studies, and a metaanalysis, all failed to demonstrate convincingly a survival benefit. Important background data from studies in patients with measurable metastatic disease clearly showed the superiority of MVAC over single-agent cisplatin on survival.[90] Randomized trials have given conflicting results, but there are now several studies that have shown a survival benefit from neoadjuvant combination chemotherapy. Do these results, however, as interesting and important as they are, effectively make the case for neoadjuvant chemotherapy as a new standard of treatment in muscularis propria–invasive bladder cancer?

The study by Grossman et al.[86] evaluated the ability of neoadjuvant chemotherapy to improve survival in patients with locally advanced bladder cancer treated with radical cystectomy. Patients with muscularis propria–invasive bladder cancer (stage T2 to T4a) were randomly assigned to radical cystectomy alone or three cycles of MVAC followed by radical cystectomy. Over an 11-year period, 317 patients were enrolled. Patients assigned to neoadjuvant chemotherapy were given three 28-day cycles of MVAC as follows: methotrexate (30 mg/m² on days 1, 15, 22), vinblastine (30 mg/m² on days 2, 15, 22), doxorubicin (30 mg/m² on day 2), and cisplatin (70 mg/m² on day 2). The authors reported that MVAC can be given safely before radical cystectomy, but not without significant side effects. One-third of patients had severe hematologic or gastrointestinal reactions, but, on the positive side, there were no drug-related deaths, and the chemotherapy did not adversely affect the performance of surgery.

Grossman et al.[86] reached the following conclusions: (1) The survival benefit associated with MVAC appeared to be strongly related to down-staging of the tumor to pT0. Of the chemotherapy-treated patients, 38% had no evidence of cancer at cystectomy, as compared with 15% of those in the cystectomy-only group ($P \leq .001$). In both groups, improved survival was associated with the absence of residual cancer in the cystectomy specimen. (2) The median survival was 77 months for the chemotherapy-treated patients compared with 46 months for the cystectomy-only group. (3) The 5-year actuarial survival was 43% in the cystectomy group, which was not significantly different from 57% in the chemotherapy-treated group ($P = .06$). The authors point out that their study is different from seven previous negative studies that used either single-agent cisplatin (demonstrated to be inferior to MVAC in measurable metastatic disease) or a two-drug combination.

It should be noted that it took 11 years to accrue 317 cases in 120 institutions, and over that lengthy duration, diagnostic standards; patient care, including supportive care during chemotherapy and surgery have all changed. Furthermore, some of the problems associated with large cooperative studies are evident. The authors state that central pathologic review was not possible in 46 cases because slides were not available and that muscle invasion could not be confirmed in central review in 17 patients. Another concern is the wide 95% confidence interval, 25 to 60 in the median survival of 46 months in the cystectomy group and 55 to 104 in the 77-month survival in the chemotherapy plus cystectomy group.

This clinical trial favors MVAC neoadjuvant chemotherapy over cystectomy only, but although this study alone does not yet make the case convincingly for neoadjuvant MVAC to be the declared standard treatment precystectomy in muscularis propria–invasive bladder cancer, it would be reasonable on the basis of these data for urologists and medical oncologists to discuss the pros and cons of neoadjuvant MVAC with their patients before cystectomy.

The Medical Research Council (MRC) and the European Organization for Research and Treatment of Cancer (EORTC), with Dr. R. R. Hall as coordinator,[91] began in 1989 a prospective randomized trial of neoadjuvant cisplatin, methotrexate, and vinblastine in patients undergoing cystectomy or full-dose external-beam radiotherapy for muscularis propria bladder cancer. The authors of the study, published in 1999, acknowledged that the equivalence of radiotherapy and cystectomy had not been proved by all the historic randomized trials. Moreover, some patients who underwent cystectomy first had a short course of preoperative radiotherapy. The type of local radical treatment, surgery or radiation treatment, was chosen by the individual doctors. Patients enrolled were those in clinical stages T2 to

T4a, considered suitable for curative treatment. The authors indicated that, although pretreatment CT scans, MRIs, or ultrasounds were recommended, none of these imaging studies were mandatory. The chemotherapy regimen used was as follows: methotrexate (30 mg/m^2 day 1), vinblastine (4 mg/m^2 day 1), and cisplatin (100 mg/m^2 day 2). Folic acid was used as "methotrexate rescue." This schedule was repeated every 21 days for three cycles.

To detect an absolute improvement in survival of 10% (50% increased to 60%), a total of 915 patients was planned. It is important, in assessing the results of this study, to note that in 6 years 976 patients were recruited from more than 100 institutions in 20 countries. The median length of follow-up was 4 years. Further, of 491 patients assigned chemotherapy, 99 did not receive all three cycles for a variety of reasons, and 26% of patients required dose decreases or delay. Of 561 patients, 76 did not undergo a planned cystectomy; 32.4% of patients underwent (optional) cystoscopy and biopsy after chemotherapy, and the biopsy confirmed endoscopic CR in 44%. The median survival for the chemotherapy group was 44 months versus 37.5 months for the cystectomy-only group, and the difference was not considered statistically significant when this study was published.

This study represents the largest randomized trial of neoadjuvant cisplatin-based chemotherapy for muscularis propria–invasive bladder cancer. The study was powered to detect a 10% improvement in survival, but the results showed only a possible 5% difference in 3-year survival, and to confirm this benefit statistically would require 3500 patients. The authors concluded, therefore, that although they observed a possible improvement in 3-year survival, "…this conclusion is not certain because this very large multicenter trial had sufficient power to detect only a larger survival benefit." The authors cannot conclude from this study—and the authors do not suggest—that neoadjuvant chemotherapy should be considered the new standard of care in the treatment of muscularis propria bladder cancer based on these data.

This MRC/EORTC study was updated in a presentation at the meeting of the American Society of Clinical Oncology in May 2002.[92] Based on their interpretation of the data as presented, Sharma and Bajorin[93] stated that a significantly improved survival was seen in all patients receiving chemotherapy. Overall survival was superior for patients who received chemotherapy at 3 years (55% vs. 50%), 5 years (50% vs. 44%), and 8 years (43% vs. 37%), with a median follow-up of 7 years. An improved disease-free survival (P = .012) and local-regional progression-free survival (P = .003) were also seen. Publication of these data will allow for critical review by oncologists to determine whether the additional years of follow-up of this large clinical trial will merit a change in the standard of care of invasive bladder cancer. This published update should clarify the extent of the benefit of neoadjuvant MCV by type of planned local therapy because cystectomy was performed in only approximately one-half of the 976 patients.

A third randomized trial, the Nordic Cystectomy Trial I, provides support for the value of neoadjuvant chemotherapy.[94] Patients were treated with two cycles of neoadjuvant doxorubicin and cisplatin. All patients received 5 days of radiation followed by cystectomy. A subgroup analysis was performed and showed a 20% difference in disease-specific survival at 5 years in patients with T3 and T4 disease, but there was neither a difference in stages T1 and T2 nor a difference when all entered patients were compared.

The Nordic Cystectomy Trial II included only stage T3 to T4a patients in an attempt to confirm the positive results in Nordic I in this subgroup of patients. This trial eliminated radiation therapy and substituted methotrexate for doxorubicin to lower toxicity.[95] In 317 patients studied, no survival benefit was noted in the chemotherapy arm.

Raghavan et al.[96] published a metaanalysis of all completed randomized trials of neoadjuvant chemotherapy for invasive bladder cancer. Their analysis, comprising 2688 patients, led the authors to the following conclusions: Single-agent neoadjuvant chemotherapy is ineffective and should not be used, and current combination chemotherapy regimens improve the 5-year survival by 5%, which reduces the risk of death by 13% compared with the use of definitive local treatment alone (i.e., from 43% to 38%). Although each of the studies cited above were adequately designed and sufficiently powered to settle the question as to whether neoadjuvant chemotherapy should be considered the new standard of care in invasive bladder cancer, a careful review of all of the published material on this subject suggests the following conclusion: Although the published data on neoadjuvant chemotherapy do not meet the required standard to declare neoadjuvant chemotherapy the new standard of care in muscularis propria bladder cancer, the data in support of benefit are sufficiently compelling that patients should be informed of the potential benefits versus the risks of neoadjuvant chemotherapy as part of the discussion leading to a decision to proceed with cystectomy. The possible role of adjuvant chemotherapy should also be discussed with these patients.

Adjuvant Chemotherapy. The obvious advantage of adjuvant, as opposed to neoadjuvant, chemotherapy is that pathologic staging allows for a more accurate selection of patients. This approach facilitates the separation of patients in stage pT2 from those in stages pT3 or pT4 or node-positive disease, all at a high risk for progression (see Table 30.2-1). The major disadvantage is the delay in systemic therapy for occult metastases while the primary tumor is being treated. It is not possible to assess response to treatment, as there is no clinical end point except for clinically detectable disease progression. Pathologic staging has been used to advantage in breast cancer and colon cancer, two diseases in which adjuvant chemotherapy has been demonstrated to increase disease-free survival. The parallel continues in that, in breast cancer, colon cancer, and bladder cancer, drugs for use in the adjuvant setting have been selected on the basis of their demonstrated activity in advanced, measurable metastatic disease.

Adjuvant chemotherapy has been studied in two major clinical settings: (1) after bladder-sparing chemoirradiation and (2) after radical cystectomy. In the former case, it became clear in the authors' early bladder-sparing studies that bladder cancer is a systemic disease and that simply rendering the bladder free of invasive cancer is not sufficient to prevent death from metastatic disease in the majority of patients whose bladders were cured of the primary tumor.[97] In our earlier studies, which used cisplatin alone as the radiosensitizing drug, the MCV combination, a total of three 28-day cycles, was used as the treatment of choice for the adjuvant phase of therapy. The adjuvant regimen of choice in the authors' later studies has consisted of four cycles of cisplatin plus gemcitabine.[73] In the authors' current study, the adjuvant regimen of choice consists of four cycles of cisplatin, gemcitabine, and paclitaxel, a potent and well-tolerated regimen in the treatment of metastatic disease.[98]

The results thus far of the contribution of adjuvant chemotherapy in affecting survival in patients undergoing bladder-sparing treatment are uncertain. No study is currently in progress prospectively comparing adjuvant chemotherapy versus no adjuvant chemotherapy in patients undergoing bladder-preserving treatment.

The place of adjuvant chemotherapy after cystectomy has been studied, but the results are not clear, as several of the reported studies were small phase II studies using a variety of chemotherapeutic regimens. Many of the early studies used drug combinations that are now little-used as combinations of newer drugs have come to the forefront. Investigators generally agree that in the face of positive nodes and even with negative nodes and high pathologic stage of the primary tumor, adjuvant chemotherapy is likely to be important in improving survival. In reviewing existing reports of adjuvant trials in bladder cancer, there are five randomized trials using adjuvant chemotherapy.[96,97,99–103]

As reviewed by Sharma and Bajorin,[93] three studies found no difference between adjuvant chemotherapy and cystectomy alone, but all three were seriously flawed in design or accrual, or both. Two of five studies[96,99–103] showed a survival benefit for cystectomy and adjuvant chemotherapy over cystectomy alone, but the first is subject to criticism for methodologic considerations and small accrual.[96,102] Unfortunately, methodology and accrual issues bear on the second study's validity as well.[103] Nonetheless, in a follow-up report by Stockle et al.,[104] an analysis of 166 patients including the 49 initially randomized patients, difference was noted in the 80 patients who received adjuvant chemotherapy as compared with 86 who underwent cystectomy alone. The extent of nodal involvement proved important, and when patients were stratified by the number of nodes involved, adjuvant chemotherapy was most effective in patients with N1 disease.

The group at M. D. Anderson Cancer Center conducted a trial comparing two cycles of neoadjuvant MVAC and three cycles of postcystectomy MVAC versus five cycles of adjuvant MVAC.[105] No difference in survival was noted, but 40% of patients given two cycles of neoadjuvant MVAC had no evidence of muscularis propria disease (pTo). The overall cancer-free survival rate was 58%, with a follow-up of 6.8 years. This trial had the largest fraction of truly poor-risk patients, as individuals with clinical stage T2 were excluded. By the study design, this clinical investigation does not provide a comparison between neoadjuvant and adjuvant treatment, as all patients received some adjuvant chemotherapy.

Several phase III trials of adjuvant chemotherapy have been reported over the past decade. The first randomized trial,[96] reported first in 1991, concluded that node-positive patients treated with the combination of cyclophosphamide, doxorubicin, and cisplatin experienced a modest disease-free survival after cystectomy. As with several other reported adjuvant studies, including those by Stockle et al.[102,103] and Freiha et al.,[101,107] these reported adjuvant studies have been hampered by small numbers of patients. The vital question of the usefulness of adjuvant chemotherapy is now being tested in an EORTC/Intergroup trial appropriately designed and powered to settle the issue. In this trial, patients will be randomized to receive adjuvant chemotherapy, standard-dose MVAC, high-dose MVAC, or gemcitabine/cisplatin after cystectomy[108] for muscularis propria–invasive bladder cancer versus observation. This study, to accrue more than 1300 patients, will evaluate four cycles of immediate chemotherapy versus therapy at the time of relapse in patients with pT3 to pT4 tumors or with node-positive disease. The chemotherapy regimens will be used at the choice of the individual investigator.

Another important adjuvant trial is under way that is an example of the convergence of biologic predictors and chemotherapy in the search for improved treatment of bladder cancer. This is a multi-institutional SWOG phase III trial, sponsored by the National Cancer Institute and led by the University of Southern California. The purpose of the study is to evaluate the therapeutic and prognostic significance of altered p53 expression by the tumor p53 after radical cystectomy in patients whose tumors are pT1 or pT2 and assessed for p53 status. For patients with p53-negative tumors, the treatment is observation. For those with p53-positive tumors, the patients are randomized to MVAC or observation. The possible significance of other genes, including p21, pRB, c-erb B-2, and others may prove to be important as relates to prognosis and possible benefit for chemotherapy after cystectomy.[44] Until the completion of a well-designed and well-executed clinical trial(s), sufficiently powered to settle the question, the place of adjuvant chemotherapy will necessarily remain uncertain. The place of newer drug combinations, already determined to be active in advanced bladder cancer, is yet to be determined.

QUALITY OF LIFE AFTER CYSTECTOMY OR BLADDER PRESERVATION. Evaluating the quality of life in long-term survivors of bladder cancer has been difficult, and only recently have attempts been made to assess this in an objective and quantitative fashion.[109–118] A number of problems arise in the interpretation of the published studies. Tools to assess quality-of-life variables were developed early for common prostate and gynecologic cancers, but no such instruments exist for bladder cancer. The instruments now used in bladder cancer are thus adaptations of uncertain validity. The published studies are all cross-sectional, and patients have follow-up of varying lengths. This may matter in a surgical series in which functional outcome improves with time and a radiation series in which it may deteriorate. All studies are hampered by incomplete accrual of all potential participants. It is never clear whether the nonparticipants are those who have had a worse outcome or are the most satisfied. Despite these limitations some conclusions can now be drawn.

Radical cystectomy causes changes in many areas of quality of life, including urinary, sexual, and social function; daily living activities; and satisfaction with body image.[110–114] Sexual function has been particularly emphasized because of the high prevalence of erectile dysfunction. Researchers have, over the last decade, concentrated on the relative merits of continent and noncontinent diversions. Available data have been mixed, with some groups, surprisingly, reporting few differences between the quality of life of those with an ileal conduit and those with continent diversions. Until recently little comparative data have been available on those who have neobladders. Hart et al.[113] have compared outcome in cystectomy patients who have either ileal conduits, cutaneous Kock pouches, or urethral Kock pouches. Of 1074 patients undergoing cystectomy for bladder cancer at the University of Southern California, 368 were eligible for study because they were alive, spoke English, and had no major health issues that could affect global quality of life; 61% of these patients completed self-reporting questionnaires. Regardless of the type of urinary diversion, the majority of patients reported good overall quality of life, little emotional distress, and few problems with social, physical, or functional activities. Problems with their diversions and with sexual function were the most commonly reported. After controlling for age no significant differences were seen among urinary diversion subgroups in any quality-of-life area. It might be anticipated that those receiving the urethral Kock diversions would be the most satisfied, and the explanation why this is not so is unclear. It may be that the subgroups were too small to detect differences, but perhaps it is more likely that each group adapts in time to the specific difficulties presented by that type of diversion.

Zietman et al.[114] have performed a study on patients treated with TURBT, chemotherapy, and radiation for muscularis propria–invasive bladder cancer at the MGH. Of 221 patients with clinical stages T2 to T4a cancer of the bladder treated at the MGH from 1986 to 2000, 71 were alive with their native bladders and disease free in 2001. These patients were asked to undergo a urodynamic study and to complete a quality-of-life questionnaire. Sixty-nine percent participated in some component of this study, with a median time from trimodality therapy of 6.3 years. This long follow-up is sufficient to capture the majority of late radiation effects. Seventy-five percent of patients had normally functioning bladders by urodynamic studies. Reduced bladder compliance, a recognized complication of radiation, was seen in 22%, but in only one-third of these patients was it reflected in distressing symptoms. The urodynamic study in 2 of 12 women showed bladder hypersensitivity, involuntary detrusor contractions, and incontinence. The questionnaire showed that bladder symptoms were uncommon, especially among men, with the exception of control problems. These were reported by 19%, with 11% wearing pads (all women). Distress from urinary symptoms was half as common as their prevalence. Bowel symptoms occurred in 22%, with only 14% recording any level of distress. The majority of men retained sexual function. Global health-related quality of life was high. The great majority of patients treated by trimodality therapy therefore retain good bladder function. It was concluded that there is a small but detectable level of lasting bowel dysfunction and distress and that this might be judged the additional price that these patients have had to pay to retain their bladders for a higher chance of sexual potency.

Two cross-sectional questionnaire studies, one from Sweden and one from Italy, have compared the outcome after radiation with the outcome after cystectomy.[115,116] The questionnaire results for urinary function after radiation were very similar to those recorded in the MGH study. More than 74% of patients reported good urinary function. Both studies compared bowel function in irradiated patients with that seen in patients undergoing cystectomy. In both, the bowel symptoms were greater for those receiving radiation than for those receiving cystectomy (10% vs. 3% and 32% vs. 24%, respectively), but in neither was this statistically significant.

In the assessment of sexual function, most women in the MGH study preferred not to answer the questions, and therefore no data were available for them. Almost all men answered the questions, however. In contrast to individuals who have been irradiated for prostate cancer, the majority of male bladder-sparing patients reported adequate erectile function (full or sufficient for intercourse), and only 8% reported dissatisfaction with their sex lives. These percentages are in line with those obtained in the Swedish and Italian series, in which 38% and 25% of men retained useful erections as compared with 13% and 8% of cystectomized controls. The MGH series allowed the use of sildenafil, probably contributing to the better outcome.

Chemotherapy for Metastatic Disease

An estimated 12,500 deaths per year in the United States are due to metastatic bladder cancer.[117] Initial spread of bladder cancer most typically is to pelvic lymph nodes. Through lymphatic and hematogenous means, bladder cancer can then metastasize to distant organs, most commonly the lungs, bones, liver, brain, and elsewhere. The prognosis of metastatic bladder cancer, as with other metastatic solid tumors, is poor, with a median survival on the order of 12 months. Nevertheless, since the discovery that platinum-containing agents have a significant antitumor effect in bladder cancer, there has been great interest in the use of chemotherapy for advanced disease.

Compared with other solid-tumor malignancies, transitional cell cancer is particularly chemosensitive. In contemporary phase II clinical trials, overall response rates are as high as 70% to 80%, and even in phase III clinical trials, response rates are on the order of 50%. This compares favorably to other solid malignancies, such as lung, colon, or breast cancer, which typically have much lower response rates in phase III studies. Moreover, a small but substantial minority of responding patients manifest a CR, and among these patients some long-term, durable responses are observed. Overall, however, the duration of response in TCC is short, with a median of 4 to 6 months, and thus the impact of chemotherapy on survival has been disappointing. The hope is that newer cytotoxic chemotherapy and biologic agents will further increase the response rates and the percentage of patients with CRs, ultimately translating into a meaningful improvement in survival among patients with advanced TCC.

CISPLATIN. In 1976, a series of 24 patients with bladder cancer treated with single-agent cisplatin was reported.[118] The investigators observed eight partial responses in addition to four minor responses. Fourteen of the subjects were chemonaïve patients, and all eight responders were in this group. Subsequent studies confirmed the activity of cisplatin in TCC, although the response rate to single-agent cisplatin has been lower than that of cisplatin-containing combination therapy.[119,120] Thus, most subsequent studies have explored combination regimens.

CISPLATIN-BASED COMBINATION CHEMOTHERAPY. The standard chemotherapy regimen for advanced bladder cancer for more than a decade was MVAC, developed at Memorial Sloan-Kettering Cancer Center in the 1980s.[121,122] MVAC is administered in 28-day cycles, with starting doses of methotrexate, 30 mg/m^2 (days 1, 15, 22); vinblastine, 3 mg/m^2 (days 2, 15, 22); doxorubicin, 30 mg/m^2 (day 2); and cisplatin, 70 mg/m^2 (day 2). Another commonly used regimen has been cisplatin, methotrexate, and vinblastine (CMV), which omits the doxoru-

TABLE 30.2-8. Standard Cisplatin-Containing Regimens for Transitional Cell Carcinoma

Agents	Regimen		Response			
		Schedule	Composite No. of Assessable Patients	CR (%)	RR (%)	Median Survival (Mo)
MVAC[120,124,125]	Methotrexate	30 mg/m² d 1, 15, 22	374	12–35	39–65	12.5–14.8
	Vinblastine	3 mg/m² d 2, 15, 22				
	Doxorubicin	30 mg/m² d 2				
	Cisplatin	70 mg/m² d 2				
CMV[190]	Cisplatin	70 mg/m² d 2	104	10	36	7
	Methotrexate	30 mg/m² d 1, 8				
	Vinblastine	4 mg/m² d 1, 8				
GC[125]	Gemcitabine	1000 mg/m² d 1, 8, 15	200	12	49	13.8
	Cisplatin	70 mg/m² d 2				

CR, complete response; RR, response rate.

bicin and has somewhat less toxicity.[123] The MVAC regimen was shown to be superior to cisplatin alone[121,122] and to other cisplatin-containing regimens.[126] The published response rate to MVAC is 40% to 65%,[122,124,125] and there is improved progression-free and overall survival compared with either single-agent cisplatin or CISCA (cisplatin, cyclophosphamide, doxorubicin). CR is seen in 15% to 25% of patients, but with an expected median survival of only 12 months.[121,123,125,126]

On the negative side, MVAC is associated with significant toxicity. This is a difficult chemotherapy regimen, and most patients require dose adjustment at some point in their treatment. Toxic effects of MVAC in significant numbers of patients include neutropenia, anemia, thrombocytopenia, stomatitis, nausea, and fatigue.[86,127] The majority of patients experience grade 3 or 4 myelosuppression, and grade 3 or 4 gastrointestinal toxicity occurs in one-third. The rate of chemotherapy-induced fatality among patients with metastatic disease may be as high as 3%, most often due to neutropenic sepsis.[127]

Three phase II studies explored the use of gemcitabine and cisplatin together (GC) in metastatic bladder cancer.[125–127] Gemcitabine (1000 mg/m²) was administered on days 1, 8, and 15 every 4 weeks. Cisplatin was given once every 4 weeks, either on day 1 or 2 (70 to 75 mg/m²) or weekly on days 1, 8, and 15 (35 mg/m²). In total, 116 patients were treated in the three studies with this doublet, with a response rate of 42% to 66% and a CR rate of 18% to 28%. The median survival was 12.5 to 14.3 months in the three studies (Table 30.2-8). Primary toxicity was hematologic and was generally easily managed, with rare hospitalizations for febrile neutropenia and no toxic deaths. The least hematologic toxicity was seen when cisplatin was administered on day 2.[127]

Because of its apparently comparable efficacy and improved tolerability, GC was compared to standard MVAC in a multicenter phase III study.[125] MVAC was administered as described earlier,[123] and GC was administered in 28-day cycles with gemcitabine, 1000 mg/m² (days 1, 8, 15), and cisplatin, 70 mg/m² (day 2). Four hundred five patients were randomized to one of the two treatment arms, and the two groups exhibited similar characteristics, with slightly more adverse factors on the GC arm. Median survival was 13.8 months with GC and 14.8 months with MVAC, which were statistically comparable. At 6, 12, and 18 months, survival rates were 82%, 58%, and 37%, respectively, with GC, and 81%, 63%, and 38% with MVAC. The response rates were 49% for the GC

arm and 46% for the MVAC arm. No significant difference was seen in time to progression or time to treatment failure.

In contrast, patients treated with GC had significantly less toxicity and improved tolerability. Toxic deaths (1% vs. 3%), neutropenic fevers (2% vs. 14%), grade 3/4 neutropenia (71% vs. 82%), grade 3/4 mucositis (1% vs. 22%), and alopecia (11% vs. 55%) were all lower in the GC group. Patients who received GC gained more weight, reported less fatigue, and had better performance status than patients receiving MVAC. As a result of this study, GC is generally considered the current standard of care for metastatic bladder cancer.

TAXANE- AND PLATINUM-CONTAINING REGIMENS. The addition of taxanes to cisplatin-based regimens has been the subject of numerous phase II trials in bladder cancer, some of which are summarized in Table 30.2-9. Many other similar studies with comparable results have been presented in abstract form. The doublets of cisplatin/paclitaxel and cisplatin/docetaxel appear to have response rates comparable to those of GC.[128–131]

In contrast, substitution of carboplatin for cisplatin may provide inferior results. At least four studies have been published of the pair of carboplatin and paclitaxel, and overall survival in each study is worse than that expected with standard chemotherapy.[132–135] In a study conducted by SWOG, 29 patients were treated every 3 weeks with paclitaxel, 200 mg/m², and carboplatin at AUC (area under the concentration-time curve) 5.[133] As expected, toxicity was primarily hematologic and neurologic, and therapy was generally well tolerated, with an average of five cycles received. However, only six partial responses were observed, for an overall response rate of 20.7%, and median survival was a dismal 9 months. These results, taken together with prior studies comparing the two,[136,137] strongly suggest that cisplatin is superior to carboplatin in the treatment of TCC.

Interestingly, omission of platinum completely with a doublet of gemcitabine and paclitaxel (GP) appears to provide a reasonable outcome. Phase II studies looking at this regimen have demonstrated response rates and survival comparable to those of GC, with minimal toxicity.[138,139] The authors have also seen instances of long-term durable CRs with GP.[140]

TRIPLET CHEMOTHERAPY. Because of the activity of each of these agents in TCC, investigators have asked whether triplet

TABLE 30.2-9. Phase II Trials of Taxane-Containing Chemotherapy Regimens

Regimen	Composite No. of Patients	Response Rate (%)	Median Survival (Mo)	Reference(s)
Carboplatin/paclitaxel	104	21–65	8.5–9.5	132–135
Cisplatin/paclitaxel	52	50	10.6	130
Cisplatin/docetaxel	129	52–60	8.0–13.6	128,129,131
Cisplatin/paclitaxel/ifosfamide	29	79	20	191
Cisplatin/gemcitabine/paclitaxel	61	78	15.8	141
Carboplatin/gemcitabine/paclitaxel	49	68	14.7	142
Cisplatin/gemcitabine/docetaxel	35	66	15.5	143
Gemcitabine/paclitaxel	94	54–60	14.4	138,139

combinations of platinum, taxanes, and gemcitabine might have increased activity. Three such published studies, with cisplatin/gemcitabine/paclitaxel,[141] carboplatin/gemcitabine/paclitaxel,[142] and cisplatin/gemcitabine/docetaxel[143] had intriguingly high CR rates of 28% to 32% and overall response rates of 66% to 78%. Part of the explanation for such favorable results might be selection bias, in that a majority of patients in these studies did not have visceral metastases. Nevertheless, the response rates were high even among patients with visceral metastases.

Equally important, the toxicity of these triplet regimens was readily manageable, with 1% to 4% febrile neutropenia in the paclitaxel studies and 14% febrile neutropenia in the docetaxel study. One toxic death in total occurred among the 145 patients in all three studies. Median survival of 14.8 to 15.8 months was longer than that seen with GC in phase III studies but again may reflect selection bias. In response to these data, an international, randomized phase III study under the auspices of the EORTC is ongoing comparing standard treatment with GC versus the triplet of GC plus paclitaxel.

TCC is among the most chemotherapy-sensitive solid tumors, and platinum-based regimens have been standard therapy for advanced disease for a number of decades. A variety of different combinations have been used, and the current standard treatments are either MVAC or GC. Addition of taxanes may provide further activity, increase the CR rate, and prolong survival. Nevertheless, overall survival remains poor in metastatic disease, and newer therapies, including rationally targeted agents against tumor-specific growth factor pathways, are needed to effect real change in our treatment of this disease.

Combined Modality Treatment of Advanced Disease

The place of combined modality therapy for advanced disease has not been settled. Dodd et al.[144] presented data demonstrating an improvement in long-term survival in selected patients undergoing resection of persistent cancer deposits after MVAC or CMV. In their original series, the group from Memorial Sloan-Kettering reported that 13 patients who had complete resection of viable tumor after chemotherapy had a median survival of 25 months, and some of those patients survived longer than 5 years. Other investigators have reported similar results.[145]

In the authors' experience, carefully selected patients with locally advanced unresectable bladder cancer, including some with pelvic nodal masses, may experience long-term survival with the combination of chemotherapy and radiation. To be selected for this combined modality treatment, patients had to have

(1) an excellent performance status, (2) locally advanced measurable disease, (3) a normal hemogram and kidney function tests, and (4) no evidence of distant metastases beyond the common iliac lymph nodes. The initial treatment consisted of four to six cycles of combination chemotherapy, usually MCV, and, less commonly, gemcitabine/cisplatin. If significant regression of tumor was achieved, radiation treatment was administered in combination with radiosensitizing chemotherapy, usually cisplatin/paclitaxel. Gemcitabine was not generally used in the program because of the problems associated with the exquisite radiosensitizing properties of gemcitabine, with severe reactions seen with the usual therapeutic doses of gemcitabine when administered concurrently with radiation. When gemcitabine was used in the neoadjuvant part of the program, the authors avoided gemcitabine-radiation interactions by using a waiting period of at least 2 months from the completion of gemcitabine treatment to the start of radiation.

These patients were carefully selected, but in the majority of individuals so treated, excellent tumor shrinkage and long-term survival were achieved in patients who would otherwise have been expected to succumb within a median time of 24 months if treatment had consisted of chemotherapy alone. These results must now be subjected to phase II and phase III studies if they are to merit wider usage.

SUMMARY

Our understanding of cancer of the urinary bladder is in a state of evolution, with important advances in our appreciation of multiple risk factors, strategies of prevention, and possibly earlier detection through screening. Superficial bladder cancer accounts for the majority of patients at presentation, and although it uncommonly progresses to muscularis propria–invasive disease, it is difficult to eradicate by local treatment. The mainstay of treatment after TURBT is by the intravesical route, either by one of several chemotherapeutic agents or BCG, with BCG the initial treatment of choice of most urologists. For muscularis propria–invasive disease, there have been improvements in surgical techniques, including continent diversions and neobladders, which have the potential of improving quality of life for patients. Bladder preservation approaches, although still under study in the interest of improving results and limiting side effects, are now moving into the mainstream of treatment, with results in comparable patients equal to those achieved by radical cystectomy and with increasing numbers of patients expressing an interest in organ-sparing treatment. Quality-of-life considerations have come to the forefront in the care of patients with bladder cancer, much as they have in other cancers, and there are now some important scientific data documenting the quality of life after cystectomy as well as with bladder-sparing treatment.

Whether bladder sparing or cystectomy is used as local treatment, combined modality approaches are essential if treatment is to be optimal. Neoadjuvant chemotherapy has been carefully studied and appears to be of value in improving survival, although further studies will be necessary before this combined approach can be considered standard treatment. For adjuvant treatment, the data are much less convincing. The results of studies recently begun using newer drug combinations may help to establish the role of adjuvant chemotherapy in improving survival. In advanced (metastatic) disease, several newer drug combinations have led to an improvement in overall and disease-specific response rates, but thus far no improvement in survival has been demonstrated.

CANCERS OF THE URETER AND RENAL PELVIS

Most tumors of the upper urinary system are TCC, but these are unusual tumors, with fewer than 3000 patients diagnosed annually in the United States. Because of the difficulty in gaining access to the tumors in the upper urinary tract and their relative rarity, the diagnostic and staging maneuvers are more problematic and less accurate than for the TCCs of the bladder. Ninety percent of these tumors are TCC, and squamous cell carcinoma accounts for most of the remaining 10%. Primary tumors of the ureter occur only half as frequently as do tumors of the renal pelvis.[16] Upper tract TCC develops in men two to three times more than in women, with the peak age of development of these tumors in the seventh and eighth decades of life.[146] As discussed earlier in Epidemiology, the majority of these tumors arise in response to, or at least associated with, environmental stresses.

CLINICAL PRESENTATION AND STAGING

Gross hematuria is the presenting symptom in 75% to 95% of all patients who present with tumors of the renal pelvis and ureter. The hematuria may be accompanied by flank pain as in renal colic if either the tumor or clotted blood causes obstruction of the upper urinary tract.[147] Patients may describe the passage of vermiform clots. Urinary cytology is an important part of the workup for an upper tract tumor, but it has only a 10% to 40% sensitivity in the detection of low-grade TCC lesions, whereas for high-grade tumors the sensitivity may be as high as 80%. Patients in whom a positive urinary cytology is found but neither diagnostic radiology nor cystoscopy identifies a bladder tumor, selective barbotage of upper tracts for cytologic analysis is performed during the endoscopic procedure.

Improvements in endoscopic technology with flexible fiber endoscopes allow the urologist to view directly and to obtain tissue in many of the TCCs of the ureter and renal pelvis. This allows pathologic confirmation of the cell type of these tumors at diagnosis.

After diagnosis careful radiographic evaluation is important in determining tumor extent and provisional tumor stage. Intravenous urography had been the mainstay of radiographic

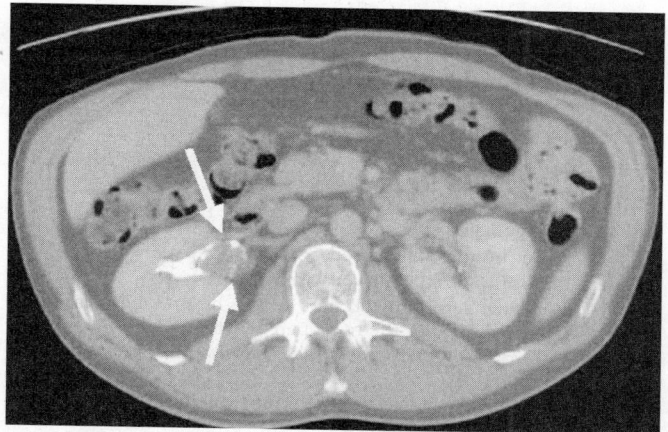

FIGURE 30.2-5. Abdominal computed tomographic scan of a stage T3 transitional cell carcinoma of the right renal pelvis, with intravenous contrast showing a large filling defect in the right renal pelvis (*arrows*).

evaluation of upper tract tumors because it gives a detailed appearance of the entire renal collecting system and the ureter, but in most major centers helical CT scan is now the preferred imaging method (Fig. 30.2-5).[148] MRI urography may also be useful in patients when sensitivity to iodinated contrast prevents the use of that agent.[149] For patients with poor renal function or in those who cannot tolerate intravenous contrast agents, retrograde pyelography is the preferred method of imaging. When a patient is found or judged to have a TCC more aggressive than a grade I and stage I tumor, more comprehensive staging of the patient is indicated. This includes chest CT as well as tomographic evaluation of the abdomen and pelvis for a possible hepatic or lymph node metastatic spread. Standard therapy is radical excision of the kidney and the ipsilateral ureter. Evaluation of the total remaining renal function after a proposed nephrectomy is indicated. Isotope renal scanning can accurately estimate the function of the uninvolved kidney.

The current American Joint Committee on Cancer TNM staging[53] for tumors of the upper urinary tract is shown in Figure 30.2-6 and in Table 30.2-10. This pathology-based staging system depends on the determination of the extent of the invasion by

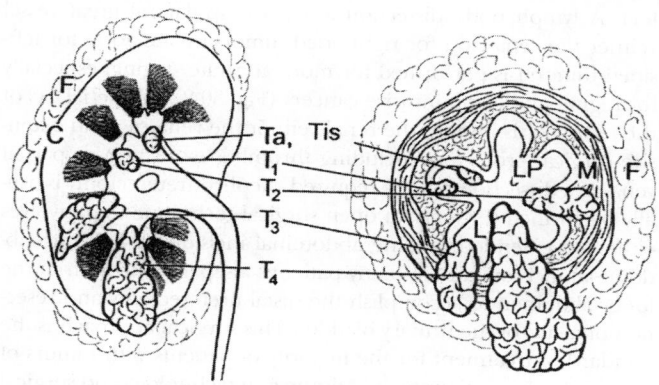

FIGURE 30.2-6. Schematic diagram of the American Joint Committee on Cancer TNM staging of cancers of the renal pelvis. C, renal capsule; F, peripelvic fat; LP, lamina propria; M, muscularis propria.

TABLE 30.2-10. American Joint Committee on Cancer 2002 TNM Staging of Renal Pelvis and Ureter Cancers: Definition of TNM

PRIMARY TUMOR (T)

TX	Primary tumor cannot be assessed
T0	No evidence of primary tumor
Ta	Papillary noninvasive carcinoma
Tis	Carcinoma *in situ*
T1	Tumor invades subepithelial connective tissue
T2	Tumor invades the muscularis
T3	(For renal pelvis only) Tumor invades beyond muscularis into peripelvic fat or the renal parenchyma
T3	(For ureter only) Tumor invades beyond muscularis into periureteric fat
T4	Tumor invades adjacent organs or through the kidney into the perinephric fat.

REGIONAL LYMPH NODES (N)[a]

NX	Regional lymph nodes cannot be assessed
N0	No regional lymph node metastasis
N1	Metastasis in a single lymph node 2 cm or less in greatest dimension
N2	Metastasis in a single lymph node more than 2 cm but not more than 5 cm in greatest dimension or multiple lymph nodes; none more than 5 cm in greatest dimension
N3	Metastasis in a lymph node, more than 5 cm in greatest dimension

DISTANT METASTASIS (M)

MX	Distant metastasis cannot be assessed
M0	No distant metastasis
M1	Distant metastasis

[a]Laterality does not affect the N classification.
(From ref. 53, with permission.)

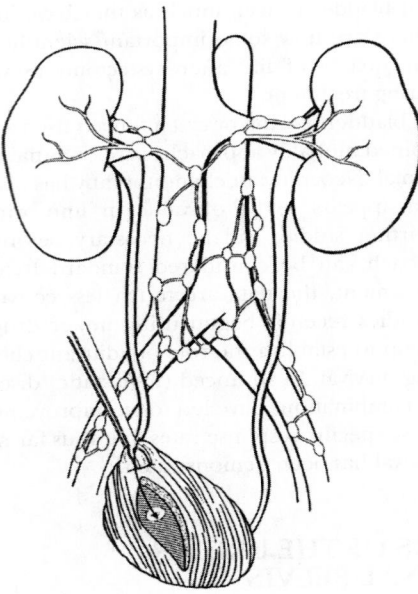

FIGURE 30.2-7. Diagram of the kidneys, ureters, bladder, and retroperitoneal lymph nodes to demonstrate that a nephroureterectomy for upper tract transitional cell carcinoma requires complete excision of the distal ureter, including the portion within the wall of the bladder. The bladder here is open to reveal the distal ureter, which tunnels within the wall of the bladder.

the resected primary tumor and by microscopic evaluation of the resected regional lymph nodes in high-grade tumors.[53]

SURGICAL TREATMENT

The standard surgical treatment for patients with invasive transitional cell cancer of the upper urinary tract is radical nephroureterectomy. This involves a complete removal of the kidney with its surrounding perirenal fat contained within Gerota's fascia and *en bloc* removal of the ureter down to and including its portion within the urinary bladder (the urethral orifice and the intramural ureter). A lymph node dissection along the ipsilateral great vessel (either the vena cava for right-sided tumors or the aorta for left-sided tumors) is performed for more accurate staging, especially for higher-grade and invasive cancers (Fig. 30.2-7). When TCC of the renal pelvis invades the renal vein or the vena cava, an extensive surgical procedure including thrombus extraction or partial vena cava dissection may be required. Nephroureterectomy is usually performed through an open surgical technique that involves either an extended midline abdominal incision or a thoracoabdominal incision and, in many patients, a separate incision in the lower abdomen to accomplish the distal ureterectomy and resection of a cuff of the urinary bladder. This surgical approach is the standard of treatment for the majority of patients with tumors of the renal pelvis and ureter.[150] Advances in technology and surgical technique have allowed a reduction in the morbidity from this procedure by using a laparoscopic surgical technique. An *en bloc* excision can be accomplished safely and effectively.[151] The operative time and blood loss with the laparoscopic technique are substantially less than with an open surgical technique without any compromise in the surgical complication rate and without any increase in problems with the pathologic tumor margins of the resected specimen except that the intravesical ureter has to be removed by a separate procedure. The hospital stay is also substantially reduced from a median of 6 days of hospitalization for the open surgery group compared to an average of 2 days for the laparoscopic surgical group.[152] Invasive TCC is known to have the capacity to seed the abdomen if spilled, allowing tumor autotransplantation, and this has led to concern among surgical oncologists about the laparoscopic approach. One group has reported three cases of laparoscopic port-site recurrence after this procedure.[153] In all three of these cases, the tumor was spilled from the operative specimen, allowing growth of the tumor tissue at the trocar sites.

In patients in whom radical excision of the tumor would result in severe renal insufficiency requiring dialysis (such as patients with a solitary kidney or patients with substantially diminished renal function), limited endoscopic therapies have been developed and have been shown, when done selectively and in experienced hands, to be effective.[154] With ureteroscopic treatment it is possible to resect small tumors of the ureter, particularly low-grade tumors, by fulguration or resection. Other TCCs of the renal pelvis and the calyceal system are more difficult to resect endoscopically because of possible associated tumor multicentricity or because the invasive tumor is associated with CIS.[153] Electrosurgical instruments or the Nd:YAG (neodymium:yttrium aluminum garnet) laser are also effective local ablative tools.

Percutaneous endoscopic management of renal pelvic and calyceal TCC has been developed as an alternative method in highly select patients who have poor renal function or who medically could not withstand an open surgical procedure.

Endoscopic access is gained percutaneously in the flank into the renal collecting system by placing a tube percutaneously into the renal pelvis. Then, using standard endoscopic tools, it is possible to resect tumors in the fashion similar to that used for bladder tumors. Because of the technical complexity of these procedures, the risk of tumor seeding, and the difficulty in resecting all the microscopic extent of the tumor, these procedures are generally limited to patients who have absolute contraindications to nephrectomy.[155] All of these endoscopic procedures require vigilant follow-up with endoscopic reevaluation on a regular schedule.

A kidney-sparing approach may be advisable in selected cases of low-stage and low-grade distal ureteral tumors because the recurrences or the multicentricity of these tumors are nearly always distal to the index lesion and it is surgically feasible to remove the entire distal ureter along with the open resection of this tumor. After this, the bladder can be advanced surgically to reach to the midureter and allow reimplantation of the midureter with reestablishment of urine flow. On the other hand, similar ureteral low-grade lesions of the upper ureter would require complete resection of the entire ureter. In this case, if the renal pelvis is free from TCC it may be possible and safe to substitute for the resected ureter a segment of small intestine and restore continuity from the renal pelvis to the bladder. Patients for whom this approach is appropriate are limited, and careful selection is mandatory.

Results of Surgical Therapy

The success rate of surgical procedures is primarily influenced by the pathologic stage of the disease at the time of resection. In a report with long follow-up from the University of Texas Southwestern Medical Center of 252 patients treated surgically for upper tract TCC, specific and overall survival was strongly influenced by the pathologic stage of the primary tumor. The 5-year actuarial disease-specific survival rates by primary tumor pathologic stage were 100% for noninvasive tumors (Ta and Tis), 92% for pathologic stage T1, 73% for pathologic stage T2, and 41% for pathologic stage T3.[150] Of those with stage T4 tumors, there were no long-term survivors (Table 30.2-11). The type of open surgical procedure used (nephroureterectomy in 77% of the patients compared to a kidney-sparing approach used in 17%) was evaluated by univariate and multivariate analysis. Patients undergoing nephroureterectomy were found to have a significantly improved recurrence-free and disease-specific survival on multivariate analysis but not on univariate analysis.[150] However, in other series patients with ureteral cancers who were selected for kidney-sparing resections did not have a poorer outcome.[156]

Adjuvant Topical Therapy after Local Excision Only

In cases in which endoscopic resection alone was the treatment of choice for individual patients, the adjuvant use of topical immunotherapy or topical chemotherapy may be important in preventing or delaying local tumor recurrence. BCG appears to be useful in this regard in carcinomas of the upper tract that are stage Tis.[157] Adriamycin given prophylactically after conservative resection of upper tract TCCs using an antegrade infusion also has been judged to be of some benefit in reducing recurrence.[158]

ADJUVANT COMBINED MODALITY THERAPY

The most appropriate treatment for invasive transitional cell cancers of the upper urinary tract is nephroureterectomy. Despite aggressive surgery, cure rates are low when the disease has spread beyond the muscularis, with 5-year survival rates varying between 0 and 34%.[155,159–163] Whether these low survival rates can be improved by adjuvant therapy depends on the pattern of failure and the efficacy of the available treatment. Metastatic relapse appears to predominate over local relapse, and systemic cisplatin-based chemotherapy has been used, extrapolating from the experience with locally advanced bladder cancer. The true rate of local-regional failure is, however, unknown because many of the published series are old and used pre-CT methods of intraabdominal evaluation. The available data suggest an overall local-regional failure of 2% to 27%, although these figures may be an underestimate.[164–166] Cozad et al.[167] report local failure rates of 50% in stage T3 disease, rising to 60% if the tumors were high grade. Brookland and Richter[168] and Ozsahin et al.[169] have reported local-regional recurrence in 45% and 62%, respectively. Most series report a close association between local failure and distant metastasis, although whether the association is causal or simply synchronous cannot be determined from the small numbers in the series.

Radiation has been used as an adjuvant therapy, with mixed results reported in the literature (Table 30.2-12). Several small phase II studies have suggested a local control and perhaps survival advantage for adjuvant radiation.[169–171] One study reported no benefit, although their treated population was diluted with 30% early-stage patients.[170] Another study showed no advantage to radiation. A criticism of this study is that the radiation doses given were inadequate.[171]

At the MGH, a more aggressive approach has been taken over the last 20 years, in which patients with high-risk disease were treated first with adjuvant radiation alone and then more recently with concomitant radiation-sensitizing chemotherapy and, if tolerable, further combination chemotherapy. Although our series of 31 patients is nonrandomized and small, the authors observed that local failure was lower if chemotherapy was combined with radiation (22% vs. 45%), and the survival rate at 5 years was higher (67% vs. 27%; *unpublished data*; see Table 30.2-12).

Very few published data exist to guide physicians managing patients with a local relapse after nephroureterectomy. If the relapse is bulky and metastases present elsewhere, palliation with chemotherapy would be the most appropriate course. When the relapse appears isolated and the patient relatively vigorous, con-

TABLE 30.2-11. Five-Year Disease-Specific Survival by Primary Tumor Pathologic Stage after Surgical Resection of Transitional Cell Carcinoma of the Upper Urinary Tract

Tumor Stage	Number	Percent
pTa/pTis	38	100
pT1	99	92
pT2	34	73
pT3	53	41
pT4	19	0

(From ref. 150, with permission.)

TABLE 30.2-12. Larger Published Series Using Surgery with or without Adjuvant Radiation for Carcinoma of the Upper Urinary Tract

	No. of Patients	Median Dose (Gy)	Local-Regional Failure % (Absolute)	Overall 5-Y Survival (%)
SURGERY + RADIOTHERAPY				
Ozsahin et al.[169]	45	50	38 (17/45)	21
Maulard-Durdux et al.[170]	26[a]	45	19 (5/26)	49 (T2, 60%; T3, 19%)
Catton et al.[171]	86[b]	35	34 (29/86)	43 (T3N0, 45%; N+, 15%)
Brookland and Richter[168]	11	50	9 (1/11)	27
Cozad et al.[167]	9	50	11 (1/9)	44
MGH (*unpublished*)	31	47	23 (7/31)	39 (67% in combined modality group)
SURGERY ONLY				
Ozsahin et al.[169]	81		65 (53/81)	33
Cozad et al.[167]	17[c]		53 (9/17)	24
Brookland and Richter[168]	11		45 (5/11)	17

MGH, Massachusetts General Hospital.
[a]Thirty percent stage T2.
[b]Twenty-seven percent stage T1 to T2.
[c]All stages ≥T3.

sideration can be given to an aggressive approach that holds out the chance for cure. The first step would be to downsize and perhaps improve the resectability of the recurrence using external radiation to a modest preoperative dose of 30 to 45 Gy along with sensitizing chemotherapy. An attempt could then be made at resection or debulking, and, if the facility were available, intraoperative radiation could then be given directly onto the tumor bed or onto an unresectable mass with the bowel and other critical organs displaced out of the field. Such an approach allows the delivery of high doses of radiation to the target without the risk of bowel injury that is present when managing such disease using external radiation treatment alone (Fig. 30.2-8). This is a paradigm that has been used with considerable success for retroperitoneal sarcomas and locally advanced rectal cancer. Such cases are unusual and require individualized treatment that follows basic oncologic principles developed for other sites in the body. Multiple modalities are usually required, and a strong case can be made for these patients to be managed in a multidisciplinary genitourinary oncology clinic.

CHEMOTHERAPY FOR METASTATIC DISEASE

Most patients with upper tract TCC have superficial disease, with a generally favorable prognosis as discussed above.[172,173] However, patients with disease that invades beyond the muscularis propria have a significantly worse prognosis. The most consistent prognostic variables for the outcome of patients with upper tract TCC, including renal pelvic and ureteral carcinomas, are tumor stage and grade.[174–177] Molecular markers have been analyzed as well, including p27, p53, MDM2, and Ki-67 labeling index. Poor outcome may be predicted by overexpression of p53 and higher Ki-67 labeling index, although not all studies support this finding.[178–183]

In a series of 252 patients with mostly localized disease, relapse occurred in 67 (27%) after a median of 12 months.[184] Survival was highly stage specific, with 5-year disease-specific survival of 92% for T1, 73% for T2, 41% for T3, and 0 for T4. In a series of 126 patients with nonmetastatic but more advanced renal pelvic or ureteral tumors, relapsed disease was noted in 81 (64%) after a median of 9 months.[185] Overall 5- and 20-year survival was 29% and 19%, respectively. The most common sites of distant metastases were liver, bone, or lung. Use of postoperative radiation therapy did not have an impact on local or distant relapse. Factors that influenced survival outcome in multivariate analysis were initial tumor stage, residual postsurgery tumor, and location of initial tumor, with renal pelvic cancer being more favorable than ureteral cancer. The role of adjuvant chemotherapy in reducing relapse has not been explored in randomized fashion in this uncommon disease.

Coronal pre treatment

Coronal post treatment

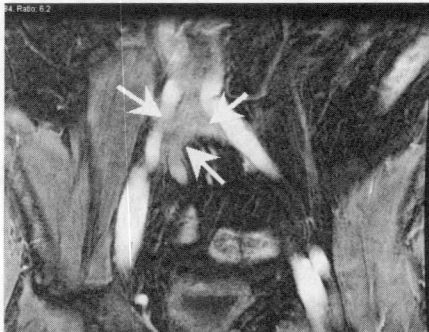
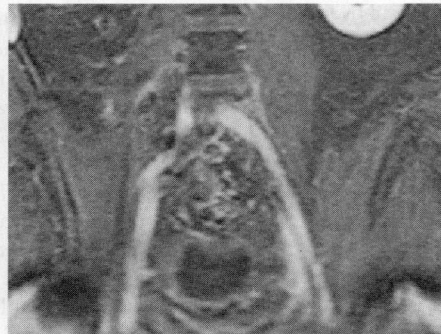

FIGURE 30.2-8. Sequential coronal magnetic resonance imaging (MRI) of a patient with an unresectable ureteral tumor mass. The mass shown on the MRI on the left was at the bifurcation of the aorta; it was initially judged unresectable due to involvement of the vessels. Partial resection, however, became possible as part of a combined modality treatment approach that included preoperative conformal external-beam radiation. Intraoperative electron-beam radiation was given to the entire tumor bed after resection. On the right is the repeat MRI 1 year after treatment without any visible tumor. (See Color Fig. 30.2-8 in the CD-ROM.)

The biology of upper tract TCC is considered to be identical to that of bladder TCC. Consequently, the chemotherapy regimens recommended for advanced or metastatic upper tract TCC are the same as those for bladder cancer, as described in Cancer of the Bladder. Standard treatment is cisplatin-based combination therapy, such as GC or MVAC. More recent studies have explored the addition of taxanes to cisplatin-based regimens, with higher response rates.[186–188] These findings have yet to be validated in large-scale multicenter studies. As with bladder cancer, upper tract TCC is highly responsive to chemotherapy but has a short median duration of response. A minority of patients may have CR to therapy, and some of these individuals may experience long-term disease remission.[189] Overall, however, the prognosis of metastatic upper tract TCC is as poor as that of metastatic bladder TCC.

SUMMARY

Tumors of the upper urinary tract are uncommon tumors and less accessible than cancers of the bladder to accurate diagnosis, surgical identification, and effective local treatment. The epidemiology of these tumors, although generally similar to that of bladder cancer, exhibits some characteristics peculiar to these tumors.

Hematuria, the most common presenting symptom, is similar to that of bladder cancer, but the location of these tumors, much less accessible than tumors of the bladder, poses special problems for urologists in their attempts to locate these tumors precisely. Because urinary cytology is less useful in upper tract tumors than in bladder cancer, improvements in endoscopic technology allowing for the direct viewing of the ureters and renal pelvis are especially important, as are evaluations of the place of molecular tumor markers in diagnosis. Advances in radiologic studies are significant, with the major improvement that of helical CT imaging.

Surgical treatment of upper tract tumors is in evolution, with new laparoscopic approaches likely to achieve wider usage as urologic surgeons in the United States and abroad master this technique. Despite aggressive surgery, cure rates of upper tract tumors are low, and radiation and chemotherapy, often used in combination, may prove to be important in lengthening survival. The place of radiation and chemotherapy, however, has yet to be established. Because there is a paucity of published data to support this approach, carefully planned studies are needed.

REFERENCES

1. Maralani S, Wood DP Jr, Grignon D, et al. Incidence of urethral involvement in female bladder cancer: an anatomic pathologic study. *Urology* 1997;50(4):537.
2. Erckert M, Stenzl A, Falk M, et al. Incidence of urethral tumor involvement in 910 men with bladder cancer. *World J Urol* 1996;14(1):3.
3. Munoz JJ, Ellison LM. Upper tract urothelial neoplasms: incidence and survival during the last 2 decades. *J Urol* 2000;164(5):1523.
4. Oldbring J, Glifbert I, Mikulowski P, et al. Carcinoma of the renal pelvis and ureter following bladder carcinoma: frequency, risk factors and clinicopathological findings. *J Urol* 1989;141:1311.
5. Rabbani F, Perrotti M, Russo P, et al. Upper-tract tumors after an initial diagnosis of bladder cancer: argument for long-term surveillance. *J Clin Oncol* 2001;19(1):94.
6. Hurle R, Losa A, Manzetti A, et al. Upper urinary tract tumors developing after treatment of superficial bladder cancer: 7-year follow-up of 591 consecutive patients. *Urology* 1999;53(6):1144.
7. Toncheval DI, Atanassova SY, Gergov TD, et al. Genetic changes in uroepithelial tumors of patients with Balkan endemic nephropathy. *J Nephrol* 2002;15(4):387.
8. Chou YH, Huang CH. Unusual clinical presentation of upper urothelial carcinoma in Taiwan. *Cancer* 1999;85(6):1342.
9. Yang MH, Chen KK, Yen CC, et al. Unusually high incidence of upper urinary tract urothelial carcinoma in Taiwan. *Urology* 2002;59(5):681.
10. Shinohara N, Koyanagi T. Ras signal transduction in carcinogenesis and progression of bladder cancer: molecular target for treatment? *Urol Res* 2002;30(5):273.
11. Primdahl H, von der Masse H, Sorenson FB, et al. Immunohistochemical study of the expression of cell cycle regulating proteins at different stages of bladder cancer. *J Cancer Res Clin Oncol* 2002;128(6):295.
12. Feldman AS, Tang Z, Kirley S, et al. Expression of CABLES, a cell cycle regulatory gene is lost in invasive transitional cell carcinoma of the bladder. Abstract #727. *J Urol* 2003;169(4)S:188.
13. Sgambato A, Migaldi M, Faraglia B, et al. Cyclin D1 expression in papillary superficial bladder cancer: its association with other cell cycle-associated proteins, cell proliferation and clinical outcome. *Int J Cancer* 2002;97(5):671.
14. Santos LL, Amaro T, Pereira SA, et al. Expression of cell-cycle regulatory proteins and their prognostic value in superficial low-grade urothelial cell carcinoma of the bladder. *Eur J Surg Oncol* 2003;29(1):74.
15. Zeegers MP, Goldbohm RA, van den Brandt PA. A prospective study on active and environmental tobacco smoking and bladder cancer risk (The Netherlands). *Cancer Causes Control* 2002;13(1):83.
16. Donat SM, Herr HW. Transitional cell carcinoma of the renal pelvis and ureter: diagnosis, staging, management, and prognosis. In: Oesterling JE, Richie JP, eds. *Urologic oncology*. Philadelphia: WB Saunders, 1997:215.
17. Mayfield MP, Whelan P. Bladder tumours detected on screening: results at 7 years. *Br J Urol* 1998;82(2):825.
18. Wakui M, Shiigai T. Urinary tract cancer screening through analysis of urinary red blood cell volume distribution. *Int J Urol* 2000;7(7):248.
19. Stampfer DS, Carpinito GA, Rodriguez-Villanueva J, et al. Evaluation of NMP22 in the detection of transitional cell carcinoma of the bladder. *J Urol* 1998;159(2):394.
20. Oeda T, Manabe D. The usefulness of urinary FDP in the diagnosis of bladder cancer: comparison with NMP22, BTA and cytology. *Nippon Hinyokika Gakkai Zasshi* 2001;92(1):1.
21. Eissa S, Swellam M, Sadek M, et al. Comparative evaluation of the nuclear matrix protein, fibronectin, urinary bladder cancer antigen and voided urine cytology in the detection of bladder tumors. *J Urol* 2002;168(2):465.
22. Ichikawa T, Nakayama Y, Yamada D, et al. Clinical evaluation of basic fetoprotein in bladder cancer. *Nippon Hinyokika Gakkai Zasshi* 2000;91(7–8):579.
23. Strefford JC, Lillington DM, Steggall M, et al. Novel chromosome findings in bladder cancer cell lines detected with multiplex fluorescence in situ hybridization. *Cancer Genet Cytogenet* 2002;135(2):139.
24. Utting M, Werner W, Dahse R, et al. Microsatellite analysis of free tumor DNA in urine, serum, and plasma of patients: a minimally invasive method for the detection of bladder cancer. *Clin Cancer Res* 2002;8(1):35.
25. Ito H, Kyo S, Kanaya T, et al. Detection of human telomerase reverse transcriptase messenger RNA in voided urine samples as a useful diagnostic tool for bladder cancer. *Clin Cancer Res* 1998;4(11):2807.
26. Boman H, Hedelin H, Holmang S. Four bladder tumor markers have a disappointingly low sensitivity for small size and low grade recurrence. *J Urol* 2002;167(1):80.
27. Young RH. Pathology of carcinomas of the urinary bladder. In: Vogelzang NJ, Scardino PT, Shipley WU, Coffey DS, eds. *Comprehensive textbook of genital urinary oncology*, 2nd ed. Philadelphia: Lippincott Williams & Wilkins, 2000:310.
28. Reuter VE. Pathology of bladder cancer: assessment of prognostic variables in response to therapy. *Semin Oncol* 1990;17:524.
29. Epstein JI, Amin MB, Reuter VE, et al. The World Health Organization/International Society of Urological Pathology consensus classification of urothelial (transitional cell) neoplasms of the urinary bladder. *Am J Surg Pathol* 1998;22:1435.
30. Young RH, Oliva E. Transitional cell carcinomas of the urinary bladder that may be underdiagnosed: a report of four invasive cases exemplifying the homology between neoplastic and nonneoplastic transitional cell legions. *Am J Surg Pathol* 1996;20:1448.
31. Younes M, Sussman J, True LD. The usefulness of the level of the muscularis mucosae in the staging of invasive transitional cell carcinoma of the urinary bladder. *Cancer* 1990;66:543.
32. Farrow GM. Pathology of carcinoma in situ of the urinary bladder and related lesions. *J Cell Biochem* 1992;161[Suppl]:39.
33. Melamed MR, Reuter VE. Pathology and staging of urothelial tumors of the kidney and ureter. *Urol Clin North Am* 1993;20:333.
34. Sidransky D, Frost P, Von Eschenbach A, et al. The clonal origin of bladder cancer. *N Engl J Med* 1992;326:737.
35. Miyao N, Tsai YC, Lerner SP, et al. Role of chromosome IX in human bladder cancer. *Cancer Res* 1993;53:4066.
36. Williams SG, Buscarini M, Stein JP. Molecular markers for diagnosis, staging and prognosis of bladder cancer. *Oncology* 2001;15:1461.
37. Markl IDC, Salem CE, Jones PA. Molecular biology of bladder cancer. In: Volgelzang NJ, Scardino PT, Shipley WU, Coffey DS, eds. *The comprehensive textbook of genitourinary oncology*, 2nd ed. Philadelphia: Lippincott Williams & Wilkins, 2000:298.
38. Raghavan D. Molecular targeting and pharmacogenomics in the management of advanced bladder cancer. *Cancer* 2003;97[Suppl 8]:2086.
39. Colquhoun CL, Jones GDD, Al-Moneef M, et al. Improving and predicting radiosensitivity in muscle invasive bladder cancer. *J Urol* 2003;169:1993.
40. Cote RJ, Esrig D, Groshen S, et al. p53 and the treatment of bladder cancer. *Nature* 1997;385:123.
41. Sarkis A, Bajorin D, Reuter V, et al. Prognostic value of p53 nuclear over expression in patients with invasive bladder cancer treated with neoadjuvant MVAC. *J Clin Oncol* 1995;13:1384.

42. Rodel C, Grabenbauer GG, Rodel F, et al. Apoptosis, p53, bcl-2, Ki-67 in invasive bladder carcinoma: possible predictors for response to radiochemotherapy and successful bladder preservation. *Int J Radiat Oncol Biol Phys* 2000;46:1213.
43. Smith ND, Rubinstein JN, Eggener SE, Kozlowski JM. The p53 tumor suppressor gene and nuclear protein: basic science review and relevance in the management of bladder cancer. *J Urol* 2003;169:1219.
44. Al-Sukhun S, Hussain M. Current understanding of the biology of advanced bladder cancer. *Cancer* 2003;97[Suppl 8]:2064.
45. Neal DE, Sharples L, Smith K, et al. The epidermal growth factor receptor and the prognosis of bladder cancer. *Cancer* 1990;65:1619.
46. Wood DP Jr, Fair WR, Chaganti RS. Evaluation of epidermal growth factor receptor DNA amplification and mRNA expression in bladder cancer. *J Urol* 1992;147:274.
47. Lipponen P, Eskelinen M. Expression of epidermal growth factor receptor in bladder cancer as related to established prognostic factors, oncoprotein (c-erbB-2, p53) expression and long-term prognosis. *Br J Cancer* 1994;69:1120.
48. Mellon JK, Lunec J, Wright C, et al. C-erbB-2 in bladder cancer: molecular biology, correlation with epidermal growth factor receptors and prognostic value. *J Urol* 1996;155:321.
49. Ciardiello F, Caputo R, Bianco R, et al. Antitumor effect and potentiation of cytotoxic drugs activity in human cancer cells by ZD-1839 (Iressa), an epidermal growth factor receptor-selective tyrosine kinase inhibitor. *Clin Cancer Res* 2000;6:2053.
50. Jimenez RE, Hussain M, Bianco FJ Jr, et al. Her-2/neu overexpression in muscle-invasive urothelial carcinoma of the bladder: prognostic significance and comparative analysis in primary and metastatic tumors. *Clin Cancer Res* 2001;7:2440.
51. Kim SI, Kwon SM, Kim YS, et al. The association of cyclooxygenase-2 expression with prognosis of stage T1 grade 3 bladder cancer. *Urology* 2002;60:816.
52. Droller MJ. Editorial comment. *J Urol* 2003;170:672.
53. American Joint Committee on Cancer. *Cancer staging manual*, 6th ed. New York: Springer-Verlag, 2002.
54. Harisinghani MG, Barentsz J, Hahn PF, et al. Noninvasive detection of clinically occult lymph-node metastases in prostate cancer. *N Engl J Med* 2003;348(25):2491.
55. Bohle A, Jocham D, Bock PR. Intravesical bacillus Calmette-Guerin versus mitomycin C for superficial bladder cancer: a formal meta-analysis of comparative studies on recurrence and toxicity. *J Urol* 2003;169(1):900.
56. Shahin O, Thalmann GN, Rentsch C, et al. A retrospective analysis of 153 patients treated with or without intravesical bacillus Calmette-Guerin for primary state T1 grade 3 bladder cancer: recurrence, progression and survival. *J Urol* 2003;169(1):96.
57. Davis JW, Sheth SI, Doviak MJ, et al. Superficial bladder carcinoma treated with bacillus Calmette-Guerin: progression-free and disease specific survival with minimum 10-year followup. *J Urol* 2002;167:494.
58. Yiou R, Patard JJ, Benhard H, et al. Outcome of radical cystectomy for bladder cancer according to the disease type at presentation. *BJU Int* 2002;89(4):374.
59. McDougal WS. Urethrectomy. In: McDougal WS, ed. *Rob & Smiths operative surgery, urology*, 4th ed. London: Butterworth, 1983:526.
60. Gschwend JE, Dahm P, Fair WR. Disease specific survival as endpoint of outcome for bladder cancer patients following radical cystectomy. *Eur Urol* 2002;41(4):440.
61. Stein JP, Cai J, Groshen S, Skinner DG. Risk factors for patients with pelvic lymph node metastases following radical cystectomy with en bloc pelvic lymphadenectomy: concept of lymph node density. *J Urol* 2003;170(1):35.
62. McDougal WS. Metabolic complications of urinary intestinal diversion. *J Urol* 1992;147:1199.
63. Srinivas S, Mahalati K, Freiha FS. Methotrexate tolerance in patients with ileal conduits and continent diversions. *Cancer* 1998;82(6):1134.
64. Chahal R, Sundaram SK, Iddenden R, et al. A study of the morbidity, mortality and long-term survival following radical cystectomy and radical radiotherapy in the treatment of invasive bladder cancer in Yorkshire. *Eur Urol* 2003;43(3):246.
65. McDougal WS. Use of intestinal segments and urinary diversion. In: Walsh PC, Retik AB, Vaughan ED Jr, Wein AJ, eds. *Campbell's urology*, 8th ed. Philadelphia: WB Saunders, 2002:3745.
66. Shipley WU, Prout GR Jr, Einstein AB Jr, et al. Treatment of invasive bladder cancer by cisplatin and irradiation in patients unsuited for surgery: a high success rate in clinical stage T2 tumors in a National Bladder Cancer Group trial. *JAMA* 1987;258:931.
67. Coppin CM, Gospodarowicz MK, James K, et al. Improved local control of invasive bladder cancer by concurrent cisplatin and preoperative or definitive radiation. *J Clin Oncol* 1996;14(11):2901.
68. Shipley WU, Prout GR Jr, Kaufman SD, Perrone TL. Invasive bladder carcinoma. The importance of initial transurethral surgery and other significant prognostic factors for improved survival with full-dose irradiation. *Cancer* 1987;60:514.
69. Dunst J, Sauer R, Schrott KM, Kuhn R, Wittekind C, Altendorf-Hofmann A. Organ-sparing treatment of advanced bladder cancer: a 10-year experience. *Int J Radiat Oncol Biol Phys* 1994;30:261.
70. Smith DC, Montie JE, Sandler HS, et al. A pilot trial of concurrent gemcitabine and radiotherapy as a bladder preserving stragedy. *Proc Am Soc Clin Oncol* 2000;19:360a(abst 1419).
71. Tester W, Porter A, Asbell S, et al. Combined modality program with possible organ preservation for invasive bladder carcinoma: results of RTOG protocol 85-12. *Int J Radiat Oncol Biol Phys* 1993;25:783.
72. Tester W, Caplan R, Heaney J, et al. Neoadjuvant combined modality program with selective organ preservation for invasive bladder cancer: results of Radiation Therapy Oncology Group phase II trial 8802. *J Clin Oncol* 1996;14:119.
73. Shipley WU, Winter KA, Kaufman DS, et al. A phase III trial of neoadjuvant chemotherapy in patients with invasive bladder cancer treated with selective bladder preservation by combined radiation therapy and chemotherapy: initial results of RTOG 89-03. *J Clin Oncol* 1998;16:3576.
74. Housset M, Dufour B, Maulard C. Concomitant 5-fluorouracil-cisplatin and bifractionated split course radiation therapy for invasive bladder cancer. *Proc Am Soc Clin Oncol* 1997;16:319a.
75. Rodel C, Grabenbauer GG, Kuhn R, et al. Combined-modality treatment and selective organ preservation in invasive bladder cancer: long-term results. *J Clin Oncol* 2002;20:3061.
76. Rodel C, Grabenbauer GG, Kuhn R, et al. Organ preservation in patients with invasive bladder cancer: initial results of an intensified protocol of transurethral surgery and radiation therapy plus concurrent cisplatin and 5-fluorouracil. *Int J Radiat Oncol Biol Phys* 2002;52(5):1303.
77. Rodel C, Grabenbauer GG, Kuhn R, et al. Invasive bladder cancer: organ preservation by radiochemotherapy. *Front Radiat Ther Oncol* 2002;36:118.
78. Shipley WU, Kaufman DS, Tester WJ, Philepich MV, Sandler HM. An overview of bladder cancer trials in the Radiation Therapy Oncology Group (RTOG). *Cancer* 2003;97[Suppl 8]:2115.
79. Shipley WU, Kaufman DS, Zehr E, et al. Selective bladder preservation by combined modality protocol treatment: long-term outcomes of 190 patients with invasive bladder cancer. *Urology* 2002;60:62.
80. Zietman AL, Grocela J, Zehr E, et al. Selective bladder conservation using transurethral resection, chemotherapy and radiation: the management and consequences of Ta, T1, Tis recurrence within the retained bladder. *Urology* 2001;58:380.
81. Turner S, Swindell R, Bowl N, et al. Bladder movement during radiation therapy for bladder cancer: implication for treatment planning. *Int J Radiat Oncol Biol Phys* 1994;30:199.
82. Moonen LM, Hornblas S, Van der Voet JC, et al. Bladder conservation in selective T1G3 and muscle invasive T2-T3a bladder carcinoma using combination therapy of surgery and iridium-192 implantation. *Br J Urol* 1994;74:322.
83. Wijkstrom H, Norning U, Lagerkvist M, et al. Evaluation of clinical staging before cystectomy transitional cell bladder carcinoma: a long-term follow-up of 276 consecutive patients. *Br J Urol* 1998;81:686.
84. Stein JP, Lieskovsky G, Kote R, et al. Radical cystectomy in the treatment of invasive bladder cancer: long-term results in 1,054 patients. *J Clin Oncol* 2001;19:666.
85. Dalbagni G, Genega E, Hashibe M, et al. Cystectomy for bladder cancer: a contemporary series. *J Urol* 2001;165:1111.
86. Grossman HB, Natale RB, Tangen CM, et al. Neoadjuvant chemotherapy plus cystectomy compared with cystectomy alone for locally advanced bladder cancer. *N Engl J Med* 2003;349:859.
87. Herr HW. Transurethral resection of muscle-invading bladder cancer. Ten-year outcome. *J Clin Oncol* 2001;19:89.
88. Scher HI, Shipley WU, Herr HW. Cancer of the bladder. In: DeVita VT Jr, Hellman S, Rosenberg SA, eds. *Cancer principles and practice of oncology*, 5th ed. Philadelphia: JB Lippincott, 1997:1300.
89. Housset M, Maulard C, Chretien Y, et al. Combined radiation and chemotherapy for invasive transitional-cell carcinoma of the bladder: a prospective study. *J Clin Oncol* 1993;11:2150.
90. Vogelzang NJ. Neoadjuvant MVAC: the long and winding road is getting shorter and straighter [Editorial]. *J Clin Oncol* 2001;19:4003.
91. Hall RR. Neoadjuvant cisplatin, methotrexate, and vinblastine chemotherapy for muscle-invasive bladder cancer: a randomized controlled trial. *Lancet* 1999;354:533.
92. Hall R. On behalf of the International Collaboration of Trialists of the MRC Advanced Bladder Cancer Group: updated results of a randomised controlled trial of neoadjuvant cisplatin (C), methotrexate (M) and vinblastine (V) chemotherapy for muscle-invasive bladder cancer. *Proc Am Soc Clin Oncol* 2002;21:178(abst).
93. Sharma P, Bajorin D. Controversies in neoadjuvant and adjuvant chemotherapy for muscle-invasive urothelial cancer and clinical research initiatives in locally advanced disease. *Am Soc Clin Oncol* 2003:478.
94. Malmstrom PU, Rintala E, Wahlqvist R, et al. Five-year follow-up of a prospective trial of radical cystectomy and neoadjuvant chemotherapy: Nordic Cystectomy Trial I. The Nordic Cooperative Bladder Cancer Study Group. *J Urol* 1996;155:1903.
95. Malmstrom PPU, Rintala E, Wahlquist R, et al. Neoadjuvant cisplatin-methotrexate chemotherapy of invasive bladder cancer: Nordic cystectomy trial 2—XIVth Congress of the European Association of Urology. *Eur Urol* 1999;35[Suppl 2]:60(abst 268).
96. Raghavan D, Quinn D, Skinner DG, et al. Surgery and adjunctive chemotherapy for invasive bladder cancer. *Surg Onc* 2002;11:55.
97. Prout GR Jr, Griffin PP, Shipley WU. Bladder carcinoma as a systemic disease. *Cancer* 1979;43:2532.
98. Bellmunt J, Guillem V, Paz-Ares L, et al. Phase I-II study of paclitaxel, cisplatin and gemcitabine in advanced transitional-cell carcinoma of the urothelium. *J Clin Oncol* 2000;18(8):3247.
99. Studer UE, Bacchi M, Biedermann C, et al. Adjuvant cisplatin chemotherapy following cystectomy for bladder cancer: results of a prospective randomized trial. *J Urol* 1994;152:81.
100. Bono AV, Benvenuti C, Reali L, et al. Adjuvant chemotherapy in advanced bladder cancer. Italian Uro-Oncologic Cooperative Group. *Prog Clin Biol Res* 1989;303:533.
101. Freiha F, Reese J, Torti FM. A randomized trial of radical cystectomy versus radical cystectomy plus cisplatin, vinblastine and methotrexate chemotherapy for muscle invasive bladder cancer. *J Urol* 1996;155:499.
102. Skinner DG, Daniels JR, Russell CA, et al. The role of adjuvant chemotherapy following cystectomy for invasive bladder cancer: a prospective comparative trial. *J Urol* 1991;145:459.
103. Stockle M, Meyenburg W, Wellek S, et al. Advanced bladder cancer (stages pT3b, PT4a, pN1 and pN2): improved survival after radical cystectomy and 3 adjuvant cycles of chemotherapy results of a controlled prospective study. *J Urol* 1992;148:302.
104. Stockle M, Meyenburg W, Wellek S, et al. Adjuvant polychemotherapy of nonorgan-confined bladder cancer after radical cystectomy revisited: long-term results of a controlled prospective study and further clinical experience. *J Urol* 1995;153:47.
105. Millikan R, Dinney C, Swanson D, et al. Integrated therapy for locally advanced bladder cancer: final report of a randomized trial of cystectomy plus adjuvant M-VAC versus cystectomy with both preoperative and postoperative M-VAC. *J Clin Oncol* 2001;19(20):4005.
106. Stockle M, Meyenburg W, Wellek S, et al. Radical cystectomy with or without adjuvant polychemotherapy for non-organ-confined transitional cell carcinoma of the urinary bladder: prognostic impact of lymph node involvement. *Urology* 1996;48:868.

107. Freiha F, Reese J, Torti FM. A randomized trial of radical cystectomy versus radical cystectomy plus cisplatin, vinblastine and methotrexate chemotherapy for muscle invasive bladder cancer. *J Urol* 1996;155:495.

108. Sternberg CN. Neo-adjuvant and adjuvant chemotherapy of bladder cancer: is there a role? *Ann Oncol* 2002;13[Suppl 4]:273.

109. Boyd SD, Feinberg SM, Skinner DG, et al. Quality of life survey of urinary diversion patients: comparison of ileal conduits versus continent Koch urinary reservoirs. *J Urol* 1987;138:1386.

110. Mansson A, Johnson G, Mansson W. Quality of life after cystectomy: comparison between patients with conduit and those with caecal reservoir urinary diversion. *Br J Urol* 1988;62:240.

111. Raleigh ED, Berry M, Monite JE. A comparison of adjustments to urinary diversions: a pilot study. *J Wound Ostomy Continence Nurs* 1995;22:58.

112. Bjerre BD, Johansen C, Steven K. Health related quality of life after cystectomy: bladder substitution compared with ileal conduit diversion. A questionnaire survey. *Br J Urol* 1995;75:200.

113. Hart S, Skinner EC, Meyerowitz BE, et al. Quality of life after radical cystectomy for bladder cancer in patients with an ileal conduit, or cutaneous or urethral Kock pouch. *J Urol* 1999;162:77.

114. Zietman AL, Sacco D, Skowronski U, et al. Organ-conservation in invasive bladder cancer treated by trans-urethral resection, chemotherapy, and radiation: results of a urodynamic and quality of life study on long-term survivors. *J Urol* 2003;170:1772.

115. Caffo O, Fellin G, Graffer U, Luciani L. Assessment of quality of life after cystectomy or conservative therapy for patients with infiltrating bladder carcinoma. *Cancer* 1996;78:1089.

116. Henningsohn L, Wijkstrom H, Dickman PW, Bergmark K, Steineck G. Distressful symptoms after radical radiotherapy for urinary bladder cancer. *Radiother Oncol* 2002;60:215.

117. Jemal A, Murray T, Samuels A, et al. Cancer statistics, 2003. *CA Cancer J Clin* 2003;53:5.

118. Yagoda A, Watson RC, Gonzalez-Vitale JC, Grabstald H, Whitmore WF. Cis-dichlorodiammineplatinum(II) in advanced bladder cancer. *Cancer Treat Rep* 1976;60:917.

119. Saxman SB, Propert KJ, Einhorn LH, et al. Long-term follow-up of a phase III intergroup study of cisplatin alone or in combination with methotrexate, vinblastine, and doxorubicin in patients with metastatic urothelial carcinoma: a cooperative group study. *J Clin Oncol* 1997;15:2564.

120. Loehrer PJ Sr, Einhorn LH, Elson PJ, et al. A randomized comparison of cisplatin alone or in combination with methotrexate, vinblastine, and doxorubicin in patients with metastatic urothelial carcinoma: a cooperative group study. *J Clin Oncol* 1992;10:1066.

121. Sternberg CN, Yagoda A, Scher HI, et al. Methotrexate, vinblastine, doxorubicin, and cisplatin for advanced transitional cell carcinoma of the urothelium. Efficacy and patterns of response and relapse. *Cancer* 1989;64:2448.

122. Sternberg CN, Yagoda A, Scher HI, et al. Preliminary results of M-VAC (methotrexate, vinblastine, doxorubicin and cisplatin) for transitional cell carcinoma of the urothelium. *J Urol* 1985;133:403.

123. Harker WG, Meyers FJ, Freiha FS, et al. Cisplatin, methotrexate, and vinblastine (CMV): an effective chemotherapy regimen for metastatic transitional cell carcinoma of the urinary tract. A Northern California Oncology Group study. *J Clin Oncol* 1985;3:1463.

124. Logothetis CJ, Dexeus FH, Finn L, et al. A prospective randomized trial comparing MVAC and CISCA chemotherapy for patients with metastatic urothelial tumors. *J Clin Oncol* 1990;8:1050.

125. von der Maase H, Hansen SW, Roberts JT, et al. Gemcitabine and cisplatin versus methotrexate, vinblastine, doxorubicin, and cisplatin in advanced or metastatic bladder cancer: results of a large, randomized, multinational, multicenter, phase III study. *J Clin Oncol* 2000;18:3068.

126. Kaufman D, Raghavan D, Carducci M, et al. Phase II trial of gemcitabine plus cisplatin in patients with metastatic urothelial cancer. *J Clin Oncol* 2000;18:1921.

127. Moore MJ, Winquist EW, Murray N, et al. Gemcitabine plus cisplatin, an active regimen in advanced urothelial cancer: a phase II trial of the National Cancer Institute of Canada Clinical Trials Group. *J Clin Oncol* 1999;17:2876.

128. Sengelov L, Kamby C, Lund B, Engelholm SA. Docetaxel and cisplatin in metastatic urothelial cancer: a phase II study. *J Clin Oncol* 1998;16:3392.

129. Dimopoulos MA, Bakoyannis C, Georgoulias V, et al. Docetaxel and cisplatin combination chemotherapy in advanced carcinoma of the urothelium: a multicenter phase II study of the Hellenic Cooperative Oncology Group. *Ann Oncol* 1999;10:1385.

130. Dreicer R, Manola J, Roth BJ, et al. Phase II study of cisplatin and paclitaxel in advanced carcinoma of the urothelium: an Eastern Cooperative Oncology Group Study. *J Clin Oncol* 2000;18:1058.

131. Garcia del Muro X, Marcuello E, Guma J, et al. Phase II multicentre study of docetaxel plus cisplatin in patients with advanced urothelial cancer. *Br J Cancer* 2002;86:326.

132. Redman BG, Smith DC, Flaherty L, Du W, Hussain M. Phase II trial of paclitaxel and carboplatin in the treatment of advanced urothelial carcinoma. *J Clin Oncol* 1998;16:1844.

133. Vaughn DJ, Malkowicz SB, Zoltick B, et al. Paclitaxel plus carboplatin in advanced carcinoma of the urothelium: an active and tolerable outpatient regimen. *J Clin Oncol* 1998;16:255.

134. Zielinski CC, Schnack B, Grbovic M, et al. Paclitaxel and carboplatin in patients with metastatic urothelial cancer: results of a phase II trial. *Br J Cancer* 1998;78:370.

135. Small EJ, Lew D, Redman BG, et al. Southwest Oncology Group Study of paclitaxel and carboplatin for advanced transitional-cell carcinoma: the importance of survival as a clinical trial end point. *J Clin Oncol* 2000;18:2537.

136. Petrioli R, Frediani B, Manganelli A, et al. Comparison between a cisplatin-containing regimen and a carboplatin-containing regimen for recurrent or metastatic bladder cancer patients. A randomized phase II study. *Cancer* 1996;77:344.

137. Bellmunt J, Ribas A, Eres N, et al. Carboplatin-based versus cisplatin-based chemotherapy in the treatment of surgically incurable advanced bladder carcinoma. *Cancer* 1997;80:1966.

138. Meluch AA, Greco FA, Burris HA III, et al. Paclitaxel and gemcitabine chemotherapy for advanced transitional-cell carcinoma of the urothelial tract: a phase II trial of the Minnie Pearl cancer research network. *J Clin Oncol* 2001;19:3018.

139. Sternberg CN, Calabro F, Pizzocaro G, et al. Chemotherapy with an every-2-week regimen of gemcitabine and paclitaxel in patients with transitional cell carcinoma who have received prior cisplatin-based therapy. *Cancer* 2001;92:2993.

140. Michaelson MD, Kaufman DS, Oh WK. Transitional cell carcinoma of the upper uroepithelial tract. *Clin Adv Hematol Oncol* 2003;1:102.

141. Bellmunt J, Guillem V, Paz-Ares L, et al. Phase I-II study of paclitaxel, cisplatin, and gemcitabine in advanced transitional-cell carcinoma of the urothelium. Spanish Oncology Genitourinary Group. *J Clin Oncol* 2000;18:3247.

142. Hussain M, Vaishampayan U, Du W, Redman B, Smith DC. Combination paclitaxel, carboplatin, and gemcitabine is an active treatment for advanced urothelial cancer. *J Clin Oncol* 2001;19:2527.

143. Pectasides D, Glotsos J, Bountouroglou N, et al. Weekly chemotherapy with docetaxel, gemcitabine and cisplatin in advanced transitional cell urothelial cancer: a phase II trial. *Ann Oncol* 2002;13:243.

144. Dodd PM, McCaffrey JA, Herr H, et al. Outcome of postchemotherapy surgery after treatment with methotrexate, vinblastine, doxorubicin and cisplatin in patients with unresectable or metastatic transitional cell carcinoma. *J Clin Oncol* 1999;17:2546.

145. Miller RS, Freiha FS, Torti FM. Surgical resection of residual tumor mass following chemotherapy for advanced transitional cell carcinoma. *Oncol Muchen Sympomed* 1994;3:370.

146. Mungan NA, Kiemeney LA, Van Dijck JA, et al. Gender differences in stage distribution of bladder cancer. *Urology* 2000;55(3):368.

147. Grabstald H, Whitmore WF, Melamed MR. Renal pelvic tumors. *JAMA* 1971;218(6):845.

148. O'Malley ME, Hahn PF, Yoder IC, et al. Comparison of excretory phase, helical computed tomography with intravenous urography in patients with painless haematuria. *Clin Radiol* 2003;58(4):294.

149. Jung P, Brauers A, Nolte-Ernsting CA, et al. Magnetic resonance urography enhanced by gadolinium and diuretics: a comparison with conventional urography in diagnosing the cause of ureteric obstruction. *BJU Int* 2000;86(9):960.

150. Hall MC, Womack S, Sagalowsky AI, et al. Prognostic factors, recurrence and survival in transitional cell carcinoma of the upper urinary tract: a 30-year experience in 252 patients. *Urology* 1998;52:594.

151. El Fettouh HA, Rassweiler JJ, Schulze M, et al. Laparoscopic radical nephroureterectomy: results of an international multicenter study. *Eur Urol* 2002;42(5):447.

152. Gill IS, Sung GT, Hobart MG, et al. Laparoscopic radical nephroureterectomy for upper tract transitional cell carcinoma: the Cleveland Clinic experience. *J Urol* 2000;164(5):1513.

153. Ong AM, Bhayani SB, Pavlovich CP. Trocar site recurrence after laparoscopic nephroureterectomy. *J Urol* 2003;170(4):1301.

154. Daneshmand S, Quek ML, Huffman JL. Endoscopic management of upper urinary tract transitional cell carcinoma: long-term experience. *Cancer* 2003;98(1):55.

155. Goel MC, Mahendra V, Roberts JG. Percutaneous management of renal pelvic urothelial tumors: long-term followup. *J Urol* 2003;169(3):925, discussion 929.

156. Heney NM, Nocks BN, Daly JJ, Blitzer PH, Parkhurst EC. Prognostic factors in carcinoma of the ureter. *J Urol* 1981;125:632.

157. Okubo K, Ichioka K, Terada N, et al. Intrarenal bacillus Calmette-Guerin therapy for carcinoma in situ of the upper urinary tract: long-term follow-up and natural course in cases of failure. *BJU Int* 2001;88(4):343.

158. See WA. Continuous antegrade infusion of adriamycin as adjuvant therapy for upper tract urothelial malignancies. *Urology* 2000;56(2):216.

159. Reitelman C, Sawczuk IS, Olsson CA, Puchner PJ, Benson MC. Prognostic variables in patients with transitional cell carcinoma of the renal pelvis and proximal ureter. *J Urol* 1987;138:1144.

160. Rubenstein MA, Walz BJ, Bucy JG. Transitional cell carcinoma of the kidney: 25 year experience. *J Urol* 1978;119:595.

161. Mills C, Vaughan ED Jr. Carcinoma of the ureter: natural history, management and 5-year survival. *J Urol* 1983;129:275.

162. Kirkali Z, Moffat LEF, Deane RF, Kyle KF, Graham AG. Urothelial tumors of the upper urinary tract. *Br J Urol* 1989;64:18.

163. Booth CM, Cameron KM, Pugh RCB. Urothelial carcinoma of the kidney and ureter. *Br J Urol* 1980;52:430.

164. Mufti GR, Gove JRW, Badenoch DF, et al. Transitional cell carcinoma of the renal pelvis and ureter. *Br J Urol* 1989;63:135.

165. Das AK, Carson CC, Bolick D, Paulson DF. Primary carcinoma of the upper urinary tract (effect of primary and secondary therapy on survival). *Cancer* 1990;66:1919.

166. Vahlensieck W Jr, Sommerkamp H. Therapy and prognosis of carcinoma of the renal pelvis. *Eur Urol* 1989;16:286.

167. Cozad SC, Smalley SR, Austenfeld M, et al. Transitional cell carcinoma of the renal pelvis or ureter: patterns of failure. *Urology* 1995;46:796.

168. Brookland RK, Richter MP. The postoperative irradiation of transitional cell carcinoma of the renal pelvis and ureter. *J Urol* 1985;133:952.

169. Ozsahin M, Zouhair A, Villa S, et al. Prognostic factors in urothelial renal pelvis and ureter tumours: a multicentre Rare Cancer Network study. *Eur J Cancer* 1999;35:738.

170. Maulard-Durdux C, Dufour B, Hennequin C, et al. Postoperative radiation therapy in 26 patients with invasive transitional cell carcinoma of the upper urinary tract: no impact on survival? *J Urol* 1996;155:115.

171. Catton CN, Warde P, Gospodarowicz MK, et al. Transitional cell carcinoma of the renal pelvis and ureter: outcome and patterns of relapse in patients treated with postoperative radiation. *Urol Oncol* 1996;2:171.

172. Guinan P, Volgelzang NJ, Randazzo R, et al. Renal pelvic transitional cell carcinoma. The role of the kidney in tumor-node-metastasis staging. *Cancer* 1992;69:1773.

173. Seaman EK, Slawin KM, Benson MC. Treatment options for upper tract transitional-cell carcinoma. *Urol Clin North Am* 1993;20:349.

174. Huben RP, Mounzer AM, Murphy GP. Tumor grade and stage as prognostic variables in upper tract urothelial tumors. *Cancer* 1988;62:2016.

175. Charbit L, Gendreau MC, Mee S, Cukier J. Tumors of the upper urinary tract: 10 years of experience. *J Urol* 1991;146:1243.

176. Corrado F, Ferri C, Mannini D, et al. Transitional cell carcinoma of the upper urinary tract: evaluation of prognostic factors by histopathology and flow cytometric analysis. *J Urol* 1991;145:1159.

177. Guinan P, Vogelzang NJ, Randazzo R, et al. Renal pelvic cancer: a review of 611 patients treated in Illinois 1975-1985. Cancer Incidence and End Results Committee. *Urology* 1992;40:393.

178. Terrell RB, Cheville JC, See WA, Cohen MB. Histopathological features and p53 nuclear protein staining as predictors of survival and tumor recurrence in patients with transitional cell carcinoma of the renal pelvis. *J Urol* 1995;154:1342.

179. Masuda M, Iki M, Takano Y, et al. Prognostic significance of Ki-67 labeling index in urothelial tumors of the renal pelvis and ureter. *J Urol* 1996;155:1877, discussion 1880.

180. Rey A, Lara PC, Redondo E, Valdes E, Apolinario R. Overexpression of p53 in transitional cell carcinoma of the renal pelvis and ureter. Relation to tumor proliferation and survival. *Cancer* 1997;79:2178.

181. Furihata M, Ohtsuki Y, Sonobe H, et al. Prognostic significance of cyclin E and p53 protein over expression in carcinoma of the renal pelvis and ureter. *Br J Cancer* 1998;77:783.

182. Jinza S, Takano Y, Iki M, Noguchi S, Masuda M. Prognostic significance of p53 protein over expression in transitional cell carcinoma of the renal pelvis and ureter. *Urol Int* 1998;60:147.

183. Kamai T, Takagi K, Asami H, et al. Prognostic significance of p27Kip1 and Ki-67 expression in carcinoma of the renal pelvis and ureter. *BJU Int* 2000;86:14.

184. Hall MC, Womack S, Sagalowsky AI, et al. Prognostic factors, recurrence, and survival in transitional cell carcinoma of the upper urinary tract: a 30-year experience in 252 patients. *Urology* 1998;52:594.

185. Ozsahin M, Zouhair A, Villa S, et al. Prognostic factors in urothelial renal pelvis and ureter tumours: a multicentre Rare Cancer Network study. *Eur J Cancer* 1999;35:738.

186. Bellmunt J, Guillem V, Paz-Ares L, et al. Phase I-II study of paclitaxel, cisplatin, and gemcitabine in advanced transitional-cell carcinoma of the urothelium. Spanish Oncology Genitourinary Group. *J Clin Oncol* 2000;18:3247.

187. Hussain M, Vaishampayan U, Du W, Redman B, Smith DC. Combination paclitaxel, carboplatin, and gemcitabine is an active treatment for advanced urothelial cancer. *J Clin Oncol* 2001;19:2527.

188. Meluch AA, Greco FA, Burris HA III, et al. Paclitaxel and gemcitabine chemotherapy for advanced transitional-cell carcinoma of the urothelial tract: a phase II trial of the Minnie Pearl cancer research network. *J Clin Oncol* 2001;19:3018.

189. Michaelson MD, Kaufman DS, Oh WK. Transitional cell carcinoma of the upper uroepithelial tract. *Clin Adv Hematol Oncol* 2003;1:102.

190. Mead GM, Russell M, Clark P, et al. A randomized trial comparing methotrexate and vinblastine (MV) with cisplatin, Methotrexate and vinblastine (CMV) in advanced transitional cell carcinoma: results and a report on prognostic factors in a Medical Research Council study. MRC Advanced Bladder Cancer Working Party. *Br J Cancer* 1998;78:1067.

191. Bajorin DF, McCaffrey JA, Hilton S, et al. Treatment of patients with transitional-cell carcinoma of the urothelial tract with ifosfamide, paclitaxel, and cisplatin: a phase II trial. *J Clin Oncol* 1998;16:2722.

HOWARD I. SCHER
STEVEN A. LEIBEL
ZVI FUKS
CARLOS CORDON-CARDO
PETER T. SCARDINO

SECTION 3

Cancer of the Prostate

STATES AND STATE TRANSITIONS

The approach to prostate cancer diagnosis and treatment is changing rapidly across the spectrum of the disease. New diagnostic algorithms are available to determine whether a cancer is clinically significant. The techniques of surgery and radiation, which are the standards for the management of localized disease, continue to be refined so that cure rates are increased while morbidity declines. More patients and physicians recognize that there are effective treatments for metastatic disease, and, analogous to the management of other malignancies, systemic therapies are finally being tested in the minimal disease setting in which they have the potential for greater benefit. The old dogma of "not treating prostate cancer because it is a slow-growing disease of the elderly" is finally falling by the wayside because we have better prognostic models to determine patients who need treatment and those who do not based on the clinical and biologic determinants of an individual's disease.

The age-specific mortality and the absolute number of deaths from prostate cancer have been decreasing since 1993. The ratio between the incidence and mortality from disease in 2004 is expected to be more than 7:1 (230,000:29,900).[1] What is uncertain is whether the decreased mortality is due to the more widespread use of early detection strategies or more effective treatment, or a combination of the two. That the proportion of patients being diagnosed with tumors confined to the prostate has increased is well recognized, whereas chemoprevention strategy was recently shown to reduce overall prostate cancer incidence. But, because many cancers recur after

therapy, and some patients still present with metastatic disease, decreasing prostate cancer mortality further requires systemic treatments that work. In 2004, for the first time, a docetaxel-based chemotherapy program was shown to prolong the lives of prostate cancer patients who had progressed on hormonal therapy. This, along with the increased understanding of the biology of the disease, makes further improvements in survival a realistic goal.

DEFINING THERAPEUTIC OBJECTIVES

Each individual is focused on himself. Men without a cancer diagnosis question whether they should undergo testing procedures to detect the disease. Those with a cancer confined to the prostate question how best to eliminate it while maintaining potency, urinary control, and bowel function or whether treatment can be safely deferred. This contrasts with men who have symptoms of metastatic disease, facing what are arguably more serious issues, including how to alleviate symptoms, prevent their reoccurrence, and how to prolong their lives. The effects of any intervention for each of these scenarios can be assessed only in the context of clinical trials with defined objectives relevant to the question at hand. Although the ultimate goal of treatment is to prolong life, therapeutic objectives in the short term differ for those in the early versus late states of the illness, for those with versus without symptoms, and according to the individual's anticipated survival or longevity if no cancer was present relative to the anticipated lifespan with the disease as it is currently manifest.

A clinical framework for prognostic assessments, therapeutic objectives, and the assessments outcomes for a disease continuum is provided by considering prostate cancer as a series of easily recognized states.[2] As shown in Figure 30.3-1, the states are initial prostate evaluation, no cancer diagnosis, clinically localized disease, rising prostate-specific antigen (PSA; noncastrate and castrate), clinical metastases noncastrate, and clinical metastases castrate disease. A patient's state is determined by the clinical assessment, physical examination, and imaging studies and whether the level of testosterone in the blood is in

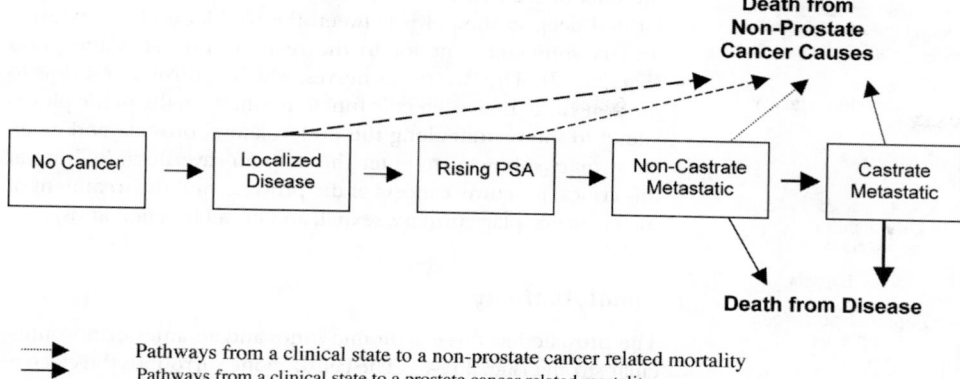

FIGURE 30.3-1. Clinical states model of prostate cancer progression. Dashed line arrows indicate pathways from a clinical state to a nonprostate cancer–related mortality; solid line arrows indicate pathways from a clinical state to a prostate cancer–related mortality. PSA, prostate-specific antigen. (Modified from ref. 2.)

noncastrate or castrate range. At any one time, a patient resides in only one state; once the state of the patient is identified, a prognostic assessment is made for a specific therapeutic objective, treatment options are considered, and a decision is made whether or not to offer an intervention. A patient who undergoes treatment having reached a given state remains in that state until he has progressed to the next state. Patients do not go backward.

In general, the more advanced the disease, the greater the need for therapy. In some cases, be it at the time of diagnosis or at the time of recurrence after treatment for localized disease, the patient may not be at risk for developing metastases or symptoms for many years, and the risk of death from non-cancer-related causes may greatly exceed that of the cancer. In such situations, it may be more appropriate to defer treatment until the disease declares itself as being more aggressive. By considering the disease in this way, therapeutic objectives can be balanced based on the morbidity and mortality of the cancer relative to the patient's noncancer-related causes of morbidity and mortality.

The therapeutic objectives for patients in each state vary. For those who do not have a cancer diagnosis but who may be harboring the disease or are at risk for developing it, the issues are early detection and prevention. For those with localized disease, the first issue is to determine whether the tumor is of such low biologic potential that it can be safely observed or whether it requires treatment. For tumors that require treatment, further issues are whether the tumor can be cured with therapies directed solely to the prostate or whether the integration of a systemic treatment will be required to achieve cure because of micrometastases that may be present. For patients who have a rising level of PSA as the sole manifestation of the disease after local therapy, the "state of a rising PSA," the objective is to determine whether the rise reflects local or systemic disease and, for the latter, to determine the probability of metastases becoming detectable clinically and in what period of time. Detectable metastases were chosen as a milestone because they represent a "transition" to a state in which death from cancer exceeds that of other causes.[3] For those who already have detectable metastases, be it at the time of diagnosis or recurrence, objectives are to delay progression and to prolong the response to medical or surgical castration. Finally, for those who have progressed on castration, the goal is to improve or to maintain quality of life, as well as to prolong it.[2]

All of the interventions currently available, be they surgical, radiation, or medical, have adverse effects that may be permanent, and none of the systemic treatments are curative. The issue for management is what risk of progression over what time frame would lead a patient to accept a given therapy or a physician to recommend it, assuming accurate predictions. There is no simple answer. Consider a 45-year-old individual with localized disease and a 10% predicted probability of cure using current predictive models. Should surgery be denied? Should radiation be offered without surgery? Should he be treated or referred for a combined local and systemic approach? Further illustrating the complexity of these issues, a study in 2004 found that men were willing to sacrifice longevity to maintain potency.[4] An area of active research is how best to assess individuals' prognoses for a specific therapeutic outcome as accurately as possible and to apply the assessment to patient counseling and clinical trial design. Outcomes can include the probability of cure, recurrence, symptoms, metastases, death from disease, or quality of life after therapy. Any factor, be it demographic, clinical, or biologic, can be considered when making the prognostic assessment.

A challenge in developing systemic treatments for prostate cancer in particular is that the most common manifestations of the disease are a rising PSA or metastases to bone. Although PSA levels can be measured accurately and quantitatively, declines do not necessarily mean that tumor growth has been slowed, and rises do not universally indicate progression.[5] This is because changes in the level do not always correlate with tumor growth. Tumor masses that can be accurately measured and assessed serially over time occur infrequently. Even when measurable masses are present, changes in soft tissue mass, such as lymph node, may not parallel the change in the tumor in bone. As a result, although posttherapy changes in PSA and regressions of a measurable mass are important outcomes for phase II investigations, they cannot be used as surrogates of clinical benefit.[6]

As is discussed in the management of the individual disease state, each intervention that is considered for a patient, be it to prevent the disease, to eliminate it, or to control it, must be considered in the context of a defined objective and outcome relevant to the state of the patient for whom it is advised. As the objectives differ by state, so must the outcomes: A uniform set of outcome criteria cannot be applied across the spectrum of the disease. Proof of clinical benefit requires randomized trials that compare the experimental approach with an established standard or

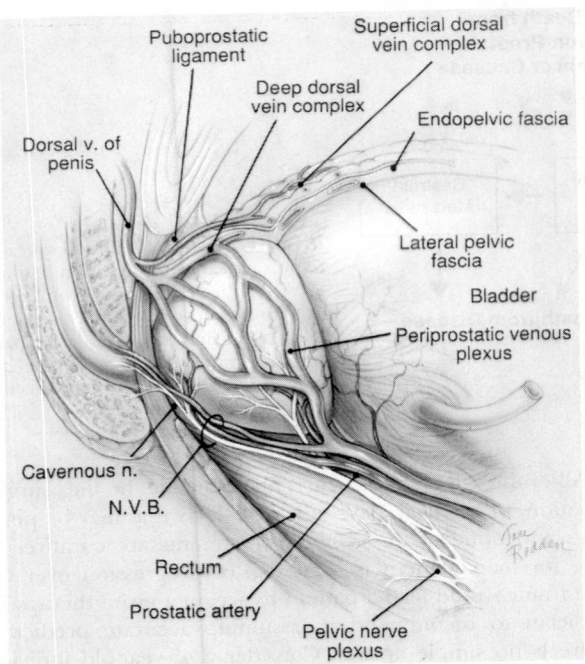

FIGURE 30.3-2. Lateral view of normal anatomy of the pelvis. NVB, neurovascular bundle. (From ref. 8, with permission.)

placebo. Before these trials are considered, there must be evidence that the agent or approach has sufficient efficacy to justify the large-scale comparison.[7]

ANATOMY OF THE PROSTATE

The prostate is an exocrine organ weighing 20 to 25 g, which consists of lobular tubuloalveolar glands that secrete fluid through ducts that empty into the prostatic urethra. The fluid comprises the bulk of seminal emissions and is rich in PSA. The prostate is located deep in the pelvis between the bladder and the external urinary sphincter, anterior to the rectum and below the pubis (Fig. 30.3-2). The cavernous nerves, which control blood flow to the penis and, hence, erectile function, run from the pelvic plexus lateral to the rectum along the posterolateral prostate and external urinary sphincter to enter the corpora cavernosa. By lying at this critical juncture, cancers of the prostate, and the treatment of such cancers, place urinary, sexual, and bowel function at risk.

Zonal Anatomy

The prostate has three anatomic zones and an anterior fibromuscular stroma (Fig. 30.3-3). The central zone surrounds the ejaculatory ducts, the transition zone surrounds the urethra, and the peripheral zone makes up the bulk of a normal gland. The posterior peripheral zone lies against the rectum and is the area palpable by digital rectal examination (DRE). These zonal boundaries are indistinct in the gland of a normal, postpubescent male, but, as men age, the transition zone enlarges from nonmalignant growth (benign prostatic hyperplasia, or BPH). The frequency of malignancy in the different zones is disproportionate to the glandular tissue present. Very few cancers originate in the central zone, and only 15% originate in the transition zone; most originate in the peripheral zone.

Patterns of Spread

Although most cancers arise near the capsule in the peripheral zone, the disease is generally multifocal, and tumors are often present throughout the gland. Spread may occur by local extension through defects in the capsule where the neurovascular structures and the ejaculatory ducts enter the gland or in the region of the bladder neck. Local invasion can progress to involve the seminal vesicles or the bladder or to invade the levator muscles. Rarely does a tumor invade the rectal wall. Tumors

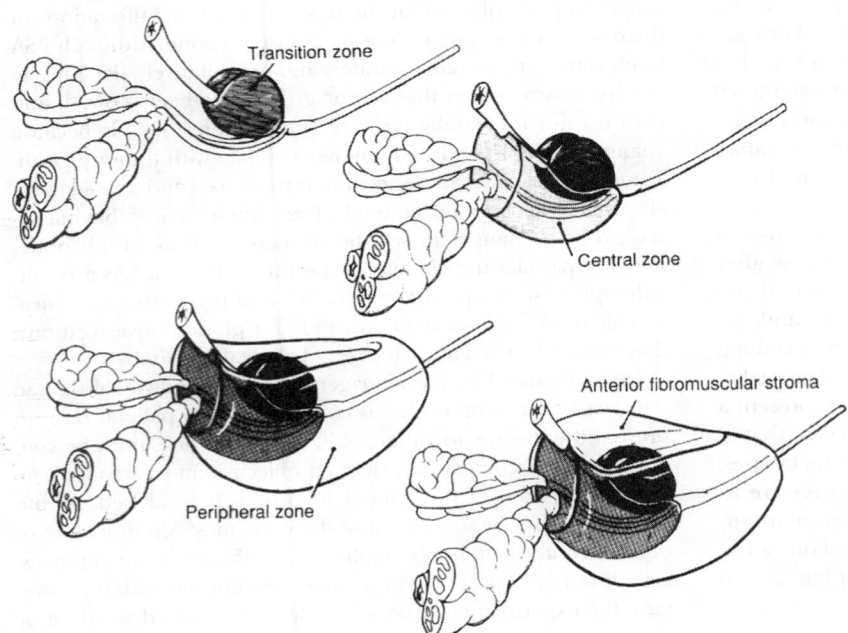

FIGURE 30.3-3. Zonal anatomy of prostate, after McNeal. The transition zone is the periurethral tissue that grows to become benign prostatic hypertrophy with age. The central zone surrounds the ejaculatory ducts and rarely gives rise to cancer. The peripheral zone remains constant with age but is the site of most cancers. The anterior stroma contains skeletal muscle in continuity with the urethral sphincter. (Adapted from refs. 9 and 10.)

TABLE 30.3-1. Comparison of the 1992, 1997, and 2002 American Joint Committee on Cancer/International Union Against Cancer TNM Staging System

Stage	1992	1997	2002
T1	Clinically inapparent, not palpable or visible by imaging		
T1a	Incidental histologic finding, ≤5% of resected tissue		
T1b	Incidental histologic finding, >5% of resected tissue		
T1c	Tumor identified by needle biopsy, for any reason (e.g., elevated PSA)		
T2	Palpable or visible tumor, confined within the prostate		
T2a	≤½ one lobe	One lobe	≤½ one lobe
T2b	One lobe	Both lobes	One lobe
T2c	Both lobes	—	Both lobes
T3	Tumor extends through the capsule		
T3a	Unilateral ECE	ECE, unilateral or bilateral	
T3b	Bilateral ECE	Seminal vesicle involvement	
T3c	Seminal vesicle involvement	—	—
T4	Tumor is fixed or invades adjacent structures		
T4a	Invades bladder neck, external sphincter or rectum		
T4b	Invades levator muscles or fixed to pelvic sidewalls		

ECE, extracapsular extension; PSA, prostate-specific antigen; TNM, tumor, node, metastasis.
(Modified from refs. 11–13, and 173.)

of the apex are prone to early extracapsular extension (ECE) due to a weakness of the capsule in this location. Systemic spread can occur via the lymphatics to involve the obturator, hypogastric, presacral, and external iliac nodes or hematogenously to involve bone, lung, or liver. Prostate cancers in particular have a predilection for bone, in part owing to a unique bidirectional interaction between tumor cells and the surrounding stroma.

Staging

Prostate cancers are staged using the TNM (tumor, node, metastasis) classification developed by the American Joint Committee on Cancer and the International Union Against Cancer. The authors recommend use of the latest version, first published in 1992 (Table 30.3-1). With the TNM system, designations for the primary tumor, regional nodes, and distant metastases are noted separately. A distinct category, T1c, is used to describe cancers that are neither palpable nor visible but were detected by a biopsy performed because of an abnormal PSA or another reason. Cancers that are not palpable but are visible by an imaging study, such as transrectal ultrasound (TRUS) or magnetic resonance imaging (MRI), are classified appropriately along with palpable cancers in the T2 to 4 categories. The previous version of the TNM classification, from 1997, is not recommended because it inappropriately combined the present T2a and T2b categories, distinctly different in pathologic features and prognosis, into a single category, T2a. The 2002 system reestablished three T2 categories—a, b, and c. The authors use the 2002 system exclusively.

BIOLOGIC CHARACTERIZATION AND PATHOLOGY

The diagnosis, management, and control of prostate cancer are major challenges. Well recognized is that, morphologically, similar tumors of a given stage may have radically different prognoses, which limits our ability to predict the clinical behavior of an individual case. Biologic markers, such as alterations of p27, PTEN, and the androgen receptor (AR), await validation studies. Prospective clinical protocols using well-characterized cohorts of patients are required to delineate the role of alterations in critical genes and pathways in the disease and its management. Clinical advances are also dependent on model systems, such as xenografts designed to mimic discrete points in the illness, and transgenic models in which critical genes are activated or inactivated in a tissue-specific manner. Integrating the results of all the studies will accelerate progress.

HISTOPATHOLOGY

Two main growth-related diseases develop in the prostate: BPH, which affects both the epithelial and mesenchymal components, and cancer.[14] There is no direct etiologic relationship between BPH and cancer. They are related only by their close anatomic site of origin and the high incidence in men older than 40 years. More than 95% of malignant tumors of the prostate are adenocarcinomas that arise in acinar and proximal ductal epithelium. Grossly, adenocarcinomas appear pale yellow or with gray flecks of tissue coalesced into a firm, poorly defined mass, which is difficult to distinguish from the surrounding normal tissue. Often, they are multifocal, heterogeneous, and follow a papillary, cribriform, comedo, or acinar pattern. Immunohistochemistry may assist the diagnosis when few abnormal areas are present in a biopsy sample and, in particular, the differentiation of high-grade prostatic intraepithelial neoplasia (PIN) and atypical adenomatous hyperplasias from well-differentiated carcinoma. Cancers tend to stain negative for basal cell markers (basal-specific cytokeratin) and p63 and positive for alpha-methylacyl-coenzyme A racemase, which is up-regulated in cancer.[15]

For adenocarcinomas, the degree of differentiation has prognostic significance and is judged primarily using the Gleason grading system. Gleason grading evaluates the architectural details of individual cancer glands under low-to-medium magnification. Cytologic features under high magnification are not considered.[16,17] Five distinct patterns of growth from well to poorly differentiated are described on a scale from 1 to 5 (Fig. 30.3-4). Pattern 1 tumors are the most differentiated, with discrete glandular formation, whereas pattern 5 lesions are the most undifferentiated, with virtually complete loss of the glandular architecture. The final Gleason score is the sum of the grades of the primary and secondary growth patterns; the Gleason score can range from 2 (1 + 1) to 10 (5 + 5). Noteworthy is that the system is not based on the highest grade within the tumor and would not account for the presence of Gleason pattern 5 disease if the dominant patterns of growth were graded as 3 or 4, or both. Nonetheless, reproducibility and reliability are high. In contemporary series, 85% of tumors are intermediate grade (Gleason 5 to 7), 11% are well differentiated (Gleason sum 2 to 4), and 4% are poorly differentiated cancers (Gleason 8 to 10).[8] Transition zone cancers tend to have higher Gleason grades than nontransition zone cancers, and are less likely to extend outside the prostate.[19] Although other grading systems have been proposed, they are not widely used.

Other tumors developing in the prostate include the intralobular acinar carcinomas, ductal carcinomas, small cell or scirrhous pattern tumors, a clear-cell variant resembling renal cell

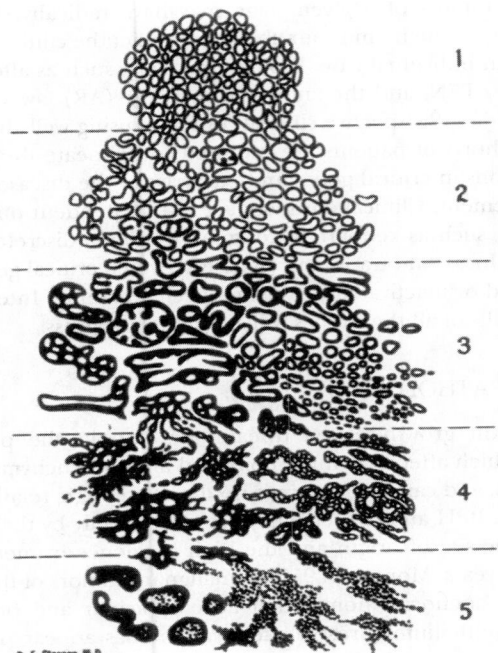

FIGURE 30.3-4.   Gleason grading system includes five histologic patterns distinguished by the glandular architecture of the cancer. (From ref. 18, with permission.)

carcinomas, and mucinous carcinoma. Ductal carcinomas comprise 1% of lesions, appear similar to comedocarcinomas of the breast, and are clinically aggressive. Small cell tumors of the prostate typically comprise small, round, and undifferentiated cells. Distinguishing these tumors from lymphomas or round cell sarcomas can be difficult without immunohistochemical analysis.[14] Ductal and small cell tumors tend to metastasize early. Transitional cell carcinoma of the prostate gland tends to be confined to periurethral ducts rather than peripheral sites. Malignant mesenchymal tumors make up less than 0.3% of prostatic neoplasms, of which rhabdomyosarcomas are most common in younger patients, and leiomyosarcomas are most common in older patients. Carcinosarcomas are defined by the coexistence of adenocarcinomas of the epithelial cells along with malignant mesenchymal elements that have differentiated into identifiable chondrosarcoma, osteosarcoma, myosarcoma, liposarcoma, or angiosarcoma.[20] They are highly resistant to therapy. Metastatic tumors to the prostate include lymphomas, leukemias, adenocarcinomas of the lung, melanoma, seminoma, and malignant rhabdoid tumors, whereas tumors of the bladder and colon may sometimes involve the gland by direct extension.

MOLECULAR PATHOGENESIS

Prostate cancers develop from the accumulation of genetic alterations that result in an increase in cell proliferation relative to cell death, arrest differentiation, and confer the ability to invade, metastasize, and proliferate in a distant site. Histologic changes are present in the prostates of men in their 20s, yet the diagnosis is typically made 3 to 4 decades later, which suggests that the development of the disease is a multistep process.[21] The alterations include somatic point mutations, gene

deletions, amplifications, chromosomal rearrangements, and changes in DNA methylation.[22] It is believed that the accumulation of changes acting synergistically is more critical than the order in which the alterations occur. Identifying and understanding the events has implications for control of the disease at the earliest stages of transformation, for progression as an invasive tumor, for prognostication, and for points of therapeutic attack. Men who are castrated or who become hypopituitary before the age of 40 years rarely develop prostate cancer.[23] The evolution of the tumor is influenced by hormonal factors; it is also influenced by environmental, infectious/inflammatory factors, and, given the long history once the diagnosis is established, the specific therapy(ies) used to treat the disease.

The phenotypic alterations that occur during prostate carcinogenesis and progression are shown in Figure 30.3-5. The alterations include a reduction in defense against carcinogen-induced damage, inflammation, and changes in androgen signalling and changes in growth-regulatory genes that contribute to cell proliferation, survival, and spread. The earliest precursor lesion is the subject of debate, as is the cell type that is actually transformed. Histologic changes begin with proliferation within ducts termed *prostatic intraepithelial neoplasia* adjacent to areas of proliferative inflammatory atrophy (PIA), followed by loss of the basal cell layer in prostatic glands, the development of an anaplastic morphology with nuclear pleomorphism and prominent nucleoli, invasion of the basement membrane, overt invasion, and metastatic spread. PIA refers to focal areas of atrophy that occur primarily in the peripheral lobe, adjacent to areas of PIN, which contain proliferative epithelial cells that do not fully differentiate (Fig. 30.3-6).[25] PIN is defined by the presence of cytologically atypical or dysplastic epithelial cells within architecturally benign-appearing glands and acini and is subdivided into low and high grade. PIA and PIN are often associated with chronic inflammation.[25] Only high-grade PIN is considered a precursor for some invasive carcinomas,[24,26] because it develops preferentially in the peripheral zone in which most cancers originate and it precedes the development of cancer by 10 years or more,[27] and prostates with extensive PIN tend to have multifocal tumors. Not all lesions progress to invasive prostatic cancer during the lifetime of the host. Atypical adenomatous hyperplasias are not considered malignant precursor lesions, although some have proposed that they may be precursors of transition zone cancers.[28]

BIOLOGIC CHARACTERIZATION

Neoplastic growth is the result of genetic, hormonal, environmental, and possibly infectious factors that modulate the expression of specific genes. The normal mutation frequency of DNA (1×10^{-10}) is too low to produce significant changes in overall gene expression, and it is now believed that tumor cells themselves have an inherent genetic instability that results in the coexistence of multiple genetically related, yet distinct, clones within a tumor mass.[29] Clones with a survival advantage continue to proliferate, whereas those that acquire changes that reduce viability undergo cell death.

The molecular genetic changes within specific tumors are being studied with a variety of techniques, each of which has limitations. One difficulty is that areas of cancer are difficult to distinguish on gross section from surrounding normal tissue, and the tumors themselves are heterogeneous histologically at

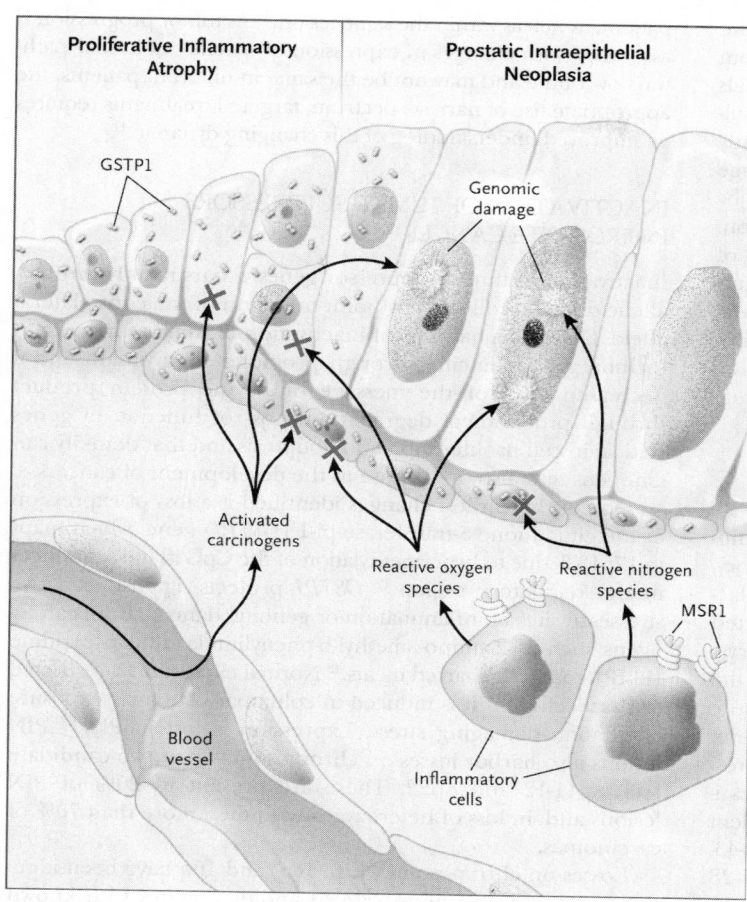

FIGURE 30.3-5. Phenotypic alterations during prostate carcinogenesis and progression. GSTP1, glutathione S-transferase pi-1; MSR1, macrophage-scavenger receptor 1. (From ref. 22, with permission.) (See Color Fig. 30.3-5 in the CD-ROM.)

the microscopic level. Most lesions also contain at least some areas of acinar/terminal duct differentiation. Classic cytogenetics is limited by the low mitotic rate of prostate cancers and the need to grow the cells in culture. Interphase fluorescence *in situ* hybridization (FISH) offers the advantage of visualizing genetic alterations in paraffin sections but is limited by the number of regions examined and the need to select specific areas of the genome to study. Nevertheless, if FISH analysis shows that cells from the patient's cancer retain both polymorphic alleles of the informative gene, then no loss of heterozygosity has occurred at that particular chromosomal region. The absence of one or both of the alleles suggests heterozygous or homozygous deletion. A difficulty is that samples rich in stroma or other normal cell populations, or both, can obscure the evidence of deletion. Comparative genomic hybridization

offers a view of losses or gain, or both, across the entire genome through a single hybridization. Using this technique, clonal cytogenetic abnormalities have been found in 25% (range, 16% to 50%) of primary tumors, whereas FISH on interphase nuclei showed changes in DNA copy number in up to 70% of primary lesions. High throughput technologies, which allow the study of multiple genes and pathways, shift the focus from single determinants to multiple markers, from single pathways to networks, and from a diagnosis-based strategy to defined molecular signatures specific to distinct disease states. These approaches represent a change in paradigm for tumor markers, because they can better interrogate the complexity of the processes under analysis.

Molecular genetic results must also be evaluated in the context of the tissue evaluated. Different results may be obtained

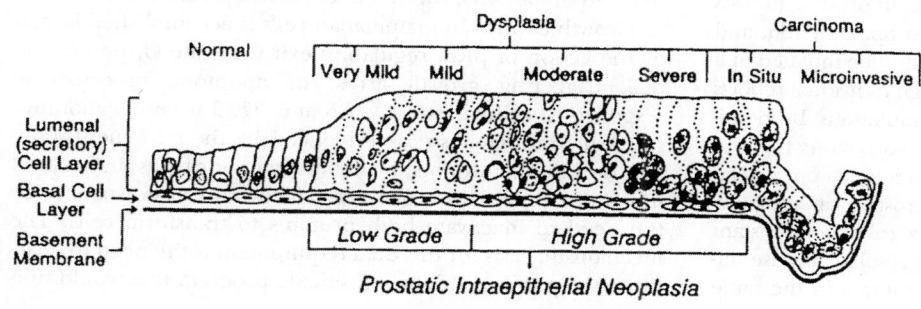

FIGURE 30.3-6. Evolution of invasive cancer from prostatic intraepithelial neoplasia, dysplasia, and normal epithelial cells. (From ref. 24, with permission.)

from primary versus metastatic and noncastrate versus castrate lesions; a larger number of alterations are found in lesions from the later states of the illness. In most cases, archival materials obtained from prostates removed by radical surgery are available. For studies on carcinogenesis, microdissection is frequently used to obtain tumor cell–enriched populations from early-stage PIN lesions. Metastatic disease is most frequently represented by lymph nodes removed at the time of surgical exploration. Depending on the question, they may not be representative of metastases from bone or visceral sites. In 2000, several groups initiated studies of tumors obtained immediately postmortem from patients with castration-resistant disease.[30] The profiles developed have been used to understand the mechanisms associated with disease development and progression, to refine prognostic assessments, and to select therapy.

GENETIC SUSCEPTIBILITY

Evidence for a genetic susceptibility is derived from epidemiologic studies showing that, relative to men with no family history, the lifetime risk of developing prostate cancer increases by factors of 2, 5, and 11 by the presence of one, two, or three affected family members.[31] Further support is provided by the observation that a monozygotic twin with prostate cancer increases the risk more than a dizygotic twin with the disease.[32] Although there is evidence of autosomal dominant and X-linked inheritance in some families, there is no cancer syndrome that includes prostate cancer. Based on family linkage analysis, eight prostate cancer susceptibility loci have been reported by independent groups: 1p36 (*CAPB*), 1p13 (*HSD3B*), 1q24-25 (HPC1), 1q42.2-43, 16q23, 17p (*HPC2/ELAC2*), 20q13 (*HPC20*), and Xq27-28 (*HPCX*).[33–35] Several interesting candidate genes emerged from these and other analyses. *HPC2/ELAC* encodes a metal-dependent hydrolase. *RNASEL*, which is linked to *HPC1*, encodes a ribonuclease that degrades viral and cellular RNA and can induce apoptosis on viral infection.[34] The macrophage-scavenger receptor 1 (*MSR1*) on 8p22 encodes a receptor responsible for cellular uptake of bacterial lipopolysaccharides and other toxins on macrophages found at sites of inflammation in the prostate.[36] Last, *SRD5A2* on 2p23 encodes the predominant prostatic isozyme of 5α-reductase, which converts testosterone to dihydrotestosterone (DHT). Despite these reports, no major susceptibility gene of clinical significance has been identified.[15]

SOMATIC CHANGES

As noted, somatic alterations can accumulate over several decades before prostate cancer appears.[37] Overall, losses of genetic material are five times more frequent than gains, implying that the loss of suppressor function may be most contributory to the malignant phenotype.[38] The most common abnormalities in prostate tumors are gains at 7p, 7q, 8q, and Xq and losses at 8p, 10q, 13q, and 16q.[15,38,39] Some of these loci have been found to be mutated in a large percentage of tumor specimens, although individual reports vary on the nature and frequency of specific mutations. By identifying changes in tumors of defined states and correlating them to the functions of known genes in the mutated region, a profile can be made of the changes that contribute to prostate carcinogenesis, progression, metastasis, and growth as a castration-resistant tumor. Caution is advised when generalizing results, because different profiles can be observed in separate tumors in the same

patient, as well as within the same lesion.[40] As tumor progression is associated with changes in expression of specific molecular pathways over time and may not be the same in different patients, the appropriate use of narrow-spectrum, targeted treatments requires an improved understanding of this changing dynamic.[41]

INACTIVATION OF TUMOR SUPPRESSORS IN PROSTATE CANCER

Inactivation of tumor suppressor genes occurs mainly through allelic deletion followed by point mutation of the contralateral allele. Other mechanisms of inactivation of tumor suppression include gene silencing through promoter methylation and a decreased level of the message or of the protein product through proteasomal degradation. Loss of function of genes critical in cell proliferation and apoptosis and that detoxify carcinogens may also predispose to the development of cancers.

One of the earliest changes identified is a loss of expression of the glutathione S-transferase pi-1 (*GSTP1*) gene, which maps to 17p13.3, due to hypermethylation of the CpG island sequences in the regulatory region.[42] *GSTP1* protects against oxidative stresses at sites of inflammation or genome damage from carcinogens such as 2-amino-l-methyl-6-phenylimidazo[4,5-6]pyridine (PhIP), found in charred meats.[43] Normal expression is restricted to basal cells, but it is induced in columnar cells after exposure to genome-damaging stress. Expression is lost in PIN.[44] PIN lesions also harbor losses on chromosome 8p at two candidate loci, 8p11-12 and 8p22. These are present in 20% of PIN lesions and, in loss of heterozygosity studies, more than 70% of carcinomas.

Losses on chromosomes 17p, 10q, and 16q have been identified in localized tumors.[38,44,45] Candidate genes with known critical functions found to be altered at a higher frequency in later relative to early states include *TP53* (17p13), *PTEN* (10q23), and the AR gene (Xq11-13). The retinoblastoma (*RB*) gene has also been implicated; pRB (retinoblastoma protein) suppresses cell division by preventing cells in the G$_1$ phase from entering the S phase. Evidence includes abnormal *RB* reported in a prostate cancer cell line, DU145, and the loss or reduction of expression in tumor samples. In addition, chromosomal losses at the *RB* locus (13q14) have been reported in 60% of primary tumors.[46]

The *TP53* gene codes for a nuclear phosphoprotein—p53—that activates apoptosis and cell-cycle arrest, among other processes. *TP53* mutations usually result in aberrant p53 products with an enhanced half-life, which in turn can be visualized by immunohistochemical assays as nuclear staining patterns. *TP53* mutations and altered p53 expression have been detected at a higher frequency in metastatic versus primary disease[40] and have been shown to be an independent prognostic marker for reduced disease-free survival after radical prostatectomy.

Growth control in mammalian cells is accomplished largely by the action of pRB, regulating exit from the G$_1$ phase, and p53, triggering growth arrest or apoptotic processes in response to cellular stress.[47] *RB* and *TP53* have collaborative roles in tumorigenesis, as evidenced by their frequent alterations in human tumors, by the many tumor types that exhibit mutations in both genes and, in oncoviral transformation, by the need to inactivate both proteins to transform cells. The mechanistic basis for this dual requirement is the need to deactivate the p53-dependent cell suicide program that would normally be brought about as a response to unchecked cellular proliferation resulting from pRB deficiency. These issues have important clinical implications, because unchecked proliferation and the failure to arrest growth or induce apoptosis contribute both to the growth advantages and the failure to respond to treatments that are hallmarks of cancer.

Cyclin-dependent kinase (CDK) inhibitors are negative regulators of cell-cycle transitions.[47] These proteins are grouped into two families, KIPs (kinase inhibitory proteins) and INKs (inhibitors of kinases), based on sequence homology and functional similarity. KIPs include p21/WAF1, p27/KIP1, and p57/KIP2; they form complexes with early cyclin-CDK subunits. INKs, including p16/INK4A, p15/INK4B, p18/INK4C, and p19/INK4D, form complexes only with D-type cyclins and CDK4. Normal prostate has abundant p27 and p27 transcripts in both epithelial and stromal cells. However, p27 protein and transcripts are almost undetectable in epithelial and stromal cells of BPH lesions. Prostatic carcinomas may contain high levels of p27 or low to undetectable levels,[48,49] and primary prostatic carcinomas displaying less p27 expression were found to be biologically more aggressive, based on their association with time to PSA failure after radical prostatectomy. The expression of p16 was undetectable in normal and benign hyperplastic tissues. However, p16 overexpression was observed in approximately 40% of prostate carcinomas.[50] Overexpression of p16 protein was found to correlate with increased p16 transcripts, and it appears to be linked to inactivation of *RB* and with a higher pretreatment PSA level, the use of neoadjuvant androgen ablation, and a shorter time to PSA relapse after radical prostatectomy. It has been, thus, concluded that p16 overexpression is associated with tumor recurrence and a poor clinical course for patients with prostate cancer.[50]

The *PTEN* (phosphatase and tensin homologue deleted from chromosome 10) tumor suppressor gene encodes a dual specificity phosphatase.[51] Loss of the 10q chromosomal region, which contains *PTEN*, is a common finding even in PIN and primary prostate cancer.[51,52] Moreover, it has been reported that 70% of primary tumors show loss or alteration of at least one *PTEN* allele, supporting the evidence for *PTEN* involvement in prostate tumor progression. Phosphatidylinositol 3,4,5-triphosphate (PIP_3), the product of phosphatidylinositol 3 kinase (PI3K) activity, is the main PTEN substrate. PTEN thus keeps levels of PIP_3 low. Accumulation of PIP_3 at the membrane allows recruitment and activation of the serine/threonine kinase Akt, a product of a protooncogene. Activated Akt is a well-established survival factor exerting antiapoptotic activity. Loss of *PTEN* function results in an increased concentration of PIP_3 and in Akt hyperactivation, leading to protection from various apoptotic stimuli and decreased levels of p27.[53]

METASTASES

Loss of genes that affect normal cell adhesion promotes detachment and can also serve to activate genes that promote invasion into the basement membrane, necessary for metastatic spread, and into blood vessels.[54] The long arm of chromosome 16 (i.e., 16q22.1) is deleted in 30% of primary and more than 70% of metastatic prostate cancer cells. This region contains the gene for E-cadherin, a Ca^{2+}-dependent cell surface glycoprotein that functions as an epithelial cell–cell adhesion molecule.[55] It is involved in the tight association between normal prostatic glandular cells. A correlation between decreased E-cadherin expres-

sion and metastatic progression has been demonstrated, making it a strong candidate for a "metastatic suppressor."[55] *Carcinoembryonic antigen–like cell adhesion molecule 1* expression is decreased in BPH and cancer. This gene, which maps to 9q13, encodes a cell adhesion molecule that promotes contact inhibition of growth.

ACTIVATION OF ONCOGENES IN PROSTATE CANCER

Activation of protooncogenes by point mutation, amplification, translocation, or insertion of noneukaryotic sequences, results in a "gain" of function. More than 70 oncogenes have been identified as participating in cellular proliferation, differentiation, senescence, and apoptosis. The normal functions can be classified into broad groups, such as growth factors and their receptors (e.g., *EGF-EGFR*), signal transducers (e.g., *ras*), and nuclear protooncogenes (e.g., AR).

Overexpression of certain growth factors, such as epidermal growth factor (EGF), basic fibroblast growth factor, and platelet-derived growth factor (PDGF), has been reported to be involved in prostate cancer as autocrine and paracrine signaling loops together with their corresponding receptors (EGFR, fibroblast growth factor receptor, and PDGFR, respectively).[56-58] The insulin-like growth factor-1 and -2 (IGF-1, IGF-2), and transforming growth factor-α and -β (TGF-α, TGF-β) and their receptors (IGFR and TGFR, respectively) have also been implicated.[59,60] IGFs are potent mitogens for human prostate cancer cells and osteoblasts via interaction with IGF receptors. Elevated levels of serum IGF-binding proteins have been reported in metastatic human prostate cancer. HER-2/neu protein is a transmembrane tyrosine kinase receptor with strong homology to EGFR. Amplification of the *HER-2/neu* gene and overexpression of the protein have prognostic significance in breast cancer and are used to select therapy. *HER-2/neu* amplification in prostate cancer is uncommon. Nevertheless, increased HER2/neu protein was found in 20% of untreated hormone-naive primary tumors, whereas overexpression was observed in 80% of metastatic cases and more than 60% of primary tumors surviving after androgen ablation. Investigators have also reported that HER2/neu overexpression is significantly associated with time to PSA relapse[61,62] and that HER2 can activate AR independent of ligand.[63] *c-myc*, also on 8p, is another candidate for amplification, and high levels have been correlated with castration-resistant disease.[64]

Another critical program dysregulated in prostate cancer is the cell cycle. The major positive regulators of cell-cycle transitions are a group of heterodimeric protein kinases comprising a cyclin as a regulatory element and a catalytic subunit known as *cyclin-dependent kinase*.[47] Cyclin D1 is a key regulator of the G_1/S phase progression of the cell cycle, acting with CDK4 to phosphorylate and inactivate pRB. Increasing evidence implicates deregulated cyclin D1 expression in the evolution of castration-resistant lesions. A cyclin D1–positive phenotype, defined as identification of positive immunoreactivity in the nuclei of 20% or more of tumor cells, was observed in approximately 10% of primary prostate carcinomas, and more than 60% of castration-resistant lesions in bone.[65]

CELL SURVIVAL PATHWAYS

Telomerase is an enzyme that prevents the normal shortening of telomeres as cells age. Increased expression has been detected in 25% of PIN lesions and in 85% of prostate cancers.[66] Telomerase expression is reduced with successful differentiation of a cell. PIN lesions also exhibit overexpression of the BCL-2 protein (18q21) and multiple copies of *c-myc*.[67] The frequency of mutations in the *ras* family of oncogenes (i.e., H-, K-, and N-*ras*) is very low in patients with localized disease. However, expression of a mutated H-*ras* oncogene in prostatic cancer cells increases genetic instability and facilitates the acquisition of a metastatic phenotype.[64] Inhibiting wild-type ras proteins can slow growth.[68]

ANGIOGENESIS

Recent studies have demonstrated that the intensity of angiogenesis within an individual tumor can predict the probability of metastasis for several human cancers, including prostatic cancer.[69] Angiogenic ability appears first in a subset of hyperplastic lesions before the onset of tumor formation. Thus, hyperplasia per se does not require angiogenesis. The microvessel density (a measure of tumor angiogenesis) is lower in histologically detected prostate cancers than in clinically manifest tumors. Normal stroma has a lower microvessel density than tumor-involved stroma. Angiogenesis is greatest in poorly differentiated prostate carcinomas, suggesting that the switch to a highly angiogenic phenotype occurs when relatively well-differentiated tumors progress to poorly differentiated tumors. Within the subset of poorly differentiated cancers, there is a significant difference in vascularity between organ-confined and metastatic cancer. Poorly differentiated histology alone is not sufficient for metastases to occur.[70]

CASTRATION RESISTANCE

The major cause of death from prostate cancer is progressive castration-resistant disease—a tumor that continues to grow despite castrate levels of testosterone. As prostate cancers evolve to castration resistance, PSA synthesis resumes. The current view is that prostatic cancers at the time of diagnosis are composed of cells with three distinct cellular phenotypes: androgen-dependent, androgen-sensitive, and androgen-independent cells. Androgen-dependent cancer cells continuously require a critical level of androgenic stimulation for maintenance and growth (i.e., without adequate androgenic stimulation, these cells die) and, in this regard, are very similar to the androgen-dependent nonneoplastic cells of the normal prostate. The growth of androgen-sensitive cancer cells slows when androgens are withdrawn and they become dormant. They do not die. In contrast, the growth of androgen-independent cells does not change after androgen deprivation, no matter how complete; these cells are completely free of androgenic effects on growth.[71,72] In contrast to what can be accomplished *in vitro* using charcoal-stripped serum to eliminate androgens completely, *in vivo* it is virtually impossible to eliminate all androgens completely.

How do resistant tumor cells emerge during androgen ablation therapy? Some researchers theorize that *selection* of intrinsically resistant cells occurs, whereas others suggest that, under the pressure of androgen-ablative therapies, cells that were sensitive only to the point at which growth was slowed without cell death *adapt* to the low androgen environment and, over time, acquire additional somatic changes that result in tumor regrowth.[73–75] Clinically, selection of resistant or insensitive cells may be more relevant immediately after androgen withdrawal and adaptation more important later. The observation that basal epithelial cells preferentially survive androgen ablation (in contrast to secretory epithelial cells) demonstrates that intrinsically resistant cells do exist even in the normal prostate gland, in line with the selection hypothesis. This is consistent with the theorized role of basal cells as the stem cells for the prostatic epithelium.[76–78] Unknown is whether the first transformed cell that ultimately develops into the self-renewing stem cell of a prostate cancer is dependent, sensitive, or insensitive to androgens. It is also difficult to determine whether the resistant/surviving cell population has a more basal or stem cell genotype, or a basal or a more differentiated cell that has been transformed. That hormonal ablation alone cannot eradicate the disease completely in either the primary site or in a metastatic focus suggests an intrinsic resistance and, at best, partial androgen sensitivity. Many pathways associated with resistance involve inhibition of proapoptotic molecules or the up-regulation of cell-survival molecules.

The AR is a member of a super-family of ligand-dependent transcription factors. The *AR* gene is located on chromosome Xq11-13 and spans eight exons, whereas the AR protein has three functional domains: a large, highly variable amino-terminal domain (NTD) encoded entirely by exon 1 that contains two regions with strong transactivation functions, AF-1 and AF-5; a DNA-binding domain encoded by exons 2 and 3; and a carboxy-terminal ligand-binding domain encoded by exons 4 through 8 that contains a highly conserved ligand-dependent transactivation function (AF-2).[79] Binding of high-affinity ligands induces conformational changes that lead to the recruitment of coregulator proteins: coactivators that enhance or corepressors that repress AR function. The N-terminal domain contains a glutamine-rich segment and a proline-rich segment, believed to play a role in transcriptional regulation. The former is coded by trinucleotide microsatellites called CAG repeats.[80] Higher numbers of repeats are associated with a decrease in transactivation activity. The average CAG repeat number among African American (20.1), white (22), and Asian American (22.4) populations in the United States is inversely proportional to risk, with African Americans having the highest risk, suggesting that repeat number and risk are linked.[81,82] Specific AR variants may prevent carcinogenesis in Japanese men by diminishing AR function.

Alterations in AR signaling that have been identified in human prostate cancer include alterations in steroid metabolism, an increase in the level of the protein, changes in coregulator profiles, and ligand-independent activation (Fig. 30.3-7). Changes in AR occur as the disease progresses from a clinically localized lesion in a noncastrate environment to a castrate metastatic lesion.[83–85] All of these mechanisms are consistent with continued signaling through the receptor in castration-resistant lesions.

STEROID METABOLISM

Among the genes up-regulated in castration-resistant tumors are several genes corresponding to enzymes in the steroid precursor synthesis pathway. These include 3-hydroxy-3-methylglutaryl-coenzyme A synthase 1 and squalene epoxidase, which are considered rate limiting in sterol synthesis.[86] Increased levels of androgenic steroids, combined with an increase in the amount of receptor protein (see Receptor Level), could contribute to maintenance of AR signaling despite castrate levels of testosterone in the blood. A recent study using laser capture mass spec-

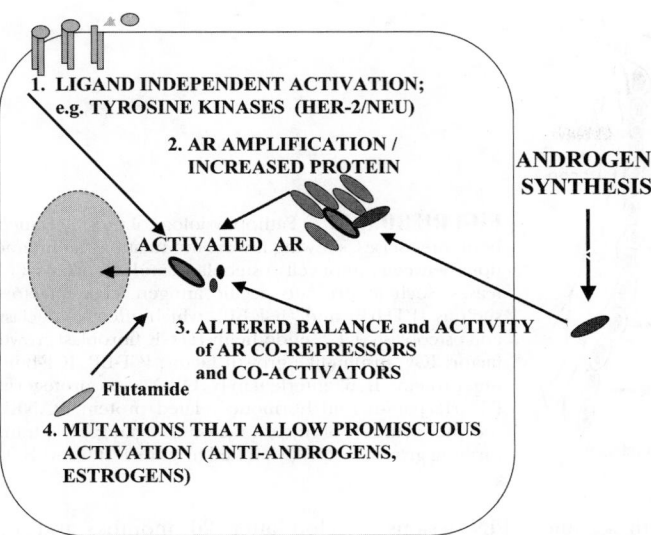

FIGURE 30.3-7. Alterations in androgen receptor (AR) signaling. (From ref. 41, with permission.) (See Color Fig. 30.3-7 in the CD-ROM.)

trometry documented levels of androgenic steroids in tumors from men with progressive disease after hormonal therapy that were sufficient to induce signaling.[87]

RECEPTOR LEVEL

The AR protein is expressed in prostate cancers of all clinical states. In upwards of 30% of cases, levels are higher in castration-resistant as opposed to noncastrate tumors.[88–90] Amplification of the *AR* gene itself has also been reported in approximately 22% of castration-resistant metastases[91] and in 23% to 28% of recurrent primary tumors and is associated with increased levels of the AR and the proteins it regulates.[92,93]

MUTATIONS IN THE ANDROGEN RECEPTOR

The most common mutations in the AR that have been identified in clinical specimens are in the ligand-binding domain. Virtually all are associated with a gain of function, as opposed to the loss of function mutations, which are most common among patients with androgen-insensitivity syndromes. Most disrupt a protein–protein interaction surface and result in an increase in the transactivation activity of the receptor in response to a range of classical and nonclassical ligands.[94] Less frequently, mutations in the amino-terminal transactivation domain are found. These tend to affect receptor structure or transactivation function. Alterations in the AF-5 domain, for example, affect the interaction of the amino- and carboxy-terminal regions and the stability of the receptor. The AF-5 region is also the site where a number of AR coactivators and corepressors interact and has been implicated in ligand-independent activation of the AR by HER-2/neu signaling through mitogen-activated protein kinase.[95]

ALTERED PROFILE OF ANDROGEN RECEPTOR COREGULATORS

A change in the ratio of AR coactivators to corepressors can alter AR transactivation activity in the presence of low concen-

trations of DHT or in the absence of circulating native ligand. For example, the coactivators ARA54, ARA55, and ARA70 can selectively enhance the ability of 17β-estradiol, hydroxyflutamide, and androst-5-ene-3β,17β-diol, a precursor to testosterone, to activate the AR.[79] Conversely, the corepressors SMRT and NCoR can inhibit AR function in a ligand-dependent manner. Overexpression of the p160 coactivators, as observed in castration-resistant tumors and CWR22 xenografts, increases AR transactivation activity at physiologic levels of nonclassic ligands, such as estradiol, progesterone, and adrenal androgens.[96] These findings may explain, in part, the agonist effects of antiandrogens and other steroid hormones and the response to their discontinuation in patients with castration-resistant tumors.

LIGAND-INDEPENDENT ACTIVATION OF THE ANDROGEN RECEPTOR

In addition to steroid hormones, growth factors, such as keratinocyte growth factor, IGF-1, and EGF; HER2; and cytokines, such as interleukin-6 (IL-6), can activate the AR independent of ligand.[63,97,98] Exactly how these factors activate signaling is an area of active study. This can also contribute to progression in castration-resistant disease.

Inhibitors of apoptosis are also implicated in the acquisition of the castration-resistant phenotype. Blocking cell death pathways that are normally induced by androgen ablation allows cells to survive. BCL-2, which inhibits the death of cancer cells without affecting their rate of proliferation, is essentially undetectable in most noncastrate lesions but is highly expressed in castration-resistant disease.[99] Similarly, survivin, a member of the class of proteins called *inhibitors of apoptosis*, is highly expressed in benign and malignant prostate neuroendocrine cells.[100] Survivin functions to inhibit effector caspases.

BONE METASTASIS

Prostate cancer cells that have gained access to the circulation have a unique predilection for bone. The establishment of a metastatic focus in bone involves multiple steps, including adhesion of the tumor cells to endothelial cells in the marrow and migration through fenestrations in the endothelial cell layer. This migration is driven, in part, by a chemoattractant gradient of marrow- and stromal-derived growth factors. Once established, tumor cells and marrow-derived cells develop a bidirectional interaction that protects the epithelial cells and promotes tumor cell survival and proliferation.[101]

Radiographically, metastatic prostate cancers are primarily osteoblastic. Osteoclast stimulation and activation are, however, still present at a histologic level. Indeed, increased levels of markers of bone turnover, such as N-telopeptide and NTX, can be detected in the blood and urine of patients with progressing disease.[102] Thus, the normal bone remodeling process is not uncoupled; rather, there is a shift in the balance in favor of bone growth. It is hypothesized that the resorptive process itself, under the direction of osteoclasts, promotes the release of factors that amplify the metastatic and invasive process[103–105] (Fig. 30.3-8). The protease action of PSA results in the activation of functional signaling molecules adjacent to tumor that further contribute to tumor cell growth and proliferation. For example, PSA cleavage of IGF, from its binding protein (IGFBP3), increases

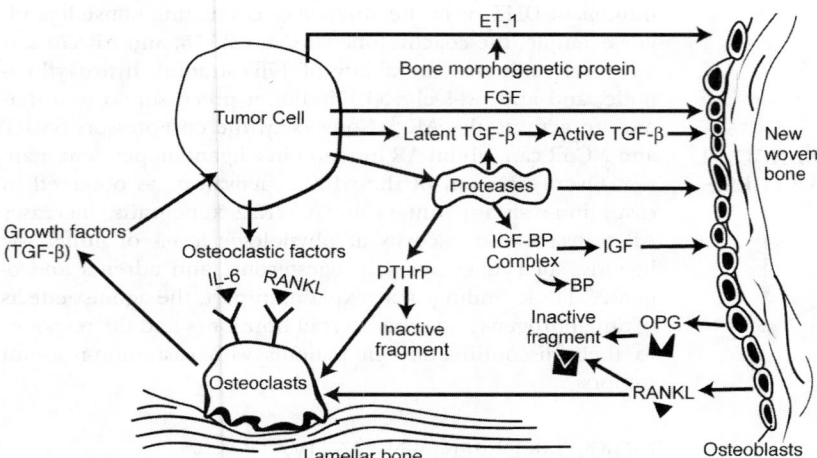

FIGURE 30.3-8.   Pathophysiology of prostate cancer bone metastases, showing factors modulating the interactions between tumor cells, osteoblasts, and osteoclasts. Proteases, such as prostate-specific antigen, cleave factors, such as (PTHrP) and (IGF-BP), which affect osteoclasts and osteoblasts. ET-1, endothelin-1; FGF, fibroblast growth factor; IGF, insulin-like growth factor; IGF-BP, IGF-binding protein; IL-6, interleukin-6; OPG, osteoprotegerin; PTHrP, parathyroid hormone–related protein; RANKL, receptor activator of nuclear factor κB ligand; TGF, transforming growth factor. (Modified from refs. 106 and 109.)

the local levels of a functional prostate cancer mitogen that is normally inactive as a bound complex.[106] PSA can also activate parathyroid hormone–related protein, which inhibits osteoblast apoptosis.[104]

Factors that contribute to cancer growth in bone are broadly divided into osteoblastic and osteolytic factors. Sources include the tumor cells themselves, normal bone cells, and reserves in the bone matrix that are released as part of the remodeling process. Many of the factors contributing to the osteoblastic phenotype, such as endothelin-1 (ET-1)[107] and IL-6 can be targeted directly. ET-1, produced by prostate cells, stimulates the differentiation of osteoblast precursors, decreases osteoclastic bone resorption and motility, and augments the mitogenic effects of IGF-1, IGF-2, and PDGF. In normal bone, osteoblasts regulate osteoclastogenesis by interacting with mononuclear hematopoietic precursors. Osteoblasts express receptor activator of nuclear factor κB ligand (RANKL) and osteoprotegerin. Osteoprotegerin level increases in patients with bone metastases.[108] IL-6 is another cytokine released by prostate cancer cells that contributes to increased bone resorption.[109] Binding of RANKL to RANK on osteoclastic precursors initiates intracellular signals that activate an osteoclastic phenotype. Osteoprotegerin regulates bone resorption by acting as a decoy receptor for RANKL; it also inhibits tumor necrosis factor–related apoptosis–inducing ligand–mediated apoptosis.[110]

MODELS OF PROSTATE CANCER

Mouse models are of primary importance in understanding cancer biology and developing novel therapies. Certain mouse models with knockouts of tumor suppressor genes, especially prostate-specific knockouts, have revealed their parallelism to human prostate cancer pathogenesis and progression. Among the most commonly used transgenic models of prostate cancer are the TRAMP series (transgenic adenocarcinoma of the mouse prostate) in which Simian virus 40 (SV40) large T and small t antigens are expressed under control of the rat probasin promoter.[111] Overexpression of the SV40 oncogene inactivates critical proteins, such as p53 and pRB, in the prostate. In the TRAMP model, PIN lesions are produced in less than 12 weeks after birth, and metastatic lesions develop at approximately 30 months. Another early model using SV40 is the so-called LADY, which expresses only the large T antigen under the control of the probasin promoter. In

these mice, PIN lesions develop after 20 months, and no metastases are identified. Other models, such as those using *c-myc* under control of a modified C3(1) promoter[112] and a knockout of *Mxi1*, produced subtle phenotypes with hyperplastic glands with signs of dysplasia. Similarly, driving *AR* expression in the prostate by the use of probasin promoter produces hyperplasia at approximately 1 year of age, and PIN was observed in some older mice. The p27 knockout produced hyperplastic glands with a certain degree of dysplasia but no tumors.[48]

The specific localization of the neoplastic lesion in the mouse prostate is important because not all of the lobes of this organ have an analogous counterpart in the human gland. For example, the mouse ventral lobe has no analogous structure in the human prostate, whereas the dorsolateral lobe corresponds to the peripheral zone in the human gland. The peripheral zone is the area undergoing transformation in approximately 80% of human prostate cancers. An important result was seen in Pten[+/−] mice: The dorsolateral prostate was involved with PIN and prostatic carcinomas in 100% of cases, as observed in human prostate cancers.[113,114] Thus, *Pten*[+/−] mice represent a faithful model in which loss of a gene relevant for human prostate cancer pathogenesis results in tumors with features recapitulating, in part, the development of human prostate lesions. Pten[+/−] × p27[−/−] mice developed a more aggressive, locally invasive prostate carcinoma with earlier onset, revealing the negative cooperative effects of these two genes in prostate cancer initiation and progression. To date, metastatic lesions have not been observed.

HIGH-THROUGHPUT TECHNOLOGIES AND PROSTATE CANCER

Microarrays constitute a group of technologies characterized by the ability to measure hundreds or thousands of items (e.g., DNA sequences, RNA transcripts, or proteins) within a single experiment using miniaturized devices.[115,116] Appropriate experimental design and the use of well-characterized *in vitro* and *in vivo* systems, and well-annotated clinical specimens, allow detailed analysis of biologic and clinical phenotypes. Thus, array technologies represent high-throughput means to identify molecular targets associated with these phenotypes by comparing samples representative of distinct disease states. Hybridization-based methods and the microarray format together constitute an extremely versatile platform, allowing both static and dynamic views of DNA structure, as well as RNA and protein expression patterns in cultured cancer cells and tumor tissues. The most widespread use of this technology to date has been the analysis of gene expression. There is an increasingly broad range of additional applications for microarrays, including genotyping polymorphisms and mutations, determining the sites of DNA-binding proteins, and identifying structural alterations using array comparative genome hybridization.

A comprehensive gene expression analysis of prostate cancer using oligonucleotide arrays with 63,175 probe sets was performed to identify genes with strong and uniform differential expression between nonrecurrent primary prostate cancers and metastatic prostate cancers.[86] Many of the differentially expressed genes found in this analysis participate in biologic processes that may contribute to the clinical phenotype. For example, high proliferation rates in metastatic cancers were strongly associated with overexpression of genes that participate in cell-cycle regulation, DNA replication, and DNA repair. Other differentially expressed genes included those involved in transcriptional regulation, signaling, signal transduction, cell structure, and motility. Prostate cancers that were removed after 3 months of androgen deprivation were also studied. In general, these tumors were not proliferating and are presumed to represent the quiescent/dormant lesions that "survive" after androgen withdrawal rather than the proliferating castration-resistant phenotype. In this study, resistance/survival to androgen withdrawal was associated with differential expression of a unique set of genes reflecting mechanisms of AR reactivation. Included was an increase in expression of the AR and key enzymes for steroid biosynthesis, consistent with an increase in sensitivity to and the endogenous synthesis of androgenic hormones. The specific pathways of reactivation provide an opportunity for refining the classification of resistant lesions based on their molecular signature and for more selected targeted treatments.

INITIAL UROLOGIC EVALUATION: NO CANCER DIAGNOSIS

Therapeutic objectives for men with no cancer diagnosis are to detect the disease at an early curable stage and to prevent its development in those men at risk. Two strategies are under evaluation: *primary prevention*, which is the use of drugs, other agents, or dietary alterations to slow the carcinogenic process before invasion and metastasis, and *secondary prevention*, which includes early detection and treatment of the cancer while it is at a curable stage.

At present, prostate cancer accounts for 29% of all male malignancies and 11% of male cancer deaths in North America, making it the most common malignant cancer and second leading cause of cancer death for men (http://www.nci.nih.gov/cancerinfo). Autopsy studies show that histologic prostate cancer occurs at a young age with an approximate 2.4-fold variation in frequency worldwide.[37] In contrast, the incidence of clinically detectable prostate cancer varies by 10.8-fold among different countries.[37,117,118] There are significant ethnic, geographic, and racial differences in incidence and mortality rates.[119]

FAMILY HISTORY

A familial component of prostate cancer risk has been identified. The risk may take two forms—a familial cancer and a less common hereditary prostate cancer. The level of risk when a family member is affected is similar as in breast and prostate cancers. Men with a first-degree relative with prostate cancer have a two- to threefold increased risk, and those with two or more first-degree relatives affected have a 5- to 11-fold increased risk compared to the general population.[120] In addition, a hereditary form of prostate cancer has been characterized.[121] It is associated with early onset of the disease and a Mendelian autosomal dominant inheritance with incomplete penetrance. Overall, hereditary prostate cancer probably accounts for less than 10% of all cases but could account for more than 40% of cases in men younger than 55 years.[122]

ETHNICITY

The incidence and frequency of clinical cancers are similar in most Western countries, with the highest age-adjusted mortality rates in Scandinavia and significantly lower rates in non-Western countries. Uncertain is whether the reason for populations having a higher incidence of clinical cancers is genetic susceptibility or exposure to causative environmental factors. There is evidence for both.

GENETIC FACTORS

The prostate requires androgens to develop. The most active intracellular androgen in the prostate is DHT, which is converted from testosterone by the enzyme 5α-reductase. There has been no consistent association between the levels of individual androgenic hormones and incidence. As noted earlier in Biologic Characterization, one study showed that the incidence of prostate cancer varied inversely with the number of CAG repeats in exon 1 of the AR gene.[123]

RACIAL FACTORS

Black men within the United States have the highest incidence of prostate cancer in the world, with striking differences in mortality relative to white men (Fig. 30.3-9). Black men are also diagnosed at a younger age and have higher tumor burdens within each stage category,[125] a twofold higher frequency of metastatic disease at presentation,[126] and lower survival rates.[127] Mortality rates among different ethnic groups and nationalities are also affected by environmental factors.[118] Asians who migrate to the United States have a higher incidence of the disease, which increases with each succeeding generation.[128]

Many epidemiologic studies have shown an association between high-fat intake and breast, colon, and prostate cancer incidence and mortality.[129,130] Higher circulating levels of β-carotene, dependent on vitamin A absorption, appear protective, and diets rich in tomato-based products, which contain high amounts of carotenoids and lycopene, may reduce the risk of prostate cancer.[131] A role for vitamin D was suggested by the decreasing geographic north-to-south incidence paralleling sunlight exposure.[132,133] Vitamin D induces differentiation of prostate cancer cells. Similarly, diets deficient in vitamin E (α-tocopherol) may also increase risk,[134] and dietary supplements of α-tocopherol have been associated with increased lifespan after prostate cancer diagnosis.[135] In a randomized intervention trial, the risk of prostate cancer for men receiving a daily supplement of 200 μg of selenium was one-third of that

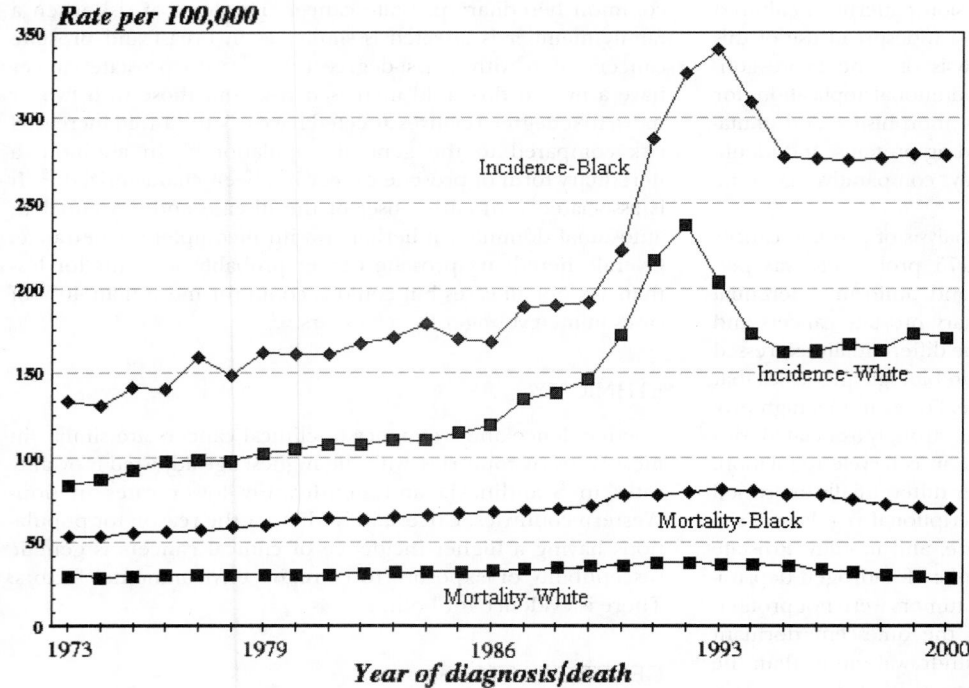

FIGURE 30.3-9. Age-adjusted mortality and incidence rates for prostate cancer by race in the United States, 1973 to 2000. [Data from the Surveillance, Epidemiology, and End Results (SEER) program.[124]]

for men receiving placebo.[136] Cigarette smoking, alcohol use, height, weight, blood group, body hair distribution, and urban versus rural residence do not affect risk.[137] There are no known data to support a viral origin of prostate cancer. Similarly, there is no convincing evidence that a vasectomy places men at increased risk for developing prostate cancer.[138]

PREVENTION

Two issues in chemoprevention trials are which patients to enter and which end points to use. Urgently needed are biomarkers to define an individual patient's risk for developing prostate cancer, to detect early premalignant lesions, to determine their risk of progression and whether they are reversible, and to monitor treatment effects. Patient groups for study can be considered on the basis of pathologic features. It is known from autopsy studies that PIN precedes the development of carcinoma by 10 years or more, and 50% of patients with high-grade PIN in a needle-biopsy specimen develop invasive tumors within 5 years, compared to 10% to 15% of control subjects (see Fig. 30.3-6).[24] Monitoring changes in PIN by serial biopsy is not possible technically, and, even if it was, the clinical significance of decreasing the number of PIN lesions is unknown. As such, most trials use the end point of clinical cancer on follow-up biopsy obtained at fixed intervals after an intervention. Another strategy is to study the pathologic effects of the agent on the prostates and prostate cancers of patients scheduled to undergo radical surgery.[139,140] This provides the entire gland for evaluation and the opportunity to evaluate molecular genetic events as well as histologic factors. Unknown at this point is whether an effect that is measured before surgery after short-term exposure will ultimately translate into a therapeutic effect in the long term. Studies in each risk group are important, as the mechanisms that underlie disease development and progression may be unique.[141] The difficulties

in designing chemoprevention trials are readily apparent when one considers the number of patients that must be enrolled and followed over the long term. An additional consideration is what preliminary data should be required to justify the testing of a particular strategy. Unfortunately, even in cases in which the study is completed, the results may be difficult to interpret.

Diet, dietary supplements, and activity level are the only risk factors that can be manipulated to prevent prostate cancer. The rationale for testing a low-fat diet was related in part to epidemiologic studies and studies of animals harboring prostate cancers fed on isocaloric diets that differed in fat content.[142] A study of men randomized to a low-fat; high-fruit, -vegetable, and -fiber diet as part of a colonic polyp prevention study showed no effect on PSA or overall incidence of prostate cancer during the observation period of the study.[143] Despite this finding, recommending a low-fat diet is reasonable pending more information about specific dietary components. There is insufficient information about the role of micronutrients in the etiology or prevention of the disease to make sound recommendations.

An important confounder is the potential contamination of the "control" group. It is possible, for example, for patients randomized to a "control" group to change their diets or to obtain interventions that are readily available, such as selenium or vitamin E, outside of the study. It is also important to be aware of and monitor the use of complementary and alternative medicines that a patient may be taking. Estimates are that between 30% and 70% of patients with cancer use some form of complementary and alternative medicine, including vitamins in 34% and herbal medicines in 13%.[144] Worse is that in one study, only 33% voluntarily reported the information, when on close questioning upwards of 80% were in fact taking them. These too may confound the results in either a favorable or unfavorable way.

TABLE 30.3-2. Possible Chemopreventive Agents for Prostate Cancer

Agent	Comments
Retinoids	Natural and synthetic analogues of vitamin A; these bind to specific nuclear receptors, regulate various biologic activities, and inhibit carcinogenesis in animal models
Finasteride	5α-Reductase inhibitor; blocks intracellular conversion of testosterone to dihydrotestosterone; ongoing Prostate Cancer Prevention Trial assesses the chemopreventive potential of this agent
Vitamin D	Reduced exposure to sunshine and low levels of vitamin D are associated with increased risk; newer analogues of vitamin D_3 that do not induce hypercalcemia may be useful chemopreventive agents
Vitamin E	Vitamin E intake may reduce the risk of prostate cancer
Selenium	Men with prostate cancer have a reduced level of selenium; dietary selenium supplements associated with reduced prostate cancer incidence

(From ref. 8, with permission.)

Current chemopreventive efforts are focused on natural and synthetic chemical agents.[145] Among the agents showing promise are finasteride, vitamin E, and selenium (Table 30.3-2). The first major clinical trial specifically designed to test whether a systemic agent could prevent prostate cancer was the Prostate Cancer Prevention Trial, a double-blind, randomized, multicenter trial that investigated the ability of finasteride, a 5α-reductase inhibitor, to prevent the development of prostate cancer in men age 55 years and older. The trial showed a 25% reduction in the rate of cancer for men on finasteride, from 24.4% to 18.6%. The benefits were confounded by the extraordinarily high rate of cancer in the control group and the absolute increase in the rate of development of high-grade (Gleason 7 through 10) cancers in the treated group or in both groups.[146] As of 2004, one cannot recommend finasteride for the prevention of prostate cancer until further analysis of this trial or other studies alleviates the concerns that cancers prevented with finasteride posed no significant risk, and growth of high-grade, potentially lethal cancers is not facilitated by the drug.[147] Nevertheless, this trial clearly showed that a widely used and safe drug, acting through the androgen axis, had a profound effect on prostate cancer, a finding that raises hope that chemoprevention of prostate cancer will eventually prove feasible.

More recent efforts are focused on vitamin E and selenium. Vitamin E, or α-tocopherol, functions as an antioxidant and can modulate AR expression. Interest as a potential chemoprevention agent in prostate cancer was derived from the Alpha Tocopherol, Beta Carotene cancer prevention study (ATBC) in which more than 29,000 male smokers were randomized to vitamin E or β-carotene. The results showed an increased incidence of lung cancer and 32% reduction in prostate cancer incidence with 41% decrease in mortality.[135] The effect may be limited to smokers, as the United States Health Professionals Follow up Study not only found no association in nonsmokers, but also at 100 IU/d the risk of prostate cancer may have increased. Smokers had a 56% reduction in lethal or advanced cancers.[134] Selenium protects against oxidative stress and promotes DNA repair. Levels in patients depend in part on the soil content of the region in which the foods that are consumed are produced.[148] The recommended daily dose is 70 μg/d. Once

again, the interest in a prostate cancer prevention approach was indirect. The Nutritional Prevention of Cancer Study randomized trial of selenium supplementation for the prevention of nonmelanoma skin cancer recurrence at a dose of 200 μg/d reduced the risk of prostate cancer by 65%.[149] The effect was limited to men with medium to low levels of selenium; men with higher levels had an increased risk. Higher doses are associated with gastrointestinal effects, nail-bed changes, hair loss, fatigue, and neurologic disorders.

In 2001, the largest ever prostate cancer prevention trial SELECT (Selenium and Vitamin E Cancer Prevention Trial) was initiated. The trial is a double-blind, 2×2 factorial study of selenium (200 μg) and vitamin E (400 mg/d) alone and in combination for men with a normal DRE and PSA less than 4 ng/mL for 7 to 12 years. The end point, unlike that of the Prostate Cancer Prevention Trial, is clinical incidence rather than biopsy finding of cancer. SELECT began enrollment in August 2001 and completely accrued 32,400 men as of the spring of 2004—ahead of the planned 5-year accrual period. The study is open to men 55 years and older and to black men 50 years and older and is accruing at more than 400 SELECT sites throughout the United States, Puerto Rico, and Canada.[150]

EARLY DETECTION AND SCREENING

Early detection refers to the use of diagnostic tests for men who seek an evaluation after being informed of the issues surrounding evaluation. *Screening* refers to the use of diagnostic procedures for a general population. Individuals considered for screening include men with enlarged prostates, a family history of prostate cancer, elevated PSA, or urologic symptoms. These men are evaluated to detect the presence of cancer at an early, curable stage. For most men, detection of a curable cancer requires periodic DREs and PSA testing. In 1983, approximately two-thirds of cancers detected were clinically localized, whereas 19% were metastatic at diagnosis (Fig. 30.3-10).[119,151] In 1995, 90% of new cancers were localized, and only 5% were metastatic. In large screening trials, PSA testing nearly doubles the detection rate possible with DRE alone; more than 90% of cancers detected by combined screening are clinically organ confined and 70% pathologically confined.[152,153]

Based on these data, PSA testing was approved by the U.S. Food and Drug Administration for screening and early detection of prostate cancer. Both the American Urological Association and the American Cancer Society recommend that healthy men should be informed of the risks and benefits of screening if they

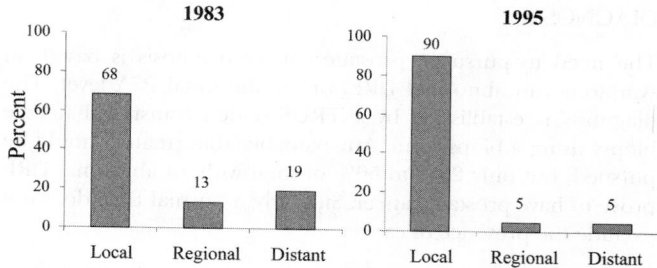

FIGURE 30.3-10. Favorable shift in stage at diagnosis from 1983 to 1995, when prostate-specific antigen testing became widespread in the United States. (Modified from ref. 127.) (See Color Fig. 30.3-10 in the CD-ROM.)

TABLE 30.3-3. Policy on Screening for Prostate Cancer from Major North American Organizations

Organization	Policy
American Cancer Society,[154–157] National Cancer Comprehensive Network,[a] and American Urological Association	DRE and PSA are offered annually, beginning at 50 y, to men who have at least a 10-y life expectancy and to younger men who are in high-risk groups, such as those with a strong familial predisposition (e.g., ≥2 affected first-degree relatives) or African Americans, who may be tested at younger ages (e.g., age 45 y).
American College of Physicians,[155] American Academy of Family Practitioners	
Canadian Preventive Services Task Force[156]	Evidence is insufficient for/against the use of DRE, PSA, and TRUS; these are not recommended for routine screening.
United States Preventive Services Task Force[157]	No current evidence supports annual PSA testing and DRE examinations for asymptomatic men >50 y old, which does not mean that men with possible prostate cancer symptoms should not be tested.

DRE, digital rectal examination; PSA, prostate-specific antigen; TRUS, transrectal ultrasound.
[a]Guidelines, 2004.

TABLE 30.3-4. Clinical Symptoms and Signs of Prostate Cancer

	Symptoms and Signs	
	Common	Uncommon
Local disease	Abnormal digital rectal examination	Rectal obstruction
	Lower urinary tract obstruction	Priapism (corporal body invasion)
	Hematuria	
	Ureteral obstruction	
Distant disease	Bone pain	Neurologic: metastases to brain, cranial nerve, temporal bone, skull base, pituitary
	Neurologic: cord compression	Visceral: lung, liver, stomach, adrenal, gastrointestinal bleeding, testes
		Cutaneous
		Paraneoplastic: Cushing's disease, SIADH, hyper- or hypocalcemia
		Hematologic: disseminated intravascular coagulopathy

SIADH, syndrome of inappropriate secretion of antidiuretic hormone. [Adapted from Davis JW, Schellhammer PF. Prostate cancer: clinical presentation in the 21st century. In: Vogelzang NV, Scardino PT, Shipley WU, et al., eds. *Comprehensive textbook of genitourinary oncology*, 3rd ed. Baltimore: Lippincott Williams & Wilkins, 2005(*in press*).]

are older than 50 years and have a life expectancy of at least 10 years. If they agree, these men should have a DRE and PSA test annually (Table 30.3-3). Those at high risk—black men and men with a family history of the disease—should begin regular examinations earlier, by age 45 years. The National Comprehensive Cancer Network (http://www.nccn.org) concurs with these policies,[158] but the U.S. Preventive Medicine Task Force disagrees.[159]

The success of screening and early detection in reducing mortality from breast and cervical cancer suggests that the same can be achieved with prostate cancer. The dramatic increase in the number of new prostate cases diagnosed between 1981 and 1992 was most likely related to the large pool of men with previously undetected, clinically significant cancers in the population. Since 1992, the age-specific mortality rate has declined by nearly 20%,[160] after rising steadily for decades. Although some attribute this to early detection and screening with PSA,[161] others question the clinical significance of the cancers being detected, because the age-adjusted incidence rate in the United States has risen far faster than the corresponding mortality rate.[159,162] Prospective trials are under way to test this hypothesis with PSA screening showing promising early results.[163]

DIAGNOSIS

The need to pursue a prostate cancer diagnosis is based on symptoms, an abnormal DRE, or an abnormal PSA level. The diagnosis is established by a TRUS-guided transrectal needle biopsy using a biopsy gun. Any palpable abnormality should be pursued, but only 25% to 50% of men with an abnormal DRE prove to have prostate cancer. Similarly, a normal DRE does not exclude the presence of cancer.

Signs and Symptoms

The most common symptom of prostatic disease in men older than 50 years is bladder outlet obstruction, including hesitancy,

nocturia, incomplete emptying, and a diminished urinary stream. Their occurrence, although more commonly related to BPH, should prompt a careful DRE and PSA determination (Table 30.3-4). The sudden development of impotence or hematuria mandates further evaluation. Today, men rarely present with symptoms of metastatic disease, such as bone pain, anemia or pancytopenia from bone marrow replacement, involvement, or disseminated intravascular coagulation.

Digital Rectal Examination

Physical findings are usually limited to the rectal examination. Special attention should be paid to detect areas of induration and to determine whether there is extension laterally to the pelvic sidewall, superiorly to the seminal vesicles, and inferiorly at the apex to the pelvic floor diaphragm. If there is urinary outlet obstruction, the bladder may be palpable. There is subjectivity to this examination, and the findings often correlate poorly with the volume of cancer and disease extent. Nevertheless, the DRE results are an integral part of the algorithms used to determine the probability of whether a tumor is confined to the gland and whether it has spread to regional sites (as discussed in Nomograms Prognostic Models).

Prostate-Specific Antigen

PSA is a 28-kD protein of the kallikrein family, a group of serine proteases whose genes are found on chromosome 19q13. PSA is abundant in seminal fluid, at concentrations up to 3.0 mg/mL, a million times more abundant than in serum.[164] The enzymatic activity of PSA induces liquefaction of seminal fluid and the release of mobile spermatozoa. PSA is synthesized in the ductal and acinar epithelium and is secreted into the lumina. PSA is organ specific and not cancer specific; normal prostatic tissue (and BPH) produces more PSA per gram than cancer, and well-differentiated cancer produces more PSA per gram than poorly differentiated cancer.[165] Under pathologic conditions, PSA reaches serum through the disrupted epithelial basement membrane, passing into capillaries and lymphatics. Each gram of cancer is thought to raise the serum PSA level by 3 ng/mL, whereas each gram of BPH contributes only 0.3 ng/mL. Thus, there is considerable overlap in values between patients with prostate cancer and those with benign conditions, such as BPH and prostatitis. Acute urinary retention and prostatic manipulation by needle biopsy or transurethral resection of the prostate (TURP) may raise serum PSA levels dramatically. Performance of DRE does not. PSA can be detected in female and male periurethral glands, anal glands, apocrine sweat glands, apocrine breast cancers, salivary gland neoplasms, and human breast milk.[166]

The normal range of PSA is less than 4 ng/mL, but levels are best considered as a continuum. The sensitivity for detecting cancer with a PSA greater than 4 ng/mL is approximately 80%: 20% of men with a normal DRE and PSA level between 2.5 and 4.0 have cancer.[167,168] For men with a PSA level of 4 to 10 ng/mL, ultrasound-guided biopsies detect cancer in 25%, of which 75% are pathologically confined. If the PSA is greater than 10 ng/

mL, 60% have cancer, but only 40% to 50% are confined.[169,170] The specificity is 15% to 20%—that is, one of five or six men without cancer will have an elevated PSA. Men with a PSA of 2 to 3 ng/mL are 5.5 times more likely to be diagnosed with cancer within 5 years than men with a PSA less than 1 ng/mL.[171]

Transrectal Ultrasound

TRUS is used to target sites for needle biopsy in the prostate, staging, and to determine prostate volume.[9] It is not used for screening. Cancers are typically hypoechoic relative to the normal peripheral zone, but there is no pathognomonic imaging finding that predicts cancer with certainty (Fig. 30.3-11).[172,173]

Needle Biopsy of the Prostate

The needle biopsy procedure is performed transrectally with a thin, 18-gauge needle mounted on a spring-loaded gun directed by ultrasound (Fig. 30.3-12).[9] All palpable or visibly abnormal areas should be sampled, along with a total of at least 6 to 12 systematic biopsies of the prostate taken from the left and right apex, middle, and base of the peripheral zone.[174] Each core should be

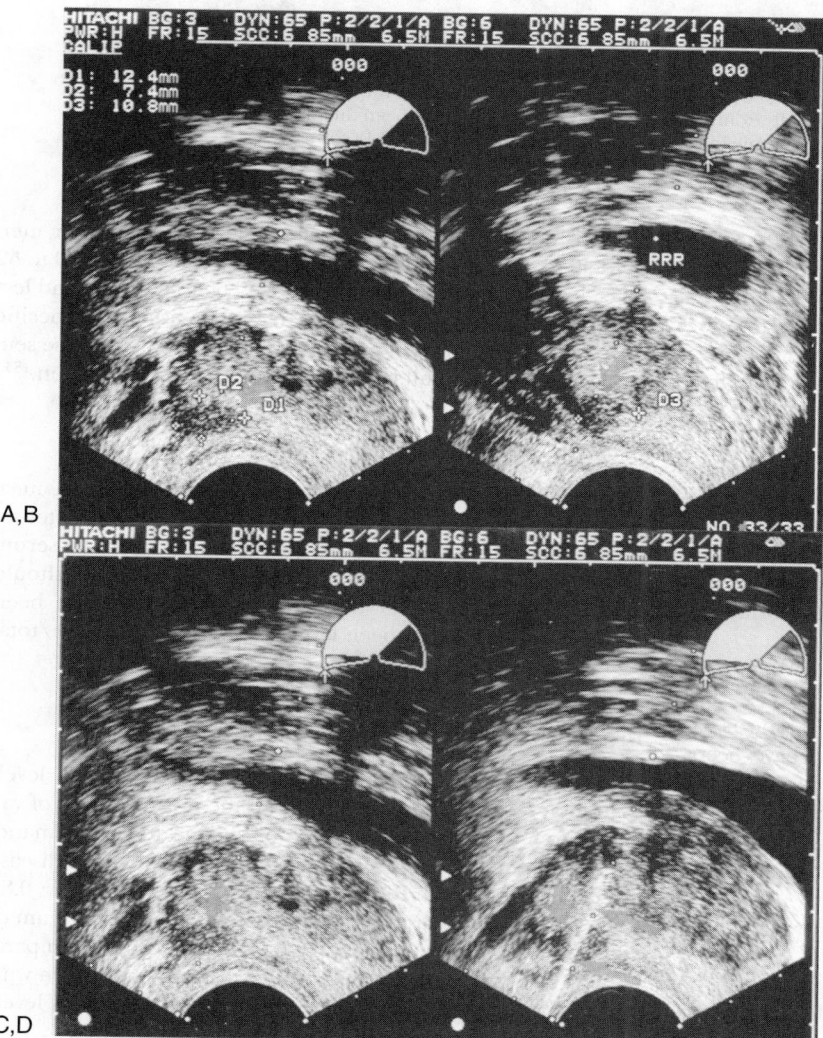

FIGURE 30.3-11. Transrectal ultrasound image of an impalpable (T1c) cancer. **A:** Axial view shows a hypoechoic tumor in right mid peripheral zone, measuring 11.3 mm in length (D1) and 3.5 mm in height (D2). **B:** A sagittal view shows the electronic needle tract through the hypoechoic tumor (*curved arrow*). **C,D:** An axial view shows the hypoechoic lesion (*curved arrow*) and the hyperechoic needle tract (*straight arrows*) through the tumor.[8] (Courtesy of Dr. Fred Lee.) (See Color Fig. 30.3-11 in the CD-ROM.)

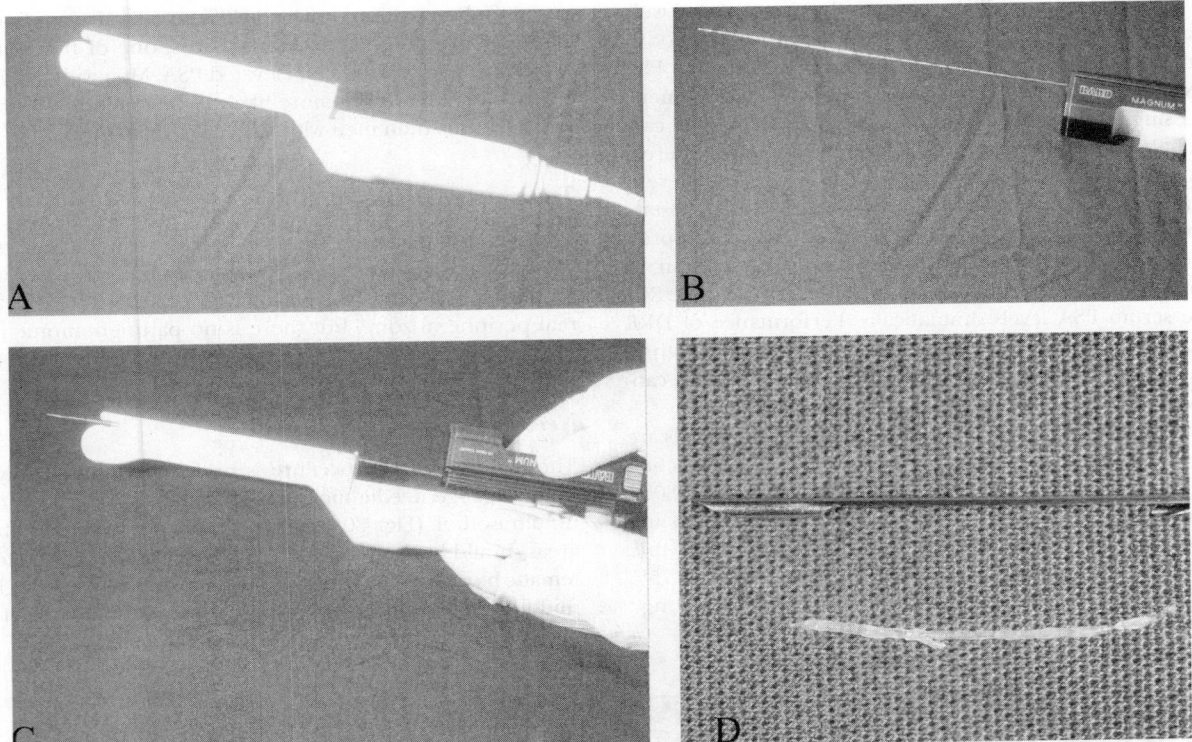

FIGURE 30.3-12. **A:** Endfire transrectal ultrasound probe. **B:** 18-Gauge needle with Biopty gun. **C:** The needle placed through the guide on the ultrasound probe. **D:** Biopsy core (17 mm) from the prostate alongside the open needle. (From ref. 8, with permission.) (See Color Fig. 30.3-12 in the CD-ROM.)

identified separately as to location and orientation, so that the pathologist can report the extent and grade of cancer in each core and the presence of any perineural invasion or ECE.[175–177]

A biopsy session that supplies six or more cores has a sensitivity of approximately 80% for the detection of a cancer.[178] Three biopsy sessions may be required to achieve 97% sensitivity for the detection of an important cancer. Transition zone biopsies are indicated in men with previously negative biopsy results and no palpable or visible lesion in the peripheral zone, especially those with a high PSA or PSA density (PSAD).[177] The presence of PIN in a biopsy increases the risk for cancer 15-fold. Consequently, patients with high-grade PIN require close follow-up. If such patients have an elevated serum PSA level, the likelihood of unsampled cancer is high, because PIN alone does not affect serum PSA levels.[179]

To improve the performance characteristics of PSA and to reduce the number of men who undergo a biopsy unnecessarily, whereas ensuring detection of clinically significant cancers, a number of modifications to the PSA measurement have been used. These include (1) age-specific reference ranges,[180] (2) PSAD determinations,[181] (3) the calculation of PSA velocity,[182] and (4) changing the lower limits of normal.[167] Catalona et al. found cancer in 17% of men with a normal DRE and a serum PSA level of 2.5 to 4.0 ng/mL.[167]

Age-Specific Prostate-Specific Antigen

PSA levels increase with age because of age-related increases in prostate volume due to BPH. In adjusting the upper limit of normal for age, PSA should be less than 2.5 ng/mL for men aged 40 to 49 years, less than 3.5 ng/mL for men aged 50 to 59 years, less than 4.5 ng/mL for men aged 60 to 69 years, and less than 6.5 for men aged 70 to 79 years.[180] The use of age-specific PSA levels has been challenged in screening trials because sensitivity is lost for a small increase in specificity in older men.[183]

Prostate-Specific Antigen Density

The ratio of PSA to gland volume is termed *PSA density*, measured in nanograms per milliliters per cubic centimeter of prostate tissue.[181] Because more PSA is released into the serum by cancer (3 ng/g) than by BPH (0.3 ng/g),[184] PSAD should help discriminate cancer from BPH. The results have been variable, and PSAD has been largely replaced by the free/total PSA ratio for diagnosis.[152,185]

Prostate-Specific Antigen Velocity

Men with cancer should have more rapid rises in PSA levels than men without cancer, even within the normal range of values. In one study, the yearly rate of change in PSA in nanograms per milliliters per year for men without prostatic disease was 0.03; for men with BPH, 0.12; and for men with cancer, 0.88 (Fig. 30.3-13).[182] With three measurements over a minimum of 18 months, a change of more than 0.75 ng/mL/y is comparable to a PSA greater than 4 ng/mL in distinguishing men with and without prostate cancer.[186] Biologic variation in PSA levels over time hamper the accuracy of the calculated result.

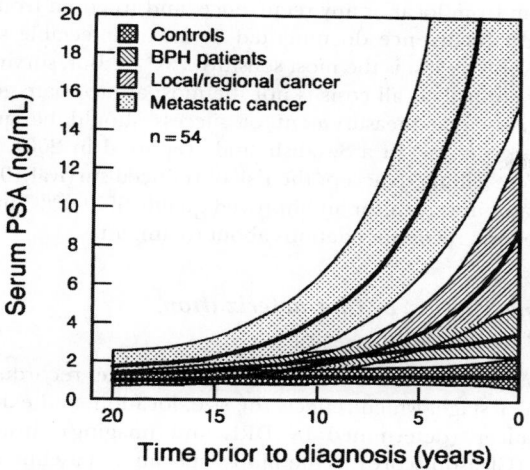

FIGURE 30.3-13. Longitudinal change in prostate-specific antigen (PSA) levels in controls, men with benign prostatic hyperplasia (BPH), and men diagnosed with local/regional or metastatic prostate cancer. Average curves (+95% confidence interval) of PSA levels, as a function of years before diagnosis, for three diagnostic groups estimated the mixed-effects model, with the assumption of an age at diagnosis of 75 years. (From ref. 182, with permission.)

Free to Total Prostate-Specific Antigen Ratio

Most (65% to 90%) measurable circulating PSA is complexed covalently (irreversibly) to the protease inhibitor α_1-antichymotrypsin, which covers a specific epitope on the kallikrein loop, allowing immunoassays for the "free" form representing 10% to 35% of the total PSA (Fig. 30.3-14).[164] The more abundant form of PSA in men with BPH is an inactivated, "clipped," form that does not interact with α_1-antichymotrypsin. Thus, the percent-free PSA in serum is higher in men with BPH than in men with a normal prostate or cancer and can be used to discriminate cancer from BPH. Percent-free PSA values less than 10% are more indicative of cancer in men with values in the 4 to 10 ng/mL range.[164,187]

LOCALIZED DISEASE

MEDICAL DECISION MAKING

Choosing Options

A man diagnosed with an apparently localized prostate cancer faces a daunting task in understanding how serious his cancer is and how it should be treated. A treatment plan should be based on the life expectancy of the patient, the nature of the cancer (stage, grade, PSA), the effectiveness and side effects of a given treatment, the experience of the treating physician, and the patient's own preferences. It can be a challenge for physicians and a heart-wrenching dilemma for patients to select the optimal therapy.

Predicting Outcomes

Definitive proof that radical prostatectomy, or any other local therapy, reduces a man's chances of dying of prostate cancer will certainly require the completion of large randomized prospective clinical trials.[188] Even if such trials were to show a ben-

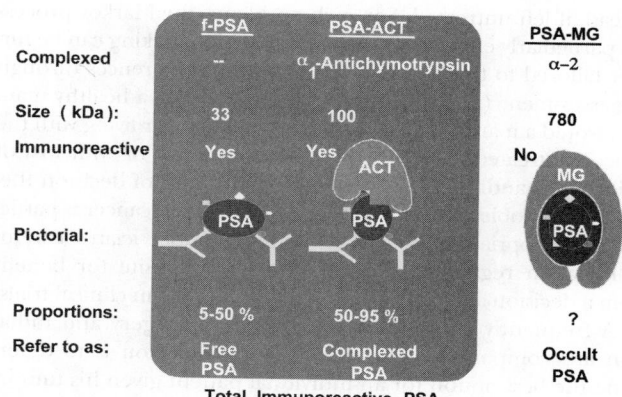

FIGURE 30.3-14. Total immunoreactive prostate-specific antigen (PSA) in the circulation consists of free and bound forms but not PSA bound to α_2-macroglobulin (PSA-MG). (From ref. 8, with permission.) (See Color Fig. 30.3-14 in the CD-ROM.)

efit for men in general, this would not determine whether some patients—depending on the characteristics of their cancer—would benefit greatly by aggressive treatment or suffer harm. More information is needed about the probability that a specific cancer type will affect the quality and quantity of a patient's survival, will cause symptoms, metastasize, or cause death.[189] Nomograms allow us to incorporate all established prognostic factors for an individual patient, so that the risk posed by a particular cancer for a specific patient can be quantified. Published nomograms include those predicting outcomes after prostate surgery,[190] external radiotherapy,[191] and brachytherapy.[192] However, we do not yet have a nomogram that would predict long-term survival or development of metastases with expectant management (watchful waiting).

Decision Analysis

The decision to observe or treat a patient involves balancing risks, benefits, and uncertainties. In addition, success with cancer treatment is not survival at any cost but rather quality-of-life survival for the patient.[193] Decision analysis can be used to develop the explicit approach to treatment for an individual patient, discriminating among the tradeoffs involved in such management problems. A decision-analytic model for clinically localized prostate cancer requires quantitative information about

- Life expectancy (age, comorbidity) of the patient
- Probability of metastases and death from prostate cancer over time for the untreated (or conservatively managed) patient
- Particular characteristics of the primary tumor (prognostic features)
- History of effectiveness of the treatment being considered
- Complication rates and side effects from the treatment
- Patient uses (values) for each health state affected by the cancer and its treatment (e.g., having rectal bleeding, living with an untreated cancer, being incontinent)

The decision about treatment of a localized prostate cancer compares the immediate risk of treatment-associated mortality and morbidity with the ongoing risk of a clinically significant event from the cancer, including local recurrence or metastatic spread, if left untreated. For such problems, the Markov process is a particularly effective model.[194,195] Decision making can be further tailored to the individual patient's life preferences through use assessment (i.e., compared to a year lived as a healthy man, how would a man with prostate cancer value a year living with the cancer untreated, or in a state of incontinence or with loss of libido from androgen ablation?).[193] Application of decision theory to the problem of clinically localized prostate cancer is particularly appropriate. The disease requires a physician's careful deliberation regarding alternatives—a prerequisite for benefit from a decision aid.[196] Any model requires proof in clinical trials.

A frequently asked question is whether surgery and radiation are comparable. The more critical question is to determine the best option for an individual patient given his tumor; comorbidities; preexisting issues with bladder, bowel, and erectile function; and preferences. Given the importance of administered radiation dose on outcome, what equipment is available can also influence the choice. Furthermore, as most patients with localized disease are destined to live for a long time, an area of active research is to understand what factors contribute to patient regret over their choice of treatment. In the past, patients referred for radiation therapy were older, sicker, and had more advanced tumors with an intrinsically worse prognosis. This negative selection, combined with limitations in staging and outcomes assessments, made surgery look better. The use of nomograms has leveled the playing field, and, in point of fact, the American Urological Association policy clearly states that surgery, radiation therapy, and watchful waiting are all potential options.[197]

LOCALIZED PROSTATE CANCER

Localized prostate cancer can be divided into two major categories, those cancers that can be cured with local therapy alone (typically cT1 to 3a N0 or X, M0 or X) and those that require a combined local and systemic approach to achieve cure. The latter are generally more locally extensive (T3b to 4, N0 to 1, M0). For the former, the objective of management is to provide long-term, symptom-free survival with minimal morbidity and maximal preservation of quality of life, recognizing that clinical stage alone cannot predict with certainty which cancers are destined to metastasize. For these tumors as well, local therapy will not suffice, and ultimate cure will require the integration of systemic therapy. For an increasing proportion of patients with clinically confined cancers, watchful waiting (deferring definitive therapy until progression) is a reasonable option. However, this depends on the nature of the cancer and the expected longevity of the patient. For those who are treated, the primary options are surgery or radiotherapy, with the latter administered by an external-beam approach, implantation of radioactive seeds, or a combination of the two with or without androgen ablation (see Radiation Therapy, later). The extent of staging studies and the selection of treatment depend on assessment of risk: How likely is a given man's cancer to progress locally, produce symptoms, or metastasize over time? What is the probability of success with treatment? What are the risks of side effects and complications? What are the individual patient's concerns and priorities?

Several end points can be used to assess the results of treatment for clinically localized prostate cancer: overall survival rate, cancer-specific survival rates, freedom from metastases, freedom from local or any recurrence, and freedom from biochemical recurrence documented by an undetectable serum PSA level. The last is the most sensitive.[13,198–200] But, survival, or cancer control, at all costs is not the most appropriate goal of treatment. The measurement of success should be quality-adjusted survival. In a Swedish study reported in 2001, some men were willing to accept the risk of reduced survival 10 to 15 years later in return for an improved quality of life.[201] This limits categoric recommendations about treatment.

Staging Studies, or Characterization, of the Local Tumor

Thorough evaluation of the local tumor includes recording the clinical T stage, which reflects the size, location, and extent of the cancer (determined by DRE and imaging), histologic grade (Gleason score) in the biopsy specimen, baseline serum PSA level, and systematic biopsy results. These factors are used to predict pathologic stage, assist treatment planning, and determine prognosis.

DIGITAL RECTAL EXAMINATION. Although not uniformly accurate[202] or reproducible,[203] DRE results are associated with pathologic stage[204] and prognosis.[173,205]

PROSTATE-SPECIFIC ANTIGEN. In general, higher values are associated with larger tumor volumes and a more advanced stage,[184] although there may be a wide range of values within any clinical T category.[190,206] Conversely, poorly differentiated cancers produce less PSA per gram than well-differentiated cancers.[165]

GLEASON GRADE AND SYSTEMATIC BIOPSY RESULTS. Higher Gleason score (see Histopathology, earlier in this chapter) is strongly associated with larger tumor volume, extension outside the prostate, probability of metastases, and duration of response to therapy.[207,208] In addition to Gleason score, the amount of cancer in each core of a systematic needle biopsy session adds important staging and prognostic information.[176,209–211] Biopsy results help to identify indolent cancers that may not require intervention.[212]

IMAGING STUDIES. Imaging studies of the prostate have been widely investigated for staging, but they have limited ability to detect small cancers or microscopic extraprostatic extension. The results depend greatly on the technique and interpretation of the examination. Currently, the best imaging study for prostate cancer is endorectal MRI (Fig. 30.3-15). MRI should include both T1- and T2-weighted, spin-echo sequences at 3- to 5-mm intervals through the gland. T1-weighted images can detect blood in the prostate, whereas T2-weighted images are most useful in demonstrating the internal architecture of the prostate and seminal vesicles and identifying low-signal intensity areas suspicious for cancer in the otherwise high-signal intensity peripheral zone. Used with MR spectroscopy, endorectal MRI more accurately identifies the presence of ECE and seminal vesicle invasion (SVI), helps to identify invasion in the area of the neurovascular bundles (NVBs), and improves staging accuracy compared to DRE and all other available staging studies.[213]

Computed tomography (CT) is rarely useful for staging. CT cannot image cancer within the prostate and lacks sensitivity

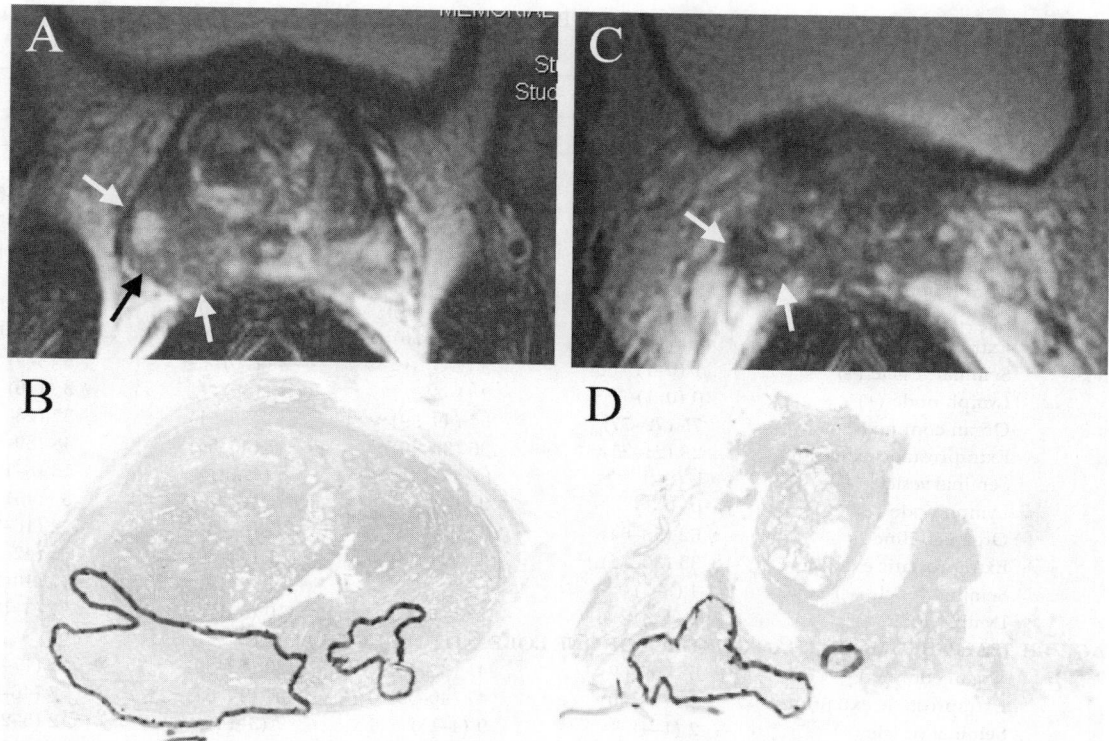

FIGURE 30.3-15. Magnetic resonance image of the prostate and seminal vesicles. **A:** Transverse T2-weighted image showing low-signal intensity areas suspicious for cancer (*arrows*) in the right peripheral zone. **B:** Corresponding pathologic section shows a large cancer in the right peripheral zone with posterolateral extracapsular extension. **C:** Transverse image shows irregular seminal vesicles with low-signal intensity. **D:** Corresponding pathologic section shows seminal vesicle invasion. (From ref. 8, with permission) (See Color Fig. 30.3-15*C,D* in the CD-ROM.)

and specificity in detecting ECE. CT scans of the abdomen and pelvis have been widely overused and are rarely indicated.

LYMPH NODE STAGING AND THE ROLE OF PELVIC LYMPH NODE DISSECTION. Prostate cancer often metastasizes first to the pelvic lymph nodes. The frequency of nodal metastases increases as clinical stage, Gleason grade, and serum PSA levels increase.[214] Preoperative staging nomograms (Table 30.3-5) use all three factors to predict the probability of positive nodes. The finding of lymph node metastases has been considered tantamount to distant spread. This dictum justified intense efforts to detect nodal metastases before definitive local therapy. If the probability of nodal metastases is high, routine pelvic lymph node dissection (PLND) is warranted. Laparoscopic PLND is attractive as a less morbid means than open PLND to find microscopic metastases in the nodes.[215]

The shift toward lower-stage disease as a result of widespread screening has markedly reduced the percentage of patients with nodal metastases found at PLND from 30% in the 1980s to 2% to 6% today.[216] The overall incidence is now so low that it is not possible to reliably identify a substantial subset of patients with a high incidence (more than 30%) of nodal metastases. Nomograms can be used to identify patients with a very low (less than 1.5%) risk of positive nodes, for whom a PLND may not be necessary. Furthermore, prostate cancer can metastasize without detectable spread to the pelvic lymph nodes, so negative nodes do not exclude preexisting metastases and eventual treatment

failure. Consequently, we do not recommend staging PLND as a separate procedure before radiotherapy.

Although most patients with positive nodes will progress (Fig. 30.3-16), some 20% remain free of recurrence 10 years after PLND and radical prostatectomy, suggesting that some patients may be cured by removal of the primary echelon of lymph nodes.[13,218] Here, the distinction between recurrence and survival becomes important as, even among patients with positive nodes, the 10-year cancer-specific survival after radical prostatectomy is more than 80%.[215] Consequently, we no longer routinely perform frozen-section examination of the nodes removed during radical prostatectomy. If a PLND is indicated, complete removal of the obturator, hypogastric, and external iliac lymph nodes is recommended (Fig. 30.3-17).

Tests to Detect Regional and Distant Metastases

BONE SCAN, COMPUTED TOMOGRAPHY, AND MAGNETIC RESONANCE IMAGING. Bone scans, although more sensitive than plain films, lack specificity for cancer; false-positive test results are common in areas of arthritis or previous injury.[220,221] If the patient has no symptoms referable to bone, the PSA is less than 8 ng/mL, and the tumor is not extensive (T3) or poorly differentiated, true positive results are rare, and the bone scan may be omitted.[222] Abnormal bone scans are often followed by plain films, which are useful to document the presence of benign conditions, such as arthritis, to explain the abnormal scan.

TABLE 30.3-5.   Predicted Probability of Each Pathologic Stage Based on Preoperative Prostate-Specific Antigen (PSA), Clinical Stage, and Gleason Grade in the Biopsy Specimen

PSA Range (ng/mL)	Pathologic Stage	Gleason Score 5–6	3 + 4 = 7	4 + 3 = 7	8–10
CLINICAL STAGE T1C (NONPALPABLE, PSA ELEVATED)					
2.6–4.0	Organ confined	84 (81–86)	68 (62–74)	58 (48–67)	52 (41–63)
	Extraprostatic extension	15 (13–18)	27 (22–33)	37 (29–46)	40 (31–50)
	Seminal vesicle (+)	1 (0–1)	4 (2–7)	4 (1–7)	6 (3–12)
	Lymph node (+)	—	1 (0–2)	1 (0–3)	1 (0–4)
4.1–6.0	Organ confined	80 (78–83)	63 (58–68)	52 (43–60)	46 (36–56)
	Extraprostatic extension	19 (16–21)	32 (27–36)	42 (35–50)	45 (36–54)
	Seminal vesicle (+)	1 (0–1)	3 (2–5)	3 (1–6)	5 (3–9)
	Lymph node (+)	0 (0–1)	2 (1–3)	3 (1–5)	3 (1–6)
6.1–10.0	Organ confined	75 (72–77)	54 (49–59)	43 (35–51)	37 (28–46)
	Extraprostatic extension	23 (21–25)	36 (32–40)	47 (40–54)	48 (39–57)
	Seminal vesicle (+)	2 (2–3)	8 (6–11)	8 (4–12)	13 (8–19)
	Lymph node (+)	0 (0–1)	2 (1–3)	2 (1–4)	3 (1–5)
>10	Organ confined	62 (58–64)	37 (32–42)	27 (21–34)	22 (16–30)
	Extraprostatic extension	33 (30–36)	43 (38–48)	51 (44–59)	50 (42–59)
	Seminal vesicle (+)	4 (3–5)	12 (9–17)	11 (6–17)	17 (10–25)
	Lymph node (+)	2 (1–3)	8 (5–11)	10 (5–17)	11 (5–18)
CLINICAL STAGE T2B (PALPABLE MORE THAN ONE-HALF OF ONE LOBE, NOT ON BOTH LOBES)					
2.6–4.0	Organ confined	63 (57–69)	41 (33–48)	30 (22–39)	25 (17–34)
	Extraprostatic extension	34 (28–40)	47 (40–55)	57 (47–67)	57 (46–68)
	Seminal vesicle (+)	2 (1–4)	9 (4–15)	7 (3–14)	12 (5–22)
	Lymph node (+)	1 (0–2)	3 (0–8)	4 (0–12)	5 (0–14)
4.1–6.0	Organ confined	57 (52–63)	35 (29–40)	25 (18–32)	21 (14–29)
	Extraprostatic extension	39 (33–44)	51 (44–57)	60 (50–68)	59 (49–69)
	Seminal vesicle (+)	2 (1–3)	7 (4–11)	5 (3–9)	9 (4–16)
	Lymph node (+)	2 (1–3)	7 (4–13)	10 (5–18)	10 (4–20)
6.1–10.0	Organ confined	49 (43–54)	26 (22–31)	19 (14–25)	15 (10–21)
	Extraprostatic extension	44 (39–49)	52 (46–58)	60 (52–68)	57 (48–67)
	Seminal vesicle (+)	5 (3–8)	16 (10–22)	13 (7–20)	19 (11–29)
	Lymph node (+)	2 (1–3)	6 (4–10)	8 (5–14)	8 (4–16)
>10	Organ confined	33 (28–38)	14 (11–17)	9 (6–13)	7 (4–10)
	Extraprostatic extension	52 (46–56)	47 (40–53)	50 (40–60)	46 (36–59)
	Seminal vesicle (+)	8 (5–11)	17 (12–24)	13 (8–21)	19 (12–29)
	Lymph node (+)	8 (5–12)	22 (15–30)	27 (16–39)	27 (14–40)

Modified from ref. 235.

A normal plain film does not exclude cancer. In some cases in which the entire skeleton is involved by tumor, the scan may be interpreted as normal. In these cases, there is no renal excretion of isotope because of extensive uptake in bone. Because the isotope is excreted by the kidneys, bone scans may provide information on the status of the upper urinary tract (e.g., unexpected hydronephrosis, congenital anomalies, and renal masses).[223]

CT scans help detect soft tissue metastases in patients with advanced prostate cancer. Metastases are most commonly found in the pelvic and retroperitoneal lymph nodes and in the lungs. However, if the patient has an MRI to evaluate the pelvic nodes, there is little need for a CT. Imaging of the pelvic lymph nodes is not necessary unless nomograms predict a more than 20% probability of nodal metastases.[224]

RADIOISOTOPIC ANTIBODY SCAN. Prostascint scan is the brand name of a technique for radioimmunoscintigraphy using an indium III–labeled monoclonal antibody (CYT-356) directed against prostate-specific membrane antigen (PSMA). In clinical trials, the scan identified metastatic deposits of prostate cancer otherwise not detectable. However, the accuracy of the scan is limited by the lack of sensitivity of the antibody to the extracellular domain of PSMA.[225]

REVERSE TRANSCRIPTASE-POLYMERASE CHAIN REACTION FOR PROSTATE-SPECIFIC ANTIGEN OR PROSTATE-SPECIFIC MEMBRANE ANTIGEN MESSENGER RNA IN CIRCULATING CELLS AND BONE MARROW. Solid tumors are well known to shed cells into the circulation at a very early stage in their growth, yet few of these cells have the capacity to lodge in a distant site, grow, and develop into a metastatic deposit. Reverse transcriptase-polymerase chain reaction assays for PSA or PSMA can identify circulating or marrow cells that contain increased copy numbers of messenger RNA (mRNA) for these protein markers of prostatic epithelial cells.[226,227] These cells are found more often in higher

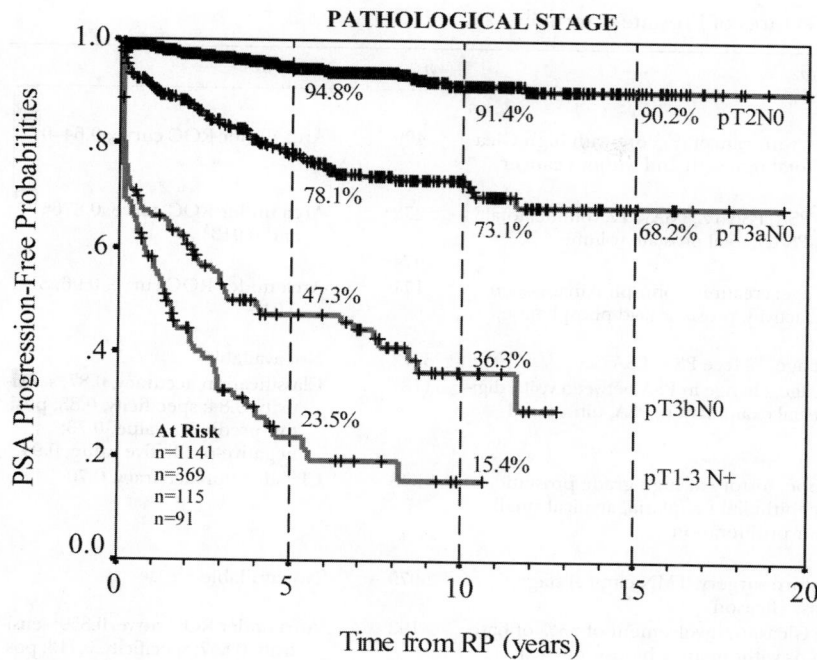

PATHOLOGICAL STAGE

94.8%   91.4%   90.2% pT2N0

78.1%   73.1%   68.2% pT3aN0

47.3%   36.3%   pT3bN0

23.5%   15.4%   pT1-3 N+

At Risk
n=1141
n=369
n=115
n=91

PSA Progression-Free Probabilities

Time from RP (years)

FIGURE 30.3-16. The actuarial probability of remaining free of progression [undetectable prostate-specific antigen (PSA), no other cancer-related therapy] over time after radical prostatectomy (RP) for pathologic stage. (From ref. 217, with permission.)

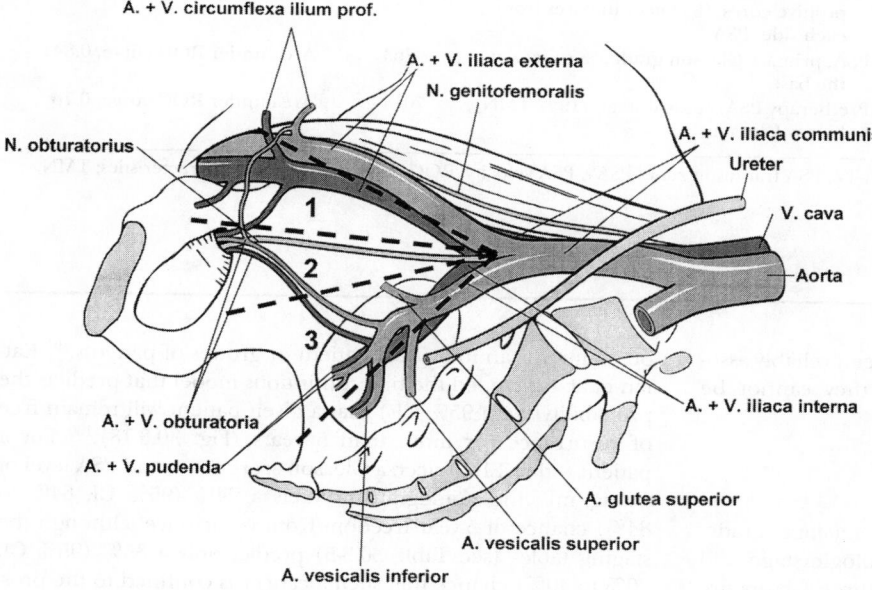

A. + V. circumflexa ilium prof.

A. + V. iliaca externa

N. genitofemoralis

A. + V. iliaca communis

Ureter

N. obturatorius

V. cava

Aorta

A. + V. obturatoria

A. + V. iliaca interna

A. + V. pudenda

A. glutea superior

A. vesicalis superior

A. vesicalis inferior

FIGURE 30.3-17. Areas that should be included in a pelvic lymph node dissection. If only area 1 is dissected, 64% of patients with pelvic lymph node metastases will be missed, compared to a complete dissection of all three areas. (From ref. 219, with permission.)

TABLE 30.3-6.   Nomograms to Predict Pathologic Features of Prostate Cancer[212]

Study	Pathologic Outcome	Predictors	n	Accuracy
IDENTIFYING INDOLENT CANCER				
Ross et al.[229]	Indolent cancer	% Cores with cancer, % core with high Gleason, total mm with and without cancer	409	Area under ROC curve, 0.64–0.79
PREDICTING CANCER DIAGNOSIS				
Djavan et al.[230]	Positive biopsy	% Free PSA, PSA-TZ, PSAV, TZ volume, total PSA, PSAD, total prostate volume	272[a] 974[b]	Area under ROC curve, 0.876[a] and 0.913[b]
Babaian et al.[231]	Positive biopsy	Patient age; creatinine phosphokinase isoenzyme activity, prostatic acid phosphatase, PSA	171	Area under ROC curve, 0.96; SD, 0.018
Carlson et al.[232]	Positive biopsy	Patient age, % free PSA, PSA	3773	Not available
Snow et al.[233]	Positive biopsy	Patient age, change in PSA between visits, digital rectal examination, PSA, ultrasound	1787	Classification accuracy, 0.87; sensitivity, 0.84; specificity, 0.88; positive-predictive value, 0.73; negative-predictive value, 0.94
Lopez-Corona et al.[234]	Positive repeat biopsy	PSA slope, history of high-grade prostatic intraepithelial neoplasia, atypical small acinar proliferation	343	Classification accuracy, 0.70
PREDICTING PATHOLOGIC STAGE				
Partin et al.[235]	Organ confined	PSA before surgery, TMN clinical stage, biopsy Gleason	5079	Not available
Badalament et al.[236]	Organ confined	Biopsy Gleason, involvement of >5% of base with or without apex biopsy, nuclear grade, PSA, total % tumor involvement	192	Area under ROC curve, 0.859; sensitivity, 0.857; specificity, 0.713; positive-predictive value, 0.729; negative-predictive value, 0.847
Ohori et al.[237]	Extracapsular extension, by side	Clinical T stage, highest biopsy Gleason, % positive cores, % cancer in cores from each side, PSA	763	Area under ROC curve, 0.788
Koh et al.[238]	Seminal vesicle invasion	PSA, primary Gleason grade, % cancer at the base	763	Area under ROC curve, 0.841
Cagiannos et al.[239]	Lymph node metastases	Pretherapy PSA, clinical stage (1992 TMN), biopsy Gleason	7014	Area under ROC curve, 0.76

PSA, prostate-specific antigen; PSAD, PSA density; PSA-TZ, PSA transition zone; PSAV, PSA velocity; ROC, receiver operating characteristics; TMN, tumor, node, metastasis.
[a]Number of patients with PSA 2.5–4.0 ng/mL.
[b]Number of patients with PSA 4–10 ng/mL.
(Modified from ref. 229.)

pathologic stages, but their presence has not been reliably associated with subsequent relapse.[228] As such, they cannot be equated with micrometastases.

Prognostic Models: Nomograms

Each of the clinical features of prostate cancer (stage, grade, and PSA level) are associated with the pathologic stage and prognosis of a localized tumor. When these three factors are combined into algorithms, predictive accuracy is much better (Tables 30.3-6 and 30.3-7). Staging tables that predict pathologic stage from the combined results of clinical T stage, Gleason grade in the biopsy specimens, and preoperative PSA levels are available and widely used (see Table 30.3-5).[214]

However, staging tables should not be used to predict prognosis or treatment outcome. Many patients whose cancer is not confined to the prostate *pathologically* can be rendered disease free for more than 10 years with surgery. Optimal treatment of prostate cancer depends on accurate assessment of risk. Most published risk stratification schemes are based on discrete cutoff values.[244,245] None of these predicts the chances of success or failure as well as a nomogram. Nomograms are graphic depictions of algorithms derived from statistic models used to predict

outcomes for an individual patient or groups of patients.[191] Kattan et al. developed the first continuous model that predicts the probability (with 95% CIs) that a given patient will remain free of recurrence for more than 5 years (Fig. 30.3-18).[190] For a patient with a T1c cancer, a Gleason score 3 + 4, and PSA level of 10 ng/mL, the nomogram predicts a 74% (95% CI, 64% to 84%) chance of 5-year freedom from recurrence, although the staging tables (see Table 30.3-5) predict only a 35% (95% CI, 30% to 40%) chance that such a cancer is confined to the prostate *pathologically*. Nomograms are widely available in computer form (Fig. 30.3-19[8]) and on the Web (http://www.mskcc.org/mskcc/html/10088.cfm) to make predictions quickly and accurately. Prognostic nomograms are being expanded to include patients treated with brachytherapy[192] and watchful waiting, as well as to incorporate additional factors, such as a quantitative analysis of the extent of cancer in systematic biopsy results.[229,246]

RADICAL PROSTATECTOMY

Radical prostatectomy is an effective way to achieve long-term control of clinically localized prostate cancer. A prospective, randomized clinical trial carried out in Sweden clearly demonstrated that surgical treatment of prostate cancer favorably

TABLE 30.3-7. Nomograms to Predict Prognosis of Prostate Cancer

Study	Predictors	End Point Predicted	At Time	Stage	Treatment
Kattan et al.[242]	Clinical TNM stage, biopsy Gleason, PSA	PSA progression-free	5 y	Local disease	Radical prostatectomy
Kattan et al.[240]	PSA, biopsy Gleason sum, ECE, SVI, LN, surgical margin	PSA progression-free	7 y	Local disease	Radical prostatectomy
Han et al.[248]	Biopsy Gleason score, clinical TNM stage, PSA	PSA progression-free	10 y	Local disease	Radical prostatectomy
Kattan et al.[242]	Clinical TNM stage, biopsy Gleason, PSA, radiation dose, neoadjuvant hormone therapy	PSA progression-free	5 y	Local disease	Radiation (3D, >70 Gy)
Kattan et al.[192]	Clinical TNM stage, biopsy Gleason, PSA, radiation dose	PSA progression-free	7 y	Local disease	Brachytherapy
Kattan et al.[242]	Clinical TNM stage, biopsy Gleason, PSA	Freedom from metastases	7 y	Local disease	Radiation (3D, >70 Gy)
Smaletz et al.[243]	KPS, HGB, ALK, albumin, and LDH	Survival	1 y, 2 y	Castrate metastases	Non-hormonal agents
Halabi et al.[618]	LDH, PSA, ALK, Gleason sum, ECOG performance status, HGB, presence of visceral disease	Survival	1 y, 2 y	Castrate metastases	Mitoxantrone, Keto-conazole, Suramin, others

3D, three-dimensional; ALK, alkaline phosphatase; ECE, extracapsular extension; ECOG, Eastern Cooperative Oncology Group; HGB, hemoglobin; KPS, Karnofsky performance status; LDH, lactate dehydrogenase; LN, lymph node; PSA, prostate-specific antigen; SVI, seminal vesicle invasion; TNM, tumor, node, metastasis.

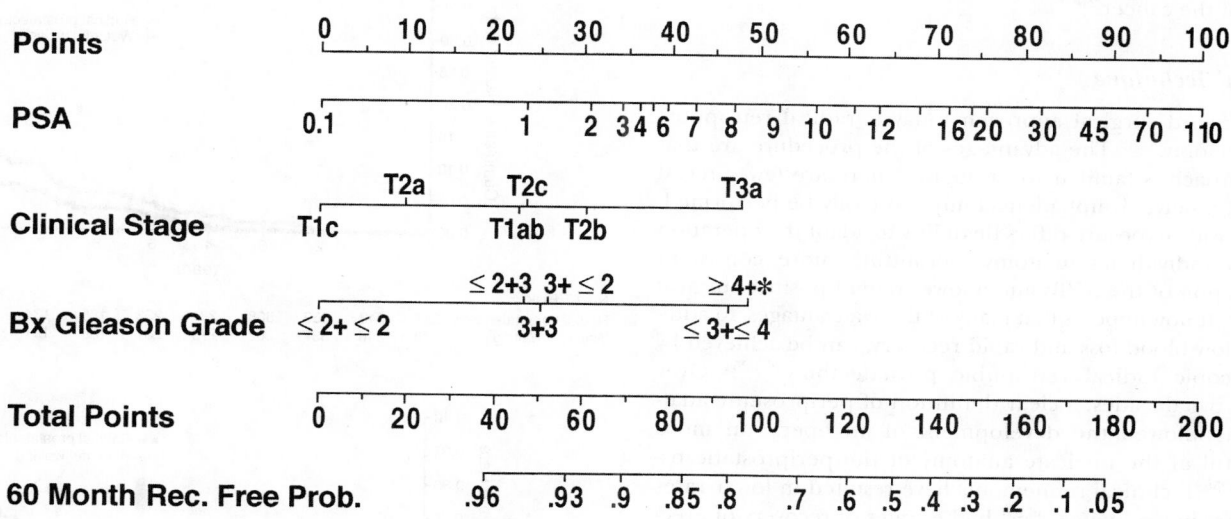

Instructions for Physician. Locate the patient's PSA on the PSA axis. Draw a line straight upwards to the **Points** axis to determine how many points towards recurrence the patient receives for his PSA. Repeat this process for the **Clinical Stage** and **Biopsy Gleason Sum** axes, each time drawing straight upward to the **Points** axis. Sum the points achieved for each predictor and locate this sum on the **Total Points** axis. Draw a line straight down to find the patient's probability of remaining recurrence free for 60 months assuming he does not die of another cause first.

Note: this nomogram is not applicable to a man who is not otherwise a candidate for radical prostatectomy. You can use this only on a man who has already had radical prostatectomy as treatment for his prostate cancer.

Instructions to Patient. "Mr. X., if we had 100 men exactly like you, we would expect between <predicted percentage from nomogram - 10%> and <predicted percentage + 10%> to remain free of their disease at 5 years following radical prostatectomy, and recurrence after 5 years is very rare."

© 1997 Michael W. Kattan and Peter T. Scardino

FIGURE 30.3-18. Nomograms to predict probability or recurrence after radical prostatectomy. Preoperative nomogram predicts 5-year probability of freedom from progression [rising prostate-specific antigen (PSA) or any cancer-related therapy] from the pretreatment PSA, biopsy Gleason grade (primary plus secondary), and clinical T stage. *4+ or any grade 5. (From ref. 190, with permission.)

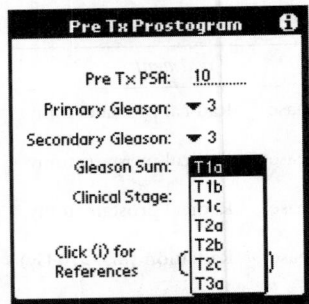

FIGURE 30.3-19. Because nomograms are mathematical algorithms, they can be programmed into desktop or handheld computers. These screens show the computation of probabilities of freedom from recurrence and of pathologic stage using a Palm Pilot. The program includes pretreatment and posttreatment predictions and uses published nomograms in prostate cancer. (From ref. 8, with permission.)

alters the natural history of the disease. In this trial, prostatectomy reduced the rate of metastases 8 years later from 27% with watchful waiting to 13% and reduced cancer-specific mortality from 13% to 7%[247] (Fig. 30.3-20). Other evidence that surgery reduces the risk of metastases and death from prostate cancer include the excellent (68% to 76%) 15-year freedom from PSA recurrence,[13,241] the findings of the multicenter analysis of metastases and cancer-specific survival after radical prostatectomy[249] compared to watchful waiting,[250] and the finding that high-grade cancers, if removed while still confined to the prostate, rarely progress.[208,251] The major advantage of radical prostatectomy in the treatment of prostate cancer is the confidence we have in the long-term eradication of the cancer.[218]

Surgical Technique

The standard surgical approach today is radical retropubic prostatectomy.[8,252] The advantages of the procedure are that the approach is familiar to urologists, there are fewer rectal injuries, a pelvic lymphadenectomy can easily be performed, and the wide exposure offers flexibility to adapt the operation to each individual's anatomy, permitting more consistent preservation of the NVBs and a lower rate of positive surgical margins. It now appears that many of these advantages, in addition to low blood loss and rapid recovery, can be achieved by laparoscopic radical retropubic prostatectomy.[253,254] Over the last two decades, a clear definition of periprostatic anatomy has allowed the development of an operation more respectful of the intricate anatomy of the periprostatic tissues.[255,256] Technical refinements have resulted in lower rates of urinary incontinence,[256,257] higher rates of recovery of erectile function,[258] less blood loss with fewer transfusions,[259] shorter hospital stays,[260] and lower rates of positive surgical margins.[255,261]

A radical prostatectomy is appropriate therapy for patients whose cancers can be resected safely with a reasonable expectation of long-term cure or local control, who are in good general health, and who have a life expectancy of at least 10 years.[13,262] It is also a major procedure with outcomes, both cancer-specific and morbidity-specific, that are highly sensitive to surgical technique.[257,263,264] Comorbid conditions must be considered before recommending the procedure,[189] as perioperative morbidity and mortality increase significantly in patients older than 75 years.[260,265] The goals of radical prostatectomy should be, in order of priority, (1) to completely excise the cancer, (2) to preserve normal urinary control, and (3) to restore erectile function to the greatest extent possible.

Achieving these goals requires careful surgical planning. As no single test provides a reliable estimate of the size, location, and extent of the cancer, we rely on the results of DRE, serum PSA levels, and a detailed analysis of the amount and grade of cancer in each individually labeled biopsy core, along with the results of the TRVS or the endorectal coil MRI with spectroscopy. The results are used to plan the steps necessary to remove the cancer completely and to assess the likelihood that one or both of the NVBs will have to be resected partially or fully to minimize the risk of a positive surgical margin.[255,266]

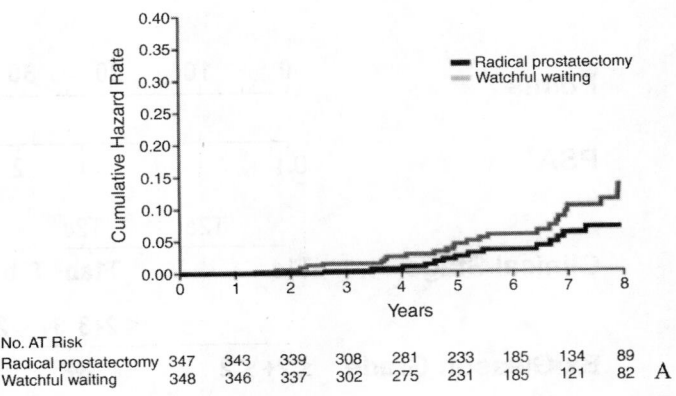

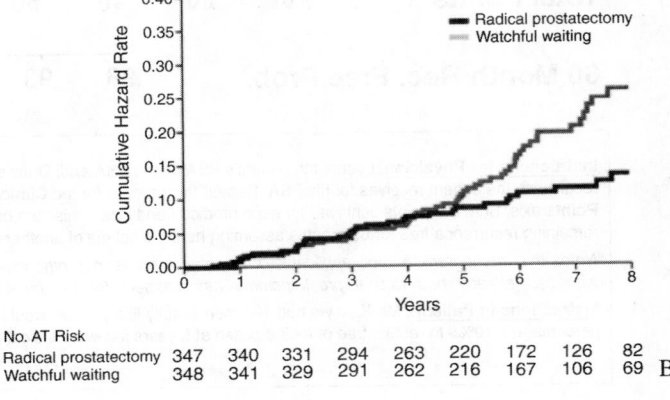

FIGURE 30.3-20. **A:** Cumulative hazard rate of death from prostate cancer. **B:** Cumulative hazard rate of development of distant metastasis. In a prospective, randomized trial of 695 patients, radical prostatectomy reduced the risk of dying of prostate cancer from 13.6% with watchful waiting to 7.1% and the risk of metastases later from 27.3% to 13.4%. (From ref. 247, with permission.)

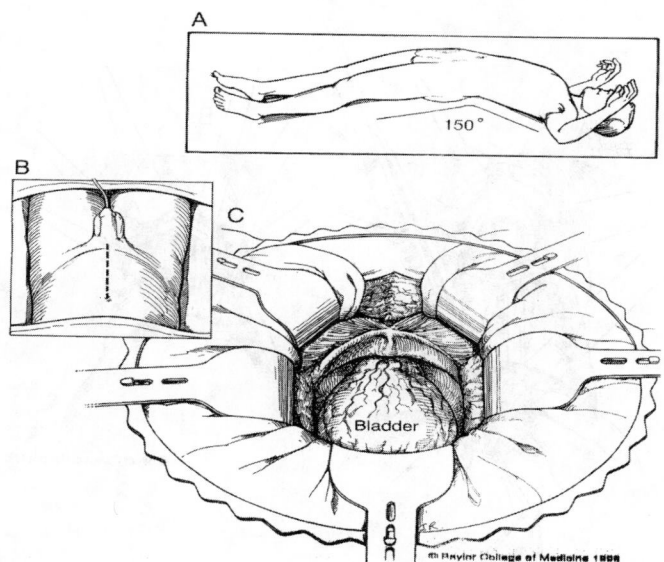

FIGURE 30.3-21. Radical retropubic prostatectomy. **A:** Patient position is supine with hyperextension of the pubis. **B:** Incision is 8 cm midline suprapubic. **C:** Cephalocaudal view of open incision with Turner-Warwick self-restraining retractor. (From ref. 8, with permission.)

The procedure is performed under general, spinal, or epidural anesthesia.

Patient Position and Pelvic Lymph Node Dissection

The patient is positioned supine with the pubis just below the break point in the table (Fig. 30.3-21). The table is flexed (approximately 150 degrees) and some Trendelenburg rotation is applied. An 8-cm suprapubic midline incision is made three fingers' breadth above the penis. Bilateral PLND should include complete removal of all fibroadipose tissue dorsal to the external iliac vein, caudal to the hypogastric artery and vein, cephalad to Cooper's ligament and the pelvic floor, medial to the muscular sidewalls of the pelvis, lateral to the bladder, and ventral to the sciatic nerve (see Fig. 30.3-17). Because the primary drainage from the prostate is to the hypogastric and obturator nodes, all node-bearing tissue above and below the obturator nerve caudal to the hypogastric vein should be removed. The commonly used dissection, limited to the nodes above the obturator nerve in the distal half of the iliac fossa, is inadequate and will detect only 36% of nodal metastases in the pelvis.[219] A frozen section of the lymph nodes is not necessary. The primary tumor should be removed unless massively enlarged nodes are found.[215]

Reducing Blood Loss

Hemorrhage is the most common serious intraoperative complication and can limit the ability to perform a meticulous anatomic dissection. To minimize blood loss requires control of (1) the dorsal vein complex (DVC) and anterior periprostatic veins, (2) the small branches from the NVBs to the prostate laterally (Fig. 30.3-22), and (3) the lateral vascular pedicles to the prostate and the seminal vesicular arteries (Fig. 30.3-23). With these considerations, combined with controlled hypotensive

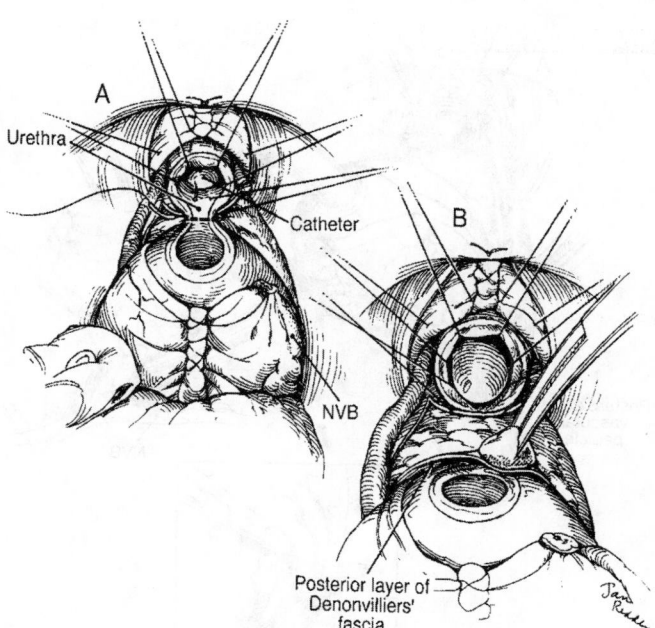

FIGURE 30.3-22. Completion of apical dissection. The catheter is withdrawn. **A:** Two posterior anastomotic sutures are placed at 5 and 7 o'clock to include the posterior layer of Denonvilliers' fascia. **B:** The urethra is transected and dissection carried posteriorly to the layer of adipose tissue anterior to the rectum, beneath the posterior layer of Denonvilliers' fascia. NVB, neurovascular bundle. (Modified from ref. 255.)

anesthesia, only 11% of the patients who did not donate preoperatively required allogeneic blood, and 30% of those who banked autologous blood were transfused.[255,259]

Preservation of the Neurovascular Bundles

Factors associated with recovery of erections are age, quality of erections before the operation, and extent of preservation of the cavernous nerves.[258] When there is little risk of posterior lateral ECE, the nerves should be preserved bilaterally. The amount of tissue that should be resected in the area of the NVB can be judged from the preoperative information and the surgeon's intraoperative assessment of the location of the NVBs in relation to the cancer. Palpable induration or dense adherence of the NVB to the prostate indicates wider dissection.[266]

Reducing Bladder Neck Contracture and Incontinence

Bladder neck contracture usually results from a tightly reconstructed bladder neck or poor mucosa-to-mucosa apposition at the time of vesicourethral anastomosis. Eversion of the bladder neck mucosa and maintenance of a wide (more than 28 French) bladder neck reduce the incidence of this complication (Fig. 30.3-24). Attempts to preserve the bladder neck increase the risk of a positive margin with no improvement in permanent continence. Recovery of continence depends principally on the integrity of the distal urethral sphincter mechanism. Dissection beyond the prostatic apex or placement of sutures deep into the urethra shortens functional length and increases the risk of incontinence.[255,257]

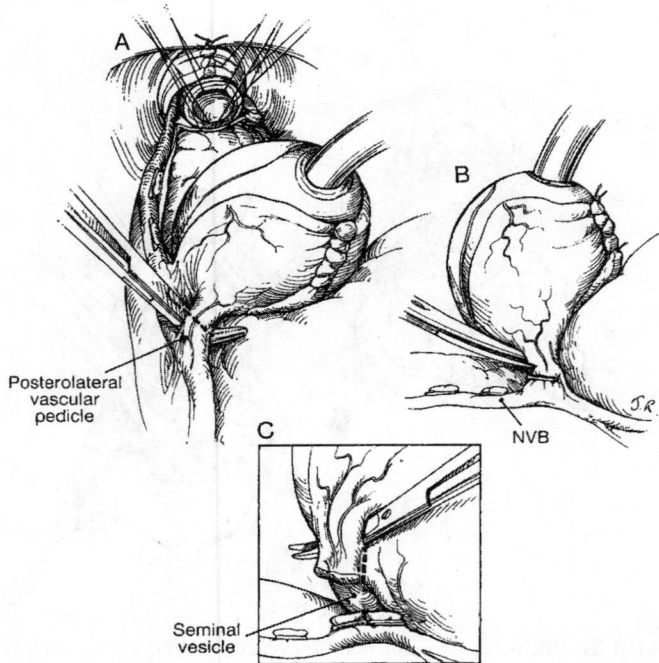

Posterolateral
vascular
pedicle

NVB

Seminal
vesicle

FIGURE 30.3-23. Mobilization of the prostate. **A:** A new catheter is placed in the bladder to allow easy manipulation of the prostate, which is mobilized from its posterolateral attachments in a side-to-side fashion. Small vessels are controlled with clips placed parallel to the neurovascular bundles (NVBs). Near the base of the prostate the NVBs again lie immediately adjacent to the capsule and are easily damaged. But dissection too close to the prostate risks a positive margin. **B:** The posterolateral vascular pedicles of the prostate are identified, isolated with a right-angled clamp, clipped, and divided. **C:** The broad vascular pedicle from the bladder to the prostate is then elevated, clipped, and divided as well. (Modified from ref. 255.)

Reducing Positive Margin Rates

A positive surgical margin indicates that the cancer may not have been completely excised and is associated with a significantly greater risk of recurrence.[13,261,267] Positive surgical margins arise from dissection into the prostatic capsule ("iatrogenic") or from dissection into extracapsular cancer.[268] The risk of both can be reduced by tailoring the dissection to conform to variations in the size and shape of the prostate and the location of the tumor, and estimating the probability of ECE by using nomograms.[237,269]

To avoid a positive margin, the key steps are (1) distal transection of the DVC; (2) wide dissection around the apex, especially posteriorly; and (3) transection of the bladder neck above the prostate. Suture ligation of the DVC distally before transecting it may force the surgeon to divide the complex too close to the anterior surface of the prostate, resulting in a positive anterior margin if the cancer is located anteriorly. Uncertain margins are confirmed with a frozen section from the distal end. The DVC is then oversewn vertically. The apical dissection should extend widely around the apex, especially posteriorly, where the distal extent of the apex beneath the urethra is highly variable.[270] A wide dissection at the bladder neck is important because there is no definitive boundary between the prostate and bladder muscle in this area.

When cancer extends through the capsule of the prostate, it does so posteriorly, over the rectum or NVBs, in 85% of cases

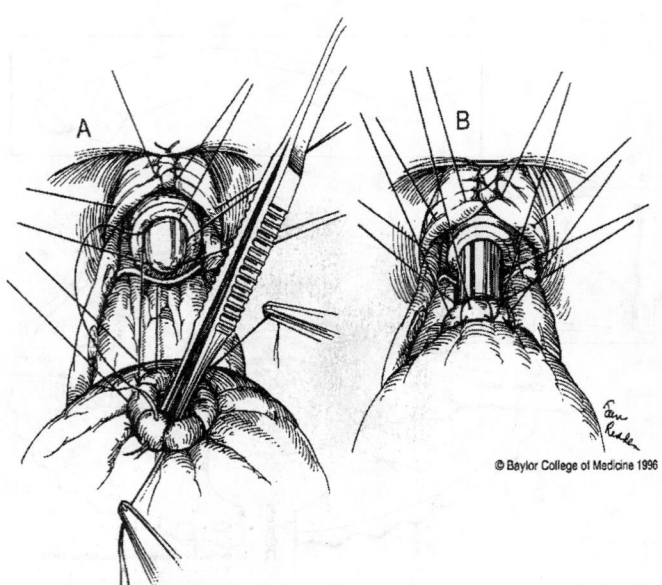

© Baylor College of Medicine 1996

FIGURE 30.3-24. Completion of the anastomosis. **A:** The four posterior anastomotic sutures are placed in corresponding positions deeply in the everted bladder neck. **B:** The catheter is then inserted into the bladder and the two anterior sutures completed. The operating table is taken out of the flex position to facilitate advancement of the reconstructed bladder neck to the urethra. Suction catheters are placed in each obturator fossa, and these are typically removed by postoperative day 3. (Modified from ref. 255.)

and posterior laterally, over the NVB, in 65% of cases[8] (Fig. 30.3-25). Although it is difficult to see or feel the cancer during the operation, the surgeon should be sensitive to areas of palpable induration or unusual adhesions between nerves and the prostate, suggesting extension of cancer. Unfortunately, frozen sections offer little help in avoiding positive margins. Although a positive margin on frozen section is invariably accurate and mandates wider resection of tissue, false-negative frozen section results are rare. More than 80% of all positive margins occur in areas completely unsuspected by the surgeon during the operation.[271] The critical technical maneuvers are a lateral approach to the apex, complete removal of Denonvilliers' fascia posteriorly (see Figs. 30.3-23 and 30.3-24), and dissection outside the posterior lateral layer of Denonvilliers' fascia that forms the medial border of the NVB in areas likely to harbor cancer. If the NVBs are preserved, the critical sites of dissection are posterior laterally at the apex and the base, where branches

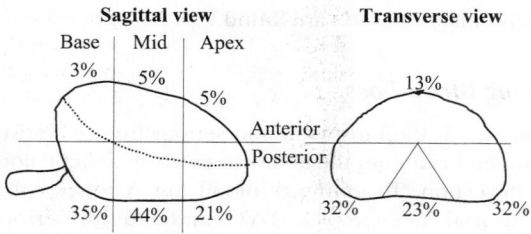

FIGURE 30.3-25. Schematic of sites of extracapsular extension (ECE) of cancer from a radical prostatectomy series. Note that 62% of patients had ECE posterior laterally directly over the area of the neurovascular bundle. (From ref. 8, with permission.)

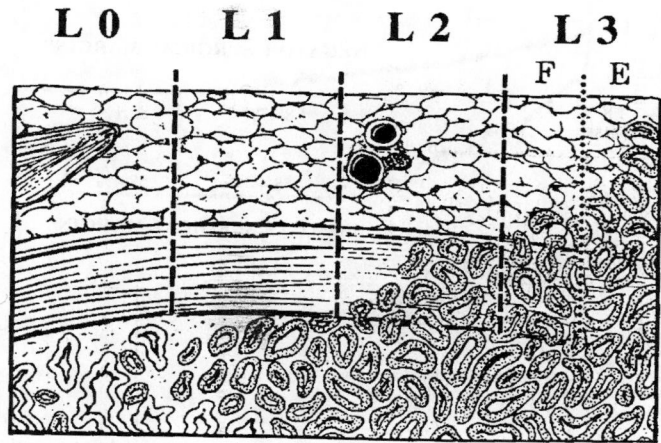

FIGURE 30.3-26. Levels of prostatic capsular invasion. Level 3 invasion (or ECE) is divided into F (focal) and E (established) based on the degree of invasion into periprostatic tissue. (From ref. 269, with permission.)

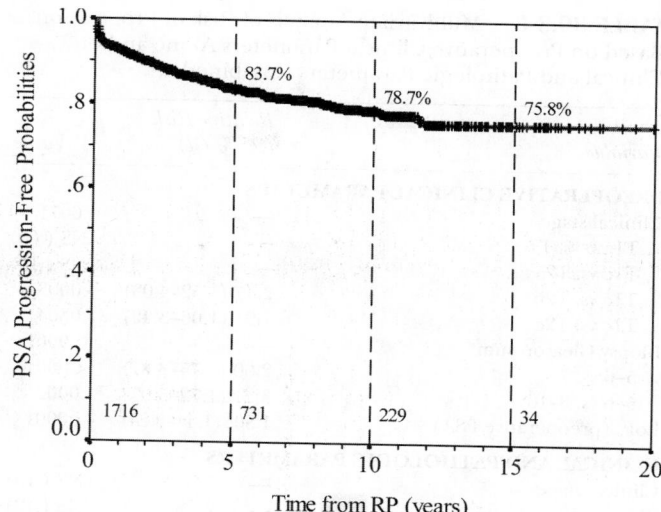

FIGURE 30.3-27. The actuarial probability of remaining free of progression [undetectable prostate-specific antigen (PSA), no other cancer-related therapy] over time after radical prostatectomy (RP) for all patients. The curve represents the overall number of patients at risk. (From ref. 217, with permission.)

from the nerves and accompanying blood vessels extend into the prostate (see Fig. 30.3-2).[272]

Pathologic Stage

Pathologic stage is determined by the histologic examination of the surgical specimen, including the seminal vesicles and the pelvic lymph nodes. The report should include the location of the primary focus of cancer and an estimate of its size, the overall Gleason primary and secondary grade and any focus of higher grade cancer, the presence and location of invasion into or through the capsule, (Fig. 30.3-26)[269] SVI,[273] the status and number of lymph nodes removed, and the status of the surgical margins, noting whether any positive margin was at the location of ECE.[13,261] The authors typically perform whole mount sections to assess the frequency of ECE and margin status, as routine processing and examination underestimates these frequencies.[274] It is also helpful to record the zone of origin of the dominant cancer.

Cancer Control

After radical prostatectomy, serum PSA levels should become unmeasurable. Depending on the preoperative level, PSA may take 6 weeks to reach a nadir. The actuarial nonprogression rates after radical prostatectomy as monotherapy, from several recent series, show that approximately 75% to 85% of patients at 5 years, 70% to 75% at 10 years, and 65% to 70% at 15 years have no evidence of cancer, documented by an undetectable PSA level, and have required no other treatment for cancer.[13,206,275,276] In our series of 4000 patients (T1 to 2 NX M0) treated with radical retropubic prostatectomy alone at Memorial Sloan-Kettering Cancer Center (MSKCC) or Baylor College of Medicine between 1983 and 2003 (Fig. 30.3-27), the actuarial 5-, 10-, and 15-year nonprogression rates were 81%, 77%, and 76%, respectively.[217] Few cancers recur after 7 years, and no patient with a PSA consistently less than 0.05 ng/mL at 10 years has had recurrence (373 patients followed for 10 years or more), so the nonprogression rate 5 years after surgery reasonably estimates the percentage of patients who will remain permanently disease free.

Pathologic stage is an important predictor of prognosis (see Fig. 30.3-16). Approximately 8% to 15% of cancers confined to the prostate pathologically do recur. Some 70% of patients with ECE but no SVI or lymph node metastases are free of cancer 10 years after radical prostatectomy. Approximately one-third of patients with SVI, in the absence of positive nodes, and 15% to 20% of patients with positive pelvic lymph nodes remain free of cancer, with an undetectable PSA and no other treatment for cancer 10 to 15 years later.[13,206,217]

The authors have developed nomograms to predict the probability of recurrence using clinical parameters (stage, grade, and PSA) before surgery and both clinical and pathologic parameters after surgery (Table 30.3-8; see Fig. 30.3-19). These nomograms are readily available and can be downloaded from the Internet at http://www.mskcc.org/mskcc/html/10088.cfm.

Surgical Margins

The primary goal of radical prostatectomy is to remove all of the cancer. Treatment failures occur either because the cancer spread before the operation (under-staging) or because the local tumor was not completely excised. Positive surgical margins, one indication of local tumor persistence, have been reported in 10% to 68% of patients.[267,277,278] In multivariable analysis, positive margins are associated with a 1.5-fold increase in the risk of progression[190] (Fig. 30.3-28). The rate of positive margins varies widely among individual surgeons, even when controlled for the pathologic features of the cancer, reflecting variations in surgical technique.[279] By estimating the location and extent of cancer in the prostate before the operation and by meticulous attention to operative technique,[203,244,280] surgeons should be able to reduce the rate of positive surgical margins to 10% or less.[261]

Adjuvant Radiation Therapy

The benefit of immediate adjuvant radiation therapy for men at increased risk of local recurrence (ECE, positive margins, SVI) has

TABLE 30.3-8. Multivariate Analysis of Risk of Progression Based on Preoperative Clinical Parameters Alone and on Clinical and Pathologic Parameters Combined

Variable	Relative Risk (95% CI)	P Value
PREOPERATIVE CLINICAL PARAMETERS		
Clinical stage	—	.0071
T1a,b vs. T1c	—	NS (.60)
T1c vs. T2a	—	NS (.10)
T1c vs. T2b	2.47 (1.52–4.03)	.0003
T1c vs. T2c	1.91 (1.06–3.42)	.0304
Biopsy Gleason sum[a]	—	<.0001
5–6 vs. 7	2.60 (1.75–3.87)	<.0001
5–6 vs. 8–10	3.21 (1.72–5.97)	.0002
Log$_2$ (preoperative PSA)	1.80[a] (1.44–2.24)	<.0001
CLINICAL AND PATHOLOGIC PARAMETERS		
Clinical stage	—	NS (.15)
Biopsy Gleason sum	—	NS (.12)
Log$_2$ preoperative PSA	—	NS (.52)
Gleason sum in prostatectomy specimen	—	.0008
5–6 vs. 7	2.48 (1.34–4.58)	.0038
5–6 vs. 8–10	4.55 (2.19–9.42)	<.0001
Extracapsular extension	—	.0019
Focal vs. none	2.17 (1.20–3.92)	.011
Established vs. none	2.72 (1.56–4.74)	.0004
Surgical margins		
Positive vs. negative	4.37 (2.90–6.58)	<.0001
Seminal vesicle involvement		
Present vs. absent	2.61 (1.70–4.01)	<.0001
Lymph node metastases		
Present vs. absent	3.31 (2.11–5.20)	<.0001

CI, confidence interval; NS, not statistically significant (*P* >.05).
[a] Each doubling of the preoperative PSA level (one unit increase in log$_2$ preoperative PSA level) resulted in an increased relative risk of progression of 1.80.
(Modified from refs. 13 and 131.)

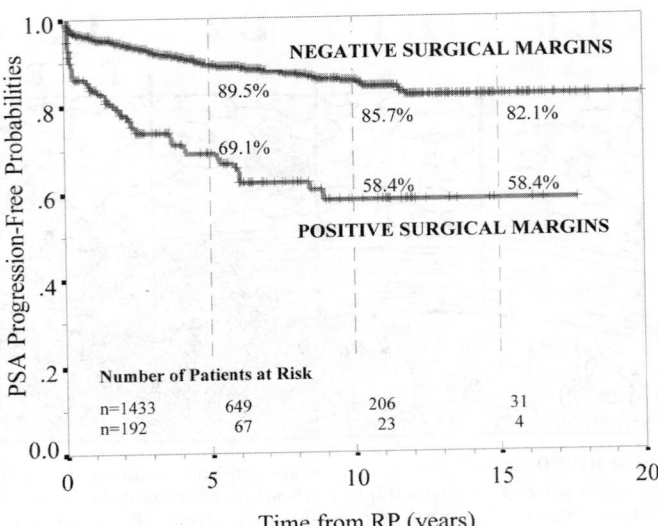

FIGURE 30.3-28. The actuarial probability of remaining free of progression [undetectable prostate-specific antigen (PSA), no other cancer-related therapy] over time after radical prostatectomy (RP) for the status of surgical margins. (From ref. 217, with permission.)

been debated for years.[281–283] In a prospective randomized trial conducted by the Radiation Therapy Oncology Group (RTOG), the risk of subsequent PSA progression was reduced substantially, but there was no effect on distant metastases or cancer-specific or overall survival.[284] Pending the outcome of other clinical trials, there is little rationale for treating microscopic ECE with adjuvant radiotherapy routinely, because 70% of such patients remain free of progression with surgery alone (see Fig. 30.3-16).[13] Those patients with SVI or lymph node metastases, especially if they also have Gleason score 8 to 10 cancers, typically develop distant metastases rather than local recurrence.[3,285]

Adjuvant radiotherapy (in those with an undetectable PSA level) seems most appropriate for patients with positive margins at the site of ECE of cancer in the absence of SVI or lymph node metastases, because the risk of progression in these patients is substantial. However, many patients with positive margins who do not receive immediate radiation therapy remain free of PSA recurrence 10 years later.[261,286] Adjuvant radiotherapy after radical prostatectomy has been associated with a small risk of incontinence and a greater risk of damaging recovery of erections. The optimal dose, target, and fields of radiation remain debatable. The authors do not routinely recommend postoperative radiotherapy if PSA is undetectable.

Morbidity

There is convincing evidence that complications after radical prostatectomy, both early and late, are related to the experience of the surgeon performing the surgery and to the surgical technique used.[264,287] Although busy surgeons generally achieve better outcomes than occasional surgeons, there is remarkable variation even among them[264] in perioperative complications, postoperative urethral strictures, and long-term incontinence. Surgeons who performed poorly by one measure were likely to perform poorly by the other measures as well, illustrating the critical role of surgical technique in this complex operation.

Early Events

With refinements in anesthesia, perioperative care and surgical technique, blood loss, and length of hospital stay, complications and mortality have decreased over time.[260] The mortality rate ranges from 0.16% to 0.66% in modern series, rising with increasing age and comorbidity.[265] Deep venous thrombosis and pulmonary embolism occur in approximately 1.1% and 1.2%, with no evidence that anticoagulants or sequential pneumatic compression are preventive. Early ambulation, a short hospital stay, and use of epidural anesthesia are probably responsible for the low rate of thromboembolic events.

Late Complications

ANASTOMOTIC STRICTURE. Anastomotic stricture has been reported in 0.5% to 9.0% of patients, with one recent survey finding patient-reported strictures in 15% of 337 patients during the first year after surgery.[288] Prior TURP, excessive intraoperative blood loss, and urinary extravasation at the anastomotic site may contribute.[289] Strictures can usually be managed successfully by simple urethral dilation in the office, or, if severe, endoscopic urethrotomy under anesthesia.

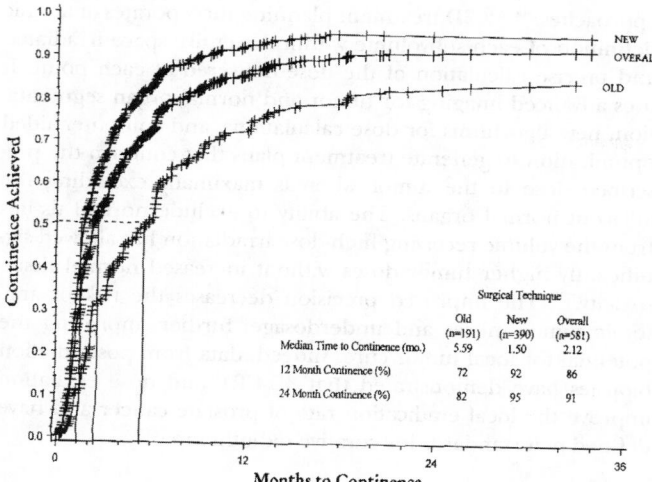

FIGURE 30.3-29. Actuarial probability of achieving continence for entire group of 581 patients and for old (n = 191) and new (n = 390) anastomotic techniques. (From ref. 257, with permission.)

INCONTINENCE. Incontinence is among the most troubling complications; incontinence rates vary widely and reflect surgical experience and technique.[201] In the National Institutes of Health–sponsored Prostate Cancer Outcomes study,[290] 8.5% of men reported "severe" incontinence 2 years or more after surgery, whereas centers with broad expertise in the procedure report some incontinence in less than 10% of patients, with severe incontinence in less than 2%.[257] Despite the relatively high rates of urinary incontinence reported in population surveys, the majority of these patients were minimally bothered by this complication and highly satisfied with their treatment.[290,291] In the authors' own series, the median time to recovery of continence was 6 weeks (Fig. 30.3-29).[257] After 1 year, 92% were dry, and, after 2 years, 95% were dry. Only 1% of patients required invasive therapy—injection of bulking agents, a sling, or an artificial sphincter. In multivariate analysis (Table 30.3-9), recovery of continence was associated with younger age, absence of a stricture, and preservation of the NVB. Spontaneous improvement in continence is common up to 1 year and may occur up to 2 years after surgery.[257]

ERECTILE FUNCTION. Recovery of erectile function after radical prostatectomy is directly related to the extent of preservation of the cavernous nerves, the patient's age, the quality of his erections before the operation, and the experience of the operating surgeon.[255,256] The probability of recovery of function is less in nationwide surveys, with only 40% of patients recovering adequate erections.[291,290] With preservation of both nerves, the average patient first experiences erections adequate for intercourse 4 months after the operation, and erections continue to improve for 2 to 3 years (Fig. 30.3-30; Table 30.3-10).[258,292,293] Approximately 50% of patients will recover normal erections, measured by an International Index of Erectile Function score of 26 or greater, 3 years after the operation. Approximately 85% recover functional erections (International Index of Erectile Function score of 17 or greater). One in five patients require oral medication, such as sildenafil, to achieve this level of function. Recovery may be facilitated by early and frequent use of oral or injectable medications to assure regular erections, at least

TABLE 30.3-9. Univariate and Multivariate Analysis of the Risk Factors for Incontinence after Radical Prostatectomy

	P Value	
Risk Factor	Univariate Analysis	Multivariate Analysis
Patient weight (continuous)	.002	Not available
Lower urinary tract symptoms (none vs. requiring treatment)		
Obstructive	.004	.111
Irritative	.624	.186
Prostate size by transrectal ultrasound (continuous)	.441	.250
Transurethral resection of prostate (yes or no)	.001	.349
Clinical stage (T1a,b/T1c/T2a/T2b/T2c/T3)	.001	.158
Tumor palpable at apex	.289	.707
Operative blood loss (continuous)	.016	.829
Postoperative bleeding (presence/absence of clinically significant bleeding)	.577	.647
Pathologic stage (confined, ECE vs. SVI, +LN)	.310	.733
Nerve resection (none vs. unilateral vs. bilateral)	.001	.015
Anastomotic stricture (yes or no)	.001	.015
Patient age (continuous)	.001	.0001
Anastomotic technique (old or new)	.001	.0001

ECE, extracapsular extension; +LN, positive lymph nodes; SVI, seminal vesicle invasion.
(From Eastham JA, Goad JR, Rogers E, et al. Risk factors for urinary incontinence after radical prostatectomy. *J Urol* 1996;156:1707, with permission.)

three times a week, in the early postoperative period.[294] Wide resection of one NVB substantially reduces recovery of erectile function.[258,293] Cavermap neurostimulation (Uromed Corporation, Boston, MA) can be used during the operation to verify functional preservation of the nerves.[295]

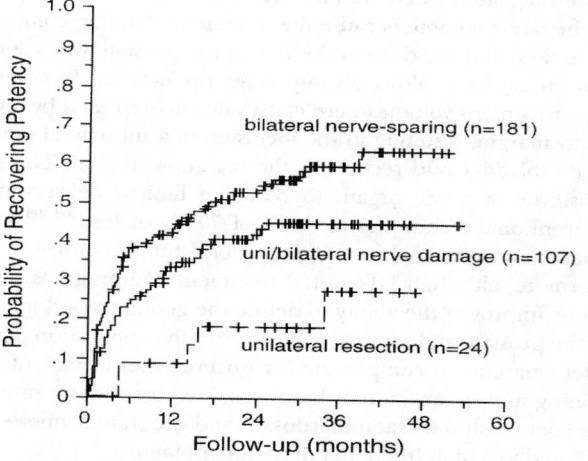

FIGURE 30.3-30. Recovery of erections for all patients, regardless of age or prior potency, after radical prostatectomy according to extent of preservation of neurovascular bundles. (From ref. 258, with permission.)

TABLE 30.3-10. Probability of Recovery of Erectile Dysfunction by 36 Months for Men with Both Nerves Preserved

	Probability (%)		
Preoperative Potency	Age 60 Y or Younger	Age 60.1–65.0 Y	Age >65 Y
Full erection	76	55	49
Full erection, recently diminished	59	39	35
Partial erection	49	31	27

(From ref. 258, with permission.)

RADIATION THERAPY

CURATIVE POTENTIAL OF RADIOTHERAPY

The goal of radiation therapy, as with surgery, is to eliminate the tumor in the prostate completely, although the prostate itself remains *in situ*, with the least possible harm to bowel, bladder, and erectile function. External-beam radiation therapy was introduced as a curative modality for localized prostate cancer in the 1950s, when megavoltage radiotherapy technology made it possible to deliver tumoricidal doses to prostate tumors without excessive damage to the skin and the normal tissues surrounding the prostate.[296,297] Incremental advances in radiation dosimetry, treatment planning, and delivery have since enabled enhanced precision, increased dose, and reduced toxicity. Consequently, the ability of radiation to cure organ-confined and locally advanced tumors has improved steadily over the past two decades.[297–300]

Evidence suggests that failure of radiotherapy to control localized disease results most frequently from tumor clonogens that are resistant to the conventional dose levels of 65 to 70 Gy—the maximum that can be delivered safely with traditional two-dimensional (2D) treatment planning and delivery techniques—and from failure to cover the entire target volume with the prescribed tumor dose. Before CT became available for treatment planning, tumor target volumes were assumed from plain-film radiographic images and were often inaccurate.[301] Dose calculations were also limited to a small number of planes in the target volume because the treatment-planning computers were slow, and the dose to the rest of the prostate was assumed from reasonable, although imprecise, projections. To compensate, treatment volumes were classically encompassed by a wide safety margin, resulting in the inclusion of a substantial portion of the bladder and rectum to the high-dose region. The high sensitivity of pelvic organs to radiation limited delivery using conventional techniques to doses of 70 Gy or less,[302,303] below what is needed to achieve maximal local tumor control.[304] Furthermore, although CT-assisted treatment planning has significantly improved the ability to define the geometry and location of the prostate and seminal vesicles,[305,306] the application of wide safety margins to compensate for uncertainties in patient positioning and organ motion have remained a common practice. The net result was that underdosage and geographic misses contributed to a high frequency of treatment failure.

Advances in computer technology have enabled the implementation of three-dimensional conformal radiation therapy (3D-CRT) to overcome the deficiencies of conventional 2D

approaches.[300,307] 3D treatment planning incorporates anatomic definition of each subvolume within the entire space irradiated and precise calculation of the dose delivered at each point. It uses advanced imaging for tumor and normal organ segmentation, new algorithms for dose calculations, and computer-aided optimization to generate treatment plans that conform the prescribed dose to the tumor whereas maximally excluding the adjacent normal organs. The ability to exclude normal tissues from the volume receiving high-dose irradiation has allowed significantly higher tumor doses without increased normal tissue toxicity.[300] The improved precision decreases the risk of anatomic tumor misses and underdosage, further improving the potential for local tumor cure. Indeed, data from postradiation biopsies have demonstrated that 3D-CRT and dose escalation improve the local eradication rate of prostate cancer and have defined new standards for curative radiotherapy.[300]

DEFINITION OF TARGET VOLUME

Carcinoma of the prostate is frequently multifocal, involving more than one lobe of the gland, and capsular involvement with or without periprostatic invasion is not infrequent in radical prostatectomy specimens even in patients with T1 and T2 lesions. As such, the clinical target volume (CTV) for irradiation must include the total prostate gland, the prostatic capsule and immediate periprostatic tissues, and the seminal vesicles, as visualized on CT. For T1 and small T2 tumors with a low PSA and Gleason score, treatment may be limited to the prostate target only, because the likelihood of seminal vesicle involvement is low. The planning target volume (PTV) encompasses the clinical target volume and an additional 1-cm margin to compensate for patient setup uncertainties and organ motion.[308,309]

The inclusion of pelvic lymph nodes in the clinical target volume is controversial. The major lymph nodes that drain the prostate—external iliac, hypogastric, presacral, and internal pudendal nodes—can be treated by fields that encompass a major portion of the pelvis.[310] Early prospective randomized studies in patients undergoing staging laparotomy[311,312] suggested that prophylactic lymph node irradiation might benefit only patients with T1 and T2 disease. This was not confirmed.[313,314] For example, the RTOG trial 77-06 randomized 449 patients with T1b to T2N0M0 tumors to receive either prostatic or prostatic plus whole pelvic irradiation after bipedal lymphangiography or staging laparotomy, or both, and reported no significant differences in local control or survival (median follow-up of 12 years).[314]

In contrast, in a trial of 201 patients with an estimated risk of lymph node involvement of more than 15% based on pretreatment profiles of PSA and Gleason scores, PSA failure rates were reduced among 117 patients who received whole pelvic irradiation, compared to 84 patients whose treatment was limited to the prostate (median PSA relapse-free survival of 34.3 vs. 21.0 months; $P = .0001$).[315] To address this further, the RTOG conducted a four-arm trial[316] in which patients with a more than 15% estimated risk of pelvic lymph node involvement were randomized to receive (1) whole pelvic radiotherapy with a boost to the prostate plus neoadjuvant and concurrent androgen deprivation therapy, (2) radiotherapy to the prostate only plus neoadjuvant and concurrent androgen deprivation therapy, (3) whole pelvic radiotherapy with a boost to the prostate plus adjuvant androgen deprivation, or (4) radiotherapy to the prostate only plus adjuvant androgen deprivation. The 4-year progression-free survival rates were 60%, 44%, 49%, and 50%, respectively (*P* = .008), suggesting an advantage to pelvic irradiation when neoadjuvant and concomitant androgen deprivation therapy are administered. This study is unique in its inclusion of androgen deprivation. Although longer follow-up is needed to confirm the trends observed thus far, the findings are likely to affect the management of high-risk patients.

SIMULATION AND TREATMENT PLANNING: CONVENTIONAL (TWO-DIMENSIONAL) EXTERNAL-BEAM RADIOTHERAPY

Much of the available long-term outcome data for radiation treatment of prostate cancer are derived from patients treated in the 1970s, before the introduction of modern cross-sectional imaging. The anatomic boundaries of the prostate and the design of treatment fields were determined by information obtained from conventional plain-film radiographic simulator techniques, using the location of the pubic bone, a Foley catheter balloon, bladder and rectal contrast media, and the DRE as landmarks.[317] Large safety margins were typically required to address uncertainties of tumor target definition. Treatment was typically administered using relatively small 6 cm × 6 cm to 8 cm × 8 cm fields applied with rotational arc techniques.[296,317] Although this approach provided satisfactory coverage for small T1 and T2a tumors,[318] reconstruction of such fields using CT imaging has since indicated that even an 8 cm × 8 cm field size did not adequately cover most bulky or locally advanced tumors.[319] Beginning in approximately 1970, treatment volumes were expanded to include the pelvic lymph node drainage of the prostate.[317]

The conventional treatment techniques currently being used are based on CT-assisted planning. Initially, radiation is given to the whole pelvis using a four-field approach, designed to include the prostate, seminal vesicles, and the regional lymph nodes.[320] The cross section of each beam is shaped using individualized Cerrobend blocks to shield the posterior wall of the rectum, the anal canal and sphincter, the small bowel, and the uninvolved bladder and urethra. Treatment is delivered in daily dose fractions of 1.8 to 2.0 Gy, given five sessions per week, to a total of 45 to 50 Gy. An additional primary target "boost," delivered with either a four-field approach[320] or a bilateral 120-degree arc rotational technique is then administered to increase the dose to the prostate and seminal vesicles (surrounded by a 1- to 2-cm "safety margin" of normal tissue).[296,317] A major drawback of rotational techniques is that shaped blocking cannot be used to shield normal tissues. Thus, a large volume of the bladder and the rectum receives the same dose as the prostatic tumor target. However, even with the four-field boost approach, effective customized shielding is difficult with conventional treatment planning methods. The standard boost dose is 20 Gy, delivered with the same fractionation schedule as used in treating the large pelvic fields, for a total dose to the prostate of 65 to 70 Gy. For T1 and small T2 tumors with a low Gleason score, treatment is limited to the prostate target volume (carried to 65 to 70 Gy), because of the small likelihood of seminal vesicle involvement and metastatic spread to the pelvic lymph nodes.[320]

THREE-DIMENSIONAL CONFORMAL RADIOTHERAPY

3D treatment planning systems vary in details but are based on common principles. CT images are used to segment the prostate and normal organs and to produce high-resolution 3D reconstructions. Modern, dedicated CT simulators incorporate traditional radiographic simulation procedures, such as establishment of the treatment isocenter and the placement of fiduciary skin marks, and CT imaging into one session. The CT data are also used in calculations of dose distribution, because modern dose calculation formalisms are based on electron density ratios of the anatomic structures included in the treatment fields.[307] Several algorithms are in use for 3D-dose calculations, but the more advanced methods, such as the pencil beam convolution algorithm with pixel-by-pixel inhomogeneity corrections,[307] are required for maximal accuracy.

Treatment is planned and delivered with the patient in the supine or prone position,[321] using individually fabricated immobilization devices to assure daily reproducibility of positioning on the treatment couch.[322] Because prostatic displacement during a course of radiotherapy is affected by rectal and bladder volumes,[323] some recommend that the patient empty his bladder and rectum before simulation and each treatment session. The prostatic target volume and the critical normal structures are segmented on every CT slice on which they appear. The PTV extends from 1 cm caudal of the apex of the prostate to 1 cm cephalad of the superior tips of the seminal vesicles and encompasses the prostate with a 1-cm margin, except posteriorly at the interface with the rectum, where some investigators have suggested the use of a 0.6-cm margin to reduce the risk of rectal toxicity.[319] The target volume and the normal organs are then reconstructed by the computer in 3D and displayed with the beam's eye view technique. The most commonly used beam arrangement consists of six coplanar fields (two lateral opposed fields and two pairs of oblique fields) shaped to conform the PTV.[324] Dose calculations are then performed, and the adequacy of target coverage by the prescription dose is evaluated on displays of isodose or color-wash distributions (Fig. 30.3-31) and by dose-volume histograms.[325] The target dose is either prescribed to the International Commission

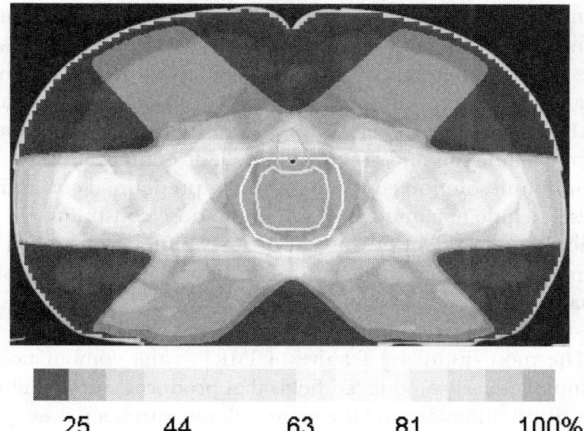

25   44   63   81   100%

FIGURE 30.3-31. Color wash displays of the dose distribution of a six-field coplanar prostate three-dimensional conformal radiation therapy plan with 15-MeV x-rays. The planned treatment consists of one pair of lateral and two pairs of oblique fields. The dose distribution is shown on axial, sagittal, and coronal computed tomography reconstructions of the prostate and surrounding normal tissue at the midplane of the planning target volume (PTV). The boundaries of the PTV are shown in yellow dots. The red region represents the prescription isodose distribution, whereas the yellow region corresponds to approximately 70% to 80%, green to 45% to 70%, and blue to 45% or less of the prescription dose. (From ref. 319, with permission.) (See Color Fig. 30.3-31 in the CD-ROM.)

on Radiation Units 50 reference point[308] or to the maximum iso-dose surface distribution that completely encompasses the PTV.[326] Some suggest restricting the rectal wall dose to no more than 30% of the prescription dose, the bladder wall dose to 50%, and the bowel dose (when bowel happens to be included in the PTV) to 65% to decrease the risk of toxicity.[327]

When radiation cannot be administered without exceeding these limits, a 3-month course of neoadjuvant androgen deprivation can effectively decrease the target volume. Nearly 90% of patients treated by this approach have shown significant reductions in PTV, allowing a reduction in the volume of normal tissue exposed to the prescription dose.[327] Beam apertures are automatically shaped by the treatment-planning computer, applying a continuously varying aperture with a margin of 0.5 cm around the outline of the tumor target to account for beam penumbra. The planned treatment fields are then shaped with Cerrobend blocks or multileaf collimators. To assure that treatment is delivered as planned, treatment verification is performed with traditional portal films or electronic portal images, produced at least once per week.

INTENSITY-MODULATED RADIATION THERAPY

Intensity-modulated radiotherapy (IMRT) is an advanced form of 3D-CRT that uses highly specialized treatment planning and delivery systems to produce dose distributions that conform to the tumor target with significantly enhanced precision. Two features that distinguish IMRT from 3D-CRT are inverse algorithms and treatment fields with varying intensities over the cross section of the beam. Inverse planning uses a mathematic approach to convert a predefined desired dose distribution into a clinically applicable treatment plan, in contrast to the trial-and-error forward planning used in 3D-CRT. A computer-aided optimization algorithm iteratively adjusts the intensity profile of each radiation beam until the planned dose distribution fulfills as closely as possible the predefined dose specifications for the tumor and normal tissue structures.[328] The outcome is a set of radiation beams with changing intensities across the treatment field. Multiple intensity-modulated beams with different profiles are used to achieve a composite homogeneous dose distribution within the PTV. The inverse algorithm at MSKCC uses a least-squares objective function and conjugate gradient minimization to find an optimum solution consistent with the predefined constraints. These include maximum and minimum dose constraints for the tumor target and both dose and dose-volume constraints for normal tissue. These constraints can be violated with a cost or penalty weighted according to the relative importance of the constraint in meeting the goals of the plan.[319]

The most distinctive feature of IMRT is the combination of multiple intensity-modulated fields that produces custom-tailored dose distributions around the target volume with steep dose gradients at the transition to normal tissue. Delivery of such beams requires multileaf collimation in either the dynamic or multisegment static (step-and-shoot) modes or tomotherapy using beams directed over a full 360-degree range, modulated by a slit, bimodal multileaf collimation in which the leaf shutters are driven in and out of the beam path. At MSKCC, a coplanar five-field IMRT technique is used to treat patients to dose levels of 81 Gy or higher.[329] The dose limit within the PTV is 110%. The dose distribution of this treatment plan is shown in Figure 30.3-32.[319] Compared to the 3D-CRT plan (see Fig. 30.3-31), the high-dose volume in the

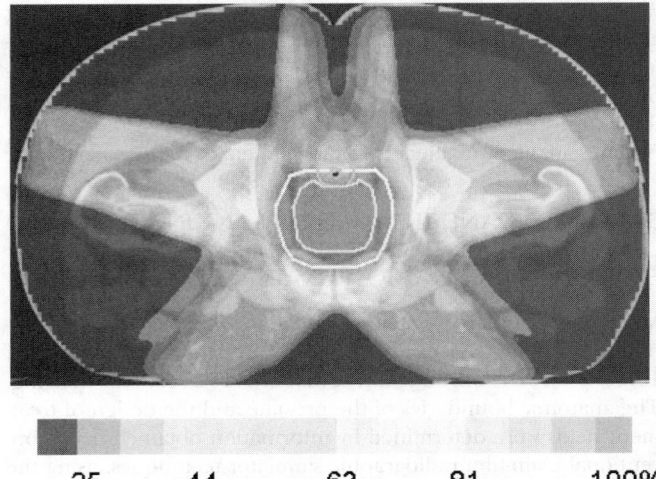

25   44   63   81   100%

FIGURE 30.3-32.   Midplane axial color wash dose distribution display of a five-field coplanar prostate intensity-modulated radiotherapy plan for 15-MeV x-rays, consisting of fields placed at angles of 0, 75, 135, 225, and 285 degrees. In this display, a band of the color spectrum corresponds to a range of doses. The prescription dose is normalized to 100%. The red region corresponds to the prescription isodose distribution (100% to 105%); yellow represents approximately 70% to 80%; green, 45% to 70%; and blue, 45% or less. The planning target volume contour is in yellow; the clinical target volume is in green, and the rectum is in magenta. (From ref. 319, with permission.) (See Color Fig. 30.3-32 in the CD-ROM.)

IMRT conforms better to the shape of the PTV and sculpts around rather than transects the adjacent rectum.

OUTCOMES: DEFINING TUMOR CONTROL AFTER RADIOTHERAPY

The specific outcomes reported after radiation therapy vary. Before the PSA era, tumor control was generally assessed by DRE, radiography, or isotope scans, or all. These methods are somewhat imprecise, especially for assessing local control. Postradiation biopsy is a more sensitive measure, but with biopsy, the time interval between the completion of radiation and the actual performance of biopsy is critical[330] because of the slow rate at which cancer cells disappear from the irradiated gland.[331] In one study, 32% of patients with a positive biopsy at 12 months after radiotherapy had a negative pathologic specimen at 24 months.[332] As a result, the American Society for Therapeutic Radiology and Oncology consensus statement recommends that biopsies be performed a minimum of 2 years after treatment.[333]

As posttreatment biopsies are not routinely performed in the absence of another indication of treatment failure, most current studies use a PSA end point. It is now recognized that PSA relapse precedes anatomic relapse by 2 years or more.[334,335] A caveat is that a rising PSA posttreatment may represent either persistent local disease or systemic failure, or both.

After pelvic irradiation, the serum PSA level typically declines over 1 to 2 years but does not reach undetectable levels, owing to normal prostate that remains when tumor is eliminated. Seventy percent of patients receiving pelvic radiotherapy for rectal and other nonprostatic tumors have PSA levels of 1 ng/mL or less for extended periods after treatment.[336] This observation led to the suggestion that a postradiation PSA value of 1 or less would be surrogate of cure[337] and that an increase of serum PSA from such postradiation nadir values would indicate relapse.[338]

Reviewing the emerging data in the field, an American Society for Therapeutic Radiology and Oncology consensus panel defined *biochemical failure* as three successive increases in the PSA value from an established nadir value.[339] The date of failure was taken as the midpoint between the last postirradiation nadir value and the first increase. Appropriately, the guideline did not stipulate a specific nadir value to be associated with a complete response. The results of several studies indicate that a PSA nadir of 1 ng/mL or less is an independent variable in predicting long-term PSA relapse-free survival.[337,340,341] In one study, the 5-year likelihood of relapse or rising PSA for patients who achieved a nadir of less than 1 ng/mL was 17% versus 70% for those with posttreatment nadirs of 1 ng/mL or greater.[340] Another study categorized patients into nadir PSA quartile groups. The 5-year freedom from failure estimates were 83%, 72%, 58%, and 33% for nadir PSA groups of less than 0.3, 0.3 to less than 0.6, 0.6 to less than 1.2, and 1.2 or less, respectively ($P < .0001$).[342] In a recent multi-institutional cohort of 4839 patients with T1 to T2 prostate cancer,[330] posttreatment PSA nadir values of 1 ng/mL or less were recorded in 65% of the patients. The 8-year PSA relapse-free survival was 70% for patients with a nadir of less than 5 ng/mL compared with 12% for those with a nadir of 4 ng/mL or greater.

This study showed that the majority of relapses occur in the first 5 years, but it did not address whether the rising PSA connotes an anatomic relapse in the prostate, a failure to respond to the radiation, or a systemic relapse. These issues were addressed by an MSKCC study that incorporated biopsies taken 2.5 years or more after treatment.[300,343] After treatment with 64.8 to 81.0 Gy, 50 of 51 patients (98%) with a posttreatment PSA nadir of 1 ng/mL or less and a nonrising PSA profile had negative biopsies, compared to only 21 of 42 (50%) of those with a similar nadir but with a rising PSA ($P < .001$). Of patients with a PSA nadir greater than 1 ng/mL, 7 of 10 (70%) with a nonrising PSA and 21 of 47 (45%) with a rising PSA profile had negative biopsy specimens ($P = .2$). Taken together, these data strongly suggest that in early-stage patients whose nadir PSA is 1 ng/mL or less, a nonrising PSA profile indicates a 95% likelihood of a permanent tumor control after radiotherapy.

LOCAL TUMOR CONTROL

True rates of local relapse after conventional radiotherapy have been difficult to assess because posttreatment biopsies are not performed routinely. Most are performed only after the patient has developed a rising PSA. Over the past three decades, 10-year rates of local control, based on DRE alone, range from 85% to 96% for T1b to T2 tumors and from 58% to 65% for T3 to T4 tumors.[126] Based on PSA, cancer control rates for T1 to T2 tumors in one series were only 49% to 53%[344] and, in a second, 59% at 5 years and 53% at 8 years for a multi-institutional pooled cohort of 4839.[345] In the latter series, the percentages were 61% and 55%, respectively, for patients who received 70 Gy or more.[345] For patients with locally advanced T3 disease, PSA relapse-free survivals were only 24%.[346] In the few studies with routine prostate biopsy after conventional radiotherapy, biopsy-proven local recurrence rates were 15% to 65% among patients with T1 to T3 tumors treated to 64 to 70 Gy.[347,348]

DOSE EFFECTS

The effects of radiation on tumor and normal tissues are dose dependent, with sigmoidal dose-response curves.[348–350] Because human tumors consist of clonogen populations heterogeneous in radiation sensitivity,[351] it was suggested that tumor control curves would be relatively shallow, representing population averages of patients with a spectrum of tumor radiosensitivities.[352,353] The validity of this notion in prostate cancer was confirmed in an MSKCC postradiation biopsy study of 103 patients who did not receive neoadjuvant androgen deprivation.[300,343] The D_{50} value was calculated to be 2.9,[354–357] significantly different from the D_{50} of approximately 4 for normal tissue complications.

Multiple studies support the notion that local tumor control is directly related to dose and indicate that more than 70 Gy is needed to control prostate cancer. For example, in a study of 624 patients with T3 prostate cancer, the actuarial 7-year clinical local recurrence rates (based on DRE findings) were 36% for patients receiving 60.0 to 64.9 Gy, 32% for 65.0 to 69.9 Gy, and 24% for 70 Gy or more.[358] An analysis from RTOG found that patients with Gleason scores of 8 to 10 who received more than 66 Gy (median, 69 Gy) had significantly better disease-specific and overall survival rates than did those treated to 66 Gy or less (median, 64 Gy). Other retrospective studies provide similar conclusions regarding a need for increased radiation doses to achieve a maximal local cure.[359,360]

Figure 30.3-33[319] shows the outcomes for 1684 stage T1c to T3 prostate cancer patients treated at MSKCC in a dose-escalation study.[300,343] The radiation dose was increased by increments of 5.4 Gy in successive groups of patients, from 64.8 Gy to 86.4 Gy. Treatment was given in daily fractions of 1.8 Gy, and the treatment volume included the prostate and seminal vesicles but not the regional lymph nodes. A total of 907 patients were treated with 3D-CRT and 777 with IMRT. The 5-year actuarial PSA relapse-free survival rate for patients with favorable prognostic indicators (stage

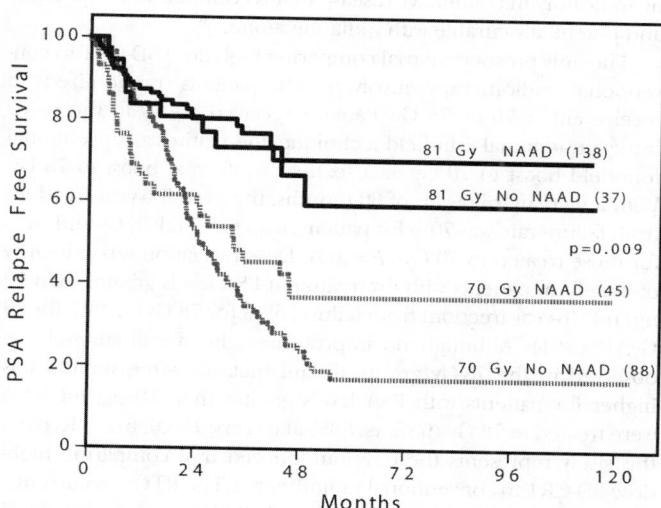

FIGURE 30.3-33. Actuarial prostate-specific antigen (PSA) relapse-free survival for unfavorable risk patients treated to 81 Gy alone or with neoadjuvant androgen deprivation (NAAD) compared with those treated to 70 Gy or less either alone or with NAAD. Within each dose level, the differences between the biochemical outcome of patients treated with radiotherapy alone or with androgen deprivation were not statistically significant. (From ref. 319, with permission.)

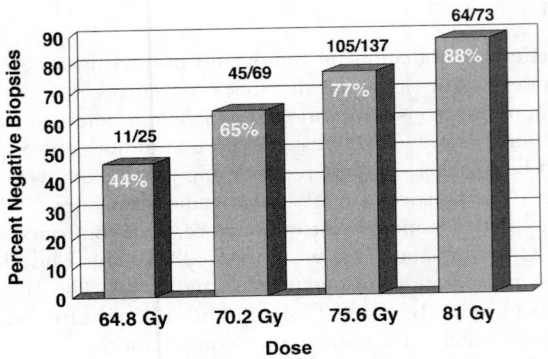

FIGURE 30.3-34. The impact of radiation dose on local control assessed by prostate biopsies in 304 patients at ≥2.5 years after three-dimensional conformal radiation therapy and intensity-modulated radiotherapy. (From ref. 319, with permission.) (See Color Fig. 30.3-34 in the CD-ROM.)

T1 to 2 pretreatment PSA, 10 ng/mL or less; Gleason score, 6 or less) who received 81.0 to 86.4 Gy was 96% compared to 86% for those treated to 75.6 Gy (*P* = .01) and 65% for patients receiving 64.8 to 70.2 Gy (*P* = .008). The corresponding rates for patients with intermediate prognosis (one of the prognostic indicators with a higher value) were 87% compared to 61% (*P* <.001) and 44%, respectively (*P* = .007). For those with unfavorable prognostic indicators (two or more of the prognostic indicators with higher values), the 5-year actuarial PSA relapse-free survival rate for 81.0 to 86.4 Gy was 69% compared to 43% for 75.6 Gy (*P* = .001) and only 22% for 64.8 to 70.2 Gy (*P* = .003). Androgen deprivation did not improve PSA relapse-free survival in any of the risk groups.[319] This study defines the critical role of dose in effecting long-term cure of prostate cancer with radiation. Combined with the results of post-treatment biopsies obtained in patients followed for 2.5 years or more (Fig. 30.3-34), these data suggest that at least 81 Gy may be required for a maximal probability of cure. It also demonstrates that a significant proportion of patients with unfavorable prognostic indicators may still have disease that is confined to the prostate and potentially curable with radiation alone.[319]

The only prospective trial comparing high-dose 3D-CRT to conventional radiotherapy involved 301 patients randomized to receive either 70 or 78 Gy. Patients received 46 Gy to the pelvis using a traditional four-field technique, then either a conventional four-field boost to 70 Gy or a six-field conformal boost to 78 Gy. With a median follow-up of 60 months, the overall 6-year freedom from failure rate was 70% for patients who received 78 Gy and 64% for those treated to 70 Gy (*P* = .03). Dose escalation was primarily of benefit in patients with pretreatment PSA levels greater than 10 ng/mL (6-year freedom from failure, 62% for 78 Gy vs. 43% for 70 Gy; *P* = .01). Although no improvement in overall survival was observed in the 78-Gy group, distant metastasis-free survival was higher for patients with PSA levels greater than 10 ng/mL who were treated to 78 Gy (98% vs. 88% at 6 years; *P* = .056).[135] To date, this study represents the only randomized trial comparing high-dose 3D-CRT to conventional radiotherapy. The RTOG is currently conducting a randomized 3D-CRT trial (P-0126) comparing 72.93 Gy with 82.28 Gy (delivered in daily fractions of 1.87 Gy).

FACTORS PREDICTIVE OF CANCER CONTROL

Long-term outcomes after radiotherapy can be predicted from baseline clinical parameters. Using proportional hazards regression analysis, most studies have identified pretreatment PSA, stage T2 by DRE, Gleason score, and dose as independent predictors. A 94% 6-year PSA relapse-free survival after radiotherapy was reported for T1 to T2 patients with PSA of 4 or less and Gleason score of 2 to 6, 70% for patients with PSA of 4 or less and Gleason score of 7 to 10 or PSA of 4 to 10 and Gleason score of 2 to 7, and 60% for patients with PSA greater than 4 and Gleason scores of 8 or greater.[335] These groups were refined further in a multi-institutional cohort of 1765 patients treated with advanced external-beam techniques to doses ranging from 63 to 79 Gy (median dose, 69.4 Gy) in which the overall 5-year PSA relapse-free survival was 65.8%. Recursive partitioning analysis of initial PSA, T stage defined by DRE, and the Gleason score yielded four prognostic groups. Patients with PSA levels less than 9.2 ng/mL had a 5-year PSA relapse-free survival rate of 81%. For patients with PSA levels between 9.2 and 19.7 ng/mL it was 69%, for a PSA of 19.7 ng/mL or greater and a Gleason score of 2 to 6 it was 47%, and for patients with a PSA greater than or equal to 19.7 ng/mL and a Gleason score of 7 to 10, the rate was 29%.[299] Other groups are also reporting outcomes based on pretreatment prognostic groups. All of these trials have to be interpreted in the context of the administered dose.

RADIATION COMPARED TO SURGERY

A true comparison of the outcomes for surgery and radiation therapy is difficult in the absence of a prospective randomized trial in which patients matched for pretreatment prognostic factors are enrolled. The difficulties associated with conducting such a trial are well recognized. The comparisons are inevitable, but, when doing so, it is important to consider the specifics of the patient population treated, the expertise of the treating team, and the end point(s)—both cancer specific and patient quality of life specific—that are reported.

Before the PSA era, it appeared that long-term outcomes with radiotherapy of T1 and T2 tumors were similar to those of radical perineal prostatectomy,[298,318,361–365] although assessment of radiotherapy outcomes in this era (by DRE, radiography, and isotope scans) was somewhat imprecise, especially for local control. Coleman et al. reported that, with the exception of very small tumors, surgery and radiotherapy resulted in a similar, constant risk of relapse throughout 20 years of follow-up.[366] Stage for stage, the survival outcome was similar for the surgical and radiation series.

It has been frequently stated that although the results of radiation and radical surgery are similar up to 10 years, at longer follow-up periods, there may be a selective rapid decrement in survival and disease-free survival for irradiated patients.[366] Despite this contention, Table 30.3-11, summarizing published long-term results with conventional external-beam irradiation, indicates outcome data for irradiated patients at 15 years similar to published outcomes for radical prostatectomy.[298,367–369]

A review of 298 stage T1 to T2 patients treated with radical prostatectomy and 253 with radiotherapy found 5-year PSA relapse-free survival rates were 43% for radiation and 57% for surgery. Multivariate analysis of time to failure showed that pretreatment PSA level and biopsy Gleason scores were independent predictors of PSA relapse. Based on these parameters, low risk (pretreatment PSA of 10 ng/mL or less and Gleason score of 6 or less) and high risk (PSA greater than 10 ng/mL or Gleason score

TABLE 30.3-11. Results of Conventional External-Beam Radiotherapy in Stage T1 through T3 Carcinoma of the Prostate

Author	Stage	No. of Patients	Survival (%)			Local Relapse-Free Survival (%)		
			5-Y	10-Y	15-Y	5-Y	10-Y	15-Y
Bagshaw et al.[382]	T1	335	85	65	40	90	85	90
	T2	242	83	55	35	80	70	65
	T3	409	68	47	20	76	63	40
Hanks et al.[367]	T1	60	84	54	51	96	96	83
	T2	312	74	43	22	83	71	65
	T3	216	56	32	23	70	65	60
Zagars et al.[369]	T1	32	76	68	—	100	100	—
	T2	82	96	70	—	97	88	—
	T3	551	72	47	27	88	81	75
Perez et al.[368]	T1	48	85	70	—	90	80	—
	T2	252	82	65	—	85	76	—
	T3	412	65	42	—	72	60	—

of 7 or greater) were defined. For low-risk patients, the 5-year PSA relapse-free survival rates for radiation versus surgery were 81% and 80%, whereas for the high-risk group the rates were 26% versus 37%, respectively.[370] A second retrospective comparison of radical prostatectomy with external-beam irradiation found that, overall, patients treated by radical prostatectomy had higher PSA relapse-free survival rates relative to those treated with radiation therapy. However, when patients receiving high-dose radiotherapy (72 Gy or greater) were compared to surgically treated patients, treatment modality was no longer an independent predictor of outcome. The investigators concluded that doses of less than 72 Gy were insufficient to control localized prostate cancer.[371] A review of the published literature on conformal radiotherapy in T1 to T2 low- and intermediate-risk prostate cancer concluded that patients who receive external irradiation should be treated using conformal radiotherapy techniques and that those with PSA levels of 10 to 20 ng/mL should receive a minimum dose of 75 to 78 Gy.[135] As is discussed in Tolerance of Treatment and Late Complications, radiation toxicities can be reduced dramatically with the application of IMRT, emphasizing the necessity of this approach when high-dose levels are administered.

TOLERANCE OF TREATMENT AND LATE COMPLICATIONS

Complication rates vary as a function of the dose and the treatment field. Doses of 70 Gy or less delivered with conventional (2D) external-beam irradiation are generally well tolerated. However, approximately 60% of patients have grade 2 (Table 30.3-12) or higher acute rectal morbidity or urinary symptoms, or both, requiring medication.[372] Symptoms typically appear during the third week of treatment and resolve within days to weeks after its completion. Acute intestinal symptoms, especially those associated with whole pelvic irradiation, are most commonly relieved with dietary manipulations. Otherwise, medications, such as loperamide hydrochloride (Imodium) or diphenoxylate hydrochloride and atropine sulphate (Lomotil), are appropriate to relieve symptoms. Internal and external hemorrhoids may become inflamed during a course of therapy. These symptoms are often best treated with sitz baths and hydrocortisone suppositories. Acute urinary symptoms are treated with phenazopyridine hydrochloride (Pyridium), nonsteroidal antiinflammatory agents, or α blockers, such as tamsulosin hydrochloride (Flomax). α Blockers have been reported to be significantly more effective than nonsteroidal antiinflammatory agents, resulting in significant resolution of urinary symptoms in 66% and moderate improvement in 22% of patients.[373]

Late complications are those that developed 3 or more months after completion of radiotherapy or that start during treatment and persist for longer than 3 months after its completion. Zelefsky et al. reported that the median time to onset of grade 2 or higher late rectal toxicity was 12 months with a range of 3 to 39 months.[300] Similarly, Teshima et al. reported median times to occurrence of grade 2 and 3 rectal toxicities of 13 and 18 months, respectively.[374] The incidence of late complications in patients receiving conventional radiotherapy doses of 70 Gy or less is low. An analysis of 1020 patients treated in two large RTOG trials demonstrated a 7.3% incidence of chronic urinary sequelae (i.e., cystitis, hematuria, urethral stricture, or bladder contracture) altering the patient's performance status or requiring hospitalization but only a 0.5% incidence of urinary complications requiring major surgical intervention. More than one-half of chronic urinary complications were urethral strictures, occurring mostly in patients who had undergone TURP before radiotherapy. The incidence of chronic intestinal or rectal sequelae (e.g., chronic diarrhea, proctitis, rectal or anal stricture, rectal bleeding, or ulcer) requiring hospitalization was 3.3%, with only 0.6% of patients experiencing bowel obstruction or perforation. Fatal complications were extremely uncommon (0.2%).

The risk of late complications increases when radiation doses exceed 70 Gy. In one study of 174 patients, 6.9% of patients treated with 70 Gy or more using conventional techniques experienced grade 3 to 4 complications versus 3.5% who received less than 70 Gy. When conventional techniques were used in a dose-escalation study, the 2-year rates of moderate to severe proctitis increased from 20% when the anterior rectal wall dose was less than 75 Gy to 60% when higher doses were administered.[303] The actuarial incidence of grade 3 to 4 rectal toxicity for patients treated with 3D-CRT who received doses of more than 68 Gy was reported as 9% at 3 years compared to 2% for those who received lower doses.[375] Among 712 patients treated with conventional or conformal radiation techniques, the risk of late toxicity strongly correlated with the central axis dose. The 5-year incidence of grade 2 to 3 late rectal toxicity was 27%, 35%, and 43% for central axis doses of 71 to 74 Gy, 74 to 77 Gy, and 77 Gy or greater, respectively ($P<.001$).[376]

TABLE 30.3-12. Radiation Therapy Oncology Group–European Organization for Research and Treatment of Cancer Scoring Scheme for Acute and Late Rectal and Bladder Morbidity

Grade	Rectal	Bladder
ACUTE DISEASE		
0	No toxicity	No toxicity
1	Increased frequency or change in quality of bowel habits not requiring medication; rectal discomfort not requiring analgesics	Frequency of urination or nocturia that is less frequent than every hour; dysuria, urgency, bladder spasm requiring local anesthetic
2	Diarrhea requiring parasympatholytic drugs [e.g., diphenoxylate (Lomotil)]; mucous discharge not necessitating sanitary pads; rectal or abdominal pain requiring analgesics	Frequency of urination or nocturia that is less frequent than every hour; dysuria, urgency, bladder spasm requiring local anesthetic
3	Diarrhea requiring parenteral support; severe mucous or bloody discharge necessitating sanitary pads; abdominal distended bowel loops	Frequency with urgency and nocturia hourly or more frequently; dysuria, pelvic pain, or bladder spasm requiring regular, frequent narcotic; gross hematuria with or without clot passage
4	Acute or subacute obstruction, fistula, or perforation; gastrointestinal bleeding requiring transfusion; abdominal pain or tenesmus requiring tube decompression or bowel diversion	Hematuria requiring transfusion; acute bladder obstruction not secondary to clot passage, ulceration, or necrosis
CHRONIC DISEASE		
0	No toxicity	No toxicity
1	Mild diarrhea; mild cramping; bowel movement 5 times daily; slight rectal discharge or bleeding	Slight epithelial atrophy; minor telangiectasia; microscopic hematuria
2	Moderate diarrhea and colic; bowel movement >5 times daily; excessive rectal mucus or intermittent bleeding	Moderate frequency; generalized telangiectasia; intermittent microscopic hematuria
3	Obstruction or bleeding requiring surgery	Severe frequency and dysuria; severe generalized telangiectasia (often with petechiae); frequent hematuria; reduction in bladder capacity (<150 cc)
4	Necrosis; perforation; fistula	Necrosis; constructed bladder (capacity <100 cc); severe hemorrhagic cystitis

Rectal complications have also been correlated with the volume of anterior rectal wall receiving a given dose (the so-called volume effect). Dose-volume patterns and their relationship with rectal bleeding were described in patients treated with 50.4-Gy whole pelvic photon beam radiotherapy followed by 25.2 Cobalt Gy equivalent (CGE) delivered via a 160-MeV perineal proton beam boost.[377] A logistic regression analysis revealed ten dose-volume combinations that were more likely associated with late rectal bleeding, ranging from 60 CGE delivered to 70% of the anterior rectal wall to 75 CGmE involving 30% of the rectal wall. When more than 40% of the anterior rectal wall was exposed to 75 CGE, the actuarial incidence of bleeding at 40 months was 61%, compared to 19% when less than 40% of the wall was exposed (*P* = .0036). In a study of patients treated with 3D-CRT to PTV doses of 70.2 and 75.6 Gy, dose-volume histograms were significantly higher in patients who developed rectal bleeding compared to those who did not.[134] Among prostate cancer patients treated to 78 Gy using a 3D-CRT boost approach, a 6-year rate of grade 2 or higher rectal toxicity of 16% was observed when 25% or less of the rectum was treated to 70 Gy or more, compared to 46% when more than 25% of the rectum was treated to 70 or more Gy (*P* = .001).[135,136] Among patients receiving PTV doses of 76 Gy or less, the use of a rectal block significantly reduced the incidence of grade 2 to 3 rectal toxicity, from 22% without a block to 7% with a block (*P* = .003).[378] These data indicated the need to maximally spare the rectal wall when high-dose therapy is used.

3D-CRT has been developed, in part, to address this issue. The ability of the 3D approach to reduce rectal and bladder toxicities has been demonstrated in several studies. The Fox Chase Cancer Center reported 34% acute grade 2 gastrointestinal or genitourinary morbidity with 3D-CRT, compared to 53% with conventional radiotherapy techniques (*P* <.001).[379] Dearnaley et al. randomized patients to receive a dose of 64 Gy with conformal or conventional techniques.[380] The rates of late grade 2 rectal toxicity were 5% for patients treated with 3D-CRT compared to 15% for those treated with the conventional plan (*P* = .01).[380] In a dose-escalation study of 1100 patients treated with 3D-CRT at MSKCC, 1% of patients developed grade 3 rectal bleeding requiring transfusion or laser cauterization, and 1% developed a grade 3 urethral stricture. All strictures occurred in patients who previously underwent TURP. The 5-year actuarial risk of grade 2 rectal bleeding for patients receiving 64.8 to 70.2 Gy was 6% compared to 17% for those treated with 75.6 to 81.0 Gy (*P* <.001).[343]

The rising rate of grade 2 rectal bleeding with increasing 3D-CRT dose indicates that dose escalation requires improved techniques to decrease the volume of exposed rectal wall and decrease the likelihood of rectal toxicity. IMRT provides this option.[343] A recent study from MSKCC compared 20 patients who were simulated and planned concomitantly with 3D-CRT and IMRT. On average, only 9% of the rectal wall would have received 75 Gy with the IMRT plan, compared to 14% with a routine six-field 3D-CRT plan (*P* <.01). With IMRT, there was also a significant improvement of the percent PTV receiving the prescription dose. To validate the decrease in toxicity expected with IMRT, 61 patients treated to 81 Gy with routine six-field 3D-CRT were compared with 171 patients treated to the same dose with IMRT. The 3-year actuarial rate of late grade 2 to 3 rectal bleeding was 3% at 81 Gy with IMRT compared to 15% for the 3D-CRT approach (*P* <.001). Only one patient in each treatment group developed grade 3 rectal bleeding.[381]

The rates of late rectal and urinary toxicity observed as of an analysis in January 2003 in 772 patients treated with IMRT are

TABLE 30.3-13. Incidence of Late Rectal and Urinary Toxicity by Grade in 772 Patients with Stage T1c-T3 Prostate Cancer Treated with Intensity-Modulated Radiotherapy to Dose Levels of 81.0 to 86.4 Gy

Grade[a]	Complication	
	Rectal, n (%)	Urinary, n (%)
None	658 (89)	570 (74)
Grade 1	97 (9)	121 (16)
Grade 2	11 (1.4)	76 (9.5)
Grade 3	6 (0.8)	5 (0.5)
Grade 4	0	0

[a]RTOG/EORTC Scoring Scheme—see Table 30.3-12.

shown in Table 30.3-13. A total of 698 patients received 81 Gy, and 74 were treated to 86.4 Gy. With a median follow-up of 36 months, only 11 patients (1.4%) developed grade 2 rectal bleeding, and six (0.8%) experienced grade 3 toxicity. Overall, the 3-year actuarial rate of late grade 2 to 3 rectal toxicity was 2.6%. The rate for the 86.4-Gy treatment group was significantly greater than that for the 81-Gy group (8% vs. 1%, $P = .008$). These findings demonstrate that the improved conformality and reduction of irradiated rectal tissue with IMRT decreased rectal toxicity compared to first-generation 3D-CRT and provided an opportunity for a safe escalation of dose to 86.4 Gy.

Sexual function is preserved in 73% to 82% of patients within the first 12 to 15 months after irradiation,[382,383] but erectile potency diminishes with time, with only 33% to 61% maintaining their potency at 5 years or longer after irradiation.[384] The radiation dose to the penile bulb appears to be an important determinant in the development of erectile dysfunction. The etiology of erectile dysfunction after radiotherapy appears to be related to vascular disruption and not cavernosal dysfunction or radiation damage to the nerve bundles, as suggested by Doppler blood-flow studies of the corporal vasculature in patients with erectile dysfunction after radiotherapy.[385] Intracavernosal prostaglandin injection therapy is effective for patients who develop impotence after radiotherapy.[386] Sildenafil citrate (Viagra) has been found to be effective in 75% of patients.[387] Responses to the medication were noted among patients with normal erectile function before radiotherapy, as compared to those with declining pretreatment function.[387]

ADJUVANT POSTOPERATIVE RADIOTHERAPY

Radiotherapy has also been used as adjuvant postoperative treatment after radical prostatectomy in patients with pathologic stage T3 to T4 disease in an attempt to eradicate microscopic residual tumor in the periprostatic tissues or adjacent pelvic lymph nodes. In an update of a Duke University series carried out in the pre-PSA era, Anscher et al. reported that this approach significantly improved local control compared with radical prostatectomy alone.[282] The actuarial local control rates at 10 and 15 years among 159 patients receiving postoperative radiation were 92% and 82%, respectively, compared to 60% and 53%, respectively, for 113 patients treated with radical prostatectomy alone ($P = .002$). There were no significant differences, however, in the rates of distant metastases and overall survival at 10 and 15 years. This trend was confirmed in a study

of patients with positive resection margins or pT3 disease, or both, who had undetectable postoperative serum PSA after radical prostatectomy.[387] Among 73 patients treated with 60- to 66-Gy adjuvant radiation therapy, the 5-year actuarial relapse-free survival, including freedom from PSA failure, was 88%, compared to 65% among 52 patients treated with surgery alone ($P <.01$). Several studies have used PSA to evaluate the outcome of this approach.[388] In a small series of 36 patients matched by preoperative PSA, Gleason score, the presence or absence of SVI, and surgical margin status, the 5-year freedom from PSA relapse rate was 89% for patients receiving adjuvant radiotherapy versus 55% for those who did not.[389] In a similar study of 76 matched pairs of patients with pT2N0 disease and a single positive margin, the 5-year freedom from PSA relapse rate was 88% for the irradiated patients and 59% for patients treated with surgery alone ($P = .005$). No patient who received postoperative irradiation had a local or distant recurrence, whereas 16% of the control group had a recurrence ($P = .015$).[390] A study from the University of California, San Francisco, showed that the actuarial 5-year PSA progression-free survival for patients receiving adjuvant radiotherapy, with or without evidence of elevated postoperative PSA, was 43% using a tumor control definition of the achievement and maintenance of a PSA of less than 0.2 ng/mL. Patients whose PSA failed to reach a nadir of less than 0.2 ng/mL after irradiation had progression with a high PSA velocity (1.5 ng/mL/yr), whereas those whose PSA reached a nadir of less than 0.2 ng/mL progressed on failure with a slower PSA velocity (0.36 ng/mL/yr).[391] Assuming that low PSA velocity is consistent with persistent local disease, these data support the notion that postoperative treatment is effective in controlling local residual disease after prostatectomy in nearly one-half of the patients. Taken together, these studies indicate that, whereas postoperative pelvic irradiation can control local disease, an impact on survival is less clear.

INTERSTITIAL BRACHYTHERAPY

Interstitial brachytherapy relies on the principle that deposition of radiation energy in tissues decreases exponentially as a square function of the distance from the radiation source. The technique is designed to deliver maximal doses of radiation to tumors infiltrated with radioactive sources, but doses fall off rapidly in surrounding normal tissues. A range of isotopes [e.g., radium 226, gold 198, iodine 125 (^{125}I), iridium 192, palladium 103 (^{103}Pd)] have been tested over the years, and the technique evolved from freehand implantation to ultrasound- and CT-guided template systems. Until the early 1990s, retropubic implantation of the prostate with ^{125}I sources was the technique of choice.[392–394] Stage for stage, failure rates were high compared to external-beam–treated patients.[330,395] Difficulties in achieving a geometrically acceptable distribution of seeds and a homogeneous dose distribution within the prostate have been regarded as major factors.

Newer approaches use diagnostic localization procedures for source placement and new methods of dosimetry and computer-aided optimization of treatment planning, improving the ability to distribute dose homogeneously within the target volume.[396–398] The most popular approach has been the TRUS-guided implantation of ^{125}I or ^{103}Pd sources with or without supplemental external-beam irradiation.[397,398] Treatment planning is based on CT or TRUS, or both, with images obtained at 5-mm intervals. Isodose distributions are provided at each 5-mm increment throughout the treatment volume to determine the precise placement of seeds and the source strength required to achieve a dose of 160 Gy with ^{125}I or 115 Gy with [103]Pd. For implantation, the patient is in a dorsal lithotomy position and under spinal anesthesia. A needle-guidance template is attached to an ultrasound apparatus and is placed against the perineum. Needles containing the radioactive sources are inserted through the template under TRUS guidance with supplemental fluoroscopy. Compliance of source placement with the pretreatment plan is determined by direct visualization on biplanar ultrasound. After implantation, 5-mm thickness CT images of the prostate are obtained and isodose contours are calculated to evaluate the dose that will actually be delivered to the prostate and the surrounding normal tissues. Wallner et al. have described a method for 3D CT–based pretreatment planning and an implantation technique using individualized template devices that permit more precise source placement within the target volume.[396,399]

The introduction of intraoperative real-time planning that uses an optimization algorithm to evaluate the dose deposited throughout the entire 3D volume for multiple seed configurations and identifies which configuration adheres best to the predetermined target, urethral, and rectal dose constraints has improved outcomes further.[400–403] The technique enables the delivery of prescribed doses to the prostate, decreased doses to the urethra and rectum to tolerance levels, and reduced toxicities.[404] Ultrasound-guided transperineal implantation has also been used in combination with external-beam radiotherapy to enhance the prostate dose in patients with unfavorable prognosis. In general, 45 to 50 Gy of external-beam radiotherapy is delivered first, followed by 110 Gy with ^{125}I implantation[405] or 90 Gy with [103]Pd sources.[406] High dose-rate brachytherapy with iridium 192 has also been used in combination with external-beam radiotherapy.[407] Patients receive pelvic irradiation to 46 Gy, followed by transperineal placement of afterloading catheters and treatment with two to three fractions of 5.5 to 10.5 Gy. Real-time intraoperative planning is performed using the intraoperative ultrasound image of each high dose-rate treatment to optimize treatment delivery.

The technologic improvements in transperineal ultrasound-based or CT-planned permanent seed implantation have enhanced the ability of this modality to target high radiation doses to the prostate more precisely than in the past. Concomitantly, treatment results have improved significantly, especially in patients with favorable-risk disease. Three- to five-year PSA relapse-free survival rates have ranged between 76% and 96%. In a study of 138 T1c to T2 patients with Gleason scores of 6 or less, PSA levels decreased gradually to less than 1 ng/mL over the first 4 years after implantation in 97%, and the actuarial PSA relapse-free survival at 5 years was 93%.[408] Beyer and Priestly reported 94% PSA relapse-free survival at 5 years for T1 patients, 70% for T2a to T2b patients, and 34% for Tic patients.[409] A dose response for ^{125}I prostate implants was shown in a study in which patients receiving a D90 (dose delivered to 90% of prostate tissue as defined by CT) of less than 140 Gy had a 4-year relapse-free survival of 68%, compared to 92% for those receiving a D90 of 140 Gy or greater (P = .02). Two-year posttreatment biopsies were negative in 70% (33 of 47) of patients with a D90 of less than 140 Gy com-

pared to 83% (24 of 29) in patients with a D90 of 140 Gy or greater (P = .2).[410]

In the absence of a randomized trial comparing 3D-CRT and permanent interstitial implantation, it is often difficult to select the most appropriate treatment for a given patient. This was addressed in part in a study that analyzed favorable-risk prostate cancer treated with either 3D-CRT to 64.8 to 81.0 Gy (137 patients) or transperineal ^{125}I implantations (145 patients). The implant dose range was 110 to 257 Gy (median, 150 Gy). The 5-year PSA relapse-free survival rates for the 3D-CRT and the implant groups were 88% and 82%, respectively (P = .09). Protracted grade 2 urinary symptoms persisting for 12 to 70 months were observed in 31% of the implant patients. In contrast, the 5-year actuarial likelihood of late grade 2 urinary toxicity for the 3D-CRT group was only 8%. The 5-year actuarial likelihood of developing a urethral stricture (grade 3 urinary toxicity) for the 3D-CRT and implant groups was 2% and 12%, respectively (P <.0002). The 5-year actuarial probabilities of rectal toxicity were not significantly different. The 5-year likelihood of posttreatment erectile dysfunction among patients who were potent before treatment was 43% for the 3D-CRT and 53% for the implant group (P = .52). These data demonstrated that 3D-CRT and transperineal ^{125}I implantation are each associated with an excellent PSA outcome, but issues of treatment toxicities may guide therapy selection for the individual patient.[411]

EXPECTANT MANAGEMENT

Watchful waiting or expectant management is a valid treatment option whenever the probability is low that the cancer will progress and produce symptoms within the patient's lifetime. In fact, nearly one in four men diagnosed with prostate cancer in this country are initially managed expectantly.[412] Studies of the natural history of localized prostate cancer managed expectantly show that within 10 years, many cancers grow locally, and some patients develop metastases, but few die of the disease.[250,413] Beyond 10 years, metastases are more likely and the risk of death from prostate cancer increases.[250] Certainly, the majority of prostate cancers detected in needle biopsy specimens in men with an abnormal DRE or elevated PSA level are clinically important cancers that should be treated actively in men expected to live at least 10 years.[117]

Formal decision analysis models that predicted a low risk of death from cancer and minimal gain in quality-adjusted life years from treatment, even in men with moderate or poorly differentiated cancers,[414] have been successfully criticized for grossly underestimating the metastatic rate of the cancer.[193] On the other hand, a growing proportion of men diagnosed today have a very small focus of low-grade (Gleason sum, 2 to 6), impalpable (T1c) cancer on biopsy, and a modest elevation of PSA (4 to 10 ng/mL). Although such patients often have more cancer in the radical prostatectomy specimen than apparent from the initial biopsy specimen (Fig. 30.3-35), a substantial minority do not. Such cancers surely pose little or no threat to a patient's life or well-being. It is worth considering whether a program of "deferred definitive therapy" would be effective, monitoring such cancers closely and postponing intervention until discrete signs of progression are observed.[415]

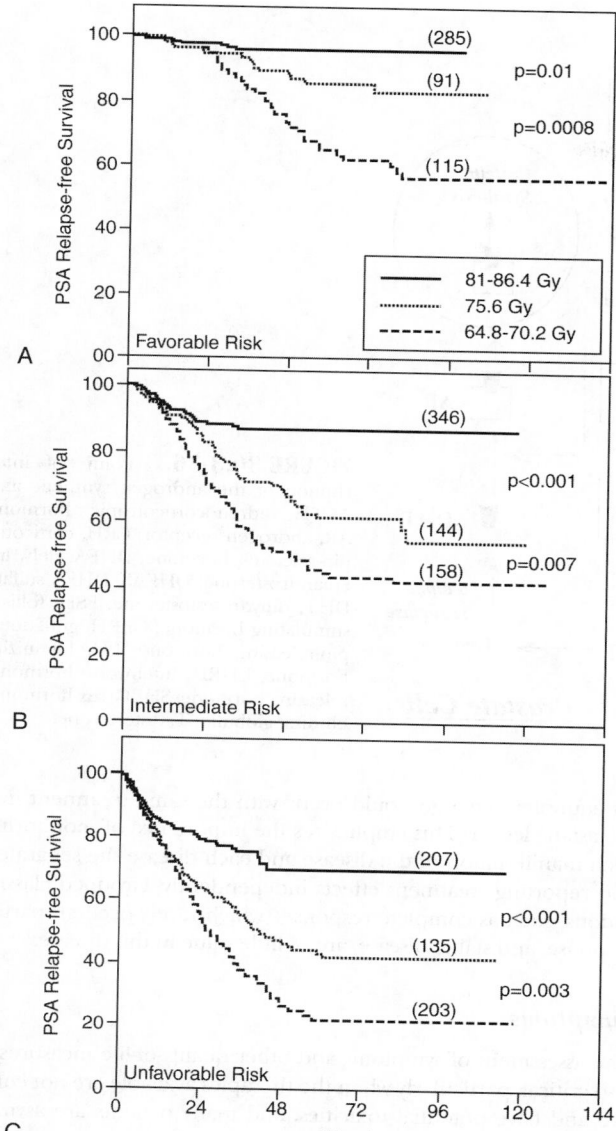

FIGURE 30.3-35. Actuarial prostate-specific antigen (PSA) relapse-free survival according to dose for patients in the favorable (**A**), intermediate (**B**), and unfavorable prognostic groups (**C**). Treated with radiation therapy. (From ref. 319, with permission.)

SYSTEMIC THERAPIES

CLINICAL METASTASIS AND RISING PROSTATE-SPECIFIC ANTIGEN: NONCASTRATE

The standard treatment for prostate cancers that have spread is to ablate the action of androgen by medical or surgical means (Fig. 30.3-36). But, before considering the antiprostate cancer effects of these and other therapies, it is essential to consider the issues in the development of systemic approaches for a disease for which the traditional measures of objective tumor regression do not apply. This has long been recognized.[416] Less recognized is that none of the systemic therapies currently in use were approved using traditional end points of tumor regression.

Drug development is traditionally divided into three phases. Phase I studies address dose and schedule, phase II studies address treatment effects, and phase III trials seek to show the efficacy and safety of a new approach in comparison to an established standard of care or placebo. Each trial is part of a sequence of studies in which the key question is whether the results justify the continued development of the approach. Important aspects of drug delivery in prostate cancer are to ensure safety and tolerance in an elderly population, and, in most contexts, to administer a drug on a long-term basis—an issue typically not addressed in phase I trials. This is because, for prostate cancer in particular, a systemic therapy that can "control or slow" the disease without eliminating the last cancer cell may be equivalent to cure for an elderly population in which the competing causes of death may be more significant than the morbidity or mortality from cancer. The second phase of development seeks to determine whether the therapy provides a treatment effect in a sufficient proportion of patients and the durability of the effect. The "effects" relevant to patients go beyond measures of tumor regression. Interest in prolongation of life is assumed, but prevention of metastatic disease, relief of pain, prevention of pain, and improving safety with equivalent anticancer effects are also important goals. In practice, treatment effects are quantified by measuring changes in disease manifestations that are present in the individual or disease state under evaluation. These changes range from a rising PSA alone to any combination of a rising PSA with recurrent/persistent local disease, nodal metastases, bone metastases, or visceral disease, or all. Symptoms of disease may or may not be present. Treatment effects can also be quantified by preventing events that are predicted to occur in the future: indicators of disease progression (e.g., new lesions on a scan or new symptoms of disease) or death from disease.

Prostate-Specific Antigen–Based End Points

Posttherapy PSA determinations are an attractive measure because they are quantitative, reproducible, and can be measured quickly and easily. For a patient with a rising PSA before treatment, the effect might be to achieve an undetectable level, a defined nadir, a decrease by a defined percentage, no change, a decline in slope, an increase in doubling time, or a rise followed by a decline as might been seen with a differentiating agent.[5] The caveat is that achieving a specific end point does not necessarily mean that the drug has affected tumor growth in a favorable or unfavorable way. To be applied clinically, a PSA-based end point must be tailored to both the disease state and the class of drug under evaluation. Examples of intervention-specific PSA-based end points are illustrated in Figure 30.3-37. Using PSA, a cytotoxic drug that does not produce a decline after treatment is likely to be of little interest, whereas a static agent that produces a prolonged period of stability without decreasing PSA might be. Similarly, a drug that inhibits angiogenesis or a drug that reduces the rate of or frequency of bony metastases could be very beneficial even if it does not kill prostate cancer cells directly and has no effect on PSA.

Bone

Assessing treatment effects in bone is problematic because bone scans assess only the secondary effects of the tumor on the skele-

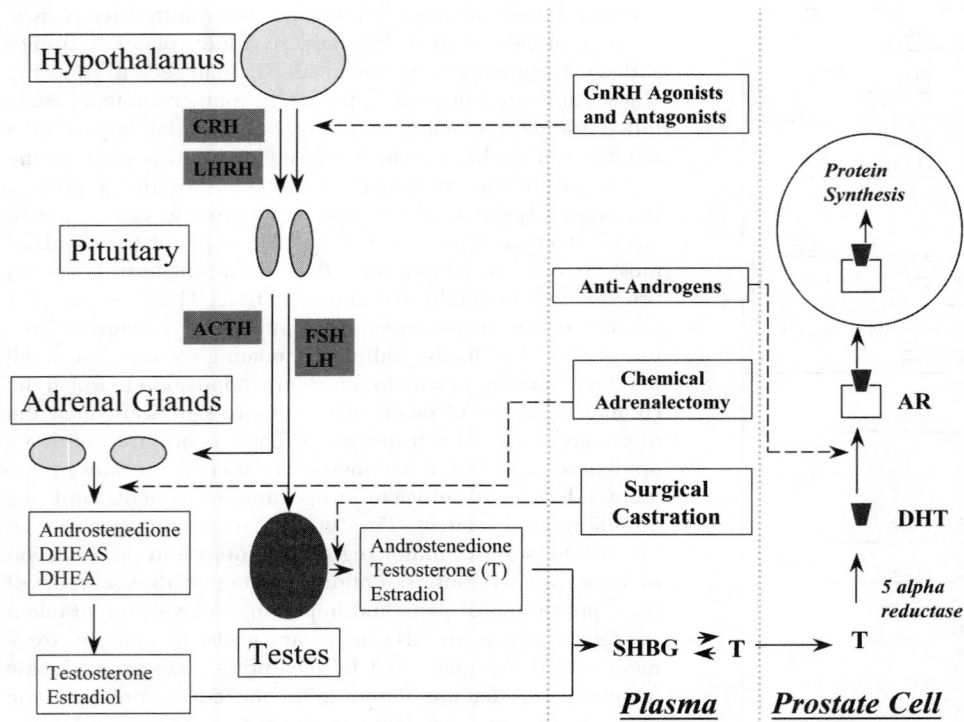

FIGURE 30.3-36. Points of interruption of the androgen synthetic axis. ACTH, adrenocorticotropic hormone; AR, androgen receptor; CRH, corticotropin-releasing hormone; DHEA, dehydroepiandrosterone; DHEAS, DHEA sulfate; DHT, dihydrotestosterone; FSH, follicle-stimulating hormone; GnRH, gonadotropin-releasing hormone; LH, luteinizing hormone; LHRH, luteinizing hormone–releasing hormone; SHBG, sex hormone–binding globulin; T, testosterone.

ton and not the tumor directly. As a result, bone healing in response to successful therapy may result in an increased intensity of preexisting lesions and, in some cases, new lesions are interpreted as progression of disease, even as PSA levels are declining and symptoms of disease abate. Visible improvements in a scan may not occur for several months, and, not infrequently, the distinction between true disease progression and pseudo-progression can be difficult.[418] In these situations, a repeat scan after a few months is often the best means to clarify whether the disease is actually responding or getting worse. We use a minimum 12-week interval between scans unless clinically indicated. When improvement in a scan is documented, it generally indicates that the treatment has had a meaningful effect on the tumor. Positron emission tomography (PET), which uses a tracer to monitor biologic events directly in the tumor, may circumvent some of the issues with bone scans. With PET, both soft tissue disease and osseous disease can be imaged simultaneously and quantitatively. Figure 30.3-38 shows PSA values, PET scans, and bone scans of a patient with osseous metastases treated with hormones. As illustrated, PSA levels declined significantly and fluorodeoxyglucose (FDG) accumulation decreased markedly, while the bone scan was unchanged.

Soft Tissue Disease

In cases in which bi-dimensionally measurable tumor masses are present, standard outcome measures, such as those outlined in the Response Criteria for Solid Tumors, should be utilized.[420] In other cases, a pathologic end point is used, such as in the preprostatectomy setting. The caveat is that tumors that have spread to different sites within the same patient may not respond in parallel, as several groups have documented differential response proportions in soft tissue versus bone, and, at present, it is unknown whether changes in the primary tumor are reliable indicators that

an equivalent change would occur with the same treatment in a metastatic lesion. This emphasizes the importance of monitoring each manifestation of the disease and each disease site separately and reporting treatment effects independently. Grouped classifications, such as complete response (which rarely occurs), partial response, and stable disease, are of little value in this disease.[421]

Symptoms

The assessment of symptoms and other quality-of-life measures is also critical, particularly when the therapies available are not curative and have potential toxicities, and many patients are asymptomatic from their cancers. Therapies that alleviate symptoms of disease are extremely valuable to patients independent of their effect on PSA. In these settings, it is important to distinguish symptoms of the disease itself from preexisting symptoms related to previous surgery and radiation (e.g., incontinence, erectile dysfunction) and symptoms from prior therapies. The patient who is progressing on hormonal therapy may already be experiencing fatigue, hot flushes, and loss of libido before a new treatment is initiated. Comorbid conditions may also confound the interpretation of treatment effects. Pain that mimics cancer may be secondary to arthritis or degenerative disease and require the same analgesics with attendant side effects that might be used to treat cancer pain. Although a detailed discussion of quality of life is beyond the scope of this chapter, another important consideration for prostate cancer patients is that symptoms of disease rarely develop in isolation. For example, the patient with pain secondary to osseous disease may also be weak, fatigued, and constipated from immobility and the analgesics necessary to control the pain. This setting requires multiple domain measures that quantitate pain relief, analgesic use, mobility, and bowel function and not simply pain alone. A number of validated scales are available

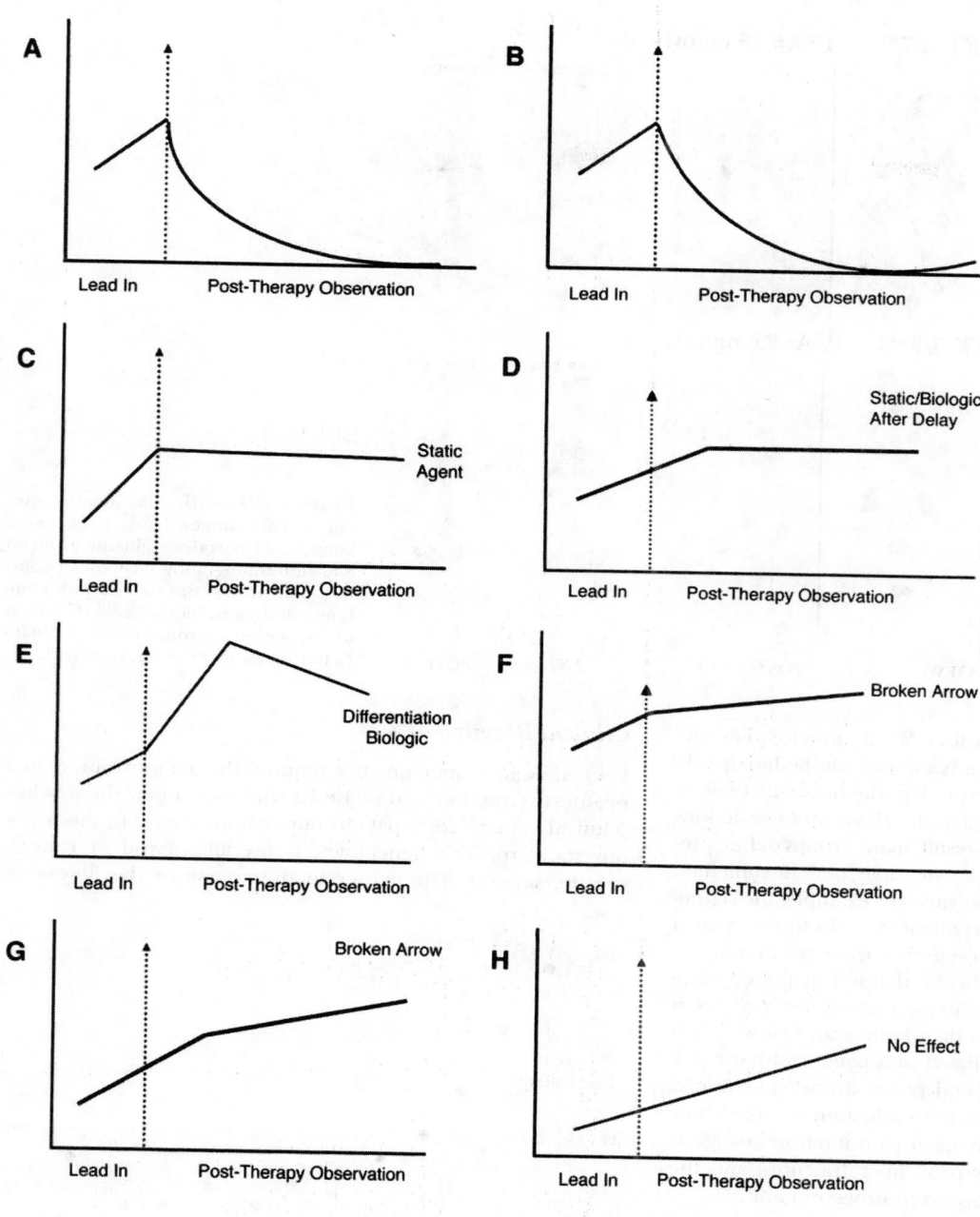

FIGURE 30.3-37. Posttherapy prostate-specific antigen (PSA) patterns after different interventions in a patient with a rising PSA: The start of treatment is indicated by the arrow. **A:** Rapid decline with no escape. **B:** Rapid decline followed by escape. **C:** A "no change" or plateau (2 days). **D:** Similar to **C** but only after a delay. **E:** An initial rise followed by decline. **F:** A "broken arrow" in which the rate of rise was slowed. **G:** Similar to **F** with a delayed effect (2 hours). **H:** A treatment with no effect on PSA. (From ref. 417, with permission)

for these assessments, such as the Functional Assessment of Cancer Therapy with Prostate Cancer Subscale or the European Organization for Research and Treatment of Cancer (EORTC) Quality of Life Thirty.[422,423] A treatment with fewer toxicities relative to a standard can also be very useful. As an example, for hormone therapies with high rates of cardiovascular or gastrointestinal toxicities, drugs with an equivalent anticancer effect with reduced toxicity would be of value.

Duration

The durability of an effect is determined in a similar fashion, with the caveat that definitions of progression and treatment failure vary by disease state and disease manifestation. Posttherapy PSA changes may be applicable to selected agents in selected contexts. PSA-based definitions that provide short-term readouts of failure/progression include an increase to a predetermined number, an increase from a nadir, an increase by an absolute percentage, a return to baseline, or a change in the postintervention rate of rise. Figure 30.3-39 shows how a change in the definition of failure can affect the assessment of durability. Using the first confirmed rise in PSA as opposed to a 50% rise from the nadir, one could conclude that therapy has short- or longer-term effect. By consensus, most use the first confirmed rise.[5,424]

A more relevant basis for assessing treatment effects is time-dependent parameters, such as survival time or the time to objective progression of disease. The latter include new lesions on bone scan, increase in size or the development of new soft tissue lesions, or new symptoms of disease. Although soft tissue disease occurs infrequently in prostate cancer, definitions of progression

FDG-PET 4/7/99   PSA= 75 ng/mL

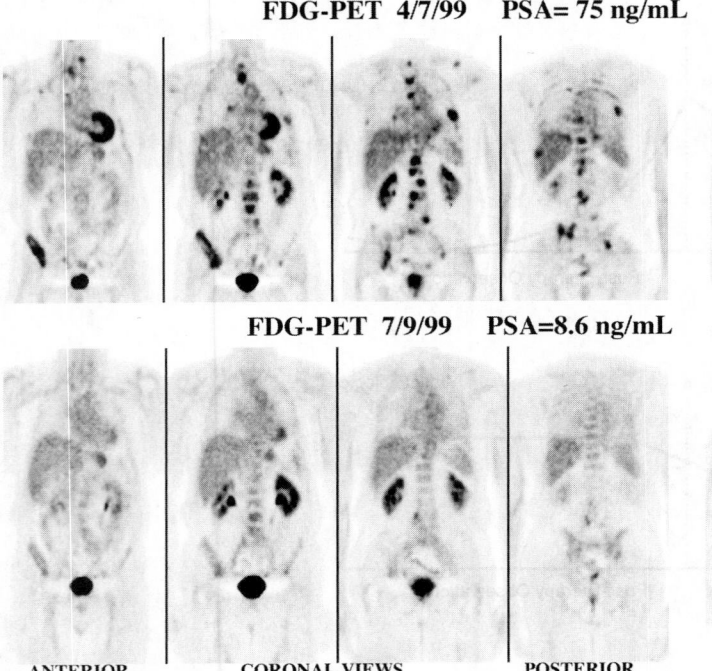

FDG-PET 7/9/99   PSA=8.6 ng/mL

ANTERIOR   CORONAL VIEWS   POSTERIOR

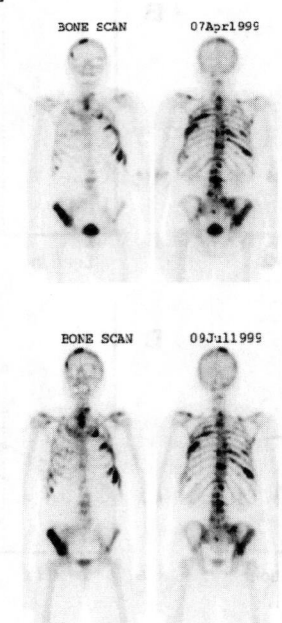

BONE SCAN   07Apr1999

BONE SCAN   09Jul1999

ANT.   POST.

FIGURE 30.3-38.   Sequential prostate-specific antigen (PSA) levels, bone scans, and fluorodeoxyglucose positron emission tomography (FDG-PET) scans in a patient who was treated with combined androgen blockage.[419] (Courtesy of Dr. Steven Larson, Memorial Sloan-Kettering Cancer Center, New York.)

in soft tissue disease are standardized.[420] As noted earlier, the interpretation of progression on a bone scan can be highly subjective. Particularly difficult is interpreting whether an increase in the intensity or an increase in area in the absence of new lesions is a sign of treatment failure. As a result, many groups define progression on a bone scan only by multiple new documented lesions. Even here, there is subjectivity—for example, the significance of a new "spot" on a rib in a patient with a history of trauma who has diffuse disease that is subjectively unchanged overall.

Progression or failure may also be defined by the development of a new manifestation of disease that was not present at the start of therapy—new lesions on a bone scan that were not present when treatment was initiated in a patient with a rising PSA. In other cases, composite end points are used. The end point of skeletal events, used in the evaluation of zoledronic acid, includes a baseline assessment of pain intensity, analgesic usage, the development of new pain, microfractures, and the time to need for additional therapy to control symptoms.[425]

In practice, once the treatment effect end point is defined, a predetermined number of patients are entered and treated and the outcome assessed. If a sufficient number show the effect, an additional number are treated to define the frequency of the effect more accurately. Enrolling more patients allows an adjustment for baseline prognostic factors with respect to the specific outcome measure being evaluated. Early readouts, such as the proportion showing a PSA change or pain relief, can form the basis for early discontinuation if no activity is observed. Assuming that a sufficient proportion of the larger cohort do show PSA declines, disease regression, or subjective improvements, or all, the next question is when to move forward. This decision is dependent on the duration of the effect, assessed with time-dependent parameters, such as treatment failure, progression, or death from disease. The use of the decision is further enhanced when the treatment effect end point in the phase II setting matches the one to be used in the phase III clinical study.

Clinical Benefit

Ultimately, to change practice requires the demonstration, in a prospective randomized phase III trial, that a new therapy has "clinical benefit" for a patient population relative to the previous standard. The benchmark is overall survival or cancer-specific survival. The earlier in the course of the illness an

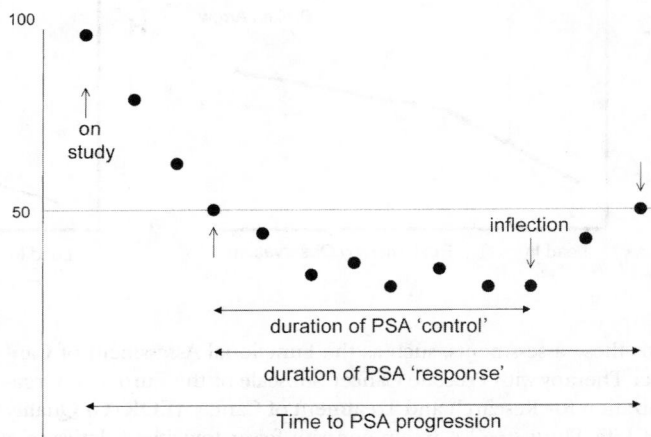

FIGURE 30.3-39.   Prostate-specific antigen (PSA)–based definitions of progression. The duration of both PSA-based reporting end points are measured from the first time point at which the PSA has declined by at least 50% (which must eventually be confirmed by a second value). The duration of PSA response is the time until PSA has increased back to 50% of the original on-study value. However, in many cases, it will be possible (in retrospect) to identify an inflection point—the point at which PSA began what became a continuous increase. Some investigators believe that this may be considered the point at which disease control could be assumed to be lost. Thus, the duration of PSA control may also be reported. Others prefer the *time to PSA progression*, which is defined as the time at which therapy started and ends when the PSA increases by 50% above the nadir. (From ref. 424, with permission.)

intervention is being evaluated, the more difficult it is to prove a survival advantage. Trials for early disease states often take 10 years or more to mature once accruals have been satisfied and often end with results that are not definitive. It is more feasible to prove benefit for patients with a high risk of prostate cancer–specific death, symptoms of disease, or metastases.

Applied to trials in localized disease, an intermediate end point might be PSA relapse-free survival at a defined period of time, using time to the development of objective evidence of local disease on an imaging study or on physical examination or detectable metastatic disease as the clinical benefit measure. For patients in the state of a rising PSA, the early end point might be a defined change in the level of PSA or PSA kinetics and the clinical benefit end point the development of disease that can be detected clinically, symptoms, or death from disease. The same principles apply to patients with noncastrate and castrate disease. In clinical scenarios in which there are established standards, the risk/reward ratio of the intervention versus no intervention might be considered. The central issue for these trials is what risk of recurrence, symptoms, or progression would lead a patient to seek and a physician to offer an alternative approach. There is no single answer.

The controversies surrounding the meaning of posttherapy changes in PSA, the rarity of "measurable" lesions, and the difficulties assessing response in bone, mandates the study of the treatment effect and clinical benefit end points early in a compound's development. It is also essential to show that the effect is superior to what is already available and by how much, so that an adequately sized and powered phase III clinical benefit trial can be designed. To address these issues, working groups are developing state-specific trial design recommendations.[417,424] Unfortunately, many of the trials in prostate cancer are underpowered and may have missed important treatment effects. With these considerations in mind, the therapies available and under evaluation for systemic disease are critically discussed.

NONCASTRATE SYSTEMIC DISEASE: RISING PROSTATE-SPECIFIC ANTIGEN AND CLINICAL METASTASES NONCASTRATE

The concept of ablating the action of androgens as a treatment for prostate cancer dates to the 1940s, when Huggins and Hodges demonstrated that a surgical orchiectomy or the administration of estrogen could reduce tumor size, decrease acid phosphatase, and palliate the symptoms of the disease.[347,426] Estimates are that 90% to 95% of androgens are synthesized in the testicles with the remainder from adrenal sources, of which DHT is the most biologically active. Subsequently, other medical approaches were developed, including estramustine,[427] steroidal and nonsteroidal antiandrogens,[428,429] synthetic adrenal steroid enzyme inhibitors (aminoglutethimide and ketoconazole),[430,431] the gonadotropin-releasing hormone (GnRH) agonist/antagonists, and pure GnRH antagonists. All of these interventions lower the level of testosterone with the exception of the nonsteroidal antiandrogens, which block the binding of testosterone to the AR. In most cases, the individual forms of hormonal ablation were approved on the basis of safety and toxicity relative to what was already available, rather than superior anticancer effects.

The adverse effects include those associated with the state of castration itself and effects unique to the specific method of blockade. The symptoms associated with castration, or *androgen deprivation syndrome*, include hot flashes, fatigue, anemia, a decrease in libido, impotence, weight gain, muscle weakness and loss of muscle mass, bone loss, memory problems, a decrease in mental acuity, mood swings and personality changes, depression, and insomnia.[432]

Not all occur in all patients, and not all occur to the same severity in different patients. Treatments for many of these symptoms are being evaluated as part of a newly characterized entity termed *andropause*, the decline in the testosterone in aging males who do not have cancer. These men, in contrast to men with cancer, can be treated with testosterone, allowing an assessment of the reversibility of the effects.[433]

Hot flashes occur in upwards of 80% of patients. They can occur at any time, even during sleep, lasting for a mean of less than 5 minutes with a range from seconds to an hour or more and are bothersome in approximately 25% of the patients who experience them. Palliation is achieved with estrogens at doses as low as 0.3 mg/d, megestrol acetate, or medroxyprogesterone (Depo-Provera).[432] The serotonin reuptake inhibitor, venlafaxine (Effexor), has also been used, which has the additional potential benefit of treating the depression that can occur. Insomnia may be the result of hot flushes or anxiety surrounding PSA.[434,435]

Fatigue may in part be related to anemia, as 90% of men on androgen ablation show a decrease in hemoglobin of 10%, and 25% show a decrease of 18% or more.[436] This anemia may persist for several months after therapy is stopped and can be reversed with erythropoietin. Impotence is almost universal for therapies that lower the level of testosterone in the blood and is exacerbated by the loss of libido that is commonly seen. Most men also experience weight gain, which exceeded 6 kg on average at 12 months in one report.[437] Contributing factors include a sedentary lifestyle, induced in part by fatigue, and an increase in appetite. Most of the weight gained is fat, as lean body mass decreased by 2.4% in one study. The decrease in lean body mass and loss of muscle tone contributes to overall weakness. Approximately 10% show an increase in cholesterol and 26% an increase in triglyceride levels. Memory problems, along with a decrease in acuity, are increasingly being recognized as an adverse effect of therapy for which there is no specific medical treatment save discontinuing the drugs.[432] The risk of fracture secondary to loss of bone mass is also increased by more than 2.5-fold, with 65% of men developing fractures at 10 years if left untreated.[438]

In a prospective trial, the loss of bone mass was documented to be 2% to 5% after 1 year of androgen ablation. The effect on bone can be assessed using changes in bone mineral density and measures of bone turnover, such as urinary N-telopeptide (a breakdown product of collagen) and bone-specific alkaline phosphatase and osteocalcin; such tests should be considered when monitoring these individuals. The etiology is in part the loss of the mitogenic effect of testosterone on IGF and osteoblasts and decreased conversion of testosterone to estrogen. Bone loss can be prevented by treatment with bisphosphonates or low doses of estrogen. Supplemental calcium (1000 to 1500 mg/d) and vitamin D (400 U) are also advised. An integral part of the maintenance of bone integrity is exercise, reduction in caffeine, and smoking cessation.

Specific Approaches to Ablate Androgen Action

Surgical orchiectomy is the "gold standard" and provides rapid palliation at a low cost, with no issues of compliance. It is, however, the least preferred by patients.[439] Estrogens inhibit production of luteinizing hormone–releasing hormone (LHRH) in the hypothalamus, producing a decrease in follicle-stimulating hormone, which acts on Sertoli cells, and in luteinizing hormone (LH), which acts on Leydig cells to control androgen production and spermatogenesis. In randomized comparisons, doses of 5 mg/d of diethylstilbestrol (DES) proved to be toxic; a dose of 3 mg/d can produce castrate levels of testosterone in 1 to 2 weeks. Estrogens may also have direct cytotoxic effects beyond the effect on testosterone.[440] The cost is low, but overall costs increase if cardiovascular complications, such as edema, thromboembolic events, myocardial infarction, and stroke, develop.[441] Even at a dose of 1 mg/d, which may not produce complete suppression in all patients, 13% of patients have vascular events.[442]

Estramustine (Emcyt), one of the first targeted agents, consists of nitrogen mustard conjugated to C17 of estrogen.[443] This agent was designed to be selectively taken up in cells with estrogen receptors, in which enzymatic cleavage would release the mustard moiety intracellularly. However, no evidence of an alkylating effect has been observed in the laboratory or the clinic, and estramustine is now known to affect the cytoskeleton and cell motility by acting on microtubules in addition to having estrogenic effects. Used alone as first-line therapy, the antiprostate cancer effects are similar to DES, as is the toxicity profile. Based on laboratory studies showing synergy, estramustine is now used most commonly for castration-resistant tumors in combination with other cytoskeletal agents [including the vinca alkaloids, vinblastine and vinorelbine (Navelbine), and the taxanes, paclitaxel and docetaxel], cytotoxics, and the podophyllotoxins (etoposide).

Progestational agents, such as megestrol acetate (Megace) and cyproterone acetate (Androcur—available only in Canada and in Europe), suppress LHRH and block the binding of DHT to the AR. They are not recommended as first-line therapy.[444,445]

GnRH agonist/antagonists are analogues of LHRH that produce an initial surge in LH along with a rise in testosterone, followed by down-regulation of LH receptors in the pituitary and inhibition of LH release. The result is a fall in testosterone 2 to 3 weeks after administration.[446] They are now the most widely used type of androgen ablation. The initial rise may result in a worsening of the disease (clinical flare), and these agents are contraindicated in patients with pain, ureteral obstruction, or impending spinal cord compromise.[447] Two approved for use in the United States—leuprolide acetate (Lupron, given intramuscularly), goserelin acetate (Zoladex, given subcutaneously in the abdominal wall)—are variably available as daily, monthly, 3-month, or 4-month depot injections. GnRH antagonists do not produce the initial LH surge and produce a rapid decline in testosterone.[448] They are, however, associated with a higher frequency of allergic reactions, and data on the long-term androgen suppressive effects are limited.

The antifungal drug, ketoconazole, at a dose of 1200 mg/d, produces castrate levels of testosterone in 24 hours through inhibition of adrenal steroidogenesis. The effects on hormone synthesis are not durable, limiting use of first-line treatment. It is useful for the patient who presents with acute spinal cord compression or disseminated intravascular coagulation, when orchiectomy or GnRH analogues are contraindicated.[431] It is used most frequently as second-line treatment, with fatigue and hepatic dysfunction being the most common side effects. Aminoglutethimide produces similar effects, but use has been largely discontinued owing to toxicities that include somnolence, rash, and hypothyroidism. Both of these agents are typically given with hydrocortisone to minimize the risk of an acute adrenal crisis.

Antiandrogens block androgen binding to the AR. There are two types. Type I, the steroidal antiandrogens, have progestational properties that suppress LH levels and lower serum testosterone. Type II nonsteroidal agents (flutamide, bicalutamide, and nilutamide) bind to ARs in the prostate as well as those in the pituitary and hypothalamus. Consequently, there is no negative feedback on LH synthesis, and testosterone levels increase over time. Of the three approved for use, flutamide has a short half-life, requiring multiple daily dosing, whereas bicalutamide and nilutamide have weekly half-lives and are administered once a day. The appeal of the type II agents is that they are relatively potency sparing, result in fewer hot flushes, and less loss of libido, muscle mass, and bone. Gynecomastia and breast pain are, however, more significant, as is the frequency of gastrointestinal toxicities, such as diarrhea (flutamide) and hepatitis (flutamide more than bicalutamide). Nilutamide in particular is associated with interstitial pneumonitis, blurred vision, difficulties with light/dark adaptation, and alcohol intolerance.[445]

Androgen blockade has been standard treatment since the 1940s; nevertheless, there are still controversies surrounding its use. Part of the controversy is the result of a PSA testing. In the past, patients tended to present with more advanced disease, and monitoring the disease was limited to insensitive techniques, such as physical examination and plain radiographs. As of 2004, more sensitive methods of detection, such as MRI and PET, can also be used. In addition, many men live and die by their PSA values and frequently demand and receive treatment based on PSA elevations when their risk of developing symptoms, metastases, or death from disease is very low.[435] Although it is true that patients with declining PSA values are less anxious than those with rising values, it is not clear that relief of anxiety is sufficient justification for treatment. In these cases in particular, the risk/reward ratio, both in terms of toxicities and of cost, is critical, raising additional questions about who to treat and when.

PSA is an androgen-responsive gene. Reducing androgen levels or blocking androgen binding to the AR results in lower PSA values. Rising values on hormonal therapy are an indication of treatment resistance that antedates the documentation of progression by physical examination, imaging, or symptoms by months or even years. Attempts to assess the effects of hormones on other disease manifestations and the durability of the effect are limited by the fact that the end points of trials initiated and completed before the use of PSA were based primarily on changes on physical examination or imaging techniques, or both, that were less sensitive than those used today. Time to progression based on insensitive measures is likely to be longer than one based on PSA. This is good in certain ways, because it allows individuals to focus on the more global question of what hormones actually provide the patient in terms of preventing or relieving symptoms and preventing disease spread and death from disease. Unfortunately, in many clinical contexts, this information is simply not available, leaving unresolved many of the questions we seem to be asking on a repeated basis including

What are the antiprostate cancer effects of hormones?
Is there an optimal form of therapy?
Will it prolong my life or at least make it better?
Am I compromising my life if I don't start right away?
Can the same results be achieved if I take hormones that are not

"castrating" in the traditional sense or if I am treated on an intermittent basis?

How much will it cost?

ANTIPROSTATE CANCER EFFECTS OF THERAPY: CHANGES IN INDIVIDUAL DISEASE MANIFESTATIONS

When first discovered, hormone therapy was primarily used in symptomatic patients with metastatic or advanced local disease: The early trials antedated the adoption of what are now considered traditional phase II end points, and many antedate the use of PSA. The specific imaging modalities, timing of their use, and follow-up algorithms used to assess outcomes have also evolved, again showing the importance of reporting outcomes based on the individual manifestations of the disease in the population enrolled and not on the basis of grouped classifications. These caveats aside, approximately 60% to 70% of patients with an abnormal PSA show a normalization to a value below 4 ng/mL after castration, 30% to 50% of measurable tumor masses regress by 50% or more, and more than 60% of patients with symptoms show palliation, be they urinary or osseous in origin. If one performs serial bone scans, 30% to 40% of scans actually show improvement, and the majority remain stable.[418] The complete elimination of disease in any site is rare, be it in bone or the prostate itself. For example, with androgen ablation used as neoadjuvant therapy before surgery for upwards of 8 months, fewer than 5% of prostates are pathologically tumor-free at prostatectomy,[449,450] suggesting that hormone therapy alone will not cure the disease.

The duration of response to androgen ablation is variably quoted as 12 to 18 months, but it is unclear where these numbers came from and on what tumor burden they are based. Well recognized by many groups is the prognostic significance of disease burden. In a Southwest Oncology Group study evaluating the role of combined androgen blockade, the prognosis of patients with disease limited to the axial skeletal differed significantly from those with disease in the axial and appendicular skeleton.[451] Groups with markedly different prognoses can be defined on the basis of the number of lesions on a bone scan.[452] The more critical issue is that once metastases are detected on physical examination or on an imaging study, clinical death rates are continuous over time, although overall survival times vary inversely by disease extent.[453–455]

Is One Form of Monotherapy That Suppresses Testosterone Levels Superior to Another?

No. In a metaanalysis of ten randomized, controlled trials that included LHRH agonists/antagonists, orchiectomy, DES, or the choice of DES or orchiectomy, outcomes were similar. All single therapy hormonal interventions that lower serum testosterone levels to castrate levels had similar overall survival times after 2 years of treatment.[445] An EORTC study, powered for a 13% difference around the medians, showed similar outcomes between DES, 1 mg, and orchiectomy.[456]

Will It Prolong My Life or Make It Better?

No one questions that hormonal therapy palliates symptoms. The question is as follows: Does it delay progression or prolong life? Prospective randomized comparisons of androgen deprivation therapy to placebo are limited. The VACURG (Veterans' Adminis-

tration Cooperative Urologic Research Group) found that DES (5 mg) compared to placebo resulted in similar 1-, 5-, and 9-year survivals for stage III and IV patients, 93% versus 91%, 71% versus 67%, and 56% versus 55%, respectively, whereas, for stage IV patients, the absolute survival difference was 12%.[457,458] The Cochrane analysis of the VACURG studies showed that, with early therapy, progression-free survival was significantly higher at 1, 2, 5, and 10 years (odds ratio = 3.99, 4.79, 3.15, and 3.48, respectively), and overall survival at 10 years was also significantly better (odds ratio = 1.5).[459] The VACURG Study 2 randomized patients with stage III or IV disease (n = 294 and 214) to placebo; DES, 0.2 mg; DES, 1 mg; or DES, 5 mg. Progression rates were similar, but mortality in the 5-mg group was too high (58% vs. 32%). Overall survival for 1 mg versus placebo at 5 years was 34% versus 20%, although the statistic significance was not reported. These trials suggest a moderate survival benefit.[459]

Would exogenous estrogens and surgical orchiectomy be approved today? Yes—based on the placebo-controlled randomized studies showing meaningful treatment effects and clinical benefits, albeit with significant toxicities for certain patients. Since the approval of DES in the 1940s, the hormone therapies currently in use were approved on the basis of trials demonstrating reduced toxicities with equivalent anticancer effects or the prevention of a specific treatment-induced adverse event. They were not approved on the basis of an improvement in cancer-specific outcomes, such as prolonging life, prolonging time to progression, or even an improved response rate. As examples, the GnRH analogues were approved on the basis of trials showing an improved safety profile relative to DES and similar anticancer effects to orchiectomy.[441] The antiandrogens were approved initially to block the flare associated with GnRH analogue administration[447] and subsequently used as part of a combined androgen blockade approach. Bicalutamide (Casodex) was approved on the basis of a comparative trial showing antitumor equivalence to flutamide and an improved safety profile, as more patients were withdrawn from flutamide for adverse events.[460]

Gonadotropin-Releasing Hormone

Abarelix is a GnRH antagonist that was recently approved by the U.S. Food and Drug Administration for patients with symptomatic prostate cancers who refuse surgical castration and who may experience a significant worsening of symptoms as a result of the testosterone surge associated with LHRH agonists. This includes patients presenting with bone pain who are at risk for pain flares and spinal cord compression, as well as those with obstructive urinary symptoms at risk for retention. Seventy percent of patients treated with abarelix achieve castrate levels of testosterone on day 8, as opposed to none in the leuprolide- and bicalutamide-treated patients. These agents have a 3% risk of hypersensitivity reactions and 0.5% risk of rapid onset hypertension or syncope.[460a,460b]

Is Combined Androgen Blockade Better than Monotherapy?

The addition of an antiandrogen to a GnRH analogue or orchiectomy has the potential to inhibit the effects of adrenal androgens on prostate cancer cell growth. Adrenal androgens can contribute 5% to 45% of the residual androgens present in tumors after surgical castration alone.[461] In one trial, the proportion of patients who showed a decline in PSA was higher using combined androgen blockade versus monotherapy, but there was no effect on time to progression or survival.[454] Several metaanalyses have been conducted that showed that antiandrogens do not add significantly to the antitumor effects of surgical castration.[462–465] One of 27 randomized trials with 8275 patients showed a 2% difference in mortality at 5 years and 72.4% for monotherapy versus 70.4% for the combined approach,[462] whereas a second metaanalysis limited to trials of a nonsteroidal antiandrogen showed a 2.9% difference—75.3% versus 72.4% at 5 years.[464] The question is whether this difference justifies the cost[466] and increased toxicities associated with combined therapy, of which gastrointestinal effects, and depending on the agent, visual complications are encountered. This controversy was increased further by a more recent analysis of 21 trials with 6871 patients that showed a significant survival difference at 5 years and a hazard ratio (HR) of 0.87 (95% CI, 0.80 to 0.94), favoring combined therapy. The analysis was most influenced by three trials that showed a median 3.7- to 7.0-month survival difference.[467]

Given that GnRH analogues do produce a rise in testosterone for the first few weeks of administration, a remaining question is whether the "superiority" of combined therapy reflects blockade of the potentially negative effect of the unopposed androgens that result from the initial LH surge or a true effect on residual adrenal androgens as postulated.[453] As a result, whether the duration of antiandrogen therapy for patients treated with GnRH agonists should be short term (1 to 3 months) or continuous remains controversial.

Do Attempts to Reduce the Toxicities of Androgen Ablation Compromise Outcomes?

The adverse effects of androgen deprivation can be quite significant, particularly to the asymptomatic patient who was diagnosed on the basis of a change in PSA and has never experienced symptoms of the disease itself. Two hormonal strategies for reducing toxicity are the use of antiandrogens (alone or in combination with finasteride) and intermittent therapy. Antiandrogen monotherapy is associated with fewer hot flashes, less loss of libido, less muscle wasting, fewer personality changes, and less bone loss relative to testosterone-lowering therapies.[468,469] Several randomized comparisons have compared antiandrogens to conventional castration. A small study of flutamide versus DES showed similar response proportions but inferior survival for flutamide (28 vs. 43 months), whereas a second study showed that bicalutamide (50 mg/d) was inferior to surgical orchiectomy.[470] Bicalutamide, 150 mg, which produces a higher frequency of PSA normalization than does the 50-mg dose (97% vs. 73% of cases), was subsequently compared to surgical castration and to observation alone. The results were paradoxic: Bicalutamide was inferior to castration for patients with metastatic disease but was equivalent for patients with M0 disease (rising PSA values with no detectable metastases on imaging studies).[469] Although a metaanalysis showed similar survivals at 2 years,[445] the long-term outcomes are inferior to those of testosterone-lowering therapies. Nevertheless, some patients may be willing to accept this risk rather than experience the impotence and other adverse effects of testosterone-lowering treatment, as long as symptoms of disease are controlled. One strategy is to use antiandrogens first and add testosterone-lowering therapy at the time of progression. This does not work universally. In one trial, only 30% of patients showed PSA declines after the addition of a GnRH analogue.[471] No formal trials evaluating sequential antiandrogens followed by testosterone-lowering

therapy at the time of progression versus testosterone-lowering therapy have been reported, nor has there been a comparative trial of an antiandrogen plus finasteride versus testosterone-lowering therapy.

A second strategy to reduce toxicities is the use of hormones on an intermittent basis. This strategy is derived from clinical observations and laboratory studies. Acknowledging the noncurative nature of the disease with androgen deprivation, intermittent therapy seeks to minimize the adaptive changes that have been documented in the AR in late-stage disease by reducing the exposure of the surviving cell population to a castrate environment. The hypothesis is that, by doing so, the sensitivity to subsequent withdrawal is retained. In practice and in the literature, reported cycling durations vary widely. Some use fixed intervals of 3 to 6 months, whereas others treat for 2 to 3 months beyond the point of maximal response, at which point all hormones are discontinued. Testosterone levels then rise, albeit at variable rates, along with the PSA. Androgen ablation is restarted at some predetermined PSA level and cycling continues. Patients on this type of intermittent therapy spend an estimated 35% to 55% of each cycle off therapy, and 90% respond to re-induction. Although patient tolerance is improved, it is not known whether cycling increases, decreases, or does not change the overall time that a tumor remains sensitive to hormonal manipulations. An ongoing international phase III trial initiated in 1995 selects patients who have responded to androgen deprivation and then randomizes them to intermittent therapy versus continuous therapy.[471a] A second trial is comparing intermittent versus continuous therapy in patients with PSA progression and no clinical metastases after radiotherapy alone, or radical prostatectomy followed by radiation therapy.[471b] The end points are time to development of hormonal resistance, quality of life, and duration of therapy.

When Should Hormone Therapy Be Initiated: Early versus Late?

There is considerable controversy regarding the timing of hormonal treatment. The central question is whether it is better to begin at the time of primary therapy based on a predicted probability of failure, at the time of PSA progression, or to wait until clinical metastases or symptoms of death from disease are documented. Methodologic differences in the trials that have attempted to address this question include the type of primary therapy (surgery; radiation, including prescription dose and field; watchful waiting; or no therapy at all), the type and duration of treatment, the imaging and follow-up schema to detect disease recurrence or progression, and the "trigger" to administer treatment to patients randomized to "no therapy" or, more appropriately, "no immediate therapy." These so-called triggers range from a rising PSA alone to metastases or symptoms. Further confounding the issue is that, in some studies, a significant proportion of the "no immediate therapy" patients never received treatment.

In this context, some advocate androgen ablation before primary treatment of a localized tumor (1) and others as an adjuvant to primary therapy (3); others are evaluating its role in lieu of or in the absence of primary treatment (2) (Fig. 30.3-40). Similarly, in the setting of a rising PSA, some advise immediate treatment (4), others defer treatment until metastases are identified on an imaging study (5), and some wait until the patient has developed symptoms of disease (5). The issue centers on the fact that many men with a localized tumor have a low risk of recurrence (detect-

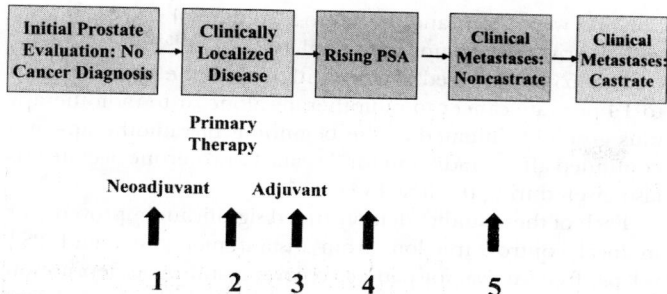

FIGURE 30.3-40. Timing of androgen deprivation. PSA, prostate-specific antigen. For description, see text.

able PSA), and these, as well as many men who have a rising PSA after surgery or radiation, still have a low risk of metastatic progression. For both groups, the risk of developing symptoms or dying from prostate cancer is low—quite low—making it difficult to justify any treatment, let alone those that are potentially toxic. The question of "early" versus "late" can be considered in the context of the primary therapy selected and the state of the patients under evaluation.

Androgen Deprivation and Watchful Waiting

Trials in patients who did not receive treatment of the primary tumor were reported by the VACURG, the Medical Research Council, and the Early Prostate Cancer Trials Group (EPC). The VACURG trials showed that DES or orchiectomy could delay the development of metastatic disease in patients with stage C disease,[458] although survival benefits were less well quantified. Staging was done primarily by DRE. The Medical Research Council trial randomized 998 patients with locally advanced or asymptomatic metastatic prostate cancer to "immediate" treatment (orchiectomy or LHRH analogue) or to the same treatment deferred until there was an "indication." Compared to those treated with deferred therapy, patients treated with early therapy were less likely to progress from M0 to M1 disease ($P < .001$, two-tailed), less likely to develop pain ($P < .001$), and less likely to die of prostate cancer.[472] In these studies, treatment was begun for local progression almost as frequently as it was for metastatic disease. An important caveat limiting the extrapolation of the results to the question of "early" versus "late" was that one-half of the men who died in the deferred arm never received therapy.[472]

The EPC included 8113 patients with localized disease who were treated by watchful waiting (trial 24), radical surgery (trial 25), or the choice of radical surgery or radiation therapy and randomized to receive bicalutamide, 150 mg, or placebo for a period ranging from 2 to 5 years.[473] The primary end point was objective clinical progression that included detectable disease in soft tissue or the documentation of bone metastases at 2 years. In trial 25, bicalutamide-treated patients showed higher frequency of metastatic progression and inferior survival relative to placebo.[474] There were too few events to assess a survival difference.

Androgen Deprivation and Surgery

Androgen deprivation has been explored both before and after radical surgery. Before surgery, androgen deprivation has the potential to reduce tumor size and improve resectability, as well as to treat micrometastatic disease. Downsizing must, however, be distinguished from down-staging, as one would not expect a tumor that has extended through the gland to involute. Most of the trials addressing this question have used a short (3 months) course of treatment, and one compared 8 months versus 3 months of therapy.[475] The results consistently show that short-term androgen deprivation can reduce the rate of positive surgical margins (from 47% to 22%), PSA levels (by 96%), and the size of the prostate (by 34%). None of the trials have shown a difference in long-term progression or survival rates.[280]

EPC trial 24, conducted in the United States, evaluated patients treated by radical surgery randomized to bicalutamide, 150 mg, or no additional therapy. There was no stratification based on risk of recurrence for entry into the trial. No difference was observed. Ultimately, however, only 6% of patients in the control group developed a recurrence, making it very difficult to demonstrate an effect, and the majority of the men enrolled did not need additional treatment beyond surgery.[473] This contrasts with a trial in which patients with node-positive disease and a higher probability of failure after radical prostatectomy were randomized to medical castration or observation. At a median follow-up of 7.1 years, 16% of men who received immediate treatment succumbed versus 36% with observation ($P = .02$). With respect to prostate cancer, 7% of the immediate and 33% of the observation group died of prostate cancer ($P < .01$), whereas, at the time of last follow-up, 77% and 18%, respectively, had no evidence of disease and an undetectable PSA level ($P < .001$).[476]

Androgen Deprivation and Radiation Therapy

Androgen deprivation before radiation therapy has the potential to improve local eradication of the tumor by reducing the size of the mass or the concurrent elimination of tumor clonogens inherently resistant to radiation therapy, or both. Decreasing the size of the prostate improves the ability to deliver maximal radiation dose levels without exceeding the tolerance of the surrounding normal tissues.[327,477,478] In one study, 3 months of leuprolide acetate and flutamide or bicalutamide reduced the prostate PTV by a mean of 25% (range, 3% to 52%).[327] Furthermore, two posttreatment biopsy series demonstrated improved local control when neoadjuvant androgen ablation was used, suggesting either an additive effect or a sensitizing effect induced by androgen deprivation. In one, a 10% (12 of 118) incidence of tumor-positive biopsy specimens among patients pretreated for 3 months with androgen deprivation was observed, compared to 36% (67 of 186) among those who received radiotherapy alone ($P < .001$; Table 30.3-14). The relative distribution of the prognostic risk groups and the prescribed dose did not differ significantly between the two groups.[319] The second, a preliminary report of a randomized trial of stage T2 to T3 prostate cancer patients biopsied at 24 months after radiotherapy, showed that patients treated for 3 months with neoadjuvant androgen deprivation (leuprolide and flutamide) followed by 64-Gy radiotherapy had a 28% incidence of positive biopsy specimens, compared with 65% in those receiving radiation alone. The positive biopsy rate when androgen deprivation was given for 3 months before and 6 months after radiotherapy to 64 Gy was only 5%, consistent with an additive rather than a radiation-sensitizing effect.[331]

TABLE 30.3-14. Impact of Neoadjuvant Androgen Deprivation and Radiation Dose on Local Control Assessed by Posttreatment Prostate Biopsies in 304 Patients at ≥2.5 Years after Three-Dimensional Conformal Radiation Therapy and Intensity-Modulated Radiotherapy

| | Number with Positive Biopsy Specimens/ Total Biopsied (%) | | |
Dose (Gy)	RT alone	NAAD + RT	P Value
64.8	14/25 (56)	ND	—
70.2	21/53 (40)	2/16 (12)	.006
75.6	25/72 (35)	7/65 (11)	<.001
81	6/36 (17)	3/37 (8)	.26
Total	67/186 (36)	12/118 (10)	<.001

NAAD, neoadjuvant androgen deprivation; ND, no data; RT, radiotherapy.

There is considerable evidence to support the use of androgen deprivation with radiotherapy in selected patients with prostate cancer, particularly those with locally advanced, unfavorable-risk disease. The results of four multi-institutional randomized trials that assessed the effect of neoadjuvant or adjuvant androgen deprivation, or both, on the outcome of radiotherapy given by conventional techniques are listed in Table 30.3-15. In each trial, the pelvic lymph nodes were treated to 45 to 50 Gy and the prostate received a total of 65 to 70 Gy. The neoadjuvant approach was tested in RTOG trial 86-10, which randomized patients with 5-cm × 5-cm or larger T2 to T4 primary tumors to either radiotherapy alone or goserelin acetate and flutamide for 2 months before and during radiotherapy.[178] Adjuvant androgen deprivation has been evaluated in three studies. RTOG trial 85-31 randomized patients with T3 to T4 tumors smaller than 5 cm × 5 cm or those with T1 to T2 disease and pelvic lymph node involvement to either goserelin beginning during the final week of radiation and continued indefinitely or until relapse or to the same treatment initiated at the time of recurrence,[153] whereas patients with T2c to T4 tumors in RTOG trial 92-02 received neoadjuvant goserelin and flutamide for 2 months before and 2 months during radiation and were then randomized to 2 additional years of androgen deprivation or no additional treatment.[154] The EORTC trial 22863 randomized patients with high-grade T1 to T2 or T3 to T4 prostate cancer to radiotherapy alone or to radiotherapy plus goserelin initiated at the beginning of radiotherapy and continued after irradiation for 3 years. Cyproterone acetate was also given during the first 4 weeks.[155]

Each of these studies demonstrated significant improvements in local control, freedom from distant metastases, and PSA relapse-free survival for patients receiving androgen deprivation therapy. Thus far, only the EORTC trial has shown a significant overall survival advantage for all patients treated with adjuvant androgen deprivation.[155] In the RTOG adjuvant therapy trials (85-31 and 92-02), survival improvements have, to date, been observed only in patients with Gleason scores of 8 to 10.[153] In contrast, a subset analysis of the RTOG neoadjuvant androgen deprivation trial (86-10) found that outcome improvements, including overall survival, occurred mainly in patients with Gleason scores of 2 to 6.[178] Combined, the data from RTOG trials 85-31 and 86-10 showed an improvement in PSA relapse-free, distant metastasis–free, and cause-specific survival in favor of long-term hormonal therapy for patients with Gleason 7 or greater tumors.[156] Longer follow-up of patients in these studies is necessary to determine whether adjuvant androgen deprivation prevents or only delays the appearance of distant metastases and whether a survival benefit will be observed for all patients.

Questions remain regarding the selection of patients for combined treatment—the sequencing of androgen deprivation with radiotherapy and the optimal length of time that androgen deprivation therapy should be administered have not, thus far, been resolved.[479,480] Whether patients with favorable and intermediate prognostic characteristics benefit from androgen deprivation is not clear. The use of neoadjuvant and concomitant androgen deprivation for patients with T1 to T2, favorable prognosis tumors was evaluated in RTOG trial 94-08, the findings of which have yet to be published. In RTOG trial 99-10, patients with intermediate prognostic risk disease are randomized to receive neoadjuvant androgen deprivation for 8 or 28 weeks. Combined adjuvant chemotherapy and conventional radiotherapy is being evaluated in unfavorable prognostic risk

TABLE 30.3-15. Five-Year Prostate-Specific Antigen (PSA) and Survival Outcomes of Four Multi-Institutional Randomized Trials Testing the Efficacy of Androgen Deprivation Combined with Conventional Radiotherapy

| | Trial[a] | | | |
	RTOG 86-10[115] (n = 471)	RTOG 85-31[116] (n = 977)	RTOG 92-02[117] (n = 1554)	EORTC 22863[118] (n = 415)
Study arm—RT plus	Neo Gos/Flu	Adj Gos	Neo Gos/Flu Adj Gos	Adj Gos
Control arm	RT alone	RT alone	RT + Neo Gos/ Flu	RT alone
Median follow-up (y)	6.7	5.6	4.8	5.5
PSA relapse-free survival (%)				
Study	28	54	46	76
Control	10	21	21	42
Overall survival (%)				
Study	72[b]	75[b]	78[b]	78
Control	68	71	79	62

Adj, adjuvant; EORTC, European Organization for Research and Treatment of Cancer; Flu, flutamide; Gos, goserelin; Neo, neoadjuvant; RT, radiotherapy; RTOG, Radiation Therapy Oncology Group.
[a]See text.
[b]Indicates differences that are not significant. All other differences are significant.

prostate cancer.[481] For example, in RTOG trial 99-02, patients receive neoadjuvant androgen deprivation for 2 months before and during radiotherapy and are then randomly assigned to an additional 2 years of androgen deprivation or four cycles of estramustine, etoposide, and paclitaxel.

Effect of Androgen Deprivation on the Outcome after High-Dose Three-Dimensional Conformal Radiation Therapy and Intensity-Modulated Radiotherapy

Because the randomized trials showing improved outcome with androgen deprivation have used exclusively conventional dose levels of 65 to 70 Gy, the question as to whether androgen deprivation would lead to similar improvements in patients receiving high-dose conformal radiotherapy remains unanswered. In an MSKCC study, shown in Table 30.3-14, 10% (12 of 118) of patients treated with neoadjuvant androgen deprivation had positive biopsy specimens at 2.5 years or more after completion of treatment, compared to 36% (67 of 186) of those who received radiotherapy alone (*P* <.001). The effect was dose dependent. Androgen deprivation significantly reduced the rate of positive biopsies for patients receiving 70.2 and 75.6 Gy (*P* = .006 and <.001, respectively). However, no benefit was observed in those treated to 81 Gy (*P* = .26). Among unfavorable prognosis patients, those who received 81 Gy with androgen deprivation had a 5-year PSA relapse-free survival of 70%, compared to 59% for those treated with radiotherapy alone (*P* = .45). In contrast, the corresponding rates for those treated to 70 Gy or less were 37% and 17%, respectively (*P* = .23). A higher administered dose improved PSA outcomes over conventional dose therapy (*P* = .009), whether neoadjuvant androgen deprivation is administered, and neoadjuvant therapy may benefit patients given higher radiation doses.

The questions of whether androgen deprivation will preclude the need for dose escalation or whether androgen deprivation may be unnecessary when higher dose levels are administered remain to be answered. In some patients, both approaches combined may further improve the outcome. However, it should be emphasized that androgen deprivation is associated with several side effects, including hot flashes, loss of libido, impotence, decreased muscle tone, osteoporosis, increased body fat, and anemia, which can strongly impair patients' quality of life. In RTOG trial 92-02, adjuvant androgen deprivation was, for reasons that are unclear, associated with a significant increase in late grade 3 and 4 bowel complications.[482] This was also observed in a second trial showing that long-term (more than 9 months) adjuvant androgen deprivation appeared to reduce rectal tolerance, whereas a shorter course of treatment did not affect the likelihood of rectal toxicity.[483] In contrast, Liu et al. found that short-term hormonal therapy increased the risk of late grade 3 toxicity.[484] In view of the apparent favorable benefit-risk ratio of high-dose IMRT when administered as a single modality, a clinical trial is being conducted at MSKCC to help reconcile some of these important questions. Patients with unfavorable prognosis tumors or those with intermediate prognosis disease and Gleason scores of 8 or higher are randomized to receive neoadjuvant and adjuvant androgen deprivation plus 75.6 Gy or 86.4 Gy alone. Radiotherapy in both treatment arms is administered using the IMRT approach.

These caveats aside, in the combined results of the three EPC trials on androgen deprivation therapy as adjuvant to watchful waiting, surgery, and radiation therapy, the propor-

tion of patients who developed osseous metastases within 2 years was 9% in the bicalutamide-treated patients and 13.8% in the placebo-treated patients (HR reduction of 0.58; *P*<.001).[473] An analysis by the Cochrane group showed that early treatment confers a small but statistically significant survival advantage and a significant improvement in progression-free survival that was durable at 10 years.[485] A recent metaanalysis of immediate androgen ablation treatment versus treatment at time of progression (variably defined) showed that, at 10 years, 74% of patients treated with immediate therapy were alive versus 62% treated with a deferred approach.[486] All of these favor early treatment.

Of interest is that the survival differences reported in these metaanalyses are similar to those reported in the European Breast Cancer Trials Cooperative Group analysis of 55 trials evaluating 30,000 women randomized to tamoxifen or no tamoxifen as an adjunct to primary treatment. In this study, the reduction in death rate was directly proportional to the duration of tamoxifen therapy (chi^2(1) = 52.0; two-sided *P*<.00001). Patients treated for 1, 2, and 5 or more years enjoyed a reduction in metastatic recurrence and mortality of 21% and 12%, 29% and 17%, and 47% and 23%, respectively, after 10 years of follow-up. The overall reduction in mortality between the breast cancer and prostate cancer treated patients, 28% and 33%, is virtually identical.[487]

Why are women treated and men not? For one, many men opt to defer treatment until the disease has declared itself as more aggressive because of the long-term side effects of androgen ablation. They are unconvinced that the outcome would be significantly different—a view shared by many physicians. But even if one accepts that long-term survival might be inferior, some prefer to enjoy their lives more completely by maintaining potency and avoiding the side effects of castration. In absence of deferment, in general, our approach is to consider treatment after local therapy and, when the PSA begins to rise, once the issue of a local versus systemic recurrence is resolved, to defer androgen ablation until the PSA begins to rise rapidly (doubling time less than 6 to 12 months) or until high levels point to imminent metastases. The recent association between PSA doubling time and survival in patients who have recurred after radiation therapy[488] has led many to base treatment decisions on PSA doubling times. A recent consensus panel on the management of patients with a rising PSA after surgery or radiation therapy, also a state of minimal disease, reached the conclusion that data were insufficient to recommend immediate androgen deprivation for this cohort of men.[417] The American Society of Clinical Oncology Prostate Cancer Practice Guidelines points out that hormone therapy is most cost effective if treatment is deferred until symptoms of the disease are documented.[489] This, however, may not be practical or realistic for many men who are continuing to watch their PSA levels rise. As such, the authors' group and others are exploring alternative approaches in patients in the state of a rising PSA.[490]

CLINICAL METASTASES: CASTRATE

There is no debate that therapies beyond hormones are needed to improve outcomes for patients with cancers that have spread and have recurred. Typically, these approaches are evaluated after failure or progression on hormones is docu-

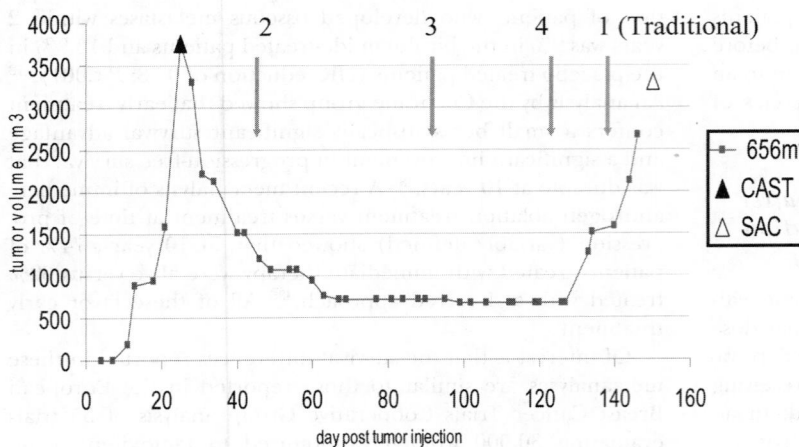

FIGURE 30.3-41. Timing of systemic interventions in relation to androgen deprivation (or cytotoxic drug therapy modeled in CWR22 xenografts. CAST, castration; SAC, sacrifice. (From ref. 491, with permission.)

mented. However, timing the integration of one therapy in relation to another may also be critical. Considered in the context of hormones, androgen deprivation produces a decline in PSA; a regression of measurable tumor masses; a period of clinical quiescence or stability in which the tumor does not change in size, followed in a variable period of time by a rise in PSA; proliferation of the tumor; and clinically detectable tumor regrowth. Assessing these changes histologically in the same patient is difficult because repeated sampling of tumor is not a part of the routine management. CWR22 human prostate cancer xenografts subject to androgen ablation show the same patterns of change in PSA, which can be grouped broadly into early, mid, or late categories (Fig. 30.3-41). Early events include a decrease in AR expression, a decrease in proliferation, and apoptosis that leads to a decrease in the size of the tumor. FDG avidity on PET changes from high to low. Mid-to-late events include and encompass the period of a stable but often abnormal PSA; an absence of proliferation or apoptosis, or both, on histologic sectioning; and no uptake of FDG on PET, whereas the period of tumor regrowth is associated with resumption of AR expression, markers of proliferation, and a return of FDG avidity.[491] How these approaches can be integrated is also shown in Figure 30.3-41 and includes strategies to (1) as is traditionally practiced, treat at the time of tumor regrowth when the resistant phenotype is fully manifest; (2) increase the initial apoptotic response after androgen ablation; (3) eliminate cells during the nonproliferating quiescent phase; or (4) prevent tumor regrowth.[419] The same considerations apply to improving outcomes with chemotherapy.

The failure of first-line androgen ablation can be manifest in several ways. In some patients, it is a rising PSA alone, others have a rising PSA and progression of osseous disease, and in others there is a visceral spread with or without osseous disease. Symptoms may or may not be present. Which pattern develops in a given patient is influenced in part by the extent of disease at the time androgen deprivation was first initiated. The patient who initially received hormones for a rising PSA alone is likely to relapse with a rising PSA and negative imaging studies. In contrast, the patient who first received hormones for symptomatic metastatic disease also shows a rising PSA but is more likely to develop symptoms in the short term and is at a higher risk of death from prostate cancer. The patient with asymptomatic metastatic disease at the start of hormone therapy is likely

to have a prognosis in between these two. Should these patients be approached differently? Should a rising PSA castrate state be defined for patients who received hormones in the state of a rising PSA and are now progressing with a rising PSA despite castrate levels of testosterone? Perhaps they should.

Regardless of the pattern, the first therapeutic consideration for patients who have not undergone surgical orchiectomy is to document that the testosterone level is in the castrate range. If it is not in the castrate range, then testosterone-lowering therapy should be administered. If the testosterone level is already in the castrate range, a variety of options are available, including second-line hormonal therapies, cytotoxic approaches, and investigational agents. There is no standard, although several groups are now consistently reporting response proportions and durations of response with cytotoxic drugs that are comparable to those in other tumor types in which a definitive survival benefit has been shown. But, independent of treatment, it is important to continue medical therapies that maintain castrate status. Allowing testosterone levels to rise in this setting may shorten survival.[492]

Tumors that are progressing despite castrate levels of testosterone have been variably classified as hormone-resistant, hormone-refractory, androgen-insensitive, and androgen-refractory, among others. These *a priori* categorizations ignore what is now known about the clinical phenotype and molecular genotype of these tumors and do not provide insights on how best to approach them therapeutically. That PSA levels rise in virtually all patients despite castrate levels of testosterone is an indication that signaling through the AR continues. The responses to secondary and tertiary hormonal manipulations that occur in many patients also argue against a categoric *hormone-refractory* classification. Many of the clinical outcomes can be explained at the molecular level, although a direct association between a given alteration and outcome has not been shown. Amplification of a wild-type AR gene producing hypersensitivity to low levels of androgen, an increase in intratumoral androgens secondary to an increase in the levels of the enzymes involved in androgen synthesis, and alterations in the ligand-binding domain and coactivator/corepressor protein interactions leading to promiscuous activation by other steroid hormones and antiandrogens are examples.[84,493] The diverse mechanisms of activation of the receptor and other mechanisms that can contribute to tumor regrowth explains why we consider these lesions as castration resistant[41,85] or simply resistant[87] rather than attempt to categorize them, often inappropriately, as androgen independent or hormone refractory. Evolving data show that the clinical phenotype and molecular genotype of resistant tumors is influenced in part by the specific therapies that have been administered in the past, under whose influence the tumor has survived and is continuing to grow. This concept of therapy-mediated selection pressure[494] has clinical significance and, if considered carefully, can increase the chance of therapeutic success with a specific intervention. It has also sparked efforts to better characterize these tumors at the molecular level. Various treatment options are considered in turn.

SECOND- AND THIRD-LINE HORMONAL THERAPIES

A proportion of patients with progressive disease and castrate levels of testosterone respond to second- and third-line hormonal manipulations. Response proportions in the literature range from 8% to 30% of patients responding for a median of 3 to 4 months, with an occasional patient showing benefit for 6 months or more.[495] Often, those who respond to a second hormonal intervention will respond to a third. Among the therapies that have shown benefit are antiandrogens, estrogens, progestational agents, inhibitors of adrenal steroid synthesis, and/or glucocorticoids.[496] Contexts that predict for a response to a specific agent, include the lack of cross resistance between different antiandrogens, in which patients previously treated with flutamide have a higher response proportion to bicalutamide relative to patients who have not been exposed to flutamide,[471,497] or the response of bicalutamide failures to nilutamide.[498]

The response to the selective discontinuation of nonsteroidal antiandrogens and other steroid hormones is another example of therapy-mediated selection pressure: Unless you have received a specific treatment, you cannot respond to its discontinuation. The phenomena of withdrawal responses was originally documented as responses to discontinuation of flutamide in patients with progressive disease on combined androgen blockade. Withdrawal responses were later shown to occur with the antiandrogens bicalutamide, nilutamide, and cyproterone acetate, as well as with other hormonal therapies that act via the AR, including estrogens, glucocorticoids, and progestational agents.[499–502] These withdrawal responses occur at approximately the same frequency as responses to second-line hormonal therapies. Consistent with the observation that a steroid hormone can have agonist effects are reports of pain flares in relapsing patients treated with megestrol acetate.[503] Discontinuation responses, if they occur, do so rapidly, but may be delayed up to 8 to 12 weeks with compounds that have a prolonged half-life, such as bicalutamide or nilutamide. It is, therefore, important to leave adequate time to assess outcomes, rather than immediately change to a different treatment.

Of the options available, estramustine phosphate is specifically approved as therapy for patients who have progressed on hormone therapy; it produced PSA declines of 50% or more in 24% of patients in a contemporary trial.[504] Responses to oral and parenteral estrogens have also been observed.[496] Other agents include the adrenal synthetic enzyme inhibitor ketoconazole, which at a dose of 1200 mg/d with or without hydrocortisone can provide responses in up to 40% of cases.[431,505] A recent trial compared simultaneous antiandrogen withdrawal plus ketoconazole and hydrocortisone to antiandrogen withdrawal alone. Although a higher proportion of patients given ketoconazole and hydrocortisone with concurrent antiandrogen withdrawal showed a decline in PSA, there was no difference in survival.[506] Similar outcomes were reported with aminoglutethimide, but use has been largely discontinued due to toxicity concerns. Both of these agents are typically administered with hydrocortisone to reduce the risk of adrenal crisis.[505,507] Varying doses of corticosteroids alone have also been studied, including prednisone, 10 to 20 mg/d; hydrocortisone, 30 to 40 mg/d; and low-dose dexamethasone (Decadron), 0.75 mg b.i.d., which has produced PSA declines in 16% to 34% of patients.[508–510]

The choice of whether to try additional hormonal manipulations or to proceed immediately to cytotoxic therapy depends in part on the patient's age, functional status and comorbidities, the duration of response to first-line hormones, current disease extent, and presence or absence of symptoms. In general, before enrolling a patient on a chemotherapy program, the authors recommend a trial of steroid hormone withdrawal if appropriate, and one additional hormonal manipulation. The relative benefit of early chemotherapy versus second-line hormone therapy followed by chemotherapy is being addressed in a randomized comparative trial of ketoconazole/hydrocortisone versus chemotherapy by the Eastern Cooperative Oncology Group (ECOG 1899). In this trial, patients with castration-resistant rising PSA are randomly assigned to either ketoconazole and hydrocortisone or docetaxel (60 mg/m² on day 2) and estramustine (two tablets twice a day on days 1 through 5). The primary end point is time to detectable metastatic disease based on serial imaging studies performed every 12 weeks.

CYTOTOXIC AGENTS

A long-held dictum in prostate cancer management is that chemotherapy should not be used because it has not been shown to prolong life in randomized comparisons. This is not only outdated but also ignores important and significant clinical benefits that can be achieved in the appropriate context with cytotoxic agents. It also shows the importance of not restricting outcomes to measures of tumor regression as the sole end point for trials and how a well-designed sequence of studies can change treatment paradigms.

Until May 2004, mitoxantrone and prednisone was the only cytotoxic therapy approved for the treatment of progressive castration-resistant prostate cancer. It is indicated for the palliation of pain of osseous metastases, based on clinical trials showing an improvement in quality of life,[511] although there was no improvement in overall survival. The studies began with an evaluation of prednisone monotherapy,[508] a phase II trial of the combination, and two phase III randomized comparisons of the combination versus prednisone monotherapy.[509,512] The first phase III trial, which enrolled 160 patients (80 patients per treatment arm), showed that a higher proportion of patients given the combination had a decrease in pain, 29% versus 12% (*P* = .011); total palliative response, 38% versus 21% (*P* = .025); and duration of palliative response, 43 weeks versus 18 weeks (*P* <.001). Consistent with the improvement in pain was a reduction in analgesic usage, improved mobility, and improved bowel function. There was no survival difference.[512] Similar results were seen in a second comparative trial,[509] establishing mitoxantrone and prednisone as a treatment standard.

Prostate cancer appears to be particularly sensitive to agents that target the cytoskeleton, such as vinblastine, vinorelbine, etoposide, paclitaxel, and docetaxel in combination with estramustine. In many of these trials, PSA declines of 50% or more in upwards of 70% of patients treated, measurable disease regression in 20% to 40%, and objective improvements in radionuclide bone scan were observed which suggests durations of response of 6 months or more.[513–518] The median survival times, historically described as being in the range of 9 to 12 months,[519] are now reported in the 16- to 24-month range.[419] Is this the result of treatment, or does it reflect a greater acceptance of chemotherapy and the referral of patients earlier in the course of the disease who have an inherently better prognosis independent of treatment? Prospective randomized trials are required to address this question, but, until recently, most of the trials reported were based on overly optimistic estimates of the potential benefit of the new therapy, and, ultimately, too few patients were enrolled. A brief history follows.

Estramustine phosphate has shown modest activity as a single agent,[504] as has vinblastine in a pre-PSA study.[520] In combination with vinblastine, higher response proportions were observed.[514,521] Subsequently, a randomized trial of estramustine and vinblastine versus vinblastine alone was conducted. It was powered to a 50% improvement in survival. The results showed measurable disease regression in 20% versus 6% ($P = .131$), PSA declines of 50% in 25% versus 3% ($P \leq .001$), and a median time to progression of 3.7 versus 2.2 months ($P \leq .001$).[522] With longer follow-up, a median survival difference of 31% was noted (median, 11.9 vs. 9.2 months), representing a trend that was not statistically significant ($P = .08$).[523] The combination of estramustine and etoposide[524] was evaluated after the activity of oral etoposide was identified,[525] and estramustine and vinorelbine[526] was evaluated after the activity of vinorelbine was reported.[527]

At present, most groups are focusing drug development efforts on the taxanes paclitaxel and docetaxel. In the first trial, paclitaxel administered as a continuous infusion showed modest activity as a single agent,[528] which increased to 40% to 50% of patients showing a response when paclitaxel was combined with estramustine.[529] Subsequently, a randomized trial of estramustine and paclitaxel versus paclitaxel was performed. Enrolling 166, the trial showed a 50% decline in PSA in 48% versus 25% of patients ($P = .01$), progression-free survival at 12 months in 29% versus 8% ($P = .083$), and a 17% difference in median survival in favor of the combination (15.1 vs. 12.9 months) that was not statistically significant ($P = .113$).[530]

In contrast, single-agent docetaxel produced PSA declines in 46% of patients on an every-3-week schedule[531] and in 41% and 46% on a weekly schedule,[532,533] with measurable disease regression in 24% to 40% of patients in whom it was manifest. In combination with estramustine, PSA declines and measurable disease regression were noted in 74% and 57%,[518] 68% and 50%,[517] and 45% and 23% of patients. The median proportion showing a PSA decline of 50% or more was 72% (range, 45% to 74%) and measurable disease regression was 50% (range, 17% to 53%).[534] The toxicities of docetaxel were acceptable and not dissimilar to what has been reported in other tumor types. The addition of estramustine, however, did produce an increase in toxicity and, in particular, an increase in cardiovascular complications—edema, phlebitis, pulmonary embolus, myocardial infarction, and stroke. Nausea and gastrointestinal discomfort are also more frequent for combination therapy.

Both single-agent docetaxel and the combination of estramustine and docetaxel were compared to mitoxantrone and prednisone in large prospective randomized trials reported in June 2004. Both were designed and powered to detect a survival improvement of 33% or more. The first, Multicenter 327, randomized 1006 patients to docetaxel (75 mg/m² every 3 weeks × 10; 30 mg/m²/wk × 5 of 6 weeks × 5 cycles) or mitoxantrone (12 mg/m² every 3 weeks × 10) treatment. Considered by treatment arm, PSA response (a 50% or greater decline) was observed in 45%, 48%, and 32% ($P = .0005$, $P = .0001$) of patients, and pain response was observed in 35% ($P = .01$), 31% ($P = .08$), and 22%, respectively. Grade 3 and 4 neutropenia was higher in the every-3-week arm. More important is that, with a median follow-up of 20.7 months, the median survivals were 18.9, 17.4, and 16.5 months, respectively, with a HR for death of 0.76 (0.62 to 0.94; $P = .009$) and 0.91 (0.75 to 1.11; $P = .36$) for the experimental arms relative to the mitoxantrone arm.[535] The results of this trial led to the FDA approval of docetaxel q3 weeks for prostate cancer patients with progressive castration resistant disease. The results established for the first time that chemotherapy can prolong life.[535] A second trial, Southwest Oncology Group 99-16, randomized 770 men to docetaxel and estramustine or mitoxantrone and prednisone. A 23% survival benefit was again shown for estramustine/docetaxel versus mitoxantone/prednisone(HR, 177; 95% CI 0.64, 0.94).[536] One issue not addressed in these trials is whether the increased response proportions observed in phase II and phase III with estramustine-based combinations justify its use on a routine basis. Unfortunately, no direct comparative trial of a taxane plus or minus estramustine of adequate size and power has been conducted.

PALLIATION OF SYMPTOMS AND BONE-DIRECTED THERAPY

A critical aspect of the management is palliation of symptoms. Supportive measures can include a TURP to relieve outlet obstruction, the placement of stents or nephrostomy tubes to improve renal function, steroids to relieve cachexia and to palliate the pain associated with osseous disease, and erythropoietin to correct the anemia related to androgen deprivation.

Pain can be one of the most debilitating and feared symptoms of the disease. Fortunately, with careful attention to the pain frequency, pattern, and precipitating factors and the early performance of appropriate diagnostic studies to establish an etiology, durable palliation of symptoms can be achieved and functional status maintained. Critical for management is a low threshold for recommending an MRI if there is back pain suggestive of neurologic compromise of the spinal cord or cauda equina; diplopia, dysarthria, difficulty swallowing, or facial weakness suggestive of involvement of the base of the skull; or numbness in the jaw or chin suggestive of mental nerve compromise, which may interfere with eating.[537] If neurologic encroachment is documented in any of these areas, radiation therapy should be administered on an urgent basis to preserve function and to maximize the chance of recovery. Corticosteroids are also administered to provide more immediate palliation and to reduce the risk of further compromise secondary to swelling that can occur after radiation therapy is initiated.

Pathologic fractures do occur, although less frequently than in other diseases owing in part to the predominantly osteoblastic nature of the lesions. Plain films are recommended, particularly of the hip, femur, and humerus to exclude this possibility. Osteoporosis, exacerbated by androgen deprivation, can increase the susceptibility to fracture either spontaneously or after trauma. Collapse of a vertebra can also occur, secondary to tumor or to bone loss.

In the absence of neurologic compromise, therapies to palliate pain can be divided broadly into those directed at the tumor itself, those directed at the tumor/bone interface with little effect on tumor, and those directed at specific cytokines and growth factors produced by tumor cells and the host that contribute to the progression and survival of prostate cancer cells in the skeleton. Reducing cytokine and growth factor production, or blocking their action, can limit the deleterious effects on the skeleton noteworthy.

TUMOR TARGETING

One of the most effective means of killing tumor cells and reducing pain is with external-beam radiation therapy. Appropriately directed in either a narrow or wide field, radiotherapy can achieve durable palliation using single or multiple fractions. Often, the overall efficacy of the approach is usually limited by the diffuse nature of the metastases such that, after successful treatment of one focal area, other areas may become symptomatic in a relatively short time.

TUMOR/BONE INTERFACE

The bone-seeking radiopharmaceuticals such as Metastron (strontium 89)[538,539] and Quadramet[540] have the potential to palliate diffuse pain. Samarium 153 phosphonic acid (1,2-ethyanediyl bis[nitrilobis (methylene)]) tetrakis-monohydrate ethylenediaminetetramethylene phosphonic acid (Quadramet)[540,541] relies on the diphosphonate moiety for targeting, whereas the radionuclide simultaneously emits gamma energies that can be imaged and short-range beta energies that can be therapeutic. Both agents are taken up rapidly in bone and localize primarily to the bone tumor interface. As a result, dosimetry to tumor is difficult to calculate, but estimated doses are significantly below those administered via an external-beam approach and are not tumoricidal. The distribution of the isotope throughout the tumor is also limited, further compromising radiation delivery.[542] These agents have been studied in a direct comparison to radiation therapy[539] or as an adjunct to radiation therapy to a dominant painful lesion versus radiation therapy alone.[543] The most common side effects are a pain flare in approximately 10% of cases that may last for several days, and myelosuppression, which varies with the extent of disease and the amount of bone marrow that has received radiation in the past. Although the palliation can last for upwards of 12 weeks, the ability to administer these agents on a repetitive basis is limited by cumulative myelosuppression and, in particular, the effect on platelets.[544]

A unique design, reported in 2001 from the M. D. Anderson Cancer Center (MDACC), evaluated a sequential bone consolidation approach in which a combination chemotherapy regimen was followed by a combination of Metastron and doxorubicin.[545] The results showed both a reduction in skeletal events and a suggestion of a survival benefit. This approach is now undergoing a large-scale phase III evaluation through the MDACC Clinical Trials Network and the Clinical Trials Support Unit (CTSU).

BONE STROMAL CELLS

Although bisphosphonates have been shown to protect against the bone loss associated with castration,[546,547] the palliative effects on existing symptoms of osseous disease have been modest even with second- and third-generation agents. In two large randomized trials, there was no difference in patient-reported bone pain intensity at 9 or 27 weeks or in overall skeletal-related events for patients receiving pamidronate versus placebo.[548] In contrast, zoledronic acid (Zometa), which had shown benefit in patients with breast cancer, lung cancer, renal cancer, and multiple myeloma, recently showed an effect on progression of established prostate cancer osseous metastases, using a composite end point of skeletal-related events. These were defined as pathologic bone fracture, spinal cord compression, surgery to the bone, radiation therapy to the bone, or a change in therapy to treat bone pain. In this trial, patients with progressive castration-resistant disease on therapy were randomized to parenteral placebo; zoledronate, 4 mg; or zoledronate, 8 mg administered every 3 weeks, but otherwise managed at the discretion of their treating physician. Most received hormonal therapy; few received chemotherapy. The adverse events at 8 mg/d proved excessive, and this arm was dropped. The results showed a reduction in skeletal-related events at 15 months from 44% to 33% (*P* = .021) and a delay to a skeletal-related event from 321 days to not yet reached (*P* = .011). Consistent with zoledronate having a limited or no direct effect on tumor cells per se, there was no difference in the time to PSA progression, although there was a trend toward an improvement in survival (*P* = .091).[549] The degree and duration of decline of both blood and urinary markers of bone turnover, such as N-telopeptides and hydroxyproline/creatinine ratios, favored bisphosphonate administered and paralleled symptom relief.

The question of whether clodronate added to first-line hormonal therapy could delay progression of disease was addressed in a trial of 311 patients randomized to androgen ablation plus clodronate versus androgen ablation plus placebo. With a median follow-up of 59 months, patients treated with clodronate were less likely to experience a deterioration of performance status (HR = 0.71; 95% CI, 0.56 to 0.92; *P* = .008), and there was a trend toward an improved bone progression-free survival (HR = 0.79; 95% CI, 0.61 to 1.02; *P* = .066) and overall survival (HR = 0.80; 95% CI, 0.62 to 1.03; *P* = .082) with early therapy. Additional studies are needed.

A question not completely answered is whether bisphosphonates add to the palliative effects of chemotherapy. In a comparative trial of mitoxantrone and prednisone with or without clodronate, no benefit was observed for the addition of the bisphosphonate.[550] Clinical trials designed to show whether a bisphosphonate can prevent metastatic disease are ongoing.

TARGETING FACTORS ASSOCIATED WITH PROGRESSION OF DISEASE IN BONE

Studies on the factors associated with progression of disease in bone have allowed more directed targeted approaches to be evaluated. ET-1, produced by prostate cancer cells and secreted in the ejaculate, is one of the mediators of the osteoblastic phenotype. *In vitro*, ET-1 is mitogenic for prostate cancer cell lines and osteoblasts and inhibits osteoclast motility and bone resorption. ET-1 is highly expressed on virtually all prostate cancer cells representing different clinical states and levels in serum-parallel disease extent. ABT-627 (atrasentan) is a potent ET-A receptor antagonist that blocks ET-1 signaling.[551] A phase I trial showed palliation of pain with adverse events, including headache, rhinitis, and lower-extremity edema.[552,553] A double-blind, placebo-controlled trial of atrasentan, 2.5 or 10 mg/d, or placebo showed a dose-dependent delay in time to progression, improvement in the development of bone-related pain, and declines in markers of bone turnover.[554] An independent monitoring committee concluded that the results were not definitive, which led to a phase III trial that recently completed accrual. Two phase III trials are ongoing, one for men with progressive metastatic disease and a second for a rising PSA after hormone therapy (rising PSA castrate disease). Another cytokine secreted by prostate cancer cells, IL-6, contributes to bone resorption. Bortezomib (Velcade), a proteosome inhibitor that blocks IL-6 inhibition of apoptosis, was recently approved for the treatment of multiple myeloma. This agent is being studied as monotherapy,[553a] in combination with glucocorticoids and in combination with chemotherapy.

STRATEGIES TO IMPROVE OUTCOMES

Strategies being evaluated to improve outcomes include three- and four-drug combinations, new agents, combinations of docetaxel with agents that have shown synergy in preclinical studies, and strategies directed toward targets and mechanisms associated with prostate cancer cell proliferation and survival.

THREE- AND FOUR-DRUG COMBINATIONS AND NEW AGENTS AS FIRST-LINE TREATMENT

The combination of paclitaxel, estramustine, and carboplatin showed a greater than 50% decline in PSA in 71% of patients (n = 55), regression of measurable disease in 56% (n = 26), and an improvement or stability in bone scan in 47%, whereas 79% (n = 24) with narcotic-dependent pain discontinued opioids. The median survival was 16 months.[515] Similar results have been reported using the same combination with docetaxel[555]; docetaxel, etoposide, and estramustine[556]; and a four-drug regimen (KAVE) in which a ketoconazole/doxorubicin doublet is alternated with estramustine/vinblastine.[557]

The epothilones have shown activity in preclinical models of prostate cancer[558] and in a spectrum of other tumors. In a phase I trial of epothilone B (BMS-247550), 11 of 12 patients (92%) showed a PSA decline of 50% or more (95% CI, 70% to 98%), with measurable partial response in three of seven patients.[559] A randomized trial of estramustine and BMS-247550 versus BMS-247550 alone was reported in June 2004. Response rates were similar, but longer follow-up is needed to assess for potential differences in durability of response between the two arms.[560]

COMBINATIONS OF DOCETAXEL WITH AGENTS THAT HAVE SHOWN ACTIVITY IN PRECLINICAL STUDIES OR POSTULATED TO HAVE INCREASED ACTIVITY BY TARGETING INDEPENDENT MECHANISMS

The combination of calcitriol and docetaxel is being studied. Calcitriol has antiproliferative effects on prostate cancer cell growth.[561,562] Effects on PSA were observed in phase I trials, and the hypercalcemia associated with continuous therapy has been ameliorated with glucocorticoids[563,564] or intermittent dosing.[565] A trial of intermittent calcitriol, 45 µg, in combination with weekly docetaxel showed PSA declines in 30 of 37 patients (81%) and measurable disease regression in 8 of 15 (53%), with a median time to progression of 11.4 months.[566] Toxicities were not increased relative to single-agent docetaxel. An ongoing randomized trial, ASCENT, is comparing docetaxel weekly for 3 out of 4 weeks versus docetaxel plus calcitriol (45 µg the day before treatment).

Antisense oligonucleotides are designed to induce the degradation of a specific mRNA, resulting in a decrease in protein expression. G3139 (Genasense), an antisense oligonucleotide that binds to mRNA of the apoptosis inhibitor BCL-2, was explored based on gene expression and immunohistochemical studies showing increased BCL-2 expression in castration-resistant metastatic disease.[567] A single-agent trial showed no responses in 23 prostate cancer patients treated at doses that produced a decrease in BCL-2 expression in peripheral blood lymphocytes.[568] In combination with mitoxantrone, significant PSA declines were observed in 2 of 26 patients (7%), whereas in combination with docetaxel, four of eight taxane-naive patients responded.[569] Subsequently, 31 patients were enrolled in a third trial at a higher dose, which produced PSA declines of more than 50% in 15 patients (48%) and measurable disease regression in 4 of 15 evaluable cases (27%). A phase III trial is planned.

ANGIOGENESIS INHIBITION

Microvessel density in a primary prostate cancer is predictive of outcome.[570] At the National Cancer Institute, the angiogenesis inhibitor thalidomide was evaluated in patients with a rising PSA and no clinical metastatic disease on the presumption that the approach would be more effective before neovascularization had occurred. PSA declines were observed in the phase I trial in 19 of 63 (27%) patients enrolled,[571] leading to a randomized phase II study of the combination of docetaxel and thalidomide versus docetaxel alone. Using a 2:1 randomization, PSA declines were noted in 50% (25 of 50) versus 27% (9 of 24) objective responses in 35% and 27%, with a median survival of 28.9 versus 14.7 months, respectively, in favor of the combination.[571] Thrombotic complications were higher in the thalidomide-treated patients.

Vascular endothelial growth factor is mitogenic for prostate cancer cells and is androgen regulated. In the clinic, higher levels of vascular endothelial growth factor are associated with an inferior outcome. In xenografts, an antibody to vascular endothelial growth factor, bevacizumab, inhibited established tumor growth by 85% ($P < .01$) during treatment, but the tumors regrew when treatment was stopped. Enhanced effects were observed in combination with paclitaxel relative to the antibody alone.[572,573]

In the clinic, no tumor regressions were observed with bevacizumab as a single agent, but, in combination with docetaxel, a higher proportion of patients showed PSA declines relative to docetaxel alone. PSA declines of 50% or more were noted in 65% of cases, with measurable disease regression in 9 of 17 (56%).[531] A phase III trial of docetaxel and prednisone plus or minus bevacizumab is planned.

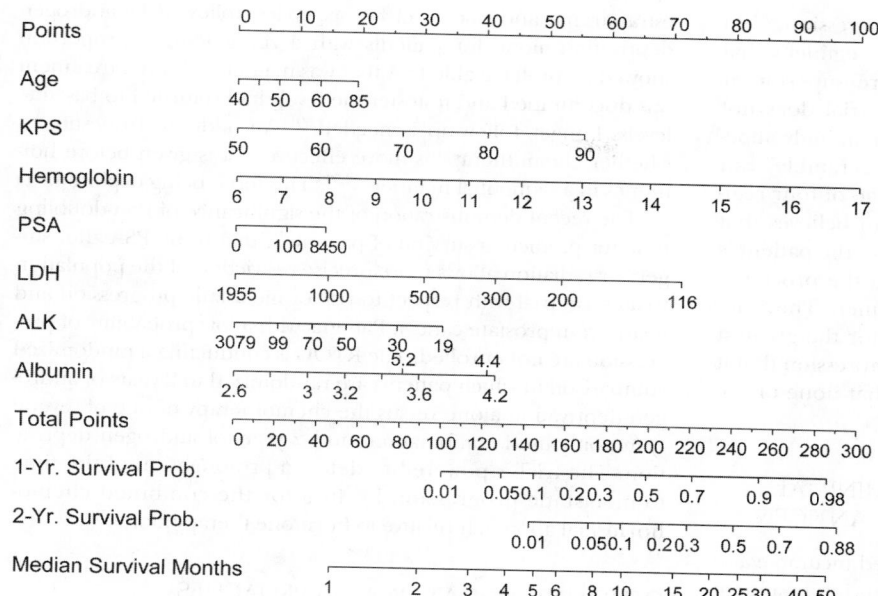

FIGURE 30.3-42. Nomogram for castrate metastatic disease. ALK, alkaline phosphatase; KPS, Karnofsky performance status; LDH, lactate dehydrogenase; PSA, prostate-specific antigen.

SIGNALING INHIBITORS

Other signaling molecules and pathways associated with prostate cancer progression are also being targeted. As discussed in Biologic Characterization, an issue for these approaches is that, not infrequently, the pattern of expression changes as the tumor progresses to the point at which a therapy for one state may not be relevant for another. Such is the case for EGFR and HER2. However, despite promising preclinical data and profiling studies showing that the specific receptors were expressed in the disease state under study, clinical results have been disappointing. An antibody to the EGFR [cetuximab (Erbitux)] showed limited activity in combination with doxorubicin, whereas an antibody to HER2 [trastuzumab (Herceptin)], showed no regressions as a single agent or in combination with paclitaxel.[574] Similarly, a small molecule inhibitor of the EGFR enzyme activity, gefitinib (Iressa), was inactive as a single agent but is also under evaluation in combination with estramustine and docetaxel and with mitoxantrone and prednisone.[575] 17-AAG is an ansamycin derivative that induces degradation of HER2, AR, and other proteins that bind to the Hsp90 (heat-shock protein 90) family of chaperones. A trial of 17-AAG recently entered the clinic, and it is also under study as a single agent and in combination with docetaxel.[576,577]

Studies of PDGF receptor expression suggest a potential role in all prostate cancer clinical states. In localized disease trials, increased *PDFGR* gene expression has been associated with recurrence in multigene models.[578] *In vivo* models of prostate cancer bone metastasis show increased expression in the tumor and the vasculature and bone healing on administration of imatinib (Gleevec), an inhibitor of PDGR signaling. With imatinib administered as a single agent, no activity was observed after 4 weeks, but responses were observed with the addition of docetaxel.[57] A decrease in the level of the receptor, both native and phosphorylated forms, was shown on tumor-involved bone biopsies. A double-blind, placebo-controlled phase III trial comparing imatinib plus docetaxel versus placebo plus docetaxel is ongoing.

WHEN IS ACTIVITY SUFFICIENT TO PROCEED TO A PHASE III TRIAL? HOW DO WE PICK THE WINNER?

That responses are observed in trials using taxane-based combinations is not surprising. Given the range and number of approaches under evaluation, limited patient resources, and the cost of conducting definitive trials, a critical question becomes how to determine which approach, if any, should be evaluated in the phase III clinical benefit setting and what the control and comparator arms should be. This can be addressed in several ways with the caveat that none are substitutes for a definitive trial. The first is to consider the results in other tumor types, because development in prostate cancer is usually behind that in other diseases. The demonstrated survival benefit with bevacizumab in patients with colon cancer is an example; the data on prostate cancer alone would not have been an indication to move forward. Another approach is to perform extended randomized phase II studies for two active regimens. This helps to ensure that the treatment groups are balanced with respect to prognostic factors, although the results in each arm are not "comparable" in the traditional sense. Using this approach, investigators at MDACC performed a randomized phase II trial of KAVE and paclitaxel, estramustine, and etoposide (TEE), which led to the conclusion that both were either too toxic or too costly (TEE), with unclear superiority to justify a phase III trial.[557,579]

Alternatively, the survival for patients given the new experimental therapy using a nomogram (Fig. 30.3-42) can be calculated and plotted with the actual survival of the patients treated. The CI around the median is then estimated, which varies as a function of the number of patients enrolled.[580] No overlap in the CIs around the median would suggest a therapy that is worthy of further study.[581] Using this approach, a study of taxane-based chemotherapy versus nontaxane-based treatment was considered justified,[580] whereas a study of the addition of platinum to taxane-estramustine-based therapy was not.

The "pick the winner" strategy is a two-stage approach in which patients are randomized to one of several regimens, and outcomes are assessed by survival or time to progression.[582] At the end of the first stage, accrual is stopped to regimens that are significantly inferior and to those that are superior or equivalent accrual continues. A new phase III trial does not have to be designed. If one regimen is overwhelmingly superior, that trial can be stopped. Alternatively, a "scramble" can be used by which patients are randomized to one of four regimens and treated with them until the physician believes that the treatment is no longer effective. At that point, the patient is randomized to one of the other regimens, and the process is repeated for the second, third, and fourth regimen. The "winning" regimen is the one that is administered for the greatest number of cycles, as surrogate for the clinical impression that it was still effective.[583] It should be emphasized that none of the strategies is a substitute for definitive trials.

SYSTEMIC THERAPY IN THE SETTING OF MINIMAL DISEASE AND RISING PROSTATE-SPECIFIC ANTIGEN

Once it is metastatic, prostate cancer is considered incurable and is approached typically as a chronic disease requiring treatment for a prolonged period of time. A critical evaluation of trials using long-term androgen ablation in the neoadjuvant or adjuvant setting, combined with either radiation therapy or surgery, suggests that a proportion of patients with micrometastatic disease at diagnosis may in fact be cured with a combined modality approach. This is consistent with reported trials in gastrointestinal,[584] thoracic, and breast cancers,[585] in which regimens with modest activity in late-stage disease can improve survival. Given the recent demonstration that chemotherapy in late-stage prostate cancers can confer a survival benefit, the question is how best to integrate chemotherapy with hormones earlier in the course of the illness.

The clinical experience to date has been limited largely to small pilot trials addressing safety and feasibility. Estramustine and vinblastine has been safely administered before radiation therapy,[481,586] and a study using estramustine/docetaxel is ongoing in the Cancer and Leukemia Group B. Pettaway et al. explored KAVE before surgery in 33 patients with high-risk disease and found that after surgery, 33% had organ-confined disease, 17% had positive margins, and 37% had disease in lymph nodes.[587] Using paclitaxel, estramustine, and carboplatin, Kelly et al. showed clinical down-staging in 39% of patients, up-staging in 36%, and a positive margin rate of 22%.[588] Docetaxel alone has also been explored as an adjuvant to radical prostatectomy, with trial entry restricted to patients with a high risk of relapse based on estimates from predictive models that incorporate baseline characteristics with the pathologic findings at surgery. Using this approach, if the observed time to PSA failure for the treated group exceeds the predicted failure time using the model, the therapy is deemed effective and studies continue.[589] Once again, given the variability in entry criteria and outcomes and that most trials are single-arm studies, it is difficult to determine which approach to take forward.

The situation is complicated further by the controversy surrounding "early" versus "late" hormonal therapy and that a proportion of men with high-risk disease (variably defined) may be cured with surgery or radiation therapy alone. An alternative is to wait until the cancer has recurred before testing cytotoxic drugs. A trial of estramustine and etoposide in this setting did not show a high complete response rate, suggesting a modest impact, and studies were not continued.[590] Taplin et al. studied the combination of estramustine and docetaxel for six cycles, followed by androgen deprivation alone for patients with a rising PSA. A proportion showed an undetectable PSA that was maintained when treatment was discontinued and testosterone levels had returned to baseline levels. Longer follow-up is needed.[591] An additional question is whether chemotherapy is more effective if it is given before hormones in a sequential manner.[592,593] This too is being explored.

The recent demonstration of the significance of PSA-doubling time for predicting survival of patients with a rising PSA after surgery or radiation allows more precise restriction of the population treated on trial with respect to risk of metastatic progression and death from prostate cancer. Patients with a low probability of progression are not enrolled. The RTOG is conducting a randomized comparison in which patients are randomized to 2 years of androgen deprivation alone versus the chemotherapy of one of several commonly used combinations and 2 years of androgen deprivation. The trial is powered to detect a prolongation of the time to metastatic progression by 40% for the combined chemo-hormonal approach relative to hormone therapy alone.[594]

OTHER INVESTIGATIONAL APPROACHES

A range of approaches are currently under evaluation. Some are directed at nonproliferating cells, whereas others aim to increase apoptotic rates, to induce differentiation, or to prevent the reemergence of a resistant phenotype. Other trials are being developed in specific disease contexts. The appeal of biotherapies is the presence of unique antigens associated with the malignant process that can be targeted, and they can be tested in a minimal disease setting in which the patients are healthy and the disease can be monitored at low tumor burdens using PSA. Targets that are prostate restricted, as opposed to prostate cancer restricted, are potentially useful, because the prostate is a nonessential gland. Biotherapies are a potential alternative to hormones, which many are reluctant to undergo owing to the side effect profile, and can be delayed without compromising outcomes. Among the antigens being targeted are PSMA; PSA; the glycolipids Lewis Y and Globo H hexa-saccharide; the gangliosides GM2, GD2, and GD3; the carbohydrate antigens TF and Tn; and the mucins MUC-1 and MUC-2.[595] Many are "self" antigens, for which a key issue in developing an immune response is breaking tolerance. Both active approaches—those designed to induce a humeral or cellular response, or both—and passive approaches—including cold and hot antibodies, antibody-toxin conjugates, synthetic antigen or whole-protein conjugate vaccines, gene therapies, and DNA immunizations—are under study. In other cases, mixtures of modified cell lines or autologous patient tumors are manipulated *ex vivo* and reinfused or injected intradermally or subcutaneously to activate cellular immune mechanisms via the skin. Some cells have been modified to secrete granulocyte-macrophage colony-stimulating factor (GM-CSF), which causes migration of dendritic cells and up-regulation of both major histocompatibility complex (MHC) and adhesion molecules on dendritic cells, and aids in antigen presentation. An antibody to CTLA-4, which functions to sustain the cellular response, has also entered clinical testing.[596]

PROSTATE-SPECIFIC MEMBRANE ANTIGEN–TARGETED THERAPY

PSMA is a 100-kD transmembrane protein expressed on prostatic epithelial cells. It is the target for a mouse monoclonal antibody, 7E11, and forms the basis for the prostascint scan to detect sites of recurrence in patients with a rising PSA after surgery or radiation therapy. Expression of PSMA is increased in higher-grade tumors and after androgen ablation. It is also expressed on the neovasculature of nonprostate solid tumors.[597] Several therapeutic strategies are under evaluation, including a cold antibody (J591), mouse and human DNA, and whole protein radiolabeled with yttrium 90 or lutetium 177[598] or as a conjugate to maytansinoid (DM-1).[598a] After DNA vaccination, the antigen is taken up by antigen-presenting cells in the skin, and portions of the protein form complexes with MHC molecules and are presented to T cells. Activated cytotoxic T cells recognized the same MHC-peptide complexes on tumor cells, which results in tumor cell death. Responses were also seen using autologous dendritic cells primed *ex vivo* with PSMA-derived peptides.[599]

OTHER SELECTED IMMUNE APPROACHES

Peptides from PSA can be found in the groove of MHC molecules on prostate cells. Pox viral vectors have been used to deliver PSA alone or in combination with GM-CSF injected at the same site. PSA-specific T cells were generated in some patients, several of who showed a change in PSA doubling time. This same gene has since been combined in a vaccinia vector also encoding the B.7 costimulatory molecule, with boosting by PSA from a fowlpox vector. GM-CSF and IL-2 are also given. The strategy is being compared to nilutamide in patients in whom first-line hormonal therapy has failed.[600,601]

An immunization approach using autologous dendritic cells pulsed with a prostatic acid phosphatase–GM-CSF fusion protein (Dendreon) is being studied. After the demonstration of PSA declines in a phase I trial, a trial was initiated in which patients were randomized on a 2:1 basis to active immunization or placebo.[602] Although no difference in time to objective progression was observed, a post hoc analysis showed a delay in time to progression for patients with tumors of Gleason grade 7 or less.[603] This observation is being tested in a phase III trial.

CV706 (Provenge) is a PSA-selective, replication-competent adenovirus that has been shown to induce regression of established human prostate cancer xenografts. A phase I dose-ranging study showed that injection into the prostates of patients with recurrent disease after radiation therapy was safe, whereas posttreatment prostatic biopsies and detection of a delayed "peak" of circulating viral copies provided evidence of replication *in vivo*. Declines in PSA were observed that correlated with the administered dose of the virus.[604,605]

GVAX (Cell Genesys) is a non–patient-specific immunization strategy in which prostate cancer cell lines are transduced with a replication-defective retrovirus encoding GM-CSF, then mixed with autologous patient mononuclear cells *ex vivo* and reinfused. The approach also showed an effect on PSA kinetics,[606] as well as an effect on bone turnover. Two phase III trials are planned. The first, for asymptomatic patients, will compare vaccine to taxane-based chemotherapy alone and the second, for symptomatic patients, will compare taxane-based chemotherapy plus vaccine to chemotherapy alone.

DIFFERENTIATION THERAPY

Putative differentiating agents, such as the histone deacetylase inhibitors[607] and phenylbutyrate,[608] are under study.[609] Ago-

nists of peroxisome proliferation–activated receptor γ, rosiglitazone and troglitazone, have been studied in a proapoptotic approach. Peroxisome proliferation–activated receptor γ is a nuclear hormone receptor integral to adipocyte differentiation, and heterozygous deletion of the gene is a common genetic alteration in prostate cancer. A trial in patients with a rising PSA highlighted the difficulty in evaluating treatments in this cohort. Although 1 of 12 (9%) showed a decrease in PSA of 50% or more and 3 of 12 (25%) a less than 50% decrease, 40% of placebo-treated patients showed PSA declines, making it difficult to determine the effects of the drug, if any. Exisulind (Aptosyn) has also been studied, and, in one trial, 96 men received oral exisulind or placebo; the treated patients showed significant suppression of increasing PSA, predominantly in the "high-risk" group.[610]

COMPLEMENTARY AND ALTERNATIVE THERAPIES

The issue of comprehensive and alternative therapies is a major one in prostate cancer management, as it is for other tumors. What is unique in prostate cancer is that these approaches often come to light on the basis of anecdotal reports of PSA declines. Particularly problematic are herbal products that are sold as dietary supplements under the Dietary Supplement Health and Education Act. These are not subject to U.S. Food and Drug Administration review before marketing. Consequently, details of the formulation, standardization, safety, contraindications, interactions, and appropriate use are often not available. Research is difficult owing to variations in the concentration of the presumed active ingredients, which may result from genetic and environmental factors, pesticides, pathogens, plant species, and extraction procedures.[611] In addition to marked inconsistencies within and between brands, upwards of 24% of the marketed products contained one or more synthetic compounds, including nonsteroidal antiinflammatory drugs, diuretics, corticosteroids, caffeine, and sildenafil.[144] An additional problem is that these alternative approaches are rarely used in isolation.

Epigallocatechin-3-gallate, a component of green tea, has been shown to inhibit metalloproteinases, acts as an oxidant, arrests growth of LNCaP and DU-145 cells,[612] and prevents cancer development in the TRAMP mouse model. No antiprostate cancer effects were observed in a phase II trial in man.[613] The soy isoflavones—genistein, daidzein, and biochanin A—have phytoestrogen effects that include differentiation, protection from DNA damage, and modulation of hormones. Soy can inhibit 5α-reductase, and genistein inhibits signaling of different tyrosine kinases. No significant anticancer effects were observed.[614]

A product that has received considerable attention is PC-SPES (*PC* for prostate cancer; *spes* is Latin for hope), which consists of eight herbs: *Ganoderma lucidum* (an adjuvant), *Scutellaria baicalensis* (an active principle), *Rabdosia rubescens, Isatis indigotica, Dendranthema morifolium* (corrective), *Serenoa repens, Panax notoginseng,* and *Glycyrrhiza uralensis* (flavors). It is intended to achieve synergy from the four attributes—active principles, adjuvants, correctives, and flavors. *S repens* (saw palmetto) relieves urinary obstruction. Although standardized by chemical analysis, the actual extract contains thousands of distinct compounds.[615] Patients who were taking PC-SPES showed declines in PSA but concurrently developed breast enlargement, vascular thrombosis, and declines in testosterone levels. This is consistent with an estrogen-like effect, which ultimately led to a randomized comparative trial of PC-SPES and DES. Also noted was significant variability in reported safety profiles, prompting further laboratory analyses that revealed synthetic compounds in varying amounts, including DES, warfarin and indomethacin, and alprazolam.[616] A recall followed, and the questions remain.

Also under-considered is how these largely unknown mixtures may interact in either a positive or negative way with primary oncolytic therapies. In addition to effects on metabolism, they may affect the safety and toxicity of any medication a patient is taking, be it for comorbid conditions or as an anticancer therapy, and these agents may neutralize the drugs we are using to treat the cancer itself. It has been shown that high levels of vitamin C can minimize the effects of the taxanes, whereas antioxidants can affect cell kill induced by radiation therapy or alkylating agents. It cannot be assumed that all comprehensive and alternative medicines are innocuous.[144]

CONCLUSION

The clinical spectrum of prostate cancer is shifting to the left: More and more patients are being diagnosed and treated at an earlier stage. This has contributed, at least in part, to the decrease in prostate cancer–specific mortality since 1996. It all seems so simple, but many issues remain. In 2004, more than 29,000 men will die from the uncontrolled growth of tumors that have spread.[1] Many of these and thousands of others will suffer considerably from symptoms related to metastatic spread.

Fortunately, there have been significant advances in the past few years. For those without a cancer diagnosis, the demonstration that a nontoxic intervention can reduce prostate cancer incidence opens the door for other interventions to change the clinical spectrum even further. For the management of early-stage tumors, we have learned that waiting and watching the "wrong" tumor can allow the window of curability to close and adversely affect both the morbidity and mortality of the disease in an individual. Fortunately, we are refining the methods to determine which tumors need an immediate intervention. The techniques of radical prostatectomy continue to be refined, and laparoscopic procedures offer the chance to reduce morbidity even further. Advances in imaging and radiation therapy delivery using IMRT and implants now permit higher doses to be administered. The result is better cancer control along with better preservation of potency, urinary control, and bowel function in both the short and long term.

The authors are also developing better decision-making models to balance the risk/reward ratio for specific interventions for an individual patient to maximize the outcome, whereas minimizing the chance that he regrets his choice of original treatment. For patients who are progressing with a rising PSA, many of who are obsessed to the point of paralysis, we now have better prognostic models to place a PSA rise in perspective, allowing patients to determine the likelihood that their disease will metastasize or cause symptoms and/or decrease the quality and quantity of survival. This allows patients to get on with their lives and to make informed decisions about whether to pursue treatment and in what form. Guidelines for the conduct of trials in this group have also been developed, so that promising agents can be identified quickly in patients who need treatment.[417]

The outlook is also changing for those with systemic disease. In 2004, it was established for the first time that chemotherapy can prolong life. We are learning that modulating the metastatic process by disrupting critical interactions between the tumor and the skeleton can improve quality-adjusted life expectancy without necessarily prolonging life. There are also more effective ways to modulate the hot flushes, anemia, and adverse effects of the hormone therapies and chemotherapies that are used to treat the disease.

Equally important are advances in the understanding of the biology of the disease. Molecular profiling studies across the spectrum of the illness have increased our understanding of the mechanisms associated with prostate cancer growth and spread. These determinants identify new targets and mechanisms for therapy; they are also being integrated into the prognostic models we are developing, refining predictions.[578] Our view of castration-resistant disease has also changed as we recognize the importance of continued signaling through the AR in the growth of these tumors and are exploring new ways to interrupt the process. Identifying which mechanism is predominant in the progression of a tumor in an individual patient offers the possibility of tailoring treatment. Specific drugs and approaches directed at a range of targets and mechanisms have also entered the clinic, with the promise of improving outcomes further. For many of these approaches, we are still on the learning curve. Simply having the target and the drug is not sufficient, and we must continue basic investigations on the mechanisms of action of these interventions and carefully design preclinical studies so we understand how best to combine them clinically.

So why don't we have more answers? Perhaps we have not asked the right questions. Clearly, the issue of combined androgen blockade occupied too many for too long. But we must also change our mindset regarding participation in trials. From 1997 to 2001, there were 107 national trials in breast cancer and 83 in prostate cancer. The similarity ended there, as 34,757 women were enrolled on these trials in contrast to only 8309 men.[617]

A paradigm in oncology is that use of an effective systemic therapy early in the course of the illness can increase cure rates. For prostate cancer in particular, by identifying high-risk patients early and through the use of drugs with proven efficacy, physicians have the opportunity to extend the window for cure even further. Now physicians are in a position to ask survival-based questions with the knowledge that early systemic therapy has worked in diseases for which the efficacy shown in advanced disease is less than that seen in patients with advanced prostate cancer. The tools are in place. The framework that divides the illness into easily recognized clinical milestones is available, placing patients and physicians on the same page with respect to prognosis, treatment selection, management, and therapeutic objectives. We are developing state-specific national standards for outcomes tailored to questions relevant to the disease state in which it is being asked. Through the integrated efforts of individuals representing the diverse disciplines, we have the potential to improve outcomes even further.

REFERENCES

1. Jemal A, Tiwari RC, Murray T, et al. Cancer statistics, 2004. *CA Cancer J Clin* 2004;54:8.
2. Scher HI, Heller G. Clinical states in prostate cancer: towards a dynamic model of disease progression. *Urology* 2000;55:323.
3. Pound CR, Partin AW, Eisenberger MA, et al. Natural history of progression to metastases

and death from prostate cancer in men with PSA recurrence following radical prostatectomy. *JAMA* 1999;281:1591.

4. Sculpher M, Bryan S, Fry P, et al. Patients' preferences for the management of non-metastatic prostate cancer: discrete choice experiment. *BMJ* 2004;328:382.
5. Scher HI, Mazumdar M, Kelly WK. Clinical trials in relapsed prostate cancer: defining the target. *J Natl Cancer Inst* 1996;88:1623.
6. Fleming TR, DeMets DL. Surrogate end points in clinical trials: are we being misled? *Ann Intern Med* 1996;125:605.
7. Fazzari M, Heller G, Scher HI. The phase II/III transition: towards the proof of efficacy in cancer clinical trials. *Control Clin Trials* 2000;21:360.
8. Ohori M, Scardino PT. Localized prostate cancer. *Curr Probl Surg* 2002;39:833.
9. Greene DR, Shabsigh R, Scardino PT. Urologic ultrasonography. In: Walsh PC, Retik AB, Stamey TA, et al., eds. *Campbell's textbook of urology,* 6th ed. Philadelphia: WB Saunders, 1992;342.
10. McNeal JE, Redwine EA, Freiha FS, et al. Zonal distribution of prostatic adenocarcinoma. *Am J Surg Pathol* 1988;12:897.
11. American Joint Committee on Cancer. *Manual for staging of cancer/American Joint Committee on Cancer,* 4th ed. Philadelphia: Lippincott, 1992.
12. Fleming ID, Cooper JS, Henson DE, et al, eds. *AJCC cancer staging manual,* 5th ed. Philadelphia: Lippincott–Raven, 1997.
13. Hull GW, Rabbani F, Abbas F, et al. Cancer control with radical prostatectomy alone in 1,000 consecutive patients. *J Urol* 2002;167:528.
14. WHO Classification of Tumors. Pathology and genetics. Tumors of the urinary system and male genital organs. In: Eble NJ, Suater G, Epstein JI, et al, eds. *Tumors of the prostate.* Lyon: IARC Press, 2004;159.
15. DeMarzo AM, Nelson WG, Isaacs WB, et al. Pathological and molecular aspects of prostate cancer. *Lancet* 2003;361:955.
16. Gleason DF. Classification of prostatic carcinomas. *Cancer Chemother Rep* 1966;50:125.
17. Gleason DF, Mellinger GT. Prediction of prognosis for prostatic adenocarcinoma by combined histological grading and clinical staging. *J Urol* 1974;111:58.
18. Gleason DF. Histologic grading and clinical staging of prostatic carcinoma. In: Tannenbaum M, ed. *Urologic pathology: the prostate.* Philadelphia: Lea & Febiger, 1977;171.
19. Noguchi M, Stamey TA, Neal JE, et al. An analysis of 148 consecutive transition zone cancers: clinical and histological characteristics. *J Urol* 2000;163:1751.
20. Ginesin Y, Bolkien M, Moskovitz B, et al. Carcinosarcoma of prostate. *Eur Urol* 1986;12:441.
21. Sakr WA, Haas GP, Cassin BF, et al. The frequency of carcinoma and intraepithelial neoplasia of the prostate in young male patients. *J Urol* 1993;150:379.
22. Nelson WG, De Marzo AM, Isaacs WB. Prostate cancer. *N Engl J Med* 2003;349:366.
23. Montie JE, Pienta KJ. Review of the role of androgenic hormones in the epidemiology of benign prostatic hyperplasia and prostate cancer. *Urology* 1994;43:892.
24. Bostwick DG. Prospective origins of prostate carcinoma. Prostatic intraepithelial neoplasia and atypical adenomatous hyperplasia. *Cancer* 1996;78:330.
25. De Marzo AM, Marchi VL, Epstein JI, et al. Proliferative inflammatory atrophy of the prostate: implications for prostatic carcinogenesis. *Am J Pathol* 1999;155:1985.
26. Bostwick DG, Brawer MK. Prostatic intra-epithelial neoplasia and early invasion in prostate cancer. *Cancer* 1987;59:788.
27. Sakr WA. Prostatic intraepithelial neoplasia: a marker for high-risk groups and a potential target for chemoprevention. *Eur Urol* 1999;35:474.
28. Doll JA, Zhu X, Furman J, et al. Genetic analysis of prostatic atypical adenomatous hyperplasia (adenosis). *Am J Pathol* 1999;155:967.
29. Sarasin A. An overview of the mechanisms of mutagenesis and carcinogenesis. *Mutat Res* 2003;544:99.
30. Rubin MA, Putzi M, Mucci N, et al. Rapid ("warm") autopsy study for procurement of metastatic prostate cancer. *Clin Cancer Res* 2000;6:1038.
31. Steinberg GD, Carter BS, Beaty TH, et al. Family history and the risk of prostate cancer. *Prostate* 1990;17:337.
32. Lichtenstein P, Holm NV, Verkasalo PK, et al. Environmental and heritable factors in the causation of cancer—analyses of cohorts of twins from Sweden, Denmark, and Finland. *N Engl J Med* 2000;343:78.
33. Tavtigian SV, Simard J, Teng DH, et al. A candidate prostate cancer susceptibility gene at chromosome 17p. *Nat Genet* 2001;27:172.
34. Carpten J, Nupponen N, Isaacs S, et al. Germline mutations in the ribonuclease L gene in families showing linkage with HPC1. *Nat Genet* 2002;30:181.
35. Nupponen NN, Carpten JD. Prostate cancer susceptibility genes: many studies, many results, no answers. *Cancer Metastasis Rev* 2001;20:155.
36. Xu J, Zheng SL, Komiya A, et al. Germline mutations and sequence variants of the macrophage scavenger receptor 1 gene are associated with prostate cancer risk. *Nat Genet* 2002;32:321.
37. Sakr WA, Grignon DJ, Crissman JD, et al. High grade prostatic intraepithelial neoplasia (HGPIN) and prostatic adenocarcinoma between the ages of 20-69; an autopsy study of 249 cases. *In Vivo* 1994;8:439.
38. Gonzalgo ML, Isaacs WB. Molecular pathways to prostate cancer. *J Urol* 2003;170:2444.
39. Visakorpi T. The molecular genetics of prostate cancer. *Urology* 2003;62:3.
40. De Marzo AM, DeWeese TL, Platz EA, et al. Pathological and molecular mechanisms of prostate carcinogenesis: implications for diagnosis, detection, prevention, and treatment. *J Cell Biochem* 2004;91:459.
41. Scher H, Shaffer D. Prostate cancer: a dynamic disease with shifting targets. *Lancet Oncology* 2003;4:407.
42. Lee WH, Morton RA, Epstein JI, et al. Cytidine methylation of regulatory sequences near the p-class glutathione-s-transferase gene accompanies human prostate cancer carcinogenesis. *Proc Natl Acad Sci U S A* 1994;91:11733.
43. Shirai T, Sano M, Tamano S, et al. The prostate: a target for carcinogenicity of 2-amino-1-methyl-6-phenylimidazo[4,5-b]pyridine (PhIP) derived from cooked foods. *Cancer Res* 1997;57:195.
44. Nakayama M, Gonzalgo ML, Yegnasubramanian S, et al. GSTP1 CpG island hypermethylation as a molecular biomarker for prostate cancer. *J Cell Biochem* 2004;91:540.
45. Gonzalez-Zulueta M, Shibata A, Ohneseit PF, et al. High frequency of chromosome 9p allelic loss and cdkn2 tumor suppressor gene alterations in squamous cell carcinoma of the bladder. *J Natl Cancer Inst* 1995;87:1383.
46. Bova GS, MacGrogan D, Levy A, et al. Physical mapping chromosome 8p22 markers and their homozygous deletion in a metastatic prostate cancer. *Genomics* 1997;35:46.
47. Cordon-Cardo C. Mutations of cell cycle regulators: biological and clinical implications regarding neoplastic processes. *Am J Pathol* 1995;147:545.
48. Cordon-Cardo C, Koff A, Drobnjak M, et al. Distinct altered patterns of p27kip1 expression in benign prostatic hyperplasia and prostatic carcinoma. *J Natl Cancer Inst* 1998;90:1284.
49. Yang RM, Naitoh J, Murphy M, et al. Low p27 expression predicts poor disease-free survival in patients with prostate cancer. *J Urol* 1998;159:941.
50. Lee C, Capodieci P, Osman I, et al. Overexpression of the cyclin-dependent kinase inhibitor p16 is associated with tumor recurrence in human prostate cancer. *Clin Cancer Res* 1999;5:977.
51. Whang Y, Wu X, Suzuki H, et al. Inactivation of the tumor suppressor PTEN/MMAC1 in advanced human prostate cancer through loss of expression. *Proc Natl Acad Sci U S A* 1998;95:5246.
52. Yang G, Ayala G, De Marzo A, et al. Elevated Skp2 protein expression in human prostate cancer: association with loss of the cyclin-dependent kinase inhibitor p27 and PTEN and with reduced recurrence-free survival. *Clin Cancer Res* 2002;8:3419.
53. Ghosh PM, Malik S, Bedolla R, et al. Akt in prostate cancer: possible role in androgen-independence. *Curr Drug Metab* 2003;4:487.
54. Umbas R, Schalken JA, Aalders TW, et al. Expression of the cellular adhesion molecular E-cadherin is reduced or absent in high-grade prostate cancer. *Cancer Res* 1992;52:5104.
55. Tomita K, van Bokhoven A, van Leenders GJ, et al. Cadherin switching in human prostate cancer progression. *Cancer Res* 2000;60:3650.
56. Scher HI, Sarkis A, Reuter V, et al. Changing pattern of expression of the epidermal growth factor receptor and transforming growth factor-α in the progression of prostatic neoplasm. *Clin Cancer Res* 1995;1:545.
57. Uehara H, Kim SJ, Karashima T, et al. Effects of blocking platelet-derived growth factor-receptor signaling in a mouse model of experimental prostate cancer bone metastases. *J Natl Cancer Inst* 2003;95:458.
58. Culig Z, Hobisch A, Cronauer MV, et al. Regulation of prostatic growth and function by peptide growth factors. *Prostate* 1996;28:392.
59. Cardillo MR, Monti S, Di Silverio F, et al. Insulin-like growth factor (IGF)-I, IGF-II and IGF type I receptor (IGFR-I) expression in prostatic cancer. *Anticancer Res* 2003;23:3825.
60. Tu WH, Thomas TZ, Masumori N, et al. The loss of TGF-beta signaling promotes prostate cancer metastasis. *Neoplasia* 2003;5:267.
61. Osman I, Scher H, Drobnjak M, et al. HER-2/neu (p185) protein expression in the natural and treated history of prostate cancer. *Clin Cancer Res* 2001;7:2643.
62. Signoretti S, Montiroini R, Manola J, et al. Her-2-neu expression and progression toward independence in human prostate cancer. *J Natl Cancer Inst* 2000;92:1918.
63. Craft N, Shostak Y, Carey M, et al. A mechanism for hormone-independent prostate cancer through modulation of androgen receptor signaling by the HER-2/neu tyrosine kinase. *Nat Med* 1999;5:280.
64. Edwards J, Krishna NS, Witton CJ, et al. Gene amplifications associated with the development of hormone-resistant prostate cancer. *Clin Cancer Res* 2003;9:5271.
65. Drobnjak M, Osman I, Scher HI, et al. Overexpression of cyclin D1 is associated with metastatic prostate cancer to bone. *Clin Cancer Res* 2000;6:1891.
66. Paradis V, Dargere D, Laurendeau I, et al. Expression of the RNA component of human telomerase (hTR) in prostate cancer, prostatic intraepithelial neoplasia, and normal prostate tissue. *J Pathol* 1999;189:213.
67. Kaur P, Kallakury BS, Sheehan CE, et al. Survivin and Bcl-2 expression in prostatic adenocarcinomas. *Arch Pathol Lab Med* 2004;128:39.
68. Sepp-Lorenzino L, Tjaden G, Moasser MM, et al. Farnesyl:protein transferase inhibitors (FTIs) as potential agents for the management of human prostate cancer. *Prostate Cancer Prostatic Dis* 2001;4:33.
69. Nicholson B, Theodorescu D. Angiogenesis and prostate cancer tumor growth. *J Cell Biochem* 2004;91:125.
70. Huss WJ, Hanrahan CF, Barrios RJ, et al. Angiogenesis and prostate cancer: identification of a molecular progression switch. *Cancer Res* 2001;61:2736.
71. Arnold JT, Isaacs JT. Mechanisms involved in the progression of androgen-independent prostate cancers: it is not only the cancer cell's fault. *Endocr Relat Cancer* 2002;9:61.
72. Isaacs JT, Lundmo PI, Berges R, et al. Androgen regulation of programmed cell death of normal and malignant prostatic cells. *J Androl* 1992;13:457.
73. Isaacs JT, Coffey DS. Adaptation versus selection as the mechanism responsible for the relapse of prostatic cancer to androgen ablation as studied in the Dunning R-3327 H adenocarcinoma. *Cancer Res* 1981;41:5070.
74. Craft N, Chhor C, Tran C, et al. Evidence for clonal outgrowth of androgen-independent prostate cancer cells from androgen-dependent tumors through a two-step process. *Cancer Res* 1999;59:5030.
75. Bruchovsky N, Rennie PS, Coldman AJ, et al. Effects of androgen withdrawal on the stem cell composition of the Shionogi carcinoma. *Cancer Res* 1990;50:2275.
76. De Marzo AM, Nelson WG, Meeker AK, et al. Stem cell features of benign and malignant prostate epithelial cells. *J Urol* 1998;160:2381.
77. Bui M, Reiter RE. Stem cell genes in androgen-independent prostate cancer. *Cancer Metastasis Rev* 1998;17:391.
78. Isaacs JT. The biology of hormone refractory prostate cancer. Why does it develop? *Urol Clin North Am* 1999;26:263.
79. Gelmann EP. Molecular biology of the androgen receptor. *J Clin Oncol* 2002;20:3001.

80. Beilin J, Ball EM, Favaloro JM, et al. Effect of the androgen receptor CAG repeat polymorphism on transcriptional activity: specificity in prostate and non-prostate cell lines. *J Mol Endocrinol* 2000;25:85.

81. Giovannucci E, Stampfer MJ, Krithivas K, et al. The CAG repeat within the androgen receptor gene and its relationship to prostate cancer. *Proc Natl Acad Sci U S A* 1997;94:3320.

82. Bennett CL, Price DK, Kim S, et al. Racial variation in CAG repeat lengths within the androgen receptor gene among prostate cancer patients of lower socioeconomic status. *J Clin Oncol* 2002;20:3599.

83. Buchanan G, Irvine RA, Coetzee GA, et al. Contribution of the androgen receptor to prostate cancer predisposition and progression. *Cancer Metastasis Rev* 2001;20:207.

84. Grossmann ME, Huang H, Tindall DJ. Androgen receptor signaling in androgen-refractory prostate cancer. *J Natl Cancer Inst* 2001;93:1687.

85. Scher H, Buchanan G, Gerald W, Butler LM, Tilley WD. Targeter of the androgen receptor: towards a complete blockade of androgen signaling in prostate cancer. *Endocr Rel Cancer* 2004;(*in press*).

86. Holzbeierlein J, Lal P, LaTulippe E, et al. Comprehensive gene expression analysis of human prostate carcinoma during hormonal therapy identifies androgen-responsive genes and multiple complementary mechanisms of therapy resistance. *Am J Pathol* 2004;164:217.

87. Mohler JL, Gregory CW, Ford OH 3rd, et al. The androgen axis in recurrent prostate cancer. *Clin Cancer Res* 2004;10:440.

88. Culig Z, Hobisch A, Hittmair A, et al. Expression, structure, and function of androgen receptor in advanced prostatic carcinoma. *Prostate* 1998;35:63.

89. Tilley WD, Buchanan G, Hickey TE, et al. Prostate cancer is associated with a high frequency of mutations in the androgen receptor gene. *Proc Am Assoc Cancer Res Special Conference on Basic and Clinical Aspects of Prostate Cancer*, 1994.

90. Pertschuk LP, Schaeffer H, Feldman JG, et al. Immunostaining for prostate cancer androgen receptor in paraffin identifies a subset of men with a poor prognosis. *Lab Invest* 1995;73:302.

91. Bubendorf L, Kononen J, Koivisto P, et al. Survey of gene amplifications during prostate cancer progression by high-throughout fluorescence in situ hybridization on tissue microarrays. *Cancer Res* 1999;59:803.

92. Koivisto P, Visakorpi T, Kallioniemi OP. Androgen receptor gene amplification: a novel molecular mechanism for endocrine therapy resistance in human prostate cancer. *Scand J Clin Lab Invest Suppl* 1996;226:57.

93. Linja MJ, Savinainen KJ, Saramaki OR, et al. Amplification and overexpression of androgen receptor gene in hormone-refractory prostate cancer. *Cancer Res* 2001;61:3550.

94. Buchanan G, Yang M, Nahm SJ, et al. Mutations at the boundary of the hinge and ligand binding domain of the androgen receptor confer increased transactivation function. *Mol Endocrinol* 2000;15:46.

95. Yeh S, Lin HK, Kang HY, et al. From HER2/Neu signal cascade to androgen receptor and its coactivators: a novel pathway by induction of androgen target genes through MAP kinase in prostate cancer cells. *Proc Natl Acad Sci U S A* 1999;96:5458.

96. Gregory CW, He B, Johnson RT, et al. A mechanism for androgen receptor-mediated prostate cancer recurrence after androgen deprivation therapy. *Cancer Res* 2001;61:4315.

97. Culig Z, Hobisch A, Cronauer MV, et al. Androgen receptor activation in prostatic tumor cell lines by insulin-like growth factor-I, keratinocyte growth factor, and epidermal growth factor. *Cancer Res* 1994;54:5474.

98. Ueda T, Mawji NR, Bruchovsky N, et al. Ligand-independent activation of the androgen receptor by interleukin-6 and the role of steroid receptor coactivator-1 in prostate cancer cells. *J Biol Chem* 2002;277:38087.

99. McDonnell TJ, Troncoso P, Brisbay SM, et al. Expression of the protooncogene bcl-2 in the prostate and its association with emergence of androgen-independent prostate cancer. *Cancer Res* 1992;52:6940.

100. Xing N, Qian J, Bostwick D, et al. Neuroendocrine cells in human prostate over-express the anti-apoptosis protein surviving. *Prostate* 2001;48:7.

101. Cher ML. Mechanisms governing bone metastasis in prostate cancer. *Curr Opin Urol* 2001;11:483.

102. Akimoto S, Okumura A, Fuse H. Relationship between serum levels of interleukin-6, tumor necrosis factor-alpha and bone turnover markers in prostate cancer patients. *Endocr J* 1998;45:183.

103. Cohen P, Graves HCB, Peehl DM, et al. Prostate-specific antigen (PSA) is an insulin-like growth factor binding protein-3 protease found in seminal plasma. *J Clin Endocrinol Metab* 1992;75:1046.

104. Sugihara A, Maeda O, Tsuji M, et al. Expression of cytokines enhancing the osteoclast activity, and parathyroid hormone-related protein in prostatic cancers before and after endocrine therapy: an immunohistochemical study. *Oncol Rep* 1998;5:1389.

105. Bryden AA, Hoyland JA, Freemont AJ, et al. Parathyroid hormone related peptide and receptor expression in paired primary prostate cancer and bone metastases. *Br J Cancer* 2002;86:322.

106. Sutkowski DM, Goode RL, Baniel J, et al. Growth regulation of prostatic stromal cells by prostate-specific antigen. *J Natl Cancer Inst* 1999;91:1663.

107. Nelson J, Bagnato A, Battistini B, et al. The endothelin axis: emerging role in cancer. *Nat Rev Cancer* 2003;3:110.

108. Jung K, Stephan C, Semjonow A, et al. Serum osteoprotegerin and receptor activator of nuclear factor-kappa B ligand as indicators of disturbed osteoclastogenesis in patients with prostate cancer. *J Urol* 2003;170:2302.

109. Keller ET, Brown J. Prostate cancer bone metastases promote both osteolytic and osteoblastic activity. *J Cell Biochem* 2004;91:718.

109a. Guise TA, Yin JJ, Mohammad KS. Role of endothelin-1 in osteoblastic bone metastases. *Cancer* 2003;97(3 Suppl):779.

110. Zhang J, Dai J, Qi Y, et al. Osteoprotegerin inhibits prostate cancer-induced osteoclastogenesis and prevents prostate tumor growth in the bone. *J Clin Invest* 2001;107:1235.

111. Foster BA, Gingrich JR, Kwon ED, et al. Characterization of prostatic epithelial cell lines derived from transgenic adenocarcinoma of the mouse prostate (TRAMP) model. *Cancer Res* 1997;57:3325.

112. Ellwood-Yen K, Graeber TG, Wongvipat J, et al. Myc-driven murine prostate cancer shares molecular features with human prostate tumors. *Cancer Cell* 2003;4:223.

113. Di Cristofano A, De Acetis M, Koff A, et al. Pten and p27KIP1 cooperate in prostate cancer tumor suppression in the mouse. *Nat Genet* 2001;27:222.

114. Trotman LC, Niki M, Dotan ZA, et al. Pten dose dictates cancer progression in the prostate. *PLoS Biol* 2003;1:E59.

115. LaTulippe E, Satagopan J, Smith A, et al. Comprehensive gene expression analysis of prostate cancer reveals distinct transcriptional programs associated with metastatic disease. *Cancer Res* 2002;62:4499.

116. Amler LC, Agus DB, LeDuc C, et al. Dysregulated expression of androgen-responsive and nonresponsive genes in the androgen-independent prostate cancer xenograft model CWR22-R1. *Cancer Res* 2000;60:6134.

117. Scardino PT, Weaver R, Hudson MA. Early detection of prostate cancer. *Hum Pathol* 1992;23:211.

118. Haenszel W, Kurihara M. Studies of Japanese migrants. I. Mortality from cancer and other diseases among Japanese in the United States. *J Natl Cancer Inst* 1968;40:43.

119. Kosary CL, Ries LAG, Miller BA, et al. *SEER cancer incidence public-use database, 1970-1980.* Bethesda, MD: National Cancer Institute, 1998.

120. Smith JR, Freije D, Carpten JD, et al. Major susceptibility locus for prostate cancer on chromosome 1 suggested by a genome wide search. *Science* 1996;274:1371.

121. Carter BS, Beaty TH, Steinberg GD, et al. Mendelian inheritance of familial prostate cancer. *Proc Natl Acad Sci U S A* 1992;89:3367.

122. Xu J, Meyers D, Freije D, et al. Evidence for a prostate cancer susceptibility locus on the X chromosome. *Nat Genet* 1998;20:175.

123. Kantoff P, Giovannucci E, Brown M. The androgen receptor CAG repeat polymorphism and its relationship to prostate cancer. *Biochim Biophys Acta* 1998;1378:C1.

124. Surveillance, Epidemiology, and End Results (SEER) Program of the National Cancer Institute. SEER 9 Registry Database (1973–2001). World Wide Web URL: http://www.seer.cancer.gov, 2004.

125. Demark-Wahnefried W, Strigo T, Catoe K, et al. Knowledge, beliefs, and prior screening behavior among blacks and whites reporting for prostate cancer screening. *Urology* 1995;46:346.

126. Polednak AP, Flannery JT. Black versus white racial differences in clinical stage at diagnosis and treatment of prostatic cancer in Connecticut. *Cancer* 1992;70:2152.

127. Greenlee RT, Hill-Harmon MB, Murray T, et al. Cancer statistics, 2001. *Ca Cancer J Clin* 2001;51:15.

128. Cook LS, Goldoft M, Schwartz SM, et al. Incidence of adenocarcinoma of the prostate in Asian immigrants to the United States and their descendants. *J Urol* 1999;161:152.

129. Correa P. Epidemiological correlations between diet and cancer frequency. *Cancer Res* 1981;41:3685.

130. Bosland MC, Oakley-Girvan I, Whittemore AS. Dietary fat, calories, and prostate cancer risk. *J Natl Cancer Inst* 1999;91:489.

131. Giovannucci E, Ascherio A, Rimm EB, et al. Intake of carotenoids and retinol in relation to risk of prostate cancer. *J Natl Cancer Inst* 1995;87:1767.

132. Schwartz GG, Hulka BS. Is vitamin D deficiency a risk factor for prostate cancer? (Hypothesis). *Anticancer Res* 1990;10:1307.

133. Skowronski RJ, Peehl D, Feldman D. Vitamin D and prostate cancer: 1,25-dihydroxyvitamin D3 receptors and actions in prostate cancer cell lines. *Endocrinology* 1993;132:1952.

134. Chan JM, Stampfer MJ, Ma J, et al. Supplemental vitamin E intake and prostate cancer risk in a large cohort of men in the United States. *Cancer Epidemiol Biomarkers Prev* 1999;8:893.

135. Heinonen OP, Albanes D, Virtamo J, et al. Prostate cancer and supplementation with alpha-tocopherol and beta-carotene: incidence and mortality in a controlled trial. *J Natl Cancer Inst* 1998;90:440.

136. Clark LC, Dalkin B, Krongrad A, et al. Decreased incidence of prostate cancer with selenium supplementation: results of a double-blind cancer prevention trial. *Br J Urol* 1998;81:730.

137. Demark-Wahnefried W, Halabi S, Paulson DF. Serum androgens: associations with prostate cancer risk and hair patterning. *J Androl* 1998;19:631.

138. Howards SS, Peterson HB. Vasectomy and prostate cancer. Chance, bias, or a causal relationship? *JAMA* 1993;269:913.

139. Carter BS, Bova GS, Beaty TH, et al. Hereditary prostate cancer: epidemiologic and clinical features. *J Urol* 1993;150:797.

140. Collinson MP, Daniel F, Tyrell CJ, et al. Response of carcinoma of the prostate to withdrawal of flutamide. *Br J Urol* 1993;72:662.

141. Kabalin JN, Hodge KK, McNeal JE, et al. Identification of residual cancer in the prostate following radiation therapy: role of transrectal ultrasound guided biopsy and prostate specific antigen. *J Urol* 1989;142:326.

142. Wang Y, Corr JG, Thaler HT, et al. Decreased growth of established human prostate LNCaP tumors in nude mice fed a low-fat diet. *J Natl Cancer Inst* 1995;87:1456.

143. Shike M, Latkany L, Riedel E, et al. Lack of effect of a low-fat, high-fruit, -vegetable, and -fiber diet on serum prostate-specific antigen of men without prostate cancer: results from a randomized trial. *J Clin Oncol* 2002;20:3592.

144. Nelson PS, Montgomery B. Unconventional therapy for prostate cancer: good, bad or questionable? *Nat Rev Cancer* 2003;3:845.

145. Kelloff GJ, Boone CW, Crowell JA, et al. Chemopreventive drug development: perspectives and progress. *Cancer Epidemiol Biomarkers Prev* 1994;3:85.

146. Thompson IM, Goodman PJ, Tangen CM, et al. The influence of finasteride on the development of prostate cancer. *N Engl J Med* 2003;349:215.

147. Scardino PT. The prevention of prostate cancer—the dilemma continues. *N Engl J Med* 2003;349:297.

148. Combs GF Jr, Combs SB. The nutritional biochemistry of selenium. *Annu Rev Nutr* 1984; 4:257.

149. Clark LC, Combs GF Jr, Turnbull BW, et al. Effects of selenium supplementation for cancer prevention in patients with carcinoma of the skin. A randomized controlled trial. Nutritional Prevention of Cancer Study Group. *JAMA* 1996;276:1957.

150. Klein EA, Thompson IM, Lippman SM, et al. SELECT: the selenium and vitamin E cancer prevention trial. *Urol Oncol* 2003;21:59.

151. Greenlee RT, Murray T, Bolden S, et al. Cancer statistics, 2000. *CA Cancer J Clin* 2000;50:7.

152. Catalona WJ, Richie JP, Ahmann FR, et al. Comparison of digital rectal examination and serum prostate specific antigen in the early detection of prostate cancer: results of a multicenter clinical trial of 6,630 men. *J Urol* 1994;151:1283.

153. Mettlin C, Murphy GP, Lee F, et al. Characteristics of prostate cancers detected in a multimodality early detection program. The investigators of the American Cancer Society-National Prostate Cancer Detection Project. *Cancer* 1993;72:1701.

154. Smart CR. The impact of the U.S. Preventive Services Task Force guidelines on cancer screening: perspective from the National Cancer Institute. *J Gen Intern Med* 1990;5:S28.

155. Screening for prostate cancer: commentary on the recommendations of the Canadian Task Force on the Periodic Health Examination. The U.S. Preventive Services Task Force. *Am J Prev Med* 1994;10:187.

156. von Eschenbach A, Ho R, Murphy GP, et al. American Cancer Society guideline for the early detection of prostate cancer: update 1997. *CA Cancer J Clin* 1997;47:261.

157. Screening for prostate cancer. American College of Physicians. *Ann Intern Med* 1997;126:480.

158. Baker LH, Hanks G, Gershenson D, et al. NCCN prostate cancer practice guidelines. The National Comprehensive Cancer Network. *Oncology (Huntingt)* 1996;10:265.

159. Woolf SH. Screening for prostate cancer with prostate-specific antigen. An examination of the evidence. *N Engl J Med* 1995;333:1401.

160. Hoeksema MJ, Law C. Cancer mortality rates fall: a turning point for the nation. *J Natl Cancer Inst* 1996;88:1706.

161. Hankey BF, Feuer EJ, Clegg LX, et al. Cancer surveillance series: interpreting trends in prostate cancer–part I: Evidence of the effects of screening in recent prostate cancer incidence, mortality, and survival rates. *J Natl Cancer Inst* 1999;91:1017.

162. Kramer BS, Brown ML, Prorok PC, et al. Prostate cancer screening: what we know and what we need to know. *Ann Intern Med* 1993;119:914.

163. Bartsch G, Horninger W, Klocker H, et al. Prostate cancer mortality after introduction of prostate-specific antigen mass screening in the Federal State of Tyrol, Austria(1). *Urology* 2001;58:417.

164. Lilja H, Piironen TP, Rittenhouse HG, et al. Value of molecular forms of prostate-specific antigen and related kallikreins, hk2, in diagnosis and staging of prostate cancer. In: Vogelzang NA, Scardino PT, Shipley WU, et al, eds. *Comprehensive textbook of genitourinary oncology*. Philadelphia: Lippincott Williams & Wilkins, 2000:638.

165. Aihara M, Lebovitz RM, Wheeler TM, et al. Prostate specific antigen and Gleason grade: an immunohistochemical study of prostate cancer. *J Urol* 1994;151:1558.

166. Graves HC. Nonprostatic sources of prostate-specific antigen: a steroid hormone-dependent phenomenon? *Clin Chem* 1995;41:7.

167. Catalona WJ, Smith DS, Ornstein DK. Prostate cancer detection in men with serum PSA concentrations of 2.6 to 4.0 ng/mL and benign prostate examination. Enhancement of specificity with free PSA measurements. *JAMA* 1997;277:1452.

168. Mettlin C, Murphy GP, Ray P, et al. American Cancer Society—National Prostate Cancer Detection Project. Results from multiple examinations using transrectal ultrasound, digital rectal examination, and prostate specific antigen. *Cancer* 1993;71:891.

169. Catalona W, Richie J, et al. Comparison of prostate specific antigen concentration versus prostate specific antigen density in the early detection of prostate cancer. *J Urol* 1994;152:2031.

170. Ohori M, Dunn JK, Scardino PT. Is prostate-specific antigen density more useful than prostate-specific antigen levels in the diagnosis of prostate cancer? *Urology* 1995;46:666.

171. Gann PH, Hennekesn CH, Stampfer MJ. A prospective evaluation of plasma prostate-specific antigen for detection of prostatic cancer. *JAMA* 1995;273:289.

172. Lee F, Gray JM, McLeary RD, et al. Transrectal ultrasound in the diagnosis of prostate cancer: location, echogenicity, histopathology, and staging. *Prostate* 1985;7:117.

173. Ohori M, Wheeler TM, Scardino PT. The New American Joint Committee on Cancer and International Union Against Cancer TNM classification of prostate cancer. *Cancer* 1994;74:104.

174. Hodge KK, McNeal JE, Terris MK, et al. Random systematic versus directed ultrasound guided transrectal core biopsies of the prostate. *J Urol* 1989;142:71.

175. Peller PA, Young DC, Marmaduke DP, et al. Sextant prostate biopsies. A histopathologic correlation with radical prostatectomy specimens. *Cancer* 1995;75:530.

176. Goto Y, Ohori M, Arakawa A, et al. Distinguishing clinically important from unimportant prostate cancers before treatment: value of systematic biopsies. *J Urol* 1996;156:1059.

177. Stamey TA. Making the most out of six systematic sextant biopsies. *Urology* 1995;45:2.

178. Catalona WJ, Smith DS, Ratliff TL, et al. Detection of organ-confined prostate cancer is increased through PSA-based screening. *JAMA* 1993;270:948.

179. Alexander EE, Qian J, Wollan PC, et al. Prostatic intraepithelial neoplasia does not appear to raise serum prostate-specific antigen concentration. *Urology* 1996;47:693.

180. Oesterling JE, Jacobsen SJ, Chute CG, et al. Serum prostate-specific antigen in a community-based population of healthy men: establishment of age-specific reference ranges. *JAMA* 1993;270:860.

181. Benson MC, Whang IS, Pantuck A, et al. Prostate specific antigen density: a means of distinguishing benign prostatic hypertrophy and prostate cancer. *J Urol* 1992;147:815.

182. Carter HB, Pearson JD, Metter EJ, et al. Longitudinal evaluation of prostate-specific antigen levels in men with and without prostate disease. *JAMA* 1992;267:2215.

183. Petteway J, Brawer MK. Age specific versus 4.0 ng/ml as a PSA cutoff in the screening population: impact on cancer detection. *J Urol* 1995;153:465A.

184. Stamey T, Yang N, Hay A, et al. Prostate-specific antigen as a serum marker for adenocarcinoma of the prostate. *N Engl J Med* 1987;317:909.

185. Ohori M, Scardino PT. Early detection of prostate cancer: the nature of cancers detected with current diagnostic tests. *Semin Oncol* 1994;21:522.

186. Smith DS, Catalona WJ. Rate of change in serum prostate specific antigen levels as a method for prostate cancer detection. *J Urol* 1994;152:1163.

187. Partin AW, Kelly CA, Subong ENP, et al. Measurement of the ratio of free PSA to total PSA improves prostate cancer detection for men with total PSA levels between 4.0 and 10.0 ng/ml. *J Urol* 1995;153:295A.

188. Wilt TJ, Brawer MB. The Prostate Cancer Intervention Versus Observation Trial (PIVOT). *Oncology* 1997;11:1133.

189. Albertsen PC, Hanley JA, Stapleton AMF, et al. Competing risk analysis of men aged 55 to 74 years at diagnosis managed conservatively for clinically localized prostate cancer. *JAMA* 1998;280:975.

190. Kattan MW, Eastham JA, Stapleton AMF, et al. A preoperative nomogram for disease recurrence following radical prostatectomy for prostate cancer. *J Natl Cancer Inst* 1998;90:766.

191. Kattan MW, Zelefsky MJ, Kupelian PA, et al. Pretreatment nomogram for predicting the outcome of three-dimensional conformal radiotherapy in prostate cancer. *J Clin Oncol* 2000;18:3352.

192. Kattan MW, Potters L, Blasko JC, et al. Pretreatment nomogram for predicting freedom from recurrence after permanent prostate brachytherapy in prostate cancer. *Urology* 2001;58:393.

193. Kattan MW, Cowen ME, Miles BJ. A decision analysis for treatment of clinically localized prostate cancer. *J Gen Intern Med* 1997;12:299.

194. Beck JR, Pauker SG. The Markov process in medical prognosis. *Med Decis Making* 1983;3:419.

195. Cowen ME, Chartrand M, Weitzel WF. A Markov model of the natural history of prostate cancer. *J Clin Epidemiol* 1994;47:3.

196. O'Connor AM, Tugwell P, Wells GA, et al. Randomized trial of a portable, self-administered decision aid for postmenopausal women considering long-term preventive hormone therapy. *Med Decis Making* 1998;18:295.

197. Panel. TAUAPCCG. *Report on the management of clinically localized prostate cancer*. Baltimore, MD: American Urological Association, Inc., 1995.

198. Zincke H, Oesterling JE, Blute ML, et al. Long-term (15 years) results after radical prostatectomy for clinically localized (stage T2c or lower) prostate cancer. *J Urol* 1994;152:1850.

199. Pound CR, Partin AW, Epstein JI, et al. Prostate-specific antigen after anatomic radical retropubic prostatectomy. Patterns of recurrence and cancer control. *Cancer* 1997;79:528.

200. D'Amico AV, Whittington R, Malkowicz SB, et al. A multivariate analysis of clinical and pathological factors that predict for prostate specific antigen failure after radical prostatectomy for prostate cancer. *J Urol* 1995;154:131.

201. Steineck G, Helgesen F, Adolfsson J, et al. Quality of life after radical prostatectomy or watchful waiting. *N Engl J Med* 2002;347:790.

202. Stamey TA, McNeal JE, Freiha FS, et al. Morphometric and clinical studies on 68 consecutive radical prostatectomies. *J Urol* 1988;139:1235.

203. Smith DS, Catalona WJ. Interexaminer variability of digital rectal examination in detecting prostate cancer. *Urology* 1995;45:70.

204. Partin AW, Yoo J, Ballentine Carter H, et al. The use of prostate specific antigen, clinical stage and Gleason score to predict pathological stage in men with localized prostate cancer. *J Urol* 1993;150:110.

205. Stamey TA, Sozen S, Yemoto CM, et al. Classification of localized untreated prostate cancer based on 791 men treated only with radical prostatectomy: common ground for therapeutic trials and TNM subgroups. *J Urol* 1998;159:2009.

206. Pound CR, Partin AW, Epstein JI, et al. Prostate-specific antigen after anatomic radical retropubic prostatectomy. Patterns of recurrence and cancer control. *Urol Clin North Am* 1997;24:395.

207. Gleason DF. Histologic grade, clinical stage, and patient age in prostate cancer. *NCI Monogr* 1988;(7):15.

208. Epstein JI, Pound CR, Partin AW, et al. Disease progression following radical prostatectomy in men with Gleason score 7 tumor. *J Urol* 1998;160:97.

209. Epstein JI, Walsh PC, Carmichael M, et al. Pathologic and clinical findings to predict tumor extent of nonpalpable (stage T1c) prostate cancer. *JAMA* 1994;271:368.

210. Ohori M, Suyama K, Maru N, et al. Prognostic significance of systemic needle biopsy findings. *J Urol* 2000;163:287A.

211. D'Amico AV, Whittington R, Malkowicz SB, et al. Clinical utility of the percentage of positive prostate biopsies in defining biochemical outcome after radical prostatectomy for patients with clinically localized prostate cancer. *J Clin Oncol* 2000;18:1164.

212. Kattan MW, Eastham JA, Wheeler TM, et al. Counseling men with prostate cancer: a nomogram for predicting the presence of small, moderately differentiated, confined tumors. *J Urol* 2003;170:1792.

213. Dhingsa R, Qayyum A, Coakley FV, et al. Prostate cancer localization with endorectal MR imaging and MR spectroscopic imaging: effect of clinical data on reader accuracy. *Radiology* 2004;230:215.

214. Partin AW, Subong ENP, Walsh PC, et al. Combination of prostate-specific antigen, clinical stage, and Gleason score to predict pathological stage of localized prostate cancer: a multi-institutional update. *JAMA* 1997;277:1445.

215. Cheng L, Zincke H, Blute ML, et al. Risk of prostate carcinoma death in patients with lymph node metastasis. *Cancer* 2001;91:66.

216. Soh S, Kattan MW, Berkman S, et al. Has there been a recent shift in the pathological features and prognosis of patients treated with radical prostatectomy? *J Urol* 1997;157:2212.

217. Bianco F, Dotan Z, Kattan MW, et al. Fifteen-year cancer-specific and PSA progression-free probabilities after radical prostatectomy. *J Urol* 2004;171:926.

218. Eastham JA, Scardino PT. Carcinoma of the prostate: radical prostatectomy. In: Walsh PC, Retik AB, Vaughan ED Jr, et al, eds. *Campbell's urology*, 8th ed. Philadelphia: W.B. Saunders, 2002.

219. Bader P, Burkhard FC, Markwalder R, et al. Is a limited lymph node dissection an adequate staging procedure for prostate cancer? *J Urol* 2002;168:514.

220. Ware JL, Maygarden SJ, Koontz WW Jr, et al. Differential reactivity with anti-c-erbB-2 antiserum among human malignant and benign prostatic tissue. *Proc Am Assoc Cancer Res* 1989;30:1737.

221. Oesterling J, Chute C, Jacobsen S, et al. Longitudinal changes in serum PSA (PSA velocity) in a community-based cohort of men. *J Urol* 1993;149:412.
222. Feneley M, McLean A, Webb J, et al. Age corrected prostate specific antigen, prostate volume and age in the benign prostate. *Br J Urol* 1994;151:312.
223. Hart IR. "Seed and soil" revisited: mechanisms of site-specific metastasis. *Cancer Metastasis Rev* 1982;1:5.
224. Scherr D, Swindle PW, Scardino PT. National Comprehensive Cancer Network guidelines for the management of prostate cancer. *Urology* 2003;61:14.
225. Rosenthal SA, Haseman MK, Polascik TJ. Utility of capromab pendetide (ProstaScint) imaging in the management of prostate cancer. *Tech Urol* 2001;7:27.
226. Moreno JG, Croce CM, Fischer R, et al. Detection of hematogenous micrometastasis in patients with prostate cancer. *Cancer Res* 1992;52:6110.
227. Katz AE, Olsson CA, Raffo AJ, et al. Molecular staging of prostate cancer with the use of an enhanced reverse transcriptase-PCR assay. *Urology* 1994;43:765.
228. Melchior SW, Corey E, Ellis WJ, et al. Early tumor cell dissemination in patients with clinically localized carcinoma of the prostate. *Clin Cancer Res* 1997;3:249.
229. Ross PL, Scardino PT, Kattan MW. A catalog of prostate cancer nomograms. *J Urol* 2001;165:1562.
230. Djavan B, Remzi M, Zlotta A, et al. Novel artificial neural network for early detection of prostate cancer. *J Clin Oncol* 2002;20:921.
231. Babaian RJ, Fritsche HA, Zhang Z, et al. Evaluation of ProstAsure index in the detection of prostate cancer: a preliminary report. *Urology* 1998;51:132.
232. Carlson GD, Calvanese CB, Partin AW. An algorithm combining age, total prostate-specific antigen (PSA), and percent free PSA to predict prostate cancer: results on 4298 cases. *Urology* 1998;52:455.
233. Snow PB, Smith DS, Catalona WJ. Artificial neural networks in the diagnosis and prognosis of prostate cancer: a pilot study. *J Urol* 1994;152:1923.
234. Lopez-Corona E, Ohori M, Scardino PT, et al. A nomogram for predicting a positive repeat prostate biopsy in patients with a previous negative biopsy session. *J Urol* 2003;170:1184.
235. Partin AW, Mangold LA, Lamm DM, et al. Contemporary update of prostate cancer staging nomograms (Partin Tables) for the new millennium. *Urology* 2001;58:843.
236. Badalament RA, Miller MC, Peller PA, et al. An algorithm for predicting nonorgan confined prostate cancer using the results obtained from sextant core biopsies with prostate specific antigen level. *J Urol* 1996;156:1375.
237. Ohori M, Kattan MW, Koh H, et al. Predicting the presence and side of extracapsular extension: a nomogram for staging prostate cancer. *J Urol* 2004;171:(*in press*).
238. Koh H, Kattan MW, Scardino PT, et al. A nomogram to predict seminal vesicle invasion by the extent and location of cancer in systematic biopsy results. *J Urol* 2003;170:1203.
239. Cagiannos I, Karakiewicz P, Eastham JA, et al. A preoperative nomogram identifying decreased risk of positive pelvic lymph nodes in patients with prostate cancer. *J Urol* 2003;170:1798.
240. Kattan MW, Wheeler TM, Scardino PT. Postoperative nomogram for disease recurrence after radical prostatectomy for prostate cancer. *J Clin Oncol* 1999;17:1499.
241. Han M, Partin AW, Zahurak M, et al. Biochemical (prostate specific antigen) recurrence probability following radical prostatectomy for clinically localized prostate cancer. *J Urol* 2003;169:517.
242. Kattan MW, Zelefsky MJ, Kupelian PA, et al. Pretreatment nomogram that predicts 5-year probability of metastasis following three-dimensional conformal radiation therapy for localized prostate cancer. *J Clin Oncol* 2003;21:4568.
243. Smaletz O, Scher HI, Small EJ, et al. Nomogram for overall survival of patients with progressive metastatic prostate cancer after castration. *J Clin Oncol* 2002;20:3972.
244. Duchesne GM, Bloomfield D, Wall P. Identification of intermediate-risk prostate cancer patients treated with radiotherapy suitable for neoadjuvant hormone studies. *Radiother Oncol* 1996;38:7.
245. Zagars GK, Pollack A, von Eschenbach AC. Prognostic factors for clinically localized prostate carcinoma: analysis of 938 patients irradiated in the prostate specific antigen era. *Cancer* 1997;24:1370.
246. Eastham JA, Kattan MW, Scardino PT. Nomograms as predictive models. *Semin Urol Oncol* 2002;20:108.
247. Holmberg L, Bill-Axelson A, Helgesen F, et al. A randomized trial comparing radical prostatectomy with watchful waiting in early prostate cancer. *N Engl J Med* 2002;347:781.
248. Reference deleted.
249. Gerber GS, Thisted RA, Scardino PT, et al. Results of radical prostatectomy in men with clinically localized prostate cancer. *JAMA* 1996;276:615.
250. Chodak GW, Thisted RA, Gerber GS, et al. Results of conservative management of clinically localized prostate cancer. *N Engl J Med* 1994;330:242.
251. Ohori M, Goad JR, Wheeler TM, et al. Can radical prostatectomy alter the progression of poorly differentiated prostate cancer? *J Urol* 1994;152:1843.
252. Eastham JA, Scardino PT. Treatment of prostate cancer: Surgery. In: DeVita VT Jr, Hellman S, Rosenberg SA, eds. *Progress in oncology, 2001.* Sudbury, MA: Jones and Bartlett, 2001.
253. Guillonneau B, Vallancien G. Laparoscopic radical prostatectomy: the Montsouris technique. *J Urol* 2000;163:1643.
254. Guillonneau B, Vallancien G. Laparoscopic radical prostatectomy: initial experience and preliminary assessment after 65 operations. *Prostate* 1999;39:71.
255. Eastham JA, Scardino PT. Radical prostatectomy for clinical stage T1 and T2 prostate cancer. In: Vogelzang NJ, Scardino PT, Shipley WU, et al, eds. *Comprehensive textbook of genitourinary oncology,* 2nd ed. Philadelphia: Lippincott Williams & Wilkins, 2000; 722.
256. Walsh PC. Anatomic radical retropubic prostatectomy. In: Walsh P, Retik A, Vaughan EJ, et al, eds. *Campbell's urology.* Philadelphia: W.B. Saunders, 1998; 2565.
257. Eastham J, Kattan MW, Rogers E, et al. Risk factors for urinary incontinence after radical prostatectomy. *J Urol* 1996;156:1707.
258. Rabbani F, Stapleton AM, Kattan MW, et al. Factors predicting recovery of erections after radical prostatectomy. *J Urol* 2000;164:1929.
259. Goad JR, Eastham JA, Fitzgerald KB, et al. Radical retropubic prostatectomy: limited benefit of autologous blood donation. *J Urol* 1995;142:332.
260. Dillioglugil O, Leibman BD, Leibman NS, et al. Risk factors for complications and morbidity after radical retropubic prostatectomy. *J Urol* 1997;157:1760.
261. Ohori M, Wheeler TM, Kattan MW, et al. Prognostic significance of positive surgical margins in radical prostatectomy specimens. *J Urol* 1995;154:1818.
262. Partin AW, Pound CR, Clemens JQ, et al. Serum PSA following anatomical radical prostatectomy: the Johns Hopkins experience after ten years. *Urol Clin North Am* 1993;20:713.
263. Walsh PC. Technique of vesicourethral anastomosis may influence recovery of sexual function following radical prostatectomy. *Atlas Urol Clin North Am* 1994;2:59.
264. Begg CB, Riedel ER, Bach PB, et al. Variations in morbidity after radical prostatectomy. *N Engl J Med* 2002;346:1138.
265. Lu-Yao GL, Albertsen P, Warren J, et al. Effect of age and surgical approach on complications and short-term mortality after radical prostatectomy—a population-based study. *Urology* 1999;54:301.
266. Scardino PT, Kim ED. Rationale for and results of nerve grafting during radical prostatectomy. *Urology* 2001;57:1016.
267. Blute ML, Bostwick DG, Seay TM, et al. Pathologic classification of prostate carcinoma: the impact of margin status. *Cancer* 1998;82:902.
268. Rosen MA, Goldstone L, Lapin S, et al. Frequency and location of extracapsular extension and positive surgical margins in radical prostatectomy specimens. *J Urol* 1992;148:331.
269. Wheeler TM, Dillioglugil O, Kattan MW, et al. Clinical and pathological significance of the level and extent of capsular invasion in clinical stage T1-2 prostate cancer. *Hum Pathol* 1998;29:856.
270. Myers RP, Goellner JR, Cahill DR. Prostate shape, external striated urethral sphincter and radical prostatectomy: the apical dissection. *J Urol* 1987;138:543.
271. Tsuboi T, Ohori M, Reuter V, et al. Are intraoperative frozen sections an efficient way to reduce positive surgical margins? 98th Annual Meeting of the American Urological Association, Chicago, IL. *J Urol* 2003;169:492 (abst).
272. Villers A, McNeal JE, Freiha FS, et al. Invasion of Denonvilliers' fascia in radical prostatectomy specimens. *J Urol* 1993;149:793.
273. Ohori M, Scardino PT, Lapin SL, et al. The mechanisms and prognostic significance of seminal vesicle involvement by prostate cancer. *Am J Clin Pathol* 1993;17:1252.
274. Grossfeld GD, Chang JJ, Broering JM, et al. Impact of positive surgical margins on prostate cancer recurrence and the use of secondary cancer treatment: data from the CaPSURE database. *J Urol* 2000;163:1171.
275. Zincke H, Oesterling JE, Blute ML, et al. Long-term (15 years) results after radical prostatectomy for clinically localized (Stage T2c or lower) prostate cancer. *J Urol* 1994;152:1850.
276. Catalona WJ, Partin AW, Slawin KM, et al. Use of the percentage of free prostate-specific antigen to enhance differentiation of prostate cancer from benign prostatic disease: a prospective multicenter clinical trial. *JAMA* 1998;279:1542.
277. Abbas F, Scardino PT. Why neoadjuvant androgen deprivation prior to radical prostatectomy is unnecessary. *Urol Clin North Am* 1996;23:587.
278. Wieder JA, Soloway MS. Incidence, etiology, location, prevention and treatment of positive surgical margins after radical prostatectomy for prostate cancer. *J Urol* 1998;160:299.
279. Eastham JA, Kattan MW, Riedel E, et al. Variations among individual surgeons in the rate of positive surgical margins in radical prostatectomy specimens. *J Urol* 2003;170:2292.
280. Klotz LH, Goldenberg SL, Jewett M, et al. CUOG randomized trial of neoadjuvant androgen ablation before radical prostatectomy: 36-month post-treatment PSA results. Canadian Urologic Oncology Group. *Urology* 1999;53:757.
281. Paulson DF, Moul JW, Robertson JE, et al. Postoperative radiotherapy of the prostate for patients undergoing radical prostatectomy with positive margins, seminal vesicle involvement and/or penetration through the capsule. *J Urol* 1990;143:1178.
282. Anscher MS, Robertson CN, Prosnitz R. Adjuvant radiotherapy for pathologic stage T3/4 adenocarcinoma of the prostate: ten-year update. *Int J Radiat Oncol Biol Phys* 1995;33:37.
283. Elias S, Parker RG, Gallardo D, et al. Adjuvant radiation therapy after radical prostatectomy for carcinoma of the prostate. *Am J Clin Oncol* 1997;20:120.
284. Bolla. [Abstract to be published by ASCO]. 2004.
285. Stephenson AJ, Shariat SF, Zelefsky MJ, et al. Salvage radiotherapy for recurrent prostate cancer after radical prostatectomy. *JAMA* 2004;291:1325.
286. Swindle PW, Ohori M, Kattan MW, et al. Do margins matter? The prognostic significance of positive surgical margins in radical prostatectomy specimens—18 year experience. 98th Annual Meeting of the American Urological Association, Chicago, IL. *J Urol* 2003;169:180 (abst).
287. Hu JC, Gold KF, Pashos CL, et al. Role of surgeon volume in radical prostatectomy outcomes. *J Clin Oncol* 2003;21:401.
288. Potosky AL, Harlan LC, Stanford JL, et al. Prostate cancer practice patterns and quality of life: the prostate cancer outcomes study. *J Natl Cancer Inst* 1999;91:1719.
289. Tomschi W, Suster G, Holtl W. Bladder neck strictures after radical retropubic prostatectomy: still an unsolved problem. *Br J Urol* 1998;81:823.
290. Stanford JL, Feng Z, Hamilton AS, et al. Urinary and sexual function after radical prostatectomy for clinically localized prostate cancer: the Prostate Cancer Outcomes Study. *JAMA* 2000;283:354.
291. Litwin MS, Hays RD, Fink A, et al. Quality-of-life outcomes in men treated for localized prostate cancer. *JAMA* 1995;273:129.
292. Quinlan DM, Epstein JI, Carter BS, et al. Sexual function following radical prostatectomy: influence of preservation of neurovascular bundles. *J Urol* 1991;145:998.
293. Catalona WJ, Carvalhal GJ, Mager DE, et al. Potency, continence and complication rates in 1,870 consecutive radical retropubic prostatectomies. *J Urol* 1999;162:433.

294. Montorsi F, Guazzoni G, Strambi LF, et al. Recovery of spontaneous erectile function after nerve-sparing radical retropubic prostatectomy with and without early intracavernous injections of alprostadil: results of a prospective, randomized trial. *J Urol* 1997;158:1408.

295. Rabbani F, Cozzi P, Scardino PT. Quantitative assessment of the response to cavermap nerve stimulation at radical prostatectomy. 97th Annual Meeting of the American Urological Association, Orlando, FL. *J Urol* 2003;167:356 (abst).

296. Bagshaw MA, Kaplan HS, Sagerman RH. Linear accelerator supervoltage therapy. VII. Carcinoma of the prostate. *Radiology* 1965;85:121.

297. Ray GR, Cassady JR, Bagshaw MA. Definitive radiation therapy of carcinoma of the prostate: a report of 15 years experience. *Radiology* 1973;106:407.

298. Perez CA, Hanks GE, Leibel SA, et al. Localized carcinoma of the prostate (stage T1b, T2, and T3); review of management with radiation therapy. *Cancer* 1993;72:156.

299. Shipley WU, Thames HD, Sandler HM, et al. Radiation therapy for clinically localized prostate cancer: a multi-institutional pooled analysis. *JAMA* 1999;281:1598.

300. Zelefsky MJ, Leibel SA, Gaudin PB, et al. Dose escalation with three dimensional conformal radiation therapy affects the outcome in prostate cancer. *Int J Radiat Oncol Biol Phys* 1998;41:491.

301. Ten Haken RK, Perez-Tamayo C, Tesser RJ, et al. Boost treatment of the prostate using shaped fixed fields. *Int J Radiat Oncol Biol Phys* 1989;16:193.

302. Lawton CA, Wong M, Pilepich MV, et al. Long-term sequelae following external beam irradiation for adenocarcinoma of the prostate: analysis of RTOG studies 7506 and 7706. *Int J Radiat Oncol Biol Phys* 1991;21:935.

303. Leibel SA, Hanks GE, Kramer S. Patterns of care outcome studies: results of the national practice in adenocarcinoma of the prostate. *Int J Radiat Oncol Biol Phys* 1984;10:401.

304. Hanks GE, Martz KL, Diamond JJ. The effect of dose on local control of prostate cancer. *Int J Radiat Oncol Biol Phys* 1988;15:1299.

305. Munzenrider JE, Pilepich M, Rene-Ferrero JB, et al. Use of body scanner in radiotherapy treatment planning. *Cancer* 1979;40:170.

306. Goitein M. The utility of computed tomography in radiation therapy: an estimate of outcome. *Int J Radiat Oncol Biol Phys* 1979;5:1799.

307. Fuks Z, Leibel SA, Kutcher GJ, et al. Three-dimensional conformal treatment: a new frontier in radiation therapy. In: DeVita Jr. VT, Hellman S, Rosenberg SA, eds. *Important advances in oncology.* Philadelphia: J.B. Lippincott, 1991;151.

308. ICRU Report 50. *Prescribing, recording, and reporting photon beam therapy.* Bethesda, MD: International Commission on Radiation Units and Measurements, 1993.

309. Kutcher GJ, Mageras GS, Leibel SA. Control, correction and modeling of setup errors and organ motion. *Semin Radiat Oncol* 1995;5:134.

310. Bagshaw MA. A technique for external beam radiotherapy for carcinoma of the prostate. In: Levitt SH, Tapley NV, eds. *Technological bias of radiotherapy: practical clinical applications.* Philadelphia: Lea & Febiger, 1984;244.

311. Bagshaw MA. Radiotherapeutic treatment of prostatic carcinoma with pelvic node involvement. *Urol Clin North Am* 1984;2:297.

312. Spaas PG, Bagshaw MA, Cox RS. The volume of extended field irradiation in surgically staged carcinoma of the prostate. *Int J Radiat Oncol Biol Phys* 1988;15:133.

313. Perez CA, Pilepich MV, Zivnuska F. Tumor control in definitive irradiation of localized carcinoma of the prostate. *Int J Radiat Oncol Biol Phys* 1986;12:523.

314. Asbell SO, Caplan RJ, Perez CA, et al. Impact of surgical staging on evaluating the radiotherapeutic outcome in RTOG #77-06. A phase III study for T1b-T2N0M0 prostatic carcinoma. *Int J Radiat Oncol Biol Phys* 1995;32:143.

315. Seaward SA, Weinberg V, Lewis P, et al. Improved freedom from PSA failure with whole pelvic irradiation for high-risk prostate cancer. *Int J Radiat Oncol Biol Phys* 1998;42:1055.

316. Ibrahim A, Zambon E, Bourhis JH, et al. High-dose chemotherapy with etoposide, cyclophosphamide and escalating dose of carboplatin followed by autologous bone marrow transplantation in cancer patients. A pilot study. *Eur J Cancer* 1993;29A:1398.

317. Bagshaw MA. Definitive megavoltage radiation therapy in carcinoma of the prostate. In: Fletcher GH, ed. *Textbook of radiotherapy,* 2nd ed. Philadelphia: Lea & Febiger, 1973;752.

318. Bagshaw MA, Kaplan ID, Cox RC. Radiation therapy for localized disease. *Cancer* 1993;71:939.

319. Leibel SA, Fuks Z, Zelefsky MJ, et al. Technological advances in external-beam radiation therapy for the treatment of localized prostate cancer. *Semin Oncol* 2003;30:596.

320. Epstein BE, Hanks GE. Radiation therapy techniques and dose selection in the treatment of prostate cancer. *Semin Radiat Oncol* 1993;3:179.

321. Zelefsky MJ, Happersett L, Leibel SA, et al. The effect of treatment positioning on normal tissue dose in patients with prostate cancer treated with three-dimensional conformal radiotherapy. *Int J Radiat Oncol Biol Phys* 1997;37:13.

322. Leibel SA, Kutcher GJ, Mohan R, et al. Three-dimensional conformal radiation therapy at the Memorial Sloan-Kettering Cancer Center. *Semin Radiat Oncol* 1992;2:274.

323. Zelefsky MJ, Crean D, Mageras GS, et al. Quantification and predictors of prostate position variability in 50 patients evaluated with multiple CT scans during conformal radiotherapy. *Radiother Oncol* 1999;50:225.

324. Leibel SA, Zelefsky MJ, Kutcher GJ, et al. Three-dimensional conformal radiation therapy in localized carcinoma of the prostate: interim report of a phase I dose escalation study. *J Urol* 1994;152:1792.

325. Drzymala RE, Mohan R, Brewster L, et al. Dose-volume histogram. *Int J Radiat Oncol Biol Phys* 1991;21:71.

326. Leibel SA, Zelefsky MJ, Kutcher GJ, et al. Three-dimensional conformal radiation therapy in localized carcinoma of the prostate: interim report of a phase I dose escalation study. *J Urol* 1994;152:1792.

327. Zelefsky MJ, Leibel SA, Burman CM, et al. Neoadjuvant hormonal therapy improves the therapeutic ratio in patients with bulky prostatic cancer treated with three-dimensional conformal radiation therapy. *Int J Radiat Oncol Biol Phys* 1994;29:755.

328. Aus G, Hugosson J, Norlen L. Long-term survival and mortality in prostate cancer treated with noncurative intent. *J Urol* 1995;154:460.

329. *Statistical abstract of the United States, 2000.* Washington, DC. Bureau of the Census 2000.

330. Kuban DA, EL-Mahdi AM. Local control after radiation for prostatic carcinoma: significance and assessment. *Semin Radiat Oncol* 1993;3:221.

331. Laverdiere J, Gomez JL, Cusan L, et al. Beneficial effect of combination hormonal therapy administered prior and following external beam radiation therapy in localized prostate cancer. *Int J Radiat Oncol Biol Phys* 1997;37:247.

332. Scardino PT, Wheeler TM. Local control of prostate cancer with radiotherapy: frequency and prognostic significance of positive results of postirradiation prostate biopsy. *NCI Monogr* 1988;7:95.

333. American Society for Therapeutic Radiology and Oncology Consensus Panel. Consensus statements on radiation therapy of prostate cancer: guidelines for prostate re-biopsy after radiation and for radiation therapy with rising prostate-specific antigen levels after radical prostatectomy. *J Clin Oncol* 1999;17:1155.

334. Pollack A, Zagars GK, Kavadi VS. Prostate specific antigen doubling time and disease relapse after radiotherapy for prostate cancer. *Cancer* 1994;74:670.

335. Zagars GK. Prostate-specific antigen as an outcome variable for T1 and T2 prostate cancer treated by radiation therapy. *J Urol* 1994;152:1786.

336. Willett CG, Zietman AL, Shipley WU, et al. The effect of pelvic radiation therapy on serum levels of prostate specific antigen. *J Urol* 1994;151:1579.

337. Zelefsky MJ, Leibel SA, Wallner KE, et al. Significance of normal serum prostate-specific antigen in the follow-up period after definitive radiation therapy for prostatic cancer. *J Clin Oncol* 1995;13:459.

338. Zietman AL, Coen JJ, Shipley WU, et al. Radical radiation therapy in the management of prostatic adenocarcinoma: the initial prostate-specific antigen value as a predictor of treatment outcome. *J Urol* 1994;151:640.

339. Consensus statement: guidelines for PSA following radiation therapy. *Int J Radiat Oncol Biol Phys* 1997;37:1035.

340. Kavadi VS, Zagars GK, Pollack A. Serum prostate-specific antigen after radiation therapy for clinically localized prostate cancer: prognostic implications. *Int J Radiat Oncol Biol Phys* 1994;30:279.

341. Schellhammer PF, El-Mahdi AM, Wright GL, et al. Prostate-specific antigen to determine progression-free survival after radiation therapy for localized carcinoma of prostate. *Urology* 1993;42:13.

342. DeWitt KD, Sandler HM, Weinberg V, et al. What does postradiotherapy PSA nadir tell us about freedom from PSA failure and progression-free survival in patients with low and intermediate-risk localized prostate cancer? *Urology* 2003;62:492.

343. Leibel SA, Fuks Z, Zelefsky MJ, et al. The treatment of localized prostate cancer with three-dimensional conformal and intensity modulated radiation therapy at the Memorial Sloan-Kettering Cancer Center. In: Purdy J, Grant III W, Palta J, et al, eds. *3D conformal radiation therapy and intensity modulated radiation therapy in the next millennium.* Madison, WI: Advanced Publishing (*in press*).

344. Kuban DA, Thames HD, Levy LB, et al. Long-term multi-institutional analysis of stage T1-T2 prostate cancer treated with radiotherapy in the PSA era. *Int J Radiat Oncol Biol Phys* 2003;57:915.

345. Zietman AL, Chung CS, Coen JJ, et al. 10-year outcome for men with localized prostate cancer treated with external radiation therapy: results of a cohort study. *J Urol* 2004;171:210.

346. Zagars GK, Pollack A, Smith LG. Conventional external-beam radiation therapy alone or with androgen ablation for clinical stage III (T3, NX/N0, M0) adenocarcinoma of the prostate. *Int J Radiat Oncol Biol Phys* 1999;44:809.

347. Huggins C, Hodges CV. Studies on prostatic cancer I. the effect of castration, of estrogen and of androgen injection on serum phosphatases in metastatic carcinoma of the prostate. *Cancer Res* 1941;1:193.

348. Barrett-Connor E, Garland C, McPhillips JB, et al. A prospective, population-based study of androstenedione, estrogens, and prostatic cancer. *Cancer Res* 1990;50:169.

349. Porter EH. The statistical dose-cure relationships for irradiated tumors. *Br J Radiol* 1980;53:336.

350. Hendry JH, Moore JV. Is the steepness of dose-incidence curves for tumor control or complications due to variation before or as a result of irradiation? *Br J Radiol* 1984;57:1045.

351. Roberts SA, Hendry JH. A realistic closed-form radiobiological model of clinical tumor-control data incorporating intertumor heterogeneity. *Int J Radiat Oncol Biol Phys* 1998;41:689.

352. Zagars GK, Schultheiss TE, Peters LJ. Inter-tumor heterogeneity and radiation dose-control curves. *Radiother Oncol* 1987;8:353.

353. Thames HD, Schultheiss TE, Hendry JH, et al. Can modest escalations of dose be detected as increased tumor control? *Int J Radiat Oncol Biol Phys* 1992;22:241.

354. Moore JV, Hendrey JH, Hunter RD. Dose-incidence curves for tumor control and normal tissue injury, in relation to the response of clonogenic cells. *Radiother Oncol* 1983;1:143.

355. Peters LJ, Fletcher GH. Causes of failure of radiotherapy in head and neck cancer. *Radiother Oncol* 1983;1:53.

356. Williams MV, Denekamp J, Fowler JF. Dose-response relationships for human tumours: implications for clinical trials of dose modifying agents. *Int J Radiat Oncol Biol Phys* 1984;10:1703.

357. Fowler JF. Potential for increasing the differential response between tumors and normal tissues: can proliferation rate be used? *Int J Radiat Oncol Biol Phys* 1986;12:641.

358. Hanks GE, Hanlon AL, Schultheiss TE, et al. Dose escalation with 3D conformal treatment: five year outcomes, treatment optimization, and future directions. *Int J Radiat Oncol Biol Phys* 1998;41:501.

359. Ohori M, Wheeler TM, Dunn JK, et al. Pathological features in prognosis of prostate cancer detectable with current diagnostic tests. *J Urol* 1994;152:1714.

360. Montie JE, Wood DP, Pontes JE, et al. Adenocarcinoma of the prostate in cystoprostatectomy specimens removed for bladder cancer. *Cancer* 1989;63:381.

361. Hanks GE, Asbell S, Kroll KM, et al. Outcome for lymph node dissection negative T1-b, T2(a-2b) prostate cancer treated with external beam therapy in RTOG 77-06. *Int J Radiat Oncol Biol Phys* 1991;21:1099.
362. Byar DP, Mostofi FK. Carcinoma of the prostate: prognostic evaluation of certain pathologic features in 208 radical prostatectomies. Examined by the step-section technique. *Cancer* 1972;30:5.
363. Stamey TA, Villers AA, McNeal JE, et al. Positive surgical margins at radical prostatectomy: importance of the apical dissection. *J Urol* 1990;143:1166.
364. Catalona WJ, Bigg SW. Nerve-sparing radical prostatectomy: evaluation of results after 250 patients. *J Urol* 1990;143:538.
365. Walsh PC. Radical prostatectomy, preservation of sexual function, cancer control: the controversy. *Urol Clin North Am* 1987;14:663.
366. Coleman CN, Beard CJ, Kantoff PW, et al. Rate of relapse following treatment for localized prostate cancer: a critical analysis of retrospective reports. *Int J Radiat Oncol Biol Phys* 1994;28:303.
367. Hanks GE, Krall JM, Hanlon AL, et al. Patterns of Care and RTOG studies in prostate cancer: long-term survival, hazard rate observations, and possibilities of cure. *Int J Radiat Oncol Biol Phys* 1994;28:39.
368. Perez CA, Lee HK, Georgiou A, et al. Technical and tumor-related factors affecting outcome of definitive irradiation for localized carcinoma of the prostate. *Int J Radiat Oncol Biol Phys* 1993;26:581.
369. Zagars GK, von Eschenbach AC, Johnson DE, et al. The role of radiation therapy in stages A2 and B adenocarcinoma of the prostate. *Int J Radiat Oncol Biol Phys* 1988;14:701.
370. Kupelian P, Katcher J, Levin H, et al. External beam radiotherapy versus radical prostatectomy for clinical stage T1-2 prostate cancer: therapeutic implications of stratification by pretreatment PSA levels and biopsy Gleason scores. *Cancer J Sci Am* 1997;3:78.
371. Kupelian PA, Elshaikh M, Reddy CA, et al. Comparison of the efficacy of local therapies for localized prostate cancer in the prostate-specific antigen era: a large single-institution experience with radical prostatectomy and external-beam radiotherapy. *J Clin Oncol* 2002;20:3376.
372. Soffen EM, Hanks GE, Hunt MA, et al. Conformal static field radiation therapy of early prostate cancer versus non-conformal techniques: a reduction in acute morbidity. *Int J Radiat Oncol Biol Phys* 1992;24:485.
373. Zelefsky MJ, Ginor RX, Fuks Z, et al. Efficacy of selective alpha-1 blocker therapy in the treatment of acute urinary symptoms during radiotherapy for localized prostate cancer. *Int J Radiat Oncol Biol Phys* 1999;45:567.
374. Teshima T, Hanks GE, Hanlon AL, et al. Rectal bleeding after conformal 3D treatment of prostate cancer: time to occurrence, response to treatment and duration of morbidity. *Int J Radiat Oncol Biol Phys* 1997;39:77.
375. Sandler HM, McLaughlin PW, Ten Haken RK, et al. Three dimensional conformal radiotherapy for the treatment of prostate cancer: low risk of chronic rectal morbidity observed in a large series of patients. *Int J Radiat Oncol Biol Phys* 1995;33:797.
376. Schultheiss TE, Lee WR, Hunt MA, et al. Late GI and GU complications in the treatment of prostate cancer. *Int J Radiat Oncol Biol Phys* 1997;37:3.
377. Benk VA, Adams JA, Shipley WU, et al. Late rectal bleeding following combined x-ray and proton high dose irradiation for patients with stages T3-T4 prostate carcinoma. *Int J Radiat Oncol Biol Phys* 1993;26:551.
378. Lee WR, Hanks GE, Hanlon A, et al. Lateral rectal shielding reduces late rectal morbidity following high dose three-dimensional conformal radiation therapy for clinically localized prostate cancer. Further evidence for a significant dose effect. *Int J Radiat Oncol Biol Phys* 1996;35:251.
379. Hanks GE, Schultheiss TE, Hunt MA, et al. Factors influencing incidence of acute grade 2 morbidity in conformal and standard radiation treatment of prostate cancer. *Int J Radiat Oncol Biol Phys* 1995;31:25.
380. Dearnaley DP, Khoo VS, Norman AR, et al. Comparison of radiation side-effects of conformal and conventional radiotherapy in prostate cancer: a randomized trial. *Lancet* 1999;353:267.
381. Zelefsky MJ, Fuks Z, Happersett L, et al. Clinical experience with intensity modulated radiation therapy (IMRT) in prostate cancer. *Radiother Oncol* 2000;55:241.
382. Bagshaw MA, Cox RS, Ray GR. Status of radiation treatment of prostate cancer at Stanford University. *Natl Cancer Inst Monogr* 1988;7:47.
383. Banker FL. The preservation of potency after external beam irradiation for prostate cancer. *Int J Radiat Biol* 1991;15:219.
384. Shipley WU, Zietman AL, Hanks GE, et al. Treatment related sequelae following external beam radiation for prostate cancer: a review with an update in patients with stages T1 and T2 tumor. *J Urol* 1994;152:1799.
385. Zelefsky MJ, Eid JF. Elucidating the etiology of erectile dysfunction after definitive therapy for prostatic cancer. *Int J Radiat Oncol Biol Phys* 1998;40:129.
386. Pierce DJ, Whittington R, Hanno PM. Pharmacologic erection with intracavernosal injection for men with sexual dysfunction following irradiation: a preliminary report. *Int J Radiat Oncol Biol Phys* 1991;21:1311.
387. Zelefsky MJ, McKee AB, Lee H, et al. Efficacy of oral sildenafil in patients with erectile dysfunction after radiotherapy for carcinoma of the prostate. *Urology* 1999;53:775.
388. Choo R, Hruby G, Hong J, et al. Positive resection margin and/or pathologic T3 adenocarcinoma of prostate with undetectable postoperative prostate-specific antigen after radical prostatectomy: to irradiate or not? *Int J Radiat Oncol Biol Phys* 2002;52:674.
389. Valicenti RK, Gomella LG, Ismail M, et al. The efficacy of early adjuvant radiation therapy for pT3N0 prostate cancer: a matched-pair analysis. *Int J Radiat Oncol Biol Phys* 1999;45:53.
390. Leibovich BC, Engen DE, Patterson DE, et al. Benefit of adjuvant radiation therapy for localized prostate cancer with a positive surgical margin. *J Urol* 2000;163:1178.
391. Nudell DM, Grossfeld GD, Weinberg VK, et al. Radiotherapy after radical prostatectomy: treatment outcomes and failure patterns. *Urology* 1999;54:1049.
392. Whitmore WF Jr, Hilaris B, Grabstald H. Retropubic implantation of iodine 125 in the treatment of prostatic cancer. *J Urol* 1972;108:918.
393. Blasko JC, Ragde H, Grimm PD. Transperineal ultrasound-guided implantation of the prostate: morbidity and complications. *Scand J Urol Nephrol Suppl* 1991;137:113.
394. Kuban DA, El-Mahdi AM, Schellhammer PF. I-125 interstitial implantation for prostate cancer. What have we learned in 10 years? *Cancer* 1989;69:2515.
395. Fuks Z, Leibel SA, Wallner KA, et al. The effect of local control on metastatic dissemination in carcinoma of the prostate: long-term results in patients treated with 125I implantation. *Int J Radiat Oncol Biol Phys* 1991;21:537.
396. Wallner K, Chiu-Tsoa S-T, Roy J, et al. An improved method for computerized tomography planned transperineal 125 iodine prostate implants. *J Urol* 1991;146:90.
397. Blasko J, Grimm PD, Ragde H. Brachytherapy and organ preservation in the management of carcinoma of the prostate. *Semin Radiat Oncol* 1993;3:240.
398. Anderson LL. Plan optimization and dose evaluation in brachytherapy. *Semin Radiat Oncol* 1993;3:290.
399. Wallner K, Roy J, Harrison L. Dosimetry guidelines to minimize urethral and rectal morbidity following transperineal I-125 prostate brachytherapy. *Int J Radiat Oncol Biol Phys* 1995;32:465.
400. Zelefsky MJ, Yamada Y, Marion C, et al. Improved conformality and decreased toxicity with intraoperative computer-optimized transperineal ultrasound-guided prostate brachytherapy. *Int J Radiat Oncol Biol Phys* 2003;55:956.
401. Kini VR, Edmundson GK, Vicini FA, et al. Use of three-dimensional radiation therapy planning tools and intraoperative ultrasound to evaluate high dose rate prostate brachytherapy implants. *Int J Radiat Oncol Biol Phys* 1999;43:571.
402. Messing EM, Zhang JB, Rubens DJ, et al. Intraoperative optimized inverse planning for prostate brachytherapy: early experience. *Int J Radiat Oncol Biol Phys* 1999;44:801.
403. Stock RG, Stone NN, Lo YC. Intraoperative dosimetric representation of the real-time ultrasound-guided prostate implant. *Tech Urol* 2000;6:95.
404. Zelefsky MJ, Yamada Y, Cohen G, et al. Postimplantation dosimetric analysis of permanent transperineal prostate implantation: improved dose distributions with an intraoperative computer-optimized conformal planning technique. *Int J Radiat Oncol Biol Phys* 2000;48:601.
405. Ragde H, Elgamal AA, Snow PB, et al. Ten-year disease free survival after transperineal sonography-guided iodine-125 brachytherapy with or without 45-gray external beam irradiation in the treatment of patients with clinically localized, low to high Gleason grade prostate carcinoma. *Cancer* 1998;83:989.
406. Dattoli M, Wallner K, Sorace R, et al. PD-103 brachytherapy and external beam irradiation for clinically localized high-risk prostatic carcinoma. *Int J Radiat Oncol Biol Phys* 1996;35:875.
407. Kestin LL, Martinez AA, Stromberg JS, et al. Matched-pair analysis of conformal high-dose-rate brachytherapy boost versus external-beam radiation therapy alone for locally advanced prostate cancer. *J Clin Oncol* 2000;18:2869.
408. Blasko JC, Wallner K, Grimm PD, et al. Prostate specific antigen based disease control following ultrasound guided 125 iodine implantation for stage T1/T2 prostatic carcinoma. *J Urol* 1996;154:1096.
409. Priestly JB Jr, Beyer DC. Guided brachytherapy for treatment of confined prostate cancer. *Urology* 1992;40:27.
410. Stock RG, Stone NN, Tabert A, et al. A dose-response study for I-125 prostate implants. *Int J Radiat Oncol Biol Phys* 1998;41:101.
411. Zelefsky MJ, Wallner KE, Ling CC, et al. Comparison of the 5-year outcome and morbidity of three-dimensional conformal radiotherapy versus transperineal permanent iodine-125 implantation for early-stage prostatic cancer. *J Clin Oncol* 1999;17:517.
412. Mettlin CJ, Murphy GP, McGinnis LS, et al. The National Cancer Data Base report on prostate cancer. American College of Surgeons Commission on Cancer and the American Cancer Society. *Cancer* 1995;76:1104.
413. Whitmore WF Jr. Expectant management of clinically localized prostatic cancer. *Semin Oncol* 1994;21:560.
414. Fleming C, Wasson JH, Albertsen PC, et al. A decision analysis of alternative treatment strategies for clinically localized prostate cancer. *JAMA* 1993;269:2650.
415. DeConcini DT, Dillioglugil O, Stapleton AMF, et al. Is deferred definitive therapy a reasonable management strategy for clinically localized prostate cancer? *J Urol* 1996; 155:649A.
416. Yagoda A, Watson RC, Natale RB, et al. A critical analysis of response criteria in patients with prostatic cancer treated with cis-diamminedichloride platinum II. *Cancer* 1979; 44:1553.
417. Scher HI, Eisenberger M, D'Amico AV, et al. Eligibility and outcomes reporting guidelines for clinical trials for patients in the state of a rising PSA: recommendations from the prostate-specific antigen working group. *J Clin Oncol* 2004;22:537.
418. Smith PH, Bono A, Calais da Silva F, et al. Some limitations of the radioisotope bone scan in patients with metastatic prostatic cancer. *Cancer* 1990;66:1009.
419. Scher HI. Prostate cancer: defining therapeutic objectives and improving overall outcomes. *Cancer* 2003;97[Suppl 3]:758.
420. Therasse P, Arbuck SG, Eisenhauer EA, et al. New guidelines to evaluate the response to treatment in solid tumors. European Organization for Research and Treatment of Cancer, National Cancer Institute of the United States, National Cancer Institute of Canada. *J Natl Cancer Inst* 2000;92:205.
421. Ettinger DS. Evaluation of new drugs in untreated patients with small-cell lung cancer: its time has come. *J Clin Oncol* 1990;8:374.
422. Osoba D, Tannock IF, Ernst DS, et al. Health-related quality of life in men with metastatic prostate cancer treated with prednisone alone or mitoxantrone and prednisone. *J Clin Oncol* 1999;17:1654.
423. Stockler MR, Osoba D, Corey P, et al. Convergent discriminative, and predictive validity of the Prostate Cancer Specific Quality of Life Instrument (PROSQOLI) assessment and

comparison with analogous scales from the EORTC QLQ-C30 and a trial-specific module. European Organisation for Research and Treatment of Cancer. Core Quality of Life Questionnaire. *J Clin Epidemiol* 1999;52:653.
424. Bubley GJ, Carducci M, Dahut W, et al. Eligibility and response guidelines for phase II clinical trials in androgen-independent prostate cancer: recommendations from the PSA Working Group. *J Clin Oncol* 1999:3461.
425. Saad F, Gleason DM, Murray R, et al. A randomized, placebo-controlled trial of zoledronic acid in patients with hormone-refractory metastatic prostate carcinoma. *J Natl Cancer Inst* 2002;94:1458.
426. Huggins C, Stevens RE Jr, Hodges CV. Studies on prostatic cancer. II. The effect of castration on advanced carcinoma of the prostate gland. *Arch Surg* 1941;43:209.
427. Mittelman A, Shukla SK, Welvaart K, et al. Oral estramustine phosphate (NSC-89199) in the treatment of advanced (stage D) carcinoma of the prostate. *Cancer Chemother Rep* 1975;59:219.
428. Geller J. Overview of enzyme inhibitors and anti-androgens in prostatic cancer. *J Androl* 1991;12:364.
429. McLeod DG, Kolvenbag GJCM. Defining the role of antiandrogens in the treatment of prostate cancer. *Urology* 1996;47:85.
430. Robinson MR. Aminoglutethimide: medical adrenalectomy in the management of carcinoma of the prostate. A review after 6 years. *Br J Urol* 1980;52:328.
431. Trachtenberg J, Pont A. Ketoconazole therapy for advanced prostate cancer. *Lancet* 1984;2:433.
432. Holzbeierlein JM, Castle EP, Thrasher JB. Complications of androgen-deprivation therapy for prostate cancer. *Clin Prostate Cancer* 2003;2:147.
433. Thompson CA, Shanafelt TD, Loprinzi CL. Andropause: symptom management for prostate cancer patients treated with hormonal ablation. *Oncologist* 2003;8:474.
434. Roth AJ, Kornblith AB, Batel-Copel L, et al. Rapid screening for psychological distress in men with prostate cancer: a pilot study. *Cancer* 1998;82:1904.
435. Lofters A, Juffs HG, Pond GR, et al. "PSA-itis": knowledge of serum prostate specific antigen and other causes of anxiety in men with metastatic prostate cancer. *J Urol* 2002;168:2516.
436. Strum SB, McDermed JE, Scholz MC, et al. Anaemia associated with androgen deprivation in patients with prostate cancer receiving combined hormone blockade. *Br J Urol* 1997;79:933.
437. Diamond TH, Higano CS, Smith MR, et al. Osteoporosis in men with prostate carcinoma receiving androgen-deprivation therapy: recommendations for diagnosis and therapies. *Cancer* 2004;100:892.
438. Morote J, Martinez E, Trilla E, et al. Osteoporosis during continuous androgen deprivation: influence of the modality and length of treatment. *Eur Urol* 2003;44:661.
439. Cassileth BR, Soloway MS, Vogelzang NJ, et al. Patients' choice of treatment in stage D prostate cancer. *Urology* 1989;33:57.
440. Scherr DS, Pitts WR Jr. The nonsteroidal effects of diethylstilbestrol: the rationale for androgen deprivation therapy without estrogen deprivation in the treatment of prostate cancer. *J Urol* 2003;170:1703.
441. Group. TLS. Leuprolide versus diethylstilbestrol for metastatic prostatic cancer. *N Engl J Med* 1984;311:1281.
442. Robinson MR, Smith PH, Richards B, et al. The final analysis of the EORTC Genito-Urinary Tract Cancer Co-Operative Group phase III clinical trial (protocol 30805).
443. Ahlgren JD. Estramustine—current status, 1983. *Semin Oncol* 1983;10:46.
444. Pavone Macaluso M, deVoogt HJ, Viggiano G, et al. Comparison of diethylstilbestrol, cyproterone acetate, medroxyprogesterone acetate, and estramustine phosphatase used for the treatment of advanced prostate cancer: final analysis of a randomized phase III trial of the EORTC. *J Urol* 1986;135:624.
445. Seidenfeld J, Samson DJ, Hasselblad V, et al. Single-therapy androgen suppression in men with advanced prostate cancer: a systematic review and meta-analysis. *Ann Intern Med* 2000;132:566.
446. Leuprolide versus diethylstilbestrol for metastatic prostate cancer. *N Engl J Med* 1984;311:1281.
447. Waxman J, Man A, Hendry WF, et al. Importance of early tumour exacerbation in patients treated with long acting analogues of gonadotrophin releasing hormone for advanced prostatic cancer. *BMJ* 1985;291:1387.
448. Trachtenberg J, Gittleman M, Steidle C, et al. A phase 3, multicenter, open label, randomized study of abarelix versus leuprolide plus daily anti-androgen in men with prostate cancer. *J Urol* 2002;167:1670.
449. Fair WR, Aprikian AG, Cohen D, et al. Use of neoadjuvant androgen deprivation therapy in clinically localized prostate cancer. *Clin Invest Med* 1993;16:516.
450. Moul JW. Neoadjuvant hormonal therapy for clinically localized prostate cancer. *Urol Annu* 1996;1046:47.
451. Eisenberger MA, Crawford ED, Wolf M, et al. Prognostic factors in stage D2 prostate cancer; important implications for future trials: results of a Cooperative Intergroup Study (INT 0036). *Semin Oncol* 1994;21:613.
452. Soloway MS, Hardeman SW, Hickey D, et al. Stratification of patients with metastatic prostate cancer based on extent of disease on initial bone scan. *Cancer* 1988;61:195.
453. Crawford ED, Eisenberger MA, McLeod DG, et al. A controlled trial of leuprolide with and without flutamide in prostatic carcinoma. *N Engl J Med* 1989;321:419.
454. Eisenberger MA, Blumenstein BA, Crawford ED, et al. Bilateral orchiectomy with or without flutamide for metastatic prostate cancer. *N Engl J Med* 1998;339:1036.
455. Schellhammer PF, Sharifi R, Block NL, et al. Clinical benefits of bicalutamide (Casodex) compared with flutamide (Eulexin) in combined androgen blockade for patients with advanced prostatic carcinoma: final report of a double-blind, randomized, multicenter trial. *Urology* 1997;50:330.
456. Robinson MRG. A phase-III trial comparing orchidectomy versus orchidectomy and cyproterone acetate and low-dose stilboestrol in the management of metastatic carcinoma of the prostate. In: Smith PH, Pavone-Macaluso M, eds. *Management of advanced cancer of prostate and bladder: EORTC genitourinary group monograph 4.* New York: Alan R. Liss, 1988;101.
457. Anonymous. Treatment and survival of patients with cancer of the prostate. The Veterans Administration cooperative Urological Research Group. *Surg Gynecol Obstet* 1967;124:1011.
458. Byar DP, Corle DK. Hormone therapy for prostate cancer: results of the Veterans Administration Cooperative Urological Research Group Studies. *NCI Monogr* 1988;7:165.
459. Nair B, Wilt T, MacDonald R, Rutks I. Early versus deferred androgen suppression in the treatment of advanced prostate cancer. *Cochrane Database Syst Rev* 2002;1:CD003506.
460. Schellhammer P, Sharifi R, Block N, et al. A controlled trial of bicalutamide versus flutamide, each in combination with luteinizing hormone-relapsing hormone analogue therapy, in patients with advanced prostate cancer. *Urology* 1995;45:745.
460a. Garnick MB, Campion M. Abarelix depot, a GnRH antagonist, v LHRH superagonists in prostate cancer: differential effects on follicle-stimulating hormone. Abarelix Depot study group. *Mol Urol* 2000;4:275.
460b. Trachtenberg J, Gittleman M, Steidle C, et al. A phase 3, multicenter, open label, randomized study of abarelix versus leuprolide plus daily anti-androgen in men with prostate cancer. *J Urol* 2002;167:1670.
461. Labrie F, Dupont A, Belanger A, et al. New approach in the treatment of prostate cancer: complete instead of partial withdrawal of androgens. *Prostate* 1983;4:579.
462. Group PCTC. Maximum androgen blockade in advanced prostate cancer: an overview of 22 randomized trials with 3283 deaths in 5711 patients. *Lancet* 1995;346:265.
463. Bennett CL, Tosteson TD, Schmitt B, et al. Maximum androgen-blockade with medical or surgical castration in advanced prostate cancer: a meta-analysis of nine published randomized controlled trials and 4128 patients using flutamide. *Prostate Cancer Prostatic Dis* 1999;2:4.
464. Caubet J, Tosteson TD, Dong EW, et al. Maximum androgen blockade in advanced prostate cancer: a meta-analysis of published randomized controlled trials using nonsteroidal antiandrogens. *Urology* 1997;49:71.
465. Schmitt B, Bennett C, Seidenfeld J, et al. Maximal androgen blockade for advanced prostate cancer. *Cochrane Database Sys Rev*, 2000.
466. Bayoumi AM, Brown AD, Garber AM. Cost-effectiveness of androgen suppression therapies in advanced prostate cancer. *J Natl Cancer Inst* 2000;92:1731.
467. Samson DJ, Seidenfeld J, Schmitt B, et al. Systematic review and meta-analysis of monotherapy compared with combined androgen blockade for patients with advanced prostate carcinoma. *Cancer* 2002;95:361.
468. Kolvenbag GJCM, Blackledge GRP, Gotting-Smith K. Bicalutamide (Casodex) in the treatment of prostate cancer: history of clinical development. *Prostate* 1998;34:61.
469. Tyrrell CJ, Kaisary AV, Iversen P, et al. A randomized comparison of 'Casodex' (bicalutamide) 150 mg monotherapy versus castration in the treatment of metastatic and locally advanced prostate cancer. *Eur Urol* 1998;33:447.
470. Iversen P, Tyrell CJ, Kaisary AV, et al. Casodex (bicalutamide) 150-mg monotherapy compared with castration in patients with previously untreated nonmetastatic prostate cancer: results from two multicenter randomized trials at a median follow-up of 4 years. *Urology* 1998;51:389.
471. Scher HI, Liebertz C, Kelly WK, et al. Bicalutamide for advanced prostate cancer: the natural vs. treated history of disease. *J Clin Oncol* 1997;15:2928.
471a. National Cancer Institute. Hormone therapy in treating patients with rising PSA levels following radiation therapy for prostate cancer. World Wide Web URL: http://cancer.gov/clinicaltrials, 2004.
471b. National Cancer Institute. Hormone therapy in treating men with stage IV prostate cancer. World Wide Web URL: http://cancer.gov/clinicaltrials, 2004.
472. The Medical Research Council Prostate Cancer Working Party Investigators Group. Immediate versus deferred treatment for advanced prostatic cancer: initial results of the medical research council trial. *Br J Urol* 1997;79:235.
473. See WA, Wirth MP, McLeod DG, et al. Bicalutamide ("Casodex") 150 mg as immediate therapy either alone or as adjuvant to standard care in patients with localized or locally advanced prostate cancer: first analysis of the early prostate cancer program. *J Urol* 2002;168:429.
474. Wirth M, Tyrrell C, Wallace M, et al. Bicalutamide (Casodex) 150 mg as immediate therapy in patients with localized or locally advanced prostate cancer significantly reduces the risk of disease progression. *Urology* 2001;58:146.
475. Gleave ME, Goldenberg SL, Chin JL, et al. Randomized comparative study of 3 versus 8-month neoadjuvant hormonal therapy before radical prostatectomy: biochemical and pathological effects. *J Urol* 2001;166:500.
476. Messing EM, Manola J, Sarosdy M, et al. Immediate hormonal therapy compared with observation after radical prostatectomy and pelvic lymphadenectomy in men with node-positive prostate cancer. *N Engl J Med* 1999;341:1781.
477. Green N, Bodner H, Broth E, et al. Improved control of bulky prostate carcinoma with sequential estrogen and radiation therapy. *Int J Radiat Oncol Biol Phys* 1984;10:971.
478. Sandler HM, Perez-Tamayo C, Ten Haken RK, et al. Dose escalation for stage C (T3) prostate cancer: minimal rectal toxicity observed using conformal therapy. *Radiother Oncol* 1992;23:53.
479. Pollack A, Zagars GK. Androgen ablation in addition to radiation therapy for prostate cancer: is there true benefit? *Semin Radiat Oncol* 1998;8:95.
480. Roach M 3rd, Lu J, Pilepich MV, et al. Predicting long-term survival, and the need for hormonal therapy: a meta-analysis of RTOG prostate cancer trials. *Int J Radiat Oncol Biol Phys* 2000;47:617.
481. Zelefsky MJ, Kelly WK, Scher HI, et al. Results of a phase II study using estramustine phosphate and vinblastine combination and high dose three-dimensional conformal radiotherapy for patients with locally advanced prostate cancer. *J Clin Oncol* 2000;18:1936.
482. Hanks GE, Pajak TF, Porter A, et al. Phase III trial of long-term adjuvant androgen deprivation after neoadjuvant hormonal cytoreduction and radiotherapy in locally advanced carcinoma of the prostate: the Radiation Therapy Oncology Group Protocol 92-02. *J Clin Oncol* 2003;21:3972.
483. Vavassori V, Cozzarini C, Bianchi C, et al. Androgen deprivation and late rectal bleeding after radiotherapy for prostate carcinoma. *Int J Radiat Oncol Biol Phys* 2002;54[Suppl 1]:109 (abst).
484. Liu M, Pickles T, Agranovich A, et al. Impact of neoadjuvant androgen ablation and other factors on late toxicity after external beam prostate radiotherapy. *Int J Radiat Oncol Biol Phys* 2004;58:59.

485. Wilt T, Nair B, MacDonald R, et al. Early versus deferred androgen suppression in the treatment of advanced prostatic cancer (Cochrane Review). In: The Cochrane Library. Chichester, UK: John Wiley & Sons, Ltd, 2004.
486. Peto R. 10-year survival in hormone adjuvant trials of breast and prostate cancer [CD]. *Proc Am Soc Clin Oncol* 2004.
487. Early Breast Cancer Trialists' Collaborative Group. Systemic treatment of early breast cancer by hormonal, cytotoxic, or immune therapy. *Lancet* 1992;339:1.
488. D'Amico AV, Moul JW, Carroll PR, et al. Cancer specific mortality following surgery or radiation for patients with clinically localized prostate cancer managed during the PSA era. *J Natl Cancer Inst* 2003;95:1376.
489. Loblaw DA, Mendelsohn DS, Talcott J, et al. American Society of Clinical Oncology recommendations for the initial hormonal management of androgen-sensitive metastatic, recurrent, or progression prostate cancer. *J Clin Oncol* (*in press*).
490. Minsky BD, Leibel SA. The treatment of hepatic metastases from colorectal cancer with radiation therapy alone or combined with chemotherapy or misonidazole. *Cancer Treat Rev* 1989;16:213.
491. Agus DB, Cordon-Cardo C, Fox W, et al. Prostate cancer cell cycle regulators: response to androgen withdrawal and development of androgen independence. *J Natl Cancer Inst* 1999;91:1869.
492. Taylor CD, Elson P, Trump DL. Importance of continued testicular suppression in hormone-refractory prostate cancer. *J Clin Oncol* 1993;11:2167.
493. Feldman BJ, Feldman D. The development of androgen independent prostate cancer. *Nat Rev Cancer* 2001;1:34.
494. Buchanan G, Greenberg NM, Scher HI, et al. Collocation of androgen receptor gene mutations in prostate cancer. *Clin Cancer Res* 2001;7:1273.
495. Scher HI, Kolvenbag GJ. The antiandrogen withdrawal syndrome in relapsed prostate cancer. *Eur Urol* 1997;31[Suppl 2]:3.
496. Small EJ, Vogelzang NJ. Second-line hormonal therapy for advanced prostate cancer: a shifting paradigm. *J Clin Oncol* 1997;15:382.
497. Joyce R, Fenton MA, Rode P, et al. High dose bicalutamide for androgen independent prostate cancer: effect of prior hormonal therapy. *J Urol* 1998;159:149.
498. Eastham JA, Sartor O. Nilutamide response after flutamide failure in post-orchiectomy progressive prostate cancer. *J Urol* 1998;159:990.
499. Kelly WK, Scher HI. Prostate specific antigen decline after antiandrogen withdrawal: the flutamide withdrawal syndrome. *J Urol* 1993;149:607.
500. Nieh PT. Withdrawal phenomenon with the antiandrogen Casodex. *J Urol* 1995;153:1070.
501. Scher HI, Kelly WK. The flutamide withdrawal syndrome: its impact on clinical trials in hormone-refractory prostate cancer. *J Clin Oncol* 1993;11:1566.
502. Wirth MP, Froschermaier SE. The antiandrogen withdrawal syndrome. *Urol Res* 1997;25 [Suppl 2]:S67.
503. Tassinari D, Fochessati F, Panzini I, et al. Rapid progression of advanced "hormone-resistant" prostate cancer during palliative treatment with progestins for cancer cachexia. *J Pain Symptom Manage* 2003;25:481.
504. Yagoda A, Petrylak DP. Cytotoxic chemotherapy for advanced hormone resistant prostate cancer. *Cancer* 1992.
505. Trump DL, Havlin KH, Messing EM, et al. High-dose ketoconazole in advanced in hormone-refractory prostate cancer: endocrinologic and clinical effects. *J Clin Oncol* 1989;7:1093.
506. Small EJ, Halabi S, Dawson NA, et al. Antiandrogen withdrawal alone or in combination with ketoconazole in androgen-independent prostate cancer patients: a phase III trial (CALGB 9583). *J Clin Oncol* 2004;22:1025.
507. Sarver RG, Dalkin BL, Ahmenn FR. Ketoconazole-induced adrenal crisis in a patient with metastatic prostatic adenocarcinoma: case report and review of the literature. *Urology* 1997;49:781.
508. Tannock I, Gospodarowicz M, Meakin W, et al. Treatment of metastatic prostatic cancer with low-dose prednisone: evaluation of pain and quality of life as pragmatic indices of response. *J Clin Oncol* 1989;7:590.
509. Kantoff PW, Halabi S, Conaway M, et al. Hydrocortisone with or without mitoxantrone in men with hormone-refractory prostate cancer: results of the Cancer and Leukemia Group B 9182 study. *J Clin Oncol* 1999;18:2506.
510. Fakih M, Johnson CS, Trump DL. Glucocorticoids and treatment of prostate cancer: a preclinical and clinical review. *Urology* 2002;60:553.
511. Moore MJ, Osoba D, Murphy D, et al. Use of palliative end points to evaluate the effects of mitoxantrone and low-dose prednisone in patients with hormonally resistant prostate cancer. *J Clin Oncol* 1994;12:689.
512. Tannock IF, Osoba D, Stockler MR, et al. Chemotherapy with mitoxantrone plus prednisone or prednisone alone for symptomatic hormone-resistant prostate cancer: a Canadian randomized trial with palliative end points. *J Clin Oncol* 1996;14:1756.
513. Pienta KJ, Coffey DS. Cell motility as a chemotherapeutic target. In: Isaacs JT, ed. *Prostate cancer.* Cold Spring Harbor Press, 1991;255.
514. Seidman AD, Scher HI, Petrylak D, et al. Estramustine and vinblastine: use of prostate specific antigen as a clinical trial endpoint in hormone-refractory prostatic cancer. *J Urol* 1992;147:931.
515. Kelly WK, Curley T, Slovin S, et al. Paclitaxel, estramustine phosphate, and carboplatin in patients with advanced prostate cancer. *J Clin Oncol* 2001;19:44.
516. Pienta KJ, Fisher EI, Eisenberger MA, et al. A phase II trial of estramustine and etoposide in hormone refractory prostate cancer: a Southwest Oncology Group Trial (SWOG 9407). *Prostate* 2001;46:257.
517. Savarese DM, Halabi S, Hars V, et al. Phase II study of docetaxel, estramustine, and low-dose hydrocortisone in men with hormone-refractory prostate cancer: a final report of CALGB 9780. Cancer and Leukemia Group B. *J Clin Oncol* 2001;19:2509.
518. Petrylak DP, MacArthur RB, O'Connor J, et al. Phase I trial of docetaxel with estramustine in androgen-independent prostate cancer. *J Clin Oncol* 1999;17:958.
519. Eisenberger MA, Simon R, O'Dwyer PJ, et al. A reevaluation of nonhormonal cytotoxic chemotherapy in the treatment of prostatic carcinoma. *J Clin Oncol* 1985;3:827.
520. Dexeus F, Logothetis CJ, Samuels ML, et al. Continuous infusion of vinblastine for advanced hormone- refractory prostate cancer. *Cancer Treat Rep* 1985;69:885.
521. Hudes GR, Greenberg R, Krigel RL, et al. Phase II study of estramustine and vinblastine, two microtubule inhibitors, in hormone-refractory prostate cancer. *J Clin Oncol* 1992;10:1754.
522. Hudes G, Einhorn L, Ross E, et al. Vinblastine versus vinblastine plus oral estramustine phosphate for patients with hormone-refractory prostate cancer: a Hoosier Group and Fox Chase Network phase III trial. *J Clin Oncol* 1999;17:3160.
523. Hudes G, Ross E, Roth B, et al. Improved survival for patients with hormone-refractory prostate cancer receiving estramustine-based antimicrotubule therapy: final report of a Hoosier Oncology Group and Fox Chase Network phase III trial comparing vinblastine and vinblastine plus oral estramustine. *Proc Am Soc Clin Oncol* 2002;21:177a.
524. Pienta KJ, Redman BG, Bandekar R, et al. A phase II trial of oral estramustine and oral etoposide in hormone refractory prostate cancer. *Urology* 1997;50:401.
525. Hussain MH, Pienta KJ, Redman BG, et al. Oral etoposide in the treatment of hormone-refractory prostate cancer. *Cancer* 1994;74:100.
526. Fields-Jones S, Koletsky A, Wilding G, et al. Improvements in clinical benefit with vinorelbine in the treatment of hormone-refractory prostate cancer: a phase II trial. *Ann Oncol* 1999;10:1307.
527. Fields S, Burris H, Wilding G, et al. Evaluating the role of Navelbine in hormone refractory prostate cancer: a clinical benefit model. *Proc Am Soc Clin Oncol* 1994;13:727.
528. Roth B, Yeap B, Wilding G, et al. Taxol (NSC 125973) in advanced, hormone-refractory prostate cancer: an ECOG phase II trial. *Proc Am Soc Clin Oncol* 1992;11:196.
529. Hudes GR, Nathan F, Khater C, et al. Phase II trial of 96-hour paclitaxel plus oral estramustine phosphate in metastatic hormone-refractory prostate cancer. *J Clin Oncol* 1997;15:3156.
530. Berry W, Gregurich M, Dakhil S, et al. Phase II randomized trial of weekly paclitaxel (Taxol) with or without estramustine phosphate in patients with symptomatic, hormone-refractory, metastatic carcinoma of the prostate (HRMCP). *Proc Am Soc Clin Oncol* 2001;20:175a (abst 696).
531. Picus J, Schultz M. Docetaxel (Taxotere) as monotherapy in the treatment of hormone-refractory prostate cancer: preliminary results. *Semin Oncol* 1999;26:14.
532. Berry W, Dakhil S, Gregurich MA, et al. Phase II trial of single-agent weekly docetaxel in hormone-refractory, symptomatic, metastatic carcinoma of the prostate. *Semin Oncol* 2001;28:8.
533. Beer TM, Pierce WC, Lowe BA, et al. Phase II study of weekly docetaxel in symptomatic androgen-independent prostate cancer. *Ann Oncol* 2001;12:1273.
534. Sinibaldi VJ, Carducci MA, Moore-Cooper S, et al. Phase II evaluation of docetaxel plus one-day oral estramustine phosphate in the treatment of patients with androgen independent prostate carcinoma. *Cancer* 2002;94:1457.
535. Eisenberger MA, de Wit R, Berry W, et al. A multicenter phase III comparison of docetaxel (D) + mitoxantrone (P) in patients with hormone-refractory prostate cancer (HRPC). *Proc Am Soc Clin Oncol* 2004;(abst 4).
536. Petrylak DF, Tangen C, Hussain M, et al. SWOG 99-16: randomized phase III trial of docetaxel (D)/estramustine (E) versus mitoxantrone (M)/prednisone (P) in men with androgen dependent prostate cancer (AIPCA). *Proc Am Soc Clin Oncol* 2004;(abst 3).
537. Cousin G, Ilankovan V. Mental nerve anesthesia as a result of mandibular metastases of prostate cancer. *Br Dent J* 1994;177:382.
538. Porter A, Order S, Caplan R, et al. Report of a multi-institutional phase I/II study to evaluate the use of strontium therapy in metastatic prostate cancer. Radiation therapy oncology group. *Proc Am Soc Clin Oncol* 1994;13:1540.
539. Quilty PM, Kirk D, Bolger JJ, et al. A comparison of the palliative effects of strontium-89 and external beam radiotherapy in metastatic prostate cancer. *Radiother Oncol* 1994;31:33.
540. Serafini AN, Houston SJ, Resche I, et al. Palliation of pain associated with metastatic bone cancer using samarium-153 lexidronam: a double-blind placebo-controlled clinical trial. *J Clin Oncol* 1998;16:1574.
541. Eary JF, Collins C, Stabin M, et al. Samarium-153-EDTMP biodistribution and dosimetry estimation. *J Nucl Med* 1993;34(7):1031.
542. Logan KW, Volkert WA, Holmes RA. Radiation dose calculations in persons receiving injection of samarium-153 EDTMP. *J Nucl Med* 1987;28:505.
543. Porter AT, McEwan AJ, Powe JE, et al. Results of a randomized phase III trial to evaluate the efficacy of strontium-89 adjuvant to local field external beam irradiation in the management of endocrine resistant metastatic prostate cancer. *Int J Radiat Oncol Biol Phys* 1993;25:805.
544. Serafini AN. Therapy of metastatic bone pain. *J Nucl Med* 2001;42:895.
545. Tu SM, Millikan RE, Mengistu B, et al. Bone-targeted therapy for advanced androgen-independent carcinoma of the prostate: a randomised phase II trial. *Lancet* 2001;357:336.
546. Smith MR, Eastham J, Gleason DM, et al. Randomized controlled trial of zoledronic acid to prevent bone loss in men receiving androgen deprivation therapy for nonmetastatic prostate cancer. *J Urol* 2003;169:2008.
547. Smith MR, McGovern FJ, Zietman AL, et al. Pamidronate to prevent bone loss during androgen-deprivation therapy for prostate cancer. *N Engl J Med* 2001;345:948.
548. Small EJ, Smith MR, Seaman JJ, et al. Combined analysis of two multicenter, randomized, placebo-controlled studies of pamidronate disodium for the palliation of bone pain in men with metastatic prostate cancer. *J Clin Oncol* 2003;21:4277.
549. Fred S, Gleason D, Murray R, et al. Zoledronic acid significantly reduces fractures in patients with hormone-refractory prostate cancer metastatic to bone. *J Urol* 2002;167:(abst703).
550. Ernst DS, Tannock IF, Winquist EW, et al. Randomized, double-blind, controlled trial of mitoxantrone/prednisone and clodronate versus mitoxantrone/prednisone and placebo in patients with hormone-refractory prostate cancer and pain. *J Clin Oncol* 2003;21:3335.
551. Nelson JB, Hedican SP, George DJ, et al. Identification of endothelin-1 in the pathophysiology of metastatic adenocarcinoma of the prostate. *Nat Med* 1995;1:944.
552. Nelson JB, Nabulsi AA, Vogelzang NJ, et al. Suppression of prostate cancer induced bone remodeling by the endothelin receptor A antagonist atrasentan. *J Urol* 2003;169:1143.

553. Nelson JB, Carducci MA, Padley RJ, et al. The endothelin-A receptor antagonist atrasentan (ABT_627) reduces skeletal remodeling activity in men with advanced, hormone refractory prostate cancer. *Proc Am Soc Clin Oncol* 2000;19(abst12).

553a. Papandreou CN, Daliani DD, Nix D, et al. Phase I trial of the proteasome inhibitor bortezomib in patients with advanced solid tumors with observations in androgen-independent prostate cancer. *J Clin Oncol* 2004;22:2108.

554. Carducci MA, Nelson JB, Bowling MK, et al. Atrasentan, an endothelin-receptor antagonist for refractory adenocarcinomas: safety and pharmacokinetics. *J Clin Oncol* 2002;20:2171.

555. Oh W, Halabi S, Kelly WK, et al. A phase II study of estramustine, docetaxel, and carboplatin (EDC) with G-CSF support in men with hormone-refractory prostate cancer (HRPC): CALGB 99813. *Proc Am Soc Clin Oncol* 2002;21:195a.

556. Smith DC, Esper PS, Todd RF III, et al. Paclitaxel, estramustine, and etoposide in patients with hormone-refractory prostate cancer (HRPC): a phase II trial. *Proc Am Soc Clin Oncol* 1997;16:310a.

557. Millikan R, Thall PF, Lee SJ, et al. Randomized, multicenter, phase II trial of two multicomponent regimens in androgen-independent prostate cancer. *J Clin Oncol* 2003;21:878.

558. Sepp-Lorenzino L, Balog A, Su DS, et al. The microtubule-stabilizing agents epothilones A and B and their desoxy-derivatives induce mitotic arrest and apoptosis in human prostate cancer cells. *Prostate Cancer Prostatic Dis* 1999;2:41.

559. Smaletz O, Galsky M, Scher HI, et al. Phase I study of epothilone B analogue (BMS-247550) and estramustine phosphate in patients with progressive metastatic prostate cancer following castration. *Ann Oncol* 2004 (*in press*).

560. Kelly WK, Galsky MD, Small E, et al. Multi-institutional trial of epothilone B analogue (BMS-247550) with or without estramustine phosphate (EMP) in patients with progressive castrate-metastatic prostate cancer (PCMPC). *Proc Am Soc Clin Oncol* 2003;22:394 (abst1584).

561. Getzenberg RH, Light BW, Lapco PE, et al. Vitamin D inhibition of prostate adenocarcinoma growth and metastasis in the Dunning rat prostate model system. *Urology* 1997;50:999.

562. Rao A, Coan A, Welsh JE, et al. Vitamin D receptor and p21/WAF1 are targets of genistein and 1,25-dihydroxyvitamin D3 in human prostate cancer cells. *Cancer Res* 2004;64:2143.

563. Yu WD, McElwain MC, Modzelewski RA, et al. Enhancement of 1,2-dihydroxyvitamin D3-mediated antitumor activity with dexamethasone. *J Natl Cancer Inst* 1998;90:134.

564. Smith DC, Johnson CS, Freeman CC, et al. A phase I trial of calcitriol (1,25-dihydroxycholecalciferol) in patients with advanced malignancy. *Clin Cancer Res* 1999;5:1339.

565. Beer TM. Development of weekly high-dose calcitriol based therapy for prostate cancer. *Urol Oncol* 2003;21:400.

566. Beer TM, Eilers KM, Garzotto M, et al. Weekly high-dose calcitriol and docetaxel in metastatic androgen-independent prostate cancer. *J Clin Oncol* 2003;21:123.

567. McDonnell TJ, Troncoso P, Brisbay SM, et al. Expression of the protooncogene bcl-2 in the prostate and its association with emergence of androgen-independent prostate cancer. *Cancer Res* 1992;52:6940.

568. Morris MJ, Tong WP, Cordon-Cardo C, et al. Phase I trial of BCL-2 antisense oligonucleotide (G3139) administered by continuous intravenous infusion in patients with advanced cancer. *Clin Cancer Res* 2002;8:679.

569. Tolcher AW. Preliminary phase I results of G3139 (bcl-2 antisense oligonucleotide) therapy in combination with docetaxel in hormone-refractory prostate cancer. *Semin Oncol* 2001;28:67.

570. Weidner N, Carrol PR, Flax J, et al. Tumor angiogenesis correlates with metastasis in invasive prostate carcinoma. *Am J Pathol* 1993;143:401.

571. Figg WD, Dahut W, Duray P, et al. A randomized phase II trial of thalidomide, an angiogenesis inhibitor, in patients with androgen-independent prostate cancer. *Clin Cancer Res* 2001;7:1888.

572. Fox WD, Higgins B, Maiese KM, et al. Antibody to vascular endothelial growth factor slows growth of an androgen-independent xenograft model of prostate cancer. *Clin Cancer Res* 2002;8:3226.

573. George DJ, Halabi S, Shepard TF, et al. Prognostic significance of plasma vascular endothelial growth factor levels in patients with hormone-refractory prostate cancer treated on Cancer and Leukemia Group B 9480. *Clin Cancer Res* 2001;7:1932.

574. Morris MJ, Reuter VE, Kelly WK, et al. HER-2 profiling and targeting in prostate carcinoma. *Cancer* 2002;94:980.

575. Blackledge G. Growth factor receptor tyrosine kinase inhibitors; clinical development and potential for prostate cancer therapy. *J Urol* 2003;170:S77.

576. Solit DB, Scher HI, Rosen N. Hsp90 as a therapeutic target in prostate cancer. *Semin Oncol* 2003;30:709.

577. Solit DB, Basso AD, Olshen AB, et al. Inhibition of heat shock protein 90 function down-regulates Akt kinase and sensitizes tumors to Taxol. *Cancer Res* 2003;63:2139.

578. Singh D, Febbo PG, Ross K, et al. Gene expression correlates of clinical prostate cancer behavior. *Cancer Cell* 2002;1:203.

579. Estey EH, Thall PF. New designs for phase 2 clinical trials. *Blood* 2003;102:442.

580. Verbel DA, Kelly WK, Smaletz O, et al. Estimating survival benefit in castrate metastatic prostate cancer: decision making in proceeding to a definitive phase III trial. *Urology* 2003;61:142.

581. Fazzari M, Heller G, Scher HI. The phase II/III transition (phase IIb): toward the proof of efficacy in cancer clinical trials. *Control Clin Trials* 2000;21:360.

582. Scher HI, Heller G. Picking the winners in a sea of plenty. *Clin Cancer Res* 2002;8:400.

583. Thall PF, Millikan RE, Sung H-G. Evaluating multiple treatment courses in clinical trials. *Stat Med* 2000;19:1011.

584. Moertel CG, Fleming TR, Macdonald JS, et al. Levamisole and fluorouracil for adjuvant therapy of resected colon carcinoma. *N Engl J Med* 1990;322:352.

585. Combination adjuvant chemotherapy for node-positive breast cancer. *N Engl J Med* 1988;319:677.

586. Khil MS, Kim JH, Bricker LJ, et al. Tumor cancer of locally advanced prostate cancer following combined estramustine, vinblastine, and radiation therapy. *Cancer J Sci Am* 1997;3:289.

587. Pettaway CA, Pisters LL, Troncoso P, et al. Neoadjuvant chemotherapy and hormonal therapy followed by radical prostatectomy: feasibility and preliminary results. *J Clin Oncol* 2000;18:1050.

588. Solit DB, Kelly WK, Fallon M, et al. Phase I/II study of intravenous (IV) estramustine (EMP), paclitaxel and carboplatin, (Hi-Tec) in patients with castrate, metastatic prostate cancer. *Proc Am Soc Clin Oncol* 2001;20;184a (abst735).

589. Partin AW, Piantadosi S, Sanda MG, et al. Selection of men at high risk for disease recurrence for experimental adjuvant therapy following radical prostatectomy. *Urology* 1999;45:831.

590. Munshi HG, Pienta KJ, Smith DC. Chemotherapy in patients with prostate specific antigen-only disease after primary therapy for prostate carcinoma: a phase II trial of oral estramustine and oral etoposide. *Cancer* 2001;91:2175.

591. Taplin ME, Bubley GJ, Rajeshkumar B, et al. Docetaxel, estramustine, and short-term androgen withdrawal for patients with biochemical failure after definitive local therapy for prostate cancer. *Semin Oncol* 2001;28:32.

592. Nordquist LT, Morris MM, Sauter N, et al. Rapid hormone cycling for prostate cancer (PC) patients: the MENS cycle. *Proc Am Soc Clin Oncol* 2003;22:415 (abst1669).

593. Hussain A, Dawson N, Amin P, et al. Docetaxel followed by hormone therapy after failure of definitive treatments for clinically localized/locally advanced prostate cancer: preliminary results. *Semin Oncol* 2001;28:22.

594. Pienta KJ, P-0014 RTOG. Radiation Therapy Oncology Group P-0014: a phase 3 randomized study of patients with high-risk hormone-naive prostate cancer: androgen blockade with 4 cycles of immediate chemotherapy versus androgen blockade with delayed chemotherapy. *Urology* 2003;62[Suppl 1]:95.

595. Slovin SF, Kelly WK, Scher HI. Immunological approaches for the treatment of prostate cancer. *Semin Urol Oncol* 1998;16:53.

596. Egen JG, Kuhns MS, Allison JP. CTLA-4: new insights into its biological function and use in tumor immunotherapy. *Nat Immunol* 2002;3:611.

597. Chang SS, Reuter VE, Heston DWD, et al. Five different anti-prostate-specific membrane antigen (PSMA) antibodies confirm PSMA expression in tumor-associated neovasculature. *Cancer Res* 1999;59:3192.

598. Bander NH, Trabulsi EJ, Kostakoglu L, et al. Targeting metastatic prostate cancer with radiolabeled monoclonal antibody J591 to the extracellular domain of prostate specific membrane antigen. *J Urol* 2003;170:1717.

598a. Galsky M, Eisenberger M, Moore-Cooper S, et al. Phase I trial of MLN2704, a PSMA antibody targeted chemotherapeutic, in patients with castrate-metastatic prostate cancer (CMPC). Submitted *Proc Am Soc Clin Oncol* 2004.

599. Murphy GP, Tjoa BA, Simmons SJ, et al. Infusion of dendritic cells pulsed with HLA-A2-specific prostate-specific membrane antigen peptides: a phase II prostate cancer vaccine trial involving patients with hormone-refractory metastatic disease. *Prostate* 1999;38:73.

600. Gulley J, Dahut WL. Novel approaches to treating the asymptomatic hormone-refractory prostate cancer patient. *Urology* 2003;62[Suppl 1]:147.

601. Gulley J, Chen AP, Dahut W, et al. Phase I study of a vaccine using recombinant vaccinia virus expressing PSA (rV-PSA) in patients with metastatic androgen-independent prostate cancer. *Prostate* 2002;53:109.

602. Burch PA, Breen JK, Buckner JC, et al. Priming tissue-specific cellular immunity in a phase I trial of autologous dendritic cells for prostate cancer. *Clin Cancer Res* 2000;6:2175.

603. Small EJ, Rini B, Higano C, et al. A randomized placebo-controlled phase III trial of APC8015 in patients with androgen-independent prostate cancer (AiPCa). *Proc Am Soc Clin Oncol* 2003;22:382 (abst).

604. Small EJ, Fratesi P, Reese DM, et al. Immunotherapy of hormone-refractory prostate cancer with antigen-loaded dendritic cells. *J Clin Oncol* 2000;18:3894.

605. DeWeese TL, van der Poel H, Li S, et al. A phase I trial of CV706, a replication-competent, PSA selective oncolytic adenovirus, for the treatment of locally recurrent prostate cancer following radiation therapy. *Cancer Res* 2001;61:7464.

606. Dummer R. GVAX (Cell Genesys). *Curr Opin Investig Drugs* 2001;2:844.

607. Kelly WK, Richon VM, Troso-Sandoval T, et al. Suberoylanilide hydroxamic acid (SAHA), a histone deacetylase inhibitor: biologic activity without toxicity. *Proc Am Soc Clin Oncol* 2001;20:87a (abst344).

608. Carducci MA, Nelson JB, Chan-Tack KM, et al. Phenylbutyrate induces apoptosis in human prostate cancer and is more potent than phenylacetate. *Clin Ca Research* 1996;2:379.

609. Galsky M, Kelly WK. The development of differentiation agents for the treatment of prostate cancer. *Semin Oncol* 2003;30:689.

610. Leibowitz SB, Kantoff PW. Differentiating agents and the treatment of prostate cancer: vitamin D3 and peroxisome proliferator-activated receptor gamma ligands. *Semin Oncol* 2003;30:698.

611. Feifer AH, Fleshner NE, Klotz L. Analytical accuracy and reliability of commonly used nutritional supplements in prostate disease. *J Urol* 2002;168:150.

612. Garbisa S, Biggin S, Cavallarin N, et al. Tumor invasion: molecular shears blunted by green tea. *Nat Med* 1999;5:1216.

613. Jatoi A, Ellison N, Burch PA, et al. A phase II trial of green tea in the treatment of patients with androgen independent metastatic prostate carcinoma. *Cancer* 2003;97:1442.

614. Jenkins DJ, Kendall CW, D'Costa MA, et al. Soy consumption and phytoestrogens: effect on serum prostate specific antigen when blood lipids and oxidized low-density lipoprotein are reduced in hyperlipidemic men. *J Urol* 2003;169:507.

615. Marks LS, DiPaola RS, Nelson P, et al. PC-SPES: herbal formulation for prostate cancer. *Urology* 2002;60:369.

616. Sovak M, Seligson AL, Konas M, et al. Herbal composition PC-SPES for management of prostate cancer: identification of active principles. *J Natl Cancer Inst* 2002;94:1275.

617. Skinner EC, Glode LM. High-risk localized prostate cancer: primary surgery and adjuvant therapy. *Urol Oncol* 2003;21:219.

618. Halabi S, Small EJ, Kantoff PW, et al. Prognostic model for predicting survival in men with hormone-refractory metastatic prostate cancer. *J Clin Oncol* 2003;21:1232.

SANJAY RAZDAN
LEONARD G. GOMELLA

SECTION **4**

Cancer of the Urethra and Penis

Penile and urethral carcinomas are uncommon malignancies with a peak incidence in the sixth decade of life. Often overshadowed by more common genitourinary cancers, such as prostate, testicular, and kidney cancers, penile and urethral cancers represent difficult treatment challenges for the treating physician. *Squamous cell carcinoma* is the most frequent histologic type of cancer in the penis and the urethra. Carcinoma of the penis is a slow-growing tumor with a well-defined pattern of dissemination, first to the inguinal lymph nodes and subsequently to the pelvic nodes. Distant spread is a late feature. This propensity of penile cancer to spread in an orderly fashion permits definitive local-regional management of the primary tumor in the majority of cases. In contradistinction, urethral carcinoma in men and in women tends to invade locally and metastasize to regional nodes early in its evolution. Depending on the site of the urethra involved and the extent of disease, a multimodal treatment approach using a combination of chemotherapy, radiation, and surgery may be required to treat this aggressive tumor.[1]

CANCER OF THE MALE URETHRA

Carcinoma of the male urethra is an uncommon malignancy. Chronic irritation and infection are the strongest associated risk factors for the development of urethral cancer. The incidence of urethral stricture in men with subsequent development of urethral cancer ranges from 24% to 76%, and most of these strictures involve the bulbomembranous urethra, which is also the most frequent portion of the urethra to be involved by tumor.[2] *Human papillomavirus-16* (HPV-16) likely has a causative role in the development of squamous cell carcinoma of the urethra.[3] No racial predisposition has been noted.

The onset of malignancy in a patient with a long-standing history of urethral stricture disease is often insidious, and a high index of suspicion is needed to diagnose these tumors early. The new onset of urethrorrhagia or urethral stricture in a man without a history of trauma or venereal disease should raise the possibility of urethral carcinoma. A palpable urethral mass associated with obstructive voiding symptoms is the most common presenting symptom.[4] Pain associated with a periurethral abscess or urethral fistula on occasion may be the harbinger of a male urethral cancer.

PATHOLOGY

Overall, 80% of male urethral cancers are squamous cell, 15% are transitional cell, and approximately 5% are adenocarcinomas or undifferentiated tumors.[5] The anatomic location of urethral cancer largely determines the histologic type of cancer. Carcinomas of the prostatic urethra are transitional cell in 90%

and squamous in 10%; conversely, carcinomas of the penile urethra are squamous in 90% and transitional in 10%. Carcinomas of the bulbomembranous urethra are squamous in 80%, transitional cell in 10%, and adenocarcinomas or undifferentiated in 10%.[6]

The *bulbomembranous urethra* is most commonly involved (60%), followed by the penile urethra (30%) and the prostatic urethra (10%). The incidence of urethral involvement associated with carcinoma of the bladder has been estimated to be approximately 6%,[7] and urethral recurrences after radical cystectomy occur in 4% to 18%.[8]

Male urethral cancer may spread locally to involve the vascular spaces of the corpus spongiosum, or it may metastasize to involve regional lymph nodes. The lymphatics of the anterior urethra drain into the superficial and deep inguinal lymph nodes and occasionally to the external iliac nodes. The lymphatics from the posterior urethra drain into the external iliac, obturator, and hypogastric nodes. Palpable inguinal nodes are found in approximately 20% of patients with urethral cancer at presentation and are almost always suggestive of metastatic disease. This is in contrast to penile cancer, in which almost 50% of palpable inguinal nodes are inflammatory. Bulbomembranous urethral cancer in particular spreads to the urogenital diaphragm, prostate, perineum, and scrotum. Hematogenous spread is rare except in advanced disease and in primary transitional cell carcinoma of the prostatic urethra.

EVALUATION AND STAGING

The American Joint Committee on Cancer (AJCC) tumor, node, metastasis (TNM) staging system (sixth edition, 2002) is based on the depth of invasion of the primary tumor and the presence or absence of regional lymph node involvement and distant metastasis (Table 30.4-1). A complete history and physical examination are essential in all patients. Examination under anesthesia with a digital rectal examination is useful in evaluating the local extent of disease. Cystoscopy and transurethral or needle biopsy of the lesion, and of the prostate if indicated, is also performed at the time of examination under anesthesia. A com-

TABLE 30.4-1.   American Joint Committee on Cancer Tumor, Node, Metastasis Classification System for Urethral Cancer

Stage Grouping			
Stage 0a	Ta	N0	M0
Stage 0is	Tis	N0	M0
	Tis pu	N0	M0
	Tis pd	N0	M0
Stage I	T1	N0	M0
Stage II	T2	N0	M0
Stage III	T1	N1	M0
	T2	N1	M0
	T3	N0	M0
	T4	N1	M0
Stage IV	T4	N0	M0
	T4	N1	M0
	Any T	N2	M0
	Any T	Any N	M1

(From AJCC. *Cancer staging manual*, 6th ed. New York: Springer-Verlag, 2002, with permission.)

plete blood count and serum chemistry coupled with urine culture and cytology are routinely obtained. Cytology is particularly helpful in patients with transitional cell carcinoma. A computed tomography (CT) scan with contrast is useful in local staging. However, a magnetic resonance imaging (MRI) scan with gadolinium is the ideal staging modality for evaluating local soft tissue, lymph node, and bone involvement.[9]

TREATMENT

Surgery forms the mainstay for treatment of carcinoma of the male urethra. In general, anterior urethral cancers are more amenable to surgical extirpation, and the prognosis is better than that of posterior urethral tumors, which are more often associated with extensive local invasion and distant metastasis.[10] Radiation therapy is reserved for selected patients with early-stage lesions of the anterior urethra who refuse surgery. Although it preserves the penis, radiation therapy may cause urethral stricture or chronic penile edema and may not prevent new tumor occurrence in the retained urethra. Multimodal treatment combining chemotherapy and radiation therapy with surgical excision for locally advanced urethral carcinomas has yielded promising results, with a disease-free survival rate of 60% in one series.[11] The median survival without treatment or with palliation is approximately 3 months.

Site-Specific Treatment

CARCINOMA OF THE DISTAL URETHRA

Superficial tumors (Ta, Tis, and T1) are adequately treated with transurethral resection and fulguration. Tumors invading the corpus spongiosum (T2) and localized to the distal half of the penis are best treated with a partial amputation with a 2-cm margin proximal to the visible or palpable tumor. If infiltrating tumor is confined to the proximal penile urethra or involves the entire urethra, total penectomy is indicated. Isolated reports of penile-sparing surgery alone consisting of urethrectomy with sparing of the corpora cavernosa have been complicated by a high incidence of local failure and distant relapse.[12] Ilioinguinal node dissection is indicated only in the presence of palpable adenopathy. Prophylactic groin dissection has no proven role in this disease site.

CARCINOMA OF THE BULBOMEMBRANOUS URETHRA.

Early superficial tumors (Ta, Tis, and T1) can be adequately treated with transurethral fulguration or segmental resection with end-to-end anastomosis; however, such cases are rare. Invasive tumors (T2, T3) are best treated with radical surgery, which usually entails a radical cystoprostatectomy with *en bloc* penectomy and pelvic lymphadenectomy. In spite of this aggressive approach, the prognosis remains dismal, with a 5-year disease-free survival of 25% in patients with invasive bulbomembranous carcinomas.[13] Isolated reports of penile preservation surgery for invasive bulbomembranous cancers have used adjuvant radiation therapy (45 Gy) and concurrent chemotherapy with 5-fluorouracil (5-FU) and mitomycin C with acceptable results.[14] Chemotherapy given concomitantly with radiation acts as a radiosensitizer and interferes with cell repair after a sublethal radiation dose.

CARCINOMA OF THE PROSTATIC URETHRA.

Primary carcinoma arising from the prostatic urethra is rare. Adenocarcinomas and transitional cell carcinomas are found. Although superficial lesions (Tis-pu, Tis-pd, T1) of the prostatic urethra can be managed by transurethral resection, such tumors are rare. Invasive transitional cell carcinoma of the prostatic stroma (T2) carries a dismal prognosis in spite of radical cystoprostatectomy and total urethrectomy, which is the treatment of choice. The overall survival is 6% to 26%.[15]

Advanced carcinoma (T3T4N1 to N3) of the prostatic urethra is best treated with a combination of neoadjuvant chemotherapy [methotrexate sodium, vinblastine sulfate, doxorubicin hydrochloride (Adriamycin), and cisplatin (M-VAC)] followed by surgery or irradiation. At Memorial Sloan-Kettering Cancer Center (MSKCC), five patients with stages T2T4N0M0 tumors of the prostatic urethra received one to four cycles of neoadjuvant M-VAC chemotherapy.[16] A clinical complete remission was obtained in three of five patients (60%) with transitional cell tumors of the prostate and prostatic urethra. The experience at MSKCC has shown that M-VAC chemotherapy preoperatively was ineffective against nontransitional cell carcinoma.

Radiation and Multimodal Therapy

Radiation therapy alone has yielded poor results in the management of male urethral carcinoma. Patients who receive radiation therapy followed by salvage surgery seem to fare worse than if surgery was performed in integrated fashion. The most common approach has been external-beam radiotherapy of 50 to 60 Gy over 6 weeks. Long-term results with radiotherapy have been best with *distal* urethral lesions.

Multimodal therapy with chemoradiation has shown the efficacy of 5-FU, mitomycin C, and cisplatin along with external-beam radiation for squamous cell carcinoma of the urethra.[17,18] Combining both modalities is conceptually appealing and is expected to lead to a better outcome.

CARCINOMA OF THE FEMALE URETHRA

Carcinoma of the female urethra is the only genitourinary neoplasm that is more common in women than in men (4:1 ratio). The peak incidence is in the sixth decade, with a predilection for white women as compared to blacks.

Chronic irritation, recurrent urinary tract infections, and a host of proliferative lesions, such as caruncles, papillomas, and polyps, are predisposing factors. The HPV may play a role in the development of female urethral carcinoma. Leukoplakia of the urethra is considered a premalignant condition. In females the urethra is approximately 4 cm long, and most of it is buried in the anterior vaginal wall. The urethra is divided into the distal one-third (anterior urethra) and the proximal two-thirds (posterior urethra).

The most common presenting symptom is urethrorrhagia, seen in more than half the patients. Urinary frequency, obstructive voiding, and a palpable urethral mass are other modes of presentation. Ulcerative lesions may produce a foul-smelling discharge. It may be difficult on initial examination to distinguish fungating tumors of the urethra from those of the vagina or vulva.

Spread of urethral carcinoma follows the anatomic subdivision. Although lymphatics of the anterior urethra drain into the superficial and deep inguinal nodes, the posterior urethra drains into the external iliac, hypogastric, and obturator lymph nodes. At presentation, one-third of patients have inguinal lymph node metastases, and 20% have pelvic node involvement. Unlike the situation in patients with penile carcinoma, palpable inguinal nodes in patients with urethral cancer invariably contain metastatic carcinoma. The most common sites of distant spread are the lungs, liver, and bone.[19]

PATHOLOGY

Stratified squamous epithelium lines the distal two-thirds of the female urethra, and transitional epithelium lines the proximal one-third. The majority (60%) of neoplasms of the female urethra are squamous cell carcinomas. Other less common histologies are transitional cell carcinoma (20%), adenocarcinoma (10%), undifferentiated tumors (8%), and melanoma (2%). Clear cell carcinoma is a distinctive clinical entity that has generated considerable interest with respect to its prognosis and relationship to urethral diverticulae.[20] Histology does not affect the prognosis, and therefore different histologic types are treated similarly. In general, carcinomas of the anterior urethra are low grade and low stage, whereas carcinomas involving the proximal or entire urethra are of a higher grade and stage.

EVALUATION AND STAGING

The workup for women with suspected urethral carcinoma includes a pelvic examination under anesthesia, cystourethroscopy, and biopsy. Radiographic evaluation includes a chest x-ray and CT of the pelvis and abdomen. MRI is particularly useful for staging of female urethral carcinoma.

The AJCC (6th edition) TNM staging has been adapted to female urethral cancer. The practical usefulness of this staging, however, is somewhat limited. On a clinical basis, it is more useful to stage, treat, and prognosticate female urethral cancers by dividing them into anterior and low-stage versus posterior or entire urethra and advanced stage.[21]

TREATMENT

The anatomic location and stage of the tumor are the most significant prognostic factors predicting local control and survival. Treatment is based on the stage at the time of initial presentation, with low-stage distal urethral tumors having a better prognosis than high-stage proximal urethral tumors. In the series of Dalbagni et al.,[22] the 5-year disease-specific survival was 46% overall, with 89% survival for low-stage tumors compared to 33% for high-stage disease.

Surgery in the form of local excision is often sufficient in selected patients with low-stage carcinoma of the distal urethra. For tumors involving the proximal urethra and for bulky locally advanced tumors, more aggressive treatment with an anterior pelvic exenteration is often needed. This treatment entails *en bloc* total urethrectomy, cystectomy with pelvic lymphadenectomy, hysterectomy with salpingectomy, and removal of the anterior wall of the vagina. Bulky tumors of the proximal urethra invading the pubic symphysis may require resection of the pubic symphysis and inferior rami. Anterior exenteration alone, however, has been reported to produce a 5-year survival rate of less than 20% in patients with invasive carcinoma of the female urethra, with a local recurrence rate of 67%.[23]

Radiation therapy is an alternative to local surgery for patients with low-stage urethral carcinoma. In such individuals, definitive radiation therapy with brachytherapy alone or combined with external-beam radiation has yielded cure rates of up to 75%. The doses in various series have ranged from 50 to 60 Gy for brachytherapy alone and 40 to 45 Gy external-beam radiation to the whole pelvis followed by a brachytherapy boost of 20 to 25 Gy over 2 to 3 days. Proximal urethral tumors with bladder neck invasion and bulky tumors require combined external-beam and brachytherapy. Large primary tumor bulk and treatment with external radiation alone (no brachytherapy) were independent adverse prognostic factors. Brachytherapy reduced the risk of local recurrence by a factor of 4.2 in one series, possibly as a result of the higher radiation dose that could be safely delivered.[24] Complications from radiation therapy occur in an average of 20% of patients and include urethral strictures and stenosis, urethrovaginal fistulas, incontinence, and bowel obstruction.

Combined modality treatment with neoadjuvant chemotherapy and preoperative radiation therapy, followed by surgery, is recommended for advanced female urethral carcinoma. In a compilation of data, Narayan and Konety[25] reported a 55% survival rate in patients with advanced urethral carcinoma treated with radiotherapy plus surgery, as compared to a rate of 34% with radiation alone. In advanced urethral carcinoma the current treatment policy at MSKCC is to deliver M-VAC chemotherapy and radiation, followed by surgery for patients with transitional cell carcinomas. Patients with squamous cell carcinoma receive combined mitomycin C and 5-FU and preoperative radiation, followed by surgery. Although long-term results from multimodal therapy are as yet unavailable, a combination of chemotherapy, irradiation, and surgery is strongly believed to be essential for local control and cure of women with larger or locally advanced urethral cancer.[22]

The overall prognosis for women with carcinoma of the urethra is poor regardless of the treatment modality used, and the median time to local recurrence for invasive carcinoma is 13 months. The majority relapse by 16 months.

Distal Urethral Carcinoma

Small superficial (Ta, Tis, and T1) tumors of the distal urethra can be safely removed surgically with little risk of urinary incontinence. Spatulation of the urethra and approximation to the adjacent vagina preserve urinary continence and prevent meatal stenosis. For small invasive tumors of the distal urethra (T2), brachytherapy alone is an excellent therapeutic option.

Proximal Urethral Carcinoma

Proximal urethral carcinoma tumors tend to be more aggressive and bulky. For advanced (T3 and T4) lesions a multimodal approach is preferred. Surgery consists of a radical cystourethrectomy or an anterior exenteration, depending on the extent of the disease. Radiation therapy with a combination of brachytherapy and external-beam irradiation is usually required. Neoadjuvant chemotherapy with 5-FU and mitomycin C has been noted to enhance the therapeutic ratio of radiation therapy.

CANCER OF THE PENIS

Carcinoma of the penis is an uncommon malignancy in Western countries, representing 0.4% of male malignancies and 3.0% of all genitourinary cancers. However, penile cancer constitutes a major health problem in many countries in Asia, Africa, and South America, where it may comprise up to 10% of all malignancies. Despite these statistics, the incidence of penile cancer has been declining in many countries, partly because of increased attention to personal hygiene.[26] It most commonly presents in the sixth decade of life but may occur in men younger than 40 years. Analysis of the Surveillance, Epidemiology, and End Results database reveals that there is no racial difference in the incidence of penile cancer among black and white men in the United States.

ETIOLOGY

Cancer of the penis has been strongly associated with phimosis and poor local hygiene. Phimosis is found in more than half the patients in most large series of penile carcinoma. The irritative effect of smegma, a by-product of bacterial action on desquamated epithelial cells within the preputial sac, is well known, although definitive evidence of its role in carcinogenesis is lacking. Neonatal circumcision as is practiced by groups such as the Jewish population virtually eliminates the occurrence of penile carcinoma. Delaying circumcision until puberty does not have the same benefit as neonatal circumcision, and adult circumcision certainly does not provide any protection against carcinoma of the penis.[27]

HPV infection, particularly HPV-16, has been implicated in the development of invasive penile cancer, as is the number of sexual partners.[27] The use of tobacco products has been shown to be an independent risk factor in the development of penile cancer on multivariate analysis.[28] Tobacco has been proposed as a promoter of malignant transformation in the setting of infection and chronic irritation. Thus, avoidance of tobacco products and HPV infection, penile hygiene, and neonatal circumcision represent important preventative strategies against penile cancer.

SYMPTOMS

Local penile symptoms and signs most often draw attention to penile cancer. The clinical spectrum of penile cancer is varied: subtle areas of erythema or induration to a frankly ulcerated, fungating, foul-smelling mass. As a rule, penile cancer is an "infected" malignancy, with infection playing an important role in the pathogenesis and ultimately in the presentation of the disease. Pain usually is not a prominent feature and is definitely not proportional to the extent of local destruction. The lesion initially involves the prepuce and glans, often under a tight phimotic ring. In late stages involvement and eventual destruction of the shaft of the penis are seen. Urethral involvement is usually a late feature, and even in advanced stages urethral obstruction is rarely seen. Instead, erosion of the urethra with development of multiple fistulas leading to the so-called watering-can perineum may be seen. Rarely, inguinal ulceration may be the presenting symptom, and in such cases the primary tumor is usually concealed within a phimotic preputial sac or the patient delays seeking medical help for social reasons. Patients with penile cancer, more than with other types of cancer, seem to delay seeking medical attention. Although earlier studies showed up to 50% of patients delayed more than 1 year in seeking medical help, more contemporary series, especially from the United States, fail to show such a trend.

PATHOLOGY

More than 95% of penile carcinomas are squamous cell in origin. Non–squamous cell carcinomas consist of melanomas, basal cell carcinomas, lymphomas, and sarcomas. Nearly 18% of patients with AIDS-related Kaposi's sarcoma have penile involvement.[29]

From a histologic standpoint, squamous cell carcinomas are graded using Broders' classification. Low-grade tumors (grade I and II), which typically are confined to the prepuce and glans penis, constitute nearly 80% of penile cancers. On the other hand most lesions involving the shaft of the penis are high grade (grade III). Thus, grade and stage are often correlated. The incidence of lymph node metastases from squamous cell carcinoma of the penis is related to histologic grade. *Verrucous carcinoma*, a particularly exuberant variant of squamous cell carcinoma, has an extremely low potential for lymph node spread and, thereby, a good prognosis. Another important predictor of lymph node metastases and, hence, prognosis is the presence of vascular invasion in the surgical specimen.[30]

PREMALIGNANT LESIONS

The description of early and premalignant lesions has been complicated by the rarity of the disease and a proliferation of eponyms.

Leukoplakia

Leukoplakia is characterized by the presence of solitary or multiple whitish plaques involving the glans or prepuce in the setting of chronic or recurrent balanoposthitis. Surgical excision in the form of circumcision or local wedge resection is usually all the treatment that is needed.

Balanitis Xerotica Obliterans

Balanitis xerotica obliterans (BXO) is an inflammatory condition of the glans and prepuce of unknown cause. BXO presents as a scaly, indurated, whitish plaque that produces significant phimosis and eventually marked meatal stenosis. Often associated with development of squamous cell carcinoma of the penis in selected reports, treatment remains controversial and consists of topical steroids and surgical excision. Although formal meatoplasty may be required for advanced meatal stenosis, early circumcision has been found to be the most effective treatment for BXO.[31]

Buschke-Löwenstein Tumor

The Buschke-Löwenstein tumor is characterized by a large exophytic mass involving the glans penis and prepuce; it is a giant condyloma acuminatum that has a good prognosis and does not metastasize. Except for unrestrained local growth, this lesion does not have any features of malignancy. A viral etiology has been proposed, with identification of HPV-6 and -11 in these tumors. Treatment consists of local conservative resection. Recurrence is common, and close follow-up is essential. Systemic interferon-α therapy combined with neodymium:yttrium aluminum garnet (Nd:YAG) laser therapy has been reported to be successful in selected cases. Radiation therapy is essentially contraindicated in this condition, as rapid malignant degeneration has been described.

DIAGNOSIS AND STAGING

The workup for penile cancer begins with a meticulous physical examination of the genitalia and inguinal nodes to ascertain the local stage of the lesion and the presence of inguinal adenopathy. Nodal status is the most significant prognostic variable predicting survival. Approximately 50% of patients with carcinoma of the penis present with palpable inguinal nodes. However, only half of these patients have metastatic disease, whereas the other half have inflammation secondary to infection of the primary lesion. Conversely, 20% of patients with a clinically negative groin are found to have metastases if prophylactic node dissection is performed. The most common distant metastatic sites are the lung, bone, and liver. The AJCC system (sixth edition) for staging penile cancer uses the TNM classification to determine the stage of the primary tumor and the extent of nodal metastases (Table 30.4-2).

After biopsy confirmation of the lesion, no further radiologic workup is generally needed in patients with early-stage disease and no inguinal adenopathy on examination. Ultrasound and gadolinium-enhanced MRI are recommended for high-grade and high-stage lesions suspected of involving the corporal bodies, especially if partial penectomy is contemplated. CT scanning is recommended in obese patients to evaluate the inguinal nodes. In patients with known inguinal metastases, CT-guided biopsy of enlarged pelvic nodes, if positive, may be an indication for neoadjuvant chemotherapy.

TREATMENT

Treatment of penile carcinoma depends on the local extent of the primary neoplasm and the status of the regional lymph nodes. For treatment of the primary lesion, a 2-cm proximal margin of resection is recommended to avoid local recurrence and is the current standard of care. Leaving the patient with inadequate penile length for hygienic upright micturition and

TABLE 30.4-2.   American Joint Committee on Cancer Tumor, Node, Metastasis Classification System for Penile Cancer

Stage Grouping			
Stage 0	Tis	N0	M0
	Ta	N0	M0
Stage I	T1	N0	M0
Stage II	T1	N1	M0
	T2	N0	M0
	T2	N1	M0
Stage III	T1	N2	M0
	T2	N2	M0
	T3	N0	M0
	T3	N1	M0
	T3	N2	M0
Stage IV	T4	Any N	M0
	Any T	N3	M0
	Any T	Any N	M1

(From AJCC. *Cancer staging manual*, 6th ed. New York: Springer-Verlag, 2002, with permission.)

sexual intercourse should be avoided. Thus, depending on the extent of the primary tumor, resection may include a partial or total penectomy. Local recurrence after a properly planned and executed partial or total penectomy is rare. In advanced cases (T4), more aggressive resections, such as an emasculation procedure, a hemipelvectomy, or even a hemicorpectomy, have been reported. Although surgery forms the mainstay for treatment of the primary lesion, radiation therapy can be considered for a select group of patients. Radiation therapy permits preservation of the penis, thereby obviating the psychosocial and physical morbidity caused by partial or total penectomy. External-beam and brachytherapy techniques have been used for treatment of the primary cancer. Circumcision is generally recommended before radiation therapy is initiated. This allows for further evaluation of the tumor extent and reduces morbidity associated with radiation, such as swelling, maceration of the prepuce, and secondary infection, all of which may eventually result in secondary phimosis. Although radiation has been shown to control early (T1 and T2) lesions with a 65% to 80% success rate, treatment of more advanced T-stage penile cancers is fraught with local recurrences (20% to 40%) and the most significant risk of tumor progression to nodal and systemic disease with loss of the window of curability.[32] Thus, radiation therapy, although attractive from a cosmesis point of view, has significant disadvantages, and in reality the number of patients for whom this treatment is appropriate is small.

Of paramount importance in treatment planning is a consideration of the lymphatic drainage of the penis. The inguinal lymph nodes constitute the first echelon of drainage. Superficial and deep inguinal nodes are involved in a stepwise manner. Bilateral drainage occurs as a result of free anastomoses and crossover at the base of the penis. The superficial inguinal nodes are located in the deep portion of Camper's fascia above the deep fascia of the thigh, the fascia lata. The superficial lymphatics drain into the deep inguinal lymphatics, which surround the femoral vessels deep to the fascia lata. Secondary drainage is to the iliac nodes, although direct drainage to these nodes (skip metastases) can occur rarely. Also, roughly 50% of patients with carcinoma of the penis present with palpable inguinal adenopathy. The presence of palpable adenopathy is associated with proven nodal metastases in 50% of cases.

Treatment of Primary Lesion

Surgery for treatment of penile carcinoma has ranged from circumcision, conservative local resection, laser ablation, and Mohs micrographic surgery to the more morbid partial and total penectomy. Radiation therapy can also be used in selected patients with early superficial lesions. Depending on the stage of the primary lesion, any of a variety of options can be used.

CARCINOMA *IN SITU* (TIS). Erythroplasia of Queyrat is a red, velvety, well-marginated lesion of the glans penis or the prepuce of uncircumcised men. After biopsy confirmation of the lesion, a conservative approach that spares penile anatomy and function is generally preferred. Preputial lesions are adequately treated with circumcision. Topical 5-FU cream has been used with excellent cosmetic results for glanular and meatal lesions. Systemic absorption of 5-FU is minimal. A prospective study using a combination of carbon dioxide and

Nd:YAG lasers has shown good local tumor control and highly satisfactory cosmetic results on long-term follow-up.[33] Mohs micrographic surgery has been described as a less deforming alternative, with local control rates up to 86% in selected patients with early penile cancer.[34] Radiation therapy has also been used successfully to eradicate these lesions with minimal morbidity.

VERRUCOUS CARCINOMA (Ta). Penile verrucous carcinoma is characterized by aggressive local growth and a low metastatic potential. In view of its rather benign course, a partial or total penectomy is usually overkill and conservative therapeutic approaches are favored. Laser ablation or Mohs micrographic surgical technique have yielded acceptable results. In one study, intraaortic infusion with methotrexate in four patients with penile verrucous carcinoma resulted in complete remission in three patients while preserving cosmetic and functional integrity of the penis.[35] However, radiation therapy in any form is contraindicated in this lesion, as it has been shown to cause subsequent rapid malignant degeneration and metastases.

INVASIVE PENILE CANCER (T1, T2, T3, AND/OR N1). Distal penile lesions in which a serviceable penis for upright micturition and sexual function can be achieved are best treated with a partial penectomy. For extensive lesions approaching the base of the penis, total penectomy with excision of both corporal bodies and creation of a perineal urethrostomy is usually required. Local recurrence after a partial penectomy in properly selected cases is rare. Patients in whom penile recurrence does develop after initial partial penectomy can be treated by further surgical salvage. Most relapses occur within the first 12 to 18 months after penectomy. Thus, close follow-up of these patients is important.

Analysis of the effectiveness of radiation therapy in the treatment of penile cancer is hindered by a lack of uniformity of radiation treatment, mostly because of different types of delivery systems and different doses of radiation. Radiation therapy, although effective for local control of small, 2- to 4-cm, T1 and T2 lesions is usually not adequate for more advanced T-stage tumors. Local recurrence is higher in those with T3 and T4 tumors, that is, 20% to 40%, but a significant percentage can be salvaged by adjuvant surgical resection.[36] Before treatment, all patients should have a circumcision to allow direct inspection and accurate staging of the tumor and to facilitate management of the acute side effects of radiation. External-beam and brachytherapy techniques have been used for the control of the primary lesion. External-beam radiotherapy can be delivered by a direct field method that uses a low-energy photon beam or an electron beam applied directly to the tumor, with a safety margin of 2 cm beyond the visible and palpable extent of the tumor. This approach is suitable only for very superficial tumors (Tis and T1). For T2 and T3 lesions, a parallel opposed field method is used. Using this approach the entire thickness of the penis can be irradiated by encasing the lesion in a wax mold to ensure uniform dosage and to negate the skin-sparing effects of supervoltage beams. A total dose of 60 Gy is recommended in most large series for tumor sterilization. A 65% to 80% local success rate has been reported with radiation therapy for small T1 and T2 tumors.[37]

Brachytherapy involves the irradiation of tumors by placement of radioactive material within the tumor (interstitial brachytherapy) or around the tumor (plesiobrachytherapy). The use of brachytherapy is usually limited to T1 and T2 tumors. Mold therapy consists of a cylindrical Perspex mold of the penis on which is loaded the radioactive source, usually iridium 192 wire. Patients with bulky tumors and obese patients with a short penis are not suitable for this form of therapy. Deeply infiltrating tumors should also not be treated with mold therapy. Interstitial therapy using iridium 192 is also used to deliver effective radiation to the primary tumor. Radiation therapy as primary treatment for invasive penile carcinoma has significant disadvantages. The acute side effects of radiation in the form of skin edema, maceration, and dysuria usually subside within 2 weeks of completion of treatment but may persist for 6 to 8 weeks. Telangiectasia and fibrosis are found in more than 90% of cases, but patients usually do not complain of these. The most serious late effects are urethral fistula, meatal stenosis, and penile necrosis. Postradiation fibrosis, scar, and necrosis may be very difficult to distinguish from recurrent cancer, and repeated biopsies may be needed. Furthermore, infection is very often associated with penile cancer and reduces the therapeutic efficacy of radiation while increasing the risk of penile necrosis. Thus, in summary, radiation therapy for primary penile cancer should be considered only in a select group of patients: young patients with small (2- to 4-cm) superficial lesions of the distal penis who wish to maintain penile integrity, patients who refuse surgery, and patients with inoperable cancer or those unsuitable for major surgery.

ADVANCED PENILE CANCER (T4, N2/N3, AND/OR M1). Primary surgery in the setting of advanced T4 penile cancer is necessarily a mutilating procedure. Large proximal shaft tumors require a total penectomy with a perineal urethrostomy. For extensive, proximal tumors with invasion of adjacent structures, total emasculation consisting of total penectomy, scrotectomy, and orchiectomy is recommended. In extreme cases, a hemipelvectomy or even a hemicorporectomy has been described. Multimodal therapy with chemoradiation and salvage surgery has also been used in this setting.

Management of Regional Lymph Nodes

The presence and extent of inguinal lymph node metastases are the most important prognostic factors in patients with penile cancer. Although 50% of patients with a penile lesion have clinically palpable inguinal nodes at presentation, in more than half of these the adenopathy is inflammatory. Thus, a 4- to 6-week course of antibiotics (e.g., cephalosporin) after treatment of the primary lesion is recommended. Patients with persistent palpable adenopathy after antibiotic therapy should undergo biopsy and definitive therapy. It should be remembered that, unlike many other genitourinary malignancies that require systemic chemotherapy, once lymph node metastases are discovered, inguinal metastases from penile cancer are potentially curable by lymphadenectomy alone, and it should be performed at the earliest suspicion of metastases.

CLINICALLY N0 PATIENTS. Although there is no controversy in the literature regarding management of the patient with clinically positive inguinal lymph nodes after a course of antibiotics, considerable controversy surrounds the management of the clinically N0 patient. Approximately, 20% of these clinically negative groins harbor occult lymphatic metastases on prophylactic lymph node dissection. Stated another way, approximately 80% of patients with clinically negative groins would be subjected to the morbidity of inguinal lymph node dissection without any benefit. To resolve this dilemma, a risk-based approach to management of the clinically negative groin has been recommended in most contemporary series. Analysis of histopathologic data from the primary penile cancer allows stratification of patients into high- and low-risk groups for lymph node metastases.[38]

Low-Risk Group. Patients with carcinoma in situ (Tis), verrucous carcinoma (Ta), and T1 tumors who have grade 1 or grade 2 tumor histology have a less than 10% chance of developing lymph node metastases and as such are best served by a policy of "watchful waiting." These patients also have a very low incidence of vascular invasion in the primary tumor, an independent predictor of lymph node metastases.[30]

High-Risk Group. Patients with invasive penile cancer (T2 and T3) with grade 3 tumors and the presence of vascular invasion have a greater than 50% incidence of inguinal lymph node metastases in various series. Vascular invasion has been shown to be strongly correlated with lymph node metastases. In pT2 patients the incidence of lymph node metastases was found to be 75% in the presence of vascular invasion and only 25% when vascular invasion was absent.[38] In this cohort of patients, a prophylactic lymphadenectomy would appear reasonable.

The timing of surgery in the clinically negative groin has also been a subject of debate in the past. However, most contemporary series have favored *early adjunctive* lymphadenectomy, especially in the high-risk group, over a policy of surveillance and *delayed therapeutic* lymphadenectomy. Sentinel lymph node biopsy as originally described by Cabanas is no longer recommended in view of the high false-negative rate. However, reports of intraoperative lymphatic mapping using dynamic scintigraphy with technetium-labeled sulfur colloid have decreased the false-negative rate considerably.[37] Further data are required before this technique can be universally accepted as a tool to direct lymphadenectomy in patients with clinically negative nodes. Superficial inguinal lymph node dissection in which the dissection is carried out superficial to the fascia lata has been found to be adequate for the N0 patient. Superficial inguinal lymph node dissection should include a frozen section, and if positive, a modified complete dissection should be carried out. Creation of thicker skin flaps, control of infection, and preservation of the areolar fat superficial to the Scarpa's fascia have greatly decreased the complications of flap necrosis, scrotal and extremity edema, lymphocele, and lymphorrhea.

CLINICALLY N1, N2, AND N3 PATIENTS. The modified inguinal lymph node dissection as described by Catalona in 1988[39] has replaced the standard complete inguinal lymphadenectomy as the procedure of choice in the patient with clinically persistent nodes after a course of antibiotics. It involves a smaller incision, limited field of inguinal dissection, and preservation of the saphenous vein in an effort to reduce the morbidity of the standard procedure while adhering to standard oncologic principles. Unlike superficial dissection the deep nodes within the fossa ovalis are also removed. In the face of synchronous unilateral N+ disease, it is standard practice to proceed with a bilateral lymph node dissection in view of the

high incidence of bilateral drainage. The exception to this rule is the patient with a clinically negative groin in whom metachronous unilateral inguinal lymphadenopathy develops some time after treatment of the primary tumor. In these patients a unilateral dissection of the clinically positive groin usually suffices. The value of pelvic lymphadenectomy in the presence of positive inguinal lymph nodes is for purposes of staging and for identifying patients who would be candidates for adjuvant chemotherapy. It has little therapeutic efficacy, with 5-year survival of patients with pelvic lymph node metastases of less than 5%.

Patients with advanced nodal disease or bulky fixed inguinal nodes (N3) may require neoadjuvant radiation or chemotherapy before any surgical intervention. The enlarged groin lymph nodes that are adherent to the skin or fungating through the skin require wide excision of the skin with use of appropriate myocutaneous flaps to cover the skin defect. The use of radiation therapy as a primary modality for inguinal node metastases has not shared the same enthusiasm as its use for treatment of the primary lesion. Current literature unequivocally favors surgical dissection as superior to radiation therapy for the treatment of inguinal lymph nodes. Other objections to the use of radiation for inguinal lymph nodes is the difficulty in clinical evaluation of the groin because of postradiation tissue changes, as well as the fact that the inguinal area tolerates radiation rather poorly and is prone to skin maceration and ulceration. Thus, radiation therapy can be used as a palliative measure in patients with fixed inoperable inguinal nodes or in those with advanced unresectable penile cancer in which the primary and the ilioinguinal region can be treated with radiation therapy.

Role of Chemotherapy and Multimodality Therapy

The role of chemotherapy in the management of penile carcinoma is still evolving, and the precise place for chemotherapy in the therapeutic armamentarium has not been established. Sufficient data are available, however, to conclude that penile cancer is sensitive to chemotherapy. Besides the use of 5-FU in the treatment of superficial penile cancer, only three other drugs have been used consistently in the management of penile cancer. Single-agent chemotherapy with cisplatin, methotrexate, and bleomycin has modest activity in advanced penile cancer. The combination of methotrexate, bleomycin, and cisplatin (MBP) is more active than cisplatin alone but is associated with marked toxicity.

The Southwest Oncology Group reported on the largest prospective clinical trial in patients with penile cancer.[40] In 40 evaluable patients treated with a combination of MBP, an overall response of 32.5% and a complete response of 12.5% were observed. The median duration of response was 16 weeks, and the median survival was 28 weeks. Toxicity was formidable, with 11% treatment-related mortality and 17% of the remaining patients experiencing life-threatening toxicity. Vincristine, bleomycin, and methotrexate (VBM) have also been studied for advanced penile cancer, with a reported response rate of 53.8%.[41]

Multimodality therapy using a combination of chemotherapy and surgery, or chemotherapy and radiation, has been used in isolated reports of advanced penile cancer. Pizzocaro et al.[41] reported responses in 7 of 13 patients treated with neoadjuvant VBM before surgery. Two of the 13 VBM-treated patients were long-term survivors without evidence of disease.[40] Bleomycin, a known radiosensitizer, has also been combined with radiation as an organ-sparing approach for patients with low-stage cancer. The 3-, 5-, and 10-year survival with this approach has been similar to surgical intervention in this favorable group of patients. In summary, chemotherapy and multimodality therapy have been used with some success in patients with advanced unresectable disease.

REFERENCES

1. Tefilli MV, Gheiler EL, Shekarriz B, et al. Primary adenocarcinoma of the urethra with metastasis to the glans penis: successful treatment with chemotherapy and radiation therapy. *Urology* 1998;52:517.
2. Donat SM, Cozzi PJ, Herr HW. Surgery of penile and urethral carcinoma. In: Walsh PC, ed. *Campbell's urology*, 8th ed. Philadelphia: Saunders, 2002:2983.
3. Weiner JS, Liu ET, Walther PJ. Oncogenic human papillomavirus type 16 is associated with squamous cell cancer of the male urethra. *Cancer Res* 1992;52:5018.
4. Fair WR, Yang CR. Urethral carcinoma in males. In: Resnick M, Kursch E, eds. *Current therapy in surgery*. Toronto: BC Decker, 1987.
5. Grabstalt H. Tumors of the urethra in men and women. *Cancer* 1973;32:1236.
6. Grigsby PW, Herr HW. Urethral tumors. In: Vogelang N, Scardino PT, Shipley WU, Coffey DS, eds. *Comprehensive textbook of genitourinary oncology*. Baltimore: Williams & Wilkins, 2000:1133.
7. Erckert M, Stenzl A, Falk M, Bartsch G. Incidence of urethral tumor involvement in 910 men with bladder cancer. *World J Urol* 1996;14:3.
8. Marino G, Marten-Perolino R. Transitional cell carcinoma of the urethra in patients after cystectomy for bladder carcinoma. *Minerva Urol Nefrol* 1992;44:209.
9. Ryu J, Kim B. MR imaging of the male and female urethra. *Radiographics* 2001;21(5):1169.
10. Zeidman EJ, Desmond P, Thompson I. Surgical treatment of carcinoma of the male urethra. *Urol Clin North Am* 1992;19:359.
11. Gheiler EL, Tefeli MV, Tiguert R, et al. Management of primary urethral cancers. *Urology* 1998;52:487.
12. Davis JW, Schellhammer PF, Schlossberg SM. Conservative surgical therapy for penile and urethral carcinoma. *Urology* 1999;53:386.
13. Krieg R, Hoffman R. Current management of unusual genitourinary cancers: Part 2: Urethral cancer. *Oncology* 1999;13:1511.
14. Christopher N, Arya M, Brown RSD, Payne CRJ, et al. Penile preservation in squamous cell carcinoma of the bulbomembranous urethra. *BJU Int* 2002;89:464.
15. Hall RR, Robinson MC. Transitional cell carcinoma of the prostate. *Eur Urol Update Series* 1998;7:1.
16. Scher HI, Yagoda A, Herr HW, et al. Neoadjuvant M-VAC (methotrexate, vinblastine, doxorubicin and cisplatin) for extravesical urinary tract tumors. *J Urol* 1988;139:475.
17. Licht MR, Klein EA, Bukowski R, et al. Combination radiation and chemotherapy treatment of squamous cell carcinoma of the male and female urethra. *J Urol* 1995;153:1616.
18. Oberfeld RA, Zinman LN, Leibenhaut M, et al. Management of invasive squamous cell carcinoma of the bulbomembranous male urethra with co-ordinated chemo-radiotherapy and genital preservation. *Br J Urol* 1996;78:573.
19. Srinivas V, Khan S. Female urethral cancer—an overview. *Int Urol Nephrol* 1987;19:423.
20. Tiguert R, Ravery V, Madjar S, Gousse AE. Acute urinary retention secondary to clear cell carcinoma of the urethra. *Prog Urol* 2001;11(1):70.
21. Sailer SL, Shipley WU, Wang CC. Carcinoma of the female urethra: a review of results with radiation therapy. *J Urol* 1988;140:1.
22. Dalbagni G, Zhang ZF, Lacombe L, Herr HW. Female urethral carcinoma: an analysis of treatment outcome and a plea for a standardized management strategy. *Br J Urol* 1998;82:835.
23. Terry P, Cookson M, Sarosdy M. Carcinoma of the urethra and scrotum. In: Raghvan D, Leibel SA, Scher HI, et al. *Principles and practice of genitourinary oncology*. Philadelphia: Lippincott–Raven, 1997:347.
24. Milosevic MF, Warde PR, Banerjee D, et al. Urethral carcinoma in women: results of treatment with primary radiotherapy. *Radiother Oncol* 2000;56(1):29.
25. Narayan P, Konety B. Surgical treatment of female urethral carcinoma. *Urol Clin North Am* 1992;19:373.
26. Yeole BB, Jussawalla DJ. Descriptive epidemiology of the cancers of male genital organs in greater Bombay. *Ind J Cancer* 1997;34:30.
27. Maden C, Sherman KJ, Beckman AM, et al. History of circumcision, medical conditions, and sexual activity and risk of penile cancer. *J Natl Cancer Inst* 1993;85:19.
28. Harish K, Ravi R. The role of tobacco in penile carcinoma. *Br J Urol* 1995;75:375.
29. Grossman H. Premalignant carcinomas of the penis and scrotum. *Urol Clin North Am* 1992;19:221.
30. Morganstern NJ, Slaton JW, Levy DA, et al. Vascular invasion and tumor stage are independent prognosticators of lymph node (LN) metastasis in squamous penile cancer (SPC). *J Urol* 1999;161:158A.
31. Depasquale I, Park AJ, Bracka A. The treatment of balanitis xerotica obliterans. *BJU Int* 2000;86:859.
32. Crook J, Grimard L, Tsihlias J, Morash C, Panzarella T. Interstitial brachytherapy for penile cancer: an alternative to amputation. *J Urol* 2002;167(2 Pt 1):506.
33. Windahl T, Andersson SO. Combined laser treatment for penile carcinoma: results after long-term followup. *J Urol* 2003;169(6):2118.
34. Mohs F, Snow S, Larson P. Mohs micrographic surgery for penile tumors. *Urol Clin North Am* 1992;19:291.
35. Sheen MC, Sheu HM, Huang CH, et al. Penile verrucous carcinoma successfully treated by intra-aortic infusion with methotrexate. *Urology* 2003;61(6):1216.
36. Krieg R, Hoffman R. Current management of unusual genitourinary cancers. Part 1: Penile cancer. *Oncology* 1999;13:1347.
37. Jakub JW, Pendas S, Reintgen DS. Current status of sentinel lymph node mapping and biopsy: fact and controversies. *Oncologist* 2003;8(1):59.
38. Slaton JW, Morgenstern N, Levy DA, et al. Tumor stage, vascular invasion and the percentage of poorly differentiated cancer: independent prognosticators for inguinal lymph node metastasis in penile squamous cancer. *J Urol* 2001;165:1138.
39. Catalona WJ. Modified inguinal lymphadenectomy for carcinoma of the penis with preservation of saphenous veins: technique and preliminary results. *J Urol* 1988;140:306.
40. Haas GP, Blumenstein BA, Gagliano RG, et al. Cisplatin, methotrexate and bleomycin for the treatment of carcinoma of the penis: a Southwest Oncology Group study. *J Urol* 1999;161:1823.
41. Pizzocaro G, Nicolai N, Piva L. Chemotherapy for cancer of the penis. In: Raghavan D, Leibel SA, Scher HI, Lange P, eds. *Principles and practice of genitourinary oncology*. Philadelphia: Lippincott–Raven, 1997:973.

George J. Bosl   Joel Sheinfeld
Dean F. Bajorin   Robert J. Motzer
R. S. K. Chaganti

CHAPTER **31**

Cancer of the Testis

Cancers of the testis comprise a morphologically and clinically diverse group of neoplasms, most of which are germ cell tumors (GCTs; Table 31-1). Approximately 90% of GCTs originate in the testis, and 10% are extragonadal in origin. The management of testicular and extragonadal GCTs (mediastinal and retroperitoneal) is discussed in this chapter.

BACKGROUND: INCIDENCE

GCTs are the most common solid tumor in men between the ages of 15 and 35 years. They have three modal peaks: infancy, ages 25 to 40, and approximately age 60. A solid testicular mass in a man aged 50 or greater is usually a lymphoma. The incidence of GCTs appears to be increasing. An estimated 8980 new cases and 360 deaths due to testicular cancer are expected in the United States in 2003.[1] The incidence of testis cancer varies significantly according to geographic area and is associated with a birth cohort effect in the United States and in Europe.[2] The reported incidence is highest in Scandinavia, Switzerland, Germany, and New Zealand; intermediate in the United States and Great Britain; and lowest in Africa and Asia.

EPIDEMIOLOGY

GCTs are seen principally in young whites and more rarely in African Americans. The published ratio between white and African American patients is approximately 4:1 to 5:1 but closer to a 40:1 ratio in the U.S. military. In African Americans, GCT behaves similarly to that of the general population.[3] Familial clustering has been observed, particularly among siblings.[4] Despite anecdotes associat-ing diethylstilbestrol exposure with the development of GCT, epidemiologic studies have failed to identify such an association.

A history of trauma is frequently noted by patients with testicular cancer. Viral orchitis, usually secondary to mumps, may result in testicular atrophy. However, epidemiologic studies have failed to identify trauma or viral infection as a cause. More recently, testicular cancer has been reported in men infected with the human immunodeficiency virus. Few data support a higher incidence of GCT in human immunodeficiency virus–infected individuals, and the results of treatment are similar.[5,6] Reports implicating vasectomy as a cause of GCT have not been confirmed in cohort analysis.[7]

Two congenital developmental defects, cryptorchidism and Klinefelter's syndrome, predispose to the disease.

CRYPTORCHIDISM

An inguinal cryptorchid testis develops a GCT in approximately 2% of cases. However, between 5% and 20% of cryptorchid patients with a GCT develop the tumor in the normally descended testis. An abdominal cryptorchid testis is more likely to develop GCT than an inguinal cryptorchid testis. Most data suggest a reduced likelihood of GCT if orchiopexy is performed before puberty.[8] If the testis is inguinal, hormonally functioning, and easily examined, surveillance is recommended. If the testis is abdominal, not amenable to orchiopexy, or cannot be adequately examined, orchiectomy is recommended.

KLINEFELTER'S SYNDROME

Characterized by testicular atrophy, absence of spermatogenesis, a eunuchoid habitus, and gynecomastia, Klinefelter's syndrome is

TABLE 31-1. Histologic Classification of Testicular Neoplasms

A. Germ cell tumors (demonstrating one or more of the following components)
  1. Seminoma
    a. Classic (typical) seminoma
    b. Spermatocytic seminoma
  2. Embryonal carcinoma
  3. Teratoma
    a. Mature
    b. Immature
    c. Mature or immature teratoma with malignant transformation
  4. Choriocarcinoma
  5. Yolk sac tumor (endodermal sinus tumor; embryonal adenocarcinoma of the prepubertal testis)
B. Sex cord–stromal (gonadal stromal) tumors
  1. Leydig cell tumor
  2. Sertoli cell tumor
  3. Granulosa cell tumor (adult and juvenile types)
C. Both germ cell and gonadal stromal elements
  1. Gonadoblastoma
D. Adnexal and paratesticular tumors
  1. Mesothelioma
  2. Soft tissue origin (e.g., sarcomas)
  3. Adnexal (e.g., adenocarcinoma) of the rete testis
E. Miscellaneous neoplasms
  1. Carcinoid
  2. Lymphoma
  3. Cysts
F. Metastatic neoplasms

diagnosed by a 47,XXY karyotype. Patients with Klinefelter's syndrome have an increased incidence of mediastinal GCT.

INITIAL PRESENTATION AND MANAGEMENT

SYMPTOMS AND SIGNS

The pathognomonic presentation of a primary testicular tumor is a painless testicular mass that may range in size from a few millimeters to several centimeters. However, the painless testicular mass occurs in only a minority of patients. The majority of patients present with symptoms consistent with infectious epididymitis or orchitis, or both, and a trial of antibiotic therapy is often required. Acute testicular pain, simulating testicular torsion, occurs less frequently and may represent intratumoral hemorrhage. If the testicular discomfort does not abate or findings do not revert to normal within 2 to 4 weeks, a testicular ultrasound is indicated. On ultrasound, the typical testicular tumor is intratesticular and may produce one or more discrete hypoechoic masses. The association between testicular microlithiasis and GCT is not clearly defined.[9,10] Higher stage at presentation has been associated with delay in diagnosis,[11] and the experience of the treatment unit with the management of GCT appears to influence survival.[12,13]

DIAGNOSIS

A radical inguinal orchiectomy, using an inguinal incision with early high ligation of the spermatic cord at the deep inguinal

ring, minimizes local tumor recurrence and aberrant lymphatic spread. It is the only acceptable therapeutic and diagnostic procedure. The vasal and vascular components are doubly clamped and divided separately; their respective stumps are pushed into the retroperitoneal space to facilitate removal of the gonadal vessels at the time of retroperitoneal lymph node dissection (RPLND). The testis and spermatic cord are removed *en bloc*, avoiding any spillage, and meticulous hemostasis is achieved. A transscrotal orchiectomy is contraindicated, because it permits the development of alternate lymphatic drainage pathways to the inguinal and pelvic lymph nodes and leaves intact the spermatic cord from the external to the internal ring. In the rare situation in which the diagnosis of a testicular tumor is in question, an inguinal incision is required for an open biopsy. The testis can then be examined *in situ* in a sterile field and an appropriate biopsy taken with minimal risk of scrotal or inguinal contamination. Regardless of the preoperative diagnosis, all potential testicular malignancies should be managed through an inguinal approach.

Extragonadal GCT comprises fewer than 10% of GCTs. The mediastinum and retroperitoneum are the most common primary sites. Pineal tumors, occurring most frequently in children, are usually GCT. Because of its unique access to the meninges, the metastatic pattern of pineal GCT includes intradural sites along the neuraxis and is less frequently systemic. In extremely rare circumstances, primary GCT has been found in unusual sites such as the sacrum, thyroid, paranasal sinuses, and soft tissues of the head and neck. In patients with extragonadal presentations of GCT, a testicular ultrasound is required. The management of extragonadal and testicular GCT is the same, and primary site is an independent factor in staging and risk classification.

HISTOLOGY

GCT is classified into two major subgroups: seminoma and nonseminoma. Two classifications are summarized in Table 31-2. Mostofi and Sesterhenn's[14] adaptation of the Dixon/Moore classification was largely adopted by the World Health Organization (WHO) and is the classification most commonly

TABLE 31-2. Comparison of Two Classifications of Germ Cell Tumors

WHO[14]	British Tumor Panel[15]
Seminoma	Seminoma
Typical (classic)	
Anaplastic	
Embryonal carcinoma	Malignant teratoma, undifferentiated
Teratoma	Malignant teratoma, differentiated
Mature	
Immature	
With malignant differentiation	
Choriocarcinoma	Malignant teratoma, trophoblastic
Yolk sac tumor	Yolk sac tumor
Mixed germ cell tumors (specify components)	Malignant teratoma, intermediate

WHO, World Health Organization.

used in North America and Europe. The British Tumor Panel's modification of the classification developed by Pugh[15] is widely used in Great Britain and Australia.

CARCINOMA *IN SITU*

Carcinoma *in situ* [CIS; intratubular germ cell (GC) neoplasia] precedes invasive testicular GCT in virtually all cases of seminoma and all nonseminomatous histologies in the adult. CIS is frequently present in retroperitoneal presentations but rarely, if ever, present in mediastinal presentations. It has not been described in spermatocytic seminoma and rarely in tumors arising in prepubertal patients. Cytologically, the CIS preceding seminoma and nonseminoma is identical. The median time for progression of CIS to invasive disease is approximately 5 years.[16] In the general population, the incidence of CIS is very low; in men with impaired fertility, it is approximately 0.5%.[17] The incidence of CIS is 2% to 5% in cryptorchid testis and the contralateral testis in patients with a documented prior testicular GCT.[18,19] Some European investigators suggest low-dose radiation therapy as management, but this is not considered standard in the United States.[20]

SEMINOMA

Seminoma accounts for approximately 50% of GCTs and most frequently appears in the fourth decade of life. The typical or classic form consists of sheets of large cells with abundant cytoplasm and round, hyperchromatic nuclei with prominent nucleoli. A lymphocytic infiltrate (and/or granulomatous reaction with giant cells) is frequently present. Trophoblastic giant cells capable of producing human chorionic gonadotropin (HCG) may be found in 15% to 20% of tumors. The presence of syncytiotrophoblastic giant cells in an otherwise pure seminoma does *not* influence prognosis or treatment. *Anaplastic seminoma* is an older term used when three or more mitotic figures are seen per high-powered field and has no clinical importance.

An "atypical" form of seminoma has been described with unusual immunohistochemical features. Although the cells cytologically resemble classic seminoma, lymphocytic infiltrate and granulomatous reaction are absent, necrosis is more common, and the nuclear-cytoplasmic ratio is higher. These tumors must be distinguished morphologically from solid variants of embryonal carcinoma and yolk sac tumor. Atypical seminoma frequently shows cytoplasmic expression of low-molecular-weight keratin or the type 1 precursor to the blood group antigens, whereas typical seminoma stains negative.[21] Electron microscopic studies have shown that the individual tumor cells acquire cytoplasmic cytokeratin intermediate filaments, suggesting epithelial differentiation. No specific association has been made of atypical seminoma with an adverse prognosis, and its management is currently the same as that of any other seminoma.

Spermatocytic seminoma is a rare histologic variant seen almost exclusively in men older than age 45. The relationship of spermatocytic seminoma to other GCTs is not clear, because it is not associated with CIS or bilaterality, does not express placental alkaline phosphatase (PLAP) (see Immunohistochemical Markers, later in this chapter), and has not been shown to have the same genetic abnormalities as other GCTs. Metastatic potential is minimal.

NONSEMINOMATOUS GERM CELL TUMORS

Nonseminomatous histology comprises approximately 50% of GCTs and most frequently presents in the third decade of life. Most tumors are mixed, consisting of two or more cell types. Seminoma may be a component, but the definition of a pure seminoma excludes the presence of any nonseminomatous cell type. The presence of any nonseminomatous cell type (other than syncytiotrophoblasts) imparts the prognosis and management of a nonseminomatous tumor.

Embryonal Carcinoma

Embryonal carcinoma is the most undifferentiated somatic cell type. Individual cells are epithelioid in appearance and may be arranged in glandular or tubular nests and cords or as solid sheets of cells. Tumor necrosis and hemorrhage are frequently observed.

Choriocarcinoma

Choriocarcinoma, by definition, consists of cytotrophoblasts and syncytiotrophoblasts. If cytotrophoblasts are not present, the diagnosis of choriocarcinoma cannot be made. Pure choriocarcinoma is an extremely rare presentation usually associated with widespread hematogenous metastases and high levels of HCG. Hemorrhage into the primary tumor may occur and is an occasional severe complication when it spontaneously occurs at a metastatic site. Elements of choriocarcinoma in a mixed tumor appear to have no prognostic importance. Syncytiotrophoblastic giant cells can be seen as a component of any GCT (including pure seminoma). They impart no prognostic value by themselves.

Yolk Sac Tumor

Yolk sac tumor (endodermal sinus tumor) is often confused with a glandular form of embryonal carcinoma. This tumor mimics the yolk sac of the embryo and produces α-fetoprotein (AFP). The cells may have a papillary, glandular, microcystic, or solid appearance and may be associated with Schiller-Duval bodies, which are perivascular arrangements of epithelial cells with an intervening extracellular space. Rarely, embryoid bodies resembling the early embryo may be seen. A pure yolk sac histology is very infrequent in the adult testis but accounts for a significant percentage of primary mediastinal nonseminomatous germ cell tumors (NSGCT).

Teratoma

Teratoma is composed of somatic cell types from two or more germ layers (ectoderm, mesoderm, or endoderm) and is derived from a totipotential, malignant precursor (embryonal carcinoma or yolk sac tumor). In a review of 41 cases of pure mature or immature teratoma of the testis, 26 (63%) displayed retroperitoneal or systemic metastases, with or without increased levels of serum tumor markers.[22] Therefore, a primary testicular tumor in a postpubertal male that displays only histologically mature or immature teratoma must be considered to be a fully malignant GCT, and management should proceed as if malignant components are present. *Mature teratoma* consists of adult-type differentiated elements such as cartilage, glandular epithelium, or nerve tissue. *Immature teratoma* generally refers to a tumor with partial somatic differentiation, similar to that seen in a fetus. Mature and immature teratoma are both histologically benign. *Teratoma with malignant transformation* refers to a form of teratoma in which one of its components, either immature or mature, develops aggressive growth and histologically resembles a non-GCT somatic cancer. These somatic cancers include acute nonlymphocytic leukemia (seen only in the context of mediastinal NSGCT), sarcomas (e.g., embryonal rhabdomyosarcoma), carcinoma (e.g., enteric-type adenocarcinoma), or neuroectodermal tumors. Somatic non-GCT malignancy arising in the context of teratoma behaves like cancer arising at its usual *de novo* site, and treatment should be directed at the transformed histology.[23]

IMMUNOHISTOCHEMICAL MARKERS

Seminoma does not display differentiation *in vitro* or *in vivo* and does not express markers of somatic differentiation, such as low-molecular-weight keratins, vimentin, or blood group antigens.[21] However, essentially all seminomas express PLAP and kit receptor (CD117).[24,25] Loss of c-kit expression in seminoma appears to be associated with a clinically more aggressive phenotype.[26] Embryonal carcinoma and yolk sac tumor display somatic differentiation. Surface expression of low-molecular-weight keratins (e.g., AE-1, CAM 5.2) and the type 1 precursor substance of the blood group antigens are invariable.[21] Most embryonal carcinomas, but not seminoma, also express the CD30 antigen, originally described as a marker of Hodgkin's disease and anaplastic large cell lymphoma.[27,28] Vimentin expression is limited to mesenchymal components of mature teratoma and interstitial and other support cells. In tumors of uncertain histogenesis, immunohistochemical studies that include PLAP, kit receptor, and low-molecular-weight keratins may be useful in establishing a diagnosis. It should be remembered that cytokeratins are expressed by all epithelial tumors, and PLAP immunoreactivity is present in a small subset of epithelial neoplasms, especially (but not limited to) those of müllerian origin.

BIOLOGY

Adult human male GCTs comprise a unique system for the study of the mechanism of totipotential GC transformation in lineage differentiation. The pluripotentiality of the tumor cells manifests as histologic differentiation into GC-like undifferentiated (seminoma), primitive zygotic (embryonal carcinoma), embryonal-like somatically differentiated (teratoma), and extraembryonally differentiated (choriocarcinoma and yolk sac tumor) phenotypes. Until recently, the molecular mechanisms of GC transformation, GCT differentiation, and GCT chemotherapy sensitivity and resistance were poorly understood. Since then, studies of GCT have suggested that (1) overexpression of cyclin D2 is a very early, possibly oncogenic, event in GC tumorigenesis; (2) differentiation in GCT may be governed by several possibly interacting pathways such as loss of GC totipotentiality regulators and of embryonic development and genomic imprinting; and (3) chemotherapy sensitivity and resistance may be rooted in part in a p53-dependent apoptotic pathway.

Mechanism of Germ Cell Transformation

Genetic analysis of male GCTs has yielded important data relevant to the mechanism of GC transformation. Virtually 100%

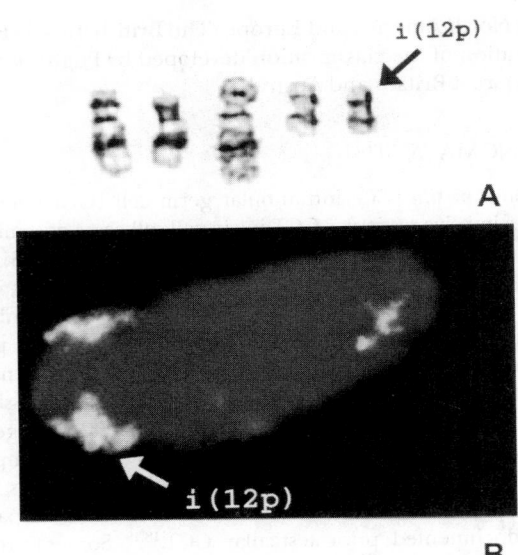

FIGURE 31-1. **A:** Partial karyotype showing four chromosomes 12 in a germ cell tumor (GCT) with the i(12p) chromosome (*arrow*) at metaphase. **B:** Fluorescence *in situ* hybridization (FISH) of a GCT cell showing three signals for 12p (*turquoise*) and three attached signals for chromosome 12 centromere (*pink*), indicating increased copy number of the 12p chromosomal arm. The large turquoise signal represents i(12p) (*arrow*), and the two small turquoise signals represent the normal chromosomes 12p. The probe used for 12p was derived from microdissection of 12pDNA from a chromosome preparation. The FISH test is now routinely used for GCT diagnosis in biopsy specimens. (See Color Fig. 31-1 in the CD-ROM.)

of tumors show increased copy number of 12p, as one or more copies of i(12p) or as tandem duplications of 12p, *in situ* or transposed elsewhere in the genome[29] (Fig. 31-1). This chromosomal marker has been observed as early as CIS, suggesting that it is among the earliest, if not the earliest, genetic change associated with the origin of these tumors.[29] A candidate gene, *CCND2*, mapped to 12p13, has been identified as the possible driver gene on 12p whose deregulated expression may lead to GCT development.[30] It is abundantly expressed in CIS as well as in many lineages of GCTs.[30] Cyclin D2 is one of the D-type cyclins that, along with the cyclin-dependent kinases cdk4, cdk6, or both, regulate the phosphorylation of pRB and control the G_1/S cell-cycle checkpoint.[31] Disruption of this checkpoint through amplification/overexpression of D-type cyclins is known to be one of the important pathways in human tumor development.

The precursor of all GCT is considered to be CIS; however, the stage in GC development at which transformation occurs is not known. Two models of CIS cell origin have been proposed. One model by Skakkebaek et al.[32,33] suggested that fetal gonocytes that have escaped normal development into spermatogonia may undergo abnormal cell division mediated by a kit receptor/SCF (stem cell factor; kit ligand) paracrine loop, leading to uncontrolled proliferation of gonocytes. Such gonocytes are postulated to be susceptible to subsequent invasive growth through the mediation of postnatal and pubertal gonadotropin stimulation. This hypothesis is based on a consideration of immunophenotypic markers expressed by gonocytes and CIS cells, types of abnormal GCs seen in developmental disorders that predispose to GCTs, and epidemiology of GCT incidence.[32]

A second model proposed by Chaganti and Houldsworth[34] takes into account four established genetic properties of GCTs—namely, increased 12p copy number, expression of cyclin D2 in CIS, consistent near triploid-tetraploid chromosome numbers, and abundant expression of wild-type p53. According to this model, aberrant chromatid exchange events during meiotic crossing-over may lead to increased 12p copy number and overexpression of cyclin D2. In a cell containing unrepaired DNA breaks (recombination associated), overexpressed cyclin D2 may block a p53-dependent apoptotic response and lead to reinitiation of cell-cycle and genomic instability.[34]

A role for cyclin D2 in the development of GCTs has also been suggested by studies of mice homozygously inactivated (mutant) for the *CCND2* gene and expression of *CCND2* messenger RNA in ovarian granulosa cell tumors and testicular GCT cell lines.[35] In GCs that have reentered the cell cycle after cyclin D2 activation, downstream events such as loss of tumor suppressor genes brought about by genomic instability may lead to neoplastic progression. Extensive molecular genetic analysis has identified loss of genomic or functional expression, or both, of several known tumor suppressor genes, such as *RB1*, *DCC*, and *NME*, and genomic loss at several previously recognized as well as novel chromosomal sites.[29,36] More recently, microarray technology has been used to identify candidate amplified and overexpressed genes on 12p that may ultimately provide a mechanistic basis for this genetic abnormality and its role in GCT development.[37,38]

Embryonal-Like Differentiation in Germ Cell Tumors

Male GCTs display, albeit in a spatially and temporally abnormal manner, patterns of differentiation that mimic stages normally undergone by the developing zygote. Among GCTs, seminoma can be viewed as transformed GCs that have retained the inhibitory mechanism for zygotic-like differentiation, a feature of GCs before fertilization. The *in vivo* expression patterns of kit receptor and SCF in GCTs are consistent with such a view. Thus, the kit receptor, which normally is expressed by spermatogonia and primary spermatocytes,[39] is expressed mainly by CIS and seminoma.[40] On the other hand, nonseminomas appear to down-regulate kit and up-regulate SCF, consistent with their loss of GC phenotype and acquisition of somatic fates.[40] The key developmental difference between seminoma and nonseminoma appears to be the loss of ability to retain GC-like totipotentiality by the former.

A great deal of effort has been directed toward understanding the mechanistic basis of decisions that determine the nature and regulation of proliferation and differentiation signals in the developing zygote.[41,42] In this context, GCTs and derived embryonal carcinoma cell lines provide a unique opportunity to study embryonal versus extraembryonal pathways of differentiation, as well as development of somatic lineage. The ability of GCTs to undergo an embryonal-like developmental program without the contribution of a maternal complement has obvious implications for genomic imprinting. Parental imprints are erased in normal GCs before meiosis, and new imprinting patterns are laid down during gametogenesis and again during embryogenesis.[43,44] Therefore, the target cell for transformation proposed in the authors' model, the meiotic spermatocyte, would be imprint-erased, which is consistent with observations of biallelic expression in GCTs of *IGF2* and *H19* genes, which normally show monoallelic expression

in postfertilization somatic tissues.[45,46] A possible mechanism by which embryonal and extraembryonal types of major differentiation paths are initiated in imprint-erased transformed GCs may be differential methylation of critical chromosomal regions. Studies have shown that promoter methylation of a number of genes indicating their functional silencing is more prevalent in nonseminomas than in seminomas.[47]

Chemotherapy Resistance of Germ Cell Tumors

Molecular genetic studies of GCTs that are clinically resistant to cisplatin-based chemotherapy have identified a subset that harbors *TP53* gene mutations,[48] a molecular alteration not normally associated with GCT.[49] Evaluation of the cellular response to cisplatin in one GCT-derived cell line with a *TP53* gene mutation indicated a relative resistance to cisplatin, in contrast to the extreme sensitivity of another GCT-derived cell line with wild-type *TP53*.[48] Presumably, the cisplatin resistance of this subset of GCTs is rooted in their inability to mount an apoptotic response after drug exposure due to an inactivating *TP53* gene mutation. On the whole, these tumors display higher than normal levels of wild-type p53,[50] with somewhat lower levels in mature teratomas.[51] Thus, somatic differentiation associated with a decline in p53 levels may comprise a cellular setting for the operation of selective pressure for *TP53* gene mutation.

A cohort of cisplatin-resistant GCTs has been analyzed for the presence of amplified DNA sequences, a genetic abnormality often associated with tumor progression and resistance to therapy. In this study, comparative genomic hybridization was performed on a panel of GCTs comprising 17 resistant and 17 sensitive tumors. High-level amplification of eight chromosomal regions (other than 12p) was detected in five resistant tumors, but in none of the sensitive group.[52] Once the identity and function of the amplified genes are determined, they may become relevant to the understanding of chemotherapy resistance of GCTs and other tumor types.

Male GCTs offer a system in which the cellular factors portending exquisite sensitivity to chemotherapy can be studied. Some studies have described a reduced ability of GCT cell lines to repair DNA lesions induced by cisplatin.[53] Although the precise biochemical link between the induction of physical damage in DNA and the cellular response to it is unclear, in general, cells treated with DNA-damaging agents respond either by induction of a delay in the cell cycle at the G_1/S phase boundary or by the induction of apoptosis, both of which are thought to be mediated by p53. It has also been suggested that the rapid apoptotic response of GCTs on exposure to chemotherapeutic agents may be due to a high ratio of the proapoptotic bax protein to the antiapoptotic bcl-2 protein, favoring apoptosis.[54] This has been substantiated in a limited number of GCT cell lines and needs to be further investigated at the *in vivo* level.[54] However, other *in vitro* studies have suggested that bcl-X_L, a bcl-2–related antiapoptotic protein, may act as the regulator of DNA damage–induced cell death in GCTs, rather than bcl-2.[55] In these studies, exogenous overexpression of bcl-2 in a GCT cell line resulted in sensitization of the cell line to DNA damage–induced cell death. Associated with this sensitization was a decreased endogenous expression of bcl-X_L, with little or no change in the level of bax expression. Other data suggest a failure of response or caspase activation, or both, as a contributor to cisplatin resistance.[56] A much attenuated apoptotic response to cisplatin has been observed in somatically differentiated GCT cell lines, reflecting the relative resistance of teratoma elements in GCT specimens.[57] The elucidation of molecular mechanisms whereby the unique apoptotic response to chemotherapeutic agents is achieved in GCT will contribute to the understanding of how such a response is achieved and suggest how resistance may be circumvented in GCTs and other tumor types.

STAGING

A comprehensive evaluation is necessary to define the extent of disease and determine the appropriate treatment. It includes pathology; physical examination; determination of serum concentrations of AFP, HCG, and lactate dehydrogenase (LDH); and radiographic studies.

ANATOMIC CONSIDERATIONS

The initial route of metastasis is lymphatic drainage to retroperitoneal lymph nodes (Fig. 31-2). Several lymphatic vessels emerge from the mediastinum testis and accompany the gonadal vessels in the spermatic cord. Where the spermatic vessels cross ventral to the ureter, some of these lymphatics diverge medially and drain into the retroperitoneal lymph node chain, whereas others follow the spermatic vessels to their origin. Lymph nodes located lateral or anterior to the inferior vena cava are called *paracaval* or *precaval nodes*, respectively. Interaortocaval nodes are those nodes between the inferior vena cava and the aorta. Nodes anterior or lateral to the aorta are preaortic or paraaortic nodes, respectively. The primary landing zone for a right testicular tumor lies in the interaortocaval nodes inferior to the renal vessels, and the ipsilateral distribution includes the paracaval, preaortic, and right common iliac. The primary landing zone for a left testicular tumor lies in the true paraaortic nodes inferior to the left renal vessels, and the ipsilateral distribution includes the paraaortic, preaortic, and left common iliac nodes. Metastatic nodal disease in more caudal areas, such as the common iliac, external iliac, or inguinal lymph nodes, is usually secondary to a large volume of disease with retro-

grade spread. If the patient has undergone a herniorrhaphy, vasectomy, or other transscrotal procedure, metastases to the pelvic and inguinal lymph nodes are more likely.

Contralateral retroperitoneal metastasis is represented by involvement of nodes usually associated with a tumor from the opposite side. For example, paraaortic lymphadenopathy in the presence of a right-sided primary tumor is considered contralateral. Contralateral spread is more common with right-sided tumors, rare with left-sided primaries, and usually occurs in the setting of large-volume disease.

Retroperitoneal lymphatics continue cephalad and empty into the cisterna chyle via the right and left lumbar trunks. Hence, lymphatic metastases above the retroperitoneal nodes may occur in the retrocrural nodes. Supradiaphragmatic spread occurs via the thoracic duct, leading to posterior mediastinal and left supraclavicular lymph node involvement. The anterior mediastinum is not part of this usual nodal hierarchy.

TUMOR IMAGING

Computed Tomography

Computed tomography (CT) is the most effective radiographic technique for identifying metastatic involvement above as well as below the diaphragm. A CT of the chest may detect pulmonary lesions, but many small lesions represent benign processes, and their clinical importance requires careful clinical judgment. In seminoma, such lesions rarely represent metastasis. A plain chest radiograph still is indicated in all patients with GCT.

CT scan with oral and intravenous contrast is the best technique for identifying retroperitoneal lymphadenopathy. The abdominal CT scan is normal in 70% of newly diagnosed seminomas and at least one-third of newly diagnosed nonseminomas. Because GCTs may grow rapidly, treatment decisions should generally be made within approximately 4 weeks of the last abdominal CT scan. Lymph nodes in a primary landing zone measuring 10 to 20 mm are involved by GCT approximately 70% of the time, and those measuring 4 to 10 mm are involved approximately 50% of the time.[58–60] Opacification of the tumor, duodenum, and proximal jejunum is often helpful

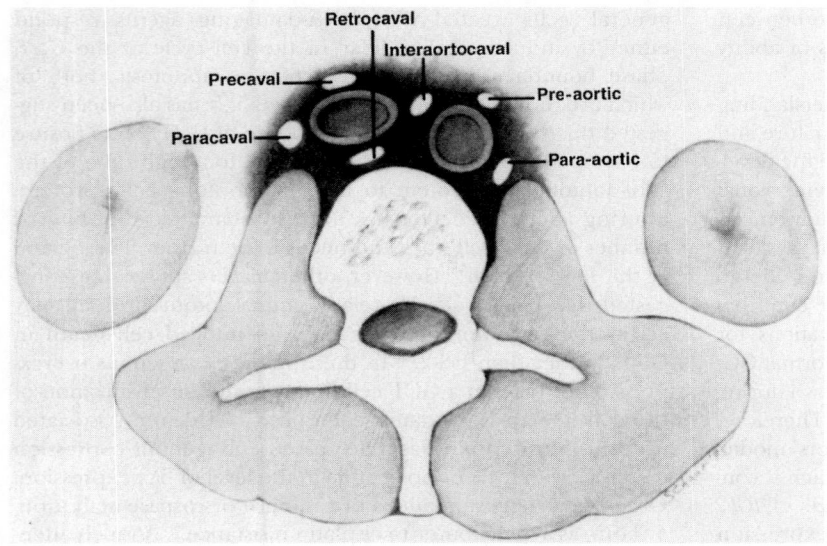

FIGURE 31-2. Retroperitoneal lymph nodes.

to distinguish bowel and the great vessels. After chemotherapy, the CT scan is unable to distinguish between residual viable tumor, teratoma, or necrosis/fibrosis; a normal postchemotherapy CT scan does not preclude the presence of disease.

Magnetic Resonance Imaging

Like CT scanning, magnetic resonance imaging (MRI) can identify enlarged lymph nodes. Although MRI occasionally provides valuable preoperative information regarding vascular anatomy and the patency of the great vessels in patients with bulky retroperitoneal disease after chemotherapy, it adds little to the management of most patients with GCT. Neither MRI nor CT can detect viable GCT after chemotherapy. Hence, MRI is generally not indicated.

Lymphangiography

Historically, lymphangiography (LAG) was used to determine the extent of retroperitoneal involvement in seminoma and nonseminoma. In most patients, CT scanning has replaced it. The role of LAG is limited to patients with stage I seminoma in which LAG is optional. LAG may reduce normal tissue irradiation by permitting more precise ports and identifying where a boost of radiation may be needed for abnormal nodes seen on LAG but not evident on CT scan.

Positron Emission Tomography

Studies have compared positron emission tomography (PET) to CT for the evaluation of patients with newly diagnosed disease or residual disease after chemotherapy. Although early studies suggest that PET may be more sensitive than CT, disease smaller than 0.5 cm was not detected.[61] In patients with NSGCT, PET has not been consistently able to identify residual viable malignant GCT and does not detect teratoma.[62,63] A study has shown that PET is useful in the detection of residual viable seminoma in patients with masses larger than 3 cm in diameter after chemotherapy.[64]

SERUM TUMOR MARKERS

α-Fetoprotein

AFP is determined by the enzyme-linked immunosorbent assay, which uses monoclonal antibodies in combination with monoclonal or polyclonal antibodies. The results of these assays are similar to those obtained by radioimmunoassay based on the binding inhibition principle. Assays are calibrated against the WHO standard code 72/225, in which 1 IU AFP corresponds to 1.21 ng. The normal adult serum concentration is usually less than 15 ng/mL. Approximately 10% to 20% of clinical stage I, 20% to 40% of low-volume clinical stage II, and 40% to 60% of advanced NSGCT will have increased AFP levels. Increased AFP levels are never seen in pure seminoma.

Human Chorionic Gonadotropin

HCG is a glycoprotein composed of two subunits and is produced by syncytiotrophoblasts. The α subunit is identical to that of luteinizing hormone (LH), follicle-stimulating hormone (FSH), and thyroid-stimulating hormone. The β subunits of HCG, LH, FSH, and thyroid-stimulating hormone are homolo-

gous but have distinct amino acid sequences. Elevated serum concentrations can be found in patients with pure seminoma as well as those with NSGCT. Most commercial methods have adopted the WHO Third International Standard (code 75/551), resulting in some uniformity in immunoassays to detect the HCG β subunit. The serum half-life of HCG β is 18 to 36 hours.

Approximately 10% to 20% of patients with clinical stage I, 20% to 30% with low-volume clinical stage II, and 40% with advanced NSGCT present with elevated serum concentrations of HCG. Approximately 15% to 20% of patients with advanced pure seminoma have increased serum concentrations of HCG.[65] False elevations of HCG secondary to either cross-reactivity of the antibody with LH; treatment-induced hypogonadism, which may resolve with testosterone replacement; or pituitary production of HCG have been reported.

Lactate Dehydrogenase

Increases in the serum concentration of LDH are a reflection of tumor burden, growth rate, and cellular proliferation. LDH comprises multiple isoenzymes, but, in practice, the combined LDH value for all isoenzymes is used for clinical decision making. Comparison of one laboratory to another is possible by using ratios of the detected level to the upper limit of normal for the individual assay. Increased serum LDH concentrations are observed in approximately 60% of NSGCT patients with advanced disease and in 80% of patients with advanced seminoma.

STAGING CLASSIFICATIONS

Revised TNM (tumor, node, metastasis) and stage groupings of the American Joint Committee on Cancer (AJCC) and the International Union Against Cancer (UICC) were adopted in 1997[66] (Table 31-3). For the first time, the serum concentrations of AFP, HCG, and LDH were incorporated into an "S" category because of their independent prognostic significance (see Factors Affecting Outcome in Advanced Disease, later in this chapter). Broadly, stage I disease is confined to the testis, stage II disease is restricted to the retroperitoneum, and stage III disease represents involvement of supradiaphragmatic or other nodal sites, visceral sites, or markedly increased serum marker levels.

Factors Affecting Staging of the Primary Tumor (T Stage)

The T stage of the primary lesion (not size), histology, and serum tumor marker concentrations predict the likelihood of retroperitoneal disease. For NSGCT, the presence of lymphovascular invasion has been associated with a higher likelihood of retroperitoneal metastasis (approximately 50%) and is now included in the definition of T2. Invasion through the tunica albuginea into the tunica vaginalis (also T2), spermatic cord (T3), or scrotum (T4) is an additional adverse feature. Prognostic factors predicting retroperitoneal disease in seminoma are controversial. Persistently elevated markers after orchiectomy imply metastatic disease.

Factors Affecting Staging of Regional (Retroperitoneal) Nodes (N Stage)

Metastatic disease to retroperitoneal lymph nodes is considered to be stage II disease. The classification of retroperitoneal

TABLE 31-3. TNM Staging of Testis Tumors: American Joint Committee on Cancer

Definition of TNM

PRIMARY TUMOR (PT)

pTX	Primary tumor cannot be assessed (if no radical orchiectomy has been performed, TX is used)
pT0	No evidence of primary tumor (e.g., histologic scar in testis)
pTis	Intratubular germ cell neoplasia (carcinoma *in situ*)
pT1	Tumor limited to the testis and epididymis without vascular/lymphatic invasion. Tumor may invade into the tunica albuginea but not the tunica vaginalis
pT2	Tumor limited to the testis and epididymis with vascular/lymphatic invasion or tumor extending through the tunica albuginea with involvement of the tunica vaginalis
pT3	Tumor invades the spermatic cord with or without vascular/lymphatic invasion
pT4	Tumor invades the scrotum with or without vascular/lymphatic invasion

REGIONAL LYMPH NODES (N)

Clinical

NX	Regional lymph nodes cannot be assessed
N0	No regional lymph node metastasis
N1	Metastasis with a lymph node mass 2 cm or less in greatest dimension; or multiple lymph nodes, none more than 2 cm in greatest dimension
N2	Metastasis with a lymph node mass more than 2 cm but not more than 5 cm in greatest dimension; or multiple lymph nodes, any one mass greater than 2 cm but not more than 5 cm in greatest dimension
N3	Metastasis with a lymph node mass more than 5 cm in greatest dimension

Pathologic (pN)

pNX	Regional lymph nodes cannot be assessed
pN0	No evidence of tumor in lymph nodes
pN1	Metastasis with a lymph node mass 2 cm or less in greatest dimension and less than or equal to 5 nodes positive, none more than 2 cm in greatest dimension
pN2	Metastasis with a lymph node mass more than 2 cm but not more than 5 cm in greatest dimension; or more than 5 nodes positive, none more than 5 cm; or evidence of extranodal extension of tumor
pN3	Metastasis with a lymph node mass more than 5 cm in greatest dimension

DISTANT METASTASES (M)

MX	Distant metastasis cannot be assessed
M0	No distant metastasis
M1	Distant metastasis
M1a	Nonregional nodal or pulmonary metastases
M1b	Distant metastasis other than to nonregional lymph nodes and lungs

SERUM TUMOR MARKERS (S)

	LDH	HCG (mIU/mL)	AFP (ng/mL)
S1	$<1.5 \times N^a$	<5000	<1000
S2	$1.5{-}10 \times N^a$	5000–50,000	1000–10,000
S3	$>10 \times N^a$	>50,000	>10,000

STAGE GROUPING

	T	N	M	S
Stage I				
IA	pT1	N0	M0	S0
IB	pT2	N0	M0	S0
	pT3	N0	M0	S0
	pT4	N0	M0	S0
IS	Any pT/Tx	N0	M0	S1–3
Stage II				
IIA	Any pT/Tx	N1	M0	S0
	Any pT/Tx	N1	M0	S1
IIB	Any pT/Tx	N2	M0	S0
	Any pT/Tx	N2	M0	S1
IIC	Any pT/Tx	N3	M0	S0
	Any pT/Tx	N3	M0	S1
Stage III				
IIIA	Any pT/Tx	Any N	M1a	S0
	Any pT/Tx	Any N	M1a	S1
IIIB	Any pT/Tx	N1–3	M0	S2
	Any pT/Tx	Any N	M1a	S2
IIIC	Any pT/Tx	N1–3	M0	S3
	Any pT/Tx	Any N	M1a	S3
	Any pT/Tx	Any N	M1b	Any S

AFP, α-fetoprotein; HCG, human chorionic gonadotropin; LDH, lactate dehydrogenase; TNM, tumor, node, metastasis.
^{a}N indicates the upper limit of normal for the LDH assay.
From ref. 66, with permission.

lymph node involvement is either pathologic based on RPLND or clinical based on CT evidence (see Table 31-3).

PATHOLOGIC STAGING. The number and size of retroperitoneal lymph nodes found at RPLND in patients with NSGCT have prognostic importance. Most retrospective studies report a low incidence of disease relapse when fewer than six nodes are involved with tumor, *and* the largest node is no larger than 2 cm, *and* no extranodal tumor extension is evident. More extensive tumor involvement is generally associated with a relapse rate of 50% or more. Once lymph node involvement is demonstrated, neither histology of the primary tumor nor the presence of vascular invasion in the primary tumor appears to add prognostic value.

CLINICAL STAGING. The transverse diameter of the largest lymph node has been used to subcategorize stage II disease. For seminoma, the size of retroperitoneal adenopathy usually dictates the treatment modality. Relapse proportions after definitive radiation therapy for seminoma increase progressively to approximately 40% to 60% for nodes larger than 5 cm. In nonseminoma, treatment decisions are based not only on retroperitoneal lymph node size and location, but also on the presence of increased serum tumor marker concentrations.

Factors Affecting Outcome in Advanced Disease

Because 70% to 80% of patients with advanced GCT are cured with modern cisplatin-based chemotherapy, it is necessary to stratify patients according to the likelihood of cure. Histology, metastatic site, primary site, and serum tumor marker concentrations are independent prognostic variables and have been shown to predict the likelihood of cure. Patients who are the most likely to be cured (the good-risk subgroup) constitute the majority of GCT patients with advanced disease and should be treated with regimens that have maximum efficacy with least toxicity. In contrast, patients who are unlikely to be cured (poor- and intermediate-risk subgroups) constitute the minority of patients. For them, more effective therapy is needed; toxicity is an important but secondary issue.

Before 1997, several classification algorithms were used to assign risk status based on the extent of disease, specific sites of disease, and/or pretreatment serum tumor marker concentrations. A comparison of several risk criteria in advanced NSGCT revealed that the allocation to either good- or poor-risk categories was in agreement in only 56% of patients. A substantial number of patients assigned good-risk status by stringent criteria were classified as poor risk by those that were less stringent. The proportion cured in the poor-risk group increased with less stringent algorithms.[67]

The International Germ Cell Cancer Collaborative Group (IGCCCG) analyzed data from more than 5000 patients treated with platinum-based chemotherapy to develop a common classification system. The IGCCCG found that pretreatment levels of LDH, HCG, and AFP; site of the primary tumor (i.e., mediastinal vs. testis or retroperitoneal); and the presence or absence of nonpulmonary visceral metastases (such as bone, brain, or liver metastases) were independent prognostic factors for progression-free survival for patients with NSGCT.[68] Nonpulmonary visceral metastasis was the only significant prognostic factor in patients with seminoma. Investigators agreed on three strata of good-, intermediate-, and poor-prognosis patients with NSGCT; no poor-risk stra-

TABLE 31-4. Germ Cell Tumor Risk Classification: International Consensus

	Seminoma	Nonseminoma
Good risk	Any HCG	AFP <1000 ng/mL
	Any LDH	HCG <5000 mIU/mL
	Nonpulmonary visceral metastases absent	LDH <1.5 × upper limit of normal
	Any primary site	Nonpulmonary visceral metastases absent
		Gonadal or retroperitoneal primary tumor
Intermediate risk	Nonpulmonary visceral metastases present	AFP 1000–10,000 ng/mL
	Any HCG	HCG 5000–50,000 mIU/mL
	Any LDH	LDH 1.5–10.0 × upper limit of normal
	Any primary site	Nonpulmonary visceral metastases absent
		Gonadal or retroperitoneal primary site
Poor risk	Does not exist	Mediastinal primary site
		Nonpulmonary visceral metastases present (e.g., bone, liver, brain)
		AFP ≥10,000 ng/mL
		HCG ≥50,000 mIU/mL
		LDH ≥10 × upper limit of normal

AFP, α-fetoprotein; HCG, human chorionic gonadotropin; LDH, lactate dehydrogenase.
From ref. 68, with permission.

tum could be defined in seminoma (Table 31-4). The marker cutoff values were incorporated into the revised TNM classification.[66] Data suggest that tumor marker half-life and IGCCCG classification are independent markers of outcome.[69] In addition, p53 and Ki67 expression and apoptotic rate in the primary tumor may be new markers.[70] More data are needed before these markers can be used in routine staging. Hence, the IGCCCG grouping should be used in all clinical trials and in treatment decision making with patients who require initial chemotherapy for advanced disease.

MANAGEMENT OF CLINICAL STAGE I DISEASE

SEMINOMA

Radiation Therapy

Radiation therapy remains the treatment of choice for patients with clinical stage I seminoma. The ipsilateral hemiscrotum does not require therapy unless gross tumor spillage has taken place. A randomized trial shows that a simple paraaortic portal excluding the ipsilateral iliac and pelvic nodes is as effective as the dog-leg portal in overall survival. Although toxicity appears less, more pelvic relapses may be seen[71] (Fig. 31-3A). Conventional fractionation for clinical stage I disease is 150 to 180 cGy/d for five sessions per week using high-energy linear accelerator beams to a total dose of 2500 to 3000 cGy. Elective, prophylactic radiation therapy to the

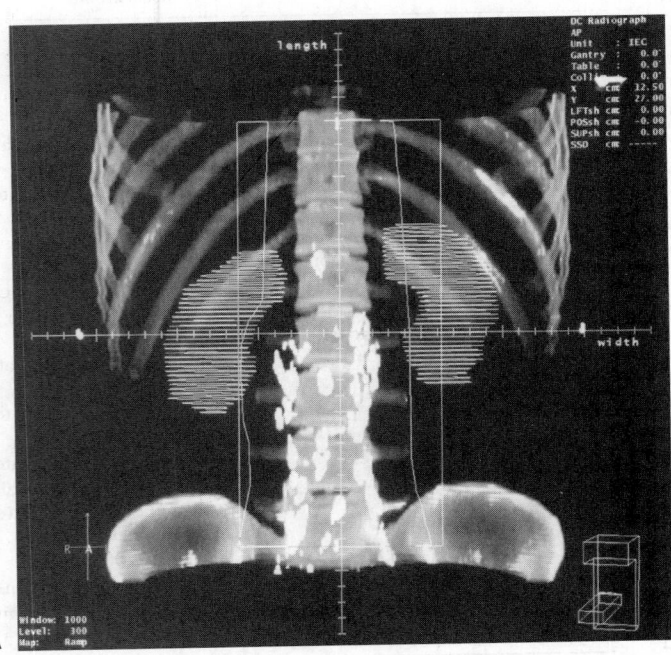

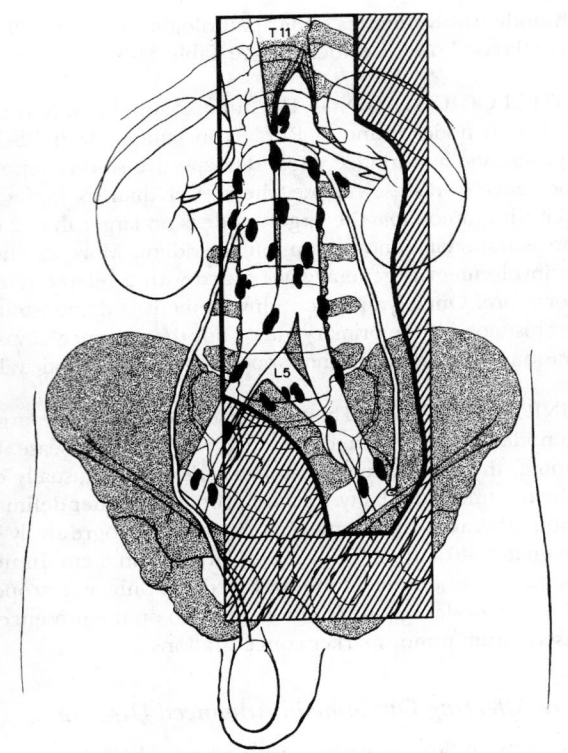

FIGURE 31-3. **A:** Paraaortic portal for clinical stage I seminoma. **B:** Contoured anterior and posterior radiation treatment fields for men with clinical stage II or IIA left testicular cancer. The diagonally shaded area is an individually made, 8-cm-thick Cerrobend block.

mediastinum is contraindicated. The contralateral testis should be shielded during treatment. Proper shielding results in an exposure of 1% or less of the total dose. For left-sided, primary testicular tumors, the left renal hilum must be encompassed. Treatment of pelvic lymph nodes is sometimes required for T4 primary tumors or for scrotal violation with tumor spillage. An involved spermatic cord margin at the internal ring may also require field extension. The relapse rate within the irradiated portal after adequate radiation therapy is negligible. The systemic relapse rate, usually presenting as a supraclavicular mass, averages 4% to 5% (Table 31-5), and the death rate is under 2%.[71–75]

Observation

Surveillance has been studied as the only management after orchiectomy, to be followed by chemotherapy at relapse[76] (Table 31-6). The relapse rate is approximately 15% to 20%, but the median time to relapse is long, with approximately 30% of relapses occurring 2 years after orchiectomy and approximately 5% occurring more than 5 years after diagnosis.[76,77] Over 5 years of follow-up, surveillance is more expensive than radiation therapy.[72] In the United States, observation for clinical stage I seminoma is not considered routine. Tumor size, rete testis invasion, and vascular invasion may be risk factors for relapse, but there is no prospective trial to test this hypothesis.[76] Risk factors for retroperitoneal relapse in seminoma remain undefined.

NONSEMINOMATOUS GERM CELL TUMORS

NSGCT is thought to be radioresistant, although one randomized trial reported no retroperitoneal relapse after radiation therapy. However, radiation therapy plays no role in its initial management, because chemotherapy for subsequent relapse might be compromised and the systemic relapse rate is higher than for seminoma.[78] If a patient has clinical stage I disease at the conclusion of initial staging, the choice of management options depends on specific histologic features and the status of serum tumor marker concentrations.

TABLE 31-6. Surveillance in the Management of Clinical Stage I Germ Cell Tumors

Tumor (Reference)	Patients (n)	Relapse (%)
Seminoma[76]	638	121 (19)
NSGCT[88–93]	996	277 (28)
T_1N_0 [90–93]	225	33 (15)
T_2N_0 [90–93]	136	68 (50)

NSGCT, nonseminomatous germ cell tumor.

TABLE 31-5. Relapse after Treatment of Seminoma with Radiation Therapy

Stage (Reference)	Patients (n)	Relapse (%)
I[71–75]	1964	79 (4)
IIA/B or "nonpalpable"[98–102]	290	17 (6)
IIC or "palpable"[98,99,102]	76	39 (51)

Retroperitoneal Lymph Node Dissection

Because of predictable lymphatic metastatic spread, the conventional approach to patients with clinical stage I NSGCT has been the modified bilateral RPLND (Fig. 31-4A). Despite refinement of radiologic imaging, 15% to 40% of patients are clinically understaged. Retroperitoneal metastasis is found in approximately 25% to 30% of patients who are judged preoperatively to have clinical stage I. Adequate exposure for RPLND can be achieved through either a thoracoabdominal or transabdominal approach. The standard bilateral infrahilar RPLND template, which remains the standard against which therapeutic alternatives are judged, includes the precaval, retrocaval, paracaval, interaortocaval, retroaortic, preaortic, paraaortic, and common iliac lymph nodes bilaterally. Because approximately 5% of these specimens harbor disease either within the gonadal vessel itself or the adjacent tissue, the ipsilateral gonadal vein and surrounding fibroadipose tissue from its insertion in the inferior vena cava (right) or left renal vein (left) to the internal ring must be completely excised. This minimizes the possibility of a late paracolic recurrence.[79]

A properly performed RPLND is a curative procedure, with rare infield recurrence and a surgical mortality of less than 1%. Infrequent major complications include pancreatitis, renal vascular or ureteral injuries, chylous ascites, aortic wall necrosis, bowel obstruction, pulmonary emboli, hemorrhage, and wound dehiscence. Minor complications include lymphocele, atelectasis, wound infection, and prolonged ileus.[80] In the past, most patients undergoing bilateral RPLND experienced retrograde ejaculation and subsequent infertility. An improved understanding of the neuroanatomy of seminal emission and ejaculation and the known pattern of retroperitoneal metastasis for right- and left-sided tumors led to modification of infrahilar surgical boundaries and techniques.

NEUROANATOMY. Antegrade ejaculation requires coordination of three separate events: (1) closure of the bladder neck, (2) seminal emission, and (3) ejaculation. The sympathetic fibers that mediate seminal emission emanate primarily from the T-12 to L-3 thoracolumbar spinal cord. In the midretroperitoneum, after leaving the sympathetic trunk, the fibers converge toward midline and form the hypogastric plexus near the aortic bifurcation. From the hypogastric plexus, sympathetic fibers travel via pelvic nerves to innervate the vas deferens, seminal vesicles, prostate, and bladder neck. Ejaculation is mediated by combined autonomic and somatic innervation originating at the sacral and lumbar spinal cord levels. Sympathetic stimulation tightens the bladder neck, whereas pudendal somatic innervation from S-2 to S-4 causes relaxation of the external urethral sphincter and rhythmic contraction of bulbourethral and perineal muscles. Preservation of ejaculatory capacity requires preservation of paravertebral sympathetic ganglia and their fibers, which converge at the superior hypogastric plexus around the aortic bifurcation. Sympathetic chains and postganglionic sympathetic fibers can be prospectively identified, meticulously dissected, and preserved.

Modified and Nerve-Sparing Retroperitoneal Lymph Node Dissection

A number of modified RPLND templates for right- and left-sided primary tumors reduce the frequency of retrograde ejaculation.

Modified templates do not identify specific nerve fibers but include a thorough resection of all interaortocaval and ipsilateral lymph nodes between the level of renal vessels and the bifurcation of the common iliac artery while limiting contralateral dissection above the level of the inferior mesenteric artery (see Fig. 31-4B,C). This approach minimizes trauma to the hypogastric plexus and contralateral postganglionic sympathetic fibers. Rates of ejaculation range between 50% and 80%. Data on reoperative surgery indicate that the paraaortic region is the most common site of surgical failure. Therefore, it is important to include a thorough dissection of the paraaortic lymph nodes in a right-sided modified RPLND template[81] (see Fig. 31-4B). Contralateral nodal involvement is higher for right-sided compared to left-sided primary tumors.

In a nerve-sparing RPLND, both sympathetic chains, the postganglionic sympathetic fibers and the hypogastric plexus, are prospectively identified, dissected, and preserved.[82] Antegrade ejaculation is reported in greater than 95% of clinical stage I patients who undergo a nerve-sparing (nerve-dissecting) RPLND. Nerve-sparing techniques can be used in the primary or postchemotherapy setting and within a standard bilateral or modified template, depending on clinical and intraoperative factors. Margins of resection should never be compromised in an attempt to preserve ejaculation.

Laparoscopic Retroperitoneal Lymph Node Dissection

Several investigators have reported that laparoscopic RPLND for clinical stage I NSGCT is technically feasible. After a lengthy learning curve, postoperative morbidity, operative blood loss, and length of hospital stay may be less compared to open surgery.[83] This approach relies on postoperative chemotherapy, because dissection is limited to areas anterior to lumbar vessels and omits the interaortocaval region for left-sided primary tumors, as well as nodes posterior to the great vessels.[83] One author reported that the dissection was limited or stopped if grossly positive nodes were found. In this study, the mean number of nodes removed for pathologic stage I and II disease (25 nodes or 14 nodes, respectively) was statistically significant ($P < .004$), raising doubts about therapeutic efficacy and therapeutic intent.[84] All patients with retroperitoneal disease, regardless of tumor volume, are treated with postoperative chemotherapy. Hence, the therapeutic efficacy of laparoscopic RPLND is difficult to assess. In addition, retroperitoneal recurrence has been reported.[83,85] Late relapses in the retroperitoneum due to inadequate dissection are potentially catastrophic.[86,87] The retroperitoneum was the most common site of late relapse in patients with clinical stage I disease (more than 2 years after initial treatment) despite adjuvant cisplatin-based chemotherapy.[87] Therefore, laparoscopic RPLND is not routine, should be considered an investigational procedure, and additional study in prospective clinical trials is necessary.

Regardless of technique, retrograde ejaculation is a potential risk with any RPLND, and preoperative sperm banking is recommended. α-Adrenergic drugs, such as ephedrine, pseudoephedrine, and imipramine, occasionally promote antegrade ejaculation in a subset of patients who are anejaculatory after RPLND. The low number of reported such cases suggests substantial case selection, and many patients will probably not respond to α-adrenergic stimulation. Transrectal electroejaculation provides an option for patients who fail sympathomimetic agents.

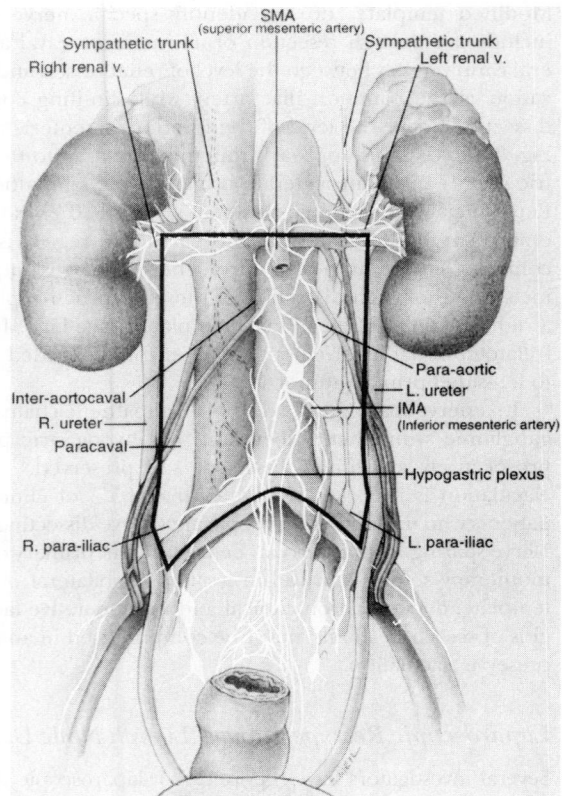

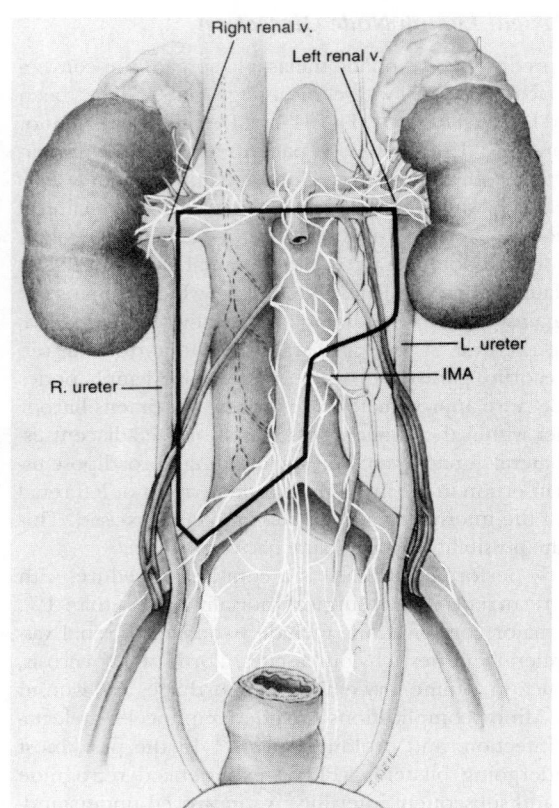

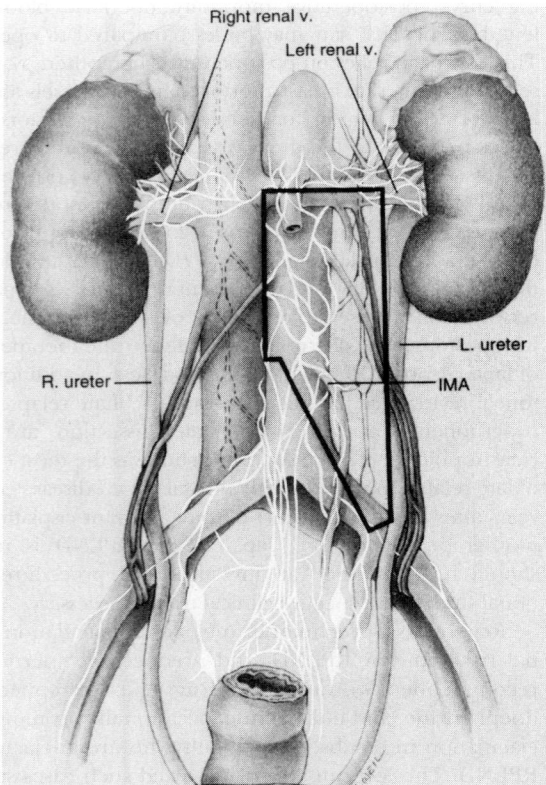

FIGURE 31-4. **A:** Standard modified bilateral retroperitoneal lymph node dissection. **B:** Modified nerve-avoiding template for right testicular tumors. **C:** Modified nerve-avoiding template for left testicular tumors.

Observation

The driving forces behind observation studies in clinical stage I patients were (1) the infertility resulting from RPLND due to retrograde ejaculation; (2) the frequent absence of therapeutic benefit from RPLND—that is, orchiectomy was a curative procedure or systemic disease occurred in the absence of retroperitoneal disease; and (3) the ability of cisplatin-based chemotherapy to cure systemic disease. Approximately 25% to 30% of patients with normal serum tumor markers relapse during surveillance[88–93] (see Table 31-6). However, approximately 50% of patients with T2 to T4 tumors relapse (T2 includes lymphatic or vascular invasion) compared to 15% of patients with T1 tumors[90–93] (see Table 31-6). Fewer than 10% of patients with NSGCT relapse more than 2 years after orchiectomy,[88,89,93] compared to approximately 30% after surveillance for seminoma.[76] Some studies suggest that a high percentage of embryonal carcinoma also predicts a higher likelihood of relapse. However, the correlation between lymphatic/vascular invasion and the presence of embryonal carcinoma is high, and general agreement on histologic criteria for relapse independent of vascular or lymphatic invasion does not exist. The retroperitoneum is the site of relapse in approximately two-thirds of patients, the lungs or markers alone in approximately one-third, and other visceral sites much less frequently. With observation, there is a slightly higher likelihood that chemotherapy and modified bilateral RPLND (not nerve sparing) will both be needed to achieve the same cure rate.

Patients with clinical stage I NSGCT with a T1 tumor and serum tumor markers that are normal or declining at half-life should be offered surgical as well as observation options. If surveillance is chosen, a possibly unnecessary RPLND is avoided, limiting therapy to orchiectomy alone in approximately 75% to 85% of the patients (i.e., those who never relapse). Patient compliance cannot be overemphasized. If RPLND is chosen, it should be of the nerve-sparing type (i.e., nerve dissection), thereby preserving ejaculatory capacity in most patients. Frequent CT scans of the abdomen are unnecessary once an RPLND has been performed. Because relapse is extremely uncommon after 2 years and rare after 5 years, periodic reevaluations may be annual in the fifth year and beyond.

Chemotherapy

Chemotherapy has been reported as initial treatment of patients with T2 to T4N0M0 stage I NSGCT. In reports of patients receiving two cycles of cisplatin-based chemotherapy, fewer than 5% relapsed and approximately 1% died of GCT.[94–96] Authors argue that this approach avoids RPLND by substituting a brief course of chemotherapy. However, all of these patients are exposed to the transient (e.g., myelosuppression), permanent (e.g., neuropathy), and delayed (i.e., cardiac events, Raynaud's phenomenon, acute leukemia) toxicities of chemotherapy. In addition, the frequency of late relapse is unknown. Thus, chemotherapy as initial treatment in patients with T2 to T4N0M0 disease is not standard in the United States.

Rarely, patients with clinical stage I disease are found to have persistently elevated serum concentrations of AFP or HCG, or both, after orchiectomy. If these markers increase or plateau at an elevated level after a period of observation, metastatic disease is present. Because the disease is often not limited to the retroperitoneum, this group of patients should receive initial systemic chemotherapy.[97] An RPLND is recommended if reevaluation after chemotherapy demonstrates new disease.

MANAGEMENT OF CLINICAL STAGE II DISEASE (LOW TUMOR BURDEN)

SEMINOMA

Low-tumor-burden stage II seminoma includes patients with retroperitoneal metastasis measuring smaller than 5 cm in maximum transverse diameter (clinical stages IIA and IIB)[98–102] (see Table 31-5). Radiation therapy is the treatment of choice for most of these patients. A dog-leg radiation portal is used. Fractionation is the same as that for patients with clinical stage I disease, except that a boost of approximately 500 to 750 rads is administered to involved lymph nodes (see Fig. 31-3B). Relapse is infrequent, and death from seminoma is rare. Prophylactic mediastinal radiation therapy is not indicated, because relapses solely in the anterior or posterior mediastinum are rare. The combination of supra- and infradiaphragmatic radiation therapy results in chemotherapy intolerance, a high rate of treatment-related mortality due to chemotherapy, and a greater-than-expected death rate from disease due to the inability to administer adequate doses of chemotherapy.[98,103]

Exceptions to the indication for radiation therapy in patients with clinical stage I and nonbulky clinical stage II seminoma include

1. Horseshoe kidney. Retroperitoneal radiation therapy in these patients will likely cause radiation-induced renal failure. Observation is preferred in clinical stage I, and primary chemotherapy is the treatment of choice for clinical stage II disease.
2. A second metachronous testicular GCT. Patients who have undergone a prior bilateral RPLND or received radiation therapy should be observed frequently if clinical stage I disease is present and undergo primary chemotherapy in the unlikely event that the disease is confined to residual retroperitoneal lymph nodes.
3. Inflammatory bowel disease. A discussion with an experienced radiation oncologist is indicated under such circumstances. If radiation therapy is not administered, the management policies noted for patients with a horseshoe kidney should be followed.

NONSEMINOMATOUS GERM CELL TUMORS

Low-tumor-burden clinical stage II NSGCT comprises disease ipsilateral to the primary tumor, at or below the renal hilum, not associated with tumor-related back pain, and limited to the primary landing zone. Ipsilateral solitary lymph nodes smaller than 3 cm are best handled by RPLND. Suprahilar or retrocrural lymphadenopathy, bilateral retroperitoneal nodal metastases, back pain, contralateral lymph nodes (even if the ipsilateral lymph nodes do not appear to be involved), nodal disease greater than 3 cm (even if solitary), or increased levels of AFP or HCG, or both, imply a higher likelihood of unresectable disease or distant metastatic disease, and initial chemotherapy generally is preferred.

Retroperitoneal Lymph Node Dissection

The standard approach to patients with clinical stage IIA and some IIB tumors and normal serum levels of AFP and HCG has been RPLND. The priority is to perform a definitive therapeutic operation, after which infield recurrence is rare. Margins of resection should not be compromised to maintain ejaculatory function. Nerve-sparing dissection may be possible, depending on the location and volume of disease.

Elevated serum tumor markers before RPLND predict for (1) relapse in patients with low-volume (pN1) retroperitoneal disease who did not receive adjuvant chemotherapy or (2) persistent NSGCT (often a persistent marker elevation after RPLND) despite complete resection of disease.[104] These patients should be considered for primary cisplatin-based chemotherapy.

Management after Retroperitoneal Lymph Node Dissection

Surveillance is a treatment choice for compliant patients with fewer than six involved nodes and none larger than 2 cm (pN1).[105] Approximately 20% of such patients relapse. Surveillance requires close monitoring and a compliant patient. Lack of patient compliance, psychological factors, occupation, geography, or other issues may make adjuvant chemotherapy the preferred choice in rare patients. Those who relapse during surveillance require three or four cycles of cisplatin-based therapy according to disease status at that time.

Adjuvant chemotherapy is a strong consideration in patients when six nodes or more are involved, any node is greater than 2 cm, or there is extranodal extension (pN2/N3).[105] A randomized trial showed that observation with standard treatment at relapse and two cycles of adjuvant chemotherapy had equivalent survival.[106] Treatment based on cisplatin and etoposide with or without bleomycin results in nearly 100% relapse-free survival.[107,108]

IDENTIFICATION OF RELAPSE

After radiation therapy for clinical stages I, IIA, and IIB seminoma, a chest radiograph; determination of serum concentrations of AFP, HCG, and LDH; and a physical examination should be performed approximately every 6 weeks to 3 months in the first year, every 3 to 4 months in the second year, and less frequently thereafter. An abdominal CT scan should be performed at the conclusion of radiation therapy. During surveillance for clinical stage I NSGCT, a physical examination, chest x-ray, and determinations of AFP, LDH, and HCG levels are required at approximately monthly intervals in the first year, every other month in the second year, and quarterly in the third year. An abdominal CT scan is required quarterly in the first year, every 4 months in the second year, and every 6 months beginning in the third year. Annual visits are sufficient in the fifth year and beyond. After RPLND, without adjuvant chemotherapy, a chest radiograph; determinations of serum concentrations of AFP, HCG, and LDH; and a physical examination are required approximately every 1 to 2 months in the first year, every 2 to 3 months in the second, and less frequently in the third year and beyond. Annual visits are sufficient to detect late relapse and second primary tumors after the fifth year. Provided that follow-up has been adequate, relapse in

these patients is nearly always "low volume" (good risk) and can be cured with chemotherapy.[109]

MANAGEMENT OF STAGE II AND STAGE III DISEASE (HIGH TUMOR BURDEN)

High-burden disease includes extensive or bulky retroperitoneal, supradiaphragmatic nodal or visceral metastases, and stage IIC seminoma, which has a high relapse rate with radiation therapy alone[98,99,102] (see Table 31-5). Cisplatin-based chemotherapy cures 70% to 80% of those patients. Adjunctive surgery is often essential to achieving a disease-free state. The commonly used standard treatment regimens are summarized in Table 31-7.

GOOD-PROGNOSIS GERM CELL TUMOR

Good-risk patients are those with the highest likelihood of complete response and cure after chemotherapy with or without surgery. Because response proportions range from 88% to 95% with favorable survival distributions, highest efficacy with least toxicity is the goal. Therefore, clinical trials have focused on eliminating bleomycin exposure, reducing the number of therapy cycles, and substituting carboplatin for cisplatin[110–115] (Table 31-8).

A randomized trial performed by Indiana University[110] examined the duration of therapy in 184 patients who received either four cycles of cisplatin, etoposide, bleomycin (PEB) administered over 12 weeks or three cycles administered over 9 weeks. Disease-free status and survival were similar in the two treatment arms. Three randomized clinical trials have evaluated the elimination of bleomycin from regimens containing etoposide and cisplatin. Etoposide and cisplatin (EP) for four cycles was compared to a five-drug, bleomycin-containing regimen in 164 evaluable patients and was found to be therapeutically equivalent.[111] No late relapses

TABLE 31-7. Commonly Used Chemotherapy Regimens for Metastatic Germ Cell Tumors

A. Previously untreated—good risk
  1. Etoposide   100 mg/m² IV daily × 5 d
     Cisplatin   20 mg/m² IV daily × 5 d
     4 cycles administered at 21-d intervals
  2. Etoposide   100 mg/m² IV daily × 5 d
     Cisplatin   20 mg/m² IV daily × 5 d
     Bleomycin   30 units IV weekly (e.g., days 2, 9, 16)
     3 cycles administered at 21-d intervals
B. Previously untreated—poor risk
     Etoposide   100 mg/m² IV daily × 5 d
     Cisplatin   20 mg/m² IV daily × 5 d
     Bleomycin   30 units IV weekly (e.g., days 2, 9, 16)
     4 cycles administered at 21-d intervals
C. Previously treated—first-line salvage therapy
  1. Ifosfamide   1.2 g/m² IV daily × 5 d
     Mesna   400 mg/m² IV every 8 h × 5 d
     Cisplatin   20 mg/m² IV daily × 5 d
     Vinblastine 0.11 mg/kg IV days 1 and 2
  2. Paclitaxel   250 mg/m² IV by continuous infusion over 24 h day 1
     Ifosfamide   1.5 g/m² IV daily days 2–5
     Cisplatin   25 mg/m² IV daily days 2–5
     Mesna   500 mg/m² IV every 8 h days 2–5

TABLE 31-8. Randomized Trials in Good-Prognosis Germ Cell Tumors

Good-Risk Criteria (Reference)	Regimen (cycles)	Complete (Favorable) Response (%)	Durable Response (%)	Conclusion
Indiana[110]	BEP (4)	97	92	Regimens equivalent
	BEP (3)	98	92	
MSKCC[111]	VAB-6 (3)	96	85	Regimens equivalent
	EP (4)	93	82	
EORTC[112]	BEP (4)	95	91	BEP superior
	E$_{360}$P (4)	87	83	Survival same
Indiana[113]	BEP (3)	94	86^a	EP (3) inferior
	EP (3)	88	69	
MSKCC[114]	EC (4)	90	87	Carboplatin inferior to cisplatin
	EP (4)	88	76	
MRC/EORTC[115]	CEB (4)	87	77^b	Carboplatin inferior to cisplatin
	BEP (4)	94	91	
GETUG[117]	BEP (3)	92	—	Regimens equivalent
	EP (4)	91	—	
Australia[118]	BE$_{360}$P	87	96	BE$_{500}$P superior to BE$_{360}$P
	BE$_{500}$P	88	84	

B, bleomycin; C, carboplatin; E, etoposide; EORTC, European Organization for Research and Treatment of Cancer; GETUG, Genito-Urinary Group of the French Federation of Cancer Centers; MRC, Medical Research Council; MSKCC, Memorial Sloan-Kettering Cancer Center; NS, not stated; P, cisplatin; VAB-6, cisplatin + vinblastine + dactinomycin + bleomycin + cyclophosphamide.
^{a}Failure-free survival.
^{b}Response defined as failure-free, 1-year survival.

were found in patients with a median follow-up of 5 years.[116] A randomized trial of cisplatin and etoposide with (BEP) and without bleomycin (EP) was performed by the European Organization for Research and Treatment of Cancer (EORTC) in 395 patients. The dose of etoposide in this study was 360 mg/m^2 per cycle with planned dose modifications for thrombocytopenia, in contrast to 500 mg/m^2 per cycle without dose attenuations in American trials. The bleomycin arm was more toxic, including Raynaud's phenomenon in 8% of patients, and two patients died of pulmonary toxicity. The complete response rate was lower in EP patients, but no differences were observed in relapses, time to progression, or survival with more than 7 years of follow-up.[112] The clinical relevance of this trial is limited because all modern regimens now use 500 mg/m^2 doses of etoposide per course.

A French trial attempted to directly compare three cycles of BEP to four cycles of EP. This trial used standard doses of bleomycin and an etoposide dose of 500 mg/m^2 per cycle in both arms.[117] The criteria for good risk were those developed by the Institute Guslave Roussy. Most patients were good risk by the IGCCCG criteria. At the primary end point of "favorable" response, BEP (92%) and EP (91%) were equivalent. With 4-year follow-up, neither the event-free survival (89% BEP vs. 84% EP, $P = .09$) or overall survival (96% BEP vs. 92% EP; $P = .1$) was statistically different.[117] The trial has been criticized for insufficient power to detect a difference or to establish noninferiority, for the use of retrospective assignment to good-risk GCT by IGCCCG criteria, and for the performance of multiple statistical analyses, increasing the possibility of a false conclusion. Hence, this trial did not definitively compare BEP for three cycles to EP for four cycles. Finally, three cycles of PEB were compared to three cycles of EP in 166 patients.[113] The number of patients with persistent or progressive carcinoma, relapse, or viable cancer at postchemotherapy surgery was greater in those treated without bleomycin.

Two randomized trials have evaluated the substitution of carboplatin for cisplatin. In a multi-institutional trial of 265 patients, four cycles of carboplatin plus etoposide (EC) were compared to four cycles of EP.[114] Patients receiving EC had an inferior event-free (incomplete response or relapse, $P = .02$) and relapse-free ($P = .005$) survival and significantly worse myelosuppression, requiring platelet transfusions and hospitalization for granulocytopenic fever. In a subset analysis, EC was inferior to EP in seminoma and in NSGCT. The Medical Research Council and EORTC conducted a confirmatory, randomized trial comparing carboplatin, etoposide, and bleomycin to BEP in 598 patients. Complete response was greater in patients allocated to BEP (94% vs. 87%, $P = .009$), and 3-year survival was better (97% vs. 90%, $P = .003$).[115] Conventional-dose carboplatin therapy has no role in the management of good-risk GCT.

The debate over etoposide dose has been resolved. A randomized trial compared three cycles of BE$_{500}$P (etoposide = 500 mg/m^2 per cycle) and four cycles of BE$_{360}$P (etoposide = 360 mg/m^2 per cycle). Disease-related mortality was higher in the BE$_{360}$P arm than in the BE$_{500}$P arm (16% vs. 4%, $P = .008$).[118] The schedule of drug administration does not appear to be clinically important.[119]

Although good-risk studies have differed in eligibility criteria, an efficacy threshold has been reached. Cisplatin-based therapy, 100 mg/m^2 per cycle, is required; there is no role for carboplatin-based therapy. Four cycles of EP or three cycles of BEP using a 500 mg/m^2 cumulative dose of etoposide per course are considered the standard of care for patients with good-prognosis GCT by IGCCCG criteria (AJCC/UICC stages I-S through IIIA).

INTERMEDIATE- AND POOR-RISK GERM CELL TUMOR

The separation of good-risk from intermediate- and poor-risk GCT is a critical assessment before starting chemotherapy. The IGCCCG criteria should be used to determine risk status.[68]

TABLE 31-9. Results of Randomized Trials in Patients with "Poor-Risk" Germ Cell Tumors

Criteria (Reference)	Treatment	No. of Patients	Complete Response (%)	Durable (%)	Benefit over Standard Arm
EORTC[120]	PEB	102	74	NS	—
	PEB/PVB	102	75	NS	No
Indiana[121]	PEB	77	73	61	—
	P(200)EB	76	68	63	No
EORTC/MRC[122]	BEP/EP	185	57	55	No
	BOP/VIP-B	186	54	53	—
Indiana[123]	PEB	141	60	57	—
	VIP	145	63	56	No

B, bleomycin; E, etoposide; EORTC, European Organization for Research and Treatment of Cancer; I, ifosfamide; MRC, Medical Research Council; NS, not stated; O, vincristine; P, cisplatin, 100 mg/m^2; P(200), cisplatin, 200 mg/m^2; V, vinblastine.

Because 75% and 45% of intermediate- and poor-risk patients, respectively, survive after treatment compared to approximately 90% of good-risk patients, clinical trials designed to increase the cure rate remain a priority. Such patients should be treated on clinical trials if at all possible.

The results of randomized studies conducted in poor-risk patients are shown in Table 31-9.[120–123] A randomized trial of bleomycin plus etoposide plus cisplatin administered at 200 mg/m^2 per cycle showed equal efficacy but greater toxicity than standard BEP.[121] Complicated multidrug regimens were not superior to BEP.[120,122] The role of ifosfamide was tested in a randomized trial. Etoposide, ifosfamide, cisplatin (VIP) had no therapeutic benefit over BEP, and VIP toxicity was more severe.[123] Therefore, in poor-risk patients, four cycles of BEP remain the standard regimen to which investigational regimens should be compared. Likewise, in nearly all intermediate-risk patients by IGCCCG criteria, four cycles of BEP are considered standard therapy.

The success of high-dose, carboplatin-containing chemotherapy in the treatment of patients with refractory disease (see Management of Relapse after Chemotherapy and Refractory Disease, High-Dose Therapy, later in this chapter) led to its incorporation into initial therapy. Poor-risk patients who were at high risk of failure based on clinical presentation were selected to receive high-dose therapy based on a prolonged clearance of serum AFP or HCG, or both, during standard induction therapy.[124,125] Hematopoietic reconstitution was rapid, only one treatment-related death was observed, and a trend to improved survival was observed in patients who received high-dose therapy when compared to historical poor-risk experience with conventional-dose, cisplatin-combination therapy.[125] Schmoll et al.[126] also reported the results of a single-arm study of high-dose chemotherapy with stem cell support as first-line therapy for advanced GCT patients with poor prognostic features. This long-term study also suggested a favorable outcome in patients receiving high-dose chemotherapy compared to a historical control of poor-risk patients treated with conventional-dose therapy.

Two large, ongoing randomized trials are designed to determine whether the higher burden of toxicity associated with high-dose therapy as first-line treatment for patients with poor-risk GCT is balanced by improved long-term survival. The phase I/II trial by Schmoll et al.[126] provided the rationale for the high-dose VIP arm in an ongoing poor-risk trial in Europe. A trial in the United States comparing BEP × 4 to two cycles of BEP plus two cycles of high-dose carboplatin, etoposide, and cyclophosphamide with stem cell support is nearing its accrual goal. In this second trial, patients deemed at intermediate risk solely on the basis of an increased LDH level 1.5 to 3.0 times the upper limit of normal were excluded because of a high complete response rate in this small subgroup.

MANAGEMENT OF RESIDUAL DISEASE

Adjunctive surgical resection of residual disease after chemotherapy is an integral part of the comprehensive management of all patients with advanced GCT.[127] In general, surgical exploration should be considered when serum tumor marker concentrations have normalized. It is generally agreed that all sites of measurable residual disease should be resected. Increased serum concentrations of AFP and HCG after chemotherapy nearly always imply unresectable, viable GCT; salvage chemotherapy is usually recommended for these patients.[128] A possible exception includes individuals with a minimal elevation of serum marker level, teratomatous elements in the primary tumor and a postchemotherapy cystic mass in the retroperitoneum. The fluid in those cysts sometimes contains elevated levels of HCG or AFP, or both, leading to minimal serum marker elevation that normalizes after surgery.[129]

Retroperitoneum

NONSEMINOMATOUS GERM CELL TUMOR. The retroperitoneal tumors resected after induction chemotherapy are necrotic/fibrotic in approximately 45% to 50% of resected specimens, teratoma in 35% to 40%, and viable GCT in the remaining 10% to 15% (Table 31-10).[130–135] The absence of teratoma in the primary site does not predict absence in a retroperitoneal metastasis.[134,136] A bilateral RPLND is often required, and retrograde ejaculation is the principal long-term consequence.

Over the past 15 years, retrospective studies have attempted to develop an accurate model to predict necrosis in the resected specimen.[134,137] Although size and shrinkage of retroperitoneal mass, preoperative marker levels, absence of teratoma in the primary site, and size of postchemotherapy mass have all been associated with a higher or lower likelihood of viable residual retroperitoneal disease, the false-negative prediction of necrosis is approximately 20%.[134,137] Moreover, the definition of a normal CT scan varies between studies and ranges from no visible mass to lymph node diameters of 10 to 20 mm.[135] Oldenburg et al.[133]

TABLE 31-10. Pathologic Findings in the Retroperitoneum after Chemotherapy in Patients with Advanced Nonseminomatous Germ Cell Tumor

Reference	Patients (n)	Necrosis (%)	Teratoma (%)	Carcinoma (%)
130	80	35 (44)	33 (41)	12 (15)
131	556	250 (45)	236 (42)	70 (13)
132	73	25 (34)	32 (44)	16 (22)
133	87	58 (67)	23 (26)	6 (7)
134	122	57 (47)	48 (39)	17 (14)
135	78	51 (65)	22 (28)	5 (6)
Total	996	476 (48)	394 (39)	126 (13)

reported that one-third of retroperitoneal postchemotherapy lesions measuring less than 2 cm contained either teratoma or viable cancer. In patients reported to have a normal CT scan after chemotherapy, either teratoma or viable GCT is present in 10% to 20% of resected specimens.[134–136] CT criteria alone are not sufficiently reliable to distinguish viable tumor or teratoma from necrosis. PET scanning has been studied as a technique to detect necrosis and fibrosis, but small size and teratoma are confounding factors.[62]

When observation is considered, the possibility of viable carcinoma, the biologic potential of teratoma, and the morbidity of RPLND are the major considerations in patients whose tumor markers have normalized and in whom the postchemotherapy CT scan is normal. If viable carcinoma is present, it is (at least) partially drug resistant and will progress. Observation of viable disease may reduce the cure rate. The cure rate of relapsed disease to vinblastine plus ifosfamide-based therapy is only 25% (see Conventional-Dose Salvage Therapy, later in this chapter), whereas complete resection of viable disease followed by two additional cycles of cisplatin-based therapy results in a cure rate between 50% and 70%.[138] In addition to viable GCT, teratoma is found in 30% of metastatic sites despite its absence in the primary tumor.[134,136] Although infrequent, the failure to resect teratoma may have at least three consequences. Mature teratoma may grow rapidly (growing teratoma syndrome),[139] become unresectable, or cause vascular or ureteral obstruction. Malignant transformation of teratoma (that is, somatic malignant elements such as sarcoma or carcinoma) is present in a minority of resected teratomas.[140,141] These elements are clonal in origin with the original GCT and do not represent second primary cancers.[142] Surgery is the only therapy for this subset of tumors that would otherwise recur and fail to respond to additional chemotherapy. Late relapse (defined as relapse occurring longer than 2 years after therapy), often manifesting as teratoma or viable GCT, is more common when teratoma is present at a metastatic site.[86,143] Late relapse of malignant GCT is often chemotherapy resistant, and chance of survival is poor.[144] Hence, RPLND remains the standard of care in management of the residual mass after chemotherapy in patients with NSGCT, and there is no subgroup of patients with retroperitoneal disease and a normal CT after chemotherapy who have a zero likelihood of either teratoma or a viable residual GCT.[134] A decision to observe in this setting should take these issues into account.

The complication rate of RPLND after chemotherapy is higher than that of primary RPLND.[80] Large-volume residual disease, postchemotherapy desmoplastic reaction, exposure to bleo-

mycin, and more extensive retroperitoneal dissection increase the technical demands of the procedure. Careful monitoring of intraoperative and postoperative oxygen concentration (particularly in patients who have received bleomycin), meticulous fluid management with strict replacement criteria, and an emphasis on colloid rather than crystalloid have reduced pulmonary toxicity and nearly eliminated perioperative death from acute respiratory distress syndrome.[128]

The best oncologic approach in NSGCT patients requiring postchemotherapy RPLND remains bilateral dissection. Ejaculatory dysfunction and sterility are common sequelae of the standard, modified bilateral RPLND, particularly after primary chemotherapy.[80] However, in selected patients without severe postchemotherapy desmoplastic changes, it is occasionally technically possible to identify individual sympathetic nerves and maintain antegrade ejaculation. Modified RPLND templates that avoid hypogastric plexus are not acceptable alternatives for residual disease after chemotherapy due to a higher risk of GCT at sites outside the limits of the nerve-avoiding template in patients with prior high-volume disease.[145]

The risk for relapse in patients with necrosis or teratoma in the retroperitoneal specimen ranges between 5% and 10%. Therefore, no additional chemotherapy is needed.[134,138] Conversely, the finding of viable GCT is associated with a high risk for relapse and decreased disease-free survival.[146] If viable disease is completely resected and two additional cycles of etoposide plus cisplatin (no bleomycin) chemotherapy are administered, the cure rate is 50% to 70%. A multicenter, retrospective study challenged the therapeutic value of additional chemotherapy in the setting of completely resected viable GCT. Additional chemotherapy appeared to benefit only those with one risk factor (complete resection or less than 10% viable malignant cells: good-risk IGC-CCG classification), but not those without risk factors or those with two or more risk factors.[147] This hypothesis has not been tested in a prospective trial. The standard of care remains two additional cycles of chemotherapy after resection of viable GCT after first chemotherapy.

Many investigators have consistently shown the adverse impact of incomplete resection. To assure complete resection in the postchemotherapy setting, it is sometimes necessary to perform adjunctive procedures, including *en bloc* nephrectomy, bowel resection, and/or *en bloc* resection of a great vessel. These patients also benefit from the experience of tertiary referral centers with surgeons who have extensive experience in postchemotherapy dissection.[81,146]

SEMINOMA. Two important features distinguish NSGCT after chemotherapy. First, teratoma in the residual mass is rare. Second, a complete RPLND after chemotherapy is often not technically feasible, secondary to severe desmoplastic reaction and obliteration of tissue planes.[148] Consequently, perioperative morbidity has been reported to be higher for seminoma than for NSGCT.

In a study of 104 patients, investigators at the Memorial Sloan-Kettering Cancer Center reported that 8 of 30 (27%) patients with a residual mass of 3 cm or larger relapsed, had residual seminoma, or harbored teratoma (2 cases), compared to only two (3%) local recurrences among 74 patients with masses smaller than 3 cm.[149] Conversely, other studies report that the size of the residual mass is not predictive of residual malignancy. Radiation therapy does not reduce the likelihood of recurrence.[150] Data have been published that clarify this debate. A 2,18 fluoro-deoxy-D-glucose (FDG)-PET scan study in 52 patients with residual masses after chemotherapy for bulky seminoma reported that all 8 positive scans and 42 of 44 negative scans were accurate.[64]

In summary, patients with residual masses smaller than 3 cm after chemotherapy for seminoma may be observed. An FDG-PET scan should be done in patients with a residual mass measuring 3 cm or larger. A negative PET scan in this setting is associated with a high likelihood of freedom from disease. A positive PET scan implies viable residual seminoma, and intervention should be considered. Surgical resection appears preferable. It should be done at centers with experienced surgeons to minimize operative morbidity.[149,150] All factors (e.g., size, site, comorbidity) must be considered in making this therapeutic decision.

Lung and Mediastinal Resections

Resection of residual disease at sites other than the retroperitoneum is less controversial. The likelihood is higher of teratoma or viable cancer, or both, occurring in a residual mass at nonretroperitoneal sites. The highest likelihood is observed in the mediastinum, probably because residual disease in the mediastinum is usually associated with primary mediastinal NSGCT.[134] Size of the pretreatment and the postchemotherapy pulmonary nodule does not correlate with final histology. Different histologies may also be present in each lung. Therefore, all sites of residual intrathoracic disease should always be resected.[151]

Other Procedures

A small percentage of patients require operation at multiple sites, usually the retroperitoneum and lung and (less frequently) the neck.[152] Again, the histology in a residual neck mass cannot be predicted based on histology at another site. When the lung and retroperitoneum are simultaneously involved, multiple, separate procedures may be required, but simultaneous bilateral thoracic and retroperitoneal resections are possible in selected cases.[153] If a primary testis tumor is present and an orchiectomy is not performed *before* chemotherapy, then it should be performed *after* chemotherapy, as that testis may harbor viable residual disease.[154] Studies repeatedly confirm that all sites of residual disease must be resected regardless of histologic findings at the initial procedure.

MANAGEMENT OF RELAPSE AFTER CHEMOTHERAPY AND REFRACTORY DISEASE

Twenty percent to 30% of patients with advanced GCT relapse or fail to achieve a complete response to conventional cisplatin-based chemotherapy. Effective second- and third-line salvage treatment options offer the possibility of cure to these patients whose disease displays a resistance to (B)EP as first therapy.

PROGNOSTIC FACTORS: SALVAGE CHEMOTHERAPY

Patients who relapse or fail to achieve a complete remission to initial (B)EP comprise a heterogeneous group with reported cure rates ranging from 0% to 78%. Prognostic factors can be used to predict which patients are most likely to benefit from conventional-dose salvage therapy and which individuals should proceed immediately to high-dose therapy. Patients with a testis or retroperitoneal primary site and a complete response to initial chemotherapy have a 35% to 40% 3-year survival with conventional-dose salvage therapy. Patients with an incomplete response to initial therapy or a relapsing mediastinal NSGCT have a less than 10% 3-year survival with conventional-dose, cisplatin-containing salvage therapy.[155] In these circumstances, a dose-intensive program, a novel treatment strategy, or a new agent should be considered.

Prognostic factors can also be used to identify patients who will most likely benefit from salvage high-dose, stem cell–supported, carboplatin-containing chemotherapy. Patients with primary mediastinal GCT refractory to initial and salvage chemotherapy, individuals with "absolute refractory" disease (rising markers or radiographic evidence of progressive disease within 4 weeks of cisplatin therapy), and patients with high HCG levels rarely achieve a complete response.[156,157] These factors should be taken into account when considering patients for a high-dose approach.

CONVENTIONAL-DOSE SALVAGE THERAPY

The combination of ifosfamide plus cisplatin, and etoposide (VIP) or vinblastine (VeIP) is a standard regimen in patients who relapse from complete remission (Table 31-11). In this heavily pretreated group, between 25% and 35% of patients achieved a complete response.[158–160] Nephrotoxicity and severe neutropenia were extremely common. Reported results suggest a markedly improved complete response rate when paclitaxel is substituted for vinblastine. Of 46 patients, 36 (78%) were progression free more than 18 months from the start of therapy.[161] The addition of

TABLE 31-11. Ifosfamide-Based Salvage Regimens for Relapsed/Refractory Germ Cell Tumors

Regimen (Reference)	No. of Prior Regimens	Evaluable	Complete Response (%)	Durable Complete Response (%)
VIP[158]	1	30	10 (33)	1 (3)
VeIP[159]	1	124	56 (45)	29 (23)
VeIP[160]	1	56	20 (36)	13 (23)
TIP[161]	1	46	—	36 (78)
VIP × 4[162] *a*	1	128	72 (56)	NS
VIP × 3[162] *a* → high dose × 1	1	135	76 (56)	NS

NS, not stated; TIP, paclitaxel, ifosfamide, and cisplatin; VeIP, vinblastine, ifosfamide, and cisplatin; VIP, etoposide, ifosfamide, and cisplatin.
*a*Randomized trial.

TABLE 31-12. High-Dose Carboplatin-Containing Chemotherapy in Patients with Refractory, Progressive Germ Cell Tumors

Institution	MSKCC[156]	Indiana[163]	Germany[164]	MSKCC[165]
No. of patients	58	40	68	37
Agents	Carboplatin, etoposide, cyclophosphamide	Carboplatin, etoposide ± ifosfamide	Carboplatin, etoposide, ifosfamide	Carboplatin, etoposide, ifosfamide, paclitaxel
% Complete response	40	30	51	57
% Alive, disease free	21	15	37	48
Median follow-up of survivors (mo)	28	>24	NS	30

MSKCC, Memorial Sloan-Kettering Cancer Center; NS, not stated.

one cycle of high-dose therapy after three standard cycles did not result in an improved survival over four standard cycles.[162]

HIGH-DOSE THERAPY

The chemosensitivity of GCT, a striking dose-response phenomena for individual drugs, the rare occurrence of bone marrow metastasis, and a young patient population permit administration of high-dose therapy. Three series of patients with refractory progressive GCT, who received carboplatin and etoposide with or without cyclophosphamide or ifosfamide, show that 15% to 37% of patients remained alive and disease free with long-term follow-up (Table 31-12).[156,163,164] The major toxicities are hematologic and infectious, with most studies reporting a 10% to 12% treatment-related death rate. In a fourth study, paclitaxel was incorporated into a four-drug regimen with three cycles of high-dose therapy, and preliminary data show that 18 of 37 patients (48%) are alive and disease free.[165] Hematopoietic growth factor support decreased the duration of neutropenia and hospitalization.[124] Peripheral blood–derived stem cells have largely replaced the use of autologous bone marrow, and randomized trials showed that peripheral blood–derived stem cells resulted not only in rapid neutrophil reconstitution, but also in faster platelet engraftment. Although these series demonstrate the curative potential of high-dose therapy, the majority of patients with cisplatin-refractory GCT die of disease, and new drugs and strategies are still needed.

High-dose chemotherapy has been studied as a treatment component for all patients who relapse after a complete response or fail to achieve complete remission to (B)EP. In one study, 57% of patients achieved a durable complete response after administration of two cycles of VeIP followed by two cycles of high-dose carboplatin and etoposide with stem cell support.[166] A study of three cycles of paclitaxel, ifosfamide, and cisplatin followed by only one cycle of high-dose therapy showed only 26% of patients achieving a durable complete remission.[167] A randomized trial of three standard cycles of etoposide plus ifosfamide plus cisplatin followed by one cycle of high-dose chemotherapy, compared to four cycles of standard therapy, reported no survival benefit in the high-dose arm.[162] Although there is no randomized trial of one versus two cycles of high-dose therapy, the data indicate that two cycles of high-dose therapy are necessary to cure refractory GCT. Three cycles of high-dose therapy are under study.[165]

NEW AGENTS

In the past decade, a number of single-agent trials have been conducted against refractory GCT. Paclitaxel, oral etoposide, gemcitabine, and oxaliplatin have demonstrated antitumor activity.[168–171] Because paclitaxel is synergistic with cisplatin and oxazaphosphorines *in vitro*, it is being studied in dose-intensive therapy with peripheral blood–derived, stem cell support,[165] and in conventional-dose therapy with ifosfamide plus cisplatin.[161] Oral etoposide plays a palliative role in refractory GCT. A report of durable complete remissions with oxaliplatin plus gemcitabine bears careful scrutiny.[172]

ROLE OF SURGERY AFTER SALVAGE CHEMOTHERAPY

Histologic findings of resected masses after salvage chemotherapy differ from those observed after primary therapy. Viable tumor occurs in approximately 50% of specimens, teratoma in 40%, and necrosis in only 10%.[138] Additional standard-dose chemotherapy confers no survival benefit in patients with viable NSGCT in the resected specimen after salvage chemotherapy, as opposed to clear benefit with two additional cycles following complete resection of NSGCT after primary chemotherapy.

In general, surgery should be avoided in patients in whom serum tumor marker concentrations remain elevated. Although this general rule holds true, surgery has curative potential in a highly select group of patients with increased marker levels and chemotherapy-refractory disease, even after salvage chemotherapy. Among three retrospective studies comprising 79 highly selected patients, 33 (42%) remain free of disease after "desperation surgery."[173–175] However, these 79 patients represent fewer than 5% of all patients with refractory disease. Hence, very few such patients are surgical candidates. Patients with a solitary retroperitoneal mass and increased AFP seem to be the best candidates. Technically difficult, this surgery should be performed at a tertiary center.

TREATMENT SEQUELAE

CHEMOTHERAPY

Control of nausea and vomiting is extremely important to maintain adequate hydration. Concurrent administration of a 5-HT$_3$ antagonist, dexamethasone, and aprepitant is superior to a 5-HT$_3$ antagonist and dexamethasone alone where cisplatin is administered in a single bolus. The role of aprepitant with 5 days of cisplatin is uncertain at this time.[176] Because cisplatin causes delayed emesis, administration of oral antiemetics is necessary for 2 to 4 days after therapy. The occasional patient in whom severe nausea and vomiting develop during chemotherapy should be hospitalized to protect renal function.

Nephrotoxicity

Nephrotoxicity from cisplatin occurs to some extent in all patients. Because of the effect of cisplatin on proximal tubules, progressive reduction in glomerular filtration and cumulative hypomagnesemia may result, associated with an increase in serum creatinine from pretreatment baseline, particularly after ifosfamide-based salvage chemotherapy. Nephrotoxicity may be severe in patients receiving high-dose chemotherapy in the salvage setting but does not appear to influence response rate or hematologic recovery.

Myelosuppression

Myelosuppression is common. Anemia occurs in virtually all patients but infrequently results in the need for red blood cell transfusions in those previously untreated. Grade 4 thrombocytopenia (platelet count smaller than 50,000) is distinctly uncommon with primary cisplatin-based therapy but frequent during salvage chemotherapy. Hematopoietic growth factors are recommended prophylactically after neutropenic fever but do not improve survival.[177] Severe anemia, neutropenia and neutropenic fever, and thrombocytopenia often accompany ifosfamide-based salvage therapy; hematopoietic growth factor support should be used prophylactically from the beginning of salvage therapy.

Peripheral Neuropathy

Peripheral neuropathy occurs in the majority of patients who receive vinblastine.[178] Replacing vinblastine with etoposide decreased the frequency of neuropathy, although cisplatin still causes symptomatic neuropathy in many patients. Auditory toxicity from cisplatin is often associated with reduced high-tone hearing and, less frequently, tinnitus.

Pulmonary Toxicity

Pulmonary toxicity from bleomycin is rare but can be fatal. In one randomized trial, it resulted in approximately half of the treatment-induced deaths.[179] In good-risk patients, a reduction in the number of bleomycin doses resulted in no bleomycin-related, treatment-related deaths.[110] Pulmonary function tests (vital capacity and diffusion capacity of carbon monoxide) have been used to dictate changes in bleomycin administration,[111] but their ability to predict clinically significant bleomycin-induced lung damage is not proven.[180]

Vascular Toxicity

Vascular toxicity is evolving as the most significant delayed toxicity of GCT chemotherapy. Raynaud's phenomenon occurs in 6% to 24% of patients receiving bleomycin administered by weekly bolus, and the substitution of etoposide for vinblastine did not reduce the incidence.[179,181] Most important, the risk of cardiac events increased two- to sevenfold over the general populations in the United Kingdom and Denmark after GCT chemotherapy.[181,182] Cardiac risk factors, including hypercholesterolemia, increased low-density and decreased high-density lipoprotein levels, and increased systolic and diastolic blood pressure were also significantly more frequent in treated patients than in the general population. Aggressive management of hypertension is warranted. Long-term attention to general health maintenance is important. Erectile dysfunction occurs and may be a sign of microvascular angiopathy.[183] Coronary artery disease resulting from mediastinal radiation therapy is well recognized and emphasizes the need to avoid mediastinal radiation therapy in the management of patients with seminoma.

Infertility

A substantial proportion of patients are subfertile or infertile at diagnosis. Reduced spermatogenesis and higher FSH levels compared to normal men are frequent in newly diagnosed patients and those with intratubular GC neoplasia.[184,185] However, paternity in patients on surveillance for clinical stage I disease does not seem to be reduced.[186] A standard, modified bilateral RPLND causes retrograde ejaculation in nearly all patients; nerve-dissecting and nerve-avoiding RPLND reduce but do not eliminate that risk. Scatter dose from radiation therapy for seminoma can affect the sperm count. The lower the scatter dose to the remaining testis, the more rapid the return of spermatogenesis.[187] Clamshell-type shields are better than pipe-cap–type shields. The mean gonadal dose in patients treated with a paraaortic field was significantly lower than that of a dog-leg field.[188] This was clinically confirmed by data from the Medical Research Council randomized trial.[71] Bieri et al.[189] showed that shielding resulted in a reduction of testis scatter even in those treated with the paraaortic field. Chemotherapy may affect the germinal epithelium directly, and Leydig cell insufficiency is frequent.[190] After chemotherapy, persistent oligospermia and abnormal forms and motility have been reported,[191] but conception may occur despite oligospermia. Therefore, cryopreservation of semen should be offered to all patients undergoing radiation, RPLND, or chemotherapy.[192]

Second Malignancies

Metachronous GCT appears in the contralateral testis in approximately 2% to 3% of all patients.[193] After the second orchiectomy, replacement testosterone is required. Etoposide causes secondary leukemia characterized by translocations involving chromosome 11q in less than 0.5% of patients receiving a total dose greater than 2000 mg/m^2,[194,195] 0.8% to 1.3% of patients receiving median cumulative etoposide doses greater than 2400 mg/m^2,[196] and as many as 6% of patients receiving total etoposide doses of greater than 3000 mg/m^2.[197] The latent period is short, averaging 2 to 4 years.

The relative risk of gastrointestinal malignancies increases after radiation therapy or radiation therapy plus chemotherapy and is greatest after 10 years.[198] Stomach cancer is the most prevalent gastrointestinal tumor. An excess of soft tissue sarcoma has also been observed.[198,199] This latent interval is long, and radiation therapy was implicated in the majority. These second malignancies do not outweigh the enormous benefits of treatment intervention. Along with the risk of recurrence, these second primary neoplasms emphasize the need for long-term follow-up of treated patients.

Sarcoidosis

Sarcoidosis appears more frequently in GCT patients.[200] Strictly speaking, it is not a sequela of therapy. It occurs before, as well as after, GCT diagnosis. Paratracheal adenopathy or pulmonary nodules without retroperitoneal adenopathy or elevated serum tumor marker levels, particularly in patients with seminoma, suggest the possible presence of sarcoidosis and should lead to biopsy.

MIDLINE TUMORS OF UNCERTAIN HISTOGENESIS

In a series of 220 patients with poorly differentiated carcinoma of unknown histogenesis and uncertain primary site, 26% achieved a complete response to cisplatin-based chemotherapy, and the 10-year actuarial survival was 16%. The cisplatin sensitivity, predominant midline tumor distribution, and occurrence in relatively young male patients suggested the possibility of an unrecognized extragonadal GCT despite the absence of increased serum concentration of AFP or HCG, or both, in most cases.[201] Molecular cytogenetic analysis for excess 12p copy number permits a diagnosis of GCT in approximately 30% of such tumors. A complete plus partial response proportion to cisplatin-based therapy is associated with the presence of a GCT genetic marker.[202] Genetic analyses also identified other tumors, such as primitive neuroectodermal tumors, lymphoma, desmoplastic small cell tumor, melanoma, and clear-cell sarcoma, indicating that this group of midline tumors has a heterogeneous histogenesis. Therefore, genetic analysis using conventional and molecular techniques has diagnostic and prognostic value.

OTHER TESTICULAR TUMORS

LEYDIG CELL TUMORS

Leydig cell (interstitial cell) tumors (LCTs) comprise approximately 2% of testicular tumors. Approximately 75% appear in adults, and the presentation is indistinguishable from GCT. A minority of patients have gynecomastia or decreased libido. The remaining 25% of cases present in children, sometimes with signs of sexual pseudoprecocity, such as pubic hair, voice change, or enlarged genitalia.[203] A testicular mass associated with virilization in a prepubertal patient is an LCT until proven otherwise. No association has been found between LCT and cryptorchidism. These tumors consist of tightly packed polygonal cells with eosinophilic granular cytoplasm and round nuclei with prominent nucleoli. Characteristic intracytoplasmic inclusion bodies (Reinke's crystals) are seen in approximately 25% to 40% of cases. A radical inguinal orchiectomy is required, and clinical staging includes a chest x-ray, CT scan of the abdomen and pelvis, and studies for urinary and serum steroids.

Most LCTs are benign. Malignant potential is difficult to predict. Vascular invasion, cellular atypia, tumor necrosis, infiltrative margins, increased mitotic rate, tumor size larger than 5 cm, and older age at presentation have been reported to predict malignant potential. Metastasis is the only reliable criterion of malignancy. The most frequent metastatic sites are the retroperitoneal lymph nodes followed by lung, liver, and bone. RPLND is reasonable in selected cases with adverse features. Metastatic LCTs are radioresistant and chemoresistant. For metastatic disease, particularly that which secretes steroids, ortho-para-DDD, a potent inhibitor of steroidogenesis, has produced responses, but cure is not possible.[204]

SERTOLI CELL TUMORS

Sertoli cell tumors (SCTs) account for fewer than 1% of primary testicular neoplasms. They are subclassified into classic, large cell calcifying (LCCSCT), and sclerosing.[205] The presentation is indistinguishable from that of GCT. LCCSCT are noted for multifocality, familial tendency, and bilaterality. An association has been reported between LCCSCT, pituitary adenoma, adrenocortical hyperplasia, cardiac myxoma, and pigmented skin and mucosal lesions. Precocious puberty is commonly noted in boys with LCCSCT. Feminization occurs in approximately 25% of classic SCT but is rare in LCCSCT.[206]

Most SCTs are benign and require RPLND only if accompanied by retroperitoneal adenopathy. Metastasis is the only reliable indicator of malignancy.[203] The most common sites for metastatic spread are the retroperitoneal lymph nodes, mediastinal nodes, lungs, liver, and bone. Sclerosing SCT and LCCSCT have minimal metastatic potential. Radiation therapy and chemotherapy are ineffective.

GRANULOSA CELL TUMORS

Granulosa cell tumors histologically resemble adult-type granulosa cell tumors of the ovary. Gynecomastia and increased estrogen secretion are common. These tumors are extremely rare; their metastatic potential appears limited. Radical orchiectomy is required. Juvenile granulosa cell tumors are the most common gonadal stromal neoplasms in early childhood, and the morphology may be confused with that of a yolk sac tumor. These patients usually present with maldescended testes, ambiguous genitalia, and an abnormal karyotype.

GONADOBLASTOMA

Gonadoblastoma are composed of sex cord elements admixed with GCs. Often bilateral, they occur in men with chromosome abnormalities and those with dysgenetic gonads. Metastasis from the GCT element may occur.

MESOTHELIOMA

Mesothelioma of the tunica vaginalis may invade the testis and frequently extends to the internal ring. Surgical intervention requires radical orchiectomy and complete excision of the spermatic cord and hemiscrotum. Retroperitoneal or inguinal metastasis may occur if the testis is invaded or if vascular invasion is present. Aggressive surgery is the only useful therapy.

SARCOMAS

Primary sarcomas may arise from the peritesticular and spermatic cord soft tissue elements and should be managed like other sarcomas (see Chapter 35.1). Radical orchiectomy is required. Subsequent adjuvant radiation therapy is occasionally required, depending on size and tumor grade.[207]

ADENOCARCINOMA OF THE RETE TESTIS

Adenocarcinoma of the rete testis is a highly malignant, very rare neoplasm that arises from the collecting system of the testis.[203] Located posteriorly, it often invades adjacent structures such as the cord and epididymis. More than one-half of patients present with metastatic disease. Survival rates are poor, with 30% to 50% dying within 1 year. These tumors generally do not respond to either radiation therapy or chemotherapy.[203] After radical orchiectomy, RPLND may be curative in some patients with minimal retroperitoneal involvement.

EPIDERMOID CYST

Epidermoid cysts of the testis usually present between the second and fourth decades. They are usually asymptomatic and discovered incidentally. These tumors are round, firm, and sharply demarcated on gross examination. Microscopically, the cyst is lined with stratified squamous epithelium. The adjacent testicular parenchyma is benign, and no CIS is present. The histogenesis of these tumors is uncertain. Their clinical behavior is uniformly benign. Testicular ultrasound may be diagnostic, in which case enucleation of the mass is sufficient treatment. Nevertheless, thorough histologic sampling must be performed to rule out a mature teratoma.

LYMPHOMA

Lymphoma is the most common secondary tumor of the testis and the most frequently occurring testicular neoplasm in men over the age of 50.[203] Approximately 40% of patients report systemic symptoms, such as fatigue, weight loss, and fever. Painless testicular enlargement is common, and bilateral involvement occurs in approximately one-third of patients. Radical orchiectomy establishes the diagnosis. Most cases are associated with systemic disease. Central nervous system as well as bone marrow disease is common. Survival is generally poor. Management of lymphoma is discussed in Chapter 41.2.

METASTATIC CARCINOMA

Metastatic carcinoma to the testis is rare and usually associated with diffuse systemic disease.[203] Bilateral involvement is noted in 15% of cases. The most common primary sites include the prostate, lung, melanoma, and kidney. Treatment may include radical orchiectomy, with further therapy dictated by the primary tumor.

REFERENCES

1. Jemal A, Tiwari RC, Murray T, et al. Cancer statistics, 2004. *CA Cancer J Clin* 2004;54:8.
2. Huyghe E, Matsuda T, Thonneau P. Increasing incidence of testicular cancer worldwide: a review. *J Urol* 2003;170:5.
3. Moul J, Schanne F, Thompson I, et al. Testicular cancer in blacks. A multicenter experience. *Cancer* 1994;73:388.
4. Forman D, Olier R, Brett A, et al. Familial testicular cancer: a report of the UK family register, estimation of risk and an HLA Class 1 sib-pair analysis. *Br J Cancer* 1992;65:255.
5. Bernardi D, Salvioni R, Vaccher E, et al. Testicular germ cell tumors and human immunodeficiency virus infection: a report of 26 cases. *J Clin Oncol* 1995;13:2705.
6. Timmerman J, Northfelt D, Small E. Malignant germ cell tumors in men infected with the human immunodeficiency virus: natural history and results of therapy. *J Clin Oncol* 1995;13:1291.
7. Moller H, Knudsen L, Lynge E. Risk of testicular cancer after vasectomy: cohort study of over 73,000 men. *Br Med J* 1994;309:295.
8. Herrinton LJ, Zhao W, Husson G. Management of cryptorchism and risk of testicular cancer. *Am J Epidemiol* 2003;157:602.
9. Peterson AC, Bauman JM, Light DE, et al. The prevalence of testicular microlithiasis in an asymptomatic population of men 18 to 35 years old. *J Urol* 2001;166:2061.
10. Rowland RG. Testicular microlithiasis: is it a benign condition with malignant potential? *Urol Oncol* 2003;21:538.
11. Bosl GJ, Vogelzang NJ, Goldman A, et al. Impact of delay in diagnosis on clinical stage of testicular cancer. *Lancet* 1981;2:970.
12. Feuer E, Frey C, Brawley O, et al. After a treatment breakthrough: a comparison of trial and population-based data for advanced testicular cancer. *J Clin Oncol* 1994;12:368.
13. Collette L, Sylvester RJ, Stenning SP, et al. Impact of the treating institution on survival of patients with "poor-prognosis" metastatic nonseminoma. *J Natl Cancer Inst* 1999;91:839.
14. Mostofi FK, Sesterhenn IA. Revised international classification of testicular tumors. In: Jones WG, Harnden P, Appleyard I, eds. *Germ cell tumors III*. Oxford: Pergamon, 1994:153.
15. Pugh RCB. *Pathology of the testis*. Oxford: Blackwell, 1976.
16. Montironi R. Intratubular germ cell neoplasia of the testis: testicular intraepithelial neoplasia. *Eur Urol* 2002;41:651.
17. Pryor J, Cameron K, Chilton C, et al. Carcinoma in situ in testicular biopsies from men presenting with infertility. *Br J Urol* 1983;55:780.
18. Berthelsen JG, Skakkebaek NE, von der Maase H, et al. Screening for carcinoma in situ of the contralateral testis in patients with germinal testicular cancer. *BMJ* 1982; 285:1683.
19. Giwercman A, Grindsted J, Hansen B, et al. Testicular cancer risk in boys with maldescended testis: a cohort study. *J Urol* 1987;138:1214.
20. Petersen PM, Giwercman A, Daugaard G, et al. Effect of graded testicular doses of radiotherapy in patients treated for carcinoma in situ of the testis. *J Clin Oncol* 2002;20:1537.
21. Motzer RJ, Reuter VE, Cordon Cardo C, et al. Blood group-related antigens in human germ cell tumors. *Cancer Res* 1988;48:5342.
22. Leibovitch I, Foster R, Ulbright T, et al. Adult primary pure teratoma of the testis. The Indiana Experience. *Cancer* 1995;75:2244.
23. Donadio AC, Motzer RJ, Bajorin DF, et al. Chemotherapy for teratoma with malignant transformation. *J Clin Oncol* 2003;21:4285.
24. Manivel J, Jessurun J, Wick M, et al. Placental alkaline phosphatase immunoreactivity in testicular germ-cell neoplasms. *Am J Surg Pathol* 1987;11:21.
25. Izquierdo M, VanDer Valk P, Van Ark-Otte J, et al. Differential expression of the c-kit proto-oncogene in germ cell tumours. *J Pathol* 1995;177:253.
26. Tickoo SK, Hutchinson B, Bacik J, et al. Testicular seminoma: a clinicopathologic and immunohistochemical study of 105 cases with special reference to seminomas with atypical features. *Int J Surg Pathol* 2002;10:23.
27. Ferreiro JA. Ber-H2 expression in testicular germ cell tumors. *Hum Pathol* 1994;25:522.
28. Hittmair A, Rogatsch H, Hobisch A, et al. CD30 expression in seminoma. *Hum Pathol* 1996;27:1166.
29. Chaganti R, Houldsworth J, Bosl G. Molecular biology of adult male germ cell tumors. In: Vogelzang N, Shipley W, Scardino P, et al., eds. *Comprehensive textbook of genitourinary oncology*. Baltimore: Williams & Wilkins, 2000:891.
30. Houldsworth J, Reuter V, Bosl GJ, et al. Aberrant expression of cyclin D2 is an early event in male germ cell tumorigenesis. *Cell Growth Differ* 1997;8:293.
31. Weinberg RA. The retinoblastoma protein and cell cycle control. *Cell* 1995;81:323.
32. Skakkebaek NE, Rajpert-de Meyts E, Jorgensen N, et al. Germ cell cancer and disorders of spermatogenesis: an environmental connection? *APMIS* 1998;106:3.
33. Skakkebaek NE, Berthelsen JG, Giwercman A, et al. Carcinoma in situ of the testis: possible origin from gonocytes and precursors of all types of germ cell tumors except spermatocytoma. *Int J Androl* 1987;10:19.
34. Chaganti RSK, Houldsworth J. The cytogenetic theory of the pathogenesis of human adult male germ cell tumors. *APMIS* 1998;106:80.
35. Sicinski P, Donaher JL, Geneg Y, et al. Cyclin D2 is an FSH-responsive gene involved in gonadal cell proliferation and oncogenesis. *Nature* 1996;384:470.
36. Murty VVVS, Chaganti RSK. A genetic perspective of male germ cell tumors. *Semin Oncol* 1998;25:133.
37. Bourdon V, Naef F, Rao PH, et al. Genomic and expression analysis of the 12p11-p12 amplicon using EST arrays identifies two novel amplified and overexpressed genes. *Cancer Res* 2002;62:6218.
38. Rodriguez S, Jafer O, Goker H, et al. Expression profile of genes from 12p in testicular germ cell tumors of adolescents and adults associated with i(12p) and amplification at 12p11.2-p12.1. *Oncogene* 2003;22:1880.
39. Loveland KL, Schlatt S. Stem cell factor and c-kit in the mammalian testis: lessons originating from Mother Nature's gene knockouts. *J Endocrinol* 1997;153:337.
40. Rajpert-de Meyts E, Skakkeback NE. Expression of the c-kit protein product in carcinoma in situ and invasive testicular germ cell tumors. *Int J Androl* 1994;17:85.
41. Conlon I, Raff M. Size control in animal development. *Cell* 1999;96:235.
42. Edlund T, Jessell TM. Progression from extrinsic to intrinsic signaling in cell fate specification: a view from the nervous system. *Cell* 1999;96:211.
43. Barlow D. Imprinting: a gamete's point of view. *Trends Genet* 1993;9:285.
44. Lyon MF. Epigenetic inheritance in mammals. *Trends Genet* 1993;9:123.
45. Van Grup RJHLM, Oosterhuis JW, Kalscheuer V, et al. Biallelic expression of the H19 and IGF2 genes in human testicular germ cell tumors. *J Natl Cancer Inst* 1994;86:1070.
46. Looijenga LHJ, Verkerk AJMH, Dekker MC, et al. Genomic imprinting in testicular germ cell tumours. *APMIS* 1998;106:187.
47. Koul S, Houldsworth J, Mansukhani MM, et al. Characteristic promoter hypermethylation signatures in male germ cell tumors. *Mol Cancer* 2002;1:8.
48. Houldsworth J, Xiao H, Murty VV, et al. Human male germ cell tumor resistance to cisplatin is linked to TP53 gene mutation. *Oncogene* 1998;16:2345.
49. Heimdal K, Lothe LA, Lystad S, et al. No germline TP53 mutations detected in familial and bilateral testicular cancer. *Genes Chromosomes Cancer* 1993;6:92.
50. Schenkman NS, Sesterhenn IA, Washington L, et al. Increased p53 protein does not correlate to p53 gene mutation in microdissected testicular germ cell tumors. *J Urol* 1995;154:617.
51. Heidenreich A, Schenkman NS, Sesterhenn IA, et al. Immunohistochemical and mutational analysis of the p53 tumor suppressor gene and the bcl-2 oncogene in primary testicular germ cell tumours. *APMIS* 1998;106:90.

52. Rao PH, Houldsworth J, Palanisamy N, et al. Chromosomal amplification is associated with cisplatin resistance of human male germ cell tumors. *Cancer Res* 1998;58:4260.
53. Masters JRW, Koberle B. Curing metastatic cancer: lessons from testicular germ cell tumors. *Nat Rev Cancer* 2003;3:517.
54. Chresta C, Masters J, Hickman J. Hypersensitivity of human testicular tumours to etoposide-induced apoptosis is associated with functional p53 and a high bax-bcl-2 ratio. *Cancer* 1996;56:1834.
55. Arriola EL, Rodriguez-Lopez AM, Hickman JA, et al. Bcl-2 overexpression results in reciprocal downregulation of Bcl-X(L) and sensitizes human testicular germ cell tumours to chemotherapy-induced apoptosis. *Oncogene* 1999;18:1457.
56. Mueller T, Voigt W, Simon H, et al. Failure of activation of caspase-9 induces a higher threshold for apoptosis and cisplatin resistance in testicular cancer. *Cancer Res* 2003;63:513.
57. Timmer-Bosscha H, de Vries EG, Meijer C, et al. Differential effects of all-trans retinoic acid, docosahexaenoic acid, and hexadecylphosphocholine on cisplatin-induced cytotoxicity and apoptosis in a cisplatin sensitive and resistant human embryonal carcinoma cell line. *Cancer Chemother Pharmacol* 1998;41:469.
58. Fernandez E, Moul J, Foley J, et al. Retroperitoneal imaging with third and fourth generation computed axial tomography in clinical stage I nonseminomatous germ cell tumors. *Urology* 1994;44:548.
59. Leibovitch I, Foster R, Kopecky K, et al. Improved accuracy of computerized tomography based clinical staging in low stage nonseminomatous germ cell cancer using size criteria of retroperitoneal lymph nodes. *J Urol* 1995;154:1759.
60. Hilton S, Herr H, Teitcher J, et al. CT detection of retroperitoneal lymph node metastases in patients with clinical stage I testicular nonseminomatous germ cell cancer: assessment of size and distribution criteria. *AJR Am J Roentgenol* 1997;169:521.
61. Albers P, Bender H, Yilmaz H, et al. Positron emission tomography in the clinical staging of patients with stage I and II testicular germ cell tumors. *Urology* 1999;53:808.
62. Stephens AW, Gonin R, Hutchins GD, Einhorn LH. Positron emission tomography evaluation of residual radiographic abnormalities in postchemotherapy germ cell tumor patients. *J Clin Oncol* 1996;14:1637.
63. Cremerius U, Effert PJ, Adam G, et al. FDG PET for detection and therapy control of metastatic germ cell tumor. *J Nucl Med* 1998;39:815.
64. De Santis M, Becherer A, Bokemeyer C, et al. 2-^{18}fluoro-deoxy-D-glucose positron emission tomography is a reliable predictor for viable tumor in postchemotherapy seminoma: an update of the prospective multicentric SEMPET trial. *J Clin Oncol* 2004;22:1034.
65. Mencel PJ, Motzer RJ, Mazumdar M, et al. Advanced seminoma: treatment results, survival, and prognostic factors in 142 patients. *J Clin Oncol* 1994;12:120.
66. Greene FL. AJCC cancer staging handbook. In: Page DL, Fleming ID, Friztz A, et al., eds. *AJCC cancer staging handbook*. New York: Springer Verlag, 2002:469.
67. Bajorin D, Katz A, Chan E, et al. Comparison of criteria for assigning germ cell tumor patients to "good risk" and "poor risk" studies. *J Clin Oncol* 1988;6:786.
68. IGCCCG. International Germ Cell Consensus classification: a prognostic factor-based staging system for metastatic germ cell cancers. *J Clin Oncol* 1997;15:594.
69. Mazumdar M, Bajorin D, Bacik J, et al. Predicting outcome to chemotherapy in germ cell tumors: the value of the rate of decline of human chorionic gonadotrophin and alpha-fetoprotein during therapy. *J Clin Oncol* 2001;19:2534.
70. Mazumdar M, Bacik J, Tickoo SK, et al. Cluster analysis of p53 and Ki67 expression, apoptosis, alpha-fetoprotein and human chorionic gonadotrophin discovers a prognostic subgroup within embryonal carcinoma germ cell tumor. *J Clin Oncol* 2003;21:2679.
71. Fossa SD, Horwich A, Russell JM, et al. Optimal planning target volume for stage I testicular seminoma: a Medical Research Council randomized trial. *J Clin Oncol* 1999;17:1146.
72. Warde P, Gospodarowicz MK, Panzarella T, et al. Long term outcome and cost in the management of stage I testicular seminoma. *Can J Urol* 2000;7:967.
73. Livsey JE, Taylor B, Mobarek N, et al. Patterns of relapse following radiotherapy for stage I seminoma of the testis: implications for follow-up. *Clin Oncol (R Coll Radiol)* 2001;13:296.
74. Santoni R, Barbera F, Bertoni F, et al. Stage I seminoma of the testis: a bi-institutional retrospective analysis of patients treated with radiation therapy only. *BJU Int* 2003;92:47.
75. Fossa S, Aass N, Kaalhus O. Radiotherapy for testicular seminoma stage I: treatment results and long-term post-irradiation morbidity in 365 patients. *Int J Radiat Oncol Biol Phys* 1989;16:383.
76. Warde P, Specht L, Horwich A, et al. Prognostic factors for relapse in stage I seminoma managed by surveillance: a pooled analysis. *J Clin Oncol* 2002;20:4448.
77. Chung P, Parker C, Panzarella T, et al. Surveillance in stage I testicular seminoma—risk of late relapse. *Can J Urol* 2002;9:1637.
78. Rorth M, Jacobsen GK, von der Maase H, et al. Surveillance alone versus radiotherapy after orchiectomy for clinical stage I nonseminomatous testicular cancer. Danish Testicular Cancer Study Group. *J Clin Oncol* 1991;9:1543.
79. Chang SS, Mohse HF, Leon A, et al. Paracolic recurrence: the importance of wide excision of the spermatic cord at retroperitoneal lymph node dissection (RPLND). *J Urol* 2002;167:94.
80. Baniel J, Foster R, Rowland R, et al. Complications of primary retroperitoneal lymph node dissection. *J Urol* 1994;152:424.
81. McKiernan JM, Motzer RJ, Bajorin DF, et al. Reoperative retroperitoneal surgery for nonseminomatous germ cell tumors: clinical presentation, patterns of recurrence and outcome. *Urology* 2003;62:732.
82. Jewett MA, Kong YS, Goldberg SD, et al. Retroperitoneal lymphadenectomy for testis tumor with nerve sparing for ejaculation. *J Urol* 1988;139:1220.
83. Janetschek G, Hobisch A, Holt L, et al. Retroperitoneal lymphadenectomy for clinical stage I nonseminomatous testicular tumor: laparoscopy versus open surgery and impact of learning curve. *J Urol* 1996;156:89.
84. Nelson JB, Chen RN, Bishoff JT, et al. Laparoscopic retroperitoneal lymph node dissection for clinical stage I nonseminomatous germ cell testicular tumors. *Urology* 1999; 54:1064.
85. Bianchi G, Beltrami P, Giusti G, et al. Unilateral laparoscopic retroperitoneal lymph node dissection for clinical stage I nonseminomatous germ cell testicular neoplasm. *Eur Urol* 1998;33:190.
86. Cespedes RD, Peretsman SJ. Retroperitoneal recurrences after retroperitoneal lymph node dissection for low-stage nonseminomatous germ cell tumors. *Urology* 1999;54:548.
87. Baniel J, Foster RS, Einhorn L, et al. Late relapse of clinical stage I testicular cancer. *J Urol* 1995;154:1370.
88. Daugaard G, Petersen PM, Rorth M. Surveillance in stage I testicular cancer. *APMIS* 2003;111:76.
89. Gels M, Hoekstra H, Sleijfer D, et al. Detection of recurrence in patients with clinical stage I nonseminomatous testicular germ cell tumors and consequences for further follow-up: a single-center 10-year experience. *J Clin Oncol* 1995;13:1188.
90. Alexandre J, Fizazi K, Mahe C, et al. Stage I non-seminomatous germ-cell tumours of the testis: identification of a subgroup of patients with a very low risk of relapse. *Eur J Cancer* 2001;37:576.
91. Roeleveld TA, Horenblas S, Meinhardt W, et al. Surveillance can be the standard of care for stage I nonseminomatous testicular tumors and even high risk patients. *J Urol* 2001;166:2166.
92. Dunphy C, Ayala A, Swanson D, et al. Clinical stage I nonseminomatous and mixed germ cell tumors of the testis. *Cancer* 1988;62:1202.
93. Sogani PC, Perrotti M, Herr HW, et al. Clinical stage I testis cancer: long-term outcome of patients on surveillance. *J Urol* 1998;159:855.
94. Pont J, DeSantis M, Albrecht W, et al. Risk-adapted management for clinical stage I nonseminomatous germ cell cancer of the testis (NSGCT) by regarding vascular invasion (VI): a 17 year experience from the Vienna Testicular Study Group. *Proc Am Soc Clin Oncol* 2003;22:388(abst).
95. Oliver RTD, Raja M, Ong J, et al. Pilot study to evaluate impact of a policy of adjuvant chemotherapy for high risk stage I malignant teratoma on overall relapse rate of stage I cancer patients. *J Urol* 1992;148:1453.
96. Cullen MH, Stenning SP, Parkinson MC, et al. Short-course adjuvant chemotherapy in high-risk stage I nonseminomatous germ cell tumors of the testis: a Medical Research Council report. *J Clin Oncol* 1996;14:1106.
97. Davis BE, Herr HW, Fair WR, et al. The management of patients with nonseminomatous germ cell tumors of the testis with serologic disease only after orchiectomy. *J Urol* 1994;152:111.
98. Thomas GM, Rider WD, Dembo AJ, et al. Seminoma of the testis: results of treatment and patterns of failure after radiation therapy. *Int J Radiat Oncol Biol Phys* 1982;8:165.
99. Willan B, McGowan D. Seminoma of the testis: a 22-year experience with radiation therapy. *Int J Radiat Oncol Biol Phys* 1985;11:1769.
100. Classen J, Schmidberger H, Meisner C, et al. Radiotherapy for stages IIA/B testicular seminoma: final report of a prospective multicenter clinical trial. *J Clin Oncol* 2003;21:1101.
101. Chung PW, Warde PR, Panzarella T, et al. Appropriate radiation volume for stage IIA/B testicular seminoma. *Int J Radiat Oncol Biol Phys* 2003;56:746.
102. Warde P, Gospodarowicz M, Panzarella T, et al. Management of stage II seminoma. *J Clin Oncol* 1998;16:290.
103. Loehrer PJ, Birch R, Williams SD, et al. Chemotherapy of metastatic seminoma: the Southeastern Cancer Study Group experience. *J Clin Oncol* 1987;5:1212.
104. Rabbani F, Sheinfeld J, Farivar-Mohseni H, et al. Low-volume nodal metastases detected at retroperitoneal lymphadenectomy for testicular cancer: pattern and prognostic factors for relapse. *J Clin Oncol* 2001;19:2020.
105. Kondagunta GV, Motzer RJ. Adjuvant chemotherapy for stage II nonseminomatous germ-cell tumors. *Semin Urol Oncol* 2002;20:239.
106. Williams SD, Stablein DM, Einhorn LH, et al. Immediate adjuvant chemotherapy versus observation with treatment at relapse in pathological stage II testicular cancer. *N Engl J Med* 1987;317:1433.
107. Behnia M, Foster R, Einhorn LH. Adjuvant bleomycin, etoposide and cisplatin in pathological stage II non-seminomatous testicular cancer. The Indiana University experience. *Eur J Cancer* 2000;36:472.
108. Kondagunta G, Sheinfeld J, Mazumdar M, et al. Relapse-free and overall survival in patients with pathologic stage II nonseminomatous germ cell cancer treated with etoposide and cisplatin adjuvant chemotherapy. *J Clin Oncol* 2004;22:464.
109. Kondagunta G, Sheinfeld J, Motzer RJ. Recommendations of follow-up after treatment of germ cell tumors. *Semin Oncol* 2003;30:382.
110. Einhorn LH, Williams SD, Loehrer PJ, et al. Evaluation of optimal duration of chemotherapy in favorable-prognosis disseminated germ cell tumors: a Southeastern Cancer Study Group protocol. *J Clin Oncol* 1989;7:387.
111. Bosl GJ, Geller NL, Bajorin D, et al. A randomized trial of etoposide + cisplatin versus vinblastine + bleomycin + cisplatin + cyclophosphamide + dactinomycin in patients with good-prognosis germ cell tumors. *J Clin Oncol* 1988;6:1231.
112. de Wit R, Stoter G, Kaye SB, et al. Importance of bleomycin in combination chemotherapy for good-prognosis testicular nonseminoma: a randomized study of the European Organization for Research and Treatment of Cancer Genitourinary Tract Cooperative Group. *J Clin Oncol* 1997;15:1837.
113. Loehrer PJ, Johnson DH, Elson P, et al. Importance of bleomycin in favorable-prognosis disseminated germ cell tumors: an Eastern Cooperative Oncology Group Trial. *J Clin Oncol* 1995;13:470.
114. Bajorin DF, Sarosdy MF, Pfister DG, et al. Randomized trial of etoposide and cisplatin versus etoposide and carboplatin in patients with good-risk germ cell tumors: a multi-institutional study. *J Clin Oncol* 1993;11:598.
115. Horwich A, Sleijfer D, Fossa S, et al. Randomized trial of bleomycin, etoposide, and cisplatin compared with bleomycin, etoposide, and carboplatin in good-prognosis metastatic nonseminomatous germ cell cancer: a multi-institutional Medical Research

Council/European Organization for Research and Treatment of Cancer trial. *J Clin Oncol* 1997;15:1844.

116. Bajorin DF, Geller NL, Weisen SF, et al. Two-drug therapy in patients with metastatic germ cell tumors. *Cancer* 1991;67:28.

117. Culine S, Kerbrat J, Bouzy C, et al. The optimal chemotherapy regimen for good-risk metastatic non seminomatous germ cell tumors (MNSGCT) is 3 cycles of bleomycin, etoposide and cisplatin: mature results of a randomized trial. *Proc Am Soc Clin Oncol* 2003; 22:382(abst).

118. Toner GC, Stockler MR, Boyer MJ, et al. Comparison of two standard chemotherapy regimens for good-prognosis germ-cell tumours: a randomised trial. Australian and New Zealand Germ Cell Trial Group. *Lancet* 2001;357:739.

119. de Wit R, Roberts JT, Wilkinson PM, et al. Equivalence of three or four cycles of bleomycin, etoposide, and cisplatin chemotherapy and of a 3- or 5-day schedule in good-prognosis germ cell cancer: a randomized study of the European Organization for Research and Treatment of Cancer Genitourinary Tract Cancer Cooperative Group and the Medical Research Council. *J Clin Oncol* 2001;19:1629.

120. de Wit R, Stoter G, Sleijfer DT, et al. Four cycles of BEP versus an alternating regimen of PVB and BEP in patients with poor-prognosis metastatic testicular non-seminoma: a randomised study of the EORTC Genitourinary Tract Cancer Cooperative Group. *Br J Cancer* 1995;71:1311.

121. Nichols CR, Williams SD, Loehrer PJ, et al. Randomized study of cisplatin dose intensity in poor-risk germ cell tumors: a Southeastern Cancer Study Group and Southwest Oncology Group protocol. *J Clin Oncol* 1991;9:1163.

122. Kaye S, Mead G, Fossa S, et al. Intensive induction-sequential chemotherapy with BOP/VIP-B compared with treatment with BEP/EP for poor-prognosis metastatic nonseminomatous germ cell tumor: a randomized Medical Research Council/European Organization for Research and Treatment of Cancer study. *J Clin Oncol* 1998;16:692.

123. Nichols CR, Catalano P, Crawford ED, et al. Randomized comparison of cisplatin and etoposide and either bleomycin or ifosfamide in treatment of advanced disseminated germ cell tumors; an Eastern Cooperative Oncology Group, Southwest Oncology Group, and Cancer and Leukemia Group B study. *J Clin Oncol* 1998;16:1287.

124. Motzer RJ, Mazumdar M, Gulati SC, et al. Phase II trial of high-dose carboplatin and etoposide with autologous bone marrow transplantation in first-line therapy for patients with poor-risk germ cell tumors. *J Natl Cancer Inst* 1993;85:1828.

125. Motzer RJ, Mazumdar M, Bajorin DF, et al. High-dose carboplatin, etoposide, and cyclophosphamide with autologous bone marrow transplantation in first-line therapy for patients with poor-risk germ cell tumors. *J Clin Oncol* 1997;15:2546.

126. Schmoll H-J, Kollmannsberger C, Metzner JT, et al. Long-term results of first-line sequential high-dose VIP-chemotherapy plus autologous stem cell support for patients with advanced metastatic germ cell cancer: an extended phase I/II study of the German Testicular Cancer Study Group. *J Clin Oncol* 2003;21:4083.

127. Sheinfeld J. The role of adjunctive postchemotherapy surgery for nonseminomatous germ-cell tumors: current concepts and controversies. *Semin Urol Oncol* 2002;20:262.

128. Sheinfeld J, Bajorin D. Management of the postchemotherapy residual mass. *Urol Clin North Am* 1993;20:133.

129. Beck S, Patel MI, Sheinfeld J. Tumor marker levels in postchemotherapy cystic masses: clinical implications for patients with germ cell tumors. *J Urol* 2004;171:168.

130. Donohue J, Rowland R, Kopecky K, et al. Correlation of computerized tomographic changes and histological findings in 80 patients having radical retroperitoneal lymph node dissection after chemotherapy for testis tumor. *J Urol* 1987;137:1176.

131. Steyerberg E, Keizer H, Fossa S, et al. Prediction of residual retroperitoneal mass histology after chemotherapy for metastatic nonseminomatous germ cell tumor: multivariate analysis of individual patient data from six study groups. *J Clin Oncol* 1995;13:1177.

132. Tait D, Peckham MJ, Hendry WF, et al. Post-chemotherapy surgery in advanced non-seminomatous germ cell testicular tumors: the significance of histology with particular reference to differentiated (mature) teratoma. *Br J Cancer* 1984;50:601.

133. Oldenburg J, Alfsen GC, Lien HH, et al. Postchemotherapy retroperitoneal surgery remains necessary in patients with nonseminomatous testicular cancer and minimal residual tumor masses. *J Clin Oncol* 2003;21:3310.

134. Toner GC, Panicek D, Heelan R, et al. Adjunctive surgery after chemotherapy for nonseminomatous germ cell tumors: recommendations for patient selection. *J Clin Oncol* 1990;8:1683.

135. Fossa SD, Qvist H, Stenwig AE, et al. Is postchemotherapy retroperitoneal surgery necessary in patients with nonseminomatous testicular cancer and minimal residual tumor masses? *J Clin Oncol* 1992;10:569.

136. Beck SD, Foster RS, Bihrle R, et al. Teratoma in the orchiectomy specimen and volume of metastasis are predictors of retroperitoneal teratoma in post-chemotherapy nonseminomatous testis cancer. *J Urol* 2002;168:1402.

137. Steyerberg EW, Keizer HJ, Fossa SD, et al. Resection of residual retroperitoneal masses in testicular cancer: evaluation and improvement of selection criteria. The ReHiT study group. Re-analysis of histology in testicular cancer. *Br J Cancer* 1996;74:1492.

138. Fox EP, Weathers T, Williams S, et al. Outcome analysis for patients with persistent germ cell nonteratomatous germ cell tumor in post-chemotherapy retroperitoneal lymph node dissections. *J Clin Oncol* 1993;11:1294.

139. Panicek DM, Toner GC, Heelan RT, et al. Nonseminomatous germ cell tumors: enlarging masses despite chemotherapy. *Radiology* 1990;175:499.

140. Motzer RJ, Amsterdam A, Prieto V, et al. Teratoma with malignant transformation: diverse malignant histologies arising in men with germ cell tumors. *J Urol* 1998;159:133.

141. Lutke Holzik MF, Hoekstra HJ, Mulder NH, et al. Non-germ cell malignancy in residual or recurrent mass after chemotherapy for nonseminomatous testicular germ cell tumor. *Ann Surg Oncol* 2003;10:131.

142. Bosl GJ, Ilson DH, Rodriguez E, et al. Clinical relevance of the i(12p) marker chromosome in germ cell tumors. *J Natl Cancer Inst* 1994;86:349.

143. Sonneveld DJA, Sleijfer DT, Koops HS, et al. Mature teratoma identified after postchemotherapy surgery in patients with dissected nonseminomatous testicular germ cell tumors. *Cancer* 1998;82:1343.

144. George DW, Foster RS, Hromas RA, et al. Update on late relapse of germ cell tumor: a clinical and molecular analysis. *J Clin Oncol* 2003;21:113.

145. Wood DPJ, Herr H, Heller G, et al. Distribution of retroperitoneal metastases after chemotherapy in patients with nonseminomatous germ cell tumors of the testis. *J Urol* 1992;148:1812.

146. Donohue JP, Lebovich I, Foster R, et al. Integration of surgery and systemic therapy: results and principles of integration. *Semin Urol Oncol* 1998;16:65.

147. Fizazi K, Tjulandin S, Salvioni R, et al. Viable malignant cells after primary chemotherapy for disseminated nonseminomatous germ cell tumors: prognostic factors and role of postsurgery chemotherapy—results from an international study group. *J Clin Oncol* 2001;19:2647.

148. Horwich A, Paluchowska B, Norman A, et al. Residual mass following chemotherapy of seminoma. *Ann Oncol* 1997;8:37.

149. Puc H, Heelan R, Mazumdar M, et al. Management of residual mass in advanced seminoma: results and recommendations from the Memorial Sloan-Kettering Cancer Center. *J Clin Oncol* 1996;14:454.

150. Duchesne GM, Stenning SP, Aass N, et al. Radiotherapy after chemotherapy for metastatic seminoma—a diminishing role. MRC Testicular Tumour Working Party. *Eur J Cancer* 1997;33:829.

151. McGuire MS, Rabbani F, Mohseni H, et al. The role of thoracotomy in managing postchemotherapy residual thoracic masses in patients with nonseminomatous germ cell tumours. *BJU Int* 2003;91:469.

152. See WA, Laurenzo JF, Dreicer R, et al. Incidence and management of testicular carcinoma metastatic to the neck. *J Urol* 1996;155:590.

153. Brenner PC, Herr HW, Morse MJ, et al. Simultaneous retroperitoneal, thoracic, and cervical resection of postchemotherapy residual masses in patients with metastatic nonseminomatous germ cell tumors of the testis. *J Clin Oncol* 1996;14:1765.

154. Geldart TR, Simmonds PD, Mead GM. Orchidectomy after chemotherapy for patients with metastatic testicular germ cell cancer. *BJU Int* 2002;90:451.

155. Motzer RJ, Geller NL, Tan CC, et al. Salvage chemotherapy for patients with germ cell tumors. the Memorial Sloan-Kettering Cancer Center experience (1979–1989). *Cancer* 1991;67:1305.

156. Motzer R, Mazumdar M, Bosl G, et al. High-dose carboplatin, etoposide, and cyclophosphamide for patients with refractory germ cell tumors: treatment results and prognostic factors for survival and toxicity. *J Clin Oncol* 1996;14:1098.

157. Beyer J, Kramar A, Mandanas R, et al. High-dose chemotherapy as salvage treatment in germ cell tumors: a multivariate analysis of prognostic variables. *J Clin Oncol* 1996; 14:2638.

158. Harstrick A, Schmoll HJ, Wilke H, et al. Cisplatin, etoposide, and ifosfamide salvage therapy for refractory or relapsing germ cell carcinoma. *J Clin Oncol* 1991;9:1549.

159. Loehrer P, Gonin R, Nichols C, et al. Vinblastine plus ifosfamide plus cisplatin as initial salvage therapy in recurrent germ cell tumor. *J Clin Oncol* 1998;15:2500.

160. McCaffrey JA, Mazumdar M, Bajorin DF, et al. Ifosfamide- and cisplatin-containing chemotherapy as first-line salvage therapy in germ cell tumors: response and survival. *J Clin Oncol* 1997;15:2559.

161. Donadio A, Sheinfeld J, Bacik J, et al. Paclitaxel, ifosfamide, and cisplatin (TIP): an effective second-line therapy for patients with related testicular germ cell tumors. *Proc Am Soc Clin Oncol* 2003;22:383(abst).

162. Rosti G, Pico J-L, Wandt H, et al. High-dose chemotherapy in the salvage treatment of patients failing first-line platinum chemotherapy for advanced germ cell tumors; first results of a prospective randomised trial of the European Group for Blood and Marrow transplantation: IT-94 study. *Proc Am Soc Clin Oncol* 2002;21:180a(abst).

163. Broun ER, Nichols CR, Kneebone P, et al. Long-term outcome of patients with relapsed and refractory germ cell tumors treated with high-dose chemotherapy and autologous bone marrow rescue. *Ann Intern Med* 1992;117:124.

164. Siegert W, Beyer J, Strohscheer I, et al. High-dose treatment with carboplatin, etoposide, and ifosfamide followed by autologous stem-cell transplantation in relapsed or refractory germ cell cancer: a phase I/II study. *J Clin Oncol* 1994;12:1223.

165. Motzer RJ, Mazumdar M, Sheinfeld J, et al. Sequential dose-intensive paclitaxel, ifosfamide, carboplatin, and etoposide salvage therapy for germ cell tumor patients. *J Clin Oncol* 2000;18:1173.

166. Bhatia S, Abonour R, Porcu P, et al. High-dose chemotherapy as initial salvage chemotherapy in patients with relapsed testicular cancer. *J Clin Oncol* 2000;18:3346.

167. Rick O, Bokemeyer C, Beyer J, et al. Salvage treatment with paclitaxel, ifosfamide, and cisplatin plus high-dose carboplatin, etoposide, and thiotepa followed by autologous stem-cell rescue in patients with relapsed or refractory germ cell cancer. *J Clin Oncol* 2001;19:81.

168. Motzer RJ, Bajorin DF, Schwartz LH, et al. Phase II trial of paclitaxel shows antitumor activity in patients with previously treated germ cell tumors. *J Clin Oncol* 1994;12:2277.

169. Einhorn L, Stender M, Williams S. Phase II trial of gemcitabine in refractory germ cell tumors. *J Clin Oncol* 1999;17:509.

170. Bokemeyer C, Gerl A, Schöffski P, et al. Gemcitabine in patients with relapsed or cisplatin-refractory testicular cancer. *J Clin Oncol* 1999;17:512.

171. Kollmannsberger C, Rick O, Derigs HG, et al. Activity of oxaliplatin in patients with relapsed or cisplatin-refractory germ cell cancer: a study of the German Testicular Cancer Study Group. *J Clin Oncol* 2002;20:2031.

172. Kollmannsberger C, Beyer J, Liersch R, et al. Combination chemotherapy with gemcitabine plus oxaliplatin in patients with intensively pretreated or refractory germ cell cancer: a study of the German Testicular Cancer Study Group (GTCSG). *J Clin Oncol* 2004;22:108.

173. Eastham J, Wilson T, Russell C, et al. Surgical resection in patients with nonseminomatous germ cell tumor who fail to normalize serum tumor markers after chemotherapy. *Urology* 1994;43:74.

174. Murphy B, Breeden E, Donohue J, et al. Surgical salvage of chemorefractory germ cell tumors. *J Clin Oncol* 1993;11:324.

175. Wood DP, Herr H, Motzer RJ, et al. Surgical resection of solitary metastases after chemotherapy in patients with nonseminomatous germ cell tumors and elevated serum tumor markers. *Cancer* 1992;70:2354.

176. Hesketh P, Grunberg S, Gralla R, et al. The oral neurokinin-1 antagonist aprepitant for the prevention of chemotherapy-induced nausea and vomiting: a multinational, randomized, double-blind, placebo-controlled trial in patients receiving high-dose cisplatin—the Aprepitant Protocol 052 Study Group. *J Clin Oncol* 2003;21:4112.

177. Fossa S, Kaye S, Mead G, et al. Filgrastim during combination chemotherapy of patients with poor-prognosis metastatic germ cell malignancy. *J Clin Oncol* 1998;16:716.

178. Stoter G, Koopman A, Vendrik C, et al. Ten-year survival and late sequelae in testicular cancer patients treated with cisplatin, vinblastine, and bleomycin. *J Clin Oncol* 1989;7:1099.

179. Williams SD, Birch R, Einhorn LH, et al. Treatment of disseminated germ-cell tumors with cisplatin, bleomycin, and either vinblastine or etoposide. *N Engl J Med* 1987;316:1435.

180. McKeage M, Evans B, Atkinson C, et al. Carbon monoxide diffusing capacity is a poor predictor of clinically significant bleomycin lung. *J Clin Oncol* 1990;8:779.

181. Meinardi MT, Gietma JA, van der Graaf WTA, et al. Cardiovascular morbidity in long-term survivors of metastatic testicular cancer. *J Clin Oncol* 2000;18:1725.

182. Huddart RA, Norman A, Shahidi M, et al. Cardiovascular disease as a long-term complication of treatment for testicular cancer. *J Clin Oncol* 2003;21:1513.

183. van Basten J, Hoekstra H, van Driel M, et al. Sexual dysfunction in nonseminoma testicular cancer patients is related to chemotherapy-induced angiopathy. *J Clin Oncol* 1997;15:2442.

184. Petersen PM, Skakkebaek NE, Vistisen K, Rorth M, Giwercman A. Semen quality and reproductive hormones before orchiectomy in men with testicular cancer. *J Clin Oncol* 1999;17:941.

185. Petersen PM, Giwercman A, Hansen SW, et al. Impaired testicular function in patients with carcinoma-in-situ of the testis. *J Clin Oncol* 1999;17:173.

186. Herr H, Bar-Chama N, O'Sullivan M, et al. Paternity in men with stage I testis tumors on surveillance. *J Clin Oncol* 1998;16:733.

187. Gordon W Jr, Siegmund K, Stanisic TH, et al. A study of reproductive function in patients with seminoma treated with radiotherapy and orchidectomy: (SWOG-8711). Southwest Oncology Group. *Int J Radiat Oncol Biol Phys* 1997;38:83.

188. Jacobsen KD, Olsen DR, Fossa K, et al. External beam abdominal radiotherapy in patients with seminoma stage I: field type, testicular dose, and spermatogenesis. *Int J Radiat Oncol Biol Phys* 1997;38:95.

189. Bieri S, Rouzaud M, Miralbell R. Seminoma of the testis: is scrotal shielding necessary when radiotherapy is limited to the para-aortic nodes? *Radiother Oncol* 1999;50:349.

190. Howell SJ, Radford JA, Ryder WDJ, et al. Testicular radiotherapy: evidence of Leydig cell insufficiency. *J Clin Oncol* 1999;17:1493.

191. Stephenson W, Poirier S, Rubin L, et al. Evaluation of reproductive capacity in germ cell tumor patients following treatment with cisplatin, etoposide, and bleomycin. *J Clin Oncol* 1995;13:2278.

192. Spermon JR, Kiemeney LA, Meuleman EJ, et al. Fertility in men with testicular germ cell tumors. *Fertil Steril* 2003;79 [Suppl 3]:1543.

193. Wanderas EH, Fossa SD, Tretli S. Risk of a second germ cell cancer after treatment of a primary germ cell cancer in 2201 Norwegian male patients. *Eur J Cancer* 1997;33:244.

194. Bajorin DF, Motzer RJ, Rodriquez E, et al. Acute nonlymphocytic leukemia in germ cell tumor patients treated with etoposide-containing chemotherapy. *J Natl Cancer Inst* 1993;85:60.

195. Nichols CR, Breeden ES, Loehrer PJ. Secondary leukemia associated with a conventional dose of etoposide: review of serial germ cell tumor protocols. *J Natl Cancer Inst* 1993;85:36.

196. Pedersen-Bjergaard J, Hansen ST, Larsen SO, et al. Increased risk of myelodysplasia and leukemia after etoposide, cisplatin, and bleomycin for germ-cell tumors. *Lancet* 1991;338:359.

197. Kollmannsberger C, Beyer J, Droz JP, et al. Secondary leukemia following high cumulative doses of etoposide in patients treated for advanced germ cell tumors. *J Clin Oncol* 1998;16:3386.

198. van Leeuwen F, Stiggelbout A, van den Belt-Dusebout A, et al. Second cancer risk following testicular cancer: a followup study of 1,909 patients. *J Clin Oncol* 1993;11:415.

199. Jacobsen G, Mellemgaard A, Engelholm S, et al. Increased incidence of sarcoma in patients treated for testicular seminoma. *Eur J Cancer* 1993;29A:664.

200. Toner GC, Bosl GJ. Sarcoidosis, "sarcoid-like lymphadenopathy," and testicular germ cell tumors. *Am J Med* 1990;89:651.

201. Hainsworth JD, Johnson DH, Greco FA. Cisplatin-based combination chemotherapy in the treatment of poorly differentiated carcinoma and poorly differentiated adenocarcinoma of unknown primary site: results of a 12-year experience. *J Clin Oncol* 1992;10:912.

202. Motzer R, Rodriguez E, Reuter V, et al. Molecular and cytogenetic studies in the diagnosis of patients with poorly differentiated carcinomas of unknown primary site. *J Clin Oncol* 1995;13:274.

203. Thrasher J, Frazier H. Non-germ cell testicular tumors. *Probl Urol* 1994;8:167.

204. Schwarzman MI, Russo P, Bosl GJ, et al. Hormone-secreting metastatic interstitial cell tumor of the testis. *J Urol* 1989;141:620.

205. Giglio M, Medica M, De Rose AF, et al. Testicular Sertoli cell tumours and relative subtypes. Analysis of clinical and prognostic features. *Urol Int* 2003;70:205.

206. Anderson G. Sclerosing Sertoli cell tumor of the testis: a distinct histological subtype. *J Urol* 1995;154:1756.

207. Russo P, Brady MS, Conlon K, et al. Adult urologic sarcoma. *J Urol* 1992;147:1032.

CHAPTER 32

Gynecologic Cancers

PATRICIA J. EIFEL
JONATHAN S. BEREK
MAURIE A. MARKMAN

SECTION 1

Cancer of the Cervix, Vagina, and Vulva

CARCINOMA OF THE CERVIX

EPIDEMIOLOGY

The American Cancer Society (ACS) estimated that 12,200 new cases of invasive cervical cancer would be diagnosed in the United States in 2003.[1] During the same year, 4100 patients were expected to die of cervical cancer; this represents approximately 1.6% of all cancer deaths in women and 15% of deaths from gynecologic cancers. However, for women aged 20 to 39 years, cervical cancer remained the second leading cause of cancer deaths after breast cancer, accounting for approximately 10% of cancer deaths.[1] In the United States, age-adjusted death rates from cervical cancer have declined steadily since statistics on the disease were first collected in the 1930s. Although this improvement is primarily due to the adoption of routine screening programs including pelvic examinations and cervical cytologic evaluation, the death rates from cervical cancer had begun to decrease before the implementation of Papanicolaou (Pap) screening, which suggests that other unknown factors may have played some role.[2] Despite the declining death rates in the United States and other developed countries, cervical cancer remains the leading cause of cancer death for women in many medically underserved countries and continues to be a serious international health problem.

Molecular and epidemiologic studies have demonstrated a strong relationship between human papillomavirus (HPV), cervical intraepithelial neoplasia (CIN), and invasive carcinomas of the cervix. Infection with HPV is now accepted as a necessary cause of most cervical cancers.[3] When sensitive primers are used, HPV DNA can be identified in more than 95% of cervical carcinomas.[4] HPV DNA transcripts and protein products have also been identified in invasive cervical carcinomas.[5,6] In high-grade CIN and invasive carcinoma, HPV DNA is typically integrated into the human genome rather than remaining in an intact viral capsid.[7] It has been theorized that integration of HPV DNA into the human genome, possibly at the E2 site, causes persistent transcription of the E6 and E7 genes. Functional inactivation of p53 by E6 protein or of Rb by E7 protein disrupts normal cell-cycle control mechanisms.[8,9] The E6 proteins of high-oncogenic-risk types of HPV (e.g., HPV-16 and HPV-18) have a greater affinity for p53 than do the E6 proteins of the low-oncogenic-risk types.[10]

More than 100 HPV subtypes have been identified, and many of these have now been isolated, sequenced, and cloned.[11] At least 35 subtypes are tropic to the genital tract mucosa. Types 6 and 11 usually cause benign genital warts (condyloma acuminata) but are occasionally associated with invasive cervical lesions. Types 16, 18, 31, 33, and 45 are commonly associated with high-grade CIN and invasive cervical cancer (Table 32.1-1).[12] HPV-18 has been associated with adenocarcinomas and poorly differentiated carcinomas and with an increased incidence of lymph node involvement and disease recurrence; HPV-16 has been associated with large cell keratinizing tumors and a lower recurrence rate.[13,14] Although the

TABLE 32.1-1. Relationship between Human Papillomavirus Type and Cervical Pathology

	Cervical Diagnosis				
Viral Type	Normal Mild Atypia (%)	Low-Grade Squamous Invasive Lesion (%)	High-Grade Squamous Invasive Lesion (%)	Cancer (%)	*Total (%)*
HPV negative	1671 (91.0)	115 (30.5)	33 (12.6)	16 (10.5)	1835 (69.8)
HPV-6, 11, 42, 43, 44, two unclassified types	80 (4.4)	111 (29.4)	26 (10.0)	8 (5.2)	225 (8.6)
HPV-16, 18, 31, 33, 35, 45, 51, 52, 56, 58	85 (4.6)	151 (40.1)	202 (77.4)	129 (84.3)	567 (21.6)
Total	1836 (100)	377 (100)	261 (100)	153 (100)	2627 (100)

HPV, human papillomavirus.
(Modified from Loricez AL, Reid R, Jenson AB, et al. Human papillomavirus infection of the cervix: relative risk associations of 15 common anogenital types. *Obstet Gynecol* 1992;79:328.)

overall prevalence of HPV DNA is similar across countries, significant variation has been found in the prevalence of some less common HPV types; for example, HPV-45 is most common in western Africa, whereas HPV-39 and HPV-59 are rarely found outside Central and South America.[15] The strong correlation between high-risk HPV subtypes and carcinoma has led to the suggestion that HPV detection and typing be incorporated into mass screening programs and has encouraged efforts to develop a prophylactic HPV vaccine.[16] In 2002, the first randomized clinical trial of a vaccine against HPV-16 yielded very encouraging results, with a significantly lower rate of persistent HPV-16 infection and HPV-related CIN in patients who received the vaccine than in patients who received a placebo.[17]

Although infection with HPV is believed to be necessary, it is probably not sufficient to cause cancer. Most HPV infections are transient, becoming undetectable within 1 to 2 years.[18] Persistent infection appears to be necessary for the development of CIN and invasive cancer. Most studies have emphasized the importance of persistent detectable HPV, although data in immunosuppressed individuals suggest that a latent state may also develop in which very small foci of cells maintain undetectable infection.[19] Investigators have suggested a number of factors that may encourage persistent infection, DNA integration, and disease progression, although the nature and importance of various cofactors remain controversial. Several studies have suggested that oral contraceptive use and high parity are associated with increased risk of neoplasia independent of HPV infection; it is possible that hormonal influences that maintain the transformation zone on the exocervix facilitate exposure to HPV or other cofactors.[20,21] Several large case-control studies have found tobacco smoking to be correlated with cervical cancer development even after controlling for HPV infection.[20,22] This may be due to direct mitogenic effects, effects on the immune system, or unknown factors. A prospective study by Giulian et al.[23] suggests that smokers maintain cervical HPV infections longer and have a lower probability of clearing the infection than nonsmokers.

As the sensitivity and specificity of tests for HPV DNA have improved, it has become increasingly apparent that most of the covariables historically associated with an increased risk of cervical cancer are surrogates for sexually transmitted HPV infection. The risk of cervical cancer is increased in prostitutes and in women who have first coitus at a young age, have multiple sexual partners, or bear children at a young age. Promiscuous sexual behavior in male partners is also a risk factor.[24] Castell-

sague et al.[25] have reported a lower incidence of HPV infection in circumcised than in uncircumcised males, with a correspondingly lower incidence of cervical cancer in their female partners.

International incidences of cervical cancer tend to reflect differences in cultural attitudes toward sexual promiscuity and the penetration of mass screening programs. The highest incidences tend to occur in populations that have low screening rates combined with a high background prevalence of HPV infection and relatively liberal attitudes toward sexual behavior.[3] Rates of invasive cervical cancer are particularly high in Latin America, southern and eastern Africa, India, and Polynesia. In many of these developing countries, cervical cancer is the leading cause of cancer deaths among women.[26] Countries that have well-advanced screening programs (e.g., the United States and Western Europe) or strict religious regulation of sexual behavior (e.g., Muslim countries of the Middle East or Asia) tend to have low rates of invasive disease. Although the overall incidence of cervical cancer is low in the United States, African American and Hispanic women have approximately twice the incidence and Vietnamese women approximately five times the incidence of white Americans.[27–29] Barriers to cervical cancer screening, including lack of insurance, low income, and cultural differences, probably contribute to higher incidence and mortality rates in these ethnic groups.[30–32] Differences in age-specific incidences between developed and medically underserved countries also illustrate the probable impact of mass screening on the development of invasive disease. For example, a comparison between data from Brazil and the United Kingdom showed similar rates in young women, suggesting similar levels of exposure to HPV, but rapidly diverging rates in older women, probably reflecting differences in the availability of mass screening in the two countries (Fig. 32.1-1).

A number of studies suggest that the incidence of cervical adenocarcinoma has been increasing, particularly among women in their twenties and thirties.[33,34] In a study based on Surveillance, Epidemiology, and End Results program (SEER) data, Smith et al.[33] found that the age-adjusted incidence of cervical adenocarcinoma in the population increased by 29.1% during a period (1973 to 1996) when the overall incidence of cervical cancer decreased by 41.9%. Several investigators have reported a correlation between cervical adenocarcinoma and prolonged oral contraceptive use.[35,36] However, the likelihood of a causative relationship is less certain because of the many potential confounding risk factors.[37] Smith et al.[33] pointed out

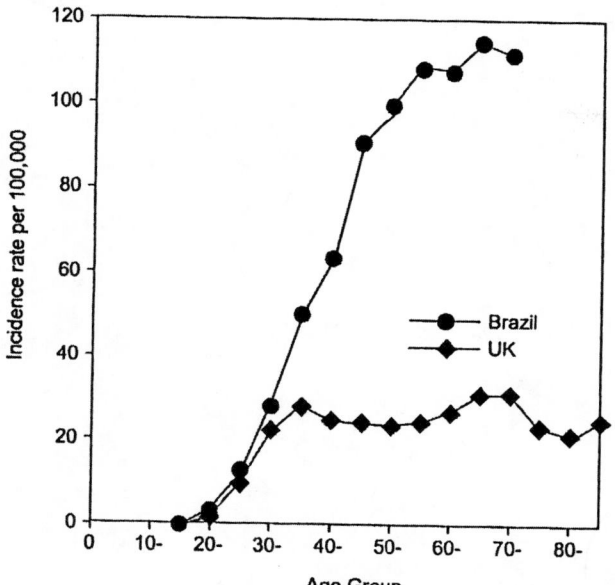

FIGURE 32.1-1. Age-specific incidences of invasive cervical cancer in Brazil and in the United Kingdom (UK). (From ref. 3, with permission.)

that the increase in adenocarcinomas of the cervix in the SEER database mirrored a decrease in the incidence of cervical cancers in "other categories" (i.e., nonsquamous and nonadenocarcinoma). These authors suggested that part of the change might reflect an increase in recognition of cases with glandular elements as adenocarcinomas. Also, cytologic screening methods may be less effective in detecting adenocarcinomas at a preinvasive stage than squamous lesions, resulting in a less dramatic reduction in the incidence of invasive adenocarcinomas in populations that display increasingly high-risk behaviors.

In 1993, the Centers for Disease Control and Prevention added cervical cancer to the list of neoplasms defining acquired immunodeficiency syndrome.[38] However, the relationship between immunosuppression (particularly human immunodeficiency virus (HIV)–related immunosuppression) and the risk of HPV-related disease is complex and incompletely understood. Current data strongly suggest that HIV-related immunosuppression is correlated with an increased risk of cervical HPV infection.[39] Several studies demonstrate an inverse correlation between CD4+ level and the risk of HPV infection, and patients with low CD4+ levels tend to have higher HPV DNA levels.[39] HIV infection also appears to be associated with a higher prevalence of CIN, with a faster rate of progression to high-grade CIN.[39,40] Iatrogenic immunosuppression (in organ transplant recipients) is also associated with an increased prevalence of CIN.[41] However, the impact of HIV infection on the risk of progression from CIN to invasive disease and on the virulence of invasive cervical cancer is less certain. In most cases, antiretroviral therapy does not appear to affect HPV levels and rarely produces regression of CIN 2 or CIN 3 lesions, even with increases in CD4+ levels.[42–44] Although several studies have suggested that the risk of progression from CIN to invasive cervical cancer is increased in HIV-positive women[39,45] and although some investigators[46,47] have suggested that cervical cancer is a more aggressive disease in immunosuppressed patients, other studies have failed to reveal an independent linkage.[48,49] Overlapping risk factors tend to confound studies of the association between HIV infection and HPV-related cancers. However, because of the increased risk of HPV infection in HIV-positive women, vigilant surveillance with Pap smears, pelvic examination, and colposcopy (when indicated) should be part of the routine care of these women.

NATURAL HISTORY AND PATTERN OF SPREAD

Most cervical carcinomas arise at the junction between the primarily columnar epithelium of the endocervix and the squamous epithelium of the ectocervix. This junction is a site of continuous metaplastic change; this change is most active *in utero*, at puberty, and during first pregnancy, and declines after menopause. The greatest risk of neoplastic transformation coincides with periods of greatest metaplastic activity. Virally induced atypical squamous metaplasia developing in this region can progress to higher-grade squamous intraepithelial lesions (SILs).

The mean age of women with CIN is approximately 15 years younger than that of women with invasive cancer, which suggests a slow progression of CIN to invasive carcinoma.[50] In a 13-year observational study of women with CIN 3, Miller[51] found that disease progressed in only 14%, whereas it remained the same in 61% and disappeared in the others. Syrjanen et al.[52] reported spontaneous regression in 38% of high-grade HPV-associated SILs. However, in a large prospective study, Richart and Barron[53] reported mean times to development of carcinoma *in situ* of 58, 38, and 12 months for patients with mild, moderate, or severe dysplasia, respectively, and predicted that 66% of all dysplasias would progress to carcinoma *in situ* within 10 years.

Once tumor has broken through the basement membrane, it may penetrate the cervical stroma directly or through vascular channels. Invasive tumors may develop as exophytic growths protruding from the cervix into the vagina or as endocervical lesions that can cause massive expansion of the cervix despite a relatively normal-appearing cervical portio. From the cervix, tumor may extend superiorly to the lower uterine segment, inferiorly to the vagina, or into the paracervical spaces by way of the broad or uterosacral ligaments. Tumor may become fixed to the pelvic wall by direct extension or by coalescence of central tumor with regional adenopathy. Although the cervix is separated from the bladder only by a thin layer of fascia and cellular connective tissue, extensive bladder involvement is uncommon; fewer than 5% of patients present with cystoscopic evidence of bladder mucosal invasion. Tumor may also extend posteriorly to the rectum, although rectal mucosal involvement is a rare finding at initial presentation.

The cervix has a rich supply of lymphatics organized in three anastomosing plexuses that drain the mucosal, muscularis, and serosal layers.[54] The lymphatics of the cervix also anastomose extensively with those of the lower uterine segment, which possibly explains the high frequency of uterine extension from endocervical primary tumors. The most important lymphatic collecting trunks exit laterally from the uterine isthmus in three groups (Fig. 32.1-2).[54] The upper branches, which originate in the anterior and lateral cervix, follow the uterine artery, are sometimes interrupted by a node as they cross the ureter, and terminate in the uppermost hypogastric nodes. The middle branches drain to deeper hypogastric (obturator) nodes. The lowest branches follow a posterior course to the inferior and superior gluteal, common iliac, presacral, and subaortic nodes.

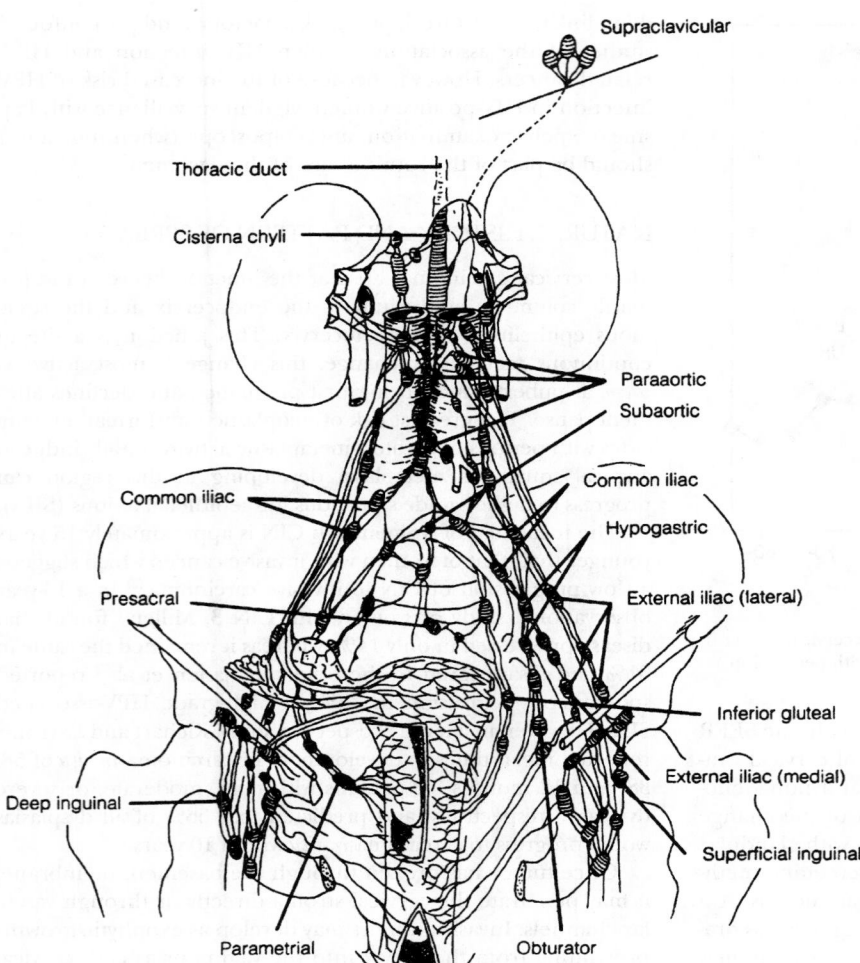

FIGURE 32.1-2. The lymphatic system of the female genital organs. (From ref. 361, with permission; adapted from Meigs JV, ed. *Surgical treatment of cancer of the cervix.* New York: Grune & Stratton, 1954:90.)

Additional posterior lymphatic channels arising from the posterior cervical wall may drain to superior rectal nodes or may continue upward in the retrorectal space to the subaortic nodes overlying the sacral promontory. Anterior collecting trunks pass between the cervix and bladder along the superior vesical artery and terminate in the internal iliac nodes.

The incidence of pelvic and paraaortic node involvement is correlated with tumor stage and with other tumor characteristics such as tumor size, histologic characteristics, depth of invasion, and presence of lymph vascular space invasion. Reported rates of regional metastasis come primarily from series of patients who underwent lymphadenectomy as part of radical surgical treatment or before radiation therapy. The incidences reported for patients who underwent radical hysterectomy vary widely, probably reflecting differences in the criteria used by surgeons to select patients for radical surgery rather than for primary radiotherapy. However, most investigators report an incidence of positive pelvic nodes of 15% to 20% for patients with stage I disease treated with radical hysterectomy; the incidence of positive paraaortic nodes is usually 1% to 5%. Reported incidences are higher for patients treated with radiation for stage I disease, with 10% to 25% reported to have positive paraaortic nodes, which reflects the more advanced stage I tumors that are usually selected for treatment with radiation. Variations in the completeness of lymphadenectomies and his-

tologic processing may lead to underestimates of the true incidence of regional spread from carcinomas of the cervix.[55,56]

Cervical cancer usually follows a relatively orderly pattern of metastatic progression, initially to primary-echelon nodes in the pelvis and then to paraaortic nodes and distant sites. Even patients with locoregionally advanced disease rarely have detectable hematogenous metastases at initial diagnosis of their cervical cancer. The most frequent sites of distant recurrence are lung, extrapelvic nodes, liver, and bone. Although early studies suggested that the lumbar spine was a relatively frequent site of skeletal metastases, more recent studies using abdominal imaging demonstrate that most patients with isolated lumbar spine involvement actually have direct extension of disease from paraaortic nodes.[57]

PATHOLOGY

Cervical Intraepithelial Neoplasia

Several systems have been developed for classifying cervical cytologic findings (Table 32.1-2). Although criteria for the diagnosis of CIN vary somewhat among pathologists, the important characteristics of this lesion are cellular immaturity, cellular disorganization, nuclear abnormalities, and increased mitotic activity. The degree of neoplasia is determined on the

TABLE 32.1-2.   Comparison of Cytology Classification Systems

Bethesda System	Dysplasia/CIN System			Papanicolaou System
Within normal limits	Normal			Class I
Infection (specify organism)	Inflammatory atypia (organism)			Class II
Reactive and reparative changes				
Squamous cell abnormalities				
Atypical squamous cells of undetermined significance	Squamous atypia			
Low-grade squamous intraepithelial lesion	Human papillomavirus atypia			Class IIR
High-grade squamous intraepithelial lesion	Mild dysplasia	CIN 1		
	Moderate dysplasia	CIN 2		Class III
	Severe dysplasia			
		CIN 3		
	Carcinoma *in situ*			Class IV
Invasive squamous carcinoma	Invasive squamous carcinoma			Class V

CIN, cervical intraepithelial neoplasia.

basis of the extent of the mitotic activity, immature cell proliferation, and nuclear atypia. If mitoses and immature cells are present only in the lower third of the epithelium, the lesion is usually designated CIN 1. Lesions involving the middle or upper third are diagnosed as CIN 2 or CIN 3, respectively.

The term *cervical intraepithelial neoplasia*, as proposed by Richart,[58] refers only to a lesion that may progress to invasive carcinoma. Although CIN 1 and CIN 2 are sometimes referred to as mild to moderate dysplasia, *CIN* is now preferred over *dysplasia*. Because the word *dysplasia* means "abnormal maturation," proliferating metaplasia without mitotic activity has sometimes erroneously been called dysplasia.

The Bethesda system of classification, designed to further standardize reporting of cervical cytologic findings, was developed after a National Cancer Institute consensus conference in 1988 and was refined in 1991.[59] This system defines SILs to include all squamous alterations in the cervical transformation zone that are induced by HPV; as such, they encompass all lesions that were classified as condyloma, dysplasia, or CIN in previous systems. The Bethesda system divides SILs into two groups—low grade and high grade. Low-grade SILs (LSILs) have nuclear crowding or atypia without frequent mitoses, parabasal cell anisokaryosis, or coarse chromatin; these lesions are usually associated with low-risk HPV subtypes and have a low likelihood of progressing to invasive cancers. These are to be distinguished from high-grade SILs (HSILs), which do have nuclear atypia in lower and upper epithelial layers, abnormal mitoses, coarse chromatin, and loss of polarity. HSILs tend to be associated with high-risk HPV types and a higher risk of progression to invasive cancer. The Bethesda system was meant to replace the Pap system and is now widely used in the United States. However, its use is still controversial. Some groups[60,61] argue that the new nomenclature has failed to improve diagnostic accuracy and believe that with dichotomization of the spectrum of atypical lesions, lesions that were formerly classified as CIN 2 (now HSIL) may be overtreated despite their relatively low risk of progression.

The Bethesda system also introduced the term *atypical squamous cells of undetermined significance* (ASCUS). This uncertain diagnosis is now the most common abnormal Pap test result in United States laboratories,[62] with 1.6% to 9% of Pap smears reported as having ASCUS. Although most cases reflect a benign process, 5% to 10% are associated with underlying HSIL, and one-third or more of HSILs are heralded by a finding of ASCUS on a Pap test smear.[63] There has been considerable controversy about the evaluation and management of patients with ASCUS, leading the National Cancer Institute to initiate the ASCUS-LSIL Triage Study.[64] This multicenter, randomized trial compared three methods of management—immediate colposcopy, cytologic follow-up, and triage by HPV DNA testing—in 5060 patients with ASCUS or LSIL. Preliminary analyses of this study[64] demonstrated that the prevalence of high-risk HPV was too high to permit useful triage of LSIL but was very helpful in evaluating patients with ASCUS, with a sensitivity comparable to that of immediate colposcopy, and thereby reduced the number of referrals for colposcopy by 50%.

Adenocarcinoma In Situ

The diagnosis of adenocarcinoma *in situ* (AIS) is made when normal endocervical gland cells are replaced by tall, irregular columnar cells with stratified, hyperchromatic nuclei and increased mitotic activity but the normal branching pattern of the endocervical glands is maintained and there is no obvious stromal invasion. Twenty percent to 50% of women with cervical AIS also have squamous CIN, and AIS is often an incidental finding in patients operated on for squamous carcinoma.[65] Because AIS is frequently multifocal, cone biopsy margins are unreliable.[66,67] Although some investigators have described a possible precursor lesion termed *endocervical glandular dysplasia*, the reproducibility and clinical value of this designation are uncertain.[67]

Microinvasive Carcinoma

Because the definition of microinvasive carcinoma is based on the maximum depth (no more than 5 mm) and linear extent (no more than 7 mm) of involvement, this diagnosis can be made only after examination of a specimen that includes the entire neoplastic lesion and cervical transformation zone. This requires a cervical cone biopsy. With the advent of cytologic screening, the proportion of invasive carcinomas that invade less than 5 mm has increased more than tenfold to approximately 20% in the United States.[68]

The earliest invasion appears as a blurring of the stromoepithelial junction with a protrusion of cells into the stroma; these cells are better differentiated than the adjacent noninvasive cells; have abundant pink-staining cytoplasm, hyperchromatic nuclei, and prominent nucleoli; and exhibit a loss of polarity at the stromoepithelial junction.[68] Early microinvasion is usually characterized by a desmoplastic response in adjacent stroma with scalloping or duplication of the neoplastic epithelium or formation of pseudoglands (nests of invasive carcinoma that can mimic crypt involvement). In a study of cone specimens, Reich et al.[69] reported that 12% of microinvasive carcinomas were multifocal. The depth of invasion should be measured with a micrometer from the base of the epithelium to the deepest point of invasion. Lesions that have invaded less than 3 mm [International Federation of Gynecology and Obstetrics (FIGO) stage IA1] rarely metastasize; 5% to 10% of tumors that invade 3 to 5 mm (FIGO stage IA2) are associated with positive pelvic lymph nodes.[70–72] Until FIGO refined its definition of microinvasive carcinoma (Table 32.1-3), most clinicians in the United States used a different definition of microinvasive carcinoma formulated by the Society of Gynecologic Oncologists: cancers that invaded less than 3 mm with no evidence of lymph–vascular space invasion (LVSI). The importance of LVSI remains somewhat controversial, although the risk of metastatic regional disease appears to be exceedingly low for any tumor that invades less than 3 mm, even in the presence of LVSI.[68] Although most clinicians have adopted the FIGO definitions, many feel that the risk of regional spread from tumors that invade 3 to 5 mm is sufficiently high to warrant treatment of the parametria and regional nodes.

Because invasive adenocarcinomas may originate anywhere along the profile of architecturally complex glands that course through the cervical stroma, no reproducible method has been found for measuring the depth of invasion of these tumors. Various authors have measured the extent of invasion from the basement membrane or from the nearest abnormal glandular epithelium; others have defined early adenocarcinomas according to the volume of tumor (in mm²).[67,73] Although these differences persist, it is apparent that a subset of patients with very small tumors have a low likelihood of lymph node metastases or recurrence.[67,74] In the absence of a consensus definition of microinvasion, decisions are usually guided by specific descriptions of the depth and extent of invasion and other features that have been correlated with increased risk, such as high grade and the presence of LVSI.[67]

Invasive Squamous Cell Carcinoma

Between 80% and 90% of cervical carcinomas are squamous. A number of systems have been used to grade and classify squamous carcinomas, but none have consistently been demonstrated to predict prognosis. One of the most commonly used systems categorizes squamous neoplasms as large cell keratinizing, large cell nonkeratinizing, or small cell carcinoma.[75] Small cell squamous carcinomas have cells with small to medium-sized nuclei, open chromatin, small or large nucleoli, and abundant cytoplasm. Most authorities believe that patients with small cell squamous carcinoma have a poorer prognosis than those with large cell neoplasms with or without keratin. However, small cell squamous carcinoma should not be confused with anaplastic small cell carcinoma (discussed in Anaplastic

TABLE 32.1-3. International Federation of Gynecology and Obstetrics Staging of Carcinoma of the Cervix (1994)

STAGE 0	Carcinoma *in situ*, intraepithelial carcinoma. *Cases of stage 0 should not be included in any therapeutic statistics for invasive carcinoma.*
STAGE I	The carcinoma is strictly confined to the cervix (*extension to the corpus should be disregarded*).
Stage IA	Invasive cancer identified only microscopically. All gross lesions, even with superficial invasion, are stage IB cancers. Invasion is limited to measured stromal invasion with a maximum depth of 5 mm and no wider than 7 mm. (*The depth of invasion should not be more than 5 mm taken from the base of the epithelium, either surface or glandular, from which it originates. Vascular space involvement, either venous or lymphatic, should not alter the staging*).
Stage IA1	Measured invasion of stroma no greater than 3 mm in depth and no wider than 7 mm.
Stage IA2	Measured invasion of stroma greater than 3 mm and no greater than 5 mm in depth and no wider than 7 mm.
Stage IB	Clinical lesions confined to the cervix or preclinical lesions greater than IA.
Stage IB1	Clinical lesions no greater than 4 cm in size.
Stage IB2	Clinical lesions greater than 4 cm in size.
STAGE II	The carcinoma extends beyond the cervix, but has not extended onto the pelvic wall; the carcinoma involves the vagina, but not as far as the lower third.
Stage IIA	No obvious parametrial involvement.
Stage IIB	Obvious parametrial involvement. The carcinoma has extended onto the pelvic wall; on rectal examination there is no cancer-free space between the tumor and the pelvic wall; the tumor involves the lower third of the vagina; all cases with a hydronephrosis or nonfunctioning kidney should be included, unless they are known to be due to another cause.
STAGE III	No extension onto the pelvic wall, but involvement of the lower third of the vagina.
Stage IIIA	Extension onto the pelvic wall or hydronephrosis or nonfunctioning kidney.
Stage IIIB	The carcinoma has extended beyond the true pelvis or has clinically involved the mucosa of the bladder or rectum.
STAGE IV	The carcinoma has extended beyond the true pelvis or has clinically involved the mucosa of the bladder or rectum.
Stage IVA	Spread of the growth to adjacent organs.
Stage IVB	Spread to distant organs.

(From ref. 104, with permission.)

Small Cell/Neuroendocrine Carcinoma, later in this chapter). Papillary variants of squamous carcinoma may be well differentiated (occasionally confused with immature condylomata) or very poorly differentiated (resembling high-grade transitional carcinoma).[68] Verrucous carcinoma is a very rare warty-appearing variant of squamous carcinoma that may be difficult to differentiate from benign condyloma without multiple biopsies or hysterectomy.[76] Sarcomatoid squamous carcinoma is another very rare variant, demonstrating areas of spindle cell carcinomatous tumor confluent with poorly differentiated squamous cell carcinoma. Immunohistochemical analysis demonstrates expression of cytokeratin as well as vimentin; the natural history of this uncommon tumor is not well understood.[77]

Adenocarcinoma

Invasive adenocarcinoma may be pure or mixed with squamous cell carcinoma (adenosquamous carcinoma). A wide variety of cell types, growth patterns, and degrees of differentiation have been observed. However, approximately 80% of cervical adenocarcinomas are of the endocervical type, made up predominantly of cells with eosinophilic cytoplasm, brisk mitotic activity, and frequent apoptotic bodies. The most common types are usually moderately differentiated with cells arranged in medium-sized glands. Endocervical-type adenocarcinomas are frequently referred to as mucinous; however, although some have abundant intracytoplasmic mucin, most have little or none.[78]

Minimal-deviation adenocarcinoma (adenoma malignum) is a rare, extremely well-differentiated adenocarcinoma that is sometimes associated with Peutz-Jeghers syndrome.[79,80] Because the branching glandular pattern strongly resembles normal endocervical glands and the mucin-rich cells can be deceptively benign appearing, minimal-deviation adenocarcinoma may not be recognized as malignant in small biopsy specimens.[78] Earlier studies reported a dismal outcome for women with this tumor, but more recently, patients have been reported to have a favorable prognosis if the disease is detected early.[81]

Young and Scully[82] have described a well-differentiated villoglandular papillary subtype of adenocarcinoma that primarily affects young women, appears to metastasize infrequently, and has a favorable prognosis. Glucksmann and Cherry[83] were the first to describe glassy cell carcinoma, a form of poorly differentiated adenosquamous carcinoma with cells that have abundant eosinophilic, granular, ground-glass cytoplasm; large round to oval nuclei; and prominent nucleoli. Other rare variants of adenosquamous carcinoma include adenoid basal carcinoma and adenoid cystic carcinoma.[84] Adenoid basal carcinoma is a well-differentiated tumor that histologically resembles basal cell carcinoma of the skin and tends to have a favorable prognosis. Adenoid cystic carcinomas consist of basaloid cells in a cribriform or cylindromatous pattern and tend to have an aggressive behavior with frequent metastases, although the natural history of these tumors may show a long course. Whether the prognoses for these rare subtypes are different from those for other adenocarcinomas of similar grade is uncertain. Rarely, primary carcinomas of the cervix are populated by endometrioid, serous, or clear cells; mixtures of these cell types may be seen, and histologically, some of these tumors are indistinguishable from those arising elsewhere in the endometrium or ovary. In a study of 17 cases of papillary serous carcinomas of the cervix, Zhou et al.[85] found that these cancers have an aggressive course, similar to that of high-grade serous tumors originating in the other müllerian sites.

Anaplastic Small Cell/Neuroendocrine Carcinoma

Anaplastic small cell carcinoma resembles oat cell carcinoma of the lung because it contains small tumor cells that have scanty cytoplasm, small round to oval nuclei, small or absent nucleoli, finely granular chromatin, and high mitotic activity.[86] Thirty percent to 50% of anaplastic small cell carcinomas display neuroendocrine features. Small cell anaplastic carcinomas behave more aggressively than poorly differentiated small cell squamous carcinomas. Most investigators report survival rates of less than 50% even for patients with early stage I disease,[87,88] although studies of aggressive multimodality treatments have been more encouraging.[89,90] Widespread hematogenous metastases are frequent, but brain metastases are rare unless preceded by pulmonary involvement.[91]

Other Rare Neoplasms

A variety of neoplasms may infiltrate the cervix from adjacent sites, and this makes differential diagnosis difficult. In particular, it may be difficult or impossible to determine the origin of adenocarcinomas involving the endocervix and uterine isthmus. Although endometrioid histology suggests endometrial origin and mucinous tumors in young patients are most often of endocervical origin, both histologic types can arise in either site.[92] Metastatic tumors from the colon, breast, or other sites may involve the cervix secondarily. Malignant mixed müllerian tumors, adenosarcomas, and leiomyosarcomas occasionally arise in the cervix but more often involve it secondarily. Primary lymphomas and melanomas of the cervix are extremely rare.

CLINICAL MANIFESTATIONS

Preinvasive disease is usually detected during routine cervical cytologic screening. Early invasive disease may not be associated with any symptoms and is also usually detected during screening examinations. The earliest symptom of invasive cervical cancer is usually abnormal vaginal bleeding, often after coitus or vaginal douching. This may be associated with a clear or foul-smelling vaginal discharge. Pelvic pain may result from locoregionally invasive disease or from coexistent pelvic inflammatory disease. Flank pain may be a symptom of hydronephrosis, often complicated by pyelonephritis. The triad of sciatic pain, leg edema, and hydronephrosis is almost always associated with extensive pelvic wall involvement by tumor. Patients with very advanced tumors may have hematuria or incontinence from a vesicovaginal fistula caused by direct extension of tumor to the bladder. External compression of the rectum by a massive primary tumor may cause constipation, but the rectal mucosa is rarely involved at initial diagnosis.

DIAGNOSIS, CLINICAL EVALUATION, AND STAGING

Diagnosis

The long preinvasive stage of cervical cancer, the relatively high prevalence of the disease in unscreened populations, and the sensitivity of cytologic screening make cervical carcinoma an ideal target for cancer screening. In the United States, screening with cervical cytologic examination and pelvic examination has led to a decrease of more than 70% in the mortality rate from cervical cancer since 1940.[93] Only nations with well-developed screening programs have experienced substantial decreases in cervical cancer death rates during this period.

In 2001, the ACS convened a consensus conference to review its 1988 recommendations concerning cervical cancer screening in the context of new technologies and information about the etiology and epidemiology of cervical cancer. In its 1988 statement, the ACS recommended annual Pap smear testing beginning at age 18 years or with the onset of sexual activity and added that, after normal findings on three or more consecutive annual examinations, the cytologic evaluation could be performed less frequently at the discretion of the physician.[94] In its new guidelines,[95] the ACS recommended that cervical cancer screening begin approximately 3 years after the onset of vaginal intercourse, but no later than 21 years of age. Screening should be performed annually using conventional cervical cytologic smear testing or every 2 years using liquid-based Pap cytologic testing, until age 30 years. Starting at age 30 years, women who have had three consecutive, technically satisfactory negative test results may be screened every 2 to 3 years. Women older than 70 years who meet these criteria and who have had no abnormal test result within 10 years and women who have had a total hysterectomy for benign gynecologic disease may cease cytologic screening. Women with a history of CIN 2 or CIN 3 before or as an indication for hysterectomy should be screened until they have had three consecutive normal test results and no abnormal test results for 10 years. Women with a history of cervical cancer, women exposed *in utero* to diethylstilbestrol (DES), and women who are immunocompromised should continue regular screening as long as they are in reasonably good health.

The rate of false-negative findings on the Pap test is 20% to 30% in women with high-grade CIN[96] and 10% to 15% in women with invasive cancer.[50,94,97] However, the sensitivity of a screening program is usually increased by repeated annual testing. The sensitivity of individual tests may be improved by ensuring adequate sampling of the squamocolumnar junction and the endocervical canal. Smears without endocervical or metaplastic cells are inadequate, and in such cases the test must be repeated. Because AIS originates near or above the transformation zone, it may be missed with conventional cervical smears. Detection of high endocervical lesions may be improved when specimens are obtained with a cytobrush. Because hemorrhage, necrosis, and intense inflammation may obscure the results, the Pap test is a poor way to diagnose gross lesions; a biopsy should always be performed on these lesions.

The U.S. Food and Drug Administration recently approved liquid-based Pap technologies for use in cervical screening. Most studies have found these methods to have greater sensitivity than conventional Pap smear tests.[95] With liquid-based Pap tests, the likelihood of drying artifact is reduced, cellular sampling tends to be better, and the cells are more evenly distributed on the slide. Greater sensitivity comes at the cost of somewhat poorer specificity, which is balanced by the less frequent need for repetition of the study to achieve adequate screening. This is the basis of the ACS recommendations for less frequent screening with liquid-based Pap methods.[95] HPV testing with cytologic analysis is currently being studied as a promising potential method of primary screening; however, clear guidelines for its use have not been established, and this approach has not yet been approved by the U.S. Food and Drug Administration.[95]

Patients with abnormal findings on cytologic examination who do not have a gross cervical lesion must be evaluated by colposcopy and directed biopsies. After application of a 3% acetic acid solution, the cervix is examined under 10- to 15-fold magnification with a bright, filtered light that enhances the acetowhitening and vascular patterns characteristic of dysplasia or carcinoma. The skilled colposcopist can accurately distinguish between low- and high-grade dysplasia,[98] but microinvasive disease cannot consistently be distinguished from intraepithelial lesions on colposcopy.[99,100]

In a patient with an atypical Pap smear result, if no abnormalities are found on colposcopic examination or if the entire squamocolumnar junction cannot be visualized, endocervical curettage should be performed. Some authorities advocate the routine addition of endocervical curettage to colposcopic examination to minimize the risk of missing occult cancer within the endocervical canal.[99,100] However, it is probably reasonable to omit this step in previously untreated women if the entire squamocolumnar junction is visible with a complete ring of unaltered columnar epithelium in the lower canal.

Cervical cone biopsy is used to diagnose occult endocervical lesions and is an essential step in the diagnosis and management of microinvasive carcinoma of the cervix. The geometry of the cone is individualized and tailored to the geometry of the cervix, the location of the squamocolumnar junction, and the site and size of the lesion. Examination of cervical cone biopsy specimens yields an accurate diagnosis and decreases the incidence of inappropriate therapy when (1) the squamocolumnar junction is poorly visualized on colposcopy and a high-grade lesion is suspected, (2) high-grade dysplastic epithelium extends into the endocervical canal, (3) the cytologic findings suggest high-grade dysplasia or carcinoma *in situ*, (4) a microinvasive carcinoma is found after directed biopsy, (5) the endocervical curettage specimens show high-grade CIN, or (6) the cytologic findings are suspicious for AIS.[94]

Clinical Evaluation of Patients with Invasive Carcinoma

All patients with invasive cervical cancer should be evaluated by taking a detailed history and performing a physical examination, with particular attention paid to inspection and palpation of the pelvic organs with bimanual and rectovaginal examinations. Standard laboratory studies should include a complete blood cell count and renal function and liver function tests. All patients should have chest radiography to rule out lung metastases and intravenous pyelography [or computed tomography (CT)] to determine the kidneys' location and to rule out ureteral obstruction by tumor. Cystoscopy and either a proctoscopy or a barium enema study should be done in patients with bulky tumors.

Many clinicians obtain CT or magnetic resonance imaging (MRI) scans to evaluate regional nodes, but the accuracy of these studies is compromised by their failure to detect small metastases and the fact that patients with bulky necrotic tumors often have enlarged reactive lymph nodes.[101,102] In a large Gynecologic Oncology Group (GOG) study that compared the results of radiographic studies with subsequent histologic findings, Heller et al.[101] found that CT detected positive paraaortic nodes in only 34% of the patients who had them. Studies suggest that positron emission tomography (PET) may be a very sensitive noninvasive method of evaluating the regional nodes of patients with cervical cancer.[103] MRI can provide useful information about the distribution and depth of invasion of tumors in the cervix but tends to yield less accurate assessments of the parametrium.[102]

Clinical Staging

FIGO has defined the most widely accepted staging system for carcinomas of the cervix.[104] The 1994 update of this system is summarized in Table 32.1-3. Since the earliest versions of the cervical cancer staging system were published, there have been numerous changes, particularly in the definition of stage I disease.[105] Preinvasive disease was not placed in a separate category until 1950, and the stage IA category for "cases with early stromal invasion" was first described in 1962. Cases of early stromal invasion and occult invasion were redistributed between stages IA$_i$, IA$_{ii}$, and IB$_{occult}$ several times until 1985, when FIGO eliminated stage IB$_{occult}$ and provided the first specific definitions of microinvasive disease (stages IA1 and IA2). In 1994, these definitions were changed again, and for the first time, stage IB tumors were subdivided according to tumor diameter (see Table 32.1-3). Although these changes have gradually improved the discriminatory value of the staging system, the many fluctuations in the definitions of stages IA and IB have complicated the ability to compare the outcomes of patients whose tumors were staged and treated during different periods.[105] Also, until recently, most gynecologic oncologists in the United States used the Society of Gynecologic Oncologists' definition of a microinvasive carcinoma—that is, tumor that "invades the stroma in one or more places to a depth of 3 mm or less below the base of the epithelium and in which lymphatic or vascular involvement is not demonstrated."[106]

FIGO stage is based on careful clinical examination and the results of specific radiologic studies and procedures. These should be performed and the stage should be assigned before any definitive therapy is administered. The clinical stage should never be changed on the basis of subsequent findings. When it is doubtful to which stage a particular case should be allotted, the case should be assigned to the earlier stage. According to FIGO,[104] "a growth fixed to the pelvic wall by a short and indurated, but not nodular, parametrium should be allotted to stage IIB." A case should be classified as stage III "only if the parametrium is nodular to the pelvic wall or if the growth itself extends to the pelvic wall." In its rules for clinical staging, FIGO states that palpation, inspection, colposcopy, endocervical curettage, hysteroscopy, cystoscopy, proctoscopy, intravenous urography, and radiographic examination of the lungs and skeleton may be used for clinical staging. Suspected bladder or rectal involvement should be confirmed by biopsy. Findings of bullous edema or malignant cells in cytologic washings from the urinary bladder are not sufficient to diagnose bladder involvement. FIGO specifically states that findings on examinations such as lymphangiography, laparoscopy, CT, and MRI are of value for planning therapy but—because these are not yet generally available and the interpretation of results is variable—should not be the basis for changing the clinical stage. Examination under anesthesia is desirable but not required. The rules and notes outlined in the FIGO staging system are integral parts of the clinical staging system and should be strictly observed to minimize inconsistencies in staging between institutions.

Although most clinicians use the FIGO classification system, a number of European groups use a staging system that divides stage IIB tumors according to the extent of parametrial involvement and divides stage III tumors according to whether there is unilateral or bilateral pelvic wall fixation. Until the mid-1980s, most reports from the University of Texas M. D. Anderson Cancer Center used a similar staging system that also categorized patients with bulky endocervical tumors into a special category.[105] Although surgically treated patients are sometimes classified according to a TNM (tumor, node, metastasis) pathologic staging system, this practice has not been widely accepted because it cannot be applied to patients who are treated with primary radiotherapy.[107]

Surgical Evaluation of Regional Spread

In the 1970s, studies of diagnostic preradiotherapy lymph node dissection used a transperitoneal approach that led to unacceptable morbidity and mortality from radiation-related bowel complications, particularly after treatment with high radiation doses and extended fields. More recently, extraperitoneal dissection, which induces fewer bowel adhesions, has been recommended. With this approach, postradiotherapy bowel complications occur in fewer than 5% of patients.[108] A number of groups are currently investigating the use of laparoscopic lymph node dissection to evaluate patients with cervical cancer.[109,110] This approach reduces the length of postoperative hospitalization. However, the rate of late complications from radiotherapy after laparoscopic lymphadenectomy has not yet been determined. The role of sentinel node evaluation in cervical cancer is also being investigated.

Although the indications for surgical staging are controversial, advocates argue that the procedure identifies patients with microscopic paraaortic or common iliac node involvement, who can benefit from extended-field irradiation. Some investigators have also suggested, on the basis of first principles and encouraging results with regard to control of pelvic disease, that debulking of large pelvic nodes before radiotherapy may improve outcome.[111,112] Because patients with radiographically positive pelvic nodes are at greatest risk for occult metastasis to paraaortic nodes, these patients may have the greatest chance of benefiting from surgical staging.

Some authors have advocated pretreatment blind biopsy of the scalene node in patients with positive paraaortic nodes and in patients with a central recurrence who are being considered for pelvic exenteration. The reported incidence of supraclavicular metastasis varies widely (5% to 20% or more) for patients with positive paraaortic lymph nodes.

PROGNOSTIC FACTORS

Although rates of survival and control of pelvic disease in cervical cancer patients are correlated with FIGO stage, prognosis is also influenced by a number of tumor characteristics that are not included in the staging system. Clinical tumor diameter is strongly correlated with prognosis for patients treated with radiation (Fig. 32.1-3)[113,114] or surgery.[115–118] For this reason,

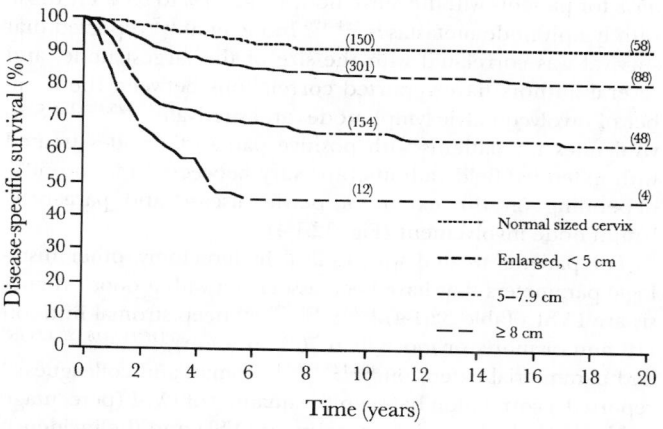

FIGURE 32.1-3. Relationship between tumor diameter and the disease-specific survival rates of 1526 patients with stage IB squamous cell carcinomas of the cervix treated with radiotherapy at M. D. Anderson Cancer Center. Numbers in parentheses represent the number of patients at risk at 10 or 20 years. (From ref. 113, with permission.)

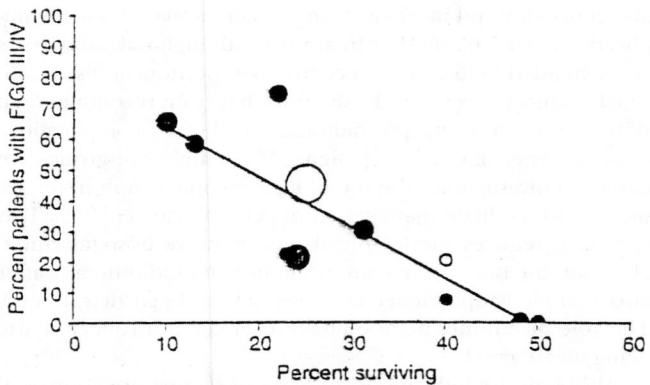

FIGURE 32.1-4. Survival rates of patients treated with radiation for biopsy-confirmed paraaortic node metastases from cervical cancer. Each point represents one series of patients; the area is proportional to the number of patients in the series (ranging from 15 to 98). Solid and open circles represent series with survival rates calculated at 5 and 3 years, respectively. FIGO, International Federation of Gynecology and Obstetrics. (From Eifel PJ. The uterine cervix. In: Cox JD, Ang KK, eds. *Radiation oncology: rationale, technique, results.* St. Louis: Mosby, 2002:692, with permission.)

FIGO recently modified the stage I category so that these tumors are subdivided according to clinical tumor diameter (i.e., 4 cm or smaller, or larger than 4 cm).[104] For patients with more advanced disease, other estimates of tumor bulk—such as the presence of medial versus lateral parametrial involvement in FIGO stage IIB tumors or the presence of unilateral versus bilateral parametrial or pelvic wall involvement—have also been correlated with outcome.[119,120] The predictive value of the staging system itself may, in part, reflect an association between the stage categories and the primary tumor volume. Operative findings often do not agree with clinical estimates of parametrial or pelvic wall involvement,[121,122] and some authors have found that the predictive power of stage diminishes or is lost when comparisons are corrected for differences in clinical tumor diameter.[123]

Lymph node metastasis is also an important predictor of prognosis. For patients treated with radical hysterectomy for stage IB disease, survival rates are usually reported as 85% to 95% for patients with negative nodes and 45% to 55% for those with lymph node metastases.[124–126] Inoue et al.[127] reported that survival was correlated with the size of the largest node, and several authors have reported correlations between the number of involved pelvic lymph nodes and survival.[117,125,126,128] Survival rates for patients with positive paraaortic nodes treated with extended-field radiotherapy vary between 10% and 50% depending on the extent of pelvic disease and paraaortic lymph node involvement (Fig. 32.1-4).

For patients treated with radical hysterectomy, other histologic parameters that have been associated with a poor prognosis are LVSI (Table 32.1-4),[117,118,125,129–134] deep stromal invasion (10 mm or more, or more than 70% invasion),[115,117,118,125,129,135] and parametrial extension.[122,129,136,137] Roman and colleagues[138] reported a correlation between the quantity of LVSI (percentage of histopathologic sections containing LVSI) and the incidence of lymph node metastases. A strong inflammatory response in the cervical stroma tends to predict a good outcome.[139] Uterine-body involvement is associated with an increased rate of distant metastases in patients treated with radiation or surgery.[140,141]

TABLE 32.1-4. Relationship between Lymph–Vascular Space Invasion, Pelvic Node Involvement, and Recurrence Rate in Patients Treated with Radical Hysterectomy

	Positive Lymph Nodes (%)		Recurrence Rate (%)	
Reference	LVSI	No LVSI	LVSI	No LVSI
Chung et al.[130]	63	13	50	6
Fuller et al.[131]	40	14	—	—
Nahhas et al.[132]	22	8	20	12
Boyce et al.[133]	32	6	36	4
Burke et al.[134]	—	—	38	9
Delgado et al.[125]	—	—	23	11
Kamura et al.[129]	—	—	18	9
Sevin et al.[118]	—	—	38	15
Kristensen et al.[117]	—	—	29	9

LVSI, lymph–vascular space invasion.

Several investigators have reported similar survival rates for patients with squamous carcinomas and those with adenocarcinomas.[142–144] However, many other investigators have drawn the opposite conclusion, noting unusually high pelvic relapse rates in patients treated surgically for adenocarcinomas and poorer survival rates among patients treated with surgery or irradiation for cervical adenocarcinomas.[145–149] In a multivariate analysis of 1767 patients treated with radiation for FIGO stage IB disease, Eifel and colleagues[146] reported a highly significant independent correlation between histologic features and survival. Using Cox regression analysis, the relative risk of death from cancer for 106 patients with adenocarcinomas 4 cm or more in diameter was determined to be 1.9 times than for patients with squamous tumors ($P < .01$) (Fig. 32.1-5). Pelvic disease control rates were similar for patients with squamous carcinomas and those with adenocarcinomas, but there was a significantly higher incidence of distant metastases in patients with adenocarcinomas. Although the prognostic significance

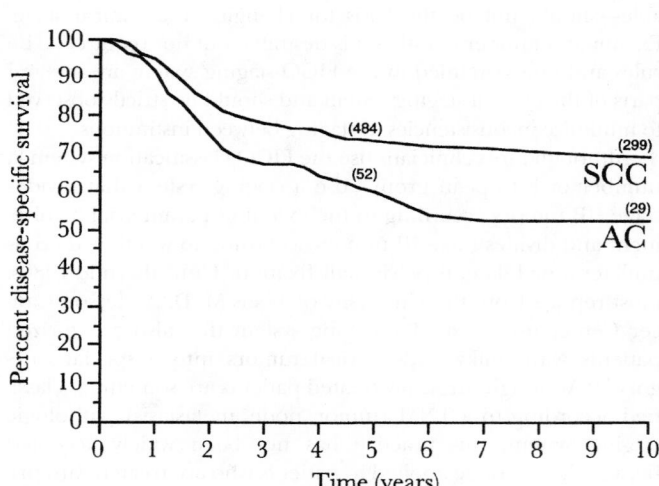

FIGURE 32.1-5. Relationship between histologic type and the disease-specific survival rates of 903 patients treated at M. D. Anderson Cancer Center for stage IB carcinomas of the cervix measuring 4 cm or greater in diameter. Numbers in parentheses represent the number of patients at risk at 10 or 20 years. AC, adenocarcinoma; SCC, squamous cell carcinoma. (From ref. 146, with permission.)

of histologic grade has been disputed for squamous carcinomas, there is a clear correlation between the degree of differentiation and the clinical behavior of adenocarcinomas.[150-152]

Several studies have demonstrated a relationship between hemoglobin level and prognosis in patients with locally advanced cervical cancer.[153-156] The strongest evidence that anemia plays a causative role in pelvic recurrence comes from a small 1978 randomized study conducted at the Princess Margaret Hospital.[153] In all patients, the hemoglobin level was maintained at at least 10 g/dL, but in patients in the treatment arm, the hemoglobin level was maintained, through the use of transfusions, at at least 12.5 g/dL. The locoregional recurrence rate was significantly higher for the 25 anemic patients in the control arm than it was for the patients who received transfusions. Other studies aimed at overcoming the theoretical radiobiologic consequences of intratumoral hypoxia with hypoxic cell sensitizers,[157,158] hyperbaric oxygen breathing,[159] or neutron therapy[160] have not been successful. Several investigators have correlated low intratumoral oxygen tension levels with a high rate of regional and distant metastases and poor survival.[161,162]

The serum concentration of squamous cell carcinoma antigen appears to correlate with the stage and size of squamous carcinomas, the presence of lymph node metastases, and the presence of recurrent disease; however, the value of this antigen as an independent predictor of prognosis and the cost effectiveness of its use as a screening modality have been disputed.[163,164] Other clinical and biologic features that have been investigated for their predictive power, with variable results, include patient age,[125,165,166] peritoneal cytologic findings,[167,168] platelet count,[169,170] tumor vascularity,[171,172] DNA ploidy or S phase,[173] cyclooxygenase-2 expression,[174] and growth factor receptors.[175,176] In two studies of patients with histologically negative lymph nodes, investigators reported higher rates of disease recurrence when a polymerase chain reaction assay of the lymph nodes was strongly positive for HPV DNA.[177,178]

TREATMENT

A number of factors may influence the choice of local treatment, including tumor size, stage, histologic features, evidence of lymph node involvement, risk factors for complications of surgery or radiotherapy, and patient preference. However, as a rule, intraepithelial lesions are managed with superficial ablative techniques; microinvasive cancers invading less than 3 mm (stage IA1) are managed with conservative surgery (excisional conization or extrafascial hysterectomy); early invasive cancers (stages IA2 and IB1 and some small stage IIA tumors) are managed with radical surgery or radiotherapy; and locally advanced cancers (stages IB2 through IVA) are managed with radiotherapy. Selected patients with centrally recurrent disease after maximum radiotherapy may be treated with radical exenterative surgery. Isolated pelvic recurrence after hysterectomy is treated with irradiation. The results of randomized trials[179-183] have led to the addition of concurrent cisplatin-containing chemotherapy to radiotherapy for patients whose cancers have a high risk of locoregional recurrence.

Preinvasive Disease (Stage 0)

Patients with noninvasive squamous lesions can be treated with superficial ablative therapy (cryosurgery or laser therapy) or with loop excision if (1) the entire transformation zone has been visualized colposcopically, (2) findings on directed biopsy specimens are consistent with Pap smear results, (3) endocervical curettage findings are negative, and (4) there is no suspicion of occult invasion on cytologic or colposcopic examination. If patients do not meet these criteria, a conization should be performed.

In cryotherapy, abnormal tissue is frozen with a supercooled metal probe until an ice ball forms that extends 5 mm beyond the lesion. Because cryonecrosis tends to be patchy and may be inadequate after a single freeze, the tissue should be frozen a second time after it has visibly thawed.[184] Another common and equally effective technique ablates tissue with a carbon dioxide laser beam. After laser ablation, there is less distortion and more rapid healing of the cervix. However, the procedure requires more training and more expensive equipment than does cryosurgery. The use of ablative therapy has declined in recent years because low-grade dysplasias are often followed without treatment and high-grade lesions are usually treated with excision to permit histologic examination.[185]

Many practitioners now consider loop diathermy excision to be the preferred treatment for noninvasive squamous lesions. In this technique, a charged electrode is used to excise the entire transformation zone and distal canal. Although control rates are similar to those achieved with cryotherapy or laser ablation,[186] loop diathermy is easily learned, is less expensive than laser excision, and preserves the excised lesion and transformation zone for histologic evaluation.[187-190] However, low-grade lesions are overtreated with this method.[185] Because loop excision may inadequately treat disease within the cervical canal and thus complicate further treatment, this technique should not be considered an alternative to formal excisional conization when microinvasive or invasive cancer is suspected or in patients with AIS.

Loop excision is an outpatient office procedure that preserves fertility. Although recurrence rates are low (10% to 15%) and progression to invasion rare (less than 2% in most series), lifelong surveillance of these patients must be maintained. The risk of recurrence may be somewhat increased in women infected with HPV type 16 or 18.[186] Treatment with vaginal or type I abdominal hysterectomy currently is reserved for women who have other gynecologic conditions that justify the procedure; invasive cancer still must be excluded before surgery to rule out the need for a more extensive operative procedure.

Microinvasive Carcinoma (Stage IA)

The standard treatment for patients with stage IA1 disease is total (type I) or vaginal hysterectomy. Because the risk of pelvic lymph node metastases from these minimally invasive tumors is less than 1%, pelvic lymph node dissection is not usually recommended.[100,136]

Selected patients with tumors that meet the Society of Gynecologic Oncologists' definition of microinvasion (FIGO stage IA1 disease without LVSI) and who wish to maintain fertility may be adequately treated with a therapeutic cervical conization if the margins of the cone are negative. In 1991, Burghardt et al.[73] reported one recurrence (which was fatal) in 93 women followed for more than 5 years after therapeutic conization for minimal (less than 1 mm) microinvasion. Morris et al.[191] reported no invasive recurrences in 14 patients followed for a mean of 26 months after conization for tumors invading 0.5 to

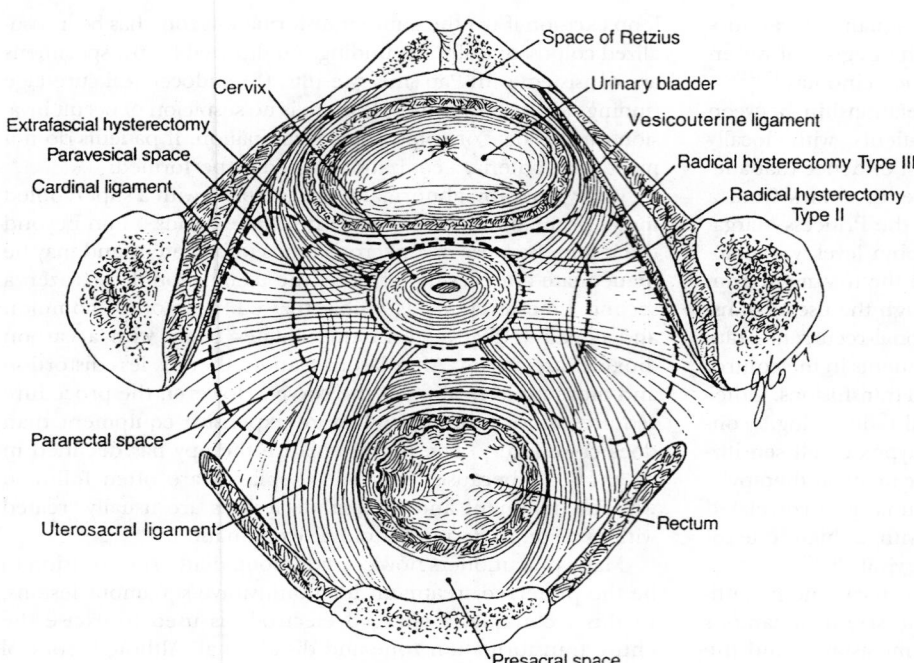

FIGURE 32.1-6. The pelvic ligaments and spaces. Dotted lines indicate the tissues removed with a type II and type III hysterectomy. (From ref. 406, with permission.)

2.8 mm. However, patients who have this conservative treatment must be followed closely with periodic cytologic evaluation, colposcopy, and endocervical curettage.

The likelihood of residual invasive disease after cone biopsy is correlated with the status of the internal cone margin and the results of an endocervical curettage performed after cone biopsy. Roman et al.[192] reported the surgical findings in 87 patients who underwent a conization that showed microinvasive squamous carcinoma, followed by either a repeat conization or hysterectomy. Residual invasion was present in 22% of the women who had dysplasia at the margin of the initial cone versus 3% of those with negative margins (*P* <.03). Residual invasion was found in only 4% of patients in whom cones had margins negative for invasion and negative findings on endocervical curettage. Residual invasion was found in 13% and 33% of women in whom cones had one or both of these features, respectively (*P* <.015), which suggests the need for a second procedure in any patient for whom one of these findings is present. The authors did not find any correlation between residual invasion and the depth of invasion or the number of invasive foci.

Diagnostic or therapeutic conization for microinvasive disease is usually performed with a cold knife or carbon dioxide laser on a patient under general or spinal anesthesia. Because an accurate assessment of the maximum depth of invasion is critical, the entire specimen must be sectioned and carefully handled to maintain its original orientation for microscopic assessment. Complications occur in 2% to 12% of patients, are related to the depth of the cone, and include hemorrhage, sepsis, infertility, stenosis, and cervical incompetence.[193] The width and depth of the cone should be tailored to produce the least amount of injury while providing clear surgical margins.

For patients whose tumors invade 3 to 5 mm into the stroma (FIGO stage IA2), the risk of nodal metastases is approximately 5%.[72,116] Therefore, a bilateral pelvic lymphadenectomy should be performed in conjunction with a modified radical (type II)

hysterectomy. Modified radical hysterectomy is a less extensive procedure than a classic radical hysterectomy (Fig. 32.1-6). The cervix, upper vagina, and paracervical tissues are removed after careful dissection of the ureters to the point of their entry to the bladder. The medial half of the cardinal ligaments and the uterosacral ligaments are also removed. With this treatment, significant urinary tract complications are rare and cure rates exceed 95%.[194]

Although surgical treatment is standard for *in situ* and microinvasive cancer, patients with severe medical problems or other contraindications to surgical treatment can be successfully treated with radiotherapy. Grigsby and Perez[195] reported a 10-year progression-free survival rate of 100% in 21 patients with carcinoma *in situ* and in 34 patients with microinvasive carcinoma treated with radiation alone. Hamberger et al.[196] reported that all patients with stage IA disease and 89 of 93 patients (96%) with small stage IB tumors (less than one cervical quadrant involved) were disease free 5 years after treatment with intracavitary irradiation alone.

Stage IB and IIA Disease

Early stage IB cervical carcinomas can be treated effectively with combined external-beam irradiation and brachytherapy or with radical hysterectomy and bilateral pelvic lymphadenectomy. The goal of both treatments is to destroy malignant cells in the cervix, paracervical tissues, and regional lymph nodes. Patients who are treated with radical hysterectomy whose tumors are found to have high-risk features may benefit from postoperative radiotherapy or chemoradiation.[179,197]

Overall survival rates for patients with stage IB cervical cancer treated with surgery or radiation usually range between 80% and 90%, which suggests that the two treatments are equally effective (Table 32.1-5).[113–115,135,198–209] However, biases introduced by patient selection, variations in the definition of stage IA disease, and variable indications for postoperative

TABLE 32.1-5. Five-Year Survival Rates for Patients with International Federation of Gynecology and Obstetrics Stage IB Carcinoma of the Cervix

| Reference | Year | Radiation Therapy | | Radical Hysterectomy | |
		Patients	5-Y Survival Rate (%)	Patients	5-Y Survival Rate (%)
Liu and Meigs[202]	1955	—	—	116	74
Volterrani et al.[203]	1983	127	91	123	89
Inoue et al.[204]	1984	59	80	362	91
Fuller et al.[135]	1989	—	—	285	86
Kenter et al.[205]	1989	—	—	178	87
Lee et al.[198]	1989	—	—	237	86
Alvarez et al.[115]	1991	—	—	401	85
Hopkins et al.[206]	1991	—	—	213	89
Burghardt et al.[207]	1992	—	—	443	83
Montana et al.[208]	1987	197	83	—	—
Horiot et al.[201]	1988	218	89	—	—
Coia et al.[209]	1990	168	74	—	—
Lowrey et al.[200]	1992	130	81	—	—
Perez et al.[114]	1992	394	85	—	—
Eifel et al.[113]	1994	1494	81	—	—
Barillot et al.[119]	1997	—	83.5	—	—
Landoni et al.[210]	1997	167[a]	74	170[a]	74

[a]Thirteen percent of patients had International Federation of Gynecology and Obstetrics stage IIA disease.

radiotherapy or adjuvant hysterectomy confound comparisons about the efficacy of radiotherapy versus surgery. Because young women with small, clinically node-negative tumors tend to be favored candidates for surgery and because tumor diameter and nodal status are inconsistently described in published series, it is difficult to compare the results reported for patients treated with the two modalities.

In 1997, Landoni and colleagues reported results from the only prospective trial comparing radical surgery with radiotherapy alone.[210] In their study, patients with stage IB or IIA disease were randomly assigned to receive treatment with type III radical hysterectomy or a combination of external-beam and low dose-rate (LDR) intracavitary radiotherapy. In the surgical arm, findings of parametrial involvement, positive margins, deep stromal invasion, or positive nodes led to the use of postoperative pelvic irradiation in 62 of 114 patients (54%) with tumors 4 cm or smaller in diameter and in 46 of 55 patients (84%) with tumors measuring more than 4 cm. Patients in the radiotherapy arm received a relatively low total dose of radiation to the cervix, with a median dose to point A of 76 Gy. With a median follow-up of 87 months, the 5-year actuarial disease-free survival rates for patients treated in the surgery and radiotherapy groups were 80% and 82%, respectively, for patients with tumors that were 4 cm or smaller and 63% and 57%, respectively, for patients with larger tumors. The authors reported a significantly higher rate of complications in the patients treated with initial surgery, and they attributed this finding to the frequent use of combined modality treatment in this group.

For patients with stage IB1 squamous carcinomas, the choice of treatment is based primarily on patient preference, anesthetic and surgical risks, physician preference, and an understanding of the nature and incidence of complications with radiotherapy and hysterectomy. For patients with similar tumors, the overall rate of major complications is similar with surgery and radiotherapy, although urinary tract complications

tend to be more frequent after surgical treatment and bowel complications are more common after radiotherapy. Surgical treatment tends to be preferred for young women with small tumors because it permits preservation of ovarian function and may cause less vaginal shortening. Radiotherapy is often selected for older, postmenopausal women to avoid the morbidity of a major surgical procedure.

Some surgeons have also advocated the use of radical hysterectomy as initial treatment for patients with stage IB2 tumors.[211–213] However, patients who have tumors measuring more than 4 cm in diameter usually have deep stromal invasion and are at high risk for lymph node involvement and parametrial extension. Because patients with these risk factors have an increased rate of pelvic disease recurrence, surgical treatment is usually followed by postoperative irradiation, which means that the patient is exposed to the risks of both treatments. Consequently, many gynecologic and radiation oncologists believe that patients with bulky (stage IB2) carcinomas are better treated with radical radiotherapy.

Two prospective randomized trials[180,183] indicate that patients who are treated with radiation for bulky central disease benefit from concurrent administration of cisplatin-containing chemotherapy. A third study suggests that patients who require postoperative radiotherapy because of findings of lymph node metastasis or involved surgical margins also benefit from concurrent chemoradiation.[179] These studies are discussed in more detail in Concurrent Chemoradiation, later in this chapter. Patients who have stage IB1 cancers without evidence of regional involvement have excellent pelvic control rates (approximately 97% at 5 years) with radiotherapy alone and probably do not require chemotherapy when they are treated with primary radiotherapy.[113,114]

RADICAL HYSTERECTOMY. The standard surgical treatment for stage IB and IIA cervical carcinomas is radical (type III) hysterectomy and bilateral pelvic lymph node dissection. This procedure involves *en bloc* removal of the uterus, cervix, and paracervical, parametrial, and paravaginal tissues to the pelvic sidewalls bilaterally, with removal of as much of the uterosacral ligaments as possible (see Fig. 32.1-6). The uterine vessels are ligated at their origin, and the proximal third of the vagina and paracolpium are resected. For women younger than 40 to 45 years, the ovaries usually are not removed. If intraoperative findings suggest a need for postoperative pelvic irradiation, the ovaries may be transposed out of the pelvis.

Intraoperative and immediately postoperative complications of radical hysterectomy include blood loss (mean, 0.8 L), ureterovaginal fistula (1% to 2% of patients), vesicovaginal fistula (less than 1%), pulmonary embolus (1% to 2%), small bowel obstruction (1% to 2%), and postoperative fever secondary to deep vein thrombosis, pulmonary infection, pelvic cellulitis, urinary tract infection, or wound infection (25% to 50%).[214] Subacute complications include lymphocyst formation and lower extremity edema, the risk of which is related to the extent of the node dissection. Lymphocysts may obstruct a ureter, but hydronephrosis usually improves with drainage of the lymphocyst.[215] The risk of complications may be increased in patients who receive preoperative or postoperative irradiation.

Although most patients have transient decreased bladder sensation after radical hysterectomy, with appropriate management severe long-term bladder complications are infrequent. However, chronic bladder hypotonia or atony occurs in 3% to 5% of patients, despite careful postoperative bladder drainage.[216,217] Bladder atony probably results from damage to the bladder's innervation and may be related to the extent of the parametrial and paravaginal dissection.[218,219] Radical hysterectomy may be complicated by stress incontinence, but reported incidences vary widely and may be influenced by the addition of postoperative radiotherapy.[220,221] Patients may also experience constipation and, rarely, chronic obstipation after radical hysterectomy.

The use of radical vaginal trachelectomy and laparoscopic lymphadenectomy has been advocated in carefully selected women with small IB1 lesions (2 cm or less) who are eager to preserve fertility. The experience, thus far, suggests that the local control and survival rates are comparable to those in women who undergo a transabdominal radical or modified hysterectomy. However, fertility is clearly compromised; the percentage of women able to become pregnant and carry a baby to term is less than half the expected rate in women without cervical cancer; and there is a significant rate of prematurity.[222]

RADIOTHERAPY AFTER RADICAL HYSTERECTOMY. The role of postoperative irradiation in patients with cervical carcinoma is still being defined. Postoperative irradiation decreases the risk of pelvic recurrence in patients whose tumors have high-risk features (lymph node metastasis, deep stromal invasion, insecure operative margins, or parametrial involvement).[223–226] However, because the patients who received postoperative radiotherapy in these studies were selected for the high-risk features of their tumors, it is difficult to determine the impact of adjuvant irradiation on survival.

In 1999, the GOG[197] reported results of a prospective trial testing the benefit of adjuvant pelvic irradiation in patients with an intermediate risk of recurrence after radical hysterectomy for stage IB carcinoma. Patients were eligible if they had at least two of the following risk factors: greater than one-third stromal invasion, LVSI, or clinical tumor diameter of at least 4 cm. Patients with involvement of the pelvic lymph nodes, parametria, or surgical margins were excluded. After radical hysterectomy, 277 patients were randomly assigned to receive 46 to 50.6 Gy of adjuvant radiotherapy to the pelvis or no further treatment. Overall, there was a 47% reduction in the risk of recurrence with adjuvant radiotherapy (P = .008). In this preliminary analysis, follow-up was too immature for a significance level to be assigned to the overall survival comparison, but there were 18 deaths (13%) in the radiotherapy arm versus 30 (21%) in the radical-hysterectomy-only arm (relative mortality rate, 0.64).[197]

Although pelvic irradiation reduces the risk of recurrence for patients with pelvic lymph node metastases or parametrial involvement, the risk of pelvic and distant recurrence remains high for these women.[223] Some authors have hypothesized that the dose of radiation that can be given safely after surgery may be inadequate to control microscopic disease in a surgically disturbed, hypovascular site.[227] To improve the results of combined modality treatment, the Southwest Oncology Group conducted a prospective trial comparing postoperative pelvic radiotherapy alone versus administration of cisplatin and 5-fluorouracil (5-FU) during and after postoperative irradiation for patients with lymph node metastases, parametrial involvement, or involved surgical margins. Initial results of this trial published in 2000 demonstrated significantly improved rates of pelvic disease control and survival for patients who received chemotherapy.[179]

The overall risk of major complications (particularly small bowel obstruction) is probably increased in patients who undergo postoperative pelvic irradiation, but inconsistencies in the methods of analysis and the relatively small number of patients in most series make studies of this subject difficult to interpret.[210,226,228] Bandy et al.[229] reported that patients who were irradiated after hysterectomy had more long-term problems with bladder contraction and instability than those treated with surgery alone.

RADICAL RADIOTHERAPY. Radiotherapy also produces excellent survival and pelvic disease control rates in patients with stage IB cervical cancer. Eifel et al.[113] reported a 5-year disease-specific survival rate of 90% for 701 patients treated with radiation alone for stage IB1 squamous tumors smaller than 4 cm in diameter. The central and pelvic tumor control rates were 99% and 98%, respectively. Disease-specific survival rates were 86% and 67% for patients with tumors measuring 4 to 4.9 cm or 5 cm or more in diameter, respectively. Pelvic tumor control was achieved in 82% of patients with tumors of 5 cm or more in diameter. Perez et al.[114] and Lowrey et al.[200] reported similar excellent disease control rates for patients with stage IB tumors treated with radiation. Survival rates for patients with FIGO stage IIA disease treated with radiation range between 70% and 85% and are also strongly correlated with tumor size.[114,119,200] For patients with bulky tumors, studies suggest that results may be improved further with concurrent administration of chemotherapy.[180,183]

As with radical surgery, the goal of radiotherapy is to sterilize disease in the cervix, paracervical tissues, and regional lymph nodes in the pelvis. Patients are usually treated with a combination of external-beam irradiation to the pelvis and brachytherapy. Clinicians balance external and intracavitary treatment in different ways for these patients, weighting one or the other component more heavily. However, brachytherapy is a critical element in the curative radiation treatment of all carcinomas of the cervix. Even relatively small tumors that involve multiple quadrants of the cervix are usually treated with total doses of 80 to 85 Gy to point A. The dose may be reduced by 5% to 10% for very small superficial tumors. Although patients with small tumors may be treated with somewhat smaller fields than patients with more advanced locoregional disease, care must still be taken to adequately cover the obturator, external iliac, low common iliac, and presacral nodes. Radiation technique is discussed in more detail in External-Beam Radiotherapy Technique, later in this chapter.

IRRADIATION FOLLOWED BY HYSTERECTOMY. In a 1969 report from M. D. Anderson Cancer Center, Durrance and colleagues[230] reported a lower pelvic recurrence rate for patients with bulky endocervical tumors (6 cm or larger) treated with external-beam and intracavitary irradiation followed by extrafascial hysterectomy than for those treated with radiation alone. Many groups subsequently adopted combined treatment as a standard approach to bulky stage IB or IIA disease. However, in a 1992 update of the M. D. Anderson experience, Thoms and colleagues[231] suggested that the differences observed in earlier reports may have resulted from a tendency to select patients with very massive tumors (8 cm or larger) or clinically positive nodes for treatment with radiation alone.

In 1991, Mendenhall et al.[232] reported no difference in pelvic disease control or survival rates for patients treated before or after the University of Florida adopted a policy (in the mid-1970s) of using combined treatment for patients with bulky tumors (6 cm or larger). In a study of 1526 patients with stage IB squamous carcinomas, Eifel and colleagues[113] reported central tumor recurrence rates of less than 10% for tumors as large as 7.0 to 7.9 cm treated with radiation alone, which suggests that the margin for possible improvement with adjuvant hysterectomy is small.

In 1991, the GOG completed a prospective randomized trial of irradiation with or without extrafascial hysterectomy in patients with stage IB tumors 4 cm or more in diameter. Results of this trial were reported by Keys et al.[233]; the study demonstrated no significant improvement in the survival rate among patients who had an adjuvant hysterectomy (relative risk of death, 0.89; 90% confidence interval, 0.65 to 1.21). These results combined with those of more recent studies demonstrating low pelvic recurrence rates after concurrent treatment with chemotherapy and radiation[180] suggest that there is little role for routine treatment with adjuvant hysterectomy. However, adjuvant hysterectomy may still play a role in selected cases in which uterine fibroids or other anatomic variations limit the dose of radiation deliverable with brachytherapy and in patients who have involvement of the uterine fundus with cancer. In these cases, a type I, extrafascial hysterectomy is usually performed, in which the cervix, adjacent tissues, and a small cuff of the upper vagina in a plane outside the pubocervical fascia are removed. This procedure involves minimal disturbance of the bladder and ureters. Intrafascial hysterectomy is not used for cervical cancer because it does not remove all cervical tissue, and radical hysterectomy is avoided after high-dose irradiation because of an increased risk of urinary tract complications.

CHEMOTHERAPY FOLLOWED BY RADICAL SURGERY. A number of researchers have investigated the use of neoadjuvant chemotherapy followed by radical surgery to treat patients with bulky stage IB or stage II cervical carcinomas. Neoadjuvant chemotherapy has usually included cisplatin and bleomycin plus one or two other drugs. The results of uncontrolled studies cannot be easily compared with the results of more traditional treatments because the series are small and often have short follow-up and the criteria for patient selection are not always clear. Some or all of the patients in each of these series underwent postoperative pelvic irradiation.

Sardi et al.[234] compared radical hysterectomy followed by postoperative radiotherapy with chemotherapy followed by surgery and irradiation; they observed similar outcomes with the two treatments for patients who had tumors smaller than 4 cm in diameter, but they reported a significantly better projected 4-year disease-free survival with neoadjuvant chemotherapy for patients who had larger tumors. In 2001, the GOG completed a similar trial; patients who underwent hysterectomy in their trial were treated with postoperative irradiation if they had high-risk features. The results of the GOG study are pending. In a somewhat different trial by Chang et al.,[235] 124 patients with bulky stage IB or IIA cervical cancer were randomly assigned to treatment with either chemotherapy followed by radical hysterectomy and radiotherapy or radical radiotherapy alone (without chemotherapy). The authors found no significant differences in disease-free or overall survival between the two treatment groups. In contrast, a similar trial by Benedetti-Panici et al.[236] suggested that, among patients with bulky IB or IIA disease, women who received neoadjuvant chemotherapy followed by surgery had a better outcome than women treated with radiotherapy alone; however, because the dose of radiation used in this trial was low and because radiotherapy was frequently protracted and administered without chemotherapy, the results are difficult to relate to current treatment standards.

Ultimately, the cost and morbidity of this triple-modality treatment may only be justified if it proves to be more effective than treatment with the current standard of concurrent chemotherapy and radiotherapy. Studies comparing these approaches have not yet been reported.

Stage IIB, III, and IVA Disease

Radiotherapy is the primary local treatment for most patients with locoregionally advanced cervical carcinoma. The success of treatment depends on achieving a careful balance between external-beam radiotherapy and brachytherapy that optimizes the dose to tumor and normal tissues and the overall duration of treatment. Five-year survival rates of 65% to 75%, 35% to 50%, and 15% to 20% are reported for patients treated with radiotherapy alone for stage IIB, IIIB, and IV tumors, respectively (Fig. 32.1-7).[104,114,119,120] With appropriate radiotherapy, even patients with massive locoregional disease have a significant chance for cure.

External-beam irradiation, often with concurrent chemotherapy, is used to deliver a homogeneous dose to the primary cervical tumor and to potential sites of regional spread. An initial course of external irradiation may also improve the efficacy of subsequent intracavitary treatment by shrinking bulky tumor and bringing it within the range of the high-dose portion of the brachytherapy dose distribution. For this reason, patients with locally advanced disease usually begin with a course of external-beam treatment. Subsequent brachytherapy exploits the inverse square law to deliver a high dose to the cervix and

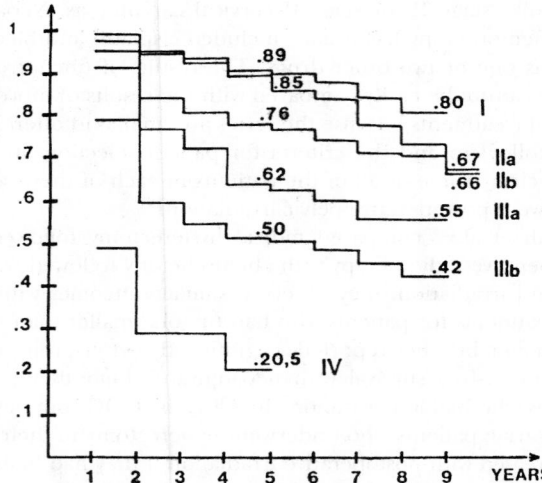

FIGURE 32.1-7. Relationship between International Federation of Gynecology and Obstetrics stage and the actuarial survival rates of 1383 patients with invasive carcinoma of the cervix treated with radiotherapy. (From ref. 201, with permission.)

paracervical tissues while minimizing the dose to adjacent normal tissues.

Although many clinicians delay intracavitary treatment until pelvic irradiation has caused some initial tumor regression, breaks between external-beam and intracavitary therapy should be discouraged, and every effort should be made to complete the entire treatment in less than 7 to 8 weeks. The favorable results documented in reports from large single-institution studies have been based on policies that dictate relatively short overall treatment durations (less than 8 weeks), and several studies of patients with locally advanced cervical cancer have suggested that longer treatment courses are associated with decreased pelvic disease control and survival rates.[237–239]

EXTERNAL-BEAM RADIOTHERAPY TECHNIQUE. High-energy photons (15 to 18 MV) are usually preferred for pelvic treatment because they spare superficial tissues that are unlikely to be involved with tumor. At these energies, the pelvis can be treated either with four fields (anterior, posterior, and lateral fields) or with anterior and posterior fields alone (Fig. 32.1-8). When high-energy beams are not available, four fields are usually used because less-penetrating 4- to 6-MV photons

often deliver an unacceptably high dose to superficial tissues when only two fields are used. However, lateral fields must be designed with great care because clinicians' estimates of the location of potential sites of disease on a lateral radiographic view may be inaccurate. In particular, "standard" anterior and posterior borders that have been described in the past may shield regions at risk for microscopic regional disease in the presacral and external iliac nodes and in the presacral and cardinal ligaments. Care must also be taken not to underestimate the posterior extent of central cervical disease in patients with bulky tumors.

The caudad extent of disease can be determined by inserting radiopaque markers in the cervix or at the lowest extent of vaginal disease. Information gained from radiologic studies such as MRI, CT, and PET can also improve estimates of disease extent and assist in localization of regional nodes and paracervical tissues that may contain microscopic disease. When all these factors are considered, differences in the volume treated with a four-field or a high-energy two-field technique may be small. For this reason, some clinicians prefer to use the simpler technique for patients with bulky tumors.

Tumor response should be evaluated with periodic pelvic examinations to determine the best time to deliver brachytherapy. Some practitioners prefer to maximize the brachytherapy component of treatment and begin it as soon as the tumor has responded enough to permit a good placement (with very bulky tumors this may still require 40 Gy or more). Subsequent pelvic irradiation is delivered with a central block. This technique may, in some cases, reduce the volume of normal tissue treated to a high dose. However, it can also result in overdoses to medial structures such as the ureters or underdosage of posterior uterosacral disease.[240] For these reasons, other clinicians prefer to give an initial dose of 40 to 45 Gy to the whole pelvis, believing that the ability to deliver a homogeneous distribution to the entire region at risk for microscopic disease and the additional tumor shrinkage achieved before brachytherapy outweigh other considerations. External-beam doses of more than 40 to 50 Gy to the central pelvis tend to compromise the dose deliverable to paracentral tissues and increase the risk of late complications.[120]

ROLE OF PARAAORTIC IRRADIATION. Results of numerous small series of patients with documented paraaortic node involvement demonstrate that 25% to 50% enjoy long-term survival after extended-field irradiation (see Fig. 32.1-4).

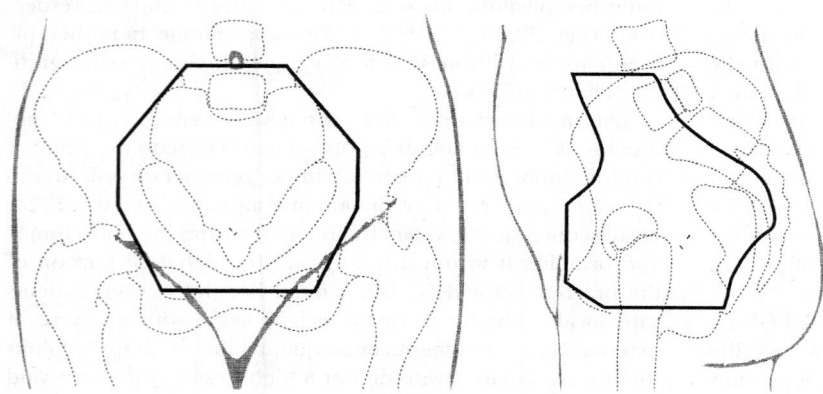

FIGURE 32.1-8. Typical fields used to treat the pelvis with a four-field technique. When lateral fields are used to treat cervical cancers, particular care must be taken to adequately encompass the primary tumor and potential sites of regional spread in the radiation fields.

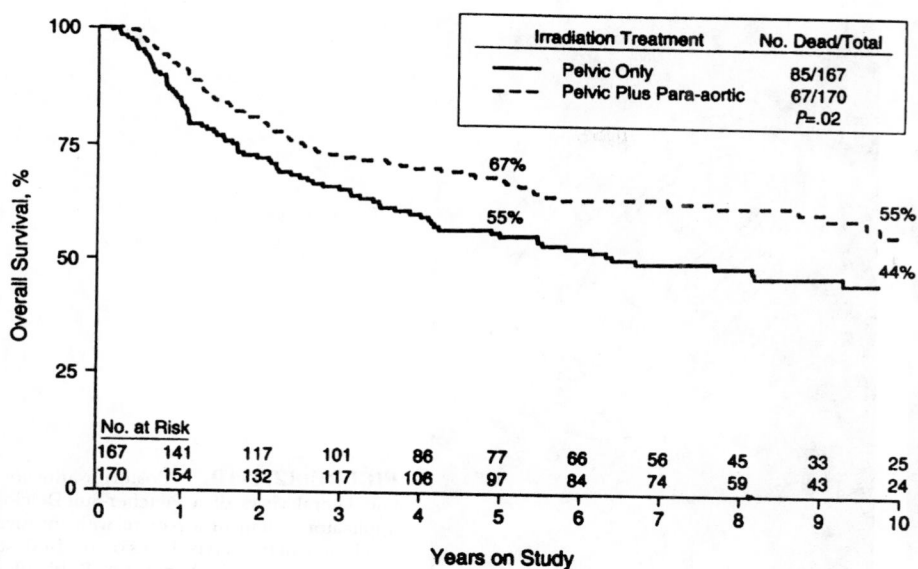

FIGURE 32.1-9. Overall survival rates for patients with stage IB, IIA, or IIB carcinoma of the cervix treated with radiation to the pelvis alone or to the pelvic and paraaortic nodes in Radiation Therapy Oncology Group study 79-20. (From ref. 242, with permission.)

Patients with microscopic involvement have a better survival than do those with gross lymphadenopathy, but even 10% to 15% of patients with gross lymphadenopathy appear to be curable with aggressive management. Survival is also strongly correlated with the bulk of central disease. A 1991 study by Cunningham et al.[241] reported a 48% 5-year survival rate in patients who had paraaortic node involvement discovered at exploration for radical hysterectomy that was then aborted. This experience with patients who had small primary disease that could be controlled with radiotherapy demonstrates that extensive regional spread can occur without distant metastases and that patients with paraaortic node metastases can often be cured if their primary disease can be sterilized.

Two randomized prospective trials have addressed the role of prophylactic paraaortic irradiation in patients without known paraaortic node involvement. In a study conducted by the Radiation Therapy Oncology Group, 367 patients with primary stage IIB tumors or stage IB or IIA tumors more than 4 cm in diameter were randomly assigned to receive either standard pelvic radiotherapy or extended-field radiotherapy before brachytherapy.[242] No consistent method was used to evaluate the paraaortic nodes. For the 337 evaluable patients, absolute survival was significantly better for those treated with extended fields than for those treated with standard pelvic radiotherapy (67% vs. 55% at 5 years; *P* = .02) (Fig. 32.1-9). There was no significant difference in disease-free survival (*P* = .56). A second trial, conducted by the European Organization for Research and Treatment of Cancer,[243] involved a similar randomization but included patients with somewhat more advanced disease. The 4-year disease-free survival rates for patients treated with pelvic fields and with extended fields were not significantly different (49.8% and 53.3%, respectively). However, the rate of paraaortic node recurrence was significantly higher in the pelvic-field group, and for patients in whom local control was achieved, the rate of distant metastases was 2.8 times greater if treatment was with pelvic irradiation only (*P* <.01). Both studies revealed an increased rate of enteric complications in patients treated with extended fields.

Taken together, these data clearly indicate that patients with occult disease can be cured if the paraaortic nodes are included

in the radiation fields. However, the recent addition of concurrent chemotherapy to the treatment regimen for many patients with locally advanced disease increases the importance of careful selection of patients for large-field irradiation because of the greater acute toxicity when chemotherapy is combined with extended-field radiotherapy.[244,245] Although studies such as PET or minimally invasive surgery add to the expense of treatment and are still infrequently performed in patients with locally advanced cervical cancer, these methods may provide better means of identifying patients with regional metastases who can benefit from extended regional irradiation.

BRACHYTHERAPY. Fletcher described three conditions that should be met for successful cervical brachytherapy: (1) the geometry of the radioactive sources must prevent underdosed regions on and around the cervix, (2) an adequate dose must be delivered to the paracervical areas, and (3) mucosal tolerance must be respected.[246] Although some clinicians have proposed a number of variations on the LDR intracavitary brachytherapy techniques practiced at M. D. Anderson, Fletcher's conditions continue to dictate the character, intensity, and timing of brachytherapy for cervical cancer.

Brachytherapy is usually delivered using afterloading applicators that are placed in the uterine cavity and vagina. A number of different intracavitary systems have been used; in the United States, variations of the Fletcher-Suit-Delclos LDR system are still used most commonly.[247] The intrauterine tandem and vaginal applicators are carefully positioned, usually with the patient under anesthesia, to provide an optimal relationship between the system and adjacent tumor and normal tissues. Vaginal packing is used to hold the tandem and colpostats in place and to maximize the distance between the sources and the bladder and rectum. Radiographs should be obtained at the time of insertion to verify accurate placement, and the system should be repositioned if positioning can be improved. Encapsulated radioactive sources are inserted in the applicators after the patient has returned to her hospital bed, which reduces exposure to personnel during applicator placement. Remote afterloading devices that further reduce personnel

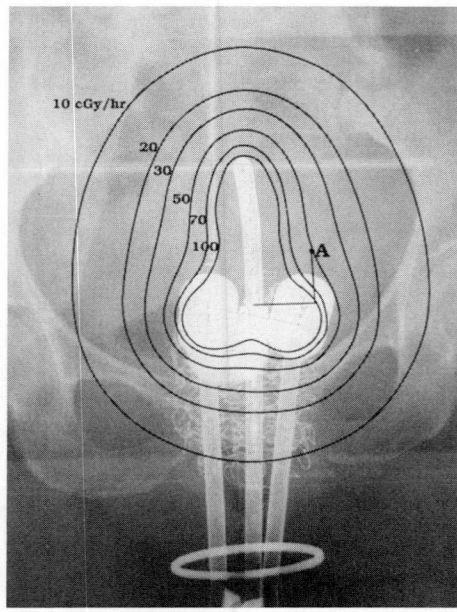
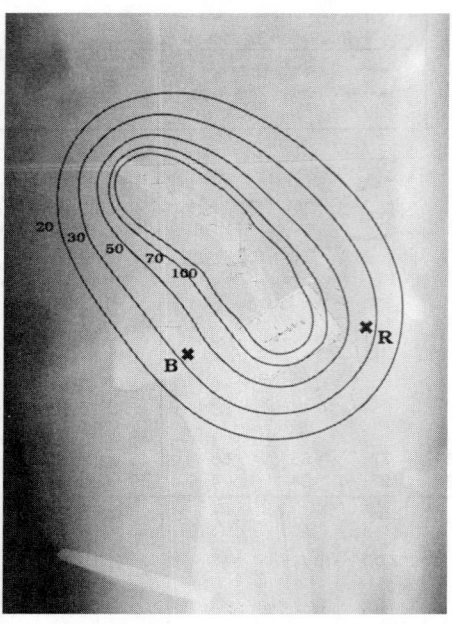

FIGURE 32.1-10.   Posterior-anterior and lateral views of a Fletcher-Suit-Delclos applicator system in a patient with invasive carcinoma of the cervix. Units on the isodose contours are cGy/h. A, point A; B, bladder reference point; R, rectal reference point.

exposure are often used in departments that treat many patients with gynecologic disease. Although radium 226 was used to treat most patients before the 1980s, it has gradually been replaced by cesium 137, which produces a similar dose distribution and avoids the radiation protection problems caused by the radon gas by-product of radium decay.

Brachytherapy Dose. Ideal placement of the uterine tandem and vaginal ovoids produces a pear-shaped distribution, delivering a high dose to the cervix and paracervical tissues and a reduced dose to the rectum and bladder (Fig. 32.1-10).

Treatment dose has been specified in a number of ways, which makes it very difficult to compare experiences. Paracentral doses are most frequently expressed at a single point, usually designated point A. This reference point has been calculated in a number of different ways. The original Manchester method defined point A as a point 2 cm lateral to the cervical collar and 2 cm above the top of the colpostats, measured at their intersection with the tandem midpoint on the lateral radiograph (see Fig. 32.1-10).[248] Although this definition continues to be used, an alternative definition places point A 2 cm lateral and vertical to the external cervical os. These different definitions can produce quite different dose estimates. Point A usually lies approximately at the crossing of the ureter and the uterine artery, but it bears no consistent relationship to the tumor or target volume. Point A was originally developed as part of the Manchester treatment system (a modification of the earlier Paris system). It was meant to be used in the context of a detailed set of rules governing the placement and loading of the intracavitary system. Today this context is often lost.

Other measures have been used to describe the intensity of intracavitary treatment. Milligram-hours (mg-hr) or milligram radium equivalent-hours (mgRaEq-hr) are proportional to the dose of radiation at relatively distant points from the system and therefore give a sense of the dose to the whole pelvis. In 1985 the International Commission on Radiation Units and Measurements recommended use of total reference air kerma—

expressed in micrograys at 1 m—as an alternative to milligram-hour that allows for the use of various radionuclides.[249] The International Commission on Radiation Units and Measurements also defined reference points for estimating the dose to the bladder and rectum. These points have been widely, although not universally, accepted. Although normal tissue reference points provide useful information about the dose to a portion of normal tissue, volumetric studies have demonstrated that they consistently underestimate the maximum dose to those tissues.[250]

Whatever system of dose specification is used, emphasis should always be placed on optimizing the relationship between the intracavitary applicators and the cervical tumor and other pelvic tissues. Source strengths and positions should be carefully chosen to provide optimal tumor coverage without exceeding normal tissue tolerance. However, optimized source placement can rarely correct for poor positioning of the applicator.

A detailed description of the characteristics of an ideal intracavitary system and of the considerations that influence source strength and position are beyond the scope of this chapter but can be found elsewhere.[249,251,252] However, an effort should always be made to deliver at least 85 Gy (with LDR brachytherapy) to point A for patients with bulky central disease. If the intracavitary placement has been optimized, this can usually be accomplished without exceeding a dose of 75 Gy to the bladder reference point or 70 Gy to the rectal reference point, doses that are usually associated with an acceptably low risk of major complications. The dose to the surface of the lateral wall of the apical vagina should not usually exceed 120 to 140 Gy. Suboptimal placements occasionally force compromises in the dose to tumor or normal tissues. To choose a treatment that optimizes the therapeutic ratio in these circumstances requires experience and a detailed understanding of factors that influence tumor control and normal tissue complications.

A total dose (external-beam and intracavitary) of 50 to 55 Gy appears to be sufficient to sterilize microscopic disease in the pelvic nodes in most patients. It is customary to boost the dose to a total of 60 to 65 Gy in lymph nodes known to contain gross disease and in heavily involved parametria.

Brachytherapy Dose Rate. Traditionally, cervical brachytherapy has been performed with sources that yield a dose rate at point A of 40 to 50 cGy/h. These low dose rates permit repair of sublethal cellular injury, preferentially spare normal tissues, and optimize the therapeutic ratio. In an effort to reduce the 3 to 4 days of hospitalization needed to deliver an appropriate dose of LDR irradiation, some investigators have explored the use of "intermediate dose-rate" brachytherapy (80 to 100 cGy/h). However, in a randomized trial, Haie-Meder et al.[253] reported a significant increase in complications when the dose rate was doubled from 40 to 80 cGy/h, which indicates that the total dose must be reduced and the therapeutic ratio of treatment may be compromised with higher dose rates. On the basis of laboratory studies, Amdur and Bedford[254] have suggested that differences in the magnitude of the dose-rate effect between tumor and normal tissues may in part reflect differences in the half-times for repair of sublethal radiation damage.

During the past two decades, computer technology has made it possible to deliver brachytherapy at very high dose rates (more than 100 cGy/min) using a high-activity cobalt 60 or iridium 192 source and remote afterloading. High dose-rate (HDR) intracavitary therapy is now being used for radical treatment of cervical cancer by many groups in Asia, Canada, and Europe[255,256]; more recently, several groups in the United States have adopted this method, although in the United States, more than 80% of patients are still treated using LDR techniques.[257] Clinicians have found HDR brachytherapy attractive because it does not require that patients be hospitalized and may be more convenient for the patient and the physician. However, unless it is heavily fractionated, HDR brachytherapy loses the radiobiologic advantage of LDR treatment, potentially narrowing the therapeutic window for complication-free cure.[258,259] Advocates of HDR treatment disagree about the number of fractions and total dose that should be delivered.[255,256] Published experiences suggest that survival rates are roughly similar to those achieved with traditional LDR treatment, but these experiences are difficult to compare because of the same potential problems of selection bias that confound other nonrandomized comparisons.[255,258] Many of the retrospective reviews provide incomplete descriptions of tumor and treatment details.[255] Three purportedly randomized trials[260–262] also have been criticized for methodologic flaws. The use of HDR brachytherapy for cervical cancer continues to be a source of controversy.

In 2000, the American Brachytherapy Society suggested guidelines for the use of HDR brachytherapy for carcinoma of the cervix.[263] The group emphasized the importance of factors that were already considered critical to successful LDR treatment—optimized applicator position, balanced use of external-beam therapy and brachytherapy, compact overall treatment duration, and delivery of an adequate dose to tumor while respecting normal tissue tolerance limits. Although cautioning clinicians about the lack of consensus in several key areas, the American Brachytherapy Society made recommendations about insertion technique, plan optimization, fractionation, dose specification, and quality assurance. Current treatment planning systems come with programs that permit clinicians to "optimize" source positions to achieve desired doses to specified points in tumor and normal tissues. Although similar programs are available for optimizing LDR treatments, the greater number of source positions used in HDR brachytherapy make these systems somewhat more flexible. However, it should be remembered that standard reference points may not accurately represent the locations of tumor and normal tissues. Most groups that use optimization programs have developed methods of forcing the distributions into fairly standard shapes that minimize the risk of underdosing or overdosing tissues that reside outside the optimization points. In the future, CT- or MRI-based volumetric treatment planning should permit more accurate delineation of target and normal tissues and improve optimization models,[264] although their validity can only be determined through careful analyses of outcome in treated patients.

Interstitial Brachytherapy. Several groups have advocated the use of interstitial brachytherapy to treat patients whose anatomy or tumor distribution make it difficult to obtain an ideal intracavitary placement. Interstitial implants are usually placed transperineally, guided by a Lucite template that encourages parallel placement of hollow needles that penetrate the cervix and paracervical spaces; needles are usually loaded with iridium 192. Advocates of the procedure describe the relatively homogeneous dose distribution achieved with this method, the ease of inserting implants into patients whose uteri are difficult to probe, and the ability to place sources directly into the parametrium. Early reports were enthusiastic, describing these theoretical advantages and high initial local control rates, but the early reports rarely included sufficient numbers of patients or had long enough follow-up to provide long-term survival rates.

In two of the larger early series, Syed and colleagues reported an encouraging projected 5-year survival rate of 53% for 26 patients with stage IIIB disease,[265] and Martinez and colleagues reported an 83% local control rate in 37 patients with stage IIB to IIIB disease.[266] However, survival results from two more recent reports have been disappointing. In a 1995 review of the combined experiences of Stanford University and the Joint Center for Radiation Therapy, the 3-year disease-free survival rates for patients with stage IIB and IIIB disease were only 36% and 18%, respectively. Local control rates were 22% and 44%, respectively, and for patients with local control, the rate of complications requiring surgical intervention was high.[267] A 1997 report of the University of California, Irvine, experience also described disappointing survival rates of 21% and 29%, respectively, for patients with stage IIB and IIIB disease, again with a high rate of major complications.

Several groups have been exploring the use of transrectal sonography, MRI, or laparoscopic guidance[268,269]; interstitial hyperthermia[270]; and HDR interstitial therapy[271] to improve local control and complication rates. However, outside of an investigational setting, interstitial treatment of primary cervical cancers should probably be limited to patients who cannot accommodate intrauterine brachytherapy and patients with distal vaginal disease that requires a boost with interstitial brachytherapy.

COMPLICATIONS OF RADICAL RADIOTHERAPY. During pelvic radiotherapy, most patients have mild fatigue and mild to moderate diarrhea that usually is controllable with antidiarrheal medications; some patients have mild bladder irritation. When extended fields are treated, patients may have nausea, gastric irritation, and mild depression of peripheral blood cell counts. Acute symptoms may be increased in patients receiving concurrent chemotherapy. Unless the ovaries have been transposed, all premenopausal patients who receive pelvic radiotherapy experience ovarian failure by the completion of treatment.

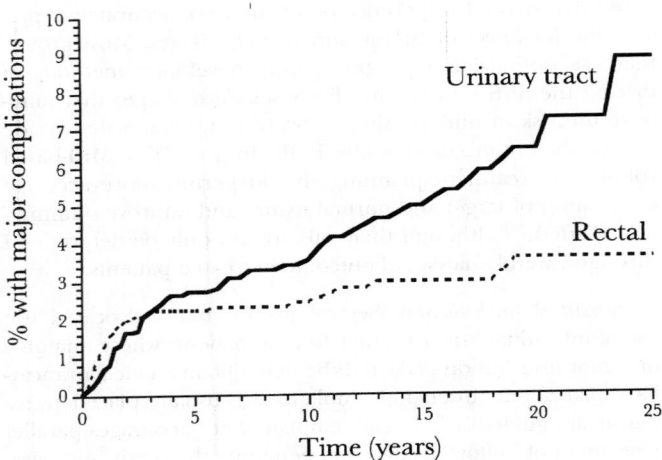

FIGURE 32.1-11. Rates of major rectal and urinary tract complications in 1784 patients with stage IB carcinomas of the cervix treated with radiotherapy. Complication rates were calculated actuarially, and patients who died without experiencing a major complication were censored at the time of death. (From ref. 274, with permission.)

Perioperative complications of intracavitary therapy include uterine perforation, fever, and the usual risks of anesthesia. Thromboembolisms are rare. In a review of 4043 patients who had 7662 intracavitary applications for cervical cancer, Jhingran and Eifel[272] reported on 11 patients (0.3%) with thromboembolisms, four of which were fatal. All four fatal pulmonary embolisms were in patients with advanced pelvic wall disease.

Estimates of the risk of late complications of radical radiotherapy vary according to the grading system, duration of follow-up, method of calculation, treatment method, and prevalence of risk factors in the study population. However, most reports quote an overall risk of major complications (requiring transfusion, hospitalization, or surgical intervention) of 5% to 15%. In a report from the Patterns of Care Study, Lanciano et al.[273] reported an actuarial risk of 8% at 3 years. In a study of 1784 patients with stage IB disease, Eifel et al.[274] reported an overall actuarial risk of major complications of 7.7% at 5 years. Although the actuarial risk was greatest during the first 3 years of follow-up, there was a continuing risk to surviving patients of approximately 0.3% per year, resulting in an overall actuarial risk of 14% at 20 years.

During the first 3 years after treatment, rectal complications are most common and include bleeding, stricture, ulceration, and fistula. In the study by Eifel and colleagues,[274] the risk of major rectosigmoid complications was 2.3% at 5 years. Major gastrointestinal complications were rare 3 years or more after treatment, but a constant low risk of urinary tract complications persisted for many years (Fig. 32.1-11). The actuarial risk of developing a fistula of any type was 1.7% at 5 years.

Small bowel obstruction is an infrequent complication of standard radiotherapy for patients without special risk factors. The risk is increased dramatically in patients who have undergone transperitoneal lymph node dissection.[108,274] However, there appears to be little added risk if the operation is performed with a retroperitoneal approach.[108] Other factors that can increase the risk of small bowel complications in patients treated for cervical cancer include pelvic inflammatory disease, thin body habitus, heavy smoking, and the use of high doses or

large volumes for external-beam irradiation, particularly with low-energy treatment beams and large daily fraction sizes.[274,275]

Most patients treated with radical radiotherapy have some agglutination and telangiectasia of the apical vagina. More significant vaginal shortening can occur, particularly in elderly, postmenopausal women and those with extensive tumors treated with a high dose of radiation.[274,276] Vaginal function can be optimized with appropriate estrogen support and vaginal dilatation.

CONCURRENT CHEMORADIATION. During the past 5 years, prospective randomized trials involving patients with locoregionally advanced cervical cancer[179–183] have provided compelling evidence that the addition of concurrent cisplatin-containing chemotherapy to standard radiotherapy reduces the risk of disease recurrence by as much as 50% and thereby improves the rates of pelvic disease control and survival (Table 32.1-6).

Individual investigators and multi-institutional groups have been exploring combinations of chemotherapy and radiotherapy in patients with cervical cancer for more than 25 years. However, until recently, studies had failed to demonstrate a clear benefit. Early trials of hydroxyurea with radiation were promising but inconclusive owing to their small size and problematic treatment technique and study design.[277] However, encouraged by these results, the GOG included hydroxyurea in the control arms of several subsequent trials.

In two studies,[181,182] the GOG randomly assigned patients with stage IIB or IVA disease to receive either hydroxyurea or cisplatin-containing chemotherapy during external-beam irradiation. All three of the cisplatin-containing regimens in these trials produced local control and survival rates superior to those for the control arms (hydroxyurea and radiation). In a third study,[183] patients with stage IB tumors measuring at least 4 cm in diameter were randomly assigned to receive radiation alone or radiation plus weekly cisplatin before extrafascial hysterectomy. Patients who received cisplatin were more likely to have a complete histologic response and were more likely to be disease free at the time of preliminary analysis. A fourth study, cosponsored by the Southwest Oncology Group and the GOG,[179] included patients who were treated with radical hysterectomy and were found to have pelvic lymph node metastases, positive margins, or parametrial involvement. Patients were randomly assigned to receive postoperative pelvic irradiation alone or combined with cisplatin and 5-FU. In a preliminary analysis, patients who received chemotherapy in this study also had a better disease-free survival rate.

During this time, the Radiation Therapy Oncology Group[180] also conducted a trial in which radiotherapy alone (including prophylactic paraaortic irradiation) was compared with pelvic irradiation plus concurrent cisplatin and 5-FU. This is the only study in which chemotherapy was administered during both the brachytherapy and external-beam components of treatment. The results of this trial were released early when highly significant differences were detected in the rates of local control, distant metastasis, overall survival, and disease-free survival favoring the treatment arm that included chemotherapy. Although acute toxic effects of treatment were greater with chemotherapy, the dose and duration of radiation were similar in the two arms, and there was no significant difference in the incidence of late treatment-related complications.[278] An update of this study demonstrates significant improvements in outcome for patients with

TABLE 32.1-6. Prospective Randomized Trials That Investigated the Role of Concurrent Radiotherapy and Cisplatin-Containing Chemotherapy for Patients with Locoregionally Advanced Cervical Cancer

Reference	Eligibility	Chemotherapy in Investigational Arm	Chemotherapy in Control Arm	Relative Risk of Recurrence (90% Confidence Interval)	P
Rose et al.[182]	FIGO IIB–IVA, PA nodes negative (dissection)	Cisplatin, 40 mg/m^2 (wks 1–6)	Hydroxyurea, 3 g/m^2 (twice weekly, weeks 1–6)	0.57 (0.42–0.78)	<.001
		Cisplatin, 50 mg/m^2 (d 1 and 29)	Hydroxyurea, 3 g/m^2 (twice weekly, weeks 1–6)	0.55 (0.40–0.75)	<.001
		5-Fluorouracil, 4 g/m^2 (96-h infusion, d 1 and 29) Hydroxyurea, 2 g/m^2 (twice weekly, wks 1–6)			
Morris et al.[180]	FIGO IB–IIA (≥5 cm), IIB–IVA, or pelvic lymph nodes positive PA nodes negative (dissection or lymphangiogram)	Cisplatin, 75 mg/m^2 (d 1 and 22, and with second brachytherapy) 5-Fluorouracil, 4 g/m^2 (96-h infusion d 1 and 22, and with second brachytherapy)	None[a]	0.48 (0.35–0.66)	<.001
Keys et al.[183]	FIGO IB (≥4 cm) PA nodes negative (computed tomography or lymphangiogram)	Cisplatin, 40 mg/m^2 (wks 1–6)[b]	None[b]	0.51 (0.34–0.75)	.001
Whitney et al.[181]	FIGO IIB–IVA, PA nodes negative (dissection)	Cisplatin, 50 mg/m^2 (d 1 and 29) 5-Fluorouracil, 4 g/m^2 (96-h infusion d 1, 29)	Hydroxyurea, 80 mg/kg (twice weekly during external-beam RT)	0.79 (0.62–0.99)	.03
Peters et al.[179]	FIGO I–IIA after radical hysterectomy with findings of: (1) Pelvic lymph node metastases (2) Positive margins (3) Parametrial involvement PA nodes negative	Cisplatin, 50 mg/m^2 (d 1 and 29) 5-Fluorouracil, 4 g/m^2 (96-h infusion d 1 and 29)	None	0.50 (0.29–0.84)	.01
Pearcey et al.[279]	FIGO IB–IIA (≥5 cm), IIB–IVA, or pelvic lymph nodes positive	Cisplatin, 40 mg/m^2 (wks 1–6)	None	—	.33

FIGO, International Federation of Gynecology and Obstetrics; PA, paraaortic; RT, radiotherapy.
[a]Patients in control arm had prophylactic paraaortic irradiation.
[b]All patients had extrafascial hysterectomy after radiotherapy.

stage III or IV disease as well as for patients with stage IB or II cervical cancers.[278]

Only one large randomized trial has failed to demonstrate a significant advantage from concurrent cisplatin-based chemotherapy in cervical cancer patients. This trial[279] was published by Pearcey et al. in 2002. The authors suggested that differences in technique could explain the difference between their results and the results of the earlier trials, although the survival rate in their control arm indicated that the margin for improvement was similar to that in the earlier trials. This trial also was the smallest of the six; thus the confidence intervals were relatively large, which may have contributed to the investigators' inability to discern a significant difference between the treatment arms.

Taken together, the randomized trials provide strong evidence that that the addition of concurrent cisplatin-containing chemotherapy to pelvic radiotherapy benefits selected patients with locally advanced cervical cancer. However, all of the studies explicitly excluded patients with evidence of paraaortic lymph node metastases, poor performance status, or impaired renal function. In the future, clinicians will be challenged to determine how these favorable results can be generalized to patients with cervical cancer who may not have been included in the prospective trials because of severe medical or social problems and to the developing nations where invasive cervical cancer is epidemic.

These studies raise other interesting questions that will undoubtedly be the subjects of future studies. Of four different cisplatin-containing regimens, only two were compared directly. It is unclear from the results which regimen achieves the most favorable therapeutic ratio and whether the inclusion of 5-FU in several of the studies contributed importantly to the results. Although North American studies have emphasized cisplatin-containing regimens, investigators in Southeast Asia have reported improved outcome when radiation was combined with epirubicin[280] or mitomycin and 5-FU.[281] Other drugs that are being studied for their radiosensitizing effects in patients with advanced disease are paclitaxel,[282] carboplatin,[283] and several biologic response modifiers. Extended-field irradiation (including the aortic nodes) has proven effective in the treatment of patients with known or suspected aortic node metastasis,[242] but the role of extended-field irradiation needs to be clarified in the context of these new results. Combinations of extended-

TABLE 32.1-7.   Results of Prospective Randomized Trials That Compared Neoadjuvant Chemotherapy Followed by Radiation Therapy with Radiation Therapy Alone in Patients with Locally Advanced Cervical Cancer

| | | | | | Survival Rate | | | |
| | | | | | Chemotherapy + Radiation Therapy (%) | Radiation Therapy Alone (%) | | |
Reference	*Year*	*Patients*	*Stages*	*Drugs*			*P*	*End Point*
Kumar et al.[288]	1994	184	IIB–IVA	BIP	38	43	.5	OS at 32 mo
Tattersall et al.[294]	1992	71	IIB–IVA	PVB	44[a]	40[a]	NS	OS at 48 mo
Chauvergne et al.[284]	1990	107	IIIB	MtxCVP	47[a]	50[a]	NS	OS at 48 mo
Tattersall et al.[289]	1995	260	IIB–IVA	EpP	50[a]	69[a]	.02	OS at 36 mo
Sundfør et al.[290]	1996	94	IIIB–IVA	PF	34[a]	37[a]	.9	OS at 48 mo
Leborgne et al.[291]	1997	96	IB2–IVA	BOP	38	45	.4	Disease-free survival at 60 mo
Souhami et al.[287]	1991	107	IIIB	BOMP	23	39	.02	OS at 60 mo

B, bleomycin; C, chlorambucil; Ep, epirubicin; F, 5-fluorouracil; I, ifosfamide; M, mitomycin C; Mtx, methotrexate; O, vincristine; OS, overall survival; P, cisplatinum; V, vinblastine.
[a]Percentages were estimated from survival curves.

field irradiation and chemotherapy appear to be feasible, but the acute toxicity is considerable, and late toxicity may be greater than with extended-field radiotherapy alone.[244,245]

NEOADJUVANT CHEMOTHERAPY WITH RADIOTHERAPY. In the late 1980s and 1990s, a number of investigators explored the use of neoadjuvant chemotherapy for locally advanced cervical carcinoma, hoping to translate the 50% to 80% response rates reported with multiple-agent, cisplatin-containing regimens in previously untreated patients[234,284–293] into improved survival rates. Seven prospective randomized trials were conducted comparing radiotherapy alone with neoadjuvant chemotherapy followed by radiotherapy (Table 32.1-7).[284,287–291,294] Unfortunately, of these seven trials, five[284,288,290,291,294] demonstrated no benefit from neoadjuvant therapy, and two[287,289] demonstrated a significantly better survival rate with radiotherapy alone. Only one small trial, published by Sardi et al.[295] in 1998, appears to have demonstrated improved survival with neoadjuvant chemotherapy in patients with stage IIIB disease. None of these trials compared neoadjuvant chemotherapy followed by radiotherapy with concurrent chemoradiation.

In summary, despite the high rate of response of locally advanced cervical cancers to neoadjuvant chemotherapy, randomized studies have demonstrated little or no improvement in outcome when neoadjuvant chemotherapy is added to radical radiotherapy. Combinations of neoadjuvant plus concurrent chemotherapy have not been tested in randomized trials; such combinations should probably be avoided outside of investigational trials because neoadjuvant chemotherapy could compromise patients' tolerance of subsequent chemoradiation. In many ways, the cervical cancer trials mirror the experience with treatment of locally advanced head and neck cancers, for which it has been hypothesized that the failure of neoadjuvant chemotherapy to influence outcome may reflect cross-resistance of tumor cells to drugs and radiation or accelerated repopulation of tumor clones induced by neoadjuvant chemotherapy.

Stage IVB Disease

Patients who present with disseminated disease are almost always incurable. The care of these patients must emphasize

palliation of symptoms with use of appropriate pain medications and localized radiotherapy. Tumors may respond to chemotherapy, but responses are usually brief.

SINGLE-AGENT CHEMOTHERAPY. Many drugs have been studied for their activity in patients with recurrent or metastatic carcinoma of the cervix. Approximately 20 have yielded response rates (partial and complete) of at least 15% and may be of therapeutic value (Table 32.1-8).[296–300]

Several of the platinum compounds have been evaluated in greater detail. Cisplatin has been studied in a variety of doses and schedules.[301–303] These studies have demonstrated activity

TABLE 32.1-8.   Cytotoxic Drugs Active against Squamous Cell Carcinoma of the Cervix (Response Rate ≥15%)

Drug	Response Rate[a] (%)
Cyclophosphamide	38/251 (15)
Chlorambucil	11/44 (25)
Dibromodulcitol	23/102 (23)
Galactitol	7/36 (19)
Ifosfamide	35/157 (22)
Melphalan	4/20 (20)
Carboplatin	27/175 (15)
Cisplatin	190/815 (23)
Doxorubicin	45/266 (17)
Porfiromycin	17/78 (22)
Baker's Antifol	5/32 (16)
5-Fluorouracil	29/142 (20)
Methotrexate	17/96 (18)
Vincristine	10/55 (18)
Vindesine	5/21 (24)
Vinorelbine	6/33 (18)
Irinotecan	36/192 (19)
Hexamethylmelamine	12/64 (19)
Razoxane	5/28 (18)
Topotecan	8/43 (19)
Paclitaxel	14/74 (19)

[a]Combined complete and partial response rate.
(Data from refs. 296–300.)

of the drug at a dose of 50 mg/m^2 given intravenously at a rate of 1 mg/min every 3 weeks. Although there appears to be a small but statistically significant increase in the response rate with a doubling of the dose to 100 mg/m^2, this has not resulted in a detectable improvement in the rates of progression-free or overall survival. More prolonged infusion of the same dose over 24 hours yields a similar response rate with less nausea and vomiting, although the recent development of more effective antiemetic agents reduces the clinical importance of this observation. The response rates with other platinum compounds (i.e., carboplatin and iproplatin) are lower than those observed with cisplatin, which remains the platinum compound of choice for patients with cervical carcinomas.

Ifosfamide has been studied as a single agent in patients with recurrent cervical cancer in at least five phase II trials.[304–308] Response rates ranged between 33% and 50% in three studies that were conducted in patients who had received no previous chemotherapy.[304,306–308] However, the response rates were much lower in two phase II trials that included patients who had received prior systemic chemotherapy, with only three partial responses (8%) seen in 36 patients.[304,305]

COMBINATION CHEMOTHERAPY. Most reports of combination chemotherapy for carcinoma of the cervix have described small, uncontrolled phase II trials of drug combinations that have included at least some agents with known activity. Although response rates have varied widely, data from these phase II studies provide no firm evidence that any of the studied combinations are superior to single-agent therapy for patients with disseminated or recurrent cervical cancer.[309] However, combinations based on ifosfamide and cisplatin and those based on 5-FU and cisplatin have attracted significant interest and deserve further discussion.

Several small phase II studies evaluated treatment with combinations of ifosfamide and either cisplatin or carboplatin in patients who had not received radiotherapy. Response rates for these combinations ranged between 50% and 62% (Table 32.1-9).[310–313] A number of investigators have combined bleomycin with ifosfamide and a platinum compound. Three studies that included patients who had not received radiotherapy reported response rates of 65% to 100%.[314–316] Reports of treatment with these drugs in previously irradiated patients have yielded mixed but generally lower response rates of between 13% and 72%.[313–317]

Combinations of cisplatin and continuous-infusion 5-FU,[318–320] cisplatin and paclitaxel,[321–323] cisplatin and vinorelbine,[324] cisplatin and gemcitabine,[325,326] and cisplatin and topotecan[327] also produce high response rates in previously untreated patients. The combination of carboplatin and liposomal doxorubicin has shown modest activity in this clinical setting.[328] Again, response rates decrease significantly if patients have had previous irradiation.[319,325,329]

In 1997, the GOG[330] reported results of a large prospective randomized trial comparing cisplatin alone with cisplatin plus ifosfamide and cisplatin plus mitolactol in patients with advanced or recurrent cervical cancers. The addition of ifosfamide to cisplatin improved the response rate (31% vs. 18%; $P = .04$) and progression-free survival (4.6 vs. 3.2 months; $P = .03$) but was associated with significantly greater toxicity (leukopenia, peripheral neuropathy, renal toxicity, and encephalopathy) and did not significantly improve the overall median survival. The addition of mitolactol did not improve the response rate or survival duration. A GOG trial revealed a higher objective response

TABLE 32.1-9. Platinum-Containing Chemotherapy Combinations Used to Treat Cervical Carcinomas: Contrast between Results in Patients Treated before or after Pelvic Irradiation

Combination	Responses (%)
No prior radiotherapy	
Cisplatin (20 mg/m^2, d 1–5), ifosfamide^a (1.5 g/m^2, d 1–5)[311]	15/24 (62)
Cisplatin (20 mg/m^2, d 1–5), ifosfamide (2.5 g/m^2, d 1–5)[310]	15/30 (50)
Carboplatin (300 mg/m^2, d 1), ifosfamide (5 g/m^2, d 1)[312]	19/32 (59)
Cisplatin (50 mg/m^2, d 1), ifosfamide (5 g/m^2, d 1), bleomycin (30 mg, d 1)[314]	17/26 (65)
Cisplatin (50 mg/m^2, d 1), ifosfamide (1 g/m^2, d 1–5), bleomycin (15 mg, d 1)[315]	9/9 (100)
Carboplatin (200 mg/m^2, d 1), ifosfamide (2 g/m^2, d 1–3), bleomycin (30 U, d 1)[316]	16/18 (89)
Cisplatin (100 mg/m^2, d 1), 5-fluorouracil (1 g/m^2/24 h, d 1–5)[319]	20/29 (69)
Cisplatin (75 mg/m^2, d 1), paclitaxel (175 mg/m^2, d 1)[321]	—
Prior radiotherapy	
Cisplatin (50 mg/m^2, d 1), ifosfamide (5 g/m^2, d 1), bleomycin (30 mg, d 1)[313]	3/24 (13)
Cisplatin (50 mg/m^2, d 1), ifosfamide (1.2 g/m^2, d 1), bleomycin (30 mg, d 1)[317]	4/14 (29)
Cisplatin (50 mg/m^2, d 1), ifosfamide (5 g/m^2, d 1), bleomycin (30 mg, d 1)[314]	26/36 (72)
Cisplatin (50 mg/m^2, d 1), ifosfamide (1 g/m^2, d 1–5), bleomycin (15 mg, d 1)[315]	5/12 (42)
Carboplatin (200 mg/m^2, d 1), ifosfamide (2 g/m^2, d 1–3), bleomycin (30 mg, d 1)[316]	5/17 (29)
Cisplatin (100 mg/m^2, d 1), 5-fluorouracil (1 g/m^2/24 h, d 1–5)[319]	3/16 (29)
Cisplatin (100 mg/m^2, d 1), 5-fluorouracil (1 g/m^2/24 h, d 1–4)^b [320]	14/52 (27)
Cisplatin (50 mg/m^2, d 1), 5-fluorouracil (1 g/m^2/24 h, d 1–5)[318]	12/55 (22)
Cisplatin (75 mg/m^2, d 1), paclitaxel (175 mg/m^2, d 1)[321]	(57)

^{a}Ifosfamide given with mesna in all combinations.
^{b}Allopurinol also given with this regimen.

rate and longer progression-free survival with a combination of cisplatin and paclitaxel than with single-agent cisplatin; however, the overall survival duration was not improved with the two-drug regimen.[331]

PALLIATIVE RADIOTHERAPY. Localized radiotherapy can provide effective relief of pain caused by metastases in bone, brain, lymph nodes, or other sites. A rapid course of pelvic radiotherapy can also provide excellent relief of pain and bleeding for patients who present with incurable disseminated disease.

Special Problems

TREATMENT OF LOCALLY RECURRENT CARCINOMA OF THE CERVIX

After Radical Surgery. Patients should be evaluated for possible recurrent disease if a new mass develops; if, in irradiated patients, the cervix remains bulky or nodular or cervical cytologic findings are abnormal 3 months or more after irradiation; or if symptoms of leg edema, pain, or bleeding develop after initial treatment. The diagnosis must be confirmed by examination of a tissue biopsy specimen, and the extent of disease should be evaluated with appropriate radiographic studies, cystoscopy, proctoscopy, and serum chemistry studies before treatment is administered.

The treatment of choice for patients who have an isolated pelvic recurrence after initial treatment with radical hysterectomy alone is aggressive radiotherapy. Treatment for patients with an isolated vaginal recurrence is similar to that for patients with a primary carcinoma of the vagina. Most patients are treated with external-beam radiotherapy with or without brachytherapy. Implants may need to be inserted under laparoscopic or laparotomy guidance. Pelvic wall recurrences are often treated with external-beam irradiation alone, although intraoperative therapy may contribute to local control in selected patients.[332,333] Reported survival rates usually range between 20% and 40% for patients treated with radical radiotherapy.[334-336] Patients with vaginal recurrence usually have a better prognosis than those with pelvic wall recurrence. Ijaz and colleagues[334] reported a survival rate of 69% 5 years after radical radiotherapy for 16 patients who had isolated vaginal recurrences that did not involve the pelvic wall. Only 18% of patients who had recurrences that were fixed to the pelvic wall or that involved pelvic lymph nodes survived 5 years. Several authors have reported significantly lower salvage rates for patients with locally recurrent adenocarcinoma.[334,337] Thomas and colleagues[338] reported encouraging results in a group of patients treated with radiation and concurrent chemotherapy, but further studies are needed to determine whether this approach is superior to radiotherapy alone.

After Definitive Irradiation. In some cases, patients who have an isolated central recurrence after radiotherapy can be cured with surgical treatment. Because the extent of disease may be difficult to evaluate and the risk of serious urinary tract complications of pelvic surgery is high after high-dose radiotherapy, surgical salvage treatment usually requires a total pelvic exenteration. Less extensive operations, such as radical hysterectomy or anterior exenteration, are reserved for selected patients with small tumors confined to the cervix or lesions that do not encroach on the rectum, respectively.[339-341]

Tumor involvement of the pelvic sidewall is a contraindication for exenteration but may be difficult to assess if there is extensive radiation fibrosis. The triad of unilateral leg edema, sciatic pain, and ureteral obstruction almost always indicates unresectable disease on the sidewall. Although advanced age is usually considered a contraindication for pelvic exenteration, Matthews and colleagues[342] reported a 5-year survival rate of 46% and an operative mortality rate of 11% for selected patients who underwent exenteration at the age of 65 years or older compared with a 5-year survival rate of 45% and an operative mortality rate of 8.5% for younger patients. In all cases, preparation for total pelvic exenteration must involve careful counseling of the patient and family regarding the extent of surgery and postoperative expectations.

The operation begins with a thorough inspection of the abdomen for evidence of intraperitoneal spread or disease in the pelvic sidewall or paraaortic lymph nodes. Despite careful preoperative evaluation, approximately 30% of operations are aborted intraoperatively.[343] Frozen-section biopsies are done of

suspicious areas. If the biopsy findings are negative, the surgeon proceeds to remove the bladder, rectum, vagina, uterus, ovaries, fallopian tubes, and all other supporting tissues in the true pelvis. A urinary conduit, a transverse or sigmoid colostomy, and a neovagina are created.

Postoperative recuperation may take as long as 3 months. The surgical mortality rate is less than 10%, with most postoperative complications and deaths related to sepsis, pulmonary thromboembolism, and intestinal complications such as small bowel obstruction and fistula formation.[344,345] Gastrointestinal complications may be reduced by using unirradiated segments of bowel and by closing pelvic floor defects with omentum, rectosigmoid colon, or myocutaneous flaps.[214] Advances in low colorectal anastomosis and techniques for creating continent urinary reservoirs have improved the quality of life for selected patients.[346-348]

Several investigators have studied the quality of patients' lives after surgical salvage treatment for recurrent cervical cancer. Hawighorst-Knapstein[349] reported on 28 patients who were prospectively assessed after surgery with periodic physical examinations, interviews, and questionnaires. Results were compared for women who had two, one, or no ostomies with or without vaginal reconstruction. At all points of evaluation, the patients' quality of life was most affected by worries about the progression of the tumor. One year after surgery, the patients with two ostomies reported a significantly lower quality of life and poorer body image than patients with no ostomy. The women with vaginal reconstruction reported fewer sexual problems and better quality of life than those without reconstruction. In another study, Ratliff et al.[350] prospectively evaluated 95 patients who underwent pelvic exenteration and gracilis myocutaneous vaginal reconstruction. Of the 40 patients who completed the study, 21 (52.5%) reported that they had not resumed sexual activity after surgery. Of the 19 patients who resumed sexual activity, 84% did so within 1 year after surgery. The most common problems were problems with adjustment to the urostomy or colostomy. Vaginal dryness and vaginal discharge were also significant problems. These findings indicate the need for adequate counseling after the exenterative surgery.

The 5-year survival rates for patients who undergo anterior and total pelvic exenteration are 33% to 60% and 20% to 46%, respectively.[346,351-353] For patients who have unresectable disease after radiotherapy, treatment options are limited. Several groups are exploring the role of intraoperative irradiation in the treatment of selected patients with recurrent disease that involves the pelvic wall.[332,333,354] However, most patients who have unresectable pelvic recurrences after radiotherapy are treated with chemotherapy alone; response rates and prognosis are generally poor.

TREATMENT AFTER SIMPLE HYSTERECTOMY WITH UNSUSPECTED INVASIVE CANCER. Every patient who undergoes a planned hysterectomy should be carefully screened before the procedure to rule out invasive cervical cancer.[355] Whenever an unexpected diagnosis of invasive cancer is made in a hysterectomy specimen, the patient should be immediately referred for additional treatment, because pelvic radiotherapy produces excellent pelvic disease control rates and survival rates for most patients in this setting.[356,357]

Patients may be classified according to the extent of disease at the time of referral for posthysterectomy treatment into the following groups: (1) those with microinvasive cancer, (2) those with tumor confined to the cervix with negative surgical margins, (3) those with positive surgical margins on resected material but no gross residual tumor, (4) those with gross residual tumor by clinical examination documented by biopsy findings, and (5) patients referred for treatment more than 6 months after hysterectomy (usually for recurrent disease). In a report of the results of radiotherapy in 123 patients, Roman et al.[357] reported 5-year survival rates of 79% and 59% for patients in groups 2 and 3, respectively. In contrast, the survival rate for 30 patients with gross disease (groups 4 and 5) was 41% (*P* = .0001).

Patients with invasion of less than 3 mm without LVSI usually require no treatment after simple hysterectomy. Patients with more extensive involvement for whom resection margins were negative require 45 to 50 Gy of pelvic radiotherapy to treat the pelvic nodes and paracolpal tissues. Most clinicians follow this with vaginal intracavitary therapy, delivering an additional vaginal surface dose of 30 to 50 Gy. Patients for whom resection margins were positive may benefit from a somewhat higher dose of external-beam irradiation through reduced fields designed to include the region at highest risk (e.g., parametria and posterior bladder wall). Patients in groups 3 and 4 reported in the series by Roman and colleagues[357] were usually treated with 65 Gy of external-beam therapy with or without intracavitary therapy. The role of interstitial therapy in this setting is not well documented. Results of studies of treatment for high-risk cervical cancer after radical hysterectomy suggest that concurrent treatment with chemotherapy and radiation should probably be considered for patients with group 3 or 4 disease.[179]

Carcinoma of the Cervical Stump. Although supracervical hysterectomy was once a popular treatment for benign uterine conditions, enthusiasm for the procedure has declined since the 1950s, and it is rarely performed today. As a result, carcinomas of the cervical stump are less common than they once were and are usually seen in elderly women. Tumors are usually subclassified as coincidental tumors (diagnosed within 2 years of supracervical hysterectomy) or true cervical stump carcinomas (diagnosed more than 2 years after hysterectomy). Tumors classified as coincidental were probably present at the time of supracervical hysterectomy and are reported to have a relatively poor prognosis, although the number of cases in most series is small.

The natural history, staging, and workup of cervical stump carcinomas are the same as for carcinomas of the intact uterus. If possible, the cervix should be probed at the beginning of treatment to determine the length of the uterine canal. MRI may be an important aid to treatment planning in these patients.

Patients with stage IA1 disease may be treated with simple trachelectomy, and selected patients with stage IA2 or small stage IB tumors may be treated with radical trachelectomy and pelvic lymph node dissection. However, most patients are treated with irradiation alone using a combination of external-beam therapy and brachytherapy. The altered geometry and short uterine canal in these patients complicate treatment planning. However, in most cases the endocervical canal is 2 cm or longer and, after a course of external-beam irradiation, patients can be adequately treated with intracavitary therapy. The endocervical canal is usually loaded with 20 to 30 mgRaEq of cesium, depending on the length of the endocervical canal, and vaginal ovoids are loaded according to their diameter and

position. Remote afterloading systems provide somewhat greater flexibility in source loading. If the endocervical canal cannot accommodate any sources, a boost dose may be delivered to the tumor with interstitial therapy, transvaginal irradiation, or reduced fields of external-beam irradiation. However, brachytherapy should be used whenever possible. Barillot et al.[358] reported a survival rate of 81.5% for patients treated with combined brachytherapy and external-beam irradiation versus 38.5% for those treated with external-beam irradiation alone. Several authors have advocated interstitial therapy, using techniques described for apical vaginal carcinomas, for patients with bulkier lesions. Vaginal ovoids alone rarely deliver an adequate dose to the cervix. In general, most investigators have reported survival rates similar to those for patients with carcinomas of the intact cervix.[358,359]

Carcinoma of the Cervix during Pregnancy. Estimates of the incidence of invasive cervical cancer during pregnancy range from 0.02% to 0.9%.[360,361] Estimates of the incidence of pregnancy in patients with invasive cervical cancer usually range between 0.5% and 5%. Hacker and colleagues[360] reported an incidence of cervical carcinoma *in situ* of 0.013% in pregnant women.

Diagnosis is often delayed because bleeding is erroneously attributed to pregnancy-related complications. All pregnant patients should have a careful pelvic examination and Pap test at their first antenatal visit. Biopsy should be performed on any suspicious lesion. If the Pap test results are positive for malignant cells and the diagnosis of invasive cancer cannot be made with colposcopy and biopsy, a diagnostic conization may be necessary. Because conization subjects the mother and fetus to complications, it should be performed only in the second trimester and only in patients with inadequate colposcopy and strong cytologic evidence of invasive cancer. Conization in the first trimester of pregnancy is associated with an abortion rate of up to 33%.[360] Conservative conization under colposcopic guidance may reduce the risk.[362]

It appears to be safe to delay definitive treatment of patients with carcinoma *in situ* or stage IA disease until the fetus has matured.[360,361,363] Patients whose disease invades less than 3 mm and shows no LVSI may be followed to term and delivered vaginally. A vaginal hysterectomy may be performed 6 weeks after childbirth if further childbearing is not desired. Patients whose disease invades 3 to 5 mm and those with LVSI may also be followed to term. The infant may be delivered by a cesarean section, which is followed immediately by modified radical hysterectomy and pelvic lymph node dissection.

Patients whose disease invades more than 5 mm should be treated as having frankly invasive carcinoma of the cervix. Treatment depends on the stage of gestation and the wishes of the patient. Modern neonatal care affords a 75% survival rate for infants delivered at 28 weeks of gestational age and 90% for those delivered at 32 weeks. Fetal pulmonary maturity can be determined by amniocentesis, and prompt treatment can be instituted when pulmonary maturity is documented. It is probably wise to avoid delays in therapy of more than 4 weeks whenever possible, although this guideline is controversial.[361,364] For most women with stage IB1 tumors, the recommended treatment is classic cesarean section followed by radical hysterectomy with pelvic lymph node dissection. There should be a thorough discussion of the risks and options with both parents before any treatment is undertaken.

Patients with stage II to IV tumors and some patients with bulky stage IB cervical cancers should be treated with radiotherapy. If the fetus is viable, it is delivered by classic cesarean section and radiotherapy is begun postoperatively. If the pregnancy is in the first trimester, external-beam irradiation can be started with the expectation that spontaneous abortion will occur before the delivery of 40 Gy. In the second trimester, a delay of therapy may be entertained to improve the chances of fetal survival. If the patient wishes to delay therapy, it is important to ensure fetal pulmonary maturity before delivery is undertaken.

Compared with other cervical cancer patients, those with cervical cancer during pregnancy have slightly better overall survival because an increased proportion have stage I disease. The diagnosis of cancer in the postpartum period tends to be associated with a more advanced clinical stage and a corresponding decrease in survival. Although studies differ in their conclusions about whether pregnancy has an independent influence on the prognosis of patients with cervical cancer,[361,365] case-matched studies have demonstrated similar survival rates for pregnant and nonpregnant patients.[366,367]

Patients who are diagnosed with invasive cervical cancer shortly after a vaginal delivery appear to be at risk for recurrence in the site of their episiotomy. At least 13 cases demonstrating this unusual pattern of failure have been reported.[368]

CARCINOMA OF THE VAGINA

Carcinomas of the vagina are rare, accounting for only 2% to 3% of gynecologic malignancies.[369] According to FIGO, cases should be classified as vaginal carcinomas only when "the primary site of the growth is in the vagina."[370] A tumor that is limited to the urethra should be classified as a primary urethral cancer, and a tumor that has extended from the vulva to involve the vagina should be classified as a primary vulvar cancer. Also, according to FIGO, any tumor that has extended to the cervical portio and has reached the area of the external os should be classified as a cervical carcinoma. For this reason, in patients with an intact uterus, it is probable that many tumors that originated in the apical vagina are actually classified as cervical cancers. This may explain why a large percentage (30% to 50%) of patients diagnosed with vaginal carcinoma have had a prior hysterectomy (preventing classification of their tumors as primary cervical cancers).[371–373]

More commonly, the vagina is a site of metastasis or direct extension from tumors originating in other genital sites, such as the cervix or endometrium, or from extragenital sites, including the rectum and bladder.

EPIDEMIOLOGY

Vaginal intraepithelial neoplasia (VAIN) often accompanies CIN and is thought to have a similar etiology.[374] VAIN lesions are more often seen in the upper third of the vagina and may be either extensions from adjacent areas of CIN or separate lesions. Kalogirou and associates[375] found 41 cases of VAIN in 993 patients followed with cytologic examination and colposcopy after hysterectomy for CIN. Most VAIN lesions were in the upper vagina, particularly in the vault angles of the suture line.

Investigators have also reported an association between vaginal carcinoma and infection with HPV—an infection rate of 60% to 65% has been found using polymerase chain reaction technology.[376,377] Because the vagina does not have a transformation zone of immature epithelial cells susceptible to HPV infection, HPV-induced vaginal lesions are thought to arise in areas of squamous metaplasia that develop during healing of mucosal abrasions caused by coitus, tampon use, or other trauma.[374] Invasive vaginal carcinoma has been associated with chronic irritant vaginitis, particularly that caused by chronic use of a vaginal pessary.[377] Schraub et al.[378] reported that 80% of vaginal cancers arising in patients who used pessaries were in the posterior fornix or posterior wall of the vagina. Pride and colleagues[379] suggested that pelvic irradiation might be a predisposing factor in some cases. However, viral and other risk factors independent of the mode of treatment undoubtedly place some of these patients at risk for multiple primary tumors.

Primary invasive carcinoma of the vagina is predominantly a disease of elderly women, with 70% to 80% of cases diagnosed in women older than 60 years.[370] However, FIGO data[370] suggest that the age of peak incidence may have decreased since the early 1960s, when the highest incidence was among women in their 80s. Except for clear cell carcinomas, which are associated with maternal DES exposure, invasive vaginal carcinomas are extremely rare in women younger than 40 years.[370,380]

In 1971, Herbst and colleagues[381] first reported a highly significant association between clear cell carcinomas of the vagina and maternal ingestion of DES during pregnancy. This led to the establishment of a registry to gather information about cases of clear cell carcinoma in the United States. The peak number of DES-associated cases occurred in 1975, when 33 were reported to the registry.[382] The peak risk period for exposed women in the United States is between the ages of 15 and 22 years; the youngest patient reported was 7 years old. The oldest patient reported so far was 42 years old at diagnosis, but the risk to women older than 40 years is still unknown because women in the first exposed cohort have not yet reached their sixth decade. Because only approximately 1 of every 1000 women exposed to DES *in utero* develops clear cell carcinoma, investigators have tried to define other risk factors for development of the disease. The risk of clear cell carcinoma has been associated with initiation of DES early during pregnancy, a maternal history of early miscarriage, and premature birth.[382] Obesity, oral contraceptive use, and pregnancy have been suggested as possible risk factors for development of clear cell carcinoma in DES-exposed women, although larger case-matched studies generally have not confirmed these associations.[383] However, Palmer et al.[383] found that women diagnosed with clear cell carcinoma before 20 years of age did appear to have a higher rate of previous pregnancy and oral contraceptive use than matched controls. Infection with HPV may be a cofactor in some cases. Among 14 cases of clear cell carcinoma studied by Waggoner and colleagues,[384] three contained HPV-31 DNA; ten of the remaining HPV-negative tumors had p53 protein detected by immunohistochemical analysis, which suggests a mutation of p53.

Although the risk of clear cell carcinoma of the vagina is small in DES-exposed women, 45% of these patients have areas of vaginal adenosis, and 25% have structural abnormalities of the uterus, cervix, or vagina. Fortunately, awareness of the risks of *in utero* DES exposure has led to a dramatic reduction in the use of high doses of estrogen to prevent miscarriage, and the number of young women who need to be followed for this problem is declining. There is as yet no evidence that DES-exposed women are at risk for malignancies other than clear cell carcinoma.[385]

NATURAL HISTORY AND PATTERN OF SPREAD

Approximately 50% of vaginal cancers arise in the upper third of the vagina.[371,373,380] Reviews have reported a fairly even distribution of lesions arising on the anterior, posterior, and lateral walls.[371,373] Tumors may exhibit an exophytic or ulcerative, infiltrating pattern of growth.

Tumors may invade directly to involve adjacent structures such as the urethra, bladder, and rectum. Despite the proximity of these structures, though, fewer than 10% of vaginal cancers are found to be stage IVA at presentation.[370,373,380,386] However, extensive infiltration of the suburethra or rectovaginal septum is common and frequently influences treatment planning. Vaginal cancers may also spread laterally to the paravaginal space and pelvic wall. Although tumors arising in the vagina undoubtedly can spread superiorly to involve the cervix and uterus, this usually leads to their classification as cervical cancers, according to FIGO convention.

The vagina is supplied with a fine anastomosing network of lymphatics in the mucosa and submucosa. Despite the continuity of lymphatic vessels within the vagina, Plentl and Friedman[387] found a regular pattern of regional drainage from specific regions of the vagina. The lymphatics of the vaginal vault communicate with those of the lower cervix, draining laterally to the obturator and hypogastric nodes. The lymphatics of the posterior wall anastomose with those of the anterior rectal wall, draining to the superior and inferior gluteal nodes. The lymphatics of the lower third of the vagina communicate with those of the vulva and drain either to the pelvic nodes or with the vulvar lymphatics to the inguinofemoral lymph nodes. Plentl and Friedman summarized their description of the lymphatic drainage of the vagina with the comment that, except for the lateral external iliac group, all lymph nodes of the pelvis may at one time or another serve as primary sites of regional drainage for vaginal lymph.[387]

Few data are available concerning the incidence of spread of vaginal cancer to the pelvic lymph nodes. In a review of early reports, Plentl and Friedman[387] quoted an overall incidence of positive nodes of 21%. More recent studies suggest that the incidence of positive pelvic nodes in patients with stage II disease is at least 25% to 30%, which emphasizes the importance of regional treatment for these patients.[388] Inguinal node metastases generally occur only in patients whose tumors involve the lower third of the vagina.[371,386]

The most frequent site of hematogenous metastasis is the lung. Less frequently, vaginal cancers may metastasize to liver, bone, or other sites.[370,371]

PATHOLOGY

Eighty percent to 90% of primary vaginal malignancies are squamous cell carcinomas.[369,370] Grossly, these tumors may be nodular, ulcerative, or exophytic plaques of any size. Histologically, they are similar to squamous tumors from other sites. Approximately one-third of these tumors are keratinizing, and more than half are nonkeratinizing, moderately differentiated lesions.

Verrucous carcinoma is an uncommon variant of squamous cell carcinoma that presents as a warty, fungating mass.[389] Histologically, verrucous carcinoma is composed of large papillary fronds covered by dense keratin. Its deep margin creates a pushing border of well-oriented rete ridges. This tumor rarely metastasizes but can extensively infiltrate into surrounding tissues, including the rectum and coccyx. Wide surgical excision is the treatment of choice in this situation.

Five percent to 10% of primary vaginal neoplasms are adenocarcinomas, although the incidence may vary with the proportion of women in the population who were exposed to DES *in utero*.[369,370] Clear cell carcinomas of the vagina, which may be associated with maternal DES exposure, are usually polypoid but may have tubulocystic or solid patterns. Adenocarcinomas not associated with DES exposure occur primarily in postmenopausal women. The differential diagnosis of adenocarcinoma occurring in the vagina is often difficult, because it must be distinguished from metastatic tumors originating in other sites. Histologic patterns include clear cell, mucinous, adenosquamous, papillary, and undifferentiated. It has been hypothesized that these tumors may arise in foci of adenosis, from mesonephric rests, or from foci of endometriosis in the vagina.[390]

Primary small cell carcinomas of the vagina are very rare; fewer than 20 cases have been reported in the literature.[391,392] They are histologically indistinguishable from neuroendocrine small cell carcinomas of the lung or cervix and like these tumors may coexist with squamous or adenocarcinoma elements.

Primary vaginal melanomas represent approximately 3% of primary vaginal cancers and fewer than 20% of genital melanomas.[369,370] Primary vaginal melanomas are thought to arise from melanocytes in areas of melanosis or atypical melanocytic hyperplasia. They usually originate in the lower third of the vagina and occur at a mean age of 55 years, with age at diagnosis ranging from 22 to 83 years. They tend to have a poorer prognosis than vulvar melanomas, with 5-year survival rates of 15% to 20% after treatment with surgery, radiation, or both.[393]

Approximately 3% of vaginal cancers are sarcomas. Approximately two-thirds of these are leiomyosarcomas, but endometrial stromal sarcomas, malignant mixed müllerian tumors, and other types have been reported.[394] Embryonal rhabdomyosarcoma (sarcoma botryoides) is a highly malignant sarcoma that occurs in children up to 6 years of age. This tumor usually forms soft nodules that fill and protrude from the vagina. The prognosis for children with this tumor has improved with the use of multimodality therapy including surgery, chemotherapy, and radiation.[395]

DIAGNOSIS, CLINICAL EVALUATION, AND STAGING

Most patients with VAIN and 10% to 20% of patients with invasive disease are asymptomatic at presentation; in these cases, carcinoma is usually diagnosed during investigation of an abnormal Pap test result. Colposcopic evaluation in the case of abnormal cytologic findings should always include a detailed examination of the entire vagina and cervix, even when there is an obvious cervical lesion, because patients can present with multiple areas of abnormality. Women who have persistent positive Pap test results after treatment of CIN should be examined carefully for VAIN.

Fifty percent to 60% of patients with invasive cancer present with abnormal vaginal bleeding, frequently after coitus or vagi-

TABLE 32.1-10. International Federation of Gynecology and Obstetrics Clinical Staging of Carcinoma of the Vagina

STAGE 0	Carcinoma *in situ*, intraepithelial carcinoma.
STAGE I	The carcinoma is limited to the vaginal wall.
STAGE II	The carcinoma has involved the subvaginal tissues but has not extended onto the pelvic wall.
STAGE III	The carcinoma has extended onto the pelvic wall.
STAGE IV	The carcinoma has extended beyond the true pelvis or has clinically involved the mucosa of the bladder or rectum. Bullous edema as such does not permit a case to be allotted to stage IV.
Stage IVA	Spread of the growth to adjacent organs and/or direct extension beyond the true pelvis.
Stage IVB	Spread to distant organs.

nal douching. Patients may also present with complaints of vaginal discharge, a palpable mass, dyspareunia, or pain in the perineum or pelvis.[380,396]

According to FIGO, the rules for clinical staging of carcinoma of the vagina are the same as those for clinical staging of cervical cancer.[370] The workup should include careful examination of the cervix and vagina and bimanual examination. All patients should have chest radiography, a complete blood cell count, and a biochemical profile. Cystoscopy and ureteroscopy are strongly recommended for patients with large tumors or tumors involving the anterior vaginal wall. Proctoscopy is indicated for lesions involving the posterior vaginal wall. A barium enema test or skeletal films may also be needed in selected cases. The kidneys should be localized and the rare case of hydronephrosis ruled out with either a classical intravenous pyelogram or a pyelogram obtained with CT. However, it should again be emphasized that the FIGO rules for clinical staging prohibit the use of other information obtained from CT, MRI, lymphangiography, or surgical staging to change clinical stage even though these studies may aid in the determination of disease extent.

The FIGO categories for staging of vaginal cancers are listed in Table 32.1-10.[370] Because this is a clinical staging system, the classification of lesions as stage I or II is probably very subjective. In general, thin (less than 0.5 cm), relatively exophytic tumors tend to be classified as stage I, and thicker, infiltrating tumors and those with obvious paravaginal nodularity tend to be classified as stage II. Perez and colleagues[386] use a modification of the FIGO system that distinguishes tumors which infiltrate the parametrium (stage IIB) from those with paravaginal submucosal extension only (stage IIA). They reported a 5-year survival rate of 55% for patients whose tumors were classified as stage IIA versus 35% for those whose tumors were classified as stage IIB.[386]

The FIGO recommendations for staging of disease associated with positive inguinal lymph nodes are somewhat ambiguous.[370] Although clinical staging is recommended, with rules similar to those used for cervical cancer, the sixth (2002) FIGO manual quoted stage groupings based on nodal involvement; the allowable methods of detection and documentation were not specified. These are further elaborated in the American Joint Committee on Cancer staging manual,[397] which suggests that nodal findings be used in a pTNM pathologic staging system. According to that system, disease associated with pelvic lymph node or unilateral inguinal lymph node involvement

should be classified as N1 and grouped with stage III, and disease associated with bilateral inguinal lymph node involvement should be classified as N2 and grouped with stage IVA. According to the American Joint Committee on Cancer, results of biopsy or fine-needle aspiration of lymph nodes may be included in the clinical staging, although FIGO states that they can be used for treatment planning only.[370] In any case, patients with inguinal metastases are sometimes cured with locoregional treatment. Kucera and Vavra[396] report uncorrected 5-year survival rates of 29% for patients with clinically suspicious inguinal nodes and 44% for patients with clinically negative groins.

PROGNOSTIC FACTORS

The rates of local control, distant metastasis, and survival in vaginal carcinoma are all correlated strongly with tumor stage (Table 32.1-11).[371,380,386,396,398-402] Tumor size also appears to be an important predictor of outcome. Chyle and colleagues[371] reported a higher rate of local and distant failure for tumors larger than 5 cm in diameter; Kirkbride and associates[380] reported a significantly better survival rate for patients with tumors smaller than 4 cm in diameter; and Stock and colleagues[373] reported better survival when disease was limited to one-third of the vaginal canal.

Most investigators have been unable to find a correlation between tumor site and outcome.[371,380,386,396,398,399,402] However, Chyle and colleagues[371] reported higher rates of local recurrence and overall relapse in patients with posterior wall lesions, and Kucera and Vavra[396] reported a better survival rate for patients whose tumors involved the upper third of the vagina. Tumors that involve the entire vagina tend to have a poorer prognosis, which probably reflects the larger size of these lesions.[371,396] Exophytic tumors may have a better prognosis than those with infiltrating or necrotic lesions.[386] Investigators disagree about the influence of histologic grade and type on outcome. Several investigators have reported a correlation between increasing grade of squamous carcinomas and recurrence,[371,403] whereas others have found no correlation.[404,405] Chyle and coinvestigators[371] reported significantly poorer survival and local control rates for patients with adenocarcinoma, but other investigators[380,388] found no difference in outcome for patients with squamous carcinoma and with adenocarcinoma.

TREATMENT

Stage 0 Disease

Patients with only HPV infection or VAIN 1 do not require treatment. These lesions often regress spontaneously, are frequently multifocal, and recur quickly after attempts at ablative therapy. VAIN 2 may be treated with observation or topical estrogen. However, VAIN 3 is more likely to harbor an invasive lesion and should be treated more aggressively. Hoffman and colleagues[374] reported finding occult invasion in upper vaginectomy specimens from 9 of 32 patients (28%) who had surgery for VAIN 3. It has been recommended that VAIN 3 lesions located in dimples of the vaginal cuff in older patients be locally excised to rule out occult invasion.[406]

VAIN 3 lesions that have been adequately sampled to rule out invasion can be treated with laser ablation. Cryosurgery

TABLE 32.1-11. Carcinoma of the Vagina: Survival Rates According to Clinical Stage

Reference	Stage I		Stage II		Stage III		Stage IV		Calculation Method
	Patients	Survival (%)	Patients	Survival (%)	Patients	Survival (%)	Patients	Survival (%)	
Pride et al.[379]	9	66	22	49	4	25	8	0	5-y, crude, uncorrected
Nori et al.[400]	14	71	6	66	3	33	13	0	5-y, disease-free
Rubin et al.[401]	12	75	29	48	13	54	12	0	5-y, crude, corrected
Macnaught et al.[399]	14	68	22	34	18	29	7	14	5-y, actuarial
Perez et al.[386]	59	80	64 (IIA)	55	20	38	15	0	10-y, actuarial, disease-free
			34 (IIB)	35					
Spiritos et al.[402]	18	94	5	80	10	50	5	0	5-y, actuarial, disease-free
Davis et al.[388]	44	82	45	53					5-y, actuarial, uncorrected
Eddy et al.[398]	25	73	39	39	15	38	12	25	5-y, actuarial, corrected
Kucera et al.[396]	73	77	110	45	174	31	77	14	5-y, crude, uncorrected
Lee et al.[412]	17	94	6 (IIA)	80	10	80	6	67	5-y, actuarial, cause-specific
			10 (IIB)	39					
Kirkbride et al.[380]	40	77	38	78	42	60	19	41	5-y, actuarial, cause-specific
Chyle et al.[371]	59	55	104	51	55	37	16	40	10-y, actuarial, uncorrected
		76		69		47		27	10-y, freedom from relapse
Stock et al.[373]	23	67	58	53	9	0	10	15	5-y, actuarial, disease-free

should not be used in the vagina because the depth of injury cannot be controlled and inadvertent injury to the bladder or rectum may occur. Superficial fulguration with electrosurgical ball cautery may be used under colposcopic control, with the epithelial tissue wiped away as it is ablated to allow observation of the depth of destruction. Local excision is an excellent method of treatment for small upper vaginal lesions. Many of these lesions are associated with vaginal atrophy in patients with a history of heavy smoking. Topical estrogen therapy may improve atrophic changes.

Although progression of stage 0 lesions to invasive disease is uncommon, the risk is sufficient to warrant close follow-up of patients treated for VAIN. In a review of 136 cases of carcinoma *in situ* of the vagina, Benedet and Saunders[407] found only 4 cases (3%) that progressed to invasive cancer with up to 30 years of follow-up. Cheng and colleagues[408] reported four cases of invasive cancer that developed in 35 patients who were followed after wide local excision for VAIN.

VAIN can also be treated effectively with intracavitary radiotherapy,[371,380,386] but this treatment is usually reserved for patients with multifocal, multiply recurrent disease or high operative risk. Treatment is usually delivered using cesium 137 loaded in a plastic vaginal cylinder 3 to 4 cm in diameter. Chyle et al.[371] reported a 17% recurrence rate at 10 years in 37 patients treated with a vaginal surface dose of 70 to 80 Gy. Perez et al.[386] reported only one recurrence (5%) in 20 patients treated with a vaginal surface dose of 60 to 70 Gy. The single vaginal recurrence was distal to the region treated with brachytherapy, and the authors emphasized the importance of treating the entire vagina to avoid marginal recurrences. More recently, some authors have reported results using fractionated

HDR intracavitary therapy to treat VAIN. MacLeod and colleagues[409] reported control of VAIN 3 in 11 of 14 patients followed for 36 to 115 months after intracavitary therapy. In these patients, the vaginal surface was treated with a total dose of 34 to 45 Gy in 4 to 10 fractions. One patient had progression to invasive disease. The authors observed no severe complications with this treatment. However, Ogino and colleagues[410] reported adhesive vaginitis and rectal bleeding in two patients in whom the entire vagina was treated with a less conservative fractionation schedule.

Stage I Disease

Radiotherapy is often the treatment of choice for stage I disease because, if surgery is used, total vaginectomy or even exenteration may be needed to obtain satisfactory resection margins. However, surgery has a definite role in selected cases.[373] Early tumors that involve the upper posterior vagina can be removed with a radical hysterectomy and partial vaginectomy (if the uterus is *in situ*) or with a radical upper vaginectomy (if the patient has had a prior hysterectomy) and bilateral pelvic lymphadenectomy. Some surgeons advocate broader indications for surgical treatment of stage I disease.[373,388] Stock and associates[373] reported a 5-year disease-free survival rate of 56% for 15 patients with stage I disease treated with surgery alone (local excision, partial vaginectomy, or radical vaginectomy). One patient in whom disease recurred had successful salvage treatment with irradiation, and two patients who received postoperative irradiation were cured of their disease. Among six patients in the series of Stock et al.[373] who were treated with definitive irradiation, the disease-free survival rate was 80%; one patient in whom disease recurred had successful salvage treatment with pelvic exenteration. For patients with a prior history of pelvic irradiation, radical surgery (usually pelvic exenteration) is indicated and is often curative.

Disease-specific survival rates for patients with stage I disease treated with definitive irradiation range from 75% to 95%.[371,386,396,402] Selected patients with small, very superficial tumors may be treated with brachytherapy alone. Perez et al.[386] achieved pelvic tumor control in 22 of 25 selected patients (88%) with stage I disease treated with brachytherapy alone. They recommended a dose of 60 to 70 Gy calculated 5 mm beyond the plane of the implant or vaginal mucosa (vaginal surface dose of 80 to 120 Gy). Thicker stage I tumors should be treated with a combination of external-beam irradiation and brachytherapy with an aim to deliver 40 to 50 Gy to the pelvic nodes and 70 to 75 Gy to the tumor.

Stage II Disease

Because investigators rarely define their criteria for distinguishing stage I from stage II disease or for selecting patients for various treatments, different institutional experiences cannot easily be compared. Reported disease-specific survival rates range from 50% to 80%. Data suggest that most patients with stage II disease require treatment with external-beam irradiation; some form of brachytherapy is usually added to supplement the dose to areas of initial gross disease. Perez and colleagues[386] achieved pelvic tumor control in only 4 of 11 selected patients (36%) with stage II tumors treated with brachytherapy alone, compared with 54 of 81 patients (67%) treated with a combination of external-beam irradiation and brachytherapy. Chyle et al.[371] reported a local recurrence rate (in the vagina) of 11% in 18 patients treated with brachytherapy (usually interstitial implant) alone but did not report the rate of pelvic wall relapse in this patient subset.

Brachytherapy should be tailored to the volume and distribution of the tumor and its response to external-beam irradiation. For tumors that flatten to less than 5 mm in thickness, the dose to the vagina may be boosted using intracavitary sources in a vaginal cylinder, although interstitial therapy may still be useful in selected cases. Because the thickness of apical vaginal tumors may be difficult to assess in patients who have had a hysterectomy, an examination under anesthesia is often needed to determine whether intracavitary therapy will cover the tumor adequately. Transvaginal sonography or MRI may also be helpful in treatment planning. When the uterus is intact, tumors high in the posterior fornix can often be treated with a tandem and ovoids. Larger tumors usually require a boost with interstitial therapy or additional external-beam irradiation. Most authors emphasize the importance of brachytherapy in the treatment of vaginal cancer.[386,402] However, brachytherapy must be designed to treat the entire vaginal tumor. Chyle and colleagues[371] argue that tumors that cannot adequately be covered with brachytherapy can often be cured with external-beam irradiation alone using carefully designed shrinking fields. They reported three (11%) vaginal recurrences in 28 patients with stage II disease treated with external-beam irradiation alone, compared with 12 (21%) recurrences in 58 patients treated with combined external-beam irradiation and brachytherapy.

Selected patients with stage II disease may be cured with radical surgery.[373] However, total radical vaginectomy or pelvic

exenteration is often required to remove the tumor, and results with radical surgery do not appear to be better than those achieved with radiotherapy alone. Primary radical surgery is usually indicated for patients who have previously had pelvic radiotherapy.

Stage III and IVA Disease

Most authors report disease-specific survival rates of between 30% and 50% for patients with stage III disease and between 15% and 30% for patients with stage IVA disease.[371,380,386,396] Stage III and IVA tumors are usually bulky, highly infiltrative lesions involving most or all of the vagina as well as the pelvic wall, bladder, or rectum. The extent of these tumors and the proximity of critical normal tissue structures make their management a formidable technical challenge. Pelvic recurrence rates are high in most series. The risk of distant metastasis is also relatively high, although distant relapse is often accompanied by locoregional recurrence.

All patients require treatment with external-beam irradiation. Most authors advocate the use of brachytherapy whenever possible. However, Chyle and colleagues[371] reported a fairly high relapse-free rate (47% at 10 years) in a series of patients with stage III disease in which the majority of patients (40 of 55) were treated with external-beam irradiation alone. Brachytherapy is undoubtedly an important part of disease management in some patients. However, in some cases interstitial therapy does not provide adequate coverage of tumors that are very large and intimately associated with critical structures. In these cases, it may be appropriate to place greater emphasis on external-beam treatment. Conformal radiotherapy techniques may help to increase the dose to tumor while limiting the treatment of critical structures; however, it is important to consider internal organ motion, particularly of the upper vagina, when planning conformal treatment.

For selected patients with relatively small, mobile stage IVA cancers who are in otherwise good medical condition, a pelvic exenteration with vaginal reconstruction using a gracilis myocutaneous flap or rectus abdominis myocutaneous flap may be the treatment of choice, particularly if a rectovaginal or vesicovaginal fistula is present.[411] Radical radiotherapy also may be curative in some cases.

RADIOTHERAPY TECHNIQUE. External-beam fields must include the primary lesion and the regional lymph nodes. Fields should be individualized according to the primary tumor site. Radiopaque markers placed at the distal edge of the tumor help to define the lower border, which often includes a portion of the introitus. Treating the patient in an open ("frog-leg") position can often reduce the severity of vulvar cutaneous reactions.

When tumors involve the lower third of the vagina, pelvic fields should be enlarged to include at least the medial inguinal lymph nodes. When four fields are used to treat the pelvis, care must be taken to cover all the draining lymph nodes. Lateral fields should adequately cover posterior perirectal nodes, particularly when the primary lesion involves the posterior vaginal wall.

Intracavitary brachytherapy is of little value in the treatment of locally advanced vaginal cancers because the dose falls off very rapidly from the surface of a vaginal cylinder. In general,

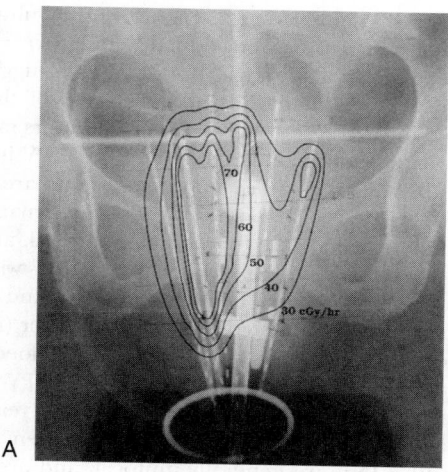

Anterior

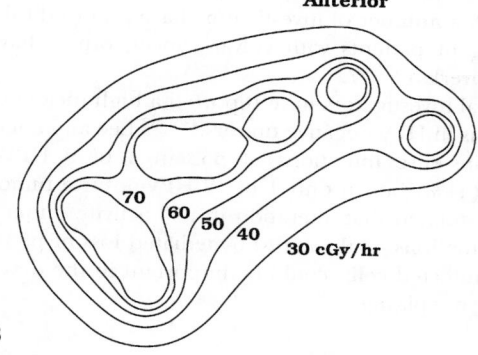

FIGURE 32.1-12. Interstitial implantation of a squamous carcinoma involving the anterior and right lateral wall of the vagina. Needles were placed transperineally while the position of the needles was monitored by fingers in the vagina and rectum. A plastic cylinder in the vagina displaced uninvolved tissues away from the needles, which were loaded with iridium 192 sources. Needles were placed and sources were selected to deliver a somewhat higher dose to the thickest portion of the tumor on the right lateral wall of the vagina. Isodose contours represent the dose rates (in centigrays per hour) delivered to tissues in a coronal plane at the approximate center of the implant (**A**) and in a transverse plane through the center of the implant (**B**).

the dose at a 5-mm depth is only 50% to 65% of the dose at the vaginal surface. Interstitial brachytherapy can provide better coverage of thick vaginal tumors. Vaginal implants can be inserted freehand, a technique that requires experience but permits excellent control of the position of sources with respect to the vaginal surface and rectal mucosa, which can be palpated as the needles are positioned (Fig. 32.1-12). Vaginal implants may also be positioned using a perineal template. This technique provides a more homogeneous dose distribution because it facilitates parallel positioning of sources, but the template interferes somewhat with the brachytherapist's ability to monitor the placement of needles with respect to the rectal and vaginal mucosa. When tumors involve the vaginal apex in patients who have had a hysterectomy, laparoscopic or laparotomy guidance may be needed to ensure accurate needle placement.

Several authors have reported a correlation between higher doses of radiation and lower rates of pelvic recurrence.[386,402] Chyle and associates[371] did not report a significant correlation

between tumor dose and outcome. However, dose-response analyses can be misleading because the total dose of radiation prescribed for a vaginal tumor is often influenced by its size, extent, and initial response to irradiation, all of which determine the feasibility of delivering high-dose brachytherapy. When good brachytherapy coverage of the tumor can be accomplished, an effort should be made to treat the tumor to a dose of 75 to 85 Gy. When brachytherapy is not possible, some patients may be cured with external-beam irradiation alone using shrinking pelvic fields to deliver a tumor dose of 60 to 66 Gy. Treatment can usually be completed in less than 6 to 7 weeks and should not be protracted unnecessarily. Lee and colleagues[412] reported a significantly lower pelvic recurrence rate in patients whose entire treatment course was completed in 9 weeks or less.

COMPLICATIONS OF RADIOTHERAPY. The close proximity of the bladder and rectum makes them vulnerable to damage when invasive vaginal cancers are treated with radiotherapy. In their review of 301 patients treated with definitive irradiation, Chyle and colleagues[371] reported a 19% actuarial incidence of serious complications at 20 years (the crude complication rate was 13%). The most frequent complications were fistulas (ten patients); rectal ulceration, proctitis, or stricture (ten patients); urethral stricture (six patients); vaginal ulceration or necrosis (eight patients); and small bowel obstruction (seven patients). Others have reported similar major complication rates.[380,386,396] There have been no comprehensive studies of vaginal function in women with vaginal cancer treated with radiotherapy. Kirkbride and colleagues[380] reported that 45 of 128 irradiated patients in their study had vaginal stenosis. The severity of vaginal morbidity is probably related to the damage to vaginal mucosa and submucosa from tumor infiltration, ulceration, and infection; the age and menopausal status of the patient; and the radiation dose and the amount of vaginal tissue treated to high doses.

ROLE OF CHEMOTHERAPY. Because primary vaginal carcinomas are rare, few reports have specifically addressed the role of chemotherapy in the treatment of this disease. Chemotherapeutic management is usually based on extrapolations from experience with the treatment of carcinomas of the cervix. For this reason, patients who have metastatic or recurrent vaginal carcinoma that is no longer amenable to locoregional treatment are sometimes treated with cisplatin-based chemotherapy even though the efficacy of this treatment is not well documented in the literature. Thigpen and colleagues[413] reported one complete and no partial responses in 16 patients with vaginal cancers treated with cisplatin 50 mg/m^2 every 3 weeks. In another GOG study, no responses were observed in 16 patients treated with etoposide for advanced vaginal cancers.[414] Reports of the use of neoadjuvant chemotherapy or concurrent chemoradiation are anecdotal.[415] However, vaginal carcinoma resembles cervical carcinoma in its location, pattern of spread, histologic appearance, relationship to HPV infection, and response to radiotherapy. It may therefore be reasonable to extrapolate from randomized trials demonstrating a benefit from concurrent chemoradiation in patients with locally advanced cervical cancer[179,180,182] to justify a similar approach in selected patients with high-risk invasive vaginal cancers.

Vaginal Clear Cell Carcinoma

The treatment of vaginal clear cell carcinoma is similar to that of squamous cell carcinoma. Conventional treatments for stage I and II disease include radical hysterectomy, vaginectomy, and lymphadenectomy with formation of a neovagina using a split-thickness skin graft; and radical radiotherapy. Because many DES-exposed women with clear cell carcinoma were young at the time of diagnosis, treatment of early lesions has emphasized preservation of vaginal and ovarian function. Senekjian and colleagues[416] reported on the use of local therapy alone in 43 patients with stage I disease who were reported to the Registry for Research on Hormonal Transplacental Carcinogenesis. Patients treated with local excision alone had a recurrence rate of more than 40% at 10 years. However, 17 patients who were treated with local irradiation (brachytherapy or transvaginal orthovoltage cone irradiation) with or without local excision had a 10-year recurrence rate of less than 10%. Of 41 assessable patients treated with local therapy in the report of Senekjian and colleagues,[416] 8 had had 15 pregnancies and 12 live births. Retroperitoneal lymphadenectomy may be indicated when local treatment is considered for stage I lesions, which are reported to have an overall rate of pelvic lymph node metastases of 17%.[417]

The overall actuarial 10-year survival rate for patients treated for vaginal clear cell carcinoma is 79%. The survival rates for patients with stage I and II tumors are 90% and 80%, respectively.[416] Most recurrences occur within 3 years of initial therapy. However, recurrences have been reported to occur as late as 10 to 20 years after treatment.[418] Approximately one-third of relapses are first detected at distant sites, most commonly the lungs or extrapelvic lymph nodes.

CARCINOMA OF THE VULVA

EPIDEMIOLOGY

Invasive vulvar carcinoma is a rare disease that accounts for approximately 4% of gynecologic cancers.[93,419] In the United States, invasive vulvar cancer occurs with an average annual age-adjusted incidence of 1.2 cases per 100,000 woman-years.[420] The median age of patients with invasive vulvar cancer at diagnosis is 65 to 70 years; the incidence peaks in women older than 75 years at approximately 20 per 100,000.[419,420] In contrast, vulvar intraepithelial neoplasia (VIN) tends to occur in younger women; the median age of women with VIN at diagnosis is 45 to 50 years. Although investigators have not demonstrated an overall increase in the incidence of invasive vulvar cancer, studies in the United States and Europe suggest that the incidence of VIN has more than doubled since the early 1970s.[420,421] This increase has been particularly marked in women younger than 55 years.[420,421] The relatively stable incidence of invasive cancer despite a steady increase in diagnoses of VIN could suggest that the etiologic factors for the two conditions are different, that diagnostic procedures have improved, or that effective treatment of VIN has prevented a significant increase in the incidence of invasive disease.

Evidence that HPV infection may play a role in the pathogenesis of cervical cancer has led investigators to look for HPV infection in patients with vulvar neoplasms. Eighty percent to 90% of VIN lesions contain HPV-16 or other HPV types. However, although more than 90% of invasive cervical cancers are associated with HPV, only 30% to 50% of invasive vulvar carcinomas are associated with evidence of HPV infection.[422–426]

Epidemiologic, histopathologic, and viral data suggest that patients with invasive squamous cell carcinomas of the vulva can be divided into at least two groups whose tumors may have different etiologies—one that is associated with HPV infection and one that is not.[420,427,428] HPV-positive tumors are usually basaloid or warty carcinomas with little keratin formation, are often associated with VIN, are frequently multifocal, and tend to occur in younger women (35 to 55 years). Patients with HPV-positive tumors are also more likely to have CIN and to have the risk factors typically associated with cervical cancer (multiple sexual partners, early age at first intercourse, low socioeconomic status, and cigarette smoking).[19,428] In contrast, HPV-negative tumors usually occur in older women (55 to 85 years), are often associated with vulvar inflammation or lichen sclerosis (but rarely with VIN), are generally unifocal, and are usually well differentiated with exuberant keratin formation.[424–426] Although a number of investigators have reported this distinct grouping of patients with vulvar cancer, others have found greater overlap.[427,429]

Several investigators have reported a high incidence of p53 mutations in HPV-negative tumors.[430–432] Lee and colleagues[430] found missense mutations of p53 in 4 of 9 HPV-negative tumors (44%) but in only 1 of 12 HPV-positive tumors (8%). They postulated that alteration in p53 activity, either through point mutations or through E6-mediated loss of p53 function in HPV-infected cells, could be important in the development of vulvar neoplasms.

NATURAL HISTORY AND PATTERN OF SPREAD

The female external genitalia include the mons pubis, labia majora, labia minora, clitoris, vestibular bulb, vestibular glands (including Bartholin's glands), and vestibule of the vagina. Together, these structures form the vulva. The region between the posterior commissure of the labia and the anus is termed the *gynecologic perineum*. Approximately 70% of vulvar squamous carcinomas involve the labia majora or minora, most frequently the labia majora. Fifteen percent to 20% involve the clitoris, and a similar proportion involve or arise in the perineum. In approximately 10% of cases, the lesion is too extensive to permit determination of the original site, and in approximately 5% of cases, the lesion is multifocal. Vulvar tumors may extend locally to invade adjacent structures, including the vagina, urethra, and anus; advanced vulvar tumors may invade adjacent pelvic bones.

A rich network of anastomosing lymphatics that frequently cross the midline drains the vulva. Even minimally invasive vulvar tumors may spread to regional lymph nodes (Table 32.1-12).[433–437] For most lateralized lesions, initial regional metastasis is to the superficial inguinal lymph nodes that are superficial to the femoral fascia; tumors may then metastasize secondarily to deeper femoral lymph nodes located along the femoral vessels and then to the pelvic lymph nodes (Fig. 32.1-13). However, more medial lesions, particularly those involving the clitoris, tend to metastasize directly to medial femoral lymph nodes; these nodes may be difficult to classify as superficial or deep because they lie in the region of the fossa ovalis, a gap in the cribriform fascia.[438,439] Theoretically, tumors involving the clitoris can also spread directly to the obturator nodes through lym-

TABLE 32.1-12. Relationship between Depth of Stromal Invasion and Inguinal Lymph Node Metastases in Patients with Squamous Cell Carcinomas of the Vulva

| Reference | Patients with Positive Lymph Nodes/Total No. of Patients by Depth of Invasion (mm) | | | | |
	≤1	1.1–2.0	2.1–3.0	3.1–5.0	>5
Binder et al.[434]	0/7	0/23	3/14	6/25	15/31
Ross and Erhmann[437]	0/17	1/9	1/13	4/15	0/1
Hoffman et al.[436]	0/24	0/19	2/17	8/15	7/13
Hacker et al.[491]	0/34	2/19	2/17	1/7	3/7
Andreasson and Nyboe[433]	0/8	1/13	3/12	5/32	19/57
Total	0/90	4/83 (5%)	11/73 (15%)	24/94 (26%)	44/109 (40%)

phatics that follow the dorsal vein of the clitoris, although evidence of this route is rarely seen in practice. Despite the extensive anastomosis of lymphatics in the region, metastasis of vulvar carcinoma to contralateral lymph nodes is uncommon in patients with well-lateralized T1 lesions.

The lungs are the most common sites of hematogenous metastasis.

PATHOLOGY

As classified by the International Society for the Study of Vulvar Disease, nonneoplastic epithelial disorders of the vulva (previously termed *vulvar dystrophies*) include lichen sclerosis, squamous hyperplasia, and other dermatoses.[440] Approximately 10% of these lesions have cellular atypia and are termed *vulvar intraepithelial neoplasia*. Histologically, VIN is characterized by disruption of the normal epithelial architecture, varying degrees of cytoplasmic and nuclear maturation, and giant cells with abnormal nuclei.[427] VIN lesions are assigned a grade from 1 to 3 according to their degree of maturation. Invasive cancers have been associated with two types of VIN.[427] The most common VINs contain nuclear atypia throughout the epithelial lay-

ers and are frequently associated with HPV. These lesions are sometimes subdivided into warty and basaloid types, which have greater and lesser degrees of differentiation, respectively.[427] In the second subset of VINs, atypia is largely confined to the basal layers of the epithelium. These lesions tend to occur in older women and are not usually associated with HPV but are commonly adjacent to areas of lichen sclerosis or hyperplasia. Buscema and Woodruff[441] estimated that approximately 4% of patients treated for VIN develop a subsequent invasive cancer.

Paget's disease of the vulva, a rare intraepithelial lesion located in the epidermis and skin adnexa, accounts for 1% to 5% of vulvar neoplasms. Histologically, vulvar Paget's disease is characterized by large, pale, mucopolysaccharide-rich cells that show a positive reaction to periodic acid–Schiff stain. The lesions are usually negative for HPV.[442] Electron microscopic studies have suggested that Paget's cells derive from apocrine cells in the stratum germinativum of the epidermis.[443] Paget's disease usually occurs in postmenopausal women, who often present with symptoms of vulvar pruritus and discomfort.[444] Grossly, Paget's lesions appear eczematoid or, when extensive, may be raised and velvety with persistent weeping. Five percent

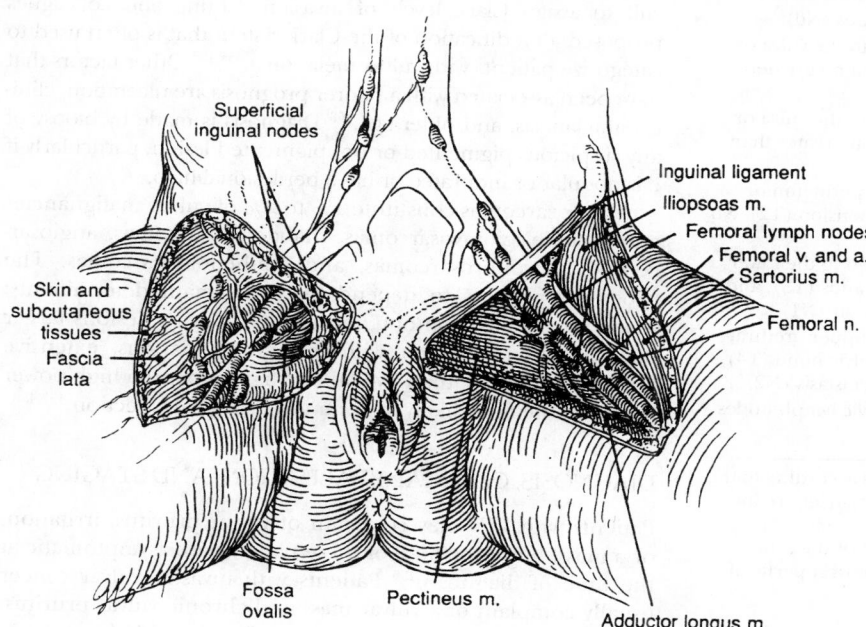

FIGURE 32.1-13. Inguinal-femoral lymph nodes. (From Hacker NF. Vulvar cancer. In: Hacker NF, Moore JG, eds. *Essentials of obstetrics and gynecology.* Philadelphia: WB Saunders, 1992:618, with permission.)

to 10% of newly diagnosed Paget's lesions are associated with underlying adenocarcinoma arising locally in a vulvar vestibular gland or skin appendage or from a distant site such as the breast or rectum.[444] It has been suggested that Paget's disease with underlying adenocarcinoma represents a different process than other types of intraepithelial Paget's disease because the other types rarely progress to invasive adenocarcinoma.[445]

The term *microinvasive carcinoma of the vulva* should be used with caution. The methods and criteria used to define microinvasive carcinoma of the cervix cannot be applied to carcinoma of the vulva. Stromal invasion by vulvar carcinomas is not measured in a uniform manner, and strict criteria for the diagnosis of microinvasive vulvar cancer have not been defined. VIN is not routinely seen adjacent to invasive vulvar cancer, and the transition from normal tissue to invasive cancer can be abrupt. Elongated rete pegs may extend 6 mm or more from the basement membrane and are sometimes misconstrued as invasive cancer. The International Society of Gynecological Pathologists recommends that the depth of stromal invasion be measured vertically from the most superficial basement membrane to the deepest tumor. Tumor thickness is defined as the distance between the granular layer of epidermis and the deepest extent of tumor. Lymph node metastases from tumors less than 1 mm in depth or thickness are extremely rare (Table 32.1-13).[433–436] For this reason, FIGO now includes a stage IA subcategory in its staging system for tumors that invade less than 1 mm (see Table 32.1-13).[419] However, the risk of inguinal lymph node metastasis rises steeply as the depth of invasion exceeds 1 mm.

More than 90% of invasive vulvar cancers are squamous cell carcinomas. Atypical keratinization is the hallmark of invasive vulvar cancer. Most squamous carcinomas are well differentiated, but mitoses may be noted. Approximately 5% of vulvar cancers are anaplastic carcinomas that may consist of large

TABLE 32.1-13. International Federation of Gynecology and Obstetrics Staging of Carcinoma of the Vulva (1994)

STAGE I	Lesions 2 cm or less in size confined to the vulva or perineum (T1).[a] No nodal metastases (N0).
Stage IA	Lesions 2 cm or less in size confined to the vulva or perineum and with stromal invasion no greater than 1 mm.[b] No nodal metastases.
Stage IB	Lesions 2 cm or less in size confined to the vulva or perineum and with stromal invasion greater than 1 mm.[b] No nodal metastases.
STAGE II	Tumor confined to the vulva and/or perineum or more than 2 cm in the greatest dimension (T2). No nodal metastasis (N0).
STAGE III	Tumor of any size with adjacent spread to the lower urethra and/or the vagina, or the anus (T3), and/or unilateral regional node metastasis (N1).
STAGE IVA	Tumor invades any of the following: upper urethra, bladder mucosa, rectal mucosa, pelvic bone (T4), and/or bilateral regional node metastasis (N2).
STAGE IVB	Any distant metastasis, including pelvic lymph nodes (M1).

[a]Equivalent tumor, node, metastasis (TNM) groupings according to the TNM Committee of the International Union Against Cancer are indicated in parentheses.[405]
[b]The depth of invasion is defined as the measurement of the tumor from the epithelial-stromal junction of the adjacent most superficial dermal papilla to the deepest point of invasion.
(Reprinted from ref. 79, with permission.)

immature cells, spindle sarcomatoid cells, or small cells. Vulvar carcinomas consisting of small cells may resemble small cell anaplastic carcinomas of the lung or Merkel-cell tumors and have demonstrated an aggressive biologic behavior in the few reported cases.[446] Verrucous carcinoma is a rare, very well-differentiated form of vulvar carcinoma that usually presents in the fifth or sixth decade of life as a large, locally invasive lesion.[447] On microscopic examination, the tumor has a papillary, exophytic appearance; tumor cells retain a normal appearance of maturation and demonstrate minimal atypia. Even with extensive local invasion, lymph node metastasis from verrucous carcinoma is very rare.

The diagnosis of Bartholin's gland carcinoma is based on clinical findings of a tumor arising in the anatomic location of Bartholin's glands and on the histologic appearance. Biopsy of a tumor arising from a Bartholin's gland usually reveals adenocarcinoma, but squamous cell carcinomas, transitional cell carcinomas (arising from the duct and histologically indistinguishable from transitional cell carcinoma of the bladder), and adenoid cystic carcinomas have also been reported.

Rare cases of primary mammary adenocarcinoma of the vulva have been reported, presumably arising in aberrant mammary tissue occurring along the embryonic milk line.[448] Other rare carcinomas that may occur in the vulva include basal cell carcinomas[449] and sebaceous carcinomas.[450]

Malignant melanomas of the vulva account for 2% to 4% of primary vulvar malignancies and 1% to 3% of melanomas arising in women.[451] Vulvar melanoma occurs most frequently in women older than 60 years of age, but 10% to 20% of vulvar melanomas occur in women younger than 40 years.[451] Approximately 50% of vulvar melanomas involve the labium majus, but tumors may also arise on the labium minus, clitoris, or perineum.[451,452] In a large Swedish series, 57% of vulvar melanomas were of the mucosal lentiginous type, 22% were nodular, and 16% were superficial spreading or lentiginous.[452] Most investigators have reported a correlation between depth of invasion or Breslow thickness and outcome.[453,454] However, because the vulvar epithelium sometimes lacks a well-developed papillary dermis, which makes it difficult to assign Clark levels of invasion, Chung and colleagues proposed a modification of the Clark system that is often used to categorize patients with vulvar melanoma.[455,456] Other factors that have been associated with a poorer prognosis are ulceration, clinical amelanosis, and older age.[453] Diagnosis is made by biopsy of any suspicious pigmented or nonpigmented lesion, particularly if it is nodular or indurated or has a perilesional halo.

Vulvar sarcomas constitute 1% to 2% of vulvar malignancies and include leiomyosarcomas, rhabdomyosarcomas, angiosarcomas, neurofibrosarcomas, and epithelioid sarcomas. The prognosis appears to depend on three main determinants: lesion size, tumor contour, and mitotic activity. Lesions larger than 5 cm in diameter with infiltrating margins, extensive necrosis, and more than five mitotic figures per ten high-power fields are the most likely to recur after surgical resection.[457,458]

DIAGNOSIS, CLINICAL EVALUATION, AND STAGING

Patients with VIN may complain of vulvar pruritus, irritation, or a mass, but up to 50% of these patients are asymptomatic at the time of diagnosis.[459] Patients with invasive vulvar cancer usually complain of a vulvar mass and chronic vulvar pruritus. Advanced lesions may bleed and are often exquisitely tender.

TABLE 32.1-14. Relative Survival by Tumor Diameter and Surgical Groin Node Status

Tumor Diameter (cm)	No. of Positive Groin Nodes									
	None		One		Two Unilateral		≥3 or Bilateral		Total	
	No.	Survival (%)	No.	Survival (%)	No.	Survival (%)	No.	Survival (%)	No.	Survival (%)
≤2	154	97.9	18	94.4	9	88.9	9	38.1	190	94.4
2.1–8.0	214	86.9	61	76.6	18	70.5	72	28.9	365	73.3
>8	13	65.8	3	66.7	3	50.0	3	0.0	22	55.7
Total	381	90.9	82	79.7	30	74.0	84	29.0	577[a]	90.9

[a]Three patients had an undetermined number of positive nodes and eight had unknown lesion diameter.
(Adapted from ref. 466.)

Because VIN can have many manifestations, biopsy of any new vulvar lesion should be performed. Once the diagnosis of VIN has been established, the entire vulva, cervix, and vagina should be carefully examined, because patients often have multifocal or multicentric involvement.[459,460] Colposcopic examination may help to define the extent of disease.

Diagnosis of invasive vulvar lesions requires a wedge biopsy of the lesion with surrounding skin and with underlying dermis and connective tissue so the pathologist can adequately evaluate the depth of stromal invasion. This procedure can usually be performed in the physician's office under local anesthesia. Excisional biopsy is preferred for lesions smaller than 1 cm in diameter.

Patients with invasive disease require additional evaluation for regional and metastatic spread. All patients with invasive disease require a careful physical examination including a detailed pelvic examination, chest radiograph, and biochemical profile. Cystoscopy and proctoscopy should be performed in patients with advanced lesions, and cystoscopy or proctoscopy should be performed in patients with tumors that are near the urethra or anus, respectively. Patients who complain of bone pain or who have tumor fixed to pelvic bones should have appropriate skeletal radiographs. CT or MRI scans can be obtained to evaluate deep inguinal and pelvic lymph nodes for possible regional metastasis. Preliminary studies of PET suggest that this study has a relatively poor sensitivity but high specificity for predicting lymph node metastases.[461]

In 1983, FIGO adopted a clinical TNM staging system for vulvar cancer. This system was based on a clinical assessment of the primary tumor and regional lymph nodes. However, the correlation between clinical assessment of the inguinal lymph nodes and pathologic findings is poor.[462–464] In a study of 588 patients with tumors that invaded 5 mm or deeper, Homesley and colleagues[463] reported that, although 93% of patients with fixed or ulcerated nodes had metastatic tumor, 24% of those with clinically negative nodes had inguinal lymph node metastases and 24% of patients with suspicious but mobile nodes had negative findings at lymphadenectomy. In 1988, the FIGO staging system was modified to incorporate the more accurate information gained from surgical assessment of regional lymph nodes. The staging system was revised again in 1994 to create a separate stage IA category for minimally invasive lesions (see Table 32.1-13).[419]

PROGNOSTIC FACTORS

The risk of regional metastases of vulvar carcinoma and the prognosis for cure after treatment are correlated with a number of clinical and pathologic features. Clinical tumor diameter is strongly predictive of outcome and has been incorporated in the FIGO staging system (see Table 32.1-13; Table 32.1-14). Other factors that have consistently been correlated with outcome include depth of invasion, tumor thickness, and the presence or absence of LVSI.[462,463,465–467] These features tend to be correlated with one another, and all are predictive of lymph node metastasis. More than 75% of patients with LVSI have positive inguinal nodes.[434,463,468] Studies of the relationship between tumor grade and outcome have drawn various conclusions, possibly reflecting the inconsistent criteria used to grade vulvar tumors.[434,463,468,469] Other factors that tend to be associated with prognosis include the amount of keratin, the mitotic rate, and the tumor growth pattern.[434,465,470,471] Aneuploid tumors appear to have a poorer prognosis than diploid tumors, but ploidy tends to be correlated with other prognostic factors and may not be an independent predictor of outcome.[472] Several authors have reported that tumors containing HPV DNA have a poorer prognosis than HPV-negative tumors.[422,426] Some investigators have reported a worse prognosis for patients aged 70 years or older, whereas others have found no correlation between prognosis and age.[463,470]

Prognosis is strongly correlated with the presence and number of inguinal node metastases (see Table 32.1-14). In a study of 586 patients treated in two GOG trials, Homesley and colleagues[466] reported 5-year survival rates of 91% for patients with negative inguinal lymph nodes and 75%, 36%, and 24%, respectively, for patients with one or two, three or four, and five or six positive nodes. None of the 16 patients with seven or more nodes involved with tumor survived. Patients with bilateral node involvement had a survival rate of 25%, compared with 71% for those with unilateral node involvement. The authors did not state whether patients with bilateral nodal disease had a poorer prognosis than did patients with a similar number of unilateral metastases. Homesley and colleagues[473] reported that patients with pelvic node metastases had a particularly poor survival rate—among patients treated with surgery alone, 3-year survival rates were 23% for patients with pelvic node metastases versus 73% for patients with only inguinal node involvement. For this reason, FIGO has categorized tumors that have spread to the pelvic nodes as stage IV. However, it should be remembered that most of the patients in these series did not receive postoperative irradiation, treatment that is now considered standard for patients who have regional metastases. It is not possible from available data to define the prognosis of patients who received multidisciplinary treatment for vulvar cancer metastatic to pelvic lymph nodes.

In 1995, van der Velden and colleagues[474] published a detailed study of nodal prognostic factors in 71 patients with inguinal node metastases from vulvar carcinomas. Patients with extranodal spread or more than two positive nodes received adjuvant radiotherapy to an unspecified dose. The most powerful predictor of outcome in their study was extranodal tumor extension: 28 of 44 patients (63%) with extranodal tumor died of disease versus three of 22 patients (14%) without this finding. In Cox regression analysis, none of the other factors studied (tumor size, number of nodes, FIGO stage, nodal size, degree of nodal replacement, or laterality) added to the predictive power of extranodal extension. Origoni and colleagues reported similar findings in a series of 53 patients with positive nodes.[475] Katz et al.[476] did not find that extracapsular extension correlated with regional recurrence. In their series, patients who had this finding received a median of 56 Gy of radiation and had a 14% rate of inguinal recurrence, versus a 9% rate for the other patients in the series with lymph node metastases.

Studying the relationship between surgical margins and tumor recurrence, Heaps and colleagues[465] reported no local failures in 91 patients whose closest tumor margin (deep or at the skin surface) was 8 mm or more in the fixed specimen. Ten of 23 patients (43%) with margins of 4.8 mm or less experienced a local recurrence, as did 8 of 13 patients (62%) with margins between 4.8 mm and 8 mm. Several studies suggest that this risk is diminished when postoperative radiotherapy is given.[477,478]

TREATMENT

The traditional operative approach to invasive carcinoma of the vulva, radical *en bloc* resection of the vulva and inguinofemoral nodes, was developed at the beginning of the twentieth century, was popularized during subsequent decades, and remained the standard of care until the early 1980s.[479] Radiotherapy was thought to have little role in the treatment of vulvar cancer. Although this surgical approach achieved 5-year survival rates of 60% to 70%, the surgery caused significant physical and psychological complications, and patients with multiple positive nodes continued to have a poor prognosis. In 1981, Hacker and colleagues[480] demonstrated that a less morbid surgical approach, operating through separate vulvar and groin incisions, achieved cure rates similar to those achieved with the traditional radical vulvectomy. Since then, there has been a continuing trend toward less radical surgery for early-stage disease. In addition, prospective and retrospective studies have established the role of radiotherapy in the curative management of locoregionally advanced disease.

Preinvasive Disease (Vulvar Intraepithelial Neoplasia)

After invasive carcinoma has been excluded by a sufficient number of excisional biopsies, the treatment of VIN should be as conservative as possible. Focal lesions can be simply excised. Multiple lesions can be excised separately or, if confluent, with a larger single excision. This approach is generally well tolerated and provides material for histologic assessment. When there is more extensive VIN, the lesions can be vaporized with a carbon dioxide laser. This method may provide an alternative to more extensive operations but does not yield a specimen for histologic inspection.

Extensive, diffuse VIN may require a wider excision, particularly if the lesion involves the perianal skin. These lesions are sometimes treated with a partial vulvectomy of the superficial skin ("skinning vulvectomy"). Whenever possible, the vulvar skin should be sutured primarily, but a split-thickness skin graft is sometimes needed to close the defect.

VIN often recurs at or near the margins of resection, even when the histopathologic analysis demonstrates that the initial lesions were completely resected. Presumably this phenomenon reflects the multifocal nature of the condition.[460] In fact, VIN can recur within the donor skin from split-thickness grafts.[406]

T1 and T2 Tumors

Invasive vulvar tumors can usually be treated effectively without the complications of *en bloc* radical vulvectomy and inguinal node dissection. Today, most gynecologic oncologists advocate an individualized approach to early invasive vulvar carcinomas.[435,481–483] Overall 5-year disease-specific survival rates for stage I (T1N0M0) and stage II (T2N0M0) disease are approximately 98% and 85%, respectively.[466]

Most T1 and selected T2 lesions can be controlled locally with a radical wide local excision. A wide and deep excision of the lesion is performed, with the incision extended down to the inferior fascia of the urogenital diaphragm. An effort should be made to remove the lesion with a 2-cm margin of normal tissue in all directions unless this would require sacrifice of the anus or urethra. The surgical defect is closed in two layers. Small T1 lesions that invade 1 mm or less can be managed with local resection alone because the risk of regional spread is very small (see Table 32.1-12). Patients with more invasive tumors must also have surgical or radiation treatment of the inguinal nodes as discussed in Treatment of Regional Disease, later in this chapter.

Larger T2 tumors may require radical vulvectomy to obtain acceptable tumor clearance with negative margins. *En bloc* resection of the vulva and inguinal nodes was once believed to be necessary to prevent recurrences in the soft tissue intervening between the vulva and regional nodes; however, most surgeons now perform the operation through separate vulvar and groin incisions. Although recurrences have been reported in this "tissue bridge," these appear to be rare, and the risk of complications is significantly decreased when separate incisions are used.[480,483,484]

Wound seroma is the most common acute complication of radical vulvectomy and inguinal node dissection, occurring in approximately 15% of cases.[435,482] Other acute complications include urinary tract infection, wound cellulitis, temporary anterior thigh anesthesia from femoral nerve injury, thrombophlebitis, and, rarely, pulmonary embolus.[435,473,482,484] The most common chronic complication is leg edema, but this risk has decreased from approximately 30% to 15% with the use of separate groin incisions.[483] Other chronic complications include genital prolapse, urinary stress incontinence, temporary weakness of the quadriceps muscle, and introital stenosis. Rare late complications include pubic osteomyelitis, femoral hernia, and rectoperineal fistula. These risks are less when separate incisions are used and are further reduced when radical local excision of the primary lesion is done instead of radical vulvectomy.[482,483,485]

TABLE 32.1-15. Concurrent Chemoradiotherapy in the Management of Locally Advanced or Recurrent Carcinoma of the Vulva

Reference	No. Patients	Chemotherapy[a]	Radiotherapy Dose (Gy)	No. with Recurrent or Persistent Local Disease after RT ± Surgery (%)	Follow-Up (Mo)
Akl et al.[493]	12	5-FU + Mito	30–36	1 (8)	8–125
Han et al.[492]	14	5-FU + Mito	40–62	6 (42)	4–273
Moore et al.[494]	73	5-FU + CDDP	47.6	15 (21)	22–72
Cunningham et al.[495]	14	5-FU + CDDP	45–50	4 (29)	7–81
Landoni et al.[496]	58	5-FU + Mito	54	13 (22)	4–48
Lupi et al.[497]	31	5-FU + Mito	54	7 (23)	22–73
Wahlen et al.[498]	19	5-FU + Mito	45–50	1 (5)	3–70
Eifel et al.[499]	12	5-FU + CDDP	40–50	5 (42)	17–30
Koh et al.[500]	20	5-FU ± CDDP or Mito	30–54	9 (45)	1–75
Russell et al.[501]	25	5-FU ± CDDP	47–72	6 (24)	4–52
Scheistroen et al.[502]	42	Bleomycin	45	39 (93)	7–60
Berek et al.[503]	12	5-FU + CDDP	44–54	0	7–60
Thomas et al.[504]	24	5-FU ± Mito	44–60	10 (42)	5–43
Iverson[505]	15	Bleomycin	15–40	11 (83)[b]	4

5-FU, 5-fluorouracil; Mito, mitomycin C; CDDP, cisplatin; RT, radiotherapy.
[a]Vulva only treated with radiation.
[b]Most patients had unresectable, stage IV lesions.

T3 and T4 Tumors

Primary tumors that involve the anus, rectum, rectovaginal septum, or proximal urethra pose a difficult problem because adequate surgical clearance can be obtained only by combining a pelvic exenteration with radical vulvectomy and bilateral groin node dissection. Although some patients may be cured with this ultraradical surgery, the risks of acute and long-term complications of the procedure are substantial.[486,487] For this reason, a number of investigators have explored the use of radiotherapy with or without surgery and chemotherapy to spare critical structures in patients with locally advanced disease.

In some cases, patients with T3 tumors that minimally involve the external urethra or anus can undergo initial vulvectomy without sacrifice of major organ function if close margins are accepted near critical structures. Postoperative radiotherapy can then be delivered to prevent local recurrence.[488] Although local recurrences are frequently successfully controlled with additional surgery, Faul and colleagues[477] reported an overall 5-year survival rate of only 40% after the first local recurrence and emphasized the importance of achieving local control. These authors reported a significant reduction in the local failure rate (from 58% to 16%) when patients whose tumors were within 8 mm of the operative margins were irradiated after surgery.[477] In such cases, the vulva may be treated with opposed anterior and posterior photon fields (if the inguinal regions also require treatment) or with an appositional perineal electron beam.[488] The vulva should receive a total dose of 50 to 65 Gy depending on the proximity of disease to the surgical margin.

In the early 1980s, several investigators[489–491] reported results of preoperative radiotherapy in small series of patients with locally advanced disease. These reports indicated that modest doses of radiation (45 to 55 Gy) produced dramatic tumor responses in some patients with T3 and T4 disease, permitting organ-sparing surgery without sacrifice of tumor control. Hacker and colleagues[491] reported that four of eight patients with T3 or T4 tumors treated preoperatively with 44 to 54 Gy had no residual tumor in the vulvectomy specimen and that seven of these eight had local control of their disease. More recently, investigators have emphasized the use of concurrent chemoradiation in this setting.

Chemoradiation in Locoregionally Advanced Disease

To reduce the need for morbid ultraradical surgery and to improve locoregional control rates, a number of investigators have explored combining chemotherapy with radiation and surgery in treatment of patients with locally advanced vulvar carcinoma.[492–505] Most studies have used combinations of cisplatin, 5-FU, and mitomycin C, extrapolating from the high response rates observed with use of this treatment for locally advanced carcinomas of the cervix and head and neck and from studies that have demonstrated the efficacy of these drugs as radiosensitizers in the treatment of carcinomas of the anus. Treatment schedules usually include a 4- to 5-day infusion of 5-FU combined with one of the other two drugs, with this course repeated every 3 to 4 weeks (Table 32.1-15). Studies have usually included small numbers of patients with very advanced local or regional disease. However, most investigators have observed impressive responses that often appear to be better than would be expected with radiation alone. Randomized trials have not been done and may be difficult to perform because of the small number of patients with locally advanced vulvar cancer. However, trials that demonstrated improved local control and survival when concurrent cisplatin-containing chemotherapy was added to radiation treatment of cervical cancers[180,182,183] and improved colostomy-free survival when mitomycin C and 5-FU were added to radiation treatment of anal cancer[506] suggest that this approach may be also be useful in the treatment of women with vulvar cancer.

Only one study has investigated the role of neoadjuvant chemotherapy in the treatment of locally advanced vulvar cancer. Benedetti-Panici and colleagues[507] treated 21 patients with stage IVA vulvar cancers with two to three cycles of cisplatin, bleomycin, and methotrexate followed by radical surgery. Two of 21 patients (10%) had partial responses of their vulvar tumors, and 14 (67%) had partial responses of regional nodes. Ninety percent of the tumors were considered operable, but the 3-year survival rate was only 24%.

Caution is warranted in designing aggressive treatment protocols for patients with vulvar cancers, who typically are elderly and often have concurrent medical problems. Serious pulmonary toxicity has been observed in a number of patients treated in studies that included bleomycin.[502,505] In the largest published series of patients treated with mitomycin C and 5-FU, hematologic tolerance was acceptable, but the administered dose of mitomycin C was somewhat lower than that generally used in the treatment of anal cancers.[504] Although chemotherapy may improve control rates, in this context its value has not been clearly defined; radiation alone can produce impressive responses and should be considered in patients who are poor surgical candidates and who cannot tolerate chemotherapy.[478]

Treatment of Regional Disease

Effective regional treatment is the single most important factor in the curative management of early vulvar cancer. Although patients with vulvar recurrences may have their disease successfully controlled with additional local treatment, patients who suffer inguinal recurrences are rarely curable.

All patients with primary tumors that invade more than 1 mm must have their inguinal nodes treated. Traditional management includes a bilateral radical inguinal lymph node dissection. Today, this is usually performed through separate groin incisions. An ellipse of skin is removed 1 cm below and parallel to the groin crease.[480] The incision is extended down to the fascia lata and 2 cm above the inguinal ligament to remove the inguinal nodes. The saphenous vein is tied off, the fascia lata is split, and the femoral nodes are dissected. A suction drain is placed, and the wound is closed in two layers.

At one time, pelvic node resection was also performed in most patients with invasive vulvar cancer. When subsequent studies demonstrated that pelvic node metastases were found only in patients with clinically suspicious or multiple positive inguinal nodes, use of the procedure was limited to patients determined intraoperatively to have positive inguinal nodes.

Then, in 1986, Homesley and colleagues[473] published results of a randomized, prospective study that compared pelvic node resection with inguinal and pelvic irradiation in patients with inguinal node metastases from carcinoma of the vulva. All patients were initially treated with radical vulvectomy and inguinal lymphadenectomy. Patient randomization was done intraoperatively after frozen-section evaluation of the inguinal nodes. This trial was closed prematurely, after 114 eligible patients had been entered, when interim analysis revealed a survival advantage for the radiotherapy arm ($P = .03$; Fig. 32.1-14). The difference was most marked for patients with clinically positive or multiple histologically positive groin nodes (Fig. 32.1-15). For patients with two or more positive nodes, the 2-year survival rates were 63% and 37% for the radiotherapy and pelvic node resection groups, respectively. Analysis of failure patterns revealed that the largest difference between treatment groups was in the number of inguinal failures (see Fig. 32.1-15). With the publication of this study, most practitioners abandoned routine pelvic node dissection, and postoperative radiotherapy became standard for most patients with inguinal node metastases.

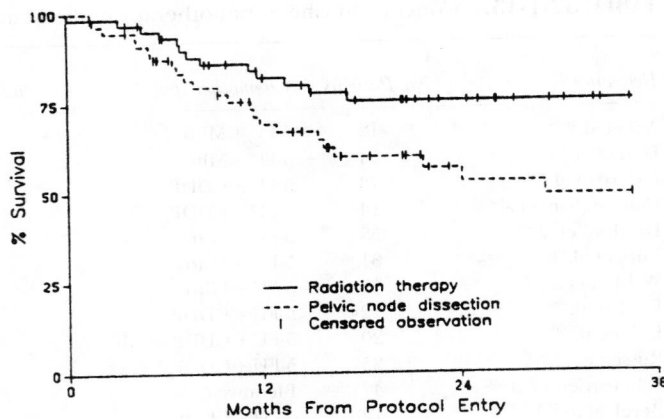

FIGURE 32.1-14. Survival rates of 114 patients with invasive squamous cell carcinoma of the vulva who were entered on a Gynecologic Oncology Group protocol in which patients with positive groin nodes after radical vulvectomy and bilateral inguinal lymphadenectomies were randomly assigned to receive pelvic lymph node dissection or postoperative irradiation to the pelvis and inguinal nodes ($P = .004$). (From ref. 473, with permission.)

Most of the serious acute and subacute complications of radical vulvectomy are related to the lymph node dissection, although these risks have decreased somewhat with the use of separate groin incisions.[508–510] Complications include wound disruption or infection in 50% to 75% of cases, chronic lymphedema in 20% to 50%, and a perioperative mortality rate of 2% to 5%. Patients who undergo vulvectomy without inguinal node dissection have significantly shorter hospital stays and fewer complications.[508,510]

Although radical inguinal lymphadenectomy has historically been considered the treatment of choice for regional management of invasive vulvar carcinoma, several retrospective studies have suggested that regional radiotherapy may be an effective and less morbid way of preventing recurrence in patients with

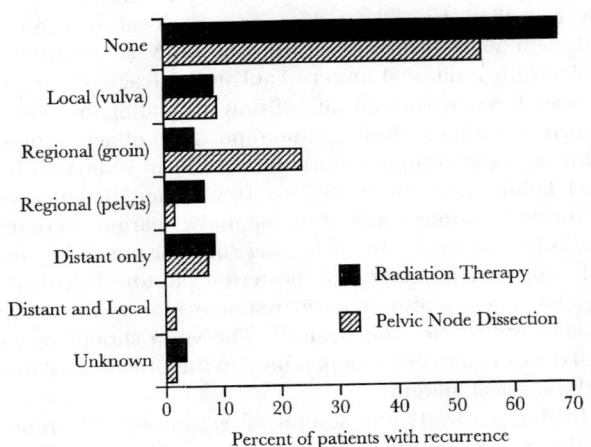

FIGURE 32.1-15. Sites of recurrence in 114 patients with invasive squamous cell carcinoma of the vulva who were entered on a Gynecologic Oncology Group protocol in which patients with positive groin nodes after radical vulvectomy and bilateral inguinal lymphadenectomies were randomly assigned to receive pelvic lymph node dissection or postoperative irradiation to the pelvis and inguinal nodes. (From ref. 473, with permission.)

clinically negative groins. In a review of 91 patients who had elective treatment of the inguinal nodes for cancers with primary drainage to the inguinal nodes, Henderson and colleagues[511] observed only two recurrences after treatment with 45 to 50 Gy over 5 weeks, and both of these occurred outside the treatment fields. In a retrospective review of 42 patients with invasive vulvar carcinomas, Petereit and colleagues[508] found no difference in the groin recurrence rate for patients with clinically negative inguinal nodes treated with radical lymphadenectomy or radiotherapy, even though the irradiated patients in their series had more advanced primary tumors. The complications of treatment, including lymphedema, wound separation, and infection, and the length of hospitalization were greater for patients who had had lymphadenectomy. More recent retrospective analyses have reported similar high regional disease control rates when radiotherapy is used to treat clinically negative groins in patients with high-risk vulvar cancers.[476,512]

In 1992, the GOG reported the results of a trial that randomly assigned patients with clinically negative inguinal nodes to receive inguinal node irradiation or radical lymphadenectomy (followed by inguinopelvic irradiation in patients with positive nodes) after resection of the primary tumor.[510] The study was closed after entry of only 58 patients, when an interim analysis demonstrated a significantly higher rate of inguinal recurrence and death in the irradiated group. The authors concluded that lymphadenectomy was the superior treatment, although the morbidity rate of lymphadenectomy was greater than that of groin irradiation. However, the radiotherapy techniques used in this study have since been criticized. CT scans were not consistently obtained to verify the position and size of inguinal nodes. Patients were treated with anterior appositional fields, the dose was prescribed at a depth of 3 cm, and the use of electrons (usually 12 MeV) was emphasized. This method of treatment can lead to significant underdosage of the inguinofemoral nodes, which frequently extend to a depth of more than 5 to 8 cm.[513,514] Because of these criticisms, the study's results and the role of radiation in the primary management of disease with clinically negative inguinal nodes remains controversial.

Some surgeons have tried to reduce surgical complications by reducing the extent of lymph node dissections. Burke and colleagues[485] reported four (5%) groin recurrences in 74 patients with T1 or T2 tumors treated with wide local excision and superficial inguinal lymphadenectomy (unilateral or bilateral depending on the location of the tumor). In a prospective study of patients with very favorable primary lesions (T1, 5 mm thick or less, no LVSI), the GOG[515] reported nine (7%) inguinal recurrences in 121 patients who had negative findings on ipsilateral superficial inguinal lymphadenectomy. However, an update of the M. D. Anderson experience had longer follow-up and demonstrated a higher recurrence risk of 16% at 5 years in patients treated with superficial lymph node dissection alone.[476] It has been suggested that the procedure used in these studies did not remove medial inguinofemoral nodes that may be the primary site of drainage of some vulvar cancers[438,516]; for this reason, many gynecologic oncologists now recommend removal of at least the superficial and medial inguinofemoral nodes. A number of investigators have explored the use of intraoperative lymphatic mapping to identify a sentinel node that would predict the presence or absence of regional metastases.[517–520] Preliminary studies suggest that a sentinel node can be identified in most patients. Further study is needed to determine whether this procedure can be used to more accurately identify patients who can be successfully treated without the morbidity of radical regional dissection.

Treatment of Metastatic Disease

A number of reports document the use of single-agent chemotherapy in patients with metastatic or recurrent squamous cell carcinomas of the vulva. Several anecdotal reports published in the 1970s suggest that bleomycin may be an active agent, but the response rate has not yet been documented in a prospective phase II trial, and the optimal dose and schedule have not been determined.[521,522] Single-agent phase II studies of cisplatin, etoposide, mitoxantrone, and piperazinedione have failed to document any objective responses.[414,523] Most data on the use of combination chemotherapy in this setting are anecdotal. In one of the largest series, Wagenaar et al.[524] observed 2 complete and 12 partial responses in 25 patients who were treated with a combination of bleomycin, lomustine, and methotrexate for locally advanced or metastatic disease; however, there were two deaths due to treatment toxicity, and the median time to progression was only 4.8 months. In the absence of reliable data specific to carcinoma of the vulva, clinicians often use combinations that have had some activity in the treatment of cervical cancer. However, there are, as yet, few data to indicate that chemotherapy can provide effective palliation for patients with metastatic or recurrent vulvar carcinoma that is not amenable to locoregional treatments.

REFERENCES

1. Jemal A, Murray T, Samuels A, et al. Cancer statistics, 2003. *CA Cancer J Clin* 2003;53:5.
2. Wingo PA, Tong T, Bolden S. Cancer statistics, 1995. *CA Cancer J Clin* 1995;45:8.
3. Bosch FX, de Sanjose S. Human papillomavirus and cervical cancer—burden and assessment of causality. *J Natl Cancer Inst Monogr* 2003:3.
4. Munoz N, Bosch FX, de Sanjose S, et al. Epidemiologic classification of human papillomavirus types associated with cervical cancer. *N Engl J Med* 2003;348:518.
5. Arends MJ, Buckley CH, Wells M. Aetiology, pathogenesis, and pathology of cervical neoplasia. *J Clin Pathol* 1998;51:96.
6. Sano T, Oyama T, Kashiwabara K, et al. Expression status of p16 protein is associated with human papillomavirus oncogenic potential in cervical and genital lesions. *Am J Pathol* 1998;153:1741.
7. Winkler B, Richart RM. Human papillomavirus and gynecologic neoplasia. *Curr Probl Obstet Gynecol Fertil* 1987;10:49.
8. Kessler I. Epidemiological aspects of uterine cervix cancer. In: Lurain JR, Sciarra J, eds. *Gynecology and obstetrics*. Philadelphia: JB Lippincott, 1990:1.
9. Scheffner M, Werness BA, Huibregtse JM, et al. The E6 oncoprotein encoded by human papillomavirus types 16 and 18 promotes the degradation of p 53. *Cell* 1990;63:1129.
10. Lechner MS, Laimins LA. Inhibition of p53 DNA binding by human papillomavirus E6 proteins. *J Virol* 1994;68:4262.
11. Harnish DG, Belland LM, Scheid EE, et al. Evaluation of human papillomavirus-consensus primers for HPV detection by the polymerase chain reaction. *Mol Cell Probes* 1999;13:9.
12. Joste NE, Rushing L, Granados R, et al. Bethesda classification of cervicovaginal smears: reproducibility and viral correlates. *Hum Pathol* 1996;27:581.
13. Burger RA, Monk BJ, Kurosaki T, et al. Human papillomavirus type 18: association with poor prognosis in early stage cervical cancer [see comments]. *J Natl Cancer Inst* 1996;88:1361.
14. Tseng CJ, Tseng LH, Lai CH, et al. Identification of human papillomavirus types 16 and 18 deoxyribonucleic acid sequences in bulky cervical cancer after chemotherapy. *Am J Obstet Gynecol* 1997;176:865.
15. Bosch FX, Manos MM, Munoz N, et al. Prevalence of human papillomavirus in cervical cancer: a worldwide perspective. International Biological Study on Cervical Cancer (IBSCC) Study Group [see comments]. *J Natl Cancer Inst* 1995;87:796.
16. Sherman ME, Schiffman MH, Strickler H, et al. Prospects for a prophylactic HPV vaccine: rationale and future implications for cervical cancer screening. *Diagn Cytopathol* 1998;18:5.
17. Koutsky LA, Ault KA, Wheeler CM, et al. A controlled trial of a human papillomavirus type 16 vaccine. *N Engl J Med* 2002;347:1645.
18. Ho GY, Bierman R, Beardsley L, et al. Natural history of cervicovaginal papillomavirus infection in young women. *N Engl J Med* 1998;338:423.
19. Schiffman M, Kjaer SK. Natural history of anogenital human papillomavirus infection and neoplasia. *J Natl Cancer Inst Monogr* 2003:14.

20. Castellsague X, Munoz N. Cofactors in human papillomavirus carcinogenesis—role of parity, oral contraceptives, and tobacco smoking. *J Natl Cancer Inst Monogr* 2003:20.

21. Meanwell CA. The epidemiology and etiology of cervical cancer. In: Blackledge GRP, Jordan JA, Shingleton HM, eds. *Textbook of gynecologic oncology*. Philadelphia: WB Saunders, 1991:250.

22. Schiffman MH. Recent progress in defining the epidemiology of human papillomavirus infection and cervical neoplasia. *J Natl Cancer Inst* 1992;84:394.

23. Giulian AR, Sedjo RL, Roe DJ, et al. Clearance of oncogenic human papillomavirus (HPV) infection: effect of smoking (United States). *Cancer Causes Control* 2002;13:839.

24. Claeys P, Gonzalez C, Gonzalez M, et al. Prevalence and risk factors of sexually transmitted infections and cervical neoplasia in women's health clinics in Nicaragua. *Sex Transm Infect* 2002;78:204.

25. Castellsague X, Bosch FX, Munoz N, et al. Male circumcision, penile human papillomavirus infection, and cervical cancer in female partners. *N Engl J Med* 2002;346:1105.

26. Ferlay J, Bray F, Pisani P, et al. *GLOBOCON 2000: cancer incidence, mortality and prevalence worldwide*, 1.0 ed. Lyon: IARC, 2001:5.

27. Ghafoor A, Jemal A, Cokkinides V, et al. Cancer statistics for African Americans. *CA Cancer J Clin* 2002;52:326.

28. Herrero R. Epidemiology of cervical cancer. *J Natl Cancer Inst Monogr* 1996;21:1.

29. O'Brien K, Cokkinides V, Jemal A, et al. Cancer statistics for Hispanics, 2003. *CA Cancer J Clin* 2003;53:208.

30. Randolph WM, Freeman DH Jr, Freeman JL. Pap smear use in a population of older Mexican-American women. *Women Health* 2002;36:21.

31. Coughlin SS, Uhler RJ, Richards T, et al. Breast and cervical cancer screening practices among Hispanic and non-Hispanic women residing near the United States-Mexico border, 1999–2000. *Fam Community Health* 2003;26:130.

32. Austin LT, Ahmad F, McNally MJ, et al. Breast and cervical cancer screening in Hispanic women: a literature review using the health belief model. *Womens Health Issues* 2002;12:122.

33. Smith HO, Tiffany MF, Qualls CR, et al. The rising incidence of adenocarcinoma relative to squamous cell carcinoma of the uterine cervix in the United States—a 24-year population-based study. *Gynecol Oncol* 2000;78:97.

34. Vizcaino AP, Moreno V, Bosch FX, et al. International trends in the incidence of cervical cancer. I. Adenocarcinoma and adenosquamous cell carcinomas. *Int J Cancer* 1998;75:536.

35. Thomas DB, Ray RM. Oral contraceptives and invasive adenocarcinomas and adenosquamous carcinomas of the uterine cervix. The World Health Organization Collaborative Study of Neoplasia and Steroid Contraceptives. *Am J Epidemiol* 1996;144:281.

36. Ursin G, Peters RK, Henderson BE, et al. Oral contraceptive use and adenocarcinoma of cervix. *Lancet* 1994;344:1390.

37. Stubblefield PG. Oral contraceptives and neoplasia. *J Reprod Med* 1984;29:524.

38. Buehler JW, Ward JW. A new definition for AIDS surveillance. *Ann Intern Med* 1993;118:390.

39. Palefsky JM, Holly EA. Immunosuppression and co-infection with HIV. *J Natl Cancer Inst Monogr* 2003:41.

40. Moscicki AB, Ellenberg JH, Vermund SH, et al. Prevalence of and risks for cervical human papillomavirus infection and squamous intraepithelial lesions in adolescent girls: impact of infection with human immunodeficiency virus. *Arch Pediatr Adolesc Med* 2000;154:127.

41. Fairley CK, Chen S, Tabrizi SN, et al. Prevalence of HPV DNA in cervical specimens in women with renal transplants: a comparison with dialysis-dependent patients and patients with renal impairment. *Nephrol Dial Transplant* 1994;9:416.

42. Heard I, Schmitz V, Costagliola D, et al. Early regression of cervical lesions in HIV-seropositive women receiving highly active antiretroviral therapy. *AIDS* 1998;12:1459.

43. Six C, Heard I, Bergeron C, et al. Comparative prevalence, incidence and short-term prognosis of cervical squamous intraepithelial lesions amongst HIV-positive and HIV-negative women. *AIDS* 1998;12:1047.

44. Lillo FB, Ferrari D, Veglia F, et al. Human papillomavirus infection and associated cervical disease in human immunodeficiency virus-infected women: effect of highly active antiretroviral therapy. *J Infect Dis* 2001;184:547.

45. Serraino D, Dal Maso L, La Vecchia C, et al. Invasive cervical cancer as an AIDS-defining illness in Europe. *AIDS* 2002;16:781.

46. Franceschi S, Dal Maso L, Arniani S, et al. Risk of cancer other than Kaposi's sarcoma and non-Hodgkin's lymphoma in persons with AIDS in Italy. Cancer and AIDS Registry Linkage Study. *Br J Cancer* 1998;78:966.

47. Serur E, Fruchter RG, Maiman M, et al. Age, substance abuse, and survival of patients with cervical carcinoma. *Cancer* 1995;75:2530.

48. Beral V, Newton R. Overview of the epidemiology of immunodeficiency-associated cancers. *J Natl Cancer Inst Monogr* 1998;23:1.

49. Goedert JJ, Cote TR, Virgo P, et al. Spectrum of AIDS-associated malignant disorders. *Lancet* 1998;351:1833.

50. Kivlahan C, Ingram E. Papanicolaou smears without endocervical cells. Are they inadequate? *Acta Cytol* 1986;30:258.

51. Miller AB. Control of carcinoma of the cervix by exfoliative cytology screening. In: Coppleson M, ed. *Gynecologic oncology fundamental principles and clinical practice*. Edinburgh: Churchill Livingstone, 1981:381.

52. Syrjanen KV, Kataja V, Vyliskoski M, et al. Natural history of cervical human papillomavirus lesions does not substantiate the biologic relevance of the Bethesda system. *Obstet Gynecol* 1992;79:675.

53. Richart RM, Barron BA. A follow-up study of patients with cervical dysplasia. *Am J Obstet Gynecol* 1969;105:386.

54. Plentl AA, Friedman EA. Lymphatics of the cervix uteri. *Lymphatic system of the female genitalia*. Philadelphia: WB Saunders, 1971:75.

55. Girardi F, Haas J. The importance of the histologic processing of pelvic lymph nodes in the treatment of cervical cancer. *Int J Gynecol Cancer* 1993;3:12.

56. Kjorstad KE, Kjolvenstvedt A, Strickert T. The value of complete lymphadenectomy in radical treatment of cancer of the cervix, stage IB. *Cancer* 1984;54:2215.

57. Kim RY, Weppelmann B, Salter MM, et al. Skeletal metastases from cancer of the uterine cervix: frequency, patterns, and radiotherapeutic significance. *Int J Radiat Oncol Biol Phys* 1987;13:705.

58. Richart RM. Cervical intraepithelial neoplasia. *Pathology annual*. East Norwalk, CT: Appleton-Century-Crofts, 1973:301.

59. Crum CP. Should the Bethesda System terminology be used in diagnostic surgical pathology? Point. *Int J Gynecol Pathol* 2003;22:5.

60. Schneider V. Should the Bethesda System terminology be used in diagnostic surgical pathology? Counterpoint. *Int J Gynecol Pathol* 2003;22:13.

61. Syrjanen KJ. Spontaneous evolution of intraepithelial lesions according to the grade and type of the implicated human papillomavirus (HPV). *Eur J Obstet Gynecol Reprod Biol* 1996;65:45.

62. Manos MM, Kinney WK, Hurley LB, et al. Identifying women with cervical neoplasia: using human papillomavirus DNA testing for equivocal Papanicolaou results [see comments]. *JAMA* 1999;281:1605.

63. Alli PM, Ali SZ. Atypical squamous cells of undetermined significance—rule out high-grade squamous intraepithelial lesion: cytopathologic characteristics and clinical correlates. *Diagn Cytopathol* 2003;28:308.

64. Schiffman M, Solomon D. Findings to date from the ASCUS-LSIL Triage Study (ALTS). *Arch Pathol Lab Med* 2003;127:946.

65. Azodi M, Chambers SK, Rutherford TJ, et al. Adenocarcinoma in situ of the cervix: management and outcome. *Gynecol Oncol* 1999;73:348.

66. Wolf JK, Levenback C, Malpica A, et al. Adenocarcinoma in situ of the cervix: significance of cone biopsy margins. *Obstet Gynecol* 1996;88:82.

67. Zaino RJ. Adenocarcinoma in situ, glandular dysplasia, and early invasive adenocarcinoma of the uterine cervix. *Int J Gynecol Pathol* 2002;21:314.

68. Kostopoulou E, Keating JT, Crum CP. Pathology. In: Eifel PJ, Levenback C, eds. *Cancer of the female lower genital tract*. London: BC Decker, Inc., 2001:9.

69. Reich O, Pickel H, Tamussino K, et al. Microinvasive carcinoma of the cervix: site of first focus of invasion. *Obstet Gynecol* 2001;97:890.

70. Creasman WT, Zaino RJ, Major FJ, et al. Early invasive carcinoma of the cervix (3 to 5 mm invasion): risk factors and prognosis. A Gynecologic Oncology Group study. *Am J Obstet Gynecol* 1998;178:62.

71. Fu YS, Reagan J. *Pathology of the uterine cervix, vagina, and vulva*. Philadelphia: WB Saunders, 1989.

72. Maiman MA, Fruchter RG, DiMaio TM, et al. Superficially invasive squamous cell carcinoma of the cervix. *Obstet Gynecol* 1988;72:399.

73. Burghardt E, Girardi F, Lahousen M, et al. Microinvasive carcinoma of the uterine cervix (International Federation of Gynecology and Obstetrics Stage IA). *Cancer* 1991;67:1037.

74. Ostor AG. Early invasive adenocarcinoma of the uterine cervix. *Int J Gynecol Pathol* 2000;19:29.

75. Robert ME, Fu YS. Squamous cell carcinoma of the uterine cervix: a review with emphasis on prognostic factors and unusual variants. *Semin Diagn Pathol* 1990;7:173.

76. Jennings RH, Barclay DL. Verrucous carcinoma of the cervix. *Cancer* 1972;30:430.

77. Brown J, Broaddus R, Koeller M, et al. Sarcomatoid carcinoma of the cervix. *Gynecol Oncol* 2003;90:23.

78. Young RH, Clement PB. Endocervical adenocarcinoma and its variants: their morphology and differential diagnosis. *Histopathology* 2002;41:185.

79. Gilks CB, Young R, Aguirre P, et al. Adenoma malignum (minimal deviation adenocarcinoma) of the uterine cervix. A clinicopathological and immunohistological analysis of 26 cases. *Am J Surg Pathol* 1989;13:717.

80. Kaku T, Enjoji M. Extremely well-differentiated adenocarcinoma ("adenoma malignum"). *Int J Gynecol Pathol* 1983;2:28.

81. Hirai Y, Takeshima N, Haga A, et al. A clinicocytopathologic study of adenoma malignum of the uterine cervix. *Gynecol Oncol* 1998;70:219.

82. Young RH, Scully RE. Villoglandular papillary adenocarcinoma of the uterine cervix. A clinicopathologic analysis of 13 cases. *Cancer* 1989;63:1773.

83. Glucksmann A, Cherry CP. Incidence, histology, and response to radiation of mixed carcinomas (adenoacanthomas) of the uterine cervix. *Am J Surg Pathol* 1956;12:134.

84. Ferry JA, Scully RE. "Adenoid cystic" carcinoma and adenoid basal cell carcinoma of the uterine cervix: a study of 28 cases. *Am J Surg Pathol* 1988;12:134.

85. Zhou C, Gilks CB, Hayes M, et al. Papillary serous carcinoma of the uterine cervix: a clinicopathologic study of 17 cases. *Am J Surg Pathol* 1998;22:113.

86. Albores-Saavedra J, Gersell D, Gilks CB, et al. Terminology of endocrine tumors of the uterine cervix: results of a workshop sponsored by the College of American Pathologists and the National Cancer Institute. *Arch Pathol Lab Med* 1997;121:34.

87. Abeler VM, Holm R, Nesland JM, et al. Small cell carcinoma of the cervix. A clinicopathologic study of 26 patients. *Cancer* 1994;73:672.

88. Sevin BU, Method MW, Nadji M, et al. Efficacy of radical hysterectomy as treatment for patients with small cell carcinoma of the cervix. *Cancer* 1996;77:1489.

89. Hoskins PJ, Swenerton KD, Pike JA, et al. Small-cell carcinoma of the cervix: fourteen years of experience at a single institution using a combined-modality regimen of involved-field irradiation and platinum-based combination chemotherapy. *J Clin Oncol* 2003;21:3495.

90. Chang TC, Lai CH, Tseng CJ, et al. Prognostic factors in surgically treated small cell cervical carcinoma followed by adjuvant chemotherapy. *Cancer* 1998;83:712.

91. Viswanathan AN, Jhingran A, Deavers MT, et al. Patterns of failure in small cell carcinoma of the cervix. *Int J Radiat Oncol Biol Phys* 2002;54[Suppl 41]:51.

92. Ross JC, Eifel PJ, Cox RS, et al. Primary mucinous adenocarcinoma of the endometrium. A clinicopathologic and histochemical study. *Am J Surg Pathol* 1983;7:715.

93. Landis SH, Murray T, Bolden S, et al. Cancer statistics, 1999. *CA Cancer J Clin* 1999;49:8.

94. American College of Obstetrics and Gynecology. *Technical Bulletin*. Washington, DC: American College of Obstetrics and Gynecology, 1987.

95. Saslow D, Runowicz CD, Solomon D, et al. American Cancer Society guideline for the early detection of cervical neoplasia and cancer. *CA Cancer J Clin* 2002;52:342.
96. Sherman ME, Schiffman M, Herrero R, et al. Performance of a semiautomated Papanicolaou smear screening system: results of a population-based study conducted in Guanacaste, Costa Rica. *Cancer* 1998;84:273.
97. Walton RJ. The task force on cervical cancer screening programs [Letter]. *Can Med Assoc J* 1976;114:981.
98. Reid R, Herschman BR, Crum CP, et al. Genital warts and cervical cancer. V. The tissue basis of colposcopic change. *Am J Obstet Gynecol* 1984;149:293.
99. Benedet JL, Anderson GH, Boyes DA. Colposcopic accuracy in the diagnosis of microinvasive and occult invasive carcinoma of the cervix. *Obstet Gynecol* 1985;65:557.
100. Kolstad P. Follow-up study of 232 patients with stage Ia1 and 411 patients with stage Ia2 squamous cell carcinoma of the cervix (microinvasive carcinoma). *Gynecol Oncol* 1989;33:265.
101. Heller PB, Malfetano JH, Bundy BN, et al. Clinical-pathologic study of stage IIB, III, and IVA carcinoma of the cervix: extended diagnostic evaluation for paraaortic node metastasis—a Gynecologic Oncology Group study. *Gynecol Oncol* 1990;38:425.
102. Bipat S, Glas AS, van der Velden J, et al. Computed tomography and magnetic resonance imaging in staging of uterine cervical carcinoma: a systematic review. *Gynecol Oncol* 2003;91:59.
103. Grigsby PW, Siegel BA, Dehdashti F. Lymph node staging by positron emission tomography in patients with carcinoma of the cervix. *J Clin Oncol* 2001;19:3745.
104. Benedet J, Odicino F, Maisonneuve P, et al. Carcinoma of the cervix uteri. *J Epidemiol Biostat* 1998;3:5.
105. Eifel PJ. Problems with the clinical staging of carcinoma of the cervix. *Semin Radiat Oncol* 1994;4:1.
106. Seski JC, Murray RA, Morley G. Microinvasive squamous carcinoma of the cervix. Definition, histologic analysis, late results of treatment. *Obstet Gynecol* 1977;50:410.
107. American Joint Committee on Cancer. Cervix uteri. In: Greene FL, Page DL, Fleming ID, et al., eds. *Manual for staging of cancer*, 6th ed. New York, NY: Springer-Verlag, 2002:259.
108. Weiser EB, Bundy BN, Hoskins WJ, et al. Extraperitoneal versus transperitoneal selective paraaortic lymphadenectomy in the pretreatment surgical staging of advanced cervical carcinoma (a Gynecologic Oncology Group study). *Gynecol Oncol* 1989;33:283.
109. Chi DS, Curtin JP. Gynecologic cancer and laparoscopy. *Obstet Gynecol Clin North Am* 1999;26:201.
110. Possover M, Krause N, Plaul K, et al. Laparoscopic para-aortic and pelvic lymphadenectomy: experience with 150 patients and review of the literature. *Gynecol Oncol* 1998;71:19.
111. Cosin JA, Fowler JM, Chen MD, et al. Pretreatment surgical staging of patients with cervical carcinoma: the case for lymph node debulking. *Cancer* 1998;82:2241.
112. Hacker NF, Wain GV, Nicklin JL. Resection of bulky positive lymph nodes in patients with cervical carcinoma. *Int J Gynecol Cancer* 1995;5:250.
113. Eifel PJ, Morris M, Wharton JT, et al. The influence of tumor size and morphology on the outcome of patients with FIGO stage IB squamous cell carcinoma of the uterine cervix. *Int J Radiat Oncol Biol Phys* 1994;29:9.
114. Perez CA, Grigsby PW, Nene SM, et al. Effect of tumor size on the prognosis of carcinoma of the uterine cervix treated with irradiation alone. *Cancer* 1992;69:2796.
115. Alvarez RD, Potter ME, Soong SJ, et al. Rationale for using pathologic tumor dimensions and nodal status to subclassify surgically treated stage IB cervical cancer patients. *Gynecol Oncol* 1991;43:108.
116. Delgado G, Bundy BN, Fowler WC, et al. A prospective surgical pathological study of stage I squamous carcinoma of the cervix: a Gynecologic Oncology Group study. *Gynecol Oncol* 1989; 36:314.
117. Kristensen GB, Abeler VM, Risberg B, et al. Tumor size, depth of invasion, and grading of the invasive tumor front are the main prognostic factors in early squamous cell cervical carcinoma. *Gynecol Oncol* 1999;74:245.
118. Sevin BU, Lu Y, Bloch DA, et al. Surgically defined prognostic parameters in patients with early cervical carcinoma. A multivariate survival tree analysis. *Cancer* 1996;78:1438.
119. Barillot I, Horiot JC, Pigneux J, et al. Carcinoma of the intact uterine cervix treated with radiotherapy alone: a French cooperative study: update and multivariate analysis of prognostics factors. *Int J Radiat Oncol Biol Phys* 1997;38:969.
120. Logsdon MD, Eifel PJ. FIGO stage IIIB squamous cell carcinoma of the uterine cervix: an analysis of prognostic factors emphasizing the balance between external beam and intracavitary radiation therapy. *Int J Radiat Oncol Biol Phys* 1999;43:763.
121. Burghardt E, Pickel H, Haas J, et al. Prognostic factors and operative treatment of stages IB to IIB cervical cancer. *Am J Obstet Gynecol* 1987;156:988.
122. Inoue T, Okumura M. Prognostic significance of parametrial extension in patients with cervical carcinoma stages IB, IIA, and IIB. A study of 628 cases treated by radical hysterectomy and lymphadenectomy with or without postoperative irradiation. *Cancer* 1984;54:1714.
123. Stehman FB, Bundy BN, Disaia PJ, et al. Carcinoma of the cervix treated with radiation therapy. I. A multivariate analysis of prognostic variables in the Gynecologic Oncology Group. *Cancer* 1991;67:2776.
124. Averette HE, Nguyen HN, Donato DM, et al. Radical hysterectomy for invasive cervical cancer. A 25-year prospective experience with the Miami technique. *Cancer* 1993;71:1422.
125. Delgado G, Bundy B, Zaino R, et al. Prospective surgical-pathological study of disease-free interval in patients with stage IB squamous cell carcinoma of the cervix: a Gynecologic Oncology Group study. *Gynecol Oncol* 1990;38:352.
126. Manusirivithaya S, Isariyodom P, Charoeniam V, et al. Risk for radical hysterectomy failure. *J Med Assoc Thai* 2001;84:791.
127. Inoue T, Chihara T, Morita K. The prognostic significance of the size of the largest nodes in metastatic carcinoma from the uterine cervix. *Gynecol Oncol* 1984;19:187.
128. Inoue T, Morita K. The prognostic significance of number of positive nodes in cervical carcinoma stages IB, IIA, and IIB. *Cancer* 1990;65:1923.
129. Kamura T, Tsukamoto N, Tsuruchi N, et al. Multivariate analysis of the histopathologic prognostic factors of cervical cancer in patients undergoing radical hysterectomy. *Cancer* 1992;69:181.
130. Chung CK, Nahhas WA, Stryker JA, et al. Analysis of factors contributing to treatment failures in stages IB and IIA carcinoma of the cervix. *Am J Obstet Gynecol* 1980;138:550.
131. Fuller AF, Elliott N, Kosloff C, et al. Lymph node metastases from carcinoma of the cervix, stages IB and IIA: implications for prognosis and treatment. *Gynecol Oncol* 1982;13:165.
132. Nahhas WA, Sharkey FE, Whitney CW, et al. The prognostic significance of vascular channel involvement and deep stromal penetration in early cervical carcinoma. *Am J Clin Oncol* 1983;6:239.
133. Boyce JG, Fruchter RG, Nicastri AD, et al. Vascular invasion in stage I carcinoma of the cervix. *Cancer* 1984;53:1175.
134. Burke TW, Hoskins WJ, Heller PB, et al. Prognostic factors associated with radical hysterectomy failure. *Gynecol Oncol* 1987;26:153.
135. Fuller AF, Elliott N, Kosloff C, et al. Determinants of increased risk for recurrence in patients undergoing radical hysterectomy for stage IB and IIA carcinoma of the cervix. *Gynecol Oncol* 1989;33:34.
136. Boyce J, Fruchter R, Nicastri A, et al. Prognostic factors in stage I carcinoma of the cervix. *Gynecol Oncol* 1981;12:154.
137. Zreik TG, Chambers JT, Chambers SK. Parametrial involvement, regardless of nodal status: a poor prognostic factor for cervical cancer. *Obstet Gynecol* 1996;87:741.
138. Roman T, Souhami L, Freeman C, et al. High dose rate afterloading intracavitary therapy in carcinoma of the cervix. *Int J Radiat Oncol Biol Phys* 1991;20:921.
139. Kainz C, Gitsch G, Tempfer C, et al. Vascular space invasion and inflammatory stromal reaction as prognostic factors in patients with surgically treated cervical cancer stage IB to IIB. *Anticancer Res* 1994;14:2145.
140. Noguchi H, Shiozawa I, Kitahara T, et al. Uterine body invasion of carcinoma of the uterine cervix as seen from surgical specimens. *Gynecol Oncol* 1988;30:173.
141. Perez CA, Camel HM, Askin F, et al. Endometrial extension of carcinoma of the uterine cervix: a prognostic factor that may modify staging. *Cancer* 1981;48:170.
142. Grigsby PW, Perez CA, Kuske RR, et al. Adenocarcinoma of the uterine cervix: lack of evidence for a poor prognosis. *Radiother Oncol* 1988;12:289.
143. Kilgore LC, Soong SJ, Gore H, et al. Analysis of prognostic features in adenocarcinoma of the cervix. *Gynecol Oncol* 1988;31:137.
144. Waldenström A-C, Hrovath G. Survival of patients with adenocarcinoma of the uterine cervix in western Sweden. *Int J Gynecol Cancer* 1999;9:18.
145. Chen RJ, Lin YH, Chen CA, et al. Influence of histologic type and age on survival rates for invasive cervical carcinoma in Taiwan. *Gynecol Oncol* 1999;73:184.
146. Eifel PJ, Burke TW, Morris M, et al. Adenocarcinoma as an independent risk factor for disease recurrence in patients with stage IB cervical carcinoma. *Gynecol Oncol* 1995;59:38.
147. Lai C-H, Hsueh S, Hong J-H, et al. Are adenocarcinomas and adenosquamous carcinomas different from squamous carcinomas in stage IB and II cervical cancer patients undergoing primary radical surgery? *Int J Gynecol Cancer* 1999;9:28.
148. Irie T, Kigawa J, Minagawa Y, et al. Prognosis and clinicopathological characteristics of Ib-IIb adenocarcinoma of the uterine cervix in patients who have had radical hysterectomy. *Eur J Surg Oncol* 2000;26:464.
149. Nakanishi T, Ishikawa H, Suzuki Y, et al. A comparison of prognoses of pathologic stage Ib adenocarcinoma and squamous cell carcinoma of the uterine cervix. *Gynecol Oncol* 2000;79:289.
150. Eifel PJ, Burke TW, Delclos L, et al. Early stage I adenocarcinoma of the uterine cervix: treatment results in patients with tumors 4 ≤ cm in diameter. *Gynecol Oncol* 1991;41:199.
151. Berek JS, Hacker NS, Fu YS, et al. Adenocarcinoma of the uterine cervix: histologic variables associated with lymph node metastasis and survival. *Obstet Gynecol* 1985;65:46.
152. Raju K, Kjorstad KE, Abeler V. Prognostic factors in the treatment of stage IB adenocarcinoma of the cervix. *Int J Gynaecol Obstet* 1991;1:69.
153. Bush R. The significance of anemia in clinical radiation therapy. *Int J Radiat Oncol Biol Phys* 1986;12:2047.
154. Girinski T, Pejovic-Lenfant M, Bourhis J, et al. Prognostic value of hemoglobin concentrations and blood transfusions in advanced carcinoma of the cervix treated by radiation therapy: results of a retrospective study of 386 patients. *Int J Radiat Oncol Biol Phys* 1989;16:37.
155. Grogan M, Thomas GM, Melamed I, et al. The importance of hemoglobin levels during radiotherapy for carcinoma of the cervix. *Cancer* 1999;86:1528.
156. Kapp KS, Poschauko J, Geyer E, et al. Evaluation of the effect of routine packed red blood cell transfusion in anemic cervix cancer patients treated with radical radiotherapy. *Int J Radiat Oncol Biol Phys* 2002;54:58.
157. Grigsby PW, Winter K, Wasserman TH, et al. Irradiation with or without misonidazole for patients with stages IIIB and IVA carcinoma of the cervix: final results of RTOG 80-05. Radiation Therapy Oncology Group. *Int J Radiat Oncol Biol Phys* 1999;44:513.
158. Overgaard J, Bentzen SM, Kolstad P, et al. Misonidazole combined with radiotherapy in the treatment of carcinoma of the uterine cervix. *Int J Radiat Oncol Biol Phys* 1989;16:1069.
159. Sundfor K, Trope C, Suo Z, et al. Normobaric oxygen treatment during radiotherapy for carcinoma of the uterine cervix. Results from a prospective controlled randomized trial. *Radiother Oncol* 1999;50:157.
160. Maor MH, Gillespie BW, Peters LJ, et al. Neutron therapy in cervical cancer: results of a phase III RTOG study. *Int J Radiat Oncol Biol Phys* 1988;14:885.
161. Fyles A, Milosevic M, Hedley D, et al. Tumor hypoxia has independent predictor impact only in patients with node-negative cervix cancer. *J Clin Oncol* 2002;20:680.
162. Sundfor K, Lyng H, Rofstad EK. Tumour hypoxia and vascular density as predictors of metastasis in squamous cell carcinoma of the uterine cervix. *Br J Cancer* 1998;78:822.
163. Duk JM, Groenier KH, de Bruijn HWA, et al. Pretreatment serum squamous cell carcinoma antigen: a newly identified prognostic factor in early-stage cervical carcinoma. *J Clin Oncol* 1996;14:111.
164. Maiman M. The clinical application of serum squamous cell carcinoma antigen level monitoring in invasive cervical carcinoma. *Gynecol Oncol* 2002;84:4.

165. Lanciano RM, Won M, Coia L, et al. Pretreatment and treatment factors associated with improved outcome in squamous cell carcinoma of the uterine cervix: a final report of the 1973 and 1978 Patterns of Care Studies. *Int J Radiat Oncol Biol Phys* 1991;20:667.
166. Rutledge FN, Mitchell MR, Munsell M, et al. Youth as a prognostic factor in carcinoma of the cervix: a matched analysis. *Gynecol Oncol* 1992;44:123.
167. Estape R, Angioli R, Wagman F, et al. Significance of intraperitoneal cytology in patients undergoing radical hysterectomy. *Gynecol Oncol* 1998;68:169.
168. Kashimura M, Sugihara K, Toki N, et al. The significance of peritoneal cytology in uterine cervix and endometrial cancer. *Gynecol Oncol* 1997;67:285.
169. Hernandez E, Heller PB, Whitney C, et al. Thrombocytosis in surgically treated stage IB squamous cell cervical carcinoma (a Gynecologic Oncology Group study). *Gynecol Oncol* 1994;55:328.
170. Lopes A, Daras V, Cross PA, et al. Thrombocytosis as a prognostic factor in women with cervical cancer. *Cancer* 1994;74:90.
171. Höckel M, Schlenger K, Mitze M, et al. Tumor vascularity—a novel prognostic factor in advanced cancer of the uterine cervix. *Proc Soc Gynecol Oncol* 1995:48.
172. Wiggins DL, Granai CO, Steinhoff MM, et al. Tumor angiogenesis as a prognostic factor in cervical carcinoma. *Gynecol Oncol* 1995;56:353.
173. Gasinska A, Urbanski K, Jakubowicz J, et al. Tumour cell kinetics as a prognostic factor in squamous cell carcinoma of the cervix treated with radiotherapy. *Radiother Oncol* 1999;50:77.
174. Gaffney DK, Holden J, Davis M, et al. Elevated cyclooxygenase-2 expression correlates with diminished survival in carcinoma of the cervix treated with radiotherapy. *Int J Radiat Oncol Biol Phys* 2001;49:1213.
175. Gaffney DK, Haslam D, Tsodikov A, et al. Epidermal growth factor receptor (EGFR) and vascular endothelial growth factor (VEGF) negatively affect overall survival in carcinoma of the cervix treated with radiotherapy. *Int J Radiat Oncol Biol Phys* 2003;56:922.
176. Oka K, Suzuki Y, Iida H, et al. Pd-ECGF positivity correlates with better survival, while iNOS has no predictive value for cervical carcinomas treated with radiotherapy. *Int J Radiat Oncol Biol Phys* 2003;57:217.
177. Ikenberg H, Wiegering I, Pfisterer J, et al. Human papillomavirus DNA in tumor-free regional lymph nodes: a potential prognostic marker in cervical cancer. *Cancer J Sci Am* 1996;2:28.
178. Kobayashi Y, Yoshinouchi M, Tianqi G, et al. Presence of human papilloma virus DNA in pelvic lymph nodes can predict unexpected recurrence of cervical cancer in patients with histologically negative lymph nodes. *Clin Cancer Res* 1998;4:979.
179. Peters WA 3rd, Liu PY, Barrett RJ 2nd, et al. Concurrent chemotherapy and pelvic radiation therapy compared with pelvic radiation therapy alone as adjuvant therapy after radical surgery in high-risk early-stage cancer of the cervix. *J Clin Oncol* 2000;18:1606.
180. Morris M, Eifel PJ, Lu J, et al. Pelvic radiation with concurrent chemotherapy compared with pelvic and paraaortic radiation for high-risk cervical cancer. *N Engl J Med* 1999;340:1137.
181. Whitney CW, Sause W, Bundy BN, et al. A randomized comparison of fluorouracil plus cisplatin versus hydroxyurea as an adjunct to radiation therapy in stages IIB–IVA carcinoma of the cervix with negative para-aortic lymph nodes: a Gynecologic Oncology Group and Southwest Oncology Group study. *J Clin Oncol* 1999;17:1339.
182. Rose PG, Bundy BN, Watkins J, et al. Concurrent cisplatin-based chemotherapy and radiotherapy for locally advanced cervical cancer. *N Engl J Med* 1999;340:1144.
183. Keys HM, Bundy BN, Stehman FB, et al. Cisplatin, radiation, and adjuvant hysterectomy for bulky stage IB cervical carcinoma. *N Engl J Med* 1999;340:1154.
184. Schantz A, Thormann L. Cryosurgery for dysplasia of the uterine ectocervix. A randomized study of the efficacy of the single- and double-freeze technique. *Acta Obstet Gynecol Scand* 1984;1984:417.
185. Alvarez RD, Helm CW, Edwards R, et al. Prospective randomized trial of LLETZ versus laser ablation in patients with cervical intraepithelial neoplasia. *Gynecol Oncol* 1994;52:175.
186. Mitchell MF, Tortolero-Luna G, Cook E, et al. A randomized clinical trial of cryotherapy, laser vaporization, and loop electrosurgical excision for treatment of squamous intraepithelial lesions of the cervix. *Obstet Gynecol* 1998;92:737.
187. Gunasekera PC, Phipps JM, Lewis BV. Large loop excision of the transformation zone (LLETZ) compared to carbon dioxide laser in the treatment of CIN: a superior mode of treatment. *Br J Obstet Gynaecol* 1990;97:995.
188. Murdoch JB, Grimshaw RN, Monaghan JM. Loop diathermy excision of the abnormal cervical transformation zone. *Int J Gynecol Cancer* 1991;1:105.
189. Burger MPM, Hollema H. The reliability of the histologic diagnosis in colposcopically directed biopsy. A plea for LETZ. *Int J Gynecol Cancer* 1993;3:385.
190. Wright TC, Richart RM, Ferenczy A, et al. Comparisons of specimens removed by CO2 laser conization and loop electrosurgical excision procedure. *Obstet Gynecol* 1992;79:147.
191. Morris M, Mitchell MF, Silva EG, et al. Cervical conization as definitive therapy for early invasive squamous carcinoma of the cervix. *Gynecol Oncol* 1993;51:193.
192. Roman LD, Felix JC, Muderspach LI, et al. Risk of residual invasive disease in women with microinvasive squamous cancer in a conization specimen. *Obstet Gynecol* 1997;90:759.
193. Luesley DM, McCrum A, Terry PB, et al. Complications of cone biopsy related to the dimensions of the cone and the influence of prior colposcopic assessment. *Br J Obstet Gynecol* 1985;92:158.
194. Magrina JF, Goodrich MA, Weaver AL, et al. Modified radical hysterectomy: morbidity and mortality. *Gynecol Oncol* 1995;59:277.
195. Grigsby PW, Perez CA. Radiotherapy alone for medically inoperable carcinoma of the cervix: stage IA and carcinoma in situ. *Int J Radiat Oncol Biol Phys* 1991;21:375.
196. Hamberger AD, Fletcher GH, Wharton JT. Results of treatment of early stage I carcinoma of the uterine cervix with intracavitary radium alone. *Cancer* 1978;41:980.
197. Sedlis A, Bundy BN, Rotman MZ, et al. A randomized trial of pelvic radiation therapy versus no further therapy in selected patients with stage IB carcinoma of the cervix after radical hysterectomy and pelvic lymphadenectomy: a Gynecologic Oncology Group study. *Gynecol Oncol* 1999;73:177.
198. Lee Y-N, Wang KL, Lin M-H, et al. Radical hysterectomy with pelvic lymph node dissection for treatment of cervical cancer: a clinical review of 954 cases. *Gynecol Oncol* 1989;32:135.
199. Morley GW, Seski JC. Radical pelvic surgery versus radiation therapy for stage I carcinoma of the cervix (exclusive of microinvasion). *Am J Obstet Gynecol* 1976;126:785.
200. Lowrey GC, Mendenhall WM, Million RR. Stage IB or IIA-B carcinoma of the intact uterine cervix treated with irradiation: a multivariate analysis. *Int J Radiat Oncol Biol Phys* 1992;24:205.
201. Horiot JC, Pigneux J, Pourquier H, et al. Radiotherapy alone in carcinoma of the intact uterine cervix according to G. H. Fletcher guidelines: a French cooperative study of 1383 cases. *Int J Radiat Oncol Biol Phys* 1988;14:605.
202. Liu W, Meigs JV. Radical hysterectomy and pelvic lymphadenectomy. A review of 473 cases including 244 for primary invasive carcinoma of the cervix. *Am J Obstet Gynecol* 1955;69:1.
203. Volterrani F, Feltre L, Sigurta D, et al. Radiotherapy versus surgery in the treatment of cervix stage Ib cancer. *Int J Radiat Oncol Biol Phys* 1983;9:1781.
204. Inoue T. Prognostic significance of the depth of invasion relating to nodal metastases, parametrial extension, and cell types. A study of 628 cases with stage IB, IIA, and IIB cervical cancer. *Cancer* 1984;54:3035.
205. Kenter GG, Ansink AC, Heintz APM, et al. Carcinoma of the uterine cervix stage I and IIA: results of surgical treatment: complications, recurrence, and survival. *Eur J Surg Oncol* 1989;15:55.
206. Hopkins MP, Morley GW. Radical hysterectomy versus radiation therapy for stage IB squamous cell cancer of the cervix. *Cancer* 1991;68:272.
207. Burghardt E, Hofmann HMH, Ebner F, et al. Results of surgical treatment of 1028 cervical cancers studied with volumetry. *Cancer* 1992;70:648.
208. Montana GS, Fowler WC, Varia MA, et al. Analysis of results of radiation therapy for stage IB carcinoma of the cervix. *Cancer* 1987;60:2195.
209. Coia L, Won M, Lanciano R, et al. The Patterns of Care Outcome Study for cancer of the uterine cervix. Results of the second national practice survey. *Cancer* 1990;66:2451.
210. Landoni F, Maneo A, Colombo A, et al. Randomised study of radical surgery versus radiotherapy for stage Ib–IIa cervical cancer. *Lancet* 1997;350:535.
211. Alvarez RD, Gelder MS, Gore H, et al. Radical hysterectomy in the treatment of patients with bulky early stage carcinoma of the cervix uteri. *Surg Gynecol Obstet* 1993;176:539.
212. Bloss JD, Berman ML, Mukhererjee J, et al. Bulky stage IB cervical carcinoma managed by primary radical hysterectomy followed by tailored radiotherapy. *Gynecol Oncol* 1992;47:21.
213. Rettenmaier MA, Casanova DM, Micha JP, et al. Radical hysterectomy and tailored postoperative radiation therapy in the management of bulky stage IB cervical cancer. *Cancer* 1989;63:2220.
214. Orr JW, Shingleton HM, Hatch KD, et al. Correlation of perioperative morbidity and conization-radical hysterectomy interval. *Obstet Gynecol* 1982;59:726.
215. Hatch KD, Parham G, Shingleton H, et al. Ureteral strictures and fistulae following radical hysterectomy. *Gynecol Oncol* 1984;19:17.
216. Green T. Ureteral suspension for prevention of ureteral complications following radical Wertheim hysterectomy. *Obstet Gynecol* 1966;28:1.
217. Mann WJ, Orr JW, Shingleton HM, et al. Perioperative influences on infectious morbidity in radical hysterectomy. *Gynecol Oncol* 1981;11:207.
218. Forney JP. The effect of radical hysterectomy on bladder physiology. *Am J Obstet Gynecol* 1980;138:374.
219. Sasaki H, Yoshida T, Noda K, et al. Urethral pressure profiles following radical hysterectomy. *Obstet Gynecol* 1982;59:101.
220. Ralph G, Tamussino K, Lichtenegger W. Urological complications after radical hysterectomy with or without radiotherapy for cervical cancer. *Arch Gynecol Obstet* 1990;248:61.
221. Farquharson DI, Shingleton HM, Soong SJ, et al. The adverse effects of cervical cancer treatment on bladder function. *Gynecol Oncol* 1987;27:15.
222. Covens A, Shaw P, Murphy J, et al. Is radical trachelectomy a safe alternative to radical hysterectomy for patients with stage IA-B carcinoma of the cervix? *Cancer* 1999;86:2273.
223. Morrow CP. Is pelvic radiation beneficial in the postoperative management of stage Ib squamous cell carcinoma of the cervix with pelvic node metastases treated by radical hysterectomy and pelvic lymphadenectomy? *Gynecol Oncol* 1980;10:105.
224. Remy JC, Di Maio T, Fruchter RG, et al. Adjunctive radiation after radical hysterectomy in stage IB squamous cell carcinoma of the cervix. *Gynecol Oncol* 1990;38:161.
225. Soisson AP, Soper JT, Clarke-Pearson DL, et al. Adjuvant radiotherapy following radical hysterectomy for patients with stage IB and IIA cervical cancer. *Gynecol Oncol* 1990;37:390.
226. Thomas GM, Dembo AJ. Is there a role for adjuvant pelvic radiotherapy after radical hysterectomy in early stage cervical cancer? *Int J Gynecol Cancer* 1991;1:1.
227. Russell AH, Tong DY, Figge DC, et al. Adjuvant postoperative pelvic radiation for carcinoma of the uterine cervix: pattern of cancer recurrence in patients undergoing elective radiation following radical hysterectomy and pelvic lymphadenectomy. *Int J Radiat Oncol Biol Phys* 1984;10:211.
228. Snijders-Keilholz A, Hellebrekers BW, Zwinderman AH, et al. Adjuvant radiotherapy following radical hysterectomy for patients with early-stage cervical carcinoma (1984–1996). *Radiother Oncol* 1999;51:161.
229. Bandy LC, Clarke-Pearson DL, Soper JT, et al. Long-term effects on bladder function following radical hysterectomy with and without postoperative radiation. *Gynecol Oncol* 1987;26:160.
230. Durrance FY, Fletcher GH, Rutledge FN. Analysis of central recurrent disease in stages I and II squamous cell carcinomas of the cervix on intact uterus. *AJR Am J Roentgenol* 1969;106:831.
231. Thoms WW, Eifel PJ, Smith TL, et al. Bulky endocervical carcinomas: a 23-year experience. *Int J Radiat Oncol Biol Phys* 1992;23:491.
232. Mendenhall WM, McCarty PJ, Morgan LS, et al. Stage IB-IIA-B carcinoma of the intact uterine cervix greater than or equal to 6 cm in diameter: is adjuvant extrafascial hysterectomy beneficial? *Int J Radiat Oncol Biol Phys* 1991;21:899.

233. Keys HM, Bundy BN, Stehman FB, et al. Radiation therapy with and without extrafascial hysterectomy for bulky stage IB cervical carcinoma: a randomized trial of the Gynecologic Oncology Group. *Gynecol Oncol* 2003;89:343.
234. Sardi JE, Giaroli A, Sananes C, et al. Long-term follow-up of the first randomized trial using neoadjuvant chemotherapy in stage Ib squamous carcinoma of the cervix: the final results. *Gynecol Oncol* 1997;67:61.
235. Chang TC, Lai CH, Hong JH, et al. Randomized trial of neoadjuvant cisplatin, vincristine, bleomycin, and radical hysterectomy versus radiation therapy for bulky stage IB and IIA cervical cancer. *J Clin Oncol* 2000;18:1740.
236. Benedetti-Panici P, Greggi S, Colombo A, et al. Neoadjuvant chemotherapy and radical surgery versus exclusive radiotherapy in locally advanced squamous cell cervical cancer: results from the Italian multicenter randomized study. *J Clin Oncol* 2002;20:179.
237. Fyles AW, Pintilie M, Kirkbride P, et al. Prognostic factors in patients with cervix cancer treated by radiation therapy: results of a multiple regression analysis. *Radiother Oncol* 1995;35:107.
238. Perez CA, Grigsby PW, Castro-Vita H, et al. Carcinoma of the uterine cervix. I. Impact of prolongation of overall treatment time and timing of brachytherapy on outcome of radiation therapy. *Int J Radiat Oncol Biol Phys* 1995;32:1275.
239. Petereit DG, Sarkaria JN, Chappell R, et al. The adverse effect of treatment prolongation in cervical carcinoma. *Int J Radiat Oncol Biol Phys* 1995;32:1301.
240. Chao C, Williamson JF, Grigsby PW, et al. Uterosacral space involvement in locally advanced carcinoma of the uterine cervix. *Int J Radiat Oncol Biol Phys* 1998;40:397.
241. Cunningham M, Dunton C, Corn B, et al. Extended-field radiation therapy in early-stage cervical carcinoma: survival and complications. *Gynecol Oncol* 1991;43:51.
242. Rotman M, Pajak M, Choi K, et al. Prophylactic extended-field irradiation of para-aortic lymph nodes in stages IIB and bulky IB and IIA cervical carcinomas. Ten-year treatment results of RTOG 79-20. *JAMA* 1995;274:387.
243. Haie C, Pejovic MH, Gerbaulet A, et al. Is prophylactic para-aortic irradiation worthwhile in the treatment of advanced cervical carcinoma? Results of a controlled clinical trial of the EORTC radiotherapy group. *Radiother Oncol* 1988;11:101.
244. Grigsby PW, Heydon K, Mutch DG, et al. Long-term follow-up of RTOG 92-10: cervical cancer with positive para-aortic lymph nodes. *Int J Radiat Oncol Biol Phys* 2001;51:982.
245. Varia MA, Bundy BN, Deppe G, et al. Cervical carcinoma metastatic to para-aortic nodes: extended field radiation therapy with concomitant 5-fluorouracil and cisplatin chemotherapy: a Gynecologic Oncology Group study. *Int J Radiat Oncol Biol Phys* 1998;42:1015.
246. Fletcher GH. Female pelvis. In: Fletcher GH, ed. *Textbook of radiotherapy*. Philadelphia, PA: Lea & Febiger, 1980.
247. Eifel PJ, Moughan J, Owen JB, et al. Patterns of radiotherapy practice for patients with squamous carcinoma of the uterine cervix. A Patterns of Care Study. *Int J Radiat Oncol Biol Phys* 1999;43:351.
248. Potish RA, Gerbi BJ, Engeler GP. Dose prescription, dose specification, and applicator geometry in intracavitary therapy. In: Williamson JF, Thomadsen BR, Nath R, eds. *Brachytherapy physics*. Madison, WI: Medical Physics Publishing, 1995.
249. International Commission on Radiation Units and Measurements. *Dose and volume specification for reporting intracavitary therapy in gynecology*. Bethesda, MD: International Commission on Radiation Units and Measurements, 1985.
250. Schoeppel SL, LaVigne ML, Martel MK, et al. Three-dimensional treatment planning of intracavitary gynecologic implants: analysis of ten cases and implications for dose specification. *Int J Radiat Oncol Biol Phys* 1994;28:277.
251. Delclos L. Gynecologic cancers: pelvic examination and treatment planning. In: Levitt S, Tapley N, eds. *Technological basis of radiation therapy: practical clinical applications*. Philadelphia: Lea & Febiger, 1984:193.
252. Eifel PJ, Morris M, Delclos L, et al. Radiation therapy for cervical carcinoma. In: Dilts PVJ, Sciarra JJ, eds. *Gynecology and obstetrics*. Philadelphia: JB Lippincott Co., 1993:1.
253. Haie-Meder C, Kramar A, Lambin P, et al. Analysis of complications in a prospective randomized trial comparing two brachytherapy low dose rates in cervical carcinoma. *Int J Radiat Oncol Biol Phys* 1994;29:1195.
254. Amdur RJ, Bedford JS. Dose-rate effects between 0.3 and 30 Gy/h in a normal and a malignant human cell line [see comments]. *Int J Radiat Oncol Biol Phys* 1994;30:83.
255. Petereit DG, Pearcey R. Literature analysis of high dose rate brachytherapy fractionation schedules in the treatment of cervical cancer: is there an optimal fractionation schedule? *Int J Radiat Oncol Biol Phys* 1999;43:359.
256. Nag S, Erickson B, Parikh S, et al. The American Brachytherapy Society recommendations for high-dose-rate brachytherapy for carcinoma of the endometrium. *Int J Radiat Oncol Biol Phys* 2000;48:779.
257. Eifel PJ, Moughan J, Erickson B, et al. Patterns of radiotherapy practice for patients with carcinoma of the cervix (1996–1999): a patterns-of-care study. *Int J Radiat Oncol Biol Phys* 2003;57:S190.
258. Eifel PJ. High dose-rate brachytherapy for carcinoma of the cervix: high tech or high risk? *Int J Radiat Oncol Biol Phys* 1992;24:383.
259. Scalliet P, Gerbaulet A, Dubray B. HDR versus LDR gynecological brachytherapy revisited. *Radiother Oncol* 1993;28:118.
260. Hareyama M, Sakata K, Oouchi A, et al. High-dose-rate versus low-dose-rate intracavitary therapy for carcinoma of the uterine cervix: a randomized trial. *Cancer* 2002;94:117.
261. Patel FD, Sharma SC, Neigi PS, et al. Low dose rate vs. high dose rate brachytherapy in the treatment of carcinoma of the uterine cervix: a clinical trial. *Int J Radiat Oncol Biol Phys* 1993;28:335.
262. Shigematsu Y, Nishiyama K, Masaki N, et al. Treatment of carcinoma of the uterine cervix by remotely controlled afterloading intracavitary radiotherapy with high-dose rate: a comparative study with a low-dose rate system. *Int J Radiat Oncol Biol Phys* 1983;9:351.
263. Nag S, Orton C, Young D, et al. The American Brachytherapy Society survey of brachytherapy practice for carcinoma of the cervix in the United States. *Gynecol Oncol* 1999;73:111.
264. Wachter-Gerstner N, Wachter S, Reinstadler E, et al. Bladder and rectum dose defined from MRI based treatment planning for cervix cancer brachytherapy: comparison of dose-volume histograms for organ contours and organ wall, comparison with ICRU rectum and bladder reference point. *Radiother Oncol* 2003;68:269.
265. Syed AMN, Puthwala AA, Neblett D, et al. Transperineal interstitial-intracavitary "Syed-Neblett" applicator in the treatment of carcinoma of the uterine cervix. *Endocurietherapy Hypertherm Oncol* 1986;2:1.
266. Martinez A, Edmundson GK, Cox RS, et al. Combination of external beam irradiation and multiple-site perineal applicator (MUPIT) for treatment of locally advanced or recurrent prostatic, anorectal, and gynecologic malignancies. *Int J Radiat Oncol Biol Phys* 1985;11:391.
267. Hughes-Davies L, Silver B, Kapp D. Parametrial interstitial brachytherapy for advanced or recurrent pelvic malignancy: the Harvard/Stanford experience. *Gynecol Oncol* 1995; 58:24.
268. Recio FO, Piver MS, Hempling RE, et al. Laparoscopic-assisted application of interstitial brachytherapy for locally advanced cervical carcinoma: results of a pilot study. *Int J Radiat Oncol Biol Phys* 1998;40:411.
269. Erickson B, Gillin MT. Interstitial implantation of gynecologic malignancies. *J Surg Oncol* 1997;66:285.
270. Gupta AK, Vicini FA, Frazier AJ, et al. Iridium-192 transperineal interstitial brachytherapy for locally advanced or recurrent gynecological malignancies. *Int J Radiat Oncol Biol Phys* 1999;43:1055.
271. Demanes DJ, Rodriguez RR, Bendre DD, et al. High dose rate transperineal interstitial brachytherapy for cervical cancer: high pelvic control and low complication rates. *Int J Radiat Oncol Biol Phys* 1999;45:105.
272. Jhingran A, Eifel PJ. Perioperative and postoperative complications of intracavitary radiation for FIGO stage I–III carcinoma of the cervix. *Int J Radiat Oncol Biol Phys* 2000;46:1177.
273. Lanciano RM, Martz D, Montana GS, et al. Influence of age, prior abdominal surgery, fraction size, and dose on complications after radiation therapy for squamous cell cancer of the uterine cervix. A Patterns of Care Study. *Cancer* 1992;69:2124.
274. Eifel PJ, Levenback C, Wharton JT, et al. Time course and incidence of late complications in patients treated with radiation therapy for FIGO stage IB carcinoma of the uterine cervix. *Int J Radiat Oncol Biol Phys* 1995;32:1289.
275. Eifel PJ, Jhingran A, Bodurka DC, et al. Correlation of smoking history and other patient characteristics with major complications of pelvic radiation therapy for cervical cancer. *J Clin Oncol* 2002;20:3651.
276. Bruner DW, Lanciano R, Keegan M, et al. Vaginal stenosis and sexual function following intracavitary radiation for the treatment of cervical and endometrial carcinoma. *Int J Radiat Oncol Biol Phys* 1993;27:825.
277. Eifel PJ. Chemoradiation for carcinoma of the cervix: advances and opportunities. *Radiat Res* 2000;154:229.
278. Eifel PJ, Winter K, Morris M, et al. Pelvic radiation with concurrent chemotherapy versus pelvic and para-aortic radiation for high-risk cervical cancer: an update of radiation therapy oncology group trial (RTOG) 90-01. *J Clin Oncol* 2004;22:872.
279. Pearcey R, Brundage M, Drouin P, et al. Phase III trial comparing radical radiotherapy with and without cisplatin chemotherapy in patients with advanced squamous cell cancer of the cervix. *J Clin Oncol* 2002;20:966.
280. Wong LC, Ngan HY, Cheung AN, et al. Chemoradiation and adjuvant chemotherapy in cervical cancer. *J Clin Oncol* 1999;17:2055.
281. Lorvidhaya V, Chitapanarux I, Sangruchi S, et al. Concurrent mitomycin C, 5-fluorouracil, and radiotherapy in the treatment of locally advanced carcinoma of the cervix: a randomized trial. *Int J Radiat Oncol Biol Phys* 2003;55:1226.
282. Chen MD, Paley PJ, Potish RA, et al. Phase I trial of Taxol as a radiation sensitizer with cisplatin in advanced cervical cancer. *Gynecol Oncol* 1997;67:131.
283. Muderspach LI, Curtin JP, Roman LD, et al. Carboplatin as a radiation sensitizer in locally advanced cervical cancer: a pilot study. *Gynecol Oncol* 1997;65:336.
284. Chauvergne J, Rohart J, Héron JF, et al. Essai randomisé de chimiothérapie initiale dans 151 carcinomes du col utérin localement étendus (T2b-N1, T3b, MO). *Bull Cancer* 1990;77:1007.
285. Sardi J, Sananes C, Giarole A, et al. Neoadjuvant chemotherapy in locally advanced carcinoma of the cervix uteri. *Gynecol Oncol* 1990;38:486.
286. Park TK, Choi DH, Kim SN, et al. Role of induction chemotherapy in invasive cervical cancer. *Gynecol Oncol* 1991;41:107.
287. Souhami L, Gil R, Allan S, et al. A randomized trial of chemotherapy followed by pelvic radiation therapy in stage IIIB carcinoma of the cervix. *Int J Radiat Oncol Biol Phys* 1991;9:970.
288. Kumar L, Kaushal R, Nandy M, et al. Chemotherapy followed by radiotherapy versus radiotherapy alone in locally advanced cervical cancer: a randomized study. *Gynecol Oncol* 1994;54:307.
289. Tattersall MHN, Larvidhaya V, Vootiprux V, et al. Randomized trial of epirubicin and cisplatin chemotherapy followed by pelvic radiation in locally advanced cervical cancer. *Am J Clin Oncol* 1995;13:444.
290. Sundfor K, Trope CG, Hogberg T, et al. Radiotherapy and neoadjuvant chemotherapy for cervical carcinoma. A randomized multicenter study of sequential cisplatin and 5-fluorouracil and radiotherapy in advanced cervical carcinoma stage 3B and 4A. *Cancer* 1996;77:2371.
291. Leborgne F, Leborgne JH, Doldán R, et al. Induction chemotherapy and radiotherapy of advanced cancer of the cervix: a pilot study and phase III randomized trial. *Int J Radiat Oncol Biol Phys* 1997;37:343.
292. Benedetti Panici P, Scambia G, Greggi S, et al. Neoadjuvant chemotherapy and radical surgery in locally advanced cervical carcinoma. Prognostic factors for response and survival. *Cancer* 1991;67:372.

293. Lai CH, Hsueh S, Chang TC, et al. Prognostic factors in patients with bulky stage IB or IIA cervical carcinoma undergoing neoadjuvant chemotherapy and radical hysterectomy. *Gynecol Oncol* 1997;64:456.
294. Tattersall MHN, Ramirez C, Coppleson M. A randomized trial comparing platinum-based chemotherapy followed by radiotherapy vs. radiotherapy alone in patients with locally advanced cervical cancer. *Int J Gynecol Cancer* 1992;2:244.
295. Sardi J, Giaroli A, Sananes C, et al. Randomized trial with neoadjuvant chemotherapy in stage IIIB squamous carcinoma cervix uteri: an unexpected therapeutic management. *Int J Gynecol Cancer* 1998;6:85.
296. Bloss JD, Thigpen JT. Chemotherapy of gynecologic cancer. In: Perry MC, ed. *The chemotherapy source book*, 3rd ed. Philadelphia: Lippincott Williams & Wilkins, 2001:732.
297. Look KY, Blessing JA, Levenback C, et al. A phase II trial of CPT-11 in recurrent squamous carcinoma of the cervix: a gynecologic oncology group study. *Gynecol Oncol* 1998;70:334.
298. Takeuchi S, Dobashi K, Fujimoto S, et al. A late phase II study of CPT-11 on uterine cervical cancer and ovarian cancer. Research Groups of CPT-11 in Gynecologic Cancers. *Gan To Kagaku Ryoho* 1991;18:1681.
299. Verschraegen CF, Levy T, Kudelka AP, et al. Phase II study of irinotecan in prior chemotherapy-treated squamous cell carcinoma of the cervix. *J Clin Oncol* 1997;15:625.
300. Kudelka AP, Winn R, Edwards CL, et al. Activity of paclitaxel in advanced or recurrent squamous cell cancer of the cervix. *Clin Cancer Res* 1996;2:1285.
301. Bonomi P, Blessing J, Stehman F, et al. Randomized trial of three cisplatin dose schedules in squamous-cell carcinoma of the cervix: a Gynecologic Oncology Group study. *J Clin Oncol* 1985;3:1079.
302. Thigpen T, Shingleton H, Homesley H, et al. Cis-platinum in treatment of advanced or recurrent squamous cell carcinoma of the cervix. *Cancer* 1981;48:899.
303. Thigpen JT, Blessing JA, DiSaia PJ, et al. A randomized comparison of a rapid versus prolonged (24 hr) infusion of cisplatin in therapy of squamous cell carcinoma of the uterine cervix: a Gynecologic Oncology Group study. *Gynecol Oncol* 1989;32:198.
304. Sutton GP, Blessing JA, Adcock L, et al. Phase II study of ifosfamide and mesna in patients with previously-treated carcinoma of the cervix: a Gynecologic Oncology Group study. *Invest New Drugs* 1989;7:341.
305. Stehman F, Perez C, Kurman R, et al. Uterine cervix. In: Hoskins W, Perez C, Young R, eds. *Principles and practice of gynecologic oncology*. Philadelphia: Lippincott, 2000:591.
306. Meanwell C, Mould J, Blackledge G, et al. Phase II study of ifosfamide in cervical cancer. *Cancer Treatment Rep* 1986;70:727.
307. Cervellino J, Araujo C, Pirisi C, et al. Ifosfamide and mesna at high doses for the treatment of cancer of the cervix: a GETLAC study. *Cancer Chemother Pharmacol* 1990;26:S1.
308. Hannigan EV, Dinh TV, Doherty MG. Ifosfamide with mesna in squamous carcinoma of the cervix: phase II results in patients with advanced or recurrent disease. *Gynecol Oncol* 1991;43:123.
309. Thigpen T, Vance R, Khansur T. Carcinoma of the uterine cervix: current status and future directions. *Semin Oncol* 1994;21[Suppl 2]:543.
310. Cervellino JC, Araujo CE, Sanchez O, et al. Cisplatin and ifosfamide in patients with advanced squamous cell carcinoma of the uterine cervix. *Acta Oncol* 1995;34:257.
311. Chiara S, Consoli R, Falcone A, et al. Cisplatin and 5-fluorouracil in advanced and recurrent cervical cancer. *Tumori* 1988;74:471.
312. Kuhnle H, Meerpohl HG, Eiermann W, et al. Phase II study of carboplatin/ifosfamide in untreated advanced cervical cancer. *Cancer Chemother Pharmacol* 1990;26:S33.
313. Ramm K, Vergote I, Kaem J, et al. Bleomycin-ifosfamide-cisplatinum (BIP) in pelvic recurrence of previously irradiated cervical carcinoma: a second look. *Gynecol Oncol* 1992;46:203.
314. Buxton EJ, Meanwell CA, Hilton C, et al. Combination bleomycin, ifosfamide, and cisplatin chemotherapy in cervical cancer. *J Natl Cancer Inst* 1989;81:359.
315. Kumar L, Bhargava V. Chemotherapy in recurrent and advanced cervical cancer. *Gynecol Oncol* 1991;40:107.
316. Murad AM, Triginelli SA, Ribalta JCL. Phase II trial of bleomycin, ifosfamide, and carboplatin in metastatic cervical cancer. *J Clin Oncol* 1994;12:55.
317. Tay SK, Lai FM, Soh LT, et al. Combined chemotherapy using cisplatin ifosfamide and bleomycin (PIB) in the treatment of advanced and recurrent cervical carcinoma. *Aust N Z J Obstet Gynaecol* 1993;32:263.
318. Bonomi P, Blessing J, Ball H, et al. A phase II evaluation of cisplatin and 5-fluorouracil in patients with advanced squamous cell carcinoma of the cervix: a Gynecologic Oncology Group study. *Gynecol Oncol* 1989;37:354.
319. Kaern J, Trope C, Kjorstad KE, et al. A phase II study of 5-fluorouracil/cisplatin in recurrent cervical cancer. *Tidsskr Nor Laegeforen* 1990;110:2759.
320. Weiss G, Green S, Hannigan E, et al. A phase II trial of cisplatin and 5-fluorouracil with allopurinol for recurrent or metastatic carcinoma of the uterine cervix: a Southwest Oncology Group trial. *Gynecol Oncol* 1990;37:354.
321. Papadimitriou CA, Sarris K, Moulopoulos LA, et al. Phase II trial of paclitaxel and cisplatin in metastatic and recurrent carcinoma of the uterine cervix. *J Clin Oncol* 1999;17:761.
322. Rose PG, Blessing JA, Gershenson DM, et al. Paclitaxel and cisplatin as first-line therapy in recurrent or advanced squamous cell carcinoma of the cervix: a gynecologic oncology group study. *J Clin Oncol* 1999;17:2676.
323. Piver MS, Ghamande SA, Eltabbakh GH, et al. First-line chemotherapy with paclitaxel and platinum for advanced and recurrent cancer of the cervix—a phase II study. *Gynecol Oncol* 1999;75:334.
324. Pignata S, Silvestro G, Ferrari E, et al. Phase II study of cisplatin and vinorelbine as first-line chemotherapy in patients with carcinoma of the uterine cervix. *J Clin Oncol* 1999;17:756.
325. Burnett AF, Roman LD, Garcia AA, et al. A phase II study of gemcitabine and cisplatin in patients with advanced, persistent, or recurrent squamous cell carcinoma of the cervix. *Gynecol Oncol* 2000;76:63.
326. Duenas-Gonzalez A, Lopez-Graniel C, Gonzalez A, et al. A phase II study of gemcitabine and cisplatin combination as induction chemotherapy for untreated locally advanced cervical carcinoma. *Ann Oncol* 2001;12:541.
327. Fiorica J, Holloway R, Ndubisi B, et al. Phase II trial of topotecan and cisplatin in persistent or recurrent squamous and nonsquamous carcinomas of the cervix. *Gynecol Oncol* 2002;85:89.
328. Verschraegen CF, Kavanagh JJ, Loyer E, et al. Phase II study of carboplatin and liposomal doxorubicin in patients with recurrent squamous cell carcinoma of the cervix. *Cancer* 2001;92:2327.
329. Brader KR, Morris M, Levenback C, et al. Chemotherapy for cervical carcinoma: factors determining response and implications for clinical trial design. *J Clin Oncol* 1998;16:1879.
330. Omura GA, Blessing JA, Vaccarello L, et al. Randomized trial of cisplatin versus cisplatin plus mitolactol versus cisplatin plus ifosfamide in advanced squamous carcinoma of the cervix: a Gynecologic Oncology Group study. *J Clin Oncol* 1997;15:165.
331. Moore DH, McQuellion RP, Blessing JA, et al. A randomized phase III study of cisplatin versus cisplatin plus paclitaxel in stage IVB, recurrent or persistent squamous cell carcinoma of the cervix: a Gynecologic Oncology Group Study. *Proc Am Clin Oncol* 2001;20:201a.
332. Mahé MA, Gérard JP, Dubois JB, et al. Intraoperative radiation therapy in recurrent carcinoma of the uterine cervix: report of the French Intraoperative Group on 70 patients. *Int J Radiat Oncol Biol Phys* 1996;34:21.
333. Stelzer KJ, Koh WJ, Greer BE, et al. The use of intraoperative radiation therapy in radical salvage for recurrent cervical cancer: outcome and morbidity. *Am J Obstet Gynecol* 1995;172:1881.
334. Ijaz T, Eifel PJ, Burke T, et al. Radiation therapy of pelvic recurrence after radical hysterectomy for cervical carcinoma. *Gynecol Oncol* 1998;70:241.
335. Potter ME, Alvarez RD, Gay FL, et al. Optimal therapy for pelvic recurrence after radical hysterectomy for early-stage cervical cancer. *Gynecol Oncol* 1990;37:74.
336. Larson DM, Copeland LJ, Stringer CA, et al. Recurrent cervical carcinoma after radical hysterectomy. *Gynecol Oncol* 1988;30:381.
337. Wang CJ, Lai CH, Huang HJ, et al. Recurrent cervical carcinoma after primary radical surgery. *Am J Obstet Gynecol* 1999;181:518.
338. Thomas GM, Dembo AJ, Black B, et al. Concurrent radiation and chemotherapy for carcinoma of the cervix recurrent after radical surgery. *Gynecol Oncol* 1987;27:254.
339. Coleman RL, Burke TW, Morris M, et al. Intra-operative radiographs to confirm the adequacy of lymph node resection in patients with suspicious lymphangiograms. *Gynecol Oncol* 1994;51:362.
340. Rutledge S, Carey MS, Prichard H, et al. Conservative surgery for recurrent or persistent carcinoma of the cervix following irradiation: is exenteration always necessary? *Gynecol Oncol* 1994;52:353.
341. Maneo A, Landoni F, Cormio G, et al. Radical hysterectomy for recurrent or persistent cervical cancer following radiation therapy. *Int J Gynecol Cancer* 1999;9:295.
342. Matthews CM, Morris M, Burke TW, et al. Pelvic exenteration in the elderly patient. *Obstet Gynecol* 1992;79:773.
343. Miller B, Morris M, Rutledge F, et al. Aborted exenterative procedures in recurrent cervical cancer. *Gynecol Oncol* 1993;50:94.
344. Orr JWJ, Shingleton HM, Hatch KD, et al. Gastrointestinal complications associated with pelvic exenteration. *Am J Obstet Gynecol* 1983;145:325.
345. Roberts WS, Cavanaugh D, Bryson SC, et al. Major morbidity after pelvic exenteration: a seven-year experience. *Obstet Gynecol* 1987;69:617.
346. Berek JS, Hacker NF, Lagasse LD. Rectosigmoid colectomy and reanastomosis to facilitate resection of primary and recurrent gynecologic cancer. *Obstet Gynecol* 1984;64:715.
347. Rowland RG, Mitchell ME, Bihrle R. Alternative techniques for a continent urinary reservoir. *Urol Clin North Am* 1987;14:797.
348. Penalver MA, Barreau G, Sevin BU, et al. Surgery for the treatment of locally recurrent disease. *J Natl Cancer Inst Monogr* 1996;21:117.
349. Hawighorst-Knapstein S, Schonefussrs G, Hoffmann SO, et al. Pelvic exenteration: effects of surgery on quality of life and body image—a prospective longitudinal study. *Gynecol Oncol* 1997;66:495.
350. Ratliff CR, Gershenson DM, Morris M, et al. Sexual adjustment of patients undergoing gracilis myocutaneous flap vaginal reconstruction in conjunction with pelvic exenteration. *Cancer* 1996;78:2229.
351. Hatch KD, Shingleton H, Soong S, et al. Anterior pelvic exenteration. *Gynecol Oncol* 1988;31:205.
352. Shingleton HM, Soong SJ, Gelder MS, et al. Clinical and histopathologic factors predicting recurrence and survival after pelvic exenteration for cancer of the cervix. *Obstet Gynecol* 1989;73:1027.
353. Stanhope CR, Webb MJ, Podratz KC. Pelvic exenteration for recurrent cervical cancer. *Clin Obstet Gynecol* 1990;33:897.
354. Höckel M, Baubmann E, Mitze M, et al. Are pelvic side-wall recurrences of cervical cancer biologically different from central relapses? *Cancer* 1994;74:648.
355. Roman L, Morris M, Eifel P, et al. Reasons for inappropriate simple hysterectomy in the presence of invasive cancer of the cervix. *Obstet Gynecol* 1992;79:485.
356. Hopkins MP, Peters WA, Anderson W, et al. Invasive cervical cancer treated initially by standard hysterectomy. *Gynecol Oncol* 1990;36:7.
357. Roman LD, Morris M, Mitchell MF, et al. Prognostic factors for patients undergoing simple hysterectomy in the presence of invasive cancer of the cervix. *Gynecol Oncol* 1993;50:179.
358. Barillot I, Horiot JC, Cuisenier J, et al. Carcinoma of the cervical stump: a review of 213 cases. *Eur J Cancer* 1993;29A:1231.
359. Miller BE, Copeland LJ, Hamberger AD, et al. Carcinoma of the cervical stump. *Gynecol Oncol* 1984;18:100.
360. Hacker NF, Berek JS, Lagasse LD, et al. Carcinoma of the cervix associated with pregnancy. *Obstet Gynecol* 1982;59:735.
361. Shingleton HM, Orr JW. *Cancer of the cervix*. Philadelphia: JB Lippincott Co., 1995.
362. Tseng CJ, Horng SG, Soong YK, et al. Conservative conization for microinvasive carcinoma of the cervix. *Am J Obstet Gynecol* 1997;176:1009.

363. Woodrow N, Permezel M, Butterfield L, et al. Abnormal cervical cytology in pregnancy: experience of 811 cases. *Aust N Z J Obstet Gynaecol* 1998;38:161.

364. Duggan B, Muderspach LI, Roman L, et al. Cervical cancer in pregnancy: reporting on planned delay in therapy. *Obstet Gynecol* 1993;82:598.

365. Hopkins MP, Morley GW. The prognosis and management of cervical cancer associated with pregnancy. *Obstet Gynecol* 1992;80:9.

366. Sood AK, Sorosky JI, Mayr N, et al. Radiotherapeutic management of cervical carcinoma that complicates pregnancy. *Cancer* 1997;80:1073.

367. van der Vange N, Weverling GJ, Ketting BW, et al. The prognosis of cervical cancer associated with pregnancy: a matched cohort study. *Obstet Gynecol* 1995;85:1022.

368. Van den Broek NR, Lopes AD, Ansink A, et al. "Microinvasive" adenocarcinoma of the cervix implanting in an episiotomy scar. *Gynecol Oncol* 1995;59:297.

369. Creasman WT, Phillips JL, Menck HR. The National Cancer Data Base report on cancer of the vagina. *Cancer* 1998;83:1033.

370. Shepherd J, Sideri M, Benedet J, et al. Carcinoma of the vagina. *J Epidemiol Biostat* 1998;3:103.

371. Chyle V, Zagars GK, Wheeler JA, et al. Definitive radiotherapy for carcinoma of the vagina: outcome and prognostic factors. *Int J Radiat Oncol Biol Phys* 1996;35:891.

372. Eddy GL, Jenrette JMI, Creasman WT. Effect of radiotherapeutic technique on local control in primary vaginal carcinoma. *Int J Gynecol Cancer* 1993;3:399.

373. Stock RG, Chen ASJ, Seski J. A 30-year experience in the management of primary carcinoma of the vagina: analysis of prognostic factors and treatment modalities. *Gynecol Oncol* 1995;56:45.

374. Hoffman MS, De Cesare LS, Roberts WS, et al. Upper vaginectomy for in situ and occult, superficially invasive carcinoma of the vagina. *Am J Obstet Gynecol* 1992;166:30.

375. Kalogirou D, Antoniou G, Karakitsos P, et al. Vaginal intraepithelial neoplasia (VAIN) following hysterectomy in patients treated for carcinoma in situ of the cervix. *Eur J Gynaecol Oncol* 1997;18:188.

376. International Agency for Research on Cancer (IARC). *Monographs on the evaluation of carcinogenic risks to humans. Human papillomaviruses.* Lyon (France): IARC, 1995.

377. Merino MJ. Vaginal cancer: the role of infectious and environmental factors. *Am J Obstet Gynecol* 1991;165:1255.

378. Schraub S, Sun XS, Maingon P, et al. Cervical and vaginal cancer associated with pessary use. *Cancer* 1992;69:2505.

379. Pride GL, Schultz AE, Chuprevich TW, et al. Primary invasive squamous carcinoma of the vagina. *Obstet Gynecol* 1979;53:218.

380. Kirkbride P, Fyles A, Rawlings GA, et al. Carcinoma of the vagina—experience at the Princess Margaret Hospital (1974–1989). *Gynecol Oncol* 1995;56:435.

381. Herbst AL, Ulfelder H, Poskanzer DC. Adenocarcinoma of the vagina: an association of maternal stilboestrol therapy with tumour appearing in young women. *N Engl J Med* 1971;284:878.

382. Herbst AL, Anderson SA, Hubby MM, et al. Risk factors for the development of diethylstilbestrol associated clear cell adenocarcinoma: a case-control study. *Am J Obstet Gynecol* 1986;154:814.

383. Palmer JR, Anderson D, Helmrich SP, et al. Risk factors for diethylstilbestrol-associated clear cell adenocarcinoma. *Obstet Gynecol* 2000;95:814.

384. Waggoner SE, Anderson SM, Van Eyck S, et al. Human papillomavirus detection and p53 expression in clear-cell adenocarcinoma of the vagina and cervix. *Obstet Gynecol* 1994;84:404.

385. Hatch EE, Palmer JR, Titus-Ernstoff L, et al. Cancer risk in women exposed to diethylstilbestrol in utero. *JAMA* 1998;280:630.

386. Perez CA, Grigsby PW, Garipagaoglu M, et al. Factors affecting long-term outcome of irradiation in carcinoma of the vagina. *Int J Radiat Oncol Biol Phys* 1999;44:37.

387. Plentl AA, Friedman EA. Lymphatics of the vagina. *Lymphatic system of female genitalia.* Philadelphia: WB Saunders, 1971:51.

388. Davis KP, Stanhope CR, Garton GR, et al. Invasive vaginal carcinoma: analysis of early-stage disease. *Gynecol Oncol* 1991;42:131.

389. Isaacs JH. Verrucous carcinoma of the female genital tract. *Gynecol Oncol* 1976;4:259.

390. Yaghesezian H, Palazzo JP, Finkel GC, et al. Primary vaginal adenocarcinoma of the intestinal type associated with adenosis. *Gynecol Oncol* 1992;45:62.

391. Joseph RE, Enghardt MH, Doering DL, et al. Small cell neuroendocrine carcinoma of the vagina. *Cancer* 1992;70:784.

392. Miliauskas JR, Leong AS. Small cell (neuroendocrine) carcinoma of the vagina. *Histopathology* 1992;21:371.

393. Buchanan DJ, Schlaerth J, Kurosaki T. Primary vaginal melanoma: thirteen-year disease-free survival after wide local excision and review of recent literature. *Am J Obstet Gynecol* 1998;178:1177.

394. Peters WA, Kumar NB, Andersen WA, et al. Primary sarcoma of the adult vagina: a clinicopathologic study. *Obstet Gynecol* 1985;65:699.

395. Andrassy RJ, Wiener ES, Raney RB, et al. Progress in the surgical management of vaginal rhabdomyosarcoma: a 25-year review from the Intergroup Rhabdomyosarcoma Study Group. *J Pediatr Surg* 1999;34:731.

396. Kucera H, Vavra N. Radiation management of primary carcinoma of the vagina: clinical and histopathological variables associated with survival. *Gynecol Oncol* 1991;40:12.

397. American Joint Committee on Cancer. Vagina. In: Greene FL, Page DL, Fleming ID, et al., eds. *Cancer staging manual,* 6th ed. New York: Springer-Verlag, 2002:251.

398. Eddy GL, Marks RD, Miller MC, et al. Primary invasive vaginal carcinoma. *Am J Obstet Gynecol* 1991;165:292.

399. Macnaught R, Symonds R, Hole D, et al. Improved control of primary vaginal tumours by combined external-beam and interstitial radiotherapy. *Clin Radiol* 1986;37:29.

400. Nori D, Hilaris B, Stanimir G, et al. Radiation therapy of primary vaginal carcinoma. *Int J Radiat Oncol Biol Phys* 1983;9:1471.

401. Rubin SC, Young J, Mikuta JJ. Squamous carcinoma of the vagina: treatment, complications, and long-term follow-up. *Gynecol Oncol* 1985;20:346.

402. Spiritos N, Doshi B, Kapp D, et al. Radiation therapy for primary squamous cell carcinoma of the vagina: Stanford University experience. *Gynecol Oncol* 1989;35:20.

403. Vavra N, Seifert M, Kucera H, et al. Die Strahlentherapie des primären Vaginalkarzinoms und der Einflub histologischer und klinischer Faktoren auf die Prognose. *Strahlenther Onkol* 1991;167:1.

404. Gallup DG, Talledo OE, Shah KJ, et al. Invasive squamous cell carcinoma of the vagina: a 14-year study. *Obstet Gynecol* 1987;69:782.

405. Peters W, Kumar N, Morley G. Carcinoma of the vagina. Factors influencing outcome. *Cancer* 1985;55:892.

406. Berek JS, Hacker NF. *Practical gynecologic oncology,* 2nd ed. Baltimore: Williams & Wilkins, 1994.

407. Benedet JL, Saunders BH. Carcinoma in situ of the vagina. *Am J Obstet Gynecol* 1984;148:695.

408. Cheng D, Ng TY, Ngan HY, et al. Wide local excision (WLE) for vaginal intraepithelial neoplasia (VAIN). *Acta Obstet Gynecol Scand* 1999;78:648.

409. MacLeod C, Fowler A, Dalrymple C, et al. High-dose-rate brachytherapy in the management of high-grade intraepithelial neoplasia of the vagina. *Gynecol Oncol* 1997;65:74.

410. Ogino I, Kitamura T, Okajima H, et al. High-dose-rate intracavitary brachytherapy in the management of cervical and vaginal intraepithelial neoplasia [see comments]. *Int J Radiat Oncol Biol Phys* 1998;40:881.

411. Benson C, Soisson AP, Carlson J, et al. Neovaginal reconstruction with a rectus abdominis myocutaneous flap. *Obstet Gynecol* 1993;81:871.

412. Lee WR, Marcus RB, Sombeck MD, et al. Radiotherapy alone for carcinoma of the vagina: the importance of overall treatment time. *Int J Radiat Oncol Biol Phys* 1994;29:983.

413. Thigpen T, Blessing J, Homesley HD, et al. Phase II trial of cisplatin in advanced or recurrent cancer of the vagina: a Gynecologic Oncology Group study. *Gynecol Oncol* 1986;23:101.

414. Slayton R, Blessing J, Beecham J, et al. Phase II trial of etoposide in the management of advanced or recurrent squamous cell carcinoma of the vulva and carcinoma of the vagina. *Cancer Treatment Reports* 1987;71:869.

415. Umesaki N, Kawamura N, Tsujimura A, et al. Stage II vaginal cancer responding to chemotherapy with irinotecan and cisplatin: a case report. *Oncol Rep* 1999;6:123.

416. Senekjian E, Frey K, Anderson D, et al. Local therapy in stage I clear cell adenocarcinoma of the vagina. *Cancer* 1987;60:1319.

417. Scully RE, Welch WR. Pathology of the female genital tract after prenatal exposure to diethylstilbestrol. In: Herbst AL, Bern HA, eds. *Developmental effects of Diethylstibestrol (DES) in pregnancy.* New York: Thieme-Stratton, 1981:26.

418. Fishman DA, Williams S, Small W Jr, et al. Late recurrences of vaginal clear cell adenocarcinoma. *Gynecol Oncol* 1996;62:128.

419. Shepherd J, Sideri M, Benedet J, et al. Carcinoma of the vulva. *J Epidemiol Biostat* 1998;3:111.

420. Sturgeon SR, Brinton LA, Devesa SS, et al. In situ and invasive vulvar cancer incidence trends (1973–1987). *Am J Obstet Gynecol* 1992;166:1482.

421. Iversen T, Tretli S. Intraepithelial and invasive squamous cell neoplasia of the vulva: trends in incidence, recurrence, and survival rate in Norway. *Obstet Gynecol* 1998;91:969.

422. Ansink AC, Krul MR, De Weger RA, et al. Human papillomavirus, lichen sclerosus, and squamous cell carcinoma of the vulva: detection and prognostic significance. *Gynecol Oncol* 1994;52:180.

423. Bloss JD, Liao SY, Wilczynski SP, et al. Clinical and histologic features of vulvar carcinomas analyzed for human papillomavirus status: evidence that squamous cell carcinoma of the vulva has more than one etiology. *Hum Pathol* 1991;22:711.

424. Crum CP. Carcinoma of the vulva: epidemiology and pathogenesis. *Obstet Gynecol* 1992;79:448.

425. Hording U, Junge J, Daugaard S, et al. Vulvar squamous cell carcinoma and papillomaviruses: indications for two different etiologies. *Gynecol Oncol* 1994;52:241.

426. Monk BJ, Burger RA, Lin F, et al. Prognostic significance of human papillomavirus (HPV) DNA in primary invasive vulvar cancer. *Obstet Gynecol* 1995;85:709.

427. Crum CP, McLachlin CM, Tate JE, et al. Pathobiology of vulvar squamous neoplasia. *Curr Opin Obstet Gynecol* 1997;9:63.

428. Trimble CL, Hildesheim A, Brinton LA, et al. Heterogeneous etiology of squamous carcinoma of the vulva. *Obstet Gynecol* 1996;87:59.

429. Haefner HK, Tate JE, McLachlin CM, et al. Vulvar intraepithelial neoplasia: age, morphological phenotype, papillomavirus DNA, and coexisting invasive carcinoma. *Hum Pathol* 1995;26:147.

430. Lee YY, Wilczanski SP, Chumakov A, et al. Carcinoma of the vulva: HPV and p53 mutations. *Oncogene* 1994;9:1655.

431. Pilotti S, D'Amato L, Della Torre G, et al. Papillomavirus, p53 alteration, and primary carcinoma of the vulva. *Diagn Mol Pathol* 1995;4:239.

432. Sliutz G, Schmidt W, Tempfer C, et al. Detection of p53 point mutations in primary human vulvar cancer by PCR and temperature gradient gel electrophoresis. *Gynecol Oncol* 1997;64:93.

433. Andreasson B, Nyboe J. Predictive factors with reference to low-risk of metastases in squamous cell carcinoma in the vulvar region. *Gynecol Oncol* 1985;21:196.

434. Binder SW, Huang I, Fu YS, et al. Risk factors for the development of lymph node metastasis in vulvar squamous cell carcinoma. *Gynecol Oncol* 1990;37:9.

435. Hacker NF, Berek JS, Lagasse LD, et al. Individualization of treatment for stage I squamous cell vulvar carcinoma. *Obstet Gynecol* 1984;63:155.

436. Hoffman JS, Kumar NB, Morley GW. Microinvasive squamous carcinoma of the vulva: search for a definition. *Obstet Gynecol* 1983;61:615.

437. Ross MJ, Ehrmann RL. Histologic prognosticators in stage I squamous cell carcinoma of the vulva. *Obstet Gynecol* 1987;70:774.

438. Micheletti L, Preti M, Zola P, et al. A proposed glossary of terminology related to the surgical treatment of vulvar carcinoma. *Cancer* 1998;83:1369.

439. Levenback C, Coleman RL, Burke TW, et al. Intraoperative lymphatic mapping and sentinel node identification with blue dye in patients with vulvar cancer. *Gynecol Oncol* 2001;83:276.

440. Ridley CM, Frankman O, Jones IS, et al. New nomenclature for vulvar disease: report of the Committee on Terminology of the International Society for the Study of Vulvar Disease. *J Reprod Med* 1990;35:483.

441. Buscema J, Woodruff JD. Progressive histobiologic alterations in the development of vulvar cancer. *Am J Obstet Gynecol* 1980;138:146.

442. Brainard JA, Hart WR. Proliferative epidermal lesions associated with anogenital Paget's disease. *Am J Surg Pathol* 2000;24:543.

443. Koss LG, Brockunier AJ. Ultrastructural aspects of Paget's disease of the vulva. *Arch Pathol* 1969;87:592.

444. Fanning J, Lambert HC, Hale TM, et al. Paget's disease of the vulva: prevalence of associated vulvar adenocarcinoma, invasive Paget's disease, and recurrence after surgical excision. *Am J Obstet Gynecol* 1999;180:24.

445. Hart WR, Millman JB. Progression of intraepithelial Paget's disease of the vulva to invasive carcinoma. *Cancer* 1977;40:2333.

446. Gil-Moreno A, Garcia-Jimenez A, Gonzalez-Bosquet J, et al. Merkel cell carcinoma of the vulva. *Gynecol Oncol* 1997;64:526.

447. Japese H, van Dinh T, Woodruff JD. Verrucous carcinoma of the vulva: study of 24 cases. *Obstet Gynecol* 1982;60:462.

448. Irvin WP, Cathro HP, Grosh WW, et al. Primary breast carcinoma of the vulva: a case report and literature review. *Gynecol Oncol* 1999;73:155.

449. Feakins RM, Lowe DG. Basal cell carcinoma of the vulva: a clinicopathologic study of 45 cases. *Int J Gynecol Pathol* 1997;16:319.

450. Carlson JW, McGlennen RC, Gomez R, et al. Sebaceous carcinoma of the vulva: a case report and review of the literature. *Gynecol Oncol* 1996;60:489.

451. Weinstock MA. Malignant melanoma of the vulva and vagina in the United States: patterns of incidence and population-based estimates of survival. *Am J Obstet Gynecol* 1994;171:1225.

452. Ragnarsson-Olding BK, Kanter-Lewensohn LR, Lagerlof B, et al. Malignant melanoma of the vulva in a nationwide, 25-year study of 219 Swedish females: clinical observations and histopathologic features. *Cancer* 1999;86:1273.

453. Ragnarsson-Olding BK, Nilsson BR, Kanter-Lewensohn LR, et al. Malignant melanoma of the vulva in a nationwide, 25-year study of 219 Swedish females: predictors of survival. *Cancer* 1999;86:1285.

454. Verschraegen CF, Benjapibal M, Supakarapongkul W, et al. Vulvar melanoma at the MD Anderson Cancer Center: 25 years later. *Int J Gynecol Cancer* 2001;11:359.

455. Chung AF, Woodruff JM, Lewis JLJ. Malignant melanoma of the vulva: a report of 44 cases. *Obstet Gynecol* 1975;45:638.

456. Tasseron EWK, van der Esch EP, Hart AAM, et al. A clinicopathological study of 30 melanomas of the vulva. *Gynecol Oncol* 1992;46:170.

457. Curtin JP, Saigo P, Slucher B, et al. Soft-tissue sarcoma of the vagina and vulva: a clinicopathologic study. *Obstet Gynecol* 1995;86:269.

458. Nirenberg A, Östör AG, Slavin J, et al. Primary vulvar sarcomas. *Int J Gynecol Pathol* 1995;14:55.

459. Bernstein SG, Kovac BR, Townsend DE, et al. Vulvar carcinoma in situ. *Obstet Gynecol* 1983;61:304.

460. Kuppers V, Stiller M, Somville T, et al. Risk factors for recurrent VIN. Role of multifocality and grade of disease. *J Reprod Med* 1997;42:140.

461. Cohn DE, Dehdashti F, Gibb RK, et al. Prospective evaluation of positron emission tomography for the detection of groin node metastases from vulvar cancer. *Gynecol Oncol* 2002;85:179.

462. Boyce J, Fruchter RG, Kasambilides E, et al. Prognostic factors in carcinoma of the vulva. *Gynecol Oncol* 1985;20:364.

463. Homesley HD, Bundy BN, Sedlis A, et al. Prognostic factors for groin node metastasis in squamous cell carcinoma of the vulva (a Gynecologic Oncology Group study). *Gynecol Oncol* 1993;49:279.

464. Sedlis A, Homesley H, Bundy BN, et al. Positive groin lymph nodes in superficial squamous cell vulvar cancer. A Gynecologic Oncology Group study. *Am J Obstet Gynecol* 1987;156:1159.

465. Heaps JM, Fu YS, Montz FJ, et al. Surgical-pathologic variables predictive of local recurrence in squamous cell carcinoma of the vulva. *Gynecol Oncol* 1990;38:309.

466. Homesley HD, Bundy BN, Sedlis A, et al. Assessment of current International Federation of Gynecology and Obstetrics staging of vulvar carcinoma relative to prognostic factors for survival (a Gynecologic Oncology Group study). *Am J Obstet Gynecol* 1991;164:997.

467. Husseinzadeh N, Wesseler T, Schellhas H, et al. Significance of lymphoplasmacytic infiltration around tumor cell in the prediction of regional lymph node metastases in patients with invasive squamous cell carcinoma of the vulva: a clinico-pathologic study. *Gynecol Oncol* 1989;34:200.

468. Husseinzadeh N, Wesseler T, Schneider D, et al. Prognostic factors and the significance of cytologic grading in invasive squamous cell carcinoma of the vulva: a clinicopathologic study. *Gynecol Oncol* 1990;36:192.

469. Hopkins MP, Reid GC, Vettrano I, et al. Squamous cell carcinoma of the vulva: prognostic factors influencing survival. *Gynecol Oncol* 1991;43:113.

470. Pinto AP, Signorello LB, Crum CP, et al. Squamous cell carcinoma of the vulva in Brazil: prognostic importance of host and viral variables. *Gynecol Oncol* 1999;74:61.

471. Smyczek-Gargya B, Volz B, Geppert M, et al. A multivariate analysis of clinical and morphological prognostic factors in squamous cell carcinoma of the vulva. *Gynecol Obstet Invest* 1997;43:261.

472. Mariani L, Conti L, Atlante G, et al. Vulvar squamous carcinoma: prognostic role of DNA content. *Gynecol Oncol* 1998;71:159.

473. Homesley HD, Bundy BN, Sedlis A, et al. Radiation therapy versus pelvic node resection for carcinoma of the vulva with positive groin nodes. *Obstet Gynecol* 1986;68:733.

474. van der Velden J, Lindert ACM, Lammes FB, et al. Extracapsular growth of lymph node metastases in squamous cell carcinoma of the vulva. The impact on recurrence and survival. *Cancer* 1995;75:2885.

475. Origoni M, Sideri M, Garsia S, et al. Prognostic value of pathological patterns of lymph node positivity in squamous cell carcinoma of the vulva stage III and IVA FIGO. *Gynecol Oncol* 1992;45:313.

476. Katz A, Eifel PJ, Jhingran A, et al. The role of radiation therapy in preventing regional recurrences of invasive squamous cell carcinoma of the vulva. *Int J Radiat Oncol Biol Phys* 2003;57:409.

477. Faul CM, Mirmow D, Huang Q, et al. Adjuvant radiation for vulvar carcinoma: improved local control. *Int J Radiat Oncol Biol Phys* 1997;38:381.

478. Jhingran A, Levenback C, Katz A, et al. Radiation therapy for vulvar carcinoma: predictors of vulvar recurrence. *Int J Radiat Oncol Biol Phys* 2003;57:S193.

479. Taussig FJ. Cancer of the vulva: an analysis of 155 cases. *Am J Obstet Gynecol* 1940;40:764.

480. Hacker NF, Leuchter RS, Berek JS, et al. Radical vulvectomy and bilateral inguinal lymphadenectomy through separate groin incisions. *Obstet Gynecol* 1981;58:574.

481. Burke TW, Stringer CA, Gershenson DM, et al. Radical wide excision and selective inguinal node dissection for squamous cell carcinoma of the vulva. *Gynecol Oncol* 1990;38:328.

482. Farias-Eisner R, Cirisano FD, Grouse D, et al. Conservative and individualized surgery for early squamous carcinoma of the vulva: the treatment of choice for stage I and II (T1-2 N0-1 M0) disease. *Gynecol Oncol* 1994;53:55.

483. Magrina JF, Gonzalez-Bosquet J, Weaver AL, et al. Primary squamous cell cancer of the vulva: radical versus modified radical vulvar surgery. *Gynecol Oncol* 1998;71:116.

484. Grimshaw RN, Murdoch JB, Monaghan JM. Radical vulvectomy and bilateral inguinal–femoral lymphadenectomy through separate incisions—experience with 100 cases. *Int J Gynecol Cancer* 1993;3:18.

485. Burke TW, Levenback C, Coleman RL, et al. Surgical therapy of T1 and T2 vulvar carcinoma: further experience with radical wide excision and selective inguinal lymphadenectomy. *Gynecol Oncol* 1995;57:215.

486. Grimshaw RN, Ghazal Aswad S, Monaghan JM. The role of ano-vulvectomy in locally advanced carcinoma of the vulva. *Int J Gynecol Cancer* 1991;1:15.

487. Hoffman MS, Cavanagh D, Roberts WS, et al. Ultraradical surgery for advanced carcinoma of the vulva: an update. *Int J Gynecol Cancer* 1993;3:369.

488. Perez CA, Grigsby PW, Chao C, et al. Irradiation in carcinoma of the vulva: factors affecting outcome. *Int J Radiat Oncol Biol Phys* 1998;42:335.

489. Boronow RC. Combined therapy as an alternative to exenteration for locally advanced vulvo-vaginal cancer: rationale and results. *Cancer* 1982;49:1085.

490. Fairey RN, MacKay PA, Benedet JL, et al. Radiation treatment of carcinoma of the vulva, 1950–1980. *Am J Obstet Gynecol* 1985;151:591.

491. Hacker NF, Berek JS, Juillard GJF, et al. Preoperative radiation therapy for locally advanced vulvar cancer. *Cancer* 1984;54:2056.

492. Han SC, Kim DH, Higgins SA, et al. Chemoradiation as primary or adjuvant treatment for locally advanced carcinoma of the vulva. *Int J Radiat Oncol Biol Phys* 2000;47:1235.

493. Akl A, Akl M, Boike G, et al. Preliminary results of chemoradiation as a primary treatment for vulvar carcinoma. *Int J Radiat Oncol Biol Phys* 2000;48:415.

494. Moore DH, Thomas GM, Montana GS, et al. Preoperative chemoradiation for advanced vulvar cancer: a phase II study of the Gynecologic Oncology Group. *Int J Radiat Oncol Biol Phys* 1998;42:79.

495. Cunningham MJ, Goyer RP, Gibbons SK, et al. Primary radiation, cisplatin, and 5-fluorouracil for advanced squamous carcinoma of the vulva. *Gynecol Oncol* 1997;66:258.

496. Landoni F, Maneo A, Zanetta G, et al. Concurrent preoperative chemotherapy with 5-fluorouracil and mitomycin C and radiotherapy (FUMIR) followed by limited surgery in locally advanced and recurrent vulvar carcinoma. *Gynecol Oncol* 1996;61:321.

497. Lupi G, Raspagliesi F, Zucali R, et al. Combined preoperative chemoradiotherapy followed by radical surgery in locally advanced vulvar carcinoma. A pilot study. *Cancer* 1996;77:1472.

498. Wahlen SA, Slater JD, Wagner RJ, et al. Concurrent radiation therapy and chemotherapy in the treatment of primary squamous cell carcinoma of the vulva. *Cancer* 1995;75:2289.

499. Eifel PJ, Morris M, Burke TW, et al. Preoperative continuous infusion cisplatinum and 5-fluorouracil with radiation for locally advanced or recurrent carcinoma of the vulva. *Gynecol Oncol* 1995;59:51.

500. Koh WJ, Wallace HJ, Greer BE, et al. Combined radiotherapy and chemotherapy in the management of local-regionally advanced vulvar cancer. *Int J Radiat Oncol Biol Phys* 1993;26:809.

501. Russell AH, Mesic JB, Scudder SA, et al. Synchronous radiation and cytotoxic chemotherapy for locally advanced or recurrent squamous cancer of the vulva. *Gynecol Oncol* 1992;47:14.

502. Scheistroen M, Trope C. Combined bleomycin and irradiation in preoperative treatment of advanced squamous cell carcinoma of the vulva. *Acta Oncol* 1992;32:657.

503. Berek JS, Heaps JM, Fu YS, et al. Concurrent cisplatin and 5-fluorouracil chemotherapy and radiation therapy for advanced-stage squamous cancer of the vulva. *Gynecol Oncol* 1991;42:197.

504. Thomas G, Dembo A, DePetrillo A, et al. Concurrent radiation and chemotherapy in vulvar carcinoma. *Gynecol Oncol* 1989;34:263.

505. Iversen T. Irradiation and bleomycin in the treatment of inoperable vulval carcinoma. *Acta Obstet Gynecol Scand* 1982;61:195.

506. Cummings B. Anal canal carcinomas. In: Meyer JL, Vaeth JM, eds. *Frontiers in radiation oncology.* Basel: Karger, 1992:131.

507. Benedetti-Panici P, Greggi S, Scambia G, et al. Cisplatin, bleomycin, and methotrexate preoperative chemotherapy in locally advanced vulvar carcinoma. *Gynecol Oncol* 1993; 50:49.
508. Petereit DG, Mehta MP, Buchler DA, et al. A retrospective review of nodal treatment for vulvar cancer. *Am J Clin Oncol* 1993;16:38.
509. Podratz KC, Symmonds RE, Taylor WF. Carcinoma of the vulva: analysis of treatment failures. *Am J Obstet Gynecol* 1982;143:340.
510. Stehman FB, Bundy BN, Thomas G, et al. Groin dissection versus groin radiation in carcinoma of the vulva: a Gynecologic Oncology Group study. *Int J Radiat Oncol Biol Phys* 1992;24:389.
511. Henderson RH, Parsons JT, Morgan L, et al. Elective ilioinguinal lymph node irradiation. *Int J Radiat Oncol Biol Phys* 1984;10:811.
512. Leiserowitz GS, Russell AH, Kinney WK, et al. Prophylactic chemoradiation of inguinofemoral lymph nodes in patients with locally extensive vulvar cancer. *Gynecol Oncol* 1997;66:509.
513. Eifel PJ. Vulvar carcinoma: radiotherapy or surgery for the lymphatics? *Front Radiat Ther Oncol* 1994;28:218.
514. Koh WJ, Chiu M, Stelzer KJ, et al. Femoral vessel depth and the implications for groin node radiation. *Int J Radiat Oncol Biol Phys* 1993;27:969.
515. Stehman FB, Bundy BN, Dvoretsky PM, et al. Early stage I carcinoma of the vulva treated with ipsilateral superficial inguinal lymphadenectomy and modified radical hemivulvectomy: a prospective study of the Gynecologic Oncology Group. *Obstet Gynecol* 1992; 79:490.
516. Levenback C, Morris M, Burke TW, et al. Groin dissection practices among gynecologic oncologists treating early vulvar cancer. *Gynecol Oncol* 1996;62:73.
517. Ansink AC, Sie-Go DM, van der Velden J, et al. Identification of sentinel lymph nodes in vulvar carcinoma patients with the aid of a patent blue V injection: a multicenter study. *Cancer* 1999;86:652.
518. Bowles J, Terada KY, Coel MN, et al. Preoperative lymphoscintigraphy in the evaluation of squamous cell cancer of the vulva. *Clin Nucl Med* 1999;24:235.
519. Levenback C, Burke TW, Morris M, et al. Potential applications of intraoperative lymphatic mapping in vulvar cancer. *Gynecol Oncol* 1995;59:216.
520. Terada KY, Coel MN, Ko P, et al. Combined use of intraoperative lymphatic mapping and lymphoscintigraphy in the management of squamous cell cancer of the vulva. *Gynecol Oncol* 1998;70:65.
521. Deppe G, Cohen C, Bruckner H. Chemotherapy of squamous cell carcinoma of the vulva: a review. *Gynecol Oncol* 1979;7:345.
522. Yahia C, Fuller AF, Cloud LP. Successful long-term palliation of stage IV vulvar carcinoma with operation and bleomycin sulfate. *Am J Obstet Gynecol* 1978;130:360.
523. Thigpen JT, Blessing JA, Homesley H, et al. Phase II trials of cisplatin and piperazinedione in advanced or recurrent squamous cell carcinoma of the vulva: a Gynecologic Oncology Group study. *Gynecol Oncol* 1986;23:358.
524. Wagenaar HC, Colombo N, Vergote I, et al. Bleomycin, methotrexate, and CCNU in locally advanced or recurrent, inoperable, squamous-cell carcinoma of the vulva: an EORTC Gynaecological Cancer Cooperative Group Study. European Organization for Research and Treatment of Cancer. *Gynecol Oncol* 2001;81:348.

SECTION 2

THOMAS W. BURKE
ARNO J. MUNDT
FRANCO M. MUGGIA

Cancers of the Uterine Body

ENDOMETRIAL CARCINOMA

CLINICAL OVERVIEW

Tumors of the uterine fundus comprise the most common group of gynecologic malignancies. Annual incidence figures for the United States have remained stable at approximately 36,000 cases during the last decade. Deaths from disease occur in 6000 women per year.[1] The large proportion of survivors with these cancers reflects a disease course characterized by early onset of symptoms and well-established diagnostic guidelines. Nevertheless, women with high-risk or advanced disease have a poor prognosis and account for the most uterine cancer deaths.

A general classification of uterine fundal cancers is provided in Table 32.2-1. Approximately 90% of tumors arise within the epithelium of the uterine lining and are categorized as endometrial carcinomas. Within this group, 90% of cancers are typical endometrial adenocarcinomas.[2] The typical endometrial carcinomas are further subdivided into three architectural grades based on the percentage of solid tumor growth: Grade 1 cancers have identifiable endometrial glands and are well differentiated, whereas grade 3 tumors demonstrate a solid growth pattern and are poorly differentiated. Rare cell types, including papillary serous carcinoma, clear cell carcinoma, papillary endometrioid carcinoma, and mucinous carcinoma, account for the remaining 10% of cases. Adenosquamous carcinomas are now classified as typical endometrial adenocarcinomas with squamous differentiation. In general, all of these uncommon cell types are associated with a later age of onset, greater risk for extrauterine metastases, and poorer prognosis when compared with typical grade 1 adenocarcinomas.[3-6]

EPIDEMIOLOGY

The normal endometrium is a hormonally responsive tissue. Estrogenic stimulation produces cellular growth and glandular proliferation, which is cyclically balanced by the maturational effects of progesterone.[7] Abnormal proliferation and neoplastic transformation of the endometrium have been associated with chronic unopposed exposure to estrogenic stimulation. It is currently believed that estrogen-associated endometrial cancers progress through a premalignant stage described as *atypical adenomatous hyperplasia*. This phase is characterized by increases in gland number and complexity as well as cytologic atypia. Although serial observations of women with adenomatous hyperplasia are scarce, it is estimated that at least one-third of such patients progress to carcinoma.[8]

The best-recognized risk factors for the development of endometrial carcinoma can be related to chronic estrogen exposure. These include oral intake of exogenous estrogen (without progestins), estrogen-secreting tumors, low parity, extended periods of anovulation, early menarche, and late menopause.[9-11] Because menarche and menopause are commonly associated with absent or irregular ovulation, women who experience early onset or late cessation of ovarian function are more likely to have additional estrogenic exposure.[12] Morbidly obese women also have a greater risk of endometrial cancer, presumably because their adipocytes are able to con-

TABLE 32.2-1. Classification of Uterine Fundal Cancer

Tumor Type	Approximate Frequency (%)
Epithelial tumors (endometrioid, papillary endometrioid, papillary serous, clear cell, mucinous)	90
Mesenchymal tumors (endometrial stromal sarcoma, leiomyosarcoma, other nonspecific sarcomas)	5
Mixed tumors (malignant mixed müllerian, adenosarcoma)	3
Secondary tumors (metastasis, direct local extension: cervix, ovary, colon)	2

TABLE 32.2-2. Epidemiologic Risk Factors for
Endometrial Carcinoma

Factors	Relative Risk
CHRONIC ESTROGENIC STIMULATION	
Estrogen replacement (no progestin)	2–12
Early menarche/late menopause	1.6–4.0
Nulliparity	2–3
Anovulation	ND
Estrogen-producing tumors	ND
DEMOGRAPHIC CHARACTERISTICS	
Increasing age	4–8
White race	2
High socioeconomic status	1.3
European/North American country	2–3
Family history of endometrial cancer	2
ASSOCIATED MEDICAL ILLNESS	
Diabetes mellitus	3
Gallbladder disease	3.7
Obesity	2–4
Hypertension	1.5
Prior pelvic radiotherapy	8

ND, no data.
(Table compiled from multiple sources.)

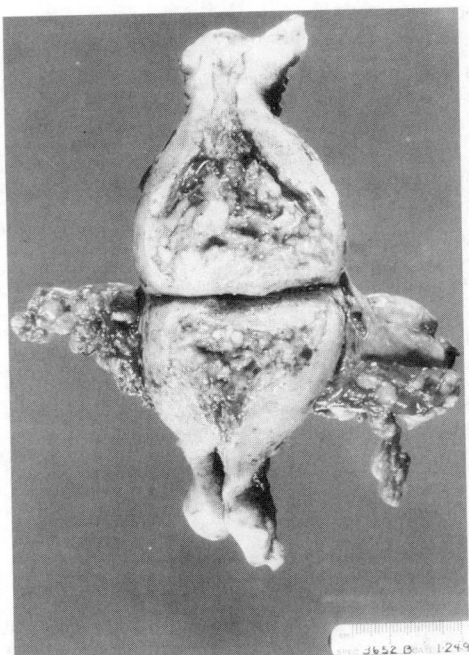

FIGURE 32.2-1. Endometrial cancers develop as polypoid lesions gradually expand to fill the uterine cavity. This well-differentiated tumor involves the anterior and the posterior uterine walls throughout the entire fundus. Scattered areas of superficial necrosis give rise to the hallmark symptom of postmenopausal bleeding.

vert androstenedione of adrenal origin to estrone, a weak circulating estrogen.

Epidemiologic studies have consistently identified women with diabetes mellitus and hypertension as having an increased risk of endometrial carcinoma. This risk remains independent of other known factors in multivariate analysis. Epidemiologic risk factors for endometrial cancer are listed in Table 32.2-2.

The potential connection between long-term tamoxifen use as adjuvant therapy for breast cancer and the development of endometrial cancers has been attributed to its estrogen agonist properties. This observation has raised concerns about the safety of such therapy in therapeutic and breast cancer prevention trials.[13–15] On the basis of current information, it seems reasonable to conclude that (1) if an association between tamoxifen and endometrial carcinoma exists, the overall risk is small compared with the risk of recurrent breast cancer, and (2) women receiving long-term tamoxifen therapy should be monitored carefully for uterine abnormalities. Any woman with abnormal vaginal bleeding should be evaluated promptly by biopsy. Exposure to adjuvant tamoxifen therapy should be limited to 5 years. The development and use of new selective estrogen receptor modulators that do not have stimulatory effects on the endometrium should eliminate all such risk for women who may benefit from antiestrogen therapy.

NATURAL HISTORY AND ROUTES OF SPREAD

Endometrial carcinoma is a disease of postmenopausal women. The average age at diagnosis is approximately 60 years. All endometrial lesions originate in the glandular component of the uterine lining. Their initial growth forms a polypoid mass within the uterine cavity (Fig. 32.2-1). This tumor mass is friable and often contains areas of superficial necrosis. Consequently, postmenopausal bleeding is the hallmark symptom for more than 90% of patients. Because most women and their

physicians recognize that this is an ominous finding, prompt diagnosis is common.

The primary tumor may extend to involve a greater proportion of the endometrial surface and ultimately extends to the lower uterine segment and cervix. Invasion into the myometrium occurs simultaneously. The uterus has a rich and complex lymphatic network. Channels draining the superior portion of the fundus parallel the ovarian vessels and empty into the paraaortic lymph nodes in the upper abdomen. Lymphatics from the middle and lower portions of the uterus travel through the broad ligaments to the pelvic nodes. A few small lymphatic vessels course through the round ligaments to the superficial inguinal nodes. As a result of this extensive network, nodal metastases can occur at any level and in any combination.[16]

Tumors that penetrate the uterine serosa may directly invade adjacent tissues, such as the bladder, colon, or adnexa, or they may exfoliate into the abdominal cavity to form implant metastases. Small tumor fragments may also gain access to the peritoneal cavity by traversing the fallopian tubes. However, the clinical importance of this potential mechanism of spread is uncertain. Hematogenous dissemination is observed but uncommon. Sites of distant spread include lung, liver, bone, and brain.

DIAGNOSIS AND PRETHERAPY EVALUATION

A diagnosis of endometrial carcinoma should be considered in postmenopausal women with any vaginal bleeding, perimenopausal women with heavy or prolonged bleeding, and premenopausal women with abnormal bleeding patterns who are obese or oligo-ovulatory. Although a formal dilatation and

TABLE 32.2-3. Frequency of Recurrence in Patients with Positive Risk Factors

Positive Risk Factor	Frequency of Recurrence[a]			Comment
	Radiation Therapy	No Radiation Therapy	Total (%)	
SPECIFIC FACTOR				
Pelvic node	4/16 (1P)	1/2 (1P)	5/18 (27.7)	—
Aortic node	0/2	2/3	2/5 (40.0)	—
Adnexa	1/5	0/2	1/7 (14.3)	—
Gross disease	1/2	0/2	1/4 (25.0)	—
Cytology	5/18 (1P)	1/14	6/32 (18.8)	2/4 With implants only
CSI	8/30	1/4	9/34 (26.5)	0/2 With implants only
Isthmus/cervix	8/65 (2P, 3V)	7/29 (4P, 1V)	15/94 (16.0)	0/8 With implants only
TOTAL[b]				
One factor	27/138 (19.6%)	12/56 (21.4%)	39/194 (20.1)	2/140 With implants only
Two factors	25/58 (4P, 1V)	6/14 (1P, 1V)	31/72 (20.1)	0/2 With implants only
Three or more factors	24/42 (5P, 1V)	13/18 (5P, 2V)	38/60 (63.3)	—

CSI, capillary-like space involvement; P, pelvic recurrence; V, vaginal recurrence.
[a]Number of cases with recurrence/total number in group.
[b]Twenty-eight patients with one positive factor did not have sufficient follow-up. Eighteen patients with two or more positive factors did not have sufficient follow-up.
(From ref. 21, with permission.)

curettage has been the standard technique for diagnosis, outpatient endometrial biopsy has replaced it in most situations.[17] A correctly performed endometrial biopsy includes an adequate amount of tissue obtained from multiple passes through the uterus, and it has a diagnostic accuracy equivalent to that of surgical curettage under anesthesia. Asymptomatic women with endometrial cancer occasionally have abnormal glandular components detected by routine cervical cytology. However, fewer than 50% of women with known endometrial cancer have an abnormal Papanicolaou smear.[18]

Endometrial carcinoma is a surgically treated and staged tumor. Consequently, the focus of the pretreatment evaluation is on the detection of unresectable disease and a determination of operative risk. For patients with disease that is clinically limited to the uterus by physical examination, a straightforward evaluation that includes laboratory studies, a chest radiograph, and an electrocardiogram is adequate. A serum CA 125 assay may be predictive of occult extrauterine disease and may be useful as a tumor marker.[19] More sophisticated imaging studies, such as ultrasound, computed tomography, intravenous pyelography, and magnetic resonance imaging, rarely provide information that is not determined after surgical exploration. These studies should be reserved for patients with advanced disease or prohibitive surgical risks. Many women with endometrial cancer are elderly and have associated medical conditions, particularly obesity, diabetes, and hypertension. The pretreatment medical evaluation should be individualized based on findings obtained from the medical history and general physical examination.

RISK FACTORS

Histopathologic risk factors have been extensively evaluated since the late 1970s.[20,21] Major prognostic factors associated with the uterine component of the tumor are grade or cell type, depth of myometrial invasion, and tumor extension to the cervix. Less important are extent of uterine cavity involvement,[22] lymph–vascular space invasion,[23] and tumor vascularity. Obvi-

ously, women whose tumors have spread beyond the uterus have a poorer prognosis. The major extrauterine risk factors are adnexal metastases, pelvic or paraaortic lymph node spread, positive peritoneal cytology, peritoneal implant metastases, and distant organ metastases.

A detailed risk analysis of nearly 1000 patients by the Gynecologic Oncology Group (GOG) is summarized in Table 32.2-3.[21] The risk for development of recurrent disease was greatest in women whose tumors had metastasized to pelvic or paraaortic lymph nodes, demonstrated gross intraperitoneal spread, or contained unequivocal lymph–vascular space invasion. An exceptionally high incidence of recurrence was noted in patients with two or more risk factors. Based on the findings of this and other surgical staging trials, the International Federation of Gynecology and Obstetrics (FIGO) adopted a surgical staging system for uterine fundal cancers in 1988.

In addition to the more classic histologic risk factors, several studies have examined archival specimens to evaluate a number of potential molecular markers. Data suggesting a prognostic role for DNA ploidy, S-phase fraction, oncogenes, tumor suppressor genes, AgNOR, and nuclear morphometric features should be considered preliminary.[24–27] Data reported by Lim et al.[28] note that some tumors are aneuploid or overexpress p53.

Endometrial tumors are a component of some of the cancer family syndromes identified and evaluated by Lynch et al.[29] Within these unique families, the risk of developing endometrial cancer may approach 50%. Endometrial cancer is also more common in women with a previous cancer of the breast, colon, or ovary. Dual neoplasms may occur simultaneously or metachronously with diagnostic time intervals as long as 10 years.[15]

STAGING

The clinical staging system used before 1988 stratified patients with early disease on the basis of a fractional biopsy specimen from the endocervix and the endometrium as well as the depth of the uterine cavity and physical examination (Table 32.2-4).

TABLE 32.2-4.   Clinical Staging of Uterine Fundal Tumors[a]

Stage	Description
I	The tumor is limited to the uterine fundus.
IA	The uterine cavity measures ≤8 cm.
IB	The length of the uterine cavity is >8 cm.
II	The tumor extends to the uterine cervix.
III	The tumor has spread to the adjacent pelvic structures.
IV	There is bulky pelvic disease or distant spread.
IVA	Tumor invades the mucosa of the bladder or rectosigmoid.
IVB	Distant metastases are present.

[a]International Federation of Gynecology and Obstetrics, 1988.

These techniques for assessment of disease volume and spread were found to be erroneous in as many as one-third of cases when compared with histopathologic findings at the time of laparotomy.[30] Women with small volume disease in retroperitoneal nodes or the peritoneal cavity were rarely identified during clinical staging. The clinical system was abandoned because the accumulating data from surgical staging reports was more accurate and allowed stratification of similar risk groups for adjuvant and adjunctive therapy trials. The surgical staging system approved at the 1988 FIGO meeting is currently used for most patients with uterine fundal cancers (Table 32.2-5). Risk factors incorporated into this system include depth of myometrial invasion, tumor extension to the cervix, tumor spread to adnexal organs, peritoneal cytology, retroperitoneal lymph node metastases, and spread to abdominal or distant sites. The clinical staging criteria have been retained for patients who do not undergo surgical exploration as a part of their initial treatment.

TREATMENT OF PRIMARY DISEASE

Surgical Resection and Operative Staging

Resection of the primary tumor by total abdominal hysterectomy and bilateral salpingo-oophorectomy is the mainstay of therapy

TABLE 32.2-5.   Surgical Staging of Uterine Fundal Tumors[a]

Stage	Description
I	The tumor is confined to the uterine fundus.
IA	The tumor is limited to the endometrium.
IB	The tumor invades less than one-half of the myometrial thickness.
IC	The tumor invades more than one-half of the myometrial thickness.
II	The tumor extends to the cervix.
IIA	Cervical extension is limited to the endocervical glands.
IIB	The tumor invades the cervical stroma.
III	There is regional tumor spread.
IIIA	The tumor invades the uterine serosa or adnexa, or there is positive peritoneal cytology.
IIIB	Vaginal metastases are present.
IIIC	The tumor has spread to pelvic or paraaortic lymph nodes.
IV	There is bulky pelvic disease or distant spread.
IVA	Tumor invades the mucosa of the bladder or rectosigmoid.
IVB	Distant metastases are present.

[a]International Federation of Gynecology and Obstetrics, 1988.

for uterine cancers. Because endometrial cancer originates in the fundus, adequate surgical margins can usually be achieved by simple extrafascial hysterectomy. Salpingo-oophorectomy is recommended because the ovary is a relatively common site of occult metastasis and because most women are already postmenopausal and no longer have hormonal function from the organ. Removal of the uterus is curative treatment for most stage I cases. The more extensive radical hysterectomy has been recommended for selected patients with gross tumor involvement of the cervix.[31] However, combined therapy, using external-beam pelvic irradiation and extrafascial hysterectomy, is more frequently used in such cases.[32] The increased expansion of endoscopic surgery has permitted its application in endometrial cancer. The staging portion of the operation is performed endoscopically followed by a transvaginal hysterectomy. Among surgical teams skilled in these techniques, the results appear to be equivalent to those obtained by open laparotomy.[33] Some evidence also suggests that aggressive cytoreduction may improve survival in women with extrauterine disease.[34]

The surgical staging system for uterine fundal tumors identifies certain histopathologic prognostic features for stage and substage assignment but does not define a specific surgical approach required to accomplish staging. The additional operative procedures associated with surgical staging produce a small, but definite, increase in operative risk. Most reported complications are related to organ injury during biopsy or hemorrhage from vascular injury during node sampling.[35,36] Patients who have extensive intraperitoneal staging procedures also have a greater risk of bowel injury if they receive postoperative external irradiation.[37]

Some advocate an extended staging procedure for all women with endometrial cancer. The authors' approach has been to limit surgical staging to patients at risk for occult disease spread. Staging procedures are routinely performed in women with grade 2 or 3 adenocarcinomas and those with variant histologic tumor types. For patients with grade 1 adenocarcinoma, the authors estimate the depth of myometrial invasion intraoperatively by making a visual estimate[38] and evaluating a frozen section (Fig. 32.2-2). Extended staging procedures are only performed when significant myometrial invasion (more than 50%) is identified. Using this stratified approach to surgical staging minimizes surgical risk for patients with low-risk tumors while maximizing the chance for detecting occult extrauterine disease in those patients at risk (Fig. 32.2-3).

An equally important question is what procedures constitute an adequate staging effort. After the collection of cytology specimens and completion of the hysterectomy, the staging assessment is focused on two general areas—the peritoneal cavity and the retroperitoneal lymph nodes. Evaluation of the peritoneal cavity begins with a careful visual and palpatory inspection. Abnormal areas from peritoneal or serosal surfaces are biopsied. Cytology or histology samples, or both, are also taken from the diaphragm. A portion of the omentum is removed. When the authors examined their peritoneal staging procedures in a group of at-risk women, they found that occult peritoneal spread is relatively uncommon.[39] Although directed biopsy of palpably suspicious areas often detected metastatic disease, random biopsies were rarely positive. Peritoneal cytology and omental biopsy, coupled with directed biopsy from abnormal sites, provided accurate and reliable information regarding intraperitoneal disease.

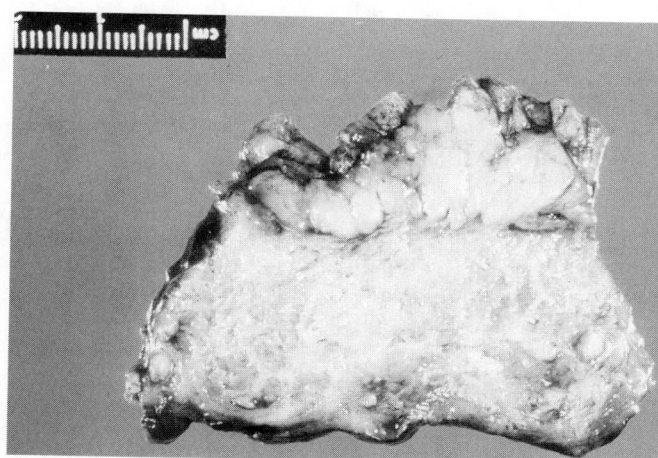

FIGURE 32.2-2. The depth of myometrial invasion can be estimated by visually examining a cut section of the uterine wall taken at the level of the tumor. A clear line distinguishes polypoid tumor growth from myometrium in this surgical specimen. The accuracy of intraoperative visual estimates can be enhanced by using frozen-section analysis in selected cases.

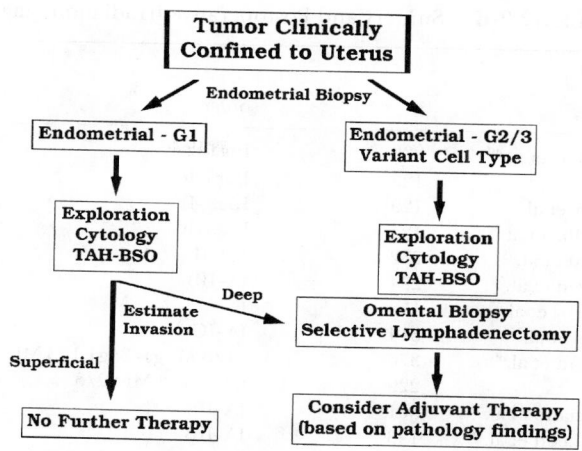

FIGURE 32.2-3. Schematic representation of a staging algorithm. Patients with grade 1 (G1) typical endometrial adenocarcinoma have an exploratory laparotomy with peritoneal cytology, total abdominal hysterectomy (TAH), and bilateral salpingo-oophorectomy (BSO). The depth of myometrial invasion and extension to the cervix are evaluated intraoperatively. Those with low-risk features have no further therapy, whereas those with high-risk features undergo an extended staging operation. All patients with high-risk features undergo an extended staging operation. All patients with grade 2 or 3 (G2/3) endometrial tumors and those with variant histologic types (papillary serous, papillary endometrioid, clear cell) undergo an extended staging procedure.

Detecting retroperitoneal lymph node spread is a potentially difficult problem. Various techniques for lymph node evaluation have been proposed, including palpation with biopsy of abnormal nodes, single lymph node biopsy, selective lymphadenectomy, and full node dissection. The authors believe that a systematic and selective approach to lymphadenectomy reliably detects occult metastases and accurately portrays the true lymph node status.[40] More limited approaches are clearly less accurate. The suggestion by Kilgore et al.[41] that complete lymphadenectomy may carry a therapeutic advantage deserves further investigation.

The primary goal of surgical staging is to provide an accurate assessment of disease spread at the time therapy is initiated. For patients with tumors confined to the uterus, those in the low-risk subgroup (grade 1 tumor with superficial myometrial invasion) are adequately treated by hysterectomy alone. Fortunately, such cases account for most women with endometrial cancer. Women with tumors demonstrating high-risk features have an incidence of recurrent disease of 25% to 40% and are excellent candidates for adjuvant therapy trials. Patients with more advanced disease warrant additional postoperative adjunct treatment.

Radiotherapy

HISTORICAL PERSPECTIVE. Once surgical therapy is complete, the patient's individual risk profile can be identified and used to design an adjuvant therapy plan. In 1935, Heyman[42] described the "Stockholm method" of radium packing in a cohort of women treated at the Radiumhemmet between 1914 and 1928. The 5-year survival rate of 58.2% reported in early-stage disease compared favorably to contemporary surgical series, demonstrating the curative potential of radiation in this disease. Radiation soon became commonplace in the treatment of endometrial cancer. Today, radiation is delivered almost exclusively after surgery in patients found to have adverse pathologic features in the hysterectomy specimen. High dose-rate brachytherapy and intensity-modulated radiotherapy are recent modifications that reduce hospitalization and treatment sequelae.[43,44]

PREOPERATIVE IRRADIATION. Arguments offered in favor of preoperative irradiation in uterine cancer include cytoreduction before hysterectomy, reduced spread of viable tumor cells at surgery, and improved treatment tolerance. Other putative benefits include irradiation of well-oxygenated tumors and better treatment delivery. Arguments against its use include overtreatment of low-risk patients and loss of prognostic pathologic information in the hysterectomy specimen. The latter concern, however, has been addressed by operating within 2 to 3 days instead of delaying surgery for 4 to 6 weeks.

Preoperative irradiation is associated with excellent pelvic control and survival rates in women with clinical stage I disease. Pelvic failure rates range from 2.3% to 9.6%.[45–47] Five-year survival rates range from 71.0% to 91.4%. Sause et al.[48] compared outcomes of clinical stage I patients treated with and without preoperative irradiation. Although no overall differences were noted, patients with grade 3 tumors treated with preoperative irradiation had a superior 5-year recurrence-free survival (76% vs. 53%) than those undergoing primary surgery.[48]

A stronger rationale exists for preoperative irradiation in stage II disease, particularly in patients with gross cervical involvement. Kinsella et al.[32] reported 5-year disease-free and overall survival rates of 83% and 75% in 40 stage II patients treated with preoperative irradiation. Patients with low-grade tumors or microscopic cervical involvement, or both, have the best outcomes.

Preoperative irradiation is delivered via intracavitary brachytherapy, pelvic radiotherapy, or both. The preferred method in stage I disease is brachytherapy alone, typically given in one insertion. Weigensberg[46] randomized stage I patients to preoperative brachytherapy or pelvic irradiation. Patients who received brachytherapy had a lower rate of residual uterine disease (50.9% vs. 70.0%) and pelvic failure (3.6% vs. 12.7%).

TABLE 32.2-6. Surgery and Postoperative Irradiation Stage I to II Endometrial Carcinoma

Study	n	Stage	Radiotherapy	Recurrence (%) Vagina	Recurrence (%) Pelvis	5-Y Survival (%)
Alektiar et al.[49]	233	IBg1–2	VB	—	4	94
Boz et al.[50]	125	IAg3–IC	P	—	4	88
Carey et al.[51]	129	IBg3–II[a]	P±VB	—	3.9	81
Chadha et al.[52]	124	IBg3–IC	VB	—	0	93
Elliott et al.[53]	232	Ig3–II	VB±P	0–10.1	—	>80
Greven et al.[54]	294	IA–IIB	±VB,VB	3.7	0.7	86
Grigsby et al.[45]	152	I	P±VB,VB	2.0	0.6	82.3[b]
Irwin et al.[55]	314	IA–IC	VB,P±VB	—	5–6	79–82
Kucera et al.[56]	376	<1/3 MI g1–3; g1 1/3 MI	VB	0.3	0.8	91.8
	229	g2–3, 1/3 MI >2/3	WP+VB	0	1.3	97.8
Lanciano et al.[57]	301	IA–IIB	P/E±VB,VB	—	4–36[c]	87–100
MacLeod et al.[58]	143	IA–IIB	VB	1.4	—	86–94
Mayr et al.[59]	115	I–II	P±VB, VB	—	2.5	65–86
Meerwaldt et al.[60]	389	IA–IC	P/E±VB,VB	—	6	67 (10-y)
Nori et al.[61]	300	I–II	VB±P	—	2	96.6
Petereit et al.[62]	191	IBg1–IC[d]	VB	0	—	95 (4-y)
Pitson et al.[63]	143	IIA–IIB	P±VB, VB	—	5.6	77[e]
Weiss et al.[64]	159	I–II	P+VB	—	0	77–92 (DFS)
Weiss et al.[68]	61	IC	P	0	1.6	86.7 (DFS)

DFS, disease-free survival; E, extended-field radiotherapy; g, grade; MI, myometrial invasion; NS, not stated; P, pelvic radiotherapy; VB, vaginal brachytherapy.
[a]Includes some patients with adenosquamous histology.
[b]Includes patients treated with preoperative irradiation.
[c]Pelvic recurrence: 4% to 12% stage I, 11% stage IIA, 36% stage IIB.
[d]Majority of patients had stage IBg1 to 2 disease.
[e]Includes some nonirradiated patients.

Toxicities were more common after pelvic irradiation.[46] In contrast, stage II patients receive pelvic radiotherapy as well as intracavitary brachytherapy.

Traditionally, preoperative brachytherapy has been performed using low dose-rate techniques, consisting of a Fletcher-Suit-Delclos tandem and ovoids, often combined with Heyman-Simon uterine capsules. A total intrauterine dose of 3000 to 5500 mg-hr is prescribed, whereas the vaginal apex receives 60 to 70 Gy. When pelvic radiotherapy (40 to 45 Gy) is administered, the intrauterine dose is reduced (2500 mg-hr).

POSTOPERATIVE IRRADIATION

Stage I to II Disease. Few issues in the management of endometrial cancer are as contentious as the role of postoperative irradiation in women with early-stage disease. When administered, controversy exists over how radiotherapy should be performed in these patients. Most investigators recommend adjuvant irradiation in early-stage patients based on pathologic features, notably myometrial invasion, grade, and cervical involvement. Numerous series have focused on early-stage patients treated with postoperative irradiation (Table 32.2-6). These reports vary greatly, with some including only patients with low-grade, minimally invasive tumors; whereas others focus on patients with high-grade disease, deep myometrial invasion, and/or cervical involvement. In some, vaginal brachytherapy is used; in others, all patients undergo pelvic irradiation. Despite such differences, pelvic/vaginal control rates exceed 95% in the great majority of reports. Five-year survival rates range from 82.3% to 98.9% for stage I and 72.0% to 85.4% for stage II disease.

Several investigators have compared outcomes of irradiated versus nonirradiated early-stage patients treated at their centers. Although fraught with potential biases, such analyses provide indirect support for adjuvant radiotherapy. In 157 stage I to II patients with high-risk features (deep invasion, grade 3, cervical involvement) treated with postoperative irradiation, Carey et al.[51] noted a local-regional recurrence rate of 3.9%. In contrast, 14.3% of patients who did not receive radiotherapy because of protocol violations had recurrence in the pelvis. Elliott et al.[53] evaluated the outcome of 927 stage I to II patients. In low-risk patients (stage I, grade 1 to 2, less than 1/3 invasion), vaginal recurrences were seen in 0% and 3.2% of women with and without brachytherapy. In high-risk patients, vaginal recurrences were noted in 1.1% and 11.7% of patients with and without adjuvant irradiation. Corresponding failure rates in stage II patients were 0% and 12.8%. In 170 stage II patients, Pitson et al.[63] noted pelvic recurrences in 5.6% and 22.2% of patients with and without postoperative irradiation.

Three prospective phase III trials have been conducted evaluating postoperative irradiation in early-stage disease. The first was performed in Norway and published in 1980.[65] Eligible patients had clinical stage I disease and underwent primary surgery without lymph node sampling. Excluding those with extrauterine disease, 540 patients received postoperative vaginal brachytherapy and were randomized to no further therapy versus pelvic radiotherapy. No difference was seen in the 5-year survival rates between the two groups. However, pelvic irradiation reduced the risk of vagina/pelvic recurrence in women with deep myometrial invasion (14.7% control, 6.6% pelvic radiotherapy) and high-grade disease (14.1% control, 3.2%

pelvic radiotherapy). Chronic toxicities were seen in 1.2% and 0.8% of patients with and without pelvic irradiation.

GOG trial No. 99 (GOG-99) was presented in 1998.[66] Four hundred forty-eight stage IB, IC, and occult II patients underwent primary surgery with pelvic and paraaortic lymph node sampling and were then randomized to pelvic radiotherapy or no further therapy. At a median follow-up of 56 months, irradiated patients had a superior 2-year relapse-free survival (96% vs. 88%, P = .004). Seventeen surgery-only patients had recurrence in the vagina/pelvis versus three in the surgery plus radiotherapy group. The 2-year pelvic relapses of patients with and without adjuvant irradiation were 2% and 12%, respectively (P = .001). Although irradiated patients had a higher 3-year survival (96% vs. 89%), this difference did not reach statistical significance (P = .09). Grade 3 to 4 complications were more common in the irradiated group (15% vs. 6%, P = .007).

Creutzberg et al.[67] reported the results of the PORTEC (Post Operative Radiation Therapy in Endometrial Carcinoma) trial. All patients underwent primary surgery without nodal sampling. Eligible women had grade 1 tumors with greater than 50% myometrial invasion, grade 2 tumors, and grade 3 tumors with less than 50% invasion. Seven hundred fifteen women were randomized to receive either pelvic irradiation or no further therapy. At a median follow-up of 52 months, irradiated patients had superior 5-year pelvic control (96% vs. 86%, P <.001). However, no difference was noted in overall survival (81% irradiated group, 85% control group). Treatment sequelae were more common in irradiated patients (25% vs. 6%, P <.001).

These trials clearly demonstrate that adjuvant irradiation reduces the risk of pelvic failure in early-stage patients with adverse pathologic features. Numerous questions remain unanswered. It is unclear whether survival is also improved. The lack of a survival benefit has led some investigators to withhold radiotherapy, even in patients with adverse pathologic features. The GOG trial *included* many low-risk patients (58% IB, 82% grade 1 to 2), whereas PORTEC *excluded* high-risk ones (stage IC grade 3, stage II). Therefore, one trial included women who were least likely to benefit from treatment, whereas the other excluded those most likely to benefit.

The optimal approach in early-stage patients who receive postoperative irradiation also remains unclear. Vaginal brachytherapy alone may be equally efficacious as pelvic radiotherapy. The more favorable toxicity profile of vaginal brachytherapy is certainly appealing. Given the large numbers needed to conduct a trial comparing vaginal brachytherapy and pelvic radiotherapy, however, such a trial is unlikely to ever be performed.

The decision as to whether to irradiate an individual patient rests on a careful assessment of the benefits and risks of treatment. The likelihood of cure and toxicity after adjuvant irradiation needs to be weighed against the likelihood of salvage and toxicity if treatment is withheld. If administered, the approach that maximizes tumor control while minimizing toxicity should be selected. The least aggressive approach should always be used if outcome is not compromised.

Stage IA and IB grade 1 to 2 patients are considered low risk and are not irradiated at most centers. Given the low risk of lymph node spread, pelvic irradiation would only expose such patients to untoward toxicity without benefit. Most investigators irradiate stage IA grade 3 patients. At some centers, vaginal brachytherapy is used; at others, patients receive pelvic radio-

therapy. Stage IB grade 2 disease is treated by some investigators with pelvic radiotherapy; others recommend vaginal brachytherapy. Given the excellent pelvic control and low toxicity associated with brachytherapy alone, it is clearly the preferred approach, particularly in surgically staged patients. Stage IB grade 3 patients are at risk for pelvic metastases and vaginal recurrence and typically undergo pelvic irradiation as well as vaginal brachytherapy. However, pelvic irradiation alone is associated with excellent pelvic control rates with less toxicity. Most radiation oncologists irradiate all stage IC patients, using pelvic radiotherapy. In a review of 541 stage I patients with deep myometrial invasion from 12 published studies, Weiss et al.[68] noted vaginal recurrences in 1.04% of patients undergoing pelvic irradiation alone versus 0.97% of patients receiving pelvic irradiation and vaginal brachytherapy.

At most centers, stage II patients receive pelvic radiotherapy and vaginal brachytherapy.[51,53,68] Stage II disease represents a heterogeneous group. Some patients have low-grade tumors with minimal myometrial invasion and only cervical glandular involvement. Excellent outcomes have been achieved in such patients with pelvic radiotherapy alone. Patients with deep myometrial invasion, high-grade tumors, and cervical stromal invasion should undergo pelvic radiotherapy and vaginal brachytherapy. In addition, promising results have been reported with brachytherapy alone in select stage II patients.[58]

An increasing number of stage I to II patients will most likely receive chemotherapy in addition to adjuvant radiotherapy. The Radiation Therapy Oncology Group is currently conducting a phase III trial (RTOG 99-05) of pelvic radiotherapy versus pelvic radiotherapy plus concurrent cisplatin (followed by cisplatin-paclitaxel) in stage IC grade 2 to 3 and stage II disease.

Pelvic radiotherapy is typically delivered via a four-field approach (anterior, posterior, and lateral fields). Doses of 45.0 to 50.4 Gy in 1.8- to 2.0-Gy fractions are prescribed, preferably with high-energy (10 to 24 mV) photons. Vaginal brachytherapy is delivered with colpostats or a vaginal cylinder. If low dose-rate techniques are used, 60 to 70 Gy is prescribed to the mucosal surface over approximately 72 hours. In women undergoing pelvic irradiation, 25 to 35 Gy is administered. Various high dose-rate approaches have been used. The American Brachytherapy Society recommended dose-fractionation schedules in patients treated with high dose-rate brachytherapy alone include 7 Gy × 3, 5.5 Gy × 4, and 4.7 Gy × 5 (specified at 0.5-cm depth). If prescribed to the vaginal surface, 10.5 Gy × 3, 8.8 Gy × 4, and 7.5 Gy × 5 are recommended. When combined with pelvic radiotherapy, 5.5 Gy × 2 or 4 Gy × 3 (at 0.5 cm) or 8 Gy × 2 or 6 Gy × 3 (at the vaginal surface) is recommended.[69]

Stage III to IV Disease. Postoperative irradiation has been used in the treatment of stage III to IV patients for many years. Patients with disease limited to the pelvis received pelvic irradiation with and without vaginal brachytherapy. Patients with more extensive disease were treated with more comprehensive volumes, including extended-field and whole abdominal irradiation. Table 32.2-7 summarizes the results of adjuvant radiotherapy studies in stage III to IV disease. These studies span the entire spectrum of locally advanced disease and treatment approaches, including phosphorus 32, extended-field, and whole abdominal radiotherapy. Some include patients also treated with chemotherapy or hormonal therapy. Outcomes vary widely, with the best results seen in stage IIIA disease. The

TABLE 32.2-7.   Surgery and Postoperative Radiotherapy, Stage III to IV Endometrial Carcinoma

Study	n	Stage	Extrauterine Site(s)[a]	Radiation Therapy	5-Y Survival (%)
Connell et al.[70]	12	IIIA	Adnexa only	P±VB	70.9 (DFS)
Corn et al.[71]	26	IIIC	PA nodes	E	46 (DFS)[b]
Greven et al.[74]	74	III	Various	P±VB	54
	42	IIIA	Adnexa only	P±VB	60
	8	IIIA	Cytology only	P±VB	60
	5	IIIC	Pelvic nodes only	P±VB	50
Greven et al.[75]	105	III	Various	P/E±VB	70
	70	IIIA	Various	P±VB	68 (DFS)
	3	IIIB	Vagina	P±VB	50 (DFS)
	32	IIIC	Pelvic/PA nodes	P/E±VB	56 (DFS)
Lee et al.[76]	11	IV	Various	W±VB	45.4 (DFS)[c]
Mundt et al.[77]	30	IIIC	Pelvic/PA nodes	P/E/W±VB	55.8
Nelson et al.[78]	17	IIIC	Pelvic nodes	P/W±VB	72
Onda et al.[79]	30	IIIC	Pelvic/PA nodes	P/E	84
Schorge et al.[80]	35	IIIA–B	Various	P±VB[d]	40
	22	IIIC	Pelvic/PA nodes	P/E±VB	50
Smith et al.[81]	22	III–IV	Various	W±VB	89 (3-y)

DFS, disease-free survival; E, extended-field radiotherapy; MS, median survival; P, pelvic radiotherapy; PA, paraaortic radiotherapy; VB, vaginal brachytherapy; W, whole abdominal radiotherapy.
[a]Predominant site of involvement (designated as solitary if specified by the author).
[b]Includes some patients with radiographic-positive involved paraaortic lymph nodes.
[c]Crude result.
[d]Some patients received a portion of the treatment before surgery.

least favorable outcomes are seen in stage III to IV patients with involvement of multiple extrauterine sites or residual disease in the upper abdomen, or both.

Positive peritoneal cytology has been considered a risk factor for abdominal relapse, leading some investigators to recommend whole abdominal irradiation. Considerable interest has also focused on intraperitoneal phosphorus 32 in this setting. Of 20 patients with positive cytology treated by Creasman et al.[72] with phosphorus 32 (15 mCi), only three had recurrences. In a subsequent article, a 2-year disease-free survival of 94% was reported by these same investigators in 43 clinical stage I patients with isolated positive cytology after phosphorus 32. Interest in these approaches has waned in light of reports refuting the prognostic significance of positive cytology in the absence of other adverse features.[82] Moreover, significant gastrointestinal toxicities have been noted in patients who receive phosphorus 32 as well as external-beam radiotherapy. Stage IIIA patients with adnexal involvement have been included in numerous irradiation series. Women with isolated adnexal involvement represent a favorable group, with survivals exceeding 70% in most reports. Due to concerns over abdominal relapse, whole abdominal irradiation has been used. However, others have reported equally favorable results using pelvic irradiation alone.[70]

Concerns over abdominal relapse have also led some investigators to recommend whole abdominal irradiation in stage IIIA patients with serosal involvement.[73,74] However, the benefit of this approach remains unclear, particularly in patients without involvement of other extrauterine sites. Stage IIIB disease is rare. These patients are usually clinically staged and undergo preoperative (or definitive) irradiation.[75]

Adjuvant irradiation in stage IIIC disease has received considerable attention. Numerous authors have reported long-term cures in women with positive paraaortic nodes after extended-field irradiation, with 5-year survivals ranging from

36.4% to 84.0%.[71,79] Patients with pelvic nodal involvement alone represent a favorable group. Nelson et al.[78] treated 17 stage IIIC patients who had positive pelvic (and negative paraaortic) nodes with pelvic or whole abdominal radiotherapy. The 5-year disease-free and overall survivals of the entire group were 81% and 72%, respectively.[78]

Patients with involvement of multiple extrauterine sites pose a therapeutic challenge. In a review of stage III patients, Greven et al.[75] noted abdominal failures in 10% and 25% of women with involvement of one versus three or more extrauterine sites ($P = .03$), supporting a role for whole abdominal radiotherapy in the latter group. Promising results have been reported using whole abdominal irradiation in these as well as in stage IV patients.[76,79] Greer and Hamberger[73] noted a 5-year survival of 80% in 27 optimally debulked stage III patients undergoing whole abdominal irradiation. In 22 stage III to IV patients treated with whole abdominal irradiation, Smith et al.[81] noted 3-year disease-free and overall survivals of 79% and 89%, respectively. The GOG conducted a phase II trial (GOG-94) of whole abdominal irradiation in stage III to IV disease. After surgery with optimal debulking, 77 stage III to IV patients received adjuvant whole abdominal irradiation. The 3-year progression-free and overall survivals of the entire group were 35% and 31%, respectively.[83]

No prospective phase III trial has been performed comparing surgery versus surgery plus postoperative irradiation in any subgroup of stage III to IV disease. Thus, the benefit of *any* form of adjuvant irradiation in these patients remains unclear. Indirect evidence supporting a role for radiotherapy in these individuals is, however, derived from nonrandomized reports. In GOG-33, Morrow et al.[21] noted a local-regional control benefit in irradiated patients with high-risk features (positive nodes, adnexal involvement, capillary lymphatic invasion, isthmus/cervical involvement, positive cytology, and/or gross extrapelvic disease). Local-regional failure was seen in 14.2% and 38.7% of women with two and three high-risk factors after surgery alone. Corresponding failure rates in irradiated patients were 8.6% and 14.2%.[21]

The benefit of adjuvant irradiation is most evident in stage III patients with nodal involvement. Rose et al.[84] noted 3-year survivals of 60% and 0% in 17 stage IIIC patients treated with and 9 patients without extended-field radiotherapy. In contrast, Schorge et al.[80] noted a significantly worse survival in stage IIIA/B patients treated with (40%) versus without (70%) adjuvant radiotherapy (*P* = .003).

Interest is shifting increasingly away from postoperative radiotherapy toward systemic chemotherapy in stage III to IV disease. The GOG has completed a large randomized trial (GOG-122) comparing adjuvant radiotherapy versus chemotherapy in these patients. Patients with optimally debulked stage III to IV received either whole abdominal irradiation or doxorubicin-cisplatin. At a median follow-up of 52 months, chemotherapy patients had better 2-year disease-free (59% vs. 46%) and overall (70% vs. 59%) survivals. Recurrences were frequent, predominantly in the pelvis and abdomen in both groups.[85] The future role of adjuvant radiotherapy in stage III to IV disease remains unclear. Although select stage III patients may benefit from radiotherapy alone, current interest focuses on combined chemoradiotherapy approaches. Promising results have been seen in small series of stage IIIC patients using the combined modality approach.[79]

Techniques and dosing of pelvic radiotherapy and vaginal brachytherapy in stage III to IV patients are identical to those used in stage I to II disease, except in those with vaginal involvement who require more comprehensive volumes. Extended-field radiotherapy is delivered with opposed anterior-posterior fields extending to the top of T10. Doses of 45.0 to 50.4 Gy are prescribed in 1.8- to 2.0-Gy fractions. Whole abdominal irradiation is administered at most centers via opposed anterior-posterior fields extending 2 cm above the diaphragm and laterally beyond the peritoneal fat strip. Posterior 5 half-value-layer kidney blocks are placed limiting the renal dose to 18 Gy. Some centers include blocks over the liver and heart. Doses of 20 to 30 Gy in 1.0- to 1.5-Gy daily fractions are used. The pelvis is boosted to 45 to 50 Gy. Higher doses to the paraaortic region, pelvis, and vagina are possible using the Martinez technique.[86]

UNFAVORABLE HISTOLOGIC TYPES. The role of radiation therapy in patients with unfavorable histologies (papillary serous, clear cell, adenosquamous) is controversial. Since the initial observation by Hendrickson et al.[5] of the propensity of papillary serous tumors to relapse in the abdomen, attention has focused primarily on whole abdominal irradiation. In a study of 26 patients (80% papillary serous), Smith et al.[81] noted a 3-year disease-free and overall survival of 87% and 87% in stage I to II and 32% and 61% in stage III to IV patients. Three had recurrences in the upper abdomen.[81]

No prospective phase III trial evaluating whole abdominal irradiation in papillary serous tumors has been conducted. Its benefit in these patients thus remains unclear. A phase II study of whole abdominal irradiation was conducted by the GOG (GOG-94) and enrolled 88 papillary serous/clear cell patients. The 5-year survivals of stage I to II and III to IV patients were 65% and 33%, respectively.[83]

The benefit of whole abdominal irradiation is particularly unclear in stage I to II papillary serous patients. In a review of 193 stage I to II patients from nine studies, Mehta et al.[87] noted abdominal failure in 6 of 68 patients (9%) treated with versus 10 of 125 patients (8%) treated without whole abdominal irradiation. A benefit in pelvic control was seen, however, with the use of pelvic or vaginal irradiation, or both.[87] Given these patients' high risk of distant failure, a reasonable approach may be chemotherapy combined with pelvic or vaginal irradiation, or both. In fact, promising results have been reported using such an approach.[88]

Fewer data are available evaluating the role of radiation therapy in clear cell carcinoma. These tumors are often simply grouped with papillary serous tumors and treated with whole abdominal irradiation, even when confined to the uterus.[81,86] Because few series report the outcome of clear cell tumors separately, the benefit of this approach remains unclear. Murphy et al.[89] reviewed the outcome of 38 clear cell patients treated with primary surgery. Pelvic recurrence was seen in 0 of 22 patients treated with versus 8 of 16 (50%) without adjuvant irradiation (*P* <.0001). Corresponding pelvic recurrence rates in stage I to II patients with and without adjuvant irradiation were 0 of 16 versus 5 of 6 (83%; *P* <.0001).

RADIOTHERAPY ALONE. Although most patients with endometrial cancer are treated with surgery, a subset of women cannot undergo surgery because of multiple medical comorbidities or advanced age, or both. These patients are often treated with radiation therapy alone, with curative intent. In addition, patients with locally advanced disease may undergo radiation alone. The most favorable results are seen in clinical stage I disease, with 5-year survival rates ranging from 51.5% to 76.8%.[90–94] Five-year cause-specific survival rates in stage II patients range from 50.2% to 88.0%. In contrast, series of clinical stage III patients report survival rates below 50%, even after controlling for intercurrent deaths. Pelvic/uterine control rates are high in most patients, particularly in stage I disease (greater than 80%).

Definitive irradiation is delivered by a variety of approaches. Early-stage patients, particularly those with low-grade disease, are treated with intracavitary brachytherapy alone due to their low risk of extrauterine involvement. Women with high-grade tumors or more advanced-stage disease, or both, receive a combination of pelvic irradiation and intracavitary brachytherapy. Brachytherapy is an essential component of definitive radiotherapy. Patanaphan et al.[94] noted 5-year survival rates of 67% and 33% in clinical stage I patients undergoing pelvic radiotherapy with and without intracavitary brachytherapy. Corresponding rates in clinical stage II disease were 43% and 0%, respectively.[94]

Definitive irradiation is often performed with low dose-rate techniques, consisting of a Fletcher-Suit-Delclos tandem, ovoids, and, except in women with small uterine cavities, Heyman-Simon uterine capsules. Doses of 5000 to 7500 mg-hr are delivered over two to three insertions. If combined with pelvic irradiation, the intrauterine dose is limited to 4000 to 4500 mg-hr. Most patients are treated today with high dose-rate brachytherapy, with comparable outcomes. Various dose-fractionation approaches have been used. The American Brachytherapy Society recommended that dose-fractionation schedules in women treated with definitive high dose-rate brachytherapy include 8.5 Gy × 4, 7.3 Gy × 5, 6.4 Gy × 6, and 5.7 Gy × 7. In patients who are also receiving pelvic radiotherapy, 8.5 Gy × 2, 6.3 Gy × 3, or 5.2 Gy × 4 can be used. All doses are specified at 2 cm from the midpoint of the intrauterine sources.

PALLIATIVE RADIATION THERAPY. Palliative radiotherapy is effective in endometrial cancer patients with bone or brain metastases. Palliation can also be achieved with hypofractionated approaches in women with symptomatic locally advanced disease. Onsrud et al.[95] administered one to three fractions of 10 Gy to the pelvis over 4 weeks in 64 patients with locally advanced disease (42% endometrial cancer). A significant benefit was achieved, with cessation of bleeding noted in 90% of women. Overall, 56% experienced no significant acute toxicities. Serious chronic sequelae developed in 6%; however, all late complications appeared 9 to 10 months after treatment.[95]

TREATMENT SEQUELAE. Although acute toxicity is common in patients with endometrial cancer who are undergoing pelvic irradiation, it is generally mild and self-limited. In a review of 317 patients receiving postoperative pelvic or vaginal irradiation, or both, Jereczek-Fossa et al.[96] noted acute toxicities in 84%. Grade 1 to 2 bowel and bladder sequelae occurred in 71.2% and 39.5% of patients. Corresponding rates of grade 3 to 4 toxicities were 5.6% and 0.8%. Six patients (2%) required premature termination of treatment. Treatment interruptions were found in 11%.[96] Weiss et al.[64] noted acute toxicity in 65.4% of 159 stage I to II patients undergoing adjuvant pelvic irradiation. Fourteen (8.8%) required treatment breaks and 8 (5%) had their treatment terminated. Acute toxicities are more common in women undergoing extended-field and whole abdominal irradiation.

Less attention has been focused on acute sequelae in patients undergoing intracavitary brachytherapy. Although preoperative and postoperative brachytherapy are well tolerated, medically inoperable patients may experience significant acute sequelae in light of their advanced age and poor health. Of 96 medically inoperable patients undergoing 150 low dose-rate intracavitary insertions, Chao et al.[97] noted life-threatening acute toxicities in four women, including two with myocardial infarction, one with congestive heart failure, and one with pulmonary embolus. Overall, the morbidity and mortality were 4.2% and 2.1%.[97] High dose-rate brachytherapy in this population may also result in significant acute toxicity.[98]

Numerous investigators have evaluated chronic toxicities in irradiated endometrial cancer patients. Corn et al.[99] noted severe chronic sequelae in 13 of 235 (6%) endometrial cancer patients treated with postoperative pelvic irradiation ± vaginal brachytherapy. The significant factors associated with late sequelae were age, lymph node sampling, and treatment with one field per day. In patients treated with multiple fields per day, lymph node sampling remained correlated with increased toxicity. Creutzberg et al.[100] evaluated chronic sequelae in patients enrolled on the PORTEC trial. Of 338 patients receiving postoperative radiotherapy, late sequelae were noted in 85 (25%); most (89%) were grade 1 to 2 and related to the gastrointestinal tract. Overall, the 5-year actuarial risk of grade 3 to 4 late sequelae was 3%.[100] Other factors correlated with chronic toxicities after pelvic irradiation include vaginal brachytherapy, pelvic lymphadenectomy, and acute sequelae. Chronic toxicities (primarily gastrointestinal) are more common and significant in patients treated with extended-field and whole abdominal irradiation.

Pre- and postoperative brachytherapy are generally well tolerated, particularly when delivered without pelvic radiotherapy. In most series, postoperative vaginal brachytherapy is associated with significant chronic sequelae in 2% or fewer of patients, using either low dose-rate or high dose-rate techniques. In high dose-rate brachytherapy, the risk of serious sequelae is highly dependent on the dose per fraction and the volume of treatment. Nori and coworkers noted 8.2% and 10.1% significant late bladder and rectal toxicity in 404 patients treated with postoperative high dose-rate vaginal brachytherapy. Late toxicities occurred in 11.2%, 24.2%, and 87.5% of patients treated with 4.5 Gy × 6, 5 Gy × 6, and 9 Gy × 4, respectively.[61] Vaginal stenosis and dyspareunia are relatively common in women treated with vaginal brachytherapy.

INTENSITY-MODULATED RADIOTHERAPY. A novel approach to treatment planning has been introduced, known as *intensity-modulated radiotherapy* (IMRT). IMRT conforms the prescription dose to the shape of the target in three dimensions, thereby sparing nearby normal tissues. Unlike conventional approaches, IMRT planning is an inverse process, whereby the target and normal tissues are delineated on a computed tomography scan. Dose-volume constraints of the target and normal tissues are entered into a computerized optimization program that generates the plan to best satisfy these goals. During the optimization process, each beam is divided into small "beamlets" whose intensity is varied to achieve the desired dose distribution. When cast into a patient, the resultant beams result in highly conformal dose distributions with rapid-dose gradients that allow considerable sparing of neighboring tissues.

Endometrial cancer therapy is an ideal application of IMRT. Conventional fields (pelvic radiotherapy, extended field, etc.) result in the irradiation of a considerable volume of normal tissues exposing patients to acute and chronic sequelae. Normal tissue sparing may allow the delivery of higher than conventional doses in select patients, a strategy that could enhance tumor control.

Several investigators have compared IMRT and conventional planning in gynecology patients undergoing pelvic irradiation. In ten patients (five endometrial cancer), Roeske and colleagues noted that IMRT planning reduced the volume of small bowel irradiated to the prescription dose by a factor of 2 and the volumes of rectum and bladder each by 23% compared with conventional techniques.[43] IMRT can also be used to spare the pelvic bone marrow, an appealing approach given the increasing use of chemotherapy in these patients.[101] Data also suggest a benefit to IMRT planning in patients undergoing extended-field[102] and whole abdominal irradiation.[103]

Mundt et al. have provided a series of detailed analyses of acute and chronic toxicity in patients treated with intensity-modulated pelvic radiotherapy. Acute sequelae were evaluated in 40 IMRT patients (40% endometrial cancer) and compared with sequelae seen in patients undergoing conventional pelvic radiotherapy.[105] IMRT patients experienced less grade 2 or greater acute gastrointestinal toxicity (60% vs. 91%; $P = .002$) than conventional patients. In a separate report, these investigators noted that reductions in the volume of pelvic bone marrow irradiated achieved with IMRT planning translates into less hematologic toxicity in patients receiving chemoradiotherapy.[104] Mundt et al.[105] have reported that patients treated with intensity-modulated pelvic radiotherapy experience less chronic gastrointestinal toxicity as well.

Although promising, gynecologic applications of IMRT are preliminary. To date, no analyses of tumor control or patterns of failure in gynecology patients treated with IMRT have been published. Clearly, more patients and longer follow-up are needed to assess pelvic control in treated patients. Standards are also needed regarding *how* IMRT is planned and delivered in these patients. A particularly important area is target design.

Postoperative Systemic Treatment (Adjuvant Therapy)

Interest is shifting increasingly away from postoperative radiotherapy toward (adjuvant) systemic chemotherapy in stage III to IV disease. Two phase III trials have been reported comparing adjuvant radiotherapy to chemotherapy. The Italian Cooperative Group trial included 340 stage IC to IIB (grade 3) and stage IIIA to C (any grade) patients. After surgery, patients were randomized to pelvic radiotherapy versus chemotherapy (cisplatin, doxorubicin, and cyclophosphamide). Although overall and progression-free survivals were not reported, no difference was seen in the overall failure rate. Although a lower rate of pelvic-only failure was noted favoring irradiated patients (5% vs. 10%), this difference failed to reach statistical significance ($P = .09$).[106]

GOG-122 randomized optimally debulked stage III to IV patients to either whole abdominal irradiation or doxorubicin-cisplatin. At a median follow-up of 52 months, chemotherapy patients had better 2-year disease-free (59% vs. 46%) and overall (70% vs. 59%) survivals. Recurrences were frequent, predominantly in the pelvis and abdomen in both groups.[107]

Combined chemoradiotherapy approaches, such as the ongoing GOG trial in optimally debulked stage III to IV patients (GOG-184) involving pelvic ± paraaortic irradiation followed by either cisplatin-doxorubicin or cisplatin-doxorubicin-paclitaxel, are gaining favor. These approaches are supported by the high local-regional failure rate seen in the chemotherapy-alone arm of GOG-122 and in earlier retrospective series of patients treated with chemotherapy alone.

The demonstration that systemic chemotherapy has the potential to improve survival (as compared to radiation in one large study by the GOG) has led to its use in stages III and IV and increasingly in the more localized stages if poor prognostic features are documented (e.g., papillary serous histology, poorly differentiated tumors). After it was shown that a combination of doxorubicin and cisplatin led to fewer recurrences than whole abdominal radiation, the GOG embarked on a trial of radiation to tumor sites followed by either the above doublet chemotherapy or the addition of paclitaxel to the doublet. Hormonal therapy, on the other hand, does not have a role in the localized stages. Reports of progestin therapy alone as primary treatment for endometrial carcinoma in an effort to preserve childbearing potential in premenopausal women have been noteworthy.[108] In the stage I postoperative setting, however, randomized studies have failed to demonstrate a benefit for medroxyprogesterone acetate (MPA), whether given by itself or with radiation, versus no adjuvant or only radiation.[109,110] This is not surprising, because tumors that are expected to benefit from progestogen therapy are primarily well differentiated and associated with low likelihood of recurrence even without adjuvant treatment.

Cytotoxic chemotherapy must also be considered as an adjuvant treatment in certain circumstances when the risk of distant recurrence exceeds 20%. These circumstances include (1) any stage II tumor, (2) clear cell or papillary serous histology, (3) absence of hormone receptors, (4) preoperative finding of elevated CA 125, and (5) selected stage I disease with deep myometrial invasion. Justification for the use of such postoperative adjuvant treatment relates to encouraging results from combination chemotherapy reported in pilot studies.[111,112] A randomized study of doxorubicin as single agent after surgery and radiation in high-risk stage I and occult stage II cancers showed no improvement in outcome from the adjuvant treatment.[113]

TREATMENT OF RECURRENT DISEASE

Treatment Failure

Treatment failure in low-risk patients is exceedingly rare. In the authors' series investigating surveillance strategies, only one failure occurred in this group.[114] Tumor recurrence is most common in women with advanced-stage disease or those with high-risk features in their primary tumor. Late recurrence is uncommon, and virtually all failures are clinically evident within 3 years of original diagnosis.[115]

One-half of patients whose tumors recur are symptomatic. A targeted examination and diagnostic evaluation should readily lead to the correct diagnosis. The remaining group with treatment failure have their recurrence detected during routine surveillance. Most recurrences are detected by physical examination. Serum CA 125 levels may be useful in monitoring patients for the development of recurrent disease, especially those who have papillary serous carcinomas or intraperitoneal disease. Follow-up intervals of 6 to 12 months coupled with prompt evaluation of symptomatic patients seem to be an appropriate approach to surveillance. Routine use of diagnostic studies beyond cytology and the selective use of CA 125 are probably not cost effective.

The patterns of recurrence depend on initial disease distribution. Patients with advanced primary disease tend to have abdominal or systemic failure. Approximately one-third of recurrences seen in women whose primary tumors were confined to the uterus are limited to the pelvis; the remaining two-thirds have some component of distant failure. It is important to identify those cases with isolated pelvic recurrence because some can be salvaged by radiotherapy or ultraradical surgery. Conversely, treatment of systemic recurrence is largely palliative.

Systemic Agents

HORMONE THERAPY

Overview of Clinical Studies. Progestogens have been used in the management of recurrent endometrial cancer after the original report by Kelley and Baker in 1961[116] used the parenterally administered hydroxyprogesterone caproate.[117,118] Beneficial results from these trials were mostly confined to a subset of patients with well-differentiated tumor, metastases to the lung, and a long disease-free interval between diagnosis of the primary tumor and the development of metastases. Subsequent trials, using MPA or megestrol acetate, explored the use of high-dose progestogen therapy on better-selected patients

TABLE 32.2-8. Selected Series of Hormonally Based Therapy in Women with Endometrial Cancer

Study	Drug	Patients (n)	Response Rate (%)	Comment
Reifenstein[117]	HPC	314	30	20-mo median survival
Thigpen et al.[119] (GOG-81)	MA, 200 mg vs.	145	25	Median PFS, 3.2; survival, 11.1 mo
	MA, 1000 mg	144	15	Median PFS, 2.5; survival, 7 mo
Thigpen et al.[120] (GOG-81F)	Tamoxifen	68	10	Median PFS, 1.9; survival, 8.8 mo
Fiorica et al.[121] (GOG-153)	Tamoxifen + MPA	56	27	Median PFS, 2.7; survival, 14 mo

GOG, Gynecologic Oncology Group; HPC, hydroxyprogesterone caproate; MA, megestrol acetate; MPA, medroxy progesterone acetate; PFS, progression-free survival.

through the study of hormone receptor content of tumors and limiting therapy to receptor-positive cases paralleling breast cancer strategies.[118,119] Overall, fewer than 30% of patients (even with the best selection) show objective responses, and the survival of patients with metastatic disease is disappointingly short, except for a rare, extremely hormone-responsive patient.

No dose-response effect for progestogens has been proven.[144] Although some responders have very long survival rates, the median duration of response in most studies does not exceed 10 months. The results of treatment with tamoxifen are generally inferior to those obtained with progestogens.[120] More recently, it has been used to sequence with megestrol acetate, yielding high response rates, presumably its estrogen agonist activity helping to modulate progesterone receptors. It remains to be seen whether tamoxifen in sequential combination with progestogens (to modulate receptors) will have an advantage over progestogen therapy alone. Selected hormonal studies are summarized in Table 32.2-8.

Other hormonal manipulations are under study. These include not only combinations of tamoxifen and MPA but also other selective estrogen receptor modulators, such as raloxifene, luteinizing hormone–releasing hormone agonists and antagonists, aromatase inhibitors, and miscellaneous other drugs such as danazol. It is likely that the same subset of patients responds to these hormonally directed therapies, and no obvious advantage of one agent over another has emerged to date. Moreover, results from small studies may be discordant, reflecting the importance of patient selection in maximizing the probability of response. In addition, distinction must be made in future trials between the primary hormonal treatment and subsequent interventions.

Biologic and Pharmacologic Considerations. The presence of estrogen and progesterone receptors in tumors has been shown to correlate with well-differentiated cancers and with response to progestogens.[7] Sequentially alternating tamoxifen and MPA or megestrol acetate regimens are based on the concept of up-regulation of progesterone receptors by the antiestrogen.[122] Other laboratory studies indicate the presence of specific binding sites for luteinizing hormone–releasing hormone and for androgen receptors.[123] Supplementing clinical observations with molecular correlates of response may bring out some differences that are currently not apparent and may also possibly lead to crossover hormonal therapies, a concept that has been useful in breast cancer treatment. The rational selection of specific hormonal manipulations from laboratory findings may become more feasible with the wider applicability of molecular immunohistochemical probes.

CYTOTOXIC CHEMOTHERAPY

Overview of Clinical Trials. Most women with recurrent or stage IV endometrial cancers must be assessed for treatment with cytotoxic chemotherapy. Doxorubicin and its analogue epirubicin have shown reproducible antitumor activity in phase II and III trials.[124,125] These phase III studies have indicated that the addition of cyclophosphamide to doxorubicin improves neither response nor survival rates and suggests that the incorporation of progestogens does not improve results[125,126] (Table 32.2-9). A number of other drugs studied by the GOG and others also have shown little efficacy but often have been used in combinations. On the other hand, cisplatin and carboplatin both show

TABLE 32.2-9. Randomized Trials of Cytotoxic Drugs in Women with Advanced or Recurrent Endometrial Carcinoma

Study	Drug(s)/Doses (mg/m²)	Patients (n)	Response Rate (%)	Major End Points
Horton et al.[126]	Dox, 40 vs.	56	27	Median survival, 27 wk
	CAF, 250/30/300	58	22[a]	Median survival, 27 wk
Thigpen et al.[125] (GOG-48)	Dox, 60 vs.	132	22	PFS, 3.2; survival, 6.9 mo
	AC, 60/500	144	30	PFS, 3.9; survival, 7.3 mo
Thigpen et al.[127] (GOG-107)	Dox, 60 vs.	137	27	PFS, 3.4; survival, 9.2 mo
	AP, 60/50	155	46[b]	PFS, 5.4[b]; survival, 8.8 mo
Fleming et al.[128] (GOG-163)	AP, 60/50 vs.	160	40	PFS, 7.2; survival, 12.4 mo
	AT,[c] 50/150	168	44	PFS, 6.0; survival, 13.6 mo
Fleming et al.[129] (GOG-177)	AP, 60/50 vs.	131	33	PFS, 5.3; survival, 12.1 mo
	TAP,[c] 160/45/50	130	57[b]	PFS, 8.3; survival, 15.3 mo[b]

AC, adriamycin/cyclophosphamide; AP, adriamycin/cisplatin; AT, adriamycin/taxol; CAF, cyclophosphamide/adriamycin/fluorouracil; dox, doxorubicin; GOG, Gynecologic Oncology Group; PFS, progression-free survival; TAP, taxol/adriamycin/cisplatin.
[a]Chemotherapy was combined with medroxyprogesterone acetate in this arm.
[b]Statistically significant difference from other arm.
[c]Regimen requires filgrastim beginning on days 3 through 12 after administration.

consistent antitumor activity,[130–134] and a phase III study combining cisplatin with doxorubicin showed superior progression-free survival over doxorubicin alone.[127] However, the overall median survival rate for patients receiving doxorubicin plus cisplatin was not improved, and subsequent trials by the GOG of circadian dose schedules for these two drugs did not improve outcome. Other agents with single-agent activity include paclitaxel,[135,136] ifosfamide,[137] and oral etoposide.[138] Paclitaxel was taken to phase III testing in combination with doxorubicin versus the cisplatin-doxorubicin doublet with no clear advantage, but when it was added to the doublet a net improvement in outcome including survival was demonstrated. Paclitaxel (250 mg/m^2) given on a 24-hour infusion schedule and requiring cytokine support with filgrastim showed remarkable activity,[139] with four complete responses and six partial responses among 28 patients. A 24-hour infusion of 150 mg/m^2 is being tested in phase III studies in combination with doxorubicin. Shorter infusions of paclitaxel have activity with less myelosuppression[140] and are often used in combination with carboplatin or in three-drug combinations.

Biologic and Pharmacologic Considerations. Laboratory and clinical studies should better define the role of systemic chemotherapy in relation to various known biologic factors in an analogous way to how pathologic features and hormone receptors have assisted in refining hormonal therapies. Endometrial cancers commonly express P-glycoprotein (P-gp). Studying the mechanisms of drug resistance mediated by multidrug resistance gene 1 (MDR1)-mediated P-gp may assist in identifying doxorubicin- and paclitaxel-resistant tumors.[141] Moreover, mutations in p53 occur somewhat concordantly with the expression of P-gp and may help to define a more resistant subpopulation. A relationship between progesterone and the expression of P-gp also has been postulated[142]; prior progestogen therapy might lead to changes in P-gp expression. The epidermal growth factor receptor and HER-2/neu are also likely to be important in determining chemosensitivity and outcome, as well as therapeutic targets.[143,144] Studies are beginning to focus on special subtypes, such as papillary serous and clear cell carcinomas, that not only have a propensity to metastasize early but may also have altered drug sensitivities. Several investigators have known that p53 mutations are more frequent in these cell types and are indicative of poor prognosis. Microsatellite instability, persistence of bcl-2191, and high proliferation indices may also be of prognostic significance.

Radiotherapy

Approximately 50% of patients with endometrial cancer who relapse after surgery have failure in the pelvis, 50% of which recurs in the vaginal vault. Patients with recurrent disease limited to the pelvis, particularly those with isolated vaginal recurrences, often undergo salvage irradiation.

Over the last 20 years, numerous investigators have reported the outcome of patients with recurrent endometrial cancer after salvage radiotherapy (Table 32.2-10). Survival rates vary considerably between the published reports, ranging from 24.1% to 71.0%. Patients with isolated vaginal recurrences represent a particularly favorable group. Pai et al.[147] evaluated the outcome of 20 patients with isolated vaginal involvement who were treated with salvage radiotherapy. The 10-year actuarial local control and cause-specific survival of the entire group

TABLE 32.2-10. Salvage Radiotherapy, Locally Recurrent Endometrial Cancer

Study	Year	n	Local Control (%)	5-Y Survival (%)
Aalders et al.[145]	1984	29	NS	24.1
Nag et al.[146]	1997	15	66.6	42.3
Pai et al.[147]	1997	20	74	71 (10-y)
Charra et al.[148]	1998	78	70.4^a	56^a
Hart et al.[149]	1998	26	65	53
Wylie et al.[150]	2000	58	65	53
Jhingran et al.[151]	2003	91	75	43

NS, not stated.
^{a}Includes 37 patients with locally recurrent cervical cancer.

were 74% and 71%, respectively.[147] In contrast, others have reported poor survivals in patients with isolated vaginal recurrences. In most reports, additional factors associated with improved survival in patients with local recurrence include long disease-free intervals, low-grade disease, adenocarcinoma histology, and no prior radiotherapy.

As seen in Table 32.2-10, local control within the treated volume is achieved in 65% to 75% of patients treated with salvage radiotherapy, with the majority of series reporting survival rates between 40% and 70%. A major determinant of local control is tumor size. Wylie et al.[150] reported 5-year local control rates of 80% and 54% in tumors of 2 cm or less and greater than 2 cm, respectively (P = .02). In a review of 26 locally recurrent patients, Hoekstra et al.[152] noted local-regional relapse in 6% of tumors of 4 cm or less versus 33% in tumors greater than 4 cm.

The optimal approach in these patients is a combination of pelvic irradiation and brachytherapy. Select small volume tumors can be treated with brachytherapy alone, especially if excised. Brachytherapy alone is used in women with prior pelvic radiotherapy. Although intracavitary approaches are typically used, interstitial brachytherapy is associated with excellent control rates and is preferable in bulky recurrent tumors.[146,148] Although low dose-rate techniques have been commonplace, equally favorable outcomes have been achieved with high dose-rate brachytherapy in recent years. High doses are required, and severe complications are seen in 3% to 12% of patients, primarily related to the gastrointestinal tract. Patients with a history of prior radiation therapy are at high risk for severe sequelae. Limited experience is available using radiotherapy in the salvage of noncentral pelvic recurrences.

Surgery

Surgery plays a limited role in the management of recurrent endometrial cancer. Although cytoreduction is probably valuable for women with advanced primary cancers, secondary cytoreduction after failure of primary therapy has no real role because of the lack of effective regional or systemic therapy. Two legitimate indications for surgical management are attempted curative resection of central pelvic recurrence by exenteration and palliative treatment in selected clinical situations.

Historically, ultraradical resection of recurrent endometrial cancer has not been recommended because of the perception that systemic spread was too common. However, reviews that have examined carefully evaluated patients have identified a subset of women whose recurrence is limited to the pelvis.[153,154] Cure rates of 40% to 50% have been obtained after resection by pelvic exenteration. Consequently, patients who have recurrent disease that is clinically limited to the central pelvis and have not been successful with radiotherapy should be considered candidates for curative resection. A diligent search for subclinical metastatic disease should be carried out before exploration and at the time of operation.

Palliative surgery is largely limited to patients with intraabdominal recurrences causing bowel obstruction or pain. Candidates for palliative operations must have realistic expectations as to the goals of surgery, and the planned procedure should have a reasonable chance of achieving the desired goal. The patient's life expectancy and clinical status should be adequate for the proposed procedure and the anticipated recovery. The operation performed should be the minimum procedure with the lowest risk capable of correcting the problem. Heroic operations attempted in patients with no chance for long-term survival are pointless.

OUTCOME AND SURVIVAL

Long-term survival of patients with endometrial cancer is clearly related to their surgical stage and substage. Representative 5-year survival rates by stage are 90% for stage I, 60% for stage II, 40% for stage III, and 5% for stage IV. Because the vast majority of patients have stage I disease and because there is a wide variation in survival based on risk profile within this stage, most research into postoperative adjuvant therapy is aimed at subsets of stage I patients. It is anticipated that the routine use of surgical staging will result in a more homogeneous subgrouping of similar-risk patients and allow a more reliable prediction of survival potential. Selected patients with advanced disease that can be encompassed by surgical resection with or without adjunctive irradiation can be cured. However, few patients meet such criteria. Although patients with disseminated disease frequently respond to cytotoxic therapy, such responses tend to be short and provide a limited improvement in progression-free survival. Posttreatment surveillance for recurrence should be used to identify candidates for clinical trials of new agents or therapeutic approaches.

UTERINE SARCOMAS

TUMOR TYPES

Tumors with a malignant mesenchymal component account for approximately 10% of uterine fundal neoplasms. Pure uterine sarcomas of the homologous type arise from native elements, as is seen in endometrial stromal sarcoma, leiomyosarcoma, and sarcomas of nonspecific supporting tissues (fibrous tissue, vessels, lymphatics). Heterologous sarcomas may contain elements with nonnative differentiation, such as skeletal muscle, bone, and cartilage.[155] The malignant mixed müllerian tumor is a combination of carcinoma and sarcoma and is now termed *carcinosarcoma*. Although any combination is possible, serous carcinoma admixed with endometrial stromal sarcoma is the most common histologic type. The adenosarcoma is a rare mixed

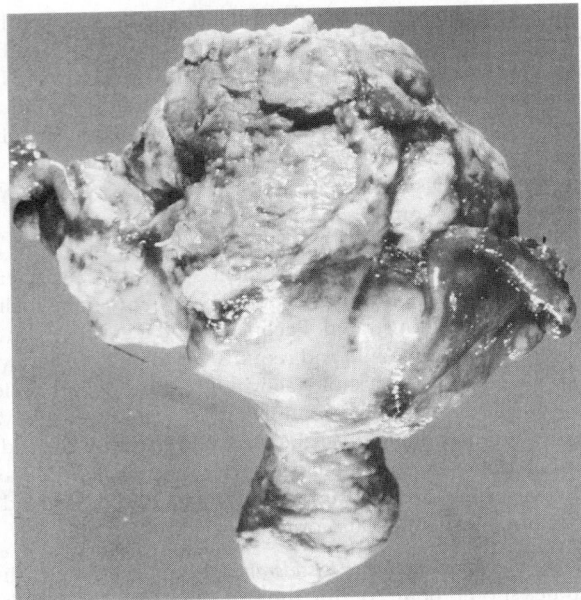

FIGURE 32.2-4. Uterine sarcomas tend to present as large, fleshy central pelvic tumors. This leiomyosarcoma has replaced most of the uterine fundus and penetrated the serosa to engulf the adnexa and directly contact intraperitoneal structures.

tumor in which a benign epithelial component is mixed with a sarcomatous element.

CLINICAL PRESENTATION

Uterine sarcomas exhibit the typical gross features of similar tumors at other sites—firm, fleshy growth with areas of hemorrhage and necrosis. The initial growth phase of most sarcomas is within the fundal portion of the uterus. If the tumor involves the endometrial cavity, postmenopausal or abnormal vaginal bleeding is common. Tumors that have a polypoid growth configuration may prolapse through the cervix to present as an upper vaginal mass. This presentation is most often seen with carcinosarcoma.

Extensive local growth is another common clinical presentation. Once the tumor has penetrated the uterine serosa, it can rapidly attach to adjacent pelvic structures or loops of bowel positioned in the pelvis (Fig. 32.2-4). This locally advanced pelvic tumor presentation is typical of leiomyosarcoma. Patients with locally advanced cancers have symptoms related to an expanding pelvic mass (fullness, pressure, pain, urinary frequency) or to entrapment and destruction of adjacent organs (hematuria, tenesmus, rectal bleeding, bowel obstruction, fistula).

As is seen for epithelial tumors of the uterus, distant spread from uterine sarcomas may occur by a variety of mechanisms. Intraabdominal and retroperitoneal nodal metastases are frequently associated with the carcinosarcoma.[156] This is not surprising because the epithelial component is usually papillary serous carcinoma and predominates within metastatic sites. Consequently, patients with advanced disease follow a clinical pattern similar to that of women with epithelial ovarian cancer. All uterine sarcomas have a propensity for hematogenous dissemination. Pulmonary metastases are most frequently observed. Other sites include liver, bone, and brain. Women with distant spread at the time of diagnosis have symptoms and examination findings based on the location of their disease.

EVALUATION

Uterine sarcoma should be suspected in any postmenopausal woman with an enlarging central pelvic mass. If the tumor projects into the uterine cavity or has partially prolapsed through the cervix, an endometrial or direct biopsy should provide a tissue diagnosis. Evaluation by an experienced pathologist is critical because uterine sarcomas are rare and the biopsy material is often fragmented or necrotic. Tumors originating within the uterine wall require exploratory laparotomy and hysterectomy to establish a diagnosis. Because primary therapy usually includes hysterectomy, the preoperative evaluation should focus on a search for disease at common metastatic sites and assessment of operative risk.

When the diagnosis of sarcoma is known or suspected, the pretreatment evaluation should include a careful history and physical examination, chest radiograph, and laboratory studies. The CA 125 level may be elevated in some cases, particularly in carcinosarcoma tumors with peritoneal spread. Other markers have not been consistently useful. Computed tomography of the abdomen and pelvis may be helpful in identifying occult extrauterine disease. Cystoscopy, proctosigmoidoscopy, and barium enema should be performed in patients with advanced pelvic disease. Brain, bone, or liver imaging should be considered in patients with abnormal physical or laboratory findings.

TREATMENT

Surgery

Patients in whom the diagnosis of uterine sarcoma is not anticipated often undergo hysterectomy for a presumed diagnosis of uterine leiomyoma or "central" pelvic mass. Although most of these cases are not surgically staged, many are apparently stage I tumors. When the diagnosis of sarcoma is established and hysterectomy is technically feasible, surgical resection of the primary tumor should be attempted. Such surgery may be curative for tumors confined to the uterus. Because of the overall poor prognosis associated with uterine sarcomas, we proceed with extended surgical staging similar to that used for patients with endometrial adenocarcinoma when disease is clinically limited to the uterus. Although a survival benefit to surgical staging has not been demonstrated, knowledge of the true extent of disease is helpful in selecting therapy options.

In more extensive disease cases, resection or debulking of the central tumor can provide important palliation of bleeding and pain. Tumor reduction may enhance the ability of postoperative adjunctive therapy to extend survival, but this concept is not as well established as in epithelial ovarian tumors. The aggressiveness of the surgical approach must include a balance between the desire to remove as much tumor as possible and the risks of additional operative procedures. Patients with widespread or bulky unresectable disease should not be subjected to high-risk operations under the guise of cytoreduction.

Occasionally, surgical intervention is indicated in women with advanced or recurrent disease, but such situations are clinically uncommon. Some women have obtained long-term survival and apparent cure after resection of an isolated pulmonary metastasis.[157] Exploration to palliate bowel obstruction or fistula is appropriate in selected refractory disease patients who have a good performance status and reasonable projected survival time. Potentially morbid palliative operations in women with terminal disease should be avoided whenever possible.

Radiotherapy

The role of radiation therapy in uterine sarcomas is controversial. Published studies have a number of limitations that render drawing definitive conclusions regarding its use difficult. First, no prospective randomized trial that uses adjuvant irradiation has been conducted. Second, considerable prognosis imbalances exist between irradiated and nonirradiated patients in most retrospective series, with radiation therapy given predominantly to those with poorer pathologic features. Finally, many reports fail to distinguish between the various sarcoma histologies (carcinosarcoma, leiomyosarcoma, endometrial stromal sarcoma) in their analysis.

Most studies that group the various histologies together note better pelvic control with adjuvant irradiation; some, but not all, report improved survivals in irradiated patients.[158,159] Ferrer et al.[159] analyzed the outcome of 103 patients with uterine sarcoma (43 leiomyosarcoma, 40 carcinosarcoma, 17 endometrial stroma sarcoma, 3 other). Irradiated patients had an improved 5-year pelvic control (76% vs. 36%; *P* <.0001) and overall survival (73% vs. 37%; *P* <.0003). Of note, radiation therapy remained correlated with improved pelvic control and survival on multivariate analysis controlling for age, stage, histology, lymphovascular invasion, chemotherapy, and grade.[159]

Hornback et al.[160] evaluated the impact of pelvic irradiation on outcome in uterine sarcoma patients enrolled on GOG-20 (a randomized trial of adjuvant adriamycin). In this study, pelvic irradiation was optional. Of 109 stage I to II patients (87% carcinosarcoma), the pelvis was the first site of failure in 10% and 23% of irradiated and nonirradiated patients, respectively. In a separate clinicopathologic study performed by the GOG, irradiated clinical stage I to II patients had a lower rate of first relapse in the pelvis (17%) than did nonirradiated patients (24%).[161]

Most studies that focus on carcinosarcoma have reported better pelvic control rates in irradiated patients, particularly those with stage I to II disease.[162,163] Impact on survival has been mixed, with a benefit seen in some, but not all, reports. Gerszten et al.[162] noted pelvic recurrences in 55% of 31 patients with stage I to II carcinosarcoma after surgery alone. In contrast, only 1 of 29 (3%) irradiated patients had recurrence in the pelvis (*P* <.001). Isolated pelvic failures occurred in 0% and 22% of irradiated and nonirradiated patients, respectively. Irradiated patients also had a better 5-year survival (85% vs. 50%, *P* = .02).

Chemotherapy and Hormonal Therapy

Differences in the management of metastatic uterine leiomyosarcomas and carcinosarcomas with respect to systemic chemotherapy have been established, and separate trials are conducted for these two entities (Tables 32.2-11 and 32.2-12). Endometrial stromal sarcomas are less common and usually not included in clinical trials. Because antitumor activity of

TABLE 32.2-11. Selected Cytotoxic Drug Trials in Uterine Leiomyosarcomas

Study	Drug	Patients (n)	Response Rate (%)	Comment
SINGLE AGENTS				
Omura et al.[164] (GOG-21)	Doxorubicin	28	25	Includes all uterine sarcomas; addition of dacarbazine did not improve outcome.
Muss et al.[165] (GOG-42)	Doxorubicin	38	8	Includes all uterine sarcomas; addition of cyclophosphamide did not improve outcome.
Thigpen et al.[166] (GOG-26C)	Cisplatin	50	—	First-line only; response duration, 3.4 mo; survival, 7.8 mo.
Sutton et al.[167] (GOG-26U)	Ifosfamide	35	17	Response duration, 3.8 mo; survival, 6 mo.
Slayton et al.[168] (GOG-26D)	Etoposide	28	11	IV d 1, 3, 5 every 3 wk.
Thigpen et al.[169] (GOG-87D)	Etoposide	—	—	IV d 1, 3, 5 every 3 wk.
Rose et al.[170] (GOG 131B)[a]	Etoposide	29	7	PO d 1–21 every 4 wk.
Sutton et al.[171] (GOG-87G)	Paclitaxel	33	10	IV 3-h infusion every 3 wk.
Gallup et al.[172] (GOG-131C)[a]	Paclitaxel	53	—	IV 3-h infusion every 3 wk.
Look et al.[173]	Gemcitabine	—	—	IV d 1, 8, 15 every 3 wk.
COMBINATION CHEMOTHERAPY				
Sutton et al.[174]	Ifosfamide + doxorubicin	33	30	Response duration, 4.1 mo; survival, 9.6 mo.
Currie et al.[175] (GOG-87C)	Hydroxyurea	38	18	Response duration, 12 mo; survival, 15 mo.
Edmondson et al.[176]	Mitomycin, doxorubicin, cisplatin	36	22	—
Hensley et al.[177]	Gemcitabine, docetaxel	34	53	Uterine primaries in 29; 16 had prior doxorubicin ± doxorubicin ± ifosfamide; survival, 18 mo.

GOG, Gynecologic Oncology Group.
[a]Previously treated with chemotherapy series.

chemotherapy regimens has been documented in advanced stages, several trials are ongoing or planned in earlier stages of disease. Evidence to support the use of chemotherapy as an adjuvant to surgery is not yet forthcoming. One randomized study of the addition of doxorubicin after surgery in stage I and II uterine sarcomas yielded no advantage for the adjuvant chemotherapy group.[164]

LEIOMYOSARCOMA. Doxorubicin was shown to be an effective drug against leiomyosarcomas arising in the uterus. Drug combinations were claimed to improve results in childhood and adult sarcomas of extrauterine origin, but the addition of dacarbazine to doxorubicin did not improve the survival of patients with metastatic uterine sarcomas beyond that obtained with doxorubicin alone.[183] A subsequent randomized study also performed by the GOG failed to show that the addition of cyclophosphamide in modest doses was advantageous over doxorubicin by itself.[165] The alkylating agent ifosfamide has modest activity[167] but does not add substantially to the therapeutic efficacy of doxorubicin.[174] Other drugs, such as cisplatin,[166] etoposide,[169] and paclitaxel,[171] also have been evaluated and have modest to minimal activity. A combination of hydroxyurea, etoposide, and dacarbazine had antitumor activity without major toxicities.[175] Another combination based on gemcitabine and docetaxel has been reported to have substantial activity in a single institution and is now being evaluated by the GOG (see Table 32.2-11).

TABLE 32.2-12. Selected Cytotoxic Drug Trials in Uterine Carcinosarcomas (Mixed Müllerian Tumors)

Study	Drug	Patients (n)	Response Rate (%)	Comment
Omura et al.[164] (GOG-21)	Doxorubicin	41	10	Includes all uterine sarcomas; addition of dacarbazine did not improve outcome.
Muss et al.[165] (GOG-42)	Doxorubicin	51	10	Includes all uterine sarcomas; addition of cyclophosphamide did not improve outcome.
Thigpen et al.[166] (GOG-26C)	Cisplatin	50	—	First-line only; response duration, 9.3 mo; survival, 7 mo.
Sutton et al.[178] (GOG-26U)	Ifosfamide	28	31	—
Sutton et al.[179]	Ifosfamide vs.	102	36	PFS, 4 mo; survival, 7.8 mo.
	Ifosfamide + cisplatin	92	54	PFS, 6 mo; survival, 9.4 mo.
Slayton et al.[180] (GOG-26D, GOG-87B)	Etoposide	31	6	IV d 1, 3, 5 every 3 wk.
Curtin et al.[181] (GOG-130B)	Paclitaxel	—	—	IV 3-h infusion every 3 wk.
Miller et al.[182] (GOG-130D)	Topotecan	—	—	—
Currie et al.[183] (GOG-87C)	Hydroxyurea, etoposide, dacarbazine	32	16	Response duration, 6.3 mo.

GOG, Gynecologic Oncology Group; PFS, progression-free survival.

CARCINOSARCOMA (MIXED MÜLLERIAN TUMOR). The sensitivity of carcinosarcomas often parallels that of epithelial endometrial and ovarian cancers, suggesting that the sarcomatous component may be a further dedifferentiated portion of the epithelial malignancy. Ifosfamide[178,179] and cisplatin have greater antitumor activity against uterine carcinosarcomas than does doxorubicin. Accordingly, the two drugs in combination have been explored in all stages and also compared with ifosfamide alone in advanced, persistent, or recurrent disease.[179] The results indicate an advantage for the combination in terms of responses and progression-free survival but nearly equivalent median survival at a cost of increasing toxicity. The combination is being administered to completely resected stage I and II mixed müllerian tumors of the uterus (GOG-117), but the assessment requires a comparison to historic controls. Taxanes, such as paclitaxel, have been evaluated, and this agent has already formed part of an active combination with the pegylated liposomal doxorubicin, Doxil.[184] Experience with a number of other platinum-based combinations has been reported in very small series. These should be regarded as leads for future trials rather than a reliable indicator of activity.

ENDOMETRIAL STROMAL SARCOMA. The systemic treatment of endometrial stromal sarcoma is guided by reports from individual institutions.[185,186] The tumor's relative rarity does not support the conduct of clinical trials. Because of the presence of hormonal receptors in low-grade (fewer than 10 mitoses per high-power field) tumors, hormonal therapy has been advocated.[187] However, high-grade tumors are usually treated with chemotherapy. Investigation of biologic and pharmacologic issues may point the way for hypothesis-driven drug trials.

BIOLOGIC AND PHARMACOLOGIC CONSIDERATIONS. The growth of benign leiomyomas is under estrogenic and progestogenic control.[188] Accordingly, the study of receptors and hormone-action inhibitors for antitumor activity may be relevant to the management of malignant smooth muscle tumors. Receptors also have been studied in endometrial stromal sarcomas[189] and justify exploration of inhibition or depletion of hormonal mediators in the management of these tumors. Overexpression in MDR2 and mutations in p53 have been noted in some uterine sarcomas, but not in leiomyomas.[190] For the development of cytotoxic therapy, the role of MDR1-mediated P-gp expression in determining resistance to doxorubicin has been investigated in a cell line from a leiomyosarcoma of the uterus and its doxorubicin-resistant derivative. Drugs that are substrates for P-gp may restore sensitivity to doxorubicin in this resistant variant. Trials of such resistance-reversing agents, including the cyclosporin analogue PSC-833, may lead to a reassessment of the potential for drugs such as doxorubicin, taxanes, and vinca alkaloids in the treatment of these traditionally refractory tumors.[191] Immunologic findings have shown concordance of certain antigens in carcinomatous and sarcomatous elements, suggesting a common origin.[192]

OUTCOME AND SURVIVAL

Stage is the most significant predictor of outcome for women with uterine sarcomas. Patients whose tumors are confined to the uterus have a survival rate of 60% to 70% after surgical resection. Major sites of failure include the pelvis, upper abdomen, and lung. Because few well-conducted prospective adjuvant therapy trials have been accomplished, a precise role for either adjuvant irradiation or chemotherapy remains undefined. As has been noted for endometrial carcinoma, adjuvant pelvic irradiation may reduce the rate of pelvic failure without improving survival if more patients succumb to distant failure. Pelvic irradiation and local tumor control may be an important issue in tumors with extension to the cervix. However, so few patients are placed in this category that meaningful treatment data are not available.

Very few patients with tumor spread outside of the uterus can be curatively treated. Some women with small volume regional disease have obtained long-term survival after external-beam irradiation. However, most patients with advanced or recurrent disease ultimately experience disease progression and die. These women are excellent candidates for new therapeutic trials.

REFERENCES

1. Jemal A, Murray T, Samuels A, et al. Cancer statistics, 2003. *CA Cancer J Clin* 2003;53:5.
2. Burke TW, Heller PB, Woodward JE, et al. Treatment failure in endometrial carcinoma. *Obstet Gynecol* 1990;75:96.
3. Kurman RJ, Scully RE. Clear cell carcinoma of the endometrium: an analysis of 21 cases. *Cancer* 1976;37:872.
4. Alberhasky RC, Connelly PJ, Christopherson WM. Carcinoma of the endometrium. IV. Mixed adenosquamous carcinoma: a clinical-pathological study of 68 cases with long-term follow-up. *Am J Clin Pathol* 1982;77:655.
5. Hendrickson M, Ross J, Eifel P, et al. Uterine papillary serous carcinoma: a highly malignant form of endometrial adenocarcinoma. *Am J Surg Pathol* 1982;6:93.
6. Sutton GP, Brill L, Michael H, et al. Malignant papillary lesions of the endometrium. *Gynecol Oncol* 1987;27:294.
7. Ehrlich CA, Young PCM, Cleary RE. Cytoplasmic progesterone and estradiol receptors in normal, hyperplastic, and carcinomatous endometrial: therapeutic implications. *Am J Obstet Gynecol* 1981;141:539.
8. Kurman RJ, Kaminski PF, Norris HJ. The behavior of endometrial hyperplasia: a long-term study of "untreated" hyperplasia in 170 patients. *Cancer* 1985;56:403.
9. Wynder EL, Escher GC, Mantel N. An epidemiological investigation of cancer of the endometrium. *Cancer* 1966;19:489.
10. Smith DC, Prentice R, Thompson DJ, et al. Association of exogenous estrogen and endometrial carcinoma. *N Engl J Med* 1975;293:1164.
11. Ziel HK, Finkle WD. Increased risk of endometrial carcinoma among users of conjugated estrogens. *N Engl J Med* 1975;297:1167.
12. McPherson CP, Sellers TA, Potter JD, et al. Reproductive factors and endometrial cancer. The Iowa Women's Health Study. *Am J Epidemiol* 1996;143:1195.
13. Fisher B, Constantino JP, Redmond CK, et al. Endometrial cancer in tamoxifen-treated breast cancer patients: findings from the National Surgical Adjuvant Breast and Bowel Project (NSABP) B-14. *J Natl Cancer Inst* 1994;86:527.
14. Barakat RR, Wong G, Curtin JP, et al. Tamoxifen use in breast cancer patients who subsequently develop corpus cancer is not associated with a higher incidence of adverse histologic features. *Gynecol Oncol* 1994;95:164.
15. Mitchell MF, Reddoch J, Atkinson EN, et al. Patients with both breast and endometrial hyperplasia or cancer. *Gynecol Oncol* 1993;49:143(abst).
16. Burke TW, Levenback C, Tornos C, et al. Intraabdominal lymphatic mapping to direct selective pelvic and paraaortic lymphadenectomy in women with high-risk endometrial cancer: results of a pilot study. *Gynecol Oncol* 1996;62:169.
17. Greenwood SM, Wright DJ. Evaluation of the office endometrial biopsy in the detection of endometrial carcinoma and atypical hyperplasia. *Cancer* 1979;43:1474.
18. Eddy GL, Wojtowycz MA, Piraino PS, Mazur MT. Papanicolaou smears by the Bethesda system in endometrial malignancy: utility and prognostic importance. *Obstet Gynecol* 1977;90:999.
19. Sood AK, Buller RE, Burger RA, et al. Value of preoperative CA 125 level in the management of uterine cancer and prediction of clinical outcome. *Obstet Gynecol* 1997;90:441.
20. Christopherson WM, Connelly PJ, Alberhasky RC. Carcinoma of the endometrium. V. An analysis of prognosticators in patients with favorable subtypes and stage I disease. *Cancer* 1983;51:1705.
21. Morrow C, Bundy B, Kurman R, et al. Relationship between surgical-pathological risk factors and outcome in clinical stage I and II carcinoma of the endometrium: a Gynecologic Oncology Group study. *Gynecol Oncol* 1991;40:55.
22. Schink JC, Lurain JR, Wallemark CB, et al. Tumor size in endometrial cancer: a prognostic factor for lymph node metastasis. *Obstet Gynecol* 1987;70:216.
23. Hanson MB, van Nagell JR Jr, Powell DE, et al. The prognostic significance of lymph-vascular space invasion in stage I endometrial cancer. *Cancer* 1985;55:1752.

24. Enomoto T, Inoue M, Perantoni AO, et al. K-ras activation in premalignant and malignant epithelial lesions of the human uterus. *Cancer Res* 1991;51:5308.
25. Hetzel DJ, Wilson TO, Kenney GL, et al. HER-2/neu expression: a major prognostic factor in endometrial cancer. *Gynecol Oncol* 1992;47:179.
26. Lukes AS, Kohler MF, Pieper DF, et al. Multivariable analysis of DNA ploidy, p53, and HER-2/neu as prognostic factors in endometrial cancer. *Cancer* 1994;73:2380.
27. Miller B, Morris M, Silva E. Nucleolar organizer regions: a potential prognostic factor in adenocarcinoma of the endometrium. *Gynecol Oncol* 1994;54:137.
28. Lim P, Aquino-Parsons CF, Wong F, et al. Low-risk endometrial carcinoma: assessment of a treatment policy based on tumor ploidy and identification of additional prognostic indicators. *Gynecol Oncol* 1999;73:191.
29. Lynch HT, Krush AJ, Larsen AL, et al. Endometrial carcinoma: multiple primary malignancies, constitutional factors and heredity. *Am J Med Sci* 1966;252:381.
30. Cowles TA, Magrina JF, Masterson BJ, et al. Comparison of clinical and surgical staging in patients with endometrial carcinoma. *Obstet Gynecol* 1985;66:413.
31. Rutledge F. The role of radical hysterectomy in adenocarcinoma of the endometrium. *Gynecol Oncol* 1974;2:331.
32. Kinsella TJ, Bloomer WD, Lavin PT, et al. Stage II endometrial carcinoma: 10-year follow-up of combined radiation and surgical treatment. *Gynecol Oncol* 1980;10:290.
33. Childers JN, Brzechffa PR, Hatch KD, et al. Laparoscopic assisted surgical staging (LASS) of endometrial carcinoma. *Gynecol Oncol* 1993;51:33.
34. Chi DS, Welshinger M, Venkatraman ES, Barakat RR. The role of surgical cytoreduction in stage IV endometrial carcinoma. *Gynecol Oncol* 1997;67:56.
35. Moore DH, Fowler WC Jr, Walton LA, et al. Morbidity of lymph node sampling in cancers of the uterine corpus and cervix. *Obstet Gynecol* 1989;74:180.
36. Orr JW, Holloway RW, Orr P, et al. Surgical staging of uterine cancer: an analysis of perioperative morbidity. *Gynecol Oncol* 1991;42:209.
37. Weiser EB, Bundy BN, Hoskins WJ, et al. Extraperitoneal versus transperitoneal selective paraaortic lymphadenectomy in the pretreatment surgical staging of advanced cervical carcinoma (a Gynecologic Oncology Group study). *Gynecol Oncol* 1989;33:283.
38. Doering DL, Barnhill DR, Weiser EB, et al. Intraoperative evaluation of depth of myometrial invasion in stage I endometrial adenocarcinoma. *Obstet Gynecol* 1989;74:930.
39. Marino BD, Burke TW, Tornos C, et al. Staging laparotomy for endometrial carcinoma: assessment of peritoneal spread. *Gynecol Oncol* 1995;56:34.
40. Chuang L, Burke TW, Tornos C, et al. Staging laparotomy for endometrial carcinoma: assessment of retroperitoneal lymph nodes. *Gynecol Oncol* 1995;58:189.
41. Kilgore L, Partridge E, Alvarez R, et al. Adenocarcinoma of the endometrium: survival comparisons of patients with and without pelvic node biopsies. *Gynecol Oncol* 1995;56:29.
42. Heyman J. The so-called Stockholm method and the results of treatment of uterine cancer at the Radiumhemmet. *Acta Radiol* 1935;22:129.
43. Roeske JC, Lujan A, Rotmensch J, et al. Intensity-modulated whole pelvic radiation therapy in patients with gynecologic malignancies. *Int J Radiat Oncol Biol Phys* 2000;48:1613.
44. Mundt AJ, Lujan AE, Rotmensch J, et al. Intensity-modulated whole pelvis radiotherapy in women with gynecologic malignancies. *Int J Radiat Oncol Biol Phys* 2002;52:1330.
45. Grigsby PW, Perez CA, Kuten A, et al. Clinical stage I endometrial cancer: results of adjuvant irradiation and patterns of failure. *Int J Radiat Oncol Biol Phys* 1991;21:379.
46. Weigensberg IJ. Preoperative radiation therapy in stage I endometrial adenocarcinoma. *Cancer* 1984;53:242.
47. Delmore JE, Wharton JT, Hamberger AD, et al. Preoperative radiotherapy for early endometrial carcinoma. *Gynecol Oncol* 1987;28:34.
48. Sause WT, Fuller DB, Smith WG, et al. Analysis of preoperative intracavitary cesium application versus postoperative external beam radiation in stage I endometrial carcinoma. *Int J Radiat Oncol Biol Phys* 1990;18:1011.
49. Alektiar KM, McKee A, Venkatraman E, et al. Intravaginal high-dose-rate brachytherapy for stage IB (FIGO grade 1,2) endometrial cancer. *Int J Radiat Oncol Biol Phys* 2002; 53:707.
50. Boz G, De Paoli A, Innocente R, et al. Postoperative radiotherapy and surgery in stage I endometrial carcinoma: a 10-year experience. *Tumori* 1998;84:52.
51. Carey MS, O'Connell GJ, Johanson CR, et al. Good outcome associated with a standardized protocol using selective postoperative radiation in patients with clinical stage I adenocarcinoma of the endometrium. *Gynecol Oncol* 1995;57:138.
52. Chadha M, Nanavanti PJ, Liu P, et al. Patterns of failure in endometrial carcinoma stage IB grade 3 and IC patients with postoperative vaginal vault brachytherapy. *Gynecol Oncol* 1999;75:103.
53. Elliott P, Green D, Coates A, et al. The efficacy of postoperative vaginal irradiation in preventing vaginal recurrence in endometrial cancer. *Int J Gynecol Cancer* 1994;4:84.
54. Greven KM, Corn BW, Case D, et al. Which prognostic factors influence the outcome of patients with surgically staged endometrial cancer treated with adjuvant radiation. *Int J Radiat Oncol Biol Phys* 1997;39:413.
55. Irwin C, Levin W, Fyles A, et al. The role of adjuvant radiotherapy in carcinoma of the endometrium—results in 550 patients with pathologic stage I disease. *Gynecol Oncol* 1998; 70:247.
56. Kucera H, Vavra N, Weghaupt K, et al. Benefit of external irradiation in pathologic stage I endometrial carcinoma: a prospective clinical trial of 605 patients who received postoperative vaginal irradiation and additional pelvic irradiation in the presence of unfavorable prognostic factors. *Gynecol Oncol* 1990;38:99.
57. Lanciano RM, Corn BW, Schultz DJ, et al. The justification for a surgical staging system in endometrial carcinoma. *Radiother Oncol* 1993;28:189.
58. Macleod C, Fowler A, Duval P, et al. High-dose-rate brachytherapy alone post-hysterectomy for endometrial cancer. *Int J Radiat Oncol Biol Phys* 1998;42:1033.
59. Mayr NA, Wen BC, Brenda JA, et al. Postoperative radiation therapy in clinical stage I endometrial cancer: corpus, cervical and lower uterine segment involvement—patterns of failure. *Radiology* 1995;196:323.
60. Meerwaldt JH, Hoekstra CJ, van Putten WL, et al. Endometrial adenocarcinoma, adjuvant radiotherapy tailored to prognostic factors. *Int J Radiat Oncol Biol Phys* 1990;18:299.
61. Nori D, Merimsky O, Batata M, et al. Postoperative high dose rate intravaginal brachytherapy combined with external irradiation for early stage endometrial cancer: a long-term follow-up. *Int J Radiat Oncol Biol Phys* 1994;30:831.
62. Petereit DG, Tannehill SP, Grosen EA, et al. Outpatient vaginal cuff brachytherapy for endometrial cancer. *Int J Gynecol Cancer* 1999;9:456.
63. Pitson G, Colgan T, Levin W, et al. Stage II endometrial carcinoma: prognostic factors and risk classification in 170 patients. *Int J Radiat Oncol Biol Phys* 2002;53:862.
64. Weiss E, Hirnle P, Arnold-Bofinger H, et al. Therapeutic outcome and relation of acute and late side effects in the adjuvant radiotherapy of endometrial carcinoma stage I and II. *Radiother Oncol* 1999;53:1999.
65. Aalders J, Abeler V, Kolstad P, et al. Postoperative external irradiation and prognostic parameters in stage I endometrial carcinoma. *Obstet Gynecol* 1980;56:419.
66. Roberts JA, Brunetto VL, Keys HM, et al. A phase III randomized trial of surgery vs surgery plus adjunctive radiation therapy in intermediate risk endometrial adenocarcinoma (GOG-99). *Gynecol Oncol* 1998;68:135(abst).
67. Creutzberg CL, van Putten WL, Koper PC, et al. Surgery and postoperative radiotherapy vs surgery alone for patients with stage-1 endometrial carcinoma: multicentre randomized trial. PORTEC Study Group, Post Operative Radiation Therapy in Endometrial Carcinoma. *Lancet* 2000;355:1404.
68. Weiss MF, Connell PP, Waggoner S, et al. External pelvic radiation therapy in stage IC endometrial carcinoma. *Obstet Gynecol* 1999;93:599.
69. Nag S, Erickson B, Parikh S, et al. The American Brachytherapy Society recommendations for high-dose-rate brachytherapy for carcinoma of the endometrium. *Int J Radiat Oncol Biol Phys* 2000;48:779.
70. Connell PP, Rotmensch J, Waggoner S, et al. The significance of adnexal involvement in endometrial carcinoma. *Gynecol Oncol* 1999;74:74.
71. Corn BW, Lanciano RM, Greven KM, et al. Endometrial cancer with para-aortic adenopathy: patterns of failure and opportunities for cure. *Int J Radiat Oncol Biol Phys* 1992;24:223.
72. Creasman WT, Disaia PJ, Blessing J, et al. Prognostic significance of peritoneal cytology in patients with endometrial cancer and preliminary data concerning therapy with intraperitoneal radiopharmaceuticals. *Am J Obstet Gynecol* 1981;141:921.
73. Greer BE, Hamberger AD. Treatment of intraperitoneal metastatic adenocarcinoma of the endometrium by the whole-abdomen moving strip technique and pelvic boost irradiation. *Gynecol Oncol* 1983;16:365.
74. Greven KM, Lanciano RM, Corn B, et al. Pathologic stage III endometrial carcinoma. *Cancer* 1993;71:697.
75. Greven KM, Curran WJ, Whittington R, et al. Analysis of failure patterns in stage III endometrial carcinoma and therapeutic implications. *Int J Radiat Oncol Biol Phys* 1989;17:35.
76. Lee SW, Russell AH, Kinney WK. Whole abdomen radiotherapy for patients with peritoneal dissemination of endometrial adenocarcinoma. *Int J Radiat Oncol Biol Phys* 2003; 56:788.
77. Mundt AJ, Murphy KT, Rotmensch J, et al. Surgery and postoperative radiation therapy in FIGO stage IIIC endometrial carcinoma. *Int J Radiat Oncol Biol Phys* 2001;50:1154.
78. Nelson G, Randall M, Sutton G, et al. FIGO stage IIIC endometrial carcinoma with metastases confined to pelvic lymph nodes: analysis of treatment outcomes, prognostic variables, and failure patterns following adjuvant radiation therapy. *Gynecol Oncol* 1999;75:211.
79. Onda T, Yoshikawa H, Mizutani K, et al. Treatment of node-positive endometrial cancer with complete node dissection, chemotherapy and radiation therapy. *Br J Cancer* 1997;75:1836.
80. Schorge JO, Molpus KL, Goodman A, et al. The effect of postsurgical therapy on stage III endometrial carcinoma. *Gynecol Oncol* 1996;63:34.
81. Smith RS, Kapp DS, Chen Q, et al. Treatment of high-risk uterine cancer with whole abdominopelvic radiation therapy. *Int J Radiat Oncol Biol Phys* 2000;48:767
82. Kadar N, Homesley HD, Malfetano JH. Positive peritoneal cytology is an adverse factor in endometrial carcinoma only if there is other evidence of extrauterine disease. *Gynecol Oncol* 1992;46:145.
83. Axelrod J, Bundy J, Roy T, et al. Advanced endometrial carcinoma (EC) treated with whole abdominal irradiation (WAI): a Gynecologic Oncology Group (GOG) study. *Gynecol Oncol* 1995;56:135(abst).
84. Rose PG, Cha SD, Tak WK, et al. Radiation therapy for surgically proven para-aortic node metastases in endometrial carcinoma. *Int J Radiat Oncol Biol Phys* 1992;24:229.
85. Randall ME, Brunetto G, Muss H, et al. Whole abdominal radiotherapy versus combination doxorubicin-cisplatin chemotherapy in advanced endometrial carcinoma: a randomized phase III trial of the Gynecologic Oncology Group. Presented at: Annual Meeting of the American Society for Clinical Oncology; May 31–June 3, 2003; Chicago, IL.
86. Martinez A, Schray M, Podratz S, et al. Postoperative whole abdomino-pelvic irradiation for patients with high risk endometrial cancer. *Int J Radiat Oncol Biol Phys* 1989;17:371.
87. Mehta N, Yamada SD, Rotmensch J, Mundt AJ. Outcome and pattern of failure in pathological stage I–II papillary serous carcinoma of the endometrium: implications for adjuvant radiation therapy. *Int J Radiat Oncol Biol Phys* 2003;57:1004.
88. Turner BC, Knisely JP, Kacinski BM, et al. Effective treatment of stage I uterine papillary serous carcinoma with high dose-rate vaginal apex radiation (192Ir) and chemotherapy. *Int J Radiat Oncol Biol Phys* 1998;40:77.
89. Murphy KT, Rotmensch J, Yamada SD, et al. Outcome and patterns of failure in pathologic stages I-IV clear-cell carcinoma of the endometrium: implications for adjuvant radiation therapy. *Int J Radiat Oncol Biol Phys* 2003;55:1272.
90. Chao CK, Grigsby PW, Perez CA, et al. Medically inoperable stage I endometrial carcinoma: a few dilemmas in radiotherapeutic management. *Int J Radiat Oncol Biol Phys* 1996;34:27.
91. Grigsby PW, Kuske KK, Perez CA, et al. Medically inoperable stage I adenocarcinoma of the endometrium treated with radiotherapy alone. *Int J Radiat Oncol Biol Phys* 1986;13:483.

92. Kucera H, Knocke TH, Kucera E, et al. Treatment of endometrial carcinoma with high-dose-rate brachytherapy alone in medically inoperable stage I patients. *Acta Obstet Gynecol Scand* 1998;77:1008.

93. Kupelian PA, Eifel PJ, Tornos C, et al. Treatment of endometrial carcinoma with radiation therapy alone. *Int J Radiat Oncol Biol Phys* 1993;27:817.

94. Patanaphan V, Salazar OM, Chougule P. What can be expected when radiation therapy becomes the only curative alternative for endometrial cancer? *Cancer* 1985;55:1462.

95. Onsrud M, Hagen B, Strickert T. 10-Gy single-fraction pelvic irradiation for palliation and life prolongation in patients with cancer of the cervix and corpus uteri. *Gynecol Oncol* 2001;82:167.

96. Jereczek-Fossa BA, Badzio A, Jassem J. Factors determining acute normal tissue reactions during postoperative radiotherapy in endometrial cancer: analysis of 317 consecutive cases. *Radiother Oncol* 2003;68:33.

97. Chao KS, Grigsby PW, Perez CA, et al. Brachytherapy-related complications for medically inoperable stage I endometrial carcinoma. *Int J Radiat Oncol Biol Phys* 1995;31:37.

98. Petereit DG, Sarkaria JN, Chappell RJ. Perioperative morbidity and mortality of high-dose-rate gynecologic brachytherapy. *Int J Radiat Oncol Biol Phys* 1998;42:1025.

99. Corn BW, Lanciano RM, Greven KM, et al. Impact of improved irradiation technique, age, and lymph node sampling on the severe complication rate of surgically staged endometrial cancer patients: a multivariate analysis. *J Clin Oncol* 1994;12:510.

100. Creutzberg CL, van Putten WL, Koper PC, et al. The morbidity of treatment for patients with stage I endometrial cancer: results from a randomized trial. *Int J Radiat Oncol Biol Phys* 2001;51:1246.

101. Lujan AE, Roeske JC, Mundt AJ. Intensity-modulated radiation therapy as a means of reducing dose to bone marrow in gynecologic patients receiving whole pelvic radiation therapy. *Int J Radiat Oncol Biol Phys* 2003;57:516.

102. Portelance L, Chao KS, Grigsby PW, et al. Intensity-modulated radiation therapy (IMRT) reduces small bowel, rectum, and bladder doses in patients with cervical cancer receiving pelvic and para-aortic irradiation. *Int J Radiat Oncol Biol Phys* 2001;51:261.

103. Hong L, Alektiar K, Chui C, et al. IMRT of large fields: whole abdomen irradiation. *Int J Radiat Oncol Biol Phys* 2002;54:278.

104. Brixey CJ, Roeske JC, Lujan AE, et al. Impact of intensity-modulated radiotherapy on acute hematologic toxicity in women with gynecologic malignancies. *Int J Radiat Oncol Biol Phys* 2002;54:1388.

105. Mundt AJ, Mell LK, Roeske JC. Preliminary analysis of chronic gastrointestinal toxicity in gynecology patients treated with intensity modulated whole pelvic radiation therapy. *Int J Radiat Oncol Biol Phys* 2003;56:1354.

106. Maggi R, Cagnazzo G, Atlante G, et al. Risk groups and adjuvant therapy in surgical staged endometrial cancer paitents. A randomized multicentre study comparing chemotherapy with radiation therapy. In: Picorelli S, Atlante G, Panici PB, et al., eds. 7th Biennial Meeting of the International Gynecologic Cancer Society, Rome, 1999:87.

107. Randall ME, Spirtos NM, Dvoretsky P. Whole abdominal radiotherapy versus combination chemotherapy with doxorubicin and cisplatin in advanced endometrial carcinoma (Phase III): Gynecologic Oncology Group Study No. 122. *J Natl Cancer Inst Monogr* 1995;19:13.

108. Kim YB, Holschneider CH, Ghosh K, Nieberg RK, Montz FJ. Progestin alone as primary treatment of endometrial carcinoma in premenopausal women. Report of seven cases and review of the literature. *Cancer* 1997;79:320.

109. Lewis GC, Slack N, Mortel R, et al. Adjuvant progestogen therapy in primary definitive treatment of endometrial cancer. *Gynecol Oncol* 1974;2:368.

110. DePalo G, Merson M, Del Vecchio M, et al. A controlled clinical study of adjuvant medroxyprogesterone acetate (MPA) therapy in pathologic stage I endometrial carcinoma with myometrial invasion. *Proc Am Soc Clin Oncol* 1985;4:121(abst).

111. Stringer CA, Gershenson DM, Burke TW, et al. Adjuvant chemotherapy with cisplatin, doxorubicin, and cyclophosphamide (PAC) chemotherapy in women with high-risk endometrial carcinoma. *Gynecol Oncol* 1990;38:305.

112. Burke TW, Gershenson DM, Morris M, et al. Postoperative adjuvant cisplatin doxorubicin and cyclophosphamide (PAC) chemotherapy in women with high-risk endometrial carcinoma. *Gynecol Oncol* 1994;55:47.

113. Morrow CP, Bundy BN, Homesley HD. Doxorubicin as an adjuvant following surgery and radiation therapy in patients with high-risk endometrial carcinoma, stage I and occult stage II: a Gynecologic Oncology Group study. *Gynecol Oncol* 1990;36:166.

114. Reddoch JM, Burke TW, Morris M, et al. Surveillance for recurrent endometrial carcinoma: development of a follow-up scheme. *Gynecol Oncol* 1995;59:221.

115. Shumsky AG, Stuart GCE, Brasher P, et al. An evaluation of routine follow-up of patients treated for endometrial carcinoma. *Gynecol Oncol* 1994;55:229.

116. Kelley RM, Baker W. Progestational agents in the treatment of carcinoma of the endometrium. *N Engl J Med* 1961;264:216.

117. Reifenstein EC. Hydroxyprogesterone caproate therapy in advanced endometrial cancer. *Cancer* 1971;27:485.

118. Lentz SS, Brady MF, Major FJ, et al. High dose megestrol acetate in advanced or recurrent endometrial cancer: a Gynecologic Oncology Group study. *J Clin Oncol* 1996;14:357.

119. Thigpen JT, Brady M, Alvarez RD, et al. Oral medroxy-progesterone acetate in the treatment of advanced or recurrent endometrial carcinoma: a dose-response study by the Gynecologic Oncology Group. *J Clin Oncol* 1999;17:1736.

120. Thigpen JT, Brady MF, Homesley HD, et al. Tamoxifen in the treatment of advanced or recurrent endometrial carcinoma: a Gynecologic Oncology Group study. *J Clin Oncol* 2001;19:364.

121. Fiorica J, Brunetto V, Hanjani P, et al. A phase II study (GOG 153) of recurrent and advanced endometrial carcinoma treated with alternating courses of megestrol acetate and tamoxifen citrate. *Proc Am Soc Clin Oncol* 2000;19379a(abst 1499).

122. Rendina GM, Donadio C, Fabri M, et al. Tamoxifen and medroxyprogesterone therapy for advanced endometrial carcinoma. *Eur J Obstet Gynecol Reprod Biol* 1984;17:285.

123. Chatzaki E, Bax CM, Eidne KA, et al. The expression of gonadotrophin-releasing hormone and its receptor in endometrial cancer, and its relevance as an autocrine growth factor. *Cancer Res* 1996;56:2059.

124. Calero F, Rodriugez-Escudero F, Jimeno J, et al. Clinical evaluation of epirubicin in endometrial adenocarcinoma and uterine cervix carcinoma. *Proc Am Soc Clin Oncol* 1989;8:156.

125. Thigpen JT, Blessing JA, DiSaia PJ, et al. A randomized comparison of doxorubicin alone versus doxorubicin plus cyclophosphamide in the management of advanced or recurrent endometrial carcinoma: a Gynecologic Oncology Group study. *J Clin Oncol* 1994;12:1408.

126. Horton J, Elson P, Gordon P, Hahn R, Creech R. Combination chemotherapy for advanced endometrial cancer. An evaluation of three regimens. *Cancer* 1982;49:2441.

127. Thigpen T, Blessing J, Homesley H, et al. Phase III trial of doxorubicin cisplatin in advanced or recurrent endometrial carcinoma: a Gynecologic Oncology Group (GOG) study. *Proc Am Soc Clin Oncol* 1993;12:261(abst 830).

128. Fleming GF, Brunetto VL, Bently R, et al. Randomized trial of doxorubicin (DOX) plus cisplatin (CIS) versus DOX plus paclitaxel (TAX) plus granulocyte colony-stimulating factor (-CSF) in patients with advanced or recurrent endometrial cancer: a report on Gynecologic Oncology Group (GOG) protocol #163. *Proc Am Soc Clin Oncol* 2000;19:3791(abst 1498).

129. Fleming GF, Brunetto VL, Mundt AJ, et al. Randomized trial of doxorubicin (DOX) plus cisplatin (CIS) versus DOX plus CIS plus paclitaxel (TAX) in patients with advanced or recurrent endometrial carcinoma: a Gynecologic Oncology Group (GOG) study. *Proc Am Soc Clin Oncol* 2002;21:202a(abst 807).

130. Thigpen JT, Blessing JA, Lagasse LD, et al. Phase II trial of cisplatin as second-line chemotherapy in patients with advanced or recurrent endometrial carcinomas: a Gynecologic Oncology Group study. *Am J Clin Oncol* 1984;7:253.

131. Long HJ, Pfeifle DM, Wieand HS, et al. Phase II evaluation of carboplatin in advanced endometrial carcinoma. *J Natl Cancer Inst* 1988;80:276.

132. Thigpen JT , Blessing JA, Homesley J, et al. Phase II trial of cisplatin as first-line chemotherapy in patients with advanced and recurrent endometrial carcinoma: a Gynecologic Oncology Group study. *Gynecol Oncol* 1989;33:68.

133. Green JB, Green S, Alberts DS, et al. Carboplatin therapy in advanced endometrial cancer. *Obstet Gynecol* 1990;75:696.

134. Burke TW, Munkarah A, Kavanagh JJ. Treatment of advanced or recurrent endometrial carcinoma with single-agent carboplatin. *Gynecol Oncol* 1993;51:397.

135. Ball HG, Blessing JA, Lentz SS, et al. A phase II trial of paclitaxel in advanced and recurrent adenocarcinoma of the endometrium: a Gynecologic Oncology Group study. *Gynecol Oncol* 1996;62:278.

136. Lincoln S, Blessing JA, Lee RB, et al. Evaluation of paclitaxel (Taxol) in the treatment of recurrent or persistent endometrial carcinoma: a Gynecologic Oncology Group study. *Gynecol Oncol* (submitted).

137. Sutton GP, Blessing JA, DeMars LR, et al. A phase II Gynecologic Oncology Group trial of ifosfamide and mesna in advanced or recurrent adenocarcinoma of the endometrium. *Gynecol Oncol* 1996;63:25.

138. Poplin EA. Phase II trial of oral etoposide in recurrent or refractory endometrial adenocarcinoma: a Gynecologic Oncology Group study. *Gynecol Oncol* 1999;74:432.

139. Price FV, Edwards RP, Kelley JL, Kunschner AJ, Hart LA. A trial of outpatient paclitaxel and carboplatin for advanced, recurrent and histologic high-risk endometrial carcinoma: preliminary report. *Semin Oncol* 1997;24[Suppl 15]:78.

140. Lissoni A, Gabriele A, Gorga G, et al. Cisplatin-, epirubicin-, paclitaxel-containing chemotherapy in uterine adenocarcinoma. *Ann Oncol* 1997;8:969.

141. Pastan I, Gottesman M. Multiple-drug resistance in human cancer. *N Engl J Med* 1987;316:1388.

142. Yang CP, DePinho SG, Greenberger LM, et al. Progesterone interacts with P-glycoprotein in multidrug-resistant cells and in the endometrium of gravid uterus. *J Biol Chem* 1989;264:782.

143. Berchuck A, Soisson AP, Olt GJ, et al. Epidermal growth factor receptor expression in normal and malignant endometrium. *Am J Obstet Gynecol* 1989;161:1247.

144. Esteller M, Garcia A, Martinez i Palones JM, Cabero A, Reventos J. Detection of c-erbB-2/neu and fibroblast growth factor-3/INT-2 but not epidermal growth factor receptor gene amplification in endometrial cancer by different polymerase chain reaction. *Cancer* 1995;75:2139.

145. Aalders JG, Abeler V, Kolstad P. Recurrent adenocarcinoma of the endometrium: a clinical and histopathological study of 379 patients. *Gynecol Oncol* 1984;17:85.

146. Nag S, Yacoub S, Copeland LJ, et al. Interstitial brachytherapy for salvage treatment of vaginal recurrences in previously unirradiated endometrial cancer patients. *Int J Radiat Oncol Biol Phys* 2002;54:1153.

147. Pai HH, Souhami L, Clark BG, et al. Isolated vaginal recurrences in endometrial carcinoma: treatment results using high-dose-rate intracavitary brachytherapy and external beam radiotherapy. *Gynecol Oncol* 1997;66:300.

148. Charra C, Roy P, Coquard R, et al. Outcome of treatment of upper third vaginal recurrences of cervical and endometrial carcinomas with interstitial brachytherapy. *Int J Radiat Oncol Biol Phys* 1998;40:421.

149. Hart KB, Han I, Shamsa F, et al. Radiation therapy for endometrial cancer in patients treated for postoperative recurrence. *Int J Radiat Oncol Biol Phys* 1998;41:7.

150. Wylie J, Irwin C, Pintilie M, et al. Results of radical radiotherapy for recurrent endometrial cancer. *Gynecol Oncol* 2000;77:66.

151. Jhingran A, Burke TW, Eifel PJ. Definitive radiotherapy for patients with isolated vaginal recurrence of endometrial carcinoma after hysterectomy. *Int J Radiat Oncol Biol Phys* 2003;56:1366.

152. Hoekstra CJ, Koper PC, van Putten WL. Recurrent endometrial adenocarcinoma after surgery alone: prognostic factors and treatment. *Radiother Oncol* 1993;27:164.

153. Morris M, Alvarez RD, Kinney WK, et al. Treatment of recurrent adenocarcinoma of the endometrium with pelvic exenteration. *Gynecol Oncol* 1996;60:288.

154. Barber HRK, Brunschwig A. Treatment and results of recurrent cancer of corpus uteri in patients receiving anterior and total pelvic exenteration, 1947–1963. *Cancer* 1968;22:949.

155. Ober WB. Uterine sarcomas: histogenesis and taxonomy. *Ann N Y Acad Sci* 1959;75:568.

156. Spanos WJ Jr, Peters LJ Oswald MJ. Patterns of recurrence in malignant mixed müllerian tumors of the uterus. *Cancer* 1986;57:155.

157. Mountain CF, McMurtrey MJ, Hermes KE. Surgery for pulmonary metastasis: a 20-year experience. *Ann Thorac Surg* 1984;38:323.

158. Vongtama V, Karlen JR, Piver SM, et al. Treatment, results and prognostic factors in stage I and II sarcomas of the copus uteri. *AJR Am J Roentgenol* 1976;126:139.

159. Ferrer F, Sabater S, Farrus B, et al. Impact of radiotherapy on local control and survival in uterine sarcomas: a retrospective study from the Grup Oncologic Catala-Occita. *Int J Radiat Oncol Biol Phys* 1999;44:47.

160. Hornback NB, Omura G, Major FJ. Observations on the use of adjuvant radiation therapy in patients with stage I and II uterine sarcoma. *Int J Radiat Oncol Biol Phys* 1986; 12:2127.

161. Majors FJ, Blessing JA, Silverberg SG, et al. Prognostic factors in early-stage uterine sarcoma. A Gynecologic Oncology Group study. *Cancer* 1993;71:1702.

162. Gerszten K, Faul C, Kounelis S, et al. The impact of adjuvant radiotherapy on carcinoma of the uterus. *Gynecol Oncol* 1998;68:8.

163. Doss LL, Llorens AS, Henriquez EM. Carcinosarcoma of the uterus: a 40-year experience from the state of Missouri. *Gynecol Oncol* 1984;18:43.

164. Omura GA, Blessing JA, Major FJ, et al. A randomized clinical trial of adjuvant Adriamycin in uterine sarcoma: a GOG study. *J Clin Oncol* 1985;3:1240.

165. Muss HB, Bundy B, Disaia PJ, et al. Treatment of recurrent or advanced uterine sarcoma. A randomized trial of doxorubicin and cyclophosphamide (a phase III trial of the Gynecologic Oncology Group). *Cancer* 1985;55:1648.

166. Thigpen JT, Blessing JA, Beecham J, et al. Phase II trial of cisplatin as first-line chemotherapy in patients with advanced or recurrent uterine sarcomas: a Gynecologic Oncology Group study. *J Clin Oncol* 1991;9:162.

167. Sutton GP, Blessing JA, Barrett RJ, et al. Phase II trial of ifosfamide and mesna in leiomyosarcoma of the uterus: a Gynecologic Oncology Group study. *Am J Obstet Gynecol* 1992;166:556.

168. Slayton RE, Blessing JA, Angel C, et al. Phase II trial of etoposide in the management of advanced or recurrent leiomyosarcoma of the uterus: a Gynecologic Oncology Group study. *Cancer Treat Rep* 1987;71:1303.

169. Thigpen T, Blessing JA, Yordan E, et al. Phase II trial of etoposide in leiomyosarcoma of the uterus: a Gynecologic Oncology Group study. *Gynecol Oncol* 1996;63:120.

170. Rose PG, Blessing JA, Soper JT, et al. Prolonged oral etoposide in recurrent or advanced leiomyosarcoma of the uterus: a Gynecologic Oncology Group study. *Gynecol Oncol* 1998; 70:267.

171. Sutton G, Blessing JA, Ball H. Phase II trial of paclitaxel in leiomyosarcoma of the uterus: a Gynecologic Oncology Group study. *Gynecol Oncol* 1999;74:346.

172. Gallup DG, Blessing JA, Andersen W, Morgan MA. Radiation therapy with and without extrafascial hysterectomy for bulky stage IB cervical carcinoma: a randomized trial of the Gynecologic Oncology Group. *Gynecol Oncol* 2003;89:343.

173. Look KY, Sandler A, Blessing J, Lucci JA, Rose PG. A phase II trial of Gemcitabine in persistent or recurrent uterine leiomyosarcoma: a gynecologic oncology group (GOG) study. *Gynecol Oncol* 2003;88:213.

174. Sutton G, Blessing JA, Malfetano HH. Ifosfamide, doxorubicin and mesna in the treatment of metastatic uterine leiomyosarcomas. *Gynecol Oncol* 1996;62:226.

175. Currie JL, Blessing JL, Muss HB, et al. Combination chemotherapy with hydroxyurea, dacarbazine (DTIC), and etoposide in treatment of uterine leiomyosarcoma: a Gynecologic Oncology Group study. *Gynecol Oncol* 1996;61:27.

176. Edmonson J, Blessing JA, Cosin JA, et al. Phase II study of mitomycin, doxorubicin, and cisplatin in the treatment of advanced uterine leiomyosarcoma: a gynecologic oncology group study. *Gynecol Oncol* 2002;85:507.

177. Hensley ML, Maki R, Venkrataman E, et al. Gemcitabine and docetaxel in patients with unresectable leiomyosarcomas: results of a phase II trial. *J Clin Oncol* 2002; 20:2824.

178. Sutton GP, Blessing JA, Rosenshein N, et al. Phase II trial of ifosfamide and mesna in mixed mesodermal tumors of the uterus (a Gynecologic Oncology Group study). *Am J Obstet Gynecol* 1989;161:309.

179. Sutton GP, Brunetto V, Kilgore L, et al. A phase III trial of ifosfamide alone or in combination with cisplatin in the treatment of advanced, persistent, or recurrent carcinosarcoma of the uterus: a Gynecologic Oncology Group study. *Gynecol Oncol* 1998;68:137(abst).

180. Slayton RE, Blessing JA, DiSaia PJ, Christopherson WA. Phase II trial of etoposide in the management of advanced or recurrent mixed mesodermal sarcomas of the uterus: a Gynecologic Oncology Group study. *Cancer Treat Rep* 1987;71:661.

181. Curtin JP, Blessing JA, Soper JT, Degeest K. Paclitaxel in the treatment of carcinosarcoma of the uterus: a gynecologic oncology group study. *Gynecol Oncol* 2001;83:268.

182. Miller DS, Blessing JA, Kilgore LC, Mannel R, Van Le L. Phase II trial of topotecan in patients with advanced, persistent, or recurrent uterine leiomyosarcomas: a Gynecologic Oncology Group Study. *Am J Clin Oncol* 2000;23:355.

183. Currie JL, Blessing JA, McGehee R, Soper JT, Berman M. Phase II trial of hydroxyurea, dacarbazine (DTIC), and etoposide (VP-16) in mixed mesodermal tumors of the uterus: a Gynecologic Oncology Group study. *Gynecol Oncol* 1996;61:94.

184. Hornreich G, Muggia FM, Wadler S, et al. Phase II combination Doxil-paclitaxel (PacliDox) in uterine carcinomas and sarcomas an active regimen. A NYGOG study. *Gynecol Oncol* 2000;76:265(abst).

185. Gadducci A, Sartori E, Landoni F, et al. Endometrial stromal sarcoma: analysis of treatment failures and survival. *Gynecol Oncol* 1996;63:247.

186. Nordal RR, Kristensen GB, Kaern J, et al. The prognostic significance of surgery, tumor size, malignancy grade, menopausal status, and DNA ploidy in endometrial stromal sarcoma. *Gynecol Oncol* 1996;62:254.

187. Scribner DR Jr., Walker JL. Low-grade endometrial stromal sarcoma preoperative treatment with Depo-Lupron and Megace. *Gynecol Oncol* 1998;71:458.

188. Hitti IF, Glasber SS, McKenzie C. Uterine leiomyosarcoma with massive necrosis diagnosed during gonadotrophin releasing hormone analog therapy for presumed uterine fibroid. *Fertil Steril* 1991;56:778.

189. Katz L, Merino M, Sakamoto H, et al. Endometrial stromal sarcoma: a clinicopathologic study of 11 cases with determination of estrogen and progestin receptor levels in three tumors. *Gynecol Oncol* 1987;26:87.

190. Hall KL, Teneriello MG, Taylor RR, et al. Analysis of Ki-ras, p53, and MDM2 genes in uterine leiomyomas and leiomyosarcomas. *Gynecol Oncol* 1997;65:330.

191. Gosland MP, Lum BL, Sikic BI. Reversal by cefoperazone of resistance to etoposide, doxorubicin, and vinblastine in multidrug resistant human sarcoma cells. *Cancer Res* 1989;49:6905.

192. Resnick MB, Sabo E, Kondratis S, et al. Cancer-testis antigen expression in uterine malignancies with an emphasis on carcinosarcomas and papillary serous carcinomas. *Int J Cancer* 2002;101:190.

FRANCO M. MUGGIA
THOMAS W. BURKE
WILLIAM SMALL, JR.

SECTION 3

Gestational Trophoblastic Diseases

Gestational trophoblastic disease affects young women and encompasses interrelated conditions spanning proliferative changes resulting from an abnormal fertilization to highly malignant lesions such as choriocarcinoma. The spectrum of disease can be subdivided into four distinct clinicopathologic entities: molar pregnancy (including complete and partial hydatidiform moles), invasive mole (chorioadenoma destruens), placental-site trophoblastic tumors, and choriocarcinoma. Although representing fewer than 1% of gynecologic malignancies, it is highly important to promote awareness of their life-threatening potential and their high curability if treated early and by experienced centers.

Earlier diagnosis of molar pregnancies has led to refinement of histopathologic criteria.[1]

EPIDEMIOLOGY

Gestational trophoblastic disease is most commonly recognized after molar pregnancy but may also occur after normal or ectopic pregnancies and spontaneous or therapeutic abortions. Its incidence varies widely among various populations, with figures as high as 1 in 120 pregnancies in some areas of Asia and South America, compared to 1 in 1200 in the United States.[2] The risk is fivefold greater in women older than 40 years[3] and is also increased in those younger than 20 years.[2] Prior molar pregnancies, lower socioeconomic status, and blood group A women married to group O men are at higher risk.[2,3] Parity, ethnicity, nutritional factors, and cigarette smoking have been examined as risk factors, but no clear association has been found. However, oral contraceptives and the number of sexual partners before the index pregnancy appear to double the risk of gestational trophoblastic tumors.[4]

PATHOLOGY AND BIOLOGY

Hydatidiform moles (complete and partial) are characterized by clusters of hydropic villi and trophoblastic hyperplasia with atypia. Partial moles show a variable amount of abnormal villus development and focal trophoblastic hyperplasia in association with identifiable fetal or embryonic tissues. Invasive moles (chorioadenoma destruens) have findings similar to those of complete moles but display a greater tendency to invade surrounding tissues. The rare placental-site trophoblastic tumors[5]—initially named *trophoblastic pseudotumors*—are derived from intermediate trophoblast cells [which secrete placental lactogen in greater amounts than human chorionic gonadotropin (HCG)[6]], and they present clinically as nodules in the endometrium and myometrium after removal of a mole. Microscopically, these tumors show no chorionic villi and are characterized by a proliferation of cells with oval nuclei and abundant eosinophilic cytoplasm. They usually arise after nonmolar abortion or a term pregnancy but occasionally after hydatidiform mole even after a metastatic gestational trophoblastic neoplasia.[6] Choriocarcinomas consist of invasive and anaplastic trophoblastic tissue made up of cytotrophoblastic and syncytiotrophoblastic elements, obligatory secretion of HCG, and rich vascularity. Commonly accompanying the trophoblastic neoplasia are one or more theca lutein ovarian cysts that are a result of HCG stimulation. Rarely, the malignancy can coexist with an intact pregnancy.[7] Treatment of choriocarcinomas has evolved based on prognostic factor risk classification and staging and not on pathologic features; this risk classification does not apply to the placental-site trophoblastic malignancies.[6]

Cytogenetics has provided clues as to the origin of hydatidiform moles: Most complete moles are diploid and have a 46XX karyotype, with the minority being 46XY. All X chromosomes are androgenetic (from paternal origin). These arise from fertilization of an empty ovum by a haploid sperm that then undergoes duplication. Occasionally, complete moles arise from fertilization of an empty ovum by two sperms. Maternally transcribed genes are lost, although one may identify maternal mitochondrial DNA.[8] On the other hand, partial moles contain maternal and paternal chromosomes and are triploid, and their sex chromosomes are typically XXY. Presumably, fertilization of a normal ovum by two sperms leads to a partial mole, whereas an extra haploid set of maternal origin results in a trisomic fetus.[9,10]

Genomic imprinting may underlie the pathophysiology of trophoblastic disease: Two paternal genomes presumably lead to trophoblastic hyperplasia[8]; this may be mediated by excess insulin-like growth factors or through immunologic mechanisms.[11] In turn, studies *in vitro* point to other alterations (e.g., expression of epidermal growth factor receptor[12] and metalloproteinases[13] with down-regulation of cad-11[14]) as modulators of malignant transformation and invasiveness. Mutations in p53 are infrequent, but overexpression of oncoproteins including mdm2 may be implicated in trophoblastic disease pathogenesis.[15]

CLINICAL DIAGNOSIS AND HUMAN CHORIONIC GONADOTROPIN

Widespread use of ultrasonography in early pregnancy is leading to a prenatal diagnosis of molar pregnancy with increasing frequency even as early as 9.5 weeks,[16] an important factor in updating our histopathologic diagnostic criteria.[17] A molar pregnancy is suspected with first-trimester bleeding, a uterus larger than expected for gestational age, and absence of fetal heart sounds and fetal parts in association with a markedly elevated HCG level. Iron-deficiency anemia is common at diagnosis because of recurrent bleeding. Other signs include hyperemesis, the passage of "prune juice–like" clots and even actual grape-like villi, toxemia during the first or second trimester, presence of ovarian enlargement with theca lutein cysts (due to overstimulation by HCG), and hyperthyroidism. In comparison with complete moles, partial moles tend to display a milder clinical course resembling a spontaneous miscarriage with recognizable fetal tissues, lack the classic "snowstorm" pattern of complete moles on ultrasound, and are often only retrospectively diagnosed.[16,17] Genetic analysis for ploidy, perhaps supplemented by molecular markers, may be helpful in confirming the histopathologic suspicion of partial moles and separating them from complete moles[18–20] or the normal placenta. Invasive moles may cause rupture of the uterus. Rupture of an ovarian cyst and metastatic disease may rarely be the presentation of an otherwise unrecognized or silent gestational trophoblastic disease. In fewer than 1% of molar pregnancies, a normal fetal (twin) pregnancy may coexist. Serial HCG determinations are of central importance in the diagnosis, treatment, follow-up, and pathogenesis of some gestational trophoblastic disease manifestations.

HCG is synthesized by syncytiotrophoblast cells of the developing placenta, and its primary function is to act on the luteinizing hormone receptors of the ovarian corpus luteum. In similarity to luteinizing hormone, follicle-stimulating hormone, and thyroid-stimulating hormone (now designated as *thyrotropin*), it is a glycoprotein consisting of an α subunit common to all four and a hormone-specific β subunit; its primary function is the maintenance of the corpus luteum during pregnancy. Normally, HCG peaks at 10 to 12 weeks of gestation, and actual levels and serial changes in β-HCG are essential to diagnose and track the outcome of trophoblastic disease. After evacuation of a molar pregnancy, β-HCG titers usually disappear in 8 to 10 weeks. Persistence of titers may indicate local and, less often, metastatic disease and occurs in 15% of women after a complete mole and 1% after a partial mole.[17] With monitoring of serum HCG, persistence is detected early; otherwise, a β-HCG level of greater than 100,000 mIU/mL, a uterine size greater than expected from gestational age, and the presence of theca lutein ovarian cysts larger than 6 cm in diameter identify women with persistent gestational trophoblastic disease, particularly after evacuation of a complete mole. The placental-site trophoblastic tumor produces low levels of HCG but may be identified by measurement of placental lactogen.[5,6]

Although short courses of methotrexate or dactinomycin eliminate persistence of trophoplastic disease without the development of invasive mole or choriocarcinoma when detected early, late presentations are associated with 8.8% metastatic (usually pulmonary) and 31% nonmetastatic manifestations.[21] Weekly HCG measurements until three nondetectable determinations, followed by monthly tests for 6 months, are advised in all instances proven to have a persistent elevation of HCG or actual trophoblastic disease. In addition, effective contraception during the entire period of follow-up is essential to avoid confusing the clinical picture. However, subsequent pregnancies have been reported as normal in more than 98% of instances.[21,22]

TABLE 32.3-1. Prognostic Scoring System for Gestational Trophoblastic Disease

Factor	Score			
	0	1	2	4
Age	—	<39 y	—	>39 y
Antecedent pregnancy	Mole	Abortion	Term	—
Interval from pregnancy (mo)	<4	4–6	7–12	>12
Serum human chorionic gonadotropin	<10^3 IU/L	10^3–10^4 IU/L	10^4–10^5 IU/L	>10^5 IU/L
Largest tumor	<3 cm	3–5 cm	>5 cm	—
Metastatic sites	Lung	Spleen, kidney	Gastrointestinal tract, liver	Brain
Number of metastases	—	1–3	4–8	>8
Prior chemotherapy	—	—	One drug	Two or more drugs

(From Bagshawe KD. Treatment of high-risk choriocarcinoma. *J Reprod Med* 1984;29:813, with permission.)

CHORIOCARCINOMA

CLINICAL FEATURES AND STAGING

Metastatic disease occurs in 4% of patients after local management of hydatidiform moles and very rarely after term pregnancies (1 in 40,000) or abortions. Rapid growth and a high propensity for hemorrhage make this tumor a medical emergency. Metastases are found in lung (80%), vagina (30%), pelvis (20%), brain (10%), and liver (10%). Other rare sites are the spleen, kidneys, and gastrointestinal tract. The lungs are often involved, with multiple lesions best detected with computed tomography during workup of persistent moles, but at times this involvement is massive. The central nervous system is seldom involved in the absence of pulmonary metastases; the presence of central nervous system metastases is usually diagnosed by magnetic resonance spectroscopy (often showing bleeding). A ratio of serum to cerebrospinal fluid β-HCG of less than 60:1[25] confirms that such metastases have not been eradicated by treatment.

Anatomic staging of choriocarcinoma (I, confined to corpus; II, metastases to pelvis and vagina; III, pulmonary metastases with or without uterine, pelvic, or vaginal involvement; and IV, other metastases, such as brain, liver, kidneys, or gastrointestinal tract) was superseded by the scoring system developed by Bagshawe et al.[3] and by the World Health Organization combined with the Federation of Gynecology and Obstetrics[24] (Table 32.3-1). The importance of using a prognostic factor–based scoring system lies in the identification of a high-risk choriocarcinoma that requires more intensive use of drug combinations to achieve cures and prevent emergence of resistance, whereas single agents or simple combinations effectively manage low-risk patients.

TREATMENT

Chemotherapy is highly effective for all forms of gestational trophoblastic disease. The curative effects of methotrexate in a disease that had previously resulted in the death of 60% of patients with disease confined to the uterus and 90% of patients with metastatic disease heralded the era of modern chemotherapy.[23] The current challenges are to provide the proper follow-up after evacuation of hydatidiform moles, to balance drug administration with surgical interventions when more invasive trophoblastic disease is present, and finally to tailor the type of chemotherapy to the risk group of gestational trophoblastic disease that has been identified. The scoring system in Table 32.3-1 assists in reaching decisions, but the expertise of a multidisciplinary team cannot be overemphasized. In particular, hysterectomy and single-agent chemotherapy must be considered in stage I disease depending on the patient's desire for future fertility. In this circumstance, chemotherapy reduces dissemination during surgery and treats any occult metastases not previously detected.

For low-risk disease, methotrexate by itself or with leucovorin rescue or dactinomycin has most commonly been used.[21] Monitoring with β-HCG to document a prompt 1 log or greater reduction in the titer in 18 days, along with continued monthly monitoring of negative values for 1 year, is standard practice. Etoposide is also effective, but its leukemogenic effect is a concern[21] in low-risk patients. Current Gynecologic Oncology Group studies for low-risk disease begun in 1999 are comparing methotrexate with dactinomycin and also assessing dactinomycin in patients not responding to methotrexate.

In high-risk patients, combination chemotherapy is the treatment of choice, and the serum EMA-CO (etoposide, dactinomycin, and folinic acid; vincristine and cyclophosphamide) combination (Table 32.3-2) is most commonly used. This combination was introduced after recognition of the activity of etoposide, even after failure of other drug regimens, including those for low risk plus cyclophosphamide, vincristine, doxorubicin, hydroxyurea, and 5-fluorouracil. Results with EMA-CO are excellent in most high-risk disease patients.[25] However, approximately 20% of patients, particularly if they have shown methotrexate resistance, do not show a complete response. These and other particularly high-risk patients (e.g., markedly elevated HCG, brain metastases) should likely begin treatment with cisplatin (P) and etoposide (E) in a weekly scheme (to avoid hazardous thrombocytopenia); a hybrid EP/EMA regimen reported excellent results in patients presenting with brain metastases,[25] in patients responding incompletely to EMA-CO, and in placental-site trophoblastic tumors. Deaths from choriocarcinoma usually result either from very late presentations leading to complications such as respiratory failure or central nervous system hemorrhage or from the development of drug resistance if the tumor burden is excessive at the outset or if treatment has not been sufficiently aggressive. Rarely, as it is for germ cell tumors and other gynecologic cancers, resistance to cisplatin is what determines an unfavorable outcome. Experimental strategies to overcome such resistance

TABLE 32.3-2. Drug Regimens for Gestational Trophoblastic Disease

LOW RISK (SINGLE AGENTS)

Methotrexate[a]: 30–50 mg/m^2 IM weekly; 0.4 mg/kg IM or IV daily for 5 d (repeat in 2 wk); or 1 mg/kg IM or IV on d 1, 3, 5, and 7 (repeat in 2 wk) plus folinic acid (leucovorin), 0.1 mg/kg or IV on d 2, 4, 6, and 8

Dactinomycin: 1.25 mg/m^2 IV (repeat in 2 wk), or 10 µg/kg (up to 0.5 mg) IV daily for 5 d (repeat in 2 wk)

HIGH RISK (DRUG COMBINATIONS)

EMA-CO consists of alternating cycles of EMA (d 1 and 2) and CO (d 8)

Day 1: EMA: *etoposide*, 100 mg/m^2 IV; *dactinomycin*, 0.5 mg IV; and *methotrexate*, 100 mg IV push followed by 200 mg/m^2 12-h IV

Day 2: EMA: *etoposide*, 100 mg/m^2 IV; *dactinomycin*, 0.5 mg IV; and *folinic acid*, 15 mg IV or PO every 12 h × 4, 24 h after start of methotrexate

Day 8: CO: *vincristine*, 1 mg/m^2 IV; and *cyclophosphamide*, 600 mg/m^2 IV

MEA consists of alternating cycles of methotrexate (d 1) with EA (d 9–11). Repeated every 19 d.

Day 1: methotrexate, 300 mg/m^2 IV; folinic acid, 15 mg every 6 h to commence 24 h after chemotherapy for 8 doses (first 4 doses to be given IV). 7-d break.

Days 9–11: etoposide, 100 mg/m^2 IV daily; dactinomycin, 0.5 mg IV daily. 7-d break and repeat methotrexate.

SALVAGE REGIMENS

VIP: etoposide, ifosfamide, and cisplatin (doses as per germ cell regimen)

EMA-EP: etoposide, methotrexate, actinomycin D–etoposide, cisplatin 25

EP: etoposide, cisplatin (doses as per germ cell regimen)

Single agents: taxanes, platinum, and vinca analogue; topoisomerase I inhibitors; ifosfamide; gemcitabine

---

[a]Requires normal renal and bone marrow function and no stomatitis.

---

include dose intensification, analogue development, and use of new drugs such as taxanes, gemcitabine, and topoisomerase I inhibitors, although experience is limited.

Radiation given concomitantly with chemotherapy (from older series) has been advocated from the outset in patients who have brain metastases.[26]

The suggested radiotherapy dose in a more recent series was 3000 cGy in 200-cGy fractions with a localized boost considered for large tumor burdens.[27] An improvement in survival in patients who present with brain metastasis and have had no prior therapy versus patients who develop brain metastasis during chemotherapy has also been emphasized. These authors also recommend the selective use of craniotomy in selected patients in whom the disease cannot be controlled by chemotherapy.[28]

Newer concepts emphasize the use of cisplatin-based regimens shortly after the diagnosis of brain metastases—particularly if this is part of the initial presentation.[25] On the other hand, symptomatic metastases occurring during chemotherapy may require radiation, as well as a change in the systemic treatment regimen and consideration of surgery.

REFERENCES

1. Paradinas FJ. The diagnosis and prognosis of molar pregnancy: the experience of the National Referral Centre in London. *Int J Gynaecol Obstet* 1998;60:S57.
2. Buckley JD. The epidemiology of molar pregnancy and choriocarcinoma. *Clin Obstet Gynecol* 1984;27:153.
3. Bagshawe KD, Dent J, Webb J. Hydatidiform mole in England and Wales 1973–1983. *Lancet* 1986;2:673.
4. Palmer JR, Driscoll SG, Rosenberg L, et al. Oral contraceptive use and risk of gestational trophoblastic tumors. *J Natl Cancer Inst* 1999;91:635.
5. Kurman RJ, Main CS, Chen HC. Intermediate trophoblast: a distinctive form of trophoblast with specific morphological, biochemical, and functional features. *Placenta* 1984;5:349.
6. Papadopoulos AJ, Foskett M, Seckl MJ, et al. Twenty five years' clinical experience with placental site trophoblastic tumors. *J Reprod Med* 2002;47:460.
7. Steigrad SJ, Cheung AP, Osborn RA. Choriocarcinoma co-existent with an intact pregnancy: case report and review of the literature. *J Obstet Gynaecol Res* 1999;25:197.
8. Fisher RA. Genetics. In: Hancock BW, Newlands ES, Berkowitz RS, eds. *Gestational trophoblastic disease.* London: Chapman & Hall, 1997:5.
9. Lawler S, Fisher RA, Dent J. A prospective genetic study of complete and partial hydatidiform moles. *Am J Obstet Gynecol* 1991;164:1270.
10. McFadden DE, Kalousek DK. Two different phenotypes of fetuses with chromosomal triploidy: correlation with parental origin of the extra haploid set. *Am J Med Genet* 1991;38:535.
11. Cross JC, Werb Z, Fisher SJ. Implantation and the placenta: key pieces of the development puzzle. *Science* 1994;266:1508.
12. Steller MA, Mok SC, Yeh J. Effects of cytokines on epidermal growth factor receptor expression by malignant trophoblast cells in vitro. *J Reprod Med* 1994;39:208.
13. Vegh GL, Tuncer ZS, Fulop V, et al. Matrix metalloproteinases and their inhibitors in gestational trophoblastic disease and normal placenta. *Gynecol Oncol* 1999;75:248.
14. MacCalman CD, Getsios S, Chen GTC, et al. Type 2 cadherins in the human endometrium and placenta: their putative roles in human implantation and placentation. *Am J Reprod Immunol* 1998;39:96.
15. Fulop V, Mok SC, Genest DR, et al. p53, p21, Rb and mdm2 oncoproteins: expression in normal placenta, partial and complete mole, and choriocarcinoma. *J Reprod Med* 1998;43:101.
16. Crade M, Weber PR. Appearance of molar pregnancy 9.5 weeks after conception: use of transvaginal ultrasound for early diagnosis. *J Ultrasound Med* 1991;10:473.
17. Sebire N, Mackydimas G, Agnantis NJ, et al. Updated diagnostic criteria for partial and complete hydatidiform moles in early pregnancy. *Anticancer Res* 2003;23:1723.
18. Genest DR. Partial hydatidiform mole: clinicopathological features, differential diagnosis, ploidy and molecular studies, and gold standards for diagnosis. *Int J Gynecol Pathol* 2001;20:315.
19. Castrillon DH, Sun D, Weremowicz S, et al. Discrimination of complete hydatidiform mole from its mimics by immunohistochemistry of the paternally imprinted gene product p57kip2. *Am J Surg Pathol* 2001;25:1225.
20. Petignat P, Billieux MH, Blouin JL, et al. Is genetic analysis useful in the routine management of hydatidiform mole? *Hum Reprod* 2003;18:243.
21. Soto-Wright V, Goldstein DP, Bernstein MR, Berkowitz RS. The management of gestational trophoblastic tumors with etoposide, methotrexate, and actinomycin D. *Gynecol Oncol* 1997;64:156.
22. Berkowitz RS, Bernstein MR, Laborde O, et al. Subsequent pregnancy experience gestational trophoblastic disease. New England Trophoblastic Disease Center, 1965–1992. *J Reprod Med* 1994;9:228.
23. Li MC, Hertz R, Spence DB. Effect of methotrexate therapy upon choriocarcinoma and chorioadenoma. *Proc Soc Exp Biol Med* 1956;93:361.
24. Kohorn EI, Goldstein DP, Hancock BW, et al. Combining the staging system of the International Federation of Gynecology and Obstetrics with the scoring system of the World Health Organization for Trophoblastic Neoplasia. *Int J Gynecol Cancer* 2000;10:84.
25. Newlands ES, Mulholland PJ, Holden L, et al. Etoposide and cisplatin/etoposide, methotrexate and actinomycin D (EMA) chemotherapy for patients with high risk gestational trophoblastic tumors refractory to EMA/cyclophosphamide and vincristine chemotherapy, and patients presenting with metastatic placental site trophoblastic tumors. *J Clin Oncol* 2000;18:854.
26. Yordan EL, Schlaerth J, Gaddis O, et al. Radiation therapy in the management of gestational choriocarcinoma metastatic to the central nervous system. *Obstet Gynecol* 1987;69:627.
27. Small W Jr, Lurain JR, Shetty RM, et al. Gestational trophoblastic disease metastatic to the brain. *Radiology* 1996;200:277.
28. Evans AC Jr, Soper JT, Clarke-Pearson DL, et al. Gestational trophoblastic disease metastatic to the central nervous system. *Gynecol Oncol* 1995;59:226.

BETH Y. KARLAN
MAURIE A. MARKMAN
PATRICIA J. EIFEL

SECTION 4

Ovarian Cancer, Peritoneal Carcinoma, and Fallopian Tube Carcinoma

OVARIAN CANCER

On the basis of distinct pathologic and clinical features, ovarian cancer can be separated into three distinct histologic subtypes: epithelial tumors, germ cell tumors, and sex cord–stromal tumors. The vast majority of ovarian cancers are epithelial in origin, with these tumors accounting for more than 90% of the estimated 25,400 new cases of ovarian cancer diagnosed in the United States in 2003.[1] Fallopian tube carcinomas and extraovarian primary peritoneal carcinomas are much less common, but because their biology and clinical characteristics are markedly similar to those of epithelial ovarian carcinomas, these tumors are also discussed in this chapter. Approximately 14,300 U.S. women died of ovarian cancer in 2003, which makes this tumor the leading cause of gynecologic cancer death.[1] Overall, ovarian cancer accounts for 4% of all cancer diagnoses and 5% of all cancer deaths. The lifetime risk of developing ovarian cancer is approximately 1.7%, and approximately 1 in 60 women will die of the disease.

The vast majority of epithelial ovarian carcinomas are diagnosed in postmenopausal women, and the median age at diagnosis is 63 years. The age-specific incidence increases from 15 to 16 per 100,000 in the 40- to 44-year-old age group to a peak rate of 57 per 100,000 in the 70- to 74-year-old age group.[2] There has been a statistically significant improvement in the 5-year survival rates over the last decades, with a rate of 37% in 1976, 41% in 1985, and 53% in 1998.[1] This improvement in survival is likely the result of more effective chemotherapies and improvements in surgery and supportive care. African American women in the United States have a lower incidence of ovarian cancer (10.3 per 100,000 women) compared with white women; however, the overall survival rate of 53% is identical. The stage distribution and stage-specific 5-year survival rates for white and African American women are also very similar.[1]

PATHOGENESIS

The common epithelial tumors account for 60% of all ovarian neoplasms and for 80% to 90% of ovarian malignancies. The remaining tumors arise from ovarian germ cells or stromal cells. The epithelial tumors arise from the surface epithelium or serosa of the ovary. During embryogenesis, the lining of the coelomic cavity consists of mesothelial cells of mesodermal origin, and the gonadal ridge is covered by serosal epithelium. Müllerian ducts, which give rise to the fallopian tubes, uterus, and vagina, are the result of invagination of the mesothelial lining. When the epithelium becomes malignant, it can express a variety of müllerian-type histologic morphologies. Serous carcinomas can resemble the fallopian tube, mucinous tumors the endocervix, and endometrioid carcinomas the endometrium. It is thought that germ cell tumors originate in cells derived from the primitive streak that ultimately migrated to the gonads. The mesenchyma gives rise to the ovarian stroma, and stromal tumors arise from this original cell type.

In the majority of cases, malignant epithelial ovarian tumors disseminate throughout the peritoneal cavity after exfoliation of malignant cells from the surface of the ovary. The typical circulation of the peritoneal fluid along the undersurface of the right hemidiaphragm facilitates the frequently observed pattern of widespread dissemination of malignant tumor cells within the peritoneal cavity. In addition, the omentum frequently attracts these malignant cells and is thus a common site of metastasis. Tumor spread also occurs via the lymphatics from the ovary. A primary source of drainage follows the ovarian blood supply in the infundibulopelvic ligament to lymph nodes around the aorta and vena cava to the level of the renal vessels. There is also lymphatic drainage through the broad ligament and parametrial channels; consequently, pelvic sidewall lymphatics, including the external iliac, obturator, and hypogastric chains, are also frequently involved. More rarely, spread may occur along the course of the round ligament, resulting in involvement of inguinal lymph nodes. Spread to lymph nodes is common. Approximately 10% of patients with ovarian cancer that appears to be localized to the ovaries have metastases to paraaortic lymph nodes, and retroperitoneal lymph node involvement is found in the majority of cases of advanced ovarian cancer. Hematogenous metastases to extraabdominal sites can occur but are relatively uncommon. There can also be direct extension of the tumor from the ovary to involve the adjacent peritoneal surfaces of the bladder, rectosigmoid, and pelvic peritoneum.

HISTOLOGIC CLASSIFICATION OF EPITHELIAL TUMORS

Table 32.4-1 details the classification of common epithelial tumors that has been developed by the World Health Organization and the International Federation of Gynecology and Obstetrics.[3] The nomenclature for these tumors reflects the cell type, location of the tumor, and degree of malignancy, ranging from benign lesions to tumors of low malignant potential (LMP) to invasive carcinomas. Tumors of LMP ("borderline malignancy") have an excellent prognosis compared with invasive carcinomas, and their clinical behavior and management are outlined later in this chapter. Tumors of LMP are characterized by epithelial papillae with atypical cell clusters, cellular stratification, nuclear atypia, and increased mitotic activity. The differentiation between these tumors and carcinomas is primarily made on the basis of pathologic architecture and the presence of stromal invasion. Overtly malignant tumors are characterized by an infiltrative destructive growth pattern, with cytologically bizarre cells growing in a disorganized pattern with dissection into stromal planes.

The invasive epithelial carcinomas are characterized by histologic cell type and the degree of differentiation (tumor grade). The histologic cell type has limited prognostic significance independent of clinical stage; however, tumor grade is an important independent prognostic factor, especially in patients with early-stage epithelial tumors. Grading systems have been based on cytologic detail or a pattern grading classi-

TABLE 32.4-1. World Health Organization Classification of Malignant Ovarian Tumors

COMMON EPITHELIAL TUMORS
Malignant serous tumor
Adenocarcinoma, papillary adenocarcinoma, papillary cystadenocarcinoma
Surface papillary carcinoma
Malignant adenofibroma, cystadenofibroma
Malignant mucinous tumor
Adenocarcinoma, cystadenocarcinoma
Malignant adenofibroma, cystadenofibroma
Malignant endometrioid tumor
Carcinoma
    Adenocarcinoma
    Adenoacanthoma
    Malignant adenofibroma, cystadenofibroma
Endometrioid stromal sarcoma
Mesodermal (müllerian) mixed tumor: homologous and heterologous
Clear cell (mesonephroid) tumor, malignant
    Carcinoma and adenocarcinoma
Brenner tumor, malignant
Mixed epithelial tumor, malignant
Undifferentiated carcinoma
Unclassified
SEX CORD–STROMAL TUMORS
Granulosa–stromal cell tumor
Granulosa cell tumor
Tumor in the thecoma-fibroma group
Fibroma
Unclassified
Androblastoma: Sertoli-Leydig cell tumor
Well differentiated
Tubular androblastoma, Sertoli cell tumor (tubular adenoma of Pick)
Tubular androblastoma with lipid storage, Sertoli cell tumor with lipid storage
Sertoli-Leydig cell tumor (tubular adenoma with Leydig cells)
Leydig cell tumor, hilus cell tumor
Of intermediate differentiation
Poorly differentiated (sarcomatoid)
With heterologous elements
Gynandroblastoma
Unclassified
Germ cell tumor
Dysgerminoma
Endodermal sinus tumor
Embryonal carcinoma
Polyembryoma
LIPID (LIPOID) CELL TUMORS
Choriocarcinoma
Teratoma
    Immature
    Mature dermoid cyst with malignant transformation
    Monodermal and highly specialized
    Struma ovarii
    Carcinoid
    Struma ovarii and carcinoid
    Others
Mixed forms
GONADOBLASTOMA
Pure
Mixed with dysgerminoma or other form of germ cell tumor

fication based on the degree to which a tumor forms papillary structures or glands versus solid tumor.

DIAGNOSIS AND SYMPTOMS

Epithelial cancers of the ovary have been described as silent killers because the overwhelming majority of patients do not present with symptoms until the disease has spread outside of the ovary and indeed outside of the pelvis. However, studies surveying ovarian cancer patients have demonstrated that 95% of these women have nonspecific abdominal symptoms many months before diagnosis.[4] Approximately 70% of patients with epithelial cancers of the ovary present with stage III or IV disease, whereas 70% of patients with germ cell ovarian malignancies present with stage I disease. Unlike epithelial cancers, ovarian germ cell malignancies tend to stretch and twist the infundibulopelvic ligament, causing severe pain while the disease is still confined to the ovary. Functioning ovarian tumors of the sex cord–stromal type may present with symptoms suggestive of excessive endogenous estrogen or androgen production. Granulosa cell tumors occurring in premenarchal girls may present with precocious puberty. Women in the reproductive years with granulosa cell tumors may present with amenorrhea or abnormal menses, and postmenopausal women may present with postmenopausal bleeding. Sertoli-Leydig cell tumors may present with symptoms of virilization, but none of these hormonal manifestations is a reliable diagnostic criterion.

Abdominal discomfort and bloating are the most common symptoms experienced by women with epithelial ovarian cancers, followed by vaginal bleeding, gastrointestinal symptoms, and urinary tract symptoms. Patients presenting with nonspecific lower abdominal discomfort and bloating require at least a prompt and careful pelvic and rectovaginal examination. The most common physical signs are ascites and a pelvic mass. The mass is frequently firm, hard, and fixed with multiple nodularities palpable in the cul-de-sac.

Level of the cancer antigen 125 (CA 125) tumor biomarker is elevated in more than 80% of serous epithelial ovarian cancers, but it can also be elevated in a variety of benign conditions and other nongynecologic malignancies. Furthermore, in early-stage ovarian cancers, CA 125 level is elevated in less than half of cases. Other tumor markers, such as CA 19-9, which is elevated in many mucinous ovarian carcinomas, and carcinoembryonic antigen, which may be elevated in 7% to 37% of patients with ovarian cancer, are less frequently used. Preoperatively, tumor marker levels are useful in predicting the potential for malignancy. During treatment for ovarian cancer, CA 125 level is a very useful barometer of disease activity and can be used to follow response to therapy and to detect an early recurrence.

Chest radiographs are routinely performed to look for malignant pleural effusions, which occur in 10% of patients, and metastatic pulmonary disease, which is very rare. Barium enema examination is not routinely performed but may be helpful in patients with blood in the stool, obstipation, or anemia to rule out a primary gastrointestinal malignancy. Results of barium enema examinations are not very useful in predicting the need for colon resection. Mammography may also be indicated preoperatively to rule out a possible metastatic or synchronous breast carcinoma.

Transvaginal ultrasonography (TVS) and abdominal ultrasonography are the most useful diagnostic examinations in the evaluation of a pelvic mass because of their ability to accurately discern the ovarian morphology and other pelvic pathology. Some of the sonographic characteristics associated with ovarian cancer include irregular ovarian cyst borders, solid elements within the cysts, papillary projections, bilateral ovarian involvement, and the presence of ascites. Color Doppler imaging evaluates blood flow to an ovarian mass and can potentially identify a malignant process based on the presence of abnormal neovascularization. Several studies suggest that color Doppler imaging may improve the specificity for detecting ovarian cancer when a mass is seen; however, Doppler imaging cannot definitively identify malignancy.[5] Three-dimensional ultrasonography has the potential benefit of improved definition of the ovarian surface and internal cyst morphology; however, its usefulness in the diagnosis of ovarian cancer is still under study.

Cross-sectional imaging, such as computed tomography (CT) and magnetic resonance imaging, may be helpful in characterizing the liver, identifying lymph node involvement, peritoneal studding, and omentum caking, and characterizing the mesentery of the bowel. CT scans may be helpful in distinguishing a gynecologic malignancy from a metastatic pancreatic neoplasm for which surgery may not be warranted. Magnetic resonance imaging in patients with an ovarian mass has not been shown to have a clear advantage over CT, except for the evaluation of adnexal masses in pregnant patients when ultrasonography is inconclusive and the desire is to avoid CT due to the radiation exposure.

Other studies such as bone and liver scintigraphy do not add any useful information. Intravenous pyelograms or renal scans may be helpful in patients with abnormal renal function or abnormal findings on ultrasonography, but they are rarely used. Positron emission tomography (PET) is a form of functional imaging that most frequently uses the positron-emitting glucose analogue, [^{18}F]fluorodeoxyglucose. Tumor masses are imaged based on their relatively increased glucose metabolism compared to normal tissues. The role of PET in preoperative evaluation for suspected recurrent ovarian carcinoma is being studied at a number of centers, and the more recent development of fusion PET-CT technologies, combining cross-sectional and functional images, has shown very promising early results.[6]

The most common complaints associated with ovarian malignancies in the pediatric population are pain, abdominal swelling, and pelvic mass. Ovarian masses in premenarchal girls require prompt evaluation and frequently an exploratory laparotomy, because functional cysts should not occur. Most premenarchal adnexal masses, however, ultimately prove to be benign.

Small ovarian cysts are often identified on ultrasonographic examinations of postmenopausal ovaries. Five percent to 10% of asymptomatic postmenopausal women may be found to have small ovarian cysts, especially in the first decade after menopause. These cysts do not need to be removed if they appear to be sonolucent and unilocular on ultrasonography and are associated with normal CA 125 levels.[8] Postmenopausal women with complex pelvic masses, simple cysts in association with elevated serum CA 125 levels, or simple cysts in association with abnormal color Doppler flow studies should undergo surgical evaluation.

Enlarged ovaries in reproductive-age women are relatively common and are frequently due to either functioning ovarian cysts, such as endometriomas and corpus luteum cysts, or to benign ovarian cysts. Women found to have such cysts may be evaluated by measurement of serum CA 125 levels. However, caution is warranted in interpreting these data because CA 125

levels can be elevated due to other benign processes in these young women. Benign conditions such as leiomyomas, adenomyosis, endometriosis, and salpingitis, to name just a few, can be associated with elevated CA 125 levels, and no absolute cutoff exists to distinguish benign from malignant pathologies.[7]

Cysts that appear by ultrasonographic criteria to be functional or simple in nature may be followed through several menstrual cycles. Often they disappear over this short observation interval. Functional cysts may also disappear when oral contraceptives are used. Neoplastic cysts do not disappear under the influence of oral contraceptives. Even in postmenopausal women, persistent unilocular ovarian cysts are very rarely associated with malignancy.[8] Rising values in serial CA 125 assays obtained during the observation period are an indication that a malignancy may be present. In turn, CA 125 values that are stable or declining generally reflect the presence of a functional cyst or other benign condition.

Diagnostic laparoscopy may be extremely useful to evaluate unexplained pelvic pain or adnexal masses of uncertain pathology. Extreme caution and sound surgical judgment are required when choosing this minimally invasive approach, however, because rupturing a malignant tumor and up-staging a stage IA ovarian cancer to a stage IC cancer may result in the need to administer chemotherapy or may even alter patient survival. Although there is no definitive evidence that rupture of an early-stage ovarian malignancy decreases survival, avoidance of rupture should be the routine when approaching ovarian masses suspicious for malignancy.

Serum CA 125 level is the gold standard for tumor markers in the evaluation of pelvic masses, particularly epithelial ovarian cancers. In younger women, serum levels of α-fetoprotein (AFP) and human chorionic gonadotropin (HCG) are helpful in recognizing the presence of an endodermal sinus tumor, embryonal carcinoma, choriocarcinoma, or mixed germ cell tumors. However, these patients often are not suspected preoperatively to have a malignancy. Measurement of AFP and HCG levels is best applied in serial monitoring of the effectiveness of therapy. Failure to identify elevations of these markers preoperatively does not preclude one from using them postoperatively in determining efficacy and duration of treatment for these diseases. Inhibin is a transforming growth factor-β–like peptide normally secreted by the ovarian stroma and functions in the feedback loop in the hypothalamic-pituitary-ovarian axis. Serum inhibin levels are useful markers for granulosa cell tumors and can aid in this diagnosis when an ovarian stromal tumor is suspected preoperatively.

Patients with a preoperative evaluation consistent with the diagnosis of ovarian cancer do best if referred to a gynecologic oncologist. Survival data suggest that those patients operated on by gynecologic oncologists for early-stage and late-stage disease have better outcomes in terms of progression-free and overall survival. This observation is at least in part due to the more complete surgical cytoreduction frequently accomplished by gynecologic oncologists, who have a better understanding of ovarian cancer biology and the nearly linear relationship between residual tumor and survival.[9,10]

SCREENING AND EARLY DETECTION

Successful early detection of ovarian cancer should decrease mortality and morbidity from the disease. However, there are no currently available tests that achieve this goal, and thus routine screening for asymptomatic ovarian cancer cannot be recommended. Successful screening for any malignancy requires detection while the disease is either precancerous or in its early stages. Although ovarian cancer's pattern of spread is well defined, the natural history of the disease is poorly understood. The time frame for progression from stage I to IV ovarian cancer remains to be established. The entire peritoneum is at risk, and peritoneal carcinomatosis may develop even after oophorectomy, or a syndrome of extraovarian peritoneal carcinomatosis may occur characterized by widespread intraperitoneal epithelial carcinoma in the presence of histologically normal ovaries. In addition, no premalignant lesion for epithelial ovarian carcinoma has been definitively identified. Borderline tumors or those with LMP do not progress to invasive malignancies in the majority of cases.

The existing screening techniques, such as ovarian palpation, TVS, and serum CA 125 determinations, are not sufficiently accurate to recommend general population screening. These tests are all limited by insufficient sensitivity and specificity. Because surgical intervention and biopsy are frequently required to make the diagnosis of ovarian cancer, the positive predictive value (PPV) of the screening test is the primary consideration. Excessive cost, morbidity, and even mortality associated with unnecessary surgeries for a false-positive screening test result have led most investigators to recommend that at least a 10% PPV be demonstrated.[11]

Although bimanual pelvic and rectovaginal examinations continue to be routinely recommended for women, ovarian palpation has not been established as a useful screening procedure. Most screening studies have used either serum tumor marker levels or ultrasonography or both. Although serum CA 125 levels correlate with progression or regression of established disease and are also useful in the preoperative evaluation of a pelvic mass, the test does not have sufficient specificity to be used as a routine screen for ovarian cancer.[12] Besides ovarian cancer, many other conditions can be associated with an elevated CA 125 level, including cirrhosis, peritonitis, pancreatitis, endometriosis, uterine leiomyomata, benign ovarian cysts, and pelvic inflammatory disease. Thus, although CA 125 is a useful marker to monitor an ovarian cancer patient's disease status, it is not an effective biomarker for early detection.

Recent advances in molecular technologies have allowed application of high-throughput techniques to ovarian cancer biomarker discovery. A number of candidate markers have been discovered that show promise for enhancing the accuracy of CA 125 levels, such as HE4 (human epididymis 4), osteopontin, mesothelin, and osteoblast-stimulating factor-2. Algorithms that define the behavior of these markers have also been developed, incorporating biologic characteristics of the tumor growth and marker behavior.[12]

In addition, other novel tumor biomarkers for ovarian cancer have been discovered, and a few hold promise for use in early detection. Lysophosphatidic acid, which had previously been shown to be elevated in malignant ascites, may also be useful as a predictive biomarker for ovarian cancer, because an elevated level was found in nine of ten patients with early-stage disease.[19] Additional studies of sensitivity and specificity are in progress. Proteomic spectral analysis of sera from ovarian cancer patients and controls using surface-enhanced laser desorption and ionization time-of-flight mass spectroscopy has been reported to distinguish between benign and malignant cases, including stage I disease, with 100% sensitivity.[13] Further confirmatory studies are under way at a number of centers.

The two best screening tests currently available are measurement of CA 125 tumor marker levels and TVS.[14] Early studies of TVS suggested a sensitivity of 100% but a specificity of 98%, which is insufficient to achieve a PPV of 10%. More recent reports suggest that use of color Doppler imaging improves the specificity of TVS, but it is unlikely that a specificity of 99.6% can be achieved. Investigators at the University of Kentucky improved the specificity of TVS by using a morphologic index. They screened 6470 women, including high-risk premenopausal women and average-risk postmenopausal women.[15] Of 90 women who underwent surgery, 6 were found to have an ovarian malignancy, which yields a PPV of 6.7%. One interval cancer was found at prophylactic oophorectomy 11 months after screening, for a sensitivity of 86%. All but one of these cancers were stage I, and no deaths due to ovarian cancer were noted in this group.

CA 125 level has been used for many years for evaluation of response to therapy and for surveillance for ovarian cancer recurrence. In 1985, Bast published the first report of a case in which CA 125 level was elevated before diagnosis of ovarian carcinoma.[15a] Since then, CA 125 level has been shown to have high sensitivity as an indicator of ovarian cancer. For all epithelial ovarian cancers, most of which are diagnosed at a late stage, the sensitivity of CA 125 is approximately 80%. More than 85% of women with advanced ovarian cancer have elevated CA 125 levels; however, only 50% of those with disease confined to the ovary have elevated levels.[11,12] Specificity is poor, however, when CA 125 level is used in this way. Nearly 6% of women without cancer have elevated levels of CA 125. Thus, the performance of CA 125 as a tumor marker does not justify its use as a stand-alone screening test, because neither its specificity nor its sensitivity for early-stage disease are acceptable.[16]

Because in 20% to 50% of cases CA 125 fails to rise in early-stage disease, complementary markers have been evaluated. Levels of OVX-1 and macrophage colony-stimulating factor have been found to be elevated in patients with clinically evident ovarian cancer but normal CA 125 levels, which suggests that these markers may be complementary to CA 125.[17] Lysophosphatidic acid level has also been reported to discriminate ovarian cancer cases, including cases with early-stage disease, from controls.[18] None of these tests has been proven to have sufficient sensitivity and specificity for routine use at the current time. Molecular discoveries by the Early Detection Research Network are likely to yield many potentially useful markers. Eventually a panel of markers will likely emerge that used together, perhaps with imaging, will yield an effective screening test for the early detection of ovarian cancer.

Two randomized controlled trials are currently under way to evaluate a multimodal screening approach using both CA 125 and TVS. In the United States, the Prostate, Lung, Colorectal, Ovarian Cancer screening trial uses measurement of CA 125 level (single threshold elevation of more than 35 U/mL) and TVS together, performed annually, as a first-line screen.[19] If either test is positive, the woman is referred for surgical consultation. In this two-arm randomized controlled trial, 74,000 women aged 55 to 74 years have been randomly assigned to the screening arm or to a standard-care control arm. Ten centers are collaborating in this 14-year trial, which will require 10 years' average follow-up.

In a second trial, in the United Kingdom, the primary focus is on ensuring high specificity. A multimodal approach was explored by Jacobs in a prevalence trial followed by a pilot randomized controlled trial using CA 125 level to select women for TVS. Jacobs et al. randomly assigned 21,935 average-risk postmenopausal women to undergo three annual screenings or no screening. The screening protocol used CA 125 level as a first-line screen and referred the woman for TVS if CA 125 level was above 30 U/mL. If the TVS revealed an ovarian mass, then the woman was referred for surgical consultation. Findings from this pilot trial were reported in 1999.[20] The trial was too small to show efficacy in terms of mortality reduction, but its results are important because they confirm the findings of the prevalence trial that an acceptable PPV is achieved by selecting women for imaging based on elevated CA 125 level. When the decision rule for surgical referral requires that results of both tests be positive, the PPV is 20%. Furthermore, there were one-half as many deaths in the screened group as there were among controls, and there was a statistically significant improvement in survival. Individuals with index cancers survived an average of 72.9 months in the screening group and 41.8 months in the control group.

This multimodal screening strategy is limited by the sensitivity of the first-line screen, CA 125 level. Accordingly, these investigators are exploring ways to improve on these results by detecting change over time in the CA 125 values. Skates et al.[21] suggested fitting an exponential model that uses data from several prior CA 125 screens; a result demonstrating an exponential rise would trigger a call-back for additional testing. Investigators in the United Kingdom are currently testing this screening strategy in a three-arm randomized controlled trial involving healthy women. The results of both the U.S. and U.K. trials will not be available for several more years.

HEREDITARY OVARIAN CARCINOMA

Genetic factors (inherited and somatic) as well as hormonal and environmental exposures all contribute to the development of ovarian cancer. Only 5% to 10% of patients with epithelial ovarian carcinoma likely have inherited a genetic predisposition to the disease; however, many studies have focused on these individuals in the hopes of gleaning additional insights into ovarian cancer biology, molecular oncogenesis, early detection, and treatment.

Hereditary ovarian cancer syndromes are linked to genetic mutations inherited in an autosomal dominant manner, and thus both maternal and paternal family histories must be obtained to determine risk. The breast-ovarian cancer syndrome accounts for approximately 90% of all hereditary ovarian cancer cases and is most frequently associated with mutations in the *BRCA1* or *BRCA2* genes.[22] The *BRCA1* gene, located on chromosome band 17q12-21, and the *BRCA2* gene, located on chromosome band 13q12-13, were identified and linked to hereditary breast and ovarian cancers in the 1990s. Emerging evidence suggests that these genes act as tumor suppressor genes and regulate cellular proliferation and DNA repair by maintaining chromosome integrity.

The presence of a BRCA-associated cancer syndrome is suspected whenever the pedigree reveals three or more affected relatives with cancer, bilateral or early-onset breast cancer, a proband with both breast and ovarian cancer, or a male relative with breast cancer. Many mutations have been described, located throughout the *BRCA1* and *BRCA2* genes, with non-

sense and frameshift mutations being predominant.[22] Nonsense mutations occur when a nucleotide substitution results in a stop codon, and frameshift mutations occur when one or more nucleotides are deleted to produce a downstream stop codon. Certain ethnic groups have higher frequencies of founder BRCA mutations. Three specific founder mutations, 185delAG BRCA1, 5382insC BRCA1, and 6174delT BRCA2, have been identified in the Ashkenazi Jewish population and are carried by 2.0% to 2.4% of this population.[23] Furthermore, 40% to 60% of epithelial ovarian cancer patients of Jewish descent carry one of these mutations (irrespective of their family histories). This is compared to a carrier frequency of approximately 5% among non-Jewish women with ovarian cancer.

The lifetime risk of ovarian cancer for patients with BRCA1 mutations is 20% to 60%, and the risk for BRCA2 mutation carriers is 10% to 35%. Ovarian cancer associated with germline mutations of BRCA1 appears to present with distinct clinical and pathologic features compared with sporadic ovarian cancer.[24,25] The vast majority of BRCA1-associated cancers are serous adenocarcinomas, with an average age at diagnosis of 48 years, whereas the mean age for BRCA2-associated ovarian cancers is 61 years. Furthermore, BRCA-associated cancers may have a more favorable course than sporadic ovarian cancer. In a study by Rubin et al.[24] a median survival of 77 months was reported for 43 patients with advanced BRCA1-associated disease compared with 29 months for matched controls. Cass et al.[26] noted a similar survival advantage for carriers in their matched cohort and went further to suggest that the improved survival in those with BRCA-associated ovarian cancers was a result of improved response to platinum-based chemotherapy compared to women who had sporadic disease. A large prospective study conducted by the Gynecologic Oncology Group (GOG) is currently in progress to compare the clinical course of sporadic ovarian cancer with that associated with BRCA1 and BRCA2 mutations.[25,27]

The hereditary nonpolyposis colorectal cancer (HNPCC) syndrome accounts for approximately 5% of all hereditary ovarian cancer cases. It is an autosomal dominant genetic syndrome in which three or more first-degree relatives have colon cancer (over 70% of cases in the proximal colon) or endometrial cancer, of whom one is a first-degree relative of the other two, and two of whom must be diagnosed with cancer before age 50 years. Four genes that are part of the DNA mismatch repair pathway have now been identified as being responsible for the HNPCC phenotype: *hMSH2* (chromosome arm 2p), *hMLH1* (chromosome arm 3p), *hPMS1* (chromosome arm 2q), and *hPMS2* (chromosome arm 7p).[22] The majority of affected patients are found to have defects in either *hMSH2* or *hMLH1*. An inherited defect in any one of these genes increases an individual's risk of developing cancer because of an impaired ability to repair somatic genetic mutations. HNPCC syndrome family members are at risk for cancers at other gastrointestinal sites as well as for tumors in the genitourinary tract and the ovary.[28] The risk of endometrial cancer among women in HNPCC syndrome families is estimated to be 40% to 60% by age 70, compared to 1.5% in the general population. Limited studies have reported a 3.5-fold increase in the risk of ovarian cancer in members of these families.

Although hereditary cancers account for only 10% of malignancies, individual risk assessment and appropriate genetic testing can identify those individuals with significant lifetime

TABLE 32.4-2.   Recommendations for Management of Women at High Genetic Risk for Gynecologic Malignancies

Method	Breast Cancer	Ovarian Cancer	HNPCC Syndrome/ Endometrial Cancer	HNPCC Syndrome/ Colon Cancer
Screening	Monthly self-examination Semiannual/annual clinical examination Annual mammography (beginning age 25–35 y)	Semiannual/annual rectovaginal pelvic examination/annual rectovaginal pelvic examination Annual/semiannual CA 125 level and TVS screening (beginning age 25–35 y)	Pelvic examination, TVS and/or endometrial biopsy every 1–2 y (beginning age 30–35 y)	Colonoscopy every 1–3 y (beginning age 20–25 y)
Chemoprevention	Consider tamoxifen	Consider OCP	Consider OCP	—
Prophylactic surgery	Counsel regarding mastectomy ± PBSO	Offer PBSO	Counsel regarding prophylactic hysterectomy/ PBSO	Counsel regarding prophylactic colectomy

CA 125, cancer antigen 125; HPNCC, hereditary nonpolyposis colorectal cancer; OCP, oral contraceptive pills; PBSO, prophylactic bilateral salpingo-oophorectomy; TVS, transvaginal ultrasonography.

risk. Genetic counseling is imperative, and the proper selection of patients for testing is very important. As genetic testing becomes more readily available to all individuals, clinicians and patients must work together to ensure that the results are used in a fashion that carefully considers the medical implications as well as any ethical, legal, and psychosocial issues that may arise. Multidisciplinary services that include pretest and posttest counseling, screening, treatment, and psychosocial counseling have been established to address each of these aspects of comprehensive care.

The American Society of Clinical Oncology updated its guidelines for genetic testing in 2003.[29] All individuals with a personal or family history suggestive of an inherited cancer susceptibility in whom the test can be adequately interpreted and for whom the results will influence medical management should be offered testing. First- and second-degree relatives of an affected individual from a breast–ovarian cancer syndrome family carrying a mutation of the BRCA1 or BRCA2 gene should be offered genetic testing. Certain ethnic groups, such as Ashkenazi Jews, are at increased risk for carrying a BRCA mutation, and a lower threshold for genetic testing may be appropriate in some of these individuals. Genetic testing for the mismatch repair genes should be considered when there is a first-degree relative with a known mutation and when the patient meets the Amsterdam or the Bethesda criteria for HNPCC syndrome.

A comprehensive family history can provide an estimate of an individual's risk of carrying a genetic mutation; however, genetic testing provides more accurate information regarding the cancer risks for an individual patient. The best way to determine if a cancer-associated mutation is present in a family is to test an affected family member, because he or she is the most likely to carry a deleterious mutation. The first family member to be tested will often need comprehensive gene sequencing. Other individuals can then be tested for the identified mutation, which may be unique to this particular family. In the Ashkenazi Jewish population, genetic testing for the three founder mutations is required because the carrier frequency in this population is high and individuals with both BRCA1 and BRCA2 mutations occasionally have been reported.

Test results may come back positive or negative for an identifiable mutation, or a mutation of indeterminate clinical sig-

nificance may be reported. When a test result is negative, interpretation will depend on the patient's family history. If an affected family member has tested positive for a mutation, then the patient with the negative result has likely not inherited the deleterious mutation, and her cancer risk approximates that of the general population. If there is no documented positive mutation in the family, it is still possible that the patient has a cancer-associated mutation that is not detectable with current testing. Approximately 12% of current test results are genetic variants or polymorphisms, reported as of indeterminate clinical significance. Further study of these genetic variants and associated cancer risks in large populations will help reduce the number of reports of "indeterminate" findings.[25]

Follow-up and management of patients with an inherited genetic predisposition to ovarian cancer are complex due to the variable penetrance of genetic alterations and the lack of effective early detection methods. Current consensus recommendations include at least annual rectovaginal pelvic examinations, serum CA 125 determinations, and TVS[14]; however, there is no conclusive evidence that mortality is reduced as a result of these interventions.[30] One prospective study of screening in high-risk women demonstrated a down-staging of the ovarian cancer cases detected; however, conclusions are limited by small patient numbers.[31] Table 32.4-2 lists the provisional recommendations for cancer surveillance for carriers of BRCA1, BRCA2, and HNPCC mutations. Screening and prophylactic surgery for patients with HNPCC-associated mutations are also based on expert opinion, although colonoscopy and stool occult blood testing have been shown in randomized clinical trials to reduce the incidence of and mortality from colon cancer.

Evidence suggests that chemoprophylaxis with oral contraceptive pills for 5 years decreases ovarian cancer risk by 50% in both the general population and in high-risk women.[32] A case-controlled study of 207 known BRCA mutation carriers and their sister controls found a 60% reduction of ovarian cancer risk with oral contraceptive use. Other risk-reducing strategies such as tubal ligation and hysterectomy have also been strated to reduce the incidence of ovarian can... high-risk women. Surgery with prophyl... oophorectomy (PBSO) is the most effe... egy for patients with BRCA mutations t...

Given that the majority of hereditary ovarian cancers occur after the age of 35 to 40 years, PBSO is an option in carefully selected patients at unequivocally high genetic risk for ovarian cancer who have completed their childbearing or are at least 35 years of age.[33,34] A laparoscopic approach is frequently possible, but the surgical options must be individualized, as must the decision for concomitant hysterectomy. In any case, the surgical pathologist must be alerted to perform a careful examination of the patient's ovaries and fallopian tubes given the frequent reports of occult ovarian and tubal carcinoma occurring in 2% to 10% of PBSO specimens.[35,36]

The efficacy of PBSO in reducing risk in hereditary breast-ovarian cancer syndrome has been evaluated in several studies. Prospective studies have documented a significant reduction with PBSO in both ovarian-peritoneal and breast carcinoma among BRCA mutation carriers. One study of 248 PBSO patients found a 98% decrease in ovarian and primary peritoneal cancers and a 50% reduction in subsequent breast cancer compared to age-matched controls.[34] Furthermore, studies have demonstrated that the risk of primary peritoneal carcinomas after PBSO is likely under 5%, and patients should be counseled regarding this potential risk. It is believed that that all coelomic epithelium, including the peritoneal covering of the entire abdominal-pelvic cavity, is prone to malignant transformation in BRCA mutation carriers. Several other significant issues remain unresolved regarding the physiologic adjustments to premature surgical menopause and the safety of hormone replacement therapy in this group, especially in those at high risk for breast cancer.

STAGING

Ovarian cancer is a surgically staged disease. Thus, it is important for physicians to be thoroughly familiar with the International Federation of Gynecology and Obstetrics (FIGO) staging system for primary carcinomas of the ovary[3] (Table 32.4-3). As described earlier in Pathogenesis, ovarian cancer most frequently spreads by direct extension to neighboring organs and by exfoliation of cells into the peritoneal cavity. It also disseminates by lymphatic spread, particularly to the pelvic sidewall lymph nodes (external iliac and obturator chains) and along the gonadal vessels to the upper common iliac and paraaortic lymph node chains (Fig. 32.4-1). Surgical staging procedures must evaluate sites to which ovarian cancer is likely to spread.

Complete surgical staging is a necessity to properly evaluate the patient and to determine whether additional therapy should be recommended. Proper surgical staging requires thorough and complete inspection of the peritoneal cavity and its contents, as well as evaluation of the retroperitoneal spaces and lymph nodes. When the peritoneal cavity is entered, any fluid present should be aspirated and sent for cytologic studies. Peritoneal fluid, even if limited to the pelvis, is more likely to yield malignant cells than are cytologic washings. If no fluid is present, however, one should routinely irrigate the pelvis and paracolic spaces and send the fluid for cytologic examination. Adhesions should be lysed to restore normal anatomy, and samples of the adhesions should be sent for pathologic examination.

If intraperitoneal carcinomatosis is not present, it may be most appropriate first to resect the ovarian tumor and then to proceed with surgical staging to help avoid rupturing of the mass. For women who desire future fertility, when the tumor is

TABLE 32.4-3. International Federation of Gynecologists and Obstetricians Stage Grouping for Primary Carcinoma of the Ovary (1998)

Stage	Description
I	Growth limited to the ovaries.
IA	Growth limited to one ovary; no ascites. No tumor on the external surface; capsule intact.
IB	Growth limited to both ovaries; no ascites. No tumor on the external surface; capsule intact.
IC[a]	Tumor either stage IA or IB but with tumor on the surface of one or both ovaries, or with capsule ruptured, or with ascites present containing malignant cells, or with positive peritoneal washings.
II	Growth involving one or both ovaries with pelvic extension.
IIA	Extension and/or metastases to the uterus and/or tubes.
IIB	Growth involving one or both ovaries with pelvic extension.
IIC[a]	Tumor either stage IIA or IIB but with tumor on the surface of one or both ovaries, or with capsule(s) ruptured, or with ascites present containing malignant cells, or with positive peritoneal washings.
III	Tumor involving one or both ovaries with peritoneal implants outside the pelvis and/or positive retroperitoneal or inguinal nodes. Superficial liver metastases equals stage III. Tumor is limited to the true pelvis but with histologically verified malignant extension to small bowel or omentum.
IIIA	Tumor grossly limited to the true pelvis with negative nodes but with histologically confirmed microscopic seeding of abdominal peritoneal surfaces.
IIIB	Tumor of one or both ovaries with histologically confirmed implants of abdominal peritoneal surfaces, none exceeding 2 cm in diameter. Nodes negative.
IIIC	Abdominal implants greater than 2 cm in diameter and/or positive retroperitoneal or inguinal nodes.
IV	Growth involving one or both ovaries with distant metastasis. If pleural effusion is present, cytologic test results must be positive to allot a case to stage IV. Parenchymal liver metastasis equals stage IV.

[a]To evaluate the impact on prognosis of the different criteria for allotting cases to stage IC or IIC, it is of value to know if rupture of the capsule was spontaneous or caused by the surgeon, and if the source of malignant cells detected was peritoneal washings or ascites.

limited to one ovary, staging may be completed without hysterectomy and complete castration. The grossly normal opposite ovary may undergo biopsy or any visible benign-appearing cysts may be excised. Preservation of fertility should be considered in any woman of reproductive age with either a borderline malignant tumor of the ovary or an invasive epithelial cancer grossly confined to one ovary. A frozen-section assessment of any abnormality involving the contralateral ovary may be helpful in guiding the extent of surgery. Pelvic and paraaortic retroperitoneal lymph nodes are removed in all patients whose tumors do not grossly extend outside of the pelvis. Any enlarged pelvic retroperitoneal lymph nodes are removed, regardless of their location, to achieve optimal cytoreduction. Lymphadenectomy is an important part of the staging of ovarian cancers, particularly when the disease is grossly limited to one ovary. In this situation, up to 20% of women have been found to have paraaortic lymph node metastases.[37]

To fully assess and resect disease in the upper abdomen, it is frequently necessary to extend the vertical incision above the umbilicus. If gross disease is not present in the omentum, an infracolic omentectomy is sufficient for diagnostic purposes.

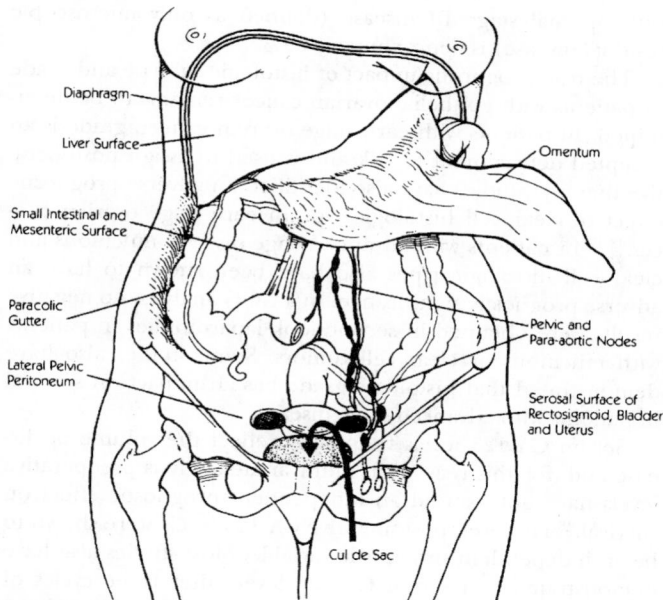

FIGURE 32.4-1. Ovarian cancer spread pattern. (From Young RC, Perez CA, Hoskins WV. Cancer of the ovary. In: DeVita VT Jr, Hellman S, Rosenberg SA, eds. *Cancer: principles and practice of oncology*, 4th ed. Philadelphia: JB Lippincott Co, 1993:1226, with permission.)

When the omentum is caked with tumor, the omentum should be excised from the greater curvature of the stomach as completely as possible (Fig. 32.4-2). The upper abdominal evaluation continues with a careful inspection of the right hemidiaphragm and liver serosa and parenchyma. The spleen is then carefully inspected, as is the left diaphragm. If splenectomy is required to achieve optimal surgical cytoreduction, then this should be con-

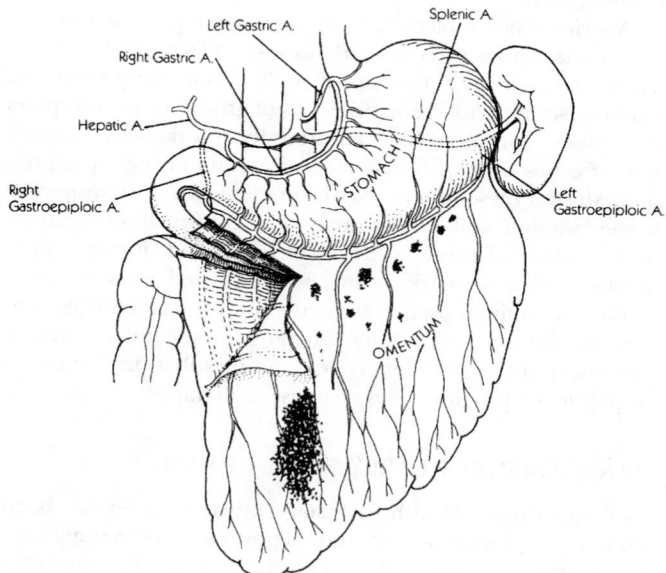

FIGURE 32.4-2. Excising omentum off stomach. (From Young RC, Perez CA, Hoskins WV. Cancer of the ovary. In: DeVita VT Jr, Hellman S, Rosenberg SA, eds. *Cancer: principles and practice of oncology*, 4th ed. Philadelphia: JB Lippincott Co, 1993:1226, with permission.)

sidered.[38] Preoperative imaging can often help predict splenic involvement so that pneumococcal vaccine (Pneumovax) can be given preoperatively. If this has not been done and splenectomy is performed, then Pneumovax should be administered postoperatively to protect against future infections with encapsulated bacteria.

The paracolic spaces and large bowel are then carefully inspected. The small intestine and its mesentery are evaluated, and any implants present are removed. If luminal narrowing, especially in the area of the terminal ileum, or any other potentially obstructing lesion is present, a small bowel resection and reanastomosis should be performed. Similarly, if tumor appears to invade the large bowel transluminally, a resection may be required, although often, with the larger diameter of the colon and the typical growth pattern of ovarian cancer, this can be avoided. In the face of advanced-stage disease, lymphadenectomy is performed only if the visible disease is less than 2 cm (stage IIIB or lower) or if grossly enlarged nodes are discovered on inspection of the retroperitoneum.[39] In postmenopausal women or in women in whom fertility is no longer desired, one should routinely perform a bilateral salpingo-oophorectomy and total abdominal hysterectomy at the time of staging. The hysterectomy is performed because the serosal surface of the uterus is a large peritoneal surface for implantation of malignant cells. In addition, field effects may occur whereby the epithelium of the fallopian tubes or uterus is involved with premalignant or malignant processes as well. These latter changes may not be grossly recognized at the time of surgery.

Under-staging occurs approximately 30% of the time, especially when the preoperative diagnosis is that of a benign process. In many cases, this leads to use of abdominal incisions that do not allow complete surgical staging even when the diagnosis of a malignancy is recognized intraoperatively. At other times, under-staging or incomplete staging is due to a lack of familiarity with accepted surgical staging procedures.[40]

The issue of inadequately staged early ovarian cancer is often a difficult one. The simplest solution for such patients is to recommend complete surgical staging via laparotomy or laparoscopy performed by a gynecologic oncologist. However, if this is not possible or practical, an alternative is to obtain a CT scan to try to identify the presence of any subclinical bulky disease. If the CT scan and CA 125 level are normal, and the tumor was of LMP and limited to one ovary, no further therapy is recommended. If there was bilateral involvement and one ovary was left *in situ*, the patient should be counseled regarding her risk for recurrence, and if fertility is no longer desired, the contralateral ovary should be removed. If the ovarian tumor is a high-grade invasive epithelial malignancy, chemotherapy is required, but the exact stage of the tumor is important in determining the number of cycles of chemotherapy that are recommended.

In the event that any gross disease is detectable on the CT scan, a surgical procedure to remove gross disease should be performed. Postoperative reevaluation and staging by laparotomy or laparoscopy may be performed.[41] Earlier papers on laparoscopic surgical staging revealed that as many as 30% to 40% of patients originally thought to have FIGO stage I or II disease actually had disease in the upper abdomen. The choice of surgical approach will be in large part dependent on the extent of disease seen on imaging, individual patient characteristics, and the skills and experience of the surgeon. Developments in laparoscopic techniques allow paraaortic lymph node dissections and omentectomies to be performed by this method.[42]

PROGNOSTIC FACTORS

At the conclusion of a comprehensive laparotomy, the clinical and pathologic findings are used to select appropriate postoperative therapy. In addition, new prognostic factors are being evaluated that may be used to identify groups of patients for whom more specific biologic treatments or more aggressive therapy is indicated.

Clinicopathologic findings determined to be clinically useful include the following:

FIGO stage
Histologic subtype
Histologic grade
Factors associated with tumor dissemination
Malignant ascites or malignant peritoneal washings
Tumor excrescences on ovarian surface or ruptured capsule
Volume of residual disease after cytoreductive surgery

The tumor stage remains the most important prognostic variable. Few trials provide an accurate assessment regarding the long-term survival of patients with early-stage ovarian cancer because earlier studies often included patients with inadequately staged disease. Patients with stage I disease with well or moderately well-differentiated tumors have a greater than 90% 5-year survival rate.[43] Patients with stage I disease with poor prognostic features are often included in treatment protocols for patients with stage II disease. This group of tumors has been termed *early-stage disease with unfavorable characteristics.* However, limited information is available regarding the actual survival impact of some of the factors used to characterize disease as having an unfavorable prognosis. Rupture of the capsule increases the stage to IC. In a Swedish series, however, no adverse effect on survival could be established for patients with early-stage disease in whom the capsule was ruptured during surgery.[44] Furthermore, the adverse effect of malignant ascites is well established; however, there is limited information regarding the prognostic significance of positive results of peritoneal cytologic examination. Dense tumor adherence to surrounding structures and the pelvic sidewall should now also be considered an adverse prognostic factor for patients with early-stage tumors because such patients have at least stage II disease.[45] Tumor size, bilaterality, and cytologically negative ascites have no prognostic significance. The most reliable long-term survival data on accurately staged early-stage ovarian cancer is derived from studies of the GOG. In these studies, patients with unfavorable-prognosis early-stage ovarian cancer have a 5-year survival rate of approximately 80%.[43]

Patients with stage III disease have a 5-year survival rate of approximately 35% that is dependent in large part on the volume of disease present in the upper abdomen. Patients with stage IV disease have less than a 10% 5-year survival rate. Volume of residual disease after cytoreductive surgery for patients with advanced ovarian cancer has a significant impact on survival. After the administration of postoperative platinum-based combination chemotherapy, 4-year survival rates for patients with optimal stage III disease (defined as only microscopic residual disease) is approximately 60%.[10,46]

The true prognostic impact of histologic subtype and grade in patients with epithelial ovarian cancer remains to be determined. In patients with early-stage ovarian cancer, grade is an accepted determinant of risk and is used to assign postoperative therapy. Studies have also identified an adverse prognostic effect of clear cell histologic type in early-stage ovarian cancer.[43,47] In patients with advanced-stage disease, mucinous and clear cell histologic types also have been shown to have an adverse prognostic significance. In a GOG analysis, no negative results were obtained in second-look laparotomies in patients with mucinous or clear cell tumors. Some studies also have demonstrated that histologic grade has an impact on survival in patients with advanced-stage disease.

Serum CA 125 levels frequently reflect the volume of disease and, for this reason, in multivariate analysis preoperative levels have not exerted an independent prognostic effect on survival.[48] However, postoperative CA 125 levels were shown to be an independent prognostic variable. Most studies also have demonstrated that serum CA 125 levels after three cycles of chemotherapy are accurate predictors of the probability that a patient will achieve a complete remission. However, the CA 125 level after three cycles of chemotherapy cannot be used as a guide for treatment decisions because of the lack of predictive power.

The prognostic significance of age on survival of patients with ovarian cancer has been recognized.[49] Median survival is at least 2 years longer in women younger than age 65 years than in those older than age 65 years.

The prognostic significance of DNA ploidy and S-phase fraction has been examined in ovarian cancer. Investigators in Europe have now included aneuploidy in their criteria for selection of patients with high-risk early-stage ovarian cancer for adjuvant therapy.[50] Controversy remains, however, as to the nature of the relationship between histologic grade and degree of aneuploidy.

A series of new molecular factors have been proposed to have prognostic significance in ovarian cancer (Table 32.4-4).[26,51–53] These factors include markers of proliferation, drug resistance markers, serum cytokine levels, levels of growth factor receptors or substances involved in signal transduction pathways, expression of genes associated with metastases, and oncogene expression. Most of these factors have been identified in retrospective studies without multivariate analysis or confirmation in larger studies. Many of these factors were discovered during experimental studies of ovarian cancer biology, and none of these markers is routinely used to select therapy for patients with ovarian cancer at the current time. Ongoing investigations are using microarray analysis to identify gene profiles that may be useful for predicting prognosis and response to therapy.[54,55]

MANAGEMENT OF EARLY-STAGE DISEASE

A subset of patients with early-stage ovarian cancer has been shown not to require any additional postoperative therapy after tumor resection and comprehensive staging. Patients with stage IA or IB disease with well or moderately well-differentiated tumors have a 5-year survival rate of more than 90% without any adjuvant treatment.[43] Patients with favorable-prognosis early-stage ovarian cancer (stage IA and IB with grade 1 and 2

TABLE 32.4-4. Experimental Prognostic Factors
in Ovarian Cancer

MORPHOMETRY
DNA PLOIDY AND S-PHASE FRACTION
DRUG RESISTANCE MARKERS
P-glycoprotein immunoreactivity
Glutathione S-transferase pi
c-erbB-2
BRCA1 and BRCA2
Multidrug resistance proteins (Lrp)
Nucleotide excision DNA repair genes ERCC1 and XPAC
BAX
ONCOGENE
Mutant p53 expression
AKT-2
MARKERS OF PROLIFERATION
Ki-67
Proliferating cell nuclear antigen
MARKERS OF TUMOR SPREAD
Metastasis-related genes (nm23-H1)
Cathepsin D
Urokinase-type plasminogen activators
Colony-stimulating factor 1
CD44 molecules
CYTOKINE LEVELS AND OTHER ACTIVE PROTEINS
Heat-shock protein
Interleukin-6
Platelet-derived growth factor

tumors) were randomly assigned in an earlier GOG study to receive no treatment or oral intermittent melphalan (0.2 mg/kg daily for 5 days) with repeat cycles every 4 to 6 weeks for a total of 12 courses or 18 months of therapy. At a median follow-up of more than 6 years, only six deaths have been reported in 81 patients: four in the observation group and two in the group receiving melphalan. Disease-free survival and overall survival is shown in Figure 32.4-3. Patients with favorable-prognosis

early-stage ovarian cancer can be spared the acute and chronic toxicities of chemotherapy, including myeloproliferative disorders such as leukemia.

The optimum treatment of early-stage ovarian cancer patients with unfavorable prognosis remains an area of controversy. Opinions differ as to not only what modality of treatment should be used (chemotherapy, external-beam radiotherapy, or intraperitoneal radioisotope therapy) but also whether treatment should be immediate or should be delayed until disease progression. Furthermore, as noted in Prognostic Factors, consensus has not been established as to the prognostic significance of some clinicopathologic features, such as positive peritoneal cytologic examination and a surgically ruptured capsule with contamination of the pelvis with cyst fluid. Clinicopathologic factors currently used by the GOG to define unfavorable-prognosis early-stage disease include FIGO stage II and IC, clear cell histology, and grade 3 tumors.

The results of two randomized European trials [International Collaborative Ovarian Neoplasm Trial 1 (ICON1) and Adjuvant ChemoTherapy in Ovarian Neoplasm Trial (ACTION)] have, for the first time, provided data demonstrating that initiation of adjuvant chemotherapy in patients with high-risk early-stage ovarian cancer can exert a favorable impact on both progression-free and overall survival.[56–58] The two studies, with a total population of 925 patients, differed somewhat in eligibility criteria, requirements for surgical staging, and the specific adjuvant chemotherapy program used. However, the trials asked the same question: Does the administration of platinum-based chemotherapy after surgery for high-risk early-stage ovarian cancer improve survival, compared to observation until objective evidence of disease progression?

The combined analysis of the trials revealed a statistically significant improvement in progression-free survival and overall survival associated with initiation of platinum-based treatment immediately after surgery. Although these data provide strong support for the conclusion that patients with high-risk early-stage ovarian cancer should be offered adjuvant chemo-

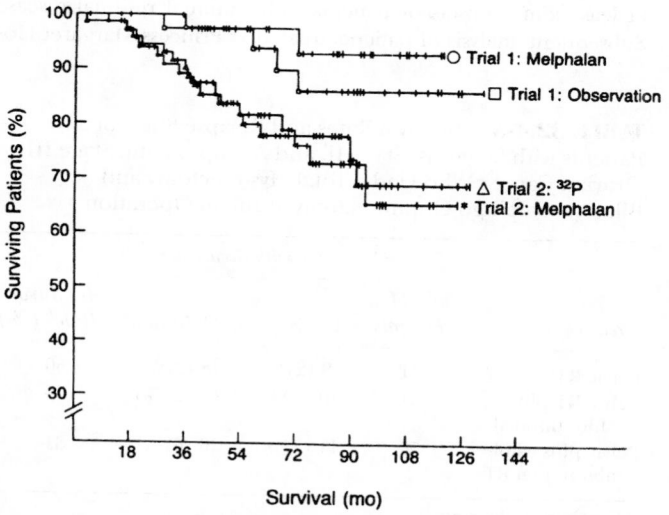

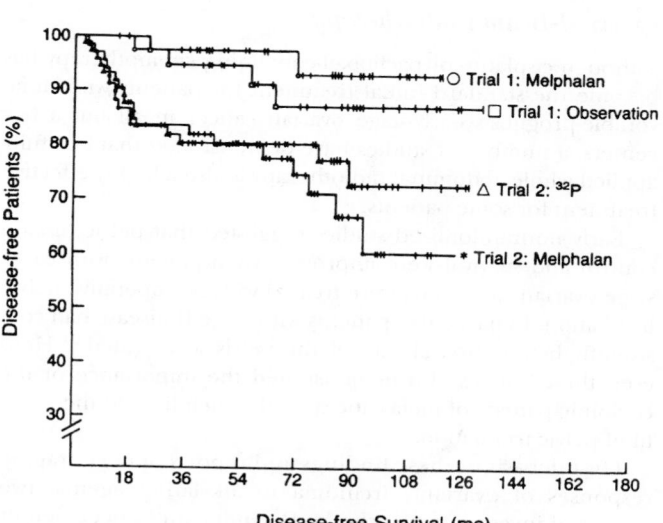

FIGURE 32.4-3. Disease-free (**A**) and overall (**B**) survival of patients with early-stage ovarian cancer. The top two curves represent patients with favorable prognoses randomly assigned to receive observation or melphalan. The lower two curves represent patients with unfavorable prognoses randomly assigned to receive either phosphorus 32 (^{32}P) or melphalan. (From ref. 43, with permission.)

therapy, some have suggested that chemotherapy may not be required in patients who have undergone optimal surgical staging. However, this conclusion is based on a retrospective analysis of a subset of patients entered into these early-stage trials, and caution is advised in drawing definitive conclusions based on any such evaluation.

The GOG trial compared three versus six cycles of carboplatin plus paclitaxel adjuvant chemotherapy in high-risk early-stage ovarian cancer in an effort to determine if the shorter treatment program may provide equivalent efficacy. Unfortunately, the preliminary results of this study suggest that a definitive answer to this question will not be provided.[59] Although there was a 33% reduction in the risk of recurrence associated with the administration of six cycles compared to three cycles, this difference did not reach the study requirement for a 50% reduction in recurrence to reach statistical significance. However, many oncologists will reasonably conclude that this level of reduction in the risk of disease recurrence with three additional cycles of carboplatin and paclitaxel justify the added time, effort, and toxicity associated with the longer treatment regimen.

The current GOG trial for patients with early-stage ovarian cancer with unfavorable prognosis compares three cycles against six cycles of a treatment with paclitaxel and carboplatin. The details of this combination are discussed later.

It is apparent that the optimum postoperative treatment for patients with early-stage ovarian cancer with unfavorable prognostic features remains to be established. Pending the results of the ongoing clinical trials, treatment options include chemotherapy with cisplatin or carboplatin, total abdominal and pelvic irradiation, and paclitaxel-based chemotherapy. In addition, a no-treatment option can be considered, although this choice has been shown to be associated with a decrease in survival in one large trial.[56–58] Second-look operations after completion of adjuvant therapy are not routinely recommended, especially for patients with early-stage disease.

External-Beam Radiotherapy

Although cisplatin- or paclitaxel-containing chemotherapy has become the standard initial treatment for patients with unfavorable-prognosis early-stage ovarian cancer in all but a few centers, a number of studies have demonstrated that carefully applied whole abdominal radiotherapy is also a highly effective treatment for some patients.

Early nonrandomized studies suggested that pelvic disease control and survival were improved when patients with early-stage ovarian carcinoma were treated with postoperative pelvic irradiation. In particular, patients with stage II disease had consistently better survival rates if the pelvis was treated.[60] However, these studies also demonstrated the importance of the coelomic pattern of metastatic spread, which limited the benefit of pelvic irradiation.

On the basis of these findings and reports of encouraging responses of ovarian carcinoma to alkylating agents, two groups of investigators at the M. D. Anderson Cancer Center and Princess Margaret Hospital[60a,61] conducted prospective trials that compared pelvic and whole abdominal irradiation with pelvic irradiation and single-agent chemotherapy. The M. D. Anderson study included patients who had stage I to III ovarian carcinomas with less than 2 cm of residual disease after surgery. Treatment was delivered with cobalt 60 using a moving strip technique, because contemporary treatment machines could not treat the entire abdomen in a single field. The authors reported that survival rates were similar for patients treated in the two arms, but the rate of serious bowel complications was higher for patients who received whole abdominal irradiation. It was concluded that chemotherapy was a superior treatment, and subsequent clinical trials at the M. D. Anderson Cancer Center and throughout the United States focused on the search for more effective chemotherapy.

Four years later, Dembo and associates[61] published the results of a similar prospective randomized study conducted at the Princess Margaret Hospital in Toronto. Patients with stage IB or II ovarian cancer were randomly assigned to one of three treatment arms: pelvic irradiation, pelvic plus whole abdominal irradiation, or pelvic irradiation plus single-agent chemotherapy. Patients with "asymptomatic" stage III disease were randomly assigned only between the last two arms. Although the treatment arms were similar to those of the M. D. Anderson trial, the details of the treatments differed significantly from that study. Patients on the chemotherapy arm received chlorambucil, an alkylating agent that has since been demonstrated to yield poorer response rates than melphalan. The total dose of abdominal strip irradiation (22.5 Gy) and the daily fraction size (2.25 Gy) were less than those used in the M. D. Anderson trial, but the liver was not shielded and particular care was taken to include the domes of the diaphragm in the treatment fields.[62]

Of 190 patients entered on the study, 132 had a hysterectomy and bilateral salpingo-oophorectomy performed at their initial laparotomy. Of these 132 (who were considered to have minimal residual disease), the 50 who received whole abdominal irradiation had significantly better rates of survival and abdominal disease control than did patients who received pelvic irradiation with chlorambucil (Table 32.4-5). Although the study has been criticized for using inconsistent surgical staging methods, it undoubtedly demonstrates the efficacy of abdominopelvic irradiation for at least some subsets of patients with minimal residual disease. Subsequent analysis of patients treated at Princess Margaret Hos-

TABLE 32.4-5. Survival Rates and Relapse Sites for 116 Patients with Stage IB, Stage II, and Asymptomatic Stage III Ovarian Cancer Who Had a Total Hysterectomy and Bilateral Salpingo-Oophorectomy at Initial Operation

| Treatment | No. of Patients | No. with Recurrence | | 4-Y Survival Rate[b] (%) |
		Pelvis	Abdomen[a]	
Pelvic RT[c]	31	8 (27%)	8 (27%)	50
Pelvic RT plus chlorambucil	51	10 (20%)	13 (25%)	55
Pelvic plus whole abdominal RT	50	11 (22%)	0 (0)	81

RT, radiation therapy.
[a] P <.01.
[b] P <.02.
[c] Stages IB and II only.

TABLE 32.4-6. Proportion of 325 Patients in Whom Disease Recurred after Treatment with Abdominopelvic Irradiation between 1971 and 1981

Stage	Gross Residual Disease	Proportion with Disease Recurrence		
		Grade 1	Grade 2	Grade 3
I	No	—	.21 (33)	.30 (27)
II	No/uncertain	.09 (32)	.29 (35)	.47 (36)
II	Yes	.17 (12)	.38 (16)	.86 (14)
III	No/uncertain	.20 (10)	.67 (18)	.67 (15)
III	Yes	.40 (15)	.79 (24)	.84 (38)

Note: Numbers in parentheses are the number of patients treated in each group.

pital demonstrated that patients who had grade 1; stage I or II, grade 2; or stage I or II, grade 3 disease and no gross residual tumor after surgery were most likely to have a prolonged disease-free interval after abdominopelvic irradiation (Table 32.4-6).[61,63]

Differences in the chemotherapy and radiotherapy techniques described earlier may explain the apparently contradictory results of the two trials. An imbalance in the proportion of stage IA patients may have favored the chemotherapy arm in the M. D. Anderson trial, but subset analysis by stage also failed to suggest an advantage for whole abdominal irradiation. The high total dose and fraction size per strip used at M. D. Anderson may explain the high rate of severe enteric complications compared with the 3% to 4% rate reported at Princess Margaret Hospital.

A number of other reports document that patients with postoperative residual disease have been cured with abdominopelvic irradiation alone; relapse-free survival rates of 40% to 60% at 10 to 15 years have been reported for patients with residual gross disease measuring less than 2 cm (Table 32.4-7).[63] Collectively, these studies demonstrate the efficacy of abdominopelvic irradiation and its superiority over pelvic radiotherapy alone. They also indicate that irradiation alone is insufficient treatment for most patients with gross residual disease, particularly when the residuum is extrapelvic.

There have been few direct comparisons between abdominopelvic irradiation and modern cisplatin- or paclitaxel-based chemotherapy. Although retrospective studies do not demonstrate a clear advantage of one treatment over the other for patients with minimal residual disease, physician biases are

TABLE 32.4-7. Evidence for Cure of Ovarian Cancer by Abdominopelvic Radiotherapy: Long-Term Outcome in Patients with Stage II and III Disease and Macroscopic Residuum

Study Center	Size of Residuum		End Point
	<2 cm	>2 cm	
Princess Margaret Hospital[63]	38 (91)	6 (91)	10-y relapse-free rate
Stanford[64]	50 (42)	14 (54)	15-y failure-free rate
Salt Lake City[65]	62 (12)	0 (10)	10-y relapse-free survival
Walter Reed Hospital[66]	42 (24)	10 (20)	10-y survival rate
Yale[67]	41 (27)	—	~6-y surviving fraction

Note: Numbers in parentheses are the number of patients treated in each group.

strong, and several multi-institutional trials addressing this question have been closed prematurely because of inadequate patient accrual. In 1993, Redman and coworkers[68] published the results of a randomized trial comparing abdominopelvic irradiation with single-agent cisplatin in 40 patients with microscopic residual disease, stages IC to III. The 5-year survival rates were 58% and 62% in the two arms, respectively, but the power of the study was weak because of the small number of patients. In 1994, Chiara and colleagues[69] reported results of a second study comparing whole abdominal radiotherapy with cisplatin and cyclophosphamide in 70 patients with high-risk stage I or II disease. This study was compromised by poor accrual and protocol violations. Eight (24%) of the 34 patients assigned to receive radiotherapy were treated with chemotherapy. Projected 5-year survival rates for those randomly assigned to receive radiation (34 patients) or chemotherapy (36 patients) were 53% and 71%, respectively ($P = .16$). In a secondary analysis, the death rates for the 44 patients who received chemotherapy and the 25 who received radiation therapy were similar (27% and 32%, respectively; $P = .7$).

These studies still leave us with an incomplete understanding of the role of radiotherapy in initial management of ovarian cancer, however. Although pelvic irradiation was routinely added to early treatments with single alkylating agents, it generally has been abandoned since platinum-containing regimens became standard. Early studies of pelvic radiation therapy alone and the success of whole abdominal plus pelvic irradiation in selected patients indicate that radiation is an active agent and suggest that pelvic irradiation may be a useful addition to chemotherapy for selected patients who have a high risk of pelvic recurrence. However, no study has ever been done to determine whether pelvic irradiation could improve the control rates achieved with modern chemotherapy.

Whole Abdominal Radiotherapy

The cobalt 60 moving strip technique was developed at the M. D. Anderson Cancer Center in the 1960s to improve the acute tolerance of patients to large whole abdominal fields of radiation. The abdomen was divided into horizontal strips of 2.5 cm each. Two to four contiguous strips were treated each day, with exposure moving down gradually until the whole abdomen had received the prescribed dose of radiation. Subsequent studies suggested that large stationary megavoltage fields could be tolerated, and they were technically less difficult to deliver. In 1983, Dembo and coworkers[69a] reported a randomized comparison of open field whole abdominal irradiation (22 Gy in 22 fractions) and the moving strip technique (22.5 Gy in 10 fractions per strip), demonstrating lower complication rates and comparable tumor control with the simpler open field technique.

The high rate of subdiaphragmatic recurrences observed after treatment with early "whole abdominal" fields that did not completely cover the diaphragm illustrates the critical importance of covering the entire peritoneal cavity. In a review of a prospective multi-institutional trial, Klaassen and colleagues[62] reported a significantly poorer survival rate for patients whose whole abdominal radiation fields were found to deviate seriously from protocol specifications. In a more recent report, Firat et al.[70] suggested that the rates of abdominal disease control and survival can be improved if patients receive more than

30 Gy to the whole abdomen, although the rate of major complications was also much higher in patients who received these higher doses.

Patients should always undergo simulation using fluoroscopy, and fields should provide a 1-cm margin on the maximum cephalad excursion of the diaphragmatic domes under quiet respiration. It is often necessary to flash the lateral abdominal wall and to include the entire bony pelvis in whole abdominal fields to avoid excluding peritoneal surfaces. In obese patients with poor abdominal tone, the fields may need to extend laterally beyond the bony pelvis. This is particularly true when the patient is treated in the prone position. The thickness of the abdominal wall should be considered in choosing the energy of the radiation beam. When fields are designed using CT scans of the whole abdomen, coverage of peritoneal surfaces can be assured. The total dose of whole abdominal irradiation varies between 22 and 30 Gy depending on the fractionation scheme, use of concurrent chemotherapy, and patient tolerance. Posterior kidney blocks are placed to limit the renal dose to 15 to 18 Gy, and a portion of the liver may be shielded during part of the treatment to limit the dose to 22 to 25 Gy. The true pelvis is usually treated to a higher dose of 45 to 50 Gy, either after whole abdominal irradiation or concurrently as a field within a field (not to exceed a total daily dose to the pelvis of 180 cGy). Martinez and coworkers[64] have suggested boosting the dose to the paraaortic nodes and medial diaphragms with a T-shaped field in selected patients. Chemotherapy that is given before or after irradiation can influence normal tissue tolerance and should be considered in estimations of organ tolerance.

Intraperitoneal Radioisotope Therapy

The characteristic transcolonic pattern of dissemination of ovarian cancer first led clinicians to treat patients with intraperitoneal isotopes in the 1950s, and this treatment is still used by some practitioners for a selected group of patients with minimal disease. The isotope that is generally used is chromic phosphate (^{32}P). ^{32}P decays with a half-life of 14.3 days, emitting β-particles with a mean energy of 0.69 MeV. Because the average penetration of these particles in soft tissue is less than 1 to 2 mm, treatment with ^{32}P is inappropriate for patients who have macroscopic residual disease. Because the goal is to distribute the isotope evenly over peritoneal surfaces, patients with intraabdominal adhesions that inhibit the flow of the isotope-containing fluid are poor candidates for this treatment. Intraabdominal distribution is usually evaluated before treatment by scanning the patient after an intraabdominal injection of technetium 99m sulfur colloid. If a good distribution is confirmed, the patient is treated with 10 to 20 mCi of ^{32}P diluted in saline and then is positioned to optimize distribution. It is estimated that this dose delivers 20 to 40 Gy of radiation to the peritoneal surface. However, nonuniform distribution can produce variations in the dose of tenfold or more.

An early GOG randomized trial,[43] reported in 1990, demonstrated 5-year survival rates of 81% and 78% for patients treated with melphalan and ^{32}P, respectively; four patients (6%) treated with ^{32}P required an operation for small bowel obstruction, and two patients (3%) treated with melphalan developed leukemia. The authors concluded that intraabdominal ^{32}P was the preferred treatment for these patients because of its limited toxicity and no known risk for causing leukemia. In a subsequent GOG study,[71] intraabdominal ^{32}P therapy was compared with three cycles of cisplatin and cyclophosphamide in patients with high-risk early-stage disease. There was no significant difference in the risk of recurrence (35% and 28%, respectively; $P = .15$) or in the probability of survival ($P = .43$) for patients treated with ^{32}P and chemotherapy. One toxicity-related death was reported in each treatment arm. Of 118 patients treated with chemotherapy, 69%, 8%, and 16% had grade 3 or 4 leukopenia, thrombocytopenia, or gastrointestinal toxicity, respectively; of 106 patients treated with ^{32}P, 3 experienced small bowel perforations during catheter insertion, which in one case may have contributed to the treatment-related death on that arm. The authors concluded that platinum-based chemotherapy should be standard because of the complications of ^{32}P administration and the trend toward a lower risk of recurrence with chemotherapy.

Two other randomized studies have compared ^{32}P with cisplatin-containing chemotherapy.[72,73] These also failed to demonstrate a significant difference in survival between the two treatments. Vergote and colleagues[72] randomly assigned 347 patients who had no gross residual disease after laparotomy to receive intraperitoneal ^{32}P (7 to 10 mCi) or cisplatin (six courses of 50 mg/m^2 each). The estimated 5-year survival rates were 83% and 81%, respectively ($P = .6$). Although the dose of ^{32}P was relatively low, 12 (9%) of 136 patients who had this treatment experienced small bowel obstructions compared with 2% of patients treated with cisplatin. For this reason, these authors also recommended platinum-based chemotherapy as standard treatment.

The most common complication of ^{32}P administration is transient abdominal pain, which occurs in 15% to 20% of patients. Chemical or infectious peritonitis is a rare complication that occurs in 2% to 3% of patients. The most serious late complication of treatment is small bowel obstruction, which has been reported in 5% to 10% of patients treated with ^{32}P alone. This risk increases to an unacceptable rate of 20% to 30% when intraperitoneal ^{32}P is combined with external-beam radiotherapy, an approach that is no longer recommended.

TREATMENT OF ADVANCED-STAGE OVARIAN CANCER

The recommended treatment strategy for patients with advanced-stage ovarian cancer (stage III or stage IV disease) is similar: optimal cytoreductive surgery to remove all visible tumor, whenever feasible, followed by platinum- and taxane-based chemotherapy.

Cytoreduction

Aggressive surgery to remove all grossly visibile tumor (i.e., cytoreductive surgery or tumor debulking surgery) has been an integral part of the initial treatment for advanced ovarian cancer for almost 30 years.[76] The theoretical benefits of cytoreductive surgery are to remove large necrotic tumors with poor blood supplies and to remove large tumors that are in a slower growth phase, which leaves behind tumors that are more sensitive to the effects of chemotherapy. *Optimal cytoreduction* has been defined differently through the years, but at the current time, cytoreduction with residual disease under 1 cm is most widely accepted. Several reports have demonstrated that the size of the largest residual disease correlates with progression-free and overall survival.[46,47,77] Theoretically, all patients with stage III and IV disease are candidates for cytoreductive surgery; however, in some cases, clinical assessment dictates that neoadjuvant chemotherapy should be initially prescribed. For example, patients with a poor performance status who cannot undergo an aggressive surgical procedure or, in some cases, stage IV patients with parenchymal liver disease, enlarged retrocrural or supraclavicular lymph nodes, mediastinal metastases, and parenchymal lung metastases may not be candidates for optimal cytoreductive surgery. Women with stage IV disease based only on the presence of malignant pleural effusion have been able to undergo optimal cytoreductive surgery. Studies have suggested that an optimal surgical cytoreductive procedure should be performed in women with stage IV disease even when parenchymal liver disease is recognized preoperatively.[74,75] In patients who underwent optimal cytoreduction with residual tumor of less than 1 to 2 cm maximum diameter, the median survival varied from 25 to 40 months, whereas among those who underwent suboptimal cytoreduction, median survival times were 10 to 18 months. Interestingly, in three of the four prospective randomized trials conducted by the GOG, the patients with stage IV disease undergoing optimal cytoreduction had survival superior to that of patients with stage III ovarian cancer who underwent optimal cytoreduction.[46]

Successful surgical management of stage III or IV ovarian cancer requires meticulous attention to surgical techniques to avoid complications and a thorough knowledge of abdominal and pelvic anatomy to allow the successful accomplishment of cytoreductive surgery. In general, it is wisest to start with an incision in the lower abdomen to free the pelvis of cancer, then work up into the upper abdomen to attempt to clear it of cancer, then complete the procedure with paraaortic and pericaval retroperitoneal lymph node sampling or resection if optimal cytoreduction has been accomplished within the peritoneal cavity. The goal of optimal cytoreductive surgery is complete removal of all palpable or visible tumor. A minimal goal of cytoreductive surgery is to reduce the residual tumor to less than 1 cm and preferably to less than 0.5 cm in maximum diameter.

When the abdominal cavity is entered, normal anatomy is restored by lysing adhesions and freeing organs from adherent tumor. Frequently the pelvis is completely filled with tumor. By identifying the round ligaments and suture ligating and dividing them, the pelvic retroperitoneum can be entered and the external iliac arteries and veins, the hypogastric arteries, and the ureters can be rapidly identified. Accomplishing this allows ligation of the infundibulopelvic ligaments with the ovarian vessels; resection of peritoneum, along with the attached vessels down to the tumor mass; and dissection of the ovarian mass off of, or with, the underlying peritoneum to elevate the mass from the pelvic sidewall. By dividing the utero-ovarian ligaments and fallopian tubes, one can then remove the mass. At times, it may be necessary to resect small bowel or sigmoid colon in continuity with the ovarian mass. An end-to-end or side-to-side anastomosis restores bowel continuity. Less frequently a colostomy is necessary. Once each of the ovaries has been removed, a hysterectomy is performed. At times, ovarian cancers infiltrate the uterus and it is necessary to take the uterus out *en bloc* with the ovarian tumor. Implants in the cul-de-sac may be resected using retroperitoneal dissection. Sigmoid colon implants usually involve epiploic appendices, which can be resected without performing a sigmoid colon resection. Retroperitoneal lymph nodes are routinely removed from the external iliac artery and vein, hypogastric arteries, and the obturator fossa. An appendectomy is routinely performed.

After resection of the pelvic disease, a complete omentectomy is performed and large masses implanting on peritoneal surfaces, including the diaphragm, are removed. Once the abdomen has been cleared of disease or the maximum residual disease is less than 1 cm, the fat pad overlying and surrounding the aorta and vena cava is removed, as are lymph nodes involved with metastatic disease in this area. In general, if large residual tumor volume is left within the peritoneal cavity, there is not much benefit in resecting retroperitoneal disease. However, when intraperitoneal disease has undergone optimal cytoreduction to less than 1 cm maximal residual tumor volume, retroperitoneal lymphadenectomies are appropriate.

Impact of Primary Cytoreductive Surgery

The clinical rationale for cytoreductive surgery has been ascribed to Griffiths,[76] who demonstrated in 1975 that survival was directly affected by the initial degree of cytoreductive surgery in women with advanced-stage ovarian cancer. In a retrospective review, patients with no residual disease had a mean survival of 39 months compared with 29 months for those with residual disease of less than 0.5 cm, 18 months for those with residual disease of 0.6 to 1.5 cm, and 11 months for those who did not have cytoreduction below 1.5 cm. None of the latter patients survived beyond 26 months. Women who underwent optimal cytoreductive surgery had survival rates similar to those of women who had minimal-size abdominal metastases at the initial surgery. Subsequent to Griffiths's report, numerous series have confirmed that aggressive cytoreductive surgery to 2 cm of residual tumor or less significantly enhances survival for patients. Most patients participated in trials in which multidrug chemotherapy was used, generally involving cisplatin-based chemotherapy. A review of nine studies in which primary cytoreductive surgery resulted in disease of less than 2 cm or greater than 2 cm demonstrated a mean survival in the group with optimal cytoreduction of 29.4 months compared with 13.4 months in the group in whom cytoreductive surgery was suboptimal[76–84] (Table 32.4-8).

Two metaanalyses gave conflicting views on the survival impact of cytoreductive surgery.[85,86] Hunter et al.[85] reviewed a total of 58 separate studies encompassing 6962 patients to determine whether maximal cytoreductive surgery benefits the survival of women with advanced ovarian cancer. These authors looked at the median survival times of groups of women with advanced ovarian cancer and used multiple linear regression techniques to analyze the effects on median survival. The variables studied were the proportion of each cohort undergoing maximal cytoreductive surgery, the use of cisplatin chemotherapy, the dose intensity of the chemotherapy, the proportion of each cohort with stage IV disease, and the year of publication of the study. The use of cisplatin chemotherapy resulted in an increased survival time of 53% [95% confidence interval (CI), 35% to 73%]. For each 0.2-U increase in dose intensity, the increase in median survival time was 11.1% (95% CI, 6% to 17%; $P = .001$). Stage IV disease had a negative impact on survival. For each 10% increase in the number of stage IV patients in the study, a negative survival increase of 2.6% (95% CI, –0.1% to –5.4%) was found. For each 10% increase in the percentage of women who underwent maximal cytoreductive surgery, the increase in survival was only 4.1% (95% CI, –0.6% to 9.1%; $P = .089$) (Fig. 32.4-4). This study concluded that cytoreductive surgery has only a small effect on the survival of women with

TABLE 32.4-8. Effect of Residual Disease at the Conclusion of Primary Cytoreductive Surgery on Survival

Investigators	Treatment	Residual Disease (cm)	Survival (Mo)
Griffiths (1975)[76]	L-PAM	0	39
		0–0.5	29
		0.6–1.5	18
		>1.5	11
Hacker et al. (1983)[77]	Varied	<0.5	40
		0.6–1.5	18
		>1.5	6
Vogl et al. (1983)[78]	CHAP	<2	>40
		>2	16
Pohl et al. (1984)[79]	Varied	<2	45
		>2	16
Delgado et al. (1984)[80]	Varied	<2	45
		>2	16
Redman et al. (1986)[83]	CAP	<3	38
		>3	26
Conte et al. (1986)[84]	CAP, CP	<2	>40
		>2	16
Neijt et al. (1991)[82]	CHAP or CP	<1	40
		>1	21
Piver et al. (1988)[81]	PAC	<2	48
		>2	21
Totals			**Mean, 36.7 (optimal)**
			Mean, 16.6 (suboptimal)

CAP, cyclophosphamide, doxorubicin(Adriamycin), and cisplatin; CHAP, cyclophosphamide, hexamethylmelamine, doxorubicin, and cisplatin; CP, cyclophosphamide and cisplatin; L-PAM, melphalan; PAC, cisplatin, doxorubicin, and cyclophosphamide.
(Modified from Young RC, Perez CA, Hoskins WV. Cancer of the ovary. In: DeVita VT Jr, Hellman S, Rosenberg SA, eds. *Cancer: principles and practice of oncology*, 4th ed. Philadelphia: JB Lippincott Co, 1993:1226, with permission.)

advanced ovarian cancer and that the type of treatment used (i.e., cisplatin) was far more important.

Three GOG studies give important insight into the impact of cytoreductive surgery in advanced ovarian cancer. The first demonstrated that removing all gross tumor defines true optimal cytoreductive surgery. Women treated with cisplatin-based chemotherapy who had no gross disease left had a progression-free interval of 42 months compared with 20 months for those with residual disease of less than 1 cm.[87] The second study revealed that women who had 1 to 2 cm of residual tumor had a significant survival improvement compared with those who had more than 2 cm of residual tumor.[88] This third study refuted early data suggesting that women undergoing optimal cytoreductive surgery have survival similar to that of patients initially found at surgery to have low-volume disease.[46] The latter study reported on 348 women with 1 cm or less residual tumor, 200 of whom initially had abdominal disease of 1 cm or less. When implants were present on parietal or visceral peritoneum, even when cytoreduction was optimal, survival rates significantly decreased. Indeed, the best survivals observed for patients with stage III disease were in those whose initial macroscopic tumor was smaller than 1 cm in the omentum and associated with either no disease or microscopic disease in other abdominal sites (P = .0001).

Those with the poorest survival had tumors initially larger than 1 cm involving omentum and had gross disease in other abdominal sites (Fig. 32.4-5). This study refutes early data suggesting that women undergoing optimal cytoreductive surgery have the same survival as those patients initially found at surgery to have low-volume disease. The study demonstrates that biologic factors responsible for bulk disease may be as important as technical ability to resect the disease.

Bristow et al.[10] performed a metaanalysis of data for 81 cohorts of patients with advanced-stage ovarian cancer (more than 6800 patients) to assess the survival effect of maximal cytoreductive surgery during the platinum-based chemotherapy era. They found a statistically significant positive correlation between percent maximal cytoreduction and log median survival time, and this correlation remained significant after controlling for all other variables (P<.001) (Fig. 32.4-6). Each 10% increase in maximal cytoreduction was associated with a 5.5% increase in median survival time. The relationship between platinum dose intensity and log median survival time was not statistically significant in this study.

Aggressive cytoreductive surgery incurs complications. Chen and Bochner[89] reported on 60 patients who underwent optimal cytoreductive surgery. These patients had a 5% operative morbidity. Blythe and Wahl[90] looked at quality of life in patients with optimal residual disease (less than 2 cm in diameter) and suboptimal residual disease (more than 2 cm in diameter) and found that 75% of the group with optimal residual disease were judged to have good or good to fair quality of life, but only 18% of the group with suboptimal residual disease achieved this quality of life. It has been argued that perhaps those women who are able to undergo optimal cytoreduction have biologically less virulent disease than those patients in whom optimal cytoreductive surgery cannot be achieved. This question has yet to be answered because there are no data from prospective randomized trials available.

CT scans have been used to identify tumor distribution and the extent of ovarian cancer metastases. In some cases, CT findings suggest metastatic disease that is not amenable to optimal surgical cytoreduction such as parenchymal liver disease and porta hepatis infiltration.[91] Although it is sometimes possible to resect tumor in these sites, many of these patients are left with a suboptimal result, and thus neoadjuvant chemotherapy has often been recommended. The initial experience with neoadjuvant chemotherapy in the management of women who have advanced disease that does not appear to be surgically resectable or who have evidence for stage IV disease suggests that it may be as effective as the conventional approach of chemotherapy after suboptimal cytoreductive surgery.[92] Interval debulking surgery is then performed after three or four cycles of chemotherapy in those patients who demonstrate response to therapy.[93] Potential advantages of neoadjuvant chemotherapy appear to be a much more rapid improvement in quality of life, a less expensive treatment program for patients, and, when surgery is ultimately performed, an easier operation requiring shorter hospitalization. Prospective randomized trials incorporating neoadjuvant chemotherapy in the management of advanced-stage ovarian cancer are definitely needed.

Chemotherapy

Chemotherapeutic agents from a wide variety of different classes have been shown to produce responses in patients with

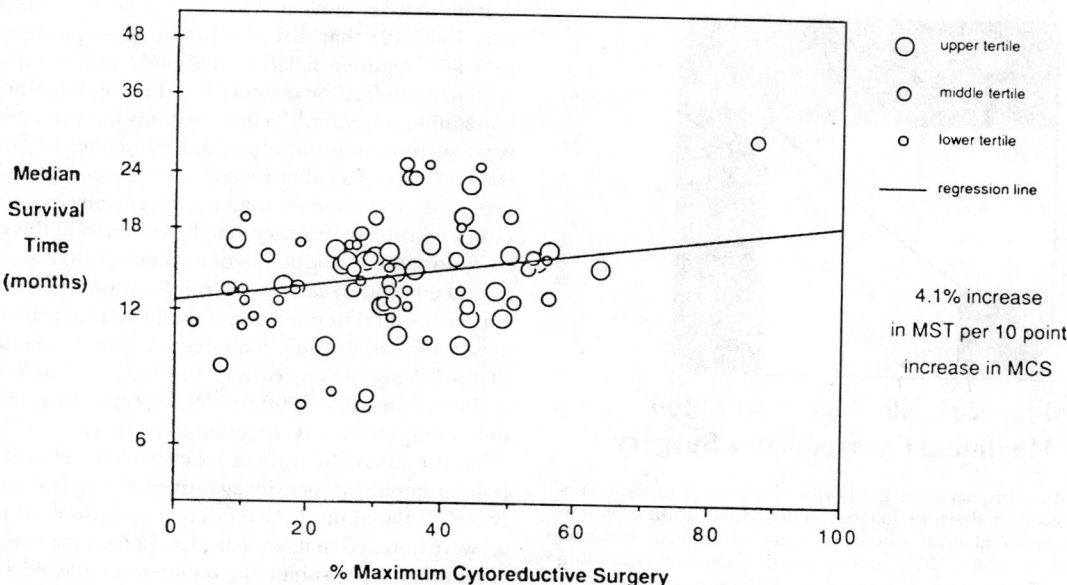

FIGURE 32.4-4.   Graph of log median survival time (MST; in months) versus percent maximal cytoreductive surgery (MCS) for 76 cohorts for which dose intensity could be calculated after adjustments for effects of dose intensity, percentage of patients with stage IV disease, and use of platinum chemotherapy. (From ref. 85, with permission.)

ovarian cancer. Numerous combination chemotherapy regimens have been studied, and individual drugs have been compared with combinations. Since the mid-1990s, the combination of a platinum agent and a taxane has been accepted as the standard of care in the United States.

The major importance of cisplatin in the management of ovarian cancer was summarized in a metaanalysis of 45 randomized trials that compared primary treatment with regimens containing this agent with regimens that did not include the drug.[94] A modest survival advantage for platinum-based combination programs compared to single-agent cisplatin was also revealed in this analysis.

The next highly relevant development in the management of ovarian cancer was the introduction of carboplatin into the

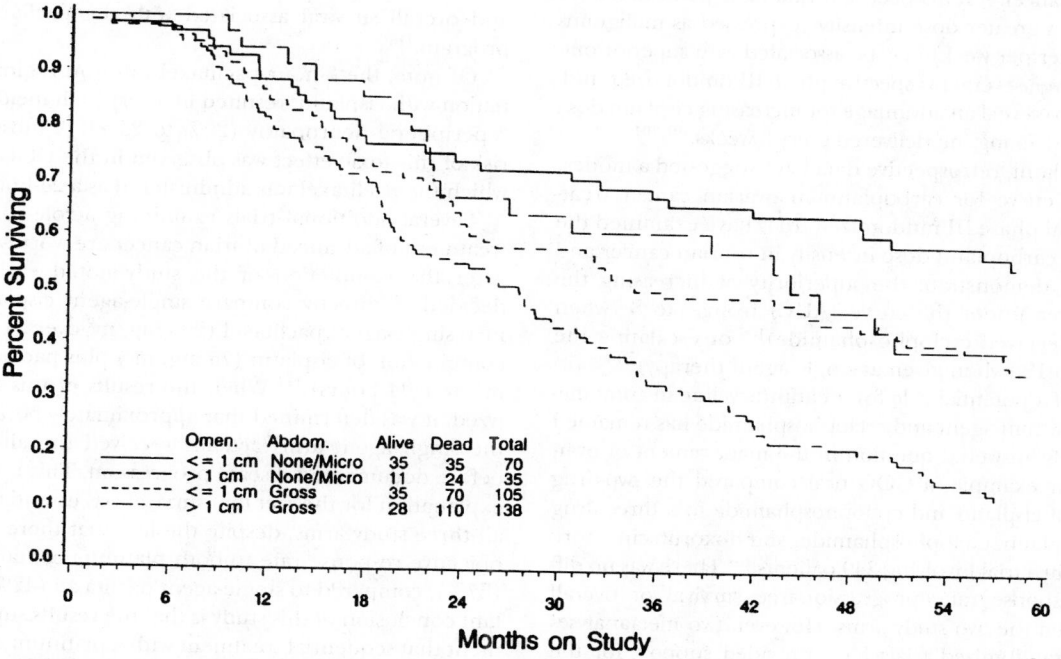

FIGURE 32.4-5.   Survival time by initial maximum omental (Omen.) and abdominal (Abdom.) tumor diameter. Micro, microscopic. (From ref. 46, with permission.)

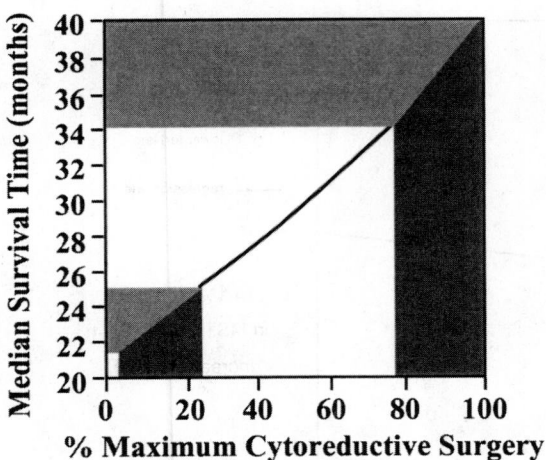

FIGURE 32.4-6. Impact of surgical cytoreduction on survival. Simple linear regression analysis: de-logged median survival time plotted against percent maximal cytoreductive surgery. Gray area, maximal cytoreductive ≤25% and >75%; crosshatched area, corresponding range of median survival times. (From ref. 10, with permission.)

oncologist's armamentarium as a less toxic analogue of cisplatin. Several prospective randomized trials, and the results of a large metaanalysis, have confirmed the equivalence of single-agent carboplatin and cisplatin, and of combination cisplatin versus carboplatin non–taxane-containing primary chemotherapy regimens in advanced ovarian cancer.[95–97]

Several trials have specifically examined the benefits of extending treatment with cisplatin-based chemotherapy beyond 5 or 6 cycles to 10 or 12 cycles.[98,99] Unfortunately, the studies only showed that such treatment increased toxicity but did not improve either progression-free or overall survival.

Other studies have examined the role of cisplatin dose intensity in ovarian cancer. A retrospective review of 33 published trials suggested that a greater dose intensity (expressed as milligrams per square meter per week) may be associated with superior outcome.[100] However, several prospective phase III randomized studies have failed to reveal an advantage for increasing cisplatin dose intensity beyond 75 mg/m^2 delivered every 3 weeks.[101–104]

As with cisplatin, retrospective data have suggested a modest dose-response curve for carboplatin in ovarian cancer treatment.[105] Several phase III randomized trials have examined the importance of carboplatin dose intensity in ovarian cancer and have failed to demonstrate the superiority of increasing the carboplatin area under the curve (AUC) from 4 to 8 (when patients also received cyclophosphamide)[106] or escalating the AUC from 6 to 12 (when given as single-agent therapy).[107]

The issue of a potential role for an anthracycline in combination with a platinum agent and cyclophosphamide has remained an incompletely answered question in the management of ovarian cancer. For example, a GOG trial compared the two-drug combination of cisplatin and cyclophosphamide to a three-drug regimen of cisplatin, cyclophosphamide, and doxorubicin (Adriamycin; PAC) in a trial involving 349 patients.[108] There was no difference in response rate, progression-free survival or overall survival between the two study arms. However, two metaanalyses of published randomized trials have provided support for the conclusion suggesting a 5% to 7% survival advantage for combination regimens that included doxorubicin compared to those

that did not contain the drug.[109,110] A large phase III randomized trial (ICON2) that directly compared single-agent carboplatin to a PAC regimen failed to demonstrate any survival advantage (progression-free or overall) for the combination doxorubicin-containing program.[111] That this study has not ended the controversy surrounding the use of anthracyclines in ovarian cancer is shown by the fact that several recently completed (but not yet reported) and ongoing trials are specifically examining a role for either epirubicin or liposomal doxorubicin in this clinical setting.

Before the introduction of paclitaxel into the management of advanced ovarian cancer, the randomized trial experience noted earlier resulted in the routine use of several primary chemotherapy regimens for this malignancy. These included either cisplatin (75 mg/m^2) or carboplatin (AUC = 5 to 7) delivered with cyclophosphamide (600 to 750 mg/m^2). In Europe, it was not uncommon for a PAC regimen to be used.

In the 1980s, the taxanes (paclitaxel, docetaxel) were shown to possess significant activity against platinum-resistant ovarian cancer.[112–114] Based on this experience, two phase III randomized trials were initiated that compared a cisplatin-paclitaxel regimen to a cisplatin-cyclophosphamide regimen (Table 32.4-9). The GOG study[115] randomly assigned patients with suboptimally resected stage III and IV ovarian cancer to one of these two chemotherapy combinations and showed that women treated with the paclitaxel-containing program experienced a statistically significantly higher objective response rate as well as improved progression-free and overall survival (38 vs. 24 months) (Fig. 32.4-7).

These impressive results were confirmed in a trial conducted in Europe and Canada that used a similar but not identical study design.[116] In this later trial the paclitaxel was delivered as a 3-hour infusion (175 mg/m^2) whereas in the GOG study the agent was administered over 24 hours (135 mg/m^2). In addition, a much larger percentage of patients in the European-Canadian study received paclitaxel as a second-line therapy than in the GOG trial. Despite this fact, this study also revealed a statistically significant improvement in both progression-free and overall survival associated with the paclitaxel-containing program.[116]

Of note, the 3-hour paclitaxel infusion regimen, in combination with cisplatin, resulted in a very high incidence of grade 3 peripheral neuropathy (20% to 25%). A substantially lower risk of this toxic effect was observed in the GOG trial (4%), in which the paclitaxel was administered as a 24-hour infusion.

Several additional trials examining a role for paclitaxel in treatment of advanced ovarian cancer are worthy of discussion. After the completion of the study noted earlier, the GOG decided to directly compare single-agent cisplatin (100 mg/m^2), single-agent paclitaxel (200 mg/m^2 over 24 hours), or the combination of cisplatin (75 mg/m^2) plus paclitaxel (135 mg/m^2 over 24 hours).[117] When the results of this trial were analyzed, it was determined that approximately 50% of patients in the single-agent arms actually received the alternative agent before documented disease progression. This is the most likely explanation for the fact that survival was essentially the same in all three study arms, despite the fact that there was a superior objective response rate to both platinum-containing regimens (67%), compared to single-agent paclitaxel (42%). One important conclusion of this study is that the results support the argument that sequential treatment with a platinum agent, followed by paclitaxel, is therapeutically equivalent to combination therapy with the two drugs in advanced ovarian cancer.

TABLE 32.4-9.   Randomized Trials of Paclitaxel plus Platinum in Advanced Ovarian Cancer

Trial and Randomization	Reference	No. of Patients/ Stage	CCR (%)	PFS Median (Mo)	OS Median (Mo)
GOG 111	115	386; Suboptimal stage II and IV			
Cisplatin (75 mg/m²) plus paclitaxel (135 mg/m² in 24 h)			51	18	38
Cisplatin (75 mg/m²) plus cyclophosphamide (750 mg/m²)			31	13	24
OV-10	116	668; Stage IIB–IV			
Cisplatin (75 mg/m²) plus paclitaxel (175 mg/m² in 3 h)			50	16	35
Cisplatin (75 mg/m²) plus cyclophosphamide (750 mg/m²)			36	12	25
GOG 132	117	—			
Cisplatin (75 mg/m²) plus paclitaxel (135 mg/m² in 24 h)			NA	14.1	26.6
Paclitaxel (200 mg/m²)			NA	11.4	26
Cisplatin (100 mg/m²)			NA	16.4	30.2
ICON3	118	2074; Stage I–IV			
Carboplatin (AUC = 5–6) plus paclitaxel (175 mg/m²)			NA	17.3	36.1
Carboplatin (AUC = 5–6) or cisplatin (50 mg/m²) plus doxorubicin (50 mg/m²) plus cyclophosphamide (500 mg/m²)			NA	16.1	35.4

AUC, area under the curve; CCR, clinical complete remission; GOG, Gynecologic Oncology Group; ICON3, International Collaborative Ovarian Neoplasm trial 3; NA, not available; OS, overall survival; PFS, progression-free survival.

A large (2000-patient) European phase III randomized trial (ICON3) compared a "control" regimen of either single-agent carboplatin or PAC to an "experimental" program of carboplatin and paclitaxel. The study failed to reveal a difference in survival between either control arm and the experimental arm.[118] A number of theories have been proposed to explain the difference in outcome between this study and the two previously mentioned trials that compared cisplatin plus cyclophosphamide and cisplatin plus paclitaxel.[115,116] Perhaps the most likely explanation is the fact that one-third of the patients on the control arms of ICON3 ultimately received paclitaxel. Thus, as in the previously mentioned three-arm GOG study,[117] this outcome provides support for the hypothesis that the sequential administration of the two active agents is therapeutically equivalent to combination drug delivery.

Due to the more favorable toxicity profile of carboplatin, compared to cisplatin, it was natural that investigators desired to use the newer platinum agent with paclitaxel,[119] assuming equivalent efficacy could be documented. Three phase III randomized trials have been reported that directly compared a carboplatin-paclitaxel regimen to cisplatin plus paclitaxel (Table 32.4-10).[120–122] As might have been anticipated, the studies have revealed equivalent progression-free and overall survival for the regimens, with a generally more favorable toxicity profile associated with the carboplatin-based programs. Of note, the studies demonstrated that it was possible to adminis-

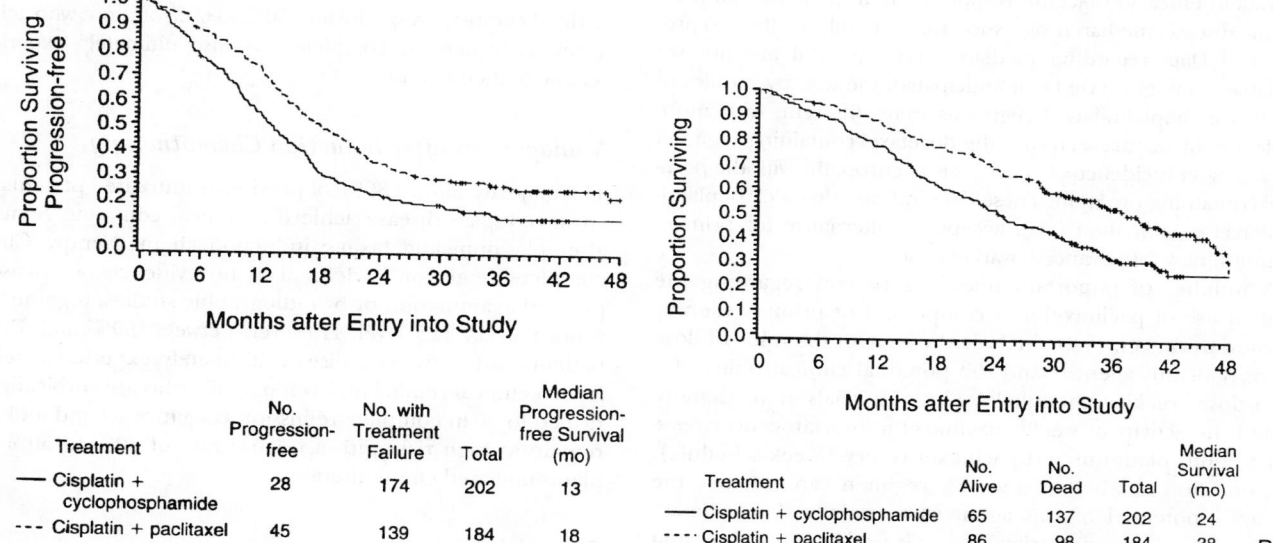

FIGURE 32.4-7.   Disease-free (**A**) and overall (**B**) survival of patients with suboptimally resected stage III and IV ovarian cancer randomly assigned to treatment with cisplatin plus cyclophosphamide (*solid line*) or cisplatin plus paclitaxel (*dotted line*). (From ref. 115, with permission.)

TABLE 32.4-10. Randomized Trials of Carboplatin plus Paclitaxel versus Cisplatin plus Paclitaxel

Trial and Randomization	Reference	No. of Patients/Stage	PFS Median (Mo)	OS Median (Mo)
GOG 158	120	792; Optimal stage III		
Carboplatin (AUC = 7.5) plus paclitaxel (175 mg/m² in 3 h)			20.7	57.4
Cisplatin (75 mg/m²) plus paclitaxel (135 mg/m²)			19.4	48.7
AGO	121	798; Stage IIB–IV		
Carboplatin (AUC = 6) plus paclitaxel (185 mg/m² in 3 h)			17.2	43.3
Cisplatin (75 mg/m²) plus paclitaxel (185 mg/m² in 3 h)			19.1	44.1
NETHERLANDS-DENMARK	122	208; Stage IIB–IV		
Carboplatin (AUC = 5) plus paclitaxel (175 mg/m² in 3 h)			ND	ND
Cisplatin (75 mg/m²) plus paclitaxel (175 mg/m² in 3 h)			ND	ND

AGO, Arbeitsgemeinschaft Gynaekologische Onkologie; AUC, area under the curve; GOG, Gynecologic Oncology Group; ND, no difference reported; OS, overall survival; PFS, progression-free survival.

ter paclitaxel over 3 hours in combination with carboplatin with an acceptable incidence of neurotoxicity, in contrast to the situation with cisplatin, in which a 24-hour infusion regimen was required.

The preceding data support the conclusion that there are two acceptable standard paclitaxel-containing combination chemotherapy regimens that may be used for primary treatment of advanced ovarian cancer: cisplatin (75 mg/m²) plus paclitaxel (135 mg/m² over 24 hours) or carboplatin (AUC = 5.0 to 7.5) plus paclitaxel (175 mg/m² over 3 hours). In general, the carboplatin-based regimen is preferred due to reduced toxicity (e.g., emesis, neutropenia, nephrotoxicity) and the ability to deliver a shorter paclitaxel infusion. In individuals for whom there is concern regarding the ability to tolerate a combination regimen (e.g., marginal performance status, significant comorbid medical conditions, advanced age) it is reasonable to initiate treatment with single-agent carboplatin and either add paclitaxel to the regimen at a later point or deliver the drugs in sequence.

The preliminary report of a randomized trial comparing a carboplatin (AUC = 5) plus paclitaxel (175 mg/m²) regimen to carboplatin (AUC = 5) plus docetaxel (75 mg/m²) has suggested equivalent efficacy (objective response rate in patients with measurable disease, median progression-free survival) for the two programs.[123] Data regarding median overall survival are not yet available. As might have been anticipated, the toxicity profiles of the two carboplatin-based regimens were different, with more grade 4 neutropenia seen with the docetaxel-containing regimen and a greater incidence of grade 2 or 3 neuropathy with the paclitaxel-containing program. These data indicate that a carboplatin-docetaxel combination is an acceptable alternative for primary chemotherapy for advanced ovarian cancer.

A number of important questions remain regarding the optimal use of paclitaxel as a component of primary therapy for ovarian cancer. These include the issue of the value of dose intensity of this agent[124] and the potential clinical utility of a lower-dose weekly schedule.[125] Phase II trials have demonstrated the activity of weekly paclitaxel in ovarian cancer resistant to both platinum and paclitaxel (every-3-week schedule). The question of whether a weekly regimen can enhance the cytotoxic potential of this agent when delivered as primary therapy for advanced ovarian cancer is worthy of examination in a randomized trial. Several novel taxane preparations that appear to produce equivalent efficacy and reduced toxicity compared to paclitaxel are currently undergoing phase I and II

testing. It is important ultimately to compare one or more of these agents with standard treatment using carboplatin and paclitaxel in phase III randomized trials.

The provocative results of a randomized trial conducted by the Southwest Oncology Group and the GOG have raised the important issue of the duration of paclitaxel therapy in advanced ovarian cancer.[126] In this trial women with advanced disease who had demonstrated a clinically defined complete response were randomly assigned to receive either 3 cycles or 12 cycles of single-agent paclitaxel (175 mg/m² over 3 hours) delivered on a schedule of every 28 days. The study was stopped early by the Data Safety Monitoring Committee when an interim analysis revealed a 50% reduction in the risk of recurrence associated with the 12-month maintenance strategy (median progression-free survival 28 months vs. 21 months in the 3-month maintenance arm; *P* = .0023). At the time of study closure there was no difference in overall survival between the two regimens, but follow-up to address this point was very limited. Further exploration in appropriately designed randomized trials of the issue of the duration of treatment for patients responding to, and tolerating, therapy is clearly indicated, because it remains the case that 70% to 80% of women with advanced ovarian cancer who achieve a clinically defined complete response and 50% to 60% of those who achieve a surgically defined complete response ultimately experience relapse of their disease.

Management after Induction Chemotherapy

The majority, almost 80%, of previously untreated patients with advanced-stage disease achieve a clinical complete remission after platinum and taxane induction chemotherapy. Clinical complete remission is defined as no evidence of disease on physical examination or by radiographic studies, together with a normal CA 125 level. However, between 50% and 75% of patients with advanced disease ultimately experience relapse from a clinical remission. Even patients who are surgically confirmed to be in complete remission (negative second look) still remain at high risk, with a relapse rate of 30% to 50% after platinum-based chemotherapy.

Second-Look Surgery

Second-look surgery is a carefully planned systematic surgical approach to evaluate patients who have completed the planned course of chemotherapy and who, by clinical examination, measurement of CA 125 level, and diagnostic imaging studies, are free of persistent cancer. The purpose of the second-look operation is to assess the pathologic or microscopic response to therapy by completely exploring the abdominal cavity and sampling any abnormalities found or performing biopsy of peritoneal surfaces where microscopic ovarian cancer is most likely to be found, or both.[127] Although the intent of second-look surgery is to improve survival by instituting additional therapy if any persistent cancer is discovered, to date, second-look procedures have not demonstrated any survival advantage and thus are no longer standard of care. In some subgroups of patients or as part of a clinical trial design, a secondary surgical assessment may still be included in the treatment management plan. In other individual cases, second-look procedures may be performed to help determine prognosis, although their therapeutic value has not been validated.

At the current time, when second-look surgery is performed, a laparoscopic approach is most frequently used. This approach allows complete visualization of the peritoneal cavity and in most cases provides sufficient ability to obtain the necessary biopsy specimens.[128] Washings of the pelvis and abdomen are performed, followed by lysis of adhesions, which are sent for histologic assessment. Sampling then begins in the pelvis with peritoneal biopsy specimens taken from the areas of the round ligaments and the infundibulopelvic ligaments, from the bladder flap peritoneum, and from the cul-de-sac peritoneum. The retroperitoneal spaces are examined, and any residual lymph node or fatty tissues surrounding the external iliac artery, vein, or hypogastric artery are sampled. Studies comparing the diagnostic accuracy of laparoscopic reassessment to reassessment via laparotomy have demonstrated equivalent ability to detect disease and predict future recurrence. Furthermore, the minimally invasive approach has proven to be more cost effective, with less associated morbidity and mortality.[128]

Radiotherapy after Chemotherapy

Numerous small phase I and II studies have used whole abdominal irradiation as salvage treatment for patients with minimal residual disease after chemotherapy. Some authors have reported 3-year progression-free survival rates as high as 25% to 35% and occasional 10- to 15-year disease-free survivors among patients treated with abdominal irradiation after an incomplete response to chemotherapy.[129–132] However, others have reported high complication rates and have been discouraged by the short duration of most remissions, particularly in patients with high-grade disease or macroscopic residual tumor.[133,134]

Although irradiation of the abdomen and pelvis may cure a small proportion of patients who have residual disease after chemotherapy, the control rates appear to be much poorer than those reported for patients treated with initial radiation for a similar volume of residual disease. A number of factors may contribute to these disappointing results. Patients who have not responded completely to chemotherapy may have disease that is inherently more aggressive than that of patients chosen for primary treatment with whole abdominal irradiation. Radiotherapy is often compromised because of poor hematologic tolerance after aggressive chemotherapy, which further decreases the probability that the tumor will be sterilized. It also has been suggested that cytoreductive treatments (surgery, irradiation, or chemotherapy) may stimulate the proliferation of clonogenic tumor cells. Consequently, to overcome rapid repopulation, higher doses of radiation may be required to sterilize tumor cells that remain after a course of chemotherapy.

Hoskins et al.[135] have reported encouraging results for a regimen that integrated whole abdominal irradiation in the initial treatment of patients with minimal residual disease after cytoreduction. In their study, radiation was given after the first three of six cycles of cisplatin and cyclophosphamide. Comparison with the results for similar patients treated during a later time with six cycles of chemotherapy alone favored the alternating regimen, particularly for patients with stage I disease ($P = .04$).

Several randomized trials have compared whole abdominal irradiation with additional consolidative chemotherapy for patients with minimal disease after surgical cytoreduction and platinum-containing chemotherapy. Bruzzone et al.[136] randomly assigned patients who had minimal or no residual disease after chemotherapy (doxorubicin, cyclophosphamide, and cisplatin or carboplatin) to receive whole abdominal irradiation or three more cycles of chemotherapy. The study was closed after accruing only 41 patients because disease progression had been observed in 55% of patients treated with radiation versus 29% of those treated with additional chemotherapy ($P = .08$). The authors recommended treatment with chemotherapy, but the small number of patients and short median follow-up weakened the conclusions of their study. In another study by Lambert et al.,[137] 254 patients with stage IIB to IV disease received five monthly courses of carboplatin and second-look laparotomy. The 117 patients who had residual disease of 2 cm or less after secondary cytoreduction were then randomly assigned to receive either five additional courses of carboplatin or whole abdominal irradiation (24 Gy in 5 weeks). The authors reported no statistical difference in survival time or disease-free survival rates between the two treatment arms. In a third trial, Pickel's group[137a] randomly assigned 64 patients who had a complete clinical response after surgery and chemotherapy (carboplatin, epirubicin, and prednimustine) to receive whole abdominal irradiation or no further treatment. No second-look laparotomy was performed. In this study, patients who had consolidation with radiation therapy had a significantly better 5-year survival than patients who had chemotherapy alone (59% vs. 33%; $P = .03$).

More recently, Sorbe et al.[138] reported results of a trial that included 172 patients with FIGO stage III ovarian carcinoma who had pathologic complete response or surgical complete response (microscopic residual only) after initial surgical cytoreduction and four cycles of chemotherapy [cisplatin (50 mg/m^2/cycle) with either doxorubicin or epirubicin]. Patients who had microscopic residual disease at second-look surgery received additional treatment with whole abdominal radiation therapy (20 Gy to the whole abdomen with an additional 20.4 Gy to the lower abdomen and pelvis) or six additional cycles of chemotherapy. The outcome for patients in this subgroup was not correlated with the type of consolidation treatment. Another group of 98 patients who had a pathologic complete response after initial therapy was then randomly assigned to receive additional chemotherapy, radiation therapy, or no further treatment. These patients had a significantly better progression-free survival rate if they had whole abdominal radiation (56%) than if they had chemotherapy (36%) or no additional treatment (33%) ($P = .03$). At 5 years, the overall survival rates were 69%, 57%, and 65% for the radiation, chemotherapy, and control arms, respectively ($P = .08$). Severe late intestinal complications occurred in 10% and 4% of patients treated with radiation and chemotherapy, respectively. This trial is the first to demonstrate a benefit from consolidation with radiation therapy. The exclusion of patients who had macroscopic residual disease probably improved the chance of demonstrating a benefit from radiation therapy and may explain the difference between the results of this trial and the results of that reported by Lambert et al.[137] However, the number of patients in this trial was small, and the overall survival comparison, although encouraging, did not achieve statistical significance. It can also be argued that more intensive initial chemotherapy (e.g., six cycles of carboplatin and paclitaxel) might have improved the relapse-free survival in the control arm, diminishing the advantage of radiation therapy. Clearly there is room to improve the outcome of this group of patients; although the results of the trial by Sorbe et al.[138] may not be definitive, they do suggest the need for further study of the question.

Although most research emphasis has been on the use of whole abdominal irradiation, several authors have reported cases of long-term disease-free survival in patients who have received radiation treatment to smaller fields for locally relapsed or persistent disease.[139,140] Although these experiences are anecdotal, they do suggest that local field radiation therapy may be of benefit to some patients.

TREATMENT OF RECURRENT OVARIAN CANCER

The selection of treatment modalities and drug regimens for patients with recurrent ovarian cancer is based on the initial chemotherapy regimen used and on the nature of the initial response to treatment. Patients with recurrent ovarian cancer can be broadly divided into two subsets with markedly different prognoses. Patients whose disease recurs after a disease-free interval of less than 6 months have a worse prognosis that approaches that of patients who progress while on their initial chemotherapeutic regimen. In contrast, patients who have a disease-free interval of longer than 6 months or 1 year have a markedly improved prognosis, primarily because of the increased efficacy of salvage chemotherapy. Among patients with a long disease-free interval, secondary cytoreductive surgery can be considered in select subsets of patients.

Secondary Cytoreductive Surgery

Primary cytoreductive surgery has well-documented benefits in the management of advanced ovarian cancer. The possibility that secondary cytoreductive surgery (i.e., surgery performed to remove known persistent or recurrent disease after initiation chemotherapy) may be beneficial to patients has been suggested by numerous authors.[141–143] Most of these reports show that a statistically significant survival advantage can be gained for patients in whom an optimal secondary surgical result is achieved. Predictive factors for achieving an optimal secondary debulking include a longer disease-free interval (more than 12 months), focal tumor distribution (one or two sites), and initial optimal cytoreduction.[141]

Berek et al.[142] reported that secondary cytoreductive surgery could be performed in 12 of 32 patients (38%), and their tumors were reduced to less than 1.5 cm of residual disease. The median survival for that group was 20 months, compared to 5 months for the 20 patients whose disease could not be optimally cytoreduced. The patients most likely to undergo optimal cytoreductive surgery were those who previously had optimal primary cytoreduction, less than 1000 mL of ascites, and a tumor size of less than 5 cm at the second operation. The interval from the primary to secondary surgery should be longer than 12 months. Factors that did not have an impact on secondary cytoreductive surgery included patient age, tumor grade, type of chemotherapy, and the presence or absence of bowel obstruction. Subsequently, Segna et al.[143] reported their experience with secondary cytoreductive surgery. They too were able to show that, if optimal secondary cytoreductive surgery could be performed, patients lived longer before succumbing to ovarian cancer. Factors that influenced successful efforts in cytoreductive surgery were a time interval of more than 1 year between the original operation and the secondary cytoreductive surgery and performance of optimal cytoreductive surgery at the initial operation.

In 1995, Vaccarello et al. reported on 57 patients with recurrent ovarian cancer.[144] This population experienced relapse a median of 33 months after documented complete surgical response to primary cytoreduction and platinum-based therapy (negative second-look laparotomy). Thirty-eight patients (67%) underwent laparotomy at the time of recurrence, of whom 36 had bulky disease (larger than 0.5 cm) before resection. Of the 23 patients in whom debulking surgery was undertaken, 14 (61%) completed surgery with optimal residual disease (smaller than 0.5 cm). The median survival for patients undergoing optimal debulking was significantly better (41 months; $P<.0001$) than that for patients undergoing suboptimal debulking (23 months) or those not undergoing exploration (9 months). In multivariate analysis, the only factor that was found significantly to affect survival was tumor debulking to less than 0.5 cm. The authors concluded that secondary cytoreductive surgery benefits those patients who had a good response to primary surgery and chemotherapy followed by a substantial disease-free interval after negative second-look laparotomy, because these qualities would predict a good response to second-line therapy.

The ideal methodology for assessing the value of secondary debulking for patients with recurrent ovarian cancer would be a prospective trial comparing results for patients randomly assigned to surgical and nonsurgical arms followed by equivalent salvage chemotherapy. Thus far, such a protocol has not been undertaken. However, a prospective trial reported by Eisenkop et al. further supports surgical debulking of recurrent disease.[145] Secondary cytoreduction was prospectively performed on 36 patients who had a minimum disease-free interval of 6 months before relapse of ovarian cancer. The mean disease-free interval was 22 months (range, 6 to 43 months). All patients had undergone a primary surgical effort and received platinum-based chemotherapy. At the time of secondary surgery, all 36 patients had recurrent disease measuring more than 1 cm (greatest dimension of largest tumor nodule), with 64% having disease larger than 6 cm. Using an aggressive surgical approach, these authors were able to remove all macroscopic disease in 30 patients (83%); however, 14 patients required a modified posterior exenteration to achieve an optimal (microscopic residual only) resection. Morbidity occurred in 30.1% of patients, and there was one postoperative mortality (2.8%). Although a control population of patients with recurrent ovarian cancer not undergoing surgery was not available for comparison, survival analysis demonstrated a dramatic advantage for patients undergoing optimal resection compared to those left with macroscopic tumor. Median survivals for these two groups were 43 and 5 months, respectively ($P = .01$). Multivariate analysis revealed that, in addition to the amount of disease after secondary cytoreductive surgery, patient performance status and a longer disease-free interval (more than 36 months) were also independently predictive of improved survival.

TABLE 32.4-11. Survival after Secondary Cytoreduction for Ovarian Cancer

Study	Median DFI (Mo)	No. of Patients	Residual Disease	Survival (Mo)	Measure	P Value
Eisenkop et al., 1995[145]	22	30	Microscopic	43	Median	<.01
		6	Macroscopic	5	Median	
Vacarello et al., 1995[144]	20	14	<0.5 cm	>41[a]	Median	<.0001
		24	>0.5 cm	23	Median	
Segna et al., 1993[143]	Not stated	61	<2 cm	27.1	Median	.0001
		39	>2 cm	9		
Janicke et al., 1992[146]	16	14	Microscopic	29	Median	.004
		12	>2 cm	9		
		4	<2 cm	3		

DFI, disease-free interval before recurrence.
[a]Median survival not reached (75% probability of surviving 41 mo).

The majority of these published reports show a statistically significant survival benefit for patients undergoing optimal debulking of recurrent ovarian cancer. Data indicate that the magnitude of this benefit is inversely proportional to the volume of "optimal" residual disease and directly related to the duration of complete clinical remission (Table 32.4-11).

Interval Cytoreduction after Neoadjuvant Chemotherapy

Neijt et al.[147] compared the survival of women who underwent optimal cytoreductive surgery with the survival of women who had an unsuccessful optimal cytoreductive procedure but in whom, generally after three cycles of cisplatin-based chemotherapy, a secondary cytoreductive surgery was attempted. Those patients who underwent optimal secondary cytoreductive surgery had a statistically better survival rate than those who were unable to undergo optimal secondary cytoreductive surgery. However, those patients who underwent optimal secondary cytoreduction did not have a survival rate comparable to that of patients who had optimal cytoreduction performed at the initial operation (Fig. 32.4-8).

Van der Burg et al.[93] reported on the experience of the European Organization for Research and Treatment of Cancer with debulking surgery after induction chemotherapy for advanced ovarian cancer. Three hundred and nineteen of 425 patients with advanced epithelial ovarian cancer who had more than 1 cm in diameter of residual tumor after primary surgery received three cycles of cyclophosphamide and cisplatin and were randomly assigned to undergo secondary cytoreductive surgery or no surgery. Both groups received additional chemotherapy. The progression-free and overall survival rates were both significantly higher in the group that underwent surgery (*P* = .01) (Fig. 32.4-9). The difference in survival was 6 months. At 2 years after initial diagnosis, 56% of those who underwent surgery were alive, as opposed to 46% of those who did not. In an update, the 5-year survival rate was found to be 23% for the surgery group and 12% for the nonsurgery group.[148] A multivariate analysis determined that debulking surgery was an independent prognostic factor for survival (*P* = .012). After adjustment for all other prognostic factors, the risk of dying was reduced by 33% (95% CI, 10% to 50%; *P* = .008). This study statistically confirmed improved survival with optimal secondary cytoreductive surgery. However, secondary cytoreductive surgery does not make up for inadequate cytoreductive surgery performed at the initial operation.

Palliative Surgery

Palliative surgery may be necessary in women with advanced ovarian cancer. This surgery may involve a colostomy for relief of a

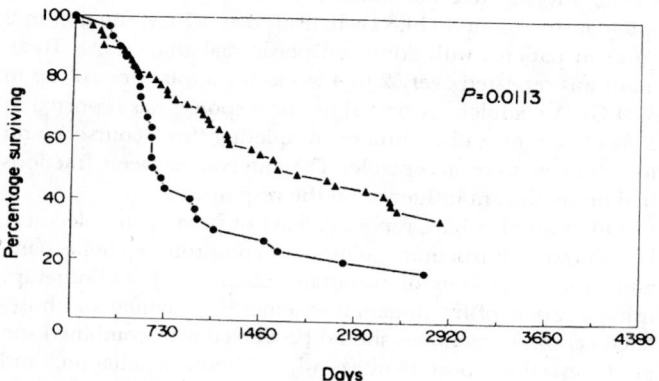

FIGURE 32.4-8. Survival after cytoreductive surgery leading to tumor residuals of 1 cm or smaller at the staging laparotomy or during chemotherapy (intervention cytoreductive surgery). (From ref. 147, with permission.)

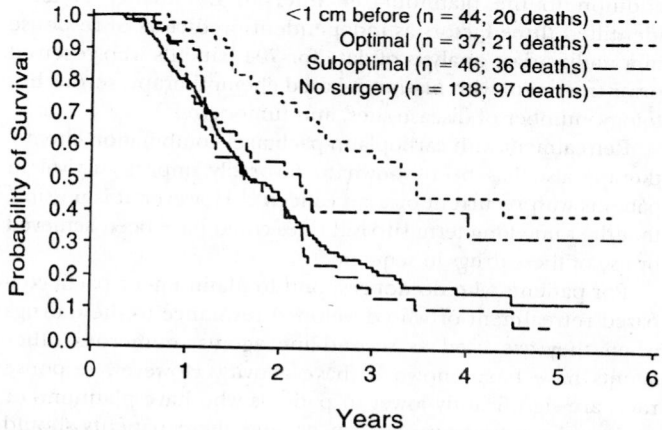

FIGURE 32.4-9. Survival of patients with advanced epithelial ovarian cancer who did not have debulking surgery and of patients who had such surgery, according to whether the lesions were smaller than 1 cm in diameter before cytoreduction, smaller than 1 cm after cytoreduction (optimal), or larger than 1 cm after cytoreduction (suboptimal). (From ref. 93, with permission.)

large bowel obstruction, lyses of adhesions, and surgical management of small bowel obstruction. Small bowel obstruction is a common complication as ovarian cancer advances and becomes refractory to chemotherapy. In considering surgery to relieve small bowel obstruction, the time from the original diagnosis and treatment of the ovarian cancer to the time of the obstruction is important, as is the adequacy of the initial cytoreductive surgery. Women who present with small bowel obstruction during the initial course of chemotherapy and who have not undergone optimal cytoreductive surgery generally have biologically aggressive tumors in the treatment of which the role of surgery of the small bowel is minimal. A palliative gastrostomy tube may be most appropriate in this situation, and frequently this can be inserted endoscopically or under radiographic (CT) guidance. In contrast, women who have had prolonged periods of freedom from disease, usually lasting more than 1 year from the original diagnosis, do benefit from small bowel surgery to relieve obstruction. However, a pseudo–small bowel obstruction pattern can be seen in women with advanced ovarian cancer with intraabdominal carcinomatosis, which occurs when ovarian cancer cells infiltrate the myenteric plexus of the small bowel. Surgery generally plays no role in management of these patients. Medical treatment with metoclopramide, which improves motility of the upper gastrointestinal tract without stimulating gastric, biliary, or pancreatic secretions, may at times be helpful. Large bowel obstruction, particularly sigmoid colon obstruction, is relieved by performing a colostomy and can provide significant prolongation of life and improved quality of life if the disease is confined to the pelvis.

Chemotherapy for Recurrent Disease

Patients with ovarian cancer who had a response to chemotherapy and then experienced relapse after a platinum-free interval of more than 6 months are considered platinum sensitive, with the likelihood of achieving a secondary response increasing as the duration of the platinum-free interval lengthens.[149] Single-agent carboplatin has a more favorable toxicity profile than cisplatin and remains the preferred platinum compound for treatment of recurrent disease. The probability of response to second-line chemotherapy is related to other clinical factors, in addition to the platinum-free interval. Eisenhauer et al.[150] identified three factors as independent predictors of response in a multivariate analysis of data for 704 patients who received prior treatment with platinum-based chemotherapy: serous histology, number of disease sites, and tumor size.

Retreatment with carboplatin-paclitaxel combination chemotherapy also has been shown to favorably impact survival in patients with recurrent ovarian cancer.[151] However, it is possible that the same long-term survival rates could have been achieved by use of these drugs in sequence.

For patients who do not respond to platinum- or paclitaxel-based retreatment or who developed resistance to these drugs when they are used as second-line agents, numerous other agents have been shown to have activity. However, response rates are significantly lower in patients who have platinum- or paclitaxel-resistant ovarian cancer, and these patients should be encouraged to enter experimental clinical trials. Drugs that have been shown to be active in patients with platinum- and paclitaxel-resistant ovarian cancer include topotecan,[152] oral etoposide,[153] gemcitabine,[154] liposomal doxorubicin,[155] vinorelbine,[156] and altretamine.[149]

Hormonal therapy has long been used in the treatment of patients with refractory ovarian cancer.[157] The overall response rate of progestational agents and antiestrogens has been 10% to 15%. Hormonal therapy continues to be a viable therapeutic option for patients who cannot tolerate or have experienced unsuccessful treatment with numerous cytotoxic regimens. Tamoxifen also has been recommended as the initial salvage therapy for patients who have a rising CA 125 level as the only manifestation of their disease. Although a rising CA 125 level in a patient in clinical complete remission is highly predictive of a symptomatic recurrence (median time to physical or radiographic evidence of recurrent disease is 4 to 6 months), there is no evidence that immediate treatment with salvage chemotherapy is more effective than reserving such treatment for the time when other manifestations of recurrent disease appear. A trial is ongoing in Europe in which patients with elevated marker levels are randomly assigned to receive immediate systemic therapy or treatment at the time of symptomatic progression.

Radiation Therapy for Recurrent Disease

Although rarely curative, radiation therapy can play an important role in palliation for patients with incurable ovarian cancer. Symptoms from a growing pelvic mass frequently dominate the final months of life for patients with terminal ovarian cancer, causing pain, bleeding, and rectal narrowing. Palliative pelvic radiotherapy can provide rapid relief and, in some cases, may prevent or delay the need for diverting colostomy.

Palliative treatment courses are designed to be convenient and to achieve rapid symptom relief. At the M. D. Anderson Cancer Center, palliation of pelvic disease has been achieved using two single-fraction treatments of 10 Gy each to the true pelvis delivered 1 month apart.[161] Treatment is delivered using 18- to 25-MeV photons. In a report of 42 patients who had advanced ovarian cancer and were treated with this approach, Adelson and coworkers[158] reported that tumors in 19% of patients partially or completely responded to irradiation after one fraction and 75% responded after two fractions. Toxicity was minimal if treatment was limited to two fractions (20 Gy). However, they reported major hemorrhagic complications in four of eight patients who survived more than 6 months after receiving three fractions. The Radiation Therapy Oncology Group investigated the efficacy of a multiple daily-fraction split-course regimen (14.8 Gy delivered at 3.7 Gy/fraction in 2 days) in patients with advanced pelvic malignancies.[159] Treatment was repeated every 2 to 4 weeks for a total dose of up to 44.4 Gy. A complete or partial tumor response was reported in 34% of patients (42% of those completing three courses), and toxic effects were acceptable. The interval between fractions had no significant influence on the response rate.

Other authors have reported relief of pelvic pain, bleeding, large bowel obstruction, pulmonary compromise, bone pain, and other symptoms of metastatic disease with radiotherapy using a variety of fractionation schemes.[139,140] Patients with isolated cerebral metastases should be treated with combined surgical resection, postoperative whole brain irradiation, and chemotherapy, if possible.[181] With this treatment, some patients survive for more than 3 years. Radiation therapy alone frequently relieves symptoms from brain metastasis but survival is usually shorter than 6 months.

TABLE 32.4-12. Pharmacokinetic Advantage Associated with Intraperitoneal Administration of Selected Cytotoxic Agents

Agent	Peak Peritoneal Cavity to Plasma Concentration Ratio
Doxorubicin	474
Mitoxantrone	620
Cisplatin	20
Carboplatin	18
Mitomycin	71
5-Fluorouracil	298
Methotrexate	92
Paclitaxel	1000

Intraperitoneal Chemotherapy

Pharmacokinetic modeling studies, based on knowledge of the anatomy and physiology of the peritoneal cavity and biologic behavior of ovarian cancer, have suggested that direct intraperitoneal antineoplastic drug delivery is a rationale management strategy for this malignancy.[160] Phase I studies have confirmed the pharmacokinetic advantage and established the local toxicity profile associated with intraperitoneal drug delivery of a number of agents with known activity in ovarian cancer (Table 32.4-12).

Thirty percent to 40% of patients with small volume disease (microscopic cancer or largest residual tumor nodule of less than 0.5 to 1.0 cm in maximum diameter) after platinum-based primary chemotherapy have been shown to achieve a surgically defined partial or complete response when treated with cisplatin-based intraperitoneal drug delivery.[161] Other agents examined for their potential clinical usefulness when delivered by the intraperitoneal route as second-line treatment of ovarian cancer include carboplatin,[162] paclitaxel,[163] interleukin-2 (IL-2),[164] interferon-α,[165] and interferon-γ.[166]

Unfortunately, there have been no randomized trials examining the second-line treatment of ovarian cancer using the intraperitoneal route of drug delivery. Thus, it remains unknown if patients treated by this technique experience better outcomes than with systemic drug administration.

Three randomized trials have now been reported, however, that directly compared intravenous to intraperitoneal cisplatin as primary therapy for ovarian cancer.[167–169]

Taken together, these data support the clinical usefulness of the intraperitoneal delivery of cisplatin as primary treatment for small-volume advanced ovarian cancer. However, the toxicity of cisplatin-based therapy, with 24-hour intravenous infusional paclitaxel, is not insignificant. A trial examining intraperitoneal administration of carboplatin with 3-hour intravenous administration of paclitaxel, compared to systemic administration of both agents, will be conducted by the GOG in the near future. It is hoped that this study will be able to provide a definitive answer to the question of whether regional drug delivery has a role in the primary chemotherapeutic management of advanced ovarian cancer.

EXPERIMENTAL THERAPIES

High-Dose Chemotherapy with Hematologic Support

Standard-dose chemotherapy produces response rates in more than 70% of patients with advanced ovarian cancer. However, most patients develop disease recurrence, at which point salvage therapy has limited curative potential. Because of the high response rate to standard-dose chemotherapy and because of retrospective studies identifying a relationship between dose intensity and response, numerous clinical studies have evaluated the use of high-dose chemotherapy with hematologic support.[170–172] To date, no role has yet been established for high-dose chemotherapy with hematologic support in the routine treatment of patients with advanced ovarian cancer. However, this remains an area of active clinical investigation.

New Drug Combinations

With the large number of active compounds available for treatment of recurrent disease, numerous new potential combinations and sequences are reasonable to evaluate. Currently, preclinical models have not been shown to be predictive in identifying the clinical activity of new combinations. Empirical phase I and phase II trials have been conducted and have been followed by prospective randomized comparisons of three-drug combinations and sequential therapy to determine if there is any clinical benefit to the combination of paclitaxel and carboplatin compared with standard treatment. The results of these trials are eagerly awaited.

Novel Drug Strategies in Treatment of Ovarian Cancer

A number of trials examining the use of highly novel biologic agents in the management of ovarian cancer have been initiated over the past few years. Ongoing trials include evaluation of monoclonal antibodies, epidermal growth factor receptor inhibitors (e.g., Iressa, C-225), immunomodulators, antiangiogenesis agents, and the addition of interferon-γ to a carboplatin-paclitaxel regimen as primary treatment of ovarian cancer.

It is important that biologic agents with potential activity against ovarian cancer be specifically evaluated in this setting before any conclusion is drawn regarding possible efficacy. For example, although the important clinical activity of trastuzumab in breast cancer has clearly been documented,[173] when this agent was tested in ovarian cancer an objective response rate of only 7% was observed.[174] Furthermore, only 11% of patients with ovarian cancer who were screened for overexpression of HER2 (2+ or 3+ by immunohistochemistry) were found even to be candidates to receive the agent.

Both systemic[175] and intraperitoneal[176] administration of IL-12 has been examined in women with advanced ovarian cancer. Although minimal objective activity was observed, a substantial percentage of patients achieved apparent stabilization of the disease process. This observation is consistent with proposed antiangiogenesis properties of IL-12.

OvaRex (MAb B43.13), a monoclonal antibody against CA 125, has been explored for its potential clinical activity in several trials.[177,178] It has been suggested that the antibody will bind to circulating CA 125 to form a complex that then elicits an immune response against CA 125–containing ovarian cancer cells.[179] It is hoped that ongoing studies will define a possible role for this antibody in the management of ovarian cancer.

TLK-286, a prodrug activated *in vivo* to become an alkylating agent, has been shown to be active (15% objective response rate) in platinum-resistant ovarian cancer.[180] The dose-limiting toxicity is bone marrow suppression. The efficacy of this drug, in comparison to standard second-line treatment of ovarian cancer, is currently being evaluated in a phase III randomized trial.

Immunotherapy and Gene Therapy in Ovarian Cancer

Genetic alterations in oncogene and suppressor gene function and the immunobiology of ovarian cancer are reviewed elsewhere in this text. Abnormalities in the function of suppressor genes, particularly TP53, are common in ovarian cancer. Cisplatin sensitivity is associated with TP53 function, with loss of function usually resulting in resistance. Loss of TP53 function may inhibit the drug-induced pathways of apoptosis. In experimental models of gene therapy, sensitivity to cisplatin can be restored in resistant cell lines by reintroduction of p53 into tumor cells.[181]

An additional potential gene therapy in ovarian cancer relates to molecular chemotherapy in which a gene product can selectively sensitize tumor cells to an agent that is not ordinarily toxic. Adenovirus-mediated delivery of herpes simplex virus thymidine kinase has been shown to selectively synthesize human ovarian cancer cells to ganciclovir, and clinical evaluation of this combination is planned.

Immunotherapy for ovarian cancer has evolved from the administration of nonspecific immunostimulants such as *Corynebacterium parvum* to more specific therapies targeting antigens and surface receptors present on tumor cells. The use of IL-2, either as a single agent administered intraperitoneally or as part of adoptive immunotherapy together with lymphokine-activated killer cells, has been studied extensively in ovarian cancer patients. In initial studies with IL-2 and lymphokine-activated killer cells, peritoneal toxicity was unacceptable. Subsequent trials with lower doses of IL-2 produced acceptable toxicity, and the preliminary report described apparent durable responses in selected patients with recurrent ovarian cancer treated with intraperitoneal IL-2.

Antibody conjugates (either with antineoplastic drug, biologic toxin, or radioisotope) also have been evaluated in early trials in ovarian cancer patients. Prolonged survival was observed in a pilot study in which patients with small volume residual disease were treated with iodine 131–labeled monoclonal antibody directed against an ovarian cancer phosphatase,[182] and a larger confirmatory trial of this conjugate is currently nearing completion.

BORDERLINE TUMORS

Epithelial tumors of LMP (borderline malignant potential tumors) are unusual in that they have the capacity to metastasize yet the required treatment seems to be limited to surgery for the overwhelming majority of patients. The different pathologic and biologic natures of these tumors were not recognized by FIGO until 1971 and by the World Health Organization until 1973.[183] Borderline malignant potential tumors are distinguished from benign mucinous and serous tumors by the presence of epithelial budding, multilayering of the epithelium, increased mitotic activity, and nuclear atypia. However, they are also associated with absence of stromal invasion. Mucinous LMP tumors are larger than their serous counterparts, and they are infrequently bilateral.[184] Mucinous tumors of borderline malignant potential tend to be larger, with a mean diameter of 17 to 20 cm, and can be associated with pseudomyxoma peritonei. One must always be certain to rule out the possibility of a synchronous appendiceal primary tumor when dealing with the latter entity.

Borderline malignant potential tumors represent 4% to 14% of all ovarian malignancies. The mean age of women developing LMP tumors is 40 years, approximately 20 years earlier than the mean age for women developing epithelial cancers of the ovary.

PATHOLOGIC CLASSIFICATION

LMP ovarian tumors have been described for all epithelial ovarian subtypes; the most common types are serous and mucinous tumors. The absence of stromal invasion is an absolute criterion for making the diagnosis. Careful examination of the tissue blocks is necessary to minimize the potential for omitting an area of invasive carcinoma in LMP tumors. Twenty percent to 30% of ovarian tumors diagnosed as borderline on frozen-section analysis prove to be carcinomas on review of the permanent section. The mean diameter of serous LMP tumors is 12 cm, and bilateral tumors are reported in 33% to 75% of patients. These tumors are usually cystic with mural clusters of papillary projections.

Mucinous LMP tumors are larger than their serous counterparts, with an average diameter of 17 to 20 cm; they are infrequently bilateral. They are characterized by multiloculated cystic masses, with smooth outer surfaces and areas of papillations and solid thickening on the inner surface. Microscopically, the epithelial lining of the cysts consists of tall, columnar, mucin-secreting cells, resembling the epithelium of the endocervix or intestine. Stratified epithelial cells may be atypical with hyperchromatic nuclei and mitotic figures, but without stromal invasion.

PSEUDOMYXOMA PERITONEI

Pseudomyxoma peritonei occurs frequently in mucinous neoplasms of the ovary and is characterized by the presence of extracellular gelatinous material in the pelvic and abdominal cavity. The primary site of origin of pseudomyxoma peritonei is debatable. Some series cite that the majority begin in the appendix, whereas others have described a synchronous origin in the ovary and appendix. Pseudomyxoma is most frequently associated with borderline or well-differentiated ovarian mucinous tumors (approximately 8% of cases) and only rarely seen in mucinous cystadenomas. The mainstay of treatment is cytoreductive surgery, and multiple treatment modalities with systemic and intraperitoneal chemotherapy have not demonstrated survival benefit. Patients have a high recurrence rate, with variable times to recurrence. Most series agree that, when patients have recurrent disease, repeat laparotomy is required to relieve symptoms. The overall 5-year survival rate is 50%, and most patients die from bowel obstruction.

Stage for stage, the 5-year survival rate for patients with LMP epithelial ovarian tumors is far better than that for patients with malignant epithelial ovarian cancer. A review of the literature by several investigators revealed a survival rate of more than 95% in patients with stage I LMP ovarian tumors. Furthermore, Kurman and Trimble[185] found that a majority of patients with LMP tumors actually died with the disease, not from it, as invasive carcinoma developed in only 8 (0.8%) of 953 patients after a mean follow-up of 7 years. The other patients died from radiation- or chemotherapy-associated complications. Recognizing that a minority of LMP tumors behave aggressively, as does an ovarian carcinoma,[186] Kurman and Trimble have challenged the current classification of LMP tumors in an attempt to develop a nomenclature that better reflects prognosis. These investigators believe that LMP tumors are actually a heterogeneous group of tumors, both histologically and clinically, that can be divided into malignant or benign phenotypes based on certain features. For serous tumors they propose that patient outcome depends on the following:

The presence or absence of micropapillary features within the ovarian tumor, or
Invasive versus noninvasive implants

In a large metaanalysis of serous LMP tumors, Kurman and Trimble report that patients with micropapillary serous carcinomas have 5- and 10-year survival rates of 81% and 71%, respectively.[186] Patients with serous borderline tumors without invasive implants (atypical proliferative serous tumors) had 5- and 10-year survival rates of more than 98%.[186] However, for those with serous borderline tumors with invasive implants, survival rates dropped to 60% to 70% at 5 and 10 years. The vast majority of patients with invasive implants, or recurrences, that progressed to invasive carcinoma were found to have micropapillary features within the primary ovarian tumor on careful sectioning. Thus, atypical proliferative serous tumors and serous borderline tumors without invasive implants follow a very benign clinical course, whereas micropapillary serous LMP tumors behave much like invasive ovarian carcinomas.

With regard to mucinous tumors, Kurman and Trimble suggest that advanced-stage mucinous LMP tumors are typically associated with pseudomyxoma peritonei, whereas apparent stage I mucinous LMP tumors are better classified to reflect their benign behavior.[186] The current category of borderline mucinous LMP tumor could then be abandoned, with the removal of pseudomyxoma peritonei–associated cases and reclassification of the remainder of cases as atypical proliferative mucinous tumors.

Micropapillary serous carcinoma is characterized by thin, elongated micropapillae with minimal or no fibrovascular support arising directly from thick, more centrally located papillary structures. Mitotic activity may be seen in some cases, ranging from one to three figures per ten high-power fields. Making the distinction between invasive and noninvasive implants may be difficult. Noninvasive implants usually have a scant epithelial component surrounded by reactive spindle cells with imperceptibly meshed epithelial and stromal cells. On the other hand, invasive implants usually have a more cellular epithelial component, with complex epithelial proliferation composed of multiple micropapillae and small, round nests that display a destructive infiltrative growth.

TREATMENT

The primary surgical treatment for patients with LMP tumors who have completed childbearing is identical to that recommended for invasive ovarian disease, including a total abdominal hysterectomy, bilateral salpingo-oophorectomy, tumor debulking, and full staging. An appendectomy should be performed in patients with mucinous LMP tumors because of the association with a synchronous primary appendiceal tumor.

In younger patients with early-stage diagnosis and a desire for future childbearing, conservative surgery with preservation of the uterus, the contralateral ovary, and in some cases the ipsilateral ovary (i.e., cystectomy) may be the appropriate treatment. Tazelaar et al.[187] found no evidence of microscopic disease in grossly normal ovaries that were bivalved in 61 patients with stage I LMP tumors of the ovary. Several studies, both cohort and observational, have reported excellent outcome with conservative management of such patients. One of the largest studies reports a 12% recurrence rate for patients treated conservatively with either unilateral salpingo-oophorectomy (n = 110) or ovarian cystectomy (n = 74) versus 2.5% for patients treated with definitive hysterectomy and bilateral salpingo-oophorectomy. Recurrences or progression to carcinoma (1.5%) were more common among patients with invasive implants or advanced-stage disease. The feasibility of performing a cystectomy for an LMP ovarian tumor and conserving the rest of the ovarian tissue in early-stage disease has been described, but requires further study.

LMP ovarian tumors have also been diagnosed during pregnancy. Conservative surgery is usually performed, and pregnancy does not appear to be deleterious in regard to the prognosis for these patients. Most patients go on to deliver at full term without any complications.

POSTOPERATIVE THERAPY

The evidence is scant to suggest that treatment beyond that of the initial surgery has any beneficial role. This is true for stage II, III, and IV disease as well as for stage I disease. Appropriate adjuvant therapy has yet to be identified in the management of women with LMP tumors. Trope et al.[188] studied the use of adjuvant therapy in 253 women with stage I and II ovarian LMP tumors in four randomized trials at the Norwegian Radium Hospital between 1970 and 1984. Adjuvant treatment regimens for the four trials consisted of (1) external radiation and intraperitoneal radioactive gold therapy, or external radiation alone; (2) intraperitoneal therapy with radioactive gold or phosphorus followed by no further treatment or thiotepa; (3) thiotepa or no further treatment; and (4) cisplatin or intraperitoneal phosphorus therapy. No differences in results could be identified for the two treatment arms in any of the four randomized studies. It was recommended that adjuvant radiation and chemotherapy not be used in patients with stage I or II ovarian LMP tumors. Barnhill et al.[189] reported on 146 women with stage I serous LMP tumors. No adjuvant therapy was offered, and at a median follow-up of 42.4 months (range, 1.6 to 108.0), no patient has developed a recurrence.

Attempts to identify women who might be at increased risk for recurrence based on flow cytometric studies have not demonstrated consistent results.[190,191] Evidence has yet to be presented confirming that routine treatment of patients whose tumors are aneuploid provides survival benefit. Surgery should be the main treatment approach for this disease. Others have suggested adjuvant chemotherapy for patients with micropapillary tumors due to their higher risk of recurrence, but there are no randomized trials to date to support this recommendation. In general, consideration of chemotherapy should be reserved for progressive or recurrent disease that does not respond to surgical management.

PRIMARY PERITONEAL CARCINOMA

The diagnosis and management of women who present with intraperitoneal carcinomatosis can present a problem. In some patients, the primary site is unknown, and peritoneal carcinomatosis can present as part of the syndrome of adenocarcinomas of unknown primary site. In other cases, although the cause is unclear, a "field effect" of malignant epithelial transformation involving multiple sites is postulated. Cases of primary peritoneal carcinoma have been described after prophylactic oophorectomy in patients with strong family histories of ovarian cancer or with documented BRCA mutations. Primary peritoneal ovarian cancer appears to be another phenotypic variant of the BRCA-associated cancer syndromes.[26]

Patients with adenocarcinomas of unknown primary site who present with peritoneal carcinomatosis can respond to chemotherapy with platinum-based regimens. In a series of 18 women treated with platinum-based chemotherapy, median survival was 23 months, and 5 patients had complete remissions and long-term survival.[192] The histologic classification and nomenclature of peritoneal carcinomatosis has been unclear and has included terms such as *mesothelioma, peritoneal papillary serous carcinoma, extraovarian serous carcinoma,* and *paraovarian cystadenocarcinoma.* Although embryologically the germinal epithelium of the ovary and the mesothelium of the peritoneal cavity are derived from the same coelomic epithelium, a subset of peritoneal tumors can be morphologically identified that have a more favorable clinical behavior in response to therapy than do peritoneal mesotheliomas.[193] It has been proposed that the former disease process be termed *peritoneal adenocarcinoma (serous) of müllerian type.* The serous type of peritoneal carcinomatosis is the most common. However, other histologic types of peritoneal carcinomatosis resulting from the common ancestry of coelomic epithelium are possible, including mucinous, endometrioid, clear cell, and mixed peritoneal adenocarcinoma of müllerian type. With the proposed terminology, when an uncommon subtype other than serous is present, it can be encompassed in the description. Malignant mesotheliomas have a different histologic pattern and, in most cases, can be separated from the müllerian-type peritoneal adenocarcinomas. Peritoneal mesotheliomas are more aggressive tumors and are associated with a survival rate of usually less than 1 year. Furthermore, in women they are relatively less common than peritoneal adenocarcinomas of müllerian type.

Most patients with extraovarian peritoneal carcinomatosis have signs and symptoms similar to those of women who present with advanced-stage ovarian cancer. At surgery, these women frequently have ascites with diffuse peritoneal carcinomatosis. Attempts at cytoreductive surgery usually are made, although no evidence supports survival benefit in those women with peritoneal carcinomatosis who undergo optimal cytoreductive surgery. This may be due to the fact that, although no tumor nodule larger than 1.5 cm is left behind, these women have innumerable such nodules throughout the peritoneal cavity, and their actual tumor burden after cytoreductive surgery remains substantial. It appears that approximately 50% of patients with peritoneal carcinomatosis can undergo successful surgical cytoreduction. Survival for patients with müllerian peritoneal adenocarcinoma is similar to that reported for advanced ovarian cancer. In a large study at the University of California, Los Angeles, the median survival time of patients who received chemotherapy after primary cytoreductive surgery was 28.4 months.[193] Patients who received cisplatin-based chemotherapy had a substantially higher survival rate (57% living longer than 23 months) than patients who were not treated with cisplatin-based regimens. Based on the pattern of metastases and

chemosensitivity to platinum-based chemotherapy, it seems prudent that current therapy for this group of patients should include cytoreductive surgery followed by chemotherapy with paclitaxel plus a platinum compound.

GERM CELL TUMORS OF THE OVARY

Germ cell tumors of the ovary are much less common than epithelial ovarian neoplasms. However, because they are highly curable and because they affect primarily young women of childbearing potential, appropriate management by specialists is exceedingly important. Germ cell tumors account for 2% to 3% of all ovarian cancers in Western countries. They almost always occur in younger women, and their peak incidence is in the early twenties. An increased incidence of germ cell tumors is found in Asian and black societies, and these tumors represent as many as 15% of all ovarian cancers in these populations.

PATHOLOGY

Table 32.4-1 provides the World Health Organization classification for germ cell tumors of the ovary.[183] The serum tumor markers HCG and AFP are useful in the diagnosis and management of these tumors. These tumors are often divided clinically into dysgerminoma and nondysgerminoma germ cell tumors.

DIAGNOSIS

Abdominal pain, pelvic fullness, and urinary symptoms are common in patients with germ cell tumors of the ovary. In a minority of patients (approximately 10%), abdominal pain can be severe, usually the result of hemorrhage, rupture, or torsion of the tumor. Abdominal distention can also be a symptom and often is associated with ascites.

Patients frequently have a palpable adnexal mass that should be ultrasonographically evaluated. Surgical exploration is usually required for masses of 8 cm or larger. Serum levels of HCG and AFP are useful in the diagnosis of some germ cell tumors.

PATTERNS OF METASTASIS

In contrast to epithelial tumors, 60% to 70% of germ cell tumors are stage I at diagnosis. Stage II and IV tumors are relatively uncommon, and stage III lesions account for 25% to 30% of tumors. Primary germ cell tumors can be very large and often are more than 20 cc in size. With the notable exception of dysgerminoma, bilateral ovarian involvement is not common. Multiple peritoneal surfaces are often involved, and lymph node involvement is frequent. These tumors also appear to have a greater tendency for hematogenous metastases than do epithelial tumors, and liver and lung involvement can be observed. Ascites is infrequent (approximately 20% of cases).

SURGICAL MANAGEMENT

The importance of initial surgical approach for the treatment of germ cell tumors of the ovary cannot be overemphasized.[194] In most patients fertility can be preserved, and the type of operative procedure is dictated by operative findings. In most cases, the contralateral ovary and the uterus can be preserved. Even in cases of dysgerminoma, in which bilaterality is more common, bilateral oophorectomy is not routinely necessary because postoperative chemotherapy is curative and fertility can be preserved. In cases in which the contralateral ovary is grossly abnormal, cystectomy or biopsy can be performed, and bilateral salpingo-oophorectomy can be undertaken in the case of a dysgenetic gonad.

The principles for surgical staging of germ cell tumors are similar to those described for epithelial tumors. After a large transverse incision is made, the entire peritoneal cavity should be carefully inspected. In the absence of ascites, peritoneal washings should be obtained, and all fluids should be histologically examined. If disease is grossly confined to the pelvis, random biopsies should be performed as in the surgical staging of early-stage epithelial ovarian carcinomas. Particular attention should be paid to paraaortic and pelvic lymph nodes, because these are more commonly involved than in epithelial tumors. Although sampling of suspicious nodes is indicated for staging, no evidence suggests that lymphadenectomy is beneficial. Cytoreductive surgery is recommended as for epithelial tumors of the ovary. However, it must be emphasized that, even in the presence of widespread metastatic disease, because of the efficacy of chemotherapy, the contralateral ovary can frequently be preserved.

There is no role for routine second-look operations in patients with germ cell tumors who are clinically free of disease after chemotherapy. In particular, if the primary tumor was completely resected and did not contain teratoma, second-look procedures after chemotherapy are of no established benefit.[194] In some patients with a teratomatous tumor, however, a second-look procedure may be beneficial. Such patients may have residual mature teratoma, particularly if the initial resection was incomplete and postchemotherapy removal of benign teratomas is beneficial. Teratomas in males with testicular cancer have been known to progress and lead to significant morbidity unless completely resected. Although experience with germ cell tumors of the ovary is not as extensive, the presumption remains that teratomas can lead to life-threatening complications and should be removed after initial chemotherapy.

MANAGEMENT OF DYSGERMINOMAS

Dysgerminomas are the most common malignant germ cell tumors of the ovary and often have been considered the female equivalent of a seminoma. In contrast to nondysgerminomatous tumors, dysgerminomas are more frequently stage I, involve both ovaries, spread to retroperitoneal lymph nodes, and are markedly sensitive to radiotherapy. Because these tumors are also exquisitely sensitive to cisplatin-based chemotherapy, the role of curative radiation therapy has decreased. Furthermore, current chemotherapy usually does not result in ovarian ablation.

The vast majority of patients with dysgerminomas are diagnosed with early-stage disease. Because preservation of fertility is an important issue for most of these women, all carefully staged patients with stage IA disease can be observed without compromising cure, because only 15% to 25% of patients experience recurrence and salvage is successful in these cases.[194,195] Until the demonstration that metastatic dysgerminoma could be cured with cisplatin-based chemotherapy, most

TABLE 32.4-13. Bleomycin, Etoposide, and Cisplatin Regimen in Germ Cell Tumors

Cisplatin	20 mg/m^2/d × 5 d
Etoposide (VP-16)	100 mg/m^2/d × 5 d
Bleomycin	20 U/m^2/wk

Note: Cycles are administered every 21 days.

patients with stage I disease and all patients with higher-stage disease were treated with radiotherapy. Virtually all patients with early-stage tumors were cured of their disease. Even in patients with stage III disease treated with radiation therapy, the 5-year survival rate was 80% to 90%, although recurrence-free survival was substantially lower.

The GOG evaluation of platinum-based chemotherapy for dysgerminomas has followed reports on the efficacy of different regimens in testicular cancer.[195] In the early 1980s, ovarian germ cell tumors were treated with the cisplatin-vinblastine-bleomycin (PVB) regimen.[196] Subsequently, based on studies in testicular cancer that demonstrated increased efficacy and less toxicity for the bleomycin, etoposide, and cisplatin (BEP) regimen, the latter regimen has been used in patients with metastatic germ cell tumors, including dysgerminoma (Table 32.4-13). At a median follow-up of more than 2 years, 17 of 18 patients with advanced-stage dysgerminoma treated with one of these platinum-based regimens were disease free.[195]

MANAGEMENT OF NONDYSGERMINOMATOUS GERM CELL TUMORS

The vast majority of nondysgerminomatous germ cell tumors of the ovary are treated with surgery followed by combination chemotherapy.

The immature teratomas are the second most common germ cell malignancy, accounting for 10% to 20% of all ovarian tumors seen in women younger than 20 years of age. The tumors rarely occur in postmenopausal women and most commonly occur between the ages of 10 and 20 years. These tumors contain elements resembling embryologically derived tissues and can occur in combination with other germ cell tumors (mixed germ cells). Occasionally, they are the source of excessive steroids, and patients can present with sexual pseudoprecocity. Tumor marker testing for AFP and HCG is negative unless a mixed germ cell tumor is present.

The most important prognostic feature, and that which is used to dictate therapy, is the grade of the lesion. For patients with stage IA, grade 1 lesions, 5-year survival rates are higher than 90%, and no evidence suggests that chemotherapy improves outcome. However, this is the only subset of patients with immature teratomas in whom chemotherapy should not be used. Even patients with stage IA, grade 2 and 3 disease have such a high relapse rate that postoperative chemotherapy is indicated.[194–196]

In patients whose tumors are confined to the ovary, unilateral oophorectomy or salpingo-oophorectomy should be performed. As noted in Patterns of Metastasis, contralateral tumor involvement is rare in germ cell tumors other than dysgerminoma. The most frequent sites of dissemination are the peritoneum and retroperitoneal lymph nodes. Widespread dissemination to lungs, liver, or brain is uncommon. Before the development of effective chemotherapy, prognosis for patients with advanced-stage germ cell tumors was poor. The same combination that was found to be curative in disseminated testicular cancer quickly replaced non-platinum regimens such as vincristine, dactinomycin, and cyclophosphamide. The PVB regimen produced a survival rate of 71% in a heterogeneous group of germ cell cancer patients.[196] The current chemotherapy regimen of choice for patients with nondysgerminomatous germ cell tumors is the BEP regimen (see Table 32.4-13). In the GOG trial, 89 of 93 patients with stage I, stage II, and stage III disease whose tumors were completely resected remained disease free after three courses of this regimen.[196]

Although no prospective comparison has been performed between PVB and BEP for treatment of patients with advanced-stage germ cell tumor of the ovary, the latter regimen is preferred because of the results of a randomized trial involving patients with advanced testicular cancer in which the superiority of BEP was established.[197] In that trial, PVB produced a 70% 4-year survival rate in patients with metastatic, far-advanced testicular tumors, which was inferior to results obtained with BEP. Furthermore, the BEP regimen was less toxic than PVB because of elimination of vinblastine-related neuromuscular toxicities.

Endodermal sinus (yolk sac) tumors are derived from the primitive yolk sac and are the third most frequent germ cell tumor of the ovary. These tumors secrete AFP, which can be used as a marker for response and recurrence. As with other germ cell tumors, a unilateral oophorectomy can be performed because the tumors are rarely, if ever, bilateral. Most patients have early-stage disease, but all patients, regardless of stage and extent of initial surgery, are treated with platinum-based chemotherapy.[198] No evidence supports a correlation between extent of initial surgery and survival. Before the development of effective chemotherapy, 2-year survival was only 20%. However, with platinum-based chemotherapy, the complete response rate is approximately 60%.

Embryonal carcinoma and nongestational choriocarcinoma of the ovary are both extremely rare. Embryonal carcinomas can secrete both AFP and HCG, whereas pure choriocarcinomas secrete only HCG. Due to the rarity of these tumors, long-term results for chemotherapy have not been specifically described. However, the recommended treatment approach consists of unilateral oophorectomy or salpingo-oophorectomy followed by combination chemotherapy using the BEP regimen.[198] Similarly, mixed germ cell tumors of the ovary that contain two or more elements should also be treated with surgery followed by combination chemotherapy. Prognosis for mixed germ cell tumors is related to the relative amount of the most aggressive malignant component. The most frequent combination consists of elements of endodermal sinus tumor and dysgerminoma. Mixed germ cell tumors may secrete any combination of markers, depending on the histologic components of the tumor.

SEX CORD–STROMAL TUMORS

Ovarian sex cord–stromal tumors represent approximately 5% of all ovarian cancers. In general, they tend to present with stage I disease and frequently are associated with hormonal effects, such as precocious puberty, amenorrhea, postmenopausal bleeding, or virilizing symptoms. Granulosa cell tumors are the most common of the sex cord–stromal tumors and may

be associated with endometrial hyperplasia and endometrial carcinoma. One cannot always tell the steroid production of the malignancies based on histologic appearance. For example, granulosa cell tumors have been reported to be associated with virilization. Sertoli-Leydig cell tumors have been associated with endometrial cancer.[199] Pascale et al.[200] have demonstrated that, in virilized women, the findings of increased serum testosterone levels with normal gonadotropin levels and gonadotropin-releasing hormone agonist suppression of gonadotropins leading to normalization of testosterone levels suggest that various ovarian androgen-secreting tumors are not autonomous but apparently depend on gonadotropin stimulation.

Willemsen et al.[201] reported on 12 patients who developed granulosa cell tumors. All patients in the series underwent ovarian hyperstimulation for the treatment of infertility. All patients received clomiphene citrate and gonadotropins or both. Willemsen et al.[201] postulated that granulosa cell tumors may already be present in the ovaries and are simply waiting for a hormone trigger or that the increased follicle-stimulating hormone concentrations used in ovulation induction are oncogenic to granulosa cells. However, it is also possible that the discovery of granulosa cells during ovarian stimulation is coincidental.

Surgical staging of sex cord–stromal tumors is the same as that for epithelial ovarian cancers (see Table 32.4-3). Surgical management of sex cord–stromal tumors is based on the stage of the tumor as well as the age of the patient. In general, premenarchal women or patients presenting in the reproductive years tend to have stage I disease in most series. A unilateral salpingo-oophorectomy is all that is routinely necessary for the management of this disease. A role for adjuvant therapy in younger women has not been demonstrated. However, in women who have completed childbearing, surgery should be more aggressive, including a bilateral salpingo-oophorectomy and total abdominal hysterectomy along with standard surgical staging. Women older than age 40 years at diagnosis are more likely to experience a recurrence of granulosa cell tumors, and for this reason adjuvant therapy is recommended by some[199] for older patients, although definitive evidence for its efficacy in preventing or delaying recurrences is lacking.

Patients with advanced-stage disease (i.e., stage II to IV) may benefit from additional therapy. Cisplatin-based combination chemotherapy has been the most frequently used treatment. However, few series have been reported, and they involve small numbers of women with granulosa cell tumors. Colombo et al.[202] demonstrated that primary treatment of six women with advanced granulosa cell tumor was effective using the PVB regimen. However, their experience with the PVB regimen in five patients with recurrent disease was complicated by significant toxicity, which led to two deaths. Pectasides et al.[203] reported on ten patients with advanced or recurrent granulosa cell tumor treated with cisplatin, doxorubicin, and cyclophosphamide. Five complete and one partial response were obtained. One of the patients showing pathologically complete response, however, experienced relapse 48 months after the onset of chemotherapy. Homesley et al.[204] reported a collaborative group experience using bleomycin, etoposide, and cisplatin combination chemotherapy in the treatment of women with sex cord–stromal tumors. Forty-eight of the 57 tumors were granulosa cell tumors. In the series as a whole, 35 patients (61.4%) receiving this combination chemotherapy regimen had complete responses. Eighteen of the 35 underwent second-look surgery. Fourteen of the 18 patients had pathologically negative second-look results, 4 patients had a partial response, 14 patients had stable disease, and 2 patients had progression of disease among the 55 patients evaluable for response. Sixteen patients received the chemotherapy after primary surgery, nine because of positive peritoneal cytologic findings and seven for the treatment of gross residual disease. Eleven of 16 patients undergoing primary treatment (68.8%) were free of progressive disease, whereas 21 of 41 patients (51.2%) who were treated only after recurrent disease was noted were free of disease.

The overall survival in two large series of granulosa cell tumors was 85% and 90%, with one series reporting 100% survival for those with stage I disease and the other reporting 94% survival for those with stage I disease at 5 years. The current recommendations for women with early-stage granulosa cell tumors are surgery only for those younger than 40 years and surgery followed by etoposide and carboplatin chemotherapy for women older than 40 years who have stage I disease. For women older than 40 years or for any woman with advanced-stage or recurrent disease, the authors recommend doxorubicin, cisplatin, and etoposide. Measurement of serum inhibin levels may be useful in monitoring for relapse.[205] However, there is at least anecdotal experience that levels may be elevated for unexplained reasons. Another tumor marker, müllerian inhibiting substance (MIS), is usually undetectable in females before puberty. Gustafson et al.[206] reported that elevated MIS levels dramatically declined in two girls with granulosa cell tumors after surgery. MIS may be an effective marker for granulosa cell tumors and Sertoli-Leydig cell tumors. Lane et al.[207] have demonstrated preoperative elevations of MIS in six of eight subjects (75%) with juvenile granulosa cell tumors and seven of nine (78%) with adult granulosa cell tumors. None of 21 women with normal or nondetectable MIS levels developed recurrent granulosa cell tumors, but incompletely resected or recurrent disease was associated with elevated MIS levels in 6 of 15 patients.

Roush et al.[208] performed flow cytometric DNA ploidy and S-phase fraction analysis on granulosa cell tumors of the ovary in 18 women. Eleven of the tumors were diploid and seven were aneuploid. Only one of ten patients (10%) with euploid tumors died of disease, whereas four out of five (80%) with aneuploid tumors died of the disease. This observation did not reach statistical correlation. Perhaps in the future flow cytometric studies may be useful in identifying which group of patients might benefit from adjuvant therapy as opposed to observation.

Sertoli-Leydig cell tumors occur much less often than granulosa cell tumors yet are the second most common sex cord–stromal tumor. Their management is the same as that of granulosa cell tumors in terms of staging, surgical management, and adjuvant chemotherapy. Rare forms of sex cord–stromal tumors include sex cord tumors with annular tubules associated with Peutz-Jeghers syndrome, which are usually confined to the ovaries and can be treated with surgery alone. Thecomas rarely are malignant. Malignant thecomas are treated in the same manner as granulosa cell tumors.

Recurrent sex cord–stromal tumors are treated with surgical resection followed by adjuvant therapy. In cases in which the recurrence is isolated and could be encompassed in a radiation field, older literature suggests that radiation therapy may be of value if the malignancy is a granulosa cell tumor. The natural history of granulosa cell tumors is characterized by slow growth.

Although late recurrences occur, it is difficult to know for certain whether it is the resection of the recurrent cancer or resection followed by the radiation therapy that has had an impact in prolonging patient survival. Patients with extensive recurrences should be treated with cisplatin-based combination chemotherapy. Evidence has yet to be presented confirming that routinely treating patients whose tumors are aneuploid provides survival benefit. Surgery should be the main treatment approach for this disease. Chemotherapy should be reserved for progressive disease that does not respond to surgical management.

FALLOPIAN TUBE CANCER

Primary malignant neoplasms of the fallopian tube are exceedingly rare, and only a few hundred new cases are diagnosed annually in the United States, which makes the fallopian tube the least common site of origin for a malignant neoplasm of the female genital tract. Most fallopian tube carcinomas present as papillary serous adenocarcinomas. Intraperitoneal dissemination of fallopian tube carcinomas is similar to that observed with epithelial ovarian cancer. However, there appears to be a higher propensity to spread outside the peritoneal cavity, especially to the retroperitoneal lymph nodes. Survival has been shown to be dependent on the depth of invasion of the tumor in the fallopian tube.[209] For patients with intermucosal lesions, 5-year survival is 91%, compared with 53% for those with tumors with mucosal wall invasion and less than 25% for patients in whom the tumor has penetrated the tubal serosa. In addition to the depth of invasion, histologic differentiation and lymphatic capillary space involvement also have been shown to be of prognostic significance.[210] In cases of metastatic disease, differentiation from metastatic ovarian carcinoma can be difficult. Criteria frequently used to confirm the diagnosis of a primary fallopian tube carcinoma include tumor in the fallopian tube and rising from the endosalpinx, histologic pattern reproducing the epithelium of the mucosa with a papillary pattern, evidence for transition between benign and malignant tubal epithelium in the wall, and less tumor in the ovaries than in the tubes. In difficult cases, tumors are at times referred to as *tubo-ovarian carcinoma*. A minority of fallopian tube carcinomas are bilateral at the time of diagnosis. In contrast to patients with ovarian cancer, a large portion of patients with tubal carcinoma are diagnosed with disease confined to the tubes and pelvic structures.

Patients with fallopian tube carcinomas appear to have a shorter history of symptoms than those with epithelial ovarian carcinoma.[210] The most common symptom is postmenopausal vaginal bleeding. Hydrops tubae profluens, characterized by colicky lower abdominal pain relieved by profuse serous yellow intermittent vaginal discharge, occurs in only a minority of cases, but intermittent abdominal pain and leukorrhea are common presentations. Tubal distention produces more intense pain than is usually reported by patients with ovarian cancer, and these symptoms may account for the fact that the number of patients presenting with earlier-stage carcinoma is higher than among patients with epithelial ovarian cancer, in whom the absence of specific symptoms may account for the higher incidence of disseminated disease. Occasionally, a Papanicolaou smear revealing abnormal glandular cells with negative cervical or endometrial findings may lead to the diagnosis of fallopian tube carcinoma.

The surgical management of patients with fallopian tube carcinoma is identical to that of patients with epithelial ovarian cancer.[210] Survival is improved in patients in whom cytoreductive surgery is successful. Similarly, postoperative chemotherapy for fallopian tube carcinoma is analogous to that for patients with epithelial ovarian cancer. Due to the rarity of fallopian tube carcinoma, the use of paclitaxel in this disease has not yet been widely studied. However, based on similar responses to platinum-based chemotherapy, it appears that the combination of paclitaxel plus a platinum compound should be considered the current chemotherapy regimen of choice for fallopian tube carcinoma.

REFERENCES

1. Jemal A, Murray T, Samuels A, et al. Cancer statistics, 2003. *CA Cancer J Clin* 2003;53:5.
2. Yancik R, Ries LG, Yates JW. Ovarian cancer in the elderly: an analysis of Surveillance, Epidemiology and End Results program data. *Am J Obstet Gynecol* 1986;154:639.
3. Scully RE. Tumors of the ovary and maldeveloped gonads, fallopian tube, and broad ligament. In: Young RH, Clement PB, eds. *Atlas of tumor pathology*, 3rd series. Washington, DC: Armed Forces Institute of Pathology, 1996:27.
4. Goff BA, Mandel L, Muntz HG, Melancon CH. Ovarian carcinoma diagnosis: results of a national ovarian cancer survey. *Cancer* 2000;89:2068.
5. Karlan BY. The status of ultrasound and color Doppler imaging for the early detection of ovarian carcinoma. *Cancer Invest* 1997;15:265.
6. Bristow RE, Simpkins F, Pannu HK, Fishman EK, Montz FJ. Positron emission tomography for detecting clinically occult surgically resectable metastatic ovarian cancer. *Gynecol Oncol* 2002;85:196.
7. Chen D, Schwartz PE, Li X, Yang Z. Evaluation of CA125 levels in differentiating malignant from benign tumors in patients with pelvic masses. *Obstet Gynecol* 1988;72:23.
8. Modesitt SC, Pavlik EJ, Ueland FR, et al. Risk of malignancy in unilocular ovarian cystic tumors less than 10 centimeters in diameter. *Obstet Gynecol* 2003;102:594.
9. Junor EJ, Hole DJ, McNulty L, Mason M, Young J. Specialist gynaecologists and survival outcome in ovarian cancer: a Scottish national study of 1866 patients. *Br J Obstet Gynaecol* 1999;106:1130.
10. Bristow RE, Tomacruz RS, Armstrong DB, Trimble EL, Montz FJ. Survival effect of maximal cytoreductive surgery for advanced ovarian carcinoma during the platinum era: a meta-analysis. *J Clin Oncol* 2002;20:1248.
11. Jacobs I. Genetic, biochemical, and multimodal approaches to screening for ovarian cancer. *Gynecol Oncol* 1994;55:S22.
12. Urban N, McIntosh MW, Andersen M, Karlan BY. Ovarian cancer screening. *Hematol Oncol Clin North Am* 2003;17:989.
13. Petricoin EF, Ardekani AM, Hitt BA, et al. Use of proteomic patterns in serum to identify ovarian cancer. *Lancet* 2002;359:572.
14. NIH consensus conference. Ovarian cancer: screening, treatment, and follow-up. *JAMA* 1995;273.
15. van Nagell JR Jr, DePriest PD, Reedy MB, et al. The efficacy of transvaginal sonographic screening in asymptomatic women at risk for ovarian cancer. *Gynecol Oncol* 2000; 77:350.
15a. Bast RC Jr, Siegal FP, Runowicz C, et al. Elevation of serum Ca 125 prior to diagnosis of an epithelial ovarian carcinoma. *Gynecol Oncol* 1985;22:115.
16. Einhorn N, Sjövall K, Knapp RC, et al. Prospective evaluation of serum CA 125 levels for early detection of ovarian cancer. *Obstet Gynecol* 1992;80:14.
17. Woolas RP, Xu FJ, Jacobs IJ, et al. Elevation of multiple serum markers in patients with stage I ovarian cancer. *J Natl Cancer Inst* 1993;85:1748.
18. Xu Y, Shen Z, Wiper DW, et al. Lysophosphatidic acid as a potential biomarker for ovarian and other gynecologic cancers. *JAMA* 1998;280:719.
19. Kramer BS, Gohagan J, Prorok PC, Smart C. A National Cancer Institute sponsored screening trial for prostatic, lung, colorectal, and ovarian cancers. *Cancer* 1993;71:589.
20. Jacobs IJ, Skates SJ, MacDonald N, et al. Screening for ovarian cancer: a pilot randomized controlled trial. *Lancet* 1999;353:1207.
21. Skates SJ, Xu FJ, Yu YH, et al. Toward an optimal algorithm for ovarian cancer screening with longitudinal tumor markers. *Cancer* 1995;76:2004(abst).
22. Boyd J, Rubin SC. Hereditary ovarian cancer: molecular genetics and clinical implications. *Gynecol Oncol* 1997;64:196.
23. Struewing JP, Hartge P, Wacholder S, et al. The risk of cancer associated with specific mutations of BRCA1 and BRCA2 among Ashkenazi Jews. *N Engl J Med* 1997;336:1401.
24. Rubin SC, Benjamin I, Behbakht K, et al. Clinical and pathological features of ovarian cancer in women with germ-line mutations of BRCA1. *N Engl J Med* 1996;335:1413.
25. King MC, Marks JH, Mandell JB. Breast and ovarian cancer risks due to inherited mutations in BRCA1 and BRCA2. *Science* 2003;302:643.
26. Cass I, Baldwin RL, Varkey T, et al. Improved survival in women with BRCA-associated ovarian carcinoma. *Cancer* 2003;97:2187.
27. Smith SA, Richards WE, Caito K, et al. BRCA1 germline mutations and polymorphisms in a clinic-based series of ovarian cancer cases: a Gynecologic Oncology Group. *Gynecol Oncol* 2001;83:586.
28. Watson P, Lin KM, Rodriguez-Bigas MA, et al. Colorectal carcinoma survival among hereditary nonpolyposis colorectal carcinoma family members. *Cancer* 1998;83:259.
29. American Society of Clinical Oncology Policy Statement update: genetic testing for cancer susceptibility. *J Clin Oncol* 2003;21:2397.
30. Karlan BY, Baldwin RL, Lopez-Luevanos E, et al. Peritoneal serous papillary carcinoma, a phenotypic variant of familial ovarian cancer: implications for ovarian cancer screening. *Am J Obstet Gynecol* 1999;180:917.
31. Kauff ND, Satagopan JM, Robson ME, et al. Risk reducing salpingo-oophorectomy in women with a BRCA1 or BRCA2 mutation. *N Engl J Med* 2002;346:1609.
32. Narod SA, Risch H, Moslehi R, et al. Oral contraceptives and the risk of hereditary ovarian cancer. *N Engl J Med* 1998;339:424.
33. Rebbeck TR, Levin AM, Eisen A, et al. Breast cancer risk after bilateral prophylactic oophorectomy in BRCA1 mutation carriers. *J Natl Cancer Inst* 1999;91:1475.
34. Grann VR, Jacobson JS, Thomason D, et al. Effect of prevention strategies on survival and quality-adjusted survival of women with BRCA1/2 mutations: an updated decision analysis. *J Clin Oncol* 2002;20:2520.
35. Lu KH, Garber JE, Cramer DW, et al. Occult ovarian tumors in women with BRCA1 or BRCA2 mutations undergoing prophylactic oophorectomy. *J Clin Oncol* 2000;18:2728.
36. Colgan TJ, Murphy J, Cole DE, Narod S, Rosen B. Occult carcinoma in prophylactic oophorectomy specimens: prevalence and association with BRCA germline mutation status. *Am J Surg Pathol* 2001;25:1283.
37. Cass I, Li AJ, Runowicz CD, et al. Pattern of lymph node metastases in clinically unilateral stage I invasive epithelial ovarian carcinomas. *Gynecol Oncol* 2001;80:56.
38. Chen LM, Leuchter RS, Lagasse LD, Karlan BY. Splenectomy and surgical cytoreduction for ovarian cancer. *Gynecol Oncol* 2000;77:362.
39. Scarabelli C, Gallo A, Zarrelli A, Visentin C, Campagnutta E. Systematic pelvic and para-aortic lymphadenectomy during cytoreductive surgery in advanced ovarian cancer: potential benefit on survival. *Gynecol Oncol* 1995;56:328.
40. McGowan L, Lesher LP, Norris HJ, Barnett M. Misstaging of ovarian cancer. *Obstet Gynecol* 1985;65:568.
41. Ozols RF, Fisher RI, Anderson T, Makuch R, Young RC. Peritoneoscopy in the management of ovarian cancer. *Am J Obstet Gynecol* 1981;140:611.
42. Childers JM, Lang J, Surwit EA, Hatch KD. Laparoscopic surgical staging of ovarian cancer. *Gynecol Oncol* 1995;59:25.
43. Young RC, Walton LA, Ellenberg SS, et al. Adjuvant therapy in stage I and stage II epithelial ovarian cancer: results of two prospective randomized trials. *N Engl J Med* 1990;322:1021.
44. Sjövall K, Nilsson B, Einhorn N. Different types of rupture of the tumor capsule and the impact of survival in early ovarian carcinoma. *Int J Gynecol Cancer* 1994;4:333.
45. Dembo AJ, Davy M, Stenwj AE, et al. Prognostic factors in patients with stage I epithelial ovarian cancer. *Obstet Gynecol* 1990;75:263.
46. Hoskins WJ, Bundy BN, Thigpen JT, Omura GA. The influence of cytoreductive surgery on recurrence-free interval and survival in small volume stage III epithelial ovarian cancer: a Gynecologic Oncology Group study. *Gynecol Oncol* 1992;47:159.
47. Omura GA, Brody MF, Homesley HD, et al. Long-term follow-up and prognostic factor analysis in advanced ovarian carcinomas: the Gynecologic Oncology Group experience. *J Clin Oncol* 1991;9:1138.
48. Fayers PM, Rustin G, Wood R, et al. The prognostic value of serum CA125 in patients with advanced ovarian carcinoma: an analysis of 573 patients by the Medical Research Council Working Party on gynaecological cancer. *Int J Gynecol Cancer* 1993;3:285.
49. Markman M, Lewis JL, Saigo P, et al. Impact of age on survival of patients with ovarian cancer. *Gynecol Oncol* 1993;49:236.
50. Kaern J, Trope CG, Kristensen GB, Tveit KM, Pettersen EO. Evaluation of deoxyribonucleic acid ploidy and S-phase fraction as prognostic parameters in advanced epithelial ovarian carcinoma: a prospective study. *Am J Obstet Gynecol* 1994;170:479.
51. Bookman MA. Factoring outcomes in ovarian cancer. *J Clin Oncol* 1996;14:325.
52. van der Zee AGJ, Hollema HH, deBruijn A, et al. Cell biological markers of drug resistance in ovarian carcinoma. *Gynecol Oncol* 1995;58:165.
53. van der Zee AGJ, Hollema H, Suurmeijer AJH, et al. Value of P-glycoprotein, glutathione S-transferase pi, c-erb B-2, and p53 as prognostic factors in ovarian carcinomas. *J Clin Oncol* 1995;13:70.
54. Schummer M, Ng WV, Bumgarner RE, Nelson PS, et al. Comparative hybridization of an array of 21,500 ovarian dDNAs for the discovery of genes overexpressed in ovarian carcinomas. *Gene* 1999;238:375.
55. Matei D, Graeber TG, Baldwin RL, et al. Gene expression in epithelial ovarian carcinoma. *Oncogene* 2002;21:6289.
56. International Collaborative Ovarian Neoplasm (ICON1) Collaborators. International Collaborative Ovarian Neoplasm Trial 1: a randomized trial of adjuvant chemotherapy in women with early-stage ovarian cancer. *J Natl Cancer Inst* 2003;95:125.
57. Trimbos JB, Vergote I, Bolis G, et al. Impact of adjuvant chemotherapy and surgical staging in early-stage ovarian carcinoma: European Organization for Research and Treatment of Cancer-Adjuvant Chemotherapy in Ovarian Neoplasm Trial. *J Natl Cancer Inst* 2003;95:113.
58. Trimbos JB, Parmar M, Vergote I, et al. International Collaborative Ovarian Neoplasm Trial 1 and Adjuvant Chemotherapy in Ovarian Neoplasm Trial: two parallel randomized phase III trials of adjuvant chemotherapy in patients with early-stage ovarian carcinoma. *J Natl Cancer Inst* 2003;95:105.
59. Bell J, Brady M, Lage J, et al. A randomized phase III trial of three versus six cycles of carboplatin and paclitaxel as adjuvant treatment in early stage ovarian epithelial carcinoma: a Gynecologic Oncology Group study. *Gynecol Oncol* 2003;88:156(abst).
60. Fuks F. External radiotherapy of ovarian cancer: standard approaches and new frontiers. *Semin Oncol* 1975;2:253.
60a. Delclos L, Smith JP. Ovarian cancer with special regard to types of radiotherapy. *Natl Cancer Inst Monogr* 1975;42:129.

61. Dembo A, Bush R, Beale F, et al. Ovarian carcinoma: improved survival following abdominopelvic irradiation in patients with a completed pelvic operation. *Am J Obstet Gynecol* 1979;134:793.

62. Klaassen D, Shelley W, Starreveld A, et al. Early stage ovarian cancer: a randomized clinical trial comparing whole abdominal radiotherapy, melphalan, and intraperitoneal chromic phosphate: a National Cancer Institute of Canada Clinical Trials Group report. *J Clin Oncol* 1988;6:1254.

63. Dembo AJ. Epithelial ovarian cancer: the role of radiotherapy. *Int J Radiat Oncol Biol Phys* 1992;22:835.

64. Martinez A, Schray MF, Howes AE, et al. Postoperative radiation therapy for epithelial ovarian cancer: the curative role based on a 24-year experience. *J Clin Oncol* 1981;3:901.

65. Fuller DB, Sause WT, Plenk HP, et al. Analysis of postoperative radiation therapy in stage I through III epithelial ovarian carcinoma. *J Clin Oncol* 1987;5:897.

66. Weiser EB, Burke TW, Heller PB, et al. Determinants of survival of patients with epithelial ovarian carcinoma following whole abdomen irradiation (WAR). *Gynecol Oncol* 1988;30:201.

67. Lindner H, Willich H, Atzinger A. Primary adjuvant whole abdominal irradiation in ovarian carcinoma. *Int J Radiat Oncol Biol Phys* 1990;19:1203.

68. Redman CWE, Mould J, Warwick J, et al. The West Midlands epithelial ovarian cancer adjuvant therapy trial. *Clin Oncol* 1993;5:1.

69. Chiara S, Conte P, Franzone P, et al. High-risk early-stage ovarian cancer. Randomized clinical trial comparing cisplatin plus cyclophosphamide versus whole abdominal radiotherapy. *Am J Clin Oncol* 1994;17:72.

69a. Dembo AJ, Bush RS, Beale FA, et al. A randomized clinical trial of moving strip versus open field whole abdominal irradiation in patients with invasive epithelial cancer of the ovary. *Int J Rad Oncol Biol Phys* 1983; 9:97.

70. Firat S, Murray K, Erickson B. High-dose whole abdominal and pelvic irradiation for treatment of ovarian carcinoma: long-term toxicity and outcomes. *Int J Radiat Oncol Biol Phys* 2003;57:201.

71. Young RC, Brady MF, Nieberg RK, et al. Adjuvant treatment for early ovarian cancer: a randomized phase III trial of intraperitoneal 32P or intravenous cyclophosphamide and cisplatin—a gynecologic oncology group study. *J Clin Oncol* 2003;21:4350.

72. Vergote IB, Vergote-De Vos LN, Abeler VM, et al. Randomized trial comparing cisplatin with radioactive phosphorus or whole-abdomen irradiation as adjuvant treatment of ovarian cancer. *Cancer* 1992;69:741.

73. Bolis G, Colombo N, Pecorelli S, et al. Adjuvant treatment for early epithelial ovarian cancer: results of two randomized clinical trials comparing cisplatin to no further treatment or chromic phosphate (^{32}P). *Am J Clin Oncol* 1995;6:887.

74. Bristow RE, Montz FJ, La Gasse LD, Leuchter RS, Karlan BY. Survival impact of surgical cytoreduction in stage IV epithelial ovarian cancer. *Gynecol Oncol* 1999;72:278.

75. Curtin JP, Mauk R, Venkatraman ES, Barakat RR, Hoskins WJ. Stage IV ovarian cancer: impact of surgical debulking. *Gynecol Oncol* 1997;64:9.

76. Griffiths CT. Surgical resection of tumor bulk in the primary treatment of ovarian carcinoma. *Natl Cancer Inst Monogr* 1975;42:101.

77. Hacker NF, Berek JS, Lagasse LD, et al. Primary cytoreductive surgery for epithelial ovarian cancer. *Obstet Gynecol* 1983;61:413.

78. Vogl SE, Pagano M, Kaplan BH, et al. Cisplatin based combination chemotherapy for advanced ovarian cancer: high overall response rate with curative potential only in women with small tumor burdens. *Cancer* 1983;51:2024.

79. Pohl R, Dallenback-Hellweg G, Plugge T, et al. Prognostic parameters in patients with advanced malignant ovarian tumors. *Eur J Gynaecol Oncol* 1984;3:160.

80. Delgado G, Oram DH, Petrilli ES. Stage III ovarian cancer: the role of a maximal surgical reduction. *Gynecol Oncol* 1984;19:293.

81. Piver MS, Lele SB, Marchetti DL, et al. The impact of aggressive debulking surgery and cisplatin chemotherapy on progression-free survival in stage III and IV ovarian carcinoma. *J Clin Obstet Gynecol* 1988;6:983.

82. Neijt JP, ten Bokkel Huinink WW, van der Burg ME, et al. Long-term survival in ovarian cancer. *Eur J Cancer* 1991;27:1367.

83. Redman JR, Petrini GR, Saigo PE, et al. Prognostic factors in advanced ovarian carcinoma. *J Clin Oncol* 1986;4:515.

84. Conte PF, Bruzzone M, Hiara S, et al. A randomized trial comparing cisplatin plus cyclophosphamide versus cisplatin, doxorubicin, and cyclophosphamide in advanced ovarian cancer. *J Clin Oncol* 1986;4:965.

85. Hunter RW, Alexander NDE, Soutter WP. Meta-analysis of surgery in advanced ovarian carcinoma: is maximum cytoreductive surgery an independent determinant of prognosis? *Am J Obstet Gynecol* 1992;166:504.

86. Allen DG, Heintz APM, Touw FW. A meta-analysis of residual disease and survival in stage III and IV carcinoma of the ovary. *Eur J Gynaecol Oncol* 1995;16:349.

87. Omura GA, Bundy BN, Berek JS, et al. Randomized trial of cyclophosphamide plus cisplatin with or without doxorubicin in ovarian carcinoma: a Gynecologic Oncology Group study. *J Clin Oncol* 1989;7:457.

88. Hoskins WJ, McGuire WP, Brady MF, et al. The effect of diameter of largest residual disease on survival after primary cytoreductive surgery in patients with suboptimal residual epithelial ovarian cancer. *Am J Obstet Gynecol* 1994;170:974.

89. Chen SS, Bochner R. Assessment of morbidity in primary cytoreductive surgery for advanced ovarian cancer. *Gynecol Oncol* 1985;20:190.

90. Blythe JG, Wahl TP. Debulking surgery: does it increase the quality of survival? *Gynecol Oncol* 1982;14:396.

91. Bristow RE, Duska LR, Lambrou NC, et al. A model for predicting surgical outcome in patients with advanced ovarian carcinoma using computed tomography. *Cancer* 2000;89:1532.

92. Schwartz PE, Chambers JT, Makuch R. Neoadjuvant chemotherapy for advanced ovarian cancer. *Gynecol Oncol* 1994;53:33.

93. van der Burg ME, van Lent M, Buyse M, et al. The effect of debulking surgery after induction chemotherapy on the prognosis in advanced epithelial ovarian cancer. Gyne- cologic Cancer Cooperative Group of the European Organization for Research and Treatment of Cancer. *N Engl J Med* 1995;332:629.

94. Stewart LA, for the Advanced Ovarian Cancer Trialists Group (AOCTG). Chemotherapy in advanced ovarian cancer: an overview of randomized clinical trials. *BMJ* 1991;303:884.

95. Aabo K, Adams M, Adnitt P, et al. Chemotherapy in advanced ovarian cancer: four systematic meta-analyses of individual patient data from 37 randomized trials. *Br J Cancer* 1998;78:1749.

96. Alberts DS, Green S, Hannigan EV, et al. Improved therapeutic index of carboplatin plus cyclophosphamide versus cisplatin plus cyclophosphamide: final report by the Southwest Oncology Group of a phase III randomized trial in stages III and IV ovarian cancer. *J Clin Oncol* 1992;10:706.

97. Swenerton K, Jeffrey J, Stuart G, et al. Cisplatin-cyclophosphamide versus carboplatin-cyclophosphamide in advanced ovarian cancer: a randomized phase III study of the National Cancer Institute of Canada Clinical Trials Group. *J Clin Oncol* 1992;10:718.

98. Hakes T, Chalas E, Hoskins WJ, et al. Randomized prospective trial of 5 versus 10 cycles of cyclophosphamide, doxorubicin and cisplatin in ovarian cancer. *Gynecol Oncol* 1992;42:284.

99. Bertelsen K, Jakobsen A, Stroyer I, et al. A prospective randomized comparison of 6 and 12 cycles of cyclophosphamide, Adriamycin, and cisplatin in advanced epithelial ovarian cancer: a Danish Ovarian Study Group trial (DACOVA). *Gynecol Oncol* 1993;49:30.

100. Levin L, Hryniuk WM. Dose intensity analysis of chemotherapy regimens in ovarian carcinoma. *J Clin Oncol* 1978;5:756.

101. McGuire WP, Hoskins WJ, Brady MF, et al. Assessment of dose-intensive therapy in suboptimally debulked ovarian cancer: a Gynecologic Oncology Group study. *J Clin Oncol* 1995;13:1589.

102. Conte PF, Bruzzone M, Carino F, et al. High dose versus low dose cisplatin in combination with cyclophosphamide and epidoxorubicin in suboptimal ovarian cancer: a randomized study of the Gruppo Oncologico Nord-Ovest. *J Clin Oncol* 1996;14:351.

103. Kay SB, Lewis CR, Paul J, et al. Randomized study of two doses of cisplatin with cyclophosphamide in epithelial ovarian cancer. *Lancet* 1992;340.

104. Kaye SB, Paul J, Cassidy J, et al. Mature results of a randomized trial of two doses of cisplatin for the treatment of ovarian cancer. *J Clin Oncol* 1996;14:2113.

105. Jodrell DI, Egorin MJ, Canetta RM, et al. Relationships between carboplatin exposure and tumor response and toxicity in patients with ovarian cancer. *J Clin Oncol* 1992;10:520.

106. Jakobsen A, Bertelsen K, Andersen JE, et al. Dose-effect study of carboplatin in ovarian cancer: a Danish Ovarian Cancer Group study. *J Clin Oncol* 1997;15:193.

107. Gore ME, Mainwaring PN, Ahern R, et al. Randomized trial of dose-intensity with single-agent carboplatin in patients with epithelial ovarian cancer. *J Clin Oncol* 1998;16:2426.

108. Omura G, Bundy B, Berek J, et al. Randomized trial of cyclophosphamide plus cisplatin with or without doxorubicin in ovarian carcinoma: a Gynecologic Oncology Group study. *J Clin Oncol* 1989;7:457.

109. Omura GA, Buyse M, Marsoni S, et al. CP versus CAP chemotherapy of ovarian carcinoma: a meta-analysis. *J Clin Oncol* 1991;9:1668.

110. A'Hern RP, Gore ME. Impact of doxorubicin on survival in advanced ovarian cancer. *J Clin Oncol* 1995;13:726.

111. The ICON Collaborators. ICON 2: randomized trial of single-agent carboplatin against three-drug combination of CAP (cyclophosphamide, doxorubicin, and cisplatin) in women with ovarian cancer. *Lancet* 1998;352:1571.

112. Thigpen JT, Blessing JA, Ball H, et al. Phase II trial of paclitaxel in patients with progressive ovarian carcinoma after platinum-based chemotherapy: a Gynecologic Oncology Group study. *J Clin Oncol* 1994;12:1748.

113. Piccart MJ, Gore M, ten Bokkel Huinink W, et al. Docetaxel: an active new drug for treatment of advanced epithelial ovarian cancer. *J Natl Cancer Inst* 1995;87:676.

114. Eisenhauer EA, ten Bokkel Huinink WW, Swenerton KD, et al. European-Canadian randomized trial of paclitaxel in relapsed ovarian cancer: high-dose versus low-dose and long versus short infusion. *J Clin Oncol* 1994;12:2654.

115. McGuire WP, Hoskins WJ, Brady MF, et al. Cyclophosphamide and cisplatin compared with paclitaxel and cisplatin in patients with stage III and stage IV ovarian cancer. *N Engl J Med* 1996;334:1.

116. Piccart MJ, Bertelsen K, James K, et al. Randomized intergroup trial of cisplatin-paclitaxel versus cisplatin-cyclophosphamide in women with advanced epithelial ovarian cancer: three-year results. *J Natl Cancer Inst* 2000;92:699.

117. Muggia FM, Braly PS, Brady MF, et al. Phase III randomized study of cisplatin versus paclitaxel versus cisplatin and paclitaxel in patients with suboptimal stage III or IV ovarian cancer: a Gynecologic Oncology Group study. *J Clin Oncol* 2000;18:106.

118. The International Collaborative Ovarian Neoplasm (ICON) Group. Paclitaxel plus carboplatin versus standard chemotherapy with either single-agent carboplatin or cyclophosphamide, doxorubicin, and cisplatin in women with ovarian cancer. The ICON3 randomized trial. *Lancet* 2002;360:505.

119. Bookman MA, McGuire WP, Kilpatrick D, et al. Carboplatin and paclitaxel in ovarian carcinoma: a phase I study of the Gynecologic Oncology Group. *J Clin Oncol* 1996;14:1895.

120. Ozols RF, Bundy BN, Greer BE, et al. Phase III trial of carboplatin and paclitaxel compared with cisplatin and paclitaxel in patients with optimally resected stage III ovarian cancer: a Gynecologic Oncology Group study. *J Clin Oncol* 2003;21:3194.

121. du Bois A, Luck H-J, Meier W, et al. A randomized clinical trial of cisplatin/paclitaxel versus carboplatin/paclitaxel as first-line treatment of ovarian cancer. *J Natl Cancer Inst* 2003;95:1320.

122. Neijt JP, Engelholm SA, Tuxen MK, et al. Exploratory phase III study of paclitaxel and cisplatin versus paclitaxel and carboplatin in advanced ovarian cancer. *J Clin Oncol* 2000;18:3084.

123. Vasey PA. CRC trials unit. Survival and longer-term toxicity results of the SCOTROC

study: docetaxel-carboplatin (DC) vs. paclitaxel-carboplatin (PC) in epithelial ovarian cancer (EOC). *Proc Am Soc Clin Oncol* 2002;21:202a(abst 804).

124. Omura GA, Brady MF, Look KY, et al. Phase III trial of paclitaxel at two dose levels, the higher dose accompanied by filgrastim at two dose levels in platinum-pretreated epithelial ovarian cancer: an intergroup study. *J Clin Oncol* 2003;21:2843.

125. Markman M, Hall J, Spitz D, et al. Phase II trial of weekly single-agent paclitaxel in platinum/paclitaxel-refractory ovarian cancer. *J Clin Oncol* 2002;20:2365.

126. Markman M, Liu PY, Wilczynski S, et al. Phase III randomized trial of 12 versus 3 months of maintenance paclitaxel in patients with advanced ovarian cancer after complete response to platinum and paclitaxel-based chemotherapy: a Southwest Oncology Group and Gynecologic Oncology Group trial. *J Clin Oncol* 2003;21:2460.

127. Schwartz PE, Smith JP. Second look operations in ovarian cancer. *Am J Obstet Gynecol* 1980;138:1124.

128. Casey AC, Farias-Eisner R, Risani AL, et al. What is the role of reassessment laparoscopy in the management of gynecologic cancers in 1995? *Gynecol Oncol* 1996;60:454.

129. Fein DA, Morgan LS, Marcus RB, Jr., et al. Stage III ovarian carcinoma: an analysis of treatment results and complications following hyperfractionated abdominopelvic irradiation for salvage. *Int J Radiat Oncol Biol Phys* 1994;29:169.

130. Morgan L, Chafe W, Mendenhall W, et al. Hyperfractionation of whole-abdomen radiation therapy: salvage treatment of persistent ovarian carcinoma following chemotherapy. *Gynecol Oncol* 1988;31:122.

131. Cmelak AJ, Kapp DS. Long-term survival with whole abdominopelvic irradiation in platinum-refractory persistent or recurrent ovarian cancer. *Gynecol Oncol* 1997;65:453.

132. Schray M, Martinez A, Howes A, et al. Advanced epithelial ovarian cancer: salvage whole abdominal irradiation for patients with recurrent or persistent disease after combination chemotherapy. *J Clin Oncol* 1988;6:1433.

133. Hoskins W, Lichter A, Wittingham, R, et al. Whole abdominal and pelvic irradiation in patients with minimal disease at second-look surgical reassessment for ovarian carcinoma. *Gynecol Oncol* 1985;20:271.

134. Fuks Z, Rizel S, Biran S. Chemotherapeutic and surgical induction of pathological complete remission and whole abdominal irradiation for consolidation does not enhance the cure of stage III ovarian carcinoma. *J Clin Oncol* 1988;6:509.

135. Hoskins PJ, Swenerton KD, Wong F, et al. Platinum plus cyclophosphamide plus radiotherapy is superior to platinum alone in "high-risk" epithelial ovarian cancer (residual negative and either stage I or II, grade III, or stage III, any grade). *Int J Gynecol Cancer* 1995;5:134.

136. Bruzzone M, Repetto L, Chiara S, et al. Chemotherapy versus radiotherapy in the management of ovarian cancer patients with pathological complete response or minimal residual disease at second look. *Gynecol Oncol* 1990;38:392.

137. Lambert HE, Rustin GJS, Gregory WM, et al. A randomized trial comparing single-agent carboplatin with carboplatin followed by radiotherapy for advanced ovarian cancer: a North Thames Ovary Group study. *J Clin Oncol* 1993;11:440.

137a. Kapp KS, Kapp DS, Poschauko J, et al. The prognostic significance of peritoneal seeding and size of postsurgical residual in patients with stage III epithelial ovarian cancer treated with surgery, chemotherapy, and high-dose radiotherapy. *Gynecol Oncol* 1999;74:400.

138. Sorbe B, Swedish-Norwegian Ovarian Cancer Study Group. Consolidation treatment of advanced (FIGO stage III) ovarian carcinoma in complete surgical remission after induction chemotherapy: a randomized, controlled, clinical trial comparing whole abdominal radiotherapy, chemotherapy, and no further treatment. *Int J Gynecol Cancer* 2003;13:278.

139. Firat S, Erickson B. Selective irradiation for the treatment of recurrent ovarian carcinoma involving the vagina or rectum. *Gynecol Oncol* 2001;80:213.

140. Fujiwara K, Suzuki S, Yoden E, et al. Local radiation therapy for localized relapsed or refractory ovarian cancer patients with or without symptoms after chemotherapy. *Int J Gynecol Cancer* 2002;12:250.

141. Bristow RE, Lagasse LD, Karlan BY. Secondary surgical cytoreduction for advanced epithelial ovarian cancer. *Cancer* 1996;78:2049.

142. Berek JS, Hacker NF, Lagasse LD, et al. Survival of patients following secondary cytoreductive surgery in ovarian cancer. *Obstet Gynecol* 1983;61:189.

143. Segna RA, Dottino P, Mandeli P, Konsker K, Cohen CJ. Secondary cytoreduction for ovarian cancer following cisplatin therapy. *J Clin Oncol* 1993;11:434.

144. Vaccarello L, Rubin SC, Vlamis V, et al. Cytoreductive surgery in ovarian carcinoma patients with a documented previously complete surgical response. *Gynecol Oncol* 1995;57:61.

145. Eisenkop SM, Friedman RL, Wang H. Secondary cytoreductive for recurrent ovarian cancer. A prospective study. *Cancer* 1995;76:1606.

146. Janicke F, Holscher M, Kuhn W, et al. Radical surgical procedure improves survival time in patients with recurrent ovarian cancer. *Cancer* 1992;70:2129.

147. Neijt J, ten Bokkel Huinink W, van der Burg ME, et al. Randomized trial comparing two combination chemotherapy regimens (CHAP-5 vs CP) in advanced ovarian carcinoma. *J Clin Oncol* 1987;5:1157.

148. van der Burg MEL, van Lent M, Kobierska A, et al. After 6 years follow-up intervention debulking surgery remains an independent prognostic factor for survival in advanced epithelial ovarian cancer. An EORTC Gynecologic Cancer Cooperative Group study. *Int J Gynecol Cancer* 1997;7[Suppl 2]:28.

149. Markman M, Bookman MA. Second-line treatment of ovarian cancer. *Oncologist* 2000;5:26.

150. Eisenhauer EA, Vermorken JB, van Glabbeke M. Predictors of response to subsequent chemotherapy in platinum pretreated ovarian cancer: a multivariate analysis of 704 patients. *Ann Oncol* 1997;8:963.

151. The ICON and AGO Collaborators. Paclitaxel plus platinum-based chemotherapy versus conventional platinum-based chemotherapy in women with relapsed ovarian cancer: the ICON4/AGO-OVAR-2.2 trial. *Lancet* 2003;361:2099.

152. Bookman MA, Malmstrom H, Bolis G, et al. Topotecan for the treatment of advanced epithelial ovarian cancer: an open-label phase II study in patients treated after prior chemotherapy that contained cisplatin or carboplatin and paclitaxel. *J Clin Oncol* 1998;16:3345.

153. Rose PG, Blessing JA, Mayer AR, Homesley HD. Prolonged oral etoposide as second-line therapy for platinum-resistant and platinum-sensitive ovarian carcinoma: a Gynecologic Oncology Group study. *J Clin Oncol* 1998;16:405.

154. Lund B, Hansen OP, Theilade K, Hansen M, Neijt JP. Phase II study of gemcitabine (2′,2′-difluorodeoxycytidine) in previously treated ovarian cancer patients. *J Natl Cancer Inst* 1994;86:1530.

155. Muggia FM, Hainsworth JD, Jeffers S, et al. Phase II study of liposomal doxorubicin in refractory ovarian cancer: antitumor activity and toxicity modification by liposomal encapsulation. *J Clin Oncol* 1997;15:987.

156. Bajetta E, DiLeo A, Biganzoli L, et al. Phase II study of vinorelbine in patients with pretreated advanced ovarian cancer: activity in platinum-resistant disease. *J Clin Oncol* 1996;14:2546.

157. Hatch KD, Beecham JB, Blessing JA, Creasman WT. Responsiveness of patients with advanced ovarian carcinoma to tamoxifen. *Cancer* 1991;68:269.

158. Adelson MD, Wharton JT, Delclos L, et al. Palliative radiotherapy for ovarian cancer. *Int J Radiat Oncol Biol Phys* 1987;13:17.

159. Spanos WJ, Perez CA, Marcus S, et al. Effect of rest interval on tumor and normal tissue response—a report of phase III study of accelerated split course palliative radiation for advanced pelvic malignancies (RTOG-8502). *Int J Radiat Oncol Biol Phys* 1993;25:399.

160. Markman M. Intraperitoneal therapy of ovarian cancer. *Semin Oncol* 1998;25:356.

161. Markman M, Reichman B, Hakes T, et al. Responses to second-line cisplatin-based intraperitoneal therapy in ovarian cancer: influence of a prior response to intravenous cisplatin. *J Clin Oncol* 1991;9:1801.

162. Speyer JL, Beller U, Colombo N, et al. Intraperitoneal carboplatin: favorable results in women with minimal residual ovarian cancer after cisplatin therapy. *J Clin Oncol* 1990;8:1335.

163. Markman M, Brady MF, Spirtos NM, et al. Phase II trial of intraperitoneal paclitaxel in carcinoma of the ovary, tube, and peritoneum: a Gynecologic Oncology Group study. *J Clin Oncol* 1998;16:2620.

164. Edwards RP, Gooding W, Lembersky BC, et al. Comparison of toxicity and survival following intraperitoneal recombinant interleukin-2 for persistent ovarian cancer after platinum: twenty-four-hour versus 7-day infusion. *J Clin Oncol* 1997;15:3399.

165. Berek JS, Markman M, Stonebraker B, et al. Intraperitoneal interferon-α in residual ovarian carcinoma: a phase II Gynecologic Oncology Group study. *Gynecol Oncol* 1999;75:10.

166. Pujade-Lauraine E, Guastalla J-P, Colombo N, et al. Intraperitoneal recombinant interferon gamma in ovarian cancer patients with residual disease at second-look laparotomy. *J Clin Oncol* 1996;14:343.

167. Alberts DS, Liu PY, Hannigan EV, et al. Intraperitoneal cisplatin plus intravenous cyclophosphamide versus intravenous cisplatin plus intravenous cyclophosphamide for stage III ovarian cancer. *N Engl J Med* 1996;335:1950.

168. Markman M, Bundy BN, Alberts DS, et al. Phase III trial of standard-dose intravenous cisplatin plus paclitaxel versus moderately high-dose carboplatin followed by intravenous paclitaxel and intraperitoneal cisplatin in small-volume stage III ovarian carcinoma: an intergroup study of the Gynecologic Oncology Group, Southwestern Oncology Group, and Eastern Cooperative Oncology Group. *J Clin Oncol* 2001;19:1001.

169. Armstrong DK, Bundy BN, Baergen R, et al. Randomized phase III study of intravenous (IV) paclitaxel and cisplatin versus IV paclitaxel, intraperitoneal (IP) cisplatin and IP paclitaxel in optimal stage III epithelial ovarian cancer (OC): a Gynecologic Oncology Group trial (GOG 172). *Proc Am Soc Clin Oncol* 2002;21:201a(abst 803).

170. Stiff PJ, Bayer R, Kerger C, Potkul RK, et al. High-dose chemotherapy with autologous transplantation for persistent/relapsed ovarian cancer: a multivariate analysis of survival for 100 consecutively treated patients. *J Clin Oncol* 1997;15:1309.

171. Aghajanian C, Fennelly D, Shapiro F, et al. Phase II study of "dose-dense" high-dose chemotherapy treatment with peripheral-blood progenitor-cell support as primary treatment for patients with advanced ovarian cancer. *J Clin Oncol* 1998;16:1852.

172. Schilder RJ, Johnson S, Gallo J, et al. Phase I trial of multiple cycles of high-dose chemotherapy supported by autologous peripheral blood stem cells. *J Clin Oncol* 1999;17:2198.

173. Cobleigh MA, Vogel CL, Tripathy D, et al. Multinational study of the efficacy and safety of humanized anti-HER2 monoclonal antibody in women who have HER2-overexpressing metastatic breast cancer that has progressed after chemotherapy for metastatic disease. *J Clin Oncol* 1999;17:2639.

174. Bookman MA, Darcy KM, Clarke-Pearson D, et al. Evaluation of monoclonal humanized anti-HER2 antibody, trastuzumab, in patients with recurrent or refractory ovarian or primary peritoneal carcinoma with overexpression of HER2: a phase II trial of the Gynecologic Oncology Group. *J Clin Oncol* 2001;21:283.

175. Hurteau JA, Blessing JA, DeCesare SL, et al. Evaluation of recombinant human interleukin-12 in patients with recurrent or refractory ovarian cancer: a Gynecologic Oncology Group study. *Gynecol Oncol* 2001;82:7.

176. Lenzi R, Rosenblum M, Verschraegen C, et al. Phase I study of intraperitoneal recombinant human interleukin 12 in patients with Mullerian carcinoma, gastrointestinal primary malignancies and mesothelioma. *Clin Cancer Res* 2002;8:3686.

177. Method MW, Gordon A, Finkler N, et al. Randomized evaluation of 3 treatment schedules to optimize clinical activity of OvaRex® Mab-B43.13 (OV) in patients (pts) with epithelial ovarian cancer (EOC). *Proc Am Soc Clin Oncol* 2002;21:21a(abst 80).

178. Berek JS, Taylor PT, Gordon AN, et al. Randomized pbo-controlled study of oregovomab (OV) for consolidation of clinical remission in pts with ovarian cancer (OC): prolonged disease-free survival (DFS) in optimal chemosensitive pts. *Proc Am Soc Clin Oncol* 2003;22:165(abst 660).

179. Baum RP, Noujaim AA, Nanci A, et al. Clinical course of ovarian cancer patients under repeated stimulation of HAMA using Mab OC125 and B43.13. *Hybridoma* 1993;12:583.

180. Kavanagh JJ, Spriggs D, Bookman M, et al. Phase 2 study of TLK286 (GSTpi-1 activated glutathione analog) in patients with platinum and paclitaxel refractory/resistant advanced epithelial ovarian cancer. *Eur J Cancer* 2002;38:A100(abst).

181. Berchuck A, Bast RC. p53-based gene therapy of ovarian cancer: magic bullet? *Gynecol Oncol* 1995;59:169.

182. Epenetos AA, Hooker G, Krausz T, et al. Antibody-guided irradiation of advanced ovarian cancer with intraperitoneally administered radiolabeled monoclonal antibodies. *J Clin Oncol* 1987;5:1980.

183. Serov SF, Scully RE, Sobin LH. *International histologic classification and staging of tumors. 9. Histologic typing of ovarian tumors.* Geneva: World Health Organization, 1973.

184. Trimble EL, Trimble CL. Epithelial ovarian tumors of low malignant potential. In: Markman M, Hoskins WJ, eds. *Cancer of the ovary.* New York: Raven Press, 1993:415.

185. Kurman RJ, Trimble CL. The behavior of serous tumors of low malignant potential: are they ever malignant? *Int J Gynecol Pathol* 1993;12:120.

186. Seidman JD, Kurman RJ. Ovarian serous borderline tumors: a critical review of the emphasis on prognostic indicators. *Hum Pathol* 2000;31:539.

187. Tazelaar HD, Bostwick DG, Ballon SC, Hendrickson MR, Kempson RL. Conservative treatment of borderline ovarian tumors. *Obstet Gynecol* 1985;66:417.

188. Trope C. Kaern J, Vergote IB, Kristensen G, Abeler V. Are borderline tumors of the ovary over treated both surgically and systemically? A review of four prospective randomized trials including 253 patients with borderline tumors. *Gynecol Oncol* 1985;51:236.

189. Barnhill OR, Kurman RJ, Brady MF, et al. Preliminary analysis of the behavior of stage I ovarian serous tumors of low malignant potential: a Gynecologic Oncology Group study. *J Clin Oncol* 1995;13:2752.

190. Friedlander ML, Hedley DW, Swanton C, Russell P. Prediction of long-term survival by flow cytometric analysis of the cellular DNA content in patients with advanced ovarian cancer. *J Clin Oncol* 1988;6:282.

191. Kaern J, Trope C, Kjorstad KE, Abeler V, Pettersen EL. Cellular DNA content as a new prognostic tool in patients with borderline tumors of the ovary. *Gynecol Oncol* 1990;38:452.

192. Strand CM, Grosh WW, Baxter J, et al. Peritoneal carcinomatosis of unknown primary site in women. *Ann Intern Med* 1989;111:213.

193. Fowler JM, Nieberg RK, Schooler TA, Berek JS. Peritoneal adenocarcinoma (serous) of mullerian type: a subgroup of women presenting with peritoneal carcinomatosis. *Int J Gynecol Cancer* 1994;4:43.

194. Williams SD. Ovarian germ cell tumors: an update. *Semin Oncol* 1998;25:407.

195. Williams SD, Blessing JA, Hatch KD, Homesley HD. Chemotherapy of advanced dysgerminoma: trials of the Gynecologic Oncology Group. *J Clin Oncol* 1991;9:1950.

196. Williams SD, Blessing JA, Moore DH, Homesley HD, Adcock L. Cisplatin, vinblastine, and bleomycin in advanced and recurrent ovarian germ-cell tumors. *Ann Intern Med* 1989;111:22.

197. Williams SD, Birch R, Einhorn L, et al. Disseminated germ cell tumors: chemotherapy with cisplatin plus bleomycin plus either vinblastine or etoposide. *N Engl J Med* 1987; 316:1435.

198. Williams S, Blessing JA, Liao SY, Ball H, Hanjani P. Adjuvant therapy of ovarian germ cell tumors with cisplatin, etoposide, and bleomycin: a trial of the Gynecologic Oncology Group. *J Clin Oncol* 1994;12:701.

199. Schwartz PE, Smith J. Management of ovarian stromal tumors. *Am J Obstet Gynecol* 1976; 125:402.

200. Pascale MM, Pugeat M, Roberts M, et al. Androgen suppressive effects of GnRH agonist in ovarian hyperthecosis and virilizing tumours. *Clin Endocrinol* 1994;41:571.

201. Willemsen W, Kruitwagen R, Bastiaans B, Hanselaar T, Rolland R. Ovarian stimulation and granulosa-cell tumour. *Lancet* 1993;341:986.

202. Colombo N, Sessa C, Landoni F, et al. Cisplatin, vinblastine, and bleomycin combination chemotherapy in metastatic granulosa cell tumor of the ovary. *Obstet Gynecol* 1986;67:265.

203. Pectasides D, Alevizakos N, Athanassiou AE. Cisplatin-containing regimen in advanced or recurrent granulosa cell tumours of the ovary. *Ann Oncol* 1992;3:316.

204. Homesley HD, Bundy BN, Hurteau JA, Roth LM. Bleomycin, etoposide and cisplatin combination therapy of ovarian granulosa cell tumors and other stromal malignancies: a Gynecologic Oncology Group study. *Gynecol Oncol* 1999;72:131.

205. Healy KL, Burger HG, Mamers P, et al. Elevated serum inhibin concentrations in postmenopausal women with ovarian tumors. *N Engl J Med* 1993;329:1539.

206. Gustafson ML, Lee MM, Asmundson L, MacLaughlin DT, Donahoe PK. Müllerian inhibiting substance in the diagnosis and management of intersex and gonadal abnormalities. *J Pediatr Surg* 1993;28:439.

207. Lane AH, Fuller AF Jr, Kehas J, Donahoe PK, MacLaughlin DT. Diagnostic utility of müllerian inhibiting substance determination in patients with primary and recurrent granulosa cell tumor. *Gynecol Oncol* 1999;73:51.

208. Roush GR, El-Naggar AK, Abdul-Karim FW. Granulosa cell tumor of the ovary: a clinicopathologic flow cytometric DNA analysis. *Gynecol Oncol* 1995;56:430.

209. Schiller HM, Silverberg SG. Staging and prognosis in primary carcinoma of the fallopian tube. *Cancer* 1971;28:389.

210. Markman M, Zaino R, Busowski J, Barakat R. Carcinoma of the fallopian tube. In: Hoskins WJ, Perez CA, Young RC, eds. *Principles and practice of gynecologic oncology.* Philadelphia: JB Lippincott Co., 1992:783.

CHAPTER **33**

Cancer of the Breast

SECTION 1

ROBERT B. DICKSON
RICHARD G. PESTELL
MARC E. LIPPMAN

Molecular Biology of Breast Cancer

GENETICS

NEW METHODOLOGIES AND GENETIC MECHANISMS

The purpose of this chapter is to provide a current perspective on the rapidly evolving, increasingly integrated study of the genetic, molecular, biochemical, and cellular bases of breast cancer. Although the roles of steroid hormones have occupied breast cancer researchers since the 1950s, the roles of growth factors did not begin to emerge until the 1980s. The 1980s also saw the discovery of many of the oncogenes and suppressor genes, driving progression of the disease, and highlighted their connections to cellular adhesion, growth factor, and steroid regulatory pathways. The 1990s witnessed the discovery of genes that cause familial forms of breast cancer. The final decade of the twentieth century also ushered in major advances in our understanding of the cell cycle, DNA repair, and cell death (apoptosis) and their regulation. As the twenty-first century begins, the field is intensely involved in elucidation of the molecular bases of processes involved in treatment failure: primary mechanisms of resistance to chemotherapy, antiestrogens, and radiation and fundamental processes of invasion, angiogenesis, and metastasis. New technologies are available for human mammary cell culture, for regulatable animal models of cancer, and for high-throughput analyses of pathologic material (tissue microarrays, laser capture microdissection, and automated immunohistochemistry readers). Other advances have been made in cytogenetics [fluorescence *in situ* hybridization (FISH) and bacterial artificial chromosome array/comparative genomic hybridization (BAC array CGH)], in gene expression analysis [complementary DNA (cDNA) chip array and real-time polymerase chain reaction (PCR) assay methods], and in proteomics analysis (a plethora of techniques). These new methods are now being applied to improve tumor diagnosis and to predict response to existing therapies. Such approaches should also result in our discovery of new targets for more biologic-based therapies and prevention strategies for the disease.

Onset and progression of breast cancer appear to be intimately, but not exclusively, tied to genetic alterations (Fig. 33.1-1). Although the possibility of direct, DNA-modifying agents from environmental exposure has been studied for many years for links to breast cancer, this etiology of the disease appears to be quite rare. One clear example, however, is the instance of radiation exposure of Japanese women in World War II. More likely to play major current etiologic roles are indirect environmental effects that enhance breast epithelial cell exposure to reactive oxygen species or to estrogenic hormones. The reader is referred elsewhere for an introduction to this large, complex area of study,[1] as this chapter focuses primarily on hormones and growth factors as they affect cellular and tissue interaction aspects of the disease.

Cell biologic studies have begun to establish that defects in cell-cycle checkpoint controls are fundamental to the accumulation of genetic damage in the mammary epithelial cell, leading to cancer.[2] The four cell-cycle transitions, from $G_1 \rightarrow S$, $G_2 \rightarrow M$, spindle formation and function (cytokinesis), and daughter cell separation post M (karyokinesis), appear to be

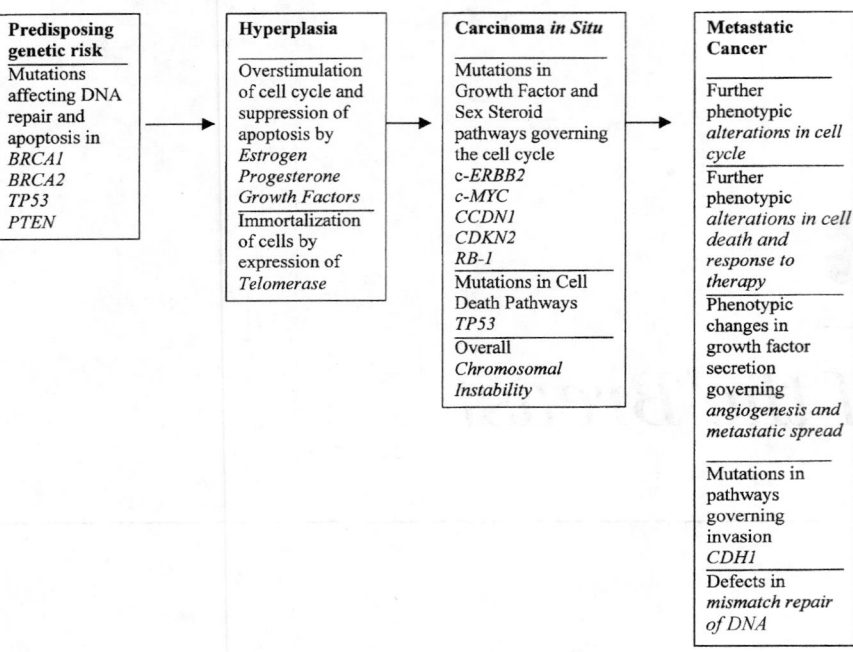

FIGURE 33.1-1. Summary of the genetic and phenotypic alterations associated with the onset and progression of familial and sporadic breast cancers.

important points of vulnerability for genetic damage. In normal cells, DNA damage and replication defects may be recognized at these and other points, resulting in cell-cycle arrest, DNA repair, and/or programmed cell death (apoptosis). Such DNA damage may be produced by environmental exposures (radiation or chemotherapy drugs), by replicative senescence (erosion of telomeres capping and protecting chromosomal ends), and by premalignancy- or malignancy-associated cellular changes. For example, direct DNA damage, aberrations in DNA methylation, mutation, or loss of expression of *BRCA1/2* or *p53* genes, deregulated expression of *c-Myc* or *cyclin D1* genes, and defects in DNA mismatch repair genes may all cause defects in DNA damage-dependent cell-cycle checkpoint controls, contributing to onset or progression, or both, of breast cancer. These concepts are further described in the next two sections.

FAMILIAL DISEASE

As noted in the previous section, significant progress has been made (Table 33.1-1) in the identification of inherited defects in somatic genes responsible for hereditary and familial breast cancers. Although several defined hereditary breast cancer syndromes are characterized by a very high penetrance of additional types of cancer, other breast cancer families may also display a lower penetrance of the disease and not be so clearly associated with elevated risk for multiple other types of cancer. In aggregate, it is estimated that 5% to 10% of breast cancer cases occur in families with significant inherited risk. A general hypothesis in the field of hereditary cancer genetics is the "two-hit" hypothesis, that a point mutation might be inherited in one allele of a candidate gene at a putative susceptibility locus and that loss of heterozygosity (LOH) or another genetic alteration might occur in the other allele of that locus later in life, leading to genomic instability and cancer.[3] This model has guided the identification of familial breast cancer genes (see Table 33.1-1).

The first triumph in identification of a gene, leading to a multicancer syndrome that includes breast cancer, was for the *TP53* gene (encoding p53, on chromosome 17p13).[3] Inherited mutations in *TP53* are responsible for the Li-Fraumeni syndrome of hereditary breast cancers, sarcomas, and other tumor types. At the time of its implication in Li-Fraumeni, mutations in this gene had already been described in the context of progression of sporadic cancers of the breast and other organs. More recently, mutations in the *PTEN* phosphatase (or *MMAC1*) gene (on chromosome 10q22-23) were described in the Cowden syndrome of hereditary breast cancers and multicutaneous lesions. The PTEN protein is discussed in Cell Cycle and Cell Death, later in this chapter, in the context of tumor suppressor genes and the cell cycle. In contrast to *TP53*, *PTEN* is not commonly mutated in sporadic breast cancers. Other studies on rarer familial diseases have implicated mutations of the *STKII/LKBI* gene (on chromosome 19 and involved in Wnt pathway signaling) in the Peutz-Jeghers syndrome of hamartomatous polyps, breast cancers, gastrointestinal cancers, and reproductive cancers and the *MLH1* or *MLH2*, or both, mismatch repair gene(s) in the Muir-Torre syndrome of gastrointestinal and genitourinary tumors and breast cancer. Finally, although initially proposed, mutations in the *ataxia-telangiectasia* gene *ATM* (ataxia-telangiectasia mutated) do not appear to contribute strongly to the risk of developing breast cancer.[3]

Two important genes that confer risk for the far more pervasive, familial forms of breast cancer have been identified: *BRCA1* and *BRCA2*.[3] Carriers of these mutant genes may display a range of cancer risk, and the mutant genes are quite prevalent in certain populations. King and coworkers first localized *BRCA1* (breast cancer and ovarian cancer-1) to chromosome 17q21. The gene was subsequently cloned and found to be novel, containing an amino-terminal, zinc- and DNA-binding "ring finger" motif; a carboxyl-terminal BCRT "domain;" and a nuclear localization sequence. Interestingly, mutations in this gene are particularly prevalent in breast cancers of Ashkenazi Jewish women and other

TABLE 33.1-1. Major Genetic Defects in Breast Cancer

ESTABLISHED FAMILIAL BREAST CANCER GENES (ALL TUMOR SUPPRESSORS)

Gene	Chromosomal Location	Familial Cancer Syndrome	Function
TP53 (*p53*)	17p13 (mutated, LOH)	Li-Fraumeni syndrome of multiple hereditary cancers	Cell-cycle/cell death/DNA repair regulator
PTEN	10q23 (mutated, LOH)	Cowden syndrome of multiple hereditary cancers	Cell survival/cell proliferation promoting phosphatase
BRCA1	17q21 (mutated, LOH)	Familial female breast and ovarian cancers	Surveillance of DNA damage
BRCA2	13q14 (mutated, LOH)	Familial female and male breast cancers	Surveillance of DNA damage

ESTABLISHED BREAST CANCER PROGRESSION GENES (ONCOGENES AND SUPPRESSOR GENES)

Gene	Chromosomal Location	Class	Function
HER-2/neu (*c-ERBB2*)	17q12	Oncogene (amplified)	Growth factor receptor subunit
c-MYC	8q24	Oncogene (amplified)	Cell-cycle/cell death regulator/protein synthesis
CCND1 (*cyclin D1*)	11q13	Oncogene (amplified)	Cell-cycle G_1 regulator
AIB-1	20q12	Oncogene (amplified)	Transcription factor sensitizes cells to estrogen/growth factor signaling
CDKN2 (*p16*)	9p21	Suppressor gene (methylated, LOH)	Cell-cycle G_1 regulator
RB-1 (*pRb*)	13q14	Suppressor gene (mutated, LOH)	Cell-cycle G_1 and G_1/S regulator
TP53 (*p53*)	17p13	Suppressor gene (mutated, LOH)	Cell-cycle/cell death/DNA repair regulator
CDH1 (*E-cadherin*)	16q22-23	Suppressor gene (methylated, LOH)	Cell-cell adhesion protein

LOH, loss of heterozygosity.

select populations. However, some families carrying *BRCA* mutations are nearly devoid of multiple afflicted members. In other studies comparing different carrier populations, *BRCA1* mutations have also been reported (but rarely) in women with no familial association of the disease. These studies emphasize the variable penetrance of inherited risk conferred by this gene. Although mutations in the *BRCA1* gene are widely prevalent in patients with familial breast and ovarian cancer, mutations are rarely detected in sporadic breast cancers. However, the BRCA1 protein is commonly down-regulated in nonfamilial (sporadic) breast cancers due to methylation of the *BRCA1* gene and other mechanisms. Consistent with these findings are observations that antisense oligonucleotides directed against the *BRCA1* messenger RNA (mRNA) enhance the proliferation of breast tumor cells and of mammary epithelial cells in culture *in vitro*. Correspondingly, other studies have demonstrated that retroviral transfer of the nonmutated *BRCA1* gene selectively inhibits the growth of non-*BRCA1*–mutated breast cancer cells *in vitro* and *in vivo* in nude mice.[3]

A separate gene, termed *BRCA2* (on chromosome 13q13), is also associated with familial cancers of the female and male breast and, to a lesser extent, the ovaries. This gene shares homology with *BRCA1*, and its encoded protein has similar biochemical functions to *BRCA1*. However, as noted above, although *BRCA2* mutation confers risk of female breast cancer, its effects on risk of ovarian cancer appear smaller than the risk conferred by *BRCA1*. Mutations of *BRCA2* confer risk of male breast cancer and (to a more limited extent) several other cancers, such as prostate cancer, pancreatic cancer, non-Hodgkin's lymphoma, basal cell carcinoma, bladder carcinoma, and fallopian tube tumors. Breast cancers of *BRCA1/2* carriers have similar prognostic significance when matched for other characteristics to the sporadic cases of breast cancer in noncarriers, although they more often also show high nuclear grade, *TP53* mutations, and amplification of the *HER2/neu* oncogene.[3] Notably, as many as two-thirds of families

with hereditary breast cancer appear to have *non-BRCA1/2* mechanisms of breast cancer initiation.[3] Current studies, using CGH and cDNA microarray analysis, suggest a distinct signature of chromosome gains and losses and gene expression for the different classes of familial breast cancers (*BRCA1, BRCA2, BRCAX*) compared to sporadic breast cancers.[4]

As noted earlier, the structure and function of the two distinct BRCA proteins appear to be similar. Each appears to serve as an important regulator of cell-cycle checkpoint control mechanisms, involving cell-cycle arrest, cell death (apoptosis), and DNA repair. BRCA1 appears to interact with the p53 protein (leading to induction of the cell-cycle inhibitor p21) directly, with the RNA polymerase holoenzyme, with the transcription factor CREB, with two proteins termed *BAP1* and *BARD1*, with the estrogen receptor-α (ER-α, suppressing its function), with the promoter of *c-MYC* (suppressing expression of this protooncogene), and with promoters of other genes. BRCA1 and BRCA2 proteins are also found in complexes with Rad51, a protein important for the cellular response to DNA damage.[3] In addition, BRCA1 is phosphorylated by the ATM kinase, in response to DNA damage. Thus, the roles of both BRCA proteins are now emerging as central gatekeepers of genomic stability.[3] In studies of mice bearing a conditional knockout of the *BRCA1* gene, its further functions have emerged: mammary ductal morphogenesis and checkpoint control in the G_1/S and G_2/M phases of the cell cycle. Perhaps most interesting among BRCA1 protein–protein interactions in mammary epithelial cells is the one with the ER-α.[5] This apparently key antiestrogenic effect may place the BRCA proteins on center stage for control of the sex steroid–regulated pathways, long suspected to induce breast cancer.

CHROMOSOMAL AND GENOMIC INSTABILITY

Breast cancers, like other forms of malignancy, are thought to progress by accumulation of a series of genetic and phenotypic changes in the pathways regulating cellular proliferation, differentiation, death (apoptosis or necrosis), DNA repair, tissue compartmentalization, and responses to therapy. Using classic cytogenetic methodologies and studies of LOH, genetic regions identified as commonly rearranged, amplified, deleted, or otherwise altered have been frequently detected on chromosomes 1, 3, 6, 7, 8, 9, 11, 13, 15, 16, 17, 18, and 20. More recently, CGH and chromosome painting followed by spectral karyotyping (SKY) have implicated additional chromosome regions, including areas of 4, 10, 12, 19, and 22. CGH has been further refined to a high-throughput array method using BACs containing the entire human genome. Using these techniques, the benign lesions termed *fibroadenomas* are observed to be largely devoid of genetic imbalances (although they do contain some chromosomal defects), premalignant epithelial tissues and near diploid tumors to contain a spectrum of genetic defects, and aneuploid breast tumors to contain large numbers of genetic mutations and chromosomal aberrations. Breast cancer, in contrast to some other common epithelial tumors, such as colon cancer, is primarily characterized by chromosomal instability, as opposed to point mutation (with *TP53* mutations, probably not an early event in the natural history of breast cancer, being a notable exception to this generality). These pervasive chromosomal changes in breast cancer may arise from defects in the centrosomes and in the associated spindle apparatus of mammary epithelial cells. However, the exact pathogenesis of these defects remains to be determined.[6,7]

SUPPRESSOR GENES AND ONCOGENES

The most common genetic abnormalities in the progression of sporadic and familial breast cancers (as in many other types of solid tumors) appear to be LOH at multiple loci (see Table 33.1-1). As noted earlier in Familial Disease, an LOH event uncovers the functional consequences of a mutation in an allele of a tumor suppressor gene by removal of the dominant, normal allele. At the present time, in addition to LOH of the *TP53* gene and the two *BRCA* loci noted earlier in Familial Disease, LOH on 13q, 9p, and 16q are known, respectively, to involve specifically the tumor suppressor genes *RB-1*, *CDKN2* (encoding the p16 protein), and *CDH1* (encoding the E-cadherin protein). *RB-1* and *CDKN2* regulate the cell cycle, whereas *CDH1* regulates differentiation and tissue compartmentalization. Other suspected tumor suppressor genes involved in the progression of breast cancer have been proposed to reside on 1p, 3p, 6q, 7q, 11p, 11q, 15q, 17q, and 22q.[7] For example, a plasma membrane inner leaflet-associated protein termed *caveolin-1* (on 7p3.1) has been proposed to be a tumor suppressor gene in breast cancer. It is notable that two types of DNA alterations can lead to suppressor gene inactivation on one allele, before LOH of the other allele. For example, although point mutation may be more common for *TP53* and possibly *Rb*, gene methylation may be more common for *CDKN2* and *CDH-1*. Additional genes that are commonly methylated in breast cancer include the gene encoding 14-3-3σ (*HME1*, a $G_2 \rightarrow M$ cell-cycle checkpoint control gene on chromosome 1p35), *GSTPI* (a carcinogen detoxification gene on chromosome 11p13), *RARβ2* (a retinoid receptor gene on chromosome 3p24), *TIMP-3* (a matrix metalloprotease inhibitor on chromosome 22q13.1), the receptor a for estrogen (*ER-α*, on 6q 25.1), and the receptor for PRA progesterone (on 11q13).[8]

In some cases, genomic areas containing tumor suppressor genes are also susceptible to complete loss or deletion of both alleles. Certain tumor suppressor gene candidates, such as the gene encoding the p27^{KIP1} cell-cycle regulatory protein, exhibit the characteristic of haploid insufficiency, whereby (in contrast to *TP53*, *BRCA1*, *BRCA2*, *PTEN*, *CDKN2*, and *CDH1*) a single normal copy of the gene is not fully suppressive of cancer. For this type of suppressor gene, mutation, deletion, and LOH are not common in breast cancer.[9]

Another common type of cytogenetic alteration in breast cancer is gene amplification. The initial step in gene amplification is thought to be the formation of extrachromosomal, self-replicating units termed *double-minute chromosomes*. These genetic elements later become permanently incorporated into chromosomal regions and are termed *homogenous staining regions*. An amplified genetic unit (amplicon) is thought to be initially much larger than the actual size of the principal gene(s) of biologic importance to tumorigenesis. Thus, silent or irrelevant genes may be detected coamplified with one or more expressed genes on an amplicon. The principal, best-established amplified and functional genes for tumorigenesis (also called *dominant oncogenes*) detected to date in breast cancer are the growth factor receptor *HER2/neu* (*c-ERBB₂*), the nuclear transcription factors *c-MYC* and *AIB-1*, and the cell-cycle kinase regulator *CCND1*. In some cases, multiple genes may be coamplified; for example, *GRB-2* and *topoisomerase II*, coamplified with *HER2/neu*, may contribute to breast cancer pathogenesis. DNA gains are common on at least 35 distinct loci in breast cancer, including 6q, 8p, 8q, 11q, 12q, 13q, and 20q, although the specific genes involved in driving the chromosome amplification process are still under active investigation. BAC array CGH, coupled with gene expression microarray, has been used to catalog the genes reproducibly, up-regulated in association with their amplification.[10] For example, a neural survival factor termed *dermocydin* (on 12q 3.1) has been proposed as an oncogene in breast cancer.[10]

STEROID AND GROWTH FACTOR PATHWAYS OF CELLULAR REGULATION

STEROID RECEPTORS

This chapter focuses on ER and progesterone receptor (PR) because of the large body of evidence supporting their importance in breast cancer. However, considerable interesting current research has been reported on other nuclear receptors that is beyond our ability to cover adequately here (androgen, peroxisome proliferator, and retinoid receptors). The ER and PR are dimeric, gene regulatory proteins. Estrogen and progesterone are well-established endocrine steroid regulators that modulate multiple aspects of mammary gland pathology. These two hormones work together to direct mammary epithelial growth, differentiation, and survival.[11,12] Although both steroids are commonly thought to be of primary importance for tumors arising in the reproductively competent years, between puberty and menopause, local aromatization of adrenal androgens provides additional estrogens in the postmenopausal years. Estrogen and progesterone act through their nuclear receptors (ER and PR, respectively, introduced in Suppressor Genes and Oncogenes, earlier in this chapter) to modulate transcription of target genes.[11–13] Genes encoding the receptors for each class of steroids are members of a single large superfamily of transcription-modulating factors. ERs may exist either in homodimeric or heterodimeric species, composed of α and β receptors. In contrast, the PR is always a heterodimeric protein (with PRA and PRB subunits). Although ER-α is of key importance in the mammary ductal elongation of puberty, PR and ER-β appear to be more involved with lactational differentiation of the lobules.[12–14]

Work with ER-α, ER-β, and PR has defined additional alternately spliced and mutated receptor forms. Steroid receptors associate with other proteins, including heat-shock proteins, and several coactivator and corepressor proteins (CBP/p300, P/CAF, SRC-1, TIF2, AIB-1, N-CoR, SMRT, NSD1), which modulate the acetylation status of receptors and histones.[11,13,38] For example, CBP/p300 acetylates ER-α at lysine residues in the ER-α hinge/ligand-binding domain. Mutation of these residues selectively enhanced ER-α transactivation activity but not mitogen-activated protein kinase (MAPK) stimulation by ER-α (a newly recognized mode of action of estrogen, described at the end of this section). These results suggest an important role of ER-α acetylation for suppression of ER activity.[15] Histone acetylation is also a critical process, thought to allow full access of the DNA to steroid receptors. DNA interaction with steroid receptors occurs through zinc finger structures of the receptors and promotes formation of a stable initiation complex to facilitate the transcription of responsive genes. Superimposed on this complexity, each receptor is able to adopt multiple conformations, depending on the characteristics of interaction of the steroid (or nonsteroid ligand) with the receptor-binding pocket. For example, the ER can adopt multiple distinct conformations, depending on the nature of the specific ligand bound. Functional roles of the other kinase effectors are still under study.

Estrogen and progesterone are well known for their abilities to modulate directly the expression of growth factor receptor pathways and downstream, cell-cycle regulatory genes known as *nuclear protooncogenes*. The nuclear protooncoproteins and other cell-cycle regulatory proteins, such as AIB-1, c-Myc, and cyclin D1, represent points of regulatory convergence of steroid and growth factor pathways in cells.[12] Of considerable interest is the observation that the cell-cycle regulator cyclin D1 (product of the *CCND1* gene) also interacts with the ER-α to promote its transcriptional activity.[16] Parallel observations have also been made with the AIB-1 protein, for sensitization of ER transactivation (as well as growth factor signal transduction).[17] An alternatively spliced variant form of AIB-1 is even more potent for these effects.[18] Amplification and expression of AIB-1 and cyclin D1 are associated with ER-positive breast cancer.[39]

ER-α activation and nuclear localization, as well as coactivator interactions, are regulated through its phosphorylation.[11,13,19] Signal transduction pathways induced by growth factors and hormones may directly or indirectly regulate steroid receptor function through these phosphorylation events. Cyclic adenosine monophosphate, epidermal growth factor (EGF), heregulin (an EGF family member), and insulin-like growth factor-1 (IGF-1) are examples of such ER regulators, in which receptor phosphorylation modulates transactivation of steroid-responsive genes, as well as the steroid specificity of receptors for gene transactivation. The ER-α is phosphorylated on serine and threonine residues by cyclin A–CDK2, c-SRC, PKA, pp90[RSK1], ERK1/2, and p38.[11,19,20] Phosphorylation by the latter kinase on Thr[311] promotes nuclear localization and coactivator interaction.[19] A very exciting discovery has been that the ER may specifically localize to the plasma membrane, bind the p85 submit of phosphoinositide 3 kinase (PI3K), and deliver promitogenic and prosurvival signaling via Akt.[21] This represents a novel, "nongenomic" mode of ER action. The nuclear ER may be localized to the cytoplasm for these nongenomic actions via multiple potential mechanisms, including interaction with a shortened, variant inform of a protein termed *metastatic tumor antigen 1 (MTA1)*. MTA1 is up-regulated in several metastatic human cancers and acts to corepress nuclear ER-α by a nuclear exclusion mechanism.[22] Cytoplasmic ER is more available than nuclear for such nongenomic, plasma membrane protein interactions, as with PI3K. Plasma membrane transfer of ER-α from the cytoplasm may involve its specific interaction (via serine 522) with calveolin.[23] Caveolin may collaborate in breast tumor suppression, although at present its inactivating mutations have been demonstrated only in the scirrhous class of human breast cancers.[24] These findings provide multiple mechanisms and complex roles for growth factor interactions with steroid receptors in the expression of progressively more malignant phenotypes by breast cancer cells and in their escape from normal hormonal control.

Because the growth of breast cancer is often regulated by the female sex steroids, determinations of the cellular concentrations of ER and PR in the tumor continue to be used to predict which patients are of good prognosis and may also benefit from antihormonal therapy. Although these assays were originally designed as radioligand techniques, they are more commonly performed today using immunohistochemistry. To improve the value of determinations of the ER for tumor prognosis, the presence of the estrogen-regulated PR protein is routinely performed. In many breast tumor cell lines and in normal, ER-containing tissues, such as the endometrium and brain, PR expression is induced by estrogen.[11] It is still not known whether ER regulates PR in normal human mammary epithelium in precisely the same subpopulation of ductal and lobular luminal cells, although this supposition is considered to be likely. It is of interest that the ER and PR appear to be strongly up-regulated in ductal carcinoma *in situ* and in hormone-dependent breast cancer, relative to normal mammary epithelium. Whereas the ER- and PR-positive epithelial cell populations are distinct from the majority of proliferative cells in the normal gland, in cancer receptor-positive cells grow rapidly. It is of interest that in carcinoma *in situ* and in histologically normal breast tissue adjacent to cancer, the epithelium also displays an aberrant, proliferative response to estrogen.[25] This result suggests that breast tumorigenesis not only involves aberrant ER/PR expression but also aberrant coupling to a proliferative response. As noted earlier, in the section Familial Disease, other studies have made a connection between the ER and the tumor suppressor BRCA1. However, it is not yet known if BRCA1 down-regulation directly contributes to the early deregulation of ER levels or responses, or both, in human breast cancer.[7]

The relationship between estrogen exposure and onset of breast cancer is thought to relate to aberrant expansion of a mammary epithelial stem cell lineage. However, although mammary epithelial stem cells have been described morphologically by Chepko and Smith, and their cell surface markers described by Dontu et al.,[26] it is unknown whether these cells are direct precursors to breast cancer. For example, it is not yet certain how ER-positive mammary epithelial cells arise in the epithelial lineage, and it is not certain how ER-positive cancers relate to their ER-negative counterparts. Several ER-negative breast cancer cell lines do not transcribe the ER mRNA, because of an extensive methylation of the 5' promoter of the gene.[8] Treatment of ER-negative breast cancer cells *in vitro* with azacytidine, an inhibitor of gene methylation, resulted in expression of a functional ER.[10] However, the physiologic relevance of this methylation mechanism to silence ER expression during the progression of clinical breast cancer is not yet certain.

Central questions in breast cancer research focus on mechanisms of desensitization of the disease to antihormonal therapy and on design of strategies to maintain antihormonal responses in patients. Mechanisms include altered ER-α isoforms, coactivators (AIB-1), signaling partners (PI3K), and aromatase expression. Tamoxifen resistance of breast cancer is associated with cellular hypersensitization to the weak estrogenic effects of the drug, perhaps due to expression of receptor-associated regulatory proteins, receptor mutation, alterations in downstream growth regulatory pathways (MAPK, PI3K), or selection for variant ER-α receptor isoforms. An exon 5–deleted variant of the ER lacks the hormone-binding domain and displays constitutively active, hormone-independent transactivational characteristics. This receptor isoform is elevated in tamoxifen-relapsing breast cancer. Expression of an exon 4–deleted ER variant correlates with low histologic grade and high PR. Expression of other variants bearing deletions in exons 2 and 4 or 3-7 are associated with high-grade tumors with high ER content.[11]

The ER cannot be clearly classified either as an oncoprotein or tumor suppressor protein. ER expressed in ER-negative cell lines functions to suppress cell growth, in spite of its apparently normal action to regulate expression of certain hormonally responsive genes. Thus, the multiple differences between ER-positive and ER-negative breast cancer appear to include incompatible growth regulatory mechanisms. Pathways of estrogen metabolism may be dysregulated in breast cancer. Aromatase, which converts adrenal androgens to estrogen in the postmenopausal breast and in other tissues, may promote breast cancer growth.[27] AIB-1 and HER2/neu up-regulation is associated with tamoxifen resistance[28]; the use of aromatase inhibitors may bypass such effects, although other mechanisms of adaptive hypersensitivity to estrogen, such as up-regulated ER, MAPK, and PI3K activation may also result.[11,20,27] Other studies have suggested that receptors for other steroids (potential cancer prevention agents; retinoids and vitamin D) may modulate ER/PR function by modulating their chromatin interactions.[29]

GROWTH FACTOR PATHWAYS IN THE NORMAL AND MALIGNANT GLAND

The natural secretory products of the mammary epithelial cell, colostrum and milk, are abundant sources of growth factors.[30] Growth factors in the normal gland probably serve multiple purposes in the development of the newborn, in mammary growth, and in mammary carcinogenesis. A large body of literature has shown that estrogen, antiestrogens, progestins, and antiprogestins strongly regulate certain growth factors and receptors of the EGF and transforming growth factor-β families, as well as growth factors, receptors, and secreted binding proteins for the IGF family (Table 33.1-2). Most recently, the powerful methodology of gene expression profiling has reconfirmed earlier literature, now bringing the total to more than 400 robustly estrogen-regulated genes

involved in cell proliferation, signal transduction, and survival (see Table 33.1-2).[31] EGF, apparently the most abundant milk-derived growth factor, is an important regulator of the proliferation and the differentiation of the mouse mammary gland *in vivo* and of mouse mammary explants *in vitro*. Circulating, mouse salivary gland–derived EGF potentiates spontaneous mammary tumor formation and growth in the mouse models. EGF, or other members of this growth factor family, is a required supplement for clonal anchorage-dependent growth *in vitro* of normal human mammary epithelial cells. In contrast, human breast cancer cells in culture are largely independent of this exogenous requirement. However, most breast cancer cell lines retain EGF receptors (EGFRs) and appear to be stimulated in their growth by either autocrine or paracrine production of this family of factors.[30]

Direct modulation of signal transduction pathways by EGF and its family members, as well as their indirect regulation by other unrelated growth factors (described in Signal Transduction and Nuclear Oncogenes, later in this chapter), are critical during mammary development. The EGF family consists of four receptors and nearly two dozen growth factors in mammals and is encoded by certain mammalian viruses. Transforming growth factor-α (TGF-α) and amphiregulin, close structural and functional homologues of EGF, can produce qualitatively the same proliferative effects as EGF in mouse mammary explants and in cultured human and mouse mammary epithelial cell lines. Each of these factors is produced in proliferative early ductal development and in the later lobuloalveolar development of pregnancy. However, the detailed localization patterns and functions of each family member differ. For example, an immunohistochemical study of the mouse gland has revealed that expression of TGF-α is highest in the basal epithelial, proliferative end-bud cap cells, whereas expression of EGF is in scattered ductal luminal secretory cells.[31] Hepatocyte growth factor (HGF), a non-EGF family factor that interacts with its cognate receptor/oncoprotein c-Met, and growth hormone/IGF-1 also appears to be involved in ductal morphogenesis (described later in this section). The EGF-related neuregulin subfamily of isoforms (including heregulin) is expressed primarily in the mammary stroma and appears to modulate the lobuloaveolar development of pregnancy. TGF-α, the heparin-binding family member termed *amphiregulin*, and its common receptor, the EGFR, are both detected *in vitro* in proliferating human mammary epithelial cells in culture. TGF-α mRNA levels are relatively low in explanted, primary cultures of resting human mammary epithelial organoids; the entire system appears tightly coupled to proliferation in the normal gland. TGF-α and amphiregulin are known to act as autocrine autostimulatory growth factors in normal and immortalized human mammary epithelial cells in mass culture; an anti-EGFR antibody or heparin (respectively) reversibly inhibited proliferation. Although the majority of work on the biology of the EGF family has focused on regulation of proliferation, it is now clear that many other aspects of mammary biology may be under its control, such as cell differentiation and survival. The complex heterodimerization pattern of the EGFR family may play a role in governing the multiple responses of this system.[30] Transgenic expression of most members of the EGF family (including TGF-α and the neuregulins) in the mouse mammary gland have been shown to lead to mammary tumorigenesis.[30,31]

Although observations of overexpression of EGF family growth factors have led to significant biologic insights into the disease, the greatest clinical impact has come from the study of

TABLE 33.1-2. Estrogen Regulation of Growth Factor Systems: Signal Transduction and Transcription Factors in Breast Cancer

Growth Factor Systems	
Family of Molecules	Receptor/Growth Factor/Binding Protein
EGF FAMILY	
Growth factors	EGF, TGF-α, amphiregulin
Receptors	EGFR, c-erbB$_2$, c-erbB$_3$
IGF FAMILY	
Growth factors	IGF-II
Receptors	IGF-IR, IGF-IIR, insulinR
Binding proteins	BP-2, BP-3, BP-4, BP-5
TGF-β FAMILY	
Growth factors	TGF-β$_1$, TGF-β$_2$, TGF-β$_3$, BMP4, inhibin βB
Receptor	TGF- βR2
PDGF FAMILY	
Growth factors	PDGF-1, PDGF-2
INTERLEUKIN FAMILY	
Growth factor	IL-4
VEGF FAMILY	
Growth factor	VEGFA
STANNIOCALCIN FAMILY	
Growth factor	Stanniocalcin 1, stanniocalcin 2
Calcitonin family receptor	CalcitoninR
OSTEOCLAST-STIMULATING FACTOR FAMILY	
Growth factor	Osteoclast-stimulating factor-1

Other Signaling Pathway Components Regulated by Estrogen		
Signal Transduction	Cell-Cycle/Survival Factors	Transcription Factors/Coregulators
SOS	Cyclin D1	c-Fos
GRB10	CDC2	c-Myc
PI3K	CDC6	c-Myb
MAPK6	CDC20	a-Myb
SMAD3	Cyclin A2	b-Myb
IRS-1	PCNA	MAD
	p130	MAD 3
	DNA polymerase α	MAD 4
	DNA polymerase ε2	Jun B
	p21	Ets 2
	Survivin	NfkB
	BC12	SRC2
	Caspase 9	SRC3 (AIB-1)
		RARα
		RXRα

EGF, epidermal growth factor; IGF, insulin-like growth factor; IL-4, interleukin-4; PDGF, platelet-derived growth factor; TGF, transforming growth factor; VEGF, vascular endothelial growth factor. (Adapted from ref. 32.)

EGF family receptors. Gene amplification and resultant overexpression of EGFR-related HER-2/neu protein occur in approximately 25% of human breast cancer cases (see Table 33.1-1; discussed in Implications of Molecular Biology for Tumor Prevention, Early Detection Prognosis, and Response to Therapy, later in this chapter), and overexpression of the EGFR occurs in the absence of gene amplification in 40% of breast tumors. Expression of each protein signifies poor prognosis for the patient. Activational mutations in the extracellular domain of the Her-2/neu oncoprotein were commonly detected in transgenic mouse mammary carcinomas. Although this type of mutation seldom occurs, an alternate splice form of extracellular domain has been described in human breast cancer. Stimulation of cells through

the EGFR family may also sensitize cells to other carcinogenic insults. For example, expression of a TGF-α transgene accelerates the progression of carcinogen-initiated mouse mammary tumors. In summary, there is compelling evidence from human pathologic studies and from transgenic mouse models for key roles of EGF family growth factors and their receptors in mammary tumorigenesis, combining many types of data.[30,31]

In humans, autocrine and paracrine functions of the EGFR ligand system may be most critical in normal gland growth and early stages of breast tumorigenesis. In more advanced disease, paracrine, tumor-host interactive functions of this family of factors (discussed in Process of Malignant Progression, later in this chapter) may dominate. Strategies using humanized, anti-

HER-2/neu (Herceptin, or trastuzumab) or humanized anti-EGFR antibodies (IMC-225), or small molecule kinase inhibitors, are in various stages of clinical trial testing at present, because a large portion of hormone-independent breast cancers express significant levels of these receptors. Antitumor action of trastuzumab appears to depend on inhibition of PI3K/Akt for effects to increase p27, to decrease cyclin D1, to slow cell-cycle progression, and to induce apoptosis.[33]

A second growth factor family of potential importance in cancer is the fibroblast growth factor (FGF) family.[30] Members of this family have also been implicated in mammary gland growth and malignant transformation. These growth factors bind to heparin, require a heparin cofactor for proper presentation to and interaction with receptors, and accumulate in the extracellular matrix after their release from cells. Some FGF isoforms do not possess a signal sequence for secretion, but all forms appear to be released by one or more mechanisms from cells. Although FGF-1 and FGF-4 are expressed during the ductal growth phase of the mouse mammary gland in luminal ductal epithelial cells, expression of FGF-2 and FGF-7 is primarily stromal. FGF-1, FGF-2, and FGF-7 have been detected in mammary preneoplasias, tumors, and cell lines but not in levels significantly elevated over normal. FGF-3 (also known in the mouse as *int-2*) is a well-known oncogenic growth factor activated in the mouse mammary gland by mouse mammary tumor virus insertional mutagenesis. FGF-4 also has been associated with metastasis of certain mouse mammary tumors. Amplification of the genes encoding FGF-3 and FGF-4 in human breast cancer is not associated with increased protein levels. This finding appears to be the result of their coamplification with other more important genes located nearby on the chromosomes (genes encoding HER-2/neu and cyclin D1, respectively). In the human mammary gland, FGF-1 and FGF-2 have been localized to myoepithelial and to epithelial cells. Although *in vitro* studies have implicated FGF-2 as an autocrine growth factor in immortalized human mammary epithelial cells, expression of FGF-2 in clinical human breast cancer is correlated with good-prognosis disease. FGF-1 has been detected in human breast cancer, localized primarily to macrophages, and may thereby contribute to inflammation and angiogenesis. FGF receptors 1 to 4 (and the gene encoding FGFR1, occasionally amplified) are overexpressed in human breast cancer. Several of the FGF family members have been shown to promote tumor growth and dissemination of metastasis in xenograft models of human breast cancer, at least partially through effects on the tumor vasculature.[30]

TGF-β, a family of at least three growth factors distinct from FGF and EGF families, is also present in the normal and malignant mammary epithelium and in human milk.[33,34] Receptors for TGF-β comprise a family of heterodimeric serine-threonine kinases, signaling through interaction with Smad family proteins. TGF-β has antiproliferative effects on the mouse mammary gland ductal epithelium *in vivo* and on most other epithelial cell types. Expression of TGF-β family members is suppressed by estrogen and progesterone. TGF-β proteins are detected at the mRNA level in the developing mouse mammary epithelium. All isoforms of TGF-β, once produced, are retained in the stromal matrix surrounding the mammary ducts, although they are absent from the matrix of growing end buds and lateral branches. Glandular production of TGF-β decreases, along with its stromal accumulation around alveoli, during midpregnancy and lactation; TGF-β suppresses lactation. However, TGF-β is again elevated as postlactational glandular regression occurs.

The roles of TGF-β have also been examined by using a transgenic mouse approach. Mammary-targeted expression of TGF-β inhibits alveolar development and lactation. All three TGF-β isoforms have been detected in the human gland, with a similar distribution in the mouse. Although TGF-β serves a growth inhibitory role in the normal gland, progression to cancer may be associated with epithelial desensitization to this growth factor. Paradoxically, TGF-β production increases with malignant progression in breast cancer, perhaps promoting the fibrous desmoplastic stroma of the disease, for tumor angiogenesis and for immune suppression. Overproduction of TGF-β may contribute to aberrant tumor-host interactions in breast cancer. At least in some cell lines *in vitro*, TGF-β may stimulate tumor cell invasion. Loss of TGF-β receptor, by mutation or by loss of expression, has been observed in colon cancer and retinoblastoma, respectively. In breast cancer, interruption of signaling occurs more distally. Thus, TGF-β signals through heterodimeric types I and II receptors and phosphorylates Smad transcription factors. In early-stage human breast cancer, lack of Smad2P expression (an element in TGF-β receptor signaling) correlated with shortened overall survival from the disease. In addition, loss of Smad4 correlated with auxiliary lymph node metastases in higher-stage breast cancers. Interestingly, type III TGF-β receptor expression, previously thought simply to present the growth factor to its functional RI/II heterodimeric receptors, may serve to modulate TGF-β responses. Loss of its expression during breast cancer progression may serve to convert TGF-β from a tumor suppressor to a tumor promoter.[35]

A complex regulatory system is also emerging from studies of the insulin-like growth factors.[36] Although the IGFIR is a heterodimeric tyrosine kinase, closely related to the insulinR, the IGFIIR is an unrelated binding protein capable of interacting with TGF-β and with cathepsin D. IGF-II production, as well as cellular responsiveness to IGFs, is stimulated by estrogen and inhibited by antiestrogens in some hormone-dependent breast cancer cell lines. Cellular responsiveness is complex; IGF extracellular growth factor–binding proteins and intracellular signal transduction–coupling proteins (IRS-1 and -2) are regulated by multiple factors.[30,36] IGF-II is thought to be a potential autocrine growth factor in breast cancer. IGF-I, in contrast, is synthesized in the tumor stroma and has important paracrine growth and survival-stimulatory actions in the disease. Transgenic mouse models have demonstrated that mammary expression of IGF-I causes ductal hypertrophy and suppression of postlactational involution and that IGF-II expression can lead further, to mammary cancer. The cellular responsiveness to IGFs appears to be modulated by estrogens and antiestrogens, as a result of regulation of both receptors (type I being induced and type II repressed); IGF-binding proteins 2, 4, and 5 (each of which is estrogen induced) and IGF-binding protein 3 (which is estrogen inhibited); and the signal transduction docking phosphoprotein IRS-1 (which is estrogen induced). The biologic functions of the IGF-binding proteins are not fully understood, although BP-1 appears inhibitory of the actions of IGF-1, even with *in vivo* models. Although BP-3 may contribute to poor prognosis of breast cancer, BP-4 and the IGFIR correlate with good prognosis. IRS-1 (but not IRS-2) is up-regulated by estrogen and down-regulated by tamoxifen. The IGFRII is under active investigation as a tumor suppressor gene in cancers of the breast and other tissues. Its gene is subject to frequent LOH and possibly mutations in breast cancer.[36]

Several dozen other growth factors have been identified in breast cancer, but their consideration is beyond the scope of the current chapter because of limitations in availability. This information is reviewed elsewhere.[30,37] In brief, prolactin might be an autocrine positive factor in breast cancer, and mammary-derived growth inhibitor and mammostatin may serve negative growth functions. HGF/scatter factor (SF) is a stromal-derived paracrine-acting stimulator of epithelial growth and of tumor angiogenesis. HGF/SF, its oncogenic receptor c-Met, the proteolytic activator of HGF/SF termed *matriptase*, and the cognate inhibitor of matriptase, HAI-1, are all correlated with poor prognosis of the disease. Finally, the vascular endothelial growth factor (VEGF) family, pleiotrophin, and platelet-derived growth factors may serve as angiogenic, vascularization-inducing factors in the disease. Expression of VEGFA correlates with poor prognosis of human breast cancer because of its proangiogenic effects, whereas VEGFC and VEGFD induce lymphangiogenesis. Many other cytokines (such as osteopontin), Wnt family members, and other growth factors are also expressed in breast cancer. Future investigations should evaluate their pathophysiologic roles and possible targeting for therapy.[30,37]

SIGNAL TRANSDUCTION AND NUCLEAR ONCOGENES

Unifying, mechanistic links between the proliferative actions of growth- and survival-modulatory steroids, growth factors, and integrins in diverse tissues are represented by the multiple classes of nuclear protooncogenes and other transcription factors (see Table 33.1-1). These transcription-regulating proteins mediate convergent pathways of regulatory stimuli, directly through steroid action, through growth factor–induced MAPK, through other cytoplasmic tyrosine kinases (Fak, Src) or phospholipase C-PKC, through cytokine-induced JAK-STAT pathways, through TGF-β family–induced Smad molecules, and through integrin-induced Fak/Src pathways. Steroid and growth factor pathways ultimately regulate gene expression through specific acetylation of histones and transcription factors. Activation of different members of the histone acetyltransferase family of enzymes causes these key acetylation reactions to proceed; specific histone deacetylases are also recruited to sites of active, regulated transcription, to allow for tight control on these processes. Components of the cell-cycle regulation apparatus are under control by acetylation and deacetylation, making this mode of regulation key to the onset, progression, and potential treatment of breast cancer.[38,39]

The MAPK pathways are central to proliferative and survival stimuli, exerted through the EGFR, HER-2/neu, and insulinR type I families. Receptors trigger this pathway through autophosphorylation and subsequent binding to SH2/SH3 or PTB domains of signal transduction adaptor proteins. After mitogenic growth factor treatment of many types of cells, including normal and malignant breast epithelial cells, a cascade of protein phosphorylations occurs. Expression of early-response genes is induced, including c-Myc, AP-1 (activator protein 1) acting (c-Fos, c-Jun, and Jun B), c-Myb, and Ets protooncogenes and ATF, EIK, SRF, and NFKB transcription factors are commonly observed to be induced. The protein products of multiple nuclear protooncogenes, *c-Myc, c-Fos, c-Jun,* and *cyclin D1* are also induced by estrogen and by progesterone in breast cancer. Progestins additionally induce JunB. Not surprisingly, tamoxifen down-modulates c-Myc expression, followed by

cyclin D1 expression, during treatment-induced regression of patient tumors. c-Myc, c-Fos, c-Jun, and cyclin D1 induction have also been shown to occur in human mammary epithelial cells *in vitro* and in the rat uterus in response to estrogen treatment *in vivo.* Cyclin D2 is a nuclear oncoprotein downstream of AP-1 and other mitogenic transcriptional controls. Not only does it regulate the G_1 phase of the cell cycle, but it also enhances ER transactivational activity.[39]

c-Fos and c-Jun proteins contain specific domains that allow them to form a heterodimeric complex that can interact with gene promoter consensus sequences termed *AP-1.* In an analogous manner, the c-Myc protein, of central importance to estrogenic stimulation of breast cancer cells, dimerizes with another protein termed *Max* to modulate genes through a different consensus sequence, termed an *E-Box* (and possibly other sequences). The cellular supply of Max that is available for productive dimerization with c-Myc depends on its interaction with its other family members, termed *Mad* and *Mxil.* The interaction of Max with either of these proteins serves to reduce its availability for interactions with Myc and may exert negative transactivation through E-box sites. Myc-Max dimers are known to induce proliferation, apoptosis, and chromosomal instability, depending on the cellular context and degree of expression. Myc-Max interaction with TATA binding protein stimulates basal transcription. Secondly, Myc-Max complexes bind promoters of genes, such as those encoding the CAD, DHFR, and ODC enzymes, through their E-boxes. However, multiple c-Myc–regulated genes do not contain E-box sequences, and these sequences are not required for c-Myc effects on proliferation and apoptosis. Several other c-Myc–interactive proteins exist in addition to TATA binding protein and Max, including TRRAP, BIN1, DAM, p107, YYI, MIZ1, and TFII-1, which contribute to transcriptional effects of c-Myc. Estrogen and progesterone induce c-Myc and cyclin D1. c-Myc may modulate the mammary epithelial cell cycle by inducing the synthesis of CDK4, triggering the degradation of p27[kip1], and suppressing p21 and p15[ink4B] transcription, possibly through interaction with Miz-1, inactivating CDK2. Activation of CDK2 inhibits pRb phosphorylation, promoting G_1/S cell-cycle progression. c-Myc induces cyclin A to activate CDK2 and induces E_2F_1 to promote S-phase cell-cycle progression. However, c-Myc can induce apoptosis through p53-dependent and possibly independent mechanisms. Thus, effects of c-Myc are highly complex and likely to depend on a multitude of environmental and other cellular factors.[39,40]

Antisense c-Myc oligonucleotides block estrogen-induced proliferation in breast cancer cells, and amplification of the *c-MYC* gene is a common genetic alteration in breast cancer; approximately one-fifth of breast cancers contain this genetic change. A putative suppressor gene (possibly *HME1*, encoding 14-3-3σ) on chromosome 1p32-pter is proposed to interact with *c-MYC* to suppress its gene amplification in breast cancer.[39,40] *c-MYC* protein has a very short half-life, and few suitable monoclonal antibodies are capable of specifically staining paraffin sections. *c-MYC* amplification is associated with poor prognosis, high S phase, and postmenopausal disease, although the latter has not been confirmed.[40] Based on several investigations in various epithelial malignancies, including those of the ovary and liver, *c-MYC* amplification is thought to cooperate with TGF-α, with EGFR overexpression, and with downstream signaling pathways (notably Ras) to activate the cell cycle and suppress apoptosis. Thus, dual stimulation of the EGFR pathway and c-Myc may serve a general cooperative function in epithelial transformation.[40]

The c-Myc protein promotes cell proliferation, inhibits differentiation, modulates cell adhesion, effects immune recognition, regulates initiation of DNA replication, and modulates DNA and energy metabolism, perhaps in part through activation of expression of telomerase.[40] Induction of apoptosis by c-Myc in mouse models depends on p19[ARF] (p14[ARF] in humans; see Cell Cycle and Cell Death) stabilization of p53 function, although a role for this mechanism in mammary cancer remains to be demonstrated. Expression of c-Myc increases with aging in multiple tissue types and has been proposed to contribute to aberrant mitogenic responses of the tissue in postmenopausal breast cancer, although increased expression of Mxil during aging may attenuate such effects.[41]

CELL CYCLE AND CELL DEATH

TUMOR SUPPRESSOR GENES AND THE CELL CYCLE

Seminal studies by Broca in the nineteenth century established that breast cancer can have a familial pattern of onset in 5% to 10% of cases. Subsequently, in studies of the inherited childhood cancer syndrome retinoblastoma, of familial cancers, Knudson[42] proposed the "two-hit model" of tumor suppressor gene function. In addition, Harris[39] demonstrated that certain chromosomes could suppress malignancy *in vitro* in cell hybrid studies. These three concepts led to the discovery of several tumor suppressor genes in breast cancer, some encoding proteins regulating the cell cycle (p16, Rb, p53) or cell death (p53, Pten), or both, and others regulating other aspects of the progression of the disease (E-cadherin). A variety of tumor suppressor–like proteins have also been described, which are down-modulated but seldom mutated in nonfamilial breast cancer (such as the gene encoding p27, BRCA1, Syk, KAI-1, Kiss1, and nm23).[39,43,44]

During the malignant progression of breast cancer to its fully metastatic state, mutation, inactivation, loss, or down-regulated expression of tumor-suppressing genes commonly occurs. Estimated incidences of these processes for the relevant, known suppressor genes are as follows: *TP53* (30% to 40%), *RB-1* (15% to 20%), *CDKN2* (20% to 30%), and *CDH1* (20% to 30%). Tumor suppressor genes appear to function in at least four major ways: as antiproliferative or antisurvival factors, as DNA-repair inducers (all in DNA damage-response pathways), and as differentiation-promoting agents. BRCA1 and BRCA2 serve roles to direct repair of damaged DNA; the ATM protein (described earlier in Familial Disease as a suspected tumor suppressor) detects the damage and transmits the signal to the BRCA proteins, whereas multiple other proteins, such as Rad51 and p53, serve roles downstream of the BRCAs.[45] E-cadherin sequesters β-catenin (a proliferation-promoting protein that regulates the T-cell factor class of transcription factors) and strengthens homotypic interactions of mammary epithelial cells to maintain their differentiated status.[46] p53, by inducing the p21 protein (Waf-1/CIP-1), also inhibits proliferation, whereas the p16 protein also serves to inhibit the cell cycle; p53 and p16 suppressor proteins ultimately promote phosphorylation and inactivation of pRb to block G_1 and G_1/S transit of the cell cycle. Although pRb is thought to be a central tumor suppressor protein in breast cancer, its inactivation is likely to occur through cyclin D1 overexpression, and pRb

mutation status remains to be fully assessed. Pten serves to suppress cell survival and proliferation by dephosphorylating phosphoinositides to prevent their activation of the three AKT signal transduction kinases.[47] Dozens of additional candidate tumor suppressor genes are reviewed elsewhere.[43]

Study of the *TP53* gene has provided remarkable insights into multiple areas of cancer biology. *TP53* is a tumor suppressor gene, but, when mutated in one of several sensitive regions, its conformation changes, its stability increases, and its regulatory properties are radically altered. Mutation can confer a loss of tumor suppressor activity or gain, or both, of tumor promotion function. The nonmutated p53 gene product is an oligomeric DNA-binding protein that functions to trigger cellular responses to DNA damage; it has been termed *guardian of the genome*. p53 functions by protein–protein interactions and by regulation of transcription. As noted under New Methodologies and Genetic Mechanisms, earlier in this chapter, the p53 protein appears to function in the context of DNA damage as a G_1/S and G_2/M checkpoint controller, to slow cell growth and induce DNA repair; cell death is triggered in a process termed *apoptosis* if damage is too severe for repair. It is of particular importance for the progression of many cancers, including breast cancer, that mutation of p53 is associated with enhanced genetic instability. Certain viral proteins, although they are probably not relevant to breast cancer, are known to inactivate p53 as a critical event in viral carcinogenesis.[50,51] Mutation of p53 not only abrogates the G_1/S checkpoint but also G_2/M and a post M spindle assembly checkpoint.[48] Two family members of p53, termed *p73* and *p63*, are under current study of their p53-like properties.[48]

It is not yet fully clear what molecular events induce (through protein stabilization) the p53 protein. However, it is well known that ultraviolet irradiation and double-strand DNA breaks are strong inducers of p53 stabilization through the DNA-dependent protein kinase and the ATM gene product. ATM is a signal transduction protein with high homology to PI3K. Inhibitors of protein kinase C, or serine-threonine phosphatases, and cyclic adenosine monophosphate can prevent p53-mediated responses. p53 induces growth arrest, in part through induction of p21, and thereby inhibition of cyclin E–CDK2–catalyzed phosphorylation of pRb (discussed in Cyclins, Cyclin-Dependent Kinases, and Inhibitors, later in this chapter). p53 regulates pRb and directly binds a partner of pRb termed *p107*. p53 induces transcription of DNA repair genes, including cyclin G, ERCC, and Gadd 45. A third general process triggered by p53 is apoptotic death. Negative regulators of p53 include phosphorylations by several kinases, acetylation by histone acetylase, its nuclear exclusion, and, most importantly, its degradation through a ubiquitin ligase called *MDM-2* (murine double-minute gene-2). MDM-2 is itself a p53-inducible protein that can function as a collaborative oncogene (at least in some cancers other than breast cancer).[48]

The nuclear tumor suppressor protein pRb is inactivated by phosphorylation and catalyzed by several cyclin-dependent protein/kinases and through binding growth regulatory proteins, including c-Myc, SP1, C/EBP, ID2, histone deacetylases, c-Abl, and many other transcription factors. pRb restricts entry into the S phase of the cell cycle. Hypophosphorylated Rb binds E_2F-1 and DP-1 family members to restrict access of these transcription factors to the chromatin. The result is a blockade of transcription from genes involved in $G_1 \rightarrow S$ progression and S phase in the cell cycle.[30,38,48,49]

CYCLINS, CYCLIN-DEPENDENT KINASES, AND INHIBITORS

As discussed earlier, growth factors, oncogenes, and tumor suppressors function to a large extent in the G_1 phase of the cell cycle. The cell cycle is directly controlled by an ordered series of cyclin-dependent kinases (CDKs), their positive regulatory subunits (cyclins), and their inhibitors (CDK inhibitors). Early G_1 is driven by the three cyclin D family members bound to CDK4 and CDK6. In the next portion of the cycle, the $G_1{\rightarrow}S$ transition is driven by cyclin E–CDK2. The S phase is driven by cyclin A–CDK2, and then the $G_2{\rightarrow}M$ transition is driven by cyclin B/A–CDC2 (CDK1).[30,38]

As important regulators of the epithelial cell cycle in breast cancer, tyrosine kinase receptor–acting growth factors and sex steroids function to induce c-Myc and cyclin D1. Thus, HER2/neu may exert its proliferative effects through a required induction of c-Myc and cyclin D1. HER2/neu (in contrast to c-Myc) fails to induce mammary tumors in mice rendered nullizygous for cyclin D1. Cyclin D1 knockout mice are also defective for lobuloalveolar development in the mammary gland. Cyclin D1–CDK4 is inhibited by the CDKI termed *p16* (*INK4a*), by the tumor-suppressive CDKI p16 (MTS1 or INK4b), and by p18 and p19, other members of the same CDKI family. Cyclin D–CDK4 and cyclin E–CDK2 are also each inhibited by the CDKI termed *p21* (*Waf-1/CIP1*, which is induced by p53), by p27 (kip1), and by p57 (kip2), which may be involved in mammary epithelial cell senescence. c-Myc has been shown to induce or inhibit cyclin D1 expression in cycling cells, to induce cyclin E (and possibly CDC 25A), and to trigger the proteosome-mediated destruction of the CDKI p27 (kip1) and activation of CDK2. c-Myc also dysregulates S phase by inducing cyclin A (to activate CDK1) and by inducing E_2F-1.[30,38,40,49,51] The synthesis of c-Myc and CDK4 is inhibited by TGF-β and CDK4; overexpression of CDK4 leads to TGF-β resistance. p27 is induced by TGF-β. As noted in the previous section, pRb is phosphorylated and inactivated by the combined actions of cyclin D–CDK4 and cyclin E–CDK2 kinases. The result of all of the multitude of common oncogenic and tumor suppressor aberrations in breast cancer seems to be similar: defective $G_1{\rightarrow}S$ transitions in the mammary epithelial cell cycle.[52] In addition, DNA damage-induced checkpoints of G_1/S, G_2/M, and post M are commonly abrogated; cells lose proliferative requirements for estrogen, growth factors, and cell substrate adhesion; and they lose inhibition by TGF-β family growth factor.[39]

APOPTOTIC MECHANISMS AND SURVIVAL SIGNALING

The mammary gland undergoes cycles of proliferation followed by programmed cell death. The menstrual cycle generates such cycles on a limited scale (with cell death occurring just after the luteal phase), and significant apoptotic death results at the end of pregnancy (involution). The latter effect has been proposed to contribute to the breast cancer–protective effects of early pregnancy in women. Regulation of members of the Bcl family of proteins is central to these cell mechanisms. Estrogen and activation of the HER-2/neu, EGFR, and insulin receptor all induce the antiapoptotic Bcl-2 and Bcl-X_L family members. These growth factors activate PI3K, creating the phospholipid IP3, which activates the Akt kinase. Akt phosphorylates the forkhead transcription faction [controlling proapoptotic Fas ligand, caspase 9, the antiapoptotic Bad protein, and the IκB kinase (Iκκα, Iκκβ),

which activates NFκB, β-catenin, and Bcl-X_L/Bcl-2]. In contrast, p53 and c-Myc up-regulate proapoptotic Bax. Thus, Bcl-2 and Bcl-X_L, induced by growth factors and other stimuli, block apoptosis; Bcl-2 is commonly expressed in p53-mutated breast cancer cells. The balance of pro- and antiapoptotic Bcl family members leads to control of mitochondrial membrane permeability to cytochrome c and other regulators of the caspase cascade (initiated by caspase 9), a protease system serving to execute death pathway signals. Bcl-2 is localized in the mitochondria, nuclear membrane, and endoplasmic reticulum. It functions, along with Bcl-X_L, to suppress the function of Bax, a death-inducing protein; the entire Bcl family acts to integrate pro- and antiapoptotic stimuli by forming mitochondrial pores of differential ionic permeability. Several other stimulatory and inhibitory family members exist, including Bcl-X_s, a promoter of apoptotic death. The apoptotic system is thought to be triggered by hypoxia or by a shift in the redox potential of the cell. A distinct set of proapoptotic signals may be initiated by ligation of death receptors on the cell surface by tumor necrosis factor, FasL, and other cytokines to initiate caspase 8–dependent death pathway signals to the same executor caspases (such as caspase 3).[53,54]

Although quite complex, the balance of life/apoptosis is critically regulated in cancer progression and response to therapy. Estrogen, progesterone, TGF-α, EGF, and insulin all appear to suppress apoptosis and promote survival of breast cancer model systems. Antiestrogens, antiprogestins, TGF-β, and the overexpressed c-Myc oncoprotein can induce apoptosis unless countered with a survival-promoting, environmental influence.

Approximately 80% of breast cancers express Bcl-2, and expression is correlated with the ER, whereas Bcl-X_L predominates in ER-negative breast cancers. Bax expression is generally low in breast cancer, and its expression has been correlated in some studies with better survival and responsiveness to chemotherapy. However, a large study has failed to associate any of these effectors of apoptosis with responsiveness of advanced human breast cancer to chemotherapy.[54]

ROLES OF ESTROGEN AND PROGESTERONE IN CELL CYCLE AND CELL DEATH

The well-orchestrated program of proliferation and apoptosis in the normal mammary gland depends on the regulated cycles of estrogen and progesterone. In breast cancer, these two steroids remain key regulators of a significant fraction of cases. In terms of cell-cycle regulation in breast cancer, estrogen induces c-Myc and cyclin D1, and cyclin D1 activates CDK4/6, and estrogen and c-Myc then activate cyclin E/CDK2. Cyclin E/CDK2 is not inhibited by p21 due to effects of estrogen (possibly through c-Myc) to block synthesis of p21. Estrogen synergizes with insulin for cell-cycle progression, potentially through p21 interactions.[55]

Estrogen induces c-Myc[55] and cyclin D1 transcription to promote S-phase entry. ER interaction with a complex containing the Src tyrosine kinase and p85-PI3K/Akt appear to be required for cyclin D1 induction.[56] Estrogen also induces Bcl-2 transcription, providing a strong antiapoptotic signal.[57] Antiestrogen suppresses transcription of c-Myc and cyclin D1, and antisense c-Myc mimics the effect of antiestrogens. Antiestrogen also promotes apoptosis of mammary tumors *in vivo*.[55]

In contrast to the actions of estrogen, progestins first transiently stimulate breast epithelial and breast cancer proliferation but then suppress proliferation. This antiproliferative effect is due to induction of p27 to block cyclin D-Cdk4/6 and p18 (INK4c) to block cyclin E–CDK2 complexes.[58]

PROCESS OF MALIGNANT PROGRESSION

Malignant progression of breast cancer involves the conversion of "benign proliferative lesions" and carcinomas *in situ* to early (stages I and II) disease, to locally advanced (stage III) disease, and then to metastasis to bone, brain, lungs, and other sites (stage IV). Fundamental to malignant progression are the heterotypic processes regulating epithelial mesenchymal transition, hypoxia, desmoplasia, and angiogenesis.[30,43,59] The development of cancer involves suppression of apoptosis and senescence, dysregulation of proliferative signaling factors, activation of oncogenes, dysregulation of growth inhibitory factors, and loss of tumor suppressor genes (see Fig. 33.1-1).[30,39]

Genetic damage is minimal in benign breast disease or premalignant atypical ductal or lobular lesions, and expression of hTERT (catalytic submit of the DNA replication-associated enzyme telomerase) is induced, suggesting that suppression of cell senescence may occur early in disease.[60] High levels of telomerase expression lead to cell immortalization, and the catalytic subunit of this enzyme (hTERT), together with three oncogenes—SV40T (a viral oncogene, which inactivates p53 and Rb), Sv40 small t (which inactivates the PP2A phosphatase), and a mutant c-Ras^H—convert human mammary epithelial cells to cancer.[61] Human and mouse cells critically differ in a signal transduction pathway activated by Ras^H that is required for transformation: The Raf/MAPK pathway is dominant in mouse cells, whereas in human cells, the key pathway is that of Ras GPS/PI3K. *c-MYC* was commonly amplified in these cells. Telomerase overexpression has been detected in the earliest stages of breast cancer, as noted earlier; it is known to be induced by estrogen and by c-Myc. Thus, telomerase dysregulation may serve a subtle, early function in breast tumorigenesis: replicative immortality.[60,61]

The subsequent steps in tumorigenesis almost entirely involve spontaneous gene amplification, LOH, methylation, and mutations, which arise as a result of overactive cell cycles, defective cell cycle checkpoints, or defective cell death responses.[62] Multiple oncogenes and tumor suppressor genes (*BRCA1*, *p53*, *c-Myc*, *Akt*, *Rb*, *p21*, *p27*) are involved. Once these types of genetic alterations begin to occur, a cascade of further genetic changes occurs, resulting from overall genomic and chromosomal instability.[6–8,62] Familial disease may bypass one or more steps in this cascade.[3] The mechanisms for genetic instability and accumulation of further mutations in other cancers, such as colon cancer, have been proposed to depend initially on overexpression of a mutator gene termed *MSH2*. To date, however, these mechanisms have not been fully evaluated for breast cancer, and mismatch repair defects appear to be associated primarily with later stages of progression metastasis of breast cancer. In contrast to colon cancer, in breast cancer centrosomal defects appear to predominate in early disease, potentially causing the chromosomal type of instability.[7,62]

Almost certainly, some of the most important consequences of these changes in genomic stability initially relate to therapeutic responses. As discussed earlier in Steroid and Growth Factor Pathways of Cellular Regulation, the mechanisms of antihormonal therapy failure in hormone receptor–positive disease may potentially relate to sensitization of the tumor to very low levels of sex hormones and to the partially estrogenic properties of the clinically used hormonal antagonists, such as tamoxifen. Chemotherapy resistance in breast cancer is also not fully understood but probably involves altered cell death responses and altered metabolism of the drugs. Resistance to radiation therapy may involve defects in the ATM pathway (including BRCA proteins and p53), leading to DNA damage–induced death. During malignant progression after treatment, additional amplifications, LOHs, and mutations occur. The cancer cells with the greatest capacity for growth, invasion, or survival undergo positive selection. Other cells may be more susceptible to necrotic or apoptotic death. Studies have detected genetic changes in histologically normal tissue surrounding breast tumors, consistent with this clonal evolution hypothesis.[62]

Certain common patterns of cytogenetic alterations and gene expression exist in breast tumors, reflecting signatures of distinct initiating lesions and pathways of progression. Acquired genetic changes may interact unfavorably with residual growth regulatory pathways operating in the normal tissue. For example, an unfavorable interaction occurs between cyclin D1 overexpression and the ER.[16] Amplified *HER-2/neu* or *c-MYC* genes synergize with the presence of an autocrine- or paracrine-activated EGFR system. *HER-2/neu* amplification associated with activation of *c-RAS^H* gene is also an unfavorable interaction. The tyrosine kinase signal transduction pathways (such as those downstream of c-Ras^H) that govern proliferation or survival, or both, enhance oncogenesis induced by c-Myc in cellular models *in vitro* and in transgenic mouse models of mammary cancer. c-Myc–induced tumors are enhanced by overexpression of apoptosis-suppressing Bcl-2. Finally, mutant p53 enhances HER-2/neu–induced tumors by blocking apoptotic pathways.[30,39]

An important approach for the future understanding of this phenomenon involves generation of the transgenic and gene knockout mouse models, which more faithfully recapitulate human disease. Investigators could harness these models to understand mechanisms of breast cancer onset and progression. Such studies may identify the biochemical and cellular bases of various patterns of malignant progressions. Future studies aimed at detailed characterization of the interaction of ER, PR, growth factors, protooncogenes, and suppressor genes with therapeutic approaches in animal models may determine molecular genetic interactions governing onset and progression of breast cancer.[30,31]

The ultimate event that leads to mortality from breast cancer is metastasis. Two separate, but apparently interactive, cellular processes seem to occur to allow metastasis of the disease: tumor angiogenesis and loss of proper tissue compartmentalization (invasion).[63] The process of tumor-stromal interactions becomes disrupted in multiple aspects in malignant progression. Loss of cell-cell attachment, altered cell substratum attachment, and altered cytoskeletal organization play a role in regulating cellular invasion. In addition, cell locomotion, proteolysis, and the ability to survive and proliferate at distant sites also must contribute. Although acquisition of this group of characteristics is responsible for a cancer to invade host tissue locally, the ability of a tumor to distribute itself to distant sites also requires the development of a tumor vasculature: the complex process of angiogenesis.[30,37] Some studies have shown that metastatic alterations may have at least some genetic basis and that distant metastases are more likely to exhibit dominance of a malignant clone than are primary tumors.

In human breast cancer, a well-established precursor of invasive disease is carcinoma *in situ* (either ductal or lobular varieties, DCIS and LCIS, respectively). DCIS and LCIS may be characteristic of hypoxic areas, indicating oxygen starvation of epithelial cells as they proliferate beyond a normal pseudostratified layer to fill the ductal and lobular structures. A normal response of such cells to hypoxia is to trigger a stress response program governed by hypoxia-inducible factor 1α.[64] This factor controls metabolic adaptation to hypoxia through regulation of glycolysis, angiogenesis (through VEGF), and proliferation/survival (through IGF-2 and c-Met transcription).[64,65] Thus, carcinomas *in situ* may be under selective pressure to use these growth factor/receptor pathways for their survival. In the case of c-Met function, cleavage of its cognate ligand HGF is required. This may involve expression of uPA/PAI-1 and matriptase/HAI-1 serine protease systems, which have been shown to be expressed in poor-prognosis, early-stage breast cancers.[66,67] As growth factors, such as VEGF and HGF, are expressed in early development of invasive breast cancers, the stroma becomes more fibrotic (desmoplastic), expressing characteristic extracellular matrix proteins (such as tenacin C and versican).[68] Angiogenesis also is a response of these developing lesions, contributing to their progression toward tumorigenesis.[69]

The E-cadherin cell-cell adhesion protein plays a central role in maintaining breast epithelial tissue structure, suppressing invasive behavior, and suppressing proliferation. In addition, it maintains a characteristic cytoskeletal organization. Loss of E-cadherin, through its genetic mutation or methylation, its expression, or its protein modification, is of central importance to progression of breast cancer. Not only does loss of E-cadherin serve to promote cell motility and invasion, but it also serves to release β-catenin, an oncogenic-transcription factor.[46] The *E-cadherin* gene promoter is under complex regulation by multiple factors, including negative regulation by the Snail zinc finger transcription factor. Interestingly, estrogen appears to down-regulate expression of E-cadherin in breast cancer cells, potentially contributing to the progression of the disease.[70] However, estrogen also may function in some respects to suppress Snail expression (through a protein termed *MTA3*), to maintain epithelial morphology of breast tumors. Loss of functional E-cadherin contributes to an "epithelial-mesenchymal transition," characterized by expression of mesenchymal cadherins (-N and −11), more fibroblastic morphology, increased motility, and increased tissue invasiveness.[71] Experimental studies targeting Rho family guanosine triphosphatase (involved in cell motility) have successfully suppressed metastatic dissemination of mammary tumor cells without modulating primary tumor growth.[72]

Malignant progression involves colonization of distant organs by the spreading tumor cells. cDNA gene expression microarray studies suggest the key genes involved in these final steps. For example, a study in bony metastasis has identified a characteristic multigenic program in such cells, involving interleukin-11, matrix metalloproteinase 1 (MMP-1), connective tissue–derived growth factor, and bone-homing chemokine receptor.[73]

IMPLICATIONS OF MOLECULAR BIOLOGY FOR TUMOR PREVENTION, EARLY DETECTION, PROGNOSIS, AND RESPONSE TO THERAPY

A major hope in the study of genetic changes in breast cancer is that they will lead to development of new prevention and early-detection strategies, therapies, and prognostic tools.[13] More rapid, accurate, and cost-effective assays of determining mutations in *BRCA1* and *BRCA2* are needed to better identify women with a familial propensity for breast cancer. In addition, the gene(s) responsible for a significant number of breast cancer families (more than half) remain to be identified, and the bases (genetic and/or environmental) for the variable penetrance of the *BRCA* genes remain to be determined. Women at high risk will undoubtedly be an important population of emphasis for future prevention trials. Although the benefits of prophylactic mastectomy and oophorectomy are now established, tamoxifen is also now known to be an effective prevention strategy. However, in the specific context of *BRCA* carriers, tamoxifen appears to be effective for prevention of breast cancer selectively initiated by *BRCA2* (but not *BRCA1*).[74] A major current trial is comparing tamoxifen to raloxifene (an antiestrogen thought to produce fewer endometrial cancers and to provide other benefits).[13] However, new pharmacologic or dietary strategies are needed, particularly to prevent ER-negative breast cancer. For example, a novel approach could use the dietary compound indole-3-carbinol to block the effects of the ER to promote breast tumorigenesis.[75]

In the area of screening and early detection, the authors now know that overproduction of growth factors such as TGF-α and HGF is very common, but they have not yet been shown to distinguish benign proliferative disease from malignant disease. It is possible that detection of telomerase expression, or the ability to detect subtle genetic alterations, will provide useful new approaches for marking the onset of cancer. Development of new nipple aspirate methodologies (such as ductal lavage), blood and urinary assays for growth factors, growth factor receptors, autoantibodies to oncoproteins, and tumor DNA are also currently under way. The new technique, made available by the rapid advancement of the field of proteomics, now renders these realistic avenues for exploration.[76,77]

In the area of prognosis and response to therapy, much hope has been vested in development of more accurate and rapid methods for immunohistochemical and fluorescent *in situ* methodologies for characterization of oncogenes, suppressor genes, and related proteins. Serum and plasma assays for growth factors are also of interest, in addition to more classic tumor markers of CA15.3 and CEA (carcinoembryonic antigen) for determining prognosis and response to therapy. Sensitive assays to detect tumor-derived cells and DNA in the blood are also under development. Again, advances in proteomic analysis of blood and tissue biopsies may lead the way for these studies in the next decade.[78] Detection of ER and PR in tumors has established the field of integration of molecular markers into clinical decisions regarding prognosis and response to therapy. Gene expression microarray studies now provide a new way to classify breast cancers, as a basal epithelial class, an HER-2/neu–overexpressing class, an ER-positive luminal epithelial class, and an ER-luminal epithelial class have been distinguished in this manner.[79] High-risk, early-stage breast cancers are also distinct in their gene expression profile from lower-risk early-stage cancers.[80] These gene expression array methods will need to be converted to methods compatible with archival tissue analysis (such as RNA extraction/real-time PCR) for general application to breast cancer diagnosis and prognosis. As described in Growth Factor Pathways in the Normal and Malignant Gland, earlier in this chapter, other studies have identified specific growth factor receptor systems (Met/HGF) and protease inhibitor systems (uPA/PAI-1 and matriptase/HAI-1) that can be applied as poor-prognosis markers for early-stage disease using antibody/histochemistry methodology.[66,67]

Pure antiestrogens and aromatase inhibitors are now in clinical trials for ER-positive relapsing tumors. Studies to detect the co-expression of cyclin D1 and AIB-1 with ER have provided new insights into mechanisms for resistance to tamoxifen.[28,87] A hope is that resistance to tamoxifen may be known prospectively and an alternate, ultimately more successful mode of hormonal therapy prescribed. The HER-2/neu oncoprotein also indicates poor-prognosis tumors and poor response to adjuvant hormonal therapy and chemotherapy. Although technically more difficult to measure, the EGFR is also of interest for future study of tumors that are likely to have a poor prognosis and poor response to hormonal therapy. Because of common expression or overexpression of these two receptors in breast cancer, they are now targets of new experimental therapies using tyrosine kinase inhibitors, antibodies to their extracellular domains, and coupling or gene-fusing these antibodies to toxic moieties.[33,81]

A large group of studies have confirmed that 20% to 30% of breast tumors contain an amplification of the *HER-2/neu* gene and overexpress the encoded receptor protein. *HER-2/neu* is also overexpressed in a very high portion of ductal carcinoma *in situ*. Expression of the HER-2/neu protein is associated with an elevated mitotic rate; it correlates with poor clinical response to certain chemotherapeutic and antihormonal drugs [5-fluorouracil, methotrexate, cyclophosphamide (Cytoxan), and tamoxifen-containing regimens] and insensitivity to tamoxifen *in vitro*. HER-2/neu expression is also associated with poor prognosis in patients who do not receive treatment with chemotherapeutic or antihormonal drugs. The *HER-2/neu* gene amplification association with poor prognosis may relate to response to treatment with chemotherapy and hormonal therapy.[82,83] Gene expression profiling is now yielding new insights into the determinants of resistance of breast cancer to chemotherapy.[84,85]

The HER-2/neu protein also holds significant interest for breast tumor immunology. Certain antibodies to the extracellular domain of this protein seem to sensitize cells to killing by *cis*-platinum, carboplatinum, and doxorubicin *in vivo*. It is thought that the mechanism of this effect is interference with DNA repair mechanisms. As noted above, the shed extracellular domain of HER-2/neu may represent a useful antigenic blood-borne marker of breast cancer burden and the protein itself a new target of immunotherapy of cancer.[33,86] Specifically, the humanized, anti–HER-2/neu antibody termed *trastuzumab* was effective in clinical trials and is now part of standard therapy regimens.[33] As noted in Growth Factor Pathways in the Normal and Malignant Gland, earlier in this chapter, results also suggest the possibility of active immunotherapy targeting the HER-2/neu protein[86]; a lymphoplasmocytic infiltrate in breast cancer was initially shown by Pupa and coworkers to indicate good prognosis for *HER-2/neu*–positive patients. This study also noted production of growth-inhibitory antibodies by peripheral lymphocytes from these patients. The EGFR is also a target for therapy, with drugs such as tyrosine kinase inhibitors and humanized antibodies. However, clinical results with these approaches have not been as successful, to date, as with HER-2/neu–directed approaches.[81]

As has been emphasized, nuclear protooncogenes are common mechanistic links between the actions of growth-promoting steroids and growth factors in diverse tissues. Study of *c-MYC* gene expression in breast cancer, using new fluorescence *in situ* and PCR methodologies, is likely to improve c-Myc studies in human breast cancer. The c-Myc protein has a very short half-life, and, until quite recently, no high-quality monoclonal antibodies were available that are capable of staining paraffin sections. Amplification of *c-MYC* gene is associated with poor prognosis. EGF family growth factors enhance c-Myc oncoprotein-induced tumorigenesis. Thus, targeting the EGFR or the HER-2/neu together with c-Myc may be useful therapeutic strategies. Other nuclear oncogenes, cyclin D1 and AIB-1, have already been discussed in association with ER function in ER-positive disease.[28] However, with ER-positive disease, a good-prognosis category, the additional presence of expression of cyclin D1 is of poor prognostic consequence.[81] More research is needed to more fully understand these complexities.

p53 protein mediates apoptotic death induced by virtually all forms of adjuvant therapy and is easily measured by immunohistochemical methodology. However, wild-type and mutant proteins are difficult to distinguish immunologically. *TP53* overexpression confers poor prognosis and likelihood of a poor response to endocrine therapy and chemotherapy. p53 is a potential agent for gene therapy trials in cancer,[48] as are the downstreams of p53. First, loss of pRb, detected by immunohistochemistry, appears to indicate poor prognosis,[88] as does expression of Bcl-2 and down-regulation of Bax.[54] However, more studies need to be carried out on *RB-1* mutation analyses and on detection of other Bcl family members. Finally, a new area of study is the identification of poor prognosis and response to therapy genes by use of high-throughput cDNA chip assay analyses. Such studies have the potential to improve tumor diagnosis and prognosis.[84,85]

Studies of metastasis have suggested that quantification of tumor angiogenesis and deposition of specific extracellular matrix proteins may be of supplementary value in prognostication with traditional lymph node biopsy measurements.[68,69] Promising new drugs are in clinical trial for blockade of angiogenesis.[69] Metastasis itself seems to depend on the elaboration of proteases, the most promising of which, for prognostic significance, are PAI-1, cognate inhibitor of urokinase, and HAI-1, cognate inhibitor of matriptase.[66,67] In addition, when tumors express uPA/PAI-1, they are more sensitive to chemotherapy.[89] Although anti-MMP drugs, such as marimastat, have not shown much promise in clinical trials,[90] blockade of other classes of proteases (such as these serine proteases) will be a very active area of future drug development. Finally, the adhesive changes that metastatic cells undergo are of major interest. Loss of expression of E-cadherin (and acquisition of a mesenchymal phenotype marked by the intermediate filament vimentin), loss of $\alpha_2\beta_1$ integrin, overexpression of a 67-kD laminin-binding protein, and overexpression of a variant form of the hyaluronic acid receptor (CD44) are all of poor prognosis or correlated with poor tumor grade in early clinical studies.[91] Much larger studies are needed to fully evaluate the clinical significance of these metastasis-associated cellular changes. Antiangiogenic drugs are now undergoing extensive testing as anticancer agents. Although angiostatin and endostatin received early attention, probably one of the most promising antiangiogenic targets now is VEGF.[69] Recent work has also found active agents to target breast cancer in the metastatic site of bone. Specifically, bis-phosphorates inhibit osteoclast-mediated bone resorption and may selectively induce through antideath growth factor effects in the metastatic site cells.[92] Thus, significant promise for antimetastatic approaches to therapy exist.

In summary, although a very large number of genetic and phenotypic alterations have been suggested in breast cancer, only a handful have been fully identified and brought to clinical study. It is quite encouraging that study of each of these genes and phenotypic changes has provided its own unique perspective to the biology of the disease. The challenge for the future, however, is to take advantage of this knowledge to improve detection of familial risk; develop prevention strategies; improve early detection, clinical diagnosis, and prediction of therapeutic outcome; and develop therapies and rapidly apply more novel biologic therapeutics. It is the authors' prediction that the next decade of discovery in breast cancer will focus on the molecular basis of treatment failure: invasion, angiogenesis, metastasis, and resistance to therapy. Central to these hopes is the development of new technologies for high-throughput analyses of pathologic material, such as laser capture microdissection techniques, FISH, and other molecular cytogenetic methods; cDNA chip array assay methods; SAGE (serial analysis of gene expression); and other cutting-edge RNA and protein analysis techniques. It is essential that new technologies be developed to improve tumor diagnosis and prediction of response to existing therapies. These approaches should also result in our discovery of new targets for more biologic-based therapies and prevention strategies for the disease. Prospects for clinical translation of basic molecular biologic results continue to be bright.

REFERENCES

1. Seifried HE, McDonald SS, Anderson DE, et al. The antioxidant conundrum in cancer. *Cancer Res* 2003;63:4295.
2. Stewart ZA, Pietenpol JA. Cell cycle checkpoints as therapeutic targets. *J Mammary Gland Biol Neoplasia* 1999;4:389.
3. De Michele A, Weber BL. Inherited genetic factors. In: Harris JR, Lippman ME, Morrow M, et al., eds. *Diseases of the breast,* 2nd ed. Philadelphia: Lippincott Williams & Wilkins, 2000:221.
4. Hedenfalk I, Ringner M, Ben-Dor A, et al. Molecular classification of familial non-BRCA1/BRCA2 breast cancer. *Proc Natl Acad Sci U S A* 2003;100:2532.
5. Fan S, Wang J, Yuan R, et al. BRCA1 inhibition of estrogen receptor signaling in transfected cells. *Science* 1999;284:1354.
6. Lingle WL, Barrett SL, Negron VC, et al. Centrosome amplification drives chromosomal instability in breast tumor development. *Proc Natl Acad Sci U S A* 2002;99:1978.
7. O'Connell P. Genetic and cytogenetic analyses of breast cancer yield different perspectives of a complex disease. *Breast Cancer Res Treat* 2003;78:347.
8. Yang X, Yan L, Davidson NE. DNA methylation in breast cancer. *Endocr Relat Cancer* 2001;8:115.
9. Fero ML, Randel E, Gurley KE, et al. The murine gene p27Kip1 is haplo-insufficient for tumour suppression. *Nature* 1998;396:177.
10. Pollack JR, Sorlie T, Perou CM, et al. Microarray analysis reveals a major direct role of DNA copy number alteration in the transcriptional program of human breast tumors. *Proc Natl Acad Sci U S A* 2002;99:12963.
11. Elledge RM, Fuqua SAW. Estrogen and progesterone receptors. In: Harris JR, Lippman ME, Morrow M, et al., eds. *Diseases of the breast,* 2nd ed. Philadelphia: Lippincott Williams & Wilkins, 2000:471.
12. Dickson RB, Russo J. Biochemical control of breast development. In: Harris JR, Lippman ME, Morrow M, et al., eds. *Diseases of the breast,* 2nd ed. Philadelphia: Lippincott Williams & Wilkins, 2000:15.
13. Jensen EV, Jordan VC. The estrogen receptor: a model for molecular medicine. *Clin Cancer Res* 2003;9:1980.
14. Palmieri C, Cheng GJ, Saji S, et al. Estrogen receptor beta in breast cancer. *Endocr Relat Cancer* 2002;9:1.
15. Wang C, Fu M, Angeletti RH, et al. Direct acetylation of the estrogen receptor alpha hinge region by p300 regulates transactivation and hormone sensitivity. *J Biol Chem* 2001;276:18375.
16. Neuman E, Ladha MH, Lin N, et al. Cyclin D1 stimulation of estrogen receptor transcriptional activity independent of cdk4. *Mol Cell Biol* 1997;17:5338.
17. Font DM, Brown M. AIB1 is a conduit for kinase-mediated growth factor signaling to the estrogen receptor. *Mol Cell Biol* 2000;20:5041.
18. Reiter R, Wellstein A, Riegel AT. An isoform of the coactivator AIB1 that increases hormone and growth factor sensitivity is overexpressed in breast cancer. *J Biol Chem* 2001;276:39736.
19. Lee H, Bai W. Regulation of estrogen receptor nuclear export by ligand-induced and p38-mediated receptor phosphorylation. *Mol Cell Biol* 2002;22:5835.
20. Levin ER. Bidirectional signaling between the estrogen receptor and the epidermal growth factor receptor. *Mol Endocrinol* 2003;17:309.
21. Simoncini T, Hafezi-Moghadam A, et al. Interaction of oestrogen receptor with the regulatory subunit of phosphatidylinositol-3-OH kinase. *Nature* 2000;407:538.
22. Kumar R, Wang RA, Mazumdar A, et al. A naturally occurring MTA1 variant sequesters oestrogen receptor-alpha in the cytoplasm. *Nature* 2002;418:654.
23. Schlegel A, Wang C, Katzenellenbogen BS, et al. Caveolin-1 potentiates estrogen receptor alpha (ERalpha) signaling. Caveolin-1 drives ligand-independent nuclear translocation and activation of ERalpha. *J Biol Chem* 1999;274:33551.
24. Hayashi K, Matsuda S, Machida K, et al. Invasion activating caveolin-1 mutation in human scirrhous breast cancers. *Cancer Res* 2001;61:2361.
25. Clarke RB, Howell A, Anderson E. Estrogen sensitivity of normal human breast tissue in vivo and implanted into athymic nude mice: analysis of the relationship progesterone receptor expression. *Breast Cancer Res Treat* 2003;45:121.
26. Dontu G, Abdallah WM, Foley JM, et al. In vitro propagation and transcriptional profiling of human mammary stem/progenitor cells. *Genes Dev* 2003;17:1253.
27. Santen RJ, Song RX, Zhang Z, et al. Adaptive hypersensitivity to estrogen: mechanism for superiority of aromatase inhibitors over selective estrogen receptor modulators for breast cancer treatment and prevention. *Endocr Relat Cancer* 2003;10:111.
28. Osborne CK, Bardou V, Hopp TA, et al. Role of the estrogen receptor coactivator AIB1 (SRC-3) and HER-2/neu in tamoxifen resistance in breast cancer. *J Natl Cancer Inst* 2003;95:353.
29. Zujewski J. Selective estrogen receptor modulators (SERMs) and retinoids in breast cancer chemoprevention. *Environ Mol Mutagen* 2002;39:264.
30. Dickson RB, Lippman ME. *Autocrine and paracrine growth factors in the normal and neoplastic breast.* In: Harris JR, Lippman ME, Morrow M, et al., eds. Philadelphia: Lippincott Williams & Wilkins, 2000:303.
31. Troyer KL, Lee DC. Regulation of mouse mammary gland development and tumorigenesis by the ERBB signaling network. *J Mammary Gland Biol Neoplasia* 2001;6:7.
32. Frasor J, Danes JM, Komm B, et al. Profiling of estrogen up- and down-regulated gene expression in human breast cancer cells: insights into gene networks and pathways underlying estrogenic control of proliferation and cell phenotype. *Endocrinology* 2003;144:4562.
33. Yakes FM, Chinratanalab W, Ritter CA, et al. Herceptin-induced inhibition of phosphatidylinositol-3 kinase and Akt Is required for antibody-mediated effects on p27, cyclin D1, and antitumor action. *Cancer Res* 2002;62:4132.
34. Roberts AB, Wakefield LM. The two faces of transforming growth factor beta in carcinogenesis. *Proc Natl Acad Sci U S A* 2003;100:8621.
35. Xie W, Mertens JC, Reiss DJ, et al. Alterations of Smad signaling in human breast carcinoma are associated with poor outcome: a tissue microarray study. *Cancer Res* 2002;62:497.
36. Gross JM, Yee D. The type-1 insulin-like growth factor receptor tyrosine kinase and breast cancer: biology and therapeutic relevance. *Cancer Metastasis Rev* 2003;22:327.
37. McLeskey S, Dickson RB. The role of angiogenesis in breast cancer progression. In: Augustin H, Rogers P, Smith S, et al., eds. *Vascular morphogenesis of the reproductive system.* New York: Springer-Verlag, 2001:41.
38. Fu M, Wang C, Wang J, et al. Acetylation in hormone signaling and the cell cycle. *Cytokine Growth Factor Rev* 2002;13:259.
39. Dickson RB, Lippman ME. Oncogenes, suppressor genes, and signal transduction. In: Harris J, Lippman ME, Morrow M, eds. *Diseases of the breast.* Philadelphia: Lippincott–Raven, 2000:281.
40. Liao DJ, Dickson RB. c-Myc in breast cancer. *Endocr Relat Cancer* 2000;7:143.
41. Schreiber-Agus N, Meng Y, Hoang T, et al. Role of Mxi1 in ageing organ systems and the regulation of normal and neoplastic growth. *Nature* 1998;393:483.
42. Knudson AG Jr. Mutation and cancer: statistical study of retinoblastoma. *Proc Natl Acad Sci U S A* 1971;68:820.
43. Debies MT, Welch DR. Genetic basis of human breast cancer metastasis. *J Mammary Gland Biol Neoplasia* 2001;6:441.
44. Coopman PJ, Do MT, Barth M, et al. The Syk tyrosine kinase suppresses malignant growth of human breast cancer cells. *Nature* 2000;406:742.
45. Rosen EM, Fan S, Pestell RG, et al. BRCA1 in hormone-responsive cancers. *Trends Endocrinol Metab* 2003;14:378.
46. Christofori G, Semb H. The role of the cell-adhesion molecule E-cadherin as a tumour-suppressor gene. *Trends Biochem Sci* 1999;24:73.
47. Weng LP, Smith WM, Dahia PL, et al. PTEN suppresses breast cancer cell growth by phosphatase activity-dependent G1 arrest followed by cell death. *Cancer Res* 1999;59:5808.
48. Agarwal ML, Taylor WR, Chernov MV, et al. The p53 network. *J Biol Chem* 1998;273:1.
49. Chellappan SP, Hiebert S, Mudryj M, et al. The E2F transcription factor is a cellular target for the RB protein. *Cell* 1991;65:1053.
50. Sheen JH, Dickson RB. Overexpression of c-Myc alters G1/S arrest following ionizing radiation. *Mol Cell Biol* 2002;22:1819.

51. Lee RJ, Albanese C, Fu M, et al. Cyclin D1 is required for transformation by activated Neu and is induced through an E2F-dependent signaling pathway. *Mol Cell Biol* 2000;20:672.

52. Nielsen NH, Loden M, Cajander J, et al. G1-S transition defects occur in most breast cancers and predict outcome. *Breast Cancer Res Treat* 1999;56:105.

53. Rosfjord EC, Dickson RB. Growth factors, apoptosis, and survival of mammary epithelial cells. *J Mammary Gland Biol Neoplasia* 1999;4:229.

54. Sjostrom J, Blomqvist C, von Boguslawski K, et al. The predictive value of bcl-2, bax, bcl-xL, bag-1, fas, and fasL for chemotherapy response in advanced breast cancer. *Clin Cancer Res* 2002;8:811.

55. Doisneau-Sixou SF, Sergio CM, Carroll JS, et al. Estrogen and antiestrogen regulation of cell cycle progression in breast cancer cells. *Endocr Relat Cancer* 2003;10:179.

56. Castoria G, Migliaccio A, Bilancio A, et al. PI3-kinase in concert with Src promotes the S-phase entry of oestradiol-stimulated MCF-7 cells. *EMBO J* 2001;20:6050.

57. Perillo B, Sasso A, Abbondanza C, et al. 17beta-estradiol inhibits apoptosis in MCF-7 cells, inducing bcl-2 expression via two estrogen-responsive elements present in the coding sequence. *Mol Cell Biol* 2000;20:2890.

58. Swarbrick A, Lee CS, Sutherland RL, et al. Cooperation of p27(Kip1) and p18(INK4c) in progestin-mediated cell cycle arrest in T-47D breast cancer cells. *Mol Cell Biol* 2000;20:2581.

59. Ellis LM, Nicolson GL, Fidler IJ. Concepts and mechanisms of breast cancer metastasis. In: Bland KI, Copeland EM, eds. *The breast*, 2nd ed. Philadelphia: WB Saunders, 1998; 564.

60. Kolquist KA, Ellisen LW, Counter CM, et al. Expression of TERT in early premalignant lesions and a subset of cells in normal tissues. *Nat Genet* 1998;19:182.

61. Elenbaas B, Spirio L, Koerner F, et al. Human breast cancer cells generated by oncogenic transformation of primary mammary epithelial cells. *Genes Dev* 2001;15:50.

62. O'Connell P, Pekkel V, Fuqua SA, et al. Analysis of loss of heterozygosity in 399 premalignant breast lesions at 15 genetic loci. *J Natl Cancer Inst* 1998;90:697.

63. Mareel M, Leroy A. Clinical, cellular, and molecular aspects of cancer invasion. *Physiol Rev* 2003;83:337.

64. Semenza GL. HIF-1 and tumor progression: pathophysiology and therapeutics. *Trends Mol Med* 2002;8[Suppl 4]:S62.

65. Pennacchietti S, Michieli P, Galluzzo M, et al. Hypoxia promotes invasive growth by transcriptional activation of the met protooncogene. *Cancer Cell* 2003;3:347.

66. Kang JY, Dolled-Filhart M, Ocal IT, et al. Tissue microarray analysis of hepatocyte growth factor/Met pathway components reveals a role for Met, matriptase, and hepatocyte growth factor activator inhibitor 1 in the progression of node-negative breast cancer. *Cancer Res* 2003;63:1101.

67. Zemzoum I, Kates RE, Ross JS, et al. Invasion factors uPA/PAI-1 and HER2 status provide independent and complementary information on patient outcome in node-negative breast cancer. *J Clin Oncol* 2003;21:1022.

68. Iacobuzio-Donahue CA, Argani P, Hempen PM, et al. The desmoplastic response to infiltrating breast carcinoma: gene expression at the site of primary invasion and implications for comparisons between tumor types. *Cancer Res* 2002;62:5351.

69. Bikfalvi A, Bicknell R. Recent advances in angiogenesis, anti-angiogenesis and vascular targeting. *Trends Pharmacol Sci* 2002;23:576.

70. Oesterreich S, Deng W, Jiang S, et al. Estrogen-mediated down-regulation of E-cadherin in breast cancer cells. *Cancer Res* 2003;63:5203.

71. Feltes CM, Kudo A, Blaschuk O, et al. An alternatively spliced cadherin-11 enhances human breast cancer cell invasion. *Cancer Res* 2002;62:6688.

72. Bouzahzah B, Albanese C, Ahmed F, et al. Rho family GTPases regulate mammary epithelium cell growth and metastasis through distinguishable pathways. *Mol Med* 2001;7:816.

73. Kang Y, Siegel PM, Shu W, et al. A multigenic program mediating breast cancer metastasis to bone. *Cancer Cell* 2003;3:537.

74. King MC, Wieand S, Hale K, et al. Tamoxifen and breast cancer incidence among women with inherited mutations in BRCA1 and BRCA2: National Surgical Adjuvant Breast and Bowel Project (NSABP-P1) Breast Cancer Prevention Trial. *JAMA* 2001;286:2251.

75. Auborn KJ, Fan S, Rosen EM, et al. Indole-3-carbinol is a negative regulator of estrogen. *J Nutr* 2003;133[Suppl 7]:2470S.

76. Sauter ER, Zhu W, Fan XJ, et al. Proteomic analysis of nipple aspirate fluid to detect biologic markers of breast cancer. *Br J Cancer* 2002;86:1440.

77. Wulfkuhle JD, Liotta LA, Petricoin EF. Proteomic applications for the early detection of cancer. *Nat Rev Cancer* 2003;3:267.

78. Hayes DF, Isaacs C, Stearns V. Prognostic factors in breast cancer: current and new predictors of metastasis. *J Mammary Gland Biol Neoplasia* 2001;6:375.

79. Sorlie T, Perou CM, Tibshirani R, et al. Gene expression patterns of breast carcinomas distinguish tumor subclasses with clinical implications. *Proc Natl Acad Sci U S A* 2001;98:10869.

80. van de Vijver MJ, He YD, van't Veer LJ, et al. A gene-expression signature as a predictor of survival in breast cancer. *N Engl J Med* 2002;347:1999.

81. de Bono JS, Rowinsky EK. The ErbB receptor family: a therapeutic target for cancer. *Trends Mol Med* 2002;8[Suppl 4]:S19.

82. Muss HB, Thor AD, Berry DA, et al. c-erbB-2 expression and response to adjuvant therapy in women with node-positive early breast cancer. *N Engl J Med* 1994;330:1260.

83. Dowsett M, Harper-Wynne C, Boeddinghaus I, et al. HER-2 amplification impedes the antiproliferative effects of hormone therapy in estrogen receptor-positive primary breast cancer. *Cancer Res* 2001;61:8452.

84. Stearns V, Singh B, Tsangaris T, et al. A prospective randomized pilot study to evaluate predictors of response in serial core biopsies to single agent neoadjuvant doxorubicin or paclitaxel for patients with locally advanced breast cancer. *Clin Cancer Res* 2003;9:124.

85. Chang JC, Wooten EC, Tsimelzon A, et al. Gene expression profiling for the prediction of therapeutic response to docetaxel in patients with breast cancer. *Lancet* 2003;362:362.

86. Bernhard H, Salazar L, Schiffman K, et al. Vaccination against the HER-2/neu oncogenic protein. *Endocr Relat Cancer* 2002;9:33.

87. Kenny FS, Hui R, Musgrove EA, et al. Overexpression of cyclin D1 messenger RNA predicts for poor prognosis in estrogen receptor-positive breast cancer. *Clin Cancer Res* 1999;5:2069.

88. Pietilainen T, Lipponen P, Aaltomaa S, et al. Expression of retinoblastoma gene protein (Rb) in breast cancer as related to established prognostic factors and survival. *Eur J Cancer* 1995;31A:329.

89. Harbeck N, Kates RE, Look MP, et al. Enhanced benefit from adjuvant chemotherapy in breast cancer patients classified high-risk according to urokinase-type plasminogen activator (uPA) and plasminogen activator inhibitor type 1 (n = 3424). *Cancer Res* 2002;62:4617.

90. Coussens LM, Fingleton B, Matrisian LM. Matrix metalloproteinase inhibitors and cancer: trials and tribulations. *Science* 2002;295:2387.

91. Rosfjord E, Dickson RB. Role of integrins in the development and malignancy of the breast. In: Bowcock A, ed. *Contemporary approaches to breast cancer*. Totowa, NJ: Humana Press, 1999:285.

92. Fromigue O, Kheddoumi N, Body JJ. Bisphosphonates antagonise bone growth factors' effects on human breast cancer cells survival. *Br J Cancer* 2003;89:178.

WILLIAM C. WOOD
HYMAN B. MUSS
LAWRENCE J. SOLIN
OLUFUNMILAYO I. OLOPADE

SECTION 2

Malignant Tumors of the Breast

After decades of increasing incidence, the rate of invasive breast cancer appears to be leveling off in Western countries, but it is still increasing in countries that until recently had low rates of the disease.[1] In 2004, estimates were that 215,990 women and approximately 1500 men in the United States would be diagnosed with invasive breast cancer.[2] There has been a decrease in age-adjusted mortality from breast cancer of 21% since 1990,[2] with the largest decrease occurring among young women, yet an estimated 40,110 women and 470 men were estimated to succumb to the disease in 2004. The decline in mortality has been attributed to early detection of the disease and the use of aggressive multimodality treatment leading to improved clinical outcomes. A further decline in breast cancer mortality is expected as a result of the tremendous advances in the understanding of the biology of the disease and its associated risk factors. Increasingly, women identified as being at high risk for breast cancer can take advantage of risk-reducing interventions that are potentially life saving.

RISK FACTORS FOR BREAST CANCER

Epidemiologic studies have provided much information on important risk factors for breast cancer.[3] These include age, family or personal history of breast cancer, reproductive history, and exposures to specific carcinogens. Although many of the established risk factors are linked to estrogens, in a series of patients presenting at an oncology clinic, Lynch and Lynch[4] documented a family history of breast cancer in 32% of 325 consecutively treated breast cancer patients. However, estimates from population-based studies suggest that only a minority of cases, 5% to 10%, are explained by inherited mutations in highly penetrant susceptibility genes such as BRCA1 and BRCA2.[5,6] These mutations are inherited in an autosomal dominant fashion with varying penetrance. Young age at diagnosis (less than 40 years); multiple affected members in a family; bilateral disease; and association with other cancers, particularly male breast cancer, ovarian cancer, and sarcoma, are features of inherited breast cancer that can aid clinicians in recognizing individuals who may be carriers of mutations in a breast cancer susceptibility gene (Tables 33.2-1A and 33.2-1B).

FAMILIAL FACTORS

Although mutations in several genes confer increased breast cancer risk, BRCA1, BRCA2, and TP53 genes appear to be the most relevant in the clinic. To date, deleterious mutations in BRCA1 and BRCA2 genes account for the largest proportion of inherited breast cancers.[7] TP53 and PTEN each account for fewer than 1% of cases.[8] Heterozygous ATM mutation carriers have an increased

TABLE 33.2-1A. Personal Characteristics Associated with an Increased Likelihood of BRCA1 or BRCA2 Mutations

Breast cancer diagnosed at an early age
Ovarian cancer diagnosed at any age
Bilateral breast cancer
A history of both breast and ovarian cancer

risk of breast cancer, but the magnitude of the risk is not quantified. Other genetic conditions with associated breast cancer risks include Muir-Torre syndrome with MLH1 mutations and Peutz-Jeghers syndrome with LKB1 and STK11 mutations. Because inherited factors are estimated to account for approximately 25% of interindividual differences in breast cancer susceptibility and only a small fraction are due to highly penetrant genes such as BRCA1 or BRCA2, a substantial proportion of cases are estimated to be due to the combined effect of polymorphisms in low penetrance genes such as CYP19, GSTP1, and GSTM1, to mention a few.[9]

Breast cancer can cluster in families purely by chance or as a result of shared environmental influences or shared lifestyle. Despite the fact that BRCA1 and BRCA2 mutations are rare, occurring in approximately 1 in 500 persons in the general population, they account for a significant proportion of breast cancer cases in young women and for approximately 10% of all cases of ovarian cancer. In addition, certain populations, such as Jews of Eastern European ancestry (Ashkenazi Jews), with a prevalence rate of 1:40 have a higher carrier rate. Individuals who are likely to benefit most from BRCA testing and who should be offered genetic counseling and testing are listed in Tables 33.2-1A and 33.2-1B.

BRCA1 is a large gene, located on chromosome band 17q12, composed of 24 coding exons encoding a protein of 1863 amino acids.[10,11] More than 700 mutations and sequence variations have been detected so far, and only a few are recurrent in unrelated families.[12] Recurrent BRCA1 mutations have been described in different European countries and in North America, but the two most common are 185delAG and 5382insC.[13,14] The BRCA2 gene is composed of 27 exons encoding a protein of 3418 amino acids. More than 300 different mutations have been described in the BRCA2 gene and only a few are recurrent.[12] One recurrent mutation 6174delT has a carrier frequency of 1.5% in Ashkenazi Jewish populations, whereas the recurrent mutation 999del5 accounts for a significant proportion of hereditary breast cancer in Iceland.[15] Mutations in BRCA1 and BRCA2 predict probabilities of breast cancer by age 70 years of 45% to 87% and 26% to 84%, respectively, which makes these the strongest predictors of breast cancer known. The lifetime risks of ovarian cancer for BRCA1 and BRCA2 mutation carriers are 16% to 63% and 10% to 27%, respectively.[7,15–17] Several other cancers appear to be part of the BRCA1 and BRCA2 spectrum, including pancreatic, prostate, fal-

TABLE 33.2-1B. Family History Characteristics Associated with an Increased Likelihood of BRCA1 or BRCA2 Mutations

Two or more family members under 50 y of age with breast cancer
Both breast and ovarian cancer in members of the family
Male breast cancer
One or more family members under the age of 50 y with breast cancer and Ashkenazi Jewish ancestry

lopian tube, laryngeal, male breast cancers, as well as adult leukemia and lymphomas. Therefore, health care providers must ask about the history of all cancers in both the paternal and maternal lineages. For patients who have already been diagnosed with a curable first primary cancer, the risk of a second primary breast or ovarian cancer is substantial and should be factored into the management of the first cancer. In addition to the family history, the histopathologic characteristics of the tumor may aid clinicians in identifying breast cancer survivors who are more likely to be carriers of BRCA1 or BRCA2 mutations.

CLINICOPATHOLOGIC FEATURES OF BRCA-ASSOCIATED TUMORS

In an attempt to understand how the BRCA proteins contribute to breast cancer, several clinical studies have addressed the clinicopathologic differences between BRCA-associated and sporadic breast and ovarian cancers.[18] Both favorable prognostic characteristics (medullary or atypical medullary carcinoma) and unfavorable characteristics (poor differentiation, high tumor grade, aneuploidy, hormone receptor negativity, p53 mutation) have been found to be associated with BRCA1-associated breast cancers.[19] Two groups described gene expression profiles of BRCA1- and BRCA2-associated cancers and have suggested that BRCA1-associated tumors have distinct patterns of gene expression, whereas BRCA2-associated tumors are indistinguishable from sporadic cases. Grushko et al.[20] have also shown that BRCA1-associated tumors are usually HER2 nonamplified. Thus, BRCA1-associated tumors are mostly estrogen receptor (ER) and HER2 negative and may express certain cytokeratins that distinguish them as arising from a basal cell of origin.[20,21] Tubular and lobular cancers are more commonly seen in BRCA2 mutation carriers, and they are more likely to be ER positive.[22] Given the early age of onset and the aggressive histopathologic features of BRCA1-related cancers, should these patients be identified and treated differently at diagnosis?

In a prospective cohort of 183 patients with invasive breast cancer treated at the Institut Curie who presented with a family history of breast or ovarian cancer, or both, and were tested for BRCA1 germline mutations, those who had a BRCA1 mutation (40 cases) had a worse overall survival than noncarriers (5-year survival rate, 80% vs. 91%; $P = .002$).[23] Similar worse outcomes have been reported in Ashkenazi Jewish women with BRCA mutations compared to noncarriers, but other studies have reported more favorable outcomes.[19,24–26] Women with BRCA mutations are at increased risk for breast cancer–related events, especially contralateral disease after breast-conservation treatment, and should be followed carefully.[27] Although the breast cancer mortality rates of BRCA1 carriers may be worse, it has been observed that ovarian cancer patients with BRCA1 and BRCA2 mutations have higher rates of disease-free survival than patients with sporadic cancer.[28,29] Thus, it is unclear from the literature whether BRCA mutations should be factored into treatment planning. Although BRCA-associated cancers may theoretically be more sensitive to therapies that promote genomic damage, such as platinum-based regimens, there have been no prospective randomized studies investigating whether conventional surgery, radiation, and chemotherapeutic treatments are more or less effective in BRCA mutation carriers than in unselected breast and ovarian cancer patients. The challenge for the future is to apply the understanding of the molecular functions of BRCA1 and BRCA2 to developing targeted therapies that are likely to be less toxic and more effective.

HORMONAL FACTORS

Many of the risk factors for breast cancer are associated with increased lifelong exposure to female reproductive hormones, including *in utero* exposure to high concentrations of estrogens.[30] The older the age at menarche, the lower a woman's risk of breast cancer, although it is not clear how much other menstrual factors such as cycle length and regularity contribute to breast cancer risk.[3] Hormone levels may be higher throughout reproductive life in women who undergo early menarche than in women with a later occurrence of menarche.[31] The age-specific incidence of breast cancer increases steeply with age, but at menopause the rate of increase is drastically reduced to approximately one-sixth the rate before menopause. Moreover, a woman with a natural menopause at age 45 years has a risk of breast cancer that is half of that for women who undergo menopause after the age of 55 years. Oophorectomy before age 50 years also provides substantial protective effect, even in women with inherited susceptibility to breast cancer such as BRCA1 and BRCA2 carriers. Thus, the total duration of exposure to endogenous estrogen or its metabolites appears to be very important in contributing to breast cancer risk.

The risk of breast cancer is increased in the period immediately after childbirth, but this risk decreases in the long term. During pregnancy, mammary cells differentiate into mature breast cells prepared for lactation. The mature breast cells have longer cell cycle, which allows more time for repair of damaged DNA and thereby reduces the rates of potentially deleterious mutations. The transient increase in breast cancer risk with pregnancy may be related to the increased proliferation of breast cells that precedes terminal differentiation before lactation. Alternatively, the increased risk may be due to the effect of high levels of hormones on subclinical cancers. The increased risk disappears after approximately 10 years, and pregnancy then provides a more durable protective effect over a lifetime.[32] Compared to nulliparous women, women who have at least one full-term pregnancy have a 25% reduction in their breast cancer risk. Furthermore, there is evidence that the more children a woman has, the greater the protection from breast cancer, and women with five or more children have 50% of the risk of nulliparous women. Late age at first full-term pregnancy also increases the risk, and women who have a first full-term pregnancy after age 30 have a twofold to fivefold greater risk than women with a first full-term pregnancy by age 18 years. Abortion does not appear to increase breast cancer risk based on multiple epidemiologic studies as well as data from a large population-based cohort comprised of 1.5 million Danish women, which show no increase in long-term risk after early termination of pregnancy.[33] Lactation, especially when total duration of breast feeding is very long, confers reduced breast cancer risk.[34]

Current users of hormonal therapy to manage the menopause are at higher risk of breast cancer than women who have never used these preparations. Hormone therapy for the menopause occurs at a time when a woman is at high and increasing background risk for breast cancer. Data from the Women's Health Initiative as well as data reanalyzed by the Collaborative Group on Hormonal Factors in Breast Cancer have shown that, among current and recent users of hormonal therapy, the risk of breast cancer increases with increasing duration of use and that this excess diminishes after cessation of use.[35,36] The Women's Health Initiative reported on 16,608 postmenopausal women aged 50 to 79 years with an intact uterus who were randomly assigned to receive combined conjugated equine estrogens (0.625 mg/d) plus medroxyprogesterone acetate (2.5 mg/d) or placebo from 1993 to 1998 at 40 clinical centers in the United States. In intent-to-treat analyses, compared with placebo, estrogen plus progestin was associated with increased total breast cancers (245 vs. 185 cases; hazard ratio, 1.24; weighted $P<.001$) and invasive breast cancers (199 vs. 150 cases; hazard ratio, 1.24; weighted $P=.003$). The invasive breast cancers diagnosed in the estrogen plus progestin group were similar in histology and grade to those diagnosed in the placebo group but were larger (mean of 1.7 cm and standard deviation of 1.1 vs. mean of 1.5 cm and standard deviation of 0.9, respectively; $P=.04$) and were at a more advanced stage (regional or metastatic, 25.4% vs. 16.0%, respectively; $P=.04$). After 1 year of hormone replacement therapy, the percentage of women with abnormal mammograms was substantially greater in the estrogen plus progestin group [716 (9.4%) of 7656] compared with the placebo group [398 (5.4%) of 7310; $P<.001$], a pattern that continued for the study duration. Based on these data, the Women's Health Initiative concluded that short-term use of combined estrogen plus progestin increases the risk of having abnormal mammograms as well as the incidence of breast cancers, which are diagnosed at a more advanced stage compared with placebo use. Interestingly, breast cancer developing in women on hormone replacement therapy is more likely to be low grade, ER positive, and therefore hormone sensitive. Nonetheless, there appears to be conclusive evidence that hormone replacement therapy increases the risk of breast cancer and cardiovascular events and should probably not be used for prolonged periods after menopause unless the potential benefit significantly justifies the risk. Use of oral contraceptive agents, especially by women with a positive family history of breast cancer, appears to increase breast cancer risk as well,[37] although use of oral contraceptive agents has been shown to reduce ovarian cancer risk.

DIETARY AND LIFESTYLE FACTORS

The large international variation in breast cancer rates, in which countries with high-fat diets have higher rates than countries like Japan and less developed countries with low-fat diets, suggested that high fat intake might be associated with increased breast cancer risk. However, pooled analysis of seven prospective epidemiologic studies does not indicate any association between fat intake and breast cancer risk in adult women in more developed countries.[38] There may be a moderate protective effect from high vegetable consumption, but results for meat, fiber, and fruit consumption have been inconsistent. However, a positive association between alcohol consumption and breast cancer risk has been consistently demonstrated, and risk appears to be linearly related to the amount of alcohol consumed.[39] Alcohol consumption may be particularly deleterious for individuals with suboptimal intake of nutrients such as folate, β-carotene, lutein and zeaxanthin, and vitamin C. The International Agency for Research on Cancer estimates that 25% of breast cancer cases worldwide are due to overweight or obesity and a sedentary lifestyle. In a study of the American Cancer Society including 495,477 women followed for 16 years, the risk of breast cancer mortality was increased significantly with increasing level of obesity. Compared to women with a body mass index (BMI) under 25.0, those with BMIs of 25 to 29.9, 30 to 34.9, 35 to 39.9, and 40 or higher had relative risks of breast cancer mortality of 1.34, 1.63, 1.7, and 2.12, respectively. The worldwide trend toward increasing obesity and reduced physical activity will lead to increased incidence of breast cancer unless large-scale population efforts are developed to counteract these effects.[40] Thus, it appears that the combination of obesity, moderate to high levels of alcohol consumption, and a sedentary lifestyle constitute a major risk factor for breast cancer.

Obesity influences the risk of breast cancer in different ways among premenopausal and among postmenopausal women. In premenopausal women, obesity is protective, possibly because it is associated with irregular menstrual periods and an increased number of anovulatory cycles. In postmenopausal women, on the other hand, obesity is associated with an increased risk of breast cancer. In the Women's Health Initiative observational study, among women who had never received hormone replacement therapy, women with BMIs of 31.1 or higher had a statistically significant 2.5 times greater risk of developing breast cancer than women whose BMIs were 22.6 or lower. The Nurses' Health Study also found that the 60% greater risk for postmenopausal breast cancer associated with overweight and obesity was limited to women who had never used hormone replacement therapy.[41,42] In postmenopausal women, androgens are aromatized to estrogen in adipose tissue, and more of this may occur in obese than in nonobese women. Obese postmenopausal women also have lower mean levels of sex hormone–binding globulin, which may contribute to higher availability of estrone at the tissue level. Hyperinsulinemia and high levels of insulin-like growth factor-1 in this situation may lead to higher ovarian androgen production, which increases the amount of substrates available for local fatty tissue aromatization.[43]

An association between physical exercise and breast cancer has been demonstrated in several cohort studies.[44] The reduction in risk ranged from 10% to 70% for the most active women and on average was 30% to 40% lower for women who exercised for 3 to 4 hours per week at moderate to vigorous levels. Lower risks associated with greater physical activity have been observed for both premenopausal and postmenopausal breast cancer. It is not clear whether adolescent activity, adult activity, or lifetime activity provides the most benefit.

RADIATION AND AGE AT EXPOSURE

Ionizing radiation exposure secondary either to nuclear explosion or to medical diagnostic and therapeutic procedures, especially if exposure was before age 40 years, increases breast cancer risk. It is estimated that approximately 1% of all breast cancers in the United States may be attributable to diagnostic mammography.[45] A high breast cancer–related mortality has been reported among U.S. radiologic technologists, especially those who had qualified 30 or more years previously. Women who received a mantle irradiation, especially when combined with chemotherapy, for the treatment of Hodgkin's disease before age 15 years have a markedly increased breast cancer risk and should be followed closely.[46]

BREAST DENSITY AND MAMMOGRAPHIC PATTERNS

Mammographic parenchymal patterns have been shown to be associated with breast cancer risk, and this risk appears to be genetically determined, as was reported in a study of twins in Australia.[47] Women in whom a greater proportion of the breasts consists of radiodense tissue are at higher risk of breast cancer than women with more radiolucent breasts. In a follow-up study of the mammograms of women in the original Breast Cancer Detection Demonstration Project, of the breast cancer risk factors assessed in the participants, high-density mammographic parenchymal patterns, as measured by the proportion of breast area composed of epithelial and stoma tissue, had the greatest impact on breast cancer risk. Of the breast cancers in this study, 28% were associated with breast densities of 50% or higher.[48]

PREMALIGNANT LESIONS

Benign breast diseases are either proliferative or nonproliferative, but the vast majority of specimens from breast biopsies done for clinical indications demonstrate nonproliferative disease. Non-proliferative lesions are generally not associated with increased breast cancer risk. However, proliferative breast diseases are further divided into proliferative lesions with or without atypia. Proliferative lesions without atypia are associated with a twofold increased risk, whereas atypical hyperplasia is associated with a fourfold to fivefold increased risk. There is marked interaction between atypia and a family history of a first-degree relative with breast cancer.[49] This subgroup of women had an 11-fold increased risk of breast cancer, which is one of the reasons why ductal lavage or random breast needle aspirates might identify such high-risk women for chemoprevention intervention studies.

DIAGNOSIS AND BIOPSY

Any area of the breast that appears suspicious by being palpably abnormal or is suspicious by radiologic criteria deserves biopsy-based diagnosis. Accuracy of diagnosis is essential for the proper management of breast lesions. Biopsy techniques

are not helpful if they fail to produce diagnostic accuracy. Sources of error include missing the lesion and obtaining a biopsy specimen of adjacent tissue, inadequately sampling a heterogeneous lesion, and misinterpreting the histopathologic or cytologic specimen. If diagnostic accuracy is the *sine qua non* of biopsies, minimal perturbation of the breast remains an important, if secondary, concern. This refers both to avoidance of invasive surgical procedures for benign breast conditions and to performance of a biopsy in such a manner that it does not compromise subsequent treatment options. Table 33.2-2A indicates preferred biopsy techniques and lists the advantages and disadvantages of each.

For a palpable lesion, fine-needle aspiration (FNA) or core-cutting needle biopsy allow office procedures. FNA is the most easily performed but requires a skilled cytopathologist for accurate interpretation of the sample obtained. The sensitivity varies from 80% to 95%, reflecting institutional experience.[50] False-positive aspirate results are extremely uncommon and occur in fewer than 1% of cases. FNA cannot reliably distinguish invasive cancer from ductal carcinoma *in situ* (DCIS). Core-cutting needle biopsy has many of the advantages of FNA and provides histologic rather than merely cytologic detail. Specimens obtained by this method are more easily interpreted by general pathologists. Both of these techniques sample a lesion and may consequently fail to accurately diagnose histologically heterogeneous lesions. Whenever a needle biopsy result fails to adequately explain the clinical findings, additional tissue should be sought, commonly by excisional biopsy. When atypical ductal hyperplasia is identified in a needle biopsy specimen, DCIS is found in 20% to 50% of cases in which excisional biopsy of the area is subsequently performed. Similarly, DCIS and lobular carcinoma *in situ* (LCIS) may be up-staged at excisional biopsy.[51]

It is ideal to have a diagnosis by needle biopsy before performing excision of a breast neoplasm. This allows procedures for axillary staging and other staging procedures to be accom-

TABLE 33.2-2A. Advantages and Disadvantages of Preferred Biopsy Techniques

Suspicious Area	Technique	Advantages	Disadvantages
Palpable	Fine-needle aspiration (FNA)	Rapid, minimal discomfort, no incision complicating local therapy, immediate results	Cannot distinguish *in situ* from invasive cancer reliably
			Some false-negatives
			Requires skilled cytopathologist
	Core-needle biopsy	Rapid, minimal to moderate discomfort, no surgical incision, interpreted by general pathologist	Some false-negatives
			Sampling error with larger lesions
Nonpalpable solid	US-guided FNA	Rapid, widely available	
	US-guided core biopsy		
	US-guided needle localization and surgical excision		
Nonpalpable microcalcifications	Stereotactic core biopsy	Requires stereotactic imaging table	Expensive
	Radiographic wire localization and surgical excision	Complete histology	More painful
		Evaluation of margins	Incision must be integrated in treatment planning
		May serve as definitive excision/lumpectomy	May perturb lymphatic pathways for sentinel lymph node mapping
			Cannot visualize faint calcifications
MRI-detected lesion	US- or MRI-guided biopsy	—	—

MRI, magnetic resonance imaging; US, ultrasonography.

TABLE 33.2-2B. Techniques of Core Biopsy by Ultrasonography or Stereotactic Guidance

CORE NEEDLES
With disposable biopsy gun
With reusable biopsy gun
VACUUM-ASSISTED CORE BIOPSY
Mammotome
Suros
AUTOMATIC BREAST BIOPSY INSTRUMENT
Mechanized single specimen
Large core excision
ELECTROSURGICAL WIRE BASKET
Single spherical specimen
Neothermia *en-bloc*

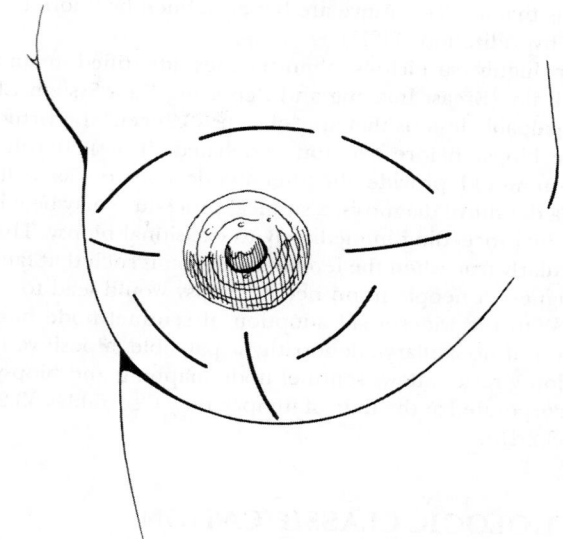

FIGURE 33.2-1. Acceptable placement of surgical incisions for breast excisions. Central tumors are best excised via circumareolar incisions. (Adapted from Spear SL. *Surgery of the breast: principles and art.* Philadelphia: Lippincott–Raven, 1998:131.)

plished at or before the time of excision. When a suspicious breast mass is excised for biopsy, a small margin of apparently normal tissue around the lesion should be removed. A 1-cm margin, as has been advocated by some authors, is not required. For smaller lesions, that could lead to removal of three or four times the volume of breast tissue actually required for the excision. Proper handling of the specimen involves orienting it for the pathologist so that margin examination not only provides the extent of margin, or lack thereof, but identification of the area where a margin may be insufficient, so that wider excision may be limited to that surface. The specimen margins should be inked to allow such analysis of margins.

Nonpalpable lesions are approached with the aid of imaging techniques. Biopsy of solid lesions may be performed by core-cutting needles or FNA under ultrasonographic guidance. Areas of clustered microcalcifications require a core biopsy performed under stereotactic mammographic guidance, or mammographically localized lesions can be needle-localized for excision. If the calcifications are highly suspicious, it may be most efficient to excise them for diagnosis. If the calcifications are of uncertain significance, a core biopsy—especially with suction core techniques that remove the majority of the calcifications—can provide effective diagnosis. Magnetic resonance imaging (MRI) can be used to perform localization. A variety of biopsy devices can be used under radiologic guidance (Table 33.2-2*B*).

When excisional biopsy with radiographic localization is used, it is essential that the localizing needle or wire be placed within the lesion. A localizing wire that appears to be only a few millimeters away from the lesion with the breast in compression may prove to be 1 or 2 cm away when compression is released. The patient should be informed that there is a 1% to 5% risk of failure to excise the mammographically identified lesion. As in any biopsy situation in which the diagnosis fails to explain the physical or radiographic findings, search for evidence of persistence of the lesion on mammogram and repeat biopsy are indicated.

Incisions for excisional biopsies should be planned with both oncologic and aesthetic considerations in mind (Fig. 33.2-1). Incisions directly over the lesion have been advocated by some authors but without evidence to support this contention. Biopsy of most areas of the breast can be performed easily via circumareolar incisions that virtually disappear with healing. For optimal cosmesis, it is especially important to avoid incisions in the upper inner quadrant of the breast when this is possible. It is

almost never helpful to excise an ellipse of skin in a breast biopsy. Even small skin ellipses draw the nipple and areola out of symmetry with the contralateral breast. A possible diagnosis of Paget's disease of the nipple or skin involvement by tumor can be made easily with a 2- or 3-mm punch biopsy without a skin ellipse.

Most surgical procedures on the breast can be performed under local anesthesia in the outpatient setting. For surgical diagnostic procedures about which the patient is anxious or which are expected to be complicated, intravenous sedation is a most helpful adjunct.

Although diagnosis based on frozen-section analysis can be performed with general reliability, its value is extremely limited. It is not uncommon for small areas of a biopsy specimen and its margins to be important in treatment planning. These should not be destroyed in the process of obtaining a frozen section. The additional delay of a few days to obtain permanent sections for histologic analysis and accurate assessment of margins is more than worthwhile. Sacchini et al. noted a discordance rate of 12% between diagnosis based on frozen sections and the final histologic diagnosis for 403 nonpalpable lesions.[52] Many of these related to *in situ* or hyperplastic lesions.

The role of the pathologist in accurate diagnosis is clearly crucial. When a lesion is borderline—for example, atypical ductal hyperplasia or a lesion with possible foci of invasion—a second opinion from a pathologist who specializes in breast disease can be most helpful. With specimen orientation and inking, the pathologic data desired include the histologic type of the neoplasm, the grade, the dimensions of the lesion, the dimensions of any invasive portion, the margin status including dimension measurements, presence of lymphatic-vascular invasion, the ER and progesterone receptor (PR) levels (reported numerically rather than as positive or negative), and HER2/*neu* analysis. An indication of HER2/*neu* negativity by immunohistochemistry (IHC) is usually sufficient for management.

Lesions that are 2+ positive are better defined by fluorescence *in situ* hybridization (FISH).

For highly suspicious abnormalities identified mammographically (Breast Imaging and Reporting Data System Class 5) or palpable lesions that are "obviously cancer," the virtue of needle biopsy before excision is debated. If a small-volume excision would provide the therapeutic excision as well as allow a definitive diagnosis, a surgical procedure may be eliminated by proceeding immediately to excisional biopsy. This is particularly true when the level of suspicion is such that failure to diagnose a neoplasm on needle biopsy would lead to excision. With the widespread adoption of sentinel node biopsy, however, if no axillary adenopathy is palpable, a positive needle biopsy result allows sentinel node mapping and biopsy to be incorporated at the time of lumpectomy (see Tables 33.2-2*A* and 33.2-2*B*).

PATHOLOGIC CLASSIFICATION OF TUMOR TYPES

The histopathologic classification of tumor types is based on conventional light-microscopic evaluation of pathologic specimens, most commonly using hematoxylin and eosin staining.[53,54] Proper classification of tumor type is essential because of its prognostic value and its role in guiding appropriate clinical management decisions. The most widely used classification is the World Health Organization classification of tumor types (Table 33.2-3).[54,55]

Breast carcinoma is conventionally divided into two major patterns: (1) ductal, which accounts for approximately 85% of breast cancer cases; and (2) lobular, which accounts for approximately 15% of breast cancer cases. These two patterns are further subcategorized on the basis of microscopic features as noninvasive (*in situ*) or invasive (infiltrating) (see Table 33.2-3).

CARCINOMA *IN SITU*

Carcinoma *in situ* is defined as the presence of malignant epithelial cells that proliferate and fill the ductules and lobular acini but remain confined by the basement membrane without invasion. Carcinoma *in situ* is subdivided into ductal carcinoma *in situ* (intraductal carcinoma) and lobular carcinoma *in situ*. DCIS and LCIS are each named descriptively according to the microanatomic spaces that the cancer cells occupy and their cytologic appearance. DCIS is most commonly detected as an abnormality on screening mammography, typically a cluster of microcalcifications, without physical examination findings. Because of the increased use of screening mammography, the rate of detection of DCIS has increased in the United States. In contrast, LCIS rarely presents with mammographic manifestations and is most often detected as an incidental finding when biopsy is performed for another reason. LCIS is considered to be a marker for increased risk for the development of breast cancer, whereas DCIS is considered to be a nonobligate precursor of invasive ductal carcinoma and thereby warrants treatment. The management of DCIS and LCIS is discussed in Ductal Carcinoma *In Situ* and Lobular Carcinoma *In Situ*, later in this chapter.

INVASIVE DUCTAL CARCINOMA

Invasive ductal carcinoma comprises the largest category of invasive carcinomas and in most series accounts for 65% to 80% of all breast malignancies. Invasive ductal carcinoma nearly always has an associated component of DCIS. On gross examination, invasive ductal carcinoma usually forms a hard, gritty (scirrhous) mass. Common invasive ductal carcinoma is designated with the modifier *NOS* (not otherwise specified) to distinguish it from special morphologic subtypes, which account for approximately 10% of all invasive ductal carcinomas and appear to have a somewhat better prognosis.[53,54,56] Important pathologic features for prognosis include tumor size, presence of axillary lymphadenopathy, grade, and lymphatic-vascular invasion.[53,54,57,58] Grading is subdivided into well differentiated (grade 1), intermediate differentiation (grade 2), and poorly differentiated (grade 3), and grade is conventionally determined using the Nottingham modification of the Bloom-Richardson system.[57]

INVASIVE LOBULAR CARCINOMA

Infiltrating lobular carcinomas comprise 5% to 10% of all invasive carcinomas. The histologic hallmark of this type of mammary carcinoma is the tendency for the tumor cells, which are typically small and monotypic, to invade the stroma in linear strands (Indian file pattern). A molecular correlate of this dyshesive growth pattern is mutation of the E-cadherin molecule.[59] These tumors tend to be detected as a mass or asymmetric density on physical examination or mammography and are not typically associated with microcalcifications on mammography. The size of the tumor is often underestimated because of the subtly diffuse, infiltrative nature of this disease. Assessment of the extent of the tumor may be improved with MRI. Because of the indistinct margins, performing a lumpectomy with clear margins may be more difficult for invasive lobular carcinoma than for invasive ductal carcinoma. An increased risk of bilaterality is associated with invasive lobular carcinoma. Lymph node metastases may grow in a subtle histologic pattern, which makes them difficult to detect, and diagnostic accuracy is improved with IHC staining for cytokeratins. The pattern of metastasis is different for invasive lobular carcinoma, with the propensity to involve less common sites of metastatic disease, such as meningeal or peritoneal surfaces.[60]

TABLE 33.2-3.   World Health Organization Classification of Carcinoma of the Breast[54,55]

NONINVASIVE CARCINOMA
Ductal carcinoma *in situ*
Lobular carcinoma *in situ*
INVASIVE CARCINOMA
Invasive ductal carcinoma
Invasive lobular carcinoma
Mucinous carcinoma
Medullary carcinoma
Papillary carcinoma
Tubular carcinoma
Adenoid cystic carcinoma
Secretory (juvenile) carcinoma
Apocrine carcinoma
Carcinoma with metaplasia (metaplastic carcinoma)
Inflammatory carcinoma
Other (specify)
PAGET'S DISEASE OF THE NIPPLE

SPECIAL SUBTYPES OF INVASIVE DUCTAL CARCINOMA

Mucinous (Colloid) Carcinoma

Mucinous (colloid) carcinomas generally comprise no more than 2% of cases, although the incidence is slightly higher in older women. The presenting symptom is commonly a mass. In this subtype, the carcinoma cells produce a variable quantity of extracellular mucin. Mucin production is visible on both gross and microscopic examination. Mucinous carcinoma tends to have a favorable prognosis, with a lower rate of axillary lymph node metastases and higher rate of survival after treatment. Invasive ductal carcinoma with a lesser amount of mucinous involvement is described as having mucinous features.

Medullary Carcinoma

Medullary carcinomas account for approximately 5% of all invasive ductal carcinomas and tend have a younger age distribution. Clinically, medullary carcinoma often presents as a well-circumscribed mass on physical examination or mammography, similar to a fibroadenoma. Medullary carcinomas have a rounded, very well circumscribed border, a florid lymphoplasmacytic infiltrate, poorly differentiated tumor cells growing in large sheets (syncytial pattern), and numerous mitoses. An invasive ductal carcinoma that has some, but not all, of the features of medullary carcinoma is referred to as atypical medullary carcinoma or a carcinoma with medullary features. Medullary carcinoma that strictly meets the pathologic criteria has a more favorable outcome with a higher rate of survival than invasive ductal carcinoma.

Papillary Carcinoma

Papillary carcinomas comprise no more than 1% to 2% of all breast cancers. Papillary carcinoma can be invasive or noninvasive (intraductal). Papillary carcinoma is characterized by a frond-like, papillary growth pattern, and may have solid and cystic components. Papillary carcinoma tends to present at a slightly older age. Invasive papillary carcinoma has a favorable prognosis in comparison to invasive ductal carcinoma.

Tubular Carcinoma

Tubular carcinomas account for no more than 1% to 2% of all invasive breast carcinomas and are the best-differentiated form of invasive ductal carcinoma. Tubular carcinomas tend to be small (generally 1 cm or less), to have associated low-grade intraductal carcinoma, and to grow as small acinar structures or tubules that mimic the normal ducts of the breast. Incidence of tubular carcinoma has increased during the era of screening mammography. The diagnosis of tubular carcinoma confers a favorable prognosis, with a low rate of axillary lymph node metastases and a high rate of survival. Coexistent tubular and lobular carcinoma (tubulolobular carcinoma) may be found in a single invasive lesion; some pathologists consider this to be a variant form of infiltrating lobular carcinoma.

Inflammatory Carcinoma

Inflammatory carcinoma is an aggressive, virulent form of carcinoma and is staged as T4d, stage III. Inflammatory carcinoma is characterized by the clinical appearance of inflammation and induration of the skin, diffuse breast enlargement, and peau d'orange. See Staging, later in this chapter.

Other Subtypes

Uncommon subtypes of invasive ductal carcinoma include adenoid cystic carcinoma, secretory (juvenile) carcinoma, apocrine carcinoma, cribriform carcinoma, and carcinoma with metaplasia (metaplastic carcinoma). Together, they account for no more than 1% of all invasive breast carcinomas. Adenoid cystic carcinoma contains both glandular (adenoid) and cystic (cylindromatous) components and resembles the salivary gland tumor of the same name. Secretory (juvenile) carcinoma tends to occur in younger adults and even children, and is notable for abundant α-lactalbumin secretion. Apocrine carcinoma resembles the apocrine (sweat) glands in the skin. Invasive cribriform carcinoma resembles the sieve-like fenestrated form of intraductal carcinoma of the same name. Carcinoma with metaplasia (metaplastic carcinoma) exhibits differentiation along lines not usually seen in the breast. For example, it can form squamous eddies, cartilage, or bone, or may grow as an undifferentiated spindle cell neoplasm (pseudosarcoma).

PAGET'S DISEASE OF THE NIPPLE

Paget's disease of the nipple is characterized by the presence of Paget cells in the epidermis of the nipple. Paget cells histologically stand out in the epidermis as large, malignant-appearing cells with pale cytoplasm and pleomorphic nuclei with prominent nucleoli. In many respects, Paget's disease is a variant of DCIS. Paget's disease is often associated with an underlying intraductal carcinoma, with or without invasive ductal carcinoma. The prognosis for Paget's disease is related to whether or not there is an associated invasive component.

STAGING OF BREAST CANCER

Staging refers to the grouping of patients according to the apparent extent of their tumors. It can be based on either clinical or pathologic findings. The most widely used staging system for breast cancer is that of the American Joint Committee on Cancer (AJCC), which is jointly sponsored by the American Cancer Society and the American College of Surgeons. The AJCC staging system includes both clinical and pathologic staging based on TNM characteristics. T refers to tumor, N to nodes, and M to metastasis. The sixth edition was published in 2002 and is tabulated in the following sections (Tables 33.2-4 through 33.2-6). It is important for publication, for maintenance of tumor registry data, and for recording of cancer information in clinic and hospital

TABLE 33.2-4. Changes in Breast Cancer Staging in the Sixth Edition of the *American Joint Committee on Cancer Staging Manual*

Micrometastases distinguished from isolated tumor cells
Identifiers added for sentinel node dissection and immunohistochemical or molecular techniques
Major lymph node classifications designated by number of involved nodes
Metastasis to supraclavicular nodes or infraclavicular nodes classified as N3
Metastasis to internal mammary chain nodes reclassified

TABLE 33.2-5. American Joint Committee on Cancer TNM Staging System for Breast Cancer

PRIMARY TUMOR (T)

Definitions for classifying the primary tumor (T) are the same for clinical and for pathologic classification. If the measurement is made by the physical examination, the examiner will use the major headings (T1, T2, or T3). If other measurements, such as mammographic or pathologic measurements, are used, the subsets of T1 can be used. Tumors should be measured to the nearest 0.1-cm increment.

TX	Primary tumor cannot be assessed
T0	No evidence of primary tumor
Tis	Carcinoma *in situ*
Tis (DCIS)	Ductal carcinoma *in situ*
Tis (LCIS)	Lobular carcinoma *in situ*
Tis (Paget's)	Paget's disease of the nipple with no tumor

Note: Paget's disease associated with a tumor is classified according to the size of the tumor.

T1	Tumor 2 cm or less in greatest dimension
T1mic	Microinvasion 0.1 cm or less in greatest dimension
T1a	Tumor more than 0.1 cm but not more than 0.5 cm in greatest dimension
T1b	Tumor more than 0.5 cm but not more than 1 cm in greatest dimension
T1c	Tumor more than 1 cm but not more than 2 cm in greatest dimension
T2	Tumor more than 2 cm but not more than 5 cm in greatest dimension
T3	Tumor more than 5 cm in greatest dimension
T4	Tumor of any size with direct extension to (a) chest wall or (b) skin, only as described below
T4a	Extension to chest wall not including pectoralis muscle
T4b	Edema (including peau d'orange) or ulceration of the skin of the breast or satellite skin nodules confined to the same breast
T4c	Both T4a and T4b
T4d	Inflammatory carcinoma

REGIONAL LYMPH NODES (N)
CLINICAL

NX	Regional lymph nodes cannot be assessed (e.g., previously removed)
N0	No regional lymph node metastasis
N1	Metastasis to movable ipsilateral axillary lymph node(s)
N2	Metastases in ipsilateral axillary lymph nodes fixed or matted, or in *clinically apparent*[a] ipsilateral internal mammary nodes in the *absence* of clinically evident axillary lymph node metastasis
N2a	Metastases in ipsilateral axillary lymph nodes fixed to one another (matted) or to other structures
N2b	Metastasis only in *clinically apparent*[a] ipsilateral internal mammary nodes and in the *absence* of clinically evident axillary lymph node metastasis
N3	Metastasis in ipsilateral infraclavicular lymph node(s) with or without axillary lymph node involvement, or in *clinically apparent*[a] ipsilateral internal mammary lymph node(s) and in the *presence* of clinically evident axillary lymph node metastasis; or metastasis in ipsilateral supraclavicular lymph node(s) with or without axillary or internal mammary lymph node involvement
N3a	Metastasis in ipsilateral infraclavicular lymph node(s)
N3b	Metastasis in ipsilateral internal mammary lymph node(s) and axillary lymph node(s)
N3c	Metastasis in ipsilateral supraclavicular lymph node(s)

PATHOLOGIC (PN)[b]

pNX	Regional lymph nodes cannot be assessed (e.g., previously removed, or not removed for pathologic study)
pN0	No regional lymph node metastasis histologically, no additional examination for isolated tumor cells
pN0(i–)	No regional lymph node metastasis histologically, negative IHC
pN0(i+)	No regional lymph node metastasis histologically, positive IHC, no IHC cluster greater than 0.2 mm
pN0(mol–)	No regional lymph node metastasis histologically, negative molecular findings (RT-PCR)[c]
pN0(mol+)	No regional lymph node metastasis histologically, positive molecular findings (RT-PCR)[c]
pN1	Metastasis in one to three axillary lymph nodes, and/or in internal mammary nodes with microscopic disease detected by sentinel lymph node dissection but not *clinically apparent*
pN1mi	Micrometastasis (greater than 0.2 mm, none greater than 2.0 mm)
pN1a	Metastasis in one to three axillary lymph nodes
pN1b	Metastasis in internal mammary nodes with microscopic disease detected by sentinel lymph node dissection but not *clinically apparent*
pN1c	Metastasis in one to three axillary lymph nodes and in internal mammary nodes with microscopic disease detected by sentinel lymph node dissection but not *clinically apparent*. (If associated with more than three positive axillary lymph nodes, the internal mammary nodes are classified as pN3b to reflect increased tumor burden.)
pN2	Metastasis in four to nine axillary lymph nodes, or in *clinically apparent* internal mammary lymph nodes in the *absence* of axillary lymph node metastasis
pN2a	Metastasis in four to nine axillary lymph nodes (at least one tumor deposit greater than 2.0 mm)
pN2b	Metastasis in *clinically apparent* internal mammary lymph nodes in the *absence* of axillary lymph node metastasis
pN3	Metastasis in ten or more axillary lymph nodes, or in infraclavicular lymph nodes, or in *clinically apparent* ipsilateral internal mammary lymph nodes in the *presence* of one or more positive axillary lymph nodes; or in more than three axillary lymph nodes with clinically negative microscopic metastasis in internal mammary lymph nodes; or in ipsilateral supraclavicular lymph nodes
pN3a	Metastasis in ten or more axillary lymph nodes (at least one tumor deposit greater than 2.0 mm), or metastasis to the infraclavicular lymph nodes
pN3b	Metastasis in *clinically apparent* ipsilateral internal mammary lymph nodes in the *presence* of one or more positive axillary lymph nodes; or in more than three axillary lymph nodes and in internal mammary lymph nodes with microscopic disease detected by sentinel lymph node dissection but not *clinically apparent*
pN3c	Metastasis in ipsilateral supraclavicular lymph nodes

Note: Isolated tumor cells are defined as single tumor cells or small cell clusters not greater than 0.2 mm, usually detected only by immunohistochemical (IHC) or molecular methods but which may be verified on hematoxylin and eosin stains. Isolated tumor cells do not usually show evidence of malignant activity, e.g., proliferation or stromal reaction.
[a]*Clinically apparent* is defined as detected by imaging studies (excluding lymphoscintigraphy) or by clinical examination or grossly visible pathologically.
[b]Classification is based on axillary lymph node dissection with or without sentinel lymph node dissection. Classification based solely on sentinel lymph node dissection without subsequent axillary node dissection is designated "(sn)" for "sentinel node" [e.g., pN0(i+) (sn)].
[c]RT-PCR, reverse transcriptase-polymerase chain reaction.

TABLE 33.2-6. Stage Grouping

Stage	Tumor (T)	Node (N)	Metastasis (M)
0	Tis	N0	M0
I	T1[a]	N0	M0
IIA	T0	N1	M0
	T1[a]	N1	M0
	T2	N0	M0
IIB	T2	N1	M0
	T3	N0	M0
IIIA	T0	N2	M0
	T1[a]	N2	M0
	T2	N2	M0
	T3	N1	M0
	T3	N2	M0
IIIB	T4	N0	M0
	T4	N1	M0
	T4	N2	M0
IIIC	Any T	N3	M0
IV	Any T	Any N	M1

Note. Stage designation may be changed if postsurgical imaging studies reveal the presence of distant metastases, provided that the studies are carried out within 4 mo of diagnosis in the absence of disease progression and provided that the patient has not received neoadjuvant therapy.
[a]T1 includes T1mic.

records. Its use facilitates research and allows comparisons among results of different studies.

As valuable as the AJCC system may be, it has several major limitations. One is change in the AJCC staging over time in different editions, which limits the ability to compare data from different studies. AJCC staging does not directly translate to an assessment of suitability for breast-conserving therapy or adjuvant systemic therapy or to prognosis or indications for postmastectomy irradiation. Staging does not distinguish patients with a long history of relatively indolent tumors from patients of similar stage with very aggressive tumors that have reached the same stage in a very brief period of time. Current research on genomic and proteomic descriptors together with newer prognostic and predictive factors offers hope of allowing better treatment planning than currently available with AJCC staging.

CLINICAL STAGING

Clinical staging includes physical examination, with careful inspection and palpation of the skin, mammary gland, and lymph nodes (axillary, supraclavicular, and cervical); imaging; and pathologic examination of the breast or other tissues as appropriate to establish the diagnosis of breast carcinoma.

PATHOLOGIC STAGING

Pathologic staging includes all data used for clinical staging, plus data from surgical exploration and resection as well as pathologic examination of the primary carcinoma, regional lymph nodes, and metastatic sites (if applicable).

HISTOLOGIC GRADING

All invasive breast carcinomas, with the exception of medullary carcinomas, should be graded. The Nottingham combined histo-

logic grade (Elston-Ellis modification of Scharff-Bloom-Richardson grading system) is recommended.[56,57] The grade for a tumor is determined by assessing morphologic features (tubule formation, nuclear pleomorphism, and mitotic count), assigning a value of 1 (unfavorable) for each feature, and adding together the scores for all three categories. A combined score of 3 to 5 points is designated as grade 1; a combined score of 6 to 7 points is grade 2; and a combined score of 8 to 9 points is grade 3.

Histologic Grade (Nottingham combined histologic grade is recommended)
GX   Grade cannot be assessed
G1   Low combined histologic grade (favorable)
G2   Intermediate combined histologic grade (moderately favorable)
G3   High combined histologic grade (unfavorable)

PROGNOSTIC AND PREDICTIVE FACTORS

The AJCC staging system reviewed here is based on established clinical and pathologic prognostic factors. The extent of axillary lymph node involvement by breast cancer is the dominant prognostic indicator for later systemic disease.[61] Although combinations of other prognostic factors have been published repeatedly that exceed the prognostic power of nodal metastases in large retrospective series, no large prospective trial has failed to find that nodal metastasis is the dominant prognostic factor. This should not be surprising, because markers of the primary tumor reflect risks that occult metastasis has already occurred. Lymph node status, on the other hand, is evidence of actual metastases growing in the regional lymph nodes. Tumor size is the second factor that predicts outcome from disease and consequently, with lymph node status and the presence or absence of distant metastases, is the basis of TNM staging.[62]

Histologic grading has clear prognostic significance in a tertiary role. The Nottingham combined histologic grade is recommended and has been well described. A criticism of the value of histologic grade has been the lack of concordance among pathologists. There is more concordance regarding grade 1 of 3 and 3 of 3. Grade 1 or its equivalent identifies a small subset of axillary lymph node–negative tumors with low risk of distant metastasis or death from breast cancer. Grade 1, stage I breast cancers (up to 2 cm in diameter) have a systemic failure rate of only 2% in some large modern series.[63]

Patient age is also an independent prognostic factor. Very young women with breast cancer have a poorer prognosis than older women. If the hazard ratio of 1.0 describes the outcome for women 40 to 45 years and 45 to 49 years of age, then it is 1.8 for women under 30 years, 1.7 for those 30 to 34 years, and 1.5 for those 35 to 39 years.[64]

ESTROGEN AND PROGESTERONE RECEPTOR EXPRESSION

A *prognostic factor* is defined as any measurement taken at the time of surgery or diagnosis that is associated with outcome (e.g., overall survival, disease-free survival, or local control). A *predictive factor* is any measurement that predicts response or lack of response to a specific treatment.[66] Currently, the vast majority of patients with invasive breast cancer receive systemic therapy. This has led to an extensive search for new and more effective predictive factors. ER and PR status are the most important and helpful predictive factors currently available. Patients with invasive breast cancer whose tumors are totally lacking in ERs and PRs do not respond to or derive benefit from hormonal manipulations.[67] More recently, the benefits of tamoxifen in DCIS have been shown to be restricted to patients with hormone receptor–positive tumors.[68] Previously, ER expression was measured in fresh or fresh frozen tissue, and complex biochemical assays were required. Moreover, results of these assays could be confounded by high endogenous levels of circulating estrogens, which increased the probability of false-negative results. Current assays are performed using IHC techniques, which have the advantages of not being confounded by endogenous estrogens, can be correlated with histologic findings to eliminate the possibility that the ER assessment was done on noncancerous tissue, can be performed on paraffin-embedded tissues, and do not have tumor size as a limiting factor for an accurate assay. Results of these IHC assays have proven to be equal or superior to biochemical assays in predicting response to adjuvant endocrine therapy.[69] It is essential that the clinician understand how ER and PR status are reported from his or her laboratory. Many laboratories still report ER and PR status as positive or negative using a cutoff point of less than 10% of cells staining for ER or PR as a definition of negative receptor status. Compelling data from the Early Breast Cancer Trialists' Collaborative Group (EBCTCG) overview analysis,[67] as well as from individual investigators, suggest that even patients whose tumors have as few as 1% of cells staining positively for hormone receptors may derive benefit from adjuvant endocrine therapy (Fig. 33.2-2).[69] For these reasons, it is most appropriate to have ER and PR expression reported as percentage of cells staining for each receptor. Numerous trials have correlated ER and PR status with prognosis. At 5 years after diagnosis, women with ER- and PR-positive tumors have a relapse rate that is 5% to 10% superior to that of patients with ER-negative tumors, but this advantage decreases and ultimately disappears with increasing time of follow-up.[70]

A review of two large databases that encompassed approximately 15,000 patients with early breast cancer confirmed the value of the PR status in addition to ER status in determining the potential benefits of tamoxifen adjuvant therapy.[71] Tamoxifen therapy significantly decreased the risk of dying of breast cancer among patients with receptor-positive tumors compared to those with ER-negative and PR-negative tumors, with decreases in the hazard ratio to 0.74 to 0.87 for patients whose tumors were ER negative and PR positive, to 0.62 to 0.68 for patients whose tumors were ER positive and PR negative, and to 0.42 to 0.53 for patients whose tumors were both ER and PR positive. These databases included both premenopausal and postmenopausal patients, and none of the patients received adjuvant chemotherapy. The data convincingly show that, when accurately measured, both ER and PR status best predict response to tamoxifen. Similar results have been previously noted for patients with metastases, with patients who have both ER- and PR-positive tumors having the best response to endocrine therapy. It is likely that this relationship between ER and PR expression and treatment outcome is true for all endocrine therapies, but further data are needed. Moreover, the percentage of cells staining positive for ER and PR has also been shown to be related to tamoxifen response in the metastatic disease setting.[72]

HER2 (HER2/*NEU*, EPIDERMAL GROWTH FACTOR RECEPTOR-2, C-ERBB-2) STATUS

HER2 is a member of the epidermal growth factor receptor (EGFR) family, which includes HER1 (EGFR-1), HER2, HER3, and HER4. Activation of the HER2 gene, located on chromosome 17 (17q21), results in synthesis of a 185-kD transmembrane glycoprotein whose intracellular domain possesses tyrosine kinase activity. Heterodimerization of the different EGFR transmembrane glycoproteins with HER2 results in activation of tyrosine pathways, with subsequent phosphorylation of cell signaling proteins that cause tumor cell proliferation. Approximately 20% of breast cancer patients have HER2 gene amplification, which results in glycoprotein overexpression. Approximately 5% of patients have overexpression without gene amplification, but otherwise gene amplification and expression are highly correlated. HER2 amplification or overexpression has been associated with higher tumor grade; lack of ERs; higher levels of indicators of tumor proliferation such as S phase, MIB-1, and Ki-67; and poorer prognosis.[73,74] HER2 status is the major predictive factor for response to trastuzumab (Herceptin), which is discussed in more detail in Trastuzumab Therapy later in this chapter. Previous measurements of HER2 have relied on IHC techniques. More recently, FISH techniques have been shown to be more reliable in characterizing gene amplification and predicting response to trastuzumab. Many investigators have found that node-positive patients whose tumors overexpress HER2 have a poorer prognosis than patients whose tumors are not overexpressors. However, in many studies, especially those in node-negative patients, IHC-defined HER2 expression was found to be either a weak or negative pure prognostic factor.[74] HER2 amplification measured by FISH analysis, however, may prove to be a helpful prognostic factor in patients with small tumors and negative nodes.[75]

HER2 amplification and overexpression may be helpful in predicting which patients are most likely to benefit from chemotherapy. Several trials have suggested that patients with tumors with HER2 overexpression are more likely to benefit from anthracycline-containing regimens than non–anthracycline-containing regimens,[76] but controversy exists.[77] Patients with HER2-negative tumors, however, appeared to receive similar benefit from anthracycline-containing and non–anthracycline-

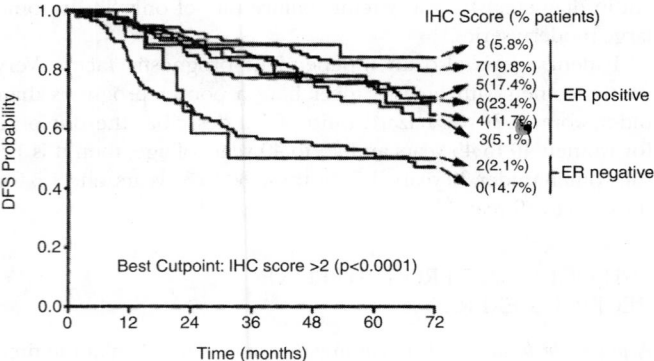

FIGURE 33.2-2. Immunohistochemical (IHC) score for estrogen receptor (ER) positivity versus relapse-free survival for patients receiving adjuvant endocrine therapy. A total score of 3 under the scoring system used in this analysis corresponds to as few as 1% to 10% weakly staining tumor cells. DFS, disease-free survival. (From ref. 69, with permission.)

containing regimens. In a trial conducted by the Cancer and Leukemia Group B (CALGB) involving patients with node-positive breast cancer, patients with HER2-positive tumors derived greater benefits from higher versus lower doses of anthracycline-based chemotherapy [cyclophosphamide (Cytoxan), doxorubicin (Adriamycin), and fluorouracil, or CAF]. Patients with HER2-positive tumors had significant improvements in both relapse-free and overall survival compared to those with HER2-positive tumors treated with lower doses of the drugs. For patients whose tumors were HER2 negative, no differences in outcome were seen for the different dosage levels of CAF.[78] Also in the adjuvant setting, patients whose tumors were HER2 positive and who were treated with cyclophosphamide, methotrexate, and fluorouracil (CMF) had lesser reductions in their risk of recurrence than CMF-treated patients whose tumors were HER2 negative.

HER2 expression may also be helpful in predicting response to endocrine therapy. In general, patients with HER2-positive tumors derive less benefit from tamoxifen or aromatase inhibitors than patients whose tumors are HER2 negative, and these observations are supported by discoveries regarding the biologic basis of endocrine therapy.[79] One randomized trial comparing neoadjuvant tamoxifen and letrozole in patients with hormone receptor–positive tumors who had locally advanced breast cancer showed that patients with HER2-positive tumors had significantly higher response rates to letrozole than to tamoxifen.[80] Correlative scientific data from trials currently in progress will clarify these results and may help explain the superiority of aromatase inhibitors compared to tamoxifen in patients with metastatic breast cancer as well as the preliminary findings showing the superiority of the aromatase inhibitor anastrozole compared to tamoxifen in the adjuvant setting.[81] However, in one large retrospective analysis of patients with node-positive breast cancer, tamoxifen was equally efficacious in patients with ER-positive and either HER2-positive or HER2-negative tumors.[82] At present, HER2 should not be used as predictive factor in the selection of patients with ER- or PR-positive tumors for endocrine therapy, whether in the adjuvant or metastatic setting. HER2 gene amplification and overexpression are the major predictive factors for the efficacy of trastuzumab and are discussed in Chemotherapy, later in this chapter.

LYMPHOVASCULAR INVASION

The prognostic significance of involvement of lymphatic or microvascular spaces in the primary tumor has been variably described. Lymphatic vessel invasion has been associated with lymph node metastases, as might be anticipated. If the terms *lymphatic invasion* and *vascular invasion* are reserved for instances in which tumor cells are present in an area outlined by endothelium, then the significance appears secure. This is an independent prognostic factor in both node-positive[83] and node-negative[84] patients.

PROLIFERATION RATE

Numerous studies have evaluated the relationship of tumor proliferative index to prognosis and treatment outcome, including ploidy [the amounts of DNA in the tumor: normal (diploid) vs. increased or decreased (aneuploid)], the number of tumor cells in S phase (S-phase fraction by flow cytometry), the percentage of cells labeling with thymidine or bromodeoxyuridine or cellular expression of Ki-67 or MIB-1 (which measure the percentage of cells in the G_1 phase of the cell cycle), and the percentage of tumor cells undergoing mitosis (mitotic index). In most studies, ploidy has not proven to be a significant prognostic factor. Several large trials have shown a significant correlation between high S phase and poorer survival,[66,85,86] but these results have not been consistent. High proliferation indices strongly correlate with poorer tumor grade, younger age, lack or ER and PR expression, and HER2 positivity. Using proliferation rates as a predictive factor, several trials have shown improved outcomes for patients with higher tumor proliferation rates given chemotherapy. A major issue, however, relates to standardization of the many available techniques, and at this time proliferative indices should not be routinely used in decision making regarding adjuvant therapy. Proliferation indices, however, may be of some value in patients with node-negative breast cancer. Patients with high proliferative indices may be better candidates for chemotherapy.

PLASMINOGEN ACTIVATOR SYSTEM

A large body of data supports a major role for the plasminogen activator system in tumor invasion and metastases. The concentrations of urokinase plasminogen activator (u-PA) and its inhibitor, plasminogen activator inhibitor-1 (PAI-1), have been shown to be strong prognostic factors.[87] In one large series of 761 patients, those with both low u-PA and low PAI-1 levels accounted for approximately 50% of patients with node-negative breast cancer and had significantly better survival than similar patients who had high levels of either u-PA or PAI-1. In a multivariate analysis that included tumor size, hormone receptor status, menopausal status, tumor grade, and u-PA and PAI-1 levels, u-PA and PAI-1 levels were the most significant prognostic indicator of relapse-free survival and were second only to grade as an indicator for overall survival. In addition, patients whose tumors expressed high-levels of u-PA or PAI-1 had significantly greater proportional reductions in relapse after adjuvant chemotherapy than patients with low levels of both u-PA and PAI-1.[88] There was no relationship between u-PA and PAI-1 levels, and endocrine therapy benefit, but in the metastatic setting high u-PA and PAI concentrations may predict resistance to tamoxifen. These data have led to the development of a prospective trial, now in progress, that uses the u-PA and PAI-1 level for selecting which patients in the trial receive adjuvant chemotherapy. Analysis of u-PA and PAI-1 has not been widely adopted because the assay requires fresh tissue. Newer assays that can be accurately performed on fresh core biopsy samples are being developed.

OTHER FACTORS

Numerous other prognostic and predictive factors have been evaluated in patients with early breast cancer. Measurements of tumor angiogenesis performed by counting the number of capillaries have generally shown that breast cancers with increased numbers of capillaries are associated with higher recurrence rates than tumors with lower numbers of capillaries. Capillaries are usually counted with IHC methods that use labeled antibodies against factor VIII in vascular endothelium. These analyses are time and labor intensive, and not all studies have shown a significant correlation between increased capillary density and poorer relapse-free survival. At present such assessment is not recommended on a routine basis. Higher capillary density, however, may ultimately prove to be a predictive factor for response to antiangiogenic agents.

The p53 gene is commonly mutated in human cancer, and numerous studies have assessed the value of p53 as either a prognostic or predictive factor with inconsistent results. Likewise, other gene mutations including BRCA1 and BRCA2, ras, myc, Rb (retinoblastoma), and ATM (ataxia telangiectasia) have not been shown to be of value as predictive or prognostic factors. Cyclins, which regulate the cell cycle, have been extensively studied as prognostic factors. Cyclin D1 has shown inconsistent results as a prognostic factor. Increased expression of a low-molecular-weight form of cyclin E, measured by Western blot analysis, has been strongly correlated with poorer relapse-free and overall survival[89]; confirmatory trials are needed. Numerous other potential prognostic factors have been explored, including cathepsin D, nm23, bcl, and bax, but none has consistently proven to be related to prognosis or helpful as a predictor of treatment outcome.

The detection of occult micrometastases in the bone marrow using IHC techniques has been evaluated as a potential prognostic indicator by numerous investigators. In a major trial of 552 patients with stage I to III breast cancer, 36% of breast cancer patients showed microscopic evidence of bone marrow metastases with cytokeratin staining of bone marrow aspirates, compared to 1% of controls.[90] Micrometastatic disease was significantly correlated with an increased risk of metastases and death from breast cancer. Moreover, an earlier metaanalysis of 20 studies that included 2494 patients with different tumor types found a small but significant correlation between bone marrow micrometastases and poorer relapse-free survival for breast cancer patients.[91] These data suggest promise for bone marrow micrometastases as a prognostic factor, but further data from larger trials, using standardized detection procedures, are needed. At present, the use of bone marrow metastases for defining prognosis should still be considered investigational. Following on this theme, there is renewed interest in defining the prognostic value of circulating tumor cells in patients with breast cancer. Newer techniques using the reverse transcriptase quantitative polymerase chain reaction[92] or magnetic antibodies[93] are capable of detecting 1 cancer cell in 10,000 cells in the peripheral blood, and several trials have suggested a correlation between increased numbers of circulating cells and the risk of relapse. Larger confirmatory trials are in progress.

MOLECULAR AND GENOMIC FACTORS

Major advances in molecular biology are now being translated to the clinic with increasing speed. In breast cancer, major efforts are under way to define gene expression signatures that can serve as prognostic and predictive factors. In a groundbreaking study, Perou and colleagues were able to classify breast cancers into tumor subtypes that had different prognoses using complementary DNA microarrays.[94] In a more recent study of 295 patients age 52 years and younger with stage I and II breast cancer followed for a median of 6.7 years, a microarray analysis using 70 genes was used to define a poor-risk and good-risk signature.[95] Multivariate analysis that included standard clinical variables as well as treatment showed that the poor-risk signature was associated with a significantly higher hazard ratio for distant metastases

(5.1) compared to the good-risk signature; mean overall 10-year relapse-free survival rates were 85% for patients with the good-prognosis signature and 55% for those with the poor-prognosis signature. More recently, microarray data were shown to predict for complete pathologic response to neoadjuvant chemotherapy using paclitaxel and FAC (fluorouracil, doxorubicin, and cyclophosphamide) in 24 patients with early-stage breast cancer.[96] Accuracy of the response prediction using the gene-prediction profile was 81%, specificity was 93%, and sensitivity was 50%. Initial microarray studies relied on frozen or fresh tumor samples, but studies suggest that accurate profiling can be done on paraffin-embedded tissues. Such technology will allow for large-scale correlative scientific studies of archival materials. The use of array technology as a prognostic and predictive tool shows great promise, and numerous trials under way should help define its role in treatment selection. It is hoped that its prognostic sorting may in time identify good-risk patients who need no adjuvant systemic therapy and allow better tailoring of adjuvant therapies, both systemic therapy and radiation treatment.

The development of new targeted therapies rests on the identification of precisely defined molecular targets that mediate breast cancer cell growth and metastases. Potential targets include enzymes and signaling proteins involved in tyrosine kinase pathways, apoptotic pathways, modulation of DNA histone deacetylation, and angiogenesis. New agents targeting these pathways have been reviewed (Table 33.2-7).[97] These

TABLE 33.2-7. Pathways Related to Cell Growth and Metastases and Targeted Agents

Pathway and Target	Agent
EPIDERMAL GROWTH FACTOR RECEPTOR PATHWAY	
Epidermal growth factor receptor	Cetuximab, ABX-EGF
Selective erbB-1 (HER1) tyrosine kinase inhibitors	Erlotinib, gefitinib
erbB-2 (HER2) inhibitors	Trastuzumab (Herceptin)
Pan-erbB inhibitors	CI-1033, GW-572016, EKB-569
RAS/RAF/MITOGEN-ACTIVATED PROTEIN KINASE PATHWAY	
Farnesyl transferase inhibitors	Tipifarnib (Zarnestra, R115777), SCH6636, BMS 214662
Raf inhibitors	BAY 43-9006, ISIS 5132
MEK inhibitors	CI-1040
PI3K/AKT AND MTOR	
Rapamycin analogs	CC-779, RAD001, AP23573
APOPTOTIC PATHWAYS	
Bcl-2 pathways	Oblimersen (G-3139, Genasense)
Tumor necrosis factor–related apoptosis ligand (TRAIL)	TRM-1
HISTONE DEACETYLASE INHIBITORS	LAQ824, suberoylanilide, depsipeptide, MS-275, CI-994, hydroxamic acid
ANGIOGENESIS INHIBITORS	
Anti–vascular endothelial growth factor (VEGF) antibody	Bevacizumab (Avastin), CP-547,632, PTK787/ZK222584
VEGF tyrosine kinase inhibitors	ZD6474, SU11248
	(Also, some chemotherapy agents being used for antiangiogenesis)

(Modified from ref. 97.)

pathways provide a wide array of targets for new chemotherapeutic agents and biologics. Potential targets, and specific agents in development or in clinical trials that have been synthesized to block these pathways, are tabulated in Table 33.2-7. In addition, specific genetic and IHC probes are available for identifying gene amplification and overexpression of numerous other potential treatment targets, including enzymes involved in chemotherapy drug activation (i.e., thymidine synthetase and phosphorylase for fluorouracil) and metabolism (i.e., dihydropyrimidine dehydrogenase for fluorouracil), and inducible enzymes that may stimulate cell proliferation [i.e., cyclooxygenase-2 (COX-2) for COX-2 inhibitors]. Analysis of specific genes and proteins involved in drug metabolism may prove to be another extremely effective way of predicting response to treatment.

ADVISING THE WOMAN AT HIGH RISK FOR BREAST CANCER

Different levels of breast cancer risk exist in the general population, and most individuals from moderate- to high-risk families overestimate their risk for breast cancer. Thus, obtaining accurate and detailed information about a patient's personal and family history of cancer or previous breast biopsy results is of paramount importance and is the first step in risk assessment. A documentation of the types of cancers in a family should be obtained from medical records, pathology reports, and death certificates whenever possible in an effort to confirm the types of cancers that have occurred in the family. It is possible for a verbal report of cervical cancer to be confirmed later as ovarian or endometrial cancer, which greatly alters the accuracy of the risk assessment. Women who have received mantle irradiation, especially in combination with chemotherapy,[46] for treatment of Hodgkin's disease and women with lesions of LCIS or atypical ductal hyperplasia on breast biopsy are also considered at high risk. By quantification of risk, patients can gain a better understanding of their personal risk, and in addition, clinicians can better advise high-risk patients regarding appropriate risk-reducing strategies.

Data from different epidemiologic studies such as the Cancer and Steroid Hormone Study (CASH) have been used to derive a woman's cumulative breast cancer risk[98] and can be readily applied to clinical situations. The CASH data take into account age at cancer onset of affected relatives, which has been shown to be a strong predictor of hereditary risk. The Gail model was developed from the Breast Cancer Detection Demonstration Project from the 1970s and uses information about well-established risk factors for breast cancer, which include number of first-degree relatives with breast cancer, age at menarche, age at first live birth, and number of previous breast biopsies.[99] These parameters are used to calculate an individual's risk of developing breast cancer but do not address mutation status. A modified Gail model is available for clinical use and can be readily accessed through the U.S. National Cancer Institute Web site at http://bcra.nci.nih.gov/brc/. Unfortunately, the Gail model may underestimate hereditary breast cancers because it does not consider paternal family history or the presence of breast cancer in second-degree relatives, nor does it take into account cases of ovarian cancer in the family. The Claus model may be more applicable to individuals with

inherited breast cancer because it incorporates age at onset of cancer in affected first- and second-degree relatives. Both models remain clinically useful tools despite their limitations. Myriad and BRACAPRO models are commonly used by genetic counselors and are derived from statistical models of penetrance based on family history; they predict the likelihood of a BRCA1 or BRCA2 mutation.[100,101] Although these models assess the likelihood that a BRCA mutation is present, they do not assess cancer risk. In considering the limitations of each model, the educated practitioner, possibly in conjunction with a genetic counselor, can determine which model or combination of models is most applicable for a particular patient. Risk assessments generated from these models can then be used to decide whether genetic testing is appropriate and which risk-reduction strategies may be beneficial whether or not genetic testing is pursued. For example, the Gail model may be most appropriate for patients who are considering taking tamoxifen for risk reduction or participating in a chemoprevention trial.

Although demand for breast cancer risk assessment and genetic testing has continued to rise in North America and Europe, there are no uniform criteria for offering genetic testing for breast cancer. Even with direct-to-consumer marketing of BRCA testing in the United States, only a small proportion of appropriate patients are being referred for genetic counseling. Although the efficacies of the different risk-reducing options are now being defined, clinicians are encouraged to provide guidance to patients during the decision-making process. The American Society of Clinical Oncology (ASCO) has updated its statement concerning genetic testing for cancer.[102,103] For patients who have already been diagnosed with a curable first primary cancer, the risks of a second primary breast or ovarian cancer are substantial and should be factored into the management of the first cancer. Current management options for high-risk women include lifestyle changes, intensive surveillance, and chemoprevention or prophylactic surgery.

LIFESTYLE MODIFICATION

Epidemiologic studies show strong evidence that excessive weight gain, a sedentary lifestyle, and moderate to high levels of alcohol use are associated with a greater risk of breast cancer.[104] A body of emerging literature suggests that behavioral modifications can substantially reduce breast cancer risk. As an example, it is likely that the population-wide adoption of greater physical activity and reduced caloric intake would result in significant reduction in overall population risk for breast cancer mortality. Individually, although women might not be able to choose age at menarche or at first full-term pregnancy, women should be counseled to engage in increased physical activity and to reduce total caloric intake so that weight remains stable over their lifetime, preferably with the BMI remaining below 25. For women who are already overweight or obese, losing weight, increasing physical activity, changing the dietary patterns, and reducing alcohol consumption could potentially reduce the risks of breast and other cancers.

INTENSIVE SURVEILLANCE AND CHEMOPREVENTION

Based on findings from the National Surgical Adjuvant Breast and Bowel Project (NSABP) Protocol P-1, tamoxifen has been approved for breast cancer prevention in women who meet a certain level of risk to justify the toxicities associated with tamoxifen use. These include women with a family history of breast cancer among first-degree relatives or biopsy-proven LCIS or atypical hyperplasia. More than 13,000 women were randomly assigned to 5 years of tamoxifen or placebo if they were 35 years of age or older and had a 5-year risk of 1.66% by the Gail model.[105] Overall, women randomly assigned to 5 years of tamoxifen therapy experienced a 49% decrease in risk of invasive breast cancer, with similar risk reduction observed in both premenopausal and postmenopausal women. The major toxicities of endometrial cancer and thromboembolic events were more commonly seen in women 50 years of age and older, which makes tamoxifen use most beneficial in younger high-risk women. Other studies of high-risk women have not observed the same degree of risk reduction for tamoxifen, and one study reported excess mortality in tamoxifen-treated patients (International Breast Cancer Intervention Study). Because raloxifene (Evista), another selective ER modulator (SERM), was shown in a randomized trial in postmenopausal women with osteoporosis to prevent breast cancer, NSABP has now embarked on a second trial, P-2 or the STAR (Study of Tamoxifen and Raloxifene) protocol, that will accrue over 19,000 women to a randomized trial of tamoxifen versus raloxifene. Raloxifene has not been used in premenopausal women, and thus the STAR trial is restricted to postmenopausal women.

Current recommendations for screening of women with BRCA mutation in the United States include monthly breast self-examination, physician breast examination every 4 to 6 months, and annual mammography beginning at age 30 years or 5 to 10 years earlier than the age at onset of the earliest case of breast cancer in the family. Because younger women, in general, have dense breast tissue, which can limit the sensitivity of mammography, and because the efficacy of intensive screening is not well known, high-risk patients who opt for intensive surveillance rather than prophylactic surgery are encouraged to enroll in clinical trials of other screening modalities. Additional modalities such as breast MRI, ultrasonography, and ductal lavage are currently under investigation. Several small studies suggest that MRI is more sensitive than mammography in this population. The state of screening for ovarian cancer is less certain. There are no known effective modalities for ovarian cancer screening in the general population or for BRCA mutation carriers. Many experts recommend yearly or twice-yearly transvaginal ultrasonography and twice-yearly measurement of CA 125 (cancer antigen 125) levels and gynecologic examinations starting at age 25 to 30 for patients who elect not to undergo prophylactic oophorectomy.[106] However, mortality benefit for these screening measures has not been established.

There are conflicting data regarding use of tamoxifen as a chemopreventive agent in BRCA mutation carriers. In an analysis of the NSABP P-1 study, among the 288 women who developed breast cancer only 19 (6.6%) were found to have BRCA1 or BRCA2 mutations, which limits interpretation of the data.[107] Of note, five of the eight BRCA1 mutation carriers with breast cancer received tamoxifen [risk ratio, 1.67; 95% confidence interval (CI), 0.32 to 10.7], whereas 3 of the 11 patients with BRCA2 mutations received tamoxifen (risk ratio, 0.38; 95% CI, 0.06 to 1.56). However, in a retrospective analysis of BRCA carriers, Narod et al. reported an odds ratio of 0.5 (95% CI, 0.28 to 0.89) for contralateral breast cancer among women who

used tamoxifen for adjuvant treatment of their first breast cancer.[108] The authors compared 209 women who had bilateral breast cancer and BRCA1 or BRCA2 mutation with 384 women who had unilateral disease and BRCA1 or BRCA2 mutation in a matched case-control study. Tamoxifen was protective against contralateral breast cancer for carriers of BRCA1 mutations (odds ratio, 0.38; 95% CI, 0.19 to 0.74) and for those with BRCA2 mutations (odds ratio, 0.63; 95% CI, 0.2 to 1.5). Tamoxifen has an acceptable toxicity profile for young women (younger than 50 years) and could be considered a reasonable agent for breast cancer risk reduction, especially in BRCA2 mutation carriers (higher rate of ER-positive tumors) and in those choosing intensive surveillance over prophylactic surgery. An argument can also be made for tamoxifen use in BRCA1 carriers, given that 20% to 30% of BRCA1-associated breast tumors are ER positive and there are no definitive data for or against its use in this group. Chemoprevention for ovarian cancer is again less certain. Prior use of oral contraceptives has been shown to be protective in a case-control study, but their potential to cause a slight increase in breast cancer has been suggested in other studies.[108]

PROPHYLACTIC MASTECTOMY

In a study in Rotterdam, a high incidence of premalignant lesions such as DCIS, LCIS, atypical lobular hyperplasia, and atypical ductal hyperplasia were observed in the prophylactic mastectomy specimens of women at hereditary risk for breast cancer, especially women who had mastectomy after the age of 40 years. Interestingly, women who had had bilateral oophorectomy before prophylactic mastectomy were less likely to have these lesions (odds ratio, 0.2; $P = .02$).[109] The occurrence of these premalignant lesions along with the known high lifetime breast cancer risk in BRCA mutation carriers argues for the clinical usefulness of prophylactic mastectomy, but timing of surgery remains difficult because prophylactic surgery may be unacceptable to young women early in their reproductive lives.

The efficacy of prophylactic mastectomy in reducing breast cancer risk has been demonstrated in several retrospective case studies as well as one large prospective study. Hartmann et al. examined 639 women with a family history of breast cancer who had undergone prophylactic bilateral mastectomy in a retrospective analysis.[110] This study was the first to demonstrate an 89.5% risk reduction for breast cancer in women at moderate risk and a greater than 90% risk reduction in the high-risk group. Although BRCA status was not examined in the initial study, it was reported in a follow-up study, which confirmed that the reduced rates of breast cancer after prophylactic mastectomy applied to BRCA mutation carriers as well as those deemed high risk by family history alone. Another large prospective study of 139 women with mutations in either BRCA1 or BRCA2 was reported in 2001.[111] The authors reported no cases of breast cancer in the 76 women who chose prophylactic mastectomy after a mean follow-up of 2.9 ± 1.4 years, whereas they found eight breast cancers in the 63 women who chose surveillance with a mean follow-up of 3.0 ± 1.5 years ($P = .003$). Of significance, four of the eight cancers were interval cancers (detected between screening sessions), and one of the patients undergoing surveillance died of cancer during the short follow-up. Rebbeck et al. have also reported on 483 women with BRCA1 or BRCA2 mutations, demonstrating a dramatic reduction in breast cancer (more than 90%) with bilateral mastectomy.[112] To date, the decrease in breast cancer risk has not produced an effect on overall survival.

PROPHYLACTIC OOPHORECTOMY

Premature menopause dramatically reduces both breast and ovarian cancer risks, but the degree of risk reduction for BRCA mutation carriers has only recently been demonstrated. Kauff et al. reported the results of a prospective study that included BRCA1 and BRCA2 gene mutation carriers who were at least 35 years of age and were offered the opportunity to enroll in a follow-up study after receiving genetic test results.[113] A statistically significant difference in 5-year cancer-free rate was observed in the oophorectomy group compared with the surveillance group (94% for the bilateral salpingo-oophorectomy group vs. 69% for the surveillance group). Three women were found to have unsuspected early-stage gynecologic cancers (two ovarian and one fallopian tube) at the time of risk-reducing salpingo-oophorectomy. Among the women who had oophorectomy, there were three cases of breast cancer, no cases of ovarian cancer, and one case of primary peritoneal cancer. In the surveillance group, there were eight cases of breast cancer, four cases of ovarian cancer, and one case of primary peritoneal cancer. The complication rate appears to be minimal, as only 4 of the 98 women (4.1%) had minor surgical complications.

Rebbeck et al. have also reported the results of a multicenter case-control study that included outcome data on the largest number of BRCA1 and BRCA2 mutation carriers published to date with a mean postoperative follow-up period of 8.2 years (range, 1 to 46 years).[114] The incidence of ovarian cancer was determined in 259 women who had undergone bilateral prophylactic oophorectomy at a mean age of 40.9 years and in 292 matched controls who had not undergone the procedure. With the exclusion of the six stage I ovarian cancers diagnosed at surgery, prophylactic oophorectomy significantly reduced the risk of epithelial ovarian and peritoneal cancers (adjusted hazard ratio, 0.04; 95% CI, 0.01 to 0.16). Of interest, there have been no cancer events in the 124 women who had oophorectomy by age 35 years, which suggests that the timing of oophorectomy may be important. Likewise, for the 241 women who had no history of breast cancer and who had not undergone mastectomy, a 53% breast cancer risk reduction was observed (adjusted hazard ratio, 0.47; 95% CI, 0.29 to 0.77). The most benefit in breast cancer risk reduction was observed in women who had prophylactic oophorectomy by age 50 years.

Thus, prophylactic bilateral salpingo-oophorectomy can be regarded as an effective risk-reducing procedure that permits early diagnosis of ovarian cancer at the time of surgery and significantly reduces the risk of breast and ovarian cancer in women with germline mutations in the BRCA1 and BRCA2 genes.

FOLLOW-UP EXAMINATIONS AFTER PRIMARY THERAPY

With improved outcomes in breast cancer treatment, there is a growing population of breast cancer survivors who are living to older ages. Most recurrences or metastases are diagnosed on the basis of symptoms and physical findings, and biochemical testing and imaging are unnecessary. For the small proportion of cancer survivors with inherited susceptibility, referral for genetic coun-

TABLE 33.2-8. Guidelines for Surveillance of Women with Operable Breast Cancer after Completion of Primary Therapy

Procedure	Frequency
Education of patient about symptoms and signs of recurrence	At the completion of therapy
History and physical examination	Every 3–6 mo for the first 3 y, every 6–12 mo for the next 2 y, then annually.
Referral for genetic counseling based on young age at diagnosis and family history	At time of diagnosis or after completion of therapy
Breast self-examination	Monthly
Mammography	
Contralateral	Annually
Ipsilateral (remaining after lumpectomy)	Semiannually or annually
Other recommended cancer screening[a]	Annually or every 2 y
Complete blood count, automated blood chemistry studies, assays for serum tumor markers [carcinoembryonic antigen, cancer antigen (CA) 27–CA 29, CA 15-3]	Not recommended
Radionuclide bone scanning, imaging of the chest, abdomen, pelvis, and brain	Not recommended

[a]Other recommended cancer screening procedures according to the American Cancer Society Screening guidelines.[115] (Modified from ref. 115.)

seling is appropriate, especially with regard to decisions about prophylactic surgery (mastectomy or oophorectomy) and intensive surveillance for other cancers. Guidelines for surveillance of asymptomatic women are shown in Table 33.2-8.

DUCTAL CARCINOMA *IN SITU*

DCIS (intraductal carcinoma, noninvasive ductal carcinoma) is defined as a proliferation of cancer cells confined to the ductal structures without invasion on conventional microscopic pathologic evaluation with hematoxylin and eosin staining. Microinvasive carcinoma is not included within the definition of DCIS and is considered to be T1a invasive carcinoma.

The pathologic classification of subtypes of DCIS is based predominately on nuclear grade (low, intermediate, and high nuclear grade) or architectural subtype or both.[116,117] Recent classifications have tended to favor nuclear grade for subclassification. Common architectural patterns include comedo, cribriform, papillary, micropapillary, solid, and sometimes clinging. Some authors have used a simple classification of comedo versus noncomedo subtype. The definition of comedo DCIS requires areas of necrosis and, for some authors, also high nuclear grade (grade 3). Only approximately two-thirds of lesions with comedo necrosis are high grade, with the remainder being intermediate grade. Finally, classifications have been proposed based on various combinations of pathologic features such as necrosis, nuclear grade architecture, or other characteristics.

Most DCIS lesions seen today are found on screening mammography in the asymptomatic patient. Reported risk factors for the development of DCIS are similar to the risk factors for invasive carcinoma, including a family history of breast cancer, previous breast biopsy, fewer pregnancies, older age at first pregnancy, and later menopause.[118] Data from the Surveillance, Epidemiology, and End Results program document a dramatic rise in the incidence of DCIS in the United States beginning in the mid-1980s associated with the increased use of screening mammography.[119] The largest increase in DCIS detection is seen for women aged 50 years and older, for whom screening mammography is recommended, with a lower increase for women aged 40 to 49 years, for whom there is controversy regarding the utility of screening mammography. Because the method of detection is predominately screening mammography for asymptomatic women, the natural history of small, mammographically detected DCIS is prolonged, and therefore long-term outcome studies are necessary to understand the effect of any given treatment on this disease.

Pathologic studies of women at high risk have evaluated the likelihood of finding previously undetected DCIS in prophylactic mastectomy specimens, but the results have not been consistent across studies. In a case-control study, Kauff et al. reported that, for 24 patients with known BRCA mutations, there was a higher likelihood of finding DCIS as well as other high-risk lesions at the time of prophylactic mastectomy.[120] Hoogerbrugge et al. reported the pathologic results for 67 high-risk women (67% BRCA positive) and found a 15% incidence of DCIS in the prophylactic mastectomy specimens, as well as other high-risk lesions.[109] In contrast, Adem et al. did not find an increased risk of DCIS or other high-risk lesions in the prophylactic mastectomy specimens from 28 women with BRCA mutations.[121]

Page et al. reported the long-term natural history for 28 patients with low-grade DCIS treated by biopsy only.[122] There were ten local recurrences (36%), nine of invasive carcinoma and one of DCIS only. Two of the local recurrences occurred more than 20 years after initial biopsy, which emphasizes the long natural history of this disease. The risk for developing invasive breast carcinoma among these patients was estimated to be nine times that of the general population. Similar findings were reported by Rosen et al.[123]

No consensus currently exists regarding the optimal management of most clinical presentations of DCIS. The different presentations of this disease, both clinically and pathologically, suggest that DCIS includes several different subsets of disease that, in turn, may require different treatments. Currently, there are three local treatment options for DCIS of the breast: (1) excision (also referred to as *lumpectomy* or *breast-conserving surgery*) plus definitive breast irradiation; (2) excision alone without definitive breast irradiation (also referred to as *observation*); and (3) mastectomy. There is now also the option of systemic therapy with tamoxifen. The optimal combination of local and systemic treatments for the individual patient with DCIS remains an area of active investigation.

The selection of patients for breast-conservation treatment for DCIS parallels that for treatment of invasive breast carcinoma. By definition, DCIS is staged according to AJCC criteria as stage TisN0M0. Although most DCIS lesions are currently detected by mammogram features only, the presence of a positive physical examination finding, such as a mass, is not a contraindication to breast-conservation treatment. Suitable candidates for breast-conservation treatment have unilateral disease at presentation, negative margins of resection, unicentric disease,

tumors of 4 to 5 cm or smaller, and no contraindications to breast-conservation treatment. Contraindications to breast-conservation treatment include diffuse suspicious microcalcifications on mammography, gross multicentric disease, prior radiation treatment, active collagen vascular disease, a large tumor size relative to breast size, or pregnancy (because of the inability to deliver radiation treatment).

The standard breast imaging for DCIS is mammography, with special views and ultrasonography as indicated. For the patient who has microcalcifications on mammography and who is a candidate for breast-conservation treatment, a postbiopsy mammogram with magnification should be performed to confirm the absence of residual microcalcifications. Specimen radiography at the time of surgical biopsy does not eliminate the need for a postbiopsy mammography. Studies have suggested the potential value of MRI for evaluating DCIS lesions.[124,125]

For patients undergoing breast-conserving treatment, the rationale for adding radiation treatment after excision for DCIS is that randomized trials have consistently shown radiotherapy to be effective in reducing the risk of local recurrence after lumpectomy by approximately half (Table 33.2-9). Arguments against the routine use of radiation after lumpectomy are as follows. First, adding radiation treatment after lumpectomy does not increase survival as demonstrated by randomized clinical trials (see Table 33.2-9). Second, in principle, there may be patients whose risk of local recurrence is sufficiently low that the reduction in local recurrence from adding radiation treatment may be so small that radiation is not warranted on a risk-benefit basis. In contrast to randomized trials, retrospective institutional studies that have attempted to identify patients suitable for lumpectomy alone (without radiation treatment) are hypothesis generating, not hypothesis testing, and the low local recurrence rates seen in many of these studies may be the result of careful selection of low-risk patients. The subgroup of patients who may avoid the increased risk of a local recurrence despite the omission of radiation therapy have not been prospectively and reproducibly identified by any clinical trial.

The randomized trial with the longest reported outcome data for patients with DCIS is the NSABP B-17 study.[126–128] This study randomly assigned 818 patients to radiation versus no radiation after lumpectomy. Patients were stratified according to age, method of detection, and the presence of LCIS associated with DCIS but were not stratified according to pathologic characteristics of the DCIS lesion. The patients studied in the NSABP B-17 trial have characteristics similar to those of patients in contemporary practice: The DCIS lesions were mammographically detected in 81% of the patients, and the tumor size was 2 cm or less in the large majority of patients. Although the protocol specifications required negative margins according to the NSABP definition of any distance between the inked surface and tumor, central pathologic review confirmed negative margins in 83% of the cases (516 of 623). At 12 years, the ipsilateral local failure rate was 31.7% without radiation compared to 15.7% with radiation ($P < .000005$). The curves for local recurrence continue to diverge through 12 years of follow-up, and therefore the reduction in local recurrence is a true reduction in local recurrence, not simply a delay in local recurrence. Statistically significant reductions also were seen at 12 years both for invasive local recurrence (16.8% vs. 7.7%, respectively; $P = .00001$) and for DCIS local recurrence (14.6% vs. 8.0%, respectively; $P = .001$).

TABLE 33.2-9. Results of Randomized Trials of Radiation after Lumpectomy for Ductal Carcinoma *In Situ*

Study	No. of Patients	Median Follow-Up (Y)	Outcome	Ipsilateral Local Recurrence				Overall Survival		
				Without Radiation (%)	With Radiation (%)	Risk Reduction (%)	P Value	Without Radiation (%)	With Radiation (%)	P Value
Fisher et al.[128]										
NSABP B-17 Trial	813	10.8	At 12 y	31.7	15.7	50	<.000005	86	87	.80
Julien et al.[130]										
EORTC 10853 Trial	1002	4.25	At 4 y	16	9	44	.005	99	99	.94
Houghton et al.[132]										
UK DCIS Trial	1030[a]	4.4	Crude incidence	14	6	57	<.0001	—	—	—

EORTC, European Organization for Research and Treatment of Cancer; DCIS, ductal carcinoma *in situ*; NSABP, National Surgical Adjuvant Breast and Bowel Project.
[a]For radiation randomization only.

Central pathologic review for the NSABP B-17 trial showed that the use of radiation reduced local recurrence for all pathologic subsets of tumor analyzed, including the most favorable lesions identified.[127] On multivariate analysis, independent variables significantly associated with a lower rate of local recurrence were clear margins, the use of radiation (compared to no radiation), and absent or slight necrosis (compared to moderate or marked necrosis); tumor type and multifocality were borderline for statistical significance. In the lowest-risk subgroup of patients with absent or slight necrosis, radiation reduced the absolute 8-year risk of local recurrence by 7%.

In the NSABP B-17 study, the overall rate of breast conservation was higher and the rate of mastectomy was lower for patients treated initially with radiation therapy. The overall mastectomy rate was 7% (29 of 411) for patients treated initially with lumpectomy plus radiation treatment, but 12% (50 of 403) for patients treated initially with lumpectomy without radiation treatment.

As in the NSABP B-17 trial, the European Organization for Research and Treatment of Cancer (EORTC) 10853 trial randomly assigned 1010 patients to receive radiation or no radiation after lumpectomy.[129,130] At a median follow-up of 4.25 years, the use of radiation was found to reduce the 4-year risk of local recurrence from 16% to 9% (P = .005). Reductions with radiation treatment were observed for invasive local recurrence (8% vs. 4%, respectively; P = .04) and DCIS local recurrence (8% vs. 5%, respectively; P = .06). Central pathologic review was performed. On multivariate analysis, independent risk factors for an increased risk of local recurrence were omission of radiation treatment (P = .009), clinical symptoms as method of detection of the primary tumor (P = .008), non-negative margins of resection (P = .0008), unfavorable architectural subtype (P = .012), and age of 40 years or younger (P = .02).

A trial in the United Kingdom used a modified two-by-two design to randomly assign 1701 patients who underwent complete local excision to radiation versus no radiation as well as to tamoxifen (20 mg daily for 5 years) versus no tamoxifen.[132] For the subset of 1030 patients randomly assigned to receive radiation treatment or no radiation treatment, the addition of radia-

tion in this trial led to a reduction in local recurrence with a magnitude of benefit similar to that in the NSABP B-17 and EORTC 10853 trials (see Table 33.2-9).

Adjuvant hormonal treatment with tamoxifen should be considered for the patient with DCIS (Table 33.2-10). The NSABP B-24 trial randomly assigned 1804 patients to receive tamoxifen (20 mg daily for 5 years) versus no tamoxifen after lumpectomy plus radiation treatment.[128,131] Although there was no difference in the 7-year rate of overall survival (95% without tamoxifen vs. 95% with tamoxifen; P = .78), there were significant reductions in the 7-year rates of ipsilateral local recurrence, contralateral breast cancer, and all breast cancer events (P ≤.02). For the subset of 1576 patients in the United Kingdom trial randomly assigned to receive tamoxifen or no tamoxifen, there was a reduction in the rate of contralateral breast cancer of borderline statistical significance (P = .07), but there was no difference in the rates of ipsilateral local recurrence or all breast cancer events.[132] Longer follow-up for these two trials will be important in assessing the value of adjuvant tamoxifen for DCIS.

Whether or not aromatase inhibitors will prove useful for DCIS remains to be established. The NSABP currently has an open trial (NSABP B-35) for postmenopausal patients that randomly assigns patients to receive either tamoxifen or anastrozole after lumpectomy plus radiation.

In the NSABP B-24 trial, Allred et al. evaluated the role of ER status in the prediction of response to adjuvant tamoxifen.[133] Patients with ER-positive tumors treated with tamoxifen had a relative risk of 0.41 for all breast cancer events compared to patients treated without tamoxifen (P = .0002). In contrast, no significant benefit for tamoxifen was seen for patients with ER-negative tumors (P = .51). However, the number of patients in the ER-negative subset was small (n = 153).

Institutional studies have attempted to identify patients who may have a sufficiently low risk of local recurrence without radiation that the marginal benefit of adding radiation after lumpectomy may be sufficiently small to consider omitting radiation treatment.[134,135] In these studies of lumpectomy alone without radiation, the actuarial rate of local recurrence was 20% to 44% at 10 years, and the actuarial rate of local

TABLE 33.2-10. Results of Randomized Trials of Tamoxifen for Ductal Carcinoma *In Situ*

Study	No. of Patients	Median Follow-Up (Y)	Local Treatment	Outcome	Ipsilateral Local Recurrence			Contralateral Breast Cancer			All Breast Cancer Events		
					Without Tamoxifen (%)	With Tamoxifen (%)	P Value	Without Tamoxifen (%)	With Tamoxifen (%)	P Value	Without Tamoxifen (%)	With Tamoxifen (%)	P Value
Fisher et al.[128] NSABP B-24 Trial	1798	6.9	Lumpectomy plus radiation	At 7 y	11.1	7.7	.02	4.9	2.3	.01	16.9	10.0	.0003
Houghton et al.[132] UK DCIS Trial	1576[a]	4.4	Local excision ± radiation	Crude local recurrence	15	13	.42	3	1	.07	18	14	.13

DCIS, ductal carcinoma *in situ*; NSABP, National Surgical Adjuvant Breast and Bowel Project.
[a]For tamoxifen randomization only.

recurrence was 22% to 49% at 15 years. In these institutional studies, favorable criteria were used to select patients to undergo excision alone—for example, small tumor size, widely negative margins of resection, mammographic detection, and favorable pathologic tumor characteristics. In a multivariate analysis of patients individually selected for the local treatment, the addition of radiation treatment was associated with a 55% reduction in local recurrence ($P = .0002$), and the risk of local recurrence was also significantly reduced for those with low tumor nuclear grade ($P = .018$), older age ($P = .0015$), smaller tumor size ($P < .0001$), and widely negative margins of resection ($P < .0001$).[134] These results are very similar to the results seen in randomized trials, as described earlier.

Multiple retrospective studies have evaluated outcomes after breast-conservation surgery and radiation treatment.[133,136,137] These studies generally show similar rates of local recurrence and survival similar to those seen in randomized trials. In a large multi-institutional collaborative study, the long-term outcomes were reported for 418 patients with 422 treated intraductal breast carcinomas (including 4 patients with bilateral DCIS at presentation).[136] With a median follow-up of 9.4 years, the 15-year actuarial outcomes after radiation treatment were as follows: overall survival 92%, cause-specific survival 98%, freedom from distant metastases 94%, local failure 60%, and contralateral breast cancer 18%.[136] The most common types of first failure after treatment were local failure (n = 41; 10%), contralateral breast cancer (n = 27; 6%), and nonbreast second malignancy (n = 17; 4%). Approximately half of the local failures were invasive cancer and half were DCIS. On multivariable analysis, younger patient age and positive margins of resection were independently associated with an increased risk for local recurrence (both $P \leq .030$).

The appropriate minimum width for negative margins of resections remains controversial. In the NSABP B-17 study, the margin was considered to be negative for any distance between the inked surface and the DCIS lesion. In most retrospective studies in which patients were treated with breast-conservation surgery followed by definitive radiation treatment, an adequate negative margin was considered to be 1 to 2 mm or more. In contrast, studies that use breast-conservation surgery alone without radiation treatment require substantially wider minimal negative margins, and a minimum negative margin width of at least 10 mm has been suggested as optimal.[135] This difference in minimum negative margin width for patients treated with radiation versus those treated without radiation must be carefully considered when selecting patients for breast-conservation treatment, particularly when omission of radiation treatment is considered. For patients undergoing breast-conservation surgery with or without radiation therapy, negative margin width may be a more important predictor of local recurrence than pathologic characteristics of the tumor.[135,138] No uniform definition of negative margins has been established in the literature, and no single definition of negative margin status has been shown to be superior to any other definition.[127]

The uncertainty as to the optimal minimum negative margin width has substantial practical implications. Margins of resection are one of the few variables that can be controlled by the treating physician, for example, by the extent of surgical resection or by the use of a reexcision. For patients undergoing breast-conservation treatment, either with or without radiation treatment, adequate surgical excision, with reexcision if indicated, is important to maximize local control. Obtaining nega-

tive margins of resection remains the goal of surgical excision or reexcision, even though the optimal extent of negative margin width remains uncertain. A large, prospective-registration Breast Intergroup study is evaluating margin and grade of small lesions in patients receiving tamoxifen therapy or no tamoxifen using central pathologic review. Accrual is completed.

Although younger patients are at increased risk for local recurrence, there is a substantial interaction between younger age and margins of resection. In retrospective studies, younger patients tend to have lower rates of negative margins of resection. Whether this is due to tumor biology or to the extent of surgical resection remains uncertain. Although results are based on small numbers of patients, younger patients with adequate excision appear to be adequately treated with breast conservation.[136,137]

Axillary lymph node staging is not indicated for pure DCIS lesions.[139] The incidence of axillary lymph node involvement is less than 1%. In the rare patient with DCIS and axillary lymph node metastasis, the probable cause is likely occult microinvasion. The recent development of the sentinel lymph node biopsy procedure, with the associated substantial reduction in morbidity compared to axillary lymph node dissection, has raised the question of whether sentinel lymph node biopsy is indicated for selected high-risk subsets of patients, such as those with larger tumors or high-grade lesions.[139–141] The use of sentinel lymph node biopsy to stage DCIS is controversial. However, sentinel lymph node biopsy is not recommended at the present time.

The technical delivery of radiation treatment for DCIS is similar to that for node-negative invasive breast carcinoma. Commonly accepted technical radiation treatment is to deliver whole breast radiation using tangential fields, generally followed by a boost to the primary tumor site. The radiation dose to the whole breast is 45 to 50 Gy using 1.8 to 2.0 Gy/fraction, with treatments delivered daily, Monday through Friday. A boost is commonly delivered to the primary tumor site to bring the total dose to 60 to 66 Gy. Negative margins of resection do not contraindicate a breast boost. However, if a boost is not used, the margins of resection must be negative. Although there is no randomized study examining breast boost in the context of DCIS, the rationale for the use of a boost is extrapolated from randomized studies of boost for invasive carcinoma, as well as from analyses of retrospective institutional studies. Acceptable local control rates were reported in the NSABP B-17 study in the radiation arm, in which the radiation dose was 50 Gy given in 2-Gy fractions, with only 9% of the patients receiving a boost. Radiation treatment to the regional lymphatics is not indicated for DCIS. However, the sentinel lymph nodes are included within standard tangent fields for the large majority of patients.

Patients currently undergoing breast-conservation treatment for DCIS without an axillary lymph node dissection should have high rates of excellent or good cosmetic outcome and low rates of complications. Mills et al. reported that the 5-year rate of excellent or good cosmetic outcome was 97% and that the risk of complications was strongly related to the use of axillary lymph node dissection, which is not the current standard of care.[142]

Mastectomy has not been compared to breast-conservation treatment in randomized trials involving DCIS patients. None of the currently accruing or completed randomized trials have a mastectomy arm. Although mastectomy has been postulated to have a potential 1% to 2% overall survival benefit compared to breast-conservation treatment, this hypothesis has not been tested in a randomized trial. Such a randomized trial would require thousands of patients with long-term follow-up and would not be acceptable to patients with contemporary management that emphasizes breast-conservation treatment. Nonetheless, there may be a small subset of patients who are likely better served with mastectomy, for example, patients with a tumor larger than 4 to 5 cm, extensive microcalcifications on mammography, or a large tumor size relative to breast size. For such patients, mastectomy, usually with immediate reconstruction, provides appropriate local treatment.

The potential role of postmastectomy radiation treatment, if any, has been poorly studied for DCIS. Chest wall recurrence after mastectomy for pure DCIS has been observed in 1% or fewer of patients in retrospective series. Little information has been reported on selection for and outcome after postmastectomy radiation treatment for DCIS.

The characteristics of DCIS at the molecular level, including biologic markers as well as proteomics, have been studied. High-grade or comedo DCIS tends to be associated with high rates of cell proliferation and biologic aggressiveness. However, the promising results of molecular biologic, genomic, and proteomic studies have not yet been integrated into routine clinical practice for the management of patients with DCIS.

LOBULAR CARCINOMA *IN SITU*

The first reference to LCIS is generally credited to Foote and Stewart in 1941.[143] They characterized LCIS as a distinct clinical entity involving a noninvasive proliferation of cells arising from the breast lobules and terminal ductal area.

LCIS is typically discovered as an incidental pathologic finding on biopsy performed for another indication. Because of the absence of distinct clinical or mammographic findings, the true incidence of LCIS is difficult to determine but is estimated to be on the order of 1% to 4% of all breast cancers. Using data from the Surveillance, Epidemiology, and End Results program, Li et al. reported that the incidence of LCIS is increasing.[144] The age distribution for LCIS tends to be slightly younger than that for women with invasive carcinoma.

For patients with an abnormal mammogram finding, LCIS is an uncommon lesion identified in 1% to 2% of core biopsy specimens obtained. When a core biopsy specimen shows only LCIS after an abnormal radiographic finding, excisional biopsy with mammographic needle localization is recommended because of the high risk of having missed an invasive carcinoma or DCIS.

The controversy regarding management of LCIS relates to whether LCIS is a precursor lesion or a marker for patients at high risk for subsequent development of invasive carcinoma. Much of the evidence suggests that LCIS is a high-risk marker, not a premalignant lesion in and of itself.

Outcome studies of patients with LCIS treated with biopsy, rather than mastectomy, have demonstrated a number of trends.[145] First, LCIS is associated with a substantially increased relative risk of developing breast cancer. Second, the diagnosis of subsequent invasive carcinoma is seen almost as frequently in the contralateral breast as in the ipsilateral breast. Third, the majority of lesions are invasive ductal carcinomas, although the incidence of invasive lobular carcinoma is greater than in patients without a prior diagnosis of LCIS.

The current management options for LCIS of the breast include careful observation and tamoxifen for chemoprevention. Unilateral mastectomy has been discarded as a rational management for LCIS because of the high risk of bilateral disease. For most patients, careful observation remains a reasonable management strategy, because the majority of such patients do not develop subsequent invasive carcinoma. Because LCIS is a marker for subsequent invasive carcinoma, negative margins of excision are not required. For the patient who elects to undergo careful observation, recommendations for screening include monthly breast self-examination by the patient, periodic physical examination by a physician (generally once or twice yearly), and yearly bilateral screening mammography. It is essential that this screening be explained as lifelong, lest negative screening results for 10 years be considered to indicate that the danger has passed. Although MRI screening may be promising for high-risk women, large-scale studies with long-term follow-up have not yet been published for women with LCIS. Radiation therapy has not been demonstrated to be effective treatment for lobular carcinoma of the breast.

In the NSABP P-1 trial, high-risk women were randomly assigned to receive tamoxifen (20 mg daily for 5 years) or placebo.[105] For the patients with LCIS, the risk reduction for invasive breast cancer was 56% in those receiving tamoxifen. Thus, tamoxifen remains a rational approach to reduce risk for women with LCIS. Patients with LCIS are currently eligible for enrollment in the NSABP STAR trial, which randomly assigns patients to receive tamoxifen 20 mg daily for 5 years or raloxifene 60 mg daily for 5 years.[146] No data on prevention are yet available for other systemic agents, for example, aromatase inhibitors.

BRCA mutation carriers are known to have an increased risk for the development of invasive breast carcinoma. The relationship of these mutations to LCIS remains uncertain. Three studies have reported the pathologic findings for high-risk patients undergoing prophylactic mastectomy. In a case-control study, Kauff et al. reported the pathologic findings for prophylactic mastectomy specimens from 24 patients with BRCA mutation, and an increased risk of LCIS as well as of other high-risk lesions was identified, with an odds ratio of 12.7.[147] Hoogerbrugge et al. reported on prophylactic mastectomy specimens from 67 high-risk women (66% with BRCA-positive mutations) and identified 25% with LCIS; the prevalence of other high-risk lesions was also increased.[109] In contrast, Adem et al. in a case-control study found no increased risk of high-risk lesions in 28 BRCA carriers.[121]

A number of studies have evaluated various molecular biologic characteristics of LCIS. LCIS tends to be associated with markers for low growth rate and proliferation as well as expression of hormone receptors. The implications of these findings for clinical practice remain to be determined.

PAGET'S DISEASE

The clinical description of Paget's disease can be found as early as the 1800s.[148] Paget's disease typically involves the nipple in its earliest stages and later can involve the areola or underlying breast. The clinical manifestations of Paget's disease include eczematoid changes, crusting, redness, irritation, erosion, discharge, retraction, and inversion. Rare manifestations of Paget's disease include bilateral Paget's disease or Paget's disease in the male patient.

Pathologically, Paget's disease represents *in situ* carcinoma in the nipple epidermis. The classic pathologic finding is the presence of Paget cells (large cells with clear cytoplasm and atypical nuclei) within the epidermis of the nipple.[149] It is uncertain whether the origin of Paget's disease is *in situ*, intra-epidermal malignancy with secondary extension to adjacent structures or migration of tumor cells into the nipple epidermis from an underlying carcinoma of the breast.[150]

The workup for the patient with Paget's disease should include mammography with attention to the subareolar region. Mammography is indicated to identify an underlying breast carcinoma, which can be seen as a mass or microcalcifications, typically in the subareolar region. Physical examination of the breast is necessary to rule out an underlying breast mass as well as to exclude axillary lymphadenopathy.

Historically, Paget's disease has been treated with mastectomy. Adverse prognostic factors include the presence of a palpable mass in the breast, associated invasive carcinoma in the breast, and pathologically involved axillary lymph nodes.[150]

Studies have focused on the potential for breast-conservation treatment, either with or without breast irradiation. The rationale for breast-conserving treatment of Paget's disease includes the success of breast-conservation treatment for DCIS of the breast and the earlier detection of Paget's disease with lower disease burden at presentation for many patients.

There are a number of series of patients who received breast-conservation treatment for Paget's disease. Marshall et al. reported on 38 patients who underwent breast-conservation surgery and definitive radiation treatment.[151] The 10- and 15-year rates of local-only first failure were 13% and 13%, respectively, and the respective rates for any local failure were 17% and 24%. Overall survival was 90% at 10 and 15 years. Four of the six local failures were invasive carcinoma and two were DCIS only. Local control was accomplished with salvage surgery for five of these six patients with local failure. Bijker et al. reported on 61 patients treated with excision followed by definitive radiation therapy.[152] The 5-year local recurrence rate was 5.2%. There were four local failures; three were invasive cancer and one was DCIS only. Fourquet et al. reported on 20 patients treated with breast-conservation surgery (3 with excisional biopsy and 17 with incisional biopsy), followed by definitive breast irradiation.[153] The 7-year recurrence-free survival was 81%, and 15% of the patients (3 of 20) had a local failure, each with Paget's disease only. Other small studies of breast-conservation treatment with radiation have been reported.

Local excision alone, without definitive radiation therapy, has been used to treat a small number of patients. In one of the largest series, Polgar et al. reported on 33 patients treated with local excision alone.[154] The local recurrence rate was 33% (11 of 33). Of the 11 local recurrences, 10 (91%) were invasive carcinoma and 1 was DCIS only. Six of the ten patients with invasive local recurrence developed subsequent distant metastatic disease. Based on these findings, Polgar et al. recommended the addition of radiation after breast-conservation surgery to obtain adequate local control. Because of the small numbers of patients treated without radiation and the high rate of local failure, such treatment must be considered as nonstandard at the present time.

The results of studies of patients with DCIS of the breast will be of great interest for the management of Paget's disease, because

these results from DCIS trials will undoubtedly be extrapolated to the setting of limited Paget's disease (i.e., Paget's disease without an associated mass and without associated invasive carcinoma). Although in published reports the largest number of patients with Paget's disease have been treated with mastectomy, breast-conservation treatment with radiation appears to be a reasonable alternative at this time, albeit with the caveats that no randomized trial has been performed and only small series of published cases have been so treated.

Various biologic markers have been studied with regard to Paget's disease of the breast. Given that the outcome after treatment for limited Paget's disease (without an associated mass or invasive carcinoma) shows very high rates of survival and freedom from distant metastases, the value of such marker studies for clinical decision making is likely limited.

EARLY-STAGE BREAST CANCER

By convention, the term *early-stage breast cancer* is applied to tumors of clinical stages I and II—clearly an arbitrary distinction, but of clinical utility. Early-stage breast cancer is best managed by considering treatment of the breast cancer (treatment of the primary); treatment of the remainder of the breast (local therapy); treatment of the regional lymph nodes of the axilla, sometimes to include the internal mammary and supraclavicular nodes (regional therapy); and systemic therapy directed to the possibility of occult metastatic disease. Today a woman with early-stage breast cancer can be approached with the assumption that her breast can be spared and that she will have all of these elements of therapy provided in a tailored and integrated fashion. Not all women are candidates for this approach, and some require mastectomy as part of their treatment. For others, one or more elements of this integrated therapy may be able to be modified or eliminated based on cost-benefit considerations. Determining the order in which these various elements are best combined involves some logistic considerations that are specific to the individual or to the institution. The order is often based on custom rather than on firm evidence of a preferable treatment sequence. Present evidence suggests that sequence is of no consequence for survival.[155–157]

SURGERY OF THE BREAST

The surgical approach to the primary breast tumor involves excision of all invasive cancer with clear margins of excision that include all DCIS that is apparent. In the easiest situation of a small tumor in a breast of adequate volume, this can be accomplished via a circumareolar incision. The incision is placed to allow direct access to the tumor while achieving the optimal cosmetic outcome. Incisions in the skin of the upper inner quadrants of the breast are best avoided for cosmetic reasons. Curvilinear incisions are of special importance in the skin of the upper breast. The preservation of subcutaneous fat is important for maintaining normal breast contour. The tumor is excised as a single block with several millimeters of apparently normal tissue surrounding it. The margins of uninvolved breast tissue acceptable for classification as "negative" vary. The NSABP requires any distance between tumor and the inked margin, some authors have required 1 to 2 mm, and still others 5 to 10 mm. Because there are no convincing data to support any specific definition of negative margins as optimal with regard to invasive breast carcinoma, 1 to 2 mm appears a useful target, provided that breast irradiation is added after surgery. Invasive lobular cancers and infiltrating ductal carcinomas with extensive intraductal components are more likely to yield histologically clear margins if 5 to 10 mm of gross margin is possible.[158,159] The specimen is oriented for the pathologist with marking sutures and its surfaces inked. Small titanium clips on the walls of the excision cavity are valuable for targeting of breast irradiation. Complete hemostasis is important. This, with avoidance of drain placement, allows a small collection of serum and fibrin to form in the cavity. Suture reapproximation of the breast parenchyma is avoided, because this tends to distort the breast shape when the patient is no longer supine. Such an excision is followed by closure of the erector areola muscle and then of the skin edges with subcuticular sutures.

If histopathologic evaluation later indicates that one or more margins are involved by invasive cancer or DCIS, outpatient reexcision of that margin under local anesthesia can minimize the risk of subsequent local failure in the breast. LCIS at a margin is not an indication for reexcision. Frozen-section examination has not proved valuable for intraoperative evaluation of margins. Treatment is best accomplished when breast imaging and localization of any suspicious microcalcifications guide the surgical excision. This assures that no suspicious areas of microcalcification in other parts of that breast are left behind. For the patient who has microcalcifications on mammography and who is a candidate for breast-conservation treatment, a postexcision mammogram should be performed to confirm the absence of residual microcalcifications. Specimen radiography at the time of surgical biopsy does not eliminate the value of a postbiopsy mammogram.

It has been repeatedly demonstrated in randomized clinical trials[160,161] that survival with such breast-conservation surgery combined with other modalities of treatment is equivalent to that with mastectomy (Table 33.2-11). Updates from the EBCTCG continue to show no advantage for either mastectomy or breast-conserving therapy with breast irradiation.[162] It is important to note that because there is no significant advantage in either direction, a woman who prefers either mastectomy or breast-conserving treatment is not opting for a more

dangerous approach to treatment. Survival for women treated with lumpectomy without radiation is inferior.

PREOPERATIVE CHEMOTHERAPY

The most common reason for performing mastectomy in treating early-stage breast cancer in the United States is the concern that the tumor is of sufficient size relative to the breast size that excision to a clear margin will leave a significant deficit in breast volume or distort the shape of the breast in such a way that a better cosmetic outcome would be achieved by skin-sparing mastectomy and reconstruction. This concern can often be addressed by preoperative (neoadjuvant) chemotherapy. This has been the standard approach for a quarter of a century for locally advanced breast cancer. Complete and partial responses are seen in 60% to 90% of women. This observation led Dr. Gianni Bonadonna to begin using preoperative chemotherapy for women with earlier-stage disease to shrink the tumors to a volume that made them acceptable for the breast-conservation program of the Istituto Nazionale Tumori of Italy.[164] The safety of this approach was demonstrated definitively by the randomized trial NSABP B-18.[165] In this trial, 1523 women with T1 to T3 and N0 or N1 breast cancer as diagnosed by needle biopsy were randomly assigned to surgery followed by four cycles of doxorubicin and cyclophosphamide or to four cycles of identical chemotherapy followed by surgery. All women over 50 years of age also received concurrent tamoxifen. Only 3% of the women receiving preoperative chemotherapy showed evidence of progression. Eighty percent showed a major response and 36% showed a complete clinical response. This led to an increase in the lumpectomy rate, albeit only from 60% to 67% in this series. A subsequent NSABP preoperative chemotherapy protocol, B-27, demonstrated a clinical response rate of 85% for the same combination of doxorubicin and cyclophosphamide and a 91% major response rate when this combination was followed by docetaxel. This approach has the advantage of allowing breast-conservation therapy in many women who would otherwise require mastectomy. In the NSABP experience, in which some of the larger tumors were moved from mastectomy to breast-conservation treatment by the chemotherapy, there was no significant increase in the local failure rate, even though the initial tumor size was larger in the patients who received neoadjuvant chemotherapy before breast-conservation treatment. Another advantage of preoperative chemotherapy for early-stage breast cancer is the identification of the small group of women who do not respond to this chemotherapy regimen. Although at present it is uncertain how such women may be best treated, their identification allows ongoing trials designed to improve their outcomes. After preoperative chemotherapy, excision to clear margins is performed in the same way as it would have been had the tumor been smaller initially. It is important to place a clip in such lesions as they shrink so that the site of their presentation can be excised at the conclusion of the chemotherapy induction. Complete clinical response is often not accompanied by complete pathologic response, and it is still important to obtain clear surgical margins to achieve local control.

Prognosis after neoadjuvant chemotherapy is based on the findings at definitive surgery. Pathologic complete response confers the greatest benefit. Neoadjuvant endocrine therapy can also produce dramatic responses in hormone receptor–expressing

TABLE 33.2-11. Breast-Sparing Surgery with Radiation versus Mastectomy: 1995 National Cancer Institute Update Conference

	Deaths/Patients		
Study	BCT with RT	Mastectomy	*Difference*
Denmark	90/430	77/429	None
EORTC	107/456	89/422	None
Institut Gustave Roussy	17/88	18/91	None
NCI—Bethesda	14/121	17/116	None
NCI—Milan	74/352	84/349	None
NSABP[a]	176/515	188/492	None
Total	478/1962	473/1899	None

BCT, breast-conserving treatment; EORTC, European Organization for Research and Treatment of Cancer; NCI, National Cancer Institute; NSABP, National Surgical Adjuvant Breast and Bowel Project; RT, radiotherapy.
[a]St. Luc Hospital data excluded.[163]

TABLE 33.2-12. Breast-Conserving Therapy Sequence without Neoadjuvant Chemotherapy

---

Core-needle biopsy

Lumpectomy and sentinel lymph node (SLN) biopsy and axillary dissection if SLN positive

Adjuvant systemic chemotherapy, if indicated

Breast irradiation

Adjuvant selective estrogen receptor modulator or aromatase inhibitor, if estrogen or progesterone receptor positive

---

cancers, but most experience has been in older women. The time course of tumor response appears slower than with cytotoxic agents. Custom has long dictated the order in which different modalities of breast cancer treatment are delivered. The use of core-needle biopsy for diagnosis has eliminated the necessity for tumor excision as the first modality. The virtue of performing sentinel lymph node biopsy before preoperative chemotherapy is based on first principles and is unproven. A case has been made for the early delivery of both systemic chemotherapy and breast irradiation. It has become conventional to deliver the adjuvant chemotherapy before the breast irradiation. Table 33.2-12 lists a common sequence for tumors small enough to be excised without preoperative chemotherapy as a consideration, and Table 33.2-13 gives the sequence for tumors for which neoadjuvant chemotherapy will be used.

INDICATIONS FOR MASTECTOMY

Treatment of the primary tumor is surgical. Treatment of the remainder of the breast tissue for control of occult disease can be accomplished by either surgery or irradiation. Although women with early breast cancer are approached with the intention of offering breast-conserving therapy, there are situations in which that is not possible. Contraindications to breast-conservation treatment include (1) presence of two or more primary tumors in separate areas of the breast, (2) diffuse malignant-appearing microcalcifications, or (3) a history of prior therapeutic irradiation to the breast that precludes full-breast irradiation for the present condition. Persistently positive margins after repeated (more than two) attempts at surgical reexcision is a relative contraindication. Pregnancy is an absolute contraindication to the delivery of breast irradiation, but the other elements of treatment may be used during pregnancy and radiation may be held until the child is delivered, as discussed later in Breast Cancer and Pregnancy. Active collagen vascular disease, particularly scleroderma

TABLE 33.2-13. Breast-Conserving Therapy Sequence with Neoadjuvant Chemotherapy

---

Core-needle biopsy

Sentinel lymph node biopsy and placement of clip at site of primary tumor

Neoadjuvant chemotherapy

Lumpectomy (and axillary dissection if sentinel lymph node positive), if feasible; otherwise, mastectomy with postmastectomy radiation treatment

Breast irradiation
   With or without further chemotherapy

Adjuvant selective estrogen receptor modulator or aromatase inhibitor (if estrogen or progesterone receptor positive)

---

or systemic lupus erythematosus, is felt to render patients intolerant of therapeutic levels of radiation because of the high risk of complications.[166] Patients with multifocal breast cancer or indeterminate calcifications require careful assessment for suitability for breast-conserving therapy. A large tumor in a small breast that does not respond to induction chemotherapy or inability to administer induction chemotherapy is a relative contraindication, if adequate excision would result in significant cosmetic deformity of the breast. Finally, breast size can be a relative contraindication in that women with very large or pendulous breasts should understand that the cosmetic outcome of the breast-conservation treatment may be less than ideal. On the other hand, mastectomy and reconstruction would also be less than ideal. For women who are not well treated by breast-conserving therapy, mastectomy is recommended. Certain situations that were once proposed as contraindications to breast-conservation treatment have subsequently been shown not to be: subareolar primary tumor, T2 tumor, clinically positive axillary lymph nodes, and extremes of age.

There are several types of mastectomy procedure. A *total mastectomy* removes the entire breast, including the nipple and areola. Flaps are elevated at a level designed to remove all of the breast tissue but not the subcutaneous fat. The thickness of the flaps is consequently specific to the individual, rather than being a fixed measurement. Optimal placement of the incision results in an oblique scar in line with the direction of least tension in the chest wall skin and ending lateral to the sternal border. The fascia of the pectoralis muscle is removed to leave no breast tissue adherent to it. The margins of the breast are just beneath the clavicle superiorly, the lateral border of the sternum medially, and the lateral border of the latissimus dorsi muscle laterally. Inferiorly, mastectomy used to be continued to the superior aspect of the rectus abdominus muscle. Today mastectomy typically ends inferiorly at the inframammary fold. *Skin-sparing mastectomy* is total mastectomy performed through a circumareolar incision removing only the skin of the nipple and areola (Fig. 33.2-3). If the breast is too large or the areola is too small to allow removal of the resected breast, the incision can be extended slightly to allow the extraction of the breast specimen. In skin-sparing mastectomy the inframammary fold is not lysed. This leaves a tiny amount of breast tissue but greatly enhances the reconstruction. If the tumor is near the inframammary fold, the fold should not be spared. The biopsy incision is excised if radiation will not be delivered. Skin-sparing mastectomy has never been evaluated in a large, prospective, randomized trial. Results from multiple series of patients treated by skin-sparing mastectomy, however, show no evidence of increased local or regional failure compared with results for patients treated concomitantly with mastectomy techniques that removed much of the breast skin.[167] Sparing the skin envelope allows immediate reconstruction and a remarkable restoration of the initial breast shape. This diminishes the number of procedures required for the reconstruction and reduces the likelihood of any tailoring, reduction, or mastopexy to the contralateral breast to make it match the shape of the reconstructed breast. The skin-sparing mastectomy is coupled with immediate reconstruction to refill the native skin envelope. If collapsed without normal tension, the skin becomes pachydermatous and will not achieve normal flexibility and appearance with delayed reconstruction. If there is any involvement of the skin, the involved skin should be removed with a margin of several centimeters of apparently normal skin. This is one time that frozen-section margin examination is helpful in breast cancer management.

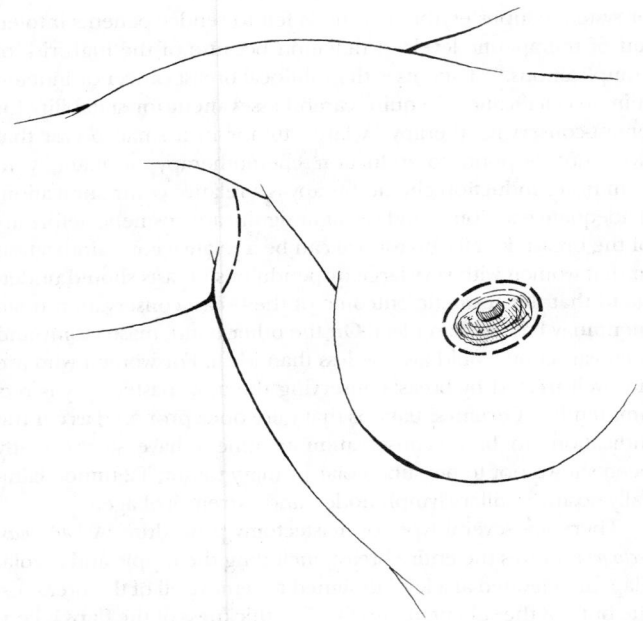

FIGURE 33.2-3. Skin-sparing mastectomy. The breast parenchyma is excised through a circumareolar incision. A transverse axillary incision may be added if required for axillary dissection. (Adapted from Spear SL. *Surgery of the breast: principles and art.* Philadelphia: Lippincott–Raven, 1998:251.)

When immediate reconstruction is not elected, it is important to remove a sufficient ellipse of skin to allow the tension of the remaining chest wall skin to be that of skin elsewhere on the trunk. Reconstruction can then be accomplished at a later date with any of the usual techniques, including implants, tissue expanders, or latissimus dorsi or transverse rectus abdominis muscle (TRAM) flaps. Less common flaps are available when required, including free flaps from the buttock, flaps from the lateral waist area, or flaps from the lateral hip. Several advantages are sometimes listed for delayed reconstruction. These include not having to irradiate a reconstructed breast. If postmastectomy irradiation is likely to be required, a reconstructive technique not requiring the use of an implant (e.g., TRAM flap) is preferred. It is probably best to construct a slightly larger breast than would otherwise be required when radiation is planned to allow for possible shrinkage. Liposuction afterward can adjust a breast that is a bit too large. Irradiating a reconstructed breast that contains a prosthesis increases the risk of excessive capsule formation requiring revision. Another advantage cited for delayed reconstruction is the time provided to grieve loss of the breast and accept the reconstructed breast as an improvement over breast absence, rather than as a disappointingly imperfect substitute for the natural breast that it replaces. Finally, when postmastectomy irradiation is anticipated, some reconstructive surgeons prefer to begin with the final results of treatment before designing optimal reconstruction.

MANAGEMENT OF REGIONAL LYMPH NODES

Attention has long been focused on the axilla as an integral aspect of breast cancer management. This attention was initially directed toward controlling cancer in the axillary lymph nodes that was believed to have escaped from the breast but not yet to have escaped from the regional lymph nodes. Today axillary lymph node metastases are considered a regional manifestation of metastatic breast cancer. Axillary lymph nodes that are suspicious by palpation for tumor can be evaluated by FNA cytologic examination when results will affect the order of therapeutic interventions. If axillary lymph nodes are matted or fixed (N2), the disease has advanced beyond "early" breast cancer. When mobile axillary lymph nodes contain tumor, an axillary dissection provides excellent local control of this axillary disease.[168] This is only the surgical aspect of such control, and there is a role for radiation and systemic therapy as well in controlling disease in the axilla.[169,170] The primary indication for axillary surgery today is the provision of pathologic staging. If the axillary lymph nodes are involved, their removal accomplishes both goals: defining prognosis and diminishing the risk of subsequent axillary recurrence.

There has long been contention about the role of axillary dissection when the axilla is clinically free of disease. For many years, axillary dissection was performed as a standard part of all early breast cancer treatment to provide this important staging information. A host of primary tumor parameters including size, grade, receptor expression, tumor markers, and certain genomic patterns also suggest the likelihood of occult systemic metastases. In prospective trials, the prognostic value of nodal staging has always exceeded that of any pattern of markers seen in the primary tumor. Such markers indicate the probability that occult metastasis has occurred in a population of similar patients. Axillary nodal metastases are outcome data establishing that metastasis has already occurred to these nodes in a given patient.

Elective axillary nodal dissection accomplishes this staging but at the cost of the complications of axillary dissection. For women found to be free of axillary nodal metastases, there is no benefit to offset this cost other than the staging information. Giuliano et al. adapted Morton's sentinel lymph node mapping and biopsy for melanoma to breast cancer.[171] The efficacy of biopsy of the sentinel lymph nodes in identifying the lymph node–negative axilla without axillary dissection has been clearly demonstrated by a host of other investigators.[172,173] Although sentinel lymph node biopsy has been widely accepted as a standard of care for women with clinically negative axillary nodes, large prospective multi-institutional studies such as NSABP B-32 and American College of Surgeons Oncology Group Z10/11 are establishing the precise efficacy of this technique.

Several techniques of sentinel lymph node mapping are in use. Lymphazurin blue dye may be injected at the border of the tumor or in the subareolar tissue.[174] The lymphatics carry the blue dye to the axilla in approximately 5 minutes with massage of the breast. The use of technetium radiocolloid injected in similar fashion 1 hour or more previously[175] or intradermally overlying the tumor allows intraoperative use of Geiger counters to identify the sentinel lymph nodes and guide the incision.[176] The incision is usually best placed transversely 1 to 2 cm above the lowest point of axillary hair-bearing skin. Blue-dyed lymphatics appear like a ballpoint pen line of bright blue. They are followed to the sentinel node, which is usually a bright blue but may be free of dye if replaced by tumor. Combining blue dye and radiocolloid improved the results in some studies. Rare instances of allergic or anaphylactic reactions to Lymphazurin have been reported. If only a single sentinel lymph node is identified, the false-negative rate is approximately 15%. If two or more sentinel lymph nodes are identified, the false-negative rate is reduced to less than 5%.[177] Before the skin is closed, it is important to palpate with a finger in the axilla for small, hard lymph nodes that might otherwise be missed. Large trials of sentinel lymph node surgery are continuing to define the optimal technique. When lymph node staging is confined to excision of a few sentinel lymph nodes, the risk of lymphedema and of injury to the intercostobrachial nerves is markedly reduced. Contraindications include clinically positive axillary lymph nodes and tumors arising in the axilla that defeat the technique for sentinel lymph node identification. Large or multiple tumors and preoperative chemotherapy are not absolute contraindications. It is not clear that sentinel lymph node biopsy is as accurate after preoperative chemotherapy,[178] and many institutions prefer to perform this technique before the administration of chemotherapy. A large trial is under way to address the need for axillary dissection when sentinel lymph nodes are positive. Until these results are available, axillary dissection for staging and control remains the customary practice for sentinel lymph node–positive women. However, radiation including the axilla is an acceptable alternative provided the decisions regarding systemic therapy would not be altered by additional information supplied by axillary lymph node dissection.[169]

Lymphoscintigraphy demonstrates alternative lymphatic drainage patterns to internal mammary chain or supraclavicular nodes on occasion. Because past trials have demonstrated that metastases to these nodal bases are rare in the absence of axillary nodal metastases, it is not customary to biopsy sentinel nodes in these locations. Drainage to an alternative lymphatic region does not in and of itself mandate radiation to this region in the absence of pathologically proven disease.

Accurate identification of the sentinel lymph node is dependent on the skill and experience of the surgeon. As the technique has been implemented, a learning curve of 10 to 20 cases with completion axillary dissection to confirm more than 90% identification and no more than one false-negative staging has been proposed for surgical credentialing.

AXILLARY DISSECTION

When axillary dissection is performed in conjunction with total mastectomy, the surgical procedure is termed *modified radical mastectomy*. The dissection is performed in continuity with the mastectomy. The level I and II axillary lymph nodes (lateral to and beneath the pectoralis minor muscle, respectively) are removed with care to spare the tissue anterior to the axillary vein, the superior cord of the intercostobrachial nerve, the thoracodorsal vessels and nerve, the long thoracic nerve, and the medial pectoral nerve. Percutaneous suction catheters are placed. The risk of seroma formation is minimized if these are left in place until the drainage is 30 mL/d or less, typically 7 days. Axillary dissection performed with breast-conservation treatment is done, if at all possible, through a separate incision from the lumpectomy for optimal cosmetic outcome.

Axillary dissection can lead to an increase in lymphedema of the breast and of the arm. Breast edema is common after breast-conservation treatment, with contributions from irradiation and axillary surgery, but is typically resolved in 18 months. Arm edema may be an early or late complication. It is seen in 3% to 5% of women with axillary level I and II dissections. It was seen in 10% to 15% of women when the level III nodes (medial to the pectoralis minor muscle) were routinely dissected with division or removal of the pectoralis minor muscle as part of the Patey technique of modified radical mastectomy. There is no evidence of benefit from removal of the level III nodes to offset this increase in morbidity, and the low frequency of skip metastases to level III is considered insufficient to justify level III dissection for most patients.[179,180] The risk of lymphedema is minimized by taking care to avoid removal of the brachial lymphatics passing anterior to the axillary vein and keeping the dissection below the vein. A single dose of perioperative antibiotics has been shown to reduce the already low risk of wound infection. Obese patients are at increased risk of lymphedema. The other morbidity associated with axillary dissection is sensory neuropathy in the distribution of the intercostobrachial nerve (posterior arm and axilla). Loss of shoulder mobility or shoulder pain has been reported after axillary dissection. Early shoulder exercises to restore mobility with physical therapy for those patients who experience early difficulty usually obviates this complication.

BREAST IRRADIATION

The goal of sparing the breast in breast-conservation treatment is substantially less likely to be accomplished without the addition of breast irradiation. NSABP B-06 demonstrated recurrence in the breast in over one-third of the women treated without irradiation over the next 10 years after breast-conserving surgery. Local failure usually leads to loss of the breast from salvage treatment with mastectomy. Data from the EBCTCG metaanalysis of randomized trials of breast-conservation treatment with or without irradiation[162] showed that the group not receiving radiation had increased mortality from breast cancer and increased overall mortality. The topic of breast irradiation as a component of breast-conservation treatment is considered separately from that of postmastectomy adjuvant irradiation.

Irradiation after lumpectomy is effective in reducing the risk of ipsilateral breast cancer recurrence. The 20-year update of NSABP B-06 reported 39.2% local failure without irradiation compared to 14.3% with irradiation.[181] Such recurrence is typically in the immediate vicinity of the lumpectomy site, termed *true recurrence* or *marginal miss*.[182] Recurrences after 5 years tend to be more distant from the initial tumor and probably include a number of new primary breast cancers. The use of whole breast irradiation with or without a boost is the standard of care at the present time. The extent of the margin of excision beyond the tumor border may limit the value of boost irradiation. A clear definition of the cosmetic and oncologic effects of wider local excision versus boost irradiation is lacking and remains an area of study. It is helpful to mark the lumpectomy site with small clips to aid in the planning of the whole breast irradiation and to ensure that the boost is delivered to the intended site. The value of adding nodal irradiation to the breast irradiation is unproven. A study by the National Cancer Institute of Canada is testing the value of such nodal irradiation. For patients with pathologically positive axillary lymph nodes, regional lymph node irradiation can be considered, particularly if there are multiple positive lymph nodes.

Technical Aspects of Radiation Treatment Delivery after Breast-Conservation Surgery

Patient positioning for radiation treatment delivery requires that the patient be in a position that is highly reproducible from day to day. A customized support system (e.g., a customized posterior upper body cast or breast board) facilitates daily treatment reproducibility. The ipsilateral arm is positioned out of the tangential radiation treatment fields, generally with the ipsilateral hand on or near the level of the head of the patient. An angle board is used to straighten the chest wall relative to the horizontal plane. The patient is typically in the supine position. For the patient with a pendulous breast, prone positioning may be considered, provided that adequate coverage of the tumor is achieved.[183]

After breast-conservation surgery, the standard initial target volume for radiation therapy is the whole breast, which is treated using tangent fields (Fig. 33.2-4). Whole breast irradiation is designed to treat the entire breast, as would be treated by a mastectomy. The tangent fields are coplanar at the posterior edge of the field to minimize dose to normal tissues. Attention should be given to the volume of heart (for left-sided tumors) and lung in the radiation fields to minimize the risk of long-term complications. Permanent small tattoos are placed to mark the fields for daily radiation treatment as well as to allow the radiation fields to be reproduced in the future, should this be required (e.g., for radiation to another field). Megavoltage irradiation is used, typically with medium-energy photons (e.g., 6 MV); however, individual patients with larger separations may require higher-photon-energy photons to improve dose homogeneity. Typical whole breast radiation doses are 45 to 50 Gy using daily fractions of 1.8 or 2.0 Gy. Radiation treatment is usually started approximately 4 weeks after the completion of adjuvant systemic chemotherapy, if used, or a minimum of 2 to 4 weeks after surgery, if adjuvant systemic chemotherapy is not used. Treatments are delivered daily, 5 days per week, Monday through Friday.

A boost may be delivered to the primary tumor site, typically to a total dose of 60 to 66 Gy. The boost treatment is most often delivered using electrons, although alternative methods are available, for example, a breast implant or cone-down photon fields. Two randomized trials have shown that adding a boost treatment to whole breast irradiation is associated with a small, but statistically significant, reduction in the rate of local failure.[184,185] When the boost is omitted, negative margins of resection from the primary tumor excision are required. However, negative margins of resection do not contraindicate using the boost.

Regional lymph node radiation remains a topic of considerable controversy. Radiation to the regional lymph nodes generally is not indicated when the surgical staging of the axilla is pathologically negative. Radiation to the full axilla is indicated when surgical staging of the axilla has not been performed. When the sentinel lymph node is positive and the choice of systemic therapy will not be altered by the findings in the remainder of the axilla, radiation to the full axilla without completion of axillary dissection is an alternative management strategy to complete axillary lymph node dissection.[169,170] Some investigators do not routinely irradiate the internal mammary lymph nodes, whereas others recommend internal mammary lymph node irradiation for patients with positive axillary lymph nodes or a primary tumor located in the inner quadrant or centrally. Of note, radiation to the internal mammary lymph node region is not mandated for the unusual circumstance in which the sentinel lymph node drainage is to the internal mammary lymph nodes.

The goal of dosimetric treatment planning for the whole breast radiation treatment is to improve the dose homogeneity to the target volume of the whole breast. Dosimetric planning may be performed adequately using a number of different techniques. The simplest technique is to obtain a contour of the treatment field in the isocentric plane and to add simple wedges to improve homogeneity in the central plane. Typically, this method does not use lung corrections. Most of the studies for which outcome data are reported in the literature used this relatively simple method of treatment planning. More recently, computed tomography (CT) has gained increasing acceptance for treatment planning. In the simplest form of planning, CT data, typically with lung corrections, are used to determine the optimal wedges for dose homogeneity. Further refinements

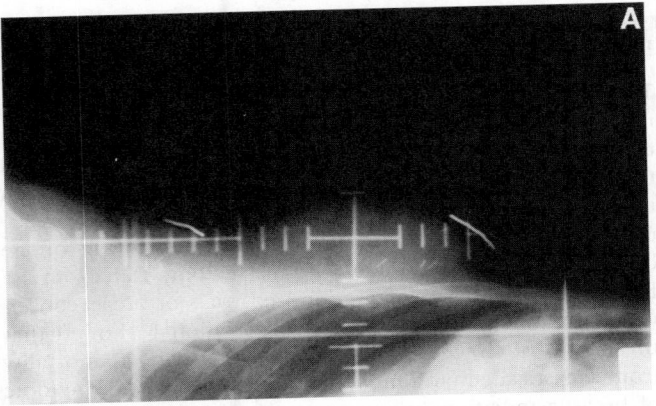

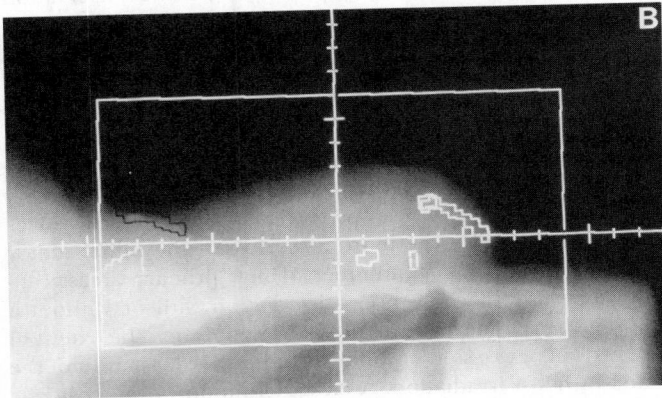

FIGURE 33.2-4.   Simulation films for definitive radiation treatment delivered to left breast tangent fields. The patient is a 37-year-old woman with a pathologic stage T1N0M0 infiltrating ductal carcinoma of the left breast. The patient had undergone surgical excision of the primary tumor with negative margins of resection, and the sentinel lymph node biopsy result was negative. **A:** Fluoroscopic simulation film. **B:** Computed tomography (CT) simulation film. For both **A** and **B**, surgical scars are delineated for both the breast incision and the axillary incision, and surgical clips are present within the respective surgical fields. Note that minimal heart volume is included within the tangent fields. Both fluoroscopic and CT simulation films are shown here for illustrative purposes only; under usual circumstances, either fluoroscopic simulation films or CT simulation films, but not both, are obtained.

can be obtained using CT data to compensate in multiple directions or even using intensity-modulated radiation treatment to optimize dose homogeneity. Such increasingly sophisticated methods of treatment planning have the theoretical appeal of improving the homogeneity of the dose delivery to the target volume of the whole breast and reducing the dose delivery to normal tissues. Decreasing hot spots to normal tissues may reduce complication rates. However, although more sophisticated treatment planning algorithms improve homogeneity, no method of treatment planning has been demonstrated to yield improved clinical outcomes in comparison to other methods.

Alternative Methods of Radiation Delivery

Alternative methods of delivering radiation treatment after breast-conservation surgery include accelerated whole breast irradiation and accelerated partial breast irradiation.[186–190] These methods of delivering radiation treatment have been developed for patient convenience, and confer no medical benefit to the patient.[191]

Accelerated whole breast irradiation has the benefit of treating the whole breast, as in conventional whole breast radiation, but delivering the radiation over a shorter period of time. In a report by Whelan et al., 1234 patients were randomly assigned to receive conventional whole breast irradiation (50 Gy in 25 fractions) or accelerated whole breast irradiation (42.5 Gy in 16 fractions) without a boost.[186] At 5 years, there was no difference between the two arms in survival, local control, cosmesis, and complications.

Accelerated partial breast irradiation delivers an accelerated course of radiation treatment to a small volume of breast tissue in and around the primary tumor site. Multiple methods of delivering accelerated partial breast irradiation have been described: (1) interstitial brachytherapy implant (high dose rate or low dose rate); (2) intracavitary brachytherapy (balloon catheter); (3) intraoperative radiation (orthovoltage or electron beam); and (4) external beam (three-dimensional conformal, intensity-modulated radiation therapy, or proton beam). The rationale for accelerated partial breast irradiation is that local recurrences tend to be primarily in and around the primary tumor site and that patient convenience may increase acceptance of radiation treatment after breast-conservation surgery. Most studies of accelerated partial breast irradiation select highly favorable patient groups for treatment, for example, those with the characteristics of older age (generally 45 years or older), small tumor size (generally 3 cm or less), lymph node–negative disease, invasive ductal carcinoma, widely negative margins of resection, negative postbiopsy mammogram, and no extensive intraductal component.

There are a number of potential disadvantages of partial breast irradiation.[191,192] Pathologic data from mastectomy specimens show a substantial risk of tumor more than 1 to 2 cm from the margin of the primary tumor.[193] Long-term studies demonstrate that, in keeping with these pathologic data, failures elsewhere (not in or near the primary tumor or boost radiation treatment volumes) continue beyond 10 years of follow-up.[194] Approximately 80% of patients treated with breast-conservation surgery currently undergo breast irradiation, and therefore a large increase in the use of radiation may be difficult to achieve. Analysis of patient preferences shows that patients consider even small differences in outcome to be important.

A randomized trial to compare accelerated partial breast irradiation to conventional breast irradiation will require thousands of patients with long-term follow-up to show whether there is a small, but meaningful, difference in outcome between study arms.[192] Randomized trials are currently accruing patients.[187,188] The NSABP and the Radiation Therapy Oncology Group have proposed a randomized trial to compare conventional whole breast radiotherapy to accelerated partial breast irradiation.

Postmastectomy Radiation Treatment

The risk of local-regional recurrence after mastectomy is directly related to the number of involved axillary lymph nodes. Postmastectomy irradiation reduces the risk of local failure by approximately two-thirds. It was a source of surprise and frustration that randomized trials of such radiation reliably demonstrated this improvement in local control but failed to show a long-term overall survival advantage. The metaanalysis of all of these randomized trials by the EBCTCG has offered an explanation. The improved local control does lead to a diminution in the risk of death from breast cancer. However, this reduction in the risk of death from breast cancer is offset by an increase in non–breast cancer mortality in the group receiving irradiation. The net effect is no benefit in overall survival at 20 years. The radiation detriment is in cardiovascular mortality. For women at low risk of local failure, the benefit is eclipsed. For women with an increased risk of recurrence, the benefit of irradiation exceeds the risks associated with it. This benefit is most apparent for women with four or more lymph nodes involved by breast cancer. Newer techniques of radiation treatment planning and delivery may lower the risk of late cardiovascular deaths and other complications.

Postmastectomy radiation treatment is defined as the delivery of adjuvant radiation treatment to the chest wall (or reconstructed chest wall) and usually to one or more regional lymph node areas. If the patient has undergone mastectomy with reconstruction, using either implant or myocutaneous flap, the reconstructed breast and chest wall are radiated.

After mastectomy without adjuvant treatment, there are four patterns of first failure: (1) distant failure only; (2) local-regional failure only; (3) both local-regional recurrence plus distant failure; or (4) no failure. Thus, patients with local-regional only first failure or local-regional plus distant first failure might, in principle, be cured of breast cancer with the addition of postmastectomy radiation treatment or postmastectomy radiation treatment plus systemic therapy, respectively. The ASCO guidelines for postmastectomy radiation treatment state that postmastectomy radiation treatment is indicated when there are four or more pathologically positive axillary lymph nodes and when the tumor is stage III (except for T3N0M0 lesions); the need for postmastectomy radiation treatment is uncertain after neoadjuvant systemic chemotherapy, with one to three pathologically positive axillary lymph nodes, for T3N0M0 tumors, for close or positive margins of resection, or for positive lymph nodes associated with extracapsular extension.[195]

The effects of postmastectomy radiation treatment include an improvement in local-regional control, a reduction in breast cancer deaths, and a potential increase in late complications, including non–breast cancer deaths. The time courses for these three effects are substantially different.

The goal of postmastectomy radiation treatment is to reduce the risk of local-regional recurrence and to increase overall survival. The improvement in local-regional control associated with postmastectomy radiation treatment has been well demonstrated in multiple randomized trials. Postmastectomy radiation treatment reduces the risk of local-regional failure by approximately two-thirds. In the EBCTCG overview analysis of randomized trials of radiation treatment (predominantly postmastectomy radiation treatment), the 20-year risk of local-regional first failure was 30.1% without radiation, but 10.4% with radiation (P <.00001).[196] Almost all of this benefit for local-regional control was seen within the first 10 years after treatment and was then maintained for 20 years after treatment. Similar reductions in local-regional recurrence have been demonstrated in virtually every randomized trial that has addressed this question for postmastectomy radiation treatment.

An overall survival benefit associated with postmastectomy radiation treatment has been more difficult to demonstrate for many reasons. In the EBCTCG overview, the absolute reduction of breast cancer deaths from postmastectomy radiation treatment was estimated as 4.8% at 20 years (53.4% vs. 48.6%; P = .0001). Three prospective randomized trials have demonstrated improvements in 10- to 15-year overall survival of approximately 10%.[197-199] In the EBCTCG overview, there was no difference in overall survival (37.1% vs. 35.9% at 20 years; P = .06), because the reduction in breast cancer deaths was offset by a 4.3% increase in non–breast cancer deaths (73.8% vs. 69.5%; P = .0003). The increase in non–breast cancer deaths was largely from cardiovascular events, including both cardiac events and other vascular, noncardiac events. The radiation treatment fields in older studies were substantially larger than the radiation treatment fields that would be used today, with substantially increased doses to the heart and mediastinum. This late toxicity will likely be substantially reduced with improvements in modern technical radiation delivery. Two metaanalyses support this hypothesis.[200,201] Evidence indicates that the use of contemporary chemotherapy regimens does not substantially alter the risk of local-regional recurrence after mastectomy when radiation is not given.[202,203]

The decision as to whether or not to recommend postmastectomy radiation must be based on the risk-benefit analysis of such treatment for the individual patient. The complications from radiation treatment (i.e., the risks) should not substantially differ from patient to patient. Assuming that the proportional decrease in local-regional recurrence from adding postmastectomy radiation is constant, the absolute benefit that the individual patient derives from postmastectomy radiation is directly related to the absolute risk of local-regional recurrence were radiation not given. Therefore, the decision-making process is largely driven by the benefit from postmastectomy radiation treatment for the individual patient. Clinicians will be aided in their decision making for individual patients by studies that define the risk of local-regional failure after mastectomy without radiation treatment based on combinations of clinically relevant factors (e.g., number of positive axillary lymph nodes plus tumor size). Recht et al. reported that the 10-year risk of local-regional recurrence without radiation varied substantially according to the combination of tumor size and number of positive axillary lymph nodes, even within the group of patients with one to three positive axillary lymph nodes.[204]

The minimum radiation volumes for postmastectomy radiation treatment are the chest wall and supraclavicular fossa.[205] Whether or not radiation should be delivered to the full axilla or internal mammary lymph nodes or both is a matter of controversy. In a 30-year update of a randomized trial examining the surgical treatment of internal mammary lymph nodes using extended radical mastectomy, Veronesi et al. found no improvement in survival with the addition of internal mammary node dissection.[206] The EORTC currently has open a randomized trial comparing regional lymphatic irradiation versus no irradiation, although the entry criteria are relatively broad. The extent of regional lymphatic irradiation in the context of postmastectomy radiation treatment remains unresolved at this time.

ADJUVANT SYSTEMIC THERAPY

The major threat of breast cancer is that of distant metastasis. Consequently, local-regional control is essential in eliminating or minimizing local recurrence and an ongoing source of metastasis, but elimination of occult metastasis with adjuvant systemic therapy is essential for optimizing the chance of cure. Systemic adjuvant therapy with hormonal treatment, chemotherapy, or both is undoubtedly related in part to the improved rates of mortality from breast cancer noted over the last decade. In a large population-based Canadian study the use of adjuvant systemic therapy was directly related to improved survival rates in women with early breast cancer. Overall survival improved by 10% for women younger than 50 years of age between 1974 and 1984, and by 4% for women aged 50 to 89 years between 1980 and 1984.[207]

Widely available hormonal and chemotherapeutic treatments used in the adjuvant setting can improve cure rates for at least one-third of patients with early-stage disease. These same treatments used in the metastatic setting are only palliative, which suggests that occult metastases from breast cancer are capable of being eradicated before the development of drug resistance. Effective adjuvant systemic therapy decreases both relapse-free (or disease-free) and overall survival, and both are important measures of effectiveness. Almost all patients with metastases die from breast cancer. Nevertheless, many patients with early-stage breast cancer survive without any adjuvant systemic treatment. In addition, coexisting illness (comorbidity) may dramatically effect survival, especially in older patients. Accurately predicting the patient's risk of metastases and the potential benefits and risks of adjuvant chemotherapy is essential in providing patients with information that leads to an appropriate and informed treatment decision. Visual aids can help convey information concerning the potential risks and benefits of adjuvant therapy.[208] In one randomized trial involving women with early-stage breast cancer, use of a decision board was compared with the standard presentation of adjuvant information. At 1 year, the women who used the decision board had a greater knowledge of the benefits of adjuvant treatment and were more satisfied with their choices, but there was no difference between the two groups in the number of patients who elected treatment.[209]

The hormonal manipulation of breast cancer cells leading to apoptosis is the most effective adjuvant systemic therapy available but is only effective in women with ER- or PR-positive tumors. Even when only a few percent of cell express ER or PR, endocrine therapy can significantly decrease the risk of metastases.[210]

The addition of chemotherapy to endocrine therapy in a patient with a hormone receptor–positive tumor can further improve the patient's chances of survival, but the overall added value of chemotherapy depends on the patient's risk of metastases. Moreover, it is becoming increasingly clear that the value of adjuvant endocrine therapy is influenced by the extent of receptor expression (patients with a greater percentages of cells that are ER or PR positive derive greater benefits[210]) and the quality of receptor expression (patients with ER- and PR-positive tumors derive greater benefits from endocrine therapy than patients with tumors that are ER positive and PR negative or ER negative and PR positive[211]). These latter data indicate that the "bystander effect," or the death of tumor cells lacking receptors caused by those responding to hormonal manipulation, can be dramatic. For women whose tumors lack both ERs and PRs, chemotherapy remains the only effective systemic adjuvant therapy.

Estimation of the Benefits of Adjuvant Systemic Therapy: The Overview Analysis

The major impact of adjuvant systemic therapy on improving survival for women with early-stage breast cancer has been demonstrated in a pioneering metaanalysis led by Sir Richard Peto and the Oxford Clinical Trials Unit. This metaanalysis was undertaken with the collaboration of virtually all of the clinical trialists worldwide under the aegis of the EBCTCG. At present, data from almost 200,000 patients entered in randomized trials comparing endocrine therapy, chemotherapy, radiation therapy, and immunotherapy have been analyzed, with the most recent analysis taking place in September 2000.[207-210] Of note, the overview analysis as well as data from large randomized trials have clearly shown that, irrespective of the risk of relapse for a given group of patients, treatment effects are associated with the same proportional reduction in risk. Thus, absolute benefits of treatment are larger in higher-risk patients. For example, a treatment that produces a relative reduction in risk of 30% (a hazard function of 0.70) compared to no treatment or another treatment has a substantially different absolute benefit for patients at different risk levels. For a population with a 10% risk of recurrence at 10 years, a 30% reduction in risk would translate into a 7% risk of recurrence with the given treatment, an absolute difference of 3%. For a population with a 50% risk of recurrence at 10 years, a 30% decrease in the risk of recurrence would translate into a 35% risk with the treatment, an absolute difference of 15%. This understanding of proportional effects on populations and subpopulations has provided a comprehensible approach to considering the benefits and risks of a given therapy. Mathematically, decreases in the annual odds of recurrence or death translate into lesser decreases over longer time periods, because for each succeeding year fewer numbers of patients are at risk for relapse or death. In the EBCTCG overview analysis, treatment effects are presented in terms of annual odds reductions in breast cancer relapse or mortality risk. Detailed data from the EBCTCG year 2000 updated analysis concerning the benefits of endocrine therapy, chemotherapy, and the combination of endocrine and chemotherapy for patients with early-stage breast cancer are presented in the following sections.

ENDOCRINE THERAPY

Tamoxifen. Key comparisons for endocrine therapy from the EBCTCG 2000 overview analysis are presented in Table 33.2-14.

TABLE 33.2-14. Key Comparisons for Endocrine Therapy from the Early Breast Cancer Trialists' Collaborative Group (Oxford 2000): Proportional Reductions in Annual Odds Relapse and Death for Systemic Adjuvant Therapy

	Reduction in Annual Odds (Standard Error)	
	Recurrence	Death
ENDOCRINE THERAPY		
Tamoxifen for 5 y vs. nil (estrogen receptor positive)	0.41 (0.03)	0.34 (0.04)
Tamoxifen 10 y vs. 5 y	0.06 (0.08)	Not reported
OVARIAN ABLATION/SUPPRESSION (OAS)		
OAS versus nil		
Younger than 40 y	0.32 (0.10)	0.32 (0.12)
40–49 y	0.25 (0.06)	0.26 (0.07)
OAS + chemotherapy versus chemotherapy		
Younger than 40 y	0.07 (0.10)	–0.01 (0.11)
40–49 y	0.07 (0.07)	–0.02 (0.08)

(Modified from ref. 162.)

Tamoxifen, a member of the SERM family, has proven to be the most effective endocrine therapy for hormone receptor–positive breast cancer patients. Other SERMs (e.g., toremifene) appear similar in efficacy to tamoxifen but offer no added benefits. Raloxifene, another SERM, has not been tested in the adjuvant setting and should not be used for adjuvant therapy. For a woman whose breast cancer expresses ERs or PRs, 5 years of adjuvant tamoxifen therapy reduces the annual risk of recurrence by approximately 40% and the annual risk of dying of breast cancer by 35%. This translates into a 15-year absolute reduction in the risk of recurrence of 12% and a reduction in the risk of dying of 9% (Fig. 33.2-5). Five years of tamoxifen therapy is more effective than 1 or 2 years and at least, and possibly more effective, than 10 years. Controversy remains, however, as to whether durations of tamoxifen therapy of longer than 5 years may ultimately prove to be more effective. Two ongoing large randomized trials, the Adjuvant Tamoxifen—Longer Against Shorter (ATLAS) trial and the Adjuvant Tamoxifen Treatment Offer More? (aTTom) trial currently in progress, should help resolve this issue. The benefits of tamoxifen are similar in premenopausal and postmenopausal women as well as in older women. Tamoxifen is generally well tolerated and has the best therapeutic index in premenopausal women, in whom it is not associated with an increased risk of endometrial cancer or venous thromboembolism. In postmenopausal women, 5 years of tamoxifen therapy is associated with a 1% risk for endometrial cancer and a 1% to 2% risk of thromboembolism. Compared to placebo, tamoxifen is not associated with an increased risk for weight gain, depression, or overall sexual dysfunction but does cause more severe sexual dysfunction, vasomotor, and gynecologic symptoms.[212] The overview also suggests no increase in non–breast cancer-related mortality in patients treated with tamoxifen. One large randomized trial has shown that, in patients who receive both chemotherapy and tamoxifen, tamoxifen should be given after completion of chemotherapy and not concurrently with chemotherapy.[213] A dosage of 20 mg/d appears optimal;

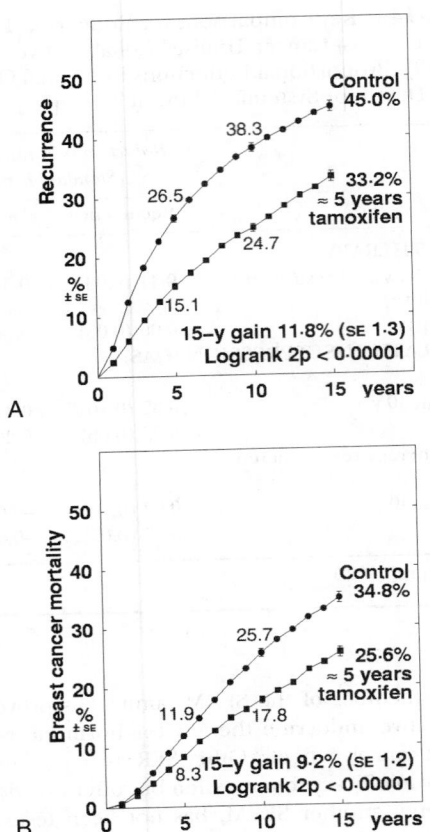

FIGURE 33.2-5.   A,B: Approximately 5-year tamoxifen therapy versus none, ER+/?: 15-year outcome (life-table curves: 10,386 women, 80% ER+, 30% N+). SE, standard error. (Data from Early Breast Cancer Trialists' Collaborative Group, to be published 2004 *Lancet.*)

higher dosages have not been associated with improved outcome and lower dosages have not been adequately tested. Hot flashes remain a major side effect of tamoxifen therapy and can be disabling in some patients. Megestrol acetate[214] can significantly ameliorate symptoms, but safety data on its long-term use in this setting are lacking. The antidepressant selective serotonin reuptake inhibitor venlafaxine has also been shown to significantly reduce the incidence and severity of hot flashes in tamoxifen-treated patients,[215] but a study with a similar selective serotonin reuptake inhibitor, paroxetine, suggests that some agents may adversely affect the metabolism of tamoxifen and diminish its effectiveness.[216] Further data are needed to resolve this issue.[217] A large retrospective analysis suggested that gene array patterns could accurately predict risk of recurrence for patients on tamoxifen and identified three distinct groups of node-negative tamoxifen-treated patients with relapse risks of 6.8%, 14.3%, and 30.5%.[218] Although these findings are exciting, other confirmatory trials are needed.

Ovarian Ablation. In premenopausal patients ovarian ablation is associated with significant reductions in risk of relapse and mortality (see Table 33.2-14). These benefits appear similar in magnitude to those of tamoxifen and can be achieved irrespective of whether ovarian ablation is accomplished by surgery, ovarian irradiation, or the use of gonadotropin hor-

mone–releasing hormone agonists (GnRH) or luteinizing hormone–releasing hormone (LHRH) agonists. Recently, the use of GnRH agonists has become more popular because the beneficial effects of ovarian ablation in decreasing relapse can be achieved with several years of treatment, yet menses resume after discontinuation in most patients, which minimizes both the short- and long-term effects of estrogen deprivation. The addition of tamoxifen to ovarian ablation may be superior to ovarian ablation alone, but much controversy exists. In addition, because aromatase inhibitors may be more effective than tamoxifen in postmenopausal women, there is interest in combining ovarian ablation with aromatase inhibition to maximize the benefits of endocrine therapy in premenopausal women. To resolve these issues, an internationally sponsored clinical trial, the Suppression of Ovarian Function Trial (SOFT), is currently under way and compares 5 years of tamoxifen alone, 5 years of tamoxifen and the GnRH agonist triptorelin, and 5 years of the aromatase inhibitor exemestane with triptorelin. Eligibility requires that patients have ER- or PR-positive tumors; chemotherapy is allowed. Because many oncologists believe that the combination of ovarian ablation and other endocrine therapies such as tamoxifen or aromatase inhibitors is superior to single-modality therapy, a second trial, the Tamoxifen/Exemestane Trial (TEXT), compares ovarian ablation (5 years of triptorelin) and tamoxifen with 5 years of triptorelin and exemestane. Both SOFT and TEXT will help answer key questions related to endocrine therapy in premenopausal women.

Ovarian ablation has been compared to CMF chemotherapy in patients with ER-positive tumors and has shown generally similar results.[219] In addition, a trial comparing goserelin and tamoxifen with CMF in premenopausal women with tumors that were ER positive or PR positive or both showed a significant improvement in 5-year relapse-free survival for the endocrine regimen (81% vs. 76%); overall survival was similar.[220] For premenopausal women at low risk for recurrence, ovarian ablation, alone or with tamoxifen, is probably similar in efficacy to chemotherapy. The major issue, however, is whether there is added value to chemotherapy in combination with endocrine therapy in premenopausal women at higher risk for recurrence. Data from the EBCTCG comparing ovarian ablation plus chemotherapy with ovarian ablation alone have not shown any added benefit from chemotherapy (see Table 33.2-14). These data are confounded by the fact that a large percentage of premenopausal women who receive chemotherapy, especially CMF, develop chemotherapy-induced ovarian ablation. Thus, these early trials comparing ovarian ablation and chemotherapy are likely underpowered because a large percentage of patients in the chemotherapy-alone arm also had ovarian ablation. Adding to this controversy are data from an ECOG trial (E5188, INT 0101) that compared CAF alone, CAF followed by ovarian ablation with goserelin (CAF-Z), and CAF, goserelin, and tamoxifen (CAF-ZT), in premenopausal women with node-positive, ER-positive breast cancer.[220] CAF-ZT significantly decreased relapse compared to CAF and CAF-Z (9-year relapse-free survival was 57%, 60%, and 68% for CAF, CAF-Z, and CAF-ZT, respectively). Subset analysis showed that goserelin added to the benefits of CAF in women who did not become amenorrheic after CAF or who had premenopausal estradiol levels after CAF. The Premenopausal Endocrine Responsive Chemotherapy (PERCHE) trial, currently in progress, will help and resolve this issue. In this trial premenopausal women all receive ovarian ablation with the GnRH agonist triptorelin and then are

TABLE 33.2-15. Key Data from the Anastrozole, Tamoxifen Alone, or in Combination Trial

	Anastrozole	Tamoxifen	Anastrozole and Tamoxifen	P Value
No. of patients (%)	3125 (100)	3116 (100)	3125 (100)	—
Median age (standard deviation)	64 (9.0)	64 (9.0)	64 (9.1)	
Node positive (%)	35	34	34	NS
First breast cancer events (no. of patients)	413	472	488	NS
Locoregional recurrence	84	101	107	—
Distant metastases	196	223	247	—
Contralateral (invasive or ductal carcinoma *in situ*)	25	40	35	—
Toxicity				—
Hot flushes (%)	34	40	40	
Fatigue/tiredness (%)	16	15	14	<.0001
Musculoskeletal disorders (%)	28	21	22	NS
Vaginal bleeding (%)	5	8	8	<.0001
Vaginal discharge (%)	3	11	12	<.0001
Endometrial cancer (%)	0.1	0.5	0.3	<.0001
Fractures (%)	6	4	5	.02
Ischemic cerebrovascular event (%)	1	2	2	.001
Any venous thromboembolic event (%)	2	4	4	.0006
				.0006

NS, not significant.
(Modified from ref. 221.)

randomly assigned to receive chemotherapy or no chemotherapy, followed by a subsequent random assignment to receive tamoxifen or exemestane.

Aromatase Inhibitors. In postmenopausal women, aromatase inhibitors represent another option for endocrine therapy. The Arimidex, Tamoxifen Alone or in Combination (ATAC) trial randomly assigned 9000 postmenopausal women with invasive breast cancer to receive anastrozole (Arimidex), tamoxifen, or the combination of both agents.[221] Among patients with receptor-positive tumors, women taking anastrozole had a significantly decreased hazard ratio (0.82; 95% CI, 0.70 to 0.96) for a breast cancer–related event (new breast cancer, local recurrence, or distant metastases) compared to patients taking tamoxifen or the combination of both agents. For patients with ER-positive tumors, relapse-free survival at 4 years was 89% and 86%, respectively, for those taking anastrozole alone and for those taking tamoxifen or the drug combination. The absolute difference in the frequency of distant metastases at 4 years was 1% for these two groups. Salient data from this trial after 4 years of follow-up are presented in Table 33.2-15. To date there have been no significant differences in overall survival. The side-effect profiles of tamoxifen and aromatase inhibitor differs substantially (see Table 33.2-15). Aromatase inhibitors are the preferred adjuvant treatment in postmenopausal women who have contraindications to tamoxifen (e.g., history of thromboembolism) or who cannot tolerate tamoxifen. Also, there are accumulating data that patients with HER2-positive tumors may derive greater benefit from aromatase inhibitors than from tamoxifen,[222] although this is controversial.[223] An analysis suggested that, compared to patients with tumors positive for both ER and PR, patients with ER-positive and PR-negative tumors derived significantly greater benefit from aromatase inhibitors than from tamoxifen.[224] Similar trials comparing tamoxifen to other aromatase inhibitors are now in progress.

More recently, the initial results of two large, randomized trials using aromatase inhibitors in women receiving tamoxifen, or just completing 5 years of tamoxifen, have been published. The Intergroup Exemestane Trial randomly assigned almost 5000 women who had received tamoxifen for 2 to 3 years to receive either 2 to 3 more years of tamoxifen therapy or to 2 to 3 years of treatment with the aromatase inhibitor exemestane. At a median follow-up of 31 months, patients receiving exemestane had a significant decrease in breast cancer–related relapse compared to those continuing on tamoxifen (hazard ratio, 0.68; P <.001).[225] In a second trial (National Cancer Institute of Canada MA-17), treatment with the aromatase inhibitor letrozole was compared with a placebo in 5000 postmenopausal women with hormone receptor–positive tumors who had received 5 years of tamoxifen therapy. This trial also showed a decrease in breast cancer–related events (new breast cancers, local-regional recurrence, and distant metastases) after a median follow-up of 28 months.[226] Key observations from this trial are presented in Table 33.2-16. No survival differences were noted in either of these trials, which are still early in follow-up.

Data from these trials as well as comparisons of the use of tamoxifen and aromatase inhibitors in patients with metastatic breast cancer (see Metastatic Breast Cancer, later in this chapter) have established a major role for aromatase inhibitors in hormone receptor–positive breast cancer. An expert panel of international breast cancer investigators selected by ASCO has concluded, after reviewing data from the ATAC trial, that tamoxifen remains the endocrine agent of choice for most postmenopausal patients.[227] However, aromatase inhibitors represent effective and attractive options to tamoxifen and may ultimately prove to be the agents of choice in this setting. Compared to tamoxifen, aromatase inhibitors are associated with an increased rate of bone loss and a higher risk of fractures. For patients who are offered adjuvant therapy with aromatase inhibitors, baseline bone density should be measured. The revised ASCO guidelines on bisphosphonates contain recommendations for maintaining bone health in this setting and should serve as a guide to management of these patients.[228]

TABLE 33.2-16. Key Data from the National Cancer Institute of Canada MA-17 Trial of Letrozole or Placebo in Postmenopausal Women Who Had Completed Five Years of Tamoxifen Therapy

	Letrozole	Placebo	P Value
No. of patients (%)	2575 (100)	2582 (100)	—
Median age (y)	62	62	NS
Node positive (%)	46	46	NS
Estrogen receptor positive (%)	98	98	NS
Prior adjuvant chemotherapy (%)	46	46	NS
Recurrence or new breast cancer (no. of patients)	75	132	—
Locoregional recurrence	14	30	
Distant metastases	47	76	
New contralateral breast cancer	14	26	
Breast cancer deaths	9	17	
Toxicity			
Hot flushes (%)	47	41	.001
Fatigue (%)	30	28	NS
Arthritis (%)	6	4	<.001
Arthralgia (%)	21	17	<.001
Myalgia (%)	12	10	.02
Fractures (%)	4	3	NS
Hypercholesterolemia (%)	12	12	NS
Vaginal bleeding (%)	4	6	.01

NS, not significant.
(Modified from ref. 226.)

TABLE 33.2-17A. Key Comparisons for Chemotherapy from the Early Breast Cancer Trialists' Collaborative Group (Oxford 2000): Proportional Reductions in Annual Odds Relapse and Death for Systemic Adjuvant Therapy

	Reduction in Annual Odds (Standard Error)	
	Recurrence	Death
POLYCHEMOTHERAPY VERSUS NONE (ALL PATIENTS)	0.23 (0.02)	0.17 (0.02)
Age <40 y	0.40 (0.06)	0.29 (0.07)
Age 40–49 y	0.36 (0.04)	0.30 (0.05)
Age 50–59 y	0.23 (0.03)	0.15 (0.04)
Age 60–69 y	0.13 (0.03)	0.09 (0.04)
Age ≥70 y and over	0.12 (0.11)	0.13 (0.12)
CHEMOTHERAPY TYPE		
Age <50 y		
Chemotherapy versus nil	0.38 (0.04)	0.29 (0.05)
CMF based	0.41 (0.04)	0.34 (0.05)
Anthracycline based	0.33 (0.08)	0.26 (0.09)
Age 50–69 y		
Chemotherapy versus nil	0.22 (0.04)	0.13 (0.04)
CMF based	0.19 (0.03)	0.10 (0.03)
Anthracycline based	0.21 (0.04)	0.17 (0.05)
ANTHRACYCLINES VERSUS CMF (ALL PATIENTS)	0.11 (0.03)	0.16 (0.03)
Age <50 y	0.10 (0.04)	0.16 (0.04)
Age 50–69 y	0.13 (0.05)	0.16 (0.06)

CMF, cyclophosphamide, methotrexate, and 5-fluorouracil.
(Modified from ref. 162.)

Several other trials comparing aromatase inhibitors with tamoxifen are in progress and should help clarify the many issues involved. Key issues still to be resolved are the following: (1) Are there enough data to establish aromatase inhibitors as the treatment of choice for all postmenopausal women with hormone receptor–positive early-stage breast cancer? (2) What is the optimal duration of aromatase inhibitor therapy? (3) What will be the future role of tamoxifen in management of patients with early-stage disease? At present, studies of aromatase inhibitors in the adjuvant setting show these agents to be superior to tamoxifen, but interpretation of these data must be tempered by the short follow-up of patients in these trials compared to the long-standing results confirming the benefits of tamoxifen.

CHEMOTHERAPY. The Oxford (EBCTCG) overview analysis has provided the best estimates for the benefits of adjuvant systemic chemotherapy. Key comparisons involving the use of chemotherapy are presented in Table 33.2-17A. It is clear from the overview that in the adjuvant setting combination chemotherapy (polychemotherapy) is superior to single-agent treatment and that the proportional benefits of chemotherapy (like those of endocrine therapy) are similar in node-negative and node-positive patients. Moreover, shorter durations of chemotherapy (3 to 6 months) are equivalent to longer durations of treatment. Adjuvant chemotherapy is also more effective in women younger than age 50 years (an age group representing premenopausal women) than in women aged 50 to 69 years. The reasons for this are probably multifactorial and include the beneficial effect of chemotherapy-induced amenorrhea in premenopausal women who receive chemotherapy alone, the more favorable endocrine profile of tumors with age that results in a greater benefit for endocrine therapy in older patients, and the increased likelihood of dosage reductions in older patients that might adversely affect the potential benefits of chemotherapy. There are still too few women aged 70 years and older in the overview analysis for accurate estimates of the value of chemotherapy, but the proportional reductions in relapse and survival for this older age group are similar to those for women aged 60 to 69 years, with this latter group showing significant reductions in relapse and mortality with chemotherapy.

After 15 years of follow-up, polychemotherapy compared to no chemotherapy significantly reduced the annual odds of recurrence by 23% and of dying of breast cancer by 17%. This translated into an absolute improvement in relapse-free survival of 12% for women younger than 50 years and 4% for women aged 50 to 69 years. Absolute improvements in survival were 10% and 3% for these groups, respectively (Fig. 33.2-6). The combination of chemotherapy and tamoxifen was also superior to either chemotherapy or tamoxifen alone. Commonly used chemotherapy regimens are presented in Table 33.2-17B.

ANTHRACYCLINES AND TAXANES. In the overview analysis, anthracyclines (doxorubicin and epirubicin) are clearly superior to CMF regimens and are associated with an 11% reduction in the annual odds of relapse and a 16% reduction in the annual odds of dying. However, certain caveats pertain to these data; large trials indicate that four cycles of doxorubicin and cyclophosphamide (AC) given every 3 weeks are similar but not superior in efficacy to six cycles of CMF (using oral

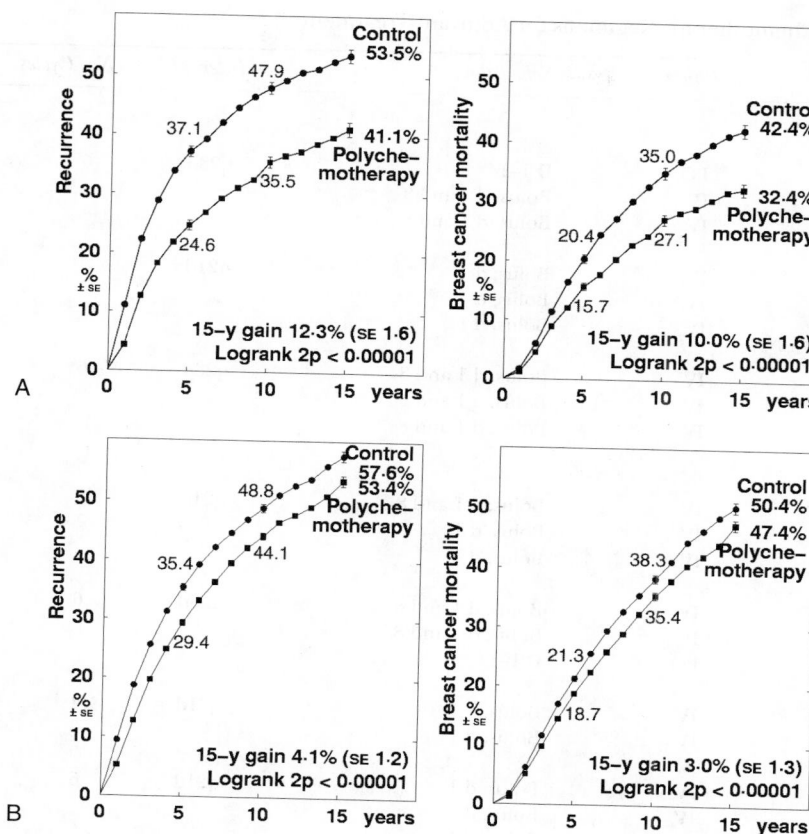

A

B

FIGURE 33.2-6. Polychemotherapy (PolyCTX) versus none: 15-year outcome (life-table curves by entry age). **A:** Entry age, less than 50 years, PolyCTX versus none (6901 women: 35% N+). **B:** Entry age, 50 to 69 years, PolyCTX versus none (18,629 women: 70% N+). SE, standard error.

cyclophosphamide), and thus the benefits of anthracyclines are associated with regimens using six or more cycles (see Tables 33.2-17*A* and 33.2-17*B*). Epirubicin and doxorubicin appear similar in efficacy, but at larger cumulative doses, epirubicin may be less cardiotoxic. The benefits of anthracycline regimens compared to CMF are similar for women younger than 50 years and women aged 50 to 69 years. Anthracycline regimens currently represent the treatment of choice for patients with high-risk node-negative and node-positive breast cancer except for patients in whom an increased risk of cardiac toxicity limits their potential usefulness. Because newer agents, especially taxanes, appear similar in efficacy to anthracyclines, clinical trials are now in progress comparing single-agent taxane therapy to anthracycline regimens, and polychemotherapy regimens that lack anthracyclines with anthracycline regimens.

Several trials have shown that anthracycline-containing chemotherapy regimens may be more effective in patients with HER2-positive tumors,[229] but these data have not been consistent.[230] Of note, at least one of these trials suggested a dose-response interaction among HER2 expression (or amplification) and relapse risk: Patients with larger percentages of tumor cells that express HER2 derived greater benefits from more dose-intense schedules of anthracyclines.[231] Several trials have also shown that CMF is less effective, but is still superior to no chemotherapy, in women with HER2-positive tumors. Although uncertainty persists, anthracycline-containing regimens should be considered the first choice for patients with HER2-positive tumors unless there are contraindications to use of these agents.

Three large randomized trials involving women with node-positive breast cancer have established the role of taxanes in the adjuvant setting. Both the CALGB 9344 and NSABP B-28 trials compared four cycles of AC alone with four cycles of AC followed by four cycles of paclitaxel. In the CALGB trial, AC plus paclitaxel (175 mg/m^2 every 3 weeks) was associated with a significant 5-year decrease in recurrence and mortality of 17% and 18%, respectively, compared to AC alone; for AC alone and AC plus paclitaxel, relapse-free survival rates were 65% versus 70%, respectively, and overall survival rates were 77% and 80%, respectively.[232] In NSABP B-28, AC plus paclitaxel (225 mg/m^2 every 3 weeks) was compared to AC alone.[233] After a median follow-up of 5 years, there was a significant 17% reduction in the relative risk of relapse for the paclitaxel arm; no significant differences in overall survival between the two regimens have yet been noted. The 5-year results of Breast Cancer International Research Group trial 001, a randomized trial comparing docetaxel, doxorubicin, and cyclophosphamide (TAC) with FAC (see Table 33.2-17*B* for treatment regimens) in patients with node-positive breast cancer, showed a significant reduction in relapse and mortality with TAC.[27,234] Compared to FAC, TAC reduced the recurrence rate by 28% and the mortality rate by 30%. At five years, relapse-free survival and overall survival for TAC versus FAC were 75% and 87% and 68% and 81%, respectively. Similar benefits for TAC compared to FAC were seen in patients with ER-positive and ER-negative, and HER2-positive and HER2-negative tumors. Moreover, this trial also suggested that use of taxanes, and not an increasing number of cycles of an anthracycline-containing regimen, is related to improved outcome.

DOSE INTENSITY AND DOSE DENSITY. Achieving optimal benefit from a chemotherapy regimen appears to be

TABLE 33.2-17B. Commonly Used Combination Chemotherapy Regimens for Adjuvant Treatment

Cytotoxic Agent	mg/m²	Route	Schedule	Interval	No. Cycles
CMF BASED					
Oral CMF			D 1–14	q28d	6
Cyclophosphamide	100	PO			
Methotrexate	40	IV	Bolus, d 1 and 8		
5-Fluorouracil	600	IV	Bolus, d 1 and 8		
IV CMF				q21d	8
Cyclophosphamide	600	IV	Bolus, d 1		
Methotrexate	40	IV	Bolus, d 1		
5-Fluorouracil	600	IV	Bolus, d 1		
or				q28d	6
Cyclophosphamide	600	IV	Bolus, d 1 and 8		
Methotrexate	40	IV	Bolus, d 1 and 8		
5-Fluorouracil	600	IV	Bolus, d 1 and 8		
ANTHRACYCLINE BASED					
CAF				q21d	6
5-Fluorouracil	500	IV	Bolus, d 1 and 8		
Doxorubicin	50	IV	Bolus, d 1		
Cyclophosphamide	500	IV	Bolus, d 1		
or				q28d	6
5-Fluorouracil	500	IV	Bolus, d 1 and 8		
Doxorubicin	25	IV	Bolus, d 1 and 8		
Cyclophosphamide	100	PO	D 1–14		
AC				q21d	4
Doxorubicin	60	IV	Bolus, d 1		
Cyclophosphamide	600	IV	Bolus, d 1		
CEF				q21d	6
5-Fluorouracil	500	IV	Bolus, d 1		
Epirubicin	100	IV	Bolus, d 1		
Cyclophosphamide	500	IV	Bolus, d 1		
FEC				q21d	6
Cyclophosphamide	75	PO	D 1–14		
Epirubicin	60	IV	Bolus, d 1 and 8		
5-Fluorouracil	500	IV	Bolus, d 1 and 8		
A to CMF				q21d	4
Doxorubicin	75	IV	Bolus, d 1		
Then				q21d	8
Cyclophosphamide	600	IV	Bolus, d 1		
Methotrexate	40	IV	Bolus, d 1		
5-Fluorouracil	600	IV	Bolus, d 1		
ANTHRACYCLINES AND TAXANES					
AC followed by paclitaxel	175	IV	Bolus, d 1	q21d	AC × 4 P × 4
AC followed by docetaxel	100	IV	Bolus, d 1	q21d	AC × 4 D × 4
ATC				q14d	A × 4
Doxorubicin	60	IV	Bolus, d 1		P × 4
Paclitaxel	175	IV	Bolus, d 1		C × 4
Cyclophosphamide	600	IV	Bolus, d 1		
TAC				q21d	6
Docetaxel	75	IV	Bolus, d 1		
Doxorubicin	50	IV	Bolus, d 1		
Cyclophosphamide	500	IV	Bolus, d 1		
Dose dense				q14d	AC × 4
AC followed by paclitaxel (all agents given at 14-d intervals with filgrastim support)	175	IV	Bolus, d 1		P × 4

related to administering a threshold dose. A retrospective review that compared the dose of CMF administered and treatment outcome showed that patients receiving higher doses of treatment had improved survival.[235] Similar analyses followed but were flawed by the inability to account for additional patient-related variables other than treatment dose that may have accounted for poorer outcome.[236] A seminal trial of the CALGB randomly assigned patients with node-positive breast cancer to four cycles of low- or high-dose CAF or six cycles of moderate-dose CAF. Patients receiving the moderate- or high-dose regimen had significantly improved relapse-free and overall survival compared to those receiving the low-dose regimen.[237] More recently, the data from CALGB 9344 showed that escalating anthracycline dose from 60 to 90 mg/m[2] as part of an AC regimen was not associated with improved outcome.[232] For epirubicin, threshold dosages of 100 mg/m[2] every 3 weeks[238] or 120 mg/m[2] every 4 weeks[32,239] appear optimal in regimens that also include cyclophosphamide and fluorouracil. Likewise, the NSABP has shown in two large trials (B-22 and B-25) that escalating doses of cyclophosphamide in an AC regimen to as high as 2400 mg/m[2] was not associated with improved outcome compared to a 600 mg/m[2] dose. In addition, several large randomized trials using high-dose chemotherapy with either autologous bone marrow or stem cell support have not shown superiority for high-dose over standard-dose therapy.

Increasing the dose density is defined as giving the same dose of an agent or the same regimen over a shorter period of time. The rationale for such a strategy, based on the Norton-Simon hypothesis, is that giving identical but effective doses of chemotherapeutic agents at more frequent intervals will be associated with increasing cell kill and a better response to treatment. Results of two randomized trials support this concept.[240] A seminal randomized trial compared four cycles of doxorubicin followed by eight cycles of CMF (the dose-dense regimen) with a sequential regimen that used the same doses in sequence (two cycles of CMF followed by one cycle of doxorubicin every 3 weeks for four cycles) in women with four or more positive lymph nodes.[241] At 10 years of follow-up, the dose-dense regimen was associated with a significant improvement in relapse-free survival of 14% (42% for the dose-dense vs. 28% for the sequential regimen) and in overall survival of 12% (58% for the dose-dense vs. 44% for the sequential regimen). More recently, the CALGB published data from a randomized trial comparing dose-dense chemotherapy with doxorubicin, cyclophosphamide, and paclitaxel with a regimen of the same agents given every 3 weeks in women with node-positive breast cancer.[242] This trial used a two-by-two factorial design that compared AC for four cycles followed by paclitaxel for four cycles (AC>T) with four cycles of doxorubicin followed by four cycles of paclitaxel followed by four cycles of cyclophosphamide (ATC) and used two different treatment schedules—an every-2-week schedule with growth factor support (the dose-dense regimen) and an every-3-week schedule (the standard treatment). After a median follow-up of 36 months, 4-year estimated disease-free survival and overall survival were both significantly improved with the dose-dense schedule compared with the standard schedule (relapse-free survival of 82% and 75%, respectively, for the dose-dense vs. the standard schedule). There was no difference in outcome among the two different chemotherapy sequences. Although severe neutropenia was less common with dose-dense therapy, other toxicities were similar for the two schedules. A Canadian trial now in progress (National Cancer Institute of Canada MA-21) comparing dose-dense therapy with standard treatment schedules will help confirm these results.

TOXICITY. Short-term toxicities differ among chemotherapy regimens and may include nausea, vomiting, stomatitis, diarrhea, myelosuppression, fatigue, bone or muscle pain, neurotoxicity, weight gain, thrombosis, and alopecia.[243] Management of these toxicities is discussed in Chapter 54 and has been extensively reviewed elsewhere.[243,244] Administration of growth factors such as filgrastim can minimize neutropenia, and criteria for the appropriate use of these agents have been developed.[245] Cardiac toxicity is a major potential complication of anthracyclines and is related to cumulative dose. It is also seen with the use of trastuzumab, especially in patients with previous anthracycline therapy. Death due to acute complications is rare, however. In the EBCTCG overview analysis, there was no significant increase in non–breast cancer-related mortality due to chemotherapy. Several cross-sectional trials have shown declines in cognitive function after chemotherapy.[246] Prospective trials are needed to further define the extent and long-term consequences of cognitive dysfunction in patients receiving chemotherapy. Longer-term complications of chemotherapy including chemotherapy-induced ovarian ablation and fatigue may also become major problems. In spite of these toxicities, long-term follow-up of patients receiving chemotherapy in the adjuvant setting has shown no major decline in quality of life compared to that of patients managed without chemotherapy.[247]

OTHER ADJUVANT SYSTEMIC THERAPIES. In addition to endocrine therapy and chemotherapy, other systemic therapies are currently being evaluated in the adjuvant setting. Trastuzumab plus chemotherapy is being tested against chemotherapy alone in patients with HER2-positive, high-risk, node-negative and node-positive tumors. These trials, currently well along, should determine the value of trastuzumab in this setting. At this time, trastuzumab should not be used in the adjuvant setting outside of a clinical trial. The oral bisphosphonate clodronate was associated with improved relapse-free and overall survival in patients with early-stage breast cancer in one trial but not others[248] and is currently being evaluated in a large randomized trial. In addition to bone preservation, bisphosphonates have been shown to have other biologic effects, including the inhibition of tumor cell growth. Newer, more potent bisphosphonates are being evaluated in the adjuvant setting for their potential in preventing bone loss in premenopausal women with treatment-related loss of ovarian function. New trials in the adjuvant setting will also address the potential role of statins, COX-2 inhibitors, and a wide array of new biologic agents. Lastly, radiation therapy, whether administered after mastectomy in node-positive patients or after lumpectomy in patients who have breast-conservation treatment, significantly decreases the risk of distant metastases and in this sense acts like other effective systemic therapies.

Selection of Adjuvant Systemic Therapy

The potential value of systemic adjuvant chemotherapy including endocrine therapy, chemotherapy, or both in decreasing the risk of distant metastases and improving overall survival can be accurately estimated using Web-based computer programs (see http://www.adjuvantonline.com or http://www.mayoclinic.com/calcs).[42–44,249–251] These programs also provide user-friendly printouts for patients that illustrate the potential benefits of adjuvant therapy for groups of women with similar tumor size, nodal involvement, and hormone-receptor status. Comparisons of

TABLE 33.2-18. Key Comparisons for Chemotherapy and Hormonal Therapy from the Early Breast Cancer Trialists' Collaborative Group (Oxford 2000): Proportional Reductions in Annual Odds of Relapse and Death for Systemic Adjuvant Therapy

	Reduction in Annual Odds (Standard Error)	
	Recurrence	Death
Chemotherapy + tamoxifen versus chemotherapy (all ages)	0.40 (0.08)	0.39 (0.09)
Chemotherapy then tamoxifen versus chemotherapy	0.31 (0.07)	0.24 (0.10)
Chemotherapy and tamoxifen versus tamoxifen (estrogen receptor positive)		
Age <50 y	0.44 (0.07)	0.31 (0.10)
Age 50–69 y	0.16 (0.07)	0.05 (0.08)

(Modified from ref. 162.)

TABLE 33.2-19A. Best Prognosis

Stage	Risk of Distant Metastatic Disease
In situ breast carcinoma	<1% at 10 y
T1a,T1bN0M0 invasive breast cancer	<2% at 10 y
T1N0M0 grade 1 invasive breast cancer	~2% at 10 y

(Adapted from ref. 65, with permission.)

potential benefits of chemotherapy and tamoxifen versus either chemotherapy or tamoxifen alone as calculated from the EBCTCG overview analysis are presented in Table 33.2-18. Guidelines regarding adjuvant systemic therapy for patients and physicians are also available from the National Comprehensive Cancer Network Web site (http://www.nccn.org), and guidelines for physicians were formulated by the St. Gallen conference.[252]

In general, almost all patients with ER- or PR-positive tumors benefit from endocrine therapy. The benefits are least for patients with tumors smaller than 1 cm that are well differentiated, node-negative and ER positive and for patients with severe comorbid illness. Likewise, low-risk, node-negative patients with hormone receptor–positive tumors derive minimal improvement in overall survival from the addition of chemotherapy (Table 33.2-19A). In some of these lower-risk patients, the potential benefits of chemotherapy are offset by the risk of the relatively rare but potentially fatal complications of myelodysplasia, acute leukemia, thromboembolism, and congestive heart failure. Nevertheless, studies have shown no major long-term declines in quality of life for patients who received adjuvant therapy compared to patients who did not,[247] and patient surveys consistently indicate that many patients are willing to undergo chemotherapy for even small benefits.[253,254] In these trials, 65% to 70% of patients were willing to undergo 6 months of chemotherapy for a 5% increase in likelihood of cancer cure.

Outside of a clinical trial, AC and CMF still represent reasonable choices for low-risk patients—those with a recurrence risk of 20% or less at 10 years. For higher-risk patients, regimens that include anthracyclines for more than four cycles [FAC or cyclophosphamide, epirubicin, and fluorouracil (FEC)], anthracyclines and taxanes (i.e., TAC or AC followed by a taxane), or dose-dense regimens are preferred (Tables 33.2-17*B* and 33.2-19*B*). Of note, when a regimen is selected, dosage modifications as defined by that regimen should be used to optimize results; a large study has shown that dosage reductions in adjuvant chemotherapy are common in the population.[255] The best decision concerning the use of adjuvant systemic therapy is one that can only be made by the patient and his or her physician after careful discussion of the risks and benefits of treatment.

LOCALLY ADVANCED AND INFLAMMATORY BREAST CANCER

Locally advanced and inflammatory breast cancer refers to a diverse and heterogeneous group of breast cancers and represents only 2% to 5% of all breast cancers in the United States. Patients with these cancers include those with operable disease at presentation (AJCC clinical stage T3N0 to N1M0), inoperable disease at presentation (AJCC clinical stage T4 or N2 to 3M0 or both), and inflammatory breast cancer (AJCC clinical stage T4dN0 to N3M0). Subdividing patients into these three broad groups (those with operable disease at presentation, inoperable disease at presentation, and inflammatory disease) facilitates clinical management. Some authors have included T3N0M0 (stage IIB) lesions and even large T2 lesions (e.g., lesions 3 cm or larger) as locally advanced disease. There have been significant changes over time in the AJCC classification,

TABLE 33.2-19B. Algorithm for Adjuvant Systemic Therapy

ER+ or PR+		ER– or PR–	
T1a,T1bN0	± Tamoxifen	T1a,T1bN0	± Combination chemotherapy
T1c–T2N0	Combination chemotherapy	T1c–T2N0	Combination chemotherapy
	Then tamoxifen × 5 y		Then tamoxifen × 5 y
Any T, N1	Combination chemotherapy	Any T, N0	Combination chemotherapy
	± Taxane		+ Taxane
	± Dose dense		± Dose dense
	Then tamoxifen × 5 y		
	± Aromatase inhibitor		

ER+/–, estrogen receptor positive/negative; PR+/–, progesterone receptor positive/negative.

particularly for nodal disease, and studies need to be carefully assessed for the definition of inoperability, particularly in relation to nodal staging. Supraclavicular lymphadenopathy is now classified as N3 disease (although it was previously classified as M1 disease), and patients with a positive supraclavicular lymph node are sometimes included in reports of locally advanced breast cancer.

Comparison of studies of locally advanced and inflammatory breast cancer is problematic for a number of reasons. First, these patients have a high degree of heterogeneity in clinical presentation, and the number of patients in each subgroup is small. Therefore, most studies tend to include a wide variety of different clinical presentations. Second, the definition of locally advanced breast cancer according AJCC staging criteria has varied over time, which makes comparison among studies difficult. Third, the subgroups of patients included in studies vary widely. For example, patients with inflammatory breast cancer or operable disease at presentation may or may not be combined with patients with locally advanced breast cancer. In addition, some studies of operable locally advanced breast cancer include larger T2 lesions (e.g., tumors 3 cm and larger). Fourth, the sequence of treatments is variable across studies, particularly with regard to local-regional treatment. Many studies select patients for mastectomy or breast-conservation treatment depending on the response to neoadjuvant chemotherapy. Fifth, the types of chemotherapy regimens used vary greatly. Further, many studies use a fixed number of cycles of neoadjuvant chemotherapy, whereas other studies deliver chemotherapy to "best response." Finally, many studies do not provide sufficient information to examine clinically relevant subgroups of patients.

The optimal method of chemotherapy delivery remains uncertain. Many studies have delivered initial, neoadjuvant chemotherapy in a flexible manner, to best clinical response with or without one or two additional cycles of chemotherapy. More recently, studies have reported using a fixed number of cycles of chemotherapy, similar to the combination chemotherapy regimens used in adjuvant studies.[256,257]

In the Aberdeen trial, patients with large tumors (3 cm or more) or locally advanced disease (T3 to T4 or N2) were initially treated with four cycles of CVAP (cyclophosphamide, vincristine, doxorubicin, and prednisone) chemotherapy.[256] Patients with a complete or partial response were then randomly assigned to four further cycles of CVAP chemotherapy or to four cycles of docetaxel chemotherapy. Nonresponding patients received four cycles of docetaxel. For the randomly assigned patients, there was an improvement in overall survival of borderline statistical significance for patients receiving cross-over chemotherapy of docetaxel compared to those receiving continued CVAP chemotherapy (88% vs. 69% estimated overall survival at 4 years; $P = .05$).

A small number of randomized studies of neoadjuvant versus adjuvant chemotherapy have been reported.[168,258–260] In these studies, no differences were seen for overall survival, local control, or breast conservation.

Given the absence of any difference in outcome for patients treated with neoadjuvant versus adjuvant chemotherapy, the decision to use preoperative versus postoperative chemotherapy must be based on other factors. Factors in favor of preoperative chemotherapy include the following: (1) patients initially presenting with tumors that historically required mastectomy can potentially be down-staged to allow for breast-conservation treatment; (2) larger tumors that require a cosmetically unsatisfactory lumpectomy at presentation can be down-staged to allow a more cosmetically favorable lumpectomy; (3) the response of individual patients to systemic chemotherapy can be assessed *in vivo*; (4) research can be facilitated, for example, by evaluating tissue specimens before and after treatment, to rapidly assess new chemotherapeutic, hormonal, or biologic agents; and (5) the pathologic response to neoadjuvant chemotherapy is a strong prognostic factor for outcome. The argument in favor of primary surgery, if possible, with adjuvant systemic therapy is the more accurate pathologic staging, both of the primary tumor as well as the axillary lymph nodes, with the valuable prognostic information acquired for prognosis and guidance of adjuvant therapy.

Numerous studies have demonstrated high rates of downstaging to breast-conservation treatment with the use of neoadjuvant chemotherapy. Although most studies have used doxorubicin- or epirubicin-containing regimens, studies have also begun to evaluate the role of taxane chemotherapy.[261,262] After neoadjuvant chemotherapy, down-staging of the tumor sufficient to allow breast-conservation treatment has been reported in 22% to 90% of patients.[202,263,264] For those patients with sufficient down-staging to permit breast-conservation surgery, definitive breast irradiation is also indicated and is delivered in a manner similar to that for patients not treated with neoadjuvant chemotherapy.

Because physical examination and mammography do not adequately predict the pathologic response to neoadjuvant chemotherapy, alternative imaging methods have been developed to attempt to more accurately predict a pathologic response and to improve breast-conservation rates. MRI is one promising modality (Fig. 33.2-7) and appears to correlate well with pathologic response.

Hormone therapy likely has a role to play as a neoadjuvant therapy, particularly when the diagnostic biopsy results confirm hormone receptor expression.[265,266] The addition of endocrine therapy to chemotherapy appears to improve outcome for patients with locally advanced breast cancer.[266]

The role of postmastectomy radiation treatment after neoadjuvant chemotherapy is in evolution. The ASCO guidelines recommend that, in general, postmastectomy radiation treatment is indicated after neoadjuvant systemic therapy, although the guidelines recognize that there may be exceptions to this recommendation.[267] The rationale for recommending postmastectomy radiation treatment is the significant down-staging associated with neoadjuvant chemotherapy, for both the primary tumor and axillary lymph nodes, and the fact that most patients who require mastectomy have presented initially with locally advanced tumors (T3 or T4 lesions) or four or more pathologically positive axillary lymph nodes. In the NSABP B-18 randomized trial, Fisher et al. reported that the number of patients with pathologically positive nodes was 41% for patients who received preoperative chemotherapy compared to 57% for patients who received postoperative chemotherapy, and the number of patients with four or more positive axillary lymph nodes was 16% versus 27%, respectively.[257] For postmastectomy radiation treatment after neoadjuvant chemotherapy followed by mastectomy, unresolved issues at this time include which patient and tumor factors (clinical and pathologic) should be used to select those patients who require treatment and the

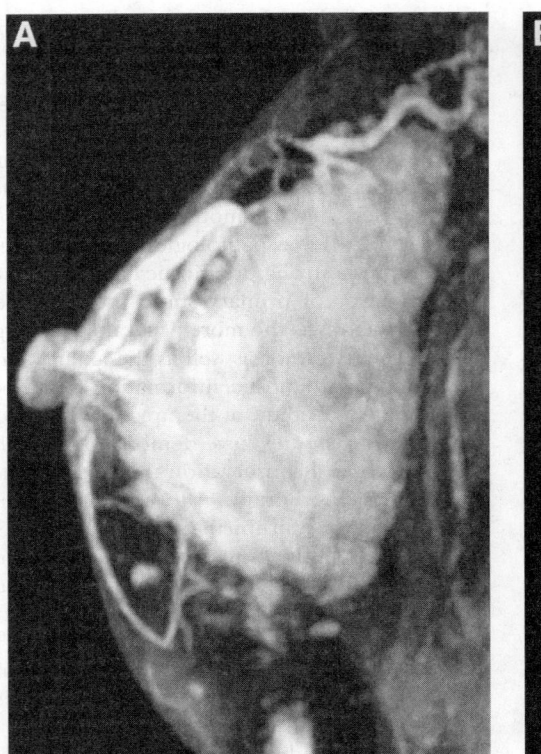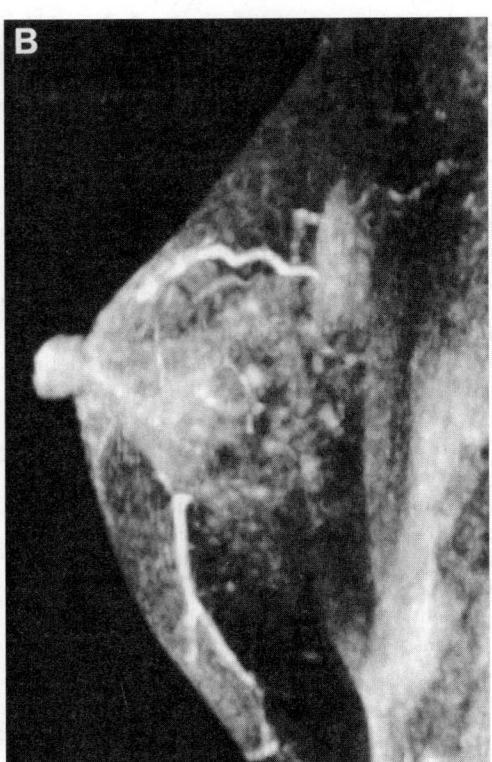

FIGURE 33.2-7. Contrast-enhanced magnetic resonance imaging (MRI) scan of the breast obtained before (**A**) and after (**B**) neoadjuvant chemotherapy. The patient is a 46-year-old premenopausal female who presented with a palpable left breast mass. Mammographic findings were negative; however, ultrasonography confirmed a mass. Core biopsy showed infiltrating lobular carcinoma. MRI study obtained before neoadjuvant chemotherapy (**A**) shows extensive enhancement throughout the majority of the breast, compatible with extensive infiltrating carcinoma. The patient received neoadjuvant doxorubicin and cyclophosphamide chemotherapy followed by paclitaxel chemotherapy. MRI study obtained after neoadjuvant chemotherapy (**B**) showed dramatic regression, with small areas of residual enhancement, possibly consistent with residual carcinoma. The patient underwent a mastectomy. Pathologic examination showed dispersed microscopic foci of residual infiltrating lobular carcinoma, with the largest focus measured as 0.2 cm. Metastatic carcinoma was found in eight axillary lymph nodes of ten evaluated.

optimal technical radiation therapy fields, including which regional lymph nodes, if any, should be treated.

LOCALLY ADVANCED BREAST CANCER OPERABLE AT PRESENTATION

The majority of patients with operable locally advanced breast cancer are treated with combined modality therapy. The options for management at presentation for this group of patients are (1) mastectomy followed by adjuvant radiation treatment and adjuvant systemic treatment as indicated based on the pathology findings; (2) neoadjuvant chemotherapy to attempt to down-stage lesions for breast-conservation treatment; most studies then add breast-conservation surgery and radiation therapy for responding patients and mastectomy for nonresponding patients, with some studies giving additional chemotherapy thereafter; or (3) initial breast-conservation surgery for selected patients for whom a cosmetically adequate lumpectomy can be performed, followed by radiation treatment to the intact breast and systemic treatment as indicated. For patients with T3 tumors treated with mastectomy, postmastectomy radiation treatment is indicated for patients with posi-

tive axillary lymph nodes and should be considered for patients with negative axillary lymph nodes.[267]

A number of studies have reported on the use of neoadjuvant chemotherapy for patients with operable, locally advanced lesions. Overall survival at 5 years has been reported as 74% to 100%, and at 10 years, 41% to 100%. The disease-free survival at 5 years has been reported as 58% to 87%, and at 10 years, 52% to 87%. In the NSABP B-18 study, 13% of the patients had T3 tumors, and the overall rate of breast conservation for these T3 tumors was increased from 8% without preoperative chemotherapy to 22% with preoperative chemotherapy.[257]

LOCALLY ADVANCED BREAST CANCER INOPERABLE AT PRESENTATION

The clinical management of patients with locally advanced, inoperable disease at presentation consists of combined modality treatment, most commonly using initial systemic chemotherapy, then local-regional treatment (generally mastectomy plus postmastectomy radiation treatment), often followed by further systemic chemotherapy. Initial systemic chemotherapy is used to address the high risk of these patients for metastatic disease, to attempt to convert an inoperable presentation to an operable state for successful local-regional treatment, and to assess *in vivo* the clinical response to chemotherapy. Historically, first-line chemotherapy regimens contained doxorubicin. However, the substantial activity of the taxanes has generated interest in taxane and even doxorubicin plus taxane regimens as first-line treatment.

For the patient who has a partial or complete response to chemotherapy and whose lesion is converted to an operable state, the next maneuver is typically mastectomy to debulk gross disease, to facilitate local-regional control, and to allow for the pathologic assessment of response. For patients with a complete or partial response, the optimal chemotherapy to use after local-regional treatment is uncertain. Specifically, it is not clear whether to continue the same chemotherapy as before after local-regional treatment or whether a cross-resistant chemotherapeutic regimen is indicated. The ASCO guidelines recommend postmastectomy radiation treatment, in general, for those patients who require a mastectomy (see earlier in Locally Advanced and Inflammatory Breast Cancer).

For the patient whose tumor remains inoperable after first-line systemic chemotherapy, the options are to proceed with second-line chemotherapy or to deliver preoperative radiation treatment. One major goal of treatment is to attempt to convert the lesion from an inoperable to an operable state, because patients without local-regional control have substantially diminished quality of life.

A number of studies have reported the outcome after neoadjuvant chemotherapy for inoperable, locally advanced breast cancer. The overall survival rates at 5 years have been reported as 44% to 88%, and at 10 years as 26% to 73%. The disease-free survival rates have been reported at 5 years as 33% to 80%, and at 10 years as 30% to 73%. Many of these studies selected local-regional treatment based on response to neoadjuvant chemotherapy; for example, breast-conservation treatment was used for responding patients, whereas mastectomy was used for non-responding patients.

Two studies have reported the outcome of patients presenting with isolated supraclavicular lymph node metastasis without other evidence of metastatic disease.[268,269] In both studies, the outcome for these patients was similar to that for patients with stage IIIB disease and better than that for patients with metastatic (stage IV) disease. These results support the classification of lesions of patients with supraclavicular metastasis at presentation as stage III, nonmetastatic disease.

INFLAMMATORY BREAST CANCER

Inflammatory breast cancer is an uncommon diagnosis in the United States and constitutes fewer than 1% of all breast cancers in the United States.[270] However, the incidence of inflammatory breast cancer is higher in less developed countries.

The clinical presentation of inflammatory breast cancer is that of heat and erythema over more than 50% of the breast surface, often with edema of the skin of the breast associated with an erysipeloid edge and peau d'orange appearance. The breast is generally enlarged, and a palpable breast mass may or may not be present. Symptoms tend to have been short in duration, typically 3 months or less. The pathologic finding often seen is the presence of dermal lymphatic invasion.[54,149] However, the diagnosis of inflammatory breast cancer is made on

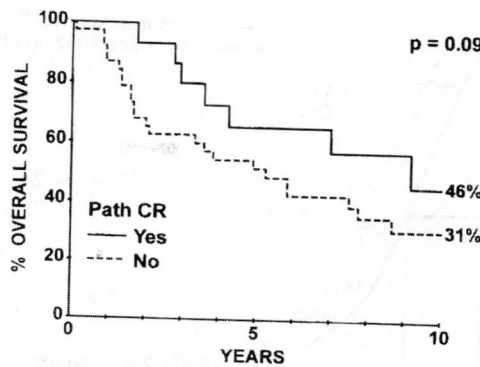

FIGURE 33.2-8. Actuarial overall survival curves for patients with inflammatory breast cancer undergoing combined modality treatment according to whether a pathologic complete response (Path CR) was achieved based on the pathologic findings at the time of mastectomy. (From Harris EE, Schultz D, Bertsch H, et al. Ten-year outcome after combined modality therapy for inflammatory breast cancer. *Int J Radiat Oncol Biol Phys* 2003;55:1200, with permission.)

clinical grounds and does not require the pathologic finding of dermal lymphatic invasion.

Because of the poor prognosis for patients with inflammatory breast cancer, the current management principles are to use aggressive combined modality therapy, starting with initial systemic chemotherapy, followed by local-regional therapy, and possibly further systemic therapy, similar to the sequencing for inoperable locally advanced breast cancer. By definition, inflammatory breast cancer renders the patient inoperable at presentation. Given the poor prognosis of these patients, doxorubicin-based regimens, taxane-containing regimens, or combined doxorubicin-taxane regimens are used initially. Hormonal therapy (tamoxifen) may improve the initial response rates for hormone receptor–positive tumors.

The reported outcomes after treatment for inflammatory breast cancer show overall survival rates at 5 years to 56%, and at 10 years of 35% to 51%. Disease-free survival rates have been reported at 5 years as 35% to 49%, and at 10 years as 34% to 38%. Although these results are poor, it is important to recognize that there is a small, but real, fraction of patients who enjoy long-term survival with contemporary combined modality treatment (Fig. 33.2-8).

METASTATIC BREAST CANCER

Approximately 40,000 women in the United States will die of metastatic breast cancer this year. In spite of major advances in screening, surgery, radiation, endocrine therapy, and chemotherapy for patients with early-stage breast cancer, there has been only modest progress in improving survival for women with metastases. The median survival for patients with metastases remains 18 to 24 months. In a classic study of 250 women with autopsy-proven untreated breast cancer, the average survival after development of symptoms was 3 years and the median survival was 2.7 years; only 2% of patients survived longer than 10 years (Fig. 33.2-9).[271] Of note, 75% of patients in this series presented with stage IV disease. Metastatic breast cancer still remains incurable, and the median survival for all patients after the discovery of metastases is still only 2 to 3

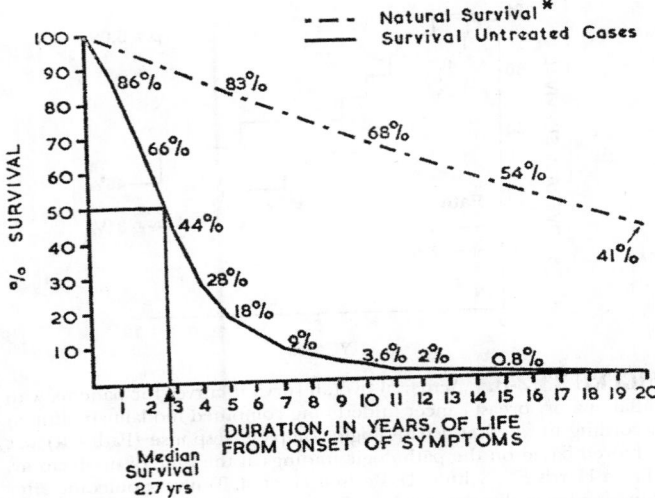

FIGURE 33.2-9. Survival over time for patients with untreated breast cancer. *Natural survival = population of similar ages without breast cancer. (From ref. 271, with permission.)

TABLE 33.2-20. Metastatic Breast Cancer: Distribution of Metastases

Site	At Time of Initial Recurrence (%)[a]	Autopsy Series (%)[b]
Bone	40–75	44–71
Locoregional	15–40	7–39[c]
Lung	5–15	59–69
Pleura	5–15	23–51
Liver	3–10	56–65
Brain	<5	9–20
Pericardium	—	19–21
Intestine	—	18
Adrenal glands	—	31–49

[a]Modified from ref. 274.
[b]Modified from ref. 275.
[c]Skin.

years. Nevertheless, with newer therapies it is estimated that approximately 10% of patients with metastases now survive for 10 years or longer. A review of data for 1581 patients treated with combination chemotherapy for metastatic breast cancer between 1973 and 1982 showed that 17% of patients achieved complete remission.[272] Approximately 20% of these patients (approximately 3% of the total group) lived for 10 years or more compared to 1% to 2% of patients with partial response or stable disease. Younger age, good performance status, and lower tumor burdens predicted a higher probability of complete response. In another series of 156 patients with metastatic disease who received no adjuvant endocrine therapy and who were treated with tamoxifen as initial therapy for metastases, 14% achieved complete response and 6% achieved partial response, and the estimated 10-year survival was 10%.[273] New treatments for metastatic breast cancer have almost certainly extended survival, but overall the improvement has been modest and some of this improvement is likely to be due to advances in imaging and the lead-time bias associated with the earlier diagnosis of metastases.

The primary sites of metastases at time of first documentation of recurrence and in representative autopsy series are presented in Table 33.2-20.[274,275] One-third of patients with recurrent breast cancer present initially with local recurrence involving regional lymph nodes or the chest wall, with the diagnosis of recurrence made on clinical examination with subsequent biopsy confirmation. However, 75% or more of such patients ultimately develop metastases at other distant sites. There is great heterogeneity in the clinical presentation of metastatic breast cancer. Nevertheless, certain characteristics can be used to predict which patients are likely to have a favorable or unfavorable course (Table 33.2-21).

The primary objective of treatment for patients with metastases is palliation, not cure. The major goals of treatment are to control the tempo of the patient's disease, to maintain quality of life, and to improve or eliminate cancer-related symptoms. Although systemic therapy with either endocrine or therapeutic agents remains the cornerstone of treatment of patients

with metastases, appropriate attention and treatment must be given to control pain, dyspnea, cachexia, depression, and other symptoms that frequently are associated with cancer spread. Thus, in addition to having an extensive knowledge of systemic therapy, the oncologist must be well grounded in the principles of supportive care to optimally manage such patients. The team approach includes participation of the nurse, the medical oncologist, the psychologist or psychiatrist, the social worker, and ultimately the home health nurse and hospice team to optimally care for patients with metastases and their families. Supporting the family and helping family members care for the patient as well as manage their own fears and concerns is fundamental in optimizing treatment for patients with metastases.

EVALUATION AND FOLLOW-UP OF PATIENTS WITH SUSPECTED OR CONFIRMED METASTASES

Patients suspected of having metastatic breast cancer should undergo a thorough history taking and physical examination; have a complete blood count and measurement of a comprehensive metabolic profile, including liver function tests; and undergo imaging focused on detecting the cause of signs or symptoms. A major decision for both the patient and oncolo-

TABLE 33.2-21. Factors That Affect Prognosis in Patients with Metastatic Breast Cancer

Favorable Clinical Course (Estimated Survival >2 Y)	Unfavorable Clinical Course (Estimated Survival <2 Y)
Long disease-free interval (at least 2 y from diagnosis; the longer the interval, the longer the estimated survival)	Short disease-free interval (<2 y from diagnosis)
Hormone receptor positivity	Hormone receptor negativity
Response to prior endocrine therapy or chemotherapy	No response to prior chemotherapy or endocrine therapy or relapse while on adjuvant chemotherapy
Single site of metastases	Multiple sites of metastases
Lack of liver, parenchymal lung, or central nervous system involvement	Bone or soft tissue as only sites of metastases

gist is whether or not to obtain a tissue diagnosis to confirm metastases. In the majority of patients, the presentation of metastases is almost certain to be related to breast cancer spread. Multiple hepatic, bone, or pulmonary lesions, regional lymph node enlargement, or pleural effusion are typical of metastatic breast cancer, especially in patients who have previously been considered at high risk for recurrence. Nevertheless, careful history taking and physical examination may suggest that other primary sites could be responsible for such findings. This is especially true with patients who have recurrences more than 5 years after their diagnosis of breast cancer or who have breast cancer in addition to another primary malignancy (e.g., colorectal cancer). Certain presentations that suggest metastasis, however, should alert the oncologist to search for another cause of malignancy, including *isolated* lung lesions (especially in smokers or those who previously smoked) and *isolated* liver and central nervous system (CNS) lesions. Biopsy confirmation of breast cancer should be obtained in these patients. Biopsy results may be helpful to confirm that a lesion in a patient who was initially found to have a hormone receptor–positive breast cancer remains hormone receptor positive and that the patient is therefore a candidate for endocrine therapy, and likewise to reevaluate patients whose tumors were initially HER2 positive for HER2 status. For some patients, even those who are almost certain to have metastatic breast cancer, a tissue diagnosis is necessary to reassure the patient that the diagnosis of metastatic breast cancer is correct. Whether additional studies should be done to evaluate the patient for other asymptomatic metastatic lesions depends on the patient's preferences, the initial site of metastatic disease, and whether such information will change treatment. Certainly, for those patients who have an initial site of metastasis that can be managed well with locally directed treatment alone (plural effusion, chest wall recurrence, and isolated bony or cerebral metastasis), the detection of other asymptomatic lesions may prompt the decision to consider systemic therapy early on. Should this be the case, CT scans of chest, abdomen, and pelvis; radionuclide bone scans; or MRI scans of specific organs such as the liver are warranted. More recently, positron emission tomography (PET) has established itself as a means of evaluating almost all sites of metastasis with a single study. PET scanning appears to have similar sensitivity to CT scanning and bone scanning for detecting metastasis in numerous sites.[276]

Serial monitoring of levels of tumor markers such as carcinoembryonic antigen, CA 15-3, and CA 27-29 may be helpful in assessing the effectiveness of systemic treatment in the metastatic setting[274,277] but should be done with caution. Patients who have been followed using tumor marker levels after early-stage disease and have progressive elevation of marker levels are likely to have metastases. Nevertheless, detection of metastases by physical examination and imaging studies is frequently delayed for as long as 3 to 6 months and occasionally longer. In these instances, most patients with elevated marker levels experience extreme psychological distress. Moreover, because of the occasional false-positive results noted in this setting, the oncologist will have great difficulty in making a treatment decision with which he or she is comfortable. Many of these patients have negative findings on imaging studies, including CT scans, bone scans, and plain radiographs. PET scanning may be helpful here and may detect metastatic disease that has not been revealed by other imaging studies. It

may ultimately become the diagnostic procedure of choice in this setting. In a patient with progressive marker levels and normal imaging studies, irrespective of methodology, neither the oncologist nor the patient can ever be certain that metastatic disease is the cause of marker elevation. Moreover, as many as one-third of patients with metastases do not have elevated marker levels. Following marker levels closely, especially after initiation of systemic therapy, can be confusing, because marker levels are well documented to increase as part of a tumor flare reaction and substantial elevations from baseline may be noted in as many as 50% of patients within the first few months of a highly successful treatment program. Following patients using tumor marker levels is probably most beneficial after several months of treatment have elapsed and in patients whose metastatic disease cannot easily be followed by physical examination or imaging. After 3 to 6 months of therapy, progressive elevation of marker levels by more than 25% on two separate occasions several weeks apart indicates disease progression in more than 75% of patients. However, whether therapy should be changed on the basis of marker findings alone, especially in patients who have excellent symptom control and relative stability of lesions on physical examination and imaging studies, is controversial. Many patients who are doing well become psychologically dependent on marker studies as an indication of their response to treatment. Using tumor marker levels as part of routine management for patients with metastatic disease is controversial, and oncologists should discuss these issues with their patients.

Monitoring the disease course in patients with metastatic disease is better done with physical examination or imaging studies that directly measure tumor size. The major exception is bone metastases. In this setting, frequently improvement in pain is the earliest and best measure of the success of systemic or locally directed therapy.[278] Bone scans may show new lesions early in the course of a successful treatment program due to healing of previously undetectable metastatic deposits. Likewise, using bone radiographs to follow radiographically visible lesions can be complicated. New blastic lesions or blastic responses in previous sites of lytic metastases may be due to healing, whereas the radiologist may attribute such findings to disease progression. The oncologist should review such films carefully with the radiologist and provide appropriate interval history to the radiologist when ordering such studies.

LOCALLY DIRECTED THERAPY

Locally directed therapy should be considered for patients with isolated sites of metastases and for patients with symptomatic metastases in skin and soft tissues, bone, pleura, liver, and the CNS. Local-regional recurrence, including ipsilateral breast tumor recurrence after breast conservation, is discussed elsewhere in this chapter and in many patients is a warning sign of impending metastatic disease. In patients with widespread metastases, locally directed therapy can be used to effectively control specific symptoms, especially in patients who have had extensive prior therapy and are not likely to respond to systemic treatment. Painful lesions in bone, symptomatic lesions in the CNS, pleural effusions, and soft tissue lesions are frequently best managed with locally directed therapy. A small percent of patients with isolated sites of metastases treated with locally directed therapy may remain disease free for long periods of time, and the role of systemic therapy in such patients is uncertain. In a randomized trial, 167 patients who had local recurrence of breast cancer that was ER or PR positive, or for which ER and PR status was unknown, and who were treated with surgery and radiation, received either tamoxifen or no tamoxifen. Tamoxifen treatment was associated with an 82-month disease-free survival compared to 26 months for observation alone ($P<.05$); median 5-year overall survival was similar for tamoxifen-treated and untreated patients (76% and 74%, respectively).[279] The role of chemotherapy in these patients is less clear, and attempts at randomized trials in this setting have been unsuccessful. In one series, the use of FAC chemotherapy in 136 patients with stage IV disease who had only one site of metastasis that was successfully treated with surgery or radiation was associated with a significantly longer disease-free and overall survival compared to historical controls.[280] FAC-treated patients had a median disease-free and overall survival of 38 and 60 months, respectively, compared to 9 and 40 months, respectively, for the control group. Of note, none of the patients in this series received adjuvant chemotherapy. Other trials have not shown similar results. At present, it appears reasonable to consider systemic therapy after isolated recurrences. In patients with ER- or PR-positive tumors, endocrine therapy is a reasonable option, especially in patients who have not received prior endocrine therapy, who have had a long disease-free interval, or who have experienced relapse 1 year or longer after completing adjuvant endocrine treatment. For those who are in otherwise good health, who have experienced relapse while on endocrine therapy or within 12 months of its cessation, or who have a short disease-free interval, chemotherapy may be worth consideration, especially in chemotherapy-naive patients. Patients should be counseled, however, that systemic therapies in this setting are of unproven value.

Locally directed therapy may also be appropriate for patients with pleural effusion, painful or solitary bone metastases, and isolated lesions in liver, lung, and CNS. A symptomatic pleural effusion is occasionally the first site of metastasis, and thoracentesis to confirm the diagnosis of breast cancer and relieve symptoms is the procedure of choice for most patients. For patients with a high likelihood of response to chemotherapy or endocrine therapy, thoracentesis can be repeated while giving systemic therapy time to achieve tumor control. When response to systemic therapy is unlikely, chest tube drainage and sclerosis should be considered early on; control of effusions is seen in 50% to 90% of patients. Symptomatic pericardial effusions, whether isolated or associated with other metastases, must be managed with pericardiocentesis or definitive surgery. Patients with isolated brain metastases should be considered for surgical resection followed by brain irradiation. Surgical resection is appropriate for those with minimal or no extracranial metastases and in most of these patients results in superior disease control compared to radiation alone. Stereotactic irradiation should also be considered for such patients, particularly when surgical resection cannot be performed. For patients who develop isolated pulmonary lesions, biopsy or resection is indicated to exclude a second primary lung cancer. An isolated pulmonary lesion is likely to be a new primary lung lesion, especially if the patient is a smoker. Isolated liver metastases in colorectal cancer have been resected with reports of long survival in a substantial percentage of patients, but in breast cancer, limited data suggest that the number of patients who benefit from such pro-

cedures is small. Other nonsurgical methods of managing single or even multiple hepatic metastases such as radiofrequency ablation, cryoablation, or tumor embolization with radioactive microspheres should be considered for patients with multiple liver metastases as the only site of recurrence.

Patients with bone metastases should be considered for bisphosphonate therapy. In patients with at least one lytic metastatic lesion on plain radiograph, randomized trials have confirmed the value of the bisphosphonate pamidronate, in addition to both chemotherapy and endocrine therapy, in decreasing skeletal complications.[281,282] Pamidronate significantly lengthened the time to an initial skeletal complication and decreased the risk of skeletal complications by approximately 12% compared to placebo but had no effect on survival. Zoledronate has been shown to be at least similar and possibly superior to pamidronate for reducing skeletal complications and can be infused in a shorter period of time. An ASCO expert panel has developed guidelines for bisphosphonate use.[283] Bisphosphonates were recommended for patients with lytic metastases on plain radiographs. For patients with an abnormal bone scan, normal plain radiographs, and MRI or CT images showing bone destruction, bisphosphonate therapy was considered "reasonable." Bisphosphonates were not recommended for patients with an abnormal bone scan, normal plain radiographs, and no evidence of bone destruction on MRI or CT. For selected patients with painful bony metastases that are unlikely to respond to systemic therapy, intravenous administration of radioactive strontium or samarium may be helpful in palliation.

ENDOCRINE THERAPY AND CHEMOTHERAPY

General Principles

Almost all patients with metastatic breast cancer are ultimately candidates for systemic therapy. The choice of therapy depends on the tempo of the metastatic disease; whether or not the patient has symptoms and, if so, the severity of symptoms; and whether the tumor is hormone receptor positive. Patients with ER- or PR-positive tumors are more likely to develop bone metastases, whereas those with ER- and PR-negative tumors are more likely to have liver and other visceral involvement. In spite of these biologic differences, all sites of metastatic disease in patients with ER- or PR-positive tumors are potentially responsive to endocrine therapy. For patients with ER- and PR-negative disease who have slowly progressive metastases and minimal symptoms, and for whom even a tumor doubling is not likely to result in a change in performance status, a trial of endocrine therapy should be considered. This is especially true for older patients for whom objective response rates of approximately 15% have been reported.[284] Conversely, because the overall response rate to chemotherapy is higher than that to endocrine therapy, patients with rapidly progressive tumors or major tumor-related symptoms should be considered for chemotherapy. If a remission is obtained, endocrine therapy can then be considered. A common concern is whether patients with hormone receptor–positive tumors and symptomatic, rapidly progressing metastatic disease should be considered for a combined modality treatment with endocrine therapy and chemotherapy. Two trials randomly assigned patients with metastatic breast cancer to receive either tamoxifen or chemotherapy.[285,286] In both, receptor studies were not routinely performed. Nevertheless, there were no differences in overall survival in either trial. Clinical trials comparing chemotherapy alone with chemotherapy plus endocrine therapy have occasionally shown a higher response rate but no survival advantage for combined treatment.[287] Moreover, there is a theoretical concern that combined modality treatment might be antagonistic. In the adjuvant setting the concurrent use of tamoxifen and CAF was inferior to the use of CAF followed by tamoxifen.[288] The authors recommend initial treatment with chemotherapy alone in almost all such patients with rapidly progressive disease.

Although the goals of systemic therapy in the metastatic setting are control of disease and maintenance or improvement in quality of life, response assessment remains an integral part of patient management. For the vast majority of patients, the cornerstone of response evaluation remains the history and physical examination, especially during the first few months of treatment and in patients with skin and soft tissue recurrence. The clinician needs to be aware of tumor flare, which occurs in a small percentage of patients and which may occur with chemotherapy as well as endocrine therapy. Tumor flare may include worsening of tumor-related symptoms, such as bone pain or worsening of soft tissue lesions, new lesions, or increased intensity of lesions on bone scan; increase in tumor marker levels; hypercalcemia; and increases in serum alkaline phosphatase levels. Tumor flare generally occurs several days to several weeks after initiation of therapy. There is no certain method to discern tumor flare from tumor progression, but the early and rapid onset of symptoms is more characteristic of tumor flare. Patients should be educated concerning the possibility of tumor flare and, should it occur, should be reassured and closely monitored. Flares generally resolve within several weeks. For the 10% to 20% of patients with metastases confined to bone, flare can be especially difficult to separate from tumor progression, but the same strategy described should be used.

For patients with measurable lesions, objective responses to systemic therapy are noted within 3 months to 4 months in the majority of patients. As noted earlier, assessing the response of bone metastases can be difficult. Improvement in bone pain remains the best indication of response and should be the major guide to continuing the patient's current treatment. Bone scans may show worsening of lesions even after 3 to 6 months of treatment, and treatment should be continued in these patients provided they have had symptomatic improvement or minimal symptoms.[289] Plain radiographs of lytic lesions may show recalcification, and new blastic lesions may be seen in bones normal on prior radiographs.[278] Such changes are usually indications of healing, and therapy should be continued. For clinical trials, the Response Evaluation Criteria in Solid Tumors criteria should be used to assess response.[290] Outside of the trial setting, imaging and laboratory studies should be judiciously used to monitor response and toxicity. It is important to note that small changes in radiologic measurements, although seemingly precise, may be clinically inaccurate, and for patients otherwise doing well, treatment changes should not be dictated on this basis. Likewise, laboratory test results, including tumor marker levels, can vary over the course of treatment. Progressive elevation of liver function test results or markers of at least 25% over baseline on two successive occasions is indicative of tumor progression in almost all patients, the exception being

in the setting of tumor flare. Although achieving an objective response is highly gratifying for both patient and physician, stabilizing metastases is also a desirable treatment goal, especially for patients who are minimally symptomatic. Patients with metastases stable for 24 weeks or longer have survival similar to that of patients with complete and partial responses[291]; indeed, it is now common in clinical trials to report the "clinical benefit response," which includes the percentage of patients with stable disease for 24 weeks or more in addition to the percentage with complete and partial responses.

Endocrine Therapy

Endocrine therapies currently available for both premenopausal and postmenopausal patients are listed in Table 33.2-22. Responses to initial endocrine therapy in both premenopausal and postmenopausal patients are seen in 30% to 50% of patients and generally last an average of approximately 1 year, usually sev-

TABLE 33.2-22. Hormonal Therapies for Patients with Breast Cancer

Patient Group and Agents	Dose and Schedule (Oral Agent Unless Specified)
PREMENOPAUSAL PATIENTS	
Selective estrogen receptor modulators (SERMs)	
Tamoxifen (Nolvadex)	20 mg daily
Toremifene (Fareston)	60 mg daily
Ovarian ablation	
Luteinizing hormone–releasing hormone agonists	
Goserelin (Zoladex)	3.6 mg SC every 4 wk
	10.8 mg SC every 12 wk
Leuprolide (Lupron)[a]	3.75 mg every 4 wk
	11.25 mg every 3 mo
Oophorectomy	Laparoscopic preferred
Ovarian irradiation	15–20 Gy in 5–10 fractions
Progestins	
Megestrol acetate (Megace)	40 mg q.i.d.
Medroxyprogesterone acetate (Provera)	400–500 mg PO daily (no FDA-approved oral dose for breast cancer in U.S.)
	500 mg IM twice weekly × 4 then weekly
Androgens	
Fluoxymesterone (Halotestin)	10–40 mg daily (in divided doses)
POSTMENOPAUSAL PATIENTS	
Aromatase inhibitors	
Anastrozole (Arimidex)	1 mg daily
Letrozole (Femara)	2.5 mg daily
Exemestane (Aromasin)	25 mg daily
SERMs (as above)	
Estrogen receptor down-regulators ("pure antiestrogens")	
Fulvestrant (Faslodex)	250 mg IM monthly
Progestins	As above
Androgens	As above
High-dose estrogens	
Diethylstilbestrol	15 mg daily

FDA, U.S. Food and Drug Administration.
[a]Not FDA approved for this indication.

TABLE 33.2-23. Selected Trials of Aromatase Inhibitors and Other Endocrine Agents in Postmenopausal
Patients with Metastatic Breast Cancer

Comparison	Reference(s)	No. Patients	CR + PR (%)	Clinical Benefit	TTP (Median, Mo)	OS (Median, Mo)
Anastrozole	69, 70	511	29	57	10.7[a]	41.0
Tamoxifen		510	27	52	6.4	41.5
Letrozole	71	453	30	49	9.5[a]	34
Tamoxifen		454	20	38	6.0	30
Fulvestrant	72	206	17.5	42.2	5.4	NA
Anastrozole		194	17.5	36.1	3.4	NA
Fulvestrant	30	313	31.6	54.3	6.8	NA
Tamoxifen		274	33.9	62.0	8.3	NA

CR, complete response; NA, not available; OS, overall survival; PR, partial response; TTP, time to progression.
[a]Statistically significant difference compared to tamoxifen.

eral months longer than responses to chemotherapy when used in the same setting.[292] In premenopausal women with metastatic breast cancer, several randomized trials have shown similar efficacy for the SERM tamoxifen and ovarian ablation. Tamoxifen, the most widely used SERM, is effective in both premenopausal and postmenopausal patients.[293] The SERM toremifene appears similar in efficacy to tamoxifen in clinical trials but offers no advantage. The choice of using tamoxifen or ovarian ablation as initial endocrine therapy in the premenopausal patient should be based on patient and physician preference. Ovarian ablation can be achieved with LHRH agonists, radiation, or surgery, with similar response rates for each modality. In premenopausal women who have received tamoxifen in the adjuvant setting and experienced relapse more than 1 year after completing tamoxifen treatment, tamoxifen is likely to be almost as effective as when used in endocrine therapy–naive patients.[294] A metaanalysis of four randomized trials that compared tamoxifen and an LHRH agonist versus an LHRH agonist alone showed a small but statistically significant improvement in response rate (39% vs. 30%), progression-free interval (hazard ratio, 0.70), and overall survival (hazard ratio, 0.78) favoring the combination.[295] Combining ovarian ablation with an aromatase inhibitor is also being explored in this setting. At present, the authors recommend sequential therapy starting with either tamoxifen or ovarian ablation for most patients. Those with extensive metastases or major symptoms should be considered for tamoxifen plus ovarian ablation as initial treatment. Almost all patients ultimately develop tumor progression after tamoxifen and ovarian ablation. Those who have had responses are most likely to benefit from further endocrine therapy. Aromatase should be considered in this setting provided that the patient has been rendered postmenopausal by ovarian ablation. Progestins are another major treatment option. For those patients who respond to several endocrine agents or who have a very slow tempo of disease progression, use of other endocrine agents such as androgens or retrial with previously used agents should be considered. Moreover, a small percentage of patients who have had disease progression on an initial endocrine regimen may respond to a second agent. Because all therapy in this setting is palliative, delaying chemotherapy, which is almost always associated with a higher toxicity profile and inferior quality of life compared to endocrine therapy, is a good strategy.

In postmenopausal patients the new aromatase inhibitors, including anastrozole, letrozole, and exemestane, have been shown to be superior to progestins and equal if not superior to tamoxifen as initial treatment for metastases.[296,297] When compared to tamoxifen as first-line endocrine therapy for metastatic breast cancer, aromatase inhibitors have shown improved complete and partial response rates, clinical benefit responses, and time to progression, but no differences in survival (Table 33.2-23). Three aromatase inhibitors are currently approved by the U.S. Food and Drug Administration for treatment of metastatic breast cancer. Two, anastrozole and letrozole, are nonsteroidal, noncompetitive inhibitors of aromatase, whereas the third, exemestane, is a steroidal compound that binds irreversibly to the aromatase binding site. In clinical trials in metastatic disease, the aromatase inhibitors appear similar in efficacy, but patients who experience tumor progression on nonsteroidal inhibitors have been shown to respond to exemestane,[298] and vice versa. More recently, the selective ER down-regulator fulvestrant has been shown to be similar in efficacy to the aromatase inhibitor anastrozole in postmenopausal women with breast cancer who experience tumor progression on tamoxifen (see Table 33.2-23). Preliminary results of a randomized trial comparing fulvestrant with tamoxifen have demonstrated similar efficacy.[299] Fulvestrant, a "pure antiestrogen" that degrades the ER, has not been tested in the premenopausal setting and should not be used in these patients outside of a clinical trial. As with premenopausal patients, postmenopausal patients should be continued on endocrine therapy until the tempo of their disease or their lack of response indicates that the tumor is refractory to endocrine therapy. There is no ideal sequence for the use of endocrine therapy, and for postmenopausal patients, tamoxifen, aromatase inhibitors, and fulvestrant are all reasonable choices for initial therapy. In responding patients, each of these agents can be used in succession. After progression on tamoxifen, aromatase inhibitors, and fulvestrant, hormone-responsive patients or those with long periods of disease stability should be considered for treatment with progestins, estrogens, or androgens.

In both premenopausal and postmenopausal patients, withdrawal responses can be seen when endocrine therapy is stopped after tumor progression.[300] Withdrawal responses include tumor regression as well as long periods of disease stability. Although historically best described in patients who discontinued high-dose estrogen therapy after tumor progression, withdrawal responses have been described after cessation of tamoxifen and progestins. Patients most likely to have a withdrawal response include patients who had previously responded to the endocrine agent they are currently taking and those with prolonged periods of disease stability. Although most patients with metastases are likely to be reluctant to be followed without an active treatment regimen, clinicians should encourage patients who are good candidates for a withdrawal response to accept a "drug holiday." In addition, patients who relapse while taking adjuvant tamoxifen, with a disease-free interval of 2 years or more, should also be considered for a drug holiday in anticipation of a withdrawal response.

The addition of several new endocrine agents to the armamentarium of hormonal therapy, coupled with the explosive scientific advances in molecular biology concerning the mechanisms of hormonal sensitivity and resistance, has led to renewed interest in endocrine therapy. In general, most investigators have found that patients with hormone receptor–positive, HER2-positive tumors are less likely to respond to endocrine therapy than are patients with hormone receptor–positive, HER2-negative tumors.[74] One randomized trial involving patients with locally advanced breast cancer has shown that, in patients with hormone receptor–positive, HER2-positive tumors, letrozole was associated with a significantly higher response rate than was tamoxifen.[80] A substantial body of preclinical evidence is emerging that is clarifying the signaling pathways and cross-talk involved in endocrine resistance.[79] Moreover, substantial preclinical data suggest that new biologic agents can modulate endocrine receptor–positive tumors to enhance or possibly even restore endocrine sensitivity in refractory tumors.[301,302] Current trials are under way combining endocrine agents with biologic agents that target the epidermal growth factor pathway, such as trastuzumab, gefitinib (ZD-1839; Iressa), and other agents in an attempt to enhance the efficacy of endocrine treatment.

Chemotherapy

Eventually, chemotherapy is considered for almost all patients with metastatic breast cancer. The median survival of patients with metastases whose disease has become refractory to endocrine therapy or who have receptor-negative tumors is 18 to 24 months. Several new agents are now available offering expanded treatment options for many patients.[292] Table 33.2-24 lists the commercial agents currently available for use. A major issue in treatment selection is whether to use sequential single-agent therapy or a combination regimen of two or more agents. Response rates to initial therapy with anthracyclines, taxanes, capecitabine, vinorelbine, and gemcitabine range on average from 25% to 60%, with the median time to progression averaging approximately 6 months. In general, response rates diminish by half for use of the agents as second- and third-line treatment, although there is great variability among trials. Although multidrug regimens of active agents consistently show improved response rates that average approximately 20% higher than those for single agents, single-agent sequential therapy is generally associated with less treatment-related toxicity, and numerous trials have shown no survival advantage for combination therapy compared to single-agent therapy. One clinical trial illustrates this principle.[303] Sledge and colleagues randomly assigned 739 patients to either doxorubicin alone, paclitaxel alone, or the combination of both agents. The response rate and time to progression for the combination regimen (47% and 8.0 months, respectively) were significantly

TABLE 33.2-24. Chemotherapeutic Agents for the Treatment of Metastatic Breast Cancer

Drug Class and Agent[a]	Dose and Schedule When Used as a Single Agent[b]
ANTHRACYCLINES AND ANTRAQUINONES	
Doxorubicin (Adriamycin)	50–60 mg/m^2 every 3 wk
	20 mg or 20 mg/m^2 weekly
Epirubicin (Ellence)	20 mg/m^2 weekly
	60–90 mg/m^2 every 3 wk
Mitoxantrone (Novantrone)	10–15 mg/m^2 every 3 wk
Liposomal doxorubicin (Doxil)	35–40 mg/m^2 every 4 wk
ALKYLATING AGENTS	
Cyclophosphamide (Cytoxan)	400–600 mg/m^2 every 3 wk
	100 mg/m^2 (maximum, 150 mg) orally for 14 d every 3 wk
Melphalan (Alkeran)	Not recommended for single-agent use
THIOTEPA (THIOPLEX)	Not recommended for single-agent use
VINCA ALKALOIDS AND RELATED DRUGS	
Etoposide (VePesid)	50 mg orally daily for 14 d every 3 wk
Vinblastine (Velban)	3–4 mg/m^2 d 1 and 8 every 3 wk
Vinorelbine (Navelbine)	30 mg/m^2 weekly
TAXANES	
Paclitaxel (Taxol)	175 mg/m^2 every 3 wk
	80–100 mg/m^2 weekly
	35 mg/m^2 weekly
Docetaxel (Taxotere)	80–100 mg/m^2 every 3 wk
ANTIMETABOLITES	
5-FLUOROURACIL (ADRUCIL) (+ LEUCO-VORIN)	500 mg/m^2 d 1–3 every 3 wk by continuous infusion (numerous other schedules)
Capecitabine (Xeloda)	1000 mg/m^2 orally b.i.d. for 14 d every 3 wk
Methotrexate	40–60 mg/m^2 d 1 and 8 every 4 wk
Gemcitabine (Gemzar)	800–1250 mg/m^2 d 1, 8, and 15 every 4 wk

[a]U.S. Food and Drug Administration approved and commercially available. All agents in table generally qualify for reimbursement in the metastatic setting and are recognized for this indication by the U.S. Pharmacopeia (see http://www.accc-cancer.org).
[b]Intravenous administration unless otherwise specified.

higher than those for single-agent doxorubicin (36% and 5.8 months, respectively) or paclitaxel (34% and 6.0 months, respectively). However, secondary responses after crossing over from paclitaxel to doxorubicin (22%) or from doxorubicin to paclitaxel (20%) compensated for the higher initial response rates and time to progression for the combination regimen. Quality of life and survival time (median of 18.9 months for initial doxorubicin treatment, 22.2 months for initial paclitaxel, and 22.0 months for paclitaxel) were similar for all groups. A similar trial was performed by Joensuu and colleagues, who compared weekly epirubicin with cyclophosphamide, epirubicin, and fluorouracil; response rates, time to progression, and survival were similar in both groups, whereas quality of life favored the less toxic, weekly epirubicin regimen.[304] Moreover, unlike combination chemotherapy, treatment with a single agent also allows the clinician to assess the benefit of the specific agent being administered. Using a novel design, Costanza and her CALGB colleagues compared four cycles of one of five sequential single agents (trimetrexate, melphalan, amonafide, carboplatin, or elsamitrucin) followed by CAF with CAF alone in patients with metastatic breast cancer previously untreated with chemotherapy.[305] There was no difference in survival (median of 20 months for the sequential arm vs. 17 months for the CAF-alone arm), and in a multivariate analysis only an increased number of previous treatment modalities, a poorer performance status, and visceral metastases were significantly correlated with poorer survival. This trial also provides support for phase II trials of new agents in chemotherapy-naive patients with metastatic breast cancer. At first glance, a well-done, randomized trial comparing docetaxel and capecitabine with docetaxel alone in 511 patients would appear to refute this strategy, because patients treated with the combination regimen has statistically superior response rates and disease-free and overall survival (14.5 months for the combination and 11.5 months for single-agent docetaxel).[306] However, in this trial only 17% of patients were treated with capecitabine after tumor progression on docetaxel, and this group had a superior overall survival compared to patients treated with the combination regimen.[307] Randomized clinical trials in metastatic breast cancer that show improved survival for a specific therapy should be reviewed critically to make certain that all patients had access to, or treatment with, all active agents, whether as part of protocol therapy or after protocol therapy was completed; if not, patients without access to other effective agents are likely to have poorer survival. Fossati and colleagues in a metaanalysis of single-agent versus combination chemotherapy found a significant survival benefit for combination therapy that translated into an absolute benefit in survival of 9% at 1 year, 5% at 2 years, and 3% at 3 years.[287] None of the individual trials included in the analysis showed a significant survival benefit for combination therapy, and no recent trials comparing single-agent taxane regimens with multidrug regimens were included. Also, it is unclear whether patients in these trials had access to all the agents used in the multidrug regimens. Most patients with metastases are still best treated using a single-agent, sequential approach. There is no evidence that any specific sequence of active agents is superior to any other. Prior chemotherapy exposure, renal and hepatic function, anticipated toxicity, and patient preference should all be taken into account. Combination regimens should be considered for patients with overwhelming symptoms or rapidly progressive or life-threatening metastases for which a combination regimen is more likely to result in a tumor response. Phase II and especially phase III trials of combination chemotherapy are certainly warranted, however. Combination regimens that show high response rates in the metastatic setting are good candidates for study in the adjuvant setting, in which these response rates may be translated into survival gains.

How long chemotherapy should be continued in patients with responding or stable disease remains a major issue, especially for patients who have high-quality responses or disease stabilization but major treatment-related toxicity. Contrary to the perception of many, quality of life is not adversely affected and may even be improved in many patients actively receiving chemotherapy. Coates and colleagues compared continuous therapy with AC or CMF with intermittent therapy using three cycles of the same regimen with reinstitution of therapy at the time of disease progression.[308] In this trial, patients receiving continuous therapy had superior response rates, time to progression, and quality-of-life scores, but no improvement in survival. Moreover, quality of life was an independent prognostic factor, and patients with higher quality of life had better treatment-related outcomes. A similar trial by the Piedmont Oncology Association randomly assigned patients who had responding or stable disease after six cycles of CAF to either CMF or observation, followed by reinstitution of CMF at disease progression.[309] Although time to progression was more than twice as long for patients on continuous therapy than for those with interrupted treatment (9.4 vs. 3.2 months, respectively), overall survival was similar. Falkson and colleagues randomly assigned 141 patients whose measurable disease showed a complete response after six cycles of CAF to receive either chemohormonal therapy or observation.[310] Time to disease progression was 19 months for patients given chemohormonal therapy and 8 months for patients on observation; overall survival was similar. These data suggest that a drug holiday is associated with a shorter time to progression but no adverse effect on survival. Physicians should share these data with patients, because some patients may wish a drug holiday whereas others, especially those with substantial tumor-related symptoms before treatment, may wish to stay on therapy. In addition, these data support newer randomized trial designs that, after remission induction with standard treatment, compare new agents with observation, or new agents with established agents. Such designs use time to progression as the major treatment end point and are especially suited for the investigation of biologic agents.

The relationship between the dose and schedule of chemotherapy administered and treatment outcome continues to be a major issue in breast cancer management. In the metastatic setting results of randomized trials comparing high-dose chemotherapy and hematopoietic support have failed to confirm the initial promising results of phase II trials of high-dose treatment. In one large randomized trial, Stadtmauer and colleagues randomly assigned 199 women who responded to four to six cycles of combination chemotherapy to receive either high-dose therapy with carboplatin, thiotepa, and cyclophosphamide or prolonged therapy with CMF.[311] The time to progression for both groups was similar (9 months). At 3 years there was no significant survival difference, with 32% of patients treated with high-dose therapy alive, compared to 38% receiving prolonged CMF. Berry et al., using data from the Autologous Blood and Marrow Transplant Registry, compared 441 women entered in phase II trials of high-dose therapy with 635 patients treated in CALGB trials of metastatic breast cancer.[312] Five-year survival was 23% for those on the high-dose trials compared to 15% for patients on CALGB trials ($P = .03$). Although this suggests a small benefit from high-dose therapy, many potential biases exist in this type of analysis, and others have shown that patients in high-dose trials are likely to have much more favorable clinical characteristics.[313,314] At present, high-dose chemotherapy with hematopoietic support has no role in the treatment of patients with metastatic breast cancer. Although there is excellent laboratory evidence to support a dose-response effect for cytotoxicity, especially with alkylating agents, the agents used in clinical trials have not proven superior to less toxic and less costly treatments.

For single-agent therapy as well as some combination regimens, higher doses and more intense schedules have frequently been associated with improvements in response rates and greater toxicity but not improved survival.[287] For CMF a higher-dose, every-3-week intravenous regimen was associated with a significantly higher response rate than a lower-dose regimen (30% vs. 11%, respectively), but dose intensity was not related to survival.[315] A second trial compared the "classic" CMF regimen using oral cyclophosphamide with an every-3-week intravenous regimen and showed a higher response rate (48% vs. 29%; P = .003), a similar duration of response (11 months), and a longer survival (17 months vs. 12 months; P = .016) for the oral-based schedule.[316] The difference in survival is hard to reconcile with the similar duration of response, but this trial has led many investigators to favor the use of "classical" CMF in the adjuvant setting. Clinical trials data suggest that a threshold dose exists for most chemotherapy agents and that doses above this threshold are associated with little to no additional benefit. Well-studied doses and schedules of active single agents are presented in Table 33.2-24. Low-dose weekly administration of anthracyclines and taxanes appears similar in efficacy to higher-dose single-agent regimens, but randomized trials addressing these issues are still in progress. Weekly schedules of treatment, although more cumbersome for many patients, allow the clinician to titrate the chemotherapy dose and minimize toxicity. This is especially true for patients with poor performance status and abnormal liver function.

Interest has been expressed in using *in vitro* assays to help select chemotherapy treatment.[317,318] Difficulties in culturing tumor cells, high cost, and differences in drug sensitivity due to tumor heterogeneity have limited the usefulness of these assays, and few oncologists currently use assays for treatment selection. Randomized trials comparing outcomes after treatment based on assay results with outcomes after standard treatment selection are needed.

TRASTUZUMAB THERAPY

Trastuzumab, a humanized monoclonal antibody directed against the extracellular domain of the transmembrane glycoprotein HER2/*neu* (c-erbB-2), provides clinicians with a valuable option in the treatment of women with HER2-positive metastatic breast cancer. HER2, a member of the EGFR family that includes HER1 (EGFR-1), HER3, and HER4, is amplified or overexpressed in the tumors of approximately 20% of all patients with metastases. Measurement of HER2 is best done using FISH techniques that accurately assesses gene amplification. IHC methods using a variety of antibodies are also useful. There is an excellent direct correlation between positivity on FISH testing and 3+ positive staining by IHC (on a scale of 0 to 3+).[319,320] Although data are lacking, it is unlikely that trastuzumab will have any benefit in patients with HER2-negative tumors, and a clinical trial testing this hypothesis (CALGB 9840) is currently in progress.

Using trastuzumab as a single agent, Vogel and colleagues reported a complete and partial response rate of 35% and a clinical benefit response rate of 48% in patients who had not received chemotherapy for metastases and whose tumors showed 3+ staining by IHC.[321] Of note, 2 of 29 patients whose tumors were 3+ HER2 positive by IHC but negative by FISH had an objective response. Fifty-seven percent of responders were progression free at 1 year, and median survival was 24 months. Two dosages were used: an 8-mg/kg loading dose followed by 4 mg/kg weekly and a 4-mg/kg loading dose followed by 2 mg/kg weekly. There was no dose-response effect. Cobleigh and col-

leagues treated 222 heavily pretreated patients with single-agent trastuzumab as second- and third-line therapy, and noted a 15% complete and partial response rate; median survival was 13 months.[322] Trastuzumab as a single agent is generally well tolerated but carries a small risk of cardiac toxicity approximating 2% in patients with minimal exposure to prior chemotherapy and approximately 5% in patients who have previously received anthracyclines or have preexisting cardiac disease. Cardiac toxicity usually manifests clinically as congestive heart failure and responds to treatment and is reversible in most patients.

In the major pivotal trial used as the basis for U.S. Food and Drug Administration approval of trastuzumab, patients with HER2-positive metastatic breast cancer were randomly assigned to receive chemotherapy alone (AC for anthracycline-naive patients and paclitaxel for patients who had previously received anthracyclines) or chemotherapy plus trastuzumab. The combination of trastuzumab and chemotherapy yielded significantly better results than chemotherapy alone in response rate (50% vs. 32%), time to progression (median of 7.4 vs. 4.6 months), and survival time (median of 25.1 vs. 20.3 months).[323] The majority of patients who progressed on chemotherapy alone were offered trastuzumab after tumor progression, which suggests that the combination of trastuzumab and chemotherapy was superior to sequential use of chemotherapy followed by trastuzumab in this setting. However, serious cardiac toxicity was noted in 19% of patients receiving AC and trastuzumab but only 5% of those receiving paclitaxel and trastuzumab, and the median overall survival in this trial for patients treated with trastuzumab and chemotherapy was similar to that of patients treated with first-line trastuzumab. The use of single-agent trastuzumab is still appropriate and may be preferred by many patients. In preclinical studies, trastuzumab, when combined with chemotherapeutic agents, has shown additive and synergistic activity.[324] Trastuzumab and other EGFR-targeted biologic agents can also reverse endocrine resistance in tumor cell cultures.[325] Trials have shown considerable activity of trastuzumab when combined with vinorelbine, taxanes given weekly, and other agents.[326]

Certain questions related to trastuzumab use remain. It is unclear how long trastuzumab administration should be continued in the stable or responding patient. Because its use is associated with minimal toxicity and because of the frequent reluctance of patients with metastatic breast cancer to stop an effective treatment, most clinicians continue therapy indefinitely. Moreover, data suggest that giving trastuzumab on a 3-week schedule is associated with efficacy similar to that of giving it on a weekly schedule,[327] which minimizes clinic visits. It is also unclear whether continuing trastuzumab administration after disease progression in patients receiving trastuzumab and chemotherapy adds to the response of subsequent chemotherapy treatment. If there is any benefit, it is likely to be small, but convincing data to resolve this issue are lacking. Pending further research, it is reasonable to continue trastuzumab in conjunction with a new chemotherapeutic agent for at least another course of therapy after initial progression on trastuzumab alone or trastuzumab plus chemotherapy. Whether trastuzumab will play a major part in improving breast cancer survival depends on whether it results in significant improvement in disease-free and overall survival when used in conjunction with chemotherapy in the adjuvant setting. In addition, new biologic agents directed at other targets in the EGFR pathway are currently in clinical trials and hold great promise.

NEW AGENTS AND CLINICAL TRIALS

The explosion of knowledge in genomics and proteomics is paving the way for the development of agents that specifically target key pathways involved in cancer cell growth and metastases. In addition to the more traditional chemotherapeutic agents, new biologic agents that target gene expression, tumor cell signaling pathways involved in cell proliferation and metastases, oncogenes, tumor-specific antigens, angiogenesis, and the cell cycle are in development. Several of these agents such as the anti–vascular endothelial growth factor receptor antibody bevacizumab, have shown modest single-agent activity but are being explored in regimens that include chemotherapy. Except for trastuzumab, none of the newer biologic agents have been approved for use in breast cancer. In addition, statins and inhibitors of COX pathways (specifically COX-2 inhibitors) have been shown to have antiproliferative effects in preclinical studies, and clinical trials of these agents are in progress. A major challenge will be how to study many of the more promising agents in trials. Standard phase II and III trials are cumbersome, which may limit testing of many of these agents. Newer designs that incorporate neoadjuvant therapy or Bayesian statistical methods may be maximizing the ability to study new agents in a timely fashion.[328,329] Patients with metastatic breast cancer should be offered participation in clinical trials whenever possible, including participation in phase I studies. Such clinical trials form the basis for exploring new and promising agents and regimens in the adjuvant setting, in which major advances have been made in improving survival with systemic therapy.

QUALITY OF LIFE AND SUPPORTIVE CARE ISSUES

Maintaining quality of life is a prime goal of treatment in metastatic breast cancer. Metastatic breast cancer is associated with profound psychological distress for many patients and families. Support groups led by trained personnel can help patients and families cope more successfully with the diagnosis. Initial trials suggested that patients participating in support groups had improved survival compared to patients who did not, but a more recent trial by Goodwin and colleagues has failed to confirm these findings.[330] In this trial, supportive-expressive group therapy was compared with standard care, and a similar median survival was noted for both groups (approximately 18 months). However, patients in the supportive-expressive care group, especially patients who were most distressed at study entry, had significant improvements in mood and pain perception. These data suggest that participation in a support group may be especially valuable for those patients who have the greatest difficulty in coping with their diagnosis. Measuring health-related quality of life (HRQOL) is difficult, but an approximation can be made using one of several validated instruments. For metastatic disease, the addition of quality-of-life measurements to clinical trials assessing the value of hormonal therapy, chemotherapy, or supportive care appear to add little to information obtained from traditional medical outcomes, including performance status, toxicity, tumor response, and survival measures.[331] HRQOL measurements, however, may be helpful in randomized trials of agents that have different toxicity profiles. Moreover, HRQOL measures may best be used in judging the effects of psychosocial interventions. As suggested by Goodwin and colleagues, future research in HRQOL should focus on the development of targeted instruments that contain items or scales capturing information not obtained by general or cancer-related measures (e.g., cognitive function).[331]

Because all therapy in the metastatic setting is palliative, making chemotherapy more acceptable to patients is an important goal of treatment. In one study of 103 patients with incurable cancer who were candidates for chemotherapy, almost 90% preferred an oral agent, but approximately 70% preferred intravenous treatment if it would result in an increased response rate or longer response duration.[332] Capecitabine has emerged as an effective oral agent in the management of metastatic disease and in small trials has appeared equal in efficacy to CMF or paclitaxel.[333] In this regard, a trial using a metronomic (low dose over a prolonged period) oral regimen of cyclophosphamide and methotrexate in 61 patients mostly pretreated with chemotherapy found a complete and partial response rate of 19% and a clinical benefit response of 32%.[334] Other potentially effective oral agents are in development and will hopefully provide even more treatment options for oral therapy.

Patients with metastases should be closely monitored for depression, pain, fatigue, nausea and vomiting, and other symptoms that frequently are associated with metastatic disease. Management of these problems is discussed elsewhere in this text. Almost all patients with breast cancer metastases will at some time become refractory to all systemic therapies, and the focus of treatment will change to end-of-life care. At this point, the oncologist should help lead a team that includes nursing and hospice professionals, as well as the patient's family and friends, with the goal of providing the most comfortable environment for the patient to experience a dignified, pain-free demise.

BREAST CANCER AND PREGNANCY

It is estimated that, among patients with breast cancer, approximately 1.5% are pregnant at the time of diagnosis and that breast cancer occurs in approximately 1 in 3000 pregnancies.[335] However, cultural changes have occurred since those estimates were made, mainly delay in childbirth, and current estimates are that breast cancer occurs in as many as 1 in 1000 pregnancies. Management of breast cancer during pregnancy remains a clinical challenge. Evidence-based guidelines grounded in an extensive literature review have been developed.[336] The diagnosis of breast cancer during pregnancy is frequently difficult and is complicated by the engorgement of breast tissue that accompanies gestation. Most breast cancers in pregnant women present as palpable masses. Mammography is safe but less sensitive during pregnancy, yet many clinicians are reluctant to order radiographic imaging in a pregnant patient. A single, unilateral medial lateral oblique mammographic view may be sufficient and minimizes x-ray exposure. Ultrasonography can be helpful in distinguishing solid and cystic masses, but biopsy of a suspicious mass should be performed to prevent delays in diagnosis. Breast MRI may also be helpful but has not been studied in this setting.

Breast cancer during pregnancy is usually detected at a later stage and is generally associated with a poorer survival than breast cancer detected in nonpregnant patients. In one large series, breast cancers diagnosed during pregnancy or lactation were more likely to be high-grade, ER and PR negative, HER2 (c-erbB-2) positive,[337] and associated with lymphovascular invasion. When adjustments are made for age and tumor stage, however, pregnant patients with breast cancer have survival similar to that of nonpregnant women.[338] Management of the pregnant patient with breast cancer should take a multidisciplinary approach that includes participation of medical, surgical, and radiation oncologists, as well as psychosocial support and integration of the obstetrics team. In addition to careful history taking and physical examination, laboratory work including complete blood count, comprehensive metabolic profile, and a chest radiograph (with appropriate shielding) should be performed. Serum alkaline phosphatase level is elevated during pregnancy and should be interpreted in conjunction with clinical findings in assessing pregnant patients for liver or bone metastases. For patients with signs or symptoms suggestive of liver metastases, an ultrasonographic examination can be safely used to further evaluate the patient. MRI appears to be safe in pregnancy and has been used to detect fetal abnormalities *in utero*. It may be helpful in defining breast lesions and evaluating patients for metastases in liver, bone, and other sites. CT scans should be avoided because of the large doses of radiation involved in such imaging.[339]

Management of breast cancer during the first trimester often leads to a discussion of termination of pregnancy. In most instances the pregnancy can be maintained without placing the patient at undue risk. Breast surgery can be performed safely during pregnancy and has not been associated with an increased risk of fetal abnormalities.[340] The efficacy and safety of the sentinel lymph node procedure in pregnancy is uncertain, but radiation exposure to the fetus is estimated to be low when radioisotope labeling is used. Nevertheless, because approximately 60% of pregnant patients are likely to have positive axillary nodes, axillary dissection remains the preferred procedure for most patients. When breast conservation is an option, the timing of radiation therapy must be carefully considered, because breast irradiation is contraindicated in the pregnant patient. A delay in breast irradiation for longer than 3 months may increase the probability of local recurrence for women who have lumpectomies in the first or second trimester of pregnancy. As a consequence, mastectomy may prove to be a more appropriate management approach, even in patients with tumors amenable to breast-conservation surgery. Because chemotherapy is likely to be a major option for the majority of women with breast cancer diagnosed during pregnancy, breast-conserving surgery and axillary dissection in the second trimester, followed by chemotherapy, with breast radiation administered after delivery, or neoadjuvant chemotherapy followed by surgery, may represent the ideal strategy for many patients. Such planning is likely to allow breast irradiation to be initiated after delivery and within several months of diagnosis and after adjuvant or neoadjuvant chemotherapy, which minimizes the potential risks for local-regional recurrence.

Adjuvant chemotherapy should be avoided during the first trimester of pregnancy. Almost all chemotherapeutic agents cross the placenta, and during the first trimester chemotherapy administration has been associated with a 15% to 20% risk of fetal malformation and an increased risk of spontaneous abor-

tion. In general, chemotherapy can be safely administered during the second and third trimesters, especially after 20 weeks' gestation. The fetal risk of malformation of 1% to 3% for patients receiving chemotherapy after the first trimester is similar to the risk of fetal malformation for healthy women. AC or AC and fluorouracil (FAC or CAF) given every 3 weeks is well tolerated by pregnant patients. In one series[341] that now includes 39 patients, the median gestational age at diagnosis of breast cancer was 20 weeks, the median gestational age at initiation of chemotherapy was 23 weeks, and the median gestation age at delivery was 38 weeks. Patients received a median of four courses of FAC (range, one to six) without major complications. Ondansetron and phenothiazines were used to control nausea and vomiting. No spontaneous abortions or stillbirths occurred, and there was no increased risk of fetal malformation. Data from this and other small series also suggest that children exposed to a wide group of chemotherapeutic agents *in utero* have normal childhood development and scholastic aptitude. There are almost no data on the safety of taxane use during pregnancy. In one case report of a single pregnant patient, there were no sequelae from its use. Tamoxifen should not be used in pregnant patients; although data are sparse, there are significant concerns regarding fetal development. The safety of growth factors such as filgrastim and erythropoietin during pregnancy is uncertain, and only small numbers of patients have been treated with no obvious deleterious effects. For patients receiving AC or CAF in standard dosages, growth factors should not be administered. The medical oncologist should work closely with the patient's obstetrician to try to minimize the probability of neutropenia at the time of delivery, and delivery should be planned 2 to 4 weeks after the last dose of chemotherapy.

Pregnancy after a diagnosis of breast cancer was previously a major concern, but data from several series have suggested no increased risk for a second breast cancer or metastatic disease for women who become pregnant after a diagnosis of breast cancer. However, in making a decision to become pregnant after a diagnosis of breast cancer, the patient's likelihood of developing metastatic disease is a major consideration. Patients with a high risk for metastasis (large primary lesions or positive lymph nodes) should have a frank discussion with their oncologist concerning the risk of recurrence. A delay of 3 to 5 years before becoming pregnant may be appropriate for these patients. Women at lower risk may also wish to wait at least 3 years before trying to conceive. With regard to the small group of patients who are carriers of the BRCA1 or BRCA2 genes, one large case-control study that compared healthy controls who were younger than 40 years of age with gene carriers found that the risk of breast cancer was 1.7 times higher in gene carriers who became pregnant than in controls.[342] Successful lactation from an irradiated breast in women who had prior lumpectomy and breast irradiation has been reported for approximately one-third of patients in a series of 11 women with 13 pregnancies; women with circumareolar biopsies were less likely to lactate successfully.[343] Nursing is possible from a single breast, however. There is also no evidence that consumption of milk from a mother previously treated for breast cancer increases the risk of breast cancer in the child. Breast feeding while receiving chemotherapy has not been studied but should be discouraged, because many chemotherapeutic agents enter breast milk.

For young women with breast cancer who desire or are contemplating pregnancy after diagnosis, major consideration should be given to protecting ovarian function. In women younger than 40 years, irreversible ovarian suppression is seen in 15% to 25% of women treated with anthracycline-containing chemotherapy regimens (AC, CAF, or a regimen of cyclophosphamide, epirubicin, and fluorouracil), and in 30% to 40% of women treated with CMF for 6 months. Data from a small series of 21 young premenopausal patients suggest that the use of LHRH analogs before and during administration of chemotherapy reversibly suppresses ovarian function.[344] Although menses recurred in 20 of these 21 patients, it is uncertain whether such treatment preserves fertility. Premenopausal breast cancer patients receiving tamoxifen should be warned against becoming pregnant while on treatment, and tamoxifen should be stopped for several months before patients attempt conception.

Metastatic breast cancer during pregnancy is fortunately a rare event. Systemic chemotherapy with AC or CAF can be safely used in most of these patients after the first trimester. Treatment for such patients must be individualized, and psychosocial and family support is essential.

BILATERAL BREAST CANCER

Bilateral breast cancer can present as carcinoma in both breasts at the same time (synchronous, concurrent, or simultaneous bilateral breast cancer) or at different times in the two breasts (metachronous or sequential bilateral breast cancer). The incidence of synchronous bilateral breast cancer has been described as up to 2% in most series, although incidence rates as high as 8.5% have been reported.[345–348] Simultaneous bilateral breast cancer may be more common in older patients.

For the patient who presents with a unilateral carcinoma of the breast, the rate of development of a metachronous contralateral breast cancer is proportional to the length of follow-up. The 10-year incidence of development of a metachronous contralateral breast cancer is 6.4% to 9.0%, with a yearly hazard function estimated at approximately 0.75% per year of follow-up.[345–348] This hazard function appears to be valid through 20 and even 30 years of follow-up. For a patient with unilateral breast cancer, the relative risk of developing a contralateral breast cancer is estimated as 1.4 to 4.5 times the risk in the normal population.[345,347,348] Population-based data from Scandinavia show a diminishing risk with increasing age, with a lifetime risk of less than 5% for women over age 60 years.[349]

A number of risk factors have been reported as associated with an increased risk of development of a contralateral breast cancer. Those risk factors most reproducibly associated with an increase in the development of a contralateral breast cancer include younger patient age, family history of breast cancer, multicentric disease, and lobular carcinoma. Most of the reported data support no increased risk of contralateral breast cancer in association with the use of radiation in the treatment of a first breast cancer, although exceptions have been noted.

For the patient who presents with an apparently unilateral carcinoma of one breast, screening of the contralateral breast should be performed to rule out a simultaneous contralateral breast carcinoma.[345,350] The standard method of screening the contralateral breast is mammography plus physical examina-

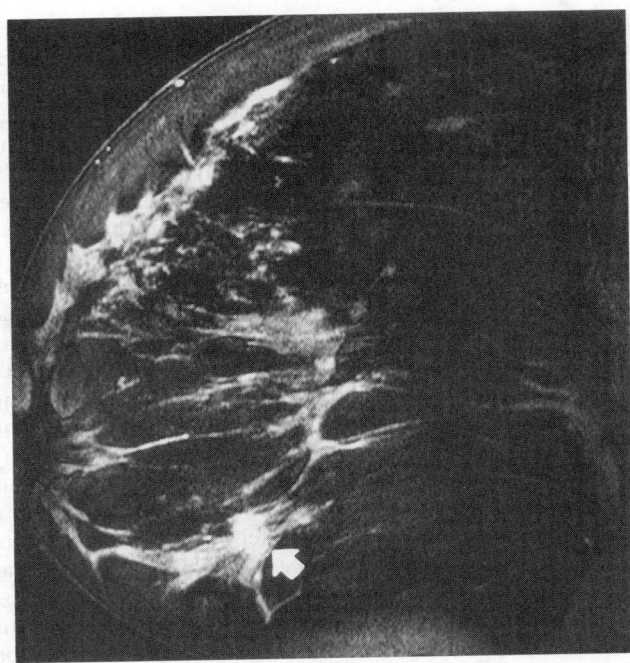

FIGURE 33.2-10. Magnetic resonance imaging (MRI) detection of a contralateral breast cancer that was not detected on mammography or physical examination. The patient presented with a newly diagnosed invasive left breast carcinoma. MRI of the right (contralateral) breast demonstrated an enhancing 1-cm mass with irregular borders (*arrow*), confirmed on subsequent directed ultrasonography (not shown). Results of MRI-guided core biopsy confirmed invasive ductal carcinoma. (From ref. 351, with permission.)

tion. MRI screening increases the detection of synchronous contralateral breast cancers[351] (Fig. 33.2-10).

Second breast cancers tend to be found at an earlier stage than first breast cancers, probably because of careful screening at the time of diagnosis of the first breast cancer as well as careful follow-up after treatment of the first breast cancer. Prognostic factors (e.g., tumor size, pathologic axillary lymph node staging, overall stage, and histologic subtype of carcinoma) for the second breast cancer tend to be more favorable than or similar to those for the first breast cancer.[345–348,350]

Most studies comparing unilateral and bilateral breast cancer have shown similar survival, although exceptions have been noted, possibly secondary to lead-time bias.[345–348,350,352] Analysis of data for patients with synchronous or metachronous bilateral breast cancer is associated with a number of difficulties. First, bilateral breast cancer must be compared to unilateral breast cancer to assess any difference in outcome. However, many studies report only patients with bilateral breast cancer, without a control population with unilateral disease. Second, the contralateral breast cancer tends to be associated with a more favorable prognosis than the first breast cancer. Thus, any decrement in outcome, such as survival, is small compared to outcome in patients with unilateral disease. Third, for patients with metachronous bilateral breast cancer, the outcome should be reported from the second breast cancer to avoid the bias that would be associated from reporting outcome from the first breast cancer, because patients would be required to live for the interval between the first and second breast cancers. Finally, data for patients with synchronous and metachronous bilateral breast cancer should be reported separately.

A number of studies have compared the treatment outcomes of patients with unilateral versus bilateral breast cancers. The reported outcomes for studies comparing patients with unilateral versus bilateral breast cancer demonstrate conflicting results. Some studies have reported no difference in survival between these two groups, whereas other studies have indicated a significant reduction in survival for patients with bilateral breast cancer.

For the management of bilateral breast cancer, each breast should be assessed separately for local treatment. Bilateral breast conservation can be performed in appropriate patients, and definitive bilateral breast radiation treatment is technically feasible.[352] Careful attention to matchline dosimetry is warranted. For the patient with bilateral breast cancer, the need for mastectomy for one breast does not preclude breast-conservation treatment for the contralateral breast.

The use of adjuvant tamoxifen for hormone receptor–positive, unilateral breast cancer has been demonstrated in multiple randomized trials to reduce the risk of a contralateral breast cancer. In the EBCTCG overview analysis, the risk of developing a contralateral breast cancer was reduced at 10 years from 32% without tamoxifen to 23% with tamoxifen (P <.0001), with a proportional risk reduction of 47% (P <.0001).[353] In the randomized ATAC trial, there was a statistically significant reduction in the rate of contralateral breast cancer for patients treated with anastrozole compared to those receiving tamoxifen or tamoxifen plus anastrozole. In comparison to tamoxifen alone, anastrozole reduced contralateral breast cancer (odds ratio, 0.42; $P = .007$).[354]

MALE BREAST CANCER

Male breast cancer typically occurs at a much lower rate than female breast cancer, but the incidence varies by geographic location, with rates being highest in some sub-Saharan countries. In the United States, approximately 1500 men are diagnosed with breast cancer each year, which represents fewer than 1% of all cancers diagnosed in men.[355] As with female breast cancer, the risk of male breast cancer appears related to increased lifelong exposure to estrogen or to reduced androgen. Thus, the risk is increased in cases of testicular injury or cirrhosis of the liver. Males with a history of mumps orchitis, undescended testes, or testicular injury are at increased risk, perhaps due to an imbalance in the estrogen-testosterone ratio. Men with Klinefelter's syndrome have a 14- to 50-fold increased risk of developing male breast cancer and may account for 3% of all male breast cancer cases. Feminization, genetically or by environmental exposure, appears to increase the risk, as reported in transsexuals receiving exogenous estrogens. Sub-Saharan countries with high rates of liver cirrhosis related to schistosomiasis also have higher incidence of male breast cancer. A family history of breast cancer is an important risk factor, and excess male breast cancer has been reported among families with BRCA1 and BRCA2 mutations. In Iceland 44% of all male breast cancers in a population-based series were explained by BRCA2 mutations.[356] Male breast cancer has also been reported among men with Cowden disease and germline *PTEN* mutations.[357] Men with male breast cancer should receive counseling regarding cancer predisposition, because sisters and daughters of male breast cancer patients have a twofold to threefold increased risk of breast cancer.

Clinical presentation of male breast cancer is similar to that of female breast cancer, but the median age of onset is later than in females (60 vs. 53 years).[358] All known histopathologic types of breast cancer have been described in men. Infiltrating ductal carcinoma is the predominant type, accounting for 70% of cases. However, the existence of invasive lobular carcinoma in men is uncertain.[53] A majority of male breast cancers are ER positive, and a few studies have examined the contribution of markers such as HER2/*neu* and p53. Stage and lymph node status appear to be the predominant prognostic indicators, although a few studies have reported a preponderance of high-grade tumors with aggressive behavior leading to poor overall outcomes compared to female breast cancer.

Primary treatment has evolved over time, and breast-conservation treatment or modified radical mastectomy can be used. Postoperative radiation therapy has been shown to reduce local-regional recurrence, and in general, guidelines for adjuvant radiation in female breast cancer may be used, in particular for patients with large tumors or involved lymph nodes. Similarly, adjuvant systemic chemotherapy is advocated in men, although no controlled trials have confirmed its value. Tamoxifen treatment, with a response rate as high as 80%, has been the mainstay for hormone therapy in ER-positive breast cancer, but aromatase inhibitors might also be used in this situation. Metastatic breast cancer in men is treated identically to metastatic disease in women.

NONEPITHELIAL NEOPLASMS

Nonepithelial neoplasms are a category of less common breast neoplasms that are troubling when diagnosed. These range from benign phyllodes tumors through the malignant variety and include metaplastic breast carcinoma and primary sarcomas of the breast.

Clinically, phyllodes tumors resemble fibroadenomas. They may be smooth or multinodular and firmer than the surrounding breast tissue, but are usually quite well demarcated. If they grow large, they can distort the breast considerably or ulcerate the skin by pressure necrosis. Histologically, they also resemble fibroadenomas with epithelial elements and connective tissue stroma. The histologic appearance may be quite benign or may show cellular atypia and mitotic activity typical of malignant sarcomas. A histologic borderline variety between the two is also seen. These classifications are not closely related to behavior. The benign-appearing lesions are commonly called *phyllodes tumors*, whereas those that look highly malignant are often termed *phyllodes sarcomas*. Phyllodes tumors may be initially treated by excision to clear margins. This dictates close follow-up, because one in five will recur locally if excised with close or absent margins. When a wider margin can be achieved with acceptable cosmesis, it is desirable.[359] Because the great majority of these tumors do not recur regardless of histologic appearance, mastectomy or excision with a very wide margin has not been shown to offer any advantage over local excision. The phyllodes sarcomas or borderline lesions that recur or behave aggressively require mastectomy or reexcision and irradiation. The use of systemic therapy is not evidence-based because of the rarity of these lesions.

Soft tissue sarcoma of the breast is poorly studied because of its rarity—fewer than 1% of malignant breast tumors are of this type. Metaplastic breast carcinoma is a biphasic lesion that contains both sarcomatous and epithelial elements. It is hormone receptor negative 80% to 90% of the time, often overexpresses HER2/*neu*, and behaves in an aggressive fashion. A histologically distinguishable low-grade variant has been identified that does not metastasize frequently but is still prone to local failure.[360] These nonepithelial lesions uncommonly metastasize to axillary nodes. When presenting in an advanced state, they are optimal candidates for neoadjuvant chemotherapy as a way of identifying agents to which they may be sensitive. Anecdotal evidence suggests that they respond to therapies associated with sarcoma treatment better than those used for carcinoma of the breast. These are sufficiently rare lesions that all such series, even from the largest institutions, are anecdotal and retrospective.

Because primary sarcoma of the breast is so rare, its identification should always raise the question of possible metastasis from a poorly differentiated lesion elsewhere. Melanoma metastases have been mistaken for a primary breast sarcoma. Primary sarcoma of the breast has not been associated with axillary metastases when modified radical mastectomy has been performed in the past. It can be treated with complete excision, which may require total mastectomy. High-grade lesions appear to benefit from adjuvant radiation in addition to complete surgical excision.[361] There are no data suggesting that primary breast sarcoma should be treated differently from soft tissue sarcomas arising in other sites.[362]

LYMPHOMA OF THE BREAST

Primary lymphoma of the breast is extremely uncommon and accounts for fewer than 0.1% of all breast malignancies.[363] As with breast carcinoma, the usual presenting symptom is a painless breast mass, and there is no specific mammographic abnormality that is predictive of lymphoma. On rare occasions lymphoma can mimic inflammatory breast cancer and is likely associated with a T-cell phenotype. Lymph node involvement is uncommon. In one review of breast lymphoma, the mean age at diagnosis was 60 years, the diagnosis was more common in women, and bilateral synchronous or metachronous breast involvement occurred in as many as 25% of patients. At diagnosis most breast lymphomas were larger than 5 cm, and B symptoms were uncommon.[364] The clinical and histologic criteria for making a diagnosis of primary breast lymphoma have been defined by Wiseman and Liao[365] and Dixon et al.[366] and include close association of breast tissue and lymphoma, no evidence of widespread lymphoma, no prior extramammary lymphoma, and documentation of the breast as the principal organ of lymphoma involvement. Although Hodgkin's disease of the breast has been reported, it is extremely rare, and the vast majority of patients have non-Hodgkin's lymphoma.

Although all histologic types of lymphoma have been described, diffuse intermediate B-cell non-Hodgkin's lymphomas are the most common. Mucosa-associated lymphoid tissue lymphomas have also been described. Core biopsy is frequently adequate for establishing a diagnosis, but incisional biopsy may be needed for classification. The Revised European American Lymphoma classification should be used for pathologic classification. Cytogenetic, immunophenotypic, and gene rearrangement studies may also be useful in diagnosis and classification. The Ann Arbor staging system developed for Hodgkin's disease is also used for non-Hodgkin's lymphoma.[367]

Staging should be based on careful history taking and physical examination; laboratory work, including lactate dehydrogenase level; performance status assessment; appropriate imaging using CT of the chest, abdomen, and pelvis; and bone marrow biopsy.[367] PET or gallium scans are also helpful in staging lymphoma and monitoring response to treatment. The treatment of breast lymphoma depends on histologic typing and immunophenotyping as well as stage.[367] Results of treatment for breast lymphomas are similar to those for stage I and II lymphomas at other sites, and treatment recommendations are the same as for primary lymphomas presenting in other nodal or extranodal areas. For patients with intermediate- and high-grade lymphoma localized to the breast (stage IE), optimum therapy includes chemotherapy and localized breast irradiation. For those with low-grade lymphoma localized to the breast, involved-field radiation alone is appropriate. The management of lymphoma is discussed in Chapter 41. Recommendations for management and staging can also be found at http://www.nccn.org.

AXILLARY LYMPH NODE PRESENTATION

Presentation with an involved axillary lymph node in a patient with an unknown primary carcinoma is unusual, and such cases represent fewer than 1% of breast cancer patients. Rarely, an axillary lymph node is the first manifestation of disease from a contralateral primary breast carcinoma.

The initial workup for the patient with an axillary lymph node presentation and unknown primary tumor site represents an important diagnostic problem. A lymph node biopsy should be performed to confirm the diagnosis of adenocarcinoma and to obtain tissue for ER and PR testing as well as other IHC staining that may help the pathologist provide guidance as to the source of the metastasis.[53,54] ER or PR expression is strongly suggestive of metastatic breast carcinoma, although negative hormone receptor test results do not exclude the breast as the primary tumor site. Special stains may also be of value. The differential diagnosis for axillary lymph node presentation includes carcinoma (e.g., lung, pancreatic, gastrointestinal, thyroid, ovarian, or renal cell carcinoma), noncarcinomatous malignancy (e.g., melanoma, lymphoma, or germ cell tumor), and nonmalignant causes (e.g., benign inflammatory changes, infection, or tuberculosis).

Mammography detects the primary breast carcinoma in 10% to 56% of cases.[150] Investigation has focused on alternative breast-imaging methods to attempt to identify an occult breast primary carcinoma in patients with negative mammographic findings. Breast MRI identifies the primary breast carcinoma in 75% to 85% (range, 25% to 100%) of patients with negative findings on mammography.[368,369] The detection of a primary breast carcinoma has substantial importance, because finding a primary breast carcinoma ends the search for other sites of primary malignancy and guides local, regional, and systemic management. The finding of a primary breast carcinoma often renders the patient eligible for breast-conservation treatment.[370]

The most common local treatment for patients with axillary lymph node presentation has been mastectomy. Pathologic findings at the time of mastectomy vary widely, with invasive carcinoma detected in 8% to 100% of cases.[150] Uncommonly, identification of noninvasive DCIS or LCIS is the only pathologic finding from mastectomy, and the inability to find invasive carcinoma may represent a sampling error. Pathologic results from occult breast carcinomas show that approximately one-third of the tumors are 1 cm or larger and approximately two-thirds are smaller than 1 cm. Approximately 40% of patients have four or more positive axillary lymph nodes. Axillary dissection provides prognostic staging information and diminishes the risk of axillary recurrence.

The reported 5-year actuarial survival after mastectomy ranges from 52% to 82%, and the 10-year actuarial survival ranges from 42% to 71%.[150] These results are generally similar to the outcomes for breast cancer patients with other similarly staged tumors and pathologically positive nodes.

A small number of studies have been reported for patients treated with breast-conservation surgery and definitive radiation therapy.[371–375] Although based on small numbers of patients treated, these studies demonstrate a number of trends. First, there is no difference in outcome (e.g., survival or freedom from distant metastases) for patients treated with breast conservation and those treated with mastectomy. Second, adding radiation after breast-conservation surgery leads to a substantial reduction in the rate of local failure. Third, the strongest prognostic factor for outcome after treatment is the number of positive axillary lymph nodes. Finally, outcome after treatment is similar to that in other studies of patients with pathologically positive nodes.

Because of the variety of treatments used and the small number of cases reported, optimal management remains uncertain. Workup should include bilateral mammography and, if results are negative, ipsilateral breast MRI because of the high rate of detection of an occult breast primary tumor, even in patients with negative mammogram findings. Axillary lymph node biopsy is necessary to confirm a diagnosis of malignancy, to allow the pathologist to aid in the search for the primary lesion, and to determine hormone receptor status. Should the pathologic examination of the lymph node confirm a likely primary breast carcinoma, a comprehensive search for other primary tumor sites generally is not warranted. Breast-conservation treatment can be considered, with recognition that only a small number of cases have been reported. Mastectomy has been the predominant surgical approach, although axillary lymph node dissection may be considered for selected cases. Additional systemic therapy and postoperative radiation therapy are then added, as dictated by the pathologic findings. When radiotherapy is delivered to the intact breast, the recommended dose is generally 45 to 50 Gy, although higher doses have been used.[371,373,375] In view of the involvement of at least one axillary lymph node, most authors recommend regional lymph node radiotherapy to the supraclavicular fossa and possibly comprehensive nodal radiation.[371,373,375]

LOCAL AND REGIONAL RECURRENCE

LOCAL RECURRENCE AFTER BREAST-CONSERVATION TREATMENT

Although local recurrence after breast-conservation treatment is uncommon, recognition of such an event is important because of the potential for salvage treatment. After breast-conservation treatment, local recurrence is the development of tumor in the ipsilateral (treated) breast that occurs after treatment of the initial breast cancer. Local recurrence can occur as the first and only evidence of recurrence of disease or can occur simultaneously with or after regional recurrence or distant metastases. Comparison of studies can be difficult because of differences in the definitions of local recurrence.

Approximately one-fourth to one-half of local recurrences are detected by routine mammography only. Both physical examination and mammography are important to detect local recurrence.[376] New or changing physical examination findings that occur more than 1 to 2 years after the completion of radiation treatment require workup to rule out local recurrence.

The location of the local recurrence is classified in relation to the primary tumor site as follows: (1) true recurrence (within the primary tumor or boost radiation treatment volumes); (2) marginal miss (near the boost radiation treatment volume, although this definition is imprecise); and (3) elsewhere (beyond the volumes for true recurrence or marginal miss).[377] Most series report that the vast majority of local recurrences can be categorized as a true recurrence or marginal miss. These two categories are usually combined, because distinguishing between them on clinical grounds is difficult and has no prognostic significance. Less common types of local recurrence include skin recurrence, inflammatory recurrence, and Paget's disease of the nipple.

Mammography remains the mainstay for breast imaging of the patient suspected of having local recurrence. A new cluster of microcalcifications, a new mass, or an increase in architectural distortion should be viewed as suspicious for the development of local recurrence, particularly if more than 1 to 2 years has elapsed since completion of treatment. Ultrasonography is a useful adjunct to mammography in many patients to characterize a clinically palpable or radiologic mass. Mammograms obtained after breast-conservation treatment frequently show a mass effect or architectural distortion in the primary tumor site that can be difficult to distinguish from local recurrence. MRI may be useful to characterize a lesion that is suspicious based on clinical or radiologic findings.

Salvage mastectomy is the current standard local treatment for patients with local recurrence after breast-conservation treatment. After salvage mastectomy, 5-year overall survival rates have been reported as 34% to 88%.[378] This large variation likely reflects substantial differences in prognostic variables between studies. However, comparison between studies is difficult, because prognostic factors are not well established after local recurrence, and therefore are often not reported in detail.

A number of factors have been reported as prognostic for outcome after local recurrence. Patients with a shorter interval to local recurrence (generally 2 years or less or 5 years or less) have a reduced survival compared to patients with a longer interval to local recurrence. In the series from the University of Pennsylvania, Doyle et al. reported that the 5-year overall survival rate was 65% for patients with an interval to local recurrence of 2 years or less, 84% for those with an interval of 2.1 to 5 years, and 89% for those with an interval of more than 5 years ($P = .03$)[379] (Fig. 33.2-11). A number of other prognostic factors have been studied. Favorable prognostic factors include smaller tumor size, node-negative disease, in-field or marginal miss as the location of the local recurrence, ER positivity, low grade, and mammographic detection. However, the impor-

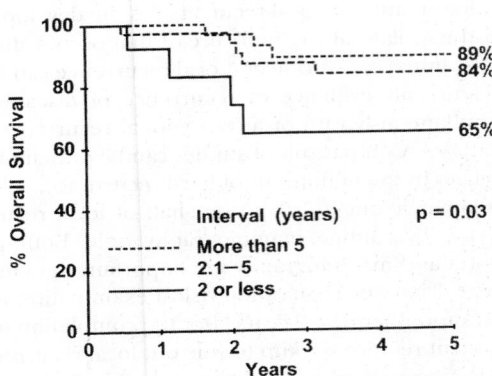

FIGURE 33.2-11. Actuarial overall survival after invasive local recurrence after breast-conservation treatment according to interval to local recurrence. (From ref. 379, with permission.)

tance of individual prognostic factors varies widely across different studies.

The vast majority of patients with local recurrence in reported studies had undergone an axillary lymph node dissection at the time of initial breast-conservation treatment. For the patient with a clinically negative axilla at the time of local recurrence, a second axillary surgical procedure is generally not warranted. However, positive axillary lymph nodes have been observed in selected patients.[379] Patients treated more recently with breast-conservation surgery are increasingly undergoing axillary staging using sentinel lymph node biopsy. Whether axillary reexploration is indicated for such patients at the time of local recurrence is unknown.

A second attempt at breast conservation (local excision) has been selectively used at the time of local recurrence.[380–382] After excision as salvage surgery, the incidence of a second local recurrence has been reported as 14% to 40%, and 5-year overall survival has been reported as 79% to 85%.[378] The risk of a second local recurrence is often cited as the rationale for using salvage mastectomy as treatment for the first local recurrence. Small numbers of patients have been treated with a second attempt at breast conservation using excision and reirradiation.

The role of systemic therapy after local recurrence remains uncertain. In most series, systemic therapy was given to patients thought to have worse prognoses, and therefore the value of systemic therapy in this setting remains difficult to determine.

LOCAL RECURRENCE AFTER MASTECTOMY

After mastectomy, local recurrence most commonly occurs as one or more asymptomatic nodules in the skin of the chest wall, typically in or around the mastectomy scar or in the area of the skin flaps. Other less common presentations include diffuse skin involvement, pruritic skin rash, skin ulceration, inflammatory recurrence, or carcinoma *en cuirasse*. Biopsy for local recurrence is required to confirm a diagnosis of malignancy, to obtain tissue for ER and PR analysis, and to rule out an unusual histologic type, such as sarcoma. Prior distant metastases occur in 20% to 30% of patients, and 20% to 30% of patients have simultaneous distant metastases at the time of local recurrence. The large majority of local recurrences (approximately 90%) occur within 5 years after mastectomy.

Because of the high risk of distant metastases, restaging evaluation should be undertaken at the time of local recurrence. CT or MRI study of the chest is useful to evaluate the location and extent of local recurrence, as well as to rule out other areas of unsuspected disease, such as regional lymph node metastases or pulmonary metastases.

The factor most reproducibly correlated with prognosis after local recurrence is interval to local recurrence, with a shorter interval (2 years or less or 5 years or less) associated with a worse prognosis.[383,384] Other factors that have been cited as prognostically important include initial surgical stage, initial lymph node status, number of sites of recurrence, location of recurrence, tumor grade, patient age, ER and PR status, and type of prior treatment.

The ability to achieve local control is strongly related to the volume and resectability of the initial tumor recurrence. Initial gross resection, smaller volume of disease (e.g., less than 3 to 4 cm), and isolated local recurrence are associated with improved local control. Rarely, chest wall resection may be indicated to excise gross disease. In patients with inflammatory local recurrence or carcinoma *en cuirasse*, local control is difficult to achieve. The ability to achieve local control is an important end point for patients, because uncontrolled local failure is associated with substantially reduced quality of life, for example, the presence of pain or ulceration with secondary infection.

Radiation treatment should be delivered to fields encompassing a minimum of the chest wall (most commonly using tangent fields) and supraclavicular fossa, followed by a boost to the area of local recurrence. Comprehensive radiation treatment achieves better local-regional control than small-field radiation treatment. Full axillary treatment and internal mammary nodal treatment are not required in the absence of involvement of these areas. The radiation dose to uninvolved sites is 45 to 50 Gy using 1.8 to 2.0 Gy daily fractions. A boost to previously resected areas of gross disease for an additional 10 Gy is optional. For areas of gross involvement, a boost to a total dose of 60 Gy or higher is indicated. Boost treatments are generally done with electrons. Full-thickness bolus is applied to uninvolved areas of the chest wall every third day or every other day; alternatively, half-thickness bolus may be applied daily. Daily bolus is applied to areas of gross disease or any biopsy scars. The matchline between the supraclavicular fossa and the chest wall tangential fields should avoid areas of gross disease or areas of previously resected gross disease, if possible. Alternative methods of radiation treatment have been described.[385]

The vast majority of patients develop distant metastases after local failure. The reported results of radiation treatment after an isolated local recurrence show 5-year overall survival rates of 35% to 82% and 10-year overall survival rates of 25% to 62%. The 5-year rate of freedom from distant metastases is 25% to 75%, and the 10-year rate of freedom from distant metastases is 7% to 49%.[378,382,383,386–388] The large variation in reported outcomes likely reflects differences in prognostic factors in the patient populations studied.

Postmastectomy radiation treatment at the time of initial mastectomy has assumed an increasing role in the initial definitive management of patients with breast cancer. Only small numbers of patients with chest wall recurrence after mastectomy followed by postmastectomy radiation treatment have been reported, and such patients are typically treated with excision (if feasible), followed by small-field radiation.

Randomized trials have compared treatment with radiotherapy to treatment with radiotherapy plus hyperthermia for chest wall recurrence.[388] Although adding hyperthermia increases the complete response rate, the long-term value of hyperthermia remains to be established.

The use of systemic therapy (chemotherapy or hormonal therapy or both) is appealing because a large fraction of patients develop distant metastatic disease. However, the efficacy of systemic therapy has not yet been reliably established. In a randomized trial of tamoxifen therapy after local recurrence, no improvement was found in overall survival.[386]

REGIONAL LYMPH NODE RECURRENCE

Regional lymph node recurrence is an uncommon manifestation of treatment failure after either breast-conservation treatment or mastectomy. Regional nodal recurrence can occur as an isolated event or concurrent with local or distant recurrence, or both. In the majority of patients, regional nodal recurrence presents as an asymptomatic mass in the axilla or supraclavicular fossa. The wide adoption of sentinel lymph node biopsy makes it likely that nodal recurrence in the dissected axilla will be detected occasionally. This makes examination of the ipsilateral axilla an important aspect of the follow-up of patients who undergo sentinel lymph node biopsy. For the patient with regional lymph node recurrence after breast-conservation treatment, careful evaluation of the ipsilateral breast, including mammography and physical examination, is indicated. Patients with an isolated axillary failure have the most favorable prognosis.[387,389,390] Gross surgical excision is associated with improved outcome.

Recommendations for management of regional lymph node recurrence must be individualized because of the substantial heterogeneity of the patient population. A biopsy is indicated to establish the diagnosis of malignancy as well as to test for ER and PR status. If feasible, surgical excision is indicated. For the patient with regional lymph node recurrence after breast-conservation treatment, the value of mastectomy in this setting is uncertain. Radiation therapy is indicated for patients without previous radiation treatment at the time of initial presentation. Although most patients develop distant metastatic disease, the value of systemic therapy is uncertain.

BREAST CANCER IN THE ELDERLY

In 2003 almost half of all women newly diagnosed with breast cancer in the United States were 65 years of age or older, and more than 50% of breast cancer deaths are in this age group. Between 1997 and 1999, 1 in 14 women aged 60 to 79 years developed breast cancer, compared to 1 in 24 women aged 40 to 59 years and 1 in 228 women younger than age 40.[1,391] Similar statistics are noted in other affluent nations, and the trend will be compounded in the future by the aging of the population. Currently in the United States, 12% of women are 65 years of age or older, whereas in 2025 one in five Americans will be in this age group. Life expectancy is also increasing: A healthy woman 65 years of age has an estimated average life expectancy of 20 more years; a healthy 75-year-old, 12 more years; and a healthy 85-year-old, 6 more years. Older and younger women have similar stage-adjusted breast cancer–

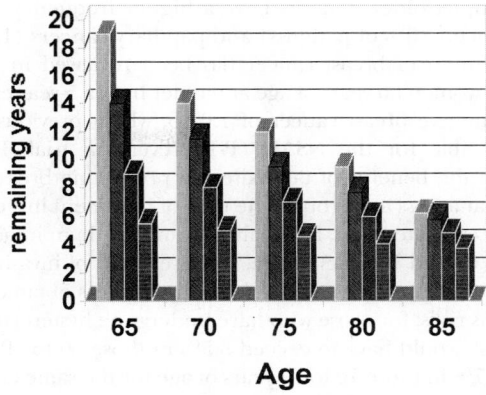

FIGURE 33.2-12. Estimates of survival time by age for normal patients and for patients with comorbid illness that have expected mortality of 10%, 25%, and 50% at 5 years. (Modified from ref. 396.) (See Color Fig. 33.2-12 in the CD-ROM.)

specific survival; the exceptions are women in whom breast cancer develops before age 40 years or at 85 years or older.[392] Even with the prevalence of breast cancer in older patients, numerous trials have shown an age bias among physicians in caring for older patients. Older women in good health and without breast cancer are less likely to undergo mammographic screening, and older women with breast cancer are less likely to be offered breast-conservation treatment, breast irradiation after breast-conservation surgery, and adjuvant systemic therapy. Several excellent reviews of breast cancer in older women are available.[393,394]

The major issue affecting management and treatment recommendations for older patients with breast cancer is coexisting illness or comorbidity. The type and frequency of comorbidity has been well defined in older women with breast cancer and may have a profound effect on survival. In one large population study of 1800 patients 55 years of age and older with breast cancer, Yancik and colleagues found that diabetes, renal failure, stroke, liver disease, a history of previous malignancy, and smoking were significant predictors of early mortality in a model that included age and breast cancer stage.[395] How serious illness affects outcome can be reasonably estimated. Welch and colleagues developed a model that predicts the effect of illnesses with different estimated 5-year survivals on life expectancy for patients in different age groups (Fig. 33.2-12).[396] Factoring comorbidity into management decisions, especially decisions regarding the use of adjuvant systemic chemotherapy, is necessary to provide optimal treatment for these patients.

The biologic characteristics of breast cancer are more favorable in older patients compared to younger patients. Older patients are more likely to have node-negative tumors, lower tumor proliferative rates (low S phase, low tritiated-thymidine labeling and low Ki-67 levels), diploid tumors, normal p53 expression, lower tumor grade, and tumor negative for EGF-1 (epidermal growth factor-1 or HER-1) and EGF-2 (HER2, c-erbB-2).[397] Moreover, in women 65 year of age and older, ER positivity is found in more than 85% of tumors. Older patients are also more likely to have favorable histologic types of tumor;

for example, older patients have a higher frequency of mucinous cancers (6% of patients) and papillary cancers (1%).

Prevention of breast cancer has been reviewed in Chapter 33.1. All women 60 years of age and older have a 5-year estimated risk of invasive breast cancer of 1.67%, which previously made them eligible for the NSABP P-1 prevention trial. However, although the benefits of tamoxifen in preventing breast cancer are similar across age groups, the risks of treatment increase with age. It is estimated that, for healthy women with an intact uterus between 60 and 79 years of age, the 5-year risk of invasive breast cancer would have to exceed 7% for the benefits of tamoxifen to exceed its risks; for those who have undergone hysterectomy, the 5-year risk would have to exceed 3.5% in those 60 to 69 years of age and 7% in those 70 to 79 years of age for the same tamoxifen benefit. Older patients who are candidates for prevention should also be considered for NSABP P-2 (STAR). As for younger women, encouraging a healthy lifestyle including weight control and exercise may also decrease breast cancer risk. Older patients are also less likely to have mammographic screening. Although data from randomized trials are sparse for women older than 75 years, data from mathematical models suggest that the benefits of annual or semiannual mammography will be seen in older women provided they have an expected survival of 5 years or longer. Mammography is more sensitive and specific in older patients. The physician's recommendation is the most important stimulus for convincing older women to undergo mammographic screening.

Older women diagnosed with DCIS or invasive breast cancer should generally be offered the same treatment options as younger women. Breast conservation should be offered when appropriate; body image and sexuality are important to older women and should not be minimized. For frail older women with ER- or PR-positive tumors, tamoxifen therapy alone can result in partial and complete response rates of 60% to 70%; alternatively, excision plus tamoxifen can be considered. The median time to response averages approximately 3 months, and the response persists for up to 5 years in approximately one-third of patients. Several randomized trials have shown similar survivals for patients treated with tamoxifen only and with surgery, but the majority of patients who survive longer than 5 years have tumor progression requiring surgery. Patients with expected survival of 5 years or longer are best treated with surgery. More recently, aromatase inhibitors have been used in this setting with impressive preliminary results.

Older patients with locally advanced breast cancer should be managed in the same way as younger patients. Preoperative chemotherapy—or, for selected patients with ER- or PR-positive tumors, endocrine therapy—frequently results in tumor shrinkage substantial enough to make patients candidates for mastectomy or breast-conservation surgery. In women offered breast conservation, breast irradiation should be considered, especially in women with estimated survivals of longer than 5 years. Lumpectomy alone, even in patients with T1 tumors, is associated with rates of ipsilateral breast tumor recurrence of approximately 2% per year; for patients with ER- or PR-positive tumors, tamoxifen therapy reduces this risk to approximately 1%. Breast irradiation is more effective than tamoxifen therapy and after lumpectomy reduces the rate of in-breast recurrence by approximately two-thirds. A Breast Intergroup trial in which women older than 70 years of age with receptor-positive, stage I disease were randomly assigned to receive radiation or no radi-

ation after lumpectomy and were given tamoxifen showed few local failures without radiation and no survival benefit for radiation treatment.[398] Long-term follow-up of patients of all ages treated with lumpectomy alone suggests that such patients have inferior survival compared to patients treated with lumpectomy and breast irradiation. Breast irradiation should generally be offered to women after lumpectomy except for those with limited expected survival.

The role of axillary dissection in older women with breast cancer is controversial. In the majority of women with clinically negative axilla and small primary tumors, axillary dissection is not likely to alter treatment decisions. In the near future, sentinel lymph node biopsy is likely to replace axillary dissection for almost all women with clinically negative axillae. In older women for whom chemotherapy would become a treatment option in the setting of positive axillary nodes, standard dissection or sentinel lymph node biopsy is indicated; this is especially true for patients with ER- and PR-negative primary tumors. For patients with small, ER- or PR-positive primary lesions and clinically negative axillae, axillary dissection or sentinel lymph node biopsy are likely to be of minimal value, because only if these patients had extensive nodal involvement would the addition of adjuvant chemotherapy provide major added value to endocrine therapy. Estimated survival based on age and comorbidity, as well the clinical characteristics of the breast cancer and axilla, play a major role in management of the axilla in older women. Among patients with clinically positive axillae in whom surgery is feasible, axillary dissection is indicated for almost all patients with the exception of the frail elderly.

Systemic adjuvant therapy should be considered for most older women with invasive breast cancer and an estimated life expectancy of 5 years or longer.[394] The EBCTCG overview analysis of 1998 clearly shows that, in women 70 years of age and older with ER-positive tumors, adjuvant tamoxifen therapy yields significant improvement in both relapse-free and overall survival. For postmenopausal patients, anastrozole offers another option for endocrine therapy[81] (see Endocrine Therapy: Aromatase Inhibitors, earlier in this chapter). Data on the value of chemotherapy in older patients are sparse and controversial. Some data suggest that women older than 70 years are likely to derive the same proportional benefits in reduction of relapse and death from breast cancer as are younger women. The EBCTCG overviews show diminishing proportional benefit with increasing age. On the other hand, a substantial amount of data indicates that standard chemotherapy regimens are almost as well tolerated in healthy older patients as in younger patients. Extermann and colleagues used a Markov model to estimate the threshold risk for breast cancer recurrence at 10 years for older women with ER-positive tumors necessary for tamoxifen therapy or chemotherapy to provide at least a 1% increase in 10-year survival (Fig. 33.2-13).[399] Of note, for patients 80 years of age and older, these estimates pertain only to 5-year survival. These data suggest that in patients 75 years and older, and especially in those with ER- or PR-positive tumors, adjuvant chemotherapy will only be of substantial benefit if the patient has a significant risk for recurrence. Patients 65 years of age and older derive greater benefits from more intense chemotherapy regimens such as doxorubicin and cyclophosphamide followed by paclitaxel, or six courses of CAF, than from less intense regimens, but have a

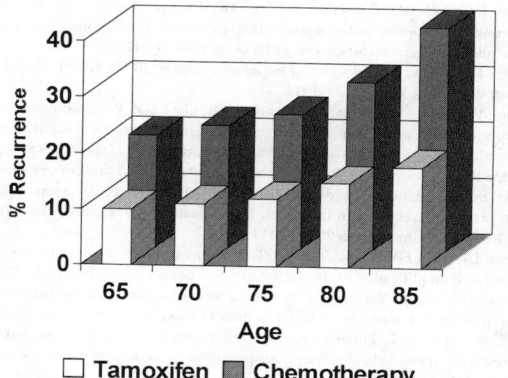

FIGURE 33.2-13. Threshold risk of recurrence at 10 years needed to achieve a 1% increase in 10-year survival with tamoxifen or chemotherapy in women with estrogen receptor–positive breast cancer. For patients 80 years of age and older, the threshold risk of recurrence is for 5 years. (Modified from ref. 399.)

treatment-related mortality rate of approximately 1%. Healthy older patients with reasonable life expectancy but at high risk for recurrence (e.g., more than 50% at 10 years) should be considered for more intensive adjuvant chemotherapy programs.[400] Recommendations for adjuvant therapy for patients older than 70 years of age are presented in Table 33.2-25.

Older patients with metastatic breast cancer should be managed using the same strategy as for younger patients (see Metastatic Breast Cancer, earlier in the chapter). Those with endocrine receptor–positive tumors should be treated until they have disease progression. Standard chemotherapy regimens are well tolerated by older patients, but the judicious use of sequential agents is preferred because this treatment approach is associated with similar periods of disease control and similar survival durations as with combination regimens.

TABLE 33.2-25. Recommendations for Adjuvant Systemic Therapy in Older Patients

Size and Node Status	10-Y Recurrence Risk (%)	ER or PR Positive	ER and PR Negative
NODE NEGATIVE			
<1 cm	≤10	No therapy or endocrine therapy	No therapy
1–3 cm	10–30	Endocrine therapy	No therapy or chemotherapy
>3 cm	>30	Endocrine therapy ± chemotherapy	Chemotherapy
NODE POSITIVE	>40	Endocrine therapy ± chemotherapy	Chemotherapy

ER, estrogen receptor; PR, progesterone receptor.
Note: Patients should be in fair to excellent general health with life expectancy of 5 y or more.

Older patients remain underrepresented in clinical trials.[401] Compared to younger patients, older patients are more likely to have comorbidity, functional impairment, less access to care, and more limited social and logistic support, which limits their ability to participate in trials. Moreover, even when these barriers are accounted for, an age bias in considering patients for trials persists, although available data suggest that, as with younger patients, approximately half of older patients offered entry into a trial will elect to participate.[402] Several new trials in both the adjuvant and metastatic settings are focused on older patients and should be offered to eligible patients by their physicians.

REFERENCES

1. Parkin DM, Pisani P, Ferlay J. Global cancer statistics. *CA Cancer J Clin* 1999;49:33.
2. Jemal A, Tiwani RC, Murray T, et al. Cancer statistics, 2004. *CA Cancer J Clin* 2004;54:8.
3. Key TJ, Verkasalo PK, Banks E, et al. Epidemiology of breast cancer. *Lancet Oncol* 2001;2:133.
4. Lynch HT, Lynch JF. Breast cancer genetics in an oncology clinic: 328 consecutive patients. *Cancer Genet Cytogenet* 1986;22:369.
5. Claus EB, Schildkraut JM, Thompson WD, et al. The genetic attributable risk of breast and ovarian cancer. *Cancer* 1996;77:2318.
6. Whittemore AS. Risk of breast cancer in carriers of *BRCA* gene mutations. *N Engl J Med* 1997;337:788.
7. Ford D, Easton DF, Stratton M, et al. Genetic heterogeneity and penetrance analysis of the *BRCA1* and *BRCA2* genes in breast cancer families. The breast cancer linkage consortium. *Am J Hum Genet* 1998;62:676.
8. Fackenthal J, Marsh D, Richardson A, et al. Male breast cancer in Cowden syndrome patients with germline PTEN mutations. *J Med Genet* 2001;38:159.
9. Dunning AM, Healey CS, Pharoah PD, et al. A systematic review of genetic polymorphisms and breast cancer risk. *Cancer Epidemiol Biomarkers Prev* 1999;8:843.
10. Miki Y, Swensen J, Shattuck ED, et al. A strong candidate for the breast and ovarian cancer susceptibility gene *BRCA1*. *Science* 1994;266:66.
11. Smith TM, Lee MK, Szabo CI, et al. Complete genomic sequence and analysis of 117 kb of human DNA containing the gene *BRCA1*. *Genome Res* 1996;6:1029.
12. *Breast Cancer Information Core*. National Humane Genome Research Institute. World Wide Web URL: http://research.nhgri.nih.gov/bic/, 2002.
13. Couch FJ, Weber BL. Mutations and polymorphisms in the familial early-onset breast cancer (BRCA1) gene. Breast Cancer Information Core. *Hum Mutat* 1996;8:8.
14. Roa BB, Boyd AA, Volcik K, et al. Ashkenazi Jewish population frequencies for common mutations in BRCA1 and BRCA2. *Nat Genet* 1996;14:185.
15. Thorlacius S, Struewing JP, Hartge P, et al. Population-based study of breast cancer in carriers of BRCA2 mutation. *Lancet* 1998;352:1337.
16. King MC, Marks JH, Mandell, JB. Breast and ovarian cancer risks due to inherited mutations in BRCA1 and BRCA2. *Science* 2003;302:643.
17. Struewing JP, Hartge P, Wacholder S, et al. The risk of cancer associated with specific mutations of *BRCA1* and *BRCA2* among Ashkenazi Jews. *N Engl J Med* 1997;336:1401.
18. Verhoog LC, Brekelmans CT, Seynaeve C, et al. Survival and tumour characteristics of breast-cancer patients with germline mutations of BRCA1. *Lancet* 1998;351:316.
19. Phillips KA, Andrulis IL, Goodwin PJ. Breast carcinomas arising in carriers of mutations in BRCA1 or BRCA2: are they prognostically different? *J Clin Oncol* 1999;7:3653.
20. Grushko TA, Blackwood MA, Schumm PL, et al. Molecular-cytogenetic analysis of HER-2/neu gene in BRCA1-associated breast cancers. *Cancer Res* 2002;62:1481.
21. Foulkes WD, Stefansson IM, Chappuis PO, et al. Germline BRCA1 mutations and a basal epithelial phenotype in breast cancer. *J Natl Cancer Inst* 2003;95:1482.
22. Lakhani SR, Van De Vijver MJ, Jacquemier J, et al. The pathology of familial breast cancer: predictive value of immunohistochemical markers estrogen receptor, progesterone receptor, HER-2, and p53 in patients with mutations in BRCA1 and BRCA2. *J Clin Oncol* 2002;20:2310.
23. Stoppa-Lyonnet D, Laurent-Puig P, Essioux L, et al. BRCA1 sequence variations in 160 individuals referred to a breast/ovarian family cancer clinic. Institut Curie Breast Cancer Group [see comments]. *Am J Hum Genet* 1997;60:1021.
24. Phillips K. Current perspectives on BRCA1- and BRCA2-associated breast cancers. *Intern Med J* 2001;31:349.
25. Robson M, Gilewski T, Haas B, et al. BRCA-associated breast cancer in young women. *J Clin Oncol* 1998;16:1642.
26. Robson M, Rajan P, Rosen PP, et al. BRCA-associated breast cancer: absence of a characteristic immunophenotype. *Cancer Res* 1998;58:1839.
27. Pierce LJ, Strawderman M, Narod SA, et al. Effect of radiotherapy after breast-conserving treatment in women with breast cancer and germline BRCA1/2 mutations. *J Clin Oncol* 2000;18:3360.
28. Boyd J, Sonoda Y, Federici MG, et al. Clinicopathologic features of BRCA-linked and sporadic ovarian cancer. *JAMA* 2000;283:2260.
29. Rubin SC, Benjamin I, Behbakht K, et al. Clinical and pathological features of ovarian cancer in women with germ-line mutations of BRCA1 [see comments]. *N Engl J Med* 1996;335:1413.
30. Ekbom A, Hsieh CC, Lipworth L, et al. Intrauterine environment and breast cancer risk in women: a population-based study. *J Natl Cancer Inst* 1997;89:71.

31. Kelsey JL, Gammon MD, John EM. Reproductive factors and breast cancer. *Epidemiol Rev* 1993;15.
32. Ewertz M, Duffy SW, Adami HO, et al. Age at first birth, parity and risk of breast cancer: a meta-analysis of 8 studies from the Nordic countries. *Int J Cancer* 1990;46:597.
33. Melbye M, Wohlfahrt J, Olsen JH, et al. Induced abortion and the risk of breast cancer. *N Engl J Med* 1997;336:81.
34. Lipworth L, Bailey LR, Trichopoulos D. History of breast-feeding in relation to breast cancer risk: a review of the epidemiologic literature. *J Natl Cancer Inst* 2000;92:302.
35. Breast cancer and hormonal contraceptives: collaborative reanalysis of individual data on 53,297 women with breast cancer and 100,239 women without breast cancer from 54 epidemiological studies. Collaborative Group on Hormonal Factors in Breast Cancer. *Lancet* 1996;347:1713.
36. Design of the Women's Health Initiative clinical trial and observational study. The Women's Health Initiative Study Group. *Control Clin Trials* 1998;19:61.
37. Grabrick DM, Hartmann LC, Cerhan JR, et al. Risk of breast cancer with oral contraceptive use in women with a family history of breast cancer. *JAMA* 2000;284:1791.
38. Hunter DJ, Spiegelman D, Adami HO, et al. Cohort studies of fat intake and the risk of breast cancer—a pooled analysis. *N Engl J Med* 1996;334:356.
39. Singletary KW, Gapstur SM. Alcohol and breast cancer: review of epidemiologic and experimental evidence and potential mechanisms. *JAMA* 2001;286:2143.
40. McTiernan A. Behavioral risk factors in breast cancer: can risk be modified? *Oncologist* 2003;8.
41. Kritz-Silverstein D, Barrett-Connor E. Long-term postmenopausal hormone use, obesity, and fat distribution in older women. *JAMA* 1996;275:46.
42. Morimoto LM, White E, Chen Z, et al. Obesity, body size, and risk of postmenopausal breast cancer: The Women's Health Initiative (United States). *Cancer Causes Control* 2002;13:741.
43. Hankinson SE, Willett WC, Colditz GA, et al. Circulating concentrations of insulin-like growth factor-I and risk of breast cancer. *Lancet* 1998;351:1393.
44. Thune I, Furberg AS. Physical activity and cancer risk: dose-response and cancer, all sites and site-specific. *Med Sci Sports Exerc* 2001;33:S530.
45. Evans JS, Wennberg JE, McNeil BJ. The influence of diagnostic radiography on the incidence of breast cancer and leukemia. *N Engl J Med* 1986;315:810.
46. Bhatia S, Yasui Y, Robison LL, et al. High risk of subsequent neoplasms continues with extended follow-up of childhood Hodgkin's disease: report from the Late Effects Study Group. *J Clin Oncol* 2003;21:4386.
47. Boyd NF, Dite GS, Stone J, et al. Heritability of mammographic density, a risk factor for breast cancer. *N Engl J Med* 2002;347:886.
48. Byrne C, Schairer C, Wolfe J, et al. Mammographic features and breast cancer risk: effects with time, age, and menopause status. *J Natl Cancer Inst* 1995;87:1622.
49. Page DL, Salhany KE, Jensen RA, et al. Subsequent breast carcinoma risk after biopsy with atypia in a breast papilloma. *Cancer* 1996;78:258.
50. Hammond S, Keyhai-Rofagha S, O'Toole R. Statistical analysis of fine needle aspiration of the breast: a review of 678 cases plus 4,265 cases from the literature. *Acta Cytol* 1987;31:276.
51. Moore MM, Hargett CW, Hanks JB, et al. Association of breast cancer with the finding of atypical ductal hyperplasia at core breast biopsy. *Ann Surg* 1997;225:726.
52. Sacchini V, Luini A, Agrest R, et al. Nonpalpable breast lesions: analysis of 952 operated cases. *Breast Cancer Res Treat* 1995;32:59
53. Rosen PP. *Rosen's breast pathology.* 2nd ed. Philadelphia: Lippincott Williams & Wilkins, 2001.
54. Rosen PP, Oberman HA. Tumors of the mammary gland. In: *Atlas of tumor pathology,* Series 3, Fascicle 7. Washington, DC: Armed Forces Institute of Pathology, 1993.
55. *Histological typing of breast tumours.* 2nd ed. Geneva, Switzerland: World Health Organization, 1981.
56. Weiss MC, Fowble BL, Solin LJ, et al. Outcome of conservative therapy for invasive breast cancer by histologic subtype. *Int J Radiat Oncol Biol Phys* 1992;23:941.
57. Elston CW, Ellis IO. Assessment of histological grade. In: Elston CW, Ellis IO, eds. *The breast.* Edinburgh: Churchill Livingstone, 1998:365.
58. Rosen PP, Groshen S, Kinne DW, et al. Factors influencing prognosis in node-negative breast carcinoma: analysis of 767 T1N0M0/T2N0M0 patients with long-term follow-up. *J Clin Oncol* 1993;11:2090.
59. Berx G, Cleton-Jansen AM, Strumane K, et al. E-cadherin is inactivated in a majority of invasive human lobular breast cancers by truncation mutations throughout its extracellular domain. *Oncogene* 1996;13:1919.
60. Harris M, Howell A, Chrissohou M, et al. A comparison of the metastatic pattern of infiltrating lobular carcinoma and infiltrating duct carcinoma of the breast. *Br J Cancer* 1984;50:23.
61. Henderson IC, Patek AJ. The relationship between prognostic and predictive factors in the management of breast cancer. *Breast Cancer Res Treat* 1998;52:261.
62. Fisher ER, et al. Pathologic findings from the National Surgical Adjuvant Breast Project (Protocol No. 4). *Am J Clin Pathol* 1987;65:1554.
63. Lundin J, et al. Omission of histologic grading from clinical decision making may result in overuse of adjuvant therapies in breast cancer: results from a nationwide study. *J Clin Oncol* 2001;19:28.
64. Bernstein V, et al. How young is too young? The impact of age on premenopausal breast cancer prognosis. *Breast Cancer Res Treat* 2002;76:A137.
65. Wood WC, Styblo TM. Clinically established prognostic factors in breast cancer. In: Bland KI, Copeland EM, eds. *The breast.* St. Louis: Saunders, 2004: Table 21-2, 452.
66. Clark GM. Interpreting and integrating risk factors for patients with primary breast cancer. *J Natl Cancer Inst Monogr* 2001;30:17.
67. Anonymous. Tamoxifen for early breast cancer: an overview of the randomised trials. Early Breast Cancer Trialists' Collaborative Group [see comments]. *Lancet* 1998;351.9114:1451.
68. Allred DC, Bryant J, Land S, et al. Estrogen receptor expression as a predictive marker of the effectiveness of tamoxifen in the treatment of DCIS: findings from NSABP protocol B-24. *Breast Cancer Res Treat* 2002;76:S36(abst).
69. Harvey JM, Clark GM, Osborne CK, Allred DC. Estrogen receptor status by immunohistochemistry is superior to the ligand-binding assay for predicting response to adjuvant endocrine therapy in breast cancer. *J Clin Oncol* 1999;17:1474.
70. Elledge RM, Fuqua SA. *Estrogen and progesterone receptors.* JR Harris, ed. Philadelphia: Lippincott Williams & Wilkins, 2000:471.
71. Bardou V J, Arpino G, Elledge RM, Osborne CK, Clark GM. Progesterone receptor status significantly improves outcome prediction over estrogen receptor status alone for adjuvant endocrine therapy in two large breast cancer databases. *J Clin Oncol* 2003;21:1973.
72. Elledge RM, Green S, Pugh R, et al. Estrogen receptor (ER) and progesterone receptor (PgR), by ligand-binding assay compared with ER, PgR and pS2, by immuno-histochemistry in predicting response to tamoxifen in metastatic breast cancer: a Southwest Oncology Group Study. *Int J Cancer* 2000;89:111.
73. Slamon DJ, Clark GM, Wong SG, et al. Human breast cancer: correlation of relapse and survival with amplification of the HER-2/neu oncogene. *Science* 1987;235:177.
74. Yamauchi H, Stearns V, Hayes DF. When is a tumor marker ready for prime time? A case study of c-erbB-2 as a predictive factor in breast cancer. *J Clin Oncol* 2001;19:2334.
75. Press MF, Bernstein L, Thomas PA, et al. HER-2/neu gene amplification characterized by fluorescence in situ hybridization: poor prognosis in node-negative breast carcinomas. *J Clin Oncol* 1997;15:2894.
76. Ravdin PM. Is Her2 of value in identifying patients who particularly benefit from anthracyclines during adjuvant therapy? A qualified yes. *J Natl Cancer Inst Monogr* 2001;30:80.
77. Sledge GW, Jr. Is HER-2/neu a predictor of anthracycline utility? No. *J Natl Cancer Inst Monogr* 2001;30:85.
78. Thor AD, Berry DA, Budman DR, et al. erbB-2, p53, and efficacy of adjuvant therapy in lymph node-positive breast cancer. *J Natl Cancer Inst* 1998;90:1346.
79. Pietras RJ. Interactions between estrogen and growth factor receptors in human breast cancers and the tumor-associated vasculature. *Breast J* 2003;9:361.
80. Ellis MJ, Coop A, Singh B, et al. Letrozole is more effective neoadjuvant endocrine therapy than tamoxifen for ErbB-1- and/or ErbB-2-positive, estrogen receptor-positive primary breast cancer: evidence from a phase III randomized trial. *J Clin Oncol* 2001;19:3808.
81. Anastrozole alone or in combination with tamoxifen versus tamoxifen alone for adjuvant treatment of postmenopausal women with early breast cancer: first results of the ATAC randomised trial. The ATAC Trialists Group. *Lancet* 2002;359:2131.
82. Berry DA, Muss HB, Thor AD, et al. HER-2/neu and p53 expression versus tamoxifen resistance in estrogen receptor-positive, node-positive breast cancer [In Process Citation]. *J Clin Oncol* 2000;18:3471.
83. Davis BW, Gelber RD, Goldhirsch A, et al. Prognostic significance of peritumoral vessel invasion in clinical trials for adjuvant therapy for breast cancer. *J Clin Oncol* 1999;17:1474.
84. deMascarel I, Bonichon F, Durand M, et al. Obvious peritumoral emboli: an elusive prognostic factor reappraised. *Eur J Cancer* 1998;34:58.
85. Bryant J, Fisher B, Gunduz N, Costantion JP, Emir B. S-phase fraction combined with other patient and tumor characteristics for the prognosis of node-negative, estrogen-receptor-positive breast cancer. *Breast Cancer Res Treat* 1998;51:239.
86. Clark GM, Dressler LG, Owens MA, et al. Prediction of relapse or survival in patients with node-negative breast cancer by DNA flow cytometry. *N Engl J Med* 1989;320:627.
87. Look MP, van Putten WL, Duffy, MJ et al. Pooled analysis of prognostic impact of urokinase-type plasminogen activator and its inhibitor PAI-1 in 8377 breast cancer patients. *J Natl Cancer Inst* 2002;94:116.
88. Harbeck N, Kates RE, Look MP, et al. Enhanced benefit from adjuvant chemotherapy in breast cancer patients classified high-risk according to urokinase-type plasminogen activator (uPA) and plasminogen activator inhibitor type 1 (n = 3424). *Cancer Res* 2002;62:4617.
89. Keyomarsi K, et al. Cyclin E and survival in patients with breast cancer. *N Engl J Med* 2002; 347:1566.
90. Braun S, Pantel K, Muller P, et al. Cytokeratin-positive cells in the bone marrow and survival of patients with stage I, II, or III breast cancer. *N Engl J Med* 2000;342:525.
91. Funke I, Schraut W. Meta-analyses of studies on bone marrow micrometastases: an independent prognostic impact remains to be substantiated. *J Clin Oncol* 1998;16:557.
92. Smith BM, Slade MJ, English J, et al. Response of circulating tumor cells to systemic therapy in patients with metastatic breast cancer: comparison of quantitative polymerase chain reaction and immunocytochemical techniques. *J Clin Oncol* 2000;18:1432.
93. Krag DN, Ashikaga T, Moss TJ, et al. Breast cancer cells in the blood: a pilot study. *Breast J* 1999;5:354.
94. Perou CM, Sorlie T, Eisen MB, et al. Molecular portraits of human breast tumours. *Nature* 2000;406:747.
95. van de Vijver MJ, He YD, van't Veer LJ, et al. A gene-expression signature as a predictor of survival in breast cancer. *N Engl J Med* 2002;347:1999.
96. Pusztai L, Ayers M, Simmans FW, et al. Emerging science: prospective validation .of gene expression profiling-based prediction of complete response to neoadjuvant paclitaxel/FAC chemotherapy in breast cancer. *Proc Am Soc Clin Oncol* 2003;22:1.
97. Syed S, Rowinsky E. The new generation of targeted therapies for breast cancer. *Oncology* 2003;17:1339.
98. Claus EB, Risch N, Thompson WD. Genetic analysis of breast cancer in the cancer and steroid hormone study. *Am J Hum Genet* 1991;48:232.
99. Gail MH, Brinton LA, Byar DP, et al. Projecting individualized probabilities of developing breast cancer for white females who are being examined annually. *J Natl Cancer Inst* 1989;81:1879.
100. Frank TS, Deffenbaugh AM, Reid JE, et al. Clinical characteristics of individuals with germline mutations in BRCA1 and BRCA2: analysis of 10,000 individuals. *J Clin Oncol* 2002;20:1480.
101. Berry DA, Iversen ES Jr, Gudbjartsson DF, et al. BRCAPRO validation, sensitivity of genetic testing of BRCA1/BRCA2, and prevalence of other breast cancer susceptibility genes. *J Clin Oncol* 2002;20:2701.

102. American Society of Clinical Oncology. Statement of the American Society of Clinical Oncology: genetic testing for cancer susceptibility. Adopted on February 20, 1996. *J Clin Oncol* 1996;14:1730.

103. American Society of Clinical Oncology. American Society of Clinical Oncology policy statement update: genetic testing for cancer susceptibility. *J Clin Oncol* 2003;21:2397.

104. McTiernan A. Behavioral risk factors in breast cancer: can risk be modified? *Oncologist* 2003;8.

105. Fisher B, Costantino JP, Wickerham DL, et al. Tamoxifen for prevention of breast cancer: report of the National Surgical Adjuvant Breast and Bowel Project P-1 Study [see comments]. *J Natl Cancer Inst* 1998;90:1371.

106. Burke W, Daly M, Garber J, et al. Recommendations for follow-up care of individuals with an inherited predisposition to cancer. II. *BRCA1* and *BRCA2*. Cancer Genetics Studies Consortium. *JAMA* 1997;277:997.

107. King MC, Wieand S, Hale K, et al. Tamoxifen and breast cancer incidence among women with inherited mutations in BRCA1 and BRCA2: National Surgical Adjuvant Breast and Bowel Project (NSABP-P1) Breast Cancer Prevention Trial. *JAMA* 2001;286:2251.

108. Narod SA, Brunet JS, Ghadirian P, et al. Tamoxifen and risk of contralateral breast cancer in BRCA1 and BRCA2 mutation carriers: a case-control study. Hereditary Breast Cancer Clinical Study Group. *Lancet* 2000;356:1876.

109. Hoogerbrugge N, Bult P, de Widt-Levert LM, et al. High prevalence of premalignant lesions in prophylactically removed breasts from women at hereditary risk for breast cancer. *J Clin Oncol* 2003;21:41.

110. Hartmann LC, Schaid DJ, Woods JE, et al. Efficacy of bilateral prophylactic mastectomy in women with a family history of breast cancer. *N Engl J Med* 1999;340:77.

111. Meijers-Heijboer H, van Geel B, van Putten WL, et al. Breast cancer after prophylactic bilateral mastectomy in women with a BRCA1 or BRCA2 mutation. *N Engl J Med* 2001;345.

112. Rebbeck TR, Friebel T, Lynch HT, et al. Bilateral prophylactic mastectomy reduces breast cancer risk in BRCA1 and BRCA2 mutation carriers: the PROSE Study Group. *J Clin Oncol* 2004;22:1055.

113. Kauff ND, Satagopan JM, Robson ME, et al. Risk-reducing salpingo-oophorectomy in women with a BRCA1 or BRCA2 mutation. *N Engl J Med* 2002;346:1609.

114. Rebbeck TR, Lynch HT, Neuhausen SL, et al. Prophylactic oophorectomy in carriers of BRCA1 or BRCA2 mutations. *N Engl J Med* 2002;346:1616.

115. American Society of Clinical Oncology. Recommended breast cancer surveillance guidelines. *J Clin Oncol* 1997;15:1868–Solin table.

116. Badve S, A'Hern RP, Ward AM, et al. Prediction of local recurrence of ductal carcinoma in-situ of the breast using five histological classifications: a comparative study with long follow-up. *Hum Pathol* 1998;29:915.

117. Consensus Conference Committee. Consensus conference on the classification of ductal carcinoma in-situ. *Cancer* 1997;1798.

118. Claus AB, Stowe M, Carter B. Breast carcinoma in-situ: risk factors in screening patterns. *J Natl Cancer Inst* 2001;93:1811.

119. Ernster VL, Barclay J, Kerlikowske K, et al. Incidence of and treatment for ductal carcinoma in situ of the breast. *JAMA* 1996;275:913.

120. Kauff ND, Brogi E, Scheuer L, et al. Epithelial lesions in prophylactic mastectomy specimens for women with BRCA mutations. *Cancer* 2003;1997:1601.

121. Adem C, Reynolds C, Soderberg CL, et al. Pathologic characteristics of breast parenchyma in patients with hereditary breast carcinoma, including BRCA1 and BRCA2 mutation carriers. *Cancer* 2003;1997:1.

122. Page DL, DuPont WD, Rogers LW. Continued local recurrence of carcinoma 15-25 years after a diagnosis of low-grade ductal carcinoma in situ of the breast treated only by biopsy. *Cancer* 1995;76:1197.

123. Rosen PP, Braun DW, Kinne DE. The clinical significance of pre-invasive breast carcinoma. *Cancer* 1980;46:919.

124. Hwang ES, Kinkel K, Esserman LJ, et al. Magnetic resonance imaging in patients diagnosed with ductal carcinoma in situ: value of diagnosis of residual disease, occult invasion, and multicentricity. *Ann Surg Oncol* 2003;10:381.

125. Tillman GF, Orel SG, Schnall MD, et al. The effect of breast magnetic resonance imaging (MRI). In clinical management of women with early-stage breast carcinoma. *J Clin Oncol* 2002;20:3413.

126. Fisher B, Dignam J, Wolmark N, et al. Lumpectomy and radiation therapy for the treatment of intraductal breast cancer: findings from National Surgical Adjuvant Breast and Bowel Project B-17. *J Clin Oncol* 1998;16:441.

127. Fisher ER, Dignam J, Tan-Chiu E, et al. Pathologic findings from the National Surgical Adjuvant Breast Project (NSABP) eight-year update of Protocol B-17: intraductal carcinoma. *Cancer* 1999;86:429.

128. Fisher B, Land S, Mamounas E, et al. Prevention of invasive breast cancer in women with ductal carcinoma in situ: an update of the National Surgical Adjuvant Breast and Bowel Project Experience. *Semin Oncol* 2001;28:400.

129. Bijker N, Peterse N, Duchateau L, et al. Risk factors for recurrence and metastasis after breast-conserving therapy for ductal carcinoma-in-situ: analysis of European Organization for Research and Treatment of Cancer trial 10853. *J Clin Oncol* 2001;19:2263.

130. Julien J, Bijker N, Fentiman IS, et al. Radiotherapy in breast-conserving treatment for ductal carcinoma in situ: first results of the EORTC randomized phase III trial 10853. *Lancet* 2000;355:528.

131. Fisher B, Dignam J, Wolmark N, et al. Tamoxifen in treatment of intraductal breast cancer: National Surgical Adjuvant Breast and Bowel Project B-24 randomized controlled trial. *Lancet* 1999;353:1993.

132. Houghton J, George WD, Cuzick J, et al. Radiotherapy and tamoxifen in women with completely excised ductal carcinoma in situ of the breast in the UK, Australia, and New Zealand: randomized controlled trial. *Lancet* 2003;362:95.

133. Allred C, et al. ER status and response to tamoxifen in ductal carcinoma in situ (DCIS). Presented at: The San Antonio Breast Conference; December 2002; San Antonio, Texas (abst).

134. Silverstein MJ, Recht A, Lagios MD, eds. *Ductal carcinoma in situ of the breast.* 2nd ed. Philadelphia: Lippincott Williams & Wilkins, 2002.

135. Silverstein MJ, Lagios MD, Groshen S, et al. The influence of margin width on local control of ductal carcinoma in-situ of the breast. *N Engl J Med* 1999;340:1455.

136. Solin LJ, Fourquet A, Vicini FA, et al. Mammographically detected ductal carcinoma in situ of the breast treated with breast-conserving surgery and definitive breast irradiation: long-term outcome and prognostic significance of patient age and margin status. *Int J Radiat Oncol Biol Phys* 2001;50:991.

137. Vicini FA, Kestin LL, Goldstein NS, et al. Impact of young age on outcome in patients with ductal carcinoma in-situ treated with breast-conserving therapy. *J Clin Oncol* 2000;18:296.

138. Boland GP, Chan KC, Knox WF, et al. Value of the Van Nuys Prognostic Index in prediction of recurrence of ductal carcinoma in situ after breast-conserving surgery. *Br J Surg* 2003;90:426.

139. Schwartz GF, Solin LJ, Olivotto IA, et al. Consensus conference on the treatment of in situ ductal carcinoma of the breast, April 22-25, 1999. *Cancer* 2000;88:946.

140. Lucci A Jr, Kelemen PR, Miller C 3rd, et al. National practice patterns of sentinel lymph node dissection for breast carcinoma. *J Am Coll Surg* 2001;192:453.

141. McMasters KM, Chao C, Wong SL, et al. Sentinel lymph node biopsy in patients with ductal carcinoma in situ: a proposal. *Cancer* 2002;95:15.

142. Mills J, Schultz DJ, Solin LJ. Preservation of cosmesis with low complication risks after conservative surgery in radiotherapy for ductal carcinoma in situ of the breast. *Int J Radiat Oncol Biol Phys* 1997;39:637.

143. Foote FW Jr, Stewart FW. Lobular carcinoma in-situ: a rare form of mammary carcinoma. *Am J Pathol* 1941;17:491.

144. Li CI, Anderson BO, Dailing JR, Moe RE. Changing incidence of lobular carcinoma in situ of the breast. *Breast Cancer Res Treat* 2002;75:259.

145. Otteson GL, Graversen HP, Blichert-Toft M, et al. Carcinoma in situ of the female breast. 10 year follow-up results of a prospective nationwide study. *Breast Cancer Res Treat* 2000;62:197.

146. Vogel VG, Costantino JP, Wickerham DL, et al. The study of tamoxifen and raloxifene: preliminary enrollment data from a randomized breast cancer risk reduction trial. *Clin Breast Cancer* 2002;3:153.

147. Kauff ND, Brogi E, Scheuer L, et al. Epithelial lesions in prophylactic mastectomy specimens for women with BRCA mutations. *Cancer* 2003;1997:1601.

148. Paget J. On disease of the mammary areola preceding cancer of the mammary gland. *St. Bartholomew's Hosp Rep* 1874;10:87.

149. Rosen PP. *Rosen's breast pathology.* 2nd ed. Philadelphia: Lippincott Williams & Wilkins, 2001.

150. Solin LJ. Special considerations. In: Fowble B, Goodman RL, Glick JH, Rosato EF, eds. *Breast cancer treatment: a comprehensive guide to management.* St. Louis: Mosby Year Book, 1991:521.

151. Marshall JK, Griffith KA, Haffty BG, et al. Conservative management of Paget disease of the breast with radiotherapy: 10- and 15-year results. *Cancer* 2003;97:2142.

152. Bijker N, Rutgers EJT, Duchoateau L, et al. Breast-conserving therapy for Paget disease of the nipple: a prospective European Organization for Research and Treatment of Cancer study in 61 patients. *Cancer* 2001;91:472.

153. Fourquet A, Campana F, Vielh P, et al. Paget's disease of the nipple without detectable breast tumor: conservative management with radiation therapy. *Int J Radiat Oncol Biol Phys* 1987;13:1463.

154. Polgar C, Orosz Z, Kovacs T, Fodor J. Breast conserving therapy for Paget disease of the nipple [Letter]. *Cancer* 2002;94:1904.

155. Bellon JR, Come SE, Gelman RS, et al. Sequencing of chemotherapy and radiation therapy for patients with early stage breast cancer: updated results of a prospective randomized trial. *Int J Radiat Oncol Biol Phys* 2001;51[Suppl 1]:2(abst).

156. Fisher B, Bryant J, Wolmark N, et al. Effect of preoperative chemotherapy on the outcome of women with operable breast cancer. NSABP B-18 study. *J Clin Oncol* 1998;16:2672.

157. Pierce LJ, Lew D, Hutchins L, et al. Patterns of recurrence by sequence of chemotherapy and radiotherapy in early stage breast cancer. *Int J Radiat Oncol Biol Phys* 2003;57[Suppl 1]:S127(abst).

158. Vicini F, Eberlein T, Connolly J, et al. The optimal extent of resection for patients with stages I or II breast cancer treated with conservative surgery and radiotherapy. *Ann Surg* 1992;214:200.

159. Clarke D, Martinez A. Identification of patients who are at high risk for locoregional breast cancer recurrence after conservative surgery and radiotherapy: a review article for surgeons, pathologists, and radiation and medical oncologists. *J Clin Oncol* 1992;10:474.

160. Veronesi U, Cascinelli N, Mariani L, et al. Twenty-year follow-up of a randomized study comparing breast-conserving surgery with radical mastectomy for early breast cancer. *N Engl J Med* 2002;347:1227.

161. Fisher B, Anderson S, Bryant J, et al. Twenty-year follow-up of a randomized trial comparing total mastectomy, lumpectomy, and lumpectomy plus irradiation for the treatment of invasive breast cancer. *N Engl J Med* 2002;347:1233.

162. Early Breast Cancer Trialists' Collaborative Group 2000 Trialists' Meeting at Oxford, September, 2000.

163. NCI issues information on falsified NSABP trials. *J Natl Cancer Inst* 1994;86:487.

164. Gianni L, Valagussa P, Zambetti M, et al. Adjuvant and neoadjuvant treatment of breast cancer. *Semin Oncol* 2001;28:13.

165. Fisher B, Bryant J, Wolmark N, et al. Effect of preoperative chemotherapy on the outcome of women with operable breast cancer. *J Clin Oncol* 1998;16:2672.

166. Morris MM, Powel SN. Irradiation in the setting of collagen vascular disease: acute and late complications. *J Clin Oncol* 1997;15:2728.

167. Carlson G, Bostwick JI, Styblo TM, et al. Skin-sparing mastectomy. Oncologic and reconstructive considerations. *Ann Surg* 1997;225:570.

168. Fisher B, Jeong JH, Anderson S, et al. Twenty-five-year follow-up of a randomized trial comparing radical mastectomy, total mastectomy, and total mastectomy followed by irradiation. *N Engl J Med* 2002;347:567.

169. Schwartz GF, Giuliano AE, Veronesi U. Consensus conference on sentinel lymph node biopsy. *Cancer* 2002;94:2542.
170. Louise-Sylvestre C, Clough K, Asselain B, et al. Axillary treatment in conservative management of operable breast cancer: dissection or radiotherapy? Results of a randomized study with 15 years of follow-up. *J Clin Oncol* 2004;22:97.
171. Giuliano AE, Kirgan DM, Guenther JM, Morton DL. Lymphatic mapping and sentinel lymphadenectomy for breast cancer. *Ann Surg* 1994;220:391.
172. Giuliano AE, Haigh PI, Brennan MB, et al. Prospective observational study of sentinel lymphadenectomy without further axillary dissection in patients with sentinel node-negative breast cancer. *J Clin Oncol* 2000;18:2553.
173. McMasters KM, Tuttle TM, Carlson DJ, et al. Sentinel lymph node biopsy for breast cancer: a suitable alternative to routine axillary dissection in multi-institutional practice when optimal technique is used. *J Clin Oncol* 2000;18:2560.
174. Bauer TW, Spitz FR, Callans LS, et al. Subareolar and peritumoral injection identify similar sentinel nodes for breast cancer. *Ann Surg Oncol* 2002;9:169.
175. Tuttle TM, Colbert M, Christensen R, et al. Subareolar injection of 99mTc facilitates sentinel lymph node identification. *Ann Surg Oncol* 2002;9:77.
176. Cox CE, Haddad F, Bass S, et al. Lymphatic mapping in the treatment of breast cancer. *Oncology* 1998;12:1283.
177. Wong SL, Edwards MJ, Chao C, et al. Sentinel lymph node biopsy for breast cancer: impact of the number of sentinel nodes removed on the false-negative rate. *J Am Coll Surg* 2001;192:684.
178. Stearns V, Ewing CA, Slack R, et al. Sentinel lymphadenectomy after neoadjuvant chemotherapy for breast cancer may reliably represent the axilla except for inflammatory breast cancer. *Ann Surg Oncol* 2002;9:235.
179. Veronesi U, Rilke F, Luini A, et al. Distribution of axillary node metastases by level of invasion: an analysis of 539 cases. *Cancer* 1987;59:682.
180. Rosen PP, Lesser ML, Kinne DW, Beattie EJ. Discontinuous or "skip" metastases in breast carcinoma; analysis of 1228 axillary dissections. *Ann Surg* 1983;197:276.
181. Fisher B, Anderson S, Bryant J, et al. Twenty-year follow-up of a randomized trial comparing total mastectomy, lumpectomy, and lumpectomy plus irradiation for the treatment of invasive breast cancer. *N Engl J Med* 2002;347:1233.
182. Recht A, Silver B, Schnitt S, et al. Breast relapse following primary radiation therapy for early breast cancer. I. Classification, frequency and salvage. *Int J Radiat Oncol Biol Phys* 1985;11:1271.
183. Grann A, McCormick B, Chabner ES, et al. Prone breast radiotherapy in early-stage breast cancer: a preliminary analysis. *Int J Radiat Oncol Biol Phys* 2000;47:319.
184. Bartelink H, Horiot JC, Poortmans P, et al. Recurrence rates after treatment of breast cancer with standard radiotherapy with or without additional radiation. *N Engl J Med* 2001;345:1378.
185. Romestaing P, Lehingue Y, Carrie C, et al. Role of a 10-Gy boost in the conservative treatment of early breast cancer: results of a randomized clinical trial in Lyon, France. *J Clin Oncol* 1997;15:963.
186. Whelan T, MacKenzie R, Julian J, et al. Randomized trial of breast irradiation schedules after lumpectomy for women with lymph node-negative breast cancer. *J Natl Cancer Inst* 2002;94:1143.
187. Polgar C, Sulyok Z, Fodor J, et al. Sole brachytherapy of the tumor bed after conservative surgery for T1 breast cancer: five-year results of a phase I-II study and initial findings of a randomized phase III trial. *J Surg Oncol* 2002;80:121.
188. Vaidya JS, Baum M, Tobias JS, et al. The novel technique of delivering targeted intraoperative radiotherapy (Targit) for early breast cancer. *Eur J Surg Oncol* 2002;28:447.
189. Kuske RR, Bolton JS, Fuhrman G, et al. Wide volume brachytherapy alone for select breast cancers: the ten-year experience of the Ochsner Clinic. *Int J Radiat Oncol Biol Phys* 2000;48[Supplement]:296(abst).
190. Vicini FA, Kestin L, Chen P, et al. Limited-field radiation therapy in the management of early-stage breast cancer. *J Natl Cancer Inst* 2003;95:1205.
191. Bartelink H. Commentary on the paper "A preliminary report of intraoperative radiotherapy (IORT) in limited-stage breast cancers that are conservatively treated." A critical review of an innovative approach. *Eur J Cancer* 2001;37:2143.
192. Coleman CN, Wallner PE, Abrams JS. Inflammatory breast issue. *J Natl Cancer Inst* 2003;95:1182.
193. Holland R, Veling SH, Mravunac M, Hendricks JH. Histologic multifocality of Tis, T1-2 breast carcinomas. Implications for clinical trials of breast-conserving surgery. *Cancer* 1985;56:979.
194. Santiago RJ, Wu L, Harris E, et al. Fifteen-year results of breast-conserving surgery and definitive irradiation for stage I and I breast carcinoma: the University of Pennsylvania experience. *Int J Radiat Oncol Biol Phys* 2004;58:233.
195. Recht A, Edge SB, Solin LJ, et al. Postmastectomy radiotherapy: clinical practice guidelines of the American Society of Clinical Oncology. *J Clin Oncol* 2001;19:1539.
196. Early Breast Cancer Trialists' Collaborative Group. Favorable and unfavorable effects on long-term survival of radiotherapy for early breast cancer: an overview of the randomized trials. *Lancet* 2000;355:1757.
197. Overgaard M, Hansen PS, Overgaard J, et al. Postoperative radiotherapy in high-risk premenopausal women with breast cancer who receive adjuvant chemotherapy. *N Engl J Med* 1997;337:949.
198. Overgaard M, Jensen MB, Overgaard J, et al. Postoperative radiotherapy in high-risk postmenopausal breast cancer patients given adjuvant tamoxifen: Danis Breast Cancer Cooperative Group DBCG 82c trial. *Lancet* 1999;353:1641.
199. Ragaz J, Jackson SM, Le N, et al. Adjuvant radiotherapy and chemotherapy in node-positive premenopausal women with breast cancer. *N Engl J Med* 1997;337:956.
200. Whelan TJ, Julian J, Wright J, et al. Does locoregional radiation therapy improve survival in breast cancer? A meta-analysis. *J Clin Oncol* 2000;18:1220.
201. Van de Steene J, Soete G, Storme G. Adjuvant radiotherapy for breast cancer significantly improves overall survival: the missing link. *Radiother Oncol* 2000;55:263.
202. Fisher B, Anderson S, Wickerham DL, et al. Increased intensification and total dose of cyclophosphamide in a doxorubicin-cyclophosphamide regimen for the treatment of primary breast cancer: findings from National Surgical Adjuvant Breast and Bowel Project B-22. *J Clin Oncol* 1997;15:1858.
203. Fisher B, Brown AM, Dimitrov NV, et al. Two months of doxorubicin-cyclophosphamide with and without interval reinduction therapy compared with 6 months of cyclophosphamide, methotrexate, and fluorouracil in positive-node breast cancer patients with tamoxifen-nonresppo nsive tumors: results from the National Surgical Adjuvant Breast and Bowel Project B-15. *J Clin Oncol* 1990;8:1483.
204. Recht A, Gray R, Davidson NE, et al. Locoregional failure 10 years after mastectomy and adjuvant chemotherapy with or without tamoxifen without irradiation: experience of the Eastern Cooperative Oncology Group. *J Clin Oncol* 1999;17:1689.
205. Recht A, Barelinek K, Fourquet A, et al. Postmastectomy radiotherapy: questions for the twenty-first century. (Special Article). *J Clin Oncol* 1998;16:2886.
206. Veronesi U, Marubini E, Mariani L, et al. The dissection of internal mammary nodes does not improve the survival of breast cancer patients: 30-year results of a randomized trial. *Eur J Cancer* 1999;35:1320.
207. Olivotto IA, Bajdik CD, Plenderleith IH, et al. Adjuvant systemic therapy and survival after breast cancer. *N Engl J Med* 1994;330:805.
208. Levine MN, Gafni A, Markham B, MacFarlane D. A bedside decision instrument to elicit a patient's preference concerning adjuvant chemotherapy for breast cancer. *Ann Intern Med* 1992;117:53.
209. Whelan T, Sawka C, Levine M, et al. Helping patients make informed choices: a randomized trial of a decision aid for adjuvant chemotherapy in lymph node-negative breast cancer. *J Natl Cancer Inst* 2003;95:581.
210. Harvey JM, Clark GM, Osborne CK, Allred DC. Estrogen receptor status by immunohistochemistry is superior to the ligand-binding assay for predicting response to adjuvant endocrine therapy in breast cancer. *J Clin Oncol* 1999;17:1474.
211. Bardou VJ, Arpino G, Elledge RM, Osborne CK, Clark GM. Progesterone receptor status significantly improves outcome prediction over estrogen receptor status alone for adjuvant endocrine therapy in two large breast cancer databases. *J Clin Oncol* 2003;21:1973.
212. Day R, Ganz PA, Costantino JP, et al. Health-related quality of life and tamoxifen in breast cancer prevention: a report from the National Surgical Adjuvant Breast and Bowel Project P-1 Study. *J Clin Oncol* 1999;17:2659.
213. Albain KS, Green SJ, Ravdin PM, et al. Adjuvant chemohormonal therapy for primary breast cancer should be sequential instead of concurrent: initial results from intergroup trial 0100 (SWOG-8814). *Proc Am Soc Clin Oncol* 2002;21:37a.
214. Loprinzi CL, Michalak JC, Quella SK, et al. Megestrol acetate for the prevention of hot flashes. *N Engl J Med* 1994;331:347.
215. Loprinzi CL, Kugler JW, Sloan JA, et al. Venlafaxine in management of hot flashes in survivors of breast cancer: a randomized controlled trial. *Lancet* 2000;356:2059.
216. Stearns V, Johnson MD, Rae JM, et al. Active tamoxifen metabolite plasma concentrations after coadministration of tamoxifen and the selective serotonin reuptake inhibitor paroxetine. *J Natl Cancer Inst* 2003;95:1758.
217. Goetz MP, Loprinzi CL. A hot flash on tamoxifen metabolism. *J Natl Cancer Inst* 2003;95:1734.
218. Paik S, Shak S, Tang G, et al. Multi-gene RT-PCR assay for predicting recurrence in node negative breast cancer patients—NSABP studies B-20 and B-14. *Breast Cancer Res Treat* 2003;82:S10.
219. Pritchard KI. The best use of adjuvant endocrine treatments. *Breast* 2003;12:497.
220. Davidson NE, O'Neill A, Vukov A, et al. Chemohormonal therapy in premenstrual node-positive, receptor-positive breast cancer: an Eastern Cooperative Oncology Group phase III intergroup trial. Proceedings of ASCO 22, 5. 2003.
221. The ATAC Trialists Group. Anastrozole alone or in combination with tamoxifen versus tamoxifen alone for adjuvant treatment of postmenopausal women with early breast cancer: first results of the ATAC randomized trial. *Lancet* 2002;359:2131.
222. Ellis MJ, Coop A, Singh B, et al. Letrozole is more effective neoadjuvant endocrine therapy than tamoxifen for ErbB-1- and/or ErbB-2-positive, estrogen receptor-positive primary breast cancer: evidence from a phase III randomized trial. *J Clin Oncol* 2001;19:3808.
223. Berry DA, Muss HB, Thor AD, et al. HER-2/neu and p53 expression versus tamoxifen resistance in estrogen receptor-positive, node-positive breast cancer. *J Clin Oncol* 2000;18:3471.
224. Dowsett SI. Comparison of anastrozole vs tamoxifen alone and in combination as neoadjuvant treatment of estrogen receptor-positive (ER+) operable breast cancer in postmenopausal women: the IMPACT trial. *Breast Cancer Res Treat* 2003;82:56.
225. Coombes RC, Hall E, Gibson LJ, et al. A randomized trial of exemestane after two to three years of tamoxifen therapy in postmenopausal women with primary breast cancer. *N Engl J Med* 2004;350:1081.
226. Goss PE, Ingle JN, Martino S, et al. A randomized trial of letrozole in postmenopausal women after five years of tamoxifen therapy for early-stage breast cancer. *N Engl J Med* 2003;349:1793.
227. Winer EP, Hudis C, Burstein HJ, et al. American Society of Clinical Oncology technology assessment working group update: use of aromatase inhibitors in the adjuvant setting. *J Clin Oncol* 2003;21:2597.
228. Hillner BE, Ingle JN, Chlebowski RT, et al. American Society of Clinical Oncology 2003 update on the role of bisphosphonates and bone health issues in women with breast cancer. *J Clin Oncol* 2003;21:4042.
229. Ravdin PM. Is Her2 of value in identifying patients who particularly benefit from anthracyclines during adjuvant therapy? A qualified yes. *J Natl Cancer Inst Monogr* 2001;80.
230. Sledge GW, Jr. Is HER-2/neu a predictor of anthracycline utility? No. *J Natl Cancer Inst Monogr* 2001;85.
231. Thor AD, Berry DA, Budman DR, et al. erbB-2, p53, and efficacy of adjuvant therapy in lymph node-positive breast cancer. *J Natl Cancer Inst* 1998;90:1346.

232. Henderson IC, Berry DA, Demetri GD, et al. Improved outcomes from adding sequential Paclitaxel but not from escalating Doxorubicin dose in an adjuvant chemotherapy regimen for patients with node-positive primary breast cancer. *J Clin Oncol* 2003;21:976.

233. Mamounas EP, Bryant J, Lembersky BC, et al. Paclitaxel (T) following doxorubicin/cyclophosphamide (AC) as adjuvant chemotherapy for node-positive breast cancer: results from NSAPB B-28. Proceedings of ASCO 22, 4. 2003.

234. Martin M, Pienkowski T, Mackey J, et al. TAC improves disease-free survival and overall survival over FAC in node-positive early breast cancer patients, BCIRG 001: 55 months follow-up. *Breast Cancer Res Treat* 2003;82[Suppl 1] (abst43).

235. Bonadonna G, Valagussa P. Dose-response effect of adjuvant chemotherapy in breast cancer. *N Engl J Med* 1981;304:10.

236. Hryniuk WM, Levine MN, Levin L. Analysis of dose intensity for chemotherapy in early (stage II) and advanced breast cancer. *NCI Monogr* 1986;87.

237. Wood WC, Budman DR, Korzun AH, et al. Dose and dose intensity trial of adjuvant chemotherapy for stage II, node positive breast carcinoma. *N Engl J Med* 1994;330:1253.

238. Bonneterre JM, Roche H, Kerbrat P, and et al. Long-term cardiac follow-up in free of disease patients (pts) after receiving 6 FEC 50 vs 6 FEC 100 (FASG-05 Trial) as adjuvant chemotherapy (CT) for node-positive (N+) breast cancer (BC). Proceedings American Society of Clinical Oncology 21. 2002.

239. Levine MN, Bramwell VH, Pritchard KI, et al. Randomized trial of intensive cyclophosphamide, epirubicin, and fluorouracil chemotherapy compared with cyclophosphamide, methotrexate, and fluorouracil in premenopausal women with node-positive breast cancer. National Cancer Institute of Canada Clinical Trials Group. *J Clin Oncol* 1998;16:2651.

240. Norton L, Simon R. The Norton-Simon hypothesis revisited. *Cancer Treat Rep* 1986;70:163.

241. Bonadonna G, Zambetti M, Valagussa P. Sequential or alternating doxorubicin and CMF regimens in breast cancer with more than three positive nodes. Ten-year results [see comments]. *JAMA* 1995;273:542.

242. Citron M , Berty D, Cirrincione C, et al. Superiority of dose-dense (DD) over conventional scheduling (CS) and equivalence of sequential (SC) vs. combination adjuvant chemotherapy (CC) for node-positive breast cancer (CALGB 9741, INT C9741). *Breast Cancer Res Treat* 2002;76[Suppl 1]:S32.

243. Shapiro CL, Recht A. Side effects of adjuvant treatment of breast cancer. *N Engl J Med* 2001;344:1997.

244. Burstein HJ, Winer EP. Primary care for survivors of breast cancer. *N Engl J Med* 2000;343:1086.

245. Ozer H, Armitage JO, Bennett CL, et al. 2000 update of recommendations for the use of hematopoietic colony-stimulating factors: evidence-based, clinical practice guidelines. American Society of Clinical Oncology Growth Factors Expert Panel. *J Clin Oncol* 2000;18:3558.

246. Olin JJ. Cognitive function after systemic therapy for breast cancer. *Oncology* 2001;15:613.

247. Goodwin PJ, Black JT, Bordeleau LJ, Ganz PA. Health-related quality-of-life measurement in randomized clinical trials in breast cancer—taking stock. *J Natl Cancer Inst* 2003;95:263.

248. Coleman RE. Bisphosphonates for the prevention of bone metastases. *Semin Oncol* 2002;29:43.

249. Loprinzi CL, Thome SD. Understanding the utility of adjuvant systemic therapy for primary breast cancer. *J Clin Oncol* 2001;19:972.

250. Thome SD, Loprinzi CL. The adjuvant therapy of breast cancer: how to translate annual proportional risk reductions into absolute 10-year benefits. *Breast Cancer Res Treat* 2000;64:64.

251. Ravdin PM, Siminoff LA, Davis GJ, et al. Computer program to assist in making decisions about adjuvant therapy for women with early breast cancer. *J Clin Oncol* 2001;19:980.

252. Goldhirsch A, Wood WC, Gelber RD, Coates AC, Thürlimann B, Senn HJ. (St. Gallen Breast Cancer Expert Consensus 2003). Meeting highlights: updated international expert consensus on the primary therapy of early breast cancer. *J Clin Oncol* 2003;21:3357.

253. Lindley C, Vasa S, Sawyer WT, Winer EP. Quality of life and preferences for treatment following systemic adjuvant therapy for early-stage breast cancer. *J Clin Oncol* 1998;16:1380.

254. Simes RJ, Coates AS. Patient preferences for adjuvant chemotherapy of early breast cancer: how much benefit is needed? *J Natl Cancer Inst Monogr* 2001;146.

255. Lyman GH, Dale DC, Crawford J. Incidence and predictors of low dose-intensity in adjuvant breast cancer chemotherapy: a nationwide study of community practices. *J Clin Oncol* 2003;21:4524.

256. Heys SD, Hutcheon AW, Sarkar TK, et al. Neoadjuvant docetaxel in breast cancer: 3-year survival results from the Aberdeen trial. *Clin Breast Cancer* 2002;3[Suppl 2]:S69.

257. Fisher B, Brown A, Mamounas E, et al. Effect of preoperative chemotherapy on local-regional disease in women with operable breast cancer: findings from the National Surgical Adjuvant Breast and Bowel Project B-18. *J Clin Oncol* 1997;15:2483.

258. Broet P, Scholl SM, de la Rochefordiere A, et al. Short and long-term effects on survival on breast cancer patients treated by primary chemotherapy: an updated analysis of a randomized trial. *Breast Cancer Res Treat* 1999;58:151.

259. van der Hage JA, van de Velde CJ, Julien JP, et al. Preoperative chemotherapy in primary optimal breast cancer: results from the European Organization for Research and Treatment of Cancer trial 10902. *J Clin Oncol* 2001;19:4224.

260. Mauriac L, MacGrogan G, Avril A, et al. Neoadjuvant chemotherapy for operable breast carcinoma larger than 3 cm: a unicentre randomized trial with a 124-month median follow-up. Institut Bergonie Bordeaux Groupe Sein (IBBGS). *Ann Oncol* 1999;10:47.

261. Buzdar AU, Singletary SE, Theriault RL, et al. Prospective evaluation of paclitaxel versus combination chemotherapy with fluorouracil, doxorubicin, and cyclophosphamide as neoadjuvant therapy in patients with operable breast cancer. *J Clin Oncol* 1999;17:3412.

262. Smith IC, Heys SD, Hutcheon AW, et al. Neoadjuvant chemotherapy in breast cancer: significantly enhanced response with docetaxel. *J Clin Oncol* 2002;20:1456.

263. Newman LA, Buzdar AU, Singletary SE, et al. A prospective trial of preoperative chemotherapy in resectable breast cancer: predictors of breast-conservation therapy feasibility. *Ann Surg Oncol* 2002;9:228.

264. Veronesi U, Bonadonna G, Zurrida S, et al. Conservation surgery after primary chemotherapy in large carcinomas of the breast. *Ann Surg* 1995;222:612.

265. Dixon JM, Love CD, Bellamy CO, et al. Letrozole as primary medical therapy for locally advanced and large operable breast cancer. *Breast Cancer Res Treat* 2001;66:191.

266. Rubens RD, Bartelink H, Engelsman E, et al. Locally advanced breast cancer: the contribution of cytotoxic and endocrine treatment to radiotherapy. An EORTC Breast Cancer Cooperative Group trial 10792. *Eur J Cancer Clin Oncol* 1989;25:667.

267. Recht A, Edge SB, Solin LJ, et al. Post mastectomy radiotherapy: clinical practice guidelines of the American Society of Clinical Oncology. *J Clin Oncol* 2001;19:1539.

268. Olivotto IA, Chua B, Allan SJ, et al. Long-term survival in patients with supraclavicular metastases at diagnosis of breast cancer. *J Clin Oncol* 2003;21:851.

269. Brito RA, Valero V, Buzdar AW, et al. Long-term results of combined-modality therapy for locally advanced breast cancer with ipsilateral supraclavicular metastases: the University of Texas, M. D. Anderson Cancer Center experience. *J Clin Oncol* 2001;19:628.

270. Chang S, Parker SL, Pham T, et al. Inflammatory breast carcinoma incidence and survival: the Surveillance, Epidemiology, and End Results program of the National Cancer Institute, 1975-1992. *Cancer* 1998;82:23662.

271. Bloom HJG, Richardson WW, Harries EJ. Natural history of untreated breast cancer (1805-1933): comparison of untreated and treated cases according to histological grade of malignancy. *BMJ* 1962;2:213.

272. Greenberg PA, Hortobagyi GN, Smith TL, et al. Long-term follow-up of patients with complete remission following combination chemotherapy for metastatic breast cancer. *J Clin Oncol* 1996;14:2197.

273. Kuss JT, Muss HB, Hoen H, Case LD. Tamoxifen as initial endocrine therapy for metastatic breast cancer: long term follow-up of two Piedmont Oncology Association (POA) trials. *Breast Cancer Res Treat* 1997;42:265.

274. Hayes DF. Evaluation after primary therapy. In: Harris JR, Lippman ME, Morrow M, Osborne CK, eds. *Diseases of the breast*. Philadelphia: Lippincott Williams & Wilkins, 2000:709.

275. Hellman S, Harris JR. Natural history of breast cancer. In: Harris JR, Lippman ME, Morrow M, Osborne CK, eds. *Diseases of the breast*. Philadelphia: Lippincott Williams & Wilkins, 2000:407.

276. Eubank WB, Mankoff DA, Vesselle HJ, et al. Detection of locoregional and distant recurrences in breast cancer patients by using FDG PET. *Radiographics* 2002;22:5.

277. Rodriguez PL, Arnaiz F, Estenoz J, et al. Study of serum tumor markers CEA, CA 15.3 and CA 27.29 as diagnostic parameters in patients with breast carcinoma. *Int J Biol Markers* 1995;10:24.

278. Hortobagyi GN. Bone metastases in breast cancer patients. *Semin Oncol* 1991;18:11.

279. Borner MM, Bacchi M, Castiglione M. Possible deleterious effect of tamoxifen in premenopausal women with locoregional recurrence of breast cancer. *Eur J Cancer* 1996;32A:2173.

280. Buzdar AU, Blumenschein GR, Montague ED, et al. Combined modality approach in breast cancer with isolated or multiple metastases. *Am J Clin Oncol* 1984;7:45.

281. Hortobagyi GN, Theriault RL, Porter L, et al. Efficacy of pamidronate in reducing skeletal complications in patients with breast cancer and lytic bone metastases. Protocol 19 Aredia Breast Cancer Study Group. *N Engl J Med* 1996;335:1785.

282. Theriault RL, Lipton A, Hortobagyi GN, et al. Pamidronate reduces skeletal morbidity in women with advanced breast cancer and lytic bone lesions: a randomized, placebo-controlled trial. Protocol 18 Aredia Breast Cancer Study Group. *J Clin Oncol* 1999;17:846.

283. Hillner BE, Ingle JN, Chlebowski RT, et al. American Society of Clinical Oncology 2003 update on the role of bisphosphonates and bone health issues in women with breast cancer. *J Clin Oncol* 2003;21:4042.

284. Vogel CL, East DR, Voigt W, Thomsen S. Response to tamoxifen in estrogen receptor-poor metastatic breast cancer. *Cancer* 1987;60:1184.

285. Taylor SG, Gelman RS, Falkson G, et al. Combination chemotherapy compared to tamoxifen as initial therapy for stage IV breast cancer in elderly women. *Ann Intern Med* 1986;104:455.

286. A randomized trial in postmenopausal patients with advanced breast cancer comparing endocrine and cytotoxic therapy given sequentially or in combination. The Australian and New Zealand Breast Cancer Trials Group, Clinical Oncological Society of Australia. *J Clin Oncol* 1986;4:186.

287. Fossati R, Confalonieri C, Torri V, et al. Cytotoxic and hormonal treatment for metastatic breast cancer: a systematic review of published randomized trials involving 31,510 women [see comments]. *J Clin Oncol* 1998;16:3439.

288. Albain KS, Green SJ, Ravdin PM, et al. Adjuvant chemohormonal therapy for primary breast cancer should be sequential instead of concurrent: initial results from Intergroup Trial 0100 (SWOG-8814). *Proc Am Soc Clin Oncol* 2002;21:37a(abst).

289. Vogel CL, Schoenfelder J, Shemano I, et al. Worsening bone scan in the evaluation of antitumor response during hormonal therapy of breast cancer. *J Clin Oncol* 1995;13:1123.

290. Therasse P, Arbuck SG, Eisenhauer EA, et al. New guidelines to evaluate the response to treatment in solid tumors. European Organization for Research and Treatment of Cancer, National Cancer Institute of the United States, National Cancer Institute of Canada. *J Natl Cancer Inst* 2000;92:205.

291. Robertson JF, Howell A, Buzdar A, et al. Static disease on anastrozole provides similar benefit as objective response in patients with advanced breast cancer. *Breast Cancer Res Treat* 1999;58:157.

292. Olin JJ, Muss HB. New strategies for managing metastatic breast cancer [In Process Citation]. *Oncology* 2000;14:629.

293. Osborne CK, Zhao H, Fuqua SA. Selective estrogen receptor modulators: structure, function, and clinical use. *J Clin Oncol* 2000;18:3172.

294. Muss HB, Smith LR, Cooper MR. Tamoxifen rechallenge: response to tamoxifen following relapse after adjuvant chemohormonal therapy for breast cancer. *J Clin Oncol* 1987;5:1556.

295. Klijn JG, Blamey RW, Boccardo F, et al. Combined tamoxifen and luteinizing hormone-releasing hormone (LHRH) agonist versus LHRH agonist alone in premenopausal advanced breast cancer: a meta-analysis of four randomized trials. *J Clin Oncol* 2001; 19:343.

296. Goss PE, Strasser K. Aromatase inhibitors in the treatment and prevention of breast cancer. *J Clin Oncol* 2001;19:881.
297. Smith IE, Dowsett M. Aromatase inhibitors in breast cancer. *N Engl J Med* 2003;348:2431.
298. Lonning PE, Bajetta E, Murray R, et al. Activity of exemestane in metastatic breast cancer after failure of nonsteroidal aromatase inhibitors: a phase II trial. *J Clin Oncol* 2000;18:2234.
299. Robertson JFR, Howell A, Abram WP, et al. Fulvestrant versus tamoxifen for first-line treatment of advanced breast cancer in postmenopausal women. *Ann Oncol* 2002;13:46(abst).
300. Howell A, Dodwell DJ, Anderson H, et al. Response after withdrawal of tamoxifen and progestogens in advanced breast cancer [see comments]. *Ann Oncol* 1992;3:611.
301. Gee J, Harper M, Hutcheson I, et al. The antiepidermal growth factor receptor agent gefitinib (ZD1839/IressaTM) improves anti-hormone response and prevents development of resistance in breast cancer in vitro. *Endocrinology* 2003;144:5105.
302. Morris C. The role of EGFR-directed therapy in the treatment of breast cancer. *Breast Cancer Res Treat* 2002;75[Suppl 1]:S51.
303. Sledge GW, Neuberg D, Bernardo P, et al. Phase III trial of doxorubicin, paclitaxel, and the combination of doxorubicin and paclitaxel as front-line chemotherapy for metastatic breast cancer: an intergroup trial (E1193). *J Clin Oncol* 2003;21:588.
304. Joensuu H, Holli K, Heikkinen M, et al. Combination chemotherapy versus single-agent therapy as first- and second-line treatment in metastatic breast cancer: a prospective randomized trial. *J Clin Oncol* 1998;16:3720.
305. Costanza ME, Weiss RB, Henderson IC, et al. Safety and efficacy of using a single agent or a phase II agent before instituting standard combination chemotherapy in previously untreated metastatic breast cancer patients: report of a randomized study—Cancer and Leukemia Group B 8642. *J Clin Oncol* 1999;17:1397.
306. O'Shaughnessy J, Miles D, Vukelja S, et al. Superior survival with capecitabine plus docetaxel combination therapy in anthracycline-pretreated patients with advanced breast cancer: phase III trial results. *J Clin Oncol* 2002;20:2812.
307. O'Shaughnessy J. Capecitabine and docetaxel in advanced breast cancer: analyses of a phase III comparative trial. *Oncology* 2002;16:17.
308. Coates A, Gebski V, Bishop JF, et al. Improving the quality of life during chemotherapy for advanced breast cancer. A comparison of intermittent and continuous treatment strategies. *N Engl J Med* 1987;317:1490.
309. Muss HB, Case LD, Richards F, et al. Interrupted versus continuous chemotherapy in patients with metastatic breast cancer. The Piedmont Oncology Association [see comments]. *N Engl J Med* 1991;325:1342.
310. Falkson G, Gelman RS, Pandya KJ, et al. Eastern Cooperative Oncology Group randomized trials of observation versus maintenance therapy for patients with metastatic breast cancer in complete remission following induction treatment. *J Clin Oncol* 1998;16:1669.
311. Stadtmauer EA, O'Neill A, Goldstein LJ, et al. Conventional-dose chemotherapy compared with high-dose chemotherapy plus autologous hematopoietic stem-cell transplantation for metastatic breast cancer. Philadelphia Bone Marrow Transplant Group [see comments]. *N Engl J Med* 2000;342:1069.
312. Berry DA, Broadwater G, Klein JP, et al. High-dose versus standard chemotherapy in metastatic breast cancer: comparison of Cancer and Leukemia Group B trials with data from the Autologous Blood and Marrow Transplant Registry. *J Clin Oncol* 2002;20:743.
313. Eddy DM. High-dose chemotherapy with autologous bone marrow transplantation for the treatment of metastatic breast cancer. *J Clin Oncol* 1992;10:657.
314. Rahman ZU, Frye DK, Buzdar AU, et al. Impact of selection process on response rate and long-term survival of potential high-dose chemotherapy candidates treated with standard-dose doxorubicin-containing chemotherapy in patients with metastatic breast cancer [see comments]. *J Clin Oncol* 1997;15:3171.
315. Tannock IF, Boyd NF, DeBoer G, et al. A randomized trial of two dose levels of cyclophosphamide, methotrexate, and fluorouracil chemotherapy for patients with metastatic breast cancer. *J Clin Oncol* 1988;6:1377.
316. Engelsman E, Klijn JC, Rubens RD, et al. "Classical" CMF versus a 3-weekly intravenous CMF schedule in postmenopausal patients with advanced breast cancer. An EORTC Breast Cancer Cooperative Group Phase III Trial (10808). *Eur J Cancer* 1991;27:966.
317. Kern DH. Heterogeneity of drug resistance in human breast and ovarian cancers. *Cancer J Sci Am* 1998;4:41.
318. Kern DH, Weisenthal LM. Highly specific prediction of antineoplastic drug resistance with an in vitro assay using suprapharmacologic drug exposures. *J Natl Cancer Inst* 1990;82:582.
319. Fornier M, Risio M, Van Poznak C, et al. HER2 testing and correlation with efficacy of trastuzumab therapy. *Oncology* 2002;16:1340.
320. Press MF, Slamon DJ, Flom KJ, et al. Evaluation of HER-2/neu gene amplification and overexpression: comparison of frequently used assay methods in a molecularly characterized cohort of breast cancer specimens. *J Clin Oncol* 2002;20:3095.
321. Vogel CL, Cobleigh MA, Tripathy D, et al. Efficacy and safety of trastuzumab as a single agent in first-line treatment of HER2-overexpressing metastatic breast cancer. *J Clin Oncol* 2002;20:719.
322. Cobleigh MA, Vogel CL, Tripathy D, et al. Multinational study of the efficacy and safety of humanized anti-HER2 monoclonal antibody in women who have HER2-overexpressing metastatic breast cancer that has progressed after chemotherapy for metastatic disease [In Process Citation]. *J Clin Oncol* 1999;17:2639.
323. Slamon DJ, Leyland-Jones B, Shak S, et al. Use of chemotherapy plus a monoclonal antibody against HER2 for metastatic breast cancer that overexpresses HER2. *N Engl J Med* 2001;344:783.
324. Pegram M, Hsu S, Lewis G, et al. Inhibitory effects of combinations of HER-2/neu antibody and chemotherapeutic agents used for treatment of human breast cancers. *Oncogene* 1999;18:2241.
325. Knowlden JM, Hutcheson IR, Jones HE, et al. Elevated levels of epidermal growth factor receptor/c-erbB2 heterodimers mediate an autocrine growth regulatory pathway in tamoxifen-resistant MCF-7 cells. *Endocrinology* 2003;144:1032.
326. Winer EP, Burstein HJ. New combinations with Herceptin in metastatic breast cancer. *Oncology* 2001;61[Suppl 2]:50.
327. Leyland-Jones B, Gelmon K, Ayoub JP, et al. Pharmacokinetics, safety, and efficacy of Trastuzumab administered every three weeks in combination with Paclitaxel. *J Clin Oncol* 2003;21:3965.
328. Estey EH, Thall PF. New designs for phase 2 clinical trials. *Blood* 2003;102:442.
329. Inoue LY, Thall PF, Berry DA. Seamlessly expanding a randomized phase II trial to phase III. *Biometrics* 2002;58:823.
330. Goodwin PJ, Leszcz M, Ennis M, et al. The effect of group psychosocial support on survival in metastatic breast cancer. *N Engl J Med* 2001;345:1719.
331. Goodwin PJ, Black JT, Bordeleau LJ, et al. Health-related quality-of-life measurement in randomized clinical trials in breast cancer—taking stock. *J Natl Cancer Inst* 2003;95:263.
332. Liu G, Franssen E, Fitch MI, Warner E. Patient preferences for oral versus intravenous palliative chemotherapy. *J Clin Oncol* 1997;15:110.
333. Gradishar WJ. Clinical status of capecitabine in the treatment of breast cancer. *Oncology* 2001;15:69.
334. Rocca A, Colleoni M, Masci G, et al. Low dose oral Methotrexate and Cyclophosphamide in metastatic breast cancer: an attempt to exploit the antiangiogenic activity of common chemotherapeutic agents (abst). *Proc Am Soc Clin Oncol* 2001;20:30a.
335. Gwyn K, Theriault R. Breast cancer during pregnancy. *Oncology* 2001;15:39.
336. Helewa M, Levesque P, Provencher D, et al. Breast cancer, pregnancy, and breastfeeding. *J Obstet Gynaecol Can* 2002;24:164.
337. Reed W, Hannisdal E, Skovlund E, et al. Pregnancy and breast cancer: a population-based study. *Virchows Arch* 2003;443:44.
338. Petrek JA. Breast cancer and pregnancy. [Review] *J Natl Cancer Inst* 1994;113.
339. Nicklas AH, Baker ME. Imaging strategies in the pregnant cancer patient. *Semin Oncol* 2000;27:623.
340. Woo JC, Yu T, Hurd TC. Breast cancer in pregnancy: a literature review. *Arch Surg* 2003;138:91.
341. Berry DL, Theriault RL, Holmes FA, et al. Management of breast cancer during pregnancy using a standardized protocol. *J Clin Oncol* 1999;17:855.
342. Jernstrom H, Lerman C, Ghadirian P, et al. Pregnancy and risk of early breast cancer in carriers of BRCA1 and BRCA2. *Lancet* 1999;354:1846.
343. Higgins S, Haffty BG. Pregnancy and lactation after breast-conserving therapy for early stage breast cancer. *Cancer* 1994;73:2175.
344. Fox KR, Scialla J, Moore H. Preventing chemotherapy-related amenorrhea using Leuprolide during adjuvant chemotherapy for early-stage breast cancer. *Proc Am Soc Clin Oncol* 2003;(abst).
345. Solin LJ. Bilateral breast cancer. In: Fowble B, Goodman RL, Glick JH, Rosato EF, eds. *Breast cancer treatment: a comprehensive guide to management.* St. Louis: Mosby Year Book, 199:507.
346. Polednak AP. Bilateral synchronous breast cancer: a population-based study of characteristics, method of detection, and survival. *Surgery* 2003;133:383.
347. Broet P, de la Rochefordiere A, Scholl SM, et al. Contralateral breast cancer: annual incidence and risk parameters. *J Clin Oncol* 1995;13:1578.
348. Bodian C, Haagensen CD. Bilateral carcinoma of the breast. In: Haagensen CD, ed. *Diseases of the breast.* 3rd ed. Philadelphia: WB Saunders, 1986:440.
349. Adami HO, Bergstrom R, Hansen J. Age at first primary as a determinant of the incidence of bilateral breast cancer. *Cancer* 1985;55:643.
350. Hungness ES, Safa M, Shaughnessy EA, et al. Bilateral synchronous breast cancer: mode of detection and comparison of histologic features between the 2 breasts. *Surgery* 2000;128:702.
351. Lee SG, Orel SG, Woo IJ, et al. MR imaging screening of the contralateral breast in patients with newly diagnosed breast cancer: preliminary results. *Radiology* 2003;226:773.
352. Fung MC, Schultz DJ, Solin LJ. Early-stage bilateral breast cancer treated with breast-conserving surgery and definitive radiation: the University of Pennsylvania experience. *Int J Radiat Oncol Biol Phys* 1997;38:959.
353. Early Breast Cancer Trialists' Collaborative Group. Tamoxifen for early breast cancer: an overview of the randomized trials. *Lancet* 1998;351:1451.
354. Baum M, Buzdar AU, Cuzick J, et al. Anastrozole alone or in combination with tamoxifen versus tamoxifen alone for adjuvant treatment of post-menopausal women with early breast cancer: first results of the ATAC randomized trial. *Lancet* 2002;359:2131.
355. American Cancer Society. *Breast cancer facts and figures: 2001–2002.* Atlanta: American Cancer Society, 2003.
356. Thorlacius S, Olafsdottir G, Tryggvadottir L, et al. A single BRCA2 mutation in male and female breast cancer families from Iceland with varied cancer phenotypes. *Nat Genet* 1996;13:117.
357. Fackenthal J, Marsh D, Richardson A, et al. Male breast cancer in Cowden syndrome patients with germline PTEN mutations. *J Med Genet* 2001;38:159.
358. Ravandi-Kashani F, Hayes TG. Male breast cancer: a review of the literature. *Eur J Cancer* 1998;34:1341.
359. Chaney AW, Pollack A, McNeese MD, et al. Primary treatment of cystosarcoma phyllodes of the breast. *Cancer* 2000;89:1502.
360. Gobbi H, Simpson JF, Borowsdy A, et al. Metaplastic breast tumors with a dominant fibromatosis-like phenotype have a high risk of local recurrence. *Cancer* 2000;85:2170-2182.
361. Barrow BJ, Janjan NA, Gutman H, et al. Role of radiotherapy in sarcoma of the breast—a retrospective review of the MD Anderson experience. *Radiother Oncol* 1999;52:173.
362. Zelek L, Llombart-Cussac A, Terrier P, et al. Prognostic factors in primary breast sarcomas: a series of patients with long-term follow-up. *J Clin Oncol* 2003:21:2583.
363. Freter C. Other cancers of the breast. In: Harris JR, Lippman ME, Morrow M, Osborne CK, eds. *Diseases of the breast.* Philadelphia: Lippincott, Williams and Wilkins, 2000:683.
364. Jardines L. Other cancers of the breast. In: Harris JR, Lippmann ME, Morrow M, Hellman S, eds. *Diseases of the breast.* Philadelphia: Lippincott–Raven, 1996:876.

365. Wiseman C, Liao KT. Primary lymphoma of the breast. *Cancer* 1972;29:1705.

366. Dixon JM, Lumsden AB, Krajewski A, et al. Primary lymphoma of the breast. *Br J Surg* 1987;74:214.

367. NCCN preliminary non-Hodgkin's lymphoma practice guidelines. *Oncology* 1997;11:281.

368. Orel SG, Weinstein SP, Schnall MD, et al. Breast MR imaging in patients with axillary node metastases in unknown primary malignancy. *Radiology* 1999;212:543.

369. Olson JA, Morris EA, Van Zee KJ, et al. Magnetic resonance imaging facilitates breast conservation for occult breast cancer. *Ann Surg Oncol* 2000;7:411.

370. Chen C, Orel SG, Harris E, et al. Outcome after treatment for patients with mammographically occult, MRI-detected breast cancer presenting with axillary lymphadenopathy. *Clin Breast Cancer* 2004;5:72.

371. Campana F, Fourquet A, Ashby MA, et al. Presentation of axillary lymphadenopathy without detectable breast primary (T0N1b breast cancer): experience at Institut Curie. *Radiother Oncol* 1989;15:321.

372. Foroudi F, Tiver KW. Occult breast carcinoma presenting as axillary metastases. *Int J Radiat Oncol Biol Phys* 2000;47:143.

373. Chen C, Orel SG, Schnall MD, et al. Breast conservation treatment for patients presenting with axillary lymphadenopathy from presumed primary breast cancer: the role of breast magnetic resonance imaging for staging. *Clin Breast Cancer* 2002;3:219.

374. Vlastos G, Jean ME, Mirza AN, et al. Feasibility of breast preservation in the treatment of occult primary carcinoma presented with axillary metastases. *Ann Surg Oncol* 2001;8:425.

375. Ellerbroek N, Holmes F, Singletary E, et al. Treatment of patients with isolated axillary nodal metastases from occult primary carcinoma consistent with breast origin. *Cancer* 1990;66:1461.

376. Chen C, Orel SG, Harris EER, et al. Relation between the method of detection of initial breast carcinoma and the method of detection of subsequent ipsilateral local recurrence and contralateral breast carcinoma. *Cancer* 2003;98:1596.

377. Recht A, Silver B, Schnitt S, et al. Breast relapse following primary radiation therapy for early breast cancer. I. Classification, frequency and salvage. *Int J Radiat Oncol Biol Phys* 1985;11:1271.

378. Solin LJ, Harris EER, Orel SG, Glick JH. Local-regional recurrence after breast conservation treatment or mastectomy. In: Harris JR, Lippman ME, Morrow M, Osborne CK, eds. *Diseases of the breast.* 3rd ed. Philadelphia: Lippincott Williams & Wilkins, 2004.

379. Doyle T, Schultz DJ, Peters C, et al. Long-term results of local recurrence after breast conservation treatment for invasive breast cancer. *Int J Radiat Oncol Biol Phys* 2001;51:74.

380. Kurtz JM, Amalric R, Brandone H, et al. Results of wide excision for mammary recurrence after breast conserving therapy. *Cancer* 1988;61:1969.

381. Voogd AC, van Tienhoven G, Peterse HL, et al. Local recurrence after breast conservation therapy for early stage breast carcinoma: detection, treatment and outcome in 266 patients. Dutch Study Group on Local Recurrence after Breast Conservation (BORST). *Cancer* 1999;85:437.

382. Deutsch M. Repeat high-dose external beam radiation for in-breast tumor recurrence after previous lumpectomy and whole breast irradiation. *Int J Radiat Oncol Biol Phys* 2002;53:687.

383. Schwaibold F, Fowble BL, Solin LJ, et al. The results of radiation therapy for isolated local regional recurrence after mastectomy. *Int J Radiat Oncol Biol Phys* 1991;21:299.

384. Halverson KJ, Perez, CA, Kuske RR, et al. Locoregional recurrence of breast cancer: a retrospective comparison of irradiation alone versus irradiation and systemic therapy. *Am J Clin Oncol* 1992;15:93.

385. Ballo MT, Strom EA, Prost H, et al. Local-regional control of recurrent breast carcinoma after mastectomy: does hyperfractionated accelerated radiotherapy improve local control? *Int J Radiat Oncol Biol Phys* 1999;44:105.

386. Borner MM, Bacchi M, Castiglione M. Possible deleterious effect of tamoxifen in premenopausal women with locoregional recurrence of breast cancer. *Eur J Cancer* 1996;32A:2173.

387. van Tienhoven G, Voogd AC, Peterse JL, et al. Prognosis after treatment for loco-regional recurrence after mastectomy or breast conserving therapy in two randomized trials (EORTC 10801 and DBCG-82TM). EORTC Breast Cancer Cooperative Group and the Danish Breast Cancer Cooperative Group. *Eur J Cancer* 1999;35:32.

388. Vernon CC, Hand JW, Field SB, et al. Radiotherapy with or without hyperthermia in the treatment of superficial localized breast cancer: results from five randomized controlled trials. International Collaborative Hyperthermia Group. *Int J Radiat Oncol Biol Phys* 1996;35:731.

389. Harris EE, Hwang W-T, Seyednejad F, Solin LJ. Prognosis after regional lymph node recurrence in patients with stage I-II breast carcinoma treated with breast conservation therapy. *Cancer* 2003;98:2144.

390. Galper S, Blood E, Gelman R, et al. Prognosis after isolated axillary nodal recurrence following conservative surgery and radiotherapy for early-stage breast carcinoma. *Int J Radiat Oncol Biol Phys* 2002;54[Suppl]:56.

391. Jemal A, Murray T, Samuels A, Ghafoor A, et al. Cancer statistics, 2003. *CA Cancer J Clin* 2003;53:5.

392. Yancik R, Ries LG, Yates JW. Breast cancer in aging women. A population-based study of contrasts in stage, surgery, and survival. *Cancer* 1989;63:976.

393. Holmes CE, Muss HB. Diagnosis and treatment of breast cancer in the elderly. *CA Cancer J Clin* 2003;53:227.

394. Kimmick GG, Muss HB. Systemic therapy for older women with breast cancer. *Oncology* 2001;15:280.

395. Yancik R, Wesley MN, Ries LA, et al. Effect of age and comorbidity in postmenopausal breast cancer patients aged 55 years and older. *JAMA* 2001;285:885.

396. Welch HG, Albertsen PC, Nease RF, et al. Estimating treatment benefits for the elderly: the effect of competing risks. *Ann Intern Med* 1996;124:577.

397. Diab SG, Elledge RM, Clark GM. Tumor characteristics and clinical outcome of elderly women with breast cancer. *J Natl Cancer Inst* 2000;92:550.

398. Hughes KS, Schnaper L, Berry C, et al. Comparison of lumpectomy plus tamoxifen with and without radiotherapy (RT) in women 70 years of age or older who have clinical stage I, estrogen receptor positive (ER+) breast carcinoma. ASCO Proceedings 2001;20:93A.

399. Extermann M, Balducci L, Lyman GH. What threshold for adjuvant therapy in older breast cancer patients? *J Clin Oncol* 2000;18:1709.

400. Muss H, Woolf SH, Berry DA, et al. Older women with node positive breast cancer get similar benefits from adjuvant chemotherapy as younger patients: the Cancer and Leukemia Group B (CALGB) experience. *Proc Am Soc Clin Oncol* 2003;22(abst).

401. Muss HB. Factors used to select adjuvant therapy of breast cancer in the United States: an overview of age, race, and socioeconomic status. *J Natl Cancer Inst Monogr* 2001;52.

402. Kemeny MM, Peterson BL, Kornblith AB, et al. Barriers to clinical trial participation by older women with breast cancer. *J Clin Oncol* 2003;21:2268.

JEANNE A. PETREK
JOSEPH J. DISA

SECTION 3

Rehabilitation after Treatment for Cancer of the Breast

Breast reconstruction after mastectomy has grown in popularity since the 1970s. The era of diagnosis with less extensive cancers has ushered in less extensive total mastectomies, including "skin sparing" with an incision only around the areola. Presently, the typical patient has many choices, not only regarding cancer management but also regarding multiple surgical options after mastectomy.

The first consideration after mastectomy is whether to reconstruct the breast. Not performing breast reconstruction is the simplest approach. The patient then faces postmastectomy appearance and the need, in most women, for an external prosthesis to restore appearance and weight balance. Mastectomy forms first began as individually made cotton fluff-filled forms. Then foam rubber forms were manufactured with holes in the back for metal weights to add stability and gravity. Now almost all weighted breast prostheses are made of solid silicone materials. The variably shaped breast forms are also available in several skin colors. It is very rare, but possible, to require custom manufacturing of the form for irregular mastectomy defects.

The external prosthesis is completely concealed in a bra with an adjustable built-in pocket specially constructed to accommodate it. Wearing the weighted prosthesis should help the body maintain its posture and balance and may prevent back and neck strain. With the concern that the prosthesis could become dislodged, even with such a specially fitted bra or swimsuit, adherent forms have now become popular. Using a variety of surgical adhesives, the form adheres to the chest wall or to a backing on the skin of the chest wall, so that the form can be removed every night while the backing can remain for a week or more. In retrospective studies,[1,2] the differences among those opting for breast reconstruction, those wearing external prostheses, and those doing neither were explored.

The American Cancer Society sponsors the program Reach to Recovery (1-800-ACS-2345), which began in 1952, a time when all volunteers had undergone mastectomy. Today, the survivor-to-patient outreach and support include volunteers who have had breast conservation and postmastectomy reconstruction. At the physician's request, trained volunteers meet with the patient to discuss several aspects of recovery, including physiologic, psychological, and cosmetic rehabilitation. Resources for the patient include breast prostheses information with knowledge of local resources, clothing suggestions, and even an exercise booklet and aids.

DELAYED VERSUS IMMEDIATE RECONSTRUCTION

If breast reconstruction is elected, the next decision is timing, immediate (at the time of the mastectomy) or delayed. The traditional concept of performing the mastectomy, proceeding with adjuvant therapy, and delaying reconstruction until the completion of adjuvant therapy is being supplanted by the increasing use of immediate reconstruction. In a mastectomy without immediate reconstruction, it is difficult to "save" any extra native breast skin because, with the volume of the breast missing, there is excess skin folding and wrinkling. The first large report of immediate reconstruction was in 1982 by Georgiade et al.[3] In their series of 62 patients, the authors concluded that immediate breast reconstruction in selected patients offered the advantages of improved aesthetic results, decreased cost, less morbidity, and no adverse effect on cancer management.

Because the mastectomy and reconstruction are performed under a single anesthetic, the total hospital costs and convalescent time are reduced when compared to mastectomy and delayed reconstruction.[4] Immediate reconstruction reduces physical morbidity by limiting the total number of anesthetics and reducing the need for a symmetry procedure on the opposite breast.[5] Critical landmarks for optimizing breast form and symmetry are the inframammary fold, which is preserved or reconstructed, and the breast skin envelope, which can be preserved and maintained in its native state with immediate reconstruction.

Current methods of reconstruction can be broadly classified into autologous tissue or prosthetic material. Autologous tissue reconstruction uses the patient's own tissue (skin, subcutaneous tissue, and muscle) from another site to reconstruct the missing breast. Prosthetic reconstruction uses a process known as *tissue expansion* to create a "pocket" for the ultimate placement of a breast implant. Occasionally, a combination of autologous tissue and an implant is indicated. The selection of the reconstructive technique is based on anatomic patient factors, including the laxity and thickness of the remaining chest-wall skin, the condition of the chest-wall musculature, the size of the opposite breast, and the availability of suitable autologous tissue donor sites. To identify the appropriate method of reconstruction, the anatomic factors are considered with cancer treatment goals and the patient's expectations, as well as, most importantly, clinical factors (smoking history, diabetes, obesity, other chronic illnesses), because operative complexity and postoperative recovery vary.

PROSTHETIC RECONSTRUCTION

Breast reconstruction using prosthetic materials involves the use of tissue expanders and permanent breast implants. Initially, implants were placed directly under the skin in the mastectomy space, but the results were limited by the available skin envelope and capsular contracture.[6,7] The development of tissue expanders allowed for greater control over the size of the skin envelope, thus resulting in the ability to use larger prostheses for symmetry. Current techniques use a complete submuscular placement of the tissue expander, with coverage by pectoralis major, serratus anterior, and occasionally the anterior rectus sheath.[6]

A biodimensional textured surface tissue expander is placed either at the time of mastectomy, which increases the operative time by approximately 1 hour, or in a delayed fashion, during a separate later operation. The area is allowed to heal for approximately 10 to 14 days, at which time tissue expansion is commenced. Using an integrated valve within the expander, saline is injected into the expander percutaneously until the appropriate size is reached (Fig. 33.3-1). Adjuvant chemotherapy can be commenced during the expansion process. The exchange to a

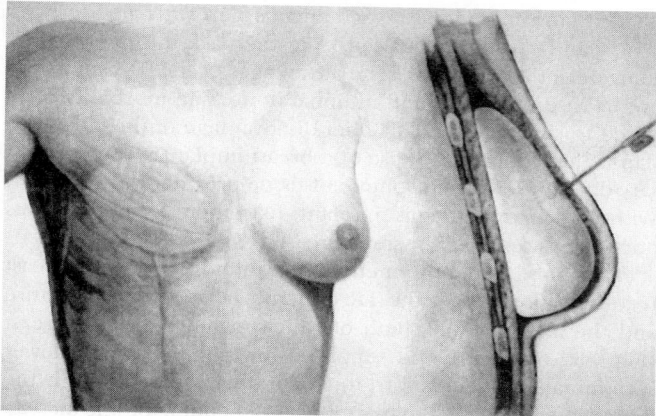

FIGURE 33.3-1. Complete submuscular placement of the tissue expander at the time of mastectomy (*left*). Percutaneous approach to expansion using a complete submuscular integrated valve tissue expander (*right*).

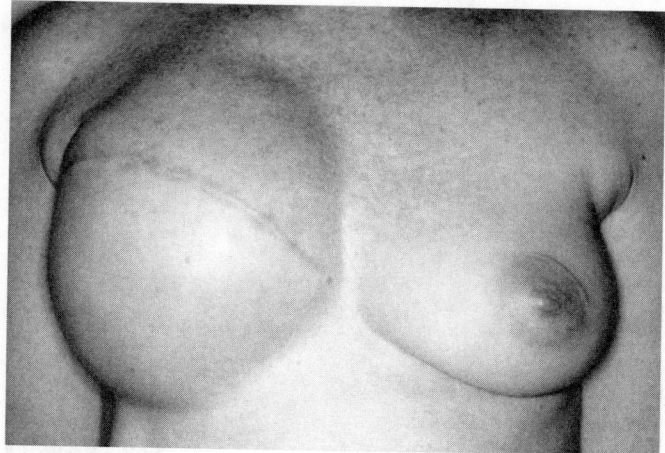

A

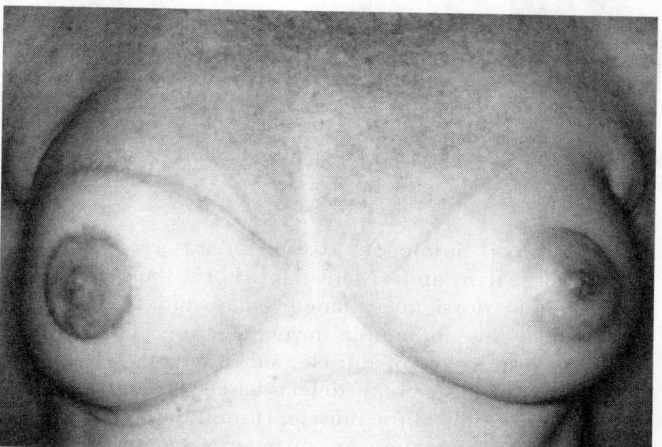

B

FIGURE 33.3-2. **A:** After expansion is complete, the pocket is over-expanded relative to the normal breast to maximize ptosis and implant projection. **B:** The same patient subsequent to exchange of the tissue expander to a permanent saline breast implant followed by nipple-areola reconstruction and tattooing.

permanent breast implant takes place after the chemotherapy course. Using a two-stage method of implant reconstruction allows for maximum control of the implant pocket and optimal symmetry with the contralateral breast (Fig. 33.3-2). When indicated, contralateral symmetry procedures, such as augmentation mammoplasty, reduction mammoplasty, or mastopexy (breast lift), are accomplished when the tissue expander is exchanged to a permanent implant (Fig. 33.3-3).

The author (J. D.) reported results with 770 consecutive patients undergoing tissue expansion over a 10-year period. In this series, premature removal of the tissue expander secondary to wound-related complications or persistent disease was necessary in only 1.8% of the patients.[8] The advantages of tissue expander implant reconstruction are the simplicity, reliability, and avoidance of donor site morbidity. The disadvantages of this technique relate to the use of prosthetic material and include infection, leakage of the implant, capsular contracture, and differences in texture and symmetry when compared to the contralateral breast, which can lead to multiple surgical procedures on the opposite breast.

Breast implants available for reconstruction vary in size, shape, surface texturing, and fill material. In general, implants are either round or anatomic in shape, with a smooth or textured surface, and are saline or silicone gel filled. Currently, saline-filled breast implants are available, and use of silicone gel implants requires enrollment in a silicone adjunct study sponsored by the implant manufacturers, the U.S. Food and Drug Administration, and the Institution Review Board where the procedure is being performed. Despite the moratorium placed on the general use of silicone gel implants, to date there is no convincing cause and effect between "human adjuvant disease" and the use of silicone gel implants.[9]

In addition to the current saline and silicone gel implants available in the United States, new implant designs and changes in filler materials are on the horizon.[10] In widespread use in Europe, and currently under investigation in the United States, are the use of cohesive gel implants. These implants have a higher-viscosity silicone gel in the lumen and therefore resist the deforming forces of the implant pocket. As a result, breast reconstruction using these implants focuses on the pro-

portions and dimensions of the patient's individual chest wall rather than on the volume of the pocket.[11] Other promising designs include dual-lumen saline/silicone gel–filled implants that are adjustable. Each implant has a fixed volume of silicone gel and a variable volume of saline that is injected either in the operating room or postoperatively much the same way a tissue expander is filled. These implants allow for simple correction of volume asymmetries and offer the promise of single-stage breast reconstruction with implants in appropriately selected patients.[10]

AUTOLOGOUS TISSUE RECONSTRUCTION

The most predictable results in breast reconstruction involve the use of autologous tissue. In general, use of the patient's own tissue results in a reconstruction that can closely match the opposite breast in size, shape, and texture. Depending on the volume of the tissue transferred and the volume of the contralateral breast, autologous tissue breast reconstruction sometimes also requires an implant.

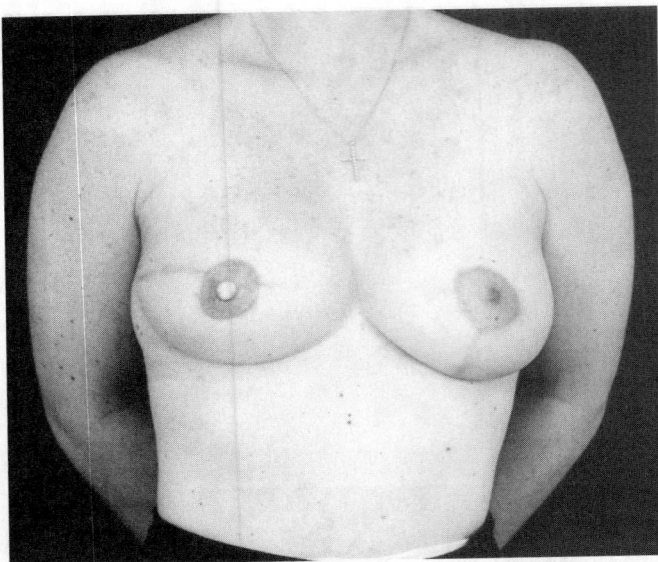

FIGURE 33.3-3. Right breast reconstruction with saline implant followed by nipple-areola reconstruction and left mastopexy for symmetry. (See Color Fig. 33.3-3 in the CD-ROM.)

Methods of autologous tissue breast reconstruction include local flaps and distant flaps. Local flaps, including the latissimus dorsi myocutaneous flap and the pedicled transverse rectus abdominus myocutaneous (TRAM) flap, rely on transposition of muscle, subcutaneous tissue, and skin into the mastectomy defect based on the attached native blood supply of the muscle. Distant flap breast reconstruction mandates the use of microvascular free-tissue transfer. The most common distant tissue donor site is the free TRAM flap.

Other distant donor sites include the deep inferior epigastric artery perforator (DIEP) flap, superficial inferior epigastric artery perforator flap, inferior gluteal flap, superior gluteal flap, superior gluteal artery perforator flap, and the Rubens flap. Reconstruction using these tissues relies on harvesting the flap with its discreet vascular pedicle. The vascular pedicle is then anastomosed using microsurgical technique to appropriate recipient vessels in the mastectomy site, usually the thoracodorsal or internal mammary vessels.

The latissimus dorsi myocutaneous flap with an overlying skin island can be transposed from the back into the mastectomy defect (Fig. 33.3-4). The advantages of the latissimus flap are its ease of harvest and minimal donor site morbidity compared to other sites.[12] The chief disadvantage of the latissimus flap is that concomitant use of a breast implant is often necessary due to the limited volume of tissue provided (Fig. 33.3-5). Without a simultaneous implant placement, the latissimus dorsi flap is reserved for small breasts.

The most common method of autologous tissue breast reconstruction is with the TRAM flap[13] because of the texture and the large volume, both of which match the other breast (Fig. 33.3-6). The blood supply to the skin island and lower abdominal fat is derived from perforating vessels through the underlying rectus abdominus muscle. Depending on the increasing volume necessary to match the other breast, the TRAM flap can be transferred on a single pedicle (either the contralateral or ipsilateral superior epigastric), double pedicle (using both rectus muscles and their associated superior epigastric vessels), or as a free flap (based on the deep inferior epigastric vessels)[14] (Fig. 33.3-7).

The TRAM flap allows the reconstructive surgeon the most versatility and design. Thus, the flap can be sculpted to closely match the contralateral breast in unilateral reconstruction, or itself in bilateral reconstruction (Fig. 33.3-8). The use of a breast implant is rarely indicated with a TRAM flap, because an ample amount of tissue exists in properly selected patients. The lower abdominal donor site scar is easily hidden with conventional clothing. Despite the obvious advantages of the TRAM flap, not everyone is a candidate. Thin patients may not have an adequate amount of tissue at the donor site, whereas obese patients have a much higher risk for local and systemic complications.[15] Total flap loss with the free TRAM flap can occur, but the risk is generally accepted to be less than 2%.[16,17] Use of the rectus abdominus muscle results in 10% loss in abdominal wall strength in unilateral reconstruction and 40% loss when both muscles are harvested.[18] Lower abdominal bulging and hernia formation occur in fewer than 10% of patients and can be minimized by surgical techniques that maximize preservation of the rectus muscles.[19]

The most recent innovation in breast reconstruction with autologous tissue involves the use of perforator flaps. The greatest experience with the DIEP flap technique involves harvesting skin and subcutaneous tissues to reconstruct the missing breast but

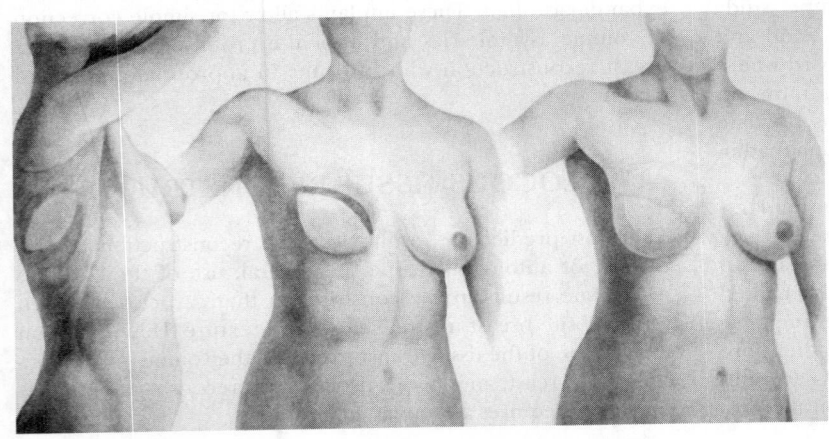

FIGURE 33.3-4. Design of the latissimus flap and skin island (*left*). Transposition of the myocutaneous latissimus dorsi flap into the mastectomy defect (*center*). Latissimus flap breast reconstruction with the placement of a breast implant underneath the latissimus dorsi flap (*right*).

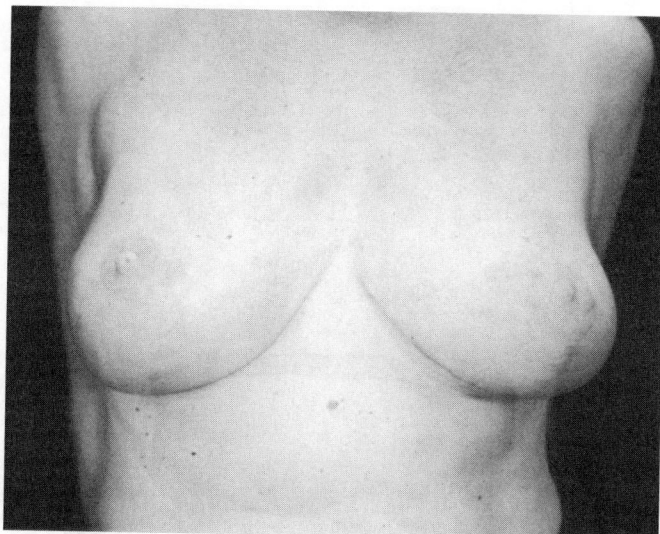

FIGURE 33.3-5. Right breast reconstruction with latissimus dorsi myocutaneous flap and permanent implant. The implant was necessary to achieve symmetry with the opposite breast. The patient has undergone a left reduction mammoplasty for symmetry. (See Color Fig. 33.3-5 in the CD-ROM.)

preserving muscle to maximize function at the donor site. With respect to the DIEP flap, the deep inferior epigastric artery vascular pedicle along with its perforators to the skin and subcutaneous tissue island are harvested while preserving the rectus abdominus muscle.[20] Although this is technically more demanding and takes more time in the operating room, this technique potentially minimizes abdominal donor site morbidity by preserving the rectus abdominus muscle.[21,22] Perforator flap technology has also been applied to the anterolateral thigh flap, the thoracodorsal artery perforator flap, and the superior gluteal artery perforator flap.[23] The quality and volume of tissue typically provided by the DIEP flap are superior to the other options. Potential downsides of the DIEP flap versus the free TRAM flap include a higher incidence of venous congestion, fat necrosis, and flap loss.[21]

POSTMASTECTOMY AFTER BREAST IRRADIATION

Breast reconstruction after local failure in the irradiated breast presents a unique challenge for the oncologic and the recon-

structive surgeon. The late effects of radiation are characterized clinically by a loss of skin elasticity, fibrosis, and decreased blood supply. The postradiation fibrosis severely limits the ability of the tissue expander to create a satisfactory pocket for the permanent implant. The incidence of infection, skin necrosis, and expander extrusion is increased when attempting to expand the irradiated skin and muscle chest wall, and there is a high rate of capsular contracture in the final result. The lack of projection of the permanent implant and capsular contracture detracts from the final aesthetic result.[24,25]

Increasing the success of breast reconstruction after prior irradiation involves the use of autologous tissue. Depending on the method, this procedure can be performed with or without a breast implant. The transfer of the ipsilateral latissimus dorsi muscle with a cutaneous skin island into the mastectomy defect delivers a large volume of healthy nonirradiated tissue into the defect. In conjunction with a tissue expander, the flap can be expanded without difficulty, and ultimately a permanent implant can be placed, with improved aesthetics and a decreased incidence of complications.[26]

In a series[27,28] of 680 consecutive patients who underwent TRAM flap breast reconstruction, 108 had had previous irradiation, and no difference was found in flap survival in the two groups. However, the incidence of infection and fat necrosis was increased in the radiated group, which detracts from the final aesthetic result. The effects of irradiation on the mastectomy flaps predispose to ischemia and may increase scar formation.[26]

SKIN-SPARING MASTECTOMY WITH IMMEDIATE RECONSTRUCTION

Although autologous tissue breast reconstruction can create a breast mound that resembles the breast in shape and consistency, one drawback is the color difference between the native breast skin and the flap skin (from the distant site), which conveys a "patch-like" appearance (Fig. 33.3-9). The technique of skin-sparing mastectomy is accomplished through one incision around the areola, with preservation of the entire breast skin envelope. When necessary, a counterincision in the axilla is used to expose blood vessels, to remove lymph nodes, or for microsurgical flap transfer. The skin island from the flap is confined to the zone of the nipple-areola complex (Fig. 33.3-10*A,B*). Subsequent nipple reconstruction covers the skin island completely, thereby virtually eliminating all visible scars

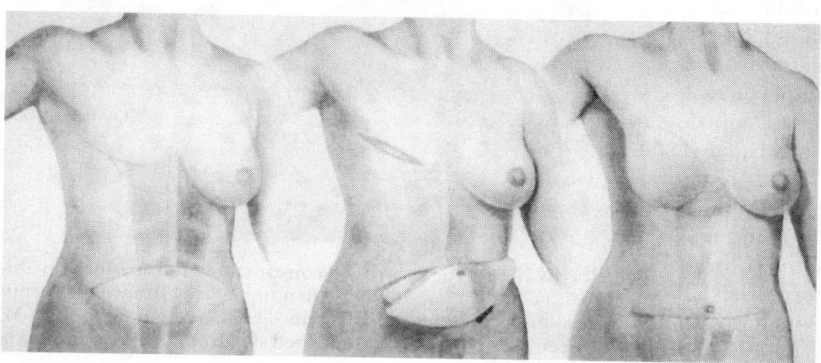

FIGURE 33.3-6. Design of a unipedicled transverse rectus abdominus myocutaneous (TRAM) flap on the lower abdomen (*left*). Elevation of the TRAM flap based on the left rectus abdominus muscle (*center*). Right breast reconstruction with unipedicled TRAM flap after closure of the donor site and inset of flap (*right*).

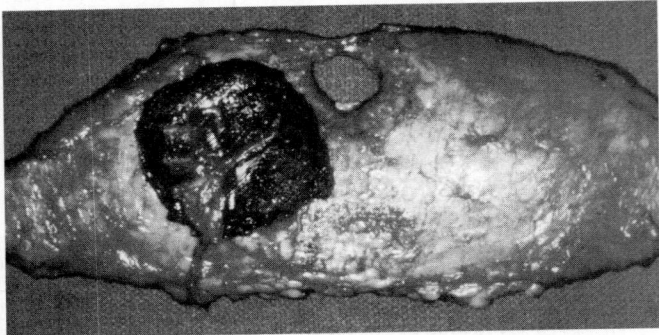

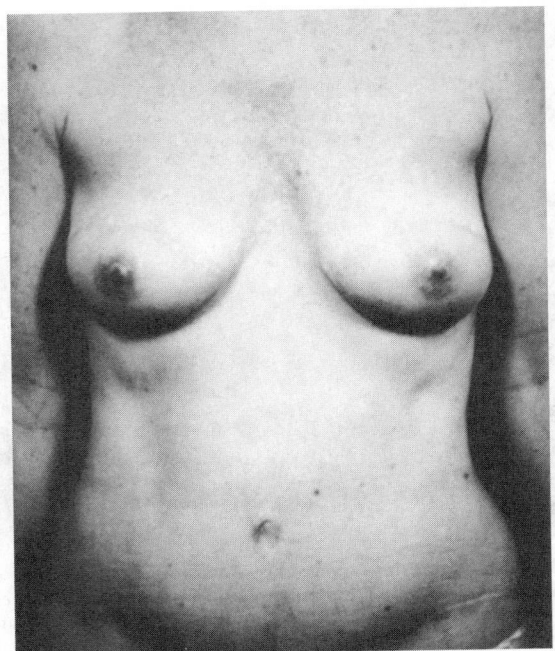

FIGURE 33.3-8. Bilateral breast reconstruction with transverse rectus abdominus myocutaneous flaps and subsequent nipple-areola reconstruction. The use of autologous tissue conveys a natural appearance to the breast reconstruction.

Although the nipple reconstruction lacks sensation and the erectile function of the natural nipple, it provides an important visual suggestion of normalcy and decreases the stigmata of mastectomy.

FIGURE 33.3-7. **A:** Anatomy of transverse rectus abdominus myocutaneous (TRAM) flap on the lower abdomen. The flap is centered over the rectus abdominus muscles and is supplied by the superior epigastric vessels and the deep inferior epigastric vessels. **B:** Posterior surface of free TRAM flap. Note: Small portion of rectus abdominus muscle with associated pedicle used to provide blood supply to the flap. (See Color Fig. 33.3-7*B* in the CD-ROM.)

(Fig. 33.3-10*C*), and the reconstructed breast is almost indistinguishable from the other. Importantly, long-term follow-up of selected patients has not shown a difference in local recurrence rates after skin-sparing mastectomy versus traditional mastectomy.[29–31] Technical advances using complete skin-sparing techniques have resulted in reconstructed breasts that are virtually indistinguishable from the native breast in terms of color, texture, and appearance.[29] In properly selected patients, skin-sparing mastectomy can be performed in previously irradiated patients with good results[23] (Fig. 33.3-11).

Nipple-areola reconstruction can be accomplished simply in the outpatient setting. One method is simply tattooing a nipple and areola onto the breast mound to imitate the color and size of the opposite nipple-areola complex. Alternatively, a local flap can be raised on the breast mound to create the nipple projection, or a skin graft can be placed (Fig. 33.3-12).

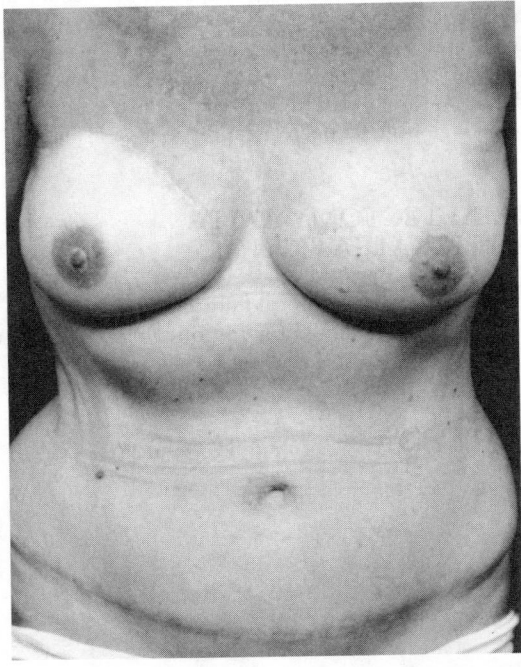

FIGURE 33.3-9. Right breast reconstruction after mastectomy for failed breast-conservation therapy with a unipedicled transverse rectus abdominus myocutaneous (TRAM) flap. The skin island on the TRAM flap has been used to replace the radiated skin from the breast mound.

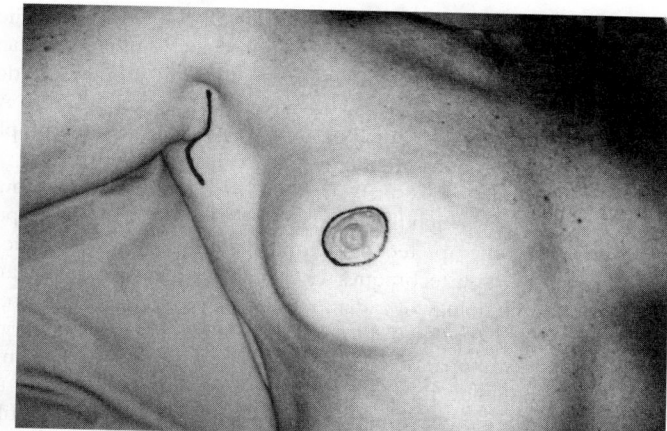

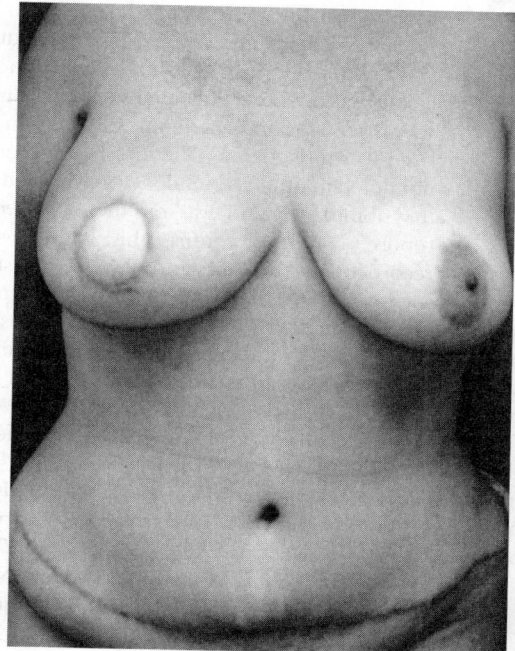

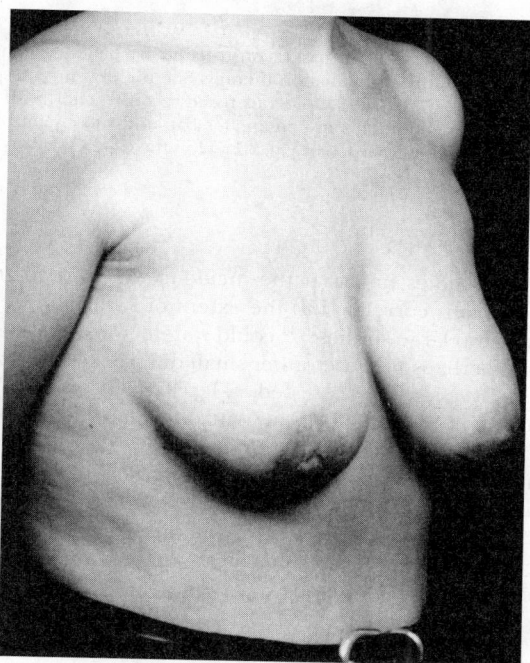

FIGURE 33.3-10.   A: Design of circumareolar incision for complete skin-sparing mastectomy and axillary counter-incision for exposure of lymph nodes and blood vessels. **B:** Complete skin-sparing mastectomy with free transverse rectus abdominus myocutaneous (TRAM) flap and reconstruction before nipple-areola reconstruction in another patient. **C:** Right breast reconstruction with a free TRAM flap after complete skin-sparing mastectomy. The patient has undergone right nipple-areola reconstruction and tattooing. Using this complete skin-sparing approach, the periareolar mastectomy incision is barely visible.

LYMPHEDEMA

Aside from recurrence, lymphedema is the most dreaded sequela of breast cancer treatment. The appearance of arm swelling is more distressing than that of a mastectomy. The disfigured arm or hand is a constant reminder of the disease to the woman herself and a subject of curiosity to others.

Lymphedema results from functional overload of the lymphatic system in which lymph volume exceeds transport capabilities. The buildup of interstitial macromolecules leads to an increase in oncotic pressure in the tissues, producing more edema. The accumulation of debris, specifically protein, triggers the recruitment of neutrophils, macrophages, and fibroblasts into the edematous area. Chronic, low-grade inflammation develops, leading to the deposition of disorganized collagen fibers and fibrosis. The resultant tethering and constriction of lymph-collecting vessels undermines their transport capacity, further aggravating lymph stasis. Stagnant protein provides an excellent culture medium for bacteria. With dilatation of the lymphatics, the valves become incompetent, causing further stasis. The overlying skin becomes metaplastic, with dermal keratinification and papillomas developing. The muscle compartments below the fascia are spared.

In a comprehensive literature review, the overall incidence of lymphedema after breast cancer treatment was estimated at 26%.[32] The incidence of the seven selected reports based on modern treatment varies from 6% to 30%.[33] In the author's study (J. A. P.)[34] based on a cohort of 20-year breast cancer survivors treated consecutively between 1977 and 1979 at Memorial Sloan-Kettering Cancer Center, the incidence of measurable lymphedema was 31%. Perhaps a half million women in the United States alone cope daily with the disfigurement, discomfort, and disability of arm and hand swelling. The reporting of lymphedema has varied greatly and depends in part on the methods used to define it, the completeness of the patient population follow-up, and the interval between axillary treatment and measurement. The denominator, the number of patients at risk for development of lymphedema in a particular population, is often imprecise or unknown.

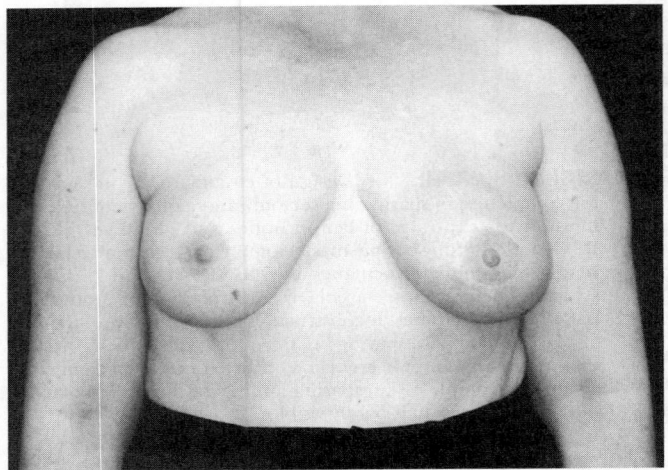

FIGURE 33.3-11. Left breast reconstruction in a patient who has had previous lumpectomy and radiation therapy. She underwent skin-sparing mastectomy and immediate autologous tissue reconstruction with a free transverse rectus abdominus myocutaneous flap and subsequent nipple-areola reconstruction. (See Color Fig. 33.3-11 in the CD-ROM.)

ETIOLOGIC FACTORS

Almost all studies find that the incidence and the degree of lymphedema is correlated to the extent of surgical dissection. However, two large studies[35,36] could not demonstrate this relationship, perhaps because rather small differences in extent of axillary dissection were assessed. A level I to II or even I-II-III dissection for staging and local control is undertaken for typical cancers with positive lymph nodes, and the scope of the dissection can be fitted to the disease. Regardless of the number of lymph nodes excised, surgeons should attempt to carefully preserve the fatty axillary tissue containing the invisible lymphatic trunks around the vein and to dissect the tissue only inferior to the axillary vein.

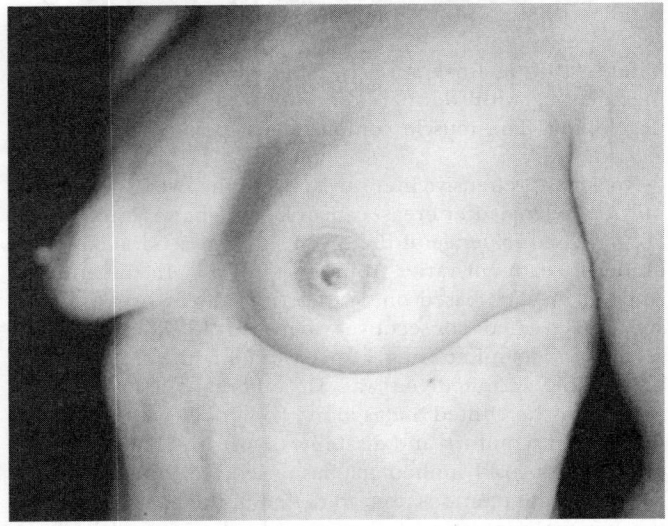

FIGURE 33.3-12. Left breast reconstruction after complete skin-sparing mastectomy with a pedicled transverse rectus abdominus myocutaneous flap and subsequent nipple-areola reconstruction using a local flap followed by tattooing.

Radiotherapy to the dissected axilla is a strong predictor of lymphedema. Although other studies have found greatly increased incidence, one report noted that axillary radiation merely doubled the risk of lymphedema over axillary dissection alone.[37] Axillary radiotherapy can usually be avoided, even in cases of multiple positive lymph nodes, after a full axillary dissection.

Nevertheless, even with only breast-field radiotherapy, some dosage may reach the dissected level I or even II area, depending on radiotherapy technique and patient anatomy. Specific breast radiotherapy techniques to avoid the dissected axilla and the pathophysiology of radiation-related lymphedema were reviewed in 1998.[38] It is helpful to indicate the extent of the axillary dissection by radiopaque clips so that the surgical boundary is marked. The radiation therapist can then more accurately avoid the dissected area, because it will be seen on the simulation films. In series reporting axillary radiotherapy but no axillary surgery at all, lymphedema incidence ranged from 2% to 5%.[38]

Beyond these two definite factors—extent of surgical dissection and radiation to the axilla—a wide range of possible etiologic factors has not been evaluated systematically. Older age at diagnosis was reported to be a significant factor in one study,[39] was unrelated to lymphedema incidence in another,[40] and, curiously, was not noted in others. A tendency to lymphedema was evident when the dominant hand was on the operated side,[41] but another report[40] could not confirm this. Patient weight (height was not recorded) was a significant factor in two studies,[35,42] but obesity, surprisingly, was not evaluated in other studies. In the author's (J. A. P.) cohort study of 20-year survivors,[43] not only obesity at diagnosis but also amount of weight gain after breast cancer treatment was significantly associated with lymphedema development. It is surprising that the incidence of lymphedema after bilateral axillary dissection is not any higher than after unilateral axillary dissection.[34,44]

Many reports have now shown very low lymphedema rates after sentinel lymph node biopsy versus axillary dissection: the Mayo Clinic,[45] 6% versus 34%; Chicago,[46] 2.6% versus 27.0%; Innsbruck, Austria,[47] 3.5% versus 27.1%; and Northwestern,[48] 3% versus 17%. Sentinel lymph node biopsy unquestionably has a small but definite risk of lymphedema. The lymphedema trunks are a bridge of lymph flow from the arm to the rest of the body. The "bridge" may be destroyed when a specific small segment is dissected, as is possible in a sentinel lymph node biopsy, if the lymph node is close to the trunk, although the chance of injuring the lymphatic trunk is higher with an extensive procedure such as axillary dissection.

PREVENTION OF LYMPHEDEMA AFTER AXILLARY TREATMENT

Because controlling lymphedema requires daily attention, and because "curing" lymphedema has not been accomplished, emphasis must be placed on prevention. Nevertheless, without evidence-based knowledge of etiologic factors, the list of posttreatment arm precautions is based on intuitive reasoning. As a background, it is important to remember that each woman has a congenitally different anatomy, which also is probably uniquely prone to degenerative and other conditions, similar to the remainder of the vascular system. This has been studied thus far in a limited fashion with lymphoscintigraphy.[49] The individual patient factors, combined with surgical and radiation treatment factors, must be the main determinants, notwithstanding the fact that lymphedema may occur several years after treatment. Events or activities, such as exercise, and hand infections have been the foundation of arm and hand precautions in the subsequent years and decades.

Arm and hand precautions are loosely based on two overarching principles: (1) Do not increase lymph production, which is directly proportional to blood flow, and (2) do not increase blockage to lymph transport. Heat (such as that in a sauna), significant infections, and vigorous arm exercise increase blood flow in the arm and thereby increase lymph production. Obstruction of lymph flow may result from tight arm garments or from infections, with ensuing fibrosis and stenosis of lymphatic vessels.

The patient is instructed as follows:

1. Avoid puncturing or injuring the skin in any way. Use meticulous skin and nail/cuticle care. Pay immediate attention and use standard first-aid care.
2. Avoid vaccinations, injections, blood pressure monitoring, blood drawing, and intravenous administration in that arm.
3. Avoid constricting sleeves or jewelry, and wear a padded bra strap (to avoid supraclavicular area compression).
4. Avoid heat, such as with sunburns or tanning, baths, and saunas.
5. Avoid violent exercises and strenuous exertion. Consider vigorous aerobic arm exercise only when compression garments support the arm.

No data exist to govern any of these recommendations. After axillary treatment patients regularly ask their clinicians about the wisdom of pursuing specific "high-risk" leisure activities or occupations with the possibility of skin injuries, such as gardening or cooking. In the author's (J. A. P.) retrospective study of lymphedema in a cohort of 20-year breast cancer survivors, high- versus low-risk occupations were not associated with lymphedema.[34] Although it may be interpreted that these activities do not have a large causative role in the group that developed measurable lymphedema, because of the study design, an effect could exist and be undetected.

More research is needed, because after axillary dissection all patients are instructed in the arm and hand care precautions, which may be too severe for those at low risk and yet not aggressive enough for those at highest risk. Because lymphedema development may occur even several decades[50] after the axillary treatment, patients are admonished to follow these demanding precautions for the remainder of their lives.

LYMPHEDEMA TREATMENTS

Therapeutic nihilism (i.e., no treatment at all) is deplorable, although common. The fact that the average clinician is ill prepared to recognize early signs of lymphedema must be remedied, because the sooner the treatment is started, the less treatment is required to prevent further progression. Treatment approaches that do not lead to the establishment of a comprehensive maintenance program will ultimately fail. Patients and family members must acquire skills for successful long-term maintenance.

Manual Lymphatic Drainage

Manual lymphatic drainage (MLD) is a highly specialized massage technique designed to decrease the sequestration and enhance transport of lymph. Specific stroke duration, orientation, pressure, and sequence characterize MLD. Through gentle, rhythmic skin distention, congested lymph is directed through residual components of the lymphatic system into intact nodal basins. MLD permits elimination of congested truncal lymph by shifting it to lymphotomes with preserved drainage. Fluid accumulating along the proximal border of bandaged limbs can be redistributed to areas with intact drainage and eventually resorbed.

From a physiologic perspective, MLD stimulates the intrinsic contractility of the lymph collectors. MLD reduces the protein concentration within the congested lymphotomes (somatic tissue drained by a particular lymph node bed) through massage techniques, such as stroking (effleurage), percussion (tapotement), or compression (pétrissage). Although European types of massage may promote improvement in overall circulatory response, they use stronger tissue pressures to manipulate superficial and deep tissues and are not selective to superficial lymphatics and regional lymph nodes. Additionally, MLD techniques emphasize drainage of lymph via lympho-lymphatic anastomoses (axillo-axillary, axillo-inguinal, inguino-inguinal) across regions of the trunk and back referred to as *watersheds*. MLD emphasizes the "clearance" of regional lymph nodal areas before massage of the cutaneous lymphatics located in the dermis of the skin. The massage is very light and superficial, limited to finger/hand pressures of, ideally, approximately 30 to 45 mm Hg.

MLD is incorporated in a sequential treatment approach to be combined with compression bandages, exercises, skin care, pressure gradient sleeves, and pneumatic pumps, depending on the severity/stage of the lymphedema. Many in the field have adopted the term *complete decongestive therapy* or *complex decongestive physiotherapy* to describe this multimodality approach to the treatment of lymphedema. A variety of health care professionals have completed courses to acquire the knowledge, skills, and ability to provide this clinical treatment. Organizations such as the American Cancer Society, National Lymphedema Network, National Cancer Institute, Lymphology Association of North America, Lymphatic Research Foundation, International Congress of Lymphology, and Oncology Nursing Society have been supportive of the clinical, research, and educational effort to promote the clinical and applied research necessary to establish the efficacy of MLD and other lymphedema management techniques.

Compression Garments/Bandaging

External compression therapy is a cornerstone of management. It increases tissue pressure, improves venous and lymphatic return, and facilitates filling of the initial lymph vessels. Compression also provides counter pressure against the muscle pump and helps mobilize protein in the tissue of fibrotic limbs.

Compression bandaging uses short-stretch "nonelastic" bandages that have a high working pressure and exert force on the underlying, working musculature[51,52] and low pressure while the musculature is resting. Long-stretch (elastic Ace bandages) do not have these characteristics and can be harmful because they can produce a tourniquet effect that obstructs blood and lymph flow.

Compression garments are essential to maintain edema reduction, skin integrity, and suppleness and to compensate for the elastic insufficiency of the skin after volume reduction. Compression garments (1) improve lymphatic flow and reduce accumulated protein, (2) improve venous return, (3) properly shape and reduce the size of the limb, (4) maintain skin integrity, and (5) protect the limb from potential trauma. Ideally, compression garments should be measured and fitted by a certified lymphedema therapist who will determine the appropriate style and compression class. Presized standard garments are less expensive but must fit well. Ill-fitted garments can worsen existing lymphedema and demoralize the patient. For upper extremity lymphedema, a class II (30 to 40 mm Hg) or III (40 to 50 mm Hg) support is generally required. A statistically significant reduction in edema has been reported in women who wore garments for 6 consecutive hours per day.[53] Use of these garments during exercise, physical activity, and air travel is strongly recommended.

Pneumatic Compression Devices

Pneumatic compression devices, sometimes called *pumps*, are commonly used. Contraindications include acute deep vein thrombosis and infection. In general, these devices function by applying either uniform pressure or multiple "graded" pressures to an extremity over a timed cycle. Pressures available range from 0 to 300 mm Hg. Results from animal studies conducted during the early 1980s suggested that experimentally induced pressures of 60 mm Hg and greater tended to promote collapse of the lymphatic vessels, and the therapeutic range is 30 to 60 mm Hg.[54] Some have argued that pumps are ineffective and harmful.[54]

The pneumatic sleeve is basically an air bladder of either single-compartment or multiple-compartment design attached to the pump. Multiple-compartment sleeves inflate in a sequential and distal to proximal manner. The intent is to promote a "pneumatic massage" effect. A few studies have investigated the physiologic effectiveness of these devices and have confirmed distal to proximal translocation of lymph.[55] Literature comparing the effectiveness of one device versus another remains scant.

MEDICATIONS

Diuretics are not effective in high-protein edemas such as lymphedema. Although the diuretics can temporarily mobilize water, the osmotic pressure from the increased protein in the interstitial space causes rapid reaccumulation of edema.

Benzopyrones belong to a group of drugs that include the bioflavonoids and the coumarins. The former occurs widely in nature, especially in fruits and vegetables. Benzopyrones may improve chronic lymphedema by stimulating macrophage activity for increased proteolysis and thereby removal of stagnant, excess protein in the tissue spaces, which results in less oncotic pressure and edema fluid. In 1993, a randomized, double-blind, placebo-controlled, crossover trial of 5,6-benzo-α-pyrone demonstrated its efficacy in an Australian study.[56] Although the effect was mild, it was statistically significant. However, in a similar study design, a larger number of breast cancer patients in an American multicenter study led by the Mayo Clinic were reported in 1999. No value was found with the benzopyrone beyond the placebo effect.[57] Furthermore, 6% of these study subjects had serious elevation of liver function tests.

REFERENCES

1. Hart SS, Meyerowitz BE, Apolone G, et al. Quality of life among mastectomy patients using external breast prostheses. *Tumori* 1997;83:581.
2. Reaby LL. Breast restoration decision making: enhancing the process. *Cancer Nurs* 1998;21:196.
3. Georgiade G, Georgiade N, McCarty KS Jr, Seigler HF. Rationale for immediate reconstruction of the breast following modified radical mastectomy. *Ann Plast Surg* 1982;8:20.
4. Khoo A, Kroll SS, Reece GP, et al. A comparison of resource costs of immediate and delayed breast reconstruction. *Plast Reconstr Surg* 1998;101:964.
5. Elliot LF, Hartrampf CR Jr. Breast reconstruction: progress in the past decade. *World J Surg* 1990;14:763.
6. Gruber RP, Kahn RA, Lash H, Maser MR. Breast reconstruction following mastectomy: a comparison of submuscular and subcutaneous techniques. *Plast Reconstr Surg* 1981;67:312.
7. Asplund O. Capsular contracture in silicone gel and saline filled breast implants after reconstruction. *Plast Reconstr Surg* 1984;73:270.
8. Disa JJ, Ad-El DD, Cohen SM, et al. The premature removal of tissue expanders in breast reconstruction. *Plast Reconstr Surg* 1999;104:1662.
9. Gabriel SE, O'Fallon WM, Kurland LT, et al. Risk of connective-tissue diseases and other disorders after breast implantation. *N Engl J Med* 1994;330:1697.
10. Spear SL, Mardini S. Alternative filler materials and new implant designs: what's available and what's on the horizon? *Clin Plast Surg* 2001;28:435.
11. Heden P, Jernbeck J, Hober M. Breast augmentation with anatomical cohesive gel implants: the world's largest current experience. *Clin Plast Surg* 2001;28:531.
12. Bostwick J III, Scheflan M. The latissimus dorsi musculocutaneous flap: a one stage breast reconstruction. *Clin Plast Surg* 1980;7:71.
13. Hartrampf CR, Scheflan M, Black PW. Breast reconstruction with a transverse abdominal island flap. *Plast Reconstr Surg* 1982;69:216.
14. Grotting JC, Urist MM, Maddox WA, Vasconez LO. Conventional TRAM flap versus free microsurgical TRAM flap for immediate breast reconstruction. *Plast Reconstr Surg* 1989; 83:828.
15. Kroll SS, Netscher DT. Complications of TRAM flap breast reconstruction in obese patients. *Plast Reconstr Surg* 1989;84:886.
16. Hidalgo DA, Disa JJ, Cordeiro PG, Hu Q. A review of 716 consecutive free flaps for oncologic surgical defects: refinement in donor-site selection and technique. *Plast Reconstr Surg* 1998;102:722.
17. Schusterman MA, Kroll SS, Miller MJ, et al. The free transverse rectus abdominus musculocutaneous flap for breast reconstruction: one center's experience with 211 consecutive cases. *Ann Plast Surg* 1994;32:234.
18. Kind GM, Rademaker AW, Mustoe TA. Abdominal-wall recovery following TRAM flap: a functional outcome study. *Plast Reconstr Surg* 1997;99:417.
19. Reece GP, Kroll SS. Abdominal wall complications: prevention and treatment. *Clin Plast Surg* 1998;25:235.
20. Craigie JE, Allen RJ, DellaCroce FJ, Sullivan SK. Autogenous breast reconstruction with the deep inferior epigastric perforator flap. *Clin Plast Surg* 2003;30:359.
21. Nahabedian MY, Momen B, Galdino G, Manson PN. Breast reconstruction with the free TRAM or DIEP flap: patient selection, choice of flap, and outcome. *Plast Reconstr Surg* 2002;110:466.
22. Futter CM, Webster MH, Hagen S, Mitchell SL. A retrospective comparison of abdominal muscle strength following breast reconstruction with a free TRAM or DIEP flap. *Br J Plast Surg* 2000;53:578.
23. Blondeel PN, Van Landuyt K, Hamdi M, Monstrey SJ. Soft tissue reconstruction with the superior gluteal artery perforator flap. *Clin Plast Surg* 2003;30:371.
24. Disa JJ, Petrek JA. Surgical management after local failure in the irradiated breast. *Semin Breast Dis* 1999;2:252.
25. Schuster RH, Kuske RR, Young VL, Fineberg B. Breast reconstruction in women treated with radiation therapy for breast cancer: cosmesis, complications, and tumor control. *Plast Reconstr Surg* 1992;90:445.
26. Kroll SS, Schusterman MA, Reece GP, et al. Breast reconstruction with myocutaneous flaps in previously irradiated patients. *Plast Reconstr Surg* 1994;93:460.
27. Williams JK, Bostwick J III, Bried JT, et al. TRAM flap breast reconstruction after radiation treatment. *Ann Surg* 1995;221:756.
28. Williams JK, Carlson GW, Bostwick J III, et al. The effects of radiation treatment after TRAM flap breast reconstruction. *Plast Reconstr Surg* 1997;100:1153.
29. Hidalgo DA, Borgen PJ, Petrek JA, et al. Immediate reconstruction after complete skin-sparing mastectomy with autologous tissue. *J Am Coll Surg* 1998;187:17.
30. Toth BA, Forley BG, Calabria R. Retrospective study of skin-sparing mastectomy in breast reconstruction. *Plast Reconstr Surg* 1999;104:77.
31. Carlson GW, Bostwick J III, Styblo TM, et al. Skin-sparing mastectomy: oncologic and reconstructive considerations. *Ann Surg* 1997;225:570.
32. Erickson VS, Pearson ML, Ganz PA, Adams J, Kahn KL. Arm edema in breast cancer patients. *J Natl Cancer Inst* 2001;93:96.
33. Petrek JA, Heelan MC. Incidence of breast carcinoma-related lymphedema. *Cancer* 1998;83:2776.
34. Petrek JA, Senie RT, Peters M, Rosen PP. Lymphedema in a cohort of breast carcinoma survivors 20 years after diagnosis. *Cancer* 2001;92:1368.
35. Werner RS, McCormick B, Petrek JA, et al. Arm edema in conservatively managed breast cancer: obesity is a major predictive factor. *Radiology* 1991;180:177.
36. Dewar JA, Sarrazin D, Benhamou E, et al. Management of the axilla in conservatively treated breast cancer: 592 patients treated at Institut Gustave-Roussy. *Int J Radiat Oncol Biol Phys* 1987;13:475.
37. Powell SN, Taghian AG, Kachnic LA, Coen JJ, Assaad SI. Risk of lymphedema after regional nodal irradiation with breast conservation therapy. *Int J Radiat Oncol Biol Phys* 2003;55:1209.
38. Meek AG. Breast radiotherapy and lymphedema. *Cancer* 1998;83:2788.
39. Delouche G, Bachelot F, Premont M, et al. Conservation treatment of early breast cancer: long term results and complications. *Int J Radiat Oncol Biol Phys* 1987;13:29.
40. Kissin MW, Querci della Rovere G, Easton D, et al. Risk of lymphoedema following the treatment of breast cancer. *Br J Surg* 1986;73:580.

41. Ivens D, Hoe AL, Podd CR, et al. Assessment of morbidity from complete axillary dissection. *Br J Cancer* 1992;66:136.

42. Larson D, Weinstein M, Goldberg I, et al. Edema of the arm as a function of the extent of axillary surgery in patients with stage I–II carcinoma of the breast treated with primary radiotherapy. *Int J Radiat Oncol Biol Phys* 1986;12:1575.

43. Petrek JA, Senie RT, Peters M, Rosen PP. Lymphedema in a cohort of breast carcinoma survivors 20 years after diagnosis. *Cancer* 2001;92:1368.

44. Mortimer PS, Bates SO, Brassington HD, et al. The prevalence of arm lymphedema following treatment for breast cancer. *QJM* 1996;89:377.

45. Blanchard DK, Donohue JH, Reynolds C, Grant CS. Relapse and morbidity in patients undergoing sentinel lymph node biopsy alone or with axillary dissection for breast cancer. *Arch Surg* 2003;138:482.

46. Martin GM, Dowlatshahi K. Sentinel lymph node biopsy lowers the rate of lymphedema when compared with standard axillary lymph node dissection. *Am Surg* 2003;69:209.

47. Haid A, Koberle-Wuhrer R, Knauer M, et al. Morbidity of breast cancer patients following complete axillary dissection or sentinel node biopsy only: a comparative evaluation. *Breast Cancer Res Treat* 2002;73:31.

48. Sener SF, Winchester DJ, Martz CH, et al. Lymphedema after sentinel lymphadenectomy for breast carcinoma. *Cancer* 2001;92:748.

49. Bourgeois P, Leduc O, Leduc A. Imaging techniques in the upper management and prevention of posttherapeutic upper limb edemas. *Cancer* 1998;83:2805.

50. Brennan MJ, Weitz J. Lymphedema 30 years after radical mastectomy. *Am J Phys Med Rehabil* 1992;71:12.

51. Partsch H. Do we need firm compression stocking exerting high pressure? *Vasa* 1984;13:52.

52. Stemmer R, Marescaux J, Furderer C. Compression therapy of the lower extremities particularly with compression stockings. *Hautarzt* 1980;31:355.

53. Bertelli G, Venturini M, Forno G, et al. An analysis of prognostic factors in response to conservative treatment of postmastectomy lymphedema. *Surg Gynecol Obstet* 1992;175:455.

54. Leduc O, Leduc A, Bourgeois P, Belgrado JP. The physical treatment of upper limb edema. *Cancer* 1998;83:2835.

55. Mridha M, Odman S. Fluid translocation measurement: a method to study pneumatic compression treatment of postmastectomy lymphoedema. *Scand J Rehabil Med* 1989;21:63.

56. Casley-Smith JR, Morgan RG, Piller NB. Treatment of lymphedema of the arms and legs with 5,6-benzo-[alpha]-pyrone. *N Engl J Med* 1993;16:1158.

57. Loprinzi CL, Kugler JW, Sloan JA, et al. Lack of effect of coumarin in women with lymphedema after treatment for breast cancer. *N Engl J Med* 1999;340:346.

CHAPTER 34

Cancer of the Endocrine System

TERRY C. LAIRMORE
JEFFREY F. MOLEY

SECTION **1**

Molecular Biology of Endocrine Tumors

The transformation of a cell from the normal to the malignant phenotype is a result of a stepwise accumulation of genetic defects that render the cell unresponsive to or independent of normal cellular growth signals. In recent years, defects in a variety of oncogenes and tumor suppressor genes have been described in endocrine neoplasms. Characterization of these specific molecular defects has yielded insight into the mechanisms of tumorigenesis in these tissues and in some cases provided clinically applicable diagnostic or prognostic information. Identification of the germline mutations associated with the multiple endocrine neoplasia (MEN) types 1 and 2 syndromes has led to the advent of direct DNA testing for individuals at risk. In patients with a hereditary form of medullary thyroid carcinoma (MTC), early thyroidectomy can be performed based on DNA mutational analysis at a time when the MTC is occult and likely curable. Finally, the molecular defects that occur in tumors arising in the familial endocrine neoplasia syndromes have been found to play an important role in tumorigenesis of sporadic neoplasms arising in the same endocrine tissues.

MULTIPLE ENDOCRINE NEOPLASIA SYNDROMES

CLINICAL FEATURES OF MULTIPLE ENDOCRINE NEOPLASIA TYPE 1

MEN type 1 (MEN 1) is characterized by the development of parathyroid neoplasms, neuroendocrine tumors of the pancreas and duodenum, and adenomas of the anterior pituitary gland.[1] In addition, bronchial and thymic carcinoids, benign thyroid and adrenocortical tumors, subcutaneous lipomas, cutaneous angiofibromas,[2] and spinal ependymomas[3] develop in affected patients with increased frequency. In greater than 90% of patients who inherit an *MEN1* gene mutation, hyperparathyroidism (HPT) develops by the second or third decade of life. Depending on the method of study, neuroendocrine tumors of the pancreas and duodenum that are frequently malignant develop in 35% to 75% of mutation carriers. The neuroendocrine tumors in patients with MEN 1 result in symptoms either due to excess secretion of a specific hormone product or the effects of the tumoral process itself. The malignant duodenopancreatic tumors and intrathoracic tumors account for the majority of the disease-related morbidity and mortality in patients affected with MEN 1.[4]

GENETICS OF MULTIPLE ENDOCRINE NEOPLASIA TYPE 1

MEN1 *Tumor Suppressor Gene*

The *MEN1* disease gene maps to chromosome 11q13.[5] *MEN1* is a classic tumor suppressor gene that requires "two hits" or inac-

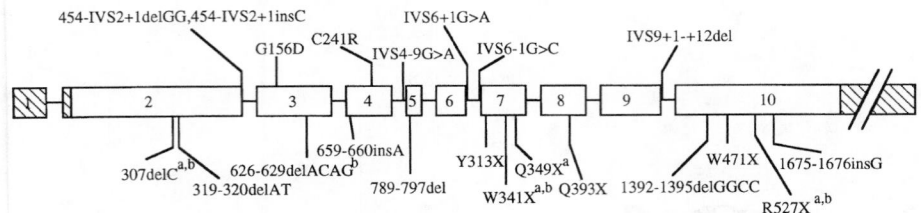

FIGURE 34.1-1. Germline mutations in the *MEN1* gene in a set of 25 independent kindreds. The mutations are distributed throughout the nine coding exons of the gene. Five splicing defects and two missense mutations are depicted above the *MEN1* gene, and seven nonsense and six frameshift mutations are depicted below the *MEN1* gene. The position of the mutation is reported as the codon in which it occurs relative to the open reading frame. The position of the splicing defects are reported as the number of bases 3' or 5' to the nearest exon [(+) indicates 3' direction and (–) indicates 5' direction relative to the exon]. For the deletions, insertions, and splicing defects, upper case letters refer to exon nucleotides and lowercase letters refer to intron nucleotides. a, previously reported mutations; b, mutations that occur in more than one family. (From ref. 10, with permission.)

tivation of both allelic copies of the gene for tumor initiation. One mutation is inherited in the germline, and a second genetic event occurs with an individual somatic cell to result in tumor formation. The frequent occurrence of chromosome deletions encompassing the 11q13 interval in tumor DNA supports the model of *MEN1* as a classic tumor suppressor gene. The multifocal involvement characteristically observed in affected endocrine tissues presumably reflects the chance occurrence of multiple "second hits."

The diverse array of reported *MEN1* mutations are distributed throughout the nine coding exons as well as the intervening intronic sequences. To date, more than 200 independent mutations have been described in the *MEN1* gene. Therefore, there are almost as many unique mutations as there are genetically independent families. The mutations may be nonsense, missense, frameshift, deletions, or even RNA splicing defects.[6–10] The *MEN1* gene mutations in a series of 33 separate kindreds with MEN 1 are depicted graphically in Figure 34.1-1. Approximately two-thirds of the reported mutations in the *MEN1* gene result in truncation of the C-terminal portion of the menin protein. No specific genotype-phenotype correlations have been established to date. Genetic testing is available in selected centers with certain limitations. The detection is simplified if the disease-associated mutation in the family of interest is known from previous research studies. In a new family with an unknown mutation, a comprehensive search of the coding sequence and intron-exon junctions is necessary, which may be more involved. Formal genetic counseling and informed consent with regard to privacy of medical information as well as how the information will be used is essential to a comprehensive program of direct genetic testing.

Cellular Biology of Menin Protein Product

The *MEN1* gene is comprised of ten exons spanning 9 kb of genomic DNA and encodes a 610 amino acid protein product termed *menin*.[6] The 2.8-kb menin messenger RNA is ubiquitously expressed in endocrine and in nonendocrine tissues. Menin is highly conserved among human, mouse (98%), and rat (97%) and more distantly among zebra fish (75%) and *Drosophila* (47%).[11–14] However, database analysis of menin protein sequence reveals no significant homology to other known protein families. No known homologue is present in the bud-

ding yeast *Saccharomyces* or the worm *Caenorhabditis elegans*. In the mouse embryo, *MEN1* expression appears as early as gestational day 7 and ultimately is detectable at high levels in diverse tissues, including the testis and the central nervous system. These findings support a broad role for the menin protein product in the regulation of cell growth that is not limited to the tissues affected in MEN 1.

Menin is predominately a nuclear protein[15] that binds to the JunD, a member of the AP-1 transcription factor family, and represses JunD-mediated transcription.[16,17] This finding seems paradoxic given the antimitogenic properties of JunD itself. In addition, menin has been shown to interact physically with a variety of other proteins (Smad3, NFκB, nm23, and others; Table 34.1-1).[18–20] The putative tumor suppressor role and predominantly nuclear localization of menin imply a role in the cell cycle. However, there have been contradicting reports about cell-cycle regulation of menin expression.[12,21] Nevertheless, the regulation of the function of menin by posttranscriptional modifications still remains a possibility.

Lymphocytes from patients with a heterozygous germline mutation in the *MEN1* gene have been shown to exhibit increased premature centromere division in cell culture when exposed to an alkylating agent.[22] The finding of increased chromosomal instability suggests that the *MEN1* gene product may normally function in part to maintain the integrity of DNA. Two groups[23,24] have explored the interaction between menin and telomeres, the latter playing an important role in chromosomal stability. Suphapeetiporn et al.[23] have demon-

TABLE 34.1-1. Menin-Interacting Proteins

Name	Nature	Reference(s)
JunD	Transcription factor	16,17
Smad3	Transcription factor	18
NFκB	Transcription factor	19
nm23	Putative tumor suppressor	20
RPA2	DNA replication	142
GFAP and vimentin	Type III IF proteins	143
NMHC II-A	Nonmuscle myosin	144
mSin3A histone deacetylase	(JunD corepressor)	145
FANCD2	DNA repair (Fanconi's anemia)	146

strated the localization of menin exclusively at telomeres of meiotic chromosomes. Interestingly, JunD does not co-localize with menin. However, menin does not specifically associate with telomeres in somatic cells and does not directly regulate telomerase activity. In contrast, Lin and Elledge[24] claim menin to be a direct repressor of telomerase. They have also demonstrated the ability of primary human fibroblasts to immortalize on depletion of menin. These immortalized cells are susceptible to transformation by the expression of SV40 T antigens and oncogenic RAS. To date, the collective studies on the function of menin have not yielded a clear picture of its role in endocrine tumorigenesis.

ANIMAL MODEL FOR MULTIPLE ENDOCRINE NEOPLASIA TYPE 1

Complete inactivation of *Men1* in mice is embryonically lethal; *Men1*−/− mice die *in utero* at embryonic days 11.5 to 12.5. However, features very similar to those of patients with the MEN 1 syndrome develop in heterozygous *Men1*+/− mice.[25] As early as 9 months, pancreatic islets develop a range of lesions from hyperplasia to insulin-producing islet cell tumors. In addition to parathyroid and pituitary adenomas that are characteristic of MEN 1, tumors of thyroid and adrenal cortex are also seen by 16 months. A high incidence of gonadal tumors of endocrine origin, such as Leydig cell tumors and ovary sex cord–stromal cell tumors, have also been noted in heterozygous *Men1* mutant mice. Importantly, loss of the wild-type *Men1* allele can be demonstrated in tumor DNA from each of these lesions, further supporting the role of *Men1* as a tumor suppressor gene.

Embryonic lethality of *Men1* null mutant mice suggests a critical role(s) for menin during development. Characterization of *Men1* null mutant embryos revealed a smaller body size, with evidence of hemorrhage and extensive edema. A significant number of animals demonstrate failure of complete closure of the neural tube. Moreover, abnormal development of the nervous system and heart was also observed in some Men1 null embryos. Furthermore, *Men1* null livers generally exhibited an altered organization of the epithelial and hematopoietic compartments associated with enhanced apoptosis.[26]

To overcome the limitations on the studies of *Men1* null mice imposed by the embryonic lethal phenotype, *Cre-lox*–mediated, tissue-specific, conditional *Men1* knockout mice have been created.[26] The loss of *Men1* alleles in the pancreatic beta cells results in the earlier development of islet tumors as compared to the *Men1* heterozygous mice. The Men1-inactivated islet cells progressively become hyperplastic, atypical, and adenomatous. The delay in tumor appearance, even with early loss of both copies of Men1, suggests the involvement of additional somatic events for adenoma formation in beta cells. Initial characterization of these mice has revealed the duplication of chromosome 11 and altered expression of E-cadherin and β-catenin.

Despite the diverse findings above, the exact mechanism(s) by which menin exerts its tumor suppressor function in neuroendocrine tissues still remains unknown. One major step in this pursuit has been the development of a near-identical mouse model. Notwithstanding the subtle differences in the tumor formation between mice and humans, these mice provide an excellent system to explore further the function(s) of menin.

CLINICAL FEATURES OF THE MULTIPLE ENDOCRINE NEOPLASIA TYPE 2 SYNDROMES

The MEN 2 syndromes include MEN 2A, MEN 2B, and familial, non-MEN MTC (FMTC). These syndromes are inherited in an autosomal dominant fashion and are caused by germline mutations in the *RET* protooncogene. The most consistent feature of MEN 2 syndromes is MTC, which is multifocal and bilateral and usually occurs at a young age (Fig. 34.1-2). Almost complete penetrance of MTC occurs in these syndromes. Other features of the syndromes are variably expressed, with incomplete penetrance. These features are summarized in Table 34.1-2.

MTCs are derived from the thyroid C cells, also called *parafollicular cells*. C cells secrete the hormone calcitonin, a specific tumor marker for MTC. Measurement of calcitonin levels is useful in the screening of individuals predisposed to the hereditary forms of the disease and in the follow-up of patients who have been treated. C cells secrete other hormones and macromolecules, including carcinoembryonic antigen.

Multifocal bilateral MTC, associated with C-cell hyperplasia, develops in patients with MEN 2A. Approximately 42% of affected patients develop pheochromocytomas, which may also be multifocal and bilateral and are usually associated with adrenal medullary hyperplasia. HPT develops in 25% to 35% of patients and is due to hyperplasia, which may be asymmetric, with one or more glands becoming enlarged. Cutaneous lichen amyloidosis (CLA) has been described in some patients with MEN 2A.[27] In this entity, macular amyloidosis presents as brownish plaques of multiple tiny papules, usually in the interscapular area. Hirschsprung's disease (HSCR) occurs in 1% to 2% of patients with MEN 2A.[28–30] This disease is characterized by absence of autonomic ganglion cells within the distal colonic parasympathetic plexus, resulting in obstruction and megacolon.

In MEN 2B, MTC develops at a very young age (infancy) and appears to be the most aggressive form of hereditary MTC, although its aggressiveness may be more related to the extremely early age of onset rather than the biologic virulence of the tumor. Pheochromocytomas develop in 40% to 50% of patients, and all individuals develop neural gangliomas, particularly in the mucosa of the digestive tract, conjunctiva, lips, and tongue. MEN 2B patients also have megacolon, skeletal abnormalities, and markedly enlarged peripheral nerves. HPT does not develop in patients with MEN 2B.

Familial FMTC is characterized by the development of MTC without any other endocrinopathies.[31] MTC in these patients has a later age of onset and a more indolent clinical course than MTC in patients with MEN 2A and MEN 2B. Occasional patients with FMTC never manifest clinical evidence of MTC (symptoms or a lump in the neck), although biochemical testing and histologic evaluation of the thyroid usually demonstrate MTC.

GENETICS OF THE MULTIPLE ENDOCRINE NEOPLASIA TYPE 2 SYNDROMES

RET *Protooncogene*

The *RET* protooncogene was first discovered based on its ability to transform mouse NIH 3T3 fibroblasts in culture.[32] The transforming *RET* sequences first identified represented a rearrangement of *RET* that occurred *in vitro* during the transfection assay.[33] Sequence analysis of the *RET* protooncogene showed that it is a

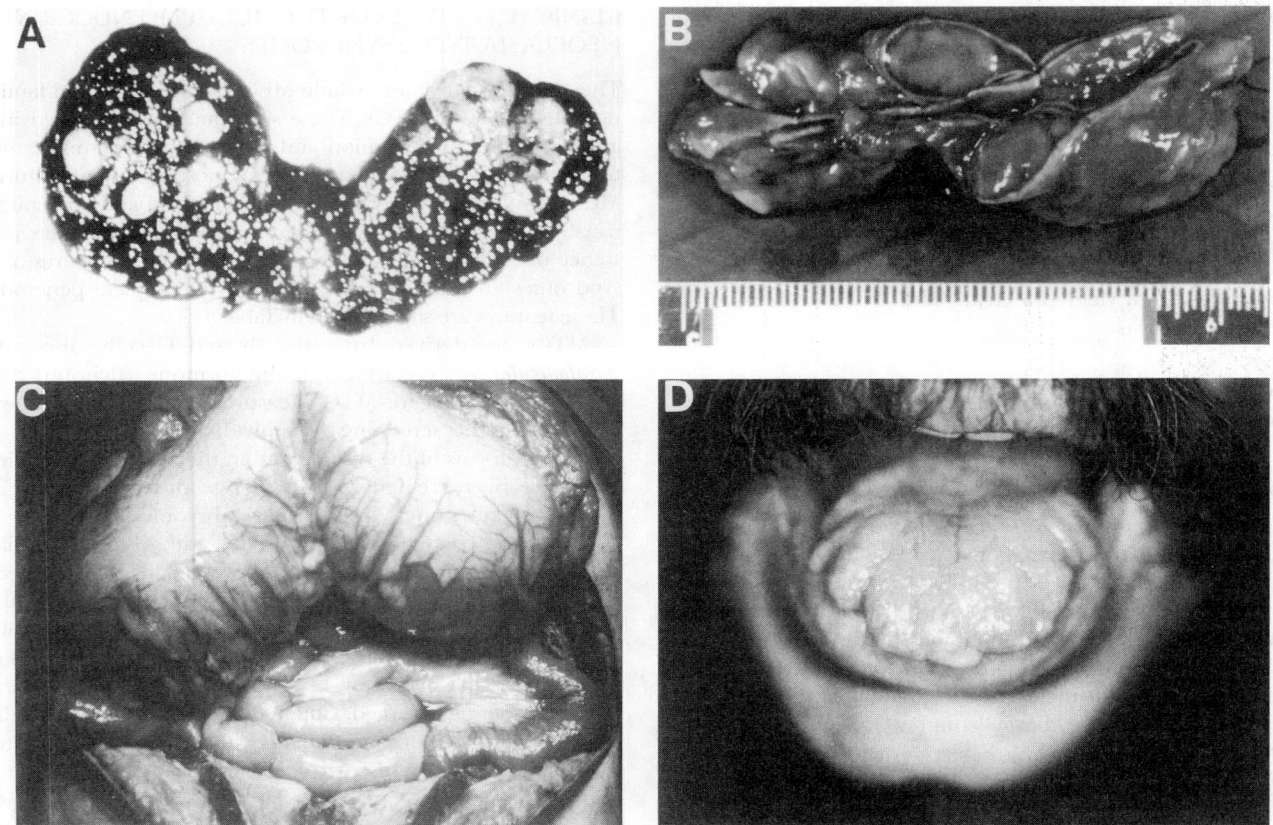

FIGURE 34.1-2.   Features of patients with hereditary medullary thyroid carcinoma (MTC). **A:** Bisected thyroid gland from a patient with multiple endocrine neoplasia (MEN) type 2A showing multicentric, bilateral foci of MTC. **B:** Adrenalectomy specimen from patient with MEN 2B demonstrating pheochromocytoma. **C:** Megacolon in patient with MEN 2B. **D:** Midface and tongue of patient with MEN 2B showing characteristic tongue notching secondary to plexiform neuromas. (**A** courtesy of Dr. S. A. Wells; **B–D** courtesy of Dr. R. Thompson.) (From Moley JF. Medullary thyroid cancer. In: Clark OH, Duh Q-Y, eds. *Textbook of endocrine surgery.* Philadelphia: WB Saunders, 1997, with permission.)

member of the receptor tyrosine kinase gene family (Fig. 34.1-3).[34] *RET* was mapped to the proximal region of the long arm of chromosome 10 in 1989[35] and was shown to be expressed at high levels in MTCs and pheochromocytomas.[36]

In 1987, the gene for MEN 2A was localized to the pericentromeric region of chromosome 10 (10q11.2) by linkage analysis.[37,38] Subsequent studies demonstrated that the predisposition gene for MEN 2B and FMTC mapped to the same region as MEN 2A.[39,40]

TABLE 34.1-2.   Clinical Features of Sporadic MTC, MEN 2A, MEN 2B, and FMTC

Clinical Setting	Features of MTC	Inheritance Pattern	Associated Abnormalities	Genetic Defect
Sporadic MTC	Unifocal	None	None	Somatic *RET* mutations in >20% of tumors
MEN 2A	Multifocal, bilateral	Autosomal dominant	Pheochromocytomas, hyperparathyroidism	Germline missense mutations in extracellular cysteine codons of *RET*
MEN 2B	Multifocal, bilateral	Autosomal dominant	Pheochromocytomas, mucosal neuromas, megacolon, skeletal abnormalities	Germline missense mutation in tyrosine kinase domain of *RET*
FMTC	Multifocal, bilateral	Autosomal dominant	None	Germline missense mutations in extracellular or intracellular cysteine codons of *RET*

FMTC, familial, non-MEN medullary thyroid carcinoma; MEN, multiple endocrine neoplasia; MTC, medullary thyroid carcinoma.
(Adapted from Moley JF. Medullary thyroid cancer. In: Clark OH, Duh Q-Y, eds. *Textbook of endocrine surgery.* Philadelphia: WB Saunders, 1997, with permission.)

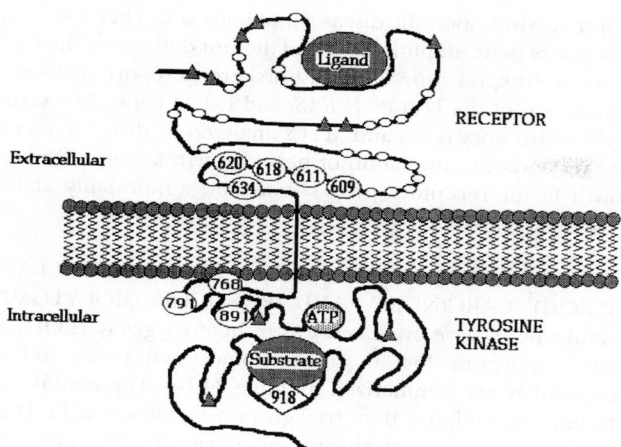

FIGURE 34.1-3. *RET* gene product. Ovals, locations of germline mutations found in multiple endocrine neoplasia (MEN) 2A and familial, non-MEN medullary thyroid carcinoma; diamonds, location of germline mutations in MEN 2B; triangles, location of mutations in hereditary Hirschsprung's disease. As mentioned in the text, the *RET* gene product is thought to form a dimer that is complexed with glial-derived neurotrophic factor receptor-α or neurturin, or both. The *RET* gene product is divided into the intracellular, transmembrane, and extracellular domains. ATP, adenosine triphosphate. (Adapted from Moley J, Kim S. *Molecular genetics in surgical oncology.* Austin: R. G. Landes, 1994.)

TABLE 34.1-3. *RET* Mutations in Hereditary Medullary Thyroid Carcinoma

Syndrome	Missense Germline Mutations in the RET Protooncogene	
	Exon	Codon
MEN 2A, FMTC	10	609
		611
		618
		620
	11	631[a]
		634
	13	790
		791
FMTC	11	630
	13	768
	14	804
		844[a]
	15	891
MEN 2B	16	918
		883

FMTC, familial, non-MEN medullary thyroid carcinoma; MEN, multiple endocrine neoplasia.

[a]Clinical features not yet characterized.

(From Moley JF, Lairmore TC, Phay JE. Hereditary endocrinopathies. *Curr Probl Surg* 1999;36:653, with permission.)

The *RET* protooncogene resides within this critical region, which made it an obvious candidate gene for the MEN 2 syndromes.

RET mutations were identified in the constitutional DNA of MEN 2A and FMTC patients in 1993 (see Fig. 34.1-3).[41,42] MEN 2A and FMTC were shown to be associated with mutations that result in substitution of cysteine residues in the extracellular portion of *RET* immediately adjacent to the transmembrane domain. Unexpectedly, the same mutations were found to characterize MEN 2A and FMTC kindreds. Mulligan et al.[41] suggested a dominant or dominant/negative mechanism for *RET* mutation in the development of MTC and pheochromocytomas in MEN 2A.[41] Subsequent investigations demonstrated mutations of *RET* in MEN 2B patients.[43,44] In 95% of cases of MEN 2B, the *RET* protooncogene mutation is a missense methionine to threonine (ATG to ACG) change at codon 918 in exon 16. This codon is positioned within the tyrosine kinase catalytic core of the intracellular domain. Two families with MEN 2B have been described that have a codon 883 mutation in the tyrosine kinase domain of *RET*.[45]

More than 30 missense mutations have been described in MEN 2A and FMTC kindreds (Table 34.1-3).[46] Most of these mutations result in nonconservative changes in cysteine residues, although changes in Glu, Val, Met, Leu, and Tyr have also been described. Several of these mutations have been shown to result in "gain of function" in the *RET* protein product, with increased intrinsic tyrosine kinase activity or alterations of substrate recognition, or both, and transforming capability.[47] The *RET* gene is expressed in a limited number of cell types in the normal individual, including the thyroid C cells, the adrenal medulla, and parts of the brain. The gene is important in the embryonic development of the enteric nervous system and the kidneys.[48] The Ret protein is a single-pass transmembrane receptor that forms receptor complexes with glycophosphati-

dylinositol–anchored glial-derived neurotrophic factor receptor-α (GFRα) co-receptors. This Ret complex mediates signals of the glial-derived neurotrophic factor family of ligands (GFLs).[49] Glial-derived neurotrophic factor is a 32-kD protein dimer that was first purified from glial cell lines and is a potent neurotrophic survival factor for motor neurons. Current evidence suggests that GFLs bind directly to GFRα and indirectly with *RET*. When triggered by ligand, wild-type *RET* dimerizes with another *RET* molecule, and this dimerization is responsible for phosphorylation and activation of the tyrosine kinase domain, with subsequent downstream signal transduction events. *RET* molecules that contain MEN 2A–type mutations are constitutively dimerized and therefore activated. The mutation responsible for MEN 2B, on the other hand, does not result in constitutive dimerization but changes the substrate specificity of the tyrosine kinase domain.[47]

Other RET *Genotype/Phenotype Correlations*

CUTANEOUS LICHEN AMYLOIDOSIS. Interscapular lesions of CLA have been described in several families with MEN 2A.[27] The total number of patients described with this entity is less than 100. A 634→Tyr mutation was reported in one family with MEN 2A and CLA, and in two other families, a 634→Arg mutation was described that segregated with *MEN2A* and CLA.[50]

HYPERPARATHYROIDISM. HPT in MEN 2A is caused by parathyroid hyperplasia, and the hypercalcemia is mild and often asymptomatic. HPT clusters in some families with MEN 2A, and there is controversy as to whether or not specific *MEN2A* mutations are associated with a higher incidence of HPT. Mulligan et al.[51] previously described a strong correlation between C634R mutation and HPT in families with MEN 2A, but other studies have not been able to definitely confirm this relationship.

HIRSCHSPRUNG'S DISEASE. HSCR is characterized by absence of autonomic ganglion cells within the distal colonic parasympathetic plexus, resulting in obstruction and proximal megacolon. Approximately 80% of HSCR cases are sporadic, and the rest are familial. A subset of familial Hirschsprung's cases have been found to be associated with germline mutations of *RET*.[29,51] Most of these mutations are inactivating and loss of function (frameshift and nonsense mutations) and not associated with the MEN 2A phenotype. Several families, however, have been described in which HSCR co-segregates with either *MEN2A* or *FMTC* (missense codon 618 or 620 mutations).[52] Additionally, a few HSCR patients have been described with missense mutations in codon 609 or 620 who have no evidence of MEN 2A or MTC.[28,51] It is interesting to note that the HSCR phenotype can be associated with either loss-of-function or gain-of-function mutations of *RET*. All patients with MEN 2B (missense codon 918 mutation) have megacolon and chronic colonic motility disturbances, although they usually do not require surgery for this (see Fig. 34.1-2*C*).[30]

RET MUTATIONS IN SPORADIC TUMORS. Mutations in the *RET* protooncogene have also been found in sporadic MTCs.[42,45,53] The most frequent mutation in sporadic MTCs is the M918T mutation found in MEN 2B. Mutations have been found in other regions of the extracellular and intracellular domains. Missense, deletions, and insertion mutations have been described.[46] Somatic *RET* mutations in sporadic pheochromocytomas are unusual but have been described.[46]

OTHER DOMINANT ONCOGENES IN MEDULLARY THYROID CARCINOMAS AND PHEOCHROMOCYTOMAS. Absence of amplification of N-myc, c-myc, and Erb B2 has been reported in MTCs and pheochromocytomas. Roncalli et al.[54] reported that N-myc expression in greater than 10% of tumor cells, as detected by immunohistochemistry, was associated with

poorer survival, sporadic disease, and male sex. They found no evidence of gene amplification and did not determine the basis for the overexpression.[54] The authors' group reported absence of mutation of the H-*RAS*, N-*RAS*, and K-*RAS* genes in a series of pheochromocytomas and MTCs analyzed by direct sequencing.[55] Likewise, examination of nerve growth factor and nerve growth factor receptor (p75) showed no abnormality at the DNA or RNA levels.

OTHER TUMOR SUPPRESSOR GENES IN MEDULLARY THYROID CARCINOMA AND PHEOCHROMOCYTOMA. Several studies have evaluated loss of heterozygosity (LOH) at tumor suppressor loci in pheochromocytomas and MTCs; these studies are summarized in Table 34.1-4. The cumulative data indicate a higher than background incidence of LOH in pheochromocytomas on chromosome arms 1p, 3p, 17p, and 22q.[56,57] In MTCs, the report by Mulligan et al.[57] suggests a significant incidence of 1p LOH; however, evaluation of other chromosomal arms yielded no consistent findings. Lack of significant LOH on 10q, at the *RET* locus, supports the hypothesis that the *RET* protooncogene acts as a dominant oncogene as opposed to a tumor suppressor gene. LOH analysis on 1p in pheochromocytomas suggests a very large region of deletion. The entire short arm of 1p is lost in pheochromocytomas from patients with MEN 2A and 2B.[56] The high rate of LOH on 3p in pheochromocytomas suggests an as yet undefined tumor suppressor locus.[57,58] LOH on 17p suggests possible involvement of the p53 gene; however, existing reports on p53 mutations in pheochromocytomas are conflicting. Two Japanese groups reported no evidence of p53 mutations in pheochromocytomas.[59,60] On the other hand, a Chinese group reported p53 mutations in five of six tumors tested.[61] Four of these mutations were in exon 4. The authors' group reported a series of 22 pheochromocytomas and 29 MTCs that were screened for LOH on 17p with four different markers.[62] Single-strand conformation variant analysis of exons 4 through 9 of the *TP53* gene was performed in 20 of the pheochromocytomas and in 22 of the MTCs. The expression of p53 was determined by

TABLE 34.1-4. Loss of Heterozygosity in Pheochromocytomas and Medullary Thyroid Carcinomas

Study	Chromosomal Arms Tested	LOH in Pheos (No. LOH/No. Informative)	LOH in MTCs (No. LOH/No. Informative)
Khosla et al.[147]	1p, 2p, 3p, 5q, 10q, 13q, 16p, 17p, 17q, 22q	1p-13/31, 2p-1/34, 3p-4/24, 10q-1/22, 17p-7/27, 22q-5/18	1p-1/11, 22-1/7
Moley et al.[56]	1p, 1q	1p-12/18 (9/9 from MEN 2A and 2B patients)	1p-3/24
Yang et al.[148]	1p	1p-5/8	
Mathew et al.[149]	1p, 1q, 5, 6, 7, 11, 12	1p-4/6	1p-3/8
Shin et al.[150]	1p, 22q	1p-12/22, 22q-8/20	
Mulligan et al.[57]	1-22, both arms	1p-15/25, 3p-10/18, 3q-9/15, 5q-1/7, 6q-1/7, 8p-1/8, 11p-3/19, 11q-2/23, 13-2/17, 17p-3/20, 17q-1/20, 22-8/20	1p-7/28, 3p-1/19, 3q-2/14, 7p-1/17, 10p-1/18, 10q-1/25, 11p-1/16, 13-2/22, 15-1/9, 21-1/8, 22-4/22
Dou et al.[58]	2-23	3q-13/13 F, 6/8 S, 21q-4/6 F, 2/7 S, 22q-7/13 F, 1/10 S, 11q-2/6 F, 3/7 S	3q-2/7 F, 1/8 S, 22q-4/15 F, 2/8 S
Herfarth et al.[62]	17p	17p-4/22	17p-0/14

F, familial (MEN 2A and 2B); LOH, loss of heterozygosity; MEN, multiple endocrine neoplasia; MTCs, medullary thyroid carcinomas; Pheos, pheochromocytomas; S, sporadic (MEN 2A and 2B).
Note: Table lists reports, chromosomal arms tested, and number of informative tumors with LOH. If arm tested is not listed in LOH column, it indicates that LOH was not found.
(Adapted from Moley J, Molecular events in the development and progression of medullary thyroid cancer and pheochromocytoma. In: Nelkin B, ed., *Genetic mechanisms in multiple endocrine neoplasia type 2*. Austin: RG Landes, 1996, with permission.)

immunohistochemistry in 19 pheochromocytomas and in 17 MTCs, using two different antibodies (D01 and D07) on frozen and paraffin-embedded tissues. Four of the 22 pheochromocytomas and none of the MTCs showed LOH on 17p. No mutations were detected in any of the tumors screened by single-strand conformation variant analysis. Immunohistochemical staining of frozen and paraffin-embedded tumor sections did not show p53 overexpression in any of the tumors examined. These findings indicate that mutations in the *TP53* gene are an uncommon event in the tumorigenesis of hereditary and sporadic pheochromocytomas and MTCs.[62]

Pheochromocytomas also occur in neurofibromatosis type 1 (NF1) and von Hippel-Lindau (VHL) disease, both of which are caused by mutations in tumor suppressor genes. NF1 gene expression was decreased or absent in 7 of 20 pheochromocytomas from patients with MEN 2 and sporadic disease.[63] Because NF1 is ubiquitously expressed, its lack of expression indicates it may play a role in the development or progression of pheochromocytomas from patients who do not have NF1. Because of the extremely large size of the NF1 gene, mutational analysis has not yet been reported. No reports have been published of the involvement of DNA repair genes (MLH1, MSH2) in development or progression of pheochromocytomas or MTCs, and replication error of repeats has not been a consistent finding in these tumors (J. F. Moley, *unpublished data*, 1999).

PREVENTATIVE SURGERY FOR *MEN2A* GENE CARRIERS

Individuals with MEN 2A, MEN 2B, and FMTC are virtually certain to develop MTC at some point in their lives (usually before age 30). Therefore, at-risk family members who are found to have inherited an *RET* gene mutation are candidates for thyroidectomy, regardless of their stimulated plasma calcitonin levels. Preventative thyroidectomies have been performed routinely in these patients since 1994. Lips et al.,[64] in a series from the Netherlands, identified 14 young members of families affected by MEN 2A who had normal calcitonin testing but who were found to be *MEN2A* gene carriers by DNA testing. Thyroidectomy was performed on 8 of these 14, and foci of MTC were identified in all 8. In a series from Washington University in St. Louis, Wells et al.[65] reported the performance of preventative surgery in 13 asymptomatic *RET* mutation carriers. In a follow-up report, Skinner et al.[66] at Washington University in St. Louis reported a series of 49 children with MEN 2A and MEN 2B. In this series, 14 children had a preventative thyroidectomy based on genetic testing. The average age of the children at the time of surgery was 10.5 years. Postoperative calcitonin levels were all undetectable, and there was no evidence of recurrent MTC with a mean follow-up of 1.3 years. In an interim report of 3-year follow-up of the earliest group of 18 patients, no recurrence of disease was noted.[67] Preventative thyroidectomy has been reported by numerous other American and international groups.

The finding of carcinoma in the thyroid glands of many of these young patients with normal stimulated calcitonin testing[66,68] indicates that the operation was therapeutic, not prophylactic. Therefore, there is some urgency to applying this genetic test to other at-risk individuals and performing thyroidectomy on those who test positive genetically. The ideal age for performance of thyroidectomy in those patients found to be genetically positive has not been determined unequivocally. Six years of age is a reasonable time to perform surgery in patients with MEN 2A and FMTC. Patients with MEN 2B should undergo thyroidectomy during infancy because of the aggressiveness and earlier age of onset of MTC in these individuals. Patient follow-up over the next decades will determine whether there is a significant rate of recurrence after preventative thyroidectomy. At present, it is advisable to follow these patients with stimulated plasma calcitonin levels every 1 to 2 years. These patients must also continue to be followed for the development of pheochromocytomas and HPT.

MOLECULAR PATHOGENESIS OF SPORADIC THYROID NEOPLASMS

The thyroid follicular cell is highly differentiated, with the ability to concentrate iodide and synthesize thyroglobulin. Thyroid-stimulating hormone (TSH) is the major regulator of differentiated function of follicular cells and also functions as a growth factor for follicular cells via a cyclic adenosine monophosphate (cAMP)–mediated signal transduction pathway. In addition, thyroid cell growth and proliferation are also influenced by a variety of growth factors and cytokines, as well as by the amount of iodine in the diet. Presumably, a host of genetic and environmental factors may result in unregulated growth or loss of differentiated function, or both, and confer a proliferative advantage to certain follicular cells, resulting in nodule formation. Progression of benign adenomatous nodules to differentiated carcinoma is speculatory at present, but good evidence exists for the development of anaplastic carcinomas from well-differentiated tumors.[69] A schematic model of the proposed events in thyroid follicular cell tumorigenesis is shown in Figure 34.1-4.

EPIDEMIOLOGIC AND GENETIC FACTORS ASSOCIATED WITH THYROID NEOPLASIA

Papillary thyroid carcinoma accounts for 85% of differentiated thyroid carcinomas in iodine-sufficient countries. In areas of iodine deficiency or endemic goiter, there is an overall increased incidence of thyroid cancer due to a higher proportion of follicular carcinomas and anaplastic thyroid carcinomas (which often arise from preexisting follicular carcinomas).[70] The incidence of thyroid neoplasia is also increased in certain hereditary syndromes, including familial adenomatous polyposis coli, Cowden disease, and MEN 1. Exposure to external radiation in childhood is a strong risk factor for the subsequent development of benign and malignant thyroid nodules.[71] Point mutations of K-*RAS* have been detected in 60% of radiation-related thyroid tumors.[72]

FOLLICULAR ADENOMAS

A local proliferative advantage may be provided to a thyroid follicular cell either by genetic mutational events, environmental factors, or the local influence of cytokines or growth factors. Clonal expansion of cells with a growth advantage leads to nodule formation.

Mutations in all three members of the *RAS* oncogene family (K-*RAS*, N-*RAS*, and H-*RAS*) have been detected in thyroid neoplasms.[73] *RAS* mutations are detected with equal frequency in

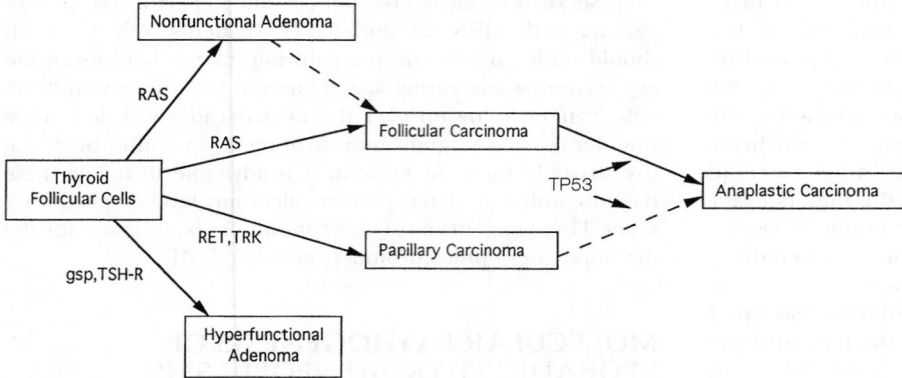

FIGURE 34.1-4. Flow diagram of proven and postulated events in thyroid follicular cell tumorigenesis. Mutations in the *RAS* oncogene are believed to be early events in the genesis of follicular neoplasms. Activation of the *RET* and *TRK* receptor tyrosine kinases is specific to papillary thyroid carcinomas. The association of mutations in the p53 tumor suppressor gene with undifferentiated thyroid tumors suggests that mutations in TP53 are critical events in the progression of follicular carcinoma to anaplastic carcinoma.

benign and malignant thyroid neoplasms[74] and are thought to represent an early event in follicular cell tumorigenesis.[75] *RAS* mutations occur predominantly in follicular thyroid carcinomas, with most of the mutations occurring at codon 61 of H-*RAS* and N-*RAS*.[74,76] It appears that *RAS* mutations are not sufficient for transformation of the thyroid cell, and additional genetic events are required. In cooperation with other oncogenes, transformation of thyroid cells *in vitro* with mutant *RAS* is associated with loss of differentiation, including decreased iodide uptake and expression of thyroid peroxidase.[77]

Mutational events affecting receptors or intermediates along the adenylate cyclase/cAMP signal transduction pathway may contribute to the formation of hyperfunctioning adenomas. A subset of hyperfunctioning adenomas have been shown to harbor somatic mutations in the gene encoding the TSH receptor (TSHR) that result in constitutive activation of downstream events.[78] Mutations in the G protein intracellular mediator of adenylate cyclase (G_s) have been detected in 25% of hyperfunctioning thyroid nodules.[79,80] Therefore, a unifying molecular theme in the pathogenesis of hyperfunctioning nodules is inappropriate activation of the TSH signal transduction pathway resulting from specific gene mutations altering a key mediator of an otherwise well-balanced cascade. Finally, deletion of chromosomal sequences from the 11q13 region has been demonstrated in 14% of follicular adenomas,[81] suggesting that inactivation of a tumor suppressor gene in this region may play a role in follicular cell tumorigenesis in a subset of tumors.

PAPILLARY THYROID CARCINOMA

Activation of receptor tyrosine kinases (*RET/PTC, NTRK1, MET*), whether by chromosomal rearrangement or gene amplification, is associated with the transformation of follicular cells into papillary thyroid carcinoma.[82,83] The *RET* protooncogene was first discovered based on its ability to transform mouse NIH 3T3 fibroblasts in culture.[32] The transforming *RET* sequences first identified represented a rearrangement of *RET* that occurred *in vitro* during the transfection assay.[33] Fusco et al.[84] subsequently demonstrated that DNAs from 25% of papillary carcinomas or their lymph node metastases were also positive in transfection assays. The transforming sequences in papillary carcinomas, originally thought to be a unique oncogene termed *PTC* (for papillary thyroid carcinoma), were shown to represent *in vivo* chromosomal rearrangements that resulted in

the juxtaposition of sequences encoding the intracellular tyrosine kinase domain of *RET* with 5' sequences from one of three unrelated genes.[82,84–87] The most frequent form of activated *RET/PTC* results from a paracentric inversion of chromosome 10q[86] that results in the gene fusion of D10S170 (H4) sequences with the catalytic domain of *RET* (Fig. 34.1-5). The frequency of *RET* rearrangements in papillary carcinomas is as high as 40% in some parts of the world,[84,88] but a lower frequency has been found in other studies,[89,90] perhaps reflecting either racial or environmental factors influencing thyroid tumorigenesis in different geographic regions.

Activation of the *NTRK1* (tropomyosin receptor kinase), which encodes a cell surface receptor for nerve growth factor, has also been detected in some papillary carcinomas.[82] The *TRK-T1* oncogene is generated by a chromosome rearrangement that juxtaposes the tyrosine kinase domain of *NTRK1* and the 5' region of the TPR gene, both mapping to chromosome 1q23-24.[91] The *MET* oncogene that also encodes a receptor tyrosine kinase is amplified and overexpressed in 70% of papillary and poorly differentiated carcinomas, but in only 25% of follicular carcinomas.[92] Activation of *MET* by amplification[92] and the presence of a rearranged, activated form of *RET* have been suggested as predictors of aggressive biologic behavior and poor prognosis in papillary carcinomas.

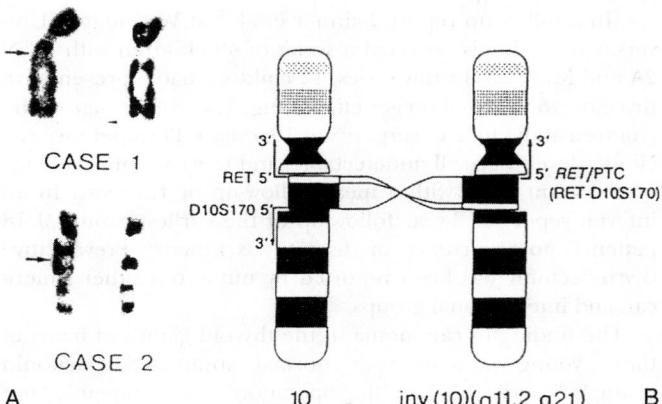

FIGURE 34.1-5. Chromosome 10q inversion in papillary thyroid carcinoma. **A:** Two representative chromosome 10 homologues from tumor cells of patients 1 and 2 showing inv(10) (q11.2q21) (*arrows*). **B:** Schematic view of the paracentric inversion of chromosome 10q generating the transforming sequence *RET/PTC*. (From ref. 86, with permission.)

Vascular endothelial growth factor is expressed at high levels in PTC and other thyroid neoplasms.[93] Vascular endothelial growth factor expression is associated with tumor size and recurrence in one study.[94] The sodium-iodide symporter is expressed in papillary and follicular thyroid neoplasms and may be associated with a lower risk of recurrence after treatment.[95]

FOLLICULAR THYROID CARCINOMA

Numerous chromosomal deletions have been detected in thyroid neoplasms, suggesting a role for multiple tumor suppressor genes in the initiation or progression of these tumors. Although sporadic follicular thyroid tumors exhibit allelic chromosomal loss of chromosome 11q13 sequences with increased frequency,[81] one study[96] failed to find accompanying mutations in the *MEN1* gene in the remaining normal allele, suggesting that a tumor suppressor gene other than *MEN1* might be involved in tumorigenesis of these neoplasms. In addition to the 11q13 deletions described in follicular adenomas, Herrmann et al.[97] have presented evidence for chromosome 3p deletions specific to follicular carcinomas and proposed that inactivation of a tumor suppressor gene on chromosome 3p is important in the progression from follicular adenoma to carcinoma.

ANAPLASTIC THYROID CARCINOMA

Point mutations in the p53 tumor suppressor gene are frequent in anaplastic thyroid carcinomas, but not in differentiated thyroid tumors.[98,99] This suggests that TP53 mutation is a critical event in the progression of follicular carcinoma to anaplastic carcinoma. Wild-type TP53 encodes a nuclear phosphoprotein that functions as a transcriptional regulator believed to influence cell-cycle arrest or programmed cell death in response to genetic damage. Disruption of this protective function appears to be relevant to the progression of thyroid neoplasms to an aggressive, undifferentiated phenotype. Codons 273[98,99] and 248[99] are hot spots for TP53 mutation in anaplastic thyroid carcinoma.

MEDULLARY THYROID CARCINOMA

The molecular genetic alterations associated with sporadic medullary carcinoma of the thyroid are discussed earlier in Genetics of the Multiple Endocrine Neoplasia Type 2 Syndromes.

GENETIC ABNORMALITIES IN PARATHYROID NEOPLASMS

BENIGN PARATHYROID NEOPLASMS

Neoplasms of the parathyroid glands are usually benign and occur with increased frequency in postmenopausal women or after neck irradiation. Approximately 5% of cases of HPT arise in the setting of one of several distinct hereditary syndromes. Benign parathyroid adenomas in patients with sporadic primary HPT have a proliferative defect (increase in cellular mass) as well as inappropriate hormone secretion or a defect in regulating parathyroid hormone (PTH) release in response to the extracellular calcium concentration ("set-point" abnormality).[100] In sporadic parathyroid tumors, frequent genetic defects have been established in two genes, including activation of an oncogene (*cyclin D1/PRAD1*) and inactivation of the *MEN1* tumor suppressor gene. The presence of clonal DNA derangements in specific subsets of parathyroid neoplasms, resulting in either *cyclin D1* overexpression or biallelic inactivation of the *MEN1* tumor suppressor gene, strongly support a primary role for each of these specific genetic alterations in the pathogenesis of sporadic parathyroid adenomas. Many questions remain unanswered, including the relationship between abnormal cell proliferation and inappropriate hormone secretion as well as the relative contributions of the primary mutation at the DNA level and additional events or subsequent facilitating genetic defects. Future studies will be aimed at uncovering potential molecular insights into the contribution of other risk factors, such as exposure to ionizing radiation, the postmenopausal state, or vitamin D deficiency.

MUTATIONS IN THE *MEN1* GENE AND ROLE OF OTHER TUMOR SUPPRESSOR GENES

Patients with the familial MEN 1 syndrome inherit one mutated copy of the *MEN1* gene in the germline and therefore require only one chance at an additional somatic event (deletion, point mutation) to result in the loss of the remaining functional copy of the gene within an individual parathyroid cell. Presumably, the relatively likely combined occurrence of these genetic events leads to the asynchronous development of multiglandular parathyroid neoplasms in affected individuals. The identification of the rare genetic defects responsible for the constellation of neoplasms in hereditary cancer syndromes prompts a search for possible identical changes relevant to sporadic varieties of identical tumor types. In fact, events presumed to result in total abrogation of the *MEN1* tumor suppressor gene have been documented in a subset of parathyroid adenomas. Inactivating defects involving both allelic copies of the *MEN1* gene have been identified in 12% to 20% of sporadic parathyroid adenomas studied.[101,102] Chromosomal deletions, or allelic LOH, occur in approximately twice (30%) this number of sporadic parathyroid adenomas.[103–105] This observed discrepancy in rate of detectable chromosome deletions raises the possibility that additional tumor suppressor gene(s) on 11q may contribute to parathyroid tumorigenesis.[106]

Transgenic mice with a germline mutation in the murine *men1* gene exhibit a phenotype including the development of hypercellular parathyroid neoplasms (without biochemical HPT), as well as the development of neuroendocrine pancreatic tumors, pituitary adenomas, and adrenocortical neoplasms, representing a close model of the spectrum of tissue involvement in the human MEN 1 syndrome.[25] Future studies in mice with an engineered *MEN1* deficiency targeted to the parathyroid glands will provide additional important information relevant to the role of menin in parathyroid cell oncosuppression.

ACTIVATION OF THE *PRAD1* PROTOONCOGENE BY CHROMOSOMAL GENE REARRANGEMENT

Overexpression of *cyclin D1*, a key regulator of G_1 progression through the cell cycle, has been implicated in approximately 20%

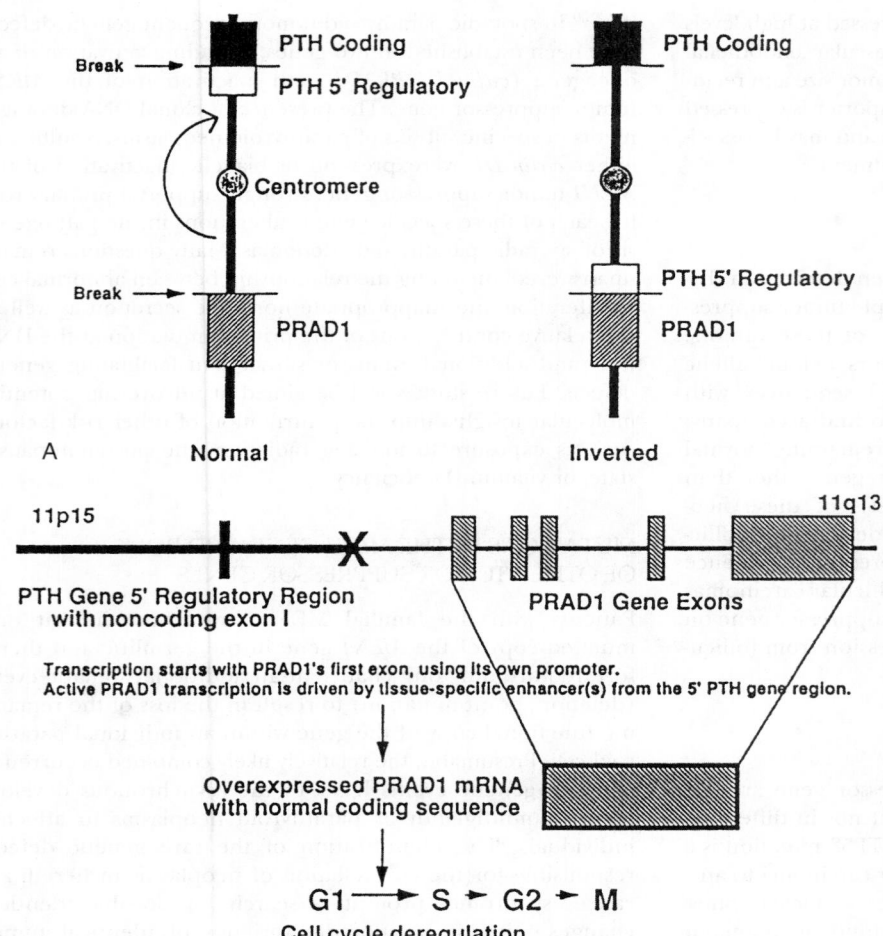

FIGURE 34.1-6. **A:** Schematic diagram illustrating the pericentromeric inversion of chromosome 11 deduced to have caused the observed rearrangement involving the parathyroid hormone (PTH) gene and the PRAD1 gene in a subset of parathyroid adenomas. The tumor's other copy of chromosome 11, which contains an intact PTH gene, is not shown. **B:** Diagram of the directly observed molecular structure of the PTH/PRAD1 DNA rearrangement in a subset of parathyroid adenomas and its functional consequences. X represents the chromosome breakpoint between the PTH gene regulatory region, plus PTH noncoding exon 1 (*solid light vertical bar*) and part of its first intron, from 11p15 (*left*), and the intact promoter and five exons of the PRAD1 gene from 11q13. mRNA, messenger RNA. (From ref. 100, with permission.)

to 40% of parathyroid adenomas. In a subset of parathyroid adenomas, chromosomal rearrangement results in a clonal activation that places tissue-specific enhancing elements of the PTH gene upstream to the *cyclin D1* oncogene. This phenomenon is most easily explained by a pericentromeric inversion. As a consequence of the breakpoint and rejoining in 11q13, the PTH transcriptional regulatory sequences and their noncoding exon 1 are placed immediately upstream of the *cyclin D1* intact promoter and its five exons (Fig. 34.1-6). The result is transcriptional activation and overexpression of *cyclin D1*.[106] Variability is present in the location of the breakpoint, and the frequency of this aberration may be underestimated by current detection techniques. Nevertheless, clear evidence of *cyclin D1* overexpression, to the extent found in patients with an identified chromosomal rearrangement, can be demonstrated in 20% to 40% of sporadic parathyroid adenomas.[106] Therefore, it is likely that multiple pathways exist for *cyclin D1* overexpression, with chromosome rearrangement responsible for only a subset. The development of a transgenic mouse model with parathyroid-targeted overexpression of cyclin D1 provides direct evidence for its primary role in parathyroid tumorigenesis.[107] The phenotype of these transgenic mice includes the gradual development of moderate biochemical HPT, hypercellular parathyroid tumors, and high rates of bone turnover. This transgenic mouse model establishes a relationship between a genetic aberration conferring abnormal parathyroid

proliferation and a primary disturbance of the regulation of hormonal secretion.

OTHER GENETIC LOCI IMPLICATED IN FAMILIAL HYPERCALCEMIC SYNDROMES

FAMILIAL BENIGN HYPERCALCEMIA (HYPOCALCIURIC HYPERCALCEMIA)

Familial benign hypercalcemia (FBH) or familial hypocalciuric hypercalcemia[108] is a dominantly inherited condition characterized by mild hypercalcemia, low urinary calcium excretion, and the absence of symptoms or the complications of hypercalcemia. The hypercalcemia in FBH begins at birth and is nonprogressive. Urinary calcium secretion is in the normal range. Recognition of hypercalcemia before the age of 10 years, relative hypocalciuria, and a familial association should alert the clinician to this infrequent familial pattern. The features of FBH are important to recognize and distinguish from those of other hypercalcemic disorders, because surgery fails to result in correction of the calcium level.[109]

Pollak et al.[110] demonstrated that mutations in the human calcium-sensing receptor gene are associated with familial benign hypocalcemia as well as neonatal severe HPT (NSHPT). Parathyroid cells from patients with FBH are characterized by an abnormally increased set point for extracellular calcium.[111]

The germline mutations that are associated with FBH are heterozygous, inactivating mutations in the calcium-sensing receptor gene.[112,113] The reported mutations[110,112–114] include point mutations, nonsense mutations, or insertions that are postulated to result in varying degrees of loss of function of the receptor's calcium-sensing function.

NEONATAL SEVERE HYPERPARATHYROIDISM

NSHPT is characterized by severe hypercalcemia, failure to thrive, dehydration, pathologic fractures and rib cage deformities, respiratory distress, and hypotonia in the newborn. The disorder usually requires urgent total parathyroidectomy in the first few weeks of life, although some have achieved a favorable outcome with intensive medical management.

In some cases, NSHPT results from homozygous mutations (mutations on both homologous alleles), resulting in loss of function of the calcium-sensing receptor gene.[114]

HEREDITARY HYPERPARATHYROIDISM–JAW TUMOR SYNDROME

The autosomal dominant inheritance of HPT without any associated features and without any apparent association to the MEN syndromes has been described in several families.[115–117] HPT–jaw tumor syndrome is an autosomal dominant disorder characterized by parathyroid neoplasms, including parathyroid carcinoma, ossifying fibromas of the maxilla and mandible that occur in approximately 30% of patients, and the variable occurrence of renal cysts and hamartomas or Wilms' tumors.[118] The onset of hypercalcemia typically occurs in childhood or the second decade of life. The association may not be recognized in many cases because the jaw lesions occur asynchronously in relation to the parathyroid tumors or may occur in some patients without HPT. The parathyroid tumors may be single or multiple but have a tendency toward recurrence after subtotal parathyroidectomy. The parathyroid adenomas in the familial HPT–jaw tumor syndrome are often cystic, and more importantly there is an approximately 15% incidence of parathyroid carcinoma. HPT–jaw tumor syndrome is associated with germline mutations in the tumor suppressor gene *HRPT2* encoding parafibromin.[119]

PARATHYROID CARCINOMA

Molecular defects with a possible role in progression to the malignant phenotype have also been sought in tumor DNA from parathyroid carcinomas. Although one study[120] failed to detect evidence of mutations in exons 5, 7, and 8 of the p53 gene in parathyroid carcinomas, another study[121] reported allelic loss of TP53 in two of six informative parathyroid carcinomas. None of 20 informative parathyroid adenomas exhibited deletions of TP53. Most recently, the retinoblastoma tumor suppressor gene has been shown to be inactivated in most parathyroid carcinomas, but not in adenomas.[122]

GENETIC ABNORMALITIES IN ADRENAL NEOPLASMS

ADRENAL CORTEX: ADRENOCORTICAL ADENOMAS AND CARCINOMAS

Solitary adrenocortical adenomas and adrenal cancers show evidence of monoclonal proliferation,[123] in contrast to the usually polyclonal processes that lead to adrenal hyperplasia. However, a sequence of accumulative genetic changes from the relatively frequent benign, nonfunctional adrenal adenoma to the very infrequent adrenocortical carcinoma has not yet been established. The finding of monoclonal proliferation in adenomas and cancers suggests the existence of specific genetic mutations within the genome that initiate tumorigenesis in the cells of the adrenal cortex. Established and candidate genes with a role in adrenocortical tumor formation include *TP53* (encoding p53), KIP2/p57, insulin-like growth factor type 2 (*IGF2*), inhibin-A, and cAMP early repressor, among others.[124] LOH for markers from 17p has been consistently demonstrated in adrenocortical carcinomas, but not in benign adrenocortical adenomas or hyperplasia.[125] Frequent LOH has also been detected for markers on chromosome 11p and 13q.[125]

Cytogenetic studies have demonstrated the relatively frequent occurrence of DNA polyploidy in benign adrenocortical lesions, especially aldosteronomas. Genes with established involvement in adrenocortical tumorigenesis are associated with chromosomes 11p (*p57/KIP2* and *IGF2*) and 17p (*TP53*). Mutations in *TP53* are typically a late event in formation of sporadic adrenal cancer, but it has been proposed that low-penetrance mutations in *TP53* might predispose to adrenal oncogenesis in the setting of facilitating genetic changes or environmental interactions.[124] Aberrations in the cAMP-dependent protein kinase A (PKA) signaling pathway, including *MC2R* (encoding the adrenocorticotropic hormone receptor) and *GNAS1* (the Gsa subunit), have also been implicated in adrenocortical tumorigenesis.[126]

The genetic basis for several hereditary syndromes associated with adrenocortical neoplasms has been described, including the Li-Fraumeni syndrome associated with germline mutations in *TP53*[127] and Beckwith-Wiedemann syndrome associated with a defect on chromosome 11p15.[128] Patients with MEN 1, caused by inactivation of the *MEN1* tumor suppressor gene, may develop bilateral nodular adrenocortical involvement that is almost always nonfunctional and with very low risk of malignant transformation. Carney complex is characterized by the association of primary pigmented nodular adrenocortical disease, myxomas, skin pigmentation and blue nevi, and diverse other endocrine neoplasms.[129] Mutations in the PKA type Iα regulatory subunit are responsible for Carney complex.[130] In primary pigmented nodular adrenocortical disease, as in other tumors associated with Carney complex, LOH of the 17q *PRKAR1A* locus and abnormal activity of PKA have been demonstrated, suggesting that *PRKAR1A* might act as a tumor suppressor.

ADRENAL MEDULLA

Sporadic Pheochromocytomas

The molecular genetic alterations associated with sporadic pheochromocytomas are discussed earlier in Genetics of Multiple Endocrine Neoplasia Type 2 Syndromes.

Familial Pheochromocytomas Arising in Patients with Multiple Endocrine Neoplasia Type 2, von Hippel-Lindau Syndrome, and Neurofibromatosis Type 1

Pheochromocytomas occur in association with the VHL and NF1 syndromes. VHL syndrome is characterized by the development of retinal, cerebellar, and spinal hemangioblastomas; pancreatic and renal cysts; renal carcinomas; pheochromocytomas; neuroendocrine tumors of the pancreas; epididymal cysts; and endolymphatic sac tumors. The original mapping of the VHL gene by positional cloning to chromosome 3p was reported in 1993.[131] The VHL tumor suppressor gene encodes a protein that regulates the transcription of DNA to messenger RNA by RNA polymerase II.[132] Clinical heterogeneity exists in patients with the VHL syndrome. In type 1, pheochromocytomas do not occur. Pheochromocytomas are associated with type 2A, but renal cell carcinomas do not occur. Finally, in type 2B, pheochromocytomas and renal cell carcinomas develop. The above classification has also been related to apparent genotype/phenotype correlations associated with mutations in the VHL gene.[133]

Mutations in the tumor suppressor gene for NF1 on chromosome 17q were identified in 1990.[134,135] Pheochromocytomas occur in approximately 1% to 2% of patients with NF1. Bilateral tumors occur with increased frequency.

Previously, it was estimated that 10% of pheochromocytomas occur as a component of the familial syndromes MEN 2, VHL disease, and NF1. More recently, dedicated hospital-based and population studies have identified germline mutations in a disease-associated gene in approximately 20% or more of patients with apparently isolated pheochromocytoma.[136] The familial occurrence of paragangliomas and carotid body tumors is associated with germline mutations in the *SDHB*, *SDHC*, and *SDHD* genes that encode subunits of the mitochondrial complex II.[137–141] Therefore, a variety of genetic abnormalities can result in neoplasia of the adrenal medulla and dispersed chromaffin cells, including *RET* protooncogene mutations, mutations in the *VHL* tumor suppressor gene, and the NF1 tumor suppressor gene. Patients who present with pheochromocytoma should be evaluated for involvement with the MEN 2 syndromes, VHL, or neurofibromatosis.

CONCLUSION

A variety of genetic abnormalities in oncogenes and tumor suppressor genes have been identified in endocrine neoplasms. The study of tumors developing in the inherited endocrine cancer syndromes has provided valuable insight into genetic events that likely play a role in the genesis of sporadic tumors developing in the same endocrine tissues. The advent of direct DNA testing for germline mutations in the *RET* protooncogene that are responsible for the MEN 2 syndromes has made early thyroidectomy possible at a time when hereditary MTC is likely occult and curable. The identification of germline mutations in the MEN 1 gene will allow direct genetic testing and an enhanced understanding of the mechanisms of tumorigenesis of related endocrine tumors.

REFERENCES

1. Marx S, Spiegel AM, Skarulis MC, et al. Multiple endocrine neoplasia type 1: clinical and genetic topics. *Ann Intern Med* 1998;129:484.
2. Darling TN, Skarulis MC, Steinberg SM, et al. Multiple facial angiofibromas and collagenomas in patients with multiple endocrine neoplasia type 1. *Arch Dermatol* 1997;133:853.
3. Kato H, Uchimura I, Morohoshi M, et al. Multiple endocrine neoplasia type 1 associated with spinal ependymoma. *Intern Med* 1996;35:285.
4. Doherty GM, Olson JA, Frisella MM, et al. Lethality of multiple endocrine neoplasia type 1. *World J Surg* 1997;22:581.
5. Larsson C, Skogseid B, Öberg K, et al. Multiple endocrine neoplasia type 1 gene maps to chromosome 11 and is lost in insulinoma. *Nature* 1988;332:85.
6. Chandrasekharappa SC, Guru SC, Manickam P, et al. Positional cloning of the gene for multiple endocrine neoplasia-type 1. *Science* 1997;276:404.
7. Lemmens I, Van de Ven WJM, Kas K, et al. Identification of the multiple endocrine neoplasia type 1 (MEN1) gene. *Hum Mol Genet* 1997;6:1177.
8. Agarwal SK, Kester MB, Debelenko LV, et al. Germline mutations in the MEN1 gene in familial multiple endocrine neoplasia type 1 and related states. *Hum Mol Genet* 1997;6:1169.
9. Bassett JHD, Forbes SA, Pannett AAJ, et al. Characterization of mutations in patients with multiple endocrine neoplasia type 1. *Am J Hum Genet* 1998;62:232.
10. Mutch MG, Dilley WG, Sanjurjo F, et al. Germline mutations in the multiple endocrine neoplasia type 1 gene: evidence for frequent splicing defects. *Hum Mutat* 1999;13:175.
11. Stewart C, Parente F, Piehl F, et al. Characterization of the mouse Men1 gene and its expression during development. *Oncogene* 1998;17:2485.
12. Guru SC, Crabtree JS, Brown KD, et al. Isolation, genomic organization, and expression analysis of Men1, the murine homolog of the MEN1 gene. *Mamm Genome* 1999;10:592.
13. Khodaei S, O'Brien KP, Dumanski J, et al. Characterization of the MEN1 ortholog in zebrafish. *Biochem Biophys Res Commun* 1999;264:404.
14. Maruyama K, Tsukada T, Honda M, et al. Complementary DNA structure and genomic organization of Drosophila menin. *Mol Cell Endocrinol* 2000;168:135.
15. Guru SC, Goldsmith PK, Burns AL, et al. Menin, the product of the MEN1 gene, is a nuclear protein. *Proc Natl Acad Sci U S A* 1998;95:1630.
16. Agarwal SK, Guru SC, Heppner C, et al. Menin interacts with the AP1 transcription factor JunD and represses JunD-activated transcription. *Cell* 1999;96:143.
17. Gobl AE, Berg M, Lopez-Egido JR, et al. Menin represses JunD-activated transcription by a histone deacetylase-dependent mechanism. *Biochim Biophys Acta* 1999;1447:51.
18. Kaji H, Canaff L, Lebrun JJ, et al. Inactivation of menin, a Smad3-interacting protein, blocks transforming growth factor type beta signaling. *Proc Natl Acad Sci U S A* 2001;98:3837.
19. Heppner C, Bilimoria KY, Agarwal SK, et al. The tumor suppressor protein menin interacts with NF-kappaB proteins and inhibits NF-kappaB-mediated transactivation. *Oncogene* 2001;20:4917.
20. Ohkura N, Kishi M, Tsukada T, et al. Menin, a gene product responsible for multiple endocrine neoplasia type 1, interacts with the putative tumor metastasis protein nm23. *Biochim Biophys Res Commun* 2001;282:1206.
21. Kaji H, Canaff L, Goltzman D, et al. Cell cycle regulation of menin expression. *Cancer Res* 1999;59:5097.
22. Sakurai A, Katai M, Itakura Y, et al. Premature centromere division in patients with multiple endocrine neoplasia type 1. *Cancer Genet Cytogenet* 1999;109:138.
23. Suphapeetiporn K, Greally JM, Walpita D, et al. MEN 1 tumor-suppressor protein localizes to telomeres during meiosis. *Genes Chromosomes Cancer* 2002;35:81.
24. Lin SY, Elledge SJ. Multiple tumor suppressor pathways negatively regulate telomerase. *Cell* 2003;113:881.
25. Crabtree JS, Scacheri PC, Ward JM, et al. A mouse model of multiple endocrine neoplasia, type 1, develops multiple endocrine tumors. *Proc Natl Acad Sci U S A* 2001;98:1118.
26. Bertolino P, Radovanovic I, Casse H, et al. Genetic ablation of the tumor suppressor menin causes lethality at mid-gestation with defects in multiple organs. *Mech Dev* 2003;120:549.
27. Gagel RF, Levy ML, Donovan DT, et al. Multiple endocrine neoplasia type 2A associated with cutaneous lichen amyloidosis. *Ann Intern Med* 1989;111:802.
28. Romeo G, Ronchetto P, Luo Y, et al. Point mutations affecting the tyrosine kinase domain of the RET proto-oncogene in Hirschsprung's disease. *Nature* 1994;367:377.
29. Edery P, Lyonnet S, Mulligan LM, et al. Mutations of the RET proto-oncogene in Hirschsprung's disease. *Nature* 1994;367:378.
30. Cohen MS, Phay JE, Albinson C, et al. Gastrointestinal manifestations of multiple endocrine neoplasia type 2. *Ann Surg* 2002;235:648.
31. Farndon JR, Leight GS, Dilley WG, et al. Familial medullary thyroid carcinoma without associated endocrinopathies: a distinct clinical entity. *Br J Surg* 1986;73:278.
32. Takahashi M, Ritz J, Cooper GM. Activation of a novel human transforming gene, ret, by DNA rearrangement. *Cell* 1985;42:581.
33. Takahashi M, Cooper GM. Ret transforming gene encodes a fusion protein homologous to tyrosine kinases. *Mol Cell Biol* 1987;7:1378.
34. Takahashi M, Buma Y, Iwamoto T, et al. Cloning and expression of the ret proto-oncogene encoding a tyrosine kinase with two potential transmembrane domains. *Oncogene* 1988;3:571.
35. Ishizaka Y, Itoh F, Tahira T, et al. Human ret proto-oncogene mapped to chromosome 10q11.2. *Oncogene* 1989;4:1519.
36. Santoro M, Rosati R, Grieco M, et al. The ret proto-oncogene is consistently expressed in human pheochromocytomas and thyroid medullary carcinomas. *Oncogene* 1990;5:1595.
37. Mathew CGP, Chin KS, Easton DF, et al. A linked genetic marker for multiple endocrine neoplasia type 2A on chromosome 10. *Nature* 1987;328:527.
38. Simpson NE, Kidd KK, Goodfellow PJ, et al. Assignment of multiple endocrine neoplasia type 2A to chromosome 10 by genetic linkage. *Nature* 1987;328:528.
39. Norum RA, Lafreniere RG, O'Neal LW, et al. Linkage of the multiple endocrine neoplasia type 2B gene (MEN2B) to chromosome 10 markers linked to MEN2A. *Genomics* 1990; 8:313.
40. Lairmore TC, Howe JR, Korte JA, et al. Familial medullary thyroid carcinoma and multiple endocrine neoplasia type 2B map to the same region of chromosome 10 as multiple endocrine neoplasia type 2A. *Genomics* 1991;9:181.

41. Mulligan LM, Kwok JBJ, Healey CS, et al. Germ-line mutations of the RET proto-oncogene in multiple endocrine neoplasia type 2A. *Nature* 1993;363:458.
42. Donis-Keller H, Dou S, Chi D, et al. Mutations in the RET proto-oncogene are associated with MEN 2A and FMTC. *Hum Mol Genet* 1993;2:851.
43. Hofstra RMW, Landsvater RM, Ceccherini I, et al. A mutation in the RET proto-oncogene associated with multiple endocrine neoplasia type 2B and sporadic medullary thyroid carcinoma. *Nature* 1994;367:375.
44. Carlson KM, Dou S, Chi D, et al. Single missense mutation in the tyrosine kinase catalytic domain of the RET protooncogene is associated with multiple endocrine neoplasia type 2B. *Proc Natl Acad Sci U S A* 1994;91:1579.
45. Smith DP, Houghton C, Ponder BAJ. Germline mutation of RET codon 883 in two cases of de novo MEN 2B. *Oncogene* 1997;15:1213.
46. Eng C, Mulligan LM. Mutations of the RET proto-oncogene in the multiple endocrine neoplasia type 2 syndromes, related sporadic tumors, and Hirschsprung disease. *Hum Mutat* 1997;9:97.
47. Santoro M, Carlomagno F, Romano A, et al. Activation of RET as a dominantly transforming gene by germline mutations of MEN2A and MEN2B. *Science* 1995;267:381.
48. Schuchardt A, D'Agati V, Larsson-Blomberg L, et al. Defects in the kidney and enteric nervous system of mice lacking the tyrosine kinase receptor Ret. *Nature* 1994;367:380.
49. Airaksinen MS, Saarma M. The GDNF family: signalling, biological functions and therapeutic value. *Nat Rev Neurosci* 2002;3:383.
50. Hofstra RM, Sijmons RH, Stelwagen T, et al. RET mutation screening in familial cutaneous lichen amyloidosis associated with multiple endocrine neoplasia. *J Invest Dermatol* 1996;107:215.
51. Mulligan LM, Eng C, Healey CS, et al. Specific mutations of the RET proto-oncogene are related to disease phenotype in MEN 2A and FMTC. *Nat Genet* 1994;6:70.
52. Borst MJ, VanCamp JM, Peacock ML, et al. Mutational analysis of multiple endocrine neoplasia type 2A associated with Hirschsprung's disease. *Surgery* 1995;117:386.
53. Marsh KJ, Learoyd DL, Andrew SD, et al. Somatic mutations in the RET proto-oncogene in sporadic medullary thyroid carcinoma. *J Clin Endocrinol* 1996;44:249.
54. Roncalli M, Viale G, Grimelius L, et al. Prognostic value of N-myc immunoreactivity in medullary thyroid carcinoma. *Cancer* 1994;74:134.
55. Moley JF, Brother MB, Wells SA, et al. Low frequency of ras gene mutations in neuroblastomas, pheochromocytomas, and medullary thyroid cancers. *Cancer Res* 1991;51:1596.
56. Moley JF, Brother MB, Fong CT, et al. Consistent association of 1p loss of heterozygosity with pheochromocytomas from patients with multiple endocrine neoplasia type 2 syndromes. *Cancer Res* 1992;52:770.
57. Mulligan LM, Gardner E, Smith BA, et al. Genetic events in tumour initiation and progression in multiple endocrine neoplasia type 2. *Genes Chromosomes Cancer* 1993;6:166.
58. Dou S, Toshima K, Liu L, et al. Identification of chromosomal loci for tumor suppressor loci implicated in progression of pheochromocytoma and medullary thyroid carcinoma. *Am J Hum Genet* 1994;55:[Suppl]A20.
59. Yoshimoto K, Iwahana H, Fukuda A, et al. Role of p53 mutations in endocrine tumorigenesis: mutation detection by polymerase chain reaction-single strand conformation polymorphism. *Cancer Res* 1992;52:5061.
60. Yana I, Nakamura T, Shin E, et al. Inactivation of the p53 gene is not required for tumorigenesis of medullary thyroid carcinoma or pheochromocytoma. *Jpn J Cancer Res* 1992;83:1113.
61. Lin SR, Lee YJ, Tsai JH. Mutations of the p53 gene in human functional adrenal neoplasms. *J Clin Endocrinol Metab* 1994;78:483.
62. Herfarth K, Wick M, Marshall H, et al. Absence of TP53 alterations in pheochromocytomas and medullary thyroid carcinomas. *Genes Chromosomes Cancer* 1997;20:24.
63. Gutmann DH, Geist RT, Rose K, et al. Loss of neurofibromatosis type I (NF1) gene expression in pheochromocytomas from patients without NF1. *Genes Chromosomes Cancer* 1995;13:104.
64. Lips CJM, Landsvater RM, Höppener JWM, et al. Clinical screening as compared with DNA analysis in families with multiple endocrine neoplasia type 2A. *N Engl J Med* 1994;331:828.
65. Wells SA Jr, Chi D, Toshima K, et al. Predictive DNA testing and prophylactic thyroidectomy in patients at risk for multiple endocrine neoplasia type 2A. *Ann Surg* 1994;220:237.
66. Skinner MA, DeBenedetti MK, Moley JF, et al. Medullary thyroid carcinoma in children with multiple endocrine neoplasia types 2A and 2B. *J Pediatr Surg* 1996;31:177.
67. Wells SA Jr, Skinner MA. Prophylactic thyroidectomy, based on direct genetic testing, in patients at risk for the multiple endocrine neoplasia type 2 syndromes. *Exp Clin Endocrinol Diabetes* 1998;106:29.
68. Lairmore TC, Frisella MM, Wells SAJ. Genetic testing and early thyroidectomy for inherited medullary thyroid carcinoma. *Ann Med* 1996;28:401.
69. Venkatesh YS, Ordonez NG, Schultz PN, et al. Anaplastic carcinoma of the thyroid: a clinicopathologic study of 121 cases. *Cancer* 1990;66:321.
70. Belfiore A, La Rosa GL, La Porta GA, et al. Cancer risk in patients with cold thyroid nodules: relevance of iodine intake, sex, age and multinodularity. *Am J Med* 1992;93:363.
71. Schneider AB, Shore-Freedman E, Ryo UY, et al. Radiation-induced tumors of the head and neck following childhood irradiation. *Medicine* 1985;64:1.
72. Wright PA, Williams ED, Lemoine NR, et al. Radiation-associated and "spontaneous" human thyroid carcinomas show a different pattern of ras oncogene mutation. *Oncogene* 1991;6:471.
73. Saurez HG, du Villard JA, Severino M, et al. Presence of mutations in all three ras genes in human thyroid tumors. *Oncogene* 1990;5:565.
74. Karga H, Lee JK, Vickery ALJ, et al. Ras oncogene mutations in benign and malignant thyroid neoplasms. *J Clin Endocrinol Metab* 1991;73:832.
75. Namba H, Rubin SA, Fagin JA. Point mutations of ras oncogenes are an early event in thyroid tumorigenesis. *Mol Endocrinol* 1990;4:1474.
76. Shi YF, Zou MJ, Schmidt H, et al. High rates of ras codon 61 mutation in thyroid tumors in an iodide-deficient area. *Cancer Res* 1991;51:2690.
77. Francis-Lang H, Zannini M, De Felice M, et al. Multiple mechanisms of interference between transformation and differentiation in thyroid cells. *Mol Cell Biol* 1992;12:5793.
78. Parma J, Duprez L, Van Sande J, et al. Somatic mutations of the thyrotropin receptor gene cause hyperfunctioning thyroid adenomas. *Nature* 1993;365:649.
79. Lyons J, Landis CA, Harsh G, et al. Two G protein oncogenes in human endocrine tumors. *Science* 1990;249:635.
80. Suarez HG, du Villard JA, Caillou B, et al. Gsp mutations in human thyroid tumors. *Oncogene* 1991;6:677.
81. Matsuo K, Tang S-H, Fagin JA. Allelotype of human thyroid tumors: loss of chromosome 11q13 sequences in follicular neoplasms. *Mol Endocrinol* 1991;5:1873.
82. Bongarzone I, Pierotti MA, Monzini N, et al. High frequency of activation of tyrosine kinase oncogenes in human papillary thyroid carcinoma. *Oncogene* 1989;4:1457.
83. Santoro M, Carlomagno F, Hay ID, et al. Ret oncogene activation in human thyroid neoplasms is restricted to the papillary cancer subtype. *J Clin Invest* 1992;89:1517.
84. Fusco A, Grieco M, Santoro M, et al. A new oncogene in human thyroid papillary carcinomas and their lymph-nodal metastases. *Nature* 1987;328:170.
85. Grieco M, Santoro M, Berlingieri MT, et al. PTC is a novel rearranged form of the ret proto-oncogene and is frequently detected in vivo in human thyroid papillary carcinomas. *Cell* 1990;60:557.
86. Pierotti MA, Santoro M, Jenkins RB, et al. Characterization of an inversion on the long arm of chromosome 10 juxtaposing D10S170 and RET and creating the oncogenic sequence RET/PTC. *Proc Natl Acad Sci U S A* 1992;89:1616.
87. Sozzi G, Bongarzone I, Miozzo M, et al. A t(10;17) translocation creates the RET/PTC2 chimeric transforming sequence in papillary thyroid carcinoma. *Genes Chromosomes Cancer* 1994;9:244.
88. Bongarzone I, Butti MG, Coronelli S, et al. Frequent activation of ret protooncogene by fusion with a new activating gene in papillary thyroid carcinomas. *Cancer Res* 1994;54:2979.
89. Wajjwalku W, Nakamura S, Hasegawa Y, et al. Low frequency of rearrangements of the ret and trk proto-oncogenes in Japanese thyroid papillary carcinomas. *Jpn J Cancer Res* 1992;83:671.
90. Zou M, Shi Y, Farid NR. Low rate of ret proto-oncogene activation (PTC/retTPC) in papillary thyroid carcinomas from Saudi Arabia. *Cancer* 1994;73:176.
91. Greco A, Pierotti MA, Bongarzone I, et al. TRK-T1 is a novel oncogene formed by the fusion of TPR and TRK genes in human papillary thyroid carcinomas. *Oncogene* 1992;7:237.
92. Di Renzo MF, Olivero M, Ferro S, et al. Overexpression of the c-MET/HGF receptor gene in human thyroid carcinomas. *Oncogene* 1992;7:2549.
93. Soh EY, Duh QY, Sobhi SA, et al. Vascular endothelial growth factor expression is higher in differentiated thyroid cancer than in normal or benign thyroid. *J Clin Endocrinol Metab* 1997;82:3741.
94. Fenton C, Patel A, Dinauer C, et al. The expression of vascular endothelial growth factor and the type 1 vascular endothelial growth factor receptor correlate with the size of papillary thyroid carcinoma in children and young adults. *Thyroid* 2000;10:349.
95. Patel A, Jhiang S, Dogra S, et al. Differentiated thyroid carcinomas that express sodium-iodide symporter have a lower risk of recurrence for children and adolescents. *Pediatr Res* 2002;52:737.
96. Nord B, Larsson C, Wong FK, et al. Sporadic follicular thyroid tumors show loss of a 200-kb region in 11q13 without evidence for mutations in the MEN1 gene. *Genes Chromosomes Cancer* 1999;26:35.
97. Herrmann MA, Hey ID, Bartelt DHJ, et al. Cytogenetic and molecular genetic studies of follicular and papillary thyroid cancers. *J Clin Invest* 1991;88:1596.
98. Fagin JA, Matsuo K, Karmarkar A, et al. High prevalence of mutations of the p53 gene in poorly differentiated human thyroid carcinomas. *J Clin Invest* 1992;91:179.
99. Ito T, Seyama T, Mizuno T, et al. Unique association of p53 mutations with undifferentiated but not with differentiated carcinomas of the thyroid gland. *Cancer Res* 1992;52:1369.
100. Arnold A. Genetic basis of endocrine disease 5. Molecular genetics of parathyroid gland neoplasia. *J Clin Endocrinol Metab* 1993;77:1108.
101. Heppner C, Kester MB, Agarwal SK, et al. Somatic mutation of the MEN1 gene in parathyroid tumours. *Nat Genet* 1997;16:375.
102. Farnebo F, Teh BT, Kytola S, et al. Alterations of the MEN1 gene in sporadic parathyroid tumors. *J Clin Endocrinol Metab* 1998;83:2627.
103. Radford DM, Ashley SW, Wells SA Jr, et al. Loss of heterozygosity of markers on chromosome 11 in tumors from patients with multiple endocrine neoplasia syndrome type 1. *Cancer Res* 1990;50:6529.
104. Byström C, Larsson C, Blomberg C, et al. Localization of the MEN1 gene to a small region within chromosome 11q13 by deletion mapping in tumors. *Proc Natl Acad Sci U S A* 1990;87:1968.
105. Friedman E, DeMarco L, Gejman PV, et al. Allelic loss from chromosome 11 in parathyroid tumors. *Cancer Res* 1992;52:6804.
106. Arnold A, Shattuck TM, Mallya SM, et al. Molecular pathogenesis of primary hyperparathyroidism. *J Bone Miner Res* 2002;17:[Suppl 2]N30.
107. Imanishi Y, Hosokawa Y, Yoshimoto K, et al. Primary hyperparathyroidism caused by parathyroid targeted overexpression of cyclin D1 in transgenic mice. *J Clin Invest* 2001;107:1093.
108. Foley TPJ, Harrison HC, Arnaud CD, et al. Familial benign hypercalcemia. *J Pediatr* 1972;81:1060.
109. Marx SJ, Attie MF, Levine MA, et al. The hypocalciuric or benign variant of familial hypercalcemia: clinical and biochemical features in fifteen kindreds. *Medicine* 1981;60:397.
110. Pollak MR, Brown EM, Chou Y-HW, et al. Mutations in the human Ca^{2+}-sensing receptor gene cause familial hypocalciuric hypercalcemia and neonatal severe hyperparathyroidism. *Cell* 1993;75:1297.
111. Khosla S, Ebeling PR, Firek AF, et al. Calcium infusion suggests a "set-point" abnormality of parathyroid gland function in familial benign hypercalcemia and more complex disturbances in primary hyperparathyroidism. *J Clin Endocrinol Metab* 1993;76:715.
112. Aida K, Koishi S, Inoue M, et al. Familial hypocalciuric hypercalcemia associated with mutation in the human Ca^{2+}-sensing receptor gene. *J Clin Endocrinol Metab* 1995;80:2594.

113. Chou Y-H, Pollak M, Brandi M, et al. Mutations in the human Ca²⁺-sensing receptor gene that cause familial hypocalciuric hypercalcemia. *Am J Hum Genet* 1995;56:1075.

114. Pearce S, Trump D, Wooding C, et al. Calcium-sensing receptor mutations in familial benign hypercalcemia and neonatal severe hyperparathyroidism. *J Clin Invest* 1995;96:2683.

115. Goldsmith RE, Sizemore GW, Chen I-W, et al. Familial hyperparathyroidism; description of a large kindred and a review of the literature. *Ann Intern Med* 1976;84:36.

116. Wassif WS, Moniz CF, Friedman E, et al. Familial isolated hyperparathyroidism: a distinct genetic entity with and increased risk of parathyroid cancer. *J Clin Endocrinol Metab* 1993;77:1485.

117. Jackson CE, Norum RA, Boyd SB, et al. Hereditary hyperparathyroidism and multiple ossifying jaw fibromas: a clinically and genetically distinct syndrome. *Surgery* 1990;108:1006.

118. Szabó J, Heath B, Hill VM, et al. Hereditary hyperparathyroidism-jaw tumor syndrome: the endocrine tumor gene HRPT2 maps to chromosome 1q21-q31. *Am J Hum Genet* 1995;56:944.

119. Carpten JD, Robbins CM, Villablanca A, et al. HRPT2, encoding parafibromin, is mutated in hyperparathyroidism-jaw tumor syndrome. *Nat Genet* 2002;32:676.

120. Hakim JP, Levine MA. Absence of p53 point mutations in parathyroid adenoma and carcinoma. *J Clin Endocrinol Metab* 1994;78:103.

121. Cryns VL, Rubio MP, Thor AD, et al. p53 abnormalities in human parathyroid carcinoma. *J Clin Endocrinol Metab* 1994;78:1320.

122. Cryns VL, Thor A, Xu H-J, et al. Loss of the retinoblastoma tumor-suppressor gene in parathyroid carcinomas. *N Engl J Med* 1994;330:757.

123. Beuschlein F, Reincke M, Karl M, et al. Clonal composition of human adrenocortical neoplasms. *Cancer Res* 1994;54:4927.

124. Stratakis CA. Genetics of adrenocortical tumors: gatekeepers, landscapers and conductors in symphony. *Trends Endocrinol Metab* 2003;14:404.

125. Yano T, Linehan M, Anglard P, et al. Genetic changes in human adrenocortical carcinomas. *J Natl Cancer Inst* 1989;7:518.

126. Reincke M. Mutations in adrenocortical tumors. *Horm Metab Res* 1998;30:447.

127. Srivastava S, Zou Z, Pirollo K, et al. Germ-line transmission of a mutated p53 gene in a cancer-prone family with Li-Fraumeni syndrome. *Nature* 1990;348:747.

128. Ping AJ, Reeve AE, Law DJ, et al. Genetic linkage of Beckwith-Wiedemann syndrome to 11p15. *Am J Hum Genet* 1989;44:720.

129. Stratakis CA, Carney JA, Lin J-P, et al. Carney complex, a familial multiple neoplasia and lentiginosis syndrome. Analysis of 11 kindreds and linkage to the short arm of chromosome 2. *J Clin Invest* 1996;97:599.

130. Kirschner LS, Carney JA, Pack S, et al. Mutations in the gene encoding the type Iα regulatory subunit of the protein kinase A (PRKARIA) in patients with Carney complex. *Nat Genet* 2000;26:89.

131. Latif F, Tory K, Gnarra J, et al. Identification of the von Hippel-Lindau disease tumor suppressor gene. *Science* 1993;260:1317.

132. Duan DR, Pause A, Burgess WH, et al. Inhibition of transcription elongation by the VHL tumor suppressor protein [see comments]. *Science* 1995;269:1402.

133. Crossey PA, Richards FM, Foster K, et al. Identification of intragenic mutations in the von Hippel-Lindau disease tumour suppressor gene and correlation with disease phenotype. *Hum Mol Genet* 1994;3:1303.

134. Cawthon RM, Weiss R, Xu G, et al. A major segment of the neurofibromatosis type 1 gene: cDNA sequence, genomic structure, and point mutations. *Cell* 1990;62:193.

135. Wallace MR, Marchuk DA, Andersen LB, et al. Type 1 neurofibromatosis gene: identification of a large transcript disrupted in three NF1 patients. *Science* 1990;249:181.

136. Neumann HP, Bausch B, McWhinney SR, et al. Germ-line mutations in nonsyndromic pheochromocytoma. *N Engl J Med* 2002;346:1459.

137. Baysal BE, Ferrell RE, Willett-Brozick JE, et al. Mutations in SDHD, a mitochondrial complex II gene, in hereditary paraganglioma. *Science* 2000;287:848.

138. Gimm O, Armanios M, Dziema H, et al. Somatic and occult germline mutations in SDHD, a mitochondrial complex II gene, in non-familial pheochromocytomas. *Cancer Res* 2000;60:6822.

139. Astuti D, Douglas F, Lennard TWJ, et al. Germline SDHD mutation in familial pheochromocytoma. *Lancet* 2001;357:1181.

140. Astuti D, Latif F, Dallol A, et al. Mutations in the mitochondrial complex II subunit SDHB cause susceptibility to familial paraganglioma and pheochromocytoma. *Am J Hum Genet* 2001;69:49.

141. Niemann S, Muller U. Mutations in SDHC cause autosomal dominant paraganglioma. *Nat Genet* 2000;26:141.

142. Sukhodolets KE, Hickman AB, Agarwal SK, et al. The 32-Kilodalton subunit of replication protein A interacts with menin, the product of the MEN1 tumor suppressor gene. *Mol Cell Biol* 2003;23:493.

143. Lopez-Egido J, Cunningham J, Berg M, et al. Menin's interaction with glial fibrillary acidic protein and vimentin suggests a role for the intermediate filament network in regulating menin activity. *Exp Cell Res* 2002;278:175.

144. Obungu VH, Lee Burns A, Agarwal SK, et al. Menin, a tumor suppressor, associates with nonmuscle myosin II-A heavy chain. *Oncogene* 2003;22:6347.

145. Kim H, Lee JE, Cho EJ, et al. Menin, a tumor suppressor, represses JunD-mediated transcriptional activity by association with an mSin3A-histone deacetylase complex. *Cancer Res* 2003;63:6135.

146. Jin S, Mao H, Schnepp RW, et al. Menin associates with FANCD2, a protein involved in repair of DNA damage. *Cancer Res* 2003;63:4204.

147. Khosla S, Patel VM, Hay ID, et al. Loss of heterozygosity suggests multiple genetic alterations in pheochromocytomas and medullary thyroid carcinomas. *J Clin Invest* 1991;87:1691.

148. Yang K-P, Nguyen CV, Castillo SG, et al. Deletion mapping on the distal third region of chromosome 1p in multiple endocrine neoplasia type IIA. *Anticancer Res* 1990;10:527.

149. Mathew CGP, Smith BA, Thorpe K, et al. Deletions of genes on chromosome 1 in endocrine neoplasia. *Nature* 1987;328:524.

150. Shin E, Fujita S, Takami K, et al. Deletion mapping of chromosome 1p and 22q in pheochromocytoma. *Jpn J Cancer Res* 1993;84:402.

TOBIAS CARLING
ROBERT UDELSMAN

SECTION 2

Thyroid Tumors

Goiter, or enlargement of the thyroid gland, has plagued humans since antiquity and was previously referred to as a *bronchocele* ("tracheal outpouch").[1] The modern name of the gland was introduced in 1656, when Thomas Wharton called it the thyroid gland, after the Greek for "shield shaped," because of the configuration of the nearby thyroid cartilage. Theodor Kocher, professor from 1871 at Berne, markedly enhanced the surgical treatment for disorders of the thyroid gland and was awarded the Nobel Prize in 1909 for his work on thyroid physiology, pathology, and surgery. His Nobel lecture entitled "Concerning Pathological Manifestations in Low-Grade Thyroid Diseases" can be read on the official Web site of the Nobel Foundation (http://www.nobel.se). Charles H. Mayo had a major interest in goiter as noted in a publication of 1904: "My first incursion into the field of thyroid surgery began on December 13, 1889, when a big Norwegian came in with an enormous goiter...."[2] The Norwegian was operated on for obstruction of the trachea by the thyroid enlargement and subsequently returned to his farm. Charles H. Mayo was not only joined in Rochester by Henry Plummer, who defined toxic multinodular goiter and was instrumental in the growth of the Mayo Clinic, but also by Edward Kendall, who succeeded in isolating bioactive crystalline material from the thyroid on Christmas Day, 1914.[2] He and his associate, A. E. Osterberg, named it *thyroxin*. At the Johns Hopkins University School of Medicine, William S. Halsted revolutionized surgical treatment and education and made enormous contribution to the operative treatment of both thyroid and parathyroid glands. Since then a number of important advances have been made in the diagnosis and management of patients with thyroid tumors, including the development of fine-needle aspiration (FNA) biopsy, radioiodine treatment, and antithyroid drugs.

THYROID TUMOR CLASSIFICATION AND STAGING SYSTEMS

The normal thyroid is composed histologically of two main parenchymal cell types. Follicular cells line the colloid follicles, concentrate iodine, and are involved in the production of thyroid hormone. These cells give rise to both well-differentiated cancers and anaplastic thyroid cancer. The second cell type, the

C or parafollicular cell, produces the hormone calcitonin and is the cell of origin for medullary thyroid carcinoma (MTC). Immune cells and stromal cells of the thyroid are responsible for lymphoma and sarcoma, respectively. Of the 20,700 new cases of thyroid cancer each year in the United States, approximately 90% are well-differentiated cancers, 5% to 9% are medullary tumors, 1% to 2% are anaplastic tumors, 1% to 3% are lymphoma, and fewer than 1% are sarcomas or other rare tumors.[3]

Within the category of well-differentiated thyroid cancers various histologic subtypes have been identified due to an improved understanding of their biology. Initial categories included papillary, follicular, and mixed tumor with variable areas of both papillary and follicular histologic features. Studies have established that these mixed tumors with areas of papillary features have a natural history and prognosis similar to those of papillary thyroid cancer without follicular features.[3] Accordingly, mixed papillary and follicular carcinoma are now grouped with papillary carcinoma. Also, the follicular variant of papillary carcinoma has cytologic characteristics of a papillary carcinoma but appears histologically to have a follicular architecture and behaves biologically as well-differentiated papillary carcinoma. The major cytologic feature shared by all members of this papillary group, regardless of the histologic pattern, is the characteristic nucleus containing Orphan Annie nuclei, nuclear grooves, and intranuclear pseudoinclusions. A third category of lesions grouped with differentiated thyroid carcinoma is Hürthle cell or oncocytic carcinoma. Analysis of the distribution of well-differentiated thyroid cancer subgroups in some reports reveals that 80% to 85% are papillary, 10% to 15% are follicular, and 3% to 5% are Hürthle cell carcinomas.[3] This distribution may not reflect adequate pathologic recognition of the recently appreciated follicular variant of papillary carcinoma. True follicular carcinoma now appears to represent 5% or fewer cases of well-differentiated thyroid cancers in countries with iodine-sufficient diets.[4]

Thyroid carcinoma can be categorized by level of clinical aggressiveness. The least aggressive are well differentiated (papillary carcinoma, follicular carcinoma), followed by intermediately or poorly differentiated (Hürthle cell carcinoma, some rare variants of papillary carcinoma including insular, columnar, and tall cell thyroid carcinoma), and the frequently incurable undifferentiated (anaplastic carcinoma).

At least nine systems have been proposed and to a lesser or greater extent validated for the staging of thyroid cancer (Table 34.2-1). None has been universally adopted, and the lack of a common staging system has impeded the development of multicenter trials and cross-institutional comparisons of thyroid cancer outcomes. In the absence of a universally accepted system, it is recommended that the TNM (tumor, node, metastasis) staging system, introduced by the International Union Against Cancer and promoted by the American Joint Committee on Cancer (AJCC), the American Cancer Society, the National Cooperative Cancer Network, and the American College of Surgeons, be adopted as the international staging system.[5] The TNM (or AJCC) classification system is outlined in Table 34.2-2.

EPIDEMIOLOGY AND DEMOGRAPHICS

Carcinomas of the endocrine glands or organs are relatively uncommon, as they account for only 1.8% of the 1.28 million

TABLE 34.2-1. Comparison of Nine Different Prognostic Classification Systems for Well-Differentiated Thyroid Carcinoma

System	Criteria	Reference
EORTC	Age, sex, cell type, invasion, metastases	124
AGES	Age, grade of tumor, extent, size	56
AMES	Age, metastases, extent, size	50
DAMES	DNA ploidy, age, metastases, size	60
MACIS	Metastases, age, completeness of resection, invasion, size	61
Ohio State	Size, cervical metastases, multiplicity, invasion, distant metastases	49
Sloan-Kettering	Age, histology, size, extension, metastases	57
NTCTS	Size, multifocality, invasion, differentiation, cervical metastases, extracervical metastases	63
TNM	Size, extension, nodal metastases, distant metastases	5

EORTC, European Organization for Research and Treatment of Cancer; NTCTS, National Thyroid Cancer Treatment Cooperative Study; TNM, tumor, node, metastasis.

new cases of non–skin cancer and 0.41% of the 555,500 cancer deaths in the United States in 2002.[6] Thyroid cancer is the most common endocrine malignancy, accounting for 91.2% of the total new endocrine cancers and 56.5% of the deaths due to endocrine cancers for 2002. In 2002, there were 20,700 new cases of thyroid cancer and 1300 deaths due to thyroid cancer. The discrepancy between the total number of cases of all endocrine cancers arising in the thyroid (91.2%) and the total proportion of endocrine cancer deaths (56.5%) reflects the relatively indolent nature of and long-term survival associated with thyroid malignancies.

Well-differentiated thyroid cancer is approximately 2.5 times as common in females versus male, and this relates to papillary and follicular thyroid carcinoma.[7,8] The median age at diagnosis is earlier in women than in men for both papillary and follicular subtypes and tends to be earlier for papillary cancer than for follicular cancer in either gender. Specifically, the median age at diagnosis in white women is between 40 and 41 years, whereas for white men, it is 44 to 45 years for papillary carcinoma.[9] For follicular thyroid carcinoma, the median age at diagnosis is 48 for white women compared with 53 for white men.[9] Well-differentiated thyroid cancer has a greater incidence in whites than in African Americans of both genders. The relative age-adjusted incidence rate is slightly more than twofold higher in whites. One significant difference in the incidence in terms of race is that the proportion of well-differentiated thyroid carcinomas that are follicular is increased greatly in African Americans compared with whites. It is reported that follicular carcinoma accounts for 15% of all well-differentiated tumors in whites compared with 34% in African Americans.[9]

ETIOLOGY AND RISK FACTORS

Radiation exposure to the thyroid gland in childhood, age, female gender, and family history are risk factors known to increase the incidence of well-differentiated thyroid cancer.

TABLE 34.2-2.   American Joint Committee on Cancer Classification of Thyroid Cancer

PRIMARY TUMOR (T)[a]

TX	Primary tumor cannot be assessed
T0	No evidence of primary tumor
T1	Tumor ≤2 cm confined to the thyroid
T2	Tumor >2 cm and <4 cm confined to the thyroid
T3	Tumor >4 cm confined to the thyroid
	or
	Tumor of any size with minimal extrathyroid extension
T4a	Tumor of any size with extrathyroid extension to subcutaneous soft tissues, larynx, trachea, esophagus, or recurrent laryngeal nerve
	or
	Intrathyroidal anaplastic carcinoma[b]
T4b	Tumor invading prevertebral fascia or encasing carotid artery or mediastinal vessels
	or
	Extrathyroidal anaplastic carcinoma[b]

REGIONAL LYMPH NODES (N) (CENTRAL COMPARTMENT, LATERAL CERVICAL, AND UPPER MEDIASTINAL)

NX	Regional lymph nodes cannot be assessed
N0	No regional lymph node metastasis
N1	Regional lymph node metastasis
N1a	Metastasis to level VI (pretracheal or paratracheal, and prelaryngeal)
N1b	Metastasis to unilateral, bilateral, or contralateral cervical or superior mediastinal lymph nodes

DISTANT METASTASIS (M)

MX	Distant metastasis cannot be assessed
M0	No distant metastasis
M1	Distant metastasis

STAGE GROUPINGS

Papillary and follicular carcinoma

Under 45 y of age

Stage I	Any T	Any N	M0
Stage II	Any T	Any N	M1

45 y of age and over

Stage I	T1	N0	M0
Stage II	T2	N0	M0
Stage III	T3	N0	M0
	T1	N1a	M0
	T2	N1a	M0
	T3	N1a	M0
Stage IVA	T4a	N0	M0
	T4a	N1a	M0
	T1	N1b	M0
	T2	N1b	M0
	T3	N1b	M0
	T4a	N1b	M0
	T4a	N1b	M0
Stage IVB	T4b	Any N	M0
Stage IVC	Any T	Any N	M1

Medullary carcinoma

Stage I	T1	N0	M0
Stage II	T2	N0	M0
	T3	N0	M0
Stage III	T1	N1a	M0
	T2	N1a	M0
	T3	N1a	M0
Stage IVA	T4a	N0	M0
	T4a	N1a	M0
	T1	N1b	M0
	T2	N1b	M0
	T3	N1b	M0
	T4a	N1b	M0
Stage IVB	T4b	Any N	M0
Stage IVC	Any T	Any N	M1

Anaplastic carcinoma

Stage IVA	T4a	Any N	M0
Stage IVB	T4b	Any N	M0
Stage IVC	Any T	Any N	M1

[a]All categories may be subdivided: (a) solitary tumor, (b) multifocal tumor (the largest determines the classification).
[b]All anaplastic carcinomas are considered T4 tumors.
(Modified from ref. 5.)

Exposure of the thyroid to radiation may occur either from external sources or from ingestion of radioactive material. External exposure of the thyroid comes primarily from medically administered external-beam irradiation and environmental exposure related to nuclear weapons attacks, testing, and power plant accidents. Internal exposure occurs by ingestion of radioisotopes of iodine that concentrate in the thyroid gland from either medical treatment with radioactive iodine or ingestion of these radioisotopes in contaminated areas.

Several studies have shown an inverse relationship between increased risk of thyroid cancer and age of exposure to radiation.[10-13] Relative risk is also linearly related to exposure dose, at least up to 2000 rad.[13] The latency period after childhood exposure is at least 3 to 5 years, and there is no apparent drop-off in the increased risk even 40 years after the radiation exposure.[13] In a comprehensive study of 4296 individuals irradiated before age 16, more than one-third developed thyroid nodules, and 309 patients were documented to have thyroid cancer.[13] The large populations studied demonstrated that the increased relative risk of thyroid carcinoma was low and thyroid cancers were rare between 5 and 10 years after radiation exposure.[12] The majority of cases occurred between 20 and 40 years after exposure. However, even after 40 years, the relative risk as compared to a nonirradiated population was still increased. For these reasons, the large cohort of patients who underwent childhood irradiation for benign medical conditions such as thymic enlargement and acne between 1920 and 1960 and are now between the ages of 40 and 80 still has an increased risk of developing thyroid carcinoma.

Although the use of irradiation for benign conditions has not been practiced since the 1960s, there is increased use of radiation treatments for neoplastic conditions in infants, children, and young adults. The majority of this population have either Hodgkin's or non-Hodgkin's lymphoma, but this group also includes long-term survivors of Wilms' tumor or neuroblastoma in the treatment of which there is some radiation scatter to the thyroid gland.[14,15] The young age at treatment for neuroblastoma and Wilms' tumor (mean ages, 2 and 3 years, respectively) and the relatively high dose of thyroid exposure (660 rad and 310 rad, respectively) has led to a dramatic increase in relative risk of 350 for neuroblastoma patients and 132 for survivors of Wilms' tumors for the development of thyroid cancer.[15] Relative risks between 16 and 80 have been reported in the patient population of adolescents and young adults treated for lymphoma.[14] In the adult patient population treated with therapeutic radiation for malignancies, there is a drop-off in risk that reflects the importance of age at exposure. In a large study of more than 150,000 women treated with radiation for cervical cancer who had an estimated thyroid exposure of 11 rad, relative risk was 2.35 compared with nonirradiated age-matched controls.[16]

Radiation exposure to the thyroid gland occurs via ingestion of radioisotopes that concentrate in the thyroid from either medical administration of radioactive iodine for diagnostic or therapeutic purposes, or environmental exposure from fallout of nuclear weapons or accidents. The most common exposure is caused by administration of iodine 131 (^{131}I) administered for diagnostic thyroid scans. In a nationwide, population-based cohort study in Sweden including all 36,792 individuals who received ^{131}I for diagnostic purposes between 1952 and 1969, there was no evidence that the diagnostic scans increased the risk of thyroid cancer.[17] In addition, therapeutic ^{131}I administered for ablation of thyroid tissue to treat hyperthyroidism seem to be associated with, at most, a very modest increased incidence ratio for thyroid cancer.[18]

A more harmful type of ingestion of radioisotopes of iodine comes from exposure to nuclear fallout. Data on the effect on thyroid cancer incidence comes from populations exposed to radioactive fallout from the nuclear power station accident at Chernobyl and the results of atomic bomb development and testing at Hanford (Washington), the Nevada test site, and the Marshall Islands.[19] The most cogent information comes from Chernobyl, where an epidemic of childhood thyroid cancer followed exposure to radioiodine that was mainly ^{131}I. Within the first decade after the Chernobyl accident, some regions of Belarus show a 100-fold increase in thyroid cancer in individuals younger than age of 15 at the time of exposure.[19] Essentially all of these radiation-induced tumors were shown to be papillary thyroid cancer, associated with more aggressive growth, a higher likelihood of local invasion and spread to regional lymph nodes, and a higher incidence of ret/PTC translocation (see Chapter 34.1).[19,20] These data reflect the importance of age at exposure in the development of radiation-associated thyroid cancer.

Although there exists an obvious association between radiation exposure and risk of well-differentiated thyroid cancer, the majority of patients who develop well-differentiated thyroid carcinoma have no history of radiation exposure. A large study indicated that 9% of thyroid cancer could be related to radiation exposure, confirming that the vast majority of cases are unrelated to radiation exposure, at least to readily identifiable exposure.[21] Other factors, including dietary influences, sex hormones, environmental exposures, or genetic susceptibility, have been studied with mixed results and no clear associations found. Studies of dietary influences have primarily focused on the level of iodine in the diet. Iodine-deficient diets or diets that include a large intake of vegetables from the crucifer family (which block iodine uptake) may lead to increased thyroid-stimulating hormone (TSH) levels and are considered goitrogenic. Increased iodine intake due to shellfish consumption occurs in the geographic areas with the highest incidence of predominantly papillary thyroid cancer, such as Iceland, Norway, and Hawaii. However, data suggest that relatively elevated levels of fish consumption do not appreciably increase thyroid cancer risk.[22]

Epidemiologic studies have demonstrated a fourfold to tenfold increased risk of well-differentiated thyroid cancer in first-degree relatives of subjects with this neoplasia.[21,23] In contrast to the well-described molecular pathology associated with MTC, the molecular and clinical genetics of thyroid follicular cell cancer have only recently been unveiled. Well-differentiated thyroid cancer can occur as the main feature in some syndromes inherited in an autosomal dominant fashion and also can show an increased incidence in those with other tumor susceptibility syndromes. The clinical and genetic characteristics of familial thyroid follicular cell carcinoma susceptibility syndromes are outlined in Table 34.2-3.[24,25] For details related to the molecular biology of these disorders, see Chapter 34.1.

TABLE 34.2-3.   Clinical and Genetic Characteristics of Familial Thyroid Follicular Cell Carcinoma Susceptibility Syndromes

Syndrome	Chromosome Linkage/ Gene	Characteristics
Papillary thyroid carcinoma with papillary renal neoplasia (PTC-RCC)	1q21/?	Associated with papillary renal neoplasia Autosomal dominant with partial penetrance
Familial nonmedullary thyroid carcinoma (fNMTC)	2q21/?	Nonmedullary thyroid carcinoma only Autosomal dominant with partial penetrance
Familial thyroid tumors with cell oxyphilia (TCO)	19p13.2/?	Benign nodules and papillary thyroid carcinoma Characteristic oxyphilic cells Autosomal dominant with partial penetrance
Papillary thyroid carcinoma without oxyphilia	19p13	Papillary thyroid carcinoma without oxyphilia Genetically linked, but clinically distinct from TCO Autosomal dominant
Familial adenomatous polyposis (FAP)	5q21-22/ APC	Papillary thyroid carcinoma with ~10× increased prevalence Colorectal carcinoma, ampullary carcinoma, hepatoblastoma, medulloblastoma Autosomal dominant
Cowden disease (multiple hamartoma syndrome)	10q23.3/ PTEN	Follicular and papillary thyroid carcinoma, benign thyroid nodules Multiple hamartomas, breast and endometrial cancer Autosomal dominant

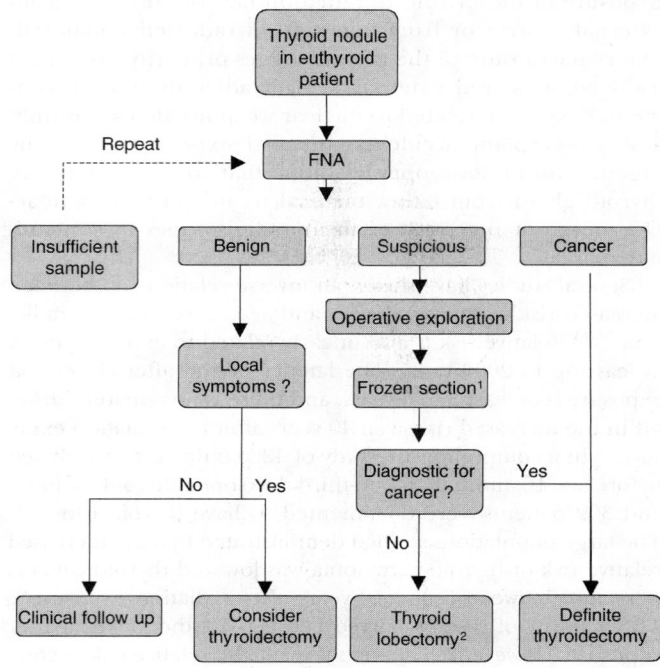

FIGURE 34.2-1.   Flow diagram for the evaluation of thyroid nodule based on the results of fine-needle aspiration biopsy. See text for special considerations in follicular, Hürthle cell, and medullary thyroid carcinoma. [1]Consider touch preparation. [2]Consider total thyroidectomy for lesions that are large and nodular, or bilateral, or both, as well as in patients with a history of radiation exposure in childhood. FNA, fine-needle aspiration.

EVALUATION OF THE THYROID NODULE

The vast majority of thyroid cancers presents as thyroid nodules detected either by the patient or clinician, or with imaging of the neck for other disorders. Because only a minority of thyroid nodules are malignant, a general discussion of the incidence, evaluation, and management of thyroid nodules precedes discussion of specific thyroid neoplasias (Fig. 34.2-1).

In iodine-replete areas, thyroid nodules are clinically detectable by physical examination in at least 4% to 7% of the general population. However, the prevalence of thyroid nodules depends on the population under study: gender, age, and history of exposure to ionizing radiation strongly influence the results in various large studies, as does the method by which nodules are detected—physical examination, intraoperative palpation, imaging techniques, histopathologic analysis, or autopsy procedure. The incidence of nodules is approximately ten times higher when based on findings at autopsy, during surgery, or by ultrasonography than when based on physical examination. There is an age-dependent increase in thyroid nodule occurrence, and in one histopathologic study, up to 90% of women older than 70 years and 60% of men older than 80 years had nodular goiter.[26] All studies show that women develop nodules more frequently than men, although reports of the female to male ratio vary from 1.2:1.0 to 4.3:1.0.[27] An increased tendency

to develop thyroid nodules is demonstrated in groups exposed to ionizing radiation, especially during childhood (see Etiology and Risk Factors, earlier in this chapter). In one large study, more than one-third of individuals receiving radiation to the neck before age 16 years developed palpable thyroid nodules.[12]

Most thyroid nodules are found in asymptomatic patients during routine physical examination or because the patient notices a neck mass. By obtaining information from the history and physical examination, the risk of malignancy in that individual can to a certain extent be assessed. In general, there is a 5% to 10% chance of malignancy in all thyroid nodules in the total population, but men and patients at the extremes of age are at higher risk for malignancy. Nodules found in a patient with a history of childhood neck irradiation carry a 33% to 37% chance of malignancy.[12] The presence of a solitary nodule is of greater concern than are multiple nodules, but a dominant nodule or a nodule that grows in the setting of a multinodular goiter should be investigated to exclude carcinoma. Patients with Graves' disease who develop a nodule may have a higher risk of cancer.[7,27] However, the occurrence of carcinoma in autonomously functioning nodules is extremely rare.[7,27]

A rapid increase in nodule size, dyspnea, dysphagia, hoarseness, or the development of Horner's syndrome, albeit not specific for malignancy, are worrisome findings. Tender nodules are more often associated with thyroiditis and are likely to be benign. A family history of thyroid cancer or history, signs, and symptoms consistent with any of the tumor susceptibility syndromes outlined in Tables 34.2-3 and 34.2-6 should prompt an extended investigation. For details, see Etiology and Risk Factors earlier and Medullary Thyroid Carcinoma, later in this chapter, and Chapter 34.1. When the neck is examined, the firmness, mobility, and size of the nodules, their adherence to surrounding structures, and the presence of lymphadenopathy are important clues to the presence of carcinoma. However, these features lack specificity for malignancy. Routine indirect or direct laryngoscopy is important not only in the preoperative evaluation but also in the assessment of a thyroid nodule, and vocal cord paralysis is generally associated with advanced thyroid malignancy.

Thyroid function testing should be performed to identify underlying thyroid pathology and not to differentiate benign from malignant nodules. Subclinical hyperthyroidism, with a suppressed TSH level, may be secondary to an autonomously functioning nodule. In this case, one can determine whether the nodule is functional with a radionuclide uptake scan. The majority of both benign and malignant thyroid nodules are hypofunctional compared to normal thyroid tissue; thus, the finding of a "cold" nodule on iodine 123 or technetium 99 scanning is nonspecific. Radionuclide scans can be helpful in determining the functional status of nodules in patients with multinodular thyroid disease to focus a biopsy on cold nodules. However, routine thyroid scanning in the initial evaluation of the thyroid nodule is not advocated because it is less cost effective, specific, and sensitive than FNA. Routine measurement of serum calcitonin level has been advocated by some authors to identify patients with medullary carcinoma of the thyroid preoperatively, although the cost effectiveness of this procedure is unknown.[28] In any case, serum calcitonin levels should be determined in all patients with a thyroid nodule and when either sporadic or familial MTC is suspected.

High-resolution ultrasonography is a useful adjunct to the clinical examination for size assessment of nodules, for the detection of multiple nodules not discerned by palpation, and for assisting in FNA.[29] Several studies have aimed at identifying sonographic criteria for distinguishing benign from malignant thyroid nodules. The presence of microcalcification, irregular margins, spotty intranodular flow, and hypervascularity are suggestive but not diagnostic of malignancy.[30] Ultrasonography can identify whether a lesion is cystic or solid, and the vast majority of purely cystic lesions are benign.

FNA, which was popularized in the 1960s by Einhorn and Franzen at the Karolinska Institute, Stockholm, has revolutionized the management of thyroid nodules, providing an extremely sensitive and cost-effective method of detecting thyroid malignancies.[29] The impact this procedure has had on clinical practice is reflected in the reduction of the total number of thyroid surgeries performed, the greater proportion of malignancies removed at surgery, and the overall reduction in the cost of managing patients with thyroid nodules.[27] The accuracy of cytologic diagnosis from FNA ranges from 70% to 97%[29] and is highly dependent on both the skill of the individual performing the biopsy and the cytopathologist examining the specimen. If an adequate sample is obtained, the results of FNA is most commonly assigned into one of the categories outlined in Table 34.2-4. Approximately 70% of samples are classified as benign (range, 53% to 90%), 4.0% as malignant (range, 1% to 10%), 10% as suspicious or indeterminate (range, 5% to 23%), and 17% as showing insufficient sampling (range, 15% to 20%).[29,31] The insufficient sample rate can be improved by performing on-site cytologic assessment of the adequacy of the sample.[29]

TABLE 34.2-4. Fine-Needle Aspiration Diagnoses for Thyroid Nodules

Benign	Suspicious	Malignant
Acute suppurative thyroiditis	Follicular neoplasm	Papillary carcinoma
Subacute thyroiditis	Hürthle cell neoplasm	Follicular variant of papillary carcinoma
Hashimoto's (lymphocytic) thyroiditis	Suspicious for papillary carcinoma	Medullary thyroid carcinoma
Nodular goiter		Anaplastic carcinoma
Adenomatoid nodule		Thyroid lymphoma
Colloid nodule		Metastatic carcinoma

The malignant potential of follicular neoplasms can rarely be determined by cytologic evaluation; thus, the biopsy findings from such lesions are generally classified as suspicious or indeterminate, and most neoplasms come to surgical resection. The cells from follicular adenomas and follicular carcinomas appear identical; only by identifying capsular or vascular invasion on histologic specimens can cancer be diagnosed. Specimens with predominantly Hürthle cells are treated in the same fashion; however, extensive Hürthle cell changes can be seen in Hashimoto's thyroiditis. Malignancy is found in approximately 20% of follicular nodules that are classified as indeterminate on FNA.[32]

A variety of molecular markers have been assessed in FNA specimens in an attempt to develop more discriminating cytologic subclassifications to improve the yield of malignancy found at surgery. These markers include telomerase activity, presence of loss of heterozygosity by polymerase chain reaction–based microsatellite analysis, as well as various patterns of protein expression by immunocytochemical analysis.[33,34] Although there is little doubt that molecular markers will prove useful in the future, currently there is no single marker or group of markers that has been adopted in routine clinical practice.

Nodules from which biopsy specimens are classified as benign or negative are safely followed nonoperatively with the caveat that false-negative results occur in 1% to 6% of cases.[29] Clinical judgment should dictate the course of action in these cases; if a large, hard nodule is fixed to surrounding tissue, surgery should be performed despite a negative FNA finding. Sampling error can occur during biopsy of large, cystic hemorrhagic nodules. False-positive results for malignancy occur in 3% to 6% of all biopsy specimens.[29] The cytologic features of Hashimoto's thyroiditis occasionally lead to these false-positive interpretations, but this can be greatly reduced with analysis by an experienced cytopathologist.

Benign thyroid nodules must be followed carefully by routine physical examination or, more precisely, by ultrasonography and do not generally require repeat biopsy. Thyroxine suppression therapy is widely used, although its efficacy is controversial.[35] A randomized, double-blind, placebo-controlled trial showed that suppressive therapy is effective in reducing solitary thyroid nodule volume and improving infraclinical extranodular changes.[36] It should be noted that the creation of a subclinical hyperthyroid state by suppressive doses of thyroxine increases the incidence of osteoporosis as well as cardiac symptoms, including tachycardia and arrhythmias.

WELL-DIFFERENTIATED THYROID CARCINOMA

PATHOLOGY

Thyroid malignancies are derived from either follicular cells (papillary, follicular, Hürthle cell, and anaplastic carcinomas) or parafollicular C cells (medullary carcinoma).

Papillary thyroid carcinomas constitute 80% to 85% of malignant epithelial thyroid tumors in developed countries where sufficient iodine is present in the diet.[3] Grossly, papillary carcinomas have a variable appearance, from minute subcapsular white scars to large tumors greater than 5 to 6 cm that grossly extend and invade contiguous structures outside the thyroid gland. Cystic change, calcification, and even ossification may be identified.

Microscopically, papillary carcinomas are characterized by the presence of papillae, but some variants contain no papillary areas, are totally follicular in pattern, and are identified as a follicular variant.[37] The term *mixed papillary and follicular carcinoma* is no longer used, because the great majority of papillary carcinomas of the thyroid do contain some follicular areas. Biologically, all these tumors, independent of their degree of follicular pattern, show similar clinical characteristics.[21,37] The World Health Organization defines papillary thyroid cancer as "a malignant epithelial thyroid neoplasm with a distinctive set of nuclear features." The nuclei of papillary carcinoma are enlarged and ovoid and contain thick nuclear membranes, small nucleoli often pressed against the nuclear membrane, intranuclear grooves, and intranuclear cytoplasmic inclusions.[38] Because the nuclei are enlarged, they frequently overlap each other, which is a helpful clue in both the cytologic preparations and histologic slides. Papillary carcinoma has a propensity to invade lymphatic spaces and therefore leads to microscopic multifocal lesions in the gland as well as a high incidence of regional lymph node metastases. The latter may be the presenting symptom of a thyroid papillary carcinoma because, in some cases, a primary tumor is very small. Papillary thyroid carcinomas smaller than 1 cm are often referred to as *microcarcinomas*.

A number of kindreds have now been identified with autosomal dominant inheritance, albeit often with partial penetrance, of a tendency to develop papillary thyroid carcinoma. The familial syndromes can typically be divided clinically into two groups. In the first group, papillary thyroid carcinoma is the predominant clinical feature of a familial tumor syndrome. In the second group of disorders, nonmedullary thyroid cancer is a relatively infrequent component of a familial tumor syndrome (see Table 34.2-3). For details, see Etiology and Risk Factors, earlier in this chapter, and Chapter 34.1. The molecular pathology of well-differentiated thyroid carcinoma is further outlined in Chapter 34.1.

True follicular thyroid carcinoma is an unusual tumor comprising 5% to 10% of thyroid malignancies in areas of the world where goiter is nonendemic.[4] Before the introduction of iodinated salt, follicular carcinoma was much more frequently diagnosed. In addition, the pathologic dictum that any tumor with a pattern that is 50% or more characteristic of follicular carcinoma should be diagnostically placed in a follicular carcinoma category has been shown to be incorrect. Indeed, most of the follicular-pattern thyroid malignancies represent the fol-

licular variant of papillary carcinoma and share the biologic features, natural history, and prognosis of papillary thyroid carcinoma.[21,37] Follicular thyroid carcinoma is unifocal and thickly encapsulated and shows invasion of the capsule or the blood vessels. Because of the diagnostic confusion, statistical data about the survival rate or the metastatic potential of true follicular carcinoma are not easily obtained. Most studies show that if capsular, but not vascular, invasion is present, the prognosis is excellent, with 85% to 100% of patients surviving at least 10 years.[39]

INTERMEDIATELY DIFFERENTIATED THYROID TUMORS

The Hürthle cell (or *oncocytic*) neoplasm is considered a variant of follicular neoplasms. Historically, all such lesions, despite the histologic features, were considered to be malignant; hence, it was recommended that they all be treated aggressively. However, many studies have evaluated the clinical pathologic features of thyroid Hürthle cell tumors and have shown that, on average, only 33% show histologic evidence of malignancy or invasive growth and may metastasize.[40] Hürthle cell tumors that do not demonstrate invasion microscopically behave as adenomas and may be treated conservatively.

A number of aggressive variants of papillary thyroid carcinoma have been identified and are generally grouped as poorly differentiated. These include the tall cell variant, in which the cells are at least twice as long as they are wide; the columnar variant, which shows a curious clear cytoplasm; and the diffuse sclerosis variant, which is found more commonly in young individuals and insular carcinoma.[41–43] These lesions all behave aggressively and are associated with an increased risk for recurrence and metastatic disease. Surgical treatment is required, and resection of adjoining structures, including strap muscles and portions of the esophagus and trachea, may be necessary. The sclerosis variant permeates the thyroid lymphatics and is reported to exhibit a 100% incidence of regional lymph node metastases at the time of diagnosis.[44] All these high-risk variants are associated with significant mortality at 5 years, ranging between 25% and 90%.[41–43,45]

NATURAL HISTORY AND PROGNOSIS

The natural history and prognosis of well-differentiated thyroid cancer has been intensively studied since the 1980s.[46,47] A clear definition of risk factors associated with poor outcome has allowed more selective and less aggressive treatment recommendations. In general, well-differentiated thyroid cancer is one of the least morbid solid carcinomas, with favorable long-term survival. However, a small proportion of patients with papillary cancer and a slightly larger proportion of patients with follicular thyroid cancer die from disease-related causes. Compared with other solid neoplasms, one major difference is that the presence of regional lymph node metastasis appears not to have a strong correlation with overall survival in most series, but does consistently correlate with local recurrence.[48,49]

At presentation, approximately two-thirds of patients have disease localized to the thyroid. The median size of tumors is between 2.0 and 2.5 cm in most large series.[49,50] Patients with papillary carcinomas smaller than 1.0 cm are considered to have minimal or occult papillary thyroid cancer (papillary microcarcinoma). In North American studies, the incidence of occult papillary tumors ranges between 0.5% and 14.0%, with a greater proportional incidence in older age groups. Studies in Scandinavia report up to one-third of patients with minimal papillary thyroid cancers.[3] There is clearly a large discrepancy between this incidence of one-fourth to one-third of patients having occult papillary thyroid cancer and the incidence of 40 per 1 million patient population of clinically significant disease. This discrepancy would argue strongly that these minimal lesions have a different biology than the clinically apparent thyroid cancers, because they tend to grow very slowly.[51] For this reason, standard practice is not to investigate or submit to biopsy nodules that are smaller than 1 cm, except in the setting of familial MTC. These patients do require follow-up. Furthermore, a proportion of patients who present with metastases to cervical lymph nodes may have a clinically occult thyroid lesion.[52]

Thirty-three percent to 61% of patients with papillary thyroid cancer have involvement of clinically apparent cervical lymph nodes at the time of diagnosis.[49] The reported incidence of positive cervical lymph node metastases in follicular thyroid cancers is lower, ranging between 5% and 20%, with a median of approximately 10%.[49,50] This is probably an overestimate, however, because many series of follicular thyroid carcinomas include follicular variants of papillary carcinoma that have the natural history of papillary thyroid cancer and metastasize to lymph nodes with a high incidence. Some argue that true lymphatic metastases from follicular thyroid carcinoma to regional lymph nodes may be extremely unusual, less than 1%,[4] although one report demonstrated a 31% incidence of nodal metastases in follicular carcinoma.[53] If patients with papillary cancer have lymph nodes studied in great detail, the incidence of micrometastases in lymph nodes increases to 80%.[3] The clinical significance of these occult micrometastases parallels the significance of the microscopic foci of intrathyroidal disease, because it is very common but does not usually progress or change clinical outcome.

Hürthle cell carcinomas generally are considered slightly more aggressive than follicular cancer,[40] and the incidence of nodal metastases is greater than that of follicular carcinomas but not as high as papillary cancers.[53] Another difference that may have an impact on outcome is that these lesions tend not to trap radioactive iodine to the same extent as either papillary or follicular thyroid carcinomas.

Only a small minority of patients have distant metastatic hematogenous disease at the time of diagnosis. In a large series 1% to 2% of papillary thyroid cancer patients and 2% to 5% of follicular thyroid cancer patients had metastases outside the neck or mediastinum at the time of diagnosis.[49] One study including 1038 patients reported that 44 patients (4.2%) presented with metastases at diagnosis, including 2.3% of patients with papillary cancer and 11% of those with follicular cancer.[54] Having distant metastases at the time of presentation is a strong predictor of very poor outcome because 43% to 90% of these patients die secondary to their thyroid malignancy.[49,54]

In the overall population with papillary thyroid cancer, there is a 90% to 95% long-term disease-free survival, and in patients with follicular cancers, a 70% to 80% long-term disease-free survival. The 20% of patients in this latter group who develop recurrent disease include a majority with local cervical recurrences either in lymph nodes or the thyroid bed and a minority of patients with distant metastases to the lung, bone,

and liver.[3,49] Once again, patients who develop distant metastases have a poorer outcome, with 50% to 90% disease-specific deaths, whereas patients with locally recurrent disease in the neck have long-term survivals between 70% and 90% even in the presence of persistent cervical disease.[3,49]

The overall 10-year survival for patients with well-differentiated papillary thyroid carcinoma ranges between 74% and 93%, whereas those with follicular cancer have a 10-year survival of 43% to 94%. Although many institutions have reported their data based on these histologic subcategories, a more meaningful system is to categorize patients according to defined risk factors more pertinent to generating prognostic information. There exist considerable databases that define prognostic risk factors for well-differentiated thyroid cancer.[49,50,55–57] The two dominant factors in these series are the age at diagnosis and the presence of distant metastases. All systems also include some measurement of the size of the lesion and other factors, such as local invasion or grade of the tumor, which have an impact on outcome. In general, younger patients with well-differentiated thyroid cancer do well. Cady and Rossi defined low-risk age categories as men younger than 40 years and women younger than 50 years.[50] Although historical data report follicular cancer as having a worse outcome than papillary thyroid cancer, Donohue et al.[58] showed that, if one corrects for age and other prognostic variables, the outcomes are similar within these two pathologic subcategories.

Patients who have distant metastatic disease either at presentation or with recurrence do much worse.[49,54,59] Similarly, patients with local invasion or high-grade lesions have a poorer prognosis. The risk categorization schema called AMES (age, metastatic disease, extrathyroidal extension, size) incorporated these components.[50] Using this system, one can identify low-risk patients, who as a group have a long-term overall survival of 98% and overall disease-free survival of 95% compared with 54% and 45%, respectively, for high-risk patients. One group added an assessment of DNA content by flow cytometry to the AMES categorization and showed that, among a small number of patients, high-risk patients with aneuploid tumors had essentially zero long-term survival.[60] The initial system developed by the Mayo Clinic group carried the acronym AGES (age, tumor grade, tumor extent, tumor size). A mathematical formula based on weighted risk factors was developed to yield a prognostic score. The scoring system showed that patients with a prognostic score of less than 4 had a 99% 20-year survival, whereas patients with a prognostic score greater than 6 had a 13% 20-year survival, with graded categories in between.[56] A more recent modification of this system is MACIS (metastasis, age at diagnosis, tumor extent subdivided into completeness of resection and invasion, and tumor size).[61] With this system, a score of less than 6 yields a 20-year survival of 99%, and a score of more than 8 results in a 20-year survival of only 24%. On the basis of these scoring systems, which have been verified by other institutions, the aggressiveness of treatment can be balanced against the possible treatment risks and costs. Clearly, if subgroups of patients with 99% 20-year survivals can be prospectively identified, aggressive therapy with potential lifelong complications cannot be justified in this subpopulation.

The Mayo Clinic group applied the AMES criteria to its long-term database, evaluating 1685 patients treated between 1940 and 1991 in the low-risk category with papillary thyroid cancer.[62] The 30-year rate for disease-specific mortality was 2%;

for those with distant metastases, it was 3% in this population. With 20-year follow-up, there was a 4% rate of local recurrence and an 8% rate of nodal recurrence. These two reports verify the criteria established much earlier for prediction of outcome in well-differentiated thyroid cancer. Age, extrathyroidal extension, and distant metastases play important roles in the AJCC staging of thyroid cancer.[5] It is important to note that all of the staging systems are based on retrospective reviews of patient outcomes.

There is no large database that has verified this adaptation of the AMES and MACIS staging system into the TNM classification used by the AJCC.[5] However, a very similar staging system was developed by the National Thyroid Cancer Treatment Cooperative Study registry, which initiated collection of data in 1987. A report of more than 1500 patients analyzed by this staging system showed that 5-year disease-specific survivals for papillary thyroid cancer in stages I and II were 100%, 93.8% for stage III, and 78.5% for stage IV.[63] The disease-free survival similarly showed a high correlation with stages I through IV papillary carcinoma, having survivals of 94.4%, 92.5%, 82.7%, and 30%, respectively (P<.0001).

TREATMENT OF WELL- AND INTERMEDIATELY DIFFERENTIATED THYROID CARCINOMA

SURGERY

The key decisions in the surgical management of thyroid nodules or cancers (or both) are on whom to operate on and how extensive a resection to perform. The development of FNA and the proven accuracy of those results since the mid-1980s have significantly decreased the number of patients who present with thyroid nodules and need to undergo surgical exploration for diagnosis.[64] Consequently, FNA has increased the proportion of nodules that are surgically excised that prove to be cancer.

Before the development and widespread use of preoperative FNA of thyroid nodules, surgeons frequently relied on frozen-section test results obtained during the procedure to guide them. The usefulness of frozen-section diagnosis for thyroid nodules is limited. The situations in which intraoperative frozen-section examination may be useful are cases in which patients have suspicious but nondiagnostic FNA results. Both the quality of the cytologic specimen and its interpretation are paramount in modern thyroid surgery. If a high-quality FNA specimen is diagnostic of malignancy, a definitive procedure can be performed in the absence of intraoperative frozen-section analysis. If the FNA result is highly suggestive but not diagnostic of papillary thyroid carcinoma, frozen-section evaluation can be beneficial, especially when touch preparation techniques are used to assess cytologic features. Most of the lesions in the indeterminate FNA result category are follicular neoplasms, the majority of which are benign. As previously discussed (see Evaluation of the Thyroid Nodule, earlier in this chapter), capsular and vascular invasion determine malignancy, and the ability to render an accurate interpretation of frozen-section analysis is very limited. A large series from Johns Hopkins University School of Medicine examined this patient population.[32] It was reported that 87% of frozen sections for follicular neoplasm of the thyroid rendered no useful informa-

tion, and 5% gave inaccurate results. The researchers' conclusions were that obtaining frozen sections did more harm than good and resulted in additional expense. The recommended approach in this group of patients is to perform excision of the thyroid lobe harboring the nodule and to wait for the definitive pathologic report. If the lesion turns out to be a follicular carcinoma with characteristics that place the patient at high risk, such as significant capsular invasion or angioinvasion, a completion total or near-total thyroidectomy is performed during a second operation to remove the contralateral thyroid lobe.[32] In cases suspicious for a follicular variant of papillary carcinoma, the presence of specific nuclear features that define papillary thyroid cancer may be identifiable by using touch preparations in addition to frozen-section analysis. For this reason, patients with FNA results that are read as follicular neoplasm with some features of papillary nuclei should undergo lobectomy and intraoperative assessment (frozen section, touch preparation) to attempt identification of a follicular variant of papillary thyroid cancer. A limited number of authors believe that frozen-section analysis in this setting of follicular neoplasm is useful. However, a randomized prospective study demonstrated a very limited role of frozen-section analysis for the vast majority of patients with follicular neoplasms.[65] This study did emphasize the importance of examining the gross specimen with a pathologist and performing selective frozen-section analyses in the setting of gross capsular invasion.

A long-standing controversy among endocrine surgeons has existed regarding the extent of surgical resection for well-differentiated thyroid cancer. This question is unlikely to be answered definitively even by a large clinical trial, because the expense and number of patients needed for trials of this indolent low-risk disease are overwhelming. A power analysis and design for such a trial has now been published.[64] Acceptable surgical procedures to remove a thyroid neoplasm include an ipsilateral lobectomy, a subtotal thyroidectomy, a near-total thyroidectomy, and a total thyroidectomy. The entire thyroid lobe on the side of the primary cancer is taken out as completely as possible in any of these procedures. The difference in procedures relates to the management of the contralateral lobe and how this choice effects both the outcome and operative morbidity. In a thyroid lobectomy, the contralateral lobe is not dissected but is simply examined for abnormalities visually and by palpation. A subtotal thyroidectomy leaves a rim of 2 to 4 g of tissue in the upper lateral portion of the contralateral thyroid lobe. By leaving thyroid tissue in this location, two things are accomplished. First, the recurrent laryngeal nerve as it enters the larynx at the ligament of Berry is not dissected and consequently is theoretically at less risk for injury. Second, the blood supply to the superior parathyroid gland on that side is less likely to be disrupted by leaving a rim of tissue in this location. A near-total thyroidectomy leaves a much smaller amount of normal tissue (less than 1 g) immediately adjacent to the ligament of Berry. This maneuver may provide some protection to the recurrent laryngeal nerve, but it offers minimal benefit in terms of preserving the blood supply of the upper parathyroid. A total extracapsular thyroidectomy implies that every effort is made to excise all thyroid tissue, with no macroscopic residual thyroid left in either lobe. The difference between a total thyroidectomy and a near-total thyroidectomy usually depends on the particular anatomy of the thyroid in any given patient. There frequently exists a small ledge of thyroid tissue, called

TABLE 34.2-5. Arguments for More Radical Surgery for Well-Differentiated Thyroid Carcinoma

---

Higher survival rate for lesions >1.5 cm in diameter
Lowest recurrence rate in all patients
Prevention of recurrence in the contralateral lobe
Reduction of the risk of developing pulmonary metastasis
Can be performed with the same morbidity and mortality as hemithyroidectomy
Improved sensitivity of serum thyroglobulin as a marker for persistent or recurrent disease
Radioactive iodine can be used to detect and treat persistent or recurrent disease
Reduces possibility of residual tumor in contralateral lobe undergoing transformation to anaplastic carcinoma

---

the *tubercle of Zuckerkandl,* near the ligament of Berry that often lies immediately superficial to the recurrent nerve. Some surgeons routinely leave this small remnant of normal thyroid tissue *in situ.*

The increased risk of performing a total thyroidectomy versus a lesser resection may be in the long-term incidence of hypocalcemia. A study at the Mayo Clinic spanning the years between 1946 and 1970 reported a 32% incidence of permanent hypocalcemia after total thyroidectomy versus only a 0.3% incidence after a subtotal procedure.[56] More recent series report much less permanent morbidity and show variable results when comparing the patients undergoing subtotal with those undergoing total thyroidectomy. Virtually all experienced surgeons should be able to perform total thyroidectomies with less than 1% recurrent nerve injuries, with the long-term risk of hypoparathyroidism of 2% to 9%.[64] It should be mentioned, however, that the surgeon's experience is strongly related to lower complication rates, especially in total thyroidectomy and when operating on malignant versus benign disease.[66] The authors advocate a more aggressive procedure (i.e., total thyroidectomy) for the vast majority of patients with well-differentiated thyroid carcinoma, and the reasons are outlined in Table 34.2-5.

The most compelling argument for performing a unilateral lobectomy or a subtotal thyroidectomy is the data that come from the definition of prognostic factors for this disease. Low-risk patients defined by the AMES criteria have a 20-year survival of 99% with a 20-year disease-free survival of more than 95%.[50] If prognostic factors can accurately diagnose patients with such excellent outcome, the added benefit of a total thyroidectomy as well as postoperative iodine therapy may not be worth the potential morbidity for the patient. However, careful medical surveillance for cancer in the contralateral lobe as well as recurrence must be maintained. Furthermore, in situations in which a small thyroid remnant is left, the true morbidity of treating the patient with ablative doses of [131]I (if indicated) is relatively minimal. In fact, it is typical in patients with a surgical report of a "total thyroidectomy" to detect normal residual thyroid tissue within the bed of the thyroid identified on the postresection diagnostic scan. This small thyroid remnant is readily ablated with postoperative ^{131}I treatments. Successful radioiodine ablation of an intact thyroid lobe is associated with considerably more difficulty.

A large review at the Mayo Clinic of 1685 patients with papillary thyroid cancer treated between 1940 and 1991 with a long-term follow-up has been reported.[61] Based on surgeons' preference, 1468 patients underwent a near-total or total thyroidectomy (87%), whereas 195 patients (12%) had a unilateral resection. With a 20-year follow-up, the incidence of local recurrence with unilateral resection was 14% and with bilateral resection it was 2%.[61] Similarly, the incidence of recurrent cervical lymph node metastases after unilateral resection was 19% compared with 6% after bilateral resection (*P* = .0001). Despite this very clear difference in recurrence rates, there was no translation of benefit in terms of disease-specific survival or distant metastases. The overall mortality at 30 years for patients with either unilateral resection or bilateral resection was approximately 2%. These results further confirm the excellent predictive outcome of the AMES low-risk criteria with long-term follow-up.[61] The authors concluded that, although no survival benefit is gained from bilateral thyroid resection, the significant improvement in local recurrence with a minimal operative morbidity in the hands of experienced surgeons leads to recommendation of near-total or total thyroidectomy for even this low-risk category of patients. Arguing the opposing viewpoint, Sanders and Cady also provided a long-term review of their personal series and came to the conclusion that there was no benefit in performing bilateral resection versus unilateral resection in low-risk patients.[67]

For patients in a high-risk category, there is much less disagreement regarding the extent of surgery, although there are still some proponents of less-than-total or near-total thyroidectomy. An analysis of 303 patients with high-risk papillary thyroid cancer showed an improvement in overall survival (relative risk ratio, 0.37) but not in cancer-specific mortality or disease-free survival.[68] In this nonrandomized study, no effect of extent of surgery was seen in patients with follicular thyroid cancer. A study of a smaller number of high-risk patients reported that 10-year disease-specific survival was 82% after total thyroidectomy, 78% after subtotal thyroidectomy, and 89% after unilateral lobectomy.[69] Again, neither of these studies was prospective or randomized and, for reasons in terms of effectiveness of adjuvant postoperative radioiodine treatments and ease of follow-up with serum thyroglobulin (Tg) measurements, the vast majority of investigators agree that a total or near-total thyroidectomy is indicated for high-risk patients. For patients with extrathyroidal extension, *en bloc* resection of invaded structures should be performed. If the tumor is on the anterior thyroid, this causes minimal morbidity, because resection of the overlying strap muscles, such as the sternothyroid, causes no symptoms postoperatively. For posterior tumors, the margins are either the trachea or esophagus. For the majority of well-differentiated thyroid cancers, tracheal or esophageal resections are not indicated. However, for gross involvement of either of these structures, resection with reconstruction may be appropriate.[70]

The surgical management of lymph node metastases from well-differentiated thyroid cancer is no longer controversial.[47] Gross cervical metastatic disease is treated by modified radical neck dissection, which results in excellent local control and minimal morbidity.[47]

As noted, the presence of metastatic disease to lymph nodes does not carry the connotation of worse prognosis as for other solid neoplasms. Although lymph node metastases correlate with increased local recurrence, they do not carry a worse prognosis in several series.[49,50] The lymph nodes typically involved are the level VI or paratracheal lymph nodes in the central compartment and the level III, IV, and V lymph nodes along the internal jugular vein in the mid and lower neck. During any thyroid resection, these lymph node areas should be palpated. Lymph nodes that are abnormal because they are firm or large should be subjected to biopsy with frozen-section pathologic evaluation. If nodes are positive for metastatic cancer, these lymph node areas should be completely dissected.

The technique of sentinel lymph node biopsy used for melanoma and breast cancer has been applied to thyroid cancer.[71] This technique does not appear applicable in patients with well-differentiated thyroid cancer because, although occult nodal metastasis are common, they convey minimal clinical significance.

Some investigators have noted a positive correlation between lymph node metastases and outcome, and have argued for more routine formal dissections. Tisell et al.,[72] who have widely promoted microdissection of all lymphatic tissue for MTC, reported their results in applying the same technique to papillary thyroid cancer. In their series of 195 patients, there was a 70% incidence of lymph node metastases in men and a 45% incidence of lymph node metastases in women. With long-term follow-up, only three patients (1.6%) of this series died, partially due to locally recurrent thyroid cancer, and all lived more than 17 years after the initial surgery. The current practice of the vast majority of endocrine surgeons with regard to well-differentiated thyroid cancer (exclusive of MTC, see Medullary Thyroid Carcinoma, later in this chapter) is to perform node dissection in the setting of imageable or palpable nodal disease. If a neck dissection is performed, the preferred approach is a modified radical neck dissection preserving the internal jugular vein, sternocleidomastoid muscle, and accessory nerve in the vast majority of patients.[47,73]

RADIOIODINE THERAPY

The postoperative treatment of patients with well-differentiated thyroid cancer, particularly relating to radioiodine therapy, is somewhat controversial. The lack of well-designed, randomized, controlled studies and the low probability that any large multicenter treatment studies will ever come to fruition force the clinician to rely on retrospective studies and surveys of practice habits.

All patients who have undergone a total or near-total thyroidectomy for a papillary or follicular carcinoma larger than 1.0 to 1.5 cm should be considered candidates for radioiodine ablation. [131]I ablation of any residual normal thyroid is important after what is thought to be complete resection of the primary tumor to aid in the detection of metastatic disease and to eradicate residual microscopic cancer. Normal thyroid tissue takes up ^{131}I more avidly than does cancer and thus prevents full visualization of the true extent of disease. Furthermore, ^{131}I ablation removes the contribution of normal thyroid tissue serum Tg, an important tumor marker in the follow-up of postoperative patients. Most importantly, many studies have documented that ^{131}I ablation decreases tumor recurrence, development of distant metastases, and cancer death.[68] Despite such data for large patient populations, some studies have failed to detect an enhanced survival with the use of radioiodine ablation, particularly in "low-risk" patients as defined by AMES criteria.[50]

The dose of ^{131}I for ablation is not standardized. Some recommend low-dose ablation with less than 30 mCi given on an outpatient basis. This approach should be reserved for low-risk young patients who may benefit from an overall lower radiation exposure and who accept the fact that several low radioiodine doses may be necessary before successful ablation. Several studies demonstrating proper diagnostic scan preparation with sufficiently elevated TSH level and adherence to a low-iodine diet describe disparate rates of successful ablations using less than 30 mCi ranging from 27% to 83%.

Higher ablative doses ranging from 100 to 150 mCi should be used for older, high-risk patients, particularly those known to have an incomplete resection of the primary tumor, an invasive primary tumor, or metastases. Some authors advocate use of dosimetry with the goal of deriving the dose of ^{131}I that will deliver no more than 200 cGy to the blood, with no more than 120 mCi retained at 48 hours or 80 mCi in the presence of pulmonary metastases. This decreases the risk of bone marrow damage and radiation fibrosis in patients with metastatic lung disease. One recommended approach is for all patients with metastatic disease treated with repeated therapeutic doses of ^{131}I to undergo dosimetric quantification of the highest safe dose, using a ceiling of 300 mCi. Other investigators recommend a standard fixed dose that may vary according to the site of uptake.[74] For example, a dose of 150 mCi is given for residual or recurrent thyroid bed carcinoma with or without metastases, up to 200 mCi for bone metastases, and a reduced dose of 75 mCi for diffuse pulmonary metastases to prevent radiation pneumonitis and fibrosis. In spite of the theoretical advantage of formal dosimetry, its use has not been embraced by most centers.

Lymph node metastases were found in up to 42% of patients at the time of initial therapy in one large study by Mazzaferri and Jhiang.[49] Radioiodine therapy is indicated in these patients to decrease recurrences that may have an impact on long-term survival.

Pulmonary metastases are frequently detected exclusively on radioiodine scanning. Schlumberger reported an increase in such cases, noting that the rate of negative chest radiograph results in patients with metastatic disease identified by radioiodine scanning has increased from 13% to 43%.[75] Earlier detection of pulmonary metastases before development of gross chest film abnormalities is thought to be due to the use of Tg screening and the enhanced sensitivity of ^{131}I scanning. This same group reported on 23 patients who had diffuse pulmonary metastases seen only on radioiodine scanning, of whom almost 90% had no further uptake and a decrease in the serum Tg after ^{131}I therapy. Bone metastases may require several modalities for adequate therapy. Surgery may be needed for orthopedic stabilization or palliation of pain. External radiation may be used in combination with radioactive iodine in difficult cases.[76]

Postoperative ablation is typically performed approximately 6 weeks after near-total or total thyroidectomy. Most, but not all, centers perform a diagnostic scan followed by ablative ^{131}I therapy. To optimize uptake by both normal residual thyroid and thyroid cancer, patients are rendered hypothyroid with a goal of increasing serum TSH. To accomplish this, thyroid replacement after thyroidectomy is often performed with the administration of triiodothyronine, because it has a much shorter half-life than thyroxine, and it is discontinued 2 weeks before treatment. In response to this hypothyroid state, TSH must achieve levels of greater than 25 to 30 µU/mL to obtain optimal uptake of radioiodine. A low-iodine diet is usually instituted 1 to 2 weeks before scanning to enhance the uptake and retention of radioiodine.

Just as there is lack of consensus regarding ablation and therapeutic doses of ^{131}I, the diagnostic scanning dose is also controversial. The ideal dose achieves high sensitivity in detecting residual thyroid tissue, thyroid cancer, and metastatic foci and reduces the potential for sublethal radiation "stunning" of thyroid tissue that prevents optimal uptake of future ^{131}I therapy. Although it is clear that higher scanning doses improve visualization of thyroid remnants and metastases, even conventional scanning doses of 4 to 5 mCi of ^{131}I were found to diminish therapeutic radioiodine uptake. Some authors suggest that diagnostic scanning with iodine 123 may prevent the stunning effect.[77] One strategy is to use a 5-mCi ^{131}I diagnostic dose followed by a whole body scan at 48 hours, with treatment following in most cases in 24 to 96 hours after whole body scanning. A posttherapy whole body scan is usually obtained after 5 to 7 days to determine the extent of disease. Follow-up diagnostic scanning is performed at outlined in Figure 34.2-2.

Medical management of malignant lesions requires thyroxine therapy to suppress TSH. The degree to which one suppresses TSH is a point of debate. It is advisable to keep the TSH at or below the normal range (0.5 to 5.0 µU/mL) in patients who are thought to be without evidence of disease and to maintain a lower TSH level (0.1 µU/mL) in patients with residual neck disease, metastases, or recurrent disease. A large review by the National Cancer Treatment Cooperative Registry of 693 patients reported that for all papillary thyroid cancer patients

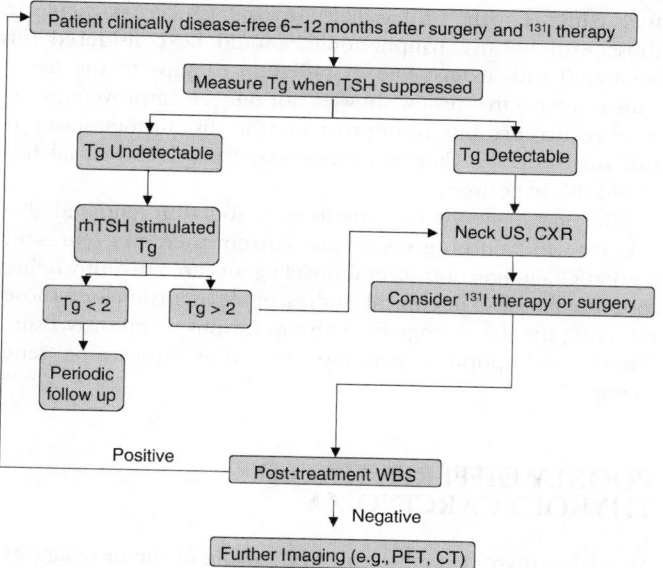

FIGURE 34.2-2. Flow diagram for follow-up after definitive thyroidectomy and remnant ablation for well-differentiated thyroid carcinoma. Note: Certain aggressive variants of well-differentiated carcinoma may not be amenable to this algorithm. Undetectable thyroglobulin (Tg) assumes that there are no Tg autoantibodies interfering with the assay. CT, computed tomography; CXR, chest radiography; PET, positron emission tomography; rhTSH, recombinant human thyroid-stimulating hormone; TSH, thyroid-stimulating hormone; US, ultrasonography; WBS, whole body scan. (Modified from ref. 81.)

TSH levels did not predict disease progression.[78] In high-risk papillary cancer, serum TSH was a predictor of risk (*P* = .03) but not when radioiodine therapy was included in the analysis (*P* = .004).[78] The degree of thyroid suppression in these cases is dictated by the need to balance the risk of recurrent thyroid cancer against the overall medical condition of patients, particularly their cardiovascular status.

The most common side effects from radioiodine therapy include sialadenitis, nausea, and temporary bone marrow suppression. Amifostine, which has been used as a radioprotector of head and neck cancer, significantly reduced sialadenitis from radiation treatment for thyroid cancer.[79] Testicular function and spermatogenesis are transiently impaired but appear to recover with time. During and immediately after ^{131}I treatment pregnancy should be avoided. There is a dose-dependent relationship between ^{131}I therapy and the development of leukemia. The incidence increases when the total cumulative dose is higher than 800 mCi and can be avoided by treating at widely spaced intervals (6 to 12 months) with activity between 100 and 200 mCi.[80] A higher incidence of bladder carcinoma has been seen in patients who have received high cumulative doses of radioiodine, and urine dilution by adequate hydration and frequent voiding can reduce the radiation exposure to the bladder wall.

FOLLOW-UP MANAGEMENT

Tg, an important tumor marker in the follow-up of thyroid cancer patients, is the protein that provides a matrix for thyroid hormone synthesis within thyroid follicles and is critical in the storage of thyroid hormone within the thyroid gland.[81] After successful thyroidectomy and ablation of residual normal or malignant thyroid tissue by radioiodine, the Tg level should be in the athyreotic range. Levels above the athyreotic range are indicative of persistent functioning thyroid tissue or carcinoma. If there is detectable serum Tg in the circumstance of suppressive thyroxine therapy, it is an indicator of persistent or recurrent thyroid carcinoma. However, thyroxine may suppress Tg in patients with metastatic disease; therefore, the test is more sensitive in the setting of thyroid hormone suppressive therapy withdrawal and frank hypothyroidism documented by an elevated TSH level.

At the time of thyroid hormone withdrawal for both initial postoperative scans and for subsequent follow-up scans, Tg level is measured in conjunction with the diagnostic whole body scan and may be more sensitive than the scan in detecting cancer.[82,83] Since the initial report,[83] there has been a great deal of debate regarding the optimal management of patients for whom results on whole body iodine scan are negative but results for Tg are positive. This debate has included discussions of the false-negative rate of Tg and alternative imaging studies, including positron emission tomography scans as well as ultrasonography, sestamibi, technetium-sestamibi, and thallium 201 scans. Without question, there are patients who have negative whole body iodine scans but have definite recurrent and metastatic well-differentiated thyroid cancer. The relatively routine use of radioiodine ablation in this population of patients who are Tg positive and whole body scan–negative has been extensively debated. Most experts agree that a selective approach incorporating prognostic features of the primary tumor (age of patient, extrathyroidal extension) should come into play in determining management of these patients. It should also be understood that a variety of patients with autoantibodies to Tg may have spurious results that are most commonly false-negative results but also have the potential to be false-positive test results. A consensus report on the role of serum Tg level as a monitoring method for low-risk patients with papillary thyroid carcinoma was published.[81] The authors emphasize the usefulness of measuring Tg levels after stimulation with recombinant human TSH (rhTSH), using a Tg cutoff of 2 µg/L (either after thyroid hormone withdrawal or 72 hours after rhTSH administration). Furthermore, they discourage routine use of diagnostic whole body scanning in the follow-up management of low-risk patients with well-differentiated thyroid carcinoma (see Fig. 34.2-2).

The success of radioiodine therapy is dependent on residual thyroid tissue's concentrating iodine avidly under the stimulation of elevated TSH. In some circumstances, stimulation by endogenous TSH is impossible, as in the case of hypopituitarism, or is contraindicated, as in patients with central nervous system metastases in whom the hypothyroid state could lead to acute intracranial swelling. The availability of rhTSH has facilitated studies comparing diagnostic whole body iodine scans after standard thyroxine withdrawal to scans obtained after administration of rhTSH.[82,84,85] In 127 patients with a diagnosis of well-differentiated thyroid cancer, rhTSH was administered 2 days before the patient received between 3 and 5 mCi of ^{131}I and underwent whole body iodine scan. This scan was compared to a subsequent scan performed after standard thyroxine withdrawal. There were 65 patients who had concordant negative scan results (51% of the patient population). In the additional 62 patients (49% of the population) who had positive scan results, both scans were positive in 41; only the standard thyroxine withdrawal study result was positive in 18, and only the rhTSH scan result was positive in 3. Although there were minor differences, rhTSH scan was equivalent to or better than the standard scan in 86% of the patients but inferior to the standard withdrawal scan in 14% ($P < .001$).[84] This difference in scan results culminated in an alteration of therapy in 13% of the patients, who were then treated with high-dose radioactive iodine based on the standard scan alone. On the other hand, there was a highly significant worsening of symptoms of hypothyroidism and dysphoric mood states after withdrawal of thyroid hormone as compared to rhTSH.[84] The rhTSH testing was shown to be safe with only some mild nausea side effects. In a review on the subject, Robbins and Robbins found that whole body iodine scans after rhTSH administration has excellent diagnostic accuracy compared with preparation by thyroid hormone withdrawal, without the need for the reduced quality of life associated with the hypothyroid state.[85]

CHEMOTHERAPY AND RADIATION THERAPY

The most effective nonsurgical treatment for well-differentiated thyroid cancer is ablation with radioiodine. Other conventional modes of neoplastic treatment—chemotherapy and external-beam radiation therapy—demonstrate poor results and, consequently, are much less studied. The best single chemotherapeutic agent for this tumor is doxorubicin (Adriamycin) with partial response rates of 30% and up to 45% in some series.[86] Combination therapy with doxorubicin and cisplatin has produced disappointing results that were no better than those with single agents, and the toxicity was worse. For surgically unresectable local disease that has not responded to radioiodine, the best treatment may be a combination of hyperfractionated radiation treatments plus doxorubicin. Response rates of more than 80% have been reported using this regimen, although even in this situation, complete responses are rare and limited in duration.[86] One retrospective study analyzed the effect of adjuvant radiation therapy for grossly resected well-differentiated thyroid cancer.[87] This study analyzed patients with T4 primary lesions (evidence of extrathyroidal extension) who underwent external-beam radiation (n = 99) compared with those who did not (n = 70).[87] Patients received a uniform treatment course of total thyroidectomy with an initial ablative radioactive iodine dose, with or without 5000 to 6000 rad of external-beam radiation therapy to the neck and mediastinum, followed by a second ablative dose of radioactive iodine. The group that had external-beam treatments had recurrent disease in 4% of cases (3 of 75 patients), whereas the group that did not receive external-beam radiation had recurrences in 26% (13 of 50 patients; $P = .0001$).[87] This benefit for external-beam radiation extended only to the subgroup of patients with lymph node–positive disease. In patients with papillary thyroid cancer who were lymph node–negative, 1 of 47 patients (2%) developed recurrence after external-beam therapy versus 2 of 21 patients (9.5%) without external-beam therapy. This difference was not statistically significant. However, among patients with T4 lesions and positive lymph nodes who received external-beam radiation, there were 2 recurrences in 28 (7.1%), whereas there were 13 recurrences in 29 (44.8%) among patients who did not receive radiation external-beam therapy ($P = .002$). These results suggest that patients with T4 papillary thyroid cancer, particularly those with positive lymph nodes, should be considered for treatment with external-beam radiation therapy to the neck. This retrospective review showed not only an improvement in local recurrence but an improvement in distant metastases in this subgroup. To date, no randomized prospective trial has tested this hypothesis.

The management of patients with well-differentiated thyroid cancers that progress despite current therapies represent a great challenge, and several novel agents are currently being tested *in vitro* and in clinical studies. Such agents include those targeting the Ras oncogenic pathway, various receptor tyrosine kinases, and apoptotic pathways, as well as those using gene therapy.[88]

POORLY DIFFERENTIATED THYROID CARCINOMA

Anaplastic thyroid carcinoma (ATC) is one of the most aggressive and difficult human malignancies to treat and is one of the most lethal. In contrast to the excellent long-term survival for well-differentiated thyroid carcinoma, ATC in most series has a median survival of 4 to 5 months from the time of diagnosis, with rare long-term survivors.[89,90]

The proportional incidence of ATC in the total number of thyroid carcinomas is variable but appears to be declining over time, and current epidemiologic studies indicate that this lethal form of thyroid cancer has decreased to between 1% and 3% of the total number of cases.[90] Institutional reviews over a distinct period suggest a real decrease in the incidence of ATC.[91] The decrease over time may be partially related to iodine prophylaxis and an overall decrease in endemic iodine-deficiency goiter in North America.

Patients with ATC differ epidemiologically from patients with well-differentiated thyroid neoplasms, with a median age two to three decades older and with a more equal gender distribution.[91] The median age at diagnosis ranges between 63 and 74 years. The largest series from the Mayo Clinic, including 134 patients, demonstrated a female to male ratio of 1.5:1.0 and a mean age of 67 years.[91] ATC is commonly related to a prior or concurrent diagnosis of well-differentiated thyroid cancer or benign nodular thyroid disease.[91] This association of ATC with well-differentiated thyroid carcinoma suggests two features of the biology of this tumor. First, ATC may arise via the dedifferentiation of formerly well-differentiated thyroid cancer, and the aggressive growth pattern of this anaplastic tumor may replace all previous evidence of well-differentiated tumor. Also, the close association between ATC and well-differentiated thyroid cancer suggests that the risk factors are similar.

The natural history, clinical presentation, and outcome of ATC reflect the biology of this tumor as an undifferentiated, rapidly growing neoplasm with invasive characteristics. The patients uniformly present with a palpable mass that is reported to be increasing in size during the period of observation. The median tumor size in patients with ATC at the Roswell Park Cancer Institute was 8 to 9 cm, with a range of 3 to 20 cm, as compared with the usual size of 2 to 3 cm for well-differentiated thyroid cancer.[90] Invasion into the trachea, larynx, or recurrent laryngeal nerve leads to obstructive symptoms, hemoptysis, dysphagia, and hoarseness, which are often present at diagnosis.

The majority of patients with ATC die from aggressive local-regional disease, primarily with upper airway respiratory failure. At the time of diagnosis, 25% to 50% of patients have synchronous pulmonary metastases.[89–91] However, it is usually the local growth causing obliteration of the airway that causes the patient's demise. For this reason, aggressive local therapy is indicated in all patients who can tolerate it and in whom it is technically possible. Unlike in well-differentiated thyroid cancer, ^{131}I plays no role in the treatment of recurrent or metastatic disease for this tumor. Therefore, total or near-total thyroidectomy is not as important in ATC, except as needed to obtain local control.[89–91]

Survival after the diagnosis of ATC is very poor. The median survival in most series is less than 5 months from the time of diagnosis. The majority of patients die due to local recurrence, although distant metastases occur, primarily in lung, bone, and liver. External radiation has been used with limited success to treat locally recurrent ATC. In the mid-1980s, Kim and Leeper[92] reported improved responses with a combination of radiation therapy and relatively low-dose doxorubicin as an apparent synergistic agent, achieving responses in eight of nine patients, although still having median survival of only 12 months. Doxorubicin is the single most effective chemotherapeutic for ATC, and it has been shown that doxorubicin plus platinum is more effective than doxorubicin alone. Early diagnosis with aggressive surgical therapy supplemented by external-beam radiation therapy and doxorubicin-based che-

motherapy is regarded by many as the most appropriate treatment. However, a prospective phase II clinical trial demonstrated one complete response and nine partial responses in 19 patients after treatment with paclitaxel, which suggests its potential role in the treatment of ATC.[93]

MEDULLARY THYROID CARCINOMA

PATHOLOGY

MTC was recognized in the 1950s by Hazard et al.[94] as a distinct clinicopathologic entity. Since this description, sequential pathologic, biochemical, and molecular genetic studies have progressed to render this one of the best characterized solid malignancies of the thyroid. In 1959, Hazard et al. described MTC as a solid thyroid neoplasm without follicular histologic features but with a high degree of lymph node metastases that accounted for 3.5% of thyroid cancers in a review at the Cleveland Clinic.[94] Over the next 10 years, investigators identified and described the parafollicular C cell that produces calcitonin and give rise to MTC. During the decade of the 1970s, Wells et al.[95] extended the measurement of calcitonin by defining a provocative test that rendered this hormonal tumor marker one of the most sensitive and specific in all of oncology. Understanding of the familial associations of MTC with corollary genetic studies reported in the 1980s and early 1990s have defined molecular changes responsible for familial forms of inherited MTC and have implications for sporadic MTC as well. For details on molecular pathogenesis of MTC, see Chapter 34.1.

MTC constitutes between 3% and 12% of most institutional series of detectible thyroid cancers.[4] Unlike well-differentiated thyroid cancer, MTC is not associated with radiation exposure, but it does occur in distinct familial syndromes (Table 34.2-6). Sporadic or nonfamilial MTC accounts for 60% to 70% of cases, with three distinct familial syndromes accounting for the remainder. MTC is the most prominent clinical diagnosis in multiple endocrine neoplasia (MEN) 2A and MEN 2B. In 1986, familial MTC in the absence of the associated features of MEN 2A or MEN 2B was described.[96] Appreciation of this syndrome

TABLE 34.2-6. Clinical and Genetic Characteristics of Familial Medullary Thyroid Cancer Syndromes

Syndrome	Characteristic Features
FMTC	MTC
MEN 2A	MTC
	Adrenal medulla (pheochromocytoma)
	Parathyroid hyperplasia
MEN 2A with cutaneous lichen amyloidosis	MEN 2A and a pruritic cutaneous lesion located over the upper back
MEN 2A or FMTC with Hirschsprung's disease	MEN 2A or FMTC with Hirschsprung's disease
MEN 2B	MTC
	Adrenal medulla (pheochromocytoma)
	Intestinal and mucosal ganglioneuromatosis
	Characteristic habitus, marfanoid

FMTC, familial medullary thyroid carcinoma; MEN, multiple endocrine neoplasia; MTC, medullary thyroid carcinoma.

has shifted the percentage of sporadic MTC in the total number of cases from 80% to 60% and even lower in some series. In addition to the presence or absence of other associated endocrine abnormalities, each of these familial forms of MTC has a unique natural history and prognosis.[97]

Parafollicular cells, or C cells, arise embryologically from the neural crest and are located primarily in the upper and middle thirds of the thyroid lobes, with a particular concentration posteriorly. This feature is important to surgical therapy, because this is in direct proximity to where the recurrent laryngeal nerve passes under the ligament of Berry and enters the larynx. Unfortunately, performance of a near-total thyroidectomy is likely to leave remnant neoplastic disease in this location.

Grossly, MTC may be circumscribed or infiltrative and is usually yellow. Histologically, this tumor demonstrates a wide variety of patterns, including glandular, solid, spindle cell, oncocytic, clear cell, papillary, small cell, and giant cell. The nuclei of MTC resemble those of neuroendocrine tumors in other areas of the body. They are usually round and have a stippled "pepper and salt" chromatin. Pathologic features associated with a poor prognosis include the presence of necrosis, a squamous pattern, oxyphil cells in the tumor and absence of cells with intermediate cytoplasm, and less than 50% calcitonin immunoreactivity.[98]

CLINICAL PRESENTATION AND DIAGNOSIS

The clinical symptoms at the time of presentation vary. Patients with familial MTC who are identified by screening with stimulation tests or with molecular analysis (detection of *RET* gene mutation) are usually identified before the development of macroscopic disease. Patients with sporadic disease typically present with an asymptomatic thyroid mass. Patients with bulky disease, local or metastatic, with extremely high levels of calcitonin may have severe secretory diarrhea as a principal symptom. Before the availability of genetic testing for familial MTC, basal and stimulated serum calcitonin levels were used to screen patients. Sequential calcitonin and carcinoembryonic antigen measurements are still important as tumor markers for following patients with MTC.

The use of various nuclear imaging studies in patients with MTC to identify gross and occult metastases has been evaluated. [131]I thyroid scans are of no utility because MTC does not concentrate iodine. Similarly, thallium as well as technetium scans have been used with minimal efficacy. [^{131}I]metaiodobenzylguanidine scans have been useful in pheochromocytoma and neuroblastoma and have been studied for MTC but do not identify a large proportion of the lesions. Several studies have used somatostatin receptor scintigraphy in the setting of MTC.[99] Like other amine precursor uptake and decarboxylation (APUD) cells, C cells may express a high level of somatostatin receptors, and pharmacologically developed radiolabeled agents, based on analogs that bind to somatostatin receptor, have been studied for use in treating MTC. Although the results are promising for this imaging technique, occult lesions smaller than 1 cm as well as liver lesions still are missed with this technique. Positron emission tomography may also prove useful in the imaging of MTC.[100]

TREATMENT

Chemotherapy and external-beam radiation therapy are, for the most part, ineffective against MTC, which rendered surgical resection the only definitive therapy. For patients with sporadic MTC who are not identified by biochemical or genetic screening, the appropriate operation in most cases is total thyroidectomy, central node dissection, and ipsilateral modified radical neck dissection. Total thyroidectomy is indicated in this sporadic setting because a small proportion of lesions may be bilateral and because it may not be clear at the time of operation whether a patient is an index case of familial disease or the disorder is a true sporadic case. Because all familial syndromes have a high propensity for bilateral tumors, total thyroidectomy is always indicated. One report of 80 patients with sporadic MTC smaller than 1 cm showed that 11% had clinically involved lymph nodes, 31% had pathologically involved lymph nodes, and 5% had distant metastases.[101] Combined with thyroid resection, a central lymph node dissection should be performed, with lymphoid tissue removed from the level of the hyoid bone superiorly to the innominate vessels inferiorly and laterally to the jugular veins. Because of the high incidence of ipsilateral nodal metastasis at presentation, formal modified radical neck "microdissections" are ideally combined with the initial exploration.

The incidence of positive lymph nodes correlates with the size of the primary lesion at the time of diagnosis. It has been reported that for lesions smaller than 1 cm, there is an 11% incidence of positive nodal disease, whereas among patients with tumors larger than 2 cm, 60% have positive cervical lymph nodes.[102]

The incidence of distant metastases at the time of diagnosis varies with the clinical setting. Twelve percent of patients with sporadic MTC have distant metastases, whereas 20% of those with MEN 2B but only 3.3% of patients with MEN 2A have metastatic spread.[103] Patients with familial non-MEN MTC tend to have even a less aggressive clinical course and approximately 2% of these patients present with distant metastases. Patients with MTC are ideally treated immediately after the diagnosis has been established. Unfortunately, patients with sporadic disease often undergo exploration without a clear diagnosis or exploration by surgeons without experience in managing this malignancy, or both. FNA specimens suggestive of MTC should be stained for calcitonin; a positive result is highly suggestive of MTC.[29] In addition, a serum calcitonin level in this setting is almost always elevated and thereby confirms the diagnosis. It is important to screen for catecholamine excess before surgical exploration, because a patient with apparent sporadic MTC may in fact have a familial syndrome with an occult pheochromocytoma.

The outcome of treatment of patients with sporadic MTC has improved. Studies show a 5-year survival between 80% and 90% and 10-year survival between 70% and 80% for combined series of familial and sporadic MTC.[104] The natural history and prognosis for the various subtypes of MTC correlate with described genetic changes. The introduction of genetic testing and prophylactic surgery has improved the prognosis in cases of familial disease (see Treatment of Familial Medullary Thyroid Carcinoma, later in this chapter).

One challenge in the surgical management of patients with MTC is the proper approach to patients who have persistently elevated basal or stimulated calcitonin levels after resection of all gross disease. In many of these cases, imaging studies fail to demonstrate areas of disease. One strategy to identify the region from which elevated calcitonin is coming is to perform selected venous sampling. Excision attempts generally do not produce normalization of calcitonin levels. Tisell et al. have advocated meticulous 12-hour neck dissections, often removing 40 to 60 additional cervical lymph nodes in patients with occult MTC.[105] In a series of 11 patients, 4 demonstrated normalization of calcitonin levels, with another 4 showing dramatic improvement in their calcitonin levels. However, even these improvements in the calcitonin levels do not necessarily translate into improved survival. Thirty-one patients were identified, all of whom had gross disease resected at initial operation at the Mayo Clinic but had documented elevated postoperative calcitonin levels.[106] With a median follow-up of almost 12 years, only 11 patients developed clinically or radiographically apparent recurrent disease, and these 11 patients were reoperated at that time. None of these patients had normalized calcitonin levels after reoperation. The overall 5- and 10-year survival rates in this population were 90% and 86%, respectively, with only two patients dying specifically from MTC.[106] More recent data suggest that 28% of these patients can achieve eucalcitonemia after aggressive re-resection.[107]

For patients with metastatic MTC, surgical resection may still offer the best chance of survival as well as long-term palliation. In 16 patients with metastatic MTC treated at the Johns Hopkins Thyroid Tumor Center, 21 palliative reoperations were performed. These procedures included neck reoperations in 11 cases but also removal of mediastinal masses and liver metastases as well as other miscellaneous lesions. All patients had clear relief of their index symptoms, typically diarrhea and fatigue, and had a median survival of 8.2 years.[108] In the setting of persistent hypercalcitonemia and negative imaging study results, remedial surgery with formal neck dissection is often indicated. However, before such an operation, it is recommended to perform a laparoscopic evaluation of the liver to rule out superficial hepatic metastases.[107] If they are present, the enthusiasm for remedial neck dissection, especially in an asymptomatic patient, is markedly reduced.

The results of MTC treatment with external-beam radiation therapy or chemotherapeutic agents are disappointing. One study in France of 59 patients reported local recurrences within the radiation field in 30% of patients,[109] and the treatment may be associated with significant local toxicity such as dysphagia and dyspnea. Chemotherapeutic agents used in the treatment of MTC include doxorubicin, dacarbazine, streptozocin, and 5-fluorouracil.[75] Single-agent response rates are poor, with aggressive doxorubicin regimens producing 20% to 30% objective responses, and combinations of chemotherapy have so far not been promising. The poor outcome of treatment of metastatic disease validates the treatment recommendation to diagnose patients with MTC early and treat with initial aggressive surgery.

TREATMENT OF FAMILIAL MEDULLARY THYROID CARCINOMA

An increasing number of patients are identified as having one of the three familial types of MTC that are diagnosed using biochemical or genetic screening for RET gene mutations. Routine use of screening to diagnose MTC led to significant decreases in both the age at diagnosis and the incidence of lymph node metastases, as well as a significant increase in the number of patients cured biochemically at these earlier opera-

tions. Wells et al.[110] used a molecular genetic screening technique to identify patients who are carriers of the MEN 2A mutation as infants or young children. Before any abnormality was seen in basal or stimulated calcitonin level, these patients underwent a total thyroidectomy and central neck dissection. Pathologic evaluation of these children's thyroid glands identified C-cell hyperplasia, microscopic, or macroscopic MTC. In the initial trial, no patients treated with this strategy had evidence of lymph node metastases, and this surgical strategy should be curative.[110]

The genetic test for the mutations in the RET gene are commercially available, and many investigators are reporting series based on early operation for patients identified by RET mutation. A review has noted that, of a total of 209 patients treated in this manner, 3.4% had normal thyroid glands with no evidence of C-cell hyperplasia or MTC. It has also been noted that in these patients undergoing prophylactic operations, there was an 8.6% incidence of lymph node metastases.[111] Based on these results, it is thought that a prophylactic central neck dissection should be performed at the time of this prophylactic thyroidectomy, based on genetic testing. Because different mutations in the RET gene are associated with variable disease aggressiveness, more recent research has attempted to correlate a certain mutation (genotype) with the patient's clinical course (phenotype), to provide genotype-specific recommendations for treatment.[112,113] Thus, individuals with RET gene mutations associated with MEN 2A and familial MTC are advised to undergo prophylactic thyroidectomy at age 5 to 6 years, whereas affected individuals in kindreds with MEN 2B should undergo thyroidectomy during infancy due to the aggressiveness and earlier age at onset of MTC in these patients.[97] At the M. D. Anderson Cancer Center, 86 patients with inherited MTC susceptibility were stratified into three RET gene mutation risk groups: level 1, low risk for MTC (mutations in codons 609, 768, 790, 791, 804, and 891); level 2, intermediate risk (mutations in codons 611, 618, 620, and 634); and level 3, highest risk (mutations in codons 883 and 918).[114] All patients in the level 3 group (all with MEN 2B) had MTC present at initial thyroidectomy performed at a median age of 13.5 years, and persistent disease. With increased knowledge of genotype-phenotype correlations, it is likely that more individualized therapy can be used in the treatment of familial variants of MTC.

THYROID LYMPHOMA

Thyroid lymphoma is a relatively rare disease constituting fewer than 1% of all lymphomas and accounting for 2% of extranodal non-Hodgkin's lymphoma.[115] Almost all these thyroid lymphomas are non-Hodgkin's lymphoma, with the majority (70% to 90%) being intermediate grade and the remainder being high grade. Many are considered mucosa-associated lymphoid tissue lymphomas or *MALTomas* and show plasmacytic differentiation and may be associated with similar lesions in extranodal sites, especially in the gastrointestinal tract.

The majority of patients with thyroid lymphoma have disease on one side of the diaphragm with a proportion confined to the thyroid (stage IE). The majority have thyroid disease plus positive cervical or mediastinal lymph nodes (stage IIE).[115]

The incidence of this disease may be changing, primarily due to improved recognition and diagnosis of thyroid lymphoma. One hypothesis to explain the increased incidence is that these patients were previously diagnosed as having ATC and, with better understanding and more sophisticated diagnostic tools, such as immunohistochemical analysis, these patients are being correctly categorized as having thyroid lymphoma.

In most series, there is a strong female predominance, ranging from 3:1 to 8:1.[116,117] The median age at diagnosis in most series places patients in the seventh decade of life, similar to the age seen for ATC and much older than patients with well-differentiated thyroid cancer. Between 10% and 30% of patients report a symptom or combination of symptoms relating to local invasion, including hoarseness, dyspnea with stridor, or dysphagia. Patients with thyroid lymphoma virtually never have hyperthyroidism but frequently have hypothyroidism. These hypothyroid patients have evidence of autoimmune thyroiditis or Hashimoto's thyroiditis, based on either the FNA sample or the pathologic specimen.[118]

The optimal treatment for thyroid lymphoma has evolved with the success of combination chemotherapy used in the treatment of non-Hodgkin's lymphoma and with the ability to obtain an accurate diagnosis without invasive surgery by large-needle or core-needle biopsy. Some argue that the role of surgery in this disease is simply to obtain adequate tissue for diagnosis and that the primary treatment should be external-beam radiation combined with a doxorubicin-based chemotherapy regimen.[116] In one publication, the 5-year survival was 70%, and the 4-year disease-free survival was also 70%.[116,118] Others have argued that in the 20% to 30% minority of patients who have no extrathyroidal extension, excellent survival is achieved by surgical excision plus postoperative radiation therapy.[115] Patients with extrathyroidal disease either by direct extension or lymph node involvement should be considered to have systemic disease. Although some surgeons argue that attempts to clear the trachea to avoid airway obstruction should be performed if at all possible in all patients, others report that the rapid use of radiation therapy (starting the day after the diagnostic biopsy procedure) produces the same beneficial results. All would agree that the efficacy and long-term survival achieved using a combination of radiation therapy and chemotherapy render aggressive surgical resection that sacrifices recurrent laryngeal nerve or possibly results in hypoparathyroidism contraindicated for thyroid lymphoma.

METASTATIC DISEASE OF THE THYROID

Clinically significant involvement of the thyroid gland by malignant metastases from other sites is rare, accounting for fewer than 1% of thyroid malignancies in most series involving surgical resection or FNA biopsies.[119,120] On the other hand, the incidence of thyroid metastases identified in autopsy series is greater and can range between 2% and 26%, probably depending on the thoroughness of the examination by the pathologist.[119] From these autopsy series, the most frequent malignancies metastatic to the thyroid are breast and lung, each accounting for 25% of the total.[119] Melanoma, renal cell carcinoma, and gastrointestinal tract malignancies each account for approximately 10% of these secondary malignancies from autopsy studies. A variety of other miscellaneous diagnoses account for the remainder.

For the more clinically relevant situation in which the thyroid metastasis is detected premortem, the most common primary site is renal cell carcinoma, which accounts for 23% of 111 such cases combined from the literature.[119,120] The next most common sites are breast (16%), lung (15%), melanoma (5%), and colon and larynx (4.5% each). Occasionally, the thyroid metastasis may be the initial presentation of an occult primary from a gastrointestinal source or a renal primary. Because FNA biopsy is the diagnostic tool used to evaluate thyroid nodules as the initial step, awareness of the potential of secondary metastases is important for interpretation of these biopsy results.

Depending on the clinical situation, some of these patients may need thyroidectomy for palliation of local symptoms. Thyroid metastases may grow at a rapid rate and can cause airway obstruction.

THYROID CARCINOMA IN CHILDREN

WELL-DIFFERENTIATED THYROID CARCINOMA

Well-differentiated thyroid carcinoma comprised only 1.4% of all newly diagnosed childhood carcinomas in the United States reported from 1975 to 1995.[121] Current treatment strategies for pediatric patients with well-differentiated thyroid carcinoma are derived from results for single-institution clinical cohorts, reports of extensive personal experience, and extrapolation of several common therapeutic practices in adults. Children with well-differentiated thyroid carcinoma more often than their adult counterparts have a history of external irradiation to the head and neck, although the majority present without such a history.[122] At presentation, pediatric patients tend to have a higher incidence of palpable cervical adenopathy, local infiltration of the primary cancer, and pulmonary metastases. The incidence of cervical nodal metastases in a series at the University of Michigan remained 88% from 1936 to 1990,[122] and the long-term mortality rate was 2.2%. Despite presenting with more advanced disease than adults, children tend to have a better prognosis.[121] Even in children with distant metastases, the survival rates are remarkably good. One study showed that at the end of a 15-year period only 14% had died from the disease.[123]

Most authors agree that aggressive initial management with total thyroidectomy and cervical lymph node dissection should be performed in most children with well-differentiated thyroid carcinoma. This is commonly followed by administration of radioiodine therapy to destroy any residual normal thyroid remnant.[121] Finally, and importantly, because the duration of follow-up is lifelong, the care of children with prior diagnosis of well-differentiated thyroid carcinoma should be transferred to an adult endocrinologist after they reach adulthood, even if they have no evidence of disease by that time.

MEDULLARY THYROID CARCINOMA

With the introduction of genetic screening for RET gene mutations, an increasing number of patients are diagnosed with inherited forms of MTC during childhood or even infancy. The current recommendations advise that individuals with RET gene mutations associated with MEN 2A and familial MTC undergo prophylactic thyroidectomy between ages 5 to 6 years, whereas affected individuals in kindreds with MEN 2B should undergo thyroidectomy during infancy due to the aggressiveness and earlier age at onset of MTC in these patients.[97] It is possible that these recommendations may be altered as more information about genotype-phenotype correlations are gathered and thus more individual recommendations based on specific genetic information can be made.

REFERENCES

1. Sawin C. Goiter. In: Kiple K, ed. *Cambridge world history of human disease.* Cambridge, England: Cambridge University Press, 1993:750.
2. Grant CS. Presidential address: boiling water to iodine—a story of unparalleled collaboration. *Surgery* 2002;132:909.
3. Jossart GH, Clark OH. Well-differentiated thyroid cancer. *Curr Probl Surg* 1994;31:933.
4. LiVolsi VA, Asa SL. The demise of follicular carcinoma of the thyroid gland. *Thyroid* 1994;4:233.
5. Greene F, Page D, Fleming I, et al. Thyroid tumors. In: Greene F, Page D, Fleming I, et al., eds. *AJCC cancer staging manual.* New York: Springer-Verlag, 2002:77.
6. Jemal A, Thomas A, Murray T, Thun M. Cancer statistics, 2002. *CA Cancer J Clin* 2002;52:23.
7. Mazzaferri EL. Management of a solitary thyroid nodule. *N Engl J Med* 1993;328:553.
8. Udelsman R. Management of thyroid cancer. *Ann Ital Chir* 2001;72:255.
9. Correa P, Chen VW. Endocrine gland cancer. *Cancer* 1995;75:338.
10. Ron E, Lubin JH, Shore RE, et al. Thyroid cancer after exposure to external radiation: a pooled analysis of seven studies. *Radiat Res* 1995;141:259.
11. Shore RE, Woodard E, Hildreth N, et al. Thyroid tumors following thymus irradiation. *J Natl Cancer Inst* 1985;74:1177.
12. Schneider AB, Fogelfeld L. Radiation-induced endocrine tumors. *Cancer Treat Res* 1997;89:141.
13. Schneider AB, Ron E, Lubin J, Stovall M, Gierlowski TC. Dose-response relationships for radiation-induced thyroid cancer and thyroid nodules: evidence for the prolonged effects of radiation on the thyroid. *J Clin Endocrinol Metab* 1993;77:362.
14. Hancock SL, Cox RS, McDougall IR. Thyroid diseases after treatment of Hodgkin's disease. *N Engl J Med* 1991;325:599.
15. Tucker MA, Jones PH, Boice JD Jr, et al. Therapeutic radiation at a young age is linked to secondary thyroid cancer. The Late Effects Study Group. *Cancer Res* 1991;51:2885.
16. Boice JD Jr, Engholm G, Kleinerman RA, et al. Radiation dose and second cancer risk in patients treated for cancer of the cervix. *Radiat Res* 1988;116:3.
17. Dickman PW, Holm LE, Lundell G, Boice JD Jr, Hall P. Thyroid cancer risk after thyroid examination with 131I: a population-based cohort study in Sweden. *Int J Cancer* 2003;106:580.
18. Ron E, Doody MM, Becker DV, et al. Cancer mortality following treatment for adult hyperthyroidism. Cooperative Thyrotoxicosis Therapy Follow-up Study Group. *JAMA* 1998;280:347.
19. Robbins J, Schneider AB. Thyroid cancer following exposure to radioactive iodine. *Rev Endocr Metab Disord* 2000;1:197.
20. Nikiforov YE, Rowland JM, Bove KE, Monforte-Munoz H, Fagin JA. Distinct pattern of ret oncogene rearrangements in morphological variants of radiation-induced and sporadic thyroid papillary carcinomas in children. *Cancer Res* 1997;57:1690.
21. Ron E, Kleinerman RA, Boice JD Jr, et al. A population-based case-control study of thyroid cancer. *J Natl Cancer Inst* 1987;79:1.
22. Bosetti C, Kolonel L, Negri E, et al. A pooled analysis of case-control studies of thyroid cancer. VI. Fish and shellfish consumption. *Cancer Causes Control* 2001;12:375.
23. Galanti MR, Ekbom A, Grimelius L, Yuen J. Parental cancer and risk of papillary and follicular thyroid carcinoma. *Br J Cancer* 1997;75:451.
24. Eng C. Familial papillary thyroid cancer—many syndromes, too many genes? *J Clin Endocrinol Metab* 2000;85:1755.
25. Malchoff CD, Malchoff DM. The genetics of hereditary nonmedullary thyroid carcinoma. *J Clin Endocrinol Metab* 2002;87:2455.
26. Denham MJ, Wills EJ. A clinico-pathological survey of thyroid glands in old age. *Gerontology* 1980;26:160.
27. Burch HB. Evaluation and management of the solid thyroid nodule. *Endocrinol Metab Clin North Am* 1995;24:663.
28. Pacini F, Fontanelli M, Fugazzola L, et al. Routine measurement of serum calcitonin in nodular thyroid diseases allows the preoperative diagnosis of unsuspected sporadic medullary thyroid carcinoma. *J Clin Endocrinol Metab* 1994;78:826.
29. Chen H, Nicol TL, Rosenthal DL, Udelsman R. The role of fine-needle aspirations in the evaluation of thyroid nodules. *Curr Probl Surg* 1997;14:1.
30. Frates MC, Benson CB, Doubilet PM, Cibas ES, Marqusee E. Can color Doppler sonography aid in the prediction of malignancy of thyroid nodules? *J Ultrasound Med* 2003;22:127.
31. Gharib H, Goellner JR, Johnson DA. Fine-needle aspiration cytology of the thyroid. A 12-year experience with 11,000 biopsies. *Clin Lab Med* 1993;13:699.
32. Chen H, Nicol TL, Udelsman R. Follicular lesions of the thyroid. Does frozen section evaluation alter operative management? *Ann Surg* 1995;222:101.
33. Zeiger MA, Smallridge RC, Clark DP, et al. Human telomerase reverse transcriptase (hTERT) gene expression in FNA samples from thyroid neoplasms. *Surgery* 1999;126:1195.
34. Takiyama Y, Saji M, Clark DP, et al. Polymerase chain reaction-based microsatellite analysis of fine-needle aspirations from Hürthle cell neoplasms. *Thyroid* 1997;7:853.
35. Castro MR, Caraballo PJ, Morris JC. Effectiveness of thyroid hormone suppressive therapy in benign solitary thyroid nodules: a meta-analysis. *J Clin Endocrinol Metab* 2002;87:4154.
36. Wemeau JL, Caron P, Schvartz C, et al. Effects of thyroid-stimulating hormone suppression with levothyroxine in reducing the volume of solitary thyroid nodules and improving extranodular nonpalpable changes: a randomized, double-blind, placebo-controlled trial by the French Thyroid Research Group. *J Clin Endocrinol Metab* 2002;87:4928.
37. Chen H, Zeiger MA, Clark DP, Westra WH, Udelsman R. Papillary carcinoma of the thyroid: can operative management be based solely on fine-needle aspiration? *J Am Coll Surg* 1997;184:605.
38. Tielens ET, Sherman SI, Hruban RH, Ladenson PW. Follicular variant of papillary thyroid carcinoma. A clinicopathologic study. *Cancer* 1994;73:424.
39. van Heerden JA, Hay ID, Goellner JR, et al. Follicular thyroid carcinoma with capsular invasion alone: a nonthreatening malignancy. *Surgery* 1992;112:1130.
40. Chen H, Nicol TL, Zeiger MA, et al. Hürthle cell neoplasms of the thyroid: are there factors predictive of malignancy? *Ann Surg* 1998;227:542.
41. Flynn SD, Forman BH, Stewart AF, Kinder BK. Poorly differentiated ("insular") carcinoma of the thyroid gland: an aggressive subset of differentiated thyroid neoplasms. *Surgery* 1988;104:963.
42. Johnson TL, Lloyd RV, Thompson NW, Beierwaltes WH, Sisson JC. Prognostic implications of the tall cell variant of papillary thyroid carcinoma. *Am J Surg Pathol* 1988;12:22.
43. Gaertner EM, Davidson M, Wenig BM. The columnar cell variant of thyroid papillary carcinoma. Case report and discussion of an unusually aggressive thyroid papillary carcinoma. *Am J Surg Pathol* 1995;19:940.
44. Fujimoto Y, Obara T, Ito Y, et al. Diffuse sclerosing variant of papillary carcinoma of the thyroid. Clinical importance, surgical treatment, and follow-up study. *Cancer* 1990;66:2306.
45. Pellegriti G, Giuffrida D, Scollo C, et al. Long-term outcome of patients with insular carcinoma of the thyroid: the insular histotype is an independent predictor of poor prognosis. *Cancer* 2002;95:2076.
46. Staunton MD. Thyroid cancer: a multivariate analysis on influence of treatment on long-term survival. *Eur J Surg Oncol* 1994;20:613.
47. Chen H, Udelsman R. Papillary thyroid carcinoma: justification for total thyroidectomy and management of lymph node metastases. *Surg Oncol Clin N Am* 1998;7:645.
48. Joensuu H, Klemi PJ, Paul R, Tuominen J. Survival and prognostic factors in thyroid carcinoma. *Acta Radiol Oncol* 1986;25:243.
49. Mazzaferri EL, Jhiang SM. Long-term impact of initial surgical and medical therapy on papillary and follicular thyroid cancer. *Am J Med* 1994;97:418.
50. Cady B, Rossi R. An expanded view of risk-group definition in differentiated thyroid carcinoma. *Surgery* 1988;104:947.
51. Ito Y, Uruno T, Nakano K, et al. An observation trial without surgical treatment in patients with papillary microcarcinoma of the thyroid. *Thyroid* 2003;13:381.
52. Allo MD, Christianson W, Koivunen D. Not all "occult" papillary carcinomas are "minimal." *Surgery* 1988;104:971.
53. Shaha AR, Shah JP, Loree TR. Patterns of nodal and distant metastasis based on histologic varieties in differentiated carcinoma of the thyroid. *Am J Surg* 1996;172:692.
54. Shaha AR, Shah JP, Loree TR. Differentiated thyroid cancer presenting initially with distant metastasis. *Am J Surg* 1997;174:474.
55. Rossi RL, Cady B, Silverman ML, Wool MS, Horner TA. Current results of conservative surgery for differentiated thyroid carcinoma. *World J Surg* 1986;10:612.
56. Hay ID, Grant CS, Taylor WF, McConahey WM. Ipsilateral lobectomy versus bilateral lobar resection in papillary thyroid carcinoma: a retrospective analysis of surgical outcome using a novel prognostic scoring system. *Surgery* 1987;102:1088.
57. Shah JP, Loree TR, Dharker D, et al. Prognostic factors in differentiated carcinoma of the thyroid gland. *Am J Surg* 1992;164:658.
58. Donohue JH, Goldfien SD, Miller TR, Abele JS, Clark OH. Do the prognoses of papillary and follicular thyroid carcinomas differ? *Am J Surg* 1984;148:168.
59. Rossi RL, Cady B, Silverman ML, et al. Surgically incurable well-differentiated thyroid carcinoma. Prognostic factors and results of therapy. *Arch Surg* 1988;123:569.
60. Pasieka JL, Zedenius J, Auer G, et al. Addition of nuclear DNA content to the AMES risk-group classification for papillary thyroid cancer. *Surgery* 1992;112:1154.
61. Hay ID, Bergstralh EJ, Goellner JR, Ebersold JR, Grant CS. Predicting outcome in papillary thyroid carcinoma: development of a reliable prognostic scoring system in a cohort of 1779 patients surgically treated at one institution during 1940 through 1989. *Surgery* 1993;114:1050.
62. Hay ID, Grant CS, Bergstralh EJ, et al. Unilateral total lobectomy: is it sufficient surgical treatment for patients with AMES low-risk papillary thyroid carcinoma? *Surgery* 1998;124:958.
63. Sherman SI, Brierley JD, Sperling M, et al. Prospective multicenter study of thyroid carcinoma treatment: initial analysis of staging and outcome. National Thyroid Cancer Treatment Cooperative Study Registry Group. *Cancer* 1998;83:1012.
64. Udelsman R, Lakatos E, Ladenson P. Optimal surgery for papillary thyroid carcinoma. *World J Surg* 1996;20:88.
65. Udelsman R, Westra WH, Donovan PI, Sohn TA, Cameron JL. Randomized prospective evaluation of frozen-section analysis for follicular neoplasms of the thyroid. *Ann Surg* 2001;233:716.
66. Sosa JA, Bowman HM, Tielsch JM, et al. The importance of surgeon experience for clinical and economic outcomes from thyroidectomy. *Ann Surg* 1998;228:320.
67. Sanders LE, Cady B. Differentiated thyroid cancer: reexamination of risk groups and outcome of treatment. *Arch Surg* 1998;133:419.
68. Taylor T, Specker B, Robbins J, et al. Outcome after treatment of high-risk papillary and non-Hürthle-cell follicular thyroid carcinoma. *Ann Intern Med* 1998;129:622.
69. Wanebo H, Coburn M, Teates D, Cole B. Total thyroidectomy does not enhance disease control or survival even in high-risk patients with differentiated thyroid cancer. *Ann Surg* 1998;227:912.

70. Talpos GB. Tracheal and laryngeal resections for differentiated thyroid cancer. *Am Surg* 1999;65:754.

71. Kelemen PR, Van Herle AJ, Giuliano AE. Sentinel lymphadenectomy in thyroid malignant neoplasms. *Arch Surg* 1998;133:288.

72. Tisell LE, Nilsson B, Molne J, et al. Improved survival of patients with papillary thyroid cancer after surgical microdissection. *World J Surg* 1996;20:854.

73. Udelsman R, Chen H. The current management of thyroid cancer. *Adv Surg* 1999;33:1.

74. Mazzaferri EL. Treating high thyroglobulin with radioiodine: a magic bullet or a shot in the dark? *J Clin Endocrinol Metab* 1995;80:1485.

75. Schlumberger M. Can iodine-131 whole-body scan be replaced by thyroglobulin measurement in the post-surgical follow-up of differentiated thyroid carcinoma? *J Nucl Med* 1992;33:172.

76. Sweeney D, Johnson G. Radioiodine therapy for thyroid cancer. *Endocrinol Metab Clin North Am* 1995;24:803.

77. Park HM, Perkins OW, Edmondson JW, Schnute RB, Manatunga A. Influence of diagnostic radioiodine on the uptake of ablative dose of iodine-131. *Thyroid* 1994;4:49.

78. Cooper DS, Specker B, Ho M, et al. Thyrotropin suppression and disease progression in patients with differentiated thyroid cancer: results from the National Thyroid Cancer Treatment Cooperative Registry. *Thyroid* 1998;8:737.

79. Bohuslavizki KH, Brenner W, Klutmann S, et al. Radioprotection of salivary glands by amifostine in high-dose radioiodine therapy. *J Nucl Med* 1998;39:1237.

80. Van Nostrand D, Neutze J, Atkins F. Side effects of "rational dose" iodine-131 therapy for metastatic well-differentiated thyroid carcinoma. *J Nucl Med* 1986;27:1519.

81. Mazzaferri EL, Robbins RJ, Spencer CA, et al. A consensus report of the role of serum thyroglobulin as a monitoring method for low-risk patients with papillary thyroid carcinoma. *J Clin Endocrinol Metab* 2003;88:1433.

82. Mazzaferri EL, Kloos RT. Is diagnostic iodine-131 scanning with recombinant human TSH useful in the follow-up of differentiated thyroid cancer after thyroid ablation? *J Clin Endocrinol Metab* 2002;87:1490.

83. Pineda JD, Lee T, Ain K, Reynolds JC, Robbins J. Iodine-131 therapy for thyroid cancer patients with elevated thyroglobulin and negative diagnostic scan. *J Clin Endocrinol Metab* 1995;80:1488.

84. Ladenson PW, Braverman LE, Mazzaferri EL, et al. Comparison of administration of recombinant human thyrotropin with withdrawal of thyroid hormone for radioactive iodine scanning in patients with thyroid carcinoma. *N Engl J Med* 1997;337:888.

85. Robbins RJ, Robbins AK. Clinical review 156: recombinant human thyrotropin and thyroid cancer management. *J Clin Endocrinol Metab* 2003;88:1933.

86. Ekman ET, Lundell G, Tennvall J, Wallin G. Chemotherapy and multimodality treatment in thyroid carcinoma. *Otolaryngol Clin North Am* 1990;23:523.

87. Farahati J, Reiners C, Stuschke M, et al. Differentiated thyroid cancer. Impact of adjuvant external radiotherapy in patients with perithyroidal tumor infiltration (stage pT4). *Cancer* 1996;77:172.

88. Braga-Basaria M, Ringel MD. Clinical review 158: beyond radioiodine: a review of potential new therapeutic approaches for thyroid cancer. *J Clin Endocrinol Metab* 2003;88:1947.

89. Nel CJ, van Heerden JA, Goellner JR, et al. Anaplastic carcinoma of the thyroid: a clinicopathologic study of 82 cases. *Mayo Clin Proc* 1985;60:51.

90. Tan RK, Finley RK 3rd, Driscoll D, et al. Anaplastic carcinoma of the thyroid: a 24-year experience. *Head Neck* 1995;17:41.

91. McIver B, Hay ID, Giuffrida DF, et al. Anaplastic thyroid carcinoma: a 50-year experience at a single institution. *Surgery* 2001;130:1028.

92. Kim JH, Leeper RD. Treatment of anaplastic giant and spindle cell carcinoma of the thyroid gland with combination Adriamycin and radiation therapy. A new approach. *Cancer* 1983;52:954.

93. Ain KB, Egorin MJ, DeSimone PA. Treatment of anaplastic thyroid carcinoma with paclitaxel: phase 2 trial using ninety-six-hour infusion. Collaborative Anaplastic Thyroid Cancer Health Intervention Trials (CATCHIT) Group. *Thyroid* 2000;10:587.

94. Hazard J, Hawk W, Crile G. Medullary (solid) carcinoma of the thyroid clinicopathologic entity. *J Clin Endocrinol Metab* 1959;19:152.

95. Wells SA Jr, Baylin SB, Linehan WM, et al. Provocative agents and the diagnosis of medullary carcinoma of the thyroid gland. *Ann Surg* 1978;188:139.

96. Farndon JR, Leight GS, Dilley WG, et al. Familial medullary thyroid carcinoma without associated endocrinopathies: a distinct clinical entity. *Br J Surg* 1986;73:278.

97. Moley JF. Medullary thyroid carcinoma. *Curr Treat Options Oncol* 2003;4:339.

98. Franc B, Rosenberg-Bourgin M, Caillou B, et al. Medullary thyroid carcinoma: search for histological predictors of survival (109 proband case analysis). *Hum Pathol* 1998;29:1078.

99. Krausz Y, Rosler A, Guttmann H, et al. Somatostatin receptor scintigraphy for early detection of regional and distant metastases of medullary carcinoma of the thyroid. *Clin Nucl Med* 1999;24:256.

100. Musholt TJ, Musholt PB, Dehdashti F, Moley JF. Evaluation of fluorodeoxyglucose-positron emission tomographic scanning and its association with glucose transporter expression in medullary thyroid carcinoma and pheochromocytoma: a clinical and molecular study. *Surgery* 1997;122:1049.

101. Evans DB, Fleming JB, Lee JE, Cote G, Gagel RF. The surgical treatment of medullary thyroid carcinoma. *Semin Surg Oncol* 1999;16:50.

102. Duh QY, Sancho JJ, Greenspan FS, et al. Medullary thyroid carcinoma. The need for early diagnosis and total thyroidectomy. *Arch Surg* 1989;124:1206.

103. O'Riordain DS, O'Brien T, Weaver AL, et al. Medullary thyroid carcinoma in multiple endocrine neoplasia types 2A and 2B. *Surgery* 1994;116:1017.

104. Modigliani E, Cohen R, Campos JM, et al. Prognostic factors for survival and for biochemical cure in medullary thyroid carcinoma: results in 899 patients. The GETC Study Group. Groupe d'etude des tumeurs a calcitonine. *Clin Endocrinol (Oxf)* 1998;48:265.

105. Tisell LE, Hansson G, Jansson S, Salander H. Reoperation in the treatment of asymptomatic metastasizing medullary thyroid carcinoma. *Surgery* 1986;99:60.

106. van Heerden JA, Grant CS, Gharib H, Hay ID, Ilstrup DM. Long-term course of patients with persistent hypercalcitoninemia after apparent curative primary surgery for medullary thyroid carcinoma. *Ann Surg* 1990;212:395.

107. Moley JF, Dilley WG, DeBenedetti MK. Improved results of cervical reoperation for medullary thyroid carcinoma. *Ann Surg* 1997;225:734.

108. Chen H, Roberts JR, Ball DW, et al. Effective long-term palliation of symptomatic, incurable metastatic medullary thyroid cancer by operative resection. *Ann Surg* 1998;227:887.

109. Nguyen TD, Chassard JL, Lagarde P, et al. Results of postoperative radiation therapy in medullary carcinoma of the thyroid: a retrospective study by the French Federation of Cancer Institutes—the Radiotherapy Cooperative Group. *Radiother Oncol* 1992;23:1.

110. Wells SA Jr, Chi DD, Toshima K, et al. Predictive DNA testing and prophylactic thyroidectomy in patients at risk for multiple endocrine neoplasia type 2A. *Ann Surg* 1994;220:237.

111. Kebebew E, Tresler PA, Siperstein AE, Duh QY, Clark OH. Normal thyroid pathology in patients undergoing thyroidectomy for finding a RET gene germline mutation: a report of three cases and review of the literature. *Thyroid* 1999;9:127.

112. Niccoli-Sire P, Murat A, Rohmer V, et al. Familial medullary thyroid carcinoma with non-cysteine RET mutations: phenotype-genotype relationship in a large series of patients. *J Clin Endocrinol Metab* 2001;86:3746.

113. Machens A, Gimm O, Hinze R, et al. Genotype-phenotype correlations in hereditary medullary thyroid carcinoma: oncological features and biochemical properties. *J Clin Endocrinol Metab* 2001;86:1104.

114. Yip L, Cote GJ, Shapiro SE, et al. Multiple endocrine neoplasia type 2: evaluation of the genotype-phenotype relationship. *Arch Surg* 2003;138:409.

115. Friedberg MH, Coburn MC, Monchik JM. Role of surgery in stage IE non-Hodgkin's lymphoma of the thyroid. *Surgery* 1994;116:1061.

116. Skarsgard ED, Connors JM, Robins RE. A current analysis of primary lymphoma of the thyroid. *Surgery* 1991;126:1199.

117. Ansell SM, Grant CS, Habermann TM. Primary thyroid lymphoma. *Semin Oncol* 1999;26:316.

118. Cha C, Chen H, Westra WH, Udelsman R. Primary thyroid lymphoma: can the diagnosis be made solely by fine-needle aspiration? *Ann Surg Oncol* 2002;9:298.

119. Rosen IB, Walfish PG, Bain J, Bedard YC. Secondary malignancy of the thyroid gland and its management. *Ann Surg Oncol* 1995;2:252.

120. Chen H, Nicol TL, Udelsman R. Clinically significant, isolated metastatic disease to the thyroid gland. *World J Surg* 1999;23:177.

121. Hung W, Sarlis NJ. Current controversies in the management of pediatric patients with well-differentiated nonmedullary thyroid cancer: a review. *Thyroid* 2002;12:683.

122. Harness JK, Thompson NW, McLeod MK, Pasieka JL, Fukuuchi A. Differentiated thyroid carcinoma in children and adolescents. *World J Surg* 1992;16:547.

123. Zimmerman D, Hay ID, Gough IR, et al. Papillary thyroid carcinoma in children and adults: long-term follow-up of 1039 patients conservatively treated at one institution during three decades. *Surgery* 1988;104:1157.

124. Byar DP, Green SB, Dor P, et al. A prognostic index for thyroid carcinoma. A study of the E.O.R.T.C. Thyroid Cancer Cooperative Group. *Eur J Cancer* 1979;15:1033.

DOUGLAS L. FRAKER

SECTION **3**

Parathyroid Tumors

Parathyroid neoplasia is a common endocrine problem, whereas parathyroid carcinoma is exceptionally rare.[1] Parathyroid carcinomas, as opposed to other endocrine tumors that become less hormonally active when malignant, are hyperfunctional and are characterized by severe elevations of serum calcium level with associated renal and bone symptoms.[2] The clinical course is variable but typically follows a pattern of local recurrence in the neck with late distant metastases to lung, bone, and liver.

The initial report of a parathyroid carcinoma was made by de Quervain in 1909.[3] He described a patient with a large, locally invasive neck mass that was parathyroid on histologic evaluation. The tumor was definitely malignant, because the patient developed lung metastases after removal of the neck mass, but no signs or symptoms of hypercalcemia were described. The initial description of severe hypercalcemia associated with parathyroid cancer was made three decades later by Armstrong.[4] The rarity of parathyroid carcinoma limits reports to primarily small institutional series with occasional reviews of all experience reported in the medical literature. Even institutions such as the Massachusetts General Hospital[5] or the Mayo Clinic[3] with extensive clinical interest in this disease have only one to two dozen cases in clinical reviews spanning four to five decades. A detailed review by Obara and Fujimoto[2] identified 270 cases of parathyroid carcinoma in the English literature between 1933 and 1991. An article drawing on the National Cancer Database in the United States identified 286 cases of parathyroid cancer reported between 1985 and 1995.[6] This single report more than doubles the number of cases in the literature for this rare disease. The epidemiology, pathology, clinical course, treatment, and prognosis of this rare malignancy are described in relation to the much more common diagnoses of parathyroid adenoma and hyperplasia.

PRIMARY HYPERPARATHYROIDISM

The vast majority of parathyroid cancers are functional with excess production of parathyroid hormone (PTH), which results in the clinical syndrome of primary hyperparathyroidism (HPT). The pathology of HPT can be grouped into three general categories: a single parathyroid adenoma (83% to 85% of cases), multiglandular hyperplasia (15%), and parathyroid cancer (0.5% to 3.0%).[7] The proportion of HPT patients who truly have parathyroid cancer is likely to be well under the 2% of cases quoted.[2] The epidemiologic and pathologic characteristics of these three general categories of HPT are shown in Table 34.3-1.

PATHOLOGY

Schantz and Castleman defined the pathologic criteria used to distinguish parathyroid carcinoma from benign parathyroid adenoma in a classic article in 1973.[8] Thick fibrous bands, pleomorphic cells in a trabecular pattern, and a high incidence of mitotic figures are the chief distinguishing features[8,9] (Fig. 34.3-1; see Table 34.3-1). Invasion of the glandular capsule and vascular invasion are also found with parathyroid carcinoma. However, as with other endocrine neoplasms, the diagnosis of parathyroid carcinoma based strictly on histologic evaluation using the criteria outlined earlier is difficult.[10] There is a spectrum of these changes present in benign adenomas, atypical adenomas, and true carcinomas.[11] Even histologic evidence of capsular or vascular invasion is not pathognomonic for parathyroid cancer, because spontaneous hemorrhage in large benign parathyroid adenomas may result in a similar histologic appearance.[12]

In addition to the histologic criteria, both the clinical course and the gross pathology observed at surgery help to define a lesion as parathyroid cancer.[12] The typical clinical presentation is discussed in greater detail later in Clinical Presentation, but parathyroid carcinoma tends to be associated with a higher serum calcium level, more marked symptoms of HPT, and lesions that are larger than those in patients with the more common benign adenomas and may be palpable in the neck. The operating surgeon finds a large lesion that is more firm than typical adenomas.[10] The color of parathyroid carcinomas is frequently gray-brown instead of the red-brown of benign lesions, reflecting the increased fibrous stroma within these tumors.[10] Most importantly, parathyroid carcinomas may locally invade into adjacent structures such as the ipsilateral thyroid gland or overlying strap muscles of the neck. This gross pathologic feature is infrequently seen with benign lesions.[8-10]

TABLE 34.3-1. Comparison of the Various Causes of Primary Hyperparathyroidism

Cause	Frequency (%)	Etiologic Factors	Gender	Age (y)	Pathology	
					Gross	Microscopic
Adenoma	83–85	Radiation exposure	F >M 2–3:1	55–61	Single enlarged soft red-brown gland	Nests of parathyroid chief cells; decreased cytoplasmic fat; possible rim at normal tissue
Hyperplasia	15	Familial in multiple endocrine neoplasia 1 and 2	M = F	25–40	Asymmetric enlargement with red-brown color of 4+ glands	Similar to adenomas; minimal intercellular fat
Carcinoma	<1	Familial? Radiation exposure?	M = F	45–50	Single large firm white-gray mass frequently invading thyroid or strap muscle	Trabecular arrangement of tumor cells divided by fibrous bands; mitotic figures present; possible capsular, vascular or adjacent structure invasion

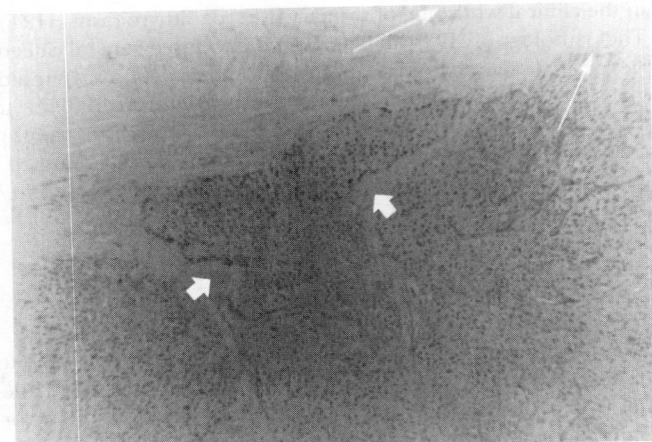

A

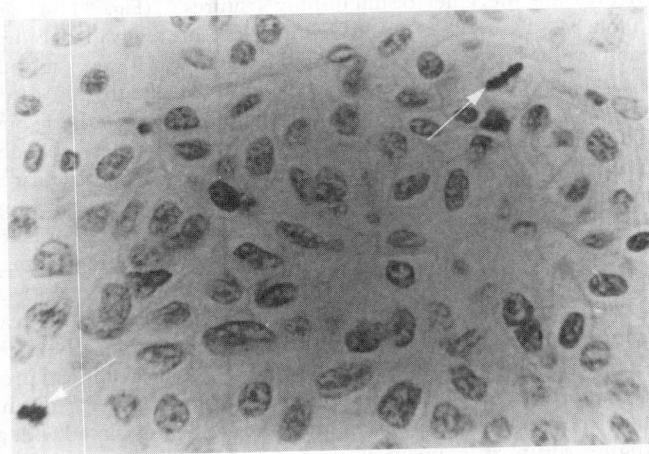

B

FIGURE 34.3-1. Pathologic characteristics used to define a lesion as a parathyroid carcinoma are shown in these two panels. **A:** A low-power view demonstrating dense fibrous bands with the cells arranged in a trabecular pattern (*arrowheads*) and evidence of capsular invasion (*arrows*). **B:** A high-power view that documents a high number of mitotic figures (*arrows*) in one single field of view.

Several groups have used flow cytometry to analyze DNA content in parathyroid carcinomas compared to adenomas. In three series, a consistent proportion between 31% and 56% of parathyroid carcinomas were documented to be aneuploid.[13–15] The DNA content of parathyroid adenomas is not as consistent, with one group reporting no aneuploidy in lesions from 32 patients[13] and other groups reporting proportions in the range of one-third aneuploidy similar to those for parathyroid carcinoma.[2] A second piece of information that these studies report is that aneuploidy is a prognostic indicator for parathyroid carcinoma. August et al. reported that four out of five patients with aneuploid parathyroid carcinoma died of disease with the fifth alive with extensive recurrence, whereas four of four patients with diploid parathyroid carcinoma were cured with no evidence of recurrence after parathyroid surgery.[15] Another interpretation of these data is that the "diploid carcinomas" were not true cancers. One study evaluated the comparative expression of human telomerase reverse transcriptase in benign and malignant parathyroid neoplasia.[16] Four parathyroid cancers, six parathyroid adenomas, and two hyperplastic glands were analyzed. One hundred percent of the cancer expressed human telomerase reverse

transcriptase, but zero of eight benign lesions did ($P = .001$), which makes this a positive test to identify carcinoma.[16] A similar study evaluated the expression of matrix metalloproteinase in malignant and benign parathyroid neoplasms.[17] Fourteen out of 18 parathyroid cancers had overexpression of gelatinase A compared with 4 of 13 atypical parathyroid adenomas.

MOLECULAR GENETICS

The study of the molecular genetics of parathyroid carcinoma is difficult because of the rarity of this disease and the inability to acquire tissue for analysis. There has been a good deal of literature regarding the overexpression of cyclin D in parathyroid adenomas. The specific genetic rearrangement of the PTH promoter enhancer to overexpress cyclin D has been defined in that benign neoplasm. There is overactivity of cyclin D noted in parathyroid carcinomas, but it is unclear whether this is a primary causative event or whether this is an epiphenomenon of the carcinoma cell. There is also a deletion in the region of chromosome 13 in parathyroid carcinomas. One study analyzed 16 specimens of parathyroid cancer from 12 patients for specific deletions or mutations of the retinoblastoma gene and BRCA2 because these known tumor suppressor genes are located on chromosome 13.[18] However, no deletions, insertions, or mutations were seen in any of the specimens.

Another study used a different investigative approach evaluating changes in the HRPT-2 gene, which is known to cause familial benign parathyroid lesions.[19] Germline mutations in HRPT-2, which codes for the parafibroma protein, cause a rare autosomal dominant syndrome characterized by parathyroid adenomas, ossifying fibromas of the jaw, including both the mandible and maxilla, and benign and malignant neoplasms of the kidney. This syndrome is known as the hereditary hyperparathyroid–jaw tumor syndrome. The HRPT-2 gene is located on chromosome bands 1q21-1q32.

Arnold's group collected 21 specimens of parathyroid carcinoma (5 primary lesions, 6 local recurrences, and 11 metastases) from around the world and analyzed them for mutations in the HRPT-2 gene.[20] A total of 15 different mutations were seen in 12 of the 21 specimens analyzed. Five mutations resulted in a truncated protein and ten gave rise to an altered reading frame, all of which resulted in dysfunctional protein. A total of 10 of the 15 patients had mutations in HRPT-2. For 11 patients, somatic tissue was available for analysis, and 3 of these 11 patients surprisingly had a germline mutation in HRPT-2 despite having no evidence of the hereditary hyperparathyroid–jaw tumor syndrome. Parathyroid carcinoma tissue is a very valuable resource, and further investigations are needed to clearly define the molecular genetics of this rare cancer.

EPIDEMIOLOGY

The incidence of parathyroid cancer is most commonly reported in the context of primary HPT. Most endocrine surgeons report 0.5% to 4.0% of all HPT as being caused by parathyroid carcinoma (Table 34.3-2). Because the estimate of the annual incidence of primary HPT is reported to be 1 per 2000,[1] then if 1% of HPT is due to parathyroid cancer, the incidence of this malignancy would be approximately 0.5 per

TABLE 34.3-2. Demographics, Proportion of Primary Hyperparathyroidism That Is Parathyroid Cancer, Tumor Size, and Calcium Levels in More Recent Institutional Series of Parathyroid Cancer

Institution	Years	Total Cases — No. of Cases	Total Cases — Total Primary Hyperparathyroidism	Percentage of Cancer	M:F	Age Mean, Range	Tumor Size (cm)	Serum Weight (g)	Ca (mg/dL)
Mayo Clinic[3]	1928–77	12	2013	0.6	4:8	51, 29–72	—	6.8	14.5
Cleveland Clinic[21]	1938–88	6	1200	0.47	4:3	47, 20–61	—	—	15.3
Lahey Clinic[37]	1942–84	9	301	3.0	3:6	48, 19–64	3.5	—	14.0
Massachusetts General Hospital[5]	1948–83	28	1200	2.3	14:14	45, 28–72	3.0	6.7	13.7
Memorial Sloan-Kettering Cancer Center[35]	1955–91	14	—	—	7:7	48, 27–81	3.3	12.0	14.8
Rochester[57]	1958–90	11	197	5.6	1:10	54, —	—	—	15.2
Emory[45]	1960–82	3	360	0.8	2:1	57, 43–69	2.9	—	16.1
M. D. Anderson[36]	1968–82	14	—	—	7:7	—, 27–61	—	—	16.8
Michigan (total)[22]	1973–90	5	1650	0.37	2:3	46, 35–61	—	—	17.5
Michigan (initial)[22,a]	1973–90	2	1450	0.14					
National Cancer Database[6]	1985–95	286	—	—	1:1	54, 14–88	3/3	—	—
Brazil[43]	1970–95	10	—	—	2:1	51, 27–74	—	—	14.3
Italy[24]	1980–96	16	290	5.2	2:1	60, 30–78	2.9	—	13.5
Dusseldorf[23]	1986–99	4	963	0.4	1:1	—	—	—	—

Ca, calcium.

[a]University of Michigan data reported as total experience and subgroup who underwent initial operation at this institution.

100,000 persons. This incidence is clearly an overestimation, because it would place the annual number of parathyroid cancers in the United States at over 1000 new cases, which greatly exceeds the actual number. Several tertiary institutions have reported their total experience with parathyroid carcinoma over several decades in the setting of over 1000 cases of primary HPT. The Mayo Clinic,[3] the Cleveland Clinic,[21] the University of Michigan,[22] and the University of Dusseldorf[23] reported an overall proportion of parathyroid cancer in HPT of 0.60%, 0.47%, 0.37%, and 0.40% (see Table 34.3-2). However, even these numbers may be overestimates, because patients with this rare diagnosis are more likely to be referred to these tertiary institutions. A review from a tertiary referral center in Padua, Italy, reported that 5.2% of all patients operated on for HPT between 1980 and 1996 had parathyroid cancers.[24] This unusually high proportion does not appear to be an overestimation due to inaccurate pathologic analysis because 13 of 16 had metastases and 2 had multiple local recurrences. Thompson's group at the University of Michigan reported an incidence of two parathyroid carcinomas in 1450 initial parathyroid operations for HPT over two decades at the University of Michigan for a percentage of 0.14%.[22] The National Cancer Database reported 286 cases of parathyroid cancer in a 10-year period. This number was believed to capture 60% to 80% of all cancers in the United States during that time interval. If that estimate is correct, then there are only 36 to 48 cases of parathyroid cancer annually in the United States. With an incidence of 0.015 per 100,000 population, parathyroid cancer is one of the most rare of all human cancers. Because of this low incidence, there is no American Joint Committee on Cancer staging system for parathyroid cancer.[6]

The gender distribution is equal or has a slight female preponderance in most series, and differs from that of benign parathyroid adenomas, which have a higher female predominance[2,6,7,9] (see Table 34.3-2). The age at diagnosis can vary between 19 and 81 years, and the median age in most series is between 45 and 51 years. The large National Cancer Database series had essentially an equivalent gender distribution (51% male and 49% female) and a mean and median age of 54.5 and 55.1 years, respectively. There was also no disproportional incidence by race in this report, with 76.2% non-Hispanic whites, 12.2% African Americans, 7.3% Hispanic Americans, and 4.2% others.[6] There are no documented causes for this malignancy, although there is a familial association in a few series. Parathyroid cancer has been reported and documented in members of kindreds with multiple endocrine neoplasia 1.[25,26] In this autosomal dominant disease, the predominant endocrine abnormality is multiglandular benign hyperplasia of the parathyroids. Familial parathyroid cancer not associated with multiple endocrine neoplasia 1 has been reported in siblings,[27] and in one report, several relatives across two generations had parathyroid carcinoma.[28] This study also reported other relatives with primary HPT who had atypical adenomas, which implies a connection between this benign pathologic entity and true parathyroid carcinoma. External radiation exposure has been correlated with parathyroid neoplasms, but virtually all reports describe an association between radiation and the more common parathyroid adenoma, although there are isolated case reports of patients with parathyroid carcinoma who had a history of radiation treatments in the distant past.[29] Patients with renal failure typically suffer from secondary HPT with nonclonal hyperplasia of all parathyroid glands, but 13 cases of parathyroid cancer have been reported in the literature in this clinical setting.[30]

CLINICAL PRESENTATION

Because virtually all parathyroid carcinomas are functional, meaning they produce high and unregulated levels of PTH, the signs and symptoms of this disease relate primarily to the consequences of this hormone excess. Specifically, various manifestations of renal disease associated with hypercalcemia and hypercalciuria such as renal stones, renal colic, nephrocalcinosis, and renal insufficiency, occur in up to 90% of cases[31,32] (Table 34.3-3). Also, the prevalence of bone disease related to calcium absorption with osteoporosis and bone pain is much greater in patients with parathyroid carcinoma than in patients with parathyroid adenoma,[33,34] with up to 70% of patients manifesting the symptoms. In nonmalignant parathyroid disease, it is unusual to have both renal and bone symptomatology documented at the time of diagnosis.[35] However, these symptoms are present simultaneously at diagnosis in up to 50% of patients with parathyroid carcinoma (see Table 34.3-3).

These amplified symptoms reflect the increased magnitude of the biochemical disturbances seen with parathyroid carcinoma. The level of total serum calcium is significantly elevated in virtually all series of parathyroid carcinoma with the mean values between 14 and 16 mg/dL compared with 11 to 12 mg/dL seen with parathyroid adenomas[2,36] (see Table 34.3-3). Similarly, the PTH level in parathyroid carcinoma is consistently higher than in benign parathyroid disease with over 70% of patients having a greater than fivefold increase over the upper limits of normal for PTH.[2,36] Because of the high degree of hypercalcemia, it is very unusual for patients to be asymptomatic at presentation with parathyroid carcinoma, whereas patients with benign causes of HPT are asymptomatic in over 50% of cases in some series.[33,34] Up to 14% of patients with parathyroid carcinoma may present with hypercalcemic crisis manifested by a depressed level of consciousness, dehydration, and extreme hypercalcemia.[5] The typical parathyroid carcinoma is much larger than benign lesions. The median maximal diameter in most series is between 3.0 and 3.5 cm compared with approximately 1.5 cm for benign adenomas[8,9] (see Table 34.3-2). Because of this large size, a significant number of patients present with a palpable neck mass, ranging between 22% and 50% of cases.[9,31,32] Again, it is extremely unusual for patients with benign lesions to have palpable abnormalities in the neck, and this is a clinical sign that

strongly suggests parathyroid carcinoma. In 10% of cases, patients with parathyroid carcinoma present with symptoms of hoarseness due to compression or invasion of the recurrent laryngeal nerve and vocal cord paresis.[2]

NATURAL HISTORY

The best information regarding the natural history of parathyroid carcinoma comes from a detailed review[2] of 163 cases reported between 1981 and 1989 (summarized in Table 34.3-4). At initial presentation, very few patients with parathyroid carcinoma have metastases either to regional lymph nodes (fewer than 5%) or distant sites (fewer than 2%). In the National Cancer Database series of 286 patients, only 16 (5.6%) had lymph node metastases noted at the time of initial surgery.[6] This report did not comment on the incidence of distant metastases and had a relatively short follow-up interval. A higher proportion of parathyroid carcinomas are locally invasive into the thyroid gland, overlying strap muscles, recurrent laryngeal nerve, trachea, or esophagus. Some patients are not identified preoperatively or intraoperatively as having parathyroid carcinoma and undergo parathyroid procedures as if to treat parathyroid adenoma. Only after review of the pathology after this resection, or when these patients experience recurrence either locally or with metastases, is a correct diagnosis of parathyroid carcinoma made. The incidence of not recognizing parathyroid carcinomas at initial operation ranges between 11% in the Lahey Clinic series (one of nine patients),[37] 36% in the M. D.

TABLE 34.3-3. Comparison of the Incidence of Signs and Symptoms at Presentation in Patients with Parathyroid Carcinoma versus Parathyroid Adenoma

	Adenoma	Carcinoma (Median Percentage, Range)
Renal	18%	60 (27–90)
Skeletal	13–20%	55 (19–64)
Renal and skeletal	<5%	32 (0–50)
Peptic ulcer disease	3–13%	18 (0–22)
Palpable neck mass	<2%	38 (22–48)
Parathyroid crisis	<2%	14 (0–27)
Asymptomatic	38–61%	3 (0–27)
Serum calcium (mg/dL)	11–12	14–16

(Data from refs. 1–3, 5, 8, 9, 31–34, 51, 56, and 58.)

TABLE 34.3-4. Clinicopathologic Features, Natural History, and Outcome in Patients with Parathyroid Carcinoma

AT INITIAL PRESENTATION[a]	
Local invasion	23%
Thyroid	15%
Recurrent laryngeal nerve	3.7%
Other (muscle, trachea, esophagus)	4.9%
Lymph node metastases	4.3%
Distant metastases	1.8%
RECURRENCE AFTER INITIAL RESECTION[a]	
Local recurrence	36%
Lymph node recurrence	17%
Cervical	14%
Mediastinal	6.1%
Distant metastases	25%
Lung	15%
Bone	6%
Liver	4%
OUTCOME AFTER SURGICAL TREATMENT[b]	
Alive	66%
No evidence of disease	42%
Mean follow-up	4.6 y
Alive with disease	24%
Mean follow-up	7 y
Dead	34%
Caused by parathyroid carcinoma	30%
Caused by unrelated causes	4%

[a]Based on 163 patients.[2]
[b]Based on 108 patients.[2]

Anderson series (5 of 14 patients),[36] and up to 86% in the Cleveland Clinic series (six of seven patients).[21]

After surgical treatment, 40% to 60% of patients have recurrent disease at some point, typically in the range of 2 to 5 years after the initial resection.[36,38] Because parathyroid carcinomas are functional, serially measured calcium or PTH levels serve as ideal tumor markers for this malignancy. In patients followed closely, hypercalcemia precedes physical evidence of recurrent disease in most cases. The most common location of recurrence is regionally either in the tissues of the neck or in cervical lymph nodes and accounts for two-thirds of the recurrent cases.[2] Often, the local recurrences in the neck are difficult to identify because they may be small and multifocal, and involve the scar from the previous procedure. Use of ultrasonography, sestamibi-thallium scanning,[39,40] and more recently positron emission tomography,[41] may aid in this difficult diagnosis. Distant metastases occur in 25% of patients primarily in the lungs but also in the bone and liver[2,42] (see Table 34.3-4). More recently published series have reported a higher incidence of recurrence than prior studies. Of nine patients with parathyroid cancer in Brazil with long-term follow-up, five had local or nodal neck recurrence (55%), three had lung metastases (33%), and one had bone metastasis (11%).[43] In a study of 16 patients in Italy, 13 had distant metastases (nine lung alone, four lung plus bone) and two others had local neck recurrences.[8] The reasons for this high incidence of recurrence of between 94% and 100% may be due to more accurate pathologic diagnosis that excludes patients with atypical adenomas.

Patients who succumb to parathyroid carcinoma typically die from metabolic consequences and not directly from malignant growth.[42] For this reason, surgical treatment to debulk parathyroid carcinoma, if possible, is indicated because medical management of the hypercalcemia of parathyroid carcinoma is difficult (see Treatment, later in this chapter). The median survival after recurrent parathyroid cancer ranges between 3 and 5 years with isolated case reports of patients surviving several decades with intermittent surgical debulking.[38]

DIFFERENTIAL DIAGNOSIS

Other non-HPT causes of hypercalcemia can be ruled out primarily by the biochemical studies of serum PTH levels simultaneous with total and ionized serum calcium levels. Secondary HPT in the setting of renal failure is clinically obvious by the concomitant renal disease. There are isolated reports of development of parathyroid carcinoma in this clinical setting as well, however.[44] Once the diagnosis of primary HPT is established, the histopathologic diagnosis of parathyroid carcinoma may be difficult as discussed in Pathology, earlier in this chapter.[10,12] Supporting evidence of malignancy comes from markedly elevated calcium levels (more than 14 mg/dL) and larger gland sizes (more than 3 cm). In most reported institutional series, it is likely that parathyroid carcinoma is overdiagnosed.[22,45] In one such study, a careful review of the pathology in the context of the clinical course identified more than half of the patients with previously diagnosed parathyroid carcinomas as more appropriate to be considered as having benign or atypical adenomas.[46] This difficulty in correctly identifying parathyroid carcinoma is also reflected by the wide variation in clinical outcome between different series. Some series report

long-term disease-free survival at rates greater than 75%. One explanation for the results of series in which outcomes are much better than the norm is that they include in their analysis patients with atypical parathyroid adenomas that were not truly malignant.[22] Other investigators take an opposite approach and include only cases in their institutional reviews that recur locally or manifest distant metastases.[35] This approach may underestimate the true cases of parathyroid carcinoma because there is a subgroup of patients with this disease who may be cured with an aggressive initial resection.

Local recurrence of parathyroid neoplasms after initial resection does not necessarily establish the diagnosis of parathyroid carcinoma. Two patterns of benign lesions that recur locally have been described. First, patients with a single parathyroid adenoma may have partial or incomplete resection of a gland such that there is an isolated regrowth after the initial procedure in the exact position where the first abnormal gland was removed.[46] The recurrent gland grows in an area of fibrosis and scar, and may very well give the gross appearance of an invasive carcinoma, but detailed pathologic analysis of the initial or recurrent specimen shows no evidence of carcinoma in terms of mitotic figures, cellular appearance, or fibrous bands. A second category of nonmalignant recurrent disease is a condition called *parathyromatosis*.[44,47] Parathyromatosis is a diffuse seeding of the cervical tissue with parathyroid cells that implant and grow. This occurs when the capsules of lesions that are being excised are ruptured and contents are spilled or when lesions are partially removed with a raw surface of the adenoma exposed to the field of dissection. This condition is much more difficult to treat than isolated local recurrence and is tantamount to a nonmetastasizing locally recurrent carcinoma, and this condition has been described for lesions that have absolutely no pathologic or clinical manifestations of parathyroid carcinoma.

TREATMENT

The only effective treatment of parathyroid cancer is surgical resection. The most important component to achieve a favorable outcome is recognition by the operating surgeon that a lesion is likely to be a parathyroid cancer, which allows performance of the appropriate *en bloc* resection of the tumor with all potential areas of invasion at the initial operation (Fig. 34.3-2).[37,38] Extremely high serum calcium levels (more than 13.5 mg/dL) should lead to suspicion of parathyroid cancer preoperatively. Other clinical features that suggest parathyroid cancer are a palpable mass and hoarseness. Intraoperatively, if a large lesion is identified, particularly if it is firm or scirrhous, then the operating surgeon should assume the lesion is parathyroid cancer and do an *en bloc* resection. The recent practice of minimally invasive parathyroidectomy, which is appropriate in the vast majority of patients with HPT, should be altered in these clinical situations.[48] Parathyroid cancer typically invades the ipsilateral thyroid lobe, and resection of the tumor with one or both thyroid lobes is frequently required to perform an adequate operation.[37] In most series, long-term results in terms of local recurrence are significantly improved when an *en bloc* excision including thyroid is done rather than removal of only the parathyroid cancer.[37,38] The recognition and diagnosis of parathyroid cancer preoperatively correlates strongly with a favorable

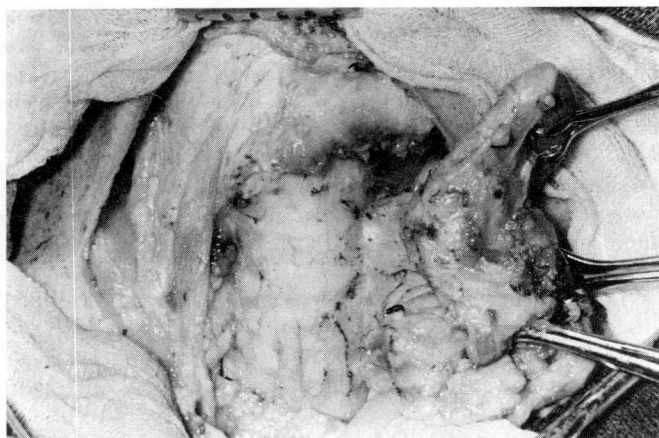

FIGURE 34.3-2. *En bloc* resection of an isolated recurrence of a parathyroid carcinoma as shown after a partial dissection. The parathyroid cancer is resected together with overlying strap muscles and the left lobe of the thyroid gland. This *en bloc* specimen is being retracted laterally in the clamps. The midline structure is the trachea, which is completely cleared of surrounding tissues. This patient is alive and well with no evidence of recurrent disease or recurrent hypercalcemia 3 years after this resection for an isolated local recurrence.

outcome. In a small series of seven patients at the Cleveland Clinic, six had parathyroid carcinomas that were not appreciated until after the procedure.[21] All of these patients had recurrence, whereas the one patient who was known to have a parathyroid cancer preoperatively underwent an *en bloc* resection and had long-term disease-free survival. An analysis of the literature from New Zealand indicated an overall 8% evidence of local recurrence after an *en bloc* resection compared to a 51% incidence after a standard parathyroidectomy.[49] The recurrent laryngeal nerve may be intimately involved or invaded by the parathyroid cancer. In these situations, patients frequently have preoperative hoarseness due to the tumor invasion of the nerve.[2] Because the nerve is at risk for loss of function due to the malignant process itself, it is appropriate to resect the recurrent laryngeal nerve if necessary to perform an *en bloc* excision during the initial procedure for parathyroid cancer. The increased potential for long-term local control achieved by this approach outweighs the complication of postoperative vocal cord paralysis, which can be improved with techniques such as Teflon injection into the paralyzed cord. Assessment of cervical lymph nodes, particularly level VI paratracheal nodes and levels III and IV internal jugular nodes, should be performed with node dissection only for enlarged or firm lesions.

For most cases of recurrent parathyroid carcinoma confined to the neck, the most appropriate treatment is aggressive re-resection. However, unlike in patients undergoing an initial procedure for whom the success rate is up to 40% to 60%, it is unusual to obtain long-term cures in patients who have to undergo re-resection.[5] In a large series from the Mayo Clinic, no patients who underwent re-resection were cured.[3] However, there are selected patients described in the literature who have disease-free intervals of more than 10 years after two or three local resections in the neck.[11,22] The benefit of sacrificing the recurrent laryngeal nerve is greatly decreased in patients undergoing re-resection for recurrent parathyroid cancer because most recurrences are multifocal. If a recurrent nodule

involves the recurrent laryngeal nerve, there are most likely other areas of parathyroid cancer that are adherent to the trachea, the esophagus, and the great vessels of the neck. Because it is impossible to remove all of these vital structures, one is unlikely to obtain a cure by taking the nerve. However, in certain circumstances in which there is an isolated local recurrence that involves the nerve, it again should be sacrificed with an *en bloc* resection, because, in rare instances, successful salvage may be accomplished for these patients by an aggressive surgical procedure (see Fig. 34.3-2).

Nonsurgical forms of therapy for parathyroid carcinoma have generally poor results, so that surgical treatment of distant metastases is appropriate in certain situations. Pulmonary metastases as well as bone metastases should be resected, if possible, primarily to debulk tumor to decrease the magnitude of the hypercalcemia.[50,51] However, occasionally long-term salvage is achieved in this group of patients with aggressive surgical treatment.

Radiation therapy, in general, does not result in meaningful antitumor responses.[52] Isolated case reports of long-term control exist, and radiation therapy should be used in patients with unresectable recurrent cervical disease.[11] Various chemotherapeutic agents alone or in combination have been used for treatment of parathyroid carcinoma with limited success.[52] Dacarbazine alone or in combination with 5-fluorouracil and cyclophosphamide has been reported to result in objective responses, including one complete response in a patient with pulmonary metastases.[52,53] Other combination therapies have resulted in rare responses. Part of the problem with the medical treatment of parathyroid carcinoma is that the rarity of this disease does not allow systematic evaluation of various combination therapies.

The second aspect of medical management for metastatic parathyroid carcinoma relates to the treatment of the hypercalcemia.[40] Acute treatment of patients with hypercalcemic crises or very high serum calcium levels is similar to that used for other causes of symptomatic hypercalcemia. Volume loading with loop diuretics causing a forced diuresis is the initial therapy. For patients with parathyroid carcinoma, the ultimate management of the hypercalcemia is directed at the tumor to decrease the level of PTH, if possible, by surgical treatment. In situations in which surgical resections are no longer possible, the treatment of hypercalcemia is very difficult, and this metabolic abnormality is the primary cause of death for the majority of these patients.[33,34,38] The most effective agents in this setting are the bisphosphonates, which inhibit osteoclast bone reabsorption.[52,54] Two agents available in the United States are etidronate and pamidronate. Other agents used in other settings of hypercalcemia such as plicamycin (formerly mithramycin) and calcitonin have limited benefit.[52] Gallium nitrate has also been used as an inhibitor of bone reabsorption, but its use is limited by nephrotoxicity.[22,55] All agents used to date in the setting of high tumor burden from parathyroid carcinoma have the limitation that patients become refractory after initial treatment. Newer generations of more potent bisphosphonates may hold some promise for symptomatic management of this group of patients.[52]

OUTCOME

The ability to achieve long-term survival in patients with parathyroid carcinoma ranges between 18% and 78% in various

TABLE 34.3-5. Five- and 10-Year Survival after Surgical Excision of Parathyroid Cancer

Institution	Time Interval	No.	5-Y Survival (%)	10-Y Survival (%)
Mayo Clinic[29]	1920–91	43	69	55
National Cancer Institute [50,a]	1933–68	46	50	13
Cleveland Clinic[15]	1938–88	7	85	57
Massachusetts General Hospital, total[5,b]	1948–83	25	80	78
Massachusetts General Hospital, recurrent[5,b]	1948–83	9	44	22
Memorial Sloan-Kettering Cancer Center[32]	1955–91	14	55	55
Columbia[28,a]	1968–81	62	50	35
M. D. Anderson[33]	1968–82	14	36	18
Karolinska, Stockholm[38,a]	1968–90	40	50	35
National Cancer Database[6]	1985–95	286	55.5	49.1
Italy[24]	1980–96	10	20	20
Total		251	57	39

[a]Series that are collective reviews from several institutions.
[b]Massachusetts General Hospital reported survival rates separately for all patients and for the subgroup that had recurrent disease.

series.[2,5,31,32,56] The 5- and 10-year overall survival rates for patients with resected parathyroid carcinoma are shown in Table 34.3-5. A summary of 251 patients analyzed shows a 5-year survival of 57% and a 10-year survival of 39%. The National Cancer Database reported a 5-year survival of 55.5% and a 10-year survival of 49.1% in 286 patients treated.[6] These two large series accounted for the majority of cases of parathyroid cancer in the literature and provide an accurate assessment of outcome. The majority of patients who have recurrence after initial surgery ultimately succumb to this disease, as there is a much lower rate of salvage after second or third procedures. Of patients with local recurrences or distant metastases, only between 0% and 15% have long-term cures after secondary resections because there is no meaningful nonsurgical therapy.

REFERENCES

1. Heath H III, Hodgson SF, Kennedy MA. Primary hyperparathyroidism: incidence, morbidity, and potential economic impact in a community. *N Engl J Med* 1980;302: 189.
2. Obara T, Fujimoto Y. Diagnosis and treatment of patients with parathyroid carcinoma: an update and review. *World J Surg* 1991;15:738.
3. van Heerden JA, Weiland LH, ReMine WH, Walls JT, Purnell DC. Cancer of the parathyroid glands. *Arch Surg* 1979;114:475.
4. Armstrong HG. Primary carcinoma of the parathyroid gland with report of a case. *Bull Acad Med (Toronto)* 1938;11:105.
5. Wang C, Gaz RD. Natural history of parathyroid carcinoma: diagnosis, treatment and results. *Am J Surg* 1985;149:522.
6. Hundahl SA, Fleming ID, Fremgen AM, Menck HR. Two hundred eighty-six cases of parathyroid carcinoma treated in the U.S. between 1985–1995. A National Cancer Database Report. *Cancer* 1999;86:538.
7. Rossi RL, ReMine SG, Clerkin EP. Hyperparathyroidism. *Surg Clin North Am* 1985;65:187.
8. Schantz A, Castleman B. Parathyroid carcinoma: a study of 70 cases. *Cancer* 1973;31: 600.
9. Fujimoto Y, Obara T. How to recognize and treat parathyroid carcinoma. *Surg Clin North Am* 1987;56:343.
10. Smith JF, Coombs RRH. Histologic diagnosis of carcinoma of the parathyroid gland. *J Clin Pathol* 1984;37:1370.
11. Levin KE, Galante M, Clark OH. Parathyroid carcinoma versus parathyroid adenoma in patients with profound hypercalcemia. *Surgery* 1987;101:649.
12. LiVolsi VA, Hamilton R. Intraoperative assessment of parathyroid gland pathology: a common view from the surgeon and the pathologist. *Am J Clin Pathol* 1994;102:365.
13. Levin KE, Chew KL, Ljung BM, et al. Deoxyribonucleic acid cytometry helps identify parathyroid carcinomas. *J Clin Endocrinol Metab* 1988;67:779.
14. Obara T, Fujimoto Y, Hirayama A, et al. Flow cytometric DNA analysis of parathyroid tumors with special reference to its diagnostic and prognostic value in parathyroid carcinoma. *Cancer* 1990;65:1789.
15. August DA, Flynn SD, Jones MA, Bagwell CB, Kinder BK. Parathyroid carcinoma: the relationship of nuclear DNA content to clinical outcome. *Surgery* 1993;113:290.
16. Kammori M, Nakamura K, Ogawa T, et al. Demonstration of human telomerase reverse transcriptase (hTERT) in human parathyroid tumours by in situ hybridization with a new oligonucleotide probe. *Clin Endocrinol* 2003;58:43.
17. Farnebo F, Svensson A, Thompson NW, et al. Expression of matrix metalloproteinase gelatinase: a messenger ribonucleic acid in parathyroid carcinomas. *Surgery* 1999;126:1183.
18. Shattuck TM, Kim TS, Costa J, et al. Mutational analyses of RB and BRCA2 as candidate tumour suppressor genes in parathyroid carcinoma. *Clin Endocrinol* 2003;59:180.
19. Wassif WS, Farnebo F, The BT, et al. Genetic studies of a family with hereditary hyperparathyroidism-jaw tumour syndrome. *Clin Endocrinol* 1999;50:191.
20. Shattuck TM, Valimaki S, Obara T, et al. Somatic and germ-line mutations of the HRPT2 gene in sporadic parathyroid carcinoma. *N Engl J Med* 2003;349:1722.
21. Hakaim AG, Esselstyn CB Jr. Parathyroid carcinoma: 50-year experience at the Cleveland Clinic Foundation. *Cleve Clin J Med* 1993;60:331.
22. Sandelin K, Thompson NW, Bondeson L. Metastatic parathyroid carcinoma: dilemmas in management. *Surgery* 1991;110:978.
23. Dotzenrath C, Goretzki PE, Sarbia M, et al. Parathyroid carcinoma: problems in diagnosis and the need for radical surgery in recurrent disease. *Eur J Surg Oncol* 2001;27:383.
24. Favia G, Lumachi F, Polistina F, D'Amico DF. Parathyroid carcinoma: sixteen new cases and suggestions for correct management. *World J Surg* 1998;22:1225.
25. Mallette LE, Bilezikian JP, Ketcham AS, Aurbach GD. Parathyroid carcinoma in familial hyperparathyroidism. *Am J Med* 1974;57:642.
26. Dionisi S, Minisola S, Pepe J, et al. Concurrent parathyroid adenomas and carcinoma in the setting of multiple neoplasia type I: presentation as hypercalcemic crisis. *Mayo Clin Proc* 2002;77:866.
27. Wassif WS, Moniz CF, Friedman E, et al. Familial isolated hyperparathyroidism: a distinct genetic entity with an increased risk of parathyroid cancer. *J Clin Endocrinol Metab* 1993;77:1485.
28. Streeten EA, Weinstein LS, Norton JA, et al. Studies in a kindred with parathyroid carcinoma. *J Clin Endocrinol Metab* 1992;75:362.
29. Takeichi N, Dohi K, Ito H, et al. Parathyroid tumors in atomic bomb survivors in Hiroshima: a review. *J Radiat Res (Tokyo)* 1991;32[Suppl]:189.
30. Takami H, Kameyama K, Nagakubo I. Parathyroid carcinoma in a patient receiving long-term hemodialysis. *Surgery* 1999;125(12):239.
31. Shane E, Bilezikian JP. Parathyroid carcinoma: a review of 62 patients. *Endocr Rev* 1982;3:218.
32. Wynne AG, van Heerden J, Carney JA, Fitzpatrick LA. Parathyroid carcinoma: clinical and pathologic features in 43 patients. *Medicine* 1992;71:197.
33. Lafferty FW. Primary hyperparathyroidism. *Arch Intern Med* 1981;141:1761.
34. Nikkila MT, Saaristo JJ, Koivula TA. Clinical and biochemical features in primary hyperparathyroidism. *Surgery* 1989;105(2):148.
35. Vetto JT, Brennan MF, Woodruf J, Burt M. Parathyroid carcinoma: diagnosis and clinical history. *Surgery* 1993;114:882.
36. Anderson BJ, Samaan NA, Vassilopoulou-Sellin R, Ordonez NG, Hickey RC. Parathyroid carcinoma: features and difficulties in diagnosis and management. *Surgery* 1983;94(6): 906.
37. Cohn K, Silverman M, Corrado J, Sedgewick C. Parathyroid carcinoma: the Lahey Clinic experience. *Surgery* 1985;98(6):1095.
38. Sandelin K, Auer G, Bondeson L, Grimelius L, Farnebo LO. Prognostic factors in parathyroid cancer: a review of 95 cases. *World J Surg* 1992;16:724.
39. Lu G, Shih WJ, Ziu JY. Technetium-99m MIBI uptake in recurrent parathyroid carcinoma and brown tumors. *J Nucl Med* 1995;36:811.
40. Al-Sobhi S, Ashari LH, Ingemansson S. Detection of metastatic parathyroid carcinoma with Tc-99m sestamibi imaging. *Clin Nucl Med* 1999;24(1):21.
41. Neumann D, Esselstyn CB, Siciliano D, et al. Preoperative imaging of parathyroid carcinoma by positron emission tomography. *Ann Otol Rhinol Laryngol* 1994;103:741.
42. Sandelin K, Tullgren O, Farnebo LO. Clinical course of metastatic parathyroid cancer. *World J Surg* 1994;18:594.

43. Cordeiro AC, Montenegro FLM, Klucsar MAV, et al. Parathyroid carcinoma. *Am J Surg* 1998;175:52.
44. Rosen IB, Young JEM, Archibald SD, Walfish PG, Vale J. Parathyroid cancer: clinical variations and relationship to autotransplantation. *Can J Surg* 1994;37(6):465.
45. McKeown PP, McGarity WC, Sewell CW. Carcinoma of the parathyroid gland: is it over-diagnosed? *Am J Surg* 1984;147:292.
46. Fraker DL, Travis WD, Merendino JJ, et al. Locally recurrent parathyroid neoplasms as a cause for recurrent and persistent primary hyperparathyroidism. *Ann Surg* 1991;213(1):58.
47. Rattner DW, Marrone GC, Kasdon E, Silen W. Recurrent hyperparathyroidism due to implantation of parathyroid tissue. *Am J Surg* 1985;149:745.
48. Norman J, Denham D. Minimally invasive radioguided parathyroidectomy in the reoperative neck. *Surgery* 1998;124(6):1088.
49. Koea JB, Shaw JH. Parathyroid cancer: biology and management. *Surg Oncol* 1999;8(3):155.
50. Flye MW, Brennan MF. Surgical resection of metastatic parathyroid carcinoma. *Ann Surg* 1981;193(4):425.
51. Obara T, Okamoto T, Ito Y, et al. Surgical and medical management of patients with pulmonary metastasis from parathyroid carcinoma. *Surgery* 1993;114(6):1040.
52. Shane E. Parathyroid carcinoma. *Curr Ther Endocrinol Metab* 1994;5:522.
53. Calandra DB, Cheijfec G, Foy BK, Lawrence AM, Paloyan E. Parathyroid carcinoma: biochemical and pathologic response to DTIC. *Surgery* 1984;96(6):1132.
54. Newrick PG, Braatvedt GD, Webb AJ, Sheffield E, Corrall RJM. Prolonged remission of hypercalcemia due to parathyroid carcinoma with pamidronate. *Postgrad Med J* 1994;70:231.
55. Warrell RP, Issacs M, Alcock NW, Bockman RS. Gallium nitrate for treatment of refractory hypercalcemia from parathyroid carcinoma. *Ann Int Med* 1987;107:683.
56. Holmes EC, Morton DL, Ketcham AS. Parathyroid carcinoma: a collective review. *Ann Surg* 1968;169(4):631.
57. Shortell CK, Andrus CH, Phillips CE, Schwartz SI. Carcinoma of the parathyroid gland: a 30-year experience. *Surgery* 1991;110(4):704.
58. Wise SR, Quigley M, Saxe AW, Zdon MJ. Hyperparathyroidism and cellular mechanisms of gastric acid secretion. *Surgery* 1990;108:1058.

SECTION 4

JEFFREY A. NORTON

Adrenal Tumors

PATHOLOGY OF THE ADRENAL CORTEX

HYPERPLASIA

The term *hyperplasia* is defined as an increased number of cells.[1] It is a pathologic change associated with increased function or compensatory change. When a pituitary tumor secretes adrenocorticotropic hormone (ACTH) and produces hypercortisolism (Cushing's disease), the adrenal gland is approximately twice normal size. The weight of each hyperplastic adrenal is between 6 and 12 g, whereas the normal adrenal weighs between 3 and 6 g. Microscopically there is a widened inner zone of the compact zona reticularis and a sharply demarcated outer zone of clear cells. Adrenal glands in ectopic ACTH syndrome are larger in size, weighing between 12 and 30 g. Macronodular adrenal hyperplasia (3-cm adrenocortical nodules weighing between 30 and 100 g) may also be a secondary response of the adrenal to ACTH but may occur with primary adrenal pathology. Primary pigmented micronodular adrenal hyperplasia (1- to 5-mm nodules with pigmented appearance and normal glandular weight) is more likely to be autonomous. It occurs in children and may be inherited.

ADRENAL CORTICAL ADENOMA

Adrenal adenoma is a benign neoplasm of adrenal cortical cells that may be functionally autonomous. An adenoma does not exceed 5 cm in diameter and 100 g in weight. Cellular pleomorphism and necrosis may be present, but are rare. It is not possible to describe the exact functional type of neoplasm based solely on histologic features, although there are consistent differences. Adenomas produce syndromes of hypercortisolism and hyperaldosteronism and seldom produce adrenogenital syndromes. Tumors larger than 6 cm that produce adrenogenital syndromes are usually carcinoma. Pleomorphism, tumor necrosis, and mitotic activity are more common in malignant tumors. The prognosis of adrenal cortical adenoma producing Cushing's syndrome is excellent, and surgical resection invariably produces cure. The prognosis of adrenal cortical adenomas producing hyperaldosteronism is not as favorable. Resection is followed by a favorable response in blood pressure and serum level of potassium; however, 30% of patients develop recurrent hypertension. Adenomas that produce the adrenogenital syndrome have the least favorable outcome, because many of these tumors are really carcinomas.

ADRENAL CORTICAL CARCINOMA

Adrenal cortical carcinoma is a malignant neoplasm of adrenal cortical cells demonstrating partial or complete histologic and functional differentiation. Adrenal cortical carcinomas are rare and compose between 0.05% and 0.20% of all cancers. This incidence translates to a rate of only 2 per million in the world population. Women develop functional adrenal cortical carcinomas more commonly than men. However, men develop nonfunctioning malignant adrenal tumors more often than women. There is a bimodal occurrence by age, with a peak incidence at less than 5 years and a second peak in the fourth and fifth decades. Adrenal cortical carcinoma has been described as part of a complex hereditary syndrome, including sarcoma, breast, and lung cancer. Studies suggest that loss of heterozygosity on the short arm of chromosome 11 (11p) may be important in the pathogenesis of adrenocortical cancer. Genetic changes are more common in malignant than benign tumors. The most frequent DNA copy number changes in adrenocortical cancers include losses of 1p21-31, 2q, 3p, 3q, 6q, 9p, and 11q14. There are also gains and amplifications of 5q12, 9q32, 9q34, 12q, and 20q.[2] Mutations in the p53 gene may occur. In adrenal cortical cancers the malignant phenotype is associated with rearrangements at the 11p15 locus and IGF-II gene overexpression.[3] Insulin-like growth factor may be a major determinant of adrenocortical tumor progression and a target for future therapies. Deficiency of 21-hydroxylase (P-450c21), an essential enzyme for zona glomerulosa and fasciculata function, has also been implicated. Prevalence of heterozygous germline mutations in the P-450c21 gene is increased in patients with adrenocortical tumors. Adrenal cortical carcinomas are larger than 6 cm and weigh between 100 and 5000 g. Areas of necrosis and hemorrhage are common. Invasion and metastases also occur. Microscopically, the appearance is variable. Cells with big nuclei, hyperchromatism, and enlarged nucleoli are all consistent with malignancy. Nuclear pleomorphism is more common in tumors larger than 500 g. Vascular invasion and many mitoses are diagnostic of malignancy. Broad desmoplastic bands are associated with metastatic potential of tumors. The diagnosis of malignancy in cortical tumors that weigh between 50 and 100 g is less certain. Predictors of survival include distant metastases; venous, capsular, and adjacent organ invasion; tumor necrosis; high mitotic rate; atypical mitosis; and mdm-2 overexpression.[4] Furthermore, the distinction between adrenal and renal carcinoma may also be difficult to make. Immunostaining for vimentin, epithelial membrane antigen, cytokeratin, and blood group antigens may be used to distinguish between the two diagnoses. Adrenal tumors stain positive for vimentin, whereas renal carcinomas are negative for vimentin, but positive for the others. Although the difference in natural history between benign and malignant adrenal cortical neoplasms is clear, it is not always possible to histologically separate one from the other. The only reliable, single criterion is the presence of nodal or distant metastases. The data used to differentiate benign from malignant adrenocortical neoplasms include whether and what type of hormone is produced, amount of tumor necrosis, fibrosis, inhibin, 21-hydroxylase deficiency, vascular invasion, mitoses, and tumor weight (Table 34.4-1). The detection of mitotic activity, aneuploidy, and venous invasion suggest a malignant tumor. Adrenal cancers may have tumor-specific mutations in p53 that serve as a marker for the tumor.[5] Mutations in the p53 gene are frequent and may be used to diagnose malignancy.[6] Quantitative nuclear analysis demonstrates that cell nuclei of adrenal cancers are larger than those of adenomas, and DNA density is diploid in adenomas and aneuploid in carcinomas. Adrenal cancer cells in culture can spontaneously transition between two subtypes by switching expression of two genes, BRG1 and Brm, at the posttranscriptional level. This mechanism allows the cell to adapt to environmental factors that may suppress growth or cause death.[7] Finally, in general carcinomas produce abnormal amounts of androgens and 11-deoxysteroids. However, this is merely suggestive of malignancy, because only 10% of malignant tumors produce masculinization, whereas the rest secrete cortisol, aldosterone, or nothing (see Table 34.4-1).

TABLE 34.4-1. Diagnosis of Malignancy in Adrenal Cortical Neoplasm

Reliability	Clinical Criteria	Pathologic and Genetic Criteria
Diagnostic of malignancy	Weight loss, feminization, nodal or distant metastases	Tumor weight >100 g, tumor necrosis, fibrous bands, vascular invasion, number of mitoses per high-power field, p53 mutations
Consistent with malignancy	Virilism, Cushing's virilism, no hormone production	Nuclear pleomorphism, aneuploidy
Suggestive of malignancy	Elevated urinary 17-ketosteroids	Capsular invasion, inhibin,[a] 21-hydroxylase deficiency[a]
Unreliable	Hypercortisolism, hyperaldosteronism	Tumor giant cells, cytoplasmic size variation, ratio between compact and clear cells

[a]Updated information (see text).

CLINICAL PRESENTATIONS OF ADRENAL CORTICAL NEOPLASMS

CUSHING'S SYNDROME (HYPERCORTISOLISM)

Signs

Cushing's syndrome, or hypercortisolism, is the result of excessive secretion of ACTH by a pituitary tumor, of cortisol by an adrenal tumor, or of ACTH by an ectopic tumor. Cushing's syndrome is rare and by itself it is associated with excessive mortality.[8] Determining the cause of the hypercortisolism involves performing multiple tests in a logical sequence (Fig. 34.4-1). Treatment aims to eliminate the hypercortisolism and tumor, while minimizing the chance of endocrine deficiency or long-term dependence on medications. The signs and symptoms of hypercortisolism are ubiquitous and diverse; nearly every organ in the body is affected. However, there is no single symptom or sign that is common to every patient. Although hypercortisolism is the most common presentation for adrenal cortical neoplasms, Cushing's syndrome is rare, with an estimated incidence of only 10 per million population. Cushing's syndrome can also rarely occur in children. The most common cause of hypercortisolism is iatrogenic administration of steroids to treat other diseases. The most common cause of endogenous hypercortisolism is a pituitary tumor that makes ACTH, or Cushing's disease. Hypercortisolism is not usually associated with multiple endocrine neoplasia type 1 (MEN 1), although it can be present in this familial syndrome. It has been reported to be present in 5% of patients with sporadic Zollinger-Ellison syndrome and 19% of patients with Zollinger-Ellison syndrome and MEN 1.

Progressive weight gain is the most universal symptom of patients with hypercortisolism. Obesity is usually truncal, and patients have thin extremities due to muscle wasting. Increased fat in the dorsal neck region combined with kyphosis secondary to osteoporosis gives the appearance of a "buffalo hump." Serial photographs show a rounding of the face. Blood pressure increases mildly secondary to excessive mineralocorticoid secretion. Striae are reliable clinical signs of Cushing's syndrome. Hirsutism consists of excessive fine hair on face, upper back, and arms. Virilization, including clitoromegaly, deep voice, and balding, suggest adrenocortical carcinoma. Glucose intolerance and hyperglycemia are common, and patients develop diabetes mellitus. Weakness secondary to muscle atrophy occurs, especially in ectopic ACTH syndrome. Menstrual irregularity or amenorrhea is common in women, whereas men have impotency. In children, the most common presenting signs are obesity and short stature. Dilatation of blood vessels and thinning of the subcutaneous tissue give the face a ruddy appearance. Mental changes vary from mild depression to severe psychosis and appear to correlate directly with serum levels of cortisol and ACTH. Hypokalemia worsens the weakness associated with Cushing's syndrome and suggests the diagnosis of adrenocortical carcinoma or ectopic ACTH syndrome. Immunosuppression results in unusual infections, including cryptococcosis, aspergillosis, nocardiosis, *Pneumocystis carinii* infection, and necrotizing fasciitis.

Workup and Diagnosis

The initial step in the workup of a patient with possible hypercortisolism is to unequivocally establish its presence. The second step is to determine if it is pituitary dependent or pituitary

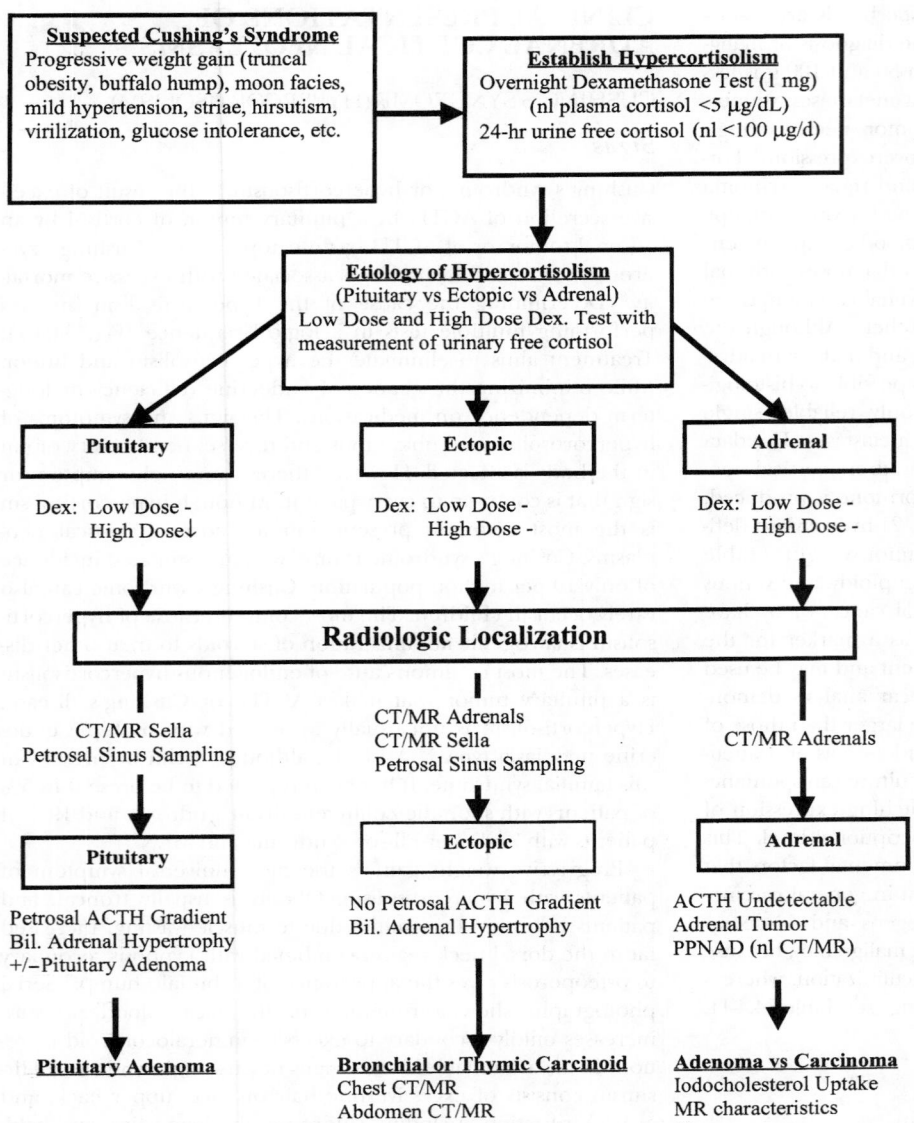

Suspected Cushing's Syndrome
Progressive weight gain (truncal obesity, buffalo hump), moon facies, mild hypertension, striae, hirsutism, virilization, glucose intolerance, etc.

Establish Hypercortisolism
Overnight Dexamethasone Test (1 mg)
(nl plasma cortisol <5 µg/dL)
24-hr urine free cortisol (nl <100 µg/d)

Etiology of Hypercortisolism
(Pituitary vs Ectopic vs Adrenal)
Low Dose and High Dose Dex. Test with measurement of urinary free cortisol

Pituitary
Dex: Low Dose -
High Dose↓

Ectopic
Dex: Low Dose -
High Dose -

Adrenal
Dex: Low Dose -
High Dose -

Radiologic Localization

CT/MR Sella
Petrosal Sinus Sampling

CT/MR Adrenals
CT/MR Sella
Petrosal Sinus Sampling

CT/MR Adrenals

Pituitary

Ectopic

Adrenal

Petrosal ACTH Gradient
Bil. Adrenal Hypertrophy
+/–Pituitary Adenoma

No Petrosal ACTH Gradient
Bil. Adrenal Hypertrophy

ACTH Undetectable
Adrenal Tumor
PPNAD (nl CT/MR)

Pituitary Adenoma

Bronchial or Thymic Carcinoid
Chest CT/MR
Abdomen CT/MR
Other Hormones produced:
(catecholamines, calcitonin, gastrin, VIP, PP, neurotensin, etc.)

Adenoma vs Carcinoma
Iodocholesterol Uptake
MR characteristics
Size

FIGURE 34.4-1. Flow diagram for evaluation of a patient with suspected hypercortisolism. ACTH, adrenocorticotropic hormone; Bil., bilateral; cal, calcitonin; CT, computed tomography; Dex, dexamethasone; MR, magnetic resonance imaging; nl, normal; PP, pancreatic polypeptide; PPNAD, primary pigmented nodular adrenocortical disease; VIP, vasoactive intestinal polypeptide.

independent, and the final step is to determine the exact cause (see Fig. 34.4-1).

ESTABLISHMENT OF HYPERCORTISOLISM. Urinary excretion of free cortisol is directly proportional to the amount of cortisol in the plasma. As the cortisol-binding globulin becomes saturated (plasma cortisol levels of 20 µg/dL), small increases in cortisol secretion produce exponential increases in urinary free cortisol. This amplification effect makes 24-hour urinary free cortisol the single best measurement to discriminate between normal and hypercortisolemic states. The overnight single-dose dexamethasone test (see Fig. 34.4-1) works because of the lack of normal feedback (Fig. 34.4-2) that occurs in all forms of hypercortisolism. Normal subjects given 1 mg of dexamethasone orally at 11:00 p.m. have plasma cortisol levels of less than 5 µg/dL at 8:00 a.m. the next day. Patients with endogenous hypercortisolism do not suppress and have cortisol levels greater than 5 µg/dL. The major disadvantage of this test is a 3% incidence of false-negative results (patients with Cushing's syndrome whose levels suppress). This test may also have false-positive results (3%) due to several causes, including depression, alcoholism, stress, and primary cortisol resistance. A normal single-dose dexamethasone test result and urinary free cortisol level (less than 100 µg/d) exclude the diagnosis of hypercortisolism.

ETIOLOGY OF HYPERCORTISOLISM. Patients with pituitary tumor (Cushing's disease) respond to 1 µg/kg corticotropin-releasing hormone (CRH) by increasing plasma ACTH and cortisol levels, whereas patients with depression or other stress diseases have a blunted ACTH response to CRH (see Figs. 34.4-1 and 34.4-2). The CRH test also distinguishes pituitary tumor from ectopic secretion of ACTH. Patients with Cushing's disease have increased plasma ACTH and cortisol levels after CRH administration, whereas patients with ectopic ACTH production

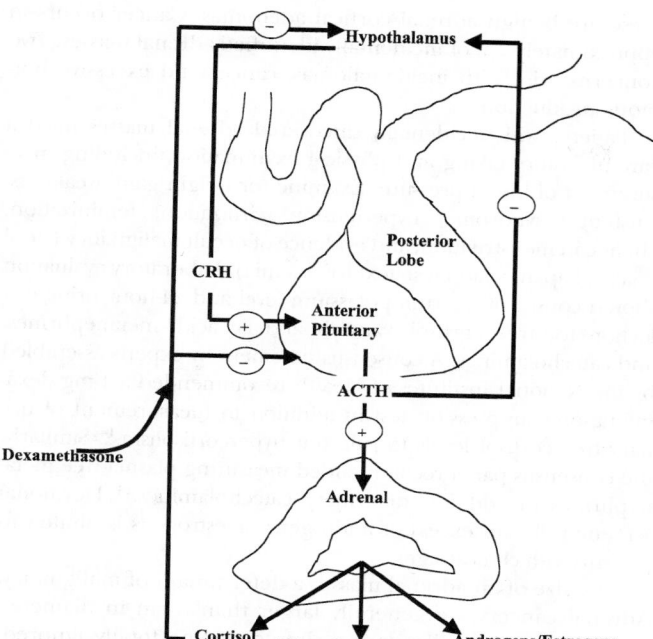

FIGURE 34.4-2. Model of cortisol secretion indicates the mechanism of dexamethasone suppression and corticotropin-releasing hormone (CRH) stimulation of normal cortisol secretion. ACTH, adrenocorticotropic hormone.

do not respond. Patients with Cushing's syndrome have abnormalities in the diurnal rhythm of plasma levels of cortisol. A low midnight cortisol level (less than 2 μg/dL) is not consistent with endogenous hypercortisolism. Determination of plasma ACTH levels may also be helpful. Patients with primary adrenal tumors or hyperplasia have undetectable or low plasma ACTH levels, those with pituitary-dependent hypercortisolism have intermediate levels, and those with ectopic ACTH-producing tumors have very high levels. Levels of urinary 17-ketosteroids can help the differential diagnosis of hypercortisolism. Low levels (less than 10 mg/d) suggest an adrenal adenoma, and very high levels (more than 60 mg/d) occur in patients with adrenal cancer and ectopic ACTH. Hypokalemia is seen most commonly with ectopic ACTH production.

The standard dexamethasone suppression test is the most useful test in establishing the cause of hypercortisolism (see Figs. 34.4-1 and 34.4-2). The expected results are that urinary free cortisol levels are markedly suppressed when normal subjects receive a low dose (2 mg) of dexamethasone, but levels do not suppress in patients with Cushing's syndrome. High-dose dexamethasone (8 mg/d) suppresses urinary levels of free cortisol to less than 50% of baseline levels in patients with pituitary-dependent hypercortisolism (Cushing's disease), but it does not suppress levels in patients with primary adrenal causes of hypercortisolism or ectopic ACTH syndrome. This single test makes the diagnosis of Cushing's syndrome and determines the cause of hypercortisolism with an accuracy rate of approximately 95%.

RADIOLOGIC EVALUATION OF HYPERCORTISOLISM. Computed tomography (CT) scans of the sella detect a tumor in only 0% to 15% of patients with pituitary-dependent Cushing's disease, and detect minor abnormalities in 23% to 60%.

Most ACTH-secreting tumors are microadenomas (less than 5 mm). Pituitary magnetic resonance imaging (MRI) studies, even with gadolinium, have similar resolution. In patients with pituitary-dependent hypercortisolism, CT and MRI scans may be normal, but bilateral petrosal sinus sampling for ACTH concentrations detects the side with a tumor in most cases.

Adrenal CT can detect normal adrenal glands in most patients. CT can reliably distinguish cortical hyperplasia from tumor. CT has great sensitivity (more than 95%); however, it lacks specificity. CT can be used to image the primary tumor plus local and distant metastases in cancer. MRI is able to distinguish among adenoma, carcinoma, and pheochromocytoma. Signal loss on chemical shift MRI occurs in adrenal cortical cancer.[9] In a study of 204 patients with adrenal masses, the sensitivity of MRI for distinguishing benign from malignant masses was 89%, specificity was 99%, and accuracy was 94%.[10] The use of [18F]fluorodeoxyglucose positron emission tomography (FDG-PET) has been studied in ten patients with adrenal cortical cancer. The sensitivity was 100% and the specificity was 95%. In 3 patients, previously unidentified lesions were seen that modified the treatment plan.[11]

INTERPRETATION OF HYPERCORTISOLISM WORKUP. Once the biochemical tests confirm endogenous hypercortisolism, the remainder of the workup can pinpoint its cause. An accurate diagnosis is made in the majority of cases.[12] In the case of an adrenal tumor, CT or MRI imaging demonstrates the tumor. There will be low plasma ACTH levels and elevated serum cortisol levels. There will be no suppression of urinary free cortisol levels with high-dose dexamethasone. In ectopic ACTH syndrome, there is enlargement of both adrenals on CT, elevated plasma ACTH levels, no suppression with high-dose dexamethasone, and no evidence of pituitary ACTH secretion. In Cushing's disease (pituitary adenoma), there is bilateral hyperplasia of the adrenal glands, normal or mildly elevated plasma ACTH levels, suppression with high-dose dexamethasone, and localization with petrosal sinus sampling.

CONN'S SYNDROME (PRIMARY ALDOSTERONISM)

Signs, Symptoms, and Diagnosis

Aldosterone overproduction with elevated plasma levels is the cause of hypertension in patients with primary aldosteronism. The most common cause of primary aldosteronism is an aldosterone-producing adenoma, next is idiopathic hyperplasia, and last is carcinoma. Secondary aldosteronism, which occurs with renal artery stenosis, is diagnosed by an increase in plasma renin activity, whereas primary aldosteronism is characterized by low plasma renin levels. Hypertension, hypokalemia, hyperaldosteronism, and decreased plasma renin levels are essential for the diagnosis of primary aldosteronism (Table 34.4-2). Primary hyperaldosteronism is also associated with weakness, muscle cramps, polyuria, and polydipsia. These clinical signs are due to hypokalemia. Hypertension is usually not severe and is mostly diastolic (diastolic pressure more than 90 mm Hg).

Adenoma versus Hyperplasia

Once the diagnosis of primary aldosteronism is established, the next important consideration is the cause: hyperplasia versus

TABLE 34.4-2. Diagnosis of Primary Aldosteronism

Measurement	Result
Blood pressure	Diastolic hypertension
Serum potassium levels	<3.5 mEq/L
Urinary potassium levels	Elevated urinary K+ excretion (>25–30 mEq/d)
Plasma aldosterone and plasma renin activity	Ratio >30 (elevated aldosterone and low renin)
Urinary aldosterone	Elevated
Captopril suppression test (25 mg orally)	After captopril, aldosterone >15 ng/mL; Aldosterone-renin ratio >50
Salt loading (9 g NaCl orally per day for 1–2 wk)	Renin suppression

adenoma (Table 34.4-3). CT can image approximately 90% of aldosteronomas but may miss small tumors. The contralateral adrenal cortex is thin. Iodocholesterol scans with iodine 131 (^{131}I)–β-iodomethyl-19-norcholesterol can distinguish between adenoma and hyperplasia. Hyperplasia has symmetric uptake in both adrenal glands and adenoma has uptake only in the tumor.[13] If the results are inconclusive, sampling of the adrenal veins for aldosterone is indicated. Adrenal venous sampling may be more sensitive than CT and iodocholesterol scans. However, the latter studies usually make the diagnosis.

Treatment

The management of primary aldosteronism depends on the cause. Hyperplasia is best managed medically with spironolactone, amiloride, or nifedipine. Aldosteronomas are best removed by laparoscopic adrenalectomy. This is associated with less pain and more rapid recovery than open procedures. Aldosterone-producing carcinomas are rare (fewer than 2% of adrenal cancers) and should be removed by open adrenalectomy.

INCIDENTAL ADRENAL MASS (INCIDENTALOMA)

High-resolution CT has resulted in a new diagnostic problem: an incidental adrenal mass detected by CT. Unexpected adrenal masses are seen in 0.6% of abdominal CT scans. The majority of

TABLE 34.4-3. Etiology of Primary Aldosteronism: Hyperplasia versus Tumor

Measurement	Hyperplasia	Tumor
Aldosterone response to upright posture	Increase (>20 ng/dL)	No response or decrease (<20 ng/dL)
Serum 18-hydroxy-corticosterone	<90 ng/dL	>100 ng/dL
High-resolution computed tomography scan	Normal adrenal glands	Tumor plus normal contralateral gland
Iodocholesterol scan	Symmetric uptake bilaterally	Uptake by benign adenoma (malignant tumors may not take up tracer)
Spironolactone	Fair response	Good response
Adrenal vein sampling	Bilateral	Unilateral

these are benign adrenal cortical adenomas. Cancer occurs in approximately 7% of incidentally identified adrenal masses. Two concerns arise with incidentalomas: cancer and excessive hormone production.

Patients with incidentally discovered adrenal masses need a careful history taking and physical examination, including measurement of blood pressure. Examine for weight gain, weakness, Cushing's syndrome, hypertension, virilization, feminization, change in menstruation, and evidence of occult malignancy (stool guaiac, Papanicolaou test, text for anemia). Laboratory evaluation should consist of a serum potassium level and 24-hour urine collection for free cortisol, vanillylmandelic acid, metanephrines, and catecholamines. A consensus statement by experts assembled by the National Institutes of Health recommended a 1-mg dexamethasone suppression test in addition to measurement of urinary free cortisol levels to rule out hypercortisolism.[14] Similarly, the consensus panel recommended measuring plasma free metanephrines in addition to urinary catecholamines.[14] Hormonal screening for an excess of androgens or estrogens is limited to patients with clinical signs.

The size of an adrenal mass is a determinant of malignancy. Adrenal cancers are generally larger than 6 cm in diameter. Nevertheless, a smaller lesion should not be totally ignored. Early diagnosis may lead to discovery of a small adrenal cortical carcinoma. Because of decreased morbidity with laparoscopic excision, some have now advocated surgery for incidentalomas of 4 cm, especially in younger patients.[14]

Fine-needle aspiration (FNA) for cytologic analysis of an adrenal mass has limited ability to differentiate benign from malignant primary adrenal lesions. False-negative results have been reported.[15] FNA may be catastrophic in a patient with an unsuspected pheochromocytoma, so biochemical results are required before needle biopsy. FNA may be complicated by hemorrhage and rupture of tumor.[16,17] In patients with suspected metastatic disease to the adrenal or lymphoma, FNA is diagnostic.

The suggested approach to an asymptomatic adrenal mass is outlined in Figure 34.4-3. Biochemical assessment should be performed to exclude hormonal function of the tumor. The size of the tumor is assessed. Size greater than 4 cm is an indication for surgical resection, especially in a younger patient. The incidence of cancer in solid adrenal masses equal to 6 cm is estimated to be between 35% and 98%. Laparoscopic excision of tumors smaller than 6 cm is recommended because of decreased pain and morbidity. Laparoscopic excision of large adrenal tumors (greater than 6 cm) is not recommended because a high proportion of these tumors are malignant. If the mass is smaller than 4 cm and nonfunctional, a repeat follow-up CT examination in 3 to 6 months is indicated to again determine size. If size increases, surgical excision is necessary.

SEX HORMONE EXCESS

Adrenocortical carcinoma may present with excessive sex hormone secretion. Virilization or feminization may be combined with hypercortisolism, or the tumor may produce only estrogen or testosterone. In children, the clinical signs of increased androgen production include increased growth, premature development of pubic and facial hair, acne, genital enlargement, increased muscle mass, and deep voice. In women, the clinical signs of excess androgen production include hirsutism, acne,

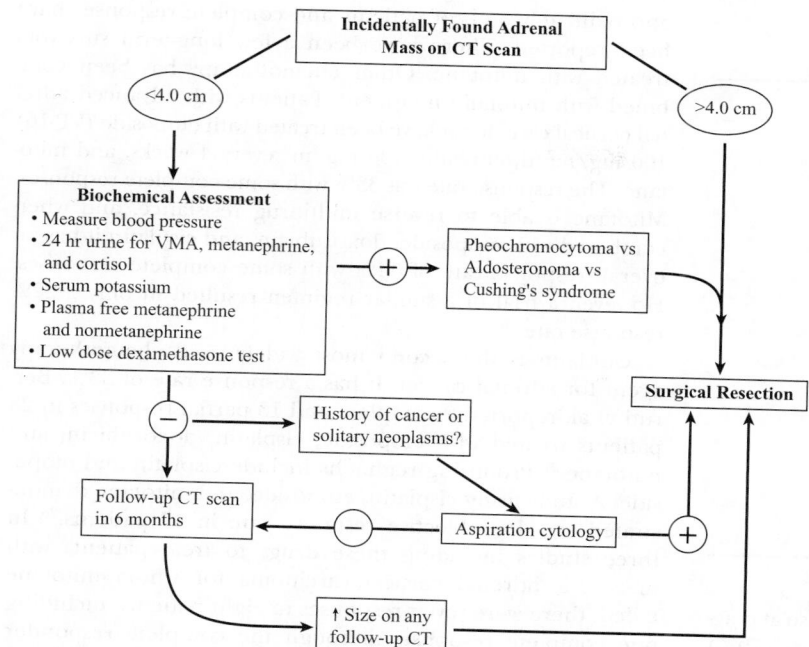

FIGURE 34.4-3. Flow diagram for management of incidentaloma. +, yes; –, no; CT, computed tomography; VMA, vanillylmandelic acid.

amenorrhea, infertility, increased muscle mass, deep voice, and temporal balding. In adult men, hyperestrogenism presents with gynecomastia, decreased sexual drive, impotence, and infertility. In adult women, hyperestrogenism presents primarily as irregular menses in premenopausal women and dysfunctional uterine bleeding or vaginal bleeding in postmenopausal women. The workup requires measurement of 24-hour urinary 17-ketosteroid levels, 17-hydroxysteroid levels, urinary free cortisol levels, and, depending on virilization or feminization, determination of serum testosterone or estrogen levels.

TREATMENT OF ADRENAL CORTICAL NEOPLASMS

ADRENAL CORTICAL ADENOMA

The definitive treatment of benign adrenal adenoma is laparoscopic surgical resection. In patients who are undergoing resection of an adrenal tumor that causes Cushing's syndrome, steroid replacement during and after surgery is necessary. Postoperative glucocorticoid replacement is indicated until complete recovery of the hypothalamic-pituitary-adrenal axis (see Fig. 34.4-2). Glucocorticoid replacement may be necessary for as long as 2 years. Surgical resection of larger adenomas weighing between 50 and 100 g requires careful long-term follow-up to exclude carcinoma.

ADRENAL CORTICAL CARCINOMA

Adrenal cancer presents with excessive glucocorticoid or mineralocorticoid secretion; however, some cancers may be nonfunctional.[18] The mainstay of treatment of adrenal cortical carcinoma is complete surgical resection. If the carcinoma is intimately associated with the adjacent organs like the kidney, concomitant nephrectomy may be necessary. CT or MRI can image the extent of disease and should include the chest to rule out pulmonary metastases. If the inferior vena cava is involved, either a cavagram

or ultrasonography is useful to assess extent of tumor. Adrenal cancer resection can be performed with acceptable morbidity and an operative mortality of 3%. Tumor size, hemorrhage, and mitotic count correlate with survival rates for patients undergoing curative resection. Tumor size less than 12 cm, mitotic rate less than six per high-power field, and absence of intratumoral hemorrhage are each associated with improved survival.[19] Radical, complete resection of all cancer is critical for prolonged survival and potential cure. There is no consensus on effective adjuvant therapy.[20] Recurrent or metastatic adrenal cortical cancer should also be resected, and reports suggest that radiofrequency ablation may be able to control recurrent tumor both inside and outside the liver.[21]

Adrenal cortical carcinoma can occur in children. It occurs in children younger than 6 years, with a higher incidence in girls than in boys. The median age at presentation for children with adrenal cancer is 4 years. Virilization is the most common presenting feature (93%), followed by Cushing's syndrome.[22] Some children may also present with precocious puberty. Approximately 65% of children can be cured by complete surgical resection of tumor. In a multivariate analysis of predictors of outcome, only primary tumor size greater than 200 cm³ independently identified a poor-prognosis group of children who may require more aggressive adjuvant therapy after surgery. The overall 5-year survival rate for children with adrenal cancer is 49%, and after complete resection it increases to 70%.

The second peak age of occurrence of adrenal cancer is between 40 and 50 years, and approximately 70% of these patients present with hormonal syndromes. The surgical staging of adrenal carcinoma is as follows:

I	Tumor smaller than 5 cm without local invasion, nodal, or distant metastases
II	Same as stage I except tumor larger than 5 cm
III	Tumor with local invasion or positive lymph nodes
IV	Tumor with local invasion and positive lymph nodes or distant metastases (Table 34.4-4)

TABLE 34.4-4.   Staging Criteria for Adrenal Cortical Carcinoma

Stage	Criteria
TUMOR	
T1	Tumor <5 cm, invasion absent
T2	Tumor >5 cm, invasion absent
T3	Tumor outside adrenal in fat
T4	Tumor invading adjacent organs
LYMPH NODES	
N0	No positive lymph nodes
N1	Positive lymph nodes
METASTASES	
M0	No distant metastases
M1	Distant metastases
STAGE GROUPING	
I	T1, N0, M0
II	T2, N0, M0
III	T1–2, N1, M0; T3, N0, M0
IV	Any T, any N, M1; T3, T4, N1

Twenty percent of patients have stage I, II, or III disease at diagnosis, whereas 80% have metastases.[20] Many patients (70%) present with stage III or IV disease.

The definitive treatment for localized disease including stage III lesions is *en bloc* resection. Even tumor thrombus within the inferior vena cava is not a contraindication to resection.[23] Surgical resection of localized disease can be curative. The median postoperative disease-free survival is only 12 months. The overall 5-year survival rate is between 20% and 35%. In one series, the 6-year survival after complete resection of all tumor was 60%.[24] Complete resection of recurrent tumor is also useful and, if achieved, is associated with a 6-year survival rate of 40%.[24,25] Patients should undergo monitoring of steroid hormone levels postoperatively. Measurement of urinary levels requires switching the glucocorticoid replacement therapy from hydrocortisone to dexamethasone. CT and MRI are also used to detect local recurrences and pulmonary metastases. If a localized recurrence is detected, it should be removed surgically. Prolonged remissions have been reported after resection of hepatic, pulmonary, and cerebral metastases from adrenal cortical carcinoma. Patients with recurrent adrenal cortical carcinoma that can be surgically resected have a 5-year survival rate of 50% versus 8% for nonoperable cases. Control of recurrent tumor can be achieved by radiofrequency ablation.[21] Palliation of bony metastases may be achieved by radiation therapy. Abdominal radiation therapy may be useful in 65% of patients with local recurrences not amenable to resection, and the treatment has even relieved bowel obstruction.

CHEMOTHERAPY

Op-DDD (mitotane) is the chemotherapy drug that is most often used for adrenal cancer. It is administered at a dosage of 2 to 6 g daily in two or three divided doses and increased until adverse reactions occur. Adverse reactions include gastrointestinal toxicity, neuromuscular toxicity, and skin rash. Mitotane is associated with prolongation of the bleeding time and abnormal platelet aggregation. A decrease in urinary 17-hydroxysteroids and 17-ketosteroids occurs in most patients due to its effect on steroid metabolism. Partial responses occur in approximately 35% of patients and complete responses have been reported. There have been a few long-term survivors treated with mitotane. Other chemotherapy has been combined with mitotane treatment. Patients with advanced adrenal cortical carcinoma have been treated with etoposide (VP-16) 100 mg/m²/d, cisplatin, 100 mg/m² every 4 weeks, and mitotane. The response rate was 33% with some complete responses. Mitotane is able to reverse multidrug resistance, and when combined with etoposide, doxorubicin, and cisplatin it has an overall response rate of 54% with some complete responses. However, a trial of a similar regimen resulted in only a 22% response rate.[26]

Cisplatin is the second most widely used chemotherapy agent for adrenal cancer. It has a response rate of 33%. Berruti et al. reported 2 complete and 13 partial responses in 28 patients treated with etoposide, cisplatin, doxorubicin, and mitotane.[27] Promising regimens include cisplatin and etoposide. A study using cisplatin, etoposide, and mitotane demonstrated an 11% objective response rate in 47 patients.[28] In three studies including these drugs to treat patients with metastatic adrenal cortical carcinoma for whom mitotane failed, there were seven responses in eight patients, including one complete response, although the complete responder had only 1 year disease free. Another active regimen includes 5-fluorouracil, doxorubicin, and cisplatin, which has produced three responses in 13 patients treated. One patient had a complete response that lasted for 42 months. Patients who have not responded to mitotane have been effectively treated with a combination of cisplatin and etoposide. Docetaxel and gemcitabine failed to demonstrate a response in two patients treated.[29]

In vitro studies in a soft agar system suggest that the new midazole tetrazirione compound 8-carbamoyl-3-methylimidazo(5,1-D)-1,2,3,5 tetrazin-4(3H)-1 (temozolomide) is very active against adrenal cortical carcinoma. Paclitaxel has been shown to be effective against the adrenocortical carcinoma cell line human NCI-H295 in *in vitro* studies. Paclitaxel also has been effective in *in vitro* studies against a steroid-secreting malignant adrenal cortical carcinoma cell line. Irinotecan (CPT-11) at 250 mg/m² has been ineffective in 12 patients with metastatic adrenal cortical carcinoma for whom other therapies failed.[30]

Gossypol has been shown in experimental studies of adrenal cancer to inhibit tumor growth and prolong survival of mice. However, in phase I human studies with metastatic adrenal cancer, it had a partial response rate of 20%. One 5-year-old child with metastatic adrenal cancer had a near-complete response to vincristine (Oncovin), cisplatin, epipodophyllotoxin, and cyclophosphamide (Cytoxan). Steroid hormone receptors have been detected *in vitro* in adrenal cortical carcinomas, which indicates dependence on progesterone and glucocorticoid. However, *in vivo* studies of therapy related to manipulation of receptors have not been done. The available chemotherapy agents and results are summarized in Table 34.4-5. A report shows that adjuvant therapy with etoposide and cisplatin may be effective after complete surgical resection of adrenal cortical carcinoma in children. Five children (aged 1 to 21 years) had adrenal carcinoma removed surgically and received etoposide 165 mg/m² and cisplatin 90 mg/m² every 3 to 4 weeks for six courses. No patient developed recurrent tumor after a median follow-up of 44 months (range, 29 to 109 months). The chemotherapy was well tolerated.[31]

TABLE 34.4-5. Chemotherapy Agents Used to Treat Adrenocortical Carcinoma

Investigation	Drug	Dosage	Frequency	No. of Patients	Efficacy
Gutierrez and Crooke, 1980[69]	Mitotane	1–12 g/d	b.i.d. or t.i.d.	37	22–33% PR
Luton et al., 1990[70]					
Van Slooten et al., 1984[71]					
Venkatesh et al., 1989[72]		7–10 g/d	b.i.d.	72	29% PR
Haak et al., 1994[73]		High dose (serum levels >14 µg/mL)			60% PR, few CR
Kornely and Schlaghecke, 1994[74]		High dose plus strepto- zotocin		2	CR with surgery plus che- motherapy
Decker et al., 1991[75]		6 g/d		36	22% PR
Stein et al., 1989[76]	Suramin	1.0–1.5 mg/m²	qwk	21	3 PR
Arit et al., 1994[77]		8–30 g		9	3 PR
LaRocca et al., 1990[78]					
Stein et al., 1989[76]	Doxorubicin	60 mg/m²	q3wk	16	19% PR
Schlumberger et al., 1991[79]	5-Fluorouracil	500 mg/m² d 1–3	q4wk	13	1 CR, 2 PR
	+ doxorubicin	60 mg/m² d 2			
	+ cisplatin	120 mg/m² d 2			
Berruti et al., 1992[80]	Etoposide	Not given		3	1 CR
	+ doxorubicin				2 PR
	+ cisplatin				
Avico et al., 1992[81]	Vincristine (Oncovin)	Not given		1	1 CR
	+ Cisplatin				
	+ Epipodophyllotoxin				
	+ Cyclophosphamide (Cytoxan)				
Berruti et al., 1998[27]	Mitotane	2–4 g/d		28	2 CR
	+ etoposide	100 mg/m² d 5–7	q4wk		13 PR
	+ doxorubicin	20 mg/m² d 1 and 8			
	+ cisplatin	40 mg/m² d 1 and 9			
Zidan et al., 1996[82]	Mitotane + cisplatin	Not given		1	1 CR
Abraham et al., 2002[26]	Mitotane	4.6 g/d	q3wk	36	1 CR
	+ doxorubicin	10 mg/m²/d			3 PR
	+ etoposide	75 mg/m²/d			
	+ vincristine	0.4 mg/m²/d			
Mekhail et al., 2003[29]	Docetaxel	20–36 mg/m²	q3wk	2	0 Responders
	+ gemcitabine	400–800 mg/m²			
Baudin et al., 2002[30]	CPT-11 (irinotecan)	250 mg/m²	q14d	12	0 Responders
Hovi et al., 2003[31]	Etoposide	165 mg/m²	q3–4wk	5 children	Postoperative without recur- rence, median 44 wk
	+ cisplatin	90 mg/m²			

CR, complete remission; PR, partial remission.

PHEOCHROMOCYTOMA

Pheochromocytomas are rare tumors that arise from chromaffin cells in the adrenal medulla and elsewhere. The tumor is estimated to occur in approximately 1 per 100,000 adults per year.[32] In autopsy series, only 0.005% to 0.1% of persons have unsuspected pheochromocytomas. When urinary catecholamines are measured in hypertensive patients, pheochromocytoma is found to be present in only 0.1% of patients. Although these tumors are rare, it is important to diagnose and localize pheochromocytomas.

Pheochromocytomas may be malignant. Earlier diagnosis and therapy may lessen the probability of death from malignancy and improve the prognosis. Incidence of malignancy in pheochromocytomas is as low as 5% and as high as 46% in different series. Extraadrenal tumors are more likely to be cancerous. Pheochromocytomas may be associated with endocrine and nonendocrine inherited disorders. Bilateral adrenal medullary pheochromocytomas are components of MEN 2A and MEN 2B. Individuals with familial pheochromocytoma have bilateral adrenal pheochromocytomas and no other manifestation of MEN. In other families, extraadrenal pheochromocytomas have also been reported. Pheochromocytomas occur in approximately 25% of patients with von Hippel-Lindau (VHL) disease and in fewer than 1% of patients with neurofibromatosis and von Recklinghausen's disease. Furthermore, studies indicate that many patients who present with nonsyndromic pheochromocytomas really have either MEN 2 or VHL. Among 271 patients with nonsyndromic pheochromocytoma, 66 (24%) were found to have mutations of VHL, RET, SDHD, and SDHB. The latter two are subtypes of VHL. This suggests that patients who present with apparently sporadic nonfamilial pheochromocytoma should be screened for RET and VHL mutations because 25% will have them.[33] Germline mutations in three of the succinate dehydrogenase subunits (SDHD, SDHB, and SDHC) cause susceptibility to head and neck paragangliomas (extraadrenal pheochromocytomas).[34,35]

Pheochromocytomas secrete catecholamines and cause intermittent, episodic, or sustained hypertension. Pheochromocytomas also cause insulin resistance and diabetes.[36] After resection of the tumor the insulin sensitivity improves.[37] Furthermore, pheochromocytomas may produce other hormones, including ectopic ACTH, and may give rise to Cushing's syndrome.

PATHOLOGY

Pheochromocytomas arise from chromaffin cells. Chromaffin cells are widespread and are associated with sympathetic ganglia during fetal life. After birth, most chromaffin cells degenerate, and the majority remain in the adrenal medulla. This may explain why approximately 90% of pheochromocytomas are in the adrenal medulla. Extraadrenal pheochromocytomas may arise anywhere, including the carotid body, intracardiac area, along the aorta (both thoracic and abdominal), and within the urinary bladder. The most common extraadrenal location is the organ of Zuckerkandl that is near the origin of the inferior mesenteric artery to the left of the aortic bifurcation. Data from series of patients with sporadic pheochromocytomas indicate that the right adrenal gland more commonly harbors a tumor than the left gland. Pheochromocytomas resected from hypertensive patients usually measure between 3 and 5 cm in diameter and weigh approximately 100 g. These tumors appear tan to gray and have a soft, smooth consistency. Larger tumors may be cystic or have necrotic areas and often have calcification. Microscopically, pheochromocytomas resemble the cell of origin. Tumors are usually arranged in cords or alveolar patterns. Tumors may be composed of cords of cells lining vascular structures that have an angiomatous appearance. Tumors are generally clearly separated from the adrenal cortex by a thin band of fibrous tissue. Extension of the pheochromocytoma into the cortex or vascular invasion may occur in benign neoplasms.

The pathologic distinction between benign and malignant pheochromocytomas is not clear. Furthermore, some reports indicate that pheochromocytomas are more often malignant than expected. Some series indicate that the tumor recurrence rate is between 10% and 46%. These results partly reflect the referral pattern of tertiary institutions, but they may also reflect a true higher malignancy rate than originally suggested. Malignant tumors tend to be larger and weigh more, although this is not an absolute criterion (Table 34.4-6). Staining for the nuclear proliferation marker MIB-1 is positive in 50% of malignant pheochromocytomas and negative in benign tumors. The only absolute criterion for malignancy is the presence of secondary tumors in sites where chromaffin cells are not usually present and visceral metastases. Benign pheochromocytomas may demonstrate marked nuclear pleomorphism, whereas, paradoxically, malignant ones demonstrate less. Malignant pheochromocytomas usually have many more mitoses than benign tumors, but capsular and vascular invasion occurs with equal frequency in both. Nuclear DNA ploidy may be a predictive indicator of malignant potential. Flow cytometry has been used to identify malignant pheochromocytomas. Tetraploidy, polyploidy, and aneuploidy are associated with malignancy. Neuropeptide Y gene expression

TABLE 34.4-6. Differentiation of Benign versus Malignant Pheochromocytomas

Characteristic	Benign	Malignant
Metastases	−	+
Weight (g)	<200	>500
Occurrence (%)	50–90	10–50
Vascular invasion	+	+
Capsular invasion	+	+
Mitoses	±	++++
Nuclear pleomorphism	+	−
Ploidy	Diploid	Hyperdiploid, triploid
Necrosis	±	++
Tumors with neuropeptide Y gene expression	+	−
Proportion of patients with elevated serum levels of neuron-specific enolase (%)	−	+

+, extent present; −, extent absent.

is more common in benign tumors. Finally, size of tumor (weight) correlates best with malignant potential (see Table 34.4-6).

CLINICAL MANIFESTATIONS AND DIAGNOSIS

Patients with pheochromocytomas can present with a range of symptoms, from mild labile hypertension to sudden death secondary to a hypertensive crisis, myocardial infarction, or cerebral vascular accident. The classic patient describes "spells" of paroxysmal headaches, pallor, palpitations, hypertension, and diaphoresis. In 50% of patients, the hypertension is intermittent, but it may be sustained. In children, hypertension is sustained. Patients may have lactic acidosis. Patients may have weight loss and hyperglycemia.

The diagnosis of pheochromocytoma is based on measurement of catecholamines and metabolites in the urine (Fig. 34.4-4). The best test is a 24-hour urine level of metanephrines and catecholamines.[38] However, levels of plasma free metanephrines and normetanephrines have also been used to diagnose pheochromocytomas.[39] Measurements of urinary total metanephrines or vanillylmandelic acid are not as reliable as plasma levels of free metanephrines and 24-hour urinary levels of fractionated normetanephrine.[40] If a pheochromocytoma is suspected, the best test is levels of fractionated plasma metanephrines.[41] Other studies suggest that urinary measurement of catecholamine, vanillylmandelic acid, and metanephrine levels is the most sensitive screening test. It is now clear that both the plasma and urinary studies are indicated in patients with suspected pheochromocytoma.

The clonidine suppression test is another study to determine whether a patient with equivocal levels of catecholamines and metabolites has a pheochromocytoma. In normal subjects and patients with idiopathic hypertension, clonidine suppresses plasma levels of catecholamines. In patients with pheochromocytoma, clonidine does not suppress levels. Levels of plasma normetanephrine in response to clonidine suppression can be used to distinguish true-positive from false-positive results.[42]

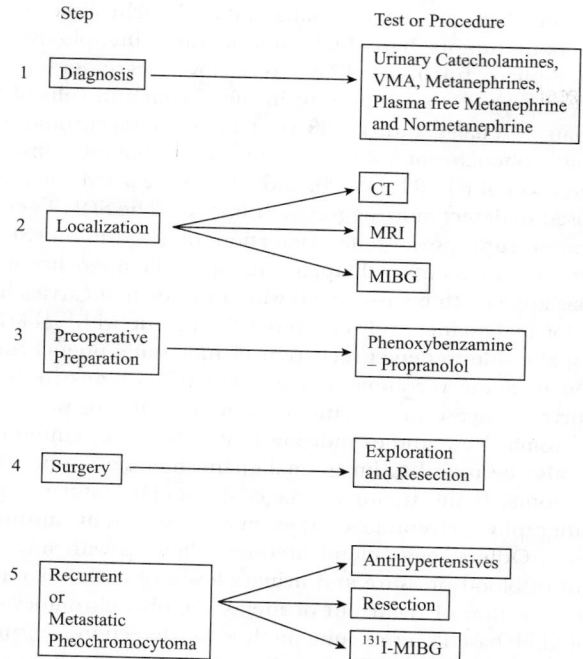

Step		Test or Procedure

1 Diagnosis → Urinary Catecholamines, VMA, Metanephrines, Plasma free Metanephrine and Normetanephrine

2 Localization → CT / MRI / MIBG

3 Preoperative Preparation → Phenoxybenzamine – Propranolol

4 Surgery → Exploration and Resection

5 Recurrent or Metastatic Pheochromocytoma → Antihypertensives / Resection / ^{131}I-MIBG

FIGURE 34.4-4. Flow diagram for diagnosis, localization, preoperative preparation, treatment, and follow-up for a patient with a pheochromocytoma. CT, computed tomography; MIBG, metaiodobenzylguanidine scanning; MRI, magnetic resonance imaging; VMA, vanillylmandelic acid.

LOCALIZATION STUDIES

CT and MRI are the two radiologic (nonnuclear medicine) procedures of choice to localize pheochromocytomas (see Fig. 34.4-4). Both are noninvasive and sensitive, and are able to detect tumors approximately 1 cm in diameter. MRI may be more specific because of findings with different sequences. Pheochromocytomas measure above 10 Hounsfield units on noncontrast CT.[17] However, low-density pheochromocytomas have been described.[43] In a Mayo Clinic study of 52 patients with pheochromocytoma, CT detected 51 of 52 tumors, including 9 of 10 bilateral tumors. In another study, unenhanced high-resolution CT detected pheochromocytomas in six of six patients who had tumors found at surgery, including two extraadrenal retroperitoneal tumors. MRI also has remarkable resolution. In seven patients with pheochromocytomas demonstrated on CT, MRI imaged all primary lesions as well as metastases to the chest, retroperitoneum, and liver. Because it involves no radiation exposure, MRI can be used to image during pregnancy.[17] In one analysis, CT imaged 16 of 19 pheochromocytomas (84%), whereas MRI imaged 12 of 15 (75%) for comparable sensitivity. In addition, MRI successfully imaged an intrapericardial pheochromocytoma and distinguished it from the cardiac chambers and surrounding great vessels, which could not be determined by CT.

Another important technique for the localization of pheochromocytomas is nuclear scanning after the administration of labeled metaiodobenzylguanidine (MIBG) (see Fig. 34.4-4). The compound is similar to norepinephrine and is taken up by vesicular monoamine transporters.[44] The use of ^{131}I-MIBG scanning to localize suspected pheochromocytoma has been studied in 400 patients. The sensitivity of MIBG scanning with ^{131}I for

pheochromocytoma is 100% and the specificity is 95%.[45] In a study of 34 patients with pheochromocytoma, ^{131}I-MIBG scanning imaged 100% of tumors.[13] It appears that MIBG scanning is safe, noninvasive, and efficacious for the localization of pheochromocytomas, including those that arise in nonadrenal sites, and malignant disease. Bone metastases from pheochromocytoma can be imaged using ^{131}I-MIBG, but bone scanning may be more sensitive. In summary, MIBG scanning images catecholamine-producing tumors with a high specificity and sensitivity. Because it is a total body study, it can image tumors wherever they are, including unusual locations.[45] Whereas CT and MRI reflect changes in morphology, scintigraphic imaging relies on tissue function. False-positive results with MIBG scintigraphy are rare, which accounts for the high specificity (98% to 100%) of the study. False-negative results can occur, which lowers sensitivity. For patients with suspected pheochromocytoma and negative MIBG findings, FDG-PET may be useful. Metastases from a predominantly dopamine-secreting pheochromocytoma that did not take up MIBG were imaged with FDG-PET.[46] Furthermore, fluorine 18 dihydroxyphenylalanine PET has imaged 17 pheochromocytomas in 17 patients. It is highly sensitive and specific and may be very useful if other studies are negative.[47] It has imaged a malignant bladder pheochromocytoma.[48] It has been shown to be superior to ^{131}I-MIBG for localization of metastatic pheochromocytoma.[49] It is not commonly available but it appears to have real utility in localizing pheochromocytomas.[50]

MANAGEMENT

Preoperative Preparation

Once the diagnosis is established and the tumor localized, preoperative preparation includes α-adrenergic blockade. Patients are started on phenoxybenzamine, 10 mg orally two or three times daily (see Fig. 34.4-4). If tachycardia develops, β-adrenergic blocking agents (propranolol) are added. Propranolol should never be started before α blockade because unopposed vasoconstriction may worsen hypertension. Phenoxybenzamine increases the total blood and plasma volume and reduces lactic acidosis. Appropriately used calcium channel antagonists and selective α$_1$-receptor blockers are also effective and safe and may have less adverse effects than nonspecific α blockade with phenoxybenzamine.[51]

Intraoperative Management

In elderly patients or those with cardiac complications, a Swan-Ganz catheter should be inserted. This allows correction of hemodynamic imbalances and optimization of cardiac performance. The morning of operation, an arterial catheter and peripheral intravenous catheters should be inserted. Arterial blood gases should be measured to rule out acidosis. During surgery, especially during manipulation of the tumor, marked increases in blood pressure may occur; hypertensive episodes should be controlled with either α-adrenergic blocking agents like phentolamine (Regitine) or agents that directly relax arterial and venous smooth muscle like sodium nitroprusside. The use of preoperative preparation with oral α-adrenergic blocking agents and intraoperative adjustment and regulation of blood pressure with nitroprusside has greatly facilitated the surgical resection of pheochromocytoma and has reduced operative morbidity and mortality.

Small (less than 6 cm) intraadrenal pheochromocytomas are removed using laparoscopic techniques.[52] However, some report that laparoscopic adrenalectomy should still be performed for large tumors (more than 6 cm). They point out that the operative time, blood loss, and length of stay is the same for either small or large adrenal tumors.[53,54] Laparoscopic procedures appear to decrease pain and shorten the time to recovery.[55] Most pheochromocytomas are well localized, which facilitates laparoscopic removal. Laparoscopic adrenalectomy for familial pheochromocytomas is especially useful because these tumors are small and within the adrenal gland.[56] Adrenal cortex–sparing surgery may be indicated for patients with familial pheochromocytomas who require bilateral adrenalectomy.[57] However, iatrogenic pheochromocytomatosis has been described as a possible complication of laparoscopic removal. Numerous tumor cells were deposited throughout the retroperitoneum near the site of the primary tumor. This may have been caused by laparoscopic excision of a malignant tumor or by spilling of benign tumor cells at the time of laparoscopic excision. Regardless of the exact cause, this is a rare complication that must be considered if it continues to occur.[58]

MALIGNANT PHEOCHROMOCYTOMAS

Malignant pheochromocytomas are present in approximately 10% of patients with pheochromocytoma, but the true incidence may be greater. Flow cytometric DNA analysis may distinguish benign from malignant pheochromocytomas. Malignant tumors have high mitotic rate, aneuploidy, and high S-phase fraction.[59] EM66 is a novel secretogranin II–derived peptide that is present in the chromaffin cells of the human adrenal gland. EM66 is at higher concentrations in benign pheochromocytomas than in malignant tumors.[60] Expression of hTERT, HSP90, and telomerase activity may also be used to detect more aggressive tumors.[61] The SDHB gene is a tumor suppressor gene. Detection of a germline SDHB mutation in patients with apparently sporadic pheochromocytomas appears to be associated with a tumor that carries high risk for malignancy and recurrence.[62] Imaging with ^{131}I-MIBG is usually able to detect recurrent or metastatic pheochromocytomas. Some recommend yearly ^{131}I-MIBG scans to detect recurrent disease in all patients after resection of pheochromocytoma. New studies indicate that octreotide scintigraphy may also be useful to image malignant, metastatic pheochromocytoma. If the tumor is imaged by somatostatin receptor scintigraphy, octreotide therapy may have potent antitumor effects. Others recommend lifetime follow-up with measurement of blood pressure and urinary levels of catecholamines. The detection of recurrent or metastatic pheochromocytoma should be based on the same methods as detection of primary or initial pheochromocytoma. These methods include measurement of urinary and serum catecholamine levels, the clonidine suppression test, CT, MRI, and ^{131}I-MIBG scanning. Careful follow-up requires some, but not necessarily all, of these studies on a yearly basis (see Fig. 34.4-4). It appears that with careful follow-up the incidence of malignant pheochromocytoma may approach 30% to 50%.

TABLE 34.4-7. Treatment of Metastatic Malignant Pheochromocytoma

Investigations	Compound	No. of Patients	Patients with Change in Catecholamine Secretion	Result of Imaging and Urine Levels of Catecholamine
Feldman et al., 1984[83]	^{131}I-MIBG	3	No change	Questionable decrease
Krempf et al., 1991[84]	^{131}I-MIBG	15	7 Partial decreases (47%) 4 Normal	5 Decreases (33%)
Nakabeppu and Nakajo, 1994[85]	^{131}I-MIBG	1	1 Normal	1 CR
Feldman 1983[86]	High-dose streptozotocin	1	Marked decrease	Marked decrease
Averbuch et al., 1988[87]	Cyclophosphamide + vincristine + dacarbazine	14	2 Normal	1 CR
			6 Partial decreases (57%)	6 PR (50%)
Noshiro et al., 1996[88]	Cyclophosphamide + vincristine + dacarbazine	2	1 Decrease	1 Marked decrease
			1 No change	
Sisson et al., 1999[89]	^{131}I-MIBG + cyclophosphamide + dacarbazine + vincristine	6	3 Decreases	2 PR
Arai et al., 1998[90]	α-Methylparatyrosine + cyclophosphamide + dacarbazine + vincristine	1	1 Partial decrease	No change
Tada et al., 1998[91]	α-Methylparatyrosine + cyclophosphamide + dacarbazine + vincristine	3	2 Decreases	No change
Rose et al., 2003[66]	^{131}I-MIBG (800 mCi)	12	3 CR	3 CR, 7 PR
Lamarre-Cliché et al., 2002[67]	LAR 20 mg q3wk	10	0 Responders	0 Responders
Nakane et al., 2003[68]	Doxorubicin (40 mg/m^2) + cyclophosphamide (750 mg/m^2) + vincristine (1, 4 mg/m^2) + dacarbazine (250 mg/m^2)	1	1 CR	1 CR

CR, complete remission; ^{131}I-MIBG, iodine 131–labeled metaiodobenzylguanidine; LAR, long-acting octreotide; PR, partial remission.

The basic principles in the treatment of malignant pheochromocytoma have been to surgically resect recurrences or metastases whenever possible and to treat hypertensive symptoms by catecholamine blockade. Even in pediatric patients, surgical resection of metastatic and recurrent pheochromocytoma has been shown to prolong survival. Painful bony metastases respond well to radiotherapy. Soft tissue masses or bony masses may be treated with radiation therapy if doses of 40 Gy or more can be administered. Doses of 6000 cGy are necessary to treat bony metastases.[63] Serum levels of chromogranin A may be used to measure response to therapy.[64] Survival data for patients with malignant pheochromocytoma are difficult to obtain because of the rarity and indolence of the tumor. The 5-year survival rate is between 36% and 60%.

The early success with streptozotocin in the treatment of neuroendocrine tumors of the gastrointestinal tract suggested that it might also be useful in the treatment of malignant pheochromocytomas. Streptozotocin has elicited mixed responses in patients with malignant pheochromocytoma. Because of the high sensitivity and specificity of ^{131}I-MIBG in imaging pheochromocytomas, its use in higher doses to treat recurrent or metastatic pheochromocytomas has been implemented. Current imaging modalities for pheochromocytoma permit relatively accurate dosimetry to the tumor on the basis of the diagnostic dose of ^{131}I-MIBG administered. If uptake by primary or metastatic tumors is high, it is possible to deliver very high radiation doses by increasing the administered activity. Specific activity of ^{131}I-MIBG of 200 mCi in 5 mg has now been achieved. A beneficial response to treatment was observed in 42% to 60% of patients. However, complete responses were not observed. Five patients had measurable partial responses to treatment, and seven had clear hormonal responses. In summary, partial remissions as measured by decrease in catecholamine secretion and tumor size have been observed in approximately one-third of patients treated. However, complete responses with ^{131}I-MIBG have been rare.[65] High-dose (800-mCi) ^{131}I-MIBG resulted in complete antitumor responses in 2 of 12 patients with skeletal and soft tissue metastases from pheochromocytoma.[66]

A combination of cyclophosphamide, vincristine, and dacarbazine has been used in patients with metastatic pheochromocytoma. Few patients have had a complete response (both biochemical and imageable) and 57% of patients have had decreases in 24-hour levels of urinary catecholamines. Biochemical response (urinary catecholamines) correlated well with response evaluated on imaging studies. All responding patients have had dramatic improvement in hypertension control and performance status. Single cases have been reported to have shown complete responses with cyclophosphamide, vincristine, and dacarbazine treatment. Long-acting octreotide has been used to treat malignant pheochromocytoma without success. Even tumors that were positive on octreotide scan did not respond to long-acting octreotide.[67] Combination chemotherapy with cyclophosphamide, vincristine, dacarbazine, doxorubicin, and epirubicin resulted in a complete response in a single patient with metastatic pheochromocytoma.[68] Table 34.4-7 lists possible treatment regimens for metastatic pheochromocytoma.

REFERENCES

1. Norton JA, Le HP. Adrenal tumors. In: DeVita VT, Hellman S, Rosenberg SA, eds. *Cancer principles and practice of oncology*, 6th ed. Philadelphia: Lippincott Williams & Wilkins 2001:1770.
2. Zhao, J, Speel E, Muletta-Feurer S, et al. Analysis of genomic alterations in sporadic adrenocortical lesions. *Am J Pathol* 1999;155:1039.
3. Logie A, Boulle N, Gaston V, et al. Autocrine role of IGF-II in proliferation of human adrenocortical carcinoma NCI H296R cell line. *J Mol Endo* 1999;23:23.
4. Stojadinovic A, Ghossein R, Hoos A, et al. Adrenocortical carcinoma: clinical, morphologic, and molecular characterization. *J Clin Oncol* 2002;20:941.
5. Hainaut P. Tumor-specific mutations in p53: the acid test. *Nat Med* 2002;8:21.
6. Barzon L, Chilosi M, Fallo F, et al. Molecular analysis of CDKN1C and TP53 in sporadic adrenal tumors. *Eur J Endocrinol* 2001;145:207.
7. Yamamichi-Nishina M, Ito T, Mizutani T, et al. SW13 cells can transition between two distinct subtype by switching expression of BRG1 and Brm genes at the post-transcriptional level. *J Bio Chem* 2003;278:7422.
8. Lindholm J, Juul S, Jorgensen JOL, et al. Incidence and late prognosis of Cushing's syndrome: a population-based study. *J Clin Endocrinol Metab* 2001;86:117.
9. Yamada T, Saito H, Moriya T, et al. Adrenal carcinoma with a signal loss on chemical shift magnetic resonance imaging. *J Comput Assist Tomogr* 2003;27:606.
10. Honigschnabl S, Gallo S, Niederle B, et al. How accurate is MR imaging in characterization of adrenal masses: update of a long-term study. *Eur J Radiol* 2002;41:113.
11. Becherer A. Vierhapper H, Potzi C, et al. FDG PET in adrenocortical carcinoma. *Cancer Biother Radiopharm* 2001;16:289.
12. Invitti C, Giraldi F, De Martin M, et al. Diagnosis and management of Cushing's syndrome: results of an Italian multicentre study. *J Clin Endocrinol Metab* 1999;84:440.
13. Maurea S, Klain M, Caraco C, et al. Diagnostic accuracy of radionuclide imaging using 131I nor-cholesterol or meta-iodobenzylguanidine in patients with hypersecreting or non-hypersecreting adrenal tumours. *Nucl Med Commun* 2002;23:951.
14. Grumbach M, Biller M, Baunstein G, et al. Management of the clinically inapparent adrenal mass. *Ann Intern Med* 2003;138:424.
15. Mesurolle B, Mignon F. False-negative results in percutaneous adrenal biopsies in oncology patients. *Clin Radiol* 2003;58:497.
16. Kardar A. Rupture of adrenal carcinoma after biopsy. *J Urol* 2001;166:984.
17. Lockhard M, Smith J, Kenney P. Imaging of adrenal masses. *Eur J Radiol* 2002;41:95.
18. Fimmano A, Pettinato G, Bonuso C, et al. Giant, nonfunctioning carcinoma of the adrenal cortex. *N Engl J Med* 2001;345:700.
19. Harrison L, Gaudin P, Brennan M. Pathologic features of prognostic significance for adrenocortical carcinoma after curative resection. *Arch Surg* 1999;134:181.
20. Langer P, Bartsch D, Moebius E, et al. Adrenocortical carcinoma-our experience with 11 cases. *Arch Surg* 2000;385:393.
21. Wood B, Abraham J, Hvizda J, et al. Radiofrequency ablation of adrenal tumors and adrenocortical carcinoma metastases. *Cancer* 2003;97:554.
22. Wajchenberg B, Pereira M, Medonca B, et al. Adrenocortical carcinoma. *Cancer* 2000;88:711.
23. Harrison LE, Gaudin PB, Brennan MF. Pathologic features of prognostic significance for adrenocortical carcinoma after curative resection. *Arch Surg* 1999;134:181.
24. Schulick R, Brennan M. Long-term survival after complete resection and repeat resection in patients with adrenocortical carcinoma. *Ann Surg Oncol* 1999;6:719.
25. Ng L, Libertino J. Adrenocortical carcinoma: diagnostic, evaluation and treatment. *J Urol* 2003;169:5.
26. Abraham J, Bakke S, Rutt A, et al. A phase II trial of combination chemotherapy and surgical resection for the treatment of metastatic adrenocortical carcinoma. *Cancer* 2002;94:2333.
27. Berruti A, Terzolo M, Angeli A, et al. Mitotane associated with etoposide, doxorubicin, and cisplatin in the treatment of advanced adrenocortical carcinoma. *Cancer* 1998;83:2194.
28. Williamson S, Lew D, Miller G, et al. Phase II evaluation of cisplatin and etoposide followed by mitotane at disease progression in patients with locally advanced or metastatic adrenocortical carcinoma. *Cancer* 2000;88:1159.
29. Mekhail T, Hutson T, Elson P, et al. Phase I trial of weekly docetaxel and gemcitabine in patients with refractory malignancies. *Cancer* 2003;97:170.
30. Baudin E, Docao C, Gicquel C, et al. Use of a topoisomerase I inhibitor (irinotecan, CPT-11) in metastatic adrenocortical carcinoma. *Ann Oncol* 2002;13:1806.
31. Hovi L, Wikstrom S, Vettenranta K, et al. Adrenocortical carcinoma in children: a role for etoposide and cisplatin adjuvant therapy? Preliminary report. 2003:324.
32. Bravo E, Tagle R. Pheochromocytoma: state-of-the-art and future prospects. *Endocr Rev* 2003;24:539.
33. Neumann H, Bausch B, McWhinney S, et al. Germ-line mutations in nonsyndromic pheochromocytoma. *N Engl J Med* 2002;346:1459.
34. Maher E, Eng C. The pressure rises: update on the genetics of phaeochromocytoma. *Hum Mol Genet* 2002;11:2347.
35. Bryant J, Farmer J, Kessler L, et al. Pheochromocytoma: the expanding genetic differential diagnosis. *J Natl Cancer Inst* 2003;95:1196.
36. La Batide-Alanore A, Chatellier G, Plouin P. Diabetes as a marker of pheochromocytoma in hypertensive patients. *J Hypertens* 2003;21:1703.
37. Wiesner T, Bluher M, Windgassen M, Paschke R. Improvement of insulin sensitivity after adrenalectomy in patients with pheochromocytoma. *J Clin Endocrinol Metab* 2003;88:3632.
38. Kudva Y, Sawka A, Young W. The laboratory diagnosis of adrenal pheochromocytoma: the Mayo experience. *J Clin Endocrinol Metab* 2003;88:4533.
39. Weise M, Merke D, Pacak K, et al. Utility of plasma free metanephrines for detecting childhood pheochromocytoma. *J Clin Endocrinol Metab* 2002;87:1955.
40. Lenders J, Pacak K, Eisenhofer G. New advances in the biochemical diagnosis of pheochromocytoma. *Ann N Y Acad Sci* 2002;970:29.
41. Sawka A, Jaeschke R, Singh R, Young W. A comparison of biochemical tests for pheochromocytoma: measurement of fractionated plasma metanephrines compared with the combination of 24-hour urinary metanephrines and catecholamines. *J Clin Endocrinol Metab* 2003;88:553.
42. Eisenhofer G, Goldstein D, McClellan R, et al. Biochemical diagnosis of pheochromocytoma: how to distinguish true-from false-positive test results. *J Clin Endocrinol Metab* 2003;88:2656.
43. Blake M, Krishnamoorthy S, Boland G, et al. Low-density pheochromocytoma on CT: a mimicker of adrenal adenoma. *Am J Radiol* 2003;181:1663.
44. Kolby L, Bernhardt P, Levin-Jakobsen A-M, et al. Uptake of meta-iodobenzylguanidine in

neuroendocrine tumours is mediated by vesicular monoamine transporters. *Br J Cancer* 2003;89:1383.

45. Jacob T, Escout J, Bussy E. Malignant diaphragmatic pheochromocytoma. *Clin Nucl Med* 2002;27:807.

46. Taniguchi K, Ishizu K, Torizuka T, et al. Metastases of predominantly dopamine-secreting phaeochromocytoma that did not accumulate meta-iodobenzylguanidine: imaging with whole body positron emission tomography using 18F-labelled deoxyglucose. *Eur J Surg* 2001;167:866.

47. Hoegerle S, Nitzsche E, Altehoefer C, et al. Pheochromocytomas: detection with 18F DOPA whole-body PET-initial results. *Radiology* 2002;222:507.

48. Hwang J, Uchio E, Pate V, et al. Diagnostic localization of malignant bladder pheochromocytoma using 6-[18F]fluorodopamine positron emission tomography. *J Urol* 2003;169:274.

49. Ilias I, Yu J, Carrasquillo J, et al. Superiority of 6-[18F]fluorodopamine positron emission tomography versus [131I]-metaiodobenzylguanidine scintigraphy in the localization of metastatic pheochromocytoma. *J Clin Endocrinol Metab* 2003;88:4083.

50. Manger W. Editorial: in search of pheochromocytomas. *J Clin Endocrinol Metab* 2003;88:4080.

51. Bravo E. Pheochromocytoma an approach to antihypertensive management. *Ann N Y Acad Sci* 2002;970:1.

52. Bentrem D, Pappas S, Ahuja Y, et al. Contemporary surgical management of pheochromocytoma. *Am J Surg* 2002;184:621.

53. MacGillivray D, Whalen G, Malchoff C, et al. Laparoscopic resection of large adrenal tumors. *Ann Surg Oncol* 2002;9:480.

54. Porpiglia F, Destefanis P, Fiori C, et al. Does adrenal mass size really affect safety and effectiveness of laparoscopic adrenalectomy? *Urology* 2002;60:801.

55. Zeh H, Udelsman R. One hundred laparoscopic adrenalectomies: a single surgeon's experience. *Ann Surg Oncol* 2003;10:1012.

56. Brunt L, Lairmore T, Doherty G, et al. Adrenalectomy for familial pheochromocytoma in the laparoscopic era. *Ann Surg* 2002;235:713.

57. Walther M. New therapeutic and surgical approaches for sporadic and hereditary pheochromocytoma. *Ann N Y Acad Sci* 2002;970:41.

58. Li M, Fitzgerald P, Price D, Norton J. Iatrogenic pheochromocytomatosis: a previously unreported result of laparoscopic adrenalectomy. *Surgery* 2001;130:1072.

59. Shah M, Karelia N, Patel S, et al. Flow cytometric DNA analysis for determination of malignant potential in adrenal pheochromocytoma or paraganglioma: an Indian experience. *Ann Surg Oncol* 2003;10:426.

60. Yon L, Guillemot J, Montero-Hadjadje M, et al. Identification of the secretogranin II-derived peptide EM66 in pheochromocytomas as a potential marker for discriminating benign versus malignant tumors. *J Clin Endocrinol Metab* 2003;88:2579.

61. Boltze C, Mundschenk J, Unger N, et al. Expression profile of the telomeric complex discriminates between benign and malignant pheochromocytoma. *J Clin Endocrinol Metab* 2003;88:4280.

62. Gimenez-Roqueplo A, Favier J, Rustin P, et al. Mutations in the *SDHB* gene are associated with extra-adrenal and/or malignant phaeochromocytomas. *Cancer Res* 2003;63:5615.

63. Naguib M, Caceres M, Thomas C, et al. Radiation treatment of recurrent pheochromocytoma of the bladder. *Am J Clin Oncol* 2002;25:42.

64. Rao F, Keiser H, O'Connor D. Malignant and benign pheochromocytoma chromaffin granule transmitters and the response to medical and surgical treatment. *Ann N Y Acad Sci* 2002;971:530.

65. Sisson J. Radiopharmaceutical treatment of pheochromocytomas. *Ann N Y Acad Sci* 2002;970:54.

66. Rose B, Matthay K, Price D, et al. High-dose [131I]-metaiodobenzylguanidine therapy for 12 patients with malignant pheochromocytoma. *Cancer* 2003;98:239.

67. Lamarre-Cliché M, Gimenez-Roqueplo A, Billaud E, et al. Effects of slow-release octreotide on urinary metanephrine excretion and plasma chromogranin A and catecholamine levels in patients with malignant or recurrent phaechromocytoma. *Clin Endocrinol* 2002;57:629.

68. Nakane M, Takahashi S, Sekine I, et al. Successful treatment of malignant pheochromocytoma with combination chemotherapy containing anthracycline. *Ann Oncol* 2003;14:1449.

69. Gutierrez ML, Crooke ST. Mitotane (o,p-DDD). *Cancer Treat Rev* 1980;7:49.

70. Luton JP, Cerdas S, Billaud L, et al. Clinical features of adrenocortical carcinoma: prognostic factors and the effect of mitotane therapy. *N Engl J Med* 1990;322:1195.

71. Van Slooten H, Moolenaar AJ, Van Seters AP, Smeek D. The treatment of adrenocortical carcinoma with o,p-DDD: prognostic implications of serum levels monitoring. *Eur J Clin Oncol* 1984;20:47.

72. Venkatesh S, Hickey RC, Sellin RV, Fernandez JF, Samoan NA. Adrenal cortical carcinoma. *Cancer* 1989;64:765.

73. Haak HR, Hermans J, van de Velde CS, et al. Optimal treatment of adrenocortical carcinoma with mitotane: results in a consecutive series of 96 patients. *Br J Cancer* 1994;69:947.

74. Kornely E, Schlaghecke R. Complete remission of metastasized adrenocortical carcinoma under o,p-DDD. *Exp Clin Endocrinol* 1994;102:50.

75. Decker RA, Elson P, Hogan TF, et al. Eastern Cooperative Oncology Group study 1989: mitotane and Adriamycin in patients with advanced adrenocortical carcinoma. *Surgery* 1991;110:1006.

76. Stein CA, LaRocca RV, Thomas R, McAtee N, Myers CE. Suramin: an anticancer drug with a unique mechanism of action. *J Clin Oncol* 1989;7:499.

77. Arit W, Reincke M, Siekmann L, Winkelmann W, Allolio B. Suramin in adrenocortical cancer: limited efficacy and serious toxicity. *Clin Endocrinol* 1994;41:299.

78. LaRocca RV, Stein CA, Danesi R, et al. Suramin in adrenal cancer: modulation of steroid hormone production, cytotoxicity *in vitro* and clinical antitumor effect. *J Clin Endocrinol Metab* 1990;71:497.

79. Raymond E, Izbicka E, Soda H, et al. Activity of temozolomide against human tumor colony-forming units. *Clin Cancer Res* 1997;10:1769.

80. Berruti A, Terzolo M, Paccotti P. Favorable response of metastatic ACC to etoposide, Adriamycin and cisplatin. *Tumori* 1992;78:345.

81. Avico M, Bossi G, Livieri C. Partial response after intensive chemotherapy in a child. *Med Pediatr Oncol* 1992;20:246.

82. Zidan J, Shpendler M, Robinson E. Treatment of metastatic adrenal cortical carcinoma with etoposide (VP-16) and cisplatin after failure with o,p'DDD. Clinical case reports. *Am J Clin Oncol* 1996;19:229.

83. Feldman JM, Frankel N, Coleman RE. Platelet uptake of the pheochromocytoma-scanning agent [131I]-meta-iodobenzylguanidine. *Metabolism* 1984;33:397.

84. Krempf M, Lumbroso J, Mornex R, et al. Use of m-[131I]iodobenzylguanidine in the treatment of malignant pheochromocytoma. *J Clin Endocrinol Metab* 1991;72:455.

85. Nakabeppu Y, Nakajo M. Radionuclide therapy of malignant pheochromocytoma with [131I]-MIBG. *Ann Nucl Med* 1994;8:259.

86. Feldman JM. Treatment of metastatic pheochromocytoma with streptozotocin. *Arch Intern Med* 1983;143:1799.

87. Averbuch SD, Steakley CS, Young RC, et al. Malignant pheochromocytoma: effective treatment with a combination of cyclophosphamide, vincristine and dacarbazine. *Ann Intern Med* 1988;109:267.

88. Noshiro T, Honma H, Shimizu K, et al. Two cases of malignant pheochromocytoma treated with cyclophosphamide, vincristine and dacarbazine in a combined chemotherapy. *Endocr J* 1996;43:279.

89. Sisson JC, Shapiro B, Shulkin BL, et al. Treatment of malignant pheochromocytomas with [131I]-MIBG (metaiodobenzylguanidine) and chemotherapy. *Am J Clin Oncol* 1999;22:364.

90. Arai A, Naruse M, Naruse K, et al. Cardiac malignant pheochromocytoma with bone metastases. *Intern Med* 1998;37:940.

91. Tada K, Okuda Y, Yamashita K. Three cases of malignant pheochromocytomas treated with cyclophosphamide, vincristine and dacarbazine combination chemotherapy and alpha-methyl-p-tyrosine to control hypercatecholaminemia. *Horm Res* 1998;49:295.

SECTION 5

H. RICHARD ALEXANDER, JR.
ROBERT T. JENSEN

Pancreatic Endocrine Tumors

Pancreatic endocrine (or neuroendocrine) tumors (PETs) are uncommon neoplasms that share a number of features.[1,2] Histologically they are classified as apudomas and share cytochemical features with melanoma, pheochromocytoma, carcinoid tumors, and medullary thyroid carcinoma.[2] All APUD (amine precursor uptake and decarboxylation) neoplasms have the capacity to synthesize and secrete polypeptide products that have specific endocrine hormone activity. Except for insulinoma, each is malignant in most cases (more than 60%) (Table 34.5-1). PETs are vascular tumors with similar radiographic appearances and metastatic patterns of spread (primarily to regional lymph nodes and liver).

PETs are considered functional if they are associated with a clinical syndrome due to ectopic hormone release and nonfunctional if they are not associated with clinical symptoms. In the latter category are pancreatic polypeptide (PP) tumors or PPomas because the hormones cause no specific symptoms.[1,3] In addition, there are PETs associated with no known hormone elevation and histologically indistinguishable from functional tumors.[1]

In general, PETs are uncommon. Functional PETs are reported to have a prevalence of 10 per million population.[4] The incidence of clinically significant PETs is 3.6 to 4.0 per million population per year. Nonfunctional PETs or PPomas are reported to account for 15% to 30% of all PETs.[3] Gastrinoma and PPomas are the most common malignant PETs, whereas insulinoma is the most common benign PET. This chapter presents information in a format that reflects the many similarities

TABLE 34.5-1. Enteropancreatic Endocrine Tumors

Tumor Name	Syndrome Name	Hormone	Percentage Malignant	Location
PPoma	PPoma	Pancreatic polypeptide	>60	Pancreas
Nonfunctioning	Nonfunctioning pancreatic endocrine tumor	None	>60	Pancreas
Symptoms due to released hormones				
Gastrinomas	Zollinger-Ellison syndrome	Gastrin	60–90	Pancreas (30–60%) Duodenum (30–43%) Other (10–20%)
Insulinoma	Insulinoma	Insulin	10–15	Pancreas (>99%)
VIPoma	Pancreatic cholera Verner-Morrison syndrome WDHA	Vasoactive intestinal peptide	80	Pancreas (90%) Adrenal gland (10%)
Glucagonoma	Glucagonoma	Glucagon	60	Pancreas (>99%)
Somatostatinoma	Somatostatinoma	Somatostatin	—	Pancreas (56%) Upper small intestine (44%)
GRFoma	GRFoma	Growth hormone–releasing peptide	30	Pancreas (33%) Lung (53%) Small intestine (10%) Other (7%)
ACTHoma	Ectopic Cushing's syndrome	ACTH	>95 (pancreatic)	Pancreas (4–16%)

ACTH, adrenocorticotropic hormone; GRF, growth hormone–releasing factor; WDHA, watery diarrhea, hypokalemia, and achlorhydria.

of PETs with specific discussions of each tumor type in detail when there are unique issues related to it.

PATHOGENESIS, PATHOLOGY, TUMOR BIOLOGY

GASTRINOMA

In 1955, Zollinger and Ellison described two patients with severe peptic ulcer disease treatable only by total gastrectomy because of extreme hypersecretion of gastric acid associated with a non–β islet cell tumor of the pancreas.[5] Analysis of tumor extracts via enzymatic degradation and amino acid analysis demonstrated that the secretagogue in the tumor was identical to human antral gastrin,[6] so these tumors are called *gastrinomas.*

Effective control of the gastric hypersecretion either medically or surgically abolishes all clinical manifestations of Zollinger-Ellison syndrome (ZES) such as peptic ulcer disease and diarrhea.[7] Along with basal gastric acid hypersecretion, hypergastrinemia causes trophic changes in the gastric mucosa with the result that patients with ZES have increased numbers of parietal cells and an increased maximal acid secretory capacity.[7,8] Many patients with ZES have diarrhea, sometimes as the sole presenting manifestation, which is due to acid hypersecretion's causing direct injury to the small intestinal mucosa, inactivation of pancreatic lipase, and precipitation of bile acids. ZES patients with diarrhea become asymptomatic when the gastric acid hypersecretion is controlled even though the hypergastrinemia remains unchanged.[9]

Gastrin has been found in a number of different molecular sizes. In ZES patients, gastrin 17 (G_{17}) is the major gastrin component, comprising 74% to 80% of the total immunoreactivity, with "big gastrin" or gastrin 34 (G_{34}) comprising most of the remainder.[7]

The proportion of gastrinomas found at surgery in the duodenum and in lymph nodes near the pancreatic head has increased to greater than 50%, so that 65% to 90% of all gastrinomas found at surgery occur in the pancreatic head–duodenal area[10,11] (Table 34.5-2). Gastrinomas have also been reported to occur in other intraabdominal sites such as the liver, stomach, jejunum, mesentery, common bile duct, and spleen.[12] In females, ovarian gastrinomas can occur and are functionally indistinguishable from other gastrinomas.[7] Extraabdominal gastrinomas in the heart (intracardiac septum) and lung (non–small cell lung cancer) have been reported.[7]

The percentage of gastrinomas that are actually malignant is unclear. No histologic criteria predict malignancy; therefore, malignancy can only be established by the presence of metastases.[2,7] The presence of necrosis and a high mitotic rate have been shown to be independent adverse prognostic factors for disease-specific and overall survival for patients with PETs.[13] Approximately one-half of patients have a malignant gastrinoma at the time of diagnosis, and metastases are usually to peripancreatic lymph nodes and to the liver.[14] Bone metastases have been reported in approximately 30% of patients with metastatic gastrinoma in the liver.[14,15] A number of cases of extrapancreatic gastrinoma localized in lymph nodes have been described with no evidence of primary tumor, and some of these cases have been apparently cured by excision of lymph nodes, which suggests that the gastrinoma was not metastatic but originated in the lymph node.[16]

Primary tumor size, but not lymph node metastases, has been shown to be an important factor in predicting liver metastases.[11] Liver metastases occurred with 4% of gastrinomas smaller than 1 cm in diameter, 28% of tumors 1.1 to 2.9 cm, and 61% of tumors larger than 3 cm.[11] Duodenal gastrinomas have been found to be malignant with metastatic spread in 48% to 75% of cases.[11,17] In one study[11] involving 90 patients with ZES with pancreatic or duodenal gastrinomas, an equal percentage had lymph node metastases (48% and 47%, respectively); however, only 5% of patients with duodenal gastrinomas had liver metastases compared with 52% of patients with pancreatic gastrinomas.[11] Because

TABLE 34.5-2. Sites of Apparent Primary Gastrinoma

Location	Frequency (%)
Duodenal	40–50
Pancreatic	30–40
Lymph node	10–15
Ectopic (nonpancreaticoduodenal or nodal)	≤5
Liver	
Common bile duct	
Cardiac	
Mesentery	
Spleen	
Ovary	
Lung (Non–small cell lung cancer)	

most duodenal gastrinomas are small (80% less than 1 cm) and most pancreatic gastrinomas are large (70% at least 3 cm), it remains unclear whether tumor size and location are independent predictors.

Some studies have attempted to use assessments of nuclear DNA to differentiate benign from malignant pancreatic or duodenal neuroendocrine tumors.[2] DNA ploidy analysis in some studies did not predict prognosis[2]; however, in one study of 59 patients with gastrinomas,[18] 54% were diploid, 15% were near diploid, 0% were pure tetraploid, 25% were nontetraploid aneuploid, and 5% were multiple stem line aneuploid. All patients with multiple stem line aneuploidy had widespread metastases, and the results of the DNA analysis correlated with disease extent.[18] Alterations in tumor suppressor genes (i.e., p53, retinoblastoma) or oncogenes (i.e., ras, myc) are uncommon in typical PETs. Studies show that alterations in INK/4a (10% to 30%), the multiple endocrine neoplasia (MEN) 1 gene (11q13) (25% to 43%), and the HER-2/*neu* gene (18% to 25%) are the most frequent. Only alterations in the HER-2/*neu* gene, epidermal growth factor receptor overexpression, or loss of heterozygosity at 1p, 3p, 3q, and 6q have been shown to be associated with malignant behavior.[19]

Approximately 20% of patients with ZES have a familial form with evidence of MEN 1.[9] MEN 1 is an autosomal dominant trait characterized by hyperplasia or tumors of multiple endocrine organs, with hyperparathyroidism being the most common abnormality. Islet cell tumors of the pancreas are the second most common, occurring in 82% of MEN 1 patients with 57% having ZES and 25% insulinomas.[20] Pituitary and adrenal adenomas are less common. Patients with MEN 1 with ZES differ from sporadic cases in that they frequently present at a younger age; their tumors are almost always multiple and frequently small, and in some studies, patients with MEN 1 have an increased survival rate compared with sporadic cases.[11,20]

Many hormones are frequently identified in a given PET by immunohistochemical analysis, but it is not possible to determine which of the hormones that stain within a tumor are clinically important. Immunohistochemically nonfunctioning PETs and PPomas can stain positively for numerous other gastrointestinal peptides. In one series of 30 nonfunctioning tumors, cells showed immunoreactivity to insulin in 50%, to glucagon in 30%, to PP in 43%, and to somatostatin in 13%; only 13% stained for no peptide.[21]

The endocrine nature of PETs is not always apparent, and a combination of clinical and biochemical data and immunocyto-chemical studies for peptides as well as for chromogranins, neuron-specific enolase, synaptophysin, and protein gene product 9.5 are frequently needed.[22] Levels of numerous plasma hormones may be elevated in a given PET, and the presence or absence of abnormal plasma levels of a particular peptide or extent of elevation does not correlate with location of tumor, extent of tumor, or the presence or absence of a particular symptom. Adrenocorticotropic hormone (ACTH) production in PETs, particularly in ZES patients, is associated with a very aggressive tumor phenotype.[23] Elevated concentrations of human chorionic gonadotropin (HCG) subunits (α or β chains) in sera or in the tumor by immunocytochemical analysis occur in some patients with PETs, but elevated plasma concentrations of α- or β-HCG are not useful in predicting malignancy.[22] Chromogranin A is a 48-kD protein that is costored and coreleased with peptide hormones from gut endocrine cells and tumors. Positive immunocytochemical staining for chromogranin A has been shown in gastrinomas, carcinoids, antral G cells, and fundic enterochromaffin-like (ECL) cells of the stomach.[22] In a study of 72 patients with PETs or carcinoid tumors, 99% had elevated plasma chromogranin A levels, 88% elevated chromogranin B levels, and 6% elevated chromogranin C levels.[24] Plasma chromogranin A levels correlate significantly with fasting serum gastrin (FSG) levels in patients with gastrinoma but do not predict stage of tumor or presence of MEN 1.[25]

Histologic studies have demonstrated the general similarity of PETs and carcinoid tumors.[2,26] Different histologic classifications have been proposed based on growth patterns, including a glandular pattern, solid nests of cells (solid pattern), a trabecular or ribbon-like structure (gyriform pattern), and unclassified pattern.[2,7,26] Similar patterns have been demonstrated in other endocrine tumors from patients, and the type of histologic pattern does not correlate with the type of hormone produced, clinical symptoms, or malignancy. Ultrastructural classifications have all been proposed based on the type of granules seen, but these also do not correlate with malignancy or clinical features.[2,7]

INSULINOMA

Insulin-secreting PETs encompass a broad range of diagnostic and therapeutic features. Insulinomas were first recognized by Whipple, who described 30 patients with hypoglycemia and pancreatic adenomas.[27] Whipple's triad consists of the characteristic symptoms of hypoglycemia associated with blood glucose levels below 50 mg/dL and immediate relief after ingestion of glucose, and these have remained the major criteria for many years for the diagnosis of insulinoma.[27] Insulinomas usually occur in patients between the ages of 20 and 75 years. The average age of presentation is between 44 and 46 years and there is a preponderance of women (60%).[28] The incidence of insulinoma is 0.8 to 0.9 cases per million population, and it is generally considered the second most common functional PET.[26]

As with other apudomas, malignancy is only defined by the presence of metastases at operation or by imaging studies. Whereas 60% to 90% of gastrinomas are malignant, only 5% to 15% of insulinomas are malignant (see Table 34.5-1).[28] Most insulinomas are found to be solitary benign pancreatic nodules, often encapsulated, with only 2% to 10% of patients having multiple tumors.[28] In patients with multiple insulinomas or PETs, MEN 1 should be suspected. Insulinomas are uniformly distributed throughout the entire pancreas and are usually less than 1.5 cm in maximal diameter.[29]

CLINICAL PRESENTATION AND DIAGNOSIS

Resection is the only curative modality for patients with PETs, and the success of operation is contingent on establishing the correct diagnosis, determining if a patient may belong to an MEN 1 kindred, performing appropriate radiographic imaging studies to assess the location of the primary tumor and the extent of regional or distant metastatic spread, and ensuring adequate medical management of the functional sequelae of excess hormone production before surgery.

GASTRINOMA

Gastrinomas are slightly more common in males (60%) than in females; the mean age at diagnosis is 45 to 50 years, and approximately 20% of patients have MEN 1.[9] The most common presentation of patients with ZES is abdominal pain in 26% to 58%, which usually cannot be differentiated from pain caused by other common acid-peptic disorders.[9] However, in some studies a significant proportion of individuals (14% to 25%) have no peptic ulcer or abdominal pain at the time of diagnosis.[9] Thirty-seven to 73% of patients have diarrhea as an initial symptom, and in 15% to 18% it is the only symptom. Esophageal symptoms, endoscopic abnormalities, or both, are present in 50% to 70% of patients.[9]

Although atypical or multiple ulcers strongly suggest the diagnosis, in 18% to 25% of patients no ulcers are present at the time of diagnosis.[26] Although the decreased severity of peptic ulcer disease at diagnosis suggests that patients with ZES are being diagnosed earlier, in almost all series there is still a delay of 3 to 6 years between the onset of symptoms and diagnosis.[9] Intestinal perforation, especially of the jejunum, is a presenting event in up to 7% of patients with ZES.[9]

The diagnosis should be suspected on the basis of the clinical presentation and established in almost all patients by demonstrating elevated basal gastric acid secretion [basal acid output (BAO)] and fasting hypergastrinemia. ZES should be suspected in the clinical setting of peptic ulcer with diarrhea, familial peptic ulcer, peptic ulcer in unusual locations, and recurrent or resistant peptic ulcer.[9] ZES should be particularly suspected in patients with peptic ulcers that persist or recur despite treatment for *Helicobacter pylori* infection or with histamine H_2-receptor antagonists, in patients with severe esophagitis, and in patients with duodenal ulcers without *H pylori*.[9] *H pylori* is present in 90% to 98% of patients with idiopathic duodenal ulcer disease and 90% heal with *H pylori* eradication; in ZES, fewer than 50% of patients have *H pylori*. In all patients who have peptic ulcer disease severe enough to require gastric

TABLE 34.5-3. Common Diagnostic Criteria for Zollinger-Ellison Syndrome

Clinical suspicion (atypical, multiple, recurrent, or refractory duodenal ulcers with no *Helicobacter pylori* infection; diarrhea; family history)

Elevated fasting serum gastrin levels (>200 pg/mL; one-third of patients have levels >1000 pg/mL)

Increased basal gastric acid secretion (≥15 mEq/h, >5 mEq/h after acid-reducing surgery)

Positive secretion stimulation test result (>200 pg/mL increase in gastrin after 2 µg/kg secretin IV bolus)

TABLE 34.5-4. Differential Diagnosis of Hypergastrinemia

INCREASED GASTRIN LEVEL AND INCREASED BASAL GASTRIC ACID SECRETION
Zollinger-Ellison syndrome
Retained gastric antrum
Antral G-cell hyperplasia
Gastric outlet obstruction
Short bowel syndrome
Helicobacter pylori infection
Chronic renal failure

INCREASED GASTRIN LEVEL AND DECREASED BASAL GASTRIC ACID SECRETION
Pernicious anemia/atrophic gastritis
Antisecretory therapy (i.e., omeprazole)
Chronic renal failure
H pylori infection
Post-vagotomy procedure

surgery, at least one measurement of preoperative FSG level should be done. To make the diagnosis of ZES it is necessary to demonstrate an elevated FSG level and an elevated BAO[7] (Table 34.5-3). Although approximately 32% of patients with ZES have an FSG of at least 1000 pg/mL, in the remaining two-thirds the FSG is elevated but less than 1000 pg/mL.[7]

Two general types of disorders other than ZES are also known to cause elevation in FSG: those associated with gastric acid hypersecretion and those associated with hypochlorhydria or achlorhydria, including chronic gastritis, gastric cancer, pernicious anemia, and postvagotomy status[4] (Table 34.5-4). One of the most common causes is drug-induced hypergastrinemia due to inhibition of acid secretion with H^+-K^+–adenosine triphosphatase inhibitors (omeprazole, lansoprazole). Similarly, *H pylori* infection can on occasion cause elevations of FSG in the range seen in ZES. No absolute level of elevation in FSG distinguishes patients with disorders of acid hypersecretion from those with hyposecretion; they can only be distinguished by directly assessing acid output. If facilities are not available to measure the BAO, then a simple determination of the pH of the gastric contents (while the patient is not taking antisecretory medications) should be performed. A pH of 2 or higher virtually excludes the diagnosis of ZES.[30]

The most commonly used secretory criteria for diagnosing ZES are a BAO of at least 15 mEq/h in patients without and at least 5 mEq/h in patients with previous acid-reducing operations.[30] The mean BAO in various series ranged from 30 to 60 mEq/h for patients without previous acid-reducing surgery.[30] A BAO of at least 15 mEq/h includes up to 87% to 90% of patients with ZES[30] and excludes 90% of patients with routine duodenal ulcers. In patients with previous acid-reducing surgery, the mean BAO exceeds 5 mEq/h in most studies, but in 0% to 45% of ZES patients is less than 5 mEq/h.[30,31] Patients with ZES also have an elevated maximal acid output (MAO) and an elevated BAO to MAO ratio that often exceeds 0.6.[30,31] However, diagnostic criteria based on the MAO or BAO to MAO ratio offer no advantage over those based on an elevated BAO alone.

If a patient has an FSG of at least 1000 pg/mL and a gastric pH of less than 2, then the diagnosis of ZES is generally established.[7,30] The only other disorder that can mimic ZES in this capacity is retained gastric antrum syndrome.[32] This is an uncommon condition that occurs in patients who have undergone a Billroth II gastroenterostomy with a portion of antrum left attached to the excluded proximal duodenal stump.[32] This diagnosis can be excluded in patients after gastric surgery by the secretin stimulation test and by gastric technetium 99m–pertechnetate scanning.[32] In patients with only moderately elevated FSGs and a gastric pH less than 2, ZES must be differentiated from retained gastric antrum syndrome,[32] *H pylori* infection, chronic gastric outlet obstruction, antral G-cell hyperplasia, massive small bowel resection, and, rarely, chronic renal failure by the use of various gastrin-provocative tests. A number of different provocative tests including the secretin test, calcium infusion test, and meal test have been developed.[7] The sensitivity of the secretin stimulation test is superior to that of the calcium and meal provocative tests. Gastrin levels after secretin increased by 110 pg/mL in 93% of patients with ZES and by more than 200 pg/mL in 87%.[7] Because of its ease, lack of side effects, high sensitivity, and very low occurrence of false-positives, the secretin test is the diagnostic provocative test of choice. A rise in gastrin level of 200 pg/mL is diagnostic.[7] The calcium infusion test should be reserved for the rare patient in whom ZES is strongly suspected but the secretin test result is negative.[7]

Antral G-cell hyperplasia is reported to mimic ZES clinically with elevated FSG and BAO.[33] This syndrome frequently occurs in patients after vagotomy, is due to increased numbers of antral G cells, is curable by antrectomy, is possibly associated with *H pylori* infections, and is differentiated from ZES by a negative secretin test and an exaggerated (at least 100% increase) postmeal serum gastrin level.[33] Antral G-cell hyperfunction is similar to antral G-cell hyperplasia except that there are normal numbers of G cells, the syndrome is frequently familial with autosomal dominant inheritance, and the syndrome is associated with hyperpepsinogenemia I.[34] This syndrome was reported to be distinguishable from ZES by a negative secretin test result and an exaggerated increase in postmeal serum gastrin level.[7,33] Of patients with ZES, only 30% have a greater than 100% increase in serum gastrin level and 10% have a greater than 150% increase.[7,33] Therefore, the meal test is actually frequently positive in patients with ZES and does not reliably differentiate ZES from antral syndromes.[7,33]

Chronic gastric outlet obstruction can be difficult to distinguish from ZES because the obstruction can be caused by ZES or it can mimic ZES and be secondary to other causes of duodenal obstruction. ZES can be differentiated from the other causes of obstruction by a secretin test and prolonged gastric suction.[33] Massive small bowel resection can cause a transient hypergastrinemia and elevation of BAO and can be distinguished from ZES by history and the secretin test.[33] Chronic renal failure and *H pylori* infections can cause hypergastrinemia, which is usually associated with acid hyposecretion, although on occasion they may be associated with acid hypersecretion,[33] and can be differentiated from ZES by the secretin test.

INSULINOMA

The clinical symptoms of insulinoma are due to hypoglycemia in almost all instances.[4,28] Most symptoms are neuroglycopenic in nature and include visual disturbances (59%), confusion (51%), altered consciousness (38%), and weakness (32%). Seizures occur but are less common (23%).[4,28] Symptoms can also occur due to excess catecholamine release (adrenergic symptoms), such as sweating (43%) and tremulousness (23%). In one study 49% of patients had both neuroglycopenic symptoms and adrenergic symptoms, 38% had neuroglycopenic symptoms only, and 12% had adrenergic symptoms only.[4] Symptoms are characteris-

TABLE 34.5-5. Common Diagnostic Criteria for Insulinoma

Symptoms of hypoglycemia (headache, lightheadedness, confusion, drowsiness, seizures)
Symptoms of catecholamine excess (tremors, palpitations)
Hypoglycemia during a monitored fast (<50 mg/dL)
Increased serum insulin (>5–10 μU/mL)
Increased proinsulin (≥25%)
Negative sulfonylurea screen
Relief of symptoms after eating
Insulin/glucose ratio >0.3

tically associated with fasting, a delayed meal, or exercise. There are numerous reports of patients with insulinoma who received erroneous psychiatric or neurologic diagnoses for several years before the correct diagnosis was made.

The diagnosis of insulinoma can only be established by documenting symptomatic hypoglycemia with inappropriately elevated serum insulin levels during a monitored fast[35,36] (Table 34.5-5). Hypoglycemia is usually defined as a blood sugar level lower than 50 mg/dL in the fasting state.[36] In healthy individuals the blood glucose value usually does not decrease to less than 70 mg/dL after an overnight fast.[36] In more than 97% of individuals a supervised fast of 48 hours or less is sufficient to diagnose insulinoma by the development of clinical symptoms and a plasma glucose level of less than 50 mg/dL.[35] In addition, patients with the diagnosis usually have serum insulin levels higher than 5 μU/mL and 97% have levels higher than 10 μU/mL. An insulin-glucose ratio greater than 0.3 is typical.[36] In some normal obese subjects, because of hyperinsulinemia due to insulin resistance, the fasting plasma insulin to glucose ratio may be elevated and mimic the pattern in insulinoma.[28] In these patients, the fasting glucose level is normal, and with prolonged fasting, blood glucose level does not decrease to less than 55 mg/dL; thus, during a prolonged monitored fast these patients can be easily differentiated from those with insulinoma.

A number of other conditions can cause fasting hypoglycemia with increased plasma insulin levels, including other causes of organic hyperinsulinism due to pancreatic islet disease besides insulinoma, factitious use of excessive insulin or hypoglycemia agents, or autoantibodies against the insulin receptor.[4,26,28,36] To differentiate insulinoma from these other conditions, additional tests are useful, including plasma determination of proinsulin level, C-peptide level, antibodies to insulin, and plasma sulfonylurea levels. Because endogenous insulin is synthesized as a precursor, proinsulin, quantification of the higher-molecular-weight component called the proinsulin-like component is useful. In patients with surreptitious use of insulin or oral hypoglycemia agents, the proinsulin level is either normal or decreased.[26,28,36] The measurement of C-peptide level has proven useful in differentiating patients with organic hypersecretion of insulin from patients surreptitiously using insulin, because commercial insulin preparations contain no C peptide. In patients with insulinoma the characteristic finding is either an elevated or a normal plasma C-peptide concentration, whereas in patients surreptitiously using insulin the plasma insulin level is high and the C-peptide level low.[26,28,36]

NONFUNCTIONING PANCREATIC ENDOCRINE TUMORS

Nonfunctioning PETs and PPomas present in the fourth and fifth decades of life.[37,38] PPomas release the hormone PP, which has no known functional sequelae.[26] Originally, it was thought that nonfunctioning PETs did not release any hormone products, but they have been shown to secrete chromogranins, α-HCG or β-HCG subunits, or other peptides that do not cause symptoms.[22] Histologically, PPomas are similar to other PETs and cannot be differentiated by immunohistochemistry. Increasingly, what in the past were thought to be nonfunctioning PETs are now appreciated to generate elevated plasma PP levels. One-half to three-fourths of PETs not associated with any clinical syndrome and classified as nonfunctioning produce detectable plasma PP levels. The elevated plasma PP level is specific for endocrine pancreatic tumors. In 53 patients with adenocarcinoma of the pancreas, none had elevated plasma PP levels.[39] There are no data to suggest that nonfunctioning PETs without elevated PP levels and PPomas differ in biologic behavior or presentation.[26,37] With these tumors, symptoms arise largely from mechanical or mass effects of the neoplasm, and therefore they are diagnosed late when they are quite large and locally invasive. They are usually solitary tumors except in patients with MEN 1 in whom multiple adenomas are seen.[2,3,26,37] The tumors are distributed throughout the pancreas in a ratio of 7:1:1.5 for pancreatic head to body to tail.[4] The malignancy rate varies from 64% to 92%.[26,37,39]

Chromogranin A and B levels are elevated in almost all patients with nonfunctioning PETs.[24] Elevated plasma levels of PP do not establish the diagnosis of a PPoma even when a pancreatic mass is present. Plasma PP levels are reported to be elevated in 22% to 71% of patients with functional PETs as well as in patients with nonpancreatic carcinoid tumors.[26] Furthermore, elevated plasma levels of PP can occur in other conditions such as old age; after bowel resection; with alcohol abuse; during certain infections; in chronic noninfective inflammatory disorders, acute diarrhea, chronic renal failure, diabetes, chronic relapsing pancreatitis, and hypoglycemia; and after eating. To increase the specificity of an elevated plasma level for a PPoma, an atropine suppression test may be used. In one study of 48 patients with elevated plasma PP levels, atropine (1 mg intramuscularly) did not suppress PP levels in any of the 18 patients with PETs but did suppress the level by 50% in all patients without tumors.

Patients present with abdominal pain in 36% of cases and with jaundice in 28% of cases; in 16% the tumors are found incidentally at surgery; and in the remaining patients a variety of symptoms due to the tumor mass are present.[26,37] The average delay from onset of symptoms until diagnosis varies from 5 months to 2 to 7 years.[26,37,39]

OTHER RARE PANCREATIC ENDOCRINE TUMORS

The VIPoma (vasoactive intestinal polypeptide tumor) syndrome was first described by Verner and Morrison in 1958[40] and the condition is also commonly called the Verner-Morrison syndrome. Because of the resemblance of the diarrheal fluid to that seen in patients with cholera, the terms *pancreatic cholera* and *endocrine cholera* and the acronym *WDHA* (watery diarrhea, hypokalemic, and achlorhydric) have also been used.[41] The tumors occur in a bimodal age distribution: The mean age for adults at diagnosis is 50 years with a range of 32 to 81 years and a female predominance; in children the mean age is 2 to 4 years with a range from 10 months to 9 years.[41]

In adults more than 80% of VIPomas are solitary pancreatic tumors.[4,26] One- to two-thirds of patients with VIPomas have metastases at the time of diagnosis or surgery.[41] Characteristically

TABLE 34.5-6. Symptoms Commonly Associated with Rare Pancreatic Endocrine Tumors

VIPoma	Glucagonoma	Somatostatinoma
Diarrhea	Weight loss	Gallbladder disease
Dehydration	Migratory necrolytic	Diabetes mellitus
Weight loss	erythema	Weight loss
Crampy abdom-	Glucose intolerance	Diarrhea
inal pain	Hypoaminoacidemia	Steatorrhea
Hypokalemia	Thromboembolic disease	Hypochlorhydria

in children younger than 10 years and rarely in adults (5% of cases) VIPoma syndrome is due to a ganglioneuroma or ganglioneuroblastoma.[26] These extrapancreatic tumors are less often malignant than pancreatic VIPomas.

Plasma levels of VIP are consistently elevated in patients with the VIPoma syndrome and appear to be responsible for the functional syndrome[26,41-43] (Table 34.5-6). The principal feature of VIPoma syndrome is the presence of severe secretory diarrhea associated with hypokalemia and dehydration.[26,41-43] The diarrhea is copious, and all patients with VIPoma pass more than 3 L/d.[41,43] A volume of less than 700 mL/d is not consistent with a diagnosis of VIPoma.[26,42] Cramping pain or colic is reported by 35% to 63% of patients.[41,43] Gross steatorrhea is usually not present but weight loss is almost universally present. Erythematous flushing of the head or trunk area is characteristic and reported in 23% of patients.[42,43] The clinical laboratory studies invariably demonstrate hypokalemia (83% to 100%) and to a lesser degree hypercalcemia (41%), hypochlorhydria (70%), and mild hyperglycemia (18%).[26,41,43] Hypokalemia is often severe, with a value of less than 2.5 mmol/L at some time in 93% of patients.[43]

The diagnosis of the VIPoma requires the documentation of an elevated plasma concentration of VIP and the presence of a large volume of secretory diarrhea.[26,41,42] A large number of possible causes for the diarrhea can be excluded by having the patient fast, because in patients with VIPomas the diarrhea persists during fasting.[26,41,42] The diarrheal fluid should be characteristic of a secretory diarrhea in which the stool electrolytes can account for all of the stool water osmolality [(sodium + potassium) × 2 = measured osmolality].[42] Other diseases can give a chronic secretory diarrhea with large volumes and can be confused with a possible VIPoma. One such syndrome is called the *pseudo-VIPoma syndrome*.[42] Other causes include ZES, chronic laxative abuse, and some cases of secretory diarrhea of unknown origin.[42]

The range of normal fasting plasma VIP level in most laboratories is 0 to 170 pg/mL and the mean value in patients with VIPoma is more than 900 pg/mL.[43] Neither the histologic studies nor electron microscopic studies can distinguish VIPomas from other PETs; however, the presence of immunoreactive VIP is strongly suggestive for VIPoma, because this is rarely found in other PETs.

Mallinson and coworkers specifically established the association of a cutaneous rash with glucagon-producing tumors of the pancreas.[44] Most glucagonomas at the time of diagnosis average in size between 5 and 10 cm with a range of 0.4 to 35 cm.[45] Glucagonomas have a predilection for arising in the pancreatic tail (50% to 80% of cases).[45,46] Most tumors are malignant and, as with other PETs, the most common site of metastatic spread is the liver. Less commonly there is spread to lymph nodes, bone, and mesentery. In most cases glucagonomas are within the pancreas; however, a glucagonoma associated with the typical clinical syndrome was found in the proximal duodenum.[46] Glucagonomas usually occur as a single tumor, although multiple tumors have been described.[45]

Glucagonomas usually occur in middle to late age, with only 16% of cases in individuals younger than 40 years of age and most in those 50 to 70 years of age. The typical dermatitis occurs in 64% to 90% of patients, diabetes mellitus or glucose intolerance in 83% to 90%, weight loss in 56% to 90%, diarrhea in 14% to 15%, abdominal pain in 12%, thromboembolic disease with venous thrombosis in 24% and with pulmonary emboli in 11%, and occasionally psychiatric disturbances[26,45,46] (see Table 34.5-6). Laboratory abnormalities include anemia in 44% to 85%, hypoaminoacidemia in 26% to 100%, hypocholesterolemia in 80%, and renal glycosuria.[26,45,46]

The pathophysiology of the glucagonoma syndrome is related to the known actions of glucagon. Glucagon stimulates glycogenolysis, gluconeogenesis, ketogenesis, lipolysis, and insulin secretion, as well as having effects on gut secretion, inhibiting pancreatic and gastric secretions, inhibiting intestinal motility, and increasing heart rate and contractility. Hyperglycemia in glucagonoma results from the increased hepatic glycogenolysis and glyconeogenesis.[26,45] Weight loss has been attributed to the known catabolic effects of glucagon.[46] It is not clearly established that the skin rash is per se due to the hyperglucagonemia; it is possible that the glucagon-induced hypoaminoacidemia that develops in 80% to 95% of patients may be involved, because correction of the hypoaminoacidemia has been shown to correct the dermatitis without changing plasma glucagon concentrations in some patients.[26,45] A prolonged infusion of glucagon in patients with tumor-induced hypoglycemia was reported to cause necrolytic migratory erythema, stomatitis, and venous thromboembolism, which suggests that the hyperglucagonemia alone is sufficient to cause these conditions.[47]

Immunocytochemical and histologic studies of glucagonomas show a number of results typical of PETs.[26,45] Glucagon is one of the most frequently seen peptides in immunocytochemical studies of PETs; however, in many cases it is not associated with any syndrome. The morphology of most glucagon-producing tumors demonstrates no general features that distinguish them from other PETs.

The presence of cutaneous lesions often precedes the diagnosis of the syndrome for long periods of time, with a mean of 6 to 8 years and a maximum of 18 years.[26,45] Typically, the rash starts as an erythematous region, usually at periorofacial or intertriginous areas such as the groin, buttocks, thighs, or perineum, and then spreads laterally.[26,45] The lesions later become raised with superficial central blistering. Healing is associated with the development of hyperpigmentation. Glossitis or angular stomatitis is reported to occur in 34% to 68% of patients.[26,45]

Once the diagnosis is suspected, it can be confirmed by establishing the presence of a marked elevation in plasma glucagon concentration.[26,45] In most laboratories the upper limit of normal for fasting glucagon concentration is 150 to 200 pg/mL. More than 90% of patients with glucagonoma have plasma levels in excess of 1000 pg/mL and almost 100% have levels greater than 500 pg/mL.[46] Hyperglucagonemia, usually less than 500 pg/mL, is reported to occur in chronic renal insufficiency, diabetic ketoacidosis, prolonged starvation, acute pancreatitis, acromegaly, hypercortisolism, septicemia, severe burns, severe stress (trauma, exercise), familial hyperglucagonemia, and hepatic insufficiency.[26,45]

Somatostatinomas release somatostatin, a hormone that inhibits numerous endocrine and exocrine functions, including the actions of insulin, glucagon, gastrin, secretin, cholecystokinin, and motilin. In addition to inhibiting endocrine secretions, somatostatin has direct effects on a number of target organs, including inhibition of gastric acid secretion, increased intestinal motility, and reduced intestinal absorption of fat. Somatostatinomas are the least common PET and fewer than 50 cases have been described.[26,48] Patients characteristically have diabetes mellitus, gallbladder disease, diarrhea, weight loss, steatorrhea, and hypochlorhydria[26,39,41] (see Table 34.5-6). The mean age of patients is approximately 50 years.[39]

Somatostatinomas occur in the pancreas in 56% to 75% of cases, and the remainder occur in the upper small intestine.[39] Tumors have a predilection for the pancreatic head and occur there two to three times as often as in the body or tail.[39] In 90%, the tumors are solitary and range from 1.5 to 10 cm in diameter. Tumors have evidence of metastatic spread at diagnosis or operation in 84% to 92% of patients.[39] The symptoms in patients with intestinal somatostatinomas are usually less severe than in those with pancreatic primary tumors presumably due to earlier diagnosis and a slightly lower incidence of metastases.[39] Diabetes mellitus, gallbladder disease, steatorrhea, and hypochlorhydria are present in more than 80% of patients with pancreatic tumors but fewer than half of those with intestinal tumors.[26,39] Metastases usually occur in the liver (75% of patients with metastases) but also in the regional lymph nodes (31%) and in bone less frequently.[39]

Electron microscopic studies reported that the secretory granules were typical of those in D cells in 89% of the tumors examined.[39] Immunocytochemical analysis shows somatostatin-like immunoreactive material in tumors and in addition 33% contained insulin, 27% calcitonin, and 13% gastrin.

GRFomas are the most recently described PET syndrome and have excessive release of the hormone growth hormone–releasing factor (GRF).[49] In reviews of GRFomas,[50] 29% to 30% originated in the pancreas, 53% in the lung, 10% in small intestine, and a rare case in the adrenal gland. Multiple pancreatic tumors have been reported in 30% of patients with GRFomas.[50] Approximately 40% of all GRFomas occur in patients with ZES, and in 40% of patients Cushing's syndrome was also present.[26,50] Tumors are generally large (more than 6 cm), varying from 1 to 25 cm in diameter.[50] On light-microscopical studies, typical neuroendocrine features are present, including trabecular or solid nests and sheets of uniform tumor cells.[48,50] Immunohistochemical studies demonstrate GRF-immunoreactive material in all tumors examined with 10% to 80% of cells possessing GRF.[48,50]

Patients are between 15 and 63 years of age with an average age of 38.[48,50] A female predominance (73%) is seen for all GRFomas. The known actions of GRF as a stimulator of growth hormone release account for the clinical presentation with acromegaly.[50] Acromegalic features are indistinguishable from those of patients with classic acromegaly and include enlargement of hands and feet, facial changes, skin changes, headache, and peripheral nerve entrapment.[48,50] The time from the onset of the acromegalic changes to the diagnosis was 5.3 years in patients with pancreatic GRFomas.[50] The diagnosis should be suspected in any patient with acromegaly without a pituitary adenoma imaged by magnetic resonance imaging (MRI) or with an abdominal mass[48] and is confirmed by measuring plasma GRF levels.

IMAGING AND LOCALIZATION OF PANCREATIC ENDOCRINE TUMORS

The nature and extent of imaging necessary to stage and treat PETs varies depending on the type of tumor and the clinical presentation. For example, relatively precise localization of gastrinoma has become an increasingly important factor in evaluating patients with ZES.[31,51] With the ability to control gastric acid hypersecretion using antisecretory drugs, the functional sequelae of the tumor can be completely controlled, which allows time to determine the location and extent of the gastrinoma. In addition, the ability for long-term control of gastric acid hypersecretion has made tumor growth and metastatic spread an increasingly important determinant of long-term survival.[7,11] Gastrinomas are frequently multiple and extrapancreatic, and accurate imaging assists in determining the nature of the operative procedure. Imaging studies identify resectable metastatic disease to the liver in up to 15% of patients.[52–54]

For patients with insulinoma the extent of preoperative imaging necessary to ensure an operative cure has not been clearly defined.[26,28,29,55] Most agree that some form of preoperative imaging to eliminate the possibility of hepatic metastases is appropriate. On the other hand, radiographic investigations are concentrated on the pancreas because, unlike gastrinomas, virtually all insulinomas are within the parenchyma of the pancreas (Fig. 34.5-1).[26,28] It is generally agreed that some preoperative localization is essential, primarily because insulinomas are frequently small (90% less than 2 cm in diameter) and to a lesser extent because of the wish to identify metastatic spread to prevent unnecessary surgery. For other PETs imaging to identify occult disease is almost never necessary, because most tumors are large at diagnosis.

A number of different techniques, including abdominal ultrasonography, computed tomography (CT), MRI, selective abdominal angiography, intraarterial secretin with hepatic venous gastrin sampling, somatostatin receptor scintigraphy (SRS), endoscopic ultrasonography (EUS) preoperatively, intraoperative ultrasonography (IOUS), and intraoperative endoscopic transillumination of the duodenum at surgery, have been reported to be helpful in localizing gastrinomas[7,10,15,51,56,57] (Fig. 34.5-2). Transabdominal ultrasonography has a low sensitivity for localizing both primary and metastatic tumors; however, it has high specificity, is noninvasive, and on occasion localizes gastrinomas not found by other modalities. CT scan detects approximately 50% of all primary PETs and metastatic liver disease; however, its ability to detect primary tumors has been shown to be directly related to tumor size, with CT detecting no tumors smaller than 1 cm, 30% between 1 and 3 cm, and 95% larger than 3 cm.[51] Frequently, small primary tumors (less than 1 cm), which are being found increasingly in the duodenum, usually are missed by CT.[17,51,58] Furthermore, CT scan is less sensitive for detecting extrahepatic, extrapancreatic gastrinomas than pancreatic gastrinomas. Selective angiography was found to detect 68% of primary tumors and 86% of hepatic metastases. Angiography has been shown to detect 20% more hepatic metastases than CT, and the combination of these modalities detected 96% of all liver metastases.[15]

Improvements in the sensitivity of MRI have made it more useful than angiography or CT for imaging metastatic disease, but it remains less sensitive than angiography for imaging pri-

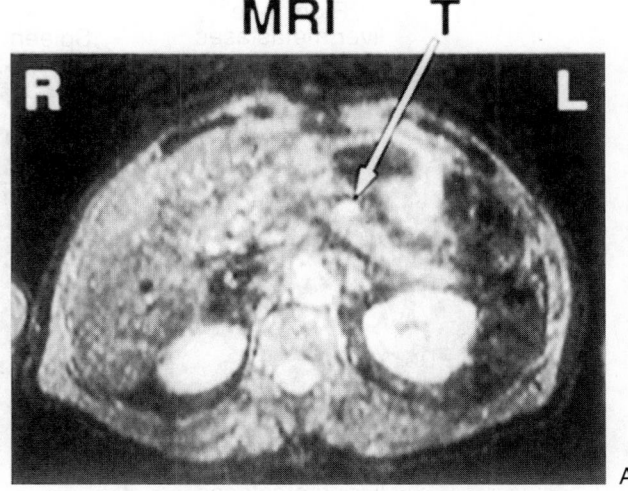

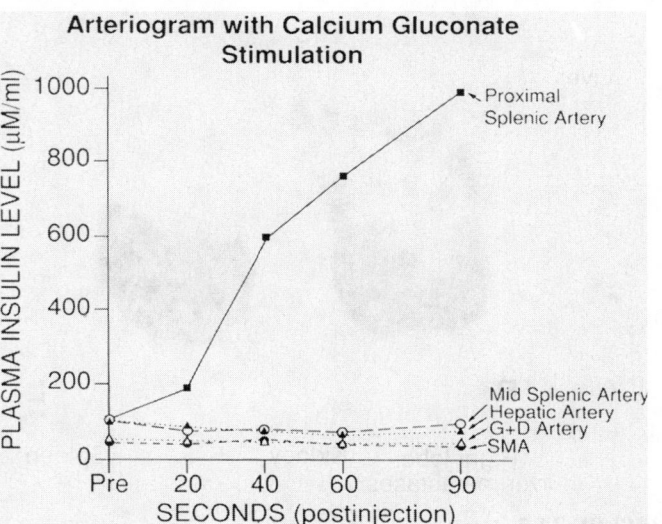

FIGURE 34.5-1. Results of hepatic venous sampling for insulin after intraarterial selective splanchnic injection with calcium. **A:** An enhancing mass is present in the proximal pancreatic body. **B:** A marked increase in hepatic vein insulin levels is seen after selective injection of calcium into the proximal splenic artery corresponding to the area of the lesion. G + D, gastroduodenal; MRI, magnetic resonance image; SMA, superior mesenteric artery; T, tumor.

mary tumors.[51] For insulinomas, ultrasonography localizes 33%, MRI 46%, CT 35%, dynamic CT 66%, selective arteriography 63%, and all imaging studies combined 80%.[26,28,57,59]

Many studies have demonstrated that gastrinomas as well as other PETs frequently have a high density of somatostatin receptors and that scanning after injection of the radiolabeled long-acting somatostatin analog octreotide localizes PETs.[57,60] This technique is one of the most sensitive methods for localizing primary or metastatic PETs except insulinomas.[56,57,60,61] It localizes 60% of primary gastrinomas and more than 90% of liver metastases[15] (see Fig. 34.5-2). The sensitivity of SRS in identifying gastrinoma in patients before operation increases with tumor size; only 30% of tumors 1.1 cm or smaller and 64% of those 1.1 to 2.0 cm are detected, compared with 96% of tumors larger than 2 cm.[56] SRS appears to be the procedure of choice to screen ZES patients for the presence of bone

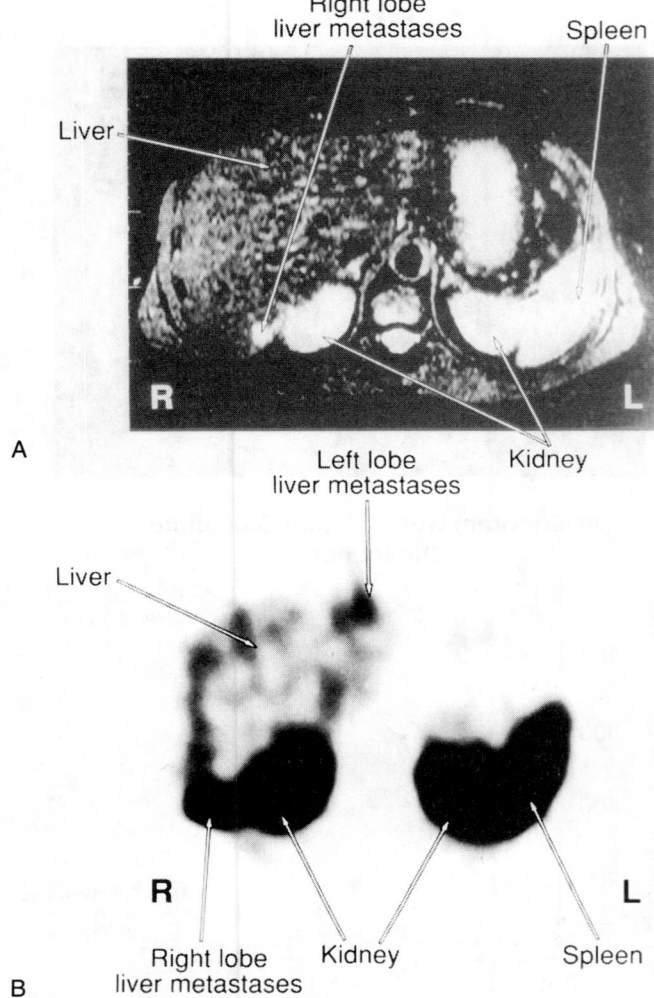

A

B

FIGURE 34.5-2. Example of somatostatin receptor scintigraphy (SRS) sensitivity in detecting gastrinoma. A patient with biochemically confirmed Zollinger-Ellison syndrome underwent imaging studies. The magnetic resonance image **(A)** demonstrated a single liver metastasis in the posterior aspect of the right lobe; however, the SRS scan **(B)** showed a second positive signal in the right lobe that was subsequently shown to be metastatic gastrinoma.

metastases. In a study of 115 patients with ZES 8 (7%) were determined to have bone metastases using SRS, whereas a false-positive bone scan was obtained in 52.[62] Because it is noninvasive, has high sensitivity, and has the ability to image the entire body for metastatic foci, SRS should be considered as the initial imaging modality for patients with all PETs except insulinomas[15,57,60,63] (see Figs. 34.5-1 and 34.5-2).

EUS is being increasingly used to localize PETs and is reported to localize 75% of primary gastrinomas, particularly within the pancreatic parenchyma.[53,64,65] However, EUS is an invasive procedure, and whether additional information is obtained beyond that provided by SRS or current MRI techniques is unproven. EUS is reported to have a high sensitivity, localizing 80% of insulinomas even though 15% were no more than 1 cm in diameter.[53,65]

Most gastrinomas (91%) demonstrate a paradoxic release of gastrin with intravenous injection of secretin.[7] This characteris-

tic has been used to localize gastrinomas selectively by injecting secretin intraarterially into various abdominal arteries and collecting venous samples from the hepatic veins for assays of gastrin.[66] Injection into the arterial supply of the tumor area causes a marked increase in gastrin level. However, whether this test can assist the surgeon in localizing gastrinomas that would not otherwise be found at surgery has not been studied prospectively.

Selective intraarterial injection of the secretagogue calcium [intraarterial injection of calcium (IAC)] into the various regions of the celiac axis during angiography with subsequent hepatic venous sampling for the peptide hormone of interest is a technique used to localize occult functional pancreatic neuroendocrine tumors, particularly insulinomas. IAC has a reported sensitivity of 94% in localizing insulinomas[29] and is also reported to have greater specificity than secretin injections in localizing gastrinomas.[67] A typical result for an insulinoma is shown in Figure 34.5-1 and illustrates the rapid increase in hepatic vein insulin concentrations after infusion of calcium into the region of the pancreas containing tumor. IAC should eliminate the need to perform blind distal pancreatectomy in patients in whom tumors are not localized by other imaging modalities.

The use of IOUS has been shown to influence the operative approach in 10% of all ZES patients at surgery either by localizing additional gastrinomas or by determining that a gastrinoma is malignant.[68] IOUS may be particularly helpful for localizing intrapancreatic lesions and determining the relationship of the tumor to pancreatic or biliary ductal anatomy.[29,69]

Even though gastrinomas frequently occur in the duodenum (see Table 34.5-2), they are rarely seen by routine upper gastrointestinal endoscopy because they are small and submucosal in location. Duodenotomy and direct palpation has been shown to be the most sensitive method of identifying primary duodenal gastrinomas.[17,58]

TREATMENT OF RESECTABLE DISEASE

GASTRINOMA

In ZES patients, gastric acid hypersecretion must be controlled, because most patients are not cured after surgical exploration.[7,10,70] If acid hypersecretion is controlled, patients have an excellent quality of life; however, long-term prognosis is being increasingly determined by the malignant nature of the gastrinoma.[11,14] As many as 90% of gastrinomas may be malignant, and therefore it is important to consider surgical therapy directed at the primary and metastatic disease if feasible (Fig. 34.5-3).

Management of Gastric Acid Hypersecretion

Numerous studies have demonstrated that gastric acid hypersecretion can now be controlled medically over the long term in every patient who reliably takes oral medication, using the H^+-K^+–adenosine triphosphatase inhibitor omeprazole or lansoprazole.[7,70–72] The availability of these agents and their long duration of action has greatly simplified management because they can be taken once or twice per day. Total gastrectomy

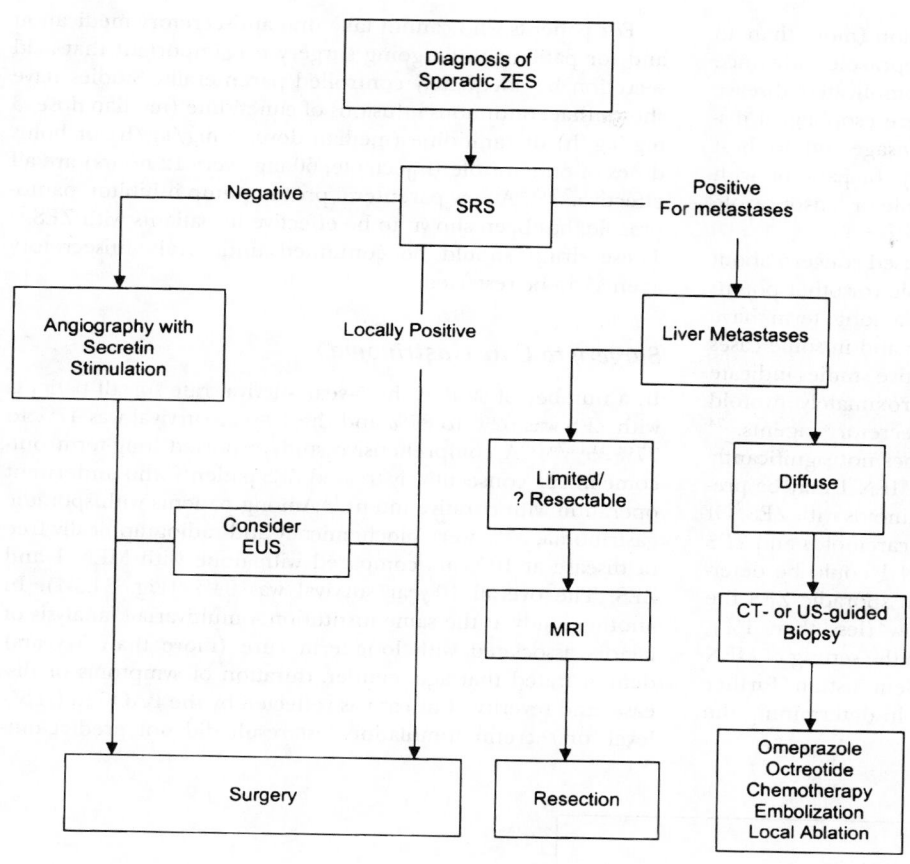

FIGURE 34.5-3. Flow diagram showing a proposed workup for patients with newly diagnosed sporadic Zollinger-Ellison syndrome (ZES). After the biochemical confirmation of disease, an initial screening study with somatostatin receptor scintigraphy (SRS) should be performed. Patients who have results positive for metastases should have additional imaging studies. If disease is confined to the liver, then resection or other therapies as shown should be considered. For those who have a locally positive result, endoscopic ultransonography (US) should be considered, after which patients undergo exploration with curative intent. If SRS results are negative, then angiography with selective secretin stimulation should be performed. CT, computed tomography; MRI, magnetic resonance imaging.

should be reserved for very specific circumstances such as those in which a patient does not have access to routine medical follow-up or cannot or will not take oral medication reliably.[7,72] Parietal cell vagotomy in ZES patients in whom no tumor was resected decreased BAO by 66%, although most patients still needed some antisecretory drug; at present, however, parietal cell vagotomy is not performed routinely.[20] In patients with ZES and the MEN 1 syndrome, correction of hyperparathyroidism reduces the FSG concentration, increases the responsiveness to a given dose of antisecretory medication, or decreases the BAO.[73] Therefore, in patients with ZES and MEN 1 with hyperparathyroidism, parathyroidectomy should be performed before any contemplated surgical procedure to control acid hypersecretion.

The results of medical treatment of gastric acid hypersecretion have been reviewed extensively.[3,7,70,72] Histamine H_2 antagonists (cimetidine, ranitidine, famotidine) alone or in combination with anticholinergic agents [propantheline (Pro-Banthine), isopropamide] and more recently the substituted benzimidazole (omeprazole), which functions as an H^+-K^+-adenosine triphosphatase inhibitor, have been used successfully in the long-term treatment of gastric hypersecretion in ZES.[7,72] The number of patients for whom medical therapy fails varies greatly in different series: from 0% to 65% for cimetidine, from 0% to 40% for ranitidine, 0% for famotidine, and from 0% to 7.5% for omeprazole and lansoprazole.[7,70–72] In general, relief of symptoms does not adequately reflect the effectiveness of antisecretory therapy. Most studies have demonstrated that to assess the adequacy

of antisecretory therapy, gastric acid secretion must be measured while the patient is taking medication.[7,72]

The amount of antisecretory medication required varies widely from patient to patient; thus the optimal dose of medication must be determined for each patient initially and must be reevaluated periodically.[7,70,72] Studies have shown that if enough antisecretory drug is used to decrease gastric acid secretion to less than 10 mEq/h for the hour before the next dose of medication in patients who did not previously undergo gastric surgery and to less than 5 mEq/h in patients who previously underwent acid-reducing procedures or have severe esophageal disease, peptic ulcers will heal and complications of peptic ulcer disease will be prevented.[7,70,72] To reduce acid output to these levels before the next dose of medication, patients frequently require more than twice the usual dose of histamine H_2 antagonist or three times the usual dose of omeprazole recommended for idiopathic peptic ulcer disease.[7,70,72] Average doses are 3.6 g/d for cimetidine, 1.2 g/d for ranitidine, 0.25 g/d for famotidine, 20 to 80 mg/d for omeprazole, and 30 to 120 mg/d for lansoprazole.[7,70,72] The long-term use of these doses of H_2 antagonists and omeprazole has proven not only effective but also safe.[7,70,72] Except for antiandrogen side effects (impotence, gynecomastia, and breast tenderness) with high-dose cimetidine in up to 60% of male patients, long-term treatment with cimetidine in females or with ranitidine, famotidine, or omeprazole in patients of either sex has been shown to be safe.[7,70,72] Most patients with ZES require histamine H_2 antagonists every 4 to 8 hours to adequately inhibit gastric secretion, whereas omeprazole or lansoprazole has a very long duration of action (more than 48 hours),[7,70,72] so that most patients take omeprazole only once or twice a day. Patients with ZES with complicated disease (previous gastric surgery, moderate to severe esophageal disease, or MEN 1) usually require a higher dosage and are best treated by starting with 40 mg twice a day. In patients with uncomplicated ZES the dosage of omeprazole or lansoprazole can be reduced with time in more than 85%.[7,72]

The long-term use of omeprazole has caused concern about toxicity because female rats given omeprazole (or other potent inhibitors of gastric acid secretion) over a long term have developed proliferation of gastric ECL cells and in some cases carcinoid tumors of the stomach.[8] Quantitative studies indicate that gastric ECL cells are increased approximately twofold independent of administration of antisecretory agents.[7,74] Omeprazole treatment for up to 4 years does not significantly increase gastric ECL cells.[7,72] Patients with MEN 1 may be predisposed to the development of gastric carcinoids with ZES. Of 15 of the 16 patients reported with gastric carcinoids and ZES in whom the presence or absence of MEN 1 could be determined, 14 had MEN 1.[7,74] In patients with sporadic ZES the incidence of gastric carcinoids is very low (less than 1%), whereas 13% to 30% of patients with ZES in the setting of MEN 1 have gastric carcinoids.[7,74] These data demonstrate further the importance of the presence of MEN 1 in determining the development of gastric carcinoids.

For patients who cannot take oral antisecretory medication and for patients undergoing surgery it is important that acid secretion be adequately controlled parenterally. Studies have shown that continuous infusions of cimetidine (median dose, 3 mg/kg/h) or ranitidine (median dose, 1 mg/kg/h) or bolus doses of omeprazole (injectable, 60 mg every 12 hours) are all effective.[7,70,72] A new parenteral proton pump inhibitor, pantoprazole, has been shown to be effective in patients with ZES.[75] These drugs should be continued until oral antisecretory agents can be restarted.

Surgery to Cure Gastrinoma

In a number of studies the 5-year survival rate for all patients with ZES was 62% to 87% and the 10-year survival was 47% to 77%.[11,14,76,77] A comprehensive study reported long-term outcome in 151 consecutively treated ZES patients who underwent operation with curative intent.[10] Among patients with sporadic gastrinoma, 34% were biochemically and radiographically free of disease at 10 years compared with none with MEN 1 and ZES. The overall 10-year survival was 94% (Fig. 34.5-4). In another study at the same institution a multivariate analysis of factors associated with long-term cure (more than 5 years) demonstrated that age, gender, duration of symptoms or disease, and severity of disease as reflected by the BAO level, FSG level, or secretin stimulation test result did not predict out-

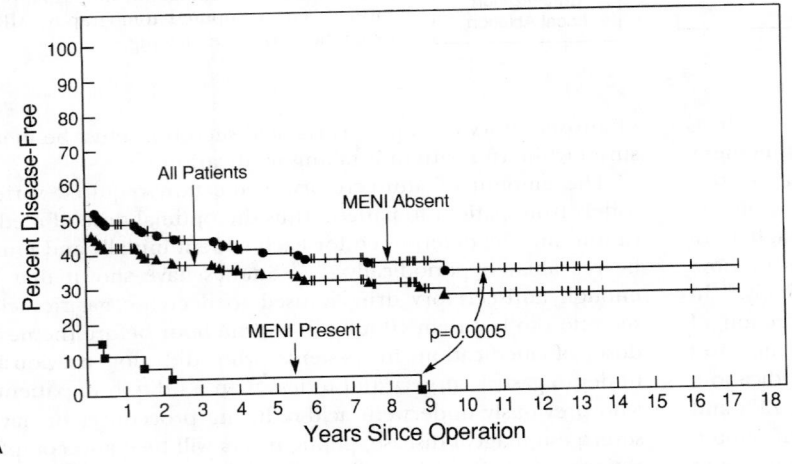

A

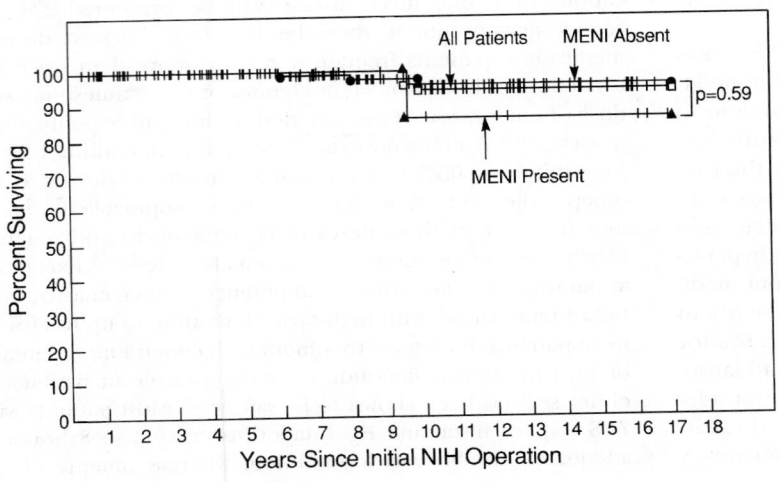

B

FIGURE 34.5-4. Disease-free (**A**) and disease-specific (**B**) survival in patients with ZES. **A:** A Kaplan-Meier plot of disease-free survival after surgical exploration to resect and potentially cure gastrinoma. Twenty-eight patients with Zollinger-Ellison syndrome (ZES) and multiple endocrine neoplasia type 1 (MEN1) underwent 32 surgical explorations, and 123 patients with sporadic ZES underwent 144 surgical explorations. Data are presented based on number of operative procedures rather than number of patients. Results show the percentage of the total number of surgical patients in each group who are disease free at the indicated time. **B:** A Kaplan-Meier plot of survival specific for ZES. There were four deaths: secondary to progressive metastatic disease in three patients and a paradoxic cerebral embolus postoperatively through a patent foramen ovale valley in one patient. NIH, National Institutes of Health. (Data from ref. 10.)

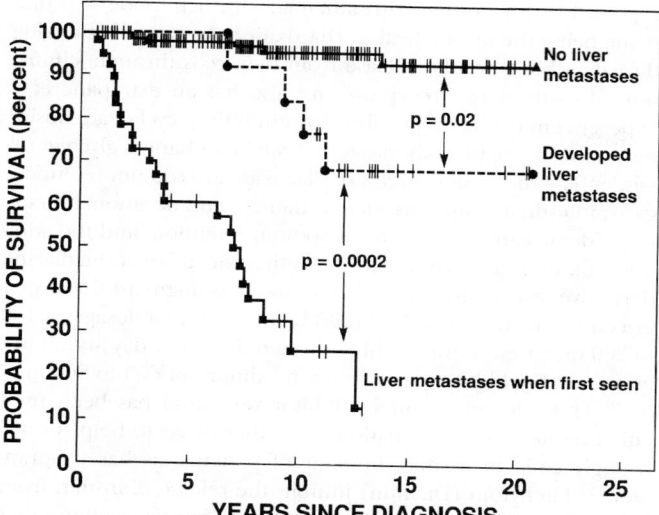

FIGURE 34.5-5. Survival based on the presence or absence of liver metastases in patients with Zollinger-Ellison syndrome (ZES). Survival rates were evaluated using death due to ZES-related causes. Six of 158 patients with no liver metastases died; 17 patients developed liver metastases during the follow-up period, of whom 4 died; and 23 of 37 patients who presented with liver metastases on initial evaluation died. (Data from ref. 10.)

come.[78] Only a diagnosis of MEN 1 was inversely correlated with cure. In addition, the status of preoperative imaging studies (either positive or negative), tumor size, and number of tumors resected did not correlate with cure. However, a normal postoperative FSG level and secretin stimulation test result did independently and significantly predict cure.

Even though the growth of gastrinoma is generally slow, in long-term studies of patients originally treated by total gastrectomy, 57% of deaths were due to tumor progression.[7] Therefore, with the ability to control gastric acid hypersecretion, the malignant potential of the tumor is an increasingly important determinant of long-term prognosis. The extent of the tumor as well as the presence of MEN 1 have been reported to determine survival rates.[14] In patients with no tumor found at laparotomy or in whom tumor is completely resected, 5- and 10-year survival rates are 90% to 100%.[10] In contrast, patients with liver metastases have a 5-year survival rate of only 53% and a 10-year survival rate of 30%[11] (Fig. 34.5-5). It is not clear whether ZES patients with MEN 1 have a better 5- and 10-year survival rate than patients without MEN 1.[7,10,79] One study[11] reported a significant difference in the percentage of patients with ZES with MEN 1 (6%) who presented with liver metastases and those without MEN 1 (22%, *P* = .03) who had metastases. For the patients without liver metastases, no difference was seen in survival rates between MEN 1 and non–MEN 1 patients. PETs that produce ACTH have a virulent biologic behavior and a poor prognosis.[14,23]

Because of the excellent prognosis of patients with gastrinoma who undergo resection and evidence of the increased importance of the malignancy in determining survival, surgical resection of gastrinoma is offered to patients with good medical risk who have ZES. One study has shown that surgical resection of gastrinoma may alter the natural history of the disease. Only 3% of patients (3 of 98) with ZES undergoing tumor resection

developed liver metastases during follow-up, whereas significantly more patients treated medically developed liver metastases (26% or 6 of 26 patients; *P* <.003).[80] Although this was not a randomized study, the two groups did not differ in clinical or laboratory characteristics or time of follow-up (15.4 ± 1.5 years from onset for those with no surgery versus 14.0 ± 0.8 years for those with surgery). The percentage of patients in whom gastrinoma can be identified and resected has increased with increasing experience and appreciation for the presence of small duodenal primary lesions.[58] The improvement in outcome after surgical exploration and resection with curative intent in most recent series is due to a number of factors. Because gastric acid hypersecretion can be managed in all patients with antisecretory agents, surgical exploration can be done electively and safely.[7,10,72] Patients can be effectively screened to eliminate occult metastatic unresectable disease and patient selection for potentially curative surgery thereby improved.[15] Furthermore, the appreciation that small duodenal primary tumors are more frequent than previously realized has resulted in higher rates of detection and resection of these frequently small lesions than in earlier studies.[10,17,58] One study[58] demonstrated that the routine use of duodenotomy significantly increases the cure rate.

At laparotomy, the entire pancreas as well as the duodenum should be dissected and exposed.[69] IOUS, duodenal transillumination, and routine duodenotomy should be performed.[17,69] Palpation alone can identify 65% of duodenal gastrinomas, endoscopic transillumination an additional 20% of tumors, and duodenotomy an additional 15% of tumors not localized by any other modality. Of duodenal tumors, 71% are in the first part of the duodenum, 21% in the second part, and 8% in the third part.[17] When this approach has been used, gastrinomas have been found in all patients undergoing operation.[10] At laparotomy, if a gastrinoma is found as a solitary lesion in the liver, it should be removed, provided the resection can be performed safely. If gastrinoma is found in the pancreatic head it should be enucleated. If extensive gastrinoma not amenable to eradication is found in the pancreatic head area, performing a pancreaticoduodenectomy (Whipple operation) for potential cure is controversial because of the possible morbidity and mortality associated with this procedure and the excellent long-term prognosis of these patients.[53] In the future, if it is possible to identify a subset of patients with a worse prognosis, then use of this procedure despite the increased risk might be justified. If no gastrinoma is found at surgery, a blind distal pancreatectomy should not be performed, because the majority of primary tumors are located in the pancreatic head or duodenum. In addition, ectopic gastrinoma can occur in a variety of other locations, including small bowel mesentery, liver, common bile duct, and ovary.[7,12,52]

At surgery the use of IOUS is recommended to localize additional lesions, to confirm the significance of a palpated mass, and to establish the relationship between the tumor and the pancreatic duct.[68,69] For either pancreatic or duodenal primaries, any abnormal or suspicious lymph nodes in that area should be excised. In some patients undergoing exploration, disease may be limited to one or more lymph nodes.[16] Despite the inability to identify a primary site of disease in the duodenum or pancreas, long-term biochemical cures can be achieved. In a study[16] with a mean follow up of 10.2 years, 10% of 138 patients had only a lymph node containing gastrinoma resected and remained cured. No chemical laboratory or lymph node characteristic at surgery was predictive of whether the lymph node was a primary tumor, which supports the conclusion that lymph nodes from the gastrinoma triangle should be routinely removed at exploration.[16]

At present, the role of surgery in the treatment of patients with ZES with MEN 1 is unclear.[53,81] Numerous studies show that in MEN 1 patients with ZES, 70% to 95% of primary tumors arise in duodenum and 10% to 25% in pancreas.[53,82] Cure is not possible in patients with MEN 1 and ZES short of pancreaticoduodenectomy, because 30% of patients have more than 20 duodenal tumors and 86% of patients have positive lymph nodes.[78,82,83] In 77 patients with MEN 1 and ZES, the only independent factor associated with the development of liver metastases was a pancreatic primary tumor larger than 3 cm.[84] However, operation with curative intent in 118 patients did not influence survival. Because biochemical relapse occurs in more than 95% of individuals within 3 to 5 years of surgery,[78] patients with MEN 1 and ZES have an excellent prognosis, acid secretion can be completely controlled medically, there are multiple other pancreatic tumors, and the morbidity of pancreaticoduodenectomy can be considerable, this procedure is not routinely recommended. There are data suggesting that MEN 1 kindreds with truncating mutations of the gene in exons 2, 9, or 10 may have tumors with a particularly aggressive biologic behavior.[85] The authors' current recommendation[10,82] is to operate on patients with MEN 1 and ZES when a tumor of at least 2.5 cm is seen on imaging studies. This policy is based on the observation that metastases to the liver correlate with tumor size.[11] If the tumor is in the pancreatic head it is enucleated if possible; if it is in the pancreatic tail it is resected and a duodenal exploration is performed.

Because most patients with sporadic ZES undergoing operation and resection have persistent or recurrent disease, the role of reoperation in these patients is an important issue that has not been well studied.[53] In a series of 17 patients who had previously undergone an operation with curative intent, 18 reoperations were performed on the basis of biochemically documented recurrent disease and one or more positive results on imaging studies.[86] In patients undergoing reoperation, it was possible to identify and resect disease in 17 of 18 cases with biochemical cures in all, although median follow-up was short (34 months). Of note, the site of recurrent disease identified at reoperation was related to the initial operative findings. For example, of those who had lymph node disease resected initially, most patients had lesions identified in the duodenum at reoperation. On the other hand, in those who had a primary duodenal or pancreatic lesion initially resected, recurrence was commonly identified in regional lymph nodes. Because of the increase in potential risk associated with reoperation in this setting, reoperation should be considered carefully.

INSULINOMA

Medical Therapy for Hypoglycemia of Insulinoma

The simplest form of nonsurgical treatment for insulinoma is dietary management. Many insulinoma patients begin consuming frequent small meals to alleviate symptoms before seeking medical evaluation, and a significant percentage report weight gain in the year before diagnosis. A number of drugs have been reported to control hyperinsulinemia, with octreotide and diazoxide being the most effective. Diazoxide, a benzthiazide analog, directly inhibits insulin release from beta cells through stimulation of α-adrenergic receptors and also has an extrapancreatic hyperglycemic effect, possibly by inhibiting cyclic adenosine monophosphate phosphodiesterase, which enhances glycogenolysis.[1,26] The major side effects of diazoxide are sodium retention, gastrointestinal symptoms such as nausea, and occasional hirsutism. Edema can result from the sodium retention, and the addition of a diuretic such as trichlormethiazide, a benzothiadiazine derivative, can correct the edema as well as augment the hyperglycemic effect. Diazoxide should be initiated at a dosage of 150 to 200 mg given in two to three divided doses per day and, if not effective, should be increased to a maximum of 600 to 800 mg/d.[1,26] The calcium channel inhibitor verapamil has been used either alone or in combination with other drugs to help control hypoglycemia in a small number of patients, as has propranolol.[1,26] Phenytoin (Dilantin) inhibits the release of insulin from beta cells and has been used successfully to treat a small number of patients with refractory hypoglycemia. Maintenance doses of 300 to 600 mg/d are used, and it is reported that in only one-third or fewer patients is the hyperglycemic effect of phenytoin of any clinical significance. Glucocorticoids (prednisone 1 mg/kg) and glucagon either alone or with diazoxide have also been used in a few patients.

Octreotide controls symptoms and hypoglycemia in 40% to 60% of patients.[1,26,87,88] Octreotide is generally well tolerated and is usually initiated at doses of 50 μg subcutaneously two or three times a day, which can be increased to 1500 μg/d.[87,88] The main side effects are gastrointestinal, such as bloating and abdominal cramping, and include long-term side effects such as malabsorption and cholelithiases.[59,87,88] Besides improving symptoms, octreotide decreases plasma insulin levels in 65% of patients with insulomas.[88] However, most patients were treated for less than 1 week before surgery, so the long-term efficacy is not known in a significant number of patients. Octreotide also decreases plasma glucagon levels and growth hormone secretion; hence, it may worsen the hypoglycemia in some patients.[59,88]

Surgery to Cure Insulinoma

All insulinomas without evidence of metastases should be surgically removed, regardless of the severity of symptoms. Of all insulinomas, 80% to 90% are benign isolated lesions that are cured by complete surgical removal.[28,55,59] The extent of preoperative imaging necessary for successful outcome for resection of presumed benign solitary pancreatic insulinoma is controversial (Fig. 34.5-6).[28,29,55] Because insulinomas are exclusively located within the pancreatic parenchyma, thorough exploration and intraoperative evaluation with inspection, palpation and IOUS can result in successful resection in the vast majority of patients undergoing operation. IOUS has been advocated as an important adjunct in operation for insulinoma not only in identifying lesions at the time of surgery but as an aid in enucleating the lesion by identifying the relationship between the tumor in the pancreatic parenchyma and the adjacent pancreatic duct.[69] This is particularly important in the case of lesions located in the head of the pancreas, where a resection other than enucleation would require pancreaticoduodenectomy. Selective arterial stimulation of the splenic vessels supplying the pancreas using the secretagogue calcium can produce a subsequent rise in insulin levels obtained

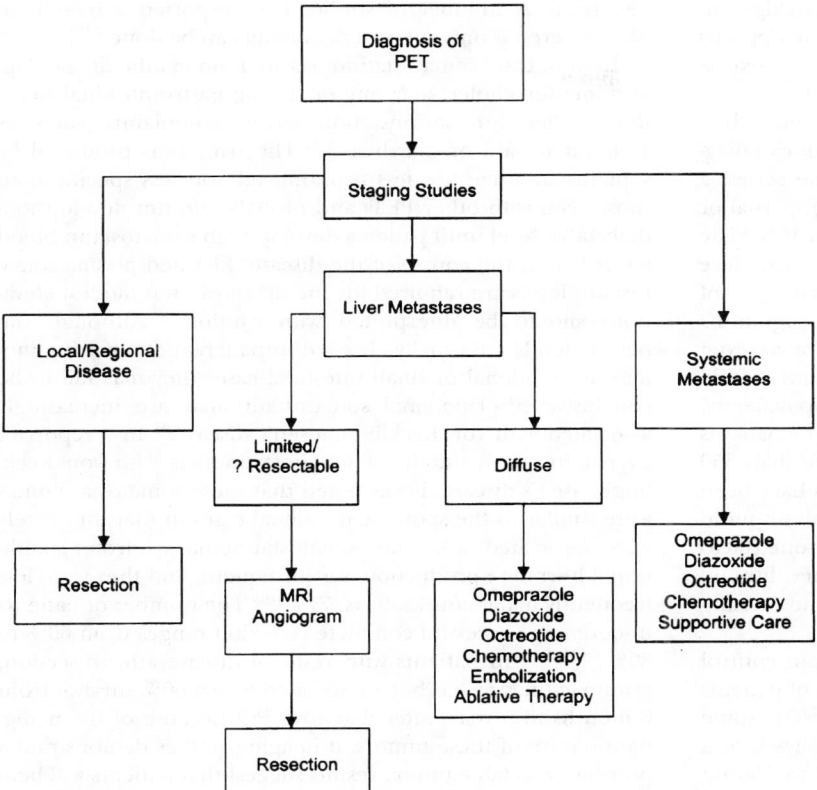

FIGURE 34.5-6. Flow diagram illustrating the general approach and management strategy for patients with pancreatic neuroendocrine tumors (PETs). Once the diagnosis has been established, initial staging studies are performed to determine the absence or presence of metastatic disease. A variety of palliative options are available to control the functional sequelae of hormone excess for increasing tumor burden. For those patients who have isolated liver metastases, resection should be performed when possible. Other regional therapies that may cause durable palliation of symptoms or disease control in the liver should be attempted. For those who have local-regional disease, resection should be considered. MRI, magnetic resonance imaging.

from catheters positioned at the orifice of the hepatic veins.[29] The sensitivity of this test is almost 90% and allows one to direct attention to a particular region of the pancreas at the time of operation. Blind distal pancreatectomy has been used in an attempt to cure insulinoma in the past in patients in whom no lesion could be identified based on the appreciation that insulinomas can be distributed anywhere in the pancreatic parenchyma and resection of a large portion of normal pancreatic tissue should therefore have a reasonable cure rate for occult disease. However, given the current status of available localization studies, this practice should be largely unnecessary. With careful inspection and the use of IOUS, the proportion of patients with occult lesions that cannot be identified at the time of operation should be fewer than 5%.[29] In this setting the authors' recommendation would be to proceed with distal pancreatectomy only in the face of a positive insulin step-up in the hepatic veins after selective intraarterial stimulation with calcium demonstrates a bona fide step-up in the splenic artery compared with the gastroduodenal or hepatic arteries.

The liver must always be explored for evidence of metastatic disease and the entire abdomen explored to rule out rare extrapancreatic tumors that primarily secrete insulinoma-related growth factors. Insulinoma-related growth factor–secreting tumors causing hypoglycemia usually are of mesodermal origin and have considerable tumor bulk by the time symptoms of hypoglycemia occur. The entire pancreas must be explored for other tumors, because multifocal tumors occur in up to 10% of all cases.[36,59] Isolated lesions of the tail may be enucleated or removed *en bloc* by distal pancreatectomy, and there are reports of this procedure's being performed laparoscopically.[53,89,90] Body and head lesions require enucleation with careful dissection to avoid damage to the main pancreatic duct and its attendant morbidity. Larger tumors of the pancreatic

neck or proximal body can be resected via a median pancreatectomy to preserve pancreatic function.[91] Even in cases of documented metastatic disease, refractory debilitating symptoms may be an indication for debulking of the pancreatic lesions, because metastases are not always secretory. Removal of peripancreatic lymph nodes may be palliative for malignant insulinoma if no liver metastases are present.[92]

The documentation of metastatic disease, either at the time of surgery or by imaging studies, is the only accurate means of diagnosing malignant insulinoma. Unlike all other PETs, malignant insulinomas are uncommon, occurring in only 5% to 15% of all cases (see Table 34.5-1). Malignant primary insulinomas are usually not occult and have a mean size of 6 cm, which is more than three times the size of benign insulinomas.[93] The median disease-free survival after curative resection of malignant insulinomas was 5 years in one series.[93] The recurrence rate was 63%, with the median interval to recurrence 2.8 years, and the median survival with recurrent tumor was 19 months. Palliative re-resection was associated with a median survival of 4 years, whereas median survival after biopsy was only 11 months.[93] Surgical resection of primary and metastatic insulinomas is desirable when possible. Malignant insulinomas, like other PETs, may respond to chemotherapy and treatment with octreotide.[87,88] The use of these agents for all malignant PETs is described later in Treatment of Metastatic Disease.

OTHER PANCREATIC ENDOCRINE TUMORS

The remainder of the PETs are relatively infrequent and include VIP-producing tumors (VIPomas), glucagonomas, ACTHomas, somatostatinomas, and GRF-producing pancreatic tumors (GRFomas). Each of these PETs is usually malignant. Interventions designed to ablate or extirpate tumor deposits are usually indicated to palliate the consequences of excess hormone production (see Fig. 34.5-6).

The treatment is surgical if possible, even in the more than 60% of cases in which metastases are present at the time of diagnosis.[3,26] Of 25 cases of nonfunctional PETs in one series, a Whipple procedure was done in five patients (20%), partial or total pancreatectomy in 25%, and tumor excision in 10%. The remaining patients had a biopsy only. The survival rates were 60% at 3 years and 44% at 5 years in this series. The cure rate of these tumors at present is low because of their late recognition.

The first treatment objective in patients with VIPomas, even before the diagnosis is considered, is the replenishment of fluid and electrolyte losses to correct the profound hypokalemia, dehydration, and acidosis that are usually present. The patients may require 5 L or more of fluid per day and more than 350 mEq/d of potassium.[26] In the past, numerous drugs have been reported to control, to varying degrees, the diarrheal output in small numbers of VIPoma patients, including prednisone (60 to 100 mg/d), clonidine, indomethacin, phenothiazines, lithium carbonate, propanolol, metoclopramide, loperamide, lidamidine, angiotensin II, and norepinephrine.[26,41]

Octreotide, a long-acting somatostatin analog, can control the diarrhea in both the short and long term in 87% of patients with VIPoma, and it is now the agent of choice.[26,41,87,88] In some patients, responses have been reported to be short-lived, or a patient may respond initially to a low dosage (50 to 100 μg three times a day) but subsequently require a larger dosage to control the diarrhea, which may even become refractory to dosages up to 1200 μg/d.[26,87,88] In nonresponsive patients or in patients whose symptoms recur, the administration of glucocorticoids concomitant with octreotide has proven effective in a small number of cases.[26,87,88] With octreotide treatment, plasma VIP concentrations decreased in 80% to 88% of patients.[26,87,88]

After imaging studies to localize the primary VIPoma and determine the extent of the tumor, in all patients without metastatic disease surgical excision for cure should be considered. Surgical resection of a pancreatic VIPoma relieves symptoms in 33% of patients.[26,87,88] Surgical resection controls symptoms in the majority of patients.[26,87,88]

For patients with glucagonomas, medical therapy with octreotide improves dermatitis and relieves diarrhea in 54% to 90% of patients, with complete disappearance in up to 30%.[26,45,87,88] Diabetes mellitus, which can be severe enough to warrant the use of oral hypoglycemic agents or insulin therapy in more than 40%, may not be improved with octreotide treatment.[26,45,87,88] Plasma glucagon levels decreased in 80% to 90% of patients with octreotide treatment but decreased into the normal range in only 10% to 20% of patients.[26,45,87,88]

In 50% to 80% of patients, metastases are already present at the time of diagnosis.[46] In patients with resectable disease, surgical resection has been successful in a number of cases,[46] but the exact percentage of cases that can be cured is not known. In one large review involving 92 cases of glucagonoma, only 16 of the malignant cases were treated by surgical resection only. Only seven patients had normal plasma glucagon levels after resection, and of the five patients who had no evidence of metastatic spread, plasma glucagon levels were normal postoperatively in two. Even if a patient eventually develops a recurrence, an extended disease-free interval may be attained that is

beneficial. A number of studies have reported a benefit to patients even if only surgical debulking can be done.[46]

In most cases somatostatinomas are found at the time of laparotomy for cholecystectomy or during gastrointestinal imaging studies for various nonspecific complaints such as abdominal pain or diarrhea.[26,39] The symptoms produced by somatostatinomas are less pronounced and less specific than those seen with other PETs and probably do not develop to a detectable level until patients develop high somatostatin blood levels late in the course of the disease. Elevated plasma somatostatin levels are required for the diagnosis, but modest elevations should be interpreted with caution.[48] Although the plasma levels are usually elevated in pancreatic somatostatinomas, in duodenal or small intestinal cases they may fail to be conclusive.[48,94] Duodenal somatostatinomas are increasingly associated with von Recklinghausen's disease.[94] In a report of 27 patients with duodenal somatostatinomas with von Recklinghausen's disease, it was noted that these somatostatinomas were similar to the sporadic duodenal cases in that they rarely were associated with the somatostatinoma syndrome, additional hormone production was infrequent, and they were less frequently malignant (30% vs. 71%).[94] The number of patients undergoing successful complete resection ranges from 60% to 80%.[26,31,38,95] In patients with residual disease after resection, cytotoxic therapy has been associated with a 60% survival from 6 months to 5 years after diagnosis.[26,39] Because of the malignant nature of these tumors, if imaging studies demonstrate a possible resectable tumor, results suggest that patients will benefit from surgical resection.

Surgical resection palliates the symptoms of patients with GRFoma.[50] Before surgery and in those patients with nonresectable lesions, various agents may reduce plasma growth hormone levels. Even though dopamine agonists such as bromocriptine are successful and widely used in patients with classical acromegaly, it is rarely possible to normalize plasma growth hormone levels in patients with GRFomas using these agents.[48,49] Octreotide significantly suppresses or normalizes growth hormone and insulin-like growth factor-1 levels, and in some cases this was associated with pituitary shrinkage.[26,87,88] In 75% of cases, octreotide decreased plasma GRF levels by more than 50%.[48,88]

In a few studies of patients with PETs secreting the peptide neurotensin, a neurotensinoma syndrome has been proposed.[3,39] Clinical features of patients with possible neurotensinomas include hypokalemia, weight loss, diabetes mellitus, cyanosis, hypotension, and flushing in a patient with a PET.[39] In a review of six cases, one-half of the patients were cured by resection of the PET and the remaining half improved with chemotherapy.[39] It is not clear if a specific neurotensinoma syndrome exists.[26]

Patients with PETs with Cushing's syndrome (ACTHoma) have been reported.[23,96] In some studies, 4% to 16% of Cushing's syndrome attributable to ectopic ACTH syndrome originated from a pancreatic tumor. Cushing's syndrome is reported in 19% of patients with ZES syndrome with MEN 1.[96] In these patients, the disease was of pituitary origin and was mild. Cushing's syndrome also is seen in 5% of sporadic cases of ZES due to ectopic ACTH production, occurs with metastatic PETs, responds poorly to chemotherapy, and is associated with a poor prognosis.[14,29,96] The occurrence of Cushing's syndrome as the only manifestation of a PET occurs in 37% to 60% of cases and it may precede any other hormonal syndrome.

Hypercalcemia due to a PET secreting a parathyroid hormone–related protein or an unknown hypercalcemic substance that mimics the action of parathyroid hormone and causes hyperparathyroidism has been reported.[97] The tumor is generally large and metastatic to the liver by the time of diagnosis, although in one case radical resection of a pancreatic tail tumor and subsequent treatment with chemotherapy resulted in a total remission for 5 years.[97]

TREATMENT OF METASTATIC DISEASE

The treatment of all metastatic PETs is considered as a unit because in most respects cytotoxic protocols and surgical approaches are generally similar. The long-term natural history of most functional PETs (malignant insulinomas, VIPomas, glucagonomas, GRFomas, somatostatinomas) is not known because, until recently, effective treatment for the functional syndrome did not exist and therefore patients often died of complications of the hormonal excess rather than the tumor per se.[14,98] In a study including 212 patients with ZES who had well-controlled gastric acid hypersecretion, 31% had died at a mean follow-up of almost 14 years.[14] One-half of these deaths were due to tumor progression, particularly in bone and liver, and to ectopic ACTH production. For patients with gastrinomas, the overall mean 10-year survival rate was 62% (range, 52% to 77%), and survival was influenced primarily by the extent of the tumor. If the tumor was not completely resectable or recurred after apparent complete resection, the mean 10-year survival rate was 30% to 67%. The development of metastatic liver disease is the primary determinant of survival in patients with PETs.[11,98,99] At present there are no data to suggest that survival of patients with other PETs will differ from that of patients with ZES, and in fact limited data for PPomas, most of which were metastatic, indicated a mean survival of 4.3 years and a 5-year survival rate of 44%, which is similar to that of patients with metastatic gastrinomas.[3,98] Treatment directed to metastatic unresectable liver disease is indicated for palliation of the functional sequelae of excess peptide hormone production and the effects of progressive or advanced tumor burden in the liver. Because of the frequently indolent nature of tumor progression, the timing of intervention should be individualized based on the rate of growth, severity of symptoms, and overall condition of the patient. Chemotherapy either alone or combined with cytoreductive surgery, hepatic arterial embolization alone or with chemotherapy, hormonal therapy with the long-acting somatostatin analog octreotide, interferon therapy, and hepatic transplantation have all been reported to be useful in small numbers of cases.[34,87,88,100–102]

CHEMOTHERAPY

In general, the efficacy of chemotherapeutic agents is presumed to be comparable for all types of metastatic PETs, although some data suggest that differences in responses rates may be observed based on histologic features or functional status.[34,101,103,104] Functioning PETs may have better response to chemotherapy than nonfunctioning tumors, and among functioning tumors, insulin- and VIP-secreting PETs may have more sensitivity to streptozotocin (STZ)-based therapies.[34,101,103] Except for STZ and chlorozotocin, single-agent chemotherapy with various other agents has had limited efficacy.[34,101,103,104] STZ, a glycosamine nitrosourea compound

originally derived from a *Streptomyces* species, was found to have cytotoxic effects on pancreatic islets and has generally been used for the treatment of metastatic PETs, most commonly in combination with other agents.[34,101,103,104]

The combination of etoposide and cisplatin has been evaluated in the treatment of 14 patients with metastatic PETs, and the results were compared with those in patients with metastatic carcinoid tumors (13 patients) and anaplastic neuroendocrine tumors (18 patients: 6, pancreas; 8, stomach or intestine; 1, lung; 3, unknown).[105] This study was performed because these two agents have activity in small cell lung cancer, which has neuroendocrine features histologically similar to those seen in PETs. Sixty-seven percent of the anaplastic neuroendocrine tumors, 14% of the PETs, and 0% of the metastatic carcinoid tumors demonstrated partial to complete regression. Other etoposide combinations including doxorubicin, cisplatin, and 5-fluorouracil have been tried in a small number of patients with limited success (i.e., response rate of 20%).[106] Glucagonomas are reported to respond frequently to dacarbazine,[1,26,34,46,101] and in some cases complete remissions have been achieved, whereas for other PETs the response rate is low.

In the first prospective randomized trial evaluating chemotherapy for metastatic islet cell cancer, which included 42 patients, the response rate to STZ alone was 36%, with 12% of patients showing a complete response, whereas the response rate to STZ plus 5-fluorouracil was 63%, with 33% of patients having a complete response.[103] A subsequent prospective randomized trial demonstrated that STZ and doxorubicin were superior to STZ and 5-fluorouracil or chlorozotocin alone (response rates of 69%, 45%, and 30%, respectively) in patients with advanced pancreatic neuroendocrine cancers.[104] Median duration of response was 18 months for the doxorubicin combination, 14 months for the 5-fluorouracil combination, and 17 months for chlorozotocin. Survival of patients treated with STZ and doxorubicin was significantly longer than that of those treated with the other regimens. In a prospective study of ten patients with progressive metastatic gastrinoma to the liver, chemotherapy with STZ, 5-fluorouracil, and doxorubicin resulted in only a 40% objective response rate, no complete remissions, and no statistical difference in survival in responders versus nonresponders.

STZ causes nausea and vomiting in almost all patients, dose-related renal dysfunction including proteinuria (20% to 70% of patients), decrease in creatinine clearance (20% to 70%), abnormalities in hepatic function (29%), and leukopenia and thrombocytopenia (6% to 9%). In one study, nine patients suffered from chronic renal failure and seven required dialysis; thus, its use must be carefully monitored.[104] The nausea and vomiting can now be controlled in almost all patients using serotonin $5-HT_3$-receptor antagonists such as ondansetron, so that renal dysfunction is the major dose-limiting toxic effect. Chlorozotocin is structurally closely related to STZ,[107] but it causes less nausea and vomiting than does STZ.

When chemotherapy should be initiated in a given patient with metastatic disease is not predictable, because the time course of tumor progression in patients with metastatic untreated PETs is highly variable. Of 19 patients with metastatic gastrinoma to the liver, 26% showed no tumor growth over a mean follow-up of 29 months, 32% had marginal progression (less than 50% increase in tumor volume), and 42% had rapid growth in less than 1 year.[108] The mean survival after diagnosis of metastatic gastrinoma is between 3 and 5 years.[7] Of the two groups with considerable experience in treating metastatic gastrinoma, one group proposed that patients be treated with chemotherapy when they become symptomatic.[103] However, if gastric acid hypersecretion is controlled adequately, symptoms due to the tumor arise only very late in the course of the disease. Another group proposed that after the initial evaluation patients be reassessed in 3 to 6 months and those patients with evidence of increasing size of hepatic metastases be treated with chemotherapy.

HORMONAL THERAPY WITH SOMATOSTATIN ANALOGS

Hormonal therapy with the long-acting somatostatin analog octreotide is effective in controlling the symptoms caused by a number of different pancreatic endocrine or carcinoid-like tumors, including VIPomas, glucagonomas, GRFomas, insulinomas, gastrinomas, and carcinoids.[26,87,88,109] More than 90% of all PETs except insulinomas possess somatostatin receptors,[26,87,88,109] and these may mediate the action of somatostatin on these tumors. Hormonal treatment with octreotide is reported to cause a decrease in tumor size in fewer than 15% of patients with malignant PETs.[26,87,88] However, octreotide results in stabilization of metastatic disease in 40% to 70% of patients,[26,87,88,109] although increased survival has not been demonstrated in these studies. These results must be extended to a larger, multicenter study, but they suggest that octreotide may have a cytostatic effect and, by decreasing the tumor growth rate, may possibly increase survival.

INTERFERON-α THERAPY

Interferon-α has been reported to be effective in controlling symptoms in patients with PETs.[101,107,110] A review of numerous new series involving 322 patients with various neuroendocrine tumors reported that 43% of patients showed a biochemical response (more than 50% decrease in hormone levels) and 12% showed a decrease in tumor size with treatment with interferon-α, either alone or in combination with other agents.[106] Of 57 patients with PETs, 47% had a biochemical response and 12% had a decrease in tumor size. The mean duration of the response was 20 months, and disease stabilization was seen in 25%. There was no difference in the response rate in patients with and without previous chemotherapy.

These results suggest that the effect of interferon-α on PETs is similar to that of octreotide in that interferon-α has minimal tumoricidal activity, with PETs rarely regressing with treatment; however, it may stabilize the disease in a significant percentage of patients. Interferon-α has been given in combination with 5-fluorouracil, octreotide, and 5-fluorouracil plus STZ[34,101,106] in some patients; however, the numbers are too small to clearly assess any advantages of these combinations.

HEPATIC ARTERY EMBOLIZATION

Hepatic artery embolization with or without postocclusion chemotherapy has been used successfully in small numbers of patients with metastatic PETs to the liver.[26,111–113] Some studies have reported that 68% to 100% of patients demonstrated symptomatic improvement.[26,112,113] In one study involving 111 patients, hepatic arterial occlusion was combined with chemotherapy using doxorubicin plus dacarbazine or STZ plus 5-fluorouracil in 64% of patients.[111] Objective remissions were observed in 60% of the patients treated with embolization

alone and in 80% of those with the chemotherapy added. Chemoembolization using doxorubicin in iodized oil combined with either gelatin powder or sponge particles has been reported in two studies to improve symptoms in 68% to 100% of patients and decrease tumor size or hormonal marker levels in 57% to 100%.[26,112,113] Side effects include abdominal pain, nausea, vomiting, and fever usually lasting 3 to 10 days. Severe complications occurring in 10% to 15% of patients include hepatic failure, infection, acute renal failure, and death. In a patient with a symptomatic PET and diffusely metastatic disease to the liver with minimal or no bone metastases in whom hormone symptoms cannot be controlled by octreotide, chemotherapy, or other medical treatment, this therapy should be considered.

SURGICAL TREATMENT

Systemic removal of all resectable tumor (debulking or cytoreductive surgery) has been recommended in general for patients with PETs (see Fig. 34.5-6).[41,48,53,54,114–116] There are no studies that have evaluated resection of metastatic disease in a controlled, prospective manner. It is important to differentiate the possible benefit of such surgery in patients with gastrinomas or nonfunctional tumors from that in patients with functional PETs, for whom medical therapy for the hormone excess state might be poor. In the former group the procedure must extend life or relieve tumor symptoms to be worthwhile, whereas in the latter group, improved ability to control the hormone excess state in situations without effective medical therapy may be a major benefit. A number of reports[53,54,99,114,116] have provided data supporting this approach. In one study 36 hepatic lobectomies or extended hepatectomies were performed and 38 nonanatomic liver resections were done.[116] Perioperative mortality was 2.7%, morbidity was 24%, and 4-year survival was 73%. Ninety percent of patients had a symptomatic improvement postoperatively. Concurrent resection of primary PETs and hepatic metastases has been reported in 23 patients, who had a median overall survival of 76 months and a median symptom-free survival of 26 months.[99] The conclusion of these studies was that resection of metastatic disease to liver should be considered in selected patients with neuroendocrine tumors. It is important to remember that such resection may be possible in only a small proportion of all patients with metastatic PETs in the liver.[53,54,114] Furthermore, at present, whether such an approach actually increases survival is not clear. This approach may be required in patients with symptomatic tumors in whom octreotide treatment or chemotherapy alone is not reducing plasma hormone levels sufficiently, so that symptoms are poorly controlled.[26,53,54,114]

LIVER TRANSPLANTATION

Liver transplantation has been attempted on small numbers of patients with metastatic PETs.[117–119] Each of the reported series included small numbers of cases. All of these studies recommend that liver transplantation be considered in selected cases, especially in patients without extrahepatic disease. In the largest series of 31 patients who underwent liver transplantation for neuroendocrine tumors, 15 were for carcinoid tumors and 16 were for PETs.[119] Survival rates were significantly higher for patients with carcinoid tumors (69% at 5 years) than for those with PETs (8% at 4 years). It appears from the small number of cases that long-term cure is uncommon, with recurrence to the liver the most frequent. It currently remains unclear whether this treatment is more effective for PETs than for other metastatic tumors and whether it appreciably prolongs survival.

RECEPTOR-TARGETED RADIONUCLIDE THERAPY

The overexpression of somatostatin receptors by PETs is now being used to direct radiolabeled somatostatin analog to the tumor for tumoricidal effects.[60,120,121] These radiolabeled analogs of somatostatin are rapidly internalized in the tumor cells similarly to native somatostatin. Indium 111–labeled compounds, which emit gamma rays; yttrium 90–coupled analogs, which emit high-energy β particles; and lutetium 177–coupled analogs, which emit both, have all been used.[60,120,121] In patients with abnormal metastatic PETs, the lutetium 177 and indium 111 compounds caused disease stabilization in 41% and 40% and decrease in tumor size in 38% and 30%, respectively. Whether these agents will extend life or have only a palliative effect is unclear at present. It is also unclear whether they potentiate the action of other antitumor agents.

REFERENCES

1. Jensen RT, Norton JA. Management of metastatic pancreatic endocrine tumors. In: Feldman M, Scharschmidt BF, Sleisenger MH, eds. *Gastrointestinal and liver disease.* Philadelphia: W.B. Saunders, 1998:871.
2. Kloppel G, Schroder S, Heitz PU. Histopathology and immunopathology of pancreatic endocrine tumors. In: Mignon M, Jensen RT, eds. *Endocrine tumors of the pancreas: recent advances in research and management.* Basel, Switzerland: S. Karger, 1995:120.
3. Eriksson B, Oberg K. PPomas and nonfunctioning endocrine pancreatic tumors: clinical presentation, diagnosis, and advances in management. In: Mignon M, Jensen RT, eds. *Endocrine tumors of the pancreas: recent advances in research and management.* Basel, Switzerland: S. Karger, 1995:208.
4. Metz DC. Diagnosis and treatment of pancreatic neuroendocrine tumors. *Semin Gastrointest Dis* 1995;6:67.
5. Zollinger RM, Ellison EH. Primary peptic ulceration of the jejunum associated with islet cell tumors of the pancreas. *Ann Surg* 1955;142:709.
6. Gregory RA, Tracy JH, Agarwal KL. Amino acid constitution of two gastrins isolated from Zollinger-Ellison tumor tissue. *Gut* 1969;10:603.
7. Jensen RT. Zollinger-Ellison syndrome. In: Doherty GM, Skogseid B, eds. *Surgical endocrinology: clinical syndromes.* Philadelphia, PA: Lippincott Williams & Wilkins, 2001:291.
8. Willems G. Trophic action of gastrin on specific target cells in the gut. In: Mignon M, Jensen RT, eds. *Endocrine tumors of the pancreas: recent advances in research and management.* Basel, Switzerland: S. Karger, 1995:50.
9. Roy PK, Venzon DJ, Shojamanesh H, et al. Zollinger-Ellison syndrome. Clinical presentation in 261 patients. *Medicine (Baltimore)* 2000;79:379.
10. Norton JA, Fraker DL, Alexander HR, et al. Surgery to cure the Zollinger-Ellison syndrome. *N Engl J Med* 1999;341:635.
11. Weber HC, Venzon DJ, Fishbein VA, et al. Determinants of metastatic rate and survival in patients with Zollinger-Ellison syndrome (ZES): a prospective long-term study. *Gastroenterology* 1995;108:1637.
12. Wu PC, Alexander HR, Bartlett DL, et al. A prospective analysis of the frequency, location, and curability of ectopic (nonpancreaticoduodenal, nonnodal) gastrinoma. *Surgery* 1997;122:1176.
13. Hochwald SN, Zee S, Conlon KC, et al. Prognostic factors in pancreatic endocrine neoplasms: an analysis of 136 cases with a proposal for low-grade and intermediate-grade groups. *J Clin Oncol* 2002;20:2633.
14. Yu F, Venzon DJ, Serrano J, et al. Prospective study of the clinical course, prognostic factors, causes of death, and survival in patients with long-standing Zollinger-Ellison syndrome. *J Clin Oncol* 1999;17:615.
15. Gibril F, Reynolds JC, Doppman JL, et al. Somatostatin receptor scintigraphy: its sensitivity compared with that of other imaging methods in detecting primary and metastatic gastrinomas. A prospective study. *Ann Intern Med* 1996;125:26.
16. Norton JA, Alexander HR, Fraker DL, et al. Possible primary lymph node gastrinoma: occurrence, natural history, and predictive factors: a prospective study. *Ann Surg* 2003;237:650.
17. Zogakis TG, Gibril F, Libutti SK, et al. Management and outcome of patients with sporadic gastrinoma arising in the duodenum. *Ann Surg* 2003;238:42.
18. Metz DC, Kuchnio M, Fraker DL, et al. Flow cytometry and Zollinger-Ellison syndrome: relationship to clinical course. *Gastroenterology* 1993;105:799.
19. Corleto VD, Delle FG, Jensen RT. Molecular insights into gastrointestinal neuroendocrine tumours: importance and recent advances. *Dig Liver Dis* 2002;34:668.
20. Marx S, Spiegel AM, Skarulis MC, et al. Multiple endocrine neoplasia type 1: clinical and genetic topics. *Ann Intern Med* 1998;129:484.
21. Heitz PU, Kasper M, Polak JM, Kloppel G. Pancreatic endocrine tumors. *Hum Pathol* 1982;13:263.
22. Eriksson B. Tumor markers for pancreatic endocrine tumors, including chromogranins, HCG-alpha and HCG-beta. In: Mignon M, Jensen RT, eds. *Endocrine tumors of the pancreas: recent advances in research and management.* Basel, Switzerland: S. Karger, 1995:121.
23. Amikura K, Alexander HR, Norton JA, et al. Role of surgery in management of adrenocorticotropic hormone-producing islet cell tumors of the pancreas. *Surgery* 1995;118:1125.
24. Stridsberg M, Oberg K, Li Q, Engstrom U, Lundqvist G. Measurements of chromogranin A, chromogranin B (secretogranin I), chromogranin C (secretogranin II) and pancreastatin in plasma and urine from patients with carcinoid tumours and endocrine pancreatic tumours. *J Endocrinol* 1995;144:49.
25. Goebel SU, Serrano J, Yu F, et al. Prospective study of the value of serum chromogranin A or serum gastrin levels in the assessment of the presence, extent, or growth of gastrinomas. *Cancer* 1999;85:1470.
26. Jensen RT, Norton JA. Pancreatic endocrine tumors. In: Feldman M, Friedman L, Sleisenger MH, eds. *Gastrointestinal and liver disease: pathophysiology, diagnosis, and management.* Philadelphia: W.B. Saunders, 2002:988.
27. Whipple AO. The surgical therapy of hyperinsulinism. *J Int Chir* 1938;3:237.
28. Grant CS. Insulinoma. *Surg Oncol Clin N Am* 1998;7:819.
29. Brown CK, Bartlett DL, Doppman JL, et al. Intraarterial calcium stimulation and intraoperative ultrasonography in the localization and resection of insulinomas. *Surgery* 1997;122:1189.
30. Roy PK, Venzon DJ, Feigenbaum KM, et al. Gastric secretion in Zollinger-Ellison syndrome. Correlation with clinical expression, tumor extent and role in diagnosis—a prospective NIH study of 235 patients and a review of 984 cases in the literature. *Medicine (Baltimore)* 2001;80:189.
31. Alexander HR Jr., Jensen RT, Doppman JL. Pancreatic endocrine tumors. In: Torosian M, ed. *Integrated cancer management: surgery, medical oncology and radiation oncology.* New York: Marcel Dekker, 1999:241.
32. Gibril F, Lindeman RJ, Abou-Saif A, et al. Retained gastric antrum syndrome: a forgotten, treatable cause of refractory peptic ulcer disease. *Dig Dis Sci* 2001;46:610.
33. Jensen RT. Treatment of pancreatic Zollinger-Ellison syndrome and other gastric hypersecretory states. In: Wolfe MM, ed. *Therapy of digestive disorders.* Philadelphia, PA: W.B. Saunders, 2000:169.
34. Rougier P, Mitry E. Chemotherapy in the treatment of neuroendocrine malignant tumors. *Digestion* 2000;62[Suppl 1]:73.
35. Hirshberg B, Livi A, Bartlett DL, et al. Forty-eight-hour fast: the diagnostic test for insulinoma. *J Clin Endocrinol Metab* 2000;85(9):3222.
36. Virally ML, Guillausseau PJ. Hypoglycemia in adults. *Diabetes Metab* 1999;25:477.
37. Hochwald SN, Conlon KC, Brennan MF. Nonfunctional pancreatic islet cell tumors. In: Doherty GM, Skogseid B, eds. *Surgical endocrinology.* Philadelphia: Lippincott Williams & Wilkins, 2001:361.
38. Thompson GB, van Heerden JA, Grant CS, Carney JA, Ilstrup DM. Islet cell carcinomas of the pancreas: a twenty-year experience. *Surgery* 1988;104:1011.
39. Vinik AI, Strodel WE, Eckhauser FE, et al. Somatostatinomas, PPomas, neurotensinomas. *Semin Oncol* 1987;14:263.
40. Verner JV, Morrison AB. Islet cell tumor and a syndrome of refractory watery diarrhea and hypokalemia. *Am J Med* 1958;29:529.
41. Matuchansky C, Rambaud JC. VIPomas and endocrine cholera: clinical presentation, diagnosis, and advances in management. In: Mignon M, Jensen RT, eds. *Endocrine tumors of the pancreas: recent advances in research and management.* Basel, Switzerland: S. Karger, 1995:166.
42. Jensen RT. Overview of chronic diarrhea caused by functional neuroendocrine neoplasms. *Semin Gastrointest Dis* 1999;10:156.
43. Long RG, Bryant MG, Mitchell SJ, et al. Clinicopathological study of pancreatic and ganglioneuroblastoma tumors secreting vasoactive intestinal polypeptide (VIPomas). *BMJ* 1981;282:1767.
44. Mallinson CN, Bloom SR, Warin AP, et al. A glucagonoma syndrome. *Lancet* 1974;2:1.
45. Chastain MA. The glucagonoma syndrome: a review of its features and discussion of new perspectives. *Am J Med Sci* 2001;321:306.
46. Guillausseas PJ, Guillausseau-Scholer C. Glucagonomas: clinical presentation, diagnosis, and advances in management. In: Mignon M, Jensen RT, eds. *Endocrine tumors of the pancreas: recent advances in research and management.* Basel, Switzerland: S. Karger, 1995:183.
47. Case CC, Vassilopoulou-Sellin R. Reproduction of features of the glucagonoma syndrome with continuous intravenous glucagon infusion as therapy for tumor-induced hypoglycemia. *Endocr Pract* 2003;9:22.
48. Sassolas G, Chayvialle JA, Fomas GR. Somatostatinomas: clinical presentation, diagnosis, and advances in management. In: Mignon M, Jensen RT, eds. *Endocrine tumors of the pancreas: recent advances in research and management.* Basel, Switzerland: S. Karger, 1995:194.
49. Guillemin R, Brazeau P, Bohlen P, et al. Growth hormone-releasing factor from a human pancreatic tumor that caused acromegaly. *Science* 1982;27:774.
50. Sano T, Asa SL, Kovacs K. Growth hormone releasing-producing tumors: clinical, biochemical and morphological manifestations. *Endocr Rev* 1988;9:357.
51. Orbuch M, Doppman JL, Strader DB, et al. Imaging for pancreatic endocrine tumor localization: recent advances. In: Mignon M, Jensen RT, eds. *Endocrine tumors of the pancreas: recent advances in research and management.* Basel, Switzerland: S. Karger, 1995:268.
52. Norton JA, Doherty GM, Fraker DL, et al. Surgical treatment of localized gastrinoma within the liver: a prospective study. *Surgery* 1998;124:1145.
53. Norton JA, Jensen RT. Resolved and unresolved controversies in the surgical management of patients with Zollinger-Ellison syndrome. *Ann Surg* (in press).

54. Sarmiento JM, Que FG. Hepatic surgery for metastases from neuroendocrine tumors. *Surg Oncol Clin N Am* 2003;12:231.

55. Hashimoto LA, Walsh RM. Preoperative localization of insulinomas is not necessary. *J Am Coll Surg* 1999;189:368.

56. Alexander HR, Fraker DL, Norton JA, et al. Prospective study of somatostatin receptor scintigraphy and its effect on operative outcome in patients with Zollinger-Ellison syndrome. *Ann Surg* 1998;228:228.

57. Gibril F, Jensen RT. Diagnostic uses of radiolabeled somatostatin receptor analogues in gastroenteropancreatic endocrine tumors. *Dig Liver Dis* 2004;36:5106.

58. Norton JA, Alexander HR, Fraker DL, Venzon D, Jensen RT. Does the use of routine duodenotomy (DUODX) affect rate of cure, development of liver metastases or survival in patients with Zollinger-Ellison Syndrome? *Ann Surg* 2004;239:617.

59. Creutzfeldt W. Insulinomas: clinical presentation, diagnosis, and advances in management. In: Mignon M, Jensen RT, eds. *Endocrine tumors of the pancreas: recent advances in research and management.* Basel, Switzerland: S. Karger, 1995:148.

60. Kwekkeboom D, Krenning EP, de Jong M. Peptide receptor imaging and therapy. *J Nucl Med* 2000;41:1704.

61. Lebtahi R, Cadiot G, Sarda L, et al. Clinical impact of somatostatin receptor scintigraphy in the management of patients with neuroendocrine gastroenteropancreatic tumors. *J Nucl Med* 1997;38:853.

62. Gibril F, Doppman JL, Reynolds JC, et al. Bone metastases in patients with gastrinomas: a prospective study of bone scanning, somatostatin receptor scanning, and magnetic resonance image in their detection, frequency, location and effect of their detection on management. *J Clin Oncol* 1998;16:1040.

63. Termanini B, Gibril F, Reynbolds JC, et al. Value of somatostatin receptor scintigraphy: a prospective study in gastrinoma of its effect on clinical management. *Gastroenterology* 1997;112:335.

64. Ruszniewski P, Amouyal P, Amouyal G, et al. Endocrine tumors of the pancreatic area: localization by endoscopic ultrasonography. In: Mignon M, Jensen RT, eds. *Endocrine tumors of the pancreas: recent advances in research and management.* Basel, Switzerland: S. Karger, 1995:258.

65. Anderson MA, Carpenter S, Thompson NW, et al. Endoscopic ultrasound is highly accurate and directs management in patients with neuroendocrine tumors of the pancreas. *Am J Gastroenterol* 2000;95:2271.

66. Strader DB, Doppman JL, Orbuch M, et al. Functional localization of pancreatic endocrine tumors. In: Mignon M, Jensen RT, eds. *Frontiers of gastrointestinal research.* Basel, Switzerland: S. Karger, 1995:282.

67. Turner JJ, Wren AM, Jackson JE, Thakker RV, Meeran K. Localization of gastrinomas by selective intra-arterial calcium injection. *Clin Endocrinol (Oxf)* 2002;57:821.

68. Norton JA, Cromack DT, Shawker TH, et al. Intraoperative ultrasonographic localization of islet cell tumors. *Ann Surg* 1988;207:160.

69. Norton JA. Surgical treatment of islet cell tumors with special emphasis on operative ultrasound. In: Mignon M, Jensen RT, eds. *Endocrine tumors of the pancreas: recent advances in research and management.* Basel, Switzerland: S. Karger, 1995:309.

70. Metz DC, Jensen RT. Advances in gastric antisecretory therapy in Zollinger-Ellison syndrome. In: Mignon M, Jensen RT, eds. *Endocrine tumors of the pancreas: recent advances in research and management.* Basel, Switzerland: S. Karger, 1995:240.

71. Metz DC, Strader DB, Orbuch M, et al. Use of omeprazole in Zollinger-Ellison: a prospective nine-year study of efficacy and safety. *Aliment Pharmacol Ther* 1993;7:597.

72. Jensen RT. Use of omeprazole and other proton pump inhibitors in the Zollinger-Ellison syndrome. In: Olbe L, ed. *Milestones in drug therapy.* Basel, Switzerland: Birkhauser Verlag AG Publishing Co., 1999:205.

73. Norton JA, Cornelius MJ, Doppman JL, et al. Effect of parathyroidectomy in patients with hyperparathyroidism and Zollinger-Ellison syndrome and multiple endocrine neoplasia type 1: a prospective study. *Surgery* 1987;102:958.

74. Peghini PL, Annibale B, Azzoni C, et al. Effect of chronic hypergastrinemia on human enterochromaffin-like cells: insights from patients with sporadic gastrinomas. *Gastroenterology* 2002;123:68.

75. Lew EA, Pisegna JR, Starr JA, et al. Intravenous pantoprazole rapidly controls gastric acid hypersecretion in patients with Zollinger-Ellison syndrome. *Gastroenterology* 2000;118:696.

76. Kisker O, Bastian D, Bartsch D, Nies C, Rothmund M. Localization, malignant potential and surgical management of gastrinomas. *World J Surg* 1998;22:651.

77. Soga J, Yakuwa Y. The gastrinoma/Zollinger-Ellison syndrome: statistical evaluation of a Japanese series of 359 cases. *J Hepatobiliary Pancreat Surg* 1998;5:77.

78. Alexander HR, Bartlett DL, Venzon DJ, et al. Analysis of factors associated with long-term (five or more years) cure in patients undergoing operation for Zollinger-Ellison syndrome. *Surgery* 1998;124:1160.

79. Jensen RT, Gardner JD. Gastrinoma. In: Go VLW, DiMagno EP, Gardner JD, et al., eds. *The pancreas: biology, pathobiology and disease.* New York, NY: Raven Press, 1993:931.

80. Fraker DL, Norton JA, Alexander HR, Venzon DJ, Jensen RT. Surgery in Zollinger-Ellison syndrome alters the natural history of gastrinoma. *Ann Surg* 1994;220:320.

81. Mignon M, Cadiot G. Diagnostic and therapeutic criteria in patients with Zollinger-Ellison syndrome and multiple endocrine neoplasia type 1. *J Intern Med* 1998;243:489.

82. Jensen RT. Management of the Zollinger-Ellison syndrome in patients with multiple endocrine neoplasia type 1. *J Intern Med* 1998;243:477.

83. MacFarlane MP, Fraker DL, Alexander HR, Norton JA, Jensen RT. A prospective study of surgical resection of duodenal and pancreatic gastrinomas. *Surgery* 1995;118:973.

84. Cadiot G, Vuagnat A, Doukhan I, et al. Prognostic factors in patients with Zollinger-Ellison syndrome and multiple endocrine neoplasia type 1. *Gastroenterology* 1999;116:286.

85. Bartsch DK, Langer P, Wild A, et al. Pancreaticoduodenal endocrine tumors in multiple endocrine neoplasia type 1: surgery or surveillance? *Surgery* 2000;128:958.

86. Jaskowiak NT, Fraker DL, Alexander HR, et al. Is reoperation for gastrinoma excision indicated in Zollinger-Ellison syndrome? *Surgery* 1996;120:1055.

87. Arnold R, Wied M, Behr TH. Somatostatin analogues in the treatment of endocrine tumors of the gastrointestinal tract. *Expert Opin Pharmacother* 2002;3:643.

88. Jensen RT. Peptide therapy: recent advances in the use of somatostatin and other peptide receptor agonists and antagonists. In: Lewis JH, Dubois A, eds. *Current clinical topics in gastrointestinal pharmacology.* Malden, MA: Blackwell Science, Inc., 1997:144.

89. Kano N, Kusanagi H, Yamada S, Kasama K, Ota A. Laparoscopic pancreatic surgery: its indications and techniques: from the viewpoint of limiting the indications. *J Hepatobiliary Pancreat Surg* 2002;9:555.

90. Iihara M, Kanbe M, Okamoto T, Ito Y, Obara T. Laparoscopic ultrasonography for resection of insulinomas. *Surgery* 2001;130:1086.

91. Sperti C, Pasquali C, Ferronato A, Pedrazzoli S. Median pancreatectomy for tumors of the neck and body of the pancreas. *J Am Coll Surg* 2000;190:711.

92. Boden G. Insulinoma and glucagonoma. *Semin Oncol* 1987;14:253.

93. Danforth DN, Gorden P, Brennan MF. Metastatic insulin secreting carcinoma of the pancreas. Clinical course and the role of surgery. *Surgery* 1984;96:1027.

94. Mao C, Shah A, Hanson DJ, Howard JM. Von Recklinghausen's disease associated with duodenal somatostatinoma: contrast of duodenal versus pancreatic somatostatinomas. *J Surg Oncol* 1995;59:67.

95. Konomi K, Chijiiwa K, Katsuta T, Yamaguchi K. Pancreatic somatostatinoma: a case report and review of the literature. *J Surg Oncol* 1990;43:259.

96. Maton PN, Gardner JD, Jensen RT. Cushing's syndrome in patients with the Zollinger-Ellison Syndrome. *N Engl J Med* 1986;315:1.

97. Mao C, Carter P, Schaefer P, et al. Malignant islet cell tumor associated with hypercalcemia. *Surgery* 1995;117:37.

98. Jensen RT. Natural history of digestive endocrine tumors. In: Mignon M, Colombel JF, eds. *Recent advances in pathophysiology and management of inflammatory bowel diseases and digestive endocrine tumors.* Paris, France: John Libbey Eurotext Publishing, 1999:192.

99. Sarmiento JM, Que FG, Grant CS, et al. Concurrent resections of pancreatic islet cell cancers with synchronous hepatic metastases: outcomes of an aggressive approach. *Surgery* 2002;132:976.

100. Miller CA, Ellison EC. Therapeutic alternatives in metastatic neuroendocrine tumors. *Surg Oncol Clin N Am* 1998;7:863.

101. Arnold R, Frank M. Systemic chemotherapy for endocrine tumors of the pancreas: recent advances. In: Mignon M, Jensen RT, eds. *Endocrine tumors of the pancreas: recent advances in research and management.* Basel, Switzerland: S. Karger, 1995:431.

102. Gibril F, Doppman JL, Jensen RT. Recent advances in the treatment of metastatic pancreatic endocrine tumors. *Semin Gastrointest Dis* 1995;6:114.

103. Moertel CG, Hanley JA, Johnson LA. Streptozotocin alone compared with streptozotocin plus fluorouracil in the treatment of advanced islet-cell carcinoma. *N Engl J Med* 1980;303:1189.

104. Moertel C, Lefkopoulo M, Lipsitz S, et al. Streptozotocin-doxorubicin, streptozotocin-fluorouracil, or chlorozotocin in the treatment of advanced islet cell carcinoma. *N Engl J Med* 1992;326:519.

105. Moertel CG, Kvols LK, O'Connell MJ, Rubin J. Treatment of neuroendocrine carcinomas with combined etoposide and cisplatin. *Cancer* 1991;68:227.

106. Eriksson B, Oberg K. Interferon therapy of malignant endocrine pancreatic tumors. In: Mignon M, Jensen RT, eds. *Endocrine tumors of the pancreas: recent advances in research and management.* Basel, Switzerland: S. Karger, 1995:451.

107. Bukowski RM, Tangen C, Lee R, et al. Phase II trial of chlorozotocin and fluorouracil in islet cell carcinoma: a Southwest Oncology Group. *J Clin Oncol* 1992;10:1914.

108. Sutliff VE, Doppman JL, Gibril F, et al. Growth of newly diagnosed, untreated metastatic gastrinomas and predictors of growth patterns. *J Clin Oncol* 1997;15:2420.

109. Shojamanesh H, Gibril F, Louie A, et al. Prospective study of the antitumor efficacy of long-term octreotide treatment in patients with progressive metastatic gastrinoma. *Cancer* 2002;94:331.

110. Oberg K. Interferon in the management of neuroendocrine GEP-tumors: a review. *Digestion* 2000;62[Suppl 1]:92.

111. Moertel CG, Johnson CM, McKusick MA, et al. The management of patients with advanced carcinoid tumors and islet cell carcinomas. *Ann Intern Med* 1994;120:302.

112. Ruszniewski P, Malka D. Hepatic arterial chemoembolization in the management of advanced digestive endocrine tumors. *Digestion* 2000;62[Suppl 1]:79.

113. Venook AP. Embolization and chemoembolization therapy for neuroendocrine tumors. *Curr Opin Oncol* 1999;11:38.

114. Pederzoli P, Falconi M, Bonora A, et al. Cytoreductive surgery in advanced endocrine tumours of the pancreas. *Ital J Gastroenterol Hepatol* 1999;31[Suppl 2]:S207.

115. Harrison LE, Brennan MF, Newman E, et al. Hepatic resection for noncolorectal, nonneuroendocrine metastases: a fifteen-year experience with ninety-six patients. *Surgery* 1997;121:625.

116. Chen H, Hardacre JM, Uzra A, Cameron JL, Choti MA. Isolated liver metastases from neuroendocrine tumors: does resection prolong survival? *J Am Coll Surg* 1998;187:88.

117. Curtiss SI, Mor E, Schwartz ME, et al. A rational approach to the use of hepatic transplantation in the treatment of metastatic neuroendocrine tumors. *J Am Coll Surg* 1995;180:184.

118. Lehnert T. Liver transplantation for metastatic neuroendocrine carcinoma. *Transplantation* 1998;66:1307.

119. Le Treut YP, Delpero JR, Dousset B, et al. Results of liver transplantation in the treatment of metastatic neuroendocrine tumors. *Ann Surg* 1997;225:355.

120. de Jong M, Kwekkeboom D, Valkema R, Krenning EP. Radiolabeled peptides for tumour therapy: current status and future directions. Plenary lecture at the EANM 2002. *Eur J Nucl Med Mol Imaging* 2003;30:463.

121. Kwekkeboom DJ, Bakker WH, Kam BL, et al. Treatment of patients with gastro-enteropancreatic (GEP) tumours with the novel radiolabeled somatostatin analogue [(177)Lu-DOTA(0),Tyr(3)]octreotate. *Eur J Nucl Med Mol Imaging* 2003;30:417.

ROBERT T. JENSEN
GERARD M. DOHERTY

SECTION **6**

Carcinoid Tumors and the Carcinoid Syndrome

PATHOLOGY AND TUMOR HISTOLOGY

Neuroendocrine tumors (NETs) are derived from the diffuse neuroendocrine system, which is made up of peptide- and amine-producing cells with different hormonal profiles depending on their site of origin.[1,2] Carcinoids are classified as NETs and share cytochemical features with melanomas, pheochromocytomas, medullary carcinomas of the thyroid, and pancreatic endocrine tumors.[1,3–6] Carcinoids are composed of monotonous sheets of small round cells with uniform nuclei and cytoplasm.[4] Mitotic figures are rare.[3,4] Oberndorfer introduced the term *carcinoid* in 1907 to describe tumors that behaved more indolently than adenocarcinomas.[1] Pathologists cannot differentiate benign from malignant carcinoids based on histologic analysis, nor can they histologically differentiate pancreatic endocrine tumors from carcinoids.[1] Malignancy can only be determined if there is invasion or distant metastases. Ultrastructurally, carcinoids possess electron-dense neurosecretory granules and they contain small clear vesicles that correspond to the synaptic vesicles of neurons.[4] Carcinoids synthesize bioactive amines and peptides, including neuron-specific enolase (NSE), 5-hydroxytryptamine (5-HT), 5-hydroxytryptophan (5-HTP), synaptophysin, and chromogranins A and C, and other peptides like insulin, growth hormone, neurotensin, adrenocorticotropic hormone (ACTH), β-melanocyte-stimulating hormone, gastrin, pancreatic polypeptide, calcitonin, substance P, other various tachykinins (neuropeptide K), growth hormone–releasing hormone, bombesin, and various growth factors such as transforming growth factor-β, platelet-derived growth factor, and fibroblast growth factor-β.[1,6,7]

Most carcinoids are tentatively identified on routine histologic analysis.[1,4,6] However, these tumors are characterized by their histologic staining patterns due to their shared secreted products and certain cytoplasmic proteins.[4] Historically, one of the most important was their staining with silver.[1,4] Characteristically, carcinoids either take up and reduce silver (argentaffin reaction) or take it up but do not reduce it (argyrophilic reaction).[1,3] The identification of chromogranin, synaptophysin, or NSE is now generally used.[1,6–8] The chromogranins (A, B, and C) are acidic polypeptides that are the major component of the secretory granules of many neuroendocrine cells.[6–8] In general, chromogranin A immunoreactivity is more specific than the argyrophilic reaction because the latter also identifies other intracellular proteins such as melanin. NSE, the γ-γ dimer of the glycolytic enzyme enolase, occurs in the cytoplasm of most neuroendocrine cells and is found in most carcinoids as well as other apudomas.[1] The advantage of NSE as a marker is that its reactivity is unrelated to secretory granule content. However, NSE can be occasionally misleading, because some tumors not considered neuroendocrine, such as fibroadenomas of the breast, carcinomas, and certain lymphomas, may contain a considerable amount of NSE activity.[1] Synaptophysin is a calcium-binding vesicle membrane glycoprotein that is expressed independently of other neuroendocrine proteins.[1]

In addition to the general histologic NET markers, specific markers for carcinoids may identify the tumor as a carcinoid.[1] Serotonin can be identified by various methods, including the use of the argentaffin reaction of Masson or the use of antibodies to serotonin.[1] In general, the argentaffin reaction of Masson is usually positive and the serotonin antibody localization is frequently weak or negative in midgut carcinoids, whereas in foregut and hindgut carcinoids, serotonin immunoreactivity is detected more often than is the argentaffin reaction.[1]

Williams and Sandler[9] proposed classifying carcinoids according to their site of origin because carcinoids with similar sites of origin frequently share functional manifestations, histochemistry, and secretory products (Table 34.6-1). Foregut carcinoids generally have a low serotonin (5-HT) content, are argentaffin negative but argyrophilic, occasionally secrete 5-HTP or ACTH, can be associated with an atypical carcinoid syndrome, are often multihormonal, and may metastasize to bone (see Table 34.6-1). Although many foregut carcinoids synthesize peptides, clinical syndromes are rarely produced and elevated plasma hormone levels are generally not detected. Midgut carcinoids are argentaffin positive, have a high serotonin content, have smaller numbers of endocrine cells than foregut tumors, most frequently cause the classic carcinoid syndrome when they metastasize, release serotonin and tachykinins (substance P, neuropeptide K, substance K), rarely secrete 5-HTP or ACTH, and uncommonly metastasize to bone (see Table 34.6-1).[10] Hindgut carcinoid tumors are argentaffin negative, often argyrophilic, rarely contain serotonin, rarely cause the carcinoid syndrome, contain numerous gastrointestinal (GI) hormones, rarely secrete 5-HTP or ACTH, and may metastasize to bone (see Table 34.6-1).[10]

Carcinoids within the same site of origin such as lung, thymus, and pancreas can differ significantly in characteristics and behavior. Therefore, it has been proposed that the term *carcinoid* be replaced by the designation *neuroendocrine tumor* and a new classification system has been devised.[4] In this proposed classification tumors are divided according to tissue of origin and subdivided by growth behavior. It is argued that this new classification system better reflects the biology of these tumors and provides better guidelines for tumors with similar behaviors in different tissues.

Carcinoids can be ubiquitous, but today most originate in three sites: bronchus, colon-rectum, and jejunoileum.[11–13] In the past carcinoids were most frequently reported in the appendix (approximately 40%); however, more recently the bronchus and lung and small intestine are the most common sites (Table 34.6-2). The distribution reported from analyses of three large National Cancer Institute databases from 1950 to 1999 are contrasted in Table 34.6-2. There are a number of trends apparent from comparison of the data from these different time periods. The percentages of gastric carcinoids increased almost threefold, whereas the percentage of appendiceal carcinoids decreased more than 16-fold. Small intestinal carcinoids remained a large group, comprising 28% of all carcinoids. Overall, GI carcinoids remain the most frequent, comprising 64% of all carcinoids, with the respiratory tract being a distant second with 28%.

The exact clinical incidence of carcinoids varies in different studies. An incidence of 7.1 per million for males and 8.7 per

TABLE 34.6-1. Classification of Carcinoid Tumors

Histochemistry and Products	Foregut[a]	Midgut[b]	Hindgut[c]
HISTOCHEMISTRY			
Silver staining	Argentaffin-negative, argyrophilic or negative	Argentaffin-positive	Argentaffin-negative (75%) or occasional argyrophilic (55%)
Neuron-specific enolase	Positive	Positive	Positive
Chromogranin A	Positive	Positive	Positive (42%)
Cytoplasmic granules (electron microscope)	Round, variable density, 180 nm	Pleomorphic, uniform density, 230 nm	Round, variable density, approximately 190 nm
PRODUCTS			
Tumor	Low 5-HT content, multihormonal[d]	High 5-HT content, multihormonal[d]	Rarely 5-HT, multihormonal[d]
Blood	5-HTP, histamine, multihormonal,[d] occasionally secrete ACTH	5-HT, multihormonal,[d] rarely secrete ACTH	Rarely release 5-HTP or ACTH
Urine	5-HTP, 5-HT, 5-HIAA, histamine, and others	5-HT, 5-HIAA	Negative
Carcinoid syndrome	Occurs but may be atypical	Occurs frequently (with metastases)	Rarely occurs
Metastasize to bone	Common	Rarely	Common

ACTH, adrenocorticotropic hormone; 5-HIAA, 5-hydroxyindoleacetic acid; 5-HT, 5-hydroxytryptamine; 5-HTP, 5-hydroxytryptophan.
[a]Respiratory tract, pancreas, stomach, proximal duodenum.
[b]Jejunum, ileum, appendix, Meckel's diverticulum, ascending colon.
[c]Includes transverse and descending colon, rectum.
[d]Multihormonal includes tachykinins (substance P, substance K, neuropeptide K), neurotensin, peptide YY, enkephalin, insulin, glucagon, gastrin, glicentin, vasoactive intestinal peptide, somatostatin, pancreatic polypeptide, ACTH, or a subunit of human chorionic gonadotropin.

TABLE 34.6-2. Carcinoid Tumor Location, Frequency of Metastases, and Association with Carcinoid Syndrome

	Location (% of Total)			Incidence of Metastases (%)		Incidence of Carcinoid Syndrome (%)
	Godwin, 1975 (1950–1971; n = 4349)	Early SEER (Modlin, 1997) (1973–1991; n = 5468)	Late SEER (Modlin, 2003) (1992–1999)	Godwin, 1975 (1950–1971)	Modlin, 1997 (1973–1991)	Godwin, 1975 (1950–1971)
FOREGUT						
Esophagus	<1	<1	<1	—	67	—
Stomach	2	3.8	5.8	22	31	9.5
Duodenum	2.6	2.1	3.8	20	—	3.4
Pancreas	<1	<1	<1	20	76	20
Gallbladder	<1	<1	<1	33	56	5
Bile duct	<1	<1	—	—	—	—
Ampulla	<1	<1	—	14	—	—
Larynx	<1	<1	—	50	0	—
Trachea/bronchi/lung	11.5	30.2	25.3	20	27	13
MIDGUT						
Jejunum	1.3	2.3	1.5	35	70	9
Ileum	23	17.6	13.4	35	—	9
Meckel's diverticulum	1	0.4	0.5	18	—	13
Appendix	38	7.6	2.4	2	35	<1
Colon	4.3	9.5	7.6	60	71	5
Liver	<1	<1	<1	—	29	—
Ovary	<1	<1	1.4	6	32	50
Testis	<1	<1	<1	—	—	50
Cervix	<1	<1	—	24	67	3
HINDGUT						
Rectum	13	10	18.5	3	14	—

SEER, Surveillance, Epidemiology, and End Results program.
(Data from refs. 11–13.)

million for females in England and Scotland and 13 cases per million population in Ireland is reported.[1] In other series, the incidence of clinically significant tumors was 7 per million population per year in Scandinavia, which was two times as common as all pancreatic endocrine tumors, seven times as common as gastrinomas, and eight times as common as insulinomas.[1] The clinical presentation of carcinoids far underestimates their occurrence, because many are asymptomatic. This is demonstrated by Surveillance, Epidemiology, and End Results program (SEER) data, which report an annual incidence rate of 2.8 per million population for small intestinal carcinoids,[1] whereas in an autopsy study at the Mayo Clinic there were 6500 cases per million.[1] The annual incidence of malignant carcinoids at autopsy was 21 per million population per year,[1] whereas in a Swedish study with calculations based on autopsy and surgical results it was 84 cases per million population.[1] The distribution of carcinoid tumors found in various surgical or clinical series differs markedly from that found at autopsy.[1] At autopsy as many as 76% of all carcinoids are found in the jejunoileum, whereas these make up approximately one-fourth of cases in clinical and surgical series.

Approximately 1 in every 200 to 300 appendectomies results in discovery of a carcinoid.[1] Most occur in the tip of the appendix. The majority (i.e., 90%) are less than 1 cm in diameter without metastases.[1] In the SEER data, of 1570 appendiceal carcinoids,[14] 62% were localized, 27% were accompanied by regional lesions, and 8% were associated with distant metastatic disease. Approximately 50% of carcinoids between 1 and 2 cm metastasize to lymph nodes.[1]

Small intestinal carcinoids may be multiple; 70% to 87% are present within the ileum and 40% to 70% are within 2 ft of the ileocecal valve.[1,15] Forty percent are smaller than 1 cm in diameter, 32% are 1 to 2 cm, and 29% are larger than 2 cm.[15] In an analysis of 12 series, 47% (range, 0% to 100%) were associated with metastases,[15] whereas 35% to 70% were associated with metastases in the National Cancer Institute studies[11–13] (see Table 34.6-2). With the carcinoid, a marked fibrotic reaction can occur that can distort the gut or mesentery and can present clinically with small bowel obstruction or venous mesenteric infarction. Distant metastases occur to the liver (22% to 60%),[13,15] to bone (3%),[15] and occasionally to lung (4%).[15] Twenty percent to 30% of patients with ileal carcinoid have one or more additional ileal primary carcinoids. The incidence of metastases from small intestinal carcinoids is dependent on tumor size.[1] If the tumor is less than 1 cm, metastases occur in fewer than 15% to 25% of cases.[1,15] If the tumor is between 1 and 2 cm in size, metastases occur in 58% to 80%.[15] If the tumor is larger than 2 cm, metastases occur in more than 70%.[15] In contrast to jejunoileal carcinoids, duodenal carcinoids are often discovered by endoscopy.[16] In two series[11,16] (see Table 34.6-2), 20% to 21% of duodenal carcinoids had metastases. Invasion into the muscularis propria, tumor size, and mitotic activity all correlated with metastatic spread, with invasion being the strongest predictor. No duodenal carcinoid smaller than 1 cm metastasized, whereas 33% of the tumors larger than 2 cm or 35% of tumors invading the muscularis mucosa metastasized.[16]

In approximately 1 in every 2500 proctoscopies, a small nodule is seen that is diagnosed as a carcinoid.[1] Nearly all rectal carcinoids occur submucosally on the anterior or lateral walls between 4 and 13 cm above the dentate line.[17] From 66% to 80% are smaller than 1 cm in diameter and rarely metastasize (5%).[17] Tumors 1 to 2 cm can metastasize (5% to 30%),[17] and tumors larger than 2 cm, which are uncommon, metastasize in more than 70% of cases.[17] Colorectal carcinoids are almost entirely limited to the sigmoid colon and rectum, with the vast majority in the rectum. Metastases occur in 10% to 22%,[17] and in most cases the tumor is larger than 2 cm in diameter and invades the muscularis propria. Invasiveness correlates with the presence of increased mitoses or atypical histologic findings. Colonic carcinoids uncommonly occur in the remainder of the colon, with almost 60% occurring in the cecum or ileocecal area. These tumors tend to be large (90% larger than 2 cm, 50% 5 cm or larger) and associated with metastases (61%).

Bronchial carcinoids resemble intestinal carcinoids and are not related to smoking.[1] Poor prognostic pathologic features include increased mitotic count, nuclear pleomorphism, vascular invasion, undifferentiated growth pattern, and lymphatic invasion.[1] The bronchus is the site of a primary carcinoid in approximately 2% of cases. The classification of bronchial carcinoids has been a subject of debate.[1] Lung NETs have been classified into four categories: the typical carcinoid (also called bronchial carcinoid, Kulchitsky cell carcinoma-I, KCC-I); atypical carcinoid (also called well-differentiated neuroendocrine carcinoma and KCC-II); intermediate small cell neuroendocrine carcinoma; and small cell neuroendocrine carcinoma (also called KCC-III).[1,18] Another proposed classification[4] includes these tumors under three general categories of lung NETs: benign or low-grade malignant (typical carcinoid); low-grade malignant (atypical carcinoid); and high-grade malignant (poorly differentiated carcinoma of the large cell or small cell type). The different categories of lung NETs have different prognosis, varying from excellent for typical carcinoids to poor for small cell neuroendocrine carcinomas.[1,18]

Gastric carcinoids account for 3 of every 1000 gastric neoplasms. Three subtypes of gastric carcinoids are proposed to occur.[1,19] These tumors originate from gastric enterochromaffin-like (ECL) cells.[19] Two subtypes are associated with hypergastrinemic states, either chronic atrophic gastritis (type I; 80%) or Zollinger-Ellison syndrome (type II; 6%), almost always as part of multiple endocrine neoplasia type 1 (MEN 1).[1,19] These tumors generally pursue a benign course, with 9% to 30% developing metastases. They are usually multiple and small, with infiltration restricted to the mucosa and submucosa. The third type of gastric carcinoid (type III; sporadic ECL tumors) occurs without hypergastrinemia, and these tumors pursue a more aggressive course, with 54% to 66% developing metastases.[19] They are often large, single tumors; 50% have atypical histologic features, and some patients develop carcinoid syndrome.[1,19]

Carcinoids can be classified by their histologic growth patterns: insular, trabecular, glandular, undifferentiated, or mixed.[1] The midgut carcinoids frequently possess the most typical morphology,[1] with insular-like formation of regular tumor cells, surrounded by fibrotic stroma. Most foregut carcinoids show a more mixed growth pattern, with a solid, ribbon-like, trabecular, or acinar pattern. Hindgut carcinoids are frequently solid or trabecular. It has been demonstrated that the histologic types have prognostic significance.[1,20] In other studies carcinoids are divided histologically into typical (well-differentiated NETs) and atypical (nuclear atypia, necrosis, increased mitotic activity),[4] and this has been shown to have prognostic significance.[1,4,20]

MOLECULAR PATHOGENESIS

Little is known about the induction of malignant growth or the factors promoting the growth of carcinoids.[1,21,22] For some gastric carcinoids, studies show that gastrin is an important growth factor.[1,19] There is an increased occurrence of gastric carcinoids in disease states that result in hypergastrinemia (pernicious anemia, atrophic gastritis, Zollinger-Ellison syndrome).[1,19] The hyperplastic effect of hypergastrinemia is restricted to gastric ECL cells. In pernicious anemia and atrophic gastritis, up to 4% to 11% of patients develop gastric carcinoids.[1,19] Patients with Zollinger-Ellison syndrome also develop gastric carcinoids, although these are much more frequent in the subgroup with MEN 1.[1] In patients with Zollinger-Ellison syndrome with MEN 1 with gastric carcinoids, there is allelic loss at the MEN 1 locus on chromosome band 11q13, and thus fundic gastric carcinoids are now included in the spectrum of MEN 1 tumors. Studies suggest that other important growth factors in some carcinoid tumors are transforming growth factor-α, transforming growth factor-β, insulin-like growth factor-1, trefoil peptides, platelet-derived growth factor, vascular endothelial growth factor, acidic and basic fibroblast growth factor, and epidermal growth factor.[1,7,22]

Limited studies have been performed of carcinoids examining the possible role of mutations of protooncogenes and alterations of tumor suppressor genes in their pathogenesis.[7,22] Mutations in common oncogenes such as K-*ras* are uncommon in GI carcinoids.[22] Overamplification of HER2/NEU, c-myc, and c-jun have been described in some cell lines derived from GI endocrine tumors and some carcinoids.[22] In bronchial carcinoids, a high expression of c-fos, c-jun, and c-met occurs early, and a high expression of c-myc and L-myc occurs late. Alterations in the common tumor suppressor gene p53 are also uncommon in carcinoids,[1,21,22] as are alterations in the retinoblastoma gene in typical carcinoids, although they may occur in atypical carcinoids.[22] MEN 1 has been shown to be due to defects in a ten-exon gene on chromosome band 11q13 that encodes for a 610–amino acid nuclear protein, MENIN.[22,23] Loss of heterozygosity at this locus has been reported in 26% to 78% of carcinoids,[22] and mutations in the MENIN gene were reported in 18% in one study.[22] Microsatellite instability is rare in carcinoids[22]; however, by comparative genomic hybridization, both frequent gains (of chromosome 5, 14, 17q, 7) and losses (especially of 9p) are reported.[22]

CLINICAL FEATURES

GENERAL CHARACTERISTICS

The age of patients ranges from 10 to 93 years, with a mean age at onset of 63 years for carcinoids of the small intestine and respiratory tract, and 66 years for those of the rectum.[12]

CARCINOID TUMORS WITHOUT SYSTEMIC FEATURES

The presentation of carcinoids that do not cause carcinoid syndrome is diverse and related to the site of origin of the tumor as well as the malignant spread of the tumor. In the appendix (see Table 34.6-2), carcinoids are usually found incidentally during surgery for suspected appendicitis. For small intestinal carcinoids, the jejunoileum is the most common location for carcinoids of clinical significance. Most small intestinal carcinoids found in autopsy studies have not caused symptoms, but these tumors can lead to fibrosis of the mesentery, which results in kinking of the bowel, intestinal obstruction, and gut infarction or intussusception. The most common presenting symptoms due to small intestinal carcinoids per se are periodic abdominal pain (51%),[15] intestinal obstruction with ileus or invagination (31%),[15] an abdominal tumor (17%),[15] and GI bleeding (11%).[1,15] Because of the vagueness of the symptoms, the diagnosis is frequently delayed, with a median time from onset from symptoms to diagnosis of approximately 2 years and a range of up to 20 years. Duodenal and gastric carcinoids are usually found incidentally during endoscopy.[16] Rectal carcinoids are frequently found incidentally during endoscopy but can be symptomatic.[17] The most common symptoms include melena and bleeding (39%), constipation (17%), and diarrhea (12%).[17] Bronchial carcinoids are frequently discovered on chest radiograph. The most common symptoms are pneumonia, hemoptysis, and cough.[1,18] Thymic carcinoids present as anterior mediastinal masses, usually on chest radiograph. Ovarian and testicular carcinoids may present as masses detected by physical examination or ultrasonography. Most carcinoids present as an isolated disease, but there are associations between foregut carcinoids and MEN 1,[19] gastric carcinoids and diseases causing hypergastrinemia,[19] ampullary somatostatin-rich carcinoids and von Recklinghausen's disease,[24] and an intestinal carcinoid and myotonic dystrophy; a gastric carcinoid was found in a patient with primary biliary cirrhosis, and duodenal carcinoid tumors have caused Zollinger-Ellison syndrome.[1] Metastatic carcinoids in the liver, presenting as hepatomegaly, may be the initial presentation in a patient who is fully active and productive with minimal symptoms and normal or near-normal liver function test results.

CARCINOID TUMORS WITH SYSTEMIC FEATURES

The most common systemic syndrome caused by carcinoids is the malignant carcinoid syndrome. As described in Pathology and Tumor Histology, carcinoids may contain and secrete a number of biologically active substances. Carcinoids may contain ACTH, gastrin, somatostatin, insulin, motilin, growth hormone, gastrin-releasing peptide, serotonin, calcitonin, neurotensin, β-melanocyte-stimulating hormone, tachykinins (substance P, substance K, neuropeptide K), glucagon, pancreatic polypeptide, vasoactive intestinal peptide, and prostaglandins.[1,15,17,20] These substances may not be released in sufficient amounts to cause symptoms. In various studies of patients with carcinoids, elevated serum concentrations of pancreatic polypeptide occur in 43%, of motilin in 14%, and of subunits of human chorionic gonadotropin in 12%; a slightly elevated level of gastrin was reported in 15%, and none were reported with an elevated vasoactive intestinal peptide level or plasma gastrin-releasing peptide level. Even though these GI peptides were present in the serum, it is not apparent that any of these peptides contributed to any clinical symptoms.

Foregut carcinoids are more likely to produce various GI peptides than midgut carcinoids.[1] Ectopic ACTH production with Cushing's syndrome is increasingly seen with foregut carcinoids, and in some studies these tumors were the most common cause of the ectopic ACTH syndrome, accounting for 64% of all patients.[1] Acromegaly due to release of growth hormone–releasing factors (GRFoma) can occur with a number of carcinoids.[24] The somatostatinoma syndrome due to somatostatin release can occur with duodenal carcinoids.[24]

CARCINOID SYNDROME

CLINICAL FEATURES

Flushing attacks occur in 23% to 65% of carcinoid syndrome patients initially and in 63% to 78% at some time during the disease course (Table 34.6-3). The typical flush is the sudden appearance of a deep red erythema of the upper part of the body, primarily the face and neck. Flushes are often associated with an unpleasant feeling of warmth, occasionally with lacrimation, itching, palpitations, facial or conjunctival edema, and diarrhea. Flushes may be spontaneous or precipitated by stress, alcohol, certain foods such as cheese, or exercise, or pharmacologically by injections of agents such as catecholamines, calcium, or pentagastrin.[1] Flushes may be brief, lasting 2 to 5 minutes, especially initially, or may be prolonged for hours, especially later. They are usually seen with carcinoids of midgut origin but can also occur in some patients with foregut tumors. With bronchial carcinoids the flushes can be frequently prolonged, lasting for hours to days, reddish, and associated with salivation, lacrimation, diaphoresis, facial swelling, palpitations, deep furrowing of the forehead, diarrhea, and hypotension. The flushing with bronchial carcinoids has a greater tendency to cause diffuse body involvement, and after repeated flushing of this type, patients may develop a constant red or cyanotic coloration. The flush associated with gastric carcinoids is also reddish but is patchy in distribution over the neck and face. It is frequently provoked by food intake or pentagas-

trin, with erythema associated with blotches and wheals with central clearing, frequently occurring around the root of the neck and on the arms, and the lesions are frequently associated with pruritus.[1]

Diarrhea is present in 32% to 73% of patients initially and in 67% to 84% at some time during the disease course (see Table 34.6-3). Diarrhea usually occurs with flushing (85% of cases), but it may occur alone (15% of cases).[1,25] The diarrhea is described as watery and less commonly as frothy or the pale bulky stool of steatorrhea; the number of stools ranges from 2 to 30 per day and 60% of patients have output of less than 1 L/d.[25] Steatorrhea is present in 67% and in 46% is more than 15 g/d.[25] Abdominal pain may be present with the diarrhea or independently, and the frequency varies from 10% to 34% (see Table 34.6-3).

Cardiac manifestations occur in 11% to 66% of patients[26,27] (see Table 34.6-3). The cardiac disease is due to fibrosis involving the endocardium, primarily of the right side of the heart, although left-side lesions can also occur.[1,26] The fibrous deposits are diffuse and are found most commonly on the ventricular aspect of the tricuspid valve and the associated chordae and less commonly on the pulmonary valve cusps. These fibrous deposits tend to cause constriction of both the tricuspid and pulmonic valves. At the pulmonic valve, stenosis is usually predominant, whereas at the tricuspid valve the constriction results in the valve's being fixed open, and tricuspid regurgitation is usually predominant.[26] In two series, 80% of the patients with cardiac lesions had evidence of heart failure.[1] Lesions on the left side are seen in 30% of autopsy studies, are less extensive, and most frequently occur on the mitral valve.[1]

Other clinical manifestations of carcinoid syndrome are wheezing or asthma-like symptoms in 3% to 18% of patients and pellagra-like skin lesions with hyperkeratosis and pigmen-

TABLE 34.6-3. Clinical Characteristics in Patients with Malignant Carcinoid Syndrome

	At Presentation		During Course of Disease			
	Davis 1973	Norheim 1987	Thorson 1958	Feldman 1987	Norheim 1987	Soga 1999
NO. OF PATIENTS	91	91	79	111	91	748
SYMPTOM OR SIGN						
Diarrhea	73%	32%	68%	73%	84%	67%
Flushing	65%	23%	74%	63%	75%	78%
Pain	—	10%	—	—	—	34%
Asthma and wheezing	8%	4%	18%	3%	15%	10%
Pellagra	2%	—	5%	—	—	—
None	12%	—	—	22%	—	—
Carcinoid heart disease present	11%	—	41%	14%	33%	33%
DEMOGRAPHICS						
Male	59%	46%	61%	—	46%	52%
Age						
Mean	57 y	59 y	52 y	—	—	54.5 y
Range	25–79 y	ND	18–80 y	—	—	9–91 y
TUMOR LOCATION						
Foregut	5%	9%	2%	—	9%	33%
Midgut	78%	87%	75%	—	87%	60%
Hindgut	5%	1%	8%	—	1%	1%
Unknown	11%	2%	15%	—	2%	6%

ND, no data.
(Data from refs. 10, 76–79.)

tation in 2% to 5% of cases (see Table 34.6-3). Rarely reported are rheumatoid arthritis, arthralgias, changes in mental state or confusion, and ophthalmic changes during flushing leading to vessel occlusion.[1] A variety of noncardiac problems secondary to increased fibrous tissue have been reported, including retroperitoneal fibrosis leading to ureteral obstruction or Peyronie's disease of the penis, intraabdominal fibrosis, and occlusion of mesenteric arteries or veins. Sexual dysfunction is a common complaint of men with carcinoid syndrome. This may be related to vascular effects of the serotonin on pelvic blood vessels.

PATHOBIOLOGY

Carcinoid syndrome developed in 8% of 8876 patients with carcinoids,[10] with an incidence of 1.7% to 18.4% in six different series.[1,10] Carcinoid syndrome occurs only when sufficient concentrations of the hormonal products released by the tumor reach the systemic circulation. Its occurrence and severity are directly related to tumor size in an area that drains into the systemic circulation. In 91% of cases this only occurs after distant metastases (especially to the liver).[1,10] Rarely, however, primary GI tumors with nodal metastases with extensive invasion retroperitoneally or drainage into the ovarian veins, pancreatic carcinoids with retroperitoneal lymph nodes, or carcinoids such as those in the lung or ovary with direct access to the systemic circulation can produce carcinoid syndrome without hepatic metastases.[10,28] All carcinoids do not have the same propensity to metastasize and to produce carcinoid syndrome (see Table 34.6-2). Because midgut tumors are the most common and frequently metastasize, midgut tumors account for 60% to 87% of cases of carcinoid syndrome, foregut tumors for 2% to 33%, hindgut tumors for 1% to 8%, and an unknown primary location for 2% to 15% (see Table 34.6-3).

Symptoms of carcinoid syndrome were originally attributed to secretion of 5-HT (serotonin) by the tumor.[1,26] In one study of 380 patients with carcinoid tumors, 56% had evidence of serotonin overproduction; 18% of 500 patients in a second study, and 88% of 103 patients with carcinoid tumors in a third study had elevated urinary levels of 5-hydroxyindoleacetic acid (5-HIAA), the major metabolite of serotonin.[1] When 44 consecutive cases were studied before any resection, 84% of the patients were found to have serotonin overproduction. In three studies, 12% to 26% of patients with evidence of serotonin overproduction did not have symptoms of carcinoid syndrome. In one study,[29] in 44 consecutively treated patients with carcinoids, platelet and urinary levels of serotonin, 5-HIAA, and seven catecholamine metabolites were measured. Platelet serotonin level was elevated in 96%, 43%, and 0% of patients with midgut, foregut, and hindgut carcinoids, respectively. Urinary levels of dopamine and catecholamine metabolites were elevated in 38% and 33% of patients with midgut carcinoids, 20% and 20% of those with foregut carcinoids, and 7% and 14% of those with hindgut carcinoids, respectively. In a large review of 748 cases of carcinoid syndrome, 92% had increased serotonin activity.[10]

Patients may develop either a typical or atypical type of carcinoid syndrome. In patients with the typical carcinoid syndrome the conversion of tryptophan to 5-HTP is the rate-limiting step. Once formed, the 5-HTP is rapidly converted to 5-HT in the tumor by dopa decarboxylase and either stored in the neurosecretory tumor granules or released into vascular compartments, and most is taken up and stored in the granules of platelets. A small amount remains in the plasma. The majority in the circulation is converted by monoamine oxidase and aldehyde dehydrogenase to 5-HIAA, which appears in large amounts in the urine.[1] This is the typical pattern in argentaffin- and argyrophil-positive tumors such as midgut carcinoids, which characteristically secrete large amounts of serotonin and which make up 60% to 87% of all cases of carcinoid syndrome (see Table 34.6-3). Some carcinoids cause an atypical carcinoid syndrome and are thought to be deficient in the enzyme dopa decarboxylase; thus, they cannot convert 5-HTP to 5-HT (serotonin), and 5-HTP is secreted into the blood stream. Plasma serotonin levels are normal in these patients, but urinary levels are usually elevated because some of the 5-HTP is decarboxylated in the kidney and excreted as serotonin (5-HT). Foregut carcinoids are more likely to excrete high levels of 5-HT and 5-HTP in the urine and give the atypical carcinoid syndrome.

The exact role of serotonin in causing the flushing in carcinoid syndrome remains unclear,[5,22,30] and several antagonists against some serotonin receptor subtypes generally have no effect on the flushing.[1,31] When a specific radioenzymatic assay was used during spontaneous flushing in patients with midgut carcinoids, increased plasma serotonin and norepinephrine levels were found, with higher levels in the external jugular than in the antecubital veins. This result suggests a possible role for these bioamines in the pathogenesis of flushing with midgut carcinoids. The exact cause of the flushing in patients with carcinoid syndrome may differ depending on the tumor type. In patients with gastric carcinoids, the red, patchy, pruritic flush is thought to be caused by histamine, because this type of flushing can be prevented by the use of H_1- and H_2-receptor antagonists.[1] In addition to serotonin, other candidates for mediators of flushing include the tachykinins (substance P, neuropeptide K), various GI peptides, and prostaglandins. However, other studies generally have concluded that prostaglandins are unlikely to be major mediators of the flushing or diarrhea.

Studies demonstrate that numerous tachykinins are stored in carcinoids and are released during flushing.[1,32] In some studies changes in plasma substance P or neuropeptide K levels did not correlate with the occurrence of flushing, which led the authors to conclude that circulating tachykinins have only a minor role, if any, in causing the flushing. In one study[1] octreotide relieved pentagastrin-induced flushing in all patients without necessarily altering the substance P response. Furthermore, pentagastrin caused flushing in some patients without rises in plasma substance P, which suggests that mediators other than substance P must be important in inducing the flushing. Even though various GI peptides have been proposed to be involved in the flushing, no changes in plasma levels of vasoactive intestinal peptide, gastric inhibitory polypeptide, neurotensin, pancreatic polypeptide, motilin, insulin, glucagon, or enteroglucagon have been detected with provocation of the flush.[1]

Patients with carcinoid syndrome have been shown to have increased colonic motility with a shortened transit time and possibly a secretory or absorptive alteration.[1,30] Serotonin is thought to be predominantly responsible for the diarrhea in some patients through its effects on gut motility and intestinal electrolyte and fluid secretion.[1,25] Serotonin receptor antagonists (especially 5-HT$_3$ receptor antagonists such as ondansetron) relieve the diarrhea.[1,31] Furthermore, alosetron, another 5-HT$_3$ receptor antagonist, decreased proximal colonic emptying in patients with carcinoid syndrome.[1] Some studies provide evidence that prostaglandin E$_2$ and tachykinins may also be important mediators of carcinoid diarrhea.[1] Patients with carcinoid syndrome had decreased absorption of Na$^+$, K$^+$, Cl$^-$ and water in the jejunum and increased intraluminal non–substance P tachykinin and prostaglandin E$_2$ concentrations compared to normal controls.[30] In combination with histamine, serotonin may be responsible for producing asthma and may be involved in the fibrotic reactions causing carcinoid-associated heart disease, Peyronie's disease, and ureteral obstruction.[1] The pathogenetic link between the carcinoid and heart disease remains a subject of controversy. No relationship between the severity of the heart disease and other common manifestations such as flushing, diarrhea, or duration of disease has been established.[1,33] Patients with heart disease have higher urinary 5-HIAA excretion[27] and higher plasma levels of neurokinin A,[33] substance P,[33] or plasma atrial natriuretic peptide[34] than those without heart disease and more frequently receive chemotherapy.[27] Studies support the role of serotonin in mediating the cardiac disease. The valvular heart disease caused by appetite-suppressant drugs such as dexfenfluramine is indistinguishable from carcinoid heart disease or cardiac disease after long exposure to 5-HT$_2$ receptor–preferring ergot drug metabolites of fenfluramine, which have high affinity for 5-HT$_2$ receptors. Furthermore, serotonin up-regulates transforming growth factor-β in aortic valve cells, which may be important in stimulating proliferation and collagen biosynthesis.[35]

DIAGNOSIS

Diagnosis of carcinoid syndrome relies on the measurement of urinary or plasma levels of serotonin or its metabolites (5-HIAA), with the measurement of 5-HIAA in a 24-hour urine sample the most commonly used test. False-positives may occur if the patient is eating serotonin-rich foods, such as bananas, plantains, pineapple, kiwi fruit, walnuts, hickory nuts, pecans, and avocados, which would falsely elevate urinary levels.[36] Medications, including cough medicine containing guaifenesin, acetaminophen, salicylates, and L-dopa, should also be avoided because they may affect urinary 5-HIAA levels.[1,36] If one properly controls dietary and medicinal intake, the normal range for urinary 5-HIAA excretion is between 2 and 8 mg/24 h, although others have suggested that using a level of 15 mg/d may reduce false-positives.[36] Many patients with serotonin-secreting carcinoids have urinary 5-HIAA excretion in the range of 8 to 30 mg/24 h. The measurement of urinary 5-HIAA levels is the current method of choice to diagnose carcinoid syndrome. In one study 5-HIAA determinations alone have a 73% sensitivity and a 100% specificity for identifying carcinoid syndrome.[1]

Most physicians rely totally on the measurement of urinary 5-HIAA for diagnosis. However, urinary and platelet measurement of serotonin itself may give additional information; thus, it has been recommended that these should also be measured.[29] In one comparative study of platelet serotonin levels,[29] urine 5-HIAA levels, and urinary serotonin levels in 44 consecutively treated carcinoid patients, the sensitivities were 50%, 29%, and 55%, respectively, in 14 patients with foregut carcinoids; 100%, 92%, and 82%, respectively, in 25 patients with midgut carcinoids; and 20%, 0%, and 60%, respectively, in 5 patients with

hindgut carcinoids. The data demonstrate the increased sensitivity of measuring platelet serotonin levels. Elevations of 5-HIAA can occur in malabsorption states and a number of other conditions.[36] It is important to remember that foregut carcinoids tend to produce an atypical carcinoid syndrome with increases in plasma 5-HTP and not serotonin, because they lack the appropriate decarboxylase, with the result that urinary 5-HIAA levels may not be markedly increased.[1]

Diagnostic difficulties may arise with patients who flush for reasons other than carcinoid syndrome, patients with carcinoid syndrome in whom flushing is not apparent, patients with certain carcinoids (especially foregut tumors) in whom 5-HIAA levels may be normal or minimally elevated, or the rare patient without metastatic disease who presents with flushing.[28] The differential diagnosis of flushing includes menopausal flushing; reactions to alcohol and glutamate; side effects of drugs like chlorpropamide, calcium channel blockers, and nicotinic acid; and other neoplastic disorders such as chronic myelogenous leukemia and systemic mastocytosis. None of these conditions causes increased urinary 5-HIAA levels, and these disorders can be distinguishable pathologically.

The diagnosis of a carcinoid may be suspected by clinical symptoms suggestive of carcinoid syndrome or by the presence of the other clinical symptoms such as abdominal pain or diarrhea, or it can be made in relatively asymptomatic patients from the pathologic report at surgery or after liver biopsy for hepatomegaly. Ileal carcinoids, which make up more than 25% of all clinically detected carcinoids, should be suspected if a patient presents with bowel obstruction, abdominal pain, flushing, or diarrhea. In one study involving 154 consecutively treated patients with GI carcinoids, 60% of those found at surgery were asymptomatic.[1] In patients with symptomatic tumors, the time from the onset of symptoms until the diagnosis is frequently delayed, varying from 1 to 2 years. Attempts are being made to identify more specific and sensitive serum markers for carcinoids, which may allow earlier diagnosis. In one study, urinary 5-HIAA level had a sensitivity of 73% and a specificity of 100%; plasma substance P level, a sensitivity of 32% and a specificity of 85%; and plasma neurotensin level, a sensitivity of 41% and a specificity of 60%. A number of studies demonstrate that serum chromogranin A levels are elevated in 56% to 100% of patients with carcinoids, and the level correlates with tumor bulk.[1,8] Serum chromogranin A elevations are not specific for carcinoids because increased levels occur with high frequency in patients with pancreatic endocrine tumors[1,8] and certain other NETs. The α or β subunit of human chorionic gonadotropin is detected frequently by immunocytochemistry in carcinoids, and elevated plasma levels of HCG are reported in 28% of patients with carcinoids and 13% of patients with carcinoid syndrome.[1] NSE is also used as a plasma marker of carcinoid tumors but it is less sensitive than chromogranin A, being positive in only 17% to 47% of patients.[1,8]

LOCALIZATION

A number of techniques, including GI endoscopy, barium radiography, chest radiography, imaging studies [ultrasonography, computed tomography (CT), magnetic resonance imaging, angiography], endoscopic ultrasonography, selective venous sampling for various hormones, positron emission tomography (PET), and various forms of radionuclide scanning [radiolabeled somatostatin receptor scintigraphy (SRS), iodinated metaiodobenzylguanidine (MIBG) scanning], have all been used to determine the location of the primary tumor as well as tumor extent.[1,37–40]

Bronchial carcinoids are usually detected by chest radiography, CT, or occasionally bronchoscopy.[18] They appear frequently (37%) as opacities with sharp or often notched margins. They are slow growing and often induce airway compression with resultant atelectasis. Enlarged hilar lymph nodes from metastasis are rare. Rectal, duodenal, colonic, and gastric carcinoids are almost always detected by GI endoscopy, with barium radiograph results being generally negative.[1,19] When barium radiograph results are positive, they show dilated loops of small bowel or extrinsic filling defects but rarely detect a mucosal lesion, whereas ileal, cecal, and right colon tumors are often diagnosed on radiographic studies.[1]

The main problem is localizing small bowel carcinoids, which may be very small and are frequently missed by barium studies, and small carcinoids in other GI tissues.[1] Some of these tumors can be localized by angiography, SRS, or CT,[1] but many are not seen with these modalities.[40,41] Liver metastases are usually detected by CT or, more recently, SRS. Angiography is more sensitive than CT for detecting liver metastases.[1] CT and SRS at present are the primary diagnostic modalities for tumor staging.[41] CT frequently misses the primary tumor, especially if it is small (less than 1.5 cm).[39] However, CT is generally helpful in evaluating the presence of liver metastases and retroperitoneal lymphadenopathy.[1,39,41]

Carcinoids possess high-affinity receptors for somatostatin in 88% to 100% of cases.[37,40,42,43] The somatostatin receptors are present in both the primary tumor and metastases. Five subtypes of somatostatin receptor (numbered sst_1 to sst_5) have been described.[42] Octreotide binds with high affinity to sst_2 and sst_5 and with a lower affinity to sst_3; it has a very low affinity for sst_1 and sst_4.[42] Studies show that almost all carcinoids (90% to 100%) possess sst_2, 50% to 60% have sst_5, 10% to 100% possess sst_3, 70% to 100% show sst_1, and 20% to 100% possess sst_4. Indium 111–diethylenetriamine pentaacetic acid–D-phenylalanyl octreotide has been approved for localizing carcinoids using radionuclide scanning.[42] SRS images the tumor in 73% to 89% of patients with carcinoids.[37,39–42] In one comparative study involving 40 patients, SRS localized tumors in 78% and CT in 82%.[1] SRS detected primary tumors in two patients whose tumors were missed on CT, and in 16% of cases it detected lesions not previously seen. Numerous other studies have demonstrated that SRS has high sensitivity for localizing carcinoids, especially the extent of metastatic spread[39–42] (Fig. 34.6-1). Studies demonstrate that SRS identifies additional bone metastases from carcinoid tumors not seen with bone scanning.[44] In general, SRS has excellent specificity, but it is important to remember that high densities of somatostatin receptors exist on a number of other normal and abnormal cells, which can lead to increased uptake and a false-positive response.[40,45] These include granulomas (sarcoid, tuberculosis, etc.), activated lymphocytes (wound infections, lymphomas), thyroid diseases (goiter, thyroiditis), pancreatic endocrine tumors, and other endocrine tumors. In one study, 12% of SRS localizations were false-positives.[40,45] Because of its sensitivity and ability to image all body areas, SRS should be the initial imaging procedure to localize and establish the extent of the carcinoid.

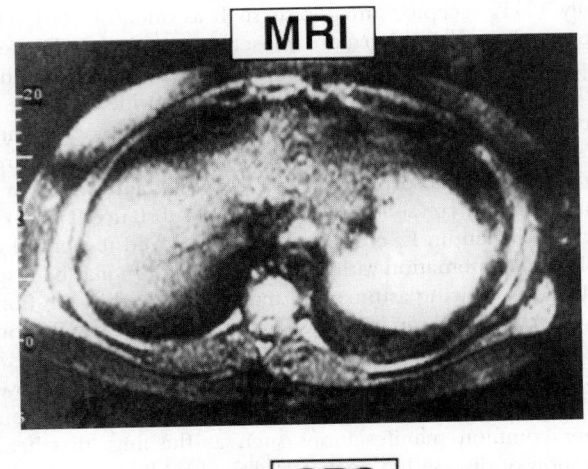

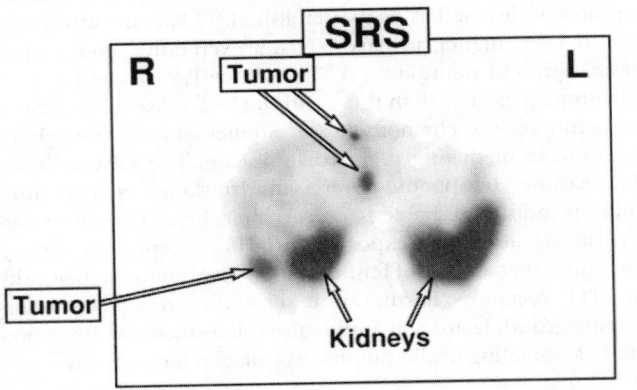

FIGURE 34.6-1. Comparison of the ability of magnetic resonance imaging (MRI) **(A)** and somatostatin receptor scintigraphy (SRS) **(B)** to localize hepatic metastases in a patient with carcinoid syndrome and metastatic gastric carcinoid to the liver. MRI was negative for tumor, whereas the SRS scan demonstrated liver metastases (labeled *Tumor*) in the left and right hepatic lobes. The imaging results in this patient demonstrate the greater sensitivity of SRS for localizing hepatic metastases from a carcinoid tumor compared with conventional imaging studies.

Bone metastases are increasingly being recognized in patients with metastatic carcinoid and other pancreatic endocrine tumors.[1,44] In general, technetium 99m bone scanning and SRS have been found to be more sensitive than conventional radiography for detecting bone metastases and can be complementary.[1,40,44]

PET scanning with carbon 111–labeled 5-HTP has been compared with CT in patients with carcinoids.[38] PET was more sensitive than CT in a number of patients.[38] During treatment there was a close correlation (r = 0.91) between changes in the PET scan transport rate constant and changes in urinary 5-HIAA level, which suggests that PET scanning may be useful for monitoring the results of therapy.[1,38]

PROGNOSIS

Clinically, carcinoid syndrome is generally a manifestation of advanced disease.[1,10] Two of three patients with carcinoid syndrome have physical signs of cancer such as an abdominal mass or hepatomegaly. There is a clear positive correlation between tumor mass and urinary 5-HIAA levels; therefore, this laboratory test is a good marker for extent of disease.

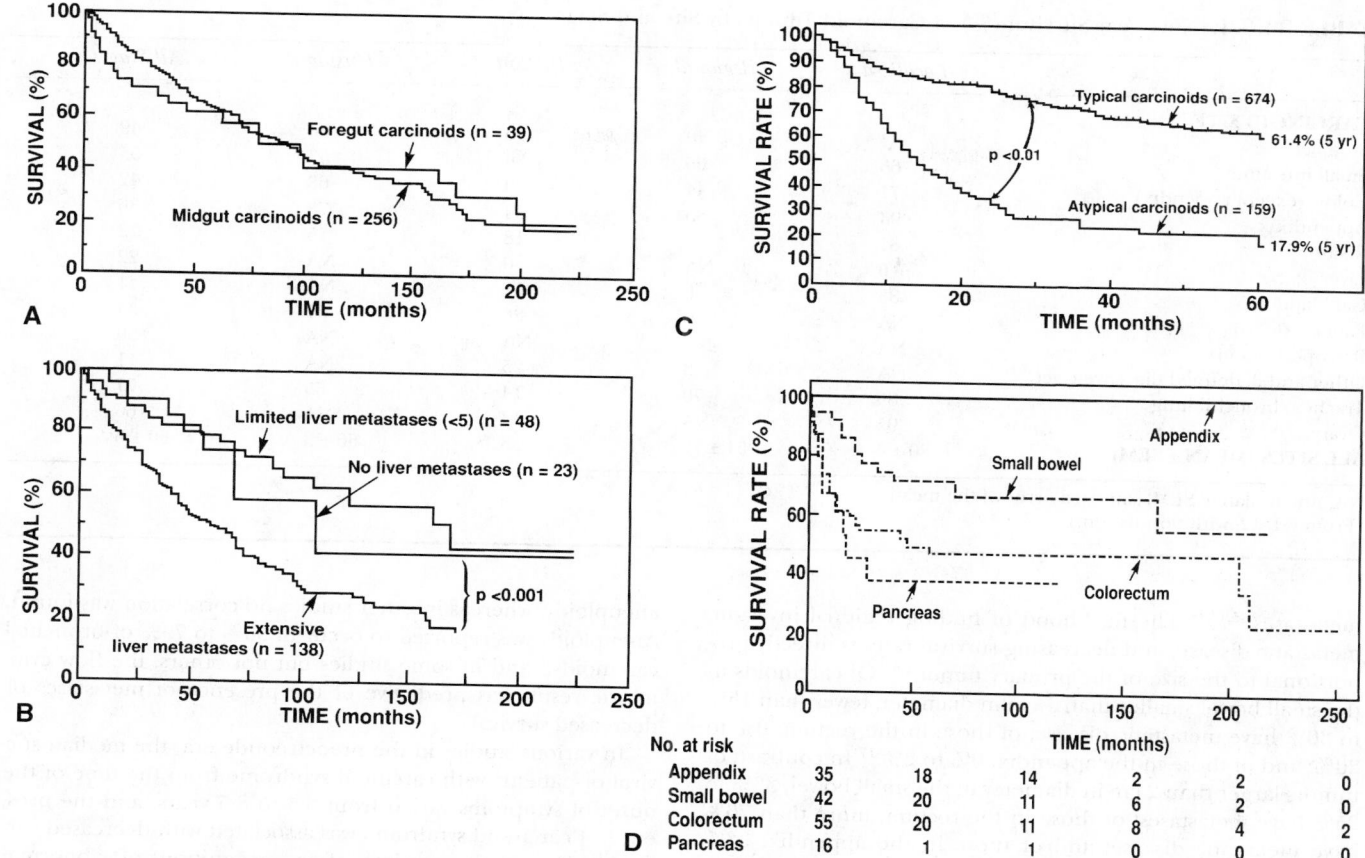

FIGURE 34.6-2. Effect of carcinoid tumor type, extent of metastases, histologic pattern, and localization of primary tumor on survival. **A:** There was no significant difference in 5-year survival for patients with foregut or midgut carcinoid tumors (60% vs. 63%).[46] **B:** The 5-year survival of patients with no liver metastases was not significantly different from that of patients with a few hepatic metastases (fewer than five) (73% vs. 79%), but was significantly greater (*P* <.001) than that of patients with extensive hepatic metastases (more than five) (47%).[46] **C:** Effect of the histologic pattern of the carcinoid tumor in 833 patients is shown, with the 5-year survival rates given for both patterns.[20] **D:** The number of patients at risk at different times is shown. Patients with an appendiceal primary had a significantly better prognosis (*P* <.01) than did those with pancreatic or colorectal carcinoids.[48]

Carcinoids in different locations not only differ in the percentage that are malignant and the percentage that produce carcinoid syndrome (see Table 34.6-2), but also in their aggressiveness.[1,13] The percentage of carcinoids in different locations characterized by localized disease, regional metastases, or distant metastases varies widely. The highest percentage of nonlocalized disease is with pancreatic (91%), colonic (77%), and small intestinal carcinoids (75%), whereas the highest percentage of localized disease is with laryngeal carcinoids (100%), followed by those of the ovary, appendix, and rectum (62% to 95%). Overall, metastases were present at the time of diagnosis in 45% of patients included in the SEER group data.[12] In one study no difference was found in the overall 5-year survival rate of patients with carcinoids of the foregut (60%) and midgut (63%)[46] (Fig. 34.6-2A).

Survival rates for patients with different carcinoids depend on both the site and the extent of tumor[1,11–13,47] (Tables 34.6-4 and 34.6-5; see Fig. 34.6-2D). For all 8305 patients represented in the SEER data[12] with local disease only, the 5-year survival rate was 80%, varying from 0% for those with liver tumors, to 65% for those with carcinoids of the small intestine and ileum, to 95%

for those with carcinoids of the ovary (see Table 34.6-4). In patients with regional involvement, 5-year survival was 51% overall, varying from 0% for carcinoids of the pancreas and gallbladder to 85% for appendix tumors. For patients with distant metastases, the overall 5-year survival was 22%, varying from 0% for the liver to 36% for the small intestine. In different studies of the common carcinoids, the 5-year survival was the highest for carcinoids of the appendix (86% to 100%),[11,14,48] followed by those of the lung (77% to 87%),[11,12] rectum (62% to 72%),[11,12,17] small intestine (42% to 73%),[1,11,12,15,48] and colon and stomach (42% to 75%)[11,12,48] (see Table 34.6-4 and Fig. 34.6-2D).

One of the main determinants of survival is the presence of liver metastases (see Tables 34.6-4 and 34.6-5 and Fig. 34.6-2).[1,12,15,17,47] In a multivariant analysis of 188 cases of patients with carcinoids,[48] the one factor independently predictive of death was the presence of metastases. Additional prognostic factors are summarized in Table 34.6-5. The extent of hepatic metastases is also an important prognostic factor (see Fig. 34.6-2B and Table 34.6-5). Female gender is associated with a better prognosis,[48] as is younger age.[46,49] The level of tissue invasion is an important predictor of the probability of developing liver

TABLE 34.6-4. Five-Year Survival (%) of Carcinoid Tumors by Site and Stage

	Localized	Regional	Distant	Unstaged	All Stages
CARCINOID SITE					
Stomach	64	40	10	66	49
Small intestine	65	66	36	53	55
Colon (except appendix)	71	44	20	68	42
Appendix	94	85	34	78	86
Rectum	81	47	18	75	72
Liver	0	NA	0	NA	22
Gallbladder	83	0	NA	NA	41
Pancreas	NA	0	26	57	34
Retroperitoneum	NA	NA	NA	NA	50
Other and ill-defined digestive tract	NA	3	25	NA	11
Trachea/bronchi/lung	85	70	14	65	77
Ovary	95	NA	13	NA	66
ALL SITES (MEAN ± SEM)	80 ± 4	51 ± 10	22 ± 3	66 ± 3	50 ± 6

NA, not available; SEM, standard error of the mean.
(From ref. 12, with permission.)

metastases.[15,17,48] The likelihood of finding regional invasion, metastatic disease, and decreasing survival rates is directly proportional to the size of the primary tumor.[1,48] Of carcinoids in the small bowel smaller than 1 cm in diameter, fewer than 15% to 30% have metastatic disease; of those in the rectum, 0% to 20%; and of those in the appendix, 0% to 2%.[17] In contrast, of tumors larger than 2 cm in diameter in the small bowel, 33% to 95% have metastases; of those in the rectum, more than 70% have metastatic disease; and of those in the appendix, 33% have metastatic disease.[1,15,17] For all patients with carcinoids, the 5-year survival varies from 11% to 86% in different studies[11,12] (see Table 34.6-4).

The histologic features as well as the stage of the carcinoid have been shown to correlate with disease-specific survival and the risk of metastases[15,16,20,48] (see Table 34.6-5 and Fig. 34.6-2C). In one study,[48] for patients with bowel tumors invading only the submucosa (T1), 5-year survival rate was 100%; for those with tumors invading the muscularis propria (T2), 81%; for those with tumors invading the subserosa (T3), 70%; and for those with tumors involving the visceral peritoneum or directly invading other structures (T4), 52%. For bronchial carcinoids,[1,18] the most important variables affecting prognosis are increasing age, tumor diameter larger than 3 cm, T stage, N stage, lymph node involvement, and number of positive lymph nodes. For all pulmonary NETs, which include typical and atypical carcinoids as well as large cell and small cell neuroendocrine carcinomas,[1] the histologic features, number of mitoses, degree of necrosis, vascular invasion, and extent of nuclear pleomorphism all had a significant effect on survival.[1] Histologic features such as necrosis, increased mitotic count, nuclear pleomorphism, vascular or lymphatic invasion, and undifferentiated growth pattern are used to classify carcinoids histologically as typical or atypical,[4] and this variable can have a marked effect on survival (see Fig. 34.6-2C; Table 34.6-5).[1,20] Measures of proliferation such as Ki-67 activity or expression of proliferative cell nuclear antigen correlate with tumor aggressiveness or survival in some studies, but not in others. Flow cytometry has been used to attempt to define the malignant potential for both GI and bronchial carcinoids.[1,50] In two studies[1,50] of GI carcinoids, the presence of metastases or decreased survival correlated with the presence of

aneuploidy, whereas in other studies no correlation was found. Aneuploidy was reported to occur in 50% to 79% of bronchial carcinoids,[1] and in some studies but not others, the flow cytometric result was predictive of the presence of metastases or decreased survival.

In various studies in the preoctreotide era, the median survival of patients with carcinoid syndrome from the time of the onset of symptoms varied from 3.5 to 8.5 years, and the presence of carcinoid syndrome was associated with decreased survival.[1] The mean survival after recognition of abnormal excretion of 5-HIAA was 23 months, and the 5-year survival rates after onset of symptoms in two studies were 30% and 67%.[1] In a number of studies the level of 5-HIAA excretion has been correlated with survival (see Table 34.6-5).[1,46] In one study patients excreting 10 to 49 mg/d had a median survival of 29 months, those excreting 50 to 149 mg/d had a survival time of 24 months, and those excreting more than 150 mg/d had a survival time of 13 months. Octreotide treatment has been proposed to extend survival. Studies show that the degree of plasma chromogranin A elevation is predictive of survival,[46] as is the plasma level of the tachykinin neuropeptide K.[46] A number of studies have provided evidence that patients with carcinoids are at increased risk for developing a synchronous adenocarcinoma (7% to 10%), with the most common site being the large intestine.[15,17] The development of a second malignancy is associated with a worse prognosis.[49]

The most immediately life-threatening complication of carcinoid syndrome, carcinoid crisis, is observed more frequently in patients who have intense symptoms from foregut carcinoids or who have greatly elevated urinary 5-HIAA levels (more than 200 mg/24 h).[1] Carcinoid crisis may occur spontaneously, or it may be associated with stress, anesthesia, chemotherapy, or even biopsy of hepatic metastases.[1,1,42,51] Patients usually develop flushing, diarrhea, and abdominal pain. Mentation is altered, ranging from light-headedness to coma. Cardiac abnormalities also occur, including tachycardia, hypertension, or profound hypotension.[1] This crisis may be successfully treated, but in some patients it is a terminal event. The value of octreotide in the treatment and prevention of carcinoid crises has been frequently reported.[1,42,51]

TABLE 34.6-5. Prognostic Factors in Carcinoid Tumors

UNIVARIATE ANALYSIS

Age ($P = .001$) (<50 y, 97%; ≥50 y, 63%)

Gender ($P<.01$) [5-y survival: female (66%) > male (47%)]

Primary tumor site ($P<.01$) (survival rate: appendix > small bowel > colorectal > pancreas)

Depth of invasion ($P<.001$)

Presence of lymph node metastases ($P<.001$) [5-y survival: no (94%) vs. yes (43%)]

Tumor size ($P<.005$) [5-y survival: 1 cm (100%) > 1.1–2.0 cm (82%) > 2.1+ cm (39%)]

Presence of liver metastases ($P<.001$) [5-y survival: no (88%) vs. yes (25%)]

Extent of hepatic metastases ($P<.001$) [extensive, 47% vs. limited (<5), 79%]

Mode of discovery ($P<.001$) (incidentally > symptomatic)

Operative intent ($P<.001$) [5-y survival: cure (91%) vs. palliative (25%)]

Presence of a second malignancy

Histologic features (typical or atypical)

Flow cytometry features (i.e., aneuploidy)

Mitotic counts ($P<.001$) (<10 per ten high-power fields vs. >10 per ten high-power fields)

Ki-67 index ($P<.05$)

Proliferative cell nuclear antigen expression

Presence of carcinoid syndrome

Laboratory results [extent of increase of serum chromogranin A ($P<.01$), urinary 5-HIAA ($P<.01$), plasma neuropeptide K ($P<.05$)]

MULTIVARIATE ANALYSIS

Death due to all causes

Gender (RR, 2.78; 95% CI, 1.2–6.5)

Death due to the disease

Presence of metastases (RR, 3.87; 95% CI, 1.0–14.5)

CI, confidence interval; 5-HIAA, 5-hydroxyindoleacetic acid; Ki-67, proliferative associated nuclear antigen recognized by monoclonal antibody Ki-67; RR, relative risk.

Note: All results are from ref. 48 except age (refs. 1, 20, 49), extent of hepatic metastases (ref. 46), histologic features (refs. 1, 20), flow cytometry results (ref. 1), presence of carcinoid syndrome (ref. 1), mitotic counts, laboratory results (refs. 1, 46), presence of a secondary malignancy (ref. 49), Ki-67 index (ref. 47), proliferative cell nuclear antigen expression (ref. 22).

TREATMENT

Many patients with hepatic metastases from carcinoid tumor remain active and well except for occasional episodes of flushing or diarrhea. Treatment of these patients includes avoiding stress and conditions or substances that precipitate flushing, and dietary supplementation with nicotinamide (Fig. 34.6-3). Heart failure may require diuretics; wheezing may require oral bronchodilators such as salbutamol, a bronchodilator that interacts with β-adrenergic receptors and does not induce flushing, or aminophylline; and mild diarrhea may respond to antidiarrheal agents such as loperamide or diphenoxylate. If patients still have carcinoid syndrome symptoms, serotonin receptor antagonists or somatostatin analogues are the drugs of choice, although a number of other drugs have also been shown to be effective in small numbers of patients.[1]

These agents act in a variety of ways, including by inhibiting the synthesis of serotonin (parachlorophenylalanine, α-methyldopa), by functioning as serotonin receptor antagonists and blocking the action of 5-HT on target tissues, or by inhibiting the release of various vasoactive substances (octreotide, interferon-α) (see Fig. 34.6-3). Parachlorophenylalanine, which blocks the hydroxylase enzyme that converts tryptophan to 5-

HTP, relieves diarrhea and improves flushing in some patients and reduces urinary 5-HIAA levels.[1] However, its side effects include hypersensitivity reactions and psychiatric disturbances, which makes it intolerable for long-term clinical use. The agent α-methyldopa blocks the conversion of 5-HTP to serotonin; however, its effect is partial. Phenoxybenzamine, an α-adrenergic antagonist, as well as the phenothiazines, possibly acting as α-adrenergic receptor antagonists, may block flushing provoked by alcohol or other agents, although patients frequently become refractory. Fourteen subclasses of serotonin (5-HT) receptors have been described.[29] The 5-HT$_1$ and 5-HT$_2$ receptor antagonists methylsergide,[29] cyproheptadine, and ketanserin[52] frequently decrease the GI symptoms but usually do not decrease the flushing.[1] In one study cyproheptadine used at a dosage of 3 to 8 mg three times a day reduced diarrhea in 50% of patients, with minimal, if any, effect on flushing or excretion of 5-HIAA. The use of methylsergide is limited because it can cause or enhance retroperitoneal fibrosis. In various studies[1,52] ketanserin diminished the frequency and severity of flushing in 6% to 100% and diarrhea in 30% to 100% of patients.[1] The 5-HT$_3$ receptor antagonists (ondansetron, tropisetron, alosetron) usually control diarrhea and nausea, and occasionally flushing.[1,29,31] A combination of histamine H$_1$- and H$_2$-receptor antagonists are effective in treating carcinoid syndrome due to gastric carcinoids. Prednisone in dosages of 20 mg/d gives relief in some patients with severe flushing; however, it is ineffective in controlling the GI symptoms. Tamoxifen was reported to cause symptomatic improvement in 2 patients with carcinoid syndrome[1]; however, in a study involving 16 patients with malignant carcinoids, no improvement or sustained reduction in 5-HIAA levels occurred.[1]

Native somatostatin reduces symptoms in patients with carcinoid syndrome. However, its use is limited by its short half-life (2.5 to 3 minutes). With the availability of the synthetic long-acting somatostatin analogues octreotide (half-life of 90 minutes) and lanreotide, treatment can be given subcutaneously every 6 to 12 hours. These drugs are now the drugs of choice to control the symptoms of patients with carcinoid syndrome.[1,7,38,42,51,53–56] These somatostatin analogues are effective at relieving symptoms and decreasing hormone levels when self-administered every 6 to 12 hours subcutaneously in patients with carcinoid syndrome.[42,51,53–56] Octreotide decreases 5-HT and neuropeptide K release and synthesis from midgut carcinoids by a direct action on tumor cells. In an analysis of 62 published studies, octreotide controlled symptoms in more than 80% of patients.[51] When doses in excess of 375 mg/d were used, diarrhea improved in more than 80%.[42,51] If more than 400 mg/d was used, flushing was controlled in more than 80%.[42,51] At least 70% of patients had a more than 50% decrease in 5-HIAA levels.[51] It was recommended that, in patients with carcinoid syndrome with mild to moderate symptoms, treatment be initiated with 100 mg subcutaneously every 8 hours.[51] Individual responses vary, and some patients require higher doses, with dosages increased as high as 3000 mg/d.[51] Forty percent of patients experienced escape from control after a median time of 4 months; the remaining patients had sustained control for up to 2.5 years, with all responding for more than 1 year and one-third for more than 2 years.

Similar results to those reported for octreotide have been described for lanreotide. In patients with life-threatening features of carcinoid syndrome or carcinoid crisis, somatostatin analogues are effective at both treating the disorders and pre-

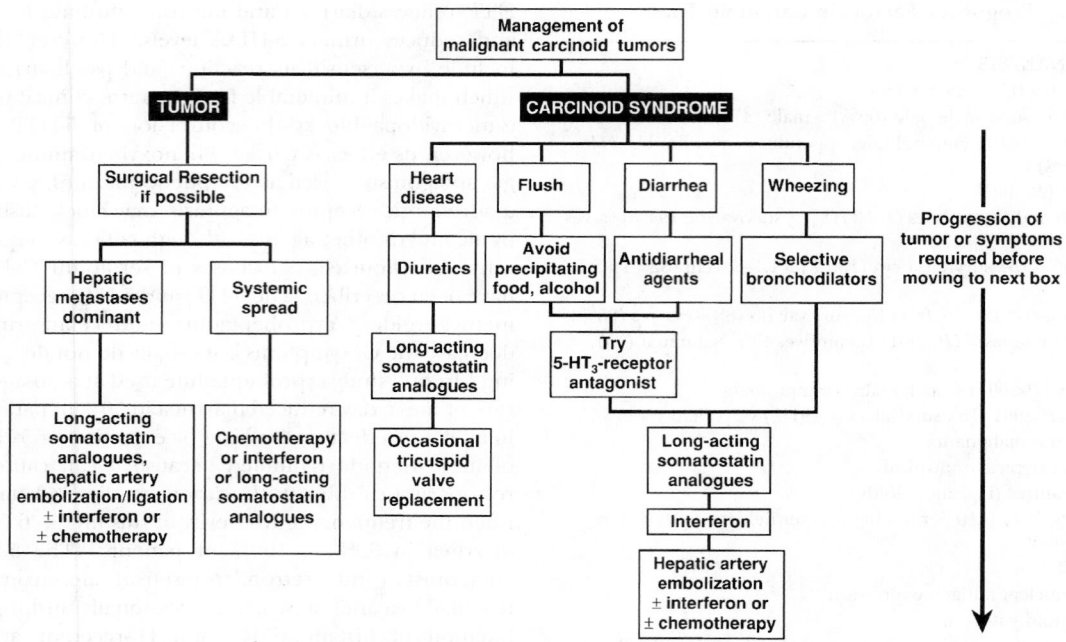

FIGURE 34.6-3. Algorithm for the treatment of malignant carcinoid tumors. *Somatostatin analogues* refers to the use of octreotide, lanreotide, or their long-acting depot formulations [octreotide LAR (long-acting release) or lanreotide SR (sustained release)].

venting their possible development during known precipitating events such as surgery, anesthesia, chemotherapy, or stress.[7,42] It has been recommended that patients with carcinoids scheduled for surgery be given 150 to 250 mg of octreotide subcutaneously every 6 to 8 hours beginning 24 to 48 hours before anesthesia. In patients receiving chemotherapy, 250 to 300 mg subcutaneously 1 to 2 hours before chemotherapy, is recommended.

Sustained-release preparations of somatostatin have been developed that facilitate treatment. These include octreotide LAR (long-acting release) given monthly and lanreotide SR (sustained release) given biweekly.[54] With octreotide LAR (30 mg/mo) a plasma level of 1 ng/mL or higher is maintained for 25 days, whereas this requires three to six injections per day of the non–sustained-release form. Like the nondepot forms, the sustained-release preparations are highly effective at controlling the symptoms of carcinoid syndrome.[54]

Short-term side effects of somatostatin analogues have been minimal, occurring in 40% to 50% of patients.[1,42] Pain at the injection site and effects related to the GI tract (discomfort in 59%; nausea, diarrhea in 15%) are the most common. Most such effects are short-lived and therapy is not interrupted.[42] Important long-term side effects include gallstone formation, steatorrhea, and deterioration in glucose tolerance.[1,42] In various studies the incidence of gallstones in patients treated long term with octreotide has varied from 5% to 80%, and in a review of 13 studies involving 213 patients with acromegaly, 29% developed gallstones.[42] In 45 patients with metastatic carcinoid or pancreatic endocrine tumors treated long term with octreotide, the overall incidence of gallstones, biliary sludge or both was 52%, with 7% having symptomatic disease requiring surgical treatment.[1]

Interferon-α is effective in carcinoid syndrome either alone[7,57,58] or combined with hepatic artery embolization.[57] In

more than 300 patients with carcinoids and carcinoid syndrome treated with interferon,[58] the overall biochemical response rate was 42%. Of 111 patients[58] at one center given interferon-α (1.5 to 7.0 mU three to seven times per week), 42% had a biochemical response (more than 50% decrease in tumor marker levels) with a median duration of 32 months. In 70% of patients an improvement in flushing or diarrhea was seen. Interferon-α has been combined with hepatic embolization[1] in 7 patients and compared with interferon given alone in 12 patients (5 mU/d) for the treatment of carcinoid syndrome.[1] Evaluation after 1 year of treatment showed that with interferon alone, 50% of patients had decreased urinary levels of 5-HIAA; when interferon was combined with embolization, 71% of patients had a decrease. With interferon alone,[1] 58% had decreased flushing and 67% had decreased diarrhea, whereas with embolization 86% had decreased flushing and 43% had decreased diarrhea.

Patients with carcinoid syndrome who have no response to octreotide or interferon-α alone have been treated with a combination of both agents.[58] In one study[58] involving 24 patients, all demonstrating increased urinary 5-HIAA levels and 19 having classical carcinoid syndrome, complete biochemical remission occurred in 18% and partial biochemical remission occurred in 59%. For a patient with severe carcinoid syndrome not responsive to other measures, hepatic artery embolization or ligation, either alone or combined with interferon or chemotherapy, may be effective[1,57] (see Fig. 34.6-3). In two studies involving 32 patients with metastatic liver disease with carcinoid syndrome, embolization or ligation resulted in at least a 50% decrease in urinary 5-HIAA levels in 63% of patients.[1] Chemoembolization,[1] which is embolization with Gelfoam and simultaneous chemotherapy (doxorubicin, mitomycin C, cisplatin, 5-fluorouracil) or interferon, was reported to result in symptomatic improvement in a significant number of patients with carcinoid syndrome. In one large study[1] involving 42 patients with carcinoid tumors, 83% had a decrease in 5-HIAA levels with chemoembolization followed by treatment with doxorubicin plus dacarbazine (DTIC) and streptozotocin plus 5-fluorouracil, and the mean decrease was 87%. Among patients responding, 98% had improvement in flushing and 88% had improvement in diarrhea. Hepatic artery occlusion or embolization can have significant side effects, with nausea, vomiting, liver pain, and fever.[1] Major complications occurred in 12% to 17% of patients, including hepatorenal syndrome, sepsis, gallbladder perforation or necrosis, upper GI bleeding, and abscess formation.[1] In two studies, 5% to 7% of patients died of a complication of hepatic artery occlusion.[1] In the literature, the mortality is reported as less than 3%, pain occurs in 100%, and pyrexia and leukocytosis are reported in 50%; occasional acute gangrenous cholecystitis from obstruction of the cystic artery, hepatic abscess, paralytic ileus, and renal failure are also reported.[1]

The approach to treatment of carcinoid syndrome at present is summarized in Figure 34.6-3. After symptomatic treatment, patients should avoid symptom-precipitating food and alcohol and use oral antidiarrheal agents for mild diarrhea and oral selective bronchodilators for wheezing. Serotonin receptor antagonists, particularly the new 5-HT$_3$ antagonists (ondansetron, tropisetron), may be effective, especially for diarrhea and nausea. Octreotide and lanreotide are the drugs of choice, self-administered by the patient or used in the newer sustained-release preparations. If tachyphylaxis develops, the dosage can be increased. If symptoms recur, are severe, and do not respond to an increased octreotide dosage, other serotonin receptor antagonists such as cyproheptadine or ketanserin should be considered, and if this approach is ineffective then interferon alone or subsequently combined with somatostatin analogues should be considered.

TREATMENT OF THE CARCINOID TUMOR

Resection of local or regional nodal metastatic disease can result in cure in some patients[1,59] (see Fig. 34.6-3). Because in the case of most carcinoids the possibility of metastatic disease is directly related to primary size, the extent of surgical resection for possible cure should be determined accordingly. In the case of appendiceal tumors smaller than 1 cm without gross metastases, which includes the majority,[14] a simple appendectomy is sufficient.[1] Of 103 such patients treated with a simple appendectomy, all of whom were followed for 5 years and 83 of whom were followed for 10 to 35 years, no patient developed a local recurrence or metastatic disease.[1] With rectal carcinoids smaller than 1 cm, local resection is usually adequate and results in cure.[1] The depth of invasion is also an important prognostic factor, and this should also be assessed in all tumors. If no invasion of the muscularis propria is present for rectal carcinoids smaller than 2 cm, local resection is adequate. Regarding small intestinal carcinoids smaller than 1 cm, there is not complete agreement. In most series 15% to 20% of tumors smaller than 1 cm have metastases.[1] However, in another series 69% of tumors smaller than 0.5 cm were associated with metastases,[60] and in a second series[15] 32% of tumors 0.6 to 1 cm had metastases, which led one group[60] to conclude that with midgut carcinoids malignancy is independent of size.[1]

This has led some to recommend a wide *en bloc* resection of the adjacent lymph node–bearing mesentery for all small intestinal carcinoids.[1] If the carcinoid is 2 cm or larger, which is uncommon in the case of carcinoids of the rectum or appendix but occurs in 40% of small bowel carcinoids, a full-scale cancer operation should be done. In the case of carcinoids of the appendix 2 cm or larger, a right hemicolectomy is the operation of choice.[1] For a tumor larger than 2 cm in the rectum or a smaller tumor with invasion through the muscularis propria, an abdominoperineal resection or a low anterior resection with primary anastomosis is recommended by some, but not by others.[1] In two studies involving patients with rectal carcinoids larger than 2 cm, all patients died from or developed metastatic disease to the liver despite abdominoperineal or low anterior resection, and the authors concluded that radical surgery is inappropriate if anorectal carcinoids can be removed by local excision.[1] In the case of a small intestinal carcinoid of 2 cm or larger, a wide resection is recommended with *en bloc* resection of the adjacent lymph node–bearing mesentery. For carcinoids of the appendix of 1 to 2 cm, simple appendectomy is recommended by some, whereas others favor more aggressive surgery such as a partial cecectomy or formal right hemicolectomy for those lesions located at the base of the appendix to ensure clear margins or in patients with invasion of the mesoappendix or vascular invasion. For carcinoids of the rectum of 1 to 2 cm, it is estimated that 11% to 47% are accompanied by metastases,[17] and thus it is recommended by some that these tumors be locally resected with a wide local full-thickness excision and that those tumors found to invade the muscularis propria be subjected to abdominoperineal or low anterior resection.[1] However, in another study 47% of these patients had metastases and 50% without metastatic disease developed metastases on follow-up, which led the authors to conclude that extensive surgery is not routinely warranted in these patients.[1] With gastric carcinoids, treatment is generally stratified by whether hypergastrinemia is present (types I and II) or not (type III).[19,61,62] Most recommend that in patients with type I or II carcinoids with lesions smaller than 1 cm, the carcinoids be removed endoscopically.[61,62] In patients with type I or II gastric carcinoids, if the tumor is larger than 2 cm or if there is local invasion, some recommend total gastrectomy, whereas others recommend that the tumor be removed surgically with resection and in type I lesions (pernicious anemia) an antrectomy be performed.[19,62] For type I or II lesions of 1 to 2 cm, there is no general agreement on treatment, with some recommending that these be treated surgically and others recommending endoscopic treatment.[62] In type III gastric carcinoids not associated with hypergastrinemia, which tend to be larger and more aggressive, if the lesion is larger than 2 cm, excision and regional lymph node clearance is recommended.[61,62] Some recommend a similar approach for any tumor larger than 1 cm, whereas others recommend that it be reserved for tumors in this size range showing histologic invasion. Most tumors smaller than 1 cm are treated endoscopically.[61]

Resection of isolated hepatic metastases may also be beneficial or curative in select patients.[1,59,60] In one study, 22% of patients had unilobar disease and could have all tumor resected, whereas in other studies fewer than 10% of patients were surgical candidates because of more disseminated disease.[1,59] In the 20% with all metastatic disease resected, 5-HIAA levels were normal and 10-year survival was 100%. The role of cytoreductive or debulking surgery in patients in whom all tumor cannot be removed is unclear. There are no prospective randomized trials that have addressed this question. There are a number of retrospective analyses that suggest such an approach should be considered in selected cases.[59] A number of studies[59,60] recommend debulking of mesenteric metastases and removal of compromised intestinal segments even in the presence of liver metastases. In one study[60] of 314 patients with midgut carcinoids, in those patients subjected to surgery with the principal aim of removing the primary and debulking mesenteric metastases, the authors concluded that this surgery provided considerable symptomatic relief and improved survival. The role of cytoreductive hepatic resection or of cryotherapy for patients with multiple hepatic metastases from carcinoids is also unclear.[1,59] In a review of data for 170 patients with metastatic GI NETs to the liver (120 of which were carcinoids) who underwent surgical exploration for possible debulking, 54% had a major hepatectomy (one lobe or more), complication rate was 14%, mortality rate was 1.2%, symptom control occurred in 96% of those undergoing resection, and survival was 61% at 5 years. Resection of hepatic metastases may relieve clinical endocrinopathies and the symptomatic response may last several months.[59,63] It was recommended that if more than 90% of the imaged tumor could be safely removed, resection should be considered.[63] Cryotherapy has also been reported to be beneficial.[1] In one study,[1] radiation therapy was used in 44 patients with symptomatic metastatic unresectable carcinoid tumors. Survival was not prolonged; however, substantial palliation was achieved in most cases, with an overall response rate of 80%, 76% (16 of 21) for abdominal tumors, 92% (12 of 13) for spinal metastases, 63% (5 of 8) for brain metastases, and 89% (8 of 9) for bone metastases. At present, radiotherapy is primarily used for symptomatic bone metastases, especially to the spine.

Because MIBG is frequently taken up by carcinoids and concentrated, the possibility of using radiolabeled MIBG therapeutically has been evaluated in a small number of patients.[1,64] Iodine 125– or iodine 131–labeled MIBG has been reported to decrease 5-HIAA urine concentrations and control symptomatic metastases in a small number of cases.[1]

CHEMOTHERAPY

There is no general agreement on when, or even if, chemotherapy should be started in patients with malignant carcinoids. Some suggest that only patients suffering significant symptoms or disability from malignant disease or syndromes or who have a poor prognosis should undergo chemotherapy.[1] Chemotherapy for metastatic carcinoids has, in general, been disappointing.[1,7,53,65] Single-agent therapy with doxorubicin, 5-fluorouracil, dacarbazine, actinomycin D, cisplatin, alkylating agents, etoposide, streptozotocin, and carboplatin has provided low tumor response rates of 0% to 30%.[1,53] In general, the duration of responses is short, usually less than a year. Combination chemotherapy for metastatic carcinoid has not been shown to have any clear advantage compared with single-agent chemotherapy. Two-dose combinations have been used of streptozotocin and 5-fluorouracil, streptozotocin and cyclophosphamide, streptozotocin and doxorubicin, etoposide and cisplatin. Dacarbazine and 5-fluorouracil, and CCNU and 5-fluorouracil, with low response rates of 0% to 40% and no apparent significant improvement over the use of single agents

alone.[1,7,53] Three-drug combinations with 5-fluorouracil, doxorubicin, and cisplatin; dacarbazine, 5-fluorouracil, and epirubicin; and streptozotocin, cyclophosphamide, and 5-fluorouracil; and four-drug combinations with streptozotocin, doxorubicin, cyclophosphamide, and 5-fluorouracil also gave low response rates of 10% to 31% and showed no additional therapeutic advantage over a single agent.[1,7,53] Remissions were short-lived with an average duration of 4 to 7 months. It can be concluded that no combination therapy has clearly had a beneficial effect in the treatment of malignant carcinoids.[1] Given the indolent nature of the tumor, the poor efficacy and undisputed toxicity of chemotherapy, and the availability of excellent symptomatic therapy (octreotide and interferon), currently chemotherapy is usually reserved for advanced tumors with evidence of progression late in the disease course.

BIOTHERAPY

Somatostatin analogues such as octreotide or lanreotide, in addition to controlling symptoms and reducing secretion of 5-HIAA or various peptides, also have been assessed for their antitumor effects.[1,7,53,66] In general, these analogues have a poor tumoricidal effect, decreasing tumor size in only 0% to 17% of patients. However, both somatostatin analogues have a tumorostatic effect, stabilizing the growth of metastatic disease and, in some studies, prolonging survival.[1,7,42,53,66] In various studies 30% to 100% of patients with metastatic disease have demonstrated tumor stabilization with treatment with somatostatin analogues.[1,7,53,54,66,67] No prospective study has proven that this tumor stabilization results in increased survival.

Numerous studies[1,66,68] show that human leukocyte interferon or interferon-α causes a decrease in tumor size in a small number (0% to 20%) of patients with metastatic tumors. However, similar to octreotide, interferon appears to have a tumorostatic effect, stopping further tumor growth and stabilizing the extent of metastatic disease, which may lead to prolonged survival.[1,58,66,68,69] In a number of studies interferon-α therapy demonstrated a more than 50% reduction in tumor size in fewer than 20% of patients with metastatic NETs while resulting in stabilization of tumor growth in 30% to 70%.[1,58,66] Interferon treatment (3 million to 9 million units three times per week) was associated with tolerable but significant side effects, including flu-like symptoms in 89%, fatigue in 70%, weight loss in 57%, reduction of blood counts in 31% (anemia in 31%, leukopenia in 3%, thrombocytopenia in 14%), increased serum levels of triglycerides in 32%, and increased liver enzyme levels in 31%.[1,58] Clinical thyroid disease developed in 76% of patients with thyroid antibodies.[1] In 22 patients it was found that the induction of the enzyme 2',5'-oligoadenylate synthetase with interferon treatment correlated with the development of a clinical response; however, it is unknown if it is predictive of changes in tumor size with interferon treatment. The optimal dosage for long-term treatment seems to be 5 to 10 mU three to five times per week; subsequently, however, it is important to titrate the dosage individually for each patient.[58] It is recommended that the leukocyte count be used as an indication of the antiproliferative effect of interferon-α, with the aim of reducing the leukocytes below $3 \times 10^9/L$.[58]

Because of their separate tumorostatic effects and ability to control symptoms, the combination of octreotide and interferon was assessed in small numbers of patients with malignant carcinoid syndrome either alone or in combination with other agents.[1,66] With octreotide and interferon,[1,66] interferon-α plus 5-fluorouracil, interferon-α and interferon-β, and streptozotocin with doxorubicin and interferon-α,[1] as with interferon-α alone, only low rates (0% to 10%) of decrease in tumor size occurred.[1]

Studies[70] demonstrate that somatostatin analogues (lanreotide, octreotide), but not interferon, can induce apoptosis in carcinoid. In contrast, treatment with interferon-α[69] induced increased expression of bcl-2 in the carcinoids, whereas treatment with somatostatin analogues did not. It was proposed this induced bcl-2 expression may contribute to keeping the malignant carcinoid cells at G_0 and therefore to the antiproliferative effects of interferon.[69]

EMBOLIZATION AND CHEMOEMBOLIZATION

Surgical hepatic artery ligation or embolization via interventional radiology has been reported to reduce hepatic tumor bulk either alone,[71] combined with interferon,[68] or as chemoembolization combined with chemotherapy with dacarbazine, cisplatin, doxorubicin, 5-fluorouracil, or streptozotocin.[1] In a review of the M. D. Anderson Cancer Center experience for 81 patients,[71] a partial response was seen in 67%, minimal response in 9%, stable disease in 16%, and progressive disease in 9%; 63% had a reduction in tumor symptoms, and the 2-year survival was 62%. Hepatic artery occlusion with chemotherapy or chemoembolization may be more effective than embolization or hepatic artery occlusion alone. In one large study,[1] the percentage of patients who had tumor regression after hepatic artery ligation alone was similar to that for patients receiving chemoembolization (treatment with dacarbazine and doxorubicin alternating with streptozotocin and 5-fluorouracil) (67% vs. 69%); however, the duration of the response was decreased (4 months vs. 18 months for the combination).[1]

In nine studies involving chemoembolization (embolization combined with doxorubicin in ethiodized oil or with 5-fluorouracil, dacarbazine, doxorubicin, cisplatin, mitomycin C, or streptozotocin),[1] a decrease in tumor size was seen in 33% to 100% of patients.[1] The average decrease in size in one study was 84%. In one study, 47% of patients survived 2 years (median survival, 17 months), and in another study the median survival time was 15 months.[1] A randomized trial[68] compared the effect of interferon-α in 69 patients with metastatic midgut carcinoids after embolization and surgery. Patients treated with interferon-α and octreotide had a reduced risk of tumor progression ($P = .008$) compared to those treated with octreotide alone; however, the 5-year survival rate was not significantly different (57% vs. 37%; $P = .13$).

LIVER TRANSPLANTATION

In contrast to other metastatic tumors to the liver for which liver transplantation has generally given poor results and has been largely abandoned, there is increased interest in liver transplantation in patients with metastatic carcinoids and pancreatic endocrine tumors.[1,24,72] In a review of 103 patients[72] with malignant NETs who underwent liver transplantation (43 carcinoids, 48 pancreatic endocrine tumors), the 2-year and 5-year survival rates were 60% and 47%, respectively. However, recurrence-free survival was less than 24%.[72] Univariate analysis

defined favorable prognostic factors as age younger than 50 years, primary tumor in lung or bowel, and pretransplantation somatostatin therapy. Multivariate analysis identified age older than 50 years and transplantation combined with upper abdominal exenteration or Whipple's resection ($P < .01$) as adverse prognostic factors. It was concluded that liver transplantation might be justified, particularly in young patients with only hepatic disease.[72]

PEPTIDE RECEPTOR RADIONUCLIDE THERAPY

The discovery that many carcinoids overexpress somatostatin receptors and internalize radiolabeled somatostatin analogues is now being used therapeutically.[7,73,74] Indium 111–, yttrium 90–, and lutetium 177–coupled somatostatin analogues are being studied.[7,73–75] Studies using indium 111 or lutetium 177 compounds reported tumor stabilization in 41% and 40% of patients with advanced metastatic NETs and a decrease in tumor size in 30% and 38%, respectively.[7,73–75] These results suggest that this novel therapy may be useful, especially in patients with advanced disease.

REFERENCES

1. Jensen RT, Doherty GM. Carcinoid tumors and the carcinoid syndrome. In: DeVita VT Jr, Hellman S, Rosenberg SA, eds. *Cancer: principles and practice of oncology,* 6th ed. Philadelphia: Lippincott Williams & Wilkins, 2001:1813.
2. DeLellis RA. The neuroendocrine system and its tumors: an overview. *Am J Clin Pathol* 2001;115:S5.
3. Langley K. The neuroendocrine concept today. *Ann N Y Acad Sci* 1994;733:1.
4. Capella C, Heitz PU, Hofler H, Solcia E, Kloppel G. Revised classification of neuroendocrine tumours of the lung, pancreas and gut. *Virchows Arch* 1995;425:547.
5. Kulke MH, Mayer RJ. Carcinoid tumors. *N Engl J Med* 1999;340:858.
6. Fenoglio-Preiser CM. Gastrointestinal neuroendocrine/neuroectodermal tumors. *Am J Clin Pathol* 2001;115:S79.
7. Oberg K. Carcinoid tumors: molecular genetics, tumor biology, and update of diagnosis and treatment. *Curr Opin Oncol* 2002;14:38.
8. Taupenot L, Harper KL, O'Connor DT. The chromogranin-secretogranin family. *N Engl J Med* 2003;348:1134.
9. Williams ED, Sandler M. The classification of carcinoid tumours. *Lancet* 1963;1:238.
10. Soga J, Yakuwa Y, Osaka M. Carcinoid syndrome: a statistical evaluation of 748 reported cases. *J Exp Clin Cancer Res* 1999;18:133.
11. Godwin JD II. Carcinoid tumors. An analysis of 2,837 cases. *Cancer* 1975;36:560.
12. Modlin IM, Sandor A. An analysis of 8305 cases of carcinoid tumors. *Cancer* 1997;79:813.
13. Modlin IM, Lye KD, Kidd M. A 5-decade analysis of 13,715 carcinoid tumors. *Cancer* 2003;97:934.
14. Sandor A, Modlin IM. A retrospective analysis of 1570 appendiceal carcinoids. *Am J Gastroenterol* 1998;93:422.
15. Soga J. Carcinoids of the small intestine: a statistical evaluation of 1102 cases collected from the literature. *J Exp Clin Cancer Res* 1997;16:353.
16. Burke AP, Sobin LH, Federspiel BH, Shekitka KM, Helwig EB. Carcinoid tumors of the duodenum. A clinicopathologic study of 99 cases. *Arch Pathol Lab Med* 1990;114:700.
17. Soga J. Carcinoids of the rectum: an evaluation of 1271 reported cases. *Surg Today* 1997;27:112.
18. Hage R, de la Riviere AB, Seldenrijk CA, van den Bosch JM. Update in pulmonary carcinoid tumors: a review article. *Ann Surg Oncol* 2003;10:697.
19. Modlin IM, Lye KD, Kidd M. Carcinoid tumors of the stomach. *Surg Oncol* 2003;12(2):153.
20. Soga J. Statistical evaluation of 2001 carcinoid cases with metastases, collected from literature: a comparative study between ordinary carcinoids and atypical varieties. *J Exp Clin Cancer Res* 1998;17:3.
21. Calender A. New insights in genetics of digestive neuroendocrine tumors. In: Mignon M, Colombel JF, eds. *Recent advances in the pathophysiology and management of inflammatory bowel diseases and digestive endocrine tumors.* Paris: John Libbey Eurotext, 1999:155.
22. Corleto VD, Delle Fave G, Jensen RT. Molecular insights into gastrointestinal neuroendocrine tumors: importance and recent advances. *Dig Liver Dis* 2002;34:668.
23. Chandrasekharappa SC, Guru SC, Manickam P, et al. Positional cloning of the gene for multiple endocrine neoplasia-type 1. *Science* 1997;276:404.
24. Jensen RT. Endocrine tumors of the pancreas. In: Yamada T, ed. *Textbook of gastroenterology.* New York: Lippincott Williams & Wilkins, 2003.
25. Jensen RT. Overview of chronic diarrhea caused by functional neuroendocrine neoplasms. *Semin Gastrointest Dis* 1999;10:156.
26. Quaedvlieg PF, Lamers CB, Taal BG. Carcinoid heart disease: an update. *Scand J Gastroenterol* 2002;236[Suppl]:66.

27. Moller JE, Connolly HM, Rubin J, et al. Factors associated with progression of carcinoid heart disease. *N Engl J Med* 2003;348:1005.

28. Feldman JM, Jones RS. Carcinoid syndrome from gastrointestinal carcinoids without liver metastasis. *Ann Surg* 1982;196:33.

29. Kema IP, deVries GE, Sloof MJH, Biesma B, Muskiet FAJ. Serotonin, catecholamines, histamine, and their metabolites in urine, platelets, and tumor tissue of patients with carcinoid tumors. *Clin Chem* 1994;40:86.

30. Makridis C, Theodorsson E, Akerstrom G, Oberg K, Knutson L. Increased intestinal non-substance P tachykinin concentrations in malignant midgut carcinoid disease. *J Gastroenterol Hepatol* 1999;14:500.

31. Wymenga AN, de Vries EG, Leijsma MK, Kema IP, Kleibeuker JH. Effects of ondansetron on gastrointestinal symptoms in carcinoid syndrome. *Eur J Cancer* 1998;34:1293.

32. Norheim I, Theodorsson-Norheim E, Brodin E, Oberg K. Tachykinins in carcinoid tumors: their use as a tumor marker and possible role in the carcinoid flush. *J Clin Endocrinol Metab* 1986;63:605.

33. Lundin L, Norheim I, Landelius J, Oberg K, Theodorsson-Norheim E. Carcinoid heart disease: relationship of circulating vasoactive substances to ultrasound-detectable cardiac abnormalities. *Circulation* 1988;77:264.

34. Zuetenhorst JM, Bonfrer JM, Korse CM, et al. Carcinoid heart disease: the role of urinary 5-hydroxyindoleacetic acid excretion and plasma levels of atrial natriuretic peptide, transforming growth factor-beta and fibroblast growth factor. *Cancer* 2003;97:1609.

35. Jian B, Xu J, Connolly J, et al. Serotonin mechanisms in heart valve disease I: serotonin-induced up-regulation of transforming growth factor-beta 1 via G-protein signal transduction in aortic valve interstitial cells. *Am J Pathol* 2002;161:2111.

36. Nuttall KL, Pingree SS. The incidence of elevations in urine 5-hydroxyindoleacetic acid. *Ann Clin Lab Sci* 1998;28:167.

37. Krenning EP, Kwekkeboom DJ, Oei HY, et al. Somatostatin-receptor scintigraphy in gastroenteropancreatic tumors. *Ann N Y Acad Sci* 1994;733:416.

38. Eriksson B, Bergstrom B, Sundin A, et al. The role of PET in localization of neuroendocrine and adrenocortical tumors. *Ann N Y Acad Sci* 2002;970:159.

39. Schillaci O, Scopinaro F, Danieli R, et al. Single photon emission computerized tomography increases the sensitivity of indium-111-pentetreotide scintigraphy in detecting abdominal carcinoids. *Anticancer Res* 1997;17:1753.

40. Gibril F, Jensen RT. Diagnostic uses of radiolabelled somatostatin receptor analogues in gastroenteropancreatic endocrine tumors. *Dig Liver Dis* 2004;36:S106.

41. Schillaci O, Spanu A, Scopinaro F, et al. Somatostatin receptor scintigraphy in liver metastasis detection from gastroenteropancreatic neuroendocrine tumors. *J Nucl Med* 2003;44:359.

42. Jensen RT. Peptide therapy. Recent advances in the use of somatostatin and other peptide receptor agonists and antagonists. In: Lewis JH, Dubois A, eds. *Current clinical topics in gastrointestinal pharmacology.* Malden, MA: Blackwell Science, 1997:144.

43. Krenning EP, Kwekkeboom DJ, Bakker WH, et al. Somatostatin receptor scintigraphy with [^{111}In-DTPA-D-Phe^1]- and [^{123}I-Tyr^3]-octreotide: the Rotterdam experience with more than 1000 patients. *Eur J Nucl Med* 1993;20:716.

44. Meijer WG, van der Veer E, Jager PL, et al. Bone metastases in carcinoid tumors: clinical features, imaging characteristics, and markers of bone metabolism. *J Nucl Med* 2003;44:184.

45. Gibril F, Reynolds JC, Chen CC, et al. Specificity of somatostatin receptor scintigraphy: a prospective study and the effects of false positive localizations on management in patients with gastrinomas. *J Nucl Med* 1999;40:539.

46. Janson ET, Holmberg L, Stridsberg M, et al. Carcinoid tumors: analysis of prognostic factors and survival in 301 patients from a referral center. *Ann Oncol* 1997;8:685.

47. Jensen RT. Natural history of digestive endocrine tumors. In: Mignon M, Colombel JF, eds. *Recent advances in pathophysiology and management of inflammatory bowel diseases and digestive endocrine tumors.* Paris: John Libbey Eurotext, 1999:192.

48. McDermott EWM, Guduric B, Brennan MF. Prognostic variables in patients with gastrointestinal carcinoid tumours. *Br J Surg* 1994;81:1007.

49. Greenberg RS, Baumgarten DA, Clark WS, Isacson P, McKeen K. Prognostic factors for gastrointestinal and bronchopulmonary carcinoid tumors. *Cancer* 1987;60:2476.

50. Tsushima K, Nagorney DM, Weiland LH, Lieber MM. The relationship of flow cytometric DNA analysis and clinicopathology in small-intestinal carcinoids. *Surgery* 1989;105:366.

51. Harris AG, Redfern JS. Octreotide treatment of carcinoid syndrome: analysis of published dose-titration data. *Aliment Pharmacol Ther* 1995;9:387.

52. Gustafsen J, Lendorf A, Raskov H, Boesby S. Ketanserin versus placebo in carcinoid syndrome. A clinical controlled trial. *Scand J Gastroenterol* 1986;21:816.

53. Oberg K, Eriksson B. Digestive endocrine tumor management; medical advanced disease. In: Mignon M, Colombel JF, eds. *Recent advances in the pathophysiology and management of inflammatory bowel diseases and digestive endocrine tumors.* Paris: John Libbey Eurotext, 1999:260.

54. Garland J, Buscombe JR, Bouvier C, et al. Sandostatin LAR (long-acting octreotide acetate) for malignant carcinoid syndrome: a 3-year experience. *Aliment Pharmacol Ther* 2003;17:437.

55. Schonfeld WH, Elkin EP, Woltering EA, et al. The cost-effectiveness of octreotide acetate in the treatment of carcinoid syndrome and VIPoma. *Int J Technol Assess Health Care* 1996;14:514.

56. Arnold R, Simon B, Wied M. Treatment of neuroendocrine GEP tumours with somatostatin analogues: a review. *Digestion* 2000;62:84.

57. Hanssen LE, Schrumpf E, Jacobsen MB, et al. Extended experience with recombinant alpha-2b interferon with or without hepatic artery embolization in the treatment of midgut carcinoid tumors. *Acta Oncol* 1991;30:523.

58. Oberg K, Eriksson B, Janson ET. The clinical use of interferons in the management of neuroendocrine gastroenteropancreatic tumors. *Ann N Y Acad Sci* 1994;733:471.

59. Sarmiento JM, Heywood M, Rubin J, et al. Surgical treatment of neuroendocrine metastases to the liver: a plea for resection to increase survival. *J Am Coll Surg* 2003;197:29.

60. Hellman P, Lundstrom T, Ohrvall U, et al. Effect of surgery on the outcome of midgut carcinoid disease with lymph node and liver metastases. *World J Surg* 2002;26:991.

61. Akerstrom G. Management of carcinoid tumors of the stomach, duodenum, and pancreas. *World J Surg* 1996;20:173.

62. Ahlman H. Surgical treatment of carcinoid tumours of the stomach and small intestine. *Ital J Gastroenterol Hepatol* 1999;31:S198.

63. Sarmiento JM, Que FG. Hepatic surgery for metastases from neuroendocrine tumors. *Surg Oncol Clin North Am* 2003;12:231.

64. Hoefnagel CA, den Hartog Jager FC, Taal BG, et al. The role of I-131-MIBG in the diagnosis and therapy of carcinoids. *Eur J Nucl Med* 1987;13:187.

65. Rougier P, Ducreux M. Systemic chemotherapy of advanced digestive neuroendocrine tumours. *Ital J Gastroenterol Hepatol* 1999;31:S202.

66. Faiss S, Pape UF, Bohmig M, et al. Prospective, randomized, multicenter trial on the antiproliferative effect of lanreotide, interferon alfa, and their combination for therapy of metastatic neuroendocrine gastroenteropancreatic tumors—the International Lanreotide and Interferon Alfa Study Group. *J Clin Oncol* 2003;21:2689.

67. Bouschey RP, Dackiw AP. Carcinoid tumors. *Curr Treat Options Oncol* 2002;3:319.

68. Kolby L, Persson G, Franzen S, Ahren B. Randomized clinical trial of the effect of interferon alpha on survival in patients with disseminated midgut carcinoid tumours. *Br J Surg* 2003;90:687.

69. Imam H, Gobl A, Eriksson B, Oberg K. Interferon-alpha induces bcl-2 proto-oncogene in patients with neuroendocrine gut tumor responding to its antitumor action. *Anticancer Res* 1997;17:4659.

70. Imam H, Eriksson B, Lukinius A, et al. Induction of apoptosis in neuroendocrine tumors of the digestive system during treatment with somatostatin analogs. *Acta Oncol* 1997;36:607.

71. Gupta S, Yao JC, Ahrar K, et al. Hepatic artery embolization and chemoembolization for treatment of patients with metastatic carcinoid tumors: the M.D. Anderson experience. *Cancer J* 2003;9:261.

72. Lehnert T. Liver transplantation for metastatic neuroendocrine carcinoma. *Transplantation* 1998;66:1307.

73. deJong M, Kwekkeboom D, Valkema R, Krenning EP. Radiolabelled peptides for tumour therapy: current status and future directions Plenary lecture at the EANM 2002. *Eur J Nucl Med Mol Imaging* 2003;30):463.

74. Buscombe JR, Caplin ME, Hilson AJW. Long-term efficacy of high-activity ^{111}In-pentetreotide therapy in patients with disseminated neuroendocrine tumors. *J Nucl Med* 2003;44:1.

75. Kwekkeboom DJ, Bakker WH, Kam BL, et al. Treatment of patients with gastro-enteropancreatic (GEP) tumours with the novel radiolabeled somatostatin analogue [(177)Lu-DOTA(0),Tyr(3)]octreotate. *Eur J Nucl Med Mol Imaging* 2003;30:417.

76. Davis Z, Moertel CG, McIlrath DC. The malignant carcinoid syndrome. *Surg Gynecol Obstet* 1973;137(4):637.

77. Feldman JM. Carcinoid tumors and syndrome. *Semin Oncol* 1987;14(3):237.

78. Norheim I, Oberg K, Theodorsson-Norheim E, et al. Malignant carcinoid tumors. An analysis of 103 patients with regard to tumor localization, hormone production, and survival. *Ann Surg* 1987;206(2):115.

79. Thorson AH. Studies on carcinoid disease. *Acta Med Scand* 1958;334[Suppl]:1.

GERARD M. DOHERTY
ROBERT T. JENSEN

SECTION 7

Multiple Endocrine Neoplasias

The multiple endocrine neoplasia (MEN) syndromes are a group of syndromes characterized by tumors of endocrine organs (Table 34.7-1). MEN 1 affects the parathyroid glands, endocrine pancreas, and pituitary gland, among other organs. MEN 2 affects the thyroid gland, parathyroid glands, and adrenal glands. Because the genetic defects responsible for these syndromes have been identified, genotype-phenotype correlations now guide the timing of interventions for some patients, specifically those with MEN 2 and its related Ret protooncogene–based syndromes.

MULTIPLE ENDOCRINE NEOPLASIA TYPE 1

Wermer first described the familial occurrence of tumors involving the pituitary gland, parathyroid glands, and pancreatic islets.[1] The syndrome was initially called *Wermer's syndrome*, subsequently called *multiple endocrine adenomatosis type 1*, and is now known as *MEN 1*. It is now clear that the parathyroid disease always affects multiple glands, that the pancreatic endocrine tumors may be malignant, and that patients can die from associated malignancies.

MEN 1 is inherited as an autosomal dominant trait. Chromosomal linkage studies localized the genetic defect to the long arm of chromosome 11 (q13 locus).[2] The gene has subsequently been identified and codes a protein called *menin*.[3] This follows the two-hit theory of neoplasia of Knudson in which an inherited mutation in one chromosome is unmasked by a somatic deletion or mutation in the other normal chromosome, which thereby removes the suppressor effect of the normal gene. These results are in contrast to those of patients without MEN 1 who develop pancreatic endocrine tumors, in whom the pancreatic neoplasms develop homozygous inactivation of the MEN 1 gene in 27% to 39% of cases.[4–6]

Asymmetric multigland primary hyperparathyroidism is the most frequent feature of MEN 1. Some studies examining the etiology of primary hyperparathyroidism in patients with MEN 1 have suggested that there is a circulating factor in the plasma that stimulates bovine parathyroid cells to proliferate.[7–9] However, other studies have demonstrated that there is a monoclonal abnormality in the enlarged parathyroid glands of patients with MEN 1, which suggests that the process in these glands may not be dependent on a circulating factor (hyperplasia) but rather occurs through inactivation of the MEN 1 gene in a precursor cell (neoplasia).[10] The relationship of asymmetry of affected glands to patient age (younger patients more frequently show asymmetric involvement, whereas older patients have involvement of all glands) and the tumor suppressor genetic basis of the syndrome favor the occurrence of multiple adenomas (neoplasia) rather than hyperplasia (Fig. 34.7-1).[11]

CLINICAL PRESENTATION

The age of peak incidence of symptoms in women with MEN 1 is during the third decade of life, whereas the peak incidence in men is during the fourth decade.[12] In individuals from known MEN 1 kindreds, the presence of the disease can usually be detected with screening by the age of 18.[13] More than one-half of patients with MEN 1 have involvement of more than one organ system, and approximately 20% have three affected endocrine glands. The frequency of glandular involvement, in descending order, is parathyroid, pancreas, pituitary, adrenal cortex, and thyroid. Both the adrenal cortex and the thyroid typically have benign, nonfunctioning adenomas. Other clinically important tumors these patients develop include gastric carcinoids,[14] bronchial carcinoids (primarily women), and carcinoid tumors of the thymus (primarily men). The clinical signs and symptoms, in descending order of frequency, are hypercal-

TABLE 34.7-1. Multiple Endocrine Neoplasia Syndromes and Familial Medullary Thyroid Cancer

Characteristics	MEN 1	MEN 2A	MEN 2B	Familial Medullary Thyroid Carcinoma
Chromosome	11q12-13	Pericentromeric 10	Pericentromeric 10	Pericentromeric 10
Genetic defect	*MEN1* mutation	RET mutation	RET mutation	RET mutation
MTC	No	Bilateral	Bilateral	Bilateral
Pheochromocytoma	No	70% bilateral	70% bilateral	No
Parathyroid disease	Hyperplasia	Hyperplasia	No	No
Phenotype	No	No	Bony abnormalities, mucosal neuromas, marfanoid habitus, bumpy lips	No
Mode of inheritance	Autosomal dominant	Autosomal dominant	Autosomal dominant	Autosomal dominant
Course of MTC	No MTC	Variable, frequently indolent	More virulent	Most indolent
Pancreatic endocrine tumors	Yes: pancreatic peptide, 80–100%; gastrinoma, 50%; insulinoma, 20%; growth hormone–releasing factor, vasoactive intestinal peptide (uncommon)	No	No	No

MEN, multiple endocrine neoplasia; MTC, medullary thyroid carcinoma.

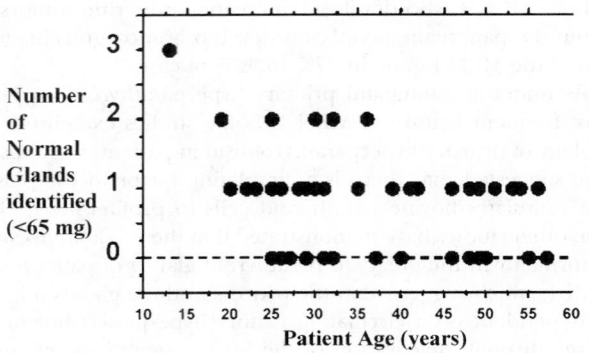

FIGURE 34.7-1. The number of normal glands identified during 44 initial operations for multiple endocrine neoplasia (MEN) 1 primary hyperparathyroidism. The number of normal glands identified during the operation declined with the age of the patient. No patient older than 40 years had more than one gland of normal weight at operation. These data support the concept of multiple parathyroid adenomas in MEN 1, as opposed to parathyroid hyperplasia. (From ref. 11, with permission.)

cemia, nephrolithiasis, peptic ulcer disease, hypoglycemia, headache, visual field loss, hypopituitarism, acromegaly, galactorrhea-amenorrhea, and rarely Cushing's syndrome. Patients with MEN 1 have a decreased life expectancy, with a 50% probability of death by age 50. One-half of the deaths are due to a malignant tumoral process or a sequela of the disease.[15–17]

PARATHYROID GLAND INVOLVEMENT

Primary hyperparathyroidism is the most common abnormality in patients with MEN 1, occurring in 88% to 97% of affected patients. The diagnosis is dependent on the detection of elevated serum levels of calcium and parathyroid hormone. Primary hyperparathyroidism is usually the initially recognized clinical manifestation of patients with MEN 1, although in prospectively screened patients, other manifestations may be biochemically detected earlier.[13,18] Occasional patients have clinical manifestations of Zollinger-Ellison syndrome (ZES) before primary hyperparathyroidism. Further, pituitary adenomas or hyperinsulinism may be identified before hypercalcemia. The pathology associated with primary hyperparathyroidism is always multiple-gland disease.

Although some glands may appear grossly normal, the likelihood of finding normal-weight glands decreases as the age of the patient increases, consistent with the development of multiple parathyroid adenomas.[11] The surgical management requires a strategy that acknowledges that all of the parathyroid glands are, or will be, abnormal, and that the patient is better served by having a smaller amount of abnormal parathyroid tissue than by having none at all. Options include removal of three and one-half glands leaving a part of one gland in the neck, or of all four parathyroid glands with immediate autograft of some of the parathyroid tissue into the musculature of the nondominant forearm. Neither strategy yields ideal results. The incidence of recurrent or persistent hyperparathyroidism is 16% to 54%, and the incidence of hypoparathyroidism is between 10% and 25%.[19,20] Reoperations are frequently necessary, and similar principles should be applied.

PANCREATIC ENDOCRINE TUMORS

Malignant pancreatic endocrine tumors are the most common MEN 1–related cause of death in MEN 1 kindreds (Table 34.7-2).[15–17] Pathologic examination of the duodenum and pancreas in patients with MEN 1 demonstrates multiple neuroendocrine tumors.[21,22] Tumors producing pancreatic polypeptide are the most common pancreatic endocrine tumor in MEN 1 patients, occurring in 80% to 100%. These tumors cause symptoms only due to the tumor mass itself and thus often present when tumor growth is advanced. Many patients develop functional pancreatic endocrine tumors, sometimes coincident with pancreatic polypeptide–producing tumors, of whom most have gastrinoma, approximately 20% insulinoma, 3% glucagonoma, and 1% vasoactive intestinal peptide–producing tumor (VIPoma) (see Table 34.7-1).

A number of studies have suggested that most gastrinomas in patients with ZES and MEN 1 are in the duodenum and not in the pancreas. The ideal treatment of the ZES tumor is surgical excision of the gastrinoma; however, in patients with MEN 1, excision of gastrinoma rarely results in normal serum gastrin levels. Because of the low probability of cure and the suggestion that the gastrinoma is less malignant in MEN 1, some have recommended that patients with MEN 1 do not undergo surgery. However, familial gastrinoma may still have a malignant course. At present, the best approach is still unclear.

TABLE 34.7-2. Multiple Endocrine Neoplasia Type 1–Related Causes of Death

	No. of Patients			
Cause of Death	Washington University Series[15]	Mayo Clinic Series[17]	Tasman-1 Family[16]	Combined Series
Malignant islet cell tumor	12	10	3	25
Malignant pituitary tumor	—	—	3	3
Malignant carcinoid tumor	6	3	4	13
Malignant adrenal tumor	—	—	2	2
Hypercalcemia and uremia	3	1	6	10
Ulcer disease	6	1	2	9
Postoperative	—	2	—	2
Total deaths in MEN 1 carriers	59	60	46	165
Fraction of total deaths in MEN 1 carriers due to MEN 1 causes	46%	28%	44%	38%

MEN, multiple endocrine neoplasia.

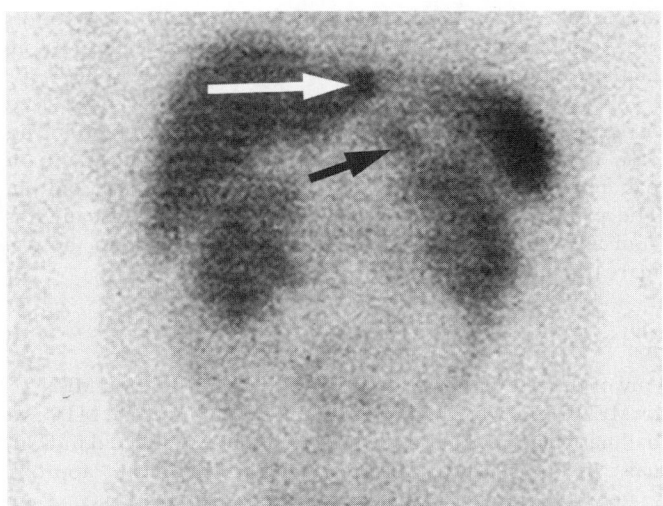

FIGURE 34.7-2. Somatostatin receptor scintigraphy can be helpful to identify sites of distant metastasis or otherwise undetected second primary tumors in the lungs or mediastinum. In this patient with a malignant nonfunctional neuroendocrine tumor in the body of the pancreas (*black arrow*), the scintigram revealed a solitary metastasis in the left lateral segment of the liver (*white arrow*) that was not demonstrated on computed tomographic scan or magnetic resonance imaging.

To date, no studies have demonstrated that surgical resection of gastrinomas in MEN 1 is beneficial. One study suggests that surgical resection of primary gastrinomas in patients with and without MEN 1 decreases the probability of the development of liver metastases, which is the most important negative predictor of survival.[23] Somatostatin receptor scintigraphy can be used to rule out distant metastases and to evaluate for other primary sites (Fig. 34.7-2). Therefore, the authors currently recommend that all patients with ZES and MEN 1 have extensive localization studies including somatostatin receptor scintigraphy. Only patients with unequivocally positive results on imaging studies and no unresectable metastases should undergo surgical exploration with intraoperative ultrasonography. Tumors larger than 1 cm identified in the pancreatic head are enucleated, the duodenum is carefully explored by duodenotomy, and solitary or multiple tumors identified are resected; large tumors in the pancreatic body or tail are removed by distal pancreatectomy and splenectomy.[24] Although some studies have shown that the primary tumor size is not correlated with the presence of lymph node metastases in MEN 1, larger studies that include patients with sporadic islet cell tumors suggest that size may be an important risk factor.[25] Resection of liver metastases from patients with MEN 1 may also be beneficial. Using this approach, although cure of ZES is unusual, resection should reduce the risk of subsequent metastatic disease. No data conclusively demonstrate that this approach increases survival, although case series are suggestive.[26]

MEN 1 is present in 20% of all patients with ZES and 4% of patients with insulinoma. The exact percentage of patients with VIPoma, glucagonoma, or somatostatinoma with MEN 1 is not known but is estimated to be low (less than 5%) (see Table 34.7-1). The surgical management of insulinoma and VIPoma in MEN 1 patients has resulted in more frequent biochemical cures than resection for gastrinoma. Medical management of the watery diarrhea in VIPoma is effective using either short-acting or depot somatostatin analogues. Hypoglycemia management in insulinoma is not reliable. Diazoxide and octreotide are available and may be useful for short-term treatment. In patients with MEN 1, insulinoma and VIPoma are frequently solitary large tumors. Resection may result in cure.[26]

PITUITARY TUMORS

Pituitary tumors occur in 54% to 80% of patients with MEN 1. Symptoms may be due to local encroachment, including headache and visual field defects. In a review of series, the most common tumor was a prolactinoma (41% to 76%), followed by growth hormone–secreting tumor, nonfunctional tumor, and rarely adrenocorticotropic hormone– or thyroid-stimulating hormone–secreting tumors.[27] Men with prolactinoma may be unable to achieve a penile erection, whereas women may have galactorrhea and infertility. Growth hormone–secreting tumors (25%) result in acromegaly. Cushing's syndrome can also result from release of adrenocorticotropic hormone–like material from a pancreatic islet cell tumor or a foregut carcinoid tumor (ectopic adrenocorticotropic hormone). Prolactinomas are generally treated by dopamine receptor agonists (bromocriptine, pergolide, cabergoline). Transsphenoidal pituitary surgery may be indicated to control any detectable pituitary mass lesion in patients with MEN 1. Incompletely resected patients may also be treated with bromocriptine.

ADRENAL AND THYROID TUMORS AND OTHER GENERALLY CLINICALLY SILENT TUMORS

Adrenal abnormalities may occur in 27% to 36% of patients with MEN 1. The most common abnormality is a benign, nonfunctional cortical adenoma, although adrenal cortical carcinomas and hyperplasia may also occur.[28] Adrenal cortical hyperfunction may rarely be found secondary to an adrenal tumor. Adrenal cortical neoplasms are usually nonfunctional in patients with MEN 1. Thyroid adenomas also occur in 5% to 30% of patients with MEN 1 and have little clinical significance. Lipomas are seen with greater frequency in patients with MEN 1, as are cutaneous angiofibromas and collagenomas.[29] Smooth muscle tumors (leiomyomas), melanomas, and central nervous system tumors (ependymomas, schwannomas, meningiomas) are also reported in patients with MEN 1.

CARCINOID TUMORS

Gastric carcinoid tumors develop in 7% to 30% of patients with MEN 1 with ZES. They arise from gastric enterochromaffin-like cells and thus are also called *ECLomas*.[30,31] Approximately 18% have metastases, the primary tumors are usually multiple, and the tumors generally pursue an indolent course. Such tumors are rare in patients with MEN 1 without ZES.

Thymic carcinoids occur in 0% to 8% of patients with MEN 1, are almost exclusively in men, are usually asymptomatic, and are not associated with Cushing's or carcinoid syndrome.[14,32] They pursue an aggressive course with distant metastases and are an increasing cause of death in older men with MEN 1. In contrast to parathyroid, pituitary, and pancreatic tumors, thymic carcinoids do not show 11q13 loss of heterozygosity and therefore likely have a different pathogenesis.

Bronchial carcinoid tumors occur in 0% to 8% of patients with MEN 1. Eighty percent are in women and 74% are benign; however, they are an occasional cause of death.

FAMILIAL MEDULLARY THYROID CARCINOMA AND MULTIPLE ENDOCRINE NEOPLASIA TYPES 2A AND 2B

HISTORY AND PATHOLOGY

In 1959, Hazard and coworkers first described medullary thyroid carcinoma (MTC) and its striking histologic characteristics of cellular argentaffin staining and amyloid production.[33] MTC is associated with three distinct familial syndromes: MEN 2A, MEN 2B, and familial non-MEN MTC, a disease characterized by hereditary MTC without associated endocrinopathies (see Table 34.7-1).

In 1961, Sipple reported an unusually high incidence of bilateral pheochromocytomas in patients with thyroid malignancy.[34] These patients were later found to have MTC, and the familial disease was inherited as a mendelian autosomal dominant trait with high gene penetrance (see Table 34.7-1). Subsequently, primary hyperparathyroidism was also noted to be part of the syndrome. In 1968, this syndrome of medullary carcinoma of the thyroid gland, pheochromocytomas, and hyperparathyroidism was termed *MEN 2*; now it is called *MEN 2A*. In 1966, Williams and Pollock called attention to the finding that some patients had multiple mucosal neuromas, with or without marfanoid habitus, puffy lips, prominent jaw, pes cavus, and medullated corneal nerves with MTC and pheochromocytomas. For this group of patients the terms *MEN 2B* and *MEN 3* were subsequently suggested. Patients with MEN 2B do not have parathyroid disease. The gene defects in patients with MEN 2A, MEN 2B, and familial MTC are each distinct germline mutations in the RET protooncogene.[35,36]

MTC is a malignant neuroendocrine tumor of the parafollicular thyroid cells or the calcitonin-secreting cells (C cells). Histologically, the MTC in patients with familial MTC, MEN 2A, and MEN 2B appears identical to the MTC occurring sporadically. However, in the familial form of MTC there is bilateral, multifocal involvement, and the cancer usually occupies a position in the superior lateral part of the thyroid lobe at the junction of the upper and middle thirds. In the sporadic setting, the MTC is usually unilateral. MTC is most malignant in MEN 2B, is malignant in MEN 2A, and is least virulent in familial MTC (see Table 34.7-1). MTC accounts for 5% to 12% of all thyroid cancers, and only 10% of all MTC is familial. In MEN 2A, 42% to 60% of patients develop pheochromocytoma.

The pheochromocytomas in patients with MEN 2A or MEN 2B usually present in the second or third decade of life and are often bilateral. The size of the tumor or tumors in patients with MEN 2A is usually less than 3 cm, whereas it is usually larger in patients with MEN 2B. Even in MEN 2A patients with apparent unilateral pheochromocytomas, the contralateral adrenal gland almost always demonstrates medullary hyperplasia on pathologic analysis. Patients with medullary hyperplasia rarely have symptoms of pheochromocytoma. Iodine 131–labeled metaiodobenzyl guanidine scans in patients with MEN 2A may be useful to predict the presence of a clinically significant pheochromocytoma and can be obtained preoperatively. Pheochromocytomas in patients with MEN 2A or MEN 2B are seldom malignant and

are usually within the adrenal gland. Histologically, these tumors are indistinguishable from those occurring sporadically in a nonfamilial setting.

The parathyroid lesions in MEN 2A consist of generalized hyperplasia and should be managed like the parathyroid disease in MEN 1 (see Table 34.7-1). Approximately 35% of patients with MEN 2A develop primary hyperparathyroidism. The primary hyperparathyroidism in MEN 2A is usually less clinically significant and causes fewer symptoms than the primary hyperparathyroidism in MEN 1.[37]

CLINICAL PRESENTATION

Any of the neoplasms that make up the syndromes of MEN 2A or MEN 2B may be the presenting problem; however, MTC is a hallmark feature that occurs in nearly 100% of affected individuals. In patients with MEN 2B, all have MTC and approximately 60% develop pheochromocytomas.[38]

In patients with MEN 2B the MTC presents at an early age and appears more aggressive, because few patients live beyond 30 years of age. In some kindreds, the MTC in MEN 2B may be less malignant and individuals may live longer. The characteristic appearance of MEN 2B patients is often the first sign of disease and may suggest the diagnosis before other clinical abnormalities. However, with investigation by measuring calcitonin, the MTC is always present at the time of clinical recognition (see Table 34.7-1).

Patients may initially seek medical advice because of episodic spells with headache, dizziness, or symptoms of irritability and nervousness. It is unusual for patients with MEN 2A to present with symptoms related to parathyroid disease.

PREOPERATIVE EVALUATION AND SCREENING

When a suspicion of familial MTC, MEN 2A, or MEN 2B exists, precise diagnosis depends on detection of missense mutations in the RET protooncogene in peripheral leukocytes. Several studies in individuals from families with MEN 2A have been able to predict the inheritance of MEN 2A by detection of missense mutations in RET, and the mutations can now be classified as to their risk of aggressive MTC, based on genotype-phenotype correlation studies (Table 34.7-3).[12,39] Screening of new patients or family members for mutations in RET involves polymerase chain reaction amplification and DNA sequence analysis for detection of known point mutations in exons 10 and 11 for MEN 2A and familial MTC and exon 16 (codon 918) for MEN 2B. If a RET mutation is detected, each individual (100%) develops MTC. Furthermore, if a RET mutation is absent, the individual does not need any additional testing. Virtually all patients with MTC have either elevated basal or stimulated plasma levels of calcitonin. Patients who present with clinically apparent disease usually have basal plasma calcitonin levels exceeding 1 ng/mL. In general, there is a direct correlation between the tumor mass of MTC and plasma calcitonin levels.

The presence of inherited MTC can be currently diagnosed in individuals from MTC kindreds before detectable elevations in plasma calcitonin levels occur. Thyroidectomy performed based solely on detection of RET mutations always demonstrates MTC or C-cell hyperplasia.[40] It is necessary in patients with MEN 2A or MEN 2B to exclude a pheochromocytoma before undertaking surgery for MTC. Pheochromocytomas can be excluded by mea-

TABLE 34.7-3.   Multiple Endocrine Neoplasia Type 2 Genotype-Phenotype Relationships

MTC Risk Group	Codons Affected	MTC Phenotypic Features	MTC Prophylactic Management
Low risk	609, 768, 790, 791, 804, 891	In general, MTC least aggressive, but variable; node metastasis and death reported for all mutations except codon 790 and 791	Thyroidectomy before age 10 y
High risk	611, 618, 620, 634	MTC reported as early as age 2 y, and lymph node metastasis as early as 5 y	Thyroidectomy before age 5 y
Highest risk	883, 918, 922	Includes MEN 2B mutations; highest risk of early MTC development and metastasis	Thyroidectomy in first month of life (6 mo at most)

MEN, multiple endocrine neoplasia; MTC, medullary thyroid carcinoma.

suring normal plasma levels of metanephrines. If an elevated level is detected, pheochromocytoma localization studies should be done. Abdominal computed tomography and magnetic resonance imaging are frequently helpful in localizing the pheochromocytoma, but additional, more sensitive studies may be needed. Metaiodobenzylguanidine is concentrated into pheochromocytoma cells and provides a means to functionally localize these tumors using scintigraphy. The sensitivity of this method varies from 79% to 91%, with a specificity of 94% to 99%.

SURGICAL MANAGEMENT

The ability to diagnose MTC in patients at risk for familial MTC allows the physician to treat this malignancy in an early preclinical stage. Should one diagnose MTC in a patient from a MEN 2A kindred, it is absolutely essential that the remainder of the family members at risk be screened. It is in this situation that RET testing has the greatest utility. Patients diagnosed by genetic testing have surgically curable C-cell hyperplasia or carcinoma confined to the thyroid gland.

MEN 2A or MEN 2B patients with pheochromocytoma merit evaluation of both adrenal glands. Pheochromocytomas in MEN 2 syndromes have not been extraadrenal, nor have they been malignant.[41] Before surgical exploration, all patients need effective α-adrenergic receptor blockade. Phenoxybenzamine should be administered 1 to 2 weeks before operation, starting with a dosage of 10 mg twice daily and increased to a usual dosage of 10 to 20 mg three times daily. The end point is normotension with mild to moderate asymptomatic postural hypotension (15 mm Hg) accompanied by symptoms of a blockade, including nasal stuffiness. β-Adrenergic blockade is usually not required except in patients with persistent sinus tachycardia. The β blocker should never be administered before the institution of α-adrenergic blockade, because this may result in unopposed α agonism with hypertensive crisis.

Solitary pheochromocytoma should be resected. In the past, some have advocated open exploration and palpation of both adrenal glands to assess for bilateral disease. Modern imaging has made this obsolete, as is the strategy of routinely resecting both adrenal glands. With imaging studies to localize the adrenal tumor, laparoscopic methods are now used to remove the abnormal gland, and careful follow-up is necessary to monitor for the metachronous development of a contralateral pheochromocytoma.[41,42] Patients with MEN 2A undergoing unilateral adrenalectomy should be followed carefully at 6-month or yearly intervals, because a second adrenal tumor may be diagnosed biochemically before it is clinically apparent.

The surgical management of familial MTC is total thyroidectomy with a central lymph node dissection.[12] It is essential that a total thyroidectomy be performed, including resection of the posterior capsule of the thyroid gland, because the MTC is always bilateral.[43]

POSTOPERATIVE FOLLOW-UP

In patients with MEN 2A and MEN 2B, MTC is the disease that is most frequently lethal. The MTC in patients with MEN 2B seems to be more virulent than that in patients with MEN 2A (see Table 34.7-1), although a group of children with MTC in the setting of MEN 2B have been reported, some of whom appear to be cured of MTC. Survival of patients with MEN 2A is dependent on the extent of MTC at initial surgical resection.

With the widespread availability of reliable radioimmunoassays for calcitonin, an individual patient can be easily followed postoperatively. Detection of an elevated basal plasma calcitonin level or the finding of an abnormal response to calcium and pentagastrin indicates recurrent or persistent disease. In patients with metastatic MTC, the best strategy is unclear. Radioactive iodine ablation, thyroid suppression, and radiation therapy have not been helpful. MTC is relatively insensitive to chemotherapy. Because of the indolent nature of the tumor, most have chosen not to aggressively treat metastatic disease but rather to rely on local (surgical and radiation) methods to address symptomatic disease.

The 10-year survival for patients with MTC is 80% to 90%. Aggressive surgical resection has been used to locally control recurrent MTC, and one-third of individuals can be rendered biochemically disease free.[44,45] However, in patients with MEN 2A, the MTC may be well tolerated. The average life expectancy of patients with MTC and MEN 2A is over 50 years. The current best therapy for familial MTC is early diagnosis and complete resection of intrathyroidal disease at the initial operation. Ablation of extrathyroidal disease when detected by persistent or recurrent elevations of plasma calcitonin levels after total thyroidectomy requires the development of effective systemic adjuvant treatment.

REFERENCES

1. Wermer P. Genetic aspects of adenomatosis of endocrine glands. *Am J Med* 1954;16:363.
2. Larsson C, Skogseid B, Öberg K, Nakamura Y, Nordenskjöld M. Multiple endocrine neoplasia type 1 gene maps to chromosome 11 and is lost in insulinoma. *Nature* 1988;332:85.
3. Chandrasekharappa SC, Guru SC, Manickam P, et al. Positional cloning of the gene for multiple endocrine neoplasia-type 1. *Science* 1997;276:404.

4. Zhuang Z, Vortmeyer AO, Pack S, et al. Somatic mutations of the MEN1 tumor suppressor gene in sporadic gastrinomas and insulinomas. *Cancer Res* 1997;57:4682.

5. Toliat MR, Berger W, Ropers HH, Neuhaus P, Wiedenmann B. Mutations in the MEN1 gene in sporadic neuroendocrine tumours of gastroenteropancreatic system. *Lancet* 1997;350:1223.

6. Goebel SU, Heppner C, Burns AL, et al. Genotype/phenotype correlation of multiple endocrine neoplasia type 1 gene mutations in sporadic gastrinomas. *J Clin Endocrinol Metab* 2000;85:113.

7. Brandi ML, Aurbach GD, Fitzpatrick LA, et al. Parathyroid mitogenic activity in plasma from patients with familial multiple endocrine neoplasia type I. *N Engl J Med* 1986;314:1287.

8. Zimering MB, Brandi ML, deGrange DA, et al. Circulating fibroblast growth factor-like substance in familial multiple endocrine neoplasia type 1. *J Clin Endocrinol Metab* 1990;70:149.

9. Zimering MB, Katsumata N, Sato Y, et al. Increased basic fibroblast growth factor in plasma from multiple endocrine neoplasia type 1: relation to pituitary tumor. *J Clin Endocrinol Metab* 1993;76:1182.

10. Thakker RV, Bouloux P, Wooding C, et al. Association of parathyroid tumors in multiple endocrine neoplasia type 1 with loss of alleles on chromosome 11. *N Engl J Med* 1989;321:218.

11. Doherty GM, Lairmore T, Moley JF, Debenedetti M. MEN-1 parathyroid adenoma development over time. *World J Surg* 2004 (*in press*).

12. Brandi ML, Gagel RF, Angeli A, et al. Guidelines for diagnosis and therapy of MEN type 1 and type 2. *J Clin Endocrinol Metab* 2001;86:5658.

13. Skogseid BS, Eriksson B, Lundqvist G, et al. Multiple endocrine neoplasia type 1: a 10-year prospective screening study in four kindreds. *J Clin Endocrinol Metab* 1991;73:281.

14. Gibril F, Chen YJ, Schrump DS, et al. Prospective study of thymic carcinoids in patients with multiple endocrine neoplasia type 1. *J Clin Endocrinol Metab* 2003;88:1066.

15. Doherty GM, Olson JA, Frisella MM, et al. Lethality of multiple endocrine neoplasia type I. *World J Surg* 1998;22:581.

16. Wilkinson S, Teh BT, Davey KR, et al. Cause of death in multiple endocrine neoplasia type 1. *Arch Surg* 1993;128:683.

17. Dean PG, van Heerden JA, Farley DR, et al. Are patients with multiple endocrine neoplasia type 1 prone to premature death? *World J Surg* 2000;24:1437.

18. Skogseid B, Oberg K. Experience with multiple endocrine neoplasia type 1 screening. *J Intern Med* 1995;238:255.

19. Hellman P, Skogseid B, Oberg K, et al. Primary and reoperative parathyroid operations in hyperparathyroidism of multiple endocrine neoplasia type 1. *Surgery* 1998;124:993.

20. Rizzoli R, Green J III, Marx SJ. Primary hyperparathyroidism in familial multiple endocrine neoplasia type I: long-term follow-up of serum calcium levels after parathyroidectomy. *Am J Med* 1985;78:467.

21. Pipeleers-Marichal M, Donow C, Heitz PU, Kloppel G. Pathologic aspects of gastrinomas in patients with Zollinger-Ellison syndrome with and without multiple endocrine neoplasia type I. *World J Surg* 1993;17:481.

22. Pipeleers-Marichal M, Somers G, Willems G, et al. Gastrinomas in the duodenums of patients with multiple endocrine neoplasia type 1 and the Zollinger-Ellison syndrome. *N Engl J Med* 1990;322:723.

23. Fraker DL, Norton JA, Alexander HR, Venzon DJ, Jensen RT. Surgery in Zollinger-Ellison syndrome alters the natural history of gastrinoma. *Ann Surg* 1994;220:320.

24. Lairmore TC, Chen VY, DeBenedetti MK, et al. Duodenopancreatic resections in patients with multiple endocrine neoplasia type 1. *Ann Surg* 2000;231:909.

25. Lowney JK, Frisella MM, Lairmore TC, Doherty GM. Islet cell tumor metastasis in multiple endocrine neoplasia type I: correlation with primary tumor size. *Surgery* 1998;124:1043.

26. Norton JA, Alexander HR, Fraker DL, et al. Comparison of surgical results in patients with advanced and limited disease with multiple endocrine neoplasia type 1 and Zollinger-Ellison syndrome. *Ann Surg* 2001;234:495.

27. Metz DC, Jensen RT, Bale AE, et al. Multiple endocrine neoplasia type 1: clinical features and management. In: Bilezekian JP, Levine MA, Marcus R, eds. *The parathyroids.* New York: Raven Press, 1994:591.

28. Skogseid B, Rastad J, Gobl A, et al. Adrenal lesion in multiple endocrine neoplasia type 1. *Surgery* 1995;118:1077.

29. Marx S, Spiegel AM, Skarulis MC, et al. Multiple endocrine neoplasia type 1: clinical and genetic topics. *Ann Intern Med* 1998;129:484.

30. Bashir S, Gibril F, Ojeaburu JV, et al. Prospective study of the ability of histamine, serotonin or serum chromogranin A levels to identify gastric carcinoids in patients with gastrinomas. *Aliment Pharmacol Ther* 2002;16:1367.

31. Bordi C, Corleto VD, Azzoni C, et al. The antral mucosa as a new site for endocrine tumors in multiple endocrine neoplasia type 1 and Zollinger-Ellison syndromes. *J Clin Endocrinol Metab* 2001;86:2236.

32. Teh BT, Zedenius J, Kytola S, et al. Thymic carcinoids in multiple endocrine neoplasia type 1. *Ann Surg* 1998;228:99.

33. Hazard JB, Hawk WH, Crile G Jr. Medullary (solid) carcinoma of the thyroid-clinicopathologic entity. *J Clin Endocrinol Metab* 1959;19:704.

34. Sipple JH. The association of pheochromocytoma with carcinoma of the thyroid gland. *Am J Med* 1961;31:163.

35. Mulligan LM, Kwok JBJ, Healey CS, et al. Germ-line mutation of the RET proto-oncogene in multiple endocrine neoplasia type 2A. *Nature* 1993;363:458.

36. Donis-Keller H, Dou S, Chi D, et al. Mutations in the RET proto-oncogene are associated with MEN 2A and FMTC. *Hum Mol Genet* 1993;2:851.

37. O'Riordain DS, O'Brien T, Grant CS, et al. Surgical management of primary hyperparathyroidism in multiple endocrine neoplasia types 1 and 2. *Surgery* 1993;114:1031.

38. Wells SA Jr. Multiple endocrine neoplasia type II: recent results. *Cancer Res* 1990;18:71.

39. Yip L, Cote GJ, Shapiro SE, et al. Multiple endocrine neoplasia type 2: evaluation of the genotype-phenotype relationship. *Arch Surg* 2003;138:409.

40. Dralle H, Gimm O, Simon D, et al. Prophylactic thyroidectomy in 75 children and adolescents with hereditary medullary thyroid carcinoma: German and Austrian experience. *World J Surg* 1998;22:744.

41. Lairmore TC, Ball DW, Baylin SB, Wells J, Samuel A. Management of pheochromocytomas in patients with multiple endocrine neoplasia type 2 syndromes. *Ann Surg* 1993;217:595.

42. Brunt LM, Lairmore TC, Doherty GM, et al. Adrenalectomy for familial pheochromocytoma in the laparoscopic era. *Ann Surg* 2002;235:713.

43. Cohen MS, Moley JF. Surgical treatment of medullary thyroid carcinoma. *J Intern Med* 2003;253:616.

44. Moley JF, Wells SA Jr, Dilley WG, Tisell LE. Reoperation for recurrent or persistent medullary thyroid cancer. *Surgery* 1993;114:1090.

45. Moley JF, Dilley WG, DeBenedetti MK. Improved results of cervical reoperation for medullary thyroid carcinoma. *Ann Surg* 1997;225:734.

CHAPTER 35

Sarcomas of the Soft Tissues and Bone

MURRAY F. BRENNAN
SAMUEL SINGER
ROBERT G. MAKI
BRIAN O'SULLIVAN

SECTION **1**

Soft Tissue Sarcoma

INCIDENCE

Approximately 10,000 new cases of soft tissue sarcoma are reported in the United States each year. The true incidence is unknown. Based on analyses of Surveillance, Epidemiology, and End Results program data, the correct incidence has been suggested to be higher. These studies include entities such as mesothelioma. A little more than 50% of patients with newly diagnosed soft tissue sarcoma go on to die of the disease.[1] The relatively small number of cases seen and the great diversity in histopathologic features, anatomic site, and biologic behavior have made comprehensive understanding of these disease entities difficult. Soft tissue sarcoma, diagnosed at an early stage, is eminently curable. When diagnosed at the time of extensive local or metastatic disease, soft tissue sarcoma is rarely curable.

Analysis of population-based data from Connecticut[2] suggests an increase in incidence in both men and women, with a greater increase in women.

ETIOLOGY AND GENETICS

MOLECULAR ABNORMALITIES

Most soft tissue sarcomas have no clearly defined cause, although multiple associated or predisposing factors have been identified

(Tables 35.1-1 and 35.1-2). Soft tissue sarcomas in which genetic alterations play a developmental role segregate into two major types. The first type consists of sarcomas with specific genetic alterations that include simple karyotypes, including fusion genes due to reciprocal translocations and specific point mutations, such as *KIT* mutations in gastrointestinal stromal tumors (GISTs) and *APC*/β-catenin mutations in desmoid tumors. The second type consists of sarcomas with nonspecific genetic alterations and typically complex unbalanced karyotypes, representing numerous genetic losses and gains. Alterations in the tumor suppressor genes Rb-1 and p53 are detected in a substantial proportion of sarcomas.[3,4] The importance of these cell-regulatory genes in the pathogenesis of sarcoma is highlighted by the high incidence of germline mutations in patients with hereditary retinoblastoma and by identification of germline mutations in p53 in Li-Fraumeni syndrome.[5] A genetic predisposition to soft tissue sarcoma has also been associated with neurofibromatosis (NF)[6] and familial adenomatous polyposis (FAP).[7]

The most common tumors in patients with NF are in the central nervous system. In a 42-year follow-up study, 47% of all malignancies were nervous system tumors.[8] This review confirms the high incidence of malignant tumors in patients with NF: Approximately 46% of all patients with this disease will develop either a malignant tumor or a benign central nervous system tumor.[8] This prevalence is slightly higher in those with a family history of NF than in those with sporadic cases, but is common in both. Relatives of such patients, whether with a family history or not, are also at risk of developing malignant tumors. Approximately 5% of patients with NF develop malignant peripheral nerve sheath tumors (MPNSTs).

Genetic predisposition to malignancy is well established in the form of an autosomal dominant gene in 8% to 9% of children with soft tissue sarcomas. Survivors of retinoblastoma with the associated Rb gene abnormality often develop tumors later in

TABLE 35.1-1. Genetic Predisposition to Soft Tissue Sarcoma

	Sarcoma	Gene	Chromosome	Reference(s)
Neurofibromatosis type I (von Reckling-hausen's disease)	Malignant peripheral nerve sheath tumor	NF-1	17q11.2	314
Retinoblastoma	Soft tissue, osteogenic	Rb-1	13q14	315
Li-Fraumeni syndrome	Soft tissue, osteogenic	TP53	17p13	5,316
Gardner's syndrome	Fibrosarcoma, desmoid tumor	APC	5q21	317
Werner's syndrome (adult progeria)	Soft tissue	WRN	8p12	318
Gorlin's syndrome (nevoid basal cell carci-noma syndrome)	Fibrosarcoma, rhabdomyosarcoma	PTC	9q22.3	2
Carney's triad	Gastrointestinal stromal tumor	Unknown	Unknown	319
Tuberous sclerosis (Bourneville disease)	Rhabdomyoma, rhabdomyosarcoma	TSC1	9q34	320,321
		TSC2	16p13.3	

life. Long-term follow-up of patients who survived treatment for retinoblastoma has demonstrated that some patients develop three or more nonocular tumors.[9] In one review of 1506 patients with neuroblastoma, 211 developed a second tumor, 142 died before an additional malignancy developed, and 28 developed a third tumor at a median of 5 to 8 years (5-year incidence, 11%). The predominant tumors were soft tissue sarcomas of the head and neck. In an examination of 1604 patients with retinoblastoma who survived longer than 1 year,[9] the incidence of subsequent cancer was increased only in the 961 patients with hereditary retinoblastoma, in whom 190 cancers developed versus 6.3 expected. Cumulative incidence of a second cancer at 50 years after diagnosis was 50% for those with hereditary retinoblastoma and 5% for those with nonhereditary retinoblastoma.

It is important to emphasize that in patients who have retinoblastoma the increased risk of a second primary is enhanced by radiotherapy in a dose-dependent fashion.[10] For soft tissue sarcoma, the relative risk showed a stepwise increase at all x-ray therapy dose categories beginning at 5 Gy and rose to a 10.7-fold at doses above 60 Gy.

FAP, a subset of which is Gardner's syndrome, is commonly associated with the development of intraabdominal desmoids. These tumors behave as low-grade fibrosarcomas, although constant debate exists as to the histopathologic classification and distinction between the desmoid tumor and aggressive fibromatosis (see Desmoid Tumor, later in this chapter). The natural history of slow growth with accompanying invasion of contiguous structures increases the risk of subsequent mortality when the tumor is managed inappropriately.

The development of soft tissue and bone sarcoma as a result of exposure to radiation has been known since 1922. There is a poor understanding of the molecular mechanisms and antecedent cause of these lesions. They are most often seen in diseases that are commonly treated with radiotherapy and in those in which a long survival period is expected. The prime candidate diseases are breast cancer, lymphomas, and cervical cancer[11] (Fig. 35.1-1), and children are at risk due to the time latency involved. An interesting feature of postirradiation-induced sarcomas is that they have a reputation for originating close to the penumbra of radiotherapy fields. The postulated explanation for this has centered on the possibility that incomplete damage in normal tissues results in mutagenic responses and disorganized reparative proliferation that can eventually trigger tumor induction.[12] Germline mutations in tumor suppressor genes or accumulated damage to DNA repair genes, or both, may lead to neoplasia but it remains unknown if most individuals have a genetic defect that underpinned the development of the first cancer, for which radiotherapy was administered, and in turn led to the induction of the irradiation-induced cancer.[13] If this is the case, it is logical to consider the possibility that there may be subgroups of individuals at considerably greater risk than is generally appreciated whereas others have relatively low risk.[13] Although uncommon, these sarcomas usually have a poor prognosis. In a review of 160 patients,[11] external radiation therapy was given to 99% of the patients, 14% of whom received additional treatment with temporary or permanent radioisotope implantation. One patient inadvertently ingested

TABLE 35.1-2. Case-Control Studies of Relationship between Exposure to Phenoxy Herbicides and Incidence of Soft Tissue Sarcoma

Location	Author	Year	No.	Relative Risk	95% Confidence Interval
North Sweden	Hardell and Sandstrom[322]	1979	46	5.3	2.4–11.5
South Sweden	Eriksson et al.[323]	1981	99	6.8	2.6–17.3
New Zealand	Smith et al.[18]	1984	82	1.6	0.7–3.3
England and Wales	Balarajan and Acheson[324]	1984	1961	1.15	0.83–1.59
New York State: Vietnam service	Greenwald et al.[325]	1984	281	0.7	0.17–2.92
Veterans' Administration patients: Vietnam service	Kang et al.[19]	1986	234	0.83	0.63–1.09
Kansas	Hoar et al.[326]	1986	133	1	0.7–1.6

(Modified from Brennan MF. Management of extremity soft tissue sarcoma. *Am J Surg* 1989;158:71.)

Antecedent Diseases [%]

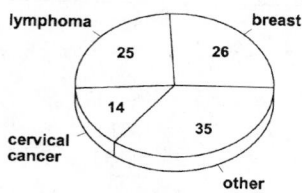

Histopathology [%]

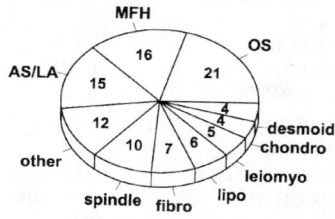

FIGURE 35.1-1.   Radiation-associated soft tissue sarcoma: antecedent disease for which radiation was given and histopathology of sarcomas that developed in 160 patients at Memorial Sloan-Kettering Cancer Center. AS, angiosarcoma; LA, lymphangiosarcoma; MFH, malignant fibrous histiocytoma; OS, osteogenic sarcoma. (From ref. 11, with permission.)

radium. The subsequent tumor that developed was most commonly an osteogenic sarcoma, followed by soft tissue tumors, particularly malignant fibrous histiocytoma (MFH) and angiosarcoma or lymphangiosarcoma. No significant difference in survival was found between patients with bone tumors and those with soft tissue sarcomas. Survival was not affected by site, latency period, or the amount of radiation received initially, nor was there any difference for patients receiving chemotherapy for their sarcoma. The three factors in the Cox multivariate analysis that had a significant unfavorable association were presentation with metastatic disease ($P = .017$), incomplete or no operative resection ($P = .004$), and tumor size of at least 5 cm ($P = .007$). Tumor grade was not significant in any analyses, but only 6% of the patients had low-grade tumors.[11]

Given the increased use of radiation therapy as a primary treatment modality for breast cancer, concern has been expressed that increased incidence of sarcoma might be expected. In one study,[14] all 122,991 women with breast cancer in Sweden from 1958 to 1992 were followed, and 116 soft tissue sarcomas were found. There were 40 angiosarcomas and 76 other sarcomas. As expected, angiosarcoma correlated with lymphedema (relative risk, 9.5; 95% confidence interval, 3.2 to 28.0), but not radiation therapy. For other sarcomas, there was a dose-response relationship with exposure to radiation therapy.

Lymphedema has long been established as a factor in the development of lymphangiosarcoma. The most well recognized association is with the postmastectomy, postirradiated lymphedematous arm, described by Stewart and Treves.[15] This is not a radiation-induced sarcoma because the lymphangiosarcoma develops both inside and outside of the irradiated field, in the edematous extremity. Similar advanced sarcomas have been seen after filarial infection and chronic lymphedema.[16]

The issue of trauma as a predisposing factor is more controversial. Often a minor episode of injury is the factor that draws attention to the presence of a mass, which implies that a causative association is not real. Abdominal desmoid tumors commonly follow parturition. However, they can occur in the extremity, both localized and multifocal, and may be associated with antecedent vigorous physical activity.[17]

Chemical agents have been implicated in the etiology of soft tissue sarcoma. There have been conflicting reports about the relationship between occupational exposure to phenoxyacetic acids found in some herbicides and chlorophenols (present in

some wood preservatives) (see Table 35.1-2).[15,18,19] Other authors have pointed to the inherent problems in occupational epidemiology in relation to the source material for soft tissue sarcoma, among which are the following: There is possible recall bias in self-reported exposure data; soft tissue sarcomas are not consistently classified in the International Classification of Diseases, which is organ based; there is variation in the operational definition of soft tissue sarcomas; and, because of their rarity, it is difficult to recruit sufficient patients for a case-control study and cohorts would have to be extremely large to identify an increase in risk. Nevertheless, some studies have suggested a link between phenoxy herbicide exposure in forestry workers, farmers, and railroad workers and subsequent development of sarcoma,[20] whereas other studies in the United States, New Zealand, and Finland have not confirmed this relationship.[18]

An increased incidence of soft tissue sarcomas was seen in a cohort of 1520 industrial workers exposed for more than 1 year to 2,3,7,8-tetrachlorodibenzo-p-dioxin,[21] but other studies did not substantiate these findings. The issue of dioxin as a risk factor remains controversial. A population-based case-control study assessed the risk of soft tissue sarcomas in Vietnam veterans, including those potentially exposed to Agent Orange, which contains dioxin, and found no increased risk among any subset of veterans compared with control groups.[22] Another study found no increased risk for Vietnam veterans compared with men who had never been in Vietnam. The risk for subgroups of veterans who were more likely to be exposed to Agent Orange, compared with their unexposed counterparts in Vietnam, was not statistically significant.

Several chemical carcinogens have an established role in the development of hepatic angiosarcomas: Thorotrast, vinyl chloride, and arsenic (including Fowler's 1% arsenic solution).[23,24] A review of pesticides and cancer[25] has again linked the phenoxy herbicides to soft tissue sarcoma and lymphoma, but questions the causal relationship of these agents.

Chemotherapy for pediatric malignancies has been associated with the subsequent development of osteogenic sarcomas; a relationship with the development of soft tissue sarcomas has not been demonstrated.

CYTOGENETIC ABNORMALITIES

It is important to emphasize that extensive cytogenetic abnormalities occur in soft tissue sarcoma (Table 35.1-3). These are usually associated with high-grade tumors, but are not consistent across tumors. For example, in an analysis of 36 tumors,[26] multiple complex karyotypes were identified and at least 24 recurrent abnormalities (defined by their presence in at least five cases) were detected. However, none of the selected rearrangements was specific for any particular subgroup. Specific changes have been identified in selected sarcomas. The best examples are the translocation in Ewing's sarcoma (primitive neuroectodermal tumor), t(11;22)(q24;q11.2-12), and the translocation in synovial sarcoma t(X;18)(p11.2;q11.2). These genetic abnormalities can be used as a diagnostic tool.

Multiple other studies of genetic abnormalities have been published.[27] Abnormalities of INK4A (coding for p16 and p19ARF on 9p21) and INK4B have been correlated with poor survival. These chromosomal alterations occur in 15% of patients with high-grade sarcomas. In myxoid and round cell liposarcomas, the presence of the TLS-CHOP fusion protein

TABLE 35.1-3. Chromosomal Changes in Soft Tissue Sarcoma

Tumor Histology	Chromosomal Alteration	Involved Gene(s)	Frequency (%)	Reference(s)
Ewing's sarcoma family[a]	t(11;22)(q24;q12)	EWS-FLI1	85	327
	t(21;22)(q22;q12)	EWS-ERG	5–10	328
	t(7;22)(p22;q12)	EVT1-EWS	Rare	329
	t(17;22)(q12;q12)	EIAF-EWS	Rare	330
	t(1;16)(q11-25;q11-24)	Unknown	~10	331,332
Myxoid or round cell liposarcoma	t(12;16)(q13;p11)	TLS (FUS)-CHOP	>75	43,44
	t(12;22)(q13;q12)	EWS-CHOP	Uncommon	333
Atypical lipomatous tumor, well-differentiated liposarcoma	12q rings and giant markers	HMGIC, CDK4 and MDM2 amplification	60	60,334,335
Alveolar rhabdomyosarcoma	t(2;13)(q35;q14)	PAX3-FKHR	~70	69,336
	t(1;13)(p36;q14)	PAX7-FKHR	~15	69,336
Malignant melanoma of soft tissues (clear cell sarcoma)	t(12;22)(q13;q12)	EWS-ATF1	>75	337
Desmoplastic small round cell tumor	t(11;22)(p13;q12)	EWS-WT1	>90	45
Synovial sarcoma	t(X;18)(p11;q11)	SYT-SSX1, SYT-SSX2	>90	42,79,80,338
Extraskeletal myxoid chondrosarcoma	t(9;22)(q22;q12)	EWS-CHN (TEC)	>75	339
Dermatofibrosarcoma protuberans	t(17;22)(q22;q13), ring chromosomes	COL1A1-PDGFB	>50; ring chromosomes >75	52
Alveolar soft parts sarcoma	Unbalanced t(X;17)(p11.2;q25)	ASPL-TFE3	>90	340
Endometrial stromal sarcoma	t(X;17)(p15;q21)	JAZF1-JJAZ1	>65	341
Congenital fibrosarcoma	t(12;15)(p13;q25)	ETV6 (TEL)-NTRK3 (TRKC)	Unknown	342
Malignant rhabdoid tumor	del 22(q11.2)	hSNF5/INI1	~50[b]	343
Uterine leiomyosarcoma (and leiomyoma)	t(12;14)(q14-15;q23-24)	Unknown	Uncommon	344
Embryonal rhabdomyosarcoma	Trisomy 2, trisomy 8	Unknown	Rare	345,346
Epithelioid sarcoma	Loss of heterozygosity (22q); t(8;22)(q22;q11)	?NF2, ?EWS	Rare	347,348
Malignant fibrous histiocytoma	Complex karyotype	Unknown	Common	26

[a]Ewing's sarcoma family includes classic Ewing's sarcoma, peripheral neuroectodermal tumor, Askin's tumor, and peripheral neuroepithelioma.
[b]Mutations seen in other cases, giving >80% with disruption of the hSNF5 gene.

has been firmly established[28] and links these two forms of liposarcoma with one another despite their strikingly different morphologic characteristics.

DISTRIBUTION

Soft tissue sarcomas can occur in any site throughout the body. Forty-three percent are in the extremities (Fig. 35.1-2) with two-thirds of extremity lesions occurring in the lower limb, and 34% are intraabdominal, divided between visceral (19%) and retroperitoneal (15%) lesions.

PATHOLOGIC CLASSIFICATION

Soft tissue tumors, although clinically often nondistinctive, form a varied and complex group that may show a wide range of differentiation[29] (Table 35.1-4). In understanding the clinical behavior of these lesions it is important to emphasize that the concept of histogenesis is not definable. Except for subcutaneous lipomas or benign smooth muscle tumors, there is very little evidence that these lesions arise from their mature (differentiated) tissue counterparts. This is emphasized by the fact that many liposarcomas arise at sites devoid of adipose tissue and most rhabdomyosarcomas develop in locations that lack

voluntary muscle. There is no evidence to support the concept of a primitive mesenchymal stem cell as the precursor of these tumors. Because all diploid cells contain the genetic information, a more likely explanation is that switching on a given set of genes that programs mesenchymal differentiation in any type of mesenchymal cell may give rise to almost any mesenchymal neoplasm.[29] Evidence from microarray and gene-chip data suggests that many histologic types of soft tissue tumors have characteristic patterns of gene expression associated with the process of neoplasia.[30–32]

Soft tissue tumors may be benign or malignant, and a variety of borderline lesions are also recognized. The ratio of benign to

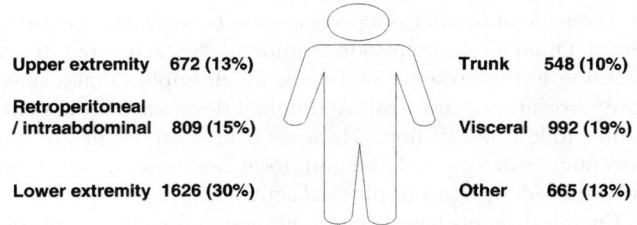

Upper extremity 672 (13%)
Retroperitoneal / intraabdominal 809 (15%)
Lower extremity 1626 (30%)
Trunk 548 (10%)
Visceral 992 (19%)
Other 665 (13%)

FIGURE 35.1-2. Distribution by site of soft tissue sarcomas in 5312 patients aged 16 years or older admitted to Memorial Sloan-Kettering Cancer Center between July 1, 1982, and December 31, 2002.

TABLE 35.1-4. Histologic Classification of Soft Tissue Sarcoma

FIBROUS TUMORS

Benign tumors

Nodular fasciitis (including intravascular and cranial types)

Proliferative fasciitis and myositis

Atypical decubital fibroplasia (ischemic fasciitis)

Fibroma (dermal, tendon sheath, nuchal)

Keloid

Elastofibroma

Calcifying aponeurotic fibroma

Fibrous hamartoma of infancy

Fibromatosis coli

Infantile digital fibromatosis

Myofibromatosis (solitary, multicentric)

Juvenile hyaline fibromatosis

Calcifying fibrous pseudotumor

Fibromatoses

Superficial fibromatoses

    Palmar and plantar (Dupuytren's contracture) fibromatoses

    Penile (Peyronie's fibromatosis)

    Knuckle pads

Deep fibromatoses

    Abdominal fibromatosis (abdominal desmoid)

    Extraabdominal fibromatosis (extraabdominal desmoid)

    Intraabdominal fibromatosis (intraabdominal desmoid)

    Mesenteric fibromatosis (including Gardner's syndrome)

    Infantile (desmoid-type) fibromatosis

Intermediate tumors

Solitary fibrous tumor

Inflammatory myofibroblastic tumor

Congenital or infantile fibrosarcoma

Malignant tumors

Fibrosarcoma

    Adult fibrosarcoma

    Inflammatory fibrosarcoma

FIBROHISTIOCYTIC TUMORS

Benign tumors

Fibrous histiocytoma

    Cutaneous fibrous histiocytoma (dermatofibroma)

    Deep fibrous histiocytoma

Juvenile xanthogranuloma

Reticulohistiocytoma

Xanthoma

Intermediate tumors

Atypical fibroxanthoma

Dermatofibrosarcoma protuberans (including pigmented form, Bednar's tumor)

Giant cell fibroblastoma

Plexiform fibrohistiocytic tumor

Angiomatoid fibrous histiocytoma

Malignant tumors

Malignant fibrous histiocytoma

    Storiform-pleomorphic

    Myxoid (myxofibrosarcoma)

    Giant cell (malignant giant cell tumor of soft parts)

    Inflammatory

LIPOMATOUS TUMORS

Benign tumors

Lipoma

    Cutaneous lipoma

    Deep lipoma

        Intramuscular lipoma

        Tendon sheath lipoma

        Intraneural and perineural fibrolipoma

Multiple lipomas

Angiolipoma

Spindle cell or pleomorphic lipoma

Myolipoma

Angiomyolipoma

Myelolipoma

Chondroid lipoma

Hibernoma

Lipoblastoma or lipoblastomatosis

Lipomatosis

    Diffuse lipomatosis

    Cervical symmetrical lipomatosis (Madelung's disease)

Intermediate tumors

Atypical lipoma

Malignant tumors

Liposarcoma

    Well-differentiated liposarcoma

        Lipoma-like liposarcoma

        Sclerosing liposarcoma

        Inflammatory liposarcoma

    Dedifferentiated liposarcoma

    Myxoid or round cell liposarcoma

    Pleomorphic liposarcoma

SMOOTH MUSCLE TUMORS

Benign tumors

Leiomyoma (cutaneous and deep)

Angiomyoma (vascular leiomyoma)

Epithelioid leiomyoma

Intravenous leiomyomatosis

Leiomyomatosis peritonealis disseminata

Malignant tumors

Leiomyosarcoma

Epithelioid leiomyosarcoma

SKELETAL MUSCLE TUMORS

Benign tumors

Adult rhabdomyoma

Genital rhabdomyoma

Fetal rhabdomyoma

Intermediate (cellular) rhabdomyoma

Malignant tumors

Rhabdomyosarcoma

    Embryonal rhabdomyosarcoma

    Botryoid rhabdomyosarcoma

    Spindle cell rhabdomyosarcoma

    Alveolar rhabdomyosarcoma

    Pleomorphic rhabdomyosarcoma

Rhabdomyosarcoma with ganglionic differentiation (ectomesenchymoma)

TUMORS OF BLOOD AND LYMPH VESSELS

Benign tumors

Papillary endothelial hyperplasia

Hemangioma

    Capillary (including juvenile) hemangioma

    Cavernous hemangioma

    Venous hemangioma

    Epithelioid hemangioma (angiolymphoid hyperplasia, histiocytoid hemangioma)

    Granulation-type hemangioma (pyogenic granuloma)

    Tufted hemangioma

Deep hemangioma (intramuscular, synovial, perineural)

Lymphangioma

Lymphangiomyoma and lymphangiomyomatosis

Angiomatosis

(continued)

TABLE 35.1-4. (*Continued*)

Lymphangiomatosis
Intermediate tumors
Endovascular papillary angioendothelioma (Dabska's tumor)
Spindle cell hemangioendothelioma
Malignant tumors
Epithelioid hemangioendothelioma
Angiosarcoma and lymphangiosarcoma
Kaposi's sarcoma
PERIVASCULAR TUMORS
Benign tumors
Glomus tumor
Glomangiomyoma
Hemangiopericytoma
Myopericytoma
Malignant tumors
Malignant glomus tumor (glomangiosarcoma)
Malignant hemangiopericytoma
SYNOVIAL TUMORS
Benign tumors
Tenosynovial giant cell tumor
    Localized tenosynovial giant cell tumor
    Diffuse tenosynovial giant cell tumor (extraarticular pigmented
      villonodular synovitis, florid tenosynovitis)
Malignant tumor
Malignant giant cell tumor of tendon sheath
NEURAL TUMORS
Benign tumors
Traumatic neuroma
Morton's neuroma
Multiple mucosal neuromas
Neuromuscular hamartoma (benign Triton tumor)
Nerve sheath ganglion
Schwannoma (neurilemoma)
    Cellular schwannoma
    Plexiform schwannoma
    Degenerated (ancient) schwannoma
    Schwannomatosis
Neurothekeoma (nerve sheath myxoma)
Neurofibroma
    Diffuse neurofibroma
    Plexiform neurofibroma
    Pacinian neurofibroma
    Epithelioid neurofibroma
Granular cell tumor
Melanotic schwannoma
Ectopic meningioma
Ectopic ependymoma
Ganglioneuroma
Pigmented neuroectodermal tumor of infancy (retinal anlage tumor,
    melanotic progonoma)
Malignant tumors
Malignant peripheral nerve sheath tumor (MPNST) (neurofibrosar-
    coma)
    Malignant Triton tumor (MPNST with rhabdomyosarcoma)

    Glandular MPNST
    Epithelioid MPNST
Malignant granular cell tumor
Primitive neuroectodermal tumor
    Neuroblastoma
    Ganglioneuroblastoma
    Neuroepithelioma (peripheral neuroectodermal tumor)
PARAGANGLIONIC TUMORS
Benign tumor
Paraganglioma
Malignant tumor
Malignant paraganglioma
EXTRASKELETAL CARTILAGINOUS AND OSSEOUS TUMORS
Benign tumors
Panniculitis ossificans and myositis ossificans
Fibroosseous pseudotumor of the digits
Fibrodysplasia (myositis) ossificans progressiva
Extraskeletal chondroma or osteochondroma
Extraskeletal osteoma
Malignant tumors
Extraskeletal chondrosarcoma
    Myxoid chondrosarcoma
    Mesenchymal chondrosarcoma
Extraskeletal osteosarcoma
PLURIPOTENTIAL MESENCHYMAL TUMORS
Benign tumor
Mesenchymoma
Malignant tumor
Malignant mesenchymoma
MISCELLANEOUS TUMORS
Benign tumors
Congenital granular cell tumor
Tumoral calcinosis
Myxoma
    Cutaneous myxoma
    Intramuscular myxoma
    Juxtaarticular myxoma
Angiomyxoma
Amyloid tumor
Parachordoma
Ossifying and nonossifying fibromyxoid tumors
Palisaded myofibroblastoma of lymph node
Malignant tumors
Alveolar soft part sarcoma
Epithelioid sarcoma
Malignant extrarenal rhabdoid tumor
Desmoplastic small cell tumor
Ewing's sarcoma—extraskeletal
Clear cell sarcoma (melanoma of soft parts)
Gastrointestinal stromal tumors
Synovial sarcoma
    Biphasic synovial sarcoma
    Monophasic synovial sarcoma
UNCLASSIFIED TUMORS

(Modified from Fletcher CDM, Unni K, Mertens K, eds. *World Health Organization classification of tumours: pathology and genetics of tumours of soft tissue and bone.* Lyon, France: International Agency for Research on Cancer, 2002.)

malignant tumors is more than 100:1. Soft tissue tumors are notorious for the ease with which benign and malignant cases may be confused, particularly in small biopsy samples.

Sarcoma histologic type is generally an important determinant of prognosis and also an important predictor of distinc-

tive patterns of behavior. Although many published series have combined all the histologic subtypes of sarcoma, the importance of such subtyping is exemplified by liposarcoma, in which the five histologic subtypes (well differentiated, dedifferentiated, myxoid, round cell, and pleomorphic) have totally

TABLE 35.1-5. Soft Tissue Sarcomas: Histologic Type and Lymph Node Metastasis

Histopathology	Weingrad and Rosenberg[349,a] No. of Nodal Metastases/All Sarcoma Patients	% of All Lesions	Mazeron and Suit[350,b] No. of Nodal Metastases/All Sarcoma Patients	% of All Lesions	Fong et al.[34,c] No. of Nodal Metastases/All Sarcoma Patients	% of All Lesions
Fibrosarcoma	55/1083	5.1	54/215	25.1	0/162	0
Malignant fibrous histiocytoma	1/30	3.3	84/823	10.2	8/316	2.5
Embryonal rhabdomyosarcoma	108/888	12.2	201/1354	14.8	12/88	13.6
Leiomyosarcoma	10/94	10.6	21/524	4	9/328	2.7
Neurofibrosarcoma, malignant peripheral nerve tumor	0/60	0	3/476	0.6	2/96	2.1
Vascular	—	—	43/376	11.4	—	—
Angiosarcoma	—	—	—	—	5/37	13.5
Lymphangiosarcoma	—	—	—	—	1/4	25.0
Osteosarcoma	20/327	6.1	—	—	0/11	0
Synovial sarcoma	91/535	17	117/851	13.7	2/145	1.4
Liposarcoma	15/288	5.2	16/504	3.2	3/403	0.7
Alveolar soft part sarcoma	6/62	9.7	3/24	12.5	0/13	0
Other	14/148	9.5	25/110	22.7	15/222	6.4
Epithelioid	—	—	14/70	—	2/12	16.7
Total	320/3515	9.1	567/5257	10.8	46/1772	2.6

[a]From a summary of 47 studies.
[b]From a summary of 122 studies.
[c]Database includes only extraskeletal osteosarcomas and chondrosarcomas.

different biologies and patterns of behavior.[29] A further clear demonstration is the importance of myogenic differentiation in pleomorphic sarcomas, which is associated with a substantially increased risk of metastasis.[33] Sarcomas are characterized by local invasiveness. The pattern of metastasis of most sarcomas is hematogenous. Lymph node metastases are uncommon, except for selected cell types usually associated with childhood sarcoma[34] (Table 35.1-5).

GRADING OF SARCOMA

After establishing the diagnosis of sarcoma, the most critical piece of information the pathologist can provide to the clinician is histologic grade. The pathologic features that define grade include cellularity, differentiation, pleomorphism, necrosis, and number of mitoses. Unfortunately, the criteria for grading are neither specific nor standardized. Several grading scales and systems are used: a four-grade system (Broders),[35] a three-grade system (low, intermediate, high) such as the National Cancer Institute (NCI) grading system[36] and that of the French Federation of Cancer Centers Sarcoma Group,[37] and a binary system (high vs. low) as is used at Memorial Hospital.[38] Even when there is agreement about the number of grades to be used, expert pathologists disagree about specific criteria for defining grade.

The clinical implications are obvious. In adjuvant chemotherapy trials high grade is defined differently at different centers, which makes comparison of results between trials, and combining results of multiple trials, hazardous. For example, tumors of 240 patients who participated in the Scandinavian Sarcoma Group adjuvant trial for high-grade extremity sarcoma were reviewed by a panel of reference pathologists. A four-grade system was used in this trial; only patients with grade III or IV sarcomas were eligible. On review, 5% of the patients were considered ineligible because their tumors were low grade.[39] Although it did not influence eligibility, there was considerable discordance between the original pathologists and the reference pathologists with regard to whether a lesion was grade III or IV. Although the adjuvant regimen did not affect survival (see Adjuvant Chemotherapy, later in this chapter), a difference in survival was noted between patients with tumors of these two grades as assigned by the reference pathologists.

Many pathologists consider mitotic activity and degree of necrosis to be the most important pathologic features. To define a practical grading system, the European Organization for Research and Treatment of Cancer (EORTC) studied the histologic features of tumors from 282 patients who participated in their adjuvant chemotherapy trial and correlated the pathologic findings with outcome.[40] In a multivariate analysis, only mitotic count (fewer than 3, 3 to 20, and more than 20 mitoses per 10 consecutive high-power fields), the presence or absence of necrosis, and tumor size predicted survival.

Mutation of p53, nuclear overexpression of p53, and a high Ki-67 proliferation index are associated with high grade and poor survival.[41] Biologic markers have not been consistently shown to be independent indicators of prognosis and cannot at present be used to grade sarcomas.

Several tumors that are considered sarcomas have no recognizable normal tissue counterpart (e.g., alveolar soft part tumor, Ewing's sarcoma, epithelioid sarcoma). These tumors often have unique clinical features and usually are not graded.

DIFFERENTIAL DIAGNOSIS

In addition to sarcoma, the differential diagnosis of a soft tissue mass includes a variety of benign lesions, as well as primary or metastatic carcinoma, melanoma, and lymphoma. Accurate diagnosis requires an adequate and representative biopsy of the tumor, and the tissue must be well fixed and well stained. Antibodies for immunohistochemical staining are available commercially, and this technique is readily applicable to paraffin-embedded tissues. The most useful immunohistochemical markers are the intermediate filaments (e.g., vimentin, keratin, desmin, leukocyte common antigen, S-100). In addition, the pathologist should be prepared to process tissue from selected cases for electron microscopy, cytogenetic studies, or molecular analysis. This implies that certain diagnoses are considered by the clinician, that the diagnostic biopsy specimen is obtained appropriately, and that the clinician and pathologist communicate before the biopsy is performed to assure that the necessary steps are taken in handling the tissue.

Cytogenetic analyses reveal specific clonal chromosomal aberrations, most commonly reciprocal translocations, in the majority of sarcomas,[39,42–45] which in a significant subset can be diagnostically and occasionally prognostically useful. The fusion gene translocations include 11 different gene fusions involving the *EWS* gene or *EWS* family members (*TLS, TAF2N*) found in five different sarcomas, and 10 other types of fusion in seven other sarcoma types. Because conventional cytogenetic analysis is labor intensive and requires short-term culture of the sarcoma cells, molecular genetic techniques [e.g., reverse transcriptase-polymerase chain reaction and fluorescence *in situ* hybridization (FISH)] may serve as useful diagnostic adjuncts, particularly for diagnosing and distinguishing among the small cell sarcomas. Oligonucleotide and complementary DNA arrays may eventually add to the sophistication of determining the diagnosis and prognosis of such tumors.[46] Table 35.1-3 describes some of the genetic changes identified in soft tissue sarcoma. FISH testing using probes to locate specific chromosomal abnormalities may become clinically useful but is unavailable for routine diagnostic use at this time. Supernumerary ring chromosomes, seen in mesenchymal neoplasms of low or borderline malignancy, such as dermatofibrosarcoma protuberans, can be identified with this technique.

As might be expected, there may be considerable disagreement among pathologists regarding the specific histologic diagnosis in individual cases. When pathologic material from 424 patients who entered into Eastern Cooperative Oncology Group (ECOG) sarcoma trials was reviewed by a panel of expert pathologists, 10% of cases were rejected as not being sarcoma, and for 14% of the remaining cases there was disagreement with respect to the histologic subtype. In the Scandinavian Sarcoma Group experience, the specific histologic diagnosis was disputed in 20%.[35] With increasing familiarity with the immunohistochemical and genetic studies needed to diagnosis soft tissue sarcoma, the rate of this discordance may be decreasing.

Overall, the three most common histopathologic subtypes are MFH, liposarcoma, and leiomyosarcoma. Some types of sarcoma occur with greater frequency in certain age groups or in specific locations, forming clinicopathologic syndromes that permit standardized treatment strategies. The distribution of common histologic types among different age groups is shown in Figure 35.1-3. Histopathologic type is anatomic site depen-

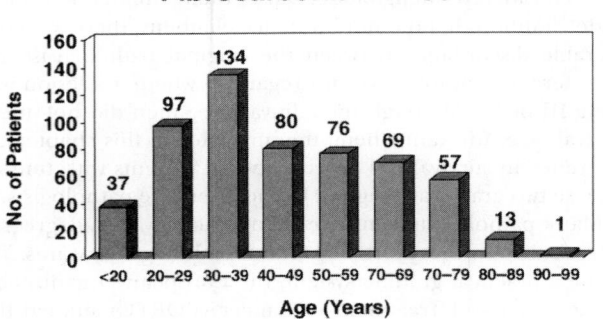

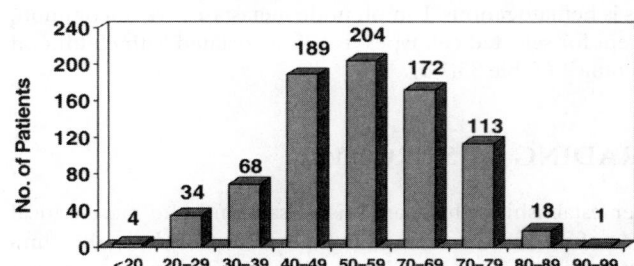

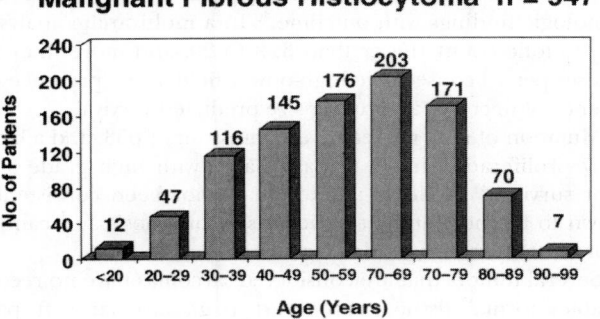

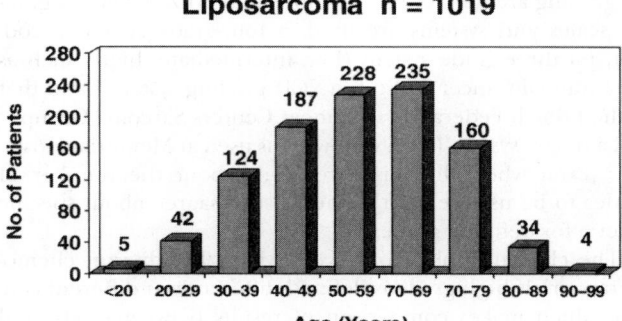

FIGURE 35.1-3. Age distribution of common histologic types of soft tissue sarcomas.

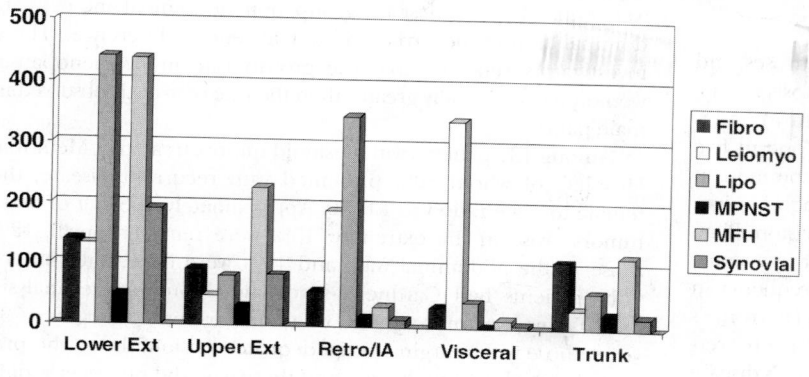

FIGURE 35.1-4. Predominant histology by site of soft tissue sarcomas in 3401 patients aged 16 years or older admitted to Memorial Sloan-Kettering Cancer Center between July 1, 1982, and December 31, 2002. MFH, malignant fibrous histiocytoma; MPNST, malignant peripheral nerve sheath tumor; Retro/IA, retroperitoneal/intraabdominal.

dent: The common subtypes in the extremities are liposarcoma, MFH, synovial sarcoma, and fibrosarcoma. In the retroperitoneal location, well-differentiated (WD) and dedifferentiated liposarcoma and leiomyosarcoma are the most common histiotypes, whereas in the visceral location, GISTs are found most commonly. The distribution of histologic type by site is shown in Figure 35.1-4.

Virtually all gastrointestinal sarcomas were previously classified as leiomyosarcomas or leiomyoblastomas. It is now recognized that many gastrointestinal sarcomas do not express markers of myogenic differentiation and are better classified as GISTs. GISTs are mesenchymal neoplasms showing differentiation toward the interstitial cells of Cajal and are typically characterized by the expression of the receptor tyrosine kinase KIT (CD117).[47] Studies have now established that activating mutations of KIT are present in up to 92% of GISTs and likely play a key role in the development of these tumors.[48] The pattern of recurrence is intraabdominal, including liver metastasis. (See Chapter 29.7.)

Overall, leiomyosarcoma is the most common type of genitourinary sarcoma in the adult and arises in the bladder, kidney, or prostate, usually in older individuals. Rhabdomyosarcoma arising in paratesticular tissues is a disease of young men. Three major types of uterine sarcoma are recognized: (1) leiomyosarcomas, tumors of the myometrium; (2) mesodermal mixed tumors (malignant mixed müllerian tumors), composed of elements of carcinoma and sarcoma; and (3) endometrial stromal sarcomas, the least common, which usually have very aggressive behavior.

Ten percent to 15% of all sarcomas occur in children. The majority of pediatric patients have small cell sarcomas, including rhabdomyosarcoma and the Ewing's sarcoma and primitive neuroectodermal tumor spectrum (see Chapter 40.2).

CLINICOPATHOLOGIC FEATURES OF SPECIFIC TYPES OF BENIGN AND MALIGNANT SOFT TISSUE TUMORS

TUMORS OF FIBROUS ORIGIN

There are a variety of benign tumors and tumor-like lesions of fibrous tissue that must be distinguished from true fibrosarcoma. These lesions are generally composed of an admixture of fibroblasts and myofibroblasts in varying proportions and may be confused with reactive or reparative processes. A variety of names have been used to designate identical or overlapping entities. In addition, there are a variety of fibrous proliferations of infancy and childhood that resemble lesions in the adult but are associated with a better prognosis. Features of lesions that may be mistaken for sarcoma are summarized in the following sections.

Nodular Fasciitis

Nodular fasciitis, also called *pseudosarcomatous fasciitis*, is a benign lesion usually seen in adults aged 20 to 40, although it has been reported in both older and younger patients. The typical lesion grows rapidly over several weeks reaching a size of 1 to 2 cm. Growth is usually self-limited, and lesions rarely are larger than 5 cm. Tenderness or soreness is a common complaint. The upper extremity is the most common site, especially the volar aspect of the forearm. Nodular fasciitis generally arises in the subcutaneous fascia or the superficial portions of the deep fascia. Histologically, the lesions are nodular, nonencapsulated masses, consisting of plump, immature fibroblasts arranged in short, irregular bundles or fascicles. Because of their cellularity, rapid growth, and high mitotic activity, these lesions may be mistaken for fibrosarcoma. In terms of clinical behavior these are all benign processes with a self-limiting clinical course. Recurrence is uncommon after simple local excision, because any residual lesional tissue undergoes spontaneous attrition by scarring.

Fibroma

The general term *fibroma* has been applied to a group of poorly defined benign lesions that arise in the skin or soft tissues. Most are effectively treated by simple excision. Fibroma of tendon sheath is a slow-growing, dense fibrous nodule that is attached to the tendon sheath, found most frequently in the hands or feet in young to middle-aged adults. Recurrence may occur after local excision.

Elastofibroma

Elastofibroma, a rare, slow-growing benign tumor, characteristically arises between the lower portion of the scapula and the chest wall of older individuals. These lesions, which typically occur in workers who have done repetitive manual tasks for years, are thought to be reactive. Elastofibromas grow as ill-defined masses, often measuring 5 to 10 cm in diameter. They may occur bilaterally and rarely have a familial association. Histologically, these lesions consist of swollen eosinophilic collagen and elastic fibers, and stain intensely for elastins. Complete excision is curative.

Superficial Fibromatosis

Superficial fibromatoses arise from the fascia or aponeuroses, and generally are small and slow-growing. Palmar fibromatosis is associated with flexion contractures (Dupuytren's contracture) and is by far the most common form, affecting as many as one in five persons aged 65 and older. This condition is more common in men than in women and tends to be familial. Although benign, these lesions have a tendency to recur after simple excision. Plantar fibromatosis (Ledderhose's disease) tends to occur in a somewhat younger age group but may occur with greater frequency in patients with palmar fibromatosis. Penile fibromatosis (Peyronie's disease), which causes pain and curvature of the penis on erection, is much less common. The fibrous mass in Peyronie's disease primarily involves fascial structures, the corpus cavernosum, and rarely the corpus spongiosum. Peyronie's disease is more common in men with palmar and plantar fibromatosis than in the general population.

Desmoid Tumor

The desmoid (deep) fibromatoses are a group of clinically diverse, deep-seated fibrous neoplasms. They are usually divided into three main biologic groups: sporadic, those associated with FAP, and those that are multicentric or familial. The desmoid was originally described as a tumor of the abdominal wall in women who had recently been pregnant, but these rare, slow-growing fibrous tumors may arise at any site in the body. The desmoids have been classified by location into three main subsets: extraabdominal (60% of cases), abdominal wall (25%), and intraabdominal (15%). As is the case for other sarcomas, site affects management, but it is unclear whether the distinction by site is biologically significant. The term *aggressive fibromatosis*, often applied to these lesions, especially when they occur in the retroperitoneum, belies their potential for invasion and progressive growth. Although desmoids do not metastasize, they tend to form large infiltrative masses that, if not widely excised, recur repeatedly. However, any attempt at complete wide excision needs to be balanced with considerations regarding preservation of function, because they may be controlled with low-dose chemotherapy or nonsteroidal antiinflammatory drugs and occasionally may even regress spontaneously. Abdominal and retroperitoneal desmoids, along with fibromas, osteomas, and epidermoid cysts, are among the extracolonic manifestations in patients with FAP coli that characterize Gardner's syndrome.[49] Some FAP patients develop desmoids at multiple sites. Multifocal desmoids of the extremity have been recognized,[17] usually in young women. The tendency to develop desmoids in the context of FAP or in a familial non-FAP setting has now been clearly linked to mutations in the APC gene on the long arm of chromosome 5.[50,51]

In a clinicopathologic study based on Finnish hospital records, the incidence of desmoid was estimated at 2 to 4 cases per 100,000. Of the 89 cases, 49% involved the abdomen. Only one patient had Gardner's syndrome, although familial bone abnormalities were noted in some patients. Four populations were defined: juvenile (aged 4.5 ± 3.5 years), fertile (27.2 ± 4.4 years), middle aged (43.9 ± 6.9 years), and old (68.1 ± 4.4 years). The juvenile desmoid was primarily an extraabdominal tumor of girls, whereas abdominal wall tumors of women were dominant in the fertile age group. Among middle-aged patients, abdominal wall tumors predominated, but the proportions of men and women were equal. In the oldest age group, both abdominal and extraabdominal tumors occurred without a gender difference. These investigators reported that the growth rate in premenopausal women was statistically greater than the rate of growth observed in male patients.

Among 131 patients with desmoid tumors treated at Memorial Hospital, of whom 39% presented with recurrent disease, the female to male ratio was 1.6:1.0. Approximately one-half of these tumors arose in the extremity; 15% were retroperitoneal, 12% arose in the abdominal wall, and 10% were chest wall tumors. Four patients had Gardner's syndrome. In univariate analysis, local failure was more common among patients aged 18 to 30 years, those with marginal or inadequate excision, those who presented with recurrent disease, and those who did not receive radiation for gross residual disease. In multivariate analysis, only presentation with recurrent disease and inadequate margins of resection were independent prognostic features. Gender had no influence on recurrence. The probability of local failure after excision was estimated at 37%. Eleven deaths were attributable to recurrent disease; none of the 11 patients had an extremity primary. Management of patients with desmoid tumors is discussed later in this chapter in Desmoids (Aggressive Fibromatoses).

Fibrosarcoma

Fibrosarcomas fall into two main groups, the adult and infantile types, both of which are very uncommon. Adult fibrosarcoma presents usually in the fourth to sixth decade as a painful, deep-seated mass. The thigh and trunk are the most common sites. Infantile fibrosarcoma usually develops within the first 2 years of life and is often congenital. The majority of these cases arise in the extremities and they rarely metastasize. Pathologically, they consist of elongated fibroblast-like cells arranged in a uniform, vesiculated growth pattern. Intersection or interlacing of the fascicles often yields a herringbone pattern on light microscopy. Electron microscopy should confirm only fibroblastic differentiation.

FIBROHISTIOCYTIC TUMORS

These tumors, originally thought to arise from histiocytes that had fibroblastic potential, almost certainly are fibroblastic in origin. Thus, the term *fibrohistiocytic* is merely descriptive of their appearance; virtually none of these lesions shows true histiocytic differentiation.

Fibrous Histiocytoma

Fibrous histiocytomas are benign tumors usually present as solitary, slow-growing nodules, although up to one-third are multiple. Histologically, they consist of fibroblastic and histiocytic cells often arranged in a cartwheel or storiform pattern. When such lesions occur in the skin, they are often called *dermatofibromas* or *sclerosing hemangiomas*. Superficially located lesions usually are cured by simple excision. Deeper lesions should be resected with a wider margin of normal tissue to prevent local recurrence.

Xanthoma

Xanthoma refers to a collection of lipid-laden histiocytes and is seen in diseases associated with hyperlipidemia. These lesions generally occur in cutaneous or subcutaneous locations but may involve deep soft tissues. Presumably, xanthomas are reactive lesions.

Dermatofibrosarcoma Protuberans

Dermatofibrosarcoma protuberans is probably best considered a low-grade sarcoma because it may recur locally but rarely metastasizes. Dermatofibrosarcoma protuberans is a relatively monomorphous, mononuclear, spindle cell lesion involving both dermis and subcutis. This lesion may occur anywhere in the body, but more than 50% occur on the trunk, 20% on the head and neck, and 30% on the extremities. This lesion typically presents in early or mid-adult life, beginning as a nodular cutaneous mass. The pattern of growth is usually slow and persistent, and as the lesion enlarges over many years, it becomes protuberant. Large lesions often are associated with satellite nodules. Dermatofibrosarcoma protuberans is histologically similar to benign fibrous histiocytoma but grows in a more infiltrative pattern, spreading along connective tissue septa in deep areas. The central portion of the tumor consists of a uniform population of plump fibroblasts arranged in a distinct ordered pattern. Unlike fibrous histiocytoma, dermatofibrosarcoma protuberans stains positive for CD34. More than 75% of these tumors have a ring chromosome, composed of translocated portions of chromosomes 17 and 22, and a consistent gene fusion product has been cloned[52] (see Table 35.1-3). This fusion gene creates an apparent platelet-derived growth factor autocrine loop, which may be sensitive to imatinib, which blocks platelet-derived growth factor receptor action.[53,54]

Up to 50% recur after simple excision. Occasionally, areas of increased pleomorphism and mitotic activity occur, especially in recurrent lesions. Metastases occur rarely to lung or to lymph nodes.[55] Because of their locally aggressive nature, these lesions may ultimately lead to amputation or even death because of extensive invasion. A variant with melanin pigmentation (Bednar's tumor) also is recognized.

Malignant Fibrous Histiocytoma

The term *malignant fibrous histiocytoma* was first introduced in 1963 to describe a group of malignant soft tissue tumors with a fibrohistiocytic appearance. Since then, this entity has become the most commonly diagnosed extremity sarcoma. A number of subtypes have been described, including myxoid, giant cell, inflammatory, angiomatoid, and pleomorphic. With advances in pathologic techniques, it has been claimed that a specific line of differentiation can be identified in the overwhelming majority of patients with pleomorphic MFH. However, oligonucleotide array analysis of MFH shows no clear subgrouping of MFH as a specific subtype, save for those MFHs that are also termed *myxofibrosarcoma*.[32] MFH characteristically is a tumor of later adult life with a peak incidence in the seventh decade, although it may occur in younger adults. MFH usually presents as a painless mass; the most common site is the lower extremity, followed by the upper extremity and the retroperitoneum.

TUMORS OF ADIPOSE TISSUE

Lipoma

Lipomas are the most common benign neoplasm and usually arise in the subcutaneous tissue. The trunk and proximal limbs are the most frequent sites. Although deep-seated benign lipomas do occur in the mediastinum or retroperitoneum, seemingly mature fatty neoplasms in the retroperitoneum should be regarded with suspicion, because most are WD liposarcoma. Most lipomas are solitary, soft, and painless, and grow slowly; however, 2% to 3% of patients have multiple lesions that are occasionally seen in a familial pattern. *Lipomatosis* is a term applied to a poorly circumscribed overgrowth of mature adipose tissue that grows in an infiltrating pattern.

Solitary lipomas are well circumscribed, lobulated lesions composed of fat cells, but are demarcated from surrounding fat by a thin fibrous capsule. Most subcutaneous, solitary lipomas show reproducible cytogenetic aberrations: translocations involving 12q13-15, rearrangements of 13q, or rearrangements involving 6p21-33.[56] In spindle cell lipoma, mature fat is replaced by collagen-forming spindle cells; this lesion typically arises in the posterior neck and shoulder in men between the ages of 45 and 65. Spindle cell lipomas show consistent chromosomal aberrations of 13q and 16q.[57] Pleomorphic lipoma is a closely related lesion. Local excision of lipoma and these variants is generally curative, with a local recurrence after simple excision in no more than 1% to 2% of cases. Intramuscular lipomas differ from their more superficial counterparts by usually being poorly circumscribed and infiltrative. These typically present in mid-adult life as slow-growing, deep-seated masses most often located in the thigh or trunk. Approximately 10% of intramuscular lipomas are noninfiltrative and well circumscribed. In a patient with a deep-seated fatty tumor, it is important to exclude an atypical lipomatous tumor (ALT; see Liposarcoma, later in this chapter), which tends to be more common than an intramuscular lipoma.

Angiolipomas present as subcutaneous nodules, usually in young adults, and in more than 50% of cases are multiple. The most common site is the upper extremity. Angiolipomas rarely reach more than 2 cm in size, but they often are painful, especially during their initial growth period. Microscopically, these tumors consist of adipocytes with interspersed vascular structures. Myxoid and fibroblastic angiolipomas are recognized.

Angiomyolipoma

The term *angiomyolipoma* is used for a nonmetastasizing renal tumor that is composed of fat, smooth muscle, and blood vessels. Angiomyolipoma is more common in women than in men and is seen in association with tuberous sclerosis. Although angiomyolipoma is usually well demarcated from normal kidney, it may extend into the surrounding retroperitoneum. Angiomyolipomas may be solitary or multicentric, and may produce abdominal pain or hematuria. Wide excision is curative. Angiomyolipomas of the liver have also been described.

Hibernoma

Hibernoma is a rare, slow-growing benign neoplasm that resembles the glandular brown fat that is found in hibernating animals. The literature consists primarily of case reports, and in most of these the tumor arises within the thorax.[58] Lesions of the trunk, retroperitoneum, and extremities also are reported. Excision is generally curative.

Lipoblastoma and Lipoblastomatosis

Lipoblastoma and lipoblastomatosis are peculiar variants of lipoma that occur almost exclusively in infancy and early childhood.[59] They differ from lipoma by their cellular immaturity and their close resemblance to the myxoid form of liposarcoma.

Liposarcoma

Liposarcoma is primarily a tumor of adults with a peak incidence between ages 50 and 65. It accounts for at least 20% of all soft tissue sarcoma in adults. Liposarcoma may occur anywhere in the body, although the most common sites are the thigh and the retroperitoneum. Liposarcoma has three principal forms: (1) WD or dedifferentiated, (2) myxoid or round cell, and (3) pleomorphic. Each of these types of adipocytic neoplasm has distinctive morphology, natural history, and karyotypic and genetic aberrations, which can be of considerable help in diagnosis. ALT-WD liposarcoma is a locally aggressive, nonmetastasizing malignant mesenchymal neoplasm composed of a mature adipocytic proliferation with significant variation in cell size and at least focal nuclear atypia. ALT-WD liposarcoma usually presents as a deep-seated, painless, enlarging mass that can slowly over many years attain a very large size. ALT-WD liposarcomas can be subdivided morphologically into four main subtypes: adipocytic (lipoma-like), sclerosing, inflammatory, and spindle cell. The supernumerary ring and giant marker chromosomes are the characteristic cytogenetic abnormality detected in most ALT-WD liposarcomas.[60] FISH combined with Southern blotting showed that MDM2, CDK4, and HMGIC was consistently amplified; all of these genes are located in the 12q14-15 region of the ring and giant marker chromosomes. Location is an important predictor of outcome in patients with ALT-WD liposarcoma. Extremity tumors rarely recur and have essentially no mortality. [In a series at Memorial Sloan-Kettering Cancer Center (MSKCC), all such cases with local recurrence recurred after 5 years and had a significant component of sclerosing morphology.[61]] In contrast, tumors in the retroperitoneum and mediastinum recur repeatedly and eventually result in the patient's death as a result of uncontrolled local effects, or they may dedifferentiate and metastasize. In a series of 177 patients with primary retroperitoneal liposarcoma, the WD histology was associated with a 5-year disease-specific survival of 83% and probability of freedom from local recurrence of only 54% at 5 years.[62]

Dedifferentiated liposarcoma is defined as an ALT-WD liposarcoma that shows abrupt transition in the primary tumor or recurrence to a nonlipogenic sarcoma (of variable histologic grade) at least several millimeters in diameter. Dedifferentiation occurs in up to 10% of ALT-WD liposarcomas, although the risk is higher in deep-seated locations such as the retroperitoneum. Approximately 90% of cases occur *de novo*, whereas 10% develop in recurrences. Radiologic imaging typically shows coexistence of both fatty and nonfatty solid components, which in the retroperitoneum may be discontiguous. Macroscopically dedifferentiated liposarcoma consists of large multinodular yellow masses containing discrete solid, often tan-gray nonlipomatous (dedifferentiated) areas. The dedifferentiated areas may also contain areas of necrosis and hemorrhage. Dedifferentiated liposarcoma appears to exhibit less aggressive clinical behavior than other high-grade pleomorphic sarcomas. In a study of primary retroperitoneal liposarcoma, 65 of 177 patients had tumors with dedifferentiated histology, which was associated with a 5-year disease-specific survival of only 20% and a local and distant recurrence–free survival at 3 years of 17% and 70%, respectively.[62] Dedifferentiated liposarcoma is also characterized by ring or giant marker chromosomes on cytogenetic analysis and by amplification of the 12q13-21 region on FISH analysis.[63]

Myxoid or round cell liposarcoma accounts for approximately 40% of all liposarcomas. The tumor consists of uniform round to oval primitive nonlipogenic mesenchymal cells and a variable number of small signet-ring lipoblasts in a prominent myxoid stroma with a characteristic branching vascular pattern. The myxoid–round cell subtype usually occurs in the deep soft tissues of the extremities, and in more than 66% of cases arises within the thigh musculature. It occasionally may arise in the retroperitoneum but rarely in the subcutaneous tissue. Myxoid–round cell liposarcoma typically has a t(12;16)(q13-14;p11) translocation, which is present in more than 90% of cases. The translocation leads to the fusion of the CHOP and TLS genes at 12q13 and 16p11, respectively, and the generation of TLS-CHOP hybrid protein. The presence of the TLS-CHOP rearrangement is highly sensitive and specific for the myxoid–round cell entity and is absent in other morphologic mimics, such as myxoid WD liposarcomas of the retroperitoneum and myxofibrosarcomas.[64] High histologic grade, often defined as greater than 5% round cell component, is a predictor of worse outcome in localized myxoid–round cell liposarcoma. In general, pure myxoid lesions (no round cell areas) are associated with a 90% 5-year survival and are considered low grade. In contrast, those lesions containing a significant (more than 5%) round cell component are associated with a 5-year survival of only 50%[65] and are thus high grade. In contrast to other liposarcoma types, myxoid–round cell liposarcomas tend to metastasize to unusual soft tissue and bone locations, with multifocal synchronous or metachronous spread to fat pad areas in the retroperitoneum and axilla occurring even in the absence of pulmonary metastasis.[65]

Pleomorphic liposarcoma, as the name implies, is a pleomorphic, high-grade, highly malignant sarcoma containing a variable number of pleomorphic lipoblasts. Mitotic activity is high, and hemorrhage or necrosis is common. Pleomorphic liposarcomas account for fewer than 5% of all liposarcomas. The majority arise in elderly patients older than 50 years of age and occur in the deep-seated soft tissue of the extremities (lower more frequently than upper limbs). Clinically, they metastasize early to lung in more than 50% of patients, and these patients usually die within a short period of time.[66] Cytogenetic analysis typically shows high chromosome counts and complex structural rearrangements.

TUMORS OF SMOOTH MUSCLE

Leiomyoma

Benign smooth muscle tumors are quite common in the uterus and in the gastrointestinal tract. Rare cutaneous leiomyomas arise from the piloerector muscles of the skin. Some occur on a familial basis. These lesions are often multiple and may be quite painful. Typically, these cutaneous leiomyomas develop in adolescence or early adult life as small, discreet papules that eventually form nodules. The extensor surfaces of the extremities are most often affected, and the nodules may follow a dermatomal distribution. Although these tumors are histologically benign, recurrences after surgical incision are seen frequently, and often the lesions are so numerous that surgical excision is not possible. Leiomyoma may also occur deep within the extremities, abdominal cavity, or retroperitoneum.

Angiomyoma is a solitary form of leiomyoma. This lesion tends to occur on the extremity in people between the fourth and sixth decades of life. Women are more commonly affected than men.

Intravenous leiomyomatosis is a rare condition in which nodules of benign smooth muscle tissue grow within the veins of the myometrium and may extend into the uterine and hypogastric veins. Rarely, these tumors extend up the inferior vena cava into the heart. Diffuse peritoneal leiomyomatosis is also recognized, often occurring in association with pregnancy. Leiomyomas in children have been associated with human immunodeficiency virus (HIV) infection.

Leiomyosarcoma

Leiomyosarcoma is a malignant tumor composed of cells showing distinct smooth muscle features. Leiomyosarcomas may arise in any location, but more than half are located in retroperitoneal or intraabdominal sites. These masses often reach quite large proportions, but present insidiously with nonspecific symptoms. Cutaneous leiomyosarcomas usually appear as small solitary extremity nodules. Deep extremity leiomyosarcomas most frequently arise in the thigh and may arise in association with medium or large veins. Although rare, leiomyosarcoma may arise in large vascular structures and present with symptoms of obstruction to the normal flow of blood. The most common arterial site is the pulmonary artery; patients present with symptoms of decreased pulmonary outflow. Leiomyosarcoma of the inferior vena cava, which may present with Budd-Chiari syndrome with obstruction of hepatic veins, is also described. Location in the middle portion of the vena cava may result in blockage of renal veins and renal dysfunction, whereas involvement of the lower portion may cause leg edema.[67]

The typical cell of leiomyosarcoma is elongated and has an abundant cytoplasm. Multinucleated giant cells are common. Epithelioid changes, in which the cells become rounded, with concomitant clear cell changes in the neoplasm, may occur in otherwise typical leiomyosarcomas. When the tumor is predominantly or exclusively epithelioid, the term *leiomyoblastoma* has been used. The term *leiomyoblastoma*, however, fails to convey any information with regard to clinical behavior.

Localization of muscle antigens by means of immunohistochemistry proves the diagnosis of leiomyosarcoma. Desmin and smooth muscle actin are the most common immunohistochemical stains. Grading of leiomyosarcoma can be quite difficult; mitotic activity appears to be the best indicator of prognosis, along with tumor location and size. Retroperitoneal leiomyosarcomas are fatal in the great majority of cases; they are typically large (more than 10 cm) and prone to both local recurrence and distant metastasis to liver and lung.

TUMORS OF SKELETAL MUSCLE

Nonmalignant tumors of striated muscle, rhabdomyomas, are rare but are clinically benign and have no great biologic significance once they have been accurately diagnosed. Several types of rhab-

domyosarcoma (malignant tumors showing skeletal differentiation) are recognized, and they represent the largest subset of soft tissue sarcomas in infants and children. Embryonal rhabdomyosarcoma is a small cell tumor showing phenotypic and biologic features of embryonic skeletal muscle that usually arises in the orbit or genitourinary tract in children. The botryoid type of embryonal rhabdomyosarcoma, which frequently originates in mucosa-lined visceral organs such as the vagina and the urinary bladder, generally grows as a polypoid tumor. These tumors may disseminate widely but are very responsive to chemotherapy and radiation. Embryonal rhabdomyosarcomas occasionally arise in adults. Although regression of tumor in response to pediatric chemotherapy regimens usually occurs, age is an important prognostic factor for survival, with worse outcomes in older patients.[68] Extremity rhabdomyosarcoma in adolescents and young adults often has an alveolar histology. Alveolar rhabdomyosarcoma is composed of ill-defined aggregates of poorly differentiated round or oval cells that frequently show central loss of cellular cohesion and formation of irregular "alveolar" spaces. They cytologically resemble lymphoma and show partial skeletal differentiation. These tumors appear to have a worse prognosis than embryonal rhabdomyosarcoma in younger children but not in adults. Specific translocations associated with alveolar rhabdomyosarcomas include t(2;13)(q35;q14) in the majority of patients, and t(1;13)(p36;q14) was noted in a smaller subset. These translocations involve the PAX3 or PAX7 gene on chromosomes 2 and 1, respectively, with the FKHR gene on chromosome 13, to generate chimeric genes that encode PAX3-FKHR and PAX7-FKHR fusion proteins.[69]

In adults, pleomorphic rhabdomyosarcoma is the most common form of rhabdomyosarcoma. The prognosis for these pleomorphic tumors is poor, and in one series 28 of 38 patients (74%) died of the disease.[70]

VASCULAR TUMORS

Hemangioma

Hemangiomas are among the most common soft tissue tumors. Most hemangiomas are present at birth and regress spontaneously. Rapid growth with impingement on vital structures may occur, however, and treatment with intralesional injection of interferon has been life-saving.[71] Pulmonary hemangiomatosis, a rare disorder of diffuse microvascular proliferation in the lung, has been treated effectively with systemic interferon. Cavernous hemangioma refers to a benign lesion consisting of large dilated blood vessels with a flattened endothelium.

Lymphangioleiomyomatosis

Pulmonary lymphangioleiomyomatosis is a disease of women of childbearing age. Patients present with cough, hemoptysis, and dyspnea. Grossly, the lungs demonstrate multiple small cystic lesions. On microscopic examination, there is proliferation of normal smooth muscle around the airways and the blood and lymphatic vessels. Tamoxifen does not appear to be useful, but responses to progestational agents have been seen.[72]

Epithelioid Hemangioendothelioma

As its name implies, epithelioid hemangioendothelioma is an angiocentric vascular tumor with metastatic potential, composed of epithelioid endothelial cells arranged in short cords and nests set in a distinctive myxohyaline background. These lesions may appear as a solitary, slightly painful mass in either superficial or deep soft tissue. Metastases to lung, regional lymph nodes, liver, and bone are reported. Another pattern is that of a diffuse bronchoalveolar infiltrate or multiple small pulmonary nodules. This entity has also been called *IBVAT* (intravascular, bronchiolar, and alveolar tumor of the lung). Patients may present with cough and hemoptysis. Epithelioid hemangioendothelioma can also arise in the liver, often presenting as an incidental finding or as part of a workup for mild elevation of liver enzymes or vague abdominal pain. Multiple liver nodules are the rule. Although these lesions can metastasize, they usually run an indolent course. Liver transplantation has been performed, even in patients with metastatic disease.[73]

Kaposi's Sarcoma

Classic Kaposi's sarcoma is an unusual vascular sarcoma that occurs in the skin of the lower extremities of elderly men of Mediterranean or Jewish extraction. The disease is usually indolent, although it can spread to the lungs and the gastrointestinal tract. Cutaneous lesions can be palliated with radiation therapy when necessary. Another form of Kaposi's sarcoma occurs in Bantu men in Africa and in African children, in whom it runs a more aggressive course. Kaposi's sarcoma has arisen in renal allograft recipients who are receiving immunosuppressant therapy. Epidemic Kaposi's sarcoma is a complication of HIV infection. In all cases of HIV-related Kaposi's sarcoma, there is an association with human herpesvirus-8 infection. (See Chapter 48.1.)

Angiosarcoma

Angiosarcomas may arise in either blood or lymphatic vessels. Cutaneous lymphangiosarcoma may develop in chronically lymphedematous extremities. The classical presentation is Stewart-Treves syndrome, lymphangiosarcoma in the chronically lymphedematous arms of women who have been treated for breast cancer with radical mastectomy and, often, axillary irradiation.[15] Hemangiosarcomas are usually located in the skin or superficial soft tissue. Multicentric angiosarcomas occur on the scalp and face of elderly men, in whom unrelenting progression can cause severe ulceration and infection. Angiosarcoma of the breast is usually an aggressive lesion that recurs locally and may metastasize, primarily to lung; histologic grade has been of prognostic value. Angiosarcomas are known to occur in sites of prior irradiation without chronic lymphedema—in particular, in the pelvis of women who have received radiation therapy for gynecologic cancers. Soft tissue angiosarcoma, often with epithelioid features, may arise on the extremities or within the abdomen.[74]

PERIVASCULAR TUMORS

Glomus Tumor

Glomus tumors mimic the modified smooth muscle cells of the glomus body, a special form of arteriovenous anastomosis that is located in the skin and participates in thermal regulation. The glomus tumor generally presents as a small, blue-red nod-

ule in subcutaneous tissue or in the subungual region of the finger. These tumors are often associated with paroxysmal pain irradiating away from the tumor. Complete excision is the appropriate management.

Hemangiopericytoma

The cells of hemangiopericytomas resemble pericytes, cells that normally are arranged along capillaries and venules. These rare tumors usually arise in adults, although an infantile hemangiopericytoma is recognized. The adult form is most common in the lower extremity, but also occurs in the pelvis, retroperitoneum, or other sites. The tumors tend to be well circumscribed and consist of tightly packed cells around thin-walled vascular channels of varying caliber. The cells of hemangiopericytoma stain immunohistochemically with factor XIIIa and HLA-DR antigen but not with factor VIII–related antigen.[75] Many hemangiopericytomas have an indolent behavior, although some behave like other high-grade sarcomas.

TUMORS OF SYNOVIAL TISSUE

Nodular Tenosynovitis

A variety of benign tumors and tumor-like lesions arise from the synovium. Nodular tenosynovitis (tenosynovial giant cell tumor) is a giant cell tumor that may occur at any age but is most commonly seen between the ages of 30 and 50. These tumors are somewhat more common in women. They occur with greatest frequency in the hand but are also seen in the ankles and knees, among other sites. These slow-growing tumors develop as circumscribed lobulated masses and are usually diagnosed when they are smaller than 5 cm in diameter. Because of their location, excision is often done with close margins, and local recurrence is seen in 10% to 20% of patients. A diffuse form occurs in and around joints, most commonly around the knee or ankle. In contrast to most giant cell tumors, this neoplasm grows in expansive sheets without a mature capsule. Treatment is surgical, including arthroscopic resection alone when intraarticular disease has not invaded beyond the joint. Multiple recurrent lesions that threaten limb integrity can be controlled with radiotherapy in both the tendon sheath and intraarticular variants.[76] However, this should be reserved for advanced local presentation of diffuse disease with bone, neurovascular, or extensive soft tissue disease, or lesions that prove refractory to surgical approaches. Malignant giant cell tumors of the tendon sheath are also recognized[77] and should be managed with the same approaches as soft tissue sarcoma elsewhere.

Synovial Sarcoma

Synovial sarcoma usually occurs in young adults.[78,79] The tumors are typically found in the paraarticular areas of the tendon sheaths and joints. At least 50% of cases are in the lower limbs (especially the knee), and most of the remainder are seen in the upper limbs. Synovial sarcoma may also be encountered in regions without apparent relationship to synovial structures, including the head and neck (fewer than 10%), thoracic and abdominal wall (fewer than 10%), or intrathoracic sites. It generally does not originate from synovial tissue, and

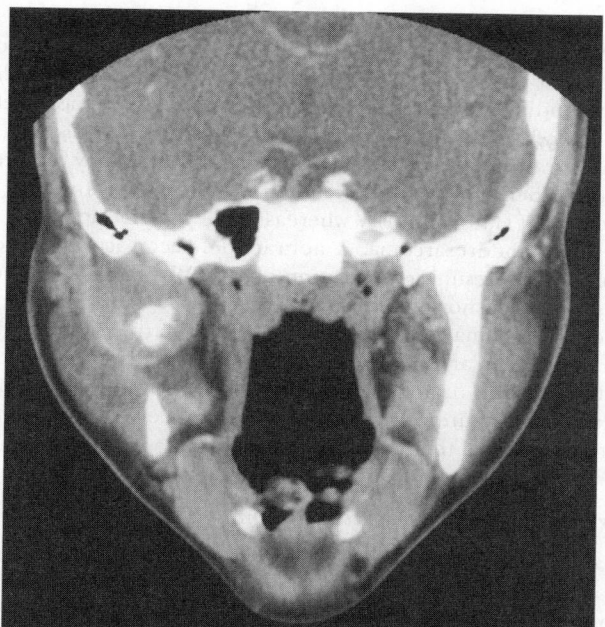

FIGURE 35.1-5. Coronal reconstruction of a computed tomography showing a synovial sarcoma arising in the right temporomandibular joint. This diagnosis was established only after the molecular characteristics were identified and the hallmark translocation confirmed. Note the prominent calcification in a lesion that was symptomatic for approximately 4 years in a young patient.

for this reason, it has been suggested that the name of this sarcoma subtype be modified. This tumor is composed of two morphologically distinct types of cells that form a characteristic biphasic pattern. The biphasic synovial sarcoma includes epithelial cells with a surrounding spindle or fibrous component. Calcification, with or without ossification, is seen in up to 10% of tumors (Fig. 35.1-5), and synovial sarcoma may be confused with other calcifying tumors (e.g., lower neck lesions need to be distinguished from thyroid neoplasms, which may also exhibit calcification). The spindle cells stain positive for keratin and epithelial membrane antigen. Vimentin is demonstrable in spindle cells but absent in epithelial cells. S-100 staining may give positive results. Monophasic synovial sarcomas of both fibrous and epithelial types are recognized, although the monophasic epithelial variant of synovial sarcoma is extremely rare. Synovial sarcomas contain a characteristic chromosomal translocation, t(X;18)(p11.2;q11.2); a hybrid transcript has been identified.[42] The type A fusion transcript (SYT-SSX) has been suggested to be of prognostic significance.[79] These hallmark translocations have become the gold standard in diagnosing synovial sarcoma[80] with the observation that 100% of biphasic and 96% of monophasic synovial sarcomas possess the specific t(X;18)(p11.2;q11.2) translocation. At the molecular level this involves the SYT gene on chromosome band 18p11 and three of the six members of the SSX gene family on chromosome band Xq11, namely, the SSX1 or SSX2 gene and less frequently the SSX4 gene. Local treatment follows the general principles of soft tissue sarcoma treatment with adequate excision and adjuvant radiotherapy when appropriate, with or without adjuvant chemotherapy. This histologic subtype exhibits more favorable responses to chemotherapy than most other

histologic subtypes, as is apparent when treating metastatic disease. The disease also has a reputation for higher risk of lymph node metastasis, although varying rates have been identified (e.g., 1.4% to 13.7%).[34]

TUMORS OF THE PERIPHERAL NERVES

Neurofibroma

Solitary neurofibromas are small, slow-growing cutaneous or subcutaneous nodules that usually arise during the third decade of life. By definition, these lesions are not associated with NF. NF type 1 (NF1; peripheral NF, von Recklinghausen's disease) is one of the most common genetic disorders, affecting approximately 1 in 3000 live births. An autosomal dominant mutation at the 17q11.2 locus has been identified.[81] The clinical features of NF1 include café au lait spots, Lisch nodules (pigmented hamartomas) of the iris, and neurofibromas of several types. Cutaneous neurofibromas—soft, fleshy growths—arise in the skin in all patients with NF1. These lesions may range in size from a few millimeters to 50 to 60 cm. Although some patients have only a few such lesions, others may have hundreds. Subcutaneous neurofibromas are firm and nodular, and may be painful. Plexiform neurofibromas are large lesions that affect large segments of a nerve, thickening and distorting the nerve into a tortuous mass. They may cause severe dysesthetic pain.

Benign Schwannoma

Also called neurilemoma, benign schwannoma occurs most commonly in people aged 20 to 50 years. Common sites include the head and neck and the flexor surfaces of the extremities. It grows slowly and is usually smaller than 5 cm when the diagnosis is made. This encapsulated nerve sheath tumor is distinguished from neurofibroma in that schwannoma consists of two components: a highly ordered cellular region (Antoni A area), and a loose, myxoid component (Antoni B area).

Cellular Schwannoma

Cellular schwannoma is more cellular than classical schwannoma. It usually presents in patients during the seventh decade of life as a painless paravertebral mass.[82] Complete excision is curative in most patients.

Granular Cell Tumor

The granular cell tumor (also called *granular cell myoblastoma*) is a rare tumor that is probably of neural origin. This tumor usually presents in adults as a small, poorly circumscribed subcutaneous nodule, although there are patients who have multiple lesions. This entity has a distinct histologic appearance and stains positively for S-100. Granular cell tumor usually runs a benign course, but metastases have been reported.

Malignant Peripheral Nerve Sheath Tumors

MPNSTs have also been called *malignant schwannoma, neurofibrosarcoma,* and *neurogenic sarcoma.* Most are associated with major nerves of the body wall and extremities and typically affect adults in the third to fifth decades of life. Tumor cells are usually elongated, with frequent mitoses, and are arranged in a hypocellular myxoid stroma; pronounced atypia and epithelioid features are also characteristic. The majority of MPNSTs are high grade and characteristically stain for the S-100 protein. These tumors originate from the nerve sheath, rather than from the nerve itself. A malignant peripheral nerve tumor with rhabdomyosarcomatous elements also exists, termed a *Triton tumor*, and the Schwann cell may be the source of a variety of heterologous elements in nerve sheath tumors.[83] The lower extremity and the retroperitoneum are the most common sites, but MPNSTs may arise anywhere in the body. Although higher estimates appear in the literature, approximately 5% of patients with NF1 develop MPNSTs, usually arising from a plexiform neurofibroma. The majority of patients with MPNST do not have NF. The malignant peripheral nerve tumor that develops in the patient with NF has historically been considered to have a poor prognosis compared with other malignant sarcomas of the extremity. However, when other factors of known risk for outcome such as grade and size are accounted for, malignant peripheral nerve tumors arising both spontaneously and in the presence of NF tend to have a similar outcome to other poor prognosis peripheral sarcomas.[84] MPNSTs tend to present with a greater preponderance of large size and high grade than other soft tissue sarcomas; hence, their reputation for aggressivity and the association appears inconsistent.[85] In a series of 18 patients with neurogenic sarcoma, 7 had NF1 and 6 of these developed distant metastases compared to 4 of 11 for patients without NF1.[85] In addition, patients with NF1 may be difficult to evaluate, independently of the features of the tumor itself. Staging and follow-up assessments are confounded by the detection of other nodules and masses that, although generally representing benign neurofibromas, need to be distinguished from recurrent local or metastatic disease or a second neurogenic sarcoma.

Because of evolving concepts and nomenclature, the literature is confusing with regard to MPNST and peripheral neuroectodermal tumor. The latter, a small cell tumor of children and young adults, is a variant of Ewing's sarcoma.

EXTRASKELETAL CARTILAGINOUS AND OSSEOUS TUMORS

Myositis Ossificans

The benign lesion myositis ossificans is a self-limiting process that usually is associated with trauma. Despite its name, myositis ossificans is not necessarily confined to the muscle, nor is inflammation a prominent feature. The condition usually presents in athletic young adults as a tender soft tissue mass. Over a period of weeks, the mass usually becomes firm to hard. Radiographs show calcification several weeks after the lesion appears. Histologically the mass consists of fibroblastic tissue, often with prominent mitotic activity. Nonetheless, this process is benign and may be managed conservatively. It is important to distinguish between myositis ossificans and sarcoma, especially extraosseous osteogenic sarcoma. The lesions can be very vascular at the time of biopsy, which suggests a more neoplastic process.

Extraskeletal Chondrosarcoma

Myxoid chondrosarcoma (also called *chordoid sarcoma*) occurs most commonly in patients older than 35 years. The tumor characteristically demonstrates a lace-like growth pattern of tumors in a myxoid matrix in which the malignant cells show round or oval nuclei and a narrow rim of dense, acidophilic, surrounding cytoplasm. In contrast to the more common skeletal chondrosarcoma of bone, mature cartilage is unexpected. The ultrastructure of these lesions is characterized by the presence of densely packed intracisternal microtubules as well as prominent mitochondria, whereas these are not apparent in skeletal chondrosarcoma. A nonrandom reciprocal translocation t(9;22), resulting in a fusion of the EWS and CHN genes, has also been shown in these tumors and is not seen in skeletal chondrosarcoma, which suggests that the two diseases have different molecular lineage. More than two-thirds occur in the extremity. This tumor usually grows slowly, but late recurrence and metastasis are common, and this rate seems to be greater for extraskeletal than for skeletal variants.[86]

Extraosseous Osteogenic Sarcoma

Extraosseous osteogenic sarcomas are rare, high-grade sarcomas defined by their production of malignant osteoid and bone. By definition, they are not attached to the skeleton. Unlike typical osteogenic sarcoma of bone, these tumors rarely occur in patients under the age of 20, and most patients are older than 50 years.[87] These high-grade tumors present like other soft tissue sarcomas. Most arise in the extremities, although osteosarcoma of other sites, including breast, retroperitoneum, urinary bladder, and other visceral organs, have been reported. There is considerable heterogeneity in the histologic appearance. Spindle cell varieties may resemble MFH, MPNST, or fibrosarcoma, whereas others have a more epithelioid appearance. Giant cells are a common feature. Some lesions that contain bone or cartilage are hard to distinguish from MFH, but bone in MFH is well differentiated. Nonetheless, extraosseous osteogenic sarcoma resembles MFH in terms of age, sites of distribution, and clinical behavior.

TUMORS OF UNCERTAIN HISTOGENESIS

Myxoma

Intramuscular myxoma is a rare tumor that occurs in adults, usually in the large muscles of the extremities. Myxomas consist of abundant mucoid material but few cells. Although these lesions often measure 5 to 10 cm, their clinical behavior is generally benign. Multiple intramuscular myxomas occur in association with fibrous dysplasia.

Aggressive angiomyxoma is a tumor that usually occurs in women, although male patients have been reported. The lesion generally presents as a mass in the perineal or pelvic area. Local recurrence can result in considerable morbidity given the location of these tumors, but distant metastases do not occur.

Mesenchymoma

Malignant mesenchymoma is defined as a malignant tumor showing at least two types of malignant mesenchymal differentiation in addition to a poorly differentiated fibrosarcomatous element. These rare tumors are generally thought to behave clinically in accordance with the predominant component, although one report suggests that their behavior is not as aggressive as might be expected.[88]

Alveolar Soft Part Tumor

Alveolar soft part tumor is a rare tumor that occurs most frequently in patients between 15 and 35 years of age. Women outnumber men, especially among patients younger than 20 years of age.[89] Prognosis is better in those patients who present at a younger age. These tumors often present in the lower extremities as a slow growing painless mass. Grossly, alveolar soft part tumors are poorly circumscribed. They typically grow in an organoid or nest-like arrangement. The alveolar spaces actually are necrotic areas. Considerable controversy regarding histogenesis persists. Neural derivation has been suggested, but other data suggest a myogenic origin.[90] Lung, brain, and bone are the most common sites of metastasis. Although this tumor tends to grow slowly, the ultimate prognosis is quite poor. Patients may remain asymptomatic over years, even with metastatic disease.

Epithelioid Sarcoma

Epithelioid sarcoma is a tumor of adolescents and young adults. This tumor usually presents as a small, firm nodule in the subcutaneous tissue of the distal extremities. Multiple recurrences, which grow along tendons and fascial planes, are a characteristic feature. Unlike with most other sarcomas, lymph node metastases are common, and the tumor may appear in the extremity in transit to the regional nodes.[34] Lung is the most common site of distant metastasis.

Clear Cell Sarcoma (Malignant Melanoma of Soft Parts)

Clear cell sarcoma, also called *clear cell sarcoma of tendons and aponeuroses*, presents as a soft tissue mass. Because of the presence of intracellular melanin and the tendency for regional nodal metastasis, it has been suggested that this entity is better considered a melanoma than a soft tissue sarcoma. Analysis by genomic profiling and cluster analysis strongly suggest that these lesions should be considered a subtype of melanoma.[91] Size is the most important prognostic factor. Treatment of the primary is similar to that of other sarcomas. There are few reported responses to chemotherapy.

Desmoplastic Small Round Cell Tumor

Desmoplastic small round cell tumor is a tumor of adolescents and young adults.[92] It usually presents in the abdomen, often with diffuse peritoneal implants. Because of its multifocal nature, complete resection is usually impossible. Chemotherapy regimens used in the treatment of Ewing's sarcoma have induced responses in patients with this disease but are rarely curative. A specific translocation between chromosomes 11 and 22 that is different from the translocation of Ewing's sarcoma has been identified.[93]

Follicular Dendritic Cell Sarcoma

Follicular dendritic cell sarcoma is an unusual lesion thought to arise from lymphatic tissue.[94] It commonly occurs in the neck but has been described in other sites.

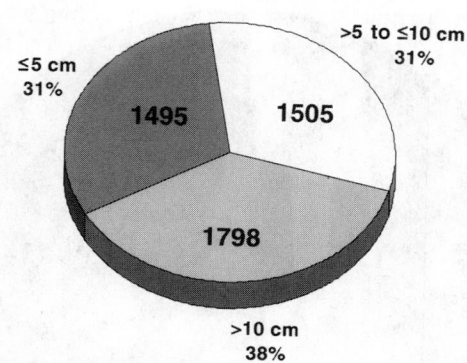

FIGURE 35.1-6.   Distribution by size of soft tissue sarcomas in 4798 patients aged 16 years or older admitted to Memorial Sloan-Kettering Cancer Center between July 1, 1982, and December 31, 2002.

CLINICAL PRESENTATION

The presence of soft tissue sarcoma almost invariably is suggested by the development of a mass. This mass is usually large, often painless, and may be associated by the patient with an episode of injury. The majority present at a size larger than 5 cm. The size distribution of soft tissue sarcomas in 4798 patients admitted to MSKCC is illustrated in Figure 35.1-6. The focus of the clinical evaluation is to determine the likelihood of a benign or malignant soft tissue tumor, the involvement of muscular or neurovascular structures, and the ease with which biopsy or subsequent excision can be performed. Size becomes an important feature (see Prognostic Factors, later in this chapter), and definitive diagnosis is dependent on biopsy results and histologic confirmation.

DIFFERENTIAL DIAGNOSIS

The major concern, when confronted with a soft tissue mass, is whether or not the lesion is benign or malignant. In most patients with small lesions, or even on occasion large lesions, the differentiation is from the most common soft tissue tumor, lipoma. Most benign lesions are located in superficial (dermal or subcutaneous) soft tissue. This may be simple but becomes more difficult as the more aggressive and underappreciated inherently benign lesions are considered. Particularly difficult is myositis ossificans. The patient often has a history of trauma and often presents with a large, firm to hard lesion that, on plain film, may have a telltale sign of intrinsic calcification. This does not preclude a malignant lesion. Tru-Cut needle biopsy or open biopsy is often accompanied by aggressive hemorrhage, which suggests a vascular neoplasm. In most cases, diagnosis can be made fairly accurately by either plain film (Fig. 35.1-7) or magnetic resonance imaging (MRI) scan (Fig. 35.1-8). Certainly, the diagnosis should be suspected when there is a significant history of trauma, the lesion is particularly hard, and there is inherent calcification.

Other difficult lesions are the angiomyolipoma, which can also be a vascular lesion; the atypical schwannoma, which can be quite large and is often invasive (Fig. 35.1-9); and the rare angiomyxoma (Fig. 35.1-10). They can often be quite destructive, causing ureteric obstruction and bone invasion. The man-

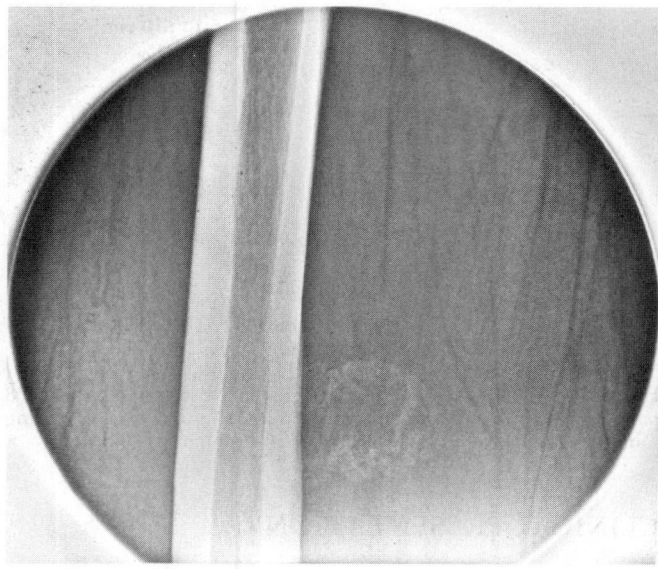

FIGURE 35.1-7. Myositis ossificans suggested by calcification on a plain film.

agement is as difficult as for any sarcoma. Conversely, unless absolutely imperative, multiple radical operations in inherently indolent lesions should be avoided.

IMAGING STUDIES

Imaging studies for soft tissue sarcoma vary, depending to some extent on the site. They involve evaluation of both the primary lesion and the potential site of metastasis. Evaluation of the primary lesion in the extremity and head and neck predominantly is either by computed tomography (CT) or by MRI, which provides some increased definition. In the hands of a knowledgeable radiologist, MRI can provide information over and above that provided by CT. Nevertheless, a Radiology Diagnostic Oncology Group study comparing these modalities has shown no benefit of MRI over CT.[95] What is clear in this era

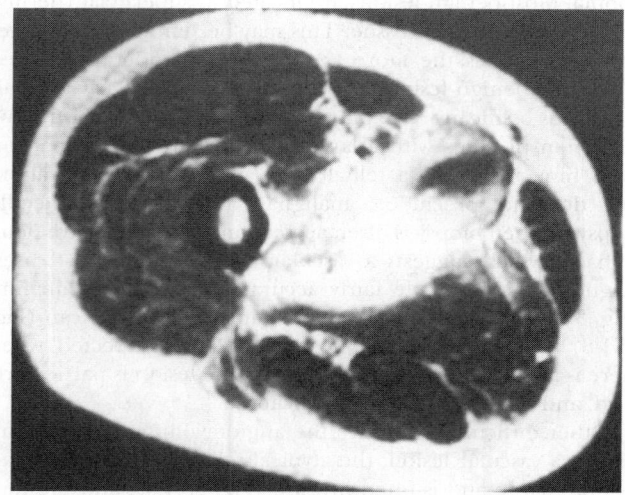

FIGURE 35.1-8. Characteristic findings of myositis ossificans on magnetic resonance imaging, including diffuse tissue expansion.

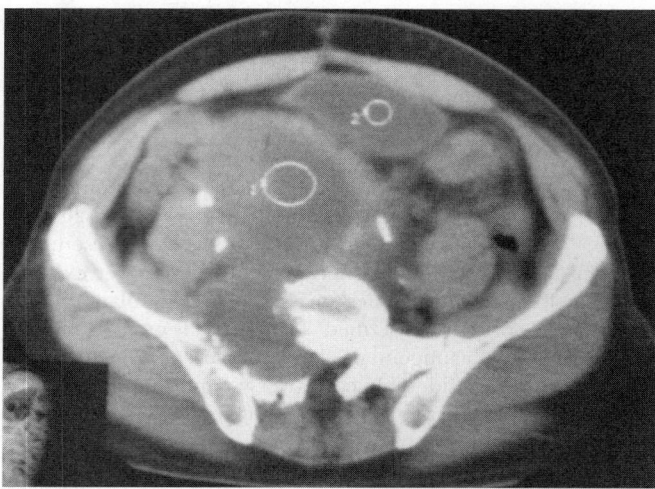

FIGURE 35.1-9. Atypical schwannoma can be quite large and often invasive, as shown here in a man with a 20-year history of having undergone multiple resections for large invasive lesions.

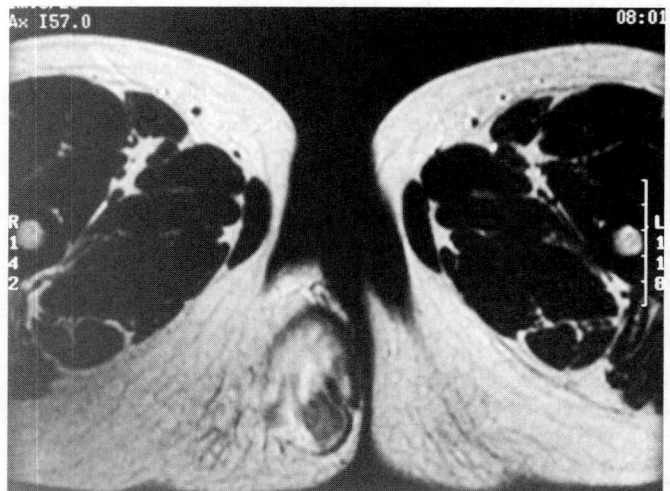

A

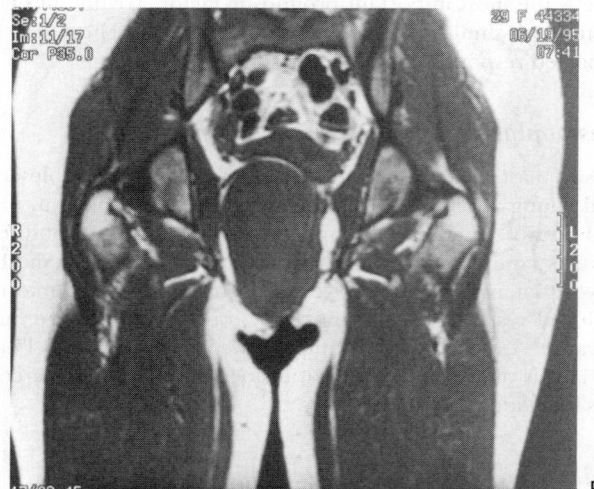

B

FIGURE 35.1-10. Another similarly difficult lesion is angiomyxoma, here seen growing as a mass in the perineum (**A**) and pelvis (**B**) in a young woman.

of cost containment is that imaging with multiple modalities, all focusing on the same entity, is not required.

An important issue for the primary clinician is identification of the relationship of the sarcoma to neurovascular structures. Angiography is rarely, if ever, of value. For the primary intraabdominal and chest sarcoma, a spiral CT scan is preferable (Fig. 35.1-11), because air-tissue interface and motion artifacts often degrade MRI quality, and both the primary and potential for metastasis is assessed in a single study.

POSITRON EMISSION TOMOGRAPHY

Although positron emission tomography (PET) has been used as an investigational modality for several years, it has yet to gain universal acceptance. It does appear in some studies that grade can be distinguished by this modality. At present it would appear that the role of PET is primarily in the identification of unsuspected sites of metastasis in patients with recurrent high-grade tumors. PET may also be useful in the future for determining responses to systemic therapy for soft tissue sarcoma and in particular for GIST, but this use remains investigational.[96]

SITES OF METASTATIC DISEASE

As important as imaging studies of the primary lesion is evaluation of possible sites of metastasis. An analysis of patients treated at MSKCC revealed the common sites of metastasis (Fig. 35.1-12). Metastatic disease from soft tissue sarcoma is site specific. For patients with extremity lesions, most metastases (70%) go to the lung.[97] For patients with retroperitoneal or visceral lesions, a much more common site for metastases is the liver, with lung only a secondary site. Nevertheless, no site is immune from soft tissue sarcoma metastasis, and other unique patterns can be identified (e.g., the unusual presentation of intraabdominal or soft tissue metastasis after an extremity myxoid or round cell liposarcoma).[98]

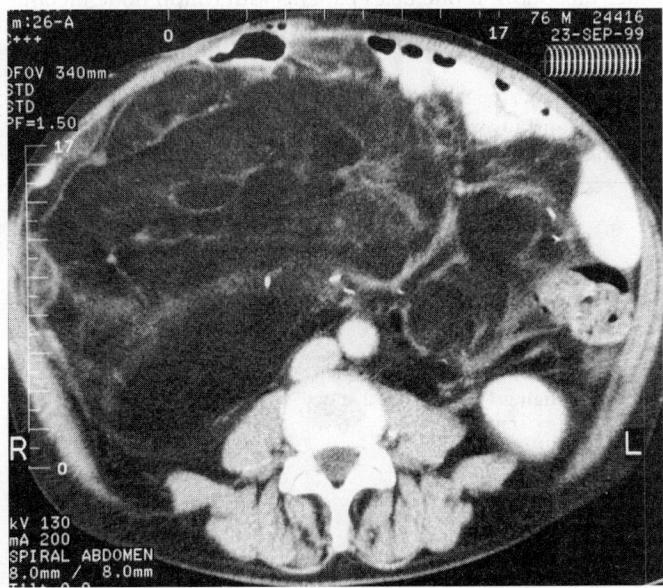

FIGURE 35.1-11.   Computed tomography of a massive intraabdominal liposarcoma.

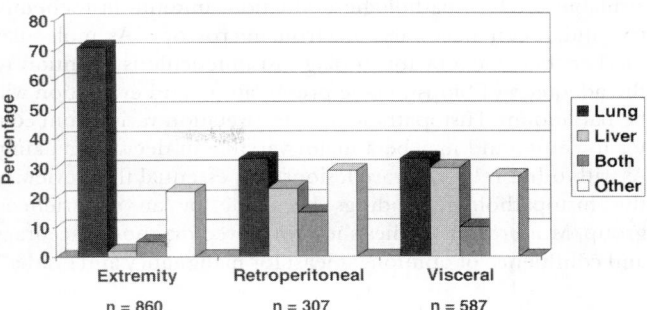

FIGURE 35.1-12.   Common sites of metastasis that can guide investigation. The primary site of metastasis for extremity lesions is the lung. Data are for patients aged 16 years or older admitted to Memorial Sloan-Kettering Cancer Center between July 1, 1982, and December 31, 2002.

For small, superficial extremity lesions, either high or low grade, evaluation for sites of metastasis is less important and simple chest radiography will suffice. Conversely, for patients with large high-grade lesions, for which the risk of metastatic disease is significant, more extensive evaluation is required. For extremity lesions (see Imaging Studies, earlier in this chapter), the primary modality is a chest radiograph followed by a CT scan of the chest. For retroperitoneal, visceral, and intraabdominal lesions, the site of metastasis that is most common (i.e., the liver) is evaluated with the modality used for evaluation of the primary lesion.

BIOPSY

The primary thrust of biopsy is to obtain adequate tissue for definitive histopathologic confirmation, to evaluate grade, and to identify prognostic factors that would alter the approach to definitive treatment. In the main, for lesions that are smaller than 5 cm, particularly those that are superficial, excisional biopsy is the preferred approach.

VALUE OF TRU-CUT BIOPSY

Several studies have examined the value of Tru-Cut biopsy, and a summary of the accuracy of Tru-Cut, incisional, and frozen-section biopsies is included in Table 35.1-6.[99] In the main, the important issue is the adequacy of the sample. Sufficient viable tissue is required that is both representative of the lesion and

TABLE 35.1-6.   Accuracy of Tru-Cut Biopsy[a]

	Tru-Cut	Incisional	Frozen Section
Number	60	45	36
Adequate tissue (%)	93	100	94
Correct malignancy (%)	95	100	88
Correct grade (%)	88	96	62[b]
Correct histology (%)	75	84	47[b]

[a]Memorial Sloan-Kettering Cancer Center, 1990 through 1995.
[b]Significance by Fisher exact test, P <.05, versus Tru-Cut.
(From Heslin MJ, Lewis JJ, Woodruff JM, Brennan MF. Core needle biopsy for diagnosis of extremity soft tissue sarcoma. *Ann Surg Oncol* 1997;4:425, with permission.)

available for histopathologic evaluation, immunohistochemistry, and, when necessary, electron microscopy. As molecular markers become a factor in diagnosis, meticulous attention to the adequacy of biopsy, tissue preservation, and evaluation will be paramount. Histopathologic interpretation varies from center to center and may be a major variable in decision making. As with other relatively rare lesions, it is essential that review of the histopathologic findings be made by an experienced group. More recent studies show improved diagnostic accuracy and confluence of opinion, at least for malignancy and grade.[99]

FINE-NEEDLE ASPIRATION CYTOLOGY

Fine-needle aspiration (FNA) cytology has been examined by a number of authors but is usually confined to the confirmation of recurrence, rather than used for the primary diagnosis.

Some authors have argued that biopsy itself is not justified if FNA is available. Rydholm[100] has suggested that no open biopsy is ever indicated, with the argument against its use being that it risks local tumor spread and increases both the magnitude of the subsequent operation and the need for adjuvant radiation therapy. Those against the procedure argue that, without biopsy, radiation therapy is not needed in the majority of cases and the need for more extensive resections is limited. Using FNA, the surgeon proceeds directly to open operation. The authors point out that this requires referral before antecedent biopsy, a relatively uncontrollable event in the United States. Other authors suggest that this approach results in the referral of ten patients with benign lesions for every sarcoma patient, certainly an untenable situation under the present system.

In addition, this approach presupposes that all that is required is a malignant sarcoma diagnosis and that the type or grade of sarcoma does not determine therapy. At MSKCC, for extremity lesions, brachytherapy (BRT) is used for high-grade lesions and external-beam radiation therapy (EBRT) is used for low-grade lesions, particularly of large size, which would preclude such an approach. The use of FNA in patients with large sarcomas who are candidates for neoadjuvant therapy to improve survival is also problematic due to difficulty in grading and subtyping these tumors accurately from such small samples. However, proponents argue that immunohistochemistry, electron microscopy, DNA cytology, and chromosomal analysis, all of which can be performed on FNA specimens, will ensure the appropriateness of this approach.[101] The authors still favor obtaining adequate tissue from Tru-Cut, excisional, or incisional biopsy to begin such a procedure.

FROZEN SECTION

In some institutions, frozen section is relied on as the diagnostic tool of choice. Results from MSKCC for frozen section are described in Table 35.1-6. For diagnosis of malignancy, frozen section is accurate, but for histopathologic subtypes and grade, it is inferior to permanent sections of either Tru-Cut or incisional biopsy.

STAGING

There have been significant changes in the staging of soft tissue sarcoma. The original 1992 staging system was based on a review published in 1977.[102] That staging system has since been consid-

TABLE 35.1-7A. Newer Approaches to Staging System of Soft Tissue Sarcoma: Stage Groupings

Stage	Grade	Tumor	Nodes	Metastasis
I	G1–2	T1a–1b, T2a–2b	N0	M0
II	G3–4	T1a–1b, T2a	N0	M0
III	G3–4	T2b	N0	M0
IV	Any G	Any T	N1	M0
	Any G	Any T	N0	M1

(From ref. 107, with permission.)

erably modified. The major difference was the inclusion in the original staging system of a subcategory grade, that is, small (less than 5 cm) lesions that were high grade were considered as stage IIIA. Several reviews, however, have suggested that such lesions (small, high grade) have a much more favorable prognosis than outlined in the original 1977 proposal. Reports from two separate institutions[103,104] suggest that survival of these patients is certainly better than 80% and in many cases reaches 90%. Consequently, size, which had been historically considered a subcategory of grade, was redefined. Clearly, size is a continuous variable, and the decision to divide tumors into those smaller than 5 cm and larger than 5 cm is clearly arbitrary.[105] An analysis of 1041 patients with localized extremity sarcoma seen at MSKCC between 1982 and 1997 has been published.[106] The staging system has now been further modified. The present 2002 staging system takes into account the relative infrequency of high-grade, large, superficial sarcomas [*American Joint Committee on Cancer* (AJCC) *cancer staging manual*, 6th edition][107] and simplifies the category of stage III tumors to represent only large, deep, high-grade sarcomas (Table 35.1-7*A* and *B*). Stage III can be further divided into tumors larger than 5 cm to 10 cm and those larger than 10 cm (Fig. 35.1-13).

Stage IV disease from lymph node metastasis is rare in the majority of adult soft tissue sarcomas and is equivalent to any other metastasis. If one takes patients with lymph node metasta-

TABLE 35.1-7B. Five-Year Local Recurrence, Disease-Free Survival, and Overall Survival in Patients with Current Staging (American Joint Committee on Cancer, 2002)

Stage		Freedom from Local Recurrence (%)	Disease-Free Survival (%)	Overall Survival (%)
I	Low grade any size, any depth	84	81	88
II	High grade <5 cm, any depth	82	66	76
	High grade >5 cm, superficial			
III	High grade >5 cm, deep	83	49	54
		$P = .53$	$P = .0001$	$P = .00001$

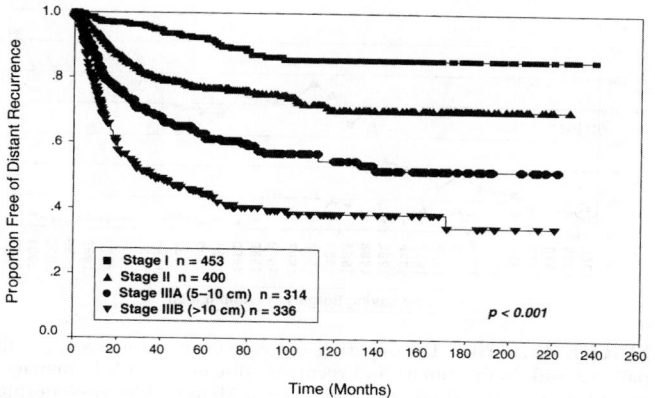

FIGURE 35.1-13. Distant metastasis-free survival for patients with primary extremity soft tissue sarcoma (n = 1503) using the American Joint Committee on Cancer 2002 staging system revised for size. Significance describes the overall difference between the curves. Data are for patients aged 16 years or older admitted to Memorial Sloan-Kettering Cancer Center between July 1, 1982, and December 31, 2002.

sis only or lymph nodes plus other metastases and contrasts them with patients with other systemic metastases, then disease-specific survival is the same (Fig. 35.1-14). It is important to emphasize that prognostic factors can vary with time. For early recurrence, it would appear that grade is predominant, whereas for late recurrence, size assumes a progressively more important role.[108]

Whether or not age should be a determinant in a staging system is unclear. When age is examined in overall survival, the older patient has a shorter survival than the younger patient. Age has been arbitrarily divided into younger than 50 years and older than 50 years, with a patient older than 50 years having a worse prognosis. Conversely, a distinction into three groups can show some separation that is disease dependent rather than age dependent (Fig. 35.1-15). Patients younger than 16 years have a different prognosis and a different response to treatment than do adults and should not be included in the current adult staging system. An analysis of the most common histopathologic

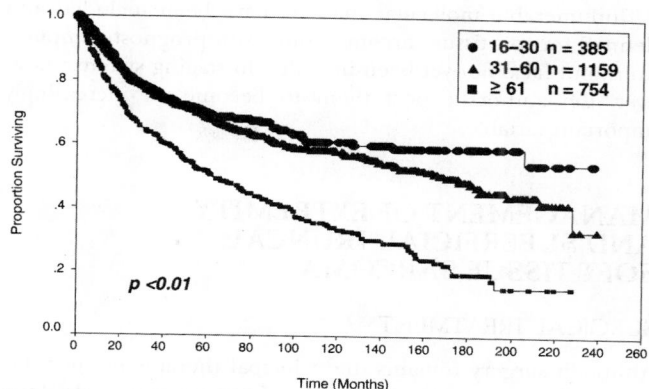

FIGURE 35.1-15. Overall survival for extremity soft tissue sarcoma by age group in 2298 patients aged 16 years or older admitted to Memorial Sloan-Kettering Cancer Center between July 1, 1982, and December 31, 2002. Significance describes the overall difference between the curves.

type in children, rhabdomyosarcoma, suggested that early-stage disease and late-stage disease are similar in children and adults, but intermediate-stage lesions have a better prognosis in children, which does not appear due to their ability to tolerate greater treatment.[68] Site is a clear determinant of outcome. Patients with retroperitoneal and visceral sarcomas certainly do worse than patients with extremity lesions (Fig. 35.1-16).

It is difficult to separate site from adequacy of treatment. Patients with retroperitoneal sarcoma can and do die of local recurrence, an uncommon event in extremity lesions. Intraabdominal visceral leiomyosarcomas still maintain a high metastatic rate as the primary cause of death.

Bone invasion and neurovascular invasion have historically been considered bad prognostic features. Because bone invasion is relatively uncommon in soft tissue sarcoma, it has not been uniformly included in any staging system but should be considered as a poor prognostic factor.

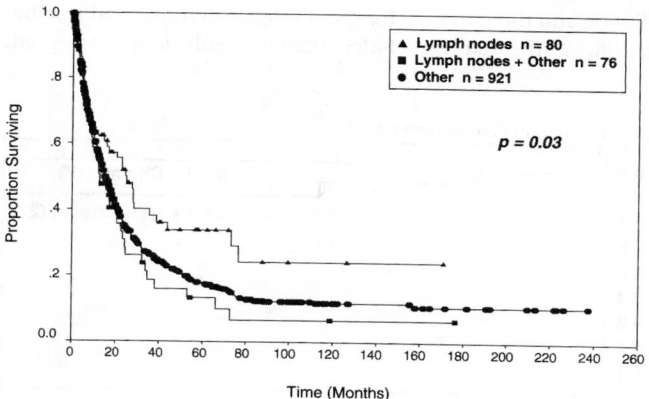

FIGURE 35.1-14. Disease-specific survival for patients with soft tissue sarcoma with metastases (n = 1077): lymph node metastases alone versus lymph node metastases with other metastases versus all other metastases. Data are for patients aged 16 years or older admitted to Memorial Sloan-Kettering Cancer Center between July 1, 1982, and December 31, 2002.

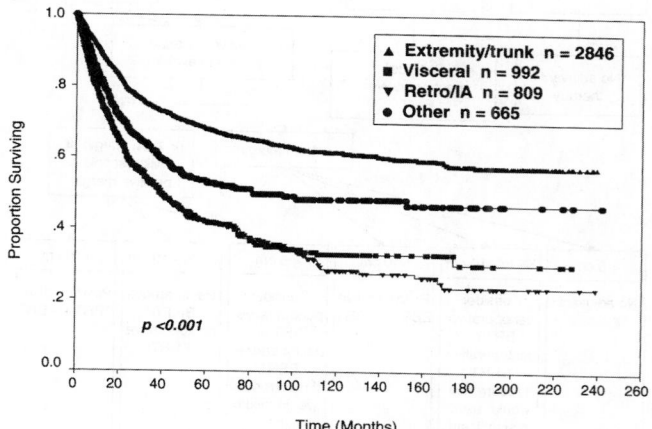

FIGURE 35.1-16. Disease-specific survival by site of soft tissue sarcoma in 5312 patients aged 16 years or older admitted to Memorial Sloan-Kettering Cancer Center between July 1982 and December 31, 2002. Patients with retroperitoneal or visceral sarcomas did worse than patients with extremity lesions. Significance describes the overall difference between the curves. Retro/IA, retroperitoneal/intraabdominal.

Innumerable molecular markers have been included and defined for soft tissue sarcoma, some with prognostic implications, but have not yet been included in staging systems; however, the authors expect them to become an increasingly important variable.

MANAGEMENT OF EXTREMITY AND SUPERFICIAL TRUNCAL SOFT TISSUE SARCOMA

SURGICAL TREATMENT

Although surgery remains the principal therapeutic modality in soft tissue sarcoma, the extent of surgery required, along with the optimum combination of radiotherapy and chemotherapy, remains controversial. Important clinical and pathologic prognostic variables should be used by the surgeon to design the most effective treatment plan for the individual patient based on the predicted patterns of spread of certain histologic types with the aim of minimizing local recurrence, maximizing function, and improving overall survival. A suggested algorithm for patient management based on sarcoma size and surgical margin is shown in Figure 35.1-17.

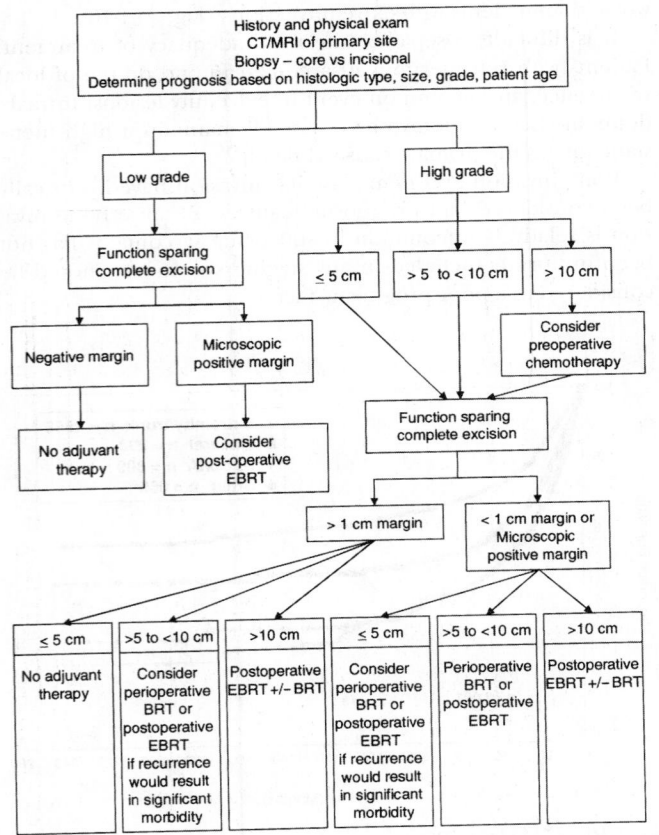

FIGURE 35.1-17. Management algorithm for extremity and superficial truncal soft tissue sarcoma. It should be noted that postoperative external-beam radiation therapy (EBRT) is mentioned in the algorithm, but preoperative EBRT could be used in the same types of patients. BRT, brachytherapy; CT, computed tomography; MRI, magnetic resonance imaging.

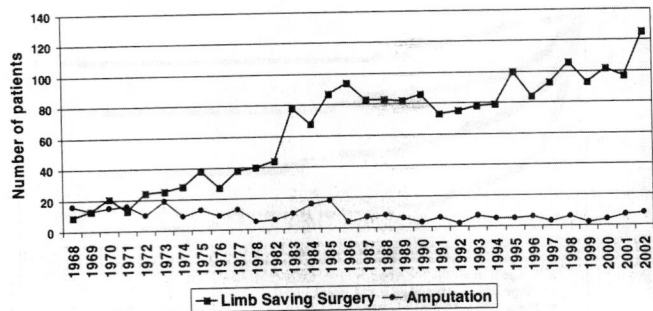

FIGURE 35.1-18. Limb-sparing surgery versus amputation for all patients, with both primary and recurrent disease. Trends in management over time based on the experience at Memorial Sloan-Kettering Cancer Center from 1968 to 2002.

Wide *en bloc* resection is used most often. Historical attempts to resect all muscle bundles from origin to exertion have now been supplanted by an encompassing resection, aiming to obtain a 2-cm margin of uninvolved tissue in all directions. The limiting factor is usually neurovascular or, occasionally, bony juxtaposition. Because most soft tissue sarcomas tend not to invade bone directly, only rarely does bone need to be resected. Soft tissue sarcomas uncommonly involve the skin, so major skin resection should be limited. In situations of primary or recurrent tumors in which skin is involved, or which the tumor is so extensive that skin is involved, then consideration of free flap or rotational flap closure becomes important, particularly in those patients who are candidates for subsequent adjuvant radiation therapy.

EXTENT OF SURGICAL RESECTION

The most extensive resection is clearly amputation. This should be only rarely indicated in soft tissue sarcoma because limb-sparing operations are possible in at least 90% of patients. Experience over the last 25 years at MSKCC indicates that the 50% amputation rate in the late 1960s is now less than 10% (Fig. 35.1-18). Amputation should be reserved for tumors not able to be resected by any other means, without evidence of metastatic disease and the potential for good long-term functional rehabilitation. This usually includes patients with large, low-grade

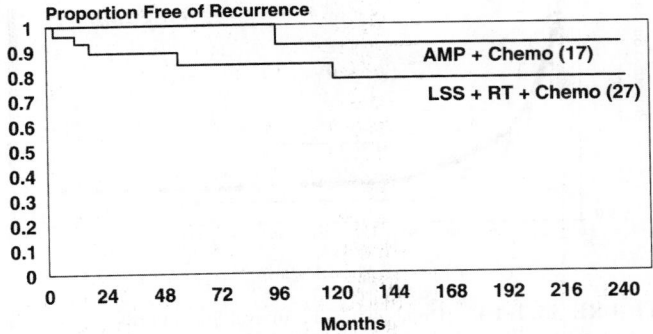

FIGURE 35.1-19. Soft tissue sarcoma, local recurrence according to treatment: limb-sparing surgery (LSS) plus irradiation (RT) compared with amputation (AMP) at the National Cancer Institute. Chemo, chemotherapy. (Courtesy of J. C. Yang and S. A. Rosenberg.)

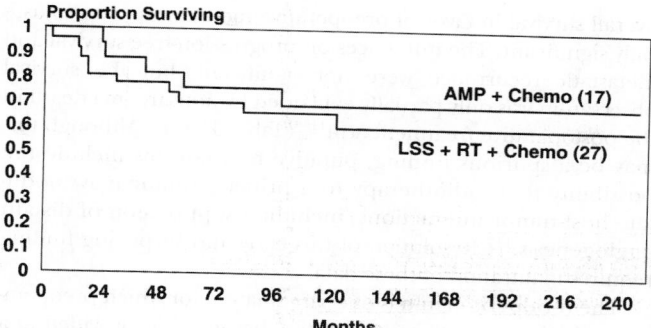

FIGURE 35.1-20. Soft tissue sarcoma, disease-free survival according to treatment: limb-sparing surgery (LSS) plus irradiation (RT) compared with amputation (AMP) at the National Cancer Institute. Chemo, chemotherapy. (Courtesy of J. C. Yang and S. A. Rosenberg.)

tumors with considerable cosmetic and functional deformity, who can be rendered symptom free by a major amputation.

Local recurrence can occur after a limb-sparing operation, and follow-up data confirm that salvage is almost invariably possible, but there is no impact on long-term survival. The issue of amputation versus limb-sparing surgery for extremity lesions has been addressed by a prospective randomized trial at the NCI. In patients in this trial, follow-up is well past 10 years. Although local recurrence is greater in those undergoing limb-sparing operation plus irradiation than in those undergoing amputation (Fig. 35.1-19), disease-free survival is not different (Fig. 35.1-20).[109]

SIZE

Because size is a prognostic factor for both local recurrence and metastatic disease, the approach to these lesions can be varied. In patients with small lesions of less than 5 cm, complete surgical excision with margins of more than 1 cm is usually sufficient; adjuvant therapy is reserved for those with recurrent lesions (see Radiation Therapy, later in this chapter). A significant subset of subcutaneous and small intramuscular sarcomas can be treated adequately by wide excision alone (without adjuvant radiotherapy) with a local recurrence rate of around 10%.[110] Given the high risk of recurrence and of systemic disease for lesions larger than 10 cm that are high grade, patients with these lesions are candidates for investigational approaches, especially neoadjuvant chemotherapy (see Preoperative Chemotherapy, later in this chapter). All patients with lesions larger than 5 cm should be considered for adjuvant radiation therapy as a proven method of limiting local recurrence.[103]

RADIATION THERAPY

The goals of adjuvant radiotherapy in the management of soft tissue sarcoma are to enhance local control, preserve function, and achieve acceptable cosmesis by contributing to tissue preservation. Radiotherapy is ordinarily combined with surgical approaches that use surgical margins of limited size to achieve these goals. The alternative, if local control is to be maintained, would be amputation or functionally debilitating surgery for limb lesions, or substantial ablation with structural, functional,

or cosmetic deficits for lesions at other anatomic sites. It should be recognized that superficial lesions and smaller, contained lesions confined to individual muscles may be managed with surgery alone in expert hands.[103,110,111] In contrast, evidence strongly suggests that, in most other situations, surgery that does not achieve wide clearance through normal tissue has a significantly higher rate of local failure, and even some small lesions may behave adversely.[104] The literature on whether there is benefit from the addition of radiotherapy for small (less than 5 cm) high-grade lesions is controversial.[112] The benefit of adjuvant radiotherapy in enhancing local control with conservative surgical resection in soft tissue sarcoma overall has been demonstrated in two randomized clinical trials, one using EBRT and the other using BRT,[113,114] with corroboration in a third trial with high local control that compared two EBRT strategies.[115] The principle of limb conservation using adjuvant radiotherapy was also demonstrated in a randomized trial at the NCI in which this approach was compared with amputation.[109] Based on the principles outlined, radiotherapy should ordinarily not be used when surgical resection alone can be performed with appropriate confidence. Ironically, this applies to opposite ends of the severity spectrum for extremity soft tissue sarcoma. On the one hand, there exist cases with favorable presentation in which conservative surgery alone is readily accomplished; on the other hand, there are rare adverse presentations that require ablative surgery (e.g., amputation) to accomplish a sufficiently wide normal tissue removal to eradicate all lesional tissue.

EXTERNAL-BEAM RADIATION THERAPY

EBRT is the most popular adjuvant radiotherapy approach, perhaps because there is less reliance on special technical and operational requirements as are needed for BRT, which include specific collaboration between surgical and radiation oncologists. EBRT requires comprehensive and multidisciplinary pretreatment consultation and accurate pathologic and radiologic assessment. Relative advantages and disadvantages exist to the use of preoperative and postoperative EBRT (Table 35.1-8). Most have

TABLE 35.1-8. Relative Advantages and Disadvantages of Postoperative and Preoperative External-Beam Radiation Therapy in the Management of Soft Tissue Sarcoma

POSTOPERATIVE RADIOTHERAPY

No potential added problems with impaired wound healing over baseline risk (approximately 15% risk for postoperative radiotherapy in a randomized trial)

Final margins available to help determine need for radiotherapy

Less requirement for preoperative multidisciplinary assessment (an operational advantage of dubious benefit)

Increased late tissue morbidity (dose and volume related) evident in a randomized trial

PREOPERATIVE RADIOTHERAPY

Well-defined treatment volume—better tissue sparing possible

Better blood supply—possibly lower dose needed to control disease

Increased risk to wound healing compared to postoperative (risk confined to lower extremity in a randomized trial)

Potential to reduce micrometastasis, may confer survival advantage

Requires preoperative multidisciplinary assessment (major benefit)

(From ref. 126, with permission.)

been validated prospectively, although confirmation of a hypothetical radiobiologic principle concerning efficacy of lower doses in preoperative radiotherapy remains elusive. This mechanism is potentially mediated by an intact vascular supply and microenvironment and a relative absence of actively proliferating tumor clonogens and radioresistant hypoxic cells, which results in a need for higher doses in postoperative radiotherapy (see Rationale for Postoperative External-Beam Radiation Therapy, later in this chapter). It remains unclear what approach is superior, because emerging clinical trial outcome data suggest competing outcomes, related to the radiotherapy strategy chosen. These outcomes include differing risks of acute wound complications, deteriorating late-response tissue sequelae, and even possible tumor outcomes. The contemporary era has brought newer techniques for radiotherapy planning and delivery that permit unprecedented accuracy in the use of both BRT and EBRT.

Rationale for Postoperative External-Beam Radiation Therapy

Postoperative EBRT was the first and remains the most widely practiced local adjuvant approach, in part because it is rational and convenient to sterilize microscopic nests of residual disease without postponing surgery. Its use is supported by numerous single-institution studies, and it has been shown to enhance local control in a randomized trial that compared conservative surgery and radiotherapy to conservative surgery alone.[114]

Postoperative radiotherapy acquired a veneer of superiority compared to preoperative radiotherapy after the first report of the Canadian Sarcoma Group randomized trial, which demonstrated that preoperative radiotherapy doubles the risk of early acute wound complication. This observation seems to apply almost exclusively to lower limb lesions.[115] Several significant limitations of postoperative EBRT remain, relating to the less precise target volumes compared to those of preoperative EBRT (see Table 35.1-8). Postoperative volumes are larger and associated with higher doses, both of which impact negatively on late tissue morbidity. Thus, with 2-year follow-up in the same trial, postoperative radiotherapy was associated with significantly deteriorating later tissue effects.[116] Substantial difficulties include increased tissue fibrosis and edema mediated by larger doses and larger irradiated volumes in the postoperative setting. Late bone fracture may be related in part to higher radiotherapy doses and larger volumes associated with the timing of radiotherapy (see Serious Complications of Primary Treatment, later in this chapter).

Rationale for Preoperative External-Beam Radiation Therapy

Preoperative EBRT is the only common local adjuvant radiotherapy strategy that has not been subjected to a randomized comparison against surgery alone, although it has been compared to postoperative radiotherapy. There are different incentives for preoperative radiotherapy than for postoperative treatment (see Table 35.1-8). Although most discussion has traditionally focussed on the anatomic outcomes governing morbidity (acute or late), an unexpected early observation concerning survival has emerged in the Canadian Sarcoma Group trial. At a median of 3.3 years of follow-up, local control was identical (93%) in both arms of the study (Fig. 35.1-21), but a small advantage in

overall survival in favor of preoperative radiotherapy was statistically significant. The influences on progression-free survival and metastatic recurrence were not significant, but the survival observation was only partially explained by nonsarcoma death in the postoperative treatment arm[115] (Table 35.1-9). Although this may be a spurious finding, putative mechanisms include the possibility that radiotherapy to a primary tumor may modulate host-tumor interactions, including suppression of distant angiogenesis.[117] Resolution of this early and surprising finding requires maturation of these data.

The retroperitoneum is one sarcoma site for which preoperative radiotherapy may be well suited, because it is provided in a setting in which the tumor has frequently displaced bowel from the target volume (Fig. 35.1-22). In contrast, postoperative radiotherapy is also frequently associated with tethering or fixation of loops of bowel within the target area. The reports of trials involving retroperitoneal sarcoma conducted at the M. D. Anderson Cancer Center[118] and the Princess Margaret Hospital[119] are instructive because the design of each trial mandated that the acute toxicity of preoperative radiotherapy be prospectively separated from overall toxicity. In the Princess Margaret Hospital study, median preoperative doses of radiotherapy of 45 Gy in 25 fractions were administered to median radiation volumes exceeding 7 L, but were associated with acute toxicity scores of 2 or less in all patients who underwent resection, and no patient was hospitalized for acute toxicity or experienced treatment interruptions or cessation of treatment because of acute toxicity.

BRT used postoperatively in selected Princess Margaret Hospital cases was associated with toxicity and also did not appear to have contributed to enhanced tumor outcome.[119] Qualitatively similar findings were apparent in the M. D. Anderson Cancer Center trial, although here the strategy also included the use of concurrent preoperative doxorubicin chemotherapy allocated to one of six sequential 1.8-Gy/fraction escalating radiotherapy protocols (from 18.0 to 50.4 Gy); intraoperative radiotherapy (IORT) with electron beam was also attempted when feasible.[118] Preoperative radiotherapy for retroperitoneal sarcomas is not a new strategy and has been retrospectively reported by the Mayo Clinic group and the Massachusetts General Hospital.[120,121] In neither study were toxicities related to preoperative radiotherapy differentiated from other toxicities (e.g., related to IORT or surgical morbidity), presumably because of their retrospective design. It remains unproven whether these approaches are more effective than postoperative radiotherapy or whether radiotherapy has any true benefit, and it is hoped that the conduct of future prospective clinical trials will address these controversies. For example, one strategy that may be examined is the concept of preoperative dose escalation using more precise methods of radiotherapy delivery as discussed in Dose and Volume Issues in External-Beam Radiation Therapy, later in this chapter.

COMBINED CHEMORADIOTHERAPY

High-risk soft tissue sarcomas (i.e., those of large size, deep location, and high tumor grade) present a significant dual threat locally and at distant anatomic sites. For this reason a dose-intensity chemoradiation strategy in the treatment of 48 patients with localized, high-grade, large (more than 8 cm) soft tissue sarcomas of an extremity was explored at the Massachusetts General Hospital.[122] Interdigitating courses of chemother-

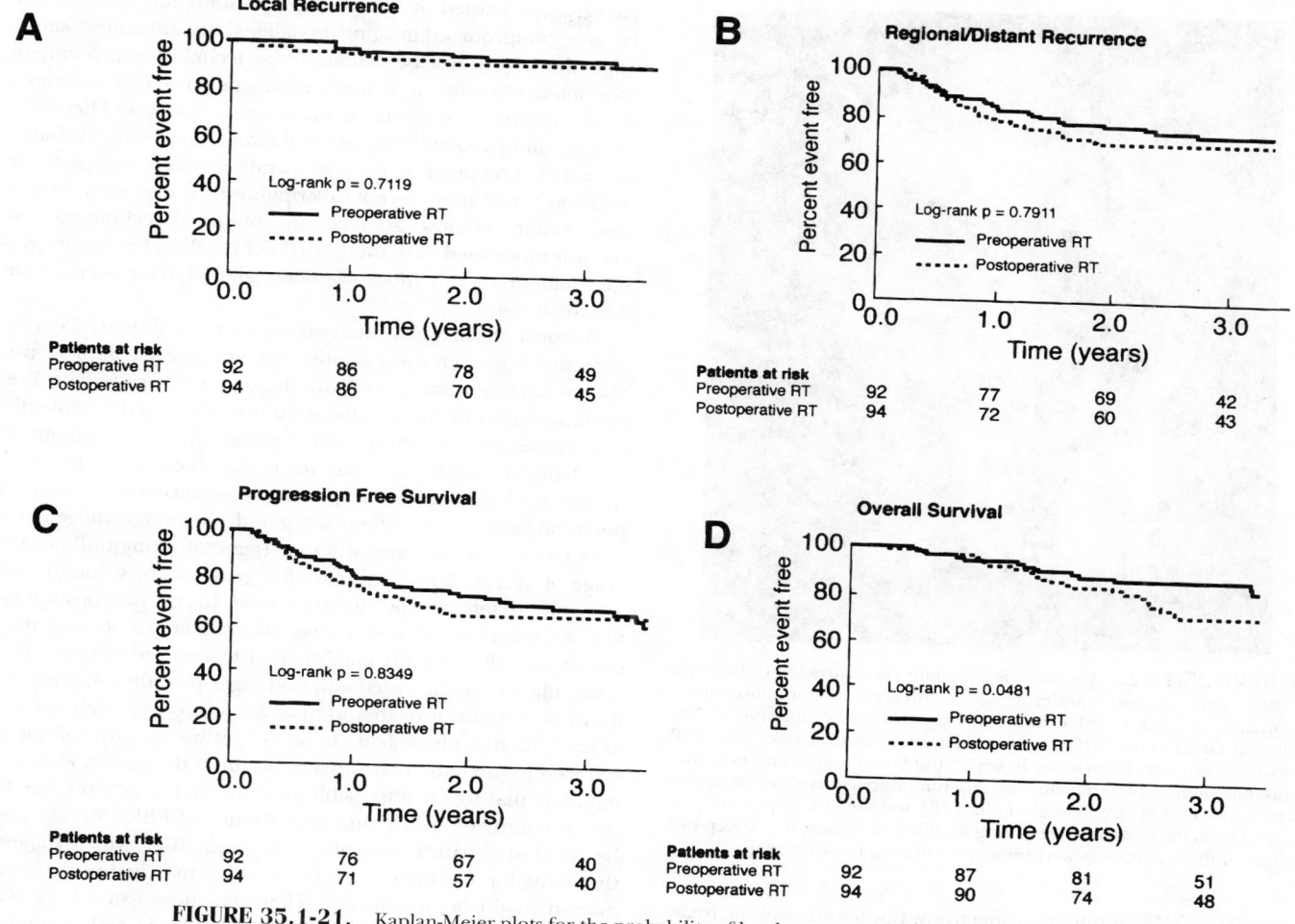

FIGURE 35.1-21. Kaplan-Meier plots for the probability of local recurrence (**A**), regional and distant recurrence (**B**), progression-free survival (**C**), and overall survival (**D**) in a randomized trial of preoperative versus postoperative radiotherapy (RT) in extremity soft tissue sarcoma. (From ref. 115, with permission.)

apy and a lower total dose of radiotherapy were used: three courses of doxorubicin, ifosfamide, mesna, and dacarbazine and two 22-Gy courses of radiation (11 fractions each) for a total preoperative radiation dose of 44 Gy. An additional 16-Gy

boost dose (in eight fractions) was delivered for microscopically positive surgical margins.

The 5-year actuarial local control, distant metastasis–free survival, and overall survival rates for the chemoradiation group

TABLE 35.1-9. Mortality and Causes of Death for All Eligible Cases (n = 186) in a Canadian Trial Comparing Preoperative and Postoperative Radiotherapy

	Preop n (%)	*Postop n (%)*	*Total n (%)*
PATIENT STATUS AT LAST CONTACT (*P* = .05)			
Alive	78 (85)	68 (72)	146 (78.5)
Dead	14 (15)	26 (28)	40 (21.5)
Total	92 (100)	94 (100)	186 (100)
CAUSE OF DEATH			
Disease	13 (93)	21 (81)	34 (85)
Other[a]	0 (0)	3 (11.5)	3 (7.5)
Other primary malignancy	1 (7)	2 (8)	3 (7.5)
Total deaths	14 (100)	26 (100)	40 (100)

Preop, preoperative radiotherapy; Postop, postoperative radiotherapy.
[a]The three "other" deaths were death due to bronchopneumonia (age 87 years) with 2-year follow-up without sarcoma; self-inflicted death without sarcoma (age 33 years) with 3-year follow-up; fatal myocardial infarction (age 77 years) near the completion of postoperative radiotherapy. (Modified from ref. 115, with permission.)

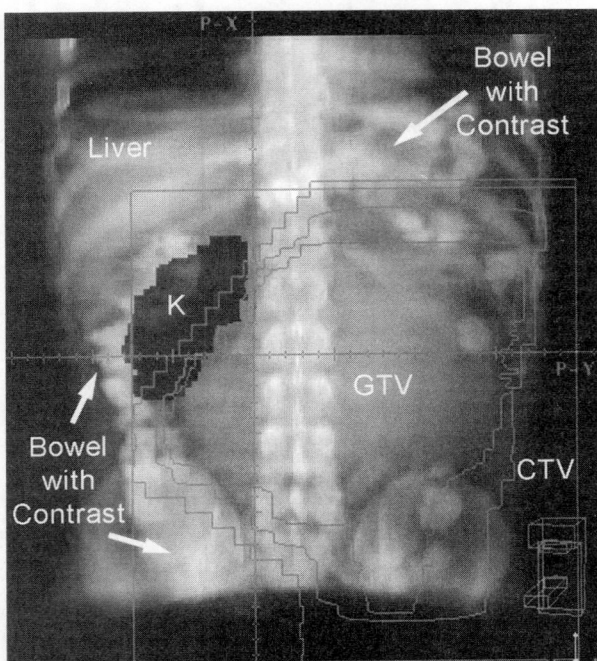

FIGURE 35.1-22. Coronal view digitally reconstructed radiograph (DRR) with soft tissue rendering taken with a computed tomographic simulator to exhibit the location of the gross tumor volume (GTV), the clinical target volume (CTV), and adjacent organs at risk. The DRR readily illustrates the manner in which the bowel containing oral contrast has been displaced from the main tumor area into more protected areas. Also evident are the right kidney (K) and the liver, which are protected from the high-dose area using multileaf collimation (see step-like edges of the radiation beam) for a conventional two-field plan.

were 92%, 75%, and 87%, respectively. Local and systemic toxicity included significant and expected wound-healing complications in the lower limbs (evident in 29%), evaluated using the Canadian Sarcoma Group criteria.[115] One patient died from late marrow dysfunction attributed to chemotherapy. Clearly the use of early neoadjuvant chemoradiotherapy delivered in this fashion is appealing in the subset of patients at very highest risk. These results in adverse cases may be explained by imbalance between the treatment and control groups and require confirmation in prospective trials, especially because of the local and systemic toxicity associated with the protocol.[123]

VOLUME ISSUES IN EXTERNAL-BEAM RADIATION THERAPY

Despite the importance of volume issues, there have been no prospective assessments of the volumes to be used in EBRT, although this may be explained by the favorable results usually evident after treatment of these lesions (i.e., local control rates that approximate the 90% range are expected with current extremity sarcoma approaches). The existing literature on this subject is vulnerable to problems of retrospective interpretation and is confounded by selection bias. Given the success of reported results, it is important to explore opportunities to lessen treatment intensity, including administered doses or volumes, in the interest of amelioration of normal tissue toxicity.

Generally, basic radiotherapy volumes of rectangular and cylindrical shapes have been the rule over recent decades because lim-

itations have existed in radiotherapy planning and delivery and because compromised imaging modalities have influenced knowledge about local disease extent. Today technical improvements have made it feasible to deliver radiotherapy volumes that more closely approximate intended ideal target volumes. Therefore, existing guidelines outlining optimal radiotherapy target volumes for either preoperative or postoperative EBRT may now be outdated[124] and more recent descriptions[125,126] may soon require modification, because advances in conformal techniques and intensity-modulated radiotherapy (IMRT) make it feasible to consider volumes that are more accurately tailored to the needs of the individual case.

By conventionally accepted principles of treatment, preoperative and postoperative radiotherapy effectively comprise two disease treatment scenarios from the standpoint of targets. Preoperative radiotherapy can focus on the extent of definable disease (generally determined using imaging), and the target is based on the anatomic location, containment by barriers to spread, and allowance for geometric uncertainty related to potential variation in patient setup and physiologic movement. Alternatively, an estimated distance (generally longitudinal coverage of at least 2 to 5 cm from the gross tumor volume) that may contain microscopic disease is used. In contrast, postoperative radiotherapy volumes are significantly larger because they encompass all surgically manipulated tissues and because anatomic planes are disrupted and no longer provide containment barriers to tumor growth and must be considered high risk for at least the first phase (e.g., to 50 Gy). Subsequently, volume is reduced to the immediate area of origin of the tumor, with recognition that this is impossible in some anatomic sites due to the proximity of critical anatomy. Results of EBRT should also be contrasted with the results of adjuvant BRT, which suggest that radiation treatment directed to the tumor bed plus a 2-cm margin might be adequate.[127] However, these issues have not been compared prospectively or in situations in which equivalent local control has been documented. Unfortunately, the only prospective evaluation of radiotherapy target volumes available was in a Canadian trial that showed a statistically clear reduction in the field sizes for upper and lower extremity lesions treated with preoperative radiotherapy.[115]

DOSE ISSUES IN EXTERNAL-BEAM RADIATION THERAPY

The dose of radiotherapy represents an additional unexplored area. The preoperative dose used in most institutions is approximately 50 Gy in daily fractions of 1.8 to 2.0 Gy over approximately 5 weeks. Generally, with preoperative radiotherapy a postoperative boost is administered only if the surgical margins are positive, although it remains unclear whether this is beneficial. Existing reports describing radiation dose response are generally unhelpful and based on underpowered retrospective studies confounded by selection. A retrospective study at the Institut Gustave Roussy, Villejuif, France, has the advantage that the investigators used a consistent approach throughout the period of study.[128] Although including only a small number of patients (n = 62), the study evaluated two postoperative radiotherapy schedules in terms of dose, fractionation, and overall treatment time. Forty-five patients received 50 Gy with conventional fractionation plus a boost dose (5 to 20 Gy) after "maximal conservative surgery" and experienced a 3-year local control

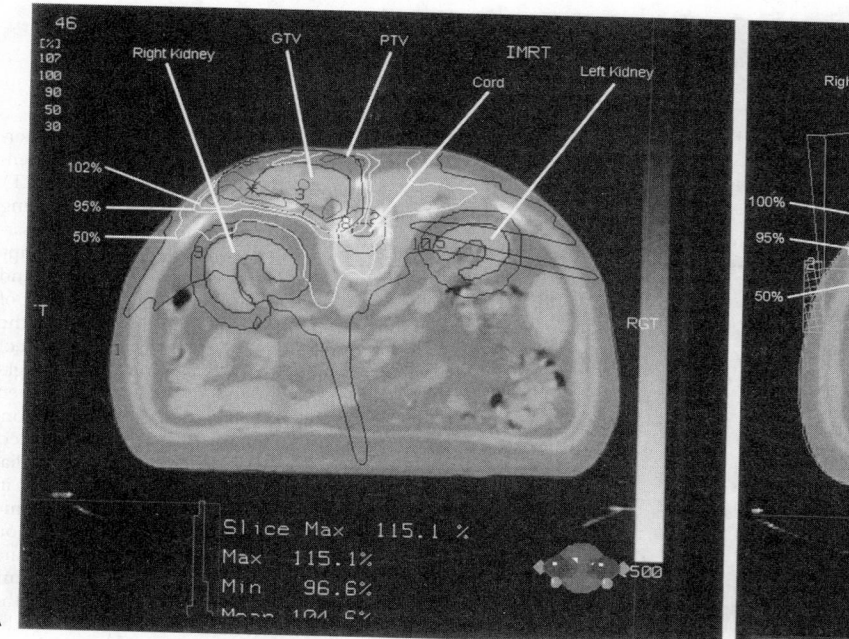
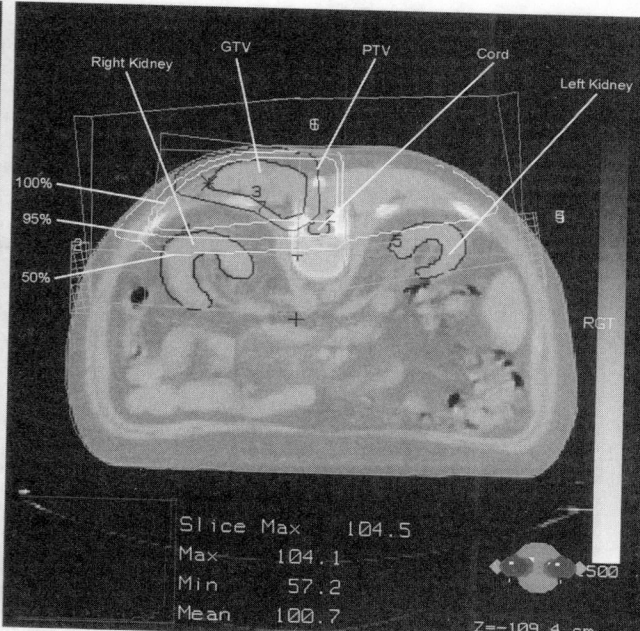

FIGURE 35.1-23. Intensity-modulated radiotherapy (IMRT) plan **(A)** to deliver preoperative radiotherapy (50 Gy) to a right paraspinal sarcoma identified as the gross tumor volume (GTV) located adjacent to the spinal cord and right kidney. The planning target volume (PTV) is the area being irradiated with a margin surrounding the GTV. Note shaping of the IMRT 50% isodose curves to conformally avoid the right and left kidney compared to a more traditional three-field conformal plan **(B)**.

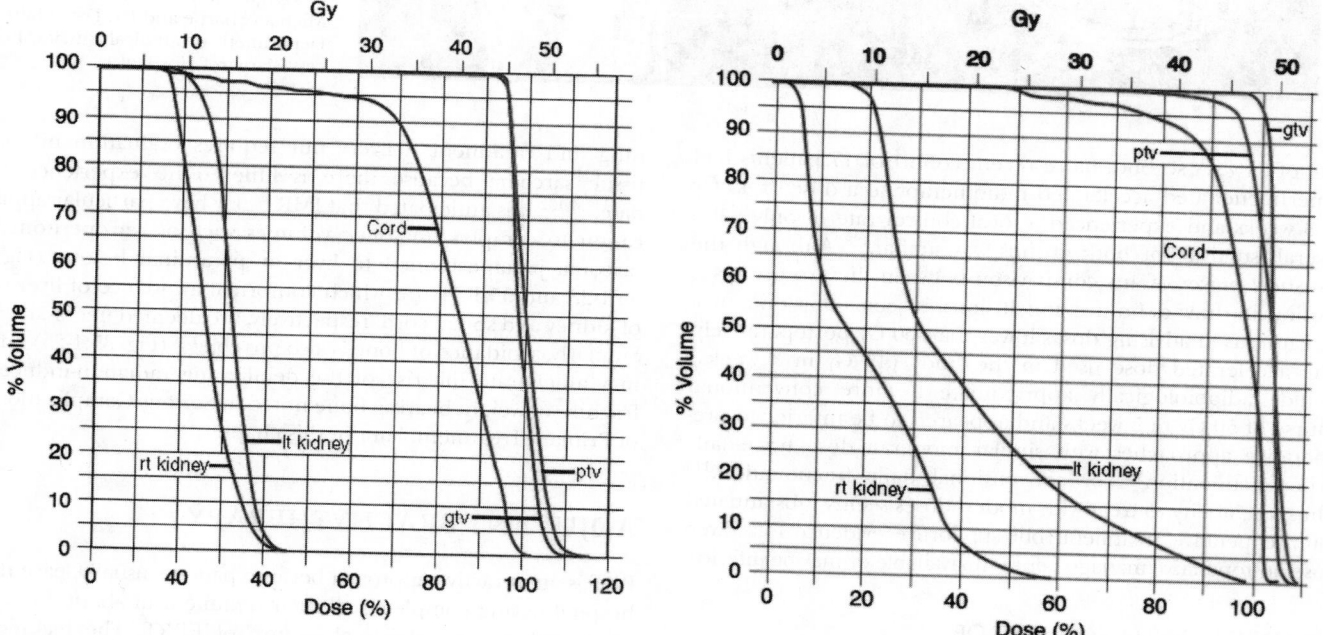

FIGURE 35.1-24. Comparison of dose-volume histograms (DVHs) for the intensity-modulated radiotherapy (IMRT) plan outlined in Figure 35.1-23*A* versus the conventional three-field conformal plan outlined in Figure 35.1-23*B*, both of which provide good coverage of the gross tumor volume (gtv) and the planning target volume (ptv). The IMRT plan illustrates reduction of dose to the spinal cord (50% of cord volume receiving 40 Gy), and the left kidney is also receiving less dose (all of the volume receiving less than 20 Gy) **(A)**. In contrast, the three-field conformal plan requires 50% of the spinal cord volume to receive approximately 47 Gy, and 40% of the left kidney volume is receiving between 20 and 50 Gy **(B)**. The DVHs indicate better protection of two critical organs at risk with IMRT while also achieving equivalent target coverage.

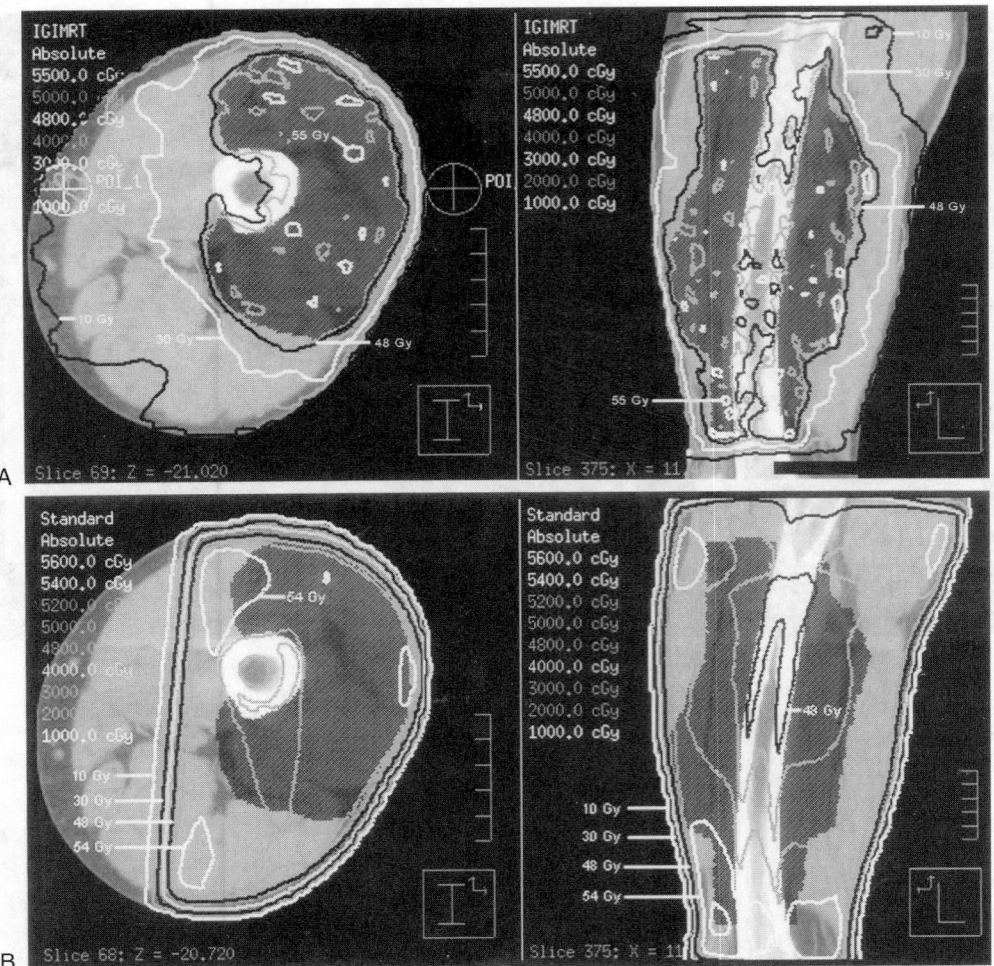

FIGURE 35.1-25. Two radiotherapy treatment plans, one using intensity-modulated radiotherapy (IMRT) (**A**) and the other conformal planning (**B**) to treat the same medial thigh sarcoma with preoperative radiotherapy to a dose of 50 Gy. In **A**, an axial and coronal depiction shows the ability of IMRT to sculpt the dose around the femur and protect a substantial part of the limb cross section from the high-dose radiotherapy volume indicated by the dark 48-Gy isodose line. As configured, there is also greater protection of the groin and proximal medial thigh by the IMRT plan as evident in the coronal view. In **B**, the 48-Gy line encompasses a much greater proportion of the volume of the limb and includes administration of a substantial dose to the bone. Note also the small, scattered "hot spots" in the IMRT plan (**A**), which are characteristic of the composite volume derived from beams of highly modulated intensity. In practice, these are not consequential, although care must be taken that they are appreciated in the plan. The dose-volume histogram (not shown) comparing these two plans clearly indicated the superiority of the IMRT plan in this situation. IGIMRT, image-guided IMRT. (Courtesy of Dr. Michael Sharpe and Dr. David Jaffray, Department of Medical Physics, Princess Margaret Hospital.)

rate of 84%. A second, more recent cohort of 17 patients had hyperfractionated accelerated radiotherapy to a dose of 45 Gy in 3 weeks and experienced a local control rate of only 64%. Overall survival for both groups was similar.[128] Although the statistical power of any comparison between the two groups is too low to draw definitive conclusions, it seems that one must be cautious in advising doses lower than 60 Gy postoperatively. The accelerated dose used in the study (45 Gy in 3 weeks) would radiobiologically approximate a more conventional course of 50 Gy in 5 weeks and appeared to be inferior to preoperative approaches with similar moderate-dose twice-daily hyperfractionation[129] or conventional daily fractionation.[115] Thus, the ability to treat with modest doses seems substantiated for preoperative treatment, but supportive evidence for lower-dose postoperative management is unavailable or may be inferior.

TECHNICAL ENHANCEMENT OF RADIOTHERAPY DELIVERY

Soft tissue sarcomas present in many ways with great variation in their patterns of local involvement, size, and three-dimensional form. The past decade has witnessed an unprecedented improvement in delivery of EBRT to complex volumes and shapes. Leading these advances is IMRT,[130] a nascent technology that uses powerful computer algorithms for inverse planning and treatment delivery but requires evaluation in soft tissue sarcoma because there is little to no experience to date.[131,132] It is anticipated that IMRT may have particular application to complex anatomic volumes such as retroperitoneal sarcoma juxtapositioned to liver or paraspinal lesions (Figs. 35.1-23 and 35.1-24) for which conformal avoidance of liver or of kidney and spinal cord, respectively, are deemed necessary.[132] Similarly, avoidance of bone is also possible[133] (Fig. 35.1-25) and may ameliorate the risk of the debilitating radiation-induced fracture of weight-bearing bone noted in Serious Complications of Primary Treatment, later in this chapter.

ADJUVANT BRACHYTHERAPY

BRT is an attractive approach because patients usually leave the hospital having completed all their treatment in about 2 weeks compared to a 6- to 7-week course of EBRT. The technical aspects of BRT are different from those of EBRT, and specific guidelines for its use and technical delivery have been published.[134] The rapid dose fall-off with BRT usually spares more normal tissue than EBRT except with the use of precision techniques such as IMRT. Of importance, the loading of the catheters takes place no sooner that the sixth postoperative day to allow enough time for wound healing.[135] Also, unlike in postop-

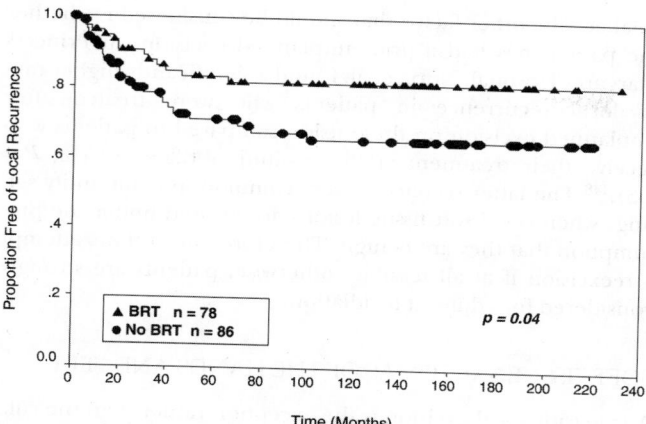

FIGURE 35.1-26. Results of a prospective randomized trial at Memorial Sloan-Kettering Cancer Center of adjuvant brachytherapy (BRT) in patients undergoing limb-sparing surgery (between July 1982 and July 1992, follow-up to December 31, 2002). Patients who received adjuvant BRT had a statistically significant improvement in local control. (Updated from ref. 13.)

erative irradiation, no attempts are made to treat large margins or to include the scar and the drainage site, although it is acknowledged that this approach has not been formally compared with EBRT in similar cases. In patients treated with BRT alone, the dose is usually 45 Gy given over 4 to 6 days, and when given as a boost the dose is usually 15 to 20 Gy plus 45 to 50 Gy with EBRT. The most commonly used isotope is low dose-rate iridium 192; however, high-activity iodine 125 is occasionally used in young patients or to protect the gonads. More recently, high dose-rate iridium 192 has been advocated by some authors to take advantage of its radiation safety aspects as well as its dose-optimization capabilities.[134] In contrasting BRT with EBRT, it is interesting to note that savings of $1000 per patient treated may be feasible, at least using one set of assumptions.[136]

Adjuvant BRT was evaluated in a randomized trial to determine its role after complete gross resection (78 patients were randomly assigned to receive adjuvant BRT and 86 patients to

receive no further therapy). With a median follow-up of 76 months, the 5-year actuarial local control rates were 82% and 69% (*P* = .04) in the BRT and no-BRT groups, respectively (Fig. 35.1-26). This improvement in local control, however, was limited to patients with histologically high-grade tumors (Fig. 35.1-27). For this group, local control was 89% and 66% (*P* = .002) in the BRT and no-BRT groups, respectively. Analysis by histologic grade did not demonstrate an impact of BRT on the development of distant metastasis or survival.[137] Even though adjuvant BRT did not lead to an improvement in local control in patients with low-grade tumors, the local recurrence rates were 22% (no BRT) and 27% (BRT), which indicates the need for adjuvant external radiation in these patients.[113] BRT is often used as a boost in combination with EBRT, but whether this combination is needed in all patients is unclear.[138–140] Alekhteyar et al. reported on 105 patients with primary or locally recurrent high-grade soft tissue sarcomas who were treated with wide local excision and BRT (87 patients) or BRT and EBRT (18 patients). At a median follow-up of 22 months, there was no statistically significant difference in the 2-year actuarial local control rates between the two groups: 82% in the BRT group and 90% in the BRT plus EBRT group (*P* = .32).[141] However, case selection was such that the groups are not completely comparable, and this may explain the difference in target volumes between the two radiotherapy approaches (EBRT and BRT). For example, at MSKCC, EBRT is added to BRT only when the geometry of the implant is suboptimal or there is a positive surgical margin.

One of the most attractive aspects of BRT is the ability to deliver further radiation in previously irradiated patients who may otherwise need amputation to obtain good local control. Pearlstone et al. reported a local control rate of 82.5% (33 of 40) and 65% (17 of 26), respectively, when using conservative surgery and reirradiation with BRT.[142] Catton et al. reported a local control rate of only 36% (4 of 11) for patients treated with conservative surgery and no further irradiation. They also reported local control rate of 100% in patients treated with further surgery and reirradiation (predominantly using BRT), with a short median follow-up of 24 months.[143]

SPECIAL CONSIDERATIONS

Although adjuvant radiation has been shown to improve local control in soft tissue sarcoma of the extremity, its impact in patients with positive microscopic margins has not been clearly defined. Data from the Princess Margaret Hospital, Massachusetts General Hospital, and MSKCC have shown higher 5-year local recurrence rates in patients with positive margins than in those with negative margins despite the use of adjuvant irradiation, although radiotherapy reduces the risk of recurrence compared to no adjuvant treatments.[106,144] In a study at MSKCC reporting actuarial local control of 71%, the group that received adjuvant radiation experienced a 5-year local control rate of 75% compared to 56% for those treated with surgery alone (*P* = .01). Adjuvant radiation also retained its significance as an independent prognostic factor for local control when multivariate analysis was performed (*P* = .01).[145] Whether one radiation modality is better than another in such cases is debatable due to the paucity of data and the problems of selection bias. Alekhteyar et al.[141] demonstrated a trend

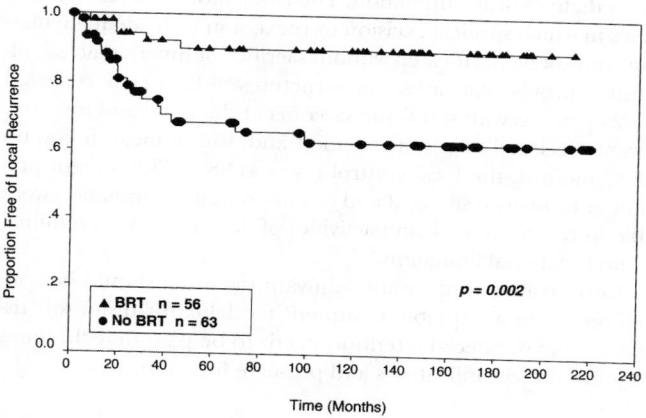

FIGURE 35.1-27. Results of a prospective randomized trial at Memorial Sloan-Kettering Cancer Center of adjuvant brachytherapy (BRT) in patients undergoing limb-sparing surgery (between July 1982 and July 1992, follow-up to December 31, 2002). This local control advantage was limited to patients with high-grade lesions. (Updated from ref. 13.)

toward improvement in local control if BRT was supplemented with EBRT in patients with positive margins (90% vs. 59%; *P* = .08). However, others showed no difference in local control between EBRT and BRT boost.[146]

Princess Margaret Hospital reported that the cause of positive margins also appears important because this has an influence on local control.[147] One cause is oncologically inadequate surgery in which positive resection margins may have been avoidable in another surgeon's hands. When this is the case, microscopically positive surgical margins can be considered a technical failure. Alternatively, positive resection margins may arise in anatomically adverse presentations in which locally advanced disease challenges the goals of conservative resection from the outset. After adjuvant radiotherapy, patients with low-grade liposarcomas and microscopically positive surgical margins have a low risk of local failure (4.2%), as do those in whom a positive margin is anticipated before surgery to preserve critical structures and radiotherapy is used to sterilize minimal residual disease (3.6%). However, in two categories of patients, positive margins are associated with a higher risk of local recurrence: (1) patients who present after a prereferral excision without adequate preoperative staging or consideration of the need to remove normal tissue around tumor (unplanned excision; see Small Soft Tissue Sarcomas later in this chapter) and who have a positive margin on subsequent reexcision (local recurrence rate of 31.6%), and (2) those with unanticipated positive margins occurring during primary sarcoma resection (recurrence rate of 37.5%).[148] The importance of this observation is that it seems to be possible, with appropriate evaluation and anticipation, to resect disease and protect critical juxtapositioned anatomy. This may result in only a minimal microscopic burden of disease residuum in a small area of positive margin that can be eradicated with adjuvant radiotherapy. For the latter cases, from a cancer control perspective, it probably does not matter whether radiotherapy is administered as BRT or as EBRT delivered preoperatively or postoperatively.

SMALL SOFT TISSUE SARCOMAS

Geer et al. described the more favorable outcome of small tumors.[103] They reported on 174 patients with primary soft tissue sarcoma of the extremity measuring 5 cm or smaller. When only patients with negative margins of resection were analyzed (159 patients), the 5-year local control rate was 77% in those selected to receive adjuvant radiation compared to 92% in those undergoing surgery alone (*P* = .08).[103] The treatment policy at MSKCC and Princess Margaret Hospital has been to omit adjuvant irradiation in patients primarily treated with small tumors and adequate margins. It is very important to consider other factors when deciding whether or not to omit radiation therapy. One such factor is the status of the surgical margin of resection. In the Geer et al. study,[103] the impact of adjuvant radiation was analyzed only in the subset of patients with negative margins. In fact, patients with positive margins in that study had a 5-year local control rate of only 56% versus 88% in those with negative margins (*P* = .01). Similar findings were reported by Fleming et al. at M. D. Anderson Cancer Center[104] and are a reminder that the burden of residuum is relevant and that adjuvant radiotherapy may not always be able to sterilize it successfully.[147] It is also the authors' policy to treat patients with positive margins even if the tumors were 5 cm or

smaller. The other factor that should be considered is whether the patient has had a prior unplanned excision. At Princess Margaret Hospital, Noria et al. found a significantly higher rate of local recurrence in patients who were treated after unplanned excision on the outside compared to patients who receive their treatment at the institution (22% vs. 7%; *P* = .03).[148] The latter scenario is very common in community settings when small soft tissue lesions are excised under the presumption that they are benign. Therefore, the authors attempt a reexcision if at all feasible; otherwise, patients are strongly considered for adjuvant irradiation.

SOFT TISSUE SARCOMAS OF THE HANDS AND FEET

A true wide local excision is the exception rather than the rule in sites of the hands and feet due to the lack of muscular bulk and the proximity to neurovascular structures and bone. In addition, the overall prognosis has been shown to be inferior to that of tumors at other sites in the extremity. At MSKCC, Brien et al. showed that, even in patients with hand tumors that are 5 cm or smaller, the survival rate was significantly lower than that of patients with tumors at other distal extremity sites (*P* = .0008).[149]

In the past, there was concern about the tolerance of the distal extremities to radiotherapy, but data suggest that conservative resections with adjuvant radiotherapy should be considered.[150] Special attention needs to be paid to radiation treatment technique to minimize complications and preserve function. Lin et al. reported the outcome of 115 patients with soft tissue sarcomas of the hand or foot treated between 1980 and 1998. The majority (95%) were referred after surgery elsewhere. Patients treated with definitive wide reexcision had a 10-year local recurrence-free survival rate of 88%, which was significantly better than the corresponding rate of patients who did not have reexcision (local control of 58%) (*P* = .05). Also, radiotherapy improved local control in patients who did not undergo reexcision but did not improve local control in the small number of patients who had definitive reexcision with negative margins. The authors concluded that limb-sparing treatment is possible in many patients with soft tissue sarcomas of the hand and foot and that there does not appear to be a survival benefit from immediate radical amputation. The latter should be reserved for cases in which surgical excision or reexcision with adequate margins cannot be performed without sacrifice of functionally significant neurovascular or osseous structures.[151] Bray et al. reported on 25 patients with soft tissue sarcoma of the hand and forearm. Twenty received adjuvant radiation and, with a mean follow-up of 37 months, the local control rate was 88%. Eighty-eight percent of those who survived and did not require amputation were able to return to work and activities of daily living with minimal or no functional limitation.[152]

Conservative surgery and adjuvant radiation should be considered as an acceptable treatment modality for distal soft tissue sarcomas. Special attention needs to be paid to techniques to minimize complications and preserve function.

DEFINITIVE RADIATION

Surgery remains the main treatment for patients with sarcoma of the extremity, and every effort should be made to attempt resection. In some patients with unresectable disease or medical contraindications to operation, definitive radiation can be considered to achieve palliation. Because sarcoma may be radiocurable in terms of cell killing but not radioresponsive in terms of shrinkage of the mass, this can be perplexing, because such masses can give the false impression that little has been accomplished whereas in reality the mass is mainly sterilized tumor cells or debris. Tepper and Suit reported on 51 patients treated with definitive photon beam irradiation to a total dose of 64 to 66 Gy. The 5-year local control and survival rates were 33% and 25%, respectively. Local control was better for tumors smaller than 5 cm (87.5%) than for tumors 5 to 10 cm (53%) or larger than 10 cm (30%).[153] Slater et al. reported similar findings in 57 patients treated with definitive photon beam irradiation to 44 to 88 Gy. The 5-year local control rate was 28%.[154] An additional 15 patients were also treated with neutrons without obvious benefit.

Other investigators have considered neutron radiotherapy either alone or in combination with photon beam irradiation. The attraction of this approach is the lower oxygen enhancement ratio compared to x-rays and the consequent possibility of eliminating hypoxic cells. Neutron irradiation results in less repair of sublethal and potentially lethal damage, and neutrons are less vulnerable than photons to the differential radiosensitivities associated with different phases of the cell cycle. Unfortunately, all these biologic features also pertain to normal tissue, which implies that late toxicity is likely to be heightened given the absence of the usual protection afforded by fractionation that occurs with more conventional photon treatment schedules. Schwarz et al. reviewed the European experience with such an approach and reported a local control rate of 50%, but the rate of severe complications ranged from 6.6% when neutron therapy was used as a boost to 50% when used alone.[155] More recently Schwartz et al. reported a North American experience of fast neutron therapy in a heterogeneous series of bone and in soft tissue sarcomas. A minority of patients had unresectable disease (n = 34), and they estimated a local relapse-free survival at 1 year of 62% for this group.[156] In ten patients (15%) requiring administration of high neutron doses or large radiotherapy fields or both, serious chronic radiation-related complications occurred. Hyperfractionated photon beam radiation has been combined with intravenous iododeoxyuridine as a radiosensitizer. Goffman et al. reported on 36 patients treated in this fashion, and with a median follow-up of 4 years the local control rate was 60%.[157]

The use of concurrent chemotherapy with definitive radiotherapy has been explored with evidence of benefit in numerous other cancers and should be considered for soft tissue sarcomas that cannot be resected, given the limited expectation of local control and the grave prognosis. The observations of high local control achieved with a reduced dose of radiotherapy delivered with concurrent mesna, doxorubicin (Adriamycin), ifosfamide, and dacarbazine (MAID) chemotherapy in the high-risk adjuvant setting was outlined in Combined Chemoradiotherapy, earlier in this chapter.[122] Potentially, higher doses of radiotherapy with concurrent dose-intensified chemotherapy regimens, possibly delivered with conformal radiotherapy volumes to further protect normal tissues, provide an opportunity to enhance local control in this setting. Preliminary data have been obtained using a concurrent ifosfamide-based protocol. This regimen appears to have acceptable morbidity, although

skin toxicity seemed to be enhanced, which makes it important to explore radiotherapy avoidance targeting in suitable patients if escalated radiotherapy doses are to be used.[158]

Further evidence on combining systemic agents with radiotherapy to enhance local control in unresectable disease was provided by Rhomberg et al. These authors evaluated the use of the radiation sensitizer razoxane on soft tissue sarcomas in a prospective randomized controlled trial. This trial had a long accrual period (1978 to 1988), a modest number of evaluable cases (130 of 144 accrued), a modest radiation dose, and some imbalance between the treatment arms. Nevertheless, among 82 patients with gross disease, radiotherapy (median dose of 56 to 58 Gy) combined with razoxane (daily oral doses of 150 mg/m^2 throughout radiotherapy) demonstrated an increased response rate compared to photon irradiation alone (74% vs. 49%). The local control rate was improved (64% vs. 30%; P <.05), although acute skin reactions were enhanced in the sensitizer arm. Late toxicity was not increased in this study.[159]

ADJUVANT CHEMOTHERAPY

Surgery remains the mainstay of therapy for soft tissue sarcoma in the control of local disease. Radiation therapy plays a role in the local control of soft tissue sarcomas. Nonetheless, as many as half of all patients with adequate local control of disease develop distant metastasis, usually to the lungs (extremity sarcomas) or liver (abdominal primary). As has been demonstrated in breast cancer, colorectal cancer, and osteosarcoma, it was hoped that adjuvant chemotherapy would help decrease the frequency of distant metastases and thus increase overall survival. More than 15 studies of adjuvant therapy for soft tissue sarcoma have been performed. Because anthracyclines are the most active agents in sarcoma therapy in the metastatic setting, they have been used in nearly all of the adjuvant trials, alone or in combination. Most of the studies have been small and lack statistical power to detect small changes in overall survival. Metaanalyses have been performed on the randomized trials for adjuvant chemotherapy in soft tissue sarcoma. Earlier in the chapter, in Randomized Studies of Adjuvant Doxorubicin Alone, the data from the individual studies and metaanalyses are examined in detail (Table 35.1-10).

RANDOMIZED STUDIES OF ADJUVANT DOXORUBICIN ALONE

One of the earliest studies to accrue patients in a randomized trial of adjuvant chemotherapy was performed by the Gynecologic Oncology Group in patients with uterine sarcomas.[160] Two hundred and twenty-five patients with stage I or II uterine sarcomas of any histopathologic subtype were treated surgically for local control. Radiation was added at the discretion of the physician for local control, then patients were randomly assigned to receive doxorubicin 60 mg/m^2 every 3 weeks for eight cycles or to observation alone. For the 156 evaluable patients, disease-free survival was no different between the two groups, nor was there a statistically significant difference in overall survival (73.7 months in the treated arm vs. 55.0 months in the control arm). The addition of radiation therapy did not affect survival, although there was a lower rate of vaginal relapse in the group treated with radiation.

TABLE 35.1-10. Adjuvant Studies in Soft Tissue Sarcoma

Study	Regimen	Doxorubicin Dose (mg/m²)	No. of Evaluable Patients	Extremity Patients	Median Follow-Up (Y)	Reported DFS Control (%)	Reported DFS Treated (%)	Reported OS Control (%)	Reported OS Treated (%)	Reference(s)
NCI extremity	CAM	50–70	65	65	7.1	54[a]	75[a]	60	83	169–171
NCI head and neck, trunk, breast	CAM	50–70	31	0	3.0	49	77	58	68	173
NCI retroperitoneal	CAM	50–70	15	0	2.4	84	50	100	47	174
GOG	Dox	60	156	0	NA	47	59	52	60	160
MDA	VACAR	60	47	43	>10	35[a]	55[a]	57	65	175,351
Mayo Clinic	VCAct/VAD	50	61	48	5.4	65	83	70	90	176
EORTC	CyVADIC	50	317	216	6.7	43[a]	56[a]	55	63	177
Intergroup	Dox	70–90	78	50	1.7	55	73	70	91	163,352
ECOG	Dox	70	30	18	>4.9	55	66	52	65	162
Boston	Dox	90	42	25	>3.8	62	67	72	71	161,353
SSG	Dox	60	181	155	3.3	NA	NA	NA	NA	164
Rizzoli	Dox	75	77	77	NA	45[a,b]	73[a,b]	70[a,b]	91[a,b]	165,354
UCLA	Dox	90	119	119	2.3	54[b]	58[b]	80[b]	85[b]	167
Fondation Bergonié	CyVADIC	50	59	36	4.4	32[a]	81[a]	54[a]	87[a]	178
RPMI	Dox	60–75	19	0	5.0	46	75	36	63	168
ISSG	I/Epi	Epi at 120	104	104	4.9	37[a]	50[a]	50[a]	69[a]	355
EORTC/NCIC	Dox/I	50	134	123	7.3	52	56	64	65	180
Austria	AI with DTIC (q2wk)	50	59	47	3.4 (mean)	57	77	>80	>80	181
1997 meta-analysis	Any	Various	1568	904	9.4	44[a]	52[a]	53	57	186

AI, doxorubicin, ifosfamide; CAM, cyclophosphamide, doxorubicin, methotrexate; CyVADIC, cyclophosphamide, vincristine, doxorubicin, dacarbazine; DFS, disease-free survival; Dox, doxorubicin; DTIC, dacarbazine; ECOG, Eastern Cooperative Oncology Group; EORTC, European Organization for Research and Treatment of Cancer; Epi, epirubicin; GOG, Gynecologic Oncology Group; I, ifosfamide; ISSG, Italian Sarcoma Study Group; MDA, M. D. Anderson Cancer Center; NA, not available; NCI, National Cancer Institute; NCIC, National Cancer Institute of Canada; OS, overall survival; RPMI, Roswell Park Memorial Institute; SSG, Scandinavian Sarcoma Group; UCLA, University of California at Los Angeles; VACAR, vincristine, doxorubicin, cyclophosphamide, dactinomycin; VCAct/VAD, vincristine, cyclophosphamide, dactinomycin alternating with vincristine, doxorubicin, dacarbazine.

Note: DFS and OS are not necessarily indicated at the median follow-up time.

[a]Survival difference reached significance.

[b]Some patients on control arm received chemotherapy.

Between 1978 and 1982, the Dana-Farber Cancer Institute, Brigham and Women's Hospital, and Massachusetts General Hospital enrolled patients with AJCC stage IIB to IVA to a study in which local therapy consisted of radical surgery or to wide *en bloc* excision followed by radiation.[181] Forty-two patients were randomly assigned to receive five doses of doxorubicin, 90 mg/m², every 3 weeks, or to observation. The timing of chemotherapy varied for patients at the Dana-Farber Cancer Institute and Brigham and Women's Hospital and for patients at Massachusetts General Hospital, with the former receiving both radiation and chemotherapy postoperatively and the latter receiving radiation and two of the five cycles of chemotherapy before surgery. There was no significant difference in local control, relapse-free survival, or overall survival in this study, although there was a trend (not statistically significant) toward better overall survival of patients with extremity sarcomas who received chemotherapy compared to the patients who did not receive chemotherapy.

The ECOG enrolled 47 patients with AJCC stage IIB to IVA disease in a study in which local therapy consisted of radical surgery or of wide *en bloc* excision followed by radiation.[162] Patients with local recurrence were permitted on the study. Patients received doxorubicin 70 mg/m² every 3 weeks for seven cycles. Thirty-two were eligible for analysis. There was no difference in local control, relapse-free survival, or overall survival in the treatment and control arms.

The Intergroup Sarcoma Study Group examined patients with AJCC stage IIB to IVA tumors treated with surgery for local control. Seventy-eight eligible patients were randomly assigned to observation or to doxorubicin at 35 mg/m² given as daily bolus doses on two consecutive days.[163] Six cycles of doxorubicin were given at 3-week intervals in the chemotherapy arm. There was no significant difference in local recurrence, disease-free survival, or overall survival in the chemotherapy arm compared to the control arm. A trend was noted toward improved disease-free survival for extremity lesions that was of borderline statistical significance ($P = .06$). Pooling of the data from the Boston, ECOG, and Intergroup studies demonstrated no survival benefit for adjuvant doxorubicin.[163]

The Scandinavian Sarcoma Group performed the largest study of doxorubicin as an adjuvant to local therapy for soft tissue sarcomas.[164] Two hundred forty patients were treated with surgery with the option of adjuvant radiation for local control. Patients were then randomly assigned either to receive doxorubicin 60 mg/m² every 4 weeks for nine cycles or to receive no chemotherapy. Chemotherapy was started within 6 weeks of surgery when radiation was not used for local control or within 10 weeks when radiation was used. One hundred eighty-one patients were evaluable. At a median follow-up of 40 months, there was no difference in local control, disease-free survival, or overall survival for the evaluable patients. Survival data were also assessed for the entire 240-patient cohort; there was no difference among treatment groups in disease-free or overall survival.

The Istituto Ortopedico Rizzoli examined a heterogeneous group of 77 patients with high-grade extremity sarcomas.[165] For local control some patients had radical surgery alone, surgery and preoperative radiation therapy, or radiation therapy and chemotherapy before surgical resection (the "conservative surgery" group). Patients were randomly assigned to receive or not to receive doxorubicin 25 mg/m² given daily as boluses on 3 consecutive days in a 21-day cycle, for a total of six cycles. Relapse-free survival was improved in the chemotherapy arm (79% vs. 45%) at a median of 28 months of follow-up. In an update,[166] disease-free and overall survival benefits were not seen in the group treated with conservative surgery and chemotherapy compared with those treated with conservative surgery alone. These data are difficult to analyze owing to the complex randomization scheme of the study as well as contamination of the control arm with patients receiving at least some chemotherapy.

Another study at University of California at Los Angeles (UCLA) treated 119 patients with high-grade extremity sarcoma with intraarterial doxorubicin for 3 days before radiation of the anatomic region and wide excision of the tumor.[167] Patients were randomly assigned to observation alone or to five cycles of doxorubicin 45 mg/m² daily as a bolus on two consecutive days, once a month. At a median follow-up time of 28 months, there was no improvement in either disease-free or overall survival in the chemotherapy arm. There was a statistically insignificant improvement in local control rates in the chemotherapy arm (3 of 21 patients vs. 9 of 27 patients in the control arm relapsed). The use of intraarterial preoperative doxorubicin in the control arm complicates comparison with the other adjuvant doxorubicin studies.

At Roswell Park Memorial Institute, 19 patients with stage I uterine sarcoma were randomly assigned to undergo surgery alone or surgery plus adjuvant doxorubicin 60 to 75 mg/m² every 4 weeks for six cycles.[168] No statistically significant difference in survival was noted. Six of the patients randomly assigned to the chemotherapy arm refused randomization and were assessed as part of the control group, instead of using an intention-to-treat analysis.

RANDOMIZED STUDIES OF ADJUVANT COMBINATION CHEMOTHERAPY

In 1983 the NCI issued the first in a series of publications on adjuvant chemotherapy for soft tissue sarcoma of different anatomic sites. A pilot study examined 26 patients with extremity sarcoma grades II and III, treated for local control with amputation or limb-sparing surgery with radiation.[169] These patients were treated postoperatively with escalating dosages of cyclophosphamide (500 to 700 mg/m²) and doxorubicin (50 to 70 mg/m²) every 28 days, with a maximum cumulative dose of 550 mg/m² doxorubicin. This combination was followed by six cycles of intermediate-dose methotrexate (50 to 250 mg/kg with dose escalation). Patients were randomly assigned to receive chemotherapy with or without *Corynebacterium parvum* adjuvant immunotherapy and were compared to historical controls. There was no effect of the immunologic adjuvant, but the overall survival at 5 years was 73%, better than the 45% seen in the historical controls.

These initial data led to examination of adjuvant chemotherapy alone in a second cohort of patients with extremity sarcomas. Sixty-five patients underwent similar local control as described earlier, then were randomly assigned to observation or to the same cyclophosphamide, doxorubicin, and methotrexate regimen of the pilot study.[170] Initial data indicated that disease-free survival and overall survival were improved in the chemotherapy arm. With longer follow-up (median, 7.1 years), 5-year disease-free survival was still improved (75% vs. 54% in the control arm), but the difference in overall survival (83% vs. 60% in the control arm) was not statistically significant.[171] Local control was improved in the chemotherapy arm. In long-term follow-up there has been non–tumor-related mortality; there continues to be no survival advantage in either treatment arm.

Fourteen of the 101 patients treated with the NCI regimen developed clinical congestive heart failure. Other patients had radioventriculograms performed confirming a subclinical decrease in cardiac ejection fraction at rest or with exercise. In all, there was an overall event rate of 46% for clinical or subclinical cardiomyopathy in the 75 evaluated patients.[172] The high rate of cardiomyopathy led to a third trial examining the same cyclophosphamide, doxorubicin, and methotrexate combination versus a regimen without methotrexate and a doxorubicin cumulative dose of 350 mg/m².[171] No difference in 5-year overall survival was observed (69% for low dose, 75% for high dose), nor was there a difference in 5-year disease-free survival. There was no clinical congestive heart failure documented in the low-dose arm, and the decrease in cardiac ejection fraction by nuclear medicine study was less pronounced than in the high-dose arm.

The NCI has also examined adjuvant chemotherapy for tumors at other sites in two other trials, using the same cyclophosphamide, doxorubicin, and methotrexate combination regimen.[173,174] In one study, some of the 37 patients with retroperitoneal sarcoma (15 of whom were prospectively randomly assigned) were given adjuvant chemotherapy.[174] Patients given chemotherapy had a trend to poorer overall survival compared to the control group ($P = .06$). Analysis of this study is difficult because of the small number of patients and lack of prospective randomization for all patients. A separate NCI study using the same chemotherapy regimen examined 31 patients with soft tissue sarcoma of the head and neck, breast, and trunk.[173] All patients had resection and postoperative radiation therapy, then were randomly assigned to receive chemotherapy or no further therapy. Six patients received *C parvum* adjuvant immunotherapy. A trend toward improved disease-free survival was seen in the chemotherapy patients, but there was no statistically significant difference in overall survival.

The M. D. Anderson Cancer Center started one of the earliest adjuvant trials for soft tissue sarcoma.[175] Because of the high local relapse rate, patients with head and neck or abdominal sarcomas all received surgery, radiation, and chemotherapy in this study. Forty-three eligible patients with trunk and extremity sarcomas were treated with local therapy (surgery and radiation) with or without chemotherapy. The chemotherapy regimen consisted of vincristine, oral cyclophosphamide, and doxorubicin every 4 weeks. After seven cycles of doxorubicin-based therapy, dactinomycin was substituted for doxorubicin in a maintenance phase to complete 2 years of chemotherapy. The initial results demonstrated poorer disease-free survival in the chemotherapy arm (76% vs. 83% for the control arm; *P* value not significant) and double the rate of metastasis in the chemotherapy arm (P >.3), and the study was stopped. The original study stratified patients by tumor histologic features, not by tumor grade. In a reanalysis of the data for patients with truncal or extremity sarcomas, disease-free survival was found to be improved in the chemotherapy arm (55% vs. 35% at 10 years; *P* = .05), although there was no difference in overall survival in the two groups.[175]

Another early study of combination chemotherapy was reported by the Mayo Clinic.[176] Sixty-one patients with sarcomas of the trunk or extremities were treated with surgery alone for local control, then randomly assigned to no further therapy or to chemotherapy. The chemotherapy alternated between cycles of vincristine, dactinomycin, and cyclophosphamide and cycles of vincristine, doxorubicin, and dacarbazine, given at 6-week intervals for eight courses. Thirteen patients (randomly selected from either group) were given bacille Calmette-Guérin methanol extraction residue as nonspecific immunotherapy, but this was discontinued owing to ulceration at the injection site. There was no benefit in overall survival in the chemotherapy arm, and there was a high local recurrence rate, likely due to the omission of radiation in the local control phase of therapy. The chemotherapy regimen used in this study had low dose intensity by today's standards.

The largest single study of adjuvant combination chemotherapy in soft tissue sarcoma was performed by the EORTC.[177] Four hundred sixty-eight patients (excluding only those with "very low grade" sarcomas) were treated with surgery for their primary sarcoma and with adjuvant radiation if surgical margins were less than 1 cm. Patients were randomly assigned to receive or not to receive combination chemotherapy with cyclophosphamide, vincristine, doxorubicin, and dacarbazine (CyVADIC; Table 35.1-11), given every 28 days for eight cycles. Disease-free survival and local control were both better in the chemotherapy arm, but overall survival was not significantly different between the two arms. Improvement in local recurrence rates was limited to patients with head, neck, and trunk sarcomas, and was not observed for patients with extremity sarcomas. Some criticism has been

TABLE 35.1-11. Combination Chemotherapy for Sarcoma: A Comparison of Formulations

Regimen	Dose	Comments
DOXORUBICIN	60–90 mg/m^2	Bolus or IVCI over 3–4 d q3wk
IFOSFAMIDE		
24-h continuous dosing	5 g/m^2	24-h IVCI with mesna q3–4wk
High dose	2–4 g/m^2/d	Bolus or IVCI with mesna for 4 d q3–4wk
AD		
Doxorubicin	60 mg/m^2	Bolus or IVCI over 3–4 d q3wk
Dacarbazine	750–1200 mg/m^2	
MAID		
Doxorubicin	60 mg/m^2	Bolus or divided over 3 d by bolus or IVCI q3–4wk
Ifosfamide with mesna	2.0–2.5 g/m^2	Daily × 3 d or IVCI q3–4wk with mesna
Dacarbazine	900–1200 mg/m^2	Bolus or over 3 d IVCI q3–4 wk
AI OR AIM		
Doxorubicin	50–90 mg/m^2	Bolus or divided over 2–3 d by bolus or IVCI q3–4wk
Ifosfamide (with mesna)	5–10 g/m^2	Daily × 3 d or IVCI q3–4wk with mesna
MAP		
Mitomycin C	8 mg/m^2	Bolus q3wk
Doxorubicin	40 mg/m^2	
Cisplatin	60 mg/m^2	
CYVADIC		
Cyclophosphamide	500 mg/m^2	—
Vincristine	1.5 mg/m^2 d 1 and 5; max 2 mg/dose	—
Doxorubicin	50 mg/m^2	Bolus q3wk
Dacarbazine	250 mg/m^2/d × 5	

IVCI, intravenous continuous infusion.

raised as to the long accrual time of the study (11 years), the inability of nearly half the patients to complete all eight cycles of chemotherapy, and the relatively large number of patients ineligible for analysis, which most commonly was due to inappropriate radiation therapy.

A smaller study by the Fondation Bergonié also examined the CyVADIC regimen as adjuvant therapy.[178] After local therapy with surgery and radiation, 59 eligible patients with AJCC stage IIB to IVA tumors were randomly assigned to receive no chemotherapy or CyVADIC chemotherapy, in dosages similar to those used in the EORTC study. In comparison to the EORTC trial, patients were treated with chemotherapy sooner after surgery and on 21-day cycles, whereas 28-day cycles were used in the EORTC study. More patients with extremity sarcomas were in the chemotherapy group, and the histologic features of tumors in the treated groups were different (e.g., more MFH and no "undifferentiated sarcoma" in the chemotherapy arm). In contrast to the EORTC trial, local control, distant metastasis-free survival (*P* = .003), and overall survival (*P* = .002) were better in the chemotherapy arm than in the control arm. However, in comparison to the EORTC study, the chemotherapy arm fared better (5-year survival 85% vs. 68% for the EORTC study), and the control group performed more poorly (5-year survival under 37%, compared to 63% in the EORTC trial).

One of the most important studies of adjuvant chemotherapy for extremity soft tissue sarcomas is that conducted using both an anthracycline (epirubicin) and ifosfamide, performed by the Italian Sarcoma Study Group.[179] After surgery with or without local radiation, 104 patients were randomly assigned to receive no chemotherapy or to receive ifosfamide (1.8 g/m² on five consecutive days) with epirubicin (60 mg/m² on two consecutive days), with filgrastim support. Interim analysis in 1996 led to early conclusion of the trial, because the study had reached its primary end point of improved disease-free survival. At a median follow-up of 36 months, overall survival in the chemotherapy arm was 72%, compared to 55% in the control arm ($P = .002$). This investigation is promising for its use of the two most active classes of agents against sarcoma in an appropriate cohort of patients. Interpretation of the study is made more difficult by the finding of equal rates of distant or local recurrence or both at 4 years as well as by subtle imbalances in the distribution of patients on the control and treatment arms of the study. With longer follow-up, overall and disease-free survival no longer reach a statistical significance level of $P = .05$, but 5-year overall survival is still significantly better with chemotherapy. These data indicate that chemotherapy may delay, but may not ultimately eliminate, metastatic disease.

The data from the Italian randomized study must also be taken into consideration with other data from two smaller studies of adjuvant chemotherapy for extremity sarcomas. The first, a randomized phase II study of the EORTC and National Cancer Institute of Canada, compared doxorubicin 50 mg/m² bolus and ifosfamide 5 g/m² 24-hour infusion every 3 weeks to no adjuvant chemotherapy in 134 evaluable patients with "high-risk" soft tissue sarcomas.[180] Overall and disease-free survival rates were not significantly different in the two treatment arms: overall survival of 64% at 5 years with no chemotherapy versus 65% with chemotherapy ±7%. The major criticism of this study is that it did not achieve the dose intensity of other studies with a similar combination of drugs.

A dose-intensive schedule of chemotherapy was examined in an Austrian study of 59 patients receiving no chemotherapy or doxorubicin 50 mg/m², dacarbazine total dose 800 mg/m², and ifosfamide 6 g/m² every 2 weeks with granulocyte colony-stimulating factor support after surgical resection of the primary sarcoma. Overall and relapse-free survival were not different in the two treatment arms at a mean follow-up of 41 months.[181]

CONCLUSIONS FROM INDIVIDUAL ADJUVANT CHEMOTHERAPY STUDIES

The small size of the adjuvant chemotherapy trials makes interpretation on an individual basis difficult, because most studies had no statistical power to detect small (e.g., 10% to 20%) changes in overall survival. In many of the studies, a significant proportion of patients were ineligible for analysis, which raises the question of selection bias. A second example of selection bias arises from the fact that patients who are enrolled on clinical trials are healthier overall than nonrandomized patients and survive longer, as demonstrated in the Mayo Clinic study.[176] Historical controls are inadequate for comparison because there continue to be advances in diagnosis, specific therapy, and supportive care that could affect outcome.[169]

Beyond general problems with randomized studies, staging and dose intensity also affect the ability to draw conclusions from individual studies. A number of patients with low-grade or small tumors are included in the trials described earlier in Randomized Studies of Adjuvant Doxorubicin Alone and Randomized Studies of Adjuvant Combination Chemotherapy. Patients with high-grade sarcomas do well as long as the primary tumor is small (less than 5 cm). The improved outcome with small, high-grade tumors has been incorporated into the 2002 staging system for sarcoma.[107] It may be most relevant to move forward with studies of adjuvant therapy for specific subtypes of sarcoma, to identify better which might benefit from the use of adjuvant chemotherapy. Furthermore, dose intensity of doxorubicin is low to moderate in many studies of adjuvant chemotherapy to date, and growth factors such as filgrastim were largely unavailable. It is reasonably clear that doxorubicin and ifosfamide show dose-dependent responses,[182,183] and with better supportive care more intensive therapy may lead to improved survival.[179] The authors believe that, if there is any benefit, it is small and merits discussions with patients on a case by case basis.

METAANALYSES OF RANDOMIZED TRIALS OF ADJUVANT CHEMOTHERAPY FOR SARCOMA

Given the lack of statistical power of the existing randomized trials, it was hoped that combining the data from individual studies of adjuvant chemotherapy for sarcoma would reveal improvement in overall survival that could not be detected in smaller studies. For example, to detect a 10% difference between control group and treatment group with a power of 0.90 would require approximately 1000 patients to be enrolled in a randomized study.

Antman and colleagues[163] pooled the data for three randomized studies (ECOG, Dana-Farber Cancer Institute and Massachusetts General Hospital, and the Intergroup studies). The 168 eligible patients examined in this study comprise a smaller group than the EORTC adjuvant trial, but were followed for up to 11 years in some cases. Patients with extremity lesions fared better than those with disease at other sites ($P = .02$), but there was no difference in overall survival in those receiving chemotherapy compared with control patients.

Zalupski et al.[184] examined overall and disease-free survival data for patients with extremity sarcoma obtained from ten of the adjuvant studies mentioned earlier in this chapter in Randomized Studies of Adjuvant Doxorubicin Alone and Randomized Studies of Adjuvant Combination Chemotherapy. Only patients eligible for the study were included in the analysis. The combined data indicated a 10% absolute improvement in overall survival (from 71% to 81%; $P = .0005$) and a 15% improvement in disease-free survival (53% vs. 68%; $P<.00001$). Criticism of this metaanalysis includes the fact that potentially inappropriate patients were being included (e.g., those in the Rizzoli and UCLA studies who received preoperative chemotherapy) and some of the data were immature, such as the EORTC and Bergonié studies.

Tierney and colleagues assessed 15 published studies 2 years later and converted the survival data into the odds of recurrence based on the latest available publication from each trial.[185] Standardization was performed to account for different lengths of follow-up. In all, 1546 patients were included in the study, which showed improved survival at 2 years and at 5 years in the 13 and 11 studies eligible for analysis at each time point, respectively. In contrast to the previous metaanalysis from

Zalupski et al.,[184] the Rizzoli data were included in this study, but not the data from UCLA.

The most rigorous metaanalysis regarding adjuvant chemotherapy for soft tissue sarcoma was published in 1997.[186] In this analysis, 23 potential studies were considered and 14 ultimately included; only 31 potential patients were omitted due to unavailability of data, which gave a cohort of 1568 patients to examine. Patient accrual had to be complete by the end of 1992, which excluded one trial. Tumor histology for each patient was recorded, but pathology review was not centralized. Median follow-up was 9.4 years. Analyses were stratified by trial, and hazard ratios were calculated for each trial and combined, which allowed for an assessment of the risk of death or recurrence in comparison to control patients. Disease-free survival at 10 years was found to be improved from 45% to 55%, and the difference was statistically significant ($P = .0001$). Local disease-free survival at 10 years also favored the chemotherapy arm, improving from 75% to 81% ($P = .016$). However, although overall survival improved at 10 years from 50% to 54%, the difference was not statistically significant ($P = .12$). The largest difference in overall survival was found in subgroup analysis of the 886 patients with extremity sarcomas: Absolute overall survival was shown to increase 7% in the group receiving chemotherapy ($P = .029$).

CONCLUSIONS: ADJUVANT CHEMOTHERAPY FOR SOFT TISSUE SARCOMAS

The data from the metaanalyses, like those from the multiple randomized studies, must be examined with caution. Although the 1997 metaanalysis[186] is a useful tool, it still combines studies with different designs, diverse criteria for enrollment, variations in pathologic assessment such as grading, different chemotherapeutic regimens, and different end points. In particular, only one-fourth of the specimens in the metaanalysis underwent review of tumor grade; approximately 60% were reviewed for histologic subtype. Of 15 published adjuvant studies included in the metaanalysis, only 2—the Rizzoli and Bergonié studies—show improved overall survival in the chemotherapy arm.

Only one small study included in the 1997 metaanalysis used ifosfamide, another active agent in sarcoma. Three studies since the 1997 metaanalysis show conflicting results regarding the benefit of anthracycline- and ifosfamide-based chemotherapy.

If there is a benefit for the adjuvant use of chemotherapy, it appears modest, based on the aforementioned data. Given the lack of a statistically significant benefit in a population of patients typically healthier than patients not enrolled on protocols, the data do not support the routine use of adjuvant chemotherapy for soft tissue sarcoma outside of the setting of a clinical trial. However, moderate to large extremity lesions represent one situation in which adjuvant chemotherapy may be considered in a case by case basis. However, knowing that disease-free survival is improved with chemotherapy may be a rationale for some physicians or patients to proceed with adjuvant chemotherapy. As the Italian Sarcoma Study Group investigation and the subset analysis of the metaanalysis of 1997 indicate, extremity soft tissue sarcomas represent one situation in which adjuvant chemotherapy can be considered. Given the lack of consensus regarding this issue, the treatment of patients with adjuvant chemotherapy remains a situation best reserved for clinical trials. The authors hope this issue can be better addressed by better analysis of patient tumors for sensitivity by gene arrays, proteomics, and other means, and by identification of new agents active against soft tissue sarcoma.

PREOPERATIVE CHEMOTHERAPY

Preoperative chemotherapy has been very successful in the management of predominantly pediatric sarcomas such as Ewing's sarcoma and osteosarcoma. With this success, the concept was extended to adult soft tissue sarcomas. Preoperative, or neoadjuvant, chemotherapy can make subsequent surgery easier and potentially treats micrometastatic disease early before acquisition of resistance. Treating with chemotherapy before surgery also leaves primary vasculature intact for drug delivery. In addition, preoperative chemotherapy can guide postoperative treatment based on pathologic review of the tissue response after chemotherapy. In experimental models, preoperative chemotherapy eliminates a postoperative surge in growth of metastases noted after resection of primary tumors.[187,188]

There is relatively little evidence concerning the use of neoadjuvant chemotherapy in the treatment of soft tissue sarcomas. Rouesse et al. retrospectively examined a group of 34 patients with locally advanced sarcomas for whom only amputation or mutilating surgery was feasible.[189] Patients received doxorubicin-based chemotherapy for two to seven cycles before resection. Postoperative radiation was offered to some patients. Partial or complete responses were noted in more than one-third of patients; not surprisingly, those patients who had a complete response by any means had a better overall survival than those who did not respond completely.

A retrospective trial of 46 patients at M. D. Anderson Cancer Center examined preoperative chemotherapy using cyclophosphamide, doxorubicin, and dacarbazine.[190] Forty percent of patients demonstrated complete, partial, or minor responses to chemotherapy and had better rates of survival than the patients who did not have an objective clinical response to chemotherapy.

A prospective trial was performed at MSKCC in which 29 patients with large, high-grade primary tumors or recurrent metastases were given two cycles of combination chemotherapy before definitive therapy with surgery and radiation.[191] Clinical and radiologic studies were performed before chemotherapy, and the specimen was assessed for response after surgical resection. Only 1 of 29 patients demonstrated a clinical partial response, although liquefaction, cystic necrosis, and hemorrhage into the tumor were noted regularly in the resected specimens, with three tumors showing more than 90% necrosis. Most patients did not elect to receive postoperative chemotherapy, and survival results for this study did not differ significantly from those for studies using adjuvant doxorubicin or no chemotherapy.

Assessing the response to preoperative chemotherapy in primary soft tissue sarcomas is difficult. Some softening or liquefaction can be noted clinically without significant change in tumor size, but in the trial at MSKCC neither CT nor MRI provided information that predicted long-term outcome. It appears that there are significantly fewer cases of complete response than with preoperative adjuvant chemotherapy for sarcoma of bone (osteosarcoma or Ewing's sarcoma), and it is difficult to objectively evaluate responses grossly or microscopically after chemotherapy. Other imaging modalities may demonstrate changes consistent with a chemotherapeutic effect

(MRI spectroscopy, PET, gallium scan, thallium scan),[192-194] but these modalities remain investigational.

In sum, preoperative chemotherapy has been given to some patients with high-grade sarcomas with poor risk features in whom the chance of recurrence well exceeds 50%. It is unclear whether distant or local control is improved with this approach, so it remains investigational. Nonetheless, preoperative chemotherapy is worth consideration during an attempt to maintain function of an extremity. Selected patients have had responses that allow for a more conservative resection or have avoided the need for amputation.

INTRAARTERIAL CHEMOTHERAPY

There have been many studies examining the role of intraarterial chemotherapy with doxorubicin, cisplatin, or both; in some situations other drugs have been used as well. This infusional approach is to be differentiated from local limb perfusion, discussed later in this chapter in Hyperthermia and Limb Perfusion. Intraarterial chemotherapy has the potential benefit of providing higher doses of chemotherapy to the limb in a first-pass effect. However, pharmacokinetic data have not shown an advantage over intravenous chemotherapy.

Intraarterial chemotherapy has been used in conjunction with radiation as well. In a neoadjuvant study at UCLA, patients received 3 days of intraarterial doxorubicin before administration of 35-Gy external-beam radiation over 10 days, or 17.5 Gy administered over 5 days.[195] Patients were then randomly assigned to receive postoperative doxorubicin intravenously or no further chemotherapy. No difference in survival or local control was noted in this study. Thereafter, a randomized trial by the same group examined preoperative intravenous versus intraarterial chemotherapy before radiation (28 Gy given over 8 days) followed by wide excision. There was no difference in local recurrence or survival between the 45 patients receiving intraarterial doxorubicin and the 54 patients receiving intravenous doxorubicin.[196]

A number of studies have examined intraarterial chemotherapy before radiation and surgery, doxorubicin alone[196] or in combination with other drugs such as cisplatin, single-agent intraarterial cisplatin, or intraarterial doxorubicin in combination with intravenous doxorubicin or other agents.[197] Doxorubicin with simultaneous radiation has also been examined.[198,199] In these studies, some patients have been able to avoid amputation. Infusional chemotherapy has its attendant complications, including arterial thromboembolism, infection, gangrene, and problems with wound healing, requiring amputation. Pathologic fractures have been reported in patients receiving chemotherapy and relatively large doses of radiation. One study[199] reported ten major complications in 13 patients treated with intraarterial chemotherapy with simultaneous radiation, which emphasizes the investigational nature of this approach. Although there are situations in which such therapy should be considered, intraarterial chemotherapy at present has a limited role in the treatment of extremity sarcomas.

HYPERTHERMIA AND LIMB PERFUSION

In contrast to systemic intraarterial chemotherapy infusion, perfusion of limbs requires isolating the arterial and venous system of the limb by means of a tourniquet and obtaining access to arteries and veins supplying the limb. The arterial and venous supply of the limb is connected to an extracorporeal circulation system to isolate the limb from the rest of the body. Recirculation of the blood from the limb is performed by a heart-lung machine to reoxygenate the blood. Care is taken after isolation of the limb to insure that there is no leakage of the circuit into the systemic circulation; technetium-labeled albumin is injected into the circuit and a probe is used over the heart to insure isolation of the bypass circuit. Because mild hyperthermia may make chemotherapy more effective in some clinical settings (as mentioned later in this section), the blood of the circuit is often warmed to 39° to 40°C.

A number of chemotherapeutic agents have been used for limb perfusion, such as melphalan, nitrogen mustard, dactinomycin, and doxorubicin. The most effective agent to date has been melphalan when given with tumor necrosis factor (TNF). The greatest experience with this technique comes from Eggermont et al.[200,201] Two hundred forty-six patients with primary or recurrent sarcomas that would otherwise require amputation or marked loss of function were treated with one and occasionally two isolated limb perfusion sessions. After isolation of the extremity, melphalan (10 to 13 mg/L limb volume) was perfused into the limb with a dose of TNF ten times the lethal dose for humans, under mild hyperthermic conditions. In early studies interferon-α was included in the regimen, but it was later dropped because it did not appear to improve results over melphalan and TNF alone. Both components of the regimen appeared important; the omission of TNF led to a decrease in tissue dose of melphalan, probably from its effects on the tumor vasculature. Surgery to remove residual tumor was performed 2 to 4 months after limb perfusion. With a median follow-up of 3 years, 71% of patients had successful limb salvage.

It is difficult to compare this approach to standard chemotherapy, given the heterogeneity of patients in the two types of studies. In aggregate, the response rate does appear higher in the perfusion studies than in the infusion studies. However, isolated limb perfusion requires substantial expertise and specialized dedicated equipment. Complications of this technique include shock (from systemic leak of TNF); infection; chronic damage to skin, muscles, and nerve; persistent edema; and arterial or venous thrombosis. Experience has led to a decrease in the incidence and severity of complications. Isolated limb perfusion does appear to hold promise for at least a subset of patients who would otherwise require amputation for local control and has been approved for such patients in Europe. Studies are under way to examine the use of regional limb infusion, which would not require bypass machines, as a simplified means of treating otherwise unresectable extremity sarcomas.

Hyperthermia has been used in other ways to enhance the effects of chemotherapy in patients with locally advanced disease. Whole body hyperthermia using extracorporeal heating of blood has been combined with ifosfamide and carboplatin intravenous chemotherapy, and responses have been seen in patients with otherwise refractory small cell sarcomas.[202] Regional hyperthermia provided through an external electromagnetic field (phased array) has been examined in combination with ifosfamide and etoposide as well as other combinations of chemotherapy.[203-205] In a series of studies over the last 20 years or more, investigators have demonstrated partial and complete responses in patients with locally advanced and metastatic soft tissue sarcoma. The hyperthermia used in these protocols is more aggressive than that used with limb perfusion; higher temperatures have led to a higher rate of local complications. Isolated limb perfusion has not been compared directly with simultaneous hyperthermia and chemotherapy. Isolated limb perfusion and hyperthermia-enhanced chemotherapy represent novel ways of attempting to preserve function of limbs in what otherwise would be situations in which amputation would be necessary. In the United States, such procedures remain investigational; the most advanced studies with this modality are being performed in Europe.

SPECIAL FEATURES OF THE MANAGEMENT OF SARCOMAS OF NONEXTREMITY SITES

MANAGEMENT OF VISCERAL OR RETROPERITONEAL SARCOMA

Clinical Presentation

Most patients present with an asymptomatic abdominal mass (Fig. 35.1-28). On occasion pain is present, and less common symptoms include gastrointestinal bleeding, incomplete obstruction, and neurologic symptoms related to retroperitoneal invasion or pressure on neurovascular structures. Weight loss is uncommon and incidental diagnosis is the norm. In one report,[206] neurologic symptoms related primarily to an expanding retroperitoneal mass were identified in 27% of patients.

On physical examination, a large abdominal mass is often present. Important issues of differential diagnosis, particularly in the young, are the presence of a germ cell tumor, lymphoma, or primary retroperitoneal tumor arising from the adrenal. Most of such lesions, however, are tumors of mesenchymal origin, either benign or malignant.

Imaging Studies

CT remains the primary modality for evaluation of retroperitoneal and visceral sarcomas. Because the most likely site of vis-

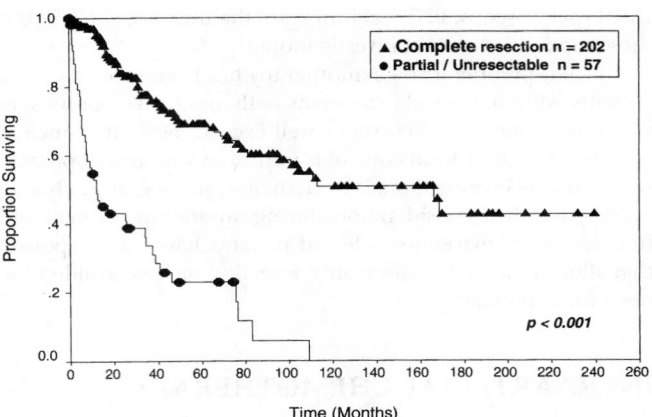

FIGURE 35.1-29. Survival after resection of primary retroperitoneal sarcoma according to resection status in 259 patients aged 16 years or older admitted to Memorial Sloan-Kettering Cancer Center between July 1982 and July 1992, follow-up to December 2002.

ceral metastasis is the liver, a CT scan of the abdomen and pelvis encompasses the primary lesion and the most likely site of metastasis.

Retroperitoneal and visceral sarcomas account for approximately 30% of all sarcomas. The most common histopathologic types in the retroperitoneum are liposarcoma (40%), leiomyosarcoma (25%), MPNST, and fibrosarcoma. In the visceral location GIST, leiomyosarcoma, and desmoid are the most common histologic types seen (see Fig. 35.1-4). Approximately 55% of retroperitoneal liposarcomas are well differentiated and low grade with tumors in roughly 40% of patients showing dedifferentiated, high-grade histologic features at primary presentation. Primary surgical resection is the dominant therapeutic modality. Preoperative bowel preparation is important, not because of tumor invasion but because of the frequent technical difficulty of performing resection without encompassing the intestine. Because many tumors involve the retroperitoneum, evaluation of renal function, particularly the establishment of contralateral adequate renal function, is important to allow nephrectomy when appropriate.

Although resection of adjacent organs is common,[206] proof that a more extensive resection of adjacent organs has impact on long-term survival seems very limited. It is clear that complete surgical resection is the primary factor in outcome (Fig. 35.1-29). Once complete resection is accounted for, the predominant factor in outcome is the grade of the lesion.

Technical Issues

The major issue in resection of visceral and retroperitoneal lesions is adequate exposure. Thoracoabdominal incisions, rectus-dividing incisions, incisions extending through the inguinal ligament into the thigh, the availability of venovenous bypass, adequate and appropriate anesthetic, and blood replacement therapy are all important issues for many of these large lesions. Resectability rates vary widely but seem independent of histologic type, grade, or size.[206]

Complete resection is usually possible in 60% to 70% of patients presenting with a second or subsequent recurrence. In two reviews,[206,207] although nephrectomy was performed in 46%

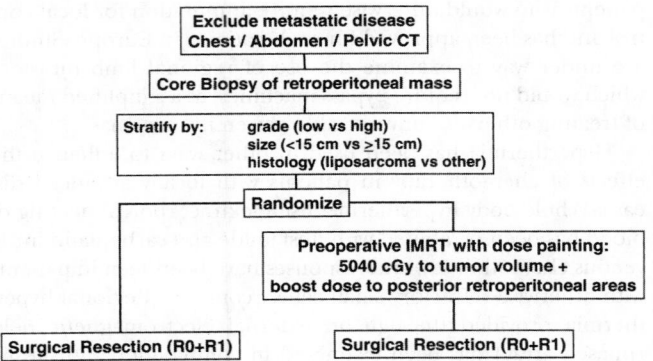

FIGURE 35.1-28. Algorithm for the management of retroperitoneal or visceral sarcoma based on a phase III randomized trial. CT, computed tomography; IMRT, intensity-modulated radiotherapy.

of cases, the kidney itself was rarely involved. In the report by Jaques and coworkers,[206] only 2 of 30 nephrectomy specimens showed true parenchymal invasion. Nevertheless, the encompassment of the kidney and the involvement of the hilar renal vasculature all make the resection of the kidney often necessary.

The overriding principle is not to be reticent about resection of adjacent organs should they be involved by tumor. Conversely, one should not resect uninvolved organs if they are not the limiting factor for the tumor margin. The resection of a kidney when the vena cava is the closest margin makes little oncologic sense. Overall, the use of debulking for recurrent lesions is of limited value in terms of long-term survival. More extended resections do not seem to improve local recurrence or survival. It is often difficult to decide how much palliation can be achieved by incomplete removal of tumor. The concept should be that, unless palliation can be achieved, operation should be reserved for those patients for whom complete resection is at least possible, if not probable. In retroperitoneal liposarcoma, there is some evidence that incomplete resection is associated with prolonged survival.[208] The basis for unresectability is usually the presence of peritoneal implants or extensive vascular involvement.

Retroperitoneal sarcomas remain a major clinical challenge. Most of these tumors are large, making it difficult to obtain adequate margins of resection. Compounding the problem, the presence of normal organs such as small bowel, large bowel, kidney, and liver make delivery of therapeutic doses of radiation therapy either difficult or impossible.

Jaques et al.[206] reported the experience at MSKCC from 1982 to 1987. Half the patients presented with liposarcoma, whereas 29% had leiomyosarcoma. Sixty-five percent of patients with primary sarcomas underwent a complete resection, whereas approximately half the patients with recurrent retroperitoneal sarcomas could have a complete resection. Despite complete resection, local recurrence developed in 40% to 50% of cases. There is a clear need for adjuvant local therapy. Importantly, local recurrence is a problem for both high-grade and low-grade lesions: The local recurrence rate is similar, but the time to recurrence differs significantly. The median time for recurrence was 15 months for high-grade and 42 months for low-grade sarcomas. Fifty-three percent of patients required adjacent organ resection, and 40% of patients required more than one adjacent organ resection, to accomplish complete removal of disease.

Adjuvant EBRT is limited because of the low tolerance of surrounding normal organs. However, there are data to suggest some improvement in local control with moderate doses of external-beam irradiation.[209,210] Tepper and associates[211] reviewed a cohort of 23 patients with retroperitoneal sarcomas treated with surgery and radiation therapy. For patients who underwent a complete resection, local control was 71%. Radiation dose appeared to influence tumor control, with only 30% of patients having local control at doses less than 5000 cGy and 83% of patients having control with doses greater than 6000 cGy. Obviously, the total dose of radiation that is possible varies with the size and location of that lesion.

With the need to deliver higher doses of radiation to the tumor and lower doses to surrounding tissue, there has been an interest in using IORT.[212,213] Petersen et al. at the Mayo Clinic reported on 87 patients who were treated with IORT, which was supplemented by external-beam radiation in 80 of 87. With a median follow-up of 3 years, the 5-year local control and survival rates were 58% and 50%, respectively.[121] Sindelar and coworkers[214] reported on a prospective, randomized clinical trial using intraoperative radiation therapy at the NCI. Thirty-five patients with surgically resected sarcomas of the retroperitoneum were randomly assigned to receive IORT (20 Gy) followed by low-dose EBRT (35 to 40 Gy) or EBRT alone (50 to 55 Gy). The study revealed a significant improvement in local control for those who received IORT. There was no impact on survival. Patients who received IORT also received misonidazole, and they had a higher incidence of peripheral neuropathy than those who received EBRT alone. On the other hand, those who received higher-dose EBRT alone, without IORT, had a higher incidence of radiation enteritis.

At MSKCC, resection was combined with EBRT and high dose-rate intraoperative BRT (HDR-IOBRT) in an attempt to optimize treatment effect and minimize toxicity to critical anatomy.[215] A phase I and II trial was reported in which 32 patients with primary and recurrent retroperitoneal sarcoma underwent resection and HDR-IOBRT (1200 to 1500 cGy). Twenty-five patients were treated with EBRT (4500 to 5040 cGy) after resection. The high dose-rate iridium 192 was delivered with a Harrison-Anderson-Mick flexible silicone applicator that readily conforms to the tumor bed. The median HDR-IOBRT procedure time was 110 minutes (range, 30 to 240 minutes). Median follow-up was 33 months and overall 5-year local recurrence–free survival was 62%. Five-year actuarial rates of local control for primary and recurrent tumors were 74% and 54%, respectively. These rates were not significantly different when analyzed according to histologic grade. Treatment-related morbidity was observed in 34% of patients. The most common complication was gastrointestinal obstruction (n = 6, 19%: 5 grade 3, 1 grade 5), followed by gastrointestinal fistula (n = 3, 9%: 2 grade 3, 1 grade 5). Peripheral neuropathy is a common complication of IORT; this developed in only 2 (6%, both grade 2) of the patients. Treatment-related mortality was 6% (n = 2).

Given the morbidity associated with IORT and its inherent limitations in large tumor beds, it is unlikely that such an approach would be applicable to most primary retroperitoneal sarcomas. The ideal radiation approach is the one that could dose-escalate preoperative radiation. With conventional radiation it is impossible to escalate preoperative radiation beyond 5040 cGy without incurring excessive toxicity. However, with a dose-painting preoperative IMRT approach, targeted dose escalation to areas at highest risk is achievable. The whole tumor volume will receive 5040 cGy and thus the tolerance is respected, while at the same time the posterior structures, where there are no intestines, will receive 6000 cGy. A report from the University of Alabama showed the feasibility of such an approach of boost within the field. In that study, 14 patients were treated with preoperative radiation to the whole target volume to 4500 cGy; then the area that was judged to be at risk for positive margin at the time of resection was separately boosted with IMRT to bring the total dose to 5750 cGy. Only one patient experienced grade 3 nausea and vomiting. Eleven patients had complete resection with negative margins. With a median follow-up of 12 months there was no late toxicity related to radiation. Further dosimetric studies showed the technical feasibility of delivering doses as high as 7520 to 8280 cGy using this technique.[216]

A prospective, randomized trial of preoperative IMRT with dose painting is now under way at MSKCC to determine whether preoperative IMRT in addition to resection improves local control and hence survival compared to resection alone in patients with primary retroperitoneal sarcoma.

MANAGEMENT OF HEAD AND NECK SARCOMA

Soft tissue sarcomas of the head and neck in adults are rare. They represent approximately 1% of all head and neck malignancies and 10% of all soft tissue sarcomas. Most of these tumors present as a painless subcutaneous or submucosal mass. Any histologic type of soft tissue sarcoma can originate in the head and neck area, but there is preponderance of angiosarcoma in the scalp. A multimodality approach is required for most soft tissue sarcomas of the head and neck. Surgery is the primary treatment, and every attempt should be made to obtain gross total resection. Unlike extremity sarcomas, head and neck sarcomas are not amenable to wide local excision with generous margins of normal tissue due to anatomical constraints. The use of adjuvant radiation is more liberal in this site, because local recurrence can be the cause of death.

Eeles et al. reported on 103 patients with soft tissue sarcoma of the head and neck area treated by surgery with or without radiation. The 5-year survival rate was 50% and the local control rate was 47%. The only independent prognostic factor for survival was surgery other than biopsy ($P = .003$). For local control the combined use of surgery and radiation as opposed to a single treatment modality was an independent prognostic factor ($P = .002$). Local tumor was the cause of death in 63% of cases.[217] Willers et al. reported on 46 patients with soft tissue sarcoma excluding angiosarcoma, who were treated by radiation with or without surgery. The 5-year survival and local control rates were 74% and 69%, respectively. On multivariate analysis survival correlated with low grade, recurrent presentation, and lack of direct extension ($P = .001, .01,$ and $.03$, respectively). For local control the only independent prognostic factor was the T stage ($P = .05$). There was a 15-fold increased risk of dying for patients whose tumor had recurred locoregionally, compared to those with controlled sarcomas ($P = .004$).[218]

Le et al. reported on 65 patients treated by surgery with or without radiation and found the 5-year survival and local control rates to be 56% and 66%, respectively. On multivariate analysis, the independent predictors of improved survival were age younger than 55 years ($P = .009$), low grade ($P = .0002$), extent of resection ($P = .008$), and negative margins ($P = .0009$). For local control, smaller tumor size ($P = .004$) and grade 1 or 2 ($P = .01$) were independent predictors.[219]

Angiosarcoma of the head and neck deserves special consideration because of its poor prognosis compared to other sarcomas.[218–220] Difficulty in management is due to the propensity to infiltrate throughout the dermis beyond what is clinically apparent, which makes wide local excision with negative margins difficult, and the high incidence of regional lymph node metastasis (10% to 15%) compared to other sarcomas.

Morrison et al. reported on 14 patients with angiosarcoma of the head and neck treated by radiation with or without surgery. The 5-year overall and distant metastasis–free survival rates were 29% and 37%, respectively. The 5-year above-clavicle local control rates were 24% with definitive radiation compared to 40% with adjuvant radiation ($P = .03$).[221] Similar findings were reported by Willers et al. for 11 patients, with 5-year overall, distant metastasis–free, and local recurrence–free survival rates of 31%, 42%, and 24%, respectively.[218]

MANAGEMENT OF BREAST SARCOMA

Primary soft tissue sarcomas of the breast are very rare, representing approximately 1% of all breast malignancies. They usually present as a painless mass with no distinctive findings on mammography. The main treatment is surgery. The extent of resection is debatable, but most authors believe that wide excision with generous negative margins is adequate.[222] North et al. reported on 25 patients treated by surgery with or without radiation. The 5-year overall survival rate was 61%, which did not vary significantly between those treated with wide excision and those who underwent mastectomy ($P = .9$). Five patients received adjuvant radiation and none of them developed local recurrence.[223]

Gutman et al. reported similar findings for 60 cases of breast sarcoma treated by surgery with or without radiation.[224] Johnstone et al. reported on ten patients treated with mastectomy and adjuvant radiation. The 5-year survival rate was 66% with no local or regional failures.[225]

SERIOUS COMPLICATIONS OF PRIMARY TREATMENT

WOUND COMPLICATIONS

It is well established that radiation and chemotherapy inhibit wound healing. Early studies defined the effects of doxorubicin and x-ray treatment on wound healing in animal models.[226] The authors demonstrated that the timing and the combination of multiple antineoplastic agents were critical to inhibiting wound healing. They suggested that radiation or antineoplastic drugs delivered more than 7 days before or after the wound creation were accompanied by minimal inhibition of wound healing. Conversely, the application of radiation or chemotherapy just before, or in close juxtaposition to, the time of wounding, resulted in significant impairment of wound healing, as demonstrated by wound-breaking strength. This appeared to be due to inhibition of newly synthesized collagen as determined by hydroxyproline assays.

Assessment of the influence of preoperative chemotherapy on the risk of wound complications is a complex topic.[227] Perhaps the most comprehensive study is that reported by the M. D. Anderson Cancer Center.[228] The authors compared morbidity of radical surgery in soft tissue sarcoma in 104 patients who received induction chemotherapy before surgery and in 204 patients who had surgery first. The most common complications were wound infections and other wound complications; more importantly, however, the incidence of surgical complications was no different for patients undergoing preoperative chemotherapy than for patients undergoing surgery alone in those with sarcomas of the limbs (34% vs. 41%) and in those with retroperitoneal or visceral sarcomas (29% vs. 34%). It must be recognized that the data are sparse, based entirely on retrospective design, and the effects of preoperative chemotherapy are often confounded by the concomitant use of radiotherapy also given preoperatively (as is the case in the concurrent radiotherapy-

MAID protocol discussed in Definitive Radiation, earlier in this chapter).[229] One of the more popular delivery methods for preoperative chemotherapy has been the intraarterial route, often combined with radiotherapy at the same time with apparently greater morbidity than when radiotherapy is given alone.[230] Therefore, there is additional complexity in inferring risk to "usual" chemotherapy delivered intravenously, and an independent effect of chemotherapy on surgical morbidity is difficult to evaluate. Although much of the data seem to suggest that chemotherapy alone does not add to the risk, one small study claims uniqueness in observing a heightened risk, although again other adjuvant approaches included EBRT and BRT.[231]

In the MSKCC studies of adjuvant BRT and wound complications, it was also demonstrated that, when particular attention is paid to the timing of delivery of radiation via afterloading catheters to beyond the fifth postoperative day, the major wound complication rate approaches that with surgery alone.[135]

More recently, wound complications (wound infection or the need for further operative intervention) were analyzed in the randomized BRT trial at MSKCC.[145] The overall complication rate was 24% in the BRT arm compared to 15% in the control arm ($P = .18$). However, the rate of reoperation was higher in the BRT group, 9% versus 1% ($P = .03$). The other covariable that contributed to wound reoperation was the width of the excised skin. If the width was more than 4 cm, the rate was 9%, but if the width was 4 cm or less, the rate was 1% ($P = .02$). These types of complications are not unique to BRT but have been shown with external-beam irradiation as well.[115,232,233] In the Canadian trial comparing preoperative and postoperative irradiation discussed in Rationale for Postoperative External-Beam Radiation Therapy, earlier in this chapter, wound complication was a primary end point of the study, which accrued 190 patients. Wound complications were defined as secondary wound surgery, hospital admission for wound care, or need for deep packing or prolonged dressings within 120 days after tumor resection (Table 35.1-12). Patients undergoing preoperative radiation had a significantly higher rate of wound complications (35% vs. 17%; $P = .01$).[115]

One of the features of the Canadian study was that the criteria for an acute wound complication were built into the study design from its inception and were prospectively applied with a specific requirement for reporting at frequently defined time points for the initial 4 months after surgery. It is also notable that, using these criteria, postoperative radiotherapy also showed an appreciable risk of wound complications (17%). The application of criteria in this way results in reporting of wound complications more frequently than is ordinarily seen in retrospective evaluations. The complications of prolonged dressings or packing (often administered to outpatients) may be overlooked in patients evaluated retrospectively at a remote interval from the time of surgery. In the actual study used to develop the wound complication criteria that the present authors later used in their randomized trial, the authors found that the wound complication rate after preoperative radiotherapy and primary direct wound closure was 16% and seemed to be lower in those treated with vascularized tissue transfer.[233] This lower rate and the rate of 29% in the retrospectively evaluated concurrent chemotherapy-MAID report[122] contrast with those found in the authors' prospective trial of adjuvant radiotherapy alone.[123]

In situations in which wound complications may be anticipated because of the magnitude of the wound, extent of the

TABLE 35.1-12. Incidence of Major Wound Complications with Criteria for 182 Evaluable Cases in the Canadian Trial Comparing Preoperative and Postoperative Radiotherapy (n = 190)

	Preoperative n (%)	Postoperative n (%)
WOUND COMPLICATION IN ALL CASES[a]		
Yes	31 (35)	16 (17)
No	57 (65)	78 (83)
CRITERIA FOR DECLARATION OF MAJOR WOUND COMPLICATION		
(1) Secondary operation (débridement, operative drainage, secondary closure, e.g., rotationplasty, free flaps, or skin grafts) for wound repair	14 (45)	5 (31)
(2) Invasive procedure for wound management without (1)	5 (16)	4 (25)
(3) Deep wound packing deep to dermis in area of wound of at least 2 cm and/or prolonged dressings >6 wk from wound breakdown without (1) or (2)	11 (35.5)	7 (44)
(4) Readmission for wound care without (1), (2), or (3)	1 (3)	0 (0)
TOTAL COMPLICATIONS	31 (100)	16 (100)
TOTAL EVALUABLE CASES	88 (100)	94 (100)

Note: Two patients required amputation due to complications (both were treated with preoperative radiotherapy).
[a]$P = .01$.
(Modified from ref. 115, with permission.)

resection, prior radiation, and so on, serious consideration should be given to bringing fresh vascularized tissue in the form of either transpositional or free grafts into the area to cover the defect before the placement or delivery of radiation therapy. With this approach, postoperative morbidity can be markedly diminished. This is difficult to prove, because selection bias often determines the use of nonprimary closure when cases can be expected to have larger tumors and more problematic resections. In the Canadian trial, when multivariate analysis was used, the only significant variables for wound complication were the timing of radiotherapy (i.e., preoperative vs. postoperative), the volume of tissue removed at surgery, and the location of the tumor (upper vs. lower extremity). The manner in which the wound was closed, comorbidity, age, smoking history, and treatment center had no apparent influence on the risk.[115]

These results merit a final comment in relation to the role of anatomic sites in the risk of wound complication. As noted, the risk of wound complication appears to be almost entirely confined to lower extremity lesions.[115,122] This observation is of interest because it implies that the choice of postoperative radiotherapy to possibly avoid a wound complication is less relevant for some anatomic sites. This may be advantageous in sites for which restriction of radiotherapy dose and volumes may be of benefit in the long term (e.g., overlying brachial plexus and lung in proximal arm lesions). Other sites to which this also applies are the head and neck, where critical anatomy often restricts the dose and volumes of radiotherapy, which may explain the inferior cancer control results that are seen. The authors have reported the outcome of a prospective series which shows that the head and neck are a site of soft tissue sarcoma with relatively low wound complication rates even in cases specifically selected for preoperative radiotherapy because of adverse anatomic presentations. Frequently these included lesions in the skull base, for which the choice was made based on the wish to avoid the optic apparatus, spine, and brainstem.[234]

OTHER COMPLICATIONS

The impact of adjuvant radiation and chemotherapy on the development of bony fracture has been reported in the literature, but the data are scant. Stinson et al. reported on 145 patients with soft tissue sarcoma who underwent limb-sparing surgery and postoperative radiation with or without chemotherapy and found a 6% fracture rate.[235] For patients treated with adjuvant BRT in the MSKCC randomized trial, the rate of fracture was 4% compared to 0% in the control arm. This difference was not statistically significant ($P = .2$).[236] Helmstedter et al. reported a fracture rate of 7% and felt that the dose, timing, and fractionation of radiation therapy were not related to the risk of fracture. A high rate of complications was seen with this series, including fracture nonunion (45%) and deep infection (20%). These authors suggest that prophylactic intramedullary fixation of the femur should be considered for patients undergoing resection of large tumors in the anterior compartment of the thigh requiring extensive periosteal stripping and adjuvant radiation therapy.[237]

Lin et al. evaluated 205 patients with soft tissue sarcoma of the thigh to determine the factors contributing to pathologic fracture of the femur in patients treated with adjuvant radiation (115 patients were treated with BRT alone, EBRT was used in 59, and 31 received a combination of EBRT and BRT). The 5-year actuarial risk was 8.6%, which on univariate analysis correlated with periosteal stripping ($P = .0001$), location in the anterior compartment ($P = .008$), female gender ($P = .01$), the use of chemotherapy ($P = .02$), age of 50 years or older ($P = .03$), and the use of EBRT instead of BRT ($P = .04$). On multivariate analysis only periosteal stripping retained significance ($P = .01$).[238]

These results can be compared with data from the Princess Margaret Hospital, where a long-term prospective series of 364 patients with lower extremity sarcomas treated with combined EBRT and limb-salvage surgery (without adjuvant chemotherapy) showed a significantly higher rate of pathologic fractures with higher radiotherapy doses (60 or 66 Gy; rate of 10%) than with lower doses (50 Gy; rate of 2%), and a higher rate of fracture when radiation therapy was given postoperatively than when it was given preoperatively.[239] It is conceivable that the use of BRT in the majority of patients in the MSKCC study, even when moderate postoperative EBRT was also used (31 of 205 patients), confers an advantage over conventional full-dose postoperative radiotherapy, which carried the highest risk in the Princess Margaret Hospital study. This advantage in reducing the risk of fracture may be exerted through better dose conformity with BRT and overall lower dose as used in preoperative EBRT.

The other complication encountered with adjuvant radiation is peripheral nerve damage. In the MSKCC randomized trial the rate was 5% in the control arm compared to 9% in the BRT arm ($P = .5$).[141] Le Pechoux et al. reported a rate of 1.6%

of peripheral nerve damage in 62 patients treated with postoperative radiation.[128] Brant et al. reported a 3.4% rate for patients treated with preoperative radiation.[240]

A common concern practitioners have about postoperative radiotherapy is the tolerance of bone grafting used during musculoskeletal reconstructions. Evidence suggests that postoperative radiotherapy can ordinarily be administered without detriment to graft union 3 to 4 weeks after grafting.[241] For soft tissue reconstruction (e.g., tissue transfer in the form of pedicle flaps, free flaps, or skin grafts) to repair surgical defects, there is theoretical risk for wound breakdown related to radiotherapy that may require reoperation. This risk has now been shown to be very low (5%), and most tissue transfers tolerate subsequent adjuvant radiation therapy well.[242] The authors did observe that more wound complications necessitating reoperation were seen in patients who received BRT. It is unclear whether this relates to the inherent susceptibility of flaps and skin grafts to breakdown in the immediate postoperative period or is a direct result of BRT. It is important that practitioners be aware of the complications that may result in the treatment of foot lesions, especially if skin grafts become infected and prolonged delayed healing may ensue.[144]

Evolving results suggest that patients treated with postoperative radiotherapy have deteriorating rates of fibrosis and peripheral edema compared to those receiving preoperative radiotherapy, and it is conceivable that their risk of fracture may ultimately be greater.

PROGNOSTIC FACTORS

An analysis of prospective data collected from 1041 patients older than 16 years with localized soft tissue sarcoma of the extremity[106] with long-term follow-up has determined the clinical and pathologic factors that influence local recurrence, distant recurrence, and disease-specific and overall survival. The 5-year survival rate was 76%, with a median follow-up of 4 years. Factors that increased the risk of local recurrence are shown in Table 35.1-13.

Factors that increased distant recurrence rates were tumor size larger than 5 cm, high histologic grade, deep location,

TABLE 35.1-13. Relative Risk Influence on Recurrence of Localized Extremity Soft Tissue Sarcoma[a]

	Local Recurrence (P)	Distant Recurrence (P)	Disease-Free Survival (P)
Age	1.6 (.001)	—	—
Recurrent presentation	2.0 (.001)	1.5 (.02)	1.5 (.033)
Fibrosarcoma	2.5 (.006)	—	—
Malignant peripheral nerve tumor	1.8 (.001)	—	1.9 (.008)
Size >5 cm	—	1.9 (.0001)	2.1 (.0001)
Margin positive	1.8 (.0001)	—	1.7 (.011)
Depth	—	2.5 (.0007)	2.8 (.0002)
High grade	—	4.3 (.0001)	4.0 (.0001)
Leiomyosarcoma	—	1.7 (.024)	1.9 (.012)

[a]Multivariate number = 1041.
(From ref. 106, with permission.)

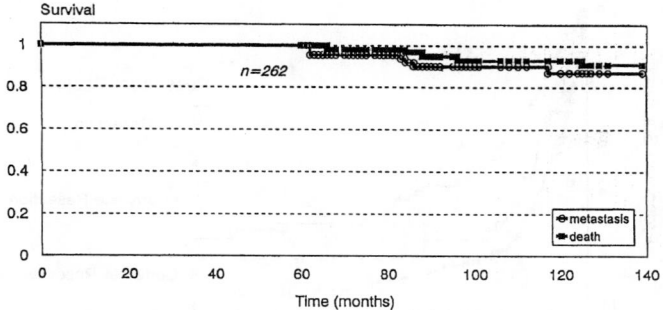

FIGURE 35.1-30. Survival in patients with extremity soft tissue sarcoma who were metastasis free at 5 years. (From Brennan MF. The surgeon as a leader in cancer care: lessons learned from the study of soft tissue sarcoma. *J Am Coll Surg* 1996;182:520, with permission.)

recurrent disease at the time of presentation, and histologic subtype of leiomyosarcoma. Histologic subtype of liposarcoma was favorable for decreased distant recurrence rate when compared with other histologic types.

For disease-specific mortality, large tumor size, high histologic grade, deep location, recurrent disease at presentation, positive histologic margins at the time of resection of the primary, lower extremity site, and the histologic types of leiomyosarcoma and malignant peripheral nerve tumor were all influential factors.

Postmetastasis survival for most patients is independent of factors involved in the primary presentation, although an association has been found with large tumor size. High-grade lesions have a much greater cumulative hazard rate of developing a distant metastasis in the first 30 months. Low-grade lesions, however, have a continued slow but inexorable progression to a continuing long-term rate of metastasis. Prognostic factors clearly vary with time. Grade is a dominant factor in early metastasis, but in late recurrence initial size becomes equally important.

In an effort to include multiple factors associated with prognosis, the authors have developed nomograms for both primary[243] and locally recurrent extremity[244] lesions. These nomograms can be readily transferred to handheld personal organizers for instant calculation of disease-specific survival probability.

Five-year survival does not guarantee cure. An analysis of patients disease free 5 years after the diagnosis and treatment of extremity lesions showed that 9% would go on to have a further recurrence in the next 5 years[245] (Fig. 35.1-30). Unfortunately, survival has not measurably improved with time when corrected for stage.[246] A review of 1261 completely resected extremity lesions by 5-year increments for 1982 to 2001 suggests that disease-specific actuarial 5-year survival is 79% and remains unchanged over 20 years. For high-risk patients (those with high-grade, larger than 10-cm, deep tumors) disease-specific survival remains at around 50%.

QUALITY OF LIFE AND FUNCTIONAL OUTCOME

Quality-of-life assessment has gained importance in many randomized trials, which are evaluating that issue either as the primary end point or secondary to outcome. This is of great significance in patients with soft tissue sarcoma of the extremity who are being treated with conservative surgery and adju-

vant therapy to preserve function and potentially improve the overall quality of life.

To determine the impact of adjuvant therapy, it is important to look at other potential contributing factors. Davis et al. reported a significantly higher level of handicap in amputated patients compared to those treated with conservative surgery.[247] Robinson et al. reported on 54 patients who were disease free 2 or more years after limb-conserving treatment for soft tissue sarcoma of the leg or pelvic girdle. The extent of surgery was not an independent prognostic factor for limb function, although univariate analysis suggested an association with range of movement ($P < .025$).[248]

Bell et al. showed that neural sacrifice performed at the time of wide local excision was associated with poorer outcome on univariate ($P = .002$) and multivariate analysis ($P = .019$).[249] Conventional chemotherapy has not been shown to impact the functional outcome of patients with extremity sarcomas.

The impact of adjuvant radiation on functional outcome has been studied more extensively. Yang et al. reported that adjuvant postoperative EBRT, compared to surgery alone, resulted in significantly worse limb strength, edema, and range of motion, but these deficits were often transient and had few measurable effects on activities of daily life or global quality of life.[114] Schupak et al. reported on a group of patients who underwent rigorous psychofunctional testing and were part of the BRT randomized trial at MSKCC. There were no significant differences in functional outcome between the BRT group and the no-BRT group. The psychofunctional scores, however, revealed a higher level of anxiety, depression, and appreciation of illness in patients who received adjuvant BRT.[250] Karasek et al. evaluated 41 patients who were treated with surgery and radiation and showed that 83% of them had good or excellent functional outcome. There was a correlation between volume irradiated to 55 Gy or higher and poorer functional score, strength, fibrosis, and skin changes.[251]

Although many of the effects noted were initially observed in retrospective analysis, prospective data now also exist. The authors have reported short-term functional outcome in the randomized trial of preoperative versus postoperative radiotherapy, and these data continue to be collected prospectively.[252] The trial design applied two validated instruments—the Toronto Extremity Salvage Score and the Short Form-36 Health Survey quality-of-life instrument—in addition to the observer-based Musculoskeletal Tumor Society Rating Scale.[252] At 6 weeks after surgery, the preoperative group had inferior function with lower bodily pain scores on all three rating instruments. For later assessments extending up to 1 year after surgery, there were no differences in these rating scores. It can be concluded that, for most of the first posttreatment year, the timing of radiotherapy has minimal impact on the function of soft tissue sarcoma patients. Thereafter, evidence suggests that additional and significant outcomes will likely be manifest. These include the deteriorating late tissue sequelae resulting from larger radiotherapy doses and volumes that result in fibrosis and edema, and potentially in bone fractures. These may override the influence of acute wound complications, although patients who do experience wound complications continue to experience impaired function.[252]

TREATMENT OF LOCAL RECURRENCE

Locally recurrent sarcomas are difficult to treat and are more likely to recur, probably as a result of prior contamination of tissue planes as well as intrinsically aggressive tumor biology. The treatment of locally recurrent soft tissue sarcoma in almost any site that is amenable to low-morbidity surgical resection is re-resection. Resection usually encompasses all palpable tumor and all potential microscopic foci present in adjacent tissues traversed during previous surgical procedures. Local recurrence remains a significant factor in long-term morbidity and mortality. When surgical resection can be achieved, then adjuvant radiation therapy should be considered in the vast majority of patients with recurrent disease.

Analyses of patients undergoing local resection of intraabdominal lesions have been extensively reviewed.[206,207] It is clear that, when complete gross resection can be achieved, operation for local recurrence should be attempted along with investigational approaches such as IMRT (see Technical Enhancement of Radiotherapy Delivery, earlier in this chapter). Intraperitoneal chemotherapy after debulking of peritoneal metastases has been advocated but remains an investigational approach.

MANAGEMENT OF ADVANCED DISEASE

Control of the primary site can be achieved in the vast majority of patients with soft tissue sarcoma, but close to one-half of patients succumb to metastatic or locally advanced disease. The most active chemotherapeutic options are of limited value and are associated with serious and potentially life-threatening toxicity. Median survival from the time metastases are recognized is 8 to 12 months, although 20% to 25% of patients with metastatic sarcoma are alive 2 years after diagnosis. Patients with metastatic sarcoma often feel well at the time that a radiograph or CT reveals metastases and may remain free of symptoms for months or years. Alleviation of symptoms is not an immediate concern in many patients, although progression is inevitable. Surgical resection can provide selected patients with prolonged periods of freedom from disease, and radiation therapy provides palliation for individual patients who have localized symptomatic metastases. Optimal treatment of patients with unresectable or metastatic soft tissue sarcoma requires an appreciation for the natural history of the disease, close attention to the individual patient, and an understanding of the benefits and limitations of the therapeutic options.

RESECTION OF METASTATIC DISEASE

Approximately 20% of patients with a soft tissue sarcoma of an extremity or the trunk develop pulmonary metastases, and in the majority, the lung remains the only clinically evident site of metastasis. The histopathology of 1643 pulmonary metastases has been described.[253] The most common primary tumors to develop pulmonary metastases are MFH (23%), synovial sarcoma (19%), and leiomyosarcoma (15%). Most metastases are detected in follow-up, because only 30% of all pulmonary metastases present synchronously, although 80% develop within 2 years of diagnosis. In retrospective series, 20% to 30% of patients who undergo metastasectomy are alive 5 years later.[254,255]

Of 716 patients with primary extremity sarcoma who were treated at MSKCC over a period of 6 years, pulmonary-only metastases occurred in 19%, or 135 patients. Of these 135 patients, 58% underwent thoracotomy and 83% of those had a

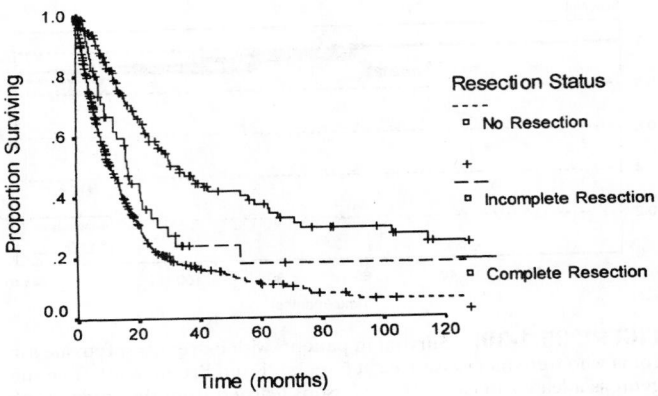

FIGURE 35.1-31. Pulmonary resection of soft tissue sarcoma metastases from the extremity. Comparison of no resection versus incomplete resection versus complete gross resection of all known metastases. [From Billingsley K, Burt M, Jara E, et al. Pulmonary metastases from soft tissue sarcoma: analysis of patterns of disease and postmetastasis survival. *Ann Surg* 1999;229(5):602, with permission.]

complete resection of their tumor. In the 65 patients who had a complete resection of their tumor, 69% had recurrence with pulmonary metastases as their only site of disease. Median survival time from complete resection was 19 months, and 3-year survival was 23% of those undergoing resection and 11% of those presenting with lung metastasis only. Patients who did not undergo thoracotomy all died within 3 years.[97] Chemotherapy had no obvious impact on survival in either the patients who did or those who did not undergo resection. Incomplete resection was no better than no operation (Fig. 35.1-31). At the M. D. Anderson Cancer Center, in contrast to the experience with primary sarcoma, response to chemotherapy administered before pulmonary resection did not predict improved outcome.[256] After curative resection 40% to 80% of patients will have recurrence in the lung. Re-resection is often possible.[257] In a series of 86 patients who underwent repeat resection, predictors of poor survival included more than three lesions, a lesion larger than 2 cm, and high-grade histology. If two or three of these factors were present, disease-specific survival was 10 months.

In patients who have pulmonary-only metastatic disease that is not amenable to resection, an innovative approach under study is isolated lung perfusion.[258] This technique of direct lung infusion can be used to administer chemotherapeutic drugs or biologic agents in a way that results in a high concentration of the agent in the lung, with no systemic exposure. It is unlikely, however, that this will become standard therapy.

SYSTEMIC THERAPY FOR ADVANCED DISEASE

The activity of individual commercially available chemotherapeutic agents in patients with soft tissue sarcoma is summarized in Table 35.1-14. Doxorubicin has been the mainstay of chemotherapy for advanced sarcoma. Whereas early studies suggested an overall response rate of 30%,[259] in more recent trials the response rate was closer to 20%, and was 11% in one study in which outside review of imaging studies was performed.[260–262]

TABLE 35.1-14. Selected Studies of Single-Agent Chemotherapy for Advanced Disease

Regimen	Dose and Schedule	Notes	No. Patients Evaluable	No. Patients Responding	Response Rate (%)	Reference
ANTIBIOTICS						
Doxorubicin	70 mg/m² q3wk	A	94	17	18	356
	70 mg/m² q3wk	A	148	26	17	357
	75 mg/m² q3wk	A	83	21	25	358
	80 mg/m² q3wk	A	90	18	20	261
Liposomal doxorubicin	75–105 mg/m² q2wk		23	3	13	359
Pegylated liposomal doxorubicin	55 mg/m² q4wk	B	35	2	6	360
Epirubicin	75 mg/m² q3wk		84	15	18	358
Epirubicin ± dexrazoxane	Epirubicin 160 mg/m² q3wk ± dexrazoxane 1000 mg/m²		34	8	24	361
Mitomycin C	12 mg/m² q3wk		34	0	0	362
Bleomycin			32	0	0	363
Dactinomycin	Combinations with phenylalanine mustard		76	1	1	364
ALKYLATING AGENTS						
Cyclophosphamide	1.5 g/m² q3wk	A	67	8	12	365
Hexamethylmelamine			40	3	7	366
Ifosfamide	5 g/m² × 24 h IVCI	A	68	12	18	365
	2 g/m² × 4 d IVB		95	17	18	367
	2 g/m² × 7 d IVB	B	72	21	29	368
	1.0 g/m² × 14–21 d IVCI		33	8	24	369
Cisplatin	50 mg/m²	C	96	13	13	370
	75 mg/m²		42	3	7	371
	200 mg/m²		40	6	15	372
Carboplatin	320–400 mg/m²		50	6	12	373
ANTIMETABOLITES						
Gemcitabine	1000 mg/m² qwk × 3–7		19	2	11	374
Methotrexate	Various		41	15	36	375
	≥5 g/m² q2wk with vincristine		14	2	14	376
5-Fluorouracil	—		8	1	12	377
MICROTUBULE TOXINS						
Docetaxel	100 mg/m² q3wk		29	5	17	378
Paclitaxel	250 mg/m² q3wk		48	6	12	379
Vinblastine	1.5 mg/m²/d × 5		≤15	0	0	380
Vinorelbine	30 mg/m² q1wk × 8		36	4	11	381
TOPOISOMERASE INHIBITORS						
Etoposide	100 mg/m²/d × 3 d q3wk	D	28	0	0	382
	50 mg/m² PO qd × 21 d q4wk	D	29	2	7	383
Topotecan	1.5 mg/m² qd × 5, q3wk		29	3	10	384
OTHER AGENTS						
Dacarbazine	Various		53	9	17	385
	1200 mg/m²		44	8	18	265
Gallium nitrate	700 mg/m²		24	0	0	386
Mitoxantrone	—		53	0	0	387
			61		2	388

A, one arm of a randomized study; B, includes soft tissue and bone sarcomas; C, uterine leiomyosarcoma and mixed mesodermal sarcoma; D, uterine leiomyosarcoma only; IVB, intravenous bolus; IVCI, intravenous continuous infusion.
Note: Only the largest series or unique studies of individual drugs are considered here.

Subset analysis of data for patients with soft tissue sarcoma enrolled in a large randomized phase II trial of different doses of doxorubicin demonstrated a dose-response relationship. These data have been confirmed in other trials of single-agent doxorubicin and trials with doxorubicin-containing combination therapy.[183] Studies have begun to examine liposomal forms of doxorubicin, which may have fewer side effects than doxorubicin itself. Response rates have been low, however, and in one randomized phase II study, the response rate to doxorubicin was very low, perhaps due to distribution of sarcoma subtypes.[263]

Ifosfamide has approximately the same efficacy as doxorubicin. In the past, ifosfamide dosing was limited by severe urothelial toxicity (hemorrhagic cystitis). The uroprotective agent mesna has markedly changed the ability to give both ifosfamide and cyclophosphamide, and ifosfamide doses as large as 14 to 18 g/m² or more over 1 to 2 weeks have been given. There has been a debate as to the relative efficacy of cyclophosphamide versus ifosfamide, in particular, whether ifosfamide is truly a different drug or whether differences in dosing of the two drugs account for the difference in response. The EORTC performed a randomized phase II trial examining the response rates for ifosfamide 5 g/m^2 and cyclophosphamide 1.5 g/m^2. There was greater myelosuppression with cyclophosphamide, but response rates were 7.5% for cyclophosphamide and 18% for ifosfamide; although suggestive, this difference did not achieve statistical significance. In addition, there is some evidence to suggest a dose-response relationship for ifosfamide.[182] This is borne out by the large number of phase II trials examining the use of high-dose ifosfamide in metastatic soft tissue sarcoma (see Table 35.1-14). Responses to higher doses of ifosfamide are occasionally seen in patients who do not respond to lower doses of alkylating agents. The similar response rates of ifosfamide and doxorubicin, even in doxorubicin-resistant patients, suggested a lack of cross-resistance in combination chemotherapy. It should be noted that synovial sarcoma appears particularly responsive to ifosfamide.[264]

The third drug with modest activity in sarcoma is dacarbazine (DTIC). Its activity was recognized more than 20 years ago and later confirmed.[265] Dacarbazine has frequently been used in combination chemotherapy with doxorubicin (see Combination Chemotherapy for Advanced Soft Tissue Sarcoma, later in this chapter). Dacarbazine is given in a variety of schedules, from intravenous continuous infusion as part of the MAID protocol (see Table 35.1-11) to one large bolus. The major side effects of dacarbazine are nausea and vomiting, which have been substantially reduced with the use of serotonin antagonist antiemetics. Antiemetic use allows for dacarbazine administration in a single treatment, rather than in divided doses. Temozolomide, the oral equivalent of dacarbazine, appears to have some activity against leiomyosarcomas as well.[266]

As for other single agents, cisplatin and carboplatin have produced occasional responses in phase II trials. However, unlike in pediatric sarcomas such as Ewing's sarcoma and rhabdomyosarcoma, other agents such as single-agent vincristine, etoposide, and dactinomycin appear to be inactive. The taxanes also show little activity in sarcomas except for angiosarcoma. More recent data indicate that gemcitabine may have minor activity depending on the administration schedule[267,268] and more activity when given with a taxane (see Combination Chemotherapy for Advanced Soft Tissue Sarcoma, later in this chapter). Vinorelbine may also have minor activity in metastatic sarcoma. Few investigational drugs have demonstrated meaningful activity in soft tissue sarcoma, except for epirubicin, a close relative of doxorubicin, now approved for commercial use. Excluding the remarkable story of the sensitivity of GIST to the tyrosine kinase inhibitor imatinib, the most significant investigational agent in soft tissue sarcomas is presently ecteinascidin (ET-743), with 14 responses in 189 patients (7% response rate) in patients with a variety of subtypes of sarcoma, in particular myxoid liposarcoma and leiomyosarcoma. When tested as first-, second-, or third-line therapy, a 7% minor response rate was also noted.[269] Ecteinascidin binds the minor groove of DNA and bends the DNA toward the major groove. It also affects transcription and appears to be dependent on intact nucleoside excision repair systems of the cell for its potency. Its toxicity is largely hematologic and hepatic, with significant increases in levels of transaminases and occasionally alkaline phosphatase and bilirubin levels after treatment; these resolve spontaneously and are likely mitigated with the use of glucocorticoids. It remains investigational as of May 2004.[269–271]

Used in some of the earliest studies in sarcoma adjuvant chemotherapy, immunotherapy for sarcoma is seeing renewed

TABLE 35.1-15. Newer Investigational Agents and Biologic Agents Used in Sarcoma Therapy

Agent	No. of Patients	Responses (Partial or Complete)	Reference
Ecteinascidin (ET-743)	189	14/189 (also 14 minor response)	269
SU5416	26	0/26	272
CT-2584	28	1/28	389
Brostallicin	42	2/42	390
Bortezomib (PS-341)	21	1/21	391
Interferon-α	16	0	392
Interferon-α$_{2b}$	64	5	393
Interferon-α$_{2b}$ with tamoxifen	7	0	394
Interferon-β	20	1/20	395
Interferon-β$_{ser}$	23	0	393
Interleukin-2	6	—	396
Liposomal muramyl tripeptide phosphatidylethanolamine	19	0	397
Tumor necrosis factor	16	0	398
Troglitazone	3	—	273

interest, although without significant success to date. Cytokines alone appear to be ineffective in sarcoma (Table 35.1-15), as does nonspecific immunotherapy with bacterial cell wall components. Studies at the NCI and elsewhere are beginning to examine vaccination of patients with peptides representing the fusion proteins observed in specific subtypes of sarcoma. Lymphokine-activated killer cell and other T-cell immunotherapy with cytokines was investigated in a very small number of patients at the NCI without any observed responses. Dendritic cell vaccines and other forms of tumor-specific immunotherapy are undergoing investigation and may be of relevance to patients with soft tissue sarcoma.

Angiogenesis inhibition has emerged as a new frontier for treatment of solid tumors of all types, including sarcoma. To date, weak angiogenesis inhibitors such as the interferons have not shown efficacy in sarcoma (see Table 35.1-15). Stronger angiogenesis inhibitors such as TNP-470 (AGM-1470) and the vascular endothelial growth factor pathway inhibitor SU5416 have been examined in phase I and phase II studies,[272] but no partial responses and only one minor response were observed in 31 patients treated in the phase II study. The antiangiogenic compound SU6668, an oral drug, was not bioavailable in humans and is no longer under active investigation. However, SU11248, a blocker of c-kit, vascular endothelial growth factor receptors 1 and 2, and flt-3, has shown early promise in GIST, other sarcomas, and other cancers as well. Thalidomide as a single agent has not been studied formally in patients with soft tissue sarcoma.

Newer biologic agents are beginning to be assessed, based on the biology of specific sarcoma subsets, in particular liposarcoma. The antidiabetic drug troglitazone binds to the peroxisome proliferator–activated receptor γ. This receptor is present on the cell surface of some liposarcomas. When peroxisome proliferator–activated receptor γ binds a ligand, it can induce differentiation of the liposarcoma toward an adipocyte, with abundant fat droplet accumulation and decreased S-phase fraction. This laboratory finding led to an ongoing trial of troglitazone in patients with advanced liposarcoma.[273] A subset of patients with liposarcoma demonstrated similar lipid accumulation *in vivo* to that noted *in vitro*. There are no data on relapse-free or overall survival of this cohort of patients.

COMBINATION CHEMOTHERAPY FOR ADVANCED SOFT TISSUE SARCOMA

A variety of combinations of chemotherapy have been developed and examined in phase II trials. The typical backbone of a combination regimen is doxorubicin (or its analog epirubicin) with an alkylating agent, with or without other agents (see Table 35.1-11). One of the earliest combinations used was doxorubicin and dacarbazine, which has been well studied by the Southwest Oncology Group. Although initial analysis noted a 41% major response rate, subsequent study of either a bolus or continuous infusion of the same regimen yielded a 17% response rate.[274]

CyVADIC (cyclophosphamide, vincristine, doxorubicin, and dacarbazine) has been widely used for sarcoma therapy in the United States and Europe. Although single-arm studies showed response rates as high as 71%, a randomized trial showed no significant difference in overall survival between patients given CyVADIC and those given doxorubicin as a single agent.[260] The two-drug combinations of doxorubicin and ifosfamide[260] or epirubicin and ifosfamide[275] have consistently given response rates above 25%. Current studies are investigating higher dosages of ifosfamide with fixed doxorubicin dosage and growth factor support.

MAID was proven effective in metastatic soft tissue sarcoma in a large phase II trial at the Dana-Farber Cancer Institute.[276] This randomized trial took place before the routine use of growth factors for aggressive chemotherapeutic regimens and examined doxorubicin and dacarbazine versus MAID. The study showed an increased response rate in the MAID arm (32% vs. 17%; $P < .002$).[277] In results that underscore the increased toxicity of aggressive chemotherapy regimens, there were eight toxicity-related deaths in the study, seven among the 170 patients treated with the 7.5-g/m^2 total dosage of ifosfamide per cycle. This dosage was decreased to 6 g/m^2 during the course of the study. All treatment-related deaths occurred in patients older than 50 years of age. In a univariate analysis, there was a survival advantage for the two-drug arm (13 months vs. 12 months for MAID); however, this difference was not significant in a multivariate analysis. As noted in Dose Intensity later in this chapter, with the introduction of growth factors, the dose intensity of this regimen has become better tolerated.

The response rates of metastatic sarcoma to cisplatin are low, and response rate to mitomycin C was zero in one study. The combination of the two drugs with doxorubicin (called *MAP*) yielded a 43% response rate in a study at the Mayo Clinic. The activity of the MAP regimen has been confirmed in an independent ECOG trial.[261,278] A metaanalysis of all of the data from seven large EORTC studies provided a very useful resource to assess response rates to combination chemotherapy in a multi-institutional setting.[279] Data for the 2185 patients with follow-up in this study were subjected to a univariate and multivariate analysis of survival based on a number of factors, including age, sex, performance status before chemotherapy, presence and site of metastatic disease, histologic subtype, histologic grade, and disease-free interval (time since initial diag-

nosis of sarcoma). The overall median survival time was 51 weeks. The predictors of overall survival included good performance status, lack of liver involvement, low histopathologic grade, long disease-free interval, and young age ($P < .005$ for all these factors in a multivariate analysis). Although absence of liver involvement, young age, and high histopathologic grade also predicted response to chemotherapy, so did liposarcoma histology ($P < .01$ for all these factors in a multivariate analysis); leiomyosarcoma histology did not qualify as a predictive factor for response to chemotherapy independent of liver metastasis. Although lesions were not stratified by site, these data provide some of the best evidence that response rate does not necessarily correlate with overall survival.

Is combination chemotherapy better than single-agent doxorubicin for overall survival? Again, the concept arises that response rates may differ from rates of overall survival. There have been several phase III trials examining the issue of combination chemotherapy versus single-agent chemotherapy in patients with metastatic disease (Table 35.1-16). Two such trials examined this question for uterine sarcoma. There were improved response rates in several of the trials with combination chemotherapy, but there was no survival advantage over single-agent doxorubicin. Complete responses were very rare during these studies and were not durable. These data argue that single agents are as effective as combination chemotherapy for patients with metastatic disease in terms of overall survival. However, some patients may be eligible for palliative resection of metastatic disease or are symptomatic from their metastases. In these situations in which aggressive therapy is contemplated, combination chemotherapy, which gives better response rates than single agents, can be considered.

Perhaps analogously to the situation with the MAP combination of chemotherapy, the combination of gemcitabine with docetaxel appears to be more than additive in terms of its benefit for patients with sarcomas. Gemcitabine and docetaxel have borderline activity in sarcoma, but the combination gave a remarkable 53% response rate in a group of patients with leiomyosarcoma, the great majority of whom had leiomyosarcoma originating in the uterus.[280] The mechanism of this apparent synergy is unclear, but it may also apply to treatment of osteogenic sarcoma, at least based on anecdotal evidence. Because each drug has some activity—in particular, some leiomyosarcomas respond to gemcitabine alone—the combination is being examined against gemcitabine in a phase III study.

DOSE INTENSITY

It is a central tenet of oncology that response to chemotherapy is a function of dose and dose intensity.[281] A dose-response effect for doxorubicin and ifosfamide has been suggested in a variety of studies. However, toxicity limits the amount of chemotherapy that can be given in any one cycle, as illustrated by the phase III trial of the MAID combination chemotherapy described in Combination Chemotherapy for Advanced Soft Tissue Sarcoma, earlier in this chapter.[277] It is argued that if dose could be increased, better responses might be seen. Better supportive care can help increase dose intensity as outlined here.

The use of hematopoietic growth factors has allowed the study of higher dosages of chemotherapy in sarcoma. Some of the aggressive regimens for treatment of metastatic sarcoma satisfy the American Society of Clinical Oncology guidelines for

TABLE 35.1-16. Selected Randomized Trials in Advanced Disease

Group	Regimen	No. of Patients	Response Rate, % (Complete Response Rate, %)	Median Survival (Mo)	Reference
GOG[a]	A	80	16 (6)	7.7	Omura[399]
	AD	66	24 (10)	7.3	
GOG[a]	A	50	19 (4)	11.6	Muss[298]
	ACy	54	19 (8)	10.9	
COG	A	41	17 (2)	8.5	Cruz[400]
	ActL	25	4	8.1	
	ActLV	26	0	11.5	
	ActLCyclo	26	0	5.1	
ECOG	A	54	30 (7)	8.6	Schoenfeld[401]
	CyAV	56	21 (5)	7.9	
	CyActV	58	12 (2)	9.5	
ECOG	A	94	18 (5)	8.0	Borden[356]
	A	88	17 (3)	8.4	
	ADTIC	92	30 (6)	8.0	
ECOG	A	148	17 (4)	9.4	Borden[357]
	AVD	143	18 (6)	9.0	
ECOG	A	90	20 (2)	<9	Edmonson[261]
	AI	88	34 (3)	11	
	MAP	84	32 (7)	9	
EORTC	A	240	23 (4)	12.0	Santoro[260]
	AI	231	28 (5)	12.6	
	CyVADIC	134	28 (8)	11.7	
CALGB/SWOG	AD	170	17 (2)	13.3	Antman[277]
	AID	170	32 (2)	11.9	
EORTC	A	112	14 (2)	10.4	Nielsen[402]
	Epi	111	15 (3)	10.8	
	Epi	111	14 (3)	10.4	
EORTC meta-analysis	Any anthracy-cline-based regimen	2185	26 (n/a)	11.8	Van Glabbeke[279]

A, doxorubicin; Act, actinomycin D; CALGB, Cancer and Leukemia and Group B; COG, Central Oncology Group; Cy, cyclophosphamide; Cyclo, cycloleucine; D, dacarbazine; DTIC, dacarbazine; Epi, epirubicin; GOG, Gynecologic Oncology Group; I, ifosfamide; L, L-PAM (L-phenylalanine mustard); M, mitomycin C; n/a, not available; P, cisplatin; SWOG, Southwest Oncology Group; V, vincristine; VD, vindesine.
[a]Uterine sarcoma only; response rates are only for subset of patients with measurable disease.

use of growth factors given their high rate of associated febrile neutropenia.[282] Granulocyte-macrophage colony-stimulating factor or GM-CSF (sargramostim), the first granulocyte growth factor used, decreased the myelosuppression seen with combinations such as CyVADIC or MAID[283] and high-dose ifosfamide. GM-CSF allowed for escalation of the dose of doxorubicin when given in combination with 5 g/m² ifosfamide, with improvement in response rate.[284] GM-CSF has also been shown to allow increased dose intensity of the MAP combination of chemotherapy, allowing addition of ifosfamide.

Similarly, granulocyte colony-stimulating factor (filgrastim) has been widely used to increase dose intensity and decrease myelotoxicity of aggressive chemotherapeutic regimens such as MAID[285] or dose-escalated doxorubicin and ifosfamide. However, with escalated doses (25% increase) in the MAID regimen, there appears to be no significant increased response rate despite use of growth factors. There may be other ways to achieve dose intensity. A study of low-dose, long-term (approximately 2-week) ifosfamide treatment showed responses in patients who did not respond to other forms of chemotherapy for sarcoma. As was seen for previous studies, it may well be that responsiveness to a particular regimen may not translate into increased survival.

Unfortunately, the cardiac toxicity of doxorubicin and the nephrotoxicity and central nervous system toxicity of ifosfamide prevent much greater dose escalation than performed in some studies today. The next logical step is to proceed to high-dose therapy with stem cell support, which is currently under study for pediatric sarcomas such as rhabdomyosarcoma and Ewing's sarcoma.[286] Such studies show long-term disease-free survival for a few patients with Ewing's sarcoma, osteosarcoma, or rhabdomyosarcoma. Even in the case of these relatively chemotherapy-sensitive tumors, the majority of patients have relapsed rapidly. Given that complete responses (and therefore chemotherapy sensitivity) are rare in the metastatic setting of adult soft tissue sarcoma, it is not surprising that the few patients with soft tissue sarcoma who undergo high-dose therapy with stem cell rescue relapse quickly. High-dose therapy with stem cell rescue should not be considered for patients with metastatic sarcoma outside the setting of a clinical trial.[287] Given the poor results of high-dose therapy, the pursuit of agents with better activity against soft tissue sarcoma remains a primary focus for treatment of relapsed disease.

RESPONSE BY HISTOLOGIC SUBTYPE AND SITE

A major focus in critical reading of the literature concerning responses of soft tissue sarcoma to chemotherapy is the variety of patient sarcoma histologic subtypes. Pediatric sarcomas are known for their relative sensitivity to chemotherapy (Ewing's sarcoma, osteosarcoma, and rhabdomyosarcoma). As for adult sarcomas, synovial sarcomas, fibrosarcomas, and round cell liposarcomas are generally responsive to chemotherapy. GISTs, alveolar soft parts sarcoma, and low- to intermediate-grade chondrosarcomas are notorious for their resistance to standard chemotherapy agents. An imbalance in the subtypes of sarcoma in various groups of patients can markedly affect overall outcome for the study in question.

Site of disease is another important factor in determination of outcome for patients with soft tissue sarcoma. For example, patients with large low-grade liposarcomas of the extremity show lower relapse rates than patients with low-grade liposarcomas of the retroperitoneum; the latter are more difficult to control locally. Similarly, most tumors formerly called leiomyosarcomas of the gastrointestinal tract are now considered GISTs, known to be less responsive to standard chemotherapy than leiomyosarcomas of other sites (see Leiomyosarcoma, later in this chapter), although remarkably sensitive to imatinib. Anatomy of metastatic disease can also affect overall response rates. For example, metastases to liver are less likely to respond to chemotherapy than metastases to another site[287]; however, this may represent the tendency of GISTs to metastasize to the liver. Variations in the site of disease or metastasis pattern may account at least in part for the different responses noted in randomized trials of chemotherapy for soft tissue sarcoma.

It is clear that specific subtypes of soft tissue sarcoma demonstrate unique biologic behavior. As diagnosis and classification of sarcomas improve, these unique features may become more evident. In the following sections are listed examples of specific sites or subtypes of sarcoma and their characteristics.

LEIOMYOSARCOMA

Leiomyosarcomas are one of the most common forms of soft tissue sarcoma. They are also easier to classify based on the presence of markers such as smooth muscle actin that are easily noted using standard immunohistochemistry, and thus there may be greater concordance of pathologists in the diagnosis of leiomyosarcoma than in diagnosis of other forms of soft tissue sarcoma. Analysis of data from a variety of randomized studies dissecting out the response rate for leiomyosarcomas versus other subtypes of sarcomas is useful to delineate the differential response of leiomyosarcoma and of other subtypes such as liposarcoma, synovial sarcoma, or MFH. It should be noted that subset analyses cannot substitute for primary trials of chemotherapy but still can be useful in generating hypotheses. Doxorubicin appears to be active against leiomyosarcomas, but ifosfamide appears to add little to the response rate of this subset of tumors.[261] This finding has been observed in other studies, but again there may be contamination of the leiomyosarcoma group with what would today be classified as GISTs. In one small study of uterine leiomyosarcomas, a modest response to ifosfamide was observed, but this finding is in the minority among studies examined in greater detail in a previous version of this text. Ifos-

famide, in contrast, appears to be effective in other subtypes of sarcoma such as synovial sarcoma and liposarcoma.

The primary site of leiomyosarcoma can have an equally important effect on survival. The difference in response rates for leiomyosarcomas of different sites is highlighted in the trials conducted by ECOG and the Southwest Oncology Group.[261,277] Although only 20% to 25% of uterine leiomyosarcomas responded to chemotherapy, uterine leiomyosarcoma was approximately twice as responsive to chemotherapy than were leiomyosarcomas arising from the GI tract (GISTs). These data are at odds with the cumulative EORTC metaanalysis of therapy for metastatic sarcomas[287]; however, in the EORTC study, leiomyosarcomas were not stratified with respect to site; poorly responding GISTs were likely grouped together with better responding leiomyosarcomas of other sites. Attention to improved histopathologic diagnosis will continue to play a important part in the design of future studies of chemotherapy in the adjuvant or metastatic setting.

SYNOVIAL SARCOMA

Synovial sarcomas demonstrate two histologic forms, a monophasic form and a biphasic form. Specific translocations in this subset of sarcoma between the SSX and SYT genes on chromosomes X and 18 may be prognostic factors for this subtype of sarcoma. Patients with tumors of the biphasic histologic form demonstrated SYT-SSX1 gene fusions. These patients fared more poorly than patients with SYT-SSX2–positive tumors that were associated with the monophasic phenotype. These data were confirmed in a multi-institutional study.[79,288] Such molecular phenotyping represents an attractive method of predicting outcome to therapy and need for more or less intensive therapy.

Patients with synovial sarcoma tend to be younger than patients with other subtypes of soft tissue sarcoma. Patients with synovial sarcoma are therefore likely to have a better performance status than patients with other subtypes of sarcoma, a positive predictor for response to chemotherapy in the EORTC database.[287] The higher response rates in such patients may therefore be due in part to patient selection factors, not just histologic diagnosis.

In patients with advanced synovial sarcomas, ifosfamide (at a high dose of 14 to 18 g/m^2) appears to be an active agent, with a 100% response rate in one study of 13 patients.[264] The EORTC metaanalysis of 2185 sarcoma patients included 115 synovial sarcomas evaluable for response to chemotherapy.[287] The response rate was 31%, not significantly different from the overall response rate of 26%; however, survival curves for patients with synovial sarcoma showed at least an initial benefit for the synovial sarcoma diagnosis, although these patients later joined the overall survival curve of those with other metastatic sarcomas. The differences between these results may be due at least in part to dose intensity. The EORTC data examined the response of metastatic sarcoma to anthracyclines, and only a portion of patients received ifosfamide (at a maximum dose of 5 g/m^2, a low dose by today's standards).

PEDIATRIC SARCOMAS IN ADULT POPULATIONS

A number of pediatric sarcomas occur in adults, including Ewing's sarcoma (in soft tissue or bone), rhabdomyosarcoma (usually embryonal), and extraskeletal osteosarcoma. These diseases differ from typical adult sarcomas in that they are considered systemic diseases despite their initial presentation. Ewing's sarcoma and rhabdomyosarcoma are typically much more sensitive to chemotherapy than adult soft tissue sarcomas.[289] In osteosarcoma, long-term survival has been achieved in pediatric patients with the use of adjuvant chemotherapy. Unfortunately, adults with osteosarcoma are generally more resistant to chemotherapy than are children. Adjuvant (or neoadjuvant) chemotherapy is the standard of care for adults with a diagnosis of rhabdomyosarcoma or Ewing's sarcoma. Also, adults with a typical osteosarcoma of bone should receive neoadjuvant or adjuvant chemotherapy in addition to therapy for local control of the tumor. However, in extraskeletal osteosarcoma, the use of chemotherapy as an adjuvant to surgical control of the primary disease remains controversial, largely due to the low response rates to chemotherapy seen in patients with metastatic soft tissue osteosarcoma.[290]

Typical regimens for small cell pediatric sarcomas, specifically rhabdomyosarcoma and Ewing's sarcoma, include the combination of vincristine, doxorubicin, and cyclophosphamide (dactinomycin, in particular, for rhabdomyosarcoma), and the combination of ifosfamide and etoposide.[291–293] The MAID regimen also shows activity in pediatric sarcomas.[294] There is debate as to whether adults do worse than pediatric patients with the same stage of disease. Adults are less likely than children to tolerate the aggressive regimens of chemotherapy used against these diseases. In addition, adults may present with advanced-stage disease relative to children or adolescents. One retrospective study showed that older patients with rhabdomyosarcoma tolerated chemotherapy as well as the pediatric population but fared worse overall.[68] Tumor size, site, and response to chemotherapy predicted outcome in another series.[269] In Ewing's sarcoma, the role of age in predicting outcome is controversial.[295,296] A high percentage of patients with pediatric sarcomas are enrolled on protocols examining new therapy in the setting of randomized trials. Adults with a diagnosis of a sarcoma usually seen in pediatric populations should be included on pediatric protocols whenever feasible to help determine appropriate care for patients with these rare diagnoses.

UTERINE SARCOMA

Uterine sarcomas are very rare, accounting for 3% to 7% of all uterine malignancies. The uterus is a unique site in that at least three different sarcomatous entities may arise from this organ, including leiomyosarcoma, endometrial stromal sarcoma, and carcinosarcoma (also known as *malignant mixed müllerian tumor* or MMMT). The most common histopathologic type is MMMT.

For localized disease surgery is the main treatment. The use of adjuvant radiation remains a controversial topic. Most studies showed some improvement in local control but not in survival. In contrast, Ferrer et al. reviewed the experience of the Grup Oncologic Catala-Occita and found that the addition of radiation to surgery improved local control as well as survival in 103 patients with stage I to IVA disease.[297] The ongoing EORTC 55874 randomized trial will hopefully determine the exact impact of adjuvant radiation in treating this malignancy.

The Gynecologic Oncology Group conducted a prospective randomized trial comparing adjuvant chemotherapy to no further therapy in patients with stage I or II uterine sarcoma. No significant improvement was noted in progression-free interval or overall survival.[160]

For advanced disease, the Gynecologic Oncology Group also compared doxorubicin alone to doxorubicin and dacarbazine in a randomized trial. Response rates and overall survival did not differ between the two arms; the response rate to doxorubicin of 28 women with leiomyosarcoma was 25%. Thereafter, doxorubicin was compared to doxorubicin plus cyclophosphamide; response rates in both arms were 19%, with a 13% response rate to doxorubicin in patients with leiomyosarcoma.[298] Uterine sarcoma overall showed a 22% to 25% response rate to chemotherapy as noted in Response by Histologic Subtype and Site, earlier in this chapter.[274]

A number of phase II studies have examined responses to various agents by specific subtypes of uterine sarcoma. Patients with carcinosarcoma (MMMT) have been treated with cisplatin or doxorubicin in the past. There were no responses in the small cohort of patients given doxorubicin alone. Ifosfamide and paclitaxel are also active agents against this subtype of uterine sarcoma.[299,300] When patients develop metastatic disease from carcinosarcoma, it is usually of the carcinomatous elements, which indicates that this is the more important characteristic of the tumor to treat. This may explain the responses of this sarcoma to therapy effective for epithelial tumors. The addition of cisplatin to ifosfamide improved the response rate, with a modest change in progression-free survival, but did not appear to affect overall survival in comparison to ifosfamide alone.[300]

Leiomyosarcoma is responsive to doxorubicin, is less sensitive to ifosfamide (see Leiomyosarcoma, earlier in this chapter), and is also relatively unresponsive to cisplatin. The combination of gemcitabine and docetaxel is particularly active against uterine leiomyosarcoma,[301] but it is not clear if the addition of a taxane to the gemcitabine is any more useful than single-agent gemcitabine.

Endometrial stromal sarcomas express estrogen and progesterone receptors, and anecdotal responses to progestins have been noted.[302] However, it is clear that frequency of positive estrogen or progesterone receptor staining is substantially greater than the response rate to hormonal therapy such as tamoxifen. In a prospective trial of tamoxifen in treatment of uterine sarcomas, only one patient (with an MMMT) responded, out of a total 29 patients treated (19 with leiomyosarcoma).[303]

DESMOIDS (AGGRESSIVE FIBROMATOSES)

Desmoid tumors belong to a family of myofibroblastic fibromatoses that are unusual in their bland histology and slow progression. Surgery remains the treatment of choice for these lesions, which cannot truly be called sarcomas due to their lack of metastatic potential.

The role of adjuvant radiation for completely resected primary desmoid tumor is controversial. Most authors agree that for patients with negative resection margins, postoperative radiation is not recommended.[304] However, for patients with positive microscopic margins the role of adjuvant radiation is more debatable. Spear et al. reported a local control rate of 61% for patients with primary tumors with positive microscopic margins treated with surgery alone.[304] Others, however, have reported lower local control rates.[305] The conclusion from these studies is that failure does not invariably occur if residual microscopic tumor from a primary lesion is left *in situ* as long as local progression would not cause significant morbidity.

When adjuvant radiation is indicated for some primary lesions or most recurrent tumors, the usual dose is on the order of 50 Gy. In advanced cases desmoids can still cause significant morbidity in proximal extremity lesions and can be fatal if they arise in the retroperitoneum, because in such sites they are difficult to resect completely.

Although the use of adjuvant radiation is becoming more restricted, definitive radiation is emerging as a reasonable alternative to radical surgery. Ballo et al. reported a 5-year local control rate of 69% for patients treated with radiation for gross disease.[306] Others have shown similar findings.[304] The recommended dose for definitive radiation is usually 56 Gy in 2 Gy per fraction to 60 Gy given at 1.8 Gy/fraction.

Desmoids classically arise in pregnancy as an abdominal mass independent of the uterus. Desmoids have been examined for hormone receptors and have binding sites for estrogens and antiestrogens in some cases. There are anecdotal accounts of responses to hormonal manipulation such as tamoxifen, gonadotropin-releasing hormone agonists, or aromatase inhibitors.[307,308] There are well-documented responses of desmoids to sulindac and other nonsteroidal antiinflammatory drugs.[309,310] Responses can take months and continue for years.

Responses have been reported to single-agent doxorubicin chemotherapy[311] as well as to combination chemotherapy at either standard or relatively low doses.[312,313] Responses can be slow, and therapy should not be abandoned for stable disease, but changes should be made for toxicity, because patients need several months or even years of therapy to achieve maximum benefit. Complete responses are exceptionally rare, so the timing of discontinuation of therapy in the setting of responding disease remains a difficult question and requires clinical judgment.

In summary, for easily resectable disease, surgery alone appears to be the optimal approach, especially in patients with negative microscopic margins. In advanced cases, a trial of nonsteroidal antiinflammatory drugs or hormonal therapy can be considered in most patients. A period of close observation is also reasonable, because some patients demonstrate regression without any therapy. However, if a patient is symptomatic and not a candidate for surgery, consideration should be given to radiation or chemotherapy to increase the chance of a response.

RECOMMENDATIONS FOR PATIENTS WITH ADVANCED DISEASE

Low-grade tumors grow very slowly and may be less responsive to chemotherapy than higher-grade lesions. Accordingly, an asymptomatic patient with stable or only slowly progressive disease can be observed only. Resection of metastatic disease, in particular lung metastases, provides some patients with long-term survival and can be considered if the lungs are the only site of remaining disease.[97]

Randomized studies have shown that combination chemotherapy can provide a better probability of a response than single-agent doxorubicin. However, overall survival for any combination chemotherapy has not been proven superior to that for doxorubicin alone as a single agent. When a clinical response is needed, for example, before potential surgery for metastases, combinations of agents such as doxorubicin and ifosfamide should be considered, especially for patients with good performance status. For patients with poorer performance status, single-agent doxorubicin remains the standard of care, because no other therapy or combination of treatments has proven superior to it for overall survival. Pegylated liposomal doxorubicin can be considered in patients in whom the toxicity of doxorubicin would not be tolerated, but the response rates to this single agent may be lower than that to standard doxorubicin.

Single-agent ifosfamide or dacarbazine can be used as a second-line agent if doxorubicin is used alone in first-line therapy. Ifosfamide is useful against synovial sarcomas and liposarcomas but less effective against leiomyosarcomas. Dacarbazine demonstrates modest activity in soft tissue sarcoma and with doxorubicin is a well-studied and well-tolerated combination in metastatic disease. Dacarbazine shows some activity against leiomyosarcomas, in particular. Patients with angiosarcoma may respond to taxanes, gemcitabine, vinorelbine, and pegylated liposomal doxorubicin, as well as standard doxorubicin or ifosfamide chemotherapy. Patients with advanced disease are candidates for enrollment in phase I and phase II studies of new therapies for sarcoma, because there are but few tools with which to treat such patients at present.

FUTURE DIRECTIONS

Metastatic sarcoma, whether at time of disease presentation or after local control of primary disease, remains an extremely difficult problem. The search for effective agents will be the focus of continuing research for patients with advanced disease. There is already a broad movement to identify and test antiangiogenic agents, specific tyrosine kinase inhibitors, and novel chemotherapeutic agents such as ecteinascidin. In the longer term, some of the results of oligonucleotide and complementary DNA arrays, proteomics, and tissue arrays may lead to a more accurate determination of which patients will benefit from a specific therapy. For example, fully half of Ewing's sarcomas express c-kit (CD117), but Ewing's sarcoma is unresponsive to imatinib, in contrast to the 60% response rate seen for GISTs using that agent. It will be necessary to identify the reason for such differences to be able to tailor therapy more accurately. It is hoped that new biologic agents for sarcoma therapy can be found that are as potent as TNF in murine models of sarcoma. TNF, interleukin-2, and cytokines appear to be toxic and largely inactive as sarcoma therapy when given systemically. Nonetheless, other biologic interventions may show promise, such as inhibitory RNA strategies or immunotherapy with vaccines, monoclonal antibodies, dendritic cells, or T cells. Characteristic fusion proteins of sarcomas (or peptides thereof) will be tested in the near future for their effectiveness in the appropriate subtypes of sarcomas, such as many pediatric sarcomas. Vaccines incorporating dendritic cells appear to be very effective immunogens in preclinical studies. Preparations of heat-shock proteins or of immunogenic glycolipids found in sarcoma cell membranes may also provide interesting agents for therapy. The first furtive steps into the realm of gene therapy for cancer are just now being taken. It is hoped that the continued strides made in understanding molecular and cell biology, such as the specific survival or growth pathways induced by translocations in Ewing's sarcoma, alveolar rhabdomyosarcoma, and synovial sarcoma, will lead to new therapies that will impact the treatment of this diverse family of tumors.

REFERENCES

1. Jemal A, Murray T, Samuels A, et al. Cancer statistics. *CA Cancer J Clin* 2003;53:5.
2. Zahm S, Fraumeni J Jr. The epidemiology of soft tissue sarcoma. *Semin Oncol* 1997;24(5):504.
3. Latres E, Drobnjak M, Pollack D, et al. Chromosome 17 abnormalities and TP53 mutations in adult soft tissue sarcomas. *Am J Pathol* 1994;145:345.
4. Cance W, Brennan M, Dudas M, et al. Altered expression of the retinoblastoma gene product in human sarcomas. *N Engl J Med* 1990;323:1457.
5. Li F, Fraumeni J Jr. Soft tissue sarcomas, breast cancer and other neoplasms. A familial syndrome? *Ann Intern Med* 1969;71:747.
6. D'Agostino A, Soule E, Miller R. Sarcomas of the peripheral nerves and somatic soft tissues associated with multiple neurofibromatosis (von Recklinghausen's disease). *Cancer* 1963;16:1015.
7. Fraumeni J Jr, Vogel C, Easton J. Sarcomas and multiple polyposis in a kindred. A genetic variety of hereditary polyposis? *Arch Intern Med* 1968;121:57.
8. Sorensen S, Mulvihill J, Nielsen A. Long-term follow-up of von Recklinghausen neurofibromatosis. *N Engl J Med* 1986;314:1010.
9. Abramson DH, Melson MR, Dunkel IJ, Frank CM. Third (fourth and fifth) nonocular tumors in survivors of retinoblastoma. *Ophthalmology* 2001;108(10):1868.
10. Wong F, Boice J Jr, Abramson D, et al. Cancer incidence after retinoblastoma. Radiation dose and sarcoma risk. *JAMA* 1997;278(15):1262.
11. Brady M, Gaynor J, Brennan M. Radiation-associated sarcoma of bone and soft tissue. *Arch Surg* 1992;127:1379.
12. Sheppard DG, Libshitz HI. Post-radiation sarcomas: a review of the clinical and imaging features in 63 cases. *Clin Radiol* 2001;56:22.
13. Spiro IJ, Suit HD. Radiation-induced bone and soft tissue sarcomas: clinical aspects and molecular biology. *Cancer Treat Res* 1997;91:143.
14. Karlsson P, Holmberg E, Samuelsson A, et al. Soft tissue sarcoma after treatment for breast cancer—a Swedish population-based study. *Eur J Cancer* 1998;34(13):2068.
15. Stewart F, Treves N. Lymphangiosarcoma in post-mastectomy lymphedema. *Cancer* 1943;1:64.
16. Muller R, Hajdu S, Brennan M. Lymphangiosarcoma associated with chronic filarial lymphedema. *Cancer* 1987;59:179.
17. Fong Y, Rosen P, Brennan M. Multifocal desmoids. *Surgery* 1993;114:902.
18. Smith A, Pearce N, Fisher D, et al. Soft tissue sarcoma and exposure to phenoxyherbicides and chlorophenols in New Zealand. *J Natl Cancer Inst* 1984;73:1111.
19. Kang H, Weatherbee L, Breslin P, et al. Soft tissue sarcoma and military service in Vietnam: a case comparison group analysis of hospital patients. *J Occup Med* 1986;28:1215.
20. Hoppin J, Tolbert P, Herrick R, et al. Occupational chlorophenol exposure and soft tissue sarcoma risk among men aged 30–60 years. *Am J Epidemiol* 1998;148(7):693.
21. Fingerhut M, Halperin W, Marlow D, et al. Cancer mortality in workers exposed to 2,3,7,8-tetrachlorodibenzo-p-dioxin. *N Engl J Med* 1991;324:212.
22. Brann E. The association of selected cancers with service in the US military in Vietnam: II. Soft tissue and other sarcomas. *Arch Intern Med* 1990;150:2485.
23. DaSilva H, Abbatt J, DaMotta L. Malignancy and other effects following the administration of thorotrast. *Lancet* 1965;2:201.
24. Creech J, Makk L. Liver disease among polyvinyl chloride production workers. *Ann N Y Acad Sci* 1973;246:88.
25. Dick J, Zahm S, Hanberg A, Adami H. Pesticides and cancer. *Cancer Causes Control* 1997;8(3):420.
26. Mertens F, Fletcher C, Dal Cin P, et al. Cytogenetic analysis of 46 pleomorphic soft tissue sarcomas and correlation with morphologic and clinical features: a report of the CHAMP Study Group. Chromosomes and Morphology. *Genes Chromosomes Cancer* 1998;22(1):16.
27. Orlow I, Drobnjak M, Zhang Z, et al. Alteration of INK4A and INK4B genes in adult soft tissue sarcomas: effect on survival. *J Natl Cancer Inst* 1999;91(1):73.
28. Sreekantaiah C, Karakousis C, Leong S, Sandberg A. Cytogenetic findings in liposarcoma correlate with histopathologic subtypes. *Cancer* 1992;69(10):2484.
29. Fletcher CD, Unni KK, Mertens F. Pathology and genetics of tumors of soft tissue and bone. In: Kleihues P, Sobin LH, eds. World Health Organization Classification of Tumors. Lyon: IARC Press, 2002.
30. Allander SV, Illei PB, Chen Y, et al. Expression profiling of synovial sarcoma by cDNA microarrays: association of ERBB2, IGFBP2, and ELF3 with epithelial differentiation. *Am J Pathol* 2002;161:1587.
31. Nielsen TO, West RB, Linn SC, et al. Molecular characterisation of soft tissue tumours; a gene expression study. *Lancet* 2002;359:1301.
32. Segal NH, Pavlidis P, Antonescu CR, et al. Classification and subtype prediction of adult soft tissue sarcoma by functional genomics. *Am J Pathol* 2003;163:691.
33. Brown FM, Fletcher CD. Problems in grading soft tissue sarcomas. *Am J Clin Pathol* 2000;114[Suppl]:S82.
34. Fong Y, Coit D, Woodruff J, et al. Lymph node metastasis from soft tissue sarcoma in adults: analysis of data from a prospective database of 1772 sarcoma patients. *Ann Surg* 1993;218:72.
35. Broders A, Hargrave R, Meyerding H. Pathological features of soft tissue fibrosarcoma with special reference to the grading of its malignancy. *Surg Gynecol Obstet* 1939;69:267.
36. Costa J, Wesley RA, Glatstein E, et al. The grading of soft tissue sarcomas. Results of a clinicohistopathologic correlation in a series of 163 cases. *Cancer* 1984;53:530.
37. Trojani M, Contesso G, Coindre JM, et al. Soft-tissue sarcomas of adults; study of pathological prognostic variables and definition of a histopathological grading system. *Int J Cancer* 1984;33:37.
38. Hajdu S. *Pathology of soft tissue tumors.* Philadelphia: Lea & Febiger, 1979.
39. Alvegard T, Berg N. Histopathology peer review of high-grade soft tissue sarcoma: the Scandinavian Sarcoma Group experience. *J Clin Oncol* 1989;7:1845.
40. van Unnik J, Coindre J, Contesso G. Grading of soft tissue sarcomas: experience of the EORTC soft tissue and bone sarcoma group. *Dev Oncol* 1988;55:7.
41. Drobnjak M, Latres E, Pollack D, et al. Prognostic implications of p53 nuclear overexpression and high proliferation index of Ki-67 in adult soft-tissue sarcomas. *J Natl Cancer Inst* 1994;86:549.
42. Clark J, Rocques P, Crew A, et al. Identification of novel genes, SYT and SSX, involved in the t(X;18)(p11.2;q11.2) translocation found in human synovial sarcoma. *Nat Genet* 1994;7:502.
43. Crozat A, Aman P, Mandahl N, et al. Fusion of CHOP to a novel RNA-binding protein in human myxoid liposarcoma. *Nature* 1993;363:640.
44. Knight J, Renwick P, Cin P, et al. Translocation t(12;16)(q13;p11) in myxoid liposarcoma and round cell liposarcoma: molecular and cytogenetic analysis. *Cancer Res* 1995;55:24.
45. Ladanyi M, Gerald W. Fusion of the EWS and WT1 genes in the desmoplastic small round cell tumor. *Cancer Res* 1994;54:2837.
46. Khan J, Wei JS, Ringner M, et al. Classification and diagnostic prediction of cancers using gene expression profiling and artificial neural networks. *Nat Med* 2001;7:673.
47. Fletcher CD, Berman JJ, Corless C, et al. Diagnosis of gastrointestinal stromal tumors: a consensus approach. *Hum Pathol* 2002;33:459.
48. Rubin BP, Singer S, Tsao C, et al. KIT activation is a ubiquitous feature of gastrointestinal stromal tumors. *Cancer Res* 2001;61:8118.
49. Gardner E. Follow up study of a family group exhibiting dominant inheritance for a syndrome including intestinal polyps, osteomas, fibromas, and epidermal cysts. *Am J Hum Genet* 1962;14:376.
50. Eccles DM, van der Luijt R, Breukel C, et al. Hereditary desmoid disease due to a frameshift mutation at codon 19234 of the APC gene. *Am J Hum Genet* 1996;59:1193.
51. Miyaki M, Konishi M, Kikuchi-Yanoshita R, et al. Coexistence of somatic and germ-line mutations of APC gene in desmoid tumors from patients with familial adenomatous polyposis. *Cancer Res* 1993;53:5079.
52. Sandberg AA, Bridge JA. Updates on the cytogenetics and molecular genetics of bone and soft tissue tumors. Dermatofibrosarcoma protuberans and giant cell fibroblastoma. *Cancer Genet Cytogenet* 2003;140:1.
53. Maki RG, Awan RA, Dixon RH, Jhanwar S, Antonescu CR. Differential sensitivity to imatinib of 2 patients with metastatic sarcoma arising from dermatofibrosarcoma protuberans. *Int J Cancer* 2002;100:623.
54. Rubin BP, Schuetze SM, Eary JF, et al. Molecular targeting of platelet-derived growth factor B by imatinib mesylate in a patient with metastatic dermatofibrosarcoma protuberans. *J Clin Oncol* 2002;20:3586.
55. Bowne WB, Antonescu CR, Leung DHY, et al. Dermatofibrosarcoma protuberans (DFSP): a clinico-pathologic analysis of patients treated and followed at a single institution. *Cancer* 2000;88:2711.
56. Willen H, Akerman M, Dal Cin P, et al. Comparison of chromosomal patterns with clinical features in 165 lipomas: a report of the CHAMP study group. *Cancer Genet Cytogenet* 1998;102:46.
57. Dal Cin P, Sciot R, Polito P, et al. Lesions of 13q may occur independently of deletion of 16q in spindle cell/pleomorphic lipomas. *Histopathology* 1997;31:222.
58. Ahn C, Harvey J. Mediastinal hibernoma, a rare tumor. *Ann Thorac Surg* 1990;50:828.
59. Mentzel T, Calonje E, Fletcher C. Lipoblastoma and lipoblastomatosis: a clinicopathological study of 14 cases. *Histopathology* 1993;23:527.
60. Mandahl N, Mertens F, Willen H, et al. Nonrandom pattern of telomeric associations in atypical lipomatous tumors with ring and giant marker chromosomes. *Cancer Genet Cytogenet* 1998;103:25.
61. Kooby D, Antonescu CR, Brennan MF, Singer S. Atypical lipomatous tumor/well-differentiated liposarcoma of the extremity and trunk wall: importance of histologic subtype with treatment recommendations. *Ann Surg Oncol* 2004;11(1):78.
62. Singer S, Antonescu CR, Riedel E, et al. Histologic subtype and margin of resection predict pattern of recurrence and survival for retroperitoneal liposarcoma. *Ann Surg* 2003;238:358.
63. Meis-Kindblom JM, Sjogren H, Kindblom LG, et al. Cytogenetic and molecular genetic analyses of liposarcoma and its soft tissue simulators: recognition of new variants and differential diagnosis. *Virchows Arch* 2001;439:141.
64. Antonescu CR, Elahi A, Humphrey M, et al. Specificity of TLS-CHOP rearrangement for classic myxoid/round cell liposarcoma; absence in predominantly myxoid well-differentiated liposarcoma. *J Mol Diagn* 2000;2:132.
65. Antonescu CR, Tschemyavsky SJ, Decuseara R, et al. Prognostic impact of P53 status, TLS-CHOP fusion transcript structure, and histological grade in myxoid liposarcoma: a molecular and clinicopathologic study of 82 cases. *Clin Cancer Res* 2001;7:3977.
66. Downes KA, Goldblum JR, Montgomery EA, et al. Pleomorphic liposarcoma: a clinicopathologic analysis of 19 cases. *Mod Pathol* 2001;14:179.
67. Hollenbeck ST, Grobmyer SR, Kent KC, et al. Surgical treatment and outcome of patients with primary inferior vena cava leiomyosarcoma. *J Am Coll Surg* 2003;197:575.
68. LaQuaglia M, Heller G, Ghavimi F, et al. The effect of age at diagnosis on outcome in rhabdomyosarcoma. *Cancer* 1994;73:109.
69. Davis R, D'Cruz C, Lovell M, et al. Fusion of PAX7 to FKHR by the variant t(1;13)(p36;q14) translocation in alveolar rhabdomyosarcoma. *Cancer Res* 1994;54(11):2869.
70. Furlong MA, Mentzel T, Fanburg-Smith JC. Pleomorphic rhabdomyosarcoma in adults: a clinicopathologic study of 38 cases with emphasis on morphologic variants and recent skeletal muscle-specific markers. *Mod Pathol* 2001;14:595.
71. White C. Treatment of hemangiomatosis with recombinant interferon alfa [Review]. *Semin Hematol* 1990;27:15.
72. Taylor J, Ryu J, Colby T, et al. Lymphangioleiomyomatosis. Clinical course in 32 patients. *N Engl J Med* 1990;323:1254.
73. Kelleher M, Iwatsuki S, Sheahan D. Epithelioid hemangioendothelioma of liver. Clinicopathological correlation of 10 cases treated by orthotopic liver transplantation. *Am J Surg Pathol* 1989;13:999.
74. Fletcher C, Beham A, Bekir S, et al. Epithelioid angiosarcoma of deep soft tissue: a distinctive tumor readily mistaken for an epithelial neoplasm. *Am J Surg Pathol* 1991;15:915.
75. Nemes Z. Differentiation markers in hemangiopericytoma. *Cancer* 1992;69:133.

76. O'Sullivan B, Cummings B, Catton C, et al. Outcome following radiation treatment for high-risk pigmented villonodular synovitis. *Int J Radiat Oncol Biol Phys* 1995;32:777.

77. Bertoni F, Unni KK, Beabout JW, et al. Malignant giant cell tumor of the tendon sheaths and joints (malignant pigmented villonodular synovitis). *Am J Surg Pathol* 1997;21:153.

78. Lewis JJ, Antonescu CR, Leung D, et al. Synovial sarcoma: a multivariate analysis of prognostic factors in 112 patients with primary localized tumors of the extremity. *J Clin Oncol* 2000;18:2087.

79. Ladanyi M, Antonescu CR, Leung DH, et al. Impact of SYT-SSX fusion type on the clinical behavior of synovial sarcoma: a multi-institutional retrospective study of 243 patients. *Cancer Res* 2002;62:135.

80. Ladanyi M. Fusions of the SYT and SSX genes in synovial sarcoma. *Oncogene* 2001;20:5755.

81. Wallace M, Marchuk D, Andersen L, et al. Type I neurofibromatosis gene: identification of a large transcript disrupted in three NF1 patients. *Science* 1990;249:181.

82. White W, Shiu M, Rosenblum M, et al. Cellular schwannoma. *Cancer* 1990;66:1260.

83. Kurtkaya-Yapicier U, Scheithauer BW, Woodruff JM, et al. Schwannoma with rhabdomyoblastic differentiation: a unique variant of malignant triton tumor. *Am J Surg Pathol* 2003;27:848.

84. Vauthey JN, Woodruff JM, Brennan MF. Extremity malignant peripheral nerve sheath tumors (neurogenic sarcomas): a 10 year experience. *Ann Surg Oncol* 1995;2:126.

85. Angelov L, Davis A, O'Sullivan B, et al. Neurogenic sarcomas: experience at the University of Toronto. *Neurosurgery* 1998;43:56.

86. Antonescu CR, Argani P, Erlandson RA, et al. Skeletal and extraskeletal myxoid chondrosarcoma: a comparative clinicopathologic, ultrastructural, and molecular study. *Cancer* 1998;83:1504.

87. Lee J, Fetsch J, Wasdhal D, et al. A review of 40 patients with extraskeletal osteosarcoma. *Cancer* 1995;76:2253.

88. Newman P, Fletcher C. Malignant mesenchymoma. Clinicopathologic analysis of a series with evidence of low-grade behavior. *Am J Surg Pathol* 1991;15:607.

89. Lieberman P, Brennan M, Kimmel M, et al. Alveolar soft-part sarcoma. A clinico-pathologic study of half a century. *Cancer* 1989;63:1.

90. Tallini G, Parham D, Dias P, et al. Myogenic regulatory protein expression in adult soft tissue sarcomas. A sensitive and specific marker of skeletal muscle differentiation. *Am J Pathol* 1994;144:693.

91. Segal NH, Pavlidis P, Noble WS, et al. Classification of clear cell sarcoma as a subtype of melanoma by genomic profiling. *J Clin Oncol* 2003;21:1775.

92. Gerald W, Miller H, Battifora H, et al. Intra-abdominal desmoplastic small round-cell tumor: report of 19 cases of a distinctive type of high-grade polyphenotypic malignancy affecting young individuals. *Am J Surg Pathol* 1991;15:499.

93. Rodriguez E, Sreekantaiah C, Gerald W, et al. A recurring translocation, t(11;22(p13;q11.2), characterizes intraabdominal desmoplastic small round-cell tumors. *Cancer Genet Cytogenet* 1993;69:17.

94. Fonesca R, Yamakawa M, Nakamura S, et al. Follicular dendritic cell sarcoma and interdigitating reticulum cell sarcoma: a review. *Am J Hematol* 1998;59(2):161.

95. Panicek D, Gatsonis C, Rosenthal D, et al. CT and MR imaging in local staging of primary malignant musculoskeletal neoplasms. Report of the Radiology Diagnostic Oncology Group. *Radiology* 1997;202(1):237.

96. Vernon CB, Eary JF, Rubin BP, et al. FDG PET imaging guided re-evaluation of histopathologic response in a patient with high-grade sarcoma. *Skeletal Radiol* 2003;32:139.

97. Gadd M, Casper E, Woodruff J, et al. Development and treatment of pulmonary metastases in adult patients with extremity soft tissue sarcoma. *Ann Surg* 1993;218:705.

98. Cheng E, Dempsey S, Springfield S, et al. Frequent incidence of extrapulmonary sites of initial metastases in patients with liposarcoma. *Cancer* 1995;75:1120.

99. Heslin MJ, Lewis JJ, Woodruff JM, et al. Core needle biopsy for diagnosis of extremity soft tissue sarcoma. *Ann Surg Oncol* 1997;4:425.

100. Rydholm A. Soft tissue lesions in adults: biopsy—yes or no? *Ann Oncol* 1992;3[Suppl 2]:S57.

101. Akerman M, Killander D, Rydholm A, et al. Aspiration of musculoskeletal tumors for cytodiagnosis and DNA analysis. *Acta Orthop Scand* 1987;58:525.

102. Russell W, Cohen J, Enzinger F, et al. A clinical and pathological staging system for soft tissue sarcoma. *Cancer* 1977;40:1562.

103. Geer R, Woodruff J, Casper E, et al. Management of small soft tissue sarcoma of the extremity in adults. *Arch Surg* 1992;127:1285.

104. Fleming J, Berman R, Cheng S, et al. Long-term outcome of patients with American Joint Committee on Cancer stage IIB extremity soft tissue sarcomas. *J Clin Oncol* 1999;17:2772.

105. Brennan MF. Staging of soft tissue sarcomas. *Ann Surg Oncol* 1999;6(1):8.

106. Pisters P, Leung D, Woodruff J, et al. Analysis of prognostic factors in 1,041 patients with localized soft tissue sarcomas of the extremities. *J Clin Oncol* 1996;14(5):1679.

107. Greene FL, Page DL, Fleming ID, et al. *AJCC cancer staging manual*, 6th ed. New York: Springer, 2002.

108. Stojadinovic A, Leung DHY, Allen P, et al. Primary adult soft tissue sarcoma: time-dependent influence of prognostic factors. *J Clin Oncol* 2002;20:4344.

109. Rosenberg S, Tepper J, Glatstein E, et al. The treatment of soft-tissue sarcoma of the extremities: prospective randomized evaluations of (1) limb-sparing surgery plus radiation therapy compared with amputation and (2) the role of adjuvant chemotherapy. *Ann Surg* 1982;196:305.

110. Baldini EH, Goldberg J, Jenner C, et al. Long term outcomes after function-sparing surgery without radiotherapy for soft tissue sarcoma of the extremities and trunk. *J Clin Oncol* 1999;17:3252.

111. Fabrizio PL, Stafford SL, Pritchard DJ. Extremity soft-tissue sarcomas selectively treated with surgery alone. *Int J Radiat Oncol Biol Phys* 2000;48:227.

112. Alektiar KM, Leung D, Zelefsky MJ, et al. Adjuvant brachytherapy for primary high-grade soft tissue sarcoma of the extremity. *Ann Surg Oncol* 2002;9:48.

113. Pisters PW, Harrison LB, Leung DH, et al. Long-term results of a prospective randomized trial of adjuvant brachytherapy in soft tissue sarcoma. *J Clin Oncol* 1996;14:859.

114. Yang JC, Chang AE, Baker AR, et al. Randomized prospective study of the benefit of adjuvant radiation therapy in the treatment of soft tissue sarcomas of the extremity. *J Clin Oncol* 1998;16:197.

115. O'Sullivan B, Davis AM, Turcotte R, et al. Preoperative versus postoperative radiotherapy in soft tissue sarcoma of the limbs: a randomised trial. *Lancet* 2002;359:2235.

116. O'Sullivan B, Davis AM. A randomized phase III trial of pre-operative compared to post-operative radiotherapy in extremity soft tissue sarcoma. Proceedings American Society of Therapeutic Radiology and Oncology. *Int J Radiat Oncol Biol Phys* 2001;51:151(abst).

117. Hartford AC, Gohongi T, Fukumura D, Jain RK. Irradiation of a primary tumor, unlike surgical removal, enhances angiogenesis suppression at a distal site: potential role of host-tumor interaction. *Cancer Res* 2000;60(8):2128.

118. Pisters PW, Ballo MT, Fenstermacher MJ, et al. Phase I trial of preoperative concurrent doxorubicin and radiation therapy, surgical resection, and intraoperative electron-beam radiation therapy for patients with localized retroperitoneal sarcoma. *J Clin Oncol* 2003;21(16):3092.

119. Jones JJ, Catton CN, O'Sullivan B, et al. Initial results of a trial of preoperative external-beam radiation therapy and postoperative brachytherapy for retroperitoneal sarcoma. *Ann Surg Oncol* 2002;9(4):346.

120. Gieschen HL, Spiro IJ, Suit HD, et al. Long-term results of intraoperative electron beam radiotherapy for primary and recurrent retroperitoneal soft tissue sarcoma. *Int J Radiat Oncol Biol Phys* 2001;50(1):127.

121. Petersen IA, Haddock MG, Donohue JH, et al. Use of intraoperative electron beam radiotherapy in the management of retroperitoneal soft tissue sarcomas. *Int J Radiat Oncol Biol Phys* 2002;52(2):469.

122. DeLaney TF, Spiro IJ, Suit HD, et al. Neoadjuvant chemotherapy and radiotherapy for large extremity soft-tissue sarcomas. *Int J Radiat Oncol Biol Phys* 2003;56(4):1117.

123. O'Sullivan B, Bell RS. Has "MAID" made it in the management of high-risk soft-tissue sarcoma? *Int J Radiat Oncol Biol Phys* 2003;56(4):915.

124. Tepper J, Rosenberg SA, Glatstein E. Radiation therapy technique in soft tissue sarcomas of the extremity—policies of treatment at the National Cancer Institute. *Int J Radiat Oncol Biol Phys* 1982;8(2):263.

125. Lartigau E, Kantor G, Taieb S, et al. Definitions of target volumes in soft tissue sarcomas of the extremities. *Cancer Radiother* 2001;5(5):695.

126. O'Sullivan B, Wunder J, Pisters PW. Target description for radiotherapy of soft tissue sarcoma. In: Gregoire V, Scalliet P, Ang KK, eds. *Clinical target volumes in conformal radiotherapy and intensity modulated radiotherapy*. Heidelberg: Springer, 2003:205.

127. Harrison LB, Franzese F, Gaynor JJ, Brennan MF. Long-term results of a prospective randomized trial of adjuvant brachytherapy in the management of completely resected soft tissue sarcomas of the extremity and superficial trunk. *Int J Radiat Oncol Biol Phys* 1993;27(2):259.

128. Le Pechoux C, Le Deley MC, Delaloge S, et al. Postoperative radiotherapy in the management of adult soft tissue sarcoma of the extremities: results with two different total dose, fractionation, and overall treatment time schedules. *Int J Radiat Oncol Biol Phys* 1999;44(4):879.

129. Virkus WW, Mollabashy A, Reith JD, et al. Preoperative radiotherapy in the treatment of soft tissue sarcomas. *Clin Orthop* 2002;(397):177.

130. Leibel SA, Fuks Z, Zelefsky MJ, et al. Intensity-modulated radiotherapy. *Cancer J* 2002;8(2):164.

131. Borden EC, Baker LH, Bell RS, et al. Soft tissue sarcomas of adults: state of the translational science. *Clin Cancer Res* 2003;9(6):1941.

132. O'Sullivan B, Ward I, Haycocks T, et al. Techniques to modulate radiotherapy toxicity and outcome in soft tissue sarcoma. *Curr Treat Options Oncol* 2003;4:453.

133. Chan MF, Chui CS, Schupak K, et al. The treatment of large extraskeletal chondrosarcoma of the leg: comparison of IMRT and conformal radiotherapy techniques. *J Appl Clin Med Phys* 2001;2(1):3.

134. Nag S, Shasha D, Janjan N, et al. The American Brachytherapy Society recommendations for brachytherapy of soft tissue sarcomas. *Int J Radiat Oncol Biol Phys* 2001;49(4):1033.

135. Ormsby MV, Hilaris BS, Nori D, et al. Wound complications of adjuvant radiation therapy in patients with soft-tissue sarcomas. *Ann Surg* 1989;210(1):93.

136. Janjan NA, Yasko AW, Reece GP, et al. Comparison of charges related to radiotherapy for soft-tissue sarcomas treated by preoperative external-beam irradiation versus interstitial implantation. *Ann Surg Oncol* 1994;1(5):415.

137. Pisters PW, Harrison LB, Woodruff JM, et al. A prospective randomized trial of adjuvant brachytherapy in the management of low-grade soft tissue sarcomas of the extremity and superficial trunk. *J Clin Oncol* 1994;12(6):1150.

138. Schray MF, Gunderson LL, Sim FH, et al. Soft tissue sarcoma. Integration of brachytherapy, resection, and external irradiation. *Cancer* 1990;66(3):451.

139. Thomas L, Delannes M, Stockle E, et al. Intraoperative interstitial iridium brachytherapy in the management of soft tissue sarcomas: preliminary results of a feasibility phase II study. *Radiother Oncol* 1994;33(2):99.

140. Delannes M, Thomas L, Martel P, et al. Low-dose-rate intraoperative brachytherapy combined with external beam irradiation in the conservative treatment of soft tissue sarcoma. *Int J Radiat Oncol Biol Phys* 2000;47(1):165.

141. Alekhteyar KM, Leung DH, Brennan MF, et al. The effect of combined external beam radiotherapy and brachytherapy on local control and wound complications in patients with high-grade soft tissue sarcomas of the extremity with positive microscopic margin. *Int J Radiat Oncol Biol Phys* 1996;36(2):321.

142. Pearlstone DB, Janjan NA, Feig BW, et al. Re-resection with brachytherapy for locally recurrent soft tissue sarcoma arising in a previously radiated field. *Cancer J Sci Am* 1999;5(1):26.

143. Catton C, Davis A, Bell R, et al. Soft tissue sarcoma of the extremity. Limb salvage after failure of combined conservative therapy. *Radiother Oncol* 1996;41(3):209.

144. Levay J, O'Sullivan B, Catton C, et al. Outcome and prognostic factors in soft tissue sarcoma in the adult. *Int J Radiat Oncol Biol Phys* 1993;27:1091.

145. Alektiar KM, Velasco J, Zelefsky MJ, et al. Adjuvant radiotherapy for margin-positive high-grade soft tissue sarcoma of the extremity. *Int J Radiat Oncol Biol Phys* 2000;48(4):1051.

146. Sadoski C, Suit HD, Rosenberg A, et al. Preoperative radiation, surgical margins, and local control of extremity sarcomas of soft tissues. *J Surg Oncol* 1993;52(4):223.

147. Gerrand CH, Wunder JS, Kandel RA, et al. Classification of positive margins after resection of soft-tissue sarcoma of the limb predicts the risk of local recurrence. *J Bone Joint Surg Br* 2001;83(8):1149.

148. Noria S, Davis A, Kandel R, et al. Residual disease following unplanned excision of soft tissue sarcoma of an extremity. *J Bone Joint Surg Am* 1996;78:650.

149. Brien EW, Terek RM, Geer RJ, et al. Treatment of soft tissue sarcomas of the hand. *J Bone Joint Surg Am* 1995;77:564.

150. Karakousis CP, De Young C, Driscoll DL. Soft tissue sarcomas of the hand and foot: management and survival. *Ann Surg Oncol* 1998;5(3):238.

151. Lin PP, Guzel VB, Pisters PW, et al. Surgical management of soft tissue sarcomas of the hand and foot. *Cancer* 2002;95(4):852.

152. Bray PW, Bell RS, Bowen CV, et al. Limb salvage surgery and adjuvant radiotherapy for soft tissue sarcomas of the forearm and hand. *J Hand Surg Am* 1997;22(3):495.

153. Tepper JE, Suit HD. Radiation therapy along for sarcoma of soft tissue. *Cancer* 1985; 56(3):475.

154. Slater JD, McNeese MD, Peters LJ. Radiation therapy for unresectable soft tissue sarcomas. *Int J Radiat Oncol Biol Phys* 1986;12(10):1729.

155. Schwarz R, Krull A, Lessel A, et al. European results of neutron therapy in soft tissue sarcomas. *Recent Results Cancer Res* 1998;150:100.

156. Schwartz DL, Einck J, Bellon J, et al. Fast neutron radiotherapy for soft tissue and cartilaginous sarcomas at high risk for local recurrence. *Int J Radiat Oncol Biol Phys* 2001;50(2):449.

157. Goffman T, Tochner Z, Glatstein E. Primary treatment of large and massive adult sarcomas with iododeoxyuridine and aggressive hyperfractionated irradiation. *Cancer* 1991;67(3):572.

158. Cormier JN, Patel SR, Herzog CE, et al. Concurrent ifosfamide-based chemotherapy and irradiation. Analysis of treatment-related toxicity in 43 patients with sarcoma. *Cancer* 2001;92(6):1550.

159. Rhomberg W, Hassenstein EO, Gefeller D. Radiotherapy vs. radiotherapy and razoxane in the treatment of soft tissue sarcomas: final results of a randomized study. *Int J Radiat Oncol Biol Phys* 1996;36(5):1077.

160. Omura GA, Blessing JA, Major F, et al. A randomized clinical trial of adjuvant adriamycin in uterine sarcomas: a Gynecologic Oncology Group study. *J Clin Oncol* 1985;3(9):1240.

161. Antman K, Suit H, Amato D, et al. Preliminary results of a randomized trial of adjuvant doxorubicin for sarcomas: lack of apparent difference between treatment groups. *J Clin Oncol* 1984;2(6):601.

162. Lerner HJ, Amato DA, Savlov ED, et al. Eastern Cooperative Oncology Group: a comparison of adjuvant doxorubicin and observation for patients with localized soft tissue sarcoma. *J Clin Oncol* 1987;5(4):613.

163. Antman K, Ryan L, Borden E, et al. Pooled results from three randomized adjuvant studies of doxorubicin versus observation in soft tissue sarcomas: 10 year results and review of the literature. In: Salmon SE, ed. *Adjuvant therapy of cancer*, 6th ed. Philadelphia: WB Saunders, 1990:529.

164. Alvegard TA, Sigurdsson H, Mouridsen H, et al. Adjuvant chemotherapy with doxorubicin in high-grade soft tissue sarcoma: a randomized trial of the Scandinavian Sarcoma Group. *J Clin Oncol* 1989;7(10):1504.

165. Gherlinzoni F, Bacci G, Picci P, et al. A randomized trial for the treatment of high-grade soft-tissue sarcomas of the extremities: preliminary observations. *J Clin Oncol* 1986;4(4):552.

166. Gherlinzoni F, Picci P, Bacci G, Cazzola A. Late results of a randomized trial for the treatment of soft tissue sarcomas (STS) of the extremities in adult patients. *Proc Am Soc Clin Oncol* 1993;12:a1633.

167. Eilber FR, Giuliano AE, Huth JF, Morton DL. Postoperative adjuvant chemotherapy (adriamycin) in high grade extremity soft tissue sarcoma: a randomized prospective trial. In: Salmon SE, ed. *Adjuvant therapy of cancer*, 5th ed. Orlando: Grune & Stratton, 1987:719.

168. Piver MS, Lele SB, Marchetti DL, Emrich LJ. Effect of adjuvant chemotherapy on time to recurrence and survival of stage I uterine sarcomas. *J Surg Oncol* 1988;38(4):233.

169. Rosenberg SA, Tepper J, Glatstein E, et al. Prospective randomized evaluation of adjuvant chemotherapy in adults with soft tissue sarcomas of the extremities. *Cancer* 1983;52(3):424.

170. Rosenberg SA, Chang AE, Glatstein E. Adjuvant chemotherapy for treatment of extremity soft tissue sarcomas: review of the National Cancer Institute experience. *Cancer Treat Symp* 1985;3:83.

171. Chang AE, Kinsella T, Glatstein E, et al. Adjuvant chemotherapy for patients with high-grade soft-tissue sarcomas of the extremity. *J Clin Oncol* 1988;6(9):1491.

172. Dresdale A, Bonow RO, Wesley R, et al. Prospective evaluation of doxorubicin-induced cardiomyopathy resulting from postsurgical adjuvant treatment of patients with soft tissue sarcomas. *Cancer* 1983;52(1):51.

173. Glenn J, Kinsella T, Glatstein E, et al. A randomized, prospective trial of adjuvant chemotherapy in adults with soft tissue sarcomas of the head and neck, breast, and trunk. *Cancer* 1985;55(6):1206.

174. Glenn J, Sindelar WF, Kinsella T, et al. Results of multimodality therapy of resectable soft-tissue sarcomas of the retroperitoneum. *Surgery* 1985;97(3):316.

175. Benjamin RS, Terjanian TO, Fenoglio CJ, et al. The importance of combination chemotherapy for adjuvant treatment of high-risk patients with soft-tissue sarcomas of the extremities. In: Salmon SE, ed. *Adjuvant therapy of cancer*, 5th ed. Orlando: Grune & Stratton, 1987:735.

176. Edmonson JH, Fleming TR, Ivins JC, et al. Randomized study of systemic chemotherapy following complete excision of nonosseous sarcomas. *J Clin Oncol* 1984;2(12):1390.

177. Bramwell V, Rouesse J, Steward W, et al. Adjuvant CyVADIC chemotherapy for adult soft tissue sarcoma—reduced local recurrence but no improvement in survival: a study of the European Organization for Research and Treatment of Cancer Soft Tissue and Bone Sarcoma Group. *J Clin Oncol* 1994;12(6):1137.

178. Ravaud A, Bui NB, Coindre J-M, et al. Adjuvant chemotherapy with CyVADIC in high risk soft tissue sarcoma: a randomized prospective trial. In: Salmon SE, ed. *Adjuvant therapy of cancer*, 6th ed. Philadelphia: WB Saunders, 1990:556.

179. Frustaci S, Gherlinzoni F, De Paoli A, et al. Adjuvant chemotherapy for adult soft tissue sarcomas of the extremities and girdles: results of the Italian randomized cooperative trial. *J Clin Oncol* 2001;19:1238.

180. Gortzak E, Azzarelli A, Buesa J, et al. A randomized phase II study on neo-adjuvant chemotherapy for 'high-risk' adult soft-tissue sarcoma. *Eur J Cancer* 2001;37:1096.

181. Brodowicz T, Schwameis E, Widder J, et al. Intensified adjuvant IFADIC chemotherapy for adult soft tissue sarcoma: a prospective randomized feasibility trial. *Sarcoma* 2000;4:151.

182. Benjamin RS, Legha SS, Patel SR, et al. Single-agent ifosfamide studies in sarcomas of soft tissue and bone: the M.D. Anderson experience. *Cancer Chemother Pharmacol* 1993;31[Suppl 2]:S174.

183. Steward WP, Verweij J, Somers R, et al. Granulocyte-macrophage colony-stimulating factor allows safe escalation of dose-intensity of chemotherapy in metastatic adult soft tissue sarcomas: a study of the European Organization for Research and Treatment of Cancer Soft Tissue and Bone Sarcoma Group. *J Clin Oncol* 1993;11(1):15.

184. Zalupski MM, Ryan JR, Hussein ME, et al. Defining the role of adjuvant chemotherapy for patients with soft tissue sarcoma of the extremities. In: Salmon SE, ed. *Adjuvant chemotherapy of cancer*, 7th ed. Philadelphia: JB Lippincott, 1993:385.

185. Tierney JF, Mosseri V, Stewart LA, et al. Adjuvant chemotherapy for soft-tissue sarcoma: review and meta-analysis of the published results of randomised clinical trials. *Br J Cancer* 1995;72(2):469.

186. Adjuvant chemotherapy for localized resectable soft-tissue sarcoma of adults: meta-analysis of individual data. Sarcoma Meta-analysis Collaboration. *Lancet* 1997;350(9092):1647.

187. Fisher B, Gunduz N, Saffer EA. Influence of the interval between primary tumor removal and chemotherapy on kinetics and growth of metastases. *Cancer Res* 1983;43(4):1488.

188. Simpson-Herren L, Sanford AH, Holmquist JP. Effects of surgery on the cell kinetics of residual tumor. *Cancer Treat Rep* 1976;60:1749.

189. Rouesse JG, Friedman S, Sevin DM, et al. Preoperative induction chemotherapy in the treatment of locally advanced soft-tissue sarcomas. *Cancer* 1987;60(3):296.

190. Pezzi CM, Pollock RE, Evans HL, et al. Preoperative chemotherapy for soft-tissue sarcomas of the extremities. *Ann Surg* 1990;211(4):476.

191. Casper ES, Gaynor JJ, Harrison LB, et al. Preoperative and postoperative adjuvant combination chemotherapy for adults with high grade soft tissue sarcoma. *Cancer* 1994;73(6):1644.

192. Menendez LR, Fideler BM, Mirra J. Thallium-201 scanning for the evaluation of osteosarcoma and soft-tissue sarcoma. A study of the evaluation and predictability of the histological response to chemotherapy. *J Bone Joint Surg Am* 1993;75(4):526.

193. Koutcher JA, Ballon D, Graham M, et al. 31P NMR spectra of extremity sarcomas: diversity of metabolic profiles and changes in response to chemotherapy. *Magn Reson Med* 1990;16(1):19.

194. Nieweg OE, Pruim J, Hoekstra HJ, et al. Positron emission tomography with fluorine-18-fluorodeoxyglucose for the evaluation of therapeutic isolated regional limb perfusion in a patient with soft-tissue sarcoma. *J Nucl Med* 1994;35(1):90.

195. Eilber FR, Giuliano AE, Huth JF, Morton DL. A randomized prospective trial using postoperative adjuvant chemotherapy (adriamycin) in high-grade extremity soft-tissue sarcoma. *Am J Clin Oncol* 1988;11(1):39.

196. Eilber F, Giuliano A, Huth J, Mirra J. Neoadjuvant chemotherapy, radiation, and limited surgery for high grade soft tissue sarcoma of the extremity. In: Ryan JR, Baker LH, eds. *Recent concepts in sarcoma treatment*. Dordrecht, The Netherlands: Kluwer, 1988:115.

197. Azzarelli A, Quagliuolo V, Casali P, et al. Preoperative doxorubicin plus ifosfamide in primary soft-tissue sarcomas of the extremities. *Cancer Chemother Pharmacol* 1993;31[Suppl 2]:S210.

198. Levine EA, Trippon M, Das Gupta TK. Preoperative multimodality treatment for soft tissue sarcomas. *Cancer* 1993;71(11):3685.

199. Mason M, Robinson M, Harmer C, Westbury G. Intra-arterial adriamycin, conventionally fractionated radiotherapy and conservative surgery for soft tissue sarcomas. *Clin Oncol (R Coll Radiol)* 1992;4(1):32.

200. Eggermont AM, Schraffordt Koops H, Lienard D, et al. Isolated limb perfusion with high-dose tumor necrosis factor-alpha in combination with interferon-gamma and melphalan for nonresectable extremity soft tissue sarcomas: a multicenter trial. *J Clin Oncol* 1996;14(10):2653.

201. Eggermont AM, de Wilt JH, ten Hagen TL. Current uses of isolated limb perfusion in the clinic and a model system for new strategies. *Lancet Oncol* 2003;4:429.

202. Wiedemann GJ, d'Oleire F, Knop E, et al. Ifosfamide and carboplatin combined with 41.8 degrees C whole-body hyperthermia in patients with refractory sarcoma and malignant teratoma. *Cancer Res* 1994;54(20):5346.

203. Wendtner CM, Abdel-Rahman S, Krych M, et al. Response to neoadjuvant chemotherapy combined with regional hyperthermia predicts long-term survival for adult patients with retroperitoneal and visceral high-risk soft tissue sarcomas. *J Clin Oncol* 2002;20:3156.

204. Issels RD, Abdel-Rahman S, Wendtner C, et al. Neoadjuvant chemotherapy combined with regional hyperthermia (RHT) for locally advanced primary or recurrent high-risk adult soft-tissue sarcomas (STS) of adults: long-term results of a phase II study. *Eur J Cancer* 2001;37:1599.

205. Westermann AM, Wiedemann GJ, Jager E, et al. A Systemic Hyperthermia Oncologic Working Group trial. Ifosfamide, carboplatin, and etoposide combined with 41.8 degrees C whole-body hyperthermia for metastatic soft tissue sarcoma. *Oncology* 2003;64:312.

206. Jaques D, Coit D, Hajdu S, Brennan M. Management of primary and recurrent soft tissue sarcoma of the retroperitoneum. *Ann Surg* 1990;212:51.

207. Bevilacqua R, Rogatko A, Hajdu S, et al. Prognostic factors in primary retroperitoneal soft tissue sarcoma. *Arch Surg* 1991;126:328.

208. Shibata D, Lewis JJ, Leung D, Woodruff J, Brennan MF. Is there a role for incomplete resection in the management of retroperitoneal liposarcomas? *J Am Coll Surg* 2001;193:373.

209. Catton C, O'Sullivan B, Kotwall C. Outcome and prognosis in retroperitoneal soft tissue sarcoma. *Int J Radiat Oncol Biol Phys* 1994;29:1005.

210. Fein D, Corn B, Lanciano R. Management of retroperitoneal sarcomas: does dose escalation impact on locoregional control? *Int J Radiat Oncol Biol Phys* 1995;31:129.

211. Tepper JE, Suit HD, Wood WC, et al. Radiation therapy of retroperitoneal soft tissue sarcomas. *Int J Radiat Oncol Biol Phys* 1984;10:825.
212. Willet C, Suit H, Tepper J. Intraoperative electron beam radiation therapy for retroperitoneal soft tissue sarcomas. *Cancer* 1991;68:278.
213. Gunderson L, Najorney D, McIlrath D. External beam and intraoperative electron irradiation for locally advanced soft-tissue sarcomas. *Int J Radiat Oncol Biol Phys* 1993;25:647.
214. Sindelar W, Kinsella T, Chen P. Intraoperative radiotherapy in retroperitoneal sarcomas. *Arch Surg* 1993;128:402.
215. Alektiar KM, Brennan MF, Hu K, Anderson L, Harrison LB. High dose rate intraoperative brachytherapy (HDR-IOBRT) for retroperitoneal sarcomas. *Int J Radiat Oncol Biol Phys* 2000;47:157.
216. Fiveash JB, Murshed H, Duan J, et al. Effect of multileaf collimator leaf width on physical dose distributions in the treatment of CNS and head and neck neoplasms with intensity modulated radiation therapy. *Med Phys* 2002;29:1116.
217. Eeles R, Fisher C, A'Hern R, et al. Head and neck sarcomas: prognostic factors and implications for treatment. *Br J Cancer* 1993;68:201.
218. Willers H, Hug E, Spiro I, et al. Adult soft tissue sarcomas of the head and neck treated by radiation and surgery or radiation alone: patterns of failure and prognostic factors. *Int J Radiat Oncol Biol Phys* 1995;33(3):585.
219. Le Q, Fu K, Kroll S, et al. Prognostic factors in adult soft-tissue sarcomas of the head and neck. *Int J Radiat Oncol Biol Phys* 1997;37(5):975.
220. Lydiatt W, Shaha A, Shah J. Angiosarcoma of the head and neck. *Am J Surg* 1994;168(5):451.
221. Morrison W, Byers R, Garden A, et al. Cutaneous angiosarcoma of the head and neck: a therapeutic dilemma. *Cancer* 1995;76:319.
222. Moore M, Kinne D. Breast sarcoma. *Surg Clin North Am* 1996;76(2):383.
223. North JH, McPhee M, Arredondo M, et al. Sarcoma of the breast: implications of the extent of local therapy. *Am Surg* 1998;64:1059.
224. Gutman H, Pollock RE, Ross MI, et al. Sarcoma of the breast: implications for extent of therapy. The MD Anderson experience. *Surgery* 1994;116:505.
225. Johnstone P, Pierce L, Merino M, et al. Primary soft tissue sarcomas of the breast: local-regional control with post-operative radiotherapy. *Int J Radiat Oncol Biol Phys* 1993;27:671.
226. Devereux D, Kent H, Brennan M. Time dependent effects of adriamycin and x-ray therapy on wound healing in the rat. *Cancer* 1980;45:2805.
227. Shamberger R, Devereux D, Brennan M. The effect of chemotherapeutic agents on wound healing. In: Murphy G, ed. *International advances in surgical oncology.* New York: Alan R. Liss, 1981:15.
228. Meric F, Milas M, Hunt KK, et al. Impact of neoadjuvant chemotherapy on postoperative morbidity in soft tissue sarcomas. *J Clin Oncol* 2000;18(19):3378.
229. Arbeit JM, Hilaris BS, Brennan MF. Wound complications in the multimodality treatment of extremity and superficial truncal sarcomas. *J Clin Oncol* 1987;5(3):480.
230. Simon MA, Nachman J. The clinical utility of preoperative therapy for sarcomas. *J Bone Joint Surg Am* 1986;68(9):1458.
231. Chmell MJ, Schwartz HS. Analysis of variables affecting wound healing after musculoskeletal sarcoma resections. *J Surg Oncol* 1996;61(3):185.
232. Bujko K, Suit HD, Springfield DS, et al. Wound healing after preoperative radiation for sarcoma of soft tissues. *Surg Gynecol Obstet* 1993;176(2):124.
233. Peat BG, Bell RS, Davis A, et al. Wound-healing complications after soft-tissue sarcoma surgery. *Plast Reconstr Surg* 1994;93(5):980.
234. O'Sullivan B, Gullane P, Irish J, et al. Preoperative radiotherapy for adult head and neck soft tissue sarcoma: assessment of wound complication rates and cancer outcome in a prospective series. *World J Surg* 2003;27(7):875.
235. Stinson S, DeLaney T, Greenberg J, et al. Acute and long-term effects on limb function of combined modality limb sparing therapy for extremity soft tissue sarcoma. *Int J Radiat Oncol Biol Phys* 1991;21:1493.
236. Alektiar KM, Zelefsky MJ, Brennan MF. Morbidity of adjuvant brachytherapy in soft tissue sarcoma of the extremity and superficial trunk. *Int J Radiat Oncol Biol Phys* 2000;47:1273.
237. Helmstedter CS, Goebel M, Zlotecki R, Scarborough MT. Pathologic fractures after surgery and radiation for soft tissue tumors. *Clin Orthop* 2001;389:165.
238. Lin PP, Schupak KD, Boland PJ, et al. Pathologic femoral fracture after periosteal excision and radiation for the treatment of soft tissue sarcoma. *Cancer* 1998;82:2356.
239. Holt GE, Wunder JS, Griffin AM, et al. Fractures following radiation therapy and limb salvage surgery for soft tissue sarcomas: high versus low dose radiotherapy. *Proc Musculoskeletal Tumor Soc* 2002:41.
240. Brant TA, Parsons JT, Marcus RB, et al. Preoperative irradiation for soft tissue sarcomas of the trunk and extremities in adults. *Int J Radiat Oncol Biol Phys* 1990;19:899.
241. Spear MA, Dupuy DE, Park JJ, et al. Tolerance of autologous and allogeneic bone grafts to therapeutic radiation in humans. *Int J Radiat Oncol Biol Phys* 1999;45:1275.
242. Spierer MM, Alektiar KM, Zelefsky MJ, et al. Tolerance of tissue transfers to adjuvant radiation therapy in primary soft tissue sarcoma of the extremity. *Int J Radiat Oncol Biol Phys* 2003;56:1112.
243. Kattan MW, Leung DHY, Brennan MF. Postoperative nomogram for 12-year sarcoma specific death. *J Clin Oncol* 2002;20:791.
244. Kattan MW, Heller G, Brennan MF. A competing-risks nomogram for sarcoma-specific death following local recurrence. *Stat Med* 2003;22:3515.
245. Lewis J, Leung D, Casper E, et al. Multifactorial analysis of long-term follow-up (more than 5 years) of primary extremity sarcoma. *Arch Surg* 1999;134:190.
246. Weitz J, Antonescu CR, Brennan MF. Localized extremity soft tissue sarcoma: improved knowledge with unchanged survival over time. *J Clin Oncol* 2003;21:2719.
247. Davis A, Devlin M, Griffin A, et al. Functional outcome in amputation versus limb sparing of patients with lower extremity sarcoma: a matched case-control study. *Arch Phys Med Rehabil* 1999;80:615.
248. Robinson MH, Spruce L, Eeles R, et al. Limb salvage following conservation treatment of adult soft tissue sarcoma. *Eur J Cancer* 1991;27:1567.
249. Bell R, O'Sullivan B, Davis A, et al. Functional outcome in patients treated with surgery and irradiation for soft tissue tumors. *J Surg Oncol* 1991;48:224.
250. Schupak K, Lane J, Weilepp A, et al. The psychofunctional handicap associated with the use of brachytherapy in the treatment of lower extremity high grade soft tissue sarcomas. Proceedings of the 35th Annual ASTRO Meeting. *Int J Radiat Oncol Biol Phys* 1993;27(1):293.
251. Karasek K, Constine L, Rosier R. Sarcoma therapy: functional outcome and relationship to treatment parameters. *Int J Radiat Oncol Biol Phys* 1992;24:651.
252. Davis AM, O'Sullivan B, Bell RS, et al. Function and health status outcomes in a randomized trial comparing preoperative and postoperative radiotherapy in extremity soft tissue sarcoma. *J Clin Oncol* 2002;20:4472.
253. Temple LK, Brennan MF. The role of pulmonary metastasectomy in soft tissue sarcoma. *Semin Thorac Cardiovasc Surg* 2002;14:35.
254. Casson A, Putnam J, Natarajan G, et al. Five-year survival after pulmonary metastasectomy for adult soft tissue sarcoma. *Cancer* 1992;69:662.
255. Verazin G, Warneke J, Driscoll D, et al. Resection of lung metastases from soft tissue sarcomas. A multivariate analysis. *Arch Surg* 1992;127:1407.
256. Lanza L, Putnam J Jr, Benjamin R, Roth J. Response to chemotherapy does not predict survival after resection of sarcomatous pulmonary metastases. *Ann Thorac Surg* 1991;51:219.
257. Weiser MR, Downey RJ, Leung DH, et al. Repeat resection of pulmonary metastases in patients with soft tissue sarcoma. *J Am Coll Surg* 2000;191:184.
258. Weksler B, Lenert J, Ng B, et al. Isolated single lung perfusion with doxorubicin is effective in eradicating soft tissue sarcoma lung metastases in a rat model. *J Thorac Cardiovasc Surg* 1994;107:50.
259. O'Bryan RM, Luce JK, Talley RW, et al. Phase II evaluation of adriamycin in human neoplasia. *Cancer* 1973;32:1.
260. Santoro A, Tursz T, Mouridsen H, et al. Doxorubicin versus CyVADIC versus doxorubicin plus ifosfamide in first-line treatment of advanced soft tissue sarcomas: a randomized study of the European Organization for Research and Treatment of Cancer Soft Tissue and Bone Sarcoma Group. *J Clin Oncol* 1995;13(7):1537.
261. Edmonson JH, Ryan LM, Blum RH, et al. Randomized comparison of doxorubicin alone versus ifosfamide plus doxorubicin or mitomycin, doxorubicin, and cisplatin against advanced soft tissue sarcomas. *J Clin Oncol* 1993;11(7):1269.
262. Lorigan PC, Verweij J, Papai Z, et al. Randomised phase III trial of two investigational schedules of ifosfamide versus standard dose doxorubicin in patients with advanced or metastatic soft tissue sarcoma (ASTS). *Proc Am Soc Clin Oncol* 2002;21:1616(abst).
263. Judson I, Radford JA, Harris M, et al. Randomised phase II trial of pegylated liposomal doxorubicin (DOXIL/CAELYX) versus doxorubicin in the treatment of advanced or metastatic soft tissue sarcoma: a study by the EORTC Soft Tissue and Bone Sarcoma Group. *Eur J Cancer* 2001;37:870.
264. Rosen G, Forscher C, Lowenbraun S, et al. Synovial sarcoma. Uniform response of metastases to high dose ifosfamide. *Cancer* 1994;73(10):2506.
265. Buesa JM, Mouridsen HT, van Oosterom AT, et al. High-dose DTIC in advanced soft-tissue sarcomas in the adult. A phase II study of the E.O.R.T.C. Soft Tissue and Bone Sarcoma Group. *Ann Oncol* 1991;2(4):307.
266. Talbot SM, Keohan ML, Hesdorffer M, et al. A phase II trial of temozolomide in patients with unresectable or metastatic soft tissue sarcoma. *Cancer* 2003;98:1942.
267. Patel SR, Gandhi V, Jenkins J, et al. Phase II clinical investigation of gemcitabine in advanced soft tissue sarcomas and window evaluation of dose rate on gemcitabine triphosphate accumulation. *J Clin Oncol* 2001;19:3483.
268. Svancarova L, Blay JY, Judson IR, et al. Gemcitabine in advanced adult soft-tissue sarcomas. A phase II study of the EORTC Soft Tissue and Bone Sarcoma Group. *Eur J Cancer* 2002;38:556.
269. Lopez-Martin JA, Verweij J, Blay J, et al. An exploratory analysis of tumor growth rate (TGR) variations induced by trabectedin (ecteinascidin-743, ET-743) in patients (pts) with pretreated advanced soft tissue sarcoma (PASTS). *Proc Am Soc Clin Oncol* 2003;22:3293(abst).
270. D'Incalci M, Jimeno J. Preclinical and clinical results with the natural marine product ET-743. *Expert Opin Investig Drugs* 2003;12:1843.
271. Garcia-Carbonera R, Supko JG, Manola J, et al. Phase II and pharmacokinetic study of ecteinascidin 743 in patients with progressive sarcomas of soft tissues refractory to chemotherapy. *J Clin Oncol* 2004;22:1480.
272. Kuenen BC, Tabernero J, Baselga J, et al. Efficacy and toxicity of the angiogenesis inhibitor SU5416 as a single agent in patients with advanced renal cell carcinoma, melanoma, and soft tissue sarcoma. *Clin Cancer Res* 2003;9:1648.
273. Demetri GD, Fletcher CD, Mueller E, et al. Induction of solid tumor differentiation by the peroxisome proliferator-activated receptor-gamma ligand troglitazone in patients with liposarcoma. *Proc Natl Acad Sci U S A* 1999;96(7):3951.
274. Zalupski M, Metch B, Balcerzak S, et al. Phase III comparison of doxorubicin and dacarbazine given by bolus versus infusion in patients with soft-tissue sarcomas: a Southwest Oncology Group study. *J Natl Cancer Inst* 1991;83(13):926.
275. Frustaci S, Foladore S, Buonadonna A, et al. Epirubicin and ifosfamide in advanced soft tissue sarcomas. *Ann Oncol* 1993;4(8):669.
276. Elias A, Ryan L, Sulkes A, et al. Response to mesna, doxorubicin, ifosfamide, and dacarbazine in 108 patients with metastatic or unresectable sarcoma and no prior chemotherapy. *J Clin Oncol* 1989;7(9):1208.
277. Antman K, Crowley J, Balcerzak SP, et al. An intergroup phase III randomized study of doxorubicin and dacarbazine with or without ifosfamide and mesna in advanced soft tissue and bone sarcomas. *J Clin Oncol* 1993;11(7):1276.
278. Edmonson JH, Long HJ, Richardson RL, et al. Phase II study of a combination of mitomycin, doxorubicin and cisplatin in advanced sarcomas. *Cancer Chemother Pharmacol* 1985;15(2):181.
279. Van Glabbeke M, van Oosterom AT, Oosterhuis JW, et al. Prognostic factors for the outcome of chemotherapy in advanced soft tissue sarcomas: an analysis of 2,185 patients treated with anthracycline containing first-line regimens—an European Organization for

Research and Treatment of Cancer Soft Tissue and Bone Sarcoma Study Group. *J Clin Oncol* 1999;17(1):150.

280. Hensley ML, Maki R, Venkatraman E, et al. Gemcitabine and docetaxel in patients with unresectable leiomyosarcoma: results of a phase II trial. *J Clin Oncol* 2002;20:2824.

281. Frei E III, Elias A, Wheeler C, et al. The relationship between high-dose treatment and combination chemotherapy: the concept of summation dose intensity. *Clin Cancer Res* 1998;4(9):2027.

282. Ozer H. American Society of Clinical Oncology guidelines for the use of hematopoietic colony-stimulating factors. *Curr Opin Hematol* 1996;3(1):3.

283. Antman KS, Griffin JD, Elias A, et al. Effect of recombinant human granulocyte-macrophage colony-stimulating factor on chemotherapy-induced myelosuppression. *N Engl J Med* 1988;319(10):593.

284. Schutte J, Mouridsen HT, Steward W, et al. Ifosfamide plus doxorubicin in previously untreated patients with advanced soft-tissue sarcoma. *Cancer Chemother Pharmacol* 1993;31 [Suppl 2]:S204.

285. Bui BN, Chevallier B, Chevreau C, et al. Efficacy of lenograstim on hematologic tolerance to MAID chemotherapy in patients with advanced soft tissue sarcoma and consequences on treatment dose-intensity. *J Clin Oncol* 1995;13(10):2629.

286. Walterhouse DO, Hoover ML, Marymont MA, et al. High-dose chemotherapy followed by peripheral blood stem cell rescue for metastatic rhabdomyosarcoma: the experience at Chicago Children's Memorial Hospital. *Med Pediatr Oncol* 1999;32(2):88.

287. Seynaeve C, Verweij J. High-dose chemotherapy in adult sarcomas: no standard yet. *Semin Oncol* 1999;26(1):119.

288. Kawai A, Woodruff J, Healey JH, et al. SYT-SSX gene fusion as a determinant of morphology and prognosis in synovial sarcoma. *N Engl J Med* 1998;338(3):153.

289. Grier HE. The Ewing family of tumors. Ewing's sarcoma and primitive neuroectodermal tumors. *Pediatr Clin North Am* 1997;44(4):991.

290. Bane B, Evans H, Ro J, et al. Extraskeletal osteosarcoma. A clinicopathologic review of 26 cases. *Cancer* 1990;76:2762.

291. Grier HE, Krailo MD, Tarbell NJ, et al. Addition of ifosfamide and etoposide to standard chemotherapy for Ewing's sarcoma and primitive neuroectodermal tumor of bone. *N Engl J Med* 2003;348:694.

292. Crist WM, Anderson JR, Meza JL, et al. Intergroup rhabdomyosarcoma study-IV: results for patients with nonmetastatic disease. *J Clin Oncol* 2001;19:3091.

293. Kolb EA, Kushner BH, Gorlick R, et al. Long-term event-free survival after intensive chemotherapy for Ewing's family of tumors in children and young adults. *J Clin Oncol* 2003;21:3423.

294. Antman K, Crowley J, Balcerzak SP, et al. A Southwest Oncology Group and Cancer and Leukemia Group B phase II study of doxorubicin, dacarbazine, ifosfamide, and mesna in adults with advanced osteosarcoma, Ewing's sarcoma, and rhabdomyosarcoma. *Cancer* 1998;82(7):1288.

295. Baldini EH, Demetri GD, Fletcher CD, et al. Adults with Ewing's sarcoma/primitive neuroectodermal tumor: adverse effect of older age and primary extraosseous disease on outcome. *Ann Surg* 1999;230(1):79.

296. Ahrens S, Hoffmann C, Jabar S, et al. Evaluation of prognostic factors in a tumor volume-adapted treatment strategy for localized Ewing sarcoma of bone: the CESS 86 experience. Cooperative Ewing Sarcoma Study. *Med Pediatr Oncol* 1999;32(3):186.

297. Ferrer F, Sabater S, Farrus B, et al. Impact of radiotherapy on local control and survival in uterine sarcomas: a retrospective study from the Grup Oncologic Catala-Occita. *Int J Radiat Oncol Biol Phys* 1999;44(1):47.

298. Muss HB, Bundy B, DiSaia PJ, et al. Treatment of recurrent or advanced uterine sarcoma. A randomized trial of doxorubicin versus doxorubicin and cyclophosphamide (a phase III trial of the Gynecologic Oncology Group). *Cancer* 1985;55(8):1648.

299. Curtin JP, Blessing JA, Soper JT, DeGeest K. Paclitaxel in the treatment of carcinosarcoma of the uterus: a Gynecologic Oncology Group study. *Gynecol Oncol* 2001;83:268.

300. Sutton G, Brunetto VL, Kilgore L, et al. A phase III study of ifosfamide with or without cisplatin in carcinosarcoma of the uterus: a Gynecologic Oncology Group study. *Gynecol Oncol* 2000;79:147.

301. Hensley ML, Maki R, Venkatraman E, et al. Gemcitabine and docetaxel in patients with unresectable leiomyosarcoma: results of a phase II trial. *J Clin Oncol* 2002;20:2824.

302. Keen CE, Philip G. Progestogen-induced regression in low-grade endometrial stromal sarcoma. Case report and literature review. *Br J Obstet Gynaecol* 1989;96(12):1435.

303. Wade K, Quinn MA, Hammond I, et al. Uterine sarcoma: steroid receptors and response to hormonal therapy. *Gynecol Oncol* 1990;39(3):364.

304. Spear M, Jennings L, Mankin H, et al. Individualizing management of aggressive fibromatoses. *Int J Radiat Oncol Biol Phys* 1998;40(3):637.

305. Goy B, Lee S, Eilber F, et al. The role of adjuvant radiotherapy in the treatment of resectable desmoid tumors. *Int J Radiat Oncol Biol Phys* 1997;39(3):659.

306. Ballo M, Zagars G, Pollack A. Radiation therapy in the management of desmoid tumors. *Int J Radiat Oncol Biol Phys* 1998;42(5):1007.

307. Wilcken N, Tattersall MH. Endocrine therapy for desmoid tumors. *Cancer* 1991;68(6):1384.

308. Lanari A. Effect of progesterone on desmoid tumors (aggressive fibromatosis). *N Engl J Med* 1983;309(24):1523.

309. Waddell WR, Kirsch WM. Testolactone, sulindac, warfarin, and vitamin K1 for unresectable desmoid tumors. *Am J Surg* 1991;161(4):416.

310. Klein WA, Miller HH, Anderson M, et al . The use of indomethacin, sulindac, and tamoxifen for the treatment of desmoid tumors associated with familial polyposis. *Cancer* 1987;60(12):2863.

311. Seiter K, Kemeny N. Successful treatment of a desmoid tumor with doxorubicin. *Cancer* 1993;71(7):2242.

312. Patel SR, Evans HL, Benjamin RS. Combination chemotherapy in adult desmoid tumors. *Cancer* 1993;72(11):3244.

313. Weiss AJ, Horowitz S, Lackman RD. Therapy of desmoid tumors and fibromatosis using vinorelbine. *Am J Clin Oncol* 1999;22(2):193.

314. Jhanwar S, Chen Q, Li F, et al. Cytogenetic analysis of soft tissue sarcomas. Recurrent chromosome abnormalities in malignant peripheral nerve sheath tumors (MPNST). *Cytogenet* 1994;78(2):138.

315. Scholz R, Kabisch H, Delling G, Winkler K. Homozygous deletion within the retinoblastoma gene in a native osteosarcoma specimen of a patient cured of a retinoblastoma of both eyes. *Pediatr Hematol Oncol* 1990;7(3):265.

316. Malkin D, Li F, Strong L, et al. Germ line p53 mutations in a familial syndrome of breast cancer, sarcomas, and other neoplasms. *Science* 1990;250(4985):1233.

317. Okamoto M, Sato C, Kohno Y, et al. Molecular nature of chromosome 5q loss in colorectal tumors and desmoids from patients with familial adenomatous polyposis. *Hum Genet* 1990;85(6):595.

318. Goto M, Miller R, Ishikawa Y, Sugano H. Excess of rare cancers in Werner syndrome (adult progeria). *Cancer Epidemiol Biomarkers Prev* 1996;5(4):239.

319. Carney J, Sheps S, Go V, Gordon H. The triad of gastric leiomyosarcoma, functioning extra-adrenal paraganglioma and pulmonary chondroma. *N Engl J Med* 1977;296(26):1517.

320. van Slegtenhorst M, de Hoogt R, Hermans C, et al. Identification of the tuberous sclerosis gene TSC1 on chromosome 9q34. *Science* 1997;277(5327):805.

321. Povey S, Burley M, Attwood J, et al. Two loci for tuberous sclerosis: one on 9q34 and one on 16p13. *Ann Hum Genet* 1994;58:107.

322. Hardell L, Sandstrom A. A case-control study: soft tissue sarcoma and exposure to chemical substances: a case referent study. *Br J Cancer* 1979;39:711.

323. Eriksson M, Hardell L, Ber N, et al. Soft tissue sarcomas and exposure to chemical substances: a case referent study. *Br J Ind Med* 1981;38:27.

324. Balarajan R, Acheson E. Soft tissue sarcomas in agriculture and forestry workers. *J Epidemiol Commun Health* 1984;38:113.

325. Greenwald P, Kovasznay B, Collins D, Therriault G. Sarcomas of soft tissue after Vietnam service. *J Natl Cancer Inst* 1984;73:1107.

326. Hoar S, Blair A, Holmes F, et al. Agricultural herbicide use and risk of lymphoma and soft tissue sarcoma. *JAMA* 1986;256:1141.

327. Turc-Carel C, Philip I, Berger MP, Philip T, Lenoir G. Chromosomal translocation in Ewing's sarcoma. *N Engl J Med* 1983;309:497.

328. Kaneko Y, Kobayashi H, Handa M, et al. EWS-ERG fusion transcript produced by chromosomal insertion in a Ewing sarcoma. *Genes Chromosomes Cancer* 1997;18:228.

329. Jeon I, David J, Braun B, et al. A variant Ewing's sarcoma translocation (7;22) fuses the EWS gene to the ETS gene ETV1. *Oncogene* 1995;10(6):1229.

330. Kaneko Y, Yoshida K, Handa M, et al. Fusion of an ETS-family gene, EIAF, to EWS by t(17;22)(q12;q12) chromosome translocation in an undifferentiated sarcoma of infancy. *Genes Chromosomes Cancer* 1996;15(2):115.

331. Mugneret F, Lizard S, Aurias A, Turn-Carel C. Chromosomes in Ewing's sarcoma. II. Nonrandom additional changes, trisomy 8 and der(16)t(1;16). *Cancer Genet Cytogenet* 1988;32(2):239.

332. Douglass E, Rowe S, Valentine M, et al. A second nonrandom translocation, der(16)t(1;16)(q21;q13), in Ewing sarcoma and peripheral neuroectodermal tumor. *Cytogenet Cell Genet* 1990;53(2–3):87.

333. Panagopoulos I, Hoglund M, Mertens F, et al. Fusion of the EWS and CHOP genes in myxoid liposarcoma. *Oncogene* 1996;12(3):489.

334. Heim S, Mandahl N, Dristoffersson U, et al. Marker ring chromosome—a new cytogenetic abnormality characterizing lipogenic tumors? *Cancer Genet Cytogenet* 1987;24(2):319.

335. Rosai J, Akerman M, Dal Cin P, et al. Combined morphologic and karyotypic study of 59 atypical lipomatous tumors. Evaluation of their relationship and differential diagnosis with other adipose tissue tumors (a report of the CHAMP Study Group). *Am J Surg Pathol* 1996;20(10):1182.

336. Kelly K, Womer R, Sorensen P, et al. Common and variant gene fusions predict distinct clinical phenotypes in rhabdomyosarcoma. *J Clin Oncol* 1997;15(5):1831.

337. Peulve P, Michot C, Vannier J, et al. Clear cell sarcoma with t(12;22)(q13-14;q12). *Genes Chromosomes Cancer* 1991;3(5):400.

338. Turc-Carel C, Dal Cin P, Limon J, et al. Translocation X;18 in synovial sarcoma. *Cancer Genet Cytogenet* 1986;23(1):93.

339. Sciot R, Dal Cin P, Fletcher C, et al. t(9;22)(q22-31;q11-12) is a consistent marker of extraskeletal myxoid chondrosarcoma: evaluation of three cases. *Mod Pathol* 1995;8(7):765.

340. Ladanyi M, Lui MY, Antonescu CR, et al. The der(17)t(X;17)(p11;q25) of human alveolar soft part sarcoma fuses the TFE3 transcription factor gene to ASPL, a novel gene at 17q25. *Oncogene* 2001;20:48.

341. Koontz JI, Soreng AL, Nucci M, et al. Frequent fusion of the JAZF1 and JJAZ1 genes in endometrial stromal tumors. *Proc Natl Acad Sci U S A* 2001;98:6348.

342. Knezevich S, McFadden D, Tao W, et al. A novel ETV2-NTRK3 gene fusion in congenital fibrosarcoma. *Nat Genet* 1998;18(2):184.

343. Versteege I, Sevenet N, Lange J, et al. Truncating mutations of hSNF5/INI1 in aggressive paediatric cancer. *Nature* 1998;394(6689):203.

344. Nibert M, Heim S. Uterine leiomyoma cytogenetics. *Genes Chromosomes Cancer* 1990;2(1):3.

345. Rodriguez E, Reuter V, Mies C, et al. Abnormalities of 2q: a common genetic link between rhabdomyosarcoma and hepatoblastoma? *Genes Chromosomes Cancer* 1991;3(2):122.

346. Dietrich C, Jacobsen B, Starklint H, Heim S. Clonal karyotypic evolution in an embryonal rhabdomyosarcoma with trisomy 8 as the primary chromosomal abnormality. *Genes Chromosomes Cancer* 1993;7(4):240.

347. Quezado M, Middleton L, Bryant B, et al. Allelic loss on chromosome 22q in epithelioid sarcomas. *Hum Pathol* 1998;29(6):604.

348. Cordoba J, Parham D, Meyer W, Douglass E. A new cytogenetic finding in an epithelioid sarcoma, t(8;22)(q22;q11). *Cancer Genet Cytogenet* 1994;72(2):151.

349. Weingrad D, Rosenberg S. Early lymphatic spread of osteogenic and soft-tissue sarcomas. *Surgery* 1978;84:231.

350. Mazeron J, Suit H. Lymph nodes as sites of metastases from sarcomas of soft tissue. *Cancer* 1987;60:1800.

351. Lindberg RD, Murphy WK, Benjamin RS, et al. Adjuvant chemotherapy in the treatment

of primary soft tissue sarcomas: a preliminary report. In: *Management of primary bone and soft tissue tumors: a collection of papers presented at the Twenty-First Annual Clinical Conference on Cancer, 1976, at the University of Texas System Cancer Center, M. D. Anderson Hospital and Tumor Institute, Houston, Texas.* Chicago: Year Book Medical, 1977:343.

352. Baker LH. Adjuvant treatment for soft tissue sarcomas. In: Ryan JR, Baker LH, eds. *Recent concepts in sarcoma treatment.* Dordrecht, the Netherlands: Kluwer, 1988:130.

353. Wilson RE, Wood WC, Lerner HL, et al. Doxorubicin chemotherapy in the treatment of soft-tissue sarcoma. Combined results of two randomized trials. *Arch Surg* 1986;121(11):1354.

354. Picci P, Bacci G, Gherlinzoni F, et al. Results of a randomized trial for the treatment of localized soft tissue tumors (STS) of the extremities in adult patients. In: Ryan JR, Baker LH, eds. *Recent concepts in sarcoma treatment.* Dordrecht, The Netherlands: Kluwer, 1988:144.

355. Frustaci S, Gherlinzoni F, De Paoli A, et al. Maintenance of efficacy of adjuvant chemotherapy (CT) in soft tissue sarcoma (STS) of the extremities. Update of a randomized trial. *Proc Am Soc Clin Oncol* 1999;18:A2108(abst).

356. Borden EC, Amato DA, Rosenbaum C, et al. Randomized comparison of three adriamycin regimens for metastatic soft tissue sarcomas. *J Clin Oncol* 1987;5(6):840.

357. Borden EC, Amato DA, Edmonson JH, et al. Randomized comparison of doxorubicin and vindesine to doxorubicin for patients with metastatic soft-tissue sarcomas. *Cancer* 1990;66(5):862.

358. Mouridsen HT, Bastholt L, Somers R, et al. Adriamycin versus epirubicin in advanced soft tissue sarcomas. A randomized phase II/phase III study of the EORTC Soft Tissue and Bone Sarcoma Group. *Eur J Cancer Clin Oncol* 1987;23(10):1477.

359. Casper ES, Schwartz GK, Sugarman A, et al. Phase I trial of dose-intense liposome-encapsulated doxorubicin in patients with advanced sarcoma. *J Clin Oncol* 1997;15(5):2111.

360. Skubitz KM. A phase II trial of pegylated liposomal doxorubicin (DOXIL) demonstrates activity in refractory sarcoma, mesothelioma, and head and neck cancer. *Proc Am Soc Clin Oncol* 1999;18:A2090(abst).

361. Lopez M, Vici P, Di Lauro K, et al. Randomized prospective clinical trial of high-dose epirubicin and dexrazoxane in patients with advanced breast cancer and soft tissue sarcomas. *J Clin Oncol* 1998;16(1):86.

362. van Oosterom AT, Santoro A, Bramwell V, et al. Mitomycin C (MCC) in advanced soft tissue sarcoma: a phase I study of the EORTC Soft Tissue and Bone Sarcoma Group. *Eur J Cancer Clin Oncol* 1985;21(4):459.

363. Amato DA, Borden EC, Shiraki M, et al. Evaluation of bleomycin, chlorozotocin, MGBG, and bruceantin in patients with advanced soft tissue sarcoma, bone sarcoma, or mesothelioma. *Invest New Drugs* 1985;3(4):397.

364. Cruz AB Jr, Thames EA Jr, Aust JB, et al. Combination chemotherapy for soft tissue sarcomas: a phase III study. *J Surg Oncol* 1979;11(4):313.

365. Bramwell VH, Mouridsen HT, Santoro A, et al. Cyclophosphamide versus ifosfamide: a randomized phase II trial in adult soft-tissue sarcomas. The European Organization for Research and Treatment of Cancer [EORTC], Soft Tissue and Bone Sarcoma Group. *Cancer Chemother Pharmacol* 1993;31[Suppl 2]:S180.

366. Borden EC, Larson P, Ansfield FJ, et al. Hexamethylmelamine treatment of sarcomas and lymphomas. *Med Pediatr Oncol* 1977;3(4):401.

367. Antman KH, Ryan L, Elias A, et al. Response to ifosfamide and mesna: 124 previously treated patients with metastatic or unresectable sarcoma. *J Clin Oncol* 1989;7(1):126.

368. Patel SR, Vadhan-Raj S, Papadopolous N, et al. High-dose ifosfamide in bone and soft tissue sarcomas: results of phase II and pilot studies—dose-response and schedule dependence. *J Clin Oncol* 1997;15(6):2378.

369. Frustaci S, Comandone A, Bearz A, et al. Efficacy and tolerability of an ifosfamide continuous infusion (IFO-C.I.) in soft tissue sarcoma (STS) patients (pts). *Proc Am Soc Clin Oncol* 1998;17:A1993(abst).

370. Thigpen JT, Blessing JA, Beecham J, et al. Phase II trial of cisplatin as first-line chemotherapy in patients with advanced or recurrent uterine sarcomas: a Gynecologic Oncology Group study. *J Clin Oncol* 1991;9(11):1962.

371. Samson MK, Baker LH, Benjamin RS, et al. Cis-dichlorodiammineplatinum(II) in advanced soft tissue and bony sarcomas: a Southwest Oncology Group Study. *Cancer Treat Rep* 1979;63(11–12):2027.

372. Budd GT, Metch B, Balcerzak SP, et al. High-dose cisplatin for metastatic soft tissue sarcoma. *Cancer* 1990;65(4):866.

373. Goldstein D, Cheuvart B, Trump DL, et al. Phase II trial of carboplatin in soft-tissue sarcoma. *Am J Clin Oncol* 1990;13(5):420.

374. Patel SR, Jenkins J, Papadopoulos NE, et al. Preliminary results of a two-arm phase 2 trial of gemcitabine in patients with gastrointestinal leiomyosarcomas and other soft-tissue sarcomas (STS). *Sarcoma* 1999;3(1):56(abst).

375. Subramanian S, Wiltshaw E. Chemotherapy of sarcoma. A comparison of three regimens. *Lancet* 1978;1(8066):683.

376. Vaughn CB, McKelvey E, Balcerzak SP, et al. High-dose methotrexate with leucovorin rescue plus vincristine in advanced sarcoma: a Southwest Oncology Group study. *Cancer Treat Rep* 1984;68(2):409.

377. Gold G, Hall T, Shnider B, et al. A clinical study of 5-fluorouracil. *Cancer* 1959;19:935.

378. van Hoesel QG, Verweij J, Catimel G, et al. Phase II study with docetaxel (Taxotere) in advanced soft tissue sarcomas of the adult. EORTC Soft Tissue and Bone Sarcoma Group. *Ann Oncol* 1994;5(6):539.

379. Balcerzak SP, Benedetti J, Weiss GR, Natale RB. A phase II trial of paclitaxel in patients with advanced soft tissue sarcomas. A Southwest Oncology Group study. *Cancer* 1995;76(11):2248.

380. Yap BS, Benjamin RS, Plager C, et al. A randomized study of continuous infusion vindesine versus vinblastine in adults with refractory metastatic sarcomas. *Am J Clin Oncol* 1983;6(2):235.

381. Fidias P, Demetri GD, Harmon DC. Navelbine shows activity in previously treated sarcoma patients: phase II results from MGH/Dana-Farber/Partners Cancer Care Study. *Proc Am Soc Clin Oncol* 1998;17:A1977(abst).

382. Thigpen T, Blessing JA, Yordan E, et al. Phase II trial of etoposide in leiomyosarcoma of the uterus: a Gynecologic Oncology Group study. *Gynecol Oncol* 1996;63(1):120.

383. Rose PG, Blessing JA, Soper JT, Barter JF. Prolonged oral etoposide in recurrent or advanced leiomyosarcoma of the uterus: a gynecologic oncology group study. *Gynecol Oncol* 1998;70(2):267.

384. Bramwell VH, Eisenhauer EA, Blackstein M, et al. Phase II study of topotecan (NSC 609 699) in patients with recurrent or metastatic soft tissue sarcoma. *Ann Oncol* 1995;6(8):847.

385. Gottlieb JA, Benjamin RS, Baker LH, et al. Role of DTIC (NSC-45388) in the chemotherapy of sarcomas. *Cancer Treat Rep* 1976;60(2):199.

386. Saiki J, Stephens R, Fabian C, et al. Phase II evaluation of gallium nitrate (NSC-15200) in soft tissue and bone sarcomas. *Proc Am Assoc Cancer Res* 1981;22:525(abst).

387. Presant CA, Gams R, Bartolucci AA. Treatment of metastatic sarcomas with mitoxantrone. *Cancer Treat Rep* 1984;68(5):813.

388. Bull FE, Von Hoff DD, Balcerzak SP, et al. Phase II trial of mitoxantrone in advanced sarcoma: a Southwest Oncology Group study. *Cancer Treat Rep* 1985;69:321.

389. Keohan ML, Taub R, Plitsas M, et al. Phase II study of CT-2584, a novel inhibitor of phosphatidylcholine biosynthesis, in patients with soft tissue sarcoma. *Proc Am Soc Clin Oncol* 2000;19:2187(abst).

390. Leahy MG, Blay J-Y, Le Cesne A, et al. EORTC 62011: Phase II trial of brostallicin for soft tissue sarcoma. *Proc Connective Tissue Oncol Soc* 2003;9:94(abst).

391. Maki RG, Kraft A, Skoog L, et al. A phase II study of bortezomib (PS-341, Velcade) in sarcomas. *Proc Connective Tissue Oncol Soc* 2003;9:148(abst).

392. Schuff-Werner P, Bartsch H, Schremi W, Nagel GA. Treatment of soft tissue sarcoma with recombinant alpha-interferon. *Antiviral Res* 1984;3:93(abst).

393. Borden EC, Kim K, Ryan L, et al. Phase II trials of interferons-alpha and -beta in advanced sarcomas. *J Interferon Res* 1992;12(6):455.

394. Jazieh AR, McIntyre W, Husain M, et al. Phase I clinical trial of tamoxifen and interferon alpha in the treatment of solid tumors. *Proc Am Soc Clin Oncol* 1999;18:A829(abst).

395. Harris J, Das Gupta T, Vogelzang N, et al. Treatment of soft tissue sarcoma with fibroblast interferon (beta-interferon): an American Cancer Society/Illinois Cancer Council study. *Cancer Treat Rep* 1986;70(2):293.

396. Rosenberg SA, Lotze MT, Muul LM, et al. A progress report on the treatment of 157 patients with advanced cancer using lymphokine-activated killer cells and interleukin-2 or high-dose interleukin-2 alone. *N Engl J Med* 1987;316(15):889.

397. Verweij J, Judson I, Steward W, et al. Phase II study of liposomal muramyl tripeptide phosphatidylethanolamine (MTP/PE) in advanced soft tissue sarcomas of the adult. An EORTC Soft Tissue and Bone Sarcoma Group study. *Eur J Cancer* 1994;6:842.

398. Rinehart J, Balcerzak SP, Hersh E. Phase II trial of tumor necrosis factor in human sarcomas: a Southwest Oncology Group study. *Proc Am Soc Clin Oncol* 1990;9:1229(abst).

399. Omura GA, Major FJ, Blessing JA, et al. A randomized study of adriamycin with and without dimethyl triazeno imidazole carboxamide in advanced uterine sarcomas. *Cancer* 1983;52:626.

400. Cruz AB Jr, Thames EA Jr, Aust JB, et al. Combination chemotherapy for soft-tissue sarcomas: a phase III study. *J Surg Oncol* 1979;11(4):313.

401. Schoenfeld DA, Rosenbaum C, Horton J, et al. A comparison of adriamycin versus vincristine and adriamycin, and cyclophosphamide versus vincristine, actinomycin-D, and cyclophosphamide for advanced sarcoma. *Cancer* 1982;50(12):2757.

402. Nielsen OS, Dombernowsky P, Mouridsen H, et al. High-dose epirubicin is not an alternative to standard-dose doxorubicin in the treatment of advanced soft tissue sarcomas. A study of the EORTC soft tissue and bone sarcoma group. *Br J Cancer* 1998;78(12):1634.

MARTIN M. MALAWER
LEE J. HELMAN
BRIAN O'SULLIVAN

SECTION **2**

Sarcomas of Bone

Malignant tumors arising from the skeletal system are rare, representing just 0.001% of all new cancers.[1] Only 400 to 600 new primary bone sarcomas are diagnosed annually in the United States. Osteosarcoma and Ewing's sarcoma, the two most common bone tumors, occur mainly during childhood and adolescence[2–4] (Fig. 35.2-1). Other mesenchymal (spindle cell) neoplasms that characteristically arise after skeletal maturity—fibrosarcoma, chondrosarcoma, and malignant fibrous histiocytoma (MFH)—are less common.[5–8] The vast majority of experience reported in the management of bone neoplasms has been obtained in patients with osteosarcomas. As a result, the surgical, chemotherapeutic, and radiotherapeutic principles developed for treatment of osteosarcomas form the basis of the management strategy for most of the spindle cell neoplasms.

Since the late 1970s, clinical knowledge and experience in the management of bone neoplasms have grown dramatically.[9–13] The development of centers of specific interest in these tumors has played an important role in the advancement of biologic understanding and surgical management of these lesions and in the development of multimodality treatment regimens.[12,14] A surgical staging system that permits standardized preoperative evaluation, analysis, and end-result reporting has been developed.[15]

Amputation had been the standard method of treatment for most bone sarcomas, but the 1980s witnessed the development of limb-sparing surgery for most malignant bone tumors.[16–20] Today, limb-sparing surgery is considered safe and routine for approximately 90% of patients with extremity osteosarcomas. Advances in orthopedics, bioengineering, radiographic imaging, radiotherapy, and chemotherapy have contributed to safer, more reliable surgical procedures.[21–25] Computed tomography (CT), developed during the early 1980s, and, more recently, magnetic resonance imaging (MRI), permit extremely accurate evaluation of the local anatomy and enhance the possibility of safe resection.[26–31] An evaluation system has been developed to determine a patient's functional status after limb-sparing surgery of the extremities as well as of the pelvic and shoulder girdle.[15] This system, for the first time, permits evaluation and comparison of the various limb-sparing procedures and types of surgical reconstructions.

Paralleling these advances has been the demonstrated effectiveness of adjuvant chemotherapy in dramatically increasing overall survival: The bleak 15% to 20% survival rate associated with surgery alone before the 1970s rose to 55% to 80% with various adjuvant treatment regimens by the 1980s.[32–37] Multiple-drug regimens are now considered essential treatment. The timing, mode of delivery, and different combinations of these agents are being investigated at many centers. Preoperative chemotherapy regimens (termed *neoadjuvant* or *induction* chemotherapy) and postoperative regimens are being evaluated to determine their effect on the tumor and their impact on the choice of operative procedure and on overall survival.[38–44]

This chapter focuses only on malignant spindle cell tumors. The topic of Ewing's sarcoma is presented in detail in Chapter 35.1. Emphasis is placed on natural history, surgical staging, tumor imaging, criteria of patient selection for amputation versus limb-sparing surgery, and technique of limb-sparing procedures. The development, role, timing, and mode of delivery of adjuvant chemotherapy and its relationship to stage of disease are discussed, along with the role of radiotherapy in specific clinical situations.

CLASSIFICATION AND TYPES OF BONE TUMOR

Bone consists of cartilaginous, osteoid, and fibrous tissue and bone marrow elements. Each tissue can give rise to benign or malignant spindle cell tumors.[2–4] Bone tumors are classified on the basis of cell type and recognized products of proliferating cells. The classification system, described by Lichtenstein and modified by Dahlin, is presented in Table 35.2-1.[2,3,45] Jaffe[4] recommends that each tumor be considered a separate clinicopathologic entity. Radiographic, histologic, and clinical data are necessary to form an accurate diagnosis and to determine the degree of activity and malignancy of each lesion.

Cartilage tumors are lesions in which cartilage is produced. They are the most common bone tumors. Osteochondroma is the most common benign cartilage tumor; some 1% to 2% of solitary osteochondromas become malignant.[46,47] Enchondroma is a benign cartilage tumor that occurs centrally; in adults, malignant transformation may occur. Chondrosarcoma, the most common malignant cartilage tumor, is either intramedullary or peripheral. Ten percent are secondary, arising from an underlying benign lesion.[2] Most chondrosarcomas are low grade, although 10% dedifferentiate into high-grade spindle cell sarcomas or, rarely, a mesenchymal chondrosarcoma.[2,47] Osteoid tumors are lesions in which the stroma produces osteoid. The benign forms are osteoid osteoma and osteoblastoma. Osteoid osteomas are never malignant. Osteoblastomas rarely metastasize; when they do, it is only after multiple local recurrences.[48] Osteosarcomas are the most common primary malignant tumors of the bone. Histologically, they are composed of malignant spindle cells and osteoblasts that produce osteoid or immature bone. Several variants are now recognized.[49] Parosteal, periosteal, and low-grade intraosseous osteosarcomas are histologically and radiographically distinct from the "classic" central medullary osteosarcomas and have a more favorable prognosis.[50,51]

Fibrous tumors of bone are rare. Desmoplastic fibroma is a locally aggressive, nonmetastasizing tumor, analogous to fibromatosis of soft tissue.[5,52] Fibrosarcoma of bone appears histologically as its soft tissue counterpart. Multiple sections must be obtained to demonstrate the lack of osteoid production. If osteoid is present, the lesion is classified as an osteosarcoma. MFH, a rare lesion and the counterpart of soft tissue MFH, has been described in bone.[6,53,54] The pathophysiologic behavior of bone and soft tissue MFH is similar, consisting of a storiform pattern with a histiocytic component. Giant cell tumors (GCTs) of unknown origin were originally described as benign but are now considered low-grade sarcomas. They have high rates of local recurrence and malignant transformation.[55,56]

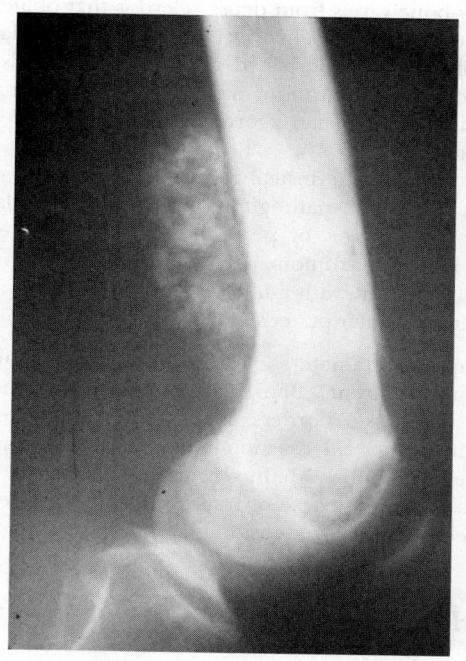
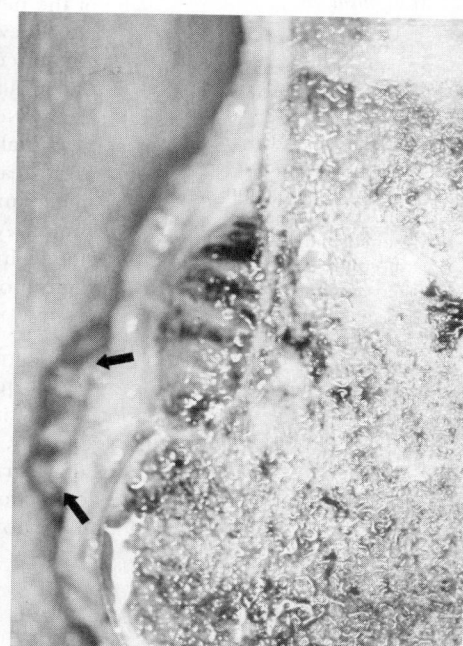
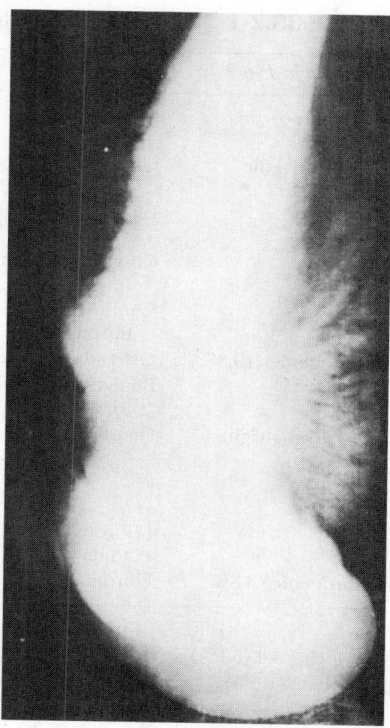

A–C

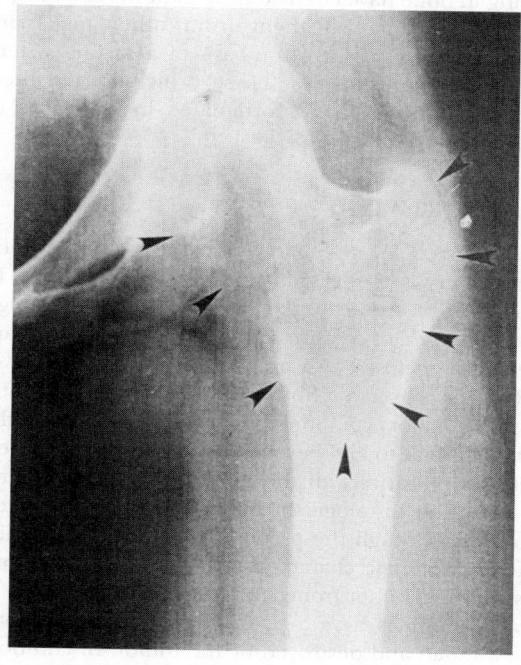
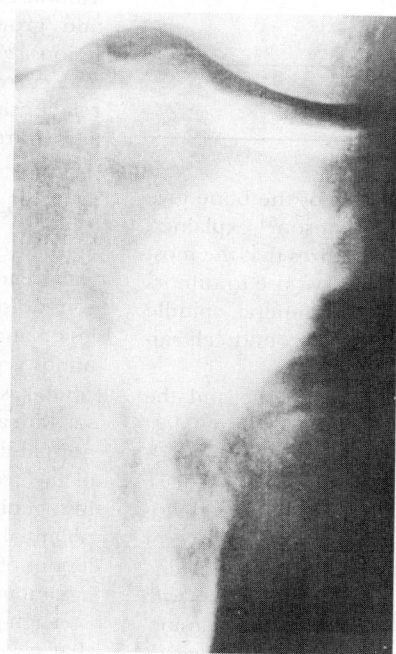

D,E

FIGURE 35.2-1. Osteosarcoma of the distal femur. **A:** Plain radiograph of a classic osteosarcoma. Marked sclerosis is present within the intramedullary canal, which represents new bone formation (malignant osteoid formation), in addition to a large posterior extraosseous component that shows osteoid formation. This is the typical appearance of a distal femoral osteosarcoma before treatment. New bone formation within the extraosseous tumor is highly suggestive of an osteosarcoma. The distal femur is the most common site of primary osteosarcoma. **B:** Gross specimen of a distal femoral osteosarcoma. The medullary canal is filled with tumor. Note that there is extraosseous extension (*arrows*) beyond the cortex. Approximately 95% of osteosarcomas have extraosseous components at the time of diagnosis. This finding necessitates accurate computed tomography, magnetic resonance imaging, and bone scan imaging before biopsy and induction chemotherapy. **C–E:** Plain radiographs demonstrate the classic variants of osteosarcoma. (See Color Fig. 35.2-1*B* in the CD-ROM.)

Tumors presumably arising from bone marrow elements are the round cell sarcomas. The two most common are Ewing's sarcoma and non-Hodgkin's lymphoma.

RADIOGRAPHIC EVALUATION AND DIAGNOSIS

Radiographic evaluation, combined with the clinical history and histologic examination, is necessary for accurate diagnosis.

Bone scan, angiography, CT, and MRI are generally not helpful in determining a diagnosis but are important in delineating the extent of local involvement. A systematic approach to the radiographic evaluation of skeletal lesions has been described by Madewell et al.,[57] who studied and correlated several hundred radiographic and pathologic specimens. They considered the radiograph as the gross specimen from which a detailed histologic interpretation could be made and biologic activity accurately diagnosed. According to their system, a bone tumor is evaluated by five radiographic parameters:

TABLE 35.2-1. General Classification of Bone Tumors

Histologic Type[a]	Benign	Malignant
Hematopoietic (41.4%)	—	Myeloma
	—	Reticulum cell sarcoma
Chondrogenic (20.9%)	Osteochondroma	Primary chondrosarcoma
	Chondroma	Secondary chondrosarcoma
	Chondroblastoma	Dedifferentiated chondrosarcoma
	Chondromyxoid fibroma	Mesenchymal chondrosarcoma
Osteogenic (19.3%)	Osteoid osteoma	Osteosarcoma
	Benign osteoblastoma	Parosteal osteogenic sarcoma
Unknown origin (9.8%)	Giant cell tumor	Ewing's tumor
	—	Malignant giant cell tumor
	—	Adamantinoma
	(Fibrous) histiocytoma	(Fibrous) histiocytoma
Fibrogenic (3.8%)	Fibroma	Fibrosarcoma
	Desmoplastic fibroma	—
Notochordal (3.1%)	—	Chordoma
Vascular (1.6%)	Hemangioma	Hemangioendothelioma
	—	Hemangiopericytoma
Lipogenic (<0.5%)	Lipoma	—
Neurogenic (<0.5%)	Neurilemoma	—

[a]Distribution based on Mayo Clinic experience.
(Adapted from ref. 2, with permission.)

1. Anatomic site. Specific anatomic sites of the bone give rise to specific groups of lesions. Johnson[58] explained this by a "field" theory, which hypothesizes that the most active cells of a certain area of bone give rise to tumors that are characteristic of that area. In general, spindle cell sarcomas are metaphyseal, whereas round cell sarcomas tend to be diaphyseal.
2. Borders. The border reflects the growth rate and the response of the adjacent normal bone to the tumor. Most tumors have a characteristic border. Benign lesions (e.g., nonossifying fibromas and unicameral bone cysts) have well-defined borders and a narrow transition area that is often associated with a reactive sclerosis. Aggressive or benign tumors (e.g., chondroblastoma and GCTs) tend to have faint borders and wide zones of transition with very little sclerosis, reflecting a faster-growing lesion. Poorly delineated or absent margins indicate an aggressive or malignant lesion.
3. Bone destruction. Bone destruction is the hallmark of a bone tumor. Three patterns of bone destruction are described[59]: geographic, moth-eaten, and permeative. In general, these patterns are found in the tubular bone rather than in the flat bone and represent a combination of cortical and cancellous destruction. These patterns reflect a progressively increasing growth rate of the underlying tumor.
4. Matrix formation. Calcification of the matrix, or new bone formation, may produce an area of increased den-

sity within the lesion. Calcification typically appears as flocculent or stippled rings or clusters. The appearance of the new bone varies from dense sclerosis that obliterates all evidence of normal trabeculae to small, irregular, circumscribed masses described as "wool" or "clouds." Calcification and ossification may appear in the same lesion. Neither type of matrix formation per se is diagnostic of malignancy.

5. Periosteal reaction. Periosteal reaction is indicative of malignancy but not pathognomonic of a particular tumor. A combination of periosteal changes is often noted. In malignant tumors, periosteal reaction is noncontinuous and thin, with multiple laminations. A parallel or a perpendicular pattern may be present.

The radiographic parameters of benign and malignant tumors are quite different. Benign tumors have round, smooth, well-circumscribed borders. No cortical destruction and, generally, no periosteal reaction are found. Malignant lesions have irregular, poorly defined margins. Evidence of bone destruction and a wide area of transition with periosteal reaction are noted. Soft tissue extension is common.

NATURAL HISTORY

Tumors arising in bone have characteristic patterns of behavior and growth that distinguish them from other malignant lesions.[60,61] These patterns form the basis of a staging system and current treatment strategies. These principles and their relationship to management, as formulated by Enneking et al.,[60,61] are described here.

BIOLOGY AND GROWTH

Spindle cell sarcomas form a solid lesion that grows centrifugally. The periphery is the least mature part of this lesion. In contradistinction to a true capsule, which surrounds a benign lesion and is composed of compressed normal cells, a malignant tumor is generally enclosed by a pseudocapsule and consists of compressed tumor cells and a fibrovascular zone of reactive tissue with an inflammatory component that interdigitates with the normal tissue adjacent to and beyond the lesion. The thickness of the reactive zone varies with the degree of malignancy and histogenic type. The histologic hallmark of sarcomas is their potential to break through the pseudocapsule to form satellite lesions of tumor cells. This characteristic distinguishes a nonmalignant mesenchymal tumor from a malignant one.

High-grade sarcomas have a poorly defined reactive zone that may be invaded and destroyed by the tumor. In addition, tumor nodules in tissue may appear to be normal and not continuous with the main tumor. These are termed *skip metastases*. Although low-grade sarcomas regularly demonstrate tumor interdigitation into the reactive zone, they rarely form tumor nodules beyond this area.

The three mechanisms of growth and extension of bone tumors are (1) compression of normal tissue, (2) resorption of bone by reactive osteoclasts, and (3) direct destruction of normal tissue. Benign tumors grow and expand by the first two mechanisms, whereas direct tissue destruction is characteristic of malignant bone tumors. Sarcomas respect anatomic borders and remain within one compartment. Local anatomy influences tumor growth by setting the natural barriers to extension. In general, bone sarcomas take the path of least resistance. Most benign bone tumors are unicompartmental; they remain confined and may expand the bone in which they arose. Malignant bone tumors are bicompartmental; they destroy the overlying cortex and go directly into the adjacent soft tissue. The determination of anatomic compartment involvement has become more important with the advent of limb-preservation surgery.

On the basis of biologic considerations and natural history, Enneking et al.[9,60] classified bone tumors into five categories, each of which shares certain clinical characteristics and radiographic patterns and requires similar surgical procedures.

1. Benign/latent: Lesions whose natural history is to grow slowly during normal growth of the individual and then to stop, with a tendency to heal spontaneously. They never become malignant and, if treated by simple curettage, heal rapidly. Surgery is not indicated unless they become symptomatic.

2. Benign/active: Lesions whose natural history is one of progressive growth. Simple curettage leaves a reactive rim with some tumor. Curettage is associated with a high recurrence rate. Wide excision through normal bone results in local control in approximately 95% of all cases.

3. Benign/aggressive: Lesions that are locally aggressive but do not metastasize. The tumor extends through the capsule into the reactive zone. Local control can be obtained only by removing the lesion with a margin of normal bone beyond the reactive zone.

4. Malignant/low grade: Lesions that have a low potential to metastasize. Histologically, a pseudocapsule, rather than a true capsule, is found. Tumor nodules exist within the reactive zone, but rarely beyond. Local control can be accomplished only by removal of all tumor and reactive tissue with a margin of normal bone. These lesions can be treated successfully by surgery alone.

5. Malignant/high grade: Lesions whose natural history is to grow rapidly and metastasize early. Tumor nodules are often found within and beyond the reactive zone and at some distance in the normal tissue. Surgery is necessary for local control, and systemic therapy is warranted to prevent metastasis.

METASTASIS

Bone tumors, unlike carcinomas, disseminate almost exclusively through the blood; bones lack a lymphatic system. Early lymphatic spread to regional nodes has only rarely been reported.[62,63] Lymphatic involvement, which has been noted in 10% of cases at autopsy, is a poor prognostic sign.[64] McKenna et al.[65] noted that 6 of 194 patients (3%) with osteosarcoma who underwent amputation demonstrated lymph node involvement. None of these patients survived 5 years. Hematogenous spread is manifested by pulmonary involvement in its early stage and secondarily by bone involvement.[65–67] Kager et al.[68] reported the findings of the Cooperative German-Austrian-Swiss Osteosarcoma Study Group (2003) that, of 1765 previously untreated, newly diagnosed osteosarcoma patients, 202 (11.4%) had proven metastases at the time of diagnosis—pulmonary (9.3%) and secondary bony sites (3.9%). Bone metastasis is occasion-

ally the first sign of dissemination (3.9%). With the use of adjuvant chemotherapy, the skeletal system has become a more common site of initial relapse.[60–71]

SKIP METASTASES

A skip metastasis, as previously defined in Biology and Growth, is a tumor nodule that is located within the same bone as the main tumor but not in continuity with it. Transarticular skip metastases are located in the joint adjacent to the main tumor.[72] Skip metastases are most often seen with high-grade sarcomas. They develop by the embolization of tumor cells within the marrow sinusoids; in effect, they are local micrometastases that have not passed through the circulation. Transarticular skips are believed to occur via the periarticular venous anastomosis. The clinical incidence of skip metastases is less than 1%.[72,73] These lesions are a prognosticator of poor survival.[72,73] Wuisman and Enneking[74] reviewed 23 cases with histologically proven skip metastases. Eleven patients received adjuvant chemotherapy. In 22 of the 23 patients, either local recurrence or distant metastases developed within 16 months of surgery. The authors compared the clinical course of these patients with that of 224 individuals without skip lesions. The overall survival rate of patients with skips was comparable to that of those with metastatic (stage III) disease. The authors concluded that patients with skip metastases should be classified as stage III and should be excluded from ongoing therapy trials. Kager at al.[68] reported their experience of 24 skip bony lesions in 1765 patients (1.4%) at the time of initial presentation.

LOCAL RECURRENCE

Local recurrence of a benign or malignant lesion is due to inadequate removal. The aggressiveness of the tumor determines which surgical procedure is required for local control. Ninety-five percent of all local recurrences, regardless of histology, develop within 24 months of attempted removal.[60,61,75] Local recurrence of a high-grade sarcoma was once thought to be independent of overall survival. Today, a local recurrence is believed to represent an inherent biologic aggressiveness and a tendency to metastasize; that is, tumors that tend to metastasize are those that are likely to recur locally. Local recurrence in patients who have undergone therapy is associated with an even poorer prognosis.[76]

STAGING BONE TUMORS

MUSCULOSKELETAL TUMOR SOCIETY CLASSIFICATION

In 1980, the Musculoskeletal Tumor Society (MSTS) adopted a surgical staging system for bone sarcomas[9] (Table 35.2-2). The system is based on the fact that mesenchymal sarcomas of bone behave similarly, regardless of histogenic type. The surgical staging system, as described by Enneking et al.,[9] is based on the "GTM" classification: grade (G), location (T), and lymph node involvement and metastases (M) (Fig. 35.2-2).

G represents the histologic grade of a lesion and other clinical data. Grade is further divided into two categories: G1 is low grade, and G2 is high grade.

TABLE 35.2-2.   Surgical Staging of Bone Sarcomas

Stage	Grade	Site
IA	Low (G1)	Intracompartmental (T1)
IB	Low (G1)	Extracompartmental (T2)
IIA	High (G2)	Intracompartmental (T1)
IIB	High (G2)	Extracompartmental (T2)
III	Any G	Any (T)
	Regional or distant metasta-sis (M1)	

G, grade; G1, any low-grade tumor; G2, any high-grade tumor; M, regional or distal metastases; M0, no metastases; M1, any metastases; T, site; T1, intracompartmental location of tumor; T2, extracompartmental location of tumor.
(From ref. 9, with permission.)

T represents the site of the lesion, which may be intracompartmental (T1) or extracompartmental (T2). Compartment is defined as "an anatomic structure or space bounded by natural barriers or tumor extension." The significance of T1 lesions is easier to define clinically, surgically, and radiographically than that of T2 lesions, and the chance is better for adequate removal of the former without amputation. In general, low-grade bone sarcomas are intracompartmental (T1), whereas high-grade sarcomas are extracompartmental (T2).

Lymphatic spread is a sign of widespread dissemination. Regional lymphatic involvement is equated with distal metastases (M1). Absence of any metastasis is designated as M0.

The surgical staging system developed by Enneking et al.[9] for surgical planning and assessment of bone sarcomas is summarized as follows:

Stage IA (G1, T1, M0): Low-grade intracompartmental lesion, without metastasis

Stage IB (G1, T2, M0): Low-grade extracompartmental lesion, without metastasis

Stage IIA (G2, T1, M0): High-grade intracompartmental lesion, without metastasis

Stage IIB (G2, T2, M0): High-grade extracompartmental lesion, without metastasis

Stage IIIA (G1 or G2, T1, M1): Intracompartmental lesion, any grade, with metastasis

Stage IIIB (G1 or G2, T2, M1): Extracompartmental lesion, any grade, with metastasis

AMERICAN JOINT COMMITTEE ON CANCER BONE TUMOR CLASSIFICATION AND INTERNATIONAL UNION AGAINST CANCER

In 1983, the American Joint Committee on Cancer (AJCC) Bone Tumor Classification recommended a staging system for the malignant tumors of bone. This system has undergone several changes and is now in its sixth edition (2002).[77] This classification is identical to that used by the International Union Against Cancer [Union Internationale Contre le Cancer (UICC)]. Cases are categorized by histologic type and grade. This system is based on the four-part "TNMG" designation: extent of the tumor (T), nodal status (N), distant metastases (M), and grade (G). The system is similar to the MSTS classification; however, the AJCC uses four stages instead of three. In the most recent version of the TNM system, it is noted that different grading systems are used in different centers and jurisdictions. Therefore, a translation of three- and four-tiered grading systems into a two-tiered system is required for TNM. In the most commonly used three-tiered classification, grade 1 is considered low grade and grades 2 and 3 high grade. In the less common four-tiered systems, grades 1 and 2 are considered low grade and grades 3 and 4 are high grade. The 2002 TNM classification contains substantial modifications from previous editions (Table 35.2-3). It considers maximum lesion size (with a breakpoint at 8 cm) in the differentiation of T1 versus T2 and the presence of discontinuous tumors in the same bone without other distant metastasis as T3 disease. Metastases to nonpulmonary sites are distinguished from M1 disease on the basis of lung involvement alone. One potential problem is that the existing stages need adjustment for the impact of grade in the stage-grouping algorithm. Thus, discontinuous tumor in the same bone that is low grade would likely have a better prognosis than if high grade, even though both tumor types are considered stage III in the new classification. A similar problem exists when considering lung versus nonpulmonary metastases. The UICC and AJCC staging system is applicable to all primary malignant tumors of bone except multiple myeloma, malignant lymphoma (both having different natural history), and juxtacortical osteosarcoma and chondrosarcoma (both with much more favorable prognosis). Although cancer registries will likely use the TNM system, at the present time most orthopedic oncologists tend to use the MSTS classification.

PREOPERATIVE EVALUATION

If the plain radiographs suggest an aggressive or malignant tumor, staging studies should be performed before biopsy. All radiographic studies are influenced by surgical manipulation of the lesion, making interpretation more difficult.[20,60] More importantly, the biopsy site may be in a location that is not optimal for subsequent *en bloc* removal or radiotherapy.[12,78] Bone scintigraphy, MRI, CT, angiography, or a combination of these

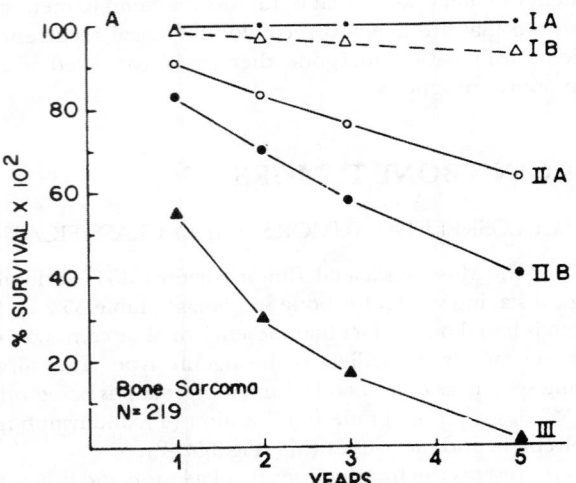

FIGURE 35.2-2.   Survival rates over a 5-year period of patients with bone sarcoma according to stage of disease. (From ref. 9, with permission.)

TABLE 35.2-3. International Union Against Cancer (UICC) and American Joint Committee on Cancer (AJCC) TNM Classification (6th Edition) of Bone Sarcomas

PRIMARY TUMOR (T)

TX	Primary tumor cannot be assessed
T0	No evidence of primary tumor
T1	Tumor (maximum dimension) ≤8 cm at time of diagnosis
T2	Tumor (maximum dimension) >8 cm at time of diagnosis
T3	Skip metastases—two discontinuous tumors in the same bone with no other distant metastases

REGIONAL LYMPH NODES (N)

NX[a]	Regional lymph nodes cannot be assessed
N0	No regional lymph node metastasis
N1	Regional lymph node metastasis to be considered equivalent to distant metastatic disease (see M1b, below)

DISTANT METASTASIS (M)

MX	Distant metastasis cannot be assessed
M0	No distant metastasis
M1	Distant metastasis
M1a	Lung-only metastases
M1b	All other distant metastases including lymph nodes

STAGE GROUPING

IA	G1, 2	T1	N0	M0
IB	G1, 2	T2	N0	M0
IIA	G3, 4	T1	N0	M0
IIB	G3, 4	T2	N0	M0
III	Any G	T3	N0	M0
IVA	Any G	Any T	N0	M1a
IVB	Any G	Any T	N0/N1	M1b

G, grade.

[a]Because of the rarity of lymph node involvement in sarcomas, the designation NX may not be appropriate and could be considered N0 if no clinical involvement is evident.

(From ref. 9, with permission.)

is required to delineate local tumor extent, vascular displacement, and compartmental localization[27,31,69,79,80] (Fig. 35.2-3). More recently, positron emission tomography (PET) imaging has been used. Its exact role has not yet been determined. Systemic staging includes a three-phase bone scan (looking for bony metastases) and chest CT (to determine the absence or presence of pulmonary metastases). Evaluation of regional lymph nodes, the abdomen, or the pelvis is not necessary.

BONE SCANS

Bone scintigraphy helps determine polyostotic involvement, metastatic disease, and intraosseous extension of tumor.[23,69,81] Malignant bone tumors, although solitary, may in rare cases present with skeletal metastasis.[24] Skip metastases are rarely detected by bone scan, because they are small and localized to the fatty marrow and do not excite cortical response.[72,73]

Appreciation of the intraosseous extension of a bone tumor is important in surgical planning. Removal of bone 3 to 4 cm beyond the area of scintigraphic abnormality has been accepted as a safe margin for limb-sparing procedures after induction chemotherapy.[18] Three-phase bone scans (flow, pool, and late-phase) are necessary to completely evaluate a bony tumor. Pre- and post-chemotherapy bone scans can be compared only when identical areas of the scan are evaluated. To eliminate uncontrolled variations in technique, the method of determining the tumor-to-nontumor ratio of uptake is important. This ratio is obtained for each of the three phases. The flow and pool phases indicate tumor vascularity, whereas the late phase is a sign of bone formation (osteoblastic activity).

COMPUTED TOMOGRAPHY

CT allows accurate determination of intra- and extraosseous extension of skeletal neoplasms.[21,81,82] It accurately depicts the transverse relationship of a tumor. By varying window settings, one can study cortical bone, intramedullary space, adjacent muscles, and extraosseous soft tissue extension. CT should include the entire bone and the adjacent joint. Infusion of intravenous contrast material permits identification of the adjacent large vascular structures. CT evaluation must be individualized. To obtain the maximum benefits from image reconstruction, the surgeon

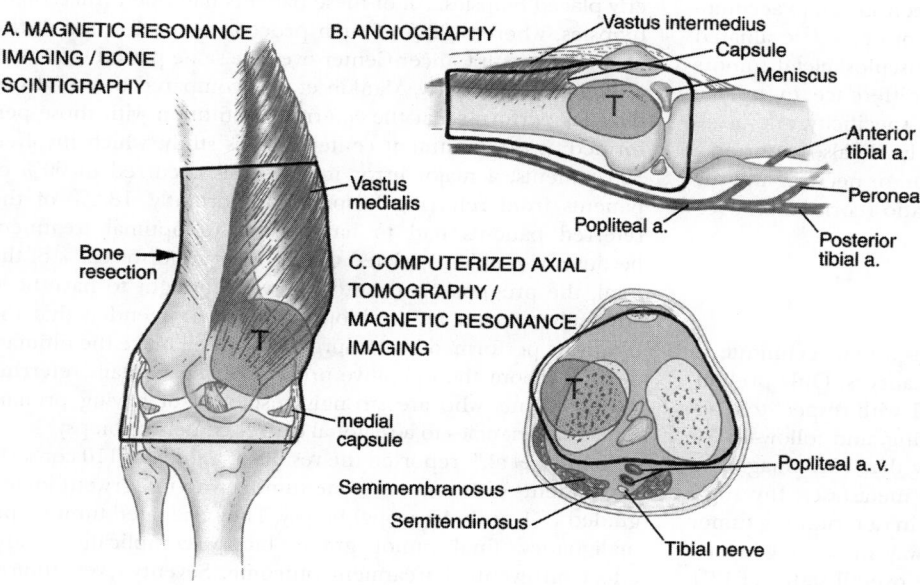

FIGURE 35.2-3. Schematic of different imaging techniques demonstrating the anatomic significance of angiography, bone scan, computed tomography scan, and magnetic resonance imaging of the distal femur in relationship to the important bony, soft tissue, and vascular anatomy. All four studies are required in the initial local staging of bony sarcomas as well as in the restaging studies after induction chemotherapy and before the definitive surgical procedure. T, tumor. (See Color Fig. 35.2-3 in the CD-ROM.)

should discuss with the radiologist what information is desired. Three-dimensional reconstruction may be useful. Today, CT and MRI are considered complementary studies for bone sarcomas. Both studies are recommended for most patients. Pulmonary CT is routinely performed to determine the presence of pulmonary disease; approximately 11% of all newly diagnosed patients with osteosarcoma have pulmonary metastases.[68]

MAGNETIC RESONANCE IMAGING AND STAGING

MRI has several advantages in the diagnoses of bone sarcomas.[27,28,75,79,80] It has better contrast discrimination than any other modality; furthermore, imaging can be performed in any plane. MRI is ideal for imaging the medullary marrow and thus for detection of tumor as well as the extraosseous component. It has proved especially helpful in several heretofore difficult clinical situations, such as detecting small lesions, evaluating a positive bone scan when the corresponding plain radiograph is negative, determining the extent of infiltrative tumors, and detecting skip metastases.[31,79,80]

ANGIOGRAPHY

The technique of angiography for bone lesions differs from that used for arterial disease. At least two views (biplane) are necessary to determine the relation of the major vessels to the tumor.[83] Because experience with limb-sparing procedures has increased, it has become essential to determine individual vascular patterns before resection. This is especially crucial for tumors of the proximal tibia, where vascular anomalies are common.[84] Angiography is the most reliable means of determining vascular anatomy and displacement, whereas MRI and CT better demonstrate extraosseous extension. The major advantage of angiography is its ability to determine residual tumor vascularity, which correlates well with chemotherapy-induced necrosis. Presently, magnetic resonance angiography (MRA) is being evaluated in the treatment of bone sarcomas.

THALLIUM SCANS

Thallium 201 chloride scintigraphy has been shown to accumulate in musculoskeletal neoplasms.[85–87] Goto et al.[87] evaluated 62 patients with malignant or benign musculoskeletal tumors and reported a statistically significant difference in uptake between the two tumor types. Sensitivity, specificity, and accuracy were 94%, 65%, and 82%, respectively. He also reported a good correlation between the extent of tumor necrosis and the percentage change in tumor-to-normal ratio (correlation coefficient, r = 0.81).

POSITRON EMISSION TOMOGRAPHY

[18F]fluorodeoxy-D-glucose (FDG)–PET is a new technique to evaluate the local and distal extents of cancers. Only preliminary data are available on the role of PET with respect to diagnosis, imaging, staging, therapy monitoring, and follow-up for osteosarcomas. These early studies show that PET imaging is not accurate in determining pulmonary metastases. Investigations of the effectiveness of PET imaging in determining tumor response to chemotherapy are under way in several institutions. Brenner et al.[88] have reviewed the overall status of PET

imaging for osteosarcoma. They concluded that too few patients have been evaluated and that further research needs to be done in larger, prospective series. PET imaging is not currently reimbursable for sarcomas.

CHOOSING A METHOD OF RADIOGRAPHIC EVALUATION

All of the studies just described are required in the preoperative evaluation [termed *restaging studies*; see later in Restaging after Induction (Preoperative) Chemotherapy] of a bone sarcoma. Each study has unique benefits. Bloem et al.[89] performed a prospective study comparing results of CT, MRI, scintigraphy, and angiography with 56 resected specimens to determine the appropriate choice of procedures. MRI, the single best study, was most accurate for determining intraosseous extent of tumor; scintigraphy and CT were often misleading. Angiography was performed only if the primary tumor was in the vicinity of the major vascular structures. Bloem et al. also reported that CT and MRI were equally accurate in evaluating cortical changes. MRI was superior to CT for detecting muscle involvement in the knee, pelvis, and shoulder. The role of newer imaging techniques, such as dynamic MRI, MRA, and PET, has not been well determined for bone sarcomas and is presently being evaluated at many institutions. MRI and CT (transverse data), combined with bone scans and angiography, allow the physician to develop a three-dimensional construct of the local tumor area before surgery and thereby formulate a detailed surgical approach.

BIOPSY TECHNIQUE AND TIMING

The biopsy of a suspected bone tumor must be performed with great care and skill.[90,91] This principle cannot be overemphasized. The consequences of a poorly executed biopsy are often the deciding factor in the choice between a limb-salvage procedure and amputation. Ayala et al.[92] from the M. D. Anderson Cancer Center judged that only 19% of patients referred to that institution for treatment of primary bone sarcomas had properly placed biopsies. All of these patients had open (incisional) biopsies, whereas 92% of such procedures performed at the M. D. Anderson Cancer Center over the same period were needle biopsies. Similarly, Mankin et al.[91] compared the results of biopsies performed at the referring institution with those performed at the treatment center. In this study, which involved 329 patients, a major error in diagnosis occurred in 60% of patients from referring hospitals. Importantly, 18.2% of the referred patients had to have less than optimal treatment because of problems related to the biopsy, and for 8.5% of the total, the prognosis and outcome were thought to have been adversely affected by the biopsy. It is recommended that the biopsy be performed by the surgeon who will make the ultimate decision about the operative procedure. This entails referring some patients who are strongly suspected of having primary bone malignancies to a regional cancer center for biopsy.

Jelinek et al.[93] reported the results of a study of 110 consecutive patients with primary bone tumors who underwent image-guided (CT or fluoroscopy) biopsy. They evaluated tumor type, malignancy, final tumor grade, biopsy complications, and effect on eventual treatment outcome. Seventy-seven tumors were malignant, and 33 were benign. Correct final diagnosis was attained in 97 (88%) of patients. In 13 patients, a definitive diagnosis could not be made. Seven of these 13 patients had tumors with large cystic components, which made biopsy difficult. Nine patients (8%) required open biopsy. No malignant tumors were called benign. The authors noted that when a core biopsy proves inconclusive, an open biopsy is likely to be associated with similar diagnostic problems. It is the surgical author's (M. M. M.) practice to proceed with an image-guided multicore biopsy for all patients with bone tumors. Open biopsy is reserved for those patients (fewer than 10%) in whom a definitive diagnosis cannot be established or those in whom a sufficient sample of pathologic tissue cannot be obtained for immunostains or cytogenetic study, or both.

RESTAGING AFTER INDUCTION (PREOPERATIVE) CHEMOTHERAPY

With the advent of preoperative chemotherapy for osteosarcoma, a need has developed for serial evaluation of the clinical and radiographic response of the tumor before surgery. The staging and preoperative clinical studies previously described are used to evaluate tumor response. These studies have been summarized.[94–96] Complete restaging studies should be obtained after the completion of induction chemotherapy. MRI, CT, thallium scans, and angiography should be evaluated before a final surgical decision is made.

CLINICAL EVALUATION

Pain often decreases after induction chemotherapy. Alkaline phosphatase (AP) levels also decrease. The tumor shrinks, especially if significant matrix is not present. Conversely, increase of pain, elevated AP values, and increasing tumor size are signs of tumor progression.

PLAIN RADIOGRAPHY

A good correlation is found between radiographic response and the amount of necrosis.[97] Smith et al.[98] described the radiographic responses seen on serial radiographs: increased ossification of tumor osteoid, marked thickening and new bone formation of the periosteum and tumor border (giving the tumor a more "benign" appearance), and decreased soft tissue mass.[98] The healing ossification is usually solid, homogeneous, and regular and is easily differentiated from tumor osteoid.[97] Less significant changes take place within the intramedullary component, which may include increased sclerosis and lysis, presumably caused by necrosis and hemorrhage.

ANGIOGRAPHY

After chemotherapy, vascularity decreases markedly. Chuang et al.[97] evaluated 53 patients and reported that those with a complete angiographic response had more than 90% necrosis; among those with a partial response, necrosis ranged from 40% to 78%. They concluded that angiographic evaluation was as reliable as pathologic evaluation and that the angiographic features were the best clinical criteria for the evaluation of tumor response.

Carrasco et al.[99] from the M. D. Anderson Cancer Center reported on their extensive experience with intraarterial chemotherapy for osteosarcoma (81 patients) and evaluated the angiographic appearance and changes after two and four cycles of preoperative chemotherapy. They developed a simple radiographic system for angiographic changes. These authors evaluated the midarterial (tumor vascularity) and parenchymal (capillary) phases and described three types of responses: (1) angiographic response: complete disappearance of tumor vascularity and stain; (2) total disappearance of tumor vascularity, with slight persistence of tumor stain (capillary phase); and (3) no response: persistence of tumor vascularity and capillary stain. They reported that 40% of the histologic responders (more than 90% tumor necrosis) and 91% of nonresponders were identified after two cycles. The number of courses was no different between the responders and nonresponders. These authors concluded that the disappearance of tumor vascularity after two courses of chemotherapy was highly suggestive of a good histologic response and was unlikely to occur in the histologic nonresponders.

COMPUTED TOMOGRAPHY

The most consistent finding in patients who respond to therapy is a decrease in soft tissue mass and the development of a rim-like calcification similar to that seen on plain radiographs.[96] Changes in marrow are not helpful in evaluating response.

BONE SCINTIGRAPHY

Bone scan changes are difficult to evaluate. A decrease in activity generally indicates a favorable response; however, reparative bone formation, signaled by increased activity, may be misleading. Dynamic (quantitative) bone scans, which are based on tumor blood flow and regional plasma clearance by bone and soft tissue, may allow more valid evaluations.[100] Regions that show a greater than 20% decrease in technetium 99m methylene diphosphonate plasma clearance are reported to be associated with necrotic tumor. To quantify bone scans, a tumor-to-nontumor ratio is obtained after bone scintigraphy. This ratio is then determined preoperatively and after induction chemotherapy on serial scans. A decrease in this ratio (usually less than 4) is an indication of a good response to chemotherapy.

MAGNETIC RESONANCE IMAGING

Monitoring of neoadjuvant chemotherapy by MRI has become the focus of many studies. Holscher et al.[101] evaluated 57 patients at the University Hospital of Leiden. T1- and T2-weighted images were obtained in longitudinal, coronal or sagittal, and axial planes. Factors evaluated were margins, homogeneity, hematoma, fibrosis, calcification liquefaction, edema, joint effusion, and fracture. The authors concluded that increased tumor volume or increased or unchanged peritumoral edema and inflammation indicated a poor response. Subjective criteria, such as improved tumor demarcation or an increase in size of area of low signal intensity (presumably necrotic tumor), were independent of tumor response. The authors concluded that subjective criteria could not predict the good responders.

THALLIUM SCINTIGRAPHY

Several studies have demonstrated that serial thallium 201 scintigraphy is an accurate way to follow the response of osteosarcoma during the course of neoadjuvant treatment and to predict tumor responses.[85,86,102] Rosen et al.[86] used this technique to evaluate tumor necrosis after preoperative chemotherapy in 27 patients. They concluded that serial thallium scans can accurately predict a good histologic response and good prognosis. Furthermore, thallium scintigraphy can identify poor responders within the first 2 weeks after the initiation of treatment. They described a simple classification of response: type I, no response; type II, discernible lesion still present; and type III, no detectable lesion. All patients with a type III classification and 67% of those with a type II classification were rated as good responders (types II and III constituted a total of nine patients).[86]

POSITRON EMISSION TOMOGRAPHY

Positron emission tomographic scans are nuclear medicine scintigraphy techniques that use 2-FDG as the radiopharmaceutical. This technique is under investigation. It is hoped that it will be able to dynamically evaluate the tumor and the percentage of tumor necrosis after chemotherapy.[103] Hawkins et al.[104] evaluated 33 patients with osteosarcoma and Ewing's-related bone tumors before and after chemotherapy and compared the FDG-PET standard uptake values (SUV1 and SUV2; "1" refers to the average value and "2" to the peak value), respectively, to the tumor response of the resected specimens. The SUV2 and SUV2:SUV1 ratio correlated with histologic response. Franzius et al.[105] reported that good responders could be distinguished from poor responders in all cases in which there was a decrease in the tumor-to-nontumor ratio of greater than 30%.

SURGICAL MANAGEMENT OF SKELETAL TUMORS

Surgical removal, including curettage, resection, and amputation, is the traditional method of managing skeletal neoplasms. Limb-sparing techniques were developed during the early 1970s.[10,11,15,16,20] Marcove et al.[106–108] have described cryosurgery for some bony tumors. Enneking et al.[9] have formulated means of classifying surgical procedures on the basis of the surgical plane of dissection in relationship to the tumor and the method of accomplishing the removal (Tables 35.2-4 and 35.2-5). The

TABLE 35.2-4.   Classification of Surgical Procedures for Bone Tumors

Margin[a]	Local	Amputation
Intralesional	Curettage or debulking	Debulking amputation
Marginal	Marginal excision	Marginal amputation
Wide	Wide local excision	Wide through bone, amputation
Radical	Radical local resection	Radical disarticulation

[a]Tumors are classified by the type of margin achieved and whether they are obtained by a local or ablative procedure.
(From ref. 9, with permission.)

TABLE 35.2-5.   Surgical Procedure, Plane of Dissection, and Residual Disease for Musculoskeletal Tumors

Type	Plane of Dissection	Result
Intralesional	Piecemeal debulking or curettage	Leaves macroscopic disease
Marginal	Shell out *en bloc* through pseudocapsule or reactive zone	May leave either satellite or skip lesions
Wide	Intracompartmental *en bloc* with cuff of normal tissue	May leave skip lesions
Radical	Extracompartmental *en bloc*, entire compartment	No residual

(From ref. 9, with permission.)

scheme, summarized below, affords meaningful comparisons of various operative procedures and gives surgeons a common language (Fig. 35.2-4).

Intralesional: An intralesional procedure passes through the pseudocapsule of the neoplasm directly into the lesion. Macroscopic tumor remains, and the entire operative field is potentially contaminated. Curettage is an intralesional procedure.

Marginal: A marginal procedure is one in which the entire lesion is removed in a single piece. The plane of dissection passes through the pseudocapsule or reactive zone around the lesion. When performed for a sarcoma, it leaves macroscopic disease.

Wide (intracompartmental): A wide excision, commonly termed *en bloc resection*, includes the entire tumor, the reactive zone, and a cuff of normal tissue. The entire structure of origin of the tumor is not removed. In patients with high-grade sarcomas, this procedure may leave skip nodules.

Radical (extracompartmental): A radical procedure involves removal of the entire tumor and the structure of origin of the lesion. The plane of dissection is beyond the limiting fascial or bony borders.

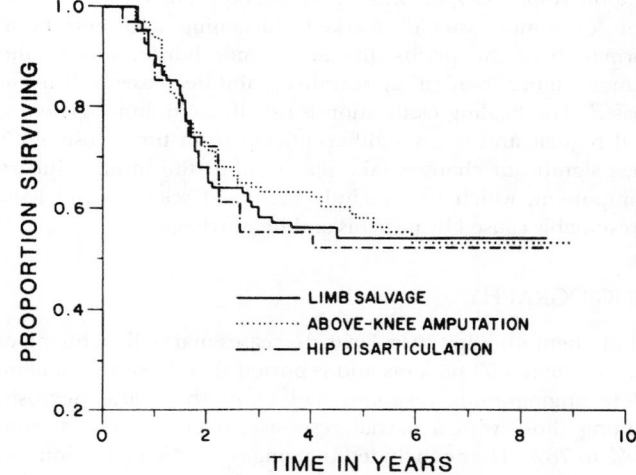

FIGURE 35.2-4.   Patient survival after three different types of surgical procedures for osteosarcoma of the distal femur.

It is important to note that any of these procedures can be accomplished by either a limb-sparing procedure or by amputation. Thus, amputation may entail a marginal, wide, or radical excision, depending on the plane through which it passes. Amputation does not necessarily remove all cancer, but it can achieve a specific margin. The local anatomy determines how such a margin can be obtained. Therefore, the aim of preoperative staging is to assess local tumor extent and important local anatomy to enable the surgeon to decide how to achieve a desired margin (i.e., to evaluate the feasibility of one surgical procedure over another). This system allows meaningful comparisons of surgical procedures, end-result reporting, and analysis of combined data. In general, benign bone tumors can be treated adequately by an intralesional procedure (curettage) or a marginal excision. Malignant tumors require either a wide (intracompartmental) or radical (extracompartmental) removal, by an amputation or an *en bloc* procedure. Today, wide excision combined with adjuvant chemotherapy is the treatment for most high-grade bone sarcomas. Radical resections are rare.

PRINCIPLES AND TECHNIQUES OF LIMB-SPARING SURGERY

Limb-salvage surgery is a safe operation for selected cases. This technique can be used for all spindle cell sarcomas, regardless of histogenesis. Approximately 90% of osteosarcomas can be treated successfully with this technique. Successful management of localized osteosarcomas and other sarcomas requires careful coordination and timing of staging studies, biopsy, surgery, and preoperative and postoperative chemotherapy or radiation therapy.

PHASES OF OPERATION

Successful limb-sparing procedures consist of three surgical phases[11]:

1. Resection of tumor: Tumor resection follows strictly the principles of oncologic surgery. Avoiding local recurrence is the criterion of success and the main determinant of how much bone and soft tissue are to be removed.
2. Skeletal reconstruction: The average skeletal defect after adequate bone tumor resection measures 15 to 20 cm. Techniques of reconstruction vary and are independent of the resection, although the degree of resection may favor one technique over another.
3. Soft tissue and muscle transfers: Muscle transfers are performed to cover and close the resection site and to restore motor power. Adequate skin and muscle coverage is mandatory. Distal tissue transfers are not used because of the possibility of contamination.

GUIDELINES FOR LIMB-SPARING RESECTION

The surgical guidelines and technique of limb-sparing surgery used by the surgical author (M. M. M.) are as follows[11]: (1) no major neurovascular tumor involvement; (2) wide resection of the affected bone, with a normal muscle cuff in all directions; (3) *en bloc* removal of all previous biopsy sites and potentially contaminated tissue; (4) resection of bone 3 to 4 cm beyond abnormal uptake, as determined by CT or MRI and bone scan; (5) resection of the adjacent joint and capsule; and (6) adequate motor reconstruction, accomplished by regional muscle transfers. Soft tissue coverage should be adequate.

TYPES OF SKELETAL RECONSTRUCTION

Large skeletal defects are reconstructed after tumor resection by several different modalities. Osteoarticular defects are most often reconstructed by segmental, modular prostheses that are fixed to the remaining intramedullary bone by polymethylmethacrylate (PMMA). The newer knee prostheses allow rotation as well as flexion and extension. This mobility decreases the forces on the bone-cement interface and thus reduces the risk of loosening.

Increasing interest has been shown in applying a porous coating to the prosthesis in the hope of obtaining long-term, perhaps even permanent, fixation.[60] In addition, titanium, a new alloy with superior metallurgic properties, has been introduced. Modular endoprosthetic replacement systems that can be assembled in the operating room are now available and avoid the problem of long delays for custom manufacturing. Alternative methods of segmental replacement include large autografts or allografts, used to obtain an arthrodesis, or osteoarticular allografts that may replace the affected joint.[17,109] Composite allograft (i.e., allograft placed over a prosthesis) has been used. In general, allografts have been used successfully for low-grade sarcomas and for GCTs of bone that do not require chemotherapy or radiotherapy. Most large cancer centers in the United States now favor the use of endoprosthetic implants for high-grade bone sarcomas. Long-term results of allograft survival in this group of patients have been extremely disappointing.[110]

Today, most surgeons prefer endoprosthetic replacements. The modular replacement systems can replace the most commonly affected bones: the proximal femur, proximal humerus, distal femur, proximal tibia, and entire femur, as well as the scapula.

CONTRAINDICATIONS TO LIMB-SPARING SURGERY

Major Neurovascular Involvement

Although vascular grafts can be used, the adjacent nerves are usually at risk, making successful resection less likely. In addition, the magnitude of resection in combination with vascular reconstruction is often prohibitive.

Pathologic Fractures

A fracture through a bone affected by a tumor spreads tumor cells via the hematoma beyond accurately determined limits. The risk of local recurrence increases under such circumstances. If a pathologic fracture heals after neoadjuvant chemotherapy, a limb-salvage procedure can be performed successfully.

Inappropriate Biopsy Sites

An inappropriate or poorly planned biopsy jeopardizes local tumor control by contaminating normal tissue planes and compartments.

INFECTION. The risk of infection after implantation of a metallic device or an allograft in an infected area is prohibitive. Sepsis jeopardizes the effectiveness of adjuvant chemotherapy.

SKELETAL IMMATURITY. The predicted leg-length discrepancy should not be greater than 6 to 8 cm, although expandable prostheses have been used with success in this situation. Upper extremity reconstruction is independent of skeletal maturity.

EXTENSIVE MUSCLE INVOLVEMENT. Enough muscle must remain to reconstruct a functional extremity.

RELATIONSHIP OF VARIOUS ASPECTS OF SURGICAL MANAGEMENT TO PROGNOSIS

Makley et al.[111] from the Children's Cancer Study Group reported a randomized study of 166 patients that examined the relationship of various aspects of surgical management to prognosis for disease-free survival. They found no advantage to the various aspects of surgical management, specifically, interval from first symptom to definitive surgery, interval from biopsy to definitive surgery, surgical sequence, type of surgery, or site of primary tumor.

LIMB-SPARING SURGERY AND PERIOPERATIVE PAIN MANAGEMENT

Pain after extensive limb-sparing resections of bone is severe, and patients require large amounts of narcotics. Pain after amputations in young people is especially difficult to control. Within the past decade, there has been increased interest in managing postoperative pain by various modalities in addition to the standard patient-controlled analgesia (PCA). Patients who have preoperative pain are more difficult to treat adequately and are at a higher risk of postoperative pain syndromes than are those with no preoperative pain.

Most patients with bone sarcomas present with pain and are under various treatment modalities. The anesthesiologist or a pain management specialist should be involved with the management of these patients as early as possible. Psychological evaluation is also important; signs of anxiety and depression should be treated early.

The aim of postoperative pain management is to eliminate or greatly attenuate pain. The use of multiple modalities is routine. Epidural anesthesia (with or without patient control), an intravenous PCA, and a regional block are ideal. We have termed this *triple-modality* pain control.

The surgical author (M. M. M.) has developed a technique of "perineural" anesthesia that is used in conjunction with an epidural and an intravenous PCA (Fig. 35.2-5). Perineural anesthesia is a form of a continuous regional block that was developed specifically for the management of patients with sarcoma.[112] Major limb-sparing procedures such as amputations expose the major nerves. This affords the surgeon the opportunity to directly catheterize all the nerves (thus the term *perineural*) within the operative field (e.g., in distal femoral resections, the sciatic nerve is exposed and catheterized, and in proximal humeral resections, the infraclavicular portion of the brachial plexus is similarly treated). Henshaw et al.[113] reported their experience with 166 patients implanted with one or more perineural catheters; there were 119 limb-

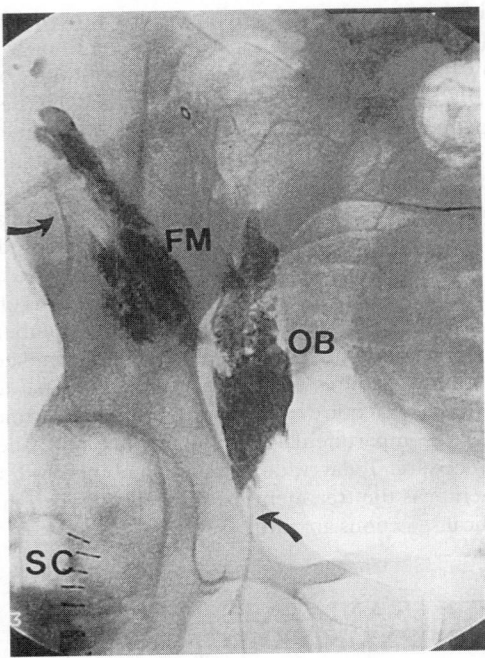

FIGURE 35.2-5. Photograph demonstrating perineural catheter placement into the femoral nerve (FM), obturator nerve (OB), and sciatic nerve (SC). Each catheter receives a 10-mL bolus of 0.25% bupivacaine during the immediate postoperative period, then 4 to 8 mL continuous infusion thereafter for local pain control. This technique may obviate the symptoms of phantom limb pain.

sparing resections, 31 amputations, and 16 other major procedures. No complications occurred related to the catheters. These authors recommend the use of triple-modality pain control for patients undergoing limb-sparing resection or amputation.

QUALITY-OF-LIFE CONSIDERATIONS: LIMB-SPARING SURGERY VERSUS AMPUTATION

During the 1990s, as the techniques of limb-sparing surgery were being developed, it had been assumed that such surgery was superior to amputation. Nonetheless, when complications occurred, many surgeons thought that an amputation might have been preferable. Despite the extensive literature on the various chemotherapy regimens, surgical techniques, and limb-sparing surgery, few studies have focused on the patients' evaluation of their overall quality of life.[114–117] Three studies that have been published are described here.

Greenberg et al.[115] from Massachusetts General Hospital and the Children's Hospital/Dana-Farber Cancer Institute evaluated 62 osteosarcoma survivors at a mean of 12 years from diagnosis. Of 89 survivors contacted, 62 patients (42 women and 20 men) agreed to be interviewed. These patients responded to a comprehensive battery of psychological questions. In general, most survivors were in good mental and physical health. The results are summarized as follows:

1. The reported rates of psychopathology among amputees and those undergoing limb-sparing surgery did not differ significantly.
2. Fertility was not a problem. Twenty-three normal progeny were born after chemotherapy to eight women and

the wives of five men. Only two women were considered infertile; both had undergone radiation therapy associated with other childhood cancers.

3. All responders who had undergone limb-sparing surgery believed that the effort to save their limb was worthwhile. Twenty patients rated the effort of limb salvage very worthwhile (mean, 4.5 out of 5.0). Those in whom the attempt at limb salvage failed rated the effort as 4.0 (not significantly different than the successful group). Those patients who were less satisfied with surgery had secondary amputations.

4. Pain was usually minimal but, when present, was associated only with lower extremity amputation. The pain pattern suggested deafferentation syndromes. No patients undergoing upper extremity limb-sparing procedures incurred pain.

5. Among patients who did not do well, multiple symptoms, family problems, and socioeconomic problems were more common than among patients who fared well.

The authors concluded that attention to the management of depression, treatment of substance abuse, and help with financial difficulties could contribute to the quality of life of patients who undergo limb-sparing surgery or amputation. Pain management, physical and vocational rehabilitation, and sexual counseling may also be beneficial, as may psychotherapeutic counseling.

Christ et al.[116] evaluated the long-term psychosocial effects of limb-sparing surgery and primary amputation for coping capacity and the degree of psychopathology. The overall incidence of emotional disturbance among these patients was no different from that in the general population. Unlike patients in other studies, those in the group with initial amputations had substantial difficulty maintaining an optimal functioning level. Their difficulty was even greater than that of limb-salvage patients with a compromised outcome, including those with late amputation. Specifically,

1. An amputee was significantly less likely to have married than a limb-spared patient.

2. Coping mechanisms of those with primary amputations were less effective than those of patients in the limb-salvage group. This deficit was still evident several years after surgery.

3. Patients who had limb salvage without later complications were very pleased with their outcome.

4. Good work experience was an important compensation for physical loss.

5. Male dependency needs were often underestimated. Some men were left to manage their own adaptation tasks, whereas for women the opposite was true. Female patients tended to become excessively dependent.

6. Patients reported no difficulty in enjoying sexual activity. The first postsurgical sexual experience was described as no more traumatic than the first experience that required showing the leg (e.g., swimming).

Despite good social support scores, the amputees had higher psychopathology scores than did patients who had undergone limb-sparing procedures. The authors concluded that patients undergoing primary amputation need more intensive support than those whose limbs are spared. They recommend an overall approach similar to that for posttraumatic stress disorder.

Nagarajan et al.[117] reported the long-term psychosocial outcome results of the Childhood Cancer Survivor Study, a cooperative study of 25 institutions. The authors evaluated 694 survivors of pediatric lower extremity bone tumors. Patients were divided into four groups on the basis of age (younger or older than 12 years) and type of surgery (limb-sparing vs. amputation). Unlike other studies, only patients with lower extremity and pelvic tumors, which are the most common site for pediatric bone cancers, were evaluated. This study analyzed education, employment, insurance, and marital status. Two-thirds of participants were married, and 97% were employed. Half had graduated from college, and 93% were high school graduates. Eighty-seven percent had health insurance. Men were less likely to be married than were women. Patients older than 12 years of age who underwent amputation had the most difficulty, especially with educational level, employment, and health insurance.

CLINICAL ANALYSIS OF LIMB-SPARING SURGERY

Rougraff et al.[114] evaluated 227 patients with nonmetastatic osteosarcoma of the distal femur treated at 26 institutions. They reported eight (11%) local recurrences in 73 patients with a limb-salvage procedure and nine (8%) local recurrences in 115 patients who had an above-knee amputation. No local recurrences were reported in the 39 patients who had a hip disarticulation.

Bacci et al.[118] retrospectively evaluated 540 patients treated over 10 years in three multicenter studies with 63 participating institutions. The rate of local recurrence was 8% for patients with a poor histologic response and 3% for those with a good histologic response. A limb-sparing procedure was performed on 84% of the 540 cases evaluated, with a local recurrence rate of 6%. The most important determinant of local recurrence was the type of surgical margin and the response to chemotherapy. Of the 540 patients, 31 had a local recurrence. The overall outcome of this group was extremely poor. All local recurrences were accompanied by metastases, and despite treatment, only one patient remains alive (3%). Local recurrence did not correlate with patient age, gender, histologic type, site and volume, pathologic fracture incidence, chemotherapy, or type of surgical procedure.

ALLOGRAFT REPLACEMENT

Allograft (cadaver bone) replacement was popular in the 1970s and mid-1980s, which were the early days of limb-sparing surgery. Allograft was used for replacement of large bony segments after limb-sparing surgery. When used in patients in conjunction with chemotherapy, allografts have a significant complication rate, including infection, fracture, nonunion, and local recurrence, which may lead to secondary amputation.[110]

PROSTHESIS SURVIVAL AND COMPLICATIONS

Prosthetic replacement is commonly used for reconstruction after resection of the proximal humerus, proximal femur, distal femur, and proximal tibia. Several studies have evaluated the long-term results, prosthetic survivorship, and complications associated with prosthetic replacement.

Ruggieri et al.[119] reported on 144 cases of nonmetastatic osteosarcoma of the extremities treated with neoadjuvant chemotherapy and limb-sparing surgery. Sixty-three percent of the patients had one or more complications. Twenty-eight complications were considered minor (i.e., no surgery was required), and 77 complications were major. The infection rate was 6.2%. Mechanical problems occurred in seven patients (5%). The average number of complications per patient was 1.3. The authors thought that the most serious problems resulting from a complication were those that required the delay of chemotherapy or deviation from the recommended dose, either of which could jeopardize survival. Such consequences were not, however, demonstrable statistically.

Campanna et al.[120] from the IOR reported on 95 distal femoral resections performed between 1983 and 1989 (average follow-up 51 months). The overall complication and infection rates were 55% and 5%, respectively. The most common complication was failure of the polyethylene bushings used with the knee component, which occurred at an average of 5.3 years after the procedure. These authors reported an overall local recurrence rate of 5% (average, 15 months). Mechanical stem breakage was rare (6%) and was associated with two factors: the use of a narrow stem and extensive quadriceps excision. The results were not related to patient age or length of resection. The tibia component caused no problems. All revisions performed for infections were unsatisfactory. The incidence of infection correlated with the extent of soft tissue resection of the quadriceps. No revisions were needed because of loosening.

In 1998, Henshaw et al.[121] reported the long-term prosthetic survival analysis of 100 patients treated with the American-designed modular replacement system (Howmedica and Osteonics, Inc., Allendale, NJ). The minimum follow-up period was 2 years. Prosthetic failure was defined as removal of the implant for any reason. Kaplan-Meier survival analysis was performed for all implants and for each site of reconstruction. The authors reported no mechanical failures of the stem, body, or taper components. No clinically significant prosthetic loosening was reported. The infection rate was 8% (four in distal femurs, three in proximal tibias, and one in proximal humerus), leading to six amputations and one prosthetic removal. The amputation rate was 7% (six infections and one local recurrence). The Kaplan-Meier survival analysis for all sites was 88% at 10 years, with a median follow-up of 64.4 months. The estimates of 10-year survival for the distal femur, proximal humerus, proximal femur, and proximal tibia were 90%, 98%, 100%, and 78%, respectively. Today, modular prostheses are forged by several manufacturers and are the standard prostheses used for most limb-sparing procedures (Figs. 35.2-6 and 35.2-7).

COST OF LIMB-SPARING SURGERY VERSUS AMPUTATION

The question of the cost effectiveness of limb-salvage surgery for bone tumors has arisen in the face of managed care, especially within the United States. The only published report on this subject is by Grimer et al.,[122] who compared the cost of a limb-sparing pro-

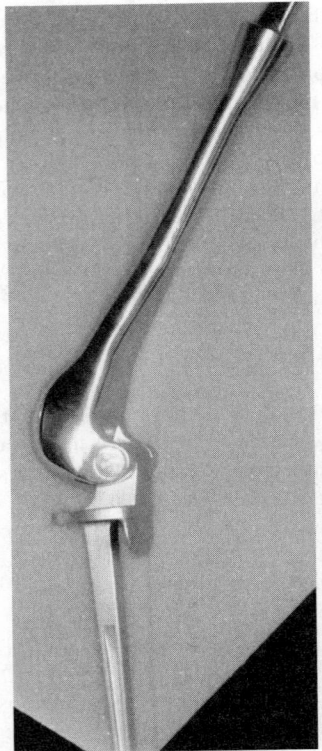

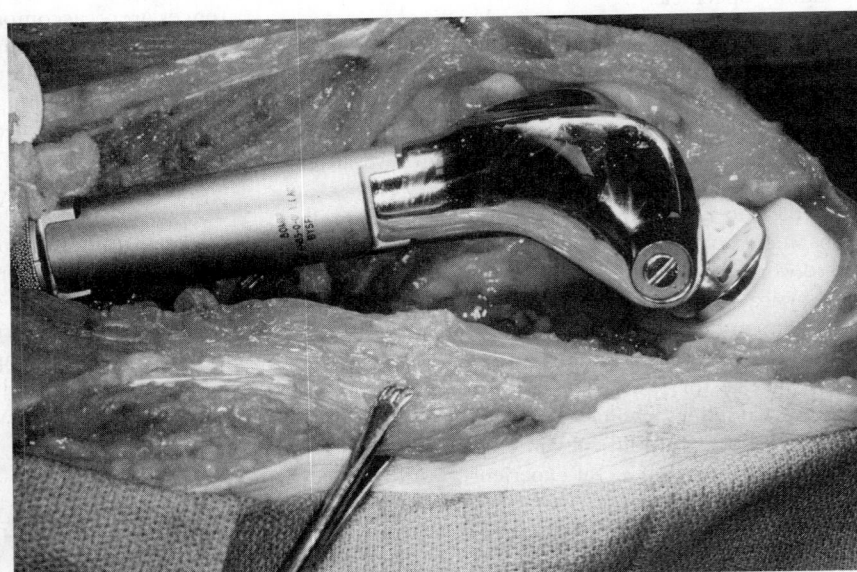

FIGURE 35.2-6. Modular replacement prosthesis. **A:** Photograph of the original segmental prosthesis, which was made as one component. The knee joint was designed as a straight hinge. The Wallidus prosthesis was the first to be used in the United States, by Dr. Kenneth Francis at New York University, in 1973. **B:** Intraoperative view of a distal femoral modular prosthesis, which reconstructs the distal femur as well as the knee joint. The knee component is a rotating hinge that has a 20-year successful record. There, prostheses have an 80% to 90% survival rate at 10 and 15 years, that is, not requiring revision. (See Color Fig. 35.2-6 in the CD-ROM.)

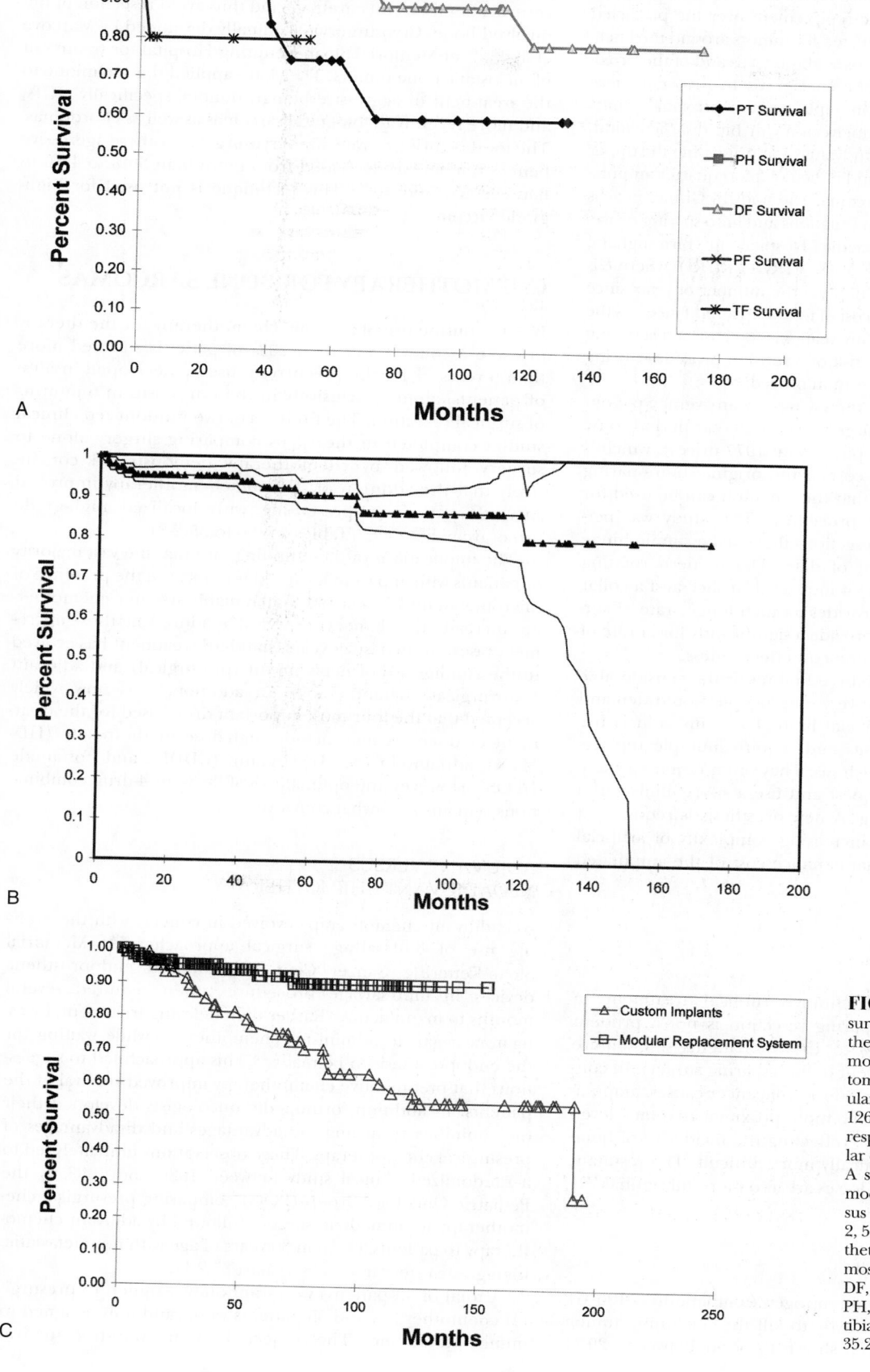

FIGURE 35.2-7. Kaplan-Meier survival curves. **A:** Long-term prosthetic survival of 126 patients with modular replacement systems by anatomic site. **B:** Overall long-term modular prosthetic survival at all sites of 126 patients at 5, 10, and 15 years, respectively. **C:** Custom versus modular endoprosthetic survival at all sites. A significant difference was seen in modular endoprosthetic survival versus custom endoprosthetic survival at 2, 5, and 10 years. Modular endoprosthetic prostheses are routinely used in most limb-sparing procedures today. DF, distal femur; PF, proximal femur; PH, proximal humerus; PT, proximal tibia; TF, total femur. (See Color Fig. 35.2-7 in the CD-ROM.)

cedure in lieu of an amputation. They developed a formula for the cost of the limb-salvage procedure versus an above-knee amputation with subsequent prosthetic replacement over the predicted life of the patient. This was calculated for tumors around the knee. They excluded tumors of the proximal humerus and of the proximal femur, because, whatever difference in cost might occur, there was a tremendous advantage in replacing the proximal femur rather than performing a hemipelvectomy or hip disarticulation. Similarly, there is a tremendous advantage in preserving the upper extremity and a functioning hand in lieu of a forequarter amputation for a proximal humeral sarcoma. The study by Grimer et al. is based on large experience of amputations and limb-sparing procedures at the Royal Orthopaedic Hospital in Birmingham, England. The formula is E + 2Fy + sSy + rRy + 3R(rRy), where E is the cost of the original procedure, y is the number of years since the original operation, F is the cost of follow-up attendance, s is the risk of a service procedure in any year, S is the cost of a servicing procedure in any year, r is the risk of a revision procedure being needed, and R is the cost of a revision procedure.

Grimer et al.[122] concluded the savings for an average patient undergoing a limb-sparing surgery over a 20-year period to be approximately 70,000 British pounds (at 1977 prices), which is approximately six times the cost of the original limb-sparing procedure. They concluded that the equation can be used for any method of limb-salvage procedure. This study was performed with distal femoral resections that used a simple hinge prosthesis, which is now out of date. The modern rotating hinged-knee prosthesis, with an improved surface and a collar coated with porous beads, provides a much longer rate of survival. These features should provide a significantly lower rate of wear and failure, thus increasing cost effectiveness.

The surprising feature of these findings is the considerable cost of amputation. Most active young people would demand and use a sophisticated artificial limb. These individuals frequently have stump problems and require multiple replacements of the socket and prosthesis. They often require a spare prosthesis as well. Many request and use a sports limb and a limb designed for swimming. A new prosthesis is required at regular intervals. With the increasing complexity of artificial limbs, it is likely that the maintenance cost of the amputated extremity will increase.

AMPUTATIONS

An amputation provides definitive surgical treatment in patients in whom a limb-sparing resection is not a prudent option. Approximately 10% to 15% of patients still require amputation, despite the advent of limb-sparing surgery. In contrast to amputations performed for noncancer causes, amputations for cancer tend to be at a more proximal anatomic level, to occur in younger people (reflecting the incidence of bone sarcomas), and to be technically more difficult. The resultant psychological and cosmetic losses are also more substantial.[123]

CRYOSURGERY

Cryosurgery is the use of liquid nitrogen (temperature, −196°C) after curettage of a tumor cavity to kill the remaining tumor cells.[106-108] Necrosis has been shown to occur between −20°C

and −40°C.[124] In general, a double freeze-thaw cycle is required. The aim of this technique is to enhance local tumor control after a careful curettage and thus avoid resection of the involved bone. Cryosurgery was initially developed by Marcove et al.[106-108] at Memorial Sloan-Kettering Hospital for treatment of metastatic bone tumors. They have applied this technique to the treatment of aggressive benign tumors, specifically GCTs, and more recently to low-grade sarcomas as well as chordomas. The local recurrence rate after cryosurgery for these aggressive benign tumors has decreased from more than 30% to 40% to between 5% and 10%. This technique is not used for high-grade sarcomas.

CHEMOTHERAPY FOR BONE SARCOMAS

Before routine use of systemic chemotherapy for the therapy of osteosarcoma, fewer than 20% of patients survived more than 5 years.[125] Further, recurrent disease developed in 50% of patients, almost exclusively in the lungs, within 6 months of surgical resection. The findings of two randomized clinical studies completed in the 1980s comparing surgery alone to surgery followed by chemotherapy demonstrated conclusively that the addition of systemic chemotherapy improved survival in patients presenting with localized high-grade osteosarcoma[37,126,127] (Tables 35.2-6 to 35.2-8).

The implications of these findings are that the vast majority of patients with apparent localized tumors have the presence of micrometastatic disease and that available systemic chemotherapy increases the chances of survival by addressing those micrometastases. In the last 20 years, standard treatment has evolved to the routine use of neoadjuvant (presurgical) and adjuvant (postsurgical/chemotherapy). In addition, it is now widely accepted that the four most important drugs used for the treatment of osteosarcoma include high-dose methotrexate (HD-MTX), adriamycin (ADM), cisplatin (CDDP), and ifosfamide (IFOS). However, the optimal use of 2-, 3-, or 4-drug combinations remains somewhat controversial.

ADJUVANT VERSUS NEOADJUVANT CHEMOTHERAPY

Neoadjuvant chemotherapy evolved in concert with the evolving use of limb-salvage surgical approaches. At Memorial Sloan-Kettering Cancer Center, customized endoprosthetic devices in limb-salvage procedures often required several months to manufacture. Rather than delaying treatment, investigators began to administer chemotherapy while waiting for the endoprosthesis to be made.[78] This approach led to suggestions that preoperative chemotherapy improved survival of the patients. In addition, orthopedic oncologists developed their own opinions regarding the advantages and disadvantages of presurgical chemotherapy. These observations ultimately led to a randomized clinical study between 1986 and 1993 by the Pediatric Oncology Group (POG) comparing presurgical chemotherapy to immediate surgery followed by adjuvant chemotherapy to patients less than 30 years of age with nonmetastatic, high-grade osteosarcoma[128] (Chart 35.2-1).

A total of 45 patients were randomly assigned to presurgical chemotherapy, and 55 patients were randomly assigned to immediate surgery. The projected 5-year event-free survival

TABLE 35.2-6. Reported Results of Representative Trials of Adjuvant Therapy for Osteosarcoma

Adjuvant Regimen	Investigators	Number of Patients	% Relapse-Free	References
HDMTX, VCR (Study I)	DFCI	12	42	323,324
HDMTX, VCR ± BCG[a]	NCI	39	38	325
DOX	CALGB	88	39	326,327
DOX ± HDMTX[a]	CALGB	62	50	328
DOX + VCR + HDMTX (Study II)	DFCI	22	59	323
DOX + VCR + HDMTX (weekly) (Study III)	DFCI	46	60	323,329
DOX + VCR + (HDMTX vs. IDMTX)[a]	CCG	166	38	330–332
COMPADRI I (CTX, VCR, DOX, PAM)	SWOG	43	49	331,332
COMPADRI II (CTX, VCR, DOX, PAM, HDMTX)	SWOG	53	35	331,332
COMPADRI III (CTX, VCR, DOX, PAM, HDMTX)	SWOG	84	38	332
DOX + HDMTX + CTX (OSTEO 72)	St. Jude	26	50	333
DOX + HDMTX + CTX (OSTEO 77)	St. Jude	50	56	333
DOX + CDDP	Roswell Park	22	61	334,335
HDMTX + VCR vs. no adjuvant therapy[b]	Mayo Clinic	38	40 (chemotherapy) 44 (no chemotherapy)	336
BCD + HDMTX + DOX + CDDP vs. no adjuvant therapy[c]	MIOS	36 randomized 165 nonrandomized	63 (chemotherapy) 12 (no chemotherapy)	337–339
BCD + HDMTX + VCR + DOX (+ intraarterial DOX + XRT) vs. no adjuvant therapy[c]	UCLA	59	55 (chemotherapy) 20 (no chemotherapy)	340
Whole lung irradiation vs. no adjuvant treatment[d]	EORTC	86	43 (with treatment) 28 (no treatment)	341,342
Whole lung irradiation (+ dactinomycin) vs. no adjuvant treatment[a]	Mayo Clinic	53	40	343
HDMTX + VCR + DOX + CTX (T4 + T5 pooled)	MSKCC	52 (<21 y)	48	344–346

BCD, bleomycin, cyclophosphamide, and dactinomycin; BCG, Calmette-Guérin bacillus; CALGB, Cancer and Acute Leukemia Group B; CCG, Children's Cancer Group; CDDP, cisplatin; CTX, Cytoxan (cyclophosphamide); DFCI, Dana-Farber Cancer Institute; DOX, doxorubicin; EORTC, European Organization for Research and Treatment of Cancer; HDMTX, high-dose methotrexate (5 g/m² or more) + leucovorin rescue; IDMTX, intermediate-dose methotrexate (750 mg/m²) + leucovorin rescue; MIOS, Multi-Institutional Osteosarcoma Study; MSKCC, Memorial Sloan-Kettering Cancer Center; NCI, National Cancer Institute; OSTEO, osteosarcoma protocol; PAM, phenylalanine mustard; SWOG, Southwest Oncology Group; UCLA, University of California, Los Angeles; VCR, vincristine; XRT, radiation therapy.
[a]Randomized study; no significant difference in relapse-free survival for patients on each treatment arm of study.
[b]Randomized study; no significant difference in relapse-free survival for patients receiving and not receiving adjuvant HDMTX (see text).
[c]Randomized study; difference in results of treatments highly significant ($P > .01$) (see text).
[d]Randomized study; difference in results of treatments significant at 6% level.

was 65% for all patients, with no difference observed among the two arms of the study. Both arms of the study also had similar rates of limb salvage (55% for immediate surgery and 50% for presurgical chemotherapy). Although this study can be criticized on numerous grounds, including the low incidence of limb-salvage surgery (most modern series report limb-salvage rates of at least 80%) and the inclusion of bleomycin, cyclophosphamide (Cytoxan), and dactinomycin (BCD) in addition to MTX, CDDP, and ADM, it is still noteworthy because the 5-year event-free survival of 65% is as good as any multi-institutional study in osteosarcoma. Thus, the inescapable conclusion is that there is no benefit to survival whether adjuvant or neoadjuvant therapy is used, and modern-era survival for nonmetastatic osteosarcoma should be at least 65%.

ASSESSMENT OF HISTOLOGIC RESPONSES TO NEOADJUVANT CHEMOTHERAPY

Although the randomized study noted above showed no survival benefit, preoperative chemotherapy has become standard practice at most centers, in large part because of the important survival implications of histologic response to such therapy. Several issues need to be considered when evaluating the predictive value of histologic response on survival. Several related but independent systems have evolved to evaluate histologic response. These include the grading system developed at Memorial Sloan-Kettering Cancer Center by Huvos et al.,[129] the system developed by Salzer-Kuntschik et al.[130] and used by the German-Austrian-Swiss Cooperative Osteosarcoma Study Group (COSS), and the system developed by Picci et al.[131] at the Istituti Ortopedico Rizzoli (IOR) in Bologna. Although each of these grading systems attempts to objectively determine the effect of chemotherapy in tumor necrosis, each has a different scale applied and is subject to observer interpretation (Table 35.2-9). In addition, the timing of surgery (i.e., the duration of preoperative chemotherapy) would be expected to impact histologic response. However, in spite of these shortcomings, a consensus has emerged that uses greater than 90% necrosis and less than 90% necrosis as separating good and poor responses, respectively. Furthermore, most current studies use 10 to 12 weeks of preoperative chemotherapy.

Using the criteria of greater than 90% as a good response and less than 90% necrosis as a poor response, several studies have reviewed 8- to 18-year experiences. The IOR reviewed

TABLE 35.2-7.   Reported Results of Representative Trials Incorporating Presurgical Chemotherapy for Osteosarcoma

Regimen	Investigators	Number of Patients	% Relapse-Free	References
HDMTX + VCR + DOX + BCD (T-7 regimen)	MSKCC	54 (younger than 21 y)	74	344,346, 347
HDMTX + VCR + DOX + BCD ± CDDP (depending on response) (T-10 regimen)	MSKCC	79 (younger than 21 y)	76	346–348
DOX + HDMTX + (BCD or CDDP) ± interferon (COSS 80)[a]	GPO	116	68	349,350
HDMTX + DOX + CDDP	Mount Sinai	25	77	351
HDMTX + VCR + DOX + BCD ± CDDP (depending on response) (CCG-782)	CCG	231	56	352
HDMTX + DOX + CDDP + IFOS (COSS 82)	GPO	125	58	353
DOX + CDDP ± HDMTX[b]	EOIS	231	63 (−HDMTX) 48 (+ HDMTX)	354
IA CDDP + (HDMTX vs. IDMTX) + DOX ± BCD (depending on response)[c]	Instituto Ortopedico Rizzoli	127	51 (overall) 58 (HDMTX) 42 (IDMTX)	355
HDMTX + DOX + IA CDDP ± etoposide, IFOS (postoperative therapy determined based on response to preoperative therapy)	Instituto Ortopedico Rizzoli	164	63	356
(IA CDDP vs. HDMTX) + DOX (postoperative therapy determined based on response to preoperative therapy) (TIOS I)	M. D. Anderson Cancer Center	43	60	357
IA CDDP + DOX ± CTX (depending on response) (TIOS III)	M. D. Anderson Cancer Center	24	—	—
HDMTX + DOX + IFOS ± CDDP	CCG (selected investigators)	95	82	—
HDMTX + DOX + CDDP BCD (POG 8651)[a]	POG	100	70 (presurgical chemotherapy) 73 (immediate surgery)	—
HDMTX + VCR + DOX + BCD + CDDP vs. DOX + CDDP	EOI	391	44	358
HDMTX + BCD + DOX + CDDP (T-12 regimen)	MSKCC	61	76	359
HDMTX + DOX + CDDP ± IFOS ± MTP-PE[d]	CCG and POG	679	67	—

BCD, bleomycin, cyclophosphamide, and dactinomycin; CCG, Children's Cancer Group; CDDP, cisplatin; COSS, Germany-Austria-Swiss Cooperative Osteosarcoma Study; CTX, cyclophosphamide; DOX, doxorubicin; EOI, European Osteosarcoma Intergroup; EOIS, First European Osteosarcoma Intergroup Study; GPO, German Society for Pediatric Oncology; HDMTX, high-dose methotrexate (12 g/m² or more) + leucovorin rescue; IA, intraarterial administration; IDMTX, intermediate-dose methotrexate (750 mg/m²) + leucovorin rescue; IFOS, ifosfamide; MTP-PE, muramyl-tripeptide phosphatidylethanolamine; MSKCC, Memorial Sloan-Kettering Cancer Center; POG, Pediatric Oncology Group; TIOS, Treatment and Investigation Osteosarcoma Study; VCR, vincristine.

[a]Randomized study; no significant difference in relapse-free survival for patients on each treatment arm of study.
[b]Randomized study; favors treatment without HDMTX (some patients treated only adjuvantly).
[c]Randomized study; difference in results of treatment significant at 7% level.
[d]Randomized study; analysis of results by randomized treatment not yet available.

TABLE 35.2-8.   Considerations for Presurgical and Postsurgical Chemotherapy

Timing of Chemotherapy	Advantages	Disadvantages
Preoperative	Early institution of systemic therapy against micrometastases Reduced chance of spontaneous emergence of drug-resistant clones in micrometastases Reduction in tumor size, increasing the chance of limb salvage Provides time for fabrication of customized endoprosthesis Less chance of viable tumor being spread at the time of surgery Individual response to chemotherapy allows selection of different risk groups	High tumor burden (not optimal for first-order kinetics) Increased probability in the selection of drug-resistant cells in primary tumor, which may metastasize Delay in definitive control of bulk disease; increased chance for systemic dissemination Psychological trauma of retaining tumor Risk of local tumor progression with loss of a limb-sparing option
Postsurgical	Radical removal of bulk tumor decreases tumor burden and increases growth rate of residual disease, making S phase–specific agents more active and optimizing conditions for first-order kinetics Decreased probability of selecting a drug-resistant clone in the primary tumor	Delay of systemic therapy for micrometastases No preoperative *in vivo* assay of cytotoxic response Possible spread of viable tumor by surgical manipulation

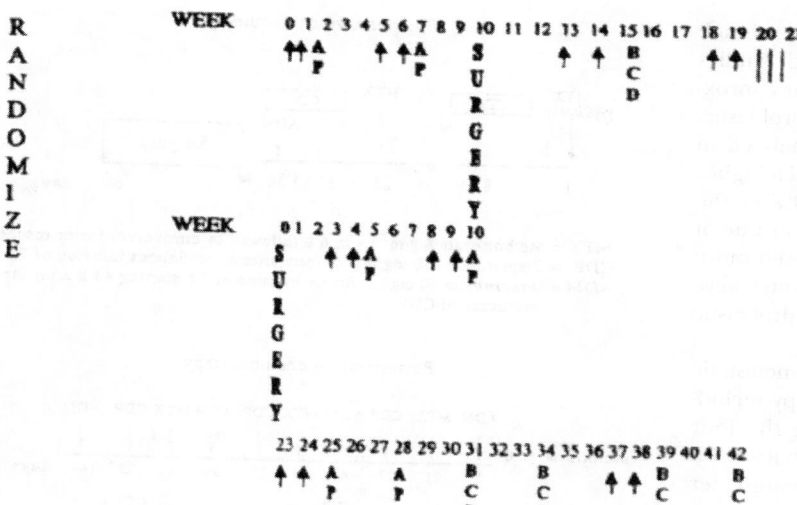

CHART 35.2-1. Chemotherapy regimen. The timing of surgery was determined by randomization to be performed at either week 0 or week 10. ↑, administration of high-dose methotrexate and leucovorin rescue; AP, doxorubicin and cisplatin administration; BCD, cyclophosphamide, bleomycin, and dactinomycin; |||, doxorubicin administration. (From ref. 128, with permission.)

data on localized-extremity osteosarcoma in patients less than 40 years of age over the 19-year period from 1983 to 2002.[132] More than 1000 patient records were analyzed. Fifty-nine percent of all patients had a good response to chemotherapy, and 41% had a poor response. Patients with a good histologic response to chemotherapy had a 5-year survival of 76%, whereas those with a poor response had a 5-year survival rate of 56%.

The COSS database was similarly reviewed and included 1700 patients entered on study between 1980 and 1998. This analysis included all sites, ages, and presence or absence of metastases.[133] The data look remarkably similar to those of the Italian study, with 55.6% of patients classified as having a good response to therapy and 44.4% having a poor response. The 5-year survival rate was 77.8% for good responders and 55.5% for poor responders. Of further note, all the patients in both of these analyses received HD-MTX, and the majority also received ADM, CDDP, ± IFOS. Also, most patients in these two analyses received preoperative chemotherapy, with surgery occurring between weeks 9 and 11 of treatment.

The European Osteosarcoma Intergroup (EOI) from the European Organization for Research and Treatment of Cancer, United Kingdom, and International Society of Paediatric Oncology (SIOP) analyzed data for two consecutive studies between 1983 and 1986 and 1986 and 1991.[134] A total of 570 patients were analyzed in the report. This analysis is notable for several differences compared to the COSS and IOR analyses. Only 28% of patients had a good histologic response, whereas 72% of

patients had a poor histologic response. Patients with a good histologic response had a 5-year survival of 75%, whereas those with a poor response had a 5-year survival of 45%. Of note, many of the patients included in the analysis did not receive HD-MTX, because many were treated on a randomized study comparing two drugs, ADM and CDDP, to more intensive therapy including HD-MTX, similar to the COSS and IOR studies. The large randomized study failed to show an advantage of multiagent therapy compared to ADM and CDDP alone.[135] However, the 5-year survival was 55% overall in this study, which is lower than that of the other studies reported above. Although the findings have continued to stir debate regarding optimal therapy, it suggests that patients who have a poor response to ADM and CDDP therapy alone (the majority of patients) have a much worse 5-year survival than those who have a poor response to three- or four-drug therapy. All three studies together strongly suggest that good responders can be expected to have a 5-year survival of approximately 75%, whereas poor responders have a 5-year survival in the range of 45% to 55%, depending on the treatment. It is important to point out that, although poor responders have a worse outcome than good responders, 45% to 55% 5-year survival is still dramatically improved compared to the less than 20% 5-year survival in the prechemotherapy era.

Another factor that could possibly influence histologic response to therapy and its predictive value on survival is the histologic subtype of the tumor. The clinical and biologic relevance of histologic subtypes has generally been believed to be minimal. In the IOR and the EOI studies discussed above,[132,134]

TABLE 35.2-9. Three Different Histologic Grading Systems for Response to Induction Chemotherapy for Osteosarcoma

Salzer-Kuntschik		*Picci*		*Huvos*	
I	No viable tumor cells	Total response	No viable tumor	IV	No histologic evidence of viable tumor
II	Single viable tumor cells or cluster <0.5 cm	Good response	90–99% tumor necrosis	III	Only scattered foci of viable tumor cells
III	Viable tumor <10%	Fair response	60–89% tumor necrosis	II	Areas of necrosis due to chemotherapy with areas of viable tumor
IV	Viable tumor 10–50%	Poor response	<60% tumor necrosis		
V	Viable tumor >50%			I	Little or no chemotherapy effect
VI	No effect of chemotherapy				

histology was characterized as osteoblastic or conventional, fibroblastic, chondroblastic, or telangiectatic. In both studies approximately 70% of cases were osteoblastic, whereas approximately 10% of cases were either chondroblastic or fibroblastic, with 6% telengiectatic, a number too small to be analyzed in the EOI study. In both studies, fibroblastic tumors had a higher rate of good histologic response (approximately 80% in the IOR study), whereas chondroblastic tumors had a lower rate of good responders (43% in the IOR study). Perhaps even more importantly, unlike other histologies, 5-year survival rates were identical for good and for poor responders in chondroblastic histology, at 68%.[132]

To summarize, treatment of patients with nonmetastatic high-grade osteosarcoma with adjuvant chemotherapy including HD-MTX and at least two other drugs among the four most-active drugs in osteosarcoma can be expected to lead to a 75% 5-year survival among good histologic responders (greater than 90% necrosis) and 55% among poor histologic responders (less than 90% necrosis). However, care should be taken when assessing histologic response in patients with chondroblastic histology, as histologic responses may not be as important a predictor of survival in this subgroup.

ADJUSTING CHEMOTHERAPY FOR POOR RESPONDERS

Another hypothetical advantage of determining histologic response to preoperative chemotherapy is the potential to alter therapy in those patients who do not have a good response to preoperative treatment. If this "tailored therapy" approach is successful, one might expect to alter the impact of poor histologic response on survival by treating such patients with different drugs and improving their outcome. This approach has indeed proven to be successful in Hodgkin's lymphoma and leukemia. This approach was initially pioneered in the early 1980s at Memorial Sloan-Kettering Cancer Center, where poor responders had CDDP substituted for HD-MTX in addition to continuing BCD and ADM.[33] Although the initial analysis of this study suggested that there was no longer a difference in survival between good and poor responders, longer follow-up data demonstrated that initial response to preoperative chemotherapy continued to be predictive of survival. Furthermore, patients who had adjustments in their postoperative chemotherapy based on poor initial response did not have improvement in survival compared to those who had no modifications.[136] More recently, the Rizzoli Institute reported long-term follow-up data on a study carried out between 1986 and 1989 on 164 patients less than 40 years of age with nonmetastatic extremity osteosarcoma[137] (Chart 35.2-2). Patients with less than 90% necrosis at the time of surgical resection had IFOS and etoposide added to HD-MTX, ADM, and CDDP, whereas patients with greater than 90% necrosis continued to receive only the three drugs. The 10-year event-free survival was 67% for patients with 90% necrosis at the time of surgical resection and 51% for those with less than 90% necrosis. Although this difference in survival did not quite reach statistical significance (*P* = .08), it still favored those patients who had an initial good histologic response to therapy. Several other reports also have failed to demonstrate an ability to rescue poor responders.[43,138,139] Thus, to date, it has not been possible to improve the outcome of poor responders by altering postoperative chemotherapy.

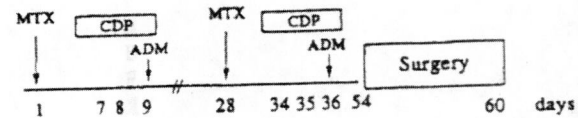

Preoperative chemotherapy

MTX = Methotrexate 8 g/m² i.v in 6 h followed by citrovorum factor rescue
CDP = Cisplatinum 120 mg/m² for intra-arterial continuous infusion of 72 h
ADM = Doxorubicin 60 mg/m² for i.v infusion of 8 h starting 48 h after the beginning of CDP

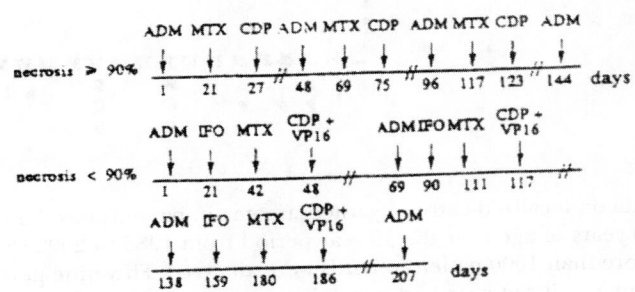

Postoperative chemotherapy

CHART 35.2-2. Pre- and postoperative chemotherapy regimens. (From ref. 137, with permission.)

CHEMOTHERAPY FOR METASTATIC DISEASE

The presence of metastatic disease at presentation continues to be an extremely poor prognostic finding, with most studies showing survival rates in the range of 20%.[133,140,141] It is therefore clear that new approaches are needed. The POG reported early data from a small phase II study for patients less than 30 years old with newly diagnosed metastatic osteosarcoma.[142] Forty-one patients were treated with two cycles of etoposide and IFOS preoperatively, followed by 32 weeks of postoperative chemotherapy, including three additional cycles of etoposide and IFOS along with standard HD-MTX, ADM, and CDDP (Chart 35.2-3). It should be noted that patients underwent surgical resection of all sites of disease whenever possible. The data are still immature, but the projected 2-year progression-free survival was 43%. In the large analysis of the COSS database that included more than 1700 consecutively treated patients, the 10-year survival probability was 40% for patients who were able to have all sites of metastatic disease resected.[133] Thus, although there is no accepted standard approach for the treatment of newly diagnosed metastatic patients, available data would suggest that such patients should be treated with currently available aggressive multiagent chemotherapy with complete surgical resection of all sites of disease if at all possible.

CHEMOTHERAPY FOR RELAPSED OSTEOSARCOMA

Similar to patients who present with primary metastatic disease, individuals in whom recurrent disease develops have an overall poor prognosis, with 5-year survival rates in the range of 20%.[143–145] As noted for metastatic disease at presentation, new salvage strategies are needed. Although there is no standard second-line chemotherapy that currently is uniformly applied,

Treatment Plan
Induction Therapy
VP/IFOS + G q 3 weeks × 2
(6 weeks)
Radiologic and Pathologic Assessment
+
Surgery
Continuation Therapy

VP = Etoposide 100 mg/m²/d × 5 days = 500 mg/m²/course × 2
courses = Total 1,000/mg/m²
IFOS = Ifosfamide 3.5 g/m²/d × 5 days = 17.5 g/m²/course × 2
courses = Total 35 g/m²

A   G = G-CSF 5 µg/kg/d, begin day 6

Week	1	2	3	4	5	6	7	8	9	10	11	12	13	14	15	16	17	18
	M	M	A			M	M	I			M	M	A			M	M	I
	T	T	P			T	T	VP			T	T	P			T	T	VP
	X	X				X	X	G*			X	X				X	X	G*

Week	19	20	21	22	23	24	25	26	27	28	29	30	31	32	33	34
			A			I		A				M	M	A		
			P			VP		P				T	T			
						G*						X	X			

VP = Etoposide 100 mg/m²/d × 5 days: 5 courses = Total 2,500 mg/m².
MTX = Methotrexate, 12 g/m² over 4 hours, plus leucovorin, 15 mg q6h × 10 doses: 10 courses = 120 g/m²
I = Ifosfamide, 2.4 g/m² + mesna/d × 5 days: 3 courses = Total 36 g/m². Total Ifosfamide = 71 g/m²
A = Doxorubicin, 37.5 mg/m²/d × 2 days: 5 courses = Total 375 mg/m²
P = CDDP, 60 mg/m²/d × 2 days: 4 courses = Total 480 mg/m²

B   *G = G-CSF 5 µg/kg/d.

CHART 35.2-3. **A:** Treatment plan for induction therapy. Patients received two courses of etoposide and ifosfamide, then radiologic assessment and surgery of primary tumor. The pathologic assessment of tumor necrosis was performed after surgery. **B:** Continuation chemotherapy regimen started 1 to 2 weeks after surgery. CDDP, cisplatin; G-CSF, granulocyte colony-stimulating factor. (From ref. 142, with permission.)

several principles have been clearly established. Most importantly, as with primary metastatic disease, complete resection of recurrent disease appears to be mandatory for long-term survival.[143–145] It also is likely that multiagent chemotherapy contributes to successful salvage of some patients. In general, patients should be treated with any of the four most active agents noted earlier in Assessment of Histologic Responses to Neoadjuvant Chemotherapy if initial therapy did not include one or more of these agents. Patients who have recurrences more than 1 year after completing prior systemic therapy may benefit from reintroduction of at least some of the same drugs in a salvage regimen. The use of high-dose chemotherapy with autologous hematopoietic stem cell rescue has been applied to salvage therapy. However, at least two small pilot studies failed to demonstrate an advantage to standard salvage therapy approaches.[146,147]

LATE EFFECTS OF SYSTEMIC THERAPY

The universal application of systemic chemotherapy for all patients with osteosarcoma has led to an increased likelihood of survival as noted earlier in the introduction to Chemotherapy for Bone Sarcomas. However, with this increase in survival has come the inevitable increase in late effects secondary to chemotherapy. The most important long-term side effects that

have now been well documented are ADM-induced cardiomyopathy, male infertility, and development of second malignant neoplasms. In a long-term follow-up report of 164 patients treated with cumulative doses of 480 mg/m² ADM, there were six documented cases of severe cardiomyopathy.[137] It is likely that subclinical cardiac damage may occur and be underestimated.[148] Although earlier reports suggested little effect on infertility, more recent inclusion of IFOS into front-line therapy has likely increased the risk of male infertility after treatment.[149] In the long-term follow-up study from the IOR noted above, 10 of 12 patients who underwent sperm analysis were noted to have azoospermia. All 10 had received chemotherapy at the time of puberty, and 9 of 10 had received IFOS. As more patients survive their primary osteosarcoma, the development of second malignant neoplasms has become of increasing concern as well. In a long-term follow-up study from St. Jude's, there were nine documented cases of second malignant neoplasms among 334 patients treated between 1962 and 1996, for an incidence of 2%. The tumors included two cases of MFH; a chondrosarcoma; carcinomas of the rectum, colon, stomach, and breast; a melanoma; and a glioblastoma.[150] Although this incidence is significantly lower than that of survivors of Hodgkin's disease, it is likely that as more patients are cured of osteosarcoma, this problem will continue to increase. Because of these late sequelae of systemic treatment, and continued reports of recurrences more than 5 years after treatment, these patients should be followed long term by the centers performing the initial curative treatment on these patients.

RADIOTHERAPY FOR BONE TUMORS

Radiation therapy is generally not used in the primary treatment of osteosarcoma, although this may change with the greater implementation of new technologies. Radiation therapy is used for patients who have refused definitive surgery, require palliation, or have lesions in axial locations. Experience with radiotherapy has been greater in the treatment of chondrosarcoma, possibly due to the lesser availability of adjuvant chemotherapy in facilitating the goals of tissue preservation. Tumors of the axial skeleton and facial bones are treated by a combination of limited surgery and radiotherapy, because the goals of treatment frequently focus more on functional and cosmesis preservation. For these reasons, radiotherapy assumes greater importance in these sites. Ewing's sarcoma and peripheral primitive neuroectodermal tumors of bone can be managed by definitive radiation treatment, complete surgical excision, or combined surgical and radiotherapy approaches and are discussed in Chapter 35.1.

TREATMENT PLANNING

Optimal radiotherapy of bone tumors requires careful technical treatment planning (Table 35.2-10) and adherence to radiobiologic principles, including treatment of all fields each day to ensure homogeneous distribution of dose to all areas of the target at every treatment session. Normal tissue should be protected from the high-dose regions wherever possible, and this is achieved using precise, three-dimensional delineation of tumor and normal tissue in the same way as for surgical evaluation (see earlier in Preoperative Evaluation).

All candidate patients should undergo simulation and must be treated with megavoltage therapy beams to maximize physical reduction in absorbed dose delivered to bone. Orthovoltage has no place in the contemporary management of primary tumors of bone because it deposits dose preferentially in bone rather than soft tissue. Today's radiotherapy is frequently planned volumetrically using computerized CT simulation

TABLE 35.2-10. Guidelines for Optimal Radiation Therapy in the Treatment of Bone Sarcomas

---

Appropriate imaging studies to define tumor location correlated with surgical pathologic findings

Physical fluoroscopic simulation or computed tomography–based virtual simulation

Patient immobilization and/or stereotactic localization

Megavoltage conventional external-beam delivery

High radiation dose with appropriate fractionation

Large radiation field/volumes with "shrinking field" techniques to reduce volumes beyond threshold doses for microscopic disease

Beam-shaping devices (mounted shielding or multileaf collimation)

Beam modifiers for contour shape—compensating filters, wedges, or dynamic wedge or beam segmentation with or without intensity modulation

Multiple fields to be treated per day

---

technologies. Patient immobilization is essential to optimal radiotherapy, especially when very precise delivery is used and the margins around the target are less than usual, particularly when avoidance of normal tissues is being undertaken.

DOSE AND VOLUME CONSIDERATIONS

Large treatment volumes that include the entire clinical and radiographic extent of tumor plus a generous margin for microscopic or subclinical extension of disease are needed. For tumors that tend to spread along the medullary canal (e.g., lymphoma, Ewing's sarcoma), the standard radiation field in the past included the entire bone, with a boost of radiation to the area of bulky disease. However, current practice suggests that radiation confined to the involved area may be sufficient for small, round cell bone tumors that have responded to induction chemotherapy. If large fields are needed, it is desirable to use an extended source-to-skin distance to enable the entire radiation field to fit into one portal. If extended distances are not possible and two radiation fields must abut, the abutment must pass through areas of microscopic, rather than gross, disease. Match lines should be routinely moved every 10 Gy. The introduction of volumetric-based planning techniques, such as three-dimensional conformal radiotherapy and intensity-modulated radiotherapy (IMRT), is an important opportunity to reevaluate many aspects of the current treatment paradigm, which had evolved under the technologic constraints of the past (see Precision Technology in Radiotherapy Delivery, later in this chapter).

The irradiated field should encompass at least the volume of tissue that would be resected, plus an allowance of approximately 2 cm in total for patient movement (the planning target volume margin of at least 5 mm) and dose falloff at the margin of the field (the beam penumbra effect measuring approximately 1 cm). Extremity fields should be planned with a strip of tissue deliberately out of the beam to allow for lymphatic and venous return and to decrease morbidity. This nonirradiated strip should, wherever possible, overlie the lymphatic drainage, which is located medially in the extremity. In volumetric planning with multiple fields, the plan should be similar to permit the same clearances for uncertainty and a reduction in the intensity of dose in the lymphatic areas (e.g., maintenance of the maximum dose in such areas to less than 40 Gy).

Because large doses often are necessary for treatment of malignant bone tumors, a shrinking field volume technique is recommended. This approach allows treatment to a large volume of tissue involved by subclinical disease with a moderate radiation dosage (e.g., 45 to 50 Gy delivered over a period of approximately 5 weeks in daily fractions), while the area of gross tumor is treated further with a larger, sterilizing dose.

Additional principles involve using multiple beam-shaping devices so that shaped fields can be designed to conform to individual tumor volume and anatomy. Multiple fields should be used to optimize the radiation dosage, and all fields must be treated every day. When necessary, beam modifiers, such as compensating filters and wedge filters, or beam segmentation with multileaf collimation, should be used to account for individual variations in patient thickness (see Table 35.2-10). Three-dimensional conformal radiation techniques using multiple fields, multileaf collimation, and intensity-modulated IMRT beams are useful aids to optimize the homogeneity of the dose within the target volume while sparing adjacent normal structures. When chemotherapy, such as ADM and BCD, and radiotherapy are used, it is important to avoid concomitant administration of drugs that may act as radiation sensitizers to normal tissue.

PRECISION TECHNOLOGY IN RADIOTHERAPY DELIVERY

Traditional radiotherapy treatment approaches used to be largely constrained by the technologies of the era when they were developed and in general have not changed substantially until recently. Thus, a typical plan used parallel opposed or relatively standard three- or four-field plans with some forward-planned beam shaping to reduce the irradiated volume as much as possible without shielding the disease-bearing target. As noted earlier, this may suffice for uncomplicated lesions. However, for many lesions, more precise targeting with conformal plans or IMRT is necessary. For IMRT, the planning objective includes two important specifications: (1) a description of the required dose to each part of the target and the normal tissues in the treated region and (2) the need to achieve that dose in relative terms compared to the other structures (target or normal tissues) as a "weighting" expressed in a mathematical equation. The result of the IMRT approach is that the delivered dose can be fitted to volumes tailored to complex shape specifications. These can be shaped externally (i.e., convex shaping), as in traditional fields; at the same time, the external "surface" of the intended RT dose region can be excavated, thereby providing concave or indented shaping ("dose sculpting")[151] that permits previously inaccessible target areas to be treated while avoiding adjacent vulnerable anatomy that may be partially surrounded by the target.

Finally, precision photon methods such as IMRT may use several forms of delivery platforms. In some situations (e.g., adjacent to the spinal cord or optic chiasm) extremely accurate delivery may demand stereotactic precision for guidance to minimize interfraction differences and ensure safety in tumor coverage and avoidance of critical anatomy. Some methods use equipment uniquely designed for this purpose but not necessarily advantageous for use in general oncology, given the ever present problem of "marginal miss," which requires extreme vigilance in quality assurance. One such method (e.g., cyberknife) uses a frameless reference system for stereotactic guidance and a robotic delivery system, permitting adaptive beam pointing to account for positional variance.[152] The absence of a frame provides great flexibility and makes it possible to treat extracranial sites with the same or better precision than other systems achieved by fixing the lesion with respect to the cranium using the frame. This seems particularly applicable to spine lesions, because it is difficult to firmly immobilize the torso, in contrast with limb or skull sites, for which customized physical immobilization systems are the rule. A tendency with very accurate delivery approaches is to forgo usual radiobiologic principles by delivering a relatively small number of large dose fractions to a precise target with extraordinary accuracy.[153,154] This has the advantage of efficiency in treatment delivery to a complex target. Long-term results are needed to assess the ultimate safety of dose fractionation regimes delivered in this fashion, in particular when the total dose administered is high.

Technologic enhancements now also permit full three-dimensional planning for brachytherapy with dose-volume histograms and other tools. Real application of brachytherapy to the treatment of primary bone tumors is awaited, although some very preliminary experience in recurrent disease is available using high dose-rate perioperative approaches.[155]

Charged particle beam also provides alternatives. In proton beam irradiation, high-dose volume treatment volumes can be made to conform precisely to the target by varying the depth and breadth of the unique "Bragg peak" characteristic of the high-energy release at the end of the beam's range. This provides theoretic and practical advantage in improved dose distribution in deep locations compared to photon irradiation.[156] Protons exert their biologic properties in a similar way to photons, and, therefore, normal tissues can be spared damage through the principles of fractionation. The major drawback to the application of proton technology is that it is only available at a handful of sites, although an increasing number of treatment units will be available in the future. Neutron radiotherapy has been emphasized by certain groups because of the lower oxygen enhancement ratio compared to x-rays and the consequent attractive possibility of overcoming the biologic phenomenon that hypoxic cells generally limit the curability of malignancy with x-rays. Compared to photons, they are also less vulnerable to the differential radiosensitivities associated with different phases of the cell cycle. However, it should be apparent that some of these repair phenomena also have a negative impact on the tolerance of normal tissues, and they suffer badly from lack of ability to target dose precisely at depth. Neutron pilot data have not suggested a substantial influence in sterilization of 12 patients with osteosarcoma, and, moreover, toxicity was apparent in the majority of patients.[157] Sterilization of disease was also apparent in a smaller osteosarcoma series reported by Carrie et al.[158] and in a series containing 14 chondrosarcomas.[159] Kamada et al.[160] reported a phase I/II dose-escalation study of carbon ion radiotherapy that included unresectable bone sarcomas. This modality combines the biologically damaging character of a high linear energy transfer particle beam with a Bragg peak, thereby achieving the potential benefits of cell-cycle and oxygen-independent irreversible damage with precision delivery. Of interest, in a selected subgroup (15 unresectable osteosarcomas, including 10 pelvic and 5 spine lesions) of their study, Kamada et al. noted a 3-year overall actuarial survival of 45% (95% confidence interval 7% to 83%), results that the authors note to be unexpectedly better than those reported in the literature.

COMPLICATIONS OF RADIATION

The complications of radiation are related directly to treatment dose and volume. Reactions that occur during the early stages of treatment usually are reversible and not of major significance. These include erythema, dry desquamation of the skin, and epilation. More serious, later reactions may include fibrosis, contracture, atrophy, impaired growth, secondary fracture, and radiation-induced neoplasm. When pelvic treatment is necessary in young women, it is important to consider ovarian transposition whenever possible. Techniques to move the small bowel out of the pelvis are useful, as is avoiding treatment of the entire bladder if cyclophosphamide or IFOS is also being used. Fibrosis and contracture can be minimized—or possibly avoided—by embarking on an active physical therapy program during radiation therapy. Such a program should be continued in the postradiation therapy follow-up period.

Whenever possible, treating across a joint space and treating an open epiphysis should be avoided. For tumors of weight-bearing bones, partial weight-bearing and protective bracing are important until reossification occurs.

MALIGNANT BONE TUMORS

CLASSIC OSTEOSARCOMA

Osteosarcoma is a high-grade, malignant spindle cell tumor that arises within a bone. Its distinguishing characteristic is the production of "tumor" osteoid or immature bone directly from a malignant spindle cell stroma.[2,3,49,161]

Clinical Characteristics

Osteosarcoma typically occurs during childhood and adolescence. An epidemiologic study from the Swedish Cancer Institute documented that the mean and median age of patients with osteosarcoma has increased since 1971.[162] Investigators evaluated 227 patients from 1971 to 1984 and reported the peak incidence to be between 10 and 19 years of age but noted the mean and median values to be 29 and 20 years, respectively. The overall incidence—2.1 cases per million people per year—has not changed. When osteosarcoma occurs in patients older than 40 years, it is usually associated with a preexisting condition, such as Paget's disease, irradiated bones, multiple hereditary exostosis, or polyostotic fibrous dysplasia.[161–164] Bones of the knee joint and the proximal humerus are the most common sites, accounting for 50% and 25%, respectively, of all osteosarcomas.[165] In general, 80% to 90% of osteosarcomas occur in the long tubular bones, and the axial skeleton is rarely affected. Fewer than 1% are found in the hands and feet.[161–164,166–168]

With the exception of serum AP (SAP) levels, which are elevated in 45% to 50% of patients, laboratory findings are usually not helpful.[167] Furthermore, elevated AP per se is not diagnostic, because it is also found in association with other skeletal disease. Pain is the most common complaint. Night pain gradually develops and becomes a hallmark of skeletal involvement. Physical examination demonstrates a firm, soft mass fixed to the underlying bone with slight tenderness. No effusion is noted in the adjacent joint, and motion is normal. Incidence of pathologic fracture is less than 1%. Systemic symptoms are rare.

Radiographic Characteristics

Typical findings are increased intramedullary radiodensity (due to tumor bone or calcified cartilage), an area of radiolucency (due to nonossified tumor), a pattern of permeative destruction with poorly defined borders, cortical destruction, periosteal elevation, and extraosseous extension with soft tissue ossification.[167–169] This combination of characteristics is not seen in any other lesion. Wilner[169] classified 600 radiographs of osteosarcoma seen at the Memorial Sloan-Kettering Cancer Center into three broad categories: sclerotic (32%), osteolytic (22%), and mixed (46%). Although no statistically significant difference was found in overall survival rates among these types, the patterns are important to recognize. The sclerotic and mixed types offer few diagnostic problems. Errors of diagnosis most often occur with pure osteolytic tumors. The differential diagnosis of osteolytic osteosarcoma includes GCT, aneurysmal bone cyst, fibrosarcoma, and MFH. In a series of 305 osteosarcoma cases, deSantos and Edeiken[170] reported that 42 (13.5%) were purely lytic. Most commonly, they presented as ill-defined lesions with a moderate to large soft tissue component. Nine of the lesions had benign radiographic features.

Clinical and Prognostic Considerations (before Adjuvant Chemotherapy and Postadjuvant Chemotherapy)

Before the era of adjuvant chemotherapy, treatment consisted of amputation. Metastasis to lungs and other bones generally occurred within 24 months. A large number of series show an overall survival of 5% to 20% at 2 years.[72,76,171] This pattern has been altered by adjuvant chemotherapy and aggressive thoracotomy for pulmonary disease.[69–71,172] Metastases may now appear at less common sites, and disease-free intervals are longer.[71] Lockshin and Higgins[172] reviewed the experience of 100 authors over 50 years and concluded that there was no significant difference between survival rates of patients with the three histogenic subtypes (osteoblastic, chondroblastic, and fibroblastic) or between patients whose lesions had a different radiographic appearance (sclerotic, osteolytic, or mixed). Likewise, tumor size, patient age, and degree of malignancy did not correlate with survival. The most significant variable was anatomic site. Patients with pelvic and axial lesions had a lower survival rate than those with tumors of the extremities, probably because of surgical inaccessibility and incomplete removal. Patients with tumors of the tibia had a significantly higher survival rate than those with tumors of the distal femur (35% vs. 16%). Larsson et al.,[173] using a multifactorial analysis of all patients from the Swedish Cancer Registry between 1958 and 1968, similarly concluded that patients with tibial lesions had a better survival rate than those with femoral lesions (38.1% vs. 15.1%), because the former were less advanced at the time of treatment.

Marcove et al.,[66] reviewing 145 patients younger than 21 years of age who underwent surgery without adjuvant chemotherapy at Memorial Sloan-Kettering Cancer Center, noted no statistically significant differences with regard to race, gender, or duration of symptoms. Younger patients developed metastases sooner, but this made no difference in overall survival. Location had no impact on the 5-year survival rate. Brostrom et al.[174] evaluated 52 patients treated by surgery alone. They studied tumor size and site and reported that patients with distal lesions measuring smaller than 10 cm had a significantly higher survival ($P<.01$) than those with proximal lesions larger than 10 cm (43% vs. 12%, respectively). More recently, Hudson et al.[175] reported on 98 patients treated at the M. D. Anderson Cancer Center with three different protocols. Tumor size ($P = .04$) and the percentage of tumor necrosis induced by induction therapy ($P = .01$) were the most important prognostic factors.

Baldini et al.[176] from the IOR have reviewed the prognostic factors of patients with osteosarcoma treated with preoperative chemotherapy. This is one of the more recent studies that attempts to determine prognostic factors when chemotherapy is administered, in contrast to older studies, which evaluated prognostic factors before chemotherapy. These authors evaluated 160 patients with stage II high-grade osteosarcomas at a single institution; 142 patients were treated by a limb-sparing procedure, and 18 underwent amputation. Tumor size was not found to be associated with a histologic response to chemotherapy. One hundred fifteen patients had a good response (greater than 90% necrosis), and 40 had a poor response. Larger tumors were not found to be associated with a lower likelihood of response to chemotherapy. No association was shown between the size of the tumor and the event-free survival of the patients, as determined by university and multivariate analysis.

Alkaline Phosphatase

SAP level is an important biologic marker of tumor activity in patients with osteosarcoma. The early studies of the relationship between AP activity and survival were performed before the introduction of adjuvant chemotherapy (i.e., in patients treated with surgery alone).

The prognostic significance of AP has more recently been evaluated in conjunction with neoadjuvant chemotherapy. Bacci et al.[177] evaluated patients treated for osteosarcoma between 1972 and 1989. The study demonstrated that for patients with osteosarcoma of the extremities, presurgical SAP levels are useful prognostic markers in those treated with adjuvant or neoadjuvant chemotherapy. Specifically, the study demonstrated that patients presenting with nonmetastatic osteosarcoma and an elevated SAP level had a worse prognosis than did those with normal values (relapse rates of 55% and 26%, respectively). Among those patients determined to have elevated pretreatment SAP levels, the higher the AP serum levels, the greater the risk for relapse. Patients with elevated pretreatment SAP who experienced relapse or recurrence had a poorer disease-free survival than did individuals who relapsed and had normal pretreatment SAP levels.

Bacci et al.[178] reported on an evaluation of the SAP levels among 560 patients with high-grade osteosarcomas of the extremity who were treated at a single institution. Forty-six percent of these patients had elevated SAP levels before treatment; such levels were most commonly found in males older than 14 years and in patients with tumors greater than 150 mL of the osteoblastic type. Only two factors by a multivariate analysis were independently correlated with 5-year event-free survival: SAP levels ($P = .002$) and grade of chemotherapy-induced tumor necrosis ($P = .0001$). The authors recommend that, in planning randomized trials, patients be stratified according to SAP levels.

Biology and Prognostic Factors

Although the etiology of osteosarcoma remains for the most part unknown, several predisposing conditions have been clearly identified. The most common known risk factor is radiation exposure, and osteosarcoma is the most common histology found in radiation-associated second malignancies.[179] Several hereditary risk factors are known to predispose toward osteosarcoma. Hereditary retinoblastoma associated with germline mutations in the RB gene is associated with a 100-fold increase in the risk of osteosarcoma, even in the absence of radiation exposure, which further increases the risk of osteosarcoma development.[180] The Li-Fraumeni syndrome is associated with germline mutations in the p53 gene and also with an increased risk for the development of osteosarcoma.[181] Rothmund-Thomson syndrome is an autosomal recessive disorder characterized by cataracts; skeletal, dental, and nail abnormalities; skin rash; and short stature and is known to be asso-

ciated with an increased risk of osteosarcoma.[182] This syndrome is now known to be associated with mutations in the DNA helicase RECQL4, and a report has demonstrated that all patients with Rothmund-Thomson syndrome in whom osteosarcomas developed had evidence of truncating mutations of the RECQL4 gene.[183] This is of particular note because alterations in a related RecQ DNA helicase in Werner's syndrome are associated with an increased risk of osteosarcoma.[184]

In view of these genetic predisposition syndromes, it is not surprising that RB1 and p53 are frequently found to be altered in patients with osteosarcoma. For p53, numerous studies have found the frequency of p53 mutations to be in the 18% to 30% range.[185–187] The presence or absence of p53 mutations at diagnosis does not appear to carry prognostic implications.[187] Alterations in the RB1 gene appear to be even more common than p53 alterations, with loss of heterozygosity reported in more than 50% of informative cases.[188] The more sensitive technique of allelotyping found high frequencies of RB1 and p53 allelic imbalances, with no association with prognosis.[189] The p53 and RB pathways are regulated by a series of activators and inhibitors, and these can be altered in tumors. In osteosarcomas, the incidence of alterations in either p15ARF or HDM2, positive and negative regulators of p53 function, respectively, is quite low.[190] In contrast, alterations in the positive regulator of RB1 function, p16^{Ink4a}, was found to be greater than 15%,[190] making overall incidence of RB pathway abnormalities in osteosarcoma likely to be even higher than 50%. No large studies of RECQL4 status in sporadic osteosarcomas have been reported.

Osteosarcomas are genetically characterized by complex karyotypes characteristic of severe disturbances in genomic stability.[191,192] This virtually invariate presence of a complex karyotype is the cytogenetic hallmark of marked telomere dysfunction.[193] A small, retrospective analysis of 62 patients with osteosarcoma revealed that 11 had no evidence of telomere maintenance. These individuals had significantly increased 5-year survival (90%) compared with the 51 patients with evidence of activation of telomere maintenance, who had a 5-year survival rate of 60%.[194] Although these data require confirmation, they raise the possibility that, although the vast majority of patients with osteosarcoma have activation of telomere maintenance mechanisms leading to chromosomal instability, a minority may have normal telomere function and may constitute a particularly favorable subset.

Initial enthusiasm was shown in regard to the prognostic significance of expression of the multidrug resistance gene, MDR1 or P-glycoprotein, in osteosarcoma. The IOR group reported that increased expression of P-glycoprotein was associated with poor prognoses.[176] However, subsequent studies have failed to confirm these observations; for example, a prospective multicenter study showed no correlation between MDR1 messenger RNA expression and disease.

In summary, although the overwhelming majority of osteosarcomas occur sporadically, there are several known hereditary risk factors for the development of this tumor. These risk factors have pointed out several key genetic alterations that occur commonly in sporadic osteosarcomas and likely play a major role in the biology of these tumors. The genetic hallmark of osteosarcoma is the presence of complex karyotypes, suggesting that chromosomal instability and mechanisms contributing to this phenotype also contribute to the biology of these tumors.

Changing Pattern of Metastasis

The classic pattern and time frame of metastatic dissemination of osteosarcoma has been somewhat modified by the use of adjuvant chemotherapy and thoracotomy. Bacci et al.[195] evaluated the pattern of metastatic spread of osteosarcoma in 193 patients at the Rizzoli Institute. Thirty patients who were treated with surgery alone were compared to 163 patients who underwent adjuvant chemotherapy. No difference was found in sites of first relapse; approximately 90% of metastases in both groups occurred in the lungs. After chemotherapy, extrapulmonary spread occurred in 10% of cases, usually to bony sites. Simultaneous bone and lung metastases occurred in approximately 2%. The time to metastasis differed (surgery alone was 13 months, and adjuvant chemotherapy was 8 months), and the number of metastatic nodules was reduced when chemotherapy was used. In general, lung metastases appeared later and were fewer in number after adjuvant chemotherapy, but with variable difference on extrapulmonary or bony spread. The authors concluded that the alteration of metastatic spread permitted surgical resection of pulmonary metastases in a larger number of patients (51% vs. 29%).

Histologic Subtype and Influence on Chemotherapy Response

Within the past decade, as more patients have been treated in cooperative studies and the number of patients treated with induction chemotherapy has increased, the question of the significance of the histologic subtype on the chemotherapy response of an osteosarcoma has begun to be examined. Bacci et al.[196] analyzed the factors that determined the rate of chemotherapy response in the subgroup of patients who attained total (100%) tumor necrosis. Of 510 patients treated between 1983 and 1995, a 100% tumor necrosis was not related to gender, age, tumor site or size, SAP, or route of CDDP administration. The histologic complete response was related to only two factors: the number of drugs used and histologic subtype. According to the drugs used, the percentage of total necrosis was 31% for a four-drug regimen, 18% for a three-drug regimen, and only 1.5% for a two-drug regimen. According to the histologic subtypes, the rates of 100% total necrosis were telangiectatic tumors (41%), fibroblastic tumors (31%), and chondroblastic tumors (3%).

Hauben et al.[134] reviewed 570 patients included in two consecutive studies of the EOI. The proportion of patients responding well to chemotherapy differed significantly between the subtypes. A higher proportion of good responders was found in the fibroblastic group and a lower percentage in the chondroblastic group. Good responders survived longer. Interestingly, despite different rates of chemotherapy response by subtype, survival did not differ by subtype. Thus, the percentage of tumor necrosis by itself, without the knowledge of subtype, may not be comparable.

Limb-Sparing Surgery and Pathologic Fracture

Traditionally, a fracture through an osteosarcoma was treated by amputation. As experience with induction chemotherapy and limb-sparing surgery has increased, however, several centers have attempted limb-sparing surgery in this high-risk patient population. The assumption has been that if the fracture can be immobilized during the induction period and the tumor shows clear signs of necrosis and secondary fracture healing, an amputation may be avoided. The earlier strategy, immediate amputation, was based on the presumed high risk of local recurrence after a limb-sparing procedure. A limb-sparing procedure can now be safely performed if the response to induction chemotherapy is good, as evidenced by fracture healing.

Steadman et al.[197] evaluated their experience with patients who had osteosarcoma-induced pathologic fractures between 1970 and 1995. Nine primary instances of limb salvage in patients with preoperative chemotherapy and eight primary cases of amputation with postoperative chemotherapy were studied. No significant difference in survival was found. One local recurrence occurred in the limb-salvage group and none in the amputation group. This retrospective analysis, combined with other reported results, makes a convincing case that a pathologic fracture does not indicate the need for an immediate amputation. The strategy today is to immobilize the extremity and proceed with induction chemotherapy. If the fracture heals and the tumor appears to respond to chemotherapy, a limb-sparing operation is warranted. Repeat staging studies after induction chemotherapy and close serial observation during the induction period are essential.

Scully et al.,[198] in the largest series evaluating the significance of pathologic fracture, reviewed 55 patients from eight institutions in a cooperative MSTS study and compared these individuals to a matched 55-patient nonfracture cohort. They concluded that patients who presented with a pathologic fracture or developed one during chemotherapy were at an increased risk of local recurrence and decreased overall survival as compared to the nonfracture group, 55% versus 77% and 75% versus 96%, respectively. Interestingly, the local recurrence rates of those patients treated by limb-sparing surgery were essentially the same as those who underwent amputation—23% and 18%, respectively. The authors concluded that a limb-sparing procedure in carefully selected patients with a fracture does not increase the risk of local recurrence or death.

Surgical Resection of Localized-Extremity Osteosarcoma

Before the early 1980s, treatment for localized osteosarcoma was amputation one joint above the tumor-containing bone or, occasionally, transmedullary amputation. Since the early 1980s, parallel developments in radiology, orthopedics, and oncology have made limb-sparing procedures an option in 50% to 80% of patients. A significant impetus for these developments was the introduction of effective chemotherapeutic agents in the early 1970s[2,3,66,67,76] (Fig. 35.2-8).

Springfield et al.[199] from the University of Florida compared limb-sparing surgery with amputation in 53 patients with stage IIB osteosarcoma. For ethical reasons, the patients were not randomized. No difference in survival was found between amputation and resection or between radical resection and a wide surgical margin. Three local recurrences were reported. The investigators concluded that a wide surgical resection was adequate for local control. In general, they recommended amputation if the major neurovascular bundle was involved. They concluded that local recurrence was due to an extremely aggressive tumor or to skip metastases.

Rougraff et al.[114] updated a combined study from the MSTS of 227 patients from 26 institutions treated for osteosarcoma of

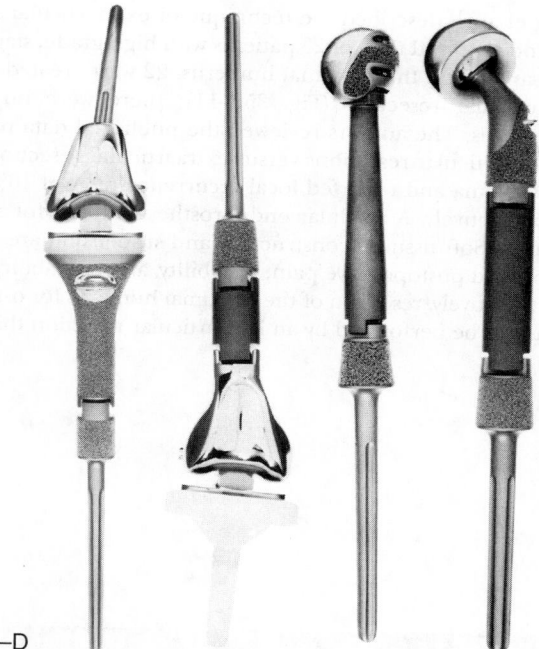

A–D

FIGURE 35.2-8. Prostheses used in selected patients for skeletal reconstruction: distal femoral prosthesis (**A**), proximal tibial prosthesis (**B**), proximal humeral prosthesis (**C**), and proximal femoral prosthesis (**D**).

the distal femur; 109 patients (48%) were alive at an average of 11 years after surgery. No differences in local recurrence, overall survival, or duration of disease-free survival were noted between amputation and limb-sparing groups. The local recurrence rate (10%) was identical for above-knee amputation and limb-sparing surgery. The most common causes of failed limb-sparing procedures were infection and local recurrence. Rougraff et al. concluded that the type of surgery did not affect outcomes. No difference was noted among patients treated with endoprostheses, allografts, composites, rotationplasties, and arthrodesis; however, the numbers of patients in those categories were small.

Bacci et al.[200] analyzed the type of surgical margin and the responses to chemotherapy and then analyzed them together; differences in outcome were dramatic. The patients with poor necrosis (fewer than 60%) and wide margins had ten times the risk of local recurrence. The worst combination was poor necrosis and less than wide margins.

Treatment by Anatomic Site

The unique features of evaluation, management, and resection of tumors of the most common anatomic areas, the shoulder and knee, are described and illustrated in this section.

SHOULDER GIRDLE. A surgical classification for shoulder girdle resections has been described.[201] This classification is useful for all limb-sparing procedures of the shoulder girdle. It is recommended that osteosarcomas arising from the proximal humerus be treated by a type VB resection (Fig. 35.2-9).

PROXIMAL HUMERUS. The proximal humerus is the third most common site for osteosarcoma. Joint involvement is common in patients with high-grade malignancies of the proximal

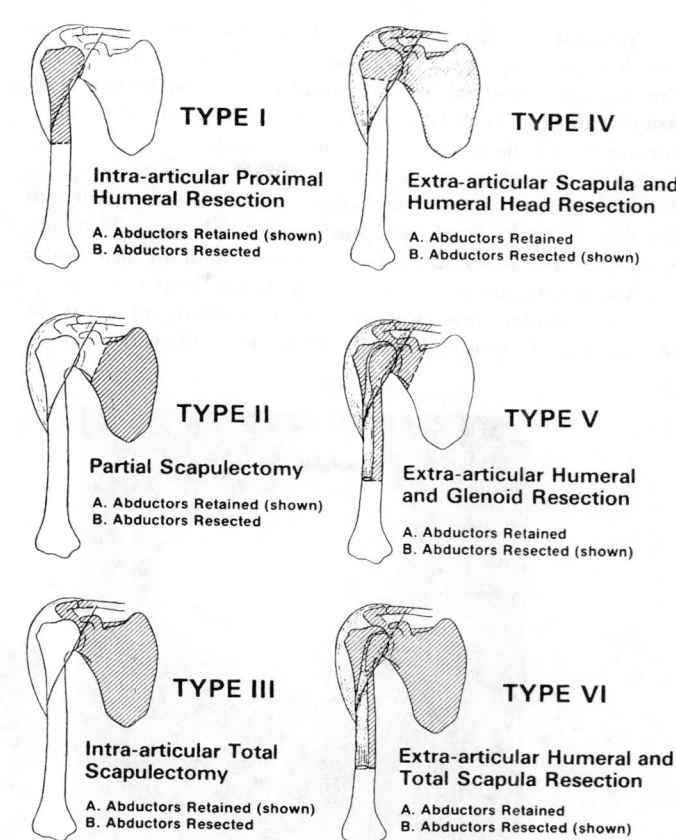

TYPE I
Intra-articular Proximal Humeral Resection
A. Abductors Retained (shown)
B. Abductors Resected

TYPE IV
Extra-articular Scapula and Humeral Head Resection
A. Abductors Retained
B. Abductors Resected (shown)

TYPE II
Partial Scapulectomy
A. Abductors Retained (shown)
B. Abductors Resected

TYPE V
Extra-articular Humeral and Glenoid Resection
A. Abductors Retained
B. Abductors Resected (shown)

TYPE III
Intra-articular Total Scapulectomy
A. Abductors Retained (shown)
B. Abductors Resected

TYPE VI
Extra-articular Humeral and Total Scapula Resection
A. Abductors Retained
B. Abductors Resected (shown)

FIGURE 35.2-9. Schematic of proposed surgical classification of shoulder girdle resections. In general, types I to III are for benign or low-grade tumors, and types IV to VI are for high-grade tumors. A and B denote the status of the abductor mechanism: A is intact, and B is partially or completely excised. Types I to III and types IV to VI are intraarticular and extraarticular resections, respectively.

humerus; for this reason, an extraarticular resection is commonly performed. Intraarticular resections are reserved for small, intraosseous (stage IIA) lesions. The aim of surgery is to create a stable new "shoulder" that permits the placement of the hand in space and enables the patient to retain elbow function (Fig. 35.2-10).

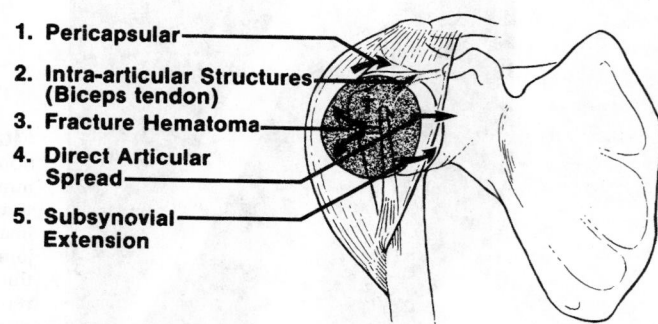

1. **Pericapsular**
2. **Intra-articular Structures (Biceps tendon)**
3. **Fracture Hematoma**
4. **Direct Articular Spread**
5. **Subsynovial Extension**

FIGURE 35.2-10. Mechanisms of local tumor spread for sarcomas of the shoulder. (From Malawer MM, Buch R, Reaman G, et al. Impact of two cycles of preoperative chemotherapy with intraarterial cisplatin and intravenous doxorubicin on the choice of surgical procedure for high-grade bone sarcomas of the extremities. *Clin Orthop* 1991;270:214, with permission.)

Proximal humeral lesions should not be biopsied through the deltopectoral interval. Biopsy under fluoroscopy through the anterior one-third of the deltoid by a trocar is preferred. Angiography is the most useful preoperative study. If the neurovascular bundle is clear, resection is feasible.

Adequate resection of the proximal humerus requires removal of 15 to 20 cm of the humerus and shoulder joint with the deltoid, rotator cuff, and portions of the biceps and triceps muscles.[202] The procedure involves suspension of the arm, motor reconstruction, and provision of adequate soft tissue coverage.

Extraarticular resection of the glenohumeral joint by medial scapulosteotomy is safer than intraarticular resection.

Wittig et al.[203] described the technique of extraarticular resection and reported that, of 23 patients with high-grade, stage IIB osteosarcoma of the proximal humerus, 22 were treated by an extraarticular resection (Fig. 35.2-11); there were no local recurrences. The authors reviewed the published data regarding intraarticular resections versus extraarticular resections for osteosarcoma and reported local recurrence rates of 16% and 4%, respectively. A modular endoprosthesis is used for reconstruction. Soft tissue reconstruction and suspension are essential to avoid postoperative pain, instability, and fatigability.

Alternatively, resection of the proximal humerus for osteosarcomas can be performed by an intraarticular resection that pre-

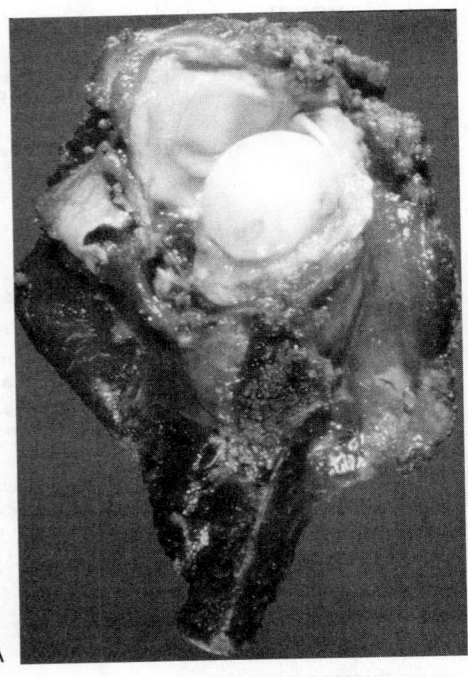

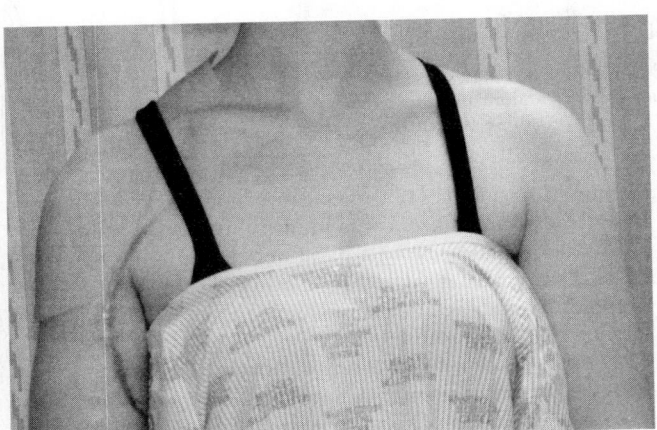

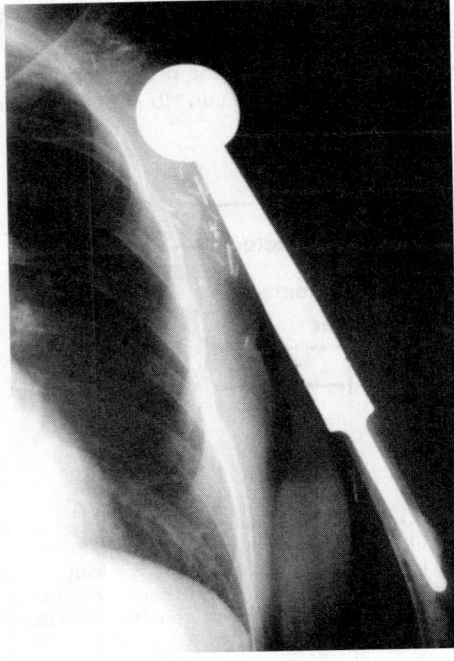

FIGURE 35.2-11.   Gross specimen after an extraarticular resection of a high-grade osteosarcoma (stage IIB) of the proximal humerus. **A:** The joint has been opened after resection. This demonstrates that adequate resection for most high-grade tumors of the proximal humerus requires an extraarticular excision of the glenohumeral joint, deltoid muscle, abductor mechanism, and approximately two-thirds of the humerus (Malawer type VB classification). Local recurrence should be less than 4%. Intraarticular resections are reserved for small, intraosseous (stage IIA) lesions (see text). Radiographic and cosmetic appearance: **B:** This patient underwent a proximal humeral replacement in lieu of a forequarter amputation. **C:** The same patient after a proximal resection is fitted with a cosmetic shoulder that is easily worn underneath bra straps or attached by Velcro. This restores the normal contour of the shoulder and improves cosmesis. (See Color Fig. 35.2-11*A* and *C* in the CD-ROM.)

serves the glenoid and the adjacent deltoid muscle. The problems associated with this procedure include significant local recurrence and instability of the reconstructed prosthesis or allograft. When the glenoid and deltoid are preserved in this procedure, minimum margins are obtained along the shoulder joint, deltoid muscle, and axillary nerve. Because of this serious drawback, this technique is not recommended by the surgical author (M. M. M.). Fewer than 5% of osteosarcomas of the proximal humerus [usually those without an extraosseous component (stage IIA)] can be treated by an intraarticular resection.

SCAPULA. The scapula is an uncommon site for osteosarcoma (less than 5%); however, it is a common site for round cell tumors (Ewing's sarcoma) and metastatic cancers in adults. A fair amount of knowledge regarding scapular prosthetic design, indications, and techniques of resection and reconstruction has been developed. Most high-grade sarcomas of the scapula involve the body as well as the glenoid. The glenoid cannot be preserved. The classic operation for high-grade tumors of the scapula has been the Tikhoff-Lindberg resection, originally described in 1928 and now identified as Malawer's classification,[201] type IVB. The Tikhoff-Lindberg resection is a complete (extraarticular) *en bloc* resection of the scapula and the proximal humerus. Reconstruction is by a hanging shoulder and some muscle transfers.

Wodajo et al.[204] reported a retrospective comparison of patients undergoing scapular resection and reconstruction with and without an endoprosthesis. Patients with endoprosthetic reconstruction had a higher MSTS score than did patients with no endoprosthesis (86% and 62%, respectively). The former group also had a larger arc of abduction (60% to 90% vs. 10% to 20%) and improved cosmesis. Most bony sarcomas of the scapula are "contained" by the two surrounding muscles, the infraspinatus posteriorly and the subscapularis muscle anteriorly. Therefore, most tumors of the scapula, irrespective of size, are amenable to endoprosthetic replacement.

DISTAL FEMUR. Adequate *en bloc* resection includes 15 to 20 cm of the distal femur and proximal tibia and portions of the adjacent quadriceps. Biplane angiography is crucial to determine popliteal vessel involvement. MRA has been used more recently. Biopsy must avoid the sartorial canal and the knee joint. Contraindications to resection are popliteal vessel involvement, massive soft tissue contamination from previous biopsy, and displaced pathologic fracture. Large tumors requiring removal of the entire quadriceps or hamstrings can be adequately reconstructed by an arthrodesis. Segmental endoprostheses are routinely used for the bony reconstruction. The use of large segmental allografts or allograft composite (with an endoprosthesis) has become less frequent within the past decade. Bickels et al.[205] reported a low prosthetic failure in 110 consecutive modular distal femoral endoprostheses. Several surgical techniques were consistently used, including routine cementation of the stem, gastrocnemius rotation flaps for adequate soft tissue coverage, and bone grafting of the prosthetic-bone junction to improve extracortical fixation. The development of extracortical fixation is thought to prevent aseptic loosening by preventing particulate debris from reaching the bone-cement interface. The 5- and 10-year survival rates of persons with distal femoral prostheses were 93% and 88%, respectively.

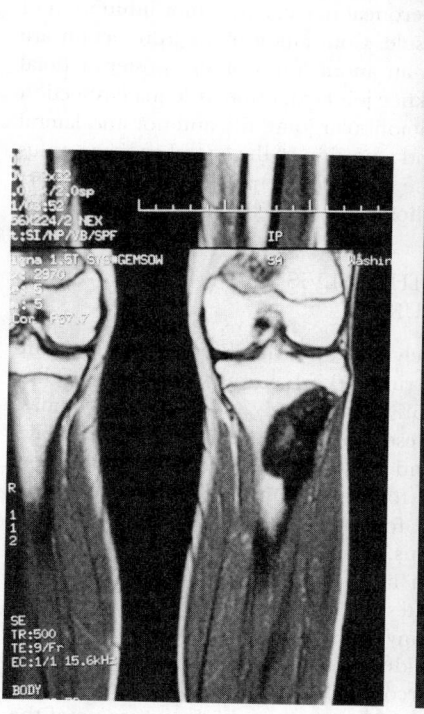
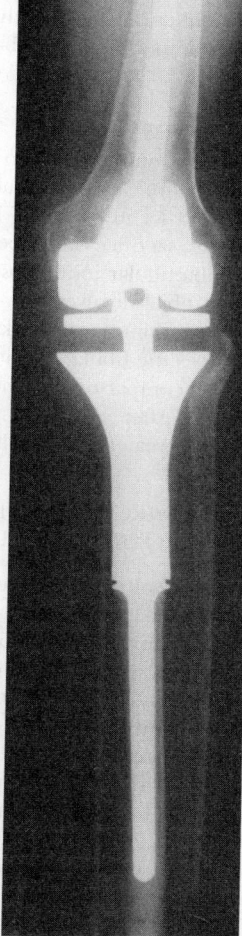

FIGURE 35.2-12. Osteosarcoma of the proximal tibia. The proximal tibia is the second most common site of osteosarcoma. **A:** Magnetic resonance imaging demonstrating the intramedullary extension of the tumor. **B:** Postoperative radiograph after proximal tibial replacement with a modular prosthesis and a kinematic rotating hinged knee joint. A portion of the fibula was excised with the tibia. An extraarticular proximal tibiofibular joint resection is routinely performed with proximal tibial resections.

PROXIMAL TIBIA. Today, limb-sparing procedures often are feasible for tumors of the proximal tibia after induction chemotherapy (Fig. 35.2-12). It is more difficult to obtain an adequate margin of resection and a good functional result with lesions of the proximal tibia and a good functional result with lesions of the proximal tibia, which tend to have a higher incidence of local complications than do distal femoral tumors. These problems are directly related to the anatomic constraints: minimal adjacent soft tissue and the normal subcutaneous location of the medial tibial border. It is extremely important that the biopsy be small and that it avoid the knee joint. A core biopsy of medial flare is preferred to avoid contamination of the anterior musculature and peroneal nerve.

Reconstruction is achieved by endoprosthetic replacement, arthrodesis, or allograft. The medial gastrocnemius is routinely transferred to provide soft tissue coverage of the reconstructed area.[206] The surgical author (M. M. M.) prefers an endoprosthetic replacement. The proximal tibia remains the most difficult site in which to perform a limb-sparing resection and reconstruction. As a result of the development of smaller, modular prostheses, which are easier to cover with muscle; the routine use of the medial gastrocnemius flaps for prosthetic coverage; and reconstruction of the extensor mechanism, limb-survival rates have almost doubled from the early 1980s (from 35% to 40% of all cases to 70% to 80%).

PROXIMAL FIBULA. Tumors of the proximal fibula require the same evaluation as do proximal tibial lesions. Unique considerations are early soft tissue extension, proximity to the lateral tibial condyle, necessity of ligation of the anterior and peroneal arteries, sacrifice of the peroneal nerve, and tumor infiltration of the tibiofibular joint capsule. Contraindications to resection are direct tibial involvement, an anomalously absent posterior tibial artery, and intraarticular knee joint extension. Adequate resection includes the fibula, the tibiofibular joint, the anterior and lateral muscle compartments, and a portion of the lateral gastrocnemius muscle. After surgery, the only functional deficit is foot drop, which is treated by an orthosis. Knee function is normal.[84]

OSTEOSARCOMA OF THE PELVIS AND PROXIMAL FEMUR

Osteosarcomas of the pelvis and proximal femur are less common than those occurring at other anatomic areas. They account for 10% and 5%, respectively, of all osteosarcomas. Tumors arising from these structures are often large, involve important structures, and are difficult to resect. Hemipelvectomy often is required for pelvic tumors, whereas modified hemipelvectomy is used for tumors of the proximal femur.[123] The limb-sparing options, when feasible, are all functionally superior to amputation at this level.[60,207] A poorly planned biopsy often contaminates the extrapelvic structures, typically making a hemipelvectomy the only safe option. Detailed anatomic and surgical considerations are discussed later in Chondrosarcoma; chondrosarcomas often arise in these sites.

Fahey et al.[208] reviewed 25 patients with osteosarcoma of the pelvis treated at the University of Florida between 1967 and 1990 and described their biologic behavior, growth, and histologic and vascular findings. Common problems included delay in diagnosis, widespread invasion into major pelvic veins, microscopic foci of tumor in otherwise normal tissue, and extension into adjacent (and other) pelvic structures.

Kawai et al.[209,210] similarly evaluated 40 patients with osteosarcoma of the pelvis treated at Memorial Sloan-Kettering Cancer Center between 1977 and 1994. Thirty of the tumors were in the ilium, five in the sacrum, four in the ischium, and one in the pubis. Fifty-eight percent of the tumors were chondroblastic. Thirty of the patients had surgery; 20 were limb-sparing procedures, and 10 were hemipelvectomies. The authors noted that it was difficult to obtain negative margins. Positive margins occurred at the sacrum (11), lumbar vertebra (1), perirectal space (1), and contralateral rami (1). Like Fahey et al., these authors reported frequently finding macroscopic tumor emboli within the regional large vessels; emboli were found in 7 of 30 (23%) of the gross specimens. The 1- and 5-year patient survival rates were 73% and 34%, respectively. Tumor size, surgical excision of the primary tumor, surgical margin, and type of surgical procedure were prognostic factors for patients with stage IIB osteosarcoma of the pelvis.

The high incidence of venous invasion requires that the iliac vessels be evaluated preoperatively and intraoperatively.

Radiographic staging studies should include a thorough evaluation of the iliac vessels. This can best be performed by CT, MRI with contrast, and pelvic venography. Survival for patients with pelvic osteosarcoma is dismal.

EXPANDABLE PROSTHESES FOR YOUNG CHILDREN

Use of endoprosthetic (or allograft) replacement in young children continues to present problems because of the effect of the procedure on subsequent bone growth. Approximately 70% of the total growth of the lower limb is a result of growth of the distal femoral and proximal tibial growth plates. Although there are techniques to avoid destroying both growth plates at the time of reconstruction, these options have varied results. Resection of the distal femur or proximal tibia in a very young patient (usually less than 10 years of age) causes significant leg-length discrepancy. Additional problems are prosthetic breakage, "collapsing" of the prosthesis, and prosthetic loosening. A new expandable prosthesis, manufactured in France and approved by the U.S. Food and Drug Administration for the lower extremity, was described at the 2002 MSTS meeting. Neel et al.[211] reported on the short and intermediate results of the Phenix (Wright Medical, Inc., Memphis, TN) prosthesis in 16 patients. Repeat surgical expansions have been avoided by a novel design. The device uses an externally applied electromagnetic field to control lengthening. This procedure does not require anesthesia. At an average of 25 months, 58 lengthening procedures have been performed, resulting in a total lengthening of 34 mm. Although this technique appears promising, more experience is required in the design and application. Today, many manufacturers and surgeons are concentrating on designing prostheses that do not require an open surgical procedure for expansion.

CLINICAL PRESENTATIONS OF OSTEOSARCOMA AND TREATMENT

Treatment Considerations

LOCALIZED-EXTREMITY DISEASE. Management of osteosarcoma requires the expertise of a multidisciplinary team familiar with the various management options. Before biopsy, patients with a suspected diagnosis of osteosarcoma (based on radiographic findings) should be referred to centers with treatment programs. The biopsy should be performed by an orthopedic surgeon familiar with the management of malignant bone tumors and experienced in the required techniques.[91] Whenever possible, this individual should be the surgeon who will ultimately perform the definitive surgical procedure, because the biopsy must be planned carefully, with a consideration of subsequent definitive surgery. A poorly conceived and poorly placed biopsy may jeopardize the subsequent treatment, especially a subsequent limb-salvage procedure.

The patient with a primary tumor of the extremity without evidence of metastases requires surgery to control the primary tumor and chemotherapy to control micrometastatic disease. The choice between amputation and limb-sparing resection must be made by an experienced orthopedic oncologist, taking into account tumor location, size, or extramedullary extent; the presence or absence of distant metastatic disease; and patient factors such as age, skeletal development, and lifestyle preference. Routine amputations are no longer performed; all patients should be evaluated for limb-sparing options. Intensive, multiagent chemotherapeutic regimens have provided the best results to date. Patients who are judged unsuitable for limb-sparing options may be candidates for presurgical chemotherapy; those with a good response may then become suitable candidates for limb-sparing operations. In addition, the possibility of radiotherapy as a treatment also exists for adverse presentations and is discussed later (see Radiotherapy in the Radical Setting). The management of these patients mandates close cooperation between the medical oncologist, radiation oncologist, and surgeon.

PELVIC TUMORS AND UNRESECTABLE DISEASE. In some pelvic and most vertebral primary tumors, complete resection often is not possible. Most pelvic osteosarcomas can be treated by hemipelvectomy; more centrally located pelvic tumors, especially those involving the sacrum, are unresectable. Only a few pelvic osteosarcomas can be treated by limb-sparing resection (internal hemipelvectomy). Contraindications to resection are unusually large extraosseous extensions with sacral plexus or major vascular involvement. On rare occasions, vertebral and sacral resections have been attempted.[212–214] In general, these tumors cannot be resected with negative margins and are best treated by radiotherapy and chemotherapy. Some success has been achieved with systemic or intraarterial chemotherapy, which is administered to convert apparently inoperable tumors into lesions that can be ablated surgically.[36] Patients with primary tumors of the axial skeleton have had a poor outcome, because local control was rare. The prognosis for these patients may improve with a more aggressive surgical approach and more effective chemotherapy.[215] Patients whose tumors can be completely resected should be approached with curative intent; radiotherapy may provide significant palliation in individuals with unresectable primary tumors.

Radiation Therapy for Osteosarcoma of the Pelvis

Ozaki et al.[216] have reported the outcome of patients who were registered in the COSS. Of 30 patients who did not undergo surgery or only intralesional surgery, 11 underwent radiotherapy (median dose, 61 Gy; range, 56 to 68 Gy), although 1 received samarium 153–ethylenediamine tetramethylene phosphonate ([153]Sm-EDTMP) therapy (see later in Bone-Seeking Targeted Radioisotopes), with an additional 60 Gy delivered by external-beam radiotherapy. The latter represents the only patient who remained disease free without relapse and who had not undergone resection.[216,217] Although the 11 patients who were treated with radiotherapy had better overall survival than the 19 who did not receive radiotherapy ($P = .0033$), the results are not provided in a manner than can attribute this specifically to the radiotherapy intervention. In essence, local control by the treatment intervention is not addressed in the report.

Metastatic Pulmonary Disease at Diagnosis

Metastatic disease detected at initial diagnosis does not preclude a curative treatment strategy, although the presence of extrathoracic metastases makes cure extremely unlikely. In general, the surgical principles outlined for the treatment of relapsing patients apply equally to the patient presenting with macroscopic

metastases. Newly diagnosed patients have not been exposed to chemotherapy and are, thus, less likely to have drug-resistant tumors. Therefore, several options are available to them. Kager et al.[68] reported that, for the patient presenting with resectable disease (i.e., usually fewer than 15 pulmonary nodules and a primary tumor of the extremity), the traditional approach has been resection of all evidence of macroscopic disease by median sternotomy and limb amputation or resection, followed by intensive adjuvant chemotherapy. The tumor burden is thereby reduced to a minimum before the application of adjuvant therapy. Some investigators have favored treatment with chemotherapy, followed weeks or months later by definitive surgery for residual macroscopic disease in primary and metastatic sites. Arguments advanced to justify this approach are similar to those used to support preoperative chemotherapy in general, and the theoretic advantages and disadvantages of this strategy as discussed for patients with nonmetastatic osteosarcoma apply here as well. The risk for the patient with metastases is that growth of tumor nodules in the face of chemotherapy may render small, operable metastases unresectable and prevent cure. Although the timing of the surgery of the primary tumor and metastatic sites has been variable, most modern approaches entail alternating chemotherapy and surgery. The initial treatment is usually a course of chemotherapy, followed by surgical resection of the primary tumor, followed by a second course of chemotherapy and surgical ablation of metastatic sites, followed by the remaining courses of chemotherapy. Patients with tumors that respond to presurgical chemotherapy are more likely to be cured. In those with inoperable metastases, primary treatment with chemotherapy is probably appropriate; metastases may respond sufficiently to allow complete resection. Because these patients usually require surgery for the primary tumor as a palliative procedure, early surgery may be recommended, despite unresectable pulmonary disease. Although improving, the outlook for patients presenting with metastatic disease remains poor.[141,218]

The presence of metastatic disease at presentation continues to be an extremely poor prognostic finding, with most studies showing survival rates in the range of 20%.[133,140] It is therefore clear that new approaches are needed. The POG reported early data from a small phase II study for patients less than 30 years old with newly diagnosed metastatic osteosarcoma.[142] Forty-one patients were treated with two cycles of etoposide and IFOS preoperatively, followed by 32 weeks of postoperative chemotherapy, including three additional cycles of etoposide and IFOS along with standard HD-MTX, ADM, and CDDP (Chart 35.2-4). It should be noted that patients underwent surgical resection of all sites of disease whenever possible. The data are still immature, but the projected 2-year progression-free survival was 43%. In the large analysis of the COSS database that included more than 1700 consecutively treated patients, the 10-year survival probability was 40% for patients who were able to have all sites of metastatic disease resected.[133] Thus, although there is no accepted standard approach for the treatment of newly diagnosed metastatic patients, available data suggest that such patients should be treated with currently available, aggressive multiagent chemotherapy with complete surgical resection of all sites of disease if at all possible.

Recurrent Disease after Curative Attempt

Historically, patients in whom recurrent disease developed had a poor prognosis and were treated palliatively; most died within 1 year of the development of metastatic disease. Because more

INDUCTION   MAINTENANCE

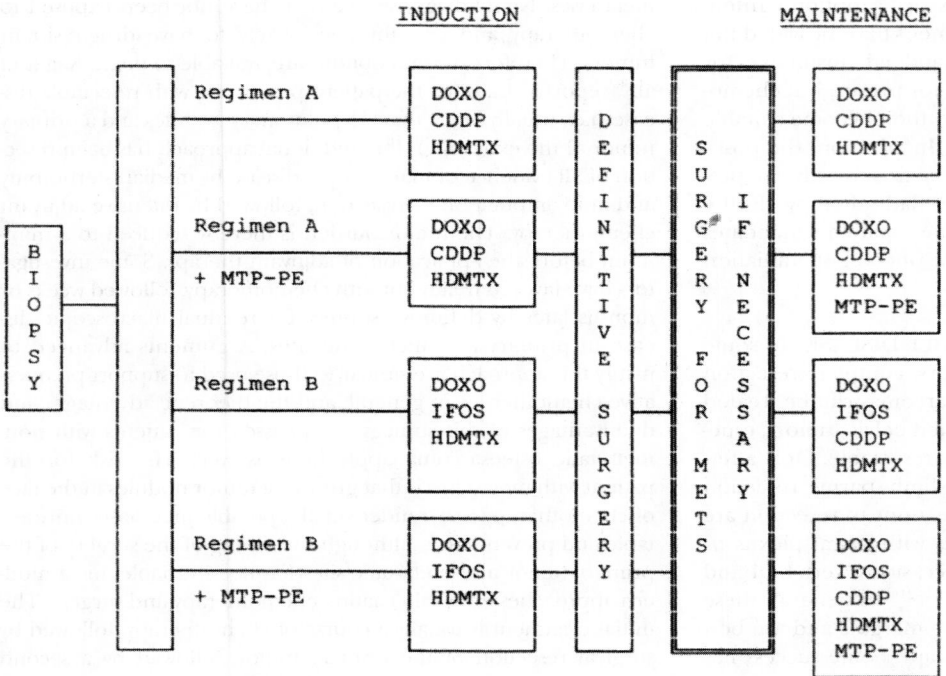

CHART 35.2-4. Typical chemotherapy protocol for pediatric osteosarcoma. CDDP, cisplatin; DOXO, doxorubicin; HDMTX, high-dose methotrexate; IFOS, ifosfamide; MTP-PE, liposomal muramyl tripeptide. (Data from Children's Oncology Group, P. Meyers, *personal communication*, with permission.)

than 85% of metastases occur in the lung, surgical resection of tumor nodules can be readily accomplished. With the advent of thoracic CT scanning, metastatic nodules can be detected when quite small and more easily resectable, although in most cases the surgeon discovers more lesions at thoracotomy than anticipated on the basis of the CT scan.[219–221] In many patients, the lungs are likely to be the only site of metastasis, especially in cases in which recurrences appear more than 1 year after diagnosis and in which the metastatic lesion is solitary. In such cases, the recurrent tumors are likely to behave more indolently and may not metastasize further. These patients have been cured by thoracotomy alone.

Surgical resection of all overt metastatic disease is a prerequisite for long-term salvage after relapse. Patients not treated by thoracotomy have little hope for cure, because complete responses of macroscopic metastases to chemotherapy are rare. The completeness of surgical resection is an important determinant of outcome, because patients left with measurable or microscopic disease at the resection margins are unlikely to be cured.[220–223]

Many investigators have recommended adjuvant chemotherapy after thoracotomy for the management of metastatic osteosarcoma to destroy residual microscopic tumor deposits.[63,70,126] For patients in whom recurrent disease develops within 1 year of initial surgery, the possibility of additional microscopic metastatic disease is quite high, and further chemotherapy is indicated. Long-term survival has been reported for some patients with recurrent osteosarcoma who were treated only with surgery.[42–44] These survivors were more likely to be patients experiencing late relapses with solitary pulmonary nodules.

If overt metastatic disease is discovered, a thorough search for all metastatic lesions is essential. The discovery of unresectable extrathoracic metastases or unresectable pulmonary disease is a contraindication to aggressive thoracotomy, and the patient should be treated palliatively. Radiotherapy may be particularly useful in this context. In some patients with unresecta-

ble disease, an aggressive approach with curative intent may still be indicated.

Patients with resectable lung disease should undergo thoracotomy to remove all evidence of disease. Bilateral disease can be approached by staged bilateral thoracotomies or a median sternotomy. The role of adjuvant chemotherapy after thoracotomy should be studied; it is probably indicated for patients with more than three lesions appearing 6 months to 1 year after initial surgery, for individuals whose metastatic disease has not been completely resected, or for those with evidence of pleural disruption by tumor. Repeat thoracotomies may be required for subsequent recurrence and should be performed if all disease can be resected.

Survival after relapse has undeniably been enhanced by approaches designed with curative intent that incorporate repeated aggressive surgery to remove overt disease. With such treatment, 30% to 40% of patients have been reported to survive beyond 5 years after relapse,[42,44,143,145,224] although not all of these patients are ultimately cured. Such considerations emphasize the value of close follow-up, with frequent chest radiographs and thoracic CT scans, to detect recurrent disease when it is still resectable. Thus, for the patient with osteosarcoma, the development of metastases is not a hopeless situation; aggressive systemic treatment offers prolonged survival for many patients and the possibility of cure for a significant fraction. Ironically, as adjuvant regimens used in front-line therapy of patients are intensified and the number of patients surviving without ever developing recurrence increases, the proportion who are likely to be salvageable after relapse may decrease, because relapsing patients are more likely to have drug-resistant recurrences. Similar to patients who present with primary metastatic disease, patients in whom recurrent disease develops have an overall poor prognosis, with 5-year survival rates in the range of 20%.[144] As noted for metastatic disease at presentation, new salvage strategies are needed. Although there is no standard second-line chemotherapy that currently is uniformly applied, several principles have been clearly established. Most importantly, as with primary metastatic disease, complete resection of recurrent disease appears to be mandatory for long-term survival.[144,145] It also is likely that multiagent chemotherapy contributes to successful salvage of some patients. In general, patients should be treated with any of the four most-active agents noted earlier in Assessment of Histologic Responses to Neoadjuvant Chemotherapy if initial therapy did not include one or more of these agents. Patients who experience recurrence more than 1 year after completing prior systemic therapy may benefit from reintroduction of at least some of the same drugs in a salvage regimen. The use of high-dose chemotherapy with autologous hematopoietic stem cell rescue has been applied to salvage therapy. However, at least two reported small pilot studies failed to demonstrate an advantage to standard salvage therapy approaches.[146,147]

New Systemic Therapeutic Approaches

Over the years, there has been interest in developing immunostimulatory agents that might be of benefit in the treatment of osteosarcoma. A randomized, double-blind study performed in spontaneous canine osteosarcoma in 1989 demonstrated that the macrophage activator, muramyl tripeptide (MTP), prolonged survival in dogs after amputation.[225] Subsequent clinical studies in patients with pulmonary metastases at M. D. Anderson showed a median time to relapse of 9 months after metastasectomy and 24 weeks of liposomal MTP (MTP-PE), compared to 4.5 months for historical control patients.[226–228] Based on these promising results, the POG and Children's Cancer Group performed a joint randomized study to determine whether the addition of MTP-PE to chemotherapy would enhance survival in newly diagnosed patients (see Chart 35.2-4). The study also evaluated whether the addition of IFOS to HD-MTX, ADM, and CDDP improved survival. The results of this study, which accrued almost 800 patients, were somewhat surprising in that the addition of MTP-PE appeared to improve survival only in the patients who received IFOS. The 4-year event-free survival in this group is 70%, compared to 57% for patients receiving IFOS but no MTP-PE. However, patients treated with the standard three-drug combination of HD-MTX, ADM, and CDDP had a 4-year disease-free survival of 65% compared to 62% for those patients who also received MTP-PE.[229] These results suggest that there may be some modest benefit to patients treated with the macrophage-activating agent MTP. However, there appears to be specific drug interactions because this benefit is only seen in patients receiving IFOS. Similarly, a group from the Karolinska Hospital have reported that the use of leukocyte interferon may enhance survival for high-risk osteosarcoma patients and suggested that this should be studied in more detail in high-risk patients.[230]

Because the overwhelming majority of metastases in osteosarcoma occur in the lung, many investigators have sought to develop therapies that target microscopic and macroscopic disease in the lungs. Toward that end, investigators at the Mayo Clinic have reported the results of early clinical studies using aerosolized granulocyte-macrophage colony-stimulating factor for patients with a variety of tumors and pulmonary metastases. The results of this study were promising, and the Children's Oncology Group is planning a phase II study for patients with osteosarcoma and pulmonary metastases.[231]

Several groups have recently reported that the expression of the Her2/neu/ErbB-2 protein occurs in osteosarcoma. In a retrospective study of 26 patients with osteosarcoma treated at the University of Tokyo, 42% of tumors expressed Her2 protein, and expression was associated with early pulmonary metastases and poor survival.[231a] Another retrospective study of 53 patients at Memorial Sloan-Kettering Cancer Center also found Her2 expression in 42% of tumors at presentation and confirmed that expression was associated with a worse event-free survival.[231b] Other groups have reported similar findings.[231c] This is of potential therapeutic interest, because breast cancers that express Her2/neu have been shown to respond to the humanized monoclonal antibody, Herceptin, directed against Her2/neu.[231d,231e] However, these data have been contradicted by several reports, one finding Her2/neu expression to be correlated with increased survival in osteosarcoma[231f] and another study finding no Her2/neu membranous staining (that is characteristic of breast cancer) in 66 osteosarcoma samples.[231g] It may be of note that none of the studies showing expression of Her2/neu found clear evidence of gene amplification, which is almost uniformly associated with overexpression in breast cancers. Nonetheless, based on the findings of expression and the promising results of the use of Herceptin in Her2-positive breast cancer, the Children's Oncology Group is conducting a study that includes the use of Herceptin in high-risk osteosarcoma patients with documented expression of Her2/neu. This has just begun to accrue patients.

Radiation Therapy in the Treatment of Osteosarcoma

BACKGROUND. Significant experience with primary radiotherapy for osteosarcomas was obtained in the 1950s and early 1960s. Primary radiotherapy with delayed amputation gained acceptance in 1955, when Cade[232] advocated initial therapy with radiation and delayed amputation for patients in whom there was no evidence of metastasis 4 to 6 months after radiotherapy. This approach was designed to circumvent amputation in the majority of patients who were destined to develop an early relapse. Radiation doses were 7000 to 8000 cGy administered over 7 to 9 weeks at 1000 cGy/wk. A few patients in Cade's series who were not subjected to delayed amputation were controlled with irradiation alone, and amputation was eventually performed. The 5-year survival rate was 21.8%. Other investigators followed a similar regime, using various radiation doses and schemes. Subsequent surgical specimens of many of the patients managed in this fashion were found to have no histologic evidence of tumor. The ability of high radiation doses to sterilize some tumors, however, was associated with significant necrosis of normal tissue.[233–235]

Radiotherapy has, however, been shown to be successful in several distinct clinical situations—facial lesions, palliation, and, possibly, as a postoperative adjuvant. High-dose combination photon and proton radiation using three-dimensional treatment planning may improve long-term local control. Guidelines for the use of radiotherapy for osteosarcoma and other malignant bone tumors are shown in Tables 35.2-10 and 35.2-11.

RADIOTHERAPY IN THE RADICAL SETTING. In previous decades, as is evident from the local management of patients on randomized trials addressing the role of adjuvant whole lung irradiation, radiotherapy, alone or as a local adjuvant, was used relatively frequently.[236,237] With the high local control expectation of

TABLE 35.2-11. Radiation Guidelines for
Malignant Bone Lesions

Tumor	Radiation Dose	Comments
Osteosarcoma	70–80 Gy	See text
Chondrosarcoma	50–70 Gy	Radiotherapy as local adjuvant treatment or if unresectable or inoperable
Giant cell tumor (osteoclastoma)	30–55 Gy	Putative sarcomatous transformation has been reported
Hemangioendothelioma	50–60 Gy	
Chordoma	74–75 CGE	Mixed photon–photon beam
Lymphoma	40–50 Gy	High local control with chemotherapy; radiotherapy may not be needed in pediatric patients

CGE, cobalt-gray equivalent.

surgery after induction chemotherapy and pathologic response assessment, the role for radiotherapy in osteosarcoma fell out of favor, and today it is restricted to selected circumstances. For the most part, these are determined by critical and life-threatening locations of primary disease where adequate surgical removal is unlikely. With little exception these are not stage-dependent situations but are represented by lesions arising in critical areas of the head and neck, spine, and pelvis where surgery has already been attempted or where it has been deemed not to be possible. In view of the lack of exemplary results with radiotherapy, notwithstanding the bias that selection of only the most adverse cases for radiotherapy may have on observed outcome, accessible lesions in other sites are generally managed with complete surgical removal, even if this results in function and cosmetic loss. In such situations, some authors have suggested novel alternative methods for the management of extremity osteosarcoma that emphasize radiotherapy (see Experimental *In Situ* Radiotherapy of Extremity Osteosarcoma). In addition, DeLaney et al.[238] have summarized the Massachusetts General Hospital data and showed that radiation therapy can provide local control of osteosarcoma in situations in which surgical resection with negative margins is not possible.

EXPERIMENTAL *IN SITU* RADIOTHERAPY OF EXTREMITY OSTEOSARCOMA. An unusual approach is the use of modern neoadjuvant chemotherapy administered with external-beam radiotherapy to achieve local control of nonmetastatic osteosarcoma. Machak et al.[239] described the largest experience of this approach in a consecutive series of 31 of 187 patients who had refused surgery and had been enrolled from 1986 to 1999 in induction chemotherapy and surgery protocols at the N. N. Blokhin Cancer Research Center, Moscow. This investigational approach used radiotherapy (median dose of 60 Gy fractionated) in place of surgery and involved informed consent. In the subgroup of one-third of patients with a pronounced imaging and biochemical (i.e., AP level) response, the 5-year survival after chemoradiotherapy was 90%. These results suggest that the disappointing effect of standard doses of radiotherapy on osteosarcoma may not apply in the setting of effective response to chemotherapy and contrasts with the experience of nonsurgical management without radiotherapy, for which control rates were much poorer.[240] Notwithstanding these promising selected results that may suggest

additional options for patients, they must still be balanced against the potential of late adverse outcomes, including local and metastatic recurrence, as well as deleterious normal tissue effects, even if the promise of this approach is better function and quality of life.

Palliation

EXTERNAL-BEAM AND RADIATION SENSITIZERS. Radiation therapy is extremely beneficial in patients requiring palliation of metastatic bony sarcomas; tumors at axial sites, which are unresectable; and advanced, inoperable lesions of the pelvis or extremities.

BONE-SEEKING TARGETED RADIOISOTOPES. A promising approach is the use of the isotope ^{153}Sm-EDTMP to target "bone-specific" radiotherapy to osteoblastic osteosarcomas.[217,241,242] The compound is administered by intravenous injection and is distributed in a very similar way to technetium 99m methylene diphosphonate in a diagnostic bone scan. Originally introduced for palliation of bone pain arising from osteoblastic bone metastasis, preliminary evidence suggests that ^{153}Sm-EDTMP has attractive possibilities to target bone-forming tumors in surgically inaccessible sites and in refractory tumors, possibly in combination with external-beam radiotherapy.[242] The therapeutic effect of this compound comes from its beta-emitting capability derived by neutron capture from ^{153}Sm. The circumstances for the use of this treatment are almost ideal, because there is rapid bone uptake and bone surface retention of ^{153}Sm-EDTMP for many months, and unbound compound undergoes rapid urinary excretion.[241] Unfortunately, the beta-emitting property can also result in myeloablation due to marrow tolerance necessitating autologous peripheral blood stem cell support. Anderson et al.[241] from the Mayo Clinic reported a dose-escalation trial of ^{153}Sm-EDTMP and showed this to be of particular risk with high doses of ^{153}Sm-EDTMP (30 mCi/kg). Of note, however, nonhematologic sequelae are mimimal, and reduction or elimination of opiates is a uniform finding in all cases.[241] These investigators showed that an additional 40 to 200 Gy can be administered to bones and osteoblastic osteosarcomas, respectively, in patients with avid technetium 99m methylene diphosphonate bone scans. Already, as noted earlier, some groups are using it as adjunctive treatment in selected cases of unfavorable osteosarcoma, with the possibility of long-term control when combined with external-beam irradiation in patients who have not undergone surgery.[216,217,243]

VARIANTS OF CLASSIC OSTEOSARCOMA

Dahlin and Unni[49] have identified 11 variants of the classic osteosarcoma. These accounted for 268 of 1021 (26%) cases reviewed at the Mayo Clinic. Osteosarcoma arising in the jawbone, the most common variant, is characterized by well-differentiated cells with a low metastatic potential. Excluding tumors arising secondary to Paget's disease, irradiation, or dedifferentiation of a chondrosarcoma, parosteal and periosteal osteosarcomas are the most common variants of classic osteosarcoma arising in the extremities. In contrast to classic osteosarcoma, which arises within a bone, parosteal and periosteal osteosarcomas arise on the surface of the bone (juxtacortical).

The three types of surface osteosarcomas are parosteal osteosarcoma, periosteal osteosarcoma, and high-grade surface osteosarcoma. The Mayo Clinic reported 518 surface osteosarcomas seen between 1926 and 1996. The incidence was 335 parosteal osteosarcomas (64.7%), 137 periosteal osteosarcomas (26.4%), and 46 high-grade surface osteosarcomas (8.9%). These 518 surface osteosarcomas were from a pool of 4365 osteosarcoma tumors (i.e., a ratio of 1.0:8.4 cases).[244]

Parosteal Osteosarcoma

CLINICAL CHARACTERISTICS. Parosteal osteosarcoma is a distinct variant of conventional osteosarcoma that accounts for 4% of all osteosarcomas.[244] It arises from the cortex of a bone and generally occurs in older individuals. It has a better prognosis than classic osteosarcoma.

RADIOGRAPHIC FINDINGS. A slight predominance of parosteal osteosarcoma is found in women. The distal posterior femur is involved in 72% of all cases; the proximal humerus and proximal tibia are the next most frequent sites. Parosteal osteosarcoma metastasizes slowly and has an overall survival rate of 75% to 85%.[49,51] Unni et al.[51] noted that all patients who died of tumor lived longer than 5 years. The natural history of parosteal osteosarcoma is progressive enlargement and late metastasis. Parosteal osteosarcoma presents a mass and occasionally is associated with pain. In contrast to conventional osteosarcoma, duration of symptoms varies from months to years. Unni et al.[51] reported that 50 of 79 patients had complaints of longer than 1 year, and one-third of this group had pain for more than 5 years. Tumor size, location, and duration of symptoms did not correlate with survival.[49,51]

PATHOLOGY AND GRADING. Parosteal osteosarcoma is characterized by well-formed lamellar or woven bone with a mature spindle cell stroma and few signs of malignancy. The cellularity of the spindle cell components varies; generally, it is not anaplastic, with few mitoses.[49,51] The differential diagnosis is osteochondroma, myositis ossificans, and conventional osteosarcoma. Cortical tumors of the posterior femur should always be suspected of being malignant; this is a rare location for a benign osteochondroma. In contrast to sarcoma, myositis ossificans is rarely attached to the underlying bone. In addition, the periphery is more mature radiographically and histologically. Ahuja et al.[50] reviewed all cases of parosteal osteosarcoma at Memorial Sloan-Kettering Cancer Center from 1934 to 1975 and described three grades: grade I (low grade), grade II (intermediate), and grade III (high grade). They emphasized the importance of evaluating the fibroblastic, cartilaginous, and osseous components independently. Of 24 patients, eight were grade I, ten grade II, and six grade III. Unni et al.[51] reviewed 79 patients and reported that 18 were grade II (23%) and 7 had high-grade foci (9%). Neither group of researchers could distinguish the three grades on plain radiographs. The survival rate of patients with grade III tumors is similar to that of those with conventional osteosarcoma.

Jelinek et al.[245] reviewed the records of the Armed Forces Institute of Pathology and evaluated 60 patients with parosteal osteosarcomas for tumor size, location, and presence of cleavage plane; intramedullary extension; soft tissue mass; and the presence and pattern of ossification. Tumors were classified as low grade or high grade. The average maximal length for low- and high-grade tumors was 7.7 and 15.0 cm, respectively. A cleavage plane was present in 20 low-grade (62%) and 19 high-grade (68%) lesions. On cross-sectional imaging, intramedullary extension was present in 13 low-grade (41%) and 14 high-grade (50%) lesions. These authors concluded that a poorly defined soft tissue component distinct from the ossified matrix is the most distinctive feature of high-grade parosteal osteosarcoma and may be the optimal site to perform a biopsy.

Intramedullary involvement does not necessarily imply a worse prognosis, although this may be the case in patients with high-grade lesions. Eleven of 24 patients (46%) reviewed by Ahuja et al.[50] had medullary involvement; moreover, the patients with medullary involvement who had a local resection all had a local recurrence.

Okada et al.[244] have updated the experience of the Mayo Clinic. They reviewed the records of 226 patients. Dedifferentiation was more common (16% of patients) than previously reported. They emphasized the usefulness of cross-sectional imaging in planning surgical resection. The tumor often had extensive intramedullary, extraosseous, and adjacent soft tissue components. Medullary involvement was present in 22% of the patients, and extraosseous, unmineralized soft tissue peripheral to the mineralized cortical mass was noted in 51% of the patients. Adjacent soft tissue extension occurred in 46% of patients. In contrast to their previous studies, intramedullary involvement was not a poor prognostic factor. The authors stressed the need for long-term follow-up. Eleven of the 67 patients managed at their institution died at an average of 14 years (range, 2 to 41 years). Ten of the 11 patients died from a dedifferentiated tumor.

TREATMENT. Wide excision of the tumor is the treatment of choice. This may be accomplished either by an amputation or a limb-sparing procedure. No experience with preoperative chemotherapy or radiotherapy has been reported. Parosteal osteosarcomas are often amenable to limb preservation due to their distal location, low grade, and lack of local invasiveness. If the adjacent neurovascular bundle is free of tumor, resection is feasible. Vascular displacement is not a contraindication for resection. The major surgical decision usually is whether to remove the entire end of the bone and the adjacent joint or to preserve the joint. Small lesions can be resected with joint preservation. If the medullary canal is involved, the joint usually cannot be preserved. A second factor mitigating against joint preservation is extensive cortical involvement. Techniques of resection and reconstruction are similar to those described for conventional osteosarcoma. The major difference is that only a small amount of soft tissue usually must be resected; consequently, a good functional result is obtained. Grade III parosteal lesions warrant systemic therapy because of the risk of metastasis.

Periosteal Osteosarcoma

Periosteal osteosarcoma is a rare cortical variant of osteosarcoma that arises superficially on the cortex, most often on the tibia shaft. Radiographically, it is a small, radiolucent lesion with some evidence of bone spiculation. The cortex is characteristically intact, with a scooped-out appearance and a Codman's triangle. Histologically, periosteal osteosarcomas are relatively high-grade chondroblastic osteosarcomas composed of a malignant cartilage with areas of anaplastic spindle cells and osteoid production. Dahlin and Unni,[49] in a report of 23 cases, found periosteal osteosarcomas to occur one-third as frequently as the parosteal variant. The largest tumor measured 2.5 by 3.5 cm. Four of the 23 patients died of metastatic disease.

One of the largest reported series was by Okada et al. from the Mayo Clinic.[244] They evaluated 46 patients and described their radiographic, clinical, and pathologic evaluation. All the tumors were broad based and attached to the underlying cortex. Nineteen of the 46 tumors (41%) showed infiltration into the cortex of the underlying bone. Medullary involvement was documented on gross or radiologic examination in 13 tumors and by microscopic examination only in 6 tumors. The authors attempted to evaluate the effectiveness of chemotherapy in this very rare subtype of osteosarcoma. Fifteen of the 21 patients receiving systemic treatment showed no response to chemotherapy. Among these 15, only 1 patient remains alive. All six patients who showed a good response to chemotherapy are alive. Medullary involvement did not affect prognosis. The survival rate was 57.5% at 3 years and 46.1% at 5 years.

Treatment is similar to that of other high-grade lesions. *En bloc* resection should be performed when feasible; amputation is rarely indicated.

Paget's Sarcoma

In approximately 1% of patients with Paget's disease, a primary bone sarcoma will develop. Greditzer et al.[164,166] reported 41 sarcomas among 4415 patients with Paget's disease followed at the Mayo Clinic; 35 were osteosarcomas, and 6 were fibrosarcomas. The average patient age was 64 years, and the most common sites were the pelvis, femur, and humerus. One-half of these lesions were osteolytic; the remainder had a mixed pattern. Cortical destruction and a soft tissue component were the most common signs noted; periosteal elevation was rare. Most patients with this condition present with pain; thus, a patient with known Paget's disease who complains of increasing pain, especially when it is well localized, should be evaluated radiographically. The diagnosis is usually made by plain radiography and confirmed by biopsy. Traditionally, fewer than 8% of patients survive, and most deaths occur within 2 years.[164,166] Treatment is similar to that recommended for adolescent patients with osteosarcoma without metastatic disease while recognizing that the characteristic older age of Paget's-associated patients often influences the intensity of treatment that can be offered.

High-Grade Surface Osteosarcoma

High-grade surface osteosarcoma (peripheral conventional osteosarcoma) is the rarest variant of surface osteosarcoma. The parosteal and periosteal osteosarcomas have a better prognosis, whereas the high-grade surface variant has the same prognosis as the conventional, intramedullary lesion. This variant was previously called *type III parosteal osteosarcoma*. Schajowicz et al.[246] studied the different surface osteosarcomas. They reported that only 7 of 80 surface osteosarcomas (9%) were considered to be the high-grade variant. Clinically, the median age was 13.5 years (younger than that of patients with other surface lesions), and almost all were located in the diaphyseal region of the bone. The femur was the most common site. This tumor may show extensive intramedullary involvement. Radiographically, it appears as a small or moderate-size lesion with slight to heavy calcification. The broad base of the lesion abuts the cortex. The radiographic features often are misleading and may suggest the periosteal variant; thus, the preoperative diagnosis may be difficult. However, the young age, the diaphyseal location and, most importantly, the highly malignant histologic features indicate the correct diagnosis. Wide excision with limb preservation has been reported. Adjuvant chemotherapy is warranted due to the high rate of metastases.

Small Cell Osteosarcoma

The small cell osteosarcoma, a rare variant of osteosarcomas, resembles a Ewing's sarcoma and is often classified as an "atypical" Ewing's sarcoma.[247,248] Characteristically, areas of osteoid and, on occasion, chondroid formation are present. The differential diagnosis includes Ewing's sarcoma, atypical Ewing's sarcoma, primitive neuroectodermal tumor, mesenchymal chondrosarcoma, lymphoma, and Askin's tumor. Differentiation from Ewing's sarcoma and the typical osteosarcoma is important, because the response of small cell osteosarcoma to treatment is poorly defined.

Devaney et al.[249] from the Bone Branch of the Armed Forces Institute of Pathology evaluated 79 round cell tumors of bone with immunohistochemistry in an attempt to distinguish small cell osteosarcoma from the other round cell tumors of bone. They noted that none reacted with cytokeratin, epithelial membrane antigen, factor VIII–related antigen, or synaptophysins, and none were Leu-M1 positive. Thus, a strong positivity of any of these studies should rule out small cell osteosarcoma. Vimentin was seen in the majority of the various tumor types. The authors concluded that immunohistochemical stains alone could not make the diagnosis.

Sim et al.[247] recommend surgery. At the Pediatric Branch of the National Cancer Institute, however, these tumors, like other pediatric round cell tumors, are treated by a combination of surgical resection, radiation therapy, and chemotherapy.

Radiation-Induced Osteosarcoma

Radiation-induced osteosarcomas arise in a previously irradiated field and meet the general criteria of a radiation-induced sarcoma [i.e., they appear after a latent period of 5 to 20 years, are documented to be secondary (different from the original one), and occur in a documented irradiated field]. Amendola et al.[250] from the University of Michigan reviewed 22,306 patients treated with radiation between 1934 and 1983 and reported 23 patients with radiation-associated sarcoma (prevalence, 0.1%). The median latent period was 13 years (range, 3 to 34 years). The radiation doses ranged from 25 to 72 Gy. The data suggest that intensive chemotherapy may have shortened the latency period.

In two nested case-control studies of 3-year cancer survivors from France and the United Kingdom,[251] the risk of osteosarcoma was found to be a linear function of radiation dose and alkylating agent chemotherapy. The 20-year risk of osteosarcoma among survivors of retinoblastoma (7.2%), Ewing's sarcoma (5.4%), and other bone tumors (2.2%) suggests a genetic influence in the induction of secondary osteosarcoma. However, the risk of developing bone sarcoma within 20 years for the majority of survivors of childhood cancer is less than 0.9%.

The treatment of radiation-associated osteosarcoma is wide resection, when possible, combined with adjuvant chemotherapy.[252] A previously irradiated field presents a unique challenge for the surgeon—choosing the best local option. The likelihood of local complications is greater in such cases. Tabone et al.[253] reported results from the French Society of Pediatric Oncology indicating that an intensive approach using chemotherapy and surgery will yield 8-year overall and event-free survival rates of 50% and 41%, respectively.

CHONDROSARCOMA

Chondrosarcomas are the second most common primary malignant spindle cell tumors of bone.[2] They form a heterogeneous

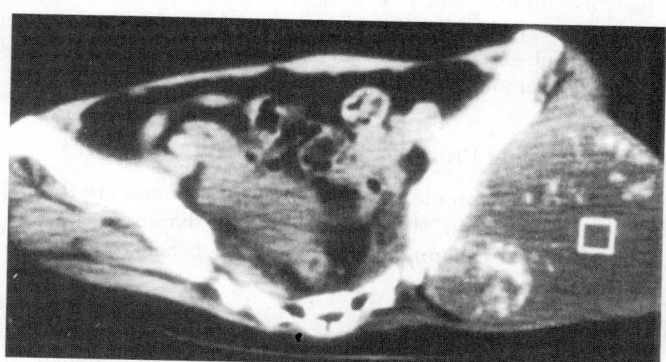

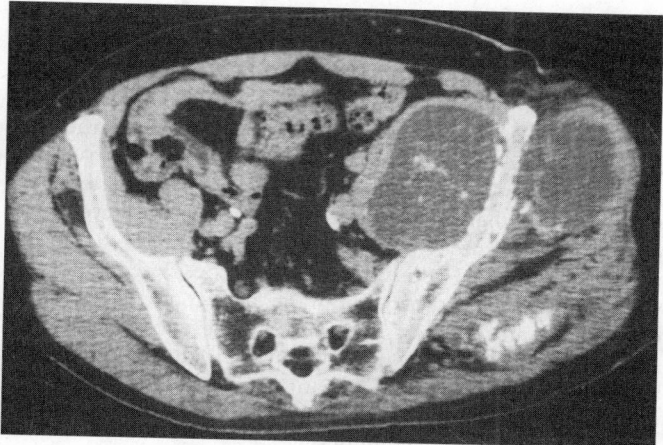

FIGURE 35.2-13. Chondrosarcoma of the pelvis. **A:** Large chondrosarcoma involving the left iliac wing with extensive buttock involvement. **B:** Typical radiograph of a large chondrosarcoma of the iliac wing with extension to the sacroiliac joint and into the abductor mechanism. This patient was treated with a type I iliac wing and partial sacral alar resection. Amputation was not required.

group of tumors whose basic neoplastic tissue is cartilaginous without evidence of direct osteoid formation.[254] Occasionally, bone formation occurs from differentiation of cartilage. If evidence is found of direct osteoid or bone production, the lesion is classified as an osteosarcoma. The five types of chondrosarcomas are central, peripheral, mesenchymal, differentiated, and clear cell.[2,7,255] The classic chondrosarcomas are central (arising within a bone) or peripheral (arising from the surface of a bone). The other three are variants and have distinct histologic and clinical characteristics.

Central and peripheral chondrosarcomas can arise as primary tumors or secondary to underlying neoplasm. Seventy-six percent of primary chondrosarcomas arise centrally.[2,7,254,255] Secondary chondrosarcomas most often arise from benign cartilage tumors. The multiple forms of benign osteochondromas or enchondromas have a higher rate of malignant transformation than the corresponding solitary lesions.[8,255]

Central and Peripheral Chondrosarcomas

CLINICAL CHARACTERISTICS. One-half of all chondrosarcomas occur in persons older than 40 years of age; only 3.8% develop in those younger than 20 years.[2] The most common sites[165] are the pelvis (31%), femur (21%), and shoulder girdle (13%).[8,165,255] Chondrosarcomas are the most common malignant tumors of the sternum and scapula. The clinical presentation varies. Peripheral chondrosarcomas may become large without causing pain, and local symptoms develop only because of mechanical irritation. Pelvic chondrosarcomas are often large and present with referred pain to the back or thigh, sciatica secondary to sacral plexus irritation, urinary symptoms from bladder neck involvement, unilateral edema due to iliac vein obstruction, or a painless abdominal mass. Conversely, central chondrosarcomas present with dull pain; a mass is rare. Pain, which indicates active growth, is an ominous sign of a central cartilage lesion. This cannot be overemphasized. An adult with a plain radiograph suggestive of a "benign" cartilage tumor but associated with pain most likely has a chondrosarcoma (Fig. 35.2-13).

HISTOLOGY AND GRADING. Chondrosarcomas are categorized as grade I, II, or III. The majority of chondrosarcomas are

either grade I or II.[256,257] The metastatic rate of moderate-grade lesions is 15% to 40%; in high-grade lesions, it is 75%. Grade III lesions have the same metastatic potential as osteosarcomas.

Because cartilage tumors are difficult to grade histologically,[256–259] some investigators have attempted to apply cytologic, histochemical, and biochemical analysis to evaluate these lesions. Sanerkin[257,260] described a combination of cytologic and histologic criteria. He emphasized that cytologic analysis evaluates nuclear abnormalities better than conventional histologic sections, whereas histologic evaluation of bone-tumor interface is the best predictor of local aggressiveness. Kreicbergs et al.[261] performed a retrospective study of DNA content of 45 chondrosarcomas as an indicator of malignancy by evaluating diploid (normal DNA content) and hyperploid (abnormal increase in DNA) cells and correlating the findings to 10-year survival. Regardless of tumor grade, size, and location, patients with diploid cells had a better prognosis than those with hyperploid cells. A preliminary report assessing the malignancy of cartilage tumor by flow cytometry to determine the percentage of diploid, tetraploid, and aneuploid cells indicates that it may be a promising method of grading chondrosarcomas.[261]

RADIOGRAPHIC DIAGNOSIS AND EVALUATION. Central chondrosarcomas have two distinct radiologic patterns.[262] One is a small, well-defined lytic lesion with a narrow zone of transition and surrounding sclerosis with faint calcification. This is the most common malignant bone tumor that may appear radiographically benign. The second type has no sclerotic border and is difficult to localize. The key sign of malignancy is endosteal scalloping. It is difficult to diagnose on plain radiographs and may go undetected for a long period. In contrast, peripheral chondrosarcoma is recognized easily as a large, calcified mass protruding from a bone. Its differential diagnosis includes large benign osteochondroma, parosteal osteosarcoma, and juxtacortical myositis ossificans. Correlation of clinical, radiographic, and histologic data is essential for accurate diagnosis and evaluation of the aggressiveness of cartilage tumor. Proximal or axial location, skeletal maturity, and pain point toward malignancy, even though the cartilage may appear benign.

PROGNOSIS. Metastatic potential tends to correlate with the histologic grade of the lesions.[7,8,255,256] Marcove et al.[256] reported on long-term follow-up of 113 chondrosarcomas of the proximal femur and the pelvis. The survival rates in patients with grade I, II, or III lesions were 47%, 38%, and 15%, respectively; the overall survival rate was 52%. No significant difference was noted between grades I and II; however, the mortality for grade III was significantly higher (*P*<.02) than for the other two. Eleven of 59 deaths occurred after 5 years. The authors emphasized that the meaningful survival interval should be considered 10 or 15 years. No relationship between grade, age, gender, or location was found, and there was no statistical difference between primary and secondary chondrosarcomas. Adequacy of surgical removal was the main determinant of recurrence. In general, chondrosarcomas occurring during childhood have a worse prognosis than those of adult onset.[263]

In the largest reported series of chondrosarcomas from one institution, Bjornsson et al.[264] from the Mayo Clinic reported the experience and the clinicopathologic profiles of 344 patients with chondrosarcomas over 80 years. They analyzed the anatomic site, clinical history, and overall survival. Survival analysis was limited to 233 patients whose primary tumors were treated at the Mayo Clinic. The minimum follow-up was 5 years. The overall 5-year survival rate was 77%. Local recurrence developed in 19.7% of patients and metastatic lesions in 13.7%. The recurrence rate was higher for tumors of the shoulder and pelvis than for tumors of long bones. Histologic tumor grade was an important predictor of local recurrence and metastases.

In general, peripheral chondrosarcomas have a lower grade than central lesions. Gitelis et al.[265] reported that 43% of peripheral lesions, compared with 13% of central lesions, were grade I. The 10-year survival rate among those with peripheral lesions was 77% and among those with central lesions was 32%. Secondary chondrosarcomas arising from osteochondromas also have a low malignant potential. Eighty-five percent are grade I. Garrison et al.[46] reported that only 3% of 75 patients with secondary chondrosarcomas from an osteochondroma developed metastases, although 12% died of local recurrence. Ahmed et al.[266] described the largest reported series of secondary chondrosarcoma. The report included a total of 107 patients. Sixty-one of the secondary lesions occurred in patients with solitary osteochondromas and 47 in patients with multiple exostoses. The 5- and 10-year local recurrence rates after surgery were 15.9% and 17.5%, respectively. The 5- and 10-year mortality was 1.6% and 4.8%, respectively. Metastases developed in only five patients. Most of the deaths were caused by the sequelae of local recurrences.

TREATMENT. The treatment of chondrosarcomas is surgical removal.[263,267] No reports of effective adjuvant chemotherapy have been published. Resection guidelines for high-grade chondrosarcomas are similar to those for osteosarcoma. The shoulder and pelvic girdle are the most common sites for chondrosarcomas. This combined with the fact that chondrosarcomas tend to be low grade, make them amenable to limb-sparing procedures. Lesions of the ribs and sternum are treated by wide excision. Cryosurgery, a technique using liquid nitrogen after thorough curettage of the lesion, has been used for central, low-grade chondrosarcomas.[107,108] A few reports have been published of effective radiation therapy for axial chondrosarcomas and, more recently, encouraging reports using fractionated proton radiation therapy for the low-grade chondrosarcomas arising at the base of the skull.[268] The

Massachusetts General Hospital group report a 5-year local control rate of 82% and a 10-year local control rate of 58% among 28 patients with low-grade base of skull chondrosarcomas treated to approximately 69 CGE (cobalt-gray equivalent) using the proton beam. High-grade chondrosarcomas warrant consideration of adjuvant chemotherapy.[269]

Limb-Sparing Procedures: Specific Anatomic Sites

The four most common sites of chondrosarcomas are the pelvis, proximal femur, shoulder girdle, and diaphyseal portions of long bones. The unique characteristics of each are described in the following sections.

PELVIS. The pelvis consists of three areas: ilium, periacetabulum, and pubic rami. Each site can be resected independent of the others.[270] Resections are classified as type I (iliac wing), type II (acetabulum), or type III (pubic rami, pelvic floor). Bone scan most accurately determines specific bony involvement, whereas CT and MRI delineate the extraosseous component. Contraindications to resection are vascular (iliac artery and vein), peritoneal, and sacroiliac joint and/or sarcoplexus involvement (Fig. 35.2-14).

The retroperitoneal space is explored first to determine resectability. Type I resection is performed by a supraacetabular osteotomy and disarticulation of the sacroiliac joint. Type II resection may require removal of the femoral head; intraarticular involvement of the hip joint by tumor is evaluated by arthrotomy before the surgical plan is finalized. Type II and III resections require mobilization of the iliac vessels and femoral nerve. Care must be taken to protect these structures. Type III procedure requires mobilization of the bladder and urethra before resection. Bilateral pelvic floor resection can be used for chondrosarcomas arising from the midline of the symphysis pubis, in which case urethral resection and reconstruction may be required. Partial cystectomy may be necessary.

Long-term results of these procedures have been published by Enneking and Dunham,[16] who reported that local recurrence was only 4% if adequate margins were obtained. Function was nearly normal if the hip joint was preserved. If the hip joint was removed and fusion was obtained, results were good. A saddle prosthesis has been developed, permitting reconstruction after periacetabular resections.[270] Pelvic allograft combined with hip arthroplasty is an alternative technique of reconstruction. In general, this approach has had a high failure rate as a result of infection, fracture, and dislocation. Langlais et al.[271] reported the results of 13

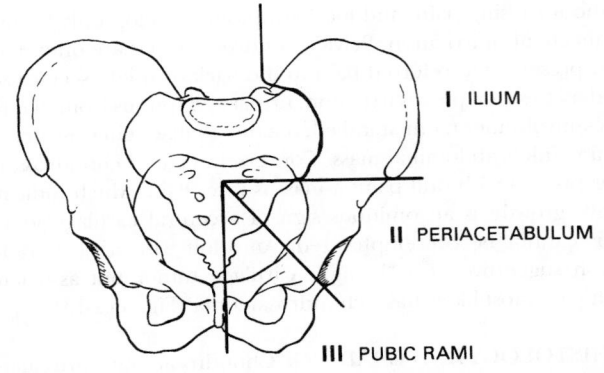

I ILIUM

II PERIACETABULUM

III PUBIC RAMI

FIGURE 35.2-14. Segmental resection for pelvic tumors.

patients treated by large pelvic allograft reconstruction combined with hip arthroplasty. The functional results were considered excellent in only two patients in whom the gluteal muscles were preserved. The mean MSTS rating was 56.4%. These authors reported follow-ups at 7, 8, 10, and 14 years. They concluded that reconstruction of the hemipelvis with allograft and arthroplasty is a demanding procedure that should be reserved for physically active patients who are in good general health and are expected to have a good response to chemotherapy.

Treatment of malignant tumors of the pelvis is one of the greatest challenges in musculoskeletal oncology. Kawai et al.[209] reviewed 102 patients with localized pelvic sarcomas who underwent surgical excision at Memorial Sloan-Kettering Cancer Center. Chondrosarcoma was the most common diagnosis. They evaluated the prognostic factors for local recurrence, metastasis, and survival. The 5-year survival rate for sarcomas of pelvic chondrosarcomas was 65%. An inadequate surgical margin was the only independent prognostic factor for local recurrence. For distant metastases, surgical stage (i.e., histologic grade and site) is an independent prognostic factor.

PROXIMAL FEMUR. Chondrosarcoma of the proximal femur can often be treated successfully by resection and prosthetic replacement. A lateral trephine or core biopsy is recommended. Care must be taken to avoid intraarticular, groin, or retrogluteal contamination. A posterior approach should be avoided because of potential contamination of the posterior flap in the event that a hemipelvectomy is required.

SHOULDER. The technique of resection of chondrosarcomas of the proximal humerus and scapula is similar to that described for osteosarcomas. In low-grade, intracompartmental (stage IA) tumors, preservation of the deltoid, rotator cuff musculature, and glenoid is possible, and alternatives for reconstruction are more variable. Endoprostheses, fibula autografts, and allografts all have a high rate of success.[19,109,272] Wittig et al.[203] have described a technique of intraarticular resection and reconstruction using a Gore-Tex sleeve as a new capsule. The use of Gore-Tex capsular reconstruction reduces the incidence of shoulder subluxation or dislocation reported for low-grade intraosseous chondrosarcomas or aggressive enchondromas. Mechanical burring combined with cryosurgery can obtain local control in all cases. Bony reconstruction with intramedullary fixation, combined with PMMA and autogenous bone graft, is required. This technique preserves the humerus and avoids resection and segmental reconstruction.

DIAPHYSEAL SEGMENTS OF THE TIBIA, FEMUR, AND HUMERUS. Central diaphyseal chondrosarcomas can be adequately treated by segmental resection without sacrificing the adjacent joint. Because the ends of the bones are not involved, function is excellent. Reconstruction is performed by allografts or autografts combined with internal fixation.

CRYOSURGERY. Marcove et al.[107,108] pioneered the technique of cryosurgery for bone tumors. This method involves thorough curettage and cryotherapy of the cavity with liquid nitrogen. With increasing experience, the indications were expanded to low-grade intramedullary cartilage tumors as well as to some high-grade lesions. With these indications, these authors have treated 30 chondrosarcomas with only one local

recurrence. The major advantages of cryosurgery are preservation of bone stock and the avoidance of resection.

Schreuder et al.[273] reported their experience with 26 benign and low-grade intramedullary chondrosarcomas treated with curettage and cryosurgery. Fourteen enchondromas and nine grade I chondrosarcomas were treated with curettage, cryosurgery, and bone grafting. After a follow-up of 26 months, no recurrences were observed. The most common complication was postoperative fracture (two cases). All bone grafts had incorporated, resulting in full weight-bearing capacity and excellent functional results. These authors emphasized that the preoperative assessment of these lesions is essential and that only low-grade cartilage tumors should be treated with a cryosurgical technique. Bickels et al.[274] have described the techniques of cryosurgery combined with internal fixation and cementation to avoid complications and to restore skeletal stability. Van Der Geest et al.[275] evaluated the functional capability and quality of life of patients treated for chondrosarcoma. The best functional results were obtained after bone graft reconstruction and cryosurgery.

Variants of Chondrosarcoma

CLEAR CELL CHONDROSARCOMA. Clear cell chondrosarcoma, the rarest form of chondrosarcoma, is a slow-growing, locally recurrent tumor resembling a chondroblastoma but with some malignant potential.[276] It generally occurs in adults. The most difficult clinical problem of this entity is early recognition. It is often confused with chondroblastoma. Metastases occur only after multiple local recurrences. Primary treatment is wide excision. Systemic therapy is not required.

MESENCHYMAL CHONDROSARCOMA. Mesenchymal chondrosarcoma is a rare, aggressive variant of chondrosarcoma characterized by a biphasic histologic pattern (i.e., small, compact cells intermixed with islands of cartilaginous matrix).[277,278] It has a predilection for flat bones; long, tubular bones are rarely affected.[277] It tends to occur in younger individuals and has high rates of metastatic potential. Harwood et al.[278] reported that 8 of 17 patients died within 1 year of diagnosis. The 10-year survival rate is 28%. This entity responds favorably to radiotherapy. It is hypothesized that the round cell component, similar to other round cell sarcomas, is relatively radiosensitive. Treatment is surgical removal combined with adjuvant chemotherapy. Radiotherapy is recommended if the tumor cannot be completely removed.[279]

DEDIFFERENTIATED CHONDROSARCOMA. Approximately 10% of chondrosarcomas may be dedifferentiated into a fibrosarcoma or osteosarcoma.[7,47] This occurs in older individuals and is highly fatal. Surgical treatment is similar to that described for other high-grade sarcomas. Adjuvant therapy is warranted.

Radiation Therapy in the Treatment of Chondrosarcoma

Unresectable or inoperable chondrosarcomas arising within the axial skeleton and pelvic or shoulder girdle, or both, can be controlled, and in some cases cured, by radiation therapy. A unique situation is chondrosarcomas of the facial bones and skull, in which a combination of radiotherapy and surgery has been shown to be successful. For reasons that are unclear, chondrosarcoma has been considered resistant to radiotherapy by numerous authors. However, although its very infrequent use is undoubtedly appropriate, we would caution that this should not be confused with lack of efficacy. In particular, when it is used the circumstances are understandably adverse and not appropriate for comparison against more usual approaches to treatment such as margin-negative surgery. Indeed, it is in these very circumstances in which the selection criteria for radiotherapy apply, being almost always in situations in which adequate surgery is either not possible to accomplish or the patient is not suitable for surgery because of medical reasons. Alternatively, the functional and cosmetic circumstances may make it undesirable to proceed with the type of ablation needed to accomplish complete resection. Although chondrosarcomas have generally been considered radioresistant, data in fact exist from several sources to show that some of these lesions are radiocurable, although it is preferable if it can be combined with surgery.

The situations in which radiotherapy is used are divided into two general groups: those that can still be managed with surgery but in which margins are not adequate and radiotherapy can play a role as an adjuvant treatment or, alternatively, the situation in which surgery is not possible to accomplish for fear of major risk to life or function. For the latter the situation of skull base or pelvic lesions with neurovascular invasion are obvious examples, and in the former, cases can be managed with postoperative radiotherapy or with preoperative radiotherapy if inadequate margin surgery can be predicted beforehand. As with sarcomas of soft tissue, advantages and disadvantages of preoperative versus postoperative radiotherapy exist, with the predominant rationale for the preoperative approach resting on the advantage provided by smaller treatment volumes and lower doses of radiotherapy. Among 38 patients undergoing radical irradiation, with or without concurrent chemotherapy, at the Princess Margaret Hospital,[279] 5- and 10-year actuarial survival rates of 41% and 36%, respectively, were achieved. Median survival was 46 months. The best results, a 48% 5-year actuarial survival rate, were obtained in the group with favorable (well and moderately differentiated) histology. Conversely, for those with unfavorable (mesenchymal and poorly differentiated) histology, the 5-year survival rate was only 22%. Radical radiotherapy was defined as a minimum of 40 Gy in 4 or more weeks of megavoltage therapy. In the 38 patients treated, local recurrence developed in 17. The authors recommend 50 Gy in 4 weeks with treatment to the whole bone if possible and, if not, at least a 5-cm margin of normal bone. These authors noted tumor regression continued slowly for 2 to 3 years after therapy. Recently, a further cohort of 31 patients at Princess Margaret Hospital with primaries arising in the extracranial skeleton was reviewed. These patients were selected for radiotherapy because of high recurrence risk and because of locations where salvage treatment would be exceptionally difficult and were generally managed with conservation surgery in addition to adjuvant radiotherapy. Local recurrence alone manifested in four patients, of whom three had gross residual and one had microscopic residual disease after surgery. Of these, one was successfully salvaged and three had stable disease at last follow-up. Disease was controlled in all patients who initially presented with recurrence. Lung metastases developed in four patients, all of whom had grade II or III tumors. The authors believe that these confirmatory, although as yet unpublished, results justify an approach to chondrosarcoma for which resection remains the cornerstone

of treatment. If this cannot be accomplished with adequate margins, the addition of radiotherapy contributes to local control in patients at high risk for local failure.

GIANT CELL TUMOR OF BONE

GCT is an aggressive, locally recurrent tumor with a low metastatic potential.[280–283] It consists of spindle-shaped and ovoid cells uniformly interspersed with multinucleated giant cells. *Giant cell sarcoma of bone* is a term that refers to the *de novo*, malignant GCT, not the tumor that arises from the transformation of a GCT previously thought to be benign. These two lesions are separate clinical entities.

Clinical Characteristics

GCTs occur slightly more often in females than in males. Pain, mass, local tenderness, and decreased motion in the adjacent joint are the most common clinical symptoms. Eighty percent of GCTs in the long bones occur after skeletal maturity, and 75% of these develop around the knee joint.[3,55] An effusion or pathologic fracture, uncommon with other sarcomas, is common with GCTs. GCTs occasionally occur in the vertebrae (2% to 5%) and the sacrum (10%).[4]

Grading and Pathologic Characteristics

Jaffe[4] attempted to grade GCTs as grade I (completely benign), grade II (borderline), and grade III (frankly sarcomatous). In general, grades I and II do not correlate well with biologic behavior. The correlation is also poor between the histologic pattern and the tendency for recurrence or malignant transformation.[280–283] Nineteen percent to 25% of GCTs have some osteoid product.[165] When osteoid formation is noted, care must be exercised in differentiating a GCT from an osteosarcoma. Conversely, an osteosarcoma with giant cells may be misinterpreted as a benign GCT. No correlation has been found between osteoid formation and increased risk of recurrence or metastasis. Necrosis or hemorrhage is often noted. Neither has a relationship to malignant potential or local recurrence rate.[55]

Natural History and Malignancy

Although GCTs are rarely malignant *de novo* (2% to 8%),[280–283] they may undergo transformation and demonstrate malignant potential histologically and clinically after multiple local recurrences. Local recurrence of a GCT is determined by the adequacy of surgical removal rather than histologic grade. Between 8.6% and 22% of known GCTs become malignant after local recurrence.[280–283] This rate decreases to less than 10% if patients who have undergone radiotherapy are excluded from the series. Hutter et al.[281] noted that 40% of malignant GCTs were malignant at the first recurrence; the remainder had become malignant by the second or third recurrence. Thus, each recurrence increases the risk of malignant transformation of typical GCT, especially if the transformation occurs after radiation therapy.

It should be recognized that cases selected for radiotherapy may also be of adverse prognosis in the first instance and therefore statements about subsequent disease behavior in comparison to that following other treatment modalities may lack validity. It is also important to consider the physical properties of the radiotherapy equipment used for treatment and the high likelihood that cases from the older literature were treated with orthovoltage radiotherapy. Such kilovoltage beams, because of predominant radiation dose absorption by the photoelectric effect, have preferential absorption of radiotherapy dose compared to soft tissue, and the risk of bone injury, including malignant induction, is consequently much larger than with beams of megavoltage energy. Earlier, in Treatment Planning, we emphasized that bone tumors should not be treated with equipment of lower energy spectra (i.e., orthovoltage). Moreover, Feigenberg et al.,[284] in their review of the University of Florida experience and the world literature, were unable to find convincing evidence that megavoltage radiotherapy with modern techniques enhanced the small risk of secondary malignancy that exists after treatment of GCTs, whether or not radiotherapy was used. Their estimate was that the incidence after megavoltage radiotherapy was 0.6% in the megavoltage context, compared to 1% or greater in those patients who did not have prior radiotherapy.

Bertoni et al.[285] reviewed all the cases of primary and secondary malignant GCTs at the Rizzoli Institute. They reported only 17 patients, 5 with primary and 12 with secondary malignant GCTs. Half of the secondary GCTs occurred after radiation. This small number of malignant GCTs attests to the rarity of this entity. They defined a primary GCT as a high-grade sarcoma that arises side-to-side with a benign GCT. A secondary malignant GCT was defined as a high-grade sarcoma that arises at a previously treated GCT site. The mean age for the primary malignant GCT was 67 years; for the secondary malignant GCT group, it was 40 years. Patients in both age groups were older than those with the typical, benign GCT, which is between 20 and 30 years. They concluded that malignancy associated with GCTs is always high grade with a poor prognosis.

Radiographic and Clinical Evaluation

GCTs are eccentric lytic lesions without matrix production. They have poorly defined borders with a wide area of transition. They are juxtaepiphyseal with a metaphyseal component. Although the cortex is expanded and appears destroyed at surgery, it is usually found to be attenuated but intact. Periosteal elevation is rare; soft tissue extension is common.

Treatment

Treatment of GCT of bone is surgical removal. Resection is curative in 90% of these tumors,[280–283] whereas curettage, with or without bone grafts, has a recurrence rate of 40% to 75%.[286] Johnson and Dahlin[282] reported a recurrence rate of 29% within 1 year of curettage and of 54.1% within 5 years. O'Donnell et al.[287] reviewed the literature from 1970 to 1990 and reported an overall recurrence rate of approximately 40%.

Although *en bloc* excision offers a reliable cure, routine resection is not recommended.[287,288] Primary resection of a joint has a significant morbidity. It is recommended for GCT of the proximal radius and fibula, distal ulna, tubular bones of the hand and foot, coccyx, sacrum, and pelvic bones. Under certain situations, a curettage is reasonable. If the lesion heals, resection is avoided. In general, curettage does not rule out a later curative resection. Curettage is accomplished through a large cortical window, equal to the length of the bony defect, using mechanical curettage and a mechanical burr. This exten-

sive technique has been termed *curettage-resection* and has decreased the rate of local recurrence to approximately 15% to 25%. Bone graft and PMMA are used to reconstruct the surgical defect. Results of a Canadian multicenter study of 186 cases shows no difference in function, health status, or recurrence rate whether cement or bone graft was used after curettage.[289]

O'Donnell et al.[287] reviewed the experience at the Massachusetts General Hospital of 60 patients with GCTs treated by curettage and packing with PMMA. The overall rate of local recurrence was 25% (15 of 60 patients), occurring at an average of 4 years. Risk factors for local recurrence were pathologic fracture, stage III disease, anatomic site, and the use of adjuvant treatment. The distal radius and the proximal tibia had the highest rate of local recurrence: 50% (5 of 10 patients) and 28% (7 of 25 patients), respectively. These authors emphasized that adjuvant treatment with a high-speed burr or PMMA, or both, after curettage decreased the local recurrence rate from 42% (8 of 19 patients) to 17% (7 of 41 patients). They concluded that PMMA alone did not reduce the rate of local recurrence but that the use of a wide curettage combined with additional curettage with a high-speed burr is necessary.

Malawer et al.,[288] in a multicenter study of 100 cases of GCTs of the extremities (treated with wide curettage, high-speed burr, and either a single or double cycle of cryosurgery with liquid nitrogen), reported a local recurrence rate of 9% (9 of 100 patients). They used the direct-pour technique as described by Marcove et al.[106] Reconstruction of the surgical defect was performed with PMMA (combined with internal fixation in most cases). The secondary fracture rate was 5%. Only two patients required a secondary resection and prosthetic replacement. These authors recommend liquid nitrogen adjuvant after curettage in the treatment of GCTs.

Amputation is reserved for massive recurrence, malignant transformation, or infection. Because of the putative biologic propensity for malignant transformation, radiation is reserved for specific lesions, usually lesions of the spine that cause bone destruction in a confined area and can lead to spinal cord compression and severe deformity.[290] Thus, treatment of GCT of the vertebrae and sacrum must be individualized. A combination of surgical excision and cryosurgery or radiotherapy is required to eradicate the tumor and prevent neurologic impairment.

Cryosurgery

Cryosurgery has been used more successfully for GCTs than for any other type of bone tumor. Marcove et al.[106] developed the technique of cryosurgery because of the high recurrence rates after curettage and the significant risk of sarcomatous degeneration in GCTs treated by irradiation. They found cryosurgery effective in eradicating the tumor while preserving joint motion and avoiding resection or amputation. These authors reported a 17-year experience of 100 GCTs treated by thorough curettage and cryosurgery. They noted a recurrence rate of 16% in the first 50 cases and 2% in the following 50 cases. The major complications of cryosurgery are necrosis of the adjacent bones, which are liable to develop a late pathologic fracture, and delayed union. The rate of secondary pathologic fracture has been decreased by a combination of PMMA, augmentation, bone graft, internal fixation of the cavity, and postoperative use of a long-leg brace with a quadrilateral socket.[124,291] Persson and Wouters[292] have reported curettage with PMMA augmentation

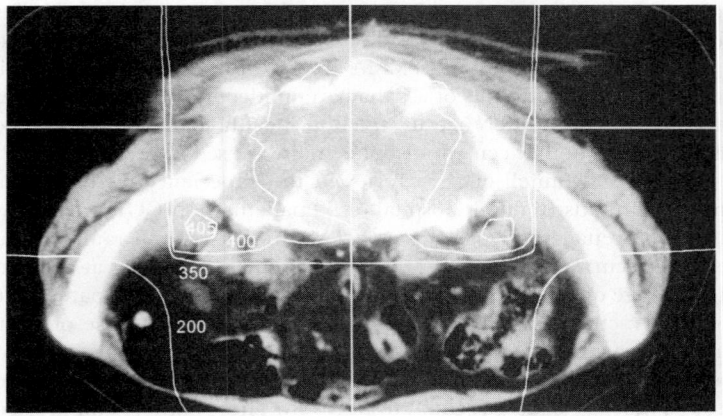
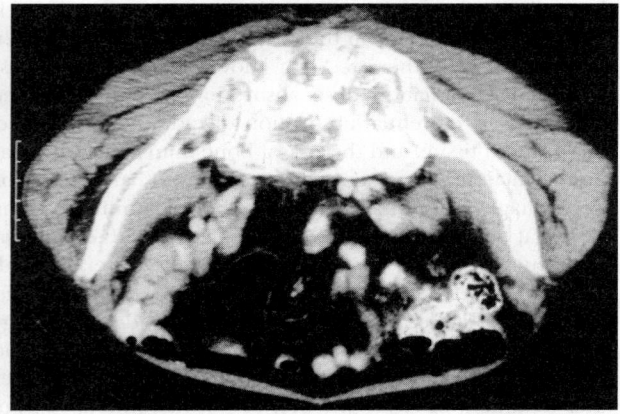

A   B

FIGURE 35.2-15. Recurrent cell tumor of the sacrum showing isodose distributions for a large lesion replacing the sacrum after surgery and grafting 12 months previously. **A:** Four-field computed tomography (CT)–based (a pair of opposed 14 × 17 cm and a second pair of opposed 16 × 17 cm fields) 6-mV photon technique to deliver 50 Gy in 25 fractions at the 400% isodose line as sole treatment for this extensive giant cell tumor (GCT) in a young woman. All four fields were treated at each daily session to maintain dose homogeneity throughout the volume at each session. At the time of presentation to the radiation oncologist (B. O'S.), this patient had severe saddle anesthesia, could not walk because of pain, and could only lie in the lateral decubitus position with extensive narcotic requirements for pain management. **B:** Axial CT images showing residual bone changes but marked resolution of GCT 10 years later. Approximately 12 months had elapsed before narcotics could be stopped and full ambulation resumed. The radiotherapy was tolerated, with minimal acute effects and no long-term sequelae with 13 years of follow-up at the time of writing. This patient is now entirely symptom free and continues annual follow-up. She represents one of the patients in the Princess Margaret Hospital series described in the text.

of the bony defect with bony necrosis due to the heat of polymerization. This technique may provide better local control than curettage alone.

Bickels et al.[274] reported 102 patients treated by curettage and cryosurgery at two institutions between 1983 and 1993. The surgical stage was I in 15 cases, II in 47 cases, and III in 40 cases. Sixteen percent of the patients had presented with local recurrences. The local recurrence rate among 86 patients treated primarily with cryosurgery was 2.3%. Six local recurrences occurred among 16 patients who were referred with recurrent disease. The overall recurrence rate was 7.9%. The most common complication was pathologic fracture (5.9%). No pathologic fractures occurred when internal fixation was used along with PMMA. This study emphasized that the overall function was good to excellent in 92% of the patients. All 102 patients were free of disease at final follow-up. Cryosurgery is a powerful physical adjunct to curettage in the treatment of GCTs of bone. Bickels et al. recommend routine use of cryosurgery for all GCTs of long bones, as well as for all aggressive benign and active bone tumors.

Giant Cell Tumors of the Sacrum

GCTs of the sacrum are difficult to treat. Patients often present with back pain, neurologic deficits, and rectal symptoms. The diagnosis is often delayed. CT, MRI, and bone scintigraphy are required for accurate local anatomic staging. Turcotte et al.[293] reviewed the treatment of 26 patients treated at the Mayo Clinic between 1960 and 1986 with an average follow-up of 7.8 years. Neurologic deficit was present in 88%. The local recurrence rate for patients treated by curettage was 33%. Twenty-one patients had radiation therapy; malignant transformation occurred in three. These authors suggested complete curettage for initial treatment. Radiation therapy is recommended for incomplete resection and

local recurrence (Fig. 35.2-15). Resection of the sacrum should be reserved for extensive recurrences. The technique of surgical resection of the sacrum is similar to the combined anterior and posterior approach described for chordomas. Cryosurgery has been used in conjunction with curettage in lieu of resections. Surprisingly, there is minimal effect on the "frozen" nerves in the operative field. Increased interest has been shown in sacral-sparing surgery, be it a combination of cryosurgery or newer techniques of radiation therapy. Although the doses of radiotherapy are usually modest and well tolerated, for example, 50 Gy in 25 fractions, it is likely that IMRT or other conformal or stereotactic approaches may be of use to minimize dose to nontarget structures.

Radiation Therapy

GCT is not radioresistant, as was once believed. Local control rates range from 75% to 85% in more recent series.[293–295] At Princess Margaret Hospital, local control was achieved in 13 of 14 patients with GCT treated with one course of megavoltage radiation. The disease in 12 patients was controlled for longer than 5 years without any malignant transformation.[294] These results have been updated with similar findings in an expanded series (n = 21) of patients selected with adverse prognosis. The only two local failures seen were subsequently salvaged, for an ultimate control rate of 100%. One of the two radiotherapy failures was a marginal failure and was subsequently salvaged with combined surgery and radiotherapy. No patient died of GCT. Radiotherapy was well tolerated, with no serious late toxicity. No cases of malignant transformation or radiation-induced cancer occurred.[296] Larsson et al.[290] reported three patients with GCT of the spine and sacrum treated by moderate doses of radiotherapy; all have done well. The specific indications for radiation include inoperable and incompletely resected lesions and lesions that occur locally despite definitive surgery. These situations are most likely to occur in the spine.[290] Doses of 35 to 50 Gy in 4.0 to 5.5 weeks using megavoltage equipment are recommended. After radiotherapy, slow radiographic resolution is common and may take many years. In some cases, bone reconstitution may never be complete.[297]

MALIGNANT FIBROUS HISTIOCYTOMA

MFH is a high-grade bone tumor that is histologically similar to its soft tissue counterpart.[6,53,54] It is a disease of adulthood. The most common sites are the metaphyseal ends of long bones, especially around the knee. AP values are normal. Pathologic fracture is common. Huvos[54] emphasized that a lytic metaphyseal lesion with a pathologic fracture in an adult with a normal SAP level suggests a primary MFH rather than an osteosarcoma or fibrosarcoma. MFH disseminates rapidly. Spanier et al.[6] reported that 9 of 11 patients died of the tumor. The average disease-free survival was 6 months. One-third of patients (three of nine) with pulmonary metastasis had lymph node dissemination. The author hypothesized that lymphatic spread was due to the histiocytic component of the tumor.

Radiographic Characteristics

MFH is an osteolytic lesion associated with marked cortical disruption, minimal cortical or periosteal reaction, and no evidence of matrix formation. The extent of the tumor routinely exceeds plain radiographic signs. McCarthy et al.,[53] reporting on 35 patients with MFH, noted that four tumors were multicentric and four were associated with bone infarcts.

Treatment

Today, MFH and osteosarcoma of bone are treated in much the same way. Data demonstrate that results of limb-sparing surgery for MFH of bone, as well as responses to chemotherapy among MFH patients, are very similar to those of patients with primary osteosarcoma. Picci et al.,[298] in the largest review to date, evaluated the effects of neoadjuvant chemotherapy of MFH of bone and extremity osteosarcomas. They reported 51 patients treated with high-grade MFH of bone and 390 patients with high-grade osteosarcoma treated with identical regimens of neoadjuvant chemotherapy at the Rizzoli Institute between 1982 and 1994. All tumors were located in the limbs. Preoperative chemotherapy was performed according to three successively activated regimens consisting of MTX and *cis*-diamminedichlorplatinum II (CDP): MTX/CDP intraarterially, MTX/CDP plus ADM, and MTX/CDP plus ADM and IFOS. Rates of limb salvage were approximately the same for MFH (92%) and osteosarcoma (85%). Although MFH showed a statistically significantly lower rate of good histologic response, the rate of tumor necrosis for MFH was 90% or more [27% vs. 67% for osteosarcoma (*P* <.001)] for all three regimens. Despite this low chemosensitivity, the disease-free survival rates for the two neoplasms were similar (67% vs. 65%). Nevertheless, the two tumors had similar prognoses when treated with chemotherapy regimens based on MTX, cisplatinum, ADM, and IFOS. The surgical procedures were similar limb-sparing procedures. This study emphasized that induction chemotherapy, followed by limb-sparing surgery and subsequent postoperative chemotherapy, was just as effective for MFH of bone as for the osteosarcomas.

Bacci et al.,[299,300] also from the Rizzoli Institute, reported on 65 patients treated with MFH of bone in the extremities with neoadjuvant chemotherapy. The limb-salvage rate was 89% (58 patients), and the amputation rate was 11% in seven patients. The histologic response to preoperative chemotherapy was good (90% or more tumor necrosis) in 16 patients (25%) and poor in 49 patients (75%). At a median follow-up of 7 years, 40 patients (62%) remained free of disease and 20 patients experienced relapse (18 metastases and 2 local recurrences followed by metastases). The rate of disease-free survival was significantly higher for patients who had a good response than for those who had a poor response (94% vs. 61%). Similarly, these authors concluded that a high percentage of patients with MFH of the extremities can be cured with neoadjuvant chemotherapy and that it is usually possible to avoid amputation. Bielack et al.[301] analyzed 125 patients with MFH of bone in a retrospective study of the European Musculoskeletal Oncology Society. Chemotherapy was used in 9 of 125 (7.2%) of the patients. The overall actuarial disease-free survival was 59%. In 22 of 66 patients in whom tumor response histologically was noted, there was a good (greater than 90%) response. Among these 23 patients, only 1 relapsed.

FIBROSARCOMA OF BONE

Clinical Characteristics

Fibrosarcoma of bone is a rare entity characterized by interlacing bundles of collagen fibers (herringbone pattern) without any evidence of tumor bone or osteoid formation.[52] Fibrosarcoma occurs in middle age. The long bones are most affected. Fifteen percent of tumors are found in the bones of the head and neck.[165] Fibrosarcomas occasionally arise in conjunction with an underlying disease, such as fibrous dysplasia, Paget's disease, bone infarcts, osteomyelitis, and postirradiation bone and GCT. Fibrosarcoma may be either central or cortical (periosteal). The histologic grade is a good prognosticator of metastatic potential. Huvos and Higinbotham[52] reported overall survival rates of 27% and 52% for central and peripheral lesions, respectively. Late metastases do occur, and 10- and 15-year survival rates vary. In general, periosteal tumors have a better prognosis than central lesions.

Radiographic Features

Fibrosarcoma is a radiolucent lesion that shows minimal periosteal and cortical reaction. The radiographic appearance closely correlates with the histologic grade of the tumor.[52] Low-grade tumors are well defined, whereas high-grade lesions demonstrate indistinct margins and bone destruction similar to those of osteolytic osteosarcoma. In general, plain radiographs underestimate the extent of the lesion. Pathologic fracture is common (30%) owing to the lack of matrix formation. Differential diagnosis includes GCT, aneurysmal bone cyst, MFH, and osteolytic osteosarcoma.[5,52]

Fibrosarcoma of bone is primarily managed surgically. Irradiation is recommended for inoperable tumors, for patients with postsurgical residual disease, and for palliation.

MALIGNANT HEMANGIOENDOTHELIOMA OF BONE

Malignant hemangioendothelioma of bone (also referred to as *epithelioid hemangioepithelioid sarcoma* or *histiocytoid hemangioma*) comprises only 0.5% to 1.0% of primary malignant bone tumors.[302–304] More than one-third of these lesions arise in the long, tubular bones, especially those of the lower extremity. Incidence peaks in the third decade of life, but the tumor can present at any age. Multicentric lesions are common. The treatment of choice has been surgery, often in combination with radiotherapy. In rare cases, radiotherapy has been the sole modality of treatment.[302–305] Radiation doses in the range of 50 to 60 Gy are associated with long-term local control.[305] Chemotherapy plays no significant role in treatment.

CHORDOMA

Chordoma is a rare neoplasm arising from notochordal remnants in the midline of the neural axis and involving the adjacent bone. The ends of the spine are the most common sites. The sacrococcus and the base of the skull (35%) near the sphenooccipital area are most commonly involved, accounting for 50% and 35%, respectively, of all chordomas.[165] Histologically, the physaliferous cell is pathognomonic. Large areas of syncytial strands of cells lying in a mass of mucus are typically present. Myxoid chondrosarcoma and metastatic carcinoma must be differentiated. This tumor is highly fatal because of the high rate of local recurrence and local complications.[306–308] Death is most commonly due to local disease. Gray et al.[308] reviewed 222 cases from the literature and noted that only two patients were disease free at 10 years. Average survival was 5.7 years. Mindell[307] emphasized that the main malignant potential of chordomas resides in their critical locations adjacent to important structures, their locally aggressive nature, and their extremely high rate of recurrence. Chordomas at the base of the skull are often described as chondroid chordomas. Patients with these lesions at this site tend to survive longer than those with the sacrococcygeal tumors. The most common complaint of patients with sacrococcygeal tumors is dull pain; constipation is an occasional symptom. Bladder and sensory loss are late complaints. Clinical suspicion is the key to early diagnosis. Rectal examination characteristically reveals a large presacral mass. Sphenooccipital tumors present with signs of cranial nerve or pituitary dysfunction, or both. CT and MRI are essential for accurate evaluation. Myelography is used to determine intraspinal extension. A transrectal biopsy should not be performed because of potential contamination. A small midline posterior incision or trocar biopsy is recommended.

Treatment

The first surgical procedure has the best chance of cure.[306,308] Inadequate surgery results in local recurrence, with little chance of subsequent surgical removal. Sacrococcygeal tumors are best removed by a combined abdominosacral approach, as described by Localio et al.[306] They emphasized wide excision of the sacrum one level higher than the lesion. A lateral position is used. The rectum can be controlled anteriorly. The rectum can be removed with the sacrum if necessary. Guterberg et al.[309] reported that if only one-half of the first sacral vertebra remains bilaterally, the pelvic girdle is still stable enough to allow immediate mobilization.

Radiation Therapy

Because local recurrence is common with chordomas, radiation therapy is an integral treatment modality, particularly for tumors of the base of the skull and sphenooccipital region. Results of conventional radiation therapy have been disappointing.

Amendola et al.[310] reported on 21 patients with a 5-year survival rate of 50% but a disappointing 10-year survival rate of only 20%. This is not surprising, because chordomas are relatively slow growing; in fact, long-term survival free of tumor regrowth over 10 years is relatively rare. Amendola et al. emphasized the importance of using CT in planning the radiation field, administering high radiation doses (i.e., 5500 to 7000 cGy with megavoltage equipment), and use of irradiation immediately after surgery to prolong local control, rather than reserving it until recurrence. The Massachusetts General Hospital experience of 48 patients is similar to that reported by others; the 5-year actuarial survival rate of all patients treated with radiotherapy was 50%.[311] Radiation doses varied from 4500 to 8040 cGy, but even with higher doses, the incidence of local recurrence was 45%. The Princess Margaret Hospital group investigated various fraction schedules in an effort to improve local control. With a median survival of 65 months, the authors concluded that external-beam radiation provided useful palliation but was rarely curative.[312,313]

SMALL ROUND CELL SARCOMAS OF BONE

Round cell sarcomas of bone behave differently than spindle cell sarcomas and require different therapeutic management.[314,315] These tumors consist of poorly differentiated small cells without matrix production. They present radiographically as osteolytic lesions. These lesions are best treated with radiation and chemotherapy; surgery is reserved for special situations. Non-Hodgkin's lymphoma and Ewing's sarcoma are the two most common small cell sarcomas. The differential diagnosis of all round cell sarcomas includes metastatic neuroblastoma, metastatic undifferentiated carcinoma, histiocytosis, small cell osteosarcoma, osteomyelitis, and multiple myeloma.

LYMPHOMAS OF BONE (DIFFUSE LARGE CELL LYMPHOMA)

Lymphoma of bone (previously called *reticulum cell sarcoma of bone*) accounts for only 5% of the primary bone tumors. In general, lymphoma presenting in bone is a sign of disseminated (stage IV) disease; occasionally, it may be a true solitary lesion defined as "involvement of single extralymphatic organ or site" (stage IE). Reimer et al.[314] at the National Cancer Institute reported that only 1 of 12 patients presenting with bone lymphomas had a true solitary lesion. Sweet et al.[315] from the University of Chicago reported that 50% of so-called solitary lesions were associated with disease elsewhere. Sweet et al. presented a useful algorithm for the evaluation and treatment of bone lymphomas. They emphasized that all patients with a presumed solitary lymphoma of bone should undergo a thorough evaluation for other involvement.[314,315]

Treatment is based on extent of disease. Stage IE lesions have traditionally been treated with radiotherapy, with a reported 90% cure rate. The role of surgery is limited to obtaining adequate tissue for diagnosis and treatment of pathologic fracture. The technique of biopsy is important to avoid secondary fracture through potentially irradiated bone. Biopsy for a suspected round cell tumor should always include a frozen section and additional material for electron microscopy, tissue culture, and immunophenotyping. Patients presenting with pathologic fractures require fixation. To prevent late fractures, all patients treated with radiotherapy should be protected with a brace until reossification occurs.

Radiation Therapy

Local control of the primary tumor with retention of good function of the affected part is commonly achieved after radiation therapy. Radiation therapy is administered to the entire bone and soft tissue extent with a dose of 4000 cGy and a boost to the original tumor area of 500 cGy. Regional lymph nodes should be included in the radiation port if they are adjacent to the area treated or if clinically involved. Mendenhall et al.[316] from the University of Florida achieved local and regional control in all irradiated sites among 21 patients with primary bone lymphomas. Two patients relapsed in apparently uninvolved regional lymph node sites that had not been included in the primary treatment portal.

Patients with lymphoma of the bone should be considered to have systemic disease; accordingly, they require chemotherapy. Patients treated with radiation and ADM-based chemotherapy have long-term survival in the 90% to 100% range. The Dana-Farber Cancer Institute reported 90% lymphoma-free survival at 8 years, with radiation and the ADM, prednisone, and vincristine (Oncovin) combination regimen.[317] Similarly, the Bone Tumor Center in Bologna, Italy, reported 88% disease-free survival at 7.5 years with radiation and ADM, vincristine, and cyclophosphamide.[318] Patients presenting with monostotic disease have a better outcome than those with polyostotic disease.[319,320] Although a randomized, controlled clinical trial testing radiation therapy and chemotherapy versus radiation therapy alone has not been performed, combined modality is commonly used in adults with primary and non-Hodgkin's lymphoma of the bone.[321,322]

REFERENCES

1. Landis SH, Murray T, Bolden S, Wingo PA. Cancer statistics, 1999. *CA Cancer J Clin* 1999;49:8.
2. Dahlin DC. *Bone tumors: general aspects and data on 6221 cases*, 3rd ed. Springfield: Charles C Thomas Publisher, 1978.
3. Lichtenstein L. *Bone tumors*, 5th ed. St. Louis: Mosby, Inc., 1977.
4. Jaffe H. *Tumors and tumorous conditions of the bone and joints*, 1st ed. Philadelphia: Lea & Febiger, 1958.
5. Wilner D. Fibrosarcoma. In: Wilner D, ed. *Radiology of bone tumors and allied disorders*. Philadelphia: Saunders, 1982:2291.
6. Spanier SS, Enneking WF, Enriquez P. Primary malignant fibrous histiocytoma of bone. *Cancer* 1975;36:2084.
7. Shives T. Chondrosarcoma and its variants. In: Sim FH, ed. *Diagnosis and treatment of bone tumors; a team approach. Mayo Clinic Monograph*. Thorofare, NJ: Slack, Inc.,1983:211.
8. Marcove RC. Chondrosarcoma: diagnosis and treatment. *Orthop Clin North Am* 1977;8:811.
9. Enneking WF, Spanier SS, Goodman MA. A system for the surgical staging of musculoskeletal sarcoma. *Clin Orthop* 1980;153:106.
10. Marcove RC, Rosen G. En bloc resections for osteogenic sarcoma. *Cancer* 1980;45:3040.
11. Malawer M. Distal femoral osteogenic sarcoma, principles of soft tissue resection and reconstruction in conjunction with prosthetic replacement. In: Chao E, ed. *Design and application of tumor prosthesis for bone and joint reconstruction*. New York: Thieme-Stratton Publisher, 1983:297.
12. Marcove RC, Lewis MM, Rosen G, Huvos AG. Total femur and total knee replacement. A preliminary report. *Clin Orthop* 1977;126:147.
13. Weisenburger TH, Eilber FR, Grant TT, et al. Multidisciplinary "limb salvage" treatment of soft tissue and skeletal sarcomas. *Int J Radiat Oncol Biol Phys* 1981;7:1495.
14. Eilber FR, Morton DL, Ekardt J, Grant T, Weisenburger T. Limb salvage for skeletal and soft tissue sarcomas. Multidisciplinary preoperative therapy. *Cancer* 1984;53:2579.
15. Enneking WF. A system for functional evaluation of the surgical management of musculoskeletal tumors. In: Enneking WF, ed. *Limb sparing surgery for musculoskeletal tumors*. New York: Churchill Livingstone, 1987:5.
16. Enneking WF, Dunham WK. Resection and reconstruction for primary neoplasms involving the innominate bone. *J Bone Joint Surg Am* 1978;60:731.
17. Mankin HJ, Fogelson FS, Thrasher AZ, Jaffer F. Massive resection and allograft transplantation in the treatment of malignant bone tumors. *N Engl J Med* 1976;294:1247.
18. Watts HG. Introduction to resection of musculoskeletal sarcomas. *Clin Orthop* 1980;153:31.
19. Chao E, Ivins JC, eds. *Design and application of tumor prosthesis for bone and joint reconstruction—the design and application*. New York: Thieme-Stratton, 1983.
20. Sim FH, Bowman W, Chao E. Limb salvage surgery and reconstructive techniques. In: Sim FH, ed. *Diagnosis and treatment of bone tumors: a team approach. A Mayo Clinic Monograph*. Thorofare, NJ: Slack, Inc.,1983.
21. Destouet JM, Gilula LA, Murphy WA. Computed tomography of long-bone osteosarcoma. *Radiology* 1979;131:439.
22. deSantos LA, Bernardino ME, Murray JA. Computed tomography in the evaluation of osteosarcoma: experience with 25 cases. *AJR Am J Roentgenol* 1979;132:535.
23. McKillop JH, Etcubanas E, Goris ML. The indications for and limitations of bone scintigraphy in osteogenic sarcoma: a review of 55 patients. *Cancer* 1981;48:1133.
24. Bacci G, Picci P, Calderoni P, Figus E, Borghi A. Full-lung tomograms and bone scanning in the initial work-up of patients with osteogenic sarcoma. A review of 126 cases. *Eur J Cancer Clin Oncol* 1982;18:967.
25. Cortes EP, Holland JF, Glidewell O. Amputation and adriamycin in primary osteosarcoma. *N Engl J Med* 1974;291:998.
26. Bohndorf K, Reiser M, Lochner B, Feaux de Lacroix W, Steinbrich W. Magnetic resonance imaging of primary tumours and tumour-like lesions of bone. *Skeletal Radiol* 1986;15:511.
27. Cohen MD, Weetman RM, Provisor AJ, et al. Efficacy of magnetic resonance imaging in 139 children with tumors. *Arch Surg* 1986;121:522.
28. Turner DA. Nuclear magnetic resonance in oncology. *Semin Nucl Med* 1985;15:210.
29. Zimmer WD, Berquist TH, McLeod RA, et al. Bone tumors: magnetic resonance imaging versus computed tomography. *Radiology* 1985;155:709.
30. Powers JA. Magnetic resonance imaging in marrow diseases. *Clin Orthop* 1986;206:79.
31. Sundaram M, McGuire MH, Herbold DR. Magnetic resonance imaging of osteosarcoma. *Skeletal Radiol* 1987;16:23.
32. Rosen G, Marcove RC, Caparros B, et al., Primary osteogenic sarcoma: the rationale for preoperative chemotherapy and delayed surgery. *Cancer* 1979;43:2163.
33. Rosen G, Caparros B, Huvos AG, et al. Preoperative chemotherapy for osteogenic sarcoma: selection of postoperative adjuvant chemotherapy based on the response of the primary tumor to preoperative chemotherapy. *Cancer* 1982;49:1221.
34. Muggia F, Catani R, Lee Y. Factor responsible for therapeutic success in osteosarcoma. In: *Adjuvant therapy for cancer*. Jones S, Salmon S, eds. New York: Grune & Stratton, 1979.
35. Cortes EP, Holland JF. Adjuvant chemotherapy for primary osteogenic sarcoma. *Surg Clin North Am* 1981;61:1391.
36. Link M. Adjuvant therapy in the treatment of osteosarcoma. In: *Important advances in oncology*. DeVita V, Hellman S, Rosenberg S, eds. Philadelphia: JB Lippincott Co.,1986:193.
37. Eilber F, Giuliana A, Eckardt J, et al. Adjuvant chemotherapy for osteosarcoma: a randomized prospective trial. *J Clin Oncol* 1987;5:21.
38. Edmonson JH, Creagan ET, Gilchrist GS. Phase II study of high-dose methotrexate in patients with unresectable metastatic osteosarcoma. *Cancer Treat Rep* 1981;65:538.
39. Dahlin DC. The problems in assessment of new treatment regimens of osteosarcoma. *Clin Orthop* 1980;153:81.
40. Goorin AM, Perez-Atayde A, Gebhardt M, et al. Weekly high-dose methotrexate and doxorubicin for osteosarcoma: the Dana-Farber Cancer Institute/the Children's Hospital—study III. *J Clin Oncol* 1987;5:1178.
41. Ettinger LJ, Douglass HO Jr, Mindell ER, et al. Adjuvant adriamycin and cisplatin in newly diagnosed, nonmetastatic osteosarcoma of the extremity. *J Clin Oncol* 1986;4:353.
42. Rosen G, Marcove RC, Huvos AG, et al. Primary osteogenic sarcoma: eight-year experience with adjuvant chemotherapy. *J Cancer Res Clin Oncol* 1983;106[Suppl]:55.
43. Winkler K, Beron G, Delling G, et al. Neoadjuvant chemotherapy of osteosarcoma: results of a randomized cooperative trial (COSS-82) with salvage chemotherapy based on histological tumor response. *J Clin Oncol* 1988;6:329.
44. Winkler K, Beron G, Kotz R, et al. Neoadjuvant chemotherapy for osteogenic sarcoma: results of a Cooperative German/Austrian study. *J Clin Oncol* 1984;2:617.
45. Lichtenstein L. Classification of primary tumors of bone. *Cancer* 1951;4:335.
46. Garrison RC, Unni KK, McLeod RA, Pritchard DJ, Dahlin DC. Chondrosarcoma arising in osteochondroma. *Cancer* 1982;49:1890.
47. Spjut H, et al. *Tumors of bone and cartilage- Atlas of Tumor Pathology Fasc. 5*, 2nd ed. Washington, DC: Armed Forces Institute of Pathology, 1971.
48. Merryweather R, Middlemiss JH, Sanerkin NG. Malignant transformation of osteoblastoma. *J Bone Joint Surg Br* 1980;62:381.
49. Dahlin DC, Unni KK. Osteosarcoma of bone and its important recognizable varieties. *Am J Surg Pathol* 1977;1:61.
50. Ahuja SC, Villacin AB, Smith J, et al. Juxtacortical (parosteal) osteogenic sarcoma: histological grading and prognosis. *J Bone Joint Surg Am* 1977;59:632.
51. Unni KK, Dahlin DC, Beabout JW, Ivins JC. Parosteal osteogenic sarcoma. *Cancer* 1976;37:2466.
52. Huvos AG, Higinbotham NL. Primary fibrosarcoma of bone. A clinicopathologic study of 130 patients. *Cancer* 1975;35:837.
53. McCarthy EF, Matsuno T, Dorfman HD. Malignant fibrous histiocytoma of bone: a study of 35 cases. *Hum Pathol* 1979;10:57.
54. Huvos AG. Primary malignant fibrous histiocytoma of bone; clinicopathologic study of 18 patients. *N Y State J Med* 1976;76:552.
55. Goldenberg RR, Campbell CJ, Bonfiglio M. Giant-cell tumor of bone. An analysis of two hundred and eighteen cases. *J Bone Joint Surg Am* 1970;52:619.
56. Johnson EJ, Dahlin DC. Treatment of giant cell tumor of bone: an evaluation of 24 cases treated at the Johns Hopkins Hospital between 1925-1955. *Clin Orthop* 1969;62:187.

57. Madewell JE, Ragsdale BD, Sweet DE. Radiologic and pathologic analysis of solitary bone lesions. Part I: internal margins. *Radiol Clin North Am* 1981;19:715.

58. Johnson L. A general theory of bone tumors. *Bull N Y Acad Med* 1953;19:164.

59. Lodwick G. The bone and joints. In: *Atlas of tumor radiology*. Chicago: Year Book Medical Publishers, 1971.

60. Enneking WF. *Musculoskeletal tumor surgery* Vol. 1. New York: Churchill Livingstone, 1983.

61. Enneking WF, Spanier SS, Malawer MM. The effect of the anatomic setting on the results of surgical procedures for soft parts sarcoma of the thigh. *Cancer* 1981;47:1005.

62. Weingrad DN, Rosenberg SA. Early lymphatic spread of osteogenic and soft-tissue sarcomas. *Surgery* 1978;84:231.

63. Tobias JD, Pratt CB, Parham DM, Green AA, Rao B. The significance of calcified regional lymph nodes at the time of diagnosis of osteosarcoma. *Orthopedics* 1985;8:49.

64. Jeffree GM, Price CH, Sissons HA. The metastatic patterns of osteosarcoma. *Br J Cancer* 1975;32:87.

65. McKenna R, et al. Sarcoma of the osteogenic series arising in abnormal bone: an analysis of 552 cases. *J Bone Joint Surg Am* 1966;48:1.

66. Marcove RC, Mike V, Hajek JV, Levin AG, Hutter RV. Osteogenic sarcoma under the age of twenty-one. A review of one hundred and forty-five operative cases. *J Bone Joint Surg Am* 1970;52:411.

67. Sweetnam R. The surgical management of primary osteosarcoma. *Clin Orthop* 1975;111:57.

68. Kager L, Zoubek A, Potschger U, et al. Primary metastatic osteosarcoma: presentation and outcome of patients treated on neoadjuvant Cooperative Osteosarcoma Study Group protocols. *J Clin Oncol* 2003;21:2011.

69. Goldstein H, McNeil BJ, Zufall E, Jaffe N, Treves S. Changing indications for bone scintigraphy in patients with osteosarcoma. *Radiology* 1980;135:177.

70. Giuliano AE, Feig S, Eilber FR. Changing metastatic patterns of osteosarcoma. *Cancer* 1984;54:2160.

71. Jaffe N, Smith E, Abelson HT, Frei E 3rd. Osteogenic sarcoma: alterations in the pattern of pulmonary metastases with adjuvant chemotherapy. *J Clin Oncol* 1983;1:251.

72. Enneking WF. Intramarrow spread of osteosarcoma. In: Enneking WF, ed. *Management of primary bone and soft tissue tumors*. Chicago: Year Book Medical Publishers, 1976.

73. Malawer MM, Dunham WK. Skip metastases in osteosarcoma: recent experience. *J Surg Oncol* 1983;22:236.

74. Wuisman P, Enneking WF. [Staging of osteosarcoma with skip metastases]. *Z Orthop Ihre Grenzgeb* 1990;128:457.

75. Simon MA, Enneking WF. The management of soft-tissue sarcomas of the extremities. *J Bone Joint Surg Am* 1976;58:317.

76. Campanacci M, Bacci G, Bertoni F, et al. The treatment of osteosarcoma of the extremities: twenty year's experience at the Istituto Ortopedico Rizzoli. *Cancer* 1981;48:1569.

77. Greene FL, et al. Bone. In: *AJCC cancer staging manual*. Greene FL, ed. New York: Springer, 2002;187.

78. Rosen G, Murphy ML, Huvos AG, Gutierrez M, Marcove RC. Chemotherapy, en bloc resection, and prosthetic bone replacement in the treatment of osteogenic sarcoma. *Cancer* 1976;37:1.

79. Easton E Jr, Powers JA. *Musculoskeletal magnetic resonance imaging*. Thorofare, NJ: Slack, Inc., 1986.

80. Pettersson H, Springfield D, Enneking WF. *Radiologic management of musculoskeletal tumors*. Philadelphia: Springer Publishers, 1999.

81. Levine E. Computed tomography of musculoskeletal tumors. *Crit Rev Diagn Imaging* 1981;16:279.

82. Rosenthal DI. Computed tomography in bone and soft tissue neoplasm: application and pathologic correlation. *Crit Rev Diagn Imaging* 1982;18:243.

83. Hudson TM, Haas G, Enneking WF, Hawkins IF Jr. Angiography in the management of musculoskeletal tumors. *Surg Gynecol Obstet* 1975;141:21.

84. Malawer MM, McHale KA. Limb-sparing surgery for high-grade malignant tumors of the proximal tibia. Surgical technique and a method of extensor mechanism reconstruction. *Clin Orthop* 1989;239:231.

85. Menendez LR, Fideler BM, Mirra J. Thallium-201 scanning for the evaluation of osteosarcoma and soft-tissue sarcoma. A study of the evaluation and predictability of the histological response to chemotherapy. *J Bone Joint Surg Am* 1993;75:526.

86. Rosen G, Loren GJ, Brien EW, et al. Serial thallium-201 scintigraphy in osteosarcoma. Correlation with tumor necrosis after preoperative chemotherapy. *Clin Orthop* 1993;293:302.

87. Goto Y, Ihara K, Kawauchi S, et al. Clinical significance of thallium-201 scintigraphy in bone and soft tissue sarcoma. *J Orthop Sci* 2002;7:304.

88. Brenner W, Bohuslavizki KH, Eary JF. PET imaging of osteosarcoma. *J Nucl Med* 2003;44:930.

89. Bloem JL, Taminiau AH, Eulderink F, Hermans J, Pauwels EK. Radiologic staging of primary bone sarcoma: MR imaging, scintigraphy, angiography, and CT correlated with pathologic examination. *Radiology* 1988;169:805.

90. Enneking WF. The issue of the biopsy. *J Bone Joint Surg Am* 1982;64:1119.

91. Mankin HJ, Lange TA, Spanier SS. The hazards of biopsy in patients with malignant primary bone and soft-tissue tumors. *J Bone Joint Surg Am* 1982;64:1121.

92. Ayala AG, Raymond AK, Ro JY, et al. Needle biopsy of primary bone lesions. M.D. Anderson experience. *Pathol Annu* 1989;24:219.

93. Jelinek JS, Murphey MD, Welker JA, et al. Diagnosis of primary bone tumors with image-guided percutaneous biopsy: experience with 110 tumors. *Radiology* 2002;223:731.

94. Hogeboom WR, Hoekstra HJ, Mooyaart EL, et al. Magnetic resonance imaging (MRI) in evaluating in vivo response to neoadjuvant chemotherapy for osteosarcomas of the extremities. *Eur J Surg Oncol* 1989;15:424.

95. Jaffe N, Knapp J, Chuang VP, et al. Osteosarcoma: intra-arterial treatment of the primary tumor with cis-diammine-dichloroplatinum II (CDP). Angiographic, pathologic, and pharmacologic studies. *Cancer* 1983;51:402.

96. Mail JT, Cohen MD, Mirkin LD, Provisor AJ. Response of osteosarcoma to preoperative intravenous high-dose methotrexate chemotherapy: CT evaluation. *AJR Am J Roentgenol* 1985;144:89.

97. Chuang VP, Benjamin R, Jaffe N, et al. Radiographic and angiographic changes in osteosarcoma after intraarterial chemotherapy. *AJR Am J Roentgenol* 1982;139:1065.

98. Smith J, Heelan RT, Huvos AG, et al. Radiographic changes in primary osteogenic sarcoma following intensive chemotherapy. Radiological-pathological correlation in 63 patients. *Radiology* 1982;143:355.

99. Carrasco CH, Charnsangavej C, Raymond AK, et al. Osteosarcoma: angiographic assessment of response to preoperative chemotherapy. *Radiology* 1989;170:839.

100. Sommer HJ, Knop J, Heise U, Winkler K, Delling G. Histomorphometric changes of osteosarcoma after chemotherapy. Correlation with 99mTc methylene diphosphonate functional imaging. *Cancer* 1987;59:252.

101. Holscher HC, van der Woude HJ, Hermans J, et al. Magnetic resonance relaxation times of normal tissue in the course of chemotherapy: a study in patients with bone sarcoma. *Skeletal Radiol* 1994;23:181.

102. Springfield D. Thallium-201 scanning for the evaluation of osteosarcoma and soft-tissue sarcoma. *J Bone Joint Surg Am* 1993;75:1880.

103. Lampreave JL, Benard F, Alavi A, Jimenez-Hoyuela J, Fraker D. PET evaluation of therapeutic limb perfusion in Merkel's cell carcinoma. *J Nucl Med* 1998;39:2087.

104. Hawkins DS, Rajendran JG, Conrad EU 3rd, Bruckner JD, Eary JF. Evaluation of chemotherapy response in pediatric bone sarcomas by [F-18]-fluorodeoxy-D-glucose positron emission tomography. *Cancer* 2002;94:3277.

105. Franzius C, Sciuk J, Brinkschmidt C, Jurgens H, Schober O. Evaluation of chemotherapy response in primary bone tumors with F-18 FDG positron emission tomography compared with histologically assessed tumor necrosis. *Clin Nucl Med* 2000;25:874.

106. Marcove RC, Lyden JP, Huvos AG, Bullough PB. Giant-cell tumors treated by cryosurgery. A report of twenty-five cases. *J Bone Joint Surg Am* 1973;55:1633.

107. Marcove RC, Stovell PB, Huvos AG, Bullough PG. The use of cryosurgery in the treatment of low and medium grade chondrosarcoma. A preliminary report. *Clin Orthop* 1977;122:147.

108. Marcove RC. A 17-year review of cryosurgery in the treatment of bone tumors. *Clin Orthop* 1982;163:231.

109. Enneking WF, Shirley PD. Resection-arthrodesis for malignant and potentially malignant lesions about the knee using an intramedullary rod and local bone grafts. *J Bone Joint Surg Am* 1977;59:223.

110. Brigman B. Allograft reconstructions in young patients with high-grade sarcomas about the knee. Presented at: American Academy of Orthopaedic Surgeons; February 13–17, 2002; Dallas, TX.

111. Makley JT, Krailo M, Ertel IJ. The relationship of various aspects of surgical management to outcome in childhood nonmetastatic osteosarcoma: a report from the Childrens Cancer Study Group. *J Pediatr Surg* 1988;23:146.

112. Malawer MM, Buch R, Khurana JS, Garvey T, Rice L. Postoperative infusional continuous regional analgesia. A technique for relief of postoperative pain following major extremity surgery. *Clin Orthop* 1991;266:227.

113. Henshaw RM, Kellar-Graney K, Levy NA. Regional postoperative analgesia via indwelling epineural catheters following major limb sparing resections and amputations: analysis of 166 patients. Connective Tissue Oncology Society; 2001; Washington, DC.

114. Rougraff BT, Simon MA, Kneisl JS, Greenberg DB, Mankin HJ. Limb salvage compared with amputation for osteosarcoma of the distal end of the femur. A long-term oncological, functional, and quality-of-life study. *J Bone Joint Surg Am* 1994;76:649.

115. Greenberg DB, Goorin A, Gebhardt MC, et al. Quality of life in osteosarcoma survivors[discussion]. *Oncology (Huntingt)* 1994;8:19.

116. Christ C, et al. Long term psychosocial adaptation of osteosarcoma survivors. *Oncology* 1993;335:1.

117. Nagarajan R, Neglia JP, Clohisy DR, et al. Education, employment, insurance, and marital status among 694 survivors of pediatric lower extremity bone tumors: a report from the childhood cancer survivor study. *Cancer* 2003;97:2554.

118. Bacci G, Ferrari S, Mercuri M, et al. Predictive factors for local recurrence in osteosarcoma: 540 patients with extremity tumors followed for minimum 2.5 years after neoadjuvant chemotherapy. *Acta Orthop Scand* 1998;69:230.

119. Ruggieri P, De Cristofaro R, Picci P, et al. Complications and surgical indications in 144 cases of nonmetastatic osteosarcoma of the extremities treated with neoadjuvant chemotherapy. *Clin Orthop* 1993;295:226.

120. Campanna R, et al. Intraepiphyseal resection of high grade bone sarcomas. In: *International Society of Limb Salvage*. 1995; Florence, Italy.

121. Henshaw RM, Jones V, Malawer M. Endoprosthetic reconstruction with the modular replacement system. Survival analysis of the first 100 implants with a minimum 2-year follow-up. In: *4th Combined meeting of the American and European musculoskeletal tumor societies*. 1998; Washington, DC.

122. Grimer RJ, Carter SR, Pynsent PB. The cost-effectiveness of limb salvage for bone tumours. *J Bone Joint Surg Br* 1997;79:558.

123. Malawer M, Baker A. Amputations for tumor. In: Evarts C, ed. *Surgery of the musculoskeletal system*. New York: Churchill Livingstone, 1990.

124. Malawer M, et al. The management of aggressive and low grade malignant bone tumors by cryosurgery: analysis of 40 consecutive cases. In: Enneking WF, ed. *Limb-sparing surgery for musculoskeletal tumors*. New York: Churchill Livingstone, 1987:498.

125. Friedman MA, Carter SK. The therapy of osteogenic sarcoma: current status and thoughts for the future. *J Surg Oncol* 1972;4:482.

126. Link MP, Goorin AM, Miser AW, et al. The effect of adjuvant chemotherapy on relapse-free survival in patients with osteosarcoma of the extremity. *N Engl J Med* 1986;314:1600.

127. Link MP, Goorin AM, Horowitz M, et al. Adjuvant chemotherapy of high-grade osteosarcoma of the extremity. Updated results of the Multi-Institutional Osteosarcoma Study. *Clin Orthop* 1991;270:8.

128. Goorin AM, Schwartzentruber DJ, Devidas M, et al. Presurgical chemotherapy compared with immediate surgery and adjuvant chemotherapy for nonmetastatic osteosarcoma: Pediatric Oncology Group Study POG-8651. *J Clin Oncol* 2003;21:1574.

129. Huvos AG, Rosen G, Marcove RC. Primary osteogenic sarcoma: pathologic aspects in 20 patients after treatment with chemotherapy en bloc resection, and prosthetic bone replacement. *Arch Pathol Lab Med* 1977;101:14.

130. Salzer-Kuntschik M, Delling G, Beron G, Sigmund R. Morphological grades of regression in osteosarcoma after polychemotherapy—study COSS 80. *J Cancer Res Clin Oncol* 1983;106[Suppl]:21.

131. Picci P, Bacci G, Campanacci M, et al. Histologic evaluation of necrosis in osteosarcoma induced by chemotherapy. Regional mapping of viable and nonviable tumor. *Cancer* 1985;56:1515.

132. Bacci G, Bertoni F, Longhi A, et al. Neoadjuvant chemotherapy for high-grade central osteosarcoma of the extremity. Histologic response to preoperative chemotherapy correlates with histologic subtype of the tumor. *Cancer* 2003;97:3068.

133. Bielack SS, Kempf-Bielack B, Delling G, et al. Prognostic factors in high-grade osteosarcoma of the extremities or trunk: an analysis of 1,702 patients treated on neoadjuvant cooperative osteosarcoma study group protocols. *J Clin Oncol* 2002;20:776.

134. Hauben EI, Weeden S, Pringle J, Van Marck EA, Hogendoorn PC. Does the histological subtype of high-grade central osteosarcoma influence the response to treatment with chemotherapy and does it affect overall survival? A study on 570 patients of two consecutive trials of the European Osteosarcoma Intergroup. *Eur J Cancer* 2002;38:1218.

135. Souhami RL, Craft AW, Van der Eijken JW, et al. Randomized trial of two regimens of chemotherapy in operable osteosarcoma: a study of the European Osteosarcoma Intergroup. *Lancet* 1997;350:911.

136. Meyers PA, Heller G, Healey J, et al. Chemotherapy for nonmetastatic osteogenic sarcoma: the Memorial Sloan-Kettering experience. *J Clin Oncol* 1992;10:5.

137. Bacci G, Ferrari S, Bertoni F, et al. Long-term outcome for patients with nonmetastatic osteosarcoma of the extremity treated at the Istituto Ortopedico Rizzoli according to the Istituto Ortopedico Rizzoli/osteosarcoma-2 protocol: an updated report. *J Clin Oncol* 2000;18:4016.

138. Saeter G, Alvegard TA, Elomaa I, et al. Treatment of osteosarcoma of the extremities with the T-10 protocol, with emphasis on the effects of preoperative chemotherapy with single-agent high-dose methotrexate: a Scandinavian Sarcoma Group study. *J Clin Oncol* 1991;9:1766.

139. Provisor AJ, Ettinger LJ, Nachman JB, et al. Treatment of nonmetastatic osteosarcoma of the extremity with preoperative and postoperative chemotherapy: a report from the Children's Cancer Group. *J Clin Oncol* 1997;15:76.

140. Harris MB, Gieser P, Goorin AM, et al. Treatment of metastatic osteosarcoma at diagnosis: a Pediatric Oncology Group Study. *J Clin Oncol* 1998;16:3641.

141. Meyers PA, Heller G, Healey JH, et al. Osteogenic sarcoma with clinically detectable metastasis at initial presentation. *J Clin Oncol* 1993;11:449.

142. Goorin AM, Harris MB, Bernstein M, et al. Phase II/III trial of etoposide and high-dose ifosfamide in newly diagnosed metastatic osteosarcoma: a Pediatric Oncology Group trial. *J Clin Oncol* 2002;20:426.

143. Saeter G, Hoie J, Stenwig AE, et al. Systemic relapse of patients with osteogenic sarcoma. Prognostic factors for long term survival. *Cancer* 1995;75:1084.

144. Duffaud F, Digue L, Mercier C, et al. Recurrences following primary osteosarcoma in adolescents and adults previously treated with chemotherapy. *Eur J Cancer* 2003;39:2050.

145. Tabone MD, Kalifa C, Rodary C, et al. Osteosarcoma recurrences in pediatric patients previously treated with intensive chemotherapy. *J Clin Oncol* 1994;12:2614.

146. Sauerbrey A, Bielack S, Kempf-Bielack B, et al. High-dose chemotherapy (HDC) and autologous hematopoietic stem cell transplantation (ASCT) as salvage therapy for relapsed osteosarcoma. *Bone Marrow Transplant* 2001;27:933.

147. Fagioli F, Aglietta M, Tienghi A, et al. High-dose chemotherapy in the treatment of relapsed osteosarcoma: an Italian sarcoma group study. *J Clin Oncol* 2002;20:2150.

148. Grenier MA, Lipshultz SE. Epidemiology of anthracycline cardiotoxicity in children and adults. *Semin Oncol* 1998;25(4 Suppl 10):72.

149. Nicholson HS, Mulvihill JJ, Byrne J. Late effects of therapy in adult survivors of osteosarcoma and Ewing's sarcoma. *Med Pediatr Oncol* 1992;20:6.

150. Pratt CB, Meyer WH, Luo X, et al. Second malignant neoplasms occurring in survivors of osteosarcoma. *Cancer* 1997;80:960.

151. Ling CC, Humm J, Larson S, et al. Towards multidimensional radiotherapy (MD-CRT): biological imaging and biological conformality. *Int J Radiat Oncol Biol Phys* 2000;47:551.

152. Adler JR Jr, Chang SD, Murphy MJ, et al., The Cyberknife: a frameless robotic system for radiosurgery. *Stereotact Funct Neurosurg* 1997;69:124.

153. Chang SD, Main W, Martin DP, Gibbs IC, Heilbrun MP. An analysis of the accuracy of the CyberKnife: a robotic frameless stereotactic radiosurgical system[discussion]. *Neurosurgery* 2003;52:140.

154. Ryu SI, Chang SD, Kim DH, et al. Image-guided hypo-fractionated stereotactic radiosurgery to spinal lesions. *Neurosurgery* 2001;49:838.

155. Koizumi M, Inoue T, Yamazaki H, et al. Perioperative fractionated high-dose rate brachytherapy for malignant bone and soft tissue tumors. *Int J Radiat Oncol Biol Phys* 1999;43:989.

156. Suit H. The Gray Lecture 2001: coming technical advances in radiation oncology. *Int J Radiat Oncol Biol Phys* 2002;53:798.

157. Li HG, Ma ZT, He Q. [Fast neutron treatment of osteosarcoma]. *Zhonghua Zhong Liu Za Zhi* 1994;16:199.

158. Carrie C, Breteau N, Negrier S, et al. The role of fast neutron therapy in unresectable pelvic osteosarcoma: preliminary report. *Med Pediatr Oncol* 1994;22:355.

159. Schwartz DL, Einck J, Bellon J, Laramore GE. Fast neutron radiotherapy for soft tissue and cartilaginous sarcomas at high risk for local recurrence. *Int J Radiat Oncol Biol Phys* 2001;50:449.

160. Kamada T, Tsujii H, Tsuji H, et al. Efficacy and safety of carbon ion radiotherapy in bone and soft tissue sarcomas. *J Clin Oncol* 2002;20:4466.

161. Dahlin DC, Coventry MB. Osteogenic sarcoma. A study of six hundred cases. *J Bone Joint Surg Am* 1967;49:101.

162. Stark A, Kreicbergs A, Nilsonne U, Silfversward C. The age of osteosarcoma patients is increasing. An epidemiological study of osteosarcoma in Sweden 1971 to 1984. *J Bone Joint Surg Br* 1990;72:89.

163. Richter MP, D'Angio GJ. The role of radiation therapy in the management of children with histiocytosis X. *Am J Pediatr Hematol Oncol* 1981;3:161.

164. Wick MR, Siegal GP, Unni KK, McLeod RA, Greditzer HG 3rd. Sarcomas of bone complicating osteitis deformans (Paget's disease): fifty years' experience. *Am J Surg Pathol* 1981;5:47.

165. Huvos A. *Bone tumors. Diagnosis, treatment, and prognosis.* Philadelphia: W.B. Saunders, 1979.

166. Greditzer HG 3rd, McLeod RA, Unni KK, Beabout JW. Bone sarcomas in Paget disease. *Radiology* 1983;146:327.

167. Francis KC, Kohn H, Malawer M. Osteogenic sarcoma. *J Bone Joint Surg Am* 1976;55:754.

168. Scranton PE Jr, DeCicco FA, Totten RS, Yunis EJ. Prognostic factors in osteosarcoma. A review of 20 year's experience at the University of Pittsburgh Health Center Hospitals. *Cancer* 1975;36:2179.

169. Wilner D. Osteogenic sarcoma (osteosarcoma). In: *Radiology of bone tumors and allied disorders.* Philadelphia: W.B. Saunders, 1982.

170. deSantos LA, Edeiken B. Purely lytic osteosarcoma. *Skeletal Radiol* 1982;9:1.

171. Brostrom LA. On the natural history of osteosarcoma. Aspects of diagnosis, prognosis and endocrinology. *Acta Orthop Scand Suppl* 1980;183:1.

172. Lockshin M, Higgins T. Prognosis in osteogenic sarcoma. *Int Orthop* 1981;5:305.

173. Larsson SE, et al. The prognosis in osteosarcoma. *Int Orthop* 1981;5:305.

174. Brostrom LA, Strander H, Nilsonne U. Survival in osteosarcoma in relation to tumor size and location. *Clin Orthop* 1982;167:250.

175. Hudson M, Jaffe MR, Jaffe N, et al. Pediatric osteosarcoma: therapeutic strategies, results, and prognostic factors derived from a 10-year experience. *J Clin Oncol* 1990;8:1988.

176. Baldini N, Scotlandi K, Barbanti-Brodano G, et al. Expression of P-glycoprotein in high-grade osteosarcomas in relation to clinical outcome. *N Engl J Med* 1995;333:380.

177. Bacci G, Picci P, Ferrari S, et al. Prognostic significance of serum alkaline phosphatase measurements in patients with osteosarcoma treated with adjuvant or neoadjuvant chemotherapy. *Cancer* 1993;71:1224.

178. Bacci G, Longhi A, Ferrari S, et al. Prognostic significance of serum alkaline phosphatase in osteosarcoma of the extremity treated with neoadjuvant chemotherapy: recent experience at Rizzoli Institute. *Oncol Rep* 2002;9:71.

179. Mark RJ, Poen J, Tran LM, et al. Postirradiation sarcomas. A single-institution study and review of the literature. *Cancer* 1994;73:2653.

180. Wong FL, Boice JD Jr, Abramson DH, et al. Cancer incidence after retinoblastoma. Radiation dose and sarcoma risk. *JAMA* 1997;278:1262.

181. Quesnel S, Verselis S, Portwine C, et al. p53 compound heterozygosity in a severely affected child with Li-Fraumeni syndrome. *Oncogene* 1999;18:3970.

182. Wang LL, Levy ML, Lewis RA, et al. Clinical manifestations in a cohort of 41 Rothmund-Thomson syndrome patients. *Am J Med Genet* 2001;102:11.

183. Wang LL, Gannavarapu A, Kozinetz CA, et al. Association between osteosarcoma and deleterious mutations in the RECQL4 gene in Rothmund-Thomson syndrome. *J Natl Cancer Inst* 2003;95:669.

184. Goto M, Miller RW, Ishikawa Y, Sugano H. Excess of rare cancers in Werner syndrome (adult progeria). *Cancer Epidemiol Biomarkers Prev* 1996;5:239.

185. Toguchida J, Yamaguchi T, Ritchie B, et al. Mutation spectrum of the p53 gene in bone and soft tissue sarcomas. *Cancer Res* 1992;52:6194.

186. Patino-Garcia A, Sierrasesumaga L. Analysis of the p16INK4 and TP53 tumor suppressor genes in bone sarcoma pediatric patients. *Cancer Genet Cytogenet* 1997;98:50.

187. Gokgoz N, Wunder JS, Mousses S, et al. Comparison of p53 mutations in patients with localized osteosarcoma and metastatic osteosarcoma. *Cancer* 2001;92:2181.

188. Feugeas O, Guriec N, Babin-Boilletot A, et al. Loss of heterozygosity of the RB gene is a poor prognostic factor in patients with osteosarcoma. *J Clin Oncol* 1996;14:467.

189. Entz-Werle N, Schneider A, Kalifa C, et al. Genetic alterations in primary osteosarcoma from 54 children and adolescents by targeted allelotyping. *Br J Cancer* 2003;88:1925.

190. Tsuchiya T, Sekine K, Hinohara S, et al. Analysis of the p16INK4, p14ARF, p15, TP53, and MDM2 genes and their prognostic implications in osteosarcoma and Ewing sarcoma. *Cancer Genet Cytogenet* 2000;120:91.

191. Helman LJ, Meltzer P. Mechanisms of sarcoma development. *Nat Rev Cancer* 2003;3:685.

192. Al-Romaih K, Bayani J, Vorobyova J, et al. Chromosomal instability in osteosarcoma and its association with centrosome abnormalities. *Cancer Genet Cytogenet* 2003;144:91.

193. Gisselsson D, Jonson T, Petersen A, et al. Telomere dysfunction triggers extensive DNA fragmentation and evolution of complex chromosome abnormalities in human malignant tumors. *Proc Natl Acad Sci U S A* 2001;98:12683.

194. Ulaner GA, Huang HY, Otero J, et al. Absence of a telomere maintenance mechanism as a favorable prognostic factor in patients with osteosarcoma. *Cancer Res* 2003;63:1759.

195. Bacci G, Avella M, Picci P, et al. Metastatic patterns in osteosarcoma. *Tumori* 1988;74:421.

196. Bacci G, Ferrari S, Bertoni F, et al. Histologic response of high-grade nonmetastatic osteosarcoma of the extremity to chemotherapy. *Clin Orthop* 2001;386:86.

197. Steadman P, Pritchard DJ, Larson D. Pathological fractures in osteosarcoma—a descriptive study 1977–1985. in International Symposium on Limb Salvage. Cairns, Australia, 1999.

198. Scully SP, Ghert MA, Zurakowski D, Thompson RC, Gebhardt MC. Pathologic fracture in osteosarcoma: prognostic importance and treatment implications. *J Bone Joint Surg Am* 2002;84-A:49.

199. Springfield DS, Schmidt R, Graham-Pole J, et al. Surgical treatment for osteosarcoma. *J Bone Joint Surg Am* 1988;70:1124.

200. Bacci G, Ferrari S, Longhi A, et al. High-grade osteosarcoma of the extremity: differences between localized and metastatic tumors at presentation. *J Pediatr Hematol Oncol* 2002;24:27.

201. Malawer MM, Meller I, Dunham WK. A new surgical classification system for shoulder-girdle resections. Analysis of 38 patients. *Clin Orthop* 1991;267:33.

202. Malawer MM, Sugarbaker PH, Lampert M, Baker AR, Gerber NL. The Tikhoff-Linberg procedure: report of ten patients and presentation of a modified technique for tumors of the proximal humerus. *Surgery* 1985;97:518.

203. Wittig JC, Bickels J, Kellar-Graney KL, Kim FH, Malawer MM. Osteosarcoma of the proximal humerus: long-term results with limb-sparing surgery. *Clin Orthop* 2002;397:156.

204. Wodajo F, et al. Reconstruction with scapular endoprostheses provides superior results after total scapular resection. In: *Musculoskeletal tumor society*. Toronto, Ontario Canada, 2002.

205. Bickels J, Wittig JC, Kollender Y, et al. Distal femur resection with endoprosthetic reconstruction: a long-term follow-up study. *Clin Orthop* 2002;400:225.

206. Malawer MM, Price WM. Gastrocnemius transposition flap in conjunction with limb-sparing surgery for primary bone sarcomas around the knee. *Plast Reconstr Surg* 1984;73:741.

207. Miller G. Opening remarks. In: Enneking WF, ed. *Limb sparing surgery for musculoskeletal tumors*. New York: Churchill Livingstone, 1987.

208. Fahey M, Spanier SS, Vander Griend RA. Osteosarcoma of the pelvis. A clinical and histopathological study of twenty-five patients. *J Bone Joint Surg Am* 1992;74:321.

209. Kawai A, Healey JH, Boland PJ, et al. Prognostic factors for patients with sarcomas of the pelvic bones. *Cancer* 1998;82:851.

210. Kawai A, Huvos AG, Meyers PA, Healey JH. Osteosarcoma of the pelvis. Oncologic results of 40 patients. *Clin Orthop* 1998;348:196.

211. Neel M, et al. Early experience with non-invasive expandable prosthesis for reconstruction following resection about the knee. In: *Musculoskeletal tumor society*. Toronto, Ontario Canada, 2002.

212. Martin NS, Williamson J. The role of surgery in the treatment of malignant tumours of the spine. *J Bone Joint Surg Br* 1970;52:227.

213. Sterner B. Total spondylectomy in chondrosarcoma arising in the seventh thoracic vertebrae. *J Bone Joint Surg Am* 1971;53B:278.

214. Sterner B, Johnson O. Complete removal of three vertebra for giant cell tumor. *J Bone Joint Surg Am* 1971;53B:278.

215. Estrada-Aguilar J, Greenberg H, Walling A, et al. Primary treatment of pelvic osteosarcoma. Report of five cases. *Cancer* 1992;69:1137.

216. Ozaki T, Flege S, Kevric M, et al. Osteosarcoma of the pelvis: experience of the Cooperative Osteosarcoma Study Group. *J Clin Oncol* 2003;21:334.

217. Franzius C, Schuck A, Bielack SS. High-dose samarium-153 ethylene diamine tetramethylene phosphonate: low toxicity of skeletal irradiation in patients with osteosarcoma and bone metastases. *J Clin Oncol* 2002;20:1953.

218. Marina NM, Pratt CB, Rao BN, Shema SJ, Meyer WH. Improved prognosis of children with osteosarcoma metastatic to the lung(s) at the time of diagnosis. *Cancer* 1992;70:2722.

219. Creagan ET, Frytak S, Pairolero P, Hahn RG, Muhm JR. Surgically proven pulmonary metastases not demonstrated by computed chest tomography. *Cancer Treat Rep* 1978;62:1404.

220. Telander RL, Pairolero PC, Pritchard DJ, Sim FH, Gilchrist GS. Resection of pulmonary metastatic osteogenic sarcoma in children. *Surgery* 1978;84:335.

221. Putnam JB Jr, Roth JA, Wesley MN, Johnston MR, Rosenberg SA. Survival following aggressive resection of pulmonary metastases from osteogenic sarcoma: analysis of prognostic factors. *Ann Thorac Surg* 1983;36:516.

222. Goorin AM, Delorey MJ, Lack EE, et al. Prognostic significance of complete surgical resection of pulmonary metastases in patients with osteogenic sarcoma: analysis of 32 patients. *J Clin Oncol* 1984;2:425.

223. Meyer WH, Schell MJ, Kumar AP, et al. Thoracotomy for pulmonary metastatic osteosarcoma. An analysis of prognostic indicators of survival. *Cancer* 1987;59:374.

224. Han MT, Telander RL, Pairolero PC, et al. Aggressive thoracotomy for pulmonary metastatic osteogenic sarcoma in children and young adolescents. *J Pediatr Surg* 1981;16:928.

225. MacEwen EG, Kurzman ID, Rosenthal RC, et al. Therapy for osteosarcoma in dogs with intravenous injection of liposome-encapsulated muramyl tripeptide. *J Natl Cancer Inst* 1989;81:935.

226. Kleinerman ES, Jia SF, Griffin J, et al. Phase II study of liposomal muramyl tripeptide in osteosarcoma: the cytokine cascade and monocyte activation following administration. *J Clin Oncol* 1992;10:1310.

227. Asano T, Kleinerman ES. Liposome-encapsulated MTP-PE: a novel biologic agent for cancer therapy. *J Immunother* 1993;14:286.

228. Kleinerman ES, Gano JB, Johnston DA, Benjamin RS, Jaffe N. Efficacy of liposomal muramyl tripeptide (CGP 19835A) in the treatment of relapsed osteosarcoma. *Am J Clin Oncol* 1995;18:93.

229. Meyers PA, et al. Addition of ifosfamide and muramyl tripeptide to cisplatin, doxorubicin and high-dose methotrexate improves event free survival (EFS) in localized osteosarcoma (OS). In: *Proceedings of the Annual Meeting of the American Society of Clinical Oncology*. 2001.

230. Strander H, Bauer HC, Brosjo O, et al. Long-term adjuvant interferon treatment of human osteosarcoma. A pilot study. *Acta Oncol* 1995;34:877.

231. Anderson PM, Markovic SN, Sloan JA, et al. Aerosol granulocyte macrophage-colony stimulating factor: a low toxicity, lung-specific biological therapy in patients with lung metastases. *Clin Cancer Res* 1999;5:2316.

231a. Onda M, et al. ErbB-2 expression is correlated with poor prognosis for patients with osteosarcoma. *Cancer* 1996;77(1):71.

231b. Gorlick R, Huvos AG, Heller G, et al. Expression of HER2/erbB-2 correlates with survival in osteosarcoma. *J Clin Oncol* 1999;17(9):2781.

231c. Zhou H, et al. Her-2/neu expression in osteosarcoma increases risk of lung metastasis and can be associated with gene amplification. *J Pediatr Hematol Oncol* 2003;25(1):27.

231d. Baselga J, Tripathy D, Mendelsohn J, et al. Phase II study of weekly intravenous recombinant humanized anti-p185HER2 monoclonal antibody in patients with HER-2/neu-overexpressing metastatic breast cancer. *J Clin Oncol* 1996;14(3):737.

231e. Pegram MD, Lipton A, Hayes DF, et al. Phase II study of receptor-enhanced chemosensitivity using recombinant humanized anti-p185 HER2/neu monoclonal antibody plus cisplatin in patient with HER2/neu-overexpressing metastatic breast cancer refractory to chemotherapy treatment. *J Clin Oncol* 1998;16:2659.

231f. Akatsuka T, et al. Loss of ErbB2 expression in pulmonary metastatic lesions in osteosarcoma. *Oncology* 2001;60(4):361.

231g. Thomas DG, et al. Absence of HER2/neu gene expression in osteosarcoma and skeletal Ewing's sarcoma. *Clin Cancer Res* 2002;8(3):788.

232. Cade S. Osteogenic sarcoma: a study based on 33 patients. *J R Coll Surg Edinb* 1955;1:79.

233. Lee E, Mackenzie D. Osteosarcoma: a study of the value of preoperative megavoltage radiotherapy. *Br J Surg* 1964;51:252.

234. Sweetnan R, Knowelden J, Seedon H. Bone sarcoma treatment by irradiation, amputation, or a combination of the two. *BMJ* 1969;2:363.

235. Phillips TL, Sheline GE. Radiation therapy of malignant bone tumors. *Radiology* 1969;92:1537.

236. Rab GT, Ivins JC, Childs DS Jr, Cupps RE, Pritchard DJ. Elective whole lung irradiation in the treatment of osteogenic sarcoma. *Cancer* 1976;38:939.

237. Burgers JM, van Glabbeke M, Busson A, et al. Osteosarcoma of the limbs. Report of the EORTC-SIOP 03 trial 20781 investigating the value of adjuvant treatment with chemotherapy and/or prophylactic lung irradiation. *Cancer* 1988;61:1024.

238. DeLaney TF, Park L, Goldberg SI, et al. Radiation therapy for local control of osteosarcoma. Proceedings of the 45th Annual ASTRO Meeting. *Int J Radiat Oncol Biol Phys* 2003;27[2 Supplement]:S449[abst 2180].

239. Machak GN, Tkachev SI, Solovyev YN, et al. Neoadjuvant chemotherapy and local radiotherapy for high-grade osteosarcoma of the extremities. *Mayo Clin Proc* 2003;78:147.

240. Jaffe N, et al. Pediatric osteosarcoma: can cure be achieved with chemotherapy (only) and elimination of surgery? *Proc Am Soc Clin Oncol* 1993;12;420:1443[abst].

241. Anderson PM, Wiseman GA, Dispenzieri A, et al. High-dose samarium-153 ethylene diamine tetramethylene phosphonate: low toxicity of skeletal irradiation in patients with osteosarcoma and bone metastases. *J Clin Oncol* 2002;20:189.

242. Bruland OS, Skretting A, Solheim OP, Aas M. Targeted radiotherapy of osteosarcoma using 153 Sm-EDTMP. A new promising approach. *Acta Oncol* 1996;35:381.

243. Ozaki T, Flege S, Liljenqvist U, et al. Osteosarcoma of the spine: experience of the Cooperative Osteosarcoma Study Group. *Cancer* 2002;94:1069.

244. Okada K, Frassica FJ, Sim FH, et al. Parosteal osteosarcoma. A clinicopathological study. *J Bone Joint Surg Am* 1994;76:366.

245. Jelinek JS, Murphey MD, Kransdorf MJ, et al. Parosteal osteosarcoma: value of MR imaging and CT in the prediction of histologic grade. *Radiology* 1996;201:837.

246. Schajowicz F, McGuire MH, Santini Araujo E, Muscolo DL, Gitelis S. Osteosarcomas arising on the surfaces of long bones. *J Bone Joint Surg Am* 1988;70:555.

247. Sim FH, Unni KK, Beabout JW, Dahlin DC. Osteosarcoma with small cells simulating Ewing's tumor. *J Bone Joint Surg Am* 1979;61:207.

248. Martin SE, Dwyer A, Kissane JM, Costa J. Small-cell osteosarcoma. *Cancer* 1982;50:990.

249. Devaney K, Vinh TN, Sweet DE. Small cell osteosarcoma of bone: an immunohistochemical study with differential diagnostic considerations. *Hum Pathol* 1993;24:1211.

250. Amendola BE, Amendola MA, McClatchey KD, Miller CH Jr. Radiation-associated sarcoma: a review of 23 patients with postradiation sarcoma over a 50-year period. *Am J Clin Oncol* 1989;12:411.

251. Le Vu B, de Vathaire F, Shamsaldin A, et al. Radiation dose, chemotherapy and risk of osteosarcoma after solid tumours during childhood. *Int J Cancer* 1998;77:370.

252. Huvos AG, Woodard HQ, Cahan WG, et al. Postradiation osteogenic sarcoma of bone and soft tissues. A clinicopathologic study of 66 patients. *Cancer* 1985;55:1244.

253. Tabone MD, Terrier P, Pacquement H, et al. Outcome of radiation-related osteosarcoma after treatment of childhood and adolescent cancer: a study of 23 cases. *J Clin Oncol* 1999;17:2789.

254. Marcove RC. *The surgery of tumors of bone and cartilage*, 2nd ed. New York: Grune & Stratton, 1984.

255. Pritchard DJ, Lunke RJ, Taylor WF, Dahlin DC, Medley BE. Chondrosarcoma: a clinicopathologic and statistical analysis. *Cancer* 1980;45:149.

256. Marcove RC, Mike V, Hutter RV, et al. Chondrosarcoma of the pelvis and upper end of the femur. An analysis of factors influencing survival time in one hundred and thirteen cases. *J Bone Joint Surg Am* 1972;54:561.

257. Sanerkin NG. The diagnosis and grading of chondrosarcoma of bone: a combined cytologic and histologic approach. *Cancer* 1980;45:582.

258. Mankin HJ, Cantley KP, Lippiello L, Schiller AL, Campbell CJ. The biology of human chondrosarcoma. I. Description of the cases, grading, and biochemical analyses. *J Bone Joint Surg Am* 1980;62:160.

259. Mankin HJ, Cantley KP, Lippiello L, Schiller AL, Campbell CJ. The biology of human chondrosarcoma. II. Variation in chemical composition among types and subtypes of benign and malignant cartilage tumors. *J Bone Joint Surg Am* 1980;62:176.

260. Sanerkin NG. Definitions of osteosarcoma, chondrosarcoma, and fibrosarcoma of bone. *Cancer* 1980;46:178.

261. Kreicbergs A, Boquist L, Borssen B, Larsson SE. Prognostic factors in chondrosarcoma: a comparative study of cellular DNA content and clinicopathologic features. *Cancer* 1982;50:577.

262. Edeiken J. Bone tumors and tumor-like conditions. In: Edeiken J, ed. *Roentgen diagnosis and disease of bone*. Baltimore: Williams and Wilkins, 1981:30.

263. Aprin H, Riseborough EJ, Hall JE. Chondrosarcoma in children and adolescents. *Clin Orthop* 1982;166:226.

264. Bjornsson J, McLeod RA, Unni KK, Ilstrup DM, Pritchard DJ. Primary chondrosarcoma of long bones and limb girdles. *Cancer* 1998;83:2105.

265. Gitelis S, Bertoni F, Picci P, Campanacci M. Chondrosarcoma of bone. The experience at the Istituto Ortopedico Rizzoli. *J Bone Joint Surg Am* 1981;63:1248.

266. Ahmed AR, Tan TS, Unni KK, et al. Secondary chondrosarcoma in osteochondroma: report of 107 patients. *Clin Orthop* 2003;411:193.

267. Steel HH. Partial or complete resection of the hemipelvis. An alternative to hindquarter amputation for periacetabular chondrosarcoma of the pelvis. *J Bone Joint Surg Am* 1978;60:719.

268. Austin-Seymour M, Munzenrider J, Goitein M, et al. Fractionated proton radiation therapy of chordoma and low-grade chondrosarcoma of the base of the skull. *J Neurosurg* 1989;70:13.

269. Scanlon PW. Split-dose radiotherapy for radioresistant bone and soft tissue sarcoma: ten years' experience. *Am J Roentgenol Radium Ther Nucl Med* 1972;114:544.

270. Aboulafia A, Faulks C, Li W. Reconstruction using the saddle prosthesis following excision of malignant periacetabular tumors. In: *International Society of Limb Salvage.* Montreal, Canada, 1991.

271. Langlais F, Lambotte JC, Thomazeau H. Long-term results of hemipelvis reconstruction with allografts. *Clin Orthop* 2001;388:178.

272. Francis K, Worcester JJ. Radical resection for tumors of the shoulder with preservation of a functional extremity. *J Bone Joint Surg Am* 1962;44:1423.

273. Schreuder HW, Pruszczynski M, Veth RP, Lemmens JA. Treatment of benign and low-grade malignant intramedullary chondroid tumours with curettage and cryosurgery. *Eur J Surg Oncol* 1998;24:120.

274. Bickels J, Meller I, Shmookler BM, Malawer MM. The role and biology of cryosurgery in the treatment of bone tumors. A review. *Acta Orthop Scand* 1999;70:308.

275. Van Der Geest IC, Servaes P, Schreuder HW, et al. Chondrosarcoma of bone: functional outcome and quality of life. *J Surg Oncol* 2002;81:70.

276. Unni KK, Dahlin DC, Beabout JW, Sim FH. Chondrosarcoma: clear-cell variant. A report of sixteen cases. *J Bone Joint Surg Am* 1976;58:676.

277. Huvos AG, Rosen G, Dabska M, Marcove RC. Mesenchymal chondrosarcoma. A clinico-pathologic analysis of 35 patients with emphasis on treatment. *Cancer* 1983;51:1230.

278. Harwood AR, Krajbich JI, Fornasier VL. Mesenchymal chondrosarcoma: a report of 17 cases. *Clin Orthop* 1981;158:144.

279. Krochak R, Harwood AR, Cummings BJ, Quirt IC. Results of radical radiation for chondrosarcoma of bone. *Radiother Oncol* 1983;1:109.

280. Dahlin DC, Cupps RE, Johnson EW Jr. Giant-cell tumor: a study of 195 cases. *Cancer* 1970;25:1061.

281. Hutter V, Worcester JJ, Francis K. Benign and malignant giant cell tumor of bone. A clinicopathological analysis of the natural history of the disease. *Cancer* 1962;15:653.

282. Johnson EJ, Dahlin DC. Treatment of giant cell tumor of bone. *J Bone Joint Surg Am* 1959;41:895.

283. Nascimento AG, Huvos AG, Marcove RC. Primary malignant giant cell tumor of bone: a study of eight cases and review of the literature. *Cancer* 1979;44:1393.

284. Feigenberg SJ, Marcus RB Jr, Zlotecki RA, et al. Radiation therapy for giant cell tumors of bone. *Clin Orthop* 2003;411:207.

285. Bertoni F, Bacchini P, Staals EL. Malignancy in giant cell tumor. *Skeletal Radiol* 2003;32:143.

286. Campanacci M, Giunti A, Olmi R. Giant cell tumors of bone: a study of 209 cases with long term follow-up in 130. *Ital J Orthop Traumatol* 1977;1:249.

287. O'Donnell RJ, Springfield DS, Motwani HK, et al. Recurrence of giant-cell tumors of the long bones after curettage and packing with cement. *J Bone Joint Surg Am* 1994;76:1827.

288. Malawer MM, Bickels J, Meller I, et al. Cryosurgery in the treatment of giant cell tumor. A long-term followup study. *Clin Orthop* 1999;359:176.

289. Turcotte RE, Wunder JS, Isler MH, et al. Giant cell tumor of long bone: a Canadian Sarcoma Group study. *Clin Orthop* 2002;397:248.

290. Larsson SE, Lorentzon R, Boquist L. Giant-cell tumors of the spine and sacrum causing neurological symptoms. *Clin Orthop* 1975;111:201.

291. Marcove RC, Weis LD, Vaghaiwalla MR, Pearson R. Cryosurgery in the treatment of giant cell tumors of bone: a report of 52 consecutive cases. *Clin Orthop* 1978;134:275.

292. Persson BM, Wouters HW. Curettage and acrylic cementation in surgery of giant cell tumors of bone. *Clin Orthop* 1976;00:125.

293. Turcotte RE, Sim FH, Unni KK. Giant cell tumor of the sacrum. *Clin Orthop* 1993;291:215.

294. Bell RS, Harwood AR, Goodman SB, Fornasier VL. Supervoltage radiotherapy in the treatment of difficult giant cell tumors of bone. *Clin Orthop* 1983;174:208.

295. Bennett CJ Jr, Marcus RB Jr, Million RR, Enneking WF. Radiation therapy for giant cell tumor of bone. *Int J Radiat Oncol Biol Phys* 1993;26:299.

296. Malone S, O'Sullivan B, Catton C, et al. Long-term follow-up of efficacy and safety of megavoltage radiotherapy in high-risk giant cell tumors of bone. *Int J Radiat Oncol Biol Phys* 1995;33:689.

297. Schwartz LH, Okunieff PG, Rosenberg A, Suit HD. Radiation therapy in the treatment of difficult giant cell tumors. *Int J Radiat Oncol Biol Phys* 1989;17:1085.

298. Picci P, Bacci G, Ferrari S, Mercuri M. Neoadjuvant chemotherapy in malignant fibrous histiocytoma of bone and in osteosarcoma located in the extremities: analogies and differences between the two tumors. *Ann Oncol* 1997;8:1107.

299. Bacci G, Springfield D, Capanna R, et al. Adjuvant chemotherapy for malignant fibrous histiocytoma in the femur and tibia. *J Bone Joint Surg Am* 1985;67:620.

300. Bacci G, Mercuri M, Ruggieri P, et al. Neoadjuvant chemotherapy for malignant fibrous histiocytoma of bone and for osteosarcoma of the limbs: a comparison between the results obtained for 21 and 144 patients, respectively, treated during the same period with the same chemotherapy protocol. *Chir Organi Mov* 1996;81:139.

301. Bielack SS, Schroeders A, Fuchs N, et al. Malignant fibrous histiocytoma of bone: a retrospective EMSOS study of 125 cases. European Musculo-Skeletal Oncology Society. *Acta Orthop Scand* 1999;70:353.

302. Larsson SE, Lorentzon R, Boquist L. Malignant hemangioendothelioma of bone. *J Bone Joint Surg Am* 1975;57:84.

303. Campanacci M, Boriani S, Giunti A. Hemangioendothelioma of bone: a study of 29 cases. *Cancer* 1980;46:804.

304. Wold LE, Unni KK, Beabout JW, et al. Hemangioendothelial sarcoma of bone. *Am J Surg Pathol* 1982;6:59.

305. Welles L, et al. Low grade malignant hemangioendothelioma of bone: a disease potentially curable with radiotherapy. *Med Pediatr Oncol* 1994;23:144.

306. Localio AS, Francis KC, Rossano PC. Abdominosacral resection of sacrococcygeal chordoma. *Ann Surg* 1980;166:394.

307. Mindell ER. Chordoma. *J Bone Joint Surg Am* 1981;63:501.

308. Gray SW, Singhabhandhu B, Smith RA, Skandalakis JE. Sacrococcygeal chordoma: report of a case and review of the literature. *Surgery* 1975;78:573.

309. Guterberg B, Romanus B, Sterner B. Pelvic strength after major amputation of the sacrum. *Acta Orthop Scand* 1976;47:635.

310. Amendola BE, Amendola MA, Oliver E, McClatchey KD. Chordoma: role of radiation therapy. *Radiology* 1986;158:839.

311. Rich TA, Schiller A, Suit HD, Mankin HJ. Clinical and pathologic review of 48 cases of chordoma. *Cancer* 1985;56:182.

312. Cummings BJ, Hodson DI, Bush RS. Chordoma: the results of megavoltage radiation therapy. *Int J Radiat Oncol Biol Phys* 1983;9:633.

313. Catton C, O'Sullivan B, Bell R, et al. Chordoma: long-term follow-up after radical photon irradiation. *Radiother Oncol* 1996;41:67.

314. Reimer RR, Chabner BA, Young RC, Reddick R, Johnson RE. Lymphoma presenting in bone: results of histopathology, staging, and therapy. *Ann Intern Med* 1977;87:50.

315. Sweet DL, Mass DP, Simon MA, Shapiro CM. Histiocytic lymphoma (reticulum-cell sarcoma) of bone. Current strategy for orthopaedic surgeons. *J Bone Joint Surg Am* 1981;63:79.

316. Mendenhall NP, Jones JJ, Kramer BS, et al. The management of primary lymphoma of bone. *Radiother Oncol* 1987;9:137.

317. Loeffler JS, Tarbell NJ, Kozakewich H, Cassady JR, Weinstein HJ. Primary lymphoma of bone in children: analysis of treatment results with adriamycin, prednisone, Oncovin (APO), and local radiation therapy. *J Clin Oncol* 1986;4:496.

318. Bacci G, Jaffe N, Emiliani E, et al. Therapy for primary non-Hodgkin's lymphoma of bone and a comparison of results with Ewing's sarcoma. Ten years' experience at the Istituto Ortopedico Rizzoli. *Cancer* 1986;57:1468.

319. Ferreri AJ, Reni M, Ceresoli GL, Villa E. Therapeutic management with adriamycin-containing chemotherapy and radiotherapy of monostotic and polyostotic primary non-Hodgkin's lymphoma of bone in adults. *Cancer Invest* 1998;16:554.

320. Rapoport AP, Constine LS, Packman CH, et al. Treatment of multifocal lymphoma of bone with intensified ProMACE-CytaBOM chemotherapy and involved field radiotherapy. *Am J Hematol* 1998;58:1.

321. Baar J, Burkes RL, Gospodarowicz M. Primary non-Hodgkin's lymphoma of bone. *Semin Oncol* 1999;26:270.

322. Christie DR, Barton MB, Bryant G, et al. Osteolymphoma (primary bone lymphoma): an Australian review of 70 cases. Australasian Radiation Oncology Lymphoma Group (AROLG). *Aust N Z J Med* 1999;29:214.

323. Goorin A, Delorey M, Lack E, et al. Prognostic significance of complete surgical resection of pulmonary metastases in patients with osteogenic sarcoma: analysis of 32 patients. *Clin Oncol* 1984;2:425.

324. Jaffe N, Frei E, Traggis D, Watts H. Adjuvant methotrexate and citrovorum factor treatment of osteogenic sarcoma. *N Engl J Med* 1974;291:994.

325. Rosenberg SA, Chabner BA, Young RC, et al. Treatment of osteogenic sarcoma. I. Effect of adjuvant high dose methotrexate after amputation. *Cancer Treat Rep* 1979;63:739.

326. Cortes EP, Holland JF, Wang JJ, et al. Amputation and Adriamycin in primary osteosarcoma. *N Engl J Med* 1974;291:998.

327. Cortes EP, Holland JP. Adjuvant chemotherapy for primary osteogenic sarcoma. *Surg Clin North Am* 1981;61:1391.

328. Cortes E, Necheles TF, Holland JF, et al. Adjuvant therapy of operable primary osteosarcoma: a Cancer and Leukemia Group B experience. In: Salmon S, Jones S, eds. *Adjuvant therapy of cancer,* vol 3. New York: Grune & Stratton, 1981:201.

329. Goorin A, Perez-Atayde A, Gebhardt M, et al. Weekly high-dose methotrexate and doxorubicin for osteosarcoma: the Dana Farber Cancer Institute/the Children's Hospital—study III. *J Clin Oncol* 1987;5:1178.

330. Sutow WW, Sullivan WP, Fernbach DJ, et al. Adjuvant chemotherapy in primary treatments of osteogenic sarcoma. A Southwest Oncology Group study. *Cancer* 1975;36:1598.

331. Sutow WW, Gehan EA, Dyment PG, et al. Multidrug adjuvant chemotherapy for osteosarcomas of the extremity: interim report of a Southwest Oncology Group study. *Cancer Treat Rep* 1978;62:265.

332. Herson J, Sutow WW, Elder K, et al. Adjuvant chemotherapy in nonmetastatic osteosarcoma: a Southwest Oncology Group study. *Med Pediatr Oncol* 1980;8:343.

333. Pratt CB, Champion JE, Fleming ID, et al. Adjuvant chemotherapy for osteosarcoma of the extremity. Long-term results of two consecutive prospective protocol studies. *Cancer* 1990;65:439.

334. Ettinger LJ, Douglas HO, Mindell ER, et al. Adjuvant Adriamycin and cisplatin in newly diagnosed, nonmetastatic osteosarcoma of the extremity. *J Clin Oncol* 1986;4:353.

335. Ettinger LJ, Douglass HO, Higby DJ, et al. Adjuvant Adriamycin and cis-diamminedichloroplatinum (cisplatinum) in primary osteosarcoma. *Cancer* 1981;47:248.

336. Edmonson JH, Green SJ, Ivins JC, et al. A controlled pilot study of high-dose methotrexate as post surgical adjuvant treatment for primary osteosarcoma. *J Clin Oncol* 1984;2:152.

337. Link MP, Goordin AM, Miser AW, et al. The effect of adjuvant chemotherapy on relapse-free survival in patients with osteosarcoma of the extremity. *N Engl J Med* 1986;314:1600.

338. Link MP, Shuster JJ, Goorin AM, et al. Adjuvant chemotherapy in the treatment of osteosarcoma: results of the Multi-Institutional Osteosarcoma Study. In: Ryan J, Baker LO, eds. *Recent concepts in sarcoma treatment.* Proceedings of the International Symposium on Sarcomas, Tarpon Springs, Florida, October 8–10, 1987. Dordrecht, The Netherlands: Kluwer Academic Publishers, 1988:283.

339. Link MP, Goorin AM, Horowitz M, et al. Adjuvant chemotherapy of high grade osteosarcoma of the extremity: updated results of the Multi-Institutional Osteosarcoma Study. *Clin Orthop* 1991;270:8.

340. Eilber F, Guiliano A, Eckardt J, et al. Adjuvant chemotherapy for osteosarcoma: a randomized prospective trial. *J Clin Oncol* 1987;5:21.

341. Breur K, Cohen P, Schweisguth O, Hart A. Irradiation of the lungs as an adjuvant therapy in the treatment of osteosarcoma of the limbs: an EORTC randomized study. *Eur J Cancer* 1978;14:461.

342. van der Scheuren E, Breur K. Role of lung irradiation in the adjuvant treatment of osteosarcoma. *Recent Results Cancer Res* 1982;80:98.

343. Rab GT, Ivins JC, Childs DS, Cupps RE, Pritchard DJ. Elective whole lung irradiation in the treatment of osteogenic sarcoma. *Cancer* 1976;38:939.

344. Rosen G, Marcove RC, Caparros B, et al. Primary osteogenic sarcoma. The rationale for preoperative chemotherapy and delayed survey. *Cancer* 1979;43:2163.

345. Rosen G, Murphy ML, Huvos AG, et al. Chemotherapy, en bloc resection and prosthetic replacement in the treatment of osteogenic sarcoma. *Cancer* 1976;37:1.

346. Rosen G, Marcove RC, Huvos AG, et al. Primary osteogenic sarcoma: 8-year experience with adjuvant chemotherapy. *J Cancer Res Clin Oncol* 1983;106[Suppl]:55.

347. Meyers PA, Heller G, Healey J, et al. Chemotherapy for non-metastatic osteogenic sarcoma: the Memorial Sloan Kettering experience. *J Clin Oncol* 1992;10:5.

348. Rosen G, Caparros B, Huvos AC, et al. Preoperative chemotherapy for osteogenic sarcoma: selection of postoperative adjuvant chemotherapy based upon the response of the primary tumor to preoperative chemotherapy. *Cancer* 1982;49:1221.

349. Winkler K, Beron G, Kotz R, et al. Neoadjuvant chemotherapy for osteogenic sarcoma. Results of a cooperative German/Austrian study. *J Clin Oncol* 1984;2:617.

350. Winkler K, Beron G, Kotz R, et al. Adjuvant chemotherapy in osteosarcoma effects of cisplatinum, BCD, and fibroblast interferon in sequential combination with HDMTX and Adriamycin. Preliminary results of the COSS 80 study. *J Cancer Res Clin Oncol* 1983;106[Suppl]:1.

351. Weiner M, Harris M, Lewis M, et al. Neoadjuvant high dose methotrexate, cisplatin, and doxorubicin for the management of patients with nonmetastatic osteosarcoma. *Cancer Treat Rep* 1986;70:1431.

352. Provisor AJ, Ettinger LJ, Nachman JB, et al. Treatment of nonmetastatic osteosarcoma of the extremity with preoperative and postoperative chemotherapy: a report from the Children's Cancer Group. *J Clin Oncol* 1997;15:76.

353. Winkler K, Beron G, Delling G, et al. Neoadjuvant chemotherapy of osteosarcoma: results of a randomized cooperative trial (COSS82) with salvage chemotherapy based on histological tumor response. *J Clin Oncol* 1988;6:329.

354. Bramwell VHC, Burgers M, Sneath R, et al. A comparison of two short intensive adjuvant chemotherapy regimens in operable osteosarcoma of limbs in children and young adults: the first study of the European Osteosarcoma Intergroup. *J Clin Oncol* 1992; 10:1579.

355. Bacci G, Picci P, Ruggieri P, et al. Primary chemotherapy and delayed surgery (neoadjuvant chemotherapy) for osteosarcoma of the extremities. The Instituto Rizzoli experience in 127 patients treated preoperatively with intravenous methotrexate (high versus moderate doses) and intraarterial cisplatin. *Cancer* 1990;65:2539.

356. Bacci G, Picci P, Ferrari S, et al. Primary chemotherapy and delayed surgery for nonmetastatic osteosarcoma of the extremities. Results in 164 patients preoperatively treated with high doses of methotrexate followed by cisplatin and doxorubicin. *Cancer* 1993;72:3227.

357. Hudson M, Jaffe MR, Jaffe N, et al. Pediatric osteosarcoma: therapeutic strategies, results and prognostic factors derived from a 10-year experience. *J Clin Oncol* 1990;8:1988.

358. Miser J, Arndt C, Smithson W, et al. Treatment of high grade osteosarcoma (OGS) with ifosamide (Ifos), MESNA, Adriamycin (ADR), and high dose methotrexate (HDMTX). *Proc Am Soc Clin Oncol* 1991;10:310.

359. Goorin A, Baker A, Gieser P, et al. No evidence for improved event-free survival [EFS] with presurgical chemotherapy [PRE] for non-metastatic extremity osteogenic sarcoma [OGS]: preliminary results of randomized Pediatric Oncology Group [POG] trial 8651. *Proc Am Soc Clin Oncol* 1995;14:444.

Harvey I. Pass   Stephen M. Hahn
Nicholas J. Vogelzang   Michele Carbone

CHAPTER **36**

Benign and Malignant Mesothelioma

Malignant mesotheliomas are highly aggressive neoplasms that arise primarily from the surface serosal cells of the pleural, peritoneal, and pericardial cavities. Epidemiologic studies have established that exposure to asbestos fibers is the primary cause of malignant mesothelioma,[1,2] and recent investigations have implicated simian virus 40 (SV40) and genetic predisposition in the etiology of some malignant mesotheliomas.[1–3] Malignant mesothelioma is characterized by a long latency from the time of exposure to asbestos to the onset of disease, suggesting that multiple somatic genetic events are required for tumorigenic conversion of a normal mesothelial cell (see Overview of Molecular Mechanisms in Mesothelioma, later in this chapter). Early evidence in support of this notion was provided by karyotypic analyses, which revealed multiple cytogenetic alterations in most human mesotheliomas (reviewed in ref. 2). Although a specific chromosomal change is not shared by all malignant mesotheliomas, several prominent sites of chromosomal loss have been identified in this malignancy. Tumor suppressor genes (TSGs) residing in these deleted chromosomal regions may be responsible for the tumorigenic conversion of mesothelial cells, and recent studies have begun to identify the specific TSGs that contribute to the development and progression of malignant mesothelioma. Here, the authors review the mechanistic role of asbestos and other potential etiologic factors, particularly SV40, and genetic predisposition in this malignancy.

MECHANISM OF ASBESTOS-INDUCED ONCOGENESIS

Presently, it is not known whether asbestos fibers act directly on mesothelial cells or indirectly via formation of reactive oxygen species and growth factors.[1,2] There are six types of asbestos: amosite, crocidolite, anthophyllite, actinolite, tremolite, and chrysotile.[2] The former five types are termed *amphibole asbestos*. Chrysotile, the latter type, is a nonamphibole mineral that has a different texture, composition, and pathogenic behavior than amphibole asbestos.[2] Numerous experimental models demonstrating asbestos carcinogenicity have been established in animals. As many as 80% of mesothelioma patients have been exposed to asbestos,[2] establishing an indisputable link between the asbestos and mesothelioma development. Although this link is well accepted, the exact proportion of mesotheliomas linked to asbestos exposure, the relative carcinogenicity of the various fiber types, a dose-response relationship, and the mechanism of its pathogenicity remain controversial.

EXPOSURE QUANTIFICATION

The proportion of mesotheliomas that are thought to be associated with asbestos varies in the literature from 16% to 90%.[4] Although this difference may reflect the distinct populations studied, it is more likely a result of the different methodologies used to determine exposure rates.[2] Rates determined by history are the most imprecise and appear to produce the greatest variation in results.[2] Even when exposure has been established in patients, such as in studies analyzing cohorts of asbestos workers, it is difficult to quantify the level of exposure by history.[5] Lung content analysis, in contrast to history, is a more reliable indicator of exposure because it allows the investigator to determine both the amount and type of exposure.[2] Nevertheless, these studies may also underestimate the number of chrysotile fibers that were originally deposited in the lungs, as chrysotile fibers, but not amphiboles, are cleared from the lungs.[6] Aside from lung content analysis, a number of studies have reported pleural fiber content, which may be most biologically relevant for mesothelioma development. As discussed by Smith and

Wright,[6] pleural content studies demonstrate that chrysotile fibers are the predominant fiber type found in the pleura of asbestos-exposed individuals.

ANIMAL MODELS OF ASBESTOS CARCINOGENICITY

Mesotheliomas and sarcomas are induced in a dose-dependent fashion after intrapleural and intraperitoneal injection of asbestos into animals.[7–10] Chronic inhalational studies are thought to be the best representation of asbestos carcinogenicity. Due to the cost of these experiments, very few have been performed.

ASBESTOS CARCINOGENICITY IN HUMANS

Although injection and inhalation studies in animals suggest that all forms of asbestos are equally carcinogenic and that there is a clear dose-response relationship between asbestos exposure and mesothelioma risk, epidemiologic studies in humans do not support these observations. Most human studies have indicated that amosite and crocidolite exposure carries a much greater risk than exposure to chrysotile,[2,11,12] but in fact chrysotile is frequently combined with tremolite, an amphibole, which may instead be responsible for mesothelioma development. It is possible that the discrepancy between chrysotile carcinogenicity in animals and humans is related to the types of exposure in each group. In animal studies, exposure is usually intense and over a short period, whereas humans tend to be exposed to asbestos in smaller concentrations over longer periods.

Overall, it is difficult to conclusively determine the relative carcinogenicities of different fiber types at this time. Results of lung content analysis studies, which are the most reliable indicators of exposure to date, are inconsistent. The question of whether different fiber types may act by different mechanisms to cause tumors is also unknown.

In humans, there is no clear dose-response curve to asbestos, and a threshold level below which mesotheliomas do not develop has not been determined, although it is generally accepted in the scientific community that background levels of exposure, such as those found in the lungs of almost all individuals, do not increase the risk of mesothelioma. It is estimated that less than 5% of asbestos miners exposed to high levels of asbestos develop mesotheliomas.[2] However, wives of some of these workers have developed mesotheliomas after they were presumably exposed to lower levels of asbestos compared to their husbands while washing their clothes.[13,14] Similarly, mesothelioma development commonly occurs in workers in occupations in which asbestos exposure is higher than in the general population but much lower than in asbestos miners. The carpenters, electricians, and construction workers who have developed mesotheliomas are a reflection of this.[15] These data suggest that high levels of exposure are not necessarily correlated with increased risk of malignancy compared to moderate asbestos exposure, arguing against a classic dose-response relationship.

MECHANISM OF ASBESTOS PATHOGENICITY

The mechanism of asbestos pathogenicity is not fully understood (reviewed in ref. 3). It is thought that when fibers reach the alveoli after inhalation, smaller fibers are phagocytized and efficiently removed from the lung. Larger fibers are not easily engulfed and can usually only be removed if solubilized. However, amphiboles are not soluble and thus remain in the lung. These fibers may eventually reach the pleura via the lymphatics or direct extension, where they may lead to pleural plaques, fibrosis, and mesothelioma. In the pleura, asbestos fibers may cause mutagenic changes through hydroxy radical and superoxide anion production during phagocytosis, leading to DNA strand breaks and deletions. In hamster cells, asbestos fibers can also mechanically interfere with mitotic segregation to alter chromosome morphology and ploidy as well as produce DNA strand breaks. In rat mesothelial cells, crocidolite asbestos was found to cause autophosphorylation of the epidermal growth factor (EGF) receptor, leading to stimulation of the extracellular regulated kinase cascade, increased AP-1 activity, and mitosis. Finally, it has been suggested that asbestos may also allow tumor development by stimulating macrophages to produce lymphokines and oxyradicals that depress immune function.[2] In short, how asbestos causes or contributes to mesothelioma development is still an enigma.

It is difficult to reconcile what is known about the carcinogenic actions of asbestos and the long latency period between asbestos exposure and mesothelioma development. Lanphear and Buncher[16] reviewed 21 studies of 1690 mesotheliomas and found that 96% occurred at least 20 years after exposure. The mean latency was 32 years. Several theories have been postulated to describe what happens during this period.[2] One theory suggests that malignant transformation of a mesothelial cell occurs soon after asbestos exposure and it then takes years for the tumor to grow. This is quite unlikely because malignant mesothelioma has no detectable preinvasive phase and is a rapidly growing tumor. A second hypothesis is that asbestos induces genetic alterations in mesothelial cells over a long period that eventually lead to a malignant cell. This may occur if a key regulatory gene, such as the INK4a/ARF locus, is deleted or silenced. With loss of key regulatory genes, additional mutations could accumulate rapidly. INK4a/ARF codes for p16 (a cyclin-dependent kinase inhibitor) and for p14ARF, which promotes MDM2 degradation, preventing MDM2 from neutralizing p53. Both p16 and p14ARF are often deleted in malignant mesotheliomas (see Alterations of Specific Tumor Suppressor Genes in Mesothelioma, later in this chapter). Occasionally, this process may allow enough mutations to accumulate and lead to malignancy. Cell growth from this point would be rapid, leading to a clinically detectable tumor.[2]

OVERVIEW OF MOLECULAR MECHANISMS IN MESOTHELIOMA

CYTOGENETIC ASSESSMENT OF MALIGNANT MESOTHELIOMAS

As previously mentioned, chromosome banding analyses have revealed that most malignant mesotheliomas have complex karyotypes. Deletions of specific chromosomal sites in the short (p) arms of chromosomes 1, 3, and 9 and long (q) arm of 6 are repeatedly observed in these tumors, and deletion mapping has defined the most common areas of abnormalities to occur at *1p22, 3p21, 6q14-q21, 6q16.6-q21, 6q21-q23.2* and *6q25, 9p21,* and *15q11.1-15.*[17] Loss of a copy of chromosome 22 is the single most consistent numerical change seen in malignant mesothelioma.

ALTERATIONS OF SPECIFIC TUMOR SUPPRESSOR GENES IN MESOTHELIOMA

p16

Cheng et al.[18] reported homozygous deletions of one or more of the three *p16* exons in 34 of 40 (85%) malignant mesothelioma cell lines and a point mutation in one cell line. Down-regulation of *p16* was observed in four of the remaining cell lines. Homozygous deletions of *p16* were identified in 5 of 23 (22%) malignant mesothelioma tumor samples. Down-regulation of *p16* in malignant mesothelioma cells may result from 5'CpG island hypermethylation, as has been demonstrated in other types of cancer, although this is not prominent in the mesothelioma methylation studies performed to date. Homozygous deletions at this locus, however, could in many cases also lead to the inactivation of another putative TSG, *p14^ARF* because *p16* and *p14^ARF* share exons 2 and 3, although their reading frames differ. These data could have translational impact as it has been reported that human mesothelioma cell lines and xenografts with wild-type p53 yet lacking p14(ARF) were successfully treated by ONYX-015 therapy or by p14(ARF) viral transfection.[19,20]

p53

Cell lines derived from murine models of asbestos-induced mesothelioma have reduced or absent expression of p53 messenger RNA (mRNA) compared to the RNA from nontumorigenic cell lines or reactive mesothelial cells.[21] In human cell lines derived from patients with malignant mesothelioma, attention has turned to specific mutations or genetic abnormalities in p53. In general, mutational analyses of p53 in mesothelioma have not revealed reasons for its inactivation. As detailed later in Simian Virus 40, a stronger candidate for such inactivation of p53 is SV40 large tumor antigen.

Wilms' Tumor Gene

The detection of Wilms' tumor gene (*WT1*) mRNA or protein provides a specific molecular or immunohistochemical marker for differentiation of mesothelioma from other pleural tumors, in particular, adenocarcinoma.[22]

Neurofibromatosis Gene

Mutations in the neurofibromatosis gene (*NF2*) coding region have been detected in 12 of 23 malignant mesothelioma cell lines,[23] and loss of heterozygosity analyses revealed that 72% of the lines showed losses at one or both of two polymorphic DNA markers residing at or near the *NF2* locus in chromosome 22q12. All cases exhibiting mutation or aberrant expression of *NF2*, or both, showed allelic losses, implying that inactivation of *NF2* in malignant mesothelioma occurs via a two-hit mechanism.

ALTERATIONS OF ONCOGENES IN MESOTHELIOMA

C-sis (Platelet-Derived Growth Factor)

Malignant mesothelioma cell lines produce numerous growth factors and cytokines, possibly as a consequence of altered oncogene status. One of the more intriguing oncogenes in malignant mesothelioma is C-sis, which codes for one of the two chains (α and β) of platelet-derived growth factor (PDGF).[24] Gerwin et al. were the first to describe elevation of RNA levels for both the α and β chains of PDGF in mesothelioma cell lines and correlated the increase with PDGF-like activity secreted by the cells.[25] It is of interest that overexpression of A chain transforms human mesothelial cells to the tumorigenic phenotype *in vitro* and that the use of antisense ODN to the A chain inhibits growth of mesothelioma cell lines.

Transforming Growth Factor

Transforming growth factor-β (TGF-β) is another growth-regulatory and immunomodulatory cytokine, and high levels of TGF-β have been described in several human and mouse malignant mesothelioma cell lines. TGF-β may have a potential role in regulation of the differential PDGF receptor expression in malignant mesothelioma and thus have an effect on proliferation as well as other events.

Insulin Growth Factor

Insulin growth factor (IGF) is another of the important autocrine loops in mesothelioma.[26] In humans, both normal mesothelium and mesothelioma cell lines express IGF-1 and IGF-1R RNAs (by Northern blot or reverse transcriptase polymerase chain reaction), and IGF-1 protein is detected in their conditioned media. These studies suggest that mesothelioma growth, both in human and animal models for the disease, may involve the IGFs.[27]

ANGIOGENIC MECHANISMS IN MESOTHELIOMA

The most relevant cytokines and growth factors in angiogenic pathways involve the interleukins (specifically IL-6 and IL-8), fibroblast growth factors (FGFs), vascular endothelial growth factors (VEGFs), platelet-derived endothelial growth factors, and IGFs. Moreover, mutational or posttranslational silencing of TSGs or their products, particularly p53 and p16, have also been associated with increased angiogenic mechanisms.

IL-6 levels are elevated in the serum and pleural effusions of patients with mesothelioma, and there have been correlations seen between the IL-6 level and the degree of thrombocytosis in these patients.[28] IL-6 expression is elevated in tissues undergoing angiogenesis, but by itself it has a limited role in proliferation of endothelial cells. IL-6, however, induces angiogenesis by elevating the expression of VEGF, a specific mitogen for vascular endothelial cells.[29] Serum VEGF and IL-6 levels are elevated in patients with mesothelioma, and their levels each correlate with platelet count.[28]

IL-8 is also an important angiogenic factor for the development of new capillaries *in vivo* and has direct growth-potentiating activity in mesothelioma. Pleural fluid from patients with mesothelioma have significantly higher IL-8 levels by enzyme-linked immunosorbent assay compared to patients with other malignant effusions.[30]

Mesotheliomas present with a high intratumoral vessel density that also has prognostic relevance,[31–33] and, immunohistochemically, VEGF, FGF-1 and -2, and TGF-β immunoreactivity are present in 81%, 67%, 92%, and 96% of mesotheliomas, and in 20%, 50%, 40%, and 10% of samples of the non-neoplastic mesothelium, respectively. Depending on the study, high immunohistochemical FGF-2 expression[33] or VEGF expression by reverse transcriptase polymerase chain reaction correlate with more tumor aggressiveness and worse prognosis for mesothelioma.[31]

SIMIAN VIRUS 40

SV40 is a DNA tumor virus that has been associated with the development of malignant mesothelioma.[2,3] Although this virus is endogenous in rhesus monkeys, epidemiologic studies have shown that it is widespread among the human population. The modes by which the virus was transferred from monkey to human are uncertain, but it is possible that the bulk of this transfer may have occurred from 1954 to 1963 through SV40-contaminated poliovaccines administered worldwide.[3] This mode alone does not fully explain the transfer, however, as many humans who could not have received those contaminated vaccines are infected with the virus.

Once inside of its host, SV40 produces two proteins associated with its oncogenesis, the large and small t antigens.[2,34] The large T antigen (Tag) is a 90-kD protein found predominantly in the nucleus of infected cells that is capable of inducing structural and numerical chromosomal alterations. Tag also induces IGF expression, inhibits p53 and the pRB family, and induces c-met activity to stimulate cell proliferation.[3,34] The small t antigen (tag) is a 17-kD protein found in the cytoplasm of infected cells where it inhibits cellular phosphatase 2A and stimulates microtubule-associated protein (MAP) kinase and AP-1 activity. The small tag also works with Tag to bind and inhibit p53 and pRB.[3] The combined activity of both the large Tag and the small tag induce Notch-1 and telomerase activity, which are required for malignant transformation and immortalization.[35,36]

Analysis of human mesotheliomas for the virus revealed that SV40 sequences were present in 29 of 48 (60%) of human mesothelioma samples. Sequence analysis confirmed that the virus detected was SV40.[37] Since this study, several other laboratories, as well as a multilaboratory study sponsored by the International Mesothelioma Interest Group (IMIG), confirmed that SV40 sequences were present in human mesotheliomas.[3,34] Although more than 60 laboratories have found SV40 in human mesotheliomas and other tumors, the virus was not detected in Finnish, Austrian, and Turkish mesothelioma specimens.[2,3,34] This suggests that the presence of SV40 in human tumors may be influenced by geographic factors. One of these factors may be related to poliovaccine distribution, as SV40-contaminated poliovaccines were not administered in Finland, Austria, and Turkey.[2,3] Three independent panels have reviewed and confirmed the association of SV40 with human tumors, especially mesothelioma.[38–40]

Overall, substantial evidence exists supporting a role for SV40 in mesothelioma pathogenesis. SV40 is present in human mesotheliomas, where it is specifically found in the tumor cells and not in the normal surrounding tissues. Within these tumor cells, SV40 binds and inactivates essential TSG products, including p53 and pRB, and stimulates met, Notch-1, and telomerase activity (Fig. 36-1). Moreover, SV40 causes promoter methylation and thus inactivation of the tumor suppressor RASSF1A, which causes a more aggressive tumor phenotype.[41] In animals, SV40 is a potent carcinogen, causing mesotheliomas in 100% of hamsters after intrapleural injection. SV40 is

closely related to the human polyomaviruses JCV and BKV, which also inhibit p53 and Rb.

Several arguments about the precise role of SV40 in the pathogenesis of all mesotheliomas remain, however. First, the possible impact of SV40 on the overall mesothelioma incidence has not been determined. This has been limited by the fact that studies comparing mesothelioma incidence in SV40-infected cohorts versus noninfected cohorts are unreliable, as it appears to be impossible to identify infected and uninfected cohorts.[40] Second, the majority of mesotheliomas develop in those who have been exposed to asbestos, some of whom are SV40 negative. It may be difficult to separate the effect of SV40 and asbestos in individuals exposed to both carcinogens. Third, SV40-infected mesothelial cells should express viral antigens that would be an easy target for the immune system. Why they would not be eliminated before tumor development is unclear, but the immunosuppressive effects of asbestos may play a role. Fourth, SV40 was not found in mesotheliomas in certain countries,[3] and it is not found in all U.S. mesotheliomas, indicating that, similarly to asbestos, it is not always necessary for mesothelioma development.

It is unlikely that SV40 acts alone in mesothelioma development (see Fig. 36-1 for a working model of how SV40 and asbestos may cooperate to cause mesothelioma), as most cancers are multifactorial, and most mesotheliomas occur in asbestos-exposed individuals. Instead, it seems more likely that asbestos and SV40 may act as co-carcinogens in the development of some mesotheliomas.

RADIATION AND MESOTHELIOMA

In the literature, there are a few studies reporting mesothelioma development in patients exposed to thorotrast (intravenously) or who had received radiation to the chest and abdomen.[2] In some of these cases, asbestos exposure could not be ruled out, and SV40 status was not investigated. However, in a few cases in which mesotheliomas developed in young adults who received radiotherapy because of Wilms' tumor, radiation was the only likely causative factor. Studies in rats support a role for radiation as a causative factor. Although it appears that radiation may cause mesotheliomas, the number of mesotheliomas for which it is responsible is probably small.

GENETIC PREDISPOSITION TO MESOTHELIOMA

Recent evidence indicates that genetic predisposition plays an important role in determining individual susceptibility to mineral fiber carcinogenesis and to the development of mesothelioma. In the villages of Karain (population, ~600), Tuzkoy (population, ~1400), and Sarihidir (this village was abandoned) in Cappadocia, a region in Central Anatolia, Turkey, 50% or more of deaths are caused by malignant mesothelioma.[42–46] Erionite is a type of fibrous zeolite commonly found in the stones of the houses of Karain, Sarihidir, and Tuzkoy.[2,46–48] When erionite was injected intrapleurally into animals, it caused mesothelioma,[49] and it was concluded that erionite was the cause of mesothelioma in these villages.[46,47,50]

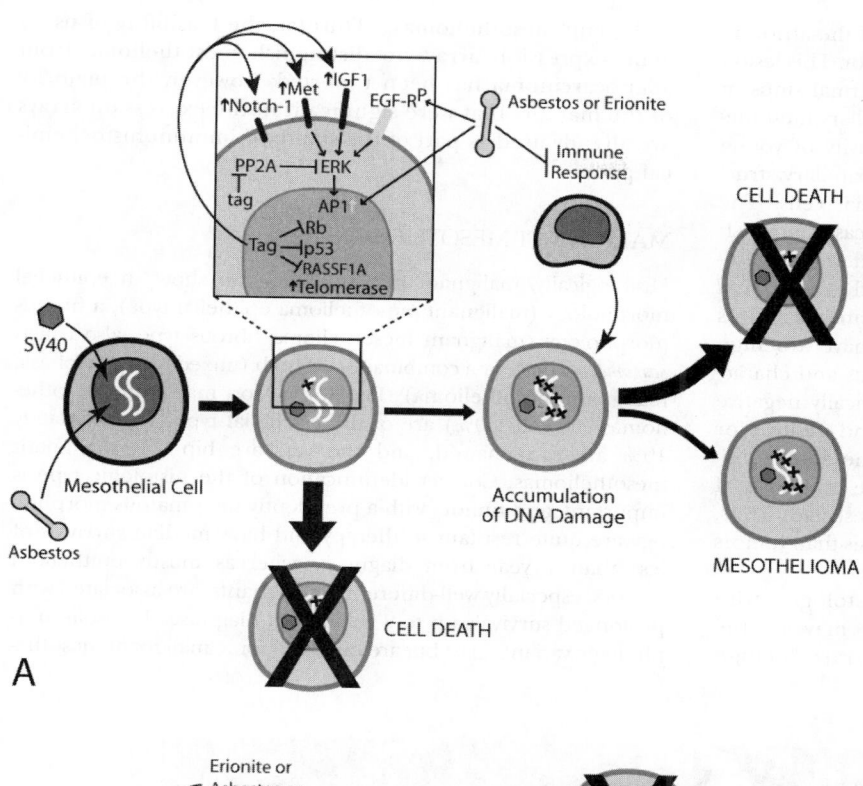

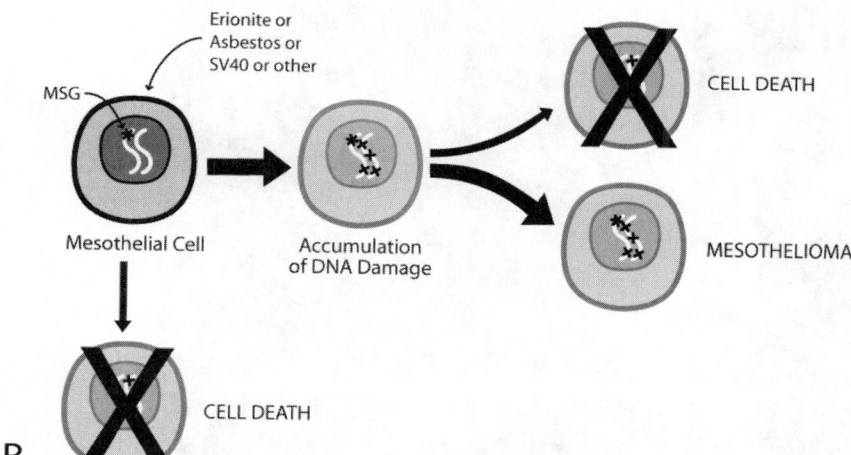

FIGURE 36-1. Mesothelioma pathogenesis. Pathogenic mechanisms of asbestos, erionite, simian virus 40 (SV40), and possible role of genetic predisposition. Arrowheads indicate a stimulatory effect. Crossed bars indicate an inhibitory effect. **A:** The presence of asbestos or erionite leads to autophosphorylation of the epidermal growth factor receptor (EGF-R), which activates the microtubule-associated protein (MAP) kinases and eventually leads to AP-1 induction, cell mitosis, and apoptosis. If the mesothelial cell is infected with SV40, SV40 large T antigen (Tag)–mediated inactivation and activation of the indicated oncogene/tumor suppressor genes cause cell mitosis and genetic alterations. Tag-induced telomerase activity promotes continuous cell growth. In addition, the SV40 small t antigen (tag) inhibits phosphatase 2A (PP2A), which normally dephosphorylates and inactivates the MAP kinases. This increases the stimulatory effect of asbestos on AP-1. Furthermore, asbestos is phagocytosed by macrophages that, in response, release numerous cytokines that interfere with the local and systemic immunity. An altered immune response may facilitate tumor cells expressing viral antigens to evade immune detection. Cells exposed to SV40 and asbestos are likely to die (apoptosis or cell lysis) because of the effects of these carcinogens and because of the DNA damage they accumulate (*X symbols in the nuclei*). Occasionally, a cell that has accumulated numerous genetic alterations escapes cell death to form a malignancy. It is postulated that individuals exposed to both asbestos and SV40 are at higher risk of mesothelioma when compared to individuals exposed to only one of these two carcinogens. **B:** It is postulated that members of certain families with high incidence of mesothelioma have a genetic predisposition to the disease, represented here by the inborn genetic alteration of a putative mesothelioma suppressor gene (MSG). When these individuals are exposed to erionite of other mesothelioma carcinogens, they have a high risk of developing malignancy. Whether this genetic predisposition can be sufficient to cause the disease in some individuals in the absence of exposure to other carcinogens is unknown. IGF, insulin growth factor. (See Color Fig. 36-1 in the CD-ROM.)

However, closer observation revealed that mesotheliomas only occurred in certain homes and not in others (homes in these areas are inhabited by multiple generations and passed down) even though all homes contained similar amounts of erionite according to recent mineralogic analysis.[2,51] Further analysis of pedigrees of families who lived in homes where mesotheliomas occurred showed that these mesotheliomas appeared to be inherited in an autosomal dominant pattern. Approximately 50% of descendants of affected parents developed mesotheliomas. When members of unaffected families married into affected families, 50% of their descendants also developed mesotheliomas.[2,51] Whether genetics alone or in conjunction with erionite is responsible for these mesotheliomas remains unknown, but clearly genetics is a key factor, as mesotheliomas do not develop in nonaffected families regardless of environmental exposure.

Familial malignant mesothelioma has been occasionally described in the United States and in Europe.[2,52] These families, however, were too small to prove genetic transmission.

PATHOLOGY OF MESOTHELIOMA

BENIGN MESOTHELIOMAS

True malignant mesothelioma is an aggressive malignancy with a dismal prognosis. There are, however, a number of benign mesothelial proliferations that must be distinguished from malignant mesothelioma. Multicystic mesothelioma, also called *multilocular peritoneal inclusion cyst*, is a benign mesothelial lesion, characteristically formed by multiple cysts arranged in grape-like clusters. Adenomatoid mesotheliomas are benign mesothelial lesions of the genital system. Mesothelioma of the atrioventricular node is neither a mesothelioma nor a tumor. This lesion represents congenital heterotopia of the endodermal sinus in the atrioventricular node. Well-differentiated papillary mesothelioma is found more often in the abdominal cavity of young women. Histologically, it is formed by multiple papillary structures covered by cytologically benign mesothelial cells. The lesion is benign, but there have been occasional cases in which several years after diagnosis the patient developed a true mesothelioma. Localized mesothelioma, better referred to as *localized fibrous tumor of the pleura* (FTP), is similar to other fibrous tumors found elsewhere in the body. The tumor cells have a benign appearance and are usually immersed in a fibrous and characteristically vascular stroma. FTPs are characteristically negative for cytokeratin (a marker of mesothelial cells) and positive for CD34, which suggests that these cells are not of mesothelial origin. The most important predictive factor in the prognosis of FTP is whether the tumor can be completely resected. Thus, pedunculated tumors have a much better prognosis than tumors that grow over a broad pleural area.

Tumor array studies comparing variant histologies with classical epithelial malignant mesothelioma may in the future provide us with tools to identify these rare "benign malignant mesotheliomas." Thus far, the feasibility of using gene expression arrays to distinguish mesothelioma from adenocarcinoma has been reported; however, the majority of the markers that were significant in the expression arrays are already used as part of the standard immunohistochemical panel.[53]

MALIGNANT MESOTHELIOMA

Histologically, malignant mesothelioma can show an epithelial morphology (malignant mesothelioma epithelial type), a fibrous morphology (malignant mesothelioma fibrous type, also called *sarcomatoid type*), or a combination of both (mixed type or biphasic malignant mesothelioma) (Fig. 36-2). Most malignant mesotheliomas (50% to 60%) are of the epithelial type, approximately 10% are sarcomatoid, and the rest are biphasic malignant mesotheliomas. Correct identification of the histologic type is important, and tumors with a prevalently sarcomatous morphology are quite resistant to therapy and have median survivals of less than 1 year from diagnosis; whereas mostly epithelioid tumors, especially well-differentiated variants, are associated with prolonged survivals up to 2 years from diagnosis. Unusual morphologic variants exist but are rare, and some malignant mesothe-

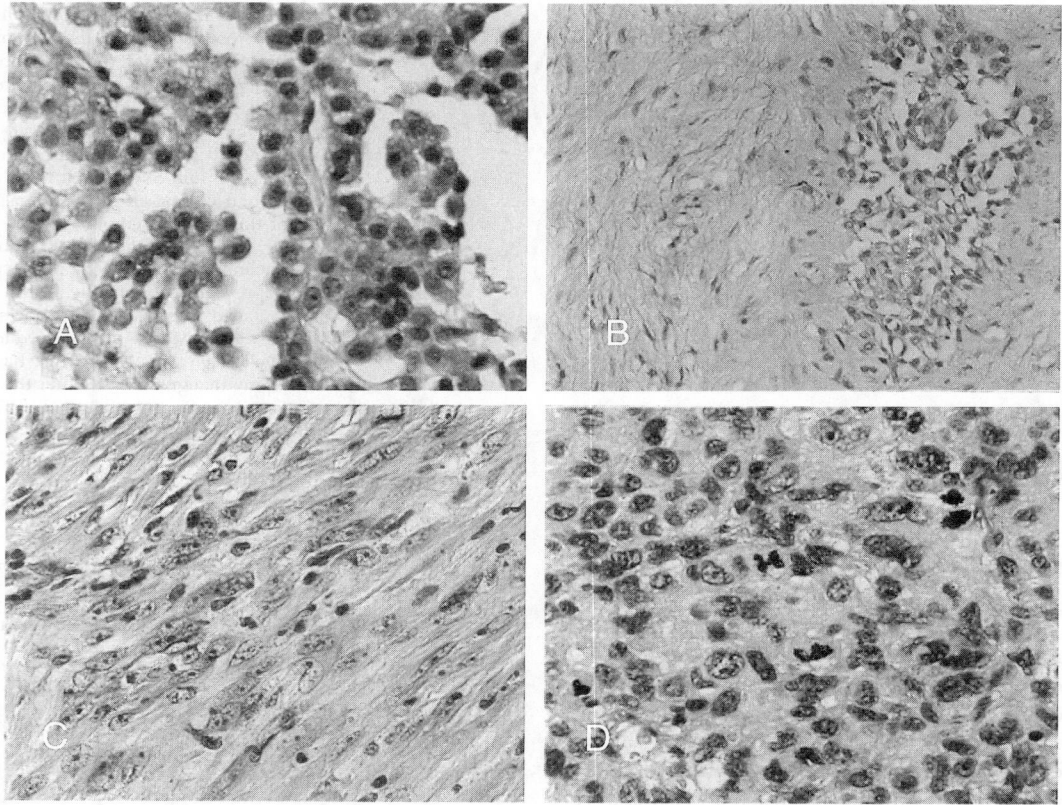

FIGURE 36-2. Histology of mesothelioma. **A:** Epithelioid mesothelioma. Note tubular structures and malignant mesothelioma cells showing a hobnail morphology with bland nuclei and abundant cytoplasm. **B:** Biphasic malignant mesothelioma, showing a nest of mesothelioma cells with epithelial differentiation within the sarcomatoid component. **C:** Sarcomatoid mesothelioma, positivity for pankeratin, and rare foci of cells suggestive of epithelioid differentiation indicated the diagnosis. **D:** High-grade sarcoma. A highly aggressive tumor that is vimentin positive but negative for over 15 different immunostains for other markers and without distinctive electron microscopic features. In this case, the diagnosis of mesothelioma could not be confirmed. Original magnification: **A, C,** and **D,** ×400; **B,** ×200. (See Color Fig. 36-2 in the CD-ROM.)

liomas cannot be subcategorized histologically and should be called *poorly differentiated malignant mesothelioma*.[54]

The diagnosis of malignant mesothelioma, in contrast to common belief, is usually straightforward, provided that the pathologist has extensive experience with this malignancy. Some epithelial mesotheliomas grow forming sheets of epithelioid cells. The experienced pathologist easily recognizes these tumors as mesothelial in origin; however, occasionally a carcinoma can look very much like a malignant mesothelioma, or a malignant mesothelioma can look so atypical that it resembles a metastatic carcinoma. Therefore, to rule out these rare mimics, the diagnosis of malignant mesothelioma should be further confirmed by immunohistochemistry, which shows that the tumor cells are positive for pankeratin, keratin 5/6, calretinin, and WT-1, and negative for the epithelial markers CEA, LeuM1, B72.3, Ber-EP4, Moc-1, TTF-1, etc. Usually, positive stainings for pankeratin and calretinin and negative stainings for three epithelial markers are considered sufficient for diagnosis. Occasionally, however, more stainings are required, because some carcinomas are positive for calretinin or are negative for some of the epithelial markers. In these difficult cases, electron microscopy showing the classic long-branching microvilli of human mesothelial cells compared to the short nonbranching microvilli of carcinomas can still be considered the gold standard for a correct diagnosis.

Fibrous mesotheliomas are more difficult to diagnose because they show a morphology that can be essentially identical to other primary or metastatic pleural sarcomas. Immunohistochemistry showing positive staining for pankeratin is useful to confirm the diagnosis. Only a fraction, which varies depending on the study, of sarcomatoid malignant mesothelioma are positive for calretinin, and some of them are positive for WT-1.

SOLITARY FIBROUS TUMORS OF PLEURA

More than 700 solitary fibrous tumors of pleura have been reported in the literature and, on presentation, are frequently confused with pleural mesothelioma. The solitary FTP is a mesenchymal growth that arises from the visceral or parietal pleura.[55] The benign variant is an encapsulated lobulated tumor that on microscopic examination may resemble a sarcomatoid mesothelioma with interweaving bundles of ovoid or spindle cells without atypia. A malignant variant characterized by high cellularity, marked pleomorphism, and a high mitotic activity is seen in approximately 10% of the cases. FTPs, unlike mesotheliomas, are immunohistochemically negative when stained for cytokeratins.[56] Sixty percent of the patients have symptoms, and both males and females with FTP can present with dyspnea from compressive atelectasis, as well as with lower extremity edema from mediastinal compression. Clubbing and osteoarthropathy are present in 20% to 50% of cases versus only 6% in malignant mesothelioma.[57] Hyponatremia attributed to inappropriate secretion of antidiuretic hormone and hypoglycemia have been described.[58,59]

Plain chest x-ray reveals a well-circumscribed lobulated tumor that is heterogeneous appearing on computed tomogram with a pedicle that is usually attached to the visceral pleura. Rarely, there are multiple tumors that are pedunculated on the visceral pleura. Effusions are rarely associated with FTPs, except with the malignant variety.

Benign FTPs can recur and transform to the malignant variant, and the malignant variants are usually not pedunculated, are larger, and present in unusual locations.

Surgical resection (Fig. 36-3) is the treatment of choice, with complete resection of the tumor and its pedunculated portion along with the site of origin.[55] Five-year survival rates as high as 97% have been reported. *En bloc* resection of the lung, chest wall, or diaphragm may be necessary. For recurrences, re-excision is the treatment of choice. Long-term survival with re-excision is possible, but with incomplete resection or malignant transformation, the median survival is 24 to 36 months.[55,60]

CLINICAL PRESENTATION OF MALIGNANT PLEURAL MESOTHELIOMA

Classically, mesothelioma affects older men in their 50s, 60s, and 70s due to the aforementioned 25- to 40-year latency period between occupational asbestos exposure and the development of the tumor. Table 36-1 lists the most common industries identified in 1048 cases of histologically confirmed mesothelioma cases reviewed by Roggli.[61] Women and children can have the disease, but the male to female ratio is approximately 3 to 5:1.[62]

SYMPTOMS

The duration of symptoms varies; however, the range can extend from 2 weeks to 2 years, with most series having a median time to diagnosis from symptoms of 2 to 3 months. As many as 25% of patients with the disease have symptoms for 6 months or more before seeking medical attention. The right side is affected more than the left side (60% vs. 40%), most likely due to the right side's greater volume.

Approximately 60% of the patients present with nonpleuritic chest pain that classically is located posterolaterally and low in the thorax. Dyspnea is present in 50% to 70% of the cases, and, indeed, 80% of the patients present with dyspnea and effusion. The presence of a pleural effusion is documented at some time in the course of the disease in 95% of patients with malignant pleural mesothelioma (MPM). Approximately 5% of patients also have metastatic disease at presentation, usually to the lungs.

PHYSICAL EXAMINATION

Physical examination usually reveals signs associated with a pleural effusion, with decreased breath sounds, dullness to percussion, or decreased motion of the involved chest wall. Failure to significantly relieve the dyspnea after thoracentesis may be an indication of fixation of a nonexpanding, contracted, and trapped lung. In the late stages of the disease, there is often dramatic cachexia, marked contraction of the involved chest with narrowed interspaces, and hypertrophy of the contralateral hemithorax. A chest wall mass occurs in up to 25% of patients, often at the site(s) of prior thoracentesis, thoracotomy, or thoracoscopy wounds.

LABORATORY EXAMINATION

The workup of the patient with mesothelioma may reveal nonspecific laboratory findings, including hypergammaglobulinemia, eosinophilia, and/or anemia of chronic disease. It has been recently noted that 14% to 15% of patients have elevated homocys-

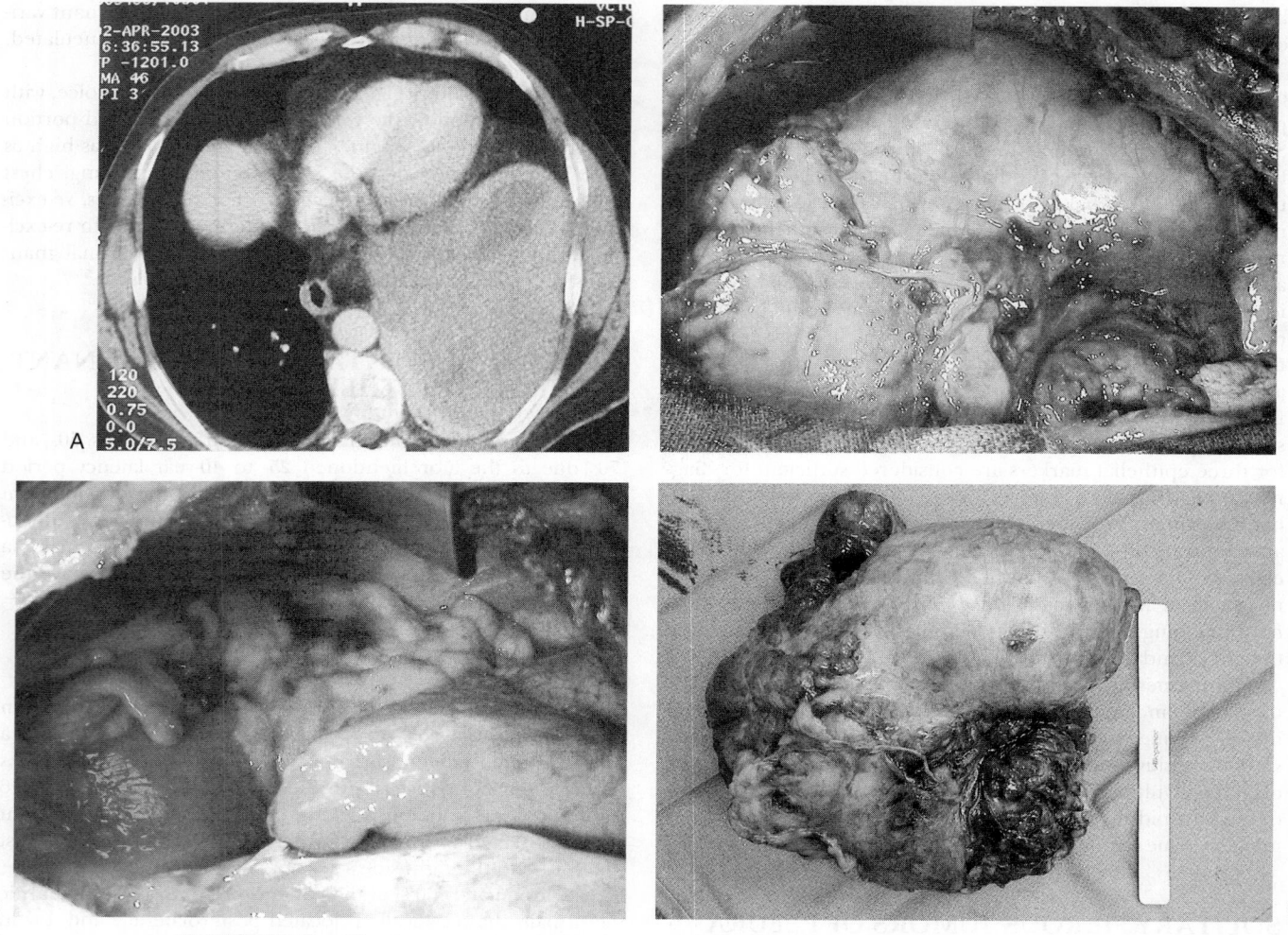

FIGURE 36-3. Fibrous tumor of pleura. **A:** Computed tomography reveals a large mass compressing the lower lobe of the lung. **B:** Intraoperative photograph. Tumor arose from a wide stalk on the diaphragm. **C:** Intraoperative photograph after resection of the mass revealing expansion of the lung and no other disease. **D:** Resected specimen. (See Color Fig. 36-3 in the CD-ROM.)

teine levels, reflecting folic acid deficiency; 17% have biochemical evidence of vitamin B$_{12}$ deficiency; and 32% have biochemical signs of vitamin B$_6$ deficiency.[63] The most striking laboratory abnormality is thrombocytosis (greater than 400,000), which is seen in 60% to 90% of patients,[64] and approximately 15% of patients have platelet counts greater than 1,000,000. At present, validated serum markers that are both sensitive and specific for mesothelioma do not exist. Recently, a dual-monoclonal forward sandwich enzyme-linked immunosorbent assay for the measurement of soluble members of the mesothelin/megakaryocyte potentiating factor family of proteins expressed by mesothelial cells has been reported to predict the development of mesothelioma in high-risk individuals as well as to reflect the influence of therapeutic efficacy in mesothelioma.[65]

RADIOLOGIC EXAMINATION

Malignant mesothelioma can have a diverse radiographic appearance. Many of the early changes are associated with a previous exposure to asbestos, consisting both of pleural and parenchymal changes, including pleural plaques or parenchymal pulmonary fibrosis.

Chest Radiography

The most common chest radiography features associated with mesothelioma progression and symptoms include the presence of a pleural effusion, diffuse pleural thickening, and nodularity. The involved hemithorax can eventually have smooth, lobular pleural masses that infiltrate the pleural space and fissures[115–117] in 45% to 60% of patients with contraction and fixation of the chest (Fig. 36-4). The lung becomes encased, and the mediastinum shifts due to volume loss. The effusion can be loculated, chiefly in the lower portion of the chest, completely obscuring a view of the diaphragm, lower lobes, and pericardium. In many of these instances, the lower lobe is viewed on computed tomography (CT) to be completely collapsed.

Chest Tomography

Chest tomography allows for density resolution that is not available with chest radiography, and these characteristics are useful not only in the evaluation of the patient with mesothelioma but also with asbestos-related diseases. Pleural changes on chest tomography include pleural plaques, diffuse pleural

TABLE 36-1. Occupational Exposure and Mesothelioma

Occupation	Single Exposure	Multiple Exposures	Percent of Total
Shipbuilding[a]	203	86	30
U.S. Navy[b]	91	84	18
Construction[c]	99	35	13
Insulation[d]	92	11	10
Oil and chemical	78	10	8
Power plant	50	10	5
Railroad	37	16	4
Automotive[e]	24	27	4
Steel/metal[f]	33	10	3
Asbestos manufacturing[g]	34	5	3
Papermill	7	0	1
Ceramics/glass	6	0	1

[a]Includes joiner, shipwright, rigger, sandblaster, shipfitter, electrician, painter, and welder.
[b]Includes merchant marine seamen.
[c]Includes construction worker, laborer, carpenter, painter, dry wall/plasterer.
[d]Includes pipecoverer, insulator, asbestos sawyer, asbestos sprayer.
[e]Includes auto mechanic, brake repair worker, brake line worker.
[f]Includes steel, aluminum, and iron foundry workers; furnace worker; potroom worker.
[g]Includes asbestos textile worker, asbestos manufacturer, asbestos plant worker.
(From ref. 103, with permission.)

thickening, and pleural effusion. Additional CT features of mesothelioma include localized nodular or plaque-like pleural thickening, possibly associated with pleural effusion. The lobulated pleural encasement frequently causes lower lobe collapse (Fig. 36-5). Intrapulmonary nodules can occur in 60% of patients, and infiltration into fissures along with enlarged

hilar and mediastinal lymph nodes may be seen. The CT allows a better view of the involved pericardium, which is irregularly thickened and associated with infiltration to the pericardial fat pad. A clear fat plane between the inferior diaphragmatic surface and the adjacent abdominal organs as well as a smooth inferior diaphragmatic contour may imply resectability.[66] CT may reveal a hemidiaphragm encased by a mass or poor definition between the liver, stomach, and inferior diaphragmatic surface.

Magnetic Resonance Imaging

Magnetic resonance imaging (MRI) is appealing due to the differential signal intensity, depending on the sequence used and the ability to image in the coronal, sagittal, and transverse planes. Studies have suggested gadolinium contrast enhancement MRI can improve tumor detection and extension (Fig. 36-6). Detection of diaphragm invasion and invasion of endothoracic fascia or a single chest wall focus may be better with MRI compared to CT.[66]

Positron Emission Tomography Imaging

There are a number of studies of positron emission tomography (PET) and the radionuclide imaging agent [18F]fluorodeoxyglucose (FDG) in mesothelioma (Fig. 36-7). Four studies have reported that FDG-PET is accurate in the diagnosis of pleural malignancies, specifically mesothelioma, and that it may be superior to CT for defining mediastinal lymph node involvement.[67–70] Moreover, the ability to define extrathoracic, otherwise occult disease in newly diagnosed patients can be as high as 10% to 45% who are followed after therapy. Moreover, in preliminary data, the standard uptake value (SUV) of the tumor before resection can discriminate longer- from shorter-

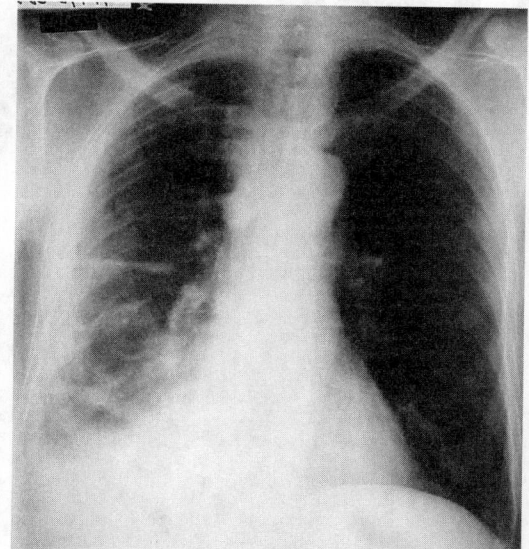

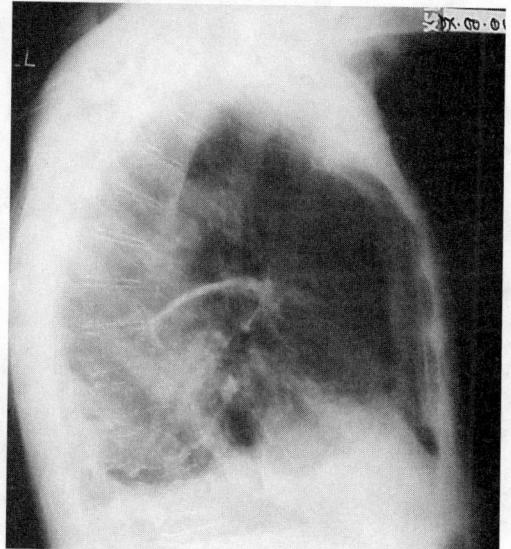

FIGURE 36-4. Chest radiography of malignant pleural mesothelioma. **A:** Anteroposterior view reveals a contracted right hemithorax with nodular scalloping of the pleura at the right base. There is fluid or tumor in the fissure, and the diaphragm and right heart border are obscured. **B:** Lateral view demonstrates fluid or tumor at the right base with thickened pleura and disease in the fissure.

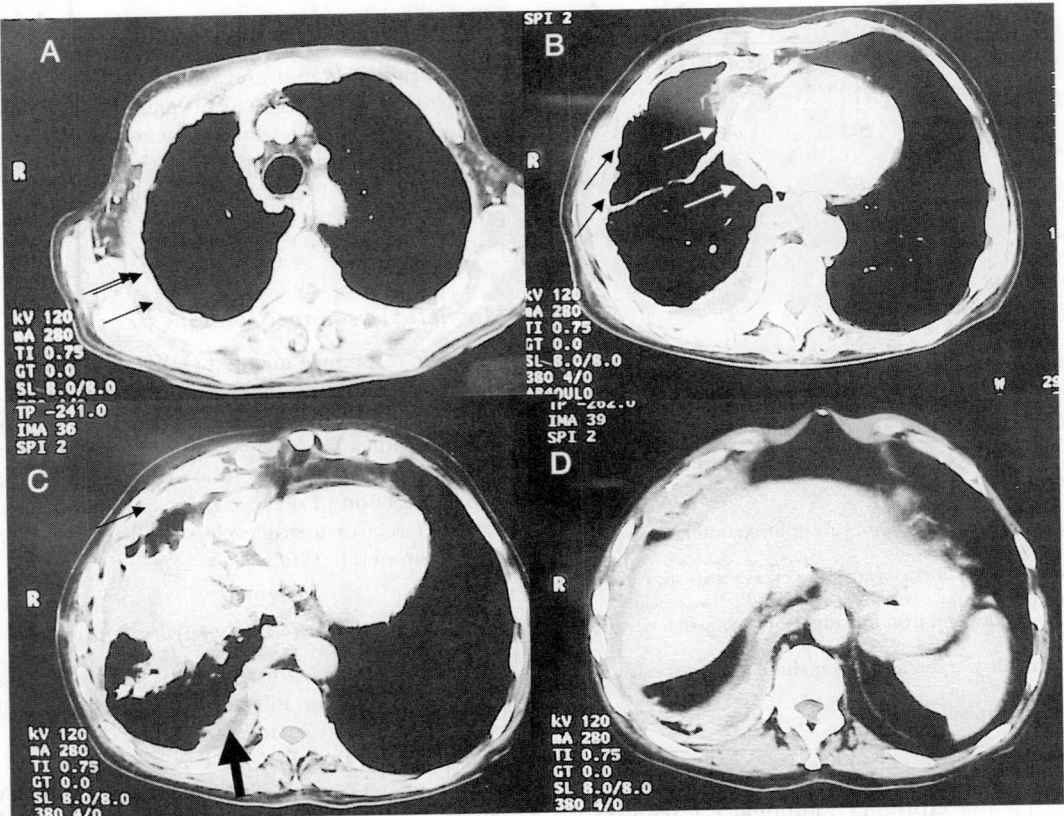

FIGURE 36-5. Computed tomography of a patient with a right-sided pleural mesothelioma. As one progresses from the apex **(A)** to the diaphragm **(D)**, loculated fluid (*bold black arrow*), thickened pleura (*thin black arrows*), and thickened pericardium (*white arrows*) can be appreciated.

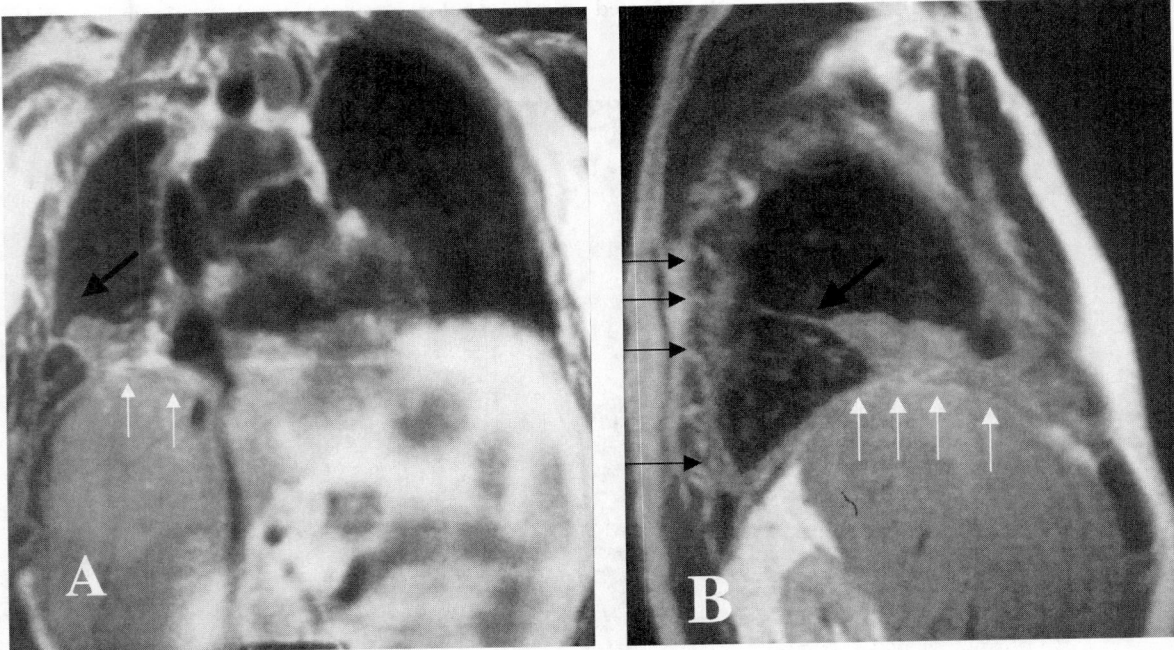

FIGURE 36-6. Magnetic resonance imaging and mesothelioma. **A:** Coronal magnetic resonance imaging of a right-sided pleural mesothelioma. White arrows indicate diaphragmatic involvement. Black arrows delineate fluid in fissure and associated mass. **B:** Sagittal magnetic resonance image of same patient reveals the thickened pleura (*thin black arrows*), involvement in the fissure (*thick black arrow*), and involvement of the diaphragm (*white arrows*).

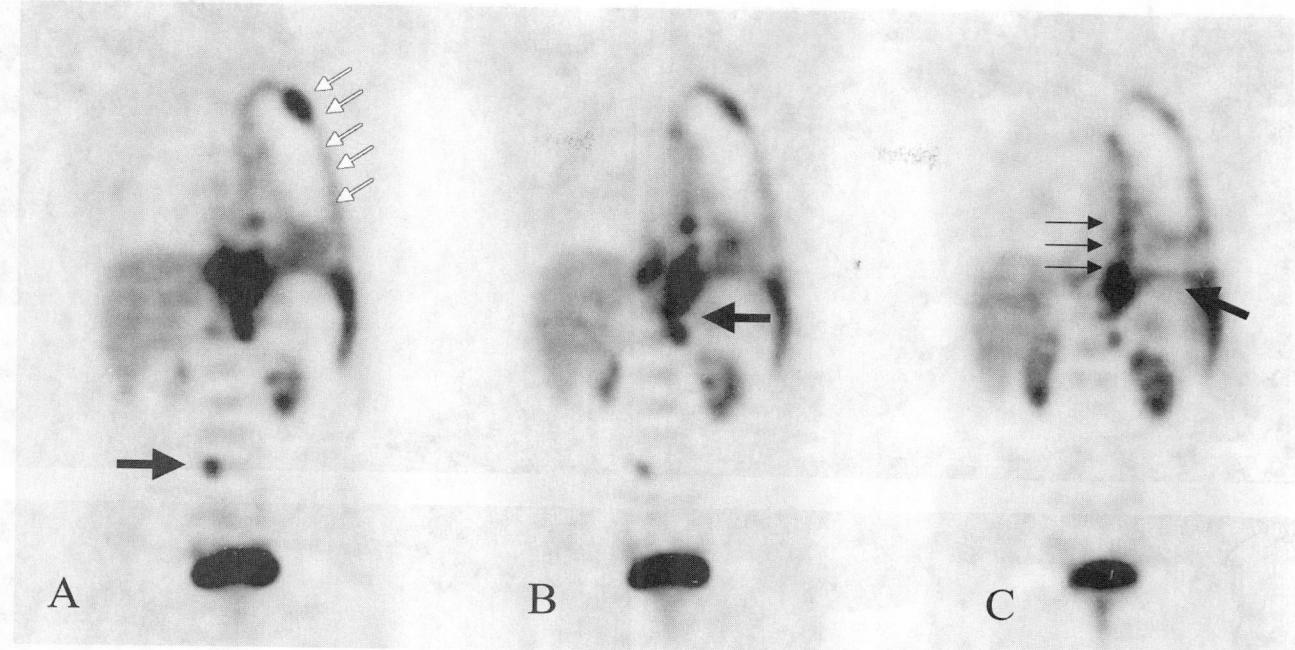

FIGURE 36-7. Positron emission tomography with [18F]fluorodeoxyglucose in a patient with an unresectable stage IV mesothelioma. **A:** Short white arrows outline the involved pleura, with an area of bulky disease superiorly. Bold black arrow points out an occult metastasis in the abdomen. **B:** Bold black arrow depicts posterior infracrural mediastinal lymph node disease. **C:** Bold black arrow points out diaphragmatic involvement. Thin black arrows depict mesothelioma medially.

surviving patients and stratify good risk versus bad risk patients. Those with low SUV and epithelial histology have the best prognosis, whereas those with high SUV and nonepithelial histology fare the worst.[71]

Follow-Up Radiologic Assessment

After extrapleural pneumonectomy (EPP), CT scanning of the resected hemithorax reveals a smooth-walled, well-defined postoperative membrane lining the pneumonectomy space, which is usually concentrically smooth. As the interval from operation to follow-up lengthens, the membrane may actually become thicker (Fig. 36-8). Unexplained, irregular focal thickening at the base of the chest should alert the clinician to a recurrence of disease. This is especially pronounced in the pleurectomy patient in whom recurrent mesothelioma may start to thicken rapidly and infiltrate the underlying lung (Fig. 36-9).

Other presentations of recurrence include the development of new mediastinal adenopathy or ascites otherwise undetectable by physical examination. The development of asymptom-

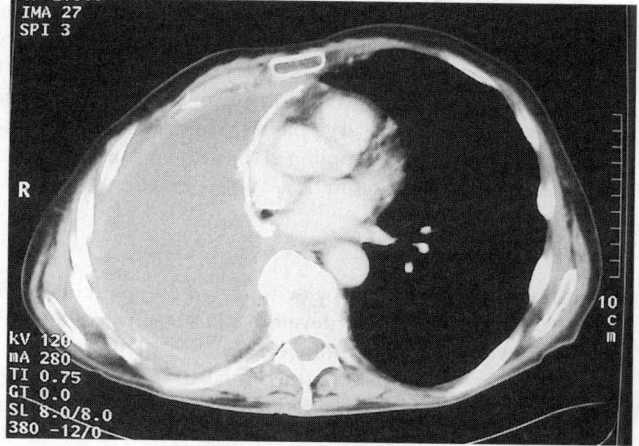
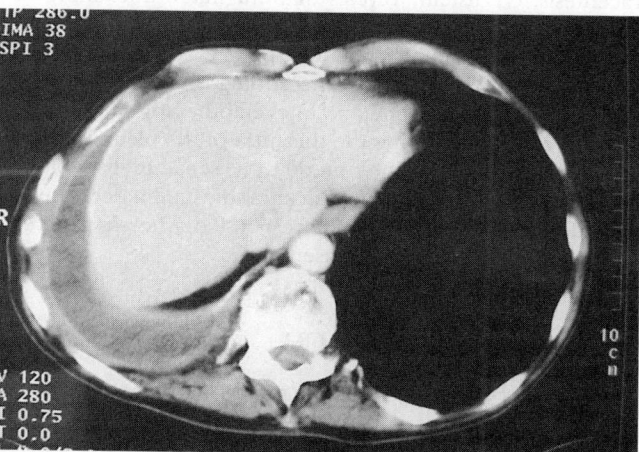

FIGURE 36-8. Appearance of computed tomogram after right extrapleural pneumonectomy. **A:** Smooth interior chest wall and intact pericardial patch. **B:** The new Gore-Tex diaphragm is seen as a white line at the edge of the liver. Note the smooth contour of the chest wall and lack of air in the hemithorax.

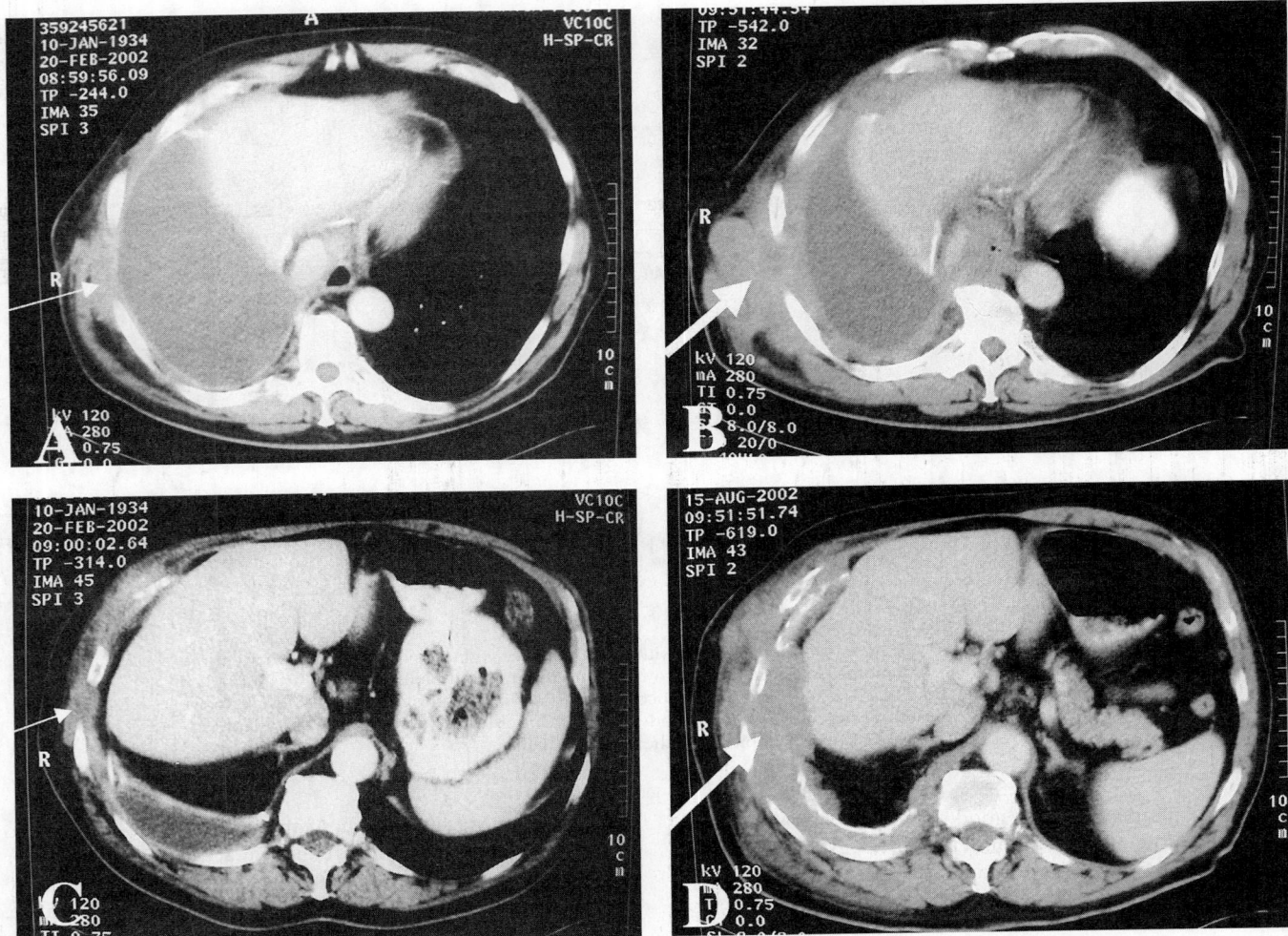

FIGURE 36-9.   Progression of mesothelioma after extrapleural pneumonectomy. **A,C:** Minimal thickening in the soft tissues in the inferior portion of the right chest (*thin arrows*). **B,D:** Massive growth of subcutaneous and retroperitoneal and pleural tumor encasing the neodiaphragm (*thick arrows*).

atic abdominal fluid after EPP is an ominous sign and calls for paracentesis. CT usually reveals diaphragmatic thickening or diffuse mesenteric infiltration in these cases (Fig. 36-10).

Besides evaluation of postoperative progression, an important role of follow-up or sequential CT scanning is in the assessment of the response of mesothelioma to chemotherapy. Multicenter protocols require measuring the thickness of the pleural rind at one to three locations on the rind on three separate slices of the CT every 6 to 9 weeks. The total thickness must then decrease by 30% to declare the patient to have responded, whereas progressive disease requires a 20% increase.[72]

DIAGNOSTIC APPROACH

THORACENTESIS AND CLOSED PLEURAL BIOPSY

Patients who present with a large, unexplained pleural effusion and minimal or moderate evidence of pleural thickening should have initial thoracentesis and pleural biopsy. In the past, due to the difficulty in distinguishing between reactive mesothelial cells and tumor cells, the diagnosis of mesothelioma was made from pleural fluid in only 33% of cases. However, by preserving a cell block from the pleural fluid and using both histochemical and immunohistochemical staining techniques along with electron microscopic analysis, the diagnosis of mesothelioma can be obtained from the pleural effusion in as high as 84% of suspected cases. In cases of a large pleural effusion, multiple closed pleural biopsies to avoid sampling error with an Abrams or Cope needle aid in the diagnoses in 30% to 50% of cases.

THORACOSCOPY

A video-assisted thoracoscopy is indicated for patients at risk for mesothelioma who (1) develop a large effusion and who have negative studies on thoracentesis and pleural biopsy or (2) who recur with effusion after initial thoracentesis. Thoracoscopy can be invaluable for estimating extent of disease with regard to the diaphragm, pericardium, chest wall, and nodes. The compulsive use of thoracoscopy by Boutin et al.[73] led to the finding that patients with exclusive involvement of the diaphragmatic pleura and parietal pleura (stage IA) had a median

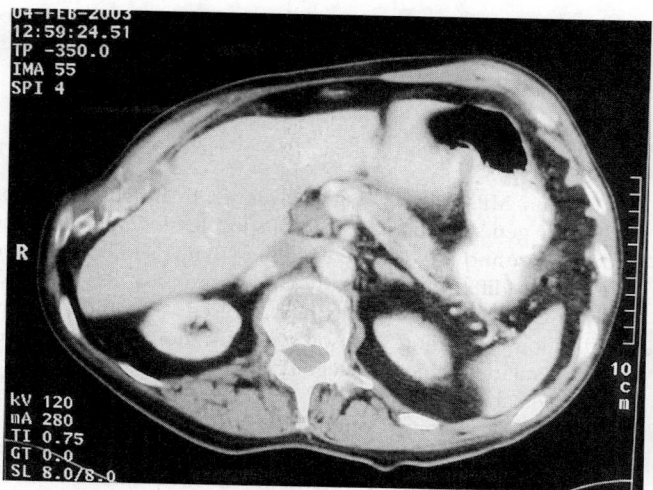
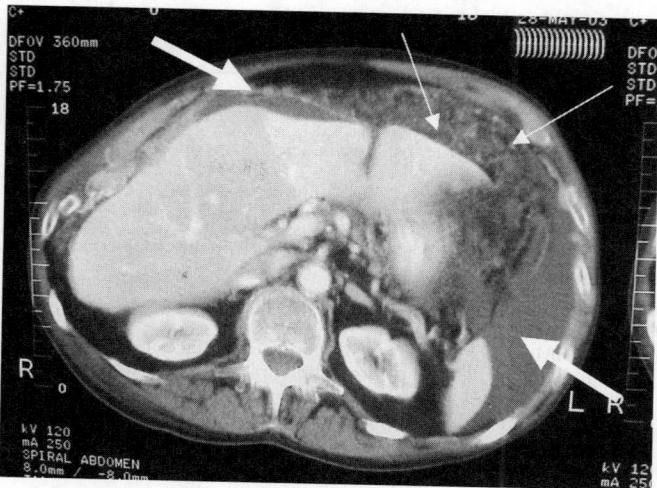

FIGURE 36-10.   Progression of mesothelioma after resection. **A:** Normal-appearing upper abdomen without ascites and normal mesenteric fat. **B:** Ascites (*thick arrows*) surrounding the spleen and liver is present 3 months later, and there is diffuse infiltration of the mesentery with disease (*thin arrows*).

survival of 31.2 months, whereas patients with visceral pleura invasion had a median survival of 6.75 months. The later development of chest wall masses from seeding of the biopsy site or surgical scar is an uncommon complication (approximately 10%) of any diagnostic procedure, but can usually be avoided by radiotherapy to the scar if appropriate.[74]

OPEN PLEURAL BIOPSY

If there is no free pleural space due to previous treatment of pleural effusion and the bulk of the disease in the hemithorax is solid, open biopsy is required. Such a biopsy should be carefully planned such that the scar could be incorporated into the definitive incision if a major resection is entertained after definitive diagnosis. When enlarged mediastinal lymph nodes are detected by CT or PET scan, a mediastinoscopy should be performed. The yield from mediastinoscopy may underestimate the extent of nodal involvement because the majority of mediastinal nodal involvement in mesothelioma is below the subcarinal level.[75]

NATURAL HISTORY

The majority of patients with pleural mesothelioma, treated or untreated, die of complications of local disease due to (1) increasing tumor bulk that eventually replaces the pleural effusion and causes progressive respiratory compromise, pneumonia, or myocardial dysfunction with arrhythmias and/or (2) unrelenting chest wall pain requiring narcotics, which leads to cachexia, and (3) dysphagia from tumor compression of the esophagus. The most important predictor of survival is performance status. The median survival of 337 patients treated in ten clinical trials by the Cancer and Leukemia Group B (all of whom were required to be performance status 0 to 2) was 7 months[64]; however, for those with performance status 0, the median survival was 13 to 14 months. In various series from single institutions, the median survival varies from 4 to 18 months (range, weeks to 16 years), but performance status was rarely reported in older series. Patients generally die of respiratory

failure or pneumonia. Small bowel obstruction from direct extension through the diaphragm develops in approximately one-third of patients, and 10% die of pericardial or myocardial involvement.[76]

Extrathoracic metastases occur late in the course of disease and are not usually the direct cause of the patient's death. In the largest series of patients with MPM who had autopsy, 54% to 82% had distant metastases, with the most frequently involved organs being the liver, adrenal gland, kidney, and contralateral lung.[77–79] Intracranial metastases are seen in approximately 3% of patients and are predominantly of the sarcomatous type.[78]

PROGNOSTIC INDICATORS

There have been a number of publications that have retrospectively analyzed variables characterizing the mesothelioma population in an attempt to weight their prognostic index.

Factors predictive of poorer survival among 337 patients with mesothelioma in Cancer and Leukemia Group B studies included poor performance status, chest pain, dyspnea, platelet count greater than 400,000/µL, weight loss, serum lactate dehydrogenase level greater than 500 IU/L, pleural involvement, low hemoglobin level, high white blood cell count, and age older than 75 years.

The molecular prognostication of mesothelioma has been explored by two groups. Using the 12,000 U95 Affymetrix gene chip, Gordon et al.[80] developed a four-gene expression ratio test that was able to predict treatment-related patient outcome in mesothelioma independent of the histologic subtype of the tumor. Using similar technology, Pass et al.[81] have reported a 27-gene expression array for mesothelioma prognostication. The groups predicted by the gene classifier recapitulated the actual time to progression and survival of the test set with 95.2% accuracy using tenfold cross validation. Clinical outcomes were independent of histology, and heterogeneity of progression and survival in early-stage patients was defined by the classifier. These data require further validation in larger prospective analyses but

TABLE 36-2. International Staging System for Diffuse Malignant Pleural Mesothelioma

T1

T1a

Tumor limited to the ipsilateral parietal ± mediastinal ± diaphragmatic pleura

No involvement of the visceral pleura

T1b

Tumor involving the ipsilateral parietal ± mediastinal ± diaphragmatic pleura

Tumor also involving the visceral pleura

T2

Tumor involving each of the ipsilateral pleural surfaces (parietal, mediastinal, diaphragmatic, and visceral pleura) with at least one of the following features:

Involvement of diaphragmatic muscle

Extension of tumor from visceral pleura into the underlying pulmonary parenchyma

T3

Describes locally advanced but potentially resectable tumor

Tumor involving all of the ipsilateral pleural surfaces (parietal, mediastinal, diaphragmatic, and visceral pleura) with at least one of the following features:

Involvement of the endothoracic fascia

Extension into the mediastinal fat

Solitary, completely resectable focus of tumor extending into the soft tissues of the chest wall

Nontransmural involvement of the pericardium

T4

Describes locally advanced technically unresectable tumor

Tumor involving all the ipsilateral pleural surfaces (parietal, mediastinal, diaphragmatic, and visceral pleura) with at least one of the following features:

Diffuse extension or multifocal masses of tumor in the chest wall, with or without associated rib destruction

Direct transdiaphragmatic extension of tumor to the peritoneum

Direct extension of tumor to the contralateral pleura

Direct extension of tumor to mediastinal organs

Direct extension of tumor into the spine

Tumor extending through to the internal surface of the pericardium with or without a pericardial effusion; or tumor involving the myocardium

N-LYMPH NODES

NX: Regional lymph nodes cannot be assessed

N0: No regional lymph node metastases

N1: Metastases in the ipsilateral bronchopulmonary or hilar lymph nodes

N2: Metastases in the subcarinal or the ipsilateral mediastinal lymph nodes, including the ipsilateral internal mammary nodes

N3: Metastases in the contralateral mediastinal, contralateral internal mammary, ipsilateral, or contralateral supraclavicular lymph nodes

M-METASTASES

MX: Presence of distant metastases cannot be assessed

M0: No distant metastasis

M1: Distant metastasis present

STAGE I

Ia: T1aN0 M0

Ib: T1bN0 M0

STAGE II

T2 N0 M0

STAGE III

Any T3 M0

Any N1 M0

Any N2 M0

STAGE IV

Any T4

Any N3

Any M1

imply that gene expression data in mesothelioma at the time of initial biopsy may predict clinical outcomes.[81]

STAGING

The original MPM staging system proposed by Butchart relies on pathologic generalizations instead of specific quantitative aspects of the disease and was designed at a time that was well before recognition of different prognostic implications of N1 and N2 nodes.[82] Other staging systems have evolved since the Butchart classification, including Mattson's classification, which defines contralateral involvement as stage II rather than stage III (this has largely been abandoned).

The American Joint Committee on Cancer (AJCC) staging system for mesothelioma (Table 36-2) was adopted from that proposed by the IMIG in 1995 and has been validated in a number of surgically based trials. The system evolved from a greater understanding of the relationships between the tumor (T) status and nodal (N) status and overall survival. There was a redefinition of the T categories, and the T1 lesions were divided into T1a (involvement of the parietal pleura only) and T1b (involvement of the visceral pleura), leading to a division of stage I into stage IA and IB. T3 is defined as a locally advanced but potentially resectable tumor, and T4 is defined as a locally advanced, technically unresectable tumor. The Brigham and Women's Staging System has also been proposed for pleural mesothelioma and differs from the AJCC by defining intrapleural adenopathy as stage II disease and extrapleural adenopathy as stage III disease.[83–85] The AJCC system classifies any nodal involvement, either intrapleural or extrapleural as stage III disease.

TREATMENT

OVERVIEW

There are no published standards of care for the treatment of resectable pleural mesothelioma, and treatment decisions are influenced not only by the functional evaluation of these often elderly individuals but also by the philosophy of the treating physician. The evolution of the use of surgery in MPM with or without intraoperative or postoperative innovative adjuvant therapies, or both, is being defined in general by centers that see more than 100 MPM patients per year, and innovative, multimodality protocols that incorporate surgery as part of the package are being explored in larger numbers of patients.

For unresectable patients who are candidates for chemotherapy, the well-powered phase III trial that showed a 3- to 4-month survival advantage for the two-drug regimen of pemetrexed and cisplatin compared to the one-drug regimen of cisplatin has defined a standard of care for 2003.[86]

SUPPORTIVE CARE

Estimates of the median survival of patients who select supportive care only range from 4[87] to 13 months.[88] This variation in quoted median survival is likely due to variations in survival as a result of differences in tumor biology, host response to tumor, detection bias, lead-time bias, and the use of ad hoc or unreported treatments by some patients and physicians.

There are a number of options for the control of pleural effusion, including repeated thoracenteses, talc pleurodesis, pleuroperitoneal shunting, or placement of a Pleurex catheter. Talc pleurodesis is performed by instilling 2 to 5 g of asbestos-free, sterile talc over the lung and the parietal surfaces. Success rates in effusion control with talc, used either via thoracoscopy or via slurry, approach 90%. Failure of these techniques are usually associated with lung trapped by the tumor, a large solid tumor mass, a long history of effusion with multiple thoracenteses leading to loculations, age older than 70 years, or poor performance status. In such cases, the Pleurex catheter, with its one-way valve, can be implanted under local anesthesia into pleural effusion and patients can drain themselves at home using the available disposable drainage kits.[89] Internal drainage from the pleura to the abdomen can be accomplished using the Denver pleuroperitoneal shunt.

The chest pain of malignant mesothelioma requires narcotics, and these patients should be seen in consultation by a dedicated pain management team to assist in the optimization of the patient's quality of life. Subcutaneous tunneling of epidural catheters for long-term out-of-hospital use has also been used in selective cases. When only local radiotherapy has been delivered solely for chest wall pain or chest wall nodules, the median survival has been reported to be 4 to 5 months.[90,91]

SURGERY

The protocols that use an aggressive approach to the treatment of mesothelioma involve the use of surgery as part of the treatment package. The operations involved in this management include thoracoscopy (usually for diagnosis and palliation only), pleurectomy/decortication, or EPP. The indications for each of these operations depend on the extent of disease, performance and functional status of the patient, and the philosophy and experience of the treating institution. Basically, operative intervention in mesothelioma falls into one of three categories: (1) for primary effusion control, as described in Supportive Care; (2) for cytoreduction before multimodal therapy; or (3) to deliver and monitor innovative intrapleural therapies.

Preoperative Surgical Considerations

The majority of patients seeking treatment for mesothelioma are middle to older aged individuals with a long latency period between asbestos exposure and tumor development. If surgical intervention is to be considered, a detailed physiologic and functional workup directed chiefly at the cardiopulmonary axis must be performed.

PULMONARY EVALUATION. Poor underlying pulmonary function in patients with malignant mesothelioma usually reflects asbestos exposure, concomitant smoking history (up to 70% of the patients have had a heavy tobacco intake), the degree of lung trapped by tumor or fluid, and patient age. In general, forced expiratory volume in 1 second (FEV_1) of less than 1 L per second, a PO_2 less than 55, or a pCO_2 greater than 45 are relative contraindications to performance of EPP. If the patient presents with an FEV_1 of less than 2 L per second, or if the predicted FEV_1 is less than 1.2 L per minute after pneumonectomy, quantitative lung perfusion scanning should be performed and correlated to the pulmonary function tests (PFTs) to estimate the individual's pulmonary reserve after operation.

CARDIAC EVALUATION. Operations for mesothelioma are associated with profound blood loss and potentially significant cardiac demands. Any patient sustaining a myocardial infarction within the past 3 months or having an arrhythmia requiring medication should not be considered for EPP. Patients without objective evidence of cardiac injury who have a history of chest pain compatible with angina or remote myocardial infarction should have nuclear medicine studies to investigate reversible perfusion defects indicative of myocardium at risk. In general, patients with an ejection fraction of less than 45% are not considered to be candidates for EPP. Patients with coronary disease may be considered for angioplasty before operative intervention for their disease and, indeed, may be better candidates after such interventions if a multimodality approach is being contemplated.

OTHER PREOPERATIVE EVALUATION. Careful scrutiny of preoperative medications must be performed; specifically, of any nonsteroidal antiinflammatory drugs that could impact on platelet function. If patients are to participate in multimodality programs that use drugs with potential renal toxicity (i.e., cisplatin), a preoperative creatinine clearance should be performed.

Staging and Operative Therapy

Patients are candidates for surgical resection in mesothelioma if a cytoreductive procedure can be performed that does not leave gross disease at its completion, or, in other words, leaves only microscopic residual disease. This would include all IMIG clinically staged individuals from stages I to III, as the T3 category of stage III patients includes invasion of the endothoracic fascia or mediastinal fat, a solitary focus of tumor invading the soft tissues of the chest wall (i.e., at an old thoracoscopy site), and/or nontransmural involvement of the pericardium. The influence of nodal status and eligibility for surgery is less defined, as only 30% to 40% of nodes involved from resected mesothelioma patients are in the upper mediastinum and thus accessible to routine mediastinoscopy.[75] In the absence of routine thoracoscopic sampling of multiple nodal stations in mesothelioma before definitive resection, mediastinoscopy may be justified in those patients with obvious (i.e., greater than 1.5 cm) nodal involvement in levels 7, 4R, 4L, 5L, or 6L, or in patients with a suspicion for contralateral nodal involvement on presentation.[92] It is possible that FDG-PET scanning, as previously discussed in Positron Emission Tomography Imaging, will help to at least define those patients with node-involved mesothelioma in the future.

Which Operation?

The majority of diffuse malignant mesotheliomas cannot be surgically removed *en bloc* with truly negative histologic margins because many of the patients have had a previous biopsy and there is invasion of the endothoracic fascia and intercostal muscles at that site and/or pleural effusion that, although cytologically negative, may be breached, leading to local permeation of tumor cells either into the residual cavity or into the abdomen. Nevertheless, in the largest series of EPPs performed for mesothelioma, 66 of 183 patients were defined as having negative resection margins after EPP. Patients with negative margins at resection who had epithelial mesothelioma were found to have 2- and 5-year survival rates of 68% and 46%, respectively, if the node dissection did not reveal tumor.[93] Because the minority of patients are able to have a margin-free resection and because those patients who have margin-free resections usually have less bulky disease, it may be justifiable to spare functioning lung if the visceral pleura is minimally involved. Such "lung-preserving surgery" can potentially be accomplished by performing a radical parietal pleurectomy instead of EPP. Minimal visceral pleural disease is, however, an undefined entity, and there are no criteria for how many sites should be involved, the size of these involved sites, or whether involvement of the fissure is worse than nonfissural involvement. Suffice it to say that individual surgeons with expertise in the management of mesothelioma have different philosophies about the use of pleurectomy in this situation, and some make the decision regarding the type of operation in an individual patient at the time of the exploration.

There is no doubt that EPP is a more extensive dissection and may serve to remove more bulk disease than a pleurectomy, chiefly in the diaphragmatic and visceral pleural surfaces (Fig. 36-11). Some surgeons, however, include diaphragmatic resection and pericardial resection with their pleurectomies to accomplish removal of "all gross disease." For EPP, it is almost a necessity to include pericardiotomy and partial pericardiectomy during the resection because the maneuver aids in the exposure of the vessels and allows intrapericardial control to prevent a surgical catastrophe. In many instances, the final decision as to whether pleurectomy and decortication or EPP is to be performed becomes an intraoperative decision unless a protocol calls specifically for one operation or the other.

Pleurectomy

MORBIDITY AND MORTALITY. When performed routinely, pleurectomy for mesothelioma can be associated with few major

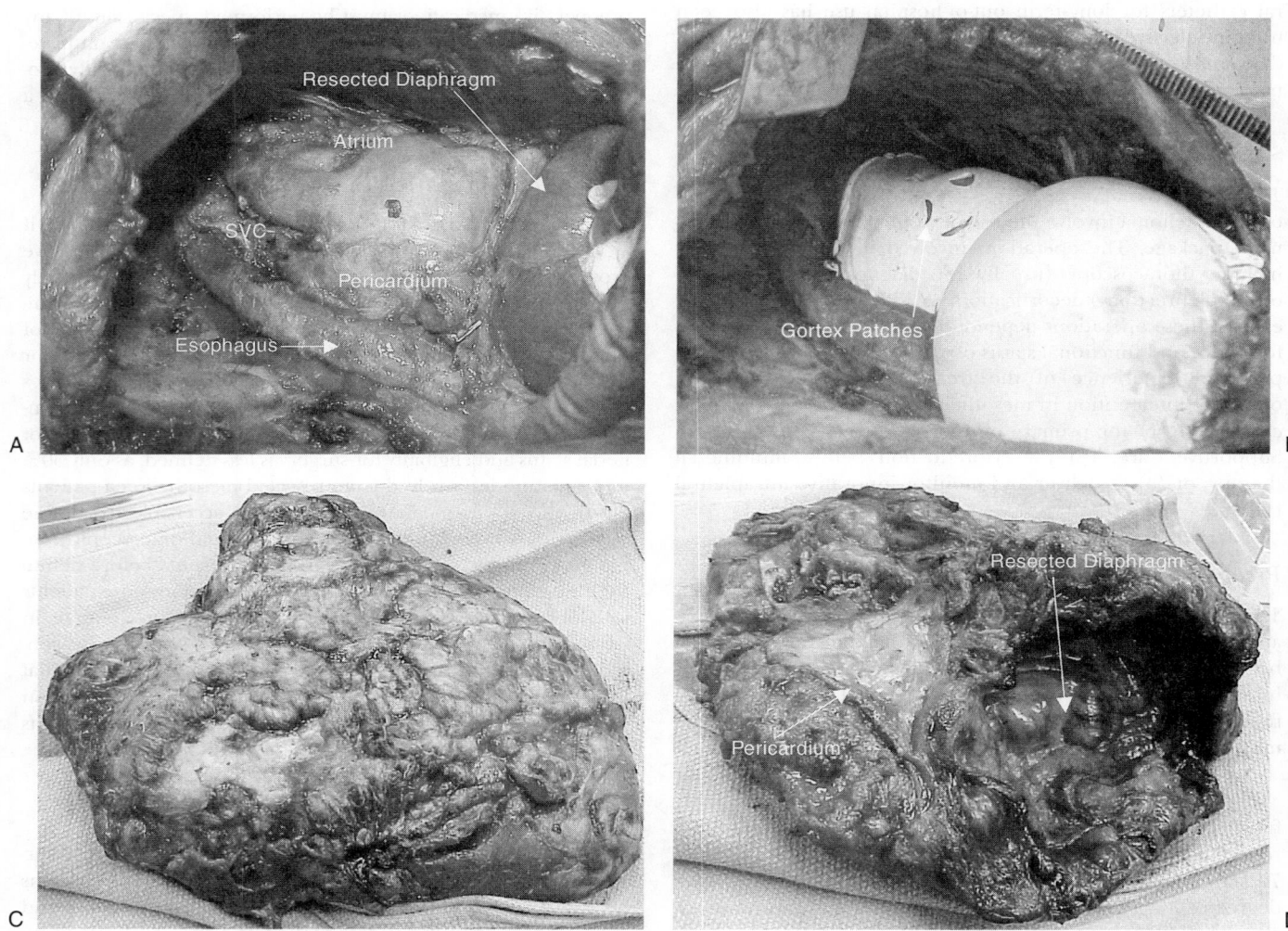

FIGURE 36-11.   Intraoperative and specimen photography of the patient whose computed tomograms are seen in Figure 36-10. **A:** Right hemithorax after resection of lung, pleura, diaphragm, pericardium, and lymph nodes. **B:** Replacement of the diaphragm and pericardium with Gore-Tex material. **C:** View of lateral aspect of specimen, which reveals the entire lung coated with thickened, mesothelioma-involved pleura. **D:** Medial view of specimen revealing the resected pericardium and diaphragm, hilar structures, and lung. SVC, superior vena cava. (See Color Fig. 36-11 in the CD-ROM.)

complications. In the series that specify postoperative morbidity, the most common complication was prolonged air leak (i.e., more than 7 days, occurring in 10% of the patients). Pneumonia and respiratory insufficiency may occur and are usually related to the burden of disease and preoperative functional status. Empyema is a rare occurrence (2%) and is managed by prolonged chest tube drainage and antibiotics. Hemorrhage requiring reexploration is rare (i.e., less than 1%). The modern-day mortality for pleurectomy for mesothelioma is generally considered to be 1.5% to 2.0%, with death either from respiratory insufficiency or hemorrhage.[94,95]

SHORT- AND LONG-TERM RESULTS. Pleurectomy and decortication are effective in controlling malignant pleural effusion. Law et al.[96] report effusion control in 88% of patients having decortication for mesothelioma. In 63 patients having partial decortication and pleurectomy, Ruffie et al.[97] reported 86% control of effusion, and Brancatisano et al.[98] reported a 98% control of effusion after pleurectomy in 50 cases of pleural mesothelioma.

Many of the published series using pleurectomy for palliative management have added therapies postoperatively in an uncontrolled, institution-related fashion. Further discussion of multimodality therapy and pleurectomy is found in Multimodality Treatment.

Extrapleural Pneumonectomy

Not all patients who are explored with the intent of undergoing an EPP are found to be truly cytoreducible at the time of the operation. In Butchart et al.'s review,[99] 29 of 46 or 63% of patients were eligible for EPP, and in a series of EPPs performed at Rush Presbyterian-St. Luke's Medical Center in Chicago, only 33 of 56 explored patients over a 27-year period had EPP (59%).[100] Sugarbaker has recently reported 50% of the patients seen at his institution are not eligible for EPP and adjuvant therapy.[84]

The Lung Cancer Study Group performed a pilot study of EPP from 1985 to 1988.[101] To be eligible for entry into the study, patients were required to have disease limited to the hemithorax by roentgenographic evaluation, a residual FEV_1 after resection of at least 1 L per second, and no significant cardiovascular illness. Only 20 of the 83 evaluated patients were resected with an EPP. The reasons that EPP could not be performed were chiefly extent of disease not allowing complete gross resection (54%), inadequate respiratory reserve (33%), stage IV disease (11%), and concurrent medical illness (10%).

COMPLICATIONS OF EXTRAPLEURAL PNEUMONECTOMY. Due to its magnitude, EPP has significantly greater morbidity than pleurectomy. The major complication rate ranges from 20% to 40%, and arrhythmia requiring medical management is the most common complication. In Sugarbaker et al.'s most recent report, major morbidity occurred in 24% of the patients having EPP and minor morbidity in 41%.[102] The rate for bronchopleural fistula is greater with right-sided EPPs, with an overall fistula rate of 3% to 20%. The bronchopleural fistula can be handled for the most part with open thoracostomy drainage with or without muscle flap interposition.

MORTALITY. The mortality rates after EPP were unacceptably high in the 1970s, with a 31% rate reported by Butchart et al.[99] Since then, however, there has been a steady decline in the operative mortality for the operation to consistent rates less than 10% in a series of 20 of more patients. Mortality occurs chiefly in older patients from respiratory failure, myocardial infarction, or pulmonary embolus. Rusch et al.[103,104] reported a perioperative mortality of 6% to 8% after EPP, and Sugarbaker et al.[93] reported a benchmark perioperative mortality of 3.8%. Mortalities were due to myocardial infarction and presumed pulmonary emboli.

RECURRENCE AFTER EXTRAPLEURAL PNEUMONECTOMY. EPP is associated with distant sites of recurrence compared to locoregional sites of recurrence in patients having biopsy only or pleurectomy-decortication, and the local control for EPP was superior to that of the other modalities. Pass et al.[95] found that the pattern of recurrence was chiefly local progression after pleurectomy and systemic failures after EPP. In Sugarbaker's series of patients, Baldini et al.[105] have reported that the sites of first recurrence were local in 35% of patients, abdominal in 26%, in the contralateral thorax in 17%, and in other distant sites in 8%.

SURVIVAL. Long-term survival rates after EPP remain disappointing, with the median survivals ranging from 9.3 to 17.0 months for the majority of series. Rusch et al.[101,103] reported a median survival of 10 months, and Pass et al.[95] reported the median survival after EPP (all histologies) to be 9.4 months. The majority of patients were pathologic stage II or III in these two series. Most recently, Sugarbaker et al.[93] have reported a 17-month median survival for all patients in a series heavily weighted with stage I epithelial patients (n = 52 of 183), whose 2- and 5-year survivals were 68% and 46%, respectively. In the series by Rusch and Venkatraman,[75] the 2- and 5-year survivals of stage I patients (n = 16 of 131) were 65% and 30%, respectively.

RADIOTHERAPY FOR MESOTHELIOMA

Curative Radiation Therapy As a Single Modality

The limitation of potentially "curative" radiotherapy for treatment of MPM is the inability to treat a large volume of disease in the chest with a curative radiation dose (greater than 60 Gy) because of the risks of severe damage to normal tissue. Law et al.[96] administered radiation using a rotational technique to deliver 5000 to 5500 cGy to the pleural space. Survival in this group of patients ranged from 3 to 10 months, with the exception of one patient who was alive and well 4 years after the completion of treatment. Ball and Cruickshank[106] treated 12 patients with 5000 cGy to the entire hemithorax. Median survival of these patients was 17 months compared to 7 months for those offered palliative treatment only. This difference is likely the result of a selection bias, with those fit enough to undergo a full course of radiation likely to have a greater survival regardless of treatment given. In addition, in these 12 patients, two had toxicity that led to their deaths—one with radiation hepatitis and one with radiation myelopathy. A larger study of 49 patients with MPM that included patients treated with definitive radiotherapy was reported by Ruffie et al.[97] with a median survival of 9.8 months in patients treated with radical radiotherapy, which was no different than those treated with palliative radiation. Alberts et al.[107] used a variable schedule, split course of radiotherapy in 13 patients who were treated with definitive radiation alone. Patients received variable schedules of radiation. Some received 1000 cGy in 1 week (five 200-cGy fractions) every 6 weeks up to a maximum of four courses. Others received 150 cGy fractions for 10 days, followed by a rest period of 2 weeks. This was followed by an additional 3000 cGy in 2 weeks, using 300-cGy fractions. The median duration of response was 133 days. Holsti et al.[108] have also reported their results with 57 patients with pleural mesothelioma having radical hemithoracic radiotherapy. The 2-year survival rate of the group overall was 21%, and the 5-year survival rate was 9%.

Combined Chemotherapy and Definitive Radiotherapy

The poor results reported for definitive radiotherapy alone have led to studies evaluating the combination of chemotherapy and radiation. Alberts et al.[109] treated patients with a variety of chemotherapy regimens, all concurrent with radiation therapy (RT). The median survival was not significantly increased over those patients who received radiation alone. Ruffie et al.[97] treated mesothelioma patients with chemotherapy consisting of doxorubicin-based regimens and other combination chemotherapy regimens. There was a significant increase in survival in those patients receiving chemotherapy (median survival time of 12.3 months vs. 7.3 months) compared to those who did not receive chemotherapy. Linden et al.[110] treated patients with hemithoracic radiotherapy (40 Gy in 20 daily fractions) followed by chemotherapy in good-performance status patients. The median survival was highest (13 months) in patients treated with combined modality therapy. The differences in survival among the different treatment groups are likely the result of a selection bias in favor of the combined modality group.

Some investigators have evaluated the addition of radiation sensitizers with definitive RT. Herscher et al.[111] from the U.S. National Cancer Institute studied the use of a 5-day continuous infusion of paclitaxel with radical radiotherapy in patients with mesothelioma and non–small cell lung cancer. In mesothelioma patients, hemithoracic radiation was delivered initially. This was followed by a boost of radiotherapy to the gross tumor volume for a total dose of 5760 to 6300 cGy. The maximally tolerated dose of paclitaxel in combination with radiation was 105 mg/m² as a 120-hour continuous infusion. The toxicities were neutropenia, nausea and vomiting, grade 2 lung injury, and persistent cough. The authors concluded that this treatment was well tolerated. Chen et al.[112] reported a 12% complete response rate and an 88% partial response rate with pulsed paclitaxel delivered during radiotherapy in a phase I trial. Although these combination approaches are interesting, it is not likely that the addition of radiation sensitizers to radical radiotherapy will be a curative, and as such definitive chemoradiotherapy should be considered experimental for patients with mesothelioma.

Combined Surgical Resection and Definitive Radiotherapy

After an EPP, radical radiotherapy can be administered without concern for damage to the underlying ipsilateral lung because it has been removed surgically (Fig. 36-12). However, radical radiotherapy after a pleurectomy continues to place the ipsilateral lung at risk for substantial loss of function.

Both Ruffie et al.[97] and Law et al.[96] reported no difference in survival when decortication or EPP was followed by RT.

Rusch and colleagues[103] at Memorial Sloan-Kettering Cancer Center completed a phase II trial of surgery followed by postoperative radiation in patients with pleural mesothelioma. Eighty-eight patients with biopsy-confirmed mesothelioma were treated. Twenty-one patients were unresectable and taken off study. The majority of patients (n = 62) underwent an EPP followed by 54 Gy delivered through anterior and posterior fields in 30 fractions of 1.8 Gy. Five patients were treated with a pleurectomy, which was followed by intraoperative RT to a dose of 15 Gy, using a high-dose iridium applicator. This was followed by 54 Gy to the hemithorax via anterior and posterior fields in the same fractionation schedule as those who underwent EPP. There were seven postoperative deaths, all primarily related to pulmonary complications in patients who had undergone an EPP. A total of 33 patients had some complications, with the most common being atrial arrhythmias (17), respiratory failure (6), pneumonia (5), and empyema (5). Only the patients who underwent EPP were considered for survival analysis. The median survival was 17 months, with an overall survival of 27% at 3 years. Only 13% had locoregional recurrence, with the majority of patients failing to respond and having distant metastases. The authors concluded that their approach of aggressive surgery with EPP followed by high-dose radiation to the entire hemithorax provided a favorable outcome for those patients who were able to complete the therapy compared to historical data.

Lee et al.[113] recently retrospectively reviewed the efficacy and toxicity of surgery with intraoperative radiotherapy followed by chemotherapy. Twenty-six patients with MPM were included in the analysis. Twenty-four patients were treated with surgery consisting of a pleurectomy/decortication followed by intraoperative radiotherapy using 4- to 9-MeV electrons to a median dose of 15 Gy (range, 5 to 15 Gy). External-beam radiation was delivered by three-dimensional conformal RT in 14 patients and intensity-modulated RT (IMRT) in 10 patients. The median dose of radiation delivered was 41.4 Gy (range, 30.1 to 48.8 Gy). Chemotherapy consisting of cisplatin, doxorubicin, and cyclophosphamide was administered to selected patients beginning 1 to 2 months after radiation was completed. The median overall survival was 18.1 months, and the median progression-free interval was 12.2 months. Locoregional relapse was the most common site of failure. The authors concluded that this approach was a potential treatment option for adjuvant radiotherapy in patients who were unable to tolerate an EPP.

IMRT offers the potential for administering higher doses of radiotherapy to the hemithorax while minimizing normal tissue toxicities. Ahamad et al.[114] and Forster et al.[115] at the M. D. Anderson Cancer Study have treated 28 patients with IMRT after EPP. The hemithorax was treated with doses of 4500 to 5000 cGy. Some regions of the hemithorax were boosted to a total dose of 6000 cGy. Radiation-dose homogeneity to the entire hemithorax was excellent. Side effects included nausea, vomiting, dyspnea, and esophagitis. The median follow-up was 9 months, and the local control rate was 100%. One-year survival was 65%. These early results are encouraging and are worthy of additional study.

Prevention of Scar Recurrences

Malignant seeding along thoracentesis tracts, biopsy tracts, chest tube sites, and surgical incisions is a common complication of procedures in patients with malignant mesothelioma.[74] The frequency of malignant seeding has been reported to occur in approximately 20% to 50% of mesothelioma patients who undergo these procedures. Boutin et al.[74] have investigated the use of radiation to prevent malignant seeding after invasive diagnostic procedures. Forty patients were randomized after an inva-

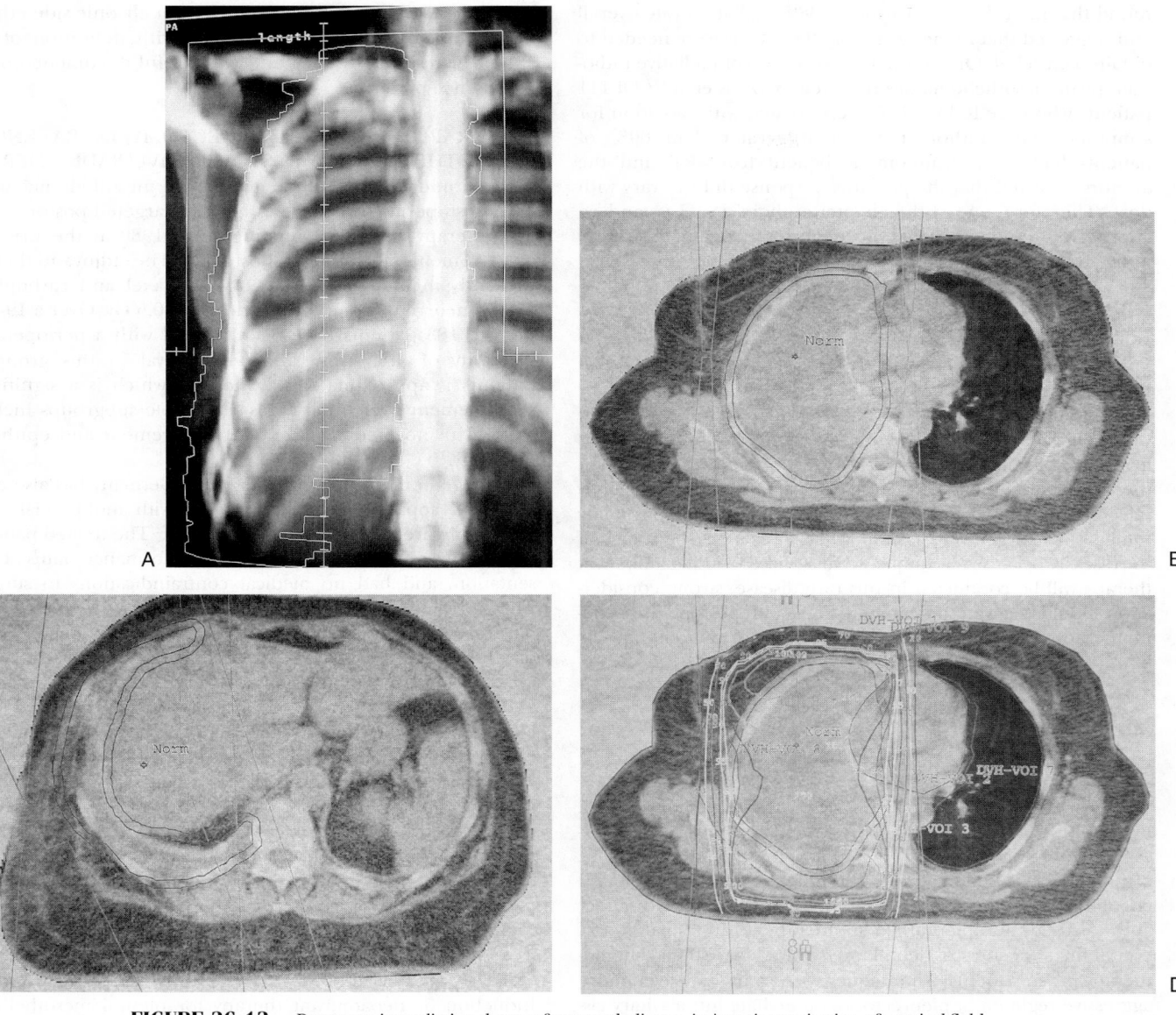

FIGURE 36-12. Postoperative radiation therapy for mesothelioma. **A:** Anterior projection of a typical field encompassing the right hemithorax. The hemithorax target volume is outlined. The target volume crosses midline and extends inferiorly to the diaphragmatic sulci. **B:** The target volume is shown on an axial projection. **C:** The complex geometry of the target volume at the inferior extent of the hemithorax is demonstrated on this axial projection. The target volume wraps around the liver. **D:** Isodose lines demonstrating the coverage of the target volume from anterior and posterior radiation fields. (See Color Fig. 36-12*B–D* in the CD-ROM.)

sive diagnostic procedure to either radiotherapy or no treatment. The radiotherapy regimen consisted of 21 Gy in 3 days delivered with electrons to healing biopsy tracts and thoracoscopic sites and was delivered 10 to 15 days after the procedure. No patient in the radiation treatment group developed subcutaneous nodules. Alternatively, 8 of 20 patients in the untreated group developed metastases.

Palliation Using Radiation Therapy

Palliation of patients with mesothelioma commonly involves the management of dyspnea and chest pain. Radiotherapy is most commonly used to palliate pain in patients with advanced mesothelioma,[90] and investigators from the Netherlands have reported using palliative radiotherapy to treat painful chest wall metastases in patients with mesothelioma. The authors reported that a total dose of 36 Gy in 400-cGy fractions provided local palliation in at least 50% of patients. Ball and Cruickshank[106] reported a 72% rate of symptom improvement using palliative courses of RT. These investigators reported that short courses of radiation (20 Gy in five fractions) were as efficacious for symptom relief as more protracted courses of radiation (30 to 40 Gy in 10 to 15 fractions). Ruffie et al.[97] reported the results of palliative RT in 85 patients with mesothelioma. When doses greater than 4500 cGy were used, pain relief was attained in more than 50% of the cases. An additional study by Gordon et al.[116] reported results that supported the dose-response relationship suggested by Ruffie et al.[97] These authors found that radiotherapy provided a 38% palliation rate overall and suggested that higher doses of 40 to 50 Gy were needed to obtain pain relief. One of the largest studies of palliative radiotherapy in mesothelioma was reported by Davis et al.[117] Of 111 patients who were followed, 71 were treated with radiation for symptoms. The authors found that greater than 60% of patients had some symptomatic benefit from RT, and the authors reported that the palliative response did not vary with dose. Therefore, one of the chapter authors' (S. H.) standard approach is to offer patients short courses of treatment (20 Gy in five fractions) rather than longer courses of radiotherapy.

ADJUVANT THERAPY FOR SURGICALLY CYTOREDUCED MESOTHELIOMA PATIENTS

Patients treated with surgery and postoperative adjuvant therapy have an apparent improved survival compared to those treated with palliative therapy alone in consecutively treated patients from single institutions. There are no phase III trials of adjuvant therapy in mesothelioma. These results may be explained by selection bias or by a number of other factors. Yet, the possibility remains that surgery and adjuvant therapy changes the course of the disease. Because it is unlikely that a phase III trial of adjuvant therapy will be conducted in this rare disease, strong consideration should be given to treating patients with postoperative chemotherapy (if pleurectomy was performed) or radiotherapy, or both (if EPP was performed).[103]

MULTIMODALITY TREATMENT

Surgery and Standard Agents

PLEURECTOMY/INTRAPLEURAL CHEMOTHERAPY ± POSTOPERATIVE CHEMOTHERAPY. There has been interest in combining debulking surgery with intracavitary treatment of pleural mesothelioma since the first reports of intrapleural chemotherapy alone for malignant mesothelioma. Rusch et al.[118,119] used intrapleural chemotherapy with cisplatin and cytarabine after surgical debulking followed by systemic chemotherapy in ten patients. A subsequent report used an even more aggressive regimen of pleurectomy, immediate intracavitary cisplatin, and mitomycin C with two cycles of systemic cisplatin and mitomycin C. In the initial trial, there was one postoperative death, and the chemotherapy complications were reversible, making such an approach feasible. The most recent trial revealed an overall survival rate of 68% at 1 year and 44% at 2 years in the 27 patients who received the therapy, with a median survival of 17 months. Recurrences, however, were chiefly locoregional. A similar regimen combining pleurectomy or EPP with cisplatin and mitomycin C resulted in a disappointing median survival of 13 months, and only 50% of the chemotherapy treatments were delivered adjuvantly. In an Italian study of 20 patients, pleurectomy and diaphragmatic or pericardial resection combined with intrapleural chemotherapy with cisplatin and cytarabine for 4 hours immediately after pleurectomy followed by systemic chemotherapy with epirubicin and mitomycin C revealed a median time to disease progression of 7.4 months and median survival of only 11.5 months.[120]

The intrapleural route with standard agents or RT remains intriguing but unanswered with regard to its efficacy. Phase II studies with the following design principles continue to be

needed: (1) a tolerable regimen without chronic side effects, (2) a standard debulking approach with definition of the extent of residual disease, and (3) careful documentation of recurrence patterns.

EXTRAPLEURAL PNEUMONECTOMY/INTRAVENOUS CHEMOTHERAPY AND POSTOPERATIVE RADIOTHERAPY. A multimodal approach to malignant mesothelioma using EPP, postoperative chemotherapy, and targeted postoperative radiotherapy has been ongoing since 1980 at the Brigham and Women's Hospital in Boston.[121] The adjuvant therapy presently includes two cycles of paclitaxel and carboplatin with concurrent radiation to a dose of 40.5 Gy. Over a 19-year period, 183 patients have been treated with a perioperative mortality of 3.8%. The median survival in this group of patients is approximately 17 months, which is a significant improvement over other trials. Favorable subgroups include those with no mediastinal nodal involvement and epithelial histology.[121]

A large nonrandomized series from Germany has also demonstrated apparent increased survival with multimodal treatment compared to best supportive care.[122] The treated patients, however, were younger, had a better performance status at presentation, and had no medical contraindications to surgery. These 93 patients chose either best supportive care or multimodal treatment. Surgery consisted of pleurectomy decortication or EPP followed by systemic chemotherapy with doxorubicin, cyclophosphamide, and vindesine. Patients in remission at the end of the chemotherapy (16 of the 57 accrued) received 45 to 60 Gy of RT to the hemithorax. Median survival was 13 months compared to 7 months for those receiving best supportive care.

In a series of 32 patients from Italy, Maggi et al.[123-125] used the Brigham and Women's protocol of EPP followed by adjuvant chemotherapy and concurrent hemithoracic radiation up to a total dose of 55 Gy. The results were encouraging, with only 6.25% operative mortality rate. However, a median survival of only 9.5 months was reported because 50% of the patients were found to be in stage III after the procedure.

INDUCTION CHEMOTHERAPY FOLLOWED BY SURGERY. Induction or neoadjuvant therapy for pleural mesothelioma followed by surgery has been patterned after such therapy with non–small cell lung cancer. With the improved efficacy of doublet chemotherapy (gemcitabine/cisplatin or pemetrexed/cisplatin), there is renewed interest in investigating a neoadjuvant approach for mesothelioma. A Swiss neoadjuvant study used three cycles of cisplatin 80 mg/m^2 on day 1 and gemcitabine 1000 mg/m^2 on days 1, 8, and 15 every 28 days followed by surgery. RT was considered after EPP to areas at risk. In all, 30 patients entered thus far have been reported. After chemotherapy, 22 (73%) underwent EPP. Histology after surgery revealed epithelioid (10), mixed (11), and sarcomatoid disease (3). There was one postoperative fatality. The median overall survival was 20 months, and the 1-year survival rate was 77%.[126] A similar trial was performed by de Perrot et al.[127] that involved induction chemotherapy, surgery, and postoperative hemithorax RT, with a 6% operative mortality and 74% 1-year survival. A neoadjuvant approach is presently being investigated in the United States as a multicenter trial of four cycles of pemetrexed and cisplatin followed by EPP and postoperative hemithorax RT.

NOVEL INTRAPLEURAL APPROACHES: NEW TECHNIQUES WITH NEW/OLD AGENTS

Intrapleural Photodynamic Therapy

Photodynamic therapy (PDT) involves the light-activated sensitization of malignant cells[128] using a photosensitizer, such as Photofrin II, which is retained by malignant tissue *in vivo* in comparison to normal tissue (Fig. 36-13). The sensitizer is activated by 630-nm light and then interacts with molecular oxygen to produce an excited reactive oxygen species. After a series of phase I and II trials, a group of 63 patients with localized mesothelioma were randomized to surgery, with or without intraoperative PDT.[128] There were no differences in median survival (14.4 vs. 14.1 months) or median progression-free time (8.5 vs. 7.7 months), and sites of first recurrence were similar. Other phase II trials of PDT and mesothelioma have not demonstrated therapeutic efficacy,[129,130] and, most recently,[131] preliminary results using intrapleural PDT with metaTetraHydroxyPhenylChlorin after EPP have revealed significant toxicities without survival benefit.[132]

PLEURAL PERFUSION

Hyperthermic chemoperfusion of the pleura after resection of mesothelioma is based on the hypothesis that the treatment will provide increased local control and avoid systemic chemotherapy toxicity (Fig. 36-14). Ratto et al.[133] delivered cisplatin to the pleural space after pleurectomy or EPP in ten patients, and other small phase II studies using cisplatin or doxorubicin with cisplatin have recorded morbidity rates of 33% to 65% using temperatures of 40° to 42°C without impacting survival.[134,135] Sugarbaker et al.[135a] presented a phase I/II trial using hyperthermic cisplatin (42°C) to perfuse both the abdomen and the pleura after pleurectomy/decortication. Operative mortality was 11%, and survival of all patients was 10.5 months; however, in the group of patients surviving surgery who received 225 mg/m^2 of cisplatin, the median survival was 22 months, and disease-free survival was 20 months.

NOVEL GENE AND CYTOKINE-RELATED THERAPIES

By transferring the herpes simplex virus thymidine kinase (HSVtk) gene to a tumor by infecting it with an adenovirus construct containing the TK gene (AdHSVtk), one essentially kills the tumor with the addition of ganciclovir. A phase I trial of intrapleural suicide gene therapy has been reported that delivered a replication-deficient adenovirus encoding HSVtk (AdHSVtk) that, in preclinical studies, was found to transduce mesothelioma cells and treat human mesothelioma xenografts in SCID mice.[136] Gene transfer was demonstrated in 17 of 25 evaluable patients and was dose-dependent. There was one partial response, 3 of the first 18 patients remained stable for up to 2 years after treatment, and one early-stage patient was tumor free for more than 31 months. The median survival of all patients was 11 months.

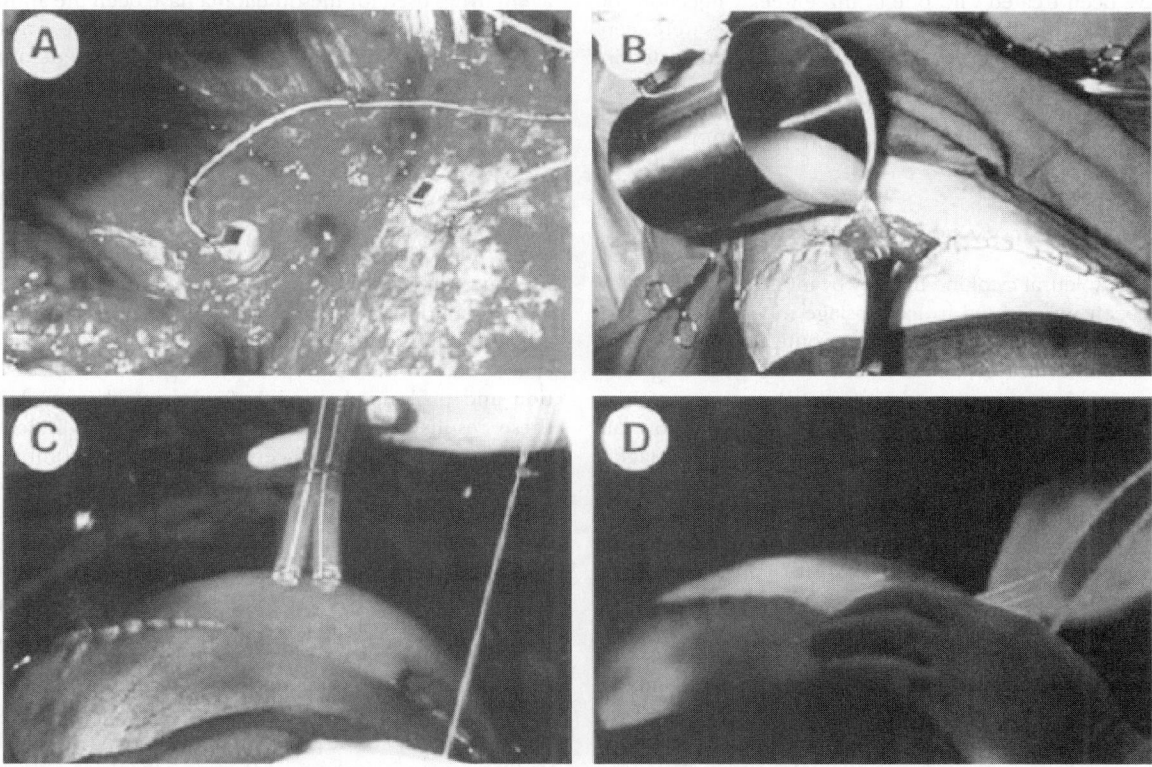

FIGURE 36-13. Intraoperative photodynamic therapy for mesothelioma. **A:** After pleurectomy or pneumonectomy, light-sensing diodes are placed in strategic areas of the chest for dosimetry measurements. **B:** Light-scattering solution, usually intralipid, is poured into the partially closed chest. **C:** Laser fibers housed in modified endotracheal tubes are then placed into the chest, illuminating the chest wall and remaining organs **(D)**, which had received the photosensitizer 48 hours previously. (See Color Fig. 36-13 in the CD-ROM.)

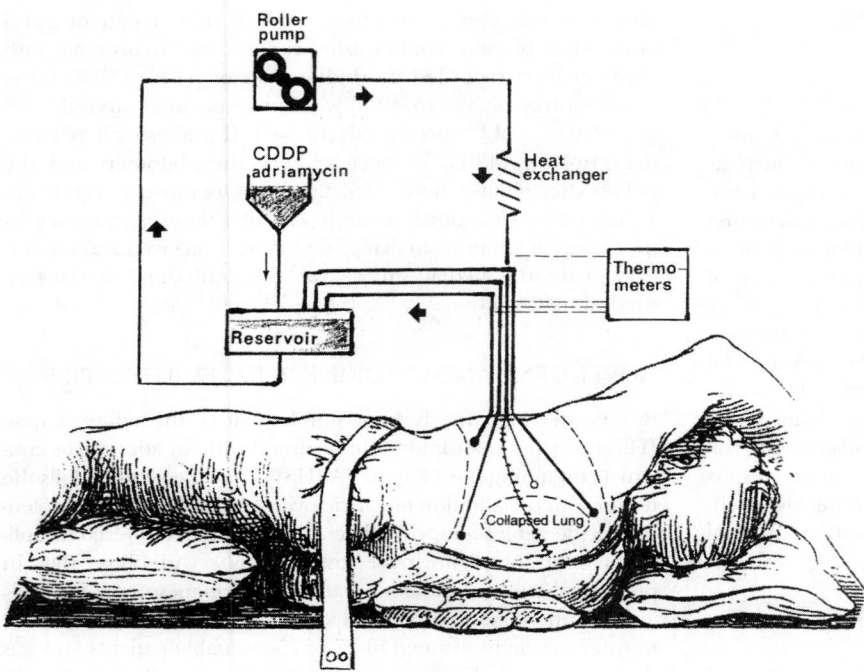

FIGURE 36-14. Intrathoracic chemoperfusion for mesothelioma. CDDP, cisplatin. (From ref. 205, with permission.)

Immunomodulatory gene therapy is also being investigated for mesothelioma by transfecting tumors with cytokine genes that can activate CD4 T cells or stimulate CD8 T cells. The IL-2 gene has been inserted into a replication-deficient vaccinia virus, and six patients have been treated with one to three weekly injections of vaccinia virus–IL-2 intratumorally. No clinical responses were seen although expression of vaccinia virus–IL-2 mRNA was detected in tumor biopsies, and a T-cell infiltrate was detected in 50% of tumor biopsies at the site of injection.[137–139] Preclinical trials of the transfection of interferon-β,[140,141] IL-4, and p14(ARF)[19,20] into mesothelioma are ongoing.

INTRAPLEURAL AND SYSTEMIC CYTOKINE THERAPY

The use of intrapleural cytokine therapy by infusional techniques has chiefly been investigated in earlier-stage mesothelioma, and the effectiveness of interferon-γ by this route has been documented by Boutin et al.[142] and Driesen et al.[143] Eight histologically confirmed complete responses and nine partial responses with at least a 50% reduction in tumor size were obtained. The overall response rate was 20%. The response rate for patients with stage I disease was 45%, with the main side effects being hyperthermia, liver toxicity, neutropenia, and catheter-related infection.

Intrapleural IL-2–based regimens have also been exploited in mesothelioma.[144] Intrapleural IL-2 [21 × 10(6) IU/m²/day for 5 days] was given to 22 patients with mesothelioma. There were 11 partial responses and 1 complete response. Stable disease occurred in three patients and disease progression in seven patients. The overall median survival time was 18 months, and the 24- and 36-month survival rates for responders were 58% and 41%, respectively. No confirmatory trials of this promising approach have been published.

CHEMOTHERAPY AND NEWER AGENTS

The rarity and dismal survival of pleural mesothelioma has precluded, until recently, phase III trials. It was not surprising, therefore, that early studies reported the results of single-agent chemotherapy drugs tested in 20 to 40 patients with the hope that a major therapeutic advance would be discovered with limited numbers of patients. In general, the most common single-agent drugs used for mesothelioma have been the anthracyclines, platinum agents, and antimetabolites.[145] The anthracyclines have had response rates of 0% to 15%, with median survivals of 4.4 to 9.5 months. Cisplatinum or carboplatinum have had response rates of 7% to 16%, with median survivals of 5 to 8 months. Antimetabolites as single agents have had response rates from 0% to 37%, the highest observed in methotrexate (37%) and gemcitabine (31%).[145] Typically, tumor regression of short duration associated with symptomatic improvement occurred in 15% of patients treated with chemotherapy, but the median survival remained at approximately 7 to 9 months. Those data led Ong and Vogelzang[146] to conclude that there was no chemotherapeutic agent(s) sufficiently active to be called "standard." Some patients experienced disease stabilization and prolonged survival after chemotherapy, but whether these results were due to the therapy or to indolent tumor behavior could not be discerned. In general, combination chemotherapies have had higher response rates and longer median survival times. Patients taking anthracycline-based combinations have had response rates from 11% to 32% and median survivals from 5.5 to 13.8 months; those taking platinum-based combinations have had response rates of 6% to 48%, with median survivals of 5.8 to 16.0 months.[145]

A 1998 report from the United Kingdom was somewhat encouraging, suggesting that clinical benefit (as measured by reduction in pain and dyspnea) occurred in up to 40% to 50% of patients treated with a regimen of three agents: mitomycin C, vinblastine, and cisplatin.[147] Recently, Steele et al.[148] reported a similar rate of clinical benefit with the single-agent vinorelbine (Navelbine). The Medical Research Council and British Thoracic Society thus are conducting a trial that will randomize more than 800 patients with malignant mesothelioma to either single-agent vinorelbine, the mitomycin/vinblastine/cisplatin combination, or active supportive care to determine whether chemotherapy improves either quality or length of life in this disease.[149]

Another encouraging report was from Byrne et al.[150] on the combination of the older chemotherapeutic agent cisplatin combined with a new antimetabolite, gemcitabine. Forty-seven percent of patients (10 of 21) had a 30% or greater reduction in the thickness of the pleural rind and improvement in symptoms. A follow-up multicenter trial from Australia with 53 patients reported a 26% rate of activity but a median survival of only 7.5 months.[151] The activity of the combination in other multicenter phase II studies[152] in patients previously treated with other chemotherapy[153] and the gemcitabine/carboplatin regimen[154] has led to its widespread use. Gemcitabine,[155,156] cisplatin,[157–160] and carboplatin[161–163] all have independent but modest single-agent activity. Whether the cisplatin/gemcitabine doublet is superior to either single agent is not known, and no phase III studies are in progress examining the question.

A role for the antifolates has been suggested since Solheim et al.[164] reported methotrexate-induced regressions in 37% of patients. Other antifolates had consistent but low activity as well.

A novel antifolate, pemetrexed (Alimta) binds with high affinity to folate transport proteins; is extensively polyglutamated; inhibits dihydrofolate reductase, thymidylate synthase, and glycinamide ribonucleotide formyltransferase; and demonstrates broad antitumor activity in phase I and II trials.[165] When combined with cisplatin, pemetrexed induced regressions in 38% of pleural mesothelioma patients (5 of 12) who entered a phase I trial in Germany.[166] A British phase I study of pemetrexed and carboplatin conducted exclusively on patients with pleural mesothelioma reported significant radiologic improvements in approximately 40% of patients.[167] These two trials led to a phase II trial of pemetrexed as a single agent

in the treatment of mesothelioma[168] in which 14% of patients responded. While that trial, the phase III mesothelioma trial, and other phase I and II trials were under way, a comprehensive multivariate analysis by Eli Lilly and Company and its clinical investigators revealed that folic acid and vitamin B_{12} deficiency states (as measured by elevated serum homocysteine and methylmalonic acid levels) were the major contributors to grade III and IV toxicity of pemetrexed.[169] Thus, beginning on 12/2/99, Eli Lilly investigators were required to use supplementation with folic acid and vitamin B_{12} in all patients receiving pemetrexed. Folic acid therapy (400 μg/day to 1000 μg/day) and vitamin B_{12} injections every 9 weeks reduced myelosuppression and gastrointestinal toxicity while preserving and possibly enhancing efficacy.

Because of the encouraging results in phase I and II trials, Eli Lilly conducted a 452-patient (448 patients evaluable) phase III trial comparing single-agent cisplatin (75 mg/m²) versus pemetrexed (500-mg/m² intravenous bolus over 10 minutes) plus the same dose of cisplatin. Both regimens were given every 3 weeks. The results showed that the two-drug regimen was clearly superior to a one-drug regimen as assessed by median survival time (12.1 months vs. 9.3 months, respectively) (Fig. 36-15). Response rates (as measured by an average 30% reduction in the thickness of the pleural rind measured at up to 9 points on the CT scan) were 41.3% versus 16.7% in the cisplatin-alone arm. Time to disease progression, pulmonary function, and quality of life also improved in a statistically significant manner in the pemetrexed/cisplatin-treated patients.

While the first 117 patients were being enrolled in the phase III trial, Eli Lilly completed a multiple regression analysis of virtually all patients treated in pemetrexed trials. Increased vitamin metabolite markers (plasma homocysteine and methylmalonic acid) was a predictor of increased risk of severe pemetrexed tox-

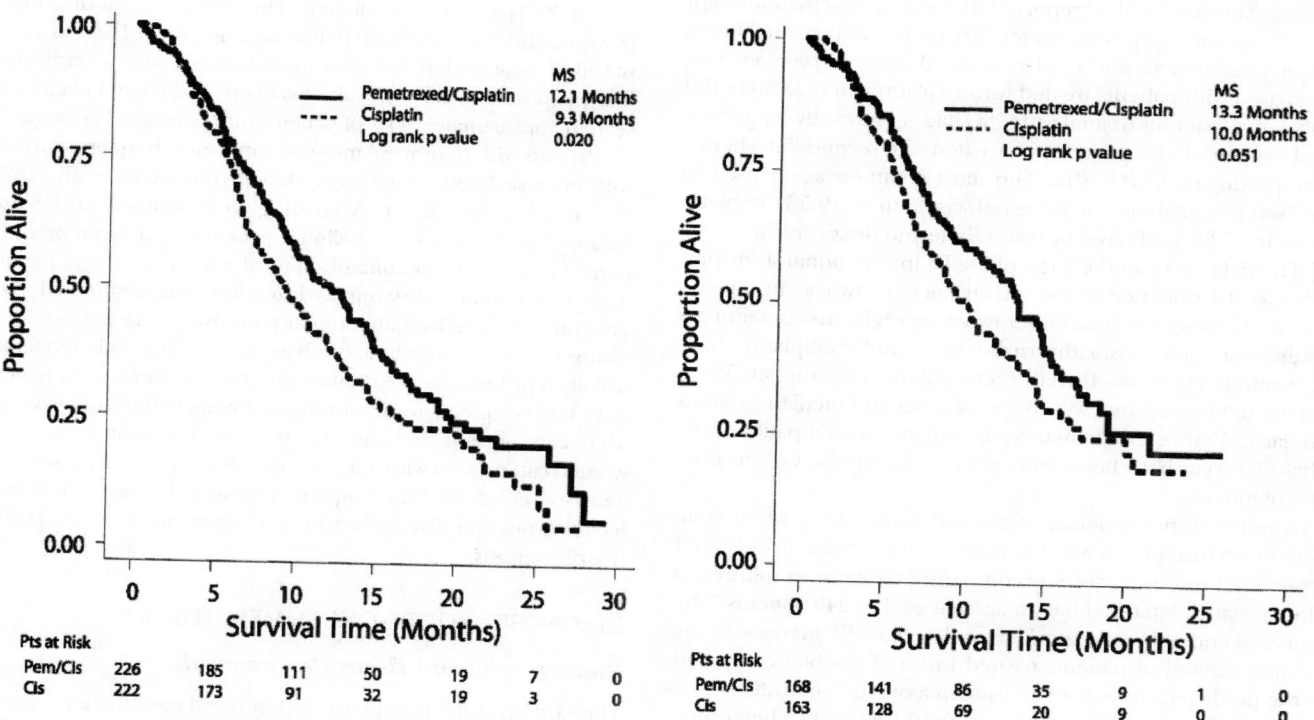

FIGURE 36-15. Results of the phase III trial of pemetrexed (Pem) and cisplatin (Cis) versus cisplatin alone. See text for details. MS, median survival; Pts, patients.

icity. Vitamin B_{12} and folic acid were subsequently added to both arms of the study. Treatment with the two-drug regimen had resulted in greater serious adverse events, including drug-related death, grade 3/4 neutropenia, thrombocytopenia, as well as nausea and vomiting relative to the cisplatin arm only; however, supplementation with folic acid and vitamin B_{12} significantly reduced the incidence of these toxicities in the pemetrexed/cisplatin arm but not in the cisplatin-alone arm of the study. These results suggest treatment with pemetrexed and cisplatin, supplemented with folic acid and vitamin B_{12}, provides an improved risk-benefit ratio in the treatment of mesothelioma.

Four additional analyses of this large database were presented in 2003. Gralla et al.[170] presented results demonstrating that the pemetrexed and cisplatin combination was associated with significantly sustained improvement in quality of life and symptom relief (including pain, dyspnea, fatigue, anorexia, and cough) when compared with cisplatin alone. By using Cox multiple regression analysis, Symanowski et al.[171] identified additional factors in the randomized trial. Powerful predictors of increased survival included good performance status ($P < .01$), epithelial subtype ($P < .01$), and early-stage disease ($P < .01$). Decreased survival was associated with elevation in white blood cells ($P < .01$) and unexpected elevation in vitamin metabolite markers of folic acid and vitamins B_{12} and B_6 (i.e., homocysteine, methylmalonic acid, and cystathione). Vitamin supplementation in this study was associated with longer survival ($P < .01$). Another correlative study[172] indicated that PFTs before each cycle of therapy (with either cisplatin alone or with doublet therapy) were improved in both the responder and stable-disease patients. Changes in slow vital capacity, forced vital capacity, or FEV_1 all correlated significantly with tumor response status. These results suggest that the commonly used objective measurement with PFTs may be particularly helpful and more sensitive than CT scanning in detecting response to treatment for patients with stable disease in mesothelioma. Manegold et al.[173] reported that post-study chemotherapy (PSC) was associated with longer survival in the mesotheliomas. Fewer pemetrexed- and cisplatin-treated patients received PSC compared with patients treated with cisplatin alone. Despite this imbalance, patients treated with PSC had significantly longer survival compared with patients not treated with second-line chemotherapy (log-rank, $P = .01$). The most common agent used in PSC was gemcitabine (pemetrexed/cisplatin in 19.5%, cisplatin alone in 17.3%) followed by vinorelbine and doxorubicin.

The data set from the large phase III international study provides level I evidence of the effectiveness of two-agent chemotherapy in mesothelioma. Other two-drug regimens containing a platinating agent (cisplatin, carboplatin, and oxaliplatin) have been studied in phase II trials (gemcitabine/cisplatin, etc.) and appear to be associated with response rates and median survivals similar to that of the pemetrexed/cisplatin-treated patients. No phase III trials have been reported comparing the various doublet regimens.

Another antimetabolite, raltitrexed (Tomudex), when combined with oxaliplatin, also has antimesothelioma activity,[174] and a phase III trial is under way comparing cisplatin to raltitrexed plus cisplatin. That trial has an accrual goal of 240 patients. The statistical end point of that trial is to detect a 50% increase in the median survival of patients treated with the doublet compared to the predicted survival after cisplatin alone of 8 months.

Another agent subjected to a phase III trial in the chemotherapy of mesothelioma was ranpirnase, which was reported in 2000. After an encouraging phase II experience,[175] the phase III trial compared the median survival of 154 patients randomized to treatment with either single-agent doxorubicin or single-agent ranpirnase (Onconase), a ribonuclease derived from frog eggs. Using an intention-to-treat analysis, there was no difference in the median survivals (7 to 8 months in each group). The randomization failed to equally distribute poor-risk patients. When those patients were omitted from the analysis, the median survival favored ranpirnase (11 vs. 8 months). The trial has been extended to compare doxorubicin to doxorubicin plus ranpirnase and will accrue a total of 250 to 300 patients. Ranpirnase has recently been granted orphan drug status for the treatment of mesothelioma by the European Union.

In spite of these modestly heartening results, effective agents with unique mechanisms of action against mesothelioma are still desperately needed. VEGF signal transduction inhibitors are being tested and have clinical activity. To optimally test the many newer agents, referral of fit patients with no prior exposure to systemic therapy in clinical trials is strongly encouraged.

In conclusion, chemotherapeutic agents have historically had little effectiveness against mesothelioma. Newer agents seem to be somewhat more effective, and the pemetrexed and cisplatin combination alters the natural history of mesothelioma. Second-line chemotherapy may also alter the natural history of mesothelioma, but phase III trials using a placebo-controlled population are needed.

MALIGNANT PERITONEAL MESOTHELIOMA

PRESENTATION

The incidence of peritoneal mesotheliomas appears to be increasing in the United States and Europe, and these now account for 25% to 33% of all mesotheliomas. The median age at diagnosis is 60 years, and there is a male to female ratio of 3:1. There is a clear statistical relationship between mesothelioma and a particularly heavy exposure to airborne asbestos fibers, and pleural plaques are seen in approximately 50% of patients with peritoneal primaries.[176]

Patients with peritoneal mesothelioma most frequently present with increased abdominal girth (49%) from ascites, pain (43%), and weight loss (22%). According to Mohamed and Sugarbaker,[177] peritoneal mesothelioma presents as a "pain-predominant" or "ascites-predominant" clinical type, and 14% of patients have concomitant abdominal distention and abdominal pain. Patients with localized abdominal pain usually have a dominant tumor mass (6%) with little or no ascites, and the abdominal mass usually represents a cake of tumor in the omentum. Most patients have had symptoms for 6 months to 2 years before the diagnosis. Men can present with an inguinal or umbilical hernia, and women can present with a pelvic mass. Some patients present with a new-onset hernia. Other signs of advanced disease include fever, leukocytosis, and thrombocytosis, and these are associated with a poor prognosis.

DIAGNOSIS OF PERITONEAL MESOTHELIOMA

Radiography and Tissue Procurement

The workup of the patient with a peritoneal mesothelioma usually includes abdominal ultrasonography, CT of the abdomen,[178–180]

MRI, and, most recently, PET scanning.[181] Definitive diagnosis requires CT-guided core biopsy of tumor masses or infiltrated omentum,[182] paracentesis with cell block for immunohistochemical staining, or, preferably, laparoscopy with biopsy.[183,184] Ultimately, definitive diagnosis requires adequate tissue sampling, preferably from laparoscopy or an open, directed biopsy. The endoscopic appearance of mesothelioma is indistinguishable from that of metastatic tumors, with nodules, plaques, and masses that involve the parietal and visceral peritoneum. The absence of hepatic parenchymal metastases should alert the physician to the possibility that the pathology is mesothelioma, and careful examination of the ovaries and the bowel to rule out nonmesothelioma neoplasms should be performed.

Peritoneal mesotheliomas must be differentiated from so-called papillary tumors of the peritoneum (also known as *well-differentiated papillary mesothelioma* or *cystic mesotheliomas of the peritoneum*) as these tumors have a completely different natural history. Asbestos exposure is much less frequently associated with these neoplasms compared to true abdominal mesotheliomas, and the papillary tumors are predominantly seen in women but can occur in men.[185] The tumor's differential diagnosis from malignant mesothelioma may be based on the lack of immunostaining for keratin 5/6 and calretinin.[186] Although the ability to diagnose cystic mesotheliomas of the peritoneum before or at the time of exploratory laparotomy is limited, there has been advocacy for the avoidance of treatment unless there is evidence of progressive disease.[187] Differential diagnosis from ovarian cancer or true mesothelioma, however, may be possible only after the pathologic examination of the surgically resected ovaries along with the tumor to document that the tumor has minimal or no superficial invasion of the ovarian cortex or through immunohistochemical methods.[188] There have been recent anecdotal reports of an aggressive approach to these tumors either by adding adjuvant platinum-based chemotherapy after resection or primary treatment with cytoreductive surgery and heated chemoperfusion.[189]

Staging and Natural History of Malignant Peritoneal Mesothelioma

There is no staging system for peritoneal mesothelioma, although suggestions have been proposed in the literature. The tumor generally remains confined to the abdomen until late in the course and even then is more likely to spread to one or both pleural cavities than to disseminate hematogenously. Most patients die without metastases or involvement of the chest. Involvement of the serosa overlying the small and large bowel, the liver, the spleen, and other organs leads to encasement of these organs in tumor tissue and repeated bowel obstructions. The median survival of untreated patients is 5 to 12 months.

TREATMENT

Due to the low response rates of systemic chemotherapy in the disease, novel approaches involving either induction therapy followed by surgery or postoperative intraperitoneal drug delivery after surgical debulking have been explored. Intraperitoneal chemotherapy with a variety of agents, including cisplatinum, mitomycin C, doxorubicin, epidoxorubicin, etoposide, and cytarabine used either singly or in combination, has been

reported, with responses up to 50% in small phase II studies.[190–194] Whole abdominal radiotherapy as an adjunct to intraperitoneal chemotherapy and surgery was first described in ten patients with peritoneal mesothelioma who were treated at the Joint Center for Radiation Therapy between 1968 and 1985. Six of the ten patients remained free of disease at 19+ to 78+ months after diagnosis. Four patients not treated with this multimodality approach died from the disease.[195]

Intraperitoneal Chemotherapy

The use of intraperitoneal chemotherapy for mesothelioma has been extensively reviewed by Antman et al.[196] and Markman.[197] Intraperitoneal cisplatin and intravenous thiosulfate protection have resulted in a 59% complete response rate. However, many patients have relapsed quickly after treatment, implying incomplete eradication of tumor using cisplatin alone.[198] Intraperitoneal cisplatin in 19 patients (with mitomycin as well in 18) resulted in two (10%) disease-free responses more than 5 years after therapy.[199] Cisplatin and etoposide resulted in one complete response in five patients with measurable disease.

Of four patients receiving cisplatin-based intraperitoneal therapy in a Dutch study, two responded, one completely. At 2 years, he developed intestinal obstruction, and laparotomy revealed only adhesions.[200] A case report noted continuing complete response at 53 months in a patient treated with intraperitoneal cisplatin and cytarabine.[201]

Evolution of Combined Modality Approaches for Peritoneal Mesothelioma

Combined modality approaches for peritoneal mesothelioma have been studied at several institutions and usually involve surgery with cytoreduction, intraperitoneal chemotherapy, intraoperative treatment with cytotoxic chemotherapy, and postoperative chemotherapy and/or RT. Taylor and Johnson[202] described the use of surgery, intraperitoneal chemotherapy, and abdominal radiation in four patients. Eltabbakh et al.,[203] in a retrospective review of 15 women with peritoneal mesothelioma, reported that the response rate to first-line chemotherapy regimens was 30% overall, but 67% to paclitaxel and cisplatin. The median survival of all patients was 12 months. The median survival, however, was longer for patients who underwent cytoreductive surgery versus biopsy only (14 vs. 6 months, *P* = .24) and chemotherapy versus none (29 vs. 1 month, *P* = .03).

The evolution of multimodality therapy has been summarized by Taub et al.[204] Three sequential series of patients (1980 to 1982, 1982 to 1985, and 1986 to 1988) were treated at the Dana Farber Cancer Institute and Joint Center for Radiation Therapy. In the initial trial, one of nine patients treated with surgery, intravenous cyclophosphamide, doxorubicin, and dimethyltriazenoimidazole carboxamide (before and after whole abdominal radiotherapy) survived longer than 10 years after diagnosis. On the second phase I trial between 1982 and 1985, 6 of 13 patients having a debulking resection of all lesions of more than 1 cm in size were treated with intraperitoneal doxorubicin (6 to 50 mg/m^2) and cisplatin (60 to 100 mg/m^2) for a total of 8 to 12 treatments. At the time of the second laparotomy for removal of the access device, all six patients had an objective decrease of at least 50% in the size of the tumor. The complete treatment package of surgical resection and chemotherapy followed by whole abdominal irradiation was completed in four patients. Four of the six patients (including three of the four who received irradiation) remained disease free for at least 36, 48, 60, and 61 months after diagnosis. In the third phase II series, patients were treated with surgical debulking and intraperitoneal cisplatin and doxorubicin every 2 weeks for 20 weeks. Patients with no visible disease at second-look laparotomy received whole abdominal external-beam radiotherapy, and patients found at second-look laparotomy with macroscopic residual disease were treated with intravenous cyclophosphamide and doxorubicin, and then RT. Thirteen patients responded to therapy (seven partially and six completely, although random biopsies were positive in all patients). Three patients with partial responses relapsed at 8, 24, and 25 months. At the time of reporting, all six patients with complete responses had remained in remission from 9 to 30 months (median, 25 months). Toxicity was generally mild; nausea and vomiting occurred secondary to cisplatin, transient elevation in creatinine was as high as 2.4, and mild to moderate hematologic toxicity was reported. Two episodes of small bowel obstructions in responding patients resolved without surgical intervention. No patient discontinued therapy due to toxicity. In a series of 17 early-stage patients between 1984 and 1999 who underwent cytoreductive surgery followed by five cycles of intraperitoneal doxorubicin (25 mg/m^2) and cisplatin (75 mg/m^2), 11 patients responded (65%) as assessed by second laparotomy or CT scan and received total abdominal radiation (30 Gy; n = 3), intravenous chemotherapy (n = 3), or both (n = 4); ten patients completed all planned treatment. Toxicity included nausea, fatigue, and myelosuppression. Median survival for this group was 27.6 months (3.6 to 66.0). Eight patients were alive at follow-up of median 24 months (3 to 49 months).

Other investigators have combined hyperthermia to 42°C with chemotherapy at the time of the cytoreduction.[205–207] Of 18 patients with primary peritoneal mesothelioma who underwent tumor debulking followed by a 90-minute continuous hyperthermic peritoneal profusion with cisplatin as part of three consecutive phase I trials conducted at the National Cancer Institute, 13 had associated ascites. Nine of ten patients had resolution of their ascites postoperatively. Three patients with recurrent ascites at 10, 22, and 27 months after initial treatment had resolution of their ascites with ongoing responses at 4, 6, and 24 months after the second perfusion. The median progression-free survival is 26 months, and the overall 2-year survival is 80% at early follow-up. In Loggie's series,[205] 12 patients underwent exploratory laparotomy with cytoreduction followed by a 2-hour hyperthermic chemoperfusion using mitomycin C. One patient died 50 days postoperatively from complications relating to small bowel perforation. Ascites was controlled in all patients and permanently in 86% of patients presenting with ascites. To date, median survival is 34.2 months, with median follow-up of 45.2 months; however, long-term follow-up is lacking, and whether any of these patients had cystic mesothelioma must be determined. Sugarbaker et al.'s[208] series of 51 patients reports an encouraging median survival of 50 to 60 months using cytoreduction and heated chemotherapy with adriamycin and cisplatinum followed by paclitaxel. Further delineation of the histology of the patients is needed.

MALIGNANT MESOTHELIOMA OF THE TUNICA VAGINALIS TESTIS

Fewer than 100 cases of gonadal mesothelioma have been reported in the literature, and although most patients are in their 50s or older, approximately 10% of the patients are younger than 25 years.[209] Asbestos exposure is documented in approximately one-half of the more recently reported cases. Patients generally present with a hydrocele or hernia. An accurate preoperative diagnosis has been reported in only two cases.

All patients with a suspected testicular malignancy should undergo a radical or high inguinal orchiectomy.

Local resection of the tumor or hydrocelectomy is associated with a high recurrence rate compared with high inguinal orchiectomy. Because preoperative diagnosis of gonadal mesothelioma is difficult, management should be as for any testicular tumor. The inguinal approach avoids interruption of the scrotal lymphatics, which would alter the metastatic pathway of the tumor, and also allows complete removal of the spermatic cord up to the internal ring. Patients with evidence of disease extending into the retroperitoneal nodes should undergo a retroperitoneal lymphadenectomy.

The overall recurrence rate (local and disseminated) for gonadal mesothelioma can be as high as 52%, with 38% of patients dying of disease progression.[210] Local recurrence occurs in 36% of patients who undergo local resection of the hydrocele wall; 10% after scrotal orchiectomy and 12% after inguinal orchiectomy.[210] More than 60% of recurrences developed within the first 2 years of the follow-up. The median survival of the patients averaged 23 months. There are little data regarding the use of adjuvant therapy after resection of gonadal mesothelioma.

MALIGNANT MESOTHELIOMA OF THE PERICARDIUM

A recent review of the primary pericardial mesothelioma has been published by Vigneswaran and Stefanacci.[211] It is a rare neoplasm with a reported incidence of 0.0022% in an autopsy series of 5,000,000 case studies[212] and a calculated annual incidence of 1 in 40 million in a Canadian epidemiologic survey.[213] An antemortem diagnosis was made in less than one-third of 150 reported cases in the literature. Pericardial mesotheliomas can occur at any age, but people in the fourth to seventh decades of life are most likely to be afflicted, and there is a 2:1 male to female ratio. Patients generally present with a pericardial effusion, congestive heart failure, an anterior mediastinal mass, or tamponade. Diagnosis can be difficult given the nonspecific presentation, and chest radiography may demonstrate only an enlarged cardiac silhouette. Echocardiography can reveal evidence of an effusion, thickening of the pericardium, or mass involvement of the myocardium.[214] CT scanning or MRI can show a thickened pericardium and may help determine invasion into myocardium.[215,216]

Currently, surgical excision is the treatment for primary pericardial mesothelioma primarily to palliate symptoms of constriction or tamponade.

REFERENCES

1. Price B. Analysis of current trends in United States mesothelioma incidence. *Am J Epidemiol* 1997;145:211.

2. Carbone M, Kratzke RA, Testa JR. The pathogenesis of mesothelioma. *Semin Oncol* 2002;29:2.

3. Gazda AF, Butel JS, Carbone M. SV40 and human tumours: myth, association or causality? *Nat Rev Cancer* 2002;2:957.

4. Walker AM, Loughlin JE, Friedlander ER, Rothman KJ, Dreyer NA. Projections of asbestos-related disease 1980–2009. *J Occup Med* 1983;25:409.

5. Sluis-Cremer GK. Linking chrysotile asbestos with mesothelioma. *Am J Ind Med* 1988;14:631.

6. Smith AH, Wright CC. Chrysotile asbestos is the main cause of pleural mesothelioma. *Am J Ind Med* 1996;30:252.

7. Smith WE, Hubert DD. The intrapleural route as a means for estimating carcinogenicity. In: Karbe E Parke JF eds. *Experimental lung cancer carcinogenesis and bioassays.* New York: Experimental Lung Cancer, Carcinogenesis and Bioassays, 2003:92.

8. Wagner JC, Berry G, Timbrell V. Mesotheliomata in rats after inoculation with asbestos and other materials. *Br J Cancer* 1973;28:173.

9. Smith WE. Asbestos, talc and nitrites in relation to gastric cancer. *Am Ind Hyg Assoc J* 1973;34:227.

10. Stanton MF, Wrench C. Mechanisms of mesothelioma induction with asbestos and fibrous glass. *J Natl Cancer Inst* 1972;48:797.

11. Mossman BT, Bignon J, Corn M, Seaton A, Gee JB. Asbestos: scientific developments and implications for public policy. *Science* 1990;247:294.

12. Robledo R, Mossman B. Cellular and molecular mechanisms of asbestos-induced fibrosis. *J Cell Physiol* 1999;180:158.

13. Vianna NJ, Polan AK. Non-occupational exposure to asbestos and malignant mesothelioma in females. *Lancet* 1978;1:1061.

14. Li FP, Lokich J, Lapey J, Neptune WB, Wilkins EW Jr. Familial mesothelioma after intense asbestos exposure at home. *JAMA* 1978;240:467.

15. Yates DH, Corrin B, Stidolph PN, Browne K. Malignant mesothelioma in south east England: clinicopathological experience of 272 cases. *Thorax* 1997;52:507.

16. Lanphear BP, Buncher CR. Latent period for malignant mesothelioma of occupational origin. *J Occup Med* 1992;34:718.

17. De Rienzo A, Testa JR. Recent advances in the molecular analysis of human malignant mesothelioma. *Clin Ter* 2000;151:433.

18. Cheng JQ, Jhanwar SC, Klein WM, et al. p16 alterations and deletion mapping of 9p21-p22 in malignant mesothelioma. *Cancer Res* 1994;54:5547.

19. Yang CT, You L, Lin YC, et al. A comparison analysis of anti-tumor efficacy of adenoviral gene replacement therapy (p14ARF and p16INK4A) in human mesothelioma cells. *Anticancer Res* 2003;23:33.

20. Yang CT, You L, Uematsu K, et al. p14(ARF) modulates the cytolytic effect of ONYX-015 in mesothelioma cells with wild-type p53. *Cancer Res* 2001;61:5959.

21. Cora E, Kane A. Expression of the tumor suppressor gene, p53, during the development of murine malignant mesotheliomas induced by asbestos fibers. *FASEB J* 1991;5:A1442.

22. Amin KM, Litzky LA, Smythe WR, et al. Wilms' Tumor 1 susceptibility (WT1) gene products are selectively expressed in malignant mesothelioma. *Am J Pathol* 1995;146:344.

23. Cheng JQ, Lee WC, Klein MA, et al. Frequent mutations of NF2 and allelic loss from chromosome band 22q12 in malignant mesothelioma: evidence for a two-hit mechanism of NF2 inactivation. *Genes Chromosomes Cancer* 1999;24:238.

24. Silver BJ. Platelet-derived growth factor in human malignancy. *Biofactors* 1992;3:217.

25. Gerwin BI, Lechner JF, Reddel RR, et al. Comparison of production of transforming growth factor-beta and platelet-derived growth factor by normal human mesothelial cells and mesothelioma cell lines. *Cancer Res* 1987;47:6180.

26. Lee TC, Zhang Y, Aston C, et al. Normal human mesothelial cells and mesothelioma cell lines express insulin-like growth factor I and associated molecules. *Cancer Res* 1993;53:2858.

27. Pass HI, Mew DJ, Carbone M, et al. Inhibition of hamster mesothelioma tumorigenesis by an antisense expression plasmid to the insulin-like growth factor-1 receptor. *Cancer Res* 1996;56:4044.

28. Salgado R, Vermeulen PB, Benoy I, et al. Platelet number and interleukin-6 correlate with VEGF but not with bFGF serum levels of advanced cancer patients. *Br J Cancer* 1999;80:892.

29. Cohen T, Nahari D, Cerem LW, Neufeld G, Levi BZ. Interleukin 6 induces the expression of vascular endothelial growth factor. *J Biol Chem* 1996;271:736.

30. Antony VB, Hott JW, Godbey SW, Holm K. Angiogenesis in mesotheliomas. Role of mesothelial cell derived IL-8. *Chest* 1996;109:21S.

31. Ohta Y, Shridhar V, Bright RK, et al. VEGF and VEGF type C play an important role in angiogenesis and lymphangiogenesis in human malignant mesothelioma tumours. *Br J Cancer* 1999;81:54.

32. Kumar-Singh S, Weyler J, Martin MJ, Vermeulen PB, Van Marck E. Angiogenic cytokines in mesothelioma: a study of VEGF, FGF-1 and -2, and TGF beta expression. *J Pathol* 1999;189:72.

33. Kumar-Singh S, Vermeulen PB, Weyler J, et al. Evaluation of tumour angiogenesis as a prognostic marker in malignant mesothelioma. *J Pathol* 1997;182:211.

34. Carbone M, Pass HI, Miele L, Bocchetta M. New developments about the association of SV40 with human mesothelioma. *Oncogene* 2003;22:5173.

35. Bocchetta M, Miele L, Pass HI, Carbone M. Notch-1 induction, a novel activity of SV40 required for growth of SV40-transformed human mesothelial cells. *Oncogene* 2003;22:81.

36. Foddis R, De Rienzo A, Broccoli D, et al. SV40 infection induces telomerase activity in human mesothelial cells. *Oncogene* 2002;21:1434.

37. Carbone M, Pass HI, Rizzo P, et al. Simian virus 40-like DNA sequences in human pleural mesothelioma. *Oncogene* 1994;9:1781.

38. Klein G, Powers A, Croce C. Association of SV40 with human tumors. *Oncogene* 2002;21:1141.

39. Wong M, Pagano JS, Schiller JT, et al. New associations of human papillomavirus, Simian virus 40, and Epstein-Barr virus with human cancer. *J Natl Cancer Inst* 2002;94:1832.

40. Stratto K, Almario DA, McCormick M. SV40 contamination of polio vaccine and cancer. The National Academy of Sciences. IOM Report 2002. Immunization Safety Review Committee. 2003.

41. Toyooka S, Carbone M, Toyooka KO, et al. Progressive aberrant methylation of the RASSF1A gene in simian virus 40 infected human mesothelial cells. *Oncogene* 2002;21:4340.

42. Baris YI, Sahin AA, Ozesmi M, et al. An outbreak of pleural mesothelioma and chronic fibrosing pleurisy in the village of Karain/Urgup in Anatolia. *Thorax* 1978;33:181.

43. Artvinli M, Baris YI. Malignant mesotheliomas in a small village in the Anatolian region of Turkey: an epidemiologic study. *J Natl Cancer Inst* 1979;63:17.

44. Baris YI, Artvinli M, Sahin AA. Environmental mesothelioma in Turkey. *Ann N Y Acad Sci* 1979;330:423.

45. Baris YI, Saracci R, Simonato L, Skidmore JW, Artvinli M. Malignant mesothelioma and radiological chest abnormalities in two villages in Central Turkey. An epidemiological and environmental investigation. *Lancet* 1981;1:984.

46. Baris I, Simonato L, Artvinli M, et al. Epidemiological and environmental evidence of the health effects of exposure to erionite fibres: a four-year study in the Cappadocian region of Turkey. *Int J Cancer* 1987;39:10.

47. Baris B, Demir AU, Shehu V, et al. Environmental fibrous zeolite (erionite) exposure and malignant tumors other than mesothelioma. *J Environ Pathol Toxicol Oncol* 1996;15:183.

48. Baris YI. *Asbestos and erionite related chest diseases.* Ankara, Turkey: Semih Ofset Matbaacilik Ltd. Co., 1987.

49. Wagner, JC, Skidmore JW, Hill RJ, Griffiths DM. Erionite exposure and mesotheliomas in rats. *Br J Cancer* 1985;51:727.

50. Emri S, Demir A, Dogan M, et al. Lung diseases due to environmental exposures to erionite and asbestos in Turkey. *Toxicol Lett* 2002;127:251.

51. Roushdy-Hammady I, Siegel J, Emri S, Testa JR, Carbone M. Genetic-susceptibility factor and malignant mesothelioma in the Cappadocian region of Turkey. *Lancet* 2001;357:444.

52. Ascoli V, Mecucci C, Knuutila S. Genetic susceptibility and familial malignant mesothelioma. *Lancet* 2001;357:1804.

53. Gordon GJ, Jensen RV, Hsiao LL, et al. Translation of microarray data into clinically relevant cancer diagnostic tests using gene expression ratios in lung cancer and mesothelioma. *Cancer Res* 2002;62:4963.

54. Battifora H, McCaughey WTE. *Atlas of tumor pathology, 3, fascicle,* 15th ed. Washington, DC: Armed Forces Institute of Pathology, 2003.

55. Magdeleinat P, Alifano M, Petino A, et al. Solitary fibrous tumors of the pleura: clinical characteristics, surgical treatment and outcome. *Eur J Cardiothorac Surg* 2002;21:1087.

56. Brozzetti S, D'Andrea N, Limiti MR, et al. Clinical behavior of solitary fibrous tumors of the pleura. An immunohistochemical study. *Anticancer Res* 2000;20:4701.

57. Briselli M, Mark EJ, Dickersin GR. Solitary fibrous tumors of the pleura: eight new cases and review of 360 cases in the literature. *Cancer* 1981;47:2678.

58. Filosso PL, Oliaro A, Rena O, et al. Severe hypoglycemia associated with a giant solitary fibrous tumor of the pleura. *J Cardiovasc Surg (Torino)* 2002;43:559.

59. Kishi K, Homma S, Tanimura S, Matsushita H, Nakata K. Hypoglycemia induced by secretion of high molecular weight insulin-like growth factor-II from a malignant solitary fibrous tumor of the pleura. *Intern Med* 2001;40:341.

60. de Perrot M, Fischer S, Brundler MA, Sekine Y, Keshavjee S. Solitary fibrous tumors of the pleura. *Ann Thorac Surg* 2002;74:285.

61. Roggli VL, Sharma A, Butnor KJ, Sporn T, Vollmer RT. Malignant mesothelioma and occupational exposure to asbestos: a clinicopathological correlation of 1445 cases. *Ultrastruct Pathol* 2002;26:55.

62. Connelly RR, Spirtas R, Myers MH, Percy CL, Fraumeni JF Jr. Demographic patterns for mesothelioma in the United States. *J Natl Cancer Inst* 1987;78:1053.

63. Vogelzang NJ, Emri S, Boyer M, et al. Effect of folic acid and vitamin b12 supplementation on risk-benefit ratio from phase III study of pemetrexed + cisplatin versus cisplatin in malignant pleural mesothelioma. *Proc Am Soc Clin Oncol* 2003;22:657(abst).

64. Herndon JE, Green MR, Chahinian AP, et al. Factors predictive of survival among 337 patients with mesothelioma treated between 1984 and 1994 by the Cancer and Leukemia Group B. *Chest* 1998;113:723.

65. Pass HI, Bones J, Hellstrom KE, et al. A sensitive serum test for monitoring of malignant pleural mesothelioma. 2003. 8-30-0003. Conference proceeding.

66. Patz EF Jr, Shaffer K, Piwnica-Worms DR, et al. Malignant pleural mesothelioma: value of CT and MR imaging in predicting resectability. *AJR Am J Roentgenol* 1992;159:961.

67. Flores RM, Akhurst T, Gonen M, Larson SM, Rusch VW. Positron emission tomography defines metastatic disease but not locoregional disease in patients with malignant pleural mesothelioma. *J Thorac Cardiovasc Surg* 2003;126:11.

68. Schneider DB, Clary-Macy C, Challa S, et al. Positron emission tomography with f18-fluorodeoxyglucose in the staging and preoperative evaluation of malignant pleural mesothelioma. *J Thorac Cardiovasc Surg* 2000;120:128.

69. Benard F, Sterman D, Smith RJ, et al. Metabolic imaging of malignant pleural mesothelioma with fluorodeoxyglucose positron emission tomography. *Chest* 1998;114:713.

70. Gerbaudo VH, Sugarbaker DJ, Britz-Cunningham S, et al. Assessment of malignant pleural mesothelioma with (18)F-FDG dual-head gamma-camera coincidence imaging: comparison with histopathology. *J Nucl Med* 2002;43:1144.

71. Flores R, Akhurst T, Gonen M, Larson SM, Rusch VW. FDG-PET predicts survival in patients with malignant pleural mesothelioma. *Proc Am Soc Clin Oncol* 2003;22:620 (abst).

72. Therasse P, Arbuck SG, Eisenhauer EA, et al. New guidelines to evaluate the response to treatment in solid tumors. European Organization for Research and Treatment of Cancer, National Cancer Institute of the United States, National Cancer Institute of Canada. *J Natl Cancer Inst* 2000;92:205.

73. Boutin C, Schlesser M, Frenay C, Astoul P. Malignant pleural mesothelioma. *Eur Respir J* 1998;12:972.

74. Boutin C, Rey F, Viallat JR. Prevention of malignant seeding after invasive diagnostic procedures in patients with pleural mesothelioma. A randomized trial of local radiotherapy. *Chest* 1995;108:754.

75. Rusch VW, Venkatraman ES. Important prognostic factors in patients with malignant pleural mesothelioma, managed surgically. *Ann Thorac Surg* 1999;68:1799.

76. Antman KH. Current concepts: malignant mesothelioma. *N Engl J Med* 1980;303:200.

77. Law MR, Hodson ME, Heard BE. Malignant mesothelioma of the pleura: relation between histological type and clinical behavior. *Thorax* 1982;37:810.

78. Falconieri G, Grandi G, DiBonito L, Bonifacio-Gori D, Giarelli L. Intracranial metastases from malignant pleural mesothelioma. Report of three autopsy cases and review of the literature. *Arch Pathol Lab Med* 1991;115:591.

79. Huncharek M, Smith K. Extrathoracic lymph node metastases in malignant pleural mesothelioma. *Chest* 1988;93:443.

80. Gordon GJ, Jensen RV, Hsiao LL, et al. Using gene expression ratios to predict outcome among patients with mesothelioma. *J Natl Cancer Inst* 2003;95:598.

81. Pass H, Liu Z, Wali A, et al. Gene expression profiles predict survival and progression of pleural mesothelioma. *Clin Cancer Res* 2004;10:849.

82. Butchart EG, Ashcroft T, Barnsley WC, Hoden MP. The role of surgery in diffuse malignant mesothelioma of the pleura. *Semin Oncol* 1981;8:321.

83. Zellos L, Sugarbaker DJ. Current surgical management of malignant pleural mesothelioma. *Curr Oncol Rep* 2002;4:354.

84. Sugarbaker DJ, Flores RM, Jaklitsch MT, et al. Resection margins, extrapleural nodal status, and cell type determine postoperative long-term survival in trimodality therapy of malignant pleural mesothelioma: results in 183 patients. *J Thorac Cardiovasc Surg* 1999;117:54.

85. Sugarbaker DJ, Norberto JJ, Swanson SJ. Surgical staging and work-up of patients with diffuse malignant pleural mesothelioma. *Semin Thorac Cardiovasc Surg* 1997;9:356.

86. Vogelzang NJ, Rusthoven JJ, Symanowski J, et al. Phase III study of pemetrexed in combination with cisplatin versus cisplatin alone in patients with malignant pleural mesothelioma. *J Clin Oncol* 2003;21:2636.

87. Edwards JG, Abrams KR, Leverment JN, et al. Prognostic factors for malignant mesothelioma in 142 patients: validation of CALGB and EORTC prognostic scoring systems. *Thorax* 2000;55:731.

88. Antman KH, Blum RH, Greenberger JS, et al. Multimodality therapy for malignant mesothelioma based on a study of natural history. *Am J Med* 1980;68:356.

89. Pien GW, Gant MJ, Washam CL, et al. Use of an implantable pleural catheter for trapped lung syndrome in patients with malignant pleural effusion. *Chest* 2001;119:1641.

90. Graaf-Strukowska L, van der ZJ, van Putten W, Senan S. Factors influencing the outcome of radiotherapy in malignant mesothelioma of the pleura—a single-institution experience with 189 patients. *Int J Radiat Oncol Biol Phys* 1999;43:511.

91. Bissett D, Macbeth FR, Cram I. The role of palliative radiotherapy in malignant mesothelioma. *Clin Oncol (R Coll Radiol)* 1991;3:315.

92. Schouwink JH, Kool LS, Rutgers EJ, et al. The value of chest computer tomography and cervical mediastinoscopy in the preoperative assessment of patients with malignant pleural mesothelioma. *Ann Thorac Surg* 2003;75:1715.

93. Sugarbaker DJ, Flores RM, Jaklitsch MT, et al. Resection margins, extrapleural nodal status, and cell type determine postoperative long-term survival in trimodality therapy of malignant pleural mesothelioma: results in 183 patients. *J Thorac Cardiovasc Surg* 1999;117:54.

94. Rusch VW. Pleurectomy/decortication in the setting of multimodality treatment for diffuse malignant pleural mesothelioma. *Semin Thorac Cardiovasc Surg* 1997;9:367.

95. Pass HI, Kranda K, Temeck BK, Feuerstein I, Steinberg SM. Surgically debulked malignant pleural mesothelioma: results and prognostic factors. *Ann Surg Oncol* 1997;4:215.

96. Law MR, Gregor A, Hodson ME, Bloom HJ, Turner-Warwick M. Malignant mesothelioma of the pleura: a study of 52 treated and 64 untreated patients. *Thorax* 1984;39:255.

97. Ruffie P, Feld R, Minkin S, et al. Diffuse malignant mesothelioma of the pleura in Ontario and Quebec: a retrospective study of 332 patients. *J Clin Oncol* 1989;7:1157.

98. Brancatisano RP, Joseph MG, McCaughan BC. Pleurectomy for mesothelioma. *Med J Aust* 1991;154:455.

99. Butchart EG, Ashcroft T, Barnsley WC, Holden MP. Pleuropneumonectomy in the management of diffuse malignant mesothelioma of the pleura. Experience with 29 patients. *Thorax* 1976;31:15.

100. Faber LP. 1986: extrapleural pneumonectomy for diffuse, malignant mesothelioma. Updated in 1994. *Ann Thorac Surg* 1994;58:1782.

101. Rusch VW, Piantadosi S, Holmes EC. The role of extrapleural pneumonectomy in malignant pleural mesothelioma. A Lung Cancer Study Group trial [see comments]. *J Thorac Cardiovasc Surg* 1991;102:1.

102. Sugarbaker PH. Management of peritoneal-surface malignancy: the surgeon's role. *Langenbecks Arch Surg* 1999;384:576.

103. Rusch VW, Rosenzweig K, Venkatraman E, et al. A phase II trial of surgical resection and adjuvant high-dose hemithoracic radiation for malignant pleural mesothelioma. *J Thorac Cardiovasc Surg* 2001;122:788.

104. Rusch VW. Indications for pneumonectomy. Extrapleural pneumonectomy. *Chest Surg Clin N Am* 1999;9:327.

105. Baldini EH, Recht A, Strauss GM, et al. Patterns of failure after trimodality therapy for malignant pleural mesothelioma. *Ann Thorac Surg* 1997;63:334.

106. Ball DL, Cruickshank DG. The treatment of malignant mesothelioma of the pleura: review of a 5-year experience, with special reference to radiotherapy. *Am J Clin Oncol* 1990;13:4.

107. Alberts AS, Falkson G, Goedhals L, Vorobiof DA, Van der Merwe CA. Malignant pleural mesothelioma: a disease unaffected by current therapeutic maneuvers. *J Clin Oncol* 1988;6:527.

108. Holsti LR, Pyrhonen S, Kajanti M, et al. Altered fractionation of hemithorax irradiation for pleural mesothelioma and failure patterns after treatment. *Acta Oncol* 1997;36:397.

109. Alberts AS, Falkson G, van Zyl L. Malignant pleural mesothelioma: phase II pilot study of ifosfamide and mesna. *J Natl Cancer Inst* 1988;80:698.

110. Linden CJ, Mercke C, Albrechtsson U, Johansson L, Ewers SB. Effect of hemithorax irradiation alone or combined with doxorubicin and cyclophosphamide in 47 pleural mesotheliomas: a nonrandomized phase II study. *Eur Respir J* 1996;9:2565.

111. Herscher LL, Hahn SM, Kroog G, et al. Phase I study of paclitaxel as a radiation sensitizer in the treatment of mesothelioma and non-small-cell lung cancer. *J Clin Oncol* 1998;16:635.

112. Chen Y, Pandya K, Keng PP, et al. Schedule-dependent pulsed paclitaxel radiosensitization for thoracic malignancy. *Am J Clin Oncol* 2001;24:432.

113. Lee TT, Everett DL, Shu HK, et al. Radical pleurectomy/decortication and intraoperative radiotherapy followed by conformal radiation with or without chemotherapy for malignant pleural mesothelioma. *J Thorac Cardiovasc Surg* 2002;124:1183.

114. Ahamad A, Stevens CW, Smythe WR, et al. Intensity-modulated radiation therapy: a novel approach to the management of malignant pleural mesothelioma. *Int J Radiat Oncol Biol Phys* 2003;55:768.

115. Forster KM, Smythe WR, Starkschall G, et al. Intensity-modulated radiotherapy following extrapleural pneumonectomy for the treatment of malignant mesothelioma: clinical implementation. *Int J Radiat Oncol Biol Phys* 2003;55:606.

116. Gordon W Jr, Antman KH, Greenberger JS, Weichselbaum RR, Chaffey JT. Radiation therapy in the management of patients with mesothelioma. *Int J Radiat Oncol Biol Phys* 1982;8:19.

117. Davis SR, Tan L, Ball DL. Radiotherapy in the treatment of malignant mesothelioma of the pleura, with special reference to its use in palliation. *Australas Radiol* 1994;38:212.

118. Rusch V, Saltz L, Venkatraman E, et al. A phase II trial of pleurectomy/decortication followed by intrapleural and systemic chemotherapy for malignant pleural mesothelioma. *J Clin Oncol* 1994;12:1156.

119. Rusch VW, Niedzwiecki D, Tao Y, et al. Intrapleural cisplatin and mitomycin for malignant mesothelioma following pleurectomy: pharmacokinetic studies. *J Clin Oncol* 1992;10:1001.

120. Colleoni M, Sartori F, Calabro F, et al. Surgery followed by intracavitary plus systemic chemotherapy in malignant pleural mesothelioma. *Tumori* 1996;82:53.

121. Zellos LS, Sugarbaker DJ. Diffuse malignant mesothelioma of the pleural space and its management. *Oncology (Huntingt)* 2002;16:907.

122. Calavrezos A, Koschel G, Husselmann H, et al. Malignant mesothelioma of the pleura. A prospective therapeutic study of 132 patients from 1981–1985. *Klin Wochenschr* 1988;66:607.

123. Maggi G, Casadio C, Giobbe R, Ruffini E. The management of malignant pleural mesothelioma. *Eur J Cardiothorac Surg* 2003;23:255.

124. Maggi G, Giobbe R, Casadio C, Rena O. Palliative surgery for malignant pleural mesothelioma. *Eur J Cardiothorac Surg* 2002;21:1128.

125. Maggi G, Casadio C, Cianci R, Rena O, Ruffini E. Trimodality management of malignant pleural mesothelioma. *Eur J Cardiothorac Surg* 2001;19:346.

126. Stahel R, Weder W, Ballabio P, et al. Neoadjuvant chemotherapy followed by pleuropneumonectomy for pleural mesothelioma: a multicenter phase II trial of the SAKK. *Lung Cancer* 2003;41:[Suppl 2]S59(abst).

127. de Perrot M, Ginsberg R, Payne D, et al. A phase II trial of induction chemotherapy followed by extrapleural pneumonectomy and high-dose hemithoracic radiation for malignant pleural mesothelioma. *Lung Cancer* 2003;41:[Suppl 2]S59(abst).

128. Pass HI, Temeck BK, Kranda K, et al. Phase III randomized trial of surgery with or without intraoperative photodynamic therapy and postoperative immunochemotherapy for malignant pleural mesothelioma. *Ann Surg Oncol* 1997;4:628.

129. Bonnette P, Heckly GB, Villette S, Fragola A. Intraoperative photodynamic therapy after pleuropneumonectomy for malignant pleural mesothelioma. *Chest* 2002;122:1866.

130. Schouwink H, Rutgers ET, van der SJ, Oppelaar H, van Zandwijk N. Intraoperative photodynamic therapy after pleuropneumonectomy in patients with malignant pleural mesothelioma: dose finding and toxicity results. *Chest* 2001;120:1167.

131. Baas P, Murrer L, Zoetmulder FA, et al. Photodynamic therapy as adjuvant therapy in surgically treated pleural malignancies. *Br J Cancer* 1997;76:819.

132. Friedberg JS, Mick R, Stevenson J, et al. A phase I study of Foscan-mediated photodynamic therapy and surgery in patients with mesothelioma. *Ann Thorac Surg* 2003;75:952.

133. Ratto GB, Civalleri D, Esposito M, et al. Pleural space perfusion with cisplatin in the multimodality treatment of malignant mesothelioma: a feasibility and pharmacokinetic study. *J Thorac Cardiovasc Surg* 1999;117:759.

134. Yellin A, Simansky DA, Paley M, Refaely Y. Hyperthermic pleural perfusion with cisplatin: early clinical experience. *Cancer* 2001;92:2197.

135. van Ruth S, Baas P, Haas RL, et al. Cytoreductive surgery combined with intraoperative hyperthermic intrathoracic chemotherapy for stage I malignant pleural mesothelioma. *Ann Surg Oncol* 2003;10:176.

135a. Sugarbaker DJ, Richards W, Zellos L, et al. Feasibility of pleurectomy and intraoperative bicavitary hyperthermic cisplatin lavage for mesothelioma: a phase I–II study. *Proc Am Soc Clin Oncol* 2003;22.

136. Sterman DH, Kaiser LR, Albelda SM. Gene therapy for malignant pleural mesothelioma. *Hematol Oncol Clin North Am* 1998;12:553.

137. Mukherjee S, Nelson D, Loh S, et al. The immune anti-tumor effects of GM-CSF and B7-1 gene transfection are enhanced by surgical debulking of tumor. *Cancer Gene Ther* 2001;8:580.

138. Mukherjee S, Haenel T, Himbeck R, Scott B, Ramshaw I. Replication-restricted vaccinia as a cytokine gene therapy vector in cancer: persistent transgene expression despite antibody generation. *Cancer Gene Ther* 2000;7:663.

139. Nowak AK, Lake RA, Kindler HL, Robinson BW. New approaches for mesothelioma: biologics, vaccines, gene therapy, and other novel agents. *Semin Oncol* 2002;29:82.

140. Odaka M, Wiewrodt R, DeLong P, et al. Analysis of the immunologic response generated by Ad.IFN-beta during successful intraperitoneal tumor gene therapy. *Mol Ther* 2002;6:210.

141. Odaka M, Sterman DH, Wiewrodt R, et al. Eradication of intraperitoneal and distant tumor by adenovirus-mediated interferon-beta gene therapy is attributable to induction of systemic immunity. *Cancer Res* 2001;61:6201.

142. Boutin C, Nussbaum E, Monnet I, et al. Intrapleural treatment with recombinant gamma-interferon in early stage malignant pleural mesothelioma. *Cancer* 1994;74:2460.

143. Driesen P, Boutin C, Viallat JR, et al. Implantable access system for prolonged intrapleural immunotherapy. *Eur Respir J* 1994;7:1889.

144. Astoul P, Picat-Joossen D, Viallat JR, Boutin C. Intrapleural administration of interleukin-2 for the treatment of patients with malignant pleural mesothelioma: a phase II study [see comments]. *Cancer* 1998;83:2099.
145. Janne PA. Chemotherapy for malignant pleural mesothelioma. *Clin Lung Cancer* 2003;5:98.
146. Ong ST, Vogelzang NJ. Chemotherapy in malignant pleural mesothelioma. A review. *J Clin Oncol* 1996;14:1007.
147. Middleton GW, Smith IE, O'Brien ME, et al. Good symptom relief with palliative MVP (mitomycin-C, vinblastine and cisplatin) chemotherapy in malignant mesothelioma. *Ann Oncol* 1998;9:269.
148. Steele JP, Shamash J, Evans MT, et al. Phase II study of vinorelbine in patients with malignant pleural mesothelioma. *J Clin Oncol* 2000;18:3912.
149. Girling DJ, Muers MF, Qian W, Lobban D. Multicenter randomized controlled trial of the management of unresectable malignant mesothelioma proposed by the British Thoracic Society and the British Medical Research Council. *Semin Oncol* 2002;29:97.
150. Byrne MJ, Davidson JA, Musk AW, et al. Cisplatin and gemcitabine treatment for malignant mesothelioma: a phase II study. *J Clin Oncol* 1999;17:25.
151. Nowak AK, Byrne MJ, Williamson R, et al. A multicentre phase II study of cisplatin and gemcitabine for malignant mesothelioma. *Br J Cancer* 2002;87:491.
152. van Haarst JM, Baas P, Manegold C, et al. Multicentre phase II study of gemcitabine and cisplatin in malignant pleural mesothelioma. *Br J Cancer* 2002;86:342.
153. Vogelzang NJ. Gemcitabine and cisplatin: second-line chemotherapy for malignant mesothelioma? *J Clin Oncol* 1999;17:2626.
154. Favaretto AG, Aversa SM, Paccagnella A, et al. Gemcitabine combined with carboplatin in patients with malignant pleural mesothelioma: a multicentric phase II study. *Cancer* 2003;97:2791.
155. van Meerbeeck JP, Baas P, Debruyne C, et al. A phase II study of gemcitabine in patients with malignant pleural mesothelioma. European Organization for Research and Treatment of Cancer Lung Cancer Cooperative Group. *Cancer* 1999;85:2577.
156. Kindler HL, van Meerbeeck JP. The role of gemcitabine in the treatment of malignant mesothelioma. *Semin Oncol* 2002;29:70.
157. Mintzer DM, Kelsen D, Frimmer D, Heelan R, Gralla R. Phase II trial of high-dose cisplatin in patients with malignant mesothelioma. *Cancer Treat Rep* 1985;69:711.
158. Zidar BL, Green S, Pierce HI, et al. A phase II evaluation of cisplatin in unresectable diffuse malignant mesothelioma: a Southwest Oncology Group Study. *Invest New Drugs* 1988;6:223.
159. Zidar BL, Pugh RP, Schiffer LM, et al. Treatment of six cases of mesothelioma with doxorubicin and cisplatin. *Cancer* 1983;52:1788.
160. Planting AS, Schellens JH, Goey SH, et al. Weekly high-dose cisplatin in malignant pleural mesothelioma. *Ann Oncol* 1994;5:373.
161. Mbidde EK, Harland SJ, Calvert AH, Smith IE. Phase II trial of carboplatin (JM8) in treatment of patients with malignant mesothelioma. *Cancer Chemother Pharmacol* 1986; 18:284.
162. Raghavan D, Gianoutsos P, Bishop J, et al. Phase II trial of carboplatin in the management of malignant mesothelioma. *J Clin Oncol* 1990;8:151.
163. Vogelzang NJ, Goutsou M, Corson JM, et al. Carboplatin in malignant mesothelioma: a phase II study of the cancer and leukemia group B. *Cancer Chemother Pharmacol* 1990;27:239.
164. Solheim OP, Saeter G, Finnanger AM, Stenwig AE. High-dose methotrexate in the treatment of malignant mesothelioma of the pleura. A phase II study. *Br J Cancer* 1992; 65:956.
165. Rusthoven JJ, Eisenhauer E, Butts C, et al. Multitargeted antifolate LY231514 as first-line chemotherapy for patients with advanced non-small-cell lung cancer: a phase II study. National Cancer Institute of Canada Clinical Trials Group. *J Clin Oncol* 1999;17:1194.
166. Thodtmann R, Depenbrock H, Dumez H, et al. Clinical and pharmacokinetic phase I study of multitargeted antifolate (LY231514) in combination with cisplatin. *J Clin Oncol* 1999;17:3009.
167. Hughes A, Calvert P, Azzabi A, et al. Phase I clinical and pharmacokinetic study of pemetrexed and carboplatin in patients with malignant pleural mesothelioma. *J Clin Oncol* 2002;20:3533.
168. Shin DM, Scagliotti G, Kindler HL, et al. A phase II trial of pemetrexed in malignant pleural mesothelioma patients: clinical outcome, role of vitamin supplementation, respiratory symptoms and lung function. *Proc Am Soc Clin Oncol* 2003:21(abst).
169. Niyikiza C, Baker SD, Seitz DE, et al. Homocysteine and methylmalonic acid: markers to predict and avoid toxicity from pemetrexed therapy. *Mol Cancer Ther* 2002;1:545.
170. Gralla R, Hollen PJ, Liepa AM, et al. Improving quality of life in patients with malignant pleural mesothelioma: results of the randomized pemetrexed + cisplatin vs. cisplatin trial using the LCSS-meso instrument. *Proc Am Soc Clin Oncol* 2003;22:621(abst).
171. Symanowski J, Rusthoven J, Nguyen P, et al. Multiple regression analysis of prognostic variables for survival from the phase III study of pemetrexed + cisplatin vs. cisplatin in malignant pleural mesothelioma. *Proc Am Soc Clin Oncol* 2003;22:647(abst).
172. Paoletti P, Pistolesi M, Rusthoven J, et al. Correlation of pulmonary function tests with best tumor response status: results from the phase III study of pemetrexed + cisplatin vs. cisplatin in malignant pleural mesothelioma. *Proc Am Soc Clin Oncol* 2003;22:659(abst).
173. Manegold C, Symanowski J, Gattini V, et al. Secondary (post-study) chemotherapy in the phase III study of pemetrexed + cisplatin vs. cisplatin in malignant pleural mesothelioma is associated with longer survival. *Proc Am Soc Clin Oncol* 2003;22:667.
174. Fizazi K, Doubre H, Le Chevalier T, et al. Combination of raltitrexed and oxaliplatin is an active regimen in malignant mesothelioma: results of a phase II study. *J Clin Oncol* 2003;21:349.
175. Mikulski SM, Costanzi JJ, Vogelzang NJ, et al. Phase II trial of a single weekly intravenous dose of ranpirnase in patients with unresectable malignant mesothelioma. *J Clin Oncol* 2002;20:274.
176. Antman KH. Clinical presentation and natural history of benign and malignant mesothelioma. *Semin Oncol* 1981;8:313.
177. Mohamed F, Sugarbaker PH. Peritoneal mesothelioma. *Curr Treat Options Oncol* 2002;3:375.
178. Puvaneswary M, Chen S, Proietto T. Peritoneal mesothelioma: CT and MRI findings. *Australas Radiol* 2002;46:91.
179. Sugarbaker PH, Acherman YI, Gonzalez-Moreno S, et al. Diagnosis and treatment of peritoneal mesothelioma: the Washington Cancer Institute experience. *Semin Oncol* 2002;29:51.
180. Guest PJ, Reznek RH, Selleslag D, Geraghty R, Slevin M. Peritoneal mesothelioma: the role of computed tomography in diagnosis and follow up. *Clin Radiol* 1992;45:79.
181. Eade TN, Fulham MJ, Constable CJ. Primary malignant peritoneal mesothelioma: appearance on F-18 FDG positron emission tomographic images. *Clin Nucl Med* 2002;27:924.
182. Pombo F, Rodriguez E, Martin R, Lago M. CT-guided core-needle biopsy in omental pathology. *Acta Radiol* 1997;38:978.
183. Stamat JC, Chekan EG, Ali A, et al. Laparoscopy and mesothelioma. *J Laparoendosc Adv Surg Tech A* 1999;9:433.
184. Piccigallo E, Jeffers LJ, Reddy KR, et al. Malignant peritoneal mesothelioma. A clinical and laparoscopic study of ten cases. *Dig Dis Sci* 1988;33:633.
185. Hafner M, Novacek G, Herbst F, Ullrich R, Gangl A. Giant benign cystic mesothelioma: a case report and review of literature. *Eur J Gastroenterol Hepatol* 2002;14:77.
186. Ordonez NG. Role of immunohistochemistry in distinguishing epithelial peritoneal mesotheliomas from peritoneal and ovarian serous carcinomas. *Am J Surg Pathol* 1998;22:1203.
187. Hoekman K, Tognon G, Risse EK, Bloemsma CA, Vermorken JB. Well-differentiated papillary mesothelioma of the peritoneum: a separate entity. *Eur J Cancer* 1996;32A:255.
188. Ordonez NG. Role of immunohistochemistry in distinguishing epithelial peritoneal mesotheliomas from peritoneal and ovarian serous carcinomas. *Am J Surg Pathol* 1998; 22:1203.
189. Sethna K, Mohamed F, Marchettini P, Elias D, Sugarbaker PH. Peritoneal cystic mesothelioma: a case series. *Tumori* 2003;89:31.
190. Markman M. Intraperitoneal chemotherapy. *Crit Rev Oncol Hematol* 1999;31:239.
191. Markman M. Intracavitary chemotherapy. *Crit Rev Oncol Hematol* 1985;3:205.
192. Langer CJ, Rosenblum N, Hogan M, et al. Intraperitoneal cisplatin and etoposide in peritoneal mesothelioma: favorable outcome with a multimodality approach. *Cancer Chemother Pharmacol* 1993;32:204.
193. Howell SB, Pfeifle CE. Peritoneal access for intracavitary chemotherapy. *Cancer Drug Deliv* 1986;3:157.
194. Howell SB, Pfeifle CL, Wung WE, et al. Intraperitoneal cisplatin with systemic thiosulfate protection. *Ann Intern Med* 1982;97:845.
195. Lederman GS, Recht A, Herman T, et al. Long-term survival in peritoneal mesothelioma. The role of radiotherapy and combined modality treatment. *Cancer* 1987;59:1882.
196. Antman KH, Pass HI, Schiff PB. Benign and malignant mesothelioma. In: DeVita VT Jr, Hellman S, Rosenberg SA, eds. *Cancer: principles and practice of oncology*, 6th ed. Philadelphia: Lippincott–Raven, 2001:1943.
197. Markman M. Intraperitoneal chemotherapy. *Crit Rev Oncol Hematol* 1999;31:239.
198. Howell SB, Pfeifle CL, Wung WE, et al. Intraperitoneal cisplatin with systemic thiosulfate protection. *Ann Intern Med* 1982;97:845.
199. Markman M, Kelsen, D. Efficacy of cisplatin-based intraperitoneal chemotherapy as treatment of malignant peritoneal mesothelioma. *J Cancer Res Clin Oncol* 1992;118:547.
200. Vlasveld LT, Taal BG, Kroon BB, et al. Intestinal obstruction due to diffuse peritoneal fibrosis at 2 years after the successful treatment of malignant peritoneal mesothelioma with intraperitoneal mitoxantrone. *Cancer Chemother Pharmacol* 1992;29:405.
201. Garcia Moore ML, Savaraj N, Feun LG, Donnelly E. Successful therapy of peritoneal mesothelioma with intraperitoneal chemotherapy alone. A case report. *Am J Clin Oncol* 1992;15:528.
202. Taylor RA, Johnson LP. Mesothelioma: current perspectives. *West J Med* 1981;134:379.
203. Eltabbakh GH, Piver MS, Hempling RE, Recio FO, Intengen ME. Clinical picture, response to therapy, and survival of women with diffuse malignant peritoneal mesothelioma. *J Surg Oncol* 1999;70:6.
204. Taub RN, Keohan ML, Chabot JC, Fountain KS, Plitsas M. Peritoneal mesothelioma. *Curr Treat Options Oncol* 2000;1:303.
205. Loggie BW. Malignant peritoneal mesothelioma. *Curr Treat Options Oncol* 2001;2:395.
206. Mohamed F, Sugarbaker PH. Peritoneal mesothelioma. *Curr Treat Options Oncol* 2002;3:375.
207. Park BJ, Alexander HR, Libutti SK, et al. Treatment of primary peritoneal mesothelioma by continuous hyperthermic peritoneal perfusion (CHPP). *Ann Surg Oncol* 1999;6:582.
208. Sugarbaker PH, Acherman YI, Gonzalez-Moreno S, et al. Diagnosis and treatment of peritoneal mesothelioma: the Washington Cancer Institute experience. *Semin Oncol* 2002;29:51.
209. Khan MA, Puri P, Devaney D. Mesothelioma of tunica vaginalis testis in a child. *J Urol* 1997;158:198.
210. Plas E, Riedl CR, Pfluger H. Malignant mesothelioma of the tunica vaginalis testis: review of the literature and assessment of prognostic parameters. *Cancer* 1998;83:2437.
211. Vigneswaran WT, Stefanacci PR. Pericardial mesothelioma. *Curr Treat Options Oncol* 2000;1:299.
212. Cohen JL. Neoplastic pericarditis. *Cardiovasc Clin* 1976;7:257.
213. McDonald AD, Harper A, McDonald JC, el Attar OA. Epidemiology of primary malignant mesothelial tumors in Canada. *Cancer* 1970;26:914.
214. Agatston AS, Robinson MJ, Trigo L, Machado R, Samet P. Echocardiographic findings in primary pericardial mesothelioma. *Am Heart J* 1986;111:986.
215. Thomason R, Schlegel W, Lucca M, Cummings S, Lee S. Primary malignant mesothelioma of the pericardium. Case report and literature review. *Tex Heart Inst J* 1994;21: 170.
216. Gossinger HD, Siostrzonek P, Zangeneh M, et al. Magnetic resonance imaging findings in a patient with pericardial mesothelioma. *Am Heart J* 1988; 115:1321.

Sumaira Z. Aasi
David J. Leffell

CHAPTER 37

Cancer of the Skin

One in five Americans develops skin cancer during his or her life, and more than 97% of these are non-melanoma skin cancer (NMSC). Although NMSC has a low mortality, it is more common than all other cancers and has a higher incidence than lung cancer, breast cancer, prostate cancer, and colon cancer combined.[1] This "epidemic" has economic significance as well: The total cost of NMSC care in the United States is more than 600 million dollars per year.[2] The rising incidence of NMSC is probably due to a combination of increased sun exposure, more frequent outdoor activities, changes in clothing style, increased longevity, and ozone depletion. Some studies suggest that development of NMSC, including basal cell carcinoma (BCC) and squamous cell carcinoma (SCC), may indicate increased risk for internal malignancy.[3,4] However, the precise relationship between skin cancer and the risk of internal malignancy is not yet completely defined, and the issue remains controversial.

DIAGNOSIS

Although many NMSCs present with classic clinical findings such as nodularity and erythema, definitive diagnosis can be made only by biopsy. Adequate tissue obtained in an atraumatic fashion is critical to histopathologic diagnosis.

Skin biopsies may be performed by shave, punch, or fusiform excision. The type of biopsy performed should be based on the morphology of the primary lesion. A shave biopsy is usually adequate for raised lesions such as nodular BCC, SCC, or tumors of follicular origin. Punch biopsy is appropriate for sampling flat, broad lesions. An excisional biopsy may be used to sample deep dermal and subcutaneous tissue. Excision is indicated when it is necessary to distinguish between a benign lesion, such as a der-matofibroma, and a malignant tumor, such as dermatofibrosarcoma protuberans (DFSP).

SHAVE BIOPSY

Basic skin biopsy techniques are demonstrated in Figure 37-1. A shave biopsy is performed under clean conditions. Local anesthetic (lidocaine 1% with epinephrine, 1:100,000, unless contraindicated) is injected with a 30-gauge needle. The use of a sterilized razor blade, which can be precisely manipulated by the operator to adjust the depth of the biopsy, is often superior to the use of a No. 15 scalpel. After the procedure, adequate hemostasis is achieved with topical application of aqueous aluminum chloride (20%) or electrocautery.

PUNCH BIOPSY

A punch biopsy is performed under local anesthesia, using a trephine or biopsy punch. The operator makes a circular incision to the level of the superficial fat, using a rotating or twisting motion of the trephine. Traction applied perpendicularly to the relaxed skin tension lines minimizes redundancy at closure. Hemostasis is achieved by placement of simple, nonabsorbable sutures that can be removed in 7 to 14 days depending on anatomic site. If the punch biopsy is small and not in a cosmetically important area, then the wound will heal well by second intention.

EXCISIONAL BIOPSY

After local anesthesia has been achieved under sterile conditions, a scalpel is used to incise a fusiform ellipse to the level of the subcutis. Hemostasis is obtained with cautery as needed, and the wound is closed in a layered fashion using absorbable and nonabsorbable sutures. In most cases, postoperative care involves daily

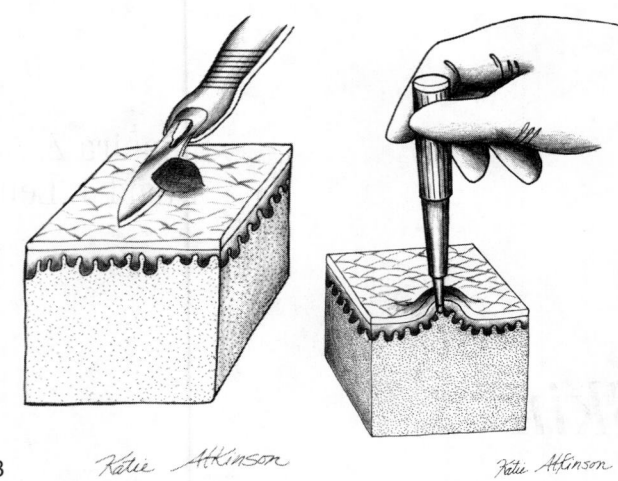

A,B

FIGURE 37-1.   Biopsy techniques. **A:** Shave biopsy. A scalpel blade is precisely manipulated by the operator to adjust the depth of the biopsy, and hemostasis is achieved with topical application of aqueous aluminum chloride (20%), ferric chloride (25%), or electrocautery. **B:** Punch biopsy. The operator makes a circular incision to the level of the superficial fat using a rotating motion of the trephine. Traction applied perpendicularly to the relaxed skin tension lines minimizes redundancy at closure. Hemostasis is achieved by placement of sutures.

cleansing with tap water followed by application of antibiotic ointment and a nonadherent dressing. Although popular in the past, it is now known that hydrogen peroxide may have an unfavorable effect on wound healing. The toxicity of hydrogen peroxide to keratinocytes has been well described.[5]

GENERAL APPROACH TO MANAGEMENT OF SKIN CANCER

The management of skin cancer is guided by the biologic and histologic nature of the tumor, the anatomic site, the underlying medical status of the patient, and whether the tumor is primary or recurrent. Because specific management varies with histologic diagnosis, an accurate interpretation of the biopsy is essential. Depending on the aggressiveness of the tumor and its histologic subtype, cancers of the skin may be excised or, in some cases of superficial tumors or precancerous lesions, eliminated in a less invasive fashion. Electrodesiccation and curettage is the most common nonexcisional approach. If a cancer requires excision, the two options are conventional excision or extirpation by Mohs micrographic surgery (MMS).

EXCISION

Excisional surgery involves removal of the cancer and a margin of clinically uninvolved tissue, followed by layered closure or second intention healing. Frozen or permanent sections interpreted by the pathologist determine adequacy of margins. Margins are assessed from representative sections of the specimen in "breadloaf" fashion, allowing for sampling of the surgical margin. This sampling may occasionally result in a false-negative assessment of clear margins in cases of infiltrating or aggressive-growth cancers. A similar misdiagnosis may result when one relies on vertically prepared frozen specimens for intraoperative margin control. Excision, especially when per-

formed in a physician's office rather than in a hospital operating room, is effective and cost-efficient when the cancer is small (less than 1 cm), nonrecurrent, or noninfiltrative.

MOHS MICROGRAPHIC SURGERY

MMS facilitates optimal margin control and conservation of normal tissue in the management of NMSC.[6] It has become the standard of care in a variety of skin cancer subtypes. Individuals specially trained in the technique perform MMS in the office setting under local anesthesia. After gentle curettage to define the clinical gross margin of the cancer, a tangential specimen of tumor with a minimal margin of clinically normal-appearing tissue is excised, precisely mapped in a horizontal fashion, and processed immediately by frozen section for microscopic examination (Fig. 37-2). Optimal margin control is obtained by examination of the entire perimeter of the specimen and contiguous deep margin. Meticulous mapping allows for directed extirpation of any remaining tumor. A key defining feature of MMS is that the surgeon excises, maps, and reviews the specimen personally, minimizing the chance of error in tissue interpretation and orientation. MMS has gained acceptance as the treatment of choice for recurrent skin cancers, as well as for primary skin cancers located on anatomic sites that require maximal tissue conservation for preservation of function and cosmesis.[7] In addition, when long-term costs of various treatment modalities are compared, MMS is significantly less expensive than radiotherapy and frozen-section–guided excisional surgery.[8]

CURETTAGE AND ELECTRODESICCATION

Common methods of skin cancer destruction include curettage and electrodesiccation (C&D)[9] and cryotherapy using liquid nitrogen.[10] C&D is performed under clean conditions with local anesthesia. Visible tumor is first removed by curettage, which is extended for a margin of 2 to 4 mm beyond the clinical borders of the cancer. Electrodesiccation is then performed to destroy another 1 mm of tissue at the lateral and deep margins. Salasche[11] recommended that C&D be performed for three cycles. Others report satisfactory results after a single cycle of C&D for tumors smaller than 1 cm. Although this leads to decreased scarring, it may lead to higher rates of recurrence of BCC, as suggested by Robins and Albom,[12] who attributed to insufficiently aggressive treatment the higher rates of recurrence observed in young women. A detailed review of primary BCC treated by C&D revealed 5-year recurrence rates of 8.6% for lesions located on the neck, trunk, and extremities and 17.5% for lesions located on the face.[13] In addition, it has been shown that tumors that recur after C&D are often multifocal.[14] C&D is thus reserved for small (less than 1 cm) superficial or nodular BCC, actinic keratoses (AKs), and SCC *in situ* without follicular involvement located on the trunk or extremities.

CRYOSURGERY

Cryosurgery exposes skin cancers to destructive subzero temperatures (Fig. 37-3). Heat transfer occurs from the skin, which acts as a heat sink. Tissue damage is caused by direct effects initially and subsequently by vascular stasis, ice crystal formation, cell membrane disruption, pH changes, hyper-

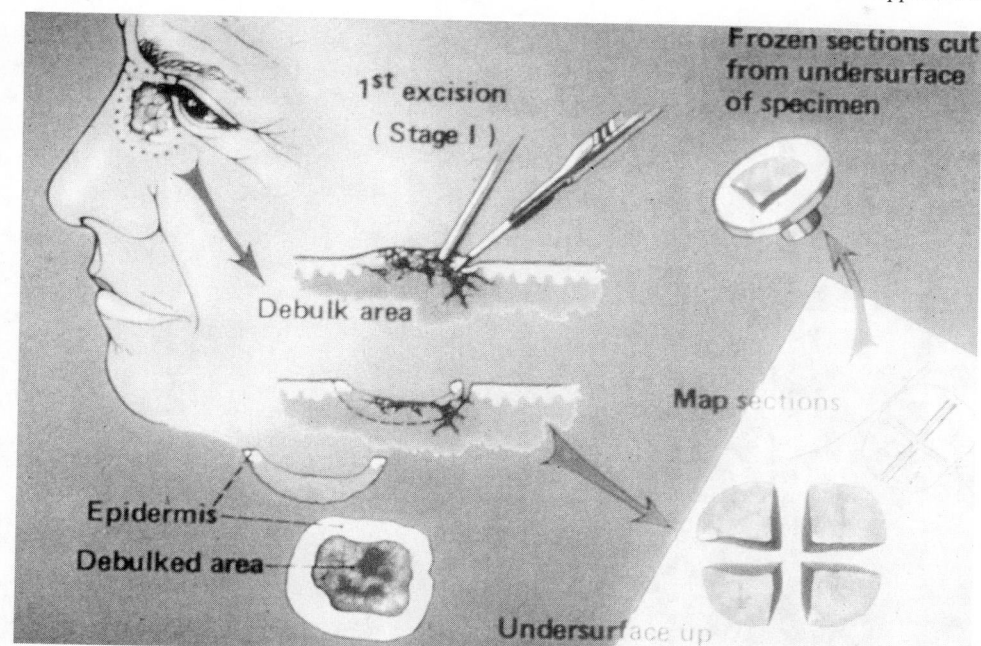

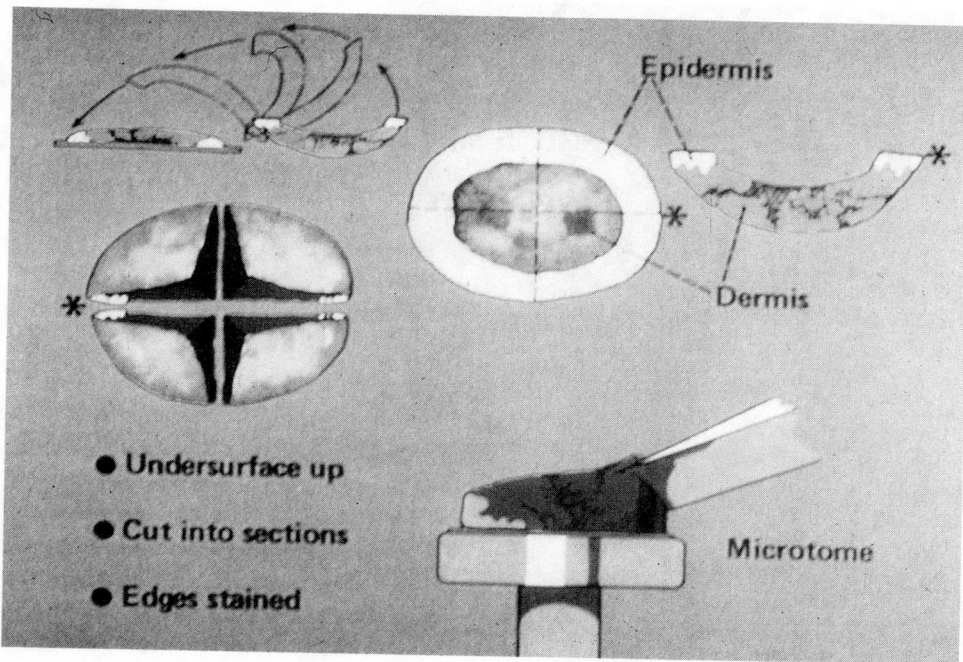

FIGURE 37-2. Mohs micrographic surgery. **A–D:** After gentle curettage, a tangential specimen of tumor with a minimal margin of clinically normal-appearing tissue is obtained, precisely mapped, and processed immediately by frozen section for microscopic examination. Superior margin control is obtained through examination of the entire perimeter of the specimen. Precise mapping allows for directed extirpation of any remaining tumor. (Courtesy of Neil A. Swanson, M.D.) (*Figure continues*)

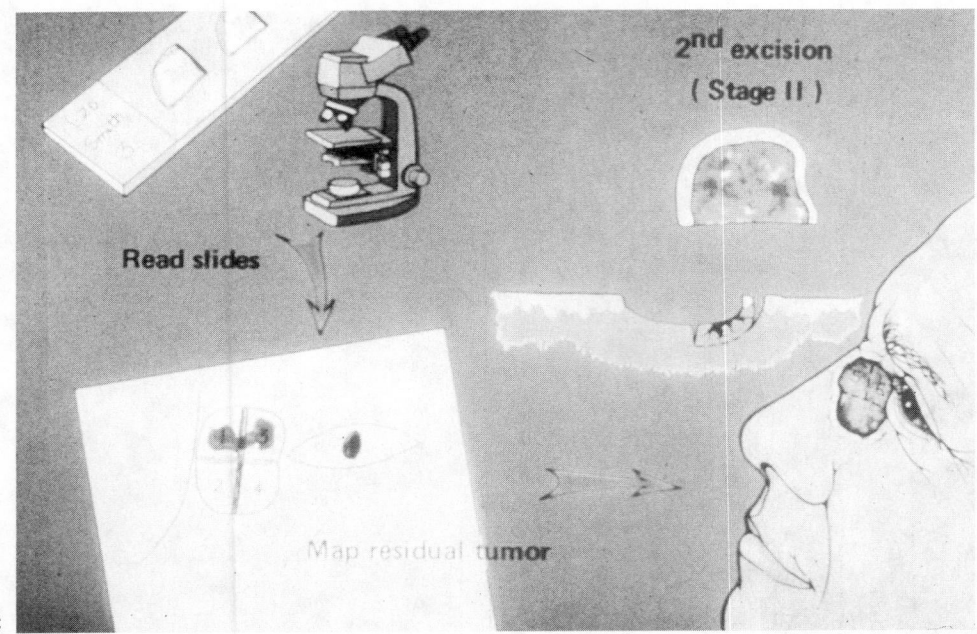

C

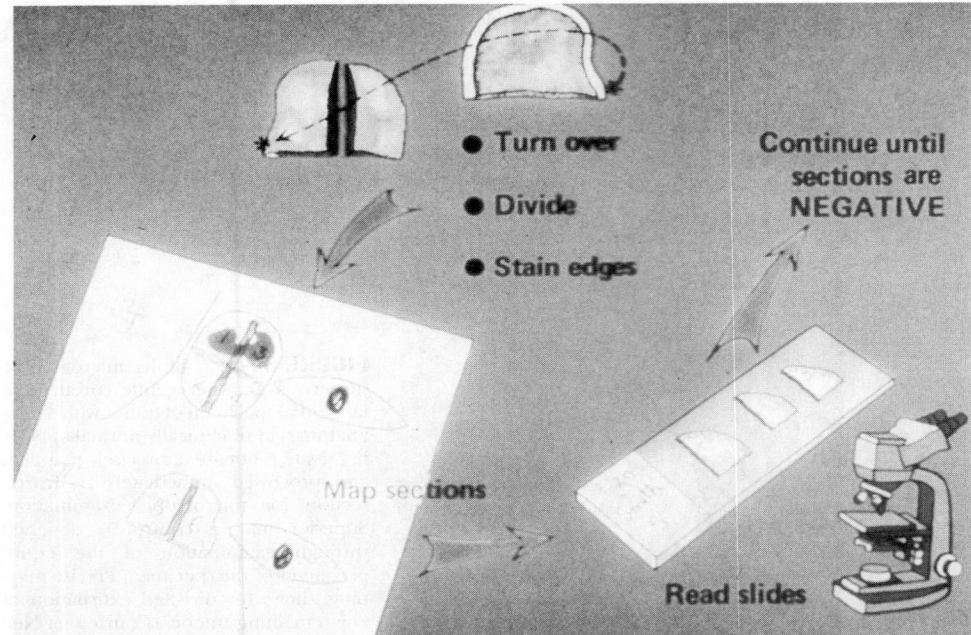

D

(*Figure continues*)

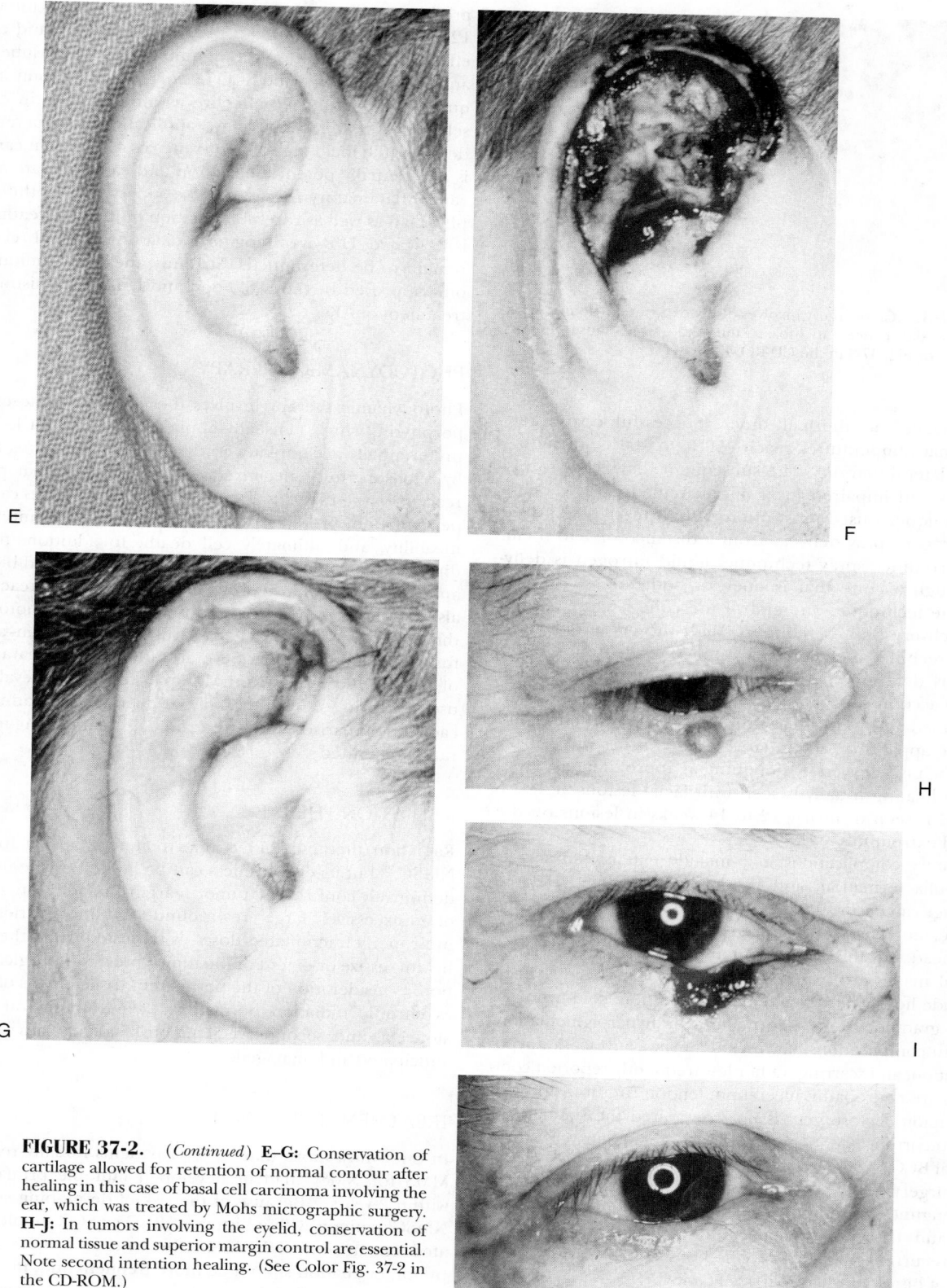

FIGURE 37-2. (*Continued*) **E–G:** Conservation of cartilage allowed for retention of normal contour after healing in this case of basal cell carcinoma involving the ear, which was treated by Mohs micrographic surgery. **H–J:** In tumors involving the eyelid, conservation of normal tissue and superior margin control are essential. Note second intention healing. (See Color Fig. 37-2 in the CD-ROM.)

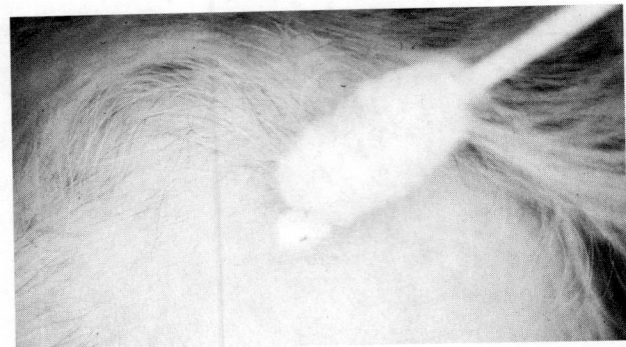

FIGURE 37-3. Cryosurgery involves direct exposure of actinic keratoses or small skin cancers to subzero temperatures to cause destruction. (See Color Fig. 37-3 in the CD-ROM.)

tonic damage, and thermal shock. Successful cryosurgery requires that temperatures reach −50°C to −60°C, including deep and lateral margins. The subsequent thaw leads to vascular stasis and impaired local microcirculation. The open-spray technique is used most often and requires pressurized liquid nitrogen spray delivery from a distance of 1 to 3 cm. With the confined-spray technique, liquid nitrogen is delivered through a cone that is open at both ends. With the closed-cone technique, one end of the cone is closed and a shorter delivery time is required. With the cryoprobe technique, a prechilled metal probe is applied to the tumor. Delivery time is determined via a depth-dose estimation, which takes into account freeze time, lateral spread, and halo thaw time. Immediately after cryosurgery, local erythema and edema are apparent. An exudative phase ensues in 24 to 72 hours, which is followed by sloughing at approximately day 7. Complete healing usually is seen with facial lesions at 4 to 6 weeks and is seen in nearly 12 to 14 weeks in lesions on the trunk and extremities.

Temporary complications may include extensive drainage, edema, bulla formation, and hypertrophic scarring. Delayed hemorrhage can occur suddenly approximately 2 weeks after the procedure, most commonly after treatment on the nose, temple, and forehead, but this is uncommon. Paresthesia may occur if superficial nerves are frozen. Other less common side effects may include headache, syncope, febrile reaction, cold urticaria, pyogenic granuloma, milia formation, or hyperpigmentation. Permanent complications may include tissue contraction, hypopigmentation, and scarring. Other less frequently reported complications are neuropathy, ulceration, tendon rupture, alopecia, and ectropion. Cryosurgery is not considered the standard of care for recurrent NMSC or any tumor other than very small, superficial BCC or SCC.

Cryosurgery and C&D are limited by the inability to evaluate thoroughness of tumor eradication. The absence of margin control and the development of dense scar, which might obscure recurrence, make these methods valuable primarily in the care of histologically superficial NMSC.

IMIQUIMOD

Imiquimod is an immune-response modifier that promotes a cell-mediated immune response through induction of cytokine production, particularly interferon-α and -γ and interleukin-12.[15] It has been shown to promote antitumor and antiviral effects. Studies with topical imiquimod for AKs,[16] superficial[17] and nodular BCC,[18] and SCC *in situ*[19] are very promising. Imiquimod appears to be effective as monotherapy in carefully selected cases and could have application postoperatively to decrease the incidence of recurrence of certain skin cancers. It is a potentially potent medication and can stimulate a significant inflammatory reaction. Close supervision by the treating physician as well as careful evaluation of the posttreatment site is indicated. However, long-term data on cure and recurrence remain to be determined. Currently, the use of imiquimod is only approved by the U.S. Food and Drug Administration for treatment of AKs.

PHOTODYNAMIC THERAPY

Photodynamic therapy involves the use of a photosensitizing porphyrin, which is usually applied topically to a lesion and preferentially accumulates in dysplastic cells. This is followed by exposure to a specific wavelength of light that produces reactive oxygen species. The reactive oxygen species cause lipid peroxidation, protein cross-linking, increased membrane permeability, and ultimately cell death. In addition, there are direct effects on blood vessels resulting in impaired blood flow and stimulation of a vigorous local inflammatory reaction that also promote tumor destruction.[20] Currently, photodynamic therapy is only U.S. Food and Drug Administration–approved for the treatment of AKs. Several studies report clearance rates of 81% to 100% for AKs.[21] Multiple studies have evaluated its use in treating BCC and SCC, but data demonstrating its efficacy in comparison with other modalities and long-term cure rates are limited.[22]

RADIATION THERAPY

Radiation therapy (RT) is one treatment option for certain NMSC,[23] but its effectiveness can be limited by the inability to definitively confirm the tumor margins. In addition, treatment of an excessively large area around the tumor carries risk. RT, in properly fractionated doses, is indicated when the patient's health or size or extent of the tumor precludes surgical extirpation. Consideration of the permanent tissue effects of RT, such as chronic radiation dermatitis, delayed radiation necrosis, alopecia, and secondary cutaneous malignancies,[24] must be anticipated and managed.

TREATMENT FOLLOW-UP

In one study, more than 39% of patients initially referred for MMS for NMSC had or developed multiple primary NMSC within 2 years.[25] Because of the risk of developing subsequent NMSC, patients with a history of BCC or SCC should be evaluated on an annual basis. In the case of a more aggressive tumor, evaluation should be more frequent and, in the case of SCC, should include examination of draining lymph nodes. Laboratory evaluation, generally not indicated in uncomplicated cases of BCC and SCC, may be necessary for other types of particularly aggressive tumors. Imaging studies may be necessary in the case of aggressive tumors or in cases of long-neglected tumors impinging on vital structures. Magnetic resonance imaging allows visualization of the soft tissues, whereas computed tomography (CT) scan may be used to evaluate involvement of bone. In general, imaging studies have not proven helpful in definitively evaluating the presence of perineural invasion by NMSC.

PRECANCEROUS LESIONS

ACTINIC KERATOSIS

AKs are very common lesions that tend to occur on sun-exposed areas in blond or red-haired, fair-skinned individuals with green or blue eyes. Although not invasive, AKs are considered by some dermatopathologists to be SCC *in situ*.[26]

AKs are caused by exposure to ultraviolet B light (UVB), and specific UVB-induced p53 mutations have been demonstrated in these precancerous lesions. Clinically, AKs have three possible behavior patterns: spontaneous regression, persistence, or progression into invasive SCC.[27] A study[28] of asymptomatic AKs, inflamed AKs, and SCCs showed a stepwise loss of differentiation manifesting as diminishing 27-kD heat-shock protein, an initial increase in lymphocytes suggesting the occurrence of an active inflammatory and immune response, a stepwise increase in the number of cells expressing detectable levels of p53 suggesting an increase in DNA damage, decreasing levels of Bcl-2, an apoptosis inhibitor, and loss of Fas antigen suggesting that these cells become less sensitive to FasL-mediated apoptosis as they progressed. All of these changes serve to demonstrate the clinical, histologic, and molecular progression from benign to malignant. The risk for transformation of a single AK has been estimated to be as low as 1 per 1000 per year.[29] However, the long-term risk of the development of invasive SCC in patients with multiple AKs has been estimated to be as high as 10%. In one study, AK was histologically present or adjacent to invasive SCC in 82% of cases.[30] Molecular characterization of the role of the p53 tumor suppressor gene in AK, and its similar finding in SCC and BCC, suggests that the AKs represent an early stage in the molecular carcinogenesis of NMSC.[31] It has recently been suggested that the term *actinic keratosis* be replaced by another term, such as *solar keratotic intraepidermal SCC*.[26]

Clinical Features

AKs are red, pink, or brown papules with a scaly to hyperkeratotic surface (Fig. 37-4). They occur on sun-exposed areas and are especially common on the balding scalp, forehead, face, and dorsal hands. AKs increase in prevalence with advancing age.

The microscopic spectrum of AK includes hyperplastic, atrophic, bowenoid, acantholytic, and pigmented subtypes. In each subtype, disordered, atypical keratinocytes with nuclear atypia are seen. In the hyperplastic variant, pronounced hyperkeratosis is intermingled with parakeratosis. Epidermal hyperplasia and downward displacement without dermal invasion are present. A thin epidermis devoid of rete ridges characterizes the atrophic variant. Atypical cells predominate in the basal layer. The bowenoid AK is indistinguishable from Bowen's disease (BD), also known as *SCC* in situ. In this variant, considerable epidermal

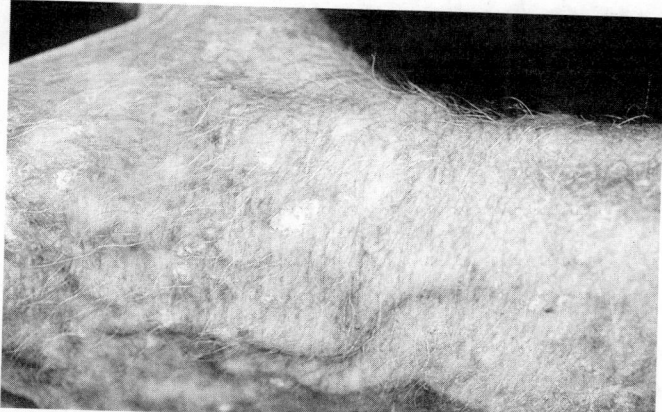

FIGURE 37-4. Actinic keratoses are characterized by erythema and rough surface. (See Color Fig. 37-4 in the CD-ROM.)

cell disorder and clumping of nuclei exist, giving a windblown appearance. The presence of suprabasal lacunae is characteristic of acantholytic AK. The acantholysis occurs secondary to cellular changes. Excessive melanin is present within the basal layer in the pigmented variant of AK.

Treatment

Prevention of disease is always preferable to the need for treatment. Use of broad-brimmed hats, sun-protective clothing, sunscreen, and judicious avoidance of sunlight can protect patients from sunlight and prevent the formation of AKs. Due to their potential to develop into invasive SCC and the inability to determine which lesions will do so, AKs should be treated. Numerous destructive options are available for the treatment of AKs, including cryosurgery, C&D, topical 5-fluorouracil (5-FU), immune modulators such as imiquimod, photodynamic therapy,[32] chemical cauterization using trichloroacetic acid, or excision (Fig. 37-5). Treatment of solitary lesions is straightforward with cryosurgery, which has been reported to have cure rates of 98%. However, management of patients with hundreds of lesions can become complicated. In this situation, initially, the largest lesions are often treated by C&D. Raised lesions of smaller size are then treated by destructive methods, especially the open-spray cryosurgery technique. When flat lesions are

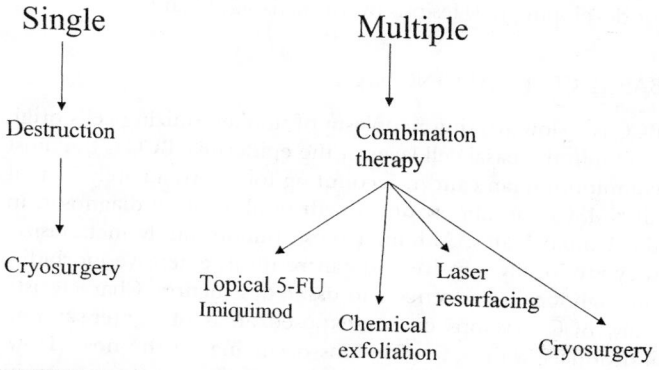

FIGURE 37-5. Management of a solitary actinic keratosis does not present a therapeutic challenge, whereas management of multiple actinic keratoses is likely to require combination therapy. 5-FU, 5-fluorouracil.

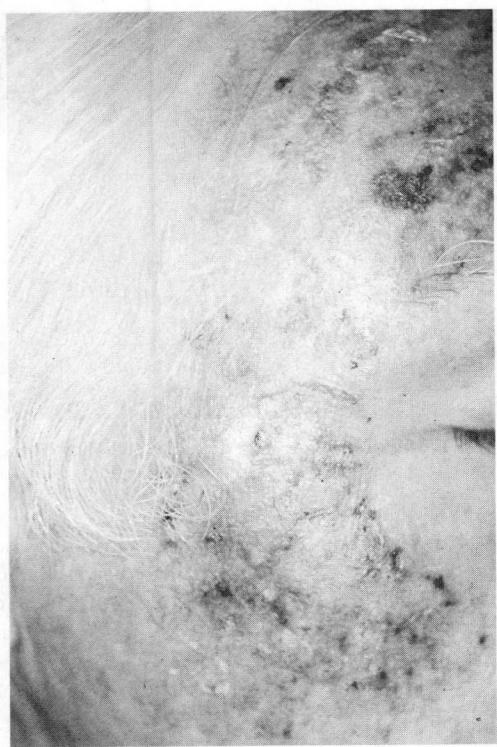

FIGURE 37-6. Erythema, crusting, and discomfort secondary to the use of topical 5-fluorouracil limit compliance with its use. (See Color Fig. 37-6 in the CD-ROM.)

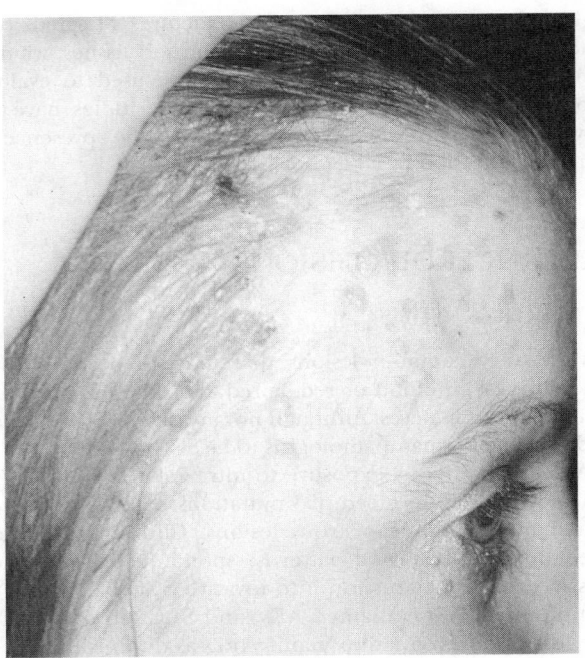

FIGURE 37-7. Nevoid basal cell carcinoma syndrome. Patients with this syndrome can present with hundreds of superficial basal cell carcinomas. (See Color Fig. 37-7 in the CD-ROM.)

extensive, topical application of 5-FU with or without topical retinoids can be effective. The clinical effects of erythema, crusting, or discomfort associated with 5-FU therapy may limit compliance with its use (Fig. 37-6). 5-FU works by blocking the methylation reaction of deoxyuridylic acid to thymidylic acid and interferes with DNA synthesis. Topical imiquimod is an alternative topical therapy option for multiple AKs. Alternative specialized de-epithelializing techniques, such as laser and chemical exfoliation, may be helpful in the patient with severe solar damage and extensive AKs. Lesions that do not respond to treatment and show signs of bleeding, induration, rapid growth, or pain suggest progression to SCC and should be biopsied. Patients also need to be informed that because AK is a clonal disease that results from exposure to UVB, the chance for developing new lesions over time is significant.

BASAL CELL CARCINOMA

BCC is a slow-growing neoplasm of nonkeratinizing cells originating in the basal cell layer of the epidermis. BCC is the most common human cancer, accounting for approximately 75% of all NMSCs and almost one-fourth of all cancers diagnosed in the United States. Although these tumors rarely metastasize, they are locally invasive and can result in extensive morbidity through local recurrence and tissue destruction. Characteristically, BCC develops on sun-exposed areas of lighter-skinned individuals, with 30% of lesions occurring on the nose. However, it must be stressed that BCC can occur anywhere, even in non–sun-exposed areas, and has been reported to occur on the vulva, penis, scrotum, and perianal area. Men are affected only slightly more often than are women, and, although once rare before the age of 50 years, BCCs are becoming more common in younger individuals.[33]

The pathogenesis of BCC most commonly involves exposure to ultraviolet light (UVL),[34] particularly rays in the UVB spectrum (290 to 320 nm), which trigger mutations in tumor suppressor genes.[31] Individuals at highest risk for BCC are white individuals with light hair and eyes who had an early history of recreational exposure to the sun—that is, intermittent, intense exposure that usually results in sunburn.[35] Other factors that appear to be involved in the pathogenesis include mutations in regulatory genes; exposure to ionizing radiation, arsenicals, polyaromatic hydrocarbons, and psoralen-plus-UVA therapy; and alterations in immune surveillance.

BCC can be a feature of inherited conditions. Included among these are the nevoid BCC syndrome (NBCCS), Bazex's syndrome, Rombo syndrome, and unilateral basal cell nevus syndrome. NBCCS is a rare autosomal dominant genetic disorder characterized by a predisposition to multiple BCC and other tumors, as well as a wide range of developmental defects. Patients with this syndrome may exhibit a broad nasal root, borderline intelligence, jaw cysts, palmar pits, and multiple skeletal abnormalities in addition to hundreds of BCCs (Fig. 37-7).[36] This syndrome has significantly helped to elucidate the molecular pathogenesis of BCC.[37] The behavior of neoplasms occurring in NBCCS suggests that the underlying defect in this disorder is a mutation in a tumor suppressor gene and that it fits the two-hit model of carcinogenesis—tumors develop in cells sustaining two genetic alterations. The first alteration or hit is inheritance of a mutation in a tumor suppressor gene, and the second hit is inactivation of the normal homologue by environmental mutagenesis or random genetic rearrangement. Sporadic BCCs would arise in cells that underwent two somatic events resulting in inactivation of the NBCCS tumor suppressor gene, known as the patched gene (PTCH). Studies of BCC have indicated an association with mutations in the PTCH regulatory gene, which maps to chromosome 9q22.3. Loss of heterozygosity at this site in both sporadic and hereditary BCC suggests that it functions as a tumor suppressor. Inactivation of the PTCH gene is probably a necessary, if not sufficient, step for BCC formation. The only known function of PTCH protein, part of a receptor complex, is participation in the hedgehog signaling pathway, a key regulator of embryonic development that controls cellular proliferation. The PTCH protein binds in a complex with smoothened, another transmembrane molecule, which together serve as a receptor for the secreted molecule hedgehog. In the absence of hedgehog, smoothened and PTCH form an inactive complex. On hedgehog binding, smoothened is released from the inhibitory effects of PTCH and transduces a signal allowing it to function as an oncogene. PTCH mutations have also been found in SCC.[38] UV-induced mutations in the p53 gene, such as CC→TT changes at dipyrimidine sites, have been reported in up to 60% of BCCs as well.[39]

Clinical Behavior of Basal Cell Cancer

BCC is associated with extremely low metastatic potential, but it does invade locally. This biologic behavior depends on angiogenic factors, stromal conditions, and the propensity for the cancer to follow anatomic paths of least resistance.[40] In addition, size may play a role, as larger primary BCCs have higher recurrence rates.[41] BCCs can elicit angiogenic factors that account for the telangiectatic vessels characteristically seen on the tumor's surface.[42] Necrosis occurs in tumors that have outgrown their blood supply. Tumor microcirculation was examined *in vivo* in 12 BCCs from the head and neck by Bedlow et al.[43] Mean blood vessel size, density, and length per unit area were increased in BCC in comparison to normal tissue. An earlier study showed that mean vessel counts were increased in SCCs versus BCCs,[42] suggesting that angiogenesis may be linked to biologic aggressiveness and that antiangiogenic factors may play a potential therapeutic role in the treatment of aggressive BCCs.

Tumor stroma is critical for both initiating and maintaining the development of BCC.[40] Transplants of neoplasms devoid of stroma usually are unsuccessful. In one study, Hernandez et al.[44] demonstrated that cultured BCC tumor cells stimulated collagenase production by fibroblasts. The concept of stromal dependence is supported by the low incidence of metastatic BCC.

BCC has a tendency to grow along the path of least resistance. Invasive BCC can migrate along the perichondrium, periosteum, fascia, or tarsal plate.[40] This type of spread accounts for higher recurrence rates noted in tumors involving the eyelid, nose, and scalp not treated by MMS. Embryonic fusion planes possibly offer little resistance and can lead to deep invasion and tumor spread, with very high rates of recurrence (Fig. 37-8). The most susceptible areas include the inner canthus, philtrum, middle to lower chin, nasolabial groove, preauricular area, and the retroauricular sulcus.[40] In a study[45] looking at risk factors for extensive subclinical spread of more than 1000 NMSCs treated by MMS, the most significant predictors were anatomic location on the nose of any type of BCC; morpheaform BCC on the cheek; recurrent BCC in men; any tumor located on the neck in men; any tumor located on the ear helix, eyelid, or temple; and increasing preoperative size.

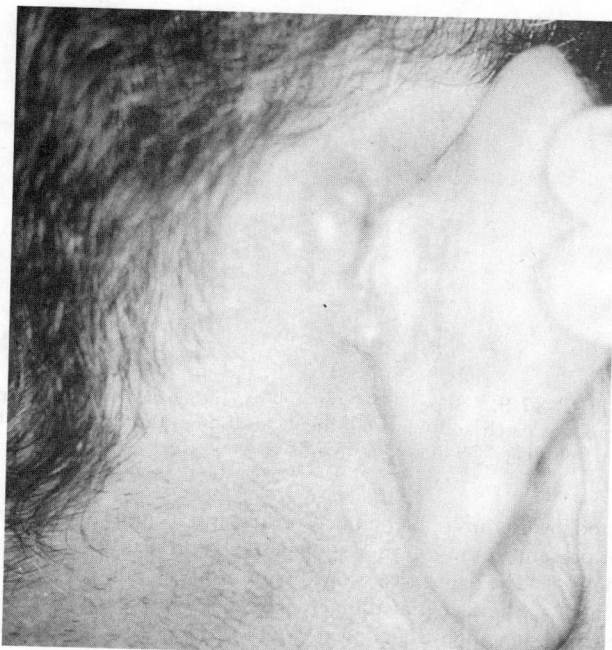

FIGURE 37-8. Recurrent nodular basal cell carcinoma. Embryonic fusion planes offer little resistance to tumor spread. (See Color Fig. 37-8 in the CD-ROM.)

Perineural spread is infrequent but occurs most often in recurrent, aggressive lesions.[46] In one series, Niazi and Lamberty[47] noted perineural invasion in 0.178% of BCC. In all cases, perineural extension was associated with recurrent tumors that were most often located in the periauricular and malar areas. Perineural invasion may present with paresthesia, pain, and weakness or, in some cases, paralysis. Involvement of the cranial nerves and, in one case, thoracic spine has been reported.[46] Metastatic BCC is rare, with incidence rates varying from 0.0028% to 0.1%.[48] Metastases, when reported, have involved the lung, lymph nodes, esophagus, oral cavity, and skin. Although long-term survival has been reported, the prognosis for metastatic BCC is generally poor, survival of 8 to 10 months after diagnosis being the norm.[49] Platinum-based chemotherapy appears to have some effect in the treatment of metastatic BCC.[50]

Basal Cell Carcinoma Subtypes

Clinical variants of BCC include nodular, superficial, morpheaform (also termed *aggressive-growth BCC* or *infiltrative BCC*), pigmented, cystic BCC, and fibroepithelioma of Pinkus (FEP) (Figs. 37-9 through 37-15). Nodular BCC presents as a raised, translucent papule or nodule with telangiectasia and has a propensity for involving sun-exposed areas of the face. Superficial BCC commonly presents as an erythematous scaly or eroded macule on the trunk and may be difficult to differentiate clinically from AK, SCC *in situ*, or a benign inflammatory lesion. Not uncommonly, superficial BCC may be mistakenly treated without response as eczema or psoriasis. Biopsy in such cases is definitive. Morpheaform BCC presents as a flat, slightly firm lesion, without well-demarcated borders, and may be difficult to differentiate from a scar. Traction on the skin often highlights the clinical extent of the lesion which otherwise might go unde-

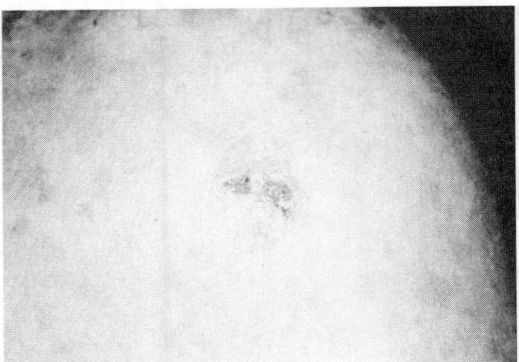

FIGURE 37-9. Superficial basal cell carcinoma presents as an erythematous patch and may be difficult to distinguish from dermatitis. (See Color Fig. 37-9 in the CD-ROM.)

tected. Symptoms of bleeding, crusting, and ulceration are often not present in these tumor subtypes and can lead to a delay in diagnosis. The aggressive growth pattern of this subtype is highlighted by the fact that the actual size of the cancer is usually much greater than the clinical extent of the tumor. Pigmented BCC is a variant of nodular BCC and may be difficult to differentiate from nodular melanoma. The presence of pigment may be of value in determining adequate margins for excision. FEP usually presents as a pink papule on the lower back.[51] It may be difficult to distinguish clinically from amelanotic melanoma.

Histologic subtypes of BCC include superficial, nodular and micronodular, and infiltrative BCC. All BCC subtypes tend to share certain histologic characteristics. These include peripheral palisading of large basophilic cells, nuclear atypia, and retraction from surrounding stroma. Nodular BCC accounts for approximately 50% of BCCs and is characterized by the presence of tumor cells in rounded masses within the dermis (see Fig. 37-14). Peripheral palisading of nuclei is prominent, and surrounding retraction artifact may be present. Groups of cells may be solid, or there may be dermal necrosis or degradation, with formation of cysts or microcysts. The stroma is characteristically coarse and myxoid. If nodules measure less than 15 μm, the tumor may be called *micronodular*. Infiltrative histology is seen in 15% to 20% of BCCs and represents that subclass of BCCs referred to as *aggressive-growth* tumors. Tumor cells manifest irregular outlines with a spiky appearance. Palisading is characteristically absent. The stroma is less myxoid than in the nodular form. In the morpheaform variant, which accounts for approximately 5% of BCCs, small groups or cords of tumor cells infiltrate a dense, collagenous stroma parallel to the skin surface (see Fig. 37-11*B*). Superficial multifocal BCC accounts for approximately 15% of BCCs and is characterized by basophilic buds extending from the epidermis. Retraction artifact is present, as is peripheral palisading within the buds. FEP, which accounts for 1% of BCCs, is characterized by a polypoid lesion in which basaloid cells grow downward from the surface in a network of anastomoses of cords of cells in loose connective tissue. Mixed histology is often apparent in BCCs.

The significance of histologic subtype lies in the correlation with biologic aggressiveness. The infiltrative and micronodular types are the most likely to be incompletely removed by conventional excision. Rates of incomplete excision vary from 5% to 17%. Incompletely excised infiltrative and micronodular BCCs may recur at rates of 33% to 39%. Recurrences after RT show a ten-

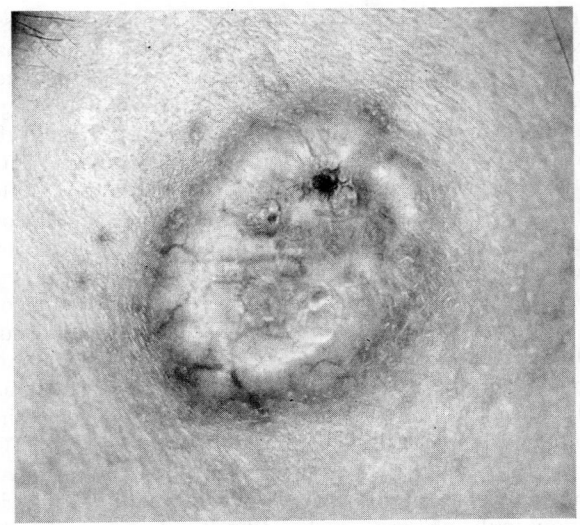

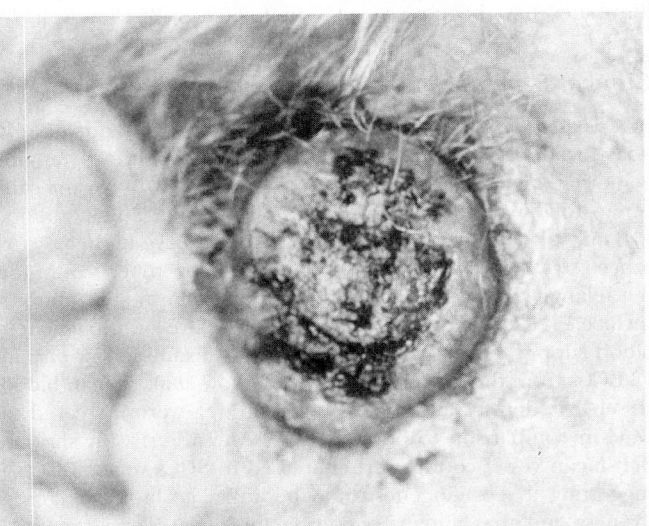

FIGURE 37-10. Nodular basal cell carcinoma. **A:** A red, translucent nodule with rolled border, as seen here, is a classic presentation of nodular basal cell carcinoma. **B:** Nodular basal cell carcinoma demonstrating ulceration. (See Color Fig. 37-10 in the CD-ROM.)

dency toward infiltrative histology and evidence of squamous transformation, and even recurrent BCC after excision or C&D may become metatypical. In general, recurrences are more frequent in BCCs with infiltrative and micronodular histology, when clear margins are less than 0.38 mm and are in the presence of squamous differentiation. Although historical reports in the literature[40] suggested that 60% of incompletely excised BCCs will not recur, none of these studies provided an appraisal of recurrence rates as a function of histologic subtype. In general, incompletely excised BCCs should be removed completely, preferably by MMS, especially if they occur in anatomically critical areas such as the central zone of the face, retroauricular sulcus, or periocular area.

On occasion, it may appear that a BCC has been adequately removed by biopsy alone, leading to the question of whether to render further treatment. In one study, 41 consecutive patients with 42 BCCs apparently removed by biopsy were treated by MMS, and blocks of tissue, sectioned consecutively until exhausted, were

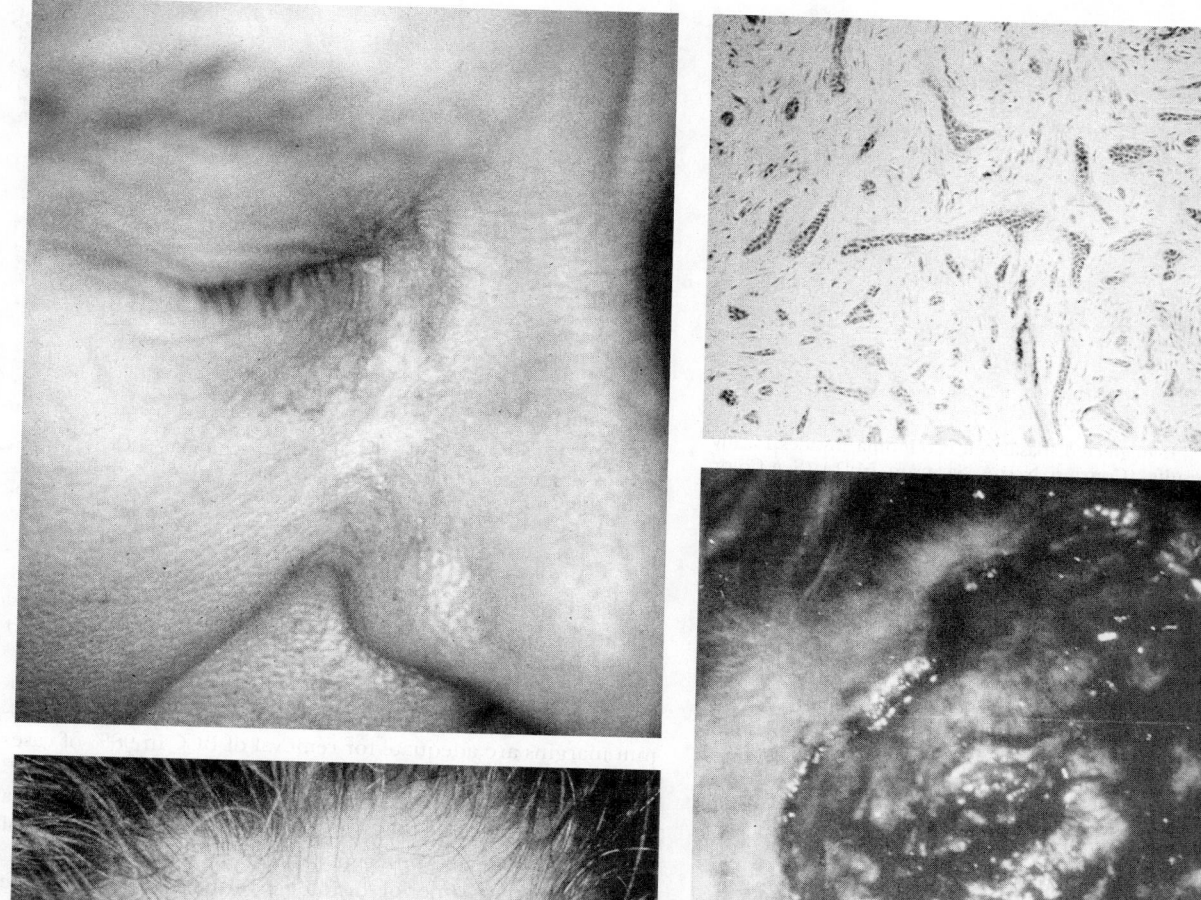

FIGURE 37-11. Morpheaform or aggressive-growth basal cell carcinoma (BCC). **A:** Morpheaform BCC may be difficult to differentiate from scar. **B:** Microscopic examination reveals strands of basaloid cells aggressively infiltrating dense collagen. **C:** BCC may recur without an obvious clinical lesion. **D:** Recurrent BCC after extirpation by Mohs micrographic surgery in the patient depicted in **C**. (See Color Fig. 37-11 in the CD-ROM.)

examined for the presence of residual tumor.[52] In 28 of 42 cases (66%), residual cancer was identified. The presence of residual cancer was not related to age, site, histologic subtype, or extent of surrounding inflammation. The results indicate that patients with small BCCs that appear to be completely removed by initial biopsy may be at risk for recurrence if not treated further.

Characteristics Related to Anatomic Site

BCCs may demonstrate unique characteristics based on anatomic site. The nose is the most common site for cutaneous malignancies (30%), and BCCs involving the nose may be aggressive. A study of 193 cases of infiltrative BCC involving the nose confirmed that the majority of infiltrating and recurrent BCCs affect the ala.[53] Analysis of the recurrences' aggressive local behavior indicated that recurrent lesions were subjected to inadequate therapy initially. In one study, 26 recurrences were identified in 71 nasal skin cancers at an average of 36 months after non-MMS excision.[54] This suggests that MMS may be the treatment of choice for all BCCs involving the nose, especially those exhibiting aggressive growth characteristics.

Periocular BCC represents a significant therapeutic challenge and is the most common tumor affecting the eyelid. In one study, periocular BCC accounted for 7.3% of 3192 BCCs treated over a 10-year period.[7] Of these, 48.5% involved the medial canthus, 22.35% involved the lower eyelid, 10.7% involved the upper eye-

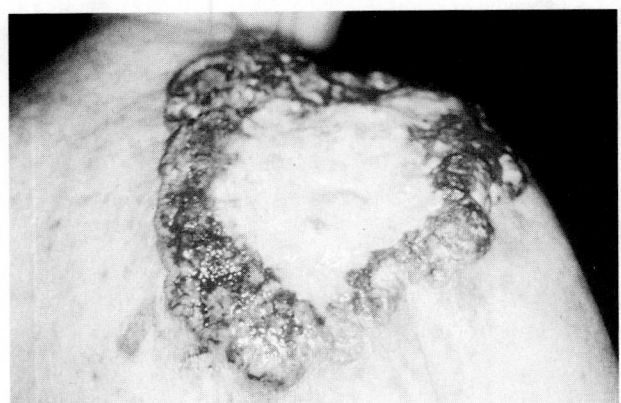

FIGURE 37-12. If neglected, basal cell carcinoma invades locally with devastating results. (Courtesy Neil A. Swanson, M.D.) (See Color Fig. 37-12 in the CD-ROM.)

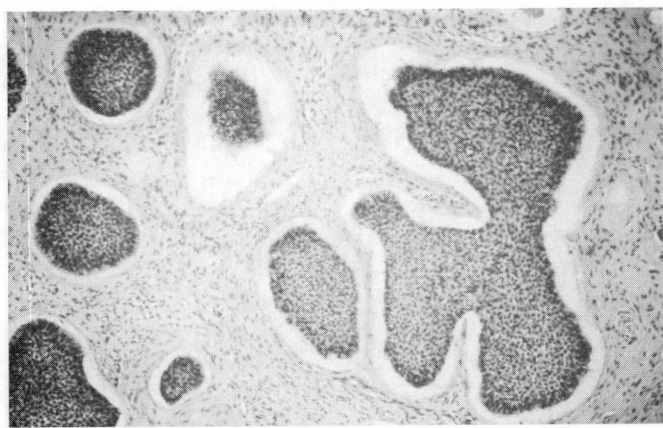

FIGURE 37-14. Nodular basal cell carcinoma (BCC). Microscopic examination of nodular BCC reveals islands of basophilic cells exhibiting typical BCC morphology. (See Color Fig. 37-14 in the CD-ROM.)

lid, and 5.6% involved the lateral canthus. In a review of 24 eyelid tumors treated by MMS, high clearance rates were shown (100%), although follow-up was short (14.6 months).[55] In addition, 50% of patients were left with intact posterior lamellae, highlighting conservation of normal tissue. The results suggest that MMS followed by oculoplastic reconstruction, if necessary, is the preferred strategy in the management of periocular BCC. In the case of small defects on the lid margin, healing by second intention may often yield an excellent cosmetic and functional result.

Approximately 6% of BCCs involve the ear, a site notable for high rates of recurrence. In a recent study, nine patients with BCC involving the conchal bowl were treated by an interdisciplinary approach.[56] In each case, tumor extirpation was accomplished by MMS, and an otolaryngologist was available in the event of temporal bone involvement. There were no cases of recurrence at mean follow-up of 1 year.

Treatment

Excisional surgery, C&D, and cryosurgery have been used to treat circumscribed, noninfiltrating BCCs (Fig. 37-16). MMS is the treatment method of choice for all recurrent and infiltrative BCCs, particularly if a tumor is located on the face.[57] RT is

best suited for older patients, particularly those with extensive lesions on the ear, lower limbs, or eyelids.[58] RT is not indicated for recurrent or morpheaform lesions.

Surgical excision offers the advantage of histologic evaluation of the excised specimen. It has been demonstrated that 4-mm margins are adequate for removal of BCC in 98% of cases of non-morpheaform BCC of less than 2 cm in diameter.[59] Extending the excision into fat generally is adequate for a small primary BCC. It should be noted that the majority of BCCs are well treated with conventional excision or C&D.

MMS permits superior histologic verification of complete removal, allows maximum conservation of tissue, and remains cost-effective as compared to traditional excisional surgery for NMSCs.[8] In a large study of treatment of primary BCC by Rowe et al.,[60] MMS demonstrated a recurrence rate of 1% over 5 years. This was superior to all other modalities, including excision (10%), C&D (7.7%), RT (8.7%), and cryotherapy (7.5%). In a similar study of treatment of recurrent BCC, treatment with MMS demonstrated a long-term recurrence rate of 5.6%.[61] Once again, this was superior to all other modalities, including excision (17.4%), RT (9.8%), and C&D (40%). MMS is the pre-

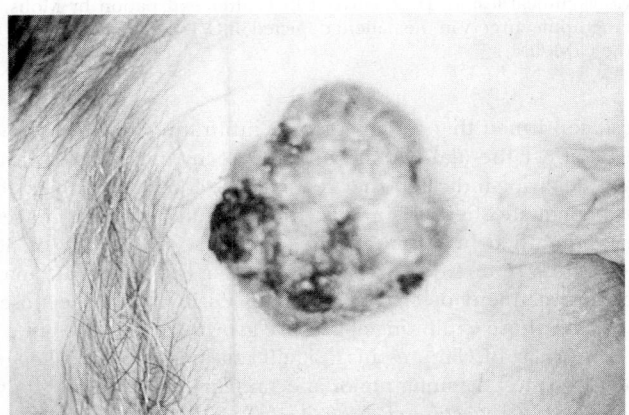

FIGURE 37-13. Pigmented basal cell carcinoma may be difficult to differentiate clinically from melanoma. (See Color Fig. 37-13 in the CD-ROM.)

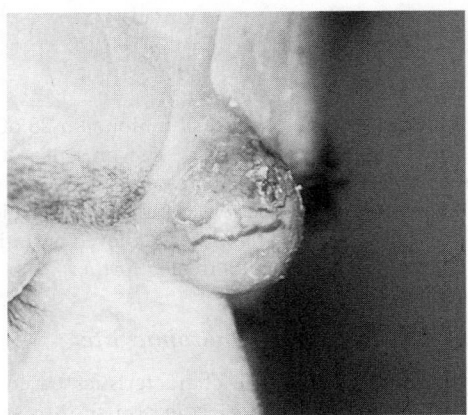

FIGURE 37-15. Cystic basal cell carcinoma. This variant may resemble an epidermal inclusion cyst. (See Color Fig. 37-15 in the CD-ROM.)

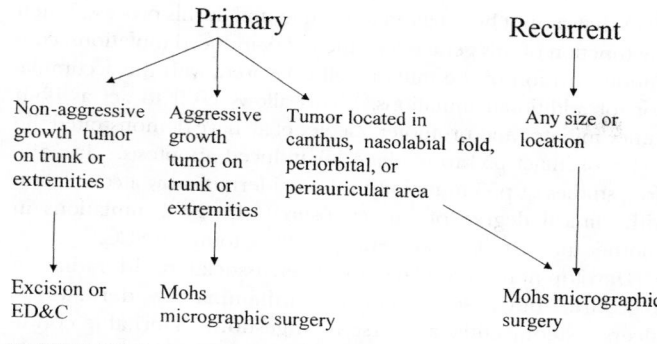

FIGURE 37-16. Primary basal cell carcinomas may be managed by electrodesiccation curettage (ED&C), excision, or Mohs micrographic surgery, depending on histology, size, and anatomic location. Recurrent basal cell carcinomas should be treated by Mohs micrographic surgery.

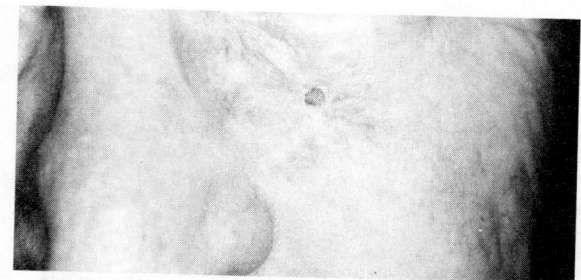

FIGURE 37-17. After radiation therapy, scar and hypopigmentation can result. (See Color Fig. 37-17 in the CD-ROM.)

ferred treatment for morpheaform; recurrent, poorly delineated, high-risk, and incompletely removed BCC; and for those sites in which tissue conservation is imperative.

C&D is frequently used by dermatologists in the treatment of BCC. Knox[62] noted cure rates as high as 98.3%, whereas Kopf et al.,[63] in an earlier study, cited a significant difference in the cure rates obtained between patients treated by private practitioners (94.3%) and those treated by trainees in the New York University Skin and Cancer Unit (81.2%). This supports the premise that although C&D is simple and cost-effective, it is dependent on operator skill. In a series of 233 patients treated by Spiller et al.,[64] an overall cure rate of 97% was reported. The highest cure rate was obtained in lesions that measured less than 1 cm (98.8%), with recurrences observed in 2 of 165 patients treated. Recurrences were noted in 2 of 45 patients with lesions that measured between 1 cm and 2 cm, for an overall cure rate of 95.5%. Recurrences were significantly higher in patients with lesions larger than 2 cm, for whom the overall cure rate was 84%. In this series, as in others, recurrences were most commonly noted on the forehead, temple, ears, nose, and shoulders. Some practitioners advocate that the procedure be repeated for three cycles, but histology, location, and behavior of the tumor should dictate the number of cycles. In another study, curettage followed by two cycles of cryosurgery was used to treat 100 NMSC, the majority being non-morpheaform, non-recurrent BCCs of the external ear resulting in one recurrence with a follow-up of 5 years.[65] C&D should be reserved for small or superficial BCCs, not located on the midface, in patients who may not tolerate more extensive surgery.

When surgery is contraindicated, RT is an option for treating primary BCC. RT may be indicated postoperatively if margins are ambiguous. Advantages of RT include minimal discomfort for the patient and avoidance of an invasive procedure in a patient who may not be able to tolerate or is unwilling to undergo surgery. Disadvantages include lack of margin control, poor cosmesis over time, a drawn-out course of therapy, and possible increased risk of future skin cancers. The recurrence rate for primary BCC treated by RT approaches 5% to 10% over 5 years. In one study by Wilder et al.,[66] local control rates among 85 patients with 115 biopsy-proven BCCs were compared. A 95% control rate was achieved for primary BCC and a 56% control rate obtained for recurrent BCC at 5 years. From the standpoint of cosmesis, scars from RT tend to worsen

over time (Fig. 37-17), as contrasted to surgical scars, which improve over time.

Cryosurgery has been used to treat BCC.[10] Two freeze-thaw cycles with a tissue temperature of $-50°C$ are required to destroy the tumor sufficiently. A margin of normal skin also should be frozen to ensure eradication of subclinical disease. Complications include hypertrophic scarring and postinflammatory pigmentary changes. Fractional cryotherapy has been used with success in treating eyelid lesions.[67] The method has been described as quick and cost-effective. A serious potential adverse outcome is recurrent BCC that can become extensive because of concealment by the fibrous scar created when aggressive cryosurgery is used.

Ablation by the CO_2 laser has been used in the treatment of BCC. In a recent study, Humphreys et al.[68] reported ablation of primary superficial BCC with the high-energy, pulsed CO_2 laser. Because of the absence of margin control and lack of large series studies, physicians familiar with laser and tumor biology should use this method only in carefully considered circumstances.

Management of BCC must be directed by the histologic nature of the tumor and the clinical context in which it presents. MMS is recommended for BCCs showing aggressive growth patterns and for BCCs occurring in high-risk anatomic sites or sites that require maximum conservation of normal tissue. For non-aggressive-growth BCCs on the trunk and extremities, fusiform excision with margins of 4 mm or C&D are appropriate. MMS may be helpful for BCC of the lower extremities where healing difficulties are anticipated. The smaller wound that results from MMS may obviate the need for complex reconstruction and facilitate healing. For patients with numerous BCCs, including patients with NBCCS, curettage and cauterization for smaller, superficial lesions is effective. Cryosurgery can be helpful in the management of multiple, small BCCs of NBCCS.

It is imperative that patients with a history of BCC receive annual full-body skin examinations. Although most recurrences appear within 1 to 5 years, they can develop later. Rowe et al.[60] found that 30% of recurrences developed within the first year after therapy, 50% within 2 years, and 66% within 3 years. Subsequent new primary BCC can present at rates of approximately 40%, with 20% to 30% of these developing within 1 year of treatment of the original lesion.

SQUAMOUS CELL CARCINOMA

SCC is a neoplasm of keratinizing cells that shows malignant characteristics, including anaplasia, rapid growth, local invasion, and metastatic potential. More than 100,000 cases of SCC are diag-

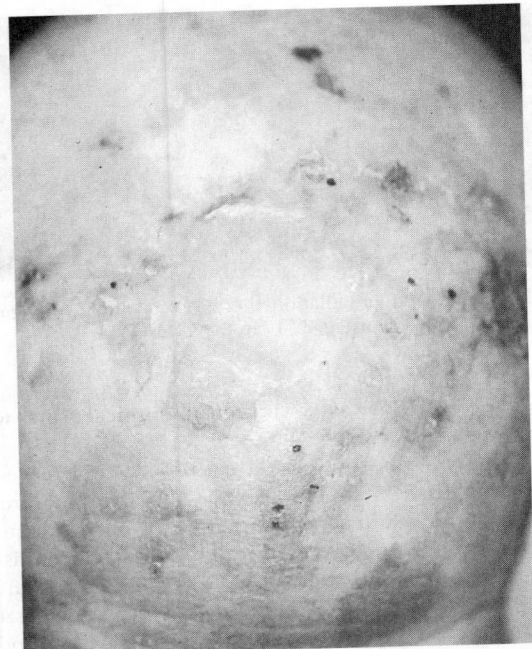

FIGURE 37-18. Extensive solar damage. Patients with this degree of solar damage are at increased risk for squamous cell carcinoma. (See Color Fig. 37-18 in the CD-ROM.)

nosed in the United States each year, making it the second most common human cancer after BCC. As with BCC, the cancer affects men more than women.[69] People of Celtic descent, individuals with fair complexions, and those with poor tanning ability and a predisposition to sunburn are at increased risk for developing SCC (Fig. 37-18). SCC in black populations arises most often on sites of preexisting inflammatory conditions, burn injuries, scars, or trauma.[70] Patients taking immunosuppressive medications after organ transplantation are also at increased risk (see Pathogenesis and Immunosuppression and Non-Melanoma Skin Cancer, later in this chapter). Another high-risk group includes patients treated with psoralens and UVA light for psoriasis.[71] Patients exposed to arsenic are at increased risk for SCC, particularly BD.[72]

Pathogenesis

Factors involved in the pathogenesis of SCC are similar to those for BCC and include exposure to UVL, genetic mutations, immunosuppression, and viral infection. The evidence for an association with UVL is even stronger for SCC than for BCC.[31,73] UVL mediates development of SCC through several mechanisms. Exposure to UVB appears to interfere with the density and antigen-processing capability of Langerhans' cells and may suppress production of the T helper 1 cytokines interleukin-2 and interferon-γ.[74] Studies have demonstrated that UVL introduces mutations into the tumor suppressor gene p53 by producing dimers of neighboring pyrimidines of the DNA that are considered UV signature mutations. The normal function of p53 protein is to induce the expression of different proteins that regulate the cell cycle and to induce apoptosis. In the epidermis, p53 is UV-inducible and its activation leads to cell-cycle arrest at G_1 phase, allowing for repair of DNA damage. It also leads to programmed death of the cell if the DNA impairment is lethal. Thus, cells having UV-damaged

DNA that cannot be repaired are eliminated by this process. When the function of this gene is lost due to UV-induced mutations, continuous division of the mutant cell is favored, with the accumulation of additional mutations.[75] This allows UVL to act as both tumor initiator and promoter. Ziegler et al. have demonstrated the ability of intact p53 to mediate UV-induced apoptosis.[76] In addition, studies of p53 mutation in the epidermis show a correlation with clinical degree of sun exposure.[77] In 2002, mutations in another tumor suppressor gene, p16, were found in SCC.[78]

Development of SCC has also been associated with radiation exposure, burn scars, chronic inflammatory dermatoses, ulcers, osteomyelitis, and arsenic ingestion.[79] Heritable conditions associated with SCC include xeroderma pigmentosum and oculocutaneous albinism. Immunosuppression also plays a role in pathogenesis. Skin cancers in immunosuppressed patients appear primarily on sun-exposed sites.[80] This suggests that immunosuppression and UVL act as cofactors in the development of SCC. Human immunodeficiency virus patients tend to have a higher incidence of SCC than the general population.[81] However, the exact nature of the relationship between human immunodeficiency virus and SCC has not yet been determined. The role of human papillomavirus (HPV) in the development of SCC has been studied. Eliezri et al.[82] found a direct correlation between the venereal spread of HPV-16 and the initiation of SCC, and others have demonstrated an association of HPV-16 with periungual SCC.[83]

Biologic Behavior

The biologic behavior of SCC is determined by a number of variables.[84] The overall invasiveness and depth of the neoplasm is important when determining the risk of recurrence. SCCs that invade the reticular dermis and subcutis tend to recur if not properly treated. Degree of cellular differentiation is also an important factor in recurrence. Poorly differentiated neoplasms show increased rates of recurrence.

SCC *in situ* is SCC limited to the epidermis and lacks invasion into the dermis. Although SCC *in situ* carries no risk of metastasis, invasive SCC can metastasize[84] and can originate in neglected SCC *in situ* (Fig. 37-19).

The tendency for regional lymph node metastasis is variable. Tumors arising in areas of chronic inflammation have a 10% to 30% rate of metastasis, whereas the incidence of metastasis from SCC that is not due to preexisting inflammatory or degenerative conditions varies from 0.05% to 16.0%.[84] Although tumors that arise on sun-damaged skin were initially thought to behave less aggressively than *de novo* SCC, all lesions have the potential to become invasive locally and to metastasize to draining lymph nodes. A study recently showed that 44% of the original lesions of cutaneous SCC that metastasized had contiguous AKs histologically and the skin adjacent to the tumors showed solar degeneration in almost all cases.[85] The large number of sun-mediated SCCs makes this clinical potential a concern. Friedman et al.[86] demonstrated that all trunk and extremity primary SCCs that later developed local or nodal recurrence were at least 4 mm deep and penetrated into the reticular dermis or subcutis. The extent of cellular differentiation also influences the metastatic potential in that tumors that invade regional lymph nodes tend to be more anaplastic than those that have not metastasized. Tumors are more likely to disseminate to regional lymph nodes than to distant sites,

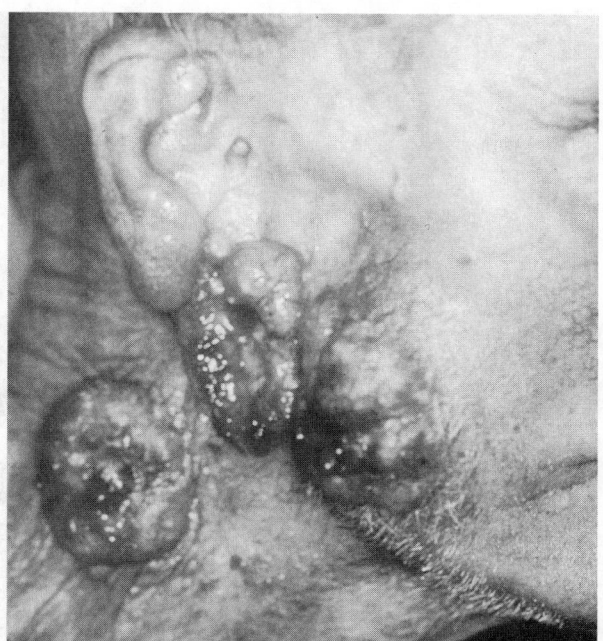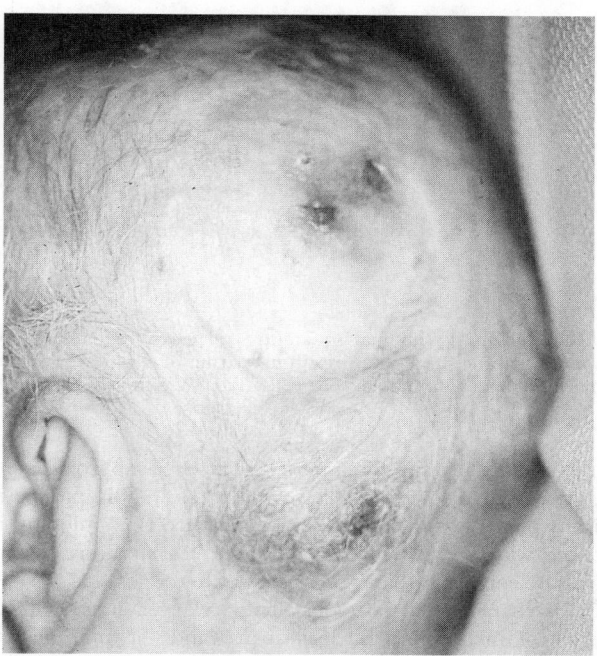

FIGURE 37-19. Metastatic squamous cell carcinoma (SCC). **A:** In this patient, primary cutaneous SCC metastasized to the parotid gland and draining lymph nodes. **B:** Metastatic SCC after multiple excisions. (See Color Fig. 37-19 in the CD-ROM.)

although intravascular metastases to viscera have appeared in as many as 5% to 10% of SCCs metastatic from skin.

Invasive SCC has the potential to involve nerves.[84] SCCs on the midface and lip are prone to neural involvement. These patients show a lower 10-year survival (23% vs. 88%) and a higher local recurrence rate (47% vs. 7.3%) than do those without neural involvement. Regional lymph node and distant metastases may increase with perineural involvement. SCCs on the skin of the head and neck may metastasize to cervical lymph nodes and distantly to the central nervous system; the latter occurs either hematogenously or via the perineural space, which directly connects to the subarachnoid space.

Clinical Features

SCC appears as a slightly raised, red, hyperkeratotic macule or papule on sun-exposed sites but may occur anywhere (Figs. 37-20 through 37-24). It can be difficult to clinically distinguish an invasive SCC from a hypertrophic actinic keratosis, a benign seborrheic keratosis, or a benign inflammatory lesion. Appropriate biopsy should be performed on any lesion suspicious for SCC, considering the potential for invasive disease. Shave biopsy is sufficient and will not lead to spread of the cancer. Verrucous carcinoma, a variant of SCC, includes oral florid papillomatosis, giant condyloma of Buschke-Löwenstein, and epithelioma cuniculatum.[87–89] A biopsy should be performed on an atypical wart or one that is unresponsive to therapy to rule out the presence of verrucous carcinoma.

BD represents SCC *in situ* with a distinctive microscopic appearance (see Fig. 37-24). Clinically, BD presents as a gradually enlarging well-demarcated erythematous plaque with an irregular border and surface crusting or scaling. Retrospective studies suggest that the risk of progression of BD to invasive SCC is approximately 3%.[90] Erythroplasia of Queyrat is BD occurring on the glans penis, usually in uncircumcised men. The risk of

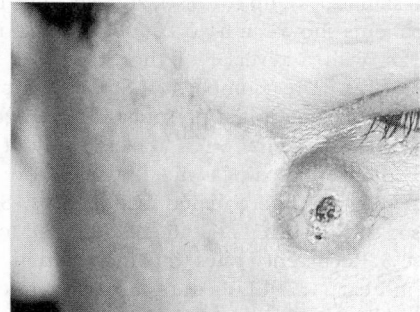

FIGURE 37-20. Recurrent squamous cell carcinoma, keratoacanthoma type, successfully treated by Mohs micrographic surgery. (See Color Fig. 37-20 in the CD-ROM.)

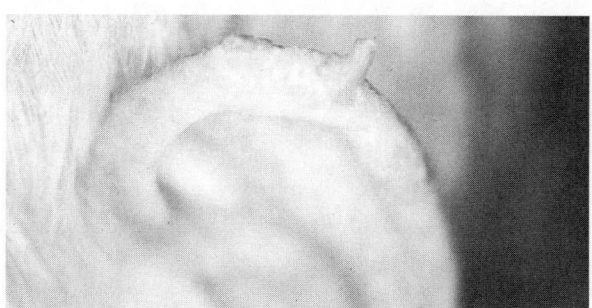

FIGURE 37-21. Squamous cell carcinoma can arise within a cutaneous horn. (See Color Fig. 37-21 in the CD-ROM.)

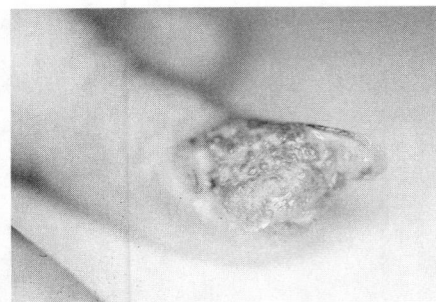

FIGURE 37-22. Periungual squamous cell carcinoma treated by Mohs micrographic surgery can result in sparing of a digit that otherwise may have been amputated. (See Color Fig. 37-22 in the CD-ROM.)

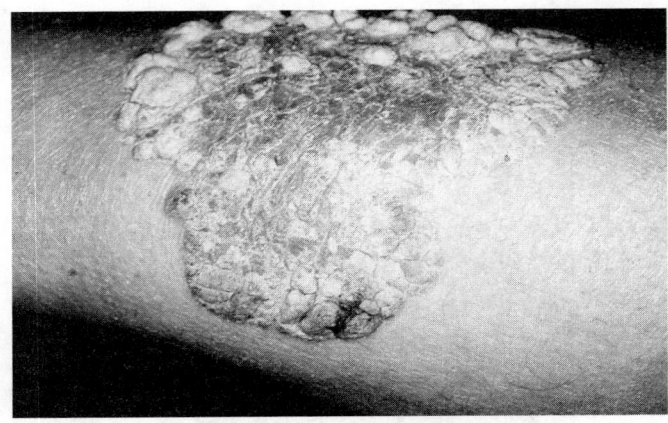

A

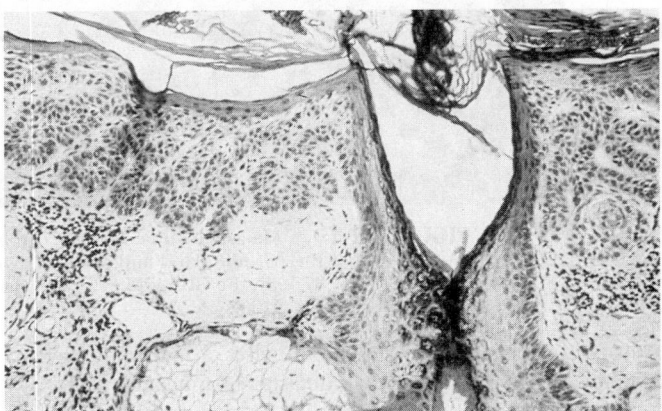

B

FIGURE 37-24. **A:** Bowen's disease presents as an erythematous plaque and can be difficult to differentiate from a benign inflammatory process. **B:** Bowen's disease is characterized by proliferation of atypical cells arranged in such a way as to suggest a windblown appearance. (See Color Fig. 37-24 in the CD-ROM.)

progression into invasive disease for genital BD is approximately 10%, greater than for typical sites of BD.[91] Bowenoid papulosis classically presents as a reddish brown verrucous papule and is associated with HPV-16[82] and -18. Bowenoid papulosis usually involves the genitals but may present elsewhere.[92]

SCC is characterized histologically by relatively large cellular size, lack of maturation, nuclear atypia, and the presence of mitotic figures (see Fig. 37-24; Fig. 37-25). Lack of dermal invasion separates SCC *in situ* from histologically invasive SCC. Verrucous carcinoma is characterized microscopically by an endophytic epidermal proliferation with atypia sufficient to distinguish it from verruca vulgaris, or the common wart.[87] Variants of BD are characterized by proliferation of atypical cells arranged in such a way as to suggest a windblown appearance. A grading system was devised to classify SCC with respect to percentage of differentiated cells. Grade 1 tumors are described as having more than 75% well-differentiated cells, whereas in grade 2 SCC, 50% to 75% of cells are described as well-differentiated and, in grade 3 SCC, 25% to 50% of cells are described this way. Primary cutaneous SCC with fewer than 25% well-differentiated cells is termed *grade 4 SCC*. Prognosis worsens with decreased degree of differentiation.[84]

Recurrence and Metastatic Risk

In a review of studies of SCCs from 1940 to 1992, Rowe et al.[84] correlated risk for local recurrence and metastasis with treat-

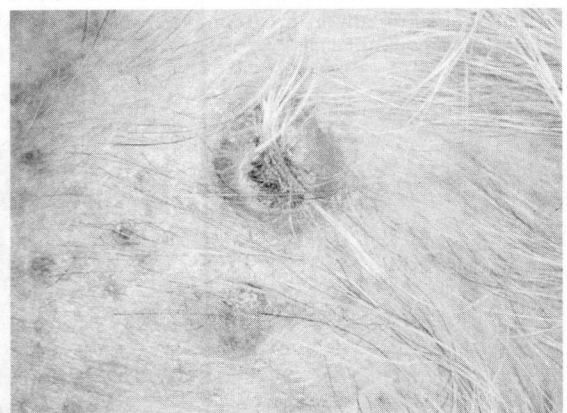

FIGURE 37-23. Squamous cell carcinoma, keratoacanthoma type. This variant of squamous cell carcinoma presents as a rapidly growing nodule. (See Color Fig. 37-23 in the CD-ROM.)

ment modality, prior treatment, location, size, depth, histologic differentiation, evidence of perineural involvement, precipitating factors other than UVL, and immunosuppression. They found that with tumors greater than 2 cm in diameter, recurrence rates double from 7.4% to 15.2%. In addition, they demonstrated that tumors less than 4 mm deep were at low risk for metastasis (6.7%) as compared with tumors deeper than 4 mm (45.7%). Locally recurrent SCCs showed an overall metastatic rate of 30%, with high rates of metastasis in the context of local recurrence in skin (25%), lip (31.5%), and ear (45%). Immunosuppressed patients showed a 5- to 20-fold increase in the incidence of SCCs, with a reversal of the SCC/BCC ratio from 0.25:1.0 to 3.0:1.0. The number of SCCs per patient was increased, and the age at initial presentation was decreased. In immunosuppressed patients, SCCs metastasized at a rate of 12.9%. Poorly differentiated SCC metastasized more frequently (32.9%) than did well-differentiated SCC (9.2%). SCC arising on sun-exposed skin recurred at a rate of 7.9% and metastasized at a rate of 5.2%. Recurrence rates were increased in SCC on the lip (10.5%) and ear (18.7%), as were metastatic rates from the lip (13.7%) and ear (11%). SCCs with perineural invasion recurred in almost one-half of cases (47.2%) and showed metastatic rate of 47.3%. Another study[93] comparing metastasizing SCC to non-metastasizing SCC also reported factors such as size

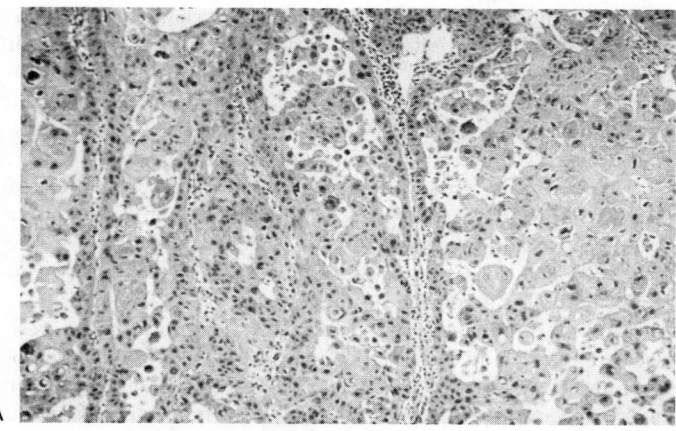
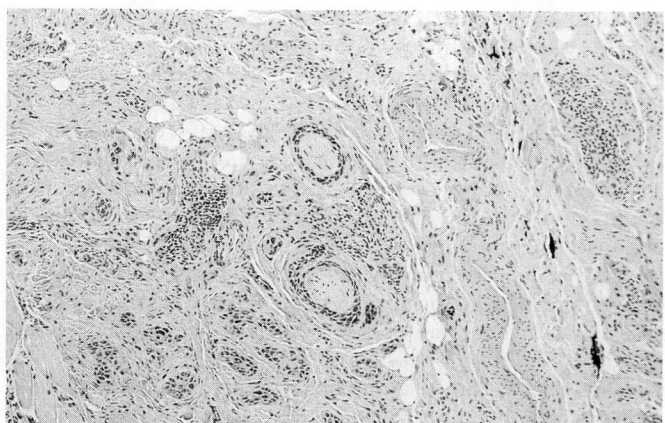

A   B

FIGURE 37-25. Squamous cell carcinoma (SCC), microscopic view. **A:** Infiltrative SCC. Note large cellular size and nuclear atypia. **B:** SCC demonstrating perineural invasion on microscopic examination. (See Color Fig. 37-25 in the CD-ROM.)

(greater than 2 cm), depth (Clark's level V), degree of differentiation, the presence of small tumor nests, infiltrative tumor strands, single-cell infiltration, perineural invasion, acantholysis, and recurrence to correlate strongly with metastasis.

Treatment of nodal disease may involve radiation or lymph-node dissection, or both. Treatment of metastatic SCC may include systemic chemotherapy or treatment with biologic response modifiers, but the efficacy of these methods has not been established. Long-term prognosis, however, for metastatic disease is extremely poor. Ten-year survival rates are less than 20% for patients with regional lymph node involvement and less than 10% for patients with distant metastases.[94]

Treatment

Many of the treatments for BCC are appropriate for SCC (Fig. 37-26). The type of therapy should be selected on the basis of size of the lesion, anatomic location, depth of invasion, degree of cellular differentiation, and history of previous treatment.[95] There are three general approaches to treatment of SCC: (1) destruction by C&D or cryosurgery, (2) removal by traditional excisional surgery or MMS, and (3) RT.

C&D can be used for small lesions arising on sun-damaged skin. Well-differentiated, primary SCCs measuring less than 1

cm in diameter are amenable to this form of therapy. Honeycutt and Jansen[96] reported a 99% cure rate for 281 SCCs after a 4-year follow-up. In this study, two recurrences were noted in lesions less than 2 cm in diameter. C&D is also frequently used for SCC *in situ*; however, with all forms of destructive therapy, extension of BD down hair follicles and clinically unrecognized foci of invasive tumor are a concern.

SCC *in situ* may be treated by cryotherapy. As with BCC, two freeze-thaw cycles with a tissue temperature of –50°C are required to destroy the tumor sufficiently. A margin of normal skin also should be frozen to ensure eradication of subclinical disease. Complications include hypertrophic scarring and postinflammatory pigmentary changes. Concealment of recurrence within dense scar tissue presents a danger. Imiquimod has demonstrated efficacy in the treatment of SCC *in situ*.[19]

Surgical excision is a well-accepted treatment modality for SCC. Brodland and Zitelli[97] have demonstrated that lesions of less than 2 cm in diameter are best treated by excision, with margins of 4 mm, whereas high-risk SCC requires 6-mm margins. These investigators found that certain characteristics were associated with a greater risk of subclinical tumor extension, thus qualifying such tumors as high-risk. These included the size of 2 cm or larger, histologic grade higher than 2, invasion of the subcutaneous tissue, and location in high-risk areas. Carcinomas of the penis, vulva, and anus usually are treated by excision because of the poor tolerance of these areas to irradiation.[98,99] Surgical excision is the treatment of choice for verrucous carcinoma.[87]

MMS is indicated in cases of large primary or recurrent SCC, as this modality allows conservation of normal tissue with preservation of function and enhanced cosmesis. MMS is also superior to other forms of treatment with regard to local recurrence.[57,95] Recurrence rates with Mohs surgery are superior to those obtained with traditional excisional surgery in primary SCC of the ear (3.1% vs. 10.9%), primary SCC of the lip (5.8% vs. 18.7%), recurrent SCC (10% vs. 23.3%), SCC with perineural invasion (0% vs. 47%), SCC larger than 2 cm (25.2 vs. 41.7%), and poorly differentiated SCC (32.6% vs. 53.6%).[84] MMS has proven useful in SCC involving the nail unit[100] and has been used as a limb-sparing procedure in cases of SCC arising in osteomyelitis.

RT may be used for head and neck cutaneous SCC in which there is no spread to bone or cartilage and there is no evidence

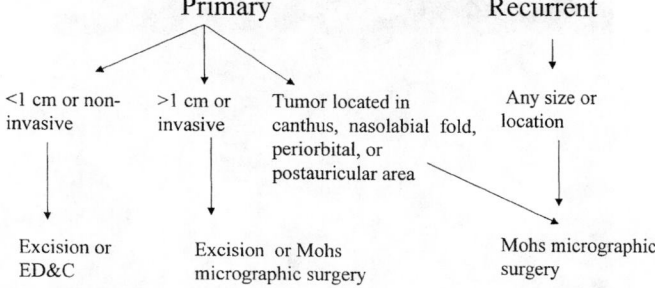

FIGURE 37-26. Primary squamous cell carcinoma may be managed by electrodesiccation and curettage (ED&C), excision, or Mohs micrographic surgery, depending on histology, tumor size, and anatomic location. Recurrent squamous cell carcinomas should be treated by Mohs micrographic surgery.

of metastasis.[101] As with BCC, RT may be indicated for elderly patients with SCC who are unwilling or unable to undergo surgery.[58] In one series, 108 patients with SCC of the lower vermilion lip were stratified into stage T1 (82.4%), T2 (15.7%), or T3 (1.9%) disease and were treated with RT. Recurrences occurred in 12.4% of patients with T1 disease and 6.7% of patients with T2 disease.[102] RT often is used as an adjuvant modality after treatment of SCC in which perineural involvement is identified, although no controlled studies have proven its usefulness.

MMS is indicated for invasive lesions, poorly differentiated lesions, and lesions occurring in high-risk anatomic sites or sites in which conservation of normal tissue is essential for preservation of function or cosmesis.

Invasive SCC can be a potentially lethal neoplasm and warrants close follow-up. In one study, approximately 30% of patients with SCC developed a subsequent SCC, with more than one-half of these occurring within the first year of follow-up.[103] Thus, it is recommended that patients with SCC be examined every 3 months during the first year after treatment, every 6 months during the second year after treatment, and annually thereafter. Evaluation should include total body cutaneous examination and palpation of draining lymph nodes. Currently, radiography, magnetic resonance imaging, and CT play no role in the routine workup of uncomplicated cutaneous SCC.

Immunosuppression and Non-Melanoma Skin Cancer

The role of the immune system in the pathogenesis of skin cancer is not completely understood. Immunosuppressed patients with lymphoma or leukemia[104] and patients with depressed cellular immunity secondary to human immunodeficiency virus infection show a higher frequency of infiltrative BCC.[81] Increasingly, the population at high risk for NMSC are patients who have undergone organ transplants.[80] These patients experience a marked increase in the incidence of SCC (65-fold greater than the general population in one study[105]) but only a slight increase in BCC. Furthermore, the SCCs in organ transplant patients occur at a younger age and tend to be more aggressive. There is an increased risk of local recurrence, regional and distant metastasis, and mortality. Other cutaneous tumors may also be increased in organ transplant recipients.[106] Here as well, UV radiation is the primary pathogenic factor for the development of NMSC, but degree and duration of immunosuppression are also significant.[107] Although organ transplant recipients have an increased incidence of viral warts, the role of HPV in skin cancer is not clearly defined. Prevention, patient education, and timely and aggressive management of skin cancers in this special population are crucial to reduce the significant potential of morbidity and mortality. Transplantation immunosuppressive medications that are more selective in impairing recipient immune system activation against the allograft are being developed and may alter the behavior of skin cancer in these patients.

MERKEL CELL CARCINOMA

Merkel cell carcinoma (MCC) is a rare and aggressive tumor of neuroendocrine cell origin with an estimated 470 new cases in the United States each year. MCC affects more men than women, whites more than blacks, and most often occurs between the seventh and ninth decades of life.[108]

The pathogenesis of MCC is incompletely characterized. UVL has been indirectly implicated in its development, as 36% of such cancers arise on the face.[109] The Merkel cell derives from the neural crest and differentiates as part of the amine precursor uptake and decarboxylation system. Merkel cells function as slowly adapting type I mechanoreceptors, and the density of Merkel cells in sun-exposed skin is much higher compared with sun-protected skin. A review of 875 cases demonstrated that 47% of cases occur on the head and neck, 40% on the extremities, and 8% on the trunk.[110] MCC/SCC[111] and, recently, MCC/BCC[112] have been reported, thus supporting the role of UVL exposure as a risk factor. A multicenter study of 1380 patients with psoriasis who were treated with oral methoxypsoralen and ultraviolet A photochemotherapy showed that the incidence of MCC was 100 times higher than expected in the general population.[113] Immunosuppression, whether through iatrogenic means, human immunodeficiency virus infection, or neoplasia, may play a role in the development of MCC, as rapid progression has been reported in the setting of immunosuppressive therapy after organ transplantation.[114] In addition, one study demonstrated an increased malignant neoplasm rate among patients with MCC.[115]

MCC usually presents as a rapidly growing, firm, red-violaceous, dome-shaped papule or plaque on sun-exposed skin (Fig. 37-27).[108,116] It is predominantly located in sun-exposed head and neck skin, extremities, and less often on the trunk. Clinical differential diagnosis includes leukemia cutis, amelanotic melanoma, metastatic carcinoma, pyogenic granuloma, and SCC.

Microscopic examination reveals sheets and cords of atypical cells in the dermis extending to the subcutaneous layer that sometimes form an interlacing trabecular or pseudoglandular pattern.[108] A grenz zone often is present, separating tumor from epidermis. Cell membranes often are indistinct, giving a syncytial appearance. Cells are round to oval and generally noncohesive. Cytoplasm tends to be scant, with round to oval nuclei containing two to three nucleoli. Special stains may prove useful in the histologic diagnosis of MCC. Cytokeratin-20 staining gives a characteristic paranuclear dot pattern. Histologic differential diagnosis includes lymphoma, BCC, metastatic oat cell carcinoma, or noncutaneous neuroendocrine tumors. Lymphoma cells are differentiated in that they are CD45-positive and cytokeratin-20–negative. Melanoma can be differentiated in that melanocytes are strongly S-100-positive. In addition to cytokeratin-20, MCC stains positively for chromogranin neuron-specific enolase, synaptophysin, and

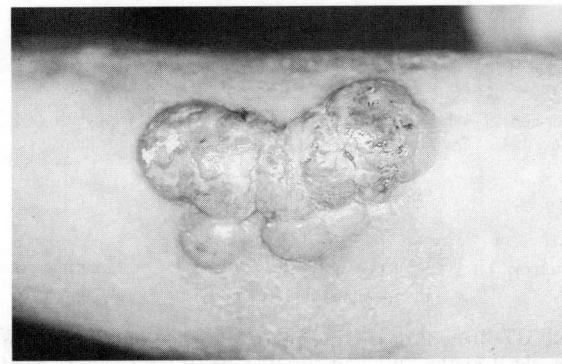

FIGURE 37-27. Merkel cell carcinoma presenting as a red to violaceous, dome-shaped papule or plaque on the sun-exposed skin of an elderly person. (See Color Fig. 37-27 in the CD-ROM.)

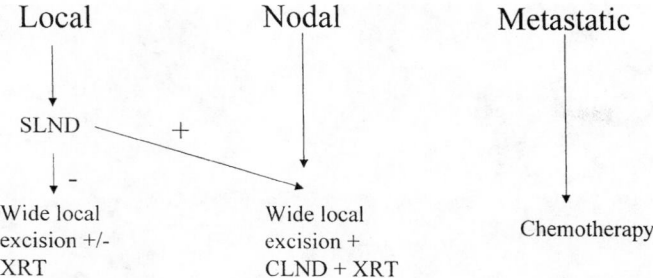

FIGURE 37-28. Merkel cell carcinoma should be treated by wide local excision followed by sentinel or complete lymph node dissection (SLND, CLND), radiation therapy (XRT), or chemotherapy, depending on stage.

may be weakly positive for S-100 protein. In 2002, it was shown that MCC may also stain for the KIT receptor tyrosine kinase (CD117) and perhaps abnormal functioning of the KIT receptor could be involved in the malignant transformation of this tumor.[117]

MCC warrants aggressive therapy (Fig. 37-28). It has a high propensity for local recurrence (20% to 75%), regional node metastases (31% to 80%), and distant metastases (26% to 75%), and approximately one-third of patients eventually die of the disease.[110,115] Evaluation must include full-body skin examination with lymph node evaluation, a complete blood cell count, and liver function tests. CT scanning of the chest, pelvis, and abdomen may be indicated to rule out the presence of small cell carcinoma of the lung. CT scanning of the head and neck may prove valuable in detection of nodal disease. Octreotide scans may be more sensitive than CT scans in diagnosing primary and metastatic MCC.[118] Management of MCC follows staging of patients according to simple classification: stage I (primary tumor alone), stage II (locoregional metastases), or stage III (metastatic disease). Some authors have recommended incorporating size as a criterion in staging, dividing stage I patients into those with IA (less than 2 cm in maximal diameter) and IB (equal to or greater than 2 cm).[128] Although MCC is a highly aggressive and potentially lethal cancer, spontaneous regression has been reported.[119] The significance of this phenomenon is unknown. Recommended management has usually been wide local excision (WLE) with 1- to 3-cm margins; however, treatment guidelines are not well defined, owing to the rarity of the tumor, which precludes randomized clinical trials. Recurrence rates after primary therapy for MCC with surgery alone are reported to be within the range of 22% to 100%. MMS has been proposed as being more successful in controlling local disease than traditional wide excision, especially in cosmetically sensitive anatomic areas such as the face.[120] Uncontrolled clinical experience is promising, but definitive clinical studies still have to be conducted.[121,122] Although a substantial benefit in both time to recurrence and disease-free survival has been demonstrated with adjuvant RT, a survival benefit has not been shown. Due to the propensity for early nodal spread and the significant negative impact nodal disease has on outcome, regional lymph node dissection or sentinel lymph node dissection may be advisable.

Many have likened MCC to melanoma because both derive from neural crest and both malignancies have a propensity for initial lymphatic, then distant spread. Given these similarities, it is suggested that perhaps depth of tumor may be more of a prognostic indicator than the actual diameter of the primary tumor.[123] In a recent study, 18 patients with stage I MCC underwent sentinel lymph node dissection. In two patients, involvement of the sentinel node was identified, resulting in complete lymph node dissection. Sentinel node–negative patients received no therapy other than wide and deep excision.[124] All patients remained free of recurrence at 7 months. Again, however, improved local and regional control can be demonstrated, but there is no impact on survival. Patients with negative sentinel nodes may be treated by WLE with margins of up to 3 cm and, possibly, adjunctive RT. Patients with positive sentinel nodes should be treated as patients with regional disease. The combination of WLE, therapeutic lymph node dissection, and RT has been suggested for treatment of regional disease.[125] Studies show that local and regional control and disease-free survival improve significantly with postoperative radiotherapy. However, there is no difference in overall survival.[126] In a study of 60 patients with head and neck MCC, of 34 patients treated with WLE alone, 44% developed local recurrence, 85% developed a regional recurrence, and 59% developed distant metastases. Of 26 patients treated with WLE followed by radiation treatment to the primary surgical site and regional lymph node basin, 12% developed a local recurrence, 27% developed a regional recurrence, and 42% developed distant metastases. Rates of survival did not differ between the two groups.[127]

MCC tends to spread in a cascade pattern, first affecting local, then regional lymph nodes, and finally progressing to fatal distant metastatic disease.[128] MCC spreads to regional lymph nodes within 2 years in up to 70% of cases. The overall 5-year survival rate for patients with this condition is only 50% to 68%. Lymph node metastases have been identified in up to 20% of cases of MCC at initial presentation. Approximately 50% of patients experience nodal disease at some point in the disease course. Distant metastases have been reported in up to 52% of patients at presentation. Metastases have been noted most commonly in skin and lymph nodes but also in the lung, liver, brain, intestine, bladder, stomach, and abdominal wall.[129] The reported median survival for stage I patients was 97 months and for stage II patients only 15 months,[116] and the median survival after the diagnosis of metastasis is in the range of 6 months.[128] MCC is chemosensitive but rarely chemocurable in patients with metastasis or locally advanced tumors. Although there is no consensus, the most common regimens used in the treatment of metastatic MCC include cyclophosphamide (Cytoxan), doxorubicin, and vincristine and cisplatin and etoposide.[130] However, brief responses have been reported recently in a small series of patients treated with carboplatin and etoposide.[131] In a review by Voog et al.,[132] overall response to first-line chemotherapy for MCC was 61%, with a 57% response in metastatic disease and a 69% response in locally advanced disease. The 3-year survival rate was 17% in metastatic disease and 35% in locally advanced disease. Forty-two regimens were used to treat these 107 reported cases.

Patients with MCC must be followed up aggressively for potential local recurrence and development of metastatic disease. Age older than 65 years, male sex, size of primary lesion greater than 2 cm, truncal site, nodal/distant disease at presentation, and duration of disease before presentation (less than or equal to 3 months) appear to be poor prognostic factors.[133] In some studies, patient gender and primary tumor location were not independent predictors of survival.[125] Allen et al. reported tumor stage as the only independent predictor of sur-

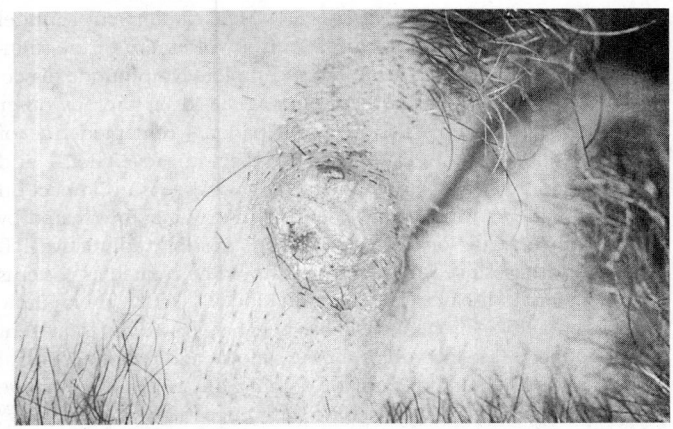
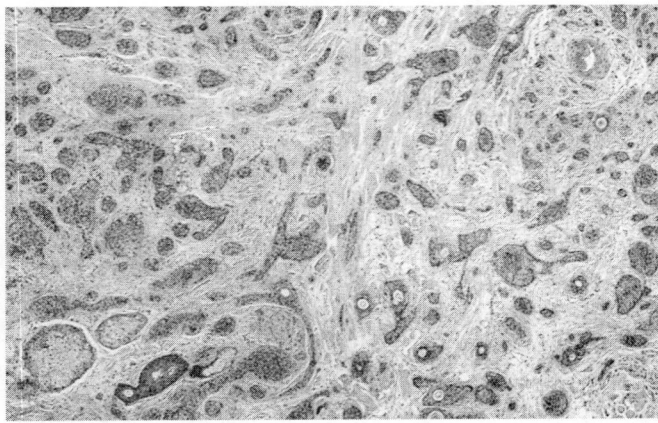

FIGURE 37-29.   Microcystic adnexal carcinoma. **A:** Classic presentation is as an indurated plaque with intact epidermis and yellow hue. **B:** On microscopic examination, the dermis shows numerous basaloid cells forming cords, nests, small ducts, and horn microcysts. (See Color Fig. 37-29 in the CD-ROM.)

vival and elective lymph node dissection as the only predictor of improved relapse-free survival in patients with stage I disease.[125] They also described three factors influencing survival after the first recurrence of disease: (1) the disease-free interval between treatment of the primary tumor and the time of first recurrence (recurrence after 8 months had better survival), (2) patients with nodal recurrence as their first recurrence had a better disease-specific survival than that of patients with local or distant failure, and (3) patients who could be rendered free of disease by surgical excision had a better survival rate than patients who could only undergo palliative treatment.

MICROCYSTIC ADNEXAL CARCINOMA

Microcystic adnexal carcinoma (MAC) was first described as a distinct entity in 1982 by Goldstein et al.[134] In this study, six cases of MAC were described. In each case, the tumor was originally misdiagnosed on initial biopsy as benign. MAC originates from pluripotent adnexal cells capable of eccrine and follicular differentiation. Synonyms for MAC include *sclerosing sweat duct carcinoma*, *sweat duct carcinoma with syringomatous features*, and *combined adnexal tumor of the skin*.

MAC is an aggressive, locally destructive cutaneous appendageal neoplasm with a high rate of recurrence. It primarily affects white, middle-aged individuals,[135] although it has been reported in children[136] and black patients.[137] Unlike the other primary cutaneous malignancies considered thus far, affected women outnumber affected men.[135] The pathogenesis of MAC is not completely understood but may involve exposure to ionizing radiation,[138] and this may precede development of MAC by as long as 40 years. Because these tumors present on the central face, UVL may also play a role.

MAC classically presents as a sclerotic or indurated plaque with an intact epidermis and yellow hue (Fig. 37-29A).[134] The tumor usually involves the central face and lip but is not limited to those anatomic sites.[134] MAC involvement of the eyelid,[139] scalp,[140] tongue,[141] and genitalia[142] have been reported. The lesion is usually asymptomatic but can manifest with numbness, tenderness, burning, anesthesia, or paresthesia due to the high frequency of perineural invasion. This tumor is often misdiagnosed clinically and histologically.

On microscopic examination, MAC may be misdiagnosed as a benign adnexal process. The dermis contains numerous basaloid cells forming cords, nests, small ducts, and horn microcysts (see Fig. 37-29B). Horn microcysts usually are present superficially, containing laminated keratin and, occasionally, small vellus hairs. Cysts may be calcified. Small ducts, either empty or filled with eosinophilic material composed of sialomucin, commonly are present. Ducts may be well differentiated, with two rows of cuboidal cells, or less differentiated, with single strands without lumina. A dense sclerotic stroma is present. Immunohistochemical analysis may be useful in differentiating MAC from desmoplastic trichoepithelioma. Wick et al. reported that MACs were reactive to hard keratin subclasses AE13 and AE14, epithelial membrane antigen, carcinoembryonic antigen, and LeuM1.[143] Desmoplastic trichoepitheliomas were positive for AE14, epithelial membrane antigen, and LeuM1 only focally and were, in contrast, negative for carcinoembryonic antigen. In addition, the absence of Merkel cells in MAC may help to distinguish it from desmoplastic trichoepithelioma, another sclerosing epithelial neoplasm that can be histologically confused with MAC.[144] Correct diagnosis of MAC is imperative, as the tumor can be highly invasive and may involve adipose, vascular adventitia, muscle, perichondrium, or bone.[145]

MAC has been treated by WLE as well as MMS.[135] Studies[146] suggest that extirpation by Mohs technique may prove beneficial in the management of MAC. However, these findings must be interpreted cautiously, as recurrences have been reported up to 30 years after surgical excision.[147] Non-Mohs surgical excision is associated with recurrence rates of 47% to 59%.[148] It appears that the tumor is resistant to RT, thus presenting difficulties in the management of MAC with perineural invasion.

After surgery for MAC, patients must be evaluated regularly for recurrence and for development of other skin cancers. Evaluation should include examination of skin and lymph nodes and, due to the potential for recurrence long after treatment, continue indefinitely.

SEBACEOUS CARCINOMA

Sebaceous carcinoma (SC) is a malignant adnexal tumor with variable sites of origin, histologic growth patterns, and clinical presentations. Ocular SC is more common and may arise from meibomian glands and, less frequently, from the glands of Zeis. The upper eyelids are most frequently involved. Approximately 50% of SCs are initially incorrectly diagnosed histologically and, in some series, all have been initially misdiagnosed clinically.[149] SC is the second most common eyelid malignancy after BCC and is the second most lethal after melanoma.[150]

Worldwide, SC affects all races, but Asians in particular.[150] Women are affected more commonly than men, at a ratio of approximately 2:1.[149] SC classically presents in the seventh to ninth decade.[149] SC is associated with sebaceous adenomas, radiation exposure, BD, and Muir-Torre syndrome. In Muir-Torre syndrome, an autosomal dominant heritable condition, SC and, more commonly, sebaceous adenoma (or sebaceous epithelioma) are associated with a second internal malignancy, usually a carcinoma of the colon or urogenital tract. SC has been reported after RT for retinoblastoma,[151] eczema,[152] and cosmetic epilation.[153] In addition, recent studies have identified HPV DNA[154] and overexpression of p53 protein in some SCs.[155]

Commonly, SC presents as a slowly growing, deeply seated nodule of the eyelid and may present as chronic diffuse blepharoconjunctivitis or keratoconjunctivitis, particularly when pagetoid or intraepithelial spread of tumor onto the conjunctival epithelium occurs.[149] The most common clinical misdiagnosis is chalazion. Upper eyelid involvement is more common. Approximately 25% of cases of SC involve extraocular sites, which may include head and neck, trunk,[156] salivary glands, and external genitalia.[154]

SC can spread by lymphatic or hematogenous routes or by direct extension. Distant metastases are reported in up to 20% of cases and may involve the lungs, liver, brain, bones, and lymph nodes.[149] The parotid gland may be involved secondarily.[157] Ocular SC may spread via the lacrimal secretory and excretory systems.

On microscopic examination, SC shows nonencapsulated tumors within the dermis.[149] Sebaceous cells exhibiting varying degrees of differentiation, nuclear pleomorphism, hyperchromatism, and locally infiltrating surrounding tissues and neurovascular spaces are observed. Special stains, including lipid stains as Oil-Red-O or Sudan IV for fresh tissue, and immunohistochemical stains such as EMA or LeuM1 are also helpful for the diagnosis of SC.

Treatment options for SC include traditional excisional surgery and extirpation by MMS. The local recurrence rate after WLE has been reported to be as high as 36%.[158] In one study of 14 cases of SC excised with frozen-section margin control, five recurrences were observed in cases with surgical margins of 1 to 3 mm, whereas no recurrences were seen with margins of 5 mm.[159] Potential difficulties arise because tumors are often multicentric with discontinuous foci of tumor, and pagetoid spread is difficult to determine even on high-quality, paraffin-embedded sections. Extirpation of SC by Mohs has yielded varying results. Folberg et al.[160] reported recurrences in two of three patients treated by the Mohs technique, with tumor noted at reconstruction in one of the three patients. Dzubow[161] reported two patients with recurrent SC who underwent MMS. One patient who underwent MMS followed by oculoplastic repair was tumor-free at 6 months. In the other patient, tumor distal to the Mohs defect was noted at reconstruction. Snow et al.[162] reported nine cases of ocular SC treated with MMS followed for 1 to 14 years, with one local recurrence at 1.5 years. They also reviewed the literature on the use of MMS for the treatment of

SC and accumulated 49 cases of ocular SC treated with a cure rate for primary tumors of 88%. A case of poorly differentiated SC successfully treated with RT has been reported.[163]

Patients with SC should be evaluated by an internist, and routine screening for internal malignancy (stool for occult blood, analysis of urine, colonoscopy) should be current. A family history for internal malignancy should be sought and family members screened, if indicated, to rule out Muir-Torre syndrome (an autosomal genodermatosis characterized by the occurrence of at least one sebaceous tumor in conjunction with at least one malignant visceral tumor and occasionally keratoacanthomas).[164] Poor prognostic indicators in SC include a duration of more than 6 months, multicentric origin, poor differentiation, infiltrative pattern, pagetoid changes, vascular invasion, lymphatic channel involvement, previous radiation, and orbital spread. After treatment for SC, patients should be followed up for recurrence or progression through regular examination of skin and lymph nodes. A mortality rate of 20% to 22% has been reported in ocular and extraocular SC.[158]

ATYPICAL FIBROXANTHOMA

Atypical fibroxanthoma (AFX) is a spindle cell tumor that occurs on the head and neck of sun-exposed individuals and on the trunk and extremities of younger patients.[165] Tumors of the head and neck characteristically present during the eighth decade, whereas tumors involving the extremities often present during the fourth decade. The ratio of affected men to affected women appears to be equal.[165]

The pathogenesis of AFX may involve exposure to UVL, ionizing radiation, or aberrant host response. In one study of ten cases of AFX, seven cases showed mutation in p53. Of the seven, all showed abnormal single-strand conformation polymorphism, with four of those showing CT mutations characteristically induced by UVL.[166] Another study detected p53 mutations in 67% of AFX tumors compared to 25% in malignant fibrous histiocytoma (MFH) and none in benign fibrous histiocytoma.[167] Exposure to ionizing radiation may play a role in the development of the tumor.[168] An increased incidence of AFX was shown in a study of 642 renal transplant patients,[169] and invasive AFX has been reported in a heart transplant patient.[170] Finally, metastatic AFX has been reported in a patient with null cell variant chronic lymphocytic leukemia.[171]

AFX usually presents as an asymptomatic papule or nodule in individuals with a fair complexion. There may be hyperpigmentation or ulceration.[172] The clinical appearance is not distinctive, and the lesion may be confused with pyogenic granuloma, SCC, or BCC.[173] The tumor characteristically presents on the head and neck of the elderly or the trunk or extremities of younger individuals but is not limited to these sites. Occurrence on the eyelid[174] and within the ethmoid sinus[175] and oral cavity[168] have been reported.

On microscopic examination, there is a dermal nodule with a dense infiltrate of bizarre spindle cells arranged in haphazard fashion without connection to the epidermis (Fig. 37-30).[172] Special stains for vimentin are positive and for CD68 are weakly positive, whereas stains for HMB-45 and S-100 are negative, distinguishing this lesion from spindle cell melanoma.[176] AFX stains negatively for LN-2, a marker present on B cells, Reed-Sternberg cells, and macrophages, which helps differentiate it from MFH.[177]

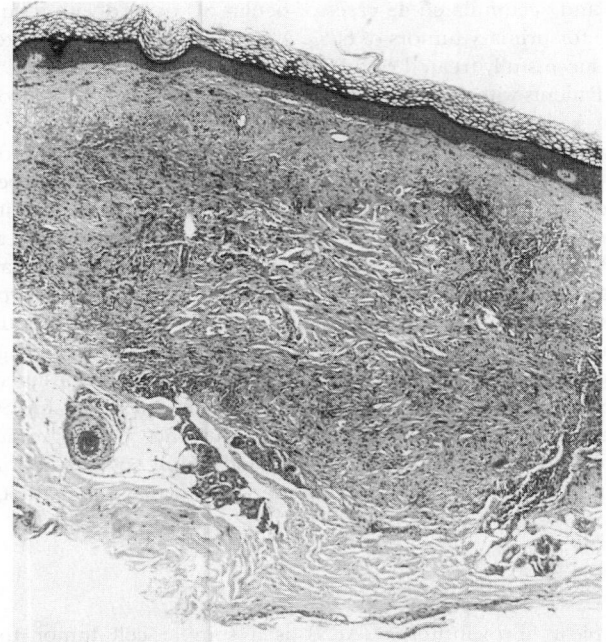

FIGURE 37-30.   Atypical fibroxanthoma. On microscopic examination, there is a dermal nodule with a dense infiltrate of atypical spindle cells arranged in haphazard fashion and associated with bizarre giant cells. (See Color Fig. 37-30 in the CD-ROM.)

Treatment options for AFX include WLE and MMS. In one large series comparing WLE with MMS,[165] recurrences were observed during a mean follow-up period of 73.6 months in 12% of 25 cases treated by WLE. Metastatic involvement of the parotid gland occurred in one of these patients, for an overall regional metastatic rate of 4%. In contrast, no recurrences or metastases were observed over a mean follow-up period of 29.6 months in any patient treated by MMS. Others have reported similarly favorable outcomes after treatment of AFX by MMS.[178] The authors favor the use of MMS for AFX because of the superior margin control and conservation of normal tissue.

Although AFX rarely metastasizes, it is a locally aggressive tumor with metastatic potential.[179] Metastases to the parotid gland,[180] lymph nodes,[181] and lung[182] have been reported. In a series of eight cases of metastatic AFX, poor prognostic indicators included vascular invasion, recurrence, deep-tissue penetration, necrosis, and impaired host resistance.[180]

MALIGNANT FIBROUS HISTIOCYTOMA

MFH is an aggressive spindle cell cancer and is the most common soft tissue tumor in the elderly, primarily affecting the extremities.[183] Peak incidence is during the seventh decade.

Although the pathogenesis of MFH is incompletely understood, there appears to be a predilection for development after radiation and in scar tissue. Inoshita and Youngberg[184] report development of MFH in an amputation site in one patient and in a hernioplasty scar in another. In both patients, the initial clinical diagnosis was subcutaneous abscess. MFH in a burn scar has also been reported.[185] A case of MFH associated with discoid lupus erythematosus has also been described.[186] Decreased immune surveillance may play a role in the development of MFH. A signifi-

cant increase in the incidence of MFH (158 per 100,000) has been reported in a large series of renal transplant patients.[169]

Clinically, MFH may present as a subcutaneous mass or ulcerative nodule. In one large series, MFH occurred principally as a mass on an extremity (lower extremity, 49%; upper extremity, 19%) or in the abdominal cavity or retroperitoneum (16%) of adults.[183] There are reports of MFH presenting on the scalp and lip.[187] Deep fascial involvement was typical (19%), as was involvement of skeletal muscle (59%). Fascial involvement was absent in only a small percentage of cases (7%).

MFH is aggressive and has high metastatic potential. In one series, a higher percentage of histologically infiltrative tumors (83% vs. 24%) were observed in subcutaneous MFH as opposed to intramuscular MFH.[188] An increased percentage of local recurrences (17% vs. 0%) were observed in the subcutaneous variant. In one large series, the local recurrence rate was 44%, and the rate of metastasis was 42%.[183] In this series, metastasis occurred most commonly in lung (82%) and lymph nodes (32%). Factors that appear to influence metastasis include depth and size of tumor, histologic grade, and inflammatory response. Small, superficially located tumors and tumors with a prominent inflammatory component metastasized less frequently.

On microscopic examination, MFH are deep tumors that are located beneath the fascia. However, the tumor occasionally occurs in the subcutaneous tissue. The tumor stains for fibroblastic-associated antigen, suggesting a fibroblastic origin. Morphologic features vary, and MFH may show transitions from areas with a highly ordered, storiform pattern to less differentiated areas with a pleomorphic appearance. Differentiation from AFX may be aided by staining with LN-2, a marker present in 90% of MFHs in one series but absent or only weakly present in AFX.[177]

Treatment options for MFH include WLE, although recurrence rates of up to 40% have been reported with this approach.[183] Some authors have reported successful treatment of subcutaneous MFH with MMS.[188] Brown and Swanson[189] reported no recurrences over a 3-year follow-up period among 17 patients with 20 tumors treated by MMS. Hafner et al.[178] reported successful treatment of MFH by MMS with margin control achieved using paraffin-embedded tissue sections. Adjuvant radiotherapy has been found to decrease local relapse rate.[190] After treatment for MFH, patients should be followed up aggressively for development of recurrent and metastatic disease.

DERMATOFIBROSARCOMA PROTUBERANS

DFSP is a low-grade cutaneous sarcoma with aggressive local behavior and low metastatic potential. DFSP classically presents as a plaque on the trunk and, less frequently, on the extremities, but it may occur anywhere.[191] The tumor most commonly presents during early or middle adulthood, although it can occur during childhood.[192] It tends to affect males more than females.[193] The Bednar tumor is a rare pigmented variant of DFSP.[194] Clinically, it may be difficult to differentiate from a dermatofibroma or a keloid.[195]

The pathogenesis of DFSP is incompletely understood but may involve factors as diverse as aberrant tumor suppressor genes or history of local trauma.[196] In one study, increased p53 protein immunoreactivity was found in DFSP but not in dermatofibroma, suggesting that expression of the protein may be important in the pathogenesis of DFSP.[197]

Microscopically, the tumor is composed of monomorphous spindle cells arranged in a storiform pattern and embedded in a sparse to moderately dense fibrous stroma.[191] The distinction between deep penetrating dermatofibroma (DPDF), which involves the subcutis, and DFSP may be challenging. In most instances, attention to the cytologic constituency of the lesions and the overall architecture is sufficient for differentiation. DPDF is typified by cellular heterogeneity. DPDF includes giant cells and lipidized histiocytes and extends deeply, using the interlobular subcuticular fibrous septa as scaffolds, or is in the form of broad fronts. In contrast, DFSP tends to be monomorphous, surrounding adipocytes diffusely or extending in stratified horizontal plates. This infiltration is characteristically eccentric, often with long, thin extensions in one direction and not another. Immunostaining for factor XIIIa and CD34 may be helpful in distinguishing DPDF from DFSP. Characteristically, DPDF is diffusely factor XIIIa–positive and CD34-negative, whereas DFSP is factor XIIIa–negative and CD34-positive.[198]

Treatment options for DFSP include WLE and MMS. Most authors advocate surgical excision with a minimal margin of 2 to 3 cm of surrounding skin, including the underlying fascia, without elective lymph node dissection.[199] The likelihood of local recurrence is related to the adequacy of surgical margins. Conservative resection can lead to recurrence rates of 33% to 60%, whereas wider excision margins (greater than or equal to 2.5 cm) have been reported to reduce the recurrent rate to 10% to 25%.[200] In one series, 58 patients with DFSP treated by MMS at three institutions showed a local recurrence rate of 2%.[201] There were no cases of regional or distant metastases. It is thought that the advantage that MMS provides is in the ability to track tumor growth patterns histologically, as the microscopic extent of these tumors is often both extensive and eccentric.[201] Caution is advised in attempting to interpret immunostains on frozen sections of DFSP because, in one study, microscopic examination of paraffin-embedded sections showed CD34-negative DFSP tumor cells with positive staining of endothelial cells.[202] For well-defined tumors located on trunk or extremities, WLE is likely to achieve tumor clearance with satisfactory cosmetic and functional result. However, extirpation of tumor by MMS, using frozen sections with confirmation by examination of paraffin-embedded sections may be beneficial in sites where maximum conservation of normal tissue is required.

Patients with DFSP should be followed closely for evidence of local or regional recurrence or metastatic disease.

DFSP has a tendency to recur locally, with an overall rate of 50%. The average time for recurrence is within the first 3 years. DFSP of the head and neck has been reported to have a higher local recurrence rate (50% to 75%) than DFSP in other locations.[203] Although metastases are rare, multiple local recurrences appear to predispose to distant metastases.[204] In one series of 19 cases of DFSP, there were 20 local recurrences in 8 patients.[200] Recurrences in this series followed narrow excision. No recurrences were noted during a mean follow-up period of 13.2 years after WLE with margins greater than 2 cm. Lymph node metastases occur in approximately 1% of cases, and distant metastases, principally to lung, occur in approximately 4% of DFSP cases. A fibrosarcomatous variant, FS-DFSP, represents an uncommon form of DFSP.[205] In a series of 41 patients with FS-DFSP, follow-up in 34 patients for a mean period of 90 months revealed a local recurrence rate of 58%. Metastases were observed at a rate of 14.7%. Thus, fibrosarcomatous

change in DFSP is indicative of a more aggressive clinical course. DFSP is a radioresponsive tumor, and combined conservative resection and postoperative radiation should also be considered in situations in which adequate wide excision alone would result in major cosmetic or functional deficits.[206]

ANGIOSARCOMA

Angiosarcoma (AS) is an aggressive, usually fatal neoplasm of vascular cells.[207] Four variants of cutaneous AS currently are recognized, including AS of the scalp and face, AS in the context of lymphedema (Stewart-Treves syndrome), radiation-induced AS, and epithelioid AS. Although these variants differ in presentation, they share key features, including clinical appearance of primary lesions, a biologically aggressive nature and, ultimately, poor outcome.

Cutaneous AS of the head and scalp usually affects the elderly, with men being affected more often than women.[208] Although no predisposing factors have been identified, exposure to UVL has been suggested as a risk factor due to the propensity for the tumor to affect sun-exposed sites of the scalp and face. Other researchers have questioned this connection because, in several series, AS has presented on scalps protected by hair as frequently as on bald scalps. Others have demonstrated that patients with AS show no significant increase in numbers of BCCs and SCCs, thus arguing against increased UVL exposure.

AS presents as a violaceous to red ill-defined plaque, often initially resembling a bruise (Fig. 37-31). The differential diagnosis may include benign vascular tumors, hematoma secondary to trauma, or an inflammatory dermatosis. Unexplained facial edema may be a presenting sign as well. AS can be associated with acute hemorrhage, anemia, or coagulopathy. As AS progresses, lesions increase in size, become indurated, and may eventually ulcerate. Satellite lesions are common.

On microscopic examination, it becomes evident that AS extends far beyond clinical margins. In well-differentiated lesions, histology shows irregularly dilated vascular channels lined by flattened endothelial cells. Less differentiated tumors show proliferation of polygonal or spindle-shaped, pleomorphic endothelial cells and anastomosing vascular channels. The state of cellular differentiation has not been shown to correlate with prognosis. Special stains may be of value in histologic diagnosis of AS, as cells stain positively for *Ulex europaeus* I

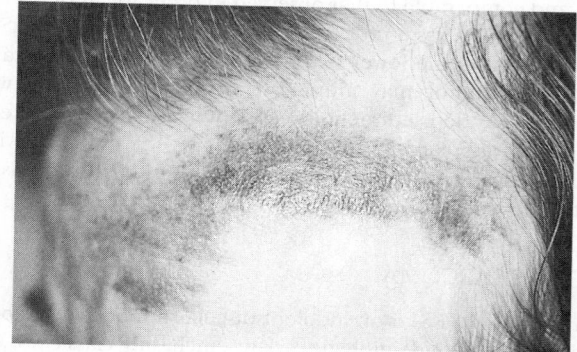

FIGURE 37-31. Angiosarcoma may present as a violaceous, ill-defined plaque on the scalp. (See Color Fig. 37-31 in the CD-ROM.)

lectin and factor VIII–related antigen. *Ulex* I is considered to be more sensitive for AS. In addition, AS cells express stem cell antigen CD34 and endothelial cell surface antigen CD31.

AS is a biologically aggressive tumor with high metastatic potential. Metastases to lung, lymph nodes, and brain are common. Prognosis for metastatic disease is poor. Although prognosis does not correlate with degree of cellular differentiation, there appears to be a correlation with lesion size at presentation: Increased survival has been demonstrated in lesions smaller than 5 cm at time of presentation.

Because of the aggressiveness and poor prognosis of AS, treatment options are limited. Radical excision is currently the treatment of choice and may be difficult to accomplish in tumors involving the face. Amputation with shoulder disarticulation or hemipelvectomy are recommended for tumors involving the extremities. As stated, AS tends to extend far beyond clinically appreciated margins, thus complicating excision. Several cases of AS have been treated by MMS in an attempt to control margins; however, the difference between AS and normal vasculature may be difficult to interpret on frozen sections, even with the use of immunohistochemical stains. Prognosis of AS is poor, with a mortality rate of 50% at 15 months after diagnosis. The 5-year survival rate is approximately 12%.

Lymphedema-associated AS (LAS) was first reported by Stewart and Treves[209] in six patients with postmastectomy lymphedema. In each case, AS developed in the ipsilateral arm and occurred several years after mastectomy. Subsequently, LAS was reported after axillary node dissection for melanoma and in the context of congenital lymphedema, filarial lymphedema, and chronic idiopathic lymphedema. The risk for developing LAS 5 years after mastectomy is approximately 5%. The most common site is the medial aspect of the upper arm.

LAS presents as a violaceous plaque or nodule superimposed on brawny, nonpitting edema. Ulceration may develop rapidly. The pathogenesis of LAS is incompletely understood and may be related to imbalances in local immune regulation or angiogenesis, leading to proliferation of neoplastic cells. The prognosis is poor, and survival rates are comparable to AS involving the scalp and face. Long-term survival has been reported after amputation of the affected limb.

Radiation-induced AS has been reported to occur after RT for benign or malignant conditions.[207] AS may occur from 4 to 40 years after RT for benign conditions, including acne and eczema, or from 4 to 25 years after RT for malignancies. Lesions appear at sites treated with radiation and are clinically and histologically similar to AS involving the scalp and face. Prognosis is poor and comparable to that observed in other forms of AS.

Epithelioid AS is a rare, recently described variant of AS. It tends to involve the lower extremities. On microscopic examination, the tumor may mimic an epithelial neoplasm, with sheets of rounded, epithelioid cells intermingled with irregularly lined vascular channels. Epithelioid AS results in widespread metastases within 1 year of presentation. Prognosis, as in other forms of AS, is poor.

KAPOSI'S SARCOMA

Kaposi's sarcoma (KS) is an indolent vascular tumor that has been subdivided into epidemiologic variants, including classic KS, African endemic KS, iatrogenic KS, and epidemic, acquired immunodeficiency syndrome–associated (AIDS-associated) KS.[207]

KS-associated herpesvirus (also known as *human herpesvirus-8*) is found in tissues from all four forms of KS and suggests a central role for the virus in the development and etiology for all KS types. The risk of developing KS in immune-deficient conditions is strictly related to the human herpesvirus-8 prevalence in each region. And, at an individual level, it has been shown that the risk of developing KS in immunosuppressed transplant recipients is related to the human herpesvirus-8 status of both recipient and donor.[210]

Classic KS affects elderly men, with increased incidence in Ashkenazi Jews and in persons of Mediterranean descent. Classic KS typically presents with asymptomatic violaceous macules on the lower extremities. Slow progression with coalescence to plaques is observed. Eventually, the disease enters a nodular phase and may ultimately progress to a hyperkeratotic or even ulcerative phase. Up to one-third of patients with classic KS develop a second primary malignancy, most often a lymphoproliferative disorder, such as non-Hodgkin's lymphoma, which may antedate or follow the appearance of KS lesions.[211]

African endemic KS can be further subdivided into three forms: indolent nodular, locally aggressive (florid and infiltrative), and disseminated aggressive. Nodular African endemic KS presents clinically and behaves similarly to classic KS. The more aggressive forms predominantly affect young black Africans, with the fulminant lymphadenopathic disease with visceral organ involvement usually without cutaneous manifestations. The prognosis is very poor, with a 100% fatality rate within 3 years.

Iatrogenic KS occurs in the context of immunosuppressive drug therapy. Iatrogenic KS is usually chronic but may be somewhat more aggressive than classic KS. Iatrogenic KS presents with lesions similar to those observed in classic KS. Tumor extension has been correlated to the degree of depression of cellular immunity, with some regression as a result of reduction or changes in immunosuppressive therapy.

Epidemic KS appears in approximately 21% of homosexual men with AIDS. It presents with pink-violaceous macules involving the face, chest, and oral mucosa. The hard palate and ocular conjunctiva are frequently involved. Epidemic KS often progresses in an orderly fashion from a few localized or widespread mucocutaneous lesions to a more generalized skin disease with lymph node involvement and gastrointestinal tract disease. Recent studies indicate that the highly active antiretroviral therapy, including at least one human immunodeficiency virus protease inhibitor, is associated with a dramatic decrease in the incidence of AIDS-KS and with a regression of KS in treated individuals.[212] Results from preclinical studies indicate that protease inhibitors have potent and direct antiangiogenic and anti-KS activities.

A classification system that is inclusive of all clinical variants of KS divides the disease into four stages: stage I, locally indolent cutaneous lesions; stage II, locally invasive lesions; and stage III and IV, disseminated and systemic KS with generalized lymphadenopathy. Each stage is further subdivided as A or B according to the absence or presence of systemic symptoms such as fever or weight loss of more than 10%. There appear to be three distinct prognostic factors: (1) the extent of the disease (tumor burden), (2) the presence or absence of systemic symptoms, and (3) the presence of opportunistic infections.

On microscopic examination, KS varies according to patch, plaque, and nodular subtypes. The histologic changes in early patch-stage KS are inconspicuous, leading to misdiagnosis of a benign inflammatory process. A superficial and deep perivascular infiltrate with increased numbers of jagged vascular spaces is observed in the dermis. The thin-walled vessels surround normal vessels and adnexal structures, resulting in the so-called promontory sign. Plasma cells may be seen surrounding the newly formed vessels. In plaque-stage KS, the entire dermis and superficial fat may be involved, with an increase in the number of spindle cells arranged in small fascicles between collagen bundles centered around proliferating vascular channels. The spindle cells outline irregular slit-like vascular spaces that contain erythrocytes. In nodular KS, the number of spindle cells increases. They are arranged in interwoven fascicles with erythrocytes scattered in the interstices. Although nuclear atypia, mitotic figures, and pleomorphism may be observed, these are not prominent. Cells that stain positively for factor VIII–related antigen and spindle cells that stain positively for *Ulex europaeus* I lectin line well-formed vessels within KS lesions.

Both local and systemic therapies have been used in the management of KS, depending on epidemiologic context, extent of disease, and concomitant disease.[207] For patients with single lesions, surgical excision often provides adequate treatment. KS has been treated successfully using cryosurgery, RT, laser ablation, and intralesional injection of interferon-α or cytotoxic agents.[212] Local infiltration with vincristine has been particularly effective in the treatment of oral lesions in epidemic AIDS-associated KS. Other, more aggressive approaches have included systemic therapy with interferon or with single- or multiagent chemotherapy. Experimental therapies, including antiangiogenesis agents TNP-470 and thalidomide, 9-*cis* retinoic acid, and human chorionic gonadotropin, may prove useful in management of KS in the future.[213]

CARCINOMA METASTATIC TO SKIN

The relative frequency of cutaneous metastases are similar to those observed with primary cancers. The most frequently observed cutaneous metastatic cancers are breast, colon, and melanoma in women and lung, colon, and melanoma in men. Cutaneous metastases may represent an opportunity to detect a potentially treatable cancer before other evidence of it is present, to modify therapy as appropriate to the tumor stage, or,

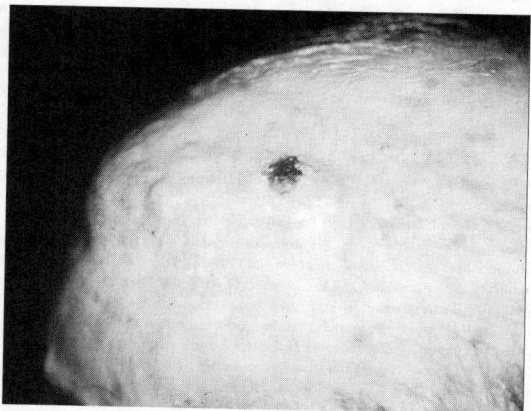

FIGURE 37-32. The scalp is a common site for cutaneous metastatic disease. (See Color Fig. 37-32 in the CD-ROM.)

MAC	MMS
Sebaceous carcinoma	Excision or MMS
AFX	MMS
MFH	WLE or MMS
DFSP	WLE or MMS with permanent section confirmation
Angiosarcoma	WLE or MMS with permanent section confirmation
Kaposi's sarcoma	Cryosurgery, intralesional, or systemic chemotherapy

FIGURE 37-33. The appropriate management of less common skin cancers may include wide local excision (WLE), Mohs micrographic surgery (MMS), cryosurgery, or intralesional or systemic chemotherapy. AFX, atypical fibroxanthoma; DFSP, dermatofibrosarcoma protuberans; MAC, microcystic adnexal carcinoma; MFH, malignant fibrous histiocytoma.

possibly, to use the cutaneous lesion as a source of easily accessible tumor cells for specific therapy. Cutaneous metastatic disease as the first sign of internal cancer is most commonly seen with cancers of the lung, kidney, and ovary. Cutaneous involvement is also seen in the leukemias, with a wide variation in morphology of lesions.[214] The scalp is a common site for cutaneous metastatic disease (Fig. 37-32). Perhaps the most widely known cutaneous manifestation of an internal carcinoma is the Sister Mary Joseph nodule.[215] Dr. William Mayo's surgical assistant, Sister Mary Joseph, noted the association of the presence of an indurated umbilical nodule in the setting of gastric cancer with poor prognosis. The discovery of cutaneous metastatic disease should result in prompt consultation with an oncologist for staging and management (Fig. 37-33).

CONCLUSION

The discovery of an atypical skin lesion should result in consultation with a dermatologist for evaluation. It is necessary that skin biopsy specimens be sent to a dermatopathologist for interpretation to minimize misdiagnosis and delayed treatment of skin cancers. Management of skin cancer is based on histopathologic analysis of a given lesion; hence, accurate interpretation of skin biopsy specimens is essential. After treatment for skin cancer, patients should be followed up regularly, through full-body skin examinations performed by a dermatologist, for the development of recurrences as well as new primary skin cancers.

REFERENCES

1. American Cancer Society. *Cancer facts and figures, 2001.* World Wide Web URL: http://www.cancer.org, 2004.
2. Chen JG, Fleischer AB, Smith ED, et al. Cost of nonmelanoma skin cancer treatment in the United States. *Dermatol Surg* 2001;27:1035.
3. Spratt JS Jr. Cancer mortality after nonmelanoma skin cancer. *JAMA* 1999;281:325.
4. Karagas MR, Greenberg ER, Mott LA, Baron JA, Ernster VL. Occurrence of other cancers among patients with prior basal cell and squamous cell skin cancer. *Cancer Epidemiol Biomarkers Prev* 1998;7:157.
5. O'Toole EA, Goel M, Woodley DT. Hydrogen peroxide inhibits human keratinocyte migration. *Dermatol Surg* 1996;22:525.

6. Shriner DL, et al. Mohs micrographic surgery. *J Am Acad Dermatol* 1998;39:79.

7. Arlette JP, et al. Basal cell carcinoma of the periocular region. *J Cutan Med Surg* 1998;2:205.

8. Cook J, Zitelli JA. Mohs micrographic surgery: a cost analysis. *J Am Acad Dermatol* 1998;39:698.

9. Sheridan AT, Dawber RPR. Curettage, electrosurgery and skin cancer. *Australas J Dermatol* 2000;41:19.

10. Nordin P. Curettage-cryosurgery for non-melanoma skin cancer of the external ear: excellent 5-year results. *Br J Dermatol* 1999;140:291.

11. Salasche SJ. Status of curettage and desiccation in the treatment of primary basal cell carcinoma [Letter]. *J Am Acad Dermatol* 1984;10:285.

12. Robins P, Albom MJ. Recurrent basal cell carcinomas in young women. *J Dermatol Surg* 1975;1:49.

13. Silverman MK, Kopf A, Grin CM, et al. Recurrence rates of treated basal cell carcinomas. Part 2: curettage-electrodesiccation. *J Dermatol Surg Oncol* 1991;17:720.

14. Wagner RF, Cottle WI. Multifocal recurrent basal cell carcinoma following primary treatment by electrodesiccation and curettage. *J Am Acad Dermatol* 1987;17:1047.

15. Hurwitz DJ, Pincus L, Kupper TS. Imiquimod: a topically applied link between innate and acquired immunity. *Arch Dermatol* 2003;139:1347.

16. Salasche S, Levine N, Morrison L. Cycle therapy of actinic keratoses of the face and scalp with 5% topical imiquimod cream: an open label trial. *J Am Acad Dermatol* 2002;47:571.

17. Marks R, Gebauer K, Shumack S, et al. Imiquimod 5% cream in the treatment of superficial basal cell carcinoma: results of a multicenter 6-week dose-response trial. *J Am Acad Dermatol* 2001;44:807.

18. Shumack S, Robinson J, Kossard S, et al. Efficacy of topical 5% imiquimod cream for the treatment of nodular basal cell carcinoma. *Arch Dermatol* 2002;138:1165.

19. Mackenzie-Wood A, de Kossard S, Launey J, Wilkinson B, Owens MI. Imiquimod 5% cream in the treatment of Bowen's disease. *J Am Acad Dermatol* 2001;44:462.

20. Kalka K, Merk H, Mukhtar H. Photodynamic therapy in dermatology. *J Am Acad Dermatol* 2000;42:389.

21. Kurwa HA, Yong-Gee SA, Seed PT, et al. A randomized paired comparison of photodynamic therapy and topical 5-fluorouracil in the treatment of actinic keratoses. *J Am Acad Dermatol* 1999;41:414.

22. Fink-Puches R, Soyer HP, Hofer A, Helmut K, Wolf P. Long-term follow-up with histological changes of superficial nonmelanoma skin cancers treated with topical delta-aminolevulinic acid photodynamic therapy. *Arch Dermatol* 1998;134:821.

23. Voss N, Kim-Sing C. Radiotherapy in the treatment of dermatologic malignancies. *Dermatol Clin* 1998;16:313.

24. Lichter MD, Karagas MR, Mott LA, et al. Therapeutic ionizing radiation and the incidence of basal cell carcinoma and squamous cell carcinoma. *Arch Dermatol* 2000;136:1007.

25. Schinstine M, Goldman GD. Risk of synchronous and metachronous second nonmelanoma skin cancer when referred for Mohs micrographic surgery. *J Am Acad Dermatol* 2001;44:497.

26. Cockerell CJ. Histopathology of incipient intraepidermal squamous cell carcinoma ("actinic keratosis"). *J Am Acad Dermatol* 2000;42:S11.

27. Schwartz RA. The actinic keratosis: a perspective and update. *Dermatol Surg* 1997;23:1009.

28. Berhane T, Halliday GM, Cooke B, Barnetson RSC. Inflammation is associated with progression of actinic keratoses to squamous cell carcinomas in humans. *Br J Dermatol* 2002;146:810.

29. Marks R, Rennie G, Selwood TS. Malignant transformation of solar keratoses to squamous cell carcinoma. *Lancet* 1988;1:795.

30. Mittelbronn MA, et al. Frequency of pre-existing actinic keratosis in cutaneous squamous cell carcinoma. *Int J Dermatol* 1998;37:677.

31. Brash DE, et al. Sunlight and sunburn in human skin cancer: p53 apoptosis and tumor promotion. *J Investig Dermatol Symp Proc* 1996;1:136.

32. Alexiades-Armenakas MR, Geronemus RG. Laser-mediated photodynamic therapy of actinic keratoses. *Arch Dermatol* 2003;139:1313.

33. Leffell DJ, et al. Aggressive-growth basal cell carcinoma in young adults. *Arch Dermatol* 1991;127:1663.

34. Leffell DJ, Brash DE. Sunlight and skin cancer. *Sci Am* 1996;275:52.

35. Zanetti R, et al. The multicentre south European study "Helios" I: skin characteristics and sunburns in basal cell and squamous cell carcinomas of the skin. *Br J Cancer* 1996;73:1440.

36. Hahn H, et al. The patched signaling pathway in tumorigenesis and development: lessons from animal models. *J Mol Med* 1999;77:459.

37. Hahn H, et al. Mutations of the human homolog of Drosophila patched in the nevoid basal cell carcinoma syndrome. *Cell* 1996;85:841.

38. Ping XL, Ratner D, Zhang H, et al. PTCH mutations in squamous cell carcinomas of the skin. *J Invest Dermatol* 2001;116:614.

39. Ziegler A, Leffell DJ, Kunula S, et al. Mutation hotspots due to sunlight in the p53 gene of nonmelanoma skin cancers. *Proc Natl Acad Sci U S A* 1993;90:4216.

40. Miller SJ. Biology of basal cell carcinoma (part I). *J Am Acad Dermatol* 1991;24:1.

41. Thissen MR, Neumann MHA, Schouten LJ. A systematic review of treatment modalities for primary basal cell carcinomas. *Arch Dermatol* 1999;135:1177.

42. Weninger W, et al. Differences in tumor microvessel density between squamous cell carcinomas and basal cell carcinomas may relate to their different biologic behavior. *J Cutan Pathol* 1997;24:364.

43. Bedlow AJ, et al. Basal cell carcinoma—an in-vivo model of human tumour microcirculation? *Exp Dermatol* 1999;8:222.

44. Hernandez AD, Hibbs MS, Postlewaite AE, et al. Establishment of basal cell carcinoma in culture: evidence for a basal cell carcinoma-derived factor(s) which stimulates fibroblasts to proliferate and release collagenase. *J Invest Dermatol* 1985;85:470.

45. Batra RS, Kelley L. Predictors of extensive subclinical spread in nonmelanoma skin cancer treated by Mohs micrographic surgery. *Arch Dermatol* 2002;138:1043.

46. Di Gregorio C, et al. Mental nerve invasion by basal cell carcinoma of the chin: a case report. *Anticancer Res* 1998;18:4723.

47. Niazi ZB, Lamberty BG. Perineural infiltration in basal cell carcinomas. *Br J Plast Surg* 1993;46:156.

48. Robinson JK, Dahiya M. Basal cell carcinoma with pulmonary and lymph node metastasis causing death. *Arch Dermatol* 2003;139:643.

49. Raszewski RL, Guyuron B. Long-term survival following nodal metastases from basal cell carcinoma. *Ann Plast Surg* 1990;24:170.

50. Pfeiffer P, Hansen O, Rose C. Systemic cytotoxic therapy of basal cell carcinoma A review of the literature. *Eur J Cancer* 1990;26:73.

51. Scherbenske JM, et al. A solitary nodule on the chest: fibroepithelioma of Pinkus. *Arch Dermatol* 1990;126:955.

52. Holmkvist KA, Rogers GS, Dahl PR. Incidence of residual basal cell carcinoma in patients who appear tumor free after biopsy. *J Am Acad Dermatol* 1999;41:600.

53. Salgarello M, Seccia A, Vricella M, Farallo E. Analysis of infiltrating epitheliomas of the nose examined from 1986 to 1995. *J Otolaryngol* 1998;27:288.

54. Evans GR, Williams JZ, Ainslie NB. Cutaneous nasal malignancies: is primary reconstruction safe? *Head Neck* 1997;3:182.

55. Kumar B, et al. A review of 24 cases of Mohs surgery and ophthalmic plastic reconstruction. *Aust N Z J Ophthalmol* 1997;25:289.

56. Glied M, Berg D, Witterick I. Basal cell carcinoma of the conchal bowl: interdisciplinary approach to treatment. *J Otolaryngol* 1998;27:322.

57. Leslie DF, Greenway HT. Mohs micrographic surgery for skin cancer. *Australas J Dermatol* 1991;32:159.

58. Halpern JN. Radiation therapy in skin cancer: a historical perspective and current applications. *Dermatol Surg* 1997;23:1089.

59. Wolf DJ, Zitelli JA. Surgical margins for basal cell carcinoma. *Arch Dermatol* 1987;123:340.

60. Rowe DE, Carroll RJ, Day CL Jr. Long-term recurrence rates in previously untreated (primary) basal cell carcinoma: implications for patient follow-up. *J Dermatol Surg Oncol* 1989;15:315.

61. Rowe DE, Carroll RJ, Day CL Jr. Mohs surgery is the treatment of choice for recurrent (previously treated) basal cell carcinoma. *J Dermatol Surg Oncol* 1989;15:424.

62. Knox JM. Treatment of skin cancer. *J Am Acad Dermatol* 1985;12:589.

63. Kopf AW, et al. Curettage-electrodesiccation treatment of basal cell carcinomas. *Arch Dermatol* 1977;113:439.

64. Spiller WF, et al. Treatment of basal cell epithelioma by curettage and electrodesiccation. *J Am Acad Dermatol* 1984;11:808.

65. Nordin P, Stenquist B. Five-year results of curettage-cryosurgery for 100 consecutive auricular non-melanoma skin cancers. *J Laryngol Otol* 2002;116:893.

66. Wilder RB, Kittelson JM, Shimm DS. Basal cell carcinoma treated with radiation therapy. *Cancer* 1991;68:2134.

67. Goncalves JC. Fractional cryosurgery. A new technique for basal cell carcinoma of the eyelids and periorbital area. *Dermatol Surg* 1997;23:475.

68. Humphreys TR, et al. Treatment of superficial basal cell carcinoma and squamous cell carcinoma in situ with a high-energy pulsed carbon dioxide laser. *Arch Dermatol* 1998;134:1247.

69. Gloster HM Jr, Brodland DG. The epidemiology of skin cancer. *Dermatol Surg* 1996;22:217.

70. Mora RG, Perniciaro C. Cancer of the skin in blacks. I. A review of 163 black patients with cutaneous squamous cell carcinoma. *J Am Acad Dermatol* 1981;5:535.

71. Stern RS, Lunder EJ. Risk of squamous cell carcinoma and methoxsalen (psoralen) and UV-A radiation (PUVA). A meta-analysis. *Arch Dermatol* 1998;134:1582.

72. Karagas MR, et al. Design of an epidemiologic study of drinking water arsenic exposure and skin and bladder cancer risk in a US population. *Environ Health Perspect* 1998;106[Suppl 4]:1047.

73. Brash DE, Ponten J. Skin precancer. *Cancer Surv* 1998;32:69.

74. Dandie GW, et al. Effects of UV on the migration and function of epidermal antigen presenting cells. *Mutat Res* 1998;422:147.

75. Ortonne JP. From actinic keratosis to squamous cell carcinoma. *Br J Dermatol* 2002;146[Suppl 61]:20.

76. Ziegler A, Jonason AS, Leffell DJ, et al. Sunburn and p53 in the onset of skin cancer. *Nature* 1994;372:773.

77. Jonason AS, Kunala S, Price GJ, et al. Frequent clones of p53 mutated keratinocytes in normal human skin. *Proc Natl Acad Sci U S A* 1996;93:14025.

78. Hodges A, Smoller BR. Immunohistochemical comparison of p16 expression in actinic keratoses and squamous cell carcinomas of the skin. *Mod Pathol* 2002;15:1121.

79. Wong SS, Tan KC, Goh CL. Cutaneous manifestations of chronic arsenicism: review of seventeen cases. *J Am Acad Dermatol* 1998;38:179.

80. Montagnino G, et al. Cancer incidence in 854 kidney transplant recipients from a single institution: comparison with normal population and with patients under dialytic treatment. *Clin Transplant* 1996;10:461.

81. Smith KJ, et al. Cutaneous neoplasms in a military population of HIV-1-positive patients. Military Medical Consortium for the Advancement of Retroviral Research. *J Am Acad Dermatol* 1993;29:400.

82. Eliezri YD, Silverstein SJ, Nuovo GJ. Occurrence of human papillomavirus type 16 DNA in cutaneous squamous and basal cell neoplasms. *J Am Acad Dermatol* 1990;23:836.

83. Moy RL, et al. Human papillomavirus type 16 DNA in periungual squamous cell carcinomas [see comments]. *JAMA* 1989;261:2669.

84. Rowe DE, Carroll RJ, Day CL Jr. Prognostic factors for local recurrence metastasis and survival rates in squamous cell carcinoma of the skin, ear, and lip. Implications for treatment modality selection. *J Am Acad Dermatol* 1992;26:976.

85. Dinehart SM, Nelson-Adesokan P, Cockerell C, Russell S, Brown R. Metastatic cutaneous squamous cell carcinoma derived from actinic keratosis. *Cancer* 1997;79:920.

86. Friedman HI, Cooper PH, Wanebo HJ. Prognostic and therapeutic use of microstaging of cutaneous squamous cell carcinoma of the trunk and extremities. *Cancer* 1985;56:1099.

87. Spiro RH. Verrucous carcinoma then and now. *Am J Surg* 1998;176:393.

88. Bouquot JE. Oral verrucous carcinoma. Incidence in two US populations. *Oral Surg Oral Med Oral Pathol Oral Radiol Endod* 1998;86:318.

89. Casanova D, et al. Plantar verrucous carcinoma: a case report and literature review. *Ann Chir Plast Esthet* 1997;42:56.

90. Kao GF. Carcinoma arising in Bowen's disease. *Arch Dermatol* 1986;122:1124.

91. Mikhail GR. Cancers, precancers, and pseudo cancers on the male genitalia. *J Dermatol Surg Oncol* 1980;6:1027.

92. Olhoffer IH, et al. Facial bowenoid papulosis secondary to human papillomavirus type 16. *Br J Dermatol* 1999;140:761.

93. Cherpelis BS, Marcusen C, Lang PG. Prognostic factors for metastasis in squamous cell carcinoma of the skin. *Dermatol Surg* 2002;28:268.

94. Dinehart SM, Pollack SV. Metastases from squamous cell carcinoma of the skin and lip: an analysis of twenty-seven cases. *J Am Acad Dermatol* 1989;21:241.

95. Goldman GD. Squamous cell cancer: a practical approach. *Semin Cutan Med Surg* 1998;17:80.

96. Honeycutt WM, Jansen GT. Treatment of squamous cell carcinoma of the skin. *Arch Dermatol* 1973;108:670.

97. Brodland DG, Zitelli JA. Surgical margins for excision of primary cutaneous squamous cell carcinoma. *J Am Acad Dermatol* 1992;27:241.

98. Wilson SM, Beahrs OH, Manson R. Squamous cell carcinoma of the anus. *Surg Annu* 1976;8:297.

99. Haberthur F, Almendral AC, Ritter B. Therapy of vulvar carcinoma. *Eur J Gynaecol Oncol* 1993;14:218.

100. Goldminz D, Bennett RG. Mohs micrographic surgery of the nail unit. *J Dermatol Surg Oncol* 1992;18:721.

101. Geisse JK. Comparison of treatment modalities for squamous cell carcinoma. *Clin Dermatol* 1995;13:621.

102. de Visscher JG, et al. Surgical treatment of squamous cell carcinoma of the lower lip: evaluation of long-term results and prognostic factors—a retrospective analysis of 184 patients. *J Oral Maxillofac Surg* 1998;56:814.

103. Frankel DH, Hanusa BH, Zitelli JA. New primary nonmelanoma skin cancer in patients with a history of squamous cell carcinoma of the skin. Implications and recommendations for follow-up. *J Am Acad Dermatol* 1992;26:720.

104. Ramsay HM, et al. Multiple basal cell carcinomas in a patient with acute myeloid leukaemia and chronic lymphocytic leukaemia. *Clin Exp Dermatol* 1999;24:281.

105. Jensen P, Hansen S, Moller B, et al. Skin cancer in kidney and heart transplant recipients and different long-term immunosuppressive therapy regimens. *J Am Acad Dermatol* 1999;40:177.

106. Harwood CA, McGregor JM, Swale VJ, et al. High frequency and diversity of cutaneous appendageal tumors in organ transplant recipients. *J Am Acad Dermatol* 2003;48:401.

107. Otley CC, Coldiron BM, Stasko T, Goldman GD. Decreased skin cancer after cessation of therapy with transplant-associated immunosuppressants. *Arch Dermatol* 2001;137:459.

108. Haag ML, Glass LF, Fenske NA. Merkel cell carcinoma. Diagnosis and treatment. *Dermatol Surg* 1995;21:669.

109. Miller RW, Rabkin CS. Merkel cell carcinoma and melanoma: etiological similarities and differences. *Cancer Epidemiol Biomarkers Prev* 1999;8:153.

110. Akhtar S, Oza KK, Wright J. Merkel cell carcinoma: report of 10 cases and review of the literature. *J Am Acad Dermatol* 2000;43:755.

111. Iacocca MV, et al. Mixed Merkel cell and squamous cell carcinoma of the skin. *J Am Acad Dermatol* 1998;39:882.

112. Simstein NL, Sduggs NK. Merkel cell tumor: two cases. *Int Surg* 1998;83:60.

113. Lunder EJ, Stern RS. Merkel cell carcinoma in patients treated with methoxsalen and ultraviolet radiation. *N Engl J Med* 1998;339:1247.

114. Williams RH, et al. Merkel cell carcinoma in a renal transplant patient: increased incidence? *Transplantation* 1998;65:1396.

115. Ott MJ, et al. Multimodality management of Merkel cell carcinoma. *Arch Surg* 1999;134:388.

116. Medina-Franco H, et al. Multimodality treatment of Merkel cell carcinoma: case series and literature review of 1024 cases. *Ann Surg Oncol* 2001;8:204.

117. Su LD, Fullen DR, Lowe L, et al. CD117 (KIT receptor) in Merkel cell carcinoma. *Am J Dermatopathol* 2002;24:289.

118. Kwekkeboom DJ, et al. Somatostatin analogue scintigraphy: a simple and sensitive method for the in vivo visualization of Merkel cell tumors and their metastases. *Arch Dermatol* 1992;128:818.

119. Yanguas I, et al. Spontaneous regression of Merkel cell carcinoma of the skin. *Br J Dermatol* 1997;137:296.

120. Boyer JD, Zitelli JA, Brodland DG, Angelo GD. Local control of primary Merkel cell carcinoma: review of 45 cases treated with Mohs micrographic surgery with and without adjuvant radiation. *J Am Acad Dermatol* 2002;47:885.

121. O'Connor WJ, Roenigk RK, Brodland DG. Merkel cell carcinoma: comparison of Mohs micrographic surgery and wide excision in eighty-six patients. *Dermatol Surg* 1997;23:929.

122. Brissett AE, et al. Merkel cell carcinoma of the head and neck: a retrospective case series. *Head Neck* 2002;24:982.

123. Pan D, Narayan D, Ariyan S. Merkel cell carcinoma: five cases reports using sentinel lymph node biopsy and a review of 110 new cases. *Plast Reconstr Surg* 2002;110:1259.

124. Hill ADK, Brady MS, Coit DG. Intraoperative lymphatic mapping and sentinel lymph node biopsy for Merkel cell carcinoma. *Br J Surg* 1999;86:518.

125. Allen PJ, Zhang ZF, Coit DG. Surgical management of Merkel cell carcinoma. *Ann Surg* 1999;229:97.

126. Eich HT, et al. Role of postoperative radiotherapy in the management of Merkel cell carcinoma. *Am J Clin Oncol* 2002;25:50.

127. Gillenwater AM, et al. Merkel cell carcinoma of the head and neck: effect of surgical excision and radiation on recurrence and survival. *Arch Otolaryngol Head Neck Surg* 2001;127:149.

128. Yiengpruksawan A, et al. Merkel cell carcinoma. Prognosis and management. *Arch Surg* 1991;126:1514.

129. Marks S, Radin DR, Chandrasoma P. Merkel cell carcinoma. *J Comput Tomogr* 1987;11:291.

130. Tai PTH, et al. Chemotherapy in neuroendocrine/Merkel cell carcinoma of the skin: case series and review of 204 cases. *J Clin Oncol* 2000;18:2493.

131. Pectasides D, et al. Chemotherapy for Merkel cell carcinoma with carboplatin and etoposide. *Am J Clin Oncol* 1995;18:418.

132. Voog E, et al. Chemotherapy for patients with locally advanced or metastatic Merkel cell carcinoma. *Cancer* 1999;85:2589.

133. Tai PT, YU E, Tonita J, Gilchrist J. Merkel cell carcinoma of the skin. *J Cutan Med Surg* 2000;4:186.

134. Goldstein DJ, Barr RJ, Santa Cruz DJ. Microcystic adnexal carcinoma: a distinct clinico-pathologic entity. *Cancer* 1982;50:566.

135. Sebastien TS, et al. Microcystic adnexal carcinoma. *J Am Acad Dermatol* 1993;29:840.

136. McAlvany JP, et al. Sclerosing sweat duct carcinoma in an 11-year-old boy. *J Dermatol Surg Oncol* 1994;20:767.

137. Park JY, Parry EL. Microcystic adnexal carcinoma. First reported in a black patient. *Dermatol Surg* 1998;24:905.

138. Borenstein A, et al. Microcystic adnexal carcinoma following radiotherapy in childhood. *Am J Med Sci* 1991;301:259.

139. Brookes JL, et al. Microcystic adnexal carcinoma masquerading as a chalazion [Letter]. *Br J Ophthalmol* 1998;82:196.

140. Chow WC, Cockerell CJ, Geronemus RG. Microcystic adnexal carcinoma of the scalp. *J Dermatol Surg Oncol* 1989;15:768.

141. Schipper JH, Holecek BU, Sievers KW. A tumour derived from Ebner's glands: microcystic adnexal carcinoma of the tongue. *J Laryngol Otol* 1995;109:1211.

142. Chiller K, Passaro D, Scheuller M, et al. Microcystic adnexal carcinoma. *Arch Dermatol* 2000;136:1355.

143. Wick MR, Cooper PH, Swanson PE, et al. Microcystic adnexal carcinoma: an immunohistochemical comparison with other cutaneous appendage tumors. *Arch Dermatol* 1990;162:189.

144. Abesamis-Cubillan E, El-Shabrawi-Caelen L, LeBoit PE. Merkel cells and sclerosing epithelial neoplasms. *Am J Dermatopathol* 2000;22:311.

145. Billingsley EM, Fedok F, Maloney ME. Microcystic adnexal carcinoma. Case report and review of the literature. *Arch Otolaryngol Head Neck Surg* 1996;122:179.

146. Snow S, et al. Microcystic adnexal carcinoma: report of 13 cases and review of the literature. *Dermatol Surg* 2001;27:401.

147. Lupton GP, McMarlin SL. Microcystic adnexal carcinoma. Report of a case with 30-year follow-up. *Arch Dermatol* 1986;122:286.

148. Bier-Lansing CM, et al. Microcystic adnexal carcinoma: management options based on long-term follow-up. *Laryngoscope* 1995;105:1197.

149. Wolfe JT, et al. Sebaceous carcinoma of the eyelid. Errors in clinical and pathologic diagnosis. *Am J Surg Pathol* 1984;8:597.

150. Tan KC, Lee ST, Cheah ST. Surgical treatment of sebaceous carcinoma of eyelids with clinico-pathological correlation. *Br J Plast Surg* 1991;44:117.

151. Rundle P, et al. Sebaceous gland carcinoma of the eyelid seventeen years after irradiation for bilateral retinoblastoma [Letter]. *Eye* 1999;13:109.

152. Rumelt S, et al. Four-eyelid sebaceous cell carcinoma following irradiation. *Arch Ophthalmol* 1998;116:1670.

153. Hood IC, et al. Sebaceous carcinoma of the face following irradiation. *Am J Dermatopathol* 1986;8:505.

154. Carlson JW, et al. Sebaceous carcinoma of the vulva: a case report and review of the literature. *Gynecol Oncol* 1996;60:489.

155. Gonzalez-Fernandez F, et al. Sebaceous carcinoma. Tumor progression through mutational inactivation of p53. *Ophthalmology* 1998;105:497.

156. Rinaggio J, McGuff HS, Otto R, Hickson C. Postauricular sebaceous carcinoma arising in association with nevus sebaceus. *Head Neck* 2002;24:212.

157. Mandreker S, Pinto RW, Usgaonkar U. Sebaceous carcinoma of the eyelid with metastasis to the parotid region: diagnosis by fine needle aspiration cytology [Letter]. *Acta Cytol* 1997;41:1636.

158. Rao NA, Hidayat AA, McLean JW, Zimmerman LE. Sebaceous carcinomas of the ocular adnexa: a clinicopathologic study of 104 patients with five year follow-up data. *Hum Pathol* 1982;13:113.

159. Dogru M, et al. Management of eyelid sebaceous carcinomas. *Ophthalmologica* 1997;211:40.

160. Folberg R, et al. Recurrent and residual sebaceous carcinoma after Mohs excision of the primary lesion. *Am J Ophthalmol* 1987;103:817.

161. Dzubow LM. Sebaceous carcinoma of the eyelid: treatment with Mohs surgery. *J Dermatol Surg Oncol* 1985;11:40.

162. Snow SN, Larson PO, Lucarelli MJ, Lemke BN, Madjar DD. Sebaceous carcinoma of the eyelids treated by Mohs micrographic surgery: report of nine cases with review of the literature. *Dermatol Surg* 2002;28:623.

163. Matsumoto CS, et al. Sebaceous carcinoma responds to radiation therapy. *Ophthalmologica* 1995;209:280.

164. Schwartz RA, Torre DP. The Muir-Torre syndrome: a 25-year retrospect [see comments]. *J Am Acad Dermatol* 1995;33:90.

165. Dahl I. Atypical fibroxanthoma of the skin: a clinico-pathological study of 57 cases. *Acta Pathol Microbiol Scand [A]* 1976;84:183.

166. Dei Tos AP, et al. Ultraviolet-induced p53 mutations in atypical fibroxanthoma. *Am J Pathol* 1994;145:11.

167. Sakamoto A, et al. Immunoexpression of ultraviolet photoproducts and p53 mutation analysis in atypical fibroxanthoma and superficial malignant fibrous histiocytoma. *Mod Pathol* 2001;14:581.

168. High AS, Hume WJ, Dyson D. Atypical fibroxanthoma of oral mucosa: a variant of malignant fibrous histiocytoma. *Br J Oral Maxillofac Surg* 1990;28:268.

169. Hafner J, Kirzi W, Weinreich T. Malignant fibrous histiocytoma and atypical fibroxanthoma in renal transplant recipients. *Dermatology* 1999;198:29.

170. Paquet P, Pierard GE. Invasive atypical fibroxanthoma and eruptive actinic keratoses in a heart transplant patient. *Dermatology* 1996;192:411.

171. Kemp JD, et al. Metastasizing atypical fibroxanthoma. Coexistence with chronic lymphocytic leukemia. *Arch Dermatol* 1978;114:1533.

172. Heintz PW, White CR Jr. Diagnosis: atypical fibroxanthoma or not? Evaluating spindle cell malignancies on sun damaged skin: a practical approach. *Semin Cutan Med Surg* 1999;18:78.

173. Fretzin DF, Helwig EB. Atypical fibroxanthoma of the skin. A clinicopathologic study of 140 cases. *Cancer* 1973;31:1541.

174. Boynton JR, Markowitch W Jr, Searl SS. Atypical fibroxanthoma of the eyelid. *Ophthalmology* 1989;96:1480.

175. Lesica A, Harwood TR, Yokoo H. Atypical fibroxanthoma of ethmoid sinus. *Arch Otolaryngol* 1975;101:506.

176. Diaz-Cascajo C, Borghi S, Bonczkowitz M. Pigmented atypical fibroxanthoma. *Histopathology* 1998;33:537.

177. Lazova R, et al. LN-2 (CD74): a marker to distinguish atypical fibroxanthoma from malignant fibrous histiocytoma. *Cancer* 1997;79:2115.

178. Hafner J, et al. Micrographic surgery (slow Mohs) in cutaneous sarcomas. *Dermatology* 1999;198:37.

179. Dzubow LM. Mohs surgery report: spindle cell fibrohistiocytic tumors: classification and pathophysiology. *J Dermatol Surg Oncol* 1988;14:490.

180. Helwig EB, May D. Atypical fibroxanthoma of the skin with metastasis. *Cancer* 1986;57:368.

181. Grosso M, et al. Metastatic atypical fibroxanthoma of skin. *Pathol Res Pract* 1987;182:443.

182. Glavin FL, Cornwell ML. Atypical fibroxanthoma of the skin metastatic to a lung. Report of case features by conventional and electron microscopy and a review of relevant literature. *Am J Dermatopathol* 1985;7:57.

183. Weiss SW, Enzinger FM. Malignant fibrous histiocytoma: an analysis of 200 cases. *Cancer* 1978;41:2250.

184. Inoshita T, Youngberg GA. Malignant fibrous histiocytoma arising in previous surgical sites. Report of two cases. *Cancer* 1984;53:176.

185. Yamamura T, et al. Malignant fibrous histiocytoma developing in a burn scar. *Br J Dermatol* 1984;110:725.

186. Farber JN, Koh HK. Malignant fibrous histiocytoma arising from discoid lupus erythematosus. *Arch Dermatol* 1988;124:114.

187. Camacho FM, et al. Malignant fibrous histiocytoma of the scalp. Multidisciplinary treatment. *J Eur Acad Dermatol Venereol* 1999;13:175.

188. Fanburg-Smith JC, et al. Infiltrative subcutaneous malignant fibrous histiocytoma: a comparative study with deep malignant fibrous histiocytoma and an observation of biologic behavior. *Ann Diagn Pathol* 1999;3:1.

189. Brown MD, Swanson NA. Treatment of malignant fibrous histiocytoma and atypical fibrous xanthomas with micrographic surgery. *J Dermatol Surg Oncol* 1989;15:1287.

190. Le Doussal V, et al. Prognostic factors for patients with localized primary malignant fibrous histiocytoma: a multicenter study of 216 patients with multivariate analysis. *Cancer* 1996;77:1823.

191. Diaz-Cascajo C, Weyers W, Borghi S. Sclerosing dermatofibrosarcoma protuberans. *J Cutan Pathol* 1998;25:440.

192. Bouyssou-Gauthier ML, et al. Dermatofibrosarcoma protuberans in childhood. *Pediatr Dermatol* 1997;14:463.

193. Gloster HM. Dermatofibrosarcoma protuberans. *J Am Acad Dermatol* 1996;35:355.

194. Elgart GW, et al. Bednar tumor (pigmented dermatofibrosarcoma protuberans) occurring in a site of prior immunization: immunochemical findings and therapy. *J Am Acad Dermatol* 1999;40:315.

195. Mbonde MP, Amir H, Kitinya JN. Dermatofibrosarcoma protuberans: a clinicopathological study in an African population. *East Afr Med J* 1996;73:410.

196. Bashara ME, Jules KT, Potter GK. Dermatofibrosarcoma protuberans: 4 years after local trauma. *J Foot Surg* 1992;31:160.

197. Lee CS, Chou ST. p53 protein immunoreactivity in fibrohistiocytic tumors of the skin. *Pathology* 1998;30:272.

198. Wick MR, et al. The pathological distinction between "deep penetrating" dermatofibroma and dermatofibrosarcoma protuberans. *Semin Cutan Med Surg* 1999;18:91.

199. Stojadinovic A, et al. Dermatofibrosarcoma protuberans of the head and neck. *Ann Surg Oncol* 2000;7:696.

200. Rutgers EJ, et al. Dermatofibrosarcoma protuberans: treatment and prognosis. *Eur J Surg Oncol* 1992;18:241.

201. Ratner D, et al. Mohs micrographic surgery for the treatment of dermatofibrosarcoma protuberans. Results of a multiinstitutional series with an analysis of the extent of microscopic spread. *J Am Acad Dermatol* 1997;37:600.

202. Garcia C, et al. Dermatofibrosarcoma protuberans treated with Mohs surgery. A case with CD34 immunostaining variability. *Dermatol Surg* 1996;22:177.

203. Barnes L, Coleman JA Jr, Johnson JT. Dermatofibrosarcoma protuberans of the head and neck. *Arch Otolaryngol* 1984;110:398.

204. Gloster HM. Dermatofibrosarcoma protuberans. *J Am Acad Dermatol* 1996;35:355.

205. Mentzel T, et al. Fibrosarcomatous ("high-grade") dermatofibrosarcoma protuberans: clinicopathologic and immunohistochemical study of a series of 41 cases with emphasis on prognostic significance. *Am J Surg Pathol* 1998;22:576.

206. Ballo MT, Zagras GK, Pisters P, Pollack A. The role of radiation therapy in the management of dermatofibrosarcoma protuberans. *Int J Radiat Oncol Biol Phys* 1998;40:823.

207. Requena L, Sangueza OP. Cutaneous vascular proliferations: III. Malignant neoplasms, other cutaneous neoplasms with significant vascular component, and disorders erroneously considered as vascular neoplasms. *J Am Acad Dermatol* 1998;38:143.

208. Kirova YM, et al. Radiation-induced sarcoma after breast cancer. Apropos of 8 cases and review of the literature. *Cancer Radiother* 1998;2:381.

209. Bisceglia M, et al. Early stage Stewart-Treves syndrome: report of 2 cases and review of the literature. *Pathologica* 1996;88:483.

210. Parravicini C, et al. Risk of Kaposi's sarcoma-associated herpes virus transmission from donor allografts among Italian posttransplant Kaposi's sarcoma patients. *Blood* 1997;90:2826.

211. Buonaguro FM, Tornesello ML, Buonaguro L, et al. Kaposi's sarcoma: aetiopathogenesis, histology, and clinical features. *J Eur Acad Dermatol Venereol* 2003;17:138

212. Toschi E, et al. Treatment of Kaposi's sarcoma—an update. *Anticancer Drugs* 2002;13:977.

213. Yarchoan R. Therapy for Kaposi's sarcoma: recent advances and experimental approaches. *J Acquir Immune Defic Syndr Hum Retrovirol* 1999;21[Suppl 1]:S66.

214. Schwartz RA. Cutaneous metastatic disease [see comments]. *J Am Acad Dermatol* 1995;33:161.

215. Quaglino D, et al. Cutaneous involvement in leukaemic patients. A review of the literature and personal experience. *Recenti Prog Med* 1997;88:415.

CHAPTER 38

Melanoma

ZHAO-JUN LIU
MEENHARD HERLYN

SECTION **1**

Molecular Biology of Cutaneous Melanoma

Cutaneous melanoma has been one of the fastest-rising malignancies over the past several decades. A yearly increase in the incidence among the white population of approximately 3% has occurred for the last 30 years. In the United States alone, 53,600 new cases and 7400 deaths were reported in 2002.[1] Unlike many other cancers, melanoma affects a relatively younger population and is notorious for its propensity to metastasize and for its poor response to current therapeutic regimens. Although representing only approximately 4% of skin cancers, melanoma accounts for approximately 79% of skin cancer deaths, with an annual mortality of 2.3 per 100,000 people. Fortunately, 95% of melanoma cases are curable if diagnosed early and surgically excised. In fact, mortality has not increased as steeply as incidence rates thanks to the early diagnosis achieved over the last decades.

Melanoma originates from pigment-producing melanocytes. In human skin, with its epidermis and dermis separated by a basement membrane, melanocytes are positioned at the epidermal-dermal junction and are interspersed among every five to ten basal keratinocytes. With their dendrites, they physically interact with keratinocytes to distribute the pigment melanin.[2] Melanin is packaged in melanosomes and provides protection against the damaging effects of ultraviolet (UV) light. Despite the dynamic nature of epidermal shedding, involving constant growth, differentiation, and vertical migration of keratinocytes,

proliferation of melanocytes is strictly controlled and rarely observed under physiologic conditions, albeit melanocytes maintain a lifelong proliferation potential. Developmentally, melanocytes are derived from their progenitor cells, melanoblasts that arise from pluripotent cells of the neural crest. Their survival, migration to the skin, and differentiation are related to spatial and temporal expression of molecules, not only on the migrating cells, but also on juxtaposed other cell types and the extracellular matrix (ECM). Genes specific for either melanocyte development or pigmentation, such as those from the *WNT* signaling pathway, microphthalmia-associated transcription factor (*MITF*), *PAX3*, and *SOX10*, are potentially important determinants for melanoma development, but a causal relationship has not yet been established. Growth factor receptor genes such as *c-KIT* or endothelin receptor-B (*EDNRB*) can also have a potential role in melanocyte transformation.

ETIOLOGY OF MELANOMA

Development of melanoma is the pathologic consequence of environmentally initiated disruptions to cellular genetic control mechanisms. Epidemiologic data support UV radiation as the major environmental carcinogen for melanoma. UV exposure at the B (UVB; 260 to 320 mm) and A (UVA; 320 to 400 mm) range is the most biologically relevant factor for sporadic melanoma.[3] The exact mechanism, however, whereby UV irradiation induces melanoma has not been determined. Several theories of UV-induced carcinogenesis have been proposed; for example, UV has been suggested to induce permanent genotoxic damage, act as a melanocyte mitogen, induce the production of tumor-promoting paracrine factors, or attenuate antitumor immune surveillance. It is now appreciated that transformation of melanocytes into malignant melanoma involves the interplay between genetic factors, UV exposure, and the tumor microenvironment. Recently, prospects for elucidating the molecular mechanisms underlying such gene-environment interactions have brightened considerably through the development of UV-responsive experimental animal models of melanoma, such as genetically engineered mice and human skin xenografts.

TYR-*RAS*/P16$^{INK4A-/-}$ AND TYR-*RAS*/P19$^{ARF-/-}$ MICE

To explore the role of neonatal UV exposure in promoting melanoma development, in particular whether UV-induced melanoma incidence is modulated by the status of the retinoblastoma (Rb) versus p53 pathways, Chin and colleagues used well-characterized murine melanoma models and have identified components of the Rb pathway as the principal targets of UV mutagenesis in murine melanoma development.[4] In a melanoma model driven by H-RAS activation and loss of p19(ARF) function (Tyr-*RAS*/p19$^{ARF-/-}$), UV exposure results in a marked acceleration in melanomagenesis, with nearly half of these tumors harboring amplification of cyclin-dependent kinase (*cdk*) *6*, whereas none of the melanomas arising in the absence of UV treatment contained *cdk6* amplification. Moreover, UV-induced melanomas show a strict reciprocal relationship between *cdk6* amplification and p16^{INK4} loss, which is consistent with the actions of UV occurring along the Rb pathway. Most significantly, UV exposure has no impact on the kinetics of melanoma driven by H-RAS activation and p16^{INK4} deficiency (Tyr-*RAS*/p16$^{INK4A-/-}$).

HEPATOCYTE GROWTH FACTOR/SCATTER FACTOR TRANSGENIC MICE

Hepatocyte growth factor/scatter factor (HGF/SF) executes its actions through its tyrosine kinase receptor c-MET. In combination with UV irradiation, aberrant HGF/SF–MET signaling can induce melanoma development. In HGF/SF transgenic mice, trunk skin melanocytes in newborns localize at or near the epidermal-dermal junction, similar to normal human skin. Spontaneous melanoma arises after a long latency in a few transgenic mice, suggesting that additional alterations are required for tumor development in most animals. Although suberythemal UV irradiation of adult HGF/SF mice does not accelerate melanoma development, a single neonatal dose of erythemal UV radiation is sufficient to induce, with high penetrance and relatively short latency, melanocytic lesions with staged progression from premalignant dysplastic foci, through radial growth phase (RGP) and vertical growth phase (VGP), and culminating in the metastatic phenotype, histopathologically resembling human melanoma.[5] It is likely that melanocytic progenitor cells, which represent a relatively high percentage of melanocytes in young mice, are the primary cellular targets of UV radiation. This response in mice is remarkable because retrospective epidemiologic studies suggest that melanoma is provoked by intense intermittent exposure to UV, particularly during childhood.[6,7] These results are the first experimental validation of epidemiologic evidence in a genetic mouse model suggesting that childhood sunburn poses a significant melanoma risk.

HUMAN SKIN XENOGRAFT MODELS

The architecture of mouse skin is different from that of human. Murine melanocytes are largely absent from the epidermis and reside in hair follicles and dermis. Hence, human skin-grafting techniques have been developed to circumvent the inadequacy of mouse melanoma models for studying the biology of the human melanoma. Human skin grafted onto immunodeficient mice preserves its unique architecture. When melanoma cells are injected into grafted human skin, they grow rapidly and spread in a similar manner to that of lesions in patients. This model is also useful for testing environmental factors, such as UV irradiation, for melanoma induction in a physiologic context. UVB treatment of immunodeficient mice engrafted with human newborn foreskin produced melanocytic hyperplasia and, in combination with DMBA initiation, infrequently induced nodular melanoma.[8] Similar melanocytic lesions are not found in most adult skin grafts.[9] However, when basic fibroblast growth factor (bFGF), a major autocrine growth factor in melanoma, is combined with UVB irradiation, pigmented lesions with hyperplastic melanocytic cells, including a lentigo maligna melanoma, are induced in adult skin grafts,[10] demonstrating a critical role for a combinative effect of gene-environment interaction on melanoma development.

GENETICS OF MELANOMA

Genetic defects affecting p53 and Rb genes occur frequently in many cancer types but appear to be rare or at least relatively late events in malignant melanoma. Although causative molecular defects intrinsic to melanocytes have not been well defined in the majority of human melanomas, epidemiologic, genetic, and genomic investigations are uncovering the spectrum of intrinsic defects that are associated with melanoma.

p16^{INK4A}

Cytogenetic studies have helped to identify the 9p21 locus, which is frequently affected in melanoma. As shown in Figure 38.1-1, this locus encodes two distinct proteins, p16INK4A and p14ARF (p19ARF in the mouse), both of which demonstrate tumor suppressor activity in genetically distinct anticancer pathways (i.e., the "Rb pathway" for p16INK4A and the "p53 pathway" for p14ARF).[11,12] At first, it was not known whether these somatic lesions target p16^{INK4A}, p14^{ARF}, both, or closely linked gene(s) such as *MTAP* or p15^{INK4B}. In a mouse model, it has been demonstrated that both tumor suppressors of the *INK4A/ARF* locus play prominent roles in melanoma formation.[11] In humans, however, further studies showed that only p16^{INK4A} is affected through germline mutations or deletions in patients with familial melanoma, which represent 8% to 10% of all melanoma cases. Approximately 50% of patients with familial melanoma have germline abnormalities at chromosome 9p21,[13] making this the most frequently abnormal locus. Of these, approximately 50% have mutations or deletions in the p16^{INK4A} gene. Thus, p16^{INK4A} abnormalities represent approximately 5% of all melanomas. They are also significant in sporadic melanomas, in which 25% to 40% of all lesions have mutations or deletions or in which the gene is transcriptionally silenced. p16INK4A has been identified initially as a CDK4-associated protein capable of inhibiting CDK4/6-mediated phosphorylation of the Rb tumor suppressor protein. Because hypophosphorylated Rb binds to and represses E2F transcriptional activity and constrains G$_1$ exit, p16^{INK4A}

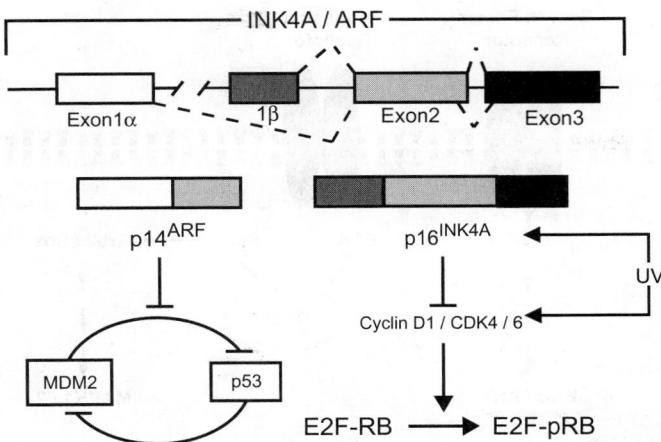

FIGURE 38.1-1. Role of p14ARF and p16INK4A in the regulation of p53, Rb, cyclin D1, and CDK4/6 in the melanoma cell. The human INK4A/ARF locus encodes p16INK4A and p14ARF. They are processed by different splicing mechanisms. p16INK4A inhibits cyclin D1/cyclin-dependent kinase (cdk) 4/6 complexes and thus suppresses Rb and antagonizes the proliferative stimulus of E2F, whereas the role of ARF is to stabilize p53 by inhibiting its murine double-minute gene-2 (MDM-2)–mediated ubiquitinylation. Ultraviolet (UV) light may induce mutations in p16INK4A and CDK4/6.

expression results in cell-cycle arrest. Besides p16^{INK4A}, the *cdk4* gene has been found mutated in familial melanoma, but only two families have been identified to date.[14]

N-RAS

Ras mutation occurs frequently in many types of cancers. In melanoma only *N-Ras* mutations have been identified in 5% to 15% of all sporadic melanomas.[15] A linkage between *N-Ras* mutations and UV irradiation has not been well established. A hypothetically UV-inducible *N-Ras* hypermutability in familial melanoma with p16^{INK4A} mutations has been observed.[16] The investigators compared *N-Ras* mutations in melanomas from patients in Swedish melanoma-prone families carrying germline p16^{INK4A} mutations with *N-Ras* mutations in melanomas from patients with sporadic melanomas. Activating *N-Ras* mutations were found in 95% of familial melanomas but in only 10% of sporadic melanomas. These data demonstrate the remarkable *N-Ras* hypermutability in familial melanoma. Besides activation through specific mutations, RAS can be constitutively activated in melanoma through as yet unknown mechanisms but likely due to constitutively produced autocrine growth factors such as bFGF and HGF.[17]

B-RAF

Activating somatic missense mutations in the B-Raf protooncogene have been discovered in as many as 66% of human melanoma samples and cell lines, but at far lower frequency in a wide range of human cancers.[18,19] Three types of mutations have thus far been identified[20] and, importantly, these point mutations are clustered in specific regions of biochemical importance. An inverse correlation is found between mutations in the *N-Ras* and *B-Raf* genes because tumors carry only one and not both at the same time.[21] The most frequently occurring mutation (accounting for 80% of total) is a single phosphomimetic substitution in the kinase-activation domain (V599E) that is known to confer constitutive activation of B-RAF. Mutated B-RAF proteins cause hyperstimulation of the mitogen-activated protein kinase (MAPK) cascade and are able to transform NIH3T3 cells *in vitro* (Fig. 38.1-2). Soon after the report, it was observed that V599E mutations are detectable in 68% of melanoma metastases, in 80% of primary melanomas, and, unexpectedly, in 82% of nevi,[22] suggesting that mutational activation of the RAS/RAF/MAPK pathway in nevi is a critical step in the initiation of melanocytic neoplasia but alone is insufficient for melanoma tumorigenesis. Functional importance of B-RAF in melanomagenesis has been demonstrated. Suppression of B-RAF(V599E) expression through RNAi in cultured human melanoma completely abrogates the transformed phenotype *in vitro*.[23] These results are specific for B-RAF, as targeted interference of C-RAF in melanoma cells does not significantly alter their biologic properties. The MAPK pathway can be activated not only through mutations in the *B-Raf* gene but also through autocrine and paracrine growth factors that stimulate proliferation and survival of the malignant cells.[17,24] Even if nevi harbor *B-Raf* mutations, ERK1/2 (extracellular signaling-regulated kinase 1/2) are not phosphorylated, suggesting that in melanoma several mechanisms are responsible for activation of this pathway.[25]

p53/APAF-1

Although p53 mutations are rarely detectable in melanoma, p53 and its downstream signal pathway seems to be kept in an inactive state. Apaf-1 (apoptotic protease cascade factor-1), a death effector that acts with cytochrome *c* and caspase 9 to mediate p53-dependent apoptosis, is often lost in metastatic melanoma cells through loss of heterozygosity or DNA methylation.[26] This may help explain why p53 is not able to modulate melanoma cells and why melanoma remains chemo and radiation resistant. Two other mechanisms can account for the functional inactivation of p53 leading to the high radiation and chemoresistance of melanoma: overexpression of the p53 inhibitor Mdm2 and suppression of p14ARF.[27,28]

PTEN/AKT

PTEN is a tumor suppressor gene mutated in some human melanomas.[29] It has emerged as a major component in regulating survival of tumor cells through its involvement in intricate cascading pathways for growth and adhesion signaling (Fig. 38.1-3). It has lipid phosphatase and protein phosphatase activity. The lipid phosphatase activity of PTEN decreases intracellular PtdIns(3,4,5)P3 level and downstream Akt activity. A mutated PTEN can constitutively activate PKB/AKT to influence downstream genes. PTEN can also up-regulate pro-apoptotic machinery involving caspases and BID and down-regulate the antiapoptotic proteins such as Bcl2. The protein phosphatase activity of PTEN is apparently less central to its involvement in tumorigenesis. It is involved in the inhibition of focal adhesion formation, cell spreading, and migration, as well as the inhibition of growth factor–stimulated MAPK signaling. Therefore, the combined effects of the loss of PTEN lipid and protein phosphatase activity may result in aberrant cell growth and escape from apoptosis, as well as abnormal cell spreading and migration. In melanoma, PTEN loss has

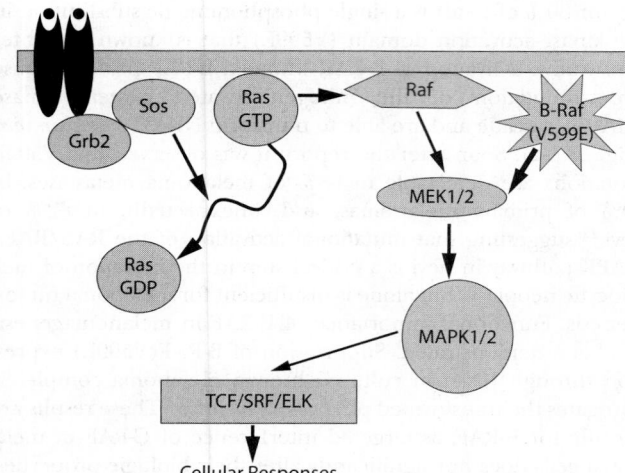

FIGURE 38.1-2. Hyperstimulation of mitogen-activated protein kinase (MAPK) pathway by B-RAF mutation. Growth factors induce dimerization of their receptors and recruitment of Grb2 and Sos to the plasma membrane. Sos then activates Ras by catalyzing guanosine diphosphate (GDP) exchange for guanosine triphosphate (GTP). Activated Ras recruits Raf to the membrane, and membrane-bound Raf is subsequently phosphorylated to activate the MEK/MAPK pathway. Activated MAPK translocates into nucleus and activates transcription factors such as T-cell factor (TCF)/SRF/ELK, which stimulate target genes to regulate cell proliferation. Mutated B-RAF can constitutively activate the MEK/MAPK pathway and is independent of upstream signals.

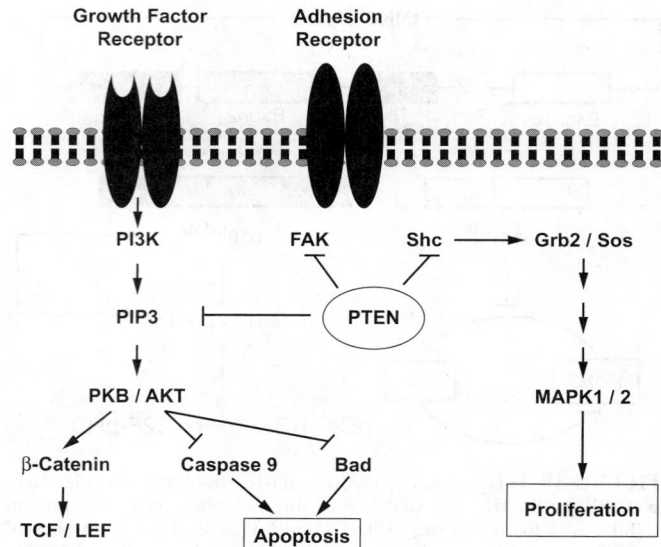

FIGURE 38.1-3. PTEN pathways in melanoma. Schematic representation of PTEN as a central molecule influencing the phosphoinositide 3 kinase (PI3K)/Akt pathway and the Ras/Raf/mitogen-activated protein kinase (MAPK) pathway to regulate cell survival and proliferation. PTEN also dephosphorylates focal adhesion kinase (FAK) to inhibit focal adhesion formation and control cell adhesion and migration. Suppressive effect of PTEN on PI3K/Akt is through decreasing intracellular PIP3 level. Inhibition of Akt activity results in down-regulation of the β-catenin pathway and up-regulation of proapoptotic machinery involving caspase 9 and Bad.

been mostly observed as a late event, although a dose-dependent loss of PTEN protein and function has been implicated in early stages of tumorigenesis as well. Similar to p53 and p16^{INK4A}, *PTEN* may be structurally normal in the vast majority of melanomas but functionally inactive, or expression is silenced due to hypermethylation.[30] In addition, loss of PTEN and oncogenic activation of RAS seem to occur in a reciprocal fashion, both of which could cooperate with p16INK4A loss in contribution to melanomagenesis.

CYCLIN D1/CDK4

As a target gene of many proliferating signaling pathways, such as the RAS/RAF/MAPK pathway, cyclin D1 is an important regulator of the G_1/S cell-cycle transition, contributing to the phosphorylation of the Rb by binding to CDK4. In melanoma, amplification of *cyclin D1* has been identified mostly in acral melanomas (44%) and less frequently in other subtypes.[31,32] Acral melanomas appear distinct from other subtypes in that they are frequently characterized by amplifications in one or two loci. Strong evidence supporting an oncogenic role for cyclin D1 comes from experiments demonstrating that antisense treatment of mice bearing melanoma xenografts overexpressing cyclin D1 leads to apoptosis and tumor shrinkage.[33] On the other hand, a point mutation in CDK4 producing an amino acid substitution of arginine to cysteine at residue 24 (R24C) has been detected in SK-MEL-29 cells,[34] as well as in three melanoma families. This mutation interferes with the binding of CDK4 to p16, but not to cyclin D. Moreover, Cdk4R24C/R24C murine models appear susceptible to melanoma development.[35]

WNT5A

WNT genes encode a family of secreted glycoproteins that modulate cell fate and behavior in embryos through activation of receptor-mediated signaling pathways. Wnt signaling is initiated on binding of a secreted Wnt molecule to its cognate receptor Frizzled (Frz), a seven-pass transmembrane protein. The two types of Wnt signaling pathways are canonical and noncanonical, depending on the particular Wnt/Frz combination. Canonical Wnt signaling (i.e., Wnt1 and Wnt3a) occurs through β-catenin/T-cell factor–mediated transcriptional activation of Wnt target genes, whereas noncanonical signaling (i.e., Wnt5a) is mediated through activation of phospholipase C, protein kinase C (PKC), and Ca^{2+}-calmodulin–dependent kinase II (Fig. 38.1-4).

It has been observed that melanomas show increased Wnt5a expression relative to skin and the increased expression of Wnt5a in melanoma tumors is localized, occurring in cells at the site of active invasion and in cells that show morphologic features associated with aggressive tumor behavior,[36] suggesting that Wnt5a may affect melanoma progression. Consistently, an increased Wnt5a gene expression has also been found in the highly aggressive metastatic melanomas in a gene expression profiling study.[37] Wnt5A determines invasive behavior of melanoma.[38] Overexpression of Wnt5a in melanoma cells induces actin reorganization and increases cell adhesion. Although no increase in β-catenin expression or nuclear translocation is observed, there is a dramatic increase in activated PKC. In direct correlation with Wnt5a expression and PKC activation, there is an increase in melanoma cell invasion. Blocking this pathway using antibodies to Frz-5

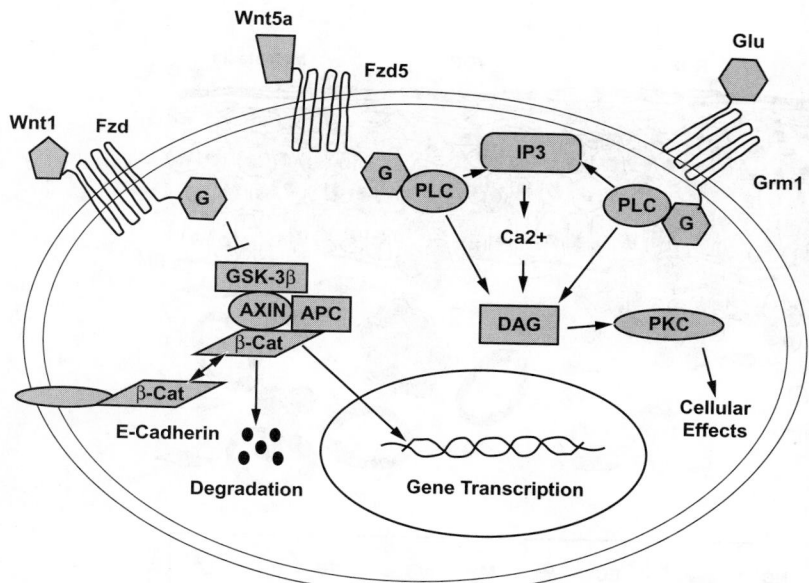

FIGURE 38.1-4. Activation of the protein kinase C (PKC) pathway by Wnt5a and metabolic glutamate receptor 1 (Grm1) stimulation is mediated by G-protein–coupled receptor. Canonical Wnt1 signaling is mediated through β-catenin (β-Cat)/T-cell factor. Wnt1 signals via Fzd to stabilize β-Cat and its subsequent nucleus translocation. Wnt5a, however, signals via Fzd-5 to activate phospholipase C (PLC), causing phospholipid turnover in the membrane, releasing calcium from intracellular stores and increasing PKC activity. Grm1 mediates glutamate signal through a similar pattern to activate the PKC pathway. GSK, glycogen synthase kinase.

inhibits PKC activity and cellular invasion. Consistently, Wnt5a expression in human melanoma biopsies directly correlates to increasing tumor grade. Thus, the Wnt5a/PKC pathway can play an important role in evoking the invasive phenotype of metastatic melanoma and the likelihood that Wnt5a may be a potential marker of tumor progression.

METABOTROPIC GLUTAMATE RECEPTOR 1

Metabotropic glutamate receptor 1 (Grm1) has been linked to the development of melanoma in a study to characterize a transgenic insertional mouse mutant, TG3.[39] Investigators have found multiple tandem insertions of the transgene into intron 3 of the *Grm1* gene with concomitant deletion of 70 kb intronic sequence. To assess the effects of this insertion on transcription regulation, they have analyzed *Grm1* and *2* flanking genes for aberrant expression in melanomas from TG3 mice. Only Grm1 shows aberrant expression. It is ectopically expressed in melanomas from TG3 mice but is not expressed in normal mouse melanocytes. The involvement of Grm1 in melanocytic neoplasia was confirmed with an additional transgenic line with Grm1 expression driven by the dopachrome tautomerase promoter. This line is also susceptible to melanoma. In contrast to human melanoma, these transgenic mice have a generalized hyperproliferation of melanocytes with limited transformation to fully malignant metastasis. Human melanoma biopsies and cell lines, but not benign nevi and melanocytes, express Grm1. This is the first study implicating metabotropic glutamate signaling in tumorigenesis. However, it remains unclear why Grm1 as an excitatory neurotransmitter in the mammalian central nervous system is involved in melanoma development. Interestingly, Grm1 is a member of the large family of seven-transmembrane-domain G protein–coupled receptors. The downstream signaling pathways link to PKC activation. Taking the Wnt5a signaling pathway into consideration, in which the G-protein–mediated PKC pathway is activated, activation of the G-protein–mediated PKC pathway perhaps plays a critical role in melanoma development and progression (see Fig. 38.1-4).

BIOLOGIC BASIS OF MELANOMA DEVELOPMENT AND PROGRESSION

Clinical and histologic studies have resulted in defining five major steps of melanoma development and progression (Fig. 38.1-5): step 1, common acquired and congenital nevi with structurally normal melanocytes; step 2, dysplastic nevi with structural and architectural atypia; step 3, RGP, nontumorigenic primary melanomas without metastatic competence; step 4, VGP, tumorigenic primary melanomas with competence for metastasis; and step 5, metastatic melanoma.[40] The progression from each stage to the next is associated with specific biologic changes, which are based on experimental models and clinical and histopathologic observations (Fig. 38.1-6). Melanoma development and progression have now been viewed as a result of disruption of normal skin homeostasis rather than just a genetic alteration. Normal skin melanocytic homeostasis is maintained by dynamic interactions between the melanocytes and their microenvironment, such as keratinocytes, fibroblasts, endothelial and immune cells, and the ECM. During transformation and progression of melanocytes to melanoma cells, there are, however, deregulated interactions between the neoplastic cells and the adjacent stromal cells (Fig. 38.1-7). The characteristics of solid tumors, that is, uncontrolled proliferation, derangement of cellular and morphologic differentiation, invasion, and colonization to distant organs, can be attributed, in part, to alterations in communications between neoplastic cells and the normal cells in their immediate microenvironment.[41]

MELANOMA–STROMAL CELL INTERACTIONS THROUGH ADHESION RECEPTORS

Melanoma cells express all major groups of adhesion receptors: integrins, cadherins, and cellular adhesion molecules of the immunoglobulin gene supergene family. During the transition from normal cells to benign and malignant lesions, then to metastatic cancer, stepwise changes in inter-

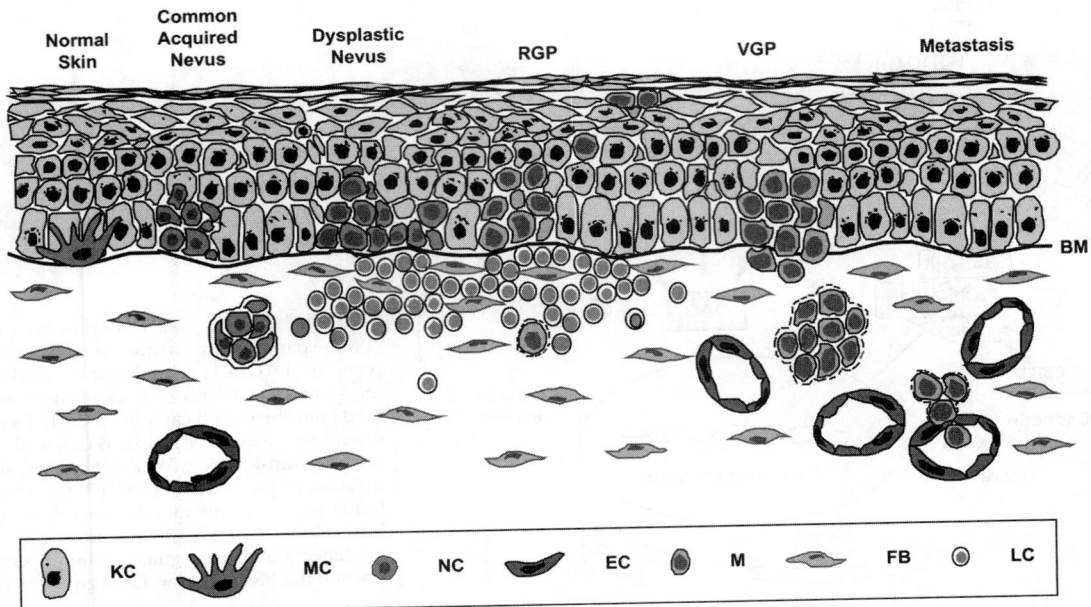

FIGURE 38.1-5. Process of melanoma development from normal melanocytes. Nevi are characterized by aberrant cell growth, consisting of enlarged, coalescent nests of nevocytes, which display different degrees of cytologic dysplasia. Further progression results in malignant cells, which grow only within or in close proximity to the epidermis [radial growth phase (RGP)]. Eventually, cells acquire the ability to invade deeply into dermis [vertical growth phase (VGP)] and then into lymphatics and blood vessels, leading to systemic dissemination (metastatic melanoma). BM, basement membrane; EC, endothelial cell; FB, fibroblast; KC, keratinocyte; LC, lymphocyte; M, melanoma cell; MC, melanocyte; NC, nevocyte. (See Color Fig. 38.1-5 in the CD-ROM.)

cellular communications provide tumor cells with the ability to overcome microenvironmental controls from the host and to invade surrounding tissues and disperse to distant locations.

CADHERIN

Cellular adhesion molecule of the cadherin is important to growth and metastasis of malignant melanoma. An E- to N-cadherin switch occurs during the process of transformation of melanocytes to melanomas, as well as a loss of E-cadherin expression and a parallel gain in N-cadherin function (Fig. 38.1-8). The expression of E-cadherin by melanocytes allows them to adhere to keratinocytes and develop gap junctions through connexin 43, whereas N-cadherin expression allows communication of melanoma cells with N-cadherin–expressing fibroblasts (Fig. 38.1-9).[42] N-cadherin mediates homotypic aggregation among melanoma cells as well as heterotypic adhesion of melanoma cells to dermal fibroblasts and vascular endothelial cells, which may improve their ability to migrate through stroma and enter the vasculature.[43] N-cadherin–mediated cell adhesion activates antiapoptotic protein PKB/AKT and subsequently stabilizes β-catenin and inactivates the proapoptotic factor Bad. Thus, cadherin subtype switching from E- to N-cadherin during melanoma development not only frees melanocytic cells from the control of keratinocytes but also provides growth and possibly metastatic advantages to melanoma cells. Keratinocytes can control the phenotype of normal melanocytes but not melanoma cells. They can regulate melanocyte growth and the expression of cell surface adhesion receptors.

MCAM

MCAM, also known as *MUC18*, *Mel-CAM*, or *CD146*, belongs to the immunoglobulin superfamily; it can mediate heterotypic adhesion between melanoma and stromal cells,[44] although the counter-receptor or ligand for MCAM has yet to be identified. The malignant potential of melanoma is directly related to the

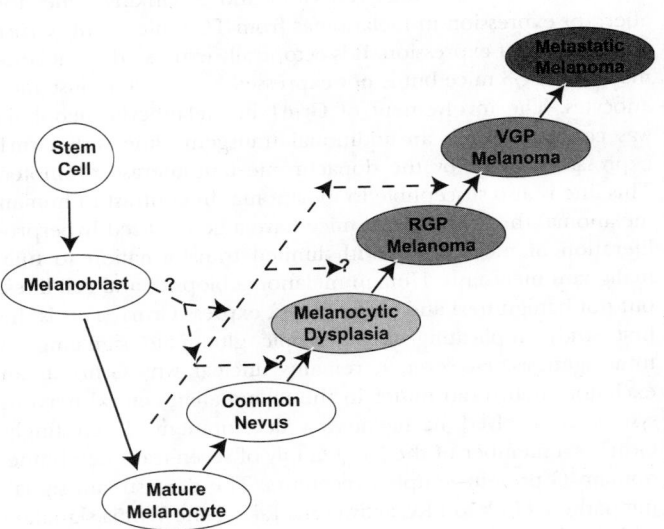

FIGURE 38.1-6. Melanoma development and progression. The model implies that melanomas develop and progress in a sequence of steps. However, malignancy can also develop *de novo*. RGP, radial growth phase; VGP, vertical growth phase.

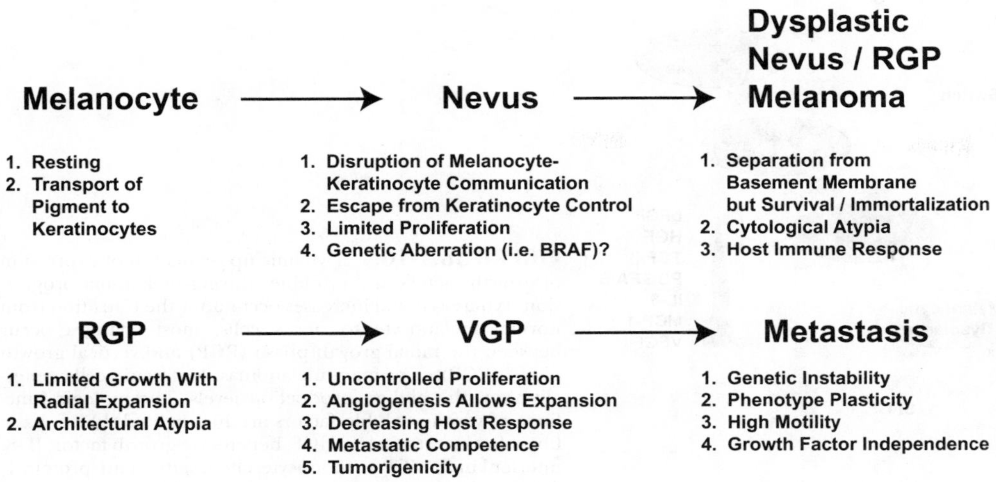

Melanocyte ⟶ **Nevus** ⟶ **Dysplastic Nevus / RGP Melanoma**

Melanocyte
1. Resting
2. Transport of Pigment to Keratinocytes

Nevus
1. Disruption of Melanocyte-Keratinocyte Communication
2. Escape from Keratinocyte Control
3. Limited Proliferation
4. Genetic Aberration (i.e. BRAF)?

Dysplastic Nevus / RGP Melanoma
1. Separation from Basement Membrane but Survival / Immortalization
2. Cytological Atypia
3. Host Immune Response

RGP ⟶ **VGP** ⟶ **Metastasis**

RGP
1. Limited Growth With Radial Expansion
2. Architectural Atypia

VGP
1. Uncontrolled Proliferation
2. Angiogenesis Allows Expansion
3. Decreasing Host Response
4. Metastatic Competence
5. Tumorigenicity

Metastasis
1. Genetic Instability
2. Phenotype Plasticity
3. High Motility
4. Growth Factor Independence

FIGURE 38.1-7. Biologic events during melanoma progression. Each transition is marked by characteristic changes in the cells. RGP, radial growth phase; VGP, vertical growth phase.

vertical thickness of the lesion. Analysis of primary melanomas indicates that, although the majority of advanced and metastatic tumors strongly express the MCAM antigen, its expression on thin tumors (less than 0.75 mm) and on benign nevi is weaker and less frequent (see Fig. 38.1-8). In addition, there is a positive correlation between MCAM expression and the ability of human melanoma cell lines to metastasize in nude mice. Ectopic expression of MCAM in RGP melanoma cell lines (MCAM negative) resulted in an increase in their tumorigenicity and metastatic potential in nude mice, whereas inhibition of MCAM expression by a specific genetic suppressor element inhibits dermal invasion of melanoma cells in a three-dimensional skin reconstruct.[45] MCAM is also expressed on endothelial cells and smooth muscle cells and thus plays a role in the molecular dialogues between tumor and host cells and may also be involved in tumor angiogenesis and metastasis.

β_3 INTEGRIN

β_3 integrin is present on almost all VGP primary and metastatic melanomas, but not on cells of earlier stages of progression, and thus is useful as one of the most specific markers that characterize VGP and metastatic cells (see Fig. 38.1-8). When the β_3 gene is transduced to RGP melanoma cells, there are no changes in growth properties *in vitro*[46]; however, the cells

become highly invasive in a skin reconstruction model and are tumorigenic in mice, two attributes of VGP melanoma cells. Apparently, β_3 integrin expression triggers the up-regulation of a variety of genes associated with invasion and tumor growth. The β_3 integrin subunit is also up-regulated by tumor-infiltrating endothelial cells, and several clinical studies have been initiated to target β_3 on endothelial or melanoma cells, or both, for therapy.

MELANOMA–STROMAL CELL INTERACTIONS BY SOLUBLE FACTORS

Normal melanocytes are relatively inactive in growth factor production, even after stimulation. Nevus cells may produce bFGF and chemoattractive cytokines such as interleukin (IL)-8 or MCP-1 (monocyte chemoattractant protein-1). With progression, melanoma cells show an increase in production of

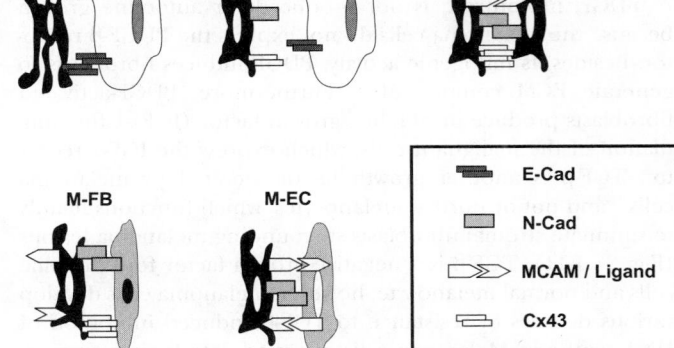

FIGURE 38.1-9. Melanocyte and melanoma cell interactions with juxtaposed cells in their environment. In normal skin, melanocytes are controlled by keratinocytes (KCs) through E-cadherin (E-Cad) and connexin 43 (Cx43). A switch from E-Cad to N-cadherin (N-Cad) during melanoma development frees the cells from KC control. Melanoma cells communicate with each other through multiple adhesions (i.e., N-Cad and MCAM) or junction receptors. Melanoma cells also interact with fibroblast (FB) and endothelial cells (EC) through N-Cad and gap junction.

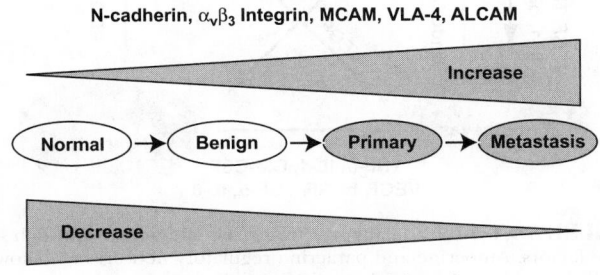

N-cadherin, $\alpha_v\beta_3$ Integrin, MCAM, VLA-4, ALCAM

Increase

Normal ⟶ Benign ⟶ Primary ⟶ Metastasis

Decrease

E-cadherin, VCAM, Desmoglein, $\alpha_6\beta_1$

FIGURE 38.1-8. Dynamic shifts in the expression of adhesion receptors and their matrix proteins by melanoma cells. The increase or decrease in expression may already start in nevi or only in vertical growth phase melanomas.

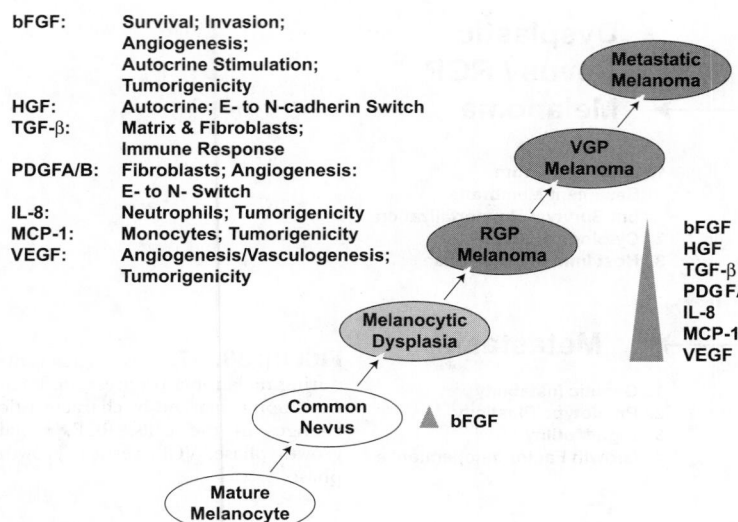

bFGF: Survival; Invasion; Angiogenesis; Autocrine Stimulation; Tumorigenicity
HGF: Autocrine; E- to N-cadherin Switch
TGF-β: Matrix & Fibroblasts; Immune Response
PDGFA/B: Fibroblasts; Angiogenesis: E- to N- Switch
IL-8: Neutrophils; Tumorigenicity
MCP-1: Monocytes; Tumorigenicity
VEGF: Angiogenesis/Vasculogenesis; Tumorigenicity

FIGURE 38.1-10. Dynamic up-regulation of expression of growth factors and cytokines during melanoma progression. Whereas initial increases occur after the transition from normal melanocyte to nevus cells, most changes occur between the radial growth phase (RGP) and vertical growth phase (VGP) of primary melanomas. Metastatic cells generally show the highest production levels. The biologic functions of various soluble factors are highlighted. bFGF, basic fibroblast growth factor; HGF, hepatocyte growth factor; IL-8, interleukin-8; MCP-1, monocyte chemoattractant protein-1; PDGF, platelet-derived growth factor; TGF, transforming growth factor; VEGF, vascular endothelial growth factor.

growth factors and cytokines. Autocrine growth factors [bFGF, IL-8, HGF, platelet-derived growth factor-A (PDGF-A)] stimulate proliferation and migration of the melanoma cell itself, whereas paracrine growth factors [PDGF, transforming growth factor (TGF)-β, bFGF, vascular endothelial growth factor (VEGF), MCP-1] modulate the microenvironment, especially stromal fibroblasts, to the benefit of melanoma growth, invasion, and metastasis (Fig. 38.1-10).

bFGF is the most significant autocrine growth factor in melanoma.[47] Blocking of bFGF production with antisense oligonucleotides stops melanoma cell proliferation. In spite of lack of a signal sequence, it can be released from cells through yet unknown mechanisms. Once released from cells, bFGF binds to matrix proteins such as heparin sulfate proteoglycan and can then stimulate fibroblasts and endothelial cells. bFGF is not only a survival factor and a growth stimulator for melanoma cells but also a motility factor. Its role in invasion comes from up-regulation of serine proteinases and metalloproteinases. Potentially, a variety of other genes are activated as well, which still need to be identified.

PDGF, in contrast, is not produced for autocrine growth because the melanoma cells do not express the PDGF-β receptor. Besides its mitogenic activity, PDGF induces fibroblasts to generate ECM components.[48] Furthermore, PDGF-activated fibroblasts produce insulin-like growth factor (IGF)-1 for stimulation of the malignant cells, which express the IGF-1 receptor. TGF-β is another growth factor secreted by melanoma cells[49] and not by normal melanocytes, which functions mainly to stimulate stromal fibroblasts surrounding melanoma lesions (Fig. 38.1-11). TGF-β is a negative growth factor for epithelial cells and normal melanocyte; however, melanoma cells develop various degrees of resistance to TGF-β–induced inhibition of DNA synthesis. Melanoma cells can modulate their surrounding stroma for their own benefits through the paracrine activity of TGF-β. Stimulation of ECM production by stromal fibroblasts provides scaffolding for the melanoma cells, which show increased survival and metastasis in SCID mice.[50]

On the other hand, fibroblasts are also a rich source of growth factors, but only after activation.[51] On stimulation, fibroblasts can produce a pool of growth factors (IGF-1, HGF, bFGF,

and endothelin-3). For normal melanocytes, benign nevus cells, and melanoma cells from the RGP and early VGP stage, IGF-1 is one of the most critical growth factors required for survival and growth of cells in chemically defined media.[52] IGF-1 receptor is expressed by all melanocytic cells, and the expression increases with progression. Melanoma cells apparently rely on IGF-1 secreted by fibroblasts because they do not produce it on their own. Data indicate that IGF-1 enhances survival, migration, and growth of cells from biologically early lesions but not from biologically late primary or metastatic lesions. Early melanoma cells are activated by IGF-1 to activate the MAPK pathway.[24] A study has shown that fibroblast-derived IGF-1 can induce IL-8 expression in melanoma cells, especially in early-stage melanomas, through the MAPK/JNK/AP-1 pathway. Antibody blockage of IL-8 signaling can abolish IGF-1–induced cell migration, suggest-

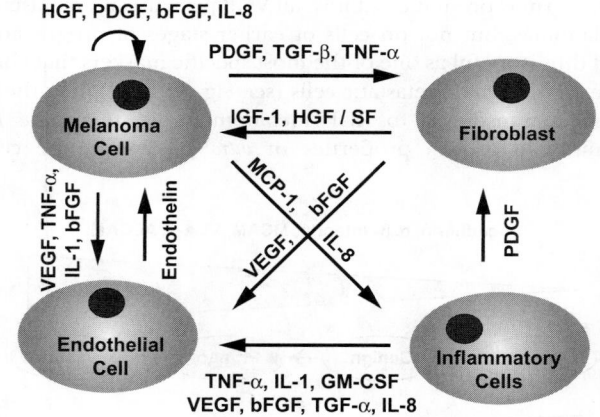

FIGURE 38.1-11. Melanoma–stroma cell interactions through soluble factors. Autocrine and paracrine regulatory networks are shown. bFGF, basic fibroblast growth factor; GM-CSF, granulocyte-macrophage colony-stimulating factor; HGF, hepatocyte growth factor; IGF, insulin-like growth factor; IL-8, interleukin-8; MCP-1, monocyte chemoattractant protein-1; PDGF, platelet-derived growth factor; SF, scatter factor; TGF, transforming growth factor; TNF, tumor necrosis factor; VEGF, vascular endothelial growth factor.

ing that the motility effect of IGF-1 on melanoma is mediated by subsequent events of IL-8 induction and autocrine stimulation. The possibility that the angiogenic effect of IGF-1 is also mediated by IL-8 induction is hinted by the discovery that VEGF expression can also be elevated by IGF-1 treatment.

Accumulating evidence has demonstrated the importance of tumor microenvironment on the behavior of malignant cells. Interactions between melanoma cells and stromal cells create a context that promotes tumor growth, migration, invasion, and angiogenesis. A better understanding of this process and developing new experimental and screening models is important for the development of effective therapeutic strategies to treat melanoma.

REFERENCES

1. American Cancer Society. *Cancer Facts & Figures*. American Cancer Society, Inc., 2002.
2. Hsu MY, Meier F, Herlyn M. Melanoma development and progression: a conspiracy between tumor and host. *Differentiation* 2002;70:522.
3. Gruijl FR. IL-40 UV carcinogenesis and melanocytes. *Pigment Cell Res* 2003;16:591.
4. Kannan K, Sharpless NE, Xu J, et al. Components of the Rb pathway are critical targets of UV mutagenesis in a murine melanoma model. *Proc Natl Acad Sci U S A* 2003;100:1221.
5. Noonan FP, Recio JA, Takayama H, et al. Neonatal sunburn and melanoma in mice. *Nature* 2001;413:271.
6. Holman CD, Armstrong BK, Heenan PJ. A theory of the etiology and pathogenesis of human cutaneous malignant melanoma. *J Natl Cancer Inst* 1983;71:651.
7. Whiteman DC, Whiteman CA, Green AC. Childhood sun exposure as a risk factor for melanoma: a systematic review of epidemiologic studies. *Cancer Causes Control* 2001;12:69.
8. Atillasoy ES, Seykora JT, Soballe PW, et al. UVB induces atypical melanocytic lesions and melanoma in human skin. *Am J Pathol* 1998;152:1179.
9. Berking C, Takemoto R, Binder RL, et al. Photocarcinogenesis in human adult skin grafts. *Carcinogenesis* 2002;23:181.
10. Berking C, Takemoto R, Satyamoorthy K, et al. Basic fibroblast growth factor and ultraviolet B transform melanocytes in human skin. *Am J Pathol* 2001;158:943.
11. Sherr CJ, Roberts JM. Inhibitors of mammalian G1 cyclin-dependent kinases. *Genes Dev* 1995;9:1149.
12. Pomerantz J, Schreiber-Agus N, Liegeois NJ, et al. The Ink4a tumor suppressor gene product, p19Arf, interacts with MDM2 and neutralizes MDM2's inhibition of p53. *Cell* 1998;92:713.
13. Cannon-Albright LA, Goldgar DE, Meyer LJ, et al. Assignment of a locus for familial melanoma, MLM, to chromosome 9p13-p22. *Science* 1992;258:1148.
14. Platz A, Hansson J, Ringborg U. Screening of germline mutations in the CDK4, CDKN2C and TP53 genes in familial melanoma: a clinic-based population study. *Int J Cancer* 1998;78:13.
15. Ball NJ, Yohn JJ, Morelli JG, et al. Ras mutations in human melanoma: a marker of malignant progression. *J Invest Dermatol* 1994;102:285.
16. Eskandarpour M, Hashemi J, Kanter L, et al. Frequency of UV-inducible NRAS mutations in melanomas of patients with germline CDKN2A mutations. *J Natl Cancer Inst* 2003; 95:768.
17. Satyamoorthy K, Li G, Gerrero MR, et al. Constitutive mitogen-activated protein kinase activation in melanoma is mediated by both BRAF mutations and autocrine growth factor stimulation. *Cancer Res* 2003;63:756.
18. Davies H, Bignell GR, Cox C, et al. Mutations of the BRAF gene in human cancer. *Nature* 2002;417:949.
19. Brose MS, Volpe P, Feldman M, et al. BRAF and RAS mutations in human lung cancer and melanoma. *Cancer Res* 2002;62:6997.
20. Tuveson DA, Weber BL, Herlyn M. BRAF as a potential therapeutic target in melanoma and other malignancies. *Cancer Cell* 2003;4:95.
21. Gorden A, Osman I, Gai W, et al. Analysis of BRAF and N-RAS mutations in metastatic melanoma tissues. *Cancer Res* 2003;63:3955.
22. Pollock PM, Harper UL, Hansen KS, et al. High frequency of BRAF mutations in nevi. *Nat Genet* 2003;33:19.
23. Hingorani SR, Jacobetz MA, Robertson GP, et al. Suppression of BRAF(V599E) in human melanoma abrogates transformation. *Cancer Res* 2003;63:5198.
24. Satyamoorthy K, Li G, Vaidya B, et al. Insulin-like growth factor-1 induces survival and growth of biologically early melanoma cells through both the mitogen-activated protein kinase and beta-catenin pathways. *Cancer Res* 2001;61:7318.
25. Dong J, Phelps RG, Qiao R, et al. BRAF oncogenic mutations correlate with progression rather than initiation of human melanoma. *Cancer Res* 2003;63:3883.
26. Soengas MS, Capodieci P, Polsky D, et al. Inactivation of the apoptosis effector Apaf-1 in malignant melanoma. *Nature* 2001;409:207.
27. Landers JE, Cassel SL, George DL. Translational enhancement of mdm2 oncogene expression in human tumor cells containing a stabilized wild-type p53 protein. *Cancer Res* 1997;57:3562.
28. Bardeesy N, Bastian BC, Hezel A, et al. Dual inactivation of RB and p53 pathways in RAS-induced melanomas. *Mol Cell Biol* 2001;21:2144.
29. Robertson GP, Herbst RA, Nagane M, et al. The chromosome 10 monosomy common in human melanomas results from loss of two separate tumor suppressor loci. *Cancer Res* 1999;59:3596.
30. Stahl JM, Cheung M, Sharma A, et al. Loss of PTEN promotes tumor development in malignant melanoma. *Cancer Res* 2003;63:2881.
31. Bastian BC, Kashani-Sabet M, Hamm H, et al. Gene amplifications characterize acral melanoma and permit the detection of occult tumor cells in the surrounding skin. *Cancer Res* 2000;60:1968.
32. Sauter ER, Yeo UC, von Stemm A, et al. Cyclin D1 is a candidate oncogene in cutaneous melanoma. *Cancer Res* 2002;63:3200.
33. Sauter ER, Takemoto R, Litwin S, et al. p53 alone or in combination with antisense cyclin D1 induces apoptosis and reduces tumor size in human melanoma. *Cancer Gene Ther* 2002;9:807.
34. Wolfel T, Hauer M, Schneider J, et al. A p16INK4a-insensitive CDK4 mutant targeted by cytolytic T lymphocytes in a human melanoma. *Science* 1995;269:1281.
35. Sotillo R, Garcia JF, Ortega S, et al. Invasive melanoma in Cdk4-targeted mice. *Proc Natl Acad Sci U S A* 2001;98:13312.
36. Iozzo RV, Eichstetter I, Danielson KG. Aberrant expression of the growth factor Wnt-5A in human malignancy. *Cancer Res* 1995;55:3495.
37. Bittner M, Meltzer P, Chen Y, et al. Molecular classification of cutaneous malignant melanoma by gene expression profiling. *Nature* 2000;406:536.
38. Weeraratna AT, Jiang Y, Hostetter G, et al. Wnt5a signaling directly affects cell motility and invasion of metastatic melanoma. *Cancer Cell* 2002;1:279.
39. Pollock PM, Cohen-Solal K, Sood R, et al. Melanoma mouse model implicates metabotropic glutamate signaling in melanocytic neoplasia. *Nat Genet* 2003;34:108.
40. Clark WH. Tumor progression and the nature of cancer. *Br J Cancer* 1991;64:631.
41. Hanahan D, Weinberg RA. The hallmarks of cancer. *Cell* 2000;100:57.
42. Hsu M, Andl T, Li G, et al. Cadherin repertoire determines partner-specific gap junctional communication during melanoma progression. *J Cell Sci* 2000;113:1535.
43. Li G, Satyamoorthy K, Herlyn M. N-cadherin-mediated intercellular interactions promote survival and migration of melanoma cells. *Cancer Res* 2001;61:3819.
44. Shih IM, Speicher D, Hsu MY, et al. Melanoma cell-cell interactions are mediated through heterophilic Mel-CAM/ligand adhesion. *Cancer Res* 1997;57:3835.
45. Satyamoorthy K, Muyrers J, Meier F, et al. Mel-CAM-specific genetic suppressor elements inhibit melanoma growth and invasion through loss of gap junctional communication. *Oncogene* 2001;20:4676.
46. Hsu MY, Shih DT, Meier FE, et al. Adenoviral gene transfer of beta3 integrin subunit induces conversion from radial to vertical growth phase in primary human melanoma. *Am J Pathol* 1998;153:1435.
47. Nesbit M, Nesbit HK, Bennett J, et al. Basic fibroblast growth factor induces a transformed phenotype in normal human melanocytes. *Oncogene* 1999;18:6469.
48. George D. Platelet-derived growth factor receptors: a therapeutic target in solid tumors. *Semin Oncol* 2001;28:27.
49. Reed JA, McNutt NS, Prieto VG, et al. Expression of transforming growth factor-beta 2 in malignant melanoma correlates with the depth of tumor invasion. Implications for tumor progression. *Am J Pathol* 1994;145:97.
50. Berking C, Takemoto R, Schaider H, et al. Transforming growth factor-beta1 increases survival of human melanoma through stroma remodeling. *Cancer Res* 2001;61:8306.
51. Halaban R. The regulation of normal melanocyte proliferation. *Pigment Cell Res* 2000; 13:4.
52. Herlyn M, Thurin J, Balaban G, et al. Characteristics of cultured human melanocytes isolated from different stages of tumor progression. *Cancer Res* 1985;45:5670.

CHARLES M. BALCH
MICHAEL B. ATKINS
ARTHUR J. SOBER

SECTION **2**

Cutaneous Melanoma

Cutaneous melanoma is the malignancy derived from the melanocyte, the cell responsible for pigmentation in humans. Once considered a rare tumor with an unpredictable natural history and a frequently lethal outcome, cutaneous melanoma is now recognized as one of the more common cancers in humans, with a reasonably predictable natural history and, when the lesion is detected early in its course, a quite favorable outcome. Because this tumor is on the cutaneous surface, most often is pigmented, and most often has certain distinct clinical features, both self-recognition and early recognition by the health care professional is possible.

Melanoma continues to exhibit rather dramatic epidemiologic changes. Its incidence is rising faster than that of any other solid tumor, and although death rates are beginning to level off, melanoma is affecting an increasingly younger population of adults, and even children, and is therefore a major threat to people in the most productive years of life. It is now the fifth most common cancer in men and the seventh most common in women.[1] It is one of the few remaining cancers for which mortality rates are increasing, especially in men older than 60 years of age. Because one of the associated risk factors, ultraviolet irradiation from natural and artificial light sources, is modifiable, greater emphasis is being placed on screening of and prevention in high-risk populations. Since the last edition of this textbook, advances have continued in the application of intralymphatic mapping and sentinel node excision; in the understanding of predictive factors, which has led to a totally revised staging system; in the availability of new agents for systemic treatment; and in the understanding of the biology and genetics of melanoma.

EPIDEMIOLOGY

Melanoma incidence has risen continuously within the United States and throughout the world in most white populations.[2] It was estimated that 55,100 cases of invasive melanoma would be diagnosed in the United States in 2004 (4% of all cancer cases) and that 7910 patients would die of the disease (1.4% of all cancer deaths).[1]

INCIDENCE AND MORTALITY RATES

The incidence of melanoma has continued to increase in the United States (Fig. 38.2-1) and in most white populations throughout the world.[2,3] Incidence rates vary dramatically, ranging from as low as 0.2 per 100,000 for females in India to 42.0 per 100,000, among females in North Queensland, Australia. Rates in males range from 0.5 per 100,000 to 49.0 per 100,000, respectively. Since the Surveillance, Epidemiology, and End Results program began collecting accurate incidence data in 1973, the incidence in the United States has risen from 6.7 per 100,000 in white males and 5.9 per 100,000 in white

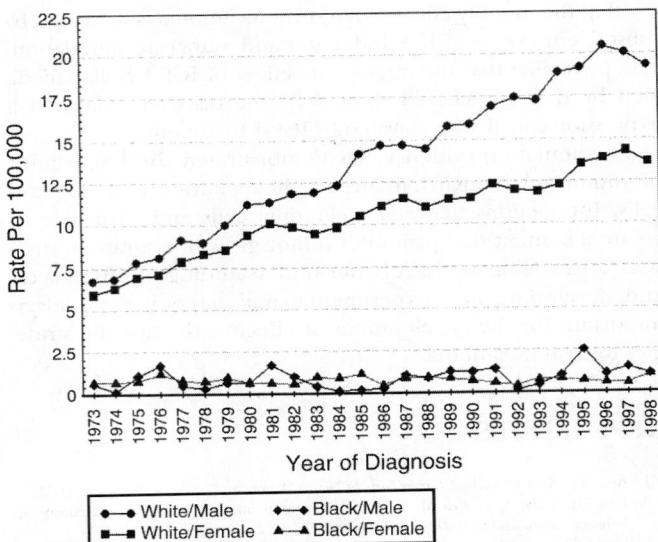

FIGURE 38.2-1. Age-adjusted melanoma incidence rates in the United States by race and gender, 1973 to 1998. (From the National Cancer Institute Surveillance, Epidemiology, and End Results program.)

females to a high in white males of 20.4 per 100,000 in 1996 and in white females of 14.3 per 100,000 in 1997 (see Fig 38.2-1). The current estimated lifetime risk of melanoma among white Americans is approximately 1 in 74; stratified according to gender, the lifetime probability of developing invasive melanoma is 1 in 58 in men and 1 in 82 in women.[2]

The increase in melanoma incidence is probably real, because the absolute number of patients dying from melanoma in the United States continues to rise even though the survival rate for melanoma overall has improved from a 40% 5-year survival rate in the 1940s to the current 5-year survival rate of approximately 89% (Fig. 38.2-2). Deaths from melanoma have also risen consistently over the past several decades, although the slope of the rise is substantially lower than that for the increase in incidence (see Figs. 38.2-1 and 38.2-2), and, in fact, mortality may already have peaked.[2,4]

For white populations in Australia, New Zealand, and Europe, similar trends are seen.[4] In all databases the mortality is higher among males than among females. The highest mortality rate in the world is noted for males in New Zealand, with 5.3 per 100,000 per year; the rate for females is 3.2 per 100,000 per year. The United States ranks seventh in the world for melanoma mortality at 2.7 per 100,000 per year for males and does not appear in the top ten countries for female mortality.

Melanoma has become one of the most survivable cancers, with an 89% 5-year survival rate for whites treated in the United States from 1992 to 1997 according to the Surveillance, Epidemiology, and End Results data.[2] Nonetheless, because melanoma affects, on average, a relatively young group of patients, it is disproportionately overrepresented when average years of life lost is considered.[5] The countries with the highest numbers of survivors of melanoma in the world are Australia and the United States.[2]

GEOGRAPHIC DIFFERENCES

Lancaster first reported an association between sun exposure and melanoma development.[6] There appears to be a latitude

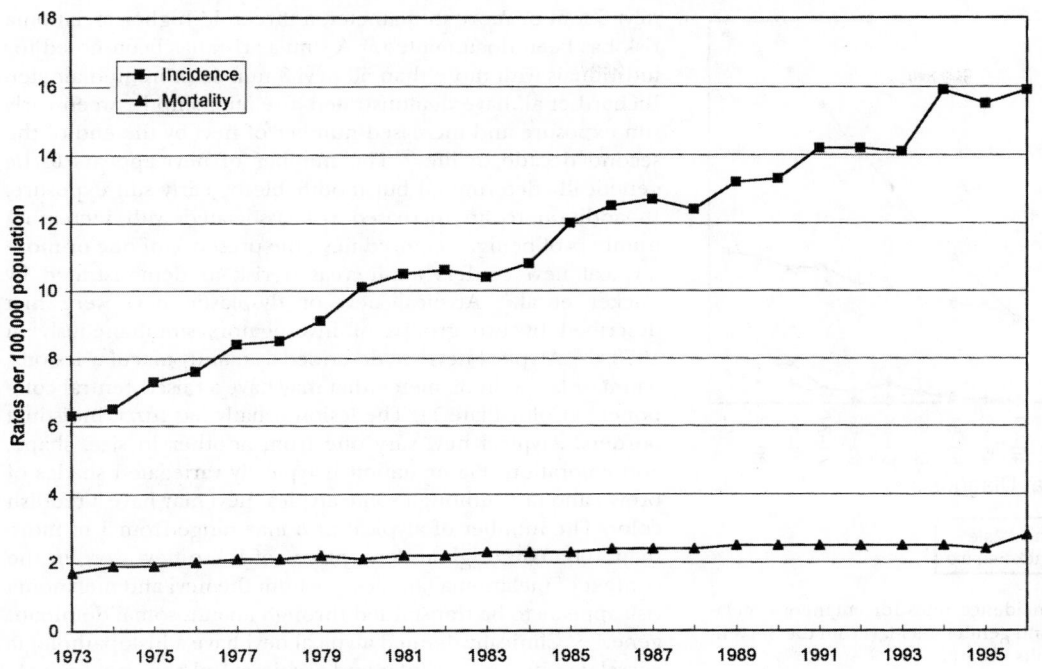

FIGURE 38.2-2. Melanoma incidence and mortality in the United States, 1973 to 1996. All rates are age-adjusted to the 1970 U.S. standard population. (Incidence data are derived from Surveillance, Epidemiology, and End Results Cancer Incidence 1973–2001 Public-Use Data.)

gradient for light-skinned whites. Those living closer to the equator have higher melanoma rates than those living farther from the equator. Such gradients have been observed within the United States and Australia; however, within Europe the incidence rates for individuals from northern European countries are higher than those in the Mediterranean area.[7,8] This paradox has been explained by differences in constitutive and facultative pigmentation phenotypes. In migrant studies it has been shown that individuals who move to sunny areas in childhood develop melanoma at rates higher than those of their country of origin and similar to those of their adopted country.[9,10]

GENDER AND AGE DISTRIBUTION

In the United States and Australia the gender ratio of melanoma is approximately 1:1. In northern Europe there has been a female predominance, but this trend appears to be diminishing. The mean age of melanoma patients is in the early fifties. Thus, melanomas occur in relatively young individuals with a mean age approximately one decade earlier than that for the more common solid tumors, such as lung, breast, colon, and prostate cancers. While melanoma in the first decade of life is rare (approximately 1 case per million per year), it is not unusual to see melanomas from the mid-teen years onward.[11] When melanoma does occur in children and young adolescents, the staging and treatment approach is generally the same as in adults with melanoma.[12,13] As a result of the relatively early median age at diagnosis, melanoma is responsible for a disproportionately large percentage of useful life years lost.[5] In fact, melanoma is the leading cause of cancer-related mortality in women 25 to 35 years of age. In the United States the increase noted in mortality from 1973 to 1997 has primarily been in age groups older than 65 years. There has been an especially alarming increase in mortality

in men older than age 60. Among males younger than age 60, rates either stabilized or declined, whereas in those older than age 60, rates have increased relative to those for comparably aged females.

RACIAL DIFFERENCES

Examination of incidence rates in nonwhite populations fails to show the increase seen in the white population,[4] although changes in the melanoma incidence rates among nonwhite populations are less reliable because the frequency of melanoma is considerably lower in these groups. Incidence rates among black Africans and African Americans are extremely low and are at least an order of magnitude lower than in whites[14] (Fig. 38.2-3). In addition, the distribution of melanoma by body site shows a preponderance of lesions on acral locations, especially the foot, as well as nail beds and mucosal surfaces. Although the incidence in black Africans and African Americans appears stable, there may be a slight increase in incidence among Hispanic individuals. Data from Puerto Rico suggest a doubling of the incidence from 1.5 per 100,000 to 3.0 per 100,000 over the past 10 years.[15]

ANATOMIC DISTRIBUTION

The anatomic sites that are most common are the back in white males and the lower leg from knee to ankle and back in females. Although melanomas can occur at almost any site on the body, they are less common in areas where the skin is doubly covered, such as the boxer short/panty area in men and women, and the breasts in women. Certain types of melanomas show a predilection for certain locations of the body. Lentigo maligna melanoma (LMM) most frequently affects the sun-damaged surfaces of the head and neck in older individuals.

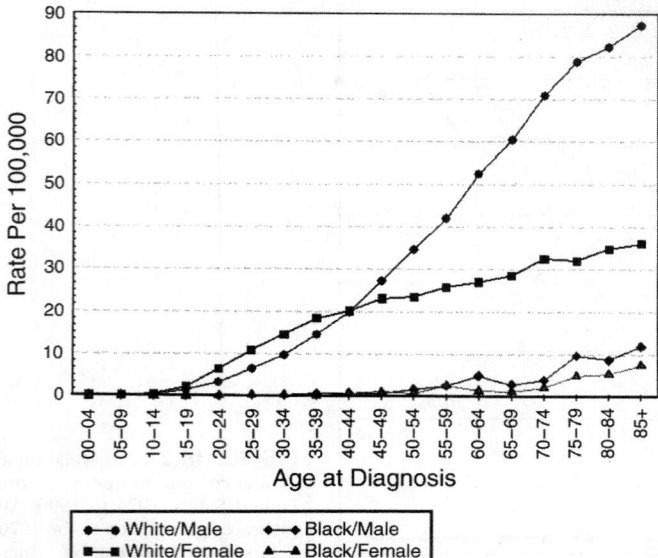

FIGURE 38.2-3.   Age-specific incidence rates for cutaneous melanoma in the United States by race and gender, 1998. (From the Surveillance, Epidemiology, and End Results program.)

Acral lentiginous melanoma (ALM), as reflected in the name, affects peripheral locations such as the palms and soles as well as the nail beds.

RISK FACTORS

SUN EXPOSURE

As noted previously in Geographic Differences, Lancaster in 1956 reported a relationship between ambient sun exposure and melanoma incidence.[6] Numerous case-control studies have been performed since then that have demonstrated a relationship between intense sun exposure early in life and an increased risk for melanoma in some individuals.[16-20] There are paradoxes, however, in that it has also been shown that individuals who develop a tan decrease their risk for melanoma. Armstrong and Kricker have estimated that approximately two-thirds of the world's cases of melanoma may be related to sun exposure.[21] There is a twofold to threefold increased risk for melanoma in those individuals who burn easily, tan poorly, and had at least one episode of traumatic sunburn before the age of 18 years. Although this may not appear as substantial as certain other relative risks—for example, the enormous relative risk associated with familial melanoma—the population-attributable fraction for those susceptible to traumatic sunburn is much larger. At the present time, sun exposure is a modifiable environmental factor; therefore, it would seem reasonable to continue to support avoidance of traumatic exposure in younger individuals especially as a preventative strategy.

NUMBER OF MOLES

The number of moles has also been identified as an important factor related to melanoma risk.[22,23] In individuals with five nevi 6 mm or more in diameter, a threefold higher melanoma risk has been documented.[24] A similar risk has been noted for individuals with more than 50 nevi 3 mm or more in diameter. Richard et al. have demonstrated a relationship between early sun exposure and increased number of nevi by the end of the second decade of life.[25] The number of nevi appears to be genetically determined but modifiable by early sun exposure. In addition to an increased risk associated with increasing numbers of benign acquired nevi, the presence of one or more atypical nevi confers an increased risk as demonstrated by Tucker et al.[26] Atypical nevi or dysplastic nevi were first described by two groups of investigators simultaneously in 1978.[27,28] Atypical nevi are described as mainly macular lesions, 5 mm or larger in diameter, that may have a raised central component (Color Plate 1). The lesion usually has fuzzy, indistinct borders. Atypical nevi vary one from another in size, shape, and coloration. Pigmentation is typically variegated shades of brown and tan, although some atypical nevi may have a reddish color. The number of atypical nevi may range from 1 to more than 100. The original descriptions of these nevi were in the context of melanoma families in whom the nevi and melanoma risk appears to be transmitted through an autosomal dominant gene.[27,28] Clinically defined atypical nevi have a histopathologic correlate with both cellular and architectural abnormalities. At present there is a lack of universal agreement on the diagnostic criteria histopathologically. The frequency of atypical moles in the population at large has been estimated to range from 5% to above 15%.[29,30] Atypical nevi appear to be both a risk factor for melanoma and at times a precursor lesion. In melanomas arising in patients with familial melanoma, the majority of melanomas appear to arise in association with atypical moles. In one study the age-adjusted incidence of melanoma was more than ten times higher for patients with atypical nevi than for the general population.[31] Increasing number of atypical nevi is associated with an increased risk for melanoma.[31-34] Tucker et al. noted that the presence of a single dysplastic nevus results in a 2.3-fold increased risk for melanoma, whereas having more than five lesions leads to a more than tenfold increased risk for developing melanoma.[26]

CONGENITAL NEVI

Congenital nevi, present in approximately 1% of the population by prevalence, have also been considered as precursor lesions for melanoma. This has been especially true for the giant congenital nevus that affects between 1 in 20,000 and 1 in 50,000 individuals. Definitions vary for what is considered a giant congenital nevus. Such definitions range from nevi that are too large to be removed by surgical excision with direct approximation of the margins without skin rotation or grafting, to nevi that cover more than 144 in.[2] of body surface area. Most individuals would consider a nevus larger than 20 cm in one dimension to fall into the giant category (see Color Plate 1*F*). Lifetime risk for melanoma development with giant congenital nevi has been estimated to be approximately 6%.[35,36] The greatest risk appears to be in the first decade of life. Although most melanomas arise at the dermoepidermal junction, melanomas arising in giant congenital nevi usually do so in the deeper reticular dermis or subcutaneous locations, which makes early detection difficult to nearly impossible. The risk for melanoma associated with the much more common, small congenital nevus is controversial, and although some papers cite a modest increase in risk, this is not accepted by all.[37]

PATIENT HISTORY OF MELANOMA

A patient history of melanoma is also associated with an increased risk of developing a second or additional primary melanoma. In one study of patients with multiple primary tumors, one-third of melanomas were noted concomitantly and two-thirds were noted sequentially.[38] Because of the concomitant occurrence of melanoma, a full body skin examination of patients in whom a melanoma has been diagnosed is recommended. The mean interval between primary diagnoses is 3 years with a range extending to 30 years.[38] It has been estimated that approximately 5% to 10% of melanoma patients will develop a second primary melanoma over their lifetime. However, within familial melanoma, the frequency of second primaries is considerably higher.[39] Eight percent of patients with multiple primary melanomas were found to have germline mutations in CDKN2A.[39]

FAMILY HISTORY

Approximately 10% of melanoma patients appear to have another close relative with cutaneous melanoma. In 1978, Clark et al. and Lynch et al. independently reported on aggregations of melanoma within families in which, in addition to melanoma, the affected family members also had multiple clinically atypical nevi.[27,28] Initial evaluations of these families suggested that there was a melanoma susceptibility gene on chromosome band 1p36.[40] Further studies, however, excluded chromosome 1 from the area of greatest concern.[41] More recent studies have suggested a linkage to chromosome 9p21.[42] Further studies resulted in the isolation of a gene termed *CDKN2A*, which is a tumor suppressor gene.[43–45] This genetic abnormality appears to represent the molecular basis for melanoma susceptibility in a subset of familial melanoma cases.[46] An abnormality at this location seems to occur in approximately one-fourth of unselected families with heritable melanoma.[47] Because of the recognized occurrence of familial melanoma, it is recommended that first-degree family members of patients with melanoma be screened by their health care providers for the possibility of melanoma. There appears to be an interaction between familial melanoma and the presence of atypical nevi. It has been estimated that the lifetime risk for melanoma development in an individual who has had two first-degree family members affected with melanoma and has atypical nevi exceeds 50%.[48] In familial melanoma the incidence of melanoma is highly concentrated in family members with atypical nevi; however, melanoma may occur in family members without atypical nevi.[49]

TRANSPLANTATION AND IMMUNOSUPPRESSION

Melanoma risk is modestly increased in patients with an organ transplant. The increased risk is estimated to be approximately threefold.[50] In a study of 38 children with renal transplants, the total body nevus counts were noted to have increased, and data suggested that this increase was associated with the duration of immunosuppression.[51] A similar increase in nevus counts has been reported in patients positive for human immunodeficiency virus,[52] although a concomitant increase in melanoma in this population has so far not been documented.

PREGNANCY AND ESTROGEN USE

Melanomas may occur during pregnancy and in women taking birth control pills or estrogen replacement therapy. However, after extensive study, no convincing evidence has been found to link melanoma occurrence with any of these factors. To date there has not been shown to be an increased frequency of melanoma during pregnancy.[53,54] Nor has there been a convincing study showing a relationship between prior oral contraceptive use or estrogen replacement therapy and an increased risk for melanoma development. The prognosis of melanoma in pregnancy appears to be similar to that of melanoma in nonpregnant women as long as the melanoma is treated promptly.[55] In one study, however, it was shown that melanomas occurring during pregnancy were thicker on average than those occurring in nonpregnant women.[55] Changes in moles during pregnancy have been observed. Consequently, women with many atypical moles or a history of melanoma should be followed closely by a dermatologist during pregnancy. If any woman develops a pigmented lesion of concern during pregnancy, prompt biopsy for histologic evaluation is indicated.

OTHER RISK FACTORS

Other factors associated with a relatively increased risk for melanoma include older age, certain phenotypic factors, and psoralen plus ultraviolet A light (PUVA) therapy. There is approximately a 100-fold difference in melanoma rates between individuals younger than age 10 and those older than age 15.[56] Melanoma incidence increases with age, as is observed for other solid tumors. Fair complexion, freckling, easy burning, poor tanning, blond or red hair color, and blue or gray eyes have all been associated with a modestly increased relative risk for melanoma in the twofold to threefold range. Individuals who have had extensive exposure (more than 250 treatment sessions) to PUVA therapy for psoriasis have been shown to have a significantly increased risk for melanoma 15 years after treatment.[57]

XERODERMA PIGMENTOSUM

Individuals with xeroderma pigmentosum have a rare genetic DNA defect in repair of ultraviolet light damage and are at a considerable increased risk for developing melanoma.[58] Not only is this group at substantial increased risk, but melanomas may occur quite early in life and may frequently be the cause of death. This ultra-high-risk group needs a special monitoring program for melanoma as well as for other types of skin cancer, and absolute protection from sunlight exposure is essential.

PREVENTION AND SCREENING

Because the treatment of late-stage melanoma is of limited efficacy, emphasis on early diagnosis and prevention remains a priority.

SUNSCREENS

As noted earlier in Sun Exposure, the one modifiable environmental factor that may lead to a lowering of melanoma risk is reduction in ultraviolet exposure from both natural and artificial sources. A three-pronged attack is recommended to avoid excessive exposure. Patients are advised to avoid the midday sun from 10:00 a.m. to 2:00 p.m. or 11:00 a.m. to 3:00 p.m. depending on the time zone and time of year. Seventy percent of the ultraviolet light in the sunburn wavelengths impacts the earth during that period. Recreational activities can frequently be scheduled either earlier or later in the day. Clothing protection is the second line of defense. Hats with broad brims, especially those covering the ears, are recommended as well as shirts with short sleeves to protect the shoulders. Although special sun-protective fabrics are being marketed, in general, clothing with a tight weave that one cannot see through is effective in blocking ultraviolet light. A third line of defense, which is somewhat more controversial, is the use of broad-spectrum sunscreens with a sun protection factor of 15 or higher. Sunscreens are demonstrably effective in reducing acute sunburn risk. It is less clear, however, whether sunscreens are beneficial in long-term use for melanoma risk reduction.[59–65] There is no conclusive epidemiologic evidence for a benefit of sunscreen use for melanoma protection, and on the other hand, paradoxical reports of an increased melanoma risk in patients with sunscreen use has been reported. Explanations for these observations include (1) increased sunscreen use by individuals susceptible to both sunburn and melanoma and (2) the inability of most sunscreens to block UVA. In fact, sunscreens, by preventing sunburn, may enable sun-sensitive individuals to extend their time in the sun, which potentially increases exposure to harmful components of sunlight, such as UVA, that are not blocked by most sunscreens.

SELF-EXAMINATION

There are two pieces of evidence to suggest that self-examination may be of value in improved melanoma detection. In a study by Koh et al., approximately one-half of melanomas were detected by the patient or family member.[66] Women are most likely to detect their own melanomas as well as those on their spouses.[66] In another study by Berwick et al., patients performing self-examination appeared to have melanomas that were detected in an earlier microstage.[67] Teaching aids for patients on how to perform skin self-examination are available from the American Cancer Society and the American Academy of Dermatology. Having a spouse, partner, or parent participate in the examination of the back may be helpful, especially in detecting melanomas in males. The ideal frequency of performing skin self-examinations remains to be established, but 6- to 8-week intervals seems reasonable at the present time.

EXCISION OF ATYPICAL MOLES

In general the routine removal of nevi is not recommended as a useful technique for melanoma risk reduction. In many instances melanoma in patients with atypical nevi arise *de novo* in normal-appearing skin. It has been estimated that only 25% to 50% of melanomas arise in nevi. In those with familial melanoma, however, as many as 70% of melanomas appear to arise in nevi. All lesions that have suspicious features reaching a certain threshold should be considered for histopathologic evaluation. The threshold for removal varies from physician to physician. Being aware of the clinical features of melanoma and having particular concern for changes in individual lesions results in the recognition of most melanomas. Processing of a biopsy specimen from a suspicious pigmented lesion should include serial sectioning, because one portion of the lesion may be benign, whereas another portion may show an associated melanoma.

DIAGNOSIS WITH NONINVASIVE TECHNIQUES

Over the past two decades numerous techniques have been proposed to improve on the unaided visual examination of the skin for the diagnosis of melanoma. A review by Marghoob et al. summarizes many of these techniques.[68] Instruments are available to access structures at four levels: subcellular elements, single cells, cellular aggregates, and gross clinical lesions. Tools that have been of definitive benefit in the evaluation of pigmented lesions include handheld magnifying lenses that magnify threefold to tenfold, Wood's light devices, epiluminescence microscopy, and lesional photography. A magnifying lens is of value in assessment of pigment pattern and distribution. In general, more irregular patterns are associated with an increased likelihood of a malignant process being present. Conversely, regular patterns are more typical of benign processes. Wood's light (long-wave ultraviolet) enhances epidermal pigmentation as well as enhancing areas where pigmentation has been lost. This tool is helpful in assessing the margins of lentigo maligna and LMM as well as in finding the residual site of a possibly regressed primary melanoma in patients who present with regional or distant metastases and no known primary tumor. The leukoderma associated with stage III melanoma[69,70] is also enhanced with the use of a Wood's light as is the evaluation of halo nevi. Individual lesional photography and total cutaneous photography has at times assisted in the early recognition of melanoma by documenting the presence of a subtle change that might not have been recognized without prior photographic documentation.[71]

Epiluminescence microscopy or dermatoscopy, although commonly used in certain European countries, is used by only a minority of dermatologists in the United States. Epiluminescence microscopy has proven beneficial in experienced hands in the assessment of pigmented lesions that are difficult to diagnose.[72,73] It is used primarily to exclude benign pigmented lesions such as seborrheic keratoses or various vascular lesions and certain dysplastic nevi from biopsy. Although the presence of certain features such as radial streaming, pseudopods, and a blue-gray veil are highly associated with the presence of melanoma, their absence does not rule out melanoma. Pehamberger et al. have demonstrated an improvement in diagnostic ability in the 10% range with epiluminescence microscopy for pigmented lesions that are difficult to diagnose.[74]

Various computerized digital imaging devices are also currently being used to analyze mathematically the likelihood that a particular pigmented lesion is malignant.[75] In addition, confocal scanning laser microscopy can be used to evaluate *in vivo* the histologic appearance of melanocytes within the epidermis and in the upper dermis.[76] These tools should be considered investigational at present, and further advances are required before their general clinical application can be considered.

COST EFFECTIVENESS OF SCREENING

Koh et al. have demonstrated that cost effectiveness of a total skin examination for skin cancer detection is at least as good as that of Papanicolaou smear testing for cervical cancer and stool guaiac testing for colon cancer.[77] Because the majority of skin examinations can be performed at the same time that the patient receives a general physical examination, the incremental cost of such an evaluation would be modest. The downstream cost of the resultant increased numbers of confirmatory dermatologic evaluations and biopsies of suspicious but ultimately benign lesions has yet to be fully assessed.

For more than a decade, the American Academy of Dermatology has performed yearly voluntary open access screening examinations for the general public. Approximately 1 individual in 300 who has presented for screening has been diagnosed with melanoma. The vast majority of these tumors have been detected quite early in their evolution, which raises the possibility that increased screening will lead to an increase in diagnosis of early (surgically curable) melanoma.[78,79]

An additional approach to evaluating the cost effectiveness of early diagnosis of melanoma is to examine the overall cost of the management of a year's worth of melanoma cases in the United States. Such a study was done by Tsao et al., who showed that the overall cost of melanoma management in the United States was $563 million dollars in 1997.[80] When the cost was apportioned by stage, the vast majority of the dollars (more than 90%) was spent on the treatment of patients with stage III or IV disease. Because patients with stage III and IV melanomas comprise fewer than 30% of the total melanoma population, considerably less than 10% of the expenditure was related to the costs associated with treatment of stage I and stage II disease. Because of the immense cost of treatment of more advanced disease, one can argue that additional efforts directed at early recognition might result in an overall cost savings by preventing melanomas in some patients from ever reaching more advanced stages.[80]

DIAGNOSIS OF MELANOMA

CHARACTERISTICS OF MELANOMA

The cardinal clinical feature of cutaneous melanoma is a pigmented skin lesion that changes visibly over a period of months to years.[81] Sometimes the change is so gradual that the patient is unaware of it. Lesions that change over the course of days are typically inflammatory in nature. However, as a general rule, any lesion noted to have changed in color, shape, size, or elevation warrants medical attention (Color Plate 2). Changes in color, shape, contour, and size are highlighted in the ABCD mnemonic (Asymmetry, Border, Color, Diameter) that was developed as an aid to identify biologically early curable lesions (Table 38.2-1). There are now suggestions for expanding this mnemonic to the letters A through F (see Table 38.2-1). Symptoms of bleeding, itching, tenderness, and ulceration can be associated with cutaneous melanomas. Imaging techniques such as dermatoscopy and *in vivo* confocal scanning laser microscopy may expand the clinician's ability to correctly diagnose a suspicious lesion in a noninvasive fashion.[81]

There are four main types of clinically recognized melanomas, each with a histopathologic correlate (see Color Plate 2). Three of the types, superficial spreading melanoma (SSM), LMM, and ALM, have a recognized period of lateral growth within the skin before deep downward growth appears. The fourth type, nodular melanoma, does not have a recognized period of lateral growth but appears to grow downward from the outset. Each subtype of melanoma has certain recognizable clinical features (see Color Plate 2).

SUPERFICIAL SPREADING MELANOMA

SSM is the most common type, representing approximately 70% of all melanomas. SSM is the most common type of cutaneous melanoma occurring in the white population and is largely responsible for the increased incidence of melanoma noted over the past few decades.[81,82] Melanoma arising in a preexisting dysplastic nevus is usually of superficial spreading type. It can occur on all body surface areas but is most common on the torso of men and on the lower legs and back of women. It has been estimated that SSM may be present from 1 to 7 years before diagnosis. The lesion presents as a plaque with a barely perceptible elevation above the plane of the skin. Typically, SSMs have irregular borders, variation in both pigment pattern and coloration, and often fulfill the ABCDs of melanoma diagnosis[83] (see Color Plate 2A, B). Development of a nodule within the plaque indicates the onset of the vertical growth phase and is associated with higher risk for metastasis and death.

TABLE 38.2-1.   ABCDs of Cutaneous Melanoma and Possible Changes as Well as Mnemonic for Subungual Melanoma

	Current	*Possible Change*			*Subungual Melanoma[a]*
A	Lesional asymmetry			A	Age (peak incidence fifth to seventh decades of life in African Americans, Asians, and Native Americans)
B	Border irregularity			B	Brown to black with a breadth of ≥3 mm; variegated borders
C	Color variation			C	Change in the nail band or lack of change in the nail morphology (despite adequate treatment)
D	Diameter >6 mm	Different		D	Digit most commonly involved (great toe or thumb)
		E	Evolution	E	Extension of pigment onto the proximal and/or lateral nail fold (Hutchinson's sign)
		E	Elevation		
		E	Enlargement		
		F	"Funny looking"	F	Family or personal history of melanoma or dysplastic nevus

[a]Ref. 86.

NODULAR MELANOMA

The nodular melanoma growth pattern is found in approximately 15% of melanomas and is the second most common type by frequency. Nodular melanoma can occur on any surface of the body. By definition, nodular melanoma arises without an apparent precursor radial growth phase. It may arise either in normal-appearing skin or in a preexisting nevus. The lesion appears as a papule or nodule, often is relatively symmetrical, and may be uniform in color. The degree of pigmentation may range from dark brown-black to blue-gray to completely amelanotic (see Color Plate 2*C*). Amelanotic lesions are usually recognized as a skin lesion that is either new or changing. These lesions may become ulcerated and commonly bleed either spontaneously or as a result of trauma. These lesions are invariably in the vertical growth phase when recognized and therefore virtually never fall into the minimal-risk group.

ACRAL LENTIGINOUS MELANOMA

ALMs comprise approximately 10% of melanomas.[84] These tumors appear on palms, soles, and mucosal surfaces, and in subungual locations (see Color Plate 2*D*).[81,82] ALM occurs mainly on the palms, soles, subungual regions, and digits of individuals of all ethnicities, including African, Hispanic, and Asian individuals. It appears to be a form of melanoma that is genetically distinct from the other growth patterns and is probably not influenced by ultraviolet irradiation from sunlight as are the other types of growth patterns. The radial growth phase presents as a macule of pigmentation with irregularity of border and irregularity of pigment distribution in the locations noted. As with other melanomas, the presence of a nodule within the macular lesion indicates the presence of vertical growth and is associated with increased likelihood of metastasis and death. Because of location, these lesions tend to be diagnosed later than other forms of melanoma. Special attention needs to be devoted to the diagnosis of subungual melanomas.[85,86] The ABCD mnemonic is also used in describing these melanomas, but with some variation in the definition (see Table 38.2-1). The most common locations are under the great toenail and, for hand lesions, under the thumbnail. Subungual melanomas arise in the nail matrix. Therefore, diagnostic biopsy must include the matrix to establish the presence of melanoma. Clinically, subungual melanoma is suspected when the nail bed contains a new or enlarging pigmented streak wider than 3 mm. The presence of pigmentation encroaching on the posterior nail fold (Hutchinson's sign) is a worrisome feature that should also suggest the possibility of a melanoma.

LENTIGO MALIGNA MELANOMA

LMMs comprise approximately 5% of melanomas and occur nearly exclusively in older individuals on chronically sun-exposed skin (see Color Plate 2*E*).[81,82] More than 75% of patients diagnosed with LMM are older than 60 years of age. These melanomas most commonly occur on the skin of the face. The radial growth phase precursor to invasive melanoma, known as *lentigo maligna* or *Hutchinson's freckle*, usually grows slowly for periods of up to 15 or more years as a pigmented macule before invasion develops (see Color Plate 1*E*). Lentigo

maligna is associated histologically with a proliferation of atypical melanocytes along the dermoepidermal junction extending down the rete and appendages. With lentigo maligna, invasion through the basement membrane has not occurred. Not all lentigo maligna lesions evolve to melanomas, and the frequency of transformation has been estimated in the range of 5% to as high as one-third.[87] Lentigo maligna has irregular borders and variations in pigmentation with shades of tan, brown, and sometimes black (see Color Plate 1*E*). Lentigo maligna and LMM may undergo partial spontaneous regression, so that a portion of the lesion may be disappearing as another area shows extension. The development of elevation within the lesion indicates the presence of invasion, and at this point, the lesion is clinically termed LMM.

DESMOPLASTIC MELANOMA

Desmoplastic melanoma, first described in 1971, is an uncommon variant that may be suspected clinically when it arises in association with a preexisting pigmented lesion such as lentigo maligna.[81,82] When the lesion is not pigmented, it is often mistaken clinically for a scar, a fibroma, or a basal cell carcinoma. One classic presentation is as a fleshy or firm nonpigmented nodule reminiscent of a scar. Desmoplastic melanoma occurs most often in the head and neck area and the upper back, but also affects acral sites and mucosae such as the vulva or gingiva.[82] Desmoplastic melanoma more commonly affects males in the sixth to eighth decades of life.[81,82,88–91] It is associated with a very high incidence of local recurrences but a very low incidence of regional lymph node metastases, either at time of presentation or during long-term follow-up.[92] This type of melanoma represents 1% to 2% of melanomas and is characterized microscopically by the presence of fibrous-appearing cells.[93–95] The malignant melanocytes in desmoplastic melanoma have a tendency to recur locally and to invade nerves (neurotropism). Clinically desmoplastic melanomas appear to present in two distinct manners. The first is as a relatively amelanotic nodule in sun-exposed areas of older individuals (see Color Plate 2*F*). Diagnosis is difficult to make clinically and may also be difficult to establish histopathologically. This type of desmoplastic melanoma may be confused clinically with a sarcoma, scar, or dermatofibroma. Immunohistochemically these lesions stain positive for S-100 positive and negative for HMB45. The second form of clinical presentation is as the vertical growth phase of a lesion arising in what appears clinically to be a typical lentigo maligna. Many desmoplastic melanomas are not recognized until they have reached a substantial thickness.

PROGNOSTIC FACTORS

The Melanoma Staging Committee of the American Joint Committee on Cancer (AJCC) used a new evidence-based methodology to propose major revisions to the tumor, node, and metastasis (TNM) staging system.[96,99] In preparation for their final recommendations to the AJCC and the International Union Against Cancer (UICC), members of the Melanoma Staging Committee and additional consultants merged prospectively accumulated melanoma outcome data obtained from 13 prospective databases into a single large database for

TABLE 38.2-2. Cox Regression Analysis of Data for 13,581 Melanoma Patients without Evidence of Nodal or Distant Metastases

Variable	DF	Chi-Square Value (Wald)	P Value	Risk Ratio	95% CL
Thickness	1	244.3	<.00001	1.558	1.473–1.647
Ulceration	1	189.5	<.00001	1.901	1.735–2.083
Age	1	45.6	<.00001	1.101	1.071–1.132
Site	1	41.0	<.00001	1.338	1.224–1.463
Level	1	32.7	<.00001	1.214	1.136–1.297
Gender	1	15.1	.001	0.836	0.764–0.915

CL, confidence limits; DF, degrees of freedom. (Modified from ref. 97.)

the purposes of validating and making final adjustments to the proposed revisions of the melanoma staging system.[97–99]

This database contained data on a total of 30,450 melanoma patients; for 17,600 of these (58%), information was available for all of the factors required for the proposed TNM classification and stage grouping analysis. Of the 17,600 patients included in this analysis, 12,837 (73%), 8633 (49%), and 2485 (14%) had at least 5 years, 10 years, or 20 years of follow-up information, respectively.

PROGNOSTIC FACTORS IN PRIMARY MELANOMA (STAGES I AND II)

In an AJCC multivariate analysis of 13,581 patients with localized primary melanoma (documented either clinically or pathologically), tumor thickness and ulceration were the two most powerful independent predictors of survival[97] (Table 38.2-2). Other statistically significant prognostic factors were patient age and gender, primary melanoma site, and Clark level of invasion.

Tumor Thickness

The AJCC classification of primary lesions is based primarily on microscopic assessment of Breslow tumor thickness.[82,100] Breslow microstaging determines the thickness of the lesion, in millimeters, using an ocular micrometer to measure its total vertical height. Breslow first established the correlation between tumor thickness and survival in 1970 when he used this measurement as a surrogate for tumor volume.[100–102] This correlation was initially confirmed in multivariate analyses performed by Balch et al.[103] and Eldh et al.[104] In a database combining results from 1786 patients treated at the University of Alabama at Birmingham (UAB) and the Sydney Melanoma Unit (SMU), tumor thickness was found to be the most statistically significant prognostic variable when both single-factor and multifactorial analyses were used.[105,106] Numerous additional studies, including the AJCC analysis, have confirmed that tumor thickness is more accurate, quantitative, and reproducible than level of invasion and represents the most important primary prognostic factor for survival in patients with stage I or II melanoma.[97]

Tumor thickness is a continuous variable for which no natural breakpoints have been identified.[97,105,107] In the AJCC analysis, a nonlinear model was used to describe the relationship between tumor thickness and survival rate. Tumor thickness is

also proportionally correlated with the risk of local recurrence, in transit metastasis, and satellites; thus it plays a role in determining surgical margins at the time of excision.[108]

Tumor Ulceration

Tumor ulceration is defined as the absence of an intact epidermis overlying a major portion of the primary melanoma based on microscopic examination of the histologic sections.[82,105,109,110] It can easily be distinguished from artifactual or traumatic disruption of the epidermis. An ulcerated melanoma (as defined histopathologically) is associated with more aggressive metastatic behavior that is independent of tumor thickness. The presence or absence of primary tumor ulceration (as documented histologically) was the second most powerful independent predictor of survival among factors analyzed by the AJCC.[97] The estimated hazard for relapse or death was twofold higher in patients with ulcerated primary tumors than in those whose tumors were not ulcerated. The only exception to this observation was thin melanomas (less than 1-mm thickness), for which the incidence of ulceration was low overall (6%), even with deeper levels of invasion. The incidence of melanoma ulceration increased as tumor thickness increased, ranging from 6% for thin lesions (less than 1 mm) to 63% for thick lesions (more than 4 mm). The duration of survival in patients with ulcerated melanomas was similar to that in patients who had nonulcerated melanomas of the next greatest AJCC tumor thickness category. This observation served as a foundation for the revised AJCC stage grouping criteria.[98,99,111] Of note, from a staging perspective, the interpretation of melanoma ulceration is one of the most reproducible of all the major histopathologic features.[112,113]

Level of Invasion

The histologic level of invasion, or Clark level, is inversely proportional to survival.[82,105,114–116] However, determination of it is variably reproducible among pathologists, and it does not correlate with survival as consistently as does tumor thickness.[97,105,114,117] For example, in a review of multiple studies in which the prognostic significance of tumor thickness was compared with that of level of invasion, tumor thickness was found to be a more significant prognostic factor with the use of multivariate analysis in 42 of 54 studies.[118] In contrast, only 8 of 48 studies demonstrated that level of invasion was a statistically significant prognostic factor.[118]

To determine the relative predictive strength of tumor thickness, ulceration, and level of invasion, a Cox multivariate analysis was performed using the AJCC melanoma database stratified according to each of the major thickness subgroups used in the melanoma T categories.[97] This analysis demonstrated that level of invasion provided more prognostic information in patients having thin lesions (1 mm or less) than did ulceration. In contrast, for all melanomas thicker than 1 mm, ulceration was clearly the most predictive factor, whereas level of invasion ranked below patient age and anatomic site of the primary melanoma. In this series, the 10-year survival rates in the 5480 patients with thin melanomas diminished with an increased level of invasion or presence of ulceration. Overall, the 10-year survival rate was significantly lower in patients who had thin melanomas with ulceration than in those who did not have ulceration (76% vs. 86%; *P* < .0001). Only 16% of the thin

TABLE 38.2-3. Five- and Ten-Year Survival Rates by Age for Patients with Stage I and II Melanomas

		Survival Rates	
Age Group	n	5-Y (% ± SE)	10-Y (% ± SE)
10–19	238	87 ± 2.6	81 ± 3.5
20–29	1400	87 ± 1.1	77 ± 1.6
30–39	2518	86 ± 0.8	77 ± 1.2
40–49	3006	85 ± 0.8	75 ± 1.2
50–59	2945	82 ± 0.9	69 ± 1.3
60–69	2805	78 ± 1.0	63 ± 1.6
70–79	1500	71 ± 1.7	56 ± 2.7
≥80	333	60 ± 5.0	43 ± 7.0

SE, standard error.
(Modified from ref. 97.)

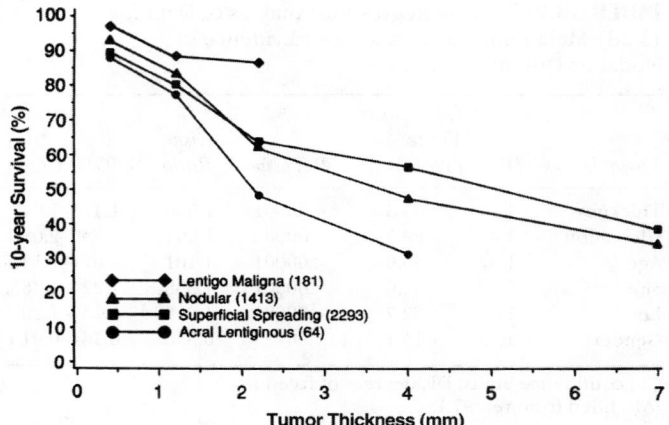

FIGURE 38.2-4. Ten-year survival rates for patients with stage I and II melanoma, according to growth pattern and tumor thickness. Among patients with melanomas of equivalent tumor thickness, those with nodular melanoma and superficial spreading melanomas had similar survival rates, those with lentigo maligna melanomas had a much more favorable prognosis, and those with acral lentiginous melanomas had the worst prognosis. Number of patients is shown in parentheses. (From ref. 105, with permission.)

melanomas had level IV invasion (less than 0.01% had level V); of these, only 8% were ulcerated.

Patient Age

In general, older patients tend to have thicker tumors. In the analysis of the AJCC melanoma database, increased patient age was also an independent prognostic factor with respect to overall survival[97] (see Table 38.2-2). This influence was observed within each of the tumor thickness groups. In addition, there was a significant, consistent decrease in survival as age increased (Table 38.2-3). More recently, an analysis of the AJCC melanoma database demonstrated that, compared to patients younger than age 60, those older than age 60 and those older than age 80 had the following adverse features: thicker melanomas that were more likely to be ulcerated and to be located on the head or neck. Elderly patients with melanoma were also more likely to be male (when comparing patients younger than 60 years vs. older than 60 years only) and had lower 5- and 10-year melanoma-specific survival rates.[105]

Anatomic Location of the Primary Tumor

In addition to patient age, the anatomic site of the primary melanoma correlated significantly with survival, with trunk and head and neck sites associated with a poorer prognosis than extremity sites.[97,105] However, because the statistical value for the anatomic site was much lower than that for melanoma thickness and ulceration (see Table 38.2-2), its impact was less than that of these other variables.

Patient Gender

The incidence of stages I and II melanoma is divided fairly equally between women and men. Although the improved survival rates seen in women are in part attributable to the higher incidence of extremity melanomas and the lower incidence of tumor ulceration, based on the analysis of the AJCC melanoma database, a small yet independent influence for gender itself may still exist.[97,105] However, when nodal status was included in the multivariate model for patients with primary melanoma, gender was no longer an independent predictor of survival,

which suggests that the impact of gender seen when only clinical and primary tumor factors were included in the model (see Table 38.2-2) could be explained, in part, by the increased frequency of occult nodal disease in men.

Growth Pattern

In the one data analysis, the melanoma growth pattern (either SSM, nodular, LMM, or ALM) was a significant prognostic indicator in univariate but not multivariate analysis.[105] After tumor thickness was accounted for, patients who had SSM and nodular melanoma had similar 10-year survival rates (Fig. 38.2-4).[105] Also, patients with LMM generally tended to have thinner lesions. In addition, patients with a thick LMM may have a better prognosis compared to patients with other histologic findings. The prognosis associated with a diagnosis of ALM is less clear. Although Gershenwald et al.[105] reported a lower 10-year survival rate, even after controlling for tumor thickness, Wells et al. did not find a significant correlation between ALM growth pattern and survival.[119]

Desmoplastic Neurotropic Melanoma Tumor Type

Desmoplastic neurotropic melanomas account for approximately 1% of all melanomas. Desmoplastic neurotropic melanomas have a high rate of local recurrence, whereas their rate of distant metastasis is believed to be similar to that of other types of melanoma. Patients with desmoplastic melanoma appear to have a lower incidence of regional metastases compared to patients with other subtypes.[89–91]

Other Prognostic Factors

As the results of new analyses from large patient data sets become available, it is likely that further refinements or adjustments of the current staging classification criteria will be considered appropriate. For example, a study of 3661 patients at the Sydney Melanoma Unit found that tumor mitotic rate was

TABLE 38.2-4. Cox Regression Analysis of Data for 1151 Patients with Stage III Melanomas (Nodal Metastases)

Variable	DF	Chi-Square Value (Wald)	P Value	Risk Ratio	95% CL
No. of metastatic nodes	1	57.616	<.00001	1.257	1.185–1.334
Tumor burden	1	40.301	<.00001	1.792	1.497–2.146
Ulceration	1	23.282	<.00001	1.582	1.313–1.906
Site	1	17.843	.0001	1.461	1.225–1.746
Age	1	13.369	.0003	1.118	1.053–1.187
Thickness	1	1.964	.1611	1.091	0.966–1.233
Level	1	0.219	.6396	1.033	0.901–1.186
Gender	1	0.006	.9407	1.007	0.836–1.213

CL, confidence limits; DF, degrees of freedom.
(From ref. 97, with permission.)

an even more powerful predictor of survival outcome than melanoma ulceration.[120] As the understanding of the angiogenic response by tumors has improved, the extent of tumor vascularity and microvessel density has been shown in a variety of solid tumors to be important for tumor progression and the metastatic process. In particular, it has been shown in a variety of neoplasms that elevated microvessel density in the tumor microenvironment correlates with poor prognosis.[121]

New approaches such as melanostatin staining and BRaf mutational status or gene expression profiling are under investigation and may eventually lead to the creation of immunohistochemical or molecularly based staging tools. Other factors such as vertical growth phase are commonly used by some centers and have been purported to have prognostic significance. These various factors are much more difficult to standardize, however, and therefore have not been incorporated into the AJCC staging system.

PROGNOSTIC FACTORS IN REGIONALLY METASTATIC MELANOMA (STAGE III): LYMPH NODE METASTASIS, SATELLITE LESIONS, AND IN TRANSIT METASTASES

American Joint Committee on Cancer Melanoma Database

Complete clinical and histopathologic data were available for 1201 patients with lymph node metastases in the AJCC melanoma database.[97,98,122] Cox multivariate analysis demonstrated that the number of metastatic nodes, tumor burden at the time of staging (i.e., microscopic vs. macroscopic), and presence or absence of ulceration of the primary melanoma were the most predictive independent factors for survival in these patients (Table 38.2-4). Although the primary tumor site and patient age were also statistically significant, they had less of an impact on survival.

Number of Metastatic Nodes

The number of nodal metastases was the most significant predictor of outcome in patients with stage III disease in the AJCC analysis (see Table 38.2-4; Table 38.2-5). Melanoma-specific survival, which was calculated from the time of the primary melanoma diagnosis, decreased significantly as nodal involvement increased (Fig. 38.2-5). The best grouping for the number of metastatic nodes that correlated with the 5-year survival rate was one versus two to three versus four or more metastatic nodes. None of the other statistical groupings, including one combining two to four metastatic nodes, delineated any greater survival differences among the cohorts analyzed.

Nodal Tumor Burden

The second most significant prognostic factor in the AJCC stage III analysis was tumor burden within the lymph nodes (microscopic or clinically occult vs. macroscopic or clinically apparent). Microscopic tumor burden was defined as nodal metastasis not detectable via clinical examination but detectable pathologically, whereas macroscopic tumor burden was defined as clinically evident and pathologically confirmed metastatic deposits. In the analysis there was a significantly lower survival duration (calculated from the time of primary melanoma diagnosis) in patients who presented with macroscopic (i.e., palpable) nodal metastases compared with patients who had microscopic (i.e., nonpalpable) nodal metastases, even after lead-time bias was accounted for.[97,123] A diminished 5-year survival rate with the increasing tumor burden was observed in all subgroups partitioned by the number of involved nodes (see Table 38.2-5).

Primary Tumor Ulceration

Ulceration was the only primary tumor feature that predicted an adverse outcome in patients with stage III disease (see Table 38.2-4). This fact implies that nodal metastasis arising from an

TABLE 38.2-5. Five-Year Survival Rates for Patients with Stage III Melanomas (Nodal Metastases) Stratified by Number of Metastatic Nodes, Ulceration, and Tumor Burden

Melanoma Ulceration	Microscopic (% ± SE)			Macroscopic (% ± SE)		
	1 Node	2 or 3 Nodes	>3 Nodes	1 Node	2 or 3 Nodes	>3 Nodes
Absent	69 ± 3.7 (n = 252)	63 ± 5.6 (n = 130)	27 ± 9.3 (n = 57)	59 ± 4.7 (n = 122)	46 ± 5.5 (n = 93)	27 ± 4.6 (n = 109)
Present	52 ± 4.1 (n = 217)	50 ± 5.7 (n = 111)	37 ± 8.8 (n = 46)	29 ± 5.0 (n = 98)	25 ± 4.4 (n = 109)	13 ± 3.5 (n = 104)

SE, standard error.
(Modified from ref. 97.)

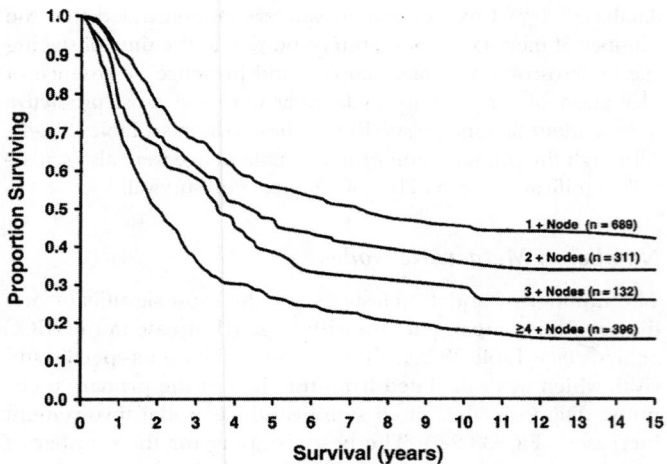

FIGURE 38.2-5. Survival curves for 1528 melanoma patients with lymph node metastases subgrouped by the actual number of metastatic nodes. (From ref. 97, with permission.)

ulcerated primary melanoma is associated with a greater capacity for metastasis to distant sites in comparison to nodal metastasis arising from a nonulcerated melanoma. This was true within each of the stage III subgroups examined, as shown by a three-way comparison that integrated subgroups according to the three most important prognostic factors—ulceration of the primary melanoma, nodal tumor burden, and number of metastatic nodes (see Table 38.2-5).

Satellites versus In Transit Metastases

The presence of clinical or microscopic satellite metastases around a primary melanoma, as well as in transit metastases between the primary melanoma and the regional lymph nodes, represents intralymphatic metastases and portends a very poor prognosis[105,124–126] (Fig. 38.2-6). Buzaid et al. assessed the definition of satellite metastases—that is, skin involvement within 2 cm of the primary lesion—to be arbitrary rather than supported by any data.[124] The M. D. Anderson Cancer Center experience, reported by Singletary et al.,[126] illustrates this point well. These investigators showed, in a multifactorial analysis of data for 135 patients with

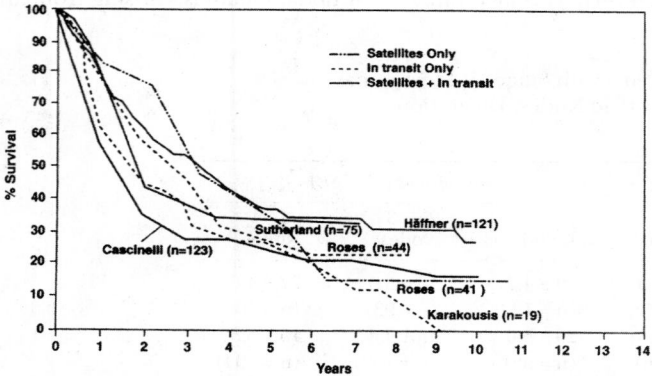

FIGURE 38.2-6. Kaplan-Meier survival curves from various series of patients with satellite, in transit, or satellite plus in transit metastases. (From ref. 124, with permission.)

regional cutaneous metastases, that classifying the lesions as satellites or in transit metastases on the basis of their distance from the primary tumor has no prognostic significance.[126] This finding is not surprising inasmuch as satellites and in transit metastases are part of the same disease process (i.e., lymphatic dissemination).

Before the revisions to the AJCC staging system,[98] stage II included both high-risk primary lesions (tumor thickness more than 4 mm) and satellite nodules (pT4b), which implies that the presence of satellite nodules has an impact on prognosis similar to that for all high-risk primary lesions. However, several studies have suggested that the prognosis in patients with satellitosis is usually worse than that in patients with thick primary lesions, and for that reason, this condition was staged in the new AJCC version in the grouping with in transit or nodal metastases (stage III).[105,124–126]

PROGNOSTIC FACTORS IN DISTANT METASTATIC MELANOMA (STAGE IV)

Patients with stage IV melanoma usually have a poor prognosis. In general the median duration of survival from the time that distant metastasis is documented is 6 to 7.5 months, and the 5-year survival rate is less than 10%.[105,127,128] Nevertheless, multivariate analyses of prognostic factors have identified several independent factors that predict survival in this group whose overall prognosis is poor.[97,128,129]

The prognostic influence of different distant metastatic sites was analyzed in 1158 patients with stage IV disease in the AJCC Melanoma Database.[97] Information regarding the number of distant metastases, serum lactate dehydrogenase (LDH) levels, and the presence or absence of intralymphatic (i.e., satellite and in transit) metastases was not sufficiently documented by the contributing institutions to permit inclusion in this analysis. Therefore, in addition to the clinical and pathologic features used in analyses for patients with stage I, II, or III disease, only the site of distant metastasis was analyzed.

Site of Distant Metastasis

The site of distant metastasis is an important independent predictor of survival in patients with stage IV disease.[97,105,127–129] Specifically, distant metastasis can be divided into two groups: visceral and nonvisceral. Overall, patients with distant nodal and soft tissue metastasis have a better survival than those with visceral metastasis.[97,105,128,129] In an analysis of the AJCC melanoma database, the greatest difference in survival was seen between patients with melanoma metastasis to visceral sites and those with metastasis to nonvisceral sites (i.e., skin, subcutaneous tissue, and distant lymph nodes) (Fig. 38.2-7).

Number of Metastatic Sites

Patients with one metastatic site have a significantly improved survival rate compared with those having two or more distant sites.[105,129,130] For example, in one large series, the number of metastatic sites was the most significant prognostic factor in patients with distant metastasis.[130]

Serum Lactate Dehydrogenase Levels

Elevated levels of serum LDH, when it has been included in multivariate analyses, is among the most predictive indepen-

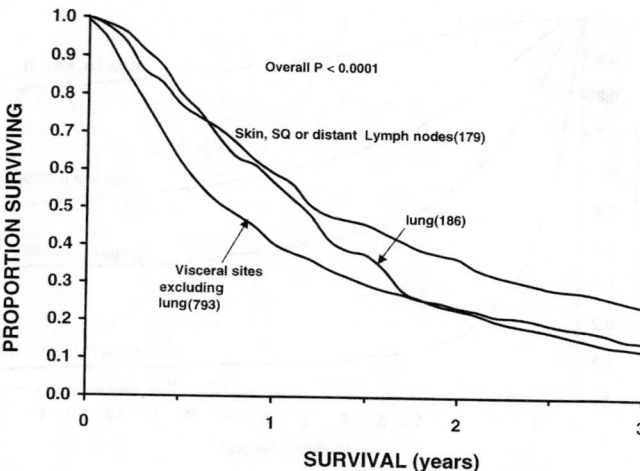

FIGURE 38.2-7. Survival curves for 1158 patients with metastatic melanoma at distant sites. Survival was significantly different for patients with skin, subcutaneous (SQ), and distant lymph node metastases compared to those with lung metastases (*P* <.003) or other visceral sites of metastases (*P* <.0001). Number of patients is shown in parentheses. (From ref. 97, with permission.)

dent factors of diminished survival for patients with stage IV melanoma, even after one accounts for site and number of metastases.[128,131–135] LDH level should be considered elevated only when level is high in two or more serum samples obtained more than 24 hours apart, because an elevated serum LDH on a single determination can be falsely positive due to hemolysis or other factors unrelated to melanoma metastases.

Performance Status

Poor performance status has been identified as another negative prognostic factor in patients with stage IV melanoma.[105,128,129,135] In a study of 1362 patients with metastatic melanoma treated in eight Eastern Cooperative Oncology Group (ECOG) melanoma trials conducted over a 25-year period, Manola et al.[128] found that, in multivariate analysis, the following factors were associated with increased risk of death: ECOG performance status score of 1 or higher [relative risk (RR), 1.49]; metastatic disease in the gastrointestinal tract (RR, 1.49), liver (RR, 1.44), pleura (RR, 1.35), or lung (RR, 1.19); and number of metastatic sites (RR, 1.12).

NEW STAGING SYSTEM FOR MELANOMA

The staging of melanoma, as of other cancers, is important to clinicians and researchers because it provides the following: (1) a nomenclature of consistent terms and definitions based on prognosis, (2) compartmentalization of patients into definable risk groups with regard to metastatic risk and survival rates, (3) criteria for stratification and reporting of results of melanoma clinical trials, (4) a critical component for comparisons of treatment results among different centers, and (5) a valuable tool for clinical decision-making.

The AJCC Melanoma Staging Committee recommended a major revision of the melanoma staging system, which was adopted by the AJCC as well as by the UICC TNM Committee, the European Organization for Research and Treatment of

TABLE 38.2-6. Melanoma TNM Classification

T Classification	Thickness (mm)	Ulceration Status
T1	≤1.0	a: Without ulceration and level II/III
		b: With ulceration or level IV/V
T2	1.01–2.0	a: Without ulceration
		b: With ulceration
T3	2.01–4.0	a: Without ulceration
		b: With ulceration
T4	>4.0	a: Without ulceration
		b: With ulceration

N Classification	No. of Metastatic Nodes	Nodal Metastatic Mass
N1	1 node	a: Micrometastasis[a]
		b: Macrometastasis[b]
N2	2 or 3 nodes	a: Micrometastasis[a]
		b: Macrometastasis[b]
		c: In transit metastasis(es)/satellite(s) *without* metastatic nodes
N3	4 or more metastatic nodes, or matted nodes, or in transit metastasis(es)/satellite(s) *with* metastatic node(s)	—

M Classification	Site	Serum LDH Level
M1a	Distant skin, subcutaneous or nodal metastasis	Normal
M1b	Lung metastases	Normal
M1c	All other visceral metastases	Normal
	Any distant metastasis	Elevated

LDH, lactate dehydrogenase; TNM, tumor, node, metastasis.
[a]Micrometastases are diagnosed after sentinel or elective lymphadenectomy.
[b]Macrometastases are defined as clinically detectable nodal metastases confirmed by therapeutic lymphadenectomy or nodal metastasis that exhibits gross extracapsular extension.
(From ref. 99, with permission.)

Cancer Melanoma Committee, and the World Health Organization (WHO) Melanoma Program.[96,98,99,111] It was implemented formally in 2003.

The new version of the melanoma TNM categories is shown in Table 38.2-6, and the stage groupings are listed in Table 38.2-7. Fifteen-year survival curves for patients with stage I to IV melanomas are shown in Figure 38.2-8. The major changes in the new (2002) version compared to the previous (1997) version of the melanoma staging system include the following[99]:

1. The new version restores the anatomic compartmentalization, consistent with staging for other cancers, that categorizes localized melanoma (i.e., without any evidence of metastases) to stages I and II, melanomas with regional metastases to stage III, and those with distant metastases to stage IV.

TABLE 38.2-7. Stage Groupings for Cutaneous Melanoma

Clinical Staging[a]				Pathologic Staging[b]			
0	Tis	N0	M0	0	Tis	N0	M0
IA	T1a	N0	M0	IA	T1a	N0	M0
IB	T1b	N0	M0	IB	T1b	N0	M0
	T2a	N0	M0		T2a	N0	M0
IIA	T2b	N0	M0	IIA	T2b	N0	M0
	T3a	N0	M0		T3a	N0	M0
IIB	T3b	N0	M0	IIB	T3b	N0	M0
	T4a	N0	M0		T4a	N0	M0
IIC	T4b	N0	M0	IIC	T4b	N0	M0
III	Any T	Any N	M0	IIIA	T1–T4a	N1a	M0
					T1–T4a	N2a	M0
				IIIB	T1–T4b	N1a	M0
					T1–T4b	N2a	M0
					T1–T4a	N1b	M0
					T1–T4a	N2b	M0
					T1–T4a,b	N2c	M0
				IIIC	T1–T4b	N1b	M0
					T1–T4b	N2b	M0
					Any T	N3	M0
IV	Any T	Any N	Any M	IV	Any T	Any N	Any M

[a]Clinical staging includes microstaging of the primary melanoma and clinical-radiologic evaluation for metastases. By convention, it should be done after complete excision of the primary melanoma with clinical assessment for regional and distant metastases.
[b]Pathologic staging includes microstaging of the primary melanoma and pathologic information about the regional lymph nodes after partial or complete lymphadenectomy. Pathologic stage 0 or stage IA tumors are the exception; they do not require pathological evaluation of the lymph nodes.
(From ref. 99, with permission.)

2. Melanoma thickness and ulceration but not level of invasion are used in the T category (except for T1 melanomas). T4 melanomas are then relocated from stage III into stage II.
3. The number of metastatic lymph nodes, rather than their gross dimensions, and the delineation of clinically occult (i.e., "microscopic") versus clinically apparent (i.e., "macroscopic") nodal metastases are used in the N category.
4. The site of distant metastases (nonvisceral vs. lung vs. all other visceral metastatic sites) and the presence of elevated serum LDH levels are used in the M category.
5. Melanomas in all patients with stage I, II, and III disease are up-staged when the primary melanoma displays histologic evidence of ulceration.
6. Merging of satellite metastases around a primary melanoma and in transit metastases into a single staging entity representing intralymphatic disease that is grouped into stage III disease.
7. A new convention is introduced for defining clinical and pathologic staging so as to incorporate pathologic information gained from lymphatic mapping and sentinel node biopsy.

CLINICAL VERSUS PATHOLOGIC STAGING

The ability to stage disease more accurately with sentinel node technology has markedly changed the understanding of the

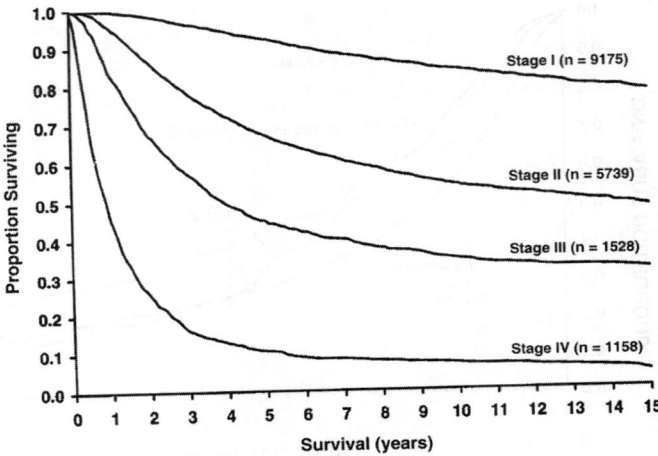

FIGURE 38.2-8. Fifteen-year survival curves comparing localized melanoma (stage I and II), regional metastases (stage III), and distant metastases (stage IV). The numbers in parentheses are the number of patients in each group from the American Joint Committee on Cancer melanoma database that were used to calculate the survival rates. The differences between the curves are significant (*P*<.0001). (From ref. 99, with permission.)

natural history of melanoma.[136,137] This powerful new staging technology has caused a significant stage migration that is now accounted for in the new AJCC staging system. Sentinel lymph node staging has had a major impact on risk assessment and treatment planning and on the conduct of clinical trials involving patients with melanoma.[98,138–141] The use of sentinel node staging has necessitated the creation of separate designations for patients who undergo clinical or radiologic staging of the regional lymph nodes and those who undergo the more accurate method of pathologic staging by means of lymphatic mapping and sentinel lymphadenectomy. The AJCC Melanoma Staging Committee addressed the issue of staging information after sentinel lymphadenectomy or elective lymph dissection through the definition of clinical and pathologic staging.[96,98,99,111] By convention, clinical staging should be performed after complete excision of the primary melanoma (including microstaging) with clinical assessment of regional lymph nodes. Pathologic staging includes information gained from both microstaging of the primary melanoma and pathologic evaluation of the nodal status after selective (i.e., sentinel node) lymphadenectomy or complete lymphadenectomy (i.e., after elective or therapeutic lymph node dissection). Significant differences among all T substages with the exception of T4b were identified when survival rates for patients with melanoma who underwent clinical staging were compared to rates for those whose nodal disease was staged pathologically (Table 38.2-8). In general, patients proven to be free of disease by sentinel lymph node biopsy had a better prognosis than patients whose nodes were evaluated by less precise techniques.

TNM STAGING CRITERIA AND STAGE GROUPINGS FOR LOCALIZED MELANOMA (STAGES I AND II)

The primary criteria for the T classification are tumor thickness (measured in millimeters) and the presence or absence of ulceration (determined histopathologically). A more clinically

TABLE 38.2-8. Five-Year Survival Rates for 5346 Patients with Clinically Negative Nodes Whose Disease Was Pathologically Staged after Either Regional Lymph Node Dissection or Sentinal Node Lymphadenectomy

T Stage	Pathologic Node Status	5-Y Survival (% ± SE)	P Value[a]
T1a	N– (n = 379)	94 ± 2.0	.0035
	N+ (n = 15)	64 ± 17.7	
T1b	N– (n = 319)	90 ± 2.5	.0039
	N+ (n = 18)	76 ± 14.9	
T2a	N– (n = 1480)	94 ± 0.8	<.0001
	N+ (n = 150)	73 ± 5.6	
T2b	N– (n = 408)	83 ± 2.3	<.0001
	N+ (n = 62)	56 ± 8.8	
T3a	N– (n = 808)	86 ± 1.6	<.0001
	N+ (n = 177)	59 ± 6.0	
T3b	N– (n = 639)	72 ± 2.1	<.0001
	N+ (n = 176)	49 ± 4.5	
T4a	N– (n = 203)	75 ± 3.9	.0116
	N+ (n = 66)	61 ± 7.4	
T4b	N– (n = 330)	53 ± 3.1	.2403
	N+ (n = 116)	44 ± 5.5	

N+/–, node positive/negative for metastasis.
[a]P value based on the comparison of survival curves using the log rank test. (From ref. 99, with permission.)

convenient and widely used threshold of 1.0 mm or less was used for the threshold of T1 melanomas, whereas T2 melanomas were defined as those measuring 1.01 to 2.0 mm in thickness. T3 melanomas were defined as those with a thickness of 2.01 to 4.0 mm and T4 melanomas as those with a thickness greater than 4.0 mm (see Table 38.2-6).

Ulceration heralds such a high risk for metastases that its presence up-stages the prognosis of all such patients compared to patients with melanomas of equivalent thickness without ulceration. Thus, survival rates for patients with an ulcerated melanoma are proportionately lower than those for patients with a nonulcerated melanoma of equivalent T category, but are remarkably similar to those for patients with a nonulcerated melanoma of the next highest T category (Table 38.2-9).

Definition of T1 Melanomas

The level of invasion, as defined by Clark et al.,[115] is an independent predictive feature for "thin" (T1) melanomas but not for thicker lesions.[97] As a result, the level of invasion is incorporated into the stage grouping definitions of T1 melanomas. In this group of T1 melanomas, the assignment of T1a is restricted to melanomas that meet the following three criteria: (1) tumor thickness 1.0 mm or less, (2) absence of ulceration, and (3) depth of invasion limited to level II or level III. T1b melanomas are defined as those with a thickness 1.0 mm or less and with the more aggressive features of level IV or V invasion, or with ulceration (regardless of level). Both conditions are associated with a significant reduction in survival rates in patients with T1 melanomas.[98,105,114,142] Approximately three-fourths of T1 melanomas are classified as T1a, with the remaining lesions being T1b (see Tables 38.2-6 and 38.2-9). Patients with T1 melanomas have approximately 95% (T1a) and 91% (T1b) 5-year survival. All T2, T3, and T4 melanomas are defined according to the thickness and ulceration criteria, as described earlier, but not the level of invasion.

Stage Grouping

Stage grouping for localized melanomas that are either clinically or pathologically staged are defined in Table 38.2-7. The sole difference in the definitions of clinical versus pathologic stage groupings is whether the regional lymph nodes are staged by clinical or radiologic examination, or by pathologic examination (after selective or complete lymphadenectomy). Because level of invasion is an independent predictive feature for "thin" (T1) melanomas, it is incorporated into the stage grouping definitions for T1 melanomas.[97,99]

TNM STAGING CRITERIA AND STAGE GROUPING FOR REGIONAL METASTATIC MELANOMA (STAGE III)

Patients with stage III melanoma include those with metastases either in the regional lymph nodes or within lymphatics manifesting as either satellite (including microsatellite) or in transit metastases. The marked diversity in the natural history of stage III melanoma is demonstrated by fivefold differences in 5-year survival rates for defined substages, ranging from 69% for patients with a nonulcerated melanoma (regardless of thickness) and a single clinically occult nodal metastasis detected by sentinel or elective lymphadenectomy to a low of 13% for patients with an ulcerated melanoma (regardless of thickness) and four or more clinically apparent nodal metastases (detected by therapeutic lymphadenectomy) (see Table 38.2-5).[97,99]

TNM Criteria

There are four major determinants of outcome for pathologic stage III melanoma: (1) the number of metastatic lymph

TABLE 38.2-9. Five-Year Survival Rates of Patients with Pathologically Staged Melanomas

	IA	IB	IIA	IIB	IIC	IIIA	IIIB	IIIC
Ta: nonulcerated	T1 95%	T2 89%	T3 79%	T4 67%	—	N1a, N2a 67%	N1b, N2b 54%	N3 28%
Tb: ulcerated	—	T1 91%	T2 77%	T3 63%	T4 45%	—	N1a, N2a 52%	N1b, N2b, N3 24%

Note. The presence of ulceration (determined histologically) in a primary melanoma (designated *Tb*) causes an up-staging by one substage compared to a nonulcerated melanoma (designated *Ta*). Five-year survival rates from the American Joint Committee on Cancer melanoma database are shown. (From ref. 99, with permission.)

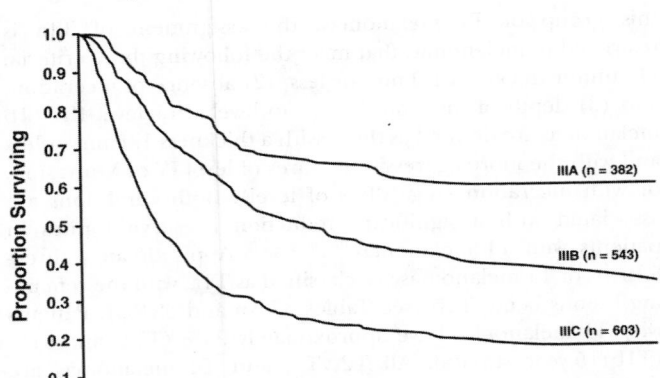

FIGURE 38.2-9. Fifteen-year survival curves for stage groupings of patients with regional metastatic melanoma (stage III) (see Table 38.2-7 for definitions of stage groupings). Numbers of patients from the American Joint Committee on Cancer melanoma database are shown in parentheses. Differences between survival curves are highly significant (*P* <.0001). (From ref. 99, with permission.)

nodes, (2) whether the tumor burden is microscopic (i.e., clinically occult and detected pathologically by sentinel or elective lymphadenectomy) or macroscopic (i.e., clinically apparent by physical or radiologic examination and verified pathologically), (3) the presence or absence of ulceration of the primary melanoma, and (4) the presence or absence of satellite or in transit metastases.[97,99] The available data thus show no substantial difference in survival outcomes for patients with either satellite or in transit metastases (see Fig. 38.2-6).[124] Therefore, melanomas with both satellite and in transit metastases are assigned to a separate N2c classification and grouped in stage IIIB in the absence of synchronous nodal metastases, because both have a prognosis equivalent to that of multiple nodal metastases (see Tables 38.2-7 and 38.2-9). Furthermore, the available data demonstrate that patients with a combination of satellite or in transit metastases plus nodal metastases have a worse outcome than patients who develop only one of these regional recurrence patterns; thus these melanomas were assigned to an N3 classification regardless of the number of synchronous metastatic nodes (see Table 38.2-7).[98,99,111,124]

Stage Grouping

The stage groupings for stage III melanoma are defined in Table 38.2-7, and survival rates for these patients are shown in Figure 38.2-9. After accounting for the prognostic features in pathologic stage III melanoma, patients can be divided into the following three definable subgroups with statistically significant differences in survival: stages IIIA, IIIB, and IIIC (see Table 38.2-9).

In summary, the stage groupings for pathologic stage III melanoma use the aforementioned four criteria to assign melanomas with regional metastases to one of three groups designated as stage IIIA, IIIB, or IIIC. Patients with pathologic stage IIIA disease have three or fewer microscopic (clinically occult) nodal metastases and a nonulcerated melanoma (T1 to 4aN1aM0 and T1 to 4aN2aM0) identified after sentinel or elective lymphadenectomy (see Table 38.2-7). Pathologic stage IIIB includes the fol-

lowing three subgroups of patients with equivalent survival rates: (1) those with three or fewer microscopic (clinically occult) nodes and an ulcerated primary melanoma (T1 to 4bN1aM0 and T1 to 4bN2aM0); (2) those with three or fewer macroscopic metastatic nodes and a nonulcerated primary lesion (T1 to 4aN1bM0 and T1 to 4aN2bM0); or (3) those with satellite or in transit metastases but no evidence of nodal or distant metastases, with or without tumor ulceration (T1 to 4a,bN2cM0) (see Table 38.2-7). Pathologic stage IIIC disease comprise the following three subgroups of patients: (1) those with four or more microscopic metastatic nodes and an ulcerated primary melanoma (T1 to 4bN2aM0), (2) those with four or more macroscopic nodes regardless of primary ulceration (T1 to 4N2bM0 and T1 to 4N3M0), or (3) any patient with any combination of satellites or in transit metastases and nodal metastases.[98,99,111]

PROGNOSIS AND STAGING OF DISTANT METASTASES (STAGE IV)

TNM Criteria

For melanomas associated with distant metastases, the site(s) of metastases and elevated serum levels of LDH are used to delineate the M categories into three groups: M1a, M1b, and M1c, with associated 1-year survival rates ranging from 40% to 60% (see Fig. 38.2-7).[99] These criteria were selected because in all studies that analyzed prognosis in patients with distant metastases by means of a Cox regression analysis, the site or number of metastases and elevated serum LDH levels were most predictive of poor survival.[98,99,111]

Melanomas with distant metastases in the skin, subcutaneous tissue, or distant lymph nodes are categorized as M1a. Melanomas with metastasis to the lung are categorized as M1b. In several studies, patients with metastasis to the lung had an "intermediate" prognosis compared to those with skin, subcutaneous, and distant nodal metastases ("better" prognosis) and all other visceral sites ("worse" prognosis).[99,98,127,128] Melanomas associated with metastases to all other visceral sites carry a relatively worse prognosis and are designated as M1c.

Although it is uncommon in staging classifications to include serum factors, an exception was made for elevated levels of serum LDH. When the patient's serum LDH level is consistently elevated above the upper limits of normal at the time of staging, a melanoma with distant metastasis is assigned to M1c, regardless of the site of the distant metastasis. An elevated serum LDH level was among the most predictive independent factors for diminished survival in all published studies when it was analyzed in a multivariate analysis, even after one accounted for site and number of metastases.[99,133,143] An elevated serum LDH level should be used only when determinations are made on two or more serum samples obtained more than 24 hours apart, because an elevated serum LDH level after a single determination can be false-positive as a result of hemolysis or other factors unrelated to melanoma metastases. Because the survival differences between the M categories are small, there are no subgroupings for stage IV melanoma.

RECOMMENDATIONS FOR CLINICAL TRIALS

The prognostic factors used to validate the melanoma staging system should be the primary stratification criteria and end results reporting criteria for melanoma clinical trials. The designs and analyses of melanoma clinical trials are dependent on the use of the most reproducible and significant independent prognostic factors, including those used to determine the melanoma TNM classifications. Otherwise, treatment differences, or lack thereof, may be influenced more by the mix of the patients' prognostic factors than by the treatment effect being studied. For example, some melanoma adjuvant therapy trials use such different stratification and patient eligibility criteria that it is difficult, if not impossible, to compare results across clinical trials conducted by cooperative groups or institutions, or even to reliably compare results of sequential trials conducted by the same investigators. The AJCC Melanoma Staging Committee therefore recommended that all melanoma patients who have clinically negative regional lymph nodes and who may be considered for later entry into surgical and adjuvant therapy clinical trials should undergo pathologic disease staging with sentinel lymphadenectomy to ensure prognostic homogeneity within assigned treatment groups. In this way, investigators will be better able to discern between the impact of natural history and treatment when interpreting results of melanoma clinical trials.

BIOPSY

Proper biopsy of a suspicious lesion is critical to proper staging. Suspicious lesions should have a full-thickness biopsy to accurately interpret the maximum tumor thickness, the presence or absence of ulceration, and the level of invasion. Excisional biopsy with a narrow margin of normal-appearing skin for small lesions is preferred; this can be performed on most lesions up to 2 cm in diameter. Orientation of an excisional biopsy should be carefully considered. The biopsy scar should be oriented to be compatible with a subsequent wide local excision should the lesion prove to be melanoma. On the extremities a longitudinal or oblique incision is preferred. On the trunk or the head and neck the biopsy scar should be oriented parallel to the skin lines.

Excisional biopsy involves complete removal of a skin lesion, usually in a fusiform shape, with a 1- to 2-mm clinical lateral margin and a deep margin in the subcutaneous fat, underneath all epithelial appendageal structures.[144] Excisional biopsy is the biopsy technique of choice whenever melanoma is suspected.[144,145]

An incisional biopsy is appropriate for lesions that are large or located at a vital anatomic site for which one would want to know the diagnosis before removing the entire lesion. The type of biopsy does not influence patient survival and the risk of metastasis. Incision into a melanoma does not promote dissemination. Incisional biopsy should be performed at the most raised area, but because it removes only part of a tumor, a repeat biopsy may be necessary if the histologic diagnosis does not agree with the clinical impression. An incisional biopsy involves removal of a portion of a skin lesion, in which the lateral margins are incomplete and therefore, by definition, positive, but the deep margin is in the subcutaneous fat, underneath all epithelial appendageal structures. Two general forms exist: the fusiform ellipse and the 6-mm punch biopsy.[144] An incisional biopsy is indicated when melanoma is highly suspected and the preferred excisional biopsy is not possible because of lesion size or loca-

tion, or logistical issues.[144,145] Final determination of the tumor thickness cannot be made until the entire lesion has been excised and examined by the pathologist. For suspicious lesions beneath nail beds, the biopsy approach is more problematic. Although digital tumors usually arise from the proximal nail fold, from which the biopsy must be procured, biopsies of subungual pigmented lesions necessitate splitting of the nail plate.

A shave biopsy involves removal of a portion of a skin lesion for diagnosis, using a shaving technique and a sharp razor blade, in which the deep margin of resection is within the dermis. Shave biopsies are inappropriate when invasive melanoma is suspected, because an incomplete Breslow depth measurement could result. However, it is a very useful biopsy technique when performed by an experienced clinician in the specific setting in which melanoma *in situ* is being considered in the differential diagnosis along with, perhaps, a benign lentigo or flat seborrheic keratosis.[146]

SURGICAL TREATMENT OF PRIMARY MELANOMA (STAGES I TO III)

Surgical excision continues to be the mainstay in the treatment of primary melanoma and consists of resecting the intact tumor or biopsy site *en bloc* with a surrounding margin of normal-appearing skin and underlying subcutaneous tissue.[147] The goals of surgical treatment are to remove all the melanoma cells at the primary site to provide durable local disease control for all patients, even when the likelihood for distant relapse is high, and to effect a cure in those patients at low risk of harboring occult metastatic disease. Without compromising these goals, efforts should be made to carry out the surgical excision in a manner that minimizes costs, functional impairment, and cosmetic disfigurement.

How wide an excision margin to use has been the center of controversy for decades. The vast majority of procedures involving narrow excision margins (1 cm) followed by primary closure of the resultant surgical defect can be accomplished under local anesthesia with minimal cost and surgical morbidity.[147–149] On the other hand, procedures involving wide excision margins (2 cm or more) not only are often performed under general anesthesia but, depending on the anatomic site, may require reconstruction with expensive and sometimes elaborate full-thickness advancement or rotation flaps or coverage with cosmetically unappealing skin grafts.[150] Narrow excisions, however, are often thought to result in a higher rate of local and regional failures, which in turn may have survival implications. Furthermore, complicated and potentially morbid treatment strategies may be necessary in the event of local recurrence.

A series of prospectively randomized surgical trials has addressed the issue of surgical margins in the treatment of primary melanoma and has provided standards of care for most clinical presentations.[147,151,152] These trials tested the following concepts:

1. Local failure is a function of both biology of the primary tumor and extent of excision.
2. Thin melanomas have a low risk for recurrence, and narrow (1 cm) margins are safe.
3. Thicker or ulcerated melanomas are associated with a higher incidence of clinically occult local metastases

that are more completely removed with wider excisions, in turn lowering the risk of subsequent local or regional recurrences, or both.

4. Increased rates of local and regional failure may or may not have an impact on survival.

Specific and unique concerns exist when interpreting results from prospective randomized clinical trials for various subsets of patients with localized melanoma. Long-term follow-up is necessary, especially for lesions that are thinner. Although thin lesions have a better overall prognosis, they have greater propensity to late recurrence.

WORLD HEALTH ORGANIZATION MELANOMA PROGRAM TRIALS

The WHO Melanoma Program formally published the first randomized trial addressing excision margins in patients with melanoma.[148,149] Its surgical protocol (Trial No. 10), compared 1-cm versus 3-cm radial margin of excision in a group of 612 patients who had melanomas limited to a thickness of 2.0 mm or less. This group of patients was selected because the predicted risk of a local recurrence was low, and therefore it was presumed safe to test a more conservative skin-sparing margin of excision. The trial was stratified and subsequently analyzed according to thickness ranges (less than 1 mm and 1 to 2 mm). Long-term results of this trial demonstrated that a 1-cm margin of excision was safe primary treatment for the thickness subsets evaluated, because no difference in survival rates was observed relative to the group undergoing excision with 3-cm radial margins.

Rates of local recurrence also were not statistically different overall between the two treatment groups. For the subset of patients who had lesions less than 1 mm in thickness, no local recurrences had been encountered at the time of the first two reports of this trial[148,149] regardless of the extent of surgical margin. By the time of the updated summary report in 1998, one patient who had a lesion less than 1 mm in thickness who was treated by a 3-cm excision had local recurrence.[152] A total of seven patients in the 1- to 2-mm thickness subset had local recurrences; five of these seven were treated with the narrower 1-cm excision. Altogether, five local recurrences in 119 patients (4.5%) were observed in patients who had primary melanoma in the thickness ranges of 1.1 to 2.0 mm and who had a 1-cm margin of excision (N. Cascinelli, *personal communication*, 2001).

The study did illustrate that the incidence of local recurrence is extremely low in this group and is primarily a function of primary tumor thickness but may also be influenced by width of excision. Because these events were so infrequent, any impact on overall survival could not be detected. Therefore the authors concluded that a 1-cm margin of excision for melanomas less than 2 mm in thickness is safe and should be the standard. Lingering concerns have been primarily a result of the trend in the WHO study (with longer follow-up reported in 1988, 1991, and 1998) toward an increase in the absolute number of local recurrences in the narrow excision group.[147]

INTERGROUP MELANOMA SURGICAL TRIAL

The Intergroup Melanoma Surgical Trial enrolled 740 patients with intermediate-thickness melanomas (i.e., 1.0 to 4.0 mm) and randomly assigned the majority of them to undergo resec-

tion with either 2- or 4-cm margins.[153–155] Two eligibility groups were established and stratified according to tumor thickness (1 to 2 mm, 2 to 3 mm, and 3 to 4 mm), anatomic site (trunk, head and neck, and extremity), and ulceration (present or absent). Eligibility in group A (n = 468) was confined to those patients who had melanomas located on the trunk or proximal extremity to ensure that the more radical 4-cm margin could be carried out if they were randomly assigned to receive such a treatment. The remaining patients, designated group B (n = 272), included those who had either head and neck or distal extremity lesions, all of whom underwent excision with 2-cm margins. All patients were also randomly assigned to undergo either an elective lymph node dissection (ELND) or observation after wide local excision.[155] More than 94% of the patients entered were eligible and evaluable. As of the latest report, 92% of patients had been followed for at least 5 years or until death. This is now a mature database with median and longest follow-up of 10 and 16 years, respectively.[155]

Among the 468 patients in group A (randomly assigned to excision with 2-cm vs. 4-cm margins), only 3 (0.6%) experienced a local recurrence as the first site of failure, and 11 (2.3%) had local recurrence overall.[155] Among the 272 patients in group B (nonrandomly assigned to excision with a 2-cm margin), a somewhat higher rate of local recurrence was observed, with 10 patients having a first local recurrence (3.7%) and a total of 17 patients (6.2%) overall experiencing a local recurrence during the course of their disease.[155] As with the patients in group A, the presence of ulceration and increasing tumor thickness correlated with an increased risk of local recurrence. Overall survival for the 28 patients who developed a local recurrence was significantly worse than that for the remaining 712 patients who did not (Fig. 38.2-10). It is interesting to note that for the entire study population no impact on rates of either local recurrence or in transit disease was observed in patients who underwent an ELND.

Results for the Randomly Assigned (Group A) Patients

There were no statistical differences in overall survival or local recurrence incidence rates in patients who were randomly

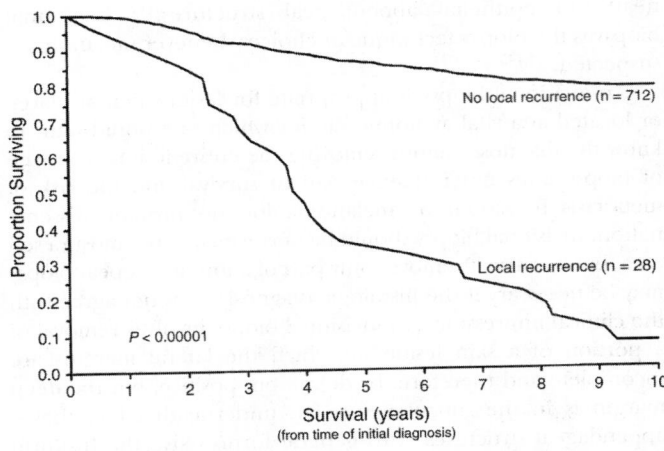

FIGURE 38.2-10. Comparison of survival for patients in the Intergroup Melanoma Surgical Trial with or without local recurrence. Number of patients is shown in parentheses. (From ref. 155, with permission.)

assigned to undergo excision with either a 2- or 4-cm surgical margin. For the 238 patients in the 2-cm margin group, the incidence of local recurrence as a first relapse was 0.4% and the incidence of local recurrence at any time was 2.1%. For those 230 patients treated with excision with a 4-cm margin, the local recurrence rates were 0.9% as a first relapse and 2.6% overall. The median time to local recurrence was 1.7 years, and the median survival time after local recurrence was only 1 year; neither time was affected by the extent of excision margin. The incidence of local recurrence was lower overall for the entire group A cohort (inclusive of all thickness groups) compared with the overlapping subset of patients with 1.0- to 2.0-mm lesions on the WHO trial who underwent excision with 1-cm margins (0.6% for the Intergroup trial vs. 4.5% for WHO Trial No. 10). Just as there was no influence of margin width on local recurrence rates, no difference in in transit disease was observed (5.2% vs. 5.9% for 4- and 2-cm excisions, respectively).

Ten-year disease-specific survival rates for the two groups demonstrated no significant differences: 70% for those in the 2-cm margin group versus 77% for those in the 4-cm margin group ($P = .074$). Furthermore, survival rates similarly were not significantly influenced by the second random assignment to ELND versus wide local excision alone, although trends in favor of treatment with ELND were noted.

Multivariate Prognostic Factors Analysis

A multifactorial stepwise regression analysis based on the Cox model was performed for the entire group of 740 patients.[155] The only two factors independently predictive of poorer local control were the presence of tumor ulceration ($P < .001$) and the head and neck site ($P = .02$). Notably, the surgical margins of excision (2 vs. 4 cm) did not correlate with local recurrence rates, after all other factors in the model were taken into account. When the analysis was performed within the two cohorts (groups A and B) separately, only melanoma ulceration was a significant and independent prognostic factor associated with an increased risk of a local recurrence in both groups.

FRENCH AND SWEDISH COOPERATIVE SURGICAL TRIALS

Two large French and Swedish randomized surgical trials had essentially the same study design comparing 2-cm versus 5-cm margins of excision and came to the same conclusions.[156,157]

The French Cooperative Group initiated a trial in the late 1970s that was only completed 16 years later. This trial included patients with stage I and II melanoma who had lesions 2 mm or less in thickness.[156] Patients were randomly assigned to undergo excision with 5- or 2-cm margins. The trial found no increased risk for local or distant recurrence among the group of patients who were treated with the narrower excision. Overall survival rates for the two treatment arms were essentially identical, which suggests that the margin of excision could be safely reduced to 2 cm for melanomas of 2 mm or less in thickness.

Nine European centers, over a period of 5 years, prospectively randomly assigned 337 patients with melanoma measuring less than 2.1 mm in thickness to undergo a local excision with either a 2- or a 5-cm margin. Data from 326 patients was eligible for statistical analysis. Excluded from the trial were patients older than 70 years; those with melanomas of the toe,

nail, or finger; and those with ALM. The median follow-up time was 192 months (16 years) for the estimation of survival and disease recurrences.[156]

The median time to disease recurrence was 43 months and 37.6 months for the groups with 2- and 5-cm margins, respectively. The 10-year disease-free survival rates were 85% for the group with a 2-cm margin and 83% for the group with a 5-cm margin. There was no difference in the 10-year overall survival rates (87% vs. 86%). The authors concluded that, for melanomas less than 2.1 mm thick, a margin of excision of 2 cm is sufficient. A larger margin of 5 cm did not have any impact on the rate of or time to disease recurrence or on survival.[156]

The Swedish Melanoma Study Group performed a prospective, randomized, multicenter study of patients with primary melanoma located on the trunk or extremities and with a tumor thickness of more than 0.8 mm and less than or equal to 2 mm.[157] Patients were allocated randomly to excision with a 2- or a 5-cm margin. In total, 989 patients were recruited between 1982 and 1991. The median follow-up was 11 years (range, 7 to 17 years) for estimation of survival and 8 years (range, 0 to 17 years) for evaluation of recurrent disease. The crude rate of local recurrence, defined as a recurrence in the scar or transplant, was less than 1% (8 of 989 patients). Twenty percent of the patients (194 of 989 patients) experienced disease recurrence of any type, and 15% (146 of 989 patients) died of melanoma. There were no statistically significant differences between the two treatment arms. In a multivariate Cox analysis with patients allocated to wide excision as the reference group, the estimated relative hazards for overall survival and recurrence-free survival among those allocated to resection with a 2-cm margin were 0.96 (95% confidence interval, 0.75 to 1.24), and 1.02 (95% confidence interval, 0.8 to 1.3), respectively. The authors concluded that local recurrences were very uncommon among patients with tumors more than 0.8 mm thick and less than or equal to 2.0 mm thick, and that because there were no differences in recurrence rate or survival between the two treatment groups, such patients can be treated with a resection margin of 2 cm as safely as with a resection margin of 5 cm.

Both the French and the Swedish cooperative trials were well-conducted phase III surgical studies with long-term follow-up, and both concluded that a 2-cm surgical margin was safe compared to a 5-cm margin. Nevertheless, neither study changed surgical practice because of the WHO Melanoma Group Trial No. 10 described earlier in World Health Organization Melanoma Program Trials, in which the same patient cohort (i.e., those with melanomas less than 2.0 mm in thickness) could safely undergo excision with a 1-cm margin.[148,152]

BRITISH COOPERATIVE GROUP TRIAL

The British randomized trial compared 1- versus 3-cm radial margins of skin excision in patients who had cutaneous melanomas with a thickness of 2 mm or more (i.e., T3, T4 melanomas).[158,159] This is the only randomized surgical trial that included patients with T4 melanomas (more than 4.0 mm thickness), which constituted 25% of the total group. A total of 900 patients with T3 and T4 melanomas were accrued; 453 were randomly assigned to undergo surgery with a 1-cm margin of excision and 447 with a 3-cm margin. Patients with melanoma on head and neck, hands, or feet locations were excluded. No patients received any surgical procedure to stage the regional nodal basins (sentinel node biopsy or ELND) or systemic adjuvant therapy. The trial was stratified according to tumor thickness (2 to 4 mm and more than 4 mm) but not according to ulceration status. A 1-cm margin of excision was associated with a significantly increased risk of locoregional recurrence. There were 168 locoregional recurrences (as first events) in the group with 1-cm margin of excision, compared with 142 in the group with a 3-cm margin (hazard ratio, 1.26; P = .05). The vast majority of locoregional recurrences occurred in the regional lymph nodes (142 events for the 1-cm group vs. 121 in the 3-cm group). There were only 57 patients who had either a local recurrence or in transit metastasis with or without simultaneous regional or distant recurrences (15% of the total locoregional events; 35 or 17% in the 1-cm group compared to 27 or 23% in the 3-cm group). Thus, the largest magnitude of difference was observed for nodal recurrence, and if these cases were excluded from the analysis, no statistical difference in local and in transit events would have been observed. There were 128 deaths attributable to melanoma in the group with a 1-cm margin, compared with 105 in the group with a 3-cm margin (hazard ratio, 1.24; P = .1). Overall survival was similar in the two groups (P = .6). A multivariate analysis of prognostic factors showed that male gender, increasing tumor thickness, and ulceration were each independent risk factors. The authors concluded that there was a greater risk of locoregional recurrence when melanomas that were at least 2 mm thick were excised with a 1-cm margin rather than a 3-cm margin.[158]

This study suggests that at least a percentage of nodal or other local or regional events may be reduced or avoided by wider excisions, which presumably remove clinically occult but potentially relevant disease more completely than a narrow excision. These data further imply that regional nodal disease can develop in part from clinically and pathologically silent local micrometastases existing in the region of skin from 1 to 3 cm beyond the primary tumor at the time of diagnosis. These results argue in favor of wider excision for the higher-risk melanoma patients (i.e., those with thicker lesions).

Although provocative, the results of this study may have limited current relevance because in U.S. surgical practices many, if not most, nodal recurrences are identified with sentinel node biopsy performed at the time of the wide local excision. Furthermore, the apparent improved locoregional control observed in this study came with a price, because the skin grafting rate and surgical morbidity were significantly greater with 3-cm excisions.

No statistical difference in overall survival has been observed between the two treatment arms. Two explanations have been offered for the lack of survival impact: (1) the number of local and regional events that were avoided by wider excision was too small to translate into a survival benefit in a study of this size and power, and (2) locoregional failures are not consistently a source of distant relapse, and therefore more complete removal of clinically occult locally metastatic disease via a wider excision does not significantly alter the natural history of the disease. Although this study established that melanomas exceeding 2 mm in thickness require surgical margins that exceed 1 cm, it does not address the question of whether a 3-cm margin is better than a 2-cm margin.

CURRENT RECOMMENDATIONS

Collectively these trials provide the basis for current recommendations for the extent of surgical margins for melanoma

TABLE 38.2-10. Recommended Surgical Margins of Excision for Primary Melanoma by Range of Melanoma Thickness

Tumor Thickness (mm)	T Stage	Excision Margin (cm)
In situ	T0	0.5–1.0
0–1	T1	1
1–2	T2	1 or 2[a]
2–4	T3	2
>4	T4	At least 2

[a]A 2-cm margin is preferable where anatomically feasible; a margin of 1–2 cm is appropriate in anatomically restricted areas, especially when a skin graft or major flap reconstruction can be avoided. (Adapted from ref. 147.)

according to tumor thickness[147] (Table 38.2-10). For melanoma *in situ*, excision of the lesion or biopsy site with a 0.5- to 1.0-cm border of clinically normal skin and a layer of subcutaneous tissue is sufficient. Although these lesions are noninvasive, a local recurrence may present as an invasive melanoma with the potential for metastasis. Margin recommendations for melanomas *in situ* are based on a consensus of the available data demonstrating excellent local control with the use of such margins. Most *in situ* melanomas are completely and easily excised with a 0.5- to 1.0-cm margin, and the surgical defect is most often closed primarily under local anesthesia. A minority, lentigo maligna type in particular, display histologically positive margins despite the removal of normal-appearing skin surrounding the gross extent of the pigmented lesion. These particular lesions may require sequential operative excisions or special techniques such as radial biopsies or *in vivo* confocal microscopy[160] to achieve adequate pathologically clear margins, and occasionally the use of a split-thickness skin graft or flap closure is necessary.

For invasive melanomas 1 mm or less in thickness (i.e., T1 melanomas), the WHO trial suggests that an excision with a 1-cm margin of clinically normal skin and underlying subcutaneous tissue is adequate. The use of this narrow margin in these low-risk patients yields excellent cosmetic and functional results in any anatomic location without compromising therapeutic efficacy. Except for the occasional lesion arising on the distal extremities, scalp, or face, essentially all excisions with 1-cm margins can be primarily closed.

The appropriate margin of excision to be used for melanomas between 1 and 2 mm in thickness cannot be resolved by the prospective trials described earlier. Because of the small number of observed events (recurrences or deaths), no reported study has the statistical power to confirm or refute equivalence in long-term clinical course for patients undergoing surgery with 1- and 3-cm margins, and no study to date has directly compared 1- and 2-cm margins. A trend toward an increased incidence of local recurrence in the narrow excision group was observed in the WHO trial. Furthermore, for the overlapping group with melanomas 1- to 2-mm thick, the incidence of local recurrence in the Intergroup Melanoma Surgical Trial for patients treated with 2-cm surgical margins was lower than that in the WHO trial for patients treated with 1-cm margins (0.6% vs. 4.5%, respectively). Of course, these are comparisons across trials, and the conclusions cannot be made definitively.[147]

In the absence of data from a randomized controlled trial, it is reasonable to perform a 2-cm surgical margin for these melanomas whenever it is anatomically feasible and when the surgical defect can be closed primarily without a skin graft.[147] However, in anatomic locations where a proposed 2-cm margin may compromise adjacent functional or cosmetic structures, or require the use of sophisticated wound reconstruction techniques or a split-thickness skin graft, a surgical margin of less than 2 cm but more than 1 cm may preferentially be used.

For melanomas between 2 and 4 mm, a 2-cm surgical margin is currently the recommended standard based on the Intergroup data. The British trial, which included a subset with 2- to 4-mm melanomas that overlapped with the Intergroup trial, demonstrated better local and regional control with a 3-cm margin than with a 1-cm margin. Although a 3-cm margin may be superior to a 1-cm margin in terms of local control (British trial), a 4-cm margin has not been demonstrated to be superior to 2-cm margin (Intergroup trial). Consequently, there are no data to support any surgical approach for this group of patients that would include margins greater than 2 cm.

Until recently, recommendations for treating thick (greater than 4 mm) melanomas have been based on retrospective analyses. Much is known from these studies about the natural history of thick melanomas in these patients. For example, patients with these tumors are at higher risk for both local recurrences (approximately 10% to 15%) and distant metastases (approximately 60%).[147,161] Prognostic variables and excision margins have been evaluated for patients who have thick melanomas through a collaborative effort of the M. D. Anderson Cancer Center and Lakeland Regional Cancer Center.[161] Patient data was retrospectively analyzed with respect to local recurrence and survival as a function of the extent of the excision margin and other prognostic factors. No increase in local recurrence rates or decrease in survival was observed for patients undergoing excision with margins of 2 cm or less compared with patients who had melanomas of similar thickness and a similar constellation of prognostic factors who underwent excision with a margin wider than 2 cm. Local recurrence appeared to be a function more of primary tumor factors than of width of excision, with the presence of primary tumor ulceration as the only factor influencing local failure identified by univariate analysis. Multivariate analysis revealed that overall survival was impacted by nodal status, tumor ulceration, and thickness greater than 6 mm but not by margin width or local recurrence.[161] Despite the retrospective nature of this study, a balance in prognostic factors was observed between the two excision groups. The inference is that 2-cm margins can be safely used for thicker lesions. Interestingly, although the local recurrence rate was, as anticipated, relatively high (11%), in contrast to findings from the Intergroup trial, such events did not appear to be associated with a poorer prognosis compared to that with absence of local failure.

The British trial is currently the only reported prospective randomized trial evaluating excision margins in the highest-risk group.[158] The authors of the British trial concluded that 3-cm margins should be considered for thicker melanomas (more than 4 mm) because of the improved locoregional control demonstrated with this wider margin. Acceptance of this conclusion has been met with reservation for the following reasons: (1) no survival differences to date have been demonstrated; (2) differences in local and regional events would not be as evident with the routine use of sentinel node biopsy; (3) statistical difference in local events is lost when nodal events are taken out of the analysis; and (4) 3-cm margins are associated with greater surgi-

cal morbidity and an increased use of skin grafts.[147] Although the data from the M. D. Anderson and Lakeland Regional cancer centers are retrospective, they do represent one of the largest reported experiences with this high-risk group (n = 278), which is not dissimilar in size to the subset of patients in this thickness group from the prospective randomized British trial (n = 300) and therefore can be used to help establish recommendations. Current recommendations call for at least 2-cm margins for this population of melanoma patients. Such an approach will remain appropriate until more data from longer follow-up of the British trial as well as results from the ongoing Swedish Melanoma Trial are available. This latter trial is currently evaluating 2-cm versus 4-cm margins in 1000 patients who have melanomas of more than 2 mm in thickness.

One could postulate that a wider surgical margin would decrease local recurrence rates by removing any retained primary melanoma tumors cells or nearby intralymphatic metastases. Alternatively, a local recurrence might be the first manifestation of circulating distant metastases homing to the surgical scar. Under the former hypothesis, one would predict that use of a wider surgical margin for an ulcerated or thick melanoma might be associated with a lower risk of a local recurrence than experienced by similar patients treated with a narrow margin. This would especially be true if a wider excision of skin and subcutaneous tissue removed lateral extensions of primary melanoma cells or microsatellites to a greater extent than a narrower surgical margin. Those patients treated with the more radical 4-cm margin of excision did not have any lower a rate of local recurrences than did those treated with a narrower 2-cm margin, both overall and compared to patients within equivalent tumor thickness and ulceration status stratification groups.

WIDE LOCAL EXCISION TECHNIQUES

Most wide local excisions can be performed as an elliptical excision with primary closure. Excision is carried down to (but not through) the underlying muscle fascia in most patients. In extremely obese patients the depth need not be all the way to the muscular fascia but should be at least to the superficial fascia. Primary closure is often facilitated by a length to width ratio of approximately 3:1. The closure is usually accomplished using a standard advancement flap, although occasionally either rotational flaps or a split-thickness skin graft may be necessary to cover the defect. On the trunk and the head and neck, the direction of the long axis of the wide local excision should usually be parallel to the skin lines. On an extremity the orientation should be either longitudinal or somewhat oblique to facilitate closure and cosmesis. Excision of melanomas on the head and neck are much more complicated because of the functional and cosmetic features of structures such as the eyelid, ear, and nose.[88,147,162] Nevertheless, appropriate surgical margins should be used and reconstruction of the defect accomplished with skin flaps or grafts.[150] Whenever a split-thickness skin graft is used to cover the defect after wide excision of a melanoma, the skin graft donor site should preferentially be chosen outside the area of any potential in transit metastases. Guidelines for wide local excision of a primary melanoma are summarized in Table 38.2-10.

Melanomas that arise on the skin or nail bed of the toes are managed with a straightforward amputation at the metatarsal-phalangeal joint.[147] The joint space can usually be covered with adequate soft tissue by raising either a plantar or dorsal soft tissue flap. A significant functional deficit is rarely produced by the total amputation of a single digit from the foot. Because the metatarsal head of the great toe is a critical structure for ambulation, its removal (i.e., a ray amputation) should be avoided when performing amputations of the great toe.

Complete amputations of fingers or thumb give rise to a more significant functional impairment. When excising melanomas on the fingers, the surgeon should preserve as much length of the digit as possible without compromising margins. The digit is preferentially amputated proximal to the distal interphalangeal joint of the fingers and the interphalangeal joint of the thumb if the extent of the nail bed or parenchymal involvement and the proximal location of the lesion's border allow.[147] Because the excision of bone offers no oncologic benefit, unless the bone is directly involved, the total amputation of a finger or ray amputation to include the metacarpal bone is not mandated for proximal finger lesions. Adequate soft tissue excisions without amputation can usually be performed for primary lesions located on the proximal portions of the fingers. Wound closure may be accomplished by full-thickness skin grafts, local rotational flaps, or full-thickness soft tissue flaps created by the amputation of an adjacent and less functionally important digit or cross-finger flap taken from a less functionally important area of an adjacent digit.

Overall, recommendations must, of course, be individualized for a given patient. The importance of other prognostic factors, the anatomic location of the primary tumor, specific factors related to wound healing, and associated medical risk factors must be considered. If these general guidelines are followed, however, overall local recurrence rates should be minimized to acceptable risk levels (less than 3%), with the overwhelming majority of patients effectively treated by relatively simple operations, usually on an outpatient basis with minimal morbidity.

LOCAL RECURRENCES

Local recurrence is not uncommon after inadequate excision of the primary lesion. This scenario typically results from a failure to obtain an accurate initial histopathologic diagnosis. In such instances, the risk of distant metastases and death may be similar to that of primary lesions with the same thickness, ulceration, and nodal status.

Local recurrence after adequate surgical excision of the primary melanoma is associated with aggressive tumor biologic features and is frequently a harbinger of metastases.[163] Local recurrence is strongly associated with the appearance of in transit metastases, lymph node metastases, and distant metastases, which suggests that the mechanisms leading to local recurrence are closely related to those leading to other types of recurrences. It is therefore not unexpected that a local recurrence portends a grave prognosis. In the Intergroup Melanoma Surgical Trial,[110,153,154] a local recurrence was associated with a high mortality rate, with a 5-year survival rate of only 9% (local recurrence as a first site of relapse) or 11% (local recurrence at any time in the disease process), compared with an 86% survival rate for those patients who did not have a local recurrence (*P* <.0001) (see Fig. 38.2-10).

Surgery remains the mainstay of treatment for local recurrences of melanoma.[163] In patients who are examined at regular intervals, local recurrences are commonly detected at a stage at which they can be managed by surgical resection. Excision with a 0.5- to 1.0-cm margin and deep dissection to the muscular fascia is appropriate. At the time when a local recurrence is surgically removed, it is generally recommended that lymphatic mapping and sentinel node excision be performed in all patients with clinically negative regional lymph nodes, because the probability of occult nodal metastases is as high as 50%.[164]

Resection is not an option in some patients because of the extensive nature of the local recurrence. Hyperthermic isolated limb perfusion is an option in these patients if the recurrence is located on an extremity.[165] Objective response rates of approximately 80% have been reported with the use of melphalan during hyperthermic isolated limb perfusion. Similarly, patients who have an unresectable local recurrence may experience significant regression after treatment with chemotherapy, biotherapy, or biochemotherapy, which may possibly enable their local recurrence to become resectable. The 5-year survival rates after hyperthermic isolated limb perfusion are approximately 61% for patients with a local recurrence or satellite lesions within 3 cm of the scar from the original melanoma excision, 30% for patients with in transit metastases, 38% for patients with lymph node metastases, and 16% for patients with both in transit and lymph node metastases.[166] However, the results of prospective randomized trials have shown no survival benefit attributable to prophylactic isolated limb perfusion administered in an effort to prevent local recurrence or in transit metastases.[167]

Local radiation therapy has been used less commonly in situations of local recurrence, with generally lower response rates.[168] It may be needed, however, in scenarios in which there is diffuse disease that would be difficult to resect. Patients are treated with 30 Gy of irradiation in 10 fractions over 2 weeks, and responses have been reported in up to 67% of the patients. This modality has a limited role but can be effective if first-line therapies fail.

Desmoplastic lesions, particularly those on the head and neck, are often associated with a high incidence of local recurrences as well as histologic evidence of perineural invasion.[88,91] Therefore, postoperative adjuvant radiation therapy to the local area is recommended for many patients with desmoplastic melanoma.[169] This is especially true when neurotropism is present, and therefore these patients in particular may benefit from prophylactic or adjuvant radiation therapy after primary excision.

Systemic treatments of melanoma produce complete responses in only a small fraction of patients who have measurable disease and therefore are rarely appropriate as the primary therapy for a local recurrence when it is the sole manifestation of relapse. For patients who have a local recurrence and clinically evident systemic disease, however, systemic treatment is often indicated.

MANAGEMENT OF REGIONAL NODES—LYMPHADENECTOMY (STAGE III)

ELECTIVE NODE DISSECTIONS

Interest in ELND grew out of the hypothesis that melanoma cells spread to regional nodal basins before metastasizing widely; thus, early removal of nodal deposits may prevent subsequent dissemination.[111,172] Four prospective trials were designed to test this hypothesis. In three trials,[123,170,171] ELND produced no significant survival benefit; in the fourth,[110] patients with intermediate-thickness melanoma did not benefit from ELND overall, but subgroup analysis showed that ELND may benefit patients younger than 60 years of age, especially those with melanomas that are non-ulcerated and between 1 and 2 mm in thickness. Debate over the merits of ELND has largely been subsumed by the emergence of sentinel node biopsy as a staging and, possibly, therapeutic procedure.

LYMPHATIC MAPPING AND SENTINEL NODE EXCISION

The technique of intraoperative lymphatic mapping and sentinel node lymphadenectomy represents a major advance in the staging and management of melanoma. It is particularly useful in informing treatment decisions for patients with clinically negative regional lymph nodes and in clarifying patient populations for clinical trials.[141,172,173] Most experts recommend lymphatic mapping and sentinel node lymphadenectomy as a staging procedure for patients with clinical stage I or II melanoma if their primary tumor is at least 1 mm thick or, if it is less than 1 mm thick, if the tumor is ulcerated or is Clark level IV or V (stage 1B). The sentinel node lymphadenectomy procedure

is best performed at the time of the wide local excision of the primary melanoma. The pathologic yield of clinically occult nodal metastases increases as the tumor thickness increases, ranging from 15% to 20% for T1b and T2 melanomas to more than 30% for T4 melanomas.[174,175] Exceptions to this finding are desmoplastic melanomas and LMMs, which have a low incidence of nodal metastases, even for thicker melanomas.[92,176] Lymphatic mapping performed after a wide excision may not be as accurate, particularly for truncal lesions or those with complicated or ambiguous drainage patterns. Although sentinel node lymphadenectomy after wide local excision may still yield accurate staging information, it often leads to sampling of more nodes and more nodal basins.[138,177–179] The use of intraoperative lymphatic mapping and sentinel node lymphadenectomy for melanoma is a highly significant and reproducible technical advance that has been validated and adopted by melanoma centers across the nation and around the world. This surgical technique has provided a precise tool that, when properly used, can stage for the presence or absence of regional metastases down to a threshold of 10^5 to 10^6 cells and with an accuracy of more than 95%[180] (Fig. 38.2-11).

The concept of the sentinel node is now well established, and the procedure should be used for all patients for whom the staging information will be useful to the patient or the physician for counseling and treatment planning. In addition, all

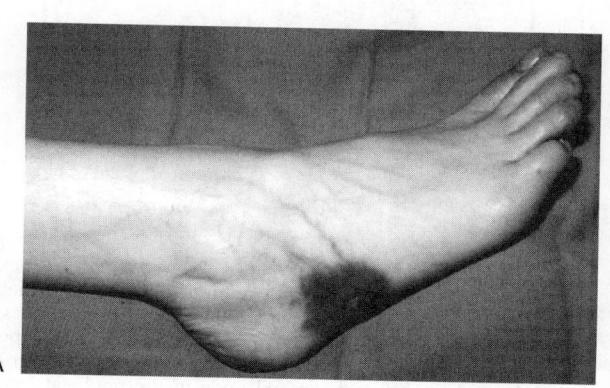

A

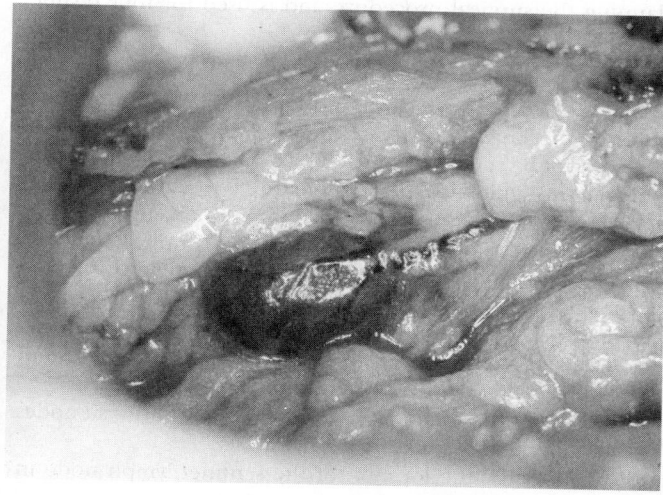

B

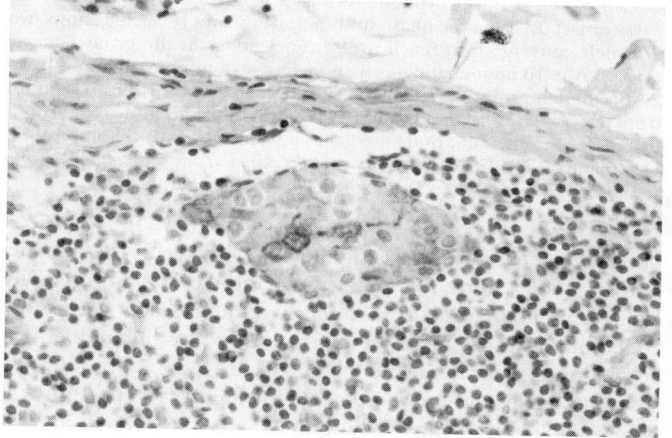

C

FIGURE 38.2-11. Technique of intraoperative lymphatic mapping and sentinel lymph node excision. Radioisotope-labeled tracer is generally injected intradermally approximately 3 hours preoperatively. **A:** At the time of surgery, 0.5 to 1.0 mL of Lymphazurin blue dye is injected intradermally. **B:** A small incision is made over the regional lymph node basin in the area with the high radioisotope counts, and the dissection is continued until one or more sentinel lymph nodes containing the blue dye and the radioisotope are identified. These are excised. **C:** Pathologic examination by serial sectioning demonstrates a subcapsular nodal metastasis. (See Color Fig. 38.2-11 in the CD-ROM.)

clinically node-negative melanoma patients being considered for possible entry into clinical trials should undergo a sentinel node staging procedure at the time of the wide local excision of the primary melanoma.

Intraoperative lymphatic mapping and sentinel node lymphadenectomy has multiple advantages in the care of the melanoma patient with clinically normal regional nodes:

1. It advances the ability to accurately stage the presence of nodal metastases by 18 to 24 months compared to clinical or radiologic assessment of the regional lymph nodes.
2. It facilitates the surgery for nodal metastases because there is no bulk disease and the treatment can be completed at the same time as that for the primary melanoma.
3. It defines a relatively homogeneous group of node-negative melanoma patients with a good prognosis who can thus be spared more radical cancer treatments.
4. It improves the accuracy, interpretability, and comparability of melanoma clinical trials.
5. It may increase cure rates among some subgroups of patients with nodal metastases.
6. It provides a new and powerful tool for examining the biologic role of lymphatic dissemination of tumor and the nodal factors that might contribute to distant spread.

Preoperative lymphoscintigraphy serves as a "road map" for planning the surgical procedure and is used for four distinct reasons:

1. To identify all nodal basins at risk for metastatic disease.[88,181,182] This is especially important with melanomas of the trunk or the head and neck, where lymphatic drainage patterns cannot be reliably predicted by clinical judgment or classical anatomic guidelines. The procedure is essential to identify all regional nodal basins at risk, including drainage to uncommon sites, such as popliteal or epitrochlear lymph nodes (Fig. 38.2-12). Existing data support the view that patients with truncal melanomas and drainage to multiple nodal basins are at increased risk for sentinel node metastases and that the histologic status of a sentinel node in a given nodal basin does not correlate with that of the other draining nodal basins.[183]
2. To identify and mark the location of any in transit nodes for subsequent harvesting.
3. To identify the location of the sentinel lymph node in relation to other nodes in the basin.
4. To estimate the number of sentinel lymph nodes in the regional basin that will have to be harvested.

Radiocolloid and vital blue dye mapping techniques are complementary. Several studies have demonstrated a significant improvement in sentinel lymph node identification rates using the combined modality approach. For example, investigators at M. D. Anderson Cancer Center compared sentinel node identification rates in 626 patients who underwent lymphatic mapping and sentinel node biopsy using isosulfan blue dye alone (n = 252) or in combination with technetium 99m–labeled sulfur colloid with tracer detection by a handheld gamma probe (n = 374).[184] In this study sentinel lymph node identification rates improved from 87% for dye alone to over 99% for the combined dye and colloid technique ($P < .0001$) for all anatomic sites examined. The mean number of sentinel lymph nodes har-

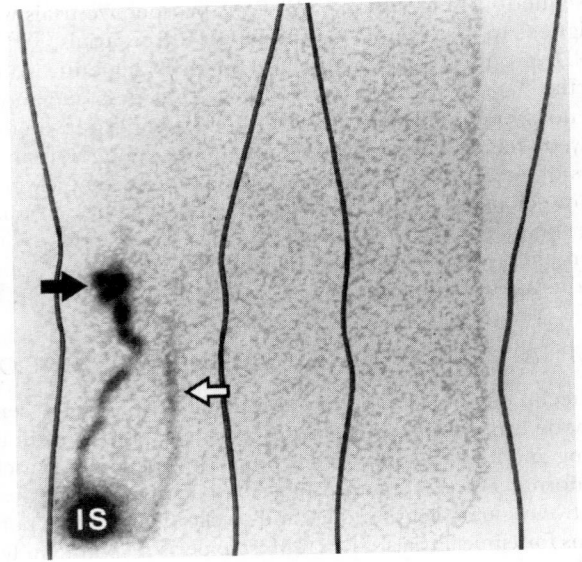

A

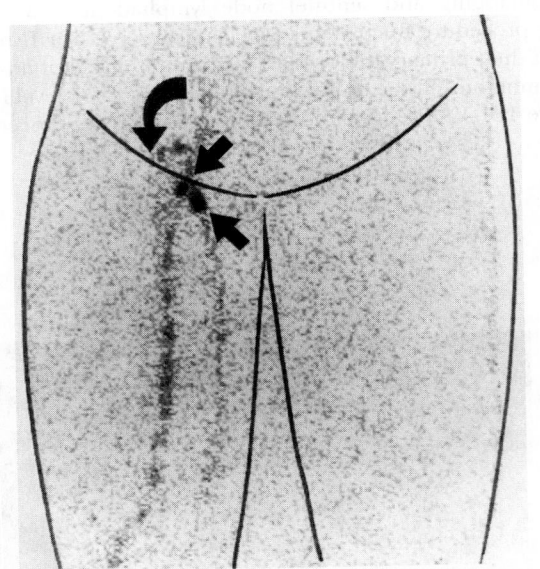

B

FIGURE 38.2-12. Cutaneous lymphoscintigraphy of a melanoma on the lower leg showing lymphatic drainage to sentinel nodes in the popliteal fossa and the inguinal area. **A:** Dynamic study in the posterior projection shows tracer in the injection site (IS) on the posterior left calf and a channel passing to a sentinel node in the popliteal fossa (*solid arrow*), as well as tracer bypassing this area to drain directly to the groin (*open arrow*). **B:** Dynamic phase study anteriorly over the groin shows two channels converging to reach two sentinel nodes in the groin (*straight arrows*). A third faint channel is seen passing to a node higher and laterally in the left groin (*curved arrow*). This is a channel that has passed on from the popliteal nodes upward to the groin; thus this node is a second-tier node, as is the faint node medial to it. (From Uren R, Thompson JF, Howman-Giles R. *Lymphatic drainage of the skin and breast: locating the sentinel nodes.* London: Martin Dunitz, 1999:65,66, with permission.)

vested from each basin was significantly greater in the patients whose nodes were mapped using the combined modality approach (1.74 vs. 1.31; $P < .0001$). In another study, the Sydney Melanoma Unit reported an 87% initial success rate in identifying sentinel lymph nodes.[181,182,185] There was a pronounced learning curve, and the success rate for the last 100 patients was 97%. Cutaneous lymphoscintigraphy was performed in 800 melanoma patients and was used to guide subsequent sentinel lymph node harvesting; 23% of patients were found to have micrometastatic disease.[181,182,185] Patients found to have a positive sentinel lymph node were returned to the operating room for completion node dissection.

When preoperative lymphoscintigraphy was followed by intraoperative mapping using vital blue dye staining in conjunction with injection of radiocolloid (technetium 99m–antimony trisulfide) and a handheld gamma probe, a 1.9% false-negative rate was reported.[184] Morton et al. published a refinement of the technique that allows for *intra*nodal mapping of the sentinel node based on intranodal compartmentalization of lymphatic flow (using injection of both Lymphazurin blue dye and carbon black dye).[180]

Once the sentinel lymph node has been harvested, it is submitted for detailed pathologic examination. Sentinel lymph nodes are bisected and submitted for both routine histologic examination and immunohistochemical staining in serial sections of the lymph node. Overall, there is still considerable variation in approach among major cancer centers. Most groups use both the S-100 and HMB45 stains and many use melanin A staining.

The findings in the studies cited earlier demonstrate that intraoperative lymphatic mapping plus sentinel lymph node biopsy yields accurate pathologic staging; does not lower standards of care; decreases morbidity (e.g., lymphedema is absent, and early return to work or normal activity is facilitated); makes possible rational, yet less aggressive, surgical and adjuvant medical approaches; and reduces costs.[141] The sentinel node staging procedure also facilitates more accurate review of the pathologic features. Because only one or two nodes are usually harvested, it is possible for the pathologist to serially section the node and perform immunohistologic staining on multiple sections. This enhances the sensitivity of melanoma detection by tenfold. The fact that most patients who exhibit regional nodal relapse after a negative sentinel lymph node evaluation can be shown to have disease in their sentinel lymph node on serial sectioning highlights the added sensitivity associated with the more intensive evaluation of the sentinel nodes.[184] In addition, the procedure has facilitated the use of molecular diagnosis and staging, especially the multimarker reverse transcriptase-polymerase chain reaction (RT-PCR) assay[180,186–188] (Fig. 38.2-13). This technology allows the reliable diagnosis of metastatic melanoma at a level of tumor burden well below that achievable with the light microscope. In one study, for example, paraffin-embedded sentinel lymph node specimens free of metastases by light-microscopical examination, including immunohistochemical staining, were reexamined by quantitative multimarker RT-PCR assay. Thirty percent of patients had RT-PCR–positive signals in their sentinel nodes, and RT-PCR positivity was associated with a significantly higher risk of disease recurrence and death than negative RT-PCR results ($P < .0001$).[180]

Reports suggest that the lymphatic mapping procedure is applicable to all primary sites of the body, including the head and neck, probably the most technically demanding area.[88,141,181,189] These reports illustrate that a combination mapping technique using both vital blue dye and colloid is especially useful in this patient population. Rates of false-negative sentinel lymph node biopsy findings in head and neck melanoma are slightly higher than when lymphatic mapping is performed in extremity and trunk melanoma (10% vs. 1% to 2%). However, these rates are not sufficiently high to outweigh the multiple other benefits associated with this staging procedure.

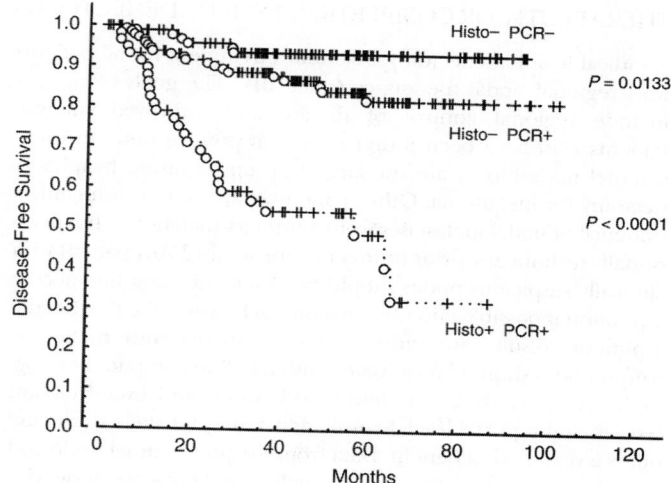

FIGURE 38.2-13. Recurrence-free survival of melanoma patients with tumor thickness greater than 0.76 mm who underwent nodal staging with lymphatic mapping, sentinel lymph node biopsy, and a detailed examination of sentinel lymph nodes that included hematoxylin and eosin staining, S-100 staining, and reverse transcriptase-polymerase chain reaction (RT-PCR) testing. Those with negative findings on all these evaluations had the best prognosis, with survival on long-term follow-up approaching 92%. Patients whose tumors were up-staged based on results of the RT-PCR assay did significantly worse than patients whose sentinel lymph nodes were negative by the three assays. Histo–/+, negative/positive results on histologic examination; PCR–/+, negative/positive results on RT-PCR testing. (From ref. 141, with permission.)

The staging value of the sentinel node technique is irrefutable. A more controversial issue is whether the earlier surgical intervention to excise all the regional lymph nodes when the sentinel node contains metastatic melanoma has any favorable impact on survival. Most studies demonstrate that there is approximately a 20% yield of additional metastases after excising additional downstream nodes with a radical lymphadenectomy.[190]

Although it is reasonable to assume that, because patients with microscopic nodal involvement (i.e., stage IIIA) have a better prognosis and overall survival than patients presenting with palpable nodes (stage IIIB or IIIC), the early identification of the sentinel lymph node and completion node dissection will produce a survival benefit. This assumption requires prospective validation. To this end, the National Cancer Institute has funded an international trial examining the role of lymphatic mapping and selective lymphadenectomy in patients with melanoma to determine if there is a survival benefit with this surgical strategy. The Multicenter Selective Lymphadenectomy Trial randomly assigned more than 2000 patients with melanomas 1.0 mm or more in thickness to either wide local excision of the primary site and observation of the regional basin or wide local excision and sentinel lymph node biopsy.[138] This trial is different from the old trials that studied the efficacy of ELND in that all patients randomly assigned to the lymphatic mapping arm of the study will undergo preoperative lymphoscintigraphy to determine all basins at risk for disease. If cutaneous lymphatic flow is confined to one or two basins, then all basins at risk are dissected for their sentinel lymph nodes. The protocol is also distinguished from the elective node dissection trials in that only those patients with disease in the sentinel lymph node will undergo a completion node dissection.

THERAPEUTIC OR COMPLETION LYMPHADENECTOMY

A radical lymphadenectomy is standard treatment for all patients with regional nodal metastases (stage III). The goals of surgery include regional control of disease and improved survival. Patients who have been found to have a positive node through sentinel node biopsy are the largest group requiring lymphadenectomy for melanoma. Other patients may present with clinical evidence of nodal metastases from a primary melanoma, but occasionally without any prior history of a melanoma. Any patient with clinically suspicious nodes should be evaluated using fine-needle aspiration if possible and using excisional biopsy if the fine-needle aspiration results are indeterminate. Patients with metastatic lymph nodes should be evaluated with baseline computed tomography (CT) scans, a complete blood count, and liver function tests, including LDH level. Lymphadenectomy for stage III disease offers a real survival benefit. Data from the pre–sentinel node and preadjuvant era show that patients with a single positive node who undergo a complete nodal dissection have approximately a 40% chance of being alive and apparently free of disease at 10 years. Those who have a single clinically occult or microscopic nodal metastasis detected by the sentinel node technology have a 5-year survival of almost 70%.

As a general principle, the lymphadenectomy should be anatomic. Nodal contents are excised in a single block within their surrounding fatty tissue, with motor nerves and muscle preserved whenever possible. Perioperative antibiotics are used routinely.

Axillary Dissection

The goal of axillary lymph node dissection for melanoma is complete resection of all lymph nodes.[191] Skeletonization of the axillary vein, thoracodorsal neurovascular bundle, and long thoracic nerve, and removal of all level I, II, and III lymph nodes should be accomplished. Although division of the pectoralis minor muscle is rarely necessary for breast cancer, it is occasionally used in melanoma patients to obtain complete exposure of level II and III nodes. The long thoracic nerve and the thoracodorsal neurovascular bundle are left intact unless they are directly invaded by tumor. A closed-suction drain is placed. Further details about surgical technique are given elsewhere.[191] Patients undergoing a radical axillary lymphadenectomy should have no appreciable loss of range of motion or motor function. A complete dissection does carry with it approximately a 10% risk of lymphedema in the upper extremity.

Inguinal and Iliac Dissection

For patients with metastatic inguinal or femoral nodes, an anatomically complete inguinofemoral dissection is performed.[192] The technical details of the operation are described elsewhere.[192] In patients with clinically detected nodal metastases, the femoral canal is opened and Cloquet's node (the lowest node in the iliac chain) is removed. This step can be omitted in patients undergoing complete nodal dissection after detection of clinically occult or microscopic nodal disease. If this lowest iliac node contains metastases, then an iliac and obturator dissection is performed through a muscle-splitting incision through the lower abdominal wall.[192]

Indications for an iliac and obturator dissection include the finding of a positive Cloquet's node intraoperatively or enlarged pelvic nodes by CT scan.[192] Iliac and obturator dissection may also be considered if four or more metastatic lymph nodes are found at the inguinofemoral level. Some patients may be cured.[173]

On closure a closed-suction drain is placed in the inguinofemoral area. Prophylactic antibiotics are usually given. The risk of lower extremity lymphedema is approximately 20%. Routine measures to reduce the risk of lymphedema include a program of wearing a fitted compression garment at 20 to 30 mm Hg during the daytime for the first 6 months postoperatively.

Cervical Dissection

The extent of cervical lymphadenectomy will depend on the location of the positive node and the presence or absence of direct invasion into the structures of the neck.[193] For a positive sentinel node, usually a comprehensive neck dissection of all five levels of neck lymph nodes, with preservation of the internal jugular vein, spinal accessory nerve, and sternocleidomastoid muscle, is generally considered to be the most appropriate lymphadenectomy procedure in that it preserves function and cosmesis.[193] When there is clinical involvement of the parotid lymph nodes, the other cervical lymph nodes are also at risk of harboring metastatic disease, even if they are clinically negative. For this reason, a neck dissection is generally performed in addition to a therapeutic parotidectomy.[193] Conversely, patients with clinically evident cervical node metastases arising from a melanoma located on the ipsilateral face, anterior scalp, or ear should have a superficial parotidectomy performed at the time of a comprehensive neck dissection, even if the parotid nodes are clinically negative, for there is a high risk of clinically occult nodal disease in the parotid area.

Even with a therapeutic neck dissection, there is still a 20% to 30% recurrence rate in the neck. Patients with multiple metastatic nodes, especially with gross extracapsular invasion into surrounding tissues, have an especially high risk of neck recurrence, even after a thorough neck dissection. When this occurs, there can be severe morbidity and debilitation. For these reasons, many centers recommend that adjuvant radiation therapy be administered postoperatively after a neck dissection for clinically palpable nodal metastases to the neck, especially when there is extranodal extension of tumor.[193–195]

RADIOTHERAPY FOR REGIONAL METASTASES (STAGE III)

Radiotherapy is used to treat melanoma involving regional lymph node basins in five clinical scenarios.[168] Radiotherapy can be therapeutic (palliative intent) for the following:

- Gross unresectable regional disease
- Gross residual disease after (intended or mistaken) debulking palliative surgery

Or radiotherapy can be adjuvant (radical intent) for suspected subclinical disease in the following circumstances:

- After initial therapeutic lymph node dissection
- After salvage lymphadenectomy for relapsed nodal disease
- As an alternative strategy to ELND in patients at high risk of locoregional relapse or to reduce the likelihood of the need for a subsequent therapeutic lymph node dissection, or both

RADIOTHERAPY FOR UNRESECTABLE NODAL DISEASE

Palliative radiotherapy for regionally recurrent disease is beneficial for many patients. The median complete response rate is 23.5% (range, 23% to 74%)[62,90–92,168] and the partial response rate is 35% to 45%, which gives an overall response rate of approximately 60%.[196,197] The duration of response is 7 months. The median duration of survival is approximately 1 year, and the 5-year survival is 8%.[168,197,198] Treatment is usually well tolerated and, given the short life expectancy of most patients, long-term morbidity is relatively limited.

ADJUVANT RADIOTHERAPY

No randomized controlled studies have addressed the role of adjuvant radiation therapy for melanoma after a therapeutic node dissection. Many physicians consider radiation in the following circumstances[168]:

- Macroscopic metastatic parotid node or multiple cervical node involvement
- Macroscopic metastatic involvement of three or more nodes in the axilla or groin
- The presence of gross extranodal metastatic invasion or matted nodes
- Metastatic nodal size larger than 3 cm
- Nodal relapse after lymphadenectomy and salvage with secondary surgery

Furthermore, in head and neck melanoma, when postoperative radiotherapy is considered for poor-prognosis primary melanoma, it is advisable also to consider including regional nodes.[168] Conversely, the primary site should be incorporated in continuity when planning regional radiotherapy if the primary was resected less than 1 year before the nodal metastases and was not located in the midline region.

Recommended radiotherapy prescriptions based on the published literature can be 30 Gy in five fractions over 2.5 weeks when optimal use of an ipsilateral electron-beam therapy technique can be undertaken for head and neck melanoma. One should ensure that critical structures such as the spinal cord (maximum of 24 Gy) and larynx do not receive more than the allowable radiation doses.[168] Otherwise, for all nodal basin sites and use of megavoltage photon techniques, more conventional regimens of 48 Gy at the depth of maximum dose in 20 fractions over 4 weeks or 50 Gy in 25 fractions over 5 weeks are advised when normal tissue tolerability is an issue and larger integral dosage is unavoidable.

Caution should be used in delivering adjuvant radiotherapy concurrently with adjuvant interferon (IFN) therapy. There is potential for increased regional toxicity, and experience in this field is limited.[168] Participation in clinical trials, when possible, is especially encouraged.

REGIONAL RELAPSES

IN TRANSIT METASTASES

In transit metastasis represents the clinical manifestation of small tumor emboli trapped within the dermal and subdermal lymphatics between the site of the primary tumor and the regional lymph node drainage basin(s). It occurs in 3% to 4% of patients with stage I and II disease and increases to 10% to 15% in patients with stage III disease.[199,200] When present, in transit metastases are usually multiple, evolve over time, and, as previously stated, are often the harbinger of subsequent systemic disease. Although previous staging systems distinguished between satellitosis (within 2 cm of the primary tumor) and in transit metastases (more than 2 cm from the primary tumor), pathophysiologically these two events represent different points on a continuum of the same biologic process. Several studies have shown that classification of regional relapse based on distance from the primary tumor site is of little prognostic value.[125,126,200]

Surgical excision is appropriate as the initial treatment for patients who present with a small number of in transit metastases. This should be accomplished with a histologically negative margin of normal surrounding skin and subcutaneous tissues, and primary closure is usually possible. Although some have suggested attempting 2-cm margins, wide radial clearance margins are probably unnecessary in the surgical management of in transit metastases.[200] Surgical excision is particularly appropriate for initial management of the solitary subcutaneous metastasis. Unfortunately, however, surgical excision alone often fails to control regional disease. One study reported that, among patients who had locoregional recurrence who underwent surgical resection, further locoregional recurrences were seen in 55% by 2 years and in 82% by 5 years.[201] At the time when an in transit metastasis is surgically removed, it is generally recommended that lymphatic mapping and sentinel node excision be performed in all patients with clinically negative regional lymph nodes, because the probability of occult nodal metastases is as high as 50%.[164] Other forms of local therapy that have been considered include intralesional injections of bacille Calmette-Guérin (BCG), laser ablation, and external-beam irradiation.[200]

When in transit metastases occur on the extremities, either isolated limb perfusion or isolated limb infusion have been recommended, especially if the lesions are multiple or recurrent.[165,200]

REGIONAL NODAL RECURRENCES

Regional nodal failure in a previously dissected basin is usually found at the periphery of the prior surgical procedure. If there is confidence that the original surgical procedure was adequate, the nodal failure should be widely excised with a histologically negative margin.[202] If concern exists that the initial surgical procedure was inadequate, then redissection of the entire nodal drainage basin is recommended. Redissection of a previously dissected basin with curative intent may be difficult and often places previously dissected and preserved structures at risk. In particular, in the axilla, the thoracodorsal neurovascular complex and the long thoracic nerve may have to be sacrificed in an attempt to regain regional control.

After resection of nodal recurrence, these patients remain at high risk for further regional and systemic recurrence. In patients who have multiple positive nodes, extensive extranodal disease, or disease that has been dissected off previously dissected vessels, the use of high-dose adjuvant radiation therapy to improve regional control should be considered.[168,200,203]

The prognosis for patients who have a nodal recurrence in a previously dissected basin is poor.[200] Five- and 10-year survival rates of 11% to 36% and 5% to 31%, respectively, are reported. In one series of 162 patients who had a recurrence in the nodal basin, only 11% survived 5 years, and only 5% survived 10 years.[204] In another series, 51 of 74 patients had recurrences in the nodal basin as a solitary first site of recurrence. Twelve of these 51 patients (11%) survived 5 years.[205] Because these patients have such a high risk of dying of distant metastases, they should be considered for adjuvant systemic therapy once surgical redissection and adjuvant irradiation for locoregional control is accomplished.

ADJUVANT SYSTEMIC THERAPY (STAGES II AND III)

More accurate staging of melanoma allows the identification of patients whose risk is sufficiently high to justify administration of adjuvant systemic treatment.[96,98,111] For the purpose of considering adjuvant therapy, patients can be divided into four risk groups according to the AJCC staging system designation: low risk (patients with stage IA disease), intermediate risk (those with stage IB and IIA melanomas), high risk (those with stage IIB, IIC, and IIIA tumors), and very high risk (those with stage IIIB and IIIC disease), which have less than 10%, 10% to 30%, 30% to 50%, and greater than 50% risk of distant recurrence and melanoma-related mortality at 10 years, respectively. In addition, patients with stage IV melanoma who have been rendered free of disease with surgery have a greater than 90% risk of distant recurrence and death at 10 years and consequently should be considered at extremely high risk. High and very high risk groups, those previously categorized as having stage IIB and III disease, have been the primary focus of studies evaluating the efficacy of adjuvant therapy. Some trials also have incorporated or examined exclusively intermediate risk patients (formerly those with stage IIA disease).

Over the past 30 years, a number of approaches have been tested in an effort to reduce the risk of melanoma recurrence. These approaches have included chemotherapy using agents such as dacarbazine[206–208]; nonspecific immune adjuvants such as BCG vaccine,[208–210] *Corynebacterium parvum*,[210–212] or levamisole[213–215]; and hormonal agents such as megestrol acetate. Despite some initial promising results, none of these agents used either alone or in combination proved beneficial when compared to observation, placebo, or each other in randomized clinical trials. In the largest trial, 761 patients with stage IIA or IIB disease (or stage I on the trunk) were randomly assigned to treatment with surgical excision alone or in combination with dacarbazine, BCG vaccine, or both.[208,216] At 3 years, the rates of disease-free survival (30% to 37%) and overall survival (42% to 50%) were similar in all groups.

At present, the most promising results have been reported with either a variety of melanoma-specific vaccines, IFN-α, or granulocyte-macrophage colony-stimulating factor (GM-CSF).

MELANOMA VACCINES

A number of different types of melanoma vaccine have been evaluated in intermediate- and high-risk patients with melanoma. These include whole cell, cell lysate, or shed antigen vaccines and ganglioside vaccines. Many of these vaccines have also been tested in patients with metastatic disease, and these results are discussed separately.

Whole Cell, Cell Lysate, or Shed Antigen Vaccines

Use of a variety of melanoma-specific vaccines comprised of whole melanoma cells or cell fractions has been investigated primarily in patients with high-risk stage III melanoma.[216,217] These include vaccines prepared from three allogeneic melanoma cell lines (with BCG as adjuvant, known as Cancer-Vax)[218,219]; from autologous tumor cells modified with the hapten dinitrophenylalanine, now known as M-VAX[220,221]; from lysates of two allogeneic melanoma cell lines (administered with Detox), the Melacine vaccine[222]; or from antigens shed from cultures of allogeneic melanoma cell lines admixed with alum, the "Bystryn" vaccine.[223]

All of these vaccines have been reported to produce responses in some patients with advanced disease and to significantly prolong survival when administered in the adjuvant setting in comparison either to historical controls or to patients who had a poor immune response to the vaccine.[216,218–221,223,224] Many of these vaccines have also shown intriguing immunogenicity that in several instances has correlated with either tumor response or relapse-free or overall survival.[218,221,225,226] Given the evolution in the technology used for melanoma staging, including high-resolution CT and positron emission tomography (PET) scans and sentinel node biopsy, and the more aggressive surgical and systemic treatment after recurrence, contemporaneous controls are essential in evaluating adjuvant treatments. Unfortunately, few large-scale randomized controlled trials of vaccine efficacy have been reported.

The randomized phase III studies reported to date are instructive in determining the true activity of melanoma vaccines and in placing the historically controlled studies in perspective. For example, although phase II studies with vaccinia melanoma cell lysates showed highly significant improvement in survival relative to both historical and nonrandomized concurrent controls,[227] this benefit could not be confirmed in subsequent randomized phase III trials performed involving patients with either stage II melanoma[228] or stage IIB and III melanoma.[229] In the latter study, 700 patients were randomly assigned either to receive the vaccine or to undergo observation. Seventy-seven percent of patients had documented lymph node metastases, including 66% with palpable nodal recurrence (current AJCC stage IIIB or IIIC disease). At a median follow-up of 8 years, median overall survival was 151 months for the vaccine-treated group versus 88 months for the control group ($P = .068$ by Cox stratified univariate analysis). The hazard ratio was 0.81 (95% confidence interval, 0.64 to 1.02) favoring treatment. Median relapse-free survival was 83 months for the vaccine treated group versus 43 months for the controls ($P = .28$). Because fewer than the anticipated number of deaths were observed on either treatment arm, more follow-up will be necessary to exclude definitively a significant survival benefit related to the vaccine.

A phase III trial comparing the Melacine vaccine to observation in 689 patients with stage II disease (primary tumors 1.5 to 4.0 mm thick with nonpalpable regional nodes) was completed by the Southwest Oncology Group.[230] At a median follow-up of 5.6 years, vaccine therapy was not found to be associated with a significant benefit in 5-year disease-free survival, which was estimated to be 65% for those receiving vaccine and 63% for those undergoing observation alone. Data were insufficiently mature to analyze any impact on overall survival. More detailed analysis of the results suggested that the Melacine vaccine might have a preferential impact in patients who were HLA-A2+ or HLA-C3+ or both. This prospectively defined subset of patients showed a significant delay in relapse and death relative to patients with other HLA types receiving the vaccine or patients on the observation arm.[231] For this subset, 5-year relapse-free survival for vaccinated and observed patients was 77% versus 64%, respectively (*P* = .004). Prospective confirmation of this intriguing result is lacking, however. Preliminary results of a phase III trial comparing Melacine vaccine plus intermediate-dose IFN-α to standard high-dose IFN-α alone suggest that the Melacine vaccine plus intermediate-dose IFN possesses similar clinical activity and less toxicity.[232]

The Bystryn polyvalent shed antigen vaccine was tested in a randomized double-blind placebo-controlled trial involving patients with stage III disease.[233] This trial was closed early due to the U.S. Food and Drug Administration (FDA) approval of IFN-α. At the time of closure, 38 patients had been enrolled, with 24 receiving the melanoma vaccine and 14 the placebo vaccine. Although the melanoma vaccine was associated with considerable improvement in median time to disease progression (1.6 vs. 0.6 years) and median overall survival (3.8 vs. 2.7 years), the survival difference was not statistically significant. Efforts to develop a new trial comparing this vaccine, either alone or in combination with IFN-α, to IFN-α alone have stalled.

Extensive phase II experience with the polyvalent allogeneic whole cell vaccine (CancerVax), largely at the John Wayne Cancer Institute, has encouraged the initiation of two randomized phase III trials of adjuvant therapy with this agent. The first trial randomly assigns patients with resected stage III disease to receive CancerVax plus BCG or BCG alone, whereas the second trial randomly assigns patients with stage IV disease who have been rendered clinically disease free with surgery to receive CancerVax or placebo.

It is hoped that these trials will clarify the benefit, if any, of these vaccine preparations. However, even if objective responses or prolongation in survival is observed with these approaches, it will be difficult to determine which components of the vaccine (i.e., which antigen-specific responses) are responsible for the therapeutic effects. Thus, although such a result might encourage further vaccine development, it may not provide sufficient information to aid in the production of increasingly effective vaccines.

Defined Melanoma Antigen Vaccines

A more specific approach has been the development of vaccines that are directed against specific tumor antigens. Two such groups of antigens are gangliosides and antigens that are recognized by T cells infiltrating melanoma lesions.

GM2 GANGLIOSIDE. Gangliosides are sialic acid–containing glycosphingolipids that are overexpressed on the cell surface of melanomas. In general, purified gangliosides have not been shown to be immunogenic. With the exception of the ganglioside GM2, for which spontaneous antibody responses have been detected in up to 5% of patients with melanoma, it has been difficult to induce antibody responses to these molecules. Two studies have demonstrated that the presence of anti-GM2 antibodies confers a relapse-free survival advantage for patients with melanoma.[234,235]

A variety of vaccine strategies involving the GM2 ganglioside have been devised. In one study, a vaccine involving purified GM2 adherent to BCG induced immunoglobulin M (IgM) antibody responses to GM2 in 85% of vaccinated patients.[235] Anti-GM2 antibody production after immunization was associated with improved prognosis compared to either antibody-negative patients or historical controls. These initial observations led to a randomized phase III trial involving 122 patients who had recently undergone resection of regional node metastases.[236] This trial, which was conducted at the Memorial Sloan Kettering Cancer Center, compared the GM2 plus BCG vaccine to BCG alone (both with cyclophosphamide pretreatment). Eighty-five percent of patients (50 of 58) treated with GM2 plus BCG developed IgM antibodies to the ganglioside, whereas six patients (5%) (five from the BCG-alone arm) had preexisting anti-GM2 antibodies. A nonsignificant increase in disease-free survival (18%) and overall survival (11%) was found for the GM2 plus BCG treatment group as a whole. However, when the six patients with preexisting anti-GM2 antibodies were excluded from the analysis, administration of the GM2 plus BCG vaccine was associated with a significant improvement in relapse-free survival (23%; *P* = .02).

This vaccine was able to be made more immunogenic by coupling the GM2 molecule to a carrier protein derived from the keyhole-limpet hemocyanin (KLH) and using QS21, a potent immunologic stimulant of the saponin class, as an immune adjuvant.[237] This new vaccine induces IgM antibodies in 100% of vaccinated patients and IgG antibodies in the majority.[237,238] The efficacy of the GM2-KLH/QS21 vaccine has been investigated in two Intergroup trials, one large-scale randomized phase III trial comparing the vaccine to high-dose IFN alone, and a second comparing the vaccine alone to the vaccine given in combination with high-dose IFN administered beginning at either week 1 or week 5. These trials have been completed and are discussed later in the context of studies involving IFN-α.

ANTIGENS RECOGNIZED BY T CELLS. Another therapeutic approach is based on identification of the HLA-restricted tumor antigens that are recognized by CD8+ T cells which infiltrate the melanoma lesions [i.e., tumor-infiltrating lymphocytes (TILs)].[239] These peptide antigens have been cloned and are currently being examined in selected HLA-compatible patients with stage IV disease, either alone or in combination with professional antigen-presenting cells (dendritic cells) or cytokines such as interleukin-2 (IL-2), IL-12, IFN, or GM-CSF.[216,217] These peptide-specific vaccine strategies are discussed in considerable detail in Chapter 61. It is hoped that the diminished tumor heterogeneity, reduced tumor-related immune suppression, and more protracted treatment time afforded by the adjuvant setting will enable these vaccines to achieve their full therapeutic potential.

INTERFERON-α

The IFNs comprise a complex family of proteins with diverse immunomodulatory and antiangiogenic properties. Immunomodulatory effects include the up-regulation of both class I

TABLE 38.2-11. Results of Eastern Cooperative Oncology Group Randomized Prospective Trials of Adjuvant High-Dose Interferon-α_{2b} Therapy in Melanoma Patients at High Risk for Recurrence (T4 and Stage III Disease)

					Hazard Ratio for RFS			
					No. of Positive Nodes			
Trial	Regimen	No.	5-Y RFS (P Value)	5-Y OS (%)	0	1	2 or 3	4+
E1684	High-dose IFN[a]	143	37% (.002)	46% (.024)	0.37	1.82	1.44[b]	NA
	Observation	137	26%	37%				
E1690	High-dose IFN	215	44% (1.28; .05)[d]	52% (1.0; .74)	1.46	1.0	1.92[b]	1.16
	Low-dose IFN[c]	215	40% (1.19; .17)	53% (1.04; .67)				
	Observation	212	35%	55%				
E1694	High-dose IFN	385	62%[e] (1.49; .0007)	78%[f] (1.38; .015)	2.07[b]	1.44	1.16	1.47
	GMK vaccine[g]	389	49%	73%				

GMK, ganglioside GM2 plus keyhole-limpet hemocyanin; IFN, interferon; NA, not applicable; OS, overall survival; RFS, relapse-free survival.
[a]20 million U/m^2/d IV 5 d/wk for 4 wk; 10 million U/m^2/d t.i.w. SC × 48 wk.
[b]P <.05 by two-sided log rank test.
[c]3 million U/d t.i.w. SC × 2 y.
[d]Hazard ratio based on intent-to-treat analysis; P value based on Cox two-sided P2.
[e]2-y RFS.
[f]2-y OS.
[g]1 mL of GMK vaccine administered via deep SC injection on days 1, 8, 15, and 22, then every 12 wk (weeks 12–96).

and class II major histocompatibility antigen expression on tumor cells and the activation of effector cells [natural killer (NK) cells, T cells, monocytes, and DCs], many of which possess tumorlytic properties. Type I IFNs (IFN-α, IFN-β) are structurally related species derived from genes on chromosome 9 that are induced by exposure of cells to virus or nucleic acids. Type II IFN (IFN-γ) is produced by T cells and NK cells and bears little structural homology to type I IFNs. Type I IFN signaling is mediated via the signal transduction and activators of transcription (STAT) family of proteins. Although both melanoma and effector cells possess IFN receptors and STATs, elegant studies by Lesinski et al. in a murine mouse melanoma model demonstrated

that IFN-α–mediated antitumor effects were dependent on a functional STAT1 signaling within the effector cells, but not the tumor cells.[240] Clinical studies of IFN-α therapy in patients with metastatic melanoma showed modest antitumor activity, whereas IFN-γ was essentially inactive in this setting. This clinical activity, together with the documented immunomodulatory properties of IFN-α, has prompted a host of clinical trials examining the merits of this agent as adjuvant therapy for patients with intermediate to very high-risk melanoma.

The results of the major randomized controlled trials evaluating IFN-α for the adjuvant treatment of patients with melanoma are summarized in Tables 38.2-11 and 38.2-12. Although results

TABLE 38.2-12. Trials of Low- and Intermediate-Dose Interferon-α for Stage II and III Disease

Trial	Year	No.	Arms	IFN Schedule	Population	Outcome Analysis
World Health Organization 16589	1994, 2001	444	IFN-α_{2a} vs. obs	3 MU SC t.i.w. × 3 y	Stage III	RFS: NS OS: NS
North Central Oncology Group	1995	262	IFN-α_{2a} vs. obs	20 MU/m^2 IM t.i.w. × 3 mo	Stage II and III	RFS: NS OS: NS
Austrian trial	1998	311	IFN-α_{2a} vs. obs	3 MU SC qd × 3 wk then 3 MU SC t.i.w. × 1 y	Stage II	RFS: P = .02 OS: NS
French trial	1998	489	IFN-α_{2a} vs. obs	3 MU SC t.i.w. × 18 mo	Stage II	RFS: P = .04 OS: NS
AIM High British trial	2004	674	IFN-α_{2a} vs. obs	3 MU SC 3 t.i.w. × 2 y	Stage IIB and III	RFS: NS OS: NS
European Organization for Research and Treatment of Cancer 18871	2001	830	IFN-α_{2b} vs. IFN-γ vs. iscador vs. obs	1 MU SC t.i.w. × 1 y	Stage IIB and III	RFS: NS OS: NS
European Organization for Research and Treatment of Cancer 18952	2002	1418	IFN-α_{2b} × 1 y vs. IFN-α_{2b} × 2 y vs. obs	A. 10 MU SC daily 5/7 d/wk × 4 wk, then 5 MU SC t.i.w. × 23 mo B. 10 MU SC daily 5/7 d/wk × 4 wk, then 10 MU t.i.w. × 11 mo	Stage IIB and III	A. RFS: NS OS: NS B. RFS: P = .01 OS: NS
Eastern Cooperative Oncology Group 1690	2000	642	IFN-α_{2b} vs. obs	3 MU SC t.i.w. × 2 y	Stage IIB and III	RFS: NS OS: NS

IFN, interferon; NS, not significant; obs, observation; OS, overall survival; RFS, relapse-free survival.

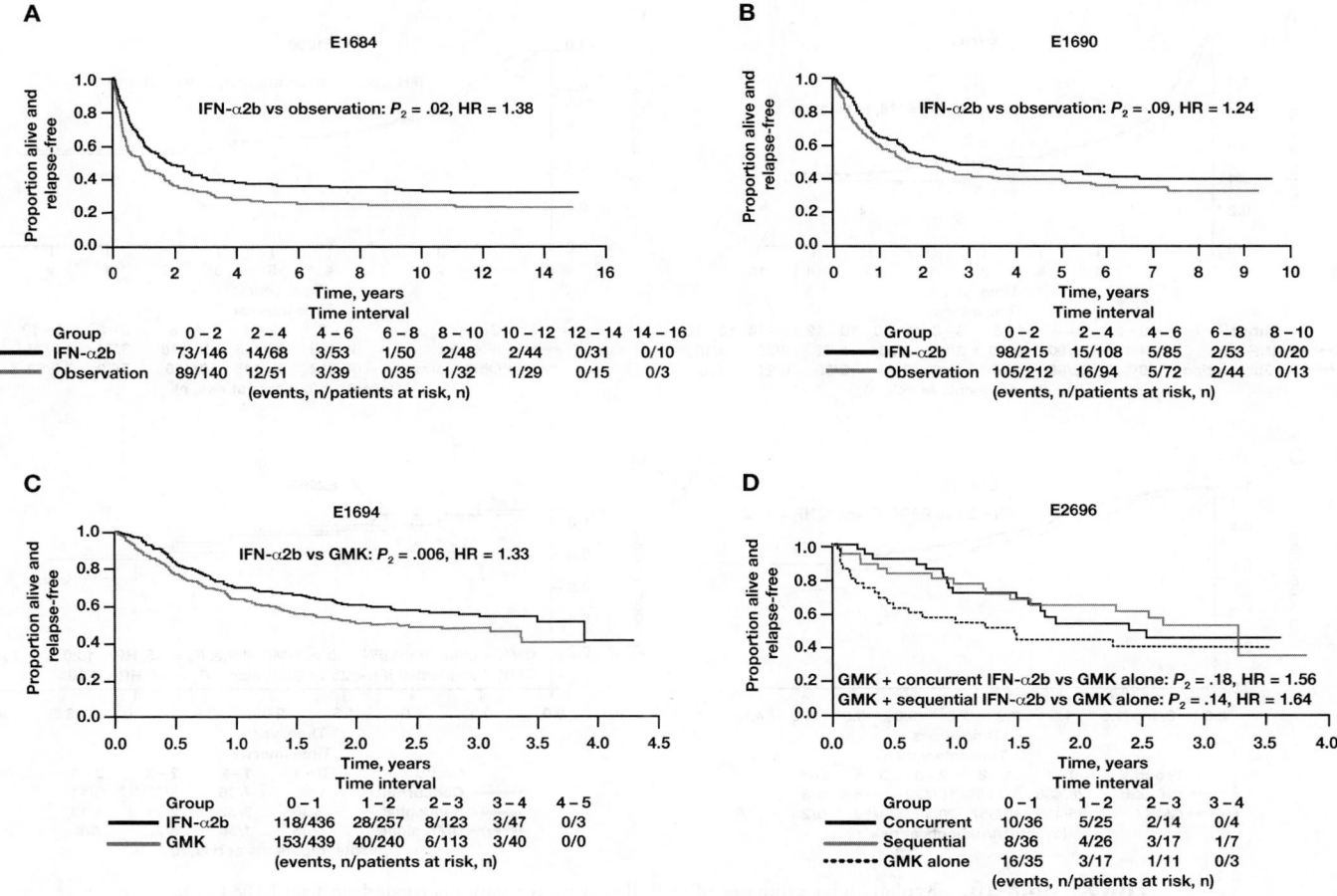

FIGURE 38.2-14. Kaplan-Meier estimates of relapse-free survival for patients treated on trial E1684 at a median follow-up of 12.6 years **(A)**, E1690 at a median follow-up of 6.6 years **(B)**, E1694 at a median follow-up of 2.1 years **(C)**, and E2696 at a median follow-up of 2.8 years **(D)**. GMK, ganglioside GM2 plus keyhole-limpet hemocyanin; HR, hazard ratio; IFN-α_{2b}, interferon-α_{2b}. (From ref. 244, with permission.)

have not always been positive, high-dose IFN-α_{2b} remains the only treatment to show reproducible disease-free and, in some instances, overall survival benefit in prospectively randomized phase III trials (see Table 38.2-11). Three U.S. Cooperative Group studies showed improvement in disease-free survival and two studies also showed significant overall survival benefit for patients receiving high-dose IFN-α_{2b} (20 million U/m^2/d intravenously, 5 days a week for 4 weeks, followed by 10 million U/m^2/d subcutaneously, 3 days a week for up to 11 months)[241–244] (Figs. 38.2-14 and 38.2-15; see Table 38.2-11). A fourth trial, E2696, involved a randomized phase II comparison of the GM2-KLH/QS21 vaccine alone to the vaccine administered in combination with high-dose IFN-α beginning either week 1 or week 5.[245] Even though this study was not designed to examine clinical end points (only 35 patients were enrolled per arm), relapse-free survival was once again significantly better for those on the two regimens containing high-dose IFN-α than for those receiving the vaccine alone. In a pooled analysis of these trials, high-dose IFN therapy appeared to improve relapse-free survival by 20% to 30% ($P = .006$) and overall survival by approximately 7% ($P = .42$).[244]

In 1996, the FDA approved high-dose IFN for the treatment of patients with primary melanomas larger than 4 mm (stage IIB or IIC) or patients with melanoma involvement of the regional lymph nodes rendered disease free by lymph node dissection (stage III). Although analyses of subsets of patients in individual studies suggested that the benefit of high-dose IFN might be restricted to certain patient populations based on number of involved nodes, no consistent pattern was observed (see Table 38.2-11). Thus, it is more reasonable to propose that the benefit of IFN-α_{2b} is proportional to the risk of melanoma recurrence and that IFN-α_{2b} therapy can therefore be considered for all patients whose chance of reduction in melanoma relapse outweighs the likely toxicity of therapy, regardless of the number of diseased nodes. In general, this would include patients with stage IIB, IIC, and III disease without significant comorbidities or major aversion to aggressive therapy and with a life expectancy exceeding 10 years.[246]

High-dose IFN-α_{2b} treatment is associated with multiple side effects, including acute flu-like constitutional symptoms, hepatic transaminitis, chronic fatigue, headaches, nausea, weight loss, myelosuppression, and depression, which are experienced to some degree by the majority of patients.[247,248] Although liver toxicity was responsible for the two treatment-related deaths in ECOG trial E1684, this has not been a cause of mortality in subsequent trials because vigilant monitoring and dose modification guidelines were mandated. Mild to moderate depression and impaired

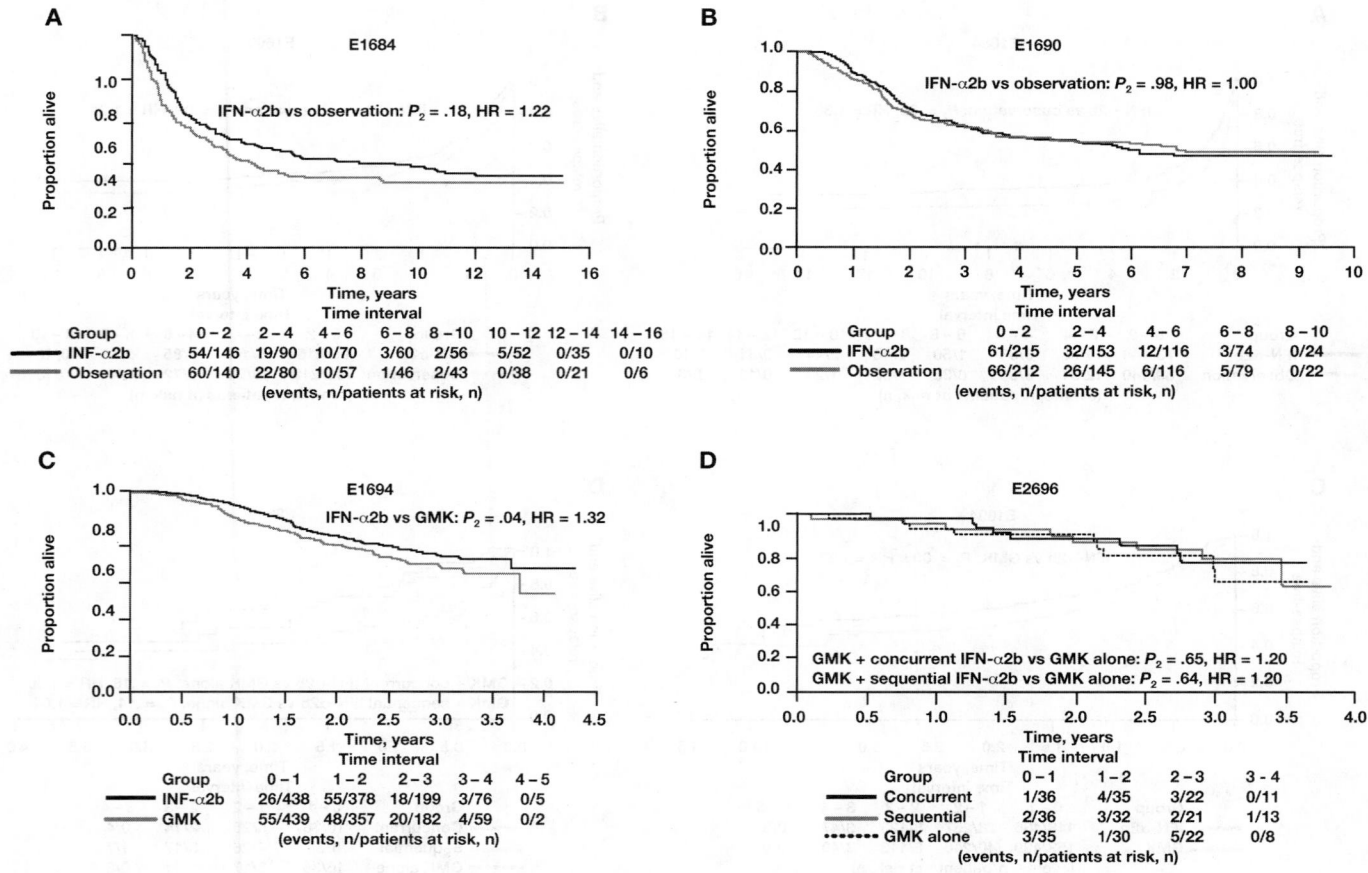

FIGURE 38.2-15. Kaplan-Meier estimates of overall survival for patients treated on trial E1684 at a median follow-up of 12.6 years (**A**), E1690 at a median follow-up of 6.6 years (**B**), E1694 at a median follow-up of 2.1 years (**C**), and E2696 at a median follow-up of 2.8 years (**D**). GMK, ganglioside GM2 plus keyhole-limpet hemocyanin; HR, hazard ratio; IFN-α_{2b}, interferon-α_{2b}. (From ref. 244, with permission.)

cognitive function is commonly reported, whereas mood instability (alternating mania and depression) occurs less often. A history of mood or psychiatric disorders is a risk factor for neuropsychiatric effects. Thyroid dysfunction, usually manifest as hyperthyroidism followed by an extended period of hypothyroidism, develops in approximately 10% of patients, typically around the third to fourth month of therapy. Although side effects can often be managed with appropriate supportive care, including oral and, if necessary, intravenous hydration, acetaminophen, nonsteroidal antiinflammatory agents, antiemetics, analgesics, and antidepressants,[247,248] 30% to 40% of patients require dose delays and dosage reductions during the course of therapy. Most adverse reactions are completely reversible with treatment discontinuation; consequently, standard management calls for withholding IFN for 1 to 4 weeks for patients experiencing severe side effects to enable their resolution, with the resumption of treatment at one-half to two-thirds of the original dose. Due to this extensive and variable toxicity profile, high-dose IFN should be administered by health care professionals experienced with its side effects. Despite the toxicity, modest efficacy, and considerable expense, retrospective analyses showed that high-dose IFN-α_{2b} therapy was associated with improvement in quality of life relative to observation[249] and was cost effective.[250] Furthermore, additional investigations have suggested that patients at high risk for melanoma recurrence prefer

high-dose IFN-α_{2b} therapy and its attendant toxicity to even a slight increase in melanoma relapse risk.[251,252]

Despite the status of high-dose IFN as the only FDA-approved adjuvant treatment for patients with high-risk melanoma, critics have raised concern over the considerable treatment toxicity and the lack of a consistent survival advantage.[253] For example, in the only study showing a significant survival advantage for IFN-α_{2b} relative to observation (E1684), that benefit no longer retained significance when reassessed at a median follow-up of over 13 years (see Fig. 38.2-15A).[241,244] Although non–melanoma-related causes of mortality may explain this narrowing of the gap between survival curves with time in E1684, especially as the relapse-free survival curves remain significantly apart (see Fig. 38.2-14A), this remains conjectural. Furthermore, many have suggested that the profound survival benefit observed in the E1694 trial may be due, in part, to a deleterious effect of the GM2-KLH/QS21 vaccine rather than a therapeutic effect of IFN-α_{2b}.[253] Mitigating this latter concern was the observation that patients developing antibodies to GM2 at day 29 had improved relapse-free survival compared to those who did not, which confirms earlier observations with GM2-based vaccines.[238] Finally, metaanalyses looking at many randomized controlled trials involving IFN at various dosages have failed to show a survival advantage for the aggregate.[254,255] Currently, this debate cannot be resolved by the extant data. Meanwhile, high-dose IFN-α therapy has yet to be accepted as a standard therapy in much of the world and is only inconsistently applied in the United States.

Regardless of one's views on the value of adjuvant high-dose IFN therapy, all agree that it remains a poor standard—possessing considerable toxicity and preventing recurrence and death in at best a minority of patients at risk. In addition, the intensity and duration of the regimen prohibits easy combination with other treatment approaches. Efforts to improve on the efficacy and toxicity profile of IFN have included use of lower-dose IFN-α regimens and combination of IFN-α with various vaccines. Low-dose IFN-α regimens have been tested extensively in Europe but relatively infrequently in the United States. Although several trials with these regimens have failed to show either relapse-free or overall survival benefits compared to observation in patients with high-risk stage II or stage III disease,[243,256–259] two trials using IFN-α$_{2a}$ did report a relapse-free survival benefit for patients with intermediate-risk melanoma[260,261] (see Table 38.2-12). This benefit has led to the approval of low-dose IFN-α$_{2a}$ in several European countries for the treatment of patients with intermediate-thickness melanomas. Nevertheless, because low-dose IFN-α regimens have yet to produce a survival advantage in a single study, they cannot currently be recommended for any subset of patients.

Other trials have evaluated IFN-α–containing regimens that omit either the high-dose intravenous induction component or the subcutaneous maintenance phase of therapy. For example, a European trial suggested a significant delay in distant relapse-free survival in patients treated with a regimen of IFN-α$_{2b}$ at 10 million U administered subcutaneously daily for 5 days for 4 weeks followed by 5 million U of IFN-α$_{2b}$ administered subcutaneously thrice weekly for 2 years.[253,262] Unfortunately, no survival benefit was observed. This delay in relapse has prompted the European melanoma research community to investigate longer durations of IFN therapy using a pegylated IFN regimen. In contrast, the early separation of the relapse-free survival and overall survival curves consistently seen with the high-dose IFN regimen has prompted investigators in the United States to examine the merits of the 4-week intravenous induction phase alone compared to observation in patients with stage IB to IIIA melanoma (E1697) or, in the case of the Sunbelt Melanoma Trial, with regional nodal disease detected only by RT-PCR for melanoma associated messenger RNA.[263]

Investigators have also attempted to improve on the efficacy of standard IFN therapy in patients with stage III disease by combining intermediate-dose IFN with the Melacine vaccine or incorporating it into a regimen including several chemotherapy drugs and IL-2 (biochemotherapy). In addition, others have studied the combination of low-dose IFN and subcutaneous IL-2. Preliminary results have suggested that the Melacine vaccine plus intermediate-dose IFN possesses similar clinical activity and less toxicity than high-dose IFN alone,[232] whereas the combination of low-dose IL-2 and low-dose IFN-α$_{2b}$ did not improve either disease-free or overall survival compared to low-dose IFN-α$_{2b}$ monotherapy.[264] Biochemotherapy, when administered before surgical resection in patients with either palpable regional nodal or in transit melanoma, produced clinically assessable partial responses in 44% of patients. Four of 62 patients had no histologic evidence of viable tumor within the surgical resection specimen.[265] At a median follow-up of 31 months, 38 of the 48 patients with stage III disease (79%) were alive, and 31 patients (65%) remained free of disease

progression.[266] A study comparing adjuvant administration of a 9-week course of intensive biochemotherapy to a year of standard high-dose IFN therapy in patients at very high risk of recurrence (stage IIIB and IIIC disease) is ongoing within the U.S. Intergroup mechanism.

Efforts to establish the value of administering radiation treatment to the regional nodal basin in conjunction with adjuvant IFN therapy have proved unrewarding due to poor protocol accrual. Nonetheless, in the absence of data to the contrary, patients with melanoma extending into the soft tissue of the regional lymph node basin (extranodal extension) should be considered for radiation treatment before the initiation of adjuvant IFN. To minimize the delay of systemic adjuvant therapy, an abbreviated radiation schedule such as 30 Gy in 5 fractions over 2.5 weeks[194] is recommended, when feasible.

Although considerable controversy exists regarding the appropriate adjuvant treatment for patients with intermediate- or high-risk melanoma, because IFN-α$_{2b}$ is the only FDA-approved therapy, it is reasonable to recommend that patients with appropriate risk should be made aware of its potential benefits and adverse effects. Patients who are unable to tolerate IFN or who prefer less toxic or more aggressive treatment should be encouraged to consider entry into controlled clinical trials. To maximize the value of these studies, they should enroll patients with melanomas adequately staged and stratified according to the AJCC staging system criteria.

GRANULOCYTE-MACROPHAGE COLONY-STIMULATING FACTOR

In vitro studies of GM-CSF indicate that it can activate macrophages to become cytotoxic for human melanoma cells[267] and mediates the proliferation, maturation, and migration of dendritic cells, which play an important role in the induction of T-cell–mediated immune responses.[268] This activity has prompted investigation of its use as adjuvant therapy for patients with high to extremely high risk melanoma.

In a preliminary single-arm study of 48 patients with stage III (more than four positive nodes) or stage IV melanoma, GM-CSF (125 μg/m^2 subcutaneously) was administered daily for 14 days followed by 14 days of rest, for a total of 1 year or until disease recurrence.[269] The outcome in these patients was compared to that in historical control patients who were treated at one institution between 1960 and 1988 and who were matched for the number of positive lymph nodes (for patients with stage III disease) or the presence or absence of visceral metastases (patients with stage IV disease). Compared with the matched controls, median survival was better for all patients (38.0 vs. 12.2 months), with observed 1- and 2-year survival rates of 89% and 69%. Although over 50% of treated patients developed transient myalgias, weakness, or mild fatigue, therapy was generally well tolerated. These results are encouraging; however, considering the previously stated concerns regarding the use of historical controls for adjuvant melanoma studies, these findings must be viewed with extreme caution. Consequently, the use of GM-CSF as adjuvant therapy for patients with melanoma cannot be recommended at this time, except as part of a clinical trial. In an effort to confirm these results, the U.S. Intergroup has begun a randomized phase III study (ECOG 4697) comparing GM-CSF to placebo in patients with either stage IV disease or regionally recurrent (stage IIIB or IIIC) disease after IFN therapy who have been rendered disease free with surgery.[270] Because GM-CSF may also have a role as a vaccine adjuvant, a second component of this study randomly assigns patients with resected melanoma who are HLA-A2+ to also receive either an HLA-A2–restricted multiepitopic peptide vaccine or placebo.

FOLLOW-UP OF MELANOMA PATIENTS (STAGES I TO III)

The risk of recurrence in patients with surgically treated melanoma is related to the thickness of the melanoma at its presentation and the presence or absence of nodal disease. The most common sites of melanoma recurrence are near the wide local excision site and in the regional node basin. Common sites of distant recurrence include cutaneous and subcutaneous sites distant from the primary, distant nodal sites, lung, liver, brain, and bone. Melanoma can have an unpredictable metastatic pattern and can spread to unusual sites such as the gastrointestinal tract and thyroid gland. For most patients with surgically treated stage I, II, or III disease, recommended follow-up is primarily with periodic history taking and physical examination. Routine performance of radiologic tests or screening blood tests has not been documented to improve survival.[202] However, periodic chest radiography is reasonable in an effort to identify lung metastases before the onset of symptoms, because early detection may increase the therapeutic options available to the patient. Although routine performance of CT scans is not indicated, directed CT scans can be very useful in evaluating patients with suspicious symptoms or physical findings, laboratory test abnormalities (anemia, or elevated LDH level), or an abnormal chest radiograph.

Among 261 patients with stage II or III melanoma followed prospectively by the North Central Cancer Treatment Group, symptoms signaled melanoma recurrence in 99 of 145 patients (68%) who had recurrences.[271] Physical examination detected recurrence in an additional 37 asymptomatic patients (26%). Altogether, 94% of recurrences were detected by history taking and physical examination. An abnormal chest radiograph identified only 9 of 145 recurrences (6%), and in no patient was an abnormal laboratory test result the sole indicator of recurrent disease. Mooney et al. assessed the impact of a surveillance program using physical examination, blood tests, and chest radiography for 1004 patients with AJCC stage I or II cutaneous melanoma.[272] Physical examination detected 72% of recurrences, constitutional symptoms indicated 17% of recurrences, and chest radiograph revealed 11% of recurrences. Thus, 76% of recurrences were diagnosed by a complete history taking and physical examination alone. Liver function tests, including LDH level, may be important screening tools for metastatic disease. An isolated elevation of serum alkaline phosphatase or LDH level is presumptive evidence of metastatic disease.[273]

The follow-up schedule for patients who have surgically resected disease is based on the depth of the primary lesion and the presence or absence of nodal disease.[202] For patients with a thin primary melanoma and negative nodes, follow-up is with clinical examination for evidence of occurrence every 6 months for the first 2 to 3 years and then yearly for 2 to 3 years beyond that. For patients with intermediate or thick melanomas and negative regional nodes, follow-up should be every 3 to 6 months for the first 2 to 3 years and every 6 to 12 months for the next 2 to 3 years. For patients with resected regional disease, follow-up should be every 3 to 4 months for the first 2 years, then

every 6 months up to year 5, and yearly beyond that. All patients must understand that they need routine lifelong dermatologic screening. Patients who have had one melanoma remain at higher-than-average risk for a second primary melanoma and also are at risk for basal cell and squamous cell carcinomas.

DIAGNOSIS OF STAGE IV MELANOMA

TIMING OF DISTANT METASTASES

The time to recurrence of metastatic tumors in patients with node-negative melanoma, stage I and II, varies inversely with tumor thickness.[274,275] Among patients with stage I and II melanoma followed by McCarthy et al., 95% of recurrence in patients with lesions thinner than 0.7 mm developed within 11 years; in contrast, 95% of recurrences in patients with lesions thicker than 3.0 mm occurred within 5 years.[276] In addition, ulceration was also identified as an important factor that influenced the timing of distant metastasis.[275,276]

Most recurrences (55% to 79%) become evident by 2 years, whereas 65% to 85% are apparent by 3 years after initial diagnosis of the primary tumor.[276,277] In general, recurrences in patients with nodal metastases, stage III, occur earlier than those in patients with negative lymph nodes.[277] In addition, age at diagnosis and adjuvant therapy can also influence timing of distant metastasis. For example, relapse has been shown to occur sooner in patients older than 50 years of age than in younger patients,[105,275] whereas adjuvant IFN treatment delays median time to recurrence by approximately 9 months.[242,244]

PATTERNS OF METASTASES

Melanoma is well known for its ability to metastasize to virtually any organ or tissue. Approximately 25% of first recurrences are at the local or regional sites The most common initial sites of distant metastases are the skin, subcutaneous tissue, and lymph nodes, which are recurrence sites for 42% to 59% of patients in various studies.[273] Visceral locations were the initial sites of relapse in approximately 25% of all melanoma patients who experienced recurrence.[276] The most common sites of visceral metastasis were the lung, brain, liver, gastrointestinal tract, and bone.[273]

DURATION OF REMISSION

The disease-free interval before the onset of distant metastasis is a significant prognostic factor.[127,130] The stage of disease preceding distant metastasis was also identified as an important prognostic factor.[127] For patients who had progressed directly from stage I or II disease, a disease-free interval of 34 months or longer was associated with prolonged survival, whereas for patients with a history of stage III melanoma, a disease-free interval of 18 months or longer was associated with prolonged survival.

CLINICAL EVALUATION OF METASTASIS

History and Physical Examination

Most melanoma metastases produce symptoms or can be discovered by physical examination. The hallmark of metastatic disease is a symptom complex that progresses in either intensity or frequency. A complete history taking and physical examination are the most important parts of the initial diagnostic evaluation.

Radiologic Studies

CT scans of the chest are useful for evaluating suspected pulmonary, pleural, or mediastinal metastases. However, even in patients with known distant metastases (stage IV disease), these scans are best suited for cases in which the presence of pulmonary metastases would alter the treatment plan or in which better definition of lesions is required for patient entry into a research protocol. For patients with suspected intraabdominal or hepatic metastases, based on abnormal findings on physical examination or abnormal liver chemistry test results, a CT scan of the abdomen should be obtained. Magnetic resonance imaging (MRI) may also be used to detect melanin as manifested by a high signal on T1-weighted images.[273] Ultrasonography may be of value in assessing hepatic, splenic, or pancreatic lesions. On ultrasonography, the lesions are usually predominantly hypoechoic. If the lesions are of heterogeneous echogenicity, hemorrhage is suspected. Contrast studies of the gastrointestinal tract, particularly upper gastrointestinal tract series with small bowel follow-through, are indicated if there are signs or symptoms suggesting metastatic disease in this area.

Radionuclide Scans

Radionuclide scans, such as brain, liver, and gallium scans, are not cost effective for routine screening for occult metastatic melanoma because of their low diagnostic yield. However, radiographic studies of the bone or a radionuclide bone scan, or both, should be obtained for specific symptoms or signs of bone disease. Other than MRI, a bone scan is probably the most sensitive test for skeletal metastatic disease, but a careful history taking and directed radiography are necessary to ensure that areas of uptake do not represent old trauma or inflammation.

Positron Emission Tomography

PET scanning using 2-[^{18}F]fluoro-2-deoxy-D-glucose (FDG) is steadily gaining acceptance as a tool for detecting metastatic melanoma and gauging the effects of therapy. Contrary to the conventional morphologic imaging, PET scanning is based on metabolic changes that could detect occult metastatic disease in high-risk patients. Studies of FDG-PET have reported a sensitivity of 78% to 100% for detecting metastatic melanoma in stage IIIB, IIIC, and IV disease but a low yield in stage I, II, and IIIA melanoma.[278–284] False-positive results have been observed in association with inflammatory response (including postoperative changes) and second primary or metastatic tumors. False-negative scans in the presence of metastases are uncommon. Metastases measuring less than 1 cm in diameter may not image well. In reported studies, use of PET for staging identified occult disease that changed treatment management for 15% to 49% of patients studied.[278–280,282,284,285]

Compared with the use of conventional diagnostics for detection of melanoma metastases, PET can be highly sensitive and specific for melanoma staging. PET scanning has been shown to detect some metastases months before conventional imaging techniques. Although PET yielded a higher sensitivity

and specificity in detecting nodal, soft tissue, and abdominal metastases, CT scan may be superior in detecting small lung metastases. PET is most useful in identifying the malignant nature of a mass detected by more conventional radiologic tests and in identifying other disease in patients with isolated stage IV disease who are being considered for major surgical resection. Except for brain imaging, one single whole body FDG-PET scan could replace the standard battery of imaging tests currently performed on high-risk melanoma patients. Although PET may prove to be an effective means of staging melanoma in high-risk patients, especially those with stage IIIB or IIIC disease, the cost effectiveness of this approach remains to be assessed. Furthermore, the enhanced sensitivity of PET scanning often leads to stage migration, which can complicate systemic treatment decisions. Hence, more data are needed about the specificity of PET and the treatment of patients whose disease is detected only on PET imaging before this test can be routinely incorporated as a staging tool.

Pathologic Tests

In a patient with a symptom, an abnormal finding on physical examination or laboratory tests, or an abnormal radiographic study, the definitive diagnosis of metastatic melanoma can be made accurately only by biopsy. An excisional or needle biopsy is relatively easy to perform when the suspected metastasis is superficially located. More deeply situated lesions may also be approached using a thin-needle biopsy.[286] Cytologic examination of urine, sputum, or cerebrospinal, peritoneal, or pleural fluid, or a bone marrow aspiration or biopsy examination also may yield a diagnosis of metastatic melanoma, especially when there are specific symptoms referable to these areas.[287,288] Laparotomy and examination of the liver and abdominal organs may be indicated occasionally to rule out occult metastatic disease before proceeding with major surgery for locally advanced or metastatic disease elsewhere. Special immunohistochemical stains are often useful in making the proper diagnosis.

Antibodies that recognize two melanoma antigens, S-100 and HMB45, are used frequently to distinguish melanomas from nonmelanocytic tumors.[273] In particular, HMB45 is a molecular marker expressed in melanosomes and is encoded by a gene called gp100/pMel17 that can determine skin color. Another set of markers, including tyrosinase and tyrosinase-related proteins, are also expressed by melanosomes and can be useful for diagnosis of melanocytic tumors, but are still considered experimental. Other markers are routinely used to identify carcinomas (cytokeratins) and lymphomas (immunoglobulin and B-cell antigens). In difficult cases, electron microscopy can be helpful. Melanoma cells contain a unique organelle, the melanosome, which is involved in the biosynthesis of pigment and can be recognized by electron microscopy in most melanoma lesions.

SURGERY AND IRRADIATION FOR DISTANT METASTASES (STAGE IV)

PATIENT SELECTION AND PROGNOSTIC FACTORS

Surgery for advanced melanoma is most effective when disease is limited to a few sites and a small number of metastases. Surgi-

TABLE 38.2-13. Median Survival (in Months) of Patients after Complete Surgical Resection of Distant Metastases

Metastatic Site[a]	John Wayne Cancer Institute[292,297]	U. of Alabama Hospitals[293]	U. of Texas M. D. Anderson Cancer Center[294]	Memorial Sloan-Kettering Cancer Center[296]	Roswell Park Memorial Institute[295]
Skin, subcutaneous	24 (36)	17 (13)	23 (65)	25 (12)	31 (25)
Lung	19 (46)	9 (17)	16 (26)	19 (17)	9 (13)
Brain	12 (17)	8 (17)	15 (16)	7.5 (5)	5 (4)
Gastrointestinal tract (nonhepatic)	10 (19)	8 (5)	18 (9)	15 (12)	8 (3)
2-y survival rate (%)	45	16	15	21	31

[a]Number of patients with metastases at each site is given in parentheses.
(Adapted from ref. 289.)

cal excision of isolated metastatic melanoma lesions can provide effective and quick palliation and, in some instances, a survival exceeding 5 or 10 years.[289–293] The favorable outcome resulting from surgical resection of distant metastases in selected patients treated at major centers is shown in Table 38.2-13.[292–297] It should be emphasized that the results of these studies cannot distinguish between the relatively more favorable biology of limited metastases and the treatment impact of surgical excision in the absence of randomized studies. In general, however, they consistently demonstrated the importance of completely resecting all distant metastases (compared to incomplete resection) with regard to survival outcome.

Surgery should only be used when the risk of perioperative morbidity is acceptable. If the initial recurrence of melanoma is a solitary lesion, surgical resection should be considered the treatment of choice after a careful diagnostic workup for metastases at other sites.[289] Surgery should also be the first consideration for patients with two or three metastases in a single organ, such as lung or skin and soft tissue. Patients with multiorgan metastases, such as to the lung, liver, and brain, are less likely candidates for resection. Surgical treatment to relieve symptoms caused by metastases is generally worthwhile, especially when the anticipated benefit from palliation exceeds the morbidity of the procedure—for example, resection of small bowel metastases to relieve bowel obstruction or gastrointestinal bleeding. Expectant (or prophylactic) palliation is used for control of disease that is likely to cause disabling symptoms. Although the survival associated with visceral metastases is generally worse than that associated with distant subcutaneous and nodal metastases when patients are treated with chemotherapy or IL-2 therapy,[97] the survival differences disappear if visceral metastases can be completely resected.[297] In addition, long-term results demonstrate the value of sequential resection of distant metastases: Ollila et al. reported a 19% rate of 5-year survival after complete resection for recurrence after initial metastasectomy (Fig. 38.2-16).[290]

SKIN, SUBCUTANEOUS TISSUE, AND LYMPH NODE METASTASES

The skin, subcutaneous tissue, and nonregional lymph nodes are among the most common sites for metastatic melanoma.[130,294] When metastases in these locations are few and isolated, surgical excision may be the safest, quickest, and most effective treatment. Lesions should be excised before they become bulky and

symptomatic, the point at which a more extensive operation would otherwise be required.[289,292,294] A rim of normal-appearing tissue (at least 1 cm, or more than 1 cm for larger lesions) should be removed to minimize the risk of local relapse. Sequential metastases in one area can be excised surgically unless they multiply rapidly or reappear concurrently with metastases to other sites. In either situation (multiple lesions or sites), radiotherapy or systemic chemotherapy, or both, may be an alternative. Excellent results have been obtained with surgical excision of skin, subcutaneous, or distant lymph node metastases, especially when there are only a few lesions. Many such patients require repeated excisions, but the median survival from the onset of these metastases averages 2 years (range, 3 to 180 months).[289] The addition of hypofractionated radiation therapy after resection of nodal and subcutaneous melanoma deposits at a variety of sites reportedly can provide excellent local control[298] but is rarely necessary if the subcutaneous metastases are resected with adequate margins.[289]

LUNG METASTASES

Pulmonary metastases are generally associated with longer survival (median, 10 to 11 months) than metastases at other vis-

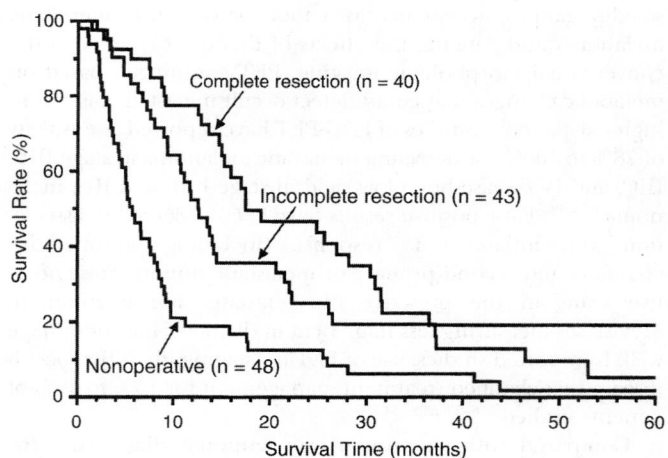

FIGURE 38.2-16. Survival after complete surgical resection, incomplete surgical resection, or nonoperative treatment of stage IV melanoma recurring after an initial complete metastasectomy. (From ref. 290, with permission.)

ceral sites.[130] Pulmonary metastases are usually multiple and bilateral, and they may be associated with hilar or mediastinal node metastases.[289]

Several institutions have demonstrated prolonged median and 5-year survival in properly selected patients undergoing a pulmonary metastasectomy.[289] The International Registry of Lung Metastases presented the long-term results of pulmonary metastasectomy in 5206 patients from 18 thoracic surgery departments worldwide.[299] These patients were considered to have undergone a complete pulmonary metastasectomy if there was no residual microscopic or macroscopic disease. The overall procedure-related mortality was 1.3%. For 282 melanoma patients undergoing a complete metastasectomy, 5-year and 10-year rates of survival were 21% and 14%, respectively, which is far superior to reported 5-year survival rates for melanoma patients managed with chemotherapy. However, selection bias for solitary metastases likely contributes significantly to these favorable results.

Resection of pulmonary metastases should be confined to patients with limited numbers and sites of disease, whose performance status and residual lung capacity are compatible with the planned procedure. Surgical resection of pulmonary metastases appears to provide a survival benefit for a small number of carefully selected patients. In most series the median survival was 16 to 19 months with a 5-year survival rate of 20% to 39%.[289,300–302] Some patients enjoyed remissions of longer than 10 years.[289]

In the experience at Duke University Medical Center, of 945 patients with pulmonary metastatic melanoma, 99 underwent partial or total pulmonary resection (Fig. 38.2-17).[302] Multivariate predictors of improved survival ($P<.001$), in order of importance, included complete resection of pulmonary disease, longer disease-free interval, presence of only one or two pulmonary nodules, treatment with chemotherapy, and lymph node negativity for metastases. When pulmonary disease was limited to a single metastatic nodule, median survival was 7.2 months without resection (142 patients) and an estimated 20 months with total resection (84 patients) ($P<.001$). Their experience clearly demonstrates that the selective use of resection for isolated pulmonary metastases can prolong survival.

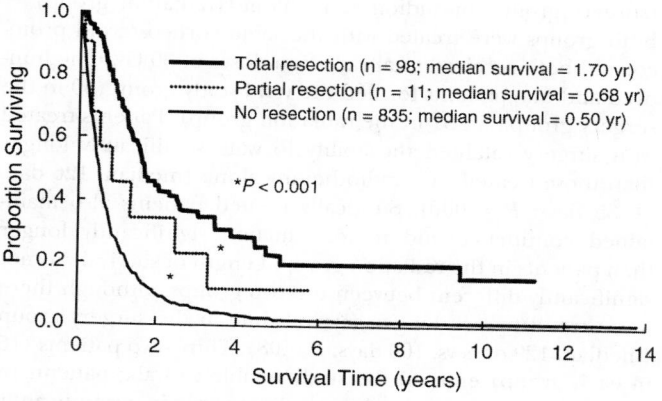

FIGURE 38.2-17. Survival data for 945 patients whose pulmonary metastases were treated at Duke University Medical Center. Survival was significantly better with complete pulmonary resection than with no resection ($P<.001$). Survival was intermediate with partial resection. (From ref. 302, with permission.)

At the University of Texas M. D. Anderson Cancer Center, 56 patients who underwent resection of pulmonary metastatic melanoma had a 5-year survival rate of 25% and a median survival of 18 months.[301] No patient died as a result of surgery. Survival after resection of pulmonary metastases was significantly longer when the initial melanoma was localized (stage I and II) rather than regional ($P = .04$). Neither the number of metastases (up to four) nor a bilateral distribution of metastases affected survival. Median survival was 30 months when disease first recurred in the lung and 17 months when locoregional recurrence preceded pulmonary metastases ($P = .03$).

In several published results from the John Wayne Cancer Institute, among 106 patients undergoing thoracotomy for metastatic melanoma, the highest 5-year survival estimate (39%) occurred in patients with solitary metastases.[291,292,303] Patients with four or fewer metastases had a better survival rate than those with five or more metastases. By multivariate analyses, a tumor-doubling time longer than 60 days and lack of extrapulmonary disease were predictive of improved survival. The median survival time and 5-year survival rate were 16 months and 0%, respectively, for a tumor-doubling time of less than 60 days, compared with 29.2 months and 20.7%, respectively, for a tumor-doubling time of 60 days or more.[290,304]

In all series, no more than 1% of patients died as a consequence of surgery. No consistent factors predicted survival after pulmonary resection except the tumor-doubling time.[304] Nevertheless, surgical resection for isolated pulmonary metastases appears justified in some patients, particularly when the time to pulmonary metastases exceeds 36 months. Criteria for resection should include an absence of metastases at other sites, control of the primary tumor, prolonged tumor-doubling time, potential for complete resection, and palliation of symptoms.[289] Normal lung parenchyma should be conserved during resection. Fortunately, most metastases occur just below the pleura, and segmental resection of a wedge of tissue usually ensures adequate tumor control. Several techniques and devices have proved useful for these procedures, including minimally invasive thoracoscopically assisted resection, newer mechanical staplers that reduce tissue damage and provide airtight staple lines, and argon cautery systems. Lobectomy is rarely needed to obtain clear margins, and pneumonectomy is usually not indicated.

BRAIN AND SPINAL CORD METASTASES

Up to 60% of patients with metastatic melanoma have clinically evident brain metastases. Cerebral metastases are among the most common causes of death from melanoma, accounting for 20% to 54% of deaths. The life span of persons with these metastases is relatively short, ranging from 2 to 7 months depending on the extent of extracranial metastatic disease and the response to treatment.[130]

Routine use of MRI for screening has increased the detection of asymptomatic central nervous system (CNS) disease. Some patients present with symptoms suggestive of increased intracranial pressure, including headaches, visual disturbances or seizures, and, less commonly, personality changes or nausea or vomiting. The mainstay of initial treatment for symptomatic disease is corticosteroid therapy. The most effective agent is dexamethasone (up to 100 mg/d). Dexamethasone reduces edema around the tumor and can provide temporary relief of symptoms.

A diagnosis of brain metastasis requires prompt attention, because median survival is about 1 month without treatment and only 2 months with corticosteroids alone.[130] Factors generally predictive of poor outcome are increased patient age (older than 50 years), more than one CNS metastasis, uncontrolled systemic disease, poor performance status, and increased intracranial pressure.[305] Patients with melanoma metastatic to the brain have a worse prognosis than patients with other solid tumors that metastasize to the brain.

With the increased use of routine MRI screening, up to 50% of patients with CNS metastases are found to have a solitary supratentorial lesion. Surgical excision is the treatment of choice for larger (more than 3.5-cm) symptomatic metastases. Rapid control of these metastases can provide effective palliation and prolong life.[289] Control rates of approximately 85% can be expected for surgery alone. Tumor excision via craniotomy has an operative mortality no greater than 5%. This approach usually alleviates symptoms and prevents further neurologic damage. Tumor resection may even be considered in some patients who have several foci of metastatic disease in the brain or at other sites, because the estimated life span of these patients can exceed 3 months and usually their neurologic status improves.[306]

Surgical excision is preferred to whole brain irradiation alone in patients who have a limited number of brain metastases, because the hemorrhagic nature of the metastatic tumor may be the major cause of symptoms. Because bleeding in and around the tumor can occur before and during surgery, laser beam excision is often safer and quicker and is accompanied by less blood loss than suction and coagulation.

Patients whose brain metastases are treated surgically survive an average of approximately 6 months postoperatively, with a range of 2 to 20 months.[289,293,307,308] The neurologic condition of the majority of symptomatic patients improves satisfactorily after surgery. The length of survival is influenced by the duration of remission, the patient's neurologic status at the time of surgery, and the presence of metastases at other sites.[309] Although long-term successes are uncommon, a few patients live 5 years or more after surgery.[307]

In a randomized trial, patients with solitary metastases from a variety of malignancies underwent surgical resection plus postoperative irradiation or whole brain irradiation alone.[310] Tumor recurrences in the brain were less frequent in the surgical group (20% vs. 52%; P <.02). Surgical patients also had a significantly longer median survival (40 weeks vs. 15 weeks; P <.01). In another series of patients whose solitary brain metastases were managed by surgery plus whole brain irradiation or whole brain irradiation alone, surgical patients had a longer duration of function and improved survival.[311]

The issue of whether adjuvant irradiation should be administered after surgical excision of melanoma brain metastases is controversial. In a multicenter randomized trial, patients with solitary metastases to the brain (from melanoma and other primary sites) underwent surgical resection with or without postoperative whole brain irradiation.[312] Although recurrence rate was lower in the radiotherapy group (18% vs. 70%), there was no difference in overall survival and duration of functional independence. However, in a retrospective analysis of the M. D. Anderson Cancer Center series, the combination of surgery and postoperative whole brain irradiation provided more effective palliation for solitary melanoma metastases in the brain

than surgical treatment alone (18-month vs. 6-month median survival; P = .002).[307] The number of brain relapses was reduced in the group receiving surgery plus radiation, which resulted in prolonged survival. Retrospective results from Memorial Sloan-Kettering Cancer Center also demonstrated significantly improved control of subsequent brain relapses if cranial irradiation was administered after surgical excision of solitary brain lesions (median interval to CNS relapse of 26.6 months compared to 5.7 months; P = .05), although overall survival was not prolonged.[313] One alternative is to administer "regional" radiation therapy to the area of the brain where the metastasis was surgically removed, because it is difficult to remove melanoma metastases to the brain with much, if any, surgical margin of normal brain tissue.

More recently, the use of stereotactic radiosurgery has gained popularity as an effective method to treat smaller (less than 3 cm) brain metastases as an alternative to craniotomy.[195,289,314–317] Linear accelerator and photon-beam gamma knife radiosurgical techniques have been used with a high tumor control rate, low morbidity and mortality, and a median survival of 9 to 10 months. The routine use of whole brain irradiation before or after stereotactic radiosurgery is controversial.[316,317] Studies favor the use of stereotactic approaches alone as initial therapy, especially when the tumor volume is small and there are only one or two lesions, and especially in younger patients with good performance status.[314,318] In one report, the local control rate for the brain metastases was 87%.[318] Patients undergoing stereotactic radiosurgery should be given prophylactic steroids and anticonvulsants.[195]

Spinal cord metastases are relatively rare and exceedingly difficult to manage.[319] Surgical decompression of obstructing spinal cord metastases is indicated in some patients, although radiotherapy might be an effective alternative.[195] High doses of corticosteroids should be given as well. Early treatment intervention is essential, because the best results for both surgery and radiation treatments occur in patients with mild neurologic symptoms. Very few treatment responses have occurred in totally paraplegic patients.

An important randomized study was reported that investigated the treatment of metastatic tumors causing spinal cord compression. Patients with cord compressions were randomly assigned to receive either surgery followed by radiotherapy (surgery group) or radiotherapy alone (radiation group).[320] Both groups were treated with the same corticosteroid protocol and both received total radiation doses of 30 Gy. One hundred and one patients formed the valid study group (50 in the surgery group and 51 in the radiation group). Patients treated with surgery retained the ability to walk significantly longer than those treated with radiotherapy alone (median, 126 days vs. 35 days; P = .006). Surgically treated patients also maintained continence and motor function significantly longer than patients in the radiation group. Length of survival was not significantly different between the two groups, although there was a trend toward longer survival time in the surgery group (median, 129 days vs. 100 days; P = .08). Thirty-two patients (16 in each group) entered the study unable to walk; patients in the surgery group regained the ability to walk in a significantly greater proportion than patients in the radiation group [9 of 16 (56%) vs. 3 of 16 (19%); P = .03]. The investigators concluded that patients with spinal cord compressions treated with radical direct decompressive surgery plus postoperative radio-

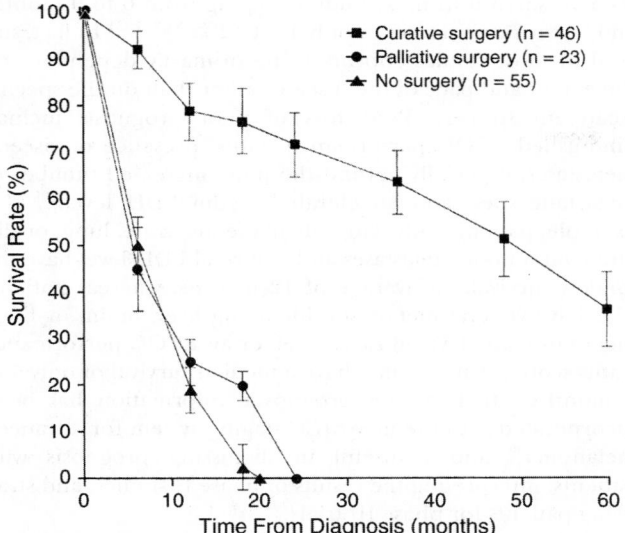

FIGURE 38.2-18. Survival curves associated with complete (potentially curative) resection, incomplete (palliative) resection, or nonsurgical intervention for melanoma metastatic to the gastrointestinal tract. (From ref. 322, with permission. Copyright 1996, American Medical Association.)

therapy regain the ability to walk more often and maintain it longer than patients treated with radiation alone.[320] Surgery permitted most patients to remain ambulatory and continent for the remainder of their lives, whereas patients treated with radiation alone spent approximately two-thirds of their remaining time unable to walk and incontinent.

GASTROINTESTINAL TRACT METASTASES

Although solitary metastases can occur in the gastrointestinal tract, each affected organ usually has multiple lesions. Moreover, gastrointestinal tract metastases usually are associated with disseminated disease and a median survival of only 5 to 11 months.[127] However, most patients with obstructive symptoms or bleeding from gastrointestinal tract metastases can be palliated by surgical intervention with minimal morbidity and mortality (Fig. 38.2-18).[321–323]

The most common presenting symptoms of gastrointestinal metastases are abdominal pain, obstruction, and bleeding. Surgery is recommended as a palliative intervention for acute complications of obstruction, bleeding, or perforation. These conditions cannot be treated by nonsurgical approaches. In anemic patients, chronic bleeding can be treated with repeated blood transfusions, but this approach is frustrating for the patient and the oncologist. Systemic therapy can be considered for patients with multiple gastrointestinal lesions, whereas surgical excision should be considered for limited gastrointestinal metastases, if the patient's performance status is acceptable.[289,321–325] The final decision regarding treatment depends on the patient's overall clinical condition, but symptoms can be successfully alleviated in most cases, and survival after surgical excision of these metastases can occasionally be quite gratifying[289,292,293,321–324] (see Fig. 38.2-18).

When there are multiple gastrointestinal metastases, only the lesions causing immediate symptoms should be excised unless all residual disease can be removed safely. Extensive operative procedures such as esophagogastrectomy or subtotal gastrectomy have

been successful but should be used only when long-term survival is expected. Survival of 2 to 20 years after excision of gastrointestinal metastases has been reported for patients who underwent complete palliative excision of symptomatic solitary gastric or intestinal metastases[289,290,292,293,321–324] (see Fig. 38.2-18).

Obstruction is usually due to large polypoid lesions that mechanically obstruct the bowel or act as a leading point for intussusception. These submucosal metastases are generally removed by means of bowel resection or occasionally through bypass, depending on the site and number of lesions. An intestinal bypass procedure may be sufficient for some patients with advanced disease who would otherwise require an extensive or risky resection with functional consequences (i.e., short bowel syndrome).[289]

Massive or repeated episodes of bleeding requiring transfusions are unusual and most commonly result from gastric metastases. Surgical treatment generally consists of segmental resection or partial gastrectomy, although more extensive operations are sometimes required.[289] When surgery is impossible or unsuccessful, the repeated transfusions required by continual bleeding tax both patient and physician. In addition, active bleeding sources make systemic therapy more difficult due to suppression of marrow erythroid response and thrombocytopenia-induced exacerbation of bleeding. Consequently, in patients with unresectable bleeding sources, a frank discussion regarding the goals of continued care is frequently required.

LIVER, BILIARY TRACT, AND SPLEEN METASTASES

Patients with liver metastases have an average life span of only 2 to 4 months.[130] Occasionally a patient has an isolated liver metastasis that can be surgically resected. Usually the duration of palliation is short, but occasional long-term survival is seen.[289,300,324] A review of the experience with 1750 prospectively followed melanoma patients with hepatic metastases reported that 34 underwent exploration with intent to resect the metastases, and 24 (71%) were able to undergo hepatic resection.[326] Eighteen of these patients (75%) underwent complete surgical resection, and the remaining six underwent only palliative or debulking procedures. Median overall survival was 28 months for patients who underwent surgical resection compared with 4 months for patients who underwent exploration only ($P<.001$).[326] The authors concluded that surgical resection of hepatic metastases should be considered if the patient could be rendered free of disease. Newer techniques for ablation of multiple liver metastases by cryosurgery or radiofrequency ablation have further extended the therapeutic options for patients with multiple metastases.

Patients with symptomatic localized gallbladder or biliary metastases may benefit from excision, bypass, or stenting.[289] For patients with localized splenic metastases who underwent complete resection, the median survival was approximately 2 years.[324,327]

BONE METASTASES

Patients with melanoma metastases involving bone have a median survival of 4 to 6 months; their survival is even shorter when other sites are also involved.[127,130] The treatment of bone metastases depends on (1) the degree of symptoms, (2) the location and magnitude of the lesions, and (3) the patient's life expectancy.[289] The goals of therapy are to relieve pain, maximize ambulation, and minimize the need for medical care. In general, patients without symptoms should be monitored to assess the progression of their lesions. Systemic treatment is also reasonable, particularly if other systemic disease is detected.

Symptomatic metastases in weight-bearing bones (e.g., the femur) require special consideration.[289] If the lesion is large, and especially if there is evidence of cortical destruction, prophylactic stabilization and irradiation are sometimes used when the patient's expected life span is at least 2 months. Stabilization techniques includes operative bone fixation (e.g., with intramedullary rods), joint replacement, repair with methyl methacrylate, or use of external braces or a cast. Radiotherapy is generally given postoperatively.[195] Alternatively, the lesion may be treated with radiation alone, in which case the patient must be monitored closely for evidence of pathologic fracture. Unless the risk of surgery is high or the patient's expected life span is extremely short, pathologic fracture of a weight-bearing bone should be stabilized to maximize the patient's quality of life and decrease hospital or nursing home costs.

Patients in whom fractures of the vertebrae have compressed the spinal cord require prompt treatment to avert paralysis.[320] The treatment may require both decompressive laminectomy and postoperative irradiation, or irradiation alone, depending on the extent of the disease and the patient's overall medical condition.

KIDNEY AND URINARY TRACT METASTASES

Kidney and urinary tract metastases generally are asymptomatic until the terminal stages of disease, and death usually occurs 1 to 4 months after the clinical diagnosis is made. Metastatic melanoma occasionally mimics primary renal or bladder carcinomas, both endoscopically and radiographically.[289] Significant bleeding, obstruction, and urosepsis can occur in patients with bladder metastases from melanoma. Only solitary or symptomatic metastatic tumors in the kidney or urinary tract should be considered for surgical excision. These bladder metastases often can be treated by transurethral resection or partial cystectomy, depending on their number, size, and location. Surgery usually relieves the symptoms, but postoperative survival averages only 3 to 6 months.[289] Rarely do patients survive longer than 1 year.

ENDOCRINE METASTASES

Solitary metastases to the endocrine organs should be excised, especially if the patient is symptomatic. Long-term surgical palliation of adrenal, thyroid, or pituitary metastases succeeds occasionally.[289,328,329] In a large series of 83 patients with adrenal metastases, median survival was 9.3 months (range, 1 to 67 months).[328] Of the 27 patients who underwent surgical exploration, 18 (67%) were rendered clinically free of disease by adrenalectomy alone (12 cases) or by adrenalectomy and resection of additional disease (6 cases). Median survival was 25.7 months after complete resection and 9.2 months after palliative resection ($P = .02$).

SYSTEMIC TREATMENT OF STAGE IV MELANOMA

The prognosis of patients with widely metastatic (stage IV) melanoma is poor. Treatment remains unsatisfactory, with median survival in most studies ranging from 6 to 9 months and 5-year survival rates of only 1% to 2%.[224,330,331] In fact, survival in most studies appears to be primarily dependent on the extent and pace of the disease rather than on the specific treatment strategy. Predictors of poor prognosis include diminished ECOG performance status, presence of visceral metastases, especially beyond the lung, increased number of metastatic sites, and an elevated serum LDH level.[128] For example, patients with skin, subcutaneous tissue, lung, or distant lymph node metastases and a normal LDH level have the longest survival, an average of 12 months, whereas patients who have visceral metastases, including liver, brain, or bone metastases, an elevated LDH level, or an ECOG performance status score greater than 1 have a median survival of only 4 to 6 months. Much of this prognostic information has been incorporated into the new AJCC staging system for advanced melanoma[99] and is useful in discussing prognosis with patients, interpreting the results of phase II studies, and stratifying patients for phase III trials.

Although the excision of limited distant metastatic disease can occasionally produce durable benefit, most patients with distant metastases require a systemic treatment approach. The major systemic treatment options for patients with metastatic melanoma include cytotoxic chemotherapy and immunotherapy, used either alone or in combination. Because most of these treatments produce durable benefits in only the rare patient, melanoma has traditionally been a disease in which novel systemic treatment options have been investigated.

IMMUNOTHERAPY

Clinical and laboratory observations suggest that host immunologic responses may occasionally influence the course of melanoma progression, which has stimulated the investigation of immunotherapeutic approaches in this disease. Primary melanomas frequently display evidence of regression, often associated with lymphocytic infiltration and pigment phagocytosis by monocytes in the subjacent tissue. Some patients also develop patches of cutaneous depigmentation remote from the primary lesion, termed *leukoderma* or *paraneoplastic vitiligo*, that appear to be a manifestation of a specific immune response directed against melanosome proteins.[332–334] Some patients develop marked vitiligo after immunotherapy, a phenomenon that is often predictive of tumor response and has frequently been used as a measure of treatment potency.[333,334]

Although immunotherapy currently is effective in only a small percentage of patients, the results can be quite dramatic. Durable complete responses are occasionally seen and can be sustained without need for additional treatment. Areas of active investigation have included use of recombinant cytokines, either alone or in combination with other biologic response modifiers, adoptive immunotherapy, vaccines, monoclonal antibodies, and gene therapy.

Recombinant Cytokines

A number of recombinant cytokines have been investigated for treatment of metastatic melanoma. The two most extensively studied are IFN-α and IL-2. These agents have sufficient activity to be incorporated into the general treatment armamentarium for this disease. Combinations of these agents, various toxicity reduction strategies, and novel cytokines with a potentially more favorable therapeutic index also have been investigated.

INTERFERON-α. IFN-α was the first recombinant cytokine to be investigated clinically for treatment of metastatic melanoma. Phase I and II trials were initiated with IFN-α alone in the 1980s and yielded an aggregate response rate of 16% in published studies.[335] Unlike with cytotoxic chemotherapy, responses could be observed with IFN-α as late as 6 months after the initiation of therapy. Up to one-third of responses were complete, and many of these were durable; however, the median duration of response was only approximately 4 months. The effective dosage of IFN-α has ranged from 10 million $U/m^2/d$ to 50 million U/m^2 three times per week. Uninterrupted treatment appears to be more effective than cyclic, interrupted schedules irrespective of the route of administration. Tumor response largely has been confined to patients with small-volume cutaneous or soft tissue disease, which limits the usefulness of IFN-α in the general metastatic melanoma population.[336] Nevertheless, this response pattern spurred the eventual successful investigation of high-dose IFN regimens in the adjuvant setting.[338]

Many phase III trials have failed to show benefit from the addition of IFN-α to cytotoxic chemotherapy or other biologic agents in the treatment of stage IV disease (see later in Interferon-α–Based Biochemotherapy Regimens). However, a metaanalysis of six published and five unpublished studies involving 1164 patients reported that the overall response rate was higher with such IFN-containing regimens (24% vs. 17%),[339] which perhaps supports a role for IFN-α in the treatment of advanced melanoma.

INTERLEUKIN-2. IL-2 was first identified in 1976 as a T-cell growth factor; isolation of the complementary DNA clone was described in 1983. Recombinant IL-2 was shown to have potent immunomodulatory and indirect antitumor activity in a number of murine tumor models. Research in animal models indicated that the response to IL-2 was dose dependent[340] and ultimately led to the development of high-dose IL-2 regimens for clinical investigation.

Initial studies used high-dose intravenous bolus IL-2 (600,000 to 720,000 IU/kg every 8 hours on days 1 to 5 and 15 to 19 with a maximum of 28 doses per course), either alone or in combination with lymphokine-activated killer (LAK) cells. This regimen produced responses in 15% to 20% of patients, with complete responses in 4% to 6%.[341–345]

Long-term follow-up of patients treated on early high-dose IL-2 trials confirmed that IL-2 monotherapy produces significant clinical benefit for a minority of patients. A retrospective analysis was conducted of data for 270 patients treated on all trials involving high-dose bolus IL-2 conducted between 1985 and 1993 and subsequently updated with follow-up through 1998 and 2002.[345–347] Response duration curves for this cohort of patients updated through December 2002 are displayed in Figure 38.2-19. The overall objective response rate was 16% and the median response duration was 8.9 months. Fifty-nine percent of patients showing complete response remained progression free at 10 years. Responses were less frequent in patients with poor performance status or those who had received prior systemic therapy, but, in contrast to

IFN-α, were seen with equal frequency in patients with visceral metastases or large tumor burdens, or both. At a minimum follow-up of 10 years, 47% of all responders remained alive, with the vast majority disease or progression free. In addition, no patient responding for longer than 30 months had progressed, which suggests that such patients may actually be "cured."

These encouraging results led to FDA approval of high-dose IL-2 therapy for patients with metastatic melanoma in 1999. No randomized studies have been performed, but in general the overall response rate, quality, and duration of response have been better with high-dose bolus IL-2 than with lower doses or alternative administration schedules or routes.[347] Comparable response rates were observed with continuous-infusion IL-2 in one study, but responses appeared to be of shorter duration.[348] Even in a group of patients who received high-dose bolus IL-2, response correlated significantly with the amount of IL-2 administered.[349]

Interleukin-2 Toxicity and Toxicity Reduction Strategies. The extensive multisystem toxicity of the high-dose IL-2 regimen has limited its use to patients with excellent organ function treated by experienced clinicians in specialized programs capable of providing care at the level of the intensive care unit. Side effects include hypotension, cardiac arrhythmias, pulmonary edema, fever, increased capillary permeability, and rarely death. Although the cause of many of these side effects is not fully understood, a protein fragment of the IL-2 molecule has been tentatively identified as playing a role in the increased vasopermeability.[350] Bacterial infection, particularly catheter-related sepsis, also has contributed significantly to the toxicity of IL-2 administration and was responsible for all six deaths reported in early high-dose IL-2 trials.[345] The use of antibiotic prophylaxis has greatly reduced the incidence of catheter-related sepsis and dramatically improved the safety of this therapy.

Even in the absence of infection, many features of IL-2 toxicity resemble bacterial sepsis. IL-2 is a potent inducer of proinflammatory cytokines such as IL-1, tumor necrosis factor-α (TNF-α), and IFN-γ.[351] These substances and others, including nitric oxide, likely play a major role in IL-2 toxicity. On the other hand, tumor responses are thought to be mediated through cellular immune function, which raises the possibility of enhancing the therapeutic index of IL-2 by dissociating its toxic effects from its antitumor effects. A number of such toxicity reduction approaches, including the coadministration of soluble receptors to TNF-α or IL-1 or inhibitors of either TNF-α or IL-1 production or signaling, have been investigated.[352–355] Unfortunately, none of these agents has successfully blocked IL-2 toxicity as measured either by the ability to administer more therapy at a given toxicity level or by induction of less toxicity with a given amount of therapy.

More recent investigation has focused on the reversal of IL-2–associated vasodilation by the administration of N-mono-methyl-L-arginine (L-NMMA), which inhibits the synthesis of nitric oxide. In a phase I study of 23 patients with renal cell cancer who became hypotensive while receiving continuous-infusion IL-2 (18 million $IU/m^2/d$), the hypotension was completely or partially reversed in all patients by administration of L-NMMA at all dose levels.[356] L-NMMA administration was accompanied by evidence of increased pulmonary vascular resistance and reversal of

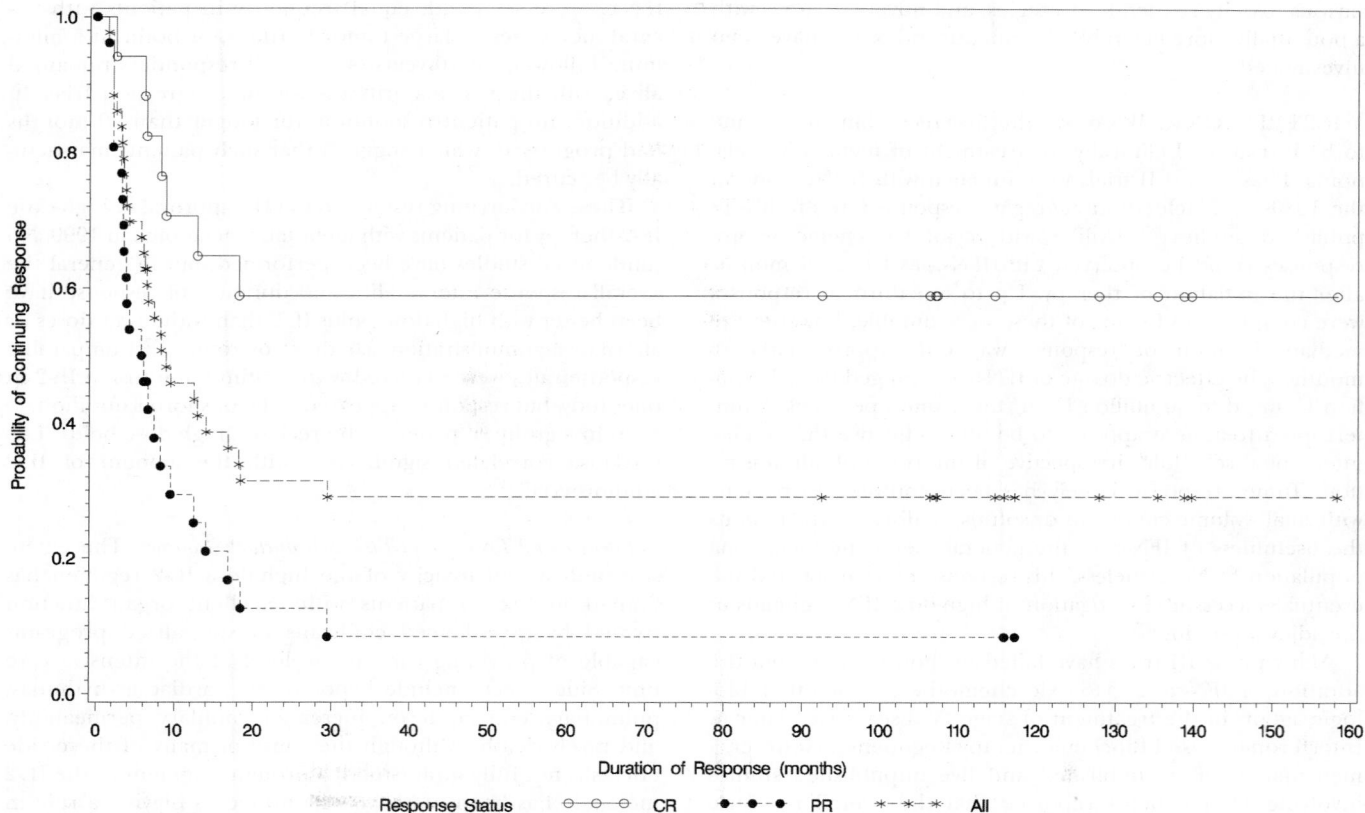

FIGURE 38.2-19. Kaplan-Meier plots of response durations for complete responses (CR), partial responses (PR), and all responses in the U.S. Food and Drug Administration submission for use of high-dose interleukin-2 in the treatment of melanoma. Updated through December 2002.

the IL-2–induced hyperdynamic cardiac output. In another approach, IL-2–associated hypotension was successfully abrogated and antitumor efficacy improved in an animal model when the superoxide dismutase mimetic M40403 was combined with IL-2.[357] These approaches require further investigation. At the moment there is no readily available means for selectively inhibiting the toxicity associated with high-dose IL-2 administration.

Predictors of Response to Interleukin-2–Based Therapy. A retrospective analysis of data for 374 patients treated with high-dose IL-2 between 1988 and 1999 revealed a correlation between sites of metastatic disease and objective response rate (54% for patients with cutaneous or subcutaneous metastasis compared to 12% for those with disease at other sites).[358] Responses to high-dose IL-2 were less common in patients who had received prior treatment with low-dose IL-2 (15%) or IFN-α (13%) than in those who had not (21%); however, these differences were not statistically significant.[359] Other analyses correlated response with Cw7 phenotype, development of vitiligo, autoimmune thyroid dysfunction, or low pretreatment serum levels of C-reactive protein.[346,347,358] A relationship between low pretreatment IL-6 levels and both enhanced response to and prolonged survival after IL-2–based therapy has also been reported.[360] More recent studies have examined pretreatment gene expression profiles within subcutaneous tumors and correlated results with treatment outcome.[361] Tumor response was associated with expression of genes related to T-cell regulation, which suggests that immune responsiveness might be predetermined by a tumor microenvironment conducive to immune recognition. Efforts to confirm and refine these response correlates and to identify additional and reproducible pretreatment predictors of response through the use of such gene expression and proteomic techniques are ongoing and raise the potential of eventually limiting this toxic therapy to those most likely to benefit.

Interleukin-2 plus Interferon-α. Preclinical data suggested that IFN-α might induce up-regulation of histocompatibility and tumor-associated antigens on tumor cells and thereby increase their susceptibility to IL-2–activated T-cell cytolysis. However, despite these promising preclinical investigations and some encouraging early clinical results, the combination of IL-2 and IFN-α has not produced major advantages over high-dose IL-2 alone.[346,347,362]

A potential exception is the "decrescendo" IL-2 and IFN-α regimen.[363] This regimen was designed to induce optimal IL-2 receptor expression while minimizing the toxicity seen with high circulating levels of secondary cytokines in conventional high-dose bolus schedules. A response rate of 31% was reported using this regimen, including 22% in patients who had progressed after dacarbazine (DTIC) therapy. A median survival of 17 months was reported. A lesser degree of benefit was reported in a second study investigating this approach. Of 21 patients who had previously received chemotherapy for advanced disease, only two

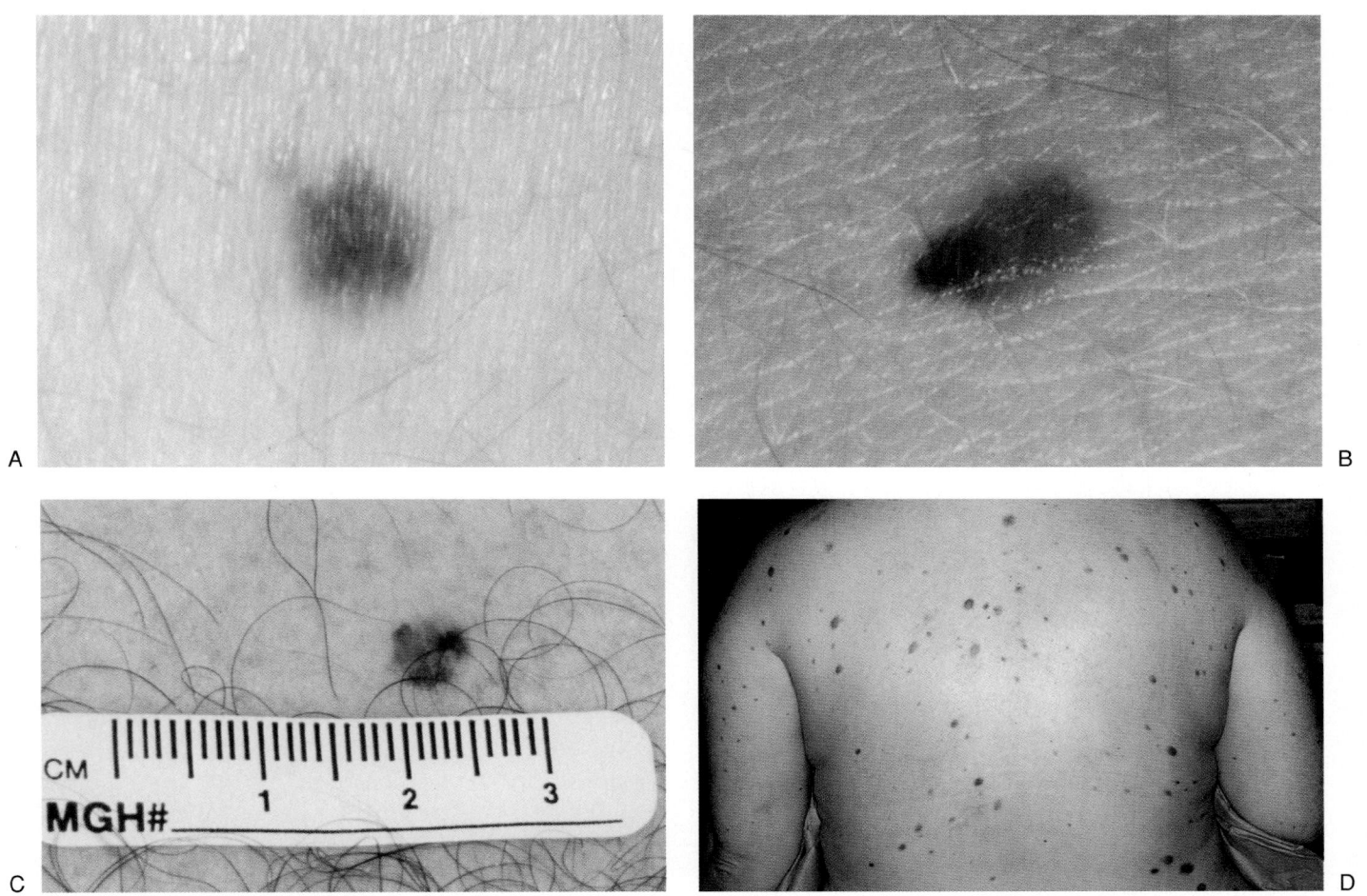

COLOR PLATE 1. Clinical presentations of melanoma precursors, markers of increased melanoma risks, and confounding lesions. **A–C:** Dysplastic nevus. **D:** Dysplastic nevi on back. (*Figure continues*)

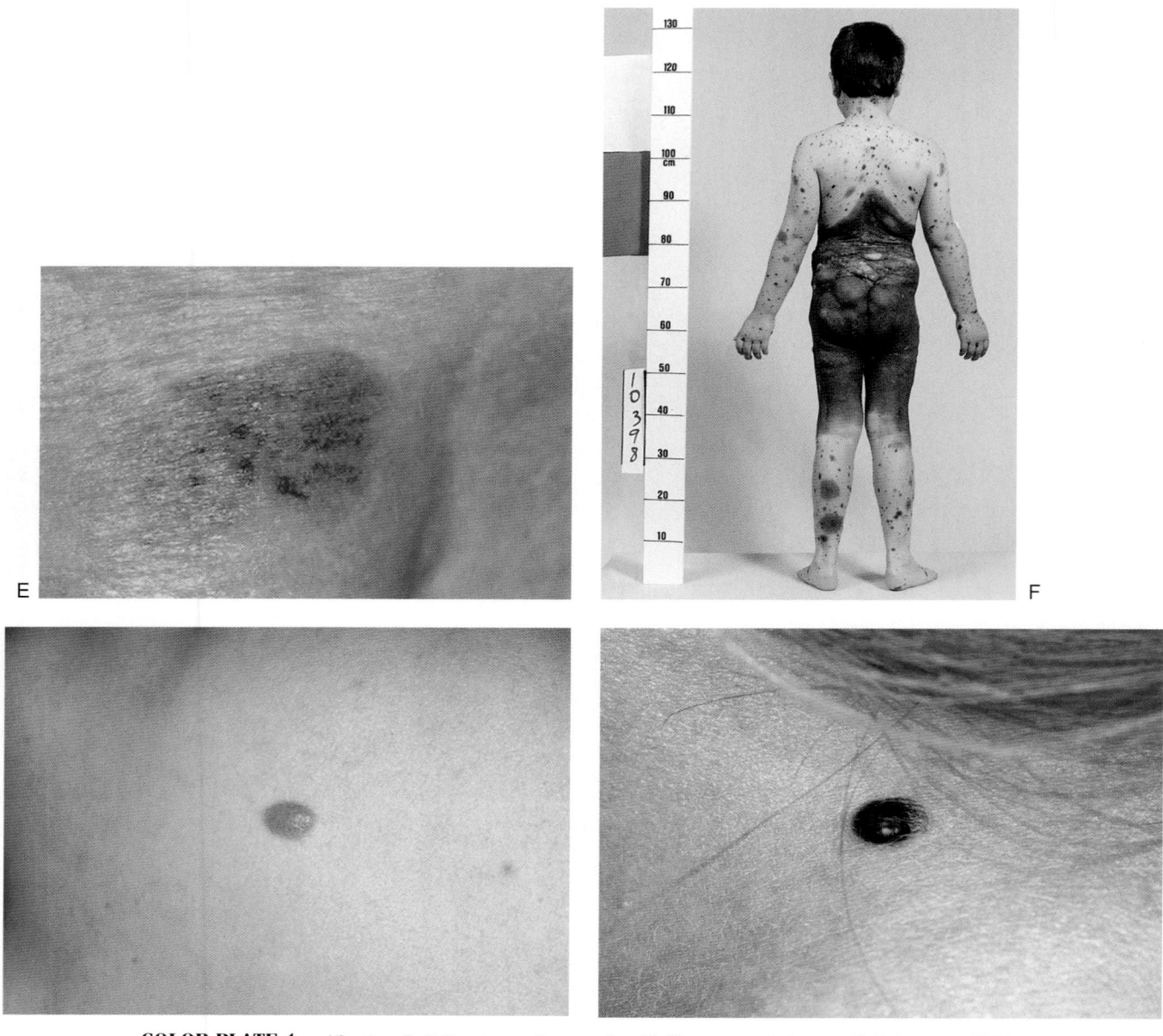

COLOR PLATE 1. (*Continued*). **E:** Lentigo maligna on face. **F:** Giant congenital nevus. **G:** Spitz nevus. **H:** Pigmented Spitz nevus. (From Balch CM, Blackwell PM, Houghton AN. *Cutaneous melanoma*, 4th ed. St. Louis, MO: Quality Medical Press, 2003, with permission.)

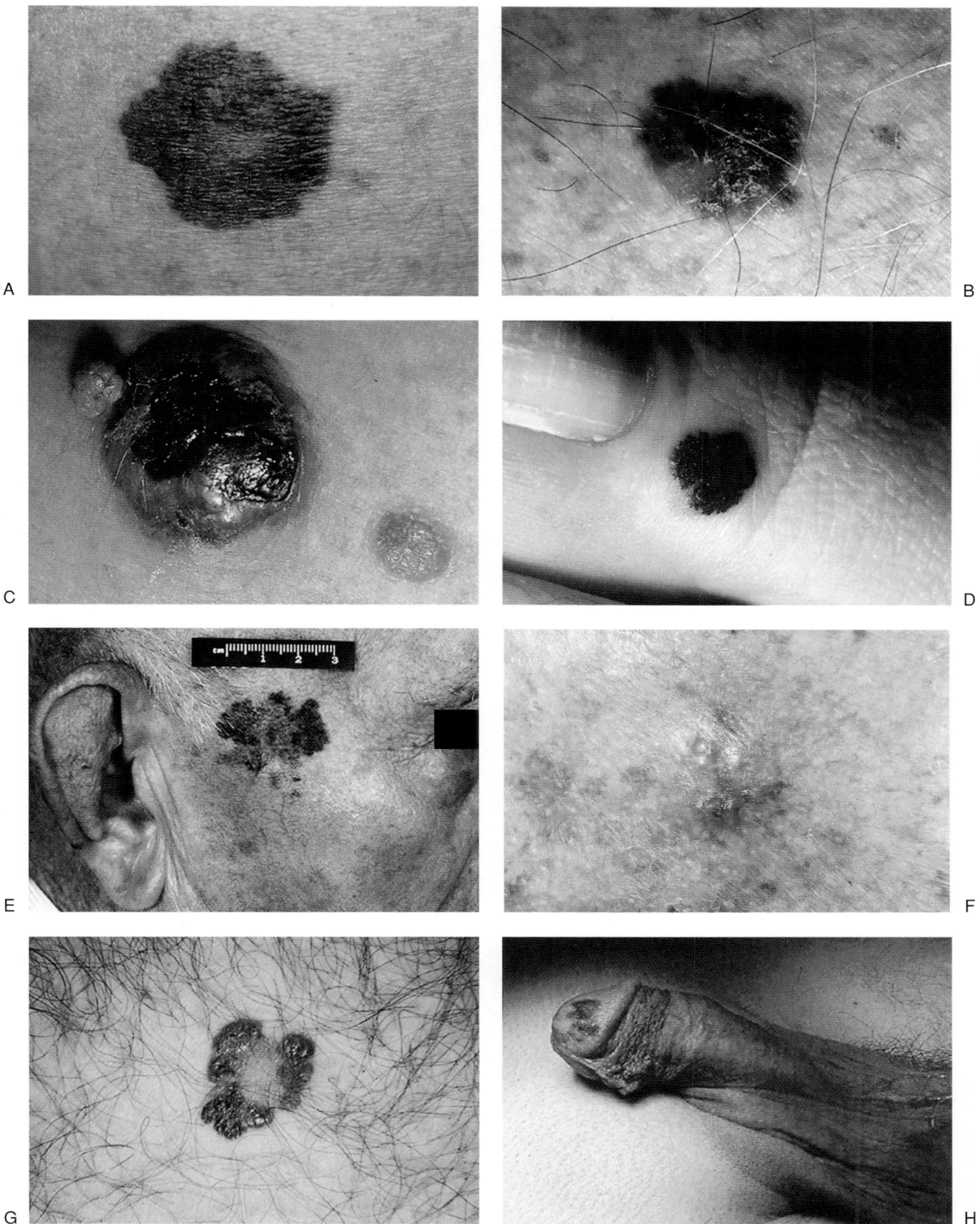

COLOR PLATE 2. Clinical presentations and growth patterns of invasive cutaneous melanoma. **A:** Superficial spreading melanoma (thin). **B:** Superficial spreading melanoma (intermediate risk). **C:** Nodular melanoma—ulcerated. **D:** Acral lentiginous melanoma. **E:** Lentigo maligna melanoma. **F:** Desmoplastic melanoma. **G:** Regressing melanoma. **H:** Penile melanoma. (From Balch CM, Blackwell PM, Houghton AN. *Cutaneous melanoma,* 4th ed. St. Louis, MO: Quality Medical Press, 2003, with permission.)

achieved durable remission, remaining alive more than 30 months after treatment.[364]

OTHER CYTOKINES. Many other recombinant cytokines have been investigated in treatment of patients with advanced melanoma. Although the results with IL-1, IL-4, IL-6, TNF-α, IFN-γ, and FLT3L have largely been disappointing,[365] some encouraging antitumor activity has been reported for GM-CSF, IL-12, and more recently IL-18.

GM-CSF, in addition having a potential role as an adjuvant to surgery in patients with resected stage IV or extensive stage III disease, has the ability to activate monocytes and dendritic cells and to induce the expression of the IL-2 receptor on T cells.[366,367] This has prompted investigation into its use as an immune adjuvant in various vaccine strategies and in combination with IL-2.[368–370] Although some antitumor activity has been reported,[370] the value of GM-CSF in these situations remains to be determined.

IL-12 produced some responses in early phase I trials. A complete remission occurred in one patient treated at the top dosage level in one report[371]; in another study, tumor shrinkage not reaching the level of partial remission occurred in 3 of 10 patients.[372] A peculiar schedule dependency associated with IL-12, whereby a single test dose increases a patient's tolerance to subsequent therapy and possibly reduces antitumor effects, has made clinical development of this agent more complicated.[373] Novel schedules of IL-12 have been explored in an effort to sustain its biologic activity.[374] These studies have shown a correlation with the ability to sustain IFN-γ production and antitumor effects. Although the addition of low-dose IL-2 to IL-12 has been able to sustain IFN-γ production in the majority of patients, the antitumor effect of the combination has remained modest.[375] IL-12 has also been shown to up-regulate Jak-STAT signaling intermediates in peripheral blood lymphocytes, perhaps potentiating IFN-α activity.[375a] This observation has led Cancer and Leukemia Group B to initiate a clinical trial evaluating combined IL-12 and IFN-α therapy in patients with advanced melanoma.

IL-18 is a novel cytokine that induces IFN-γ production and Fas- and T-cell–dependent killing and possesses antitumor activity in a variety of preclinical tumor models. Initial phase I studies with this agent have shown tumor regression in patients with advanced melanoma treated at tolerable dosage levels, which raises the potential that IL-18 may eventually play a role in the treatment of this disease.[376]

Adoptive Immunotherapy

Early research in animal models indicated that the activity of IL-2 was optimal when high doses were combined with IL-2–activated peripheral blood lymphocytes (LAK cells). However, randomized and sequential clinical trials comparing IL-2 plus LAK cells with high-dose IL-2 alone failed to show sufficient benefit from the addition of LAK cells to justify their use.[377,378] Clinical trials of IL-2 in combination with autologous TILs showed responses in 29 of 86 patients (34%).[344,379] Responses were seen in some patients who had received prior IL-2 treatment, which perhaps indicates enhanced potency for the IL-2 plus TILs combination. Only five responses were complete, and all except one partial response was of less than 10 months' duration. A total of 121 patients were enrolled to treat the 86

patients; thus, the true response rate for IL-2 plus TILs is closer to 24% for all entrants. Considering all of these factors, it is unlikely that the simple addition of TILs to IL-2 is sufficiently superior to use of IL-2 alone to justify the increased complexity and expense of this approach. Current studies have focused on *in vitro* selection of the most potent TIL populations and their administration after efforts to modulate immunosuppressive effects within the tumor microenvironment. One report demonstrated that transfer of highly avid TILs into patients after a lymphodepleting chemotherapy resulted in objective responses in 46% of patients with metastatic melanoma.[404] When this approach was used, up to 75% of circulating CD8+ lymphocytes had antitumor activity lasting months after the adoptive cell transfer. Further discussion of this approach is provided in Chapter 62. Others have attempted to expand the applicability of adoptive cell transfer therapy by transfecting T cells with a gene encoding the GD2 antibody linked to the T-cell receptor complex.[380] In theory, these "designer" T cells could bind tumors via their modified T-cell receptor, triggering the T-cell cytolytic machinery. Clinical trials with this novel approach have just been initiated.

Vaccines

Vaccination therapy with a variety of melanoma cell preparations has been pursued over the past several decades. Efforts to develop effective vaccines have been hindered by a combination of poor immunogenicity of relevant antigens, tumor-reinforced tolerance, antigen shedding, and tumor heterogeneity. Early vaccines included autologous tumor cells, allogeneic whole cells, cell lysates, and shed antigens. Although tumor responses were observed with some of these approaches, and some have shown potential benefit in prolonging relapse-free survival compared to that in historical controls when used in the adjuvant setting, recent advances in molecular biology and understanding of immunologic recognition have prompted greater emphasis on studying defined-antigen and dendritic cell–based melanoma vaccines. These investigations have been the major focus of research in patients with stage IV disease. This topic is discussed in detail in Chapter 61.

Overcoming of Immune Suppression

Resistance to immune therapy in tumor-bearing hosts has been postulated to be due to a number of probably interrelated factors, including physiologic down-modulation of immune response mediated by interactions of B7 and cytotoxic T lymphocyte-associated antigen-4,[381] CTLA-4 tumor-induced immune suppression via the FAS/fas ligand interactions,[382,383] T-cell receptor dysfunction evidenced by diminished ζ chain expression,[384] preferential Th2 T helper cell responses to tumor antigens,[385] the inability of tumor-specific CD8+ T cells to express cytokines on stimulation or lyse melanoma targets,[386,387] selective loss of antigen-specific cytotoxic T lymphocytes,[388] and the presence of regulatory CD4+/CD25+ T cells.[389] T-cell receptor abnormalities have been variably reported to be induced by monocyte arginase secretion leading to arginine depletion[390,391] or oxygen free radical production leading to T-cell apoptosis.[392] Reversal of T-cell receptor abnormalities has been seen with IL-2 immunotherapy and may correlate with tumor response.[337] Correlative laboratory studies performed in conjunction with current and future clinical trials will be necessary to sort out the importance of these various phenomena to the immunologic potency and antitumor effects of various immune therapies. Nonetheless, the extent of immune suppression in tumor-bearing hosts has fueled interest in testing vaccination strategies in the high-risk adjuvant setting, in which the enhanced ability to assess vaccine potency outweighs the loss of tumor response as an end point.

Reversal of immune suppression has been a major focus of recent immunotherapy research with some encouraging initial results. The administration of antibody against CTLA-4 together with a multiepitopic peptide vaccine has been reported to enhance vaccine immunogenicity and induce a variety of autoimmune phenomenon, including vitiligo.[393] In some studies immune potency has correlated with clinical outcome. Histamine hydrochloride has been shown to inhibit the formation of oxygen radicals, which sustains local NK and T-cell immune function as well as their responsiveness to IL-2.[392] Treatment of melanoma-bearing mice with histamine was shown to enhance the antitumor effects of IL-2, and phase II studies of IL-2, IFN, and histamine produced encouraging results (median survivals of 13.3 and 15.1 months) for the combination.[394,395] A phase III multicenter randomized trial involving 305 patients with melanoma and comparing histamine plus low-dose subcutaneous IL-2 to subcutaneous IL-2 alone showed a trend toward improved survival favoring the combination treatment in overall intent-to-treat population (9.1 months vs. 8.2 months; $P = .125$) and a significant difference in survival with combination therapy in a prospectively identified subset of patients with liver metastases (9.4 months vs. 5.1 months; $P = .004$).[396] A similar benefit for the IL-2 and histamine combination was seen in patients with M1c melanoma ($P = .02$),[397] which suggests that the protective effect of histamine was not restricted to the macrophage-rich hepatic environment. A follow-up survival analysis at 2 years after completion of accrual confirmed the benefit of histamine in the liver metastasis subset ($P = .0028$) but also now showed a significant benefit for the overall population ($P = .0464$).[398] Furthermore, an analysis of immunomodulatory effects of the combination in a phase II study showed significant increases in ζ chain expression and reductions in peripheral blood mononuclear cells IL-6 secretion with treatment.[399] Because few tumor responses were observed with either treatment approach and the hepatic metastases patient population was not prospectively stratified, these results require confirmation. A phase III trial comparing the same treatments but restricted to patients with hepatic metastases has completed accrual and results should be analyzed shortly. Of concern, a phase II trial combining histamine with IL-2 and IFN produced a median survival of only 7.8 months,[400] and a European trial comparing IFN, IL-2, and histamine to dacarbazine failed to show a significant survival difference within either the overall patient population or the liver metastasis subset, which calls into question the value of the histamine effect.[401]

Lymphodepletion has been shown to markedly enhance the efficacy of T-cell transfer therapy in murine tumor models.[402] More recently, this effect has been attributed to the elimination of the CD4+/CD25+ population of regulatory T cells.[403] To test this hypothesis clinically, Dudley et al. treated HLA-A2+ melanoma patients with immunodepleting cyclophosphamide and fludarabine chemotherapy 7 days before the administration of highly selected tumor-reactive T cells and high-dose IL-2.[404] T cells were derived from TILs generated in response to HLA-A2–restricted MART-1 (melanoma antigen recognized by T cell-1) peptide antigen vaccination that were selected for reactivity to either HLA-A2+ melanoma or an autologous melanoma cell line and then rapidly expanded *in vitro*. Patients were refractory to standard therapies including high-dose IL-2, cytotoxic chemotherapy, or biochemotherapy. Six of 13 patients exhibited at least partial tumor regression and 5 of these responding patients demonstrated signs of autoimmune melanocyte destruction, including 4 patients with vitiligo and 1 patient with anterior uveitis. All patients recovered hematopoietic function by day 11 after cell infusion, and several patients demonstrated persistence of a large clonal T-cell population in their circulation, which indicated that the *in vivo* expansion of tumor-reactive T cells had occurred. Although these results suggest the clinical usefulness of overcoming immune suppression, much investigation is necessary before this complex and expensive approach can be applied to the general population of patients with advanced melanoma.

Monoclonal Antibodies

Monoclonal antibodies have been investigated either alone (unconjugated) or conjugated to various substances as potential therapy for metastatic melanoma. Several potential target antigens have been identified; however, most efforts have focused on the ganglioside system. Melanoma cells are rich in gangliosides, two of which, GD2 and GD3, appear to be up-regulated by transformation of melanocytes.[405]

UNCONJUGATED MONOCLONAL ANTIBODIES. Phase I trials of unconjugated monoclonal antibodies have shown that they can reach tumor sites after systemic administration.[406] Some responses have been observed in phase I trials with R24 (anti-GD3), 3F8 (anti-GD2), and other mouse monoclonal antibodies administered intravenously or regionally. Combinations of monoclonal antibodies, despite theoretical advantages, have not proven to be clinically advantageous. Clinical investigation with murine monoclonal antibodies has been hampered by human anti–mouse antibody responses that limit retreatment capabilities. Although one study reported a tumor response to intralesional injection of a human IgM monoclonal antibodies against GD2,[407] human antibodies have been difficult to produce in large quantities, which limits systemic investigations involving these agents. Chimeric human-mouse antibodies (which combine the antigen-binding fab fragment of the mouse monoclonal antibody with the heavy and light chains of a human immunoglobulin molecule) have been developed in an effort to circumvent the latter problem. The chimeric 14:18 antibody (human-mouse chimeric version of the anti-GD2 Mab 14.G.A.) and the KM871 antibody (human-mouse chimeric version of the anti-GD3 monoclonal antibody) have shown some antitumor activity in phase I trials.[408,409] Investigators also have explored combinations of unconjugated monoclonal antibodies with cytokines (IL-2, GM-CSF, TNF, and IFN) in an effort to enhance either tumor antigen expression or antibody-dependent cellular cytotoxicity.[406] For the most part, these combinations have not proven superior to the use of the antibodies alone.

CONJUGATED MONOCLONAL ANTIBODIES AND FUSION PROTEINS. Monoclonal antibodies have been conjugated to cytokines, radionuclides, and immunotoxins in an effort to enhance their potency. Clinical trials with murine antimelanoma antibodies either conjugated to ricin A or radiolabeled with iodine 131 have been initiated, with rare tumor responses and generally mild toxicity observed.[406] Attempts to increase the dosage of these radiolabeled antibodies, however, have been hindered by bone marrow toxicity. In an effort to enhance antibody-dependent cellular cytotoxicity at the tumor site, investigators have linked IL-2 to the carboxy-terminal of the ch14.18 molecule.[410] Testing in animal models using this fusion protein showed it to be superior to either IL-2 or ch14.18 alone, or both in combination at comparable doses.[411] Phase I trials of this fusion protein have produced responses in patients with neuroblastoma, but little antitumor activity has been observed in patients with melanoma.[412]

Gene Therapy

Gene therapy approaches in melanoma have primarily focused on injecting genes that will enhance the immunogenicity of melanoma, analogous to the vaccine approaches described previously. In animal models, immunization with tumor cells transfected with one of several cytokines (particularly GM-CSF) or the T-cell costimulatory molecules (B7-1) protected animals from subsequent challenge by wild-type tumor cells and, in some instances, induced regression of established tumor cells.[413] Clinical trials using vaccinations with autologous melanoma cells transfected with these various gene products have been initiated, but limited clinical benefit has been observed to date. As an example, vaccination with irradiated, autologous melanoma cells engineered to secrete GM-CSF by retroviral-mediated gene transfer produced potent antitumor immunity as assessed at tumor sites on which serial biopsies were performed.[414] A follow-up trial using adenovirally mediated GM-CSF transfer yielded similar immune responses at vaccination of tumor sites and tumor regressions in 3 of 26 assessable patients.[415] Although these approaches shed light on the biology underlying immune recognition, it is unclear whether they offer any advantage over the administration of the protein itself or the other vaccine strategies mentioned previously in Chapter 61.

Others have injected melanoma lesions of HLA-B7– patients with plasmid DNA containing the HLA-B7 gene (Allovectin-7) in an attempt to enhance the immunogenicity of the tumor.[416] This foreign protein, if expressed, should trigger a potent local inflammatory response, which in theory could promote melanoma antigen–specific immune responses through the process of epitope spread. In initial clinical trials, HLA-B7 expression by injected tumors was documented, and partial regression was observed in 10% to 15% of injected lesions.[416,417] In a few patients, regression also occurred at distant sites[417] (Fig. 38.2-20). Another study using a plasmid containing both HLA-B7 and β₂-microglobulin produced tumor regressions in 4 of 52 injected lesions.[418] A phase III trial comparing Allovectin-7 plus dacarbazine to dacarbazine alone[419] and a phase II trial using higher dosages of Allovectin-7 alone[420] have been completed with only preliminary results available. The extent to which such local, presumably alloreactive reactions can be generalized remains to be determined.

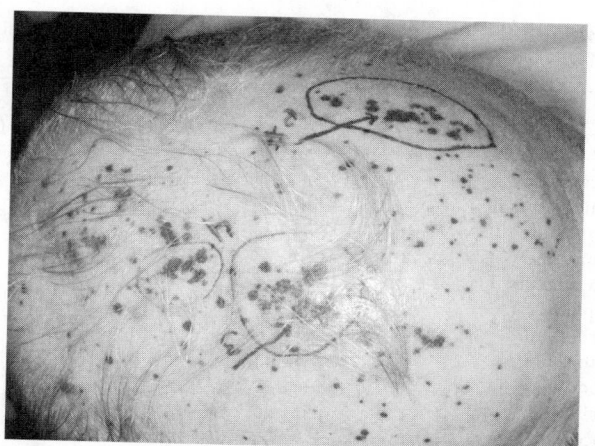

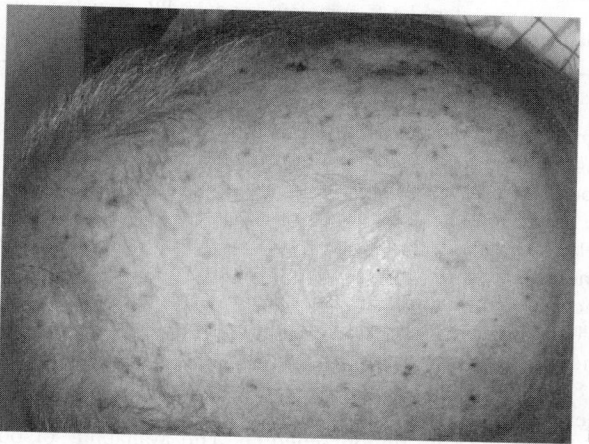

FIGURE 38.2-20. Near complete regression of multiple scalp melanoma metastases after intratumoral injection of Allovectin-7. Four of the largest lesions in **A** were injected weekly × 6 every 10 weeks for four cycles. Regression was seen in uninjected lesions and continued after cessation of intratumoral injections (**B**).

CYTOTOXIC CHEMOTHERAPY

Chemotherapy produces response rates of approximately 15% to 20% in patients with metastatic melanoma, but there is no documented associated increase in median survival time. In a metaanalysis of 83 studies involving 6322 patients, the median survival of patients treated with cytotoxic chemotherapy in the studies published since 1985 was 8.9 months.[421] Long-term survival was 13.6% at 2 years and only 2.3% at 5 years.

Single Agents

The chemotherapeutic agents that have been most widely used in patients with metastatic disease are dacarbazine, nitrosoureas, platinum analogs, and microtubular toxins. The activities of these various agents are summarized in Table 38.2-14.

DACARBAZINE AND TEMOZOLOMIDE. Dacarbazine, which produces response rates in 10% to 20% of patients and complete responses in up to 5%,[224,331] remains the benchmark. Responses have been observed mainly in soft tissues (i.e., skin, subcutaneous tissue, lymph node, and lung metastases) and are usually partial and of short duration, ranging from 3 to 6 months. Although

TABLE 38.2-14. Active Single-Agent Chemotherapy for Patients with Metastatic Melanoma

Agent	No. of Evaluable Patients	No. of CR + PR (%)	95% CI (%)
Dacarbazine	1936	382 (20)	18–22
Temozolomide	200	33 (17)	12–22
Carmustine (BCNU)	122	22 (18)	11–25
Lomustine (CCNU)	270	35 (13)	9–17
Fotemustine	153	37 (24)	17–31
Cisplatin	188	43 (23)	17–29
Carboplatin	43	7 (16)	5–27
Vinblastine	62	8 (13)	5–21
Vindesine	273	39 (14)	10–18
Paclitaxel	53	7 (13)	4–22
Docetaxel	83	13 (15)	9–21

CI, confidence interval; CR, complete response; PR, partial response. (Adapted from ref. 422.)

approximately one-fourth of complete responders experience long-term remissions,[330] fewer than 2% of all patients are expected to survive for 6 years.[224] Although dacarbazine remains the only cytotoxic agent approved for the treatment of advanced melanoma, there are no phase III trial data to support a survival benefit for dacarbazine compared to other treatments or even to a no-treatment control.[422] Dacarbazine is generally well tolerated, and major side effects are limited to nausea and vomiting. Typical schedules for dacarbazine are 200 mg/m² intravenously for 5 days or 850 mg to 1000 mg/m² intravenously over 1 hour every 3 to 4 weeks. Response rates and response durations do not appear to be affected by administration schedule. The availability of potent antiemetic agents has permitted outpatient administration of dacarbazine at a dose of 1000 mg/m² on a convenient schedule of 1 day every 3 to 4 weeks.

Temozolomide is an imidotetrazine derivative that, at physiologic pH, spontaneously converts to methyl-triazemoimidazole carboxamide, the active metabolite of dacarbazine. Temozolomide has the advantages of being absorbed orally and possessing significant CNS penetration.[423] This latter property contributed to its approval by the FDA for the treatment of anaplastic astrocytoma.[424] In a phase III trial comparing temozolomide to dacarbazine in patients with metastatic melanoma without brain metastases,[425] temozolomide produced apparent improvement in median progression-free survival (1.9 months vs. 1.5 months) and health-related quality of life relative to dacarbazine, but had no significant impact on response rate (13.5% vs. 12.1%) or overall survival (7.7 months vs. 6.4 months). Of note, in a subset of patients in this study who had regularly scheduled head CT scans, fewer CNS relapses were observed in the patients receiving temozolomide.[426] Despite its more convenient route of administration and potential for improved CNS control relative to dacarbazine, the overall clinical data were not sufficiently compelling for temozolomide to receive FDA approval for the treatment of metastatic melanoma. Investigations with temozolomide are continuing using novel dosing schedules and combinations. Regimens involving multiple doses per day or prolonged daily exposure have been studied in an effort to circumvent DNA repair processes and more optimally coordinate with radiation therapy schedules.[427,428] Initial studies have also suggested that the combination of temozolomide and thalidomide may be

superior to temozolomide alone[428,429] and may be particularly effective in patients with CNS metastasis[430]; however, data supporting the superiority of these approaches to standard therapy have yet to be produced.

NITROSOUREAS. The antitumor activity of the nitrosoureas currently available in the United States—carmustine (BCNU) and lomustine (CCNU)—is similar to that of dacarbazine, with response rates ranging from 10% to 20%.[422] Patients previously exposed to dacarbazine are less likely to respond than untreated patients.[431] Alopecia is more severe with these agents, and hematologic toxicity, particularly thrombocytopenia, is more prolonged. Fotemustine is a novel chloroethyl nitrosourea that is now commercially available in Australia and some European countries. Its mechanism of action involves the rapid metabolic conversion and consequent alkylation of thioenzymes involved in DNA synthesis. It appears to cross the blood–brain barrier more rapidly than the other nitrosoureas, possibly through an amino acid transport system.[432] Encouraging response rates were seen in phase II trials,[433] which prompted the performance of a large multicenter European phase III trial comparing fotemustine to dacarbazine.[434] This study showed trends in response rate (17% vs. 7%), median survival (7.4 months vs. 5.8 months), and median time to occurrence of brain metastases (22.7 months vs. 7.2 months), all favoring fotemustine, but none of these differences achieved statistical significance. Consequently, although fotemustine is considered standard therapy in some countries, it remains unavailable in the United States.

PLATINUM ANALOGS. Cisplatin and carboplatin have shown modest activity in patients with metastatic melanoma. Cisplatin has been more extensively studied, with response rates averaging 10% to 20%.[422] In one study, cisplatin administered at doses of up to 150 mg/m² in combination with amifostine, a thiol derivative with protective effects on bone marrow and renal tissue, produced tumor responses in 53% of patients.[435] However, all responses were partial, and the median response duration was only 4 months. In a subsequent trial within ECOG, this regimen displayed only modest antitumor activity, while causing unacceptable renal toxicity, gastrointestinal toxicity, and ototoxicity.[422,436]

OTHER AGENTS. Microtubule toxins such as vinblastine and agents that interfere with microtubule disassembly such as the taxanes have also shown modest antitumor activity in patients with metastatic melanoma. Paclitaxel administered by a variety of schedules in phase II studies encompassing over 100 melanoma patients produced an aggregate response rate of around 15%.[437,438] Docetaxel has produced similar response rates, with 13 responders observed among 83 patients studied.[439–441] When combined with temozolomide, docetaxel produced responses in 17 of 62 previously untreated patients (27%) including five complete responses,[442] which suggests a potential value for this combination. A regimen involving weekly paclitaxel (150 mg/m² over 1 hour for 6 weeks followed by 2-week rest) was well tolerated and produced responses in 2 of 15 patients (13%) who had progressed after first-line cytotoxic chemotherapy.[443] These results suggest that taxanes may be useful as second-line cytotoxic agents. In contrast, BMS-184476, a novel taxane, and the epothilones, a new class of nontaxane tubulin polymerization agents—both with activity against paclitaxel-resistant cell lines *in vitro*—have shown lim-

TABLE 38.2-15. Pivotal Randomized Controlled Trials of Chemotherapy, Tamoxifen, and Interferon for Treatment of Stage IV Melanoma

Study	Regimen	No. Evaluable Patients	Response Rate (%) (% CR/PR, If Available)	Median Survival (Mo)
TRIALS OF COMBINATION CHEMOTHERAPY VS. DACARBAZINE (DTIC)				
Costanzi et al.	Bleomycin/hydroxyurea/DTIC ±BCG	256	29	ND
	DTIC/BCG	130	18	
Buzaid et al.	Cisplatin/vinblastine/DTIC	46	24	6
	DTIC	45	11	5
Chapman et al.	Cisplatin/DTIC/BCNU/tamoxifen	108	18	7
	DTIC	118	10	7
TRIALS OF TAMOXIFEN AND/OR INTERFERON				
Cocconi et al.	DTIC/tamoxifen	60	28 (7/21); P = .03	10.7; P = .02
	DTIC	52	12 (6/6)	6.4
Rusthoven et al.	Cisplatin/DTIC/BCNU/tamoxifen	98	30 (3/27)	6.4 males
				6.9 females
	Cisplatin/DTIC/BCNU	97	21 (6/14)	6.4 males
				7.1 females
Falkson et al.	DTIC/IFN	30	53 (40/13)	17.6; P <.01
	DTIC	30	18 (7/13)	9.6
Falkson et al.	DTIC/IFN ± tamoxifen	126	16 (2.3/13.5)	9.5 tamoxifen
				9.3 no tamoxifen
	DTIC ± tamoxifen	129	20.5 (5.5/15)	8 tamoxifen
				10 no tamoxifen
Kirkwood et al.	DTIC/IFN	21	4 (19)	ND
	DTIC	24	5 (21)	
Thomson et al.	DTIC/IFN	87	18 (21)	ND
	DTIC	83	14 (17)	
Bajetta et al.	DTIC/high-dose IFN	76	21 (28)	ND
	DTIC/low-dose IFN	84	19 (23)	
	DTIC	82	16 (20)	

BCG, bacille Calmette-Guérin 2; BCNU, carmustine; CR, complete response; IFN, interferon; ND, no difference; OS, overall survival; PR, partial response.
Note: Full references for each trial are available in ref. 98.

ited activity when administered to patients with melanoma after failure of first-line cytotoxic therapy.[444,445]

Combination Cytotoxic Chemotherapy

A variety of combination chemotherapy regimens have produced response rates of 30% to 50% in single-institution phase II trials involving patients with metastatic melanoma. Pivotal phase III trials comparing cytotoxic chemotherapy regimens are highlighted in Table 38.2-15. Two of the most active combinations reported are the three-drug combination of cisplatin, vinblastine, and dacarbazine (CVD) developed by Legha et al.,[446] and the four-drug combination of cisplatin, dacarbazine, BCNU, and tamoxifen (CDBT) developed by Del Prete et al. and frequently referred to as the Dartmouth regimen.[447]

The CVD regimen produced responses in 40% of 50 patients with 4% complete responses and a median response duration of 9 months.[446] In an initial report of a randomized, multi-institutional trial comparing CVD to dacarbazine alone, the CVD treatment was associated with increases in response rate, response duration, and survival[448]; however, in a subsequent as yet unpublished analysis encompassing approximately 150 patients, there were no differences in either response rate (19% vs. 14%) or survival (A. Buzaid et al., *personal communication*, 2002).

Initial phase II studies with the CDBT regimen noted response rates as high as 46%, with one-fourth of the responses being complete responses.[449] The inclusion of tamoxifen appeared to be essential, because response rates fell to 10% when the tamoxifen was omitted.[450] However, other studies have not confirmed these high response rates. For example, a phase II study within the Southwest Oncology Group reported only a 15% response rate,[451] and two phase III trials comparing CDBT to either CDB or the Melacine vaccine reported response rates of 30% and 13% for the CDBT treatment arm.[452,453] Finally, two completed phase III trials involving 240 and 100 patients showed no benefit for CBDT compared to dacarbazine alone.[454,455] The response rates were approximately 15% and the median survival after randomization was 7 months in both studies. No difference was seen between the two treatment arms, although bone marrow suppression, nausea, vomiting, and fatigue were significantly more frequent with the CDBT therapy. Taken together, phase III trials to date have shown no compelling evidence to support the value of combination chemotherapy in patients with metastatic melanoma.

Combinations of Cytotoxic Agents and Tamoxifen

Since the report by Fisher et al.[456] in 1976 demonstrating the presence of estrogen-binding activity in metastases of human melanoma, a number of clinical trials have examined the activity of tamoxifen and other antihormonal agents in patients with metastatic melanoma. Although the antiestrogens were ultimately shown to have negligible single-agent antitumor activity in advanced melanoma, some investigators reported potential benefit when tamoxifen was combined with cytotoxic chemotherapy.[457] The potential benefit in this setting was attributed to the potentiation of the cytotoxic chemotherapy rather than to direct antiestrogenic effects.

The results of randomized studies comparing chemotherapy regimens with and without tamoxifen are summarized in Table 38.2-15.[452,458–461] Only one prospective randomized study, an Italian study that compared dacarbazine alone to dacarbazine plus tamoxifen, showed an improvement in response rate and survival.[458] In this report, the response rate was improved from 12% to 28% and median survival was improved from 23 weeks to 41 weeks with the addition of tamoxifen. All the other studies failed to show any differences in either response rate or survival. Of particular importance are the two large multicenter trials reported by ECOG and the National Cancer Institute of Canada evaluating the benefit of adding tamoxifen to either dacarbazine alone, in a fashion analogous to the Italian study, or dacarbazine plus IFN-α in a two-by-two factorial design (E3690)[461] or to the combination of cisplatin, dacarbazine, and BCNU.[452] Taken together, these studies clearly demonstrate that tamoxifen does not significantly enhance the antitumor effects of dacarbazine-based chemotherapy.

INTERFERON-α–BASED BIOCHEMOTHERAPY REGIMENS

Most phase II studies combining IFN-α with either single-agent or combination chemotherapy showed response rates and median survivals roughly comparable to those reported for the chemotherapy alone.[422] Although Pyrhonen et al.[464] reported an encouraging 63% response rate including 6 (13%) complete remissions with a combination of bleomycin, vincristine, CCNU, dacarbazine, and IFN-α, a multicenter phase II study of this combination showed a more modest 33% response rate.[465] Several groups have performed phase III trials examining the value of adding IFN-α to single-agent dacarbazine[461–463,466,467] (see Table 38.2-15). In a small single-institution trial, Falkson et al. observed 12 complete and 4 partial responses in 30 patients on the combination arm compared to 2 complete and 4 partial responses in 30 patients treated with dacarbazine alone.[466] Median response durations were 2.5 months with dacarbazine alone and 9.0 months with dacarbazine plus IFN-α; median survival was extended from 9.6 months in the group receiving dacarbazine alone to 17.6 months in those given the drug combination. Unfortunately, the other four randomized trials, including a trial performed within ECOG (E3690)[461] that investigated the same IFN-α treatment schedule that was used in the initial Falkson trial, showed no significant improvement in terms of response rate, time to progression, or survival associated with the addition of IFN-α to dacarbazine. Taken collectively, the bulk of the data suggest that the addition of IFN-α does not significantly enhance the antitumor activity of cytotoxic chemotherapy.

INTERLEUKIN-2–BASED BIOCHEMOTHERAPY REGIMENS

Combinations of IL-2 plus dacarbazine have resulted in considerably more toxicity than seen with dacarbazine alone while yielding response rates of only 13% to 33% (mean, 25%).[422]

These results are not clearly superior to those for dacarbazine alone. More encouraging results have been observed in studies that combined cisplatin-based chemotherapy with either high-dose IL-2 or lower doses of IL-2 combined with IFN-α.[422,468–473] Composite results from a variety of inpatient regimens showed a response rate of approximately 50% with 10% to 20% complete responses and median survival of approximately 11 to 12 months. Although partial responses were frequently of short duration (median of 4 to 6 months in most studies) and were not associated with prolonged survival, in some studies up to 50% of patients obtaining a complete response remained free from progression over the long term.[469] Overall, approximately 10% of patients were disease free for more than 2 years.[422] As with regimens of high-dose IL-2 alone, relapses beyond 2 years were extremely uncommon.[446]

Unlike with chemotherapy alone, responses were seen in all disease sites with equal frequency, and no clear dose-response relationship for IL-2 was apparent. Although some investigators reported partial regressions of preexisting small CNS metastases,[474] most trials excluded such patients, and the CNS was actually a common site of initial relapse.[471] Responses were seen in patients who had received prior chemotherapy[472] and appeared to be associated with the development of vitiligo, which suggests an autoimmune mechanism.[473] Cisplatin appeared to be required for synergy,[472] and activity appeared greatest when the chemotherapy was administered first.[468] Early studies documented that cytotoxic chemotherapy did not interfere with ongoing responses to immunotherapy,[470] which allowed closer integration of these two modalities. Novel regimens involving the concurrent administration of IL-2 and chemotherapy, rapidly tapered decrescendo IL-2 schedules, and lower doses of IL-2 compatible with administration in an outpatient setting produced similar antitumor activity, while reducing the toxicity and complexity of this treatment approach.[475–478] These phase II data as well as two metaanalyses[135,479] suggesting that biochemotherapy might be superior to either chemotherapy or immunotherapy alone prompted the initiation of several phase III trials.

Multiple phase III trials involving biochemotherapy have now been completed with at best mixed results (Table 38.2-16). A single-institution phase III trial comparing CVD to sequentially administered CVD plus IL-2 and IFN showed that the biochemotherapy combination produced a doubling of the response rate (48% vs. 25%) and median time to progression (4.9 months vs. 2.4 months) and an approximate 3-month prolongation in median survival (11.9 months vs. 9.2 months) (P = .06).[480] Although these results confirmed the phase II data in many respects, the fact that the median time to progression for responding patients was no different in the two treatment arms (6 months) and that few durable responses were seen was disappointing and called into question the contribution of the immunotherapy component to the overall tumor response. Furthermore, several other phase III trials failed to show significant benefit for biochemotherapy. For example, both a National Cancer Institute Surgery Branch study comparing cisplatin, dacarbazine, and tamoxifen with or without high-dose IL-2 and IFN-α, and a European Organization for Research and Treatment of Cancer trial comparing cisplatin-based biochemotherapy to IL-2 and IFN-α alone produced improved response rates for the biochemotherapy arms, but no overall survival benefit.[481,482] Similarly, another European Organization for Research and

TABLE 38.2-16. Pivotal Randomized Controlled Trials of Interleukin-2– and Cisplatin-Based Biochemotherapy for Stage IV Melanoma

Study	Regimen	No. Evaluable Patients	RR (%)	Median Survival (Mo)	Comment
Keilholz et al.	IL-2 (decrescendo regimen)/IFN	66	18	9	Improvement in RR but not in survival
	Cisplatin + IL-2/IFN	60	35	9	
Rosenberg et al.	Cisplatin/DTIC/tam	52	27	15.8	Improvement in RR, but survival worse
	Cisplatin/DTIC/tam + HD IL-2/IFN	50	44	10.7	
Eton et al.	CVD	92	25	9.5	Improved RR and TTP; borderline significant change in survival
	CVD + IL-2 (9 MU/m² IV × 96 h)/IFN (sequential)	91	48	11.8	
Keilholz et al.	Cisplatin/DTIC/IFN	180	22.8	9.0	No significant difference in RR or OS
	Cisplatin/DTIC/IFN + IL-2	183	20.8	9.0	
Atkins et al.	CVD	201	11	8.7	No significant difference in RR or OS
	CVD + IL-2/IFN (concurrent)	204	17	8.4	

CVD, cisplatin, vincristine, dacarbazine; DTIC, dacarbazine; HD, high dose; IFN, interferon; IL-2, interleukin-2; OS, overall survival; RR, response rate; tam, tamoxifen; TTP, time to progression.
(Adapted from ref. 422.)

Treatment of Cancer trial evaluating cisplatin, dacarbazine, and IFN-α with or without IL-2 showed no benefit for the addition of IL-2 in terms of either response rate or survival.[483] Finally a U.S. Intergroup study comparing CVD to concurrent administration of CVD, IL-2, and IFN revealed only insignificant increases in response rate and time to progression for the biochemotherapy regimen, but no difference in overall survival.[484]

Attempts to improve on prior biochemotherapy approaches have included (1) substituting temozolomide for dacarbazine in an effort to reduce the incidence of isolated CNS relapse, (2) using maintenance IL-2 and GM-CSF therapy in an attempt to delay disease progression in patients exhibiting partial response or stable disease after four more cycles of biochemotherapy, and (3) moving treatment into the high-risk adjuvant setting in an attempt to reduce the incidence of CNS relapse as well as the tumor resistance and immune suppression typically associated with more advanced disease. In a phase II trial in which temozolomide was substituted for dacarbazine, the CNS was the initial site of progression in only 2 of 21 responding patients compared to 12 of 19 who had received a similar dacarbazine-containing regimen.[485] Although these data suggested a significant reduction in the rate of initial CNS relapse, median response duration (3 months) and median survival (7.5 months) were disappointingly short. Furthermore, a second multicenter study of concurrent biochemotherapy incorporating temozolomide produced only 12 objective responses (1 complete response and 11 partial responses) in 60 evaluable patients (20% response rate), while producing greater than anticipated toxicity.[486] Consequently, despite the potential to improve the control of CNS disease, biochemotherapy regimens involving the substitution of temozolomide for dacarbazine cannot be recommended at present. O'Day et al.[370] explored the role of maintenance cytokine therapy for patients with stable disease or partial response after biochemotherapy.[422] The maintenance regimen consisted of daily outpatient injections of low-dose IL-2 and GM-CSF with intermittent pulses of inpatient high-dose IL-2. The median time to progression and overall survival were extended to 8.1 and 18.5 months, respectively, and 15% of patients achieved a complete response with this approach. A multicenter confirmatory trial has been completed and results await analysis. Finally, the role of biochemotherapy in the high-risk

adjuvant setting is being explored in the U.S. Intergroup protocol S0008 that compares a year of standard high-dose IFN-α to three cycles (9 weeks) of a biochemotherapy regimen of concurrent CVD plus IL-2 and IFN in patients with stage IIIB and IIIC melanoma. This protocol hopes to reach its accrual goal of 410 patients by 2005. Although these various approaches might yet establish a role for biochemotherapy in patients with high-risk or advanced melanoma, the use of this toxic combination in routine clinical practice can no longer be justified.

NOVEL THERAPEUTIC APPROACHES

Antiangiogenic Therapy

A number of agents with putative antiangiogenic properties have been investigated in treatment of patients with stage IV melanoma. Results have been disappointing to date. Although thalidomide has shown some activity when combined with temozolomide, it has been inactive as a single agent.[487] A derivative of thalidomide, CC 5013, with more potent antiangiogenic and immunomodulatory properties produced partial responses in 3 of 21 patients with melanoma in a phase I trial.[488] A large-scale multicenter trial comparing two doses of CC 5013 in an effort to establish its activity is ongoing, as are studies combining this agent with cytotoxic chemotherapy.

Expression of vascular endothelial growth factor has been postulated by some to have prognostic significance in patients with advanced melanoma.[489] However, agents that inhibit vascular endothelial growth factor signaling, such as SU5146[490] or bevacizumab, either alone or combined with thalidomide[491] or low-dose IFN-α,[492] have failed to show significant clinical activity. Ongoing studies include efforts to block fibroblast growth factor secretion with chronic low-dose IFN-α administration and to inhibit endothelial cell proliferation with combinations of low-dose paclitaxel and celecoxib.

Molecularly Targeted Therapy

Advances in melanoma biology have determined that many tumors exhibit methylation of the *APAF-1* gene,[493] sustained

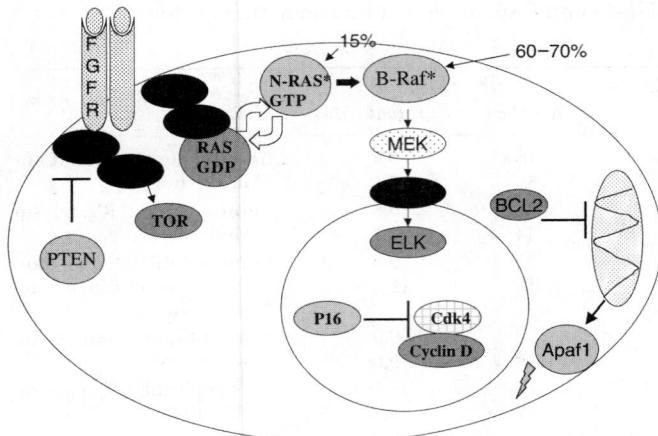

FIGURE 38.2-21. Various molecular pathways that are disturbed in melanoma and are potential targets for novel molecularly based therapy. (Adapted with permission of Lynn Schuchter, M.D.)

expression of Bcl-2 and caspase 1,[494] and activating mutations of the *BRAF* gene,[495] all serving to make these cells resistant to chemotherapy-induced apoptosis (Fig. 38.2-21). Investigations that combine chemotherapeutic drugs with agents that either suppress Bcl-2 (antisense oligonucleotides), demethylate DNA (decitabine), or block RAF function (BAY 43-9006) have been initiated with some encouraging early results. For example, preliminary results from a multicenter randomized phase III trial comparing the use of G3139, an antisense oligonucleotide that inhibits Bcl-2 protein production by binding to Bcl-2 messenger RNA, followed by dacarbazine to the use of dacarbazine alone in previously untreated patients with advanced melanoma showed higher response rates (11.7% vs. 6.8%) and longer overall survival (9.1 months vs. 7.9 months; $P = .184$) for the combination.[496] When the analysis was limited to patients who had been receiving therapy for longer than 12 months, overall survival was significantly longer (10.1 months vs. 8.1 months; $P < .05$) for the combination treatment. Preliminary studies with BAY 43-9006, an orally active inhibitor of RAF kinase, showed this agent to be inactive when administered as monotherapy[497]; however, when BAY 43-9006 was combined with carboplatin and paclitaxel, partial responses were produced in 50% of patients, many of whom had exhibited disease progression on prior cytotoxic therapies.[498] Efforts are under way to confirm these results, study this agent in combination with dacarbazine, and correlate tumor response with the presence of the activating mutations in the melanoma cells.

Expression of c-kit has also been documented in up to 50% of primary melanoma specimens.[499] However, a phase II trial of imatinib mesylate (Gleevec) produced no responses in 25 patients,[500] which suggests that, unlike in chronic myelogenous leukemia and gastrointestinal stromal tumors, c-kit by itself is not an important mediator of melanoma progression. Imatinib has yet to be tested in combination with cytotoxic chemotherapy.

It is hoped that this better understanding of the biology of melanoma and the mechanisms underlying tumor-induced immune suppression will lead to more active treatment approaches and rational treatment selection. Given the promise of these new approaches and the limited value of current standard therapies, patients with advanced disease are best managed in ongoing clinical trials, and participation should be encouraged.

REFERENCES

1. Cancer Facts and Figures. Atlanta: American Cancer Society, 2004.
2. Berwick M, Weinstock MA. Epidemiology current trends, in cutaneous melanoma. In: Balch CM, et al., eds. *Cutaneous melanoma*, 4th ed. St. Louis: Quality Medical Publishing, 2003:15.
3. Mikkilineni R, Weinstock MA. Epidemiology in skin cancer. In: Sober AJ, Haluska FG, eds. *Skin cancer*. Hamilton, Ontario: BC Decker, 2001:1.
4. Bulliard JL, Cox B. Cutaneous malignant melanoma in New Zealand: trends by anatomical site, 1969–1993. *Int J Epidemiol* 2000;29:416.
5. Albert VA, et al. Years of potential life lost: another indicator of the impact of cutaneous malignant melanoma on society. *J Am Acad Dermatol* 1990:23:308.
6. Lancaster HO. Some geographical aspects of the mortality from melanoma in Europeans. *Med J Aust* 1956;43:1082.
7. deVries E, Bray FI, Coebergh JW, Parkin DM. Changing epidemiology of malignant cutaneous melanoma in Europe 1953–1997. *Int J Cancer* 2003;20:119.
8. Berwick MW. Epidemiology: current trends in cutaneous melanoma. In: Balch CM, Sober AJ, Soong SJ, eds. *Cutaneous melanoma*, 4th ed. St. Louis: Quality Medical Publishing, 2003:15.
9. Khlat M, et al. Mortality from melanoma in migrants to Australia: variation by age at arrival and duration of stay. *Am J Epidemiol* 1992;135:1103.
10. Mack TM, Floderus B. Malignant melanoma risk by nativity, place of residence at diagnosis, and age at migration. *Cancer Causes Control* 1991;2:401.
11. Pearce M, Cotterill SJ, Gordan PM, Craft AW. Skin cancer in children and young adults. *Melanoma Res* 2003;13:421.
12. Gibbs P, et al. Pediatric melanoma: are recent advances in the management of adult melanoma relevant to the pediatric population? *J Pediatr Hematol Oncol* 2000;22:428.
13. Shaw HM, Thompson JF. Prognosis in children with melanoma. *N Z Med J* 2001;114:75.
14. Bellows CF, et al. Melanoma in African-Americans: trends in biological behavior and clinical characteristics over two decades. *J Surg Oncol* 2001;78:10.
15. Gonzalez-Fernandez M, Sanchez JL. Malignant melanoma in Puerto Rico: an update. *P R Health Sci J* 1999;18:95.
16. Green A. Sun exposure and the risk of melanoma. *Australas J Dermatol* 1984;25:99.
17. Elwood JM, et al. Cutaneous melanoma in relation to intermittent and constant sun exposure—the Western Canada melanoma study. *Int J Cancer* 1985;35:427.
18. Elwood JM, Jopson J. Melanoma and sun exposure: an overview of published studies. *Int J Cancer* 1997;73:198.
19. Holman CD, Armstrong BK, Heenan PJ. Relationship of cutaneous malignant melanoma to individual sunlight-exposure habits. *J Natl Cancer Inst* 1986;76:403.
20. Osterlind A, et al. The Danish case-control study of cutaneous malignant melanoma. II. Importance of UV-light exposure. *Int J Cancer* 1988;42:319.
21. Armstrong BK, Kricker A. How much melanoma is caused by sun exposure? *Melanoma Res* 1993;3:395.
22. Grob JJ, et al. Count of benign melanocytic nevi as a major indicator of risk for nonfamilial nodular and superficial spreading melanoma. *Cancer* 1990;66:387.
23. Bataille V, et al. Risk of cutaneous melanoma in relation to the numbers, types and sites of naevi: a case-control study. *Br J Cancer* 1996;73:1605.
24. Mansfield PF, Lee JE, Balch CM. Cutaneous melanoma: current practice and surgical controversies. *Curr Probl Surg* 1994;31:253.
25. Richard MA, et al. Role of sun exposure on nevus. First study in age-sex phenotype-controlled populations. *Arch Dermatol* 1993;129:1280.
26. Tucker MA, et al. Clinically recognized dysplastic nevi. A central risk factor for cutaneous melanoma. *JAMA* 1997;277:1439.
27. Lynch HT, Frichot BC III, Lynch JF. Familial atypical multiple mole-melanoma syndrome. *J Med Genet* 1978;15:352.
28. Clark WH Jr, et al. Origin of familial malignant melanomas from heritable melanocytic lesions. 'The B-K mole syndrome.' *Arch Dermatol* 1978;114:732.
29. Augustsson A, et al. Common and dysplastic naevi as risk factors for cutaneous malignant melanoma in a Swedish population. *Acta Derm Venereol* 1991;71:518.
30. Halpern AC, et al. Dysplastic nevi as risk markers of sporadic (nonfamilial) melanoma. A case-control study. *Arch Dermatol* 1991;127:995.
31. Halpern AC, et al. A cohort study of melanoma in patients with dysplastic nevi. *J Invest Dermatol* 1993;100:346S.
32. MacKie RM, McHenry P, Hole D. Accelerated detection with prospective surveillance for cutaneous malignant melanoma in high-risk groups. *Lancet* 1993;341:1618.
33. Rigel DS, et al. Dysplastic nevi. Markers for increased risk for melanoma. *Cancer* 1989;63:386.
34. Tiersten AD, et al. Prospective follow-up for malignant melanoma in patients with atypical-mole (dysplastic-nevus) syndrome. *J Dermatol Surg Oncol* 1991;17:44.
35. Rhodes AR, et al. Nonepidermal origin of malignant melanoma associated with a giant congenital nevocellular nevus. *Plast Reconstr Surg* 1981;67:782.
36. Lorentzen M, Pers M, Bretteville-Jensen G. The incidence of malignant transformation in giant pigmented nevi. *Scand J Plast Reconstr Surg* 1977;11:163.
37. Rhodes AR, et al. The malignant potential of small congenital nevocellular nevi. An estimate of association based on a histologic study of 234 primary cutaneous melanomas. *J Am Acad Dermatol* 1982;6:230.
38. Kang S, et al. Multiple primary cutaneous melanomas. *Cancer* 1992;70:1911.

39. Blackwood M, Holmes R, Synnestvedt M, et al. Multiple primary melanomas revisited. *Cancer* 2002;94:2248.

40. Bale SJ, et al. Mapping the gene for hereditary cutaneous malignant melanoma-dysplastic nevus to chromosome 1p. *N Engl J Med* 1989;320:1367.

41. van Haeringen A, et al. Exclusion of the dysplastic nevus syndrome (DNS) locus from the short arm of chromosome 1 by linkage studies in Dutch families. *Genomics* 1989;5:61.

42. Cannon-Albright LA, et al. Assignment of a locus for familial melanoma, MLM, to chromosome 9p13-p22. *Science* 1992;258:1148.

43. Masback A, Olsson H, Westerdahl J, et al. Clinical and histological features of malignant melanoma in germline CDKN2A mutation families. *Melanoma Res* 2002;12:549.

44. Tucker M, Goldstein AM. Melanoma etiology: where are we? *Oncogene* 2003;22:3042.

45. Serrano M, Hannon GJ, Beach D. A new regulatory motif in cell-cycle control causing specific inhibition of cyclin D/CDK4. *Nature* 1993;366:704.

46. Hussussian CJ, et al. Germline p16 mutations in familial melanoma. *Nat Genet* 1994;8:15.

47. FitzGerald MG, et al. Prevalence of germ-line mutations in p16, p19ARF, and CDK4 in familial melanoma: analysis of a clinic-based population. *Proc Natl Acad Sci U S A* 1996;93:8541.

48. Kraemer KH, et al. Dysplastic naevi and cutaneous melanoma risk. *Lancet* 1983;2:1076.

49. Carey WP Jr, et al. Dysplastic nevi as a melanoma risk factor in patients with familial melanoma. *Cancer* 1994;74:3118.

50. Jensen P, et al. Skin cancer in kidney and heart transplant recipients and different long-term immunosuppressive therapy regimens. *J Am Acad Dermatol* 1999;40:177.

51. Smith CH, et al. Excess melanocytic nevi in children with renal allografts. *J Am Acad Dermatol* 1993;28:51.

52. Grob JJ, et al. Excess of nevi related to immunodeficiency: a study in HIV-infected patients and renal transplant recipients. *J Invest Dermatol* 1996;107:694.

53. Daryanani D, Plukker JT, DeHullu JA, et al. Pregnancy and early-stage melanoma. *Cancer* 2003;97:2130.

54. MacKie R. Pregnancy and hormones in cutaneous melanoma. In: Balch CM, Sober AJ, Soong SJ, eds. *Cutaneous melanoma*, 4th ed. St. Louis: Quality Medical Publishing, 2003:319.

55. Travers RL, et al. Increased thickness of pregnancy-associated melanoma. *Br J Dermatol* 1995;132:876.

56. Rhodes AR, et al. Risk factors for cutaneous melanoma. A practical method of recognizing predisposed individuals. *JAMA* 1987;258:3146.

57. Stern RS, Nichols KT, Vakeva LH. Malignant melanoma in patients treated for psoriasis with methoxsalen (psoralen) and ultraviolet A radiation (PUVA). The PUVA Follow-Up Study. *N Engl J Med* 1997;336:1041.

58. Kraemer KH, Lee MM, Scotto J. Xeroderma pigmentosum. Cutaneous, ocular, and neurologic abnormalities in 830 published cases. *Arch Dermatol* 1987;123:241.

59. Dennis L, Beane Freeman LE, VanBeek MJ. Sunscreen use and the risk for melanoma: a quantitative review. *Ann Intern Med* 2003;139:966.

60. Autier P, et al. Melanoma and use of sunscreens: an EORTC case-control study in Germany, Belgium and France. The EORTC Melanoma Cooperative Group. *Int J Cancer* 1995;61:749.

61. Naldi L, et al. Sunscreens and cutaneous malignant melanoma: an Italian case-control study. *Int J Cancer* 2000;86:879.

62. Weinstock MA. Do sunscreens increase or decrease melanoma risk: an epidemiologic evaluation. *J Investig Dermatol Symp Proc* 1999;4:97.

63. Westerdahl J, et al. Sunscreen use and malignant melanoma. *Int J Cancer* 2000;87:145.

64. Westerdahl J, et al. Is the use of sunscreens a risk factor for malignant melanoma? *Melanoma Res* 1995;5:59.

65. Wolf P, et al. Phenotypic markers, sunlight-related factors and sunscreen use in patients with cutaneous melanoma: an Austrian case-control study. *Melanoma Res* 1998;8:370.

66. Koh HK, et al. Who discovers melanoma? Patterns from a population-based survey. *J Am Acad Dermatol* 1992;26:914.

67. Berwick M, et al. Screening for cutaneous melanoma by skin self-examination. *J Natl Cancer Inst* 1996;88:17.

68. Marghoob AA, et al. Instruments and new technologies for the in vivo diagnosis of melanoma. *J Am Acad Dermatol* 2003;49:777.

69. Nordlund JJ, et al. Vitiligo in patients with metastatic melanoma: a good prognostic sign. *J Am Acad Dermatol* 1983;9:689.

70. Koh HK, et al. Malignant melanoma and vitiligo-like leukoderma: an electron microscopic study. *J Am Acad Dermatol* 1983;9:696.

71. Wang SQ, et al. Detection of melanomas in patients followed up with total cutaneous examinations, total cutaneous photography, and dermoscopy. *J Am Acad Dermatol* 2004;50:15.

72. Binder M, et al. Epiluminescence microscopy. A useful tool for the diagnosis of pigmented skin lesions for formally trained dermatologists. *Arch Dermatol* 1995;131:286.

73. Binder M, et al. Epiluminescence microscopy of small pigmented skin lesions: short-term formal training improves the diagnostic performance of dermatologists. *J Am Acad Dermatol* 1997;36:197.

74. Pehamberger H, et al. In vivo epiluminescence microscopy: improvement of early diagnosis of melanoma. *J Invest Dermatol* 1993;100:356S.

75. Elbaum M, et al. Automatic differentiation of melanoma from melanocytic nevi with multispectral digital dermoscopy: a feasibility study. *J Am Acad Dermatol* 2001;44:207.

76. Langley RG, et al. Confocal scanning laser microscopy of benign and malignant melanocytic skin lesions in vivo. *J Am Acad Dermatol* 2001;45:365.

77. Koh H, Caruso A, Gage I, et al. Evaluation of melanoma/skin cancer screening in Massachusetts. *Cancer* 1990;65:375.

78. Koh HK, et al. Evaluation of the American Academy of Dermatology's national skin cancer early detection and screening program. *J Am Acad Dermatol* 1996;34:971.

79. Geller AC, et al. The first 15 years of the American Academy of Dermatology skin cancer screening programs: 1985-1999. *J Am Acad Dermatol* 2003;48:34.

80. Tsao H, Rogers GS, Sober AJ. An estimate of the annual direct cost of treating cutaneous melanoma. *J Am Acad Dermatol* 1998;38:669.

81. Halpern A, Marghoob AA, Sober AJ. Clinical characteristics in cutaneous melanoma. In: Balch CM, Sober AJ, Soong SJ, eds. *Cutaneous melanoma*, 4th ed. St. Louis: Quality Medical Publishing, 2003:1352.

82. Crowson AN, Barnhill RL, Mihm MC Jr. Pathology, in cutaneous melanoma. In: Balch CM, Sober AJ, Soong SJ, eds. *Cutaneous melanoma*, 4th ed. St. Louis: Quality Medical Publishing, 2003:171.

83. Friedman RJ, Rigel DS, Kopf AW. Early detection of malignant melanoma: the role of physician examination and self-examination of the skin. *CA Cancer J Clin* 1985;35:130.

84. Arrington JH 3rd, et al. Plantar lentiginous melanoma: a distinctive variant of human cutaneous malignant melanoma. *Am J Surg Pathol* 1977;1:131.

85. Blessing K, Kernohan NM, Park KG. Subungual malignant melanoma: clinicopathological features of 100 cases. *Histopathology* 1991;19:425.

86. Levit EK, et al. The ABC rule for clinical detection of subungual melanoma. *J Am Acad Dermatol* 2000;42:269.

87. Weinstock MA, Sober AJ. The risk of progression of lentigo maligna to lentigo maligna melanoma. *Br J Dermatol* 1987;116:303.

88. Fisher S, O'Brien CJ. Head and neck melanoma in cutaneous melanoma. In: Balch CM, Sober AJ, Soong SJ, eds. *Cutaneous melanoma*, 4th ed. St. Louis: Quality Medical Publishing, 2003:275.

89. Beenken S, Byers R, Smith JL, et al. Desmoplastic melanoma. Histologic correlation with behavior and treatment. *Arch Otolaryngol Head Neck Surg* 1989;115:374.

90. Carlson J, Dickersin GR, Sober AJ, et al. Desmoplastic neurotropic melanoma. *Cancer* 1995;75:478.

91. Quinn MJ, et al. Desmoplastic and desmoplastic neurotropic melanoma: experience with 280 patients. *Cancer* 1998;83:1128.

92. Gyorki DE, et al. Sentinel lymph node biopsy for patients with cutaneous desmoplastic melanoma. *Ann Surg Oncol* 2003;10:403.

93. Tsao H, Sober AJ, Barnhill RL. Desmoplastic neurotropic melanoma. *Semin Cutan Med Surg* 1997;16:131.

94. Skelton HG, et al. Desmoplastic malignant melanoma. *J Am Acad Dermatol* 1995;32:717.

95. Bruijn JA, Mihm MC Jr, Barnhill RL. Desmoplastic melanoma. *Histopathology* 1992;20:197.

96. Balch CM, et al. A new American Joint Committee on Cancer staging system for cutaneous melanoma. *Cancer* 2000;88:1484.

97. Balch CM, Soong SJ, Gershenwald JE, et al. Prognostic factors analysis of 17,600 melanoma patients: validation of the AJCC melanoma staging system. *J Clin Oncol* 2001;19:3622.

98. Balch CM, Buzaid AC, Cascinelli N, Soong SJ. Staging and classification, in cutaneous melanoma. In: Balch CM, Sober AJ, Soong SJ, eds. *Cutaneous melanoma*, 4th ed. St. Louis: Quality Medical Publishing, 2003:55.

99. Balch CM, Buzaid AC, Soong SJ, et al. Final version of the American Joint Committee on Cancer staging system for cutaneous melanoma. *J Clin Oncol* 2001;19:3635.

100. Breslow A. Thickness, cross-sectional areas and depth of invasion in the prognosis of cutaneous melanoma. *Ann Surg* 1970;172:902.

101. Breslow A. Problems in the measurement of tumor thickness and level of invasion in cutaneous melanoma. *Hum Pathol* 1977;8:1.

102. Breslow A, et al. Stage I melanoma of the limbs: assessment of prognosis by levels of invasion and maximum thickness. *Tumori* 1978;64:273.

103. Balch CM, et al. A multifactorial analysis of melanoma: prognostic histopathological features comparing Clark's and Breslow's staging methods. *Ann Surg* 1978;188:732.

104. Eldh J, Peterson LE. Prognostic factors in cutaneous malignant melanoma in stage I. A clinical, morphological and multivariate analysis. *Scand J Plast Reconstr Surg Hand Surg* 1978;12:243.

105. Gershenwald JE, Soong SJ, Thompson JF. Prognostic factors and natural history in cutaneous melanoma. In: Balch CM, Sober AJ, Soong SJ, eds. *Cutaneous melanoma*, 4th ed. St. Louis: Quality Medical Publishing, 2003:25.

106. Balch CM, Milton GW, Shaw HM, et al. A comparison of prognostic factors and surgical results in 1,786 patients with localized (stage I) melanoma treated in Alabama, USA, and New South Wales, Australia. *Ann Surg* 1982;196:677.

107. Day CL Jr, et al. The natural break points for primary-tumor thickness in clinical stage I melanoma. *N Engl J Med* 1981;305:1155.

108. Balch CM, Sober AJ, Soong SJ. *Cutaneous melanoma*, 4th ed. St. Louis: Quality Medical Publishing, 2003.

109. Balch CM, et al. The prognostic significance of ulceration of cutaneous melanoma. *Cancer* 1980;45:3012.

110. Balch CM, et al. Long-term results of a multi-institutional randomized trial comparing prognostic factors and surgical results for intermediate thickness melanomas (1.0 to 4.0 mm.). *Ann Surg Oncol* 2000;7:87.

111. Balch CM. Cutaneous melanoma. In: *AJCC cancer staging manual*, 6th ed. New York: Springer-Verlag, 2002.

112. Corona R, et al. Interobserver variability on the histopathologic diagnosis of cutaneous melanoma and other pigmented skin lesions. *J Clin Oncol* 1996;14:1218.

113. Larsen TE. International pathologists congruence survey on quantitation of malignant melanoma. *Pathology* 1980;12:245.

114. Morton DL, et al. Multivariate analysis of the relationship between survival and the microstage of primary melanoma by Clark level and Breslow thickness. *Cancer* 1993;71:3737.

115. Clark WH Jr, From L, Bernardino EA, Mihm MC. The histogenesis and biological behavior of primary human malignant melanoma of the skin. *Cancer Res* 1969;29:705.

116. Scolyer R, Shaw HM, Thompson JF, et al. Interobserver reproducibility of histopathological prognostic variables in primary cutaneous melanoma. *Am J Surg Pathol* 2003;27:1571.

117. Buttner P, Garbe C, Bertz J, et al. Primary cutaneous melanoma. Optimized cutoff points of tumor thickness and importance of Clark's level for prognostic classification. *Cancer* 1995;75:2499.

118. Vollmer R. Malignant melanoma. A multivariate analysis of prognostic factors. *Pathol Ann* 1989;24:383.

119. Wells K, Reintgen DS, Cruse CW. The current management and prognosis of acral lentiginous melanoma. *Ann Plast Surg* 1992;28:100.

120. Azzola M, Shaw HM, Thompson JF, et al. Tumor mitotic rate is a more powerful prognostic indicator than ulceration in patients with primary cutaneous melanoma. An analysis of 3661 patients from a single center. *Cancer* 2003;97:1488.

121. Kashani-Sabet M, Sagebiel R, Ferreira C, Nosrati M, Miller J. Tumor vascularity in the prognostic assessment of primary cutaneous melanoma. *J Clin Oncol* 2002;20:1826.

122. Balch C. Surgical treatment of advanced melanoma in cutaneous melanoma. In: Balch CM, Houghton AN, Sober AJ, Soong SJ, eds. *Cutaneous melanoma*, 3rd ed. St. Louis: Quality Medical Press, 1998:373.

123. Cascinelli N, et al. Immediate or delayed dissection of regional nodes in patients with melanoma of the trunk: a randomized trial. WHO Melanoma Programme. *Lancet* 1998;351:793.

124. Buzaid A, Ross M, Balch C, et al. Critical analysis of the current American Joint Committee on Cancer staging system for cutaneous melanoma and proposal of a new staging system. *J Clin Oncol* 1997;15:1039.

125. Cascinelli N, et al. Regional non-nodal metastases of cutaneous melanoma. *Eur J Surg Oncol* 1986;12:175.

126. Singletary SE, Tucker S, Boddie A. Multivariate analysis of prognostic factors in regional cutaneous metastases of extremity melanoma. *Cancer* 1988;61:1437.

127. Barth A, Wanek LA, Morton DL. Prognostic factors in 1,521 melanoma patients with distant metastases. *J Am Coll Surg* 1995;181:193.

128. Manola J, et al. Prognostic factors in metastatic melanoma: a pooled analysis of Eastern Cooperative Oncology Group trials. *J Clin Oncol* 2000;8:3782.

129. Unger J, Flaherty LE, Liu PY, et al. Gender and other survival predictors in patients with metastatic melanoma on Southwest Oncology Group trials. *Cancer* 2001;91:1148.

130. Balch CM, et al. A multifactorial analysis of melanoma. IV. Prognostic factors in 200 melanoma patients with distant metastases (stage III). *J Clin Oncol* 1983;1:126.

131. Sirott MN, Wong GYC, Tao YT, et al. Prognostic factors in patients with metastatic malignant melanoma. A multivariate analysis. *Cancer* 1993;72:3091.

132. Finck SJ, Giuliano AE, Morton DL. LDH and melanoma. *Cancer* 1983;51:840.

133. Deichmann M, et al. S100-Beta, melanoma-inhibiting activity, and lactate dehydrogenase discriminate progressive from nonprogressive American Joint Committee on Cancer stage IV melanoma. *J Clin Oncol* 1999;17:1891.

134. Eton O, et al. Prognostic factors for survival of patients treated systemically for disseminated melanoma. *J Clin Oncol* 1998;16:1103.

135. Keilholz U, et al. Results of interleukin-2-based treatment in advanced melanoma: a case record-based analysis of 631 patients. *J Clin Oncol* 1998;16:2921.

136. Essner R, et al. Efficacy of lymphatic mapping, sentinel lymphadenectomy, and selective complete lymph node dissection as a therapeutic procedure for early-stage melanoma. *Ann Surg Oncol* 1999;6:442.

137. Morton DL, et al. Improved long-term survival after lymphadenectomy of melanoma metastatic to regional nodes. Analysis of prognostic factors in 1134 patients from the John Wayne Cancer Clinic. *Ann Surg* 1991;214:491.

138. Morton DL, et al. Validation of the accuracy of intraoperative lymphatic mapping and sentinel lymphadenectomy for early-stage melanoma: a multicenter trial. Multicenter Selective Lymphadenectomy Trial Group. *Ann Surg* 1999;230:453.

139. Gershenwald JE, Mansfield PF, Lee JE, Ross MI. The role for lymphatic mapping and sentinel lymph node biopsy in patients with thick (>4 mm) primary melanoma. *Ann Surg Oncol* 2000;7:160.

140. Gershenwald JE, et al. Multi-institutional melanoma lymphatic mapping experience: the prognostic value of sentinel lymph node status in 612 stage I or II melanoma patients. *J Clin Oncol* 1999;17:976.

141. Reintgen D, Thompson JF, Gershenwald JE. Intraoperative mapping and sentinel node technology in cutaneous melanoma. In: Balch CM, Sober AJ, Soong SJ, eds. *Cutaneous melanoma*, 4th ed. St. Louis: Quality Medical Publishing, 2003:353.

142. McKinnon J, Yu XQ, McCarthy WH, Thompson JF. Prognosis for patients with thin cutaneous melanoma. *Cancer* 2003;98:1223.

143. Franzke A, et al. Elevated pretreatment serum levels of soluble vascular cell adhesion molecule 1 and lactate dehydrogenase as predictors of survival in cutaneous metastatic malignant melanoma. *Br J Cancer* 1998;78:40.

144. Miller S, Balch CM. Biopsy in cutaneous melanoma. In: Balch CM, Sober AJ, Soong SJ, eds. *Cutaneous melanoma*, 4th ed. St. Louis: Quality Medical Publishing, 2003:163.

145. Sober A, Chuang TY, Duvic M, et al. Guidelines of care for primary cutaneous melanoma. *J Am Acad Dermatol* 2001;45:579.

146. Bolognia J. Biopsy techniques for pigmented lesions. *Dermatol Surg* 2000;26:89.

147. Ross M, Balch CM, Cascinelli N, Edwards MJ. Excision of primary melanoma in cutaneous melanoma. In: Balch CM, Sober AJ, Soong SJ, eds. *Cutaneous melanoma*, 4th ed. St. Louis: Quality Medical Publishing, 2003:209.

148. Veronesi U, Cascinelli N. Narrow excision (1-cm margin). A safe procedure for thin cutaneous melanoma. *Arch Surg* 1991;126:438.

149. Veronesi U, et al. Thin stage I primary cutaneous malignant melanoma. Comparison of excision with margins of 1 or 3 cm. *N Engl J Med* 1988;318:1159. [Published erratum appears in *N Engl J Med* 1991;325:292].

150. Nahabedian M, Wagner JD. Complex closures of melanoma excisions, in cutaneous melanoma. In: Balch CM, Sober AJ, Soong SJ, eds. *Cutaneous melanoma*, 4th ed. St. Louis: Quality Medical Publishing, 2003:231.

151. Soong SJ, et al. Factors affecting survival following local, regional, or distant recurrence from localized melanoma. *J Surg Oncol* 1998;67:228.

152. Cascinelli N. Margin of resection in the management of primary melanoma. *Semin Surg Oncol* 1998;14:272.

153. Karakousis CP, et al. Local recurrence in malignant melanoma: long-term results of the multiinstitutional randomized surgical trial. *Ann Surg Oncol* 1996;3:446.

154. Balch CM, et al. Efficacy of 2-cm surgical margins for intermediate-thickness melanomas (1 to 4 mm). Results of a multi-institutional randomized surgical trial [see comments]. *Ann Surg* 1993;218:262.

155. Balch C, Soong SJ, Smith T, et al. Long term results of a prospective surgical trial comparing 2 cm. vs 4 cm. incision margins for 740 patients with 1–4 mm melanomas. *Ann Surg Oncol* 2001;8:101.

156. Khayat D, et al. Surgical margins in cutaneous melanoma (2 cm versus 5 cm for lesions measuring less than 2.1-mm thick). *Cancer* 2003;97:1941.

157. Cohn-Cedermark G, et al. Long-term results of a randomized study by the Swedish Melanoma Study Group on 2-cm versus 5-cm resection margins for patients with cutaneous melanoma with a tumor thickness of 0.8–2.0 mm. *Cancer* 2000;89:1495.

158. Thomas J, Newton-Bishop JA, A'Hern R, et al. Excision margins in high-risk melanoma. *N Engl J Med* 2004;350:757.

159. Thomas J, Newton-Bishop JA. Surgical margin excision width in high risk cutaneous malignant melanoma: a randomized trial of 1cm versus 3cm excision margins in 900 patients. *Proc Am Soc Clin Oncol* 2002;1358:340.

160. Busam KJ, et al. Detection of intraepidermal malignant melanoma in vivo by confocal scanning laser microscopy. *Melanoma Res* 2002;12:349.

161. Heaton KM, et al. Surgical margins and prognostic factors in patients with thick (>4mm) primary melanoma. *Ann Surg Oncol* 1998;5:322.

162. Pockaj BA, et al. Changing surgical therapy for melanoma of the external ear. *Ann Surg Oncol* 2003;10:689.

163. Tanabe K, Reintgen DS, Balch CM. Local recurrences and their management in cutaneous melanoma. In: Balch CM, Sober AJ, Soong SJ, eds. *Cutaneous melanoma*, 4th ed. St. Louis: Quality Medical Publishing, 2003:263.

164. Yao KA, et al. Is sentinel lymph node mapping indicated for isolated local and in-transit recurrent melanoma? *Ann Surg* 2003;238:743.

165. Fraker DL, et al. Hyperthermic regional perfusion for melanoma of the limbs, in cutaneous melanoma. In: Balch CM, Sober AJ, Soong SJ, eds. *Cutaneous melanoma*, 4th ed. St. Louis: Quality Medical Publishing, 2003:473.

166. Krementz E, Carter RD, Sutherland CM. Regional chemotherapy for melanoma. A 35-year experience. *Ann Surg* 1994;220:520.

167. Lens MB, Dawes M. Isolated limb perfusion with melphalan in the treatment of malignant melanoma of the extremities: a systematic review of randomized controlled trials. *Lancet Oncol* 2003;4:359.

168. Ainslie J, Peteres LJ, McKay MJ. Radiotherapy for primary and regional melanoma in cutaneous melanoma. In: Balch CM, Sober AJ, Soong SJ, eds. *Cutaneous melanoma*, 4th ed. St. Louis: Quality Medical Publishing, 2003:449.

169. Vongtama R, Safa A, Gallardo D, Calcaterra T, Juillard G. Efficacy of radiation therapy in the local control of desmoplastic malignant melanoma. *Head Neck* 2003;125:423.

170. Veronesi U, et al. Inefficacy of immediate node dissection in stage 1 melanoma of the limbs. *N Engl J Med* 1977;297:627.

171. Sim FH, et al. Lymphadenectomy in the management of stage I malignant melanoma: a prospective randomized study. *Mayo Clin Proc* 1986;62:697.

172. Balch CM. Randomized surgical trials involving elective node dissection for melanoma. *Adv Surg* 1999;32:255.

173. Balch CM, Ross MI. Melanoma patients with iliac nodal metastases can be cured [Editorial; comment]. *Ann Surg Oncol* 1999;6:230.

174. Carlson GW, Hestley A, Staley CA, Lyles RH, Cohen C. Sentinel lymph node mapping for thick (>or= 4 mm.) melanoma. *Ann Surg Oncol* 2003;10:408.

175. Wagner JD, et al. Patterns of initial recurrence and prognosis after sentinel lymph node biopsy and selective lymphadenectomy for melanoma. *Plast Reconstr Surg* 2003;112:486.

176. Urist MM, et al. Head and neck melanoma in 534 clinical stage I patients. A prognostic factors analysis and results of surgical treatment. *Ann Surg* 1984;200:769.

177. Evans HL, et al. Lymphoscintigraphy and sentinel node biopsy accurately stage melanoma in patients presenting after wide local excision. *Ann Surg Oncol* 2003;10:416.

178. Morton DL. Sentinel lymphadenectomy for patients with clinical stage I melanoma. *J Surg Oncol* 1997;66:267.

179. Morton DL, et al. Technical details of intraoperative lymphatic mapping for early stage melanoma. *Arch Surg* 1992;127:392.

180. Morton DL, et al. Lymphatic mapping and sentinel lymphadenectomy for early-stage melanoma: therapeutic utility and implications of nodal microanatomy and molecular staging for improving the accuracy of detection of nodal micrometastases. *Ann Surg* 2003;238:538.

181. Thompson J, Uren RF, Coventry BJ, Chatterton BE. Lymphoscintigraphy, in cutaneous melanoma. In: Balch CM, Sober AJ, Soong SJ, eds. *Cutaneous melanoma*, 4th ed. St. Louis: Quality Medical Publishing, 2003:329.

182. Thompson JF, et al. Location of sentinel lymph nodes in patients with cutaneous melanoma: new insights into lymphatic anatomy. *J Am Coll Surg* 1999;189:195.

183. Porter G, Ross MI, Berman RS et al. Significance of multiple nodal basin drainage in truncal melanoma patients undergoing sentinel lymph node biopsy. *Ann Surg Oncol* 2000;7:256.

184. Gershenwald JE, et al. Patterns of recurrence following a negative sentinel lymph node biopsy in 243 patients with stage I or II melanoma. *J Clin Oncol* 1998;16:2253.

185. Thompson JF. The Sydney Melanoma Unit experience of sentinel lymphadenectomy for melanoma. *Ann Surg Oncol* 2001;8[Suppl 9]:44S.

186. van der Velde-Zimmermann D, et al. Sentinel node biopsies in melanoma patients: a protocol for accurate, efficient, and cost-effective analysis by preselection for immunohistochemistry on the basis of Tyr-PCR. *Ann Surg Oncol* 2000;7:51.

187. van der Velde-Zimmermann D, et al. Molecular test for the detection of tumor cells in blood and sentinel nodes of melanoma patients. *Am J Pathol* 1996;149:759.

188. Bostick PJ, et al. Prognostic significance of occult metastases detected by sentinel lymphadenectomy and reverse transcriptase-polymerase chain reaction in early-stage melanoma patients. *J Clin Oncol* 1999;17:3238.
189. Morton DL, et al. Intraoperative lymphatic mapping and selective cervical lymphadenectomy for early-stage melanomas of the head and neck. *J Clin Oncol* 1993;11:1751.
190. McMasters KM, et al. Sentinel lymph node biopsy for melanoma: controversy despite widespread agreement. *J Clin Oncol* 2001;19:2851.
191. McMasters K, Wong SL, Tyler DS, Balch CM. Axillary and epitrochlear lymph node dissection in cutaneous melanoma. In: Balch CM, Sober AJ, Soong SJ, eds. *Cutaneous melanoma*, 4th ed. St. Louis: Quality Medical Publishing, 2003:397.
192. Coit D, Balch CM. Groin and popliteal dissections: technique and complications in cutaneous melanoma. In: Balch CM, Sober AJ, Soong SJ, eds. *Cutaneous melanoma*, 4th ed. St. Louis: Quality Medical Publishing, 2003:405.
193. O'Brien C, Fischer SR, Pathak I. Neck dissection and parotidectomy, in cutaneous melanoma. In: Balch CM, Sober AJ, Soong SJ, eds. *Cutaneous melanoma*, 4th ed. St. Louis: Quality Medical Publishing, 2003:419.
194. Ang K, Peters LJ, Weber RS, et al. Postoperative radiotherapy of cutaneous melanoma of the head and neck. *Int J Radiat Oncol Biol Phys* 1994;30:795.
195. McKay M, Peters LJ, Ainslie J. Radiotherapy for distant metastases and clinical radiobiology of melanoma in cutaneous melanoma. In: Balch CM, Sober AJ, Soong SJ, eds. *Cutaneous melanoma*, 4th ed. St. Louis: Quality Medical Publishing, 2003:573.
196. Sause WT, Rush S, et al. Fraction size in external beam irradiation in the treatment of melanoma. *Int J Radiat Oncol Biol Phys* 1999;20:429.
197. Corry J, Bishop M, Ainslie J. Nodal radiation therapy for metastatic melanoma. *Int J Radiat Oncol Biol Phys* 1999;44:1065.
198. Burmeister B, Smithers BM, Poulsen M, et al. Radiation therapy for nodal disease in malignant melanoma. *World J Surg* 1995;19:369.
199. Balch CM, et al. New TNM melanoma staging system: linking biology and natural history to clinical outcomes. *Semin Surg Oncol* 2003;21:43.
200. Coit D, Ferrone CR. Recurrent regional metastases in cutaneous melanoma. In: Balch CM, Sober AJ, Soong SJ, eds. *Cutaneous melanoma*, 4th ed. St. Louis: Quality Medical Publishing, 2003:439.
201. Dong X, Tyler D, Johnson JL et al Analysis of prognosis and disease progression after local recurrence of melanoma. *Cancer* 2000;88:1063.
202. Coit D, Ferrone CR. Metastatic surveillance and follow-up in cutaneous melanoma. In: Balch CM, Sober AJ, Soong SJ, eds. *Cutaneous melanoma*, 4th ed. St. Louis: Quality Medical Publishing, 2003:511.
203. Strom E, Ross MI. Adjuvant radiation therapy after axillary lymphadenectomy for metastatic melanoma: toxicity and local control. *Ann Surg Oncol* 1995;2:445.
204. Calabro A, Singletary SE, Balch CM. Patterns of relapse in 1001 consecutive patients with melanoma nodal metastases. *Arch Surg* 1989;124:1051.
205. Gadd M, Coit DG. Recurrence patterns and outcome in 1019 patients undergoing axillary or inguinal lymphadenectomy for melanoma. *Arch Surg* 1992;127:1412.
206. Karakousis CP, Emrich LJ. Adjuvant treatment of malignant melanoma with DTIC + estracyt or BCG. *J Surg Oncol* 1987;36:235.
207. Banzet P, et al. Adjuvant chemotherapy in the management of primary malignant melanoma. *Cancer* 1978;41:1240.
208. Veronesi U, et al. A randomized trial of adjuvant chemotherapy and immunotherapy in cutaneous melanoma. *N Engl J Med* 1982;307:913.
209. Morton DL, et al. BCG immunotherapy of malignant melanoma: summary of a seven-year experience. *Ann Surg* 1974;180:635.
210. Lipton A, et al. Corynebacterium parvum versus BCG adjuvant immunotherapy in human malignant melanoma. *Cancer* 1983;51:57.
211. Lipton A, et al. Corynebacterium parvum versus bacille Calmette-Guerin adjuvant immunotherapy of stage II malignant melanoma. *J Clin Oncol* 1991;9:1151.
212. Balch CM, et al. A randomized prospective clinical trial of adjuvant C. parvum immunotherapy in 260 patients with clinically localized melanoma (stage I): prognostic factors analysis and preliminary results of immunotherapy. *Cancer* 1982;49:1079.
213. Loutfi A, et al. Double blind randomized prospective trial of levamisole/placebo in stage I cutaneous malignant melanoma. *Clin Invest Med* 1987;10:325.
214. Parkinson DR. Levamisole as adjuvant therapy for melanoma: quo vadis? *J Clin Oncol* 1991;9:716.
215. Spitler LE. A randomized trial of levamisole versus placebo as adjuvant therapy in malignant melanoma. *J Clin Oncol* 1991;9:736.
216. Wolchok J, et al. *Melanoma vaccines in cutaneous melanoma.* In: Balch CM, Sober AJ, Soong SJ, eds. *Cutaneous melanoma*, 4th ed. St. Louis: Quality Medical Publishing, 2003.
217. Spitler LE. Noninterferon-based adjuvant therapy for high-risk melanoma. *Expert Rev Anticancer Ther* 2002;2:547.
218. Chung MH, et al. Humoral immune response to a therapeutic polyvalent cancer vaccine after complete resection of thick primary melanoma and sentinel lymphadenectomy. *J Clin Oncol* 2003;21:313.
219. Morton DL, et al. Polyvalent melanoma vaccine improves survival of patients with metastatic melanoma. *Ann N Y Acad Sci* 1993;690:120.
220. Lotem M, et al. Autologous cell vaccine as a post operative adjuvant treatment for high-risk melanoma patients (AJCC stages III and IV). The new American Joint Committee on Cancer. *Br J Cancer* 2002;86:1534.
221. Berd D. M-Vax: an autologous, hapten-modified vaccine for human cancer. *Expert Opin Biol Ther* 2002;2:335.
222. Mitchell MS. Perspective on allogeneic melanoma lysates in active specific immunotherapy. *Semin Oncol* 1998;25:623.
223. Bystryn JC. Clinical activity of a polyvalent melanoma antigen vaccine. *Recent Results Cancer Res* 1995;139:337.
224. Hill GJ 2nd, Krementz ET, Hill HZ. Dimethyl triazeno imidazole carboxamide and combination therapy for melanoma. IV. Late results after complete response to chemotherapy (Central Oncology Group protocols 7130, 7131, and 7131A). *Cancer* 1984;53:1299.
225. Reynolds SR, et al. Vaccine-induced CD8+ T-cell responses to MAGE-3 correlate with clinical outcome in patients with melanoma. *Clin Cancer Res* 2003;9:657.
226. Mitchell MS, Darrah D, Stevenson L. Therapy of melanoma with allogeneic melanoma lysates alone or with interferon-alfa. *Cancer Invest* 2002;20:759.
227. Hersey P. Active immunotherapy with viral lysates of micrometastases following surgical removal of high risk melanoma. *World J Surg* 1992;16:251.
228. Wallack MK, et al. Surgical adjuvant active specific immunotherapy for patients with stage III melanoma: the final analysis of data from a phase III, randomized, double-blind, multicenter vaccinia melanoma oncolysate trial. *J Am Coll Surg* 1998;187:69.
229. Hersey P, et al. Adjuvant immunotherapy of patients with high-risk melanoma using vaccinia viral lysates of melanoma: results of a randomized trial. *J Clin Oncol* 2002;20:4181.
230. Sondak VK, et al. Adjuvant immunotherapy of resected, intermediate-thickness, node-negative melanoma with an allogeneic tumor vaccine: overall results of a randomized trial of the Southwest Oncology Group. *J Clin Oncol* 2002;20:2058.
231. Sosman JA, et al. Adjuvant immunotherapy of resected, intermediate-thickness, node-negative melanoma with an allogeneic tumor vaccine: impact of HLA class I antigen expression on outcome. *J Clin Oncol* 2002;20:2067.
232. Mitchell MS, et al. Interim analysis of a phase III stratified randomized trial of Melacine + low-dose intron-a versus high-dose intron-a for resected stage III melanoma. *Proc Am Soc Clin Oncol* 2003;22:709(abstr 2851).
233. Bystryn JC, et al. Double-blind trial of a polyvalent, shed-antigen, melanoma vaccine. *Clin Cancer Res* 2001;7:1882.
234. Jones PC, et al. Prolonged survival for melanoma patients with elevated IgM antibody to oncofetal antigen. *J Natl Cancer Inst* 1981;66:249.
235. Livingston PO, et al. Vaccines containing purified GM2 ganglioside elicit GM2 antibodies in melanoma patients. *Proc Natl Acad Sci U S A* 1987;84:2911.
236. Livingston PO, et al. Improved survival in stage III melanoma patients with GM2 antibodies: a randomized trial of adjuvant vaccination with GM2 ganglioside. *J Clin Oncol* 1994;12:1036.
237. Helling F, et al. GM2-KLH conjugate vaccine: increased immunogenicity in melanoma patients after administration with immunological adjuvant QS-21. *Cancer Res* 1995;55:2783.
238. Livingston PO, et al. Phase 1 trial of immunological adjuvant QS-21 with a GM2 ganglioside-keyhole limpet haemocyanin conjugate vaccine in patients with malignant melanoma. *Vaccine* 1994;12:1275.
239. Hom SS, et al. Common expression of melanoma tumor-associated antigens recognized by human tumor infiltrating lymphocytes: analysis by human lymphocyte antigen restriction. *J Immunother* 1991;10:153.
240. Lesinski GB, et al. The antitumor effects of IFN-alpha are abrogated in a STAT1-deficient mouse. *J Clin Invest* 2003;112:170.
241. Kirkwood JM, et al. High-dose interferon alfa-2b significantly prolongs relapse-free and overall survival compared with the GM2-KLH/QS-21 vaccine in patients with resected stage IIB-III melanoma: results of intergroup trial E1694/S9512/C509801. *J Clin Oncol* 2001;19:2370.
242. Kirkwood JM, et al. Interferon alfa-2b adjuvant therapy of high-risk resected cutaneous melanoma: the Eastern Cooperative Oncology Group Trial EST 1684. *J Clin Oncol* 1996;14:7.
243. Kirkwood JM, et al. High- and low-dose interferon alfa-2b in high-risk melanoma: first analysis of intergroup trial E1690/S9111/C9190. *J Clin Oncol* 2000;18:2444.
244. Kirkwood JM, et al. A pooled analysis of Eastern Cooperative Oncology Group and Intergroup trials of adjuvant high-dose interferon for melanoma. *Clin Cancer Res* 2004;10(5):1670.
245. Kirkwood JM, et al. High-dose interferon alfa-2b does not diminish antibody response to GM2 vaccination in patients with resected melanoma: results of the Multicenter Eastern Cooperative Oncology Group Phase II Trial E2696. *J Clin Oncol* 2001;19:1430.
246. Dubois RW, et al. Developing indications for the use of sentinel lymph node biopsy and adjuvant high-dose interferon alfa-2b in melanoma. *Arch Dermatol* 2001;137:1217.
247. Kirkwood JM, et al. Mechanisms and management of toxicities associated with high-dose interferon alfa-2b therapy. *J Clin Oncol* 2002;20:3703.
248. Musselman DL, et al. Paroxetine for the prevention of depression induced by high-dose interferon alfa. *N Engl J Med* 2001;344:961.
249. Cole BF, et al. Quality-of-life-adjusted survival analysis of interferon alfa-2b adjuvant treatment of high-risk resected cutaneous melanoma: an Eastern Cooperative Oncology Group study. *J Clin Oncol* 1996;14:2666.
250. Hillner BE, et al. Economic analysis of adjuvant interferon alfa-2b in high-risk melanoma based on projections from Eastern Cooperative Oncology Group 1684. *J Clin Oncol* 1997;15:2351.
251. Kilbridge KL, et al. Patient preferences for adjuvant interferon alfa-2b treatment. *J Clin Oncol* 2001;19:812.
252. Kilbridge KL, et al. Quality-of-life-adjusted survival analysis of high-dose adjuvant interferon alpha-2b for high-risk melanoma patients using intergroup clinical trial data. *J Clin Oncol* 2002;20:1311.
253. Eggermont AM. The role interferon-alpha in malignant melanoma remains to be defined. *Eur J Cancer* 2001;37:2147.
254. Lens MB, Dawes M. Interferon alfa therapy for malignant melanoma: a systematic review of randomized controlled trials. *J Clin Oncol* 2002;20:1818.
255. Wheatley K, et al. Interferon as adjuvant therapy for melanoma: a meta-analysis of the randomized trial. *Proc Am Soc Clin Oncol* 2001.
256. Cascinelli N, et al. Effect of long-term adjuvant therapy with interferon alpha-2a in patients with regional node metastases from cutaneous melanoma: a randomized trial. *Lancet* 2001;358:866.
257. Creagan ET, et al. Randomized, surgical adjuvant clinical trial of recombinant interferon alfa-2a in selected patients with malignant melanoma. *J Clin Oncol* 1995;13:2776.
258. Hancock BW, et al. Adjuvant interferon in high-risk melanoma: the AIM HIGH Study—United Kingdom Coordinating Committee on Cancer Research randomized study of

adjuvant low-dose extended-duration interferon alfa-2a in high-risk resected malignant melanoma. *J Clin Oncol* 2004;22:53.
259. Kleeberg UR, Brocker EB, LeJeune FJ. Adjuvant trial in melanoma patients comparing rIFN-a to rIFN-g to Iscador to a control group after curative resection of high risk primary (>3 mm) or regional lymph node metastasis (EORTC 18871). *Eur J Cancer* 1999;35[Suppl 4]:S82.
260. Pehamberger H, et al. Adjuvant interferon alfa-2a treatment in resected primary stage II cutaneous melanoma. Austrian Malignant Melanoma Cooperative Group. *J Clin Oncol* 1998;16:1425.
261. Grob JJ, et al. Randomized trial of interferon alpha-2a as adjuvant therapy in resected primary melanoma thicker than 1.5 mm without clinically detectable node metastases. French Cooperative Group on Melanoma. *Lancet* 1998;351:1905.
262. Eggermont AMM, Gore M. A critical appraisal of the role of interferon-alpha in the treatment of malignant melanoma. In: *Principles and practice of biologic therapy of cancer updates.* Philadelphia: Lippincott Williams & Wilkins, 2002:3.
263. McMasters KM. The sunbelt melanoma trial. *Ann Surg Oncol* 2001;8[Suppl 9]:41S.
264. Hauschild A, et al. Prospective randomized trial of interferon alfa-2b and interleukin-2 as adjuvant treatment for resected intermediate- and high-risk primary melanoma without clinically detectable node metastasis. *J Clin Oncol* 2003;21:2883.
265. Buzaid AC, et al. Phase II study of neoadjuvant concurrent biochemotherapy in melanoma patients with local-regional metastases. *Melanoma Res* 1998;8:549.
266. Gibbs P, et al. A phase II study of neoadjuvant biochemotherapy for stage III melanoma. *Cancer* 2002;94:470.
267. Grabstein KH, et al. Induction of macrophage tumoricidal activity by granulocyte-macrophage colony-stimulating factor. *Science* 1986;232:506.
268. Szabolcs P, Moore MA, Young JW. Expansion of immunostimulatory dendritic cells among the myeloid progeny of human CD34+ bone marrow precursors cultured with c-kit ligand, granulocyte-macrophage colony-stimulating factor, and TNF-alpha. *J Immunol* 1995;154:5851.
269. Spitler LE, et al. Adjuvant therapy of stage III and IV malignant melanoma using granulocyte-macrophage colony-stimulating factor. *J Clin Oncol* 2000;18:1614.
270. Lawson D, Kirkwood JM. Granulocyte-macrophage colony-stimulating factor: another cytokine with adjuvant therapeutic benefit in melanoma? *J Clin Oncol* 2000;18:1603.
271. Weiss M, Creagan ET, Dalton RJ, Novotny P, O'Fallon JR. Utility of follow-up tests for detecting recurrent disease in patients with malignant melanomas. *JAMA* 1995;274:1703.
272. Mooney MM, Michalek AM, Petrelli NJ, Kraybill WG. Life-long screening of patients with intermediate-thickness cutaneous melanoma for asymptomatic pulmonary recurrences detection in stage I and II cutaneous melanoma. *Ann Surg Oncol* 1998;5:54.
273. Hwu W, Balch CM, Houghton AN. Diagnosis of stage IV disease, in cutaneous melanoma. In: Balch CM, Sober AJ, Soong SJ, eds. *Cutaneous melanoma,* 4th ed. St. Louis: Quality Medical Publishing, 2003:523.
274. McGovern VJ. The classification of melanoma and its relationship with prognosis. *Pathology* 1970;2:85.
275. Schultz S, Roush R, Miller V, et al. Time to recurrence varies inversely with thickness in clinical stage I cutaneous melanoma. *Surg Gynecol Obstet* 1990;171:393.
276. McCarthy WH, Thompson JF, Milton GW. Time and frequency of recurrence of cutaneous stage I malignant melanoma with guidelines for follow-up study. *Surg Gynecol Obstet* 1988;166:497.
277. Poo-Hwu W-J, Lamb L, Papac R, et al. Follow-up recommendations for patients with American Joint Committee on cancer stage I-III malignant melanoma. *Cancer* 1999;86:2252.
278. Stas M, et al. 18-FDG PET scan in the staging of recurrent melanoma: additional value and therapeutic impact. *Melanoma Res* 2002;12:479.
279. Swetter SM, et al. Positron emission tomography is superior to computed tomography for metastatic detection in melanoma patients. *Ann Surg Oncol* 2002;9:646.
280. Valk PE, Johnson DL, Pounds TR, et al. Cost-effectiveness of whole-body FDG PET imaging in metastatic. *J Nucl Med* 1997;38:90p.
281. Tyler DS, et al. Positron emission tomography scanning in malignant melanoma. *Cancer* 2000;89:1019.
282. Holder WD, Zuger JH, Easton EJ, Greene FL. Effectiveness of positron emission tomography for the detection of melanoma metastases. *Ann Surg* 1998;227:764.
283. Gulec SA, et al. The role of fluorine-18 deoxyglucose positron emission tomography in the management of patients with metastatic melanoma: impact on surgical decision making. *Clin Nucl Med* 2003;28:961.
284. Acland KM, et al. Comparison of positron emission tomography scanning and sentinel node biopsy in the detection of micrometastases of primary cutaneous malignant melanoma. *J Clin Oncol* 2001;19:2674.
285. Tatlidil R, et al. FDG-PET in the detection of gastrointestinal metastases in melanoma. *Melanoma Res* 2001;11:297.
286. Rodrigues LK, Ljung B-M, Sagebiel RW, et al. Fine needle aspiration in the diagnosis of metastatic melanoma. *J Am Acad Dermatol* 2000;42:735.
287. Khoddami M. Cytologic diagnosis of metastatic malignant melanoma of the lung in sputum and bronchial washings. *Acta Cytol* 1993;37:403.
288. Jaffer S, et al. Fine-needle aspiration biopsy of axillary lymph nodes. *Cytopathology* 2002;26:69.
289. Morton D, Essner R, Balch CM. Surgical excision of distant metastases in cutaneous melanoma. In: Balch CM, Sober AJ, Soong SJ, eds. *Cutaneous melanoma,* 4th ed. St. Louis: Quality Medical Publishing, 2003:547.
290. Ollila D, Hsueh EC, Stern SL, Morton DL. Metastasectomy for recurrent stage IV melanoma. *J Surg Oncol* 1999;71:209.
291. Tafra L, Dale PS, Wanek LA, Ramming KP, Morton DL. Resection and adjuvant immunotherapy for melanoma metastatic to the lung and thorax. *J Thorac Cardiovasc Surg* 1995;110:119.
292. Wong JH, et al. The role of surgery in the treatment of nonregionally recurrent melanoma. *Surgery* 1993;113:389.
293. Wornom ILD, et al. Surgery as palliative treatment for distant metastases of melanoma. *Ann Surg* 1986;204:181.
294. Feun L, Gutterman J, Burgess MA, et al. The natural history of resectable metastatic melanoma (stage IVA melanoma). *Cancer* 1982;50:1656.
295. Karakousis CP, Driscoll DL, Takita H. Metastasectomy in malignant melanoma. *Surgery* 1994;115:295.
296. Overett T, Shin MH. Surgical treatment of distant metastatic melanoma. Indications and results. *Cancer* 1985;56:1985.
297. Hsueh EC, et al. Prolonged survival after complete resection of disseminated melanoma and active immunotherapy with a therapeutic cancer vaccine. *J Clin Oncol* 2002;20:4549.
298. Morris K, Marquez CM, Holland JM, Vetto JT. Prevention of local recurrence after surgical debulking of nodal and subcutaneous melanoma deposits by hypofractionated radiation. *Ann Surg Oncol* 2000;7:680.
299. Pastorino U, et al. Long-term results of lung metastasectomy: prognostic analyses based on 5206 cases. *J Thorac Cardiovasc Surg* 1997;113:37.
300. Hena M, Emrich LJ, Nambisan RN, et al. Effect of surgical treatment of stage IV melanoma. *Am J Surg* 1987;153:270.
301. Gorenstein L, Pumam JB, Natarajan G, et al. Improved survival after resection of pulmonary metastases from malignant melanoma. *Ann Thorac Surg* 1991;52:204.
302. Harpole DJ, Johnson CM, Wolfe WG, et al. Analysis of 945 cases of pulmonary metastatic melanoma. *J Thorac Cardiovasc Surg* 1992;103:743.
303. Wong JH, Euhus DM, Morton DL. Surgical resection for metastatic melanoma to the lung. *Arch Surg* 1988;123:1091.
304. Ollila D, Stern SL, Morton DL. Tumor doubling time: a selection factor for pulmonary resection of metastatic melanoma. *J Surg Oncol* 1998;69:206.
305. Lagerwaard F, Levendag PC, Nowak PJ, et al. Identification of prognostic factors in patients with brain metastases: a review of 1292 patients. *Int J Radiat Oncol Biol Phys* 1999;43:795.
306. Brega K, Robinson WA, Winston K, Wittenberg W. Surgical treatment of brain metastases in malignant melanoma. *Cancer* 1990;66:2105.
307. Skibber JM, et al. Cranial irradiation after surgical excision of brain metastases in melanoma patients. *Ann Surg Oncol* 1996;3:118.
308. Wronski M, Arbit E. Surgical treatment of brain metastases from melanoma: a retrospective study of 91 patients. *J Neurosurg* 2000;93:9.
309. Galicich J, Sundaresan N, Arbit E, Passe S. Surgical treatment of single brain metastasis: factors associated with survival. *Cancer* 1980;45:381.
310. Patchell R, Tibbs P, Walsh JW, et al. A randomized trial of surgery in the treatment of single metastases to the brain. *N Engl J Med* 1990;322:494.
311. Vecht C, Haaxma-Reiche H, Noordijk EM, et al. Treatment of single brain metastasis: radiotherapy alone or combined with neurosurgery? *Ann Neurol* 1993;33:583.
312. Patchell R, Tibbs PA, Regine WF, et al. Postoperative radiotherapy in the treatment of single metastases to the brain. *JAMA* 1998;280:1485.
313. Hagen N, Cirrincione C, Thaler HT, DeAngelis LM. The role of radiation therapy following resection of single brain metastasis from melanoma. *Neurology* 1990;40:158.
314. Lavine S, Petrovich Z, Cohen-Godol AA, et al. Gamma knife radiosurgery for metastatic melanoma. An analysis of survival, outcome, and complications. *Neurosurgery* 1999;44:59.
315. Mori Y, Kondziolka D, Flickinger JC, et al. Stereotactic radiosurgery for cerebral metastatic melanoma. Factors affecting local disease control and survival. *Int J Radiat Oncol Biol Phys* 1998;42:581.
316. Varlotto J, Flickinger JC, Niranjan A, et al. Analysis of tumor control and toxicity in patients who have survived at least one year after radiosurgery for brain metastases. *Int J Radiat Oncol Biol Phys* 2003;57:452.
317. Jawahar A, Willis BK, Smith DR, et al. Gamma knife radiosurgery for brain metastases: do patients benefit from adjuvant external-beam radiotherapy? *Stereotact Funct Neurosurg* 2002;79:262.
318. Hasegawa T, et al. Brain metastases treated with radiosurgery alone: an alternative to whole brain radiotherapy? *Neurosurgery* 2003;52:1318.
319. Gokaslan Z, Aladag MA, Ellerhorst JA. Melanoma metastatic to the spine: a review of 133 cases. *Melanoma Res* 2000;10:78.
320. Patchell R, Tibbs PA, Regine WF, et al. A randomized trial of direct decompressive surgical resection in the treatment of spinal cord compression caused by metastasis. *Proc Am Soc Clin Oncol* 2003;22:1(abst 2).
321. Gutman H, et al. Surgery for abdominal metastases of cutaneous melanoma. *World J Surg* 2001;25:750.
322. Ollila DW, et al. Surgical resection for melanoma metastatic to the gastrointestinal tract. *Arch Surg* 1996;131:975.
323. Agrawal S, Yao T-J, Coit DG. Surgery for melanoma metastatic to the gastrointestinal tract. *Ann Surg Oncol* 1999;6:336.
324. Wood TF, Rose DM, et al. Does the complete resection of melanoma metastatic to solid intra-abdominal organs improve survival? *Ann Surg Oncol* 2001;8:658.
325. Al-Sheneber I, Meterissian SH, Loutfi A, Watters AK, Shibata HR. Small-bowel resection for metastatic melanoma. *Can J Surg* 1996;39:199.
326. Rose D, Essner R, Hughes TMD, et al. Surgical resection for metastatic melanoma to liver: the John Wayne Cancer Institute and Sydney Melanoma Unit Experience. *Arch Surg* 2001;136:136.
327. de Wilt JH, McCarthy WH, Thompson JF. Surgical treatment of splenic metastases in patients with melanoma. *J Am Coll Surg* 2003;197:38.
328. Haigh P, Essner R, Wardlaw JC, et al. Long-term survival after complete resection of melanoma metastatic to the adrenal gland. *Ann Surg Oncol* 1999;6:633.
329. Branum G, Epstein RE, Leight GS, Seigler HF. The role of resection in the management of melanoma metastatic to the adrenal gland. *Surgery* 1991;109:127.
330. Ahmann DL, et al. Complete responses and long-term survivals after systemic chemotherapy for patients with advanced malignant melanoma. *Cancer* 1989;63:224.
331. Anderson CM, Buzaid AC, Legha SS. Systemic treatments for advanced cutaneous melanoma. *Oncology (Huntingt)* 1995;9:1149.

332. Nathanson L. Spontaneous regression of malignant melanoma: a review of the literature on incidence, clinical features, and possible mechanisms. Conference on spontaneous regression of cancer. *Natl Cancer Inst Monogr* 1976;44:67.
333. Rosenberg SA, White DE. Vitiligo in patients with melanoma: normal tissue antigens can be targets for cancer immunotherapy. *J Immunother Emphasis Tumor Immunol* 1996;19:81.
334. Yee C, et al. Melanocyte destruction after antigen-specific immunotherapy of melanoma: direct evidence of T cell-mediated vitiligo. *J Exp Med* 2000;192:1637.
335. Agarwala SS, Kirkwood JM. Interferons in melanoma. *Curr Opin Oncol* 1996;8:167.
336. Creagan ET, et al. Phase II trials of recombinant leukocyte A interferon in disseminated malignant melanoma: results in 96 patients. *Cancer Treat Rep* 1986;70:619.
337. Rabinowich H, et al. Expression and activity of signaling molecules in T lymphocytes obtained from patients with metastatic melanoma before and after interleukin 2 therapy. *Clin Cancer Res* 1996;2:1263.
338. Agarwala SS, Kirkwood JM. Adjuvant interferon treatment for melanoma. *Hematol Oncol Clin North Am* 1998;12:823.
339. Hernberg M, Pyrhonen S, Muhonen T. Regimens with or without interferon-alpha as treatment for metastatic melanoma and renal cell carcinoma: an overview of randomized trials. *J Immunother* 1999;22:145.
340. Rosenberg SA, et al. Regression of established pulmonary metastases and subcutaneous tumor mediated by the systemic administration of high-dose recombinant interleukin 2. *J Exp Med* 1985;161:1169.
341. Dutcher JP, et al. A phase II study of interleukin-2 and lymphokine-activated killer cells in patients with metastatic malignant melanoma. *J Clin Oncol* 1989;7:477.
342. Parkinson DR, et al. Interleukin-2 therapy in patients with metastatic malignant melanoma: a phase II study. *J Clin Oncol* 1990;8:1650.
343. Rosenberg SA, et al. Durability of complete responses in patients with metastatic cancer treated with high-dose interleukin-2: identification of the antigens mediating response. *Ann Surg* 1998;228:307.
344. Rosenberg SA, et al. Treatment of patients with metastatic melanoma with autologous tumor-infiltrating lymphocytes and interleukin 2. *J Natl Cancer Inst* 1994;86:1159.
345. Atkins M, Lotze M, Dutcher J. High-dose recombinant interleukin-2 therapy for patients with metastatic melanoma: analysis of 270 patients treated between 1985 and 1993. *J Clin Oncol* 1999;17:2105.
346. Atkins MB, et al. High-dose recombinant interleukin-2 therapy in patients with metastatic melanoma: long-term survival update. *Cancer J Sci Am* 2000;6[Suppl 1]:S11.
347. Atkins MB, Shet A, Sosman JA. *IL-2 clinical applications; melanoma in biologic therapy of cancer principles and practice.* DeVita VT Jr, Hellman S, Rosenberg SA, eds. Philadelphia: JB Lippincott Company, 2000:50.
348. Legha SS, et al. Evaluation of interleukin-2 administered by continuous infusion in patients with metastatic melanoma. *Cancer* 1996;77:89.
349. Royal RE, et al. Correlates of response to IL-2 therapy in patients treated for metastatic renal cancer and melanoma. *Cancer J Sci Am* 1996;2:91.
350. Epstein AL, et al. Identification of a protein fragment of interleukin 2 responsible for vasopermeability. *J Natl Cancer Inst* 2003;95:741.
351. Mier JW, et al. Induction of circulating tumor necrosis factor (TNF alpha) as the mechanism for the febrile response to interleukin-2 (IL-2) in cancer patients. *J Clin Immunol* 1988;8:426.
352. Margolin K, et al. Prospective randomized trial of lisofylline for the prevention of toxicities of high-dose interleukin 2 therapy in advanced renal cancer and malignant melanoma. *Clin Cancer Res* 1997;3:565.
353. Du Bois JS, et al. Randomized placebo-controlled clinical trial of high-dose interleukin-2 in combination with a soluble p75 tumor necrosis factor receptor immunoglobulin G chimera in patients with advanced melanoma and renal cell carcinoma. *J Clin Oncol* 1997;15:1052.
354. McDermott DF, et al. A two-part phase I trial of high-dose interleukin 2 in combination with soluble (Chinese hamster ovary) interleukin 1 receptor. *Clin Cancer Res* 1998;4:1203.
355. Atkins MB, et al. A phase I study of CNI-1493, an inhibitor of cytokine release, in combination with high-dose interleukin-2 in patients with renal cancer and melanoma. *Clin Cancer Res* 2001;7:486.
356. Kilbourn RG, et al. Strategies to reduce side effects of interleukin-2: evaluation of the antihypotensive agent NG-monomethyl-L-arginine. *Cancer J Sci Am* 2000;6[Suppl 1]:S21.
357. Samlowski WE, et al. A nonpeptidyl mimic of superoxide dismutase, M40403, inhibits dose-limiting hypotension associated with interleukin-2 and increases its antitumor effects. *Nat Med* 2003;9:750.
358. Phan GQ, et al. Factors associated with response to high-dose interleukin-2 in patients with metastatic melanoma. *J Clin Oncol* 2001;19:3477.
359. Weinreich DM, Rosenberg SA. Response rates of patients with metastatic melanoma to high-dose intravenous interleukin-2 after prior exposure to alpha-interferon or low-dose interleukin-2. *J Immunother* 2002;25:185.
360. Soubrane C, et al. Pretreatment serum IL-6 level as predictive factor of survival in metastatic malignant melanoma patients (MMM). *Proc Am Soc Clin Oncol* 2003.
361. Wang E, et al. Prospective molecular profiling of melanoma metastases suggests classifiers of immune responsiveness. *Cancer Res* 2002;62:3581.
362. Sparano JA, et al. Randomized phase III trial of treatment with high-dose interleukin-2 either alone or in combination with interferon alfa-2a in patients with advanced melanoma. *J Clin Oncol* 1993;11:1969.
363. Keilholz U, Scheibengogen C, Brossart P. Interleukin-based immunotherapy and chemoimmunotherapy in metastatic melanoma. *Recent Results Can Res* 1995;139:383.
364. Eton O, et al. A phase II study of "decrescendo" interleukin-2 plus interferon-alpha-2a in patients with progressive metastatic melanoma after chemotherapy. *Cancer* 2000;88:1703.
365. Atkins MB. Immunotherapy and experimental approaches for metastatic melanoma. *Hematol Oncol Clin North Am* 1998;12:877.
366. Ho AD, et al. Activation of lymphocytes induced by recombinant human granulocyte-macrophage colony-stimulating factor in patients with malignant lymphoma. *Blood* 1990;75:203.
367. Crispino S, et al. Effects of granulocyte-macrophage colony stimulating factor on soluble interleukin-2 receptor serum levels and their relation to neopterin and tumor necrosis factor-alpha in cancer patients. *J Biol Regul Homeost Agents* 1993;7:92.
368. Schiller JH, et al. Clinical and immunological effects of granulocyte-macrophage colony-stimulating factor coadministered with interleukin 2: a phase IB study. *Clin Cancer Res* 1996;2:319.
369. Smith IJ, et al. Immune effects of escalating doses of granulocyte-macrophage colony-stimulating factor added to a fixed, low-dose, inpatient interleukin-2 regimen: a randomized phase I trial in patients with metastatic melanoma and renal cell carcinoma. *J Immunother* 2003;26:130.
370. O'Day SJ, et al. Maintenance biotherapy for metastatic melanoma with interleukin-2 and granulocyte macrophage-colony stimulating factor improves survival for patients responding to induction concurrent biochemotherapy. *Clin Cancer Res* 2002;8:2775.
371. Atkins MB, et al. Phase I evaluation of intravenous recombinant human interleukin 12 in patients with advanced malignancies. *Clin Cancer Res* 1997;3:409.
372. Bajetta E, et al. Pilot study of subcutaneous recombinant human interleukin 12 in metastatic melanoma. *Clin Cancer Res* 1998;4:75.
373. Leonard JP, et al. Effects of single-dose interleukin-12 exposure on interleukin-12-associated toxicity and interferon-gamma production. *Blood* 1997;90:2541.
374. Gollob JA, et al. Phase I trial of twice-weekly intravenous interleukin 12 in patients with metastatic renal cell cancer or malignant melanoma: ability to maintain IFN-gamma induction is associated with clinical response. *Clin Cancer Res* 2000;6:1678.
375. Gollob JA, et al. Phase I trial of concurrent twice-weekly recombinant human interleukin-12 plus low-dose IL-2 in patients with melanoma or renal cell carcinoma. *J Clin Oncol* 2003;21:2564.
375a. Lesinski GB, Badgwell B, Zimmerer J, et al. IL-12 pretreatments enhance IFN-alpha-induced Janus kinase-STAT signaling and potentiate the antitumor effects of IFN-alpha in a murine model of malignant melanoma. *J Immunol* 2004;172:7368.
376. Robertson MJ, Mier J, Logan T. Tolerability and anti-tumor activity of recombinant human IL-18 (rhIL-18) administered as five daily intravenous infusions in patients with solid tumors. *Proc Am Soc Clin Oncol* 2004.
377. Rosenberg SA, et al. A progress report on the treatment of 157 patients with advanced cancer using lymphokine-activated killer cells and interleukin-2 or high-dose interleukin-2 alone. *N Engl J Med* 1987;316:889.
378. Rosenberg SA, et al. Prospective randomized trial of high-dose interleukin-2 alone or in conjunction with lymphokine-activated killer cells for the treatment of patients with advanced cancer. *J Natl Cancer Inst* 1993;85:622.
379. Rosenberg SA. Keynote address: perspectives on the use of interleukin-2 in cancer treatment. *Cancer J Sci Am* 1997;3[Suppl 1]:S2.
380. Ma Q, Gonzalo-Daganzo RM, Junghans RP. Genetically engineered T cells as adoptive immunotherapy of cancer. *Cancer Chemother Biol Response Modif* 2002;20:315.
381. Hodi FS, et al. Biologic activity of cytotoxic T lymphocyte-associated antigen 4 antibody blockade in previously vaccinated metastatic melanoma and ovarian carcinoma patients. *Proc Natl Acad Sci U S A* 2003;100:4712.
382. Hahne M, et al. Melanoma cell expression of Fas(Apo-1/CD95) ligand: implications for tumor immune escape. *Science* 1996;274:1363.
383. Saito T, et al. Spontaneous apoptosis of CD8+ T lymphocytes in peripheral blood of patients with advanced melanoma. *Clin Cancer Res* 2000;6:1351.
384. Zea AH, et al. Alterations in T cell receptor and signal transduction molecules in melanoma patients. *Clin Cancer Res* 1995;1:1327.
385. Tatsumi T, et al. Disease-associated bias in T helper type 1 (Th1)/Th2 CD4(+) T cell responses against MAGE-6 in HLA-DRB10401(+) patients with renal cell carcinoma or melanoma. *J Exp Med* 2002;196:619.
386. Lee PP, et al. Characterization of circulating T cells specific for tumor-associated antigens in melanoma patients. *Nat Med* 1999;5:677.
387. Lee KH, et al. Increased vaccine-specific T cell frequency after peptide-based vaccination correlates with increased susceptibility to in vitro stimulation but does not lead to tumor regression. *J Immunol* 1999;163:6292.
388. Tatsumi T, et al. MAGE-6 encodes HLA-DRbeta1*0401-presented epitopes recognized by CD4+ T cells from patients with melanoma or renal cell carcinoma. *Clin Cancer Res* 2003;9:947.
389. Javia LR, Rosenberg SA. CD4+CD25+ suppressor lymphocytes in the circulation of patients immunized against melanoma antigens. *J Immunother* 2003;26:85.
390. Taheri F, et al. L-Arginine regulates the expression of the T-cell receptor zeta chain (CD3zeta) in Jurkat cells. *Clin Cancer Res* 2001;7[Suppl 3]:958s.
391. Rodriquez PC, et al. L-Arginine consumption by macrophages modulates expression of T cell CD3Z chain in T lymphocytes. *J Immunol* 2003;26:S281.
392. Hellstrand K. Histamine in cancer immunotherapy: a preclinical background. *Semin Oncol* 2002;29[Suppl 7]:35.
393. Weber JS. et al. Phase I trial of antibody to CTLA-4 (MDX-010) with melanoma peptides/Ifa for resected stages III/IV melanoma. ASCO 2003.
394. Hellstrand K, et al. Histamine in immunotherapy of advanced melanoma: a pilot study. *Cancer Immunol Immunother* 1994;39:416.
395. Hellstrand K. Melanoma immunotherapy: a battle against radicals? *Trends Immunol* 2003;24:232.
396. Agarwala SS, Hellstrand K, Naredi P. Interleukin-2 and histamine dihydrochloride in metastatic melanoma. *J Clin Oncol* 2002;20:3558.
397. Whitman ED, Glaspy J, O'Day S. Histamine dihydrochloride (HDC) administered with interleukin-2 (IL-2) increases survival duration in patients with AJCC stage M1c melanoma. *Proc Am Soc Clin Oncol* 2002.
398. Agarwala SS, et al. Results from a randomized phase III study comparing combined treatment with histamine dihydrochloride plus interleukin-2 versus interleukin-2 alone in patients with metastatic melanoma. *J Clin Oncol* 2002;20:125.
399. Whiteside T, Agarwala SS, Gooding W. Immunomodulatory effects of combination therapy with histamine dihydrochloride (HDC) and interleukin-2 (IL-2) in patients (pts) with metastatic melanoma. *Proc Am Soc Clin Oncol* 2002.

400. Schmidt H, Larsen S, Bastholt L. A phase II study of outpatient subcutaneous histamine dihydrochloride, interleukin-2 and interferon-a in patients with metastatic melanoma. *Proc Am Soc Clin Oncol* 2002.
401. Hauschild A. First analysis of international M-02 trial: histamine, interferon alpha-2b (IFN), interleukin (IL)-2 vs. dacarbazine (DTIC). *European Conference: perspectives in melanoma management.* Amsterdam, The Netherlands, 2003.
402. Rosenberg SA, Spiess P, Lafreniere R. A new approach to the adoptive immunotherapy of cancer with tumor-infiltrating lymphocytes. *Science* 1986;233:1318.
403. Poehlein CH, et al. Reconstitution of lymphopenic mice with CD25-depleted spleen cells from tumor-bearing mice, eliminates tumor-induced suppression, restores the tumor-specific response to vaccination and therapeutic efficacy of adoptive immunotherapy. *J Immunol* 2003;26:S44.
404. Dudley ME, et al. Cancer regression and autoimmunity in patients after clonal repopulation with antitumor lymphocytes. *Science* 2002;298:850.
405. Thurin J, et al. GD2 ganglioside biosynthesis is a distinct biochemical event in human melanoma tumor progression. *FEBS Lett* 1986;208:17.
406. Houghton AN, Chapman PB. *Melanoma in biologic therapy of cancer.* DeVita VT Jr, Hellman S, Rosenberg SA, eds. JB Lippincott Company, 2003:576.
407. Irie RF, Morton DL. Regression of cutaneous metastatic melanoma by intralesional injection with human monoclonal antibody to ganglioside GD2. *Proc Natl Acad Sci U S A* 1986;83:8694.
408. Saleh MN, et al. Phase I trial of the chimeric anti-GD2 monoclonal antibody ch14.18 in patients with malignant melanoma. *Hum Antibodies Hybridomas* 1992;3:19.
409. Scott AM, et al. Specific targeting, biodistribution, and lack of immunogenicity of chimeric anti-GD3 monoclonal antibody KM871 in patients with metastatic melanoma: results of a phase I trial. *J Clin Oncol* 2001;19:3976.
410. Gillies SD, et al. Antibody-targeted interleukin 2 stimulates T-cell killing of autologous tumor cells. *Proc Natl Acad Sci U S A* 1992;89:1428.
411. Becker JC, et al. T cell-mediated eradication of murine metastatic melanoma induced by targeted interleukin 2 therapy. *J Exp Med* 1996;183:2361.
412. King D, Albertine M, Schalch H. Phase I/IB trial of the immunocytokine hu14.18-IL-2 in patients with metastatic melanoma. *Proc Am Soc Clin Oncol* 2002.
413. Dranoff G, et al. Vaccination with irradiated tumor cells engineered to secrete murine granulocyte-macrophage colony-stimulating factor stimulates potent, specific, and long-lasting anti-tumor immunity. *Proc Natl Acad Sci U S A* 1993;90:3539.
414. Soiffer R, et al. Vaccination with irradiated autologous melanoma cells engineered to secrete human granulocyte-macrophage colony-stimulating factor generates potent antitumor immunity in patients with metastatic melanoma. *Proc Natl Acad Sci U S A* 1998;95:13141.
415. Soiffer R, et al. Vaccination with irradiated, autologous melanoma cells engineered to secrete granulocyte-macrophage colony-stimulating factor by adenoviral-mediated gene transfer augments antitumor immunity in patients with metastatic melanoma. *J Clin Oncol* 2003;21:3343.
416. Bergen M, Chen R, Gonzalez R. Efficacy and safety of HLA-B7/beta-2 microglobulin plasmid DNA/lipid complex (Allovectin-7((R))) in patients with metastatic melanoma. *Expert Opin Biol Ther* 2003;3:377.
417. Atkins MB, Bearden J, Blum R. Phase II trial of HLA-B7 plasmid on DNA/lipid (Allovectin-7) immunotherapy in patients with metastatic melanoma (MM). *Proc Am Soc Clin Oncol* 2000;(abst 1801).
418. Stopeck AT, et al. Phase II study of direct intralesional gene transfer of allovectin-7, an HLA-B7/beta2-microglobulin DNA-liposome complex, in patients with metastatic melanoma. *Clin Cancer Res* 2001;7:2285.
419. Richards J, Thompson J, Atkins MB. A controlled, randomized phase III trial comparing the response to dacarbazine with and without Allovectin-7 (A) in patients with metastatic melanoma. *Proc Am Soc Clin Oncol* 2002;(abst 1380).
420. Bedikian AY, Gonzalez R, Richards J. A phase II study of high-dose allovectin-7 in patients with advanced metastatic melanoma. *Proc Am Soc Clin Oncol* 2003.
421. Lee ML, Tomsu K, Von Eschen KB. Duration of survival for disseminated malignant melanoma: results of a meta-analysis. *Melanoma Res* 2000;10:81.
422. Atkins MB, Buzaid AC, Houghton AN. Chemotherapy and biochemotherapy in cutaneous melanoma. In: Balch CM, Sober AJ, Soong SJ, eds. *Cutaneous melanoma,* 4th ed. St. Louis: Quality Medical Publishing, Inc., 2003:589.
423. Patel M, et al. Plasma and cerebrospinal fluid pharmacokinetics of intravenous temozolomide in non-human primates. *J Neurooncol* 2003;61:203.
424. Friedman HS, Kerby T, Calvert H. Temozolomide and treatment of malignant glioma. *Clin Cancer Res* 2000;6:2585.
425. Middleton MR, et al. Randomized phase III study of temozolomide versus dacarbazine in the treatment of patients with advanced metastatic malignant melanoma. *J Clin Oncol* 2000;18:158.
426. Summers Y, et al. Effect of temozolomide (TMZ) on central nervous system (CNS) relapse in patients with advanced melanoma. *Proc Am Soc Clin Oncol* 1999;(abst).
427. Brock CS, et al. Phase I trial of temozolomide using an extended continuous oral schedule. *Cancer Res* 1998;58:4363.
428. Danson S, et al. Randomized phase II study of temozolomide given every 8 hours or daily with either interferon alfa-2b or thalidomide in metastatic malignant melanoma. *J Clin Oncol* 2003;21:2551.
429. Hwu WJ, et al. Phase II study of temozolomide plus thalidomide for the treatment of metastatic melanoma. *J Clin Oncol* 2003;21:3351.
430. Hwu WJ, et al. Treatment of metastatic melanoma in the brain with temozolomide and thalidomide. *Lancet Oncol* 2001;2:634.
431. Ahmann DL, Hahn RG, Bisel HF. Evaluation of 1-(2-chloroethyl-3-4-methylcyclohexyl)-1-nitrosourea (methyl-CCNU, NSC 95441) versus combined imidazole carboxamide (NSC 45338) and vincristine (NSC 67574) in palliation of disseminated malignant melanoma. *Cancer* 1974;33:615.
432. Khayat D, Avril MF, Auclerc G. Clinical value of the nitrosourea fotemustine in disseminated malignant melanoma: overview on 1022 patients including 144 patients with cerebral metastases. *Proc Am Soc Clin Oncol* 1993.
433. Jacquillat C, et al. Final report of the French multicenter phase II study of the nitrosourea fotemustine in 153 evaluable patients with disseminated malignant melanoma including patients with cerebral metastases. *Cancer* 1990;66:1873.
434. Aamdal S, Avril MF, Grob JJ. A phase III randomized trial of fotemustine (F) versus dacarbazine (DTIC) in patients with disseminated malignant melanoma with or without brain metastases. *Proc Am Soc Clin Oncol* 2002.
435. Glover D, et al. WR-2721 and high-dose cisplatin: an active combination in the treatment of metastatic melanoma. *J Clin Oncol* 1987;5:574.
436. Bedikian AY, Papadopoulos N, Plager C. Phase II evaluation of short IV infusion of paclitaxel in metastatic melanoma. *Proc Am Soc Clin Oncol* 2002.
437. Einzig AI, et al. A phase II study of taxol in patients with malignant melanoma. *Invest New Drugs* 1991;9:59.
438. Legha SS, et al. A phase II trial of taxol in metastatic melanoma. *Cancer* 1990;65:2478.
439. Einzig AI, Schuchter LM, Wadler S. Phase II trial of taxotere (RP 56976) in patients with metastatic melanoma previously untreated with cytotoxic chemotherapy. *Proc Am Soc Clin Oncol* 1994.
440. Bedikian AY, et al. Phase II trial of docetaxel in patients with advanced cutaneous malignant melanoma previously untreated with chemotherapy. *J Clin Oncol* 1995;13:2895.
441. Aamdal S, et al. Docetaxel (Taxotere) in advanced malignant melanoma: a phase II study of the EORTC Early Clinical Trials Group. *Eur J Cancer* 1994;30A:1061.
442. Bafaloukos D, et al. Temozolomide in combination with docetaxel in patients with advanced melanoma: a phase II study of the Hellenic Cooperative Oncology Group. *J Clin Oncol* 2002;20:420.
443. Zonder JA, et al. Phase II trial of weekly Paclitaxel as 2nd line treatment of metastatic malignant melanoma. *Proc Am Soc Clin Oncol* 2000.
444. Spriggs D, Soignet S, Bienvenu S, et al. Phase I first-in-man study of the epothilone B analog BMS-247550 in patients with advanced cancer. *Proc Am Soc Clin Oncol* 2001 (abst).
445. Gonzalez R, Bajetta E, Buzaid AC. Phase II study of novel taxane BMS-184476 in previously treated patients with metastatic non-choroidal melanoma (MM). *Proc Am Soc Clin Oncol* 2002.
446. Legha SS, et al. A prospective evaluation of a triple-drug regimen containing cisplatin, vinblastine, and dacarbazine (CVD) for metastatic melanoma. *Cancer* 1989;64:2024.
447. Del Prete SA, et al. Combination chemotherapy with cisplatin, carmustine, dacarbazine, and tamoxifen in metastatic melanoma. *Cancer Treat Rep* 1984;68:1403.
448. Buzaid AC, et al. Cisplatin (C), vinblastine (V), and dacarbazine (D) (CVD) versus dacarbazine alone in metastatic melanoma: preliminary results of a phase II cancer community oncology program (CCOP) trial. *ASCO* 1993.
449. Mastrangelo MJ, Berd D, Bellet R. Aggressive chemotherapy for melanoma. *PPO Updates* 1991;5:1.
450. McClay EF, et al. Effective combination chemo/hormonal therapy for malignant melanoma: experience with three consecutive trials. *Int J Cancer* 1992;50:553.
451. Margolin KA, et al. Phase II study of carmustine, dacarbazine, cisplatin, and tamoxifen in advanced melanoma: a Southwest Oncology Group study. *J Clin Oncol* 1998;16:664.
452. Rusthoven JJ, et al. Randomized, double-blind, placebo-controlled trial comparing the response rates of carmustine, dacarbazine, and cisplatin with and without tamoxifen in patients with metastatic melanoma. National Cancer Institute of Canada Clinical Trials Group. *J Clin Oncol* 1996;14:2083.
453. Mitchell M, Von Eschen KB. Phase III trial of melanocine melanoma theracine versus combination chemotherapy in the treatment of stage IV melanoma. *Proc Am Soc Clin Oncol* 1997.
454. Chapman PB, et al. Phase III multicenter randomized trial of the Dartmouth regimen versus dacarbazine in patients with metastatic melanoma. *J Clin Oncol* 1999;17: 2745.
455. Middleton MR, et al. A randomized phase III study comparing dacarbazine, BCNU, cisplatin and tamoxifen with dacarbazine and interferon in advanced melanoma. *Br J Cancer* 2000;82:1158.
456. Fisher RI, Neifeld JP, Lippman ME. Oestrogen receptors in human malignant melanoma. *Lancet* 1976;2:337.
457. McClay EF, McClay ME. Tamoxifen: is it useful in the treatment of patients with metastatic melanoma? *J Clin Oncol* 1994;12:617.
458. Cocconi G, et al. Treatment of metastatic malignant melanoma with dacarbazine plus tamoxifen. *N Engl J Med* 1992;327:516.
459. Legha SS, Ring S, Bedikian A. Lack of benefit from tamoxifen added to a regimen of cisplatin (C), vinblastine (V), DTIC (D) and alpha interferon (IFN) in patients with metastatic melanoma. *Proc Am Soc Clin Oncol* 1993.
460. Agarwala SS, et al. A phase III randomized trial of dacarbazine and carboplatin with and without tamoxifen in the treatment of patients with metastatic melanoma. *Cancer* 1999;85:1979.
461. Falkson CI, et al. Phase III trial of dacarbazine versus dacarbazine with interferon alpha-2b versus dacarbazine with tamoxifen versus dacarbazine with interferon alpha-2b and tamoxifen in patients with metastatic malignant melanoma: an Eastern Cooperative Oncology Group study. *J Clin Oncol* 1998;16:1743.
462. Bajetta E, et al. Multicenter randomized trial of dacarbazine alone or in combination with two different doses and schedules of interferon alfa-2a in the treatment of advanced melanoma. *J Clin Oncol* 1994;12:806.
463. Thomson DB, et al. Interferon-alpha 2a does not improve response or survival when combined with dacarbazine in metastatic malignant melanoma: results of a multi-institutional Australian randomized trial. *Melanoma Res* 1993;3:133.
464. Pyrhonen S, Hahka-Kemppinen M, Muhonen T. A promising interferon plus four-drug chemotherapy regimen for metastatic melanoma. *J Clin Oncol* 1992;10:1919.

465. Vuoristo MS, et al. Intermittent interferon and polychemotherapy in metastatic melanoma. *J Cancer Res Clin Oncol* 1995;121:175.

466. Falkson CI, Falkson G, Falkson HC. Improved results with the addition of interferon alfa-2b to dacarbazine in the treatment of patients with metastatic malignant melanoma. *J Clin Oncol* 1991;9:1403.

467. Kirkwood JM, et al. Interferon alpha-2a and dacarbazine in melanoma. *J Natl Cancer Inst* 1990;82:1062.

468. Buzaid AC, Legha SS. Combination of chemotherapy with interleukin-2 and interferon-alfa for the treatment of advanced melanoma. *Semin Oncol* 1994;21[Suppl 14]:23.

469. Legha SS, et al. Development and results of biochemotherapy in metastatic melanoma: the University of Texas M.D. Anderson Cancer Center experience. *Cancer J Sci Am* 1997;3[Suppl 1]:S9.

470. Demchak PA, et al. Interleukin-2 and high-dose cisplatin in patients with metastatic melanoma: a pilot study. *J Clin Oncol* 1991;9:1821.

471. Atkins MB, et al. Multiinstitutional phase II trial of intensive combination chemoimmunotherapy for metastatic melanoma. *J Clin Oncol* 1994;12:1553.

472. Antoine EC, et al. Salpetriere Hospital experience with biochemotherapy in metastatic melanoma. *Cancer J Sci Am* 1997;3[Suppl 1]:S16.

473. Richards JM, et al. Combination of chemotherapy with interleukin-2 and interferon alfa for the treatment of metastatic melanoma. *J Clin Oncol* 1999;17:651.

474. Mousseau M, Khayat D, Benhammouda A. Feasibility study of chemo-immunotherapy (Ch-IM) with cisplatin (CDDP) interleukin-2 (IL-2) and interferon alpha 2a (IFNa) on 14 melanoma brain metastases patients (pts). *Proc Am Soc Clin Oncol* 1997.

475. Ron IG, et al. A phase II study of combined administration of dacarbazine and carboplatin with home therapy of recombinant interleukin-2 and interferon-alpha 2a in patients with advanced malignant melanoma. *Cancer Immunol Immunother* 1994;38:379.

476. Atzpodien J, et al. Chemoimmunotherapy of advanced malignant melanoma: sequential administration of subcutaneous interleukin-2 and interferon-alpha after intravenous dacarbazine and carboplatin or intravenous dacarbazine, cisplatin, carmustine and tamoxifen. *Eur J Cancer* 1995;31A:876.

477. Thompson JA, et al. Updated analysis of an outpatient chemoimmunotherapy regimen for treating metastatic melanoma. *Cancer J Sci Am* 1997;3[Suppl 1]:S29.

478. Flaherty LE, et al. Outpatient biochemotherapy with interleukin-2 and interferon alfa-2b in patients with metastatic malignant melanoma: results of two phase II cytokine working group trials. *J Clin Oncol* 2001;19:3194.

479. Allen IE, et al. Efficacy of interleukin-2 in the treatment of metastatic melanoma. *Cancer Therapeutics* 1998;1:168.

480. Eton O, et al. Sequential biochemotherapy versus chemotherapy for metastatic melanoma: results from a phase III randomized trial. *J Clin Oncol* 2002;20:2045.

481. Keilholz U, et al. Interferon alfa-2a and interleukin-2 with or without cisplatin in metastatic melanoma: a randomized trial of the European Organization for Research and Treatment of Cancer Melanoma Cooperative Group. *J Clin Oncol* 1997;15:2579.

482. Rosenberg SA, et al. Prospective randomized trial of the treatment of patients with metastatic melanoma using chemotherapy with cisplatin, dacarbazine, and tamoxifen alone or in combination with interleukin-2 and interferon alfa-2b. *J Clin Oncol* 1999;17:968.

483. Keilholz U, et al. Dacarbazine, cisplatin and IFN-a2b with or without IL-2 in advanced melanoma: final analysis of EORTC randomized phase III trial 18951. *ASCO* 2003.

484. Atkins MB, et al. A prospective randomized phase III trial of concurrent biochemotherapy (BCT) with cisplatin, vinblastine, dacarbazine (CVD), IL-2 and interferon alpha-2b (IFN) versus CVD alone in patients with metastatic melanoma (E3695): an ECOG-coordinated intergroup trial. *ASCO* 2003.

485. Atkins MB, et al. A phase II pilot trial of concurrent biochemotherapy with cisplatin, vinblastine, temozolomide, interleukin 2, and IFN-alpha 2B in patients with metastatic melanoma. *Clin Cancer Res* 2002;8:3075.

486. Gibbs P, O'Day S, Richards J. A multicenter phase II study of modified biochemotherapy (BCT) for stage IV melanoma incorporating temozolomide, descrescendo interleukin-2 (IL-2) and GM-CSF. *Proc Am Soc Clin Oncol* 2000.

487. Eisen T, et al. Continuous low dose thalidomide: a phase II study in advanced melanoma, renal cell, ovarian and breast cancer. *Br J Cancer* 2000;82:812.

488. Sharma RA, Marriott JB, Clarke I. Tolerability of the novel oral thalidomide analog CC-5013 demonstrating extensive immune activation and clinical response. *Proc Am Soc Clin Oncol* 2003.

489. Osella-Abate S, et al. VEGF-165 serum levels and tyrosinase expression in melanoma patients: correlation with the clinical course. *Melanoma Res* 2002;12:325.

490. Peterson AC, Swiger S, Stadler W. Phase II study of the Flk-1 TK inhibitor SU5416 in patients with advanced melanoma. *Proc Am Soc Clin Oncol* 2003.

491. Forero L, Rowinsky EK, Izbicka E. A phase II, pharmacokinetic (PK) and biologic study of SU5416 and thalidomide in patients with metastatic melanoma. *Proc Am Soc Clin Oncol* 2003.

492. Carson WE, Biber J, Shah N. A phase 2 trial of a recombinant humanized monoclonal anti-vascular endothelial growth factor (VEGF) antibody in patients with malignant melanoma. *Proc Am Soc Clin Oncol* 2003.

493. Soengas MS, et al. Inactivation of the apoptosis effector Apaf-1 in malignant melanoma. *Nature* 2001;409:207.

494. Soubrane C, Mouawad R, Gil-Delgado M. Study of Bcl-2 expression on tumor cells and peripheral lymphocytes in metastatic malignant melanoma patients: relationship with caspase-1 level and clinical response. *Proc Am Soc Clin Oncol* 2002.

495. Davies H, et al. Mutations of the BRAF gene in human cancer. *Nature* 2002;417:949.

496. Emery C, Hirschler B. Update-Genta, Aventis drug improved skin cancer survival. R.-G.I.N.G.-. News), Editor. Sept. 2003.

497. Ratain MJ, Stadler W, Smith H. A phase II study of BAY 43-9006 using the randomized discontinuation design in patients with advanced refractory cancer. *Clin Cancer Res* 2003;9:6265S.

498. Flaherty KT, et al. Phase I trial of BAY 43-9006 in combination with carboplatin (C) and paclitaxel (P). *ASCO* 2003.

499. Janku F, Tomancova V, Novotny J. Expression of c-Kit was found in more than 50% of early stages malignant melanoma. A retrospective study of 261 patients. *Proc Am Soc Clin Oncol* 2003.

500. Wyman K, Atkins MB, Hubbard F. A phase II trial of Imatinab Mesylate (Gleevec) at 800 mg daily in metastatic melanoma: lack of clinical efficacy with significant toxicity. *Proc Am Soc Clin Oncol* 2002.

ROBERT B. AVERY
MINESH P. MEHTA
RICHARD M. AUCHTER
DANIEL M. ALBERT

SECTION 3

Intraocular Melanoma

Melanomas are the most common primary intraocular malignancy in adults. They arise from uveal melanocytes (i.e., mature melanin-producing and melanin-containing cells) residing in the uveal stroma and originating from the neural crest. Whereas reactive or neoplastic proliferations of pigmented cells can occur in the epithelia of the iris, ciliary body, and retina—forming adenomas or adenocarcinomas—this chapter deals exclusively with uveal melanomas. Ocular and cutaneous melanomas are quite different and contrast in their systemic symptoms, metastatic patterns, and susceptibility to treatments.[1] Ocular melanoma accounts for approximately 13% of all melanoma deaths.* Recent years have seen important advances in our understanding of this disease at the molecular level, and results of large, randomized clinical trials have helped to clarify management options.

EPIDEMIOLOGY

The incidence of ocular melanomas in the United States has been tracked by the Surveillance, Epidemiology, and End Results (SEER) program. During 1974 to 1998, the incidence for whites was 0.69 per 100,000 person-years for males and 0.54 for females.[2] Similar figures were reported from studies in France (0.73 per 100,000), the Swedish west coast (0.72 per 100,000), and Iceland (0.7 per 100,000 in males, 0.5 in females). The incidence is several-fold lower for blacks and Hispanics.[2]

In the Third National Cancer Survey, melanoma accounted for 70% of all primary ocular malignancies, followed in frequency by the childhood tumor retinoblastoma (13%). In persons older than 20 years, melanoma was the reported diagnosis for 80% of all primary ocular cancers. In the SEER, 79% of ocular melanomas arose from the choroid or ciliary body and 5% from the conjunctiva; the primary location of the rest was not specified. Approximately two-thirds of noncutaneous melano-

*Here and elsewhere, it should be noted that, although the recent references have been incorporated, owing to a reference limit, the reader may wish to refer to earlier editions for complete references.

mas arise in the eye. The annual age-adjusted incidence of ocular melanomas is approximately one-eighth that of skin melanomas in the United States. The recently observed increase in the incidence of cutaneous melanomas has not been reported for uveal melanomas.

The incidence of ocular melanoma increases steadily by decade, with a peak in the seventh decade. Most studies show a median age at diagnosis between 55 and 65, with rates dropping after age 70. In the Collaborative Ocular Melanoma Study (COMS), the mean age of eligible patients was 60 years in the large tumor trial[3] and 59 years in the medium-sized trial.[4] Cases do occur before the age of 20 years, as illustrated by 101 of the 6359 cases on file at the Registry of Ophthalmic Pathology at the Armed Forces Institute of Pathology (AFIP) and by 40 of 3706 consecutive patients seen at Wills Eye Hospital.

A lower incidence of uveal melanoma in African Americans has been noted in several series. In the SEER registries, the incidence of ocular melanomas is approximately one-tenth that of whites (0.08 per 100,00 person-years for males and 0.03 for females). Hispanic whites also have a much lower incidence than non-Hispanic whites (0.15 per 100,000 person-years for males and 0.21 for females).

Some studies have reported a male preponderance, but this has not been consistent. In the COMS large tumor trial, 56% of eligible patients were male, and 51% were male in the medium-sized trial. Ocular and skin melanoma show similar age patterns, with more women affected at younger ages and more men later in life.

MORTALITY

The most complete long-term survival studies after enucleation were performed in Finland by Raivio and in Denmark by Jensen. In the Finnish study, the 5-, 10-, and 15-year survival rates were 65%, 52%, and 46%, respectively. In the Danish study, survival rates were similar; at the end of the 25-year period, 51% of patients had died from metastasis. McCurdy et al.,[5] in a review of 3432 cases from the AFIP, found that the overall mortality from metastasis 15 years after enucleation was 46%. In the COMS, 42 patients who qualified for randomization into the medium-sized tumor arm refused treatment but did enroll in a natural history ancillary arm. The Kaplan-Meier estimate for 5-year mortality was 30%, corresponding to a relative risk of death of 1.54 compared to treated patients.[6]

In a series of studies, McLean, Foster, and Zimmerman found that most deaths from metastatic disease occurred in the first 5 years after enucleation, with a peak mortality in the second and third years (approximately 8% per year). They compared these data with the natural course of untreated melanomas and reached a conclusion that remains controversial: Enucleation *decreased* survival. Two mechanisms have been suggested: (1) dissemination of tumor cells during traumatic operations, as demonstrated by Fraunfelder and others, and (2) decreased host resistance to disseminated tumor cells. Several investigators have challenged Zimmerman and McLean's findings. Seigel et al.[7] suggested that the statistical data could be interpreted to show that enucleation is not harmful. Others have pointed out that most melanomas are diagnosed only when they have reached a

relatively large size and concomitantly given rise to metastases, and only then are they enucleated.

The similarity in mortality among different treatments or even patients without treatment is thought to reflect micrometastases at the time of diagnosis. Once metastatic disease is found clinically, median survival is short: 2 to 5 months.[8]

NATURAL HISTORY

DOUBLING TIME

Little is known about the natural history of uveal melanomas. Until recent decades, all patients underwent enucleation immediately on diagnosis. Growth appears to occur exponentially, with doubling times from 2 months to several years. In rapidly growing tumors, a high mitotic activity and the presence of epithelioid cells have been documented. Spontaneous regression of choroidal melanoma has been described but is extremely rare.

INTRAOCULAR SPREAD

Small melanomas grow from a discoid to a hemispheric shape. They progressively obliterate the choriocapillaris and displace Bruch's membrane and the retina inward. When Bruch's membrane is disrupted, the tumor usually grows in the subretinal space in a mushroom-like configuration. The retinal pigment epithelium overlying the tumors undergoes early changes called *tumor-associated retinal pigment epitheliopathy*, which includes drusen formation and orange pigment (lipofuscin) accumulation. The neurosensory retina is frequently detached and, in some instances, infiltrated by tumor cells, which can seed into the vitreous.

Anterior tumors are more likely to affect the lens and to involve the posterior chamber. A secondary glaucoma may result from obstruction of the outflow pathways by tumor cells, cell debris, and phagocytic cells swollen with ingested cell debris. The tumor may infiltrate through the scleral spur into the anterior chamber.

Although the sclera is thought to be an effective barrier against extraocular extension, scleral infiltration by tumor cells along ciliary vessels and nerves and along the vortex veins is frequent (32.3% of large melanomas in one series).[9] Approximately 5% of melanomas grow diffusely in the plane of the uvea or circumferentially along the root of the iris. They induce a slight thickening of the uvea (approximately 3 to 5 mm) and are often unsuspected or diagnosed late when secondary glaucoma or extraocular spread occurs.

EXTRAOCULAR EXTENSION

Although extrascleral extension may be observed with small tumors, it is more likely to occur when the tumor has reached a larger size. Approximately 15% of ocular melanomas demonstrate extrascleral extension. Other less common paths of extraocular spread include the optic nerve and the lumen of vortex veins.

METASTASES

Hematogenous dissemination to the liver is the most frequent form of metastatic spread. Metastases to other sites (lung, heart, gastrointestinal tract, lymph nodes, pancreas, skin, central nervous system, bones, spleen, adrenal, kidneys, ovaries, thyroid) generally occur in association with liver metastases. Lymphatic spread has not been demonstrated, consistent with the absence of lymphatics in the eye. This is in contrast to cutaneous melanomas.

MULTIPLE CHOROIDAL MALIGNANT MELANOMA

It has been estimated that bilateral choroidal melanomas will develop in 1 in 500 million people. No evidence of an inherited genetic predisposition for bilateral primary uveal melanoma has been found. It can be associated with ocular melanocytosis. Unilateral, multifocal intraocular malignant melanoma appears to be even rarer than bilateral intraocular melanoma. It has been associated with ocular melanocytosis, iris melanoma with invasion of the ciliary body, iris or choroidal nevus (or both), and systemic malignant neoplasm. However, other cases of double melanoma do not show any such associations. It is unknown whether the prognosis differs in patients with multiple versus unifocal primary uveal melanoma.

ETIOLOGY AND PATHOGENESIS

The specific causes of ocular melanomas are unknown. Familial occurrence of uveal melanoma is rare. It was first mentioned by Silcock in 1892 and has since been reported several times. Because of an insufficient number of families with more than two affected individuals, it is impossible to identify modes of inheritance or environmental factors as causes of familial aggregation.

PREDISPOSING CONDITIONS

Yanoff and Zimmerman have provided evidence that nevi are the origin of most choroidal melanomas. Yet, a nevus-like configuration associated with choroidal melanoma may, in some cases, be explained by other mechanisms, such as (1) flattening of normal uveal melanocytes or of tumor cells, (2) a secondary proliferative effect of the malignancy, or (3) common oncogenic stimuli.

Data on the occurrence of uveal melanocytic tumors in patients with the dysplastic nevus syndrome are controversial but generally support the value of periodic ophthalmoscopic examination of patients with atypical nevi. Patients with uveal melanoma have an increased prevalence of (1) numerous common nevi (i.e., 100), (2) four or more atypical nevi, (3) pigmented iris nevi, and (4) the atypical mole syndrome.

Ocular and oculodermal melanocytosis (i.e., nevus of Ota) clearly predispose to the development of uveal melanomas. In 4.6% of reported cases of nevus of Ota, malignant transformation was reported. Rare cases of uveal melanomas have been reported in patients with type 1 neurofibromatosis. The neural tumor cells in neurofibromatosis have their origin in the neural crest, in common with melanocytes.

Holly et al.[10] showed that light skin color and easily sunburned skin increase by twofold the risk of uveal melanoma. It has been suggested that cutaneous freckles (25 or more) or iris freckles and nevi may be risk factors for uveal melanomas. Evidence suggests an association between light iris color and melanocytic lesions and is supported by studies of patients with xeroderma pigmentosum.

The association between uveal melanomas and other cancers is still a matter of controversy. Turner and coworkers[11] found that the overall prevalence of non–basal cell cancers in uveal melanoma patients was twice the expected prevalence based on an age- and gender-matched population, but others have concluded that the association of prior malignancies with uveal melanomas is weak. In a study of 407 uveal melanoma patients from the western United States with 870 control subjects, Holly et al. found no excess prior cancer.

Paraneoplastic uveal melanocytic proliferations have been observed in association with various systemic malignancies, such as ovary and lung. These appear as diffuse multinodular infiltration of the uveal tract by predominantly diploid nevoid cells as well as more anaplastic cells. In addition, an association between bilateral uveal melanoma and a proliferation-associated antigen (Ki-67) has been described. The pathogenesis of paraneoplastic uveal melanocytic proliferation remains speculative. Hamartomatous paraneoplastic proliferation and stimulation of a preexisting tumor are possibilities.

ONCOGENIC STIMULI

Investigators disagree on the role of solar radiation in the development of uveal melanomas. In Australia, the higher incidence of uveal melanoma in men, rural areas, subjects with more time outside on weekdays, and light-pigmented eyes has been taken as evidence implicating solar radiation, but other studies have found no such association. A study from France[12] identified artificial ultraviolet radiation (welders) but not outdoor sunlight as a causal agent of melanoma. Similarly, there are conflicting data regarding effects of radiofrequency devices, such as mobile phones. In the United States, there has been a slight *decrease* in the incidence of ocular melanoma from 1992 to 1998, despite sharply increasing cellular phone use.

In a study of a single population of chemical workers, a higher-than-expected incidence of ocular melanomas was found. Various chemicals, including nickel bisulfamide, platinum, methylcholanthrene, ethionine, N-2-fluorenylacetamide, radium, and N-methyl-N-nitrosourea, have been reported to induce ocular melanocytic tumors in animals. An exploratory study of various occupational associations provided elevated odds ratios for agriculture and farming work, several industrial operations, and exposure to inks, insecticides, gases, radioactive substances, polybromated phenyls, and chemical solvents.[13]

The role of hormonal factors and pregnancy has been suggested in many reports. Hartge et al.[14] reported a case-control study comparing 238 women with uveal melanoma with 223 matched control women. They showed that women with a history of pregnancy or hormonal substitutive treatment with estrogens had an increased risk, whereas those with oophorectomies had a decreased risk. Oral contraceptives had no influence on relative risk.[14] Uveal melanoma growth during pregnancy is well noted. Whether the enlargement is secondary to cellular growth or other factors (e.g., fluid retention or vascular engorgement) is unclear. At least two studies have failed to detect any estrogen or progesterone receptors in choroidal melanomas.

GENETICS

Changes on chromosomes 1, 2, 3, 6 and 8, 10, and 16 have been associated with ocular melanoma. Studies have emphasized monosomy 3 and multiplication of chromosome 8q. Losses on 1p appear to increase the severity of the disease.[15]

A role for the *c-myc* oncogene, located in the region 8q2.1-qter, in uveal melanoma formation and progression is supported by cytogenetic and immunohistochemical studies. Several groups have demonstrated abnormalities of the p53 gene. The coexistence of ocular and cutaneous melanoma in some patients suggests a predisposition to both types and may imply mutations in the CDKN2A gene on chromosome 9. An association between ocular melanoma and breast or ovarian cancer (or both) has also been reported, implicating BRCA2 on chromosome 13.

CELLULAR MECHANISMS

Deregulated expression of G_1 and alterations in their interactions with cyclin-dependent kinases appear to contribute to malignant transformation.[16] Histone deacetylase inhibitors have been shown to inhibit growth of primary and metastatic melanoma cell lines *in vitro*, perhaps through the Fas/FasL signaling pathway.

Haynie et al.[17] noted significant differences in the peripheral blood lymphocytes in two subgroups of patients with clinically less favorable choroidal melanoma; ciliary body involvement was related to a reduction in natural killer (NK) cells, and patients with extrascleral extension had an increased number of activated T cells. A role for infiltrating lymphocytes in the regression of animal models of tumors has been shown for NK cell–mediated lysis and for CD8+ cytotoxic T lymphocytes. Conversely, human uveal melanoma cells produce macrophage migration-inhibitory factor to prevent NK-mediated cell lysis. NK-cell depletion fosters the development of hepatic metastases in a mouse model.[18]

Evidence has been found for down-regulation of HLA expression in metastatic human uveal melanoma cell lines.[19] MDR1 gene and its gene product, P-glycoprotein, which are known to cause drug resistance in cancer cells, are expressed in ocular melanoma. Dunne et al.[20] reported a statistically significant association between MDR1 expression by tumor cells and shorter survival times. Whether P-glycoprotein is a marker for tumor aggressiveness, for clinical chemotherapy resistance, or perhaps for both remains to be clarified.

Immunohistochemistry and cell culture assays have identified abnormalities in the transforming growth factor-β pathway in melanoma cells. Calcium-binding proteins, somatostatin receptor subtypes, epidermal growth factor receptor, and plasminogen activation have also been implicated.

ANGIOGENESIS

In 1978, Zimmerman et al.[21] postulated that enucleation might worsen the prognosis of patients with uveal melanoma. Although this hypothesis has served to stimulate major clinical trials, it is also relevant to the recent interest in the role of angiogenesis in tumor biology. Subtractive complementary DNA hybridization has been used to identify the differential expression of angiogenic factors Cyr61 and tissue factor in melanoma versus melanocyte cell lines. Vascular endothelial growth factor levels are elevated in eyes enucleated for uveal melanoma. Angiostatic agents such as anecortave acetate (a steroid) inhibit intraocular tumor growth in mouse models.

EXPERIMENTAL MODELS

Uveal melanoma cells and normal uveal melanocytes can now be passaged in tissue culture. Cells derived from human uveal melanomas can be injected into the eyes of mice, where they form tumors. Migration to the liver ensues, resulting in metastatic lesions and death.[22] This provides a particularly powerful tool for studying control mechanisms of metastasis. Transgenic models using the promoter region of the tyrosinase gene to expression oncogenes in pigment-producing cells have also been described.

HISTOPATHOLOGY

HISTOLOGIC IDENTIFICATION

Experienced pathologists are generally accurate in diagnosing uveal melanoma based on the microscopic appearance. It can be difficult to differentiate between primary and metastatic choroidal melanomas. Immunohistochemical labeling with monoclonal antibodies to S-100, HMB-45, and melan-A immunostaining can help to differentiate between melanocytic and nonmelanocytic lesions. These tests cannot distinguish between primary and metastatic choroidal melanoma or other neural crest–derived tumors (schwannomas, neurofibromas, and leiomyomas).

CYTOLOGIC CLASSIFICATION

In 1931, Callender recognized distinct cell types in the spectrum of cells composing uveal melanomas. The cell types correlate with prognosis after enucleation, making it the most common classification in use. Classification is based on cell size, shape, cytoplasmic features, nuclear and nucleolar characteristics, and loss of cohesion, as outlined in Table 38.3-1.[23]

According to Callender's cytologic characterization, uveal melanomas are divided into three categories:

- Spindle cell melanomas (type A, B, or both), accounting for 30% of intraocular tumors, composed of spindle cells
- Mixed-cell melanomas, when fewer than one-half of the tumor sections examined are composed of epithelioid cells
- Epithelioid cell melanomas (accounting for 5% of intraocular tumors), when greater than one-half are composed of epithelioid cells.

The Callender classification carries prognostic significance. Spindle cell tumors have the best prognosis and epithelioid cell tumors the worst. In the COMS series, large tumors contain more epithelioid cells than small tumors; small tumors contain a higher percentage of spindle cell types.[24]

The major cell types described by Callender are part of a continuous spectrum and the pathologist's identification of a particular cell type involves subjective judgment. Sorensen et al.[25] have attempted a more objective method of histologically assessing uveal melanomas. Their technique uses computed cytomorphometry and entails evaluating the inverse of the standard deviation of the nucleolar area with measurements made of the mean of the ten largest nucleoli and stereologic estimates produced of the volume-weighted mean nucleolar volume.[25]

TABLE 38.3-1. Designation of the Cell Type Based on the Armed Forces Institute of Pathology Modification of the Callender Classification

Callender Cell Type	Cell Size and Description	Cytoplasm	Nucleus	Nucleolus	Other
Spindle A	Elongated spindle or small and round, depending on plane of section; cell membrane not distinct; may appear more distinct in cross section	Usually sparse but may be relatively abundant	Elongated, fine chromatin pattern; chromatin line characteristic but not necessary for diagnosis; plumper than in nevus cells	Indistinct or none	Cohesive; mitoses extremely rare
Spindle B	Plumper spindle or round, depending on plane of section; cell membrane not typically distinct (syncytial) but may be identified in cross section	Relatively sparse	Larger, plumper than spindle A; coarser chromatin pattern; chromatin clumping	Sharper definition; deeply stained, small, and round; often eccentric	Less cohesive than spindle A; may form fascicular arrangements; occasional mitoses
Epithelioid	Larger, more pleomorphic, often polygonal; distinct cell border	Abundant; may be eosinophilic	Largest, round; pleomorphic; chromatin margination, often marked; can be multinucleated	Largest, may be multiple; eosinophilic; usually central; distinct	Loss of cohesiveness; cells possibly separated easily in sectioning; more mitoses

(From ref. 24, with permission.)

EXTRACELLULAR MATRIX PATTERNS

Folberg et al.[26] have identified specific staining patterns using periodic acid–Schiff (PAS). More than one pattern may exist in a single tumor. Although originally thought to represent tumor vasculature, the exact nature of the stained structures remains controversial. For now, it is probably safest to describe the staining as extracellular matrix patterns. These staining patterns also appear in foci of metastasis, regardless of the site of dissemination. The nine patterns that they observed are

- Normal vessels
- Silent (avascular) zones
- Straight with randomly distributed vessels
- Parallel-oriented straight vessels without cross-linking
- Parallel with cross-linking between vessels
- Arcs that are incomplete loops
- Arcs with branching
- Loops that represent fibrovascular septa that completely surround lobules of tumor
- Networks that are composed of at least three back-to-back loops

Two of these patterns (networks, parallel with cross-linking) show a very strong correlation with metastatic disease; two other patterns (silent, parallel without cross-linking) correlate with a more favorable outcome.[27] The presence of epithelioid cells is associated with the presence of networks, and the absence of epithelioid cells is associated with avascular zones.

HISTOPATHOLOGIC EFFECTS OF RADIATION

The histopathology of radiation-treated globes is of value in understanding the therapeutic mode of action. The aim of treatment is to kill all tumor cells or to render them incapable of sustained proliferation. It is thought that this can be achieved through direct tumor necrosis or hypoxia secondary to blood supply damage. Unfortunately histopathologic analysis of eyes enucleated for radiation-induced complications or poor tumor control may not reflect the radiation response of most treated cases. In the COMS, preenucleation radiation significantly reduced, but did not eliminate, mitotic activity. In successfully treated tumors, mitotic figures persist only for the first 30 months after treatment. Not surprisingly, tumor regrowth is correlated with significant mitotic activity. Good tumor response is linked with fewer mitotic figures and tumor and blood vessel damage. Other significant features of irradiated tumors include necrosis, fibrosis, and balloon cell formation.

DIAGNOSIS

The diagnosis of choroidal and ciliary body melanomas has reached a high degree of accuracy at eye centers where experienced clinicians and modern ancillary testing facilities are available. This is well illustrated by a comparison of the misdiagnosis rates among the eyes on file at the AFIP: 19% (of 529 eyes) until 1962, 20% (of 208 eyes) between 1963 and 1970, and 6.4% (of 744 eyes) between 1970 and 1980. The diagnostic accuracy of 99.7% in the COMS exceeds previously documented rates.[28] It reflects the value of rigorous and standardized ophthalmic and systemic evaluations.

In a series of 400 consecutive patients referred to the oncology unit of the Wills Eye Hospital with an incorrect diagnosis of melanoma, the most commonly encountered conditions mimicking a melanoma included suspicious choroidal nevi (26.5%), peripheral disciform degeneration (11%), congenital hypertrophy of the retinal pigment epithelium (9.5%), and choroidal hemangioma (8%).[29] In a review of 51 consecutive patients who had undergone enucleation for a choroidal melanoma and 50 patients with simulating lesions, Char et al.[30] found that the ophthalmoscopic examination was the most accurate diagnostic modality, allowing correct diagnosis of choroidal melanomas in all patients with clear media. In 82% of

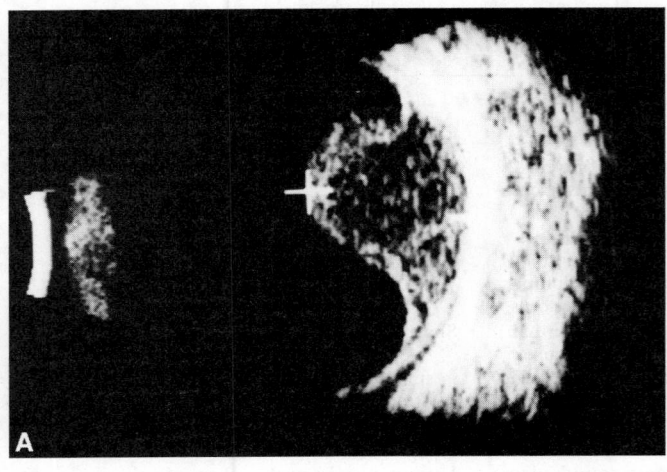

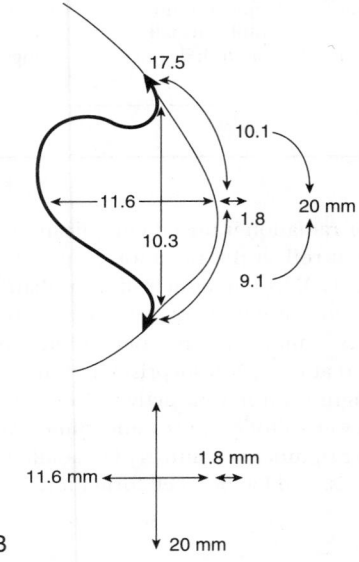

FIGURE 38.3-1. **A:** Ultrasonographic appearance of choroidal tumor. **B:** Tumor dimensions correspond to schematic drawing.

melanoma patients, A- and B-mode ultrasonography was diagnostic; in 63%, fluorescein angiography was diagnostic.[30]

CLINICAL EXAMINATION

The cornerstone of diagnosis of posterior uveal melanoma remains clinical examination, including indirect ophthalmoscopy through a dilated pupil. Fundus contact lens examination and the use of a three-mirror lens can be extremely useful. Clinical transillumination is helpful but is dependent on tumor characteristics. Transillumination can be more difficult in patients with amelanotic tumors, ocular melanocytosis, dark pigmentation, or tumors associated with hemorrhage. Pigmented conjunctival lesions, such as conjunctival melanoma, staphylomas, scleral ectasia, hematoma, cellular blue nevi, and ocular melanocytosis, may mimic extraocular extension of uveal melanomas.

It may be particularly important to diagnose ocular melanomas early to provide treatment before micrometastasis. Toward this end, the Oncology Service at Wills Eye Hospital has identi-

fied five clinical characteristics that predict the growth of pigmented lesions: thickness greater than 2 mm, subretinal fluid, symptoms, orange pigment, and margin touching the optic nerve head. At 5 years, lesions with none of these characteristics have a 3% chance of growth. In contrast, growth is seen in more than 50% of cases with two or more risk factors.[31]

ULTRASONOGRAPHY

The combined use of A- and B-mode ultrasonographic techniques is of great value in confirming the clinical diagnosis of choroidal melanoma, especially in the presence of opaque media. The A-scan mode typically reveals a solid tumor with low to medium internal reflectivity. The B-mode ultrasonographic characteristics useful in differentiating melanomas from metastases or hemangiomas are acoustic hollowness, choroidal excavation, and orbital shadowing[32] (Fig. 38.3-1). Small tumors elevated less than 2 to 3 mm cannot be evaluated accurately. A difference between ultrasonographic and histopathologic measurements of tumor thickness has been demonstrated, probably consecutive to tumor shrinkage after laboratory preparation.[33] In larger tumors, ultrasonography provides valuable size data for serial measurements and is a very important follow-up tool after conservative treatment. Ultrasound is more sensitive than magnetic resonance imaging (MRI) or computed tomography (CT) for the detection of extraocular extension of choroidal malignant melanomas.[34]

Three-dimensional ultrasonography is a promising imaging technique for evaluating the accurate position of radioactive plaques secured beneath intraocular tumors.[35] It can be used as well to observe extrascleral extension of a choroidal melanoma, to quantify the tumor volume, and for post-treatment follow-up. Color-coded Doppler imaging is also promising in the characterization and follow-up of melanomas, particularly for detection of characteristic pulsatile ocular blood flow at the tumor base.

PHOTOGRAPHY

Fluorescein angiography and monochromatic photography have proved useful in differentiating subretinal or choroidal hemorrhage and hemangioma from melanoma. Although no angiographic pattern is pathognomonic, features of value include early mottling fluorescence, orange pigment over the margin of the tumor, progressive fluorescence of the lesion with late staining, and multiple pinpoint leaks that increase in size. Breaks in Bruch's membrane and retinal invasion can be detected from abnormalities such as a double circulation pattern (simultaneous visualization of retinal and choroidal circulation). However, this double circulation pattern is often difficult to recognize, particularly when the overlying retinal pigment epithelium is intact.

Indocyanine green videoangiography with high-resolution fundus digital imaging systems has proven useful in documenting retinal vascular and choroidal diseases.[36] It can also be helpful in further differentiating amelanotic choroidal tumors (nevi or melanomas) from hemangiomas or metastases. Indocyanine green angiography using a confocal scanning laser ophthalmoscope can be used to image microvascular patterns. The angiographically seen microvascularization patterns are similar to patterns identified histologically with PAS staining that have prognostic significance in choroidal melanomas.[37] At least in theory, *in vivo* imaging of these microvascularization patterns offers noninvasive prognostic assessment of choroidal melanomas.

OTHER DIAGNOSTIC TOOLS

Radiologic examination, including CT, is useful in evaluating the presence and size of extraocular extension of tumor. It does not, however, add significant information to ultrasonography. Images of uveal melanoma have been obtained by MRI. Pigmented melanomas are hyperintense on T1-weighted images with enhancement by gadolinium and hypointense on T2-weighted images when compared to the brightness of the vitreous. This method is promising in the detection and characterization of tumors in difficult cases as well as in the differentiation of associated serous retinal detachments.

In some problematic cases, fine-needle aspiration biopsy has been used. Biopsies obtained through a transocular approach have been reported to provide informative specimens in almost 90% of cases, with accuracy greater than 95%. However, the interpretation of aspirates may be difficult even in the hands of an experienced pathologist, and subsequent tumor cell seeding in the needle track has been reported.

METASTATIC WORKUP

Patients with suspected intraocular melanoma should undergo a physical examination and metastatic workup. Clinical laboratory studies should include routine blood studies and liver enzyme measurements. Liver ultrasonography or tomography, chest radiography, and CT of the head are useful in the initial workup and surveillance.

PROGNOSTIC ASSESSMENT

Because a diagnosis of uveal melanoma traditionally led to enucleation, most prognostic algorithms make use of a combination of histopathologic and clinical factors. Tumor size and cell-type classification are the most important predictors. The location of the anterior margin of the tumor, invasion of the line of transsection, and the degree of pigmentation follow this, according to Seddon et al.[38] Extracellular matrix patterns can be powerful histologic prognostic parameters. Shammas and Blodi,[9] in a study of 253 choroidal and ciliary body melanomas, identified nine factors that significantly influenced prognosis: age of the patient at enucleation; location of the tumor; location of its anterior border; largest tumor diameter in contact with the sclera, or largest tumor dimension; height of the tumor; integrity of Bruch's membrane; cell type; pigmentation; and scleral infiltration by tumor cells. Char et al.,[30] using a multivariate analysis, reached similar conclusions for small melanomas. Parameters that significantly influenced prognosis were cell type, largest dimension, scleral extension, and mitotic activity.

SIZE

Tumor size may be the most useful prognostic factor, because tumor measurements are available at the time of diagnosis. A size classification taking into account tumor thickness and basal diameter is currently in use in most centers and in the COMS (Table 38.3-2). The current TNM (tumor, node, metastasis) staging by the American Joint Committee on Cancer[39] draws somewhat different boundary lines for small, medium, and large tumors. The COMS classification is probably more useful, because it carries with it the results of the large randomized clinical studies.

TABLE 38.3-2. Classification of Tumor Size According to Boundary Lines

Type	Apical Height	Largest Basal Diameter
Small	1.0–2.5 mm	5 mm
Medium	2.5–10.0 mm	5–16 mm
Large	10 mm	16 mm

(Adapted from ref. 45.)

Maximum tumor size is believed to be an important predictor of outcome. Diener-West et al.,[8] using selected data published during the period from 1966 to 1988, performed a metaanalysis of 5-year mortality among enucleated patients, providing weighed estimates of 5-year mortality after enucleation: 16% for small tumors, 32% for medium-sized tumors, and 53% for large tumors.

Mehaffey and coworkers[40] have showed that it is possible to separate choroidal melanomas into three prognostic groups by cross-sectional area measured from histologic sections: small (tumor area less than 16.0 mm^2), medium (tumor area greater than 16.0 mm^2 but less than 61.4 mm^2), and large (greater than 61.4 mm^2). Tumor volume has been related to outcome, but the correlation fails for small tumors (measuring less than 1.344 mm^3).

CELL TYPE

Cell type, as determined by the Callender classification, is predictive of outcome.[41] Paul et al.[42] reviewed 2652 cases accessioned at the AFIP by 1959 and found that 95% of patients with spindle A tumors, 85% of those with spindle B tumors, 60% of those with mixed tumors, and 83% with epithelioid tumors were alive 5 years after enucleation. At 15 years after enucleation, the survival rates were 85% for spindle A, 80% for spindle B, 46% for mixed, and 34% for epithelioid. In Jensen's series[43] of 302 patients reported from Denmark who had been observed for 25 years, 150 (50%) died of metastatic melanoma. Fewer than 1% of patients with spindle A tumors died of metastatic disease; 63% with mixed tumors and 71% with epithelioid tumors died from metastatic melanoma.

Computer-assisted measures of nucleoli, in conjunction with largest tumor diameter, is one of the best objective cytologic measures of a tumor's malignant potential. Counting nucleolar-organizing regions yields similar prognostic information.

EXTRACELLULAR MATRIX PATTERNS

Certain extracellular matrix patterns, as identified by PAS staining, are an independent risk factor for the growth and metastatic behavior of choroidal melanomas (see description of patterns under Histopathology, earlier in this chapter). In the absence of loops or networks, or parallel with cross-linking vascular patterns, the survival rate is 80% at 20 years but only 40% when these patterns were present. A Cox proportional hazards model has been generated with the conventional prognostic factors (including the largest tumor dimension in contact with the sclera, cell type, tumor-infiltrating lymphocytes, mitotic figures, gender, and location of the tumor within the eye) and the presence or absence of each of the nine microcirculatory patterns. The most important variable is the network pattern. However, in a study by Foss et al.,[44] the parallel with cross-linking pattern did not carry a poor prognosis; in this series, a poor prognosis was associated with absence of the normal pattern and the presence of arcs, arcs with branches, loops, and networks.

OTHER PROGNOSTIC FACTORS

Tumors involving the ciliary body have a worse prognosis than those located entirely in the choroid. In the COMS Report No. 4, older patients with a history of diabetes and patients with more anteriorly located tumors were at increased risk for death.[45] Patients with blue or gray irises show light to moderate tumor pigmentation and appear to be at increased risk of metastatic death, independent of other risk factors.

Attempts to evaluate the growth and malignant potential of uveal melanomas have been made using DNA cell-cycle studies (e.g., bromodeoxyuridine uptake or Ki-67 antibody as a marker of cycling cells, proliferating cell nuclear antigen, or DNA or RNA content by flow cytometry).[46] Reports of DNA ploidy analysis in uveal melanomas show a progressive predominance of diploid over aneuploid tumors moving from spindle to epithelioid cell type and worsening prognosis. The value of this technique as a diagnostic and prognostic tool in combination with fine-needle aspiration biopsy needs further confirmation. Uveal melanomas with higher MLN (mean of largest nuclei) and PC10 immunostaining counts have a worse prognosis.

High expression of HLA-A (and, to a lesser extent, of HLA-B) antigens on the primary uveal melanoma has been strongly correlated with poor patient survival.[47] T-lymphocytic infiltration is associated with death from metastasis.[48]

Several studies have established a correlation between rapid tumor regression after radiation therapy and a poorer life prognosis. Rapid regression may correlate with a less differentiated cell type of fast-regressing tumors. However, such a hypothesis is difficult to probe for several reasons: (1) Cytologic study of melanomas is rarely performed before radiation therapy, (2) needle biopsy often does not provide a reliable characterization of the cell type, and (3) the study of enucleated eyes after radiation therapy may not accurately reflect features of the tumor before radiation therapy, particularly in mixed or epithelioid tumors.

In summary, the prognosis for a patient enucleated for uveal melanoma is most adversely affected by the following factors:

- Largest tumor dimension exceeding 10 mm
- Tumor containing epithelioid cells (or related cytologic features)
- Tumor containing loops, networks, or parallel with cross-linking vascular patterns
- Anterior tumor border anterior to equator, especially if involving the ciliary body
- Tumor extending to the scleral surface
- Presence of numerous mitotic figures

THERAPEUTIC APPROACHES

SURGICAL

After the invention of the ophthalmoscope in 1880, most newly diagnosed melanomas were treated by enucleation. It has been suggested that the "no-touch" technique of Fraunfelder should

be considered.[49] This method was designed to minimize the possibility of seeding of tumor cells into the blood vessels during enucleation. Cryotherapy is used to minimize the flow of fluid and blood to or from the tumor during the manipulation necessary for enucleation. Although most surgeons do not use the no-touch technique, it is increasingly recognized that a person skilled and experienced in the procedure should carry out enucleation and that surgery should be done with a minimum of manipulation.

Peyman and coworkers[50] pioneered a technique of local sclerochorioretinal resection for choroidal melanomas. One-third of the eyes required enucleation because of complications, including vitreous hemorrhage and retinal detachment. Damato et al.[51] have reported the results of a technique combining lamellar scleral flap for eye closure, hypotensive anesthesia for hemostasis, and ocular decompression by pars plana vitrectomy with adjunctive ruthenium 106 (^{106}Ru) brachytherapy. Low recurrence rates and good visual results have been reported, especially for nasal tumors and for tumors located more than 1 disc diameter from the optic nerve and fovea.[51] Char et al.[52] have also claimed reasonable success with eye-wall resection. Because most patients treated by local resection are also amenable to radiation therapy and early vision loss is more frequent after surgical resection than with radiation, local resection has not been widely adopted.

Endoresection of choroidal melanoma is technically challenging but may help to conserve central vision after removal of juxtapapillary tumors. Preliminary results are encouraging in terms of visual outcome despite a high rate of complication, including retinal detachment and cataract. The risk of tumor cell release during surgery warrants long-term assessment of this procedure.

Iridocyclectomy has proven useful in the treatment of ciliary body melanomas in several series. A surprising feature is the low incidence of recurrence even when tumor extends to the margins of the resection. In contrast to resection of choroidal melanomas, iridocyclectomy is widely accepted for the treatment of ciliary body melanomas.

NONSURGICAL

Some success with photocoagulation has been documented. Shields[53] has suggested the following criteria for selecting patients with melanoma for photocoagulation treatment:

1. The diagnosis of melanoma and evidence of growth should be documented thoroughly.
2. The tumor should not be greater than 5 diopters in elevation and 6 disc diameters at its greatest diameter.
3. The tumor must be surrounded completely without damaging the fovea or the optic disc.
4. The patient must have clear ocular media and a sufficient mydriasis to enable photocoagulation to be performed.
5. The tumor surface should not have large retinal vessels.

Long-term complications of photocoagulation include retinal vascular obstruction, visual field defect, macular pucker, cystoid macular edema, choroid neovascularization, vitreous hemorrhage, and retinal detachment. Recurrences may appear, usually within 2 years of treatment. Shields[53] reported that among 35 patients treated between 1976 and 1979, 25 retained useful vision, 5 had poor vision, and 5 subsequently underwent enucleation. No tumor-related deaths occurred. Photocoagulation seems best suited for small posterior melanomas located within 3 mm of the optic disc or fovea. In such lesions, radiation-induced retinopathy may cause vision loss. The patient's wish to avoid radiation therapy or enucleation may be the deciding factor. Phototherapy can also be used as an adjunct to brachytherapy. Reports using photosensitizing compounds are still preliminary.

Transpupillary thermotherapy (TTT) is a technique that uses infrared light (diode laser, 810 mm) delivered as heat to induce necrosis in tumor tissues. In a consecutive series of 256 patients treated initially with TTT (mean of 3 treatments), Shields et al.[54] estimated tumor recurrence in 10% of cases at 3 years, with visual acuity worse than 20/200 in 32%. Other reports have also raised concerns about recurrence. Longer follow-up is necessary to assess the actual rate of local recurrence, survival, and visual outcome. The addition of indocyanine green does not appear to enhance the efficacy of TTT.

RADIATION THERAPY

Ocular melanomas have been successfully treated by a variety of radiotherapeutic modalities, including external-beam radiation using photons or charged particles (protons and helium ions); stereotactic radiosurgery with modified linear accelerators and multisource cobalt units; brachytherapy (plaque) techniques using a wide variety of isotopes; and hyperthermia in combination with brachytherapy. The techniques with the most widely reported clinical experience to date include charged-particle beam therapy and plaque therapy.

CHARGED-PARTICLE BEAM THERAPY

Charged-particle beams (protons or helium ions), produced by a cyclotron or synchrotron, are available at only a few sites around the world. They have specific dosimetric advantages in the delivery of a high dose of radiation to very precisely localized targets. Treatment of ocular melanoma requires an extremely high degree of accuracy to limit dose to the adjacent retina, optic nerve, lens, and brain. High-energy charged particles travel a fixed distance in tissue, depending on the energy of the particles and the nature of the tissue. Near the end of their path, they deposit the bulk of their energy within a well-defined, highly localized volume, referred to as the *Bragg peak*. A high and relatively uniform dose can be achieved within this small volume, thereby sparing adjacent normal tissues.

Proton beam therapy is available at approximately 30 facilities in ten countries, and helium and other ion beams at even fewer sites. Charged-particle beam therapy is generally delivered in four or five treatment sessions over 1 to 2 weeks. The treatment requires sophisticated planning techniques, precise tumor mapping, immobilization of the head, and fixation of the eye at a reproducible and verifiable gaze angle. Surgical placement of inert, radiopaque rings on the sclera assists in reproducibly identifying the target volume. Patients are treated in a seated position, with a face mask and bite-block to immobilize the head. The correct gaze angle, chosen so that the beam enters the sclera and minimizes radiation therapy of the ante-

rior chamber, is verified by an infrared camera with the patient's vision focused on a fixation light. The treatment portal (beam diameter) ranges from 1 to 4 cm. Daily setup of the patient is accomplished in 10 minutes, and the duration of radiation therapy is only 1 to 2 minutes.[55]

Long-term data on the experience with helium ion therapy for ocular melanoma have been reported.[56] This retrospective review of 218 patients treated with helium ion irradiation, with a minimum follow-up period of 10 years, demonstrated 95% local control. Twenty-two percent of patients required enucleation, most often for anterior segment complications rather than tumor recurrence. The 10-year overall survival was 53%, with half of the deaths from metastatic melanoma. Significant impairment of visual acuity was noted for tumors 6 mm thick or greater and located within 3 mm of the optic nerve and fovea.

Proton beam treatment centers report similar local control rates of 90% to 95%. Risk of distant metastasis also appears comparable to the helium ion–treated patients, at approximately 20% at 5 years. Randomized studies comparing proton beam therapy and enucleation have not been reported, and retrospective comparisons are difficult because of the need to balance the known prognostic factors (tumor size, tumor location, ocular structures involved, patient age, rate of tumor growth, etc.) between the treatment groups. A large single-institution retrospective comparison of proton beam–treated patients with those undergoing enucleation showed no apparent difference in long-term survival; an update on 1922 patients with a median follow-up of 5.2 years showed 5- and 10-year local failure rates of 3.2% and 4.3%. Approximately one-half of the failures were marginal, suggesting possible treatment planning or delivery errors.[57]

Vision preservation is one of the goals of eye-conserving therapies for ocular melanoma. Radiation maculopathy and papillopathy are major causes of vision loss after successful treatment of melanoma with charged-particle beams. Although preservation of peripheral vision and ambulatory vision has been satisfactory, visual acuity of 20/200 or better at 5 years was observed in only 55% of proton beam–treated patients at one center[58] and was 20/200 or better in only 36% of patients treated with helium ion therapy. Both of these studies also clearly demonstrated that posttreatment visual acuity is greatly affected by tumor location (in terms of proximity to the optic disc and fovea), tumor size, pretreatment visual acuity, and treatment-specific parameters. In proton beam–treated patients with the tumor edge more than 3 mm from the optic disc and fovea, 67% retained useful vision (20/200 or better), whereas for tumors located within 3 mm of these structures, only 39% maintained useful vision.

To analyze the long-term results of eye retention after conservative treatment of uveal melanoma with proton beam radiotherapy and the causes leading to enucleation after this conservative treatment approach, Egger et al.[59] undertook a prospective, noncomparative, interventional, consecutive case series analysis of 2645 patients (2648 eyes) with uveal melanoma treated between 1984 and 1999 with proton beam radiotherapy. The overall eye retention rate at 5, 10, and 15 years after treatment was 89%, 86%, and 84%, respectively. In total, 218 eyes had to be enucleated. Enucleation was related to larger tumor size, mainly tumor height; proximity of posterior tumor margin to the optic disc; male gender; high intraocular pressure; and a large degree of retinal detachment at treatment time. After optimization of the treatment technique, the eye retention rate at 5 years was increased from 97% to 100% for small tumors, from 87% to 100% for medium, and from 71% to 90% for large tumors. These findings demonstrate the positive impact of experience and quality control–based efforts for treatment technique optimization.[59]

Ocular inflammation after proton beam therapy may be a potentially underreported sequela. In one series, ocular inflammation developed in 28% of patients (with a median follow-up of 62 months). Risk factors were essentially tumor related and were correlated with larger lesions (height greater than 5 mm, diameter greater than 12 mm, volume greater than 0.4 cm[3]). Multivariate analysis identified initial tumor height and irradiation of a large volume of the eye as the two most important risk factors. Ocular inflammation usually consisted of mild anterior uveitis, resolving rapidly after topical steroids and cycloplegics. Inflammation associated with uveal melanoma has previously been described and seems to be associated with tumor necrosis, either spontaneous or after irradiation. The appearance of transient inflammation during the follow-up of these patients may be related to the release of inflammatory cytokines during tumor necrosis.

One further issue that deserves some discussion is dose selection. To determine if a reduction in proton radiation dose from the standard dose of 70 to 50 cobalt-gray equivalents (CGE) would decrease radiation-induced complications, thereby improving visual prognosis, without compromising local tumor control for patients with uveal melanoma at high risk of these complications, a randomized, double-blind clinical trial of 188 patients with small or medium-sized choroidal melanomas (less than 15 mm in diameter and less than 5 mm in height) near the optic disc or macula (within 4 disc diameters of either structure) was conducted. Patients were treated with proton beam therapy at doses of either 50 or 70 CGE between October 1989 and July 1994 and were followed up biannually through April 1998. The proportions of patients retaining visual acuity of at least 20/200 were similar in the two dose groups at 5 years after radiation (approximately 55%). Similar numbers of patients in each group experienced tumor regrowth (two patients at 50 CGE vs. three patients at 70 CGE; $P >.99$) and metastasis (seven patients at 50 CGE vs. eight patients at 70 CGE; $P = .79$). Five-year rates of radiation maculopathy also were similar (for both groups, approximately 75% for tumors within 1 disc diameter and 40% for tumors greater than 1 disc diameter from the macula). Rates of radiation papillopathy were nonsignificantly decreased in the 50-CGE treatment group. Patients treated with the lower dose also experienced significantly less visual field loss.[60]

EPISCLERAL PLAQUE RADIATION THERAPY

Episcleral plaque therapy, a highly specialized multidisciplinary treatment approach, is more widely available than charged-particle beam therapy for ocular melanoma. A concave plaque is constructed to house several small radioactive sources (or seeds) based on preoperative tumor measurements. This requires integration of data from clinical examination, ultrasonography, and occasionally CT or MRI scan. The custom-designed plaque is temporarily sutured to the sclera overlying the tumor, usually under general, but occasionally under retrobulbar, anesthesia. Operative localization of the

plaque placement is guided by transillumination, ophthalmoscopic observation, or ultrasonography. The plaque remains in place for 2 to 5 days, depending on the type and activity of the radioactive source, and is then removed under similar operative conditions.

Iodine 125 (^{125}I) is the most commonly used radioisotope in the United States and was the only isotope permitted in the COMS trial. ^{106}Ru is frequently used in Europe; other isotopes include cobalt 60 and palladium 103 (^{103}Pd). Isotopes with lower photon and electron radiation (^{125}I, ^{106}Ru, ^{103}Pd) are more easily shielded to reduce the exposure to adjacent normal tissues in the patient, with a concomitant reduction in potential exposure dose to medical personnel. The choice of radioisotope has historically been based on availability, institutional experience, and physician preference. Newer isotopes have been used after detailed dosimetric study and computer modeling. ^{103}Pd has dosimetric advantages based on its lower photon energy as compared to ^{125}I. Clinical trials of ^{103}Pd have been favorable.[61] A nonrandomized comparison of ^{125}I and ^{106}Ru plaques showed better tumor control with the ^{125}I.[62]

Preservation of useful vision, at least for a period of time, is one of the anticipated benefits of plaque therapy. However, the documentation and analysis of visual outcomes after eye-conserving therapies have been limited by a number of factors. Acuity may decrease with time after radiation therapy, and follow-up data may be incomplete for patients referred to distant tertiary eye care centers. Data from the various retrospective series are not always directly comparable. Visual acuity has been expressed as useful vision, reading vision, ambulatory vision, Snellen chart line decrement, and other measures. As noted with particle beam treatment, loss of acuity is a complex interaction of tumor size, location, and treatment effects. In the updated report by Gunduz et al.,[58] final visual acuity was better than 20/200 for 44% of patients. A factor contributing to visual deterioration that has not been well studied is the dose-rate effect. In a retrospective review of 63 patients, Jones et al.[63] demonstrated that macula dose rates of 111.0 ± 11.1 cGy/h were associated with a 50% risk of significant vision loss, and on multivariate analysis, higher macula dose rate ($P = .003$) best predicted visual decline.

Table 38.3-3 summarizes some of the retrospective data available for a variety of plaque therapy approaches. Survival rates at

TABLE 38.3-3. Retrospective Data on Radioactive Episcleral Plaque Therapy

	Gunduz et al., 1999[58]	*Finger et al., 2002*[61]	*Lommatzsch et al., 2000*[64]
Eyes treated (n)	630	80	140
Isotope	Iodine 125 (61%), cobalt 60, iridium 192	Palladium 103	Rhodium 106
Follow-up (y)	Minimum = 7	Mean = 4.6	Median = 17.3
Enucleation	11%	10%	34% at 15 y
Local control	5 y = 91%, 10 y = 88%	4.6 y = 96%	63% at 15 y
Overall survival	5 y = 87%	3 y = 92%	15 y = 48%
Metastatic disease	5 y = 12%, 10 y = 22%	3 y = 5%	15 y = 34%

5 years range from 80% to 88%. The rate of metastatic disease is approximately 10% at 5 years but appears to increase to close to 20% for studies reporting 10-year data. Enucleation has been required for either tumor progression or severe radiation complication (neovascular glaucoma, vitreous hemorrhage, ocular pain) in 10% to 17% of patients. In Table 38.3-4, clinical outcomes for charged-particle beam treatments and plaque therapy are compared, with no apparent significant differences between any of the modalities. None of these modalities, however, has been compared in a prospective randomized setting.

EPISCLERAL PLAQUE RADIATION THERAPY WITH NONIODINE ISOTOPES

Finger et al.[61] described 11 years of experience with [103]Pd ophthalmic plaque brachytherapy in 100 patients with uveal melanoma treated with [103]Pd since 1990. A mean apical radiation dose of 80.5 Gy was delivered during 5 to 7 days of continuous treatment. At a mean follow-up of 55 months, the local control rate was 96%, with six secondary enucleations. Including the enucleated patients, the visual acuity evaluations revealed that 35% lost six or more lines of vision and 73% had vision of 20/200 or better.

Long-term follow-up data with the use of other plaque isotopes, such as ruthenium, are also now becoming available. In a retrospective descriptive study in 140 patients with choroidal or ciliochoroidal melanoma treated with [106]Ru/rhodium 106 applicator radiotherapy between 1964 and 1976, median follow-up duration among surviving patients was 17.3 years. The 15-year survival rate based on all causes of death was 48%. The cumulative 15-year rates of local treatment failure and secondary enucleation were 37% and 34%, respectively. The cumulative 10-year rates of visual acuity loss to less than 20/200 and no light perception were 63% and 41%, respectively. Although a high proportion of treated eyes eventually lost a great deal of vision, and although many treated eyes ultimately underwent secondary enucleation, a substantial number of patients treated by plaque radiotherapy in this series survived for well over 10 years and retained the tumor-containing eye with a visual decrease of varying severity.[64] A systematic review generated five similarly structured case series, including survival data for 1066 patients treated by ruthenium plaque radiotherapy for uveal melanoma. After the interstudy clinical heterogeneity was assessed, data were weighed for study size and pooled. Patient and radiotherapy characteristics were largely homogeneous, but tumor size varied considerably between studies. The 5-year melanoma-related mortality was 6% for small and medium tumors (T1/T2) and 26% for large (T3) tumors. The 5- and 10-year melanoma-related mortality for a balanced set of tumors with small, medium, and large tumors being present in similar proportions were 14% and 22%, respectively. This estimate of survival after ruthenium plaque radiotherapy compares favorably with previously summarized data of survival after enucleation for similarly sized tumors.[65] However, other studies have suggested a higher local failure rate with ruthenium. To compare the efficacy of ^{125}I and [106]Ru episcleral plaque radiation therapy and proton beam radiation therapy in the treatment of choroidal melanoma, a retrospective, nonrandomized comparative study was undertaken. A total of 597 patients were identified ([125]I = 190, [106]Ru = 140, protons = 267). Patients treated with [106]Ru had a significantly greater risk of local tumor recurrence than did patients treated with either [125]I (*P* = .0133) or protons (*P* = .0097).

COLLABORATIVE OCULAR MELANOMA STUDY GROUP TRIALS

The COMS group randomized trial compared standardized ^{125}I plaque therapy to enucleation for medium-sized melanomas. Each plaque consists of a flexible inner plastic shell and a rigid outer gold shielding plate. Six different plaque sizes are available, and the size selected covers a 2- to 3-mm margin around the base of the tumor. [125]I seeds are sandwiched between the gold and plastic shells. The activity and number of seeds are selected to achieve an apical dose rate between 42 and 105 cGy/h to the prescription height. Treatment duration is calculated to deliver a total dose of 85 Gy to the prescription point.

The COMS group has published 5-year results of this landmark randomized trial comparing enucleation to ^{125}I plaque radiotherapy for medium-sized melanoma (2.5- to 10.0-mm apical height and less than 16-mm basal diameter). The accrual goal was achieved in July 1998, with 1317 patients from 43 centers in the United States and Canada randomly assigned to enucleation (660 patients) or ^{125}I plaque brachytherapy (657 patients). The unadjusted 5-year survival was 81% in the enucleation arm and 82% in the brachytherapy arm. The 5-year rate of death with confirmed melanoma metastasis was 11% and 9% after enucleation and plaque therapy, respectively (Table 38.3-5). No clinically or statistically significant difference was found in any survival- or melanoma-specific end point.

For the brachytherapy patients, additional data were prospectively collected on visual acuity and ultimate need for enucleation. Forty-three percent of patients experienced substantial impairment of visual acuity (acuity of 20/200 or worse) after plaque therapy. Tumor height and location near the fovea were the factors most strongly associated with loss of visual acuity, in addition to poor baseline acuity, diabetes, and tumor-associated retinal detachment.[66] At 5 years, 12.5% of all patients initially treated with brachytherapy required enucleation, most often

TABLE 38.3-4. Clinical Outcomes from Three Different Radiotherapy Techniques

Treatment	Local Control (%)	Enucleation (%)	5-Y Overall Survival (%)	Distant Metastasis Rate (%)	Visual Acuity 20/200 or Better (%)
Proton beam[55]	95	10	80	16	49
Helium ion beam[56]	95	22	80	24	36
Plaque therapy[58,60,61,64,65]	82–94	6–17	83–87	5–22	44

TABLE 38.3-5. Collaborative Ocular Melanoma Study Group Randomized Trial of Preenucleation Radiotherapy for Large Choroidal Melanomas

	Enucleation	Preenucleation Radiation Therapy	Statistic
Patients randomized (n)	506	497	—
Acute complications	4%	8%	P =.03
Severe ptosis	10%	5%	P =.007
Orbital recurrence	5 Patients	None	P =.03
5-y overall survival	57% (CI, 52–62%)[a]	62% (CI, 57–66%)[a]	—
Death from metastatic melanoma (at 5 y)	26%	28%	—

[a]CI = 95% confidence interval.
(From refs. 3 and 73, with permission.)

because of treatment failure (82% of the enucleations). Most treatment failures were detected within 3 years. Beyond 3 years, ocular pain was the most common reason for enucleation. Risk factors for treatment failure and enucleation included greater tumor thickness, proximity to the fovea, and older age.[67]

In summary, this authoritative trial has shown that medium-sized ocular melanomas can be treated with ^{125}I brachytherapy with survival equal to enucleation. The globe is preserved in seven of eight patients. Visual acuity preservation is maintained in approximately half the patients, with the rest experiencing deterioration in acuity to 20/200 or worse.

PLAQUE THERAPY FOR LARGE UVEAL MELANOMA

In general, these patients undergo enucleation as the standard approach; there are, however, now some initial reports comparing ^{125}I plaque brachytherapy with transscleral tumor resection of large uveal melanomas. Bechrakis et al.[68] treated and compared uveal melanoma patients with ^{125}I brachytherapy or transscleral resection. Patients were matched according to age, tumor size, and tumor location. Eighteen patients treated with ^{125}I brachytherapy and 36 patients treated with resection were eligible for the matched group comparison. Mean tumor height was 9.4 mm, and mean largest tumor diameter was 14.5 mm. Visual acuity of 20/200 or better was retained in 61% of patients after resection and 6% of patients after ^{125}I brachytherapy (P <.0009). The incidence of secondary glaucoma was higher after ^{125}I brachytherapy (33%) than after resection (6%; P = .03). No difference was found with respect to eye retention and mortality. The authors concluded that patients with large melanomas eligible for resection retain better visual function and have a lower incidence of secondary glaucoma than those treated by ^{125}I brachytherapy.[68]

Shields et al.[69] have also reported treatment complications and tumor control after plaque radiotherapy for large posterior uveal melanomas measuring 8 mm or greater in thickness. The final visual acuity in 354 patients was poor in 57% at 5 years and 89% at 10 years' follow-up. The most important risk factors for poor visual acuity included retinal invasion by mela-

noma, increasing patient age, ^{125}I isotope, and less than 2 mm distance to the optic disc. Treatment-related complications at 5 years included proliferative retinopathy (25%), maculopathy (24%), papillopathy (22%), cataract (66%), neovascular glaucoma (21%), vitreous hemorrhage (23%), and scleral necrosis (7%). Enucleation was necessary in 24% at 5 years and 34% at 10 years' follow-up. The risk factors for enucleation included left eye, peripheral tumor margin anterior rather than posterior to the equator, increasing tumor thickness, and [106]Ru isotope. Local tumor recurrence was found in 9% at 5 years and 13% at 10 years' follow-up. Risk factors for tumor recurrence included [106]Ru radioisotope and ciliary body involvement with tumor. Tumor-related metastases were found in 30% at 5 years and 55% at 10 years' follow-up. Risk factors for metastases included inferotemporal meridian, anterior extension of the tumor to the iris root, increasing tumor base, and posterior margin less than 2 mm from the optic nerve. The authors concluded that plaque radiotherapy provided tumor control at 10 years in 87% of patients with selected large posterior uveal melanomas (greater than 8 mm thick) that otherwise would have been managed with enucleation. The large intraocular mass and associated features and radiation complications led to poor visual acuity in most patients. At 10 years' follow-up, enucleation was necessary in 34% of patients, and metastasis developed in 55%.[69]

AMERICAN BRACHYTHERAPY SOCIETY RECOMMENDATIONS

Members of the American Brachytherapy Society with expertise in choroidal melanoma have formulated brachytherapy guidelines based on a literature review and clinical experience. This document serves as an important source of guidelines, and the principal recommendations include the following[70]:

Episcleral plaque brachytherapy is a complex procedure and should only be undertaken in specialized medical centers with expertise.
Most patients with very small uveal melanomas (less than 2.5 mm height and less than 10 mm in largest basal dimension) should be observed for tumor growth before treatment. Small melanomas may be candidates for plaque therapy if there is documented growth.
Patients with medium-sized choroidal melanoma (between 2.5 and 10.0 mm in height and less than 16 mm basal diameter) are candidates for episcleral plaques if the patient is otherwise healthy and without metastatic disease.
Histopathologic verification is not required for plaque therapy.
Some patients with large melanomas (greater than 10 mm height or greater than 16 mm basal diameter) may also be candidates for plaque therapy.
Patients with large tumors or with tumors at peripapillary and macular locations have a poorer visual outcome and lower local control that must be taken into account in the patient decision-making process.
Patients with gross extrascleral extension, ring melanoma, and tumor involvement of more than half of the ciliary body are not suitable for plaque therapy.
For plaque fabrication, the ophthalmologist must provide the tumor size (including basal diameters and tumor height) and a detailed fundus diagram.

The minimum recommended tumor ^{125}I dose is 85 Gy at a dose rate of 0.60 to 1.05 Gy/h using American Association of Physicists in Medicine TG-43 formalism for the calculation of dose.

One item not specifically recommended by the American Brachytherapy Society that we routinely use is intraoperative plaque localization. In a retrospective study, 117 patients with medium-sized choroidal melanoma underwent ^{125}I episcleral plaque radiotherapy with intraoperative echographic verification of plaque placement. After initial plaque placement using standard localization techniques, intraoperative echography demonstrated satisfactory tumor-plaque apposition in 76% of eyes. In 24% of eyes (28 total), repositioning of the plaque was necessitated as a consequence of intraoperative ultrasonographic findings; the extent of misplacement was less than 1 mm in ten eyes, less than 3 mm in six eyes, and greater than 3 mm in eight eyes. Repositioning was necessary in 1 eye with an anteriorly located tumor (1 of 13, 7.7%) and in 20 eyes with peripapillary or posterior pole tumors (20 of 67, 29.9%). The most commonly misaligned margins were the lateral (35%) and posterior margins (26%). In no case was an anterior marginal misalignment documented. Intraoperative echography is therefore an effective adjunct for localization and confirmation of tumor-plaque relationship. This technique facilitates the identification and correction of suboptimal plaque placement at the time of surgery, potentially minimizing treatment failures.

POSTTREATMENT QUALITY OF LIFE

Posttreatment quality of life has only been studied to a limited extent in patients undergoing plaque therapy. To investigate psychological reactions and quality of life among patients with posterior uveal melanoma, 99 consecutive patients with uveal melanoma, referred to a single institution from 1995 to 1996 and treated either with ruthenium plaque radiotherapy (n = 50) or enucleation (n = 49), were included in a nonrandomized prospective comparative study. Questionnaires were completed before treatment [Hospital Anxiety and Depression Scale (HAD scale)] and 2 and 12 months after diagnosis, including the HAD scale, the Impact of Event Scale, and the European Organization for Research and Treatment of Cancer Quality of Life Questionnaire-C30. A disease-specific questionnaire was included 12 months after diagnosis. Differences between the two groups were analyzed by chi-square, Student's t-test, and ANOVA (analysis of variance). A majority of the patients reported reduced "quality of life" (72% to 85%), "emotional functioning" (60% to 74%), and "cognitive functioning" (51% to 61%). "Fatigue" was the most frequently reported symptom (61% to 72%), followed by "insomnia" (43% to 58%). Anxiety and depressive symptoms were relatively frequent up to 1 year after treatment, but the levels of anxiety decreased during the first year after treatment. Disease and treatment-related problems were reported in both treatment groups 1 year after diagnosis. Enucleated patients had more problems with appearance and judging distances, whereas those treated with radiotherapy reported vision impairment to a higher extent. This study showed that enucleated patients reported high levels of emotional distress, problems with appearance, and judging distances during the first year after treatment. Patients treated with radiotherapy reported similar levels of quality-of-life and emotional problems but more prob-

lems with visual impairment. These differences that impact disease-related functioning should be taken into account when treatment options are discussed.[71]

In another study, patients treated for choroidal melanoma at five Midwest centers, including 65 participants treated with enucleation and 82 treated with radiation therapy, underwent quality-of-life assessment using the Medical Outcome Study Short Form 36 and the National Eye Institute Visual Function Questionnaire and by the Time-Tradeoff interview method. After adjusting for age, gender, length of follow-up, and the number of chronic conditions, few differences were seen in any of the quality-of-life measures by treatment status. Participants in the group treated with radiation therapy were more likely to have better scores on the Vitality and Mental Component subscales of the Medical Outcome Study Short Form 36 than participants treated with enucleation.

Because patients with uveal melanoma can be treated by a number of modalities and as none of the different treatments offer a survival advantage, a key factor in choosing among treatments is their differential impact on patients' quality of life. Foss et al.[72] developed a short, patient-based questionnaire and validated it for evaluating outcomes after treatment for uveal melanoma. The 21-item Measure of Outcome in Ocular Disease (MOOD) assesses the patient's view of outcome in terms of visual function and the impact of treatment. The reliability and validity of the three MOOD scores (total, vision, impact) were evaluated in 176 patients who had been treated for uveal melanoma (75 brachytherapy, 78 proton beam radiotherapy, 23 enucleation). Additionally, 165 patients also completed the SF-36. All three MOOD scales met standard criteria for acceptability, reliability, and validity. The proportion of missing data was low, and responses to all items were well distributed across response categories. All three summary scores met accepted criteria for internal consistency. Test-retest correlations for all three summary scores were excellent. Construct validity was demonstrated by high intercorrelations between the vision and impact scores and the total scale; higher scores for patients who reported being very satisfied compared with those who were not very satisfied and for those who reported persistent red eye compared with those who did not have this complication; moderate correlations between the MOOD and the SF-36 and visual acuity; and low correlations between the MOOD and age and sex. MOOD is therefore a practical and scientifically sound patient-based measure, which can be used to evaluate outcomes after treatment for uveal melanoma.[72]

PREENUCLEATION ORBITAL RADIATION THERAPY

For the treatment of larger melanomas, for which enucleation is the accepted standard treatment, COMS has published results of a randomized comparison of preoperative orbital radiation therapy (20 Gy in 5 fractions) followed immediately by enucleation versus enucleation alone. The hypothesis tested was that preoperative orbital radiation might reduce the risk of seeding of viable tumor cells during surgery and thereby improve survival through reduction in the incidence of distant metastasis. With the sponsorship of the National Eye Institute of the National Institutes of Health, the COMS Group enrolled 1003 patients from 1986 through closure in December 1994. Five-year outcome data on the first 800 patients have been published.[73]

As shown in Table 38.3-6, no advantage in overall survival or prevention of melanoma metastasis was seen with the use of

TABLE 38.3-6. Collaborative Oncology Melanoma Study Group Randomized Trial Data for Medium-Sized Melanoma: Iodine 125 Plaque Brachytherapy versus Enucleation

	Iodine 125 Plaque Brachytherapy	Enucleation
Eyes treated	657	660
Follow-up (y)	Minimum = 2; 81% of patients = 5; 32% of patients =10	Minimum = 2; 81% of patients = 5; 32% of patients = 10
Enucleation	13%[a]	100%
Local control at 5 y	90%	100%
Visual acuity better than 20/200 (treated eye, at 3 y)	57%	0%
Overall survival	5 y = 82%	5 y = 81%
Death with metastatic disease	5 y = 9%	5 y = 11%

[a]Includes enucleations for plaque treatment failure and complications. (Data from refs. 4, 66, and 67.)

preenucleation orbital radiation therapy at the dose and fractionation studied. The trial had 90% statistical power to detect a 20% relative difference in survival between the two arms. Acute complications (occurring 1 to 6 weeks after enucleation) were slightly more common in irradiated patients, but all complications were minor. For late complications (greater than 6 months after enucleation), no increase in cosmetic or functional complications was seen after radiation therapy. In fact, severe ptosis was observed less frequently in patients receiving radiation therapy (5% vs. 10%).

Preoperative radiation did appear to lower the risk of orbital recurrence, although this was a rarely noted event (local relapse developed in less than 1% of the total study population). No local recurrences were noted in the preenucleation radiation therapy arm, and five biopsy-proven recurrences were documented in the enucleation-only arm. The five patients with orbital recurrence had metastatic melanoma diagnosed before diagnosis of the orbital recurrence and died less than 1 year after presentation of the local recurrence.

Because no survival benefit was noted from routine preoperative orbital radiation therapy, as administered in the COMS, such therapy should not be considered standard. The COMS patients continue to have follow-up assessments, but any late difference in survival is unlikely, as 46% of patients in the study had died at the time of the last analysis. Preoperative or postoperative orbital radiation therapy can still be considered for selected patients who are at high risk for incomplete tumor excision or perioperative tumor seeding.

INVESTIGATIONAL RADIOTHERAPEUTIC TECHNIQUES

Radiosurgery and Fractionated Stereotactic Radiation Therapy

High-dose, conformally focused radiation therapy for small target lesions (less than 2 cm) can be accomplished by either gamma knife radiosurgery (multiple fixed, precisely aimed cobalt teletherapy beams) or stereotactic radiation therapy (multiple rotational arcs of photon beams from a linear accelerator). The techniques

are similar in their use of standard energy photon beams for therapy and rely on meticulous patient immobilization to deliver treatment to a precisely localized target within a coordinated mapping system. These techniques have been widely used and well described for the treatment of intracranial neoplasms (meningiomas, acoustic neuromas, and metastatic tumors) and for the ablation of arteriovenous malformations. Several series have examined the application of these techniques for the treatment of ocular melanomas, in the context of nonrandomized institutional reports.

The use of high-dose single-fraction Leksell gamma knife radiosurgery has been reported in a few small retrospective series. This technique has been marked by significant adverse radiation reactions, including retinopathy, optic neuropathy, and glaucoma after treatment with 50 to 70 Gy in a single fraction. One retrospective, nonrandomized report compared gamma knife radiosurgery to enucleation.[74] Tumor location (particularly ciliary body) and tumor volume were significant variables influencing survival. Using multivariate analysis to control for these variables, the authors concluded that metastasis-free survival after radiosurgery (74% at 5 years) was comparable to similar cases treated with enucleation, although the patient numbers and lack of randomization call this conclusion into question.

Linear accelerator (photon) fractionated stereotactic radiosurgery has been studied to use the radiologic advantage of multiple- rather than single-fraction treatment. Reproducible immobilization of the head and eye is required, and active optical fixation systems, similar to proton beam techniques, have been described. In these studies, 35 to 70 Gy has been delivered in two to eight fractions. One study used five-fraction, eye movement–controlled stereotactic radiotherapy to treat high-risk uveal melanoma.[75] Tumors were either unfavorably located (less than 3 mm from the macula and optical disc) or were greater than 7 mm in thickness. Local control at 20 months' median follow-up was 98%. During this short follow-up, the rate of developing metastatic disease was 3.3% and secondary enucleation was performed in 8% of patients. Significant adverse effects included retinopathy (25%), optic neuropathy (20%), cataract (19%), and neovascular glaucoma (9%).

To reduce these complications, dosimetric analysis of more conformal approaches have been performed. Use of the micromultileaf collimator has been dosimetrically compared with circular arc planning, with static conformal or dynamic arcing methods, and with intensity-modulated planning. Four treatment plans were generated with these various techniques for 40 patients with uveal melanoma (conventional arc, static conformal, dynamic arc plan, and intensity-modulated radiotherapy). The goal of treatment planning was to fully encompass the planning target volume by the 80% isodose while minimizing doses to the optic nerve and lens. This "virtual clinical trial" suggested that the conformal micromultileaf collimator and dynamic arc stereotactic radiotherapy are the treatment options of choice for uveal melanoma if one is contemplating the use of external-beam techniques.[76] Use of these techniques outside of the investigational setting is not recommended, except for patients who cannot be treated with proton beam or plaque therapy.

Hyperthermia and Episcleral Plaque Radiation Therapy

Hyperthermia has been investigated in conjunction with radiation therapy to treat a variety of tumors. Preclinical experiments have demonstrated that neoplastic cell lethality is proportional to temperature increase in the target tissue and that the combination of hyperthermia and radiation produces enhanced antitumor effects. Ocular tumor heating has been achieved by a variety of techniques, including microwave applicators, ultrasonic applicators, or ferromagnetic seeds.

One of the primary objectives for combining hyperthermia and radiation is to reduce the radiation dose, which is expected to result in fewer visual complications with a comparable rate of tumor control. An initial report of combined hyperthermia and episcleral plaque therapy used a 30% reduction in radiation dose (72 Gy, as compared to the prior standard dose of 100 Gy). In this phase I study of 25 patients, 22 showed decrease in tumor height, and ambulatory vision (greater than 5/200) was maintained in 20 patients. Two patients had severe complications (hemorrhagic retinal detachment and vitreous hemorrhage). Evaluation of long-term efficacy and late effects requires additional follow-up.[77] Shields et al.[78] reported encouraging results in patients with choroidal melanoma treated with plaque radiotherapy followed by three sessions of TTT (700 mW) provided at plaque removal and at 4-month intervals. Two hundred seventy patients with median basal tumor diameter of 11 mm (range, 4 to 21 mm) and median thickness of 4 mm (range, 2 to 9 mm), with most tumors located in the posterior pole with a median proximity of 2 mm to the foveola and 2 mm to the optic disc, were treated to a median tumor apex dose of 90 Gy. The tumor decreased in thickness to a median of 2.3 mm by 1 year and 2.1 mm by 2 years' follow-up with stable findings thereafter. Actuarial tumor recurrence was 2% at 2 years and 3% at 5 years. Actuarial treatment-related complications at 5 years included maculopathy in 18% of the participants, papillopathy in 38%, macular retinal vascular obstruction in 18%, vitreous hemorrhage in 18%, hematogenous retinal detachment in 2%, cataract in 6%, and neovascular glaucoma in 7%. Enucleation for radiation complications was necessary in three cases (1%). Plaque radiotherapy combined with TTT therefore provides excellent local tumor control, with only 3% recurrence at 5 years' follow-up.[78]

MANAGEMENT

In the last two decades, enucleation has been reassessed as the standard means of treating malignant uveal melanomas. This reassessment has resulted from (1) the development of newer and more precise diagnostic tests for recognizing malignant melanomas and the serial documentation of their size, (2) more information about clinical and pathologic features that determine survival, (3) additional observations about the natural course of untreated melanomas, and (4) therapeutic developments other than enucleation to treat tumors without destroying the eye.

The primary goal of treating uveal melanoma should be to provide the patient with the best prognosis for life possible. Secondary goals include inactivation of the neoplasm, maintenance of useful vision in the involved eye, and minimization of treatment-related side effects. The selection of treatment is based on the specific findings in each case with regard to tumor size, location, growth rate, the preferences of the ophthalmologist, and the desires of the patient. As previously noted in Posttreatment Quality of Life, treatment choice does not seem to be associated with large differences in quality of life.[79]

SMALL MELANOMAS

Despite ancillary examinations, the differential diagnosis of small tumors may be difficult. Careful follow-up of such patients at short intervals with ultrasonography, photography, and fluorescein angiography is advocated to identify tumor growth. The choices open to the physician treating a small choroidal or ciliary body melanoma include (1) observation; (2) local treatment, such as laser photocoagulation, TTT, or local resection; and (3) enucleation.

An accumulating body of evidence indicates that the risk in observing most melanomas is low. Serial examination every 3 months without intervention seems appropriate if the tumor is asymptomatic and appears dormant or the diagnosis is equivocal and no growth is seen on serial examinations. Observation is also indicated for elderly or seriously ill patients or for tumors in the patient's only useful eye, particularly if the tumor is growing slowly. If the tumor shows progression (especially rapid growth or an increase in size beyond 10 mm in diameter and 3 mm in elevation) or if the lesion results in significant impairment of vision, treatment is indicated.

In the case of patients with a healthy second eye, enucleation is advised if the tumor shows evidence of rapid progression and invasion of the optic nerve or if extraocular extension is suspected. Other considerations, including loss of central vision, failure of previous conservative treatment, and the patient's desire for complete surgical removal of the tumor, may make enucleation a reasonable choice.

MEDIUM-SIZED TUMORS

It is generally accepted that some form of treatment is necessary for medium-sized tumors. Globe-sparing therapies have become increasingly popular, especially in light of the results of the COMS medium-sized tumor trial, which found no survival difference between enucleation and ^{125}I episcleral plaque therapy. (See extensive discussion under Radiation Therapy, earlier in this chapter.) Patient and physician preferences dictate the choice of treatment for these tumors.

LARGE MELANOMAS

It is generally inadvisable to treat cases of large melanoma by methods other than enucleation. Possible exceptions include patients with only one sighted eye, rare patients in whom vision can be salvaged, and patients who refuse enucleation. Local radiation therapy is an option in these difficult cases. External-beam radiation therapy before enucleation was evaluated in the COMS. This randomized study found no survival difference in the preenucleation irradiated group.

METASTATIC DISEASE

No established treatments are available for metastatic disease. A report of patients treated with fotemustine, interferon-α_2, and interleukin-2 suggested a mean survival of 1 year, but there was no control group. Despite a promising earlier report, a multicenter trial in Europe found no objective responses to bleomycin, vincristine, lomustine, dacarbazine (BOLD) plus interferon-α_{2b} in 24 patients with metastatic uveal melanoma. For isolated metastases, a combination of surgical resection and systemic chemotherapy may prove helpful. Patients treated for advanced melanoma from an ocular primary have approximately the same survival as those with melanomas from other primary sites, approximately 5 months.[80]

FUTURE DIRECTIONS

Much still remains to be learned about the malignant transformation of uveal melanocytes and subsequent metastases. Genes and their products that are uniquely expressed in melanoma cells can be identified by one of several new approaches, including differential display, subtractive hybridization, two-dimensional gel electrophoresis–mass spectrometry, and DNA chip arrays. The contribution of these molecules, as well as aberrant functioning of traditional pathways, is now testable through the use of recently developed animal models. It will also be informative to compare detailed molecular findings with outcome data for patients made available through the collection of archival specimens.

Advancements in diagnosis should focus on confirming clinically suspicious lesions and earlier detection of metastatic disease. Noninvasive confirmation of clinically suspected melanomas may come from new imaging modalities, such as functional MRI, single photon emission CT, and positron emission tomography. As more molecular prognostic markers are identified, fine-needle aspiration may prove worth the theoretic risks. Identification of subclinical metastatic disease is a clear priority and may be aided by techniques that identify circulating melanocytes or by immunocytochemical screening of bone marrow.[81]

The COMS trials have helped to clarify treatment decisions using well-established local modalities. The long-term results of those trials will be important. In the absence of survival differences among treatments, quality-of-life issues become paramount in managing the disease. Thus, the results of the quality-of-life component of the COMS are eagerly awaited by the ophthalmic community.

Importantly, it remains unclear that any of today's treatments significantly alter the natural course of ocular melanoma. Improvements in this regard will likely require systemic therapies that prevent or contain metastases. To date, there are *no* effective treatments for metastatic disease. Melanoma-specific treatments, such as immunotargeting strategies, should supplant traditional chemotherapies.

Ocular melanoma and cutaneous melanoma are very different diseases. They diverge in their pathogenesis, systemic symptoms, metastatic patterns, and response to treatment. It is incorrect to extrapolate research on the more prevalent skin disorder to ocular melanoma. The advent of new molecular and biochemical techniques, coupled with availability of eye-specific cell lines and animal models, now renders it possible to advance our understanding of ocular tumors.

REFERENCES

1. Albert DM, Ryan LM, Borden EC. Metastatic ocular and cutaneous melanoma: a comparison of patient characteristics and prognosis. *Arch Ophthalmol* 1996;114:107.

2. Inskip PD, Devesa SS, Fraumeni JF. Trends in the incidence of ocular melanoma in the United States, 1974–1998. *Cancer Causes Control* 2003;14:251.

3. Collaborative Ocular Melanoma Study Group. The Collaborative Ocular Melanoma Study (COMS) randomized trial of pre-enucleation radiation of large choroidal melanoma. I: Initial mortality findings. COMS Report No. 10. *Am J Ophthalmol* 1998;125:779.

4. Collaborative Ocular Melanoma Study Group. The COMS randomized trial of iodine 125 brachytherapy for choroidal melanoma. III: Initial mortality findings. *Am J Ophthalmol* 2001;119:969.

5. McCurdy J, Gamel JW, McLean I. A simple, efficient, and reproducible method for estimating the malignant potential of uveal melanoma from routine H and E slides. *Pathol Res Pract* 1991;187:1025.

6. Straatsma BR, Diener-West M, Caldwell R, et al. Mortality after deferral of treatment or no treatment for choroidal melanoma. *Am J Ophthalmol* 2003;136:47.

7. Seigel D, Myers M, Ferris F III, et al. Survival rates after enucleation of eyes with malignant melanomas. *Am J Ophthalmol* 1979;87:761.

8. Diener-West M, Hawkins BS, Markowitz JA, Schachat AP. A review of mortality from choroidal melanoma. II: A meta-analysis of 5-year mortality rates following enucleation, 1966 through 1988. *Arch Ophthalmol* 1992;110:245.

9. Shammas HF, Blodi FC. Prognostic factors in choroidal and ciliary body melanomas. *Arch Ophthalmol* 1977;95:63.

10. Holly EA, Ashton DA, Ahn DK, et al. No excess prior cancer in patients with uveal melanoma. *Ophthalmology* 1991;98:608.

11. Turner BJ, Statkowski RM, Ausberger JJ, et al. Other cancers in uveal melanoma patients and their families. *Am J Ophthalmol* 1989;107:601.

12. Guenel P, Laforest L, Cyr D, et al. Occupational risk factors, ultraviolet radiation, and ocular melanoma: a case-control study in France. *Cancer Causes Control* 2001;5:451.

13. Ajani UA, Seddon JM, Hsieh CC, et al. Occupation and risk of uveal melanoma. An exploratory study. *Cancer* 1992;70:2891.

14. Hartge P, Tucker MA, Shields JA, et al. Case-control study of female hormones and eye melanoma. *Cancer Res* 1989;49:4622.

15. Sisley K, Parsons MA, Garnham J, et al. Association of specific chromosome alterations with tumor phenotype in posterior uveal melanoma. *Br J Cancer* 2000;82:330.

16. Coupland SE, Bechrakis N, Schüler A, et al. Expression patterns of cyclin D1 and related proteins regulating G_1-S phase transition in uveal melanoma and retinoblastoma. *Br J Ophthalmol* 1998;82:961.

17. Haynie GD, Shen TT, Gragoudas ES, Young LUH. Flow cytometric analysis of peripheral blood lymphocytes in patients with choroidal melanoma. *Am J Ophthalmol* 1997;124:357.

18. Dithmar SA, Rusciano DA, Armstrong CA, et al. Depletion of NK cell activity results in growth of hepatic micrometastases in murine ocular melanoma model. *Curr Eye Res* 1999;19:426.

19. Hurks HM, Metzelaar-Blok JA, Mulder A, et al. High frequency of allele-specific down-regulation of HLA class I expression in uveal melanoma cell lines. *Int J Cancer* 2000;85:697.

20. Dunne BM, McNamara M, Clynes M, et al. MDR1 expression is associated with adverse survival in melanoma of the uveal tract. *Hum Pathol* 1998;27(6):594.

21. Zimmerman LE, McLean IW, Foster WD. Does enucleation of the eye containing malignant melanoma prevent or accelerate the dissemination of tumor cells? *Br J Ophthalmol* 1978;62:420.

22. Diaz CE, Rusciano D, Dithmar S, Grossniklaus HE. B16LS9 melanoma cells spread to the liver from the murine ocular posterior compartment (PC). *Curr Eye Res* 1999;18:125.

23. McLean IW, Foster WD, Zimmerman LE. Modifications of Callender's classification of uveal melanoma at the Armed Forces Institute of Pathology. *Am J Ophthalmol* 1983;96:502.

24. Collaborative Ocular Melanoma Study Group. Histopathologic characteristic of uveal melanomas in eyes enucleated: COMS Report No. 6. *Am J Ophthalmol* 1998;125:745.

25. Sorensen FB, Gamel JW, McCurdy J. Stereologic estimation of nucleolar volume in ocular melanoma: a comparative study of size estimators with prognostic impact. *Hum Pathol* 1993;24:513.

26. Folberg R, Rummelt V, Parys-Van Ginderdeuren R, et al. The prognostic value of tumor blood vessel morphology in primary uveal melanoma. *Ophthalmology* 1993;100:1389.

27. Rummelt V, Folberg R, Rummelt C, et al. Microcirculation architecture of melanocytic nevi and malignant melanomas of the ciliary body and choroid. A comparative histopathologic and ultrastructural study. *Ophthalmology* 1994;101:718.

28. Collaborative Ocular Melanoma Study Group. Accuracy of diagnosis of choroidal melanoma in the Collaborative Ocular Melanoma Study. COMS report. *Arch Ophthalmol* 1990;108:1268.

29. Shields JA, Shields CL, Ehya H, et al. Fine-needle aspiration biopsy of suspected intraocular tumors. The 1992 Urwick Lecture. *Ophthalmology* 1993;100:1677.

30. Char DH, Stone RD, Irvine AR, et al. Diagnosis modalities in choroidal melanoma. *Am J Ophthalmol* 1980;89:223.

31. Shields CL, Cater J, Shields JA, et al. Combination of clinical factors predictive of growth of small choroidal melanocytic tumors. *Arch Ophthalmol* 2000;118:360.

32. Van Gool CA, Thijssen JM, Verbeek AM. B-mode echography of choroidal melanoma; echographic and histological aspects of choroidal excavation. *Int Ophthalmol* 1991;15:327.

33. Collaborative Ocular Melanoma Study Group. Comparison of clinical, echographic, and histopathological measurements from eyes with medium-sized choroidal melanomas in the collaborative ocular melanoma study: COMS Report No 21. *Arch Ophthalmol* 2003; 121:1163.

34. Scott IU, Murray TG, Randall Hughes J. Evaluation of imaging technics for detection of extraocular extension of choroidal melanoma. *Arch Ophthalmol* 1998;116:897.

35. Tabandeh H, Chaudhry NA, Murray TG, et al. Intraoperative echographic localization of iodine-125 episcleral plaque for brachytherapy of choroidal melanoma. *Am J Ophthalmol* 2000;129:199.

36. Shields CL, Shields JA, De Potter P. Patterns of indocyanine green videoangiography of choroidal tumours. *Br J Ophthalmol* 1995;79:237.

37. Mueller AJ, Bartsch DU, Folberg R, et al. Imaging the microvasculature of choroidal melanoma with confocal indocyanine green scanning laser ophthalmoscopy. *Arch Ophthalmol* 1998;116:31.

38. Seddon JM, Gragoudas ES, Egan KM, et al. Relative survival rates after alternative therapies for uveal melanoma. *Ophthalmology* 1990;97:769.

39. Augsburger JJ. Size classification of posterior uveal malignant melanomas. *Year Book Ophthalmology*. St. Louis: Mosby, 1993;155.

40. Mehaffey MG, Folberg R, Meyer M, et al. Relative importance of quantifying area and vascular patterns in uveal melanomas. *Am J Ophthalmol* 1997;123:798.

41. McLean IW, Keefe KS, Burnier MN. Uveal melanoma. Comparison of the prognostic value of fibrovascular loops, mean of the ten largest nucleoli, cell type, and tumor size. *Ophthalmology* 1997;104:777.

42. Paul EV, Parnell BL, Fraker M. Prognosis of malignant melanomas of the choroid and ciliary body. *Int Ophthalmol Clin* 1968;5:387.

43. Jensen QA, Prause JU. Malignant melanomas of the human uvea in Denmark: incidence and a 25-year follow-up of cases diagnosed between 1943 and 1952. In: Lommatzsch PK, Blodi FC, eds. *Intraocular tumors*. Berlin: Springer-Verlag, 1983;85.

44. Foss AJE, Alexander RA, Hungerford JL, et al. Reassessment of the PAS patterns in uveal melanoma. *Br J Ophthalmol* 1997;81:240.

45. Collaborative Ocular Melanoma Study Group. Mortality in patients with small choroidal melanoma: COMS Report no. 4. *Arch Ophthalmol* 1997;115:886.

46. Pe'er J, Gnessin H, Shargal Y, Livni N. PC-10 immunostaining of proliferating cell nuclear antigen in posterior uveal melanoma. Enucleation versus enucleation postirradiation groups. *Ophthalmology* 1994;101:56.

47. Blom DJR, Schurmans LRHM, De Waard-Siebinga I, et al. HLA expression in a primary uveal melanoma, its cell line, and four of its metastases. *Br J Ophthalmol* 1997;81:989.

48. de la Cruz PO, Specht CS, McLean IW. Lymphocytic infiltration in uveal malignant melanoma. *Cancer* 1990;65:112.

49. Fraunfelder FT, Boozman FW, Wilson RS, et al. No-touch technique for intraocular malignant melanomas. *Arch Ophthalmol* 1977;95:1616.

50. Peyman GA, Apple DJ. Local excision of a choroidal malignant melanoma: full-thickness eyewall resection. *Arch Ophthalmol* 1974;92:216.

51. Damato BE, Paul J, Foulds WS. Predictive factors of visual outcome after local resection of choroidal melanoma. *Br J Ophthalmol* 1993;77:616.

52. Char DH, Miller T, Crawford JB. Uveal tumor resection. *Br J Ophthalmol* 2001;85:1213.

53. Shields JA. The expanding role of laser photocoagulation for intraocular tumors. The 1993 H. Christian Zweng Memorial Lecture. *Retina* 1994;14:310.

54. Shields CL, Shields JA, Perez N, et al. Primary transpupillary thermotherapy for small choroidal melanoma in 256 consecutive cases: outcomes and limitations. *Ophthalmology* 2002;109:225.

55. Munzenrider JE. Proton therapy for uveal melanomas and other eye lesions. *Strahlenther Onkol* 1999;175:68.

56. Char DH, Kroll SM, Castro JR. Ten-year follow-up of helium ion therapy for uveal melanoma. *Am J Ophthalmol* 1998;125:81.

57. Gragoudas ES, Lane AM, Munzenrider J, et al. Long-term risk of local failure after proton therapy for choroidal/ciliary body melanoma. *Trans Am Ophthalmol Soc* 2002;100:43.

58. Gunduz K, Shields CL, Shields JA, et al. Radiation complications and tumor control after plaque radiotherapy of choroidal melanoma with macular involvement. *Am J Ophthalmol* 1999;127:579.

59. Egger E, Zografos L, Schalenbourg A, et al. Eye retention after proton beam radiotherapy for uveal melanoma. *Int J Radiat Oncol Biol Phys* 2003;55:867.

60. Gragoudas ES, Lane AM, Regan S, et al. A randomized controlled trial of varying radiation doses in the treatment of choroidal melanoma. *Arch Ophthalmol* 2000;118:773.

61. Finger PT, Berson A, Ng T, Szechter A. Palladium-103 plaque radiotherapy for choroidal melanoma: an 11-year study. *Int J Radiat Oncol Biol Phys* 2002;54:1438.

62. Wilson MW, Hungerford JL. Comparison of episcleral plaque and proton beam radiation therapy for the treatment of choroidal melanoma. *Ophthalmology* 1999;106:1579.

63. Jones R, Gore E, Mieler W, et al. Posttreatment visual acuity in patients treated with episcleral plaque therapy for choroidal melanomas: dose and dose rate effects. *Int J Radiat Oncol Biol Phys* 2002;52:989.

64. Lommatzsch PK, Werschnik C, Schuster E. Long-term follow-up of Ru-106/Rh-106 brachytherapy for posterior uveal melanoma. *Graefes Arch Clin Exp Ophthalmol* 2000;238:129.

65. Seregard S. Long-term survival after ruthenium plaque radiotherapy for uveal melanoma. A meta-analysis of studies including 1,066 patients. *Acta Ophthalmol Scand* 1999;77:414.

66. Collaborative Ocular Melanoma Study Group. The Collaborative Ocular Melanoma Study Group (COMS) randomized trial of I-125 brachytherapy for medium choroidal melanoma. I: Visual acuity after 3 years. COMS Report No. 16. *Ophthalmology* 2001;108:348.

67. Collaborative Ocular Melanoma Study Group. The Collaborative Ocular Melanoma Study Group (COMS) randomized trial of iodine-125 brachytherapy for choroidal melanoma. IV: Local treatment failure and enucleation in the first 5 years after brachytherapy. COMS Report No. 19. *Ophthalmology* 2002;109:2197.

68. Bechrakis NE, Bornfeld N, Zoller I, Foerster MH. Iodine 125 plaque brachytherapy versus transscleral tumor resection in the treatment of large uveal melanomas. *Ophthalmology* 2002;109:1855.

69. Shields CL, Naseripour M, Cater J, et al. Plaque radiotherapy for large posterior uveal melanomas (> or = 8-mm thick) in 354 consecutive patients. *Ophthalmology* 2002;109:1838.

70. Nag S, Quivey JM, Earle JD, et al. The American Brachytherapy Society recommendations for brachytherapy of uveal melanomas. *Int J Radiat Oncol Biol Phys* 2003;56:544.

71. Brandberg Y, Kock E, Oskar K, et al. Psychological reactions and quality of life in patients with posterior uveal melanoma treated with ruthenium plaque therapy or enucleation: a one-year follow-up study. *Eye* 2000;14:839.

72. Foss AJ, Lamping DL, Schroter S, Hungerford J. Development and validation of a patient based measure of outcome in ocular melanoma. *Br J Ophthalmol* 2000;84:347.

73. Collaborative Ocular Melanoma Study Group. The Collaborative Ocular Melanoma Study Group (COMS) randomized trial of pre-enucleation radiation of large choroidal melanoma. III: Local complications and observations following enucleation. COMS Report No. 11. *Am J Ophthalmol* 1998;126:362.

74. Cohen VM, Carter MJ, Kemeny A, et al. Metastasis-free survival following treatment for uveal melanoma with either stereotactic radiosurgery or enucleation. *Acta Ophthalmol Scand* 2003;81:383.

75. Dieckmann K, Georg D, Zehetmayer M, et al. LINAC based stereotactic radiotherapy of uveal melanoma: 4 years clinical experience. *Radiother Oncol* 2003;67:199.

76. Georg D, Dieckmann K, Bogner J, et al. Impact of a micromultileaf collimator on stereotactic radiotherapy of uveal melanoma. *Int J Radiat Oncol Biol Phys* 2003;55:881.

77. Petrovich Z, Pike M, Astrahan MA, et al. Episcleral plaque thermoradiotherapy of posterior uveal melanomas. *Am J Clin Oncol* 1996;19:207.

78. Shields CL, Cater J, Shields JA, et al. Combined plaque radiotherapy and transpupillary thermotherapy for choroidal melanoma: tumor control and treatment complications in 270 consecutive patients. *Arch Ophthalmol* 2002;120:933.

79. Cruickshanks KJ, Fryback DG, Nondahl DM, et al. Treatment choice and quality of life in patients with choroidal melanoma. *Arch Ophthalmol* 1999;117:461.

80. Flaherty LE, Unger JM, Liu PY, et al. Metastatic melanoma from intraocular primary tumors: the Southwest Oncology Group experience in phase II advanced melanoma clinical trials. *Am J Clin Oncol* 1998;21:568.

81. Schadendorf D, Dorn-Bieke A, Borelli S, et al. Limitations of the immunocytochemical detection of isolated tumor cells in frozen samples of bone marrow obtained from melanoma patients. *Exp Dermatol* 2003;12:165.

CHAPTER 39

Neoplasms of the Central Nervous System

SECTION **1**

DAVID N. LOUIS
WEBSTER K. CAVENEE

Molecular Biology of Central Nervous System Neoplasms

Neoplastic transformation in the nervous system is a multistep process in which the normal controls of cell proliferation and cell-cell interaction are lost, thus transforming a normal cell into a tumor cell. This tumorigenic process has been found to involve an interplay between different classes of genes, including oncogenes, tumor suppressor genes, DNA repair genes, and cell death genes.[6,13,19,22,39] This knowledge is improving our understanding of how brain tumors develop and progress and is also impacting clinical diagnosis and management[18,19,25,27,28] as well as enabling the development of increasingly faithful animal models of brain tumors.[13,22,37,39] For example, analysis of genomic DNA can be helpful in predicting chemosensitivity and prognosis in oligodendroglial tumors and for the differential diagnoses among different malignant gliomas as well as between medulloblastoma and atypical teratoid/rhabdoid tumors. At the RNA level, expression profiling promises to add further sensitivity to the classification of malignant gliomas as well as embryonal brain tumors such as medulloblastoma. Significant advances are being made in the establishment of mouse models of brain tumors. These models have allowed *in vivo* confirmation of the biologic role of particular genes in brain tumor formation and the dissection of tumorigenic pathways. Such models also allow inquiries into the cells of origin of brain tumors, with most data suggesting that these experimental tumors arise from progenitor cells at different stages of development.[1,9]

Insight into the etiologies underlying brain tumor initiation remains poor.[20] With the exception of hereditary predisposition (see Neurologic Tumor Syndromes, later in this chapter) and exposure to ionizing radiation, no definite etiologies have been determined. Attention to agents such as cell phone use or SV40 virus exposure has not yielded conclusive evidence that such exposures are related to brain tumor formation. Nonetheless, increased knowledge of the biologic basis of brain tumors and correlations between molecular and clinicopathologic parameters are important footholds to begin addressing tumor etiologies. This chapter reviews the molecular basis of brain tumorigenesis, covering primary tumors of the brain as well as other primary intracranial neoplasms that commonly affect the central nervous system.

DIFFUSE, FIBRILLARY ASTROCYTOMAS

FORMATION OF LOW-GRADE ASTROCYTOMA

Diffuse, fibrillary astrocytomas are the most common type of primary brain tumor in adults. These tumors are divided histopathologically into three grades of malignancy: World Health Organization (WHO) grade II diffuse astrocytoma, WHO grade III anaplastic astrocytoma, and WHO grade IV glioblastoma (GBM). WHO grade II diffuse astocytomas are the most indolent of the spectrum. Nonetheless, these low-grade tumors are infiltrative and have a marked potential for malignant progression.[22]

p53, a tumor suppressor encoded by the TP53 gene on chromosome 17p, has an integral role in a number of cellular processes, including cell-cycle arrest, response to DNA damage, apoptosis, angiogenesis, and differentiation. TP53 mutations and allelic loss of chromosome 17p are observed in at least one-third of all three grades of adult astrocytomas,[22] and high-grade astrocytomas with homogeneous TP53 mutations evolve clonally from subpopulations of similarly mutated cells present in initially low-grade tumors. Such mutational analyses are complemented by studies that have underscored the functional importance of p53 inactivation in the early stages of astrocytoma formation. For instance, cortical astrocytes from mice without functional p53 appear immortalized when grown *in vitro* and rapidly acquire a transformed phenotype. Cortical astrocytes from mice with one functional copy of TP53 behave more like wild-type astrocytes and only show signs of immortalization and transformation after they have lost the one functional TP53 copy.[3] Mouse models have also demonstrated that p53 inactivation contributes to astrocytoma tumorigenesis.[29] Thus, the abrogation of astrocytic p53 function appears to facilitate the development of other genetic lesions that are integral to further malignant progression. In addition, in higher-grade astrocytomas, the p53 pathway may be deregulated by alterations of other components, including amplification of murine double-minute gene (MDM)-2 or MDM-4 and 9p deletions that result in loss of the ARF product of the CDKN2A gene.

Many growth factors and their receptors are overexpressed in astrocytomas, including platelet-derived growth factor (PDGF), fibroblast growth factors, and vascular endothelial growth factor (VEGF). PDGF ligands and receptors are overexpressed approximately equally in all grades of astrocytoma, occurring in the majority of cases, suggesting that such overexpression is also important in the initial stages of astrocytoma formation. Tumors often overexpress cognate PDGF ligands and receptors suggesting autocrine stimulation. Significantly, loss of chromosome 17p in the region of the TP53 gene is closely correlated with PDGF-α receptor overexpression, implying that TP53 mutations have an oncogenic effect only in the presence of PDGF-α receptor overexpression. This interdependence is highlighted by observations that mouse astrocytes without functional p53 become transformed only in the presence of specific growth factors.[3]

Astrocytomas display a remarkable tendency to infiltrate the surrounding brain, confounding therapeutic attempts at local control. These invasive abilities are often apparent in low-grade as well as high-grade tumors, implying that the invasive phenotype is acquired early in tumorigenesis. Investigations into astrocytoma invasion have highlighted the complex nature of cell-cell and cell–extracellular matrix interactions.[6] A variety of cell surface and extracellular matrix molecules, such as CD44 glycoproteins, gangliosides, and integrins, are differentially expressed in astrocytomas. Many of the growth factors expressed in astrocytomas, such as fibroblast growth factor, EGF, and VEGF, also stimulate migration. Such growth factors, cell surface receptors, and extracellular molecules most likely are involved in a dynamic interplay between cell–cell adhesion, remodeling of the extracellular matrix, and cell motility.[6]

PROGRESSION TO ANAPLASTIC ASTROCYTOMA

The transition from WHO grade II astrocytoma to WHO grade III anaplastic astrocytoma is accompanied by a marked increase in malignant behavior. Whereas patients with grade II astrocytomas may survive for 5 or more years, those with anaplastic astrocytomas often die within 2 or 3 years and frequently show transformation to GBM. Histologically, the major differences between grade II and grade III tumors are increased cellularity and the presence of mitotic activity, implying that higher proliferative activity is the hallmark of the progression to anaplastic astrocytoma.

A number of molecular abnormalities have been associated with anaplastic astrocytoma, and studies have suggested that most of these abnormalities converge on one critical cell-cycle regulatory complex, which includes the p16, cyclin-dependent kinase-4 (cdk4), cdk6, cyclin D1, and retinoblastoma (Rb) proteins. The simplest schema suggests that p16 inhibits the cdk6/cyclin D1 or cdk4/cyclin D1 complex, preventing these complexes from phosphorylating pRB, and thus ensuring that pRB maintains its brake on the cell cycle. Individual components in this pathway are altered in up to 50% of anaplastic astrocytomas and in the great majority of GBMs.

Chromosome 9p loss occurs in approximately 50% of anaplastic astrocytomas and GBMs, with 9p deletions primarily affecting the region of the CDKN2A gene, which encodes the p16 and ARF proteins. The CDKN2A gene is inactivated either by homozygous deletion or, less commonly, by point mutations or hypermethylation, thereby affecting p16 and ARF expression. The role of p16 in glioma progression has been confirmed in mouse glioma models, in which the presence of a p16 null background is sufficient to change the resulting phenotype from low grade to anaplastic.[9,36,37]

Loss of chromosome 13q occurs in one-third to one-half of high-grade astrocytomas, with the RB1 gene preferentially targeted by losses and inactivating mutations. RB1 and CDKN2A alterations in primary gliomas are inversely correlated and rarely occur together in the same tumor. Inactivation of pRB in mouse astrocytes has been shown to lead to anaplastic astrocytomas.[38] Amplification of the CDK4 gene, located on chromosome 12q13-14, provides an alternative to subvert cell-cycle control and facilitate progression to GBM in 15% of malignant gliomas. CDK4 amplification, CDK6 amplification, and cyclin D1 overexpression appear to represent alternative events to CDKN2A deletions and RB1 alterations, because these genetic changes only rarely occur in the same tumors. Allelic losses of chromosome 19q have been observed in up to 40% of anaplastic astrocytomas and GBMs, indicating a progression-associated glial tumor suppressor gene that maps to 19q13.3, but it is yet to be identified.[12]

PROGRESSION TO GLIOBLASTOMA

GBM is the most malignant grade of astrocytoma, with survival times of less than 2 years for most patients. Histologically, these tumors are characterized by dense cellularity, high proliferation indices, microvascular proliferation, and focal necrosis. The highly proliferative nature of these lesions is no doubt the result of multiple mitogenic effects. As mentioned above, at least one such effect is deregulation of the p16-cdk4–cyclin D1–pRB pathway of cell-cycle control. The vast majority of, if not all, GBMs have alterations of this system, whether they be inactivation of p16 or pRB or overexpression of cdk4.

Chromosome 10 loss is a frequent finding in GBM, occurring in 60% to 95% of GBMs but far less commonly in anaplastic astrocytomas. At least two tumor suppressor loci are present on the long arm of chromosome 10, and there may be a third locus on the short arm. The PTEN/MMAC1/TEP-1 gene at 10q23.3 is one of these genes, with PTEN mutations identified in approximately 20% of GBMs and downstream activation of AKT/PKB in the vast majority of GBMs.[14] PTEN functions as a protein tyrosine phosphatase and also has 3' phosphoinositol phosphatase activity; in addition, PTEN has an amino-terminal domain with homologies to tensin and auxilin.[6] Thus, PTEN may regulate cell migration by dephosphorylating the focal adhesion kinase (FAK) protein or other phosphoprotein targets and may regulate cell proliferation through modulation of the phosphoinositide 3 kinase (PI3-kinase) signaling pathway.[10] Indeed, introduction of wild-type PTEN into glioma cells with inactivated endogenous PTEN leads to growth suppression, and alterations in the PTEN pathway facilitate glioma formation in mouse models.[14,38] DMBT1 is a candidate for a second glioma gene on 10q, but this remains controversial.[31]

In contrast to genetic loss, other genes have increases of their copy number or levels of expression, or both. Epidermal growth factor receptor (EGFR) is a transmembrane receptor tyrosine kinase, whose ligands include EGF and transforming growth factor-α. The EGFR gene is the most frequently amplified oncogene in astrocytic tumors, being amplified in approximately 40% of all GBMs but in few anaplastic astrocytomas. Those GBMs that exhibit EGFR gene amplification have almost always lost genetic material on chromosome 10 and often have CDKN2A deletions. GBMs with EGFR gene amplification display overexpression of EGFR at both the messenger RNA and protein levels, suggesting that activation of this growth signal pathway is integral to malignant progression to GBM. Approximately one-third of those GBMs with EGFR gene amplification also have specific EGFR gene rearrangements, which produce truncated molecules that are constitutively activated in the absence of ligand and that cause dramatic enhancements of tumorigenic properties *in vivo*.[6] Overexpression of another truncated version of EGFR, v-ErbB, in glial cells of transgenic mice results in gliomas.[37] The downstream targets of EGFR activation in GBMs include the Shc-Grb2-ras pathway, involving EGFR in a cascade that facilitates mitogenesis and decreases apoptosis in tumor cells.[24] Less commonly amplified oncogenes include MYCN, PDGF-α receptor, MYCC, GLI, MYB, CDK4, CDK6, MDM-2, and MDM-4.

As mentioned above, one of the hallmarks of GBM is microvascular proliferation. A host of angiogenic growth factors and their receptors are found in GBMs.[6] For example, VEGF and PDGF are expressed by tumor cells, whereas their respective tyrosine kinase receptors, VEGF receptors 1 and 2 and PDGF-β receptor, are expressed on endothelial cells. VEGF and its receptors, in particular, appear to play a major role in GBM angiogenesis.[4] A paracrine mechanism has been suggested in which VEGF is secreted by tumor cells and bound by the VEGF receptors on endothelial cells. Interestingly, VEGF is preferentially up-regulated by tumor cells surrounding regions of necrosis, perhaps as a result of necrosis-induced hypoxia, because hypoxia can up-regulate VEGF. Related mechanisms may also be responsible for tumoral edema in GBM, because some of these angiogenic molecules, such as VEGF, may also cause vascular permeability and, hence, tumoral edema.

SUBSETS OF GLIOBLASTOMA

It is an oversimplification to say that all astrocytomas progress through identifiable genetic stages in a linear fashion. Indeed, it

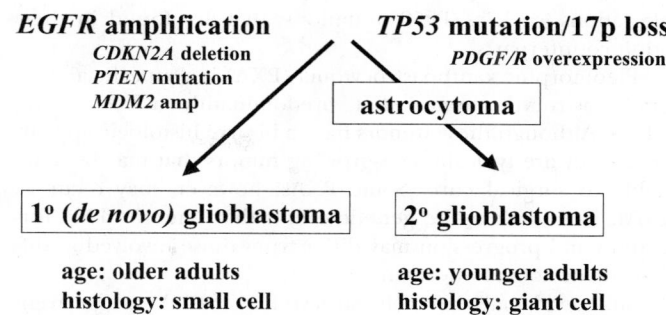

FIGURE 39.1-1. Molecular genetic subsets of glioblastoma (see text for details). EGFR, epidermal growth factor receptor; PDGFR, platelet-derived growth factor receptor.

appears as if there are biologic subsets of astrocytomas that may reflect the clinical heterogeneity observed in these tumors[18] (Fig. 39.1-1). For instance, approximately one-third of GBMs have TP53/chromosome 17p alterations, one-third have EGFR gene amplification, and one-third have neither change.[34] Experimental data also support this distinction by showing that p53-deficient cells are not transformed when cultured in the presence of EGF, whereas they are transformed in the presence of other growth factors.[3] Primary GBMs with TP53 mutations may therefore not be expected to select for cells with EGFR gene amplification if EGFR overexpression does not produce a growth advantage in such cells.[26]

The genetic pathway involving TP53 mutations often involves progression from a lower-grade astrocytic lesion, so-called secondary GBM.[17–19] On the other hand, those GBMs with EGFR amplification may arise either *de novo* or rapidly from a preexisting tumor, without a clinically evident, preceding lower-grade astrocytoma.[17–19] Interestingly, younger age at initial diagnosis has been an important prognostic parameter among patients with GBM, with younger patients faring better than older patients. In turn, those GBMs with loss of chromosome 17p occur in patients younger than those characterized by EGFR gene amplification. The predominance of tumors with 17p loss in a younger population of astrocytoma patients may therefore explain the age-based difference in prognosis.[32] Furthermore, there are sometimes striking histologic differences between GBM with different genetic makeups: Those with TP53 mutations may have a giant cell appearance, whereas those with EGFR gene amplification may have a small cell phenotype.[18,19]

OTHER GLIOMAS

OTHER ASTROCYTOMAS

Pilocytic astrocytoma is the most common astrocytic tumor of childhood and differs clinically and histopathologically from the diffuse, fibrillary astrocytoma that affects adults. These tumors do not have the same genomic alterations as diffuse, fibrillary astrocytomas and frequently affect patients with neurofibromatosis type 1 (NF1). Correspondingly, allelic loss of the NF1 gene region on chromosome 17q occurs in one-fourth of cases, and some pilocytic astrocytomas have reduced NF1 gene expression. Other pediatric astrocytic tumors are histologically similar to adult diffuse astrocytomas, anaplastic astrocytomas, and GBMs; some of these are associated with genetic alterations, such as TP53 mutations, that are found in their adult counterparts.

Pleomorphic xanthoastrocytoma (PXA) is a superficial, low-grade astrocytic tumor that predominantly affects young adults. Although these tumors have a bizarre histologic appearance, they are typically slow-growing tumors that may be amenable to surgical cure. Some PXAs, however, may recur as GBM. Nonetheless, the genetic events that underlie PXA formation and progression may differ from those involved in diffuse astrocytoma tumorigenesis.

Subependymal giant cell astrocytomas (SEGA) are periventricular, low-grade astrocytic tumors that are usually associated with tuberous sclerosis (TS) and are histologically identical to the so-called candle gutterings that line the ventricles of TS patients. Similar to the other tumorous lesions in TS, these are slow growing and may be more akin to hamartomas than true neoplasms. The association of SEGA with TS leads to the prediction that the TS genes, TSC1 on chromosome 9q and TSC2 on chromosome 16p (see Neurologic Tumor Syndromes, later in this chapter), are involved in SEGA formation. Consistent with this prediction, loss of heterozygosity studies have shown allelic loss of chromosome 9q and 16p loci in some SEGAs, particularly of the TSC2 locus on 16p. Interestingly, the gene products of TSC1 and TSC2, hamartin and tuberin, function in the regulatory pathway that involves PTEN (see Progression to Glioblastoma, earlier in this chapter),[23] suggesting that deregulation of the PI3-kinase pathway in this way may play a role in SEGA formation.

OLIGODENDROGLIOMAS AND OLIGOASTROCYTOMAS

Oligodendrogliomas and oligoastrocytomas (mixed gliomas) are diffuse, usually cerebral tumors that are clinically and biologically most closely related to the diffuse, fibrillary astrocytomas. The tumors, however, are less common than diffuse astrocytomas and have generally better prognoses. Patients with WHO grade II oligodendrogliomas, for instance, may have mean survival times of 10 years. In addition, oligodendroglial tumors appear to be differentially chemosensitive when compared with the diffuse astrocytomas.

Allelic losses in oligodendrogliomas and oligoastrocytomas occur preferentially on chromosomes 1p and 19q, affecting 40% to 80% of these tumor types.[28] Because of the frequent loss of these loci in low-grade as well as anaplastic oligodendrogliomas and oligoastrocytomas, the 1p and 19q tumor suppressors are probably important early in oligodendroglial tumorigenesis. Although genes have not yet been identified, chromosome 1p and 19q losses are closely associated. Oligodendroglial tumors with 1p loss typically also have loss of 19q, suggesting that these two putative tumor suppressor genes may be involved in biologically distinct pathways. In fact, microdissection of the oligodendroglial and astrocytic components in oligoastrocytomas has shown that, despite the histologic differences, the molecular changes are identical in these two components. Oligoastrocytomas may also suffer allelic losses of chromosome 17p, although these losses are not often associated with TP53 mutations. Oncogene amplification has only rarely been observed in oligodendroglial tumors.

Oligodendrogliomas and oligoastrocytomas may progress to WHO grade III anaplastic oligodendroglioma or anaplastic oligoastrocytoma, and sometimes to higher-grade tumors with

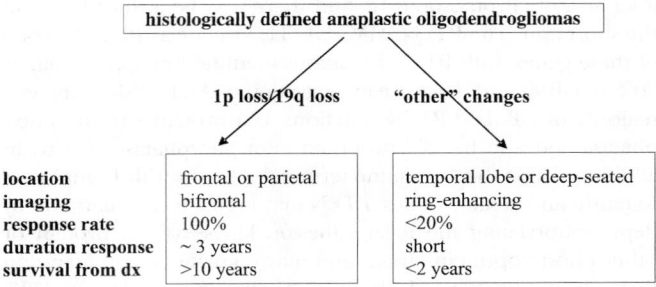

FIGURE 39.1-2.   Molecular genetic subsets of anaplastic oligodendroglioma (see text for details). dx, diagnosis.

histologic features similar to those of GBM. Anaplastic oligodendrogliomas and oligoastrocytomas may display allelic losses of chromosomes 9p involving CDKN2A and chromosome 10 involving PTEN.[28]

Anaplastic oligodendrogliomas have proved to be the first brain tumor for which molecular genetic analysis has had practical clinical ramifications: Anaplastic oligodendrogliomas that have allelic losses of chromosomes 1p and 19q follow different clinical courses from tumors that do not have these genetic changes (Fig. 39.1-2). Anaplastic oligodendrogliomas that have 1p and 19q loss are essentially always sensitive to procarbazine, CCNU, and vincristine (PCV) chemotherapy, with nearly 50% of such tumors demonstrating complete neuroradiologic responses; correspondingly, patients whose tumors have 1p and 19q loss have median survivals of approximately 10 years.[5] These tumors also appear to have better responses to radiation therapy[28] as well as to temozolamide.[7] On the other hand, anaplastic oligodendrogliomas that lack 1p and 19q loss are only PCV sensitive approximately 25% of the time and only rarely have complete neuroradiologic responses; as a result, patients whose anaplastic oligodendrogliomas lack 1p and 19q loss have median survivals of approximately 2 years.[5] Thus, molecular genetic analysis of 1p/19q allelic status has already become a clinically useful test in neurooncology.[15]

At the present time, molecular diagnostic testing is recommended for patients diagnosed with anaplastic oligodendrogliomas, for small cell malignant tumors in which the differential diagnosis is anaplastic oligodendroglioma versus small cell GBM, and for patients with grade II oligodendrogliomas for whom therapeutic decisions might be influenced by additional knowledge of probable tumor behavior.[28] Such observations further suggest that molecular analyses may eventually guide therapeutic decisions for other types of malignant glioma.

EPENDYMOMAS AND CHOROID PLEXUS TUMORS

Ependymomas are a clinically diverse group of gliomas that vary from aggressive intraventricular tumors of children to benign spinal cord tumors in adults. Chromosome 22q loss is common in ependymomas, and spinal ependymomas are associated with mutations and deletions of the neurofibromatosis type 2 (NF2) gene that resides on this chromosome. For cerebral ependymomas, the paucity of NF2 mutations suggests that another, as yet unidentified, chromosome 22q gene will probably be a more integral ependymoma locus.

Choroid plexus tumors are also a varied group of tumors that preferentially occur in the ventricular system, ranging

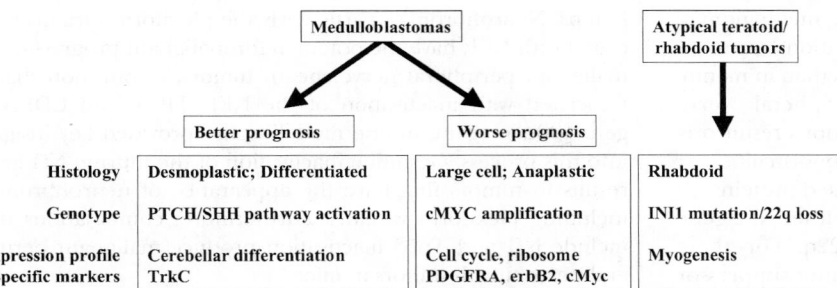

FIGURE 39.1-3. Molecular genetic subsets of pediatric embryonal brain tumors (see text for details). SHH, sonic hedgehog protein.

from aggressive supratentorial intraventricular tumors of children to benign cerebellopontine angle tumors of adults. Choroid plexus tumors have been reported occasionally in patients with Li-Fraumeni syndrome and von Hippel-Lindau (VHL) disease (as well as in Aicardi syndrome, which does not predispose to cancer), raising the possibility that the TP53 gene on chromosome 17p, responsible for Li-Fraumeni syndrome, or the VHL gene on chromosome 3p is involved in choroid plexus neoplasia. Studies of human choroid plexus tumors have not shown TP53 mutations, but choroid plexus neoplasms may be induced in transgenic mice by disrupting p53 and pRB function.[37] VHL mutations have also not been found in choroid plexus tumors, and some reported "choroid plexus" tumors in VHL patients may instead reflect papillary tumors of the middle ear (endolymphatic sac tumors), which occur in higher frequency in VHL patients and which histologically resemble choroid plexus neoplasms.

MEDULLOBLASTOMAS

Medulloblastomas are highly malignant, primitive tumors that arise in the posterior fossa, primarily in children. One-third to one-half of all medulloblastomas have an isochromosome 17q on cytogenetic analysis, and corresponding allelic loss of chromosome 17p has been noted on molecular genetic analysis. TP53 mutations, however, are rare in medulloblastomas, and 17p losses occur preferentially at regions that are telomeric to the TP53 locus, implying the presence of a second, more distal chromosome 17p tumor suppressor gene. Allelic losses of chromosome 6q, 8p, 10q, 11, and 16q have also been noted in these tumors. Oncogene amplification has not been found frequently in medulloblastomas; only MYCC is amplified in significant numbers of cases, and this change appears more common in the more aggressive large cell and anaplastic medulloblastomas. Comparative genomic hybridization studies have demonstrated amplification of chromosome bands 5p15.3 and 11q22.3 and gains of chromosomes 17q and 7.

The discovery of genes underlying two hereditary tumor syndromes has directed attention to two pathways involved in medulloblastoma tumorigenesis. Gorlin's syndrome (also termed *nevoid basal cell carcinoma syndrome*), a condition characterized by multiple basal cell carcinomas, bone cysts, dysmorphic features, and medulloblastomas, arises from defects in PTCH (a homologue of the *Drosophila* patched gene) on the long arm of chromosome 9. Medulloblastomas, particularly the nodular desmoplastic variants that are characteristic of Gorlin's syndrome, can show allelic loss of chromosome 9q and PTCH mutations, and mice that have only one functional copy of the murine Ptch gene are

predisposed to the development of tumors that are histologically identical to medulloblastomas.[35] The protein encoded by PTCH functions in the pathway regulated by the sonic hedgehog protein (SHH). Other molecules in this pathway include smoothened mutation (SMO), and rare SMO mutations have been documented in sporadic medulloblastomas. Intriguingly, germline and somatic mutations, along with allelic loss, have been identified in SUFU, another member of the SHH pathway that maps to 10q.[30,33] In the presence of SUFU mutations, the downstream GLI transcription factor may be unable to leave the nucleus, resulting in the activation of the SHH signaling pathway. Alterations in various members of the SHH pathway likely account for the majority of desmoplastic medulloblastomas. Turcot syndrome, a condition characterized by colonic tumors and brain tumors, is also associated with medulloblastoma; adenomatous polyposis may develop in patients with the phenotype medulloblastomas, and these individuals often have mutations of the APC gene on chromosome 5q. The Apc protein operates in the Wnt signaling pathway that includes β-catenin and axin-1, and rare mutations of these genes have been found in sporadic medulloblastomas. It is likely that other components of this pathway will also be implicated in medulloblastoma tumorigenesis.

The question of whether molecular analyses can provide ancillary information for the management of patients with medulloblastoma has received substantial attention (Fig. 39.1-3). Intriguing evidence has suggested that the level of expression of the trkC receptor may relate to prognosis, with those tumors showing high trkC expression after a more favorable course, and that MYCC amplification correlates with more anaplastic histology and poor prognosis. Expression profiling has been applied to the pediatric embryonal tumors of the brain, including medulloblastoma.[27] Expression profiles of medulloblastomas appear distinct from those of other embryonal brain tumors, and those of desmoplastic medulloblastomas are different from those of classic medulloblastomas; as predicted, the desmoplastic tumors display evidence of SHH pathway activation. Furthermore, expression profiling can distinguish different prognostic groups of medulloblastoma, suggesting that such analyses may play a role in future management of these tumors.

MENINGIOMAS

Meningiomas are common intracranial tumors that arise in the meninges and compress the underlying brain. Meningiomas are usually benign, but some "atypical" meningiomas may recur locally, and some meningiomas are frankly malignant. Monosomy for chromosome 22 and the NF2 gene on chromosome 22q is frequently mutated in meningiomas, clearly implicating it in meningothelial tumorigenesis.[21] In sporadic meningiomas, chromosome 22q allelic loss and NF2 gene mutations are more common in fibroblastic and transitional subtypes than in meningothelial forms. As in schwannomas (see Peripheral Nerve Tumors, later in this chapter), NF2 gene alterations result predominantly in immediate truncations, splicing abnormalities, or altered reading frames, producing grossly truncated proteins.

Approximately 40% of meningiomas have neither NF2 gene mutations nor allelic loss of chromosome 22q. For these tumors, it is likely that a second meningioma tumor suppressor gene is involved. This putative second gene may also be on chromosome 22q or on chromosomes 1p and 3p, but this is a complicated issue because allelic losses in meningiomas have also been reported for a variety of other chromosomes, including 1p, 3p, 5p, 5q, 11, 13, and 17p. The DAL-1 gene may be involved in meningioma pathogenesis, but its role remains unproven.

Atypical and malignant meningiomas are not as common as benign meningiomas. Atypical meningiomas often show allelic losses for chromosomal arms 1p, 6q, 9q, 10q, 14q, 17p, and 18q, suggesting the presence of progression-associated genes there. More frequent losses of chromosomes 6q, 9p, 10, and 14q also occur in anaplastic meningiomas. Chromosome 10 loss, in particular, has been associated with those meningiomas with morphologic features of malignancy, rather than meningiomas that are designated as malignant on the basis of brain invasion alone. Although brain invasion has been considered a histologic indicator of malignancy in meningiomas, molecular genetic analyses have shown that histologically benign meningiomas that invade brain do not have the molecular hallmarks of higher-grade meningiomas.[21] These observations provide another example of how molecular genetic investigations have clarified grading issues in neurooncology.

PERIPHERAL NERVE TUMORS

Schwannomas are benign tumors that arise on peripheral nerves. Schwannomas may arise on cranial nerves, particularly the vestibular portion of the eighth cranial nerve (vestibular schwannomas, acoustic neuromas), where they present as cerebellopontine angle masses. NF2 patients are defined by the presence of bilateral vestibular schwannomas, although unilateral vestibular schwannomas are common in the general population as well. Schwannomas occur frequently in patients with NF2, have frequent loss of chromosome 22q, and harbor NF2 gene mutations in at least 50% of cases, in vestibular tumors as well as schwannomas from other sites. Furthermore, loss of the NF2 gene-encoded merlin protein occurs in all schwannomas, consistent with an integral and universal role for NF2 gene inactivation in schwannoma formation. Thus, inactivation of NF2 is a common feature underlying inherited as well as sporadic forms of schwannoma. Mouse models have now recapitulated Schwann cell tumorigenesis by specifically inactivating the murine Nf2 gene in Schwann cells.[11]

Neurofibromas are also benign tumors of peripheral nerve that most often arise on distal, superficial nerves. Multiple neurofibromas are associated with NF1, suggesting that the NF1 gene on chromosome 17q is involved in the genesis of these benign nerve sheath lesions. Unfortunately, the large size of the NF1 gene has precluded extensive mutational analysis in these

lesions. Neurofibromas, particularly the plexiform variants associated with NF1, have the potential for malignant progression to malignant peripheral nerve sheath tumors, a transition that is associated with inactivation of the NF1, TP53, and CDKN2A genes. Once again, mouse modeling has provided key insights into this process. Germline inactivation of the murine Nf1 gene results in tumors that have the appearance of neurofibromas, including plexiform variants. Furthermore, combinations that include Nf1 and Tp53 inactivation produce malignant peripheral nerve sheath tumors in mice.[8]

MISCELLANEOUS TUMORS

HEMANGIOBLASTOMAS

Hemangioblastomas are tumors of uncertain origin that are composed of endothelial cells, pericytes, and so-called stromal cells. These benign tumors most frequently occur in the cerebellum and spinal cord of young adults. Multiple hemangioblastomas are characteristic of VHL, an inherited tumor syndrome in which patients have a tendency to develop tumors, particularly hemangioblastomas, retinal angiomas, renal cell carcinomas, and pheochromocytomas.[16] Allelic loss occurs in hemangioblastomas in the region of the VHL gene on chromsosome 3p, and the VHL gene is also mutated in sporadic hemangioblastomas, suggesting that it acts as a classic tumor suppressor. The mechanism of action of the VHL protein appears to be complex, with evidence suggesting that it participates in regulation of angiogenic molecules such as VEGF, thus beginning to explain the highly vascular nature of hemangioblastomas and other VHL-associated tumors.[16]

ATYPICAL TERATOID/RHABDOID TUMORS

Atypical teratoid/rhabdoid tumors (AT/RhTs) are uncommon lesions that preferentially affect young children, often in the first few years of life. In the past, these tumors were confused with medulloblastomas. This distinction is of substantial importance, because the prognosis and treatment of the two tumor types differ markedly. Significantly, AT/RhTs are associated with mutations of the INI1/SNF5 gene and loss of the remaining copy of 22q.[2] Occasionally, INI1/SNF5 mutations are found in the germline, including in affected families. The INI1/SNF5 gene is part of a complex of proteins involved in chromatin remodeling. The close genetic relationship of alterations of INI1/SNF5 and chromosome 22q with AT/RhT creates a useful molecular assay, with loss of 22q used as a diagnostic criterion for AT/RhT. Expression profiles of AT/RhTs also differ from those of medulloblastoma,[27] suggesting that other molecular markers may further help in this important differential diagnosis.

NEUROLOGIC TUMOR SYNDROMES

Hereditary neurologic tumor syndromes, in which patients are at risk for development of multiple nervous system tumors, have provided important clues to the genetic basis of brain tumors. Neurologic tumor syndromes include the so-called neurocutaneous syndromes, such as NF1, NF2, TS, and VHL, and other tumor conditions, such as Li-Fraumeni, Turcot, Gorlin's, and Cowden syndromes. Each syndrome is accompanied by a characteristic panoply of neurologic and nonneurologic tumors. A catalog of only the major primary brain tumors would feature optic nerve gliomas and other astrocytomas in NF1; ependymomas in NF2; subependymal giant cell astrocytomas in TS; various malignant gliomas in Li-Fraumeni syndrome, Turcot syndrome, and the hereditary glioma pedigrees; and medulloblastomas in Gorlin's, Turcot, and Li-Fraumeni syndromes. Linkage studies have provided powerful means for tracking the genes associated with these tumor syndromes and have assigned the NF1 gene to chromosome 17q, the NF2 gene to chromosome 22q, the TS genes to chromosomes 9q and 16p, and Turcot genes to chromosome 5q (APC gene) and to the DNA mismatch repair genes on various chromosomes. The NF1 gene codes for a guanosine triphosphatase–activating protein termed *neurofibromin*. Neurofibromin interacts with the p21 product of the *ras* oncogene and is important in growth factor–mediated signal transduction. The NF2 gene codes for a protein, termed *merlin*, which most likely functions by facilitating signal transduction from the cell surface via the cytoskeleton. The TS gene products, tuberin from TSC2 on chromosome 16p and hamartin from the TSC1 gene on 9q, bind one another and function in a single cellular pathway that involves PTEN and AKT/PKB. For the Li-Fraumeni syndrome, mutational analyses have implicated the TP53 gene on 17p and the hCHK2 gene on 22q. Although uncommon, the benign cerebellar lesion known as *Lhermitte-Duclos disease* or *dysplastic gangliocytoma* is sometimes associated with the Cowden syndrome, a hereditary condition in which breast cancer and skin tumors also develop and which results from germline mutations of the PTEN gene. Indeed, mouse models in which PTEN inactivation has been accomplished in the cerebellum have resulted in lesions similar to those seen in Lhermitte-Duclos.

CONCLUSION

Human brain tumors have molecular alterations that are characteristic of each type of tumor and of most stages of progression. For instance, the formation of low-grade astrocytoma and the subsequent progression to anaplastic astrocytoma and GBM involve alterations of distinct tumor suppressor genes and oncogenes. Furthermore, molecular genetic analysis has been used to distinguish subsets of astrocytomas. For instance, one type of GBM, characterized by TP53 gene mutations, is more common in younger patients, may feature giant cells, and can be associated with slower progression from lower-grade astrocytoma; another type of GBM, characterized by EGFR gene amplification or mutation, is more common in older patients, can have a small cell phenotype, and may be associated with more rapid progression or *de novo* growth. In the case of anaplastic oligodendrogliomas, molecular genetic subtyping has already provided practical information for the management of patients, because tumors with chromosome 1p and 19q loss are differentially chemosensitive and more indolent.

For the less common gliomas and for other primary tumors, such as medulloblastomas, molecular genetic studies have defined sets of genetic alterations that may have clinical relevance. For meningiomas and schwannomas, the NF2 gene has been clearly implicated, although other genetic alterations must underlie the formation of some meningiomas as well. For those tumors associated with hereditary tumor syndromes, such as the SEGAs in TS and the hemangioblastomas in VHL, the same genes appear responsible for the syndromes when mutated in the germline, and for sporadic tumors when mutated on a somatic basis. At the present time, however, these molecular data are incomplete. Mouse models, based on alterations of genes involved in the human tumors, have gone a long way toward recapitulating some of the cardinal features of human brain tumors. In the future, these models may be useful for preclinical trials of therapeutic agents. In the short term, such models will certainly help elucidate the key pathways involved in tumorigenesis. Once the molecular pathways are completely understood, such knowledge will no doubt contribute to the development of more effective therapies for many of these tumors.

REFERENCES

1. Bachoo RM, Maher EA, Ligon K, et al. Epidermal growth factor receptor and Ink4a/Arf: convergent mechanisms governing terminal differentiation and transformation along the neural stem cell to astrocyte axis. *Cancer Cell* 2002;1:269.
2. Biegel JA, Tan L, Zhang F, et al. Alterations of the hSNF5/INI1 gene in central nervous system atypical teratoid/rhabdoid tumors and renal and extrarenal rhabdoid tumors. *Clin Cancer Res* 2002;8:3461.
3. Bogler O, Huang H-JS, Cavenee WK. Loss of wild-type p53 bestows a growth advantage on primary cortical astrocytes and facilitates their in vitro transformation. *Cancer Res* 1995;55:2746.
4. Brat DJ, Van Meir EG. Glomeruloid microvascular proliferation orchestrated by VPF/VEGF: a new world of angiogenesis research. *Am J Pathol* 2001;158:789.
5. Cairncross JG, Ueki K, Zlatescu MC. Specific chromosomal losses predict chemotherapeutic response and survival in patients with anaplastic oligodendrogliomas. *J Natl Cancer Inst* 1998;90:1473.
6. Cavenee WK, Furnari FB, Nagane M. Diffuse astrocytomas. In: Kleihues P, Cavenee WK, eds. *Pathology and genetics of tumours of the nervous system*. Lyon: International Agency for Research on Cancer, 2000.
7. Chahlavi A, Kanner A, Peereboom D. Impact of chromosome 1p status in response of oligodendroglioma to temozolomide: preliminary results. *J Neurooncol* 2003;61:267.
8. Cichowski K, Shih TS, Schmitt E, et al. Mouse models of tumor development in neurofibromatosis type 1. *Science* 1999;286:2172.
9. Dai C, Celestino JC, Okada Y, et al. PDGF autocrine stimulation dedifferentiates cultured astrocytes and induces oligodendrogliomas and oligoastrocytomas from neural progenitors and astrocytes in vivo. *Genes Dev* 2001;15:1913.
10. Furnari FB, Lin H, Huang HS, et al. Growth suppression of glioma cells by PTEN requires a functional phosphatase catalytic domain. *Proc Natl Acad Sci U S A* 1997;94:12479.
11. Giovannini M, Robanus-Maandag E, van der Valk M, et al. Conditional biallelic Nf2 mutation in the mouse promotes manifestations of human neurofibromatosis type 2. *Genes Dev* 2000;14:1617.
12. Hartmann C, Johnk L, Kitange G, et al. Transcript map of the 3.7-Mb D19S112-D19S246 candidate tumor suppressor region on the long arm of chromosome 19. *Cancer Res* 2002;62:4100.
13. Holland EC. Gliomagenesis: genetic alterations and mouse models. *Nat Rev Genet* 2001;2:120.
14. Holland EC, Celestino J, Dai C, et al. Combined activation of Ras and Akt in neural progenitors induces glioblastoma formation in mice. *Nat Genet* 2000;25:55.
15. Ino Y, Betensky RA, Zlatescu MC, et al. Molecular subtypes of anaplastic oligodendroglioma: implications for patient management at diagnosis. *Clin Cancer Res* 2001;7:839.
16. Kaelin WG Jr. Molecular basis of the VHL hereditary cancer syndrome. *Nat Rev Cancer* 2002;2:673.
17. Kleihues P, Cavenee WK. *World Health Organization classification of tumours of the nervous system*. Lyon: WHO/IARC, 2000.
18. Louis DN, Holland EC, Cairncross JG. Glioma classification: a molecular reappraisal. *Am J Pathol* 2001;159:779.
19. Louis DN, Pomeroy SL, Cairncross JG. Focus on CNS neoplasia. *Cancer Cell* 2002;1:125.
20. Louis DN, Posner JB, Jacobs T, et al. Report of the brain tumor progress review group. World Wide Web URL: http://prg.nci.nih.gov/brain/finalreport.html, 2004.
21. Louis DN, Scheithauer BW, von Deimling A, et al. Meningiomas. In: Kleihues P, Cavenee WK, eds. *World Health Organization classification of tumours of the central nervous system*. Lyon: IARC/WHO, 2000.
22. Maher EA, Furnari FB, Bachoo RM, et al. Malignant glioma: genetics and biology of a grave matter. *Genes Dev* 2001;15:1311.
23. Manning BD, Tee AR, Logsdon MN, et al. Identification of the tuberous sclerosis complex-2 tumor suppressor gene product tuberin as a target of the phosphoinositide 3-kinase/akt pathway. *Mol Cell* 2002;10:151.
24. Nagane M, Coufal F, Lin H, et al. A common mutant epidermal growth factor receptor confers enhanced tumorigenicity on human glioblastoma cells by increasing proliferation and reducing apoptosis. *Cancer Res* 1996;56:5079.
25. Nutt CL, Mani DR, Betensky RA, et al. Gene expression-based classification of malignant gliomas correlates better with survival than histological classification. *Cancer Res* 2003;63:1602.

26. Okada Y, Hurwitz EE, Esposito JM. Selection pressures of TP53 mutation and microenvironmental location influence EGFR gene amplification in human glioblastomas. *Cancer Res* 2003;63:413.

27. Pomeroy SL, Tamayo P, Gaasenbeek M, et al. Prediction of central nervous system embryonal tumour outcome based on gene expression. *Nature* 2002;415:436.

28. Reifenberger G, Louis DN. Oligodendroglioma: toward molecular definitions in diagnostic neuro-oncology. *J Neuropathol Exp Neurol* 2003;62:111.

29. Reilly KM, Loisel DA, Bronson RT, et al. Nf1;Trp53 mutant mice develop glioblastoma with evidence of strain-specific effects. *Nat Genet* 2000;26:109.

30. Rubin JB, Rowitch DH. Medulloblastoma: a problem of developmental biology. *Cancer Cell* 2002;2:7.

31. Sasaki H, Betensky RA, Cairncross JG, et al. DMBT1 polymorphisms: relationship to malignant glioma tumorigenesis. *Cancer Res* 2002;62:1790.

32. Simmons ML, Lamborn KR, Takahashi M, et al. Analysis of complex relationships between age, p53, epidermal growth factor receptor, and survival in glioblastoma patients. *Cancer Res* 2001;61:1122.

33. Taylor MD, Liu L, Raffel C, et al. Mutations in SUFU predispose to medulloblastoma. *Nat Genet* 2002;31:306.

34. von Deimling A, von Ammon K, Schoenfeld D, et al. Subsets of glioblastoma multiforme defined by molecular genetic analysis. *Brain Pathol* 1993;3:19.

35. Wechsler-Reya R, Scott MP. The developmental biology of brain tumors. *Annu Rev Neurosci* 2001;24:385.

36. Weiss WA, Burns MJ, Hackett C, et al. Genetic determinants of malignancy in a mouse model for oligodendroglioma. *Cancer Res* 2003;63:1589.

37. Weiss WA, Israel M, Cobbs C, et al. Neuropathology of genetically engineered mice: consensus report and recommendations from an international forum. *Oncogene* 2002;21:7453.

38. Xiao A, Wu H, Pandolfi PP, et al. Astrocyte inactivation of the pRb pathway predisposes mice to malignant astrocytoma development that is accelerated by PTEN mutation. *Cancer Cell* 2002;1:157.

39. Zhu Y, Parada LF. The molecular and genetic basis of neurological tumours. *Nat Rev Cancer* 2002;2:616.

HOWARD A. FINE
FRED G. BARKER II
JAMES M. MARKERT
JAY S. LOEFFLER

SECTION 2

Neoplasms of the Central Nervous System

GENERAL CONSIDERATIONS

EPIDEMIOLOGY OF BRAIN TUMORS

Incidence and Prevalence

Studies using data from the Surveillance, Epidemiology, and End Results (SEER) registry report that the incidence of primary tumors of the central nervous system (CNS) is between 2 and 19 per 100,000 per year depending on age.[1] From birth to age 4 years the incidence of primary brain tumors is approximately 3.1 per 100,000 and then slowly declines to a nadir of 1.8 per 100,000 in persons aged 15 to 24 years. The incidence then rises again to a relative plateau around age 65 years with an incidence of approximately 18 cases per 100,000 persons.

The epidemiology of primary brain tumors is complex, because a large number of histologic subtypes of tumors arise within the CNS, reflecting the diversity of cell types found there. Few tumor registries or databases contain detailed information on histologic subtype of CNS tumors, a situation aggravated by frequent changes in classification schemas for CNS tumors. Nevertheless, based on informal reviews of the literature and case series from the neuropathologic literature, an estimate of the approximate frequency of 15 major subgroups of CNS tumors can be made (Table 39.2-1). Such percentages can be misleading because the frequency of particular subtypes of tumors is highly dependent on age. For example, although gliomas are the most common type of primary brain tumor—accounting for nearly 50% of all primary CNS neoplasms—gliomas represent a minority of primary brain tumors in children. By contrast, primitive neuroectodermal tumors (PNETs) represent the most common primary brain tumor in the pediatric population but are relatively uncommon in adults. Estimating the incidence and prevalence for any given tumor

subtype is further complicated because age is a continuous variable, not truly separable into discrete categories such as childhood and adulthood. Thus, whereas PNETs are generally considered pediatric brain tumors, a fair number of young adults are also affected, although the frequency of the diagnosis falls rapidly in middle-aged and older persons. Similarly, the frequency of glioma subtypes is age dependent: Low-grade tumors are much more prevalent in children and young adults, whereas malignant tumors (particularly glioblastomas) are increasingly more common in the elderly populations.

Another factor that complicates assessment of primary brain tumor incidence is that tumor registries only include cases with a histologic diagnosis. Many primary brain tumors, however, are never histologically confirmed. These tumors are diagnosed based on their radiographic appearance and clinical presentation because resection or biopsy would be too dangerous (infiltrating pontine gliomas) or because the diagnosis

TABLE 39.2-1. Frequency of Primary Intracranial Central Nervous System (CNS) Tumors

Histopathology	Primary Brain Tumors (%)	Gliomas (%)
Glioblastoma multiforme	21.7	47
Malignant astrocytomas	16.6	36
All oligodendroglioma	3.1	6.7
All ependymomas	2.3	5.1
Low-grade astrocytoma	1.8	3.9
Meningioma and other mesenchymal tumors	26.7	—
Pituitary	9.7	—
Nerve sheath (e.g., schwannoma)	7.3	—
CNS lymphoma	3.5	—
Medulloblastoma and other primitive neuroectodermal tumors	1.7	—
All neuron and neuron/glial tumors	1.0	—
Craniopharyngioma	1.0	—
Germ cell	0.5	—
Choroid plexus	0.3	—
Other tumors	2.7	—

(Data from ref. 1.)

TABLE 39.2-2. Distribution of Primary Spinal Tumors[a]

Histology	Sloof et al.[451]	Preston-Martin[456]
Schwannoma	29.0	22.0
Meningioma	25.5	42.0
Ependymoma	12.8	15.1
Sarcomas	11.9	—
Astrocytoma	6.5	11.2
Other gliomas	—	1.9
Vascular tumors	6.2	—
Chordomas	4.0	—
Epidermoids	1.4	—
Other	2.7	5.6

[a]Lipoma and subarachnoid seeding from primary intracranial tumor.

based on imaging is secure and no immediate therapeutic intervention is required (meningiomas, acoustic neuromas). Finally, many tumor registries, including SEER, have historically excluded low-grade CNS tumors such as pituitary adenomas and meningiomas from data collection because they are not truly cancer. A bill passed by Congress in 2002, however, overturned this practice, and since 2003 the SEER registry has collected data on all histologically diagnosed meningiomas.

Specific CNS tumor types differ in incidence based on anatomic location. Approximately 15% of all primary CNS tumors arise in the spinal cord, where the distribution of tumor types is significantly different from that in the brain (Table 39.2-2). Tumors of the lining of the spinal cord and nerve roots predominate (50% to 80% of all spinal tumors); schwannomas and meningiomas are most common, followed by ependymomas. Unlike in the brain, primary gliomas of the spinal cord are uncommon.

Given the problems in determining the true prevalence of CNS tumors, it is not surprising that it has been difficult to estimate whether the incidence of CNS tumors is changing. A 1990 study reported a very large increase in the incidence of malignant gliomas in the elderly.[2] These and other similar findings have been partially attributed to the greater availability of diagnostic imaging tests such as computed tomography (CT) and magnetic resonance imaging (MRI) over the last two decades, which potentially causes screening artifact.

Etiologic Factors

There are few proven etiologic risk factors for the development of brain tumors. The clearest risk factor for the development of a primary brain tumor is the presence of a hereditary tumor syndrome associated with such tumors. The most common genetic syndromes associated with CNS tumors are the neurofibromatoses. Neurofibromatosis type 1 (NF1) is an autosomal dominant disorder affecting 1 in 3000 individuals that causes intracranial and extracranial benign Schwann cell tumors. Other CNS tumors such as optic gliomas, astrocytomas, and meningiomas also occur at significantly higher frequency in patients with NF1. NF2 is far less common than NF1, occurring in only approximately 1 in 35,000 individuals, and is characterized by bilateral acoustic neuromas and meningiomas. Although systemic schwannomas also occur in NF2, there does not appear to be an increased frequency of other

systemic tumors. Other hereditary tumor syndromes affecting the CNS include Li-Fraumeni syndrome (germline mutation in one p53 allele; malignant gliomas); von Hippel-Lindau syndrome (germline mutation of the VHL gene; cerebral and spinal hemangioblastomas), and Turcot's syndrome (germline mutations of the adenomatous polyposis gene; medulloblastoma). The nevoid basal cell carcinoma syndrome (Gorlin's syndrome) is associated with medulloblastomas (and possibly an increased risk of meningiomas) and represents mutations in the PTCH gene or other members of the sonic hedgehog signaling pathway.[3,4]

Besides these hereditary cancer syndromes, there are few well-established risk factors for primary brain tumors. Meningiomas and schwannomas are more common in females, whereas gliomas, medulloblastomas, and most other CNS tumors are more common in males.[5–7] Meningiomas are more common in African Americans and gliomas and medulloblastomas in whites.[7] Finally, it has been suggested that there is a lower incidence of meningiomas and a higher incidence of gliomas and vestibular schwannomas in higher socioeconomic groups.[5,7–14]

Environmental and occupational risk factors for brain tumors have also been sought. The Radiation Epidemiology Branch of the National Cancer Institute has completed one of the largest case-control studies of such factors to date. Although data analysis continues, several interesting findings have already emerged. No association between the development of brain tumors and cellular telephone use was found.[15] A history of allergies or autoimmune diseases was protective for the development of primary brain tumors.[16] Handedness was shown to be a risk factor, with individuals describing themselves as left-handed or ambidextrous having a reduced risk of glioma.[17] Finally, there was no increased risk of developing a brain tumor associated with previous polio vaccination, which discredits claims that simian virus 40 (or other viruses) contaminating older polio vaccine preparations cause brain tumors.[18]

CLASSIFICATION

The pathologic classification of CNS tumors is complicated because of the many cell types that constitute the CNS, any of which can transform into a neoplastic phenotype. The frequency of individual tumor types roughly parallels the relative frequency of cell types within the CNS and their normal proliferative capacity. Astrocytes are among the most common cell types in the CNS and are mitogenically competent; thus astrocytomas are the most common primary CNS tumor. In contrast, although neurons are also numerous in the CNS, they are postmitotic, and therefore neuronally derived tumors are uncommon.

CNS tumors can be divided into tumors derived from glial cells, neuronal cells, cells that surround or insulate the CNS, and cells that form specialized anatomic structures. Glial cells that are thought to give rise to specific tumor types include astrocytes (astrocytomas), oligodendrocytes (oligodendrogliomas), and ependymal cells (ependymomas). Neuronal cells identified as the precursors for specific tumors include the cerebellar external granular cells (medulloblastoma) and neuroblasts (PNETs). In PNETs, the cell of origin does not entirely specify the transformed tumor phenotype, because the anatomic location is also pivotal. Thus, transformation of neuroblasts in the cortex leads to cortical PNETs, transformation of retinal neuroblast leads to retinoblastoma, and transformation of pineal gland neuroblasts causes pineoblastomas. Transformation of cells lining the CNS cause meningiomas (derived from arachnoid cells) and schwannomas (derived from Schwann cells). Specialized anatomic structures within the CNS and the tumors arising there include the pituitary gland (pituitary adenomas), pineal gland (pineocytomas), notochord remnants (chordomas), endothelial or stromal vascular cells (hemangioblastomas), primitive germ cells (all subtypes of germ cell tumors), and choroidal epithelial cells (choroid plexus papillomas and carcinomas).

Although the classical description of the cell of origin depicted previously is satisfyingly straightforward, this schema remains speculative, sometimes based on scanty phenotypical and immunohistochemical evidence. For example, oligodendrogliomas are diagnosed based on cellular morphology, including prominent nuclei surrounded by a cytoplasmic halo with a characteristic "fried egg" appearance. However, no definitive markers for oligodendrogliomas currently exist; these tumors can stain both for glial fibrillary acidic protein, an astrocytic marker, and for synaptophysin, a presumptive neuronal marker.[19] Indeed, as many as a third of all gliomas have morphologic characteristics of both astrocytoma and oligodendroglioma (i.e., mixed glioma). Evidence suggesting that some oligodendrocytes derive from a neuronal lineage whereas some neuron-derived tumors (embryonal tumors) can show significant areas of glial differentiation demonstrates the uncertainly within the field.[20,21]

Thus, it is possible that the long-accepted dogma that specific CNS tumor types are derived from specific normal differentiated cell types within the CNS may in fact be incorrect. An alternative view is that because all neuroepithelial cells are derived from a common precursor cell (i.e., a multipotent neural stem cell), all neuroepithelial tumors are derived from neural stem cells or their committed progeny.[22] This theory holds that tumors of neural stem cell origin might exhibit phenotypic characteristics of a terminally differentiated cell either because the neural stem cell of origin had undergone partial differentiation before the transforming event(s) or through the partial induction of the differentiation process through genetic perturbations responsible for transformation itself.

Proper and complete classification of tumors is important, because tumor subtyping can affect prognosis and treatment recommendations as much as does the general tumor category. Specific pathologic subtypes of clinical importance are described in this chapter within the sections covering the individual tumor types. Tumor location and patient age are also relevant in tumor classification. For instance, astrocytomas of the spine, brainstem, and cortex may portend very different prognoses. Whether the different natural histories reflect different neuroanatomic constraints or diverse biologic properties of these tumors in various locations, or both, is not known. Finally, patient age may not only influence prognosis but may actually predict a totally different tumor type. For example, tumors in many young adults with glioblastomas (the most aggressive type of astrocytoma) have the genetic and behavioral characteristics of tumors derived from lower-grade gliomas ("secondary glioblastomas"), whereas almost all older patients have *de novo* ("primary") glioblastomas.[22]

ANATOMIC AND CLINICAL CONSIDERATIONS

The clinical presentation of the various tumors is best appreciated by considering the relation of signs and symptoms to anatomy.[23]

INTRACRANIAL TUMORS

Intracranial tumors produce two kinds of symptoms: general symptoms related to intracranial pressure (ICP) and local symptoms that are specific to the tumor's location. Essentially all brain tumors can produce headache. The brain itself is not pain sensitive, and tumor headache is thought to arise from the dura and intracranial vessels. Meningiomas and other slow-growing tumors may grow remarkably large without producing headache, whereas more rapidly growing tumors can cause headache early in their course. Other mechanisms through which small tumors can cause headache include growth within an enclosed space, such as the cavernous sinus, or obstructive hydrocephalus, in which the ventricles rather than the tumor are the bulk of the extra mass. Nausea and vomiting, personality changes, and slowing of psychomotor function or even somnolence may be present with increased ICP.

Headaches can be mild and intermittent or constant and severe. Because ICP increases with recumbency and hypoventilation during sleep, early morning headache is typical. Focal headache location can be misleading; frontal and temporal tumors may produce headache in frontal, retroorbital, or temporal regions. Hydrocephalus can also produce similar headaches. Sometimes the only presenting symptoms are changes in personality, mood, or mental capacity, or slowing of psychomotor activity. These changes often are apparent to the family and the examiner but not to the patient; they may be confused with depression, especially in older patients.

Although fewer than 6% of first seizures result from brain tumors, almost one-half of patients with supratentorial brain tumors present with seizures. The value of a focal seizure in localizing tumors is so high that an MRI is almost always indicated in an adult patient with a first seizure. The distribution of primary glial brain tumors is proportional to the volume of the lobes. Frontal tumors are more common than parietal tumors, followed by temporal and occipital lobe tumors in order of frequency. Tumors in particular locations do not produce classic neurologic syndromes as reliably as do strokes, but focal syndromes do help to localize the tumor or at least can suggest the diagnosis.

The frontal lobe syndrome varies with tumor location. Anterior tumors cause changes in personality, loss of initiative, and abulia and may be quite large at presentation. Posterior frontal lobe tumors involve motor cortex and produce contralateral weakness, with expressive aphasia in the dominant (usually left) frontal lobe. Bifrontal disease, as from infiltrative "butterfly" gliomas and primary CNS lymphomas, typically causes impairment of memory, lability of mood, urinary incontinence, and frank dementia, with prominent grasp, suck, and snout reflexes.

Temporal lobe syndromes range from symptoms detectable only on careful testing of perception and spatial judgment to severe memory impairment. Homonymous superior quadrantanopsia, auditory hallucinations, and abnormal behavior can occur with tumors in either temporal lobe. Nondominant temporal lobe tumors can cause minor perceptual problems and spatial disorientation. Dominant temporal lobe tumors can present with dysnomia, impaired perception of verbal commands, and ultimately a fluent (Wernicke's-like) aphasia.

Parietal lobe tumors affect sensory and perceptual functions more than motor modalities. Tumors in either parietal lobe can produce sensory disorders ranging from mild sensory extinction or stereoagnosis, observable only by testing, to a more severe sensory loss such as hemianesthesia. Poor proprioception in the affected limb is common. Homonymous inferior quadrantanopsia, an incongruent hemianopsia, or visual inattention also may occur. Nondominant parietal lobe tumors cause contralateral neglect and, in severe cases, anosognosia and apraxia for self-dressing. Dominant parietal lobe tumors lead to alexia, dysgraphia, and certain types of apraxia. Occipital lobe tumors can produce contralateral homonymous hemianopsia or complex visual aberrations affecting perception of color, object size, or location. Bilateral occipital disease, rarely seen at presentation, can produce cortical blindness.

The classic corpus callosum disconnection syndromes are rare in brain tumor patients, even though infiltrative gliomas often cross the corpus callosum in the region of the genu or the splenium. Interruption of the anterior part of the corpus callosum can cause a failure of the left hand to carry out spoken commands. Lesions in the posterior corpus callosum interrupt visual fibers connecting the right occipital lobe to the left angular gyrus, causing an inability to read or name colors.

Thalamic tumors cause both local effects and obstructive hydrocephalus. Tumors in the thalamus and, less often, in the basal ganglia can reach 3 to 4 cm in diameter before symptoms attract attention. Headaches from generalized hydrocephalus or trapping of one lateral ventricular horn are common. Either sensory or motor syndromes or, on the dominant side, aphasia is possible. "Thalamic" pain disorders or motor syndromes from basal ganglia involvement also occur.

The brainstem, composed of the midbrain, pons, and medulla, has both nuclear groups and traversing axons. Tumors can be primarily intrinsic, intrinsic with exophytic components in the fourth ventricle or basal cisterns, or extraaxial. Cranial nerve involvement can be at the nuclear level or from involvement as the nerve leaves the brainstem or traverses the basal cerebrospinal fluid (CSF) cisterns. The most common brainstem tumor is the pontine astrocytoma (glioma), which presents with cranial nerve VI and VII palsies on one side in 90% of patients. Long tract signs usually follow, with hemiplegia, unilateral limb ataxia, ataxia of gait, paraplegia, hemisensory syndromes, gaze disorders, and occasionally hiccups.

The midbrain, juxtaposed between the pons and the cerebral hemispheres, encompasses the tectum, the cerebral peduncles, and the cerebral aqueduct. Tectal involvement causes Parinaud's syndrome, peduncular lesions cause contralateral motor impairment, and obstruction of the aqueduct causes hydrocephalus.

Tumors in the medulla can have a fulminant course, including deficits in cranial nerves VII, IX, and X, dysphagia, and dysarthria. Involvement of the medullary cardiac and respiratory centers can result in a rapidly progressive course. Unlike with the other tumors of the posterior fossa, headache, vomiting, and papilledema occur late. Fourth ventricular tumors, because of their location, cause symptomatic obstructive hydrocephalus at a relatively small size, with associated disturbances of gait and balance. Rapidly enlarging lesions may end in cerebellar herniation.

Cerebellar tumors have valuable localizing presentations. Midline lesions in and around the vermis cause truncal and gait ataxia, whereas more lateral hemispheric lesions lead to unilateral appendicular ataxia, usually worst in the arm. Abnormal head position, with the head tilting back and away from the side of the tumor, is seen often in children but rarely in adults. Bilateral sixth cranial nerve palsies are uncommon and reflect hydrocephalus.

Mass lesions within or abutting the brain or spinal cord can cause displacement of vital neurologic structures. This can lead, in the brain, to herniation syndromes with respiratory arrest and death and, in the spine, to paraplegia or quadriplegia. Intracranial tumors can cause herniation of various types: subfalcine, transtentorial, or through the foramen magnum (tonsillar). Subfalcine herniation, usually from a unilateral frontal tumor, is often asymptomatic. In transtentorial (temporal lobe) herniation, the medial temporal lobe shifts into the tentorial notch, compressing cranial nerve III and the ipsilateral cerebral peduncle. Coma usually follows. Rapidly increasing supratentorial mass effect leading to herniation has many causes, of which tumor growth is one. More common is a dramatic increase in peritumoral edema, especially resulting from hyponatremia or hypoosmolarity. The injudicious use of parenteral hypoosmolar 5% dextrose in water can lead to herniation. Seizures, which are associated with hypoventilation, can produce a resultant increase in brain edema and herniation. In tonsillar herniation, increasing posterior fossa mass effect displaces one or both cerebellar tonsils into the foramen magnum, causing posturing, coma, and respiratory arrest.[24]

Both tonsillar and transtentorial herniation are rapidly fatal without prompt intervention. Immediate treatment may include ventriculostomy placement and intravenous administration of mannitol. Intubation with induced hyperventilation is usually necessary. Large doses of synthetic glucocorticoids, such as dexamethasone, should also be given to reduce edema, although their action is not immediate. Usually surgical decompression is necessary.

Hemorrhage into a tumor can also cause acute neurologic deterioration. This is often associated with iatrogenic coagulopathies such as thrombocytopenia due to chemotherapy or anticoagulation therapy for deep venous thrombosis. Primary tumors that most often bleed *de novo* are glioblastoma and oligodendrogliomas; of the metastatic tumors, lung cancer, melanoma, renal cell cancer, thyroid cancer, and choriocarcinoma most often show hemorrhage. Treatment for intratumoral hemorrhage may include reversal of anticoagulation and administration of osmotic agents and glucocorticoids, but if it is extensive and life threatening, surgical decompression is needed.

Lumbar puncture should never be performed in any of the acute herniation syndromes or when herniation is imminent. In fact, lumbar puncture should never be done in the setting of significantly elevated ICP from a brain tumor. The indications for lumbar puncture are discussed later in this chapter in Neurodiagnostic Tests.

SPINAL AXIS TUMORS

For the clinical presentation of tumors of the spinal axis to be understood, the local anatomy must be appreciated (Fig. 39.2-1).

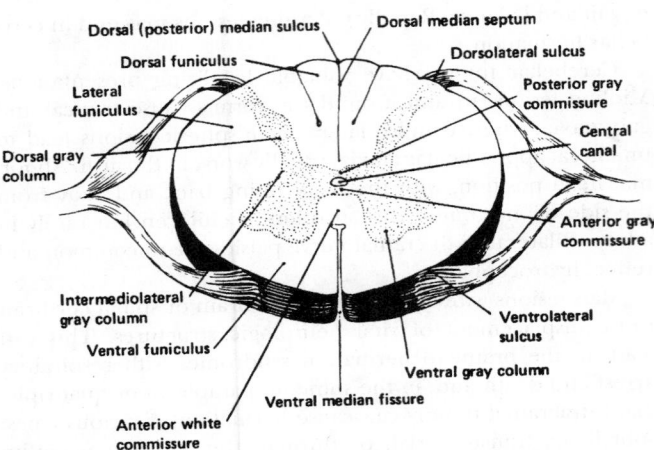

FIGURE 39.2-1. Cross section of thoracic spinal cord shows relation of spinal nerves to intraspinal tracts.

Intracranially the dura is adherent to the skull and there is normally no extradural space. In the spinal canal the extradural space contains fat and blood vessels. Through the intervertebral foramina, the extradural space communicates with the mediastinum and the retroperitoneum. Nearly all extradural tumors are metastases, arising from hematogenous spread, direct extension from adjacent vertebral bodies, or through the foramina.

Intradural spinal tumors arise from the spinal cord (intramedullary) or from surrounding structures (extramedullary). The two common extramedullary intradural tumors, schwannoma and meningioma, arise from nerve roots and from the dura, respectively, and involve the spinal cord by compression. A spinal tumor can produce local (focal) and distal (remote) symptoms, or both. Local effects indicate the tumor's location along the spinal axis, and distal effects reflect involvement of motor and sensory long tracts within the cord. Table 39.2-3 summarizes the clinical findings useful in localizing a spinal cord tumor.

Distal effects are common to all spinal tumors sooner or later, and symptoms and signs are confined to structures inner-

TABLE 39.2-3. Clinical Manifestations of Spinal Cord Tumors

Location	Findings
Foramen magnum	11th and 12th cranial nerve palsies; ipsilateral arm weakness early; cerebellar ataxia; and neck pain
Cervical	Ipsilateral arm weakness with leg and opposite arm in time; wasting and fibrillation of ipsilateral neck, shoulder girdle, and arm; decreased pain and temperature sensation in upper cervical regions early; and pain in cervical distribution
Thoracic	Weakness of abdominal muscles; sparing of arms; unilateral root pains; and sensory level with ipsilateral changes early and bilateral with time
Lumbosacral	Root pain in groin region or sciatic distribution, or both; weakened proximal pelvic muscles; impotence; bladder paralysis; and decreased knee jerk and brisk ankle jerks
Cauda equina	Unilateral pain in back and leg becoming bilateral when the tumor is quite large; and bladder and bowel paralysis

vated below the level of the tumor. Neurologic manifestations often begin unilaterally, with weakness and spasticity, if the tumor lies above the conus medullaris, or weakness and flaccidity, if at or below the conus. Impairment of sphincter and sexual function occurs later unless the tumor is in the conus. The upper level of impaired long tract function usually is several segments below the tumor's actual site. Local manifestations may reflect involvement of bone (with axial pain) or spinal roots, with radicular pain and loss of motor and sensory functions of the root or roots.

Occasionally, a cervical intramedullary tumor mimics syringomyelia, with dissociated sensory loss, weakness, and wasting in the arms and hands with variable long tract involvement. In most instances, the clinical presentation of a spinal tumor does not indicate if it is extradural or intradural. Axial pain preceding paraplegia with a history of previously diagnosed cancer suggests metastasis, and appropriate imaging of any cancer patient with new axial back pain is axiomatic.

NEURODIAGNOSTIC TESTS

NEUROIMAGING

Neuroimaging has many important roles in the care of brain tumor patients. These include refinement of the differential diagnosis based on imaging characteristics and anatomic site; precise anatomic localization for surgical or radiotherapeutic planning; measurement of residual tumor size after surgery, radiation or chemotherapy; and detection of late effects of therapy. MRI and CT are the major neuroimaging techniques used to demonstrate intracranial and spinal lesions. Both modalities produce cross-sectional images. CT images reflect tissue attenuation of x-rays. MRI pixel intensity is based on proton density, T1 and T2 relaxation times, and blood flow. For most tumors, gadolinium-enhanced MRI is the modality of choice because of higher sensitivity to pathologic alterations in brain tissue and superior anatomic resolution. Vasogenic edema associated with brain tumors involves fluid that has leaked through an incompetent blood–brain barrier (BBB). On CT scan it is hypodense (dark) compared with normal brain tissue. On MRI, edema appears as an area of low signal intensity on T1-weighted images and high signal intensity on T2-weighted images.

MRI is superior to CT in evaluating hydrocephalus and its causes, because all three orthogonal planes can be reviewed. Selective dilatation of one or both lateral ventricles suggests obstruction at the foramen of Monro, as from colloid cysts or gliomas. Dilatation of a temporal horn of the ventricular system suggests a tumor in the ventricular atrium *trapping* the temporal horn. Dilatation of only the lateral and third ventricles points to a lesion of the aqueduct; when all the ventricles are dilated, communicating hydrocephalus caused by tumor seeding to the meninges or by the reaction to previous therapy should be considered.

Brain tumors occasionally bleed. Acute hemorrhage appears as high attenuation on CT, but subacute hemorrhage is isodense to brain and harder to detect. On MRI, acute hemorrhage is of low signal intensity on T2; the subacute hemorrhage poorly seen on CT produces a bright signal on both T1- and T2-weighted MRI scans.

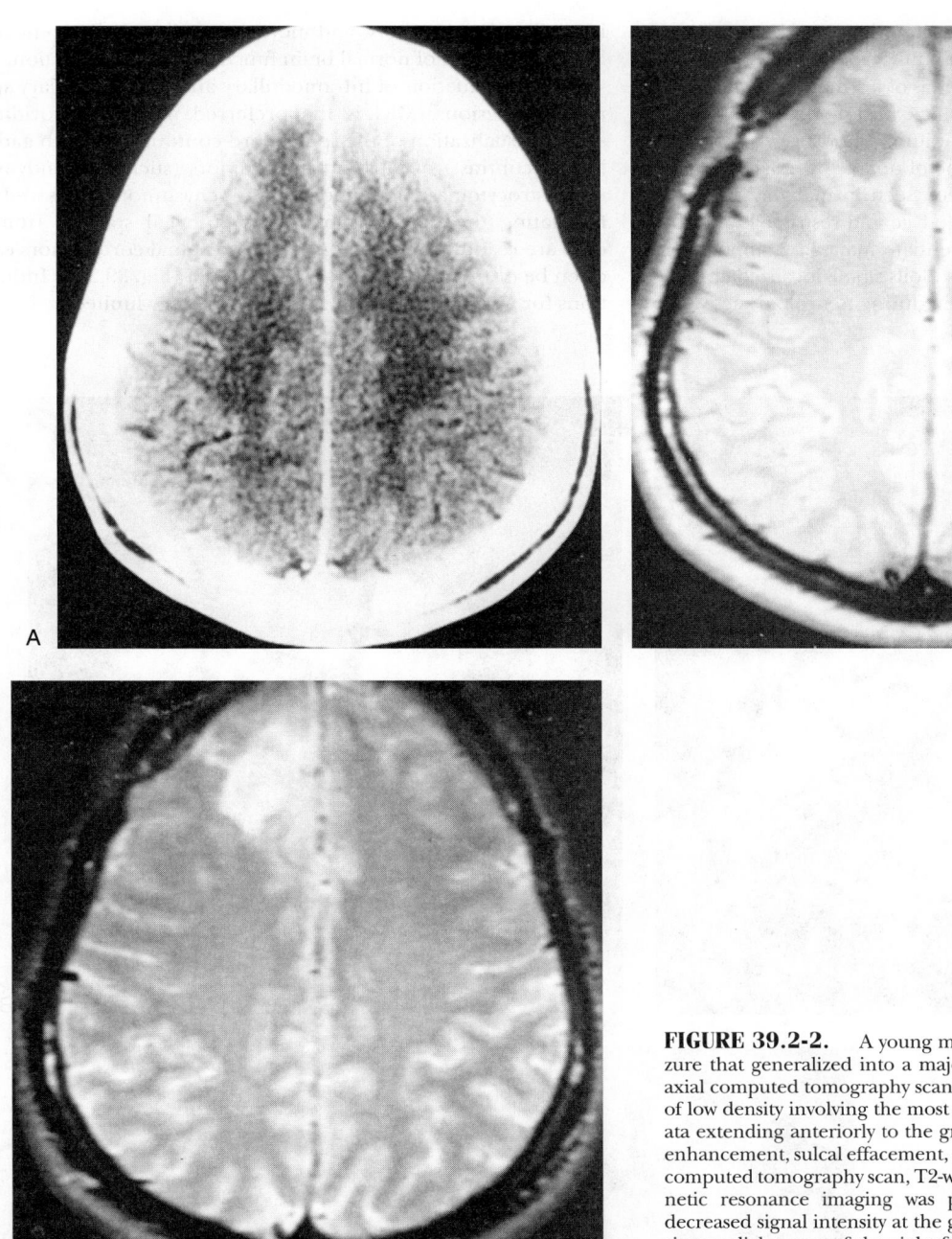

FIGURE 39.2-2. A young man presented with a single focal seizure that generalized into a major motor seizure. **A:** A postcontrast axial computed tomography scan demonstrates a poorly defined area of low density involving the most anterior portion of the corona radiata extending anteriorly to the gray matter on the right. No contrast enhancement, sulcal effacement, or mass effect is present. **B:** After this computed tomography scan, T2-weighted (TR 2000, TE 20) axial magnetic resonance imaging was performed that shows an area of decreased signal intensity at the gray-white junction at the most anterior medial aspect of the right frontal lobe. **C:** On the second echo (TR 2000, TE 60), the lesion exhibits high signal intensity. On biopsy, the tumor was found to be a well-differentiated astrocytoma.

Tumors are contrast enhancing when the BBB is disrupted. Contrast-enhanced CT and MRI scanning provides an improved ability to discern tumors from other pathologic entities, one tumor type from another, and even higher-grade from lower-grade malignancies. With few exceptions (e.g., in cases of contrast allergy, nephropathy, pregnancy) contrast agents should be included in all routine brain tumor imaging. Most low-grade gliomas (except pilocytic astrocytomas) do not enhance on CT or MRI scan and may not be detected on CT because they are isodense with brain. The MRI scan is significantly more sensitive in discerning such lesions (Fig. 39.2-2). Although almost all enhancing lesions are high grade, many nonenhancing gliomas are also high grade contrary to common dogma.

Newer MRI techniques such as magnetic resonance spectroscopy (MRS), dynamic contrast-enhanced MRI, diffusion-perfusion MRI, and functional MRI can provide additional information. MRS images the regional distribution of chemicals associated with tumor metabolism. This can distinguish tumor cells from necrosis or treatment effect.[25] MRS is now used for radiation treatment planning in investigational settings. In 45% of low-grade glioma patients studied, tumor cells were identified outside the T2 imaging abnormality with a median treatment volume increase of 2.3 cc.[26] In high-grade gliomas, MRS was found to both underestimate and overestimate the volume of microscopic residual tumor. Some areas of edema did not contain tumor and some areas of normal-appearing brain tissue did contain disease.[27] Dynamic contrast-enhanced MRI, by quantitating the uptake of gadolinium contrast agent into the lesion, can distinguish the slow rate of uptake of radiation injury from the rapid rate of uptake often seen in malignant tumors. Diffusion-perfusion MRI can image free and restricted water diffusion in the brain to help differentiate malignant tumor from radiation effect. Functional MRI exploits small, localized changes in blood flow that occur in the brain during neurologic activity to image language, sensory, and motor areas directly. This enables better protection of normal brain function during a resection.

In the evaluation of intramedullary and extramedullary spinal cord lesions, MRI is the preferred modality, providing superb visualization of the spinal cord contour and (with gadolinium contrast) of most intrinsic tumors (such as ependymomas, astrocytomas, meningiomas, and schwannomas), as well as facilitating the diagnosis of leptomeningeal spread. Tumor cysts are readily identified on MRI, and spinal cord tumors can often be distinguished from syringomyelia (Fig. 39.2-3). Indications for myelography currently are extremely limited.

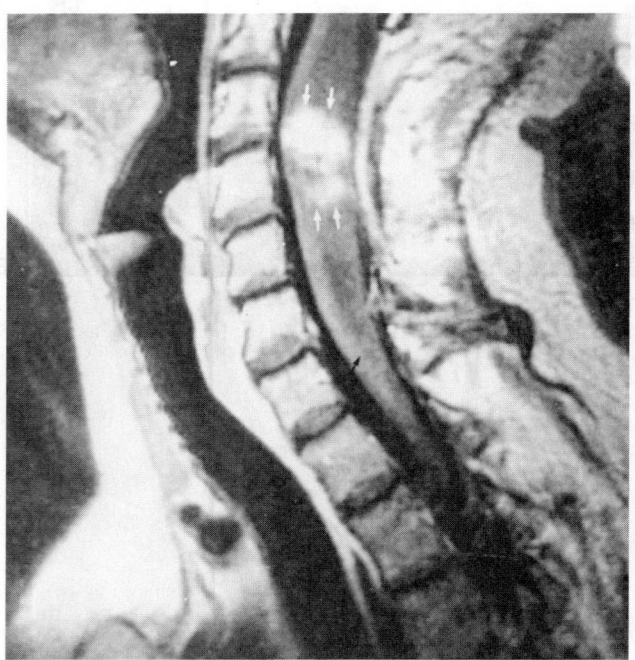

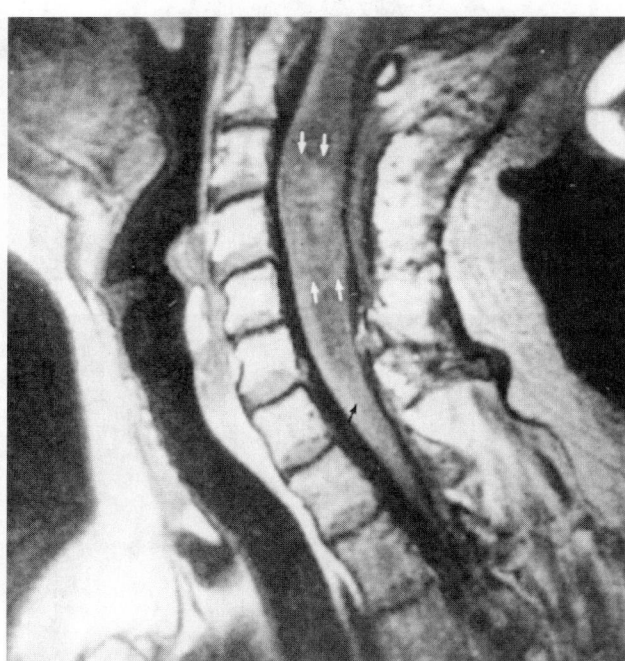

A   B

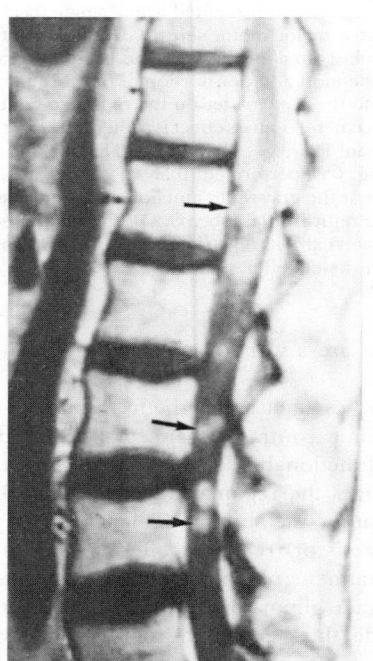
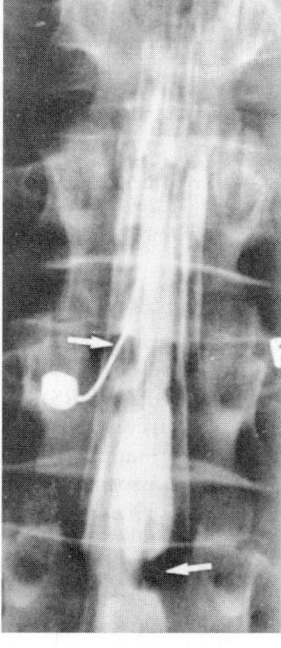

C,D

FIGURE 39.2-3.   A 39-year-old man with a known cerebral glioblastoma multiforme developed spinal cord symptoms. **A:** A T1-weighted (TR 600, TE 20) sagittal scan of the thoracolumbar spine shows mild heterogeneity of signal near the conus but is otherwise normal. **B:** A T2-weighted (TR 2000; SE 35, 70) sagittal scan provides no additional information. **C:** A T1-weighted (TR 600, SE 20) image after gadolinium–diethylenetriamine pentaacetic acid administration clearly shows high signal-enhancing tumor (*black arrows* show some of the lesions) immediately caudad to the conus resulting in a high-grade partial block and multiple additional drop metastases. **D:** A water-soluble contrast myelogram demonstrates the drop metastases (*white arrows* show some of the lesions) and incompletely delineates the mass adjacent to the conus. (Courtesy of G. Sze, Department of Radiology, Yale University School of Medicine, New Haven, CT.)

Although bedside testing for visual dysfunction is part of the standard neurologic examination, formal visual field testing using tangent screen perimetry or automated field testing is more accurate and sensitive. Visual-evoked potential testing is less often used in evaluating brain tumors but can help distinguish multiple sclerosis from tumor. Hearing is tested using audiometry, speech discrimination testing, and auditory evoked response testing. This can be helpful in the diagnosis of acoustic neuromas. Electroencephalography is used to diagnose seizure activity, especially when subclinical seizures are suspected as the cause of neurologic deterioration.

INDICATIONS FOR AND INTERPRETATION OF CEREBROSPINAL FLUID EXAMINATION

Lumbar puncture in a patient with headache, papilledema, and a presumed diagnosis of tumor is risky, because it increases the possibility of a fatal tonsillar or transtentorial herniation. Lumbar puncture should follow rather than precede appropriate neuroimaging. The examination of CSF is helpful in assessing for tumor spread through the CSF pathways. Typically, medulloblastoma, ependymoma, choroid plexus carcinoma, and some embryonal pineal and suprasellar region tumors have a high enough likelihood of spread to justify CSF examinations. In these patients, it is important to perform a lumbar puncture for CSF to examine for malignant cells (cytology) and specific markers such as human chorionic gonadotropin-β and α-fetoprotein. Other CSF findings are less helpful and do not often justify lumbar puncture. A high protein concentration with normal glucose levels and normal cytologic results is seen in tumors of the base of the skull, such as acoustic neurinoma, and in spinal cord tumors obstructing the subarachnoid space and producing stasis of the CSF in the caudal lumbar sac.

FACTORS THAT MAY PRODUCE CLINICAL DETERIORATION

The most common causes of neurologic deterioration in brain tumor patients are growth of the tumor and increased peritumoral edema, either of which can cause progressive impairment of functioning brain with resultant neurologic deficits. These manifestations may include signs and symptoms of increased ICP and temporal lobe or cerebellar herniation.

Neurologic deterioration not directly due to tumor growth can occur for any of the following reasons: hydrocephalus; hemorrhage into the tumor; increased edema due to hyponatremia, hypertension, or radiation therapy; seizures (which can be subclinical); and fever of any cause. Radiation effects can cause a clinical and imaging picture indistinguishable from tumor progression. This is most common between 6 and 18 months after treatment, although both earlier and much later occurrences are seen. In addition, an *early delayed* syndrome after radiation occurs in approximately 15% to 40% of patients.[28] This encephalopathy responds to corticosteroids and resolves within several weeks without specific sequelae.

GLUCOCORTICOID USE

Administration of glucocorticoids is often begun before surgery for brain tumor unless lymphoma is suspected. After surgi-cal decompression, the corticosteroid dose can usually be tapered to discontinue within a week or two after surgery. Some patients require corticosteroid maintenance because a large volume of tumor remains, because tumor occupies the brainstem or spinal cord, or because of corticosteroid dependence resulting from long-term prior usage. Some patients who do not require corticosteroids after surgery may need them during or after radiation therapy because of reactive edema. Signs and symptoms usually resolve within a few weeks; observation of the subsequent clinical course is often the only way to differentiate these reactions from tumor progression.

The lowest glucocorticoid dosage that maintains patients at their maximum levels of comfort and function should be sought. This is determined empirically by decreasing the dosage until symptoms increase or become apparent, then increasing the dosage until they subside.

SURGERY

GENERAL CONSIDERATIONS

The major objective of brain tumor surgery is to resect and potentially cure the tumor. For many tumors surgical cure is not possible; here, maximal tumor bulk reduction with minimal risk to the patient becomes the objective. Surgery can rapidly reduce tumor bulk with potential benefits in terms of secondary tumor mass effects, such as edema and hydrocephalus. An additional surgical goal is to provide tissue for pathologic study. Although developments in diagnostic imaging, such as MRI, and developments in treatment, including stereotactic radiosurgery, have lessened the absolute need for histopathologic confirmation of diagnosis in certain settings, in most circumstances, a tissue diagnosis is still required to determine the appropriate treatment course. Technologic advances in surgical approaches, techniques, and instrumentation have rendered most tumors amenable to resection; however, for some tumor histologic subtypes or anatomic locations, the risk of open operation supports the choice of biopsy for obtaining diagnostic tissue. Biopsy techniques include stereotactic biopsy (with or without a stereotactic frame) using CT or MRI, or both, to choose the target. Metabolic imaging, such as MRS, can be superimposed over CT or MRI anatomic images to choose targets that may be of higher biologic aggressiveness within a tumor that appears homogeneous on standard imaging. In certain settings, an approach using simple ultrasonic guidance can also be considered for obtaining diagnostic tissue, especially via needle biopsy.

ANESTHESIA AND POSTIONING

Patients with supratentorial tumors should always be given anticonvulsants before surgery if they are undergoing an operation solely under local anesthetic with sedation, to minimize the possibility of a seizure during the operation. If general anesthesia is to be used, many surgeons prescribe postoperative anticonvulsants in the immediate postoperative period to reduce seizure risk. The routine use of postoperative anticonvulsants remains controversial. Unless lymphoma is being considered, patients are given corticosteroids, usually dexamethasone, immediately preoperatively and often for several days before surgery to reduce cerebral edema and thus minimize secondary brain injury from cerebral retraction. Steroids are then continued in the immediately postoperative period and tapered as quickly as possible. Antibiotics are given just before incision to decrease the risk of wound infection.

Either general endotracheal anesthesia or local anesthesia with sedation can be used for craniotomies; patients may recuperate more quickly, which allows earlier patient discharge, if local anesthesia is used. Specific techniques to reduce patient discomfort during the surgery are required when local anesthesia is used. These include thorough preoperative discussion of the procedure with the patient (and assessment of the patient's likely tolerance of the procedure), careful patient positioning and use of sedation, and adequate local anesthetic including the use of regional blocks. Most craniotomies today are performed under general anesthesia. Isoflurane is in general use as the volatile agent for neuroanesthesia. However, it may have unfavorable effects on ICP in patients with tumors if used at higher concentrations.

Ordinarily, cranial fixation is used to minimize inadvertent patient movement during dissection. Steps are taken during the procedure to minimize ICP, which may be high due to tumor bulk. The patient's head is placed slightly above the level of the heart to increase venous drainage, and jugular vein compression is avoided. Mild hyperventilation is used. At the start of surgery, mannitol (between 0.25 and 1.0 g/kg of body weight) is given. Furosemide may be given just after the mannitol to potentiate its action. Minimizing ICP allows minimal brain retraction during the resection. In extreme cases, high ICP can produce brain herniation on dural entry.

CRANIOTOMY FOR SUPRATENTORIAL TUMORS

The bony opening is designed to be generous enough to facilitate surgery. The bone flap is centered over the tumor or positioned to give access to the route of approach. The scalp flap is designed to surround the bone flap fully; the scalp's vascular supply is given careful consideration in the design. An image-guided surgical navigation device can be used to minimize the size of the bone and scalp flaps by precisely locating the desired entry point for the procedure. After the scalp flap is reflected, burr holes are drilled and connected with an air-powered saw, or craniotome. The bone flap can then be removed. The dura is opened and reflected, and the approach to the tumor is made. A peripherally located lesion may be immediately seen. However, when the lesion is subcortical the exposed field may appear normal. If critical functional cortex is in the field, motor and speech function can be mapped intraoperatively using electrical cortical stimulation.[29] A preoperative functional MRI scan or magnetoencephalography can serve as a guide. Motor mapping can be done under general anesthesia if muscle relaxants are avoided. Glioma resections in the dominant hemisphere are often done under local anesthesia to allow speech mapping.[29]

Localization of subcortical tumors can often be accomplished using intraoperative ultrasonography, but frameless image-guided neuronavigation systems are now widely used.[30] For this technique, a preoperative MRI or CT scan is done with fiducial markers placed on the patient's scalp. During surgery the fiducial markers are used to map the images onto real space in the operative area. During surgery the system can display the actual location of a handheld probe against the background of the preoperative images in real time. Neuronavigation is used to design the craniotomy flap, to localize subcortical tumors, and to estimate progress during tumor resection. Because preoperative images are used, "brain shift" that occurs during the operation can cause discrepancy between the preoperative images and the actual brain after a portion of the tumor has been resected. Intraoperative imaging with ultrasonography, CT, and MRI can now be used to provide an immediate estimate of the progress of the resection and can be used to update the navigation system. Although neuronavigation systems do increase the degree of resection achieved, the impact on patient outcome has not yet been clarified.

Tumor removal is usually done with grasping instruments, bipolar coagulation, and suction, but removal of firm, adherent, or calcified tumor tissue can require use of the Cavitron Ultrasonic Surgical aspirator, which ultrasonically disrupts the tumor at its tip and sucks it away. In locations where access is limited (e.g., the third ventricle), some surgeons prefer using the carbon dioxide laser, which can vaporize tumor tissue *in situ*. Tumor removal with a laser is slow, however, and is reserved for special circumstances.

In the rare situations in which brain swelling is worrisome at the time of closure, a catheter is left in the ventricle to measure the ICP and drain CSF. Patients are monitored in the intensive care unit overnight after surgery, and an MRI scan is done within 24 to 48 hours to evaluate the extent of any remaining tumor.

CRANIOTOMY FOR POSTERIOR FOSSA TUMORS

Patient may be positioned prone, three-quarters prone, or lateral, depending on lesion location, surgeon preference, and patient body habitus. A linear incision is used for a midline approach, and a paramedian linear incision is used for more laterally located lesions. With larger and more caudal lesions, it is common to open the foramen magnum and even to remove the arch of C-1 to allow room for postoperative brain swelling, which otherwise can cause tonsillar herniation through the foramen magnum. A low exposure allows drainage of CSF from the cisterna magna to relax the brain. After tumor resection, the dura is closed in a watertight fashion, generally using a dural patch.

STEREOTACTIC TUMOR BIOPSY

For deeply situated intrinsic tumors, or for diffuse nonfocal tumors, resection is not practical. In these situations, needle biopsy is used for diagnosis. Open biopsy is reserved for unusual situations, such as a lesion abutting a large blood vessel or the brainstem; such lesions are often simply resected. Although tissue can be obtained through a needle directed by hand through a burr hole under ultrasonographic, CT, or MRI guidance, nothing is as simple or accurate as CT- or MRI-directed stereotactic biopsy.

Many image-guided stereotactic systems are available.[31,32] Typically, the patient undergoes a CT or MRI scan with a rigid array of fiducial bars fixed tightly to the skull to minimize movement. For cooperative adults, local anesthesia is used; for children, general anesthesia is usually required. The images show both the fiducial bars and the desired target, and a computer-guided frame is used to guide the needle through a small hole in the skull to the target point. With the advent of neuronavigation systems, stereotactic biopsy can be done without a frame. Fiducial markers are placed on the scalp and a CT or MRI scan is obtained. The target is chosen, and the system guides the needle using the known location of the fiducials and the position of the target on the preoperative image. Whether or not a frame is used, a small tissue core is obtained from the target using a side-biting needle. Frozen-section pathologic examination confirms the acquisition of diagnostic tissue and often suggests a working diagnosis. Experienced surgeons obtain diagnostic tissue in more than 95% of patients. An overnight stay or day surgery is the rule. Hemorrhage at the biopsy site, the principal risk of the surgery, occurs in few patients. Occasionally, cerebral edema is exacerbated by biopsy.

RADIATION THERAPY

GENERAL CONSIDERATIONS

Most common brain tumors, such as low-grade and malignant astrocytomas, are infiltrative into surrounding normal brain tissue many centimeters from the primary lesion. Radiation treatment volumes for these tumors generally include the enhancing volume (which contains solid tumor tissue), surrounding edema (which is comprised of normal brain infiltrated by microscopic tumor), and a margin of normal brain. Thus, even with the use of very conformal techniques, a substantial amount of "normal" brain is included in the full-dose volume. The tolerance of normal brain (and spinal cord in the case of cord tumors) is a major limiting factor in achieving local control and cure.

TOLERANCE OF THE BRAIN

Adverse reactions associated with cranial irradiation differ in their pathogenesis and can be temporally classified into (1) acute reactions that occur during or shortly after radiation therapy, (2) early delayed reactions that appear within a few weeks to 4 months after irradiation, and (3) late delayed injuries that develop several months to years after treatment.[33]

Late radiation injuries are the most serious complications of therapeutic brain irradiation and vary in severity from asymptomatic white matter changes to potentially fatal necrosis. Late radiation injury may be due to vascular endothelial injury or to a direct effect on oligodendroglial cells; multiple mechanisms are probably involved.[33] The late delayed reaction presents as a focal or diffuse white matter injury, or both. The clinical presentation depends on the site and volume of the brain exposed. Patients with *focal radiation necrosis* present with localizing neurologic signs, often accompanied by symptoms of increased ICP. Focal hypodensity or a contrast-enhancing mass with surrounding vasogenic edema may be seen on images. *Diffuse white matter injury* typically occurs after large-volume or whole brain irradiation. Clinical features range from seizure disorders and varying degrees of neuropsychological impairment to incapacitating dementia. Diffuse white matter hypodensity is seen on CT scan, often accompanied by a focal enhancing mass, whereas T2-weighted MRI shows diffuse periventricular white matter hyperintensity. Cerebral cortical atrophy, probably related to diffuse white matter injury, is observed in 17% to 39% of patients who receive whole brain irradiation with chemotherapy for malignant gliomas. Enlarged cerebral sulci and ventricles are seen on images.[34] The pathogenesis of this form of radiation damage is uncertain.[34] Uncommonly, therapeutic irradiation causes an intracranial vessel-occlusive vasculopathy, neovascular formation, or secondary neoplasia.

The tolerance of the brain depends on the size of the dose per fraction, total dose given, overall treatment time, volume of brain irradiated, host factors, and adjunctive therapies. The probability of injury increases with larger daily doses (2.2 Gy/fraction) and doses in excess of 60 Gy delivered in 30 fractions over approximately 6 weeks.

Approximately 4% to 9% of patients treated to 50 to 60 Gy with conventional fractionated radiation for brain tumors develop clinically detectable focal radiation necrosis, but this form of injury may be found in as many as 10% to 22% of patients at autopsy. A review by Marks and colleagues of 139 patients who received irradiation for primary brain tumors to at least 45 Gy in daily dose fractions of 1.8 to 2.0 Gy disclosed 7 patients (5%) with brain necrosis.[35]

Corticosteroids may improve or stabilize neurologic symptoms associated with the effects of radiation. Resection is often beneficial to patients with favorably situated, focal radiation-induced lesions who deteriorate neurologically and become corticosteroid dependent.[36] Although anticoagulation and hyperbaric oxygen have been suggested as treatment when surgery is not feasible, clinical trials demonstrating efficacy are lacking.

Cranial irradiation can lead to intellectual impairment in adults. Unlike the situation for children, however, only a limited amount of quantitative information is available, especially for patients treated with radiation therapy alone. Patients in whom a substantial portion of the brain is irradiated frequently develop recent memory loss and difficulty attending to tasks, which may prevent their return to gainful employment. Patients irradiated with partial brain fields had superior memory function and better employment histories than those treated with whole brain fields. Decrements in tests of new learning ability, recent memory, abstraction, and problem solving have been seen in patients who decline from their premorbid social or occupational level of function.[37] Early return to work after treatment may lead to improvement in neuropsychological function.

Radiation therapy may cause hypothalamic-pituitary dysfunction, and the incidence and degree of hormone suppression appear to be dose related.[28,38] Growth hormone deficiency, the most frequent endocrine dysfunction observed after radiation, can occur after doses as low as 18 Gy. Deficiencies of gonadotrophins, thyroid-stimulating hormone, and adrenocorticotrophins as well as hyperprolactinemia can be seen with doses in excess of 40 Gy.[28] Patients at risk for neuroendocrinologic sequelae should be evaluated for pituitary function before, and periodically after, irradiation. Early detection of a deficiency permits appropriate hormonal replacement therapy before clinical endocrinopathies develop.

TOLERANCE OF THE SPINAL CORD

Radiation myelopathy may present as a transient early delayed reaction or as a more ominous late delayed reaction. Transient radiation myelopathy is clinically manifested by momentary, electric shock–like paresthesias or numbness radiating from the neck to the extremities on neck flexion (Lhermitte's sign). The syndrome develops after an average latent period of 3 to 4 months and gradually resolves over the ensuing 3 to 6 months without the need for specific therapy. Not only are there the obvious neurologic sequelae of irradiation, but nearly 50% of patients die from secondary complications.[39] The latent period between the completion of radiation therapy and the onset of symptoms is bimodal in distribution, with the first peak occurring at 12 to 14 months and the second occurring at 24 to 28 months. Demyelination and white matter necrosis due to a direct effect on oligodendroglial cells and intramedullary microvascular injury each play a role in the pathogenesis. The signs and symptoms that accompany radiation myelopathy are irreversible. No laboratory tests or imaging studies distinguish radiation myelopathy from other spinal cord lesions. MRI findings include swelling of the cord with decreased intensity in T1-weighted and hyperintensity in T2-weighted images.[40] The diagnosis is often one of exclusion.

A dose of 45 Gy in 22 fractions over 5 weeks usually is considered to be safe, with the risk of myelopathy being less than 0.2%.[41,42] It is estimated that, with conventionally fractionated irradiation (1.8 to 2.0 Gy/fraction, five fractions per week), the incidence of myelopathy is 5% for doses in the range of 57 to 61 Gy and 50% for doses of 68 to 73 Gy.[41]

TUMOR TARGET VOLUME AND TREATMENT TECHNIQUES

The appropriate volume to encompass within the radiation treatment portal varies with the specific histopathologic tumor type and, with certain histologies, is controversial. Benign tumors typically do not infiltrate beyond the lesional borders seen by MRI. Certain tumors, such as benign meningiomas, pituitary adenomas, craniopharyngiomas, and acoustic neuromas, may be treated with narrow margins of surrounding normal tissue. In contrast, the astrocytic gliomas require larger margins because of their tendency to infiltrate beyond the imaged tumor border. Limited radiation portals are now used rather than whole brain irradiation for malignant gliomas. Comparisons of CT and MRI studies with clinical and pathologic findings have shown that

1. Malignant gliomas are localized, and microscopic invasion of the perilesional brain is limited at the time of initial diagnosis.[43]
2. Only 1.1% of patients present with multiple lesions.[44]
3. After initial treatment, most of these lesions, when they recur, do so at their original location.[45]
4. Isolated tumor cell infiltration may extend to the periphery of T2-weighted MRI abnormalities.[46]

The radiation beam energy and field arrangements are selected after consideration of the location of the tumor within the brain and the geometry of the target volume. The across-target volume is defined as a three-dimensional reconstruction of the tumor contour based on operative findings and data from CT and MRI studies. The planning target volume consists of the volume of tissue that must be irradiated to encompass the tumor volume with a margin of surrounding tissue considered to be at risk for microscopic tumor spread and to account for patient movement and daily setup uncertainties. Three-

dimensional conformal radiation therapy and the advanced technique of intensity-modulated radiation therapy are new methods of treatment planning and delivery designed to enhance the conformation of the dose to the target volume, while maximally restricting the dose delivered to the normal tissue outside the treatment volume. Megavoltage equipment with energies ranging from 4- to 15-MV photons is used to administer radiation therapy. Treatment is generally given in daily fractions of 1.8 to 2.0 Gy/d five times per week. In this chapter, the total doses referred to assume that a *conventional* fractionation scheme is used unless otherwise specified.

Certain neoplasms, such as medulloblastomas and other PNETs as well as some ependymomas and germ cell tumors, require treatment to the entire craniospinal axis. Patients are treated prone in an immobilization cast to ensure daily positional reproducibility. The intracranial contents, including the upper one or two segments of the cervical cord, are treated through parallel opposed lateral fields. The spine is treated through one or two posterior fields, depending on the size of the patient. The cranial and posterior spinal fields may be abutted, but a gap of 0.5 to 1.0 cm is often left between the fields. When two posterior spinal fields are used, as is usually the case, a gap is calculated so that the 50% isodose lines meet at the level of the spinal cord. All junction lines are moved 0.5 to 1.0 cm daily or at least every 10 Gy to avoid overdosing or underdosing segments of the cord. Several modifications of this approach are used in clinical practice.

Radiosurgery is being used to treat a diverse group of intracranial lesions, including small arteriovenous malformations, pituitary adenomas, acoustic neuromas, meningiomas, gliomas, and brain metastases. Radiosurgery is a method of highly focal, closed-skull external irradiation that uses an imaging-compatible stereotactic device for precise target localization. The relationship between the stereotactic coordinate system and the radiation source(s) allows accurate delivery of radiation to the target volume. Radiosurgery can be administered by gamma knife units, made up of multiple cobalt beams, and by modified linear accelerators. This technique is designed to deliver a high radiation dose to an intracranial target in a single session without delivering significant radiation to adjacent normal tissues. Stereotactic radiation may be delivered in a fractionated dose schedule using stereotactic radiosurgery hardware and software and head frames that can be relocalized daily in a reproducible fashion. This approach is referred to as *stereotactic radiotherapy* or *fractionated stereotactic radiotherapy*. More recently, frameless image-guided fractionated therapy has become available coupled with an orthogonal pair of x-ray cameras.[47] This allows a dynamically manipulated robot-mounted linear accelerator to guide therapy to treatment sites such as the brain and spine. Early results are encouraging.[48] Because fractionating the radiation dose improves the therapeutic ratio, larger tumors and those located within or adjacent to critical intracranial structures are suitable for this treatment technique. This approach is being applied to the treatment of malignant gliomas, craniopharyngiomas, pituitary adenomas, small optic tract tumors, and as a boost for medulloblastomas.

Implantation of radioactive sources into tumors and tumor beds has enjoyed renewed interest in neurooncology. This can be accomplished with radioactive sources placed stereotactically or freehand. More recently, a liquid-filled balloon brachytherapy source has been used in a multicenter study for recurrent glioma patients.[49] The temporary balloon system delivered 40 to 60 Gy over 3 to 6 days. There were no cases of radiation necrosis, and the median survival measured from the time of the procedure was 12.7 months.

CHEMOTHERAPY

Although advances in intraoperative imaging and other neurosurgical techniques now allow the safe resection of many tumors that were previously inaccessible, many tumors still remain only partially resectable or nonresectable because of their location in important areas of the brain (i.e., brainstem, base of the skull). Furthermore, some of the most common CNS tumors are never totally resectable because of their highly infiltrative nature (glial tumors) or their tendency to disseminate along CSF pathways (embryonal tumors). Although most CNS tumors are partially responsive to radiotherapy, neural tissue toxicity usually prevents administration of curative doses of radiation. Thus, there is a significant need for additional treatment modalities.

Chemotherapy offers the theoretical advantage of reaching all tumor cells, regardless of their gross or microanatomic location within the CNS, because all tumor cells must be within the perfusion zone of preexisting or tumor-associated microvasculature. Furthermore, many chemotherapeutic agents have minimum neurotoxic effects, so toxicity concerns are largely confined to systemic toxicity. Finally, because the vast majority of normal cells within the CNS are postmitotic, chemotherapeutic agents that are preferentially toxic to dividing cells should have a high therapeutic index within the CNS. Despite these theoretic arguments, the fact is that chemotherapy is used as primary therapy for few types of CNS tumors (i.e., primary CNS lymphoma), is at most an adjunct to surgery and radiation for some CNS tumors, and is totally ineffective for others.

There are several reasons for the largely disappointing results of chemotherapy. As with systemic tumors, intrinsic and acquired drug resistance at doses attainable with acceptable systemic toxicity remains a primary reason for chemotherapy failure. The challenges for successful use of chemotherapy for CNS tumors, however, are even greater than they are for systemic tumors. Central to this difference is the issue of drug delivery. The CNS is protected from toxic substances in the blood by the BBB. The BBB is a physiologic and functional barrier that results from the architectural features of the CNS microvasculature.[50] The CNS microvasculature has several unique features, including the lack of fenestrations between adjacent endothelial cells and relatively fewer pinocytotic and endocytotic endothelial vesicles. Additionally, adjacent BBB endothelial cells are connected by a continuous extension of tight junctions, which significantly limits passive diffusion between endothelial cells and through capillary structures. Tight junctions within the BBB are also enveloped by astrocytic foot processes, which increase the barrier to passive diffusion across the BBB. These unique tight junctions result in a high transendothelial electric resistance and diminished paracellular resistance.[51]

To compensate for the limited passive diffusion across the BBB, brain microvasculature selectively transports nutrients (i.e., amino acids) into the brain through 20 or more active or facilitated carrier transport systems expressed on the BBB endothelial surface.[52] The BBB endothelium is also rich with efflux pumps, including the MDR (multidrug resistance gene)-encoded P-glycoprotein and MRP (multidrug resistance protein).[53] These and other efflux pumps actively secrete substrate molecules that have somehow passed the BBB. The efficiency of the BBB for excluding molecules from the CNS is exemplified by the 8–log-unit higher rate at which an immunoglobulin crosses a liver capillary compared to a brain capillary.[54] Similarly, the hydraulic conductivity of brain capillaries, and thus the oncotic pressure driving protein influx across endothelium, is 500, 1000, and 3000 times less than it is in heart, muscle, and intestinal capillaries, respectively.[55] Thus, the BBB presents a formidable obstacle for the passage of drugs into the brain.

Ever since the blush of dye extravasation was first seen in tumors on cerebral angiography, it was appreciated that the blood–tumor barrier (BTB) was different than the BBB. The microvascular differences between the BTB and the normal BBB range from a subtle increase in endothelial fenestrations to a dramatic breakdown of tight junctions, enlargement of the perivascular space, and swelling of the basal lamina.[54,56] These tumor-induced changes have multiple causes, including aberrant angiogenic stimulation from the tumor, extracellular matrix remodeling and destruction by tumor-induced metalloproteinases, and physical disruption of the normal architecture of the BBB through loss of normal supporting cells such as astrocytes. Different tumors display different degrees of disruption of the BTB. For example, most low-grade gliomas do not have contrast enhancement on CT or MRI scans and have BTBs that are quite similar to the normal BBB. In contrast, highly malignant tumors such as glioblastoma may have nearly total disruption of most barrier functions within the avidly contrast-enhancing portion of the tumor. Even in these tumors, however, drug delivery is not normal because the tumor-induced neovasculature is often poorly perfused or not patent, and there is a relatively long distance between tumor-induced angiogenic vessels and individual tumor cells. Furthermore, even in these highly malignant and angiogenic tumors, the leading front of infiltrating tumor cells is located in normal brain parenchyma with a relatively intact BBB. The limited access of most chemotherapeutic drugs to the tumor decreases the chance that cytotoxic concentrations of the drug will be delivered to all or even most of the infiltrating tumor cells, and results in tumor cell exposure to sublethal concentrations of the drug, which increases the chances of acquired drug resistance.

Physicochemical characteristics largely determine a drug's ability to cross the BBB. Smaller, ionically neutral, lipophilic drugs, with a high octanol/water coefficient, are more likely to penetrate the BBB and BTB.[57] Unfortunately, most drugs lack these characteristics and are excluded by the barrier. For this reason, and because only a tiny portion of any systemically delivered drug finds its way into a relatively small tumor regardless of permeability issues, there are significant problems both in obtaining homogeneous, pharmacologically active concentrations of drugs throughout a brain tumor and in limiting systemic toxicity. This has led to the development of alternate drug administration techniques that either disrupt the BBB and BTB or deliver drugs directly to the region.

The first and still most widely used method for disrupting the BBB is through an intravascular osmotic load using mannitol, which results in cerebral endothelial shrinkage and disruption of endothelial tight junctions.[58] More refined attempts to disrupt the BBB have focused on specific drugs that selectively target cerebral endothelial cellular signaling pathways, such as the bradykinin pathway, and result in transient BBB disruption.[59] Although preclinical studies of such BBB disruption strategies have demonstrated enhancement of drug delivery into the CNS, clinical studies have not demonstrated convincing improvements in antitumor effect or patient outcome. Although the reasons for this failure are not entirely clear, intrinsic tumor drug resistance is probably partially responsible. Additionally, because BBB disruption affects both tumor and nontumor vasculature, the therapeutic index of chemotherapeutic agents may not improve with BBB disruption. Because the BBB disruption within the tumor is usually partial, iatrogenic BBB disruption tends to cause a relatively greater increase in the drug delivery to normal brain tissue than to tumor. This has led to significant neurotoxicity in many clinical trials of BBB disruption.

Another strategy that has been used over the last two decades to enhance drug delivery to brain tumors while minimizing systemic exposure is intraarterial administration. Intraarterial drug administration results in high local concentrations of drug by infusing the agent directly into the limited blood volume of selected brain arteries. After the first pass of the drug through the brain, it then becomes diluted into the total body blood volume. As with BBB disruption, however, this approach delivers proportionately higher levels of drug to adjacent normal brain as well as to the tumor. This has proven to be problematic, with most clinical experience suggesting that slightly higher response rates may occasionally be seen but at the expense of significant neurotoxicity.[56,60,61] Another drawback of selective arterial drug delivery is that tumors often obtain their vascular supply from multiple arteries. Finally, intraarterial drug delivery has been associated with significant morbidity, including strokes from arterial dissection and embolism. Thus, there is currently limited enthusiasm for this strategy.

Another strategy to circumvent the BBB has been to deliver drugs directly into the brain through local administration. One way to do this is the surgical placement of biodegradable synthetic polymers impregnated with a drug. The prototype implantable polymer is the Gliadel wafer, which contains carmustine (BCNU).[62] After surgical debulking of a malignant glioma the surgeon lines the surgical cavity with Gliadel wafers that are left in place. Over the next several weeks the BCNU diffuses out of the wafers into the surrounding brain, providing very high local concentrations of BCNU with little systemic exposure to the drug. Although theoretically attractive, this approach has pharmacologic constraints. BCNU is highly lipid soluble and crosses the BBB readily in both directions. BCNU that diffuses out of the polymer therefore passes into the local blood stream, where the BCNU concentration is low. This carries the drug away from the brain, a phenomenon known as the *sink effect*. Another limitation is that drug penetrates the surrounding brain only by passive diffusion, a slow and inefficient process. High concentrations of BCNU are thus found only within a few millimeters of the wafers, which makes it unlikely that cytotoxic drug concentrations will reach distant infiltrating tumor cells.[63] Despite these limitations of BCNU-impregnated polymers, it is possible that polymers containing drugs with more suitable pharmacokinetics (i.e., nonlipophilic drugs that do not cross the BBB) may prove to be more efficacious.

Convection-enhanced delivery (CED) is another strategy for local drug delivery. In contrast to polymer-based delivery strategies that depend on diffusion to move macromolecules through the interstitial space, CED uses bulk fluid flow. CED requires the implantation of catheters directly into the brain tissue followed by continuous infusion of the drug under a constant pressure gradient. CED offers several theoretic advantages over polymer-based diffusion such as the ability to move very large molecules (i.e., immunoglobulins, liposomes, small virions) through the interstitial space and the ability to achieve homogeneous concentrations of the drug even at the leading edge of the infusate, as compared to the steep fall-off in drug concentration across distance seen with diffusion.[64,65] This results in much larger volumes of distribution with CED than are achieved with diffusion.[66] CED also theoretically offers the ability to target a specific anatomic zone of cerebral tissue for treatment while sparing other areas, something nearly impossible to achieve using diffusion methods. CED is a promising approach for drug delivery but remains investigational. Current research focuses on optimizing convection parameters (i.e., volume, infusion rate, pressure) and finding methods to allow the imaging of the convected infusate. As with diffusion, the efficiency of CED is ultimately dependent on the physicochemical characteristics of the administered drug, and because an invasive procedure is required, multiple drug administrations may be impractical.

Another drug delivery approach is direct administration of the agent into the CSF. Because the CSF has the pharmacokinetic characteristics of a closed (albeit dynamic) compartment, drugs given directly into the CSF can reach high levels. Because this compartment is separate from the systemic circulation, however, drugs given in this way must be in their active form without the need for hepatic or other systemic metabolic activation. Given the high CSF drug levels that can be attained through direct administration, intra-CSF treatment can be highly effective in treating tumor cells that are in the CSF and are lining the leptomeninges. Unfortunately, there is a significant delay in equilibration between the CSF and extracellular space of the brain even for small soluble molecules given directly into the CSF. For larger, less diffusible molecules, equilibrium between the two compartments never occurs. This pharmacologic phenomenon, called the CS–brain barrier, is why intra-CSF drug administration is a very inefficient and ineffective delivery strategy for intraparenchymal brain tumors.[67] Additionally, intra-CSF drug delivery is limited by the potential for significant neurologic morbidity. With a few exceptions (i.e., methotrexate, cytarabine, thiotepa), most compounds cause unacceptable neurologic toxicity, including death, when given into the CSF. Because of these limitations, intrathecal chemotherapy is used principally to treat leptomeningeal metastases from systemic tumors and for CNS prophylaxis for high-risk leukemia.

In addition to drug delivery issues, other special pharmacokinetic challenges are presented by the brain tumor patient. Many antiepileptic agents used in brain tumor patients, including phenytoin, carbamazepine, and phenobarbital, induce the cytochrome P-450 isoenzyme system. The specific isoenzymes induced by these drugs are often also capable of metabolizing many chemotherapeutic agents. This can have dramatic consequences on chemotherapy drug levels achieved with standard dosing. For example, standard paclitaxel (Taxol) doses commonly result in subtherapeutic serum levels in patients also using phenytoin.[68] In fact, the maximally tolerated paclitaxel dose in patients using enzyme-inducing P-450 antiepileptics is nearly threefold higher than in patients not using such agents. Similar observations have been made with regard to 9-amino-campothecin, vincristine, teniposide, and irinotecan.[69–72] For this reason, most phase I clinical trials in brain tumor patients now use separate evaluation arms for patients who are and are not taking enzyme-inducing antiepileptic drugs. Oncologists using standard chemotherapeutic agents for patients who take enzyme-inducing antiepileptic agents must be aware that standard doses may be subtherapeutic. It may be preferable to change the patient over to a non–enzyme-inducing antiepileptic agent [e.g., levetiracetam (Keppra)], although it takes weeks to make the switch and another few weeks for the P-450 enzyme induction to resolve. If time or the neurologic state of the patient does not allow transition to a non–enzyme-inducing antiepileptic, the practitioner may need to consider carefully escalating the chemotherapy dose with subsequent cycles of treatment if expected toxicities (i.e., myelosuppression) are not observed in the first few cycles.

A final pharmacologic consideration in treating brain tumor patients is that they are often given long-term high-dose steroids, which causes significant adipose weight gain. Using body weight to calculate body surface area for drug dosing can therefore cause a substantial overdose if the drug or its active metabolites, or both, are water-soluble and do not efficiently equilibrate into fat. For drugs that do ultimately equilibrate into fat to some extent, dosing based on ideal body weight can lead to substantial underdosing. Thus, determining optimal drug doses for brain tumor patients is a significant challenge.

CEREBRAL ASTROCYTOMAS

PATHOLOGIC CLASSIFICATION

Astrocytomas are the most common primary brain tumors in adults, although embryonal tumors are more common in children. It is believed that tumors classified as astrocytomas are all derived from a common cell of origin, the astrocyte. The fact that astrocytes are a heterogeneous population of cells may partially explain why such a large spectrum of tumors with dramatically different natural histories fall under the classification of astrocytoma.

There has been significant controversy over the pathologic classification of astrocytic tumors. Generally speaking, slower growing and less aggressive tumors have been designated as low grade, and faster growing, more aggressive tumors have been designated as high grade. The first widely used system was devised by Kernohan and coworkers, who proposed a four-tier system with grades 1 and 2 defined as lower-grade tumors and grades 3 (*anaplastic astrocytoma*) and 4 (*glioblastoma multiforme*) as high-grade gliomas. Although there were significant differences in the prognosis of patients with grade 1 and 2 tumors compared to those with grade 3 and 4 tumors, there was little reproducible prognostic significance among the four individual grades. Recognizing the difficulty in differentiating grade 1 from grade 2 tumors in the Kernohan system, Ringertz and colleagues established a three-tier system that categorized grade 1 astrocytic tumors as astrocytomas, and grade 3 tumors as glio-

blastoma.[73,74] Grade 2 tumors were considered anaplastic or high-grade tumors that were slightly more differentiated than glioblastomas and did not have necrosis. Although this system allowed for the easy distinction between low- and high-grade tumors, the system suffered from significant intraobserver variability in differentiating grade 2 from grade 3 tumors. In contrast, the first World Health Organization (WHO) three-tier astrocytic tumor classification designated anaplastic astrocytomas as grade 3 tumors, whereas glioblastomas were considered primitive, undifferentiated tumors that were grouped with embryonal tumors.[75] A more useful approach was suggested by Daumas-Duport and coworkers, who developed a four-tier system based on a small set of objective criteria: nuclear pleomorphism, mitoses, endothelial proliferation, and necrosis.[76] Grade 1 tumors had none of these features, grade 2 tumors had one feature, grade 3 tumors had two features, and grade 4 tumors had three or four. Although the classification initially appeared to demonstrate good separation in survival among patients with all four grades of tumor, the system did not adequately differentiate between prognoses of patients with tumors designated as grades 2 and 3 in one single-center validation study.[77]

To resolve these controversies, the WHO convened an international consensus panel of neuropathologists to define a new classification system, which has since garnered worldwide acceptance.[78] In this revised WHO schema, astrocytic tumors are divided into three categories: astrocytoma (including fibrillary, gemistocytic, and protoplasmic), anaplastic astrocytoma, and glioblastoma (including giant cell glioblastoma and gliosarcoma). Juvenile pilocytic astrocytomas and pleomorphic xanthoastrocytomas, two tumors with unique histologic and clinical features, are considered as separate entities in this schema.

CLINICAL CONSIDERATIONS

As already noted in Anatomic and Clinical Considerations, anatomic location and rapidity of growth are the main determinants of a brain tumor patient's signs and symptoms. Because different histologic CNS tumor types have different growth rates and predilections for specific anatomic sites, histologic type influences the patient's likely clinical presentation. Patients with astrocytic tumors can present with focal or generalized neurologic signs and symptoms. Focal neurologic symptoms are related to the area of the brain involved by the tumor and result directly from tumor impingement on involved pathways or focally increased ICP caused by associated cerebral edema. Astrocytomas may also cause focal deficits by releasing glutamate and other potentially neurotoxic molecules.[79] Generalized symptoms of astrocytomas usually result from increased ICP: headache, often worse in the morning and exacerbated by actions that increase ICP, such as coughing. Such headaches have little localizing value. More advanced symptoms of high ICP include nausea, vomiting, generalized seizures, and progressive somnolence, ultimately leading to death.

RATIONALE FOR SURGERY

There are several reasons for performing a resection of gliomas in adults whenever it is thought to be safe. First, resection (rather than stereotactic biopsy) provides the best opportunity to obtain an accurate diagnosis. Gliomas are notoriously heterogeneous, and therapy is guided by the most aggressive histologic type detected in the specimen. Studies have shown that more complete resections are more likely to provide a high-grade diagnosis[80] and to detect an oligodendroglial component in the tumor.[81] Second, resection relieves symptoms from mass effect in many patients, and more extensive resections are associated with greater chances of neurologic improvement. Third, response to postoperative radiation therapy is more favorable and deterioration during treatment is less likely after resection.[82] Finally, it is likely that resection has a modest survival benefit through cytoreduction. Only one randomized trial of resection of malignant gliomas has been published; survival was approximately twice as long with resection.[83] Many retrospective studies of both low-grade[84] and high-grade glioma[85] have shown longer survival with resection, after adjustment for age, performance score, tumor histologic type, and other prognostic factors. Although selection bias accounts for some of the difference in survival, most surgeons believe resection is beneficial, especially in patients who have mass effect at presentation.

SURGICAL PRINCIPLES

The ideal goal of every craniotomy for a cerebral astrocytoma is gross total resection, and adequate exposure should be accomplished for this purpose, even though aggressive resection may prove impossible at the time of the operation. Tumors are approached through an incision in the crest of an overlying gyrus or through a sulcus. The selection of the entry site is aided by intraoperative ultrasonographic images and the frameless image-guided stereotactic system, or with intraoperative MRI. Self-retaining retractors are placed to retract gently both sides of the cortical incision (generally approximately 3 cm in length for deep tumors, or circumferentially around the mass when it presents superficially). The operating microscope is used for the approach through the subcortical white matter to the tumor. The tumor is resected with suction, two-point coagulation forceps, grasping instruments, the carbon dioxide laser, or an ultrasonic aspiration device, with the resection proceeding from the inside out, so that surrounding normal white matter is disturbed minimally. The glistening peritumoral white matter is seen easily through the microscope as each of the tumor's margins are reached, and at this interface the resection is stopped. Hemostasis is sometimes difficult to achieve but must be perfect. If implantation of wafers containing BCNU is planned, they are placed now against the walls of the cavity. Hemispheric tumor cysts can be drained and, when possible, fenestrated into an adjacent ventricle to prevent reaccumulation. For tumors not resectable because of their location or diffuseness, biopsy can be performed stereotactically using frameless or frame-based technique. There is usually no need for a craniotomy when the purpose is merely to perform biopsy (and not resection) on a tumor, although the need to sample multiple areas of these heterogeneous tumors is recognized.

The use of intraoperative cortical stimulation mapping facilitates the resection of tumors in or adjacent to functionally critical areas. Motor functions can be mapped even under general anesthesia; sensory and speech-associated cortex can be mapped during an awake craniotomy. Safe routes to deep-lying tumors and resection limits for superficial tumors can be determined. Preoperative mapping of functional areas using MRI-based techniques can now delineate both cortical areas and important subcortical white matter tracts that subserve speech and motor function.[86]

Reoperation for resection of recurrent cerebral astrocytomas can be modestly efficacious.[87] The rationale for the aggressive initial resection of cerebral astrocytomas cited earlier in Rationale for Surgery seems to fit equally well the prospect for resection at recurrence. In addition, when the initial tumor was low grade, histologic resampling may be necessary to guide further treatment with chemotherapy or radiation. Younger patients, patients who had gross total resections at initial surgery, and patients with high functional status are the most likely to be chosen for reoperation at recurrence and to have longer survival after reoperation.[87] As with initial operations, reoperation offers a chance to implant polymer wafers containing BCNU or to administer experimental agents, such as gene therapy agents or immunotoxins. Smaller volume of disease at the initiation of chemotherapy predicts longer survival,[84] so that reoperation may promote adjuvant treatment effectiveness as well as relieving mass effect in some patients.

RADIATION THERAPY

Many astrocytomas are not amenable to total resection and others promptly recur despite apparently total removals. Radiation treatment has long been used after resection of most astrocytomas. Its current status is summarized here.

Low-Grade Gliomas

The 5-year recurrence-free survival rates of patients with infiltrative astrocytomas or mixed oligoastrocytomas who undergo total or radical subtotal tumor resection range from 52% to 95%.[88] This variation may reflect prognostic differences related to age, the inclusion of patients with less than total resection, and the reliance on surgeons' impressions of extent of resection in the era before CT and MRI studies. Because recurrences are infrequent in children with completely resected astrocytomas, postoperative irradiation is generally not recommended. The outcome of adult patients after total or radical subtotal resection has been found in some series to be similar to that of patients undergoing less extensive surgery.[88] Thus, in adults, postoperative irradiation has been recommended after complete resection by some authors,[88] although most advise that radiation therapy be withheld until there is evidence of tumor recurrence.[89]

Radiotherapy should be given immediately to patients with radiographic evidence of tumor growth, intractable seizures, progressive neurologic impairment, or documented malignant transformation. The optimal timing of postoperative irradiation for patients with low-grade gliomas that are asymptomatic (except possibly for occasional seizures) is presently uncertain. This issue was addressed in a randomized trial conducted by the European Organization for Research and Treatment of Cancer (EORTC) and British Medical Research Council Brain Tumour Working Party. Patients with low-grade astrocytomas (65%), oligodendrogliomas (25%), or mixed tumors (10%) were randomly assigned to receive immediate postoperative irradiation to a dose of 54 Gy or no further treatment until neurologic and CT scan evidence of disease progression. Among those in the control arm, 65% of patients received subsequent radiotherapy; 19% underwent surgery, chemotherapy, or both; and the remainder received only supportive care. A preliminary analysis of the study demonstrated that, although immediate irradiation improved the 5-year progression-free survival (44% vs. 37%; *P* = .02), there was no improvement in overall 5-year survival (63% vs. 66%).[90]

Limited radiation fields are used in the treatment of low-grade astrocytomas. A lesion defined by CT scan is encompassed with a 2-cm margin of normal tissue, whereas the T2-weighted MRI abnormality, which tends to be larger than the CT-defined lesion, is given a margin of 1 to 2 cm. Complex treatment planning should be used whenever appropriate to minimize the risk of long-term sequelae. The standard dose is 54 Gy, given using daily fractions of 1.8 to 2.0 Gy. Two studies indicate that higher radiation doses do not improve the outcome (at least at 5 years) and suggest that lower doses may be preferable. In a trial conducted by the EORTC, patients were randomly assigned to receive 45 Gy in 25 fractions or 59.4 Gy in 33 fractions. No difference in survival was observed between the two dose levels. The 5-year survival rates were 58% for 45 Gy and 59% for 59.4 Gy. Progression-free rates were also similar (47% vs. 50%). Minimal surgery, poor neurologic status, large tumors, advanced age, and unfavorable histologic features were adverse prognostic factors.[91] Similarly, a combined trial of the North Central Cancer Treatment Group, Radiation Therapy Oncology Group (RTOG), and Eastern Cooperative Oncology Group trial randomly assigned adult patients with supratentorial astrocytomas to receive 50.4 Gy in 28 fractions or 64.8 Gy in 36 fractions. As in the EORTC study, the 5-year survival rates were similar for the two dose levels studied, 73% for 50.4 Gy and 68% for 64.8 Gy (*P* = .57). Age of 40 years or older and astrocytoma-dominant histology were poor prognostic features.[92] An increase in functional sequelae[93] and radiation necrosis[92] was observed in patients treated in the high-dose arms of these studies. Lo et al. reviewed results in 67 patients treated using various radiation doses after resection of low-grade glioma.[94] Twenty-seven patients received 55.2 Gy, 24 patients received 59.4 Gy and 16 patients received 63.75 Gy. Progression-free survival and overall survival were similar in all three dose arms. However, complication rates were related to total dose delivered. In another attempt to improve outcome with dose escalation, hyperfractionated radiotherapy (1.1 Gy twice daily) to a total dose of 72.6 Gy was delivered to 37 patients with low-grade gliomas.[95] The 10-year progression-free survival was 62%. Brain necrosis was not seen in this study, which will require confirmation.

Two studies evaluated the effect of fractionated, limited-field radiotherapy on neurocognitive function in patients with low-grade gliomas. Brown et al. reviewed the results of the Folstein Mini-Mental Status Examination for 203 adults irradiated for low-grade gliomas.[96] Most patients maintained a stable neurocognitive status after focal radiotherapy, and patients with abnormal baseline examination results were more likely to have improvement in cognitive abilities than to deteriorate after receiving therapy; few patients showed cognitive decline. This measure is a relatively unsophisticated assessment of neurocognitive function. Klein et al. studied 195 patients with low-grade gliomas (of whom 104 received focal radiotherapy) using objective and self-reported cognitive testing and compared them to 100 low-grade hematologic patients and 195 healthy controls.[97] Results suggested that the tumor itself had the most deleterious effect on cognitive function and that

radiotherapy resulted in long-term cognitive decline principally when large fraction sizes (more than 2 Gy) were used.

Malignant Gliomas

Partial brain fields (also called *limited fields*), defined using the extent of tumor on neuroimaging studies, are used for the treatment of malignant gliomas.[98] The target volume is defined as a 2- to 3-cm margin of tissue surrounding the perimeter of the MRI-defined contrast-enhancing lesion. RTOG protocols use a shrinking field approach. Initially, the treatment volume includes the contrast-enhancing lesion and surrounding edema on the preoperative MRI study with a 2-cm margin. Subsequently (after 46 Gy of a 60-Gy course), the target volume is reduced to include the enhancing lesion only (without edema) with a 2.5-cm margin.

With conventional radiation therapy, the median survival time for patients with anaplastic astrocytoma is 36 months, and the 3-year survival rate is approximately 55%.[99] In contrast, the median survival time for patients with glioblastoma multiforme is 10 months; only 6% live 3 years.[98] The response of malignant gliomas to standard radiation therapy techniques is limited both by their striking inherent radioresistance and by the radiosensitivity of the surrounding normal brain tissue. Both factors have prompted much study—of radiosensitizers to protect adjacent brain, and of dose-escalation schemes using altered fractionation, interstitial brachytherapy, radiosurgery and three-dimensional conformal radiotherapy, boron neutron capture therapy, and proton radiotherapy. Unfortunately, these approaches have not led to survival improvement.

A phase II trial of an allosteric modifier of hemoglobin (RSR13) and concurrent radiotherapy was reported.[100] RSR13 increases oxygen unloading in areas of hypoxia. Median survival in 50 glioblastoma patients treated in this manner was 12.3 months with an 18-month survival of 24%. When compared to appropriate historic data, these results have not been considered particularly promising. Temozolomide is a novel oral alkylating agent with known activity in patients with malignant gliomas. In a phase II study of concurrent radiation plus temozolomide followed by adjuvant temozolomide, the treatment was well tolerated in 64 glioblastoma patients. Median survival was 16 months and the 2-year survival was 31%.[101] Based on these results, the RTOG is conducting a phase III trial comparing radiation with BCNU to radiation with temozolomide.

Hyperfractionated irradiation is the use of two or more treatments per day with smaller-than-conventional dose fractions, so that a higher dose is delivered in the same overall treatment time. With hyperfractionation, tumor control probabilities should improve without increasing the risk of late complications. Furthermore, with a 6-hour interval between doses, there is greater probability that rapidly proliferating tumor cells will be irradiated during more radiosensitive phases of the cell cycle and become *self-sensitized* by redistribution. The RTOG conducted a randomized phase II dose-escalation study in which patients received 64.8, 72.0, 76.8, or 81.6 Gy in 1.2-Gy twice-daily fractions. Patients receiving 72 Gy had the longest median survival time, and no further improvement in outcome was observed at the higher dose levels.[102]

A phase II trial was reported by the Massachusetts General Hospital in which accelerated fractionated proton-photon therapy was used to escalate total dose. A total dose of 90 cobalt-gray equivalents (CGE; the dose in proton grays multiplied by 1.1, the relative biologic effectiveness for protons compared with cobalt 60) was given at 1.5 CGE twice daily to 23 patients with good performance status.[103] The median survival was 20 months, and only one patient experienced treatment failure in the high-dose volume. However, the development of significant radiation necrosis requiring reoperation or prolonged steroid therapy, or both, curtailed the trial despite the impressive interim results.

Three-dimensional conformal photon radiation therapy is a mode of treatment planning and delivery designed to enhance the conformation of the radiation dose to the target volume while minimizing dose delivered to normal tissue outside the treatment volume. Conformal treatment planning techniques, when applied to brain tumors, have permitted a 30% to 50% reduction in normal brain tissue volume receiving high doses.[104] This new approach to treatment planning may not only decrease the risk of normal tissue injury but also allow higher than traditional radiation doses to be safely given to patients with malignant gliomas. In an ongoing study at the University of Michigan, doses as high as 80 Gy have been given using three-dimensional techniques, and escalation to higher dose levels is planned. Results from this group suggest that, despite these high delivered doses, 89% of recurrences are in the full-dose region.

Another way to increase radiation dose is with interstitial brachytherapy. Iodine 125 and iridium 192 sources have been used in clinical practice. Well-circumscribed, peripheral, solitary supratentorial lesions of up to 5 cm are best suited for implantation. Early phase II studies showed promising survival in patients with glioblastoma multiforme treated with external irradiation combined with brachytherapy. Brain Tumor Cooperative Group Trial 87-01 evaluated the use of interstitial implantation (60 Gy at 10 Gy/d) preceding external irradiation (60.2 Gy at 1.72 Gy/fraction) and BCNU versus external irradiation and BCNU alone in a randomized trial involving 270 patients with newly diagnosed glioblastoma. Median survival in the group receiving brachytherapy was 68 weeks versus 58 weeks for those receiving external-beam radiation alone. The difference in survival was not statistically significant, and the authors concluded that there is no role for high-activity brachytherapy in patients with newly diagnosed glioblastoma.[105] In another randomized trial, Laperriere and colleagues found no difference in outcome in patients randomly assigned to receive either external-beam radiation alone to 50 Gy (median survival, 14 months) or external-beam radiation with an iodine 125 implant that delivered a minimum tumor dose of 60 Gy (13 months).[106] Thus, despite the survival advantage suggested in early trials, two randomized trials do not support the use of brachytherapy to treat newly diagnosed glioblastoma. Brachytherapy has also been suggested to improve the survival and quality of life of patients with recurrent malignant gliomas who meet criteria for implantation.[107] The use of less invasive highly conformal radiation techniques (i.e., radiosurgery) appears to provide results equivalent to those of brachytherapy in patients with recurrent gliomas, and this has become the radiation treatment of choice for patients with small recurrences.[108]

As was the case for brachytherapy, several small single-center trials suggest a benefit for stereotactic radiosurgery when used as a boost to conventional radiotherapy in patients with newly diagnosed malignant gliomas. The RTOG tested radiosurgery followed by external-beam radiation and BCNU versus external-beam radiation and BCNU alone (trial 93-05). Eligibility criteria required patients to be at least 18 years of age, have a Karnofsky performance score (KPS) of at least 60%, and have a histologically proven supratentorial unifocal glioblastoma. Two hundred and three patients were treated between 1994 and 2000. At a median follow-up of 44 months, the median survival was 14.1 months for the radiosurgery arm and 13.7 months for the conventional arm.[109] The 2-year survival rates were 22% and 16%, respectively. This trial does not support the routine use of radiosurgery in newly diagnosed patients with glioblastoma.

Gliomatosis cerebri, a diffuse involvement of the CNS (involving more than two lobes) by a malignant glioma that permeates the brain extensively without destroying the neural architecture, was once considered rare. In the MRI era this diagnosis is no longer uncommon. The pathology of gliomatosis can be high or low grade. Although radiotherapy appears to have a survival and performance status benefit for patients with low-grade gliomatosis, the volumes of radiotherapy required are near whole brain fields.[110] In these patients, it is reasonable to begin treatment with chemotherapy in an attempt to delay large-volume radiotherapy as long as possible.

Elderly glioblastoma patients with poor performance status require special consideration. Barker et al. showed that these patients are less likely to have a good response to radiotherapy than are their younger counterparts.[82] Hypofractionated treatment regimens (36 to 50 Gy in 3 to 4 weeks) appear to produce results equivalent to those of schedules requiring 6 to 7 weeks of therapy.[111]

CHEMOTHERAPY

Before the mid-1990s there was little consensus on standards for clinical trials in neurooncology. The era of controlled clinical trials for malignant astrocytomas began with the inception of the Brain Tumor Study Group in 1967. The EORTC then established a comparable group. The Brain Tumor Study Group has subsequently been replaced by three National Cancer Institute–sponsored brain tumor clinical trials consortia for the phase I and phase II evaluation of new therapeutic agents for gliomas (North American Brain Tumor Consortium, New Approaches to Brain Tumor Therapy, and Pediatric Brain Tumor Consortium). These groups can conduct rapid evaluation of new drugs and, along with other cooperative groups (i.e., RTOG), have defined modern standards for conducting and evaluating results of clinical trials involving patients with primary brain tumors. Many conclusions from clinical trials conducted before the mid-1990s must now be interpreted cautiously. The most reliable past reports are the randomized phase III trials; however, even some of these older studies require careful scrutiny. For instance, many early studies did not stratify patients using prognostic variables that are now known to have significant influence on patient survival, such as patient age, grade of tumor, performance status, and extent of resection for newly diagnosed tumors.[112,113] Because these factors may have a stronger influence on patient prognosis than the treatment being tested, they must be carefully accounted for in study design. Unfortunately, many early phase III trials (and still many phase II trials) did not adequately control for these factors. Furthermore, the reporting of these prognostic variables is often confusing. For instance, some groups report survival or time to tumor progression (TTP) from initiation of therapy, whereas others use the original surgery date for untreated patients. Some researchers define histologic groups and separate glioblastoma multiforme from anaplastic astrocytoma, whereas others combine the two groups under the heading of malignant glioma, a practice to be deplored.

The difficulty in interpreting the results of older phase I and II trials of brain tumor treatment is still greater. Not only are important variables such as age, histologic type, and performance status often poorly described, but the definition of "response" is highly variable across trials. Many older trials incorporated neurologic status, isotope brain scan, or CT scan results in the response definition, contrary to present practice. Even in the MRI era, there has been significant variability in defining radiographic response. Some investigators have proposed the uniform adoption of objective measurements of tumor size as is done for other solid tumors.[114] Others, however, contend that objective criteria of this kind are inappropriate for MRI assessments of brain tumor response given the complex three-dimensional shapes that gliomas assume as they grow within the brain, often with associated areas of cystic change, and the difficulty in distinguishing tumor margins from associated areas of cerebral necrosis, edema, and leukoencephalopathy. Given these uncertainties, many investigators have argued that TTP or progression-free survival is a more reliable measures of therapeutic effect than either objective or subjective imaging evidence of tumor shrinkage.

The use of TTP or progression-free survival, however, demands a reliable historic comparison group to which one can compare the results in treated patients. To this end, Wong and colleagues described the natural history of tumors in a large group of patients with recurrent malignant gliomas who were treated in prospective studies of agents shown to be largely ineffective.[115] This allows assessment of the TTP and progression-free survival of recurrent high-grade glioma patients who were essentially untreated as a comparison group for new phase II trials. It is expected that as the National Institute of Cancer–sponsored brain tumor consortia and cooperative groups continue to accrue patients to phase I and II trials, even larger and hence more dependable historical databases will become available.

Despite the large number of trials of chemotherapy for glioma conducted in the last 30 years, relatively little can be said about the proven benefit of individual agents or even of chemotherapy in general because of discrepancies and inconsistencies in clinical trial design, interpretation, and reporting. This section does not summarize all of the published literature, but rather highlights the few studies that support the current standard of care for chemotherapy for patients with astrocytomas.

Low-Grade Astrocytomas

Low-grade gliomas have historically been considered chemotherapy resistant. With the recent demonstration of the chemotherapy responsiveness of some low-grade oligodendrogliomas, however, has come renewed interest in assessing chemotherapy treatment for low-grade astrocytomas. Chemotherapy can be used after radiotherapy as it is for high-grade gliomas or as initial postoperative therapy. This treatment sequence is receiving increasing attention because low-grade gliomas have often infil-

trated large portions of the brain by the time they come to clinical attention. Radiotherapy for these tumors requires very large treatment fields, which increases the risk of substantial long-term neurotoxicity in patients who may live for many years. Effective chemotherapy might not only improve tumor-related symptoms and increase survival but also forestall the need for radiotherapy. This is particularly important in young children with any type of brain tumor.

It has been clearly demonstrated that low-grade gliomas in children can be highly responsive to chemotherapy.[116] Various regimens including dactinomycin and vincristine as well as regimens containing nitrosoureas have shown high response rates.[116,117] Possibly the most impressive results, however, have been seen with platinum-containing regimens, with or without vincristine, which result in radiographically determined response rates of between 50% and 75%.[118,119] Some of these responses can last for years, although nearly half of all children treated with chemotherapy ultimately require radiotherapy for tumor progression. It should be noted, however, that most of the chemotherapy responses seen in children with low-grade gliomas are for contrast-enhancing masses that probably represent pilocytic astrocytomas. Nonenhancing, diffusely infiltrating astrocytomas in children appear to be much less responsive to chemotherapy.

Data on the use of chemotherapy for low-grade astrocytomas in adults are scarce, both because of the rarity of the tumor and because historically most such patients have been treated with initial radiotherapy. When such tumors recur, more often than not they do so as high-grade tumors. There are few trials demonstrating benefit for nitrosoureas in low-grade astrocytomas. In a small Southwest Oncology Group trial, adult patients with incompletely excised low-grade gliomas were randomly assigned to receive radiation therapy alone or radiation therapy and lomustine (CCNU). There was no difference in survival between the two treatment arms.[118] The role of adjuvant procarbazine, CCNU, and vincristine (PCV) for "high-risk" patients (less than total resection, age older than 40 years) with low-grade gliomas was evaluated in RTOG trial 98-02, which has now completed accrual. In this trial, patients received 54 Gy to the tumor and a 2-cm margin and then were randomly assigned to receive either postradiation PCV chemotherapy or observation. Follow-up for this study is still early. The most convincing demonstration of a potential role for chemotherapy in adult low-grade astrocytomas is a trial of temozolomide treatment in 16 patients with progressive low-grade astrocytomas. There were five complete responses (31%) and six partial responses (38%), and four patents had stable disease (25%). Only two patients (13%) progressed on initial treatment; 73% were progression free at 1 year.[119] Although these early results are encouraging, the number of patients treated was small, and there are some questions regarding the criteria used for inclusion in this trial for radiographic response. Nevertheless, the reported response rate, which is higher than that reported for high-grade tumors, suggests that further evaluation of temozolomide for progressive low-grade astrocytomas is warranted.

It is clear that additional studies involving both children and adults with low-grade gliomas are needed to better define the role of chemotherapy. Nevertheless, given the morbidity of large-field radiotherapy and the lack of apparent impact of the timing of radiotherapy on overall survival, the preliminary data suggest that both platinum-based chemotherapy for contrast-enhancing low-grade gliomas in children and temozolomide for adults with progressive low-grade astrocytomas are reasonable options to forestall radiotherapy or to treat progressive tumor after radiation therapy.

High-Grade Gliomas

ADJUVANT CHEMOTHERAPY. Because chemotherapy has generally had the greatest impact on cancer patient survival when given in the adjuvant setting, there has been a long-term interest in exploring the role of chemotherapy as an adjunct to radiotherapy as part of the initial treatment in patients with newly diagnosed high-grade gliomas. There have been nearly 30 randomized trials exploring the efficacy of postradiation chemotherapy for high-grade gliomas, but conclusions from those trials have been ambiguous and often contradictory. One of the principal reasons for this ambiguity is the heterogeneity of the patient population included in each of these studies. As previously discussed, most of these trials did not control for important prognostic factors such as age, histologic type, or performance status, and the few studies that did control for these variables were generally underpowered to observe a modest therapeutic effect even if present. To address these concerns, two metaanalyses have investigated the role of postradiation chemotherapy for high-grade gliomas.[120,121] The two analyses used different methodologies. The study by Fine et al.[120] was a metaanalysis of published results of 16 randomized trials including over 3000 patients. The analysis by Stewart et al.[121] used primary patient data from 12 studies, also involving approximately 3000 patients. Despite the difference in methodology, differences in the trials that were included in the analyses, and the fact that the studies were published nearly a decade apart, there was a striking similarity in the findings. Both analyses demonstrated a modest survival increase both at 1 year (10% and 6% in Fine et al. and Stewart et al., respectively) and 2 years (8% and 5% in Fine et al. and Stewart et al., respectively) for patients who were treated with radiation plus chemotherapy compared to patients treated with radiation alone. Both studies found significant survival advantages for patients treated with chemotherapy whether they had a glioblastoma or an anaplastic glioma and regardless of the type of chemotherapy, although nearly all treatment regimens in these trials included a nitrosourea. The main difference between the metaanalyses was in the assessed benefit of chemotherapy for patient subgroups based on known prognostic factors. Stewart et al. found no impact of age, performance status, or extent of resection on the benefit afforded by adjuvant chemotherapy. By contrast, Fine and coworkers found that, although patients with anaplastic gliomas continued to demonstrate a survival advantage from chemotherapy for several years after treatment, the majority of benefit from chemotherapy in patients with glioblastomas occurred at 18 months after diagnosis. Because most patients with glioblastomas do not live 18 months, these data were interpreted to mean that patients with glioblastomas who live the longest (i.e., have the most favorable prognostic factors) are the ones who benefit the most from chemotherapy. Thus, it is clear that young, healthy patients with high-grade gliomas who have had maximal surgical debulking and who have excellent performance status should be offered postradiation chemotherapy. At the other end of the spectrum are older patients with large glioblastomas who could not undergo surgical debulking and who have multiple neurologic deficits and a poor performance status. For these patients, post-radiation chemotherapy is unlikely to extend significantly their expected short survival.

If chemotherapy is to be used, which are the most appropriate drugs? As mentioned earlier, most of the randomized trials used nitrosoureas (BCNU, CCNU) either alone or in combination with other drugs of uncertain activity. So use of single-agent nitrosoureas is a reasonable treatment option for patients with glioblastoma. For more than a decade, however, the standard of care for patient with newly diagnosed anaplastic gliomas has been the three-drug combination PCV. This practice was based on a randomized study of postradiation BCNU compared to PCV.[121a] In that study, the median survival of patients with anaplastic gliomas treated with PCV was 157 weeks compared to only 82 weeks for BCNU-treated patients (*P* = .009). The twenty-fifth percentile survival was even better for patients treated with PCV (7.7 years) than for those treated with BCNU (4.1 years). Although these data appear to be definitive, the conclusions may be suspect because they represent a subgroup analysis of a larger study that enrolled patients with both glioblastoma and other anaplastic gliomas. As a whole, the study was a negative trial showing no apparent advantage to either chemotherapy regimen. In an analysis of the small anaplastic glioma subgroup, however, a survival benefit was observed. Unfortunately, the number of patients with anaplastic gliomas in this trial was so small that there was no stratification for known prognostic factors, which makes interpretation of the data difficult. A more recent retrospective analysis of data for over 400 patients with anaplastic astrocytomas treated on various RTOG protocols compared the outcomes of 257 patients treated with postradiation BCNU with the outcomes of 175 patients treated with postradiation PCV.[122] Although there were more patients with excellent performance status in the PCV-treated group (KPS of 90% to 100% in 73% of PCV-treated patients and 61% of BCNU-treated patients), the overall survival in the two groups was equivalent. When 133 sets of patients matched exactly for relevant prognostic factors (age, KPS, extent of surgery) were analyzed separately, there was again no difference between BCNU and PCV treatment. These data favor the conclusion that BCNU and PCV are equivalent for anaplastic astrocytomas. In practical terms, it may be reasonable to use either regimen in young healthy patients with anaplastic gliomas. Given the potential for greater toxicity with the PCV regimen, however, one should maintain a low threshold for switching to single-agent nitrosoureas in the face of significant PCV toxicity. There are no good data to support the use of PCV over single-agent nitrosoureas for patients with glioblastoma.

A new standard of care for patients with newly diagnosed glioblastoma may be on the horizon. Stupp and coworkers treated 64 patients with newly diagnosed glioblastoma in a phase II trial of low-dose temozolomide (75 mg/m^2/d for 7 days) given during conventional fractionated radiotherapy, followed by six cycles of standard-dose temozolomide (200 mg/m^2/d for 5 days every 28 days) after radiotherapy.[101] Treatment was well tolerated, and the median survival of the group was an impressive 16 months, with 1- and 2-year survival rates of 58% and 31%, respectively. An EORTC randomized trial is currently comparing this treatment regimen to radiation alone. If the promising findings of the phase II study are confirmed by this trial, then low-dose temozolomide during radiotherapy followed by standard-dose adjuvant temozolomide will become the new standard of care for glioblastoma. A phase III multi-center trial of temozolomide versus BCNU for patients with newly diagnosed anaplastic astrocytomas is planned by the RTOG.

CHEMOTHERAPY FOR RECURRENT ASTROCYTOMAS. Although there is growing consensus on the benefit of adjuvant chemotherapy for high-grade astrocytomas at diagnosis, the evidence favoring chemotherapy use in the recurrent setting is much less compelling. To date there is no convincing demonstration of a survival benefit for patients with recurrent astrocytomas treated with chemotherapy, although few controlled trials have examined the question. One difficulty in designing phase III trials of chemotherapy at recurrence is the lack of active "standard" agents to use in a control arm (because nitrosoureas probably would have been used in the adjuvant setting), and physicians might hesitate to place patients with progressive malignant brain tumors on trials with a placebo arm. However, the most important reason for the small number of recurrent tumor phase III trials is the lack of agents with reasonable activity in phase II trials. Here again, an uncritical review of past literature (as previously discussed) could give the impression that multiple single agents and combinations of agents have significant antitumor activity. In fact, the prior edition of this text included a table that listed a large number of agents and combinations with combined response and stable disease rates from 21% to 73%. Yet, of the 32 agents or combinations listed as having moderate to high response rates in individual trials, only 5 agents are now ever clinically used in patients with recurrent gliomas. In addition, even those agents have minimal to moderate activity at best (temozolomide, BCNU, procarbazine, tamoxifen, Gliadel).

Clearly, the agent with the most proven activity against recurrent astrocytomas is temozolomide, an orally administered, second-generation imidazotetrazine prodrug with excellent bioavailability; wide tissue distribution, including the ability to cross the BBB; and alkylating activity principally at the O^6 position of guanine.[123] After phase I trials revealed activity in glioma patients, a pivotal open-label multicenter phase II trial of temozolomide in patients with anaplastic gliomas at first relapse was conducted.[124] There were 97 evaluable patients with anaplastic astrocytoma and 14 patients with anaplastic oligoastrocytoma. The overall objective radiographic response rate was 35% (8% complete response and 27% partial response); 26% had stable disease. Unfortunately, median progression-free survival was relatively short (5.4 months), and 12-month progression-free survival was only 12%. A parallel trial accrued 225 patients with glioblastoma at first relapse to a multicenter randomized phase II trial of temozolomide versus procarbazine.[125] Patients treated with temozolomide had statistically significantly longer median progression-free survival than patients treated with procarbazine (12.4 vs. 8.3 weeks; P <.006). Health-related quality-of-life assessments revealed improved quality-of-life scores for patients with stable disease being treated with temozolomide, whereas there was a decline in scores in patients with stable disease treated with procarbazine. Radiographic response rates, however, were disappointing: 5.4% in temozolomide-treated patients and 5.3% in procarbazine-treated patients. Based on the relatively high response rate for anaplastic astrocytomas and improved quality of life, the U.S. Food and Drug Administration (FDA)

approved temozolomide for use in recurrent anaplastic gliomas but not glioblastoma.

Gliadel, a BCNU-impregnated wafer, is the first biodegradable polymer drug delivery system to be approved for tumor treatment by the FDA. The wafers, which are approximately a centimeter in diameter, are placed against the walls of the surgical cavity at the end of a tumor resection (see Chemotherapy, earlier). For 2 or 3 weeks, as the polymer degrades, high concentrations of drug are delivered locally and spread by diffusion for a short distance into the adjacent brain. Phase III trials of Gliadel wafers after resections of both primary[126,127] and recurrent[128] malignant gliomas have shown a minimal, although statistically significant, prolongation of median survival of approximately 8 weeks in treated patients. The drug has been approved for these uses in the United States. Toxicities associated with Gliadel use include increased brain edema and seizures and possible increased problems with wound healing. Efforts to improve the effectiveness of polymer-based drug delivery to brain tumors include the evaluation of higher BCNU doses, which may penetrate surrounding brain tissue for greater distances.[129] Because systemic BCNU levels are negligible after Gliadel implantation, trials of concurrent use of O^6-benzylguanine (an inhibitor of acetyl guanine transferase, a principal enzyme involved in nitrosourea resistance) have also been initiated. This combination of agents may enhance local efficacy without increasing systemic toxicity.[130]

Unfortunately, few other agents have proven activity against recurrent high-grade astrocytomas. Although nitrosoureas (BCNU, CCNU) have historically been the mainstay of treatment at recurrence, many patients are treated with nitrosoureas in the adjuvant setting. Thus, both acquired tumor drug resistance and cumulative end-organ toxicity, particularly to the bone marrow and lungs, limit the utility of these drugs in the recurrent setting. Whether nitrosoureas are active against tumors previously treated with or resistant to temozolomide is not known. Furthermore, it remains unclear how much activity nitrosoureas truly have in the recurrent setting even in chemotherapy-naive patients, because the only relevant studies were conducted in the pre-MRI era.[131,132]

Procarbazine has also been historically considered an active drug for recurrent tumor; however, like nitrosoureas, most of the positive data comes from studies conducted before the MRI era or when the drug was used in combination with nitrosoureas (i.e., PCV).[133,134] A randomized phase II trial of procarbazine versus temozolomide demonstrated that procarbazine has minimal activity against glioblastoma at first recurrence (radiographic response rate of only 5%) with a very short median TTP. Given the significant toxicities associated with procarbazine, there seems to be little indication for its use except in the context of a more proven regimen like PCV.

Cisplatin and carboplatin have some activity against recurrent gliomas, although the radiographic response is usually stable disease at best, and median TTP is relatively short.[135,136] This may reflect relatively poor penetration of the platinum compounds across the BBB and BTB. Added to this pharmacokinetic disadvantage, experimental data in rodent tumors suggest that dexamethasone can reduce cisplatin penetration into the brain adjacent to tumor where infiltrative tumor cells reside.[137]

Tamoxifen, an estrogen receptor agonist-antagonist, has been demonstrated to have some activity against recurrent gliomas when given at very high dosages (180 to 240 mg/d).[138–142]

Because gliomas do not express estrogen or progesterone receptors, the mechanism of action of tamoxifen is unclear, although it has been suggested that at very high doses tamoxifen can block protein kinase C signaling, which does have antiproliferative effects in some tumor cells. Even at these very high dosages, tamoxifen appears to be as well tolerated as it is at standard dosages (10 to 20 mg/d). Combining ease of administration with excellent tolerability, tamoxifen represents a reasonable option for patients with multiply recurrent gliomas who value quality of life yet still want some active treatment.

An early single-center report suggested significant activity for irinotecan against recurrent glioma, when the standard doses for colorectal and non–small cell lung carcinoma were used.[29] This prompted both the North American Brain Tumor Consortium and New Approaches to Brain Tumor Therapy to perform phase I and II multicenter trials of irinotecan in patients with recurrent gliomas. Both groups found that irinotecan is a P-450 substrate and that the dosages being used in the single-institution experience were significantly lower than maximally tolerated doses in patients using enzyme-inducing antiepileptics.[29,30] When the appropriate phase II dosages were used, data from the consortia and a modestly sized European trial demonstrated that irinotecan is both toxic and relatively inactive in patients with recurrent gliomas.[29,31] Thus, although clinical trials continue to explore the use of irinotecan in combination with other agents (i.e., temozolomide) in treatment of gliomas, currently available evidence does not support the use of single-agent irinotecan in glioma treatment.

Biologic therapies have also proved disappointing to date. Interferons have been extensively evaluated in patients with recurrent gliomas. Although several studies have reported modest response rates with type I interferons, particularly interferon-β, other studies have shown completely negative results.[143,144] In general, TTP has been short even in patients who respond to interferons, and treatment has often been associated with significant constitutional toxicity or neurotoxicity (i.e., seizures, encephalopathy) or both.

Given that few drugs have significant single-agent activity against recurrent glioma, it is not surprising that few drug combinations have shown even modest antitumor activity in this setting, with the possible exception of PCV. One regimen that showed initial promise was a combination of BCNU and cisplatin given by continuous infusion. The initial phase II trial of this regimen included 52 patients with newly diagnosed high-grade gliomas treated with two or three cycles of preradiation BCNU and cisplatin. The objective response rate was an impressive 42% and the stable disease rate was 53%.[145] This regimen was then tested in a phase III Eastern Cooperative Oncology Group trial in which patients were randomly assigned to preradiation infusional BCNU and cisplatin or to radiation with standard postradiation BCNU.[146] Unfortunately the experimental regimen proved significantly toxic and had no clinical benefit. Median survival of patients treated with the BCNU and cisplatin combination was 11.0 months, compared to 11.2 months for patients treated with standard postradiation BCNU.

Despite the modest benefits afforded by radiation therapy and alkylating agent chemotherapy, it is clear that more effective treatments are desperately needed. Space does not permit a review of all the new strategies against malignant gliomas now being tested; however, at least two areas are worth noting. New

local delivery strategies such as CED allow one for the first time to circumvent the BBB and BTB and deliver even large molecules to discrete areas of the brain and spinal cord at very high concentrations. Therapeutic agents such as antibodies, never before a realistic candidate for treating brain tumors because they do not penetrate the BBB and BTB, can now be seriously considered in the context of CED. Proof of principle for the CED approach can be found in the study by Oldfield's group, in which an antitransferrin antibody–diphtheria toxin immunoconjugate was delivered by CED into the brains of patients with recurrent malignant brain tumors.[147] This study both demonstrated that CED can be safely performed in patients with brain tumors and showed early hints of efficacy, with 9 of 15 patients (60%) experiencing an objective response.

Possibly the most promising approach for the treatment of gliomas in the near future is the use of rationally developed targeted small molecules. As the genetic and molecular pathogenesis of gliomas become better understood, new therapeutic targets are being identified and small-molecule inhibitors of associated signaling pathways are being developed. One example is the identification of the epidermal growth factor receptor as a frequently deregulated key signaling molecule in glioblastomas. This finding prompted phase I and II trials of two small-molecule inhibitors of epidermal growth factor receptor, erlotinib (Tarceva) and gefitinib (Iressa), for treatment of recurrent high-grade gliomas.[148,149] Both drugs have shown single-agent activity. Other promising molecular targets for malignant gliomas are downstream effectors of phosphatidylinositol 3 kinase such as AKT and mTOR. A rapamycin analogue, CCI-779, targets mTOR and has some activity in recurrent high-grade gliomas.[150] Finally, farnesyl transferase inhibitors such as R115777 (Zarnestra) have shown objective responses in some patients with high-grade gliomas.[151] Although none of these agents has induced high single-agent response rates, it is unrealistic to think that interruption of a single transduction pathway would cause a complete tumor response given the multiple molecular aberrations found within genetically complex tumors such as gliomas. The hope, however, is that simultaneous inhibition of several different key signal transduction pathways will ultimately cause significant tumor responses. Clinical trials of combination signal transduction inhibitors in treatment of gliomas are just beginning.

BRAINSTEM GLIOMAS

CLINICAL AND PATHOLOGIC CONSIDERATIONS

The majority of brainstem tumors are astrocytomas, although ependymomas can also occur here. Brainstem gliomas can be diffusely or focally infiltrative with or without an exophytic component; the latter carry a better prognosis. Cranial nerve involvement can be at the nuclear or cranial nerve level as it leaves the brainstem. The initial manifestations of a brainstem glioma are unilateral palsies of cranial nerves VI and VII in approximately 90% of patients. Cranial nerve involvement is usually followed by long tract signs, such as hemiplegia, unilateral limb ataxia, ataxia of gait, paraplegia, hemisensory syndromes, gaze disorders, and, occasionally, hiccups. Less often, long tract signs precede the cranial nerve abnormalities; this is more likely with confined central intrinsic lesions.

On MRI, pediatric pontine gliomas demonstrate diffuse enlargement of the pons, indistinct margins, and no enhancement. Cystic changes and calcifications are rare. Cervicomedullary lesions are nonenhancing, well-circumscribed lesions with an exophytic component. Tectal gliomas are nonenhancing lesions that enlarge the tectal plate, often expanding this structure into the supracerebellar cistern with associated hydrocephalus. In young adult patients with brainstem gliomas, the lesions are diffuse and usually low-grade–appearing lesions without enhancement.[152] In older adults, contrast enhancement often heralds malignant pathology. For these tumors as a group, the prognosis is poor, with 5-year survival rates varying between 0% and 38% and a median survival of less than 1 year in most series.[153–155] Patients with low-grade exophytic tumors do better than those with higher-grade anaplastic tumors.

SURGERY

For pediatric or adult brainstem gliomas that have typical MRI characteristics, diffuse concentric pontine enlargement, with T2 hyperintensity and variable enhancement that is not marked or focal, treatment is usually initiated without a biopsy.[156] When a biopsy is felt to be necessary because atypical imaging findings or clinical characteristics suggest another diffuse brainstem disorder such as encephalitis or demyelination, stereotactic needle biopsy is used, usually with an entry point on the frontal convexity or over the lateral cerebellar convexity if the lesion is accessible via the middle cerebellar peduncle without crossing pial planes. Resection has no place in the treatment of diffuse pontine gliomas in children or adults.

For the more rare focal astrocytic lesions of the adult or pediatric brainstem, surgery may play a larger role. Tectal gliomas have a typical imaging appearance, and biopsy is neither necessary nor safe. However, the accompanying noncommunicating hydrocephalus (from compression of the aqueduct of Sylvius) can be treated with CSF diversion, either by third ventriculocisternostomy or by ventriculoperitoneal shunting.[157] Dorsally exophytic astrocytomas within the fourth ventricle or at the cervicomedullary junction are often resectable with low morbidity and excellent long-term results, if a complete removal is achieved.[158] Intrinsic astrocytomas or ependymomas at the cervicomedullary junction can often be completely removed by splitting the neuraxis in the posterior midline to access the tumor.[159] Whenever possible, attempted resection of brainstem gliomas should be performed by experienced neurosurgeons.

RADIATION THERAPY

Radiation therapy, the primary treatment for brainstem tumors, improves survival and can stabilize or reverse neurologic dysfunction in 75% to 90% of patients.[155] Traditionally, brainstem gliomas have been treated with doses of 54 Gy, given in daily fractions of 1.8 Gy, through parallel opposed portals with the tumor dose calculated at the midline on the central axis of the beam. In a multi-institutional survey by Freeman and Suissa,[154] the 1-, 2-, and 5-year survival rates of children treated with conventional radiation therapy techniques were 50%, 29%, and 23%, respectively.

Because of these relatively poor results and the observation that these tumors recur locally, hyperfractionated irradiation, designed to deliver higher tumor doses, was evaluated by several investigators. Early reports demonstrated consistent, although modest, improvements in outcome when results for patients treated with hyperfractionation regimens to doses of up to 70.2 to 72.0 Gy (1.0 to 1.17 Gy twice daily) were compared with those for historic control patients treated with conventional or low-dose hyperfractionated irradiation.[160,161] The Pediatric Oncology Group (POG) conducted a dose-escalation trial of 66.0, 70.2, and 75.6 Gy in twice-daily fractions of 1.10, 1.17, and 1.26 Gy, respectively, in children with diffuse brainstem gliomas. No difference in the median time to progression (7 to 8 months) and median survival time (10 months) for the three dose schedules was found. The highest dose was associated with steroid dependency in 62% of patients and a 45% incidence of intralesional necrosis.[162] The 70.2-Gy dose level was considered to have the best therapeutic ratio and was tested by the POG in a randomized trial comparing hyperfractionated radiotherapy with 54 Gy given in conventional fractionation. Both treatment arms included cisplatin during radiotherapy.[162] Hyperfractionation did not improve event-free survival ($P = .96$) or overall survival compared to the conventional regimen (median survival, 8.5 vs. 8.0 months for conventional and hyperfractionated regimens, respectively; $P = .65$).

Based on the results of the POG randomized trial, the current standard for the treatment of diffuse intrinsic brainstem gliomas consists of conventionally fractionated radiotherapy given to a dose of 54.0 to 59.4 Gy. The role of concurrent or preirradiation chemotherapy or radiosensitizers remains investigational. The availability of MRI and three-dimensional conformal radiotherapy treatment planning approaches offers improved target definition and allows the high-dose radiation volume to be better tailored to the contour of the lesion. Dorsal exophytic and cervicomedullary tumors that are completely resected do not require routine postoperative irradiation.[163]

CHEMOTHERAPY

The use of adjuvant chemotherapy in clinical trials involving children with brainstem gliomas has been infrequent. The Children's Cancer Group (CCG) randomly compared radiation therapy with radiation therapy followed by CCNU, PCV, and prednisone.[164] The mean survival was 11 months, with no difference between the two groups. In another trial, treatment with 5-fluorouracil and CCNU before radiation therapy and with hydroxyurea and misonidazole during radiation therapy were evaluated,[165] but TTP (32 weeks) and survival (44 weeks) were no better than in the initial CCG study. Another CCG study randomly assigned 32 patients to preradiation chemotherapy with three courses of carboplatin, etoposide, and vincristine; and 31 patients to preradiation cisplatin, etoposide, cyclophosphamide, and vincristine.[166] Response rates after chemotherapy and hyperfractionated radiation, event-free survival, and overall survival were not substantially different in either arm compared to standard radiation therapy alone. Thus, no agent used either during or after radiation treatment has been shown to have benefit over radiation alone.

There are few data to suggest that any chemotherapeutic agent truly has any significant activity in the setting of recurrent brainstem gliomas. Temozolomide, the most active agent for adult gliomas, has been evaluated in patients with recurrent brainstem gliomas and has demonstrated minimal activity with objective response rates of approximately 6%.[167] Because other pediatric high-grade recurrent cerebral gliomas were found to be temozolomide resistant in the same study (response rate, 12%), temozolomide resistance may be characteristic of pediatric gliomas in general rather than of brainstem gliomas specifically.[167] A Children's Oncology Group phase II trial of postradiation adjuvant temozolomide has now been completed, and preliminary results suggest that the drug has little clinical benefit.

CEREBELLAR ASTROCYTOMAS

CLINICAL AND PATHOLOGIC CONSIDERATIONS

Astrocytomas arising in the cerebellum are considered separately, because their prognosis is consistently better than that of astrocytomas arising in the cerebrum or brainstem. These tumors, which occur most often during the first two decades of life, arise in the vermis or more laterally in a cerebellar hemisphere. Cerebellar astrocytomas usually are well circumscribed and can be cystic, solid, or some combination of both.

Histologically, most cerebellar astrocytomas are low grade and lack anaplastic features. The majority are juvenile pilocytic astrocytomas. In a series involving 451 children reported by the Hospital for Sick Children of Toronto, cerebellar astrocytomas accounted for 25% of all posterior fossa tumors; 89% of the 111 cerebellar astrocytomas were low grade.[168] Approximately 75% of these tumors are located only in the cerebellum, with the remainder involving the brainstem as well. Because these tumors usually arise in the vermis or median cerebellar hemisphere, the clinical presentation is similar to that of medulloblastoma, with truncal ataxia, headache, nausea, and vomiting. In infants, head enlargement from hydrocephalus is seen.

SURGERY

Cystic cerebellar astrocytomas are exposed through a posterior fossa craniectomy. Early cyst drainage allows immediate brain relaxation. The cyst is located with ultrasonography or stereotaxy, cannulated, and then exposed by an incision through the cerebellar folia. With use of the operating microscope, the cyst is examined and the vascular, firm mural module is identified, dissected, and removed. The nonneoplastic cyst wall is not excised. Solid cerebellar astrocytomas are separated carefully from surrounding white matter, again using the improved visualization offered by the operating microscope. Ordinarily, the tumor has a distinctive appearance and is easily separated from surrounding white matter; the only barriers to complete resection are penetration of the tumor into the dentate nucleus, cerebellar peduncles, or brainstem. Gross total resection is tantamount to a cure for these lesions.[169]

RADIATION THERAPY

Most completely resected cerebellar astrocytomas do not require postoperative radiation therapy. The management of partially resected pilocytic astrocytomas remains controversial, because many of these tumors remain stable for years without additional treatment. Even when such tumors do progress, repeat resection is a reasonable option if a majority of the tumor can be removed and if there has been a relatively long interval between the time of the last surgery and progression. The overall prognosis for diffuse cerebellar astrocytomas in children tends to be poorer than it is for pilocytic tumors, with only 30% to 40% of patients progression free at 5 years.[170] Thus, local radiation is often used after surgery for children with partially resected diffuse cerebellar astrocytomas. Total doses of 50 to 60 Gy are delivered, depending on the histologic features and the age of the patient. Rarely, craniospinal radiation with a boost to the cerebellum has been used in patients with partially resected, diffuse astrocytomas thought to be at high risk for dissemination (i.e., anaplastic features). For young children with progressive pilocytic astrocytomas in whom one wishes to forestall irradiation for as long as possible, the use of systemic chemotherapy is a viable option (see Chemotherapy).

CHEMOTHERAPY

Because surgery alone or surgery followed by radiation often results in long-term disease-free progression, the use of chemotherapy has been limited to patients with recurrent tumor or to those rare patients with anaplastic cerebellar astrocytomas in the postradiation adjuvant setting. Historically, the most commonly used drugs have been the nitrosoureas, although reports of their effectiveness are largely anecdotal. Other drugs have been used on an ad hoc basis. One report cited the palliative potential of oral etoposide in the treatment of juvenile pilocystic astrocytomas, with 50% of patients (6 of 12) responding or having stable disease and a 7-month median progression-free survival.[171] Although it was hoped that temozolomide would be useful in this setting, the activity of the drug in high-grade childhood gliomas has been disappointing to date.[167] Its usefulness for recurrent or diffusely infiltrative cerebellar astrocytomas remains speculative. The regimen with the most proven success in treatment of recurrent pilocytic astrocytomas is carboplatin and vincristine,[172] which also has the potential for allowing one to forestall the use of radiation therapy for a period of time in some very young children.

OPTIC, CHIASMAL, AND HYPOTHALAMIC GLIOMAS

CLINICAL AND PATHOLOGIC CONSIDERATIONS

Nearly all gliomas of the optic nerve and chiasm are discovered in patients younger than 20 years of age, and most occur before the age of 10 years.[173] In some patients there is a family history of NF1. Lewis et al. found that gliomas along the anterior visual pathway occurred in 15% of NF1 patients and were occasionally bilateral.[174] Sixty-seven percent of these tumors were neither suspected clinically nor obvious on ophthalmologic examination.

With respect to tumor location, Housepian and associates reported that 25% involved one optic nerve, 73% the chiasm, and 3% the optic tracts.[175] In another series, 25% involved the chiasm alone, 33% the chiasm and hypothalamus, and 42% the chiasm and optic nerves or tracts.[176] Clinically, these tumors produce loss of visual acuity (70%), strabismus and nystagmus (33%), visual field impairment (bitemporal hemianopsia, 8%), developmental delay, macrocephaly, ataxia, hemiparesis, proptosis, and precocious puberty. Funduscopic evaluation demonstrates a range of findings from normal optic disks through venous engorgement to disk pallor due to atrophy. Chiasmal tumors often grow to involve the hypothalamus, causing a diencephalic syndrome characterized by emaciation (especially in children between 3 months and 2 years of age), motor overactivity, and euphoria.

Pathologically, these tumors range from primarily piloid and stellate astrocytes (most common), with or without oligodendroglia, through the gamut of malignant astrocytomas to glioblastoma multiforme (rare). Typically, optic gliomas appear as fusiform expansions of any part of the nerve. They may bridge through the optic foramen and expand as dumbbell-shaped tumors within the skull. The nerve can be infiltrated by tumor originating in the chiasm, the walls of the third ventricle, or the hypothalamus. The tumors found in NF patients often affect a single optic nerve, which is grossly normal in appearance, although infiltrated by tumor and surrounded by a fibrous stroma.

Diagnosis is best made by MRI, which demonstrates enlargement of the affected optic pathway structure, often with contrast enhancement. T2 bright signal may extend posteriorly along optic tracts as far as the visual cortex. This extension may represent tumor infiltration or edema. Cysts and calcification are not common within the optic nerve and chiasm, but the hypothalamic component can be cystic.[177]

NEED FOR TREATMENT

In general, children with asymptomatic lesions of the optic pathways found by MRI are not treated unless clinical or radiographic progression is documented. Tumors in children with NF1 tend to be more indolent than sporadic tumors. Only one-third to one-half of children with NF1 with asymptomatic optic pathway tumors found on screening MRIs require treatment for increasing visual symptoms.[178] Most children with sporadic tumors undergo imaging because of symptoms and should be treated. Sporadic tumors often present with advanced findings such as hydrocephalus, decreased visual acuity, and endocrinopathies.[179] Rarely, both sporadic and NF-associated optic pathway gliomas can regress spontaneously.[180]

SURGERY

Surgery is indicated only for some optic pathway gliomas. In appropriate patients, surgery may decrease the recurrence rate and increase the time to recurrence. Patients treated with surgery, followed by radiation and chemotherapy, appear to have the highest rate of long-term disease control,[181] although selection bias may have influenced these results. Regardless, in patients with progressive symptoms (e.g., severe visual loss and proptosis), unilateral anterior tumors that do not involve the optic chiasm may be resected. Biopsy or subtotal resection can be performed for posterior optic pathway gliomas that involve the hypothalamus and optic tract, particularly if they are symptomatic because of local compression and mass effect.

A transcranial approach to orbital tumors allows sparing of the globe and improves the cosmetic result without any apparent change in prognosis. The involved nerve is resected from the chiasm to the posterior globe. Initially a craniotomy is performed ipsilateral to known tumor and the nerve and chiasm

are examined directly. If the tumor is limited to the nerve, then the nerve can be sectioned just anterior to the chiasm. The orbit is unroofed, and the remainder of the nerve extending into the globe is resected. Resection of the chiasm is not indicated due to resultant blindness.

If the tumor involves the chiasm and the MRI study raises suspicion of another tumor type, such as an optic nerve sheath meningioma or another parasellar mass, a confirmatory biopsy can be performed. This is rarely needed in patients with NF1, in whom there is a high index of suspicion for an optic nerve glioma, with a typically indolent course, due to the known association with this disease. Subtotal resection is indicated if mass effect from the tumor produces dysfunction of adjacent structures such as the hypothalamus or the nerve itself. Hydrocephalus can be produced by more posteriorly situated tumors and may be alleviated by debulking. If hydrocephalus persists after tumor debulking, CSF shunting (which may need to be biventricular or require fenestration of the septum) becomes necessary.

RADIATION THERAPY

Treatment of optic nerve and chiasmal gliomas is controversial, because some patients with incomplete resections have been followed for 10 to 20 years without progression.[173] The literature suggests, however, that untreated optic gliomas, especially those involving the chiasm or extending into the hypothalamus or optic tracts, progress locally or are fatal in 75% of patients. Tenny and coworkers found that only 21% of patients who were followed after biopsy or exploration survived compared with 64% of those who received radiation therapy.[182] In general, optic nerve gliomas have a better prognosis than those involving the chiasm, and tumors confined to the anterior chiasm have a better outcome than those that involve adjacent structures (posterior chiasmal tumors).[183–185]

Routine postoperative irradiation is not indicated for most gliomas confined to the optic nerve, which can be completely resected.[185] In contrast, radiation therapy can prevent tumor progression, improve disease-free survival, and stabilize or improve vision in patients with chiasmal lesions, for whom postoperative residual is the rule. Wong and colleagues reported that 6 of 7 chiasmal gliomas (86%) that were not treated with radiation therapy progressed locally, whereas treatment failure occurred for 9 of 20 (45%) that were subjected to radiation therapy.[184] Furthermore, control was achieved in 87% of the irradiated patients who received a dose of 50 to 55 Gy compared with 55% of those who received 46 Gy or less. Hypopituitarism is common after radiotherapy, with a need for lifelong endocrine follow-up and appropriate replacement therapy. The prognosis for patients with optic pathway tumors may be somewhat better than for those with chiasmal-hypothalamic lesions. In a literature review, local control was found to be achieved for 154 of 189 irradiated anterior chiasmal tumors (81%), whereas 92 of 142 posterior tumors (65%) were controlled. Vision improved in 61 of 210 evaluable patients (29%) and remained stable in 118 of 210 patients (56%).[183] For hypothalamic tumors, radiation therapy produced radiographic improvement in 11 of 24 (46%) with a median progression-free survival of 70 months compared with 30 months for patients who did not receive radiation therapy.[186] Age and tumor location were important prognostic factors, with younger children (younger than 3 years) and children with lesions posterior to the chiasm faring less well after radiotherapy than older children and children with anterior tumors.[181]

Three-dimensional conformal, intensity-modulated radiotherapy and stereotactic radiotherapy techniques are used to minimize the dose to adjacent structures. A report by Debus et al. summarized results in patients treated with fractionated stereotactic radiosurgery (52.2 Gy median dose at 1.8 Gy/d).[187] All patients remained disease free, and no significant complications or marginal failures were seen despite highly conformal radiation dosing. Because these tumors are often focal, techniques like stereotactic radiotherapy can offer both excellent local control and decreased late effects compared to conventional techniques. A dose of 50 to 54 Gy in daily 1.8-Gy fractions is used.

CHEMOTHERAPY

The published chemotherapy trials for this group of patients represent small series. Chemotherapy has been used successfully to delay the initiation of radiation therapy in young children. Packer and associates treated 24 children (median age, 1.6 years) with optic pathway–hypothalamic tumors with a combination of dactinomycin and vincristine.[188] At a median follow-up of 4.3 years, 38% of patients had disease that progressed.

Petronio and coworkers reported on 19 infants or children with chiasmatic and hypothalamic gliomas treated with chemotherapy after diagnosis.[117] The chemotherapy included one of three regimens: dactinomycin and vincristine; BCNU, 5-fluorouracil, hydroxyurea, and 6-mercaptopurine; or the combination of 6-thioguanine, procarbazine, dibromodulcitol, CCNU, and vincristine. Fifteen of 18 patients treated with chemotherapy showed a response or stabilization of disease. The median follow-up period exceeded 1.5 years (range, 1.4 months to 5.8 years).

In another study, Prados and colleagues treated 42 children with low-grade gliomas who had either progressive neurologic symptoms or radiographic tumor enlargement with a combination of 6-thioguanine, procarbazine, dibromodulcitol, CCNU, and vincristine.[189] The group included 33 patients with hypothalamic-chiasmatic gliomas. Multivariate analysis demonstrated no difference between outcomes for this group and for those with low-grade gliomas in other sites. The median progression-free survival for the entire group was 2.5 years, and the 5-year median survival was 78%. Single-agent carboplatin has been used in newly diagnosed patients with optic pathway lesions. Aquino et al. treated 12 children with once-monthly carboplatin.[190] Six patients had stable disease, four had a partial response, and two had disease progression. Overall progression-free survival was 83%, and the median duration of response was 38.6 months. In summary, although chemotherapy is not curative, it can stabilize tumor growth in some young children and delay the use of radiotherapy until further tumor progression.

OLIGODENDROGLIOMAS

CLINICAL AND PATHOLOGIC CONSIDERATIONS

Oligodendrogliomas tend to occur in young to middle-aged adults. They are quite uncommon in the very young or the elderly. Grossly, oligodendrogliomas are often well demarcated, with 20% being cystic. Like astrocytomas, oligodendrogliomas display various degrees of clinical aggressiveness,

although they are more likely to spread along CSF pathways. Although multilevel grading systems for oligodendrogliomas have been proposed, a two-level classification of differentiated (grade 2) or anaplastic (grade 3) appears to be as useful. Oligodendrogliomas often display areas of astrocytic or, much more rarely, ependymal differentiation. Such tumors, referred to as oligoastrocytomas or mixed gliomas, are also classified as low grade (grade 2) or high grade (grade 3 or anaplastic). Although it is likely that all cellular components of mixed gliomas are derived from a common progenitor cell, it is unclear whether the percentage of the mixed glioma that is oligodendroglioma or astrocytoma carries prognostic implications. Clinically, oligodendrogliomas present in a fashion typical of cortical astrocytomas, but with a more indolent course, a longer antecedent history of symptoms (often over many years), and a higher frequency of seizures. Many are calcified on CT scan. Patients with well-differentiated tumors survive much longer than those with anaplastic tumors (median survival of 9.0 vs. 2.2 years for low-grade and high-grade oligodendrogliomas, respectively).[88,191,192] Most data suggest that patients with pure oligodendrogliomas have better prognoses than those with mixed gliomas. Shaw and colleagues found that the 5- and 10-year survival rates for patients with oligodendrogliomas were 72% and 46%, respectively, whereas the survival rates for mixed oligoastrocytomas were 63% and 33%.[192]

SURGERY

The resection of hemispheric oligodendrogliomas follows the same principles as discussed earlier for cerebral astrocytomas in Cerebral Astrocytomas: Surgical Principles, with gross total removal being the goal when consistent with good neurologic outcome. The margins of oligodendrogliomas can appear to be more distinct than those of astrocytomas, but generally the tumors are infiltrative. Because of this, surgical cure is unlikely; but the indolent course of many low-grade oligodendrogliomas can allow such a long progression-free interval after an aggressive resection that some patients never need further treatment. When oligodendrogliomas do recur, it often is in the previous operative site, and reoperation may be advisable, particularly when followed by radiation therapy or chemotherapy or both.

RADIATION THERAPY

The highly variable and often indolent natural history of differentiated oligodendrogliomas makes it difficult to evaluate the effect of radiation therapy. The problems in evaluating retrospective reports for oligodendrogliomas are similar to those discussed previously for astrocytomas in Cerebellar Astrocytomas: Chemotherapy. Most retrospective studies comparing surgery alone with surgery and radiation therapy do not contain analyses to ensure that the distribution of patients in the two treatment groups are comparable with respect to prognostic variables such as age,[193] completeness of resection,[194,195] neurologic signs and symptoms,[193,196] and histopathologic features.[191,193,195,196] Furthermore, treatment selection criteria are either not stated or unknown. It is likely that many retrospective studies in which the pathologic material was not independently reviewed contain patients with both differentiated and anaplastic oligodendrogliomas.

Generally speaking, the 5-year survival rates for patients undergoing radiation therapy range from 36% to 83%, and 10-

year rates vary from 30% to 46%. In contrast, 5-year survival rates for subtotally resected, nonirradiated tumors range from 25% to 55% and 10-year rates vary from 13% to 25%.[88,196–200] Although some authors recommend immediate postoperative irradiation for patients with incompletely resected lesions,[196,198–200] most suggest that radiation therapy be deferred until there is evidence of tumor progression for well-differentiated tumors.[197] Gannett and colleagues[196] found a significant improvement in survival with postoperative irradiation. Patients treated with surgery alone had 5- and 10-year survival rates of 51% and 36%, respectively, compared to 83% and 46% for patients receiving radiation therapy (*P* = .032). Shaw and colleagues found a survival advantage in irradiated patients with incompletely resected tumors who received at least 50 Gy.[192] Shimizu and colleagues performed a metaanalysis on reports from the current literature and concluded that postoperative irradiation conferred a 14% improvement in 5-year survival (*P*<.01).[198]

Taken together, these data suggest that there may be a benefit to radiation therapy for patients with incompletely resected tumors during the first 5 years after treatment, but this effect appears to diminish over time. As is the case for low-grade astrocytomas, it is difficult to take a categorical position regarding the role of radiation therapy in the treatment of low-grade oligodendrogliomas.[197] Some small tumors that are asymptomatic (except for controlled seizures) can be carefully observed, with surgical or radiotherapeutic intervention delayed until there is tumor progression or uncontrolled symptoms. If feasible, large, symptomatic, or progressive tumors should be resected. Patients with completely resected or small asymptomatic incompletely resected low-grade oligodendrogliomas can be observed, with radiotherapy reserved for recurrence.[197] Because of the poor long-term prognosis without treatment and the data tentatively suggesting benefit from radiotherapy, patients with large, symptomatic unresectable or incompletely resected tumors should receive radiation therapy.[197]

Radiation therapy is given using fields that encompass the tumor volume with a 2-cm margin. A dose of 54 to 60 Gy is used in adults, and the dose is reduced to 50 Gy in children. Chemotherapy (see Chemotherapy, later) may be useful in some patients as initial treatment, in combination therapy, or to reduce the size of large tumors before radiotherapy is begun.[201,202] In the latter situation, reducing the volume of brain irradiated may decrease risk of treatment-related adverse effects.

Regardless of the extent of resection, patients with pure and mixed *anaplastic* oligodendrogliomas receive postoperative irradiation to a dose of 60 Gy in conventional daily fractions of 1.8 to 2.0 Gy using an approach similar to that used for malignant gliomas. Clinical trials are currently testing whether combining PCV with radiotherapy improves the outcome for patients with these tumors.[203]

CHEMOTHERAPY

One of the major advances in neurooncology over the last 5 years has been the recognition of the chemosensitivity of many oligodendrogliomas. Thus, the role of chemotherapy in the treatment of these tumors is now in evolution. After several anecdotal reports of chemotherapy responsiveness in oligodendrogliomas, several phase II trials of PCV involving chemotherapy-naive patients with recurrent oligodendrogliomas were performed (Table 39.2-4). The combined results of these three

TABLE 39.2-4. Status of Phase II Studies of Lomustine, Procarbazine, and Vincristine for Recurrent Oligodendroglioma and Oligoastrocytoma

Reference	Complete Response % (MTP, mo)	Partial Response % (MTP, mo)	Stable Disease % (MTP, mo)
457	17 (25)	46 (12)	19 (7)
458	12 (45)	50 (24)	31 (32)
459	33 (25)	40 (16)	20 (7)
Total	18 (31)[a]	46 (16)[a]	23 (14)[a]

MTP, median time to progression.
[a]Weighted mean of three medians.

trials demonstrated a complete response rate of 19%, a partial response rate of 45%, and stable disease in 22% of patients. Patients experiencing complete and partial responses had a median TTP of 31 months and 14 months, respectively. Thus, the majority of patients (86%) treated with PCV at recurrence should either experience either response or stabilization for more than 1 year. In addition to PCV, temozolomide has been shown to give a high response rate in chemotherapy-naive patients with recurrent and newly diagnosed oligodendrogliomas (response rate, 53%; median time to progression, 10.4 months).[204] Furthermore, approximately 44% of patients with recurrent oligodendrogliomas previously treated with chemotherapy have a complete or partial response and another 40% have stable disease with temozolomide treatment.[205]

Like pure oligodendrogliomas, mixed gliomas can also be highly responsive to PCV and temozolomide in both the new diagnosis and recurrent disease settings.[124,206,207] Although initial reports were limited to high-grade oligodendrogliomas and mixed gliomas, newer data demonstrate that many low-grade oligodendrogliomas and mixed gliomas also respond well to chemotherapy.[119,204,206,207] Despite these high response rates, the exact role of chemotherapy in the management of oligodendrogliomas and mixed gliomas remains ill defined. An intergroup trial being coordinated by RTOG will address the role of neoadjuvant PCV plus radiation versus radiation alone, testing whether initial chemotherapy has an advantage over reservation of chemotherapy until tumor progression. Unfortunately this trial will not answer one of the most pressing questions in the field: whether chemotherapy can be used as sole initial therapy for oligodendrogliomas and thus forestall large-volume irradiation.[202] Thus, for a patient with a low-grade infiltrating oligodendroglioma or a mixed glioma, options include radiation with or without chemotherapy or possibly primary chemotherapy.

To help with this decision for a given patient, it would be useful to have markers to estimate both the likely biologic aggressiveness and chemotherapy responsiveness of the patient's specific tumor. Proliferation markers, such as the MIB-1 index, have been shown to reflect the ultimate aggressiveness of oligodendrogliomas and mixed gliomas regardless of grade.[208] A clinical, pathologic review of data for 180 patients with low-grade gliomas indicated that older age and high Ki-67 index are correlates of poorer outcome.[209] Complementing the predictive value of the proliferative index, specific chromosomal anomalies within the tumor cells of oligodendrogliomas and mixed gliomas have been demonstrated to predict both overall prognosis and responsiveness to radiation and chemotherapy. It has been reported that allelic loss of the short arm of chromosome 1 (1p) predicts both radiographic response to chemotherapy and long overall survival in patients with anaplastic oligodendroglioma. A retrospective analysis of data for 50 patients with anaplastic oligodendrogliomas found that patients who had combined, but isolated, deletions in chromosome arms 1p and 19q had marked, durable chemotherapy responses and long overall survival.[210] Tumors that harbored only 1p alterations also responded to chemotherapy, although response durations and overall survival were much shorter. Tumors without alterations in chromosome arm 1p but with p53 mutations had generally short responses to chemotherapy, and tumors with no alterations in 1p and wild-type p53 were poorly responsive to chemotherapy. These data must be considered preliminary, however. Indeed, an analysis of a series of pediatric gliomas found that 32 tumors (29.9%) had loss of heterozygosity of 1p, 27 (28%) had loss of heterozygosity of 19q, and 13 had both (rates consistent with the adult glioma experience), but there was no association between 1p or 19q chromosomal status and clinical outcome.[211] Although these contradictory findings may be a result of a different biology in pediatric gliomas compared to adult gliomas, a phase II trial of PCV treatment in adult patients with newly diagnosed low-grade oligodendrogliomas and mixed gliomas confirmed the high response rate to PCV but did not confirm the relationship between chemotherapy sensitivity and chromosome 1p and 19q status.[207] Although the lack of association between chromosomal status and clinical outcome in these trials may have been due to low statistical power, these results do reinforce the need to test the 1p and 19q association in a prospective trial before it can be used in making routine clinical decisions.

Thus, until there is more information from ongoing trials, when faced with a patient with a low-grade, unresectable oligodendroglioma or mixed glioma that involves a large amount of brain and has a high MIB-1 index (particularly if it harbors the 1p and 19q deletions), it would be reasonable to attempt a trial of upfront chemotherapy (PCV or temozolomide) in an attempt to forestall large-field irradiation for as long as possible. For patients with anaplastic oligodendrogliomas or mixed gliomas, however, radiation and adjuvant chemotherapy remain the standard.

EPENDYMOMAS

CLINICAL AND PATHOLOGIC CONSIDERATIONS

Ependymomas arise from the ependymal cells that line the cerebral ventricles and the vestigial central canal of the spinal cord. As a result, these tumors arise in the periventricular area, as intramedullary spinal cord tumors, and in the filum terminale. Approximately 60% of intracranial ependymomas are infratentorial, and 40% are supratentorial.[212] The most frequent location is in the fourth ventricle. Plastic extension of the tumor through the narrow foramina of Luschka or Magendie into the broad basal cisterns is characteristic. The spinal cord is the next most common site of origin, with other locations including the walls of the lateral ventricles and third ventricle. Half of supratentorial ependymomas are intraventric-

ular and half are parenchymal, likely arising from embryonic ependymal rests retained within white matter.[78]

Multiple classification schemes for ependymomas exist. Grade 2 or differentiated ependymomas include cellular, papillary, clear cell, and tanycytic subtypes. These make up the majority of ependymomas, and subtype does not appear to determine survival. Less often, ependymomas may have anaplastic features (WHO grade 2). The difference in prognosis between differentiated ependymomas and anaplastic ependymomas is not clear, and histologic features of malignancy do not always imply short survival. Individual ependymomas do not tend to progress from grade 2 to grade 3 as do other types of gliomas.[78] Seeding of CSF pathways has been reported to occur more frequently with anaplastic tumors and heralds a poor prognosis.[213] Myxopapillary ependymomas are WHO grade 1 lesions that arise in the conus, cauda equina, or filum terminale, and resection is often curative.

As usual with gliomas, clinical presentation depends on tumor location. Tumors with ventricular involvement often cause increased ICP and hydrocephalus by obstruction of CSF pathways. Headaches, nausea and vomiting, papilledema, ataxia, and vertigo are frequent signs and symptoms found in patients at presentation. Focal neurologic signs and symptoms are seen with supratentorial ependymomas that involve the parenchyma.

Although MRI is favored for making anatomic diagnoses before surgery, the presence of calcium in a fourth ventricular tumor on CT scan is very suggestive of an ependymoma. Supratentorial parenchymal tumors cannot be readily distinguished from other gliomas by imaging. Surgical resection is essential, both to make the diagnosis and to maximize survival. For anaplastic ependymomas, a staging spinal MRI with gadolinium and CSF cytologic examination are essential.

In a literature review, Vanuytsel and Brada found that the overall incidence of spinal seeding in ependymomas was 6.9%.[214] Infratentorial lesions were more likely to seed (9.7%) than were supratentorial lesions (only 1.6%), and anaplastic ependymomas seeded at a higher rate (8.4%) than low-grade tumors (4.5%). In total, 15.7% of those with high-grade infratentorial tumors developed spinal dissemination, whereas none with supratentorial anaplastic lesions did. For low-grade tumors, 2.7% of supratentorial lesions showed seeding compared with 5.5% of infratentorial lesions. Spinal seeding was directly related to local tumor progression, regardless of tumor grade. The incidence of spinal dissemination was 3.3% in patients with locally controlled primary lesions and 9.5% in those with uncontrolled primary lesions.[214] Ependymoblastomas, an aggressive subtype of embryonal cell neoplasm, are distinct from anaplastic ependymomas. These tumors tend to disseminate throughout the neuraxis, and inclusion of these tumors in series evaluating leptomeningeal spread of ependymomas tends to overestimate the risk of seeding.[161,213]

Subependymomas are benign tumors that histologically resemble ependymomas, with an admixture of fibrillary subependymal astrocytes. They are distinct from subependymal giant cell astrocytomas, which occur in the lateral ventricles in tuberous sclerosis syndrome. Subependymomas occur most often in the floor or walls of the fourth ventricle in older men. Most are asymptomatic and slow growing, and treatment is rarely needed except for hydrocephalus or demonstrated growth. They are often incidentally found at autopsy.

SURGERY

Several retrospective studies support the relationship between postsurgical residual ependymoma and a poorer outcome, and therefore maximal safe resection is the surgical goal.[215] Ependymomas arising from the floor of the fourth ventricle are approached through a bilateral suboccipital craniectomy and laminectomy of C-1. The inferior subarachnoid space is occluded with cotton patties to minimize the possibility of CSF dissemination of tumor cells to the spine. The tumor is exposed by retracting the cerebellar tonsils laterally and splitting the inferior vermis or by opening the cerebellomedullary fissure on one or both sides. Often a tongue of tumor is visible over the dorsal aspect of the medulla and upper cervical spinal cord before the tonsils are retracted. The dorsal tumor surface is seen as the vermis is divided, and its attachment to the floor of the fourth ventricle can then be exposed and evaluated. Firm attachment precludes complete removal, because the floor of the fourth ventricle must be carefully protected from injury. Tumor is removed to the extent possible using illumination and magnification afforded by the operating microscope. Residual tumor is often simply amputated flush with the floor. These tumors may also extend through the foramen of Luschka, entangling the cranial nerves in the basal cisterns, which also precludes a complete resection. A pericranial graft is used for dural closure. The less common supratentorial tumors are removed as with any glioma. Avoidance of bleeding into the ventricular system is important to prevent postoperative hydrocephalus.

RADIATION THERAPY

It is well established that postoperative irradiation improves the survival of patients with intracranial ependymomas, and 5-year survival rates with doses of 45 Gy or more range from 40% to 87%.[216] Tumor grade has been considered to be the most important determinant of tumor behavior and prognosis. The 5-year survival rate for patients with low-grade tumors ranges from 60% to 80%, whereas for patients with anaplastic ependymomas it is only 10% to 47%.[216] Most series fail to distinguish patients with malignant ependymomas from those with ependymoblastomas. It appears that when ependymoblastomas are excluded from the data set, tumor grade may have less prognostic value than initially thought.[213]

The amount of normal CNS tissue to include in the treatment volume and the need for prophylactic irradiation to the entire craniospinal axis are major areas of controversy. In their literature review, Vanuytsel and Brada found that risk of seeding was independent of whether prophylactic spinal irradiation was given.[214] For high-grade lesions, spinal dissemination occurred in 9.4% of patients receiving craniospinal axis irradiation (CSI) and in 6.7% of those treated with local radiation therapy only. Similarly, for low-grade tumors, spinal seeding occurred in 9.3% after craniospinal irradiation, whereas 2.2% developed seeding without prophylactic treatment.

The treatment volumes recommended for low-grade supratentorial ependymomas vary from generous local fields to fields encompassing the whole brain, whereas for low-grade infratentorial tumors they include local fields, the whole brain with cervical spine extension, and the craniospinal axis. Wallner and coworkers reviewed data for 20 patients with supratentorial and infratentorial low-grade ependymomas treated with partial or whole brain postoperative irradiation. Of 16 patients, only 1, who was eventually found to have a local recurrence, developed spinal dissemination.[217] The 5- and 10-year survival rates for those who received more than 45 Gy (approximately 50 Gy in most instances) were 67% and 57%, respectively. Because local failure dominated the recurrence patterns, whole brain treatment was thought unnecessary. Based on this series and others,[161,165,214] low-grade supratentorial ependymomas are treated using partial brain fields with a dose of at least 54 Gy. Low-grade infratentorial ependymomas are also treated using limited fields. The craniospinal axis is irradiated only if pretreatment CSF cytologic studies reveal malignant cells or if radiographic studies show evidence of tumor spread.

Many authors recommend CSI in the treatment of anaplastic ependymomas,[217–219] whereas others recommend only whole brain irradiation with an additional boost to the tumor for supratentorial lesions located away from the CSF pathways.[161] A dose of 54 Gy is given to the primary tumor site and 36 Gy to the remainder of the axis if CSI is to be given. If spread within the brain is demonstrated, the entire brain receives 54 Gy. Spinal imaging studies are routinely performed, and any area of gross involvement is boosted to 50 Gy. Despite the apparent usefulness of CSI, local recurrence is the primary pattern of failure with high-grade ependymomas.[161,165,217,219] Subarachnoid seeding is uncommon in the absence of local recurrence. Furthermore, the patterns of failure are similar in patients treated with local fields or with CSI, and prophylactic treatment may not prevent spinal metastases.[161,214] In one series of 28 patients with anaplastic ependymomas, 12 received CSI, 2 received treatment to the whole brain, and 14 received treatment to limited fields.[220] Actuarial 5- and 10-year survival rates were 56% and 38%, respectively. All 19 radiotherapy failures were local, and in one of these cases CSF seeding also developed. A benefit from CSI could not be demonstrated. Based on these and other data, CSI is generally not recommended for patients with anaplastic (high-grade) ependymomas unless CSF seeding is pathologically or radiographically documented.[161,165,220] There still, however, is an argument for prophylactic CSI for patients with infratentorial high-grade lesions.[165]

Because local recurrence is the most common pattern of failure,[219] clinical trials are examining more aggressive local therapies to improve local tumor control, both in low- and high-grade ependymomas. These include the use of boosts with stereotactic radiotherapy or conformal radiotherapy techniques as well as hyperfractionated dose schedules.[165] There is no evidence thus far that the addition of chemotherapy to radiotherapy improves the outcome.[221]

CHEMOTHERAPY

Ependymomas are rare tumors, and reported chemotherapy series are few. The CCG used monthly carboplatin in a pediatric brain tumor trial and found a rate of response or stable disease of 28% (4 of 14 ependymomas) with durations of 6+, 17+, 12, and 15 months.[222] In a CCG evaluation of cisplatin treatment in eight pediatric ependymoma patients included in a larger trial, despite several radiographic responses, the overall median time to progression was only 3.8 months.[135] A small trial of etoposide in ten adult patients with recurrent spinal cord ependymoma showed a 20% response rate, a median time to progression of 15 months, and overall survival of 17.5

months.[223] A multicenter trial conducted by the French Society of Pediatric Oncology used alternating courses of three different regimens (procarbazine plus carboplatin, etoposide plus cisplatin, vincristine plus cyclophosphamide) as adjuvant postsurgical treatment in 72 children younger than 5 years of age with ependymomas. Forty percent of patients had been spared radiotherapy 2 years after treatment, and 23% 4 years after treatment. The authors concluded that chemotherapy has a potential role in deferring radiotherapy, although patients spared radiation with this strategy might also have been progression-free with surgery alone. Suggesting this is that no chemotherapy responses were seen in patients with measurable disease after surgery.[224] Studies using temozolomide in ependymomas are still pending. Thus, to date, few if any drugs have shown even modest consistent activity in ependymomas.

MENINGIOMAS

CLINICAL AND PATHOLOGIC CONSIDERATIONS

Meningiomas arise from arachnoidal cells in the meninges, especially in areas of the arachnoid villi. In some series, meningiomas constitute 27% of primary CNS tumors.[225] The most frequent locations of these tumors are along the sagittal sinus and over the cerebral convexity. Table 39.2-5 summarizes the frequency of these tumors according to location.[226] Meningiomas are extraaxial, intracranial, and sometimes spinal tumors that produce symptoms and signs through compression of adjacent brain tissue and cranial nerves. They often also produce hyperostosis; bony invasion does not indicate malignancy. Table 39.2-6 summarizes the symptoms and signs associated with these tumors. Most meningiomas are sporadic and are most common in older women. Some occur after exposure to radiation or hormonal treatment. They may be multiple, especially in NF2 but also in sporadic cases through subarachnoid seeding. They rarely metastasize except after multiple resections when they may spread to the lung, where growth is typically slow.

TABLE 39.2-5. Sites of Predilections of Meningiomas within the Intracranial Regions

Site	No.
Parasagittal	65
Convexity	54
Sphenoidal ridge	53
Olfactory groove	29
Suprasellar	28
Posterior fossa	23
Spinal	18
Periocular	12
Temporal fossa	8
Falx	7
Choroidal	6
Gasserian	5
Multiple	2
Combined with neurinomas	2
Intraorbital	1

(From ref. 226, with permission.)

TABLE 39.2-6. Neurologic Findings Associated with Meningiomas as a Function of Their Location

Site	Presentation
Sphenoidal ridge	Nonpulsating, painless unilateral exophthalmos; unilateral vision loss; ophthalmoplegia; ICP
Cerebral convexity	Altered mentation; ICP; seizures
Intraventricular	Hydrocephalus; headache; mental changes; visual field abnormalities
Olfactory groove	Central scotoma; ipsilateral optic atrophy; contralateral papilledema; ipsilateral loss of smell; altered mentation; focal motor abnormalities
Tuberculum sellae	Loss of vision; bitemporal hemianopsia; papilledema or optic atrophy
Cerebellar convexity	ICP; cerebellar findings
Cerebellar-pontine angle	Cerebellar findings; hearing loss
Foramen magnum	No findings; spastic paresis and sensory findings in upper extremities

ICP, increased intracranial pressure.

Histologically, most meningiomas are well differentiated, with low proliferative capacity and limited invasiveness. Less often, meningiomas are anaplastic with a higher proliferative capacity and invade the brain.[78] In the 2000 WHO grading scheme, most meningiomas are grade 1 (benign). Some histologic subtypes are higher grade: clear cell and chordoid meningiomas are grade 2 (atypical), and rhabdoid and papillary meningiomas are grade 3 (malignant). Meningiomas of other normally benign histologic types can reach higher grades if they display certain histologic criteria. A grade 2 meningioma must have four or more mitoses per ten high-power microscopic fields or meet three of the following five criteria: necrosis, sheeting, high cellularity, high nucleus to cytoplasm ratio, or prominent nucleoli. A grade 3 meningioma has 20 or more mitoses per ten high-power fields or the histologic appearance of carcinoma, sarcoma, or melanoma.[78]

SURGERY

Although many meningiomas are surgically resectable, others pose formidable challenges even though histologically benign. Meningiomas usually are well circumscribed and do not normally invade adjacent brain. However, surgical access to some of their common sites requires deep brain retraction. Meningiomas may be extremely vascular and can surround cranial nerves and major arteries at the skull base, which often precludes a safe, total removal. In a classic paper, Simpson reported a 9% recurrence rate after apparently total excisions that included the dural attachment; recurrence was more frequent after subtotal resection.[227] A more modern series shows that a *total resection* is followed by 7% recurrence rate at 5 years, 20% at 10 years, and 32% at 15 years.[228]

The ideal goal of meningioma surgery is total resection, because this is often curative for benign tumors. Meningiomas should be completely resected during the first attempt if possible. Subsequent operations are complicated by adherence of the tumor to surrounding structures. The risk of removing meningiomas in many locations, however, must be balanced against the advantages of less aggressive removal, because meningiomas are typically slow growing, and the patients are often elderly. Observation alone is appropriate for many meningiomas, especially small tumors that are incidentally discovered. In older patients, partial removal with observation or radiation treatment of the residual mass is sometimes best.

Preoperative Planning

Meningioma surgery requires a detailed knowledge of surgical anatomy. A preoperative angiogram to assess tumor vascularity and to identify or embolize surgically inaccessible feeding arteries is sometimes indicated. Embolization is done within 24 to 96 hours of surgery so that collateral vascular supply to the tumor does not develop. Normally only the vascular supply from the external carotid artery can be embolized safely.

Surgical Principles

The arterial supply to the tumor is addressed first at the operation if accessible. The tumor capsule is then carefully dissected from surrounding normal structures as the central portion of the tumor is removed by the use of an ultrasonic aspirator, an electrocautery cutting loop, or a laser. Meningiomas at individual sites pose special surgical problems.

At the cerebral convexity, a large bone flap is made around the tumor's dural base, which is then circumscribed with a dural incision. Microdissection frees the tumor from surrounding brain as the tumor is lifted away. Overlying hyperostotic bone, which contains tumor cells, can be replaced with a cranioplasty.

Parasagittal meningiomas abut the midline. Critical draining veins from adjacent brain, invasion or occlusion of the sagittal sinus by the tumor, and massive overlying bony erosion or hyperostosis are the surgical challenges. Preoperative vascular imaging defines sagittal sinus patency and relations between cerebral veins and the tumor. A patent sagittal sinus cannot be transected for a complete tumor removal except in its anterior one-third. Further posteriorly, the involved sagittal sinus may be opened to remove tumor within, or the involved sinus wall may be resected and replaced by a graft. Because recurrence-free survival after subtotal resection of these lesions can be lengthy[228] and because residual tumor may grow to occlude the sinus completely, which makes complete resection possible later with a lesser risk, subtotal resection is also an option. Small tumor remnants can be observed or treated with conventional conformal radiation or radiosurgery.

Falx meningiomas do not involve the sagittal sinus but occupy the falx below, often becoming bilateral. Surgical interruption of adjacent cerebral veins can cause cerebral edema and venous infarction. Overzealous retraction of the adjacent brain to provide a surgical access corridor can also cause postoperative neurologic deficits.

Olfactory groove meningiomas typically grow extremely large before personality change or headache leads to their discovery. Anosmia is the rule but is rarely noted by the patient. Surgery is carried out through a large bifrontal exposure. The broad sessile tumor base is divided first to interrupt feeding arteries from the skull base. The tumor's bulk is then reduced by internal coring and dissection, while the optic nerves,

carotid arteries, and anterior cerebral arteries on the tumor's posterior aspect are protected.

Tuberculum sellae meningiomas become symptomatic at a smaller size through compression of optic nerves and chiasm. Attention to the safety of the optic apparatus and the anterior cerebral and carotid arteries is axiomatic.

The approach to sphenoid ridge meningiomas varies with their origin on the lateral, middle, or medial third of the sphenoid bone. Lateral-third tumors can present as an intracranial tumor, as massive temporal bone hyperostosis, or often as both. Removal of the intracranial mass through a frontotemporal craniotomy can be complicated by adherence to sylvian veins and the middle cerebral artery. Bony hyperostosis of the sphenoid wing can cause proptosis, requiring removal and orbital reconstruction. Middle-third tumors grow intracranially in a globular fashion. Surgical cure through a frontotemporal craniotomy is likely. Medial-third tumors arise from the anterior clinoid process, compress the optic nerve, and encase the carotid and middle cerebral arteries. They can grow diffusely into the cavernous sinus and optic canal, and even the orbit proper. Only when the tumor presents early because of optic nerve compression is total removal feasible; for larger tumors, the surgeon stops when the risk of further removal exceeds the potential benefit. Many tumors occupy the cavernous sinus with little or no tumor mass in the temporal fossa itself. Few surgeons advocate radical resection for these lesions; they may be observed or, if growing or symptomatic, treated with radiosurgery or fractionated stereotactic radiotherapy.

Cerebellopontine angle meningiomas arise from the petrous bone and if small and laterally situated are exposed through a posterior fossa craniectomy, with the cerebellum retracted medially. Tumors arising more ventrally, from the petroclival junction or clivus, require a combined approach above and below the tentorium, which affords better exposure with less brain retraction.[229] Posterior fossa meningiomas may engulf critical blood vessels and cranial nerves and may adhere to the brainstem, so surgical removal must proceed cautiously.

RADIATION THERAPY

The need for adjunctive radiation therapy is determined by the extent of surgical resection and the histopathologic grade of the tumor (benign, atypical, or malignant). The risk of recurrence for completely resected benign meningiomas is small, and postoperative irradiation is ordinarily not recommended. In contrast, the risk of relapse after subtotal resection ranges from 33% to 60% at 5 years to more than 90% at 15 years.[228,230,231] Several reports provide evidence that postoperative irradiation prolongs the interval to recurrence, prevents tumor regrowth in some patients, and improves the survival of patients with incompletely resected meningiomas. Barbaro and associates compared the outcome of 54 patients who were treated with subtotal resection and radiation therapy with that of a group of 30 patients who underwent subtotal resection alone.[232] Sixty percent of the patients not receiving radiation therapy developed recurrence, whereas 32% of those given radiation treatment experienced recurrence. The median time to recurrence was 10.4 years for the irradiated patients and 5.5 years for the nonirradiated group ($P <.05$). Irradiated patients had a more favorable outcome even though they more frequently had tumors located in surgically unfavorable sites.

Goldsmith and colleagues reported the results for 140 patients (117 with benign and 23 with malignant tumors) treated at the University of California, San Francisco (UCSF), with subtotal resection and postoperative irradiation. The median tumor dose was 54 Gy.[233] For patients with benign meningiomas, the 5- and 10-year progression-free survival rates were 89% and 77%, respectively. Patients who received at least 52 Gy had a 20-year progression-free survival rate of more than 90%. The 5-year progression-free survival of patients treated after 1980 was 98%, compared with 77% for those treated before 1980. This improvement was attributed to the availability of CT scanning and MRI for tumor localization and treatment planning.

A multivariate analysis identified that, for benign meningiomas, improved progression-free survival was not related to tumor size but was associated with younger age (*P* = .01) and treatment after 1980 with innovative technologies (*P* = .002).[234] Condra and coworkers found that at 15 years 70% of their patients had experienced relapse after subtotal excision alone, whereas only 13% of those treated with subtotal excision and postoperative irradiation experienced recurrence (*P* = .0001). The 15-year cause-specific survival rate was 86% for patients treated with combined therapy compared with 51% for nonirradiated patients (*P* = .0003). Among patients undergoing complete resection, 24% relapsed after 15 years, and the 15-year cause-specific survival was 88%.[235] The actuarial 5-, 10-, and 15-year relapse-free survival rates for patients undergoing subtotal resection and irradiation reported by Graholm and colleagues were 78%, 67%, and 56%, respectively.[236] These results and those of Goldsmith and coworkers compare favorably with the relapse-free survival rates of 63%, 45%, and 9% reported by Mirimanoff and associates for incompletely resected, nonirradiated patients.[228]

The size of the residual meningioma affects the outcome of radiotherapy. Connell and colleagues showed that, for tumors 5 cm or larger, the 5-year progression-free survival rate was 40%, significantly lower than the 93% observed for smaller tumors.[237] Among patients irradiated for unresectable tumors and in those with residual disease, the volume of visible tumor on imaging studies rarely decreases by more than 15% and often only after many years.[234]

It is controversial whether radiation should be used immediately after an initial subtotal resection or only if progression is documented. Some clinicians find that patients with benign meningiomas do equally well with either approach, but others suggest that initial postoperative irradiation is preferred because recurrence has an adverse influence on outcome.[234] Postoperative irradiation often is deferred in elderly patients and in those in poor medical condition until there is evidence of progression. When a resection is not feasible, radiation therapy may relieve symptoms and substantially decrease the rate of tumor growth.[236]

Malignant meningiomas behave more aggressively. Chan and Thompson found that the median survival of six patients treated with surgery alone was only 7.2 months, compared with 5.1 years for 12 patients treated with surgery and postoperative irradiation.[238] Six of the nine patients with malignant histology reported by Graholm and coworkers died within 5 years.[236] Goldsmith and colleagues reported a 5-year progression-free survival of 48% for 23 patients treated by subtotal resection and irradiation.[233] The recurrence rate among 53 patients with malignant meningiomas collected from six series in the litera-ture was 49%. The recurrence rates were 33% for patients treated with complete resection alone, 12% for those undergoing complete resection and radiation therapy, 55% for patients treated by subtotal resection and irradiation, and 100% for those treated by subtotal resection alone.[230] These data suggest that all patients with atypical and malignant meningiomas should be offered postoperative irradiation, regardless of the extent of resection, although patients with completely resected atypical lesions may also be managed with observation.[234,239]

For benign meningiomas, the planning target volume consists of the residual tumor with a 1- to 2-cm margin of normal tissue, defined by CT scan or MRI and modified by the neurosurgeon's description of the site of residual disease. Extensive tumors of the base of the skull and malignant meningiomas require more generous margins. The preoperative tumor volume is used for planning for completely resected malignant lesions. A dose of 54 Gy in daily fractions of 1.8 to 2.0 Gy is recommended for benign meningiomas, and 60 Gy for atypical and malignant tumors. Complex three-dimensional conformal treatment planning and delivery techniques and intensity-modulated radiotherapy are used to restrict the dose to normal tissues.

Radiosurgery is another option for meningioma treatment. Kondziolka et al. found that 93% of their patients treated with radiosurgery and followed for 5 to 10 years required no further therapy for their tumors.[240] Nearly 85% of patients treated by Hakim and coworkers experienced tumor control at a median follow-up of 22.9 months.[241] In a more recent study of 85 patients, 53% of patients experienced a decrease in the size of their meningiomas; 40% showed no change; and 6% required reoperation for tumor growth or persistent symptoms.[242] Complications, including cranial neuropathies, transient neurologic deficits, radiation necrosis, and malignant edema, have been reported in 6% to 42% of radiosurgically treated patients.[243,244] Complications are more frequent in patients with large or deep-seated tumors and in those treated with high single doses,[242,245] which suggests that radiosurgery should be reserved for small lesions. Fractionated radiotherapy may be preferable for larger tumors. Although tumor control rates for small meningiomas appear promising, several more years of follow-up are required to fully evaluate the efficacy of radiosurgery in comparison with surgery and conventional radiotherapy.

CHEMOTHERAPY

There is currently no defined role for chemotherapy for newly diagnosed or nonirradiated meningiomas. Chemotherapy has been generally reserved for meningioma recurrences that are not amenable to further surgery or radiotherapy. Unfortunately, reports of chemotherapy responses are anecdotal, with no clear drug or combination regimen giving consistent responses. Because meningiomas have estrogen and progesterone receptors, there have been unsuccessful attempts to use hormonal agents such as tamoxifen. Grunberg and colleagues reported the use of mifepristone (RU 486), an antiprogesterone, in 14 patients with recurrent meningiomas. Five of 14 patients reportedly showed objective response after 6 to 12 months of daily oral therapy.[246] A subsequent Southwest Oncology Group phase III trial of incompletely resected meningiomas treated with or without mifepristone, however, showed no benefit of the drug.

Kaba and colleagues reported on six patients with either a recurrent malignant meningioma or an unresectable meningioma who were treated with interferon-α at a dosage of 4 mU/m²/d, 5 days per week.[247] Five of six patients exhibited positive response to treatment, with stabilization of tumor size in four patients and slight regression in one for 6 to 14 months. In addition, there are anecdotal cases of disease stabilization with interferon-α at much lower doses.

Lastly, there are preliminary data suggesting that hydroxyurea may have activity in patients with unresectable and recurrent meningiomas.[248] Mason and coworkers have reported disease stabilization with a median duration of treatment of 122 weeks in 12 patients with unresectable or progressive meningiomas treated with hydroxyurea.[249] There do not appear to be any data suggesting activity for hydroxyurea in atypical or malignant meningiomas.

PRIMITIVE NEUROEPITHELIAL TUMORS

CLINICAL AND PATHOLOGIC CONSIDERATIONS

The treatment of PNETs is controversial and complex. Much of the controversy is based on the ignorance of whether these tumors are the same entity, just located in different areas of the brain, or whether they are really different tumor types. This has caused significant controversy over the years regarding the classification of PNETs.[250] Primitive, undifferentiated, small round cells with pockets of varying degrees of neuronal or glial differentiation, or both, are the hallmark of the PNET. Historically, small round cell tumors arising in the posterior fossa were called medulloblastomas. Given the cytologic similarity between all these types of tumors regardless of anatomic location (i.e., posterior fossa, pineal, cortex), however, it was suggested in the 1980s that they all be designated as PNETs. Although still controversial, the current WHO classification retains medulloblastoma as a distinct type of PNET within the larger group of "embryonal" tumors that includes medulloepithelioma, neuroblastoma, and ependymoblastoma. Pineoblastoma, historically considered as a PNET and treated as such, also retains a separate position within the category of pineal parenchymal tumors. Regardless of their formal classification, these tumors can be viewed conceptually as developmentally aberrant early neural (glial or neuronal or both) progenitor or stem cells. With the exception of medulloblastoma, PNETs are rare.

PNETs share several important clinical features. They are highly proliferative and malignant tumors that tend to spread throughout the neuraxis through CSF pathways, although hematogenous metastasis is also seen. As a result, contrast-enhanced MRI scans of the entire brain and spine and a lumbar puncture for CSF evaluation, including cytologic examination, should be performed before treatment starts. Except for medulloblastoma, there are few prospective data regarding the treatment of these relatively rare tumors. Thus, treatment recommendations must be gleaned from small retrospective and anecdotal series. Treatment considerations for medulloblastoma, which are more solidly grounded, are considered separately.

SURGERY

The initial therapy for PNETs is surgical bulk reduction whenever feasible. Surgical principles are the same as those for cerebral astrocytomas described earlier in Cerebral Astrocytomas: Surgical Principles.

RADIATION THERAPY

There is general consensus that patients with PNETs should receive postoperative irradiation. Although radiation therapy appears to improve survival time, the outcome is generally poor, and most patients develop local or regional recurrences. Because of their propensity toward CSF seeding, PNETs are treated with CSI. The primary tumor is given 54 to 60 Gy and the remainder of the axis receives 36 Gy. Chemotherapy is usually a part of the treatment program. PNETs are less radiocurable than medulloblastomas. In some series 1-year survival rates are as low as 10%,[251] whereas other investigators report 5-year survival rates of 20% to 25%.[252] The disparity in outcome data may reflect the heterogeneity of malignancies that are classified as PNETs. For example, in a series of 14 patients reported on by Gaffney and coworkers, the 3-year survival rate was 29%. None of the patients with tumors containing more than 90% undifferentiated elements was alive at 3 years, whereas 60% of those with less primitive tumors survived 3 years.[253] In another study, Mikaeloff and colleagues reported a 37% 3-year survival rate in 30 patients with CNS PNETs other than medulloblastoma who were considered good risks; 16 of 30 had gross tumor resections.[254] In a more recent series, Paulino and Melian reported a 5-year survival rate of 47% in a small group of patients treated for supratentorial PNETs.[255]

Cerebral neuroblastomas are biologically distinct from other PNETs. They tend to be less malignant, have a better outcome, and are less likely to disseminate throughout the craniospinal axis.[256] These tumors may be cystic with a mural nodule or a solid mass. The morphologic appearance is related to prognosis. Berger and colleagues found that 7 of 11 patients treated with local irradiation to an average of 52 Gy were alive with no evidence of tumor progression.[257] None of six cystic tumors recurred, whereas four of five solid tumors showed treatment failure. The only patient with a solid lesion who did not have a recurrence received adjuvant chemotherapy. Although subarachnoid dissemination is found in autopsied cases,[258] this pattern of spread does not represent a significant clinical problem. Thus, localized cerebral neuroblastomas are treated with involved-field irradiation to 54 Gy. The craniospinal axis is included only if there is evidence of CSF dissemination on imaging or CSF cytologic examination.

CHEMOTHERAPY

PNETs are uncommon, and there are no controlled chemotherapy trials. Reports of isolated cases and small series indicate that drugs active against medulloblastoma have activity in PNETs (see Medulloblastomas: Chemotherapy, later in this chapter).

MEDULLOBLASTOMAS

CLINICAL AND PATHOLOGIC CONSIDERATIONS

Medulloblastoma is the most common childhood malignant brain tumor, accounting for 16% of all pediatric brain tumors.[259] The peak incidence of medulloblastoma is between 3 and 4 years of age, and the tumor is rare in adults; it comprises approximately 1% of all primary brain tumors. For adult medulloblastoma the peak age is between 20 and 35 years, after which the incidence steadily declines.[260] Approximately 1% to 2% of medulloblastomas occur in association with Gorlin's syndrome (the nevoid basal cell carcinoma syndrome), which indicates the importance of the sonic hedgehog signaling pathway in the pathogenesis of this tumor.

Like other embryonal tumors or PNETs, medulloblastomas consist of sheets of small round blue cells with scant cytoplasm. Frequent mitoses reflect a high proliferative index. They often contain areas of glial or neuronal differentiation, or both. Two important variants are desmoplastic and multinucleated giant or large cell medulloblastomas. Large cell medulloblastoma is a particularly aggressive form of medulloblastoma with a very high proliferative and apoptotic index and large areas of necrosis. These tumors display amplification of the MYC oncogene, a known negative prognostic factor.[261] The desmoplastic variant has large areas of reticulin staining interspersed with reticulin-free areas that contain both glial and neuronal differentiation. This variant is associated with deregulation of the sonic hedgehog pathway, often through PTCH mutations.[262,263] The desmoplastic variant accounts for nearly 50% of adult medulloblastomas but only 15% of pediatric medulloblastomas.[260,262]

The typical location for childhood medulloblastoma is in the midline and posterior vermis of the cerebellum (Fig. 39.2-4). In this location, tumor progression leads to encroachment into the brainstem, the cisterna magna, and the fourth ventricle, often leading to hydrocephalus. In older patients, tumors in the lateral cerebellar hemispheres become more common (50% in adults compared to 10% in children). Regardless of location, the tendency for CSF seeding is relatively high. Many patients present with, or ultimately develop, positive cytologic or radiographic evidence of spinal metastasis.[264,265] Metastasis outside the CNS is less common and occurs in fewer than 5% of patients at presentation.[264] Most recurrences occur within 2 years of diagnosis in children. Late recurrences are much more frequent in adults (29% recurrence after 5 years), which possibly reflects a more aggressive tumor variant in children.[260,266] Metastasis outside the CNS can affect bone, lymph nodes, liver, and lung and generally occurs in the setting of end-stage disease.

The clinical signs and symptoms of medulloblastoma are related to its anatomic location in the posterior fossa. Midline tumors, as in pediatric patients, usually present with signs of increased ICP, including headache, nausea and vomiting, papilledema, irritability, and lethargy, due to progressive hydrocephalus from fourth ventricle compression. Adults often present with ataxia and unilateral dysmetria because a lateral origin is more frequent. On CT scan, medulloblastoma appears as a well-circumscribed cerebellar mass that may be calcified. MRI reveals a T1-dark lesion that usually enhances, although often inhomogeneously and occasionally not at all. CSF dissemination is identified on MRI scans as nodules that show contrast enhancement or high fluid-attenuated inversion recovery signal, or both, along the surface of the brain or spinal cord, or as a covering of the leptomeninges.

Staging is critical in treatment planning for patients with medulloblastoma. A modified version of the Chang staging system is currently the standard.[267] In the modified system, T stage is no longer considered relevant because it is poorly predictive of outcome, and therefore M stage is the critical factor. M0 is designated as no signs of tumor dissemination, whereas M1 represents the presence of tumor cells in the CSF. M2 is assigned for the presence of gross tumor nodules in the subarachnoid or ventricular space in the cerebral cortex, whereas M3 represents gross tumor nodules in the spinal subarachnoid space. M4 represents systemic metastasis. Clinical staging therefore requires the assessment of these sites for tumor dissemination and includes a complete brain and spinal MRI scan with gadolinium as well as CSF cytologic examination. This assessment is obtained before surgery (if safe) or at least 10 to 14 days after surgery to avoid a false-positive finding from surgical cellular debris.[268]

Patients with medulloblastomas are currently classified as of "average risk" or "high risk" based on three factors: age, Chang M stage, and extent of resection.[269] Of these, extent of resection is the most controversial. Several studies suggest that gross total resection is important for a favorable prognosis, whereas at least one prospective trial indicates that patients undergoing subtotal resection treated with both chemotherapy and radiation do just as well as those undergoing total resection.[260,270,271] It is clear, however, that extent of resection has no prognostic significance in patients with disseminated disease. Clearly, age and presence of disseminated disease are powerful prognostic predictors. Patients under the age of 3 years have particularly poor prognoses, either because they tend to have more primitive tumors, because they present at more advanced stages, or because radiotherapy is often withheld from the treatment regimen to avoid profound neurocognitive and physical developmental sequelae in this age group.[272]

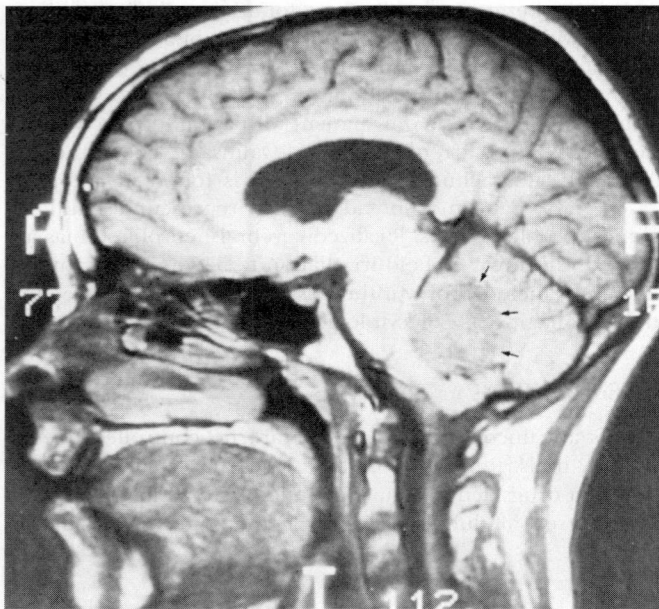

FIGURE 39.2-4.   This young girl presented with headache and gait ataxia. A T1-weighted sagittal magnetic resonance imaging scan (TR 600, TE 20) demonstrated a large, low-intensity mass involving the inferior aspect of the cerebellum in the midline and extending to and filling the fourth ventricle. There is arcuate stretching and displacement of the medulla and secondary hydrocephalus. The well-circumscribed nature and location of the tumor is fairly characteristic for medulloblastoma.

Tumor dissemination at diagnosis is the most powerful predictor of patient survival, although interestingly, the presence of tumor cells within the CSF (M1 stage) does not confer a worse prognosis.[273,274] Patients with M2 to M4 disease, however, have substantially worse outcomes, as demonstrated by the CCG experience in which 58% of patients with localized tumor were disease free at 54 months compared to only 32% of patients with disseminated tumor.[153,275,276] Overall, the assignment of average versus high risk is a powerful predictor of patient outcome. For instance, the disease-free survival of high-risk patients treated with CSI with or without chemotherapy is 25% to 30%.[277] Average-risk patients, on the other hand, have historically had a 5-year disease-free survival of 66% of 70%, which has increased to 70% to 80% in more recent reports.[278–280]

The site of first recurrence is the posterior fossa in more than 50% of patients, the frontal lobe in nearly 20%, bone in 10% to 15%, and other cerebral and suprasellar regions in 10% to 15%.[264,279] The incidence of systemic metastasis varies between 10% and 30%. Median time to systemic metastasis varies from 10 to 18 months.[277,281,282] In one study, 17% of patients with ventriculoperitoneal shunts developed systemic metastases, whereas only 4% of unshunted patients did so. In another series, 30% of patients developed systemic metastases, and none had previously had shunts. These reports suggest that except in patients with rampant disease there is little association between CSF shunting and systemic metastasis.

SURGERY

Although hydrocephalus associated with medulloblastoma obstructing the fourth ventricle can be relieved with a preresection CSF shunt, it is more usual to defer shunting and control increased ICP with corticosteroids. In up to 60% of patients, aggressive tumor resection relieves hydrocephalus. An occipital burr hole is commonly placed at surgery, before the posterior fossa is exposed, to allow cannulation of the ventricles for drainage of CSF to lower the increased ICP so that the dura can be opened safely.

Surgery for medulloblastoma is usually carried out with the patient prone. The incision and bony exposure are usually in the midline, but a paramedian incision and unilateral bony removal are done when the tumor is limited to one hemisphere, particularly in adults. The more common midline craniectomy includes the ring of the foramen magnum, and a laminectomy of C-1 (and rarely C-2) is performed to decompress herniated cerebellar tonsils or to remove a caudally extending tongue of tumor.

After dural opening the cerebellar tonsils are retracted laterally. The purplish gray tumor is usually first seen in the foramen of Magendie. The floor of the fourth ventricle is separated from the tumor by a cottonoid pledget. The pledget is advanced to protect the floor of the fourth ventricle as the tumor is resected. The thinned cerebellar vermis is progressively incised in the midline as the dorsum of the tumor is exposed. Alternatively, the naturally occurring corridor through the cerebellomedullary fissure between the tonsils and medulla is opened and exploited for exposure on one or both sides. The tumor is usually soft and moderately vascular and is readily removed under the operating microscope with suction, ultrasonic aspirator, or laser. Dissection is continued laterally to remove tumor from the cerebellar hemispheres and ventrally to remove tumor from

the fourth ventricle. When the obstructive hydrocephalus has been relieved, CSF can be seen flowing from the aqueduct of Sylvius superiorly. It is uncommon for medulloblastoma to invade the floor of the fourth ventricle. Watertight closure is obtained. Postoperative CSF shunting for hydrocephalus is necessary in approximately 35% of patients.[282a] Evidence suggests that an aggressive (gross total) removal is associated with an improved prognosis.[281]

RADIATION THERAPY

Given the propensity of medulloblastomas for CSF seeding, radiation therapy is directed to the entire craniospinal axis. Doses of 54 to 55 Gy to the primary tumor site and 35 to 36 Gy to the remainder of the neuraxis are generally recommended. These doses usually are reduced by approximately 10 Gy for children younger than 2 or 3 years of age, if radiation therapy is to be used at all in this young age group. Survival and patterns of relapse in adults with medulloblastoma are similar to those reported for children.[260] Although medulloblastoma is considered to be one of the most radiosensitive CNS tumors, local recurrence remains the primary mode of failure.[216,283] Modern radiation therapy techniques have greatly improved the prognosis for patients with medulloblastoma, but the maximal benefit that can be achieved with conventional radiation therapy has probably been reached. Adjunctive chemotherapy programs are being pursued actively to further improve the outcome (see Chemotherapy, later in this section).

Studies are also being directed at improving local tumor control. Wara and colleagues used a hyperfractionation schedule (1.0 Gy twice a day) to treat the craniospinal axis to 30 Gy and to boost the posterior fossa to 72 Gy.[284] Poor-risk patients also received chemotherapy. An excess of failures occurred outside of the primary site in good-risk patients, and there was no improvement in survival over that observed with conventional regimens in either risk group.[285] Investigators are currently exploring the use of stereotactic radiosurgery and three-dimensional conformal radiotherapy techniques to deliver an incremental increase in dose to the primary tumor site.[283,284] Proton radiotherapy has been used to treat patients with medulloblastoma.[286] With no exit dose in the spinal field, late toxicity to the organs of the chest, abdomen, and pelvis should be reduced. The posterior fossa boost can be delivered while reducing the cochlear dose to lower the risk of hearing loss. This is particularly important for children receiving platinum-based chemotherapy. Early results with craniospinal radiotherapy show promise for reducing the risk of treatment-related complications.

CHEMOTHERAPY

Use of adjuvant chemotherapy in high-risk patients clearly improves survival. The benefits of chemotherapy in these patients were first shown in randomized trials conducted by the International Society of Pediatric Oncology (SIOP)[278] and the CCG.[279] Each study compared radiation therapy plus chemotherapy with radiation therapy alone. The SIOP study used a regimen of weekly vincristine during radiation therapy followed by eight courses of vincristine and CCNU, cycled every 6 weeks. Patients in the CCG study received similar chemotherapy plus prednisone. Neither trial demonstrated an overall improvement in outcome with the addition of chemotherapy. The 5-year disease-free survival rates in the CCG and SIOP studies were 59% and 55%, respectively, for radiation therapy plus chemotherapy, and 50% and 43%, respectively, for radiation therapy alone. In a subgroup analysis, however, chemotherapy did appear to benefit patients with more advanced disease, including those with postoperative residual tumor, brainstem involvement, or advanced T (T3 and T4) and M (M1 to M3) stages. Additional evidence favoring chemotherapy was provided by a single-arm trial of 63 evaluable patients with either metastatic tumor or brainstem involvement treated with concurrent radiotherapy and weekly vincristine followed by postradiation cisplatin, CCNU, and vincristine. The overall 5-year progression-free survival rate was 83%, with 67% of patients with metastatic disease remaining progression free at 5 years.[271]

Early trials involving patients with average-risk disease failed to demonstrate a survival benefit for adjuvant chemotherapy, probably because the outcome of these patients treated with conventional-dose CSI was already good. Nevertheless, the long-term neurocognitive and endocrine sequelae of standard-dose CSI in children are significant, particularly in the very young.[287] The POG conducted a randomized trial to assess the effects of lowering the CSI dose from the conventional 36 Gy to 23.4 Gy. Patients receiving the lower dose had a higher rate of early relapse, lower 5-year event-free survival (67% vs. 52%), and lower overall survival.[288] Furthermore, the event-free survival of the average-risk patients treated with conventional-dose CSI (36 Gy) in this trial was suboptimal. Thus, a major clinical question that has been explored in average-risk patients over the last decade is whether the use of chemotherapy will allow lower, and hopefully less harmful, CSI doses. To this end, the CCG completed a large single-arm trial involving average-risk patients treated with CSI to 23.4 Gy (55.8 Gy to the posterior fossa) and weekly vincristine followed by postradiotherapy cisplatin, vincristine, and CCNU. The trial results were encouraging (79% of patients progression free at 5 years).[280] A larger trial has been completed by the CCG using the same radiation and chemotherapy regimens, except that patients are randomly assigned to receive either cyclophosphamide or CCNU after radiation therapy. A pilot trial used the same chemotherapy regimen of weekly vincristine with 18 Gy of radiation, followed by cisplatin, vincristine, and CCNU.[289] Seven of the ten treated patients were disease free 6 years after treatment and showed normal intelligent quotient test results. Thus, future trials may focus on the use of even lower CSI doses in average-risk patients.

Current approaches for patients with newly diagnosed high-risk medulloblastoma focus primarily on dose-intensive chemotherapy. For example, a trial of 53 patients, 19 of whom were high risk, used four consecutive cycles of high-dose cyclophosphamide with stem cell support and demonstrated the feasibility of dose-intensive chemotherapy in the period immediately after CSI.[290] The early data from this trial are encouraging, although it is not clear whether the outcomes will be superior to those for standard dose chemotherapy.

The treatment of very young children with medulloblastomas remains difficult given the profound neurocognitive, endocrine, and physical developmental morbidity of CSI. Upfront chemotherapy is used in an attempt to forestall radiotherapy until the child is older, when radiation might be better

TABLE 39.2-7. Efficacy of Single-Agent Chemotherapy for Recurrent and Progressive Central Nervous System Medulloblastoma

Treatment (Reference)	n	Response Rate[a] (%)
Doxorubicin[294]	6	0
PCNU[295]	4	0
Etoposide[296]	4	0
AZQ[153,291]	21	28
Bischloroethylnitrosourea[292,297]	6	33
Carboplatin[222,298]	34	35
Methotrexate, IV[299–301]	13	38
Cisplatinum[302–304]	27	40
Melphalan, IV[305]	12	50
Dibromodulcitol[293]	29	51
Vincristine[306–311]	15	73
Procarbazine[133]	4	75
Lomustine[132,312–314,460]	15	80
Cyclophosphamide[315]	7	100

AZQ, aziridinylbenzoquinone; PCNU, [1-(2-chloroethyl)-3-(2,5-dioxo-3-piperidyl)-1-nitrosourea].
[a]Response = (complete response + partial response + stable disease)/ total patients.

tolerated. Several small series using various treatment regimens have been reported, but in general, upfront chemotherapy results in response rates between 20% and 40%, with progression-free survival at 2 to 3 years of 15% to 40%.[269]

Recurrent medulloblastomas are responsive to a variety of antineoplastic agents, including vincristine, nitrosoureas, procarbazine, cyclophosphamide, etoposide, platinum compounds, and various drug combinations. Table 39.2-7 lists some of the single agents and their observed response rates for medulloblastoma when the patient is treated at recurrence or for progressive disease.[104,133,153,222,256,291–315]

Although single-agent and combination regimens can yield relatively high response rates at the time of recurrence, it is not possible to compare the durability of reported responses. Some reports pool PNETs with medulloblastoma, whereas others do not provide individual lengths of response, a median time to progression, or Kaplan-Meier curves. In general, however, the data suggest a range in median time to progression of 10 to 19 months for the more active single-agent and combination chemotherapy regimens.[316]

Whichever agent or combination is used, few if any patients with recurrent or progressive medulloblastoma appear to be cured by conventional chemotherapy, and thus better treatments are needed. One avenue of investigation has been dose-intensive chemotherapy with bone marrow or peripheral stem cell support, or both. Several studies have demonstrated the feasibility of this approach in patients with recurrent medulloblastoma.[317] Several studies now have consistently shown long-term progression-free survival in a minority of patients treated with high-dose chemotherapy and stem cell support after recurrence.[317] For example, the CCG conducted a trial involving 23 patients with recurrent medulloblastoma treated with high-dose carboplatin, etoposide, and thiotepa with autologous bone marrow support. At a median of 54 months after transplantation, 30% of patients were event free.[318] This supports a role for dose-intensive chemotherapy in patients with recurrent medulloblastoma. It appears clear, however, that the chance for long-term progression-free survival is greatest when patients have chemosensitive tumors and when transplantation is performed at a time of minimal residual disease.

PINEAL REGION TUMORS

CLINICAL AND PATHOLOGIC CONSIDERATIONS

The pineal gland is located in the posterior third ventricle. Tumors in this region are rare, accounting for fewer than 1% of intracranial tumors, although in children they constitute 3% to 8% of intracranial tumors.[319] In all series, germinomas are the most common histologic type, accounting for 33% to 50% of pineal tumors. The peak incidence of germ cell tumors is in the second decade, and few present after the third decade. Gliomas are the next most common pineal region tumor (approximately 25%). Pineal parenchymal tumors are nearly as common as glial tumors and are called pineocytomas if benign and pineoblastomas (a variant of PNET) if malignant; a rare intermediate form also exists.[78]

Neurologic signs and symptoms are caused by obstructive hydrocephalus and involvement of ocular pathways. Major symptoms are headache, nausea and vomiting, lethargy, and diplopia. Signs are primarily ocular but can include ataxia and hemiparesis. The major ocular manifestation is paralysis of conjugate upward gaze (Parinaud's syndrome), although pupillary and convergence abnormalities are seen, as are skew deviation and papilledema.

Germinomas occur in two midline sites, the suprasellar and pineal regions. On CT, these lesions are hyperdense. On MRI the mass is hypointense on T2-weighted sequences (due to the high cellularity of the mass) and shows robust enhancement with gadolinium. Calcification and fat may be seen in teratomas or mixed malignant germ cell tumors. Useful in distinguishing between germinomas and pineal parenchymal tumors is the fact that germinomas tend to surround a calcified pineal gland, whereas pineal parenchymal tumors tend to disperse the calcification into multiple small foci. The potential for leptomeningeal dissemination requires gadolinium-enhanced imaging of the entire neuraxis before surgery. Determination of tumor histology, tumor cell markers, and extent of disease is critical for optimal management of pineal region tumors. The prognosis for these tumors varies depending on the histologic type, the size of the tumor, and the extent of disease at presentation.

SURGERY

Because pineal tumors are near the center of the brain, they are among the most difficult brain tumors to remove. However, the application of modern surgical technology with superb illumination, magnification, surgical guidance, and neuroanesthesia to pineal surgery has made this region much more accessible. Surgeons can choose from several accepted approaches depending on personal preference and the tumor's position and extent.[320] The current recommendation is to obtain a tissue diagnosis when a diagnosis cannot be made from CSF markers, cytologic examination, or both. Whenever possible the tumor is completely excised, except when a germinoma is found at open surgery; here a biopsy suffices, because germinomas respond so well to radiation.[321] Resection is especially important when tumors are radioresistant or when excision may be curative (teratomas, arachnoid cysts, and pineal parenchymal tumors). Although large meningiomas must be resected, smaller ones may be suitable for treatment with stereotactic radiosurgery.

The most commonly used microsurgical approaches are currently the infratentorial supracerebellar approach, in which the surgical corridor is in the midline between the tentorium above and the superior surface of the cerebellum below, and the occipital transtentorial approach, under the occipital lobe and through an incision in the tentorium to reach the pineal region from above and to the side.[320] Both have been associated with low morbidity and mortality in experienced hands.

The place of stereotactic biopsy in the diagnosis of pineal region tumors is unclear. Although such biopsies have been described as relatively safe, particularly for large tumors,[322] some authors avoid the procedure because of the risk of damaging the large veins that flank and surround the pineal. In addition, there is a risk that tissue sampling of these heterogeneous tumors may not depict accurately the correct histologic nature of all parts of the tumor.[323] Without an accurate histologic diagnosis, treatment planning may be erroneous or inadequate. In favor of biopsy are the advantages of a rapid tissue diagnosis and shortened hospital stay. Transventricular endoscopic biopsy can also be performed, which potentially reduces the risk of hemorrhage because the trajectory is for the most part traversed under direct vision.

In patients with a pineal region mass and obstructive hydrocephalus from blockage of the aqueduct of Sylvius, endoscopic surgery can play a special role. Through a frontal burr hole, the endoscope can be passed through the foramen of Monro into the third ventricle. An endoscopic third ventriculostomy is performed by making a fenestration in the floor of the third ventricle, which relieves the hydrocephalus, and through a steerable flexible endoscope the mass in the posterior third ventricle can be viewed and biopsy performed. Alternatively, a rigid endoscope can be safely used by placing a second burr hole for the biopsy. CSF for cytologic analysis and marker studies can also be obtained and the walls of the third ventricle inspected for tumor studding, as with germinomas. There is a small risk of intraventricular hemorrhage from the biopsy of the tumor.[324]

RADIATION THERAPY

With certain exceptions, such as in benign teratomas, radiation therapy has an established role in the curative treatment of pineal germ cell and parenchymal tumors. The location and infiltrative nature of these lesions often does not allow complete resection. In the past, the risk of biopsy or attempted resection with older surgical techniques often led to the use of radiation therapy without histologic confirmation. In such instances, response to low-dose radiation therapy, measurement of levels of α-fetoprotein and human chorionic gonadotropin-β, and CSF cytologic analysis were used to provide diagnostic information. There has been a tendency to increase the use of biopsy, and resection and treatment without histologic confirmation is now less common.

Five-year survival rates with radiation therapy range from 44% to 78% and vary with histologic type and extent of disease, age, radiation volume, and dose to the primary site.[216] In a multi-institutional survey by Wara and Evans, the survival of patients with pineal parenchymal cell tumors or malignant teratomas was 21% (3 of 14) compared with 72% (26 of 36) for those with germinomas.[325] More recently, Wolden and colleagues reported 5-year disease-free survival rates of 91% for germinomas, 63% for unbiopsied tumors, and 60% for nongerminomatous germ cell tumors irradiated to doses of 50 to 54 Gy to the local tumor site with or without additional treatment to the whole brain or ventricular system.[326] Patients younger than 25 to 30 years of age have survival rates of 65% to 80% compared with 35% to 40% for older patients.[325,327] This finding may reflect the increased incidence of germinomas in younger patients.

Germinomas are infiltrative tumors that tend to spread along the ventricular walls or throughout the leptomeninges. The incidence of CSF seeding ranges from 7% to 12%. For this reason, the use of fields encompassing the entire ventricular system, the whole brain, and even the entire craniospinal axis has been recommended. The appropriate treatment volume for pineal germinomas was addressed by Haas-Kogan et al.[328] Ninety-three patients were treated at the UCSF or at Stanford. The UCSF group favored whole ventricular irradiation, whereas the Stanford group included CSI. Five-year overall survival for the combined cohort was 93%, with no difference in survival or distant CSF failure regardless of whether CSI or whole ventricular radiation was given. Current recommendations at the Massachusetts General Hospital are to deliver 25.5 Gy (1.5 Gy/d) of whole brain or whole ventricular system radiation followed by a stereotactic radiotherapy boost to the primary for a total dose of 45 to 50 Gy. CSI is reserved for patients with disseminated disease at presentation.

Treatment with neoadjuvant chemotherapy and low-dose (30- to 40-Gy) focal irradiation is being studied in some centers.[329,330] Chemotherapy might be useful in the rare young child to defer irradiation. For disseminated or multiple midline germinomas, systemic chemotherapy or CSI is given. CSI doses of 20 to 35 Gy have been used when CSF cytologic results are positive. When response to primary chemotherapy treatment is incomplete or the tumor recurs, salvage radiotherapy yields good results.[331]

Nongerminomatous malignant germ cell tumors, whether localized or disseminated, are treated with systemic chemotherapy followed by restaging studies. After restaging, localized tumors receive focal radiation therapy (20 to 24 Gy to the ventricular system with a tumor boost to 54 to 60 Gy), and disseminated tumors receive CSI (54 to 60 Gy to the primary tumor, 45 Gy to the ventricular system, 35 Gy to the spinal cord, and 45 Gy to any localized spinal cord lesions).[326]

Tumors that tend not to metastasize to the spinal cord, such as teratomas, pineocytomas, and low-grade gliomas, are treated by resection, with localized radiotherapy reserved for patients with postoperative residual disease.[332] For selected patients with small residual disease after surgery, radiosurgery has been shown to be effective.[333] CSI is reserved for tumors that have a strong tendency toward CSF seeding (such as pineoblastoma) and for those with documented seeding (by positive results on CSF cytologic analysis or imaging evidence). A German study confirmed the role of CSI in patients with pineoblastomas.[334] Sixty-three patients with supratentorial PNET were treated using chemotherapy before or after radiation (35-Gy CSI with a boost to the primary lesion of 54 Gy). The overall 3-year survival was 49.3% in those in whom treatment was delivered as prescribed, but only 6.7% in those with major protocol violations. This study clearly indicates the importance of CSI in pineoblastoma patients, as in those with medulloblastoma.

CHEMOTHERAPY

Chemotherapy for glial neoplasms is similar to that for gliomas elsewhere. The chemotherapy for germ cell tumors is in flux, but results are encouraging. Adjuvant multidrug therapy with agents such as cisplatin, etoposide, and bleomycin together with high-dose radiotherapy has produced encouraging disease-free and overall survival rates.[335] Finlay and coworkers used high-dose chemotherapy alone (carboplatin, etoposide, and bleomycin), deferring radiotherapy.[336] Their results also appear promising.

For germinomas, complete responses before radiation therapy or at recurrence have been observed with various drugs and combinations, including cisplatin and bleomycin; carboplatin; cyclophosphamide; a combination of cyclophosphamide, vinblastine, and bleomycin; a combination of cisplatin and etoposide; and a combination of dactinomycin, methotrexate, vinblastine, and cisplatin.[337,338] This has led to attempts to reduce or defer radiotherapy. Newly diagnosed germinomas treated with two courses of high-dose cyclophosphamide showed a complete response rate of 91%.[339] Building on this experience, Allen and coworkers reduced the radiation dose and volume. Of the ten patients with a complete response treated with reduced radiation, only 10% of patients had experienced treatment failure 5 years later. A comparable approach using carboplatin produced an 88% response rate and a radiation dose reduction in five of eight patients.[340] More recently, Bouffet and colleagues reported a trial using four courses of alternating etoposide-carboplatin and etoposide-ifosfamide followed by 40 Gy of localized radiation therapy for nonmetastatic cases and CSI for metastatic cases.[329] Of 57 patients registered, 47 had biopsy proof of germinoma. Median follow-up was 42 months. The 3-year event-free survival was 96%. Given the historically poor outcome of patients with nongerminoma primary CNS germ cell tumors after radiotherapy alone, there is significant interest in the use of primary chemotherapy. A study tested primary chemotherapy in 20 patients (adults and children) with newly diagnosed intracranial nongerminomatous germ cell tumors.[341] Alternating regimens of cisplatin, etoposide, cyclophosphamide, and bleomycin followed by carboplatin, etoposide, and bleomycin were used. Some patients received postchemotherapy radiation in first remission outside of the protocol. The chemotherapy response rate was 94%, 5-year overall survival was 75%, and 36% of patients were event free.

The results of high-dose chemotherapy with autologous stem cell rescue have been reported.[342] Twelve patients with pineoblastomas were treated with preradiation induction chemotherapy followed by CSI with a pineal region boost (36-Gy CSI, 59.4 Gy to primary), then with high-dose chemotherapy with stem cell support. Nine of the 12 patients remained disease free, including two infants who never received radiation. The actuarial 4-year progression-free and overall survivals were 69% and 71%, respectively. Although still considered investigational, the survival results are impressive. The use of high-dose chemotherapy and autologous bone marrow support has not been as promising for patients with recurrent tumors, although reported data are few.[343]

Given the rarity of CNS germ cell tumors and the similarity of the small trials reported in the literature, it seems clear that cooperative group trials are needed to determine which of the existing chemotherapy combinations are most active.

PITUITARY ADENOMAS

CLINICAL AND PATHOLOGIC CONSIDERATIONS

Approximately 10% of intracranial tumors are pituitary tumors. Pituitary tumors present either through local mass effect, as a result of their neuroendocrine effects, or incidentally (incidentaloma). Pituitary adenomas almost always arise from the anterior portion of the pituitary, or adenohypophysis. The tumor mass initially compresses the pituitary gland and, at a larger size, the optic chiasm and nerves superiorly. Tumors smaller than 10 mm (microadenomas) rarely compress the optic apparatus. Larger tumors are called *macroadenomas*. Further growth can involve the cavernous sinus bilaterally, the third ventricle (sometimes producing hydrocephalus), and sometimes the middle, anterior, or even posterior fossae. The classic ophthalmologic finding is visual loss, typically starting with bitemporal hemianopsia and loss of color discrimination. Automated visual field testing is more sensitive than simple confrontation in detecting the deficits. Occasionally, extraocular palsies can result from compression or invasion of the nerves of the cavernous sinus. Tumors that present with mass effect are often nonsecreting adenomas, but prolactin-, growth hormone–, thyrotropin-, and gonadotropin-producing tumors may also present in this way.

Neuroendocrine abnormalities usually indicate an endocrinologically active tumor that oversecretes pituitary hormones but can also result from tumor compression of the pituitary gland. The most common endocrinologically active tumors secrete prolactin, adrenocorticotropic hormone (ACTH), or growth hormone. Less common are thyrotropin- and gonadotropin-secreting tumors. Sexual impotence in men and amenorrhea and galactorrhea in women are hallmarks of a prolactin-secreting tumor. Hypogonadism, infertility, and osteopenia are also common.[344] Growth hormone hypersecretion causes acromegaly or, in the rare patient with a tumor occurring before epiphyseal closure, gigantism. The secondary production of insulin-like growth factor-1 (IGF-1) or somatomedin C produces a host of skeletal overgrowth changes (increased hand and foot size, macroglossia, frontal bossing, etc.). Soft tissue swelling, peripheral nerve entrapment syndromes, and arthropathies occur. More importantly, hypertension, cardiomyopathy, diabetes, and an increased risk of colon cancer are also prevalent with acromegaly. *Cushing's syndrome* refers simply to hypercortisolism, which can be produced by ectopic ACTH production, ectopic or increased corticotropin-releasing hormone levels, adrenal tumor, or pituitary tumor. Only ACTH hypersecretion by pituitary tumor results in *Cushing's disease*, with weight gain, hypertension, purple striae, hyperglycemia, infertility, osteoporosis, increased skin pigmentation, and psychiatric symptoms. Elements of hypothyroidism, adrenal insufficiency, and growth hormone deficiency may follow compression of the pituitary gland by an adenoma. Pituitary adenomas rarely present with diabetes insipidus, and other diagnoses need to be entertained in patients with this finding.

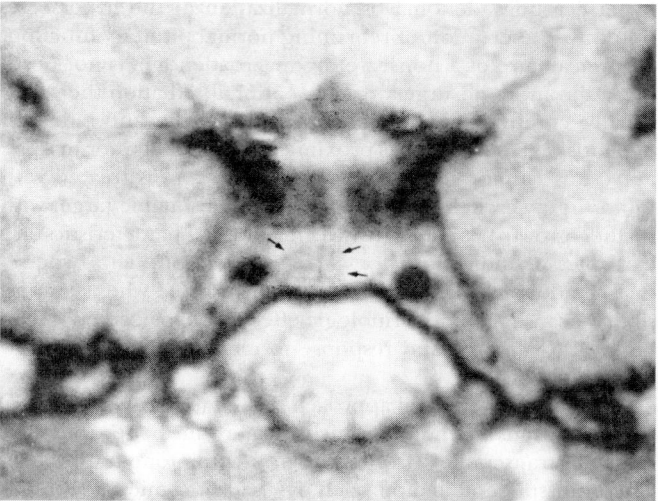

FIGURE 39.2-5. A woman 30 years of age presented with hyperprolactinemia. Coronal T1-weighted (TR 600, TE 20) 3-mm-thick section scan of the pituitary gland demonstrates a low-intensity lesion 9 mm in diameter (*arrows*) involving the right side of the pituitary fossa and displacing the gland and the stalk to the left. Findings are typical of a pituitary microadenoma.

In addition to mass effect and neuroendocrine symptoms, less common presentations of pituitary tumors include headache or CSF leak from skull base invasion.

Today, pituitary adenomas are most often diagnosed by MRI, particularly if patients present solely with symptoms from local mass effect or headache. Patients with symptomatic endocrine abnormalities may be diagnosed through sensitive serum radioimmunoassay; an MRI should be performed and results are often positive. Figure 39.2-5 shows an MRI scan of a pituitary adenoma before surgery.

The reported incidence of the various types of pituitary adenoma depends on the institution's referral patterns. In 800 patients operated on at UCSF between 1970 and 1981, 630 of 800 pituitary adenomas (79%) were endocrine active. Of these 630, 52% were prolactin secreting, 27% growth hormone secreting, 20% corticotropin secreting, and only 0.3% thyroid-stimulating hormone secreting.[345]

On imaging, pituitary microadenomas are located within the gland according to the distribution of normal cells. For example, prolactinomas tend to be located laterally within the sella. On MRI, microadenomas show subtle hypointensity to the normal gland on T1-weighted sequences and are often more difficult to detect on T2 sequences.[346] Immediately after administration of gadolinium, adenomas show less enhancement than adjacent normal gland. On delayed views, the tumor enhances more than the normal gland. Indentation of the sellar floor, stalk deviation, and mass effect on adjacent structures also provide evidence of the presence of tumor. Macroadenomas can be distinguished from other sellar masses, in part, by effects on the sella. Sellar enlargement is frequent with macroadenomas but is rare with meningiomas.

SURGERY

The goal of surgery for macroadenomas is to decompress the visual pathways and reduce tumor bulk, whereas the goal for hypersecreting adenomas is normalization of the hypersecretion with preservation of remaining normal pituitary function. If surgical cure of a nonsecreting macroadenoma is not possible, adjuvant radiosurgery or conventional radiation therapy is usually curative. Timing and choice of adjuvant radiation depends on factors such as proximity of residual tumor to optic apparatus (tumor residual approaching 3 mm is treated with radiosurgery earlier, as it may not remain a suitable target with further growth), and aggressive histologic characteristics are examples of indications for early intervention. The hypersecreting adenoma should be completely resected whenever possible, because the endocrinologic effects of hypersecretion can be life threatening, and response to radiation therapy is slow and less predictable.

The standard surgical approach for the majority of pituitary tumors is transsphenoidal, which is safer and better tolerated than the transcranial (frontotemporal craniotomy) approach. The transsphenoidal approach is used for microadenomas occupying the sella turcica and for many macroadenomas. Even when the majority of tumor is actually suprasellar, transsphenoidal resection can be safely accomplished if the tumor consistency is soft (and tumor aspiration and curettage can thus easily be performed) and if the tumor is situated so that it can drop into the sella with progressive resection. Tough, fibrous suprasellar tumors and those that extend laterally into the middle fossa, anteriorly beneath the frontal lobes, or into the posterior fossa may require a craniotomy for resection.[347] Tumor invading the cavernous sinus is generally not removed. The role of endoscopic transsphenoidal surgery for pituitary adenomas is currently being expanded. Potential advantages include a less invasive surgical approach with a wider field of view and quicker postoperative recovery.[347]

Current surgical cure rates for hormonally active adenomas are 80% to 90% if there is no involvement of the cavernous sinus, suprasellar region, or clivus.[348] Patients with microadenomas have a higher surgical cure rate than patients with macroadenomas.[349] Patients cured of their endocrine disease can expect to have a normal life span.[350] In patients not biochemically cured with initial surgery, tumor is often found at the time of second surgery just next to the original site. Growth through the dura into the adjacent cavernous sinus is often found at repeat surgery even when no tumor is seen preoperatively on MRI.[351]

RADIATION THERAPY

When a microadenoma, usually diagnosed because of endocrine hypersecretion, is totally resected, there is no indication for radiation therapy unless there is persistent hormone elevation. Radiation therapy may be indicated for hormone-secreting adenomas of any size that are not surgically cured and are refractory to pharmacologic management (see Medical Therapy, later in this section). After subtotal resection of a macroadenoma, more than 50% of patients demonstrate radiographic evidence of progression over a 5-year period.[352] Younger patients (less than 50 years old) with residual disease have faster tumor regrowth than their older counterparts. Ki-67 antigen labeling of more than 1.5% predicts more rapid growth of residual disease but not a higher incidence of invasiveness.[353] For these patients, postoperative radiotherapy rather than observation is recommended.

Radiation therapy is less effective in controlling endocrine hypersecretion than in controlling the growth of pituitary adenomas. Radiation therapy decreases serum growth hormone concentrations to normal levels in 80% to 85% of acromegalic patients.[354] Growth hormone levels decrease at a rate of 10% to 30% per year, so several years may be required for the levels to normalize.[354] The probability of endocrine cure is highest for tumors with relatively small pre–radiation therapy growth hormone elevations (30 to 50 ng/mL); response is less reliable for tumors producing higher growth hormone levels.[355] In contrast, serum IGF-1 levels remain elevated after radiotherapy,[356] and long-term treatment with somatostatin or its analogues may be required.[357] Radiation therapy controls hypercortisolism in 50% to 75% of adults and 80% of children with Cushing's disease. Response occurs within 6 to 9 months of treatment.[358]

Pituitary adenomas may be treated using several different techniques. For large tumors, a three-field technique with lateral opposed wedged portals and an anterior superior-oblique field may be used. Three-dimensional conformal radiotherapy, intensity-modulated radiotherapy, fractionated stereotactic radiotherapy, and treatment with charged-particle beams have also been advocated.[359,360] With conventional radiotherapy techniques, the total dose for nonfunctioning lesions is carried to 45 to 50 Gy in 25 to 28 fractions of 1.8 Gy, calculated at the 95% isodose line. Slightly higher total doses are recommended for secretory lesions. This combination of fraction size and total dose controls tumor growth in 90% of cases at 10 years.[361–363] Radiation-induced injury to optic apparatus or adjacent brain with this dose-fractionation scheme is rare, whereas larger fractions or greater total doses lead to a higher incidence of injury. Hypopituitarism may develop, often years after radiation treatment.[361] It is more common in patients who have had both surgery and radiation therapy than in those treated with either modality alone.[361] Hypopituitarism is largely correctable by hormone replacement therapy, and patients treated for pituitary adenomas should have lifelong endocrine follow-up. One publication suggests that patients treated with surgery and radiation have an elevated risk for late cerebrovascular mortality.[364] Possible contributing factors include hypopituitarism, radiotherapy, and extent of initial surgery. The risk of developing a radiation-induced brain tumor after treatment is 1.3% to 2.7% at 10 years and 2.7% at 30 years.[365,366]

There is a growing interest in treating patients with persistent or recurrent disease with radiosurgery. Pituitary treatment has been reported with linear accelerator techniques, proton therapy, and gamma knife.[359,367] In general, patients are eligible for radiosurgery only if the superior extent of the lesions is more than 3 to 5 mm from the optic chiasm. Doses of more than 10 Gy in a single fraction to the optic pathways can cause visual loss.[368] Radiosurgery results indicate excellent tumor control and appear to show a more rapid biochemical normalization than is seen with conventional radiation therapy.[369] In a comparison of radiosurgery with fractionated radiotherapy, Landolt et al. found the median time to normalize IGF-1 levels in acromegaly was 1.4 years after radiosurgery and 7.1 years after fractionated therapy.[370] Cranial nerve injury after radiosurgery was seen in fewer than 5% of the cases treated.[371] If the radiographic abnormality alone is treated and not the entire contents of the sella, the risk of secondary pituitary dysfunction may be reduced.[372]

Reirradiation can be considered for patients with recurrent pituitary adenomas when there has been a long interval after the first course of radiotherapy and when other therapeutic methods have been unsuccessful. Schoenthaler and colleagues reported the outcomes of 15 patients who were retreated (median dose, 42 Gy) after a median of 9 years from the initial course of radiation therapy (median dose, 40.8 Gy). At a median follow-up of 10 years, 80% of patients had local control. No visual complications were observed, but all patients developed hypopituitarism and two sustained temporal lobe injury.[373]

MEDICAL THERAPY

Medical therapy has become increasingly important and effective in the management of patients with hormone-secreting pituitary tumors.[374] Dopamine agonists (e.g., bromocriptine or cabergoline) are the most effective therapy for prolactinomas and are used as primary treatment; surgery or radiation therapy, or both, is reserved for the uncommon patient who either cannot tolerate or does not respond to a dopamine agonist. A somatostatin analogue (either short acting or long acting) is effective medical therapy for patients with acromegaly and is usually given if there is persistent growth hormone hypersecretion after resection. If radiation is delivered to patients not cured at the time of surgery, administration of somatostatin analogues (e.g., octreotide and lanreotide) continues until the radiation effects are documented in the months or years after therapy. Control rates with octreotide are approximately 50%; dopamine agonists can control growth hormone production in 10% to 34%.[375] The FDA has now approved a growth hormone receptor antagonist (pegvisomant) that can be used for patients for whom somatostatin analogues fail. Rates of IGF-1 level normalization as high as 97% have been reported with this agent.[376] Medical therapy for patients with Cushing's disease is directed at the adrenal glands to reduce cortisol hypersecretion (ketoconazole). Unfortunately, no known drug effectively reduces pituitary corticotropin production.

CRANIOPHARYNGIOMAS

CLINICAL AND PATHOLOGIC CONSIDERATIONS

Craniopharyngiomas are the most common nonglial brain tumors in children, occurring primarily in the late first and second decades, although they can present at any age.[377] Craniopharyngiomas arise from epithelial cell rests that are remnants of Rathke's pouch at the juncture of the infundibular stalk and the pituitary gland. Most have a significant associated cyst, with only 10% being purely solid. Most craniopharyngiomas become symptomatic due to effects of the combined tumor and cyst on the optic apparatus or hypothalamus or both. They may also compress the pituitary gland or extend superiorly into the third ventricle. Cyst fluid is proteinaceous, and this can be seen on MRI. CT shows calcification in 30% to 50% of cases.

Clinically, craniopharyngiomas produce increased ICP and pituitary-hypothalamic-chiasmal dysfunction. Common presenting symptoms include headache, visual complaints, nausea, vomiting, and intellectual dysfunction (especially memory loss). Specific visual signs include optic atrophy, papilledema, hemianopsia, unilateral or total blindness, and diplopia with associated cranial nerve palsies. Endocrine abnormalities at presentation can include growth retardation, menstrual abnormalities, and disorders of sexual development or regression of secondary sexual characteristics (or both). Diabetes insipidus is found in 8% of patients at presentation.[378]

SURGERY

Craniopharyngiomas are generally resected using a microsurgical subfrontal or pterional approach. Larger tumors may require bifrontal or skull base approaches, including supraorbital craniotomy. Endoscopically assisted surgery is sometimes used, although outcome advantages have not yet been clearly shown. The optic apparatus and hypothalamus must be protected during resection. Large cysts that enter and enlarge the sella turcica can be drained through a transsphenoidal approach.

Although complete resection of craniopharyngioma remains the optimal surgical outcome, the risk of devastating long-term effects on hypothalamic function and quality of life cannot be ignored. In some cases, there is no clearly defined plane between tumor and surrounding hypothalamus, which makes aggressive resection dangerous. Aggressive removal nearly guarantees some injury to the pituitary stalk, with subsequent temporary or permanent diabetes insipidus and elements of hypopituitarism. Patients injured in this manner require lifelong replacement hormones and inhaled desmopressin acetate spray for the control of diabetes insipidus. However, except in extreme cases, patients with preoperative visual loss can expect improvement after surgery. The reported mortality rates for craniopharyngioma resection range from 2% to 43% with severe morbidity in 12% to 61%.[379] Complications are less likely with experienced surgeons. A study of craniopharyngioma resections conducted at the Mayo Clinic between 1974 and 1991 showed a good outcome rate of 60% at 10 years.[380]

Predominantly cystic craniopharyngiomas can be treated with stereotactic or endoscopic instillation of colloidal therapeutic radioisotopes, particularly yttrium 90 (predominantly used in Europe)[381] or phosphorus 32 (predominantly used in the United States).[382] The short penetrance of the β-particles emitted by these isotopes allows the epithelial cells lining the cyst to be safely treated without significant dose to neighboring structures. Intracystic therapy may have a role in treating cysts that recur after conventional external-beam irradiation, or even as a primary cyst treatment. Although most cysts shrink with intracystic therapy, one-third of patients later require further surgery.[382]

RADIATION THERAPY

Although debate exists regarding the extent to which total excision should be attempted, numerous reports demonstrate that subtotal removal (either extensive resection or biopsy and cyst aspiration) and irradiation produces local tumor control and survival rates comparable to those after radical excision.[383–385] The local control rates after complete resection, subtotal resection alone, and subtotal resection with postoperative irradiation are 70%, 26%, and 75%, respectively.[385] A study at Children's Memorial Hospital in Chicago found 32% recurrence after complete resection and none after subtotal resection and adjuvant radiotherapy.[386] Ten-year survival rates range from 24% to 100% for complete resection, 31% to 52% for subtotal resection, 62% to 86% for incomplete resection and irradiation,[383,384,387] and

100% after radiotherapy alone.[387] Patients receiving only radiotherapy are those with small tumors at presentation. Patients undergoing conservative treatment including biopsy and cyst drainage and irradiation appear to enjoy a better quality of life and demonstrate less psychosocial impairment than those initially treated with more extensive resections.[384] Furthermore, conservative therapy is associated with less hypothalamic and pituitary dysfunction and a lower incidence of persistent diabetes insipidus than when a total or near total excision is attempted. More extensive resections using a subfrontal approach may be associated with frontal lobe and visual perceptual dysfunction. Evidence suggests that the negative impact on intelligence quotient is greater in patients treated with aggressive resection than in those treated with conservative surgery and postoperative irradiation.[388] The radiation treatment volume is based on CT and MRI scans, with relatively small margins around demonstrated tumor. The technique varies according to the size and location of residual tumor, but more sophisticated three-dimensional conformal radiotherapy and intensity-modulated radiotherapy approaches and stereotactic radiotherapy techniques are increasingly being used to spare surrounding normal tissues.[387] One report showed excellent tumor control (100%) with minimal late toxicity when fractionated stereotactic radiotherapy (mean dose, 52.2 Gy in 29 fractions) was used.[389] No significant effect on cognition or visual injury was reported. The total dose is 50 to 55 Gy, given in daily 1.8-Gy increments. One review suggested better local control when doses of 55 Gy or more are delivered.[390]

The use of radiosurgery is limited by the proximity of most lesions to the optic chiasm and brainstem. In a long-term analysis by the Karolinska Hospital, 9 of 11 children treated (82%) ultimately experienced recurrence after radiosurgery.[391] This was felt to be due to the required low marginal dose of 6 Gy to parts of the tumor abutting the optic chiasm. These results suggest that radiosurgery plays a limited role in the treatment of most craniopharyngiomas and should be reserved for those uncommon tumors confined to the pituitary fossa and away from the chiasm and hypothalamus.[392] In children younger than 3 years of age, radiation treatment should be deferred, whenever possible, until the child is older.

ACOUSTIC NEUROMAS (VESTIBULAR SCHWANNOMAS)

CLINICAL AND PATHOLOGIC CONSIDERATIONS

The most frequent tumors occurring in the cerebellopontine angle are acoustic neuromas and meningiomas. Acoustic neuromas, also referred to as *vestibular schwannomas*, arise from the vestibular division of cranial nerve VIII at the transition point between central and peripheral myelin located near the medial end of the internal auditory canal (IAC). Slow growth characterizes these tumors, and they can reach substantial size before clinical symptoms lead to diagnosis. They usually grow to occupy the entire IAC before expanding into the posterior fossa. By compression, they can affect cranial nerves V, VII, and, less often, IX and X, alone or in combination, as well as the adjacent brainstem. They can cause hydrocephalus by compressing the fourth ventricle, or communicating hydrocephalus, presumably due to high CSF protein levels.

Acoustic neuromas present most commonly in the fifth decade and affect women more often than men. Histologically, they are virtually always benign. When associated with NF2, they occur earlier, in late childhood and adolescence, and are typically bilateral. The most common initial symptom of sporadic acoustic neuromas is unilateral hearing loss, often noticed when using the telephone with the affected ear. This is because speech discrimination is more affected than pure tone hearing. Tinnitus and loss of balance are common early symptoms. Facial numbness is usually next, indicating that the tumor is large enough to compress the trigeminal nerve; trigeminal neuralgia is a more rare presentation. Facial weakness is unusual, and its presence should suggest the much more rare facial nerve schwannoma. Diagnosis is usually made with gadolinium-enhanced MRI. Audiometry and measurement of brainstem auditory evoked responses are essential in evaluating the hearing in both ears before treatment.

Decision making for patients with acoustic neuromas is complex. All patients with acoustic neuromas need to consider three options: simple observation, surgical removal (total or subtotal, potentially through any of three different surgical approaches), and stereotactic irradiation (single-dose radiosurgery or multiple fractionated doses). Consultation with a specialist surgeon, radiation oncologist, or both is essential.

OBSERVATION

Acoustic neuromas are slow-growing tumors; only approximately one-third grow measurably in a 5-year observation interval.[393] Neither surgery nor radiation therapy will restore hearing once it is lost due to an acoustic neuroma, and both pose risks to cranial nerve function. Thus, watchful waiting, with annual or biannual MRI, is the course selected at diagnosis by many patients with small acoustic neuromas (not compressing the brainstem)—especially older patients. Patients with useful hearing at presentation risk sudden hearing loss during observation, but there is little other risk for patients who comply with a regular imaging regimen. Active treatment is pursued when growth is shown.

SURGERY

The aim of surgery for acoustic neuromas is complete resection when possible, and recurrences after complete resection are unusual. There are three surgical approaches: middle fossa, suboccipital, and translabyrinthine.[394,395] The middle fossa approach is used only for small tumors (within the IAC or with a small cerebellopontine extension) when hearing preservation is intended. The suboccipital approach and the translabyrinthine approach can be used for tumors of any size, but only the suboccipital approach offers the possibility of preserving hearing. Most surgical teams prefer either the suboccipital or the translabyrinthine approach, but there is little difference in outcomes between the two approaches in experienced hands.

The middle fossa approach starts with a supraauricular incision and temporal craniotomy. The middle fossa floor is exposed and drilled to reveal the IAC, which is opened for tumor removal. In the translabyrinthine approach, the petrous bone is removed with a high-speed drill through a retroauricular incision. This approach destroys hearing because the labyrinth is violated. The facial nerve is identified in the lateral IAC and separated from the tumor. The dura of the posterior fossa is exposed and opened to remove the intradural tumor portion. The suboccipital approach uses a unilateral posterior fossa craniectomy, dural opening, and medial retraction of the cerebellum to expose the cerebellopontine angle. The lower cranial nerves are protected while tumor is removed, and the IAC is unroofed with a drill. Once the facial nerve is identified at the lateral end of the IAC and at the brainstem, the remainder of the tumor is removed. If hearing is to be preserved, the auditory nerve is also identified and preserved. Through any approach, separation of the tumor from the facial nerve, brainstem, and other structures is a usually lengthy and involved operation best done by an experienced team.

Although complete removal of acoustic neuromas can almost always be achieved, in modern practice subtotal removal is often done when a complete removal appears to the surgeon to be likely to cause permanent facial paralysis. Small tumor residua can be followed with serial MRI and treated with radiosurgery if they grow. Completion of the removal in a second operation, with acceptance of the likelihood of facial nerve sacrifice or palsy, is also an option. Life-threatening complications of acoustic neuroma resections are rare except in patients with extremely large tumors, especially at specialist centers.[396] Hearing preservation is achieved, at best, in approximately half of cases. Postoperative facial nerve function is strongly dependent on tumor size and surgeon experience. Good to excellent results can be achieved in approximately 95% of cases, especially when the patient has expressed a preference for subtotal excision if necessary to protect facial function. Bilateral acoustic tumors present difficult problems in surgical decision making.[397] In general, a conservative approach is taken in which the largest tumor is treated when symptoms absolutely require it. Bilateral aggressive tumor resections can lead to complete deafness and carry the risk of bilateral facial paralysis, a cosmetic and significant functional problem.

RADIATION THERAPY

Stereotactic radiosurgery and fractionated stereotactic radiotherapy have been used as an alternative to surgery in selected patients with small acoustic neuromas. In a long-term follow-up study Kondziolka and colleagues reported that 98% of 162 patients treated to a median dose of 16 Gy had tumor control.[398] Only four patients required subsequent surgical treatment. Normal facial function was preserved in 79% of patients after 5 years, and normal trigeminal function was preserved in 73%. New incomplete trigeminal and facial cranial neuropathies typically develop at approximately 6 months after radiosurgery. These tend to be mild and usually improve within a year after onset. Approximately half of patients with useful hearing before radiosurgery maintain their pretreatment hearing level, and hearing lost before treatment is not regained.[398–400] The risk of treatment-induced cranial neuropathy is directly related to the volume of the lesion, the dose given, and the length of nerve irradiated.[401] Efforts are being directed at decreasing the complication rates while maintaining the high control rates with more sophisticated planning and treatment techniques and reduction of dose levels.[402]

There is a growing interest and experience in treating patients with acoustic neuromas using fractionated stereotactic radiotherapy. Fractionated therapy should reduce cranial neuropathy rates while maintaining the excellent rates of local control seen after radiosurgery. Sawamura et al. reported the results of stereotactic radiotherapy in 101 patients with vestibular schwannoma.[403] The median diameter of treated tumors was 19 mm, with 27 tumors larger than 25 mm. The actuarial rate of local control at 5 years was 91.4%. There were no cases of permanent facial nerve injury. Of patients with useful hearing before treatment, 71% maintained useful hearing at a median observation period of 45 months. Eleven patients, all with larger tumors, developed communicating hydrocephalus that required placement of a shunt. These results are consistent with the experience other large studies using fractionated radiotherapy.[404,405] It is clear that for larger lesions stereotactic radiotherapy reduces cranial neuropathy rates compared to radiosurgery. For small lesions located in the IAC, both treatments offer a viable alternative to resection. Excisions performed for tumor regrowth after either form of radiation (radiosurgery or fractionated radiotherapy) carry a higher risk of permanent facial nerve injury. This must be clearly explained to any patient considering radiation treatment, as must the very small risk of secondary tumor formation.[406]

GLOMUS JUGULARE TUMORS

CLINICAL AND PATHOLOGIC CONSIDERATIONS

Glomus jugulare tumors (paragangliomas) arise from glomus tissue in the adventitia of the jugular bulb (glomus jugulare) or along Jacobson's nerve in the temporal bone, sometimes multifocally. The tumor invades the temporal bone diffusely, but growth is characteristically slow. Sometimes these tumors are endocrine active, with a carcinoid- or pheochromocytoma-like syndrome.[407] Because glomus jugulare tumors occur in the jugular foramen, they commonly cause lower cranial nerve palsies and early symptoms of hoarseness and difficulty swallowing. Facial weakness, hearing loss, and atrophy of the tongue from hypoglossal palsy can follow. Pulsating tinnitus also may be a presenting symptom, and a red pulsating mass is often visible behind the eardrum. A presumptive diagnosis of glomus tumor can be made by CT or MRI scanning, with jugular schwannoma and meningioma being the main differential diagnoses. On CT, glomus tumors show a characteristic salt-and-pepper appearance in involved bone; MRI often discloses large blood vessels within the mass. Glomus tumors give positive results on octreotide scintigraphy. These tumors incite a tremendous blood supply, particularly by way of the ascending pharyngeal artery. Angiography provides the definitive diagnosis. Because preoperative tumor embolization is essential to surgical removal of glomus tumors, the diagnostic angiogram should be taken just before surgery. Histopathologically, numerous vascular channels are distinctive. The background is composed of clear cells clumped in a fibrous matrix. A small percentage of glomus tumors are malignant. There is a familial form in which the tumors are multiple.

SURGERY

The treatment of glomus jugulare tumors is controversial, with advocates for radiation, surgery, and the combination. Although surgery can often provide a cure for these benign tumors, especially for small lesions, radiation avoids the morbidities that may follow surgical removal (lower cranial nerve and facial palsies). Surgery for glomus tumors is most often performed by a neurosurgeon and a head and neck surgeon together after preoperative embolization, which may decrease intraoperative blood loss during resection of these extremely vascular tumors. Because these tumors often have an intracranial and extracranial component, the surgery is conducted in two parts. The base of the skull in the region of the jugular foramen is first exposed, and neurovascular structures are identified and mobilized through a high transverse cervical incision. When the incision is extended behind the pinna and a mastoidectomy is completed, the facial nerve can be identified and protected, and the entire tumor bulb, jugular bulb, and internal jugular vein can be seen passing through the base of the skull. Finally, suboccipital craniectomy is performed, which allows the sigmoid sinus above and the jugular vein to be ligated, and the segment between them excised with the attached tumor. Complications of this procedure can include swallowing and aspiration problems, CSF leak, and facial palsy.

RADIATION THERAPY

Even though glomus tumors are histologically benign, radiation therapy is effective and has been recommended for symptomatic lesions that cannot be totally resected or as primary treatment.[408,409] These tumors regress slowly after irradiation, and the success of radiation therapy is measured by the amelioration of symptoms and the absence of disease progression. A review of the literature demonstrated local control rates with radiation in excess of 90% with or without surgery.[410] A dose of 45 Gy in 5 weeks is recommended. Although a dose of 50 Gy has been advocated for more advanced tumors, there is no evidence that such lesions require higher doses.[409]

CHORDOMAS AND CHONDROSARCOMAS

Chordomas and chondrosarcomas are rare malignant bone tumors that can arise in the skull base or spine. Although skull base chordomas and chondrosarcomas are sometimes pooled together in reported series, more recent study has shown important differences between these tumors with respect to diagnosis, treatment, and prognosis. Chordomas and chondrosarcomas affecting the nervous system are the subject of a monograph.[411]

CLINICAL AND PATHOLOGIC CONSIDERATIONS

Chordomas occur along the pathway of the primitive notochord, which extends, in human embryos, from the tip of the dorsum sellae to the coccyx. Chordomas are extradural, multilobulated tumors, varying in consistency from soft and friable to woody and cartilaginous. They are pseudoencapsulated and may invade through the basal dura.

The typical chordoma is composed of cord-like rows of "physaliferous" cells with multiple round, clear cytoplasmic vacuoles that impart a bubbly appearance to the cytoplasm. Two pathologic variants have been described. The *chondroid chordoma* has areas that resemble low-grade hyaline chondrosarcoma and may be less aggressive.[412] The *dedifferentiated chordoma* contains areas of typical chordoma admixed with components that resemble high-grade or poorly differentiated spindle cell sarcoma. Increased cellular and nuclear pleomorphism, nuclear inclusions or multinucleation, and mitotic figures may be noted. These rare tumors can arise *de novo* or after recurrence of a previously treated typical chordoma. They are biologically aggressive and carry a poor prognosis.[413,414] In typical chordomas, higher mitotic rate is associated with shorter survival.[415]

Chondrosarcomas can arise in any of the many complex synchondroses in the skull base, but the most common sites of origin are the temporooccipital synchondrosis (66%), the sphenoocciput (28%), and the sphenoethmoid complex (6%).[416] Thus, chondrosarcomas predominantly originate in lateral skull base structures, unlike most chordomas, which originate in the midline. Chondrosarcomas can be difficult to differentiate from chordomas on pathologic examination. Of 200 chondrosarcomas reviewed at the Massachusetts General Hospital, 99% stained positive for S-100 and 0% for keratin, with faint staining for epithelial membrane antigen in 8%.[416] These immunohistochemical studies allow a chondrosarcoma to be differentiated from a chordoma, which is reactive for keratin and epithelial membrane antigen. Of interest, 37% of the patients with chondrosarcomas seen at the Massachusetts General Hospital during this period were referred by outside pathologists as having chordomas. Chondrosarcomas are graded based on cellularity, cytologic atypia, and degree of mitotic activity. In one large series, approximately half of skull base chondrosarcomas were grade 1, with the remainder nearly evenly divided between mixed grade 1 and 2 and pure grade 2.[416] There were no examples of grade 3 tumors in this series. Skull base chordomas and chondrosarcomas cannot be diagnosed without radiologic tests, which often are delayed because symptoms are nonspecific and vague. At onset there is usually headache and, with upper clivus tumors, intermittent diplopia. These vague symptoms often are not reported, which can allow the tumor to grow to an enormous size before the diagnosis is made. Gradually, headache (upper clivus tumors) and neck pain (lower clivus tumors) worsen. Superiorly placed tumors can cause diplopia (from abducens palsies) and facial numbness as the cavernous sinus and Meckel's cave are invaded. Lower clivus tumors can produce symptoms by compression of the lower cranial nerves and later the brainstem.

The differential diagnosis of cranial chordoma and chondrosarcoma includes basal meningioma, schwannoma (neurilemoma), nasopharyngeal carcinoma, pituitary adenoma, and craniopharyngioma. On MRI scanning, both chordomas and chondrosarcomas are hyperintense on T2-weighted sequences, with variegated enhancement. The location of tumor origin is important in distinguishing chordomas (midline clivus) from chondrosarcomas (petrous apex).

SURGERY

Surgery for cranial chordomas is obligatory to obtain diagnostic tissue, to enhance the effectiveness of subsequent radiation therapy, and to improve the patient's clinical condition. With an aggressive resection, alleviation of the severe headaches and neurologic deficits associated with chordomas can be anticipated.

Intracranial chordomas occur at the base of the skull, a region relatively remote from surgical access. Approaches to skull base chordomas and chondrosarcomas often involve teams that include both neurosurgeons and otolaryngologists.[411] For chordomas in the upper clivus that extend into the sella or sphenoid sinus, or both, a transseptal, transsphenoidal approach (as for pituitary tumors) is best. Large, compressive, transdural extensions of these upper clivus tumors into the interpeduncular cistern can be removed using a transcranial, subtemporal, intradural approach. For more lateralized upper clival tumors and some lateralized midclival tumors, an approach through a sphenoethmoidectomy (to which may be added a maxillectomy) is useful. For midline tumors of the midclivus and lower clivus, a transoral resection is often used. The palate or mandible and tongue can be split if upward or downward extension of the approach is necessary. A combination of exposures and procedures can be used for extremely large tumors. One goal of surgery is to remove as much tumor away from the optic system and brainstem as possible so that very high doses of radiation can be delivered safely. Optimal treatment of these lesions is complete resection, if possible.

A potentially serious complication of the transsphenoidal, transsphenoethmoid, and transoral approaches is CSF leakage into the nose or oropharynx and consequent meningitis. Therefore, every attempt is made to keep the dura intact during these procedures. Because dural invasion by cranial chordomas may occur 50% of the time, dural entry during tumor resection is sometimes unavoidable. Careful intraoperative patching of the leak with fat and muscle grafts followed by postoperative spinal CSF drainage should be undertaken to decrease the risk of infection in these cases.

Approaches for chondrosarcomas are different because of the paramedian location of the tumors.[411] Like chordomas, chondrosarcomas begin as extradural tumors, and maintaining the intact dural barrier is paramount. Most commonly, a variation of the subtemporal middle fossa approach to the upper clivus is used to approach the petroclival synchondrosis. Extradural tumors can be removed through both the middle fossa and presigmoid avenues combined with a presigmoid and retrosigmoid approach. Complete tumor excision, which is paramount in chordoma surgery, is less critical for chondrosarcomas, because tumor control rates with adjuvant high-dose radiation are high. Surgery is often tailored to emphasize removal of tumor portions abutting critical structures such as the chiasm or brainstem to allow adequate radiation treatment.

Cranial chordomas often recur after surgery and radiation therapy. In this situation, reoperation directed toward symptomatic improvement is the only treatment option. Reoperations are complicated by surgical scarring and tissue compromise from irradiation, and CSF leaks and other complications are frequent.[417]

RADIATION THERAPY

Chordomas and low-grade chondrosarcomas of the base of the skull, clivus, and axial skeleton are not often amenable to complete resection, even grossly, and adjuvant radiotherapy is frequently recommended to prevent recurrence or progression of residual tumor. Chordomas and chondrosarcomas have very different response rates to radiation. With conventional megavoltage irradiation (median dose, 50 Gy), the local control rate for chordomas is only 27%.[418] A review of results for 18 patients treated with a median dose of 60 Gy using conventional techniques indicated a 5-year progression-free survival rate of only

23%.[419] Higher doses appear to improve the local control rate, but surrounding dose-limiting critical structures, such as the optic nerves, chiasm, other cranial nerves, brainstem, temporal lobes, and spinal cord, limit the dose that can be delivered safely to skull base chordomas. Charged-particle beams such as proton beams, which feature sharp lateral beam edges and have a finite range in tissue, can deliver higher doses than are possible with conventional photon irradiation while keeping the dose to neighboring critical structures at a safe level. The depth of penetration can be tailored to fit the planned target by varying beam energy or by interposing spacing material in the beam path. Proton beams can be made to stop in front of a critical structure, and by the use of several beams a target volume can be wrapped around a critical structure. Precise identification of tumor and normal tissue as well as precise beam-delivery techniques, highly reproducible patient positioning, and accurate compensation for tissue inhomogeneities in the beam path are required.

Available data suggest that the higher doses that are achievable with charged-particle irradiation result in higher local control rates for chordomas than have been observed with conventional radiation therapy techniques. These improved results are related not to a biologic advantage of protons over photons but to the superior dose distribution of protons that allows for a higher dose to be delivered to the skull base. Munzenrider and coworkers reported the outcomes of 132 patients with nonchondroid and chondroid skull base chordomas treated postoperatively at the Harvard Cyclotron Laboratory at Massachusetts General Hospital with a 160-MeV proton beam. Patients received a median dose of 69 CGE, with a range of 36 to 79 CGE, and 95% received 67 CGE (70% to 100% of dose given with a proton beam). Median follow-up was 46 months. Local control was achieved in 70% of patients (93 of 132). Local control was more common in men than in women (77% vs. 40%) and more frequent in those with chondroid chordomas than in those with nonchondroid tumors (83% vs. 66%). The 5-year actuarial local control and disease-specific survival rates were 59% and 80%, respectively.[420] Complications included functional and anatomic abnormalities in the brain and brainstem, visual and auditory deficits, and pituitary insufficiency requiring hormone replacement. The probability of recurrence of skull base chordomas depends on the gender (results better for males than for females), target volume (those with larger volumes do less well), and the level of target dose inhomogeneity (results are better when a higher percent of the tumor receives the prescribed dose).[421] Younger patients appear to fare best.[422,423]

Skull base chondrosarcomas treated with proton therapy have a much better prognosis than chordomas. Rosenberg and colleagues reported a 5- and 10-year local control rate of 99% and 98% (median dose, 70 CGE), respectively.[416]

HEMANGIOBLASTOMAS

CLINICAL AND PATHOLOGIC CONSIDERATIONS

Hemangioblastomas account for 1% to 2% of intracranial tumors, arising most often in the cerebellar hemispheres and vermis. Although usually solitary, these tumors can be multiple and may also occur in the brainstem, spinal cord, and, less often, the cerebrum. Cerebellar hemangioblastoma can be sporadic or occur as part of the autosomal dominant von Hippel-Lindau complex, which is transmitted with greater than 90% penetrance.[424] Other entities associated with von Hippel-Lindau disease are retinal angiomatosis, polycystic kidneys, pancreatic cysts, pheochromocytoma, and renal cell carcinoma. Identification of the VHL gene on chromosome band 3p25-26 now allows individuals who are at risk for the syndrome, or who have some of its components as an apparent sporadic case, to undergo genetic testing with a high degree of accuracy.[425]

Cerebellar hemangioblastomas usually are recognized in the third decade in patients with von Hippel-Lindau disease and in the third or fourth decade in patients with sporadic tumors. These tumors can cause symptoms and signs of cerebellar dysfunction, especially gait disturbance and ataxia, and hydrocephalus from obstruction of CSF pathways. These tumors tend to enlarge extremely slowly, but patients may become symptomatic from tumor cysts, which can grow quickly.[426]

Hemangioblastomas are composed of capillary and sinusoidal channels lined with endothelial cells. Interspersed are groups of polygonal stromal cells with lipid-laden cytoplasm and hyperchromatic nuclei. Immunohistochemical study of these cells shows expression of neuron-specific enolase, vimentin, and S-100 protein but not epithelial membrane antigen or glial fibrillary acidic protein.[427] Grossly, the tumor is often cystic, containing proteinaceous, xanthochromic fluid, with an orange-red, vascular, firm mural nodule. The cyst wall is a glial nonneoplastic reaction to fluid secreted by the nodule. Some hemangioblastomas lack cysts, especially in the brainstem and spinal cord, but cystic lesions are more often symptomatic, at least in patients with von Hippel-Lindau disease.[426]

The natural history of CNS hemangioblastomas has been described.[426] The authors reviewed the clinical records and MRIs of 160 consecutively treated patients with 331 spinal hemangioblastomas. Most lesions were located in the posterior cord. Cysts were commonly associated with the lesions, often showing faster growth than the solid portion of the tumor. When symptoms appeared, the mass effect derived more from the cyst than from the tumor. These tumors often have alternating periods of tumor growth and stability, and some remain stable in size for many years. These factors have to be considered in the timing and choice of treatment.

SURGERY

Complete resection of a hemangioblastoma is often curative. Although angiograms have been used in the past to evaluate suspected hemangioblastomas before surgery, frequently an MRI suffices. Hemangioblastomas are very vascular lesions, and biopsy of a suspected hemangioblastoma, either through an open approach or stereotactically, is usually ill-advised due to the high risk of hemorrhage. Surgical resection should be carried out *en bloc* with avoidance of entry into the lesion, which can result in fierce bleeding reminiscent of that of an arteriovenous malformation. Embolization is rarely safe. Fortunately, these lesions can be resected with minimal bleeding if resection is carried out entirely in the gliotic plane that surrounds the mass. This is straightforward in most cerebellar tumors, for which a margin of gliotic tissue can be resected with the lesion with little neurologic risk. In contrast, brainstem hemangioblastomas are immediately adjacent to critical structures. Even dissection immediately adjacent to the tumor can cause significant bleeding from vessels passing from the brainstem parenchyma to feed the lesion. Attempts to control the bleeding, although unavoidable, have a high risk of inducing neurologic deficits. A report of results for 12 patients with von Hippel-Lindau disease confirmed that brainstem hemangioblastomas can be safely resected in some instances.[428]

Often these tumors are associated with significant cysts that sometimes dwarf the small mural nodule of tumor. Surgery is the optimal treatment, due to rapid relief of mass effect. The cyst wall is not lined with tumor tissue, and drainage, rather than excision of the cyst lining, is required. The mural tumor nodule must be entirely resected to avoid cyst recurrence. Cysts can be drained before opening the dura completely to provide brain relaxation, but great care must be taken not to disturb the tumor nodule during this maneuver to avoid inducing significant bleeding. The risk of hemorrhage during the resection is minimized by coagulating and dividing arterial feeders before tumor removal.

Finally, hemangioblastomas occurring in patients known to have von Hippel-Lindau disease need not be resected or otherwise treated unless they have demonstrated active growth or are symptomatic from mass effect or hydrocephalus. Because many of these patients harbor multiple tumors, other approaches including radiosurgery should also be considered, although surgery remains a viable option.

RADIATION THERAPY

Radiation therapy is recommended for patients with unresectable, incompletely excised, and recurrent hemangioblastomas and for those patients who are medically inoperable. Smalley and associates reported the outcomes of 25 patients treated with radiation therapy for hemangioblastoma.[429] Nineteen patients had gross residual disease after initial surgery or recurrent tumors; six had only microscopic disease. The overall 5-, 10-, and 15-year survival rates were 85%, 58%, and 58%, respectively, and the recurrence-free survival rates were 76%, 52%, and 42%, respectively. In-field disease control rates were significantly higher in patients who received at least 50 Gy of radiation ($P = .06$) than in those who received lower doses. Based on these data, doses of at least 50 to 55 Gy in 5.5 to 6.0 weeks appear to be warranted. Due to the noninvasive nature of these lesions, conformal radiotherapy is indicated.

Radiosurgery has also been used to treat hemangioblastomas. Patrice and colleagues summarized the outcomes for 38 lesions in 22 patients who received radiosurgery as definitive treatment or for recurrent tumors after surgery with or without conventional radiotherapy. The median tumor volume was 0.97 cc (range, 0.05 to 12.0 cc), and the median radiation dose was 15.4 Gy (range, 12 to 20 Gy). With a median follow-up time of 24.5 months (range, 6 to 77 months), 31 of 36 evaluable tumors (86%), including all tumors treated definitively with radiosurgery, remained locally controlled. The five lesions that relapsed after radiosurgery had all been treated for recurrence after initial surgery. Better control rates were associated with higher doses and smaller tumor volumes. The 3-year actuarial progression-free survival rate was 86%.[430] Of 29 hemangioblastomas treated by Chang and coworkers, only one (3%) progressed. Five tumors (17%) regressed completely, 16 (55%) regressed partially, and 7 (24%) remained unchanged in size.[431] Jawahar et al. reported treatment of 29 lesions in 27 patients.[432] The actuarial control rate was 84.5% at 2 years and 75.2% at 5 years. In multivariate analysis, smaller tumor volume and higher dose (more than 18 Gy) were favorable. Radiosurgery should be considered for surgically unresectable hemangioblastomas, as adjuvant treatment for incompletely excised tumors, as definitive treatment for multifocal disease, and as salvage therapy for discrete recurrences after surgery.[430,431]

Because stromal cells in hemangioblastomas secrete vascular endothelial growth factor, there is much interest in evaluating small-molecule inhibitors of the vascular endothelial growth factor-2 (KDR, FLK-1) receptor as medical management for these tumors, especially for patients with von Hippel-Lindau disease, who routinely harbor multiple hemangioblastomas. Unfortunately, the extreme heterogeneity of tumor growth, with periods of spontaneous stability and a slow overall growth rate, makes it extremely difficult to design trials to test rigorously the efficacy of any systemic therapy.

CHOROID PLEXUS PAPILLOMAS AND CARCINOMAS

CLINICAL AND PATHOLOGIC CONSIDERATIONS

Choroid plexus papilloma and carcinoma are rare tumors that occur most often in children younger than 12 years of age, although they can occur at any age. The tumor is an irregularly lobulated reddish mass, which on histopathologic examination is apparently normal choroid plexus, with increased cellular crowding and elongation. Rarely, these tumors show malignant features such as increased mitotic activity, loss of typical cellular architecture, and brain invasion, and are then classified as choroid plexus carcinoma. Malignant histology is more common in children and infants.

In children, choroid plexus papillomas most often occur in the lateral ventricles. In adults, the fourth ventricular papilloma is most common. Third ventricle tumors are exceedingly rare. Because papillomas tend to grow slowly within ventricles, they expand to fill the ventricle and block CSF flow. In addition, papillomas can secrete CSF. Choroid plexus papillomas and carcinomas can produce hydrocephalus secondary to obstruction of the CSF, CSF overproduction by the tumor; or damage to the CSF resorptive bed from recurrent hemorrhages. As a result, increased ICP without focal findings is the most common presentation. Fourth ventricular tumors can also be associated with focal findings of ataxia and nystagmus. Although choroid plexus papillomas rarely seed throughout the CSF spaces, seeding from carcinomas is frequent and often symptomatic.

Choroid plexus tumors are seen easily by CT scan or MRI. Imaging demonstrates a lobulated, well-circumscribed, enhancing, intraventricular lesion, often with associated hydrocephalus. Calcification is not common. Choroid carcinoma may show areas consistent with necrosis and brain invasion.[433] Evidence suggests that MRS can distinguish choroid plexus papillomas from carcinomas through biochemical profiling.[434] Staging of the craniospinal axis with brain and spinal MRI scans and CSF cytologic analysis is recommended for patients with choroid tumors with anaplastic features.

Therapy for anaplastic tumors should be approached as for medulloblastoma and malignant ependymomas. Because of the aggressive nature of the more anaplastic tumors, therapy must be equally aggressive; postoperative radiation therapy and, in some instances, intraventricular chemotherapy is required.

SURGERY

The treatment of choroid plexus papillomas is total surgical excision. Tumors in the lateral ventricle are approached through the ventricular trigone using a high parietal incision or a low temporal approach, depending on the degree of cortical mantle thinning and the location of the tumor. The predilection of these tumors for the left (usually dominant) side can make the approach worrisome. Hydrocephalus is the rule and simplifies the exposure once the ventricle is opened. Tumor vessels are coagulated and divided. Smaller tumors are removed intact and larger tumors piecemeal. Perioperative CSF drainage is used to prevent subdural hygromas. In one-half of patients, hydrocephalus is relieved by tumor resection, but persistent hydrocephalus requires shunting. Although endoscopy is increasingly used for intraventricular surgery, its role in surgery for these vascular tumors is not yet established. A review of 75 cases treated between 1985 and 2000 showed 84% survival in patients who had complete resections, compared to 18% survival in those undergoing less than a gross resection.[435] This significant survival difference was seen regardless of adjuvant therapies. Unfortunately, total resection is not possible in many patients. The ability to perform a complete resection depends on histologic type, with nearly a 100% complete resection rate for papillomas versus only a 33% complete resection rate for choroid plexus carcinoma.[436] Often, tumor hypervascularity is the limiting surgical factor, especially in infants, who have small total blood volumes. When carcinoma is suspected before surgery, the tumor can be embolized or neoadjuvant chemotherapy given to shrink it and reduce its vascularity, which facilitates resection.[437]

RADIATION THERAPY

Because choroid plexus papillomas are often cured by complete resection, there is little information regarding their response to radiation.[256] Radiation therapy may be beneficial in patients with choroid plexus carcinomas even after gross total resection.[438,439] Because CSF seeding occurs in up to 44% of cases,[440] consideration must be given to treating the entire craniospinal axis. However, data to support CSI are unavailable. Chow and colleagues recommend that patients with completely excised localized choroid plexus carcinomas be treated with either chemotherapy or limited field irradiation if their spinal MRI and CSF cytologic study results are negative. They advise both chemotherapy and CSI for those with incompletely excised tumors or evidence of leptomeningeal spread.[439] A review of 566 choroid plexus tumors suggested that adjuvant radiotherapy increased survival in patients with choroid plexus carcinoma regardless of the extent of surgery.[441] All of the long-term survivors had complete resection and adjuvant radiation therapy.

CHEMOTHERAPY

Chemotherapy is not used for choroid plexus papillomas, although it is frequently used for choroid plexus carcinomas.

As with many of the less common CNS tumors, there are no firm chemotherapeutic guidelines. Anecdotal reports have cited moderate responses in choroid plexus carcinomas, particularly to the platinum compounds, as well as to alkylating agents, etoposide, methotrexate, and possibly anthracyclines. A POG study involving eight infants with choroid plexus carcinoma suggests that radiation can be forestalled by using chemotherapy in some infants with these tumors.[442]

SPINAL AXIS TUMORS

CLINICAL AND PATHOLOGIC CONSIDERATIONS

Clinical features of spinal axis tumor localization and diagnosis have been discussed previously in Anatomic and Clinical Considerations. Most primary spinal axis tumors produce symptoms and signs as a result of spinal cord and nerve root compression rather than because of parenchymal invasion. The reported frequency of primary spinal cord tumors is between 10% and 19% of all primary CNS tumors. The majority of neoplastic conditions that affect the spine are extradural metastases. Most primary spinal axis tumors are intradural. Of these, the intradural extramedullary schwannomas and meningiomas are the most common. Schwannomas and meningiomas are normally intradural, but occasionally they may present as extradural tumors. Other intradural extramedullary tumors are vascular tumors, chordomas, and epidermoids.

Intramedullary tumors have the same cellular origins as brain tumors. Ependymomas comprise approximately 40% of intramedullary tumors; the remainder are astrocytomas, oligodendrogliomas, gangliogliomas, medulloblastomas, and hemangioblastomas.

Table 39.2-8 classifies spinal axis tumors by location. Although different tumor types exhibit a predilection for certain spinal regions, taken together, spinal tumors are distributed almost evenly along the spinal axis. Approximately half of spinal tumors involve the thoracic spinal canal (the longest spinal segment), 30% involve the lumbosacral spine, and the remainder involve the cervical spine, including the foramen magnum. Schwannomas occur with greatest frequency in the thoracic spine, although they can be found at other levels. They often extend through an intervertebral foramen in a dumbbell configuration. Meningiomas are dural based and arise preferentially at the foramen magnum and in the thoracic spine. Most patients are women. Astrocytomas are distrib-

TABLE 39.2-8. Classification of Spinal Tumors by Their Location in Relation to the Spinal Cord and Dura Mater

Location	Usual Tumor Histologies
Extradural	Metastatic (carcinoma, lymphoma, melanoma, sarcoma) chordoma
Intradural	
Extramedullary	Schwannoma,[a] meningioma[a]
Intramedullary	Astrocytoma, ependymoma[b]

[a]May extend along nerve root into extradural and extraspinal spaces.
[b]Ependymomas originating from the filum terminale and involving the cauda equina, not intramedullary in the strictest sense, are included here by custom.

uted throughout the spinal cord, and most ependymomas involve the conus medullaris and the cauda equina. Spinal chordomas are characteristically sacral and only rarely affect the cervical region or the rest of the mobile spine.

Clinically, patients with spinal axis tumors present with a sensorimotor spinal tract syndrome, a painful radicular spinal cord syndrome, or a central syringomyelic syndrome. In the sensorimotor presentation, symptoms and signs reflect compression of the spinal cord. The onset is gradual over weeks to months, initial presentation is asymmetric, and motor weakness predominates. The level of impairment determines the muscle groups involved. Because of external compression, dorsal column involvement occurs with paresthesia and abnormalities of pain and temperature on the side contralateral to the motor weakness.

Radicular spinal cord syndromes occur because of external compression and infiltration of spinal cord roots. The main symptom is sharp, radicular pain in the distribution of a sensory nerve root. The intense pain is often of short duration, with pain that is more aching in nature persisting for longer periods. Pain may be exacerbated by coughing and sneezing or other maneuvers that increase ICP. Local paresthesia and numbness are common, as are weakness and muscle wasting. These findings often precede cord compression by months. Many times the pain is difficult for the clinician to differentiate from ordinary musculoskeletal symptoms, which causes diagnostic delay.

Spinal tumors, particularly intramedullary tumors, can give rise to syringomyelic dysfunction by destruction and cavitation within the central gray matter of the cord. This produces lower motor neuron destruction with associated segmental muscle weakness, atrophy, and hyporeflexia. There is also a dissociated sensory loss of pain and temperature sensation with preservation of touch. As the syrinx increases in size, all sensory modalities are affected.

SURGERY: GENERAL CONSIDERATIONS

The operating microscope is essential for spinal cord tumor surgery. Other surgical adjuncts, such as intraoperative ultrasonography, the carbon dioxide laser, and the ultrasonic aspirator, are equally valuable for the safe resection of spinal cord tumors. Ultrasonography is particularly useful for examining the spinal cord through either intact or open dura to find the level of maximum tumor involvement or to differentiate tumor cysts from solid tumor masses. Intraoperative monitoring of somatosensory evoked potentials is commonly used, although some surgeons feel that changes in somatosensory evoked potentials may occur only after irretrievable damage has occurred. Motor evoked potentials are used in some centers to guide resection, and use of intraoperative stimulation to locate motor tracts has also been reported.[443]

MRI is invaluable for the diagnosis, localization, and characterization of spinal tumors (see Fig. 39.2-3). For extremely vascular tumors, notably hemangioblastoma, angiography may provide important preoperative delineation of the tumor blood supply. CT scanning is useful for tumors of the bony spinal axis. Determination of the spinal level of the tumor and its exact relation to the spinal cord is important in planning. Corticosteroids are given before, during, and after spinal cord tumor surgery to help control spinal cord edema.

Meningiomas and schwannomas occur in the intradural extramedullary spinal compartment. Most of these tumors can be completely resected through a laminectomy. They are straightforward to separate away from the spinal cord, which is displaced but not invaded by tumor. Schwannomas arise from spinal rootlets (most often dorsal rootlets), and their removal includes section of the rootlets involved. They can grow along the nerve root in a dumbbell fashion through a neural foramen. Some of these extraspinal tumor extensions can be removed by extending the initial laminectomy exposure laterally, whereas others require a separate operation (thoracotomy, costotransversectomy, or a retroperitoneal approach). Strictly anteriorly situated cervical tumors can successfully be removed via an anterior approach using corpectomy of the appropriate vertebral levels, followed by strut grafting after the tumor resection.

The most common intramedullary tumors are ependymoma and astrocytoma. Hemangioblastomas are much less frequent. Except for malignant astrocytomas, resection is the principal treatment for these tumors. Intramedullary tumors are approached through a laminectomy. After dural opening, a longitudinal myelotomy is made, usually in the midline or dorsal root entry zone. The incision is deepened several millimeters to the tumor surface. Dissection planes around the tumor are sought microsurgically and, in the case of ependymomas, usually found and extended gradually around the tumor's surface, whereas removal of the central tumor bulk (by carbon dioxide laser or ultrasonic aspirator) causes the tumor to collapse. Usually, such tumors are completely removed, with good long-term outcome.[444] Some patients later develop spinal deformity requiring stabilization procedures.[445] Tumors without clear dissection planes (usually astrocytomas) cannot be removed completely, but bulk reduction can cause long-term palliation. If frozen-section analysis shows a tumor to be a malignant glioma, surgery is aborted, and radiation therapy is the treatment. For these tumors, even with adjuvant therapies the outcome is dismal, often with spread up and down the spinal axis through CSF.

RADIATION THERAPY

Radiation therapy is recommended for unresectable and incompletely resected neoplasms of the spinal axis. As a rule, doses of 50 to 54 Gy (1.8 Gy/d) are used so that the risk of injury to the cord from radiation is less than that from the neoplasm itself. If higher doses are to be delivered, the authors recommend that hyperfractionated radiotherapy be considered, with fraction sizes of 1.0 to 1.2 Gy twice daily. Low-grade tumors and meningiomas are treated at the lower dose level and malignant tumors to the higher level.[446] When lesions involve only the cauda equina or when complete, irreversible myelopathy already has occurred, higher doses are permissible. Ependymomas of the cord have a longer natural history than astrocytomas. Although most astrocytomas that recur do so within 3 years of treatment, recurrence of ependymomas may be delayed for as long as 12 years.[447,448] Adjunctive radiation therapy is not necessary when ependymomas are removed completely in an *en bloc* fashion.[444] All seven nonirradiated patients with incompletely excised lesions reported on by Barone and Elvidge[449] and by Schuman and coworkers[450] experienced recurrence. Postoperative irradiation appears to improve tumor control when ependymomas are incompletely resected. Sloof and colleagues found that irradiated patients survived nearly twice as long as those who were not irradiated.[451] Five- and 10-year survival rates in irradiated patients with localized ependymomas range from 60% to 100% and 68% to 95%, respectively, whereas 10-year relapse-free survival rates vary from 43% to 61%.[447,452] Tumor grade has a significant effect on outcome. Waldron and colleagues found that for patients with well-differentiated tumors the 5-year cause-specific survival was 97% compared with 71% for patients with intermediate or poorly differentiated tumors ($P = .005$).[447] Myxopapillary ependymomas that arise in the conus medullaris and filum terminale have a better prognosis than the cellular ependymomas that arise in the cord.[453] Local recurrence is the predominant pattern of treatment failure, occurring in 25% of irradiated patients.[447]

The 5- and 10-year survival rates for irradiated patients with low-grade astrocytomas of the spinal cord vary from 60% to 90% and 40% to 90%, respectively; 5- and 10-year relapse-free survival rates range from 66% to 83% and 53% to 83%, respectively.[446,448] Fifty percent to 65% of astrocytomas are controlled locally. Good neurologic condition at the time of irradiation, lower tumor histologic grade, and younger age are favorable factors.[454] Patterns of recurrence for malignant astrocytomas of the spine have been analyzed by MRI.[455] Despite surgery and full-dose radiation, spinal or brain dissemination is the predominant mode of failure. This argues against more aggressive surgical and radiotherapeutic management of the primary lesion.

CHEMOTHERAPY

There have been no reports of controlled clinical trials of chemotherapy for primary spinal axis tumors. Drugs active against intracranial astrocytomas, oligodendrogliomas, ependymomas, medulloblastoma, and germ cell tumors logically may be assumed to be equally efficacious against histologically identical tumors in the spinal cord. Unfortunately, the authors' experience suggests that primary spinal cord tumors (i.e., astrocytomas) respond less well than their intracranial counterparts.

REFERENCES

1. Davis FG, Preston-Martin S. Epidemiology. Incidence and survival. In: Bigner DD, McLendon RE, Bruner JM, eds. *Russell and Rubinstein's pathology of tumors of the central nervous system.* London: Arnold, 1999:7.
2. Greig NH, Ries LG, Yancik R. Increasing annual incidence of primary malignant brain tumors in the elderly. *J Natl Cancer Inst* 1990;82:1621.
3. Evans DGR, Farndon PA, Burnell LD. The incidence of Gorlin syndrome in 173 consecutive cases of medulloblastoma. *Br J Cancer* 1991;64:959.
4. Springate JE. The nevoid basal cell nevoid basal cell carcinoma syndrome. *J Pediatr Surg* 1986;21:908.
5. Schoenberg BS, Christine BW, Whisnant JP. The descriptive epidemiology of primary intracranial neoplasms: the Connecticut experience. *Am J Epidemiol* 1976;104:499.
6. Barker DJ, Weller RO, Garfield JS. Epidemiology of primary tumours of the brain and spinal cord: a regional survey in southern England. *J Neurol Neurosurg Psychiatry* 1976;39:290.
7. Preston-Martin S. Descriptive epidemiology of primary tumors of the brain, cranial nerves and cranial meninges. *Neuroepidemiology* 1989;8:283.
8. Wrensch M, et al. Environmental risk factors for primary malignant brain tumors: a review. *J Neurooncol* 1993;17:47.
9. Inskip PD, Linet MS, Heineman EF. Etiology of brain tumors in adults. *Epidemiol Rev* 1995;17:382.
10. Preston-Martin S, Mack WJ. Neoplasms of the nervous system. In: Schottenfeld D, Fraumeni JFJ, eds. *Cancer epidemiology and prevention.* New York: Oxford University Press, 1996:1231.
11. Demers PA, Vaughan TL, Schommer RR. Occupation, socioeconomic status, and brain tumor mortality: a death certificate-based case-control study. *J Occup Med* 1991;33:1001.
12. Preston-Martin S, et al. Descriptive epidemiology of primary cancer of the brain, cranial nerves and cranial meninges in New Zealand. *Cancer Causes Control* 1993;4:529.

13. Grayson JK. Radiation exposure, socioeconomic status, and brain tumor risk in the US Air Force: a nested case-control study. *Am J Epidemiol* 1996;143:480.
14. Faggiano F, et al. *Socioeconomic differences in cancer incidence and mortality.* IARC Scientific Publication. Lyon, France: IARC Press, 1997:138:65.
15. Inskip PD, et al. Cellular-telephone use and brain tumors. *N Engl J Med* 2001;344(2):79.
16. Brenner AV, et al. History of allergies and autoimmune disease and risk of brain tumors in adults. *Int J Cancer* 2002;10:252.
17. Inskip PD, et al. Handedness and risk of brain tumors in adults. *Cancer Epidemiol Biomarkers Prev* 2003;12:223.
18. Brenner AV, et al. Polio vaccination and risk of brain tumors in adults: no apparent association. *Cancer Epidemiol Biomarkers Prev* 2003;12:177.
19. Fujisawa H, et al. Genetic differences between neurocytoma and dysembryoplastic neuroepithelial tumor and oligodendroglial tumors. *J Neurosurg* 2002;97(6):1350.
20. Lu QR, et al. Common developmental requirement for Olig function indicates a motor neuron/oligodendrocyte connection. *Cell* 2002;109(1):75.
21. McLendon RE, Provenzale J. Glioneuronal tumors of the central nervous system. *Brain Tumor Pathol* 2002;19(2):51.
22. Maher EA, et al. Malignant glioma: genetics and biology of a grave matter. *Genes Dev* 2001;15(11):1311.
23. Levin VA, Wilson CB. Clinical characteristics of cancer in the brain and spinal cord. In: Crook ST, Prestaydo A, eds. *Cancer and chemotherapy: introduction to neoplasia and antineoplastic chemotherapy.* New York: Academic Press, 1981:167.
24. Adams R, Victor M. *Principles of neurology.* New York: McGraw-Hill, 1977.
25. Rabinov JD, Lee PL, Barker FG. In vivo 3-T MR spectroscopy in the distinction of recurrent glioma versus radiation effects initial experience. *Radiology* 2002;225:871.
26. Pirzkall A, Nelson SJ, McKnight TR. Metabolic imaging of low-grade gliomas with three-dimensional magnetic resonance spectroscopy. *Int J Radiat Oncol Biol Phys* 2002;53:1254.
27. Pirzkall A, McKnight TR, Graves EE. MR spectroscopy guided target delineation for high-grade gliomas. *Int J Radiat Oncol Biol Phys* 2001;50:915.
28. Sklar CA, Constine LS. Chronic neuroendocrinological sequelae of radiation therapy. *Int J Radiat Oncol Biol Phys* 1995;31:1113.
29. Berger MS, Kincaid J, Ojemann GA. Brain mapping techniques to maximize safety, and seizure control in children with brain tumors. *Neurosurgery* 1989;25(5):786.
30. McDermott MW, Gutin PH. Image-guided surgery for skull base neoplasms using the ISG viewing wand. Anatomic and technical considerations. *Neurosurg Clin N Am* 1996;7:285.
31. Heilbrun MP. Computed tomography-guided stereotactic systems. *Clin Neurosurg* 1984; 31:564.
32. Apuzzo ML, Chandrasoma PT, Cohen D. Computed imaging stereotaxy: experience and perspective related to 500 procedures applied to brain masses. *Neurosurgery* 1987;20:930.
33. Leibel SA, Sheline GE. Tolerance of the brain and spinal cord to conventional irradiation. In: Gutin PH, Leibel SA, Sheline GE, eds. *Radiation injury to the nervous system.* New York: Raven Press, 1991:211.
34. Posner JB. Side effects of radiotherapy. In: *Neurologic complications of cancer.* Philadelphia: FA Davis, 1995:311.
35. Marks JE, Baglan RJ, Prassad SC. Cerebral radio-necrosis: incidence and risk in relation to dose, time, fractionation and volume. *Int J Radiat Oncol Biol Phys* 1981;7:243.
36. Gutin PH. Treatment of radiation necrosis of the brain. In: Gutin PH, Leibel SA, Sheline GE, eds. *Radiation injury to the nervous system.* New York: Raven Press, 1991:271.
37. Mulhern RK, Ochs J, Kun LE. Changes in intellect associated with cranial radiation therapy. In: Gutin PH, Leibel SA, Sheline GE, eds. *Radiation injury to the nervous system.* New York: Raven Press, 1991:325.
38. Pai HH, Thornton A, Katznelson L. Hypothalamic/pituitary function following high-dose conformal radiotherapy to the base of the skull: demonstration of a dose-effect relationship using dose-volume histogram analysis. *Int J Radiat Oncol Biol Phys* 2001;49:1079.
39. Schultheiss TE, Stephens LC, Peters LJ. Survival in radiation myelopathy. *Int J Radiat Oncol Biol Phys* 1986;12:1765.
40. Wang PY, Shen WC, Jan JS. Magnetic resonance imaging in radiation myelopathy. *Am J Neuroradiol* 1992;13:1049.
41. Schultheiss TE, Kun LE, Ang KK. Radiation response of the central nervous system. *Int J Radiat Oncol Biol Phys* 1995;31:1093.
42. Marcus RBJ, Million RR. The incidence of myelitis after irradiation of cervical spinal cord. *Int J Radiat Oncol Biol Phys* 1990;19:3.
43. Burger PC, Dubis PJ, Schold SCJ. Computerized tomographic and pathologic studies in untreated, quiescent, and recurrent glioblastoma multiforme. *J Neurosurg* 1983;58:159.
44. Choucair AK, Levin VA, Gutin PH. Development of multiple lesions during radiation therapy and chemotherapy in patients with gliomas. *J Neurosurg* 1986;65:654.
45. Hochberg FH, Pruitt A. Assumptions in the radiotherapy of glioblastomas. *Neurology* 1980;30:907.
46. Kelly PJ, Daumas-Duport C, Kispert DB. Imaging-based stereotaxic serial biopsies in untreated intracranial glial neoplasms. *J Neurosurg* 1987;66:865.
47. Chang SD, Adler JR. Robotics and radiosurgery—the Cyberknife. *Stereotact Funct Neurosurg* 2001;76:203.
48. Ryu SI, Chang SD, Kim DH. Image-guided hypofractionated stereotactic radiosurgery to spinal lesions. *Neurosurgery* 2001;49:838.
49. Tatter SB, Shaw EG, Rosenblum ML. An inflatable balloon catheter and liquid 1251 radiation source for treatment of recurrent malignant glioma: multicenter safety and feasibility trial. *J Neurosurg* 2003;99:297.
50. Nag S. Morphology and molecular properties of cellular components of normal cerebral vessels. *Methods Mol Med* 2003;89:3.
51. Huber, JD, Egleton RD, Davis TP. Molecular physiology and pathophysiology of tight junctions in the blood-brain barrier. *Trends in Neurosci* 2001;24(12):719.
52. Smith QR, Fisher C, Allen DD. The role of plasma protein binding in drug delivery to brain. In: D Kobiler, ed. *Blood-brain barrier.* New York: Kluwer Academic/Plenum Publishers, 2001.
53. Toth K, Vaughn MM, Peress NS. MDR1 P-glycoprotein is expressed by endothelial cells of the neovasculature in central nervous system tumors. *Brain Tumor Pathol* 1999;16:23.
54. Groothuis DR. The blood-brain and blood-tumor barriers: a review of strategies for increasing drug delivery. *Neuro-oncology* 2000;2:45.
55. Bart J, et al. The blood-brain barrier and oncology: new insights into function and modulation. *Cancer Treat Rev* 2000;26:449.
56. Dropcho EJ, et al. Phase II study of intracarotid or selective intracerebral infusion of cisplatin for treatment of recurrent anaplastic gliomas. *J Neurooncol* 1998;36:1991.
57. Greig NH, et al. Optimizing drugs for brain action. In: D Kobiler, ed. *Blood-brain barrier.* New York: Kluwer Academic/Plenum Publishers, 2001.
58. Kroll RA, Neuwelt EA. Outwitting the blood-brain barrier for therapeutic purposes: osmotic opening and other means. *Neurosurgery* 1998;42:1083.
59. Emerich DF, et al. The development of the bradykinin agonist labradimil as a means to increase the permeability of the blood-brain barrier: from concept to clinical evaluation. *Clin Pharmacokinet* 2001;40(2):105.
60. Arafat T, et al. Toxicities related to intraarterial infusion of cisplatin and etoposide in patients with brain tumors. *J Neurooncol* 1999;42:73.
61. Hirano Y, et al. Therapeutic results of intra-arterial chemotherapy in patients with malignant glioma. *Int J Oncol* 1998;13:537.
62. Brem H, et al. Interstitial chemotherapy with drug polymer implants for the treatment of recurrent gliomas. *J Neurosurg* 1991;74:441.
63. Strasser JF, et al. Distribution of 1,3-bis(2-chloroethyl)-1-nitrosourea and tracers in the rabbit brain after interstitial delivery by biodegradable polymer implants. *J Pharmacol Exp Ther* 1995;275(3):1647.
64. Rustamzadeh E, et al. Immunotoxin therapy for CNS tumor. *J Neurooncol* 2003;64:101.
65. Lieberman DM, et al. Convection-enhanced distribution of large molecules in gray matter during interstitial drug infusion. *J Neurosurg* 1995;82:1021.
66. Bobo RH, et al. Convection-enhanced delivery of macromolecules in the brain. *Proc Natl Acad Sci U S A* 1994;91:2076.
67. Siegal T. Strategies for increasing drug delivery to the brain. In: D Kobiler, ed. *Blood-brain barrier.* New York: Kluwer Academic/Plenum Publishers, 2001.
68. Fetell MR, et al. Preirradiation paclitaxel in glioblastoma multiforme: efficacy, pharmacology, and drug interactions. New Approaches to Brain Tumor Therapy Central Nervous System Consortium. *J Clin Oncol* 1997;15:3121.
69. Prados MD, et al. Phase I trial of irinotecan (CPT-11) in patients with recurrent malignant glioma: a North American Brain Tumor Consortium Study. *Neuro-oncology* 2004;6(1):44.
70. Grossman SA, et al. Increased 9-aminocamptothecin dose requirements in patients on anticonvulsants. *Cancer Chemother Pharmacol* 1998;42:118.
71. Villikka K, Kivisto KT, Maenpaa H. Cytochrome P450-inducing antiepileptics increase the clearance of vincristine in patients with brain tumors. *Clin Pharmacol Ther* 1999;66:589.
72. Baker DK, Relling MV, Pui CH. Increased teniposide clearance with concomitant anticonvulsant therapy. *J Clin Oncol* 1992;10:311.
73. Kleihues P, Burger PC, Scheithauer BW. *Histological typing of tumors of the central nervous system.* Berlin: Springer-Verlag, 1993.
74. Ringertz N. Grading of gliomas. *Acta Pathol Microbiol Scand* 1950;27:51.
75. Zauulich KJ. *Histological typing of tumors of the central nervous system.* No. 21. Geneva: World Health Organization, 1979:15.
76. Daumas-Duport C, Scheithauer BW, O'Fallon J. Grading of astrocytomas, a simple and reproducible method. *Cancer* 1988;62:2152.
77. Kim TS, Halliday AL, Hedley-Whyte ET. Correlates of survival and the Daumas-Duport grading system of astrocytomas. *J Neurosurg* 1991;74:27.
78. Kleihues P, Cavance WK, eds. *Pathology and genetics of tumors of the central nervous system. World Health Organization Classification of Tumors.* Lyon, France: IARC Press, 2000.
79. Ye ZC, Sontheimer H. Glioma cells release excitotoxic concentrations of glutamate. *Cancer Res* 1999;59:4383.
80. Jackson RJ, Fuller GN, Abi-Said D. Limitations of stereotactic biopsy in the initial management of gliomas. *Neuro-oncology* 2001;3:193.
81. Perry A, Jenkins RB, O'Fallon JR. Clinicopathologic study of 85 similarly treated patients with anaplastic astrocytic tumors. An analysis of DNA content (ploidy), cellular proliferation, and p53 expression. *Cancer* 1999;86:672.
82. Barker FG, et al. Age and radiation response in glioblastoma multiforme. *Neurosurgery* 2001;49:1288.
83. Vuorinen V, et al. Debulking or biopsy of malignant glioma in elderly people—a randomised study. *Acta Neurochir Wien* 2003;145:5.
84. Keles GE, Lamborn KR, Berger MS. Low-grade hemispheric gliomas in adults: a critical review of extent of resection as a factor influencing outcome. *J Neurosurg* 2001;95:735.
85. Hess KR. Extent of resection as a prognostic variable in the treatment of gliomas. *J Neurooncol* 1999;42:227.
86. Henry RG, et al. Subcortical pathways serving cortical language sites: initial experience with diffusion tensor imaging fiber tracking combined with intraoperative language mapping. *Neuroimage* 2004;21:616.
87. Barker FG, et al. Survival and functional status after resection of recurrent glioblastoma multiforme. *Neurosurgery* 1998;42:709.
88. Berger MS, Leibel SA, Bruner JM. Primary central nervous system tumors of the supratentorial compartment. In: Levin VA, ed. *Cancer in the nervous system.* New York: Churchill Livingstone, 1995:57.
89. Berger MS, Deliganis AV, Dobbins J. The effect of extent of resection on recurrence in patients with low-grade cerebral hemisphere gliomas. *Cancer* 1994;74:1784.
90. Karim ABMF, Cornu P, Bleeham N. Immediate postoperative radiotherapy in low-grade glioma improves progression free survival but not overall survival: preliminary results of an EORTC/MRC randomized phase III trial. *Proc Am Soc Clin Oncol* 1998;17: 400a.
91. Karim AB, Maat B, Hatlevoll R. Randomized trial on dose-response in radiation therapy

of lwo-grade cerebral glioma: European Organization for Research and Treatment of Cancer (EORTC) Study 22844. *Int J Radiat Oncol Biol Phys* 1996;36:549.

92. Shaw E, Arusell R, Scheithauer BW. A prospective randomized trial of low- versus high-dose radiation therapy in adults with supratentorial low-grade glioma: initial report of a NCCG-RTOG-ECOG study. *Proc Am Soc Clin Oncol* 1998;17:401a.
93. Kiebert GM, Curran D, Aaronson NK. Quality of life after radiation therapy of cerebral low-grade gliomas of the adult: results of a randomized phase III trial on dose response (EORTC trial 22844). EORTC Radiotherapy Co-operative Group. *Eur J Cancer* 1998;34:1902.
94. Lo SS, Hall WA, Cho KH. Radiation response for supratentorial low-grade glioma—institutional experience and literature review. *J Neurol Sci* 2003;214:43.
95. Jeremic B, Milicic B, Grujicic D. Hyperfractionated radiation therapy for incompletely resected supratentorial low-grade glioma: a 10-year update of a phase II study. *Int J Radiat Oncol Biol Phys* 2003;57:465.
96. Brown PD, Buejner JC, O'Fallon J. Effects of radiotherapy on cognitive function in patients with low-grade glioma measured by the Folstein Mini-Mental State Examination. *J Clin Oncol* 2003;21:2519.
97. Klein M, Heimans JJ, Aaronson NK. Effect of radiotherapy and other treatment-related factors and mid-term and long-term cognitive sequelae in low-grade gliomas: a comparative study. *Lancet* 2002;360:1361.
98. Leibel SA, Scott CB, Loeffler JS. Contemporary approaches to the treatment of malignant gliomas with radiation therapy. *Semin Oncol* 1994;21:198.
99. Prados MD, Scott C, Curran WJ. Procarbazine, CCNU, and vincristine (PCV) chemotherapy for anaplastic astrocytoma: a retrospective review of Radiation Therapy Oncology Group protocols comparing survival with carmustine or PCV adjuvant chemotherapy. *J Clin Oncol* 1999;17:3389.
100. Kleinberg L, Grossman SA, Carson K. Survival of patients with newly diagnosed glioblastoma multiforme treated with RSR13 and radiotherapy: results of a phase II new approaches to brain tumor therapy consortium safety and efficacy study. *J Clin Oncol* 2002;20:3149.
101. Stupp R, et al. Promising survival for patients with newly diagnosed glioblastoma multiforme treated with concomitant radiation plus temozolomide followed by adjuvant temozolomide. *J Clin Oncol* 2002;20(5):1375.
102. Nelson DF, Curran WJ, Nelson JS. Hyperfractionation in malignant glioma, report on a dose-search phase I/II protocol of the radiation therapy oncology group (RTOG). *Proc Am Soc Clin Oncol* 1990;9:A350.
103. Fitzek MM, Thornton AF, Rabinov JD. Accelerated fractionated proton/photon irradiation to 90 cobalt gray equivalent for glioblastoma multiforme: results of a phase II prospective trial. *J Neurosurg* 1999;91:251.
104. Thornton AF. Three-dimensional treatment planning of astrocytoma, a dosimetric study of cerebral irradiation. *Int J Radiat Oncol Biol Phys* 1991;20:1309.
105. Selker RG, Shapiro WR, Burger P. The Brain Tumor Cooperative Group NIH Trial 87-01: a randomized comparison of surgery, external beam radiotherapy, and carmustine versus surgery, interstitial radiotherapy boost, external radiation therapy, and carmustine. *Neurosurgery* 2002;51:343.
106. Laperriere NJ, Leung PM, McKenzie S. Randomized study of brachytherapy in the initial management of patients with malignant astrocytoma. *Int J Radiat Oncol Biol Phys* 1998;41:1005.
107. Leibel SA, Gutin PH, Wara WM. Survival and quality of life after interstitial implantation of removable high-activity iodine-125 sources for the treatment of patients with recurrent malignant gliomas. *Int J Radiat Oncol Biol Phys* 1989;17:1129.
108. Shrieve DC, Alexander E, Wen PY. Comparison of stereotactic radiosurgery and brachytherapy in the treatment of recurrent glioblastoma multiforme. *Neurosurgery* 1995;36:275.
109. Roberge D, Souhami L. Stereotactic radiosurgery in the management of intracranial gliomas. *Technol Cancer Res Treat* 2003;2:117.
110. Perkins GH, Schomer DF, Fuller GN. Gliomatosis cerebri: improved outcomes with radiotherapy. *Int J Radiat Oncol Biol Phys* 2003;56:1137.
111. Chang EL, Yi W, Allen PK. Hypofractionated radiotherapy for elderly or younger low-performance status glioblastoma patients: outcomes and prognostic factors. *Int J Radiat Oncol Biol Phys* 2003;56:519.
112. Salcman M. Malignant glioma management. *Neurosurg Clin N Am* 1990;1:49.
113. Byar DP, Green SB, Strike TA. Prognostic factors for malignant glioma. In: Walker MD, ed. *Oncology of the nervous system.* Boston: Martinus Nijhoff, 1983:379.
114. MacDonald D, et al. Response criteria for phase II studies of supratentorial malignant glioma. *J Clin Oncol* 1990;8:1277.
115. Wong ET, et al. Outcomes and prognostic factors in recurrent glioma patients enrolled onto phase II trials. *J Clin Oncol* 1999;17:2572.
116. Packer RJ, et al. Treatment of chiasmatic/hypothalamic gliomas of childhood with chemotherapy: an update. *Ann Neurol* 1988;23:79.
117. Petronio J, Edwards MS, Prados MD. Management of chiasmal and hypothalamic gliomas of infancy and childhood with chemotherapy. *J Neurosurg* 1990;74:701.
118. Shaw EG, Wisoff JH. Clinical trials of intracranial low-grade glioma in adults and children. *Neuro-oncology* 2003;5(3):153.
119. Quinn JA, et al. Phase II trial of temozolomide in patients with progressive low-grade glioma. *J Clin Oncol* 2003;21(4):646.
120. Fine HA, et al. Meta-analysis of radiation therapy with and without adjuvant chemotherapy for malignant gliomas in adults. *Cancer* 1993;71(8):2585.
121. Stewart LA. Chemotherapy in adult high-grade glioma: a systematic review and meta-analysis of individual patient data from 12 randomised trials. *Lancet* 2002;359(9311):1011.

121a. Levin VA, Silver P, Hannigan J, et al. Superiority of post-radiotherapy adjuvant chemotherapy with CCN, procarbazine, and vincristine (PVC) over BCNU for anaplastic gliomas: NCOG 6G61 final report. *Int J Rad Onc Biol Phys* 1990;18:321.

122. Prados MD, et al. Procarbazine, lomustine, and vincristine (PCV) chemotherapy for anaplastic astrocytoma: a retrospective review of radiation therapy oncology group protocols comparing survival with carmustine or PCV adjuvant chemotherapy. *J Clin Oncol* 1999;17(11):3389.
123. Clark AS, Deans B, Stevens MF. Antitumor imidazotetrazines: 32. Synthesis of novel imidazotetrazinones and related dicyclic heterocycles to probe the mode of action on the antitumor drug temozolomide. *J Med Chem* 1995;38:1493.
124. Yung WKA, et al. Multicenter phase II trial of temozolomide in patients with anaplastic astrocytoma or anaplastic oligoastrocytoma at first relapse. Temodal Brain Tumor Group. *J Clin Oncol* 1999;17(9):2762.
125. Yung WK, et al. A phase II study of temozolomide vs. procarbazine in patients with glioblastoma multiforme at first relapse. *Br J Cancer* 2000;83(5):588.
126. Valtonen S, et al. Interstitial chemotherapy with carmustine-loaded polymers for high-grade gliomas: a randomized double-blind study. *Neurosurgery* 1997;41:44.
127. Westphal M, et al. A phase 3 trial of local chemotherapy with biodegradable carmustine (BCNU) wafers (Gliadel wafers) in patients with primary malignant glioma. *Neuro-oncology* 2003;5:79.
128. Brem H, et al. Placebo-controlled trial of safety and efficacy of intraoperative controlled delivery by biodegradable polymers of chemotherapy for recurrent gliomas. The Polymer-Brain Tumor Treatment Group. *Lancet* 1995;345:1008.
129. Olivi A, et al. Dose escalation of carmustine in surgically implanted polymers in patients with recurrent malignant glioma: a New Approaches to Brain Tumor Therapy CNS Consortium trial. *J Clin Oncol* 2003;21:1845.
130. Rhines LD, et al. 06-benzylguanine potentiates the antitumor effect of locally delivered carmustine against an intracranial rat glioma. *Cancer Res* 2000;60:6307.
131. Levin VA. Chemotherapy of primary brain tumors. *Neurol Clin* 1985;3:855.
132. Wilson CB, Gutin PH, Boldrey EB. Single-agent chemotherapy of brain tumors. A five-year review. *Arch Neurol* 1976;33:739.
133. Kumar ARV, Renaudin J, Wilson CB. Procarbazine hydrochloride in the treatment of brain tumors. *J Neurosurg* 1974;40:365.
134. Rodriguez L, Prados M, Silver P. Re-evaluation of procarbazine for the treatment of recurrent malignant CNS tumors. *Cancer* 1989;64:2420.
135. Bertolone SJ, Baum ES, Krivit W. A phase II study of cisplatin therapy in recurrent childhood brain tumors. *J Neurooncol* 1989;7:5.
136. Yung WK, Mechtler L, Gleason MJ. Intravenous carboplatin for recurrent malignant gliomas: a phase II study. *J Clin Oncol* 1991;9:860.
137. Straathof CS, van den Bent MJ, Ma J. The effect of dexamethasone on the uptake of cisplatin in 9L glioma and the area of brain around tumor. *J Neurooncol* 1998;37:1.
138. Ben Arush MW, Postovsky S, Goldsher D. Clinical and radiographic response in three children with recurrent malignant cerebral tumors with high-dose tamoxifen. *Pediatr Hematol Oncol* 1999;16:245.
139. Couldwell WT, Weiss MH, DeGiorgio CM. Clinical and radiographic response in a minority of patients with recurrent malignant gliomas treated with high-dose tamoxifen. *Neurosurgery* 1993;32:485.
140. Couldwell WT, Hinton DR, Surnock AA. Treatment of recurrent malignant gliomas with chronic oral high-dose tamoxifen. *Clin Cancer Res* 1996;2:619.
141. Chamberlain MC, Kormanik PA. Salvage chemotherapy with tamoxifen for recurrent anaplastic astrocytomas. *Arch Neurol* 1999;56:703.
142. Goodwin W, Crowley J. A retrospective comparison of high-dose BCNU with autologous marrow rescue plus radiotherapy vs IV BCNU plus radiation therapy in high grade gliomas: a Southwest Oncology Group review. *Proc Am Soc Clin Oncol* 1989;8:A352.
143. Allen J, et al. Recombinant β-interferon A phase I/II dose finding trial in pediatric brain tumor patients. *J Neurooncol* 1989;7:S4(abst).
144. Yung WK, Prados M, Levin VA. Intravenous recombinant interferon beta in patients with recurrent malignant gliomas: a phase I/II study. *J Clin Oncol* 1991;9:1945.
145. Grossman SA, et al. Phase II study of continuous infusion carmustine and cisplatin followed by cranial irradiation in adults with newly diagnosed high-grade astrocytoma. *J Clin Oncol* 1997;15(7):2596.
146. Grossman SA, et al. Phase III study comparing three cycles of infusional carmustine and cisplatin followed by radiation therapy with radiation therapy and concurrent carmustine in patients with newly diagnosed supratentorial glioblastoma multiforme: Eastern Cooperative Oncology Group Trial 2394. *J Clin Oncol* 2003;21(8):1485.
147. Laske DW, Youle RJ, Oldfield EH. Tumor regression with regional distribution of the targeted toxin TF-CRM107 in patients with malignant brain tumors. *Nat Med* 1997;3(12):1362.
148. Lieberman FS, et al. Phase I-II study of ZD-1839 for recurrent malignant gliomas and meningiomas progressing after radiation therapy. *Proc Am Soc Clin Oncol* 2003;22:105(abst 421).
149. Prados M, et al. Phase I study of OSI-774 alone or with temozolomide in patients with malignant glioma. *Proc Am Soc Clin Oncol* 2003;22:99(abst 394).
150. Chang S, et al. Phase II/pharmacokinetic study of CCI-779 in recurrent glioblastoma multiforme. Paper presented at the Eighth Annual Meeting of the Society for Neuro-Oncology. *Neuro-oncology* 2003;5:349(abst TA-09).
151. Cloughesy TF, et al. Phase II trial or R115777 (Zarnestra) in patients with recurrent gliomas not taking enzyme inducing antiepileptic drugs (EIAED): a North American Brain Tumor Consortium (NABTC) report. *Proc Am Soc Clin Oncol* 2002;21(abst 317).
152. Guillamo J-S, Doz F, Delattre J-Y. Brainstem gliomas. *Curr Opin Neurol* 2001;14:711.
153. Allen JC, et al. Brain tumors in children: current cooperative and institutional chemotherapy trials in newly diagnosed and recurrent disease. *Semin Oncol* 1986;13:110.
154. Freeman CR, Suissa S. Brain stem tumors in children: results of a survey of 62 patients treated with radiotherapy. *Int J Radiat Oncol Biol Phys* 1986;12:1823.
155. Eifel PJ, Cassady JR, Belli JA. Radiation therapy of tumors of the brainstem and midbrain in children: experience of the Joint Center for Radiation Therapy and Children's Hospital Medical Center (1971–1981). *Int J Radiat Oncol Biol Phys* 1987;13:847.
156. Albright AL. Diffuse brainstem tumors: when is a biopsy necessary? *Pediatr Neurosurg* 1996;24(5):252.
157. Daglioglu E, Cataltepe O, Akalan N. Tectal gliomas in children: the implications for natural history and management strategy. *Pediatr Neurosurg* 2003;38(5):223.

158. Khatib ZA, et al. Predominance of pilocytic histology in dorsally exophytic brain stem tumors. *Pediatr Neurosurg* 1994;20(1):2.
159. Weiner HL, et al. Intra-axial tumors of the cervicomedullary junction: surgical results and long-term outcome. *Pediatr Neurosurg* 1997;27(1):12.
160. Cairncross JG, MacDonald DR. Chemotherapy for oligodendroglioma: progress report. *Arch Neurol* 1991;48:225.
161. Goldwein JW, Corn BW, Finlay JL. Is craniospinal irradiation required to cure children with malignant (anaplastic) intracranial ependymomas? *Cancer* 1991;67:2766.
162. Freeman CR, Krischer JS. Final results of a study of escalating doses of hyperfractionated radiotherapy in brain stem tumors in children: a Pediatric Oncology Group study. *Int J Radiat Oncol Biol Phys* 1993;27:197.
163. Freeman CR, Farmer JP. Pediatric brain stem gliomas: a review. *Int J Radiat Oncol Biol Phys* 1998;40:265.
164. Levin VA, Edwards MS, Wright DC. Modified procarbazine, CCNU, and vincristine (PCV3) combination chemotherapy in the treatment of malignant brain tumors. *Cancer Treat Rep* 1980;64:237.
165. McLaughlin MP, Marcus RBJ, Buatti JM. Ependymoma: results, prognostic factors and treatment recommendations. *Int J Radiat Oncol Biol Phys* 1998;40:845.
166. Jennings MT, et al. Preradiation chemotherapy in primary high-risk brainstem tumors: phase II study CCG-9941 of the Children's Cancer Group. *J Clin Oncol* 2002;20(16):3431.
167. Lashford LS, et al. Temozolomide in malignant gliomas of childhood: a United Kingdom Children's Cancer Study Group and French Society for Pediatric Oncology Intergroup Study. *J Clin Oncol* 2002;20(24):4684.
168. Humphreys RP. Posterior cranial fossa brain tumors in children. In: Appuzzo M, ed. *Third ventricular tumors.* Baltimore: Williams & Wilkins, 1987:838.
169. Bowers DC, et al. Study of the MIB-1 labeling index as a predictor of tumor progression in pilocytic astrocytomas in children and adolescents. *J Clin Oncol* 2003;21:2698.
170. Hayostek CJ, et al. Astrocytomas of the cerebellum: a comparative clinicopathologic study of pilocytic and diffuse astrocytomas. *Cancer* 1993;72(3):856.
171. Chamberlain MC. Recurrent cerebellar gliomas: salvage therapy with oral etoposide. *J Child Neurol* 1997;12(3):200.
172. Packer RJ, et al. Carboplatin and vincristine for recurrent and newly diagnosed low-grade gliomas of childhood. *J Clin Oncol* 1993;11(5):850.
173. Walsh FB, Hoyt WF. *Clinical neuro-ophthalmology.* Baltimore: Williams & Wilkins, 1969:2076.
174. Lewis RA, Gerson LP, Axelson KA. von Recklinghausen neurofibromatosis. II. Incidence of optic gliomata. *Ophthalmology* 1984;91:929.
175. Housepian EM, Trokel SL, Jakobiec FO. Tumors of the orbit. In: Youman JR, ed. *Neurological surgery.* Philadelphia: WB Saunders, 1982:3024.
176. Ettinger LJ, Ru N, Krailo M, et al. A phase II study of diaziquone in children with recurrent or progressive primary brain tumors; a report from the Children's Cancer Study Group. *J Neurooncol* 1990;9:69.
177. Kornreich L, Blaser S, Schwarz M. Optic pathway glioma: correlation of imaging findings with the presence of neurofibromatosis. *Am J Neuroradiol* 2001;22:1963.
178. Grill J, Laithier V, Radriquez D. When do children with optic pathway tumours need treatment? An oncological perspective in 106 patients in a single center. *Eur J Pediatr* 2000;9:692.
179. Czyzyk E, et al. Optic pathway gliomas in children with or without neurofibromatosis 1. *J Child Neurol* 2003;18:471.
180. Parsa CF, Hoyt CS, Lesser RL. Spontaneous regression of optic gliomas: thirteen cases documented by serial neuroimaging. *Arch Ophthalmol* 2001;4:516.
181. Khafaga Y, et al. Optic gliomas: a retrospective analysis of 50 cases. *Int J Radiat Oncol Biol Phys* 2003;56(3):807.
182. Tenny RT, Laws ER, Young BR. The neurosurgical management of optic gliomas: results in 104 patients. *J Neurosurg* 1982;57:452.
183. Bataini JP, Delanian S, Ponvert D. Chiasmal gliomas: results of irradiation management and review of literature. *Int J Radiat Oncol Biol Phys* 1991;21:615.
184. Wong JYC, Uhl V, Wara WM. Optic gliomas: a re-analysis of the University of California, San Francisco experience. *Cancer* 1987;60:1847.
185. Jenkin D, et al. Optic glioma in children: surveillance, resection, or irradiation? *Int J Radiat Oncol Biol Phys* 1993;25:215.
186. Rodriguez LA, Edwards MS, Levin VA. Management of hypothalamic gliomas in children: an analysis of 33 cases. *Neurosurgery* 1990;26:242.
187. Debus JM, et al. Fractionated stereotactic radiotherapy (FSRT) for optic glioma. *Int J Radiat Oncol Biol Phys* 1999;44:243.
188. Packer RJ, Sutton LN, Bilaniuk LT. Treatment of chiasmatic/hypothalamic. *Ann Neurol* 1988;23:79.
189. Prados MD, Edwards MS, Rabbit J. Treatment of pediatric low-grade gliomas with a nitrosourea-based multiagent chemotherapy regimen. *J Neurooncol* 1997;32:235.
190. Aquino VM, Fort DW, Kamen BA. Carboplatin for the treatment of children with newly diagnosed optic chiasm gliomas: a phase II study. *J Neurooncol* 1999;41:255.
191. Ludwig CL, Smith MT, Godfrey AD. A clinicopathologic study of 323 patients with oligodendrogliomas. *Ann Neurol* 1986;19:15.
192. Shaw EG, Scheithauer BW, O'Fallon JR. Oligodendrogliomas: the Mayo Clinic Experience. *J Neurosurg* 1992;76:428.
193. Buckner JC, Brown LD, Kugler JW. Oligodendroglioma: an analysis of the value of radiation therapy. *Cancer* 1987;60:2179.
194. Mirk SJ, Lindegaard K-F, Halvorsen TB. Oligodendroglioma: incidence and biological behavior in a defined population. *J Neurosurg* 1985;63:881.
195. Mirk SJ, Halvorsen TB, Lindegaard K-F. Oligodendroglioma: histologic evaluation and prognosis. *J Neuropathol Exp Neurol* 1986;45:65.
196. Gannett DE, Wisbeck WM, Silbergeld DL. The role of postoperative irradiation in the treatment of oligodendroglioma. *Int J Radiat Oncol Biol Phys* 1994;30:567.
197. MacDonald DR, Low-grade gliomas, mixed gliomas, and oligodendrogliomas. *Semin Oncol* 1994;21:236.
198. Shimizu KY, Tran LM, Mark RJ. Management of oligodendrogliomas. *Radiology* 1993; 186:569.
199. Wallner K, Gonzales M, Sheline GE. Treatment of oligodendrogliomas with or without postoperative irradiation. *J Neurosurg* 1988;68:684.
200. Lindegaard K-F, Mork SJ, Eide GE. Statistical analysis of clinicopathological features, radiotherapy, and survival in 170 cases of oligodendroglioma. *J Neurosurg* 1987;67:224.
201. Allison RR, Schulsinger A, Vongtama V. Radiation and chemotherapy improve outcome in oligodendroglioma. *Int J Radiat Oncol Biol Phys* 1997;37:399.
202. Mason WP, Krol GS, DeAngelis LM. Low-grade oligodendroglioma responds to chemotherapy. *Neurology* 1996;46(1):203.
203. Jeremic B, Shibamoto Y, Grujicic D. Combined treatment modality for anaplastic oligodendroglioma: a phase II study. *J Neurooncol* 1999;43:179.
204. van den Bent MJ, et al. Phase II study of first-line chemotherapy with temozolomide in recurrent oligodendroglial tumors: the European Organization for Research and Treatment of Cancer Brain Tumor Group Study 26971. *J Clin Oncol* 2003;21(13):2525.
205. Chinot OL, et al. Safety and efficacy of temozolomide in patients with recurrent anaplastic oligodendrogliomas after standard radiotherapy and chemotherapy. *J Clin Oncol* 2001;19(9):2249.
206. Kim L, et al. Procarbazine, lomustine, and vincristine (PCV) chemotherapy for grade III and grade IV oligoastrocytomas. *J Neurosurg* 1996;85(4):602.
207. Buckner JC, et al. Phase II trial of procarbazine, lomustine, and vincristine as initial therapy for patients with low-grade oligodendroglioma or oligoastrocytoma: efficacy and association with chromosomal abnormalities. *Clin Oncol* 2003;21(2):251.
208. Schiffer D, et al. Prognostic factors in oligodendroglioma. *Can J Neurol Sci* 1997;24(4):313.
209. Fisher BJ, Naumova E, Leighton CC. Ki-67: a prognostic factor for low-grade glioma? *Int J Radiat Oncol Biol Phys* 2002;52:996.
210. Ino Y, et al. Molecular subtypes of anaplastic oligodendroglioma: implications for patient management of diagnosis. *Clin Cancer Res* 2001;7(4):839.
211. Pollack IF, et al. Association between chromosome 1p and 19q loss and outcome in pediatric malignant gliomas: results from the CCG-945 cohort. *Pediatr Neurosurg* 2003;39(1):114.
212. Schiffer D, et al. Histologic prognostic factors in ependymoma. *Childs Nerv Syst* 1991;7(4):177.
213. Ross GW, Rubinstein LJ. Lack of histopathological correlation of malignant ependymomas with postoperative survival. *J Neurosurg* 1989;70(1):31.
214. Vanuytsel L, Brada M. The role of prophylactic spinal irradiation in localized intracranial ependymoma. *Int J Radiat Oncol Biol Phys* 1991;21:825.
215. Healey EA, Barnes PD, Kupsky WJ. The prognostic significance of postoperative residual tumor in ependymoma. *Neurosurgery* 1991;28:666.
216. Leibel SA, Sheline GE. Radiation therapy for neoplasms of the brain. *J Neurosurg* 1987;66:1.
217. Wallner KE, Wara WM, Sheline GE. Intracranial ependymomas: results of treatment with partial or whole brain irradiation without spinal irradiation. *Int J Radiat Oncol Biol Phys* 1986;12:1937.
218. Salazar OM, Castro-Vita H, Van Houtte P. Improved survival in cases of intracranial ependymoma after radiation therapy: late report and recommendations. *J Neurosurg* 1983;59:652.
219. Vanuytsel LJ, Bessell EM, Ashley SE. Long-term results of a policy of surgery and radiotherapy. *Int J Radiat Oncol Biol Phys* 1992;23:313.
220. Merchant TE, Haida T, Wang MH. Anaplastic ependymoma: treatment of pediatric patients with or without craniospinal radiation therapy. *J Neurosurg* 1997;86:943.
221. Robertson PL, Zeltzer PM, Boyett JM. Survival and prognostic factors following radiation therapy and chemotherapy for ependymomas in children: a report of the Children's Cancer Group. *J Neurosurg* 1998;88:695.
222. Gaynon PS, Ettinger LJ, Baum ES. Carboplatin in childhood brain tumors. a Children's Cancer Study Group phase II trial. *Cancer* 1990;66:2465.
223. Chamberlain MC. Salvage chemotherapy for recurrent spinal cord ependymoma. *Cancer* 2002;95(5):997.
224. Grill J, Le Deley M-C, Gambarelli D. Postoperative chemotherapy without irradiation for ependymoma in children under 5 years of age: a multicenter trial of the French Society of Pediatric Oncology. *J Clin Oncol* 2001;19:1288.
225. Spallone A, Gagliardi FM, Vagnozzi R. Intracranial meningiomas related to external cranial irradiation. *Surg Neurol* 1979;12:153.
226. Cushing H, Eisehardt L. *Meningiomas: their classification, regional behavior, life history and surgical end results.* Springfield, IL: Charles C Thomas, 1938:73.
227. Simpson D. The recurrence of intracranial meningiomas after surgical treatment. *J Neurol Neurosurg Psychiatry* 1957;20:22.
228. Mirimanoff RO, Dosoretz DE, Linggood RM. Meningioma: analysis of recurrence and progression following neurosurgical resection. *J Neurosurg* 1985;62:18.
229. Jackler RK, Sim DW, Gutin PH. Systematic approach to intradural tumors ventral to the brainstem. *Am J Otol* 1995;16:39.
230. Karlsson UL, Leibel SA, Wallner K. Brain tumors. In: Perez CA, Brady LW, eds. *Principles and practice of radiation oncology,* 2nd ed. Philadelphia: JB Lippincott, 1992:515.
231. Stafford SL, Perry A, Suman VJ. Primarily resected meningiomas: outcome and prognostic factors in 581 Mayo Clinic patients, 1978–1988. *Mayo Clin Proc* 1998;73:936.
232. Barbaro NM, Gutin PH, Wilson CB. Radiation therapy in the treatment of partially resected meningiomas. *Neurosurgery* 1987;20:525.
233. Goldsmith BJ, Wara WM, Wilson CB. Postoperative irradiation for subtotally resected meningiomas. A retrospective analysis of 140 patients treated from 1967 to 1990. *J Neurosurg* 1994;80:195.
234. Wilson C. Meningiomas: genetics, malignancy, and the role of radiation in induction and treatment. *J Neurosurg* 1994;81:666.
235. Condra KS, Buatti JM, Mendenhall WM. Benign meningiomas: treatment selection affects survival. *Int J Radiat Oncol Biol Phys* 1997;39:427.
236. Graholm JH, Bloom JG, Crow JH. The role of radiotherapy in the management of intra-

cranial meningiomas: the Royal Marsden Hospital experience in 186 patients. *Int J Radiat Oncol Biol Phys* 1990;18:755.

237. Connell PP, Macdonald RL, Mansur DB. Tumor size predicts control of benign meningiomas treated with radiotherapy. *Neurosurgery* 1999;44:1194.
238. Chan RC, Thompson GB. Morbidity, mortality, and quality of life following surgery for intracranial meningiomas. *J Neurosurg* 1984;60:52.
239. Milsosevic MF, Frost PJ, Laperriere NJ. Radiotherapy for atypical or malignant meningioma. *Int J Radiat Oncol Biol Phys* 1996;34:817.
240. Kondziolka D, Levy EI, Niranjan A. Long-term outcomes after meningioma radiosurgery: physician and patient perspectives. *J Neurosurg* 1999;91:44.
241. Hakim R, Alexander E, Loeffler JS. Results of linear accelerator-based radiosurgery for intracranial meningiomas. *Neurosurgery* 1998;42:446.
242. Kondiziolka D, et al. Long-term results after radiosurgery for benign intracranial tumors. *Neurosurgery* 2003;53(4):815.
243. Engenhart R, Kimming BN, Hover KH. Stereotactic single high dose radiation therapy of benign intracranial meningiomas. *Int J Radiat Oncol Biol Phys* 1990;19:1021.
244. Kondiziolka D, Lunsford LD, Coffey RJ. Stereotactic radiosurgery for meningiomas. *J Neurosurg* 1991;74:552.
245. Morita A, Coffey RJ, Foote RL. Risk of injury to cranial nerves after gamma knife radiosurgery for skull base meningiomas: experience in 88 patients. *J Neurosurg* 1999;90:42.
246. Grunberg SM, Weiss MH, Spitz IM. Treatment of unresectable meningiomas with the antiprogesterone agent mifepristone. *J Neurosurg* 1991;74:861.
247. Kaba SE, DeMonte F, Bruner JM. The treatment of recurrent unresectable and malignant meningiomas with interferon alpha-2B. *Neurosurgery* 1997;40:271.
248. Schrell UM, Rittig MG, Anders M. Hydroxyurea for treatment of unresectable and recurrent meningiomas. II. Decrease in the size of meningiomas in patients with hydroxyurea. *J Neurosurg* 1997;86:840.
249. Mason WP, et al. Stabilization of disease progression by hydroxyurea in patients with recurrent or unresectable meningioma. *J Neurosurg* 2002;97(2):341.
250. McComb RD, Burger PC. Pathologic analysis of primary brain tumors. *Neurol Clin* 1985;3:711.
251. Kosnick EJ, Boesel CP, Bay J. Primitive neuroectodermal tumors of the central nervous system in children. *J Neurosurg* 1978;48:741.
252. Humphrey GB, Dehner LP, Kaplan RJ. Overview on the management of primitive neuroectodermal tumors. In: Humphrey GB, Dehner LP, eds. *Pediatric oncology,* vol I. The Hague: Martinus Nijhoff, 1981:289.
253. Gaffney CC, Sloane JP, Bradley NJ. Primitive neuroectodermal tumors of the cerebrum: pathology and treatment. *J Neurooncol* 1985;4:63.
254. Mikaeloff Y, Raquin MA, Lellouch-Tubiana A. Primitive cerebral neuroectodermal tumors excluding medulloblastomas: a retrospective study of 30 cases. *Pediatr Neurosurg* 1998;29:170.
255. Paulino AC, Melian E. Medulloblastoma and supratentorial primitive neuroectodermal tumors: an institutional experience. *Cancer* 1999;86:142.
256. Cohen ME. Primitive neuroectodermal tumors, oligodendrogliomas, choroid plexus papillomas. In: *Brain tumors of childhood: principles of diagnosis and treatment.* New York: Raven Press, 1984:273.
257. Berger MS, Edwards MS, Wara WM. Primary cerebral neuroblastoma. Long-term follow-up review and therapeutic guidelines. *J Neurosurg* 1983;59:418.
258. Horten BC, Rubinstein LJ. Primary cerebral neuroblastoma: a clinicopathological study of 35 cases. *Brain* 1976;99:735.
259. Central Brain Tumor Registry of the United States. *1995–1999 Statistical Report: Primary Brain Tumors in the United States.* Chicago: Central Brain Tumor Registry of the United States, 2002.
260. Chan AW, et al. Adult medulloblastoma: prognostic factors and patterns of relapse. *Neurosurgery* 2000;47:623, discussion 631.
261. Giangaspero F, Bigner S, Kleihues P, eds. Medulloblastomas. In: Kleihues P, Cavenee W, ed. *Pathology and genetics: tumors of the nervous system.* World Health Organization Classification of Tumours. Lyon, France: IARC Press, 2000:129.
262. Pietsch T, et al. Medulloblastomas of the desmoplastic variant carry mutations of the human homologue of Drosophila patched. *Cancer Res* 1997;57:2085.
263. Pomeroy SL, Tamayo P, Gaasenbeek M. Prediction of central nervous system embryonal tumour outcome based on gene expression. *Nature* 2002;415:436.
264. Bloom HJG. Medulloblastoma in children: increasing survival rates and further prospects. *Int J Radiat Oncol Biol Phys* 1982;8:2023.
265. Deutsch M. The impact of myelography on the treatment results for medulloblastomas. *Int J Radiat Oncol Biol Phys* 1984;10:999.
266. Bloom HJ. Medulloblastoma: prognosis and prospects. *Int J Radiat Oncol Biol Phys* 1977;2:1031.
267. Chang CH, Housepian EM, Herbert CJ. An operative staging system and a mega-voltage radiotherapeutic technic for cerebellar medulloblastomas. *Radiology* 1969;93:1351.
268. Kramer ED, et al. Staging and surveillance of children with central nervous system neoplasms: recommendations of the Neurology and Tumor Committee of the Children's Cancer Group. *Pediatr Neurosurg* 1994;20(4):254, discussion 262.
269. Packer RJ, Cogen P, Vezina LB. Medulloblastoma: clinical and biologic aspects. *Neurooncology* 1999;1(3):232.
270. Albright AL, Wisoff JH, Zeltzer PM. Effects of medulloblastoma resections on outcome in children: a report from the Children's Cancer Group. *Neurosurgery* 1996;38:265.
271. Packer RJ, et al. Outcome for children with medulloblastoma treated with radiation and cisplatin, CCNU, and vincristine chemotherapy. *J Neurosurg* 1994;81(5):690.
272. Saran PH, et al. Survival of very young children with medulloblastoma (primitive neuroectodermal tumor of the posterior fossa) treated with craniospinal irradiation. *Int J Radiat Oncol Biol Phys* 1998;42:959.
273. Bouffet E, et al. Metastatic medulloblastoma: the experience of the French Cooperative M7 Group. *Eur J Cancer* 1994;10:1478.
274. Zeltzer PM, et al. Metastasis stage, adjuvant treatment, and residual tumor are prognostic factors for medulloblastoma in children: conclusions from the Children's Cancer Group 921 randomized phase III study. *J Clin Oncol* 1999;17:832.
275. Choux M, Lena G, Hassoun J. Prognosis and long-term follow-up in patients with medulloblastomas. *Clin Neurosurg* 1983;30:246.
276. Deutsch M. Medulloblastoma staging and treatment outcome. *Int J Radiat Oncol Biol Phys* 1988;14:1103.
277. Lowery GS, Kimball JC, Patterson RB. Extraneural metastases from cerebellar medulloblastoma. *Am J Pediatr Hematol Oncol* 1982;4:259.
278. Tait DM, Thorton-Jones H, Bloom HJG. Adjuvant chemotherapy for medulloblastoma: the first multi-centre control trial of the International Society of Pediatric Oncology (SIOP I). *Eur J Cancer* 1990;26:464.
279. Evans AE, Jenkin RD, Sposto R. The treatment of medulloblastomas: results of a prospective randomized trial of radiation therapy with and without CCNU, vincristine and prednisone. *J Neurosurg* 1990;72:572.
280. Packer RJ, et al. Treatment of children with medulloblastomas with reduced-dose craniospinal radiation therapy and adjuvant chemotherapy: a Children's Cancer Group study. *J Clin Oncol* 1999;17(7):2127.
281. Park TS, Hoffman HJ, Hendrick EB. Medulloblastoma: clinical presentation and management experience at the hospital for sick children Toronto, 1950. *J Neurosurg* 1983;58:543.
282. Chamberlain MC, Silver P, Edwards MS. Treatment of extraneural metastatic medulloblastoma with a combination of cyclophosphamide, adriamycin, and vincristine. *Neurosurgery* 1988;23:476.

282a. Culley DJ, Berger MS, Shaw D, Geyer R. An analysis of factors determining the need for ventriculoperitoneal shunts after posterior fossa tumor surgery in children. *Neurosurgery* 1994;34:402.

283. Merchant TE, Wang MH, Haida T. Medulloblastoma: long-term results for patients treated with definitive radiation during the computed tomography era. *Int J Radiat Oncol Biol Phys* 1996;36:29.
284. Wara WM, Le QT, Sneed PK. Pattern of recurrence of medulloblastoma after low-dose craniospinal radiotherapy. *Int J Radiat Oncol Biol Phys* 1994;30:551.
285. Prados MD, Edwards MS, Chang SM. Hyperfractionated craniospinal radiation therapy for primitive neuroectodermal tumors: results of a phase II study. *Int J Radiat Oncol Biol Phys* 1999;43:279.
286. Tarbell NJ, et al. The challenge of conformal radiotherapy in the curative treatment of medulloblastoma. *Int J Radiat Oncol Biol Phys* 2000;46:265.
287. Radcliffe J, et al. Three- and four-year cognitive outcome in children with noncortical brain tumors treated with whole-brain radiotherapy. *Ann Neurol* 1992;32(4):551.
288. Thomas PR, et al. Low-stage medulloblastoma: final analysis of trial comparing standard-dose with reduced-dose neuraxis irradiation. *J Clin Oncol* 2000;18(16):3004.
289. Goldwein JW, et al. Updated results of a pilot study of low dose craniospinal irradiation plus chemotherapy for children under five with cerebellar primitive neuroectodermal tumors (medulloblastoma). *Int J Radiat Oncol Biol Phys* 1996;34(4):899.
290. Strother D, et al. Feasibility of four consecutive high-dose chemotherapy cycles with stem-cell rescue for patients with newly diagnosed medulloblastoma or supratentorial primitive neuroectodermal tumor after craniospinal radiotherapy: results of a collaborative study. *J Clin Oncol* 2001;19(10):2696.
291. Schold SCJ, Friedman HS, Bjornsson TD. Treatment of patients with recurrent primary brain tumors with AZQ. *Neurosurgery* 1984;34:615.
292. Fewer D, Wilson CB, Boldrey EB. Chemotherapy of brain tumors: clinical experience with carmustine and vincristine. *JAMA* 1972;222:549.
293. Levin VA, Edwards MS, Gutin PH. Phase II evaluation of dibromodulcitol in the treatment of recurrent medulloblastoma, ependymoma, and malignant astrocytoma. *J Neurosurg* 1984;61:1063.
294. Benjamin RS, Wiernick PH, Bachur NR. Adriamycin chemotherapy: efficacy, safety, and pharmacologic basis of an intermittent single high-dose schedule. *Cancer* 1974;74:1784.
295. Hancock C, Allen J, Tan CT. Phase II trial of PCNU in children with recurrent brain tumors and Hodgkin's disease. *Cancer Treat Rep* 1984;68:441.
296. Bleyer WA, Krivit W, Chard RL. Phase II study of VM26 in leukemia, neuroblastomas, and other refractory childhood malignancies: a report from the Children's Cancer Study Group. *Cancer Treat Rep* 1979;63:977.
297. Shapiro WR. Chemotherapy of primary malignant brain tumors in children. *Cancer* 1975;35:965.
298. Allen JC, Walker R, Luks E. Carboplatin and recurrent childhood brain tumors. *J Clin Oncol* 1987;5:459.
299. Rosen G, Ghavimi F, Nirenberg A. High-dose methotrexate with citrovorum factor rescue for the treatment of central nervous system tumors in children. *Cancer Treat Rep* 1977;61:681.
300. Djerassi I, Kim JS, Shulman K. High-dose methotrexate-citrovorum factor rescue in the management of brain tumors. *Cancer Treat Rep* 1977;61:691.
301. Mooney C, Souhami R, Pritchard J. Recurrent medulloblastoma: lack of response to high-dose methotrexate. *Cancer Chemother Rep* 1983;10:135.
302. Walker RW, Allen JC. Treatment of recurrent primary intracranial childhood tumors with cis-diamine-dichloroplatinum. *Ann Neurol* 1983;14:371.
303. Bertolone SJ, Baum E, Krivit W. Phase II trial of cisplatinum diaminodichlorida (CPDD) in recurrent childhood brain tumors: a CCSG trial. *Proc Ann Am Assoc Cancer Res* 1983;2:72.
304. Sexauer CL, Kahn A, Burger PC. MD+UL-platinum in recurrent pediatric brain tumors: a POG phase II study. *Cancer* 1985;56:1497.
305. Friedman HS, Schold SCJ, Mahaley MSJ. Phase II treatment of medulloblastoma and pineoblastoma with melphalan: clinical therapy based on experimental models of human medulloblastoma. *J Clin Oncol* 1989;7:904.
306. Haddy TB, Ferbach DJ, Watkins WL. Vincristine in uncommon malignant disease in children. *Cancer Chemother Rep* 1964;41:41.
307. Lassman LP, Pearce GW, Gang J. Effect of vincristine sulfate on the intracranial gliomata of childhood. *Br J Surg* 1966;53:774.
308. Lampkin BC, Maurer AM, McBride BH. Response of medulloblastomas to vincristine sulfate: a case report. *Pediatrics* 1967;39:761.

309. Smart CR, Ottoman RE, Rochlin DB. Clinical experience with vincristine in tumors of the central nervous system and other malignant diseases. *Cancer Chemother Rep* 1968;52:733.
310. Afra D. Vincristine therapy in malignant glioma recurrences. *Neurochirurgia* 1973;16:189.
311. Rosenstock JG, Evans AE, Schut L. Response to vincristine of recurrent brain tumors in children. *J Neurosurg* 1976;45:135.
312. Ward HWC. Central nervous system tumors of childhood treated with CCNU, vincristine and radiation. *Med Pediatr Oncol* 1978;4:315.
313. Garrett MJ, Hughs HJ, Ryall RDH. CCNU in brain tumors. *Clin Radiol* 1974;25:183.
314. Ward HWC. CCNU in the treatment of recurrent medulloblastoma. *BMJ* 1974;1:642.
315. Allen JC, Helson L. High-dose cyclophosphamide chemotherapy for recurrent CNS tumors in children. *J Neurosurg* 1981;55:749.
316. Lefkowitz IB, Packer RJ, Siegel KR. Results of treatment of children with recurrent medulloblastoma/primitive neuroectodermal tumors with lomustine, cisplatin, and vincristine. *Cancer* 1990;65:412.
317. Finlay JL. The role of high-dose chemotherapy and stem cell rescue in the treatment of malignant brain tumors: a reappraisal. *Pediatr Transplant* 1999;3[Suppl 1]:87.
318. Dunkel IJ, et al. High-dose carboplatin, thiotepa, and etoposide with autologous stem-cell rescue for patients with recurrent medulloblastoma. Children's Cancer Group. *J Clin Oncol* 1998;16(1):222.
319. Hoffman HJ. Pineal region tumors. *Prog Exp Tumor Res* 1987;30:281.
320. Apuzzo MLJ, ed. *Surgery of the third ventricle*, 2nd ed. Baltimore: Williams & Wilkins, 1998.
321. Sawamura Y, et al. Management of primary intracranial germinomas: diagnostic surgery or radical resection? *J Neurosurg* 1997;87:262.
322. Regis J, Bouillot P, Rouby-Volot F. Pineal region tumors and the role of stereotactic biopsy: review of the mortality, morbidity and diagnostic rates in 370 cases. *Neurosurgery* 1996;39:907.
323. Pecker J, Scarabin JM, Vallee B. Treatment in tumor of the pineal region: value of stereotaxic biopsy. *Surg Neurol* 1979;12:341.
324. Pople IK, et al. The role of endoscopic biopsy and third ventriculostomy in the management of pineal region tumours. *Br J Neurosurg* 2001;15:305.
325. Wara WM, Evans A. Tumors of the pineal and suprasellar region: Children's Cancer Study Group. *Cancer* 1979;43:698.
326. Wolden SL, Wara WM, Larson DA. Radiation therapy for primary intracranial germ-cell tumors. *Int J Radiat Oncol Biol Phys* 1995;32:943.
327. Jenkin RDT, Simpson WJK, Keen CW. Pineal and suprasellar germinomas: results of radiation treatment. *J Neurosurg* 1978;48:99.
328. Haas-Kogan DA, Missett BT, Wara WM. Radiation for intracranial germ cell tumors. *Int J Radiat Oncol Biol Phys* 2003;56:511.
329. Bouffet E, Baranzelli MC, Patte C. Combined treatment modality for intracranial germinomas: results of a multicentre SFOP experience. *Br J Cancer* 1999;79:1199.
330. Buckner JC, Peethambaram PP, Smithson WA. Phase II trial of primary chemotherapy followed by reduced-dose radiation for CNS germ cell tumors. *J Clin Oncol* 1999;17:933.
331. Merchant TE, Davis DL, Sheldon JM. Radiation therapy for relapsed CNS germinoma after primary chemotherapy. *J Clin Oncol* 1998;16:204.
332. Fuller BG, Kapp DS, Cox R. Radiation therapy of pineal region tumors: 25 new cases and a review of 208 previously reported cases. *Int J Radiat Oncol Biol Phys* 1993;28:229.
333. Kondziolka D, et al. The role of radiosurgery for the treatment of pineal parenchymal tumors. *Neurosurgery* 2002;51:880.
334. Timmermann B, Kortmann RD, Kuhl J. Role of radiotherapy in the treatment of supratentorial primitive neuroectodermal tumors in childhood: results of the prospective German brain tumor trials HIT 88/89 and 91. *J Clin Oncol* 2002;20:842.
335. Patel SR, Buckner JC, Smithson WA. Cisplatin-based chemotherapy in primary central nervous system germ cell tumors. *J Neurooncol* 1992;12:47.
336. Finlay J, et al. Chemotherapy without irradiation (XRT) for primary central nervous system (CNS) germ cell tumors (GCT): a report of international study. *Proc Am Soc Clin Oncol* 1992;11:A420.
337. Matsutani M, Takakura K, Sano K. Primary intracranial germ cell tumors: pathology and treatment. *Prog Exp Tumor Res* 1987;30:307.
338. Edwards MSB. Chemotherapy of third ventricle tumors. In: Appuzzo M, ed. *Third ventricular tumors.* Baltimore: Williams & Wilkins, 1987:838.
339. Allen JC, Kim JH, Packer RJ. Neoadjuvant chemotherapy for newly diagnosed germ-cell tumors of the central nervous system. *J Neurosurg* 1987;67:65.
340. Allen JC, DaRosso RC, Donahue B. A phase I trial of preirradiation carboplatin in newly diagnosed germinoma of the central nervous system. *Cancer* 1994;74:940.
341. Kellie SJ, et al. Primary chemotherapy for intracranial nongerminomatous germ cell tumors: results of the second international CNS germ cell study group protocol. *J Clin Oncol* 2004;22(5):846.
342. Gururangan S, et al. High-dose chemotherapy with autologous stem-cell rescue in children and adults with newly diagnosed pineoblastomas. *J Clin Oncol* 2003;21(11):2187.
343. Broniscer A, et al. High-dose chemotherapy with autologous stem-cell rescue in the treatment of patients with recurrent non-cerebellar primitive neuroectodermal tumors. *Pediatr Blood Cancer* 2004;42(3):261.
344. Mah PM, Webster J. Hyperprolactinemia: etiology, diagnosis, and management. *Semin Reprod Med* 2002;20(4):365.
345. Wilson CB. Surgical management of endocrine-active pituitary adenomas. In: Walker MD, ed. *Oncology of the nervous system.* Boston: Martinus-Nijhoff, 1983:117.
346. Rand T, Kink E, Sator M. MRI of microadenomas in patients with hyperprolactinemia. *Neuroradiology* 1996;38:744.
347. Jane JAJ, et al. Pituitary surgery: transsphenoidal approach. *Neurosurgery* 2002;51(2):435.
348. Swearingen B, Biller BM, Barker FG. Long-term mortality after transsphenoidal surgery for Cushing disease. *Ann Intern Med* 1999;130:821.
349. Krieger MD, Coudwell WT, Weiss MH. Assessment of long-term remission of acromegaly following surgery. *J Neurosurg* 2003;98:719.
350. Swearingen B, Barker FG, Katznelson L. Long-term mortality after transsphenoidal surgery and adjunctive therapy in acromegaly. *J Clin Endocrinal Metab* 1998;83:3419.
351. Dickerman RD, Oldfield EH. Basis of persistent and recurrent Cushing disease: an analysis of findings at repeat pituitary surgery. *J Neurosurg* 2002;97:1343.
352. Greenman Y, Ouaknine G, Veshchev I. Postoperative surveillance of clinically nonfunctioning pituitary macroadenomas: markers of tumour quiescence and regrowth. *Clin Endocrinol* 2003;58:763.
353. Honegger J, Prettin C, Feuerhaje F. Expression of Ki-67 in non-functioning pituitary adenomas: correlation with growth velocity and invasiveness. *J Neurosurg* 2003;99:674.
354. Malmed S. Acromegaly. *N Engl J Med* 1990;322:966.
355. Sheline GE. Pituitary tumors. In: Perez CA, ed. *Principles and practice of radiation oncology.* Philadelphia: JB Lippincott, 1987:1108.
356. Barkan AL, Halasz I, Dornfeld KJ. Pituitary irradiation is ineffective in normalizing plasma insulin-like growth factor I in patients with acromegaly. *J Clin Endocrinol Metab* 1997;82:3187.
357. Suliman M, Jenkin R, Ross R. Long-term treatment of acromegaly with somatostatin analogue SR-lanreotide. *J Endocrinol Invest* 1999;22:409.
358. Jennings AS, Liddle GW, Orth DN. Results of treating childhood Cushing's disease with pituitary irradiation. *N Engl J Med* 1977;297:957.
359. Mitsumori M, Shrieve DC, Alexander EI. Initial clinical results of LINAC-based stereotactic radiosurgery and stereotactic radiotherapy for pituitary adenomas. *Int J Radiat Oncol Biol Phys* 1998;3:573.
360. Levy RP, Schulte PWM, Slater JD. Stereotactic radiosurgery—the role of charged particles. *Acta Oncol* 1999;38:165.
361. Zierhut D, Flentje M, Adolph J. External radiotherapy of pituitary adenomas. *Int J Radiat Oncol Biol Phys* 1995;33:307.
362. McCord MW, Buatti JM, Fennell EM. Radiotherapy for pituitary adenoma: long term outcome and sequelae. *Int J Radiat Oncol Biol Phys* 1997;39:437.
363. Tsang RW, Brierley JD, Panzarella T. Role of radiation therapy in clinical hormonally active pituitary adenomas. *Radiother Oncol* 1996;41:45.
364. Brada M, Ashley S, Ford D. Cerebrovascular mortality in patients with pituitary adenoma. *Clin Endocrinol* 2002;57:713.
365. Breen P, Flickenger JC, Kondziolka D. Radiotherapy for nonfunctional pituitary adenomas: analysis of long-term tumor control. *J Neurosurg* 1998;89:933.
366. Brada M, Ford D, Ashley S. Risk of second brain tumor after conservative surgery and radiotherapy for pituitary adenoma. *BMJ* 1992;304:1343.
367. Loeffler JS, Smith AR, Suit HD. The potential role of proton beams in radiation oncology. *Semin Oncol* 1997;24:686.
368. Tishler RB, Loeffler JS, Lunsford LD. Tolerance of cranial nerves of the cavernous sinus to radiosurgery. *Int J Radiat Oncol Biol Phys* 1993;27:215.
369. Attanasio R, Epaminonda P, Motti E. Gamma-knife radiosurgery in acromegaly: a 4 year follow-up study. *J Clin Endocrinol Metab* 2003;88:3105.
370. Landolt AM, Haller D, Lomax N. Stereotactic radiosurgery for recurrent surgically treated acromegaly: comparison with fractionated radiotherapy. *J Neurosurg* 1998;88:1002.
371. Petrovich Z, Yu C, Giannotta SL. Gamma knife radiosurgery for pituitary adenoma: early results. *Neurosurgery* 2003;53:51.
372. Mahmoud-Ahmed AS, Suh JH. Radiation therapy for Cushing's disease: a review. *Pituitary* 2003;5:175.
373. Schoenthlar R, Albright NW, Wara WM. Reirradiation of pituitary adenoma. *Int J Radiat Oncol Biol Phys* 1992;24:307.
374. Vance ML. Medical treatment of functional pituitary tumors. *Neurosurg Clin N Am* 2003;14:81.
375. Melmed S, Vance, ML, Barkan AL. Current status and future opportunities for controlling acromegaly. *Pituitary* 2002;5:185.
376. Kinson C, Scarlett JA, Trainer PJ. Pegvisomant in the treatment of acromegaly. *Adv Drug Deliv Rev* 2003;55(10):1303.
377. Surawicz TS, et al. Descriptive epidemiology of primary brain and CNS tumors: results from the Central Brain Tumor Registry of the United States. *Neuro-oncology* 1999;1(1):14.
378. Larijani B, et al. Presentation and outcome of 93 cases of craniopharyngioma. *Eur J Cancer* 2004;13(1):11.
379. Chiou SM, et al. Stereotactic radiosurgery of residual or recurrent craniopharyngioma, after surgery, with or without radiation therapy. *Neuro-oncology* 2001;3(3):159.
380. Duff JM, et al. Long-term outcomes for surgically resected craniopharyngiomas. *Neurosurgery* 2000;46(2):291.
381. Coffey RJ, Lunsford LD. The role of stereotactic techniques in the management of craniopharyngiomas. In: Rosenblum ML, ed. *The role of surgery in brain tumor management.* Philadelphia: WB Saunders, 1991:161.
382. Pollock BE, et al. Phosphorous-32 intracavitary irradiation of cystic craniopharyngiomas: current technique and long-term results. *Int J Radiat Oncol Biol Phys* 1995;33(2):437.
383. Richmond IL, Wara WM, Wilson CB. Role of radiation therapy in the management of craniopharyngiomas in children. *Neurosurgery* 1980;6:513.
384. Fischer EG, Welch K, Belli JA. Treatment of craniopharyngiomas in children. *J Neurosurg* 1985;62:496.
385. Wen B-C, Hussey DH, Staples J. A comparison of the roles of surgery and radiation therapy in the management of craniopharyngiomas. *Int J Radiat Oncol Biol Phys* 1989;16:17.
386. Kalapurakal JA, Goldman S, Hsieh YC. Clinical outcome in children with craniopharyngioma treated with primary surgery and radiotherapy deferred until relapse. *Med Pediatr Oncol* 2003;40:214.
387. Hetelekidis S, Barnes PD, Tao ML. 20 year experience in childhood craniopharyngioma. *Int J Radiat Oncol Biol Phys* 1993;27:189.
388. Merchant TE, Kiehna EN, Sanford RA. Craniopharyngioma: the St. Jude Children's Research Hospital experience 1984–2001. *Int J Radiat Oncol Biol Phys* 2002;53:533.
389. Schulz-Ertner D, Frank C, Herfarth KK. Fractionated stereotactic radiotherapy for craniopharyngioma. *Int J Radiat Oncol Biol Phys* 2002;54:1114.
390. Varlotto JM, Flickinger JC, Kondiziolka D. External beam irradiation of craniopharyngiomas: long-term analysis of tumor control and morbidity. *Int J Radiat Oncol Biol Phys* 2002;54:492.

391. Ulfarsson E, Lindquist C, Roberts M. Gamma knife radiosurgery for craniopharyngiomas: long-term results in the first Swedish patients. *J Neurosurg* 2002;97:613.

392. Jackson AS, et al. Stereotactic radiosurgery, XVII: recurrent intrasellar craniopharyngioma. *Br J Neurosurg* 2003;17:138.

393. Charabi S, et al. Vestibular schwannoma growth: the continuing controversy. *Laryngoscope* 2000;110:1720.

394. Jackler RK, Brackmann DE, eds. *Neurotology.* St. Louis: Mosby, 1994.

395. Ojemann RG. Management of acoustic neuromas (vestibular schwannomas) (honored guest presentation). *Clin Neurosurg* 1993;40:498.

396. Barker FG, et al. Surgical excision of acoustic neuroma: patient outcome and provider caseload. *Laryngoscope* 2003;113:1332.

397. Flexon PB, et al. Bilateral acoustic neurofibromatosis (neurofibromatosis 2): a disorder distinct from von Recklinghausen's neurofibromatosis (neurofibromatosis 1). *Ann Otol Rhinol Laryngol* 1991;100:830.

398. Kondziolka D, Lunsford LD, McLaughlin MR. Long-term outcomes after radiosurgery for acoustic neuromas. *N Engl J Med* 1998;339:1426.

399. Tsao MN, Wara WM, Larson DA. Radiation therapy for benign central nervous system disease. *Semin Oncol* 1999;9:120.

400. Flickenger JC, Lunsford LD, Linskey ME. Gamma knife radiosurgery for acoustic tumors: multivariate analysis of 4-year results. *Radiother Oncol* 1993;27:91.

401. Linskey ME, Flickenger JC, Lunsford LD. Cranial nerve length predicts the risk of delayed facial and trigeminal neuropathies after acoustic tumor stereotactic radiosurgery. *Int J Radiat Oncol Biol Phys* 1993;25:227.

402. Miranjan A, Lunsford LD, Flickenger JC. Dose reduction improves hearing preservation rates after intercanalicular acoustic tumor radiosurgery. *Neurosurgery* 1999;45:762.

403. Sawamura Y, Shirato H, Sakamoto T. Management of vestibular schwannoma by fractionated stereotactic radiotherapy and associated cerebrospinal fluid malabsorption. *J Neurosurg* 2003;99:685.

404. Lederman G, Arbit E, Lowry J. *N Engl J Med* 1999;340:1119.

405. Fuss M, DeBus J, Lohr F. Conventionally fractionated stereotactic radiotherapy (FSRT) for acoustic neuromas. *Int J Radiat Oncol Biol Phys* 2000;48:1381.

406. Loeffler JS, Niemierko A, Chapman PH. Second tumors after radiosurgery: tip of the iceberg or a bump in the road? *Neurosurgery* 2003;52:1436.

407. Farriro JBI, Hymas VL, Benke RH. Carcinoid apudoma arising in glomus jugulare tumors. *Laryngoscope* 1980;90:110.

408. Springate SC, Weichselbaum RR. Radiation or surgery for the chemodectoma of the temporal bone: a review of local control and complications. *Head Neck* 1990;12:303.

409. Million RR, Cassisi NJ, Mancuso AA. Chemodectomas (glomus body tumors). In: Million RR, Cassisi NJ, eds. *Management of head and neck cancer.* Philadelphia: JB Lippincott, 1994:765.

410. Hinerman RW, et al. Definitive radiotherapy in the management of chemodectomas arising in the temporal bone, carotid body, and glomus vagale. *Head Neck* 2001;23:363.

411. Harsh G, et al., eds. *Chordomas and chondrosarcomas of the skull base and spine.* New York: Thieme, 2003.

412. Heffelfinger MJ, Dahlin DC, MacCarty CS. Chordomas and cartilaginous tumors at the skull base. *Cancer* 1973;32:410.

413. Rosenberg AE, Pathology of chordoma and chondrosarcoma of the axial skeleton. In: Harsh G, et al., eds. *Chordomas and chondrosarcomas of the skull base and spine.* New York: Thieme, 2003:8.

414. Meis JM, et al. "Dedifferentiated" chordoma: a clinicopathologic and immunohistochemical study of three cases. *Am J Clin Pathol* 1987.

415. Holton JL, Steel T, Luxsuwong M. Skull base chordomas: correlation of tumour doubling time with age, mitosis and K167 proliferation index. *Neuropathol Appl Neurobiol* 2000;26:497.

416. Rosenberg AE, Nielsen GP, Keel SB. Chondrosarcoma of the base of the skull: a clinicopathologic study of 200 cases with emphasis on its distinction from chordoma. *Am J Surg Pathol* 1999;23:1370.

417. Gay E, et al. Chordomas and chondrosarcomas of the cranial base: results and follow-up of 60 patients. *Neurosurgery* 1995;36:887, discussion 896.

418. Phillips T, Newman H. Chordomas. In: Deeley T, ed. *Modern radiotherapy and oncology: central nervous system tumors.* Boston: Butterworth, 1974:184.

419. Zorlu F, Gurkaynak M, Yildiz F. Conventional external radiotherapy in the management of clivus chordomas with overt residual disease. *Neurol Sci* 2000;21:203.

420. Munzenrider JE, Hug E, McManus P. Skull base chordomas: treatment outcome and prognostic factors in adult patients following conformal treatment with 3D planning and high dose fractionated combined proton and photon radiation therapy. *Int J Radiat Oncol Biol Phys* 1995;32:209.

421. Terahara A, Niemierko A, Goitein M. Analysis of the relationship between tumor dose in homogeneity and local control in patients with skull base chordoma. *Int J Radiat Oncol Biol Phys* 1999;45:351.

422. Noel G, Habrand JL, Jauffret E. Radiation therapy for chordoma and chondrosarcoma of the skull base and the cervical spine. Prognostic factors and patterns of failure. *Strahlenther Onkol* 2003;179:241.

423. Hug EB, Sweeney RA, Nurre PM. Proton radiotherapy in management of pediatric base of skull tumors. *Int J Radiat Oncol Biol Phys* 2002;52:1017.

424. Maher ER, et al. Clinical features and natural history of von Hippel-Lindau disease. *QJM* 1990;77(283):1151.

425. Singh AD, Shields CL, Shields JA. von Hippel-Lindau disease. *Surv Ophthalmol* 2001;46(2):117.

426. Wanebo JE, et al. The natural history of hemangioblastomas of the central nervous system in patients with von Hippel-Lindau disease. *J Neurosurg* 2003;98(1):82.

427. Acikalin MF, et al. Supratentorial hemangioblastoma: a case report and review of the literature. *Arch Pathol Lab Med* 2003;127(9):e382.

428. Weil RJ, et al. Surgical management of brainstem hemangioblastomas in patients with von Hippel-Lindau disease. *J Neurosurg* 2003;98(1):95.

429. Smalley SR, Schomberg PJ, Earle JD. Radiotherapeutic considerations in the treatment of hemangioblastomas of the central nervous system. *Int J Radiat Oncol Biol Phys* 1990;18:1165.

430. Patrice SJ, Sneed PK, Flickenger JC. Radiosurgery for hemangioblastomas: results of a multiinstitutional experience. *Int J Radiat Oncol Biol Phys* 1996;35:493.

431. Chang SD, Meisel JA, Hancock SL. Treatment of hemangioblastomas in von Hippel-Lindau disease with linear accelerator-based radiosurgery. *Neurosurgery* 1998;43:28.

432. Jawahar A, Kondiziolka D, Garces YI. Stereotactic radiosurgery for hemangioblastoma of the brain. *Acta Neurochir* 2000;142:641.

433. Pencalet P, Sainte-Rose C, Lellouch-Tubiana A. Papillomas and carcinomas of the choroid plexus in childhood. *J Neurosurg* 1998;88:521.

434. Tzikaa AA, Cheng LL, Goumnerova L. Biochemical characterization of pediatric brain tumors by using in vivo and ex vivo magnetic resonance spectroscopy. *J Neurosurg* 2002;96:1023.

435. Fitzpatrick LK, Aronson LJ, Cohen KJ. Is there a requirement for adjuvant therapy for choroid plexus carcinoma that has been completely resected? *J Neurooncol* 2002;57:123.

436. McEvoy AW, Harding BN, Phipps KP. Management of choroids plexus tumours in children: 20 years experience at a single neurosurgical center. *Pediatr Neurosurg* 2000;32:192.

437. Souweidane MM, Johnson JHJ, Lis E. Volumetric reduction of a choroid plexus carcinoma using preoperative chemotherapy. *J Neurooncol* 1999;43:167.

438. Wolff JE, Sajedi M, Coppes MJ. Radiation therapy and survival in choroid plexus carcinoma. *Lancet* 1999;353:2126.

439. Chow E, Reardon DA, Shah AB. Pediatric choroid plexus neoplasms. *Int J Radiat Oncol Biol Phys* 1999;44:249.

440. Ausman JI, Schrontz C, Chason J. Aggressive choroid plexus papilloma. *Surg Neurol* 1984;22:472.

441. Wolff JE, Sajedi M, Brant M. Choroid plexus tumours. *Br J Cancer* 2002;87:1086.

442. Duffner PK, et al. Postoperative chemotherapy and delayed radiation in infants and very young children with choroid plexus carcinomas: The Pediatric Oncology Group. *Pediatr Neurosurg* 1995;22(4):189.

443. Quinones-Hinojosa A, et al. Spinal cord mapping as an adjunct for resection of intramedullary tumors: surgical technique with case illustrations. *Neurosurgery* 2002;51(5):1199.

444. Epstein FJ, Farmer JP, Freed D. Adult intramedullary spinal cord ependymomas: the result of surgery in 38 patients. *J Neurosurg* 1993;79(2):204.

445. Jallo GI, Freed D, Epstein F. Intramedullary spinal cord tumours in children. *Childs Nerv Syst* 2003;19:641.

446. Linstadt DE. Spinal cord. In: Leibel SA, Phillips TL, eds. *Textbook of radiation oncology.* Philadelphia: WB Saunders, 1998:401.

447. Waldron JN, Laperriere NJ, Jaakkimainen L. Spinal cord ependymomas: a retrospective analysis of 59 cases. *Int J Radiat Oncol Biol Phys* 1993;27:223.

448. Linstadt D, Wara WM, Leibel SA. Postoperative radiotherapy of primary spinal cord tumors. *Int J Radiat Oncol Biol Phys* 1989;16:1397.

449. Barone B, Elvidge A. Ependymomas: a clinical survey. *J Neurosurg* 1970;33:428.

450. Schuman R, Alvord E, Leech R. The biology of childhood ependymomas. *Arch Neurol* 1975;32:731.

451. Sloof JL, Kernohan JW, MacCarty CS. *Primary intramedullary tumors of the spinal cord and filum terminale.* Philadelphia: WB Saunders, 1964.

452. Whitaker SJ, Bessell EM, Ashly SE. Postoperative radiotherapy in the management of spinal cord ependymoma. *J Neurosurg* 1991;74:720.

453. Wen B-C, Hussey DH, Hitchon PW. The role of radiation therapy in the management of ependymomas of the spinal cord. *Int J Radiat Oncol Biol Phys* 1991;20:781.

454. Lee HK, Chang EL, Fuller GN. The prognostic value of neurological function in astrocytic spinal cord tumors. *Neuro-oncology* 2003;5:208.

455. Santi M, Mena H, Wong K. Spinal cord malignant astrocytomas. Clinicopathological features in 36 cases. *Cancer* 2003;98:554.

456. Preston-Martin S. Descriptive epidemiology of primary tumors of the spinal cord and spinal meninges. *Neuroepidemiology* 1990;9:106.

457. van den Bent MJ, Kros JM, Heimans JJ. Response rate and prognostic factors of recurrent oligodendroglioma treated with procarbazine, CCNU, and vincristine chemotherapy. Dutch Neuro-Oncology Group. *Neurology* 1998;51:1140.

458. Soffietti R, Ruda R, Bradac GB. PCV chemotherapy for recurrent oligodendrogliomas and oligoastrocytomas. *Neurosurgery* 1998;43:1066.

459. Cairncross G, et al. Chemotherapy for anaplastic oligodendroglioma. National Cancer Institute of Canada Clinical Trials Group. *J Clin Oncol* 1994;12:2013.

460. Fewer D, Wilson CB, Boldrey EB. Phase II study of 1-(2-choloroethyl)-3-cyclohexyl-1-nitrosourea (CCNU) in the treatment of brain tumors. *Cancer Chemother Rep* 1972;56:421.

CHAPTER 40

Cancers of Childhood

SECTION **1**

LEE J. HELMAN
DAVID MALKIN

Molecular Biology of Childhood Cancers

The biologic nature of tumors of childhood is clinically, histopathologically, and biologically distinct from that of adult-onset malignancies. Childhood cancers tend to have short latency periods, are often rapidly growing and aggressively invasive, are rarely associated with exposure to carcinogens implicated in adult-onset cancers, and are generally more responsive to standard modalities of treatment, in particular chemotherapy. Most childhood tumors occur sporadically in families with at most a weak history of cancer. In approximately 10% to 15% of cases,[1,2] however, a strong familial association is recognized or the child has a congenital or genetic disorder that imparts a higher likelihood of specific cancer types. Examples of genetic disorders that render a child at increased risk of tumor development include xeroderma pigmentosa, Bloom's syndrome, or ataxia-telangiectasia, which predisposes to skin cancers, leukemias, or lymphoid malignancies, respectively. In all three cases, constitutional gene alterations that disrupt normal mechanisms of genomic DNA repair are blamed for the propensity to cell transformation. Other hereditary disorders, including Beckwith-Wiedemann syndrome (BWS), von Hippel-Lindau disease, Rothmund-Thomson syndrome, and the multiple endocrine neoplasias types 1 and 2, are thought to be associated with their respective tumor spectra through constitutional activation of molecular pathways of deregulated cellular growth and proliferation. The cancers that occur in these syndromes are generally secondary phenotypic manifestations of disorders that have distinctive recognizable physical stigmata. On the other hand, some cancer predisposition syndromes are recognized only by their malignant manifestations, with nonmalignant characteristics being virtually absent. These include hereditary retinoblastoma, Li-Fraumeni syndrome (LFS), familial Wilms' tumor, and familial adenomatous polyposis coli. Each of these presents with distinct cancer phenotypes, and for each the identified molecular defect is unique (Table 40.1-1).

The study of pediatric cancer and rare hereditary cancer syndromes and associations has led to the identification of numerous cancer genes, including dominant oncogenes and tumor suppressor genes. These genes are important not only in hereditary predisposition but also in the normal growth, differentiation, and proliferation pathways of all cells. Alterations of these genes have been consistently found in numerous sporadic tumors of childhood and led to studies of their functional role in carcinogenesis. The numerous properties of transformed malignant cells in culture or *in vivo* can be explained by the complex abnormal interaction of numerous positive and negative growth-regulatory genes. Pediatric cancers offer unique models in which to study these pathways in that they are less likely to be disrupted by nongenetic factors. The embryonic ontogeny of many childhood cancers suggests that better understanding of the nature of the genetic events leading to these cancers will also augment the understanding of normal embryologic growth and development. This chapter begins with an outline of tumor suppressor genes—the most frequently implicated class of cancer genes in childhood malignancy. This leads into a discussion of molecular features of retinoblastoma, the para-

TABLE 40.1-1. Hereditary Syndromes Associated with Childhood Cancers

Hereditary Syndrome	Predominant Neoplasms	Germline Mutation
Hereditary retinoblastoma	Retinoblastoma, osteosarcoma	Rb
Familial Wilms' tumor	Wilms' tumor	WT1, WT2, WT3
Beckwith-Wiedemann syndrome	Wilms' tumor, hepatoblastoma, rhabdomyosarcoma, adrenocortical carcinoma	11p15
Li-Fraumeni syndrome	Sarcomas, brain tumor, leukemia, adrenocortical carcinoma, choroid plexus carcinoma	p53
Ataxia-telangiectasia	Lymphoma, brain tumors, leukemia	ATM
Neurofibromatosis type 1	Sarcoma, glioma	NF1
Neurofibromatosis type 2	Meningioma, acoustic neuroma	NF2
Multiple endocrine neoplasia, types 1 and 2	Adenomas/carcinomas of endocrine organs	MEN 1, RET
Familial polyposis coli	Intestinal polyps, colon carcinoma, hepatoblastoma	APC
Gorlin's syndrome	Medulloblastoma, basal cell nevi	PTCH
Bloom's syndrome	Leukemia	BLM
Rothmund-Thomson syndrome	Osteosarcoma	REQL4

TABLE 40.1-2. Common Cytogenetic Rearrangements in Solid Tumors of Childhood

Solid Tumor	Cytogenetic Rearrangement	Genes[a]
Ewing's sarcoma	t(11;22)(q24;q12), +8	EWS(22) FLi-1(11)
Neuroblastoma	del1p32-36, DMs, HSRs, +17q21-qter	N-MYC
Retinoblastoma	del13q14	Rb
Wilms' tumor	del11p13, t(3;17)	WT1
Synovial sarcoma	t(X;11)(p11;q11)	SSX(X) SYT(18)
Osteogenic sarcoma	del13q14	?
Rhabdomyosarcoma	t(2;13)(q37;q14), t(2;11),3p-,11p-	PAX3(2) FKHR(13)
Peripheral neuroepithelioma	t(11;22)(q24;q12), +8	EWS(22) FLi-1(11)
Astrocytoma	i(17q)	?
Meningioma	delq22, -22	MN1, NF2, ?
Atypical teratoid/rhabdoid tumor	delq22.11	SNF 5
Germ cell tumor	i(12p)	?

[a]Chromosomal location in parentheses.

digm of cancer genetics, followed by analysis of the molecular pathways associated with other common pediatric cancers. Evaluations of the importance of molecular alterations in familial cancers, as well as new approaches in molecular therapeutics, are also addressed.

TUMOR SUPPRESSOR GENES

Faulty regulation of cellular growth and differentiation leads to neoplastic transformation and tumor initiation. Many inappropriately activated growth-potentiating genes, or *oncogenes*, have been identified through the study of RNA tumor viruses and the transforming effects of DNA isolated from malignant cells. However, activated dominant oncogenes themselves do not readily explain a variety of phenomena related to transformation and tumor formation. Among these is the suppression of tumorigenicity by fusion of malignant cells with their normal counterparts. If these malignant cells carried an activated dominant oncogene, it would be expected that such a gene would initiate transformation of the normal cells, likely leading to either embryonic or fetal death. The observation is more readily explained by postulating the existence of a factor in the normal cell that acts to suppress growth of the fused malignant cells. Malignant cells commonly exhibit specific chromosomal deletions (Table 40.1-2). The best example of this occurs in retinoblastoma, a rare pediatric eye tumor in which a small region

of the long arm of chromosome 13 is frequently missing.[3,4] The presumed loss of genes in specific chromosomal regions argues strongly against the concept of a dominantly acting gene being implicated in the development of the tumor. Hereditary forms of cancer are also not readily explained by altered growth-potentiating genes. Comparisons between the frequencies of familial tumors and their sporadic counterparts led Knudson[5] to suggest that the familial forms of some tumors could be explained by constitutional mutations in growth-limiting genes. The resulting inactivation of these genes would facilitate cellular transformation.[6] Such growth-limiting genes were termed *tumor suppressor genes.*

Whereas acquired alterations of dominant oncogenes most commonly occur in somatic cells, mutant tumor suppressor genes may be found either in germ cells or somatic cells. In the former, they may arise *de novo* or be transmitted from generation to generation within a family. The diversity of functions, cellular locations, and tissue-specific expression of the tumor suppressor genes suggest the existence of a complex, yet coordinated, cellular pathway that limits cell growth by linking nuclear processes with the intra- and extracytoplasmic environment. This discussion is limited to those genes for which pediatric tumors are frequently associated.

RETINOBLASTOMA: THE PARADIGM

Retinoblastoma is the prototype cancer caused by mutations of a tumor suppressor gene. It is a malignant tumor of the retina that occurs in infants and young children, with an incidence of approximately 1 in 20,000.[7] Approximately 40% of retinoblastoma cases are of the heritable form,[8] in which the child inherits one mutant allele at the retinoblastoma susceptibility locus (Rb1) through the germline and a somatic mutation in a single retinal cell causes loss of function of the remaining normal allele, leading to tumor formation. Tumors are often bilateral and multifocal. The disease is inherited as an autosomal dominant trait, with a penetrance approaching 100%.[9] The remaining 60% of retinoblastoma cases are sporadic (nonheritable),[10] in which both Rb1 alleles in a single retinal cell are inactivated by somatic mutations. As one can imagine, such an event is rare, and these patients usually have only one tumor that presents itself later than in infants with the heritable form. Fifteen percent of unilateral retinoblastoma is heritable[9] but by chance develops in only one eye. Survivors of heritable retinoblastoma have a several-100–fold increased risk of developing mesenchymal tumors such as osteogenic sarcoma, fibrosarcomas, and melanomas later in life.[10,11] It is thought that several genetic mechanisms may be involved in elimination of the second wild-type Rb1 allele in an evolving tumor. These mechanisms include chromosomal duplication or nondisjunction, mitotic recombination, or gene conversion.[12]

The Rb1 gene was eventually mapped to chromosome 13q14.[13] Using Southern blot analysis, it was then possible to demonstrate that the second target gene that led to disease was actually the second copy of the Rb1 locus. Reduction to homozygosity of the mutant allele [or loss of heterozygosity (LOH) of the wild-type allele] would lead to the loss of functional Rb1 and account for tumor development.

Using classic cloning techniques, a 4.7-kb complementary DNA fragment was isolated from retinal cells.[14] This gene, Rb1, consisted of 27 exons and encoded a 105-kD nuclear phosphoprotein. As well as being altered in retinoblastoma, this gene and its protein product have been found to be altered in osteosarcomas, small cell lung carcinomas, and bladder, breast, and prostate carcinomas.[14,15] Rb1 plays a central role in the control of cell-cycle regulation, particularly in determining transition from G_1 through S (DNA synthesis) phase in virtually all cell types.

Although it is clear that Rb1 and its protein product play some role in growth regulation, the precise nature of this role remains obscure. In the developing retina, inactivation of the Rb1 gene is necessary and sufficient for tumor formation.[16] Although the Rb1 gene is expressed in virtually all mammalian tissues, only in the retina is its inactivation sufficient for tumor initiation. On the other hand, some Rb1 mutations appear to lead to an attenuated form of the disease, an observation that highlights the variable penetrance in families.[17,18] Outside the retina, Rb1 inactivation is often a rate-limiting step in tumorigenesis generated by multiple genetic events. The molecular characteristics and potential functional activities of Rb1 are outlined in detail elsewhere in this volume.

The patterns of inheritance and presentation of retinoblastoma have been well described and the responsible gene identified. Although the basic mechanisms by which the gene is inactivated are understood, much still remains to be determined about the biologic function of the gene and its protein product.

WILMS' TUMOR: THREE DISTINCT LOCI

Wilms' tumor, or nephroblastoma, is an embryonal malignancy of the kidney that arises from remnants of immature kidney. It affects approximately 1 in 10,000 children, usually before the age of 6 years (median age at diagnosis, 3.5 years). Five percent to 10% of children present with either synchronous or metachronous bilateral tumors.[19] A peculiar feature of Wilms' tumor is its association with nephrogenic rests, foci of primitive but nonmalignant cells whose persistence suggests a defect in kidney development. These precursor lesions are found within the normal kidney tissue of 30% to 40% of children with Wilms' tumor. Nephrogenic rests may persist, regress spontaneously, or grow into a large mass that simulates a true Wilms' tumor and presents a difficult diagnostic challenge.[20] Another interesting feature of this neoplasm is its association with specific congenital abnormalities, including genitourinary anomalies, sporadic aniridia, mental retardation, and hemihypertrophy. The WT1 tumor suppressor gene is reduced to homozygosity,[21] at least in part, in a small but highly informative set of sporadic Wilms' tumors. In addition, sporadic and hereditary Wilms' tumors have been described in which WT1 is specifically altered.

A genetic predisposition to Wilms' tumor is observed in two distinct disease syndromes with urogenital system malformations: the WAGR (Wilms' tumor, aniridia, genitourinary abnormalities, mental retardation) syndrome and the Denys-Drash syndrome (DDS),[22] as well as in BWS, a hereditary overgrowth syndrome characterized by visceromegaly, macroglossia, and hyperinsulinemic hypoglycemia.[23] These congenital disorders have now been linked to abnormalities at specific genetic loci implicated in Wilms' tumorigenesis.

The WAGR syndrome has been correlated with constitutional deletions of chromosome 11q13.[24] Whereas it is now known that the WAGR deletion encompasses a number of contiguous genes, including the aniridia gene *Pax6*,[25] the cytogenetic observation in patients with WAGR was also important in the cloning of the WT1 gene at chromosome 11p13.[26–28] Characterization of WT1 demonstrated that this gene spans approximately 50 kb of DNA and contains ten exons. The WT1 protein is a transcription factor.[29] However, the identity of the gene(s) targeted by WT1 during normal kidney development is not known.

The second syndrome closely associated with this locus was initially described by Denys in 1967 and recognized as a syndrome by Drash 3 years later.[30,31] DDS is a rare association of Wilms' tumor, intersex disorders, and progressive renal failure.[31] It has been demonstrated that virtually all patients with DDS carry WT1 point mutations in the germline.[32]

WT1 is altered in only 10% of Wilms' tumors.[21] This observation implies the existence of alternative loci in the etiology of this childhood renal malignancy. One such locus also resides on the short arm of chromosome 11, telomeric of WT1, at 11p15. This gene, designated *WT2*, is associated with BWS. Patients with BWS are at increased risk of developing Wilms' tumor, as well as other embryonic malignancies, including rhabdomyosarcoma (RMS), neuroblastoma, and hepatoblastoma.[33] The putative BWS gene maps to chromosome 11p15[34] and is tightly linked to the Ha-*ras* oncogene homologue *HRAS-I* and the insulin-like growth factor-2 gene (*IGF2*). Whether the BWS gene and *WT2* are one and the same or two distinct yet closely linked genes remains to be determined. Other genes, including CDKN1C (p57KIP2), a maternally expressed gene that encodes a cyclin-dependent kinase inhibitor and negatively regulates cell proliferation,[35] show aberrant methylation in tumors that are associated with cell-cycle deregulation. However, CDKN1C is rarely mutated in Wilms' tumors.[36] Thus, the search for other genes linked to Wilms' tumor continues.

Although linkage studies have indicated that the gene for familial Wilms' tumor must be distinct from WT1 and WT2, and from the gene that predisposes to BWS, to date, this gene has been neither cytogenetically localized nor isolated. Whether, of course, the gene for familial Wilms' tumor interacts with the gene product of either of the two Wilms' tumor suppressor genes has yet to be determined.

Finally, loss of the long arm of chromosome 16 has been observed in approximately 20% of Wilms' tumor samples.[37] This observation implicates yet another genetic locus in Wilms' tumor. Linkage studies have generally also excluded this locus as the "familial" Wilms' tumor gene.[38] However, it is plausible that alterations at 16q can initiate tumorigenesis or be implicated in subsequent steps in the progression of malignancy.

Although both tumors represent classic models of the Knudson "two-hit hypothesis" of tumor development, the spectrum of genetic alterations in Wilms' tumor is quite different from that in retinoblastoma. In the latter, there is strong evidence that a single gene is involved, whereas a series of genetic alterations, or at least distinct genetic events, is required for Wilms' tumorigenesis.

NEUROFIBROMATOSES

The neurofibromatoses (NFs) comprise two similar entities. NF1 is one of the most common autosomal dominantly inherited disorders, affecting approximately 1 in 3500 people[39]; one-half of them arise from new spontaneous mutations. Carriers of mutant NF1 are predisposed to a variety of tumors, including optic nerve glioma, neurofibroma and neurofibrosarcoma, malignant schwannoma, astrocytoma, and pheochromocytoma.[40,41] Occurring with less frequency are leukemias, osteosarcoma, RMS, and Wilms' tumor.

Using standard linkage analysis, the NF1 gene was mapped to chromosomal band 17q11 and subsequently cloned.[42,43] The NF1 gene is unusual in that it contains three embedded genes—OMGP, EV12A, and EV12B—in a single intron.[44] This gene encodes a 2818 amino acid protein, termed *neurofibromin*, which is ubiquitously expressed. One region of the gene shows extensive structural homology to the guanosine triphosphatase–activating domain of mammalian guanosine triphosphatase–activating proteins: Loss of the protein's activity results in failure of hydrolysis of guanosine triphosphate to guanosine diphosphate by the ras oncoprotein. Loss of neurofibromin function usually results from mutations in one allele of the gene, leading to premature truncation of the protein, followed by absence or mutations of the second allele in tumors. This loss of function is thought to lead to elevated levels of the guanosine triphosphate–bound RAS protein that transduces signals for cell division. More than one mechanism appears to exist whereby malignant tumors develop in patients with NF. In addition to structural alterations of both alleles of the NF1 gene, alternative splicing leading to dysregulation at the level of transcription has also been demonstrated. It appears that the two types of resulting protein may modify the modulation of RAS-regulated signal transduction.

NF type 2, NF2, is much less frequent than NF1, occurring in only one in one million persons. Although it is also inherited as an autosomal dominant disorder with high penetrance, the new mutation rate in NF2 is low.[45] It is clinically characterized by bilateral acoustic neuromas, spinal nerve root tumors, and meningiomas.

The NF2 locus was mapped to chromosome 22, band q12,[46] and its 69-kD encoded protein, termed *merlin*, has been shown to be expressed in various tissues, including brain, although not as ubiquitously as NF1.[47,48] The mechanism of tumor formation in NF2 appears to be in concordance with the Knudson two-hit model, although the mechanism of action of the NF2 protein has not yet been elucidated. Merlin is a member of the ERM (ezrin-radixin-moesin) family of proteins that link cell surface proteins to the cytoskeleton.[49] Although ezrin expression has been linked to metastatic behavior,[50] merlin appears to compete with ezrin activation,[49] and merlin deficiency seems to enhance metastases and promote tumorigenesis through destabilization of adherens junctions.[51]

NEUROBLASTOMA

Nonrandom chromosomal abnormalities are observed in more than 75% of neuroblastomas,[52] and many of these are also found in neuroblastoma-derived cell lines. The most common of these is deletion or rearrangement of the short arm of chromosome 1, although loss, gain, and rearrangements of chromosomes 10, 14, 17, and 19 have also been reported. The allelic losses indicate loss of function of as yet unknown tumor suppressor genes in these regions. It is believed that a tumor suppressor gene that lies on band p36 of chromosome 1 is critically important in the pathogenesis and aggressive nature of neuroblastoma. It has been shown that the loss of chromosome 1p is a strong prognostic factor in patients with neuroblastoma, independent of age and stage.[53,54] Two other unique cytogenetic rearrangements are highly characteristic of neuroblastoma.[55,56] These structures, homogeneous staining regions and double-minute chromosomes, contain regions of gene amplification. The N-myc gene, an oncogene with considerable homology to the cellular protooncogene c-myc, is amplified within homogeneous staining regions and double-minute chromosomes. Virtually all neuroblastoma tumor cell lines demonstrate amplified and highly expressed N-myc,[57] and N-myc amplification is thought to be associated with rapid tumor progression. Expression of N-myc is increased in undifferentiated tumor cells compared with much lower (or single-copy) levels in more differentiated cells (ganglioneuroblastoma and ganglioneuroma). N-myc expression is diminished in association with the *in vitro* differentiation of neuroblastoma cell lines.[58] This observation formed the basis for current therapeutic trials demonstrating a survival advantage to patients treated with cis-retinoic acid.[59] Furthermore, a close correlation exists between N-myc amplification and advanced clinical stage.[60]

Although it is clear that altered expression of N-myc contributes to the development of malignancy, it is not yet apparent which cellular functions are altered. The molecular mechanisms underlying regulation of neuroblastoma differentiation may be explained in part through the contribution of other genes and proteins. This is currently under intense investigation through the use of gene expression profiling of N-myc–positive versus –negative tumors.

Neuroblastoma cells that express the high-affinity nerve growth factor receptor trkA[61] can be terminally differentiated by nerve growth factor and may demonstrate morphologic changes typical of ganglionic differentiation. Tumors showing ganglionic differentiation and trk gene activation have a favorable prognosis.[61] In contrast, trkB receptor expression is associated with poor-prognosis tumors and appears to mediate resistance to chemotherapy.[62,63] Resistance to multidrug chemotherapeutic regimens (multidrug resistance) is characteristic of aggressive, poorly responsive N-myc–amplified neuroblastomas. It is interesting to note that expression of the multidrug resistance–associated protein, found to confer multidrug resistance *in vitro*, is increased in neuroblastomas with N-myc amplification and decreased after differentiation of tumor cells *in vitro*.[64] It has in fact been demonstrated that high levels of multidrug resistance–associated protein expression are significantly associated with poor outcome, independent of N-myc amplification.[64] Gain of chromosome segment 17q21-qter has been shown to be the most powerful prognostic factor yet.[65] However, no gene has yet been implicated at this site.

EWING'S SARCOMA FAMILY OF TUMORS

Ewing's sarcoma (ES) is one of the first examples in which the application of molecular diagnostics led to improved tumor classification. ES was first described by James Ewing[66] as a bone tumor characterized by small, blue round cells and minimal mitotic activity. Turc-Carel et al.[67] identified a recurring reciprocal t(11;22) chromosomal translocation in these tumors in 1983. Investigators subsequently demonstrated a cytogenetically identical t(11;22) in adult neuroblastoma or peripheral primitive neuroectodermal tumor (pPNET), so named because of its histologic similarity to neuroblastoma.[68] Based on the presence of the identical translocation, it was hypothesized that pPNET was related to ES. This translocation breakpoint has been molecularly characterized as an in-frame fusion between a new ES gene, EWS, on chromosome 22 and an ETS transcription family member, FLI-1, on chromosome 22.[69–71]

In addition to this fusion transcript being identified in pPNET, other variants, notably the chest-wall Askin's tumor and soft tissue ES—previously treated as an RMS because of its location in soft tissue—were also shown to bear the identical fusion transcript. Several variant translocations have also been identified, invariably fusing the EWS gene to an ETS family member.[72,73] Greater than 90% of the ES family of tumors (ESFTs) carry the EWS-ETS fusion gene, and a search for EWS-ETS by either reverse transcriptase-polymerase chain reaction or fluorescence *in situ* hybridization should be considered standard practice in the diagnostic evaluation of suspected ESFTs. Interestingly, it has been suggested that the specific fusion protein expressed in ESFT has prognostic significance.[74,75] The nature of the novel fusion transcription factor and its downstream targets is currently under intense investigation. One target of the EWS-ETS fusion is repression of the transforming growth factor-β type II receptor,[76] a putative tumor suppressor gene. Expression profiling analysis has also revealed that p53 is transcriptionally up-regulated by the EWS-ETS fusion gene.[77] This is of particular interest because it is now known that expression of EWS-ETS can lead to apoptosis and that additional alterations such as loss of p53 or p16 signaling, or both, appear to be necessary components of EWS-ETS–induced transformation.[78]

RHABDOMYOSARCOMA

The two major histologic subtypes of RMS, embryonal and alveolar, have unique histologic appearances as well as distinctive molecular genetic abnormalities, while sharing a common myogenic lineage. Embryonal tumors comprise two-thirds of all RMS and are histologically characterized by a stroma-rich spindle cell appearance. Alveolar tumors comprise approximately one-third of RMS and are histologically characterized by densely packed, small round cells, often lining a septation reminiscent of a pulmonary alveolus, giving rise to its name. Both histologic subtypes express muscle-specific proteins, including α-actin, myosin, desmin, and MyoD,[79–81] and they virtually always express high levels of IGF-2.[82,83]

At the molecular level, embryonal tumors are characterized by LOH at the 11p15 locus, which is of particular interest because this region harbors the IGF-2 gene.[84,85] The LOH at 11p15 occurs by loss of maternal and duplication of paternal chromosomal material.[86] Although LOH is normally associated with loss of tumor suppressor gene activity, in this instance LOH with paternal duplication may result in activation of IGF-2. This occurs because IGF-2 is now known to be normally imprinted; that is, this gene is normally transcriptionally silent at the maternal allele, with only the paternal allele being transcriptionally active.[87,88] Thus, LOH with paternal duplication potentially leads to a twofold gene-dosage effect of the IGF-2 locus. Furthermore, in alveolar tumors in which LOH does not occur, the normally imprinted maternal allele has been shown to be reexpressed.[89,90] Thus, LOH and loss of imprinting may in this case lead to the same functional result—namely, biallelic expression of the normally monoallelically expressed IGF-2. However, loss of an as yet unidentified tumor suppressor activity due to LOH also remains a possibility.

Alveolar RMS is characterized by a t(2;13)(q35;q14) chromosomal translocation.[91] Molecular cloning of this translocation has identified the generation of a fusion transcription factor, fusing the 5' DNA-binding region of PAX-3 on chromosome 2 to the 3' transactivation domain region of FKHR gene on chromosome 13.[92,93] A variant t(1;13)(q36;q14) has been identified in a small number of alveolar RMS tumors that fuse the 5' DNA-binding region of the PAX-7 gene on chromosome 1 with the identical 3' transactivation domain of the FKHR gene.[94] Fluorescence *in situ* hybridization or reverse transcriptase-polymerase chain reaction can be used to identify these PAX-FKHR fusions in approximately 90% of tumors and are diagnostic of alveolar RMS. The nature of this fusion-derived novel transcription factor and its downstream targets is the subject of active investigation. It has also been suggested that, like ESFT, in which the specific expressed fusion transcript has prognostic significance, the PAX-3–FKHR and the PAX-7–FKHR fusions lead to distinct clinicopathologic entities.[95] To date, attempts to generate mouse models of alveolar RMS using knock-in of the PAX-3–FKHR fusion have led to developmental abnormalities but not to tumor formation.[96]

Of particular interest is the association of the PAX-3–FKHR fusion with increased expression of c-met expression.[97,98] Met is the receptor tyrosine kinase for hepatocyte growth factor/scatter factor and is overexpressed in embryonal and alveolar RMS.[99] A mouse model of embryonal RMS has been generated by expressing a hepatocyte growth factor transgene in Ink4a/Arf[−/−] mice. The tumors appear to arise from hyperplastic satellite cells (myoblastic precursor cells).[100] The putative role of satellite cells in the pathogenesis of embryonal RMS is supported by a report demonstrating high PAX-7 expression in embryonal RMS compared to alveolar RMS and the association of PAX-7 expression with satellite cells.[101] Other frequently reported genetic alterations that may be common to embryonal and alveolar RMS include activated forms of N- and K-RAS,[102,103] inactivating p53 mutations,[104] and amplification and overexpression of MDM2, CDK-4, and N-MYC.[104]

HEREDITARY SYNDROMES ASSOCIATED WITH TUMORS OF CHILDHOOD

LI-FRAUMENI SYNDROME

A few hereditary cancer syndromes are associated with the occurrence of childhood as well as adult-onset neoplasms. The paradigm Li-Fraumeni familial cancer syndrome (LFS) was first described in 1969 from an epidemiologic evaluation of more than 600 medical and family history records of patients with childhood sarcoma.[105,106] The original description of a kindred with a spectrum of tumors that includes soft tissue sarcomas, osteosarcomas, breast cancer, brain tumors, leukemia, and adrenocortical carcinoma (ACC) has been overwhelmingly substantiated by numerous subsequent studies,[107] although other cancers, usually of particularly early age of onset, are also observed.[108] Germline alterations of the *p53* tumor suppressor gene are associated with LFS.[109–111] These are primarily missense mutations that yield a stabilized mutant protein. The spectrum of mutations of p53 in the germline are indistinct from somatic mutations found in a wide variety of tumors. Carriers are heterozygous for the mutation, and in tumors derived from these individuals, the second (wild-type) allele is frequently deleted or mutated, leading to functional inactivation.[112–114] Several comprehensive databases document all reported germline (and somatic) p53 mutations and are of particular value in evaluating novel mutations as well as phenotype-genotype correlations.[115] Only 60% to 80% of "classic" LFS families have detectable alterations of the gene. It is not yet determined whether the remainder is associated with the presence of modifier genes, promoter defects yielding abnormalities of p53 expression, or simply the result of weak genotype-phenotype correlations (i.e., the broad clinical definition encompasses families that are not actual members of LFS). Other candidate predisposition genes, such as p16, p15, p21, BRCA1, BRCA2, and PTEN, associated with multisite cancer associations have generally been ruled out as potential targets. The role of the hCHK2 checkpoint kinase as an alternative mechanism for functional inactivation of p53 in LFS has been suggested,[116] although its place as a major contributor to the phenotype has been controversial.[117]

Germline p53 alterations have also been reported in some patients with cancer phenotypes that resemble the classic LFS phenotype. Between 3% and 10% of children with apparently sporadic RMS or osteosarcoma have been shown to carry germline p53 mutations.[118,119] These patients tend to be younger than those who harbor wild-type p53. It appears as well that more than 75% of children with apparently sporadic ACC carry germline p53 mutations, although in some of these cases, a family history develops that is not substantially distinct from LFS.[120,121] A striking genotype-phenotype correlation has been observed in a unique subgroup of ACC patients in Brazil in whom the same germline p53 mutation at codon 337 has been observed in 35 unrelated kindreds.[122] Other cancers typical of LFS are not observed in these families, and the functional integrity of the

mutant protein appears to be regulated by alterations in cellular pH,[123] which suggests potential biologic mechanisms in ACC cells by which the p53 mutation leads to malignant transformation. All these observations suggest that germline p53 alterations may be associated with early-onset development of the childhood component tumors of the syndrome.[124] It is not clear what clinical significance these findings have in that no studies of prognostic significance or potential impact on anticancer treatment modalities are reported. Nevertheless, in light of the critical role played by p53 in the initiation and potentiation of gamma irradiation or chemotherapy-induced DNA damage repair, studies into the effect of such germline mutations on the potentiation of tumor development related to therapeutic interventions would be important.

BECKWITH-WIEDEMANN SYNDROME

BWS occurs with a frequency of 1 in 13,700 births. More than 450 cases have been documented since the original reported associations of exomphalos, macroglossia, gigantism, and other congenital anomalies. With increasing age, phenotypic features of BWS become less pronounced. Laboratory findings may include, at birth, hypoglycemia (extremely common), polycythemia, hypocalcemia, hypertriglyceridemia, hypercholesterolemia, and high serum α-fetoprotein levels. Early diagnosis of the condition is crucial to avoid deleterious neurologic effects of neonatal hypoglycemia and to initiate an appropriate screening protocol for tumor development.[125] The increased risk for tumor formation in BWS patients is estimated at 7.5% and is further increased to 10% if hemihyperplasia is present. Tumors occurring with the highest frequency include Wilms' tumor, hepatoblastoma, neuroblastoma, and ACC.[23,126]

The genetic basis of BWS is complex. Various 11p15 chromosomal or molecular alterations have been associated with the BWS phenotype and its tumors.[127] It is unlikely that a single gene is responsible for the BWS phenotype. Because it appears that abnormalities in the region impact an imprinted domain, it is more likely that normal gene regulation in this part of chromosome 11p15 occurs in a regional manner and may depend on various interdependent factors or genes. These include the paternally expressed genes IGF2 and KCNQ10T1 and the maternally expressed genes H19, CDKN1C, and KCNQ1. Chromosomal abnormalities associated with BWS are extremely rare, with only 20 cases having been associated with 11p15 translocations or inversions. The chromosomal breakpoint in each of these cases is always found on the maternally derived chromosome 11.[128] This parent-of-origin dependence in BWS suggests that the chromosome translocations disrupt imprinting of a gene in the 11p15 region. On the other hand, BWS-associated 11p15 duplications (approximately 30 reported cases) are always paternally derived, and the duplication breakpoints are heterogeneous.[129] Paternal uniparental disomy, in which two alleles are inherited from one parent (the father), has been reported in approximately 15% of sporadic BWS patients.[130] It is interesting that the insulin/IGF2 region is always represented in the uniparental disomy, although the extent of chromosomal involvement is highly variable. Alterations in allele-specific DNA methylation of IGF2 and H19 reflect this paternal imprinting phenomenon.[130] A minority of BWS patients have demonstrable constitutional DNA sequence alterations, the most common of these being CDKN1C mutations.[131] Twenty-five percent to 50% of BWS patients exhibit biallelic rather than monoallelic expression of IGF2. Another 50% have epigenetic mutations resulting in loss of imprinting of KCNQ10T0. Of interest, epigenetic changes, such as methylation and chromatin modification, occur in many pediatric and adult cancers,[132] indicating the value of the BWS model in understanding the broad scope of molecular changes in cancer. Despite the associated cytogenetic and molecular findings for some patients, no single diagnostic test exists for BWS. This observation is not unlike that described for LFS, or perhaps for other multisite cancer phenotypes, in which the clarity of the phenotype is often weak, making the genetic link cloudy and the likelihood of multiple pathways to tumor formation strong.

GORLIN'S SYNDROME

Nevoid basal cell carcinoma syndrome, or Gorlin's syndrome, is a rare autosomal dominant disorder characterized by multiple basal cell carcinomas, developmental defects including bifid ribs and other spine and rib abnormalities, palmar and plantar pits, odontogenic keratocysts, and generalized overgrowth.[133] The sonic hedgehog (SHH) signaling pathway directs embryonic development of a spectrum of organisms. Gorlin's syndrome appears to be caused by germline mutations of the tumor suppressor gene PTCH, a receptor for SHH.[134,135] Medulloblastoma develops in approximately 5% of patients with Gorlin's syndrome. Furthermore, approximately 10% of patients diagnosed with medulloblastoma by the age of 2 are found to have other phenotypic features consistent with Gorlin's syndrome and also harbor germline PTCH mutations.[136] Although Gorlin's syndrome develops in individuals with germline mutations of PTCH, a subset of children with medulloblastoma harbor germline mutations of another gene, SUFU, in the SHH pathway, with accompanying LOH in the tumors.[137] Of further note, mice with heterozygous PTC deletions develop RMS.[138] Although RMS is not associated with Gorlin's syndrome, the mouse studies suggest a possible link between PTC signaling and RMS.[139]

MALIGNANT RHABDOID TUMORS

Malignant rhabdoid tumors are unusual pediatric tumors that occur as primary renal tumors but have also been described in lung, liver, soft tissues, and the central nervous system, where they are often termed *atypical and teratoid rhabdoid tumors*.[140,141] Recurrent chromosomal translocations of chromosome 22 involving a breakpoint at 22q11.2, as well as complete or partial monosomy 22, have been observed, strongly suggesting the presence of a tumor suppressor gene in this area. The hSNF5/INI1 gene has been isolated and has been shown to be the target for biallelic, recurrent inactivating mutations.[142] The encoded gene product is thought to be involved in chromatin remodeling. Studies have not only demonstrated the presence of inactivating mutations in the majority of malignant rhabdoid tumors (renal or extrarenal) but also in chronic myelogenous leukemia,[143] as well as in a wide variety of other childhood and adult-onset malignancies.[144,145] An intriguing feature in some individuals with malignant rhabdoid tumors is the observation of germline mutations, suggesting that this family of tumors may occur as a result of a primary inherited defect in one allele of the INI1 gene.[146] Further studies of the function of this gene will be important in determining its role in tumorigenesis of this wide spectrum of neoplasms.

PREDICTIVE TESTING FOR GERMLINE MUTATIONS AND CHILDHOOD CANCERS

Several important issues have arisen as a result of the identification of germline mutations of tumor suppressor genes in cancer-prone individuals and families. These include ethical questions of predictive testing in such families and in unaffected relatives and selection of patients to be tested, as well as the development of practical and accurate laboratory techniques, the development of pilot testing programs, and the role of clinical intervention based on test results. This chapter was not meant to discuss these problems in detail, but one would be remiss to ignore their significance.

For several reasons, testing cannot as yet be offered to the general pediatric population, particularly in light of the demonstrably low carrier rate of the abnormal tumor suppressor genes and the general lack of standardized methods of preclinical screening of carriers. Exceptions to these limitations include screening of gene carriers in families with retinoblastoma, BWS, multiple endocrine neoplasia, von Hippel-Lindau disease, and multiple melanoma. In general, it has been demonstrated that genetic testing does not lead to clinical levels of anxiety, depression, or other markers of psychological distress in the children who are tested or their parents.[147,148] However, certain circumstances or personality traits are associated with a greater likelihood of an individual experiencing psychological distress after a positive result.[147] Therefore, whether predictive testing studies are initiated in high-risk families or surveys are carried out in cancer populations likely to harbor germline mutations in tumor suppressor genes, the investigations should be undertaken in a research setting involving expertise in oncology, psychiatry, psychology, genetics and genetic counseling, medical ethics, and molecular genetics. The development of screening programs should address aspects of cost, informed consent (particularly where it affects children), socioeconomic impact on the individual tested, consistency in providing results, and counseling.[149,150] Concerns of risk of employment, health, or life insurance discrimination exist but may be alleviated by congressional legislation to ban such practices.[151]

MOLECULAR THERAPEUTICS

With the identification of alterations in a variety of molecular signaling pathways, including activated growth factor signaling pathways (e.g., IGF-2) and altered tumor suppressor pathways (e.g., retinoblastoma), it has become increasingly apparent that these alterations may potentially represent the "Achilles heel" for these tumors. New agents targeting the tyrosine kinase enzymes that transduce growth factor signals are at various stages of development in early clinical studies. Agents blocking the growth hormone IGF-1 pathway are currently being tested in clinical trials in osteosarcoma and breast cancer. Farnesyltransferase inhibitors, blockers of the RAS pathway, have been developed and are also currently in clinical testing. Of note, the activity of farnesyltransferase inhibitors against NF is under investigation, because activation of RAS signaling has been observed in NF-associated tumors (see Neurofibromatoses, earlier in this chapter). As targets of mutant transcription factors generated are identified, it is hoped that they may represent additional targets for therapeutic intervention.

Finally, fusion proteins derived from tumor-specific translocations may themselves represent potential neoantigens that could be targeted by cytotoxic T cells. It is likely that the molecular characterization of pediatric tumors will lead to novel and perhaps more effective treatment approaches in the near future. It is also likely that some of these innovative approaches will at least initially be integrated into standard therapeutic protocols.

REFERENCES

1. Knudson AG Jr. Hereditary cancers disclose a class of cancer genes. *Cancer* 1989;63:1888.
2. Li FP. Cancer families: human models of susceptibility to neoplasia—the Richard and Hinda Rosenthal Foundation Award lecture. *Cancer Res* 1988;48:5381.
3. Balaban G, Gilbert F, Nichols W, et al. Abnormalities of chromosome #13 in retinoblastomas from individuals with normal constitutional karyotypes. *Cancer Genet Cytogenet* 1982;6:213.
4. Benedict WF, Banerjee A, Mark C, et al. Nonrandom chromosomal changes in untreated retinoblastomas. *Cancer Genet Cytogenet* 1983;10:311.
5. Knudson AG Jr. Mutation and cancer: statistical study of retinoblastoma. *Proc Natl Acad Sci U S A* 1971;68:820.
6. Comings DE. A general theory of carcinogenesis. *Proc Natl Acad Sci U S A* 1973;70:3324.
7. Devesa SS. The incidence of retinoblastoma. *Am J Ophthalmol* 1975;80:263.
8. Francois J, Matton MT, De Bie S, et al. Genesis and genetics of retinoblastoma. *Ophthalmologica* 1975;170:405.
9. Knudson AG Jr, Hethcote HW, Brown BW. Mutation and childhood cancer: a probabilistic model for the incidence of retinoblastoma. *Proc Natl Acad Sci U S A* 1975;72:5116.
10. Abramson DH, Ellsworth RM, Kitchin FD, et al. Second nonocular tumors in retinoblastoma survivors. Are they radiation-induced? *Ophthalmology* 1984;91:1351.
11. Smith LM, Donaldson SS, Egbert PR, et al. Aggressive management of second primary tumors in survivors of hereditary retinoblastoma. *Int J Radiat Oncol Biol Phys* 1989;17:499.
12. Cavenee WK, Dryja TP, Phillips RA, et al. Expression of recessive alleles by chromosomal mechanisms in retinoblastoma. *Nature* 1983;305:779.
13. Squire J, Dryja TP, Dunn J, et al. Cloning of the esterase D gene: a polymorphic gene probe closely linked to the retinoblastoma locus on chromosome 13. *Proc Natl Acad Sci U S A* 1986;83:6573.
14. Friend SH, Bernards R, Rogelj S, et al. A human DNA segment with properties of the gene that predisposes to retinoblastoma and osteosarcoma. *Nature* 1986;323:643.
15. Bookstein R, Shew JY, Chen PL, et al. Suppression of tumorigenicity of human prostate carcinoma cells by replacing a mutated RB gene. *Science* 1990;247:712.
16. Gonzalez-Fernandez F, Lopes MB, Garcia-Fernandez JM, et al. Expression of developmentally defined retinal phenotypes in the histogenesis of retinoblastoma. *Am J Pathol* 1992;141:363.
17. Matsunaga E. Hereditary retinoblastoma: penetrance, expressivity and age of onset. *Hum Genet* 1976;33:1.
18. Schubert EL, Strong LC, Hansen MF. A splicing mutation in RB1 in low penetrance retinoblastoma. *Br J Cancer* 1986;53:661.
19. Montgomery BT, Kelalis PP, Blute ML, et al. Extended followup of bilateral Wilms tumor: results of the National Wilms Tumor Study. *J Urol* 1991;146:514.
20. Beckwith JB, Kiviat NB, Bonadio JF. Nephrogenic rests, nephroblastomatosis, and the pathogenesis of Wilms' tumor. *Pediatr Pathol* 1990;10:1.
21. Little M, Holmes G, Walsh P. WT1: what has the last decade told us? *Bioessays* 1999;21:191.
22. Mueller RF. The Denys-Drash syndrome. *J Med Genet* 1994;31:471.
23. Sotelo-Avila C, Gonzalez-Crussi F, Fowler JW. Complete and incomplete forms of Beckwith-Wiedemann syndrome: their oncogenic potential. *J Pediatr* 1980;96:47.
24. Riccardi VM, Sujansky E, Smith AC, et al. Chromosomal imbalance in the Aniridia-Wilms' tumor association: 11p interstitial deletion. *Pediatrics* 1978;61:604.
25. Ton CC, Hirvonen H, Miwa H, et al. Positional cloning and characterization of a paired box- and homeobox-containing gene from the aniridia region. *Cell* 1991;67:1059.
26. Call KM, Glaser T, Ito CY, et al. Isolation and characterization of a zinc finger polypeptide gene at the human chromosome 11 Wilms' tumor locus. *Cell* 1990;60:509.
27. Gessler M, Poustka A, Cavenee W, et al. Homozygous deletion in Wilms tumours of a zinc-finger gene identified by chromosome jumping. *Nature* 1990;343:774.
28. Bonetta L, Kuehn SE, Huang A, et al. Wilms tumor locus on 11p13 defined by multiple CpG island-associated transcripts. *Science* 1990;250:994.
29. Rauscher FJ III. The WT1 Wilms tumor gene product: a developmentally regulated transcription factor in the kidney that functions as a tumor suppressor. *Faseb J* 1993;7:896.
30. Drash A, Sherman F, Hartmann WH, et al. A syndrome of pseudohermaphroditism, Wilms' tumor, hypertension, and degenerative renal disease. *J Pediatr* 1970;76:585.
31. Jadresic L, Leake J, Gordon I, et al. Clinicopathologic review of twelve children with nephropathy, Wilms tumor, and genital abnormalities (Drash syndrome). *J Pediatr* 1990;117:717.
32. Coppes MJ, Liefers GJ, Higuchi M, et al. Inherited WT1 mutation in Denys-Drash syndrome. *Cancer Res* 1992;52:6125.
33. Koufos A, Grundy P, Morgan K, et al. Familial Wiedemann-Beckwith syndrome and a second Wilms tumor locus both map to 11p15.5. *Am J Hum Genet* 1989;44:711.
34. Ping AJ, Reeve AE, Law DJ, et al. Genetic linkage of Beckwith-Wiedemann syndrome to 11p15. *Am J Hum Genet* 1989;44:720.
35. Matsuoka S, Edwards MC, Bai C, et al. p57KIP2, a structurally distinct member of the p21CIP1 Cdk inhibitor family, is a candidate tumor suppressor gene. *Genes Dev* 1995; 9:650.
36. Hartmann W, Waha A, Koch A, et al. p57(KIP2) is not mutated in hepatoblastoma but shows increased transcriptional activity in a comparative analysis of the three imprinted genes p57(KIP2), IGF2, and H19. *Am J Pathol* 2000;157:1393.
37. Maw MA, Grundy PE, Millow LJ, et al. A third Wilms' tumor locus on chromosome 16q. *Cancer Res* 1992;52:3094.
38. Huff V, Reeve AE, Leppert M, et al. Nonlinkage of 16q markers to familial predisposition to Wilms' tumor. *Cancer Res* 1992;52:6117.
39. Huson SM, Compston DA, Harper PS. A genetic study of von Recklinghausen neurofibromatosis in south east Wales. II. Guidelines for genetic counseling. *J Med Genet* 1989;26:712.
40. Lynch TM, Gutmann DH. Neurofibromatosis 1. *Neurol Clin* 2002;20:841.
41. Halliday AL, Sobel RA, Martuza RL. Benign spinal nerve sheath tumors: their occurrence sporadically and in neurofibromatosis types 1 and 2. *J Neurosurg* 1991;74:248.
42. Marchuk DA, Saulino AM, Tavakkol R, et al. cDNA cloning of the type 1 neurofibromatosis gene: complete sequence of the NF1 gene product. *Genomics* 1991;11:931.
43. DeClue JE, Cohen BD, Lowy DR. Identification and characterization of the neurofibromatosis type 1 protein product. *Proc Natl Acad Sci U S A* 1991;88:9914.
44. Viskochil D, Buchberg AM, Xu G, et al. Deletions and a translocation interrupt a cloned gene at the neurofibromatosis type 1 locus. *Cell* 1990;62:187.
45. Martuza RL, Eldridge R. Neurofibromatosis 2 (bilateral acoustic neurofibromatosis). *N Engl J Med* 1988;318:684.
46. Trofatter JA, MacCollin MM, Rutter JL, et al. A novel moesin-, ezrin-, radixin-like gene is a candidate for the neurofibromatosis 2 tumor suppressor. *Cell* 1993;72:791.
47. Rouleau GA, Merel P, Lutchman M, et al. Alteration in a new gene encoding a putative membrane-organizing protein causes neuro-fibromatosis type 2. *Nature* 1993;363:515.
48. Hara T, Bianchi AB, Seizinger BR, et al. Molecular cloning and characterization of alternatively spliced transcripts of the mouse neurofibromatosis 2 gene. *Cancer Res* 1994;54:330.
49. Sun CX, Robb VA, Gutmann DH. Protein 4.1 tumor suppressors: getting a FERM grip on growth regulation. *J Cell Sci* 2002;115:3991.
50. Khanna C, Wan X, Bose S, et al. The membrane-cytoskeleton linker ezrin is necessary for osteosarcoma metastasis. *Nat Med* 2004;10:182.
51. Lallemand D, Curto M, Saotome I, et al. NF2 deficiency promotes tumorigenesis and metastasis by destabilizing adherens junctions. *Genes Dev* 2003;17:1090.
52. Brodeur GM, Sekhon G, Goldstein MN. Chromosomal aberrations in human neuroblastomas. *Cancer* 1977;40:2256.
53. Maris JM, White PS, Beltinger CP, et al. Significance of chromosome 1p loss of heterozygosity in neuroblastoma. *Cancer Res* 1995;55:4664.
54. Caron H, van Sluis P, de Kraker J, et al. Allelic loss of chromosome 1p as a predictor of unfavorable outcome in patients with neuroblastoma. *N Engl J Med* 1996;334:225.
55. Biedler JL, Ross R, Sharske S, et al. Human neuroblastoma cytogenetics: search for significance of homogeneously staining regions in double minute chromosomes. In: Evans AE, ed. *Advances in neuroblastoma research.* New York: Raven, 1980.
56. Biedler JL, Spengler BA. A novel chromosome abnormality in human neuroblastoma and antifolate-resistant Chinese hamster cell lives in culture. *J Natl Cancer Inst* 1976;57:683.
57. Schwab M, Alitalo K, Klempnauer KH, et al. Amplified DNA with limited homology to myc cellular oncogene is shared by human neuroblastoma cell lines and a neuroblastoma tumour. *Nature* 1983;305:245.
58. Thiele CJ, Reynolds CP, Israel MA. Decreased expression of N-myc precedes retinoic acid-induced morphological differentiation of human neuroblastoma. *Nature* 1985;313:404.
59. Matthay KK, Villablanca JG, Seeger RC, et al. Treatment of high-risk neuroblastoma with intensive chemotherapy, radiotherapy, autologous bone marrow transplantation, and 13-cis- retinoic acid. Children's Cancer Group. *N Engl J Med* 1999;341:1165.
60. Schwab M, Ellison J, Busch M, et al. Enhanced expression of the human gene N-myc consequent to amplification of DNA may contribute to malignant progression of neuroblastoma. *Proc Natl Acad Sci U S A* 1984;81:4940.
61. Nakagawara A, Arima-Nakagawara M, Scavarda NJ, et al. Association between high levels of expression of the TRK gene and favorable outcome in human neuroblastoma. *N Engl J Med* 1993;328:847.
62. Ho R, Eggert A, Hishiki T, et al. Resistance to chemotherapy mediated by TrkB in neuroblastomas. *Cancer Res* 2002;62:6462.
63. Jaboin J, Kim CJ, Kaplan DR, et al. Brain-derived neurotrophic factor activation of TrkB protects neuroblastoma cells from chemotherapy-induced apoptosis via phosphatidylinositol 3'-kinase pathway. *Cancer Res* 2002;62:6756.
64. Norris MD, Bordow SB, Marshall GM, et al. Expression of the gene for multidrug-resistance-associated protein and outcome in patients with neuroblastoma. *N Engl J Med* 1996;334:231.
65. Bown N, Cotterill S, Lastowska M, et al. Gain of chromosome arm 17q and adverse outcome in patients with neuroblastoma. *N Engl J Med* 1999;340:1954.
66. Ewing J. Classics in oncology. Diffuse endothelioma of bone. Proceedings of the New York Pathological Society, 1921. *CA Cancer J Clin* 1972;22:95.
67. Turc-Carel C, Philip I, Berger MP, et al. Chromosomal translocation (11; 22) in cell lines of Ewing's sarcoma. *C R Seances Acad Sci III* 1983;296:1101.
68. Whang-Peng J, Triche T, Knutsen T, et al. Chromosome translocation in peripheral neuroepithelioma. *New Engl J Med* 1984;311:584.
69. Delattre O, Zucman J, Plougastel B, et al. Gene fusion with an ETS DNA binding domain caused by chromosome translocation in human cancers. *Nature* 1992;359:162.
70. Zucman J, Delattre O, Desmaze C, et al. Cloning and characterization of the Ewing's sarcoma and peripheral neuroepithelioma t(11;22) translocation breakpoints. *Genes Chromosomes Cancer* 1992;5:271.
71. May WA, Gishizky ML, Lessnick SL, et al. Ewing sarcoma 11;22 translocation produces a chimeric transcription factor that requires the DNA-binding domain encoded by FLI1 for transformation. *Proc Natl Acad Sci U S A* 1993;90:5752.
72. Sorensen PH, Lessnick SL, Lopez-Terrada D, et al. A second Ewing's sarcoma translocation, t(21;22), fuses the EWS gene to another ETS-family transcription factor, ERG. *Nat Genet* 1994;6:146.
73. Jeon IS, Davis JN, Braun BS, et al. A variant Ewing's sarcoma translocation (7;22) fuses the EWS gene to the ETS gene ETV1. *Oncogene* 1995;10:1229.
74. Zoubek A, Dockhorn-Dworniczak B, Delattre O, et al. Does expression of different EWS chimeric transcripts define clinically distinct risk groups of Ewing tumor patients? *J Clin Oncol* 1996;14:1245.

75. deAlava E, Kawai A, Healey J, et al. EWS-FLI1 fusion transcript structure is an independent determinant of prognosis in Ewing's sarcoma. *J Clin Oncol* 1998;16:1.
76. Hahm KB, Cho K, Lee C, et al. Repression of the gene encoding the TGF-beta type II receptor is a major target of the EWS-FLI1 oncoprotein. *Nat Genet* 1999;23:222.
77. Lessnick SL, Dacwag CS, Golub TR. The Ewing's sarcoma oncoprotein EWS/FLI induces a p53-dependent growth arrest in primary human fibroblasts. *Cancer Cell* 2002;1:393.
78. Deneen B, Denny CT. Loss of p16 pathways stabilizes EWS/FLI1 expression and complements EWS/FLI1 mediated transformation. *Oncogene* 2001;20:6731.
79. Parham DM, Webber B, Holt H, et al. Immunohistochemical study of childhood rhabdomyosarcomas and related neoplasms. Results of an Intergroup Rhabdomyosarcoma study project. *Cancer* 1991;67:3072.
80. Dodd S, Malone M, McCulloch W. Rhabdomyosarcoma in children: a histological and immunohistochemical study of 59 cases. *J Pathol* 1989;158:13.
81. Dias P, Parham DM, Shapiro DN, et al. Myogenic regulatory protein (MyoD1) expression in childhood solid tumors: diagnostic utility in rhabdomyosarcoma. *Am J Pathol* 1990; 137:1283.
82. El-Badry OM, Minniti C, Kohn EC, et al. Insulin-like growth factor II acts as an autocrine growth and motility factor in human rhabdomyosarcoma tumors. *Cell Growth Differ* 1990; 1:325.
83. Minniti CP, Tsokos M, Newton WA Jr, et al. Specific expression of insulin-like growth factor-II in rhabdomyosarcoma tumor cells. *Am J Clin Pathol* 1994;101:198.
84. Scrable H, Witte D, Lampkin B, et al. Chromosomal localization of the human rhabdomyosarcoma locus by mitotic recombination mapping. *Nature* 1987;329:645.
85. Scrable H, Witte D, Shimada H, et al. Molecular differential pathology of rhabdomyosarcoma. *Genes Chromosomes Cancer* 1989;1:23.
86. Scrable H, Cavenee W, Ghavimi F, et al. A model for embryonal rhabdomyosarcoma tumorigenesis that involves genome imprinting. *Proc Natl Acad Sci U S A* 1989;86:7480.
87. Rainier S, Johnson LA, Dobry CJ, et al. Relaxation of imprinted genes in human cancer. *Nature* 1993;362:747.
88. Ogawa O, Eccles MR, Szeto J, et al. Relaxation of insulin-like growth factor II gene imprinting implicated in Wilms' tumour. *Nature* 1993;362:749.
89. Zhan S, Shapiro DN, Helman LJ. Activation of an imprinted allele of the insulin-like growth factor II gene implicated in rhabdomyosarcoma. *J Clin Invest* 1994;94:445.
90. Zhan S, Shapiro D, Zhang L, et al. Concordant loss of imprinting of the human insulin-like growth factor II gene promoters in cancer. *J Biol Chem* 1995;270:27983.
91. Douglass EC, Valentine M, Etcubanas E, et al. A specific chromosomal abnormality in rhabdomyosarcoma [published erratum appears in *Cytogenet Cell Genet* 1988;47: following 232]. *Cytogenet Cell Genet* 1987;45:148.
92. Barr FG, Galili N, Holick J, et al. Rearrangement of the PAX3 paired box gene in the paediatric solid tumour alveolar rhabdomyosarcoma. *Nat Genet* 1993;3:113.
93. Shapiro DN, Sublett JE, Li B, et al. Fusion of PAX3 to a member of the forkhead family of transcription factors in human alveolar rhabdomyosarcoma. *Cancer Res* 1993;53:5108.
94. Davis RJ, D'Cruz CM, Lovell MA, et al. Fusion of PAX7 to FKHR by the variant t(1;13)(p36;q14) translocation in alveolar rhabdomyosarcoma. *Cancer Res* 1994;54:2869.
95. Kelly KM, Womer RB, Sorensen PH, et al. Common and variant gene fusions predict distinct clinical phenotypes in rhabdomyosarcoma. *J Clin Oncol* 1997;15:1831.
96. Lagutina I, Conway SJ, Sublett J, et al. Pax3-FKHR knock-in mice show developmental aberrations but do not develop tumors. *Mol Cell Biol* 2002;22:7204.
97. Epstein J, Shapiro D, Cheng J, et al. Pax3 modulates expression of the c-Met receptor during limb muscle development. *Proc Natl Acad Sci U S A* 1996;93:4213.
98. Ginsberg JP, Davis RJ, Bennicelli JL, et al. Up-regulation of MET but not neural cell adhesion molecule expression by the PAX3-FKHR fusion protein in alveolar rhabdomyosarcoma. *Cancer Res* 1998;58:3542.
99. Ferracini R, Olivero M, Di Renzo MF, et al. Retrogenic expression of the MET proto-oncogene correlates with the invasive phenotype of human rhabdomyosarcomas. *Oncogene* 1996;12:1697.
100. Sharp R, Recio JA, Jhappan C, et al. Synergism between INK4a/ARF inactivation and aberrant HGF/SF signaling in rhabdomyosarcomagenesis. *Nat Med* 2002;8:1276.
101. Tiffin N, Williams RD, Shipley J, et al. PAX7 expression in embryonal rhabdomyosarcoma suggests an origin in muscle satellite cells. *Br J Cancer* 2003;89:327.
102. Chardin P, Yeramian P, Madaule P, et al. N-ras gene activation in the RD human rhabdomyosarcoma cell line. *Int J Cancer* 1985;35:647.
103. Stratton MR, Fisher C, Gusterson BA, et al. Detection of point mutations in N-ras and K-ras genes of human embryonal rhabdomyosarcomas using oligonucleotide probes and the polymerase chain reaction. *Cancer Res* 1989;49:6324.
104. Merlino G, Helman LJ. Rhabdomyosarcoma—working out the pathways. *Oncogene* 1999;18:5340.
105. Li FP, Fraumeni JF Jr. Rhabdomyosarcoma in children: epidemiologic study and identification of a familial cancer syndrome. *J Natl Cancer Inst* 1969;43:1365.
106. Li FP, Fraumeni JF Jr. Prospective study of a family cancer syndrome. *JAMA* 1982;247:2692.
107. Li FP, Fraumeni JF Jr, Mulvihill JJ, et al. A cancer family syndrome in twenty-four kindreds. *Cancer Res* 1988;48:5358.
108. Nichols KE, Malkin D, Garber JE, et al. Germ-line p53 mutations predispose to a wide spectrum of early-onset cancers. *Cancer Epidemiol Biomarkers Prev* 2001;10:83.
109. Malkin D, Li FP, Strong LC, et al. Germ line p53 mutations in a familial syndrome of breast cancer, sarcomas, and other neoplasms. *Science* 1990;250:1233.
110. Srivastava S, Zou ZQ, Pirollo K, et al. Germ-line transmission of a mutated p53 gene in a cancer-prone family with Li-Fraumeni syndrome. *Nature* 1990;348:747.
111. Malkin D. Li-Fraumeni syndrome. In: Vogelstein B, Kinzler KW, eds. *The genetic basis of human cancer.* New York: McGraw-Hill, 1998.
112. Sedlacek Z, Kodet R, Seemanova E, et al. Two Li-Fraumeni syndrome families with novel germline p53 mutations: loss of the wild-type p53 allele in only 50% of tumours. *Br J Cancer* 1998;77:1034.
113. Varley JM, Thorncroft M, McGown G, et al. A detailed study of loss of heterozygosity on chromosome 17 in tumours from Li-Fraumeni patients carrying a mutation to the TP53 gene. *Oncogene* 1997;14:865.
114. Frebourg T, Kassel J, Lam KT, et al. Germ-line mutations of the p53 tumor suppressor gene in patients with high risk for cancer inactivate the p53 protein. *Proc Natl Acad Sci U S A* 1992;89:6413.
115. Olivier M, Eeles R, Hollstein M, et al. The IARC TP53 database: new online mutation analysis and recommendations to users. *Hum Mutat* 2002;19:607.
116. Bell DW, Varley JM, Szydlo TE, et al. Heterozygous germ line hCHK2 mutations in Li-Fraumeni syndrome. *Science* 1999;286:2528.
117. Bougeard G, Limacher JM, Martin C, et al. Detection of 11 germline inactivating TP53 mutations and absence of TP63 and HCHK2 mutations in 17 French families with Li-Fraumeni or Li-Fraumeni-like syndrome. *J Med Genet* 2001;38:253.
118. Diller L, Sexsmith E, Gottlieb A, et al. Germline p53 mutations are frequently detected in young children with rhabdomyosarcoma. *J Clin Invest* 1995;95:1606.
119. McIntyre JF, Smith-Sorensen B, Friend SH, et al. Germline mutations of the p53 tumor suppressor gene in children with osteosarcoma. *J Clin Oncol* 1994;12:925.
120. Wagner J, Portwine C, Rabin K, et al. High frequency of germline p53 mutations in childhood adrenocortical cancer. *J Natl Cancer Inst* 1994;86:1707.
121. Varley JM, McGown G, Thorncroft M, et al. Are there low-penetrance TP53 alleles? Evidence from childhood adrenocortical tumors. *Am J Hum Genet* 1999;65:995.
122. Ribeiro RC, Sandrini F, Figueiredo B, et al. An inherited p53 mutation that contributes in a tissue-specific manner to pediatric adrenal cortical carcinoma. *Proc Natl Acad Sci U S A* 2001;98:9330.
123. DiGiammarino EL, Lee AS, Cadwell C, et al. A novel mechanism of tumorigenesis involving pH-dependent destabilization of a mutant p53 tetramer. *Nat Struct Biol* 2002;9:12.
124. Olivier M, Goldgar DE, Sodha N, et al. Li-Fraumeni and related syndromes: correlation between tumor type, family structure, and TP53 genotype. *Cancer Res* 2003;63:6643.
125. Clericuzio CL, Johnson C. Screening for Wilms tumor in high-risk individuals. *Hematol Oncol Clin North Am* 1995;9:1253.
126. Weksberg R, Teshima I, Williams BR, et al. Molecular characterization of cytogenetic alterations associated with the Beckwith-Wiedemann syndrome (BWS) phenotype refines the localization and suggests the gene for BWS is imprinted. *Hum Mol Genet* 1993;2:549.
127. Mannens M, Hoovers JM, Redeker E, et al. Parental imprinting of human chromosome region 11p15.3-pter involved in the Beckwith-Wiedemann syndrome and various human neoplasia. *Eur J Hum Genet* 1994;2:3.
128. Henry I, Jeanpierre M, Barichard F, et al. Duplication of HRAS1, INS, and IGF2 is not a common event in Beckwith-Wiedemann syndrome. *Ann Genet* 1988;31:216.
129. Henry I, Bonaiti-Pellie C, Chehensse V, et al. Uniparental paternal disomy in a genetic cancer-predisposing syndrome. *Nature* 1991;351:665.
130. Reik W, Brown KW, Schneid H, et al. Imprinting mutations in the Beckwith-Wiedemann syndrome suggested by altered imprinting pattern in the IGF2-H19 domain. *Hum Mol Genet* 1995;4:2379.
131. Li M, Squire J, Shuman C, et al. Imprinting status of 11p15 genes in Beckwith-Wiedemann syndrome patients with CDKN1C mutations. *Genomics* 2001;74:370.
132. Feinberg AP. Genomic imprinting and gene activation in cancer. *Nat Genet* 1993;4:110.
133. Gorlin RJ. Nevoid basal-cell carcinoma syndrome. *Medicine (Baltimore)* 1987;66:98.
134. Gailani MR, Stahle-Backdahl M, Leffell DJ, et al. The role of the human homologue of Drosophila patched in sporadic basal cell carcinomas. *Nat Genet* 1996;14:78.
135. Hahn H, Wicking C, Zaphiropoulous PG, et al. Mutations of the human homolog of Drosophila patched in the nevoid basal cell carcinoma syndrome. *Cell* 1996;85:841.
136. Cowan R, Hoban P, Kelsey A, et al. The gene for the naevoid basal cell carcinoma syndrome acts as a tumour-suppressor gene in medulloblastoma. *Br J Cancer* 1997;76:141.
137. Taylor MD, Liu L, Raffel C, et al. Mutations in SUFU predispose to medulloblastoma. *Nat Genet* 2002;31:306.
138. Hahn H, Wojnowski L, Zimmer AM, et al. Rhabdomyosarcomas and radiation hypersensitivity in a mouse model of Gorlin syndrome. *Nat Med* 1998;4:619.
139. Zhan S, Helman LJ. Glimpsing the cause of rhabdomyosarcoma. *Nat Med* 1998;4:559.
140. Parham DM, Weeks DA, Beckwith JB. The clinicopathologic spectrum of putative extrarenal rhabdoid tumors. An analysis of 42 cases studied with immunohistochemistry or electron microscopy. *Am J Surg Pathol* 1994;18:1010.
141. Rorke LB, Packer RJ, Biegel JA. Central nervous system atypical teratoid/rhabdoid tumors of infancy and childhood: definition of an entity. *J Neurosurg* 1996;85:56.
142. Versteege I, Sevenet N, Lange J, et al. Truncating mutations of hSNF5/INI1 in aggressive paediatric cancer. *Nature* 1998;394:203.
143. Grand F, Kulkarni S, Chase A, et al. Frequent deletion of hSNF5/INI1, a component of the SWI/SNF complex, in chronic myeloid leukemia. *Cancer Res* 1999;59:3870.
144. Sevenet N, Sheridan E, Amram D, et al. Constitutional mutations of the hSNF5/INI1 gene predispose to a variety of cancers. *Am J Hum Genet* 1999;65:1342.
145. Sevenet N, Lellouch-Tubiana A, Schofield D, et al. Spectrum of hSNF5/INI1 somatic mutations in human cancer and genotype-phenotype correlations. *Hum Mol Genet* 1999;8:2359.
146. Biegel JA, Zhou JY, Rorke LB, et al. Germ-line and acquired mutations of INI1 in atypical teratoid and rhabdoid tumors. *Cancer Res* 1999;59:74.
147. Grosfeld FJ, Beemer FA, Lips CJ, et al. Parents' responses to disclosure of genetic test results of their children. *Am J Med Genet* 2000;94:316.
148. Michie S, Bobrow M, Marteau TM. Predictive genetic testing in children and adults: a study of emotional impact. *J Med Genet* 2001;38:519.
149. Knoppers BM, Chadwick R. The Human Genome Project: under an international ethical microscope. *Science* 1994;265:2035.
150. Malkin D, Knoppers BM. Genetic predisposition to cancer—issues to consider. *Semin Cancer Biol* 1996;7:49.
151. Roth MT, Painter RB. Genetic discrimination in health insurance: an overview and analysis of the issues. *Nurs Clin North Am* 2000;35:731.

DAVID H. EBB
DANIEL M. GREEN
ROBERT C. SHAMBERGER
NANCY J. TARBELL

SECTION 2

Solid Tumors of Childhood

Malignant solid tumors account for 30% of all cases of childhood cancer. Collaborative, multimodality treatment efforts undertaken in the context of pediatric cooperative group clinical trials have produced a remarkable improvement in survival since the 1970s. In addition to improvements in survival and functional outcome, the cooperative group studies have facilitated rapid growth in our understanding of cancer genetics and tumor biology. Prospective studies are currently under way to validate new risk group stratification schemes that integrate classic tumor staging information with prognostically significant features of tumor biology detectable with molecular diagnostics. The authors review the epidemiology, pathology, clinical presentation, evaluation, treatment, and prognosis of the common malignant solid tumors of children and adolescents.

EPIDEMIOLOGY

Approximately 12,400 children and adolescents younger than 20 years were diagnosed with cancer in 1998.[1] Malignant neoplasms are a major cause of mortality in children between 1 and 14 years old. In 2001, the most recent year for which statistics are available, accidents and congenital anomalies were responsible for more deaths in the age group 1 to 4 years, whereas only accidents were a more frequent cause of death in the age group 5 to 14 years.[2]

The most common malignant neoplasms diagnosed in pediatric patients are acute leukemia, non-Hodgkin's lymphoma, Hodgkin's disease, and primary tumors of the central nervous system. Among pediatric solid tumors, the most common malignancies are neuroblastoma, Wilms' tumor, rhabdomyosarcoma (RMS), and retinoblastoma[1] (Table 40.2-1).

Since 1980, important advances have been made in elucidating germline and somatic mutations that are uniquely associated with many of these neoplasms. The molecular genetics of pediatric solid tumors are extensively reviewed in Chapter 40.1.

MANAGEMENT OF CHILDHOOD CANCER

Childhood malignant solid tumors are unique owing to their responsiveness to many chemotherapeutic agents. Effective combination chemotherapy regimens have been identified and evaluated through cooperative group multi-institutional trials. The dramatic improvements in survival of pediatric patients with cancer since the 1970s are the result of treatment by multidisciplinary teams with experience in the evaluation, staging, surgical management, radiation treatment, and administration of intensive chemotherapy regimens to these children.

Surgery plays two roles in the management of solid tumors. The first role is establishing a histologic diagnosis and staging the tumor; the second is resection of the primary site of disease. It is increasingly important that the surgeon work in a collaborative fashion with the pediatric oncologist and radiation oncologist, because resection may be best accomplished after initial chemotherapy and radiotherapy. These initial treatments may decrease both the potential risks of resection and the long-term morbidity. Similarly, it is critical that the surgeon be involved from the outset in the care of a child presenting with a solid tumor because an inappropriately performed biopsy of the tumor may complicate later resection efforts. Questions regarding timing and feasibility of resection should only be considered by surgeons who are facile in reconciling the sometimes competing demands of durable local control and optimal functional outcome in a growing child. In light of the exquisite radiosensitivity of most pediatric solid tumors, all deliberations concerning timing and extent of resection efforts must recognize the importance of radiotherapy as an effective adjunct in efforts to secure local control.

Significant advances in surgical and anesthetic management and postoperative supportive care have been complemented by substantial improvements in radiation planning and delivery. Conformal radiotherapy using three-dimensional treatment planning to spare normal tissues has had a salutary effect on functional outcome. Advances in our knowledge of radiation dosing and planning techniques are discussed separately under each specific tumor type.

WILMS' TUMOR

Wilms' tumor is the most common primary malignant renal tumor of childhood. The striking success of national cooperative studies in improving survival and decreasing treatment-related morbidity mark this disease as the paradigm for multimodal treatment of a pediatric malignant solid tumor.

EPIDEMIOLOGY AND GENETICS

Among North American white children less than 15 years of age, the incidence rate of Wilms' tumor is 8.1 cases per 1 mil-

TABLE 40.2-1. Annual Incidence Rates and Percentage Distribution of Malignant Diseases in U.S. Children

Disease	Incidence[a]	
	White	African American
Acute lymphoblastic leukemia	32.9 (23.6%)	16.9 (15.6%)
Astrocytoma	17.9 (12.8%)	14.3 (13.2%)
Neuroblastoma	10.2 (7.3%)	7.8 (7.2%)
Non-Hodgkin's lymphoma	9.1 (6.5%)	5.4 (5.0%)
Wilms' tumor	8.3 (5.9%)	9.4 (8.7%)
Hodgkin's disease	7.3 (5.2%)	4.7 (4.3%)
Primitive neuroectodermal	6.8 (4.9%)	5.9 (5.4%)
Acute myeloid leukemia	5.8 (4.2%)	4.8 (4.4%)
Rhabdomyosarcoma	4.7 (3.4%)	4.1 (3.8%)
Retinoblastoma	3.9 (2.8%)	4.5 (4.1%)
Osteosarcoma	3.4 (2.4%)	3.9 (3.6%)
Ewing's sarcoma	3.3 (2.4%)	0.3 (0.3%)
All histologic types	139.5 (100%)	108.3 (100%)

[a]Per million children younger than 15 years.

lion.[1] The incidence rate is approximately three times higher for African Americans in the United States and blacks in Africa than for East Asians, with rates for white populations in Europe and North America between these extremes.[3]

Wilms' tumor in the United States is slightly less frequent in boys than in girls. Unilateral tumors are typically diagnosed in the fourth year of life, whereas bilateral tumors present at a slightly younger age.

Children with Wilms' tumor may have associated anomalies, including aniridia, hemihypertrophy (as an isolated abnormality, or as a component of the Beckwith-Wiedemann syndrome), cryptorchidism, and hypospadias.[4] Although children with Beckwith-Wiedemann syndrome have a higher incidence of bilateral disease, their prognosis remains excellent with long-term survival secured in 89% of affected children.[5] Children with pseudohermaphroditism and renal disease (glomerulonephritis or nephrotic syndrome) who develop Wilms' tumor may have Denys-Drash syndrome, which is associated with mutations within the same gene implicated in the Wilms' tumor, aniridia, genitourinary malformations, and mental retardation (WAGR) syndrome.[6]

PATHOLOGY

Wilms' tumor is characterized by tremendous histologic diversity and is thought to be composed of, or derived from, primitive metanephric blastema. Most Wilms' tumors are unicentric lesions, although a substantial number arise multifocally in the kidney. Among 1905 National Wilms' Tumor Study Group (NWTSG) cases, approximately 5% involved both kidneys either at initial presentation or subsequent to diagnosis. An additional 7% of reported cases were multicentric unilateral tumors.[3] There is no predilection for either side. The tumor may arise anywhere within the kidney, which is usually markedly distorted by the neoplasm.

The most distinctive microscopic feature of Wilms' tumor is its structural diversity. The classic nephroblastoma is made up of varying proportions of three cell types (i.e., blastemal, stromal, and epithelial), but they are not all present in every case.[7] Anaplasia is marked by the presence of gigantic polyploid nuclei within the tumor sample. The new definition of focal anaplasia emphasizes distribution, requiring that cells with anaplastic nuclear changes be confined to sharply restricted foci within the primary tumor. By definition, focally anaplastic disease must not be identifiable in any site outside the renal parenchyma.[8]

Clear cell sarcoma of the kidney is an important primary renal tumor associated with a significantly higher rate of relapse and death than favorable histology Wilms' tumor.[9] Tumors with this histology have a wider distribution of metastases than favorable histology Wilms' tumor.

Rhabdoid tumor of the kidney was identified for the first time in 1978 by NWTSG pathologists. The neoplasm, previously confused with Wilms' tumor, is a monomorphous tumor like clear cell sarcoma of the kidney. The cell of origin for this distinctive tumor remains unknown.[10] Rhabdoid tumor of the kidney tends to metastasize to the lung and brain. Several studies have reported that separate primary neuroectodermal tumors of the brain have apparently developed in children with this neoplasm.[11] Primary rhabdoid tumors of the kidney and brain (atypical teratoid/rhabdoid tumors) share deletions of chromosome band 22q11.2.[12] This deleted locus appears to be the site of INI1, a putative tumor suppressor gene.[13]

The existence of precursor lesions to Wilms' tumor has been recognized for many years.[14] These precursor lesions, or nephrogenic rests, take the form of small, usually microscopic clusters of blastemal cells, tubules, or stromal cells that are generally situated at the periphery of the renal lobe. Intralobar or perilobar nephrogenic rests are identified in the renal parenchyma of approximately 30% of Wilms' tumor cases. Nephroblastomatosis describes kidneys with multifocal or diffuse nephrogenic rests. Children with nephroblastomatosis have a heightened risk of developing Wilms' tumor and require close monitoring for the development of renal tumors.[15]

Congenital mesoblastic nephroma is important to recognize because it is usually curable by nephrectomy alone.[16] These tumors are typically identified in the first months of life, with a median age at diagnosis of 2 months.

CLINICAL PRESENTATION AND NATURAL HISTORY

Most children with Wilms' tumor come to medical attention because of abdominal swelling or the presence of an abdominal mass. This feature is usually noticed by a parent while bathing or dressing the child. Abdominal pain, gross hematuria, and fever may be present at diagnosis. Hypertension, present in approximately 25% of cases, has been attributed to an increase in renin activity.[17]

During the physical examination, it is important to note the location and size of the abdominal mass and its movement with respiration. A varicocele secondary to obstruction of the spermatic vein may be associated with the presence of a tumor thrombus in the renal vein or inferior vena cava. It is also important to note specifically any signs of the Wilms' tumor–associated syndromes marked by the presence of aniridia, partial or complete hemihypertrophy, and genitourinary abnormalities, such as hypospadias and cryptorchidism.

STAGING

The current staging system, which was developed by the NWTSG, is shown in Table 40.2-2.

EVALUATION

Laboratory evaluation should include a complete blood cell count, differential white blood cell count, platelet count, liver function tests, renal function tests, serum calcium, and urinalysis. Elevation of the serum calcium may occur in children with rhabdoid tumor of the kidney or congenital mesoblastic nephroma.[18]

DIAGNOSTIC IMAGING

Imaging studies initially should be restricted to those necessary to establish the presence of an intrarenal space-occupying lesion. These studies should also be directed at identifying the presence of a contralateral kidney, which must be assessed for possible tumor involvement. In addition, imaging of the affected kidney must look for evidence of tumor thrombus in the renal vein and measure its proximal extent.

The initial radiographic study often selected is an abdominal ultrasound examination. This demonstrates whether the

TABLE 40.2-2. National Wilms' Tumor Study Group Staging System for Renal Tumors

Stage	Description
I	The tumor was limited to the kidney and was completely excised. The renal capsule has an intact outer surface. The tumor was not ruptured or biopsied before removal (fine-needle aspiration biopsies are excluded from this restriction). The vessels of the renal sinus are not involved. There is no evidence of tumor at or beyond the margins of resection.
II	The tumor extended beyond the kidney, but was completely excised. There may be regional extension of tumor (i.e., penetration of the renal capsule or extensive invasion of the renal sinus). The blood vessels outside the renal parenchyma, including those of the renal sinus, may contain tumor. The tumor was biopsied (except for fine-needle aspiration), or there was spillage of tumor before or during surgery that is confined to the flank and does not involve the peritoneal surface. There must be no evidence of tumor at or beyond the margins of resection.
III	Residual nonhematogenous tumor is present and confined to the abdomen. Any one of the following may occur: 1. Lymph nodes within the abdomen or pelvis are found to be involved by tumor (renal hilar, paraaortic, or beyond). (Lymph node involvement in the thorax or other extraabdominal sites would be a criterion for stage IV.) 2. The tumor has penetrated through the peritoneal surface. 3. Tumor implants are found on the peritoneal surface. 4. Gross or microscopic tumor remains postoperatively (e.g., tumor cells are found at the margin of surgical resection on microscopic examination). 5. The tumor is not completely resectable because of local infiltration into vital structures. 6. Tumor spill not confined to the flank occurred either before or during surgery.
IV	Hematogenous metastases (lung, liver, bone, brain, and so forth) or lymph node metastases outside the abdominopelvic region are present.
V	Bilateral renal involvement is present at diagnosis. An attempt should be made to stage each side according to the previously mentioned criteria on the basis of the extent of disease before biopsy or treatment.

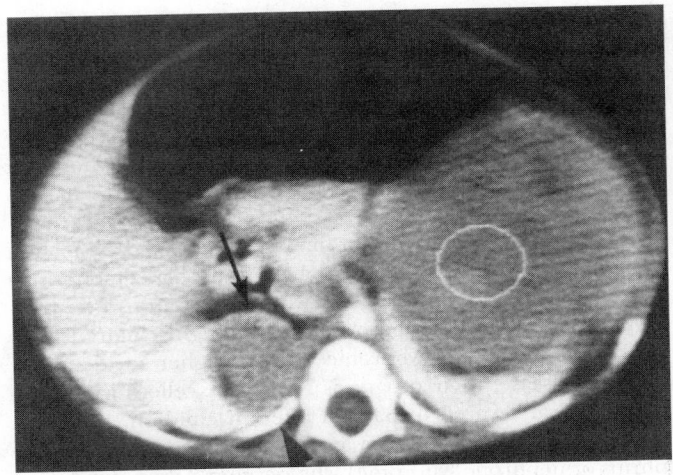

FIGURE 40.2-1. Computed tomography scan of abdomen demonstrating bilateral renal tumors (*arrows*).

abdominal mass is solid or cystic and may allow identification of the mass's organ of origin and measurement of the maximum diameter of the mass. Contrast-enhanced computed tomography (CT) of the abdomen, performed to further evaluate the nature and extent of the mass, may suggest apparent extension of the tumor into adjacent structures such as the liver, spleen, and colon (Fig. 40.2-1). Most children believed to have invasion of the liver on CT, however, are found to have hepatic compression at the time of surgery, rather than hepatic invasion. CT of the abdomen is also used to look for evidence of hematogenous metastases to the liver and pathologically enlarged lymph nodes.

The patency of the inferior vena cava may be demonstrated relatively inexpensively using real-time ultrasonography. When tumor is identified within that vessel, the proximal extent of the thrombus must be established before operation. Extension of the thrombus to the right atrium may produce few, if any, clinical signs and may not be suspected preoperatively.[19]

The results of the radiographic studies and real-time ultrasonography provide sufficient information to support proceeding with a laparotomy in most children, although no imaging

study unequivocally establishes the histologic diagnosis of Wilms' tumor.

Plain chest radiographs should be obtained to determine whether pulmonary metastases are present. Insufficient data are currently available to firmly establish the need for CT of the chest in the initial evaluation of children with Wilms' tumor. Substantial interobserver variation exists in the interpretation of chest CT scans of children with Wilms' tumor.[20] The available data suggest that, in many cases, nodules identified are not metastatic tumor. Thus, at least one nodule should be biopsied to confirm the stage pathologically.

A radionuclide bone scan and skeletal survey should be obtained postoperatively on all children with clear cell sarcoma of the kidney and all children, regardless of histologic type, with pulmonary or hepatic metastases who have suggestive symptomatology. Both of these studies are necessary owing to the potential of clear cell sarcoma of the kidney to cause lytic bony lesions, which may be evident on plain radiographs but undetectable on bone scan.[21]

In light of the association of intracranial metastases with both clear cell sarcoma and rhabdoid tumor of the kidney, children with either of these histologies should undergo brain imaging.[10,22]

TREATMENT

Surgery

Resection is the primary means of achieving local control in Wilms' tumor, with radiotherapy reserved for locally advanced or metastatic disease. Accurate surgical staging is critical, as it determines subsequent requirements for chemotherapy and radiotherapy based on penetration of renal capsule by tumor, regional lymph node involvement, and residual tumor. These factors cannot be determined radiographically with sufficient sensitivity for treatment planning. A review of children treated in NWTS-4 demonstrated an increased incidence of local recurrence in those cases in which lymph node biopsies were not obtained.[23] Presumably, these children were under-staged and thus, undertreated. The increased incidence of local recurrence in these cases highlights the need for complete surgical staging.

Initial resection of the tumor has been the policy supported by the NWTSG through all of its protocols. Despite the presentation of most Wilms' tumors as a large mass, resection is generally feasible. In contrast to neuroblastoma, attempted resections of Wilms' tumors are less likely to be complicated by tumor invasion of surrounding organs. Close surveillance of children undergoing initial nephrectomy in the NWTS-3 cohort demonstrated an operative complication rate of 19.8% in a group closely followed and evaluated.[24] The most frequent complications were intestinal obstruction (6.9%) and extensive intraoperative hemorrhage, which occurred in 5.8% of cases.[25] Factors that correlated with increased risk of surgical complications included advanced local stage, intravascular extension of the tumor, and resection of other organs. Resected adjacent organs were often found to be merely compressed or distorted by the tumor rather than directly infiltrated. Extensive resection involving removal of other organs or procedures that may carry a high risk of morbidity or mortality should be avoided. In such cases of extensive disease, initial surgery should be limited to a biopsy, followed by administration of chemotherapy. Resection can be more readily performed after the tumor has regressed.

The International Society of Pediatric Oncology (SIOP) has promoted the use of preoperative treatment of children with Wilms' tumor with radiotherapy or chemotherapy, without histologic confirmation of the diagnosis before therapy is initiated. They report a lower surgical complication rate of 8% by following this policy.[26] This approach has several risks, including (1) the potential for administration of chemotherapy for benign disease, (2) modification of the tumor histology, (3) loss of staging information, and (4) delivering treatment that is inappropriate for a particular histology (e.g., rhabdoid tumor of the kidney). Treatment without an initial diagnosis is difficult to support when NWTSG and SIOP studies have both demonstrated a 7.6% to 9.9% rate of benign or other malignant diagnosis in children with a prenephrectomy diagnosis of Wilms' tumor.[27,28]

A major driving factor for the use by SIOP of preoperative therapy was the high rate of operative tumor rupture in their early series. This rate decreased from 33% to 4% in the SIOP series when prenephrectomy abdominal radiation was given. Operative rupture occurred in NWTS-1 and NWTS-2 in 22% and 12% of children, respectively. In NWTS-4, operative rupture occurred in 14% of cases.[27,29] A subsequent randomized SIOP study reported that the rate of rupture was essentially the same for children receiving abdominal radiation and dactinomycin (8%) and those receiving vincristine and dactinomycin (6%).[30,31] In two consecutive nonrandomized studies, the proportion of stage II lymph node–negative children versus stage II lymph node–positive and stage III changed from 45% to 32% and 33% to 19%, suggesting that the preoperative treatments significantly decreased the apparent stage of the children's disease.[32] Evaluation of NWTS-4 clearly demonstrates that operative rupture, whether localized to the renal fossa or diffuse in the peritoneal cavity, is associated with an increased incidence of local recurrence.[29] This supports the need to avoid rupture by use of an adequate abdominal or thoracoabdominal incision to safely remove the tumor.

Adequate biopsy of lymph nodes in the renal hilum and along the vena cava or aorta is critical for staging. The surgeon must always consider the possibility of stage III disease and obtain adequate tissue for its diagnosis. Although grossly involved lymph nodes are generally resected, this approach should not be extrapolated into a recommendation for an extensive retroperitoneal lymph node dissection because this has not been shown to improve local control.[33]

The histologic diagnosis after preoperative treatment in a group of children followed by the NWTSG did not appear to have been distorted by treatment. It is less certain, however, that the pathologic findings that would determine staging were not altered by preoperative therapy.[34] A SIOP study randomized the use of local radiotherapy (20 Gy) in children treated preoperatively with chemotherapy who had stage II node-negative disease at resection. The study was terminated after randomization of 123 children because of an increased incidence of abdominal recurrence during the first year of follow-up in the children not receiving radiation (six vs. zero).[31] This difference in outcome suggested that prenephrectomy treatment altered the pathologic findings that would otherwise have led to a diagnosis of stage III disease (i.e., lymph node involvement or capsular penetration) and inclusion of local radiation.

Preoperative treatment of Wilms' tumor is generally accepted in certain circumstances. These include the occurrence of Wilms' tumor in children with a solitary kidney, bilateral renal tumors, tumor in a horseshoe kidney, and respiratory distress from extensive pulmonary metastases. In most instances, pretreatment biopsy should be obtained. In children with bilateral disease or involvement of a solitary kidney, preoperative chemotherapy is intended to permit maximal conservation of uninvolved renal parenchyma. Studies on pretreatment of children with unilateral tumors have demonstrated that, in most instances, a complete nephrectomy is still required owing to extensive involvement with the kidney at presentation.[35]

In the bilateral cases, preservation of normal renal tissue is a more critical issue. In these children, the contralateral tumor often is smaller and more amenable to a partial nephrectomy after treatment with chemotherapy. Concerns about long-term renal impairment after removal of more than one-half of the renal parenchyma have resulted in a less radical surgical approach to the treatment of these children.[36]

The goal of therapy in bilateral cases is first, to eradicate all tumor, and second, to preserve as much renal tissue as possible to minimize the frequency of chronic renal failure.[37,38] The management presently recommended is initial bilateral renal biopsy and staging. Children then receive combination chemotherapy based on the stage and histology. A reevaluation is performed after 5 weeks to determine whether there has been sufficient response of the tumors to allow tumor resection, with preservation of a substantial amount of normal renal tissue. Additional chemotherapeutic agents, such as doxorubicin, with or without radiation therapy, may be necessary for the management of children whose tumors respond poorly to the combination of vincristine and dactinomycin.

The absence of radiographic response or evidence of radiographic progression does not always imply lack of histologic response. Fetal rhabdomyomatous nephroblastoma is being recognized with increasing frequency as an entity with a favorable prognosis that may be misinterpreted as chemotherapy-resistant tumor in the absence of histologic confirmation.[39] This potential lack of concordance between radiographic and histologic response mandates that changes in chemotherapy or the addition of radiation therapy, or both, in the management of children with bilateral or inoperable tumors should only be made after evaluation of a posttreatment biopsy.

In NWTS-4, the 4-year survival was 81.7% for patients with bilateral disease who underwent nephron-sparing surgery. Although this approach has been very successful from the standpoint of survival and functional outcome, it is important to note that approximately 10% of bilateral tumors contain anaplastic elements. A recent retrospective review of patients with bilateral disease revealed only 25% survival for this subset, indicating that bilateral tumors with anaplasia are poor candidates for limited, kidney-sparing surgery.[40]

Intracaval or intraatrial extension of a tumor thrombus is an uncommon event, occurring in 4% of children with Wilms' tumor. Identification of vascular extension by preoperative radiographic studies or by palpation early in the surgical exploration is critical to avoid embolization during mobilization of the kidney. In one NWTSG report, 23 children with vascular extension were treated initially with chemotherapy after biopsy of the renal mass. Complete resolution of the tumor thrombus occurred in seven children, and all lesions except one decreased in size.[19] Of the 14 children with tumor initially extending into the atrium, only 4 had residual atrial involvement at resection requiring sternotomy and bypass. Tumor embolism did not occur during chemotherapy. This study suggests that children with atrial or caval involvement generally require less extensive resection after initial treatment with combination chemotherapy. A recent review of surgical management of patients with intravascular extension on NWTS-4 revealed no significant difference in complication rates between patients who underwent primary versus delayed resection. The authors note, however, that patients with atrial extension may be good candidates for neoadjuvant chemotherapy.[41]

Gross hematuria in children with Wilms' tumor is infrequent but should lead to suspicion of extensive involvement of the renal pelvis with possible extension into the ureter. Cystoscopy should be considered in these children to identify extension of the tumor into the bladder and avoid transection of the tumor with division of the ureter. Ureteral extension that is recognized and entirely resected does not increase the stage of the tumor.

Exploration of the contralateral kidney has been recommended by the NWTSG based on the 5% occurrence of synchronous lesions. A review of children with bilateral tumors treated on NWTS-4 identified 9 of 122 children in whom the diagnosis of bilateral disease was missed by the preoperative imaging studies [CT, ultrasonography, or magnetic resonance imaging (MRI)].[42]

The role of surgery in the treatment of pulmonary relapse has been evaluated by the NWTSG in 211 patients. Although diagnostic confirmation of relapse may be required, there was no therapeutic benefit identified to resection of a solitary pulmonary metastasis in addition to pulmonary radiotherapy and chemotherapy alone.[43] Four-year survival rates were identical in the two groups.

Radiation Therapy

Pioneering radiation oncologists first noted that Wilms' tumors were responsive to radiation therapy in the 1950s. Initially, the radiation treatment volume was extended across the midline to include the entire circumference of the implicated vertebral bodies.[44] This approach was taken to equalize the growth suppression. Irradiation of only one side of a vertebra had been shown to lead to an obligatory scoliosis convex away from the irradiated side.

The original radiation therapy concepts have since been modified as the result of the clinical trials conducted by the NWTSG. For example, the age-adjusted dosages were shown to be unnecessary in tumors of favorable histology. The advent of effective drugs had a profound effect, not only on the general management of these children but also on the indications for the administration of postnephrectomy abdominal irradiation. Presumed microscopic residual disease in the tumor bed of children with stage I favorable histology Wilms' tumor can be successfully treated with combination chemotherapy rather than flank irradiation. This was demonstrated in the first two NWTSG randomized clinical trials that indicated the overall relapse-free survival rate in all patients, regardless of age, was similar to that of irradiated patients in NWTS-1 who had received chemotherapy with only dactinomycin. Retrospective analyses of the data accumulated in NWTS-1 and NWTS-2 were conducted to determine the patterns of relapse and to evaluate the relationship between abdominal radiation therapy dose and intraabdominal tumor recurrence.[45] In NWTS-3—the unirradiated and the irradiated (20 Gy) stage II—favorable histology patients had similar relapse-free survival percentages, as did those with stage III favorable histology, who received nominal doses of 10 versus 20 Gy. Meanwhile, excellent results continued to be recorded for stage I favorable histology patients, none of who received radiation therapy.[46] In summary, NWTS-1, NWTS-2, and NWTS-3 demonstrated that stage I and II patients with favorable histology tumors who receive vincristine and dactinomycin do not require postoperative irradiation. A dose of 1000 cGy is sufficient for local control in stage III favorable histology patients if they also received chemotherapy with vincristine, dactinomycin, and doxorubicin.[47]

Whole lung irradiation (12 Gy) is recommended for patients who present with pulmonary metastases visible on plain chest radiography. Chemotherapy doses given immediately after the completion of whole lung irradiation are decreased by 50%.

A pilot study conducted by investigators from SIOP produced results similar to those of the NWTSG in stage IV favorable histology patients after treatment with nephrectomy and chemotherapy only.[48] Patients with persistent or recurrent lung nodules received whole lung radiation therapy or surgical removal of the metastatic lesions, or both. Using a similar approach, the United Kingdom Children's Cancer Study Group reported results inferior to those of the NWTSG in this group of patients.[49]

The potential adverse effects of whole lung irradiation and chemotherapy (which includes vincristine, dactinomycin, and doxorubicin as used in the NWTSG treatment regimens) include radiation pneumonitis or *Pneumocystis carinii* pneumonitis, or both. These complications are an important cause of morbidity and mortality in patients with stage IV Wilms' tumor.[50]

Patients with pulmonary lesions identified only on CT of the chest should undergo biopsy of one or more lesions to confirm that they are due to metastatic Wilms' tumor if treatment with whole lung irradiation and doxorubicin is planned. A report from St. Jude Children's Research Hospital suggested that such patients have an increased risk of pulmonary recurrence after treatment with chemotherapy only.[51] A review of the experience with such patients treated on NWTS-3 and NWTS-4 did not demonstrate a clear benefit of whole lung irradiation for such patients. The 4-year relapse-free survival rate was 89% among 53 irradiated patients and 80% among 37 unirradiated patients.[52,53] This improvement in relapse-free survival must be balanced against the increase in potential side effects of therapy, leaving the use of whole lung irradiation as a continued source of debate.

Chemotherapy

Wilms' tumor was the first pediatric malignant solid tumor found to be responsive to the systemic chemotherapeutic agent, dactinomycin.[54] Other active agents were subsequently identified, including vincristine, doxorubicin, and cyclophosphamide.[17]

FAVORABLE HISTOLOGY WILMS' TUMOR

NATIONAL WILMS' TUMOR STUDY-3

Patients with stage I Wilms' tumor were successfully treated using an 11-week regimen composed of vincristine and dactinomycin without abdominal irradiation. The 4-year relapse-free percentage and overall survival percentage with this regimen were 89.0% and 95.6%, respectively.[46]

Patients with stage II Wilms' tumor were randomized to receive vincristine and dactinomycin or these two drugs and doxorubicin. They were also randomized to receive tumor bed irradiation (20 Gy) or no radiation therapy. The 4-year relapse-free percentage and overall survival percentage for patients who were treated with vincristine and dactinomycin and no abdominal irradiation were 87.4% and 91.1%, respectively. There was no statistically significant difference between these results and those for the remaining three treatment regimens for patients with stage II favorable histology tumors.[46]

Patients with stage III Wilms' tumor were randomized to treatment with vincristine and dactinomycin or these two drugs and doxorubicin. They were also randomized to receive 10 or 20 Gy of abdominal irradiation. This study demonstrated that these patients benefited from the addition of doxorubicin to the two-drug combination of vincristine and dactinomycin. There was no statistically significant difference in the frequency of intraabdominal relapse among those treated with 10 Gy compared with 20 Gy. Although there was no statistically significant difference in the frequency of intraabdominal relapse in any of the subgroups, there appeared to be a higher frequency among those treated with vincristine and dactinomycin with 10 Gy (7 of 61), compared with those receiving vincristine and dactinomycin with 20 Gy (3 of 68) or vincristine, dactinomycin, and doxorubicin with 10 Gy (3 of

70).[47] The 4-year relapse-free percentage and overall survival percentage of those children treated with vincristine, dactinomycin, doxorubicin, and 10 Gy of abdominal irradiation were 82.0% and 90.9%, respectively.[46] Although improvement in relapse-free survival was achieved with the three-drug regimen, this did not result in an improvement in overall survival.

Patients with stage IV Wilms' tumor were randomized to receive vincristine, dactinomycin, and doxorubicin or these three drugs and cyclophosphamide (Cytoxan). All underwent immediate nephrectomy, and all received abdominal irradiation (20 Gy) and whole lung irradiation (12 Gy). The 4-year relapse-free percentage and overall survival percentage for the patients treated with vincristine, dactinomycin, and doxorubicin were 79.0% and 80.9%, respectively. There was no statistically significant improvement in the 4-year relapse-free percentage or overall survival percentage from the addition of cyclophosphamide to the three-drug regimen.[46]

NATIONAL WILMS' TUMOR STUDY-4

Previous success in treatment strategies allowed the design of a unique study, NWTS-4, with the primary aims of continuing to improve treatment results while decreasing the cost of therapy through modification of the schedule of drug administration. This study was based on experimental and clinical data demonstrating the safety and efficacy of dactinomycin when administered in a single, moderately high dose.[55]

The design of NWTS-4 allowed the results of pulse-intensive chemotherapy regimens using single doses of dactinomycin and doxorubicin to be compared with treatment regimens using divided-dose regimens of each drug. In addition, treatment durations of 6 and 15 months were compared in patients with stages II to IV favorable histology tumors.

Toxicity analyses confirmed that the pulse-intensive regimens not only delivered greater dose intensity but also produced less hematologic toxicity than the standard regimens. In addition, there were no statistically significant differences in the 2-year or 4-year relapse-free percentages or overall survival percentage of patients treated with pulse-intensive, compared with standard, modes of chemotherapy administration.[56]

TREATMENT

The following recommendations are based on the results of the NWTSG, which advocates early surgery without preoperative therapy and modulates therapy according to stage and histology (see Fig. 40.2-2 for current guidelines in NWTS-5). For stage I favorable or anaplastic histology and stage II favorable histology tumors, combination chemotherapy with vincristine and dactino-

Stage	Favorable Histology	Focal Anaplasia	Diffuse Anaplasia	Clear Cell Sarcoma
I	Regimen EE-4A	Regimen EE-4A	Regimen EE-4A	Regimen I
II	Regimen EE-4A	Regimen DD-4A	Regimen I	Regimen I
III	Regimen DD-4A	Regimen DD-4A	Regimen I	Regimen I
IV	Regimen DD-4A	Regimen DD-4A	Regimen I	Regimen I

FIGURE 40.2-2.   Current treatment regimens for patients entered on National Wilms' Tumor Study-5. Treatment guidelines by stage and histology.

mycin is recommended. No abdominal radiation therapy is necessary for these patients. Atrial nephrectomy alone, without chemotherapy (NWTS-5) for children younger than 24 months with small (less than 550 g) stage I favorable histology tumors was stopped early due to a recurrence rate that barely surpassed the 10% stopping threshold. All but one of these patients ultimately went into remission with salvage therapy.[57] Until this question is further assessed, the current North American approach continues to include an abbreviated 18-week course of adjuvant chemotherapy for this group of children. For stage III favorable histology tumors, combination chemotherapy with vincristine, dactinomycin, and doxorubicin and postnephrectomy abdominal radiation therapy are recommended. For stage IV favorable histology disease, combination chemotherapy with vincristine, dactinomycin, and doxorubicin and postnephrectomy abdominal radiation therapy if renal tumor is stage III are recommended. All patients with pulmonary metastases should receive whole lung radiation therapy. For stages II through IV anaplastic tumors, combination chemotherapy with dactinomycin, vincristine, doxorubicin, and cyclophosphamide is recommended. These more advanced-stage anaplastic patients should all receive abdominal radiation therapy. Patients with pulmonary metastases should undergo whole lung radiation therapy. For stages I through IV clear cell sarcoma of the kidney, combination chemotherapy with vincristine, dactinomycin, and doxorubicin is recommended. All of these patients should receive abdominal radiation therapy. As with favorable and anaplastic histologies, whole lung radiation therapy is reserved for patients with pulmonary metastases.

PROGNOSTIC FACTORS

Tumor size, age of the patient, histology, lymph node metastases, and local features of the tumor, such as capsular or vascular invasion, have been predictive of outcome. Modern treatments have been so successful that some of these factors no longer pertain.

The results of the first three NWTS were evaluated using logistic regression analysis. Children entered on NWTS-1 who were younger than 24 months had a significantly better prognosis than those who were older. The relapse rate was 14.8% for those younger than 2 years of age, compared with 34.7% for those between 2 and 4 years old, and 27.6% for those older than 4 years.[58]

The histology of Wilms' tumor was identified as the most important determinant of prognosis. More recent analyses have confirmed the importance of histopathology and lymph node involvement, whereas the prognostic significance of other factors, such as age and tumor size, changes as treatment efficacy improves.[58–60] As the survival for most children with Wilms' tumor now approaches 90% for patients with favorable histology, current and future challenges include identification of novel therapies for anaplastic tumors and validation of recently identified adverse biologic features that may facilitate improved risk group stratification for the small percentage of patients who fail despite favorable tumor histology.

NEUROBLASTOMA

EPIDEMIOLOGY AND GENETICS

Neuroblastoma is the most common malignant intraabdominal tumor in children. Based on the most recent epidemiologic survey compiled in 1995, neuroblastoma (including ganglioneuroblastoma) occurs at an annual rate of 9.1 cases per 1 million U.S. children younger than 15 years.[1] Neuroblastoma occurs more frequently in boys than in girls. The median age at diagnosis is 2 years for both boys and girls.[17] The majority of cases are diagnosed by 5 years of age. Metastatic disease is often present at initial presentation, affecting approximately 70% of newly diagnosed children.

Neuroblastoma has been pathologically documented in additional members of immediate and extended families, including parents, siblings, twins, and cousins.[17] Mediastinal or cervical neuroblastoma is associated with heterochromia and Horner's syndrome.[61] Patients with neuroblastoma have been diagnosed with several other conditions, including neurofibromatosis, Beckwith-Wiedemann syndrome, and Hirschsprung's disease.[62]

Neuroblastoma *in situ* was identified in 0.37% to 2.58% of infants younger than 3 months who died of other causes and underwent autopsy examination.[17] This finding suggests that the frequency of neuroblastoma may be higher than indicated by figures derived from death certificate diagnoses or clinical (pathologic) diagnoses. Many *in situ* neuroblastomas may undergo involution or maturation, or both.

PATHOLOGY

The microscopic features of a typical neuroblastoma include the presence of nests of tumor cells separated by fibrovascular septa, with additional areas of hemorrhage, calcification, and necrosis. The tumor cells are uniform round cells with a round hyperchromatic or densely speckled nucleus. Mitoses are not frequent. Homer-Wright rosettes, with a central fibrillar core, may be present.[63] Lymphocytic infiltration may be observed. Neuroblastoma may contain mature elements, including ganglion cells.

Histochemical stains may aid in the differentiation of neuroblastoma from other common pediatric solid tumors. The periodic acid–Schiff stain result is generally negative, and neuron-specific enolase is generally positive.[64]

Shimada and colleagues[65] developed a histologic classification of neuroblastomas that segregates tumors into two large groups: stroma-rich and stroma-poor tumors based on the presence or absence of schwannian spindle cell stroma. These histopathologic features were evaluated along with other characteristics, including patient age and the mitotic-karyorrhexis index for their importance in predicting prognosis. Patients with nodular, stroma-rich histology and undifferentiated, stroma-poor histology had a poor prognosis. The International Neuroblastoma Pathology Committee has developed a modification of the Shimada system[65] that was validated in a case-cohort sample of 227 neuroblastic tumors.[66] The International Neuroblastoma Pathology Classification (the Shimada system) is proposed for international use in assessing neuroblastic tumors. In a 2001 analysis[67] of 644 patients treated between 1995 and 1999, this histopathologic classification scheme was found to strongly correlate with other prognostic variables, including age at diagnosis, stage, primary tumor site, and biologic variables (i.e., N-myc copy number and DNA ploidy). The combination of the international neuroblastoma staging system and pathology classification has now been validated as a statistically significant prognostic tool and forms the basis of current strategies for risk group allocation in the management of newly diagnosed children with neuroblastoma.[67–69]

CLINICAL PRESENTATION AND NATURAL HISTORY

Neuroblastoma may originate from any sympathetic nervous system tissue in the body (Fig. 40.2-3). The most common site of origin of neuroblastoma is within the abdomen. The adrenal gland is the primary tumor site in 38% of cases. Other intraabdominal sites include the paravertebral sympathetic ganglia, celiac ganglion, superior mesenteric ganglion, and inferior mesenteric ganglion. The remaining patients with neuroblastoma have tumors that originate in the thorax or neck.[17]

Infants and children with neuroblastoma come to medical attention with a variety of signs and symptoms, most commonly the presence of abdominal swelling or an abdominal mass.

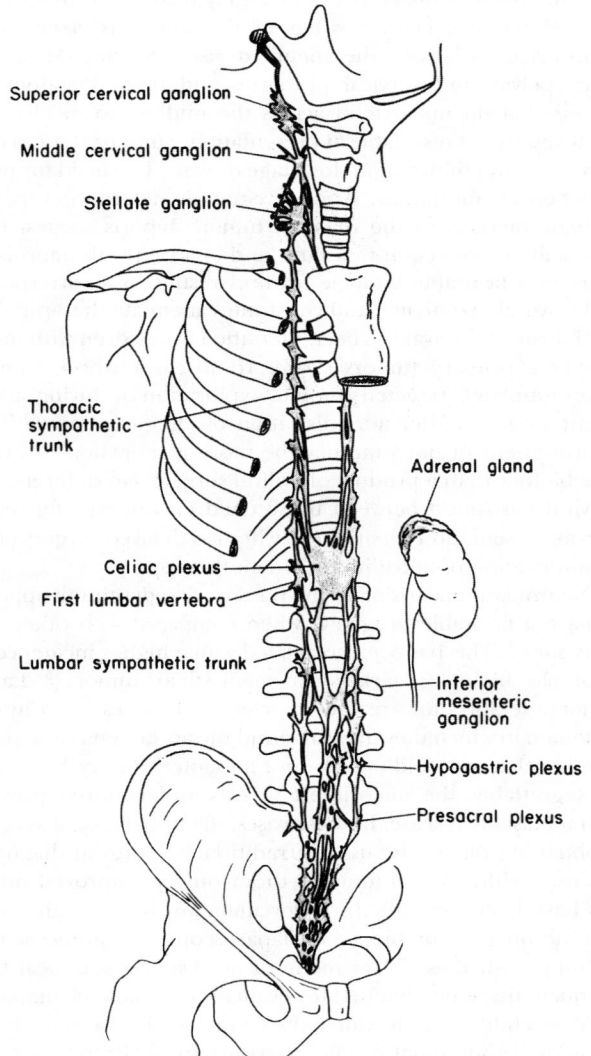

Superior cervical ganglion

Middle cervical ganglion

Stellate ganglion

Thoracic sympathetic trunk

Adrenal gland

Celiac plexus

First lumbar vertebra

Lumbar sympathetic trunk

Inferior mesenteric ganglion

Hypogastric plexus

Presacral plexus

FIGURE 40.2-3. Neuroblastoma may originate from the adrenal gland or any sympathetic nervous system plexus. (From House EL, Pansky B. General visceral efferent system. In: *A functional approach to neuroanatomy*, 2nd ed. New York: McGraw-Hill, 1967:281, with permission.)

Abdominal or thoracic paravertebral tumors frequently cause symptoms referable to the central nervous system. Children with hematogenous metastases may complain of pain in one or more bones or present with periorbital swelling or ecchymoses. Fever is present in 23% of patients at diagnosis. Uncommon clinical presentations include hydrops fetalis,[61] chronic diarrhea due to secretion of vasoactive intestinal polypeptide by the tumor,[70] and myoclonus-opsoclonus, a movement disorder often accompanied by significant cognitive impairment.[71] Hypertension is an uncommon presenting sign in children with neuroblastoma.[72]

Infants and children with neuroblastoma frequently present with hematogenous metastases. These have been identified in 62% of patients. The most frequently involved sites are bones, liver, bone marrow, and skin.[62]

Normal sympathetic tissues secrete the catecholamines epinephrine and norepinephrine. Most patients with neuroblastoma have increased urinary excretion of vanillylmandelic acid, homovanillic acid, dihydroxyphenylalanine, dopamine, and norepinephrine at the time of diagnosis.[62]

Mass screening of infants at 4 months of age has been used in Kyoto, Japan, since 1974 and throughout Japan since 1985. A similar screening program was undertaken in Canada and Germany. Mass screening in all three series has led to the preclinical identification of increased numbers of infants with favorable tumor biology who would have had an excellent prognosis with little, if any, therapy. Neither screening effort has had any effect on the number of children identified with clinically advanced disease and unfavorable tumor biology. To date, newborn screening has had a negligible impact on survival and may have led to overtreatment of children with good prognostic features.[73,74]

STAGING

Local features of neuroblastoma that can be related to treatment success include the extent of the primary tumor and the presence or absence of lymph node metastases. Dissemination of tumor to the liver, subcutaneous tissue, bone marrow, and bones can also influence prognosis.

Evans and colleagues developed a staging system—first reported in 1971—that considered the extent of the primary tumor, the presence or absence of regional lymph node tumor metastases, and the presence or absence of hematogenous metastases in determining the tumor stage. This system recognized the existence of a unique group of infants with small primary tumors and liver, skin, and bone marrow metastases but without positive findings in the skeletal survey (stage IVS). This system demonstrated the favorable prognosis of patients with localized primary tumors but did not consider the possible independent effects of lymph node involvement or surgical excision on prognosis.[75]

A new staging system, the International Neuroblastoma Staging System, was proposed in 1988.[76] Because of ambiguity regarding the classification of tumors originating near the midline and having a favorable prognosis,[77] the staging system was revised in 1993.[78] This staging system, shown in Table 40.2-3, is currently used in North American and European cooperative group studies.

CLINICAL EVALUATION

The evaluation of a child suspected to have neuroblastoma begins with a careful history. The review of systems should

TABLE 40.2-3. International Neuroblastoma Staging System

Stage	Description
I	Localized tumor with complete gross excision, with or without microscopic residual disease; representative ipsilateral lymph nodes negative for tumor microscopically (nodes attached to and removed with the primary tumor may be positive).
IIA	Localized tumor with incomplete gross excision; representative ipsilateral nonadherent lymph nodes negative for tumor microscopically.
IIB	Localized tumor with or without complete gross excision, with ipsilateral nonadherent lymph nodes positive for tumor. Enlarged contralateral lymph nodes must be negative microscopically.
III	Unresectable unilateral tumor infiltrating across the midline (defined as the vertebral column), with or without regional lymph node involvement; or localized unilateral tumor with contralateral lymph node involvement; or midline tumor with bilateral extension by infiltration (unresectable) or by lymph node involvement.
IV	Any primary tumor with dissemination to distant lymph nodes, bone, bone marrow, liver, skin, or other organs (except as defined for stage IVS).
IVS	Localized primary tumor (as defined for stage I, IIA or IIB), with dissemination limited to skin, liver, or bone marrow (<10% of nucleated cells identified as malignant), limited to infants younger than 1 y of age.

include careful questioning regarding symptoms, such as diarrhea and ataxia. The physical examination should include a careful examination of the skin. Subcutaneous metastases from neuroblastoma are reddish-purple, raised lesions that may be solitary. Periorbital ecchymoses are a frequent finding in children with disseminated tumor and orbital involvement. Owing to the paraspinal location of many tumors, a careful neurologic examination should be performed.

The laboratory examination of a child suspected to have a neuroblastoma should include a complete blood cell count, urinalysis, liver and renal function tests, sedimentation rate, serum ferritin, and a urine sample for quantitation of the excretion of vanillylmandelic acid and total catecholamines.

Radiographic evaluation of a child with an abdominal mass suspected to be a neuroblastoma begins with a plain supine examination of the abdomen that may demonstrate the presence of a soft tissue mass frequently having calcification. Abdominal ultrasonography demonstrates the presence of a solid mass that may contain cystic areas. CT and MRI provide information regarding the extent of intraabdominal disease that is not obtained with the plain radiography or abdominal ultrasound. Patients with thoracic neuroblastomas typically have a posterior mediastinal mass demonstrated on plain chest radiography. Calcification is present within this mass less frequently than within primary intraabdominal neuroblastomas. Detailed films of the ribs and vertebral bodies may demonstrate erosion of the adjacent ribs, transverse processes, and widening of the intervertebral foramina.

Patients with paraspinal primary tumors may have asymptomatic extension of the tumor through the spinal foramina. In view of the increased risk of neurologic compromise with paraspinal tumors, patients with tumors in this location should undergo careful evaluation of the spinal canal using MRI with gadolinium.

All patients should have a conventional skeletal survey, including the long bones, spine, ribs, and skull, and a technetium 99m methylene diphosphonate bone scan. Although most bone metastases are identified using the radionuclide bone scan, occasional lesions, especially in the metaphyses of long bones, are identified only on the conventional skeletal survey.[79]

Bilateral trephine bone marrow biopsies and bone marrow aspirates should be performed. The biopsy is positive in 11% to 30% of children with negative bone marrow aspirate results.[80] Bone marrow replacement by tumor is occasionally so extensive that the microscopic picture resembles acute leukemia.

TREATMENT

Surgery

Surgery plays a major role in the treatment of low-stage neuroblastoma. The surgical approach varies depending on the stage and site of the primary. It is now widely recognized that defining the biologic characteristics of the tumor is essential to appropriate, risk-based therapeutic decision making. Most thoracic, pelvic, and cervical primaries and limited abdominal lesions that do not extend across the midline to involve the great vessels are resectable at presentation. Surgery alone is curative in many children with low-stage disease. The need for postresection chemotherapy is now frequently determined by the biologic markers of the resected tumor. Reports suggest that even subtotal resection in infants and children with neuroblastoma with favorable biologic features results in a correspondingly favorable outcome and constitutes adequate therapy.[81,82]

Improved survival has been identified in children with more extensive primary tumors (stage III disease) whose tumors were completely resected at initial exploration or during subsequent surgeries after administration of chemotherapy.[83] This improvement in outcome may be more a reflection of favorable biology than a product of skillful surgery. No difference in survival was found between those children undergoing resection at presentation versus those who had delayed surgery after administration of neoadjuvant chemotherapy.

Neuroblastoma arising in the posterior mediastinum appears to have a favorable prognosis when compared with other primary sites.[84] This has been correlated with a higher incidence of favorable biologic markers in mediastinal tumors.[85] Large tumors are also more readily resected in the chest than in the abdomen in which they may surround the aorta, vena cava, renal vessels, celiac axis, and the superior mesenteric artery.[86]

Regrettably, the majority of infants and children present with metastatic disease. In these cases, the initial role of surgery is obtaining diagnostic tissue. Traditionally, surgical diagnosis has used either laparotomy or thoracotomy. Improved methods have been developed for percutaneous biopsy with radiographic imaging or biopsy via laparoscopic or thoracoscopic techniques. If these latter methods are used, it is critical that adequate tissue be obtained for evaluation of biologic markers.

Most children with widely disseminated disease have large primaries. Abdominal primaries arising from adrenal or paravertebral sites often encircle the celiac axis and the superior mesenteric vessels. Several studies have demonstrated that resection of these extensive lesions can be best accomplished after initial treatment with chemotherapy. In addition to reducing tumor volume, preoperative chemotherapy decreases the vascularity and friability of the tumor. This neoadjuvant approach has also contributed to decreased operative morbidity,[87] including a lower complication rate with nephrectomy.[88]

Postoperative diarrhea may complicate resections of extensive tumors surrounding the superior mesenteric or celiac arteries.[89] This increased stool output is presumably produced by disruption of the autonomic nerve supply to the gut and is not related to the timing of surgery. Several studies have demonstrated an apparent decrease in the frequency of local recurrences after resection of the primary in stage IV tumors.[90,91] Improved survival, however, has not been achieved because the majority of these advanced-stage patients ultimately succumb to relapse at distant sites.[92] As systemic therapy improves, local control will become more critical.

Attempts should be made to preserve the ipsilateral kidney during resection of the primary tumor in children with stage IV neuroblastoma.[93] Many of these children receive either a bone marrow transplant or nephrotoxic agents, making maximal preservation of renal function an important goal. Children with adrenal or paravertebral primaries generally have metastatic tumor in lymph nodes that wraps around the renal vessels. These must be dissected free to preserve the kidney. The risk of nephrectomy is greatest in children undergoing resection before the administration of chemotherapy.[87]

Infants with stage IVS disease require exploration or a percutaneous biopsy for diagnosis. In most cases, resection is not necessary unless the most readily obtained tissue for diagnosis is a small, easily resected primary.[94] There is no convincing evidence that resection of the primary will accelerate or ensure resolution of metastatic disease.[95] In fact, one review of 110 infants with stage IVS disease treated by members of the Pediatric Oncology Group (POG) showed that there was no statistical difference in survival rate for patients with complete resection of their primary tumor compared with those who underwent partial resection or biopsy only.[96] Decreased survival was associated with age younger than 2 months, diploid DNA complement, amplification of the N-myc protooncogene, or tumors with unfavorable histology. If a mass remains at the primary site after resolution of the distant disease, resection is often performed and frequently demonstrates a ganglioneuroma or neuroblastoma with extensive maturation. Surgical techniques have been developed for abdominal expansion for infants presenting with extensive hepatomegaly that impairs respiratory function. The abdominal fascia is divided, and prosthetic material is inserted to increase the volume of the abdominal cavity.[97]

Antenatal diagnosis of neuroblastoma appears to identify a particularly good risk population of infants. The biologic markers on these tumors are favorable. In keeping with their less aggressive biology, infants have done well after resection of the primary tumor.[98] It is not known whether spontaneous regression would occur if these infants were observed, but a report of four infants with antenatal diagnosis of adrenal masses (two solid and two cystic) demonstrated resolution of the abnormalities by 2.5 to 8.0 weeks of age.[99]

Radiation Therapy

Radiation therapy has been used in the treatment of patients with neuroblastoma both to decrease the frequency of local tumor recurrence and to eradicate microscopic or macro-

scopic distant metastases. Wyatt and Farber systematically treated patients with neuroblastoma with local irradiation. They suggested radiation therapy should be instituted in every case once the diagnosis is established.[100] Although neuroblastoma is very sensitive to ionizing radiation, this modality is currently used much more selectively in low-stage patients with uniquely favorable biology and infants with stage 4S disease.[101]

Reports have demonstrated that patients with stage I (International Neuroblastoma Staging System) neuroblastoma have a 4-year relapse-free survival percentage of 89% when treated with surgery only.[102] Children with stage II (Evans') neuroblastoma with microscopic residual disease may benefit from local irradiation.[103] The POG randomized patients with stage C neuroblastoma to treatment with postoperative chemotherapy or postoperative chemotherapy and local irradiation (24 to 30 Gy). The 3-year event-free survival (EFS) percentage was 32% for patients with stage III (Evans') randomized to treatment with combination chemotherapy, compared with 59% for those randomized to the same chemotherapy and local radiation therapy ($P = .009$).[104] Thus, in patients with residual disease or positive lymph nodes, the addition of radiation therapy appears to improve the prognosis. Refinements of these recommendations may be necessary in the future as newer studies that use biologic markers for treatment stratification identify subsets that do or do not benefit from local radiation therapy.

Chemotherapy

Although three published studies offer a glimmer of hope for metastatic patients treated with dose-intensive regimens incorporating stem cell support,[105–107] prospects for long-term survival in advanced-stage disease remain poor despite increasingly toxic therapies. At the other end of the spectrum, trials conducted in patients without evidence of gross residual disease after tumor resection have not demonstrated a survival advantage for adjuvant chemotherapy. For patients with more advanced disease or unfavorable tumor biology, combination chemotherapy has improved survival. The relatively small proportion of low-risk patients who require adjuvant therapy and all intermediate-risk patients are currently treated with regimens that include carboplatinum, cyclophosphamide, doxorubicin, and etoposide. High-risk patients are treated with a similar array of agents, augmented by the addition of ifosfamide and high-dose cisplatinum, followed by a variety of dose-intensive consolidation regimens.

The poor response of patients with metastatic neuroblastoma to aggressive combination chemotherapy programs stimulated clinical trials that incorporated autologous bone marrow transplantation (ABMT) or peripheral blood stem cell rescue. Reports of EFS 2 years after ABMT have ranged from 6% to 64% among progression-free patients with advanced neuroblastoma who received single or tandem bone marrow transplants.[105–110] The spectrum of results may reflect patient selection. A retrospective analysis by the POG showed no significant prognostic benefit of changing, in remission, from conventional therapy to bone marrow transplant.[111] The Children's Cancer Group (CCG) reported the results of a randomized trial comparing the outcome after intensive chemotherapy without bone marrow transplant to that after ABMT. The 3-year EFS was 34% ± 4% for those randomized to ABMT, compared with 22% ± 4% for those randomized to continuation chemo-

TABLE 40.2-4.   Risk Group and Protocol Assignment Schema: Pediatric Oncology Group and Children's Cancer Group

International Neuroblastoma Staging System Stage	Age (Y)	N-myc Status	Shimada Histology	DNA Ploidy	Risk Group/Study
1	0–21	Any	Any	Any	Low
2A and 2B	<1	Any	Any	Any	Low
	≥1–21	Nonamplified[a]	Any	NA	Low
	≥1–21	Amplified[b]	Favorable	NA	Low
	≥1–21	Amplified	Unfavorable	NA	High
3	<1	Nonamplified	Any	Any	Intermediate
	<1	Amplified	Any	Any	High
	≥1–21	Nonamplified	Favorable	NA	Intermediate
	≥1–21	Nonamplified	Unfavorable	NA	High
	≥1–21	Amplified	Any	NA	High
4	<1	Nonamplified	Any	Any	Intermediate
	<1	Amplified	Any	Any	High
	≥1–21	Any	Any	NA	High
4S	<1	Nonamplified	Favorable	>1	Low
	<1	Nonamplified	Any	1	Intermediate
	<1	Nonamplified	Unfavorable	Any	Intermediate
	<1	Amplified	Any	Any	High

NA, not applicable.
[a]N-myc copy number ≤10.
[b]N-myc copy number >10.

therapy (P = .034). A secondary randomization involving a 6-month course of 13-*cis*-retinoic acid after completion of treatment produced a 3-year relapse-free survival rate of 46% ± 6% for those who received the drug. This outcome compared favorably with the 29% ± 5% relapse-free survival for patients who were not randomized to treatment with *cis*-retinoic acid (P = .027).[105] Current treatment protocols used by the Children's Oncology Group (COG) stratify patients into low-, intermediate-, and high-risk cohorts by stage, age, N-myc status, Shimada histology, and DNA ploidy (Table 40.2-4). Overall 3-year survival for children with low-risk neuroblastoma (stages 1, 2, and 4S; favorable histology; no N-myc amplification; typically hyperdiploid) is excellent, exceeding 90% in large cooperative group studies. Intermediate-risk patients include children with stage 3 and 4 disease without N-myc amplification. High-risk patients typically have higher-stage disease with N-myc amplification, which is frequently accompanied by unfavorable histology. This latter group of patients has a much poorer prognosis, with 3-year survival typically approaching 20% to 30% in most published series.

Low-Risk Patients

Children with stage I neuroblastoma have an extremely good prognosis after excision of the primary tumor without adjuvant therapy. Children with stage II disease with a single copy of N-myc, regardless of histology, have an excellent prognosis after tumor excision alone. Stage II patients with more than ten copies of N-myc and favorable Shimada histology also have a good prognosis after tumor resection. Despite the amplification of N-myc in this subset of children with localized disease, the favorable Shimada histology has sufficient predictive power that radiation and chemotherapy are not recommended unless recurrence is documented. Perhaps the most unique cohort of low-risk patients consists of asymptomatic infants with dissemi-

nated stage IVS neuroblastoma and hyperdiploidy (DNA index greater than 1.0). Since many of these infants spontaneously improve, they should be observed without treatment.

Intermediate-Risk Patients

Among children without N-myc amplification, those with stage III neuroblastoma who are younger than 12 months, stage III patients with favorable Shimada histology who are older than 12 months, and those with stage IV neuroblastoma who are younger than 12 months all have a moderate risk of disease recurrence. Their treatment may include local radiation therapy and combination chemotherapy. As noted earlier in Surgery, infants with stage IVS neuroblastoma require supportive care only. Those younger than 6 weeks at diagnosis may have feeding intolerance or respiratory insufficiency due to massive hepatomegaly, mandating a brief course of chemotherapy.

High-Risk Patients

All children with N-myc amplification, regardless of stage, and all children older than 1 year with stage IV neuroblastoma have a substantial risk of disease progression. These children should be treated using study regimens being evaluated by the national or international pediatric clinical trials groups. The role of consolidation with high-dose chemotherapy with peripheral blood stem cell rescue (with or without total body irradiation) is being evaluated in the subgroup of patients who have a favorable response to combination chemotherapy. Single, tandem, and even triple courses of consolidation therapy are currently under investigation.[112,113]

In an effort to improve the unsatisfactory results of high-dose chemoradiotherapy, several groups of investigators have explored strategies targeted at minimal residual disease. These include the use of the anti-G_{D2} monoclonal antibody 3F8 that targets the ganglioside G$_{D2}$, which is uniquely expressed at high levels on the surface of neuroblastoma cells.[114] In an alternative approach, metaiodobenzylguanidine, a guanethidine derivative that is concentrated in catecholamine-producing cells (including neuroblastoma) has been conjugated to iodine 131 to target residual disease.[115] Both of these approaches show promise in pilot studies but must be further investigated in larger clinical trials.

PROGNOSTIC FACTORS

Breslow and McCann evaluated the interaction between age at diagnosis, stage (Evans'), and probability of survival. These investigators confirmed the adverse effect of increasing age at diagnosis and advanced stage on the probability of survival.[116]

Look and coworkers reported that patients with hyperdiploid tumor cells had a more favorable response to combination chemotherapy than did patients with diploid tumor cells.[117] Brodeur and colleagues demonstrated the relationship between advanced tumor stage and increased copy number of N-myc.[118] Approximately one-third of patients with advanced-stage disease have tumors characterized by amplification of the N-myc protooncogene. Nakagawara and associates have reported that increased expression of Trk A is associated with a favorable prognosis.[119] In addition to the prognostic value of Trk A, expression levels of another neurotrophin receptor, Trk B, have been shown to be predictive of outcome, albeit in a more complex fashion. Whereas high levels of the full-length Trk B receptor are correlated with aggressive tumor biology, high levels of a truncated form of Trk B are strongly correlated with good prognosis, particularly when associated with low levels of full-length Trk B expression. Deletion of the short arm of chromosome 1 (1p⁻) is associated with a poor prognosis, particularly when associated with gains of chromosomal material on the long arm of chromosome 17 (17q gain). Gains of chromosome arm 17q are the most frequent genetic perturbation identified in neuroblastoma, affecting 50% of all tumors that have been interrogated using the technique of comparative genomic hybridization.[120] As noted earlier, current treatment programs use a complex risk group stratification algorithm that includes age, stage, histology, N-myc status, and ploidy.[62,121] Although this classification scheme has great predictive value, the additional biologic characteristics just described may further refine our ability to appropriately calibrate our therapeutic interventions.

RETINOBLASTOMA

Retinoblastoma is the most frequent malignant ocular tumor in pediatric patients. It is also one of the most curable neoplasms affecting young children, with survival exceeding 90%.

EPIDEMIOLOGY AND GENETICS

The incidence rate per year is 3.7 cases per 1 million U.S. children younger than 15 years of age.[1] Approximately 70% to 75% of all cases are unilateral. Among children with unilateral disease, 10% to 15% have hereditary germline deletions of chromosome 13, band q14, which contains the RB1 tumor suppressor gene locus. Germline mutations of 13q14 uniformly affect the 25% to 30% of children with bilateral disease. Retin-

oblastoma occurs slightly more frequently in boys than in girls, especially among those who have bilateral retinoblastoma. The median age at diagnosis was 2 years for boys and 1 year for girls with unilateral retinoblastoma. In cases of bilateral disease, the median age at diagnosis is less than 12 months for both boys and girls.[17]

Whereas the majority of new cases of retinoblastoma arise spontaneously from new somatic mutations, a significant, and possibly increasing, fraction of retinoblastoma cases are hereditary. The familial pattern may demonstrate direct transmission of retinoblastoma from parent to child or the presence of two or more affected offspring from unaffected parents who have affected first-degree relatives. Retinoblastoma is transmitted in each of these situations as a highly penetrant, autosomal dominant trait.[122] An analysis of the offspring of patients with sporadic, bilateral retinoblastoma demonstrated that 49.2% of the offspring developed the disease. This suggests that essentially all patients with sporadic, bilateral retinoblastoma had a germinal mutation that was transmitted in an identical manner as in families with a positive history of retinoblastoma. Approximately 5.5% of the offspring of patients with sporadic, unilateral retinoblastoma developed the disease, suggesting that 9.9% to 12.3% of patients with sporadic, unilateral retinoblastoma actually have a germinal mutation that may be transmitted to their offspring.[123]

A more complex problem in genetic counseling arises when one is asked to estimate the risk of an unaffected member of a sibship with a positive family history for retinoblastoma who carries the retinoblastoma gene. It is also difficult to estimate the risk for recurrence of retinoblastoma in a sibship from unaffected parents with one affected sibling. Nussbaum and Puck have analyzed these situations and developed equations for estimating these various probabilities.[124]

The parents and siblings of all patients with retinoblastoma should have a thorough ophthalmoscopic examination. Retinoblastomas may undergo spontaneous regression, leaving characteristic retinal changes.[125] Margo and associates suggested such lesions were benign at their outset. These lesions indicated the presence of the same mutation found in patients with retinoblastoma, although they occurred in a more mature retinal cell.[126]

PATHOLOGY

The gross appearance of retinoblastoma is that of a chalky white, friable tumor with dense foci of calcification. Those arising from cells in the internal nuclear layer, nerve fiber layer, ganglion cell layer, or external nuclear layer grow toward the subretinal space, pushing the retina inward and frequently causing retinal detachment. Multiple foci of tumor are usually present.[127]

Retinoblastoma is composed of uniform small, round, or polygonal cells, which have scanty, poorly staining cytoplasm. The sparse cytoplasm is located at one side of the cell, suggesting the appearance of an embryonal retinal cell. The nucleus is large and deeply staining. Three types of cellular arrangements may be identified: the Homer-Wright rosette (a radial arrangement of cells surrounding a tangle of fibrils), the Flexner-Wintersteiner rosette (a radial arrangement of cuboidal to short columnar cells about a lumen, with the nuclei displaced basally, away from the lumen), and the fleurette (areas composed of pale-appearing cells, with abundant, pale eosinophilic cytoplasm and small, hyperchromatic nuclei; the cells are arranged in a *fleur-de-lis* pattern). Calcification and necrosis are often observed in retinoblastomas.[128]

CLINICAL PRESENTATION

Patients with retinoblastoma come to medical attention most frequently because of the presence of leukokoria. Strabismus, conjunctival erythema, or decreased visual acuity are other common presenting complaints. The tumor may be diagnosed during a routine examination performed because of a family history of retinoblastoma or during an examination for an unrelated complaint in patients without a family history of retinoblastoma.

The physical examination reveals the presence of a white pupillary reflex. Tumors located near the macula may be readily apparent with direct ophthalmoscopy, whereas those located at the periphery of the retina may not be detected unless the patient looks in a particular direction. Esotropia or exotropia may be identified. The eye may be red and painful due to uveitis after spontaneous necrosis of a retinal tumor or due to glaucoma. Decreased visual acuity may be due to involvement of the macula by the tumor or the presence of cells and debris in the vitreous.[127]

EVALUATION

The diagnosis of retinoblastoma is based on the clinical history of the patient (including the family history) and the results of an examination of both eyes under general anesthesia. In addition to meticulous inspection of both eyes, the staging evaluation of a child with suspected retinoblastoma may include CT of the orbit or orbital ultrasonography.[129] CT may be used to define the extent of the intraocular tumor and to determine the presence and extent of extraocular disease. Calcification was identified in orbital CT scans of 48% of patients with retinoblastoma confined to the globe, compared with 13% of patients with tumor extension beyond the globe.[130] Head CT or MRI may identify intracranial extension in patients who have normal plain radiographs of the bones adjacent to the orbit. Retinoblastoma may metastasize to the central nervous system, bones, or bone marrow.[131] The risk of such dissemination is related to the extent of the ocular tumor. A diagnostic lumbar puncture with examination of the cerebrospinal fluid after cytocentrifugation should be performed on all patients with involvement of the choroid, ora serrata, ciliary body, or anterior chamber. It should also be performed on patients with involvement of other extraocular structures, including the orbit or optic nerve, or when symptoms, signs, or diagnostic imaging studies suggest involvement of bones, soft tissues, or the central nervous system.[132]

Radionuclide bone scans should be obtained only for patients with extensive ocular involvement, symptoms suggesting the presence of a bone metastasis, and bone marrow involvement by retinoblastoma.[133]

STAGING

Martin and Reese proposed the first staging system for patients with retinoblastoma in 1942. The classification segregated patients into large treatment groups and established four catego-

TABLE 40.2-5.   Staging System for Retinoblastoma (Reese and Ellsworth)[136]

Group	Description
GROUP I	
A	Solitary tumor, <4 disc diameters in size, at or behind the equator
B	Multiple tumors, 4–10 disc diameters in size, all at or behind the equator
GROUP II	
A	Solitary tumor, 4–10 disc diameters in size, at or behind the equator
B	Multiple tumors, 4–10 disc diameters in size, behind the equator
GROUP III	
A	Any lesion anterior to the equator
B	Solitary tumors >10 disc diameters behind the equator
GROUP IV	
A	Multiple tumors, some >10 disc diameters
B	Any lesion extending anteriorly to the ora serrata
GROUP V	
A	Massive tumors involving more than one-half the retina
B	Vitreous seeding

ries: (1) unilateral tumors not extending outside of globe, (2) bilateral tumors, (3) residual tumors in the optic nerve or orbit at the time of enucleation or recurrent tumors after enucleation, and (4) widely disseminated retinoblastoma.[134] These investigators recognized the more favorable prognosis of patients with a small flat tumor and the ominous nature of tumors that extended toward the vitreous or into the choroid.[135] Subsequently, those patients with anteriorly located tumors were shown to have an unfavorable prognosis.[136] These factors were considered in developing a more detailed staging system (Table 40.2-5).

A useful staging system for patients with retinoblastoma must incorporate those features known to influence prognosis or therapy, or both. Simplicity would allow easy adoption of the system by investigators at many treatment centers. The system adopted by the St. Jude Children's Research Hospital incorporates many of these features (Table 40.2-6).[137,138]

TREATMENT: SURGICAL CONSIDERATIONS

In view of the excellent response of this tumor to vision-sparing interventions, including photocoagulation, cryotherapy, hyperthermia, plaque radiotherapy, and chemotherapy, enucleation of the involved eye must be undertaken very selectively. Given the high percentage of long-term survivors, treatment decisions must carefully weigh the functional outcome and potential long-term sequelae of local and systemic therapies.[139] The indications for enucleation include (1) unilateral retinoblastoma that completely fills the globe or that has damaged and disrupted the retina so extensively that restoration of useful vision is not possible, (2) bilateral retinoblastoma in which the previously mentioned conditions exist in only one eye, (3) a tumor present in the anterior chamber, (4) painful glaucoma with loss of vision after rubeosis iridis, (5) extensive bilateral retinoblastoma in which there is no potential for restoration of useful vision, (6) retinoblastoma unresponsive to other forms of local therapy, and (7) cases with permanent vision loss in which intraocular tumor is suspected.[140]

TABLE 40.2-6. Staging System for Retinoblastoma (St. Jude Children's Research Hospital)

Stage	Description
STAGE I	Tumor (unifocal or multifocal) confined to retina
A	Occupying one quadrant or less
B	Occupying two quadrants or less
C	Occupying more than 50% of retinal surface
STAGE II	Tumor (unifocal or multifocal) confined to globe
A	With vitreous seeding
B	Extending to optic nerve head
C	Extending to choroid
D	Extending to choroid and optic nerve head
E	Extending to emissaries
STAGE III	Extraocular extension of tumor (regional)
A	Extending beyond cut end of optic nerve (including subarachnoid extension)
B	Extending through sclera into orbital contents
C	Extending to choroid and beyond cut end of optic nerve (including subarachnoid extension)
D	Extending through sclera into orbital contents and beyond cut end of optic nerve (including subarachnoid extension)
STAGE IV	Distant metastases
A	Extending through optic nerve to brain
B	Blood-borne metastases to soft tissues and bones
C	Bone marrow metastases

ADVANCED UNILATERAL DISEASE

Patients with suspected retinoblastoma should be referred to a pediatric ophthalmologist experienced with the treatment of retinoblastoma. The standard surgical technique is modified to allow excision of the longest possible segment of optic nerve in continuity with the globe. The surgeon must be careful not to perforate the globe when the extraocular muscles are divided. The globe and optic nerve are inspected for evidence of extraocular extension of the tumor. Orbital biopsies should be obtained when extraocular extension is suspected to be present. After the globe is enucleated, a plastic implant is placed in the muscle funnel. Although the presence of the ocular prosthesis may prevent early detection of an orbital recurrence of tumor, the cosmetic result and promotion of normal development of the bony orbit are considerably improved with the use of a prosthesis.[141]

The importance of including a sufficient (10 to 15 mm) length of optic nerve in the surgical specimen is emphasized by reports of inferior survival rates among patients with extension of retinoblastoma to the margin of the excised optic nerve.[142]

The survival rate reported for patients with retinoblastoma confined to one or both globes, treated only with enucleation, was 86% for those with unilateral disease and 97% for those with bilateral disease.[17]

LIMITED UNILATERAL OR LIMITED BILATERAL DISEASE

Patients with limited unilateral or bilateral residual or recurrent disease after radiation therapy may benefit from photocoagulation or cryotherapy. Photocoagulation was reported to have successfully eradicated retinoblastomas in 80% of the patients treated. Hopping and Meyer-Schwickerath stated that suitable cases for this technique included solitary or multiple tumors, less than four to five disc diameters in size, situated at or posterior to the equator. Tumors located near the macula or papillary area and those with a mushroom shape should not be treated with photocoagulation.[143]

Cryotherapy was first used for the treatment of a patient with retinoblastoma in 1963.[144] Subsequent reports that included some patients treated sequentially with local irradiation and cryotherapy suggested long-term control of retinoblastoma was possible using this technique. Abramson and colleagues reported long-term control of retinoblastoma with one cryotherapy session in 80% of patients with previously untreated tumors, 59% of new postirradiation tumors, and 56% of recurrent tumors after irradiation. Tumors arising from the vitreous base were not responsive to cryotherapy. These investigators stated that previously untreated patients with tumors located anterior to the equator and those with recurrent or new tumors after irradiation were candidates for cryotherapy.[145] Cryotherapy is generally effective for tumors up to 2.5 mm in diameter and 1.0 mm thick that are confined to the sensory retina.[146]

BILATERAL DISEASE

Historically, external-beam irradiation was used for the treatment of the less involved eye after enucleation of the more involved eye of a patient with bilateral retinoblastoma. The decision to irradiate or enucleate the remaining eye was based on consideration of the location of the tumor, the presence of multiple foci of the tumor or vitreous seeding with tumor, and the size of the tumor.

The development of megavoltage radiation allowed the design of treatment plans that could irradiate the retinal surface to a uniform dose, whereas relatively sparing the posterior surface of the lens. All current techniques require meticulous attention to daily field placement. Treatment can be administered reproducibly with the use of general anesthesia. Many radiation oncologists prefer to use a single, temporal field, moving the edge of the field anteriorly in patients who are at high risk of anterior recurrence of tumor.[147]

Many new techniques have been proposed for a more conformal dose distribution in retinoblastoma.[148] Proton beam therapy or stereotactic techniques offer significant advantages in sparing normal tissues. For example, even with the conventional small fields used, the posterior field edge frequently encompasses the hypothalamic and pituitary area. This may lead to the late occurrence of endocrine dysfunction. Proton beam techniques avoid such an exit dose to normal structures.[149]

Increased awareness of the risk of retinoblastoma among the siblings and offspring of retinoblastoma patients resulted in the diagnosis of tumors when they were small. Abramson and coworkers reported on the treatment of patients with early, bilateral retinoblastoma using bilateral irradiation.[150] The radiation dose used for the treatment of the majority of the patients was 35 Gy. Residual tumors were present in 37% of the eyes when treatment was completed, and additional tumors developed in 16% of the eyes treated. All patients had group I, II, or III tumors. The risk of developing a second, nonocular malignancy in this group of irradiated patients is significant.[150] Overall, the cumulative risk of developing a second malignancy in patients with bilateral retinoblastoma is 51% at 50 years of age. This stands in striking contrast to the 5% incidence of second cancers observed in patients with unilateral disease, most of who do not carry germline mutations. Among children treated with external-beam radiation therapy (EBRT), the incidence of second malignancies has been reported to be as high as 35% at 30 years from initial diagnosis.[151]

Patients presenting with group IV and V bilateral retinoblastoma have been treated with radiation doses of 35 to 60 Gy. Enucleation was subsequently required for persistent or recurrent tumors in 67% of the treated eyes. The survival rate of the combined series of patients treated with bilateral irradiation was 82%, compared with a survival rate of 71% among a group of patients treated only with bilateral enucleation.[152] Although the risk of a radiation-related second malignant tumor developing in a patient with bilateral retinoblastoma is considerable, the data available suggest the long-term survival of patients treated with bilateral irradiation is not worse than that of patients treated with bilateral enucleation only. The preservation of some useful vision in these patients is an obvious advantage of such a treatment approach, but prolonged follow-up of patients so treated is necessary to thoroughly evaluate the effect of radiation-related second malignant tumors on long-term survival.[151]

Local irradiation, after enucleation, is recommended for all patients with extension of retinoblastoma into the orbit. Presentation with exophthalmos or a palpable mass through the eyelids suggests the presence of orbital extension of the tumor. The identification of an encapsulated or unencapsulated extraocular mass, enlargement of the cut end of the optic nerve at the time of enucleation, or rupture of the globe during removal is associated with orbital contamination with the tumor. These findings are confirmed histologically by the identification of an episcleral mass of tumor tissue or tumor at the margin of the cut end of the optic nerve. Patients with orbital retinoblastoma should receive irradiation to a volume that includes the entire orbit and the optic nerve up to the optic chiasm. The recommended dose is 44 Gy in 4 weeks to 50 Gy in 4.5 to 5.0 weeks.[153]

CHEMOTHERAPY

Although EBRT is an effective adjunct or alternative to enucleation of localized retinoblastoma, there is significant morbidity associated with this therapy. In addition to the heightened risk of second malignancies noted earlier, EBRT uniformly causes orbital hypoplasia and frequently contributes to cataract formation. In view of the morbidity and risk of second cancers in patients treated with EBRT, investigators have pursued alternative means of local control, increasingly in combination with chemotherapy. The use of adjuvant chemotherapy in treating intraocular and bilateral disease has been prompted by success in salvaging patients with recurrent extraocular disease with chemotherapy-based regimens. Since the earliest studies of adjuvant chemotherapy for retinoblastoma in the 1980s, most efforts at chemoreduction have included a platinating agent (cisplatinum or carboplatinum) in various combinations with vincristine, etoposide, cyclophosphamide, and doxorubicin,

with or without cyclosporin A as an multidrug-resistant reversal agent. Although platinum-based regimens appear to have significant activity in retinoblastoma, chemotherapy alone rarely achieves durable disease control.[154]

Because tumor shrinkage may decrease the need for enucleation, the goal of early trials was preservation of vision, primarily in children with bilateral disease. Since 2000, there have been a series of studies documenting promising rates of vision-sparing therapy without EBRT in intraocular unilateral disease.[155,156] The benefits of chemotherapy were most pronounced in patients with Reese-Ellsworth group I to IV tumors, allowing globe preservation in more than two-thirds of patients. Unfortunately, current chemotherapy-based regimens have been much less successful in group V patients, the majority of who require enucleation despite adjuvant therapy.[157,158]

RHABDOMYOSARCOMA

EPIDEMIOLOGY AND GENETICS

RMS is the most common malignant tumor of the soft tissues in infants and children. The incidence rate per year is 5 cases per 1 million U.S. children younger than 15 years, accounting for 4% of all cancers in this age group.[1] The annual incidence is lower for Asian children than for whites or African American children. RMS occurs slightly more frequently in boys. The median age at diagnosis of children with RMS is approximately 4 years, with girls presenting at slightly older ages than boys.[17]

RMS is a frequent tumor in families affected by the Li-Fraumeni syndrome. This syndrome is defined by familial clustering of cancers that include RMS and adrenocortical carcinoma in children and breast cancer in young adults. Affected relatives share germline mutations in the p53 tumor suppressor gene, which maps to chromosome 17p13.[159] In addition to p53 mutations, which have been associated with nearly 50% of RMS cases, mutations in the NF1 gene occurring in children with neurofibromatosis confer an increased risk for developing RMS.[160,161]

RMS may arise anywhere in the body, although the head and neck region is most frequently involved, accounting for 35% of all cases[162] (Fig. 40.2-4). The most common primary site for RMS is the orbit, accounting for 29% of the RMS in the head and neck and 13% of all RMS in children.[162]

The remaining primary tumor sites in the head and neck are divided into parameningeal and nonparameningeal locations. The parameningeal sites, including the nasopharynx, paranasal sinuses, middle ear, mastoid, pterygopalatine fossa, and infratemporal fossa, account for 40% of the RMS that originate in the head and neck. Additional primary tumor sites in the head and neck include the scalp, oral cavity, oropharynx, larynx, parotid gland, and neck.

The second most frequently involved regions include the abdomen and genitourinary tract, which account for the location of 29% of primary tumor sites in children with RMS. These tumors originate most frequently from the paratesticular tissues. Other primary tumor sites include the bladder, prostate, vagina, uterus, cervix, and bile ducts.[17] RMS arising in the genitourinary tract tends to affect young children, particularly the vaginal botryoid variant, which commonly presents in infancy.

The third group of tumor sites for RMS originates within the thorax or from the soft tissues of the trunk or extremities.

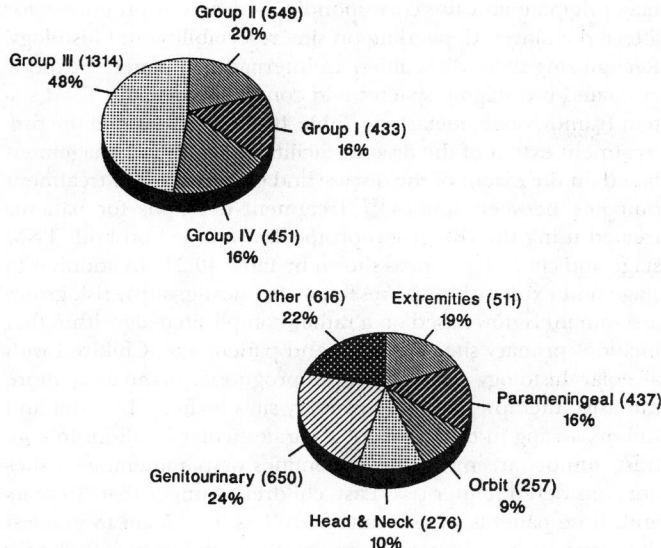

FIGURE 40.2-4. Overall distribution of patients in major Intergroup Rhabdomyosarcoma Study clinical trials according to clinical group and primary site. (From ref. 162, with permission.)

Most common, this subset of tumors involves the lower extremities, with 22% originating in the thigh or groin.[35] In contrast to the predilection for genitourinary tumors to develop in young children, RMS arising in the extremities is more likely to be identified in the second decade of life. Almost one-half of these extremity primaries contain alveolar elements that are associated with a more aggressive tumor biology.

Overall, nearly 25% of all newly diagnosed cases of RMS are metastatic at initial presentation. The most common sites of dissemination include lung, bone marrow, bone, and lymph nodes, in approximate order of frequency.[163]

PATHOLOGY

RMS has been traditionally classified into three histologies, consisting of embryonal (including botryoid), alveolar, and pleomorphic subtypes. As noted earlier, tumor histology is strongly correlated with the primary tumor site. Alveolar histology is uncommon except in primary tumors of the trunk and extremity, whereas embryonal histology is most common in RMS of the head and neck and tumors of the genitourinary system. Slightly more than one-half of all cases are characterized by favorable embryonal histology, with an additional 6% demonstrating the uniquely favorable botryoid architecture. The prognostically unfavorable alveolar histology constitutes only 21% of all cases of RMS.[163]

Various histologic classification schemes have been proposed since Horn and Enterline first categorized RMS as either embryonal or alveolar in 1958.[164–166] A revised classification of childhood RMS was proposed in 1995, based on the results of an international collaborative study. This system recognizes six subtypes: botryoid RMS, spindle cell RMS, embryonal RMS, alveolar RMS, undifferentiated sarcoma, and RMS with rhabdoid features. Application of this system has been shown to have greater reproducibility than prior classification schemes, separating patients into prognostically significant groups.[167]

Histologic classification of childhood RMS can be difficult, however, because individual tumors may have areas consistent with two or more histologic subtypes. Although immunohistochemical staining for desmin may be useful for the identification of RMS, some tumors lack distinguishing microscopic characteristics and cannot be further categorized.

In light of the limitations of immunohistochemical assessment, molecular diagnostics are gaining importance in identifying biologically less favorable subsets of patients for stratification to more intensive treatment regimens. Embryonal RMS is characterized by loss of heterozygosity at the chromosome 11p15 locus. Although chromosomal translocations are rarely associated with embryonal histology, alveolar tumors are characterized by rearrangement of the PAX3 gene on the long arm of chromosome 2 or the PAX7 gene on chromosome 1 with the FKHR gene on the long arm of chromosome 13. Rearrangement of these genes produces the characteristic translocations t(2;13)(q35;q14) and t(1;13)(p36;q14).[168,169] The fusion transcripts of these chimeric genes are thought to contribute to dysregulated transcriptional activation, culminating in transformation.[162] Using reverse transcriptase-polymerase chain reaction methodology, these signature translocations can now be identified with great sensitivity. In addition to being highly specific for alveolar histology, discriminating between these two translocations appears to have significant potential as a prognostic tool. A recently published study from the COG demonstrated substantially better survival in metastatic patients with the PAX7-FHKR fusion transcript compared to metastatic patients with the PAX3-FHKR fusion product. These provocative findings suggest that characterization of specific gene rearrangements in alveolar RMA may prove to be an important instrument in stratifying patients into risk groups for future clinical trials.[169]

CLINICAL PRESENTATION AND EVALUATION

Because RMS may originate from nearly any anatomic site, the radiographic examination of the primary tumor must be individualized. Evaluation of children with RMS requires expert radiographic interpretation, competent pathologic examination of surgical specimens, and knowledge of distant sites to which RMS may spread (Table 40.2-7 from McDowell[170]).

The staging evaluation should include a chest CT, radionuclide bone scan, CT or MRI of the primary site, and bilateral bone marrow sampling.

Pulmonary nodules identified in children with RMS are frequently benign,[171] suggesting that solitary nodules identified on a chest radiograph of a child with RMS should be examined pathologically.

The bone marrow may be involved by RMS in the absence of bone or pulmonary metastases. The bone marrow aspirate was positive at the time of diagnosis in approximately 10% of patients and may be the only definite site of identifiable disease.[172]

In addition to the aforementioned sites of hematogenous dissemination, lymph node involvement has been documented in 10% to 20% of cases of RMS.[173] These nodal sites may be evaluated radiographically or pathologically. Results from the Intergroup Rhabdomyosarcoma Study-IV (IRS-IV) suggest that radiographic staging of retroperitoneal sites may underestimate the frequency of nodal disease in this location, resulting in improper stage and risk group assignments.

TABLE 40.2-7. Clinical Presentation of Rhabdomyosarcoma

Site	Common Clinical Symptoms of Rhabdomyosarcoma
Head-neck	Asymptomatic mass, may mimic enlarged lymph node
Orbit	Proptosis, chemosis, ocular paralysis, eyelid mass
Nasopharynx	Snoring, nasal voice, epistaxis, rhinorrhea, local pain, dysphagia, CN palsies
Paranasal sinuses	Swelling, pain, sinusitis, obstruction, epistaxis, cranial nerve palsies
Middle ear	Chronic otitis media, hemorrhagic discharge, CN palsies, extruding polypoid mass
Larynx	Hoarseness, irritating cough
Trunk	Asymptomatic mass
Biliary tract	Hepatomegaly, jaundice
Retroperitoneum	Painless mass, ascites, gastrointestinal or genitourinary obstruction, spinal cord symptoms
Bladder/ prostate	Hematuria, urinary retention, abdominal mass, constipation
Female genital tract	Polypoid vaginal extrusion of mucosanguineous tissue, vulval nodule
Male genital tract	Painful or painless scrotal mass
Extremity	Painless mass, may be very small but present with lymph node involvement
Metastatic	Nonspecific symptoms associated with the diagnosis of leukemia

CN, cranial nerve.
(From ref. 170, with permission.)

STAGING

Staging and risk group stratification of children with RMS is complicated by the many potential sites from which the tumor may originate and the correspondingly different prognoses for affected children depending on site, resectability, and histology. Recognizing these difficulties, an international panel of experts evaluated two staging systems and concluded that the TNM system (tumor, node, metastasis; Table 40.2-8) best defined the pretreatment extent of the disease, facilitating patient management based on the extent of the disease and comparisons of treatment outcome between studies.[174] Treatment decisions for patients treated using the IRS group protocols are based on both TNM stage and clinical group, as shown in Table 40.2-9. In addition to stage and extent of initial resection (clinical group), risk group assignment is now based on a rather complicated algorithm that includes primary site, histology, and patient age. Children with alveolar histology have a poorer prognosis, mandating more intensive therapy. Favorable primary sites include the orbit and tumors arising in the vagina or a paratesticular location. In contrast, tumors arising in the extremities or parameningeal sites are considered higher risk. Last, children younger than 10 years and those patients whose tumors are less than 5 cm in greatest diameter have a better prognosis than children with larger tumors or more advanced age.

TREATMENT

Surgery

Surgical considerations for RMS are site specific. Although biopsy is required of tumors in all locations, progressive improvements in the response to chemotherapy and radiotherapy have obviated the need for immediate surgical resection, particularly of orbital primaries. Surgery is more frequently used at other sites where resection does not produce major functional impairment (e.g., paratesticular and extremity lesions).

TABLE 40.2-8. Tumor (T), Node (N), Metastasis (M) Pretreatment Staging for Rhabdomyosarcoma

Stage	Sites	T	Size	N	M
1	Orbit Head and neck (excluding parameningeal) Genitourinary: nonbladder/nonprostate	T1 or T2	a or b	N0 or N1 or N2	M0
2	Bladder/prostate Extremity Cranial parameningeal Other	T1 or T2	a	N0 or Nx	M0
3	Bladder/prostate Extremity Cranial parameningeal Other	T1 or T2	a b	N1 N0 or N1 or Nx	M0 M0
4	All	T1 or T2	a or b	N0 or N1	M1

Note:
T1: Confined to anatomic site of origin
    a: Less than 5 cm in diameter
    b: Greater than 5 cm in diameter
T2: Extension, fixation, or both to surrounding tissue
    a: Less than 5 cm in diameter
    b: Greater than 5 cm in diameter
N0: Regional lymph nodes not clinically involved
N1: Regional lymph nodes clinically involved by tumor
Nx: Clinical status of regional lymph nodes unknown
M0: No distant metastases
M1: Metastases present

TABLE 40.2-9. Intergroup Rhabdomyosarcoma Study Group Grouping System for Rhabdomyosarcoma

Group	Description
GROUP I	Localized disease, completely resected. Regional lymph nodes not involved; lymph node biopsy or dissection is required except for head and neck lesions.
A	Confined to muscle or organ of origin.
B	Contiguous involvement; infiltration outside the muscle or organ of origin, as through fascial planes. This includes both gross inspection and microscopic confirmation of complete resection. Any lymph nodes that may be inadvertently removed with the specimen must be negative. If the lymph nodes are involved microscopically, the patient is placed in group IIb or IIc (see following discussion).
GROUP II	Total gross resection with evidence of regional spread.
A	Grossly resected tumor with microscopic residual disease. Surgeon believes that all of the tumor has been removed, but the pathologist finds tumor at the margin of resection *and* additional resection to achieve a negative margin is not feasible. No evidence of gross residual tumor. No evidence of regional lymph node involvement. Once radiotherapy or chemotherapy have been started, reexploration and removal of the area of microscopic residual does not change the patient's group.
B	Regional disease with involved lymph nodes, completely resected with no microscopic residual.
C	Regional disease with involved lymph nodes, grossly resected but with evidence of microscopic residual and histologic involvement of the most distal regional lymph node (from the primary site) in the dissection.
GROUP III	Incomplete resection with gross residual disease.
A	After biopsy only.
B	After gross or major resection of the primary (less than 50%).
GROUP IV	Metastatic disease present at onset (lung, liver, bones, bone marrow, brain, and distant muscle and lymph nodes). The presence of positive cytology in the cerebrospinal fluid, pleural, or peritoneal fluid as well as implants on the pleural or peritoneal surfaces are regarded as indications for placing the patient in group IV.

In most cases, an initial incisional biopsy should be performed. The biopsy site and direction of the incision should always be planned with future excision in mind. Unsuccessful attempts at initial resection of an extremity lesion, leaving positive margins, can greatly complicate future resection.

Lymph node biopsy should be considered based on the primary site. Children presenting without distant metastases have an overall 10% incidence of lymphatic spread. Lymph node involvement is most frequent for tumors arising in the prostate (41%), paratesticular (26%), and genitourinary sites (24%). Extremity lesions had an intermediate frequency of 12%, whereas orbit (0%), nonorbital head and neck sites (7%), and truncal sites (3%) had the lowest frequency of lymphatic dissemination.[173] In the extremity and genitourinary sites, assessment of lymph node involvement is essential to ensure that radiation fields are appropriately designed and sufficiently inclusive.

Radiation Therapy

Cassady and colleagues demonstrated in 1968 that embryonal RMS of the orbit could be controlled locally with irradiation.[175]

In fact, orbital irradiation was proven to be superior to exenteration for the treatment of orbital RMS.[176]

Local irradiation is necessary for all patients with known microscopic or gross residual disease, representing the vast majority of patients affected by RMA. The role of local irradiation in the treatment of patients who have undergone complete resections with negative margins (group I disease) was examined in the first IRS study.[177] After complete tumor excisions, all patients received adjuvant chemotherapy with vincristine, dactinomycin, and cyclophosphamide (VAC). One-half of these patients were randomized to receive tumor bed irradiation. This study demonstrated that radiation did not confer a survival advantage to clinical group I patients. In light of these findings, radiation was not included in the treatment of group I patients enrolled on IRS-II, with the notable exception of extremity lesions with alveolar histology.

IRS-III accrued 1062 patients from 1984 through 1991. All patients received postoperative radiation therapy except those with group I favorable histology tumors and selected special pelvic sites who had pathologic confirmation of complete remission after primary chemotherapy. The dose for microscopic residual disease was 41.4 and 50.4 Gy for gross residual disease. The overall survival in IRS-III improved to 73%, a significant improvement from the results of IRS-I and -II (Fig. 40.2-5).[178]

IRS-IV opened in 1991, completing accrual in 1997. This study used the TNM staging system to determine the chemotherapy regimen and the IRS clinical group system to determine radiation therapy. Group III patients were randomized between hyperfractionated radiation therapy (110 cGy twice a day to a total dose of 59.4 Gy) and conventional radiation therapy (180 cGy once a day to a total dose of 50.4 Gy).[179] A recently published analysis of this randomized study failed to demonstrate any advantage of hyperfractionated radiotherapy over conventional fractionation in the control of neither local, regional, or metastatic disease nor any improvement in overall 5-year EFS (73%).[179]

Chemotherapy

Development of combination chemotherapy programs for children with RMS has paralleled the identification of new chemotherapeutic agents with significant activity. The first combination reported to be active in RMS was VAC. This regimen remains the internationally recognized standard 30 years after its introduction in IRS-I in 1972. The inclusion of adjuvant combination chemotherapy has been a powerful contributor to the dramatic improvement in EFS from 25% in the early 1970s to 70% 5-year EFS documented in contemporary cooperative group studies. Since the inaugural IRS trial in 1972, a total of four generations of IRS studies have been completed, with a fifth cycle of studies now under way under the aegis of the COG. These studies have failed to demonstrate any clear survival advantage from the addition of doxorubicin or cisplatinum or any advantage in the substitution of ifosfamide for cyclophosphamide. Although identification of more effective chemotherapy regimens has proven elusive, these studies have defined and validated prognostic factors that now form the basis for risk group assignments in current and proposed clinical trials.

The current IRS-V study, which opened in 1995, focuses on improving survival in the intermediate- and high-risk subsets of patients. An attempt at dose-escalating cyclophosphamide in

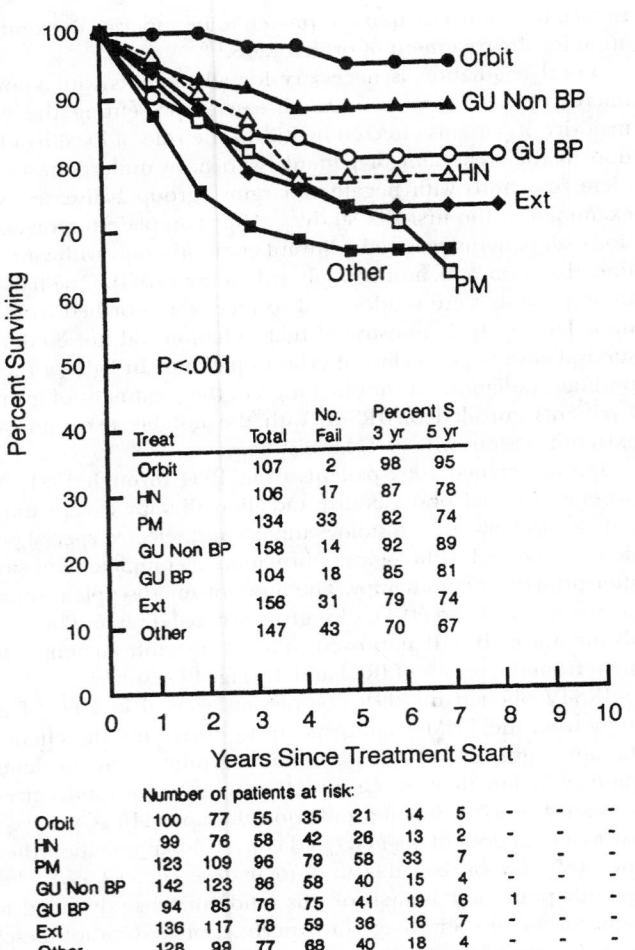

FIGURE 40.2-5. Survival (S) by primary site for all patients treated in Intergroup Rhabdomyosarcoma Study-III. BP, bladder/prostate; Ext, extremities; GU, genitourinary tract; HN, head and neck; PM, parameningeal sites. (From ref. 178, with permission.)

one of these pilots was proven to be prohibitively toxic. Because all three agents in the VAC regimen are currently delivered at maximal dose intensity, improvements in survival require identification of new active agents. Based on encouraging pilot data from treatment of metastatic patients with VAC plus topotecan,[180] this combination is being evaluated in a phase III study in intermediate-risk patients. Eligible patients are randomized to VAC alone versus VAC alternating with vincristine, topotecan, and cyclophosphamide.

In contrast to the striking improvement in survival of nonmetastatic patients over the past three decades, survival for metastatic (stage IV) patients has only marginally increased from 20% to 32% since the inception of the IRS in 1972. Current efforts to improve survival in this very high-risk subset of children include a series of phase II window studies to assess novel therapies in newly diagnosed patients. Children with metastatic RMS are now being treated with an induction regimen that combines vincristine with irinotecan. Like topotecan, irinotecan is a camptothecin analogue that exerts its cytotoxic effect by inhibition of topoisomerase I. Irinotecan has demonstrated impressive antitumor activity in preclinical studies with murine xenografts. Subsequent pilot studies for metastatic

patients may revisit the therapeutic potential of anthracyclines including Doxil, a liposomally encapsulated analogue of doxorubicin, for which a phase I study was recently completed.[181] It is hoped that the liposomal delivery system will minimize cardiotoxicity, permitting more dose-intensive application of anthracyclines to sarcoma therapy.

SPECIFIC PRIMARY TUMOR SITES

Head and Neck

ORBIT. Children with orbital RMS present with proptosis due to a retrobulbar tumor, or swelling of the eyelid. The radiographic evaluation must demonstrate whether the tumor is confined to the orbit or has extended inferiorly into the maxillary sinus or posteriorly into the ethmoid sinus and cranial cavity. CT provides excellent definition of the soft tissue mass and can demonstrate the presence of bone destruction.

Surgery. Although biopsy is required before beginning treatment of orbital tumors, surgical efforts should be constrained to diagnostic tissue sampling only. Owing to the excellent response to radiation and chemotherapy, orbital exenteration is not indicated except for the unusual cases of recurrent disease in this site.

Radiation Therapy. The technique of local irradiation should include treatment of a volume that includes the entire soft tissue mass, demonstrated radiographically, with a margin of normal tissue. The dose given to the macroscopic tumor should be 45 to 55 Gy, administered over 5 to 6 weeks. Historically, a wedged lateral and anterior or three-field treatment plan was used. Three-dimensional treatment planning yields a superior dose distribution and can potentially avoid irradiation of the pituitary gland.

Chemotherapy. Children with group II or III RMS of the orbit have a 5-year progression-free survival of approximately 90% when treated with local radiation therapy and chemotherapy that includes vincristine and dactinomycin.[177,178] These patients do not benefit from the addition of either doxorubicin or cyclophosphamide to the chemotherapy regimen.

PARAMENINGEAL SITES. The parameningeal sites include the middle ear, nasopharynx, and adjacent areas. Children with a primary tumor in the middle ear present with a peripheral facial nerve palsy or a mass in the external auditory canal and may have been misdiagnosed as having chronic otitis media or Bell's palsy. Those patients with an RMS of the nasopharynx present with signs of upper-airway obstruction, which is frequently associated with cranial nerve palsies. On examination, they are found to have a soft tissue mass that is depressing the palate and extending into the retropharyngeal space.

The radiographic evaluation of a patient with a parameningeal RMS must document the presence and extent of bone destruction and identify local or intracranial extension of the tumor.

Surgery. Surgical resection is infrequently required at this site because of the excellent response to chemotherapy and radiotherapy. In children who have persistent disease after completion of radiotherapy or who have tumor recurrence, surgery should be considered.[182] Modern methods of resection and reconstruction of these sites make surgery much less mutilating than in the past, with improved long-term functional outcomes. Before the initiation of therapy, the staging evaluation should include a lumbar puncture to look for tumor cells in the cerebrospinal fluid.

Radiation Therapy. Parameningeal RMS progresses locally by destruction of the adjacent bones and by growth along nerves.[183] To achieve local control of this tumor, a generous margin of these tissues must be included within the volume of irradiation.[184] The tumor mass must receive a radiation dose of at least 50 Gy. Meticulous treatment planning is necessary to deliver adequate therapy to the tumor without causing excessive or unnecessary damage to adjacent normal tissues including the brain and eye.

RMS of the middle ear may recur as diffuse meningeal disease. This occurred in 17.5% of patients with a parameningeal primary tumor entered on IRS-I.[185] The high rate of primary meningeal relapse in this study may have been related to inadequate radiation technique. Although these investigators recommended the administration of craniospinal irradiation to prevent meningeal recurrence, others reported isolated meningeal relapse in 5.4% to 7.4% of patients with parameningeal RMS.[184,186]

This suggests that the rate of meningeal recurrence is related to the adequacy of the volume and dose of irradiation to the primary tumor. Current guidelines in IRS-V for parameningeal disease do not recommend craniospinal irradiation. Treatment is confined to the tumor volume plus a 2-cm margin for parameningeal tumors without intracranial extension. In cases of documented intracranial extension and positive cerebrospinal fluid cytology, the skull and whole brain are included in the radiated target volume.

Chemotherapy. Approximately one-half of children with parameningeal primary tumors have group III tumors. These children require treatment with the combination of VAC. The 3-year progression-free survival percentage for all children with parameningeal primary tumors on IRS-IV was 72%, a result similar to that reported for IRS-II and IRS-III.[187] Patients with intracranial extension had a 3-year EFS of 70%, compared with 78% for those without any evidence of meningeal involvement.[186] VAC remains the therapy of choice for parameningeal disease.[187]

Other Head and Neck Sites

RMS may originate in several nonorbital and nonparameningeal sites, including the parotid region, larynx, soft and hard palate, tonsil, tongue, cheek, nose, scalp, and neck. Children with a parotid RMS present with unilateral swelling at the angle of the mandible and local pain. Those with RMS of the larynx present with hoarseness or signs of airway obstruction.

Although radical excision of tumor in these sites has been reported in a few cases, local infiltration of the tumor usually precludes gross total excision. Despite the prohibitions of surgical morbidity, local tumor control can be achieved with irradiation. The volume of irradiation should include a margin of normal tissue. Direct tumor extension along the extracranial portions of the adjacent cranial nerves may occur. These areas should be included within the treatment volume. The dose to gross residual disease should be 45 to 50 Gy. These patients should receive combination chemotherapy with VAC. The 5-year

progression-free survival percentage for these children was 78% on IRS-IV, similar to the outcomes of IRS-II and IRS-III.[178,188]

Trunk

RMS of the thorax may arise from the soft tissues of the chest wall or within the thoracic cavity. Primary tumors of the chest wall present as a localized swelling.

The radiographic evaluation of a patient with a primary tumor of the chest wall should include plain chest radiography and CT.

SURGERY. Lesions in the trunk, arising in the chest or abdominal wall and paraspinal or retroperitoneal sites, should be resected if possible because of their less favorable response to chemotherapy and radiotherapy. Complete surgical removal is often not feasible owing to the large size of these lesions at diagnosis as well as their involvement of vital structures within the abdomen or chest. Resections of the chest or abdominal wall often require prosthetic mesh reconstruction. Primary reexcision should be considered if pathologic examination of the initial specimen demonstrates microscopic residual disease.[189] In a review of IRS studies II and III, there were 84 patients with thoracic sarcomas.[190] Although 71% of these patients achieved an initial complete response, 58% ultimately died, with an average survival of 1.1 years.

RMS arising in the abdominal wall is rare, accounting for only 1% of all cases of this disease. A review of patients with abdominal wall primaries treated on IRS-I through -IV demonstrated a substantial advantage to complete versus partial resection of localized tumors (100% vs. 62%).[191]

Biliary tract primaries appear to be more responsive to chemotherapy than other truncal sites.[192] Affected children typically present with symptoms of biliary tract obstruction. Diagnostic biopsy followed by chemotherapy is appropriate, with resection reserved for those children with persistent disease.

Initial biopsy followed by chemotherapy and radiation has also been standard therapy for bulky tumors of the retroperitoneum and nongenitourinary pelvic sites. These tumors make up approximately 10% of all RMS. All of the patients with tumors in these locations in IRS-III and -IV were either group III (gross residual) or group IV (metastatic). Nearly one-half of these patients were metastatic at diagnosis. Children with embryonal histology had a 4-year failure-free survival of 56% versus only 33% for children with alveolar or undifferentiated histology. This survival advantage for children with embryonal histology may reflect the more aggressive surgical approach (debulking vs. biopsy) applied to these patients. The apparent advantage to debulking is being prospectively analyzed in IRS-V.[193]

RADIATION THERAPY. When complete tumor excision is not possible, local control is established with the use of radiation therapy. The volume must include the grossly apparent tumor with a margin of normal tissue. A radiation dose of 40 Gy is adequate for microscopic residual disease, whereas 50 Gy is required for gross residual disease. The pleural space is considered contaminated if there is a malignant pleural effusion or if the tumor is cut across and the pleural space is opened at the time of surgery. The entire pleural surface must be irradiated when pleural contamination with tumor cells has occurred. Failure to do so may result in disease recurrence on the pleural surface not included within the volume of irradiation.

CHEMOTHERAPY. Embryonal RMS of the trunk should be treated using the chemotherapy regimens appropriate for the clinical group. Group I tumors are treated with the combination of vincristine and dactinomycin, whereas groups II, III, and IV are managed with the combination of VAC.[187] Primary tumors of the trunk frequently consist of alveolar elements.[194] As in other sites, alveolar tumors in the trunk do not respond to chemotherapy as favorably as embryonal disease. Children with intermediate- or high-risk disease arising in these sites are currently being evaluated for response to VAC plus one of the camptothecin analogues.

Extremity Sites

Patients with RMS of an extremity usually present with localized swelling. On occasion, a child with RMS of an extremity comes to medical attention owing to symptoms caused by metastases, such as spinal cord compression secondary to vertebral body metastases, or pain due to other bone metastases. Nearly 25% of extremity primaries are metastatic at the time of diagnosis.

Radiographic evaluation of a patient with an RMS of the extremity should include plain radiographs of the primary tumor site and a bone scan. The presence of increased radionuclide uptake in the adjacent bone, although generally not associated with frank invasion of the bone by tumor, is correlated with the presence of inflammatory adhesions between the tumor and adjacent bone. Local recurrence of the tumor is likely if the tumor is not removed *en bloc* with the adjacent bone.[195] CT and MRI are useful for defining the extent of the soft tissue mass and the presence of bone destruction.

SURGERY. Complete resection of the tumor with negative microscopic margins is the goal in extremity sarcomas.[195] There is no advantage to amputation or muscle group excision compared with local excision with an adequate surrounding rim of normal tissue, provided the resection results in negative microscopic margins. The extent of the resection is often tempered by attempts to minimize functional impairment. In extremity tumors, consideration of the initial biopsy site and the direction of the incision are particularly important, because an inappropriate biopsy can greatly complicate later resection. Extremity lesions should rarely be resected without an initial biopsy owing to significant differences in the surgical approach when resecting a malignant lesion versus a benign process.

Extensive local lesions with invasion of vital structures are often treated first with chemotherapy and subjected to delayed surgical resection. The goal of delayed resection is to render the child free of gross residual disease and accept microscopic residual disease that can be controlled with a lower dose of radiotherapy than the dose required for gross residual disease (40 vs. 55 Gy). This multidisciplinary approach results in good local control, whereas minimizing the potential morbidity of a more extensive initial resection or amputation.

Lymph node sampling is important in extremity RMS owing to the significant risk of lymphatic involvement. Nearly 25% of all extremity tumors demonstrated regional nodal infiltra-

tion.[163] A representative sample of lymph nodes from the draining nodal group should be biopsied. A lymph node resection should not be performed because of the risks of producing lymphedema, which may complicate radiotherapy and subsequent surgical resection of the primary lesion.

Analysis of data from IRS-III has shown that the estimated 5-year survival was directly related to the clinical group, with a 95% survival in group I versus 67% in group II, 58% in group III, and 33% in group IV. Survival was independent of histology or site. Multivariate analysis of pretreatment factors showed that lymph node metastasis, age older than 10 years, and distant metastasis predicted worse survival. In IRS-IV, the failure-free survival rate was 55%, with an overall survival rate of 70%. Again, the 3-year failure-free survival was closely related to group (groups I, 91%; II, 72%; III, 50%; IV, 23%). In this cohort, clinical group and stage were both highly predictive of outcome. None of the other variables was predictive of failure-free survival in multivariate analysis.[196]

RADIATION THERAPY. Postoperative irradiation must be to a volume that includes a generous margin around the tumor. The radiation dose should be 50 Gy to areas of gross residual disease. Patients with histologic confirmation of regional lymph node involvement should receive similar treatment to a volume that includes the involved lymph nodes.

CHEMOTHERAPY. Embryonal RMS of the extremity should be treated using the chemotherapy regimens, described in Trunk, for RMS of the trunk. Approximately one-half of extremity RMSs have alveolar histology and require chemotherapy appropriate for this histologic subtype with a poorer prognosis.[194]

Genitourinary

Patients with RMS of the paratesticular tissue present with painless enlargement of the testis. The age distribution is bimodal, with peaks at 5 and 16 years of age.[17] Children with RMS of the prostate present most frequently with acute urinary retention or with difficulty in voiding. Hematuria, dysuria, and abdominal swelling are also observed. Those with RMS of the bladder usually present because of hematuria, urinary frequency, or dysuria. The physical examination of children with a prostate tumor is unremarkable except for the presence of a mass between the bladder and rectum that is palpable on rectal examination. Radiographic evaluation should include a voiding cystourethrogram or CT of the abdomen and pelvis.

Children with sarcoma botryoids of the vagina frequently present with a polypoid mass protruding from the vaginal orifice or with vaginal bleeding. These children should have an α-fetoprotein (AFP) level obtained before tumor biopsy or excision, because yolk sac tumors may also present as a vaginal mass.

SURGERY. Anterior pelvic exenteration is rarely required today. Bladder, prostate, and vaginal primaries are first biopsied, and lymph node extension is defined. Chemotherapy and radiotherapy are then used to eradicate residual disease. The mean age of children with vaginal tumors is younger than 2 years. Over the course of the first four IRS studies spanning 25 years, the percentage of children undergoing resections of vaginal tumors has steadily decreased from 90% to 13%. Despite the limitation of surgical intervention to biopsy, survival in this group remains excellent, exceeding 90% with minimal surgical morbidity.[197]

In contrast to vaginal lesions, uterine primary tumors tend to arise in older children and demonstrate a greater propensity for local recurrence. As with vaginal lesions, initial surgical intervention is limited to biopsy in most cases. Hysterectomy is reserved for those patients who fail to achieve a complete response to chemotherapy and radiation. Survival in children with uterine disease approaches 90%.[198]

Preservation of the bladder and prostate was one of the primary goals of the IRS-II study in which surgical therapy was shifted from initial resection to primary biopsy with subsequent radiotherapy or surgery.[199] The percentage of children with bladder and prostate tumors in IRS-II who retained their bladder and were alive at 3 years from diagnosis were 33% and 22%, respectively. Although sequential treatment on this protocol yielded disappointing survival and failed to improve bladder salvage, subsequent efforts that included more intensive chemotherapy and radiation have proved much more successful. More than one-half of the patients with bladder and prostate tumors enrolled on IRS-III were alive with functional bladders 4 years from diagnosis. The 3-year survival in this poor-risk cohort also dramatically improved to 90% with this more intensive therapeutic regimen.[200]

Successful treatment of paratesticular RMS first requires a transinguinal radical orchiectomy. Testicular masses should never be approached through the scrotum owing to the risk of inducing spread into the pelvis via the inguinal lymphatics. In addition, the desired high inguinal ligation of the spermatic cord cannot be accomplished by the scrotal approach. A total of 121 boys with paratesticular RMS treated on IRS-III had retroperitoneal lymph node dissection to evaluate nodal status.[201] Lymph nodes were radiographically negative based on CT in 81% of the boys, 14% of whom had positive nodes when biopsy or retroperitoneal lymph node dissection was performed. Although CT was accurate if lymph node abnormalities were identified, it was not extremely sensitive in identifying nodal involvement. In this regard, it is important to note that adolescent boys with group I tumors experienced lower failure-free survival than those with group II tumors on IRS-IV. This unexpected outcome is most likely explained by the mistaken assignment of patients with group II tumors to the less intensive group I treatment regimen, owing to failure of CT imaging to identify nodal pathology. These data suggest that adolescents should have ipsilateral retroperitoneal lymph node dissection as part of their routine staging. Patients with positive lymph nodes require intensified chemotherapy, as well as nodal irradiation.

RADIATION THERAPY. The IRS reported that there was no obvious benefit from prophylactic retroperitoneal lymph node irradiation among patients with paratesticular RMS who had negative pathologic staging of retroperitoneal nodes.[202]

Tumors of the bladder and prostate were initially managed with radical resections, including cystectomy.[203] Although excellent survival was achieved with this approach, the extensive surgical morbidity of this strategy prompted subsequent efforts at tissue-sparing treatment designs. Current IRS guidelines recommend early introduction of radiation in combination with chemotherapy after a minimally invasive biopsy.[204] Using this multimodal approach on IRS-III produced improved progression-free survival of approximately 75%, while maintaining partial or complete bladder function.[178]

CHEMOTHERAPY. Patients with group II paratesticular primary tumors of embryonal histology have an excellent prognosis when treated with the combination of vincristine and dactinomycin, with a 5-year progression-free survival percentage of 81%.[178] All patients with group III (biopsy only) genitourinary tumors are treated with VAC.

PROGNOSTIC FACTORS

As noted earlier in Rhabdomyosarcoma: Staging, the favorable prognostic factors for children and adolescents with RMS include tumor status (T1, tumor localized in the organ or tissue of origin) and primary tumor site (orbit, genitourinary nonbladder, or prostate).[205] Although alveolar histology predicts a poorer outcome with standard therapy, the difference in survival between alveolar and embryonal cases partially resolves when more intensive therapy is applied to alveolar tumors. Despite improvements in therapy, however, children with metastatic disease still fare poorly, with a 5-year survival between 20% and 30%. Most of these metastatic patients have alveolar tumors. In a noteworthy departure from the dismal prognosis for children with disseminated RMS, there is a subset of younger children (younger than 10 years) with embryonal histology with a 50% rate of failure-free survival. Identification of this relatively favorable subset of metastatic patients reinforces the importance of histology in predicting the behavior of this disease. Unfortunately, efforts at maximal dose intensification of chemotherapy with stem cell support have failed to improve the prognosis for children with metastatic disease.[206] Improved survival requires identification of new active cytotoxic agents in conjunction with efforts to target the unique genetic perturbations that are ubiquitous features of alveolar disease.

EWING'S SARCOMA AND PERIPHERAL PRIMITIVE NEUROECTODERMAL TUMOR

EPIDEMIOLOGY AND GENETICS

Ewing's sarcoma and primitive neuroectodermal tumor are closely related, if not identical, malignancies that may occur as osseous or soft tissue tumors.[207] Ewing's sarcoma is the second most common primary bone tumor in pediatric patients, accounting for approximately 4% of pediatric malignancies. The incidence rate per year is 3.4 cases per 1 million U.S. white children younger than 19 years. For reasons that remain to be elucidated, African American children are rarely affected by this cancer.[1] The vast majority of these tumors arise in the second decade, primarily among white children.

The femur is the most frequent primary site for Ewing's sarcoma, accounting for approximately 20% to 25% of all cases. Lower-extremity tumors may also arise in the tibia, fibula, or the bones of the feet. Combining all potential sites of lower-extremity disease, these tumors account for 45% of newly diagnosed Ewing's sarcomas.[208] The pelvis is the second most common primary site for Ewing's sarcoma, accounting for an additional 20% of new cases. Pelvic tumors may arise in the ilium, ischium, pubic bone, or sacrum. Upper-extremity sites comprise another 12% to 16% of new diagnoses, with the humerus accounting for the majority of these cases. The remainder of Ewing's sarcomas originates from the vertebrae, ribs, clavicle, mandible, and skull. These axial lesions account for nearly 13% of all newly diagnosed cases.[208]

PATHOLOGY

Ewing's sarcoma and primary neuroectodermal tumors are counted among the small blue round cell tumors of childhood. Based on readily apparent features noted on light microscopy, this grouping includes neuroblastoma, RMS, and non-Hodgkin's lymphoma. Tumors of the Ewing's sarcoma family are characterized by the presence of highly cellular aggregates of tumor cells compartmentalized by widely separated strands of fibrous tissue.

Within the Ewing's family of tumors, primary neuroectodermal tumors are characterized by significant neuroectodermal differentiation. These tumors typically demonstrate Homer-Wright pseudorosettes on light microscopy and positive immunohistochemical staining for synaptophysin and neuron-specific enolase. In contrast to primary neuroectodermal tumors, Ewing's sarcomas are poorly differentiated tumors that do not form pseudorosettes and do not stain positively for neural markers.[209] Regardless of the extent of neural differentiation, nearly all tumors within the Ewing's sarcoma family express the MIC2 gene product (CD99) on their cell membranes.[210] Approximately 95% of all Ewing's family tumors contain translocations consisting of either t(11;22) or t(21;22). These gene rearrangements combine the N-terminal region of the EWS gene on chromosome 22 with the C-terminal region of one of two closely related genes on chromosome 11 (FLI1) or chromosome 21 (ERG). Both FLI1 and ERG are members of the Ets gene family of transcriptional activators. The majority of these translocations involve EWS and FLI1, t(11;22), producing a fusion transcript that is presumed to contribute to dysregulated cell growth and transformation.[211] Although the mechanism of tumorigenesis mediated by EWS-FLI1 remains uncertain, one study implicates the transforming growth factor-β (TGF-β) type II receptor as a target. TGF-β is a putative tumor suppressor gene. Levels of TGF-BR2 are reduced when EWS-FLI1 is introduced into embryonic stem cells. Antisense oligonucleotides to EWS-FLI1 restore TGF-β sensitivity and block tumorigenicity in cell lines containing the fusion gene.[212]

Studies of EWS-FLI1 have demonstrated a variety of genomic breakpoints within the rearranged genes. Differences in the resulting fusion transcripts are thought to contribute to the clinical heterogeneity of Ewing's sarcoma. The most common rearrangement, designated *type 1*, consists of the first seven exons of EWS fused to exons 6 to 9 of FLI1. This fusion gene accounts for nearly two-thirds of all cases. The type 2 rearrangement, constituting an additional 25% of cases, fuses EWS to exon 5 of FLI1. Type 2 appears to be a more potent transactivator, which may account for the poorer prognosis associated with this fusion product.[213–216]

Rapid identification of EWS gene rearrangement using fluorescence *in situ* hybridization on frozen-section specimens has been described.[217] Application of this diagnostic tool may facilitate prompt discrimination between the Ewing's family tumors and other morphologically similar small round cell tumors, expediting the initiation of appropriate therapy.

CLINICAL PRESENTATION AND NATURAL HISTORY

Localized pain is typically the first symptom reported by pediatric patients with bone tumors. The pain progresses from intermittent to more constant, often awakening the patient from sleep. Depending on the location of the tumor, the patient may develop a limp, have pain that increases with respiration, or experience pain that is radicular in character. Local swelling is often noticed by the patient. This finding is more readily identified when the tumor is located in an extremity. Paraplegia secondary to vertebral disease is present at the time of diagnosis in approximately 3% of patients.

The clinical presentation of patients with Ewing's sarcoma is similar to that of patients with osteomyelitis.[218] Fever is present in 28% of patients with Ewing's sarcoma at the time of diagnosis.[17]

Metastases are present in approximately 26% of patients at initial diagnosis. The most frequent sites of metastases are the lungs and other bones. Patients may seek medical attention because of symptoms related to metastatic disease, rather than the primary tumor. Multiple pulmonary metastases may produce respiratory insufficiency. Paraplegia may develop secondary to a vertebral body metastasis.

Evaluation of a patient suspected of having Ewing's sarcoma includes radiographic examinations of the primary tumor site, documentation of the presence or absence of hematogenous metastases, and additional laboratory studies that correlate with prognosis or exclude the presence of other possible diagnoses.

Lesions that originate in the long bones characteristically involve the diaphysis, with extension toward the metaphyses. A lytic or mixed lytic-sclerotic lesion is identified in the bone. Parallel, lamellated periosteal new bone formation (onion skin) or, less frequently, radiating bone spicules may be present. A soft tissue mass is frequently identified on CT or gadolinium-enhanced MRI.

Plain radiographs of tumors that originate in the pelvic bones frequently demonstrate a mixed lytic and blastic lesion. CT and MRI of the pelvis are required to adequately delineate the presence and extent of any associated soft tissue mass.

Radionuclide bone scans should be obtained, both to define more precisely the extent of disease at the primary site and to determine whether bone metastases are present.

STAGING

Ewing's sarcoma can metastasize to the lungs, other bones, and bone marrow. As with other sarcomas, nodules identified on plain chest radiography or CT of the chest in patients with Ewing's sarcoma are not always malignant. Biopsy of solitary pulmonary nodules should be strongly considered before defining patients as metastatic.

Radionuclide bone scans demonstrated disease in additional bones in approximately 10% of patients with Ewing's sarcoma.[219]

Patients with Ewing's sarcoma may have disseminated bone marrow disease in the absence of radiographically detectable bone metastases. Bilateral bone marrow sampling is required to complete the staging of all patients regardless of primary site or tumor size.

TREATMENT

Surgery

Local control must be achieved by either high-dose radiotherapy or resection. Larger tumor size (more than 8 cm) or volume (more than 100 cm^3) has correlated with decreased success in achieving durable local control.[220,221] No randomized study has been performed to define whether local control is better accomplished with surgical resection or radiotherapy. In nonrandomized trials, the improved survival in the surgical resection group has been attributed to the allocation of larger tumors with correspondingly poorer prognosis to the radiation group. Not all series have reported better survival among patients treated surgically than among those treated with radiation therapy.[222] In the German Cooperative Ewing's Sarcoma Study, survival with resection was better, although this relative advantage of surgery lost statistical significance when tumor size was considered.[223] The 3-year relapse-free survival was 78% for patients whose tumor volume was less than 100 mL, compared with 17% for patients with tumor volumes greater than 100 mL. Extraosseous extension has also been associated with an increased risk of distant relapse.[224]

The long-term morbidity produced by radiotherapy versus surgery is often the deciding factor when selecting the most appropriate modality for local control. In addition to analyses of resectability and functional outcome, deliberations about local control must also consider the risk of late-onset second malignancies in tissues treated with intensive radiotherapy. Central pelvic or spinal lesions are frequently treated with radiation alone. Extremity lesions amenable to limb-sparing resections are treated predominantly with resection after an initial 12- to 15-week phase of induction chemotherapy. It is critical for the surgeon performing the diagnostic biopsy to place the incision appropriately to avoid complicating future resection.

Chest wall lesions make up 6.5% of primary Ewing's sarcomas, representing the most frequent chest wall tumor in children. They often present with large lesions extending into the thoracic cavity. Traditionally, these have been biopsied by open techniques that can be difficult because of the extremely vascular nature of this tumor and the limited surgical exposure. Percutaneous biopsy, which can provide adequate material for histologic and cytogenetic testing, may be a preferable approach in many cases.[225]

Preoperative chemotherapy can greatly reduce the size, vascularity, and friability of the tumor, facilitating resection and decreasing the risk of intraoperative tumor rupture.[225] Analysis of the 53 patients with nonmetastatic chest wall primaries treated on the first Intergroup Ewing's Sarcoma Study (IESS; POG/CCG) demonstrated a decreased incidence of residual tumor in those patients resected after induction chemotherapy, in contrast to those who underwent resections before treatment with chemotherapy.[226] Current practice mandates the addition of radiotherapy for all patients with microscopic or gross residual disease after resection. Because surgical outcome was improved in patients receiving preoperative chemotherapy, they were less likely to require postoperative chest wall radiotherapy with its well-established risks of cardiac and pulmonary damage and the risk of radiation-induced second malignancies.[227] As noted in the previous section on surgery, the inclusion of 12 to 15 weeks of systemic chemotherapy before introduction of local control measures has become standard practice, regardless of tumor size, location, or stage.

Radiation Therapy

Radiation responsiveness was one of the cardinal diagnostic features of the bone tumor first described by Ewing in 1921.[208] Unfortunately, the long-term survival rate of patients with Ewing's sarcoma after treatment with local radiation alone was only 9%. The vast majority of these patients ultimately succumbed to metastatic disease, suggesting the presence of occult metastatic tumor foci in most affected children.[17] These findings presaged the routine inclusion of systemic chemotherapy in the treatment of this disease, leading to a marked improvement in survival since the 1970s.

Local control of Ewing's sarcoma with radiation is dependent on the delivery of a sufficient dose of irradiation to an adequate volume of tissue. Both the requisite minimum dose and the optimal treatment volume continue to be debated. Although dose-response information is limited for modern studies that use adjuvant chemotherapy, local control rates have been fairly similar, ranging from 75% to 90% at radiation doses varying from 45 to 65 Gy.[228]

Local control rates have improved with the introduction of adjuvant chemotherapy. In an early study assessing combined modality therapy, Chan and colleagues reported local tumor recurrence in only 2.8% of patients treated with 60 Gy and adjuvant chemotherapy.[229] Local disease recurrence was identified in 33.3% of patients who received identical local irradiation but no adjuvant chemotherapy.

The IESS examined the relation of primary tumor site, radiation therapy dose, treatment volume, and adjuvant chemotherapy regimen to local tumor control. Local tumor recurrence occurred in 22.6% of patients with primary tumors in the humerus, 15.3% of those with tumors originating in the pelvis, 10.3% of patients with tibial primaries, and 6.7% of those whose tumor originated in the femur. A dose-response relationship was not apparent when local control was evaluated in patients who had received treatment to an adequate volume.[230]

Improved local control of tumor with irradiation followed the identification of a target volume encompassing the entire medullary cavity to moderately high-dose levels. Suit summarized the experience of the 1950s and 1960s in recommending irradiation to the entire involved bone with a higher dose boost to the primary tumor site, noting few instances of marginal or distant intramedullary recurrence with such treatment.[231] Such large treatment volumes are no longer used.

Assessment of the primary target volume requires detailed attention to both intraosseous and adjacent soft tissue tumor extent.

Local or tailored fields encompassing the primary tumor with a 3- to 5-cm margin, rather than treatment of the entire bone, have been evaluated.[232,233] Marcus et al. reported excellent local control using tailored fields, noting the ability to spare a component of the long bones in tumors less than 8 cm in diameter, whereas frequently requiring whole bone irradiation to achieve a 4-cm margin around larger tumors.[233]

The POG prospectively evaluated whole bone (conventional) irradiation compared with tailored treatment fields, ultimately collapsing a planned randomized study to a single-arm trial using only tailored fields. A published analysis of this trial supports the efficacy of more limited treatment volume as defined by prechemotherapy tumor extent.[232] There was no difference in local control rates between patients receiving whole bone versus involved-field radiation. This more tailored field with a 1.5- to 2.0-cm margin has become the standard strategy used in the most recent North American Ewing's sarcoma trials.

The data available in the literature, and those accumulated by the IESS, have not demonstrated a strong relationship between the radiation dose and the local control rate when doses greater than 40 Gy were used. Radiation doses greater than 60 Gy did not appear to significantly increase the local control rate and were associated with considerable long-term morbidity. Although the available data did not suggest that doses exceeding 40 Gy were essential for adequate local control rates in patients treated with adjuvant chemotherapy, comparisons between this dose and higher doses should be conducted in controlled trials. The current standard dose prescription is 55.8 Gy for gross and 45 Gy for microscopic residual disease.

The comparable outcome achieved with smaller, tailored fields is most provocative when considered in the context of the late sequelae of radiation therapy. The risk of secondary sarcomas arising in irradiated bone is variously reported as ranging from 5% to 10% at 20 years from diagnosis. Although no clear therapeutic advantage can be attributed to radiation doses in excess of 60 Gy, analysis of the long-term outcome in patients treated with doses greater than or equal to 60 Gy demonstrated an unacceptable excess risk of secondary bone sarcomas. In marked contrast to the late complications seen in patients receiving very high-dose radiation, the risk of developing a secondary bone tumor in the irradiated field was negligible at doses below 48 Gy.[234]

Chemotherapy

The availability of chemotherapeutic agents active against macroscopic deposits of Ewing's sarcoma suggested that improved relapse-free survival rates might be achieved with the use of these agents in patients with microscopic residual disease.

In 1973, the IESS initiated a trial (IESS-I) to evaluate the potential additional benefit of adding doxorubicin and prophylactic whole lung irradiation to standard treatment of patients with nonmetastatic Ewing's sarcoma with VAC. The patients treated with the four-drug regimen that included doxorubicin had superior relapse-free survival.[235] In a subsequent study (IESS-II), the efficacy of administration of high-dose (1400 mg/m²) cyclophosphamide every 6 weeks was compared with administration of cyclophosphamide (500 mg/m²) weekly for 6 weeks. The regimen that included high-dose cyclophosphamide also included a higher dose of doxorubicin (75 mg/m²) than did the weekly cyclophosphamide schema. The 5-year relapse-free survival was 73% for the high-dose cyclophosphamide, high-dose doxorubicin regimen, compared with 56% for the weekly cyclophosphamide regimen ($P = .03$).[236,237]

The POG and CCG completed an intergroup study comparing the combination of vincristine, doxorubicin, cyclophosphamide, and dactinomycin to the combination of these four drugs plus ifosfamide and etoposide. The 5-year EFS was 69%

for those who received the six-drug regimen, compared with 54% for those who received the four-drug regimen ($P = .0005$).[238] Similar improvements in survival with the addition of ifosfamide have been reported in studies by the National Cancer Institute and multiple European cooperative groups.[239–241]

Standard chemotherapy for nonmetastatic disease in North America consists of a five-drug regimen including the three-drug combination of vincristine, doxorubicin, and cyclophosphamide, alternating with the two-drug combination of ifosfamide and etoposide for a total of 48 weeks. The intergroup POG/CCG study for nonmetastatic Ewing's sarcoma compared this 48-week, five-drug combination with a dose-intensified 30-week schedule using the same agents at identical cumulative doses. The experimental arm in this study increased the dose intensity of alkylating agents by 25%. Preliminary statistic analysis of this study reveals no evidence of improved EFS with the dose-intensified regimen (L. Granowetter, *personal communication*, April 2000). Although the Kaplan-Meier plots for EFS may yet diverge, current data from this randomized study suggest that new treatment strategies will be required if further improvements in survival are to be achieved.

In contrast to the improvement in survival for nonmetastatic patients treated with the addition of ifosfamide and etoposide, no comparable benefit could be demonstrated for metastatic patients. Previous studies, however, had shown improved survival with the addition of radiation to metastatic sites of disease. Patients with hematogenous metastases entered on IESS-II were treated with irradiation to the primary tumor in addition to whole lung radiation (18 Gy) for patients with pulmonary metastases and local bone irradiation for bone metastases. This strategy yielded a progression-free survival of 39%, demonstrating that some patients with hematogenous metastases can be successfully treated.[243]

Several groups have explored the feasibility and efficacy of maximally dose-intensive chemotherapy regimens in combination with total body irradiation and peripheral blood stem cell rescue in an effort to improve the prognosis for high-risk patients.[244–248] Analysis of these studies is complicated by the nonstandardized inclusion of both metastatic and nonmetastatic patients in some of the high-risk cohorts. One study reported a 3-year relapse-free survival of 43% after megatherapy with chemotherapy, total body irradiation, and stem cell rescue.[249] Unfortunately, longer follow-up of this cohort revealed a disappointing decline in EFS to 27%.[250] None of these results is clearly superior to the outcome reported for similar patients treated on IESS-II without intensive chemotherapy or total body irradiation. Although the early response data from several of these dose-intensive regimens appears promising, their small size and short follow-up mandate a guarded approach to their therapeutic potential. Further substantial improvements in survival for both metastatic and nonmetastatic patients will require identification of new non–cross-resistant cytotoxic agents and translation of our growing understanding of the unique molecular derangements of this disease into targeted biologic therapies.[251]

PROGNOSTIC FACTORS

Historically, the prognosis for children and young adults with Ewing's family tumors has been assessed based on tumor size, location, and extent. Aside from the poor prognosis associated with metastatic disease, large tumor size (greater than 8 cm in diameter) and volume (greater than 100 mL) have correlated with adverse outcome. Children with nonmetastatic pelvic primary sites also have a poorer prognosis than children with extremity primaries, although this difference may be related to the larger size and more difficult resectability of pelvic tumors.[252-254] High serum lactate dehydrogenase levels at diagnosis have been shown to predict a poorer prognosis in several studies.

Although not true prognostic factors assessable at the time of diagnosis, radiographic and histologic response to initial chemotherapy appear to be strong predictors of treatment outcome. Poor histologic response correlates with a poor prognosis, whereas complete or near complete tumor necrosis strongly correlates with good outcome, with a 5-year EFS of 84% to 95%.[255-257] Researchers in Vienna and New York have independently identified the type of EWS-FLI1 fusion transcript as a strong predictor of outcome in nonmetastatic patients. Both studies reported remarkably congruent results, with a predicted 5-year EFS of approximately 70% for type 1 transcripts versus 20% for all other types of fusion transcripts.[213,214] Nearly two-thirds of all patients in both studies were found to have type 1 fusion transcripts. Although the prognostic significance of this finding appears to be substantial, these findings must be prospectively validated before they are used to stratify patients for therapeutic purposes. All upcoming North American pediatric cooperative group studies conducted by the COG (POG/CCG) require submission of diagnostic tissue for molecular analyses that include determination of EWS-FLI1 gene rearrangement status.

PRIMARY HEPATIC TUMORS

EPIDEMIOLOGY AND GENETICS

Approximately 60% to 70% of all primary liver tumors in children are malignant, with hepatoblastoma and hepatocellular carcinoma (HCC) representing the vast majority of malignancies arising in this location. Hemangiomas and hamartomas constitute the majority of nonmalignant liver tumors in the pediatric population.[258]

Hepatoblastoma accounts for slightly more than one-half of hepatic malignancies, occurring at an annual rate of 2.0 cases per 1 million children younger than 15 years. In contrast, HCC occurs less frequently in children, accounting for only one-third of all malignant hepatic tumors in the pediatric age group. In addition to the significant difference in incidence, hepatoblastoma and HCC are distinguished by age at diagnosis. Hepatoblastoma tends to affect young children, with a median age at diagnosis of 1 year. HCC is typically identified in older children, with a median age of 12 years. Both tumors demonstrate a male predominance.[259]

Children diagnosed with hepatoblastoma have had additional anomalies, including hemihypertrophy, Meckel's diverticulum, congenital absence of the kidney, congenital absence of the adrenal gland, and umbilical hernia.[258] Infants and children with incomplete or complete forms of the Beckwith-Wiedemann syndrome have an increased risk of developing hepatoblastoma, suggesting a link between loss of heterozygosity at chromosome 11p15.5 and the pathogenesis of both diseases.[260] Loss of heterozygosity for 11p15.5 has been identified in nearly one-third of all cases of hepatoblastoma.[261] Familial

adenomatous polyposis has been identified in the mothers and maternal relatives of several patients with hepatoblastoma.[262] The risk of hepatoblastoma arising in children from kindreds with the adenomatous polyposis coli (APC) gene on the long arm of chromosome 5 is 1000 to 2000 times higher than the risk in sporadic cases with no family history of familial adenomatous polyposis.[263] Other cytogenetic abnormalities associated with the pathogenesis of hepatoblastoma include LOH of 1p and 1q, trisomies of 2 and 20, and activating mutations of the β-catenin gene.[264] In addition to these chromosomal derangements, children with a history of prematurity and very low birth weight appear to be at increased risk for hepatoblastoma.[265] In a study based on the Japanese Children's Cancer Registry, hepatoblastoma accounted for 58% of the cancer diagnoses in children with a history of extremely low birth weight (less than 1000 g).[265] The authors suggest that this association points to a combination of aberrant genetic endowments and prenatal events or exposures that contribute to disruptions in normal organogenesis, culminating in transformation of hepatocytes.

HCC is strongly associated with infection with hepatitis B virus, both in the presence and absence of pathologic evidence of cirrhosis in nontumorous hepatic tissue. Hepatitis B virus can be acquired via vertical transmission from seropositive mothers or through exposure to contaminated blood products.[266] Several studies have documented a near 100% rate of seropositivity for hepatitis B surface antigen in children who develop HCC. Efforts to reduce the incidence of hepatitis B infection with universal hepatitis B vaccination in Taiwan have produced a corresponding decrease in the risk of developing HCC.[267]

In addition to the association with hepatitis B, HCC has been diagnosed in pediatric patients with several other underlying diseases, including tyrosinemia, galactosemia, biliary atresia, progressive familial cholestatic cirrhosis, giant cell hepatitis of infancy, Fanconi's anemia, type I glycogen storage disease, hepatic glycogenosis with Fanconi's syndrome, α_1-antitrypsin deficiency (MZ phenotype), Sotos' syndrome, and neurofibromatosis.[17,268] Hemochromatosis has not been associated with HCC in pediatric patients, although it is frequently associated with this disease in adult populations.

PATHOLOGY

Hepatoblastoma may be divided into two broad histologic subsets of uncertain prognostic significance. The pure epithelial type consists of either fetal or embryonal elements or a combination of both cell types. Alternatively, the tumor may consist of a mixture of epithelial cells with mesenchymal elements.[264] Pure fetal histology is prognostically favorable in patients with completely resected hepatoblastoma.[269] Hepatoblastoma tends to occupy a single site within the liver, most commonly arising in the right lobe.

In contrast to hepatoblastoma, HCC is often multicentric at diagnosis, substantially limiting the feasibility of complete resection.[259]

CLINICAL PRESENTATION

Infants and children with hepatoblastoma are most frequently identified by the discovery of an abdominal mass or abdominal distention. Symptoms such as weight loss, anorexia, or fever may also be present, although jaundice is infrequent.

The presenting physical findings in children with HCC are quite similar to the characteristic features of hepatoblastoma. Children with HCC typically present with an abdominal mass or abdominal distention.

EVALUATION AND STAGING

The history of pediatric patients suspected of having a malignant hepatic tumor should be reviewed for any history of jaundice or hepatitis. Laboratory data obtained in the perinatal period for the evaluation of hyperbilirubinemia should be reviewed. The maternal prenatal history should be evaluated for the use of steroidal hormones. Previous exposures to hepatotoxic agents should be recorded. The family history should be reviewed for prior cases of hepatic or biliary disease in siblings or parents.

Laboratory evaluation should include a complete blood count, white blood cell differential, tests of renal and hepatic function, and a urinalysis. The serum levels of total bilirubin, alkaline phosphatase, and glutamic-oxaloacetic acid transaminase are not generally useful for the differential diagnosis of malignant hepatic tumors in children.

The serum level of AFP is increased in approximately 90% of patients with hepatoblastoma and 78% of adult patients with HCC.[270,271] Once the diagnosis of HCC is established, additional studies should include hepatitis B surface antigen, hepatitis B antibody, serum iron, total iron-binding capacity, serum ferritin, and α_1-antitrypsin phenotyping.

Abdominal radiographic examination should include CT and MRI imaging. Malignant hepatic tumors are rarely calcified.

Abdominal ultrasonography demonstrates the presence and extent of a solid mass. Sonography assesses both kidneys and the inferior vena cava, providing information useful for differential diagnosis and surgical management. The proximal extent of tumor thrombus within the inferior vena cava may be determined by echocardiography or cardiac angiography.

Pulmonary metastases are identified on plain chest radiography in approximately 10% of patients with hepatoblastoma and HCC.[270] The additional yield of chest CT in pediatric patients with hepatoblastoma or HCC has not yet been fully evaluated, although there appears to a trend toward poorer survival in patients with lung metastases evident on CT only (negative chest x-ray).[272]

The grouping system used in the therapeutic studies of children with malignant hepatic tumors conducted by the CCG and POG segregates patients according to the resectability of the primary tumor, a criterion that may vary among treatment centers. This staging system also accounts for the presence of lymph node or hematogenous metastases (Table 40.2-10).[273] In contrast to the postoperative staging system used in the North American cooperative group studies, the first clinical trial conducted by the European International Society of Pediatric Oncology Liver Tumor Study group (SIOPEL) used the Pretreatment Extent of Disease (PRETEXT) staging system (Fig. 40.2-6).[274] This preoperative classification scheme divides the liver into four sectors and characterizes tumors by the number of sectors involved. The PRETEXT system was devised to facilitate assessment of the efficacy of neoadjuvant chemotherapy in rendering tumors resectable. Based on the first SIOPEL study,

TABLE 40.2-10. Clinical Staging System for Childhood Hepatic Tumors

Stage	Description
STAGE I	Patient had complete resection of tumor by wedge resection, lobectomy, or extended lobectomy, as the initial procedure.
STAGE II	Patient has microscopic residual disease after surgical resection. There is no evidence of regional lymph node involvement by tumor. There was no spillage of tumor.
STAGE III	Gross residual disease or regional lymph node involvement by tumor or tumor spilled.
A	Regional lymph node involvement by tumor or tumor spill, but primary tumor completely resected.
B	Gross tumor not completely resected.
STAGE IV	Distant metastases are present.
A	Primary tumor completely resected.
B	Primary tumor not completely resected.

the PRETEXT system appears to have substantial prognostic value.[274]

TREATMENT

Surgery

Resection is the cornerstone of treatment for hepatoblastoma and HCC. Long-term survival is rare for patients who have not undergone a successful resection.[273] Hepatoblastoma is gener-

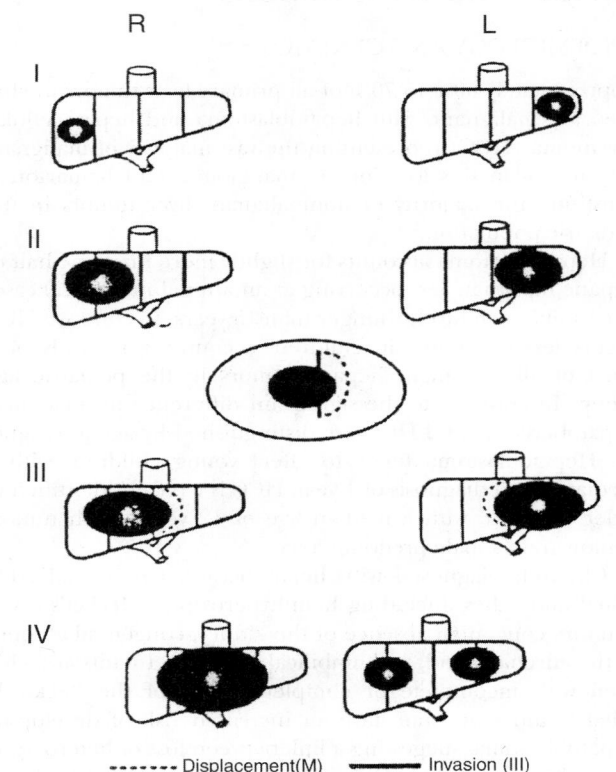

------- Displacement(M)   —— Invasion (III)

FIGURE 40.2-6. Pretreatment Extent of Disease (PRETEXT) grouping system for hepatoblastoma. (From ref. 274, with permission.)

ally unifocal, arising at one site within the liver parenchyma, whereas HCC is frequently multifocal. HCC has an invasive pattern of spread across anatomic planes and is generally unresponsive to current forms of chemotherapy.[275] Complete resection of HCC is frequently difficult owing to its multifocality and invasiveness. Approximately one-half of all hepatoblastomas are resectable at initial presentation, whereas only 30% of HCCs can be fully resected at diagnosis.[258]

Radiographic imaging (MRI with MR angiography) before surgical exploration is critical to the surgeon. It defines the critical relationship between the tumor and associated vasculature. Ultimately, the feasibility of resection can only be determined by direct surgical exploration. Factors that render a liver tumor unresectable include involvement of both lobes of the liver and lymph node involvement in the porta hepatis or mediastinum. Additional features that preclude resection include direct extension into the inferior vena cava, a central lesion that involves the left and right hepatic arteries or the portal vein, or lesions that involve all branches of the hepatic vein.

A large hepatoblastoma grossly distorts the normal anatomy and relationships of the vessels. Hepatoblastoma, in contrast with HCC, does not invade surrounding liver segments as much as it distorts them. It is as if a balloon is placed within the liver parenchyma and is progressively inflated. The vessels to the uninvolved segments may be tightly drawn over a massively enlarged segment, making safe dissection and preservation difficult. As the tumor responds to chemotherapy, it does not regress from areas of involvement, although its decreased volume permits identification of the normal uninvolved segments. Treatment with chemotherapy before definitive surgery has permitted complete resections in children whose hepatoblastomas were initially deemed unresectable.[276,277] Regrettably, HCC has been much less responsive to chemotherapy, limiting the effectiveness of preoperative pharmacologic intervention. When feasible, aggressive attempts at initial resection of HCC should be pursued.

Although complications from hepatectomy persist, perioperative mortality has significantly decreased. Bile leaks, strictures, subphrenic or subhepatic abscesses, and intraoperative hemorrhage are the most frequent complications. In the SIO-PEL study, which delivered preoperative chemotherapy to all stages of disease, complete resections were achieved in 80% of cases.[274] This compares very favorably to historic resection rates of 30% to 50%.

Hepatic transplantation has been used by several centers for children with unresectable liver tumors, with a survival rate of 50.0% to 87.5% reported for children with hepatoblastoma.[278,279] Success with this treatment approach for patients with HCC has been extremely limited, although a recent study reported promising results with a 5-year EFS of 70% in a small series of selected patients without extrahepatic disease. None of the patients with major intrahepatic venous invasion survived.[280]

Cryoablation or radiofrequency ablation of hepatic malignancies has been increasingly used in adults, particularly for metastatic lesions in the liver.[281] Although these techniques have been used in treatment of recurrent disease, their overall role in treatment of pediatric neoplasms remains to be defined.

Long-term evaluation of infants and children after hepatic resection has demonstrated normal synthetic and degradative function of the liver. Liver volumes assessed by MRI are near normal, despite prior anatomic lobectomies or trisegmentecto-mies. Sequential studies have shown that hepatic volumes continue to increase as the children grow after completion of their treatment.[282]

Radiation Therapy

Radiation therapy has a limited role in the treatment of hepatoblastoma or HCC. Generally, combination chemotherapy is given preoperatively to patients with large, unresectable tumors. Postoperative radiation therapy may be valuable in the treatment of children with residual disease after resection.[283] Doses of 25 to 40 Gy are recommended for treatment of limited volumes.

Chemotherapy

After initial biopsy, combination chemotherapy has been administered to children with malignant hepatic tumors to facilitate subsequent surgical excision. In addition to its role in reducing the size of tumors before attempted resections, chemotherapy has been used as a postoperative adjuvant after complete excision of the primary tumor. Initially reported by single institutions, these results led to the design of much larger cooperative group trials of combination chemotherapy in children with hepatoblastoma and HCC.[284–286]

Evans and coworkers reported the results of sequential studies conducted by two pediatric cooperative groups in patients with malignant hepatic tumors.[273] Patients with hepatoblastoma and HCC were evaluated together. Those patients with completely resected disease (group 1) entered on the first study received no therapy after surgery. Those entered on the second study received adjuvant chemotherapy consisting of doxorubicin, cyclophosphamide, vincristine, and 5-fluorouracil. Comparison of these sequential studies demonstrated a significant survival advantage for those patients who received adjuvant chemotherapy compared with patients treated only with surgery.[273]

Based on pilot data that demonstrated the activity of the combination of doxorubicin and cisplatin and of the combination of cisplatin, vincristine, and 5-fluorouracil in patients with malignant liver tumors, the CCG and POG conducted a randomized comparison of these two combinations.[283,287] The results of this trial demonstrated that the two combinations produced similar relapse-free and overall survival percentages within stages. The combination of cisplatin, vincristine, and 5-fluorouracil produced substantially less severe myelosuppression, less need for prolonged hyperalimentation, and fewer toxic deaths. EFS rates for patients treated with the three-drug regimen were 85% for stage I, 100% for stage II, 62% for stage III, and 23% for stage IV.[288] Similar results have been reported by investigators in Toronto,[289] Japan,[290] and Europe.[291–293] The recently published SIO-PEL study revealed 5-year EFS rates of 100%, 83%, 56%, and 46% for patients with PRETEXT stages I to IV. For patients with lung metastases, however, these investigators reported a disappointing 5-year EFS of only 28%, similar to prior North American studies.[292] These studies have consistently demonstrated that a substantial number of initially unresectable tumors can be surgically removed at second exploration after treatment with variations on either of the two-drug combinations.[294] Despite the remarkable similarity in outcomes between these various studies, there was a significant difference in survival for children who underwent initial complete resection, reflecting divergent approaches to postoperative management. The Toronto group reported a 100% EFS for children with complete resections treated with postoperative chemotherapy versus 72% survival for a similar group of children on the POG/CCG study who received no chemotherapy after definitive surgery.[289] Although the numbers in the comparison groups are small, the more favorable outcome with inclusion of chemotherapy suggests that this approach should be prospectively examined.

Japanese investigators have reported successful application of transarterial chemoembolization using cisplatinum and doxorubicin in combination with iodized oil in treatment of a small number of children with inoperable hepatoblastoma.[295] Although the results of this limited series are provocative, the role of this more invasive technique is uncertain given the efficacy of systemic, intravenous administration of the same chemotherapeutic agents.

PROGNOSIS

For both hepatoblastoma and HCC, resectability of the primary tumor and disease extent at diagnosis remain the strongest predictors of survival. Prospects for long-term survival are extremely poor for both histologies in cases of widely metastatic disease.[296]

In contrast to 5-year EFS rates of 70% to 90% for patients with localized, resectable hepatoblastoma, only 25% of patients with metastatic disease are long-term survivors. Despite aggressive efforts at surgical management of HCC, however, long-term survival remains dismal even for patients with fully resected tumors. A North American Pediatric Cooperative Group study demonstrated only 13% survival for children with totally resected HCC.[297] Results for patients with HCC treated on the European SIOPEL study were also quite discouraging, with a 5-year EFS of only 17%.[298] Although improvements in survival for children with hepatoblastoma have been dramatic and gratifying, it is clear that new therapies are required to treat advanced-stage hepatoblastoma and all stages of HCC.

GERM CELL TUMORS

Germ cell tumors arising in gonadal or extragonadal sites constitute a remarkably heterogeneous group of tumors that account for approximately 3% of all pediatric malignancies. Although extragonadal germ cell tumors are relatively infrequent in adults, accounting for only 5% to 10% of all cases, extragonadal tumors make up nearly two-thirds of all germ cell tumors in children.[299] The sacrococcygeal region represents the most common site for germ cell tumors in children, constituting 40% of all childhood germ cell tumors,[300] and 78% of all extragonadal disease.[301] Less common, extragonadal disease arises in the mediastinum, retroperitoneum, vagina, and pineal region. Biologic behavior among this diverse grouping of tumors varies from the benign mature teratoma to the highly malignant embryonal carcinoma and choriocarcinoma. Fortunately, the introduction of platinum-based chemotherapy by Einhorn and Donohue in the 1970s has greatly improved survival for most children affected by these highly chemosensitive tumors (Table 40.2-11).[302] For the vast majority of children affected by malignant germ cell tumors, survival is now so good that current clinical trials are focusing on strategies to decrease the morbidity of platinum-based therapies. These endeavors include withholding chemotherapy for localized, fully resected tumors, shortening treatment courses for selected intermediate-risk tumors and substitution of less toxic platinum analogues.[303,304]

EMBRYOLOGY

Primordial germ cells arise in the embryonic yolk sac endoderm. These cells migrate through the wall of the midgut to the genital ridge at 4 to 5 weeks' gestation. Migration along this paravertebral gonadal ridge proceeds in a caudal to cranial direction. Arrested migration of these germ cells along this pathway has been proposed as an explanation for the near midline location of most extragonadal germ cell tumors, including the sacrococcygeal region, retroperitoneum, mediastinum, and intracranial sites, which primarily consist of the pineal and suprasellar regions.[299,301,305]

PATHOLOGY

Pediatric germ cell tumors include an enormously diverse array of histologies. The majority of extragonadal tumors arising in infancy are benign teratomas. Similarly, most ovarian germ cell tumors are benign lesions. In contrast, the vast majority of germ cell tumors developing in the testis contain malignant yolk sac elements. Although many of these tumors contain a mixture of

TABLE 40.2-11.   Relative Incidence According to Age and Pathology

Site	Relative Incidence (%)	Age	Pathology
Sacrococcyx	35	Neonate	Teratoma: mature 65%, immature 5%, malignant 10–30%
Ovary	25	Early teens	Teratoma: mature 65%, immature 5%, malignant 30% (pure yolk sac 30%, mixed 30%)
Testis	20	Infant and adolescent	Teratoma: mature 20%, malignant 80% (yolk sac 90%, germinoma 10%, embryonal carcinoma 1–5%)
Cranium	5	Child	Germinoma: 20–50%, embryonal carcinoma 20–50%, mature teratomas 20–30%
Mediastinum	5	Adolescent	Teratoma: mature 60%, mixed 20%, embryonal carcinoma 20%
Retroperitoneum	5	Infant	Teratoma: mature or immature, rarely malignant
Head and neck	3	Infant and neonate	Usually mature teratoma, immature rarely malignant
Vagina	2	Infant	Usually yolk sac

(From ref. 305, with permission.)

benign and malignant elements, their clinical behavior and therapeutic management are determined by the most malignant component identified on extensive sectioning.[301] In the following sections, the authors review the various histopathologic subtypes of germ cell tumors most frequently seen in children.

Teratoma

Teratomas contain elements derived from more than one of the three primary germ layers (ectoderm, mesoderm, entoderm) frequently arranged in a haphazard manner. The tissues are immature to well differentiated and foreign to the anatomic site. Mature teratomas are either cystic or solid, although the cystic presentation predominates in gonadal sites. Immature teratomas are graded according to the amount of immature tissue present on light microscopic assessment of sampled tissue. Grade 1 immature teratomas have neuroepithelium or other immature elements limited to only one low-power field per slide. Grade 3 immature teratomas contain abundant immature tissue that is identifiable on greater than or equal to four low-power fields per slide.[306] Nearly all mature teratomas are diploid with normal karyotypes. In contrast, chromosomal derangements are frequently identified in immature teratomas and malignant germ cell tumors. Mature and immature teratomas are treated with surgical excision alone. Adjuvant chemotherapy is reserved for the infrequent recurrence of immature teratomas after resection.[307]

Yolk Sac Tumor (Endodermal Sinus Tumor)

Intracellular and intercellular hyaline droplets are present in typical yolk sac tumors. This material is periodic acid–Schiff positive and resists digestion with diastase. Several groups of investigators have shown that these droplets contain AFP as well as other proteins.[308] Teilum and colleagues suggested that the presence of AFP in these tumors supported the theory that such tumors contained or originated from the yolk sac endoderm.[309]

Several studies of chromosomal abnormalities in childhood germ cell tumors have documented deletions of the distal portion of the short arm of chromosome 1 (1p36), in addition to gains of 1q, +3, +8, +14, and +21. Older children with mediastinal tumors and gonadal tumors arising in teenage girls and boys demonstrate gain of an isochrome 12p.[310] The deletion of 1p noted in yolk sac tumors maps to the same locus identified in neuroblastoma, another embryonal malignancy that typically affects young children.[311] The prognostic importance of this finding remains uncertain. Several putative tumor suppressor genes have been mapped within or adjacent to this locus, however, suggesting a role of this deletion in the pathogenesis of these tumors.

Embryonal Carcinoma

Embryonal carcinoma is composed of cells that resemble epithelial cells. There is considerable variation in their size, shape, and arrangement. The cells may occur as solid sheets. Frequently, small or large acinar, tubular, and papillary structures are formed. Hemorrhage and necrosis are frequent.[312]

Seminoma

Seminomas arising outside the testis are referred to as *germinomas* or *dysgerminomas* (ovarian). Typical seminoma is composed of uniform cells supported by a delicate connective tissue stroma. Characteristically, the seminoma cell is large, polyhedral, or round, with a distinct cell border. Tumor giant cells may be seen. Lymphocytic infiltration is present in most seminomas, with a granulomatous reaction identifiable in approximately one-half of cases.[312] As is commonly found in adult testicular tumors, isochrome 12p (two copies of the short arm of chromosome 12) is frequently identified in adolescent testicular germinomas.[313] This chromosomal abnormality is rarely seen in malignant testicular tumors of infancy in which yolk sac tumor is the predominant histology.

Choriocarcinoma

Choriocarcinoma consists of two distinct cell types: syncytiotrophoblast and cytotrophoblast. The syncytiotrophoblast is a large, multinucleated cell with many hyperchromatic, irregular nuclei and cytoplasm usually eosinophilic or amphophilic. Cytotrophoblast cells are medium sized and closely packed with clear cytoplasm, distinct cell borders, and a single, uniform, moderate-sized vesicular nucleus.[312]

Teratocarcinoma

Teratocarcinomas contain derivatives of more than one of the three primary germ cell layers (entoderm, mesoderm, ectoderm), consistent with the diagnosis of teratoma and areas of embryonal carcinoma. In addition, areas of seminoma, endodermal sinus tumor, and choriocarcinoma may be identified within the tumor.[312]

LABORATORY MARKERS

AFP and the β subunit of human chorionic gonadotropin (β-HCG) are oncofetoproteins that are found at elevated serum levels in association with a variety of germ cell tumors. These proteins are clinically useful both as diagnostic tools and in surveillance of children on or off treatment for tumors that secrete these markers. AFP is a glycoprotein that is produced in the liver, gastrointestinal tract, and yolk sac of the human fetus. The serum concentration of AFP reaches a maximum at 13 weeks of gestation. It is readily detectable at birth, when high physiologic levels confound its diagnostic use in infants with suspected germ cell tumors. Owing to its long serum half-life of 7 days, the level of AFP may remain elevated in healthy infants as old as 6 months.[314] Abelev and colleagues reported in 1967 that patients with testicular tumors that contained elements of embryonal carcinoma had elevated levels of AFP in their serum.[315] Other investigators have reported that children with embryonal carcinomas and malignant teratomas have elevated serum levels of AFP. Most common, high serum levels of AFP are identified in pediatric patients with testicular, ovarian, presacral, and vaginal primary yolk sac tumors.[316]

HCG is a glycoprotein that is secreted by the placenta. Patients with a pure yolk sac tumor do not have detectable serum levels of HCG. Patients with malignant germ cell tumors of the ovary or embryonal carcinoma of the ovary or testis may have elevated serum HCG levels.[317] HCG has a much shorter serum half-life than AFP, lasting only 24 to 36 hours. Thus, a decline in the serum level of this marker occurs much more rapidly with successful therapeutic intervention than is seen in management of tumors that secrete AFP.

CLINICAL PRESENTATION AND TREATMENT BY ANATOMIC SITE

SACROCOCCYGEAL TUMORS

Presacral and sacrococcygeal teratomas are usually diagnosed at birth or during the first month of life. Four types have been defined on the basis of the extent of pelvic and abdominal extension of the teratoma and the presence or absence of external extension of the teratoma (Fig. 40.2-7).[318]

Only 2% of presacral and sacrococcygeal teratomas diagnosed before 6 months of age were malignant, compared with 65% of those diagnosed after 6 months of age. Both benign and malignant teratomas are more frequent in girls. Children with presacral or sacrococcygeal teratomas frequently have congenital anomalies of the vertebrae, genitourinary system, or anorectum.[318,319]

Malignant presacral or sacrococcygeal teratomas may arise *de novo* or at the site of a previously excised benign teratoma.[320]

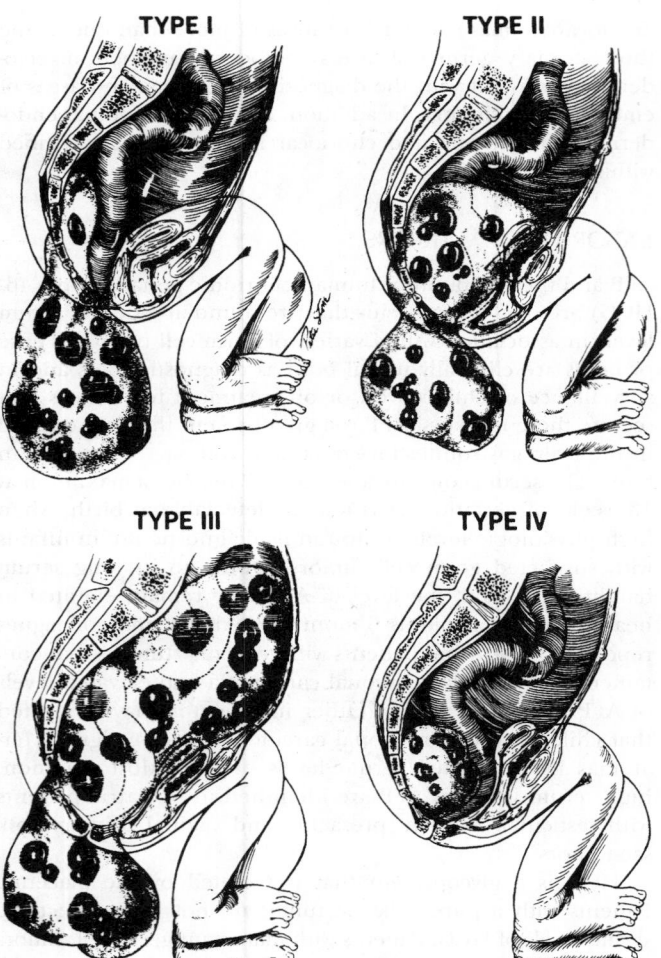

FIGURE 40.2-7. The types of presacral teratomas. Malignancy rates are as follows: type I, 8%; type II, 21%; type III, 34%; and type IV, 38%. (From ref. 318, with permission.)

The frequency of malignancy depends on the type of teratoma, ranging from 8% for patients with type I to 38% for those with type IV lesions.[318] The much higher rate of malignancy in type IV tumors may reflect inadequate or delayed treatment of infants with foci of endodermal sinus tumor within a mature or immature sacrococcygeal teratoma.[321]

Clinical Presentation and Evaluation of Sacrococcygeal Teratomas

Children with malignant pelvic teratomas present with an abdominal or buttock mass or signs of urinary and fecal obstruction. Rectal examination reveals the presence of a mass between the rectum and the sacrum. The mass may extend through the sciatic notch deep into the gluteal muscles.

Staging of the patient with a sacrococcygeal teratoma requires a radionuclide bone scan, plain radiographs of any positive area on the scan and any symptomatic bone, and plain chest radiography and CT of the chest, abdomen, and pelvis (Table 40.2-12).

Yolk sac tumor accounts for the vast majority of malignant presacral and sacrococcygeal teratomas. In marked contrast to the predominance of benign teratomas in neonates with type I tumors, nearly 90% of children with type IV anatomy have tumors consisting of malignant elements.[322] Before the inclusion of cisplatinum in chemotherapy regimens for pelvic yolk sac tumors, survival was poor, barely exceeding 10%.[323] Since the advent of modern, platinum-based chemotherapy in the late 1970s, however, more than 80% of patients with malignant sacrococcygeal teratomas are survivors.[299]

Surgery

Before surgical resection, the upper limit of the tumor should be assessed by rectal examination and either ultrasonography or MRI. In the vast majority of cases, the tumor can be resected by a perineal approach in which an incision is placed around the periphery of the protruding teratoma, preserving the maximum amount of skin. In approximately 10% of infants, a combined perineal and abdominal approach is required.[318] If the tumor is identified in an older child or there is suspicion of malignancy, a preliminary biopsy should be performed. Preoperative chemotherapy should be administered if malignancy is confirmed. A complete resection of malignant teratomas can rarely be achieved without prior treatment with combination

TABLE 40.2-12. Pediatric Oncology Group/Children's Cancer Group Staging for Malignant Extragonadal Germ Cell Tumors

Stage	Description
I	Complete resection at any site; coccygectomy for sacrococcygeal site; negative tumor margins; tumor markers positive or negative
II	Microscopic residual; lymph nodes negative; tumor markers positive or negative
III	Gross residual or biopsy only; retroperitoneal nodes negative or positive; tumor markers positive or negative
IV	Distant metastases, including liver

(From ref. 299, with permission.)

chemotherapy. This approach allows maximum preservation of normal structures, including the rectum, anus, and the sacral plexus, which is critical for bladder and bowel function.

Radiation Therapy

Radiation therapy is not necessary for those children who undergo a complete excision or who have a complete response to combination chemotherapy.[324] In patients who have residual disease after treatment with chemotherapy and second-look surgery, local control with irradiation is poor.[325] If irradiation is indicated, the dose required for extragonadal germ cell tumors is 45 to 50 Gy.

Chemotherapy

As noted previously, malignant pelvic yolk sac tumors are highly responsive to chemotherapy regimens that include cisplatinum.[326–328] Children with pelvic yolk sac tumors should be treated aggressively, with the expectation that such an approach will result in long-term tumor control. Recent publications from the North American and German pediatric cooperative groups have documented survival in excess of 80% even for children with advanced-stage disease. Both studies supported the use of neoadjuvant chemotherapy for locally advanced or metastatic disease.[329,330] Table 40.2-13 contains an algorithm for the inclusion of chemotherapy in the treatment of germ cell tumors based on the risk-group stratification currently used by the North American pediatric cooperative group, COG.

TESTICULAR TUMORS

Testicular tumors make up approximately 10% of all pediatric germ cell tumors. The vast majority of these tumors are malignant (80%), characteristically containing yolk sac elements. In contrast to adult testicular tumors, which are frequently metastatic at initial diagnosis, 90% of pediatric testicular germ cell tumors are localized.[309] Malignant germ cell tumors of the tes-

TABLE 40.2-13. Management Schema for Pediatric Germ Cell Tumors

Group	Treatment
LOW RISK	Surgery and observation
Stage I gonadal	
Stage I extragonadal	
All immature teratomas	
INTERMEDIATE RISK	Surgery and PEB × 3 cycles[a]
Stage II–IV gonadal	
Stage II extragonadal	
HIGH RISK	Surgery and HD-PEB × 4 cycles[a]
Stage III–IV extragonadal	
Recurrent stage I extragonadal (stage III–IV at recurrence)	

B, bleomycin; E, etoposide; P, cisplatin; HD-PEB, high-dose cisplatin with etoposide and bleomycin.
[a]Patients with initial biopsy or incomplete resection have surgical resection of residual disease after completion of initial therapy. Patients who are complete responders (no viable tumor) receive no further therapy, and those with partial response receive additional chemotherapy.

tis occur at an annual incidence of approximately 1 case per 1 million American children younger than 15 years. Testicular germ cell tumors follow a bimodal age distribution, occurring in very young children and adolescent boys. Yolk sac tumor, or *endodermal sinus tumor*, is the most common malignant germ cell tumor of the testis in prepubertal boys, with a median age at diagnosis of 24 months. Testicular tumors in adolescent boys have histologic features similar to those of adults.[305]

Children with yolk sac tumors of the testis have been diagnosed with additional anomalies, including inguinal hernia, double ureter, ectopic kidney, hypospadias, and renal agenesis.[331]

Clinical Presentation and Evaluation

Most children with primary testicular tumors present with painless testicular enlargement. In the relatively infrequent cases of metastatic disease, patients present with abdominal swelling due to malignant ascites, inguinal lymphadenopathy, or acute abdominal pain.

Physical examination reveals testicular enlargement. Yolk sac tumor occurs with equal frequency in the right and left testis. Less than 1% of cases have bilateral testicular involvement at the time of initial presentation.[17]

The preoperative evaluation of a child suspected to have a malignant tumor of the testis should include a plain chest radiograph and serum AFP and HCG levels. Additional studies, including CT of the abdomen, pelvis, and chest, are not necessary before orchiectomy, although they are ultimately required for complete staging of testicular tumors containing malignant elements.

Staging

Once the histologic diagnosis is established, the patient must be staged. Although the majority of pediatric testicular germ cell tumors are nonmetastatic, the tumors may spread to retroperitoneal lymph nodes, liver, lungs, and rarely to bones or brain.

As noted in Clinical Presentation and Evaluation, earlier, staging must include CT of the chest, abdomen, and pelvis, in addition to a radionuclide bone scan.

The retroperitoneal lymph nodes may be evaluated by CT or MRI. Absence of significant retroperitoneal fat in these young children and the inability of a CT to identify normal-sized lymph nodes that contain tumor may limit the sensitivity of CT for staging these patients. Because 90% of malignant testicular germ cell tumors in young children elaborate AFP, adjuvant chemotherapy is reserved for advanced-stage disease and the small percentage of children with occult metastatic disease whose AFP fails to decline after orchiectomy (Table 40.2-14).

Treatment Planning

SURGERY. Preoperative diagnostic studies of a scrotal mass may include ultrasonography that can define the solid or cystic nature of the mass and its relationship to the testicle. All scrotal masses should be explored through an inguinal incision. A transscrotal biopsy contaminates the scrotum and its lymphatic drainage to the inguinal lymph nodes and prevents high ligation of the spermatic cord. If the tumor is clearly malignant, high ligation of the spermatic cord should be performed at the internal ring.

TABLE 40.2-14.   Pediatric Oncology Group/Children's Cancer Group Staging System for Testicular Germ Cell Tumors

Stage	Description
I	Limited to testis: tumor markers normal after appropriate half-life decline (α-fetoprotein, 5 d; human chorionic gonadotropin, 16 h)
II	Transscrotal orchiectomy: microscopic disease in scrotum or high in spermatic cord (<5 cm from proximal end); retroperitoneal lymph node involvement (>2 cm), increased tumor markers after appropriate half-life decline, or both
III	Retroperitoneal lymph node involvement (>2 cm) but no visceral or extraabdominal involvement
IV	Distant metastases, including liver

(From ref. 299, with permission.)

TABLE 40.2-15.   Staging System for Yolk Sac Tumor of the Testis

Stage	Description
STAGE I	Tumor limited to one (or both) testes, which are removed by high inguinal orchiectomy; no clinical, radiographic, or histologic evidence of residual disease beyond the testis; serum α-fetoprotein negative postoperatively.
STAGE II	Transscrotal tumor aspiration, biopsy of tumor within the scrotal sac or scrotal orchiectomy; microscopic residual disease within the scrotum or high in the spermatic cord (<5 cm from the proximal end); microscopic retroperitoneal lymph node involvement (lymph nodes <2 cm in diameter, but histologically positive for tumor) or serum α-fetoprotein positive >4 weeks after orchiectomy.
STAGE III	Gross retroperitoneal lymph node involvement (lymph nodes >2 cm in diameter and histologically positive for tumor).
STAGE IV	
A	Extraabdominal lymph node metastases.
B	Extranodal metastases are present (e.g., liver, lung, peritoneum, bones, bone marrow, or brain).

Increasingly, effective cisplatin-based chemotherapy for nonseminomatous germ cell tumors has decreased the role of surgical resection of the retroperitoneal lymph nodes as a therapeutic modality. Infants have a predominance of early-stage lesions that are primarily endodermal sinus tumors (yolk sac tumors), in contrast with teenage boys in whom the embryonal carcinoma or mixed germ cell tumors predominate. Teenagers frequently delay seeking medical attention, resulting in a higher proportion of advanced-stage disease at initial presentation. In most series, infants with clinical stage I (Table 40.2-15) endodermal sinus tumors are treated by radical orchiectomy and then close follow-up. In the United Kingdom Children's Cancer Group Study of malignant germ cell tumors, 87% of the boys presented with stage I testicular tumors that were treated by orchiectomy alone.[332,333] The pathology of these lesions was predominantly yolk sac tumors (57 of 61). In seven boys, a rising serum AFP was the only evidence for incomplete resection. All responded well to chemotherapy. Survival using this protocol was 100%.

The clinical behavior of testicular embryonal carcinomas is similar in teenagers and adults. Studies have demonstrated that adults with clinical stage I embryonal carcinoma of the testes have positive retroperitoneal lymph nodes in approximately 30% of cases.[334] This earlier finding is supported by reports of a 28% relapse rate in adults with stage I disease who were initially observed after radical orchiectomy.[335] A similar approach to localized disease in children was used at the St. Jude Children's Research Hospital where relapse with a pulmonary metastasis was seen in one of eight boys.[336] In many current protocols, children with clinical stage I disease (i.e., no radiographically identifiable retroperitoneal tumor and falling serum markers) are followed after radical orchiectomy. Children with identifiable retroperitoneal tumor frequently receive initial chemotherapy, with surgery reserved for residual masses or persistently elevated markers. Resection of postchemotherapy residual masses in adults demonstrated that 45.0% had necrosis, 42.5% had teratoma, and 12.5% had viable germ cell tumor.[337] The North American and European pediatric cooperative groups currently use this strategy of surgery alone followed by close surveillance in children with stage I germ cell tumors, regardless of site or histology. This watch and wait approach for localized, fully resected germ cell tumors of all histologies was further validated by the United Kingdom Children's Cancer Group second germ cell study. In this 2000 study, British investigators reported

100% survival in the 22 stage I patients who relapsed after initial treatment with surgery. All of these patients were salvaged with platinum-based chemotherapy at relapse.[304]

Children with yolk sac tumors of the testis rarely require bilateral retroperitoneal lymph node dissection for adequate staging. Because this diagnostic procedure carries substantial potential morbidity and infrequently provides information that will change the stage or influence therapy, retroperitoneal lymphadenectomy should be avoided.

CHEMOTHERAPY. Current therapeutic practice reserves chemotherapy for children with either advanced-stage disease, recurrent localized tumors, or children with stage I disease whose tumor markers fail to decline after orchiectomy. Inclusion of chemotherapy in the treatment of children with stage I disease has not provided a statistically significant advantage in relapse-free survival.

The application of combination chemotherapy to the treatment of children with advanced stage or recurrent yolk sac tumor has proceeded from the use of similar programs for the management of adults with nonseminomatous germ cell tumors of the testis. The first effective combinations included dactinomycin, chlorambucil, and methotrexate or dactinomycin, vincristine, and cyclophosphamide. Unfortunately, neither of these regimens significantly increased the number of patients with advanced abdominal or pulmonary metastatic disease who achieved long-term, disease-free survival.

Subsequent identification of bleomycin and cisplatinum as active agents against testicular germ cell tumors, however, has substantially improved survival for patients with disseminated disease. The Einhorn regimen, consisting of cisplatin, vinblastine, and bleomycin (PVB), was developed at the Indiana University Medical Center in 1974. It has been active against embryonal carcinoma, teratocarcinoma, choriocarcinoma, and yolk sac tumor of the testis.[302] The activity of this three-drug combination has been confirmed by several groups of North American and European investigators. Increasing the dose intensity of cisplatin does not improve the response rate or survival rate but does increase the toxicity of the PVB regimen.[338] Substitution of etoposide for vinblastine in the PVB regimen did not change the response rate and substantially decreased the toxicity of the chemotherapy regimen.[339] In light of the pulmonary toxicity of bleomycin, multiple studies have been conducted to assess the value of continued inclusion of this agent in platinum-based regimens. Although several randomized adult studies suggest that bleomycin may be deleted from the cisplatin, etoposide, and bleomycin combination based on comparable response rates with and without this agent, there were sufficient differences in overall and relapse-free survival to recommend its continued use.[340,341] In view of impressive responses to alternative regimens using ifosfamide and etoposide and a United Kingdom study that effectively substituted carboplatinum for cisplatinum, there are now several potentially less toxic chemotherapy options that need to be prospectively tested.[304,342–344]

The same guidelines for management of young children with yolk sac tumors of the testis should be applied to adolescents with malignant germ cell tumors. Teenagers with stage I nonseminomatous germ cell tumors may be managed with close surveillance.[345] Those with more advanced-stage disease should receive platinum-based combination chemotherapy.

OVARY

Ovarian tumors account for approximately 25% of all pediatric germ cell tumors. The majority of these tumors arise later in childhood, with a peak incidence at 10 years of age. Most of these tumors are benign mature cystic teratomas, although nearly one-third contain malignant elements. In contrast to adult ovarian tumors, malignancies of the epithelial or stromal cell origin are uncommon in children. The most common pediatric ovarian neoplasias are dysgerminomas and yolk sac tumors. Immature teratomas account for approximately 10% of ovarian masses.[300,305]

Clinical Presentation

Patients with ovarian tumors present with abdominal pain or an abdominal mass. The pain may be severe owing to torsion of the ovarian pedicle by the ovary and tumor.[346] Fever is present in 24% of patients at the time of diagnosis.

Preoperative radiographic evaluation should include studies that localize the mass to the ovary. A plain abdominal radiograph should be obtained and examined for the presence of calcification. Abdominal ultrasonography demonstrates whether the mass is cystic in nature. CT provides more detailed information about the site of origin of the tumor. In patients with suspected ovarian germ cell tumors, serum levels of AFP and HCG should be assayed before diagnostic or therapeutic surgical intervention. Once the tissue diagnosis is established, the potential sites of metastatic disease should be examined. Possible sites of dissemination include peritoneal implants, retroperitoneal lymph nodes, lung, liver, and bone. There has been considerable controversy regarding the proper risk-group stratification and treatment of patients with immature teratomas and gliomatosis peritonei (peritoneal seeding with mature glial tissue). In general, immature teratomas are treated with surgery alone. The controversy resides in questions about the

TABLE 40.2-16. Pediatric Oncology Group/Children's Cancer Group Staging System for Pediatric Ovarian Germ Cell Tumors

Stage	Description
I	Limited to ovary (ovaries) peritoneal washings negative; tumor markers normal after appropriate half-life decline (α-fetoprotein, 5 d; human chorionic gonadotropin, 16 h)
II	Microscopic residual or positive lymph nodes (<2 cm); peritoneal washings negative for malignant cells, tumor markers positive or negative
III	Lymph node involvement (>2 cm); gross residual or biopsy only; contiguous visceral involvement (omentum, intestine, bladder); peritoneal washings positive for malignant cell; tumor markers positive or negative
IV	Distant metastases, including liver

appropriateness of surgery alone for immature teratomas that have extensively seeded the omentum and peritoneal surfaces. In a report by POG/CCG documenting 135 cases of childhood immature teratomas, 22 of 86 cases of ovarian immature teratoma were characterized by gliomatosis peritonei. Investigators on this study found that this feature had no adverse effect on outcome in patients treated with surgery alone.[347] Only the finding of microscopic foci of malignant yolk sac tumor in immature teratomas correlated with poor prognosis, mandating inclusion of adjuvant chemotherapy for this small subset of children. These same authors note that although modest elevations of AFP (less than 60) may be recorded in children with immature teratomas without malignant elements, nearly all patients with AFP greater than 100 have occult foci of malignant yolk sac tumor.[347]

Staging

Staging evaluation should include a CT of the chest, abdomen, and pelvis, in addition to bone scintigraphy with technetium 99m pertechnetate. Ovarian tumors are staged using the POG/CCG staging system, which represents a simplified derivation of the International Federation of Gynecology and Obstetrics staging system (Table 40.2-16).[299]

Treatment Planning

SURGERY. Surgical exploration of an ovarian mass must accomplish two goals: resection of the primary tumor and adequate staging. Peritoneal fluid should be aspirated for cytology. If no fluid is present, peritoneal washings should be obtained. Any peritoneal seeding should be biopsied and a partial or complete omentectomy performed. Ipsilateral lymph nodes should be examined and biopsies taken from the iliac, low periaortic, or pericaval nodes and the periaortic or pericaval nodes at the level of the renal vessels. The contralateral ovary should be examined closely, and if nodules are present, particularly in dysgerminomas or teratomas, a biopsy should be obtained. With current techniques available for *in utero* fertilization, increasing efforts are taken to preserve the fallopian tube and uterus in cases in which both ovaries must be resected.[348]

CHEMOTHERAPY. Combination chemotherapy with VAC was used in the 1970s in two small series of pediatric patients with ovarian yolk sac tumor. These early studies demonstrated that improved survival could be achieved with inclusion of chemotherapy in treatment of patients with stage I and II disease.[349,350] Results of these pediatric trials were consistent with the outcomes of studies in adults with ovarian yolk sac tumor that documented similar improvements in survival with adjuvant VAC chemotherapy.[351] Neither study reported the response rate of women with advanced ovarian yolk sac tumor to VAC.

Closely paralleling the chronology and evolution of chemotherapy for testicular germ cell tumors, subsequent clinical trials for ovarian germ cell tumors used the combination of PVB in the treatment of women with advanced ovarian germ cell tumors. Current pediatric practice uses the cisplatin, etoposide, and bleomycin regimen for treatment of primary nonlocalized or recurrent ovarian germ cell tumors. This regimen has produced survival rates exceeding 90% for localized and advanced-stage ovarian germ cell tumors in children.[299]

RADIATION THERAPY. With the advent of such effective chemotherapy for ovarian germ cell tumors, the current role of radiation therapy is uncertain. No radiation therapy is given for histologies other than dysgerminoma if surgery and chemotherapy render the child free of disease.[305] In the unusual situation in which there is persistent disease after initial surgery, chemotherapy, and a second-look operation, 40 Gy is recommended.

Treatment options for ovarian dysgerminoma are more complex. Dysgerminomas are curable with irradiation, with one small pediatric study documenting a 5-year overall survival of 94%. Unfortunately, this same study described extensive late sequelae to radiation therapy, including infertility, dysmenorrhea, hypogonadism, and pelvic fibrosis.[352] Given the morbidity of pelvic irradiation and the exquisite chemosensitivity of this tumor, radiation should be reserved for second-line therapy in patients who have relapsed after surgery and chemotherapy. In those rare cases in which radiation therapy is indicated, doses required for dysgerminoma are 20 to 25 Gy, with a boost to gross residual disease to a total dose of 35 to 40 Gy.[348]

MEDIASTINUM

Germ cell tumors of the thoracic cavity typically arise in the anterior mediastinum of adolescent boys. Although the majority of these tumors are benign teratomas, malignant yolk sac tumor and choriocarcinoma have been identified in this location.[353] Several patients with Klinefelter's syndrome have developed yolk sac tumors.[354] The clinical presentation is characterized by a brief history of cough, dyspnea, and chest pain due to tracheobronchial compression.

Routine chest radiographs may demonstrate an incidental anterior mediastinal mass. The diagnosis is established by biopsy of the primary tumor at thoracotomy or mediastinoscopy or by biopsy of an involved supraclavicular lymph node. Staging studies, including a bone scan, skeletal survey, bone marrow aspirate, and biopsy, should be performed immediately after tissue diagnosis is established.

The application of cisplatin-containing chemotherapy regimens to children with malignant mediastinal germ cell tumors has produced a dramatic improvement in survival. Recent publications from the German and British cooperative groups document 5-year survival rates in excess of 80%. These results are only slightly higher than the 71% 4-year survival

reported in a contemporary North American cooperative group study.[307,329,355]

Given that therapeutic failure is frequently due to local progression of the tumor, the ultimate extent of surgical resection, whether primary or delayed, has emerged as a strong prognostic factor.[355] Because achieving complete surgical excision in this site may be difficult, therapeutic morbidity may be minimized by treating malignant tumors with neoadjuvant chemotherapy followed by delayed resection. Based on the very encouraging results of the German, British, and North American cooperative group studies, it appears that the prognosis for children with mediastinal germ cell tumors is nearly equivalent to the excellent prognosis reported for histologically similar tumors arising in other sites.

REFERENCES

1. U.S. Cancer Statistics Working Group. *United States cancer statistics: 2000 incidence.* Atlanta: Department of Health and Human Services, Centers for Disease Control and Prevention and National Cancer Institute, 2003.
2. Arias E, MacDorman M, Strobino D, Guter B. Annual summary of vital statistics—2002. *Pediatrics* 2003;112:1215.
3. Breslow N, Olshan A, Beckwith JB, Green DM. Epidemiology of Wilms tumor. *Med Pediatr Oncol* 1993;21:172.
4. Miller RW, Fraumeni JF Jr, Manning MD. Association of Wilms' tumor with aniridia, hemihypertrophy and other congenital malformations. *N Engl J Med* 1964;270:922.
5. Porteus M, Narkool P, Neuberg D, et al. Characteristics and outcome of children with Beckwith-Wiedemann syndrome and Wilms' tumor: a report from the National Wilms' Tumor Study Group. *J Clin Oncol* 2000;18:2026.
6. Coppes MJ, Huff V, Pelletier J. Denys-Drash syndrome: relating a clinical disorder to genetic alterations in the tumor suppressor gene WT1. *J Pediatr* 1993;123:673.
7. Murphy WM, Beckwith JB, Farrow GM. *Atlas of tumor pathology. 3rd Series. Fascicle 11. Tumors of the kidney, bladder, and related urinary structures.* Washington, DC: Armed Forces Institute of Pathology, 1994.
8. Faria P, Beckwith JB, Kishra K, et al. Focal versus diffuse anaplasia in Wilms tumor: new definitions with prognostic significance. A report from the National Wilms Tumor Study Group. *Am J Surg Pathol* 1996;20:909.
9. Schmidt D, Harms D, Evers KG, Bliesener JA, Beckwith JB. Bone metastasizing renal tumor (clear cell sarcoma) of childhood with epithelioid elements. *Cancer* 1985;56:609.
10. Weeks DA, Beckwith JB, Mierau GW, Luckey DW. Rhabdoid tumor of kidney. *Am J Surg Pathol* 1989;13:439.
11. Bonnin JM, Rubinstein LJ, Palmer NF, Beckwith JB. The association of embryonal tumors originating in the kidney and in the brain. *Cancer* 1984;54:2137.
12. White FV, Dehner LP, Belchis DA, et al. Congenital disseminated malignant rhabdoid tumor: a distinct clinicopathologic entity demonstrating abnormalities of chromosome 22q11. *Am J Surg Pathol* 1999;23:249.
13. Biege JA, Zhou JY, Rourke LB, et al. Germline and acquired mutations of INI1 in atypical teratoid and rhabdoid tumors. *Cancer Res* 1999;59:74.
14. Bove KE, McAdams AJ. The nephroblastomatosis complex and its relationship to Wilms' tumor: a clinicopathological treatise. *Perspect Pediatr Pathol* 1976;3:185.
15. Bergeron C, Iliescu P, Thiesse R, et al. Does nephroblastomatosis influence the natural history and relapse rate in Wilms' tumor? A single centre experience over 11 years. *Eur J Cancer* 2001;37:385.
16. Bolande RP, Brough AJ, Izant RJ Jr. Congenital mesoblastic nephroma of infancy. *Pediatrics* 1967;40:272.
17. Green DM. *Diagnosis and management solid tumors in infants and children.* Boston: Martinus Nijhoff, 1985.
18. Jayabose S, Iqbal K, Newman L, et al. Hypercalcemia in childhood renal tumors. *Cancer* 1988;61:788.
19. Ritchey ML, Kelalis PP, Haase GM, et al. Preoperative therapy for intracaval and atrial extension of Wilms tumor. *Cancer* 1993;71:4104.
20. Wilimas JA, Kaste SC, Kauffman WM, et al. Use of chest computed tomography in the staging of pediatric Wilms' tumor: interobserver variability and prognostic significance. *J Clin Oncol* 1997;15:2631.
21. Feusner JH, Beckwith JB, D'Angio GJ. Clear cell sarcoma of the kidney: accuracy of imaging methods for detecting bone metastases. Report from the National Wilms' Tumor Study. *Med Pediatr Oncol* 1990;18:225.
22. Green DM, Breslow NE, Beckwith JB, et al. The treatment of children with clear cell sarcoma of the kidney. A report from the National Wilms Tumor Study Group. *J Clin Oncol* 1994;12:2132.
23. Shamberger RC, Guthrie KA, Ritchey ML, et al. Surgery-related factors and local recurrence of Wilms' tumor in National Wilms' Tumor Study 4. *Ann Surg* 1999;229:292.
24. Ritchey ML, Etzioni R, Breslow N, et al. Surgical complications following nephrectomy for Wilms' tumor. A report of NWTS-3. *Surg Gynecol Obstet* 1992;175:507.
25. Ritchey ML, Kelalis PP, Etzioni R, et al. Small bowel obstruction following nephrectomy for Wilms tumor: a report of NWTS-3. *Ann Surg* 1993;218:654.

26. Godzinski J, Tournade MF, deKraker J, et al. Rarity of surgical complications after post-chemotherapy nephrectomy for nephroblastoma. Experience of the International Society of Paediatric Oncology—trial and study "SIOP-9." *Eur J Pediatr Surg* 1998;8:83.

27. D'Angio GJ, Evans AE, Breslow N, et al. The treatment of Wilms' tumor. *Cancer* 1976;38:633.

28. Lemerle J, Voute PA, Tournade MF, et al. Preoperative versus post-operative radiotherapy, single versus multiple courses of actinomycin D in the treatment of Wilms' tumor. *Cancer* 1976;38:647.

29. Shamberger RC, Guthrie KA, Ritchey ML, et al. Surgery related factors and local recurrence of Wilms' tumor in National Wilms' Tumor Study 4.6. *Ann Surg* 1999;229:292.

30. Lemerle J, Voute PA, Tournade MF, et al. Effectiveness of preoperative chemotherapy in Wilms' tumor: results of an International Society of Paediatric Oncology (SIOP) clinical trial. *J Clin Oncol* 1983;1:604.

31. Tournade MF, Com-Hougue C, Voute PA, et al. Results of the sixth International Society of Pediatric Oncology Wilms tumor trial and study: a risk-adapted therapeutic approach in Wilms tumor. *J Clin Oncol* 1993;11:1014.

32. Godzinski J, Tournade MF, deKraker J, et al. The role of preoperative chemo in the treatment of nephroblastoma: the SIOP experience. *Semin Urol Oncol* 1998;17:28.

33. Othersen HB Jr, DeLorimier A, Hrabovsky E, et al. Surgical evaluation of lymph node metastases in Wilms' tumor. *J Pediatr Surg* 1990;25:330.

34. Zuppan CW, Beckwith JB, Weeks DA, Luckey DW, Pringle KC. Effect of preoperative therapy on the histologic features of Wilms' tumor. An analysis of cases from the Third National Wilms' Tumor Study. *Cancer* 1991;68:385.

35. Moorman-Voestermans CGM, Staalman CR, Delamarre JFM. Partial nephrectomy in unilateral Wilms tumor is feasible without local recurrence. *Med Pediatr Oncol* 1994;23:218(abst).

36. Novick AC, Gephardt G, Guz B, Steinmuller D, Tubbs RR. Long-term follow-up after partial removal of a solitary kidney. *N Engl J Med* 1991;325:1058.

37. Montgomery BT, Kelalis P, Blute ML, et al. Extended follow-up of bilateral Wilms' tumor: results of the National Wilms' Tumor Study. *J Urol* 1991;146:514.

38. Ritchey ML, Green DM, Thomas PRM, et al. Renal failure in Wilms tumor patients: a report from the National Wilms Tumor Study Group. *Med Pediatr Oncol* 1996;26:75.

39. Maes P, Delamarre J, deKraker J, Ninane J. Fetal rhabdomyomatous nephroblastoma: a tumor of good prognosis but resistant to chemotherapy. *Eur J Cancer* 1999;35:1356.

40. Cooper CS, Jaffe WI, Huff DS, et al. The role of renal salvage procedures for bilateral Wilms' tumor: a 15 year review. *J Urol* 2000;163:265.

41. Shamberger RC, Ritchey ML, Haase GM, et al. Intravascular extension of Wilms' tumor. *Ann Surg* 2001;234:116.

42. Ritchey ML, Green DM, Breslow N, Moksness J, Norkool P. Accuracy of current imaging modalities in the diagnosis of synchronous bilateral Wilms tumor: a report from the National Wilms Tumor Study Group. *Cancer* 1995;75:600.

43. Green DM, Breslow N, Ii Y, et al. The role of surgical excision in the management of relapsed Wilms' tumor patients with pulmonary metastases. *J Pediatr Surg* 1991;26:728.

44. Neuhauser EBD, Wittenborg MH, Berman CZ, Cohen J. Irradiation effects of roentgen therapy on the growing spine. *Radiology* 1952;59:637.

45. Thomas PRM, Tefft M, Farewell VT, et al. Abdominal relapses in irradiated second national Wilms' tumor study patients. *J Clin Oncol* 1984;2:1098.

46. D'Angio GJ, Breslow N, Beckwith JB, et al. The treatment of Wilms' tumor. Results of the Third National Wilms' Tumor Study. *Cancer* 1989;64:349.

47. Thomas PRM, Tefft M, Compaan PJ, et al. Results of two radiation therapy randomizations in the third National Wilms' Tumor Study. *Cancer* 1991;68:1703.

48. de Kraker J, Lemerle J, Voute PA, et al. Wilms' tumor with pulmonary metastases at diagnosis. The significance of primary chemotherapy. *J Clin Oncol* 1990;8:1187.

49. Pritchard J, Imeson J, Barnes J, et al. Results of the United Kingdom Children's Cancer Study Group (UKCCSG) first Wilms' tumor study (UKW-1). *J Clin Oncol* 1995;13:124.

50. Green DM, Finkelstein JZ, Tefft M, Norkool P. Diffuse interstitial pneumonitis after pulmonary irradiation for metastatic Wilms' tumor. A report from the National Wilms' Tumor Study. *Cancer* 1989;63:450.

51. Wilimas JA, Douglass EC, Magil HL, Fitch S, Hustu HO. Significance of pulmonary computed tomography at diagnosis in Wilms' tumor. *J Clin Oncol* 1988;6:1144.

52. Green DM, Fernbach DJ, Norkool P, Kollia G, D'Angio GJ. Treatment of Wilms' tumor patients with pulmonary metastases detected only with computerized tomography. *J Clin Oncol* 1991;9:1776.

53. Meisel JA, Guthrie KA, Breslow NE, Donaldson SS, Green DM. Significance and management of computed tomography detected pulmonary nodules: a report from the National Wilms' Tumor Study Group. *Int J Radiat Oncol Biol Phys* 1999;44:579.

54. Farber S. Chemotherapy in the treatment of leukemia and Wilms' tumor. *JAMA* 1966;198:826.

55. Green DM. Evaluation of single-dose vincristine, actinomycin D and cyclophosphamide in childhood solid tumors. *Cancer Treat Rep* 1978;62:1517.

56. Green D, Breslow N, Beckwith J, et al. Comparison between single-dose and divided-dose administration of dactinomycin and doxorubicin for patients with Wilms' tumor: a report from the National Wilms' Tumor Study Group. *J Clin Oncol* 1998;16:237.

57. Green D, Breslow NE, Beckwith B, et al. Treatment with nephrectomy only for small, stage I/favorable histology Wilms' tumor: a report from the National Wilms' Tumor Study Group. *J Clin Oncol* 2001;19:3719.

58. Breslow NE, Palmer NF, Hill LR, Buring J, D'Angio GJ. Wilms' tumor: prognostic factors for patients without metastases at diagnosis. *Cancer* 1978;41:1577.

59. Breslow N, Churchill G, Beckwith JB, et al. Prognosis for Wilms' tumor patients with nonmetastatic disease at diagnosis—results of the Second National Wilms' Tumor Study. *J Clin Oncol* 1985;3:521.

60. Breslow N, Sharples K, Beckwith JB, et al. Prognosis in nonmetastatic, favorable histology Wilms' tumor: results of the Third National Wilms' Tumor Study. *Cancer* 1991;68:2345.

61. Brown N. Neuroblastoma tumor genetics: clinical and biological aspects. *J Clin Pathol* 2001;54:897.

62. Brodeur GM. Neuroblastoma: biological insights into a clinical enigma. *Nat Rev Cancer* 2003;3:203.

63. Triche TJ, Askin FB. Neuroblastoma and the differential diagnosis of small-, round-, blue cell tumors. *Hum Pathol* 1983;14:569.

64. Tsokos M, Linnoila RL, Chandra RS, Triche TJ. Neuron-specific enolase in the diagnosis of neuroblastoma and other small, round-cell tumors in children. *Hum Pathol* 1984;15:575.

65. Shimada H, Ambros IM, Dehner LP, et al. Terminology and morphologic criteria of neuroblastic tumors. Recommendations by the International Neuroblastoma Pathology Committee. *Cancer* 1999;86:349.

66. Shimada H, Abros IM, Dehner LP, et al. The International Neuroblastoma Pathology Classification (the Shimada system). *Cancer* 1999;86:364.

67. Shimada H, Umehara S, Monobe Y, et al. International neuroblastoma pathology classification for prognostic evaluation of patients with peripheral neuroblastic tumors. *Cancer* 2001;92:2451.

68. Goto S, Umehara S, Gerbing RB, et al. Histopathology (international neuroblastoma pathology classification) and MYCN status in patients with peripheral neuroblastic tumors. *Cancer* 2001;92:2699.

69. Ikeda H, Iehara T, Tsuchida Y, et al. Experience with the international neuroblastoma staging system and pathology classification. *Br J Cancer* 2002;86:1110.

70. Schiebel E, Rechnitzer C, Fahrenkrug J, Hertz H. Vasoactive intestinal polypeptide (VIP) in children with neutral crest tumours. *Acta Paediatr Scand* 1982;71:721.

71. Koh PS, Raffensperger JG, Berry S, et al. Long-term outcome in children with opsoclonus-myoclonus and ataxia and coincident neuroblastoma. *J Pediatr* 1994;125:712.

72. Weinblatt ME, Heisel MA, Siegel SE. Hypertension in children with neurogenic tumors. *Pediatrics* 1983;71:947.

73. Woods WG, Gao R, Shuster J, et al. Screening of infants and mortality due to neuroblastoma. *N Engl J Med* 2002;346:1041.

74. Schilling FH, Spix C, Berthold F, et al. Neuroblastoma screening at one year of age. *N Engl J Med* 2002;346:1047.

75. Evans AE, D'Angio GJ, Randolph J. A proposed staging for children with neuroblastoma. *Cancer* 1971;27:374.

76. Brodeur GM, Seeger RC, Barrett A, et al. International criteria for diagnosis, staging, and response to treatment in patients with neuroblastoma. *J Clin Oncol* 1988;6:1874.

77. Evans AE, D'Angio GJ, Sather HN, et al. A comparison of four staging systems for localized and regional neuroblastoma: a report from the Children's Cancer Study Group. *J Clin Oncol* 1990;8:678.

78. Brodeur GM, Pritchard J, Berthold F, et al. Revisions of the international criteria for neuroblastoma diagnosis, staging, and response to treatment. *J Clin Oncol* 1993;11:1466.

79. Kaufman RA, Thrall JH, Keyes JW Jr, Brown ML, Zakem JF. False negative bone scans in neuroblastoma metastatic to the ends of long bones. *AJR Am J Roentgenol* 1978;130:131.

80. Franklin IM, Pritchard J. Detection of bone marrow invasion by neuroblastoma is improved by sampling at two sites with both aspirates and trephine biopsies. *J Clin Pathol* 1983;36:1215.

81. Kushner BH, Cheung NKV, LaQuaglia MP, et al. Survival from locally invasive or widespread neuroblastoma without cytotoxic therapy. *J Clin Oncol* 1996;14:373.

82. Kaneko M, Iwakawa M, Ikebukuro K, et al. Complete resection is not required in patients with neuroblastoma under 1 year of age. *J Pediatr Surg* 1998;33:1690.

83. Haase GM, Wong KY, deLorimier AA, Sather HN, Hammond GD. Improvement in survival after excision of primary tumor in stage III neuroblastoma. *J Pediatr Surg* 1989;24:194.

84. Adams GA, Shochat SJ, Smith EI, et al. Thoracic neuroblastoma: a Pediatric Oncology Group study. *J Pediatr Surg* 1993;28:372.

85. Morris JA, Shochat SJ, Smith EI, et al. Biological variables in thoracic neuroblastoma: a Pediatric Oncology Group study. *J Pediatr Surg* 1995;30:296.

86. Azizkhan RG, Shaw A, Chandler JG. Surgical complications of neuroblastoma resection. *Surgery* 1985;97:514.

87. Shamberger RC, Allarde-Segundo A, Kozakewich HPW, Grier HE. Surgical management of stage III and IV neuroblastoma: resection before or after chemotherapy? *J Pediatr Surg* 1991;26:1113.

88. Shamberger RC, Smith EI, Joshi VV, et al. The risk of nephrectomy during local control in abdominal neuroblastoma. *J Pediatr Surg* 1998;33:161.

89. Rees H, Markley MA, Kiely EM, et al. Diarrhea after resection of advanced abdominal neuroblastoma: a common management problem. *Surgery* 1998;123:568.

90. Ikeda H, August CS, Goldwein JW, et al. Sites of relapse in patients with neuroblastoma following bone marrow transplantation in relation to preparatory "debulking" treatments. *J Pediatr Surg* 1992;27:1438.

91. Tsuchida Y, Yokoyama J, Kaneko M, et al. Therapeutic significance of surgery in advanced neuroblastoma: a report from the Study Group of Japan. *J Pediatr Surg* 1992;27:616.

92. Kiely EM. The surgical challenge of neuroblastoma. *J Pediatr Surg* 1994;29:128.

93. Hata Y, Uchino J, Sasaki F, et al. Kidney-preserving radical tumor resection in advanced neuroblastoma. *J Pediatr Surg* 1989;24:382.

94. Evans AE, Chatten J, D'Angio GJ, et al. A review of 17 IV-S neuroblastoma patients at the Children's Hospital of Philadelphia. *Cancer* 1980;45:833.

95. Gugielmi M, DeBernardi B, Rizzo A, et al. Resection of primary tumor at diagnosis in stage IV-S neuroblastoma: does it affect the clinical course? *J Clin Oncol* 1996;14:1537.

96. Katzenstein HM, Bowman LC, Brodeur GM, et al. Prognostic significance of age, MYCN oncogene amplification, tumor cell ploidy, and histology in 110 infants with stage D(S) neuroblastoma: the Pediatric Oncology Group experience—a Pediatric Oncology Group study. *J Clin Oncol* 1998;16:2007.

97. McGahren ED, Rodgers BM, Waldron PE. Successful management of stage 4S neuroblastoma and severe hepatomegaly using absorbable mesh in an infant. *J Pediatr Surg* 1998;33:1554.

98. Ho PTC, Estroff JA, Kozakewich H, et al. Prenatal detection of neuroblastoma: a ten year experience from the Dana Farber Cancer Institute and Children's Hospital. *Pediatrics* 1993;92:358.

99. Holgersen LO, Subramaniam S, Kirpekar M, Mootabar H, Marcus JR. Spontaneous resolution of antenatally diagnosed adrenal masses. *J Pediatr Surg* 1996;31:153.

100. Wyatt GM, Farber S. Neuroblastoma sympatheticum. *AJR Am J Roentgenol* 1941;46:485.

101. Paulino AC, Mayr NA, Simon JH, et al. Locoregional control in infants with neuroblastoma: role of radiation therapy and late toxicity. *Int J Radiat Oncol Biol Phys* 2002;52:1025.

102. Nitschke R, Smith EI, Shochat S, et al. Localized neuroblastoma treated by surgery: a Pediatric Oncology Group study. *J Clin Oncol* 1988;6:1271.

103. Matthay KK, Sather HN, Seeger RC, Haase GM, Hammond GD. Excellent outcome of stage II neuroblastoma is independent of residual disease and radiation therapy. *J Clin Oncol* 1989;7:236.

104. Castleberry RP, Kun LE, Shuster JJ, et al. Radiotherapy improves the outlook for patients older than 1 year with Pediatric Oncology Group stage C neuroblastoma. *J Clin Oncol* 1991;9:789.

105. Matthay KK, Villablanca JG, Seeger RC, et al. Treatment of high-risk neuroblastoma with intensive chemotherapy, radiotherapy, autologous bone marrow transplantation, and 13-cis-retinoic acid. *N Engl J Med* 1999;341:1165.

106. Frappaz D, Michou J, Coze C, et al. LMCE3 treatment strategy: results in 99 consecutively diagnosed stage 4 neuroblastomas in children older than 1 year at diagnosis. *J Clin Oncol* 2000;18:468.

107. Grupp S, Stern J, Bunin N, et al. Tandem high-dose therapy in rapid sequence for children with high risk neuroblastoma. *J Clin Oncol* 2000;18:2567.

108. Sawaguchi S, Kaneko M, Uchino J-I, et al. Treatment of advanced neuroblastoma with emphasis on intensive induction chemotherapy. A report from the Study Group of Japan. *Cancer* 1990;66:1879.

109. Kushner BH, Gulati SC, Kwon J-H, et al. High-dose melphalan with 6-hydroxydopamine-purged autologous bone marrow transplantation for poor-risk neuroblastoma. *Cancer* 1991;68:242.

110. Matthay KK, Seeger RC, Reynolds CP, et al. Allogeneic versus autologous purged bone marrow transplantation for neuroblastoma: a report from the Children's Cancer Group. *J Clin Oncol* 1994;12:2382.

111. Shuster JJ, Cantor AB, McWilliams N, et al. The prognostic significance of autologous bone marrow transplant in advanced neuroblastoma. *J Clin Oncol* 1991;9:1045.

112. De Bernardi B, Nicolas B, Boni L, et al. Disseminated neuroblastoma in children older than one year at diagnosis: comparable results with three consecutive high-dose protocols adopted by the Italian co-operative group for neuroblastoma. *J Clin Oncol* 2003;21:1592.

113. Kletzel M, Katzenstein HM, Haut PR, et al. Treatment of high-risk neuroblastoma with triple-tandem high-dose therapy and stem-cell rescue: results of the Chicago Pilot II study. *J Clin Oncol* 2002;20:2284.

114. Kushner BH, Kramer K, Cheung N-K. Phase II trial of the anti-GD2 monoclonal antibody 3F8 and granulocyte-macrophage colony-stimulating factor for neuroblastoma. *J Clin Oncol* 2001;19:4189.

115. Yanik GA, Levine JE, Matthay KK, et al. Pilot study of iodine 131 metaiodobenzylguanidine in combination with myeloablative chemotherapy and autologous stem-cell support for the treatment of neuroblastoma. *J Clin Oncol* 2002;20:2142.

116. Breslow N, McCann B. Statistical estimation of prognosis for children with neuroblastoma. *Cancer Res* 1971;31:2098.

117. Look AT, Hayes FA, Nitschke R, McWilliams NB, Green AA. Cellular DNA content as a predictor of response to chemotherapy in infants with unresectable neuroblastoma. *N Engl J Med* 1984;311:231.

118. Brodeur GM, Seeger RC, Schwab M, Varmus HE, Bishop JM. Amplification of N-myc in untreated human neuroblastomas correlates with advanced disease stage. *Science* 1984;224:1121.

119. Nakagawara A, Arima-Nakagawara M, Scavarda NJ, et al. Association between high levels of expression of the TRK gene and favorable outcome in human neuroblastoma. *N Engl J Med* 1993;328:847.

120. Look AT, Hayes FA, Shuster JJ, et al. Clinical relevance of tumor cell ploidy and N-myc gene amplification in childhood neuroblastoma: a Pediatric Oncology Group study. *J Clin Oncol* 1991;9:581.

121. Joshi VV, Cantor AB, Brodeur GM, et al. Correlations between morphologic and other prognostic markers of neuroblastoma. A study of histologic grade, DNA index, N-myc gene copy number, and lactic dehydrogenase in patients in the Pediatric Oncology Group. *Cancer* 1993;71:3173.

122. Matsunaga E. Hereditary retinoblastoma. Penetrance, expressivity and age at onset. *Hum Genet* 1976;33:1.

123. Vogel F. Genetics of retinoblastoma. *Hum Genet* 1979;51:1.

124. Nussbaum R, Puck J. Recurrence risks for retinoblastoma: a model for autosomal dominant disorders with complex inheritance. *J Pediatr Ophthalmol* 1976;13:89.

125. Sanborn GE, Augsburger JJ, Shields JA. Spontaneous regression of bilateral retinoblastoma. *Br J Ophthalmol* 1982;66:685.

126. Margo C, Hidayat A, Kopelman J, Zimmerman LE. Retinocytoma. A benign variant of retinoblastoma. *Arch Ophthalmol* 1983;101:1519.

127. Ellsworth RM. The practical management of retinoblastoma. *Trans Am Ophthalmol Soc* 1969;67:462.

128. Sang DN, Albert DM. Retinoblastoma: clinical and histopathologic features. *Hum Pathol* 1982;13:133.

129. Shields JA, Leonard BC, Michelson JB, Sarin LK. B-scan ultrasonography in the diagnosis of atypical retinoblastomas. *Can J Ophthalmol* 1976;11:42.

130. Danziger A, Price HI. CT findings in retinoblastoma. *AJR Am J Roentgenol* 1979;133:783.

131. Freeman CR, Esseltine D-L, Whitehead VM, Chevalier L, Little JM. Retinoblastoma: the case for radiotherapy and for adjuvant chemotherapy. *Cancer* 1980;46:1913.

132. Pratt CB, Meyer D, Chenaille P, Crom DB. The use of bone marrow aspirations and lumbar punctures at the time of diagnosis of retinoblastoma. *J Clin Oncol* 1989;7:140.

133. Pratt CB, Crom DB, Magill L, Chenaille P, Meyer D. Skeletal scintigraphy in patients with bilateral retinoblastoma. *Cancer* 1990;65:26.

134. Martin H, Reese AB. Treatment of retinoblastoma (retinal glioma) surgically and by irradiation. *Arch Ophthalmol* 1942;27:40.

135. Martin H, Reese AB. Treatment of bilateral retinoblastoma (retinal glioma) surgically and by irradiation. *Arch Ophthalmol* 1945;33:429.

136. Reese AB, Ellsworth RM. The evaluation and current concept of retinoblastoma therapy. *Trans Am Acad Ophthalmol Otolaryngol* 1963;67:164.

137. Howarth C, Meyer D, Hustu HO, et al. Stage-related combined modality treatment of retinoblastoma. *Cancer* 1980;45:851.

138. Pratt CB, Fontanesi J, Lu X, et al. Proposal for a new staging scheme for intraocular and extraocular retinoblastoma based on an analysis of 103 globes. *Oncologist* 1997;2:1.

139. Shields CI, Honavar SG, Meadows AT, et al. Chemoreduction for unilateral retinoblastoma. *Arch Ophthalmol* 2002;120:1653.

140. Cassady JR. Retinoblastoma: questions in management. In: Carter SK, Glatstein E, Livingston RB, eds. *Principles of cancer treatment.* New York: McGraw-Hill, 1982:891.

141. Howard RD, Ellsworth RM. Findings in the peripheral fundi of patients with retinoblastoma. *Am J Ophthalmol* 1966;62:243.

142. Stannard C, Lipper S, Sealy R, Sevel D. Retinoblastoma: correlation of invasion of the optic nerve and choroid with prognosis and metastasis. *Br J Ophthalmol* 1979;63:560.

143. Hopping W, Meyer-Schwickerath G. Light coagulation treatment in retinoblastoma. In: Boniuk M, ed. *Ocular and adnexal tumors.* St. Louis: Mosby, 1964:192.

144. Lincoff H, McLean J, Long R. The cryosurgical treatment of intraocular tumors. *Am J Ophthalmol* 1967;63:389.

145. Abramson DH, Ellsworth RM, Rozakis GW. Cryotherapy for retinoblastoma. *Arch Ophthalmol* 1982;100:1253.

146. Shields JA, Parsons H, Shields CL, Giblin ME. The role of cryotherapy in the management of retinoblastoma. *Am J Ophthalmol* 1989;108:260.

147. Donaldson SS. Retinoblastoma. In: Levine AS, ed. *Cancer in the young.* New York: Masson, 1982:683.

148. McCormick B, Ellsworth R, Abramson D, et al. Radiation therapy for retinoblastoma: comparison of results with lens-sparing versus lateral beam techniques. *Int J Radiat Oncol Biol Phys* 1988;15:567.

149. Kooy HM, Dunbar SF, Tarbell NJ, et al. Adaptation and verification of the relocatable Gill-Thomas-Cosman frame in stereotactic radiotherapy. *Int J Radiat Oncol Biol Phys* 1994;30:685.

150. Abramson DH, Ellsworth RM, Tretter P, Javitt J, Kitchin FD. Treatment of bilateral groups I through IV retinoblastoma with bilateral radiation. *Arch Ophthalmol* 1981;99:1761.

151. Wong FL, Boice JD, Abramson D, et al. Cancer incidence after retinoblastoma. Radiation dose and sarcoma risk. *JAMA* 1997;278:1262.

152. Abramson DH, Ronner HJ, Ellsworth RM. Second tumors in nonirradiated bilateral retinoblastoma. *Am J Ophthalmol* 1979;87:624.

153. Halperin EC, Constine LS, Tarbell NJ, Kun LE. *Pediatric radiation oncology,* 2nd ed. New York: Raven Press, 1994:140.

154. Rodriguez-Galindo C, Wilson MW, Barrett GH, et al. Treatment of intraocular retinoblastoma with vincristine and carboplatinum. *J Clin Oncol* 2003;21:2019.

155. Beck MN, Balmer A, Dessing C, et al. First-line chemotherapy with local treatment can prevent external-beam irradiation and enucleation in low stage intraocular retinoblastoma. *J Clin Oncol* 2000;18:2881.

156. Friedman DL, Himelstein B, Shields CL, et al. Chemoreduction and local ophthalmic therapy for intraocular retinoblastoma. *J Clin Oncol* 2000;18:12.

157. Gallie BL, Budning A, DeBoer G, et al. Chemotherapy with focal therapy can cure intraocular retinoblastoma. *Arch Ophthalmol* 1996;114:1321.

158. Kingston JE, Hungerford JL, Madreperla SA, Plowman PN. Results of combined chemotherapy and radiotherapy for advanced intraocular retinoblastoma. *Arch Ophthalmol* 1996;114:1339.

159. Rubnitz JE, Crist WM. Molecular genetics of childhood cancer: implications for pathogenesis, diagnosis and treatment. *Pediatrics* 1997;100:101.

160. Felix CA, Kappel CC, Mitsudo I. Frequency and diversity of p53 mutations in childhood rhabdomyosarcoma. *Cancer Res* 1992;52:2247.

161. Matsui I, Tanimura M, Kobayashi N, et al. Neurofibromatosis type 1 and childhood cancer. *Cancer* 1993;72:2746.

162. Pappo AS, Shapiro DN, Crist WM, et al. Biology and therapy of pediatric rhabdomyosarcoma. *J Clin Oncol* 1995;13:2123.

163. Wexler LH, Crist WM, Helman LJ. Rhabdomyosarcoma and the undifferentiated sarcomas. In: Pizzo PA, Poplack DG, eds. *Principles and practice of pediatric oncology,* 4th ed. Philadelphia: Lippincott, 2002:939.

164. Horn RC Jr, Enterline HT. Rhabdomyosarcoma: a clinicopathological study and classification of 39 cases. *Cancer* 1958;11:181.

165. Tsokos M, Webber BL, Parham DM, et al. Rhabdomyosarcoma. A new classification scheme related to prognosis. *Arch Pathol Lab Med* 1992;116:847.

166. Asmar L, Gehan EA, Newton WA, et al. Agreement among and within groups of pathologists in the classification of rhabdomyosarcomas and related childhood sarcomas. *Cancer* 1994;74:2579.

167. Newton WA Jr, Gehan EA, Webber BL, et al. Classification of rhabdomyosarcomas and related sarcomas. Pathologic aspects and proposal for a new classification—an Intergroup Rhabdomyosarcoma Study. *Cancer* 1995;76:1073.

168. Arndt CA, Crist WM. Medical progress: common musculoskeletal tumors of childhood and adolescence. *N Engl J Med* 1999;341:342.

169. Sorensen PH, Lynch JC, Qualman SJ, et al. PAX3-FKHR and PAX7-FKHR gene fusions are prognostic indicators in alveolar rhabdomyosarcoma: a report from the Children's Oncology Group. *J Clin Oncol* 2002;20:2672.

170. Mcdowell HP. Update on childhood rhabdomyosarcoma. *Arch Dis Child* 2003;88:354.

171. Cohen M, Smith WL, Weetman R, Provisor A. Pulmonary pseudometastases in children with malignant tumors. *Radiology* 1981;141:371.

172. Kuttesch JF Jr, Parham DM, Kaste SC, et al. Embryonal malignancies of unknown primary origin in children. *Cancer* 1995;75:115.
173. Lawrence W Jr, Hays DM, Moon TE. Lymphatic metastases with childhood rhabdomyosarcoma. *Cancer* 1977;39:556.
174. Rodary C, Flamant F, Donaldson SS. An attempt to use a common staging system in rhabdomyosarcoma: a report from an international workshop initiated by the International Society of Pediatric Oncology (SIOP). *Med Pediatr Oncol* 1989;17:210.
175. Cassady JR, Sagerman RH, Tretter P, Ellsworth RM. Radiation therapy for rhabdomyosarcoma. *Radiology* 1968;91:116.
176. Loeffler JS, Leslie NT, Cassady JR. Case 10-1984: orbital rhabdomyosarcoma [Letter]. *N Engl J Med* 1984;311:262.
177. Maurer HM, Gehan EA, Beltangady M, et al. The Intergroup Rhabdomyosarcoma Study-I. *Cancer* 1993;71:1904.
178. Crist W, Gehan EA, Ragab AH, et al. The third Intergroup Rhabdomyosarcoma Study. *J Clin Oncol* 1995;13:610.
179. Donaldson SH, Meza J, Breneman JC, et al. Results from the IRS-IV randomized trial of hyperfractionated radiotherapy in children with rhabdomyosarcoma—a report from the IRSG. *Int J Radiat Oncol Biol Phys* 2001;51:718.
180. Pappo AS, Lyden E, Breneman J, et al. Up-front window trial of Topotecan in previously untreated children and adolescents with metastatic rhabdomyosarcoma: an Intergroup Rhabdomyosarcoma Study. *J Clin Oncol* 2001;19:213.
181. Marina NM, Cochrane D, Harney E, et al. Dose escalation and pharmacokinetics of pegylated liposomal doxorubicin (Doxil) in children with solid tumors: a Pediatric Oncology Group study. *Clin Cancer Res* 2002;8:413.
182. Weiner ES. Head and neck rhabdomyosarcoma. *Semin Pediatr Surg* 1994;3:203.
183. Gerson JM, Jaffe N, Donaldson MH, Tefft M. Meningeal seeding from rhabdomyosarcoma of the head and neck with base of skull invasion: recognition of the clinical evolution and suggestions for management. *Med Pediatr Oncol* 1978;5:137.
184. Berry MP, Jenkin RDT. Parameningeal rhabdomyosarcoma in the young. *Cancer* 1981;48:281.
185. Tefft M, Fernandez C, Donaldson M, Newton W, Moon TE. Incidence of meningeal involvement by rhabdomyosarcoma of the head and neck in children. *Cancer* 1978;42:253.
186. Raney RB Jr, Tefft M, Newton WA, et al. Improved prognosis with intensive treatment of children with cranial soft tissue sarcomas arising in nonorbital parameningeal sites. A report from the Intergroup Rhabdomyosarcoma Study. *Cancer* 1987;59:147.
187. Crist WM, Anderson JR, Meza JL, et al. Intergroup Rhabdomyosarcoma Study-IV: results for patients with nonmetastatic disease. *J Clin Oncol* 2001;19:3091.
188. Pappo AS, Meza JL, Donaldson SS, et al. Treatment of localized nonorbital, nonparameningeal head and neck rhabdomyosarcoma: lessons learned from Intergroup Rhabdomyosarcoma Studies III and IV. *J Clin Oncol* 2003;21:638.
189. Hays DM, Lawrence W Jr, Wharam M, et al. Primary reexcision for patients with "microscopic residual" tumor following initial excision of sarcomas of the trunk and extremity sites. *J Pediatr Surg* 1989;24:5.
190. Andrassy RJ, Wiener ES, Raney RB, et al. Thoracic sarcomas in children. *Ann Surg* 1998;227:170.
191. Beech TR, Moss RL, Anderson JA, et al. What constitutes appropriate therapy for children/adolescents with rhabdomyosarcoma in the abdominal wall? A report from the IRS. *J Pediatr Surg* 1999;34:668.
192. Spunt SL, Lobe TE, Pappo AS, et al. Aggressive surgery is unwarranted for biliary tract rhabdomyosarcoma. *J Pediatr Surg* 2000;35:309.
193. Blakely ML, Lobe TE, Anderson JR, et al. Does debulking improve survival rate in advanced-stage retroperitoneal embryonal rhabdomyosarcoma? *J Pediatr Surg* 1999;34:736.
194. Newton WA Jr, Soule EH, Hamoudi AB, et al. Histopathology of childhood sarcomas, Intergroup Rhabdomyosarcoma Studies I and II: clinicopathologic correlation. *J Clin Oncol* 1988;6:67.
195. LaQuaglia MP. Extremity rhabdomyosarcoma. Biological principles, staging, and treatment. *Semin Surg Oncol* 1993;9:510.
196. Neville HL, Andrassy RJ, Lobe TE, et al. Preoperative staging, prognostic factors and outcome in extremity rhabdomyosarcoma: a preliminary report from the Intergroup Rhabdomyosarcoma study IV (1991–97). *J Pediatr Surg* 2000;35:317.
197. Andrassy RJ, Wiener ES, Raney RB, et al. Progress in surgical management of vaginal rhabdomyosarcoma: a 25 year review from the Intergroup Rhabdomyosarcoma Study Group. *J Pediatr Surg* 1999;34:731.
198. Corpron CA, Andrassy RJ, Hays DM, et al. Conservative management of uterine pediatric rhabdomyosarcoma: a report of the Intergroup Rhabdomyosarcoma Study III and IV pilot. *J Pediatr Surg* 1995;30:942.
199. Raney RB Jr, Gehan EA, Hays DM, et al. Primary chemotherapy with or without radiation therapy and/or surgery for children with localized sarcoma of the bladder, prostate, vagina, uterus, and cervix. *Cancer* 1990;66:2072.
200. Heyn R, Newton WA, Raney RB, et al. Preservation of the bladder in patients with rhabdomyosarcoma. *J Clin Oncol* 1997;15:69.
201. Wiener ES, Lawrence W, Hays D, et al. Retroperitoneal node biopsy in paratesticular rhabdomyosarcoma. *J Pediatr Surg* 1994;29:171.
202. Tefft M, Hays D, Raney RB Jr, et al. Radiation to regional nodes for rhabdomyosarcoma of the genitourinary tract in children: is it necessary? *Cancer* 1980;45:3065.
203. Hays DM, Raney RB Jr, Lawrence W, et al. Bladder and prostatic tumors in the Intergroup Rhabdomyosarcoma Study (IRS-I). *Cancer* 1982;50:1472.
204. Hays DM, Raney RB Jr, Lawrence W, et al. Primary chemotherapy in the treatment of children with bladder-prostate tumors in the Intergroup Rhabdomyosarcoma Study (IRS-II). *J Pediatr Surg* 1982;17:812.
205. Rodary C, Gehan EA, Flamant F, et al. Prognostic factors in 951 nonmetastatic rhabdomyosarcoma in children: a report from the International Rhabdomyosarcoma Workshop. *Med Pediatr Oncol* 1991;19:89.
206. Walterhouse DO, Hoover ML, Marymount MA, Kletzel M. High-dose chemotherapy followed by peripheral blood stem cell rescue for metastatic rhabdomyosarcoma: the experience at Chicago Children's Memorial Hospital. *Med Pediatr Oncol* 1999;32:88.
207. Dehner LP. Primitive neuroectodermal tumor and Ewing's sarcoma. *Am J Surg Pathol* 1993;17:1.
208. Grier HE. The Ewing family of tumors. *Pediatr Clin North Am* 1997;44:991.
209. Dekner LP. Primitive neuroectodermal tumor and Ewing's sarcoma. *Am J Surg Pathol* 1993;17:1.
210. Ambros IM, Ambros PF, Strehl S, et al. MIC2 is a specific marker for Ewing's sarcoma and peripheral primitive neuroectodermal tumors. Evidence for a common histogenesis of Ewing's sarcoma and peripheral primitive neuroectodermal tumors from MIC2 expression and specific chromosome aberration. *Cancer* 1991;67:1886.
211. Delattre O, Zucman J, Melot T, et al. The Ewing family of tumors—a subgroup of small-round-cell tumors defined by specific chimeric transcripts. *N Engl J Med* 1994;331:294.
212. Hahm KB, Cho K, Lee C, et al. Repression of the gene encoding the TGF-beta type II receptor is a major target of the EWS-FLI1 oncoprotein. *Nat Genet* 1999;23:222.
213. Zoubek A, Dockhorn-Dwarniak B, Delattre O, et al. Does expression of different EWS chimeric transcripts define clinically distinct risk groups of Ewing tumor patients? *J Clin Oncol* 1996;14:1245.
214. deAlva E, Kawai A, Healey JH, et al. EWS-FLI1 fusion transcript structure is an independent determinant of prognosis in Ewing's sarcoma. *J Clin Oncol* 1998;16:1248.
215. Lin PP, Brody RI, Hamelin AC, et al. Differential transactivation by alternative EWS-FLI1 fusion proteins correlates with clinical heterogeneity in Ewing's sarcoma. *Cancer Res* 1999;59:1428.
216. Burchill SA. Ewing's sarcoma: diagnostic, prognostic, and therapeutic implications of molecular abnormalities. *J Clin Pathol* 2003;56:96.
217. Monforte-Munoz H, Lopez-Terrada D, Affendie H, et al. Documentation of EWS gene rearrangements by fluorescence in-situ hybridization (FISH) in frozen sections of Ewing's sarcoma—peripheral primitive neuroectodermal tumor. *Am J Surg Pathol* 1999;23:309.
218. Durbin M, Randall RL, James M, et al. Ewing's sarcoma masquerading as osteomyelitis. *Clin Orthop* 1998;357:176.
219. Goldstein H, McNeil BJ, Zufall E, Treves S. Is there still a place for bone scanning in Ewing's sarcoma? *J Nucl Med* 1980;21:10.
220. Hayes FA, Thompson EI, Meyer WH, et al. Therapy for localized Ewing's sarcoma of bone. *J Clin Oncol* 1989;7:208.
221. Arai Y, Kun LE, Brooks MT, et al. Ewing's sarcoma: local tumor control and patterns of failure following limited volume radiation therapy. *Int J Radiat Oncol Biol Phys* 1991;21:1501.
222. Scully SP, Temple HT, O'Keefe RJ, et al. Role of surgical resection in pelvic Ewing's sarcoma. *J Clin Oncol* 1995;13:2336.
223. Göbel V, Jürgens H, Etspuler G, et al. Prognostic significance of tumor volume in localized Ewing's sarcoma of bone in children and adolescents. *J Cancer Res Clin Oncol* 1987;113:187.
224. Mendenhall CM, Marcus RB Jr, Enneking WF, et al. The prognostic significance of soft tissue extension in Ewing's sarcoma. *Cancer* 1983;51:913.
225. Shamberger RC, Tarbell NJ, Perez-Atayde AR, Grier HE. Malignant small round cell tumor (Ewing's-PNET) of the chest wall in children. *J Pediatr Surg* 1994;29:179.
226. Shamberger RC, LaQuaglia MP, Krailo MD, et al. Ewing's sarcoma of the rib: results of an intergroup study with analysis of outcome by timing of resection. *J Thorac Cardiovasc Surg* 2000;119:1154.
227. Shamberger RC, LaQuaglia MP, Gebhardt MC, et al. Ewing sarcoma/primitive neuroectodermal tumor of the chest wall. *Ann Surg* 2003;238:563.
228. Horowitz ME, Malawer MM, Woo SY, et al. Ewing's sarcoma family of tumors: Ewing's sarcoma of bone. In: Pizzo PA, Poplack DG, eds. *Principles and practice of pediatric oncology*, 3rd ed. Philadelphia: Lippincott–Raven, 1997:831.
229. Chan RC, Sutow WW, Lindberg RD, et al. Management and results of localized Ewing's sarcoma. *Cancer* 1979;43:1001.
230. Perez CA, Tefft M, Nesbit M, et al. The role of radiation therapy in the management of non-metastatic Ewing's sarcoma of bone. Report of the intergroup Ewing's sarcoma study. *Int J Radiat Oncol Biol Phys* 1981;7:141.
231. Suit HD. Role of therapeutic radiology in cancer of bone. *Cancer* 1975;35:930.
232. Donaldson S, Torrey M, Link M, et al. A multidisciplinary study investigating radiotherapy in Ewing's sarcoma: end results of POG #8346. *Int J Radiat Oncol Biol Phys* 1998;42:125.
233. Marcus RB Jr, Graham-Pole JR, Springfield DS, et al. High-risk Ewing's sarcoma: end-intensification using autologous bone marrow transplantation. *Int J Radiat Oncol Biol Phys* 1988;15:53.
234. Kuttesch JF, Wexler LH, Marcus RB, et al. Second malignancies after Ewing's sarcoma: radiation dose-dependency of secondary sarcomas. *J Clin Oncol* 1996;14:2818.
235. Nesbit ME Jr, Gehan EA, Burgert EO, et al. Multimodal therapy for the management of primary, nonmetastatic Ewing's sarcoma of bone: a long-term follow-up of the first intergroup study. *J Clin Oncol* 1990;8:1664.
236. Burgert EO Jr, Nesbit ME, Garnsey LA, et al. Multimodal therapy for the management of nonpelvic, localized Ewing's sarcoma of bone: Intergroup Study IESS-II. *J Clin Oncol* 1990;8:1514.
237. Smith MA, Ungerleider RS, Horowitz ME, Simon R. Influence of doxorubicin dose intensity on response and outcome for patients with osteogenic sarcoma and Ewing's sarcoma. *J Natl Cancer Inst* 1991;83:1460.
238. Grier H, Krailo M, Tarbell N, et al. Adding ifosfamide and etoposide to standard chemotherapy for Ewing's sarcoma and primitive neuroectodermal tumor of bone. *N Engl J Med* 2003;348:694.
239. Wexler LH, Delaney TF, Tsokos M, et al. Ifosfamide and etoposide plus vincristine, doxorubicin, and cyclophosphamide for newly diagnosed Ewing's sarcoma family of tumors. *Cancer* 1996;78:901.
240. Craft A, Cotterill S, Malcolm A, et al. Ifosfamide-containing chemotherapy in Ewing's sarcoma: the second United Kingdom Children's Cancer Study Group and the Medical Research Council Ewing's tumor study. *J Clin Oncol* 1998;16:3628.

241. Bacci G, Mercuri M, Longhi A, et al. Neoadjuvant chemotherapy for Ewing's tumor of bone: recent experience at the Rizzoli Orthopaedic Institute. *Eur J Cancer* 2002; 38:2243.

242. Reference deleted.

243. Cangir A, Vietti TJ, Gehan EA, et al. Ewing's sarcoma metastatic at diagnosis. Results and comparisons of two Intergroup Ewing's Sarcoma Studies. *Cancer* 1990;66:887.

244. Madero L, Munoz A, Sanchez deToledo J, et al. Megatherapy in children with high risk Ewing's sarcoma in first complete remission. *Bone Marrow Transplant* 1998;21:795.

245. Ozkaynek MF, Matthay K, Cairo M, et al. Double alkylator non-total-body irradiation regimen with autologous hematopoietic stem-cell transplantation in pediatric solid tumors. *J Clin Oncol* 1998;16:937.

246. Meyers PA, Krailo MD, Ladanyi M, et al. High-dose melphalan, etoposide, total body irradiation, and autologous stem-cell reconstitution as consolidation therapy for high-risk Ewing's sarcoma does not improve prognosis. *J Clin Oncol* 2001;19:2812.

247. Thomson B, Hawkins D, Felgenhauer J, Radick JP. RT-PCR evaluation of peripheral blood, bone marrow and peripheral blood stem cells in children and adolescents undergoing VACIME chemotherapy for Ewing's sarcoma and alveolar rhabdomyosarcoma. *Bone Marrow Transplant* 1999;24:527.

248. Pinkerton CR, Bataillard A, Guillo S, et al. Treatment strategies for metastatic Ewing's sarcoma. *Eur J Cancer* 2001;37:1338.

249. Burdach S, Jurgens H, Peters C, et al. Myeloablative radiochemotherapy and hematopoietic stem-cell rescue in poor-prognosis Ewing's sarcoma. *J Clin Oncol* 1993;11:1482.

250. Burdach S, van Kaick B, Laws HJ, et al. Allogeneic and autologous stem-cell transplantation in advanced Ewing tumors. *Ann Oncol* 2000;11:1451.

251. Tanaka K, Iwakuma T, Harimaya K, et al. EWS-FLI1 antisense oligodeoxynucleotide inhibits proliferation of human Ewing's sarcoma and primitive neuroectodermal tumor cells. *J Clin Invest* 1997;99:239.

252. Sucato DJ, Rougraff B, McGrath BE, et al. Ewing's sarcoma of the pelvis: long-term survival and functional outcome. *Clin Orthop* 2000;373:193.

253. Paulussen M, Ahrens S, Dunst J, et al. Localized Ewing tumor of bone: final results of the Cooperative Ewing's Sarcoma Study CESS 86. *J Clin Oncol* 2001;19:1818.

254. Cotterill SJ, Ahrens S, Paulussen HF, et al. Prognostic factors in Ewing's tumor of bone: analysis of 975 patients from the European Intergroup Cooperative Ewing's Sarcoma Study Group. *J Clin Oncol* 2000;18:3108.

255. Picci P, Bohling T, Bacci G, et al. Chemotherapy-induced tumor necrosis as a prognostic factor in localized Ewing's sarcoma of the extremities. *J Clin Oncol* 1997;15:1553.

256. Wunder JS, Paulian G, Huvos AG, et al. The histological response to chemotherapy as a predictor of the oncological outcome of operative treatment of Ewing sarcoma. *J Bone Surg Am* 1998;80:1020.

257. Oberlin O, Deley MC, Bui BN, et al. Prognostic factors in localized Ewing's tumours and peripheral neuroectodermal tumours: the third study of the French Society of Pediatric Oncology (EW88 study). *Br J Cancer* 2001;85:1646.

258. Reynolds M. Pediatric liver tumors. *Semin Surg Oncol* 1999;16:159.

259. Greenberg H, Filler RM. Hepatic tumors. In: Pizzo PA, Poplack DG, eds. *Principles and practice of pediatric oncology*, 3rd ed. Philadelphia: Lippincott–Raven, 1997.

260. Sotelo-Avila C, Gonzalez-Crussi F, Fowler JW. Complete and incomplete forms of Beckwith-Wiedemann syndrome: their oncogenic potential. *J Pediatr* 1980;96:47.

261. Albrecht S, von Scheinitz D, Waha A, et al. Loss of maternal alleles on chromosome arm 11p in hepatoblastoma. *Cancer Res* 1994;54:5041.

262. Kingston JE, Herbert A, Draper GJ, Mann JR. Association between hepatoblastoma and polyposis coli. *Arch Dis Child* 1983;58:959.

263. Oda H, Imai Y, Nakatsura Y, et al. Somatic mutations of the APC gene in sporadic hepatoblastomas. *Cancer Res* 1996;56:3320.

264. Schnater JM, Kohler SE, Lamers WH, et al. Where do we stand with hepatoblastoma? *Cancer* 2003;98:668.

265. Ideda H, Matsuyama S, Tauimura M. Association between hepatoblastoma and very low birth weight: a trend or a chance? *J Pediatr* 1997;130:557.

266. Leuschner I, Harms D, Schmidt D. The association of hepatocellular carcinoma in childhood with hepatitis B virus infection. *Cancer* 1988;62:2363.

267. Chang M-H, Chen C-J, Lai M-S, et al. Universal hepatitis B vaccination in Taiwan and the incidence of hepatocellular carcinoma in children. *N Engl J Med* 1997;336:1855.

268. Eriksson S, Carlson J, Velez R. Risk of cirrhosis and primary liver cancer in alpha1-antitrypsin deficiency. *N Engl J Med* 1986;314:736.

269. Haas JE, Muczynski KA, Krailo M, et al. Histopathology and prognosis in childhood hepatoblastoma and hepatocarcinoma. *Cancer* 1989;64:1082.

270. Lack EE, Neave C, Vawter GF. Hepatoblastoma. A clinical and pathologic study of 54 cases. *Am J Surg Pathol* 1982;6:693.

271. Pritchard J, da Cunha A, Cornbleet MA, Carter CJ. Alpha feto (AFP) monitoring of response to adriamycin in hepatoblastoma. *J Pediatr Surg* 1982;17:429.

272. Perilongo G, Brown J, Shafford E, et al. Hepatoblastoma presenting with lung metastases. Treatment results of the first cooperative, prospective study of the international society of paediatric oncology on childhood liver tumors. *Cancer* 2000;89:1845.

273. Evans AE, Land VJ, Newton WA, et al. Combination chemotherapy (vincristine, adriamycin, cyclophosphamide and 5-fluorouracil) in the treatment of children with malignant hepatoma. *Cancer* 1982;50:821.

274. Schnater JM, Aronson DC, Plaschkes J, et al. Surgical view of the treatment of patients with hepatoblastoma. Results from the first prospective trial of the International Society of Paediatric Oncology Liver Tumor Study Group (SIOPEL-1). *Cancer* 2002;94:1111.

275. Ni Y-H, Chang M-H, Hsu H-Y, et al. Hepatocellular carcinoma in childhood. *Cancer* 1991;68:1737.

276. Stringer MD, Hennayake S, Howard ER, et al. Improved outcome for children with hepatoblastoma. *Br J Surg* 1995;82:386.

277. Takahiko S, Ando H, Watanabe Y, et al. Treatment of hepatoblastoma: less extensive hepatectomy after effective preoperative chemotherapy with cisplatin and adriamycin. *Surgery* 1998;123:407.

278. Bilik R, Superina R. Transplantation for unresectable liver tumors in children. *Transplant Proc* 1997;29:2834.

279. Srinivasan P, McCall J, Pritchard J, et al. Orthotopic liver transplantation for unresectable hepatoblastoma. *Transplantation* 2002;74:652.

280. Reyes JD, Carr B, Dvorchik I, et al. Liver transplantation and chemotherapy for hepatoblastoma and hepatocellular cancer in childhood and adolescence. *J Pediatr* 2000;136:795.

281. Curley SA, Izzo F, Delrio P, et al. Radiofrequency ablation of unresectable primary and metastatic hepatic malignancies. *Ann Surg* 1999;230:1.

282. Shamberger RC, Leichtner AM, Jonas MM, LaQuaglia MP. Long-term hepatic regeneration and function in infants and children following liver resection. *J Am Coll Surg* 1996;182:515.

283. Ortega JA, Krailo MD, Haas JE, et al. Effective treatment of unresectable or metastatic hepatoblastoma with cisplatin and continuous infusion doxorubicin chemotherapy: a report from the Children's Cancer Study Group. *J Clin Oncol* 1991;9:2167.

284. Quinn JJ, Altman AJ, Robinson HT, et al. Adriamycin and cisplatin for hepatoblastoma. *Cancer* 1985;56:1926.

285. Filler RM, Ehrlich PF, Greenberg ML, Babyn PS. Preoperative chemotherapy in hepatoblastoma. *Surgery* 1991;110:591.

286. Ninane J, Perilongo G, Stalens J-P, et al. Effectiveness and toxicity of cisplatin and doxorubicin (PLADO) in childhood hepatoblastoma and hepatocellular carcinoma: a SIOP pilot study. *Med Pediatr Oncol* 1991;19:199.

287. Douglass EC, Reynolds M, Finegold M, Cantor AB, Glicksman A. Cisplatin, vincristine, and fluorouracil therapy for hepatoblastoma: a Pediatric Oncology Group study. *J Clin Oncol* 1993;11:96.

288. Ortega JA, Douglass E, Feusner J, et al. Randomized comparison of cisplatin/vincristine/fluorouracil and continuous infusion doxorubicin for treatment of pediatric hepatoblastoma: a report from the Children's Cancer Group and the Pediatric Oncology Group. *J Clin Oncol* 2000;18:2665.

289. Ehrlich PF, Greenberg ML, Filler RM. Improved long-term survival with preoperative chemotherapy for hepatoblastoma. *J Pediatr Surg* 1997;32:999.

290. Uchiyama M, Iwafuchi M, Naito M, et al. A study of therapy for pediatric hepatoblastoma: prevention and treatment of pulmonary metastasis. *Eur J Pediatr Surg* 1999;9:142.

291. von Schweinitz D, Byrd DJ, Hecker H, et al. Efficiency and toxicity of ifosfamide, cisplatin and doxorubicin in the treatment of childhood hepatoblastoma. *Eur J Cancer* 1997;33:1243.

292. Brown J, Perilongo G, Shafford E, et al. Pretreatment prognostic factors for children with hepatoblastoma—results from the International Society of Paediatric Oncology (SIOP) Study SIOPEL 1. *Eur J Cancer* 2000;36:1418.

293. Fuchs J, Rydzynski J, Von Schweinitz D, et al. Pretreatment prognostic factors and treatment results in children with hepatoblastoma. A report from the German cooperative pediatric liver tumor study HB 94. *Cancer* 2002;95:172.

294. Reynolds M, Douglass EC, Finegold M, Cantor A, Glicksman A. Chemotherapy can convert unresectable hepatoblastoma. *J Pediatr Surg* 1992;27:1080.

295. Han Y-M, Park H-H, Lee J-M, et al. Effectiveness of preoperative transarterial chemoembolization in presumed inoperable hepatoblastoma. *J Vasc Intervent Radiol* 1999;10:1275.

296. von Schweinitz D, Hecker H, Schmidt-von-Arndt G, et al. Prognostic factors and staging systems in childhood hepatoblastoma. *Int J Cancer* 1997;74:593.

297. Douglas E, Ortega J, Feusner J, et al. Hepatocellular carcinoma in children and adolescents. Results from the Pediatric Intergroup Study (CCG 8881/POG 8945). *Proc Am Soc Clin Oncol* 1994;13:420(abst 1439).

298. Czauderna P, Mackinlay G, Perilongo G, et al. Hepatocellular carcinoma in children: results of the first prospective study of the International Society of Pediatric Oncology Group. *J Clin Oncol* 2002;20:2798.

299. Rescorla FJ. Pediatric germ cell tumors. *Semin Surg Oncol* 1999;16:144.

300. Göbel V, Calaminus G, Engert J, et al. Teratomas of infancy and childhood. *Med Pediatr Oncol* 1998;31:8.

301. Cushing B, Perlman E, Marina N, Castleberry R. Germ cell tumors. In: Pizzo PA, Poplack DG, eds. *Principles and practice of pediatric oncology*, 4th ed. Philadelphia: Lippincott–Raven, 2002:1091.

302. Einhorn LH, Donohue J. Cis-diamminedichloroplatinum, vinblastine and bleomycin combination chemotherapy in disseminated testicular cancer. *Ann Intern Med* 1977;87:293.

303. Stern JW, Bunin N. Prospective study of carboplatin-based chemotherapy for pediatric germ cell tumors. *Med Pediatr Oncol* 2002;39:163.

304. Mann JR, Raafat F, Robinson K, et al. The United Kingdom Children's Cancer Study Group's Second Germ Cell Tumor Study: carboplatin, etoposide, and bleomycin are effective treatment for children with malignant extracranial germ cell tumors, with acceptable toxicity. *J Clin Oncol* 2000;18:3809.

305. Pinkerton CR. Malignant germ cell tumors in childhood. *Eur J Cancer* 1997;33:895.

306. Dehner LP. Gonadal and extragonadal germ cell neoplasms: teratomas in childhood. In: Finegold MJ, Bennington J, eds. *Pathology of neoplasia in children and adolescents*. Philadelphia: WB Saunders, 1986:282.

307. Marina NM, Cushing B, Giller R, et al. Complete surgical excision is effective treatment for children with immature teratomas with or without malignant elements: a Pediatric Oncology Group/Children's Cancer Group intergroup study. *J Clin Oncol* 1999;17:2137.

308. Shirai T, Itoh T, Yoshiki T, et al. Immunofluorescent demonstration of alpha-fetoprotein and other plasma proteins in yolk sac tumors. *Cancer* 1976;38:1661.

309. Teilum G, Albrechtsen R, Norgaard-Pedersen B. The histogenetic-embryologic basis for reappearance of alpha-fetoprotein in endodermal sinus tumors (yolk sac tumors) and teratomas. *Acta Pathol Microbiol Scand* 1975;83:80.

310. Bussey KJ, Lawce HJ, Olson SB, et al. Chromosome abnormalities of eighty-one pediatric germ cell tumors: sex-, age-, site-, and histopathology-related differences—a Children's Cancer Group study. *Genes Chromosomes Cancer* 1999;25:134.

311. Perlman EJ, Valentine MB, Griffin CA, Look AT. Deletion of 1p36 in childhood endodermal sinus tumors by two-color fluorescence in situ hybridization: a Pediatric Oncology Group study. *Genes Chromosomes Cancer* 1996;16:15.

312. Mostofi FK, Price EB Jr. *Atlas of tumor pathology. Second Series. Fascicle 8. Tumors of the male genital system.* Washington, DC: American Registry of Pathology, 1973.

313. Hoffner L, Deka R, Chakravarti A, Surti V. Cytogenetics and origins of pediatric germ cell tumors. *Cancer Genet Cytogenet* 1994;74:54.

314. Wu JT, Book L, Sudar K. Serum alpha fetoprotein (AFP) levels in normal infants. *Pediatr Res* 1981;15:50.

315. Abelev GI, Assecritova IV, Kraevsky NA, Perova SD, Perevodchikova NI. Embryonal serum alpha-globulin in cancer patients: diagnostic value. *Int J Cancer* 1967;2:551.

316. Mann JR, Lakin GE, Leonard JC, et al. Clinical applications of serum carcinoembryonic antigen and alpha-fetoprotein levels in children with solid tumors. *Arch Dis Child* 1978;53:366.

317. Morinaga S. Ojima M, Sasano M. Human chorionic gonadotropin and alpha-fetoprotein in testicular germ cell tumors: an immunohistochemical study in comparison with tissue concentrations. *Cancer* 1983;52:1281.

318. Altman RP, Randolph JG, Lilly JR. Sacrococcygeal teratoma: American Academy of Pediatrics Surgical Section survey—1973. *J Pediatr Surg* 1974;9:389.

319. Fraumeni JF Jr, Li FP, Dalager N. Teratomas in children: epidemiologic features. *J Natl Cancer Inst* 1973;51:1425.

320. Ein SH, Adeyeimi SD, Mancer K. Benign sacrococcygeal teratomas in infants and children. A 25 year review. *Ann Surg* 1980;191:382.

321. Hawkins E, Isaacs H, Cushing B, Rogers P. Occult malignancy in neonatal sacrococcygeal teratomas. A report from a combined Pediatric Oncology Group and Children's Cancer Group study. *Am J Pediatr Hematol Oncol* 1993;15:406.

322. Ein SH, Mancer K, Adeyemi SD. Malignant sacrococcygeal teratoma—endodermal sinus, yolk sac tumor—in infants and children. A 32 year review. *J Pediatr Surg* 1985;20:473.

323. Schropp KP, Lobe TE, Rao B, et al. Sacrococcygeal teratoma: the experience of four decades. *J Pediatr Surg* 1992;27:1075.

324. Ablin AR, Krailo MD, Ramsay NKC, et al. Results of treatment of malignant germ cell tumors in 93 children. A report from the Children's Cancer Study Group. *J Clin Oncol* 1991;9:1782.

325. Kersh CR, Constable WC, Hahn SS, et al. Primary malignant extragonadal germ cell tumors. An analysis of the effect of radiotherapy. *Cancer* 1990;65:2681.

326. Green DM, Brecher ML, Grossi M, et al. The use of different induction and maintenance chemotherapy regimens for the treatment of advanced yolk sac tumors. *J Clin Oncol* 1983;1:111.

327. Pinkerton CR, Pritchard J, Spitz L. High complete response rate in children with advanced germ cell tumors using cisplatin-containing combination chemotherapy. *J Clin Oncol* 1986;4:194.

328. Hawkins EP, Finegold MJ, Hawkins HK, et al. Nongerminomatous malignant germ cell tumors in children. A review of 89 cases from the Pediatric Oncology Group, 1971–1984. *Cancer* 1986;58:2579.

329. Billmire D, Vinocur C, Rescorla F, et al. Malignant retroperitoneal and abdominal germ cell tumors: an intergroup study. *J Pediatr Surg* 2003;38:315.

330. Gobel U, Schneider DT, Calaminus G, et al. Multimodal treatment of malignant sacrococcygeal germ cell tumors: a prospective analysis of 66 patients of the German Cooperative Protocols MAKEI 83/86 and 89. *J Clin Oncol* 2001;19:1943.

331. Birch JM, Marsden HB, Swindell R. Pre-natal factors in the origin of germ cell tumours of childhood. *Carcinogenesis* 1982;3:75.

332. Mann JR, Pearson D, Barrett A, et al. Results of the United Kingdom Children's Cancer Study Group's malignant germ cell tumor studies. *Cancer* 1989;63:1657.

333. Flamant F, Nihoul-Fekete C, Patte C, Lemerle J. Optimal treatment of stage I yolk sac tumor of the testis in children. *J Pediatr Surg* 1986;21:108.

334. Staubitz WJ. Surgical treatment of nonseminomatous germinal testis tumors. In: Johnson DE, Samuels ML, eds. *Cancer of the genitourinary tract.* New York: Raven Press, 1979:135.

335. Hoskin P, Dilly S, Easton D, et al. Prognostic factors in stage I non-seminomatous germ-cell testicular tumors managed by orchiectomy and surveillance: implications for adjuvant chemotherapy. *J Clin Oncol* 1986;4:1031.

336. Marina N, Fontanesi J, Kun L, et al. Treatment of childhood germ cell tumors: review of the St. Jude experience from 1979 to 1988. *Cancer* 1992;70:2568.

337. Aprikian AG, Herr HW, Bajorin DF, Bosl GJ. Resection of postchemotherapy residual masses and limited retroperitoneal lymphadenectomy in patients with metastatic testicular nonseminomatous germ cell tumors. *Cancer* 1994;74:1329.

338. Nichols CR, Williams SD, Loehrer PJ, et al. Randomized study of cisplatin dose intensity in poor-risk germ cell tumors. A Southwestern Cancer Study Group and Southwest Oncology Group protocol. *J Clin Oncol* 1991;9:1163.

339. Wozniak AJ, Samson MK, Shah NT, et al. A randomized trial of cisplatin, vinblastine, and bleomycin versus vinblastine, cisplatin, and etoposide in the treatment of advanced germ cell tumors of the testis: a Southwest Oncology Group study. *J Clin Oncol* 1991;9:70.

340. Levi JA, Raghavan D, Harvey V, et al. The importance of bleomycin in combination chemotherapy for good-prognosis germ cell carcinoma. *J Clin Oncol* 1993;11:1300.

341. Loehrer PJ Sr, Johnson D, Elson P, Einhorn LH, Trump D. Importance of bleomycin in favorable-prognosis disseminated germ cell tumors: an Eastern Cooperative Oncology Group trial. *J Clin Oncol* 1995;13:470.

342. Wheeler BM, Loehrer PJ, Williams SD, Einhorn LH. Ifosfamide in refractory male germ cell tumors. *J Clin Oncol* 1986;4:28.

343. Bokemeyer C, Kohrman O, Tischler J, et al. A randomized trial of cisplatin, etoposide and bleomycin (PEB) versus carboplatin, etoposide and bleomycin (CEB) for patients with "good risk" metastatic non-seminomatous germ cell tumors. *Ann Oncol* 1996;7:1015.

344. Frazier AL, Grier HE, Green DM. Treatment of endodermal sinus tumor in children using a regimen that lacks bleomycin. *Med Pediatr Oncol* 1996;27:69.

345. Fung CY, Garnick MB. Clinical stage I carcinoma of the testis. *J Clin Oncol* 1988;6:734.

346. Breen JL, Maxson WS. Ovarian tumors in children and adolescents. *Clin Obstet Gynecol* 1977;20:607.

347. Heifetz SA, Cushing B, Giller R, et al. Pathologic considerations: a report from the combined Pediatric Oncology Group/Children's Cancer Group. *Am J Surg Pathol* 1998;22:1115.

348. Buskirk SJ, Schray MF, Podratz KC, et al. Ovarian dysgerminoma: a retrospective analysis of results of treatment, sites of treatment failure and radiosensitivity. *Mayo Clin Proc* 1987;62:1149.

349. Cangir A, Smith J, van Eys J. Improved prognosis in children with ovarian cancers following modified VAC (vincristine sulfate, dactinomycin and cyclophosphamide) chemotherapy. *Cancer* 1978;42:1234.

350. Ungerleider RS, Donaldson SS, Warnke RA, Wilbur JR. Endodermal sinus tumor. The Stanford experience and the first reported case arising in the vulva. *Cancer* 1978;41:1627.

351. Slayton RE, Hreshchyshyn MM, Silberberg SG, et al. Treatment of malignant ovarian germ cell tumors. *Cancer* 1978;42:390.

352. Teinturier C, Gelez J, Flamant F, et al. Pure dysgerminoma of the ovary in childhood: treatment results and sequelae. *Med Pediatr Oncol* 1994;23:1.

353. Norohna PA, Noronha R, Rao DS. Primary anterior mediastinal endodermal sinus tumors in childhood. *Am J Pediatr Hematol Oncol* 1985;7:312.

354. Flamant F, Schwartz L, Delons E, et al. Nonseminomatous malignant germ cell tumors in children. Multidrug therapy in stages III and IV. *Cancer* 1984;54:1687.

355. Schneider DT, Calaminus G, Reinhard H, et al. Primary mediastinal germ cell tumors in children and adolescents: results of the German Cooperative Protocols MAKEI 83/86, 89, and 96. *J Clin Oncol* 2000;18:832.

CHAPTER **41**

Lymphomas

SECTION **1**

HOWARD J. WEINSTEIN
NANCY J. TARBELL

Leukemias and Lymphomas of Childhood

LEUKEMIAS

The remarkable success in the treatment of children with acute lymphoblastic leukemia (ALL) can be attributed to a series of prospective clinical studies that clarified the natural history of ALL and demonstrated the importance of combination chemotherapy, central nervous system (CNS) preventive therapy, and supportive care.[1] Acute myelogenous leukemia (AML) proved to be more resistant to chemotherapy, and this led to the development of treatment strategies that include dose-intensified chemotherapy and bone marrow transplantation (BMT) in first remission.[1] In parallel with these clinical advances, we have also greatly advanced our knowledge of leukemia cell biology, most notably in the area of molecular pathogenesis. DNA microarray analyses have been a powerful tool for identifying new genetic pathways involved in ALL and AML. The gene profiling data has already been of prognostic importance and hopefully will identify new targets for novel therapies.[2] The improvement in long-term survival for children with acute leukemia has been gratifying but also has been associated with significant late effects that underscore the need for vigilant follow-up and for designing risk-adapted therapies.[3]

EPIDEMIOLOGY

Leukemia is the most common form of cancer in children. Approximately 2500 new cases of childhood leukemia are diagnosed each year in the United States.[4] ALL and AML are diagnosed in 75% and 20% of the cases, respectively, and chronic myeloid leukemia is diagnosed in fewer than 5%. The well-established peak incidence of childhood leukemia at age 4 years is due to ALL. ALL affects males and whites more often than females and African Americans. Nearly a threefold higher incidence of ALL at 2 to 3 years of age occurs for white children compared to African American children. The incidence of AML is constant during childhood, except for a slight peak in infancy and late adolescence.[4]

The causes of acute leukemia remain unknown, but recent studies have shed light on the origins of some cases of leukemia. Intriguing results of molecular genetic studies using stored neonatal blood spots from children with ALL suggest a prenatal origin for the disease.[5] For patients with ALL and TEL-AML1 fusion transcripts, the long latency until the diagnosis of leukemia suggests that additional genetic changes are required for leukemic transformation. Prenatal origin of ALL is also supported by studies of monozygotic twins with concordant leukemia. In this situation, the initial chromosome translocation occurred *in utero* with subsequent transfer of the leukemia clone from one twin to the other via the shared blood supply.[6]

A small number of children are at increased risk to develop leukemia because of an inherited predisposition. For example, children with Down syndrome have a 10- to 20-fold increased risk of leukemia during the first 10 years of life.[7] The types of leukemia in children with Down syndrome follow the usual distribution of childhood leukemia, except at younger than 3 years of age when AML (mostly FAB M7) is more likely to occur than

ALL. Neonates with Down syndrome or trisomy 21 mosaicism may also develop a transient myeloproliferative disorder (TMD) that is indistinguishable from congenital AML. This disorder is usually diagnosed within the first 2 weeks of life, and the incidence is unknown. Peripheral blood or bone marrow blasts from infants with TMD have features of the megakaryocytic and erythroid lineages and, in some cases, have been shown to be clonal in origin. In more than 90% of these infants, however, the blasts spontaneously disappear, and normal blood counts recover within the first several weeks to months after diagnosis of TMD. One retrospective study reported that up to 30% of infants with TMD eventually developed either a myelodysplastic syndrome or AML before the age of 3 years.[8] Results of a prospective study are lending support to this retrospective observation.[8a] It has been reported that acquired mutations in the GATA-1 gene, an erythroid/megakaryocytic transcription factor, are present in blast cells from patients with TMD as well as patients with Down syndrome and AML (FAB M7). It is not clear whether this mutation is enough for the development of TMD and what other mutations are necessary for the subsequent development of AML.[9] Because the majority of infants with TMD never develop leukemia, neonates with Down syndrome and a hematologic picture consistent with AML should be observed for 4 to 10 weeks before chemotherapy is initiated. However, there is a small subgroup of infants with TMD who have severe liver dysfunction and early death. Optimal therapy in this setting is not known, but low-dose cytarabine has been successful in several cases. If chemotherapy is eventually needed, the outcome for these children has been surprisingly favorable.[1]

Children with neurofibromatosis are predisposed to develop myeloid malignancies, especially myelodysplastic and myeloproliferative syndromes. In patients with neurofibromatosis who develop leukemia, evidence indicates loss of both neurofibromatosis (NF1) alleles in bone marrow cells. These data provide evidence that NF1 may function as a tumor suppressor gene in children with NF1.

In general, most studies have not found a consistent association between common infectious or environmental exposures and an increased risk of childhood leukemia.[5,12] Population-based studies of polymorphisms of drug-metabolizing enzymes suggest an association between several of these polymorphisms and an increased risk for either ALL or AML.[1] For example, infant leukemia has been associated with polymorphic variants of NQO1, an enzyme that detoxifies benzene metabolites and quinone-containing substances, including flavonoids. ALL and AML in infants is characterized by 11q23 MLL gene rearrangements that are similar to those seen in secondary AML after exposure to topoisomerase II inhibitors.[10] It is therefore of interest that maternal exposure to quinine-containing topoisomerase II inhibitors has been proposed as a risk factor for infant AML.

CLONALITY AND CELL OF ORIGIN

Within the hierarchy of hematopoietic development, there are many potential targets for leukemic transformation. *In vitro* culture of blasts combined with immunophenotyping and molecular techniques has helped to identify the cell of origin, clonality, and heterogeneity of the acute leukemias. The detection of lymphoid lineage antigens in the cytoplasm or on the surface of lymphoblasts plus an analysis of immunoglobulin (Ig) and T-cell receptor gene rearrangements indicates that ALL derives from either a precursor T- or precursor B-cell lymphoid stem cell.[11] The cell of origin for AML has been postulated to be either a multipotent or committed myeloid progenitor (e.g., CFU-GEMM or granulocyte-macrophage colony-forming unit), but some data indicate that the AML stem cell may be more primitive than previously postulated.[11]

CLASSIFICATION

Morphology

In the 1970s, a morphologic classification system was developed for the acute leukemias by a French-American-British (FAB) Cooperative Working Group and has since gained wide acceptance. The FAB system divides ALL into three morphologic subtypes (L1, L2, and L3). L1 lymphoblasts, the most common FAB types in children, have scanty cytoplasm and inconspicuous nucleoli. Blasts in the L2 category account for 10% of cases; they are larger and more pleomorphic in size, with abundant cytoplasm and prominent nucleoli, and they may be difficult to distinguish by morphology alone from FAB subtype M0 AML.

L3 blasts, the most rare subtype (1% to 2%) of ALL, have a very basophilic, vacuolated cytoplasm. These L3 blasts have the same immunophenotype and chromosomal translocations as the tumor cells in Burkitt's lymphoma[1,16] (see Non-Hodgkin's Lymphoma, later in this chapter).

The FAB classification recognizes eight subtypes of AML (M0 to M7).[12] Table 41.1-1 presents a distribution of FAB subtypes for 180 cases of AML in children younger than 18 years of age studied at St. Jude Children's Research Hospital from 1984

TABLE 41.1-1.   French-American-British Classification of Acute Myelogenous Leukemia (AML) in Children

Morphology	Frequency (%)	Associations
M0: large agranular blasts; negative myeloperoxidase	2	Blasts may express CD34 and TdT
M1: poorly differentiated myeloblasts	13	—
M2: myeloblasts with differentiation and frequent Auer rods	28	Granulocytic sarcomas (myeloblastomas) with t(8;21)
M3: hypergranular abnormal promyelocytes with multiple Auer rods	6	Disseminated intravascular coagulation
M4: myeloblastic and monoblastic differentiation (>20% monoblasts); M4E$_0$ variant associated with dysplastic eos	19	Age <2 y, EM (especially leukemia cutis)
M5: monoblastic	21	Age <2 y, EM (especially leukemia cutis)
M6: erythroleukemia with bizarre dyserythropoiesis and megaloblastic features	1	—
M7: megakaryoblastic (occasional myelofibrosis)	10	Down syndrome

EM, extramedullary leukemia; TdT, terminal deoxynucleotidyl transferase. (Based on 180 cases of AML in children studied at St. Jude Children's Research Hospital from 1984–1992.)

to 1992. Most children younger than 2 years of age with AML have either the M4 or M5 subtypes.[12] Although the M7 subtype may have several characteristic morphologic features, the diagnosis of M7 AML requires confirmation either by ultrastructural histochemistry (platelet peroxidase granules on electron microscopy) or monoclonal antibody positivity for specific megakaryocyte or platelet glycoproteins (i.e., IIB\IIIA or IB). The FAB M7 subtype most often is seen in children younger than 3 years of age with Down syndrome.

Immunophenotype

By using a panel of lineage-associated monoclonal antibodies, most cases of ALL can be broadly divided into precursor B- and precursor T-cell subgroups.[11] Precursor B-cell ALL is further subdivided into early pre-B and pre-B, and the T-cell cases are subtyped according to level of thymocyte differentiation (e.g., early, mid-, or late thymocyte).[13] The expression of several antigens, such as CD10 and CD34, are not lineage-specific and, in some studies, were of prognostic importance. Most infants with ALL have a CD10-negative, early pre-B immunophenotype.[14] The proportion of children with specific immunophenotypes of ALL is shown in Table 41.1-2 according to age group.

Compared to early pre–B-cell ALL, the pre-B (cytoplasmic Ig) immunophenotype develops more often in African Americans, is associated with a higher initial leukocyte count and hemoglobin level, and is more likely to have a DNA index lower than 1.16 and a pseudodiploid karyotype.[15] The previously known adverse outcome associated with pre-B ALL was due to the subgroup with the t(1:19)(q23;p13). The clinical features of T-cell ALL have long been recognized and include an adolescent male with a high leukocyte count, bulky lymphadenopathy (especially mediastinal), and extramedullary leukemia (CNS, skin, testes).[13] In the past, these children had a poor prognosis. However, the prognostic distinctions among ALL immunophenotypes have been lost by improvements in therapy with risk-directed protocols.[1]

Mature B-cell (surface Ig positive) ALL is associated with L3 morphology, male predominance, and bulky extramedullary disease (e.g., intraabdominal masses).[16] Many children with mature B-cell ALL come to medical attention because of a mass in the abdomen or head and neck area, which on biopsy is consistent with Burkitt's lymphoma.[16] However, further staging reveals extensive replacement of the bone marrow with L3 lymphoblasts. If the marrow has more than 25% blasts, these children are considered to have mature B-cell ALL rather than stage 4 Burkitt's lymphoma, but they are treated on identical protocols and now enjoy a favorable prognosis.[16]

There has been limited clinical use for a classification of AML based on immunophenotype.[17] The primary value of cell surface antigen analysis in most cases of AML is distinguishing between AML and ALL (FAB L2 vs. M0) and diagnosing FAB M7 AML.

Hybrid or Acute Mixed-Lineage Leukemias

Blasts from approximately 5% to 20% of children with acute leukemia have either morphologic, cytochemical, immunophenotypic, or genetic markers suggesting derivation from both myeloid and lymphoid lineages.[11,17] In these biphenotypic, hybrid, or acute mixed-lineage leukemias, individual blasts usually coexpress markers of more than one lineage, but, in rare instances, two distinct populations of blasts are present. Whether these cases represent aberrant gene expression or transformation of a multipotent stem cell is unknown. Hybrid leukemias appear to be more common in patients with prior myelodysplastic syndromes, secondary leukemias, leukemias associated with 11q23 [especially t(4;11)] translocations, and the Philadelphia (Ph) chromosome.

Myeloid-antigen expression (blasts reactive with two or more myeloid-specific monoclonal antibodies) is detected in fewer than 10% of cases of childhood ALL, and lymphoid-antigen expression is noted in approximately 15% of AML.[11] Mixed-lineage expression in AML lacks prognostic significance, and patients should be treated on AML protocols.[17] Myeloid-antigen–positive ALL is not associated with a poor prognosis if patients are treated on intensive, risk-adapted ALL protocols.[18] Leukemias with two distinct leukemic clones (one lymphoid and the other myeloid) are rare. No specific treatment recommendations have been established for these patients, but most oncologists favor a hybrid ALL/AML protocol in this situation.

CYTOGENETICS AND MOLECULAR GENETICS

The combination of cytogenetics, fluorescence *in situ* hybridization, and molecular methods identify chromosomal abnormalities in approximately 80% of cases of childhood acute leukemia.[19] Identification of numerous chromosomal abnormalities in leukemia blasts, including translocations, deletions, and inversions, have enabled molecular geneticists to clone the genes that ultimately have been shown to be important in the malignant transformation of hematopoietic cells. The genetic abnormalities also have been proved valuable as diagnostic and prognostic tools. For example, the TEL-AML1 is a fusion gene that is detected in approximately 25% of children with precursor B ALL. The fusion gene results from a cryptic t(12;21) translocation and identifies a group of patients with a favorable prognosis[20,21] (Fig. 41.1-1).

Many of the chromosomal translocations in ALL involve Ig or T-cell receptor genes and transcription factors. The prototype translocation is the t(8;14) in L3 ALL and Burkitt's lymphoma (see Burkitt's Lymphoma, later in this chapter).[16] The t(1;19) is seen in approximately one-fourth of patients with pre-B-cell ALL and fuses the E2A gene on chromosome 19 with the PBX1 gene on chromosome 1.[15] Approximately 2% to 5% of children with ALL have the t(9;22)(9q34;q11) or Ph chro-

TABLE 41.1-2. Percentage Distribution of Immunophenotypes of Acute Lymphoblastic Leukemia by Age Group

Immunophenotype	Infants (<1.5 Y)	Children (1.5–10.0 Y)	Adolescents (>10 Y)
Early pre-B	64	68	58
CD10 (CALLA)	49	94	87
Pre-B (cIgM)	26	18	18
T	6	13	23
B	4	1	1

cIgM, cytoplasmic immunoglobulin M.
Note. Numbers shown are weighted means from eight different studies. (Modified from Rivera G, Crist W. Blood: principles and practice of hematology. In: Handin R, Stossel T, Lux S, eds. *Acute lymphoblastic leukemia.* Philadelphia: JB Lippincott, 1995:747.)

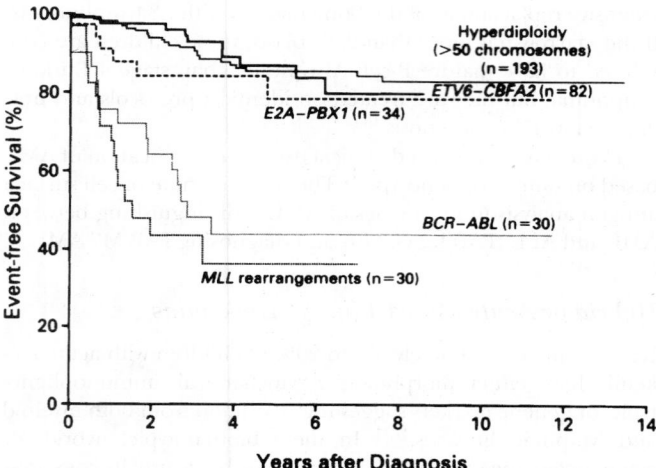

FIGURE 41.1-1. Kaplan-Meier analysis of event-free survival (EFS) according to genetic features of blast cells in 369 children with acute lymphoblastic leukemia treated at St. Jude Children's Research Hospital from 1984 to 1997. The relatively good survival of patients with BCR-ABL fusion reflects successful treatment of a subgroup with low leukocyte counts at diagnosis. The E2A-PBX1 abnormality, once associated with poor survival, now is associated with the same favorable prognosis as the ETV6-CBFA2 (TEL-AML1) abnormality. [From Pui CH, Evans WE. Acute lymphoblastic leukemia. *N Engl J Med* 1998;339(9):605, with permission.]

mosome.[1,22] In Ph-positive chronic myelogenous leukemia, the translocation results in a bcr-abl fusion gene product of 210-kD, whereas in most cases of Ph-positive ALL, the breakpoint within the bcr region is more centromeric, yielding a smaller fusion protein (185 kD). The presence of the Ph chromosome in ALL usually indicates high-risk leukemia warranting a stem cell transplantation in first remission. Children with Ph-positive ALL with a low leukocyte count or good early response to prednisone have a somewhat more favorable prognosis but are still candidates for BMT in first remission.[23] The genetic abnormalities associated with T-cell ALL are discussed in Lymphoblastic Lymphoma, later in this chapter.[24] Genes involved in cell-cycle control (e.g., p53, p16) also have been implicated in the pathogenesis of ALL.

Childhood ALL can also be classified by the number of chromosomes (or DNA content) per leukemic cell. Hyperdiploidy with a DNA index greater than 1.16 (greater than 50 chromosomes) is associated with the precursor B-cell phenotype and a highly favorable prognosis, especially if there are trisomies of chromosomes 4, 10, and 17.[25] It is not known why patients with a DNA index greater than 1.16 respond well to chemotherapy, but it may be related either to a favorable intracellular metabolism of methotrexate or the marked propensity for hyperdiploid blasts to undergo apoptosis. On the other hand, hypodiploidy (less than 45 chromosomes) is associated with a poor prognosis.[26]

Many of the chromosomal abnormalities in AML are associated with specific FAB subtypes.[27] These include t(8;21)(q22:q22) and FAB M2; t(15;17)(q22;q11-21) and acute promyelocytic leukemia (FAB M3); translocations involving chromosome band 11q23 and various partner chromosomes [e.g., t(9;11) and FAB M4 and M5]; and inv(16)(p13;q22) and FAB M4eo. The t(8;21) and t(15;17) translocations are extremely rare in patients younger than 2 years of age, whereas translocations involving 11q23 are

quite common in this age group.[12] Translocations of 11q23 almost always involve the MLL gene and are also the most frequent karyotypic change in infants with ALL. Infants with t(4;11)(q21;q23) or molecular rearrangements of MLL have an almost fivefold higher risk of relapse compared with other infants.[28] As previously mentioned, the MLL gene is also rearranged in most cases of secondary AML induced by topoisomerase II inhibitors. The t(1;22)(p13,q13), a unique but rare chromosomal translocation, has been detected in infants with FAB M7 AML. Monosomies or partial deletions of chromosomes 5 or 7 are commonly observed in adults with AML and patients with secondary AML (postalkylating agent therapy or myelodysplastic syndromes) but are unusual in *de novo* childhood AML.[19] The critical genes involved in leukemic transformation on chromosomes 5 and 7 have not yet been identified.

Clinical and Laboratory Manifestations and Diagnosis

The most common presenting signs and symptoms in children with acute leukemia are fever or infection, fatigue, pallor, and bleeding. These symptoms result from decreased normal hematopoiesis secondary to bone marrow infiltration by leukemic blasts, leading to neutropenia, anemia, and thrombocytopenia. Bone or joint pain (or both) are initial complaints in approximately 25% of children with acute leukemia and are more commonly observed in ALL than AML.[29] Bone pain is usually due to periosteal elevation but may be secondary to microfractures or bone necrosis. The classic radiologic findings in acute leukemia include metaphyseal lucent bands (growth arrest lines), periosteal elevation, and lytic lesions. These changes are best seen in the long bones near the knees, ankles, or wrists.

Moderate to massive lymphadenopathy and hepatosplenomegaly are associated with T-cell ALL and infant acute leukemias.[13] Nonspecific abdominal pain is relatively common and may be secondary to hepatosplenomegaly, gastrointestinal bleeding, or, rarely, leukemic infiltration of the bowel wall. Most of the gastrointestinal lesions encountered in patients with leukemia are secondary to complications of treatment and include oral mucositis, esophagitis, gastritis, typhlitis or neutropenic enterocolitis, lactose malabsorption, and hepatitis or cholestasis.

Extramedullary Leukemia

Extramedullary spread of leukemia at either the time of diagnosis or relapse is important because it can cause local problems, represent a sanctuary site of disease, or herald bone marrow relapse. At diagnosis, clinically detectable extramedullary leukemia of the CNS, skin, and testes is rare, except in infants. Therefore, the major treatment strategies are aimed at eradication of subclinical disease.[1] In the past, the most common sites of extramedullary relapse included the CNS and testes.[30]

Symptomatic CNS leukemia (e.g., increased intracranial pressure or cranial nerve palsies) is extremely rare, but between 4% and 10% of children with acute leukemia have blasts present in the cerebrospinal fluid (CSF) at diagnosis. The diagnosis of CNS leukemia is made by examining a cytocentrifuged preparation of CSF. Traditionally, CNS leukemia was defined by the presence of at least five leukocytes per microliter of CSF with blasts. However, more recent data indicates that the presence of blasts in CSF samples with fewer than five leukocytes per microliter or a traumatic lumbar puncture may be of prognostic significance.[31]

The most common signs of CNS leukemia include headache, nausea and vomiting, lethargy, or cranial nerve palsies (sixth and seventh being the most common). Neurologic symptoms in children with acute leukemia may also be due to epidural masses causing cord compression or myeloblastomas of the cerebral cortex or cerebellum, hemorrhage, or leukostasis (plugging of vessels by aggregates of leukemic blasts). Patients with AML and initial leukocyte counts greater than 200,000 cells per μL are at highest risk for leukostasis.[32]

Leukemia cutis is a rare finding seen most often in AML (FAB M4 and M5) and T-cell ALL. Infants with AML are at particularly high risk for leukemia cutis.[12] The lesions of leukemia cutis are typically subcutaneous nodules that are blue-gray or salmon in color. The skin nodules in babies with AML have been observed to spontaneously regress for short periods before progressive leukemia ensues.

Overt testicular leukemia is extremely unusual at diagnosis, and, with current effective chemotherapy regimens, it is rarely encountered as a site of relapse.[30] Clinically, it presents as a firm, painless, unilateral or bilateral testicular swelling. The diagnosis should be confirmed by testicular biopsy. Enlarged kidneys from infiltration of leukemia are not uncommon but are usually asymptomatic. The rare cases of renal failure in newly diagnosed children with acute leukemia are either secondary to uric acid nephropathy or ureteral obstruction from retroperitoneal lymphadenopathy.

Leukemic infiltration of the pericardium/myocardium or lungs is also extremely rare at diagnosis or during treatment. Congestive heart failure during therapy is much more likely due to sepsis or anthracycline cardiac toxicity rather than leukemic infiltration. Diffuse pulmonary infiltrates are most often secondary to an infection, but leukemic infiltration, diffuse alveolar hemorrhage, and pulmonary leukostasis should be considered in the differential diagnosis.

The most common ocular findings in patients with acute leukemia include retinal hemorrhages secondary to either thrombocytopenia or vessel infiltration or papilledema from CNS leukemia. Leukemic involvement of the anterior chamber (hypopyon) or retinal infiltration are both infrequent.

Myeloblastomas are also referred to as *chloromas* or *granulocytic sarcomas* and occur in fewer than 5% of children with AML.[12,33] These solid tumors of myeloid leukemia cells can appear simultaneously with bone marrow infiltration or may be the initial clinical manifestation of leukemia, occurring weeks to months before an increase in bone marrow blasts occurs. Myeloblastomas have a predilection for the CNS (brain or epidural) and the bones and soft tissues of the head and neck (especially the orbits).[33]

LABORATORY FEATURES AND DIFFERENTIAL DIAGNOSIS. The peripheral blood findings in patients with acute leukemia often include a normocytic anemia with teardrop or nucleated red blood cells, thrombocytopenia with platelet counts averaging between 20,000 and 50,000 cells per μL, and leukocyte counts between 5000 and 50,000 cells per μL (Table 41.1-3).[29] Approximately 20% of patients, however, have leukocyte counts greater than 100,000 cells per μL. The white blood cell (WBC) differential usually reveals neutropenia (absolute neutrophil count less than 1000 cells per μL) and circulating blasts, especially if the leukocyte count is greater than 5000 cells per μL.

TABLE 41.1-3. Initial Clinical and Laboratory Features in Children with Acute Lymphoblastic Leukemia According to Major Immunophenotypes

	Precursor B (%)	T Cell (%)
Leukocyte count/mm³		
<10,000	50	20
10,000–50,000	35	30
>50,000	15[a]	50
Platelet count/mm³		
<20,000	25	15
Hemoglobin (g/dL)		
<7.5	50	25
Hepatomegaly	8	13
Splenomegaly	10	20
Mediastinal mass	1–2	50
Lymphadenopathy (moderate/marked)	25	50

[a]Twenty-five percent of patients with pre-B subtype of precursor B acute lymphoblastic leukemia have leukocytes greater than 50,000.
(Data from Crist W, Rivera G, Pullen J, Weinstein H. The leukemias of childhood. In: Rosenthal DS, Feinstein DI, Goodnight S, McArthur JR, eds. *Hematology, 1985.* Washington, DC: American Society of Hematology, 1985.)

The bone marrow biopsy in most cases of acute leukemia is hypercellular, with blasts accounting for the majority of nucleated cells. The numbers of normal granulocyte/monocyte, erythroid, and megakaryocytic precursors are markedly decreased. To establish the diagnosis of acute leukemia, the bone marrow aspirate or biopsy must have more than 25% and 20% blasts,[34] respectively, in ALL and AML. Most cases of childhood acute leukemia can be readily diagnosed and classified by routine bone marrow morphology and histochemistry. Additional laboratory tests, such as genetics and immunophenotyping, are important for risk assignment and are sometimes necessary for distinguishing ALL from AML.

Other significant laboratory findings at diagnosis may include metabolic derangements (see Burkitt's Lymphoma, later in this chapter) and disseminated intravascular coagulation or fibrinolysis. Disseminated intravascular coagulation usually is associated with acute promyelocytic leukemia (FAB M3) or FAB M5 AML, but it may be seen in other children with newly diagnosed acute leukemia.[35]

The differential diagnosis in a child suspected of having acute leukemia includes juvenile myelomonocytic leukemia, myelodysplastic syndromes, metastatic tumors with marrow involvement (neuroblastoma and rhabdomyosarcoma), idiopathic thrombocytopenic purpura, juvenile rheumatoid arthritis, aplastic anemia, sepsis and other conditions that might result in neutropenia, infectious diseases associated with lymphocytosis, and the TMD in neonates with Down syndrome.[7]

TREATMENT

Acute Lymphoblastic Leukemia

Most children with acute leukemia are referred to tertiary care hospitals, in which they are treated by pediatric oncologists according to institutional or cooperative group protocols [e.g., Children's Oncology Group (COG), Berlin-Frankfort-Munster (BFM), Medical Research Council]. Therapy for childhood ALL

TABLE 41.1-4. Acute Leukemia: Favorable Prognostic Factors

ACUTE LYMPHOBLASTIC LEUKEMIA
Age, 1–9 y
White blood cell count <50,000/μL
DNA index >1.16 (trisomies for chromosomes 4, 10, and 17)
Chromosomal translocation t(12;22) or TEL-AML1
CNS-1
Rapid response to induction chemotherapy
ACUTE MYELOGENOUS LEUKEMIA
White blood cell count <100,000/μL
Core binding factor transcription complex [t(8;21) or inv 16]
Acute promyelocytic leukemia t(15;17)
Down syndrome
One course to complete response

has been based on risk classification systems because it has become clear that outcome of treatment varies substantially among different subsets of children with the disease. The philosophy behind this approach has been to use less toxic therapy for children with a lower risk of relapse and to treat high-risk patients with experimental and potentially more aggressive regimens. Because no single best protocol has been established for either low- or high-risk patients with ALL, enrollment in clinical trials is still encouraged.

PROGNOSTIC FACTORS. Numerous prognostic factors (Table 41.1-4) have been identified for children with ALL, and some of these have been incorporated into risk classification systems used to assign treatment. These prognostic factors include combinations of presenting clinical and laboratory parameters, biologic features of the leukemia blast, and early response to chemotherapy. Because prognostic factors are treatment-dependent, improvements in therapy may abrogate a previously accepted prognostic variable. In an effort to compare the results of various clinical trials worldwide, a uniform risk classification for treatment assignment was accepted at a National Cancer Institute workshop.[36] The agreed on standard risk category includes patients who are 1 to 9 years of age with precursor B ALL and have a WBC count at diagnosis of less than 50,000 cells per μL. The remaining patients are classified as high risk. The EFS rate for children in the standard-risk category is approximately 80% at 4 years and approximately 65% for the high-risk patients.[1,30]

Some investigators continue to classify T-cell ALL as an independent high-risk feature, and others assign risk to these children based on age and WBC criteria.[1,13] The prognosis for patients with T-cell ALL has significantly improved during the 1990s with the advent of multiagent dose-intensified ALL protocols.[30,31] Children with mixed-lineage or myeloid antigen–positive ALL are no longer considered high risk based on immunophenotype alone.

In addition to age and WBC count, other important prognostic variables established in the workshop include hyperdiploidy, cytogenetics, early response to treatment, and CNS status. The prognosis for patients with blasts with additional copies of whole chromosomes (hyperdiploidy) has been very favorable.[25] Hyperdiploidy can be measured by DNA content (DNA index) of leukemic cells, fluorescence *in situ* hybridization, and by karyotyping. A DNA index of more than 1.16 with extra copies of chromosomes 4, 10, and 17 is associated with an extremely favorable prognosis. The majority of children with hyperdiploid blasts have standard-risk age and WBC features. In some studies, DNA

index and trisomies of chromosomes 4, 10, and 17 are used to change risk assignment independent of age and WBC criteria.

Early response to chemotherapy as measured by bone marrow morphologic findings within 7 to 14 days of induction or peripheral blood blast response to corticosteroids on day 8 of treatment is associated with outcome. A more rapid clearing of blasts from either the blood or bone marrow confers a more favorable prognosis.[38] In one study, an augmented postinduction therapy for children with high-risk ALL and a slow response to induction has improved their long-term outcome.[39] Measurement of minimal residual disease by flow cytometric detection of aberrant immunophenotypes or by polymerase chain reaction analysis are more sensitive and specific than morphology and are proving to be highly prognostic.[40] New ALL clinical trials propose to stratify patients based on minimal residual disease at end of induction.

Patients with the Ph chromosome [t(9;22)] and a high initial WBC count or slow early response to prednisone and infants with t(4;11) continue to be at high risk for treatment failure.[23,28,30] Aggressive therapies, such as allogeneic stem cell transplantation in first remission, are recommended for some of these very high-risk patients.[23,28] Studies have shown that the poorer response associated with t(1;19) can be overcome by more intensive therapy.[15]

The TEL-AML1 fusion gene occurs in approximately 25% to 30% of cases of pediatric precursor B ALL and in most studies defines a subgroup with a favorable prognosis.[20] However, a few studies report initial long remissions but late relapse in these children.[21] Gene expression profiling studies are identifying genetic changes in leukemic blasts that were previously not detectable by other molecular probes.[2] These studies are now defining new genetic subtypes of leukemia that may have prognostic significance.[2]

Other factors in the past that were shown to independently affect prognosis included race, sex, blast cell morphology, lymphomatous presentations, and serum lactic dehydrogenase. African American race is no longer considered an adverse prognostic factor. These children tend to have high-risk features but enjoy a similar prognosis to whites when balanced for prognostic factors.[41] In most studies, males have a higher risk of bone marrow relapse compared to females.[42] Long-term follow-up data also indicate that females have an increased risk for some late effects, especially CNS and cardiac effects.[43,44]

It is becoming apparent that pharmacodynamic and pharmacogenomic factors exert a strong influence on the effectiveness and toxicity of leukemia therapy.[1,30] For example, patients with ALL and the null GSTM1 and GSTT1 genotypes of glutathione S-transferase enzymes have a lower rate of relapse. Another report indicated that homozygous GSTT1 deletion was associated with excess toxicity from intensive AML chemotherapy. The homozygous TT mutant of the MTHFR gene has been associated with an increased risk of methotrexate-induced oral mucositis. Other studies have correlated poor outcome in ALL with low systemic exposure to methotrexate and 6-mercaptopurine.

REMISSION INDUCTION. The achievement of a complete remission is a prerequisite for the long-term survival of patients with acute leukemia. In 1948, Sidney Farber demonstrated the first remissions in ALL using amethopterin, an analogue of methotrexate.[45] Vincristine and prednisone are effective in inducing remissions in 85% to 90% of children with ALL, without unduly suppressing normal bone marrow function. Daunorubicin and L-asparaginase were subsequently identified as active drugs in the treatment of ALL. The addition of either one of these drugs to vincristine and prednisone increased the complete remission rate in childhood ALL to more than 95%. The combination of vincristine, prednisone, and L-asparaginase is one of the standard remission induction regimens in childhood ALL.[1,1,30] PEG–L-asparaginase is an alternative form of L-asparaginase in which the *Escherichia coli* enzyme is modified by the covalent attachment of polyethylene glycol. PEG–L-asparaginase has a much longer half-life compared to standard L-asparaginase and is associated with more rapid clearance of blasts, a lower incidence of neutralizing antibodies, and is now being used more commonly in ALL induction therapy.[46] Dexamethasone has been shown to be superior to prednisone during induction for children with standard risk ALL due to fewer CNS and bone marrow relapses.[47] However, dexamethasone should be used with caution in children receiving intensive chemotherapy because it appears to increase the frequency and severity of infectious complications.[48] The use of additional drugs, such as the anthracyclines (daunorubicin or doxorubicin) or cyclophosphamide, are often reserved for children with high-risk ALL.

Data from both experimental models and human clinical trials indicate that maximum leukemia cell kill during induction decreases the likelihood for the emergence of drug-resistant clones and results in higher cure rates. Therefore, maximum tolerated doses of all active agents are delivered as early as possible during treatment. A more rapid response to induction chemotherapy as measured by day 8 peripheral blast count or day 14 marrow aspirate or minimal residual disease less than 1% at the end of induction predicts for a favorable outcome.

It has been estimated that approximately two to three logs of leukemic blasts are killed during the induction phase of therapy, leaving a residual leukemic burden of approximately 100 million cells. Therefore, additional treatment is necessary to prevent relapse. In the past, children with ALL relapsed within a median of 4 to 6 months when treatment was not continued beyond the remission induction phase. In the late 1960s, investigators at St. Jude Children's Research Hospital developed a "total therapy" approach for the treatment of children with ALL.[30] The model included remission induction, continuation chemotherapy with or without intensification, and preventive CNS therapy. The choice of continuation therapy was empiric. The early St. Jude studies evaluated 6-mercaptopurine, methotrexate, cyclophosphamide, and cytarabine in various doses and combinations. The best outcome was achieved in patients who received 2 to 3 years of daily oral 6-mercaptopurine and weekly methotrexate. Long-term follow-up of patients treated with this latter combination show a 42% disease-free survival rate for children with initial WBC counts of fewer than 25,000 cells per μL, whereas it was only 16% for all other patients.

Before the observation that the intensity of treatment required for a successful outcome varied substantially among subsets of patients, investigators in the BFM group at Memorial Sloan-Kettering Cancer Center and the Dana-Farber Cancer Institute treated all children with ALL with up-front intensive multiagent chemotherapy.[49,50] The Memorial Sloan-Kettering Cancer Center protocols used a cell kinetic rationale that combined eight cell-cycle–specific and –nonspecific agents. The Dana-Farber Cancer Institute protocols emphasized the intensive use of L-asparaginase

and doxorubicin, and the BFM group used 4 months of intensive multidrug therapy (induction, consolidation, and intensification).[37] CNS prophylaxis varied between the groups (see Central Nervous System Prophylaxis, later in this chapter). Children with high-risk ALL benefited most from these protocols. The advantage of these regimens compared to antimetabolite-based protocols for children with lower-risk ALL was less obvious. However, more recent clinical trials have shown the importance of intensive re-induction therapy or dose-intensified antimetabolite therapy, even for patients with favorable risk features.[1,30]

Other successful approaches for patients with high-risk ALL have included the use of alternating non–cross-resistant pairs of active agents. For example, investigators at St. Jude Children's Research Hospital reported encouraging results with the combination of VM-26 and cytarabine in refractory ALL and subsequently introduced those drugs into front-line protocols.[30] Most protocols for high-risk patients include the use of four or more drugs during remission induction, followed by intensification therapy for a brief period, CNS prophylaxis, and re-induction and continuation therapy. With this approach, the cure rates for these very high-risk patients have reached levels of 70% to 80%.[1,30] BMT from a related histocompatible donor is reserved for select groups of very high-risk patients (e.g., Ph-positive ALL) in first remission.

Because children with mature B-cell ALL (Burkitt's or L3 type) had such a poor prognosis after treatment with ALL protocols, an entirely different treatment approach was developed.[51] These children were treated according to regimens that were designed for patients with advanced-stage Burkitt's lymphoma. The protocols for B-cell ALL and advanced-stage Burkitt's lymphoma feature short duration (less than 6 months), dose-intensive chemotherapy with a backbone that includes cyclophosphamide, high-dose methotrexate, and cytarabine plus intensive intrathecal (IT) chemotherapy. The long-term disease-free survival rates increased from less than 10% to more than 80% with this approach.[16,51]

The duration of continuation chemotherapy for ALL has gradually been shortened from 5 years to approximately 2 to 3 years without undue risk of relapse.[1,30] The risk of relapse after cessation of therapy is highest in the first year and tapers off to 2% to 3% in the second and third years.[30] Very late relapse, after 5 years or more in remission, is rare but reported. There is an increased risk of relapse off therapy for males compared to females.

PREVENTIVE OR PROPHYLACTIC CENTRAL NERVOUS SYSTEM THERAPY. Treatment of subclinical or overt CNS leukemia is an important component of treatment and led to major increments in cure rates for ALL.[52] The early clinical trials at St. Jude Children's Research Hospital established that the risk for CNS relapse could be reduced to less than 5% by the early use of 24 Gy of craniospinal irradiation or 24 Gy of cranial irradiation plus IT methotrexate. Cranial irradiation plus IT methotrexate replaced craniospinal irradiation because of the toxicities of craniospinal irradiation.

The target volume for cranial irradiation includes the entire intracranial subarachnoid space. By convention, the caudal margin of the field extends to the bottom of the second cervical vertebra. Standard guidelines for preventive cranial irradiation also include the posterior retina and orbital apex, encompassing the extension of the subarachnoid space along the optic nerves. A subacute somnolence syndrome that follows cranial irradiation has been well described.[53] Approximately 50% of children develop some degree of lethargy, irritability, or low-grade fever at a median onset of 4 to 8 weeks after cranial irradiation.

The neurologic and cognitive sequelae of 24-Gy cranial irradiation led to treatment modifications.[52,54] In an effort to further reduce toxicity, the dose of cranial irradiation was reduced to 18 Gy and was further safely reduced by the BFM to 12 Gy.[30,52]

An alternative strategy for preventing CNS relapse has been the use of IT chemotherapy alone, starting during induction and continuing for an extended period throughout therapy.[52] Many protocols using repetitive doses of IT chemotherapy also include cycles of intravenous moderate- to high-dose methotrexate. This approach has been successful in preventing CNS relapse in children with standard-risk ALL, as well as intermediate- and high-risk patients in some studies, but it is also associated with neurotoxicity.[55]

In some protocols, select subgroups of children with ALL at high risk of CNS relapse (e.g., WBC greater than 100,000 per μL, T-cell ALL, and CNS-3) continue to be treated with cranial irradiation (12 to 18 Gy) plus IT chemotherapy. More than 85% of children with ALL do not receive cranial irradiation as part of CNS preventive therapy.[30]

Fewer than 5% of children with ALL have leukemic blasts detected in the CSF at diagnosis. Three categories of CNS leukemia have been defined according to CSF findings: CNS-1 (no blasts), CNS-2 (fewer than 5 WBCs per μL with blasts), and CNS-3 (more than 5 WBCs per μL with blasts or cranial nerve palsy). Patients with CNS-3 status have a higher frequency of isolated CNS relapse and a lower long-term survival rate than patients with CNS-1 status. Patients with CNS-2 are at increased risk of CNS and may require more IT therapy.[20]

THERAPY AFTER RELAPSE. The two most important prognostic factors for the duration of second remission are the length of the initial remission and the site of relapse.[56] Children with late relapse have a better prognosis than those with early relapse, but the definition of early and late relapse is variable. An initial remission duration of less than 3 years is considered to represent an early relapse. Relapse in extramedullary sites compared to bone marrow is also more favorable in terms of survival.[30,57]

Second complete remission rates are approximately 80%. The question of whether to perform a BMT or to continue chemotherapy has been one of the more controversial issues in second remission.[30,58] The likelihood of long-term survival after chemotherapy alone is less than 10% to 15% for patients with early relapse. This finding is in contrast to a 40% to 50% leukemia-free survival rate for children whose first remission was longer than 3 years.[56] Children who relapse also require a second course of CNS-preventive therapy. BMTs from HLA-identical sibling donors compared with chemotherapy result in fewer relapses and better leukemia-free survival rates for the early-relapse group and, in some studies, for all risk groups[58] (Fig. 41.1-2).

Autologous BMT for children with ALL in second remission who lack histocompatible family donors is no longer generally recommended because the recent results of matched unrelated stem cell transplantation are comparable to those after matched sibling BMTs.[59] The relapse rates are higher after autologous compared to allogeneic marrow transplantation owing to the lack of a graft-versus-leukemia effect.

Isolated CNS relapse occurs in 5% to 10% of children treated for ALL on current protocols despite CNS-directed therapy. In the

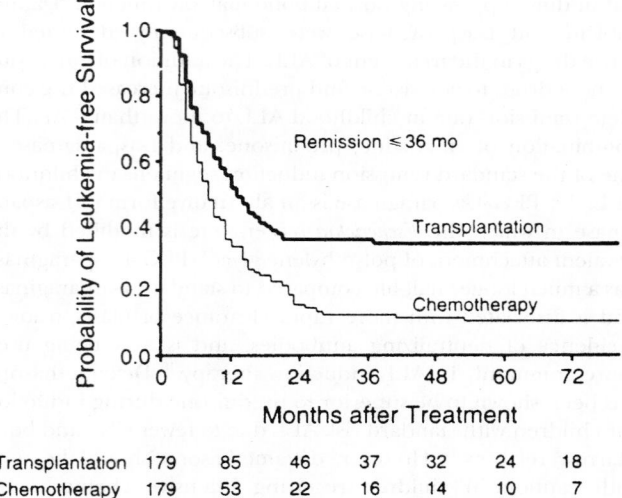

Transplantation 179 85 46 37 32 24 18
Chemotherapy   179 53 22 16 14 10   7

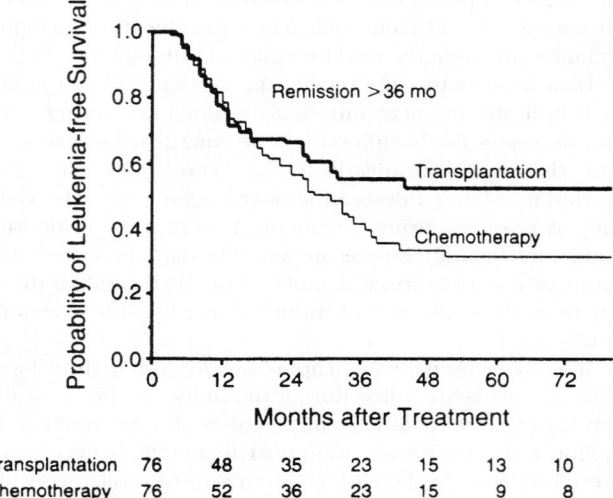

Transplantation 76 48 35 23 15 13 10
Chemotherapy   76 52 36 23 15   9   8

FIGURE 41.1-2.   Actuarial probability of leukemia-free survival in matched cohorts of children receiving chemotherapy or undergoing transplantation, according to the duration of the first remission. The numbers below the figure indicate the numbers of children at risk. (From ref. 58, with permission.)

past, CNS relapse was associated with a very poor long-term prognosis, and the few survivors had serious long-term neurotoxicity. Salvage therapies included cranial or craniospinal irradiation plus IT or intraventricular chemotherapy. In the early trials, hematologic relapse rather than a subsequent CNS event was the main obstacle to a long-term second remission. Current approaches for these children include intensified re-induction and consolidation chemotherapy, IT chemotherapy, and delayed cranial or craniospinal irradiation.[51] The delay in CNS irradiation allows for intensive chemotherapy to be administered during the early phases of therapy. The 5-year disease-free survival estimates are approximately 70% with this strategy. However, a very high rate of relapse still occurs in children whose initial duration of remission was less than 18 months. BMT should be considered for the very high risk patients with an isolated CNS relapse.

Reports of ALL treatment in the 1970s indicated that 5% to 16% of boys had a testicular relapse during hematologic remission.[30] Males with T-cell ALL were at highest risk for testicular leukemia. Testicular relapse was early during treatment for patients with T-cell ALL and usually was after cessation of therapy for precursor B ALL. These data led to trials of prophylactic testicular irradiation in T-cell ALL and testicular biopsies at completion of chemotherapy for patients with precursor B ALL. Prophylactic testicular irradiation significantly reduced the incidence of testicular relapse but did not influence overall survival. As therapy for children with ALL has improved, testicular relapse has become a rare event. Similar to other patterns of relapse, patients with early testicular relapse have a worse prognosis than those with a late relapse.[60] Treatment for testicular relapse should include re-induction chemotherapy followed by testicular radiation (24 Gy to both testes) and continuation chemotherapy. The target volume for radiation therapy includes the entire scrotal region, encompassing both the testes and epididymis bilaterally. Patients with late isolated testicular relapse have a 75% long-term disease-free survival rate. However, hormonal dysfunction usually is seen after these doses of gonadal irradiation.

COMPLICATIONS. The most concerning late complications of leukemia therapy include second cancers, adverse effects on growth and development, cardiotoxicity, and neurocognitive and neuroendocrine dysfunction.[3,43,44] The cumulative risk of second neoplasms in children treated for ALL is less than 4% 15 to 20 years after diagnosis, but is substantially higher (20.9% ± 3.9%) at 20 years for those children who received cranial or craniospinal irradiation. Most of the tumors were benign or low-grade cancers. Therefore, the long-term survival was minimally impacted. Patients treated intensively for ALL with the epipodophyllotoxins are at high risk for developing secondary AML.[10]

Short stature and obesity are common in children who received cranial irradiation, especially girls who were treated at a very young age. Many of these patients, however, have had satisfactory growth after growth hormone replacement therapy. The chemotherapeutic agents used in the treatment of the acute leukemias have been associated with many acute and chronic toxicities. The prolonged use of corticosteroids may induce osteoporosis and pathologic fractures. Avascular necrosis of long bones and foot bones also has been observed in patients with ALL who have received steroid treatment and is worse with dexamethasone compared to prednisone.[61] The antimetabolites (e.g., methotrexate, 6-mercaptopurine, and cytarabine) induce cholestatic and hepatotoxic changes in the liver but are associated with few documented long-term toxicities in this population of patients. L-Asparaginase is associated with significant acute toxicity, including allergy, pancreatitis, and deep venous thrombosis, but has not been associated with long-term complications. The anthracycline antibiotics, doxorubicin and daunorubicin, have been associated with cardiomyopathy, especially when the cumulative doses administered are more than 300 mg/m^2 of body surface area. Studies indicate that a very high percentage of long-term survivors of childhood cancer who received doxorubicin have subclinical echocardiographic abnormalities, including impaired contractility and increased afterload. Risk factors for doxorubicin cardiac toxicity include female gender, young age at treatment, cumulative dose, and dose intensity.[43] The long-term clinical significance of these findings remains to be determined, but late congestive heart failure and death have been reported. ALL regimens that do not include alkylating agents appear not to impair reproductive function.

The neurologic and cognitive sequelae of CNS-directed therapy for children with acute leukemia have been a major concern and an intensively investigated area.[52] It was once thought that cranial irradiation produced a greater impairment in cognitive function (e.g., impairment of verbal memory and coding and IQ declines) than did chemotherapy. Because of those concerns, many investigators eliminated cranial radiation from therapeutic protocols. However, studies indicate that prednisone and high doses of intravenous or IT methotrexate are associated with neurotoxicity and that 18 Gy of cranial irradiation may not be an independent toxic agent for cognitive outcome.[52,54] High-dose intravenous methotrexate is particularly toxic if it follows cranial irradiation.

Acute Myelogenous Leukemia

In contrast to ALL, only a modest improvement has been made in the long-term survival of children with AML since the late 1970s.[1,12] The complete remission rate has increased from less than 50% to approximately 85%, but only 30% to 50% of patients are long-term survivors.[62–64] The survival rate is somewhat better for those children with HLA-matched family donors who receive an allogeneic BMT early in first remission.[62]

INDUCTION. The most commonly used remission induction regimen for children with AML, excluding those with Down syndrome and FAB M3, includes a 5- to 7-day course of cytosine arabinoside, plus 2 to 3 days of daunorubicin, with or without thioguanine or etoposide.[1,63,64] The Children's Cancer Group (CCG) intensified the timing of their dexamethasone, cytosine arabinoside, thioguanine, etoposide, and rubidamycin (daunomycin) (DCTER) induction regimen in an effort to improve outcome. The intensive timing arm (second cycle on day 10) compared to standard timing did not result in a higher complete remission rate but had a very favorable impact on remission duration.[62] The high complete remission rate with all-*trans*-retinoic acid (ATRA) in patients with acute promyelocytic leukemia (FAB M3) led to prospective randomized trials testing the value of ATRA in the overall treatment plan.[65] Results of these studies clearly show that the combined use of ATRA and chemotherapy is superior to chemotherapy alone for patients with acute promyelocytic leukemia. Induction therapy for all patients with acute promyelocytic leukemia now includes ATRA combined with an anthracycline (daunorubicin or idarubicin) and cytarabine. Chemotherapy for children with Down syndrome and AML needs to be less intensive than standard AML therapy because of the increased risk of toxicity in these patients. Despite dose modifications, the outcome of children with Down syndrome and AML is excellent.[1]

CENTRAL NERVOUS SYSTEM PROPHYLAXIS. Isolated CNS relapse occurs in approximately 20% of children with AML.[1,12,63] IT chemotherapy in combination with high-dose systemic cytosine arabinoside is effective in lowering the CNS relapse rate. Data from the BFM studies using historical comparisons suggests that cranial irradiation plus IT chemotherapy in children with standard-risk AML improves outcome.[64]

POSTREMISSION THERAPY. The intensity and duration of postremission chemotherapy and the role of allogeneic and autologous BMT in first remission have been under active investigation.[1] The improvement in overall survival rates to approximately 40% to 50% at 5 years is a result of more effective remission induction and postremission chemotherapy. There is no proven role for maintenance chemotherapy if it follows several courses of high-dose cytarabine–based consolidation chemotherapy. Most pediatric AML protocols include one to three cycles of consolidation chemotherapy after remission is achieved. Patients with acute promyelocytic leukemia benefit from ATRA in both induction and maintenance.[65]

BONE MARROW TRANSPLANTATION IN FIRST REMISSION. Allogeneic BMT was first applied to children and young adults with AML in first remission as an alternative to continued chemotherapy in the mid-1970s.[1,62] The early results were favorable compared with chemotherapy, but the transplants were done in a selected group of patients. The CCG initiated the first cooperative group study comparing allogeneic BMT to chemotherapy in children with AML in first remission.[62] Long-term follow-up of that study, plus data from most other large cooperative group trials show a disease-free and survival advantage for allogeneic BMT compared to chemotherapy and autologous BMT.[1] However, fewer than one-fourth of children have a fully histocompatible family donor. Because of improving results of chemotherapy and the morbidity and mortality associated with BMT, the German BFM and Medical Research Council cooperative groups are not recommending allogeneic BMT in first remission for patients with favorable prognostic factors.[63,64] Marrow transplantation is reserved for second remission in this group of patients.

For patients who lack histocompatible family donors, autologous BMT became an attractive option in first remission after it was reported to be efficacious (30% to 40% survival) in second remission of AML.[66] The results of the early studies were controversial because they were not prospectively controlled. Beginning in the mid-1980s, both the adult and pediatric AML cooperative groups initiated prospective randomized studies to compare autologous BMT and intensive postremission chemotherapy.[12,66] In the pediatric trials, no event-free or survival advantage was found for autologous BMT compared with chemotherapy. The majority of failures after autologous BMT are due to recurrent leukemia.

PROGNOSTIC FACTORS. In contrast to childhood ALL, very few clinical or laboratory factors are consistently related to prognosis[1,12] (see Table 41.1-4). A leukocyte count of more than 100,000 cells per µL, monosomy 7, and secondary AML are associated with lower remission rates and decreased overall survival. The lower remission rates associated with hyperleukocytosis are only partially accounted for by early deaths secondary to leukostasis. In the German BFM AML studies, two risk groups were identified.[67] Standard-risk patients included FAB subtypes M1 or M2 with Auer rods, M3 or M4eo, rapid response to initial induction chemotherapy, and Down syndrome. Cytogenetics of the myeloid blasts have proven to be the most powerful prognostic factor in AML. Chromosomal translocations or inversions involving the core binding factor transcription complex t(8;21) and inv(16) and the t(15;17) in acute promyelocytic leukemia are associated with the most favorable outcome.[1,19,27] The standard-risk BFM group included these patients. EFS rates for the favorable risk patients ranges from 50% to 70% and is approximately 30% to 40% for all other patients.[63,64] In 2001 and 2003, activating mutations of the Flt3 receptor tyrosine kinase emerged as another important independent prognostic variable.[1,68]

MANAGEMENT OF THE RELAPSED PATIENT. The prognosis for children with AML who do not enter complete remission or who relapse is poor.[1,68] The likelihood of achieving a second complete remission ranges from 20% to 70%, and long-term survival is unusual unless a bone marrow transplant is performed after remission is achieved. The 5-year EFS ranges from 30% to 50% for those patients who receive an allogeneic (related or unrelated marrow donor) marrow transplant in second or subsequent remission. Autologous BMT in second remission for patients who lack suitable marrow donors offers some hope for long-term survival, but it has become a less attractive option because of the expanding unrelated marrow and cord blood banks and the opportunity to find a matched unrelated donor for an allogeneic transplant. Antibody-targeted therapy has shown promise in the treatment of relapsed AML. Second complete remissions have been achieved in approximately 30% of patients using the drug Mylotarg, which is a monoclonal antibody to CD33 coupled to the antitumor antibiotic calicheamicin.[69]

FUTURE DIRECTIONS

The major challenge for the future is to develop new targeted therapies for patients who have a poor prognosis and to minimize toxicity for those children who are successfully treated.[69] For example, Flt3 inhibitors have been effective in *in vitro* models of AML that contain the Flt3 mutation, and these drugs are in early clinical trial. Arsenic trioxide has been very effective in the situation of relapsed APL and is being tested as a consolidation agent in first remission. Other strategies such as use of multidrug reversal inhibitors have been disappointing.[1] The various hematopoietic growth factors have reduced the myelosuppressive complications from intensive chemotherapy but have not increased overall survival.

The wider availability of stem cell transplants from unrelated marrow or cord blood donors has enabled many more patients to successfully undergo marrow transplantation. Recent studies are exploring non-myeloablative marrow transplantation in an effort to achieve mixed chimerism that will hopefully achieve a more favorable balance of the graft-versus-host and graft-versus-leukemia reactions. Biologic response modifiers, such as interleukin-2, are under study for their potential to enhance the host response to tumor.

NON-HODGKIN'S LYMPHOMA

The lymphomas are the third most common childhood malignancy and account for approximately 10% of cancers in children.[16] Approximately two-thirds of the lymphomas diagnosed in children are non-Hodgkin's lymphoma (NHL), and the remainder are Hodgkin's disease. The spectrum of NHL seen in pediatric patients differs significantly from that seen in adults. The four major histologic subtypes of NHL in children are precursor B and precursor T lymphoblastic lymphoma, Burkitt's lymphoma, anaplastic large cell lymphoma, and large B-cell lymphoma (Table 41.1-5). In adults, Burkitt's and lymphoblastic lymphoma are rare, but follicular center cell and other low-grade B-cell lymphomas that are infrequently seen in children predominate. No sharp age peak (median age, 11 years) occurs in children with NHL, and the male to female ratio approaches 3:1.

TABLE 41.1-5. Pediatric Non-Hodgkin's Lymphoma: Correlation of Histology, Presenting Sites, and Immunophenotype

WHO/Updated REAL Classification	Frequency (%)	Major Anatomic Sites by Stage	Immunophenotype
Precursor B lymphoblastic	5	Neck nodes, Waldeyer's ring, scalp or other cutaneous, bone	CD10, 19; HLA-DR, TdT
Precursor T lymphoblastic	25	Anterior mediastinum, pleural effusions, bone marrow, bone, peripheral lymphadenopathy, CNS	CD2, 5, 7 ± 4, ± 8; TdT
Burkitt's or atypical Burkitt's	40–50	Stage 1/2: Waldeyer's ring, neck nodes, jaw, epidural, "limited ileocecal"	sIgM, κ or λ light chains; CD ± 10, 19, 20, 22
		Stage 3/4: Unresectable abdominal, ascites, ovary, kidney, bone marrow, CNS, bone	
Diffuse large B cell	15	Waldeyer's ring	CD19, 20, 22; sIg ±
		Anterior mediastinum, gastrointestinal tract, bone, peripheral lymphadenopathy	
Anaplastic large cell	10	Cutaneous, soft tissue, bone, mediastinal or abdominal adenopathy, CNS and marrow (rare)	CD30 (T or null) ALK positive

CNS, central nervous system; REAL, Revised European-American Lymphoma; sIgM, surface immunoglobulin M; TdT, terminal deoxynucleotidyl transferase; WHO, World Health Organization.

Therapy is best delivered by a team of pediatric oncologists, surgeons, and radiation oncologists at a major medical center with expertise in treating children. Before the use of multiagent leukemia regimens for children with all stages and histologic subtypes of NHL, fewer than 20% of children were cured. The survival of children with NHL, especially those with advanced-stage disease, has markedly improved during the past decade.[16] The 5-year EFS rate is approximately 90% to 95% for children with early-stage NHL and 70% to 90% for those with advanced-stage disease.

RISK FACTORS

Most children who develop NHL have been previously healthy, but there are several known risk factors. Children with severe combined immunodeficiency syndrome, Wiskott-Aldrich syndrome, common variable immunodeficiency, ataxia-telangiectasia, and the X-linked lymphoproliferative syndrome are at increased risk for developing a lymphoma.[70] Acquired immunodeficiency secondary to human immunodeficiency virus infection or immunosuppressive therapy, especially after solid organ transplantation or BMT, also places individuals at greater risk for developing a lymphoproliferative disorder or malignant lymphoma.[71,72] Most of the lymphomas that occur in these high-risk groups are diffuse large B-cell and Burkitt's lymphomas. Epstein-Barr virus (EBV) DNA has been identified in tumor tissue from many of these patients, indicating an important and early role for the virus in tumor development.[72] It has been postulated that the immunodeficient host does not generate an adequate T-lymphocyte response (EBV-specific cytotoxic T cells) against B cells that are latently infected with EBV.

EBV has long been associated with endemic Burkitt's lymphoma and, more recently, with hairy leukoplakia, nasopharyngeal carcinoma, and leiomyosarcomas in children with human immunodeficiency virus.[73] The exact role of EBV in the pathogenesis of Burkitt's lymphoma and other malignancies is under active investigation (see Burkitt's Lymphoma, later in this chapter).

CLASSIFICATION

The four major categories of childhood NHL in the Revised European-American Lymphoma (REAL) and World Health Organization (WHO) classifications are precursor B and T lymphoblastic, Burkitt's and atypical Burkitt's, diffuse large B-cell, and anaplastic large cell lymphoma.[74]

STAGING

The Ann Arbor staging classification is not well suited for childhood NHL for several reasons. It does not adequately reflect prognosis because there is early widespread, noncontiguous dissemination of disease, especially in Burkitt's and lymphoblastic lymphomas (e.g., mediastinal lymphoblastic lymphoma would be stage 1 or 2 in Ann Arbor but is stage 3 in Murphy) and extensive extranodal disease. In view of these deficiencies, an alternative staging system (Table 41.1-6) was developed at St. Jude Children's Research Hospital.[75] The St. Jude, or Murphy, staging system considers both primary site and extent of tumor in assigning a clinical stage, and it has been widely accepted. Pathologic staging is not helpful in the overall management of children with NHL because the mainstay of treatment is systemic chemotherapy with a very limited role for irradiation of involved sites of disease.

LYMPHOBLASTIC LYMPHOMA

Lymphoblastic lymphomas account for 30% of childhood NHL and share many clinical and biologic features with ALL. The distinction between lymphoblastic lymphoma and ALL is arbitrary (see Table 41.1-2) and has not been based on clinical presentation. If the staging bone marrow aspirate has more than 25% lymphoblasts, the patient is considered to have ALL rather than stage 4 lymphoblastic lymphoma.

The morphologic features of lymphoblastic lymphoma and precursor B and precursor T ALL are indistinguishable.[76] The cells have round or convoluted nuclei, finely dispersed chromatin, inconspicuous nucleoli, and scant cytoplasm. The precursor T-cell lymphoblastic lymphomas are usually thymic in origin with an immunophenotype that most often correlates with the middle or late stage of thymocyte maturation.[16] The cells express various combinations of the CD1, CD2, CD5, and CD7 antigens and, in many cases, express both CD4 and CD8. The CD3 antigen and associated T-cell receptor molecule are not commonly expressed. The CD10 antigen is variably present. Significant

TABLE 41.1-6.   St. Jude Children's Research Hospital Staging System for Pediatric Non-Hodgkin's Lymphoma

Stage	Description
I	A single tumor (extranodal) or single anatomic area (nodal), with the exclusion of mediastinum or abdomen
II	A single tumor (extranodal) with regional node involvement Two or more nodal areas on the same side of the diaphragm Two single (extranodal) tumors with or without regional node involvement on the same side of the diaphragm A primary gastrointestinal tract tumor, usually in the ileocecal area, with or without involvement of associated mesenteric nodes only[a]
III	Two single tumors (extranodal) on opposite sides of the diaphragm Two or more nodal areas above and below the diaphragm All the primary intrathoracic tumors (mediastinal, pleural, thymic) All extensive primary intraabdominal disease[a] All paraspinal or epidural tumors, regardless of other tumor sites
IV	Any of the above with initial central nervous system or bone marrow involvement[b]

[a]Stage II abdominal disease typically is limited to a segment (usually distal ileum) of the gut plus or minus the associated mesenteric nodes only, and the primary tumor can be completely removed grossly by segmental excision. Stage III abdominal disease typically exhibits spread to paraaortic and retroperitoneal areas by implants and plaques in mesentery or peritoneum, or by direct infiltration of structures adjacent to the primary tumor. Ascites may be present, and complete resection of all gross tumor is not possible.
[b]If bone marrow involvement is present at diagnosis, the percent blasts or abnormal cells must be 25% or less to be classified as stage IV non-Hodgkin's lymphoma. If there are more than 25% blasts, the patient is classified as having acute leukemia (either precursor B or T acute lymphoblastic leukemia or L3 acute lymphoblastic leukemia).

overlap of the immunophenotype is found in many cases of lymphoblastic lymphoma and T-cell ALL, suggesting a common cell of origin.[13] The majority of early-stage lymphoblastic lymphomas have a precursor B immunophenotype that is identical to that seen in precursor B ALL.[77]

In more than one-half of the cases of T-cell lymphoblastic lymphoma/leukemia, recurrent nonrandom chromosomal translocations involving the α, β, and γ chains of the T-cell receptor have been identified. Many of these translocations arise in error during the normal process of rearrangement of the T-cell receptor genes, a situation that is analogous to the Ig rearrangements noted in Burkitt's lymphoma.[16] Several of the partner genes involved in these translocations include the transcription factors TAL1 and HOX11, and the cysteine-rich (LIM) proteins RHOMB1 and RHOMB2. In the t(1;14)(p32;q11) detected in 3% of patients with T ALL, the TAL1 gene is rearranged in its 5' regular sequence by its translocation into the T-cell receptor α/δ chain locus. A submicroscopic deletion in the same region of TAL1 is detected in up to 25% of patients with T-cell ALL/lymphoblastic lymphoma, making it the most common genetic change in this disease.

Clinical Presentation and Staging

Most children with lymphoblastic lymphoma present with rapidly enlarging neck and mediastinal lymphadenopathy, although subdiaphragmatic nodal presentations are occasionally seen.[16,75] A typical presentation is that of an adolescent male with respiratory distress due to a large anterior mediastinal mass with or without pleural effusions. Cough, wheezing, or shortness of breath and facial swelling (evidence of superior vena cava syndrome) are frequent complaints in these patients. Other common presenting sites of disease include cervical nodes, Waldeyer's ring, cutaneous lesions, bone marrow, and single- or multiple-site bone disease. The majority of children have advanced-stage disease (see Table 41.1-5).

Because the pace of the disease is usually rapid, diagnostic studies and institution of therapy should proceed quickly. The least invasive procedure should be used to establish the diagnosis. Because bone marrow is frequently involved and patients with T-cell ALL often present with an anterior mediastinal mass, a close examination of the peripheral blood and bone marrow should be undertaken before proceeding to a more invasive procedure. A complete serum chemistry profile should be obtained, including lactate dehydrogenase. Pleural effusions should be tapped because they are often positive for malignant cells. If the bone marrow and pleural fluid are nondiagnostic, a lymph node outside of the mediastinum should be biopsied, if possible. Sufficient tissue should be obtained for histopathology, genetic studies, and immunophenotyping. A chest computed tomography (CT) scan should be obtained before any invasive procedure is undertaken to assess the major airways. Biopsy under general anesthesia should be avoided if at all possible, especially if there is significant airway narrowing (less than 50% of tracheal cross-sectional diameter) or symptoms of respiratory distress.[78] The prebiopsy use of irradiation or steroids for respiratory distress results in rapid shrinkage of the mediastinal mass and may jeopardize establishing a tissue diagnosis. The remainder of the workup should include a lumbar puncture with a cytocentrifuged examination of cerebral spinal fluid, and a CT scan of the abdomen and pelvis. Gallium and positron emission tomography (PET) scans have not been routinely evaluated in these patients.

Treatment

Historically, children with lymphoblastic lymphoma had less than a 10% survival rate after careful pathologic staging followed by extended-field radiotherapy. Within several months from the start of mantle radiation therapy, disease progression to a leukemic phase that was indistinguishable from ALL was noted in most patients. This finding suggested that widespread dissemination of lymphoma already existed at the time of diagnosis, especially to the bone marrow and meninges. Based on these observations, investigators at St. Jude Children's Research Hospital added chemotherapy that was effective against childhood ALL to local irradiation.[75] This systemic treatment approach dramatically improved the outcome for children with lymphoblastic lymphoma. Similar treatment strategies were adopted for the other histologic types of childhood NHL.

The use of chemotherapy without irradiation and with modified ALL maintenance therapy was very successful for children with stage 1 and 2 lymphoblastic lymphoma.[79] The regimen included three cycles of cyclophosphamide, doxorubicin, Oncovin, and prednisone (CHOP) followed by 24 weeks of 6-mercaptopurine and methotrexate. This therapy resulted in an EFS of 50% but a survival of 90% due to successful salvage of relapsed patients.

In contrast to the excellent results for early-stage lymphoblastic lymphoma, less than 40% of patients with stages 3 and 4 disease were long-term survivors using antimetabolite-based standard-risk ALL regimens (e.g., vincristine, steroid, L-asparaginase, methotrexate, and 6-mercaptopurine) or cyclophosphamide, Oncovin, methotrexate, and prednisone (COMP) therapy.[75] The addition of drugs such as the anthracyclines, cyclophosphamide, cytosine arabinoside, or the epipodophyllotoxins to ALL regimens substantially improved the prognosis for these children.[80]

Early preventive CNS therapy is an integral component in the treatment of children with stage 3 and 4 lymphoblastic lymphoma. Intrathecal chemotherapy and systemic high-dose methotrexate or cranial irradiation plus intrathecal methotrexate has been the mainstay of CNS preventive therapy.[80]

Relapse at any site is a significant obstacle to long-term survival for children with advanced-stage lymphoblastic lymphoma. Most of the relapses occur within 2 years of diagnosis, but occasional late relapse is observed. In contrast to relapse for early-stage disease, the outcome after a second course of chemotherapy is poor. However, these patients have a 30% to 50% survival rate after allogeneic BMT.

BURKITT'S LYMPHOMA

After Dennis Burkitt's original description of the African lymphoma, Burkitt's lymphoma was subsequently recognized worldwide and accounts for approximately 40% of childhood NHL.[81] The endemic form is common (100 per 1 million children) and is nearly always associated with EBV (95%), whereas the sporadic form is rare (1 to 2 per 1 million children) and uncommonly associated with EBV (15%). In endemic areas, involvement of the jaw and other facial bones is frequent, whereas extensive intraabdominal disease and bone marrow involvement are commonly seen in sporadic cases.

The REAL classification and WHO recognize both Burkitt's and atypical Burkitt's lymphoma.[74,76] The Burkitt's type is characterized by homogeneous cells with round to oval nuclei with multiple nuclei and intensely basophilic vacuolated cytoplasm that contains neutral fat. Atypical Burkitt's has a greater degree of nuclear pleomorphism compared to the Burkitt's type. The atypical Burkitt's type may be difficult to distinguish on a morphologic basis from some large B-cell lymphomas. In children, no obvious differences in biology or natural history are found between the two types, and, therefore, they are considered the same for treatment purposes.[16,51]

Burkitt's lymphoma is a B-cell tumor based on expression of cell surface Ig heavy chains (usually IgM) and either κ or λ light chains.[16] Approximately 50% of cases are also CD10 (CALLA)-positive. L3 lymphoblasts have a similar immunophenotype and are cytologically indistinguishable from Burkitt's cells. Because many patients with L3 ALL also have tumor masses, it is likely that these represent a spectrum of the same disease. EFS rates of 80% to 90% have been achieved for children with mature B-cell ALL (FAB L3) using treatment programs developed for advanced-stage Burkitt's lymphoma.[51]

Chromosomal translocations involving the c-myc locus on chromosome 8q24 and Ig receptor genes are characteristic of Burkitt's lymphoma. These translocations appear to result from errors in the normal process of recombination that drives Ig gene rearrangement during B-cell development. The majority of cases have a t(8;14)(q24;q32) translocation in which c-myc is translocated into the Ig heavy-chain gene on chromosome 14q32. Two variant translocations, t(2;8)(p12;q24) and t(8;22)(q24;q11), occur with less frequency. In these translocations, c-myc is fused with the κ or λ light-chain genes located on chromosomes 2 and 22, respectively. These translocations juxtapose Ig transcriptional regulatory sequences adjacent to the c-myc gene, leading to its dysregulated activity. In endemic and sporadic cases, the breakpoints on chromosome 14 involve the Ig heavy-chain joining region and switch region, respectively, suggesting that the translocation in the sporadic cases occurs at a later stage of B-cell development.[82] Up-regulation of c-myc influences the ratio between myc/max complexes in favor of transcriptional activation and B-cell proliferation. In transgenic mice, the translocation-induced dysregulation of c-myc has been shown to directly induce B-cell lymphomas.

The role of EBV in the pathogenesis of endemic Burkitt's lymphoma is unknown, but recent studies are providing new insights.[73] EBV latent membrane protein 2A (LMP2A) plays an important role in viral persistence and in the development of lymphomas. The role of malarial infection in endemic Burkitt's remains unknown but may result in a relative T-cell immunodeficiency.

Clinical Presentation

The abdomen is the most common presenting site in sporadic cases of Burkitt's lymphoma (see Table 41.1-5).[81] Approximately one-third of children with an abdominal primary tumor present with a right, lower-quadrant mass or with an acute abdomen secondary to an ileocecal intussusception. This presentation is typically seen in boys between 5 and 10 years of age. An exploratory laparotomy is indicated for diagnostic purposes. If a tumor is discovered, it is invariably a Burkitt's lymphoma that is limited in extent to the distal ileum or cecum. Complete surgical resection of the involved segment of gut with its associated mesentery, followed by an end-to-end anastomosis, is the proper treatment. Children with completely resected Burkitt's lymphoma (stage 2) of the intestinal tract have an excellent prognosis after treatment with a limited course of chemotherapy (discussed in Treatment, later in this chapter). The majority of patients with Burkitt's lymphoma of the abdomen, however, have unresectable disease that may involve the mesentery, retroperitoneum, kidneys, ovaries, and peritoneal surfaces (often associated with malignant ascites). Surgical debulking is not feasible or appropriate for this latter group of patients.[83]

The head and neck region is the second most common site of disease presentation. Patients in nonendemic areas present with tonsillar enlargement, cervical lymphadenopathy, and, occasionally, a soft tissue facial mass associated with involvement of the jaw or other facial bones.[81] Less common presenting sites include an epidural mass, skin nodules, bone, and bone marrow.

The least invasive procedure should be used to establish the diagnosis, and the staging evaluation should be expedited because these patients usually have rapidly growing tumors with significant electrolyte imbalance as well as impaired renal function. This is especially true for children with massive abdominal disease. Effusions are usually malignant in these children and contain sufficient numbers of tumor cells for diagnostic studies. Imaging should include a CT scan or magnetic resonance imaging of the primary site. Patients with head and neck primary tumors may have clinically nondetectable disease in the abdomen (especially of the kidneys) and, therefore, should also have abdominal imaging studies.

Particular attention to kidney function, and the serum levels of uric acid, potassium, calcium, and phosphorus, is critical in children with advanced-stage Burkitt's lymphoma.[81] These patients are at high risk for the *tumor lysis syndrome* and uric acid nephropathy.[84] Measures should be taken to reduce the likelihood of uric acid nephropathy, including vigorous intravenous hydration, alkalinization of urine with either sodium bicarbonate or acetazolamide (Diamox), administration of allopurinol, and careful monitoring of serum electrolytes. Rasburicase, a recombinant urate oxidase, has been shown in several clinical trials to rapidly lower serum uric acid levels and prevent the metabolic problems associated with tumor lysis, including hyperphosphatemia and renal failure.[84]

Treatment

Historically, cyclophosphamide was the single most active agent for the treatment of African children with Burkitt's lymphoma.[81] Patients with facial tumors (early stage) had sustained remissions with single- or multiple-dose cyclophosphamide, whereas the majority of children with abdominal tumors relapsed with systemic and CNS disease. Successor protocols used combination chemotherapy and IT methotrexate. The use of cyclophosphamide and vincristine with methotrexate or cytarabine was associated with higher remission rates and more durable remissions compared to single-agent cyclophosphamide.[81]

Early clinical trials in the United States demonstrated that the complete response rate, relapse frequency, and survival in American patients were similar to results in Africa.[81] Approximately 85% of patients with early-stage Burkitt's lymphoma were cured using as little as 9 weeks of CHOP chemotherapy.[79] Similar results were achieved after 6 months of COMP therapy.[151] The addition of radiotherapy did not influence outcome.[79] In 2001, results using 6 weeks of LMB chemotherapy showed 90% to 98% survival for stage 1 and stage 2 patients.[85]

More intensive chemotherapy is required for patients with advanced-stage Burkitt's lymphomas and mature B-cell ALL.[85] Several groups of investigators began to evaluate dose-intensified systemic and intrathecal chemotherapy for these high-risk patients. Cyclophosphamide, methotrexate, and cytarabine were administered in high doses with or without anthracyclines and the epipodophyllotoxins. Treatment courses were repeated at early signs of bone marrow recovery in an attempt to prevent regrowth of lymphoma between cycles of chemotherapy. Hematopoietic growth factors were used in some protocols to enhance bone marrow recovery. CNS prophylaxis included systemic chemotherapy that penetrated the CNS (high-dose methotrexate and cytarabine) and intensive IT chemotherapy. Radiation therapy was reserved for patients who presented with initial CNS involvement. The duration of treatment ranged from 2 months to 1 year. With this approach, EFS increased from 50% to 90% for stage 3 and from less than 20% to more than 80% for patients with stage 4 Burkitt's lymphoma and L3 ALL (Table 41.1-7). Patients with CNS disease at diagnosis fare less well but still have a 70% EFS and do not appear to benefit from CNS irradiation.

The management of patients with relapsed Burkitt's lymphoma is problematic. Relapse tends to occur early, while the

TABLE 41.1-7.   Recommended Protocols by Histology and Stage for Pediatric Non-Hodgkin's Lymphoma

WHO/REAL Classification	Regimen	EFS (%)	Ref.
Precursor B lymphoblastic	CHOP	60	79
	BFM	90	77
Precursor T lymphoblastic	BFM	90	80
	DFCI	80	49
Burkitt (stages 3, 4, and L3 ALL)	LMB	80–90	85
	LMB (CNS+)	70	85
Large B cell			
Stages 1 and 2	LMB	90–95	85
	CHOP	85–90	79
Stages 3 and 4	LMB	80	88
	APO	70	89
Anaplastic large cell			
Stages 1 and 2	SFOP	94	87
	CHOP	85	79
Stages 3 and 4	APO	70	89
	SFOP	55	87

APO, Adriamycin, prednisone, Oncovin; BFM, Berlin-Frankfort-Munster; CHOP, cyclophosphamide, doxorubicin, Oncovin, and prednisone; CNS, central nervous system; COMP, cyclophosphamide, Oncovin, methotrexate, and prednisone; DFCI, Dana-Farber Cancer Institute; EFS, event-free survival; LMB #89, French Pediatric Society B Non-Hodgkin's Lymphoma Trials; REAL, Revised European-American Lymphoma; SFOP, French Pediatric Oncology Society; WHO, World Health Organization.

patient is still on therapy. BMT offers the only realistic hope of long-term survival for these children.[86] The outcome is more favorable for patients who achieve a second remission before proceeding to BMT. However, second remissions are difficult to induce in these patients, especially for those with advanced-stage disease.

LARGE B-CELL LYMPHOMA AND ANAPLASTIC LARGE CELL LYMPHOMA

The large cell lymphomas constitute approximately 30% of childhood NHL.[16] Approximately 30% of pediatric large cell lymphomas are classified as ALCL in the Revised European-American Lymphoma classification. The remainder is diffuse large B-cell lymphoma, primary mediastinal large B-cell lymphoma, and the rare peripheral T-cell lymphoma. ALCL in children tends to involve lymph nodes and extranodal sites, including the skin, soft tissues, lung, and bone. Lymphomatoid papulosis and the primary cutaneous form of ALCL are rare in childhood. The majority of the cases of ALCL studied in children have had a T-cell phenotype, but some are null cell. The majority of ALCL in children have the t(2;5)(p23;q35) or variant translocations.[87] The chromosomal breakpoints involved in the t(2;5) have been cloned and involve the gene that encodes *nucleophosmin* (NPM), a nonribosomal nuclear phosphoprotein on chromosome 5, and a gene that encodes a novel transmembrane tyrosine-specific protein kinase (ALK) located on chromosome 2. The translocation results in the fusion of these genes, producing a chimeric NPM-ALK gene and message. Cases of ALCL with cytogenetic evidence of the t(2;5) or variant translocations are positive by immunohistochemistry for the ALK protein.

Clinical Presentation

The clinical presenting features of large cell lymphoma in children are more varied than those for lymphoblastic or Burkitt's lymphoma. As mentioned earlier, ALCL involves nodal and extranodal sites especially skin, bone, and soft tissues. The most common sites of diffuse large B-cell lymphoma (DLBCL) include the peripheral nodes, anterior mediastinum, bone, and abdomen. The bone marrow and CNS are rarely infiltrated in ALCL and DLBCL (see Table 41.1-5). DLBCL of the mediastinum is a unique subgroup with histologic evidence of sclerosis and is somewhat more refractory to chemotherapy.

Evaluation and Treatment

The workup and staging of the child with large cell lymphoma is similar to that recommended for children with the other histologic subtypes of NHL. Unlike Burkitt's and lymphoblastic lymphomas, both gallium and PET scans are helpful as diagnostic tools and for identifying residual disease after completion of induction chemotherapy. The treatment of large cell lymphoma (ALCL and DLBCL) in children has evolved from local radiotherapy to primarily combination chemotherapy.[85,89] Because of the relative rarity of large cell lymphoma in children, many of the treatment strategies and protocols derive from adult studies.

In some pediatric clinical trials, children with all subtypes of large cell lymphoma have been treated on a uniform protocol. Other groups have treated children with DLBCL on B-cell protocols that include Burkitt's lymphoma and have designed separate regimens for ALCL. In either case, children with localized ALCL or DLBCL have a very favorable prognosis. For example, three cycles of CHOP result in a greater than 85% survival for these children (see Table 41.1-7)[79] without the need for irradiation.

The use of an APO (Adriamycin, prednisone, and Oncovin) regimen resulted in approximately 70% EFS for children with stage 3 or 4 large cell lymphoma that included both ALCL and DLBCL.[89] Other combination chemotherapy regimens for advanced-stage ALCL result in similar survivals.[87] It appears that B-cell regimens may offer children with advanced-stage DLBCL a survival benefit over regimens such as APO and CHOP.[85] Based on the results of adult trials for DLBCL, future pediatric trials for DLBCL will test whether the addition of targeted therapy such as rituximab to chemotherapy improves outcome. CNS preventive therapy has been included in the pediatric large cell protocols, although the risk of an isolated CNS event is quite low.

There have been no consistently reported prognostic factors for children with advanced-stage ALCL and DLBCL. Gene profiling analyses and other biologic studies are under investigation.

HODGKIN'S DISEASE

Approximately 10% to 15% of all cases of Hodgkin's disease occur in patients younger than 16 years.[90] The natural history of Hodgkin's disease and outcome of treatment is similar in children and young adults 20 to 50 years of age.[91] However, treatment decisions are more complex in young children because of the adverse effects of irradiation on growth of bone and soft tissues and the risk of secondary malignancies.[92–94] The preceding concerns led to the development in the 1970s of combined modality therapy with reduced doses and volumes of irradiation for children with early and advanced stages of Hodgkin's disease.[95,96] The following sections focus on the unique aspects of the treatment of Hodgkin's disease in children.

EPIDEMIOLOGY

In industrialized countries, the age of Hodgkin's incidence is bimodal, with a first peak in adults 20 to 30 years of age and a second peak in late adulthood. Hodgkin's is uncommon before age 5 years, and the majority of pediatric cases are in children older than 11 years.[90] Before age 10, the male to female ratio is approximately 3:1; this ratio approaches 1:1 by adolescence.

The etiology of Hodgkin's disease remains unknown. An increased risk of Hodgkin's disease is noted in children with inherited immunodeficiency syndromes. Genetic susceptibility and environmental factors probably both play a role in the pathogenesis of Hodgkin's disease. A casual association between infectious mononucleosis and the EBV-positive subgroup of Hodgkin's lymphomas is likely in young adults[97] (discussed in detail in Chapter 41.5).

CLINICAL PRESENTATION, STAGING, AND WORKUP

Hodgkin's disease usually presents in supradiaphragmatic lymph nodes, with cervical, anterior mediastinal, and axillary nodes occurring in decreasing frequency. Mediastinal adenopathy may produce symptoms such as dyspnea, cough, or superior vena cava syndrome.[98] Approximately 90% of children present with painless neck adenopathy, and 60% have involvement of anterior mediastinal, paratracheal, or hilar lymph nodes. Isolated infradiaphragmatic Hodgkin's disease is rare. Approximately one-third of children have B symptoms [unexplained fever (exceeding 100.4°F), drenching night sweats, more than 10% weight loss]. The Ann Arbor staging system is used for all age groups of patients with Hodgkin's disease and is described in detail in Chapter 41.5.

Although not included in the staging system, a precise measurement of the size of the anterior mediastinal mass is important. If the ratio of the width of the mediastinal mass over the maximum transthoracic diameter is greater than one-third, this is considered large mediastinal adenopathy and is an adverse prognostic variable.[99] The diagnosis of Hodgkin's disease must be established by lymph node or tissue biopsy. The lymphocyte-predominant subtype is closely associated with stage I and II Hodgkin's disease, and lymphocyte depletion is extremely rare in children.[98] Given the unique biology and natural history of lymphocyte-predominant Hodgkin's disease, the treatment options may be more difficult in this group and range from the same stage-appropriate treatment to surgical excision only for stage I with close follow-up.[100,101] The pathology and immunobiology of Hodgkin's disease is reviewed in detail in Chapter 41.5.

Once the diagnosis is established, the pretherapy evaluation begins with "clinical" staging.[102] Clinical staging should include a history and physical examination with particular emphasis on defining lymphadenopathy by palpating the major lymph node chains. The size of the nodes should be measured and recorded for staging and follow-up. Laboratory studies include complete blood cell count with platelets, erythrocyte sedimentation rate, and kidney and liver function studies. Patients with

B symptoms or stage III or IV disease should have bone marrow biopsies from two separate sites.

Imaging studies should include a chest radiograph with a posteroanterior and lateral view and neck, thoracic, and abdominal CT scans. Lower extremity lymphangiography is no longer routinely performed in most centers because it does not visualize the upper abdominal nodes and spleen and sometimes requires general anesthesia in children. High-dose gallium scanning or PET scans, or both, in children with Hodgkin's disease, similar to the situation in adults, is most helpful for following response to therapy if the tumor is gallium or PET avid.[103]

The thoracic CT scan is useful for detecting minimal mediastinal disease, pulmonary parenchymal and hilar disease, pericardial involvement, paracardiac nodes, and chest wall extension. No optimal method has been developed for detecting abdominal involvement of Hodgkin's disease. The false-positive and false-negative rates for abdominal CT scans were 14% and 22%, respectively, in a pediatric series.[102] More than 90% of children who are upstaged by laparotomy have evidence of splenic involvement that is not detected by CT scanning or lymphangiograms. In a Pediatric Oncology Group (POG) study, models based on clinical and radiographic findings were developed to predict for splenic involvement and upstaging with laparotomy. Risk factors, such as B symptoms, an erythrocyte sedimentation rate of more than 70, histology other than nodular sclerosis or lymphocyte predominant, more than four sites of involvement, and an enlarged spleen (based on spleen CT index), were predictive for abdominal disease but still were associated with 25% to 30% false-negative and false-positive rates, respectively.[102] Because all pediatric patients with Hodgkin's disease now receive chemotherapy, staging laparotomy is no longer routinely performed.[98]

Among 2238 consecutive patients with Hodgkin's disease treated at Stanford University, 4% were 10 years old or younger and 11% were 11 to 16 years old. Stage I and II disease was present in approximately 60% of children. Stage I disease was slightly more common in younger children (18%) than in adolescents (8%); stage II disease occurred in 40% to 50% of all age groups; and stage IV disease was less common in younger children (3%) than in adolescents (15%). B symptoms occurred in 19% of younger children and in 30% of adolescents.[90]

As the treatment of Hodgkin's disease has improved, previously identified prognostic factors have diminished in importance. However, the stage of disease, tumor bulk, and constitutional symptoms continue to influence the success and certainly the choice of therapy.[98,99,104] In the German Pediatric Oncology and Hematology Group GPOH-95 study, B symptoms, histology, and male sex were significant adverse prognostic factors for EFS.[105] In a report from three institutions on 320 children, male sex; stage IIB, IIIB or IV disease; WBC of 11.5/mm[3] or greater; and hemoglobin of 11 g/dL or less were all significant predictors for an inferior EFS and overall survival.[99,105] Because prognostic factors are generally similar for adults and children with Hodgkin's disease, the reader is referred to Chapter 41.5 for an in-depth discussion of this topic.

SELECTION OF THERAPY

The cure rate for children with all stages of Hodgkin's disease is approximately 90%.[98] As the cure rate has increased, an increasing focus has been placed on the late complications of therapy. In the pediatric patient, especially the prepubescent child, treat-

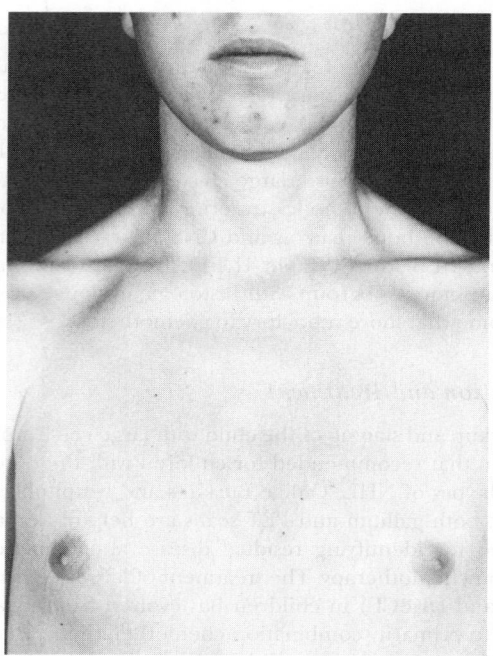

FIGURE 41.1-3. Frontal view of patient several years after mantle irradiation with 4-MeV linear accelerator for Hodgkin's disease. Note the infraclavicular narrowing and hypodevelopment of neck musculature.

ment decisions must be weighed in view of the toxicities of radiation therapy on growth and development. For example, the use of high-dose (40 Gy) extended-field radiotherapy alone in children and adults with pathologic stage I or II Hodgkin's disease results in 85% to 90% 10-year survival.[106] However, this therapy has serious late effects on musculoskeletal growth in the prepubescent child. In this young age group, the effect on bone and soft tissue is manifest by intraclavicular narrowing, shortened sitting height, decreased mandibular growth, and decreased muscle development in the treated volume (Fig. 41.1-3). Other well-known late complications of irradiation, including hypothyroidism and second neoplasms, are not unique in patients treated for Hodgkin's disease in childhood (discussed in Complications, later in the chapter).[92,93,107–109]

In an attempt to decrease the late effects of high-dose extended-field irradiation, alternative treatments have been developed. These have included chemotherapy combined with lower doses and less extensive fields of irradiation and chemotherapy alone.[99,104,110–112]

A Stanford study was one of the first to demonstrate that combined modality therapy with mechlorethamine (Mustargen), vincristine (Oncovin), procarbazine, and prednisone (MOPP) and low-dose radiation to involved regions was highly effective and associated with fewer adverse effects on musculoskeletal growth and development than had been observed with high-dose radiation alone.[113] In this study, patients were surgically staged and treated with six cycles of MOPP chemotherapy and an age-adjusted radiation dose of 15 to 25 Gy. Boost doses of 10 Gy were used in select patients. The projected 10-year survival rate was 89% for all patients. However, the long-term side effects included the development of secondary leukemia, as well as azoospermia in males tested. Therefore, the Stanford successor study alternated MOPP with doxorubicin, bleomycin, vinblastine, and dacarbazine (ABVD) for six cycles in combination with a 15- to 25-Gy radiation dose to involved fields.[95] The projected 10-year survival rates are 96%, and growth and development have progressed normally. There were no secondary leukemias, and only one solid tumor was noted. Approximately one-third of patients had asymptomatic changes noted on pulmonary function tests.

Similar treatment strategies with the goal of decreasing the risk of secondary leukemia, solid tumors, and gonadal failure have been reported by other groups. The French Society of Pediatric Oncology randomized patients with clinical stage I and IIA Hodgkin's disease to four cycles of ABVD, or two cycles of MOPP and two cycles of ABVD, plus low-dose (20-Gy) involved-field radiation therapy.[96] Children with advanced disease (stages IB, IIIB, III, and IV) were given three cycles of MOPP and three cycles of ABVD plus extended-field, low-dose radiotherapy. Patients with a poor response to chemotherapy received full doses of irradiation. The disease-free survival rate is 88%, and the actuarial survival for the entire group is 95%. The German-Austrian multicenter studies also have developed successful combined modality treatment programs for children with all stages of Hodgkin's disease.[105–110] In DAL-HD-90 (German-Austrian Hodgkin's trials), chemotherapy was limited to two cycles for stages I and IIA. Boys received vincristine, etoposide, prednisone, and doxorubicin (Adriamycin) (OEPA), and girls were given two cycles of vincristine, procarbazine, prednisone, and Adriamycin (OPPA). Radiation was applied to involved sites (25 Gy). The 5-year EFS rate is 95%. Patients with more advanced-stage disease received two cycles of OPPA or OEPA and an additional two cycles (stages IIB and IIIA) or four cycles (stages IIIB and IV) of cyclophosphamide, Oncovin, procarbazine, and prednisone (COPP) plus involved-field irradiation. Five-year EFS rates were 90% to 95% for intermediate stages and 84% to 89% for stages IIIB and IV. Testicular function was normal in the regimens without procarbazine.[110] These studies have served as a paradigm for the risk-adapted treatment approach currently used at most centers.

In the past, there had been only limited experience using chemotherapy as the only treatment modality in children with Hodgkin's disease. Ekert and colleagues reported treating children with stage I to IV Hodgkin's disease with either MOPP or chlorambucil, vinblastine, procarbazine, and prednisone (ChlVPP) therapy.[111] The EFS rate was 92% at a median follow-up of 45 months.[111,114] Twenty-eight of 32 patients with stage I or II disease and 14 of 15 patients with stage III or IV were disease-free. Although the outcome was excellent, these children were exposed to multiple cycles of alkylating agents with the high risk of secondary leukemia and infertility in males.

Several large pediatric trials have evaluated the role of low-dose involved-field radiotherapy in the treatment of Hodgkin's disease. POG showed that no benefit existed for low-dose total nodal or subtotal nodal radiation after eight cycles of MOPP alternating with ABVD in children with advanced-stage Hodgkin's disease.[115] The CCG study compared outcome in patients who achieved an initial complete response to chemotherapy followed by low-dose radiation therapy or no further therapy. Patients received risk-adapted therapy using a COPP/ABV regimen. Results indicated inferior 3-year EFS in patients with advanced-stage disease or B symptoms who were randomized to receive chemotherapy only (93% vs. 85%).[112]

The German study eliminated radiation therapy for all patients achieving a complete response after chemotherapy.[105]

Overall, EFS was 93% for patients receiving radiation and 89% for those without radiation ($P = .09$). Excluding stage I and IIA patients, the EFS was 92% with radiation and 81% for no radiation ($P = .01$). Overall survival, however, was excellent at 97%. The benefit to radiation was greater in patients with advanced-stage disease at presentation.

The combined modality approach using limited doses of both radiation (15 to 30 Gy) and chemotherapy for children with all stages of Hodgkin's disease produces an excellent outcome with significant reduction in the risk of serious late effects.[104,105,112] As the doses of irradiation are safely lowered in combined modality treatments, future studies will undoubtedly test whether chemotherapy alone can achieve these excellent results. In addition, less toxic and equally effective chemotherapy regimens are being tested.

COMPLICATIONS

The risk of infertility, secondary cancers, and late cardiopulmonary complications of newer-generation combined modality therapies in young children with Hodgkin's disease remains to be determined.[104,105] A 2003 report provides evidence that the risk of breast cancer is increased approximately three to eight times in long-term survivors of Hodgkin's disease and is related to radiation dose and ovarian damage.[116]

Based on these data, efforts to lower the doses and volumes of radiation and limit exposure to alkylating agents are steps in the right direction. Newer approaches also advocate for therapy that is response based.[117]

REFERENCES

1. Ravindranath Y. Recent advances in pediatric acute lymphoblastic and myeloid leukemia. *Curr Opin Oncol* 2003;15:23.
2. Ross ME, Zhou X, Song G, et al. Classification of pediatric acute lymphoblastic leukemia by gene expression profiling. *Blood* 2003;102:2951.
3. Pui CH, Cheng C, Leung W, et al. Extended follow-up of long-term survivors of childhood acute lymphoblastic leukemia. *N Engl J Med* 2003;349:640.
4. Smith MA, Ries LAG, Gurney JG, Ross JA. Cancer incidence and survival among children and adolescents: United States SEER Program 1975–1995. In: Ries L, Smith M, Gurney J, et al., eds. Leukemia (ICCC I). National Institutes of Health publication no. 99-4649. Bethesda, MD: National Cancer Institute SEER Program, 1999:17.
5. Wiemels JL, Daniotti M, Eden OB, et al. Prenatal origin of acute lymphoblastic leukemia in children. *Lancet* 1999;354:1499.
6. Mori H, Colman SM, Xiao Z, et al. Chromosome translocations and covert leukemic clones are generated during normal fetal development. *Proc Natl Acad Sci U S A* 2002;99:8242.
7. Zipursky A, Poon A, Doyle J. Leukemia in Down syndrome: a review. *Pediatr Hematol Oncol* 1992;9:139.
8. Homans AC, Verissimo AM, Vlacha V. Transient abnormal myelopoiesis of infancy associated with trisomy 21. *Am J Pediatr Hematol Oncol* 1993;15:392.
8a. Massey G, Zipursky A, Doyle J, et al. A prospective study of the natural history of transient leukemia (TL) in neonates with Down syndrome. *Blood* 2002;100:321(abst).
9. Xu G, Nagano M, Kanezaki R, et al. Frequent mutations in the GATA-1 gene in the transient myeloproliferative disorder of Down syndrome. *Blood* 2003;102:2960.
10. Pui C-H, Relling MV. Topoisomerase II inhibitor-related acute myeloid leukaemia. *Br J Haematol* 2000;109:13.
11. Pui CH, Raimondi SC, Head DR, et al. Characterization of childhood acute leukemia with multiple myeloid and lymphoid markers at diagnosis and at relapse. *Blood* 1991;78:1327.
12. Ebb DH, Weinstein HJ. Diagnosis and treatment of childhood acute myelogenous leukemia. *Pediatr Clin North Am* 1997;44:847.
13. Uckun FM, Gaynon PS, Sensel MG, et al. Clinical features and treatment outcome of childhood T-lineage acute lymphoblastic leukemia according to the apparent maturational stage of T-lineage leukemic blasts: a Children's Cancer Group study. *J Clin Oncol* 1997;15:2214.
14. Biondi JE, Link MP, Shuster JJ, et al. Frequency and prognostic significance of HRX rearrangements in infant acute lymphoblastic leukemia: a Pediatric Oncology Group study. *Blood* 2000;96:24.
15. Uckun FM, Sensel MG, Sather HN, et al. Clinical significance of translocation t(1;19) in childhood acute lymphoblastic leukemia in the context of contemporary therapies: a report from the Children's Cancer Group. *J Clin Oncol* 1998;16:527.

16. Sandlund JT, Downing JR, Crist WM. Non-Hodgkin's lymphoma in childhood. *N Engl J Med* 1996;334:1238.

17. Creutzig U, Harbott J, Sperling C, et al. Clinical significance of surface antigen expression in children with acute myeloid leukemia: results of study AML-BFM-87. *Blood* 1995; 86:3097.

18. Putti MC, Rondelli R, Cocito MG, et al. Expression of myeloid markers lacks prognostic impact in children treated for acute lymphoblastic leukemia: Italian experience in AIEOP-ALL 88-91 studies. *Blood* 1998;92:795.

19. Rowley JD. The critical role of chromosome translocations in human leukemias. *Annu Rev Genet* 1998;32:495.

20. McLean TW, Ringold S, Neuberg D, et al. TEL/AML-1 dimerizes and is associated with a favorable outcome in childhood acute lymphoblastic leukemia. *Blood* 1996;88:4252.

21. Loh ML, Rubnitz JE. TEL/AML1-positive pediatric leukemia: prognostic significance and therapeutic approaches. *Curr Opin Hematol* 2002;9:345.

22. Schrappe M, Arico M, Harbott J, et al. Philadelphia chromosome–positive (Ph+) childhood acute lymphoblastic leukemia: good initial steroid response allows early prediction of a favorable treatment outcome. *Blood* 1998;92:2730.

23. Aricò M, Valsecchi MG, Camitta B, et al. Outcome of treatment in children with Philadelphia chromosome-positive acute lymphoblastic leukemia. *N Engl J Med* 2000;342:998.

24. Schneider NR, Carroll AJ, Shuster JJ, et al. New recurring cytogenetic abnormalities and association of blast cell karyotypes with prognosis in childhood T-cell acute lymphoblastic leukemia: a Pediatric Oncology Group report of 343 cases. *Blood* 2000;96:2543.

25. Heerema NA, Sather HN, Sensel MG, et al. Prognostic impact of trisomies of chromosomes 10, 17, and 5 among children with acute lymphoblastic leukemia and high hyperdiploidy (> 50 chromosomes). *J Clin Oncol* 2000;18:1876.

26. Heerema NA, Nachman JB, Sather HN, et al. Hypodiploidy with less than 45 chromosomes confers adverse risk in childhood acute lymphoblastic leukemia: a report from the Children's Cancer Group. *Blood* 1999;94:4036.

27. Raimondi SC, Chang MN, Ravindranath Y, et al. Chromosomal abnormalities in 478 children with acute myeloid leukemia: clinical characteristics and treatment outcome in a cooperative Pediatric Oncology Group study—POG 8821. *Blood* 1999;94:3707.

28. Pui CH, Gaynon PS, Boyett JM, et al. Outcome of treatment in childhood acute lymphoblastic leukaemia with rearrangements of the 11q23 chromosomal region. *Lancet* 2002; 359:1909.

29. Choi S, Simone JV. Acute nonlymphocytic leukemia in 171 children. *Med Pediatr Oncol* 1976;2:119.

30. Pui Ch, Campana D, Evans WE. Childhood acute lymphoblastic leukaemia—current status and future perspectives. *Lancet Oncol* 2001;2:597.

31. Bürger B, Zimmermann M, Mann G, et al. Diagnostic cerebrospinal fluid examination in children with acute lymphoblastic leukemia: significance of low leukocyte counts with blasts or traumatic lumbar puncture. *J Clin Oncol* 2003;21:184.

32. Bunin NJ, Pui CH. Differing complications of hyperleukocytosis in children with acute lymphoblastic or acute nonlymphoblastic leukemia. *J Clin Oncol* 1985;3:1590.

33. Reinhardt D, Creutzig U. Isolated myelosarcoma in children—updated and reviewed. *Leuk Lymphoma* 2002;43:565.

34. Vardiman JW, Harris NL, Brunning RD. The World Health Organization (WHO) classification of the myeloid neoplasms. *Blood* 2002;100:2292.

35. Warrell RP Jr, de The H, Wang ZY, Degos L. Acute promyelocytic leukemia. *N Engl J Med* 1993;329:177.

36. Smith M, Arthur D, Camitta B, et al. Uniform approach to risk classification and treatment assignment for children with acute lymphoblastic leukemia. *J Clin Oncol* 1996;14:18.

37. Schrappe M, Reiter A, Ludwig WD, et al. Improved outcome in childhood acute lymphoblastic leukemia despite reduced use of anthracyclines and cranial radiotherapy: results of trial ALL-BFM 90. German-Austrian-Swiss ALL-BFM Study Group. *Blood* 2000;95:3310.

38. Gajjar A, Ribeiro R, Hancock ML, et al. Persistence of circulating blasts after 1 week of multiagent chemotherapy confers a poor prognosis in childhood acute lymphoblastic leukemia. *Blood* 1995;86:1292.

39. Nachman JB, Sather HN, Sensel MG, et al. Augmented post-induction therapy for children with high-risk acute lymphoblastic leukemia and a slow response to initial therapy (Comments). *N Engl J Med* 1998;338:1663.

40. Panzer-Grümayer ER, Schneider M, Panzer S, et al. Rapid molecular response during early induction chemotherapy predicts a good outcome in childhood acute lymphoblastic leukemia. *Blood* 2000;95:790.

41. Pui CH, Sandlund JT, Pei D, et al. Results of therapy for acute lymphoblastic leukemia in black and white children. *JAMA* 2003;290:2001.

42. Pui CH, Boyett JM, Relling MV, et al. Sex differences in prognosis for children with acute lymphoblastic leukemia. *J Clin Oncol* 1999;17:818.

43. Lipshultz S, Lipsitz S, Mone S, et al. Female sex and higher drug dose as risk factors for late cardiotoxic effects of doxorubicin therapy for childhood cancer. *N Engl J Med* 1995;33:1738.

44. Waber D, Tarbell N, Fairclough D, et al. Cognitive sequelae of treatment in childhood acute lymphoblastic leukemia: cranial radiation requires an accomplice. *J Clin Oncol* 1995;13:2490.

45. Farber S, Diamond LK, Mercer RD, Sylvester RF, Wolff JA. Temporary remission in acute leukemia in children produced by folic acid antagonist, 4 amino pteroylglutamic acid (Aminopterin). *N Engl J Med* 1948;238:787.

46. Avramis VI, Sencer S, Periclou AP, et al. A randomized comparison of native Escherichia coli asparaginase and polyethylene glycol conjugated asparaginase for treatment of children with newly diagnosed standard-risk acute lymphoblastic leukemia: a Children's Cancer Group study. *Blood* 2002;99:1986.

47. Bostrom BC, Sensel MR, Sather HN, et al. Dexamethasone versus prednisone and daily oral versus weekly intravenous mercaptopurine for patients with standard-risk acute lymphoblastic leukemia: a report from the Children's Cancer Group. *Blood* 2003;101:3809.

48. Hurwitz CA, Silverman LB, Schorin MA, et al. Substituting dexamethasone for prednisone complicates remission induction in children with acute lymphoblastic leukemia. *Cancer* 2000;88:1964.

49. Silverman LB, Gelber RD, Dalton VK, et al. Improved outcome for children with acute lymphoblastic leukemia: results of Dana-Farber Consortium Protocol 91-01. *Blood* 2001; 97:1211.

50. Gaynon PS, Desai AA, Bostrom BC, et al. Early response to therapy and outcome in childhood acute lymphoblastic leukemia: a review. *Cancer* 1997;80:1717.

51. Reiter A, Schrappe M, Tiemann M, et al. Improved treatment results in childhood B-cell neoplasms with tailored intensification of therapy: a report of the Berlin-Frankfurt-Munster Group Trial NHL-BFM 90. *Blood* 1999;94:3294.

52. Clarke M, Gaynon P, Hann I, Harrison G, Masera G, et al. CNS-directed therapy for childhood acute lymphoblastic leukemia: childhood ALL collaborative group overview of 43 randomized trials. *J Clin Oncol* 2003;21:1798.

53. Freeman AI, Johnston PG, Voke JM. Somnolence after prophylactic cranial irradiation in children with acute lymphoblastic leukemia. *BMJ* 1973;4:523.

54. Waber D, Tarbell N, Fairclough D, et al. Cognitive sequelae of treatment in childhood acute lymphoblastic leukemia: cranial radiation requires an accomplice. *J Clin Oncol* 1995;13:2490.

55. Mahoney DH Jr, Shuster JJ, Nitschke R, et al. Acute neurotoxicity in children with B-precursor acute lymphoid leukemia: an association with intermediate-dose intravenous methotrexate and intrathecal triple therapy—a Pediatric Oncology Group study. *J Clin Oncol* 1998;16:1712.

56. Gaynon PS, Qu RP, Chappell RJ, et al. Survival after relapse in childhood acute lymphoblastic leukemia: impact of site and time to first relapse—the Children's Cancer Group Experience. *Cancer* 1998;82:1387.

57. Ritchey AK, Pollock BH, Lauer SJ, et al. Improved survival of children with isolated CNS relapse of acute lymphoblastic leukemia: a Pediatric Oncology Group study. *J Clin Oncol* 1999;17:3745.

58. Barrett AJ, Horowitz MM, Pollock BH, et al. Bone marrow transplants from HLA-identical siblings as compared with chemotherapy for children with acute lymphoblastic leukemia in a second remission. *N Engl J Med* 1994;331:1253.

59. Bunin N, Carston M, Wall D, et al. Unrelated marrow transplantation for children with acute lymphoblastic leukemia in second remission. *Blood* 2002;99:3151.

60. Wofford MM, Smith SD, Shuster JJ, et al. Treatment of occult or late overt testicular relapse in children with acute lymphoblastic leukemia: a Pediatric Oncology Group study. *J Clin Oncol* 1992;10:624.

61. Mattano LA Jr, Sather HN, Trigg ME, et al. Osteonecrosis as a complication of treating acute lymphoblastic leukemia in children: a report from the Children's Cancer Group. *J Clin Oncol* 2000;18:3262.

62. Nesbit M, Buckley J, Feig S, et al. Chemotherapy for induction of remission of childhood acute myeloid leukemia followed by marrow transplantation or multiagent chemotherapy: a report from the Children's Cancer Group. *J Clin Oncol* 1994;12:127.

63. Stevens RF, Hann IM, Wheatley K, et al. Marked improvements in outcome with chemotherapy alone in paediatric acute myeloid leukemia: results of the United Kingdom Medical Research Council's 10th AML trial. MRC Childhood Leukemia Working Party. *Br J Haematol* 1998;101:130.

64. Creutzig U, Ritter J, Zimmermann M, et al. Improved treatment results in high-risk pediatric acute myeloid leukemia patients after intensification with high-dose cytarabine and mitoxantrone: result of Study Acute Myeloid Leukemia-Berlin-Frankfurt-Münster 93. *J Clin Oncol* 2001;19:2705.

65. Tallman MS, Andersen JW, Schiffer CA, et al. All-*trans* retinoic acid in acute promyelocytic leukemia: long-term outcome and prognostic factor analysis from the North American Intergroup protocol. *Blood* 2002;100:4298.

66. Ravindranath Y, Yeager AM, Chang MN, et al. Autologous bone marrow transplantation versus intensive consolidation chemotherapy for acute myeloid leukemia in childhood. *N Engl J Med* 1996;334:1428.

67. Creutzig U, Ritter J, Schellong G. Identification of two risk groups in childhood acute myelogenous leukemia after therapy intensification in study AML-BFM-83 as compared with study AML-BFM-78. *Blood* 1990;75:1932.

68. Meshinchi S, Woods WG, Stirewalt DL, et al. Prevalence and prognostic significance of Flt3 internal tandem duplication in pediatric acute myeloid leukemia. *Blood* 2001;97:89.

69. Clark JJ, Smith FO, Arceci RJ. Update in childhood acute myeloid leukemia: recent developments in the molecular basis of disease and novel therapies. *Curr Opin Hematol* 2003;10:31.

70. Filipovich AH, Mathur A, Kamat D, Shapiro RS. Primary immunodeficiencies: genetic risk factors for lymphoma. *Cancer Res* 1992;52[Suppl]:5465S.

71. Pollock BH, Jenson HB, Leach CT, et al. Risk factors for pediatric human immunodeficiency virus-related malignancy. *JAMA* 2003;289:2393.

72. Green M, Michaels MG, Webber SA, Rowe D, Reyes J. The management of Epstein-Barr virus associated post-transplant lymphoproliferative disorders in pediatric solid-organ transplant recipients. *Pediatr Transplant* 1999;3:271.

73. Thorley-Lawson DA. Epstein-Barr virus: exploiting the immune system. *Nat Rev Immunol* 2001;1:75.

74. Harris N, Jaffe E, Stein H, et al. A revised European-American classification of lymphoid neoplasms: a proposal from the International Lymphoma Study Group. *Blood* 1994;84:1361.

75. Murphy S, Fairclough D, Hutchison R, et al. NHL of childhood. An analysis of the histology, staging and response to treatment of 338 cases at a single institution. *J Clin Oncol* 1989;7:186.

76. Harris NL, Jaffe ES, Diebold J, et al. World Health Organization classification of neoplastic diseases of the hematopoietic and lymphoid tissues: report of the Clinical Advisory Committee meeting–Airlie House, Virginia, November 1997. *J Clin Oncol* 1999;17:3835.

77. Neth O, Seidemann K, Jansen P, et al. Precursor B-cell lymphoblastic lymphoma in child-

hood and adolescence: clinical features, treatment, and results in trials NHL-BFM 86 and 90. *Med Pediatr Oncol* 2000;35:20.

78. Shamberger RC, Holzman RS, Griscom NT, et al. Prospective evaluation by computed tomography and pulmonary function tests of children with mediastinal masses. *Surgery* 1995;118:468.

79. Link MP, Donaldson SS, Berard CW, et al. Results of treatment of childhood localized non-Hodgkin's lymphoma with combination chemotherapy with or without radiotherapy. *N Engl J Med* 1990;322:1169.

80. Reiter A, Schrappe M, Ludwig WB, et al. Intensive ALL type therapy without local radiotherapy provides a 90% event free survival for children with T-cell lymphoblastic lymphoma: a BFM Group report. *Blood* 2000;95:416.

81. Ziegler JL. Burkitt's lymphoma. *N Engl J Med* 1981;30:735.

82. Shiramizu B, Barriga F, Neeguaye J, et al. Patterns of chromosomal breakpoint locations in Burkitt's lymphoma: relevance to geography and Epstein-Barr virus association. *Blood* 1991;77:1516.

83. Shamberger R, Weinstein HJ. The role of surgery in abdominal Burkitt's lymphoma. *J Pediatr Surg* 1992;27:236.

84. Pui CH. Rasburicase. A potent uricolytic agent. *Expert Opin Pharmacother* 2002;3:433.

85. Patte C, Auperin A, Michon J, et al. The Société Française d'Oncologie Pédiatrique LMB89 protocol: highly effective multiagent chemotherapy tailored to the tumor burden and initial response in 561 unselected children with B-cell lymphomas and L3 leukemia. *Blood* 2001;97:3370.

86. Ladenstein R, Pearce R, Hartmann O, et al. High-dose chemotherapy with autologous bone marrow rescue in children with poor-risk Burkitt's lymphoma: a report from the European Lymphoma Bone Marrow Transplantation Registry. *Blood* 1997;90:2921.

87. Brugieres L, LeDeley MC, Pacquement H, et al. CD30+ anaplastic large-cell lymphoma in children: analysis of 82 patients enrolled in two consecutive studies of the French Society of Pediatric Oncology. *Blood* 1998;92:3591.

88. Raetz E, Perkins S, Davenport V, Cairo MS. B large-cell lymphoma in children and adolescents. *Cancer Treat Rev* 2003;29:91.

89. Laver JH, Mahmoud H, Pick TE, et al. Results of a randomized phase III trial in children and adolescents with advanced stage diffuse large cell non Hodgkin's lymphoma: a Pediatric Oncology Group study. *Leuk Lymphoma* 2001;42:399.

90. Cleary S, Link M, Donaldson S. Hodgkin's disease in the very young. *Int J Radiat Oncol Biol Phys* 1994;28:77.

91. Ng AK, Bernardo MP, Weller E, et al. Long-term survival and competing causes of death in patients with early-stage Hodgkin's disease treated at age 50 or younger. *J Clin Oncol* 2002;20:2101.

92. William K, Cox R, Donaldson S. Radiation induced height impairment in pediatric Hodgkin's disease. *Int J Radiat Oncol Biol Phys* 1994;28:85.

93. Tarbell NJ, Gelber RD, Weinstein HJ, Mauch P. Sex differences in risk of second malignant tumors after Hodgkin's disease in childhood. *Lancet* 1993;341:1428.

94. Travis LB, Hill DA, Dores GM, et al. Breast cancer following radiotherapy and chemotherapy among young women with Hodgkin's disease. *JAMA* 2003;290:465.

95. Hunger S, Link M, Donaldson S. Long-term results of ABVD/MOPP and low dose involved field radiotherapy (LDFRT) in pediatric Hodgkin's disease: the Stanford Experiences. *J Clin Oncol* 1993;12:386.

96. Oberlin O, Leverger G, Pacquement H, et al. Low dose radiation therapy and reduced chemotherapy in childhood Hodgkin's disease: the experience of the French Society of Pediatric Oncology. *J Clin Oncol* 1992;10:1602.

97. Hjalgrim H, Askling J, Rostgaard K, et al. Characteristics of Hodgkin's lymphoma after infectious mononucleosis (Comment). *N Engl J Med* 2003;349:1324.

98. Hudson MM, Donaldson SS. Treatment of pediatric Hodgkin's lymphoma. *Semin Hematol* 1999;36:313.

99. Smith RS, Chen Q, Hudson MM, et al. Prognostic factors for children with Hodgkin's disease treated with combined-modality therapy. *J Clin Oncol* 2003;21:2026.

100. Sandoval C, Venkateswaran L, Billups C, et al. Lymphocyte-predominant Hodgkin's disease in children. *J Pediatr Hematol Oncol* 2002;24:269.

101. Pellegrino B, Terrier-Lacombe MJ, Oberlin O, et al. Lymphocyte predominant Hodgkin's lymphoma in children: therapeutic abstention after initial lymph node resection—a study of the French Society of Pediatric Oncology. *J Clin Oncol* 2003;21:2948.

102. Mendenhall N, Cantor A, Williams J, et al. With modern techniques, is staging laparotomy necessary in pediatric Hodgkin's disease? A Pediatric Oncology Group study. *J Clin Oncol* 1993;11:2218.

103. Hueltenschmidt B, Sauter-Bihl ML, Lang O, et al. Whole body positron emission tomography in the treatment of Hodgkin's disease. *Cancer* 2001;91:302.

104. Donaldson SS, Hudson MH, Weinstein HJ, et al. VAMP and low dose involved field radiation for children and adolescents with favorable early stage Hodgkin's disease: results of a prospective clinical trial. *J Clin Oncol* 2002;20:3081.

105. Ruhl U, Albrecht M, Diekmann K, et al. Response-adapted radiotherapy in the treatment of Hodgkin's disease: an interim report at 5 years of the German GPOH-HD 95 trial. *Int J Radiat Oncol Biol Phys* 2001;51:1209.

106. Mauch PM, Weinstein H, Botnick L, Belli J, Cassady JR. An evaluation of long-term survival and treatment complications in children with Hodgkin's disease. *Cancer* 1988; 51:925.

107. Constine LS, Donaldson SS, McDougall IR, et al. Thyroid dysfunction after radiotherapy in children with Hodgkin's disease. *Cancer* 1984;53:878.

108. Bhatig S, Robison L, Oberlin O, et al. Breast cancer and other second neoplasms after childhood Hodgkin's disease. *N Engl J Med* 1996;334:745.

109. Sankila R, Garwicz S, Olsen JH, et al. Risk of subsequent malignant neoplasms among 1,641 Hodgkin's disease patients diagnosed in childhood and adolescence: a population-based cohort study in the five Nordic countries. *J Clin Oncol* 1996;14:1442.

110. Schellong G, Potter R, Bramswig J, et al. High cure rate and reduced long-term toxicity in pediatric Hodgkin's disease: the German-Austrian Multicenter Trial DAL-HD-90. *J Clin Oncol* 1999;17:3736.

111. Ekert H, Waters KD, Smith PF, Toogood I, Mauger D. Treatment with MOPP and CHIVPP chemotherapy only for all stages of childhood Hodgkin's disease. *J Clin Oncol* 1988;6:1845.

112. Nachman JB, Sposto S, Herzog P, et al. Randomized comparison of low dose involved field radiotherapy and no radiotherapy for children with Hodgkin's disease who achieve a complete response to initial chemotherapy. *J Clin Oncol* 2002;20:3765.

113. Donaldson SS, Link MP. Combined modality treatment with low-dose radiation and MOPP chemotherapy for children with Hodgkin's disease. *J Clin Oncol* 1987;5:742.

114. Ekert H, Toogood I, Downie P, et al. High incidence of treatment failure with vincristine, etoposide, epirubicin, and prednisolone chemotherapy with successful salvage in childhood Hodgkin's disease. *Med Pediatr Oncol* 1999;32:255.

115. Weiner MA, Leventhal B, Brecher ML, et al. Randomized study of intensive MOPP-ABVD with or without low-dose total-nodal radiation therapy in the treatment of stages IIB, IIIA2, IIIB, and IV Hodgkin's disease in pediatric patients: a Pediatric Oncology Group study. *J Clin Oncol* 1997;15:2769.

116. Travis LB, Hill DA, Dores GM, et al. Breast cancer following radiotherapy and chemotherapy among young women with Hodgkin disease. *JAMA* 2003;290:465.

117. Schwartz CL. The management of Hodgkin disease in the young child. *Curr Opin Pediatr* 2003;15:10.

RICHARD I. FISHER
PETER M. MAUCH
NANCY LEE HARRIS
JONATHAN W. FRIEDBERG

SECTION 2

Non-Hodgkin's Lymphomas

It has been known for more than 30 years that some patients with non-Hodgkin's lymphoma (NHL) can be cured using chemotherapy. In the past decade, advances in molecular medicine have provided exciting insights into the biology of NHL. The viral and bacterial etiology of certain lymphomas has now been well established. Cell surface antigens have been defined that provide targets for therapy with monoclonal antibodies and radioimmunotherapy. Moreover, knowledge of critical cell signaling pathways and the results of gene expression analyses have provided opportunities for targeted therapy with novel small molecules. With these advances, improved survival has been observed in patients with aggressive NHL, and there is great optimism for patients with indolent histologies.

EPIDEMIOLOGY

The NHLs and Hodgkin's disease are the most commonly occurring hematologic malignancies in the United States. They now represent 4% to 5% of all new cancer cases and are the fifth leading cause of cancer death in the United States and the second fastest growing cancer in terms of mortality. International NHL incidence rates vary as much as fivefold. The highest reported incidence rates are in the United States, and also Europe and Australia; the lowest rates have generally been reported in Asia.[1] In 2004, it is estimated that there will be 54,370 new cases of NHL diagnosed in the United States and that 19,450 people will die with this diagnosis.[2]

Overall survival (OS) for adult patients with indolent lymphoma has not changed in the last 20 years. Survival for adult patients with aggressive lymphoma has remained stable for the last decade, although studies now suggest that the combination of chemotherapy with rituximab may represent an improvement in survival of elderly patients.[3] Among children, lymphomas are the third most frequent malignancy, representing 15% of pediatric malignancies with 1700 new cases each year.

A striking increase in NHL incidence rates has occurred over the last four decades that has been referred to as an epidemic of NHL. The reasons for this are not entirely clear. Although there have been increases in most histologies, the largest increases have occurred in patients with aggressive lymphomas. This increase in primary central nervous system (CNS) lymphoma is in part related to the occurrence of primary CNS lymphomas in patients with acquired immunodeficiency syndrome (AIDS),[4] although the increase in incidence began before the AIDS epidemic, and incidence rates have increased in non-AIDS populations.[5] Geographic differences in histologic subtypes of NHL have been noted. Examples include the endemic form of Burkitt's lymphoma, which is seen most commonly in children in equatorial Africa.[6] Higher rates of gastric lymphoma have been reported to occur in Northern Italy.[7] Other examples include nasal T-cell lymphomas, which are most common in China; certain small intestinal lymphomas, which are most common in the Middle East; and adult T-cell leukemia/lymphoma (ATL), which is most common in southern Japan and the Caribbean. Several reports have shown a lower incidence of follicular lymphomas in Asia and in developing countries.[8] The incidence of follicular lymphomas is lower in Asian immigrants to the United States as compared with later generations, suggesting an environmental influence.[9] Geographic differences in the distribution of mantle cell lymphoma, certain T-cell lymphomas, and the incidence of primary extranodal lymphomas have also been described.[8]

Even when factors such as accuracy and completeness of diagnosis, the effect of human immunodeficiency virus (HIV), and occupational exposures are considered, the reason for most of the increase in NHL incidence is unexplained.[10] Of note, over the past few years, the increased incidence has been less striking. Many investigators have postulated that a ubiquitous environmental or toxic exposure may be responsible.[11]

ETIOLOGY

The cause of most cases of NHL is unknown, although several genetic diseases, environmental agents, and infectious agents have been associated with the development of lymphoma. Although the existence of a familial NHL risk is debated, familial aggregations of NHL have been described, and some studies have shown a higher risk of NHL in siblings or first-degree relatives of people with lymphoma or other hematologic malignancies.[10]

Several rare inherited immunodeficiency states are associated with as much as a 25% risk of developing lymphoma.[12] These disorders include severe combined immunodeficiency, hypogammaglobulinemia, common variable immunodeficiency, Wiskott-Aldrich syndrome, and ataxia-telangiectasia. Lympho-

mas associated with these disorders are often associated with Epstein-Barr virus (EBV) and vary in appearance from initial polyclonal B-cell hyperplasia to monoclonal lymphomas.

In addition to these inherited immunodeficiency states, a number of acquired conditions are associated with an increased risk of NHL. The occurrence of NHL in patients with AIDS and after solid organ transplantation is discussed later in Special Clinical Situations. Patients with a variety of autoimmune disorders, including rheumatoid arthritis,[13] psoriasis,[14] and Sjögren's syndrome,[15] also have an increased risk of developing NHL. For example, the risk of developing NHL in association with Sjögren's syndrome is increased approximately 30- to 40-fold; these are usually marginal zone lymphomas that most commonly occur in salivary glands and other extranodal sites such as the stomach and lung.[16] Celiac sprue is associated with poor-prognosis lymphomas that are now classified as enteropathy-type intestinal T-cell lymphomas.[17]

INFECTIOUS AGENTS

EBV DNA is associated with 95% of endemic Burkitt's lymphomas and less commonly with sporadic Burkitt's lymphoma.[18] Type A and type B EBV strains are both observed.[60] Because EBV is not seen in all cases of Burkitt's lymphoma, the actual relationship and the mechanism by which EBV might contribute to the development of Burkitt's lymphoma is unknown. It is hypothesized that early EBV infection and environmental factors may increase the numbers of EBV-infected precursors and the risk of genetic error; additionally, the EBV virus may contain tumor survival factors.[19]

EBV is also linked to posttransplant lymphoproliferative disorders (PTLDs), some AIDS-associated lymphomas, and some lymphomas associated with congenital immunodeficiency. Virtually all AIDS-associated primary CNS lymphomas have EBV in the tumor clone, although EBV is associated with other AIDS-associated lymphomas less frequently.[20] After EBV infection, normal host immune responses mediated by T lymphocytes suppress EBV-induced proliferation. In patients with depressed T-cell immunity, clones of EBV-transformed B cells can proliferate, leading to the development of lymphoma. The pattern of EBV-associated nuclear proteins in AIDS-associated Burkitt's lymphomas differs from that of large cell lymphomas.[20] C-myc activation in the absence of EBV infection can occur in AIDS-associated lymphomas.[21] The EBV latent membrane protein 1 is a viral analogue of the tumor necrosis factor receptor. The activity of this protein is similar to activated CD40 and is essential for *in vitro* transformation of B cells by EBV.[22] In EBV-positive AIDS-associated NHL and PTLD, it appears that latent membrane protein 1 binds to members of the tumor necrosis factor receptor–associated factor family and activates the NFκB transcription factor, leading to cellular proliferation.[22] EBV is also seen in association with human herpesvirus-8 (HHV-8) in primary effusion lymphomas.

The human T-cell lymphotropic virus type 1 (HTLV-1) was the first human retrovirus associated with a malignancy. HTLV-1 is a type C RNA virus that is responsible for ATL in addition to HTLV-1–associated myelopathy/tropical spastic paraparesis and other disorders.[23] HTLV-1 is primarily transmitted by means of breast feeding, sexual contact, and blood transfusion. The latent period between infection and development of ATL is several decades. HTLV-1 seropositivity and ATL are most prevalent in southern Japan, South America, Africa, and the Caribbean,[24] although ATL is sometimes seen in the United States.[25] In endemic areas more than 50% of all NHL cases are ATL, although the risk of developing disease is only approximately 5% in infected patients. The HTLV-1 genome contains the regulatory *tax* gene, whose product is a potent transcriptional activator of several genes and is thought to be responsible for the transforming features of HTLV-1.[26] The receptor-binding domains of HTLV-1 and -2 envelope glycoproteins inhibit glucose transport by interacting with GLUT-1, the ubiquitous vertebrate glucose transporter.[27] Perturbations in glucose metabolism resulting from interactions of HTLV envelope glycoproteins with GLUT-1 are likely to contribute to HTLV-associated disorders.

A third virus associated with NHL is HHV-8. This virus was originally discovered in Kaposi's sarcoma lesions from AIDS patients and was called *Kaposi's sarcoma–associated herpesvirus*.[28] The virus is also associated with multicentric Castleman's disease. An analysis of 193 lymphoma specimens from patients with and without AIDS identified the presence of virus in only eight specimens, all of which were from patients with primary effusion lymphomas.[29] The virus was subsequently shown to be a member of the gamma herpesvirus subfamily and was named *HHV-8*. Subsequent studies have demonstrated that primary effusion lymphomas are EBV associated, lack c-myc gene rearrangements, and have distinct clinical and phenotypic features.[30] The mechanism of HHV-8 growth stimulation is unknown, although several potential mechanisms have been proposed.[31] It has been suggested that HHV-8 may be necessary for EBV-induced transformation in these patients.

Evidence also links hepatitis C virus (HCV) infection with NHL, especially in Italy. Infection with HCV is strongly associated with essential mixed cryoglobulinemia, which is itself associated with low-grade NHL. Several analyses have demonstrated significantly higher rates of HCV infection when patients with B-cell NHL were compared with controls. In Italy, there appears to be a threefold increased risk for B-NHL in HCV-infected patients, and 1 in 20 cases of B-NHL may be attributable to HCV.[32] This association is less apparent in countries with a lower incidence of HCV.[33] The association appears strongest for patients with monocytoid B-cell lymphoma and lymphoplasmacytoid lymphomas.[34] Neoplastic transformation is probably related to chronic antigen stimulation of B cells by HCV. HCV sequences have been detected in lymph node biopsy specimens from patients with B-NHL, and the presence of HCV-associated proteins within lymphoma cells has been demonstrated.

Finally, reports have suggested that simian virus 40 (SV40) may have a role in the development of NHL.[35] SV40, a monkey polyoma virus confirmed as a viable contaminant of the Salk polio vaccine, has demonstrated oncogenic potential in laboratory animals.[36] Although early epidemiologic studies demonstrated no apparent risk of cancer among cohorts likely to be exposed to SV40 contaminated vaccine, reports suggesting that the virus may be transmitted horizontally as well as vertically to nonimmune individuals were disconcerting. Although controversial, several investigations reported the presence of SV40 DNA in more than 40% of NHL tumor specimens examined.[37,38] Studies to further evaluate the role of SV40 in specific subtypes of NHL are ongoing.

Bacterial infections have also been associated with the development of lymphoma. Several lines of evidence link the bacteria *Helicobacter pylori* to gastric mucosa-associated lymphoid tissue (MALT) lymphomas. *H pylori* can be found in the gastric mucosa of patients with gastric MALT lymphoma, and patients with gastric lymphoma are more likely than controls to have serologic evidence of past *H pylori* infection.[39] It is hypothesized that development of gastric MALT lymphomas is a multistep process beginning with *H pylori* colonization. This leads to chronic antigenic stimulation and gastritis and the subsequent development of malignant B-cell clones.[40] Stimulation by *H pylori*–associated antigens appears to be strain specific and T cell mediated. *Campylobacter jejuni* has been found in specimens of patients with immunoproliferative small intestinal disorder (α chain disease).[41] In addition, a relationship between *Borrelia burgdorferi* and primary cutaneous B-cell lymphoma has been confirmed after demonstration of the organism in lesional skin of patients with this lymphoma, presumably implicating chronic antigen stimulation in the skin in response to *B burgdorferi* infection.[42] Preliminary results suggest that patients with ocular adnexal lymphoma (marginal zone phenotype) display a high prevalence of *Chlamydia psittaci* infection, which is highly specific and does not reflect a subclinical infection widespread among the general population. Unlike the situation with *H pylori*, sequencing analysis suggests that these lymphoma specimens have variable strains of *C psittaci*.[43]

ENVIRONMENTAL AND OCCUPATIONAL EXPOSURES

Studies of occupational and environmental NHL risk are frequently inconsistent and contradictory. Difficulties in estimating risk are often related to sample size and other methodologic difficulties in addition to difficulties in quantifying exposure. The risk of NHL is increased in several occupations, including farmers, forestry workers, and agricultural workers.[10] Several studies have shown an increased risk of NHL in relation to herbicide exposure, especially phenoxy herbicides such as 2,4-dichlorophenoxyacetic acid,[93,96,97] although this is controversial.[44] The development of NHL has also been linked to hair dyes, especially darker and permanent colors used before 1980.[45] Furthermore, NHL has been associated with organic solvents[46] and high levels of nitrates in drinking water.[47]

DIET AND OTHER EXPOSURES

Cohort and case-control studies suggest that the risk of NHL is increased approximately twofold in association with higher intake of meats and dietary fat.[10] Recreational drug use has been associated with increased NHL risk, and tobacco use has been associated with a higher risk in some studies, particularly of follicular lymphoma.[48] The risk of NHL may be increased more than 20-fold after treatment for Hodgkin's disease.[49,50] Studies examining the relative risk of combined modality treatment have been inconsistent, although the risk of NHL in association with ionizing radiation is minimal. Solar ultraviolet exposure has been associated with NHL in some studies.[51] Although some analyses have shown that the risk of NHL is increased after blood transfusion, other studies have failed to identify a significantly increased risk.[52]

BIOLOGIC BACKGROUND FOR CLASSIFICATION OF LYMPHOID NEOPLASMS

Although the normal counterpart of the neoplastic cell is not known for all types of lymphoid neoplasms, it can be postulated for many of them. Understanding the normal counterpart of neoplastic cells can provide a useful framework for understand-

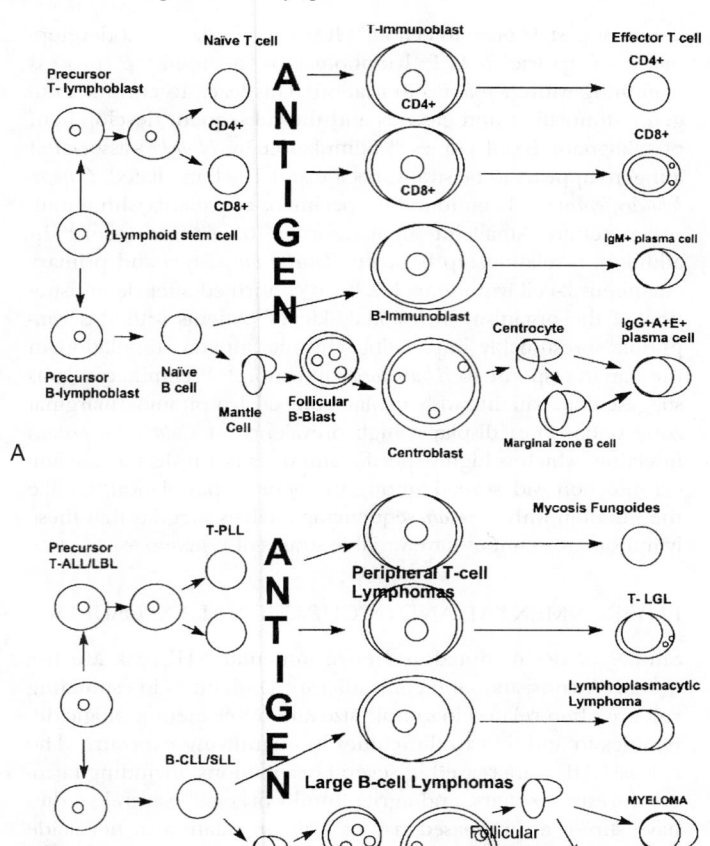

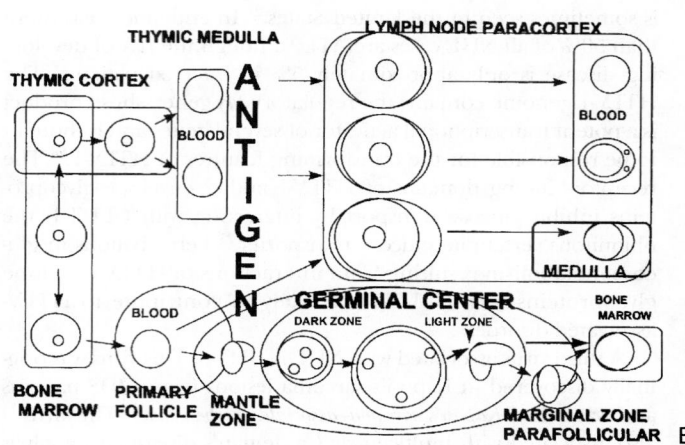

FIGURE 41.2-1. **A:** Hypothetical scheme of lymphocyte differentiation, showing anatomic locations of different stages of T- and B-cell differentiation. T cells are shown at top; B cells are at bottom. **B:** Differentiation scheme, showing nomenclature for various types of T cells (*top*) and B cells (*bottom*). **C:** Differentiation scheme, showing postulated normal counterpart of many of the T- and B-cell neoplasms that can currently be recognized. B-ALL, B-cell acute lymphoblastic leukemia; B-CLL, B-cell chronic lymphocytic leukemia; Ig, immunoglobulin; LBL, lymphoblastic lymphoma; MALT, mucosa-associated lymphoid tissue; SLL, small lymphocytic lymphoma; T-LGL, T-cell large granular lymphocyte; T-PLL, T-cell prolymphocytic leukemia.

ing the morphology, immunophenotype, and, to some extent, the clinical behavior of the neoplasms (Fig. 41.2-1).

ANATOMY AND MORPHOLOGY OF NORMAL LYMPHOID TISSUES

Lymphoid tissues can be divided into two major categories: (1) the central or primary lymphoid tissues, in which lymphoid precursor cells mature to a stage at which they are capable of performing their function in response to antigen, and (2) the peripheral or secondary lymphoid tissue, in which antigen-specific reactions occur.

PRIMARY (CENTRAL) LYMPHOID TISSUES

Bone Marrow (Bursa Equivalent)

Many of the early experiments that elucidated the basic biology of the lymphoid system used chickens and other avian species; an organ known as the *bursa of Fabricius* was the source of antibody-producing cells. Thus, these cells were termed *B cells*, for bursa-derived cells. In mammals, the bursa does not exist, and the precursors of antibody-producing cells come from the bone marrow.

Thymus

The thymus is the site at which immature T-cell precursors (prethymocytes), which migrate from the bone marrow, undergo mat-

uration and selection to become mature, naive T cells, which are capable of responding to antigen. The thymus is divided into a cortex and a medulla, each of which is characterized by specialized epithelium and accessory cells, which provide the milieu for T-cell maturation.

SECONDARY (PERIPHERAL) LYMPHOID TISSUES

Lymph Nodes

Lymph nodes are strategically placed at sites throughout the body to process antigens present in lymph drained from most organs via the afferent lymphatics. Lymph nodes have a capsule, a cortex, a medulla, and sinuses (subcapsular, cortical, and medullary). The sinuses contain macrophages, which take up antigens and process them into peptides, which are then presented to lymphocytes in the pocket of the major histocompatibility complex (MHC) molecules. The cortex contains B-cell follicles and paracortical T-cell zones, and the medulla contains medullary cords and sinuses. The paracortex contains high endothelial venules, through which T and B lymphocytes enter the node, and specialized antigen-presenting cells (APCs), the interdigitating dendritic cells, related to the cutaneous Langerhans cell, which present antigen to T cells. The follicles also contain a specific type of accessory cells, follicular dendritic cells (FDC), which bind antigen-antibody complexes and help regulate the differentiation of B cells in response to antigen. Memory B cells, plasma cells, and effector T cells generated by immune reactions accumulate in the medullary cords and exit via the medullary sinuses.

Spleen

The spleen has two major compartments: the red pulp, which functions as a filter for particulate antigens and for the formed elements of the blood, and the white pulp, which is identical in its compartments to the lymphoid tissue of the lymph node. Follicles and germinal centers are found in the malpighian corpuscles, whereas T cells and interdigitating dendritic cells are found in the adjacent periarteriolar lymphoid sheath. Plasma cells accumulate in the red pulp.

Mucosa-Associated Lymphoid Tissue

Specialized lymphoid tissue is found in association with certain epithelia, in particular the naso- and oropharynx (Waldeyer's ring: adenoids, tonsils), the gastrointestinal tract (gut-associated lymphoid tissue: Peyer's patches of the distal ileum, mucosal lymphoid aggregates in the colon and rectum), and lung (bronchus-associated lymphoid tissue). Collectively, this is known as *MALT*. These tissues tend to have prominent B-cell follicles with broad marginal zones but also may have discrete T-cell zones, similar to the paracortex of lymph nodes. MALT is thought to function in responding to intraluminal antigens and the generation of mucosal immunity. Lymphoid cells that respond to antigen in the MALT acquire homing properties that enable them to return to these tissues.

B- AND T-CELL DIFFERENTIATION

T cells and B cells undergo two major phases of differentiation: antigen independent and antigen dependent. Antigen-independent differentiation occurs in the primary lymphoid organs without exposure to antigen and produces a pool of lymphocytes that are capable of responding to antigen (naive or virgin T and B cells). The early stages are stem cells and lymphoblasts (also known as *precursor T* and *B cells*), which are self-renewing, whereas the later stages are resting cells with a finite life span ranging from weeks to years. On exposure to antigen, the naive lymphocyte undergoes "blast transformation" and becomes a large, proliferating cell, which gives rise to progeny that are capable of direct activity against the inciting antigen: antigen-specific effector cells. The early stages of antigen-dependent differentiation are proliferating cells, whereas the fully differentiated effector cells are less mitotically active. Thus, neoplasms that correspond to proliferating stages of either antigen-independent or antigen-dependent differentiation are likely to be aggressive, whereas those that correspond to naive or mature effector stages are likely to be indolent. Neoplasms corresponding to precursor cells tend to be more common in children (lymphoblastic lymphoma/leukemia), whereas those corresponding to mature effector or memory cells tend to be seen more often in adults (lymphoplasmacytic lymphoma, mycosis fungoides).

Antigen-Independent B-Cell Differentiation

PRECURSOR B CELLS. B-cell differentiation begins with rearrangements of the genes involved in immunoglobulin (Ig) production.[53] Precursor B cells have rearranged Ig heavy-chain genes but lack surface Ig (sIg). Later, they have cytoplasmic μ heavy chain, but no light chain, and still lack sIg. Both types of cells are lymphoblasts, with dispersed chromatin and small nucleoli. They contain the nuclear enzyme, terminal deoxynucleotidyl transferase (TdT), and express CD34, a glycoprotein present on immature cells of lymphoid and myeloid lineage, HLA-DR (class II MHC antigens) and the common acute lymphoblastic leukemia antigen (CD10).[54] Expression of class II MHC antigens persists throughout the life of the B cell and is important in interactions with T cells. Pan-B-cell antigens are sequentially expressed on precursor B cells: CD19, CD79a, and cytoplasmic CD22, followed by surface CD20 and CD45.

Fetal early B-cell development occurs in the liver, bone marrow, and spleen, whereas in adults it is restricted to the bone marrow. Cells with the morphologic and immunologic features of precursor B cells can be found in normal and regenerating bone marrow, where they correspond to the lymphocyte-like cells known as *hematogones*.[55] Neoplasms of precursor B cells usually involve bone marrow and peripheral blood and are known as *common or precursor B acute lymphoblastic leukemia*; rarely, they present as solid tumors (precursor B lymphoblastic lymphoma).

NAIVE B CELLS. The end stage of antigen-independent B-cell differentiation is the mature, naive (virgin) B cell, which expresses surface IgM and IgD, lacks TdT and CD10, and is capable of responding to antigen. Naive B cells have rearranged but unmutated Ig genes.[56] In addition to sIg, naive B cells express pan-B-cell antigens (CD19, CD20, CD22, CD40, and CD79a), HLA class II molecules, complement receptors (CD21 and CD35), CD44, Leu-8 (L-selectin), and CD23; some express the pan-T-cell antigen, CD5, whereas others do not.[57] Resting B cells also express Bcl-2, which promotes survival in the resting state.[58] CD5-positive naive B cells have sIg that often has broad specificity [cross-reactive idiotypes (Ids)] and reactivity with self-antigens (autoantibodies).

Naive B cells are small resting lymphocytes. In adults, they circulate in the blood and comprise a minor fraction of the B cells in primary lymphoid follicles and follicle mantle zones (so-called recirculating B cells).[59] Studies of single cells picked from the mantle zones of reactive follicles show that they are clonally diverse and contain unmutated Ig genes, consistent with naive B cells. Two neoplasms may correspond in part to CD5-positive naive B cells: B-cell chronic lymphocytic leukemia (B-CLL; 40% of the cases) and mantle cell lymphoma (80% of the cases).[60]

Antigen-Dependent B-Cell Differentiation

IMMUNOBLASTIC/PLASMA CELL REACTION. On encountering antigen, the naive B cell transforms into a proliferating cell, which ultimately matures into an antibody-secreting plasma cell. In T-cell–independent reactions, and in the early primary immune response, naive B cells transform into IgM+ blast cells (B blasts or immunoblasts) in the T-cell zones, proliferate, and differentiate into IgM-secreting plasma cells, producing the IgM antibody of the primary immune response.[61] Surface IgD is lost during blast transformation, and antigens associated with activation are up-regulated. With maturation to plasma cells, most surface antigens are lost, including pan-B-cell antigens except for CD79, HLA-DR, and the leukocyte common antigen CD45, and secretory cytoplasmic IgM accumulates. The immunoblastic reaction occurs in the lymph node paracortex, and IgM-producing plasma cells accumulate in the medullary cords. Lymphoplasmacytic lymphoma, associated with Waldenström's macroglobulinemia, may correspond to the IgM-producing plasma cell; however, these tumors typically show low levels of variable region gene mutation and may thus derive from memory B cells.

GERMINAL CENTER REACTION. Later in the primary immune response (within 3 to 7 days of antigen challenge in experimental animals) and in secondary responses, the T-cell–dependent germinal center reaction occurs. Each germinal center is formed from between three and ten naive B cells and ultimately contains approximately 10,000 to 15,000 B cells.[61] Proliferating IgM-positive B blasts formed from naive B cells that have encountered antigen in the paracortex migrate into the center of the primary follicle and fill the FDC meshwork, forming a germinal center.[62] These B blasts differentiate into centroblasts, which appear at approximately 4 days and accumulate at one pole of the germinal center, forming the "dark zone." Centroblasts are large proliferating cells with vesicular nuclei, one to three peripheral nucleoli, and a narrow rim of basophilic cytoplasm. They express no or low levels of sIg and also switch off the gene that encodes the bcl-2 protein; thus, they and their progeny are susceptible to death through apoptosis.[58] Germinal center B cells express nuclear bcl-6 protein, a zinc finger transcription factor that is expressed by centroblasts and centrocytes but not by naive or memory B cells, mantle cells, or plasma cells.[63] Centroblasts undergo somatic mutation of the Ig gene variable (V) region, which alters the affinity for antigen of the antibody that will be produced by the cell.[64] The bcl-6 gene also undergoes somatic mutation of the 5' noncoding promoter region, at a lower frequency than is seen in the Ig genes.[65,66] Thus, Ig gene mutation and bcl-6 mutation serve as markers of cells that have experienced the germinal center.

Centroblasts mature to nonproliferating medium-sized cells with irregular nuclei, inconspicuous nucleoli, and scant cytoplasm, called *centrocytes* (cleaved follicular center cells), which accumulate in the opposite pole of the germinal center, known as the *light zone*, and which also contain a high concentration of FDCs. Centrocytes reexpress sIg, which has an altered antibody-combining site, because of somatic mutations in the variable region. This process results in marked diversity of antibody-combining sites in a population of cells derived from only a few precursors.

Centrocytes whose variable region gene mutations result in an inability to produce a complete Ig molecule or those with *decreased* affinity for antigen rapidly die by apoptosis (programmed cell death); the prominent "starry sky" pattern of phagocytic macrophages seen in germinal centers at this stage is a result of the apoptosis of centrocytes. In contrast, centrocytes whose mutations have resulted in *increased* affinity are able to bind to antigen trapped in antigen-antibody complexes on the processes of FDCs. The centrocytes present the antigen to T cells in the light zone of the germinal center. The activated T cells express CD40 ligand (CD40L), which engages CD40 on the B cell. Ligation of the antigen receptor by antigen and ligation of CD40 on the surface of germinal center B cells "rescues" them from apoptosis.[62,67] Interaction with surface molecules expressed by FDCs, such as CD23, directs differentiation of the centrocytes into plasma cells and stimulates class switching from IgM to IgG or IgA production,[68] whereas interaction with T cells via CD40–CD40 ligand appears to be important in the generation of memory B cells.[61] In addition, antigen receptor ligation and CD40 ligation switch off bcl-6 messenger RNA produc-

tion and bcl-6 protein expression.[69] Through the mechanisms of Ig variable region mutation and class switching, the germinal center reaction gives rise to the better-fitting IgG or IgA antibody of the late primary or secondary immune response.[70]

Follicular lymphomas are tumors of germinal center B cells, in which centrocytes fail to undergo apoptosis because they have a chromosomal translocation, t(14;18), that prevents the normal switching off of bcl-2.[58] Most large B-cell lymphomas are composed of cells that at least in part resemble centroblasts and have mutated Ig V-region genes and are therefore thought to derive from the germinal center stage of differentiation. Finally, it is thought that Burkitt's lymphoma corresponds to the early sIgM+ B blast found in the early germinal center reaction in experimental animals.[71]

MARGINAL ZONE AND MONOCYTOID (PARAFOLLICULAR) B CELLS. When the germinal center polarizes into a dark and a light zone, the mantle zone becomes better defined and eccentric, with the broader portion surrounding the light zone. Antigen-specific B cells generated in the germinal center reaction leave the follicle and reappear in the outer mantle zone to form a "marginal zone"; this is particularly prominent in mesenteric lymph nodes, Peyer's patches, and the spleen. Marginal zone B cells have slightly irregular nuclei, resembling those of centrocytes, but with more abundant, pale cytoplasm. The term *centrocyte-like* has been applied to similar neoplastic cells. Marginal zone B cells from spleen and Peyer's patches have mutated Ig variable region genes, consistent with post–germinal center cells.[72] On rechallenge with antigen, splenic marginal zone B cells rapidly give rise to antigen-specific plasma cells, consistent with memory B cells. Memory B cells are also detectable in the peripheral blood, where they may be IgM+ and even CD5+.[73]

Monocytoid B lymphocytes are cells that resemble marginal zone B cells but with even more nuclear indentation and abundant cytoplasm. These are found in clusters adjacent to subcapsular and cortical sinuses of some reactive lymph nodes. In contrast to marginal zone B cells, monocytoid B cells in reactive lymph nodes have either unmutated variable region genes or show only a small number of randomly distributed mutations that do not suggest selection by antigen.[72] Nodal and splenic tumors resembling normal marginal zone and monocytoid B cells have been described, but analysis of Ig genes from the tumors suggests that most of these have mutations consistent with germinal center exposure and antigen selection.[74] Thus, the relationship of normal to neoplastic monocytoid B cells is not clear.

BONE MARROW PLASMA CELLS. IgG- and IgA-producing plasma cells accumulate in the lymph node medulla, but it is thought that the immediate precursor of the bone marrow plasma cell leaves the node and migrates to the bone marrow. Bone marrow plasma cells lack sIg and pan-B-cell antigens other than CD79, HLA-DR, CD40, and CD45 and contain cytoplasmic IgG or IgA but usually not IgM. Plasma cells also express CD38 and CD138; the latter may be important in adhesion to bone marrow stroma. They have rearranged and mutated Ig genes but do not have the ongoing mutations seen in follicle center cells. Tumors of these marrow-homing plasma cells correspond to plasmacytoma and plasma cell myeloma.

MUCOSA-ASSOCIATED LYMPHOID TISSUE. A subset of B cells, including all the differentiation stages listed above in the section Antigen-Dependent B-Cell Differentiation, is programmed for gut-associated rather than nodal lymphoid tissue. In these tissues (Waldeyer's ring, Peyer's patches, and mesenteric nodes), similar responses occur to antigen, but the intermediate and end-stage B cells that originate in the gut or mesenteric lymph nodes preferentially return there, rather than to peripheral lymph nodes or bone marrow. Thus, the plasma cells generated in gut-associated lymphoid tissue home preferentially to the lamina propria rather than to the bone marrow. MALT is characterized by reactive follicles with germinal centers and prominent marginal zones, as well as numerous plasma cells in the lamina propria. Marginal zone B cells in normal MALT typically infiltrate the overlying epithelium, forming a lymphoepithelium.

Many extranodal B-cell lymphomas are thought to arise from MALT. Because most MALT lymphomas contain prominent marginal zone type B cells, in addition to small B lymphocytes and plasma cells, and because similar lymphomas occur in non-MALT sites, the term *extranodal marginal zone lymphoma of MALT type* has been proposed for these tumors.[75] MALT-type lymphomas have somatically mutated Ig genes, consistent with an antigen-selected post–germinal center B-cell stage.

T-CELL DIFFERENTIATION

Antigen-Independent T-Cell Differentiation

CORTICAL THYMOCYTES. The exact site at which precursor cells become committed to the T lineage is not known because the thymus contains cells that can differentiate into either T cells or natural killer (NK) cells, but not B cells. Cortical thymocytes are lymphoblasts, which contain the intranuclear enzyme TdT, like B lymphoblasts. Within the thymus they sequentially acquire CD1a, CD2, CD5, and cytoplasmic CD3 (cyCD3) and first the CD4 "helper" and then the CD8 "suppressor" antigen ("double positive"). T-cell antigen receptor gene rearrangement occurs during T-cell differentiation. This gene begins with the γ and δ chains, followed by the β and then the α chain genes; these proteins are then expressed on the cell surface. Surface CD3 expression appears at the same time as expression of the T-cell antigen receptor β chain, with which it is closely associated and participates in signal transduction. Cortical thymocytes, like germinal center B cells, lack the antiapoptosis protein bcl-2[58] and are thus susceptible to apoptosis.

In addition to providing a pool of mature T cells through proliferation of precursor cells, the thymus is involved in the selection of T cells, so that the resulting mature T cells recognize self-MHC molecules (positive selection) and do not react to "self"-antigens (negative selection). Thymocytes that have anti-self specificity bind strongly via their T-cell receptor (TCR) complex to self-antigens presented by the MHC on thymic dendritic cells and die by apoptosis. Those that lack anti–self-reactivity but bind strongly to MHC molecules undergo positive selection on thymic epithelial cells; they then express increased levels of surface CD3, lose CD1 and either CD4 or CD8, and express bcl-2, to become mature, naive T cells.[76] The tumor that corresponds to the stages of T-cell differentiation in the thymic cortex is precursor T-lymphoblastic lymphoma/leukemia; the variety of immunophenotypes and antigen receptor gene rearrangements found in precursor T-cell neoplasia correspond to the variety of stages of intrathymic T-cell differentiation.

NAIVE T CELLS. Mature, naive T cells are small lymphocytes with a low proliferation fraction that lack TdT and CD1 and express either (but not both) CD4 or CD8, as well as surface CD3 and CD5 and bcl-2. These cells are found in the thymic medulla, in the circulation, and in the paracortex of lymph nodes. Some cases of T-cell prolymphocytic leukemia and peripheral T-cell lymphoma may correspond to naive T cells.

Antigen-Dependent T-Cell Differentiation

In contrast to B cells, which can recognize unprocessed antigen free in the tissues, T cells can only recognize antigen after it has been processed by phagocytes and presented on the surface of APCs in the "pocket" of the MHC molecule. On the T cell, the CD4 or CD8 molecules bind to MHC class II or class I molecules, respectively, on the APC. The T cell is then activated via CD40–CD40L and binding of CD28 and CTLA4 on the T cell to B7-1 and B7-2 (CD80/86) on the APC.[77]

T IMMUNOBLASTS. On encountering antigen, mature T cells transform into immunoblasts, which are large cells with prominent nucleoli and basophilic cytoplasm that are indistinguishable from B immunoblasts. T immunoblasts, in contrast to T lymphoblasts, are TdT and CD1a negative, strongly express pan-T-cell antigens, and continue to express either CD4 or CD8, not both. Antigen-dependent T-cell reactions occur in the paracortex of lymph nodes and the periarteriolar lymphoid sheath of the spleen, as well as at extranodal sites of immunologic reactions. Some mature T-cell lymphomas probably correspond to T immunoblasts.

EFFECTOR T CELLS. Antigen-specific effector T cells of either CD4 or CD8 type, as well as memory T cells, evolve from the T-cell reaction to antigen. Effector T cells of the CD4 type typically act as helper cells and those of the CD8 type as suppressor cells *in vitro*, but both types can be cytotoxic.[78] CD4 cells recognize antigen complexed with MHC class II antigens on antigen-presenting macrophages, dendritic cells, and B cells, whereas CD8 cells recognize MHC class I antigen on infected epithelial cells.[79] Cytotoxic T cells contain cytoplasmic granule-associated proteins that attack target cells (TIA-1, perforin, Granzyme B) and that can be used to identify cytotoxic cells in tissue sections. CD4+ helper T cells produce cytokines that affect the function of B cells and APCs and modulate the immune response; two major types have been described: T helper 1 (Th1) and T helper 2 (Th2). Th1 T cells produce interleukin-2 and interferon-γ, which activate macrophages and cytotoxic T cells to kill infected cells, whereas Th2 cells produce interleukin-4, -5, -6, and -10, which help B cells to produce antibodies.[79]

Fully differentiated T effector cells are small lymphocytes, morphologically similar to other nonproliferating lymphocytes of either T or B type. In addition to differences in subset antigen (CD4 vs. CD8 or double negative) expression, peripheral T cells may differ in their TCR expression (γδ vs. αβ). The majority of T cells in the circulation and in most lymphoid tissues are αβ+; γδ T cells are more numerous in mucosa and in the spleen.

Some cases of peripheral T-cell lymphomas are thought to correspond to effector T cells. For example, mycosis fungoides corresponds to a mature, effector CD4+ cell, hepatosplenic T-cell lymphoma to γδ T cells that reside in the spleen, T-cell large granular lymphocytic leukemia (LGL) to a mature effector CD8+ cell, and many extranodal T-cell lymphomas to cytotoxic T cells. However, the relationship between neoplastic and normal T cells is not nearly as well understood as in the B-cell system. The systemic symptoms, such as fever, skin rashes, and hemophagocytic syndromes associated with some peripheral T-cell lymphomas, may be a consequence of cytokine production by the neoplastic T cells.

NATURAL KILLER CELLS. A third line of lymphoid cells, called *NK cells* because they can kill certain targets without sensitization and without MHC restriction, appears to derive from a common progenitor with T cells. NK cells recognize self–class I MHC molecules on the surfaces of cells and kill cells that lack these antigens, such as virally infected and malignant cells; they also have Fc receptors and can kill antibody-coated targets. Immature NK cells have cytoplasmic CD3, but these cells do not rearrange their TCR genes or express TCRs or surface CD3. They are characterized by certain NK cell–associated antigens (CD16, CD56, and CD57), which can also be expressed on some T cells, and express some T-cell–associated antigens as

well (CD2, CD7, and CD8). NK cells appear in the peripheral blood as a small proportion of circulating lymphocytes; they are usually slightly larger than most normal T and B cells, with abundant pale cytoplasm containing azurophilic granules—so-called LGL. Extranodal NK/T-cell lymphoma and some types of LGL leukemias appear to correspond to immature and mature NK cells, respectively.

IMMUNOPHENOTYPING OF LYMPHOID CELLS

Individual B and T lymphoid cells as well as accessory cells of the mononuclear phagocyte system can be recognized in cell suspensions or tissue sections by the presence of surface or cytoplasmic molecules (antigens) that can be detected using antibodies labeled with either fluorescence or enzymatic (immunohistochemical) methods. A series of international workshops have developed a standardized nomenclature for many of the antigens detected by more than one monoclonal antibody (Table 41.2-1). Immunophenotyping with mono-

TABLE 41.2-1. Cluster Designations of Antigens Useful in the Classification of Lymphoid Neoplasms

CD	Normal Cells	Neoplasms
1a	Cortical thymocytes (strong), Langerhans cells	Precursor T-lymphoblastic lymphoma/leukemia, Langerhans cell neoplasms
2	T cells, NK cells	T-cell neoplasms
3	T cells, immature NK cells (cytoplasm)	T-cell neoplasms, some NK cell neoplasms
4	T subset (MHC class II restricted), monocytes	Some T-cell neoplasms
5	T cells, naive B cells	T-cell neoplasms, B-CLL, mantle cell lymphoma
7	T cells, NK cells	T-cell neoplasms, NK cell neoplasms
8	T subset (MHC class I restricted), NK subset, splenic sinus lining cells	Some T-cell neoplasms, some NK cell neoplasms
10	Precursor B cells, germinal center B cells, granulocytes, fibroblasts, kidney epithelium	Precursor B lymphoblastic lymphoma/leukemia, Burkitt's lymphoma, follicular lymphoma, diffuse large B-cell lymphoma (25%)
11c	Monocytes, granulocytes, activated CD8+ T cells, NK cells, B-cell subset	B-CLL (some cases); hairy cell leukemia
15	Granulocytes, monocytes	Reed-Sternberg cells of classic HL
16	NK cells, granulocytes, macrophages	NK cell neoplasms, some T-cell neoplasms
19	B cells, including precursor B	B-cell neoplasms
20	Mature B cells (not plasma cells), T-cell subset	Mature B-cell neoplasms, lymphocyte predominance HL, some classic HL
21	Mature B-cell subset, FDC	Mature B-cell neoplasms, FDCs in some lymphomas and FDC neoplasms
22	B cells (cytoplasm), B-cell subset (surface)	B-cell neoplasms
23	IgE Fc receptor: activated B cells, monocytes, FDC	B-CLL/SLL, FDCs in some lymphomas
25	IL-2 receptor: activated T cells, activated B cells, activated monocytes	Hairy cell leukemia, Reed-Sternberg cells, ALCL, some T-cell neoplasms
30	Activated T cells, B cells, NK cells, monocytes	Reed-Sternberg cells in classic HL, ALCL, some DLBCL
43	T cells, B subset, NK cells, monocytes, plasma cells, and myeloid cells	T-cell neoplasms, some B-cell neoplasms, myeloid neoplasms
45	Leukocyte common antigen, all leukocytes except plasma cells	Lymphoid and myeloid neoplasms
45RA	B cells, naive T cells, NK cells	B-cell neoplasms, some T-cell neoplasms
45RO	T cells (most), granulocytes, monocytes	T-cell neoplasms
56	Neural cell adhesion molecule: NK cells, activated T cells	NK cell neoplasms, some T-cell neoplasms
57	T-cell and NK cell subset, neural tissue	NK cell neoplasms, some T-cell neoplasms
68	Monocytes, macrophages, activated T cells	Myeloid and histiocytic neoplasms, some T-cell neoplasms
79a	B cells, including precursor B and plasma cells	B-cell neoplasms, rare T-lymphoblastic neoplasms, lymphocyte predominant HL, rare classic HL
95	Fas (apoptosis receptor): activated T cells, B cells	Some B- and T-cell neoplasms, HL
99	Cortical thymocytes	Precursor B- and T-cell neoplasms, Ewing's sarcoma
103	Mucosal intraepithelial lymphocytes	Hairy cell leukemia; enteropathy-type T-cell lymphoma
138	Syndecan-1 (stromal binding): plasma cells	Plasma cell neoplasms, plasmablastic lymphomas

ALCL, anaplastic large cell lymphoma; B-CLL, B-cell chronic lymphocytic leukemia; CD, cluster designations; DLBCL, diffuse large B-cell lymphoma; FDC, follicular dendritic cells; HL, Hodgkin's lymphoma; IgE, immunoglobulin E; IL-2, interleukin-2; MHC, major histocompatibility complex; NK, natural killer; SLL, small lymphocytic lymphoma.

TABLE 41.2-2. Genetic Abnormalities in Lymphoid Neoplasms

Genetic Abnormality	Genes	Lymphoid Neoplasms	Detection
TRANSLOCATIONS INVOLVING IG GENES (ACTIVATION BY IG PROMOTER)			
t(8;14)(q23;q32)	c-MYC/IgH	Burkitt's lymphoma (30–100%)	CG, Southern blot, FISH (c-MYC)
t(2;8)(p12;q23)	c-MYC/Igκ	—	—
t(8;22)(q23;q11)	c-MYC/Igλ	Large B-cell lymphoma (~10%)	—
t(11;14)(q13;32)	BCL1(CCND1)/IgH	Mantle cell lymphoma, plasma cell myeloma[a]	CG, PCR, FISH
t(14;18)(q32;q21)	BCL2/IgH	Follicular lymphoma (90%), large B-cell lymphoma (20%)	CG, Southern blot, PCR, FISH
t(14;19)(q32;q13)	BCL3/IgH	CLL/B-SLL	CG
t(3;14)(q27;q32) and t(V;3q27)[b]	BCL6/IgH, variable/BCL6	Large B-cell lymphoma (30%), follicular lymphoma (15%)	CG, Southern blot, FISH
t(1;14)(p22;q32)	BCL10/IgH	MALT lymphoma, large B-cell lymphoma	CG
t(9;14)(p13;q32)	PAX5(BSAP)/IgH	Lymphoplasmacytic lymphoma (~50%), plasma cell myeloma (rare)	CG
t(4;14)(p16;q32)	MMSET(FGFR)/IgH	Plasma cell myeloma	Southern blot, FISH
t(6;14)(p25;q32)	IRF4(MUM1)/IgH	—	Southern blot, FISH
t(14;16)(q32;q23)	IgH/c-MAF	—	Southern blot, FISH
t(1;14)(q21;q32)	NUM2/IgH	—	CG, FISH
TRANSLOCATIONS INVOLVING THE T-CELL RECEPTOR GENES (ACTIVATION BY TCR PROMOTERS)			
t(1;14)(p32;q11)[c,d]	TAL1/TCRβ	Precursor T-lymphoblastic lymphoma/leukemia	CG
t(8;14)(q24;q11)	cMYC/TCRβ	—	CG, FISH (c-MYC)
t(11;14)(p15;q11)[e]	RBTN1(TTG2)/TCRβ	—	CG
t(10;14)(q24;q11)	HOX11/TCRβ	—	CG
inv(14)(q11;q32)	TCRα/unknown	T-PLL (70%)	CG
t(14;14)(q11;q32)		T-PLL (10%)	
TRANSLOCATIONS PRODUCING FUSION GENES/PROTEINS (ACTIVATION OR INACTIVATION)			
t(9;22)(q34;q11)	BCR/ABL	Precursor B-lymphoblastic lymphoma/leukemia	CG, FISH
t(V)(11q23)	MLL	—	CG, PCR
t(12;21)(p12;q22)	TEL/AML1	—	CG, FISH
t(1;19)(q23;p13)	PBX/E2A	—	CG
t(11;18)(q21;q21)	API2/MLT	MALT lymphoma	CG, RT-PCR, FISH
t(2;5)(p23;q35)	NPM/ALK	ALCL	CG, RT-PCR, FISH (ALK)
CHROMOSOMAL ADDITIONS AND DELETIONS			
i(7q)(q10)	Unknown	Hepatosplenic T-cell lymphoma	CG
+3	Unknown	MALT lymphoma, large B-cell lymphoma	CG, FISH
6q23-26	Unknown	B-cell lymphomas (10–40%)	CG
+8	Unknown	PTCL	—
+3 +5 + X	Unknown	Angioimmunoblastic T-cell lymphoma	CG, FISH
+12	Unknown	CLL/B-SLL (30%)	CG, FISH
13q deletions	Unknown	CLL/B-SLL (25%)	CG, FISH
−13, 13q14 deletions	Unknown	Plasma cell myeloma	CG, FISH

ALCL, anaplastic large cell lymphoma; ALK, anaplastic lymphoma kinase; B-SLL, B-cell small lymphocytic lymphoma; CG, cytogenetics; CLL, chronic lymphocytic leukemia; FISH, fluorescence *in situ* hybridization; IgH, immunoglobulin H; MALT, mucosa-associated lymphoid tissue; PCR, polymerase chain reaction; PLL, prolymphocytic leukemia; PTCL, peripheral T-cell lymphoma; RT-PCR, reverse transcriptase-PCR.
[a]In myeloma, translocation is into switch region of IgH; in mantle cell, into joining region.
[b]Promoters other than IgH activate BCL6.
[c]May involve 7q34 (TCRγ) instead of 14q11.
[d]Deletions in the 5' regulatory region of TAL1 may also be seen.
[e]May involve RBTN2 at 11p13.

clonal antibodies can be done using viable cell suspensions, frozen-tissue sections, or paraffin-embedded tissue sections.

CHROMOSOMAL TRANSLOCATIONS AND ONCOGENE REARRANGEMENTS

Lymphoid neoplasms frequently have specific chromosomal translocations, which result in activation of oncogenes or inactivation of tumor suppressor genes (Table 41.2-2). Most translocations in lymphoid neoplasms place a gene that is normally silent in that cell type under the influence of a promoter associated with either an Ig or TRC, resulting in activation of the gene

and giving the cell either a growth or survival advantage. Examples include the t(8;14)(q24;q32) in Burkitt's lymphoma, which places the *cMYC* gene under the Ig heavy-chain promoter[80]; the t(14;18)(q32;q32) of follicular lymphoma, which places the *BCL2* gene on chromosome 18 under the Ig promotor[81]; and the t(11;14)(q13;q32) in mantle cell lymphoma, which places the cyclin D1 gene (associated with the BCL1 breakpoint) on chromosome 11 under the Ig promotor.[82]

In some lymphoid neoplasms, a translocation results in a fusion of two genes, resulting in an abnormal protein, which can be activated or inactivated as a consequence of the fusion. Examples include the t(2;5)(p23;q35) and its variants in anaplastic

TABLE 41.2–3A. Immunohistologic and Genetic Features of Common B-Cell Neoplasms

Neoplasm	sIg; CIg	CD5	CD10	CD23	CD43	CD103	Cyclin D1	Genetic Abnormality	Immunoglobulin Genes[a]
B-SLL/CLL	+; –/+	+	–	+	+	–	–	Trisomy 12; 13q	R, U (50%); M (50%)
Lymphoplasmacytic lymphoma	+; +	–	–	–	+/–	–	–	t(9;14); del 6(q23)	R, M
Hairy cell leukemia	+;–	–	–	–	+	++	+/–	None known	R, M
Splenic marginal zone lymphoma	+; –/+	–	–	–	–	+	–	None known	R, M
Follicular lymphoma	+; –	–	+/–	–/+	–	–	–	t(14;18); bcl-2	R, M, O
Mantle cell lymphoma	+; –	+	–	–	+	–	+	t(11;14); bcl-1	R, U
MALT lymphoma	+; +/–	–	–	–/+	–/+	–	–	trisomy 3; t(11;18)	R, M, O
Diffuse large B-cell lymphoma	+/–; –/+	–	–/+	NA	–/+	NA	–	t(14;18), t(8;14), 3q; bcl-2, myc, bcl-6	R, M
Burkitt's lymphoma	+; –	–	+	–	–	NA	–	t(8;14), t(2;8), t(8;22); c-myc; EBV –/+	R, M

+, >90% positive; +/–, >50% positive; –/+, <50% positive; –, < 10% positive; CIg, intracytoplasmic immunoglobulin; CLL, chronic lymphocytic leukemia; M, mutated; MALT, mucosa-associated lymphoid tissue; NA, not available; O, ongoing mutations; R, rearranged; sIg, surface immunoglobulin; SLL, small lymphocytic lymphoma; TCR, T-cell receptor gene; U, unmutated.
[a]Mutations in the Ig gene V region indicate exposure to antigen.

large cell lymphoma (ALCL), which result in activation of the ALK (anaplastic lymphoma kinase) tyrosine kinase[83] and the t(11;18)(q21;q21) in MALT lymphoma, which produces an API2-MLT fusion protein.[84]

Using polymerase chain reaction (PCR), cells carrying a given translocation can be detected by using probes that span the breakpoint or using a reverse transcriptase technique to detect RNA produced by an altered or fused gene (RT-PCR).

PCR can be used to detect minimal residual disease in patients whose tumors carry a translocation.[85] Both numeric abnormalities of chromosomes and translocations can be detected by fluorescence *in situ* hybridization on suspended nuclei, imprints, or tissue sections, using probes to specific chromosomes or segments.[86] Finally, many translocations result in abnormal protein expression, which can be detected by immunohistochemistry.[87]

TABLE 41.2-3B. Immunohistologic and Genetic Features of Common T-Cell Neoplasms

Neoplasm	CD3 S;C	CD5	CD7	CD4	CD8	CD30	TCR	NK (16, 56)	Cytotox Granule[a]	EBV	Genetic Abnormality	T-Receptor Genes
T-PLL	+	–	+,+	+/–	–/+	–	αβ	–	–	–	inv 14; trisomy 8q	R
T-LGL	+	–	+,+	–	+	–	αβ	+,–	+	–	None known	R
NK-LGL	–	–	+,–	–	+/–	–	–	–,+	+	+	None known	G
Extranodal NK/T-cell lymphoma	–;+	–	–/+	–	–	–	–	NA,+	+	++	None known	G
Hepatosplenic T-cell lymphoma	+	–	+	–	–	–	γδ>αβ	+,–/+	+	–	Iso 7q	R
Enteropathy-type T-cell lymphoma	+	+	+	–	+/–	+/–	αβ>>γδ	–	+	–	None known	R
Mycosis fungoides	+	+	–/+	+	–	–	αβ	–	–	–	None known	R
Cutaneous ALCL	+	+/–	+/–	+/–	–	++	αβ	–	–/+	–	None known	R
Subcutaneous panniculitis-like T-cell lymphoma	+	+	+	–	+	–/+	αβ>γδ	–,+/–	+	–	None known	R
PTCL-NOS	+/–	+/–	+/–	+/–	–/+	–/+	αβ>γδ	–/+	–/+	–/+	inv 14; complex	R
Angioimmunoblastic	+	+	+	+/–	–/+	–	αβ	–	NA	+/–	None known	R
Primary systemic ALCL	+/–	+/–	NA	–/+	–/+	++	αβ	–	+	–	t(2;5); NPM/ALK	R

+, >90% positive; +/–, >50% positive; –/+, <50% positive; –, < 10% positive; ALCL, anaplastic large cell lymphoma; G, germline; LGL, large granular lymphocytic leukemia; M, mutated; NA, not available; NK, natural killer; NOS, not otherwise specified; PLL, prolymphocytic leukemia; PTCL, peripheral T-cell lymphoma; R, rearranged; TCR, T-cell receptor gene; U, unmutated.
[a]Cytotox granule = TIA-1, perforin, and/or granzyme.

USE OF IMMUNOPHENOTYPING AND GENETIC STUDIES IN THE DIAGNOSIS OF LYMPHOID NEOPLASMS

Each of the lymphoid neoplasms has a characteristic morphology, which is often sufficient to permit diagnosis and classification if well-prepared sections are available. However, there are many pitfalls in the histologic diagnosis of malignant lymphoma, and immunophenotyping and genetic studies can be useful in resolving differential diagnostic problems. The major immunophenotypic and genetic features of the more common B- and T-cell neoplasms are listed in Tables 41.2-3A and 41.2-3B.

Problems that can be resolved by these techniques include (1) reactive versus neoplastic lymphoid infiltrates, (2) lymphoid versus nonlymphoid malignancies, and (3) subclassification of lymphoma. If the morphology is typical of a given entity but the immunophenotypic or genetic features are unusual, the histologic sections should be reexamined; however, the case may still be accepted as an example of the entity suggested by morphologic features. If the morphology is atypical but the immunophenotype and genetic features are classic for a given entity, these features may override morphology in classification. If the morphology and the immunophenotype are atypical, the case is best regarded as unclassifiable or borderline.

PRINCIPLES OF THE REVISED EUROPEAN-AMERICAN CLASSIFICATION OF LYMPHOID NEOPLASMS/WORLD HEALTH ORGANIZATION CLASSIFICATION OF LYMPHOID NEOPLASMS

In 1994, the International Lymphoma Study group developed a consensus on a list of diseases that could be recognized by pathologists and that appeared to be distinct clinical entities. In this approach to classification, all available information—morphology, immunophenotype, genetic features, and clinical features—is used to define a disease entity. The relative importance of each of these features varies among diseases, and there is no one "gold standard" for classification. Morphology is always important, and some diseases are primarily defined by morphology, with immunophenotype as backup in difficult cases. Some diseases have a virtually specific immunophenotype, such that one would hesitate to make the diagnosis in the absence of the immunophenotype. In a few lymphomas a specific genetic abnormality is an important defining criterion, whereas most lack specific genetic abnormalities. Still others require knowledge of clinical features as well, particularly nodal versus extranodal presentations. Experience after publication of this classification showed that it can be used by most pathologists and that the entities it describes have distinctive clinical features, making it a useful and practical classification despite its apparent complexity.

Members of the European and American Hematopathology societies published a new World Health Organization (WHO) classification of hematologic malignancies (Table 41.2-4).[75] This uses an updated version of the Revised European-American Lymphoma (REAL) classification for lymphoid neoplasms and applies the principles of the REAL classification to the classification of myeloid and histiocytic neoplasms. The project included a Clinical Advisory Committee of international expert hematologists and oncologists. Proponents of prior classifications—Working Formulation, Kiel, REAL, and French-American-British—are in agreement that the WHO consensus classification should replace existing classifications. Thus, it represents the first true international consensus on the classification of hematologic malignancies.

CATEGORIES OF LYMPHOID NEOPLASMS

The REAL and WHO classifications recognize three major categories of lymphoid neoplasms based on a combination of morphology and cell lineage: B-cell neoplasms, T/NK-cell neoplasms, and Hodgkin's disease/Hodgkin's lymphoma. Lymphomas and lymphoid leukemias are included, because solid and circulating phases are present in many lymphoid neoplasms and distinction between them is artificial. Thus, B-CLL and B-cell small lymphocytic lymphoma (SLL) are simply different manifestations of the same neoplasm, as are lymphoblastic lymphomas and acute lymphoid leukemias and Burkitt's lymphoma and Burkitt's cell leuke-

TABLE 41.2-4.   Revised European-American Lymphoma/World Health Organization Classification of Lymphoid Neoplasms

---

B-CELL NEOPLASMS
Precursor B-cell neoplasm
Precursor B-lymphoblastic leukemia/lymphoma (precursor B-cell acute lymphoblastic leukemia)
Mature (peripheral) B-cell neoplasms[a]
Chronic lymphocytic leukemia/B-cell small lymphocytic lymphoma
B-cell prolymphocytic leukemia
Lymphoplasmacytic lymphoma
Splenic marginal zone B-cell lymphoma (splenic lymphoma with villous lymphocytes)
Hairy cell leukemia
Plasma cell myeloma/plasmacytoma
Extranodal marginal zone B-cell lymphoma (MALT lymphoma)
Nodal marginal zone B-cell lymphoma
Follicular lymphoma
Mantle cell lymphoma
Diffuse large B-cell lymphomas
Burkitt's lymphoma/leukemia
T- AND NK-CELL NEOPLASMS
Precursor T-cell neoplasm
Precursor T-lymphoblastic leukemia/lymphoma (precursor T-cell acute lymphoblastic leukemia)
Blastoid NK cell lymphoma
Mature (peripheral) T-cell neoplasms
T-cell prolymphocytic leukemia
T-cell large granular lymphocytic leukemia
Aggressive NK cell leukemia
Adult T-cell lymphoma/leukemia (HTLV-1+)
Extranodal NK/T-cell lymphoma, nasal type
Enteropathy-type T-cell lymphoma
Hepatosplenic T-cell lymphoma
Subcutaneous panniculitis-like T-cell lymphoma
Mycosis fungoides/Sézary syndrome
Primary cutaneous anaplastic large cell lymphoma
Peripheral T-cell lymphoma, not otherwise specified
Angioimmunoblastic T-cell lymphoma
Primary systemic anaplastic large cell lymphoma

HTLV, human T-cell lymphotropic virus; MALT, mucosa-associated lymphoid tissue; NK, natural killer.
[a]B- and T/NK-cell neoplasms are grouped according to major clinical presentations (predominantly disseminated/leukemic, primary extranodal, predominantly nodal).

mia. Although the vast majority of cases of Hodgkin's lymphoma are of B-cell origin, their distinctive histologic and clinical features warrant a separate category.

The WHO classification of lymphoid neoplasms includes more than 30 distinct entities. These diseases are, in most cases, unrelated to one another; that is, "lymphoma" or "NHL" can no longer be considered as a single disease with a range of histologic grade and clinical aggressiveness. One of the corollaries of defining distinct lymphoma entities is that it is neither possible nor helpful to sort them precisely according to histologic grade or clinical aggressiveness. For example, although it is true that many lymphomas composed of relatively small cells with a low proliferation fraction generally have an indolent course, at least one of them—mantle cell lymphoma—is rather aggressive. In addition, each has a distinctive set of presenting features and, often, different treatments; for example, hairy cell leukemia, chronic lymphocytic leukemia, and MALT lymphoma, although all indolent, are treated quite differently with different expectancy for survival. Several lymphomas have within themselves a range of histologic grade (number of large cells or proliferation fraction) and clinical aggressiveness, for example, follicular lymphoma. Thus, histologic grade is applied within a disease entity, not across the whole range of lymphoid neoplasms.

The Clinical Advisory Committee for the WHO classification agreed that clinical groupings were neither necessary nor desirable for clinical practice.[75] Pathologists and oncologists must "get to know" each disease entity and its spectrum of morphology and clinical behavior. In practice, treatment of a specific patient is determined not by which broad "prognostic group" the lymphoma falls into but by the specific histologic type of lymphoma, with the addition of grade within the tumor type, if applicable, and clinical features such as stage, age, performance status, and the International Prognostic Index (IPI).[88]

Because of the impracticality of arranging the list of B and T/NK-cell lymphoid neoplasms according to prognostic groups, the final WHO classification lists them first according to differentiation stage and secondarily according to predominant clinical presentation. Two major differentiation stages are recognized: precursor neoplasms, corresponding to the earliest stages of differentiation, and peripheral or mature neoplasms, corresponding to more differentiated stages. Three broad categories of clinical presentation are recognized: predominantly disseminated diseases that often involve bone marrow and may be leukemic, primary extranodal lymphomas, and predominantly nodal diseases that are often disseminated and may also involve extranodal sites.[75] This approach is intended for convenience and ease of learning only, by placing diseases that are likely to resemble one another clinically and histologically in proximity to one another in the list and in a text. It also has some biologic relevance, because there appear to be important biologic differences between primary nodal and primary extranodal lymphomas, particularly in the T/NK-cell diseases. However, any principle of sorting these neoplasms is artificial, and the lists can be regrouped in different ways for different purposes.

CLINICAL RELEVANCE OF THE REVISED EUROPEAN-AMERICAN LYMPHOMA/WORLD HEALTH ORGANIZATION CLASSIFICATION

An international group of oncologists and pathologists devised a clinical study of the classification, in which five expert pathol-

TABLE 41.2-5. Reproducibility of Lymphoma Diagnosis

Reproducibility	Contribution of Immunophenotype (%)
>85% (86–96%)	
B-cell chronic lymphocytic leukemia/small lymphocytic lymphoma	3
Mantle cell lymphoma	10
Follicular lymphoma	0
Marginal zone/mucosa-associated lymphoid tissue	2
Diffuse large B-cell lymphoma	15
T-lymphoblastic lymphoma	40
Anaplastic large cell lymphoma	39
Peripheral T-cell lymphoma, unspecified	41
Mycosis fungoides	—
80%	
Angioimmunoblastic T-cell lymphoma	—
Extranodal natural killer/T-cell lymphoma	—
<50%	
Burkitt-like lymphoma	6
Lymphoplasmacytic lymphoma	—

(Data from ref. 89.)

ogists reviewed more than 1300 cases of NHL at centers around the world.[89] The aims of the study were (1) to see whether the classification could be used in practice, (2) to test its interobserver reproducibility, (3) to determine the need for immunophenotyping in diagnosis, (4) to determine whether the categories of disease identified in the classification were clinically distinctive either at presentation or in outcome, and (5) to determine the relative frequency of these diseases in the populations studied.

This study found that more than 95% of the cases with adequate material could be classified into one or another of the categories (Table 41.2-5). The interobserver reproducibility was substantially better than that for other classifications and was greater than 85% for most diseases. Immunophenotyping had been done in all cases as a requirement for entry into the study, to confirm the diagnosis of lymphoma, and to identify lineage (B, T, NK). Immunophenotyping was helpful in improving interobserver reproducibility in some diseases, such as mantle cell lymphoma and diffuse large B-cell lymphoma (DLBCL), for which it improved accuracy by 10% to 15%, and was essential for all types of T-cell lymphoma, improving reproducibility from approximately 50% to more than 90%. It was not required for many diseases, such as follicular lymphoma, B-cell SLL, and MALT lymphoma.[90]

The relative frequency of the different B- and T/NK-cell lymphomas in the study population was similar to previous patterns reported in the literature (Table 41.2-6). The most common lymphoma was DLBCL, followed by follicular lymphoma; together, these comprised 50% of the lymphomas in the study. New entities not specifically recognized in the Working Formulation accounted for 27% of the cases. These results confirm that the majority of the cases encountered by oncologists and pathologists will be only a few subtypes, with which they are already familiar. They underscore the need for recognizing the more recently described entities, which, although less common, have important clinical differences. The study also found

TABLE 41.2-6. Frequency and Presenting Features of Common B- and T-cell Neoplasms in the REAL Classification

Neoplasm	Frequency[a]	Age	Male	Stage				BSx	EN[b]	BM	GI	IPI		
				I	II	III	IV					0/1	2/3	4/5
Large B-cell	31	64	55	25	29	13	33	33	71	16	18	35	46	9
Mediastinal	2	37	34	10	56	3	31	38	56	3	0	52	37	11
Follicular	22	59	42	18	15	16	51	28	64	42	4	45	48	7
SLL/CLL	6	65	53	4	5	8	83	33	80	72	3	23	64	13
MALT	8	60	48	39	28	2	31	19	98	14	50	44	48	8
Mantle cell	6	63	74	13	7	9	71	28	81	51	9	23	54	23
Peripheral T-cell	7	61	55	8	12	15	65	50	82	36	15	17	52	31
ALCL	2	34	69	19	32	10	39	53	59	13	9	61	18	21

ALCL, anaplastic large cell lymphoma; BM, bone marrow; BSx, B symptoms; CLL, chronic lymphocytic leukemia; EN, any extranodal site, including bone marrow; GI, gastrointestinal tract; IPI, International Prognostic Index; MALT, mucosa-associated lymphoid tissue; SLL, small lymphocytic leukemia.

[a]All numbers are percent of cases in the international study.
[b]Extranodal disease.
(From ref. 89, with permission.)

differences in geographic distribution of the lymphoma types, with follicular lymphoma being more common in North America and western Europe, T-cell lymphomas more common in Hong Kong, and mediastinal large B-cell lymphoma and mantle cell lymphoma more common in Switzerland.[8]

CLINICAL FEATURES OF LYMPHOID NEOPLASMS IN REVISED EUROPEAN-AMERICAN LYMPHOMA CLASSIFICATION

The different entities recognized by the classification had significantly different clinical presentations and survivals. Entities that would have been lumped together as "low grade" or "intermediate/high grade" in the Working Formulation showed marked differences in survival, confirming that they need to be recognized and treated as distinct entities.

The study also found that pathologic classification is not the only predictor of clinical outcome. Patients with any diseases could be stratified into better and worse prognostic groups according to the IPI.[88] Thus, to plan treatment for an individual patient, the oncologist must know not only the diagnosis but also the clinical prognostic factors that will influence that patient's course.

PRINCIPLES OF MANAGEMENT OF NON-HODGKIN'S LYMPHOMA

The phases of patient management include obtaining an adequate biopsy for an accurate diagnosis, a careful history and physical examination, appropriate laboratory studies, imaging studies, and possibly further biopsies to determine an accurate stage and to plan therapy. Finally, taking into account factors related to the patient, type of lymphoma, and stage and pace of disease, a treatment recommendation must be made.

HISTORY AND PHYSICAL EXAMINATION

A careful history and physical examination are the basis for subsequent studies to determine the extent of the disease and a key factor in the therapeutic decision. The duration of symptoms and the pace of progression of the illness should be documented. The physician should not discount the possibility that waxing and waning lymphadenopathy could be related to the lymphoma. Especially in follicular lymphomas, spontaneous regressions are not infrequent. The presence of specific symptoms known to have an adverse prognosis in patients with some types of lymphoma should be ascertained. These include fevers, night sweats, and unexplained weight loss. Symptoms referable to a particular organ system, such as pain in the chest, abdomen, or bones, might lead to identification of specific sites of involvement. For example, symptoms of CNS lymphoma include headache, lethargy, focal neurologic symptoms, seizures, or paralysis.

History of a concurrent illness such as diabetes or congestive heart failure might modify therapeutic decisions. A careful physical examination can lead to important observations that will direct subsequent care. Obviously, examination of all lymph node–bearing areas and a search for hepatomegaly or splenomegaly are important. Pharyngeal involvement, a thyroid mass, evidence of pleural effusion, abdominal mass, testicular mass, or cutaneous lesions are all examples of findings that might direct further investigations and subsequent therapy.

LABORATORY EVALUATION

Laboratory studies should include complete blood count and screening chemistry studies to include renal and hepatic function studies, serum glucose, calcium, albumin, lactate dehydrogenase (LDH), and β_2-microglobulin level. Serum protein electrophoresis is frequently appropriate. The purpose of these studies is to aid in determining the prognosis (e.g., LDH, β_2-microglobulin, albumin) and identifying abnormalities in other organ systems that might complicate therapy (e.g., renal or hepatic dysfunction).

In addition to the diagnostic biopsy, almost all patients should have a bone marrow aspirate and biopsy performed. The chance of finding bone marrow involvement varies considerably among different subtypes of lymphoma. It is present in approximately 70% of patients with SLL, lymphoplasmacytoid lymphoma, and mantle cell lymphoma. Patients with follicular lymphoma have bone marrow involvement approximately 50%

of the time, whereas it is seen in approximately 15% of patients with DLBCL.[90]

In certain situations, cytologic evaluation of the cerebrospinal fluid is indicated. Patients with paranasal sinus, testicular involvement, epidural lymphoma, and possibly bone marrow involvement with large cells are especially prone to meningeal spread and should have a diagnostic lumbar puncture. In addition, a lumbar puncture is often recommended for highly aggressive histologies and lymphoma in the setting of immunocompromise, including HIV infection.

IMAGING STUDIES

Chest Radiography and Computed Tomography Scans

Chest radiography and computed tomography (CT) scans of the chest, abdomen, and pelvis should be performed at the initial evaluation in almost all patients with NHL. Although the chest radiograph is abnormal in fewer than 50% of patients, identification of hilar or mediastinal adenopathy, parenchymal lesions, or pleural effusions is important and provides an easy method for reevaluation. CT scanning can identify nodal and extranodal sites of involvement and provides an important approach to monitoring the response to therapy. Involvement of intraabdominal organs, such as kidney, ovary, spleen, and liver, can be identified on CT scans.

Magnetic Resonance Imaging

The value of magnetic resonance imaging (MRI) in the staging of NHL is limited. MRI is particularly useful in identifying bone and CNS involvement. MRI can suggest leptomeningeal involvement when gadolinium has been used. MRI can also identify bone marrow involvement[91]; however, it is not acceptable as a substitute for bone marrow biopsy.

Nuclear Medicine Studies

Nuclear scintigraphy may improve staging at the time of diagnosis, particularly through the detection of otherwise occult abdominal or splenic disease. Perhaps more important, nuclear scintigraphy may help to characterize a residual mass on anatomic imaging after therapy as either fibrosis or residual active lymphoma. Historically, gallium 67, which binds to transferrin receptors in the tumor, has been the most widely used nuclear tracer in the evaluation of lymphoma.[92] The major limitations of this technique include relatively low sensitivity and accuracy, particularly in the abdomen and extranodal sites.[93] Bone scans can sometimes be useful in patients who present with or develop back pain during the course of their lymphoma, looking for vertebral involvement and potential spinal cord compression.

Positron emission tomography (PET) is a novel functional imaging technique that can use a glucose analogue [2-fluoro-2-deoxy-D-glucose (FDG)] radiolabeled with the positron emitter fluorine 18 to evaluate glycolytic activity, which is increased in malignancies, including lymphoma.[94] PET provides several inherent advantages compared with other nuclear imaging techniques. The short half-life of FDG allows patient convenience and improved imaging characteristics. With modern dedicated PET machines, a resolution of approximately 5 mm can be achieved and the ability to coregister PET with anatomic CT imaging allows for ease of interpretation.

The majority of studies evaluating FDG-PET in NHL include patients with diffuse large cell NHL. Limited data are available on the role of PET in other histologies. A retrospective review of 172 patients with various types of lymphoma who underwent FDG-PET imaging revealed that FDG-PET accurately detected disease in patients with diffuse large B-cell NHL, mantle cell lymphoma, and follicular lymphoma.[95] PET was less reliable at detecting marginal zone lymphoma, a finding that has been confirmed by other groups, particularly in the case of extranodal marginal zone lymphomas.[96] Every published study to date has suggested increased sensitivity of PET when compared with other imaging modalities, including gallium, when used for lymphoma staging.[93,94] PET may have particular utility in the evaluation of the spleen.

Persistently positive PET scans during and after chemotherapy have high sensitivity for predicting subsequent relapse of aggressive lymphoma.[97,98] Several studies have suggested that a negative PET scan is more informative than a positive result in the evaluation of a residual mass after therapy for lymphoma due to a high false-positive rate.[99,100] Therefore, persistently positive PET scans at the end of therapy, or in follow-up, warrant close follow-up or additional diagnostic procedures, because some of these patients may remain in prolonged remission.

STAGING AND PROGNOSTIC SYSTEMS

The goal of the initial evaluation of a patient with lymphoma is to provide information that allows intelligent planning of therapy, imparting the prognosis to the patient, and making possible comparisons between patients in clinical trials. The studies to accomplish these goals can be aimed at identifying sites of involvement, characteristics of the patient (i.e., age, performance status, and so forth), or characteristic of the lymphoma (serum LDH, serum β_2-microglobulin, growth fraction, and so forth) that predict treatment outcome.

The Ann Arbor Staging System was developed for patients with Hodgkin's disease. This system (Table 41.2-7)[101] identifies anatomic sites of involvement by lymphoma and assigns patients into four categories based on the extent of disease dissemination. Patients are also subcategorized by the presence of

TABLE 41.2-7. Ann Arbor Staging System

Stage	Description[a]
I	Involvement of a single lymph node region or a single extra-lymphatic organ or site (IE)
II	Involvement of two or more lymph node regions on the same side of the diaphragm (II) or localized involvement of an extralymphatic organ or site (IIE)
III	Involvement of lymph node regions on both sides of the diaphragm (III) or localized involvement of an extralymphatic organ or site (IIIE) or spleen (IIIS) or both (IIISE)
IV	Diffuse or disseminated involvement of one or more extralymphatic organs with or without associated lymph node involvement. Bone marrow and liver involvement are always stage IV

[a]Identification of the presence or absence of symptoms should be noted with each stage designation: A, asymptomatic; B, fever, sweats, weight loss greater than 10% of body weight.

TABLE 41.2-8.   International Prognostic Index for Diffuse Large Cell Lymphoma

Number of Risk Factors	Percentage of Patients	Complete Response Rate (%)	5-Y Disease-Free Survival (%)	5-Y Survival (%)
All patients (adverse risk factors, age >60 y, performance status ≥2, lactate dehydrogenase greater than normal, Ann Arbor stage III or IV, ≥2 extranodal sites)				
0, 1	35	87	70	73
2	27	67	50	51
3	22	55	49	43
4, 5	16	44	40	26
Patients <60 y old (adverse risk factors, Ann Arbor stage III or IV, lactate dehydrogenase greater than normal, performance status ≥2)				
0, 1	22	92	86	83
2	32	78	66	69
3	32	57	53	46
4, 5	14	46	58	32

unexplained fevers, night sweats, or weight loss. This system has a significant effect on prognosis and is important in treatment planning.

At present, the most valuable and widely used system to stratify patients with lymphoma is the IPI (Table 41.2-8).[88] It was developed by investigators throughout the world for use in predicting outcome for patients with diffuse aggressive NHLs treated with an anthracycline-containing combination chemotherapy regimen. Five features were found to have approximately an equal and independent effect on survival. These included age greater than 60, serum LDH greater than upper limit of normal, performance status greater than 2, advanced-stage disease, and more than two extranodal sites. Because of the approximately equal effect on outcome, the number of abnormalities were simply summed to develop the prognostic index. Thus, patients might have a score of 0 to 5. This system was initially developed only for patients with diffuse aggressive lymphoma. However, it is clear that it applies to patients with almost all subtypes of NHL.[89]

The one area in which the IPI appears less useful is in the follicular lymphomas, where it fails to identify a significant subset of poor-prognosis patients. Other clinical predictive models for indolent lymphoma have been reported more recently.[102,103]

RESTAGING

After patients have completed the entire planned treatment regimen, reevaluation should be done to determine the response to therapy. Achieving a complete remission to therapy is the most important single prognostic factor in patients with NHL. It is particularly true because salvage treatment such as high-dose therapy and autologous or allogeneic bone marrow transplantation can sometimes cure disease in patients who fail to respond to initial therapy.[104]

A restaging evaluation typically involves repeating all previous studies with abnormal results to document their current normal results. However, especially in sites of bulky disease, masses do not always completely regress. This does not necessarily mean that patients will have persisting lymphoma. Correlation with nuclear studies, and possibly rebiopsy under these circumstances, is required to determine whether or not persistent disease is present. An international workshop has established response criteria for use in clinical trials.[105]

SPECIFIC DISEASE ENTITIES

B-CELL NEOPLASMS

Precursor B-Lymphoblastic Leukemia and Lymphoma (Precursor B-Cell Acute Lymphoblastic Leukemia/ Precursor B-Lymphoblastic Lymphoma)

Precursor B-cell acute lymphoblastic leukemia/B-lymphoblastic lymphoma is a neoplasm of lymphoblasts committed to the B-cell lineage, typically composed of small to medium-sized blast cells with scant cytoplasm, moderately condensed to dispersed chromatin and indistinct nucleoli, involving bone marrow and blood (acute lymphocytic leukemia), and occasionally presenting with primary involvement of nodal or extranodal sites (lymphoblastic lymphoma). This disease is described in detail in Chapter 42.

B-Cell Chronic Lymphocytic Leukemia/ Small Lymphocytic Lymphoma

B-CLL/SLL is a neoplasm of monomorphic, small, round B lymphocytes in the peripheral blood and lymph nodes, admixed with prolymphocytes and paraimmunoblasts forming pseudofollicles in lymph nodes, usually expressing CD5 and CD23. B-SLL is defined as a tissue infiltrate with the morphology and immunophenotype of B-CLL. The morphologic, immunophenotypic, and genetic features of the disease are described in detail in Chapter 43.2.

CLINICAL FEATURES. In the International Non-Hodgkin's Lymphoma Classification Project, 6.7% of 1378 cases were diagnosed as B-CLL/SLL. The median age was 65 years, and 83% had stage IV disease, 73% with bone marrow involvement. Generalized lymphadenopathy, hepatosplenomegaly, and extranodal infiltrates may occur. Sixty-four percent had an IPI score of 2/3. The 5-year overall actuarial survival was 51%, with a failure-free survival of 25%; for those patients with an IPI of 0/1, the overall actuarial survival was 76%, whereas for those with an IPI of 4/5 it was only 38%. Thus, the extent of the disease at the time of the diagnosis is the best predictor of survival; however, chromosomal abnormalities, immunophenotype, and somatic mutation status clearly have prognostic importance, as detailed in Chapter 43.2.[106,107]

Patients with SLL can present with hypogammaglobulinemia or develop it over the course of the illness. The presence of hypogammaglobulinemia is associated with an increased incidence of infections and can be managed in some patients with intermittent gammaglobulin injections. Polyclonal or monoclonal hypergammaglobulinemia can also be seen. Autoimmune hemolytic anemias can be seen in patients with SLL and are particularly likely to develop in patients treated with fludarabine.[108] Autoimmune thrombocytopenia is not rare. Autoimmune neutropenia and pure red cell aplasia are unusual.

THERAPY. Localized SLL is unusual and was seen in only 4% of patients in a large series.[89] The rare patient who presents in this manner could be treated with local radiotherapy. Such patients should have their slides reviewed to make certain they do not have a MALT lymphoma.

Some patients with disseminated SLL/CLL have a slowly progressive or stable disorder that does not require therapy. The traditional treatment for this lymphoma has been oral chlorambucil or oral cyclophosphamide. However, it is now clear that fludarabine is the most active single agent.[109] Several randomized trials have been completed. One study with 59 patients randomized received fludarabine, chlorambucil, or a combination of both drugs. The combination arm was closed early due to excessive toxicity. Patients who failed to respond to an individual drug were crossed over to the other arm. The overall response rate (70% vs. 43%), complete response (CR) rate (27% vs. 3%), and remission duration favored fludarabine over chlorambucil.[110] Although progression-free survival (PFS) also favored fludarabine, there was no difference in OS. Another randomized trial studied 695 patients and compared fludarabine with anthracycline-containing combinations. Fludarabine had a superior response rate.[111] It appears that combinations, including fludarabine and cyclophosphamide or rituximab,[112,113] are also active and might be more active than fludarabine alone.

Patients with SLL/CLL can respond to monoclonal antibody therapy using rituximab (anti-CD20) and Campath-1 (anti-CD52). However, the response rate to single-agent rituximab appears to be on the order of 20%, perhaps because of the lower level of expression of CD20 than seen in follicular lymphoma. Increased response rates, of relatively short duration, have been observed with higher doses of rituximab therapy than are used in follicular lymphoma.[114] Combination chemotherapy using CHOP (cyclophosphamide, doxorubicin, vincristine, prednisone) or FND (fludarabine, mitoxantrone, dexamethasone)[115] produces significant response rates in SLL, but the patients almost always relapse. High-dose therapy and autologous transplantation and allogeneic transplantation[116] have been used in fairly small numbers of patients. It appears that allogeneic transplantation can probably be curative. In general, principles of therapy of SLL apply to patients with lymphoplasmacytic lymphoma.

Lymphoplasmacytic Lymphoma (with or without Waldenström's Macroglobulinemia)

Lymphoplasmacytic lymphoma is a neoplasm of small B lymphocytes, plasmacytoid lymphocytes, and plasma cells, involving bone marrow, lymph nodes, and spleen, lacking CD5, usually with a serum monoclonal protein with hyperviscosity or cryoglobulinemia. Plasmacytoid variants of other neoplasms are excluded.

MORPHOLOGY. The tumor contains small lymphocytes, plasmacytoid lymphocytes, and plasma cells, with variable numbers of immunoblasts. Cells may contain intranuclear inclusions of periodic acid–Schiff–positive IgM (Dutcher bodies). By definition, features of other lymphomas—particularly marginal zone lymphomas and SLL—that may have plasmacytoid differentiation are absent. The bone marrow infiltrate may be either diffuse or nodular and is often interstitial and rather subtle. Peripheral blood involvement is less prominent than in CLL, and the cells often have a plasmacytoid appearance.

IMMUNOPHENOTYPE AND GENETIC FEATURES. The cells have surface and cytoplasmic (some cells) Ig, usually of IgM type; usually lack IgD; and strongly express B-cell–associated antigens (CD19, CD20, CD22, CD79a). The cells are CD5–, CD10–, CD23–, and CD43+/–; CD25 or CD11c may be faintly positive in some cases. Lack of CD5 and CD23, strong sIg and CD20, and the presence of cytoplasmic Ig are useful in distinction from B-CLL.

Ig heavy- and light-chain genes are rearranged, and variable region genes show a small load of somatic mutations, suggesting that these cells arise from a population of B cells that have been exposed to antigen.[117] Translocation t(9;14)(p13;q32) and rearrangement of the PAX-5 gene are reported in some cases.[118] PAX-5 encodes a protein, B-cell–specific activator protein, which is important in early B-cell development. Expression of B-cell–specific activator protein is restricted to B cells and is independent of the translocation; however, it is usually absent in plasma cells lacking the translocation.[119]

POSTULATED NORMAL COUNTERPART. The postulated normal counterpart is a peripheral B lymphocyte stimulated to differentiate to a plasma cell, possibly corresponding to the primary immune response to antigen or to a post–germinal center cell that has undergone somatic mutation but not heavy-chain class switch.

CLINICAL FEATURES AND THERAPY. Lymphoplasmacytic lymphoma made up only 1.2% (16 of 1378) of the cases in the REAL clinical study.[89] Similar to B-CLL/SLL, the median age was 63 years and 53% were men; most (73%) had bone marrow involvement. Sixty-nine percent had an IPI of 2/3. Lymph node and splenic involvement are common. A monoclonal serum paraprotein of IgM type, with or without hyperviscosity syndrome (Waldenström's macroglobulinemia), is present in most patients[120]; as with B-CLL, the paraprotein may have autoantibody or cryoglobulin activity.

Most cases of mixed cryoglobulinemia have been shown to be related to HCV infection, even in patients who have demonstrable B-cell lymphoma in the bone marrow.[121] Treatment of patients with HCV and cryoglobulinemia with interferon to reduce viral load has been associated with regression of the lymphoma.[208]

The clinical course of LPL is indolent; in some European series it has been reported to be more aggressive than typical B-CLL,[122] but in the REAL clinical study, 5-year overall actuarial survival (58%) and failure-free survival (25%) were identical to that of CLL/SLL.[89] The traditional therapy for this disorder has been chlorambucil with or without prednisone.[120] Anthracycline-based combination chemotherapy has not been shown to be more effective. However, purine analogues are frequently used as initial therapy for this disorder.[123] The response rate of lymphoplasmacytic lymphoma to rituximab is lower than that of follicular lymphoma[124]; however, combinations of chemotherapy and rituximab are currently under investigation. Two biologic agents have been approved for the treatment of multiple myeloma and have demonstrated clinical activity in patients with lymphoplasmacytic lymphoma. These include thalidomide (and immunomodulatory agent derivatives) and bortezomib, a proteosome inhibitor.[125]

In patients who require therapy, the authors suggest a purine analogue–containing regimen as initial therapy for most patients. Young patients with refractory disease should be considered for high-dose therapy with autologous or allogeneic stem cell support.

Extranodal Marginal Zone B-Cell Lymphoma (Low-Grade B-Cell Lymphoma of Mucosa-Associated Lymphoid Tissue)

Extranodal marginal zone B-cell lymphoma of MALT is an extranodal lymphoma consisting of heterogeneous small B cells, including marginal zone (centrocyte-like) cells, monocytoid cells, and small lymphocytes in varying proportions, and scattered immunoblast- and centroblast-like cells, with plasma cell differentiation in 40% of the cases. The infiltrate is in the marginal zone of reactive B-cell follicles and extends into the interfollicular region.

MORPHOLOGY. Extranodal marginal zone B-cell (MALT) lymphoma reproduces the morphologic features of normal MALT, with a polymorphous infiltrate of small lymphocytes, marginal zone (centrocyte-like) B cells, monocytoid B cells, and plasma cells, as well as rare centroblast- or immunoblast-like cells. Reactive follicles are usually present, with the neoplastic cells occupying the marginal zone or the interfollicular region, or both; occasional follicles may be "colonized" by marginal zone or monocytoid cells. In epithelial tissues, neoplastic cells typically infiltrate the epithelium, forming so-called lymphoepithelial lesions. Blast cells are typically present but are by definition in the minority.

Clusters or sheets of blasts sufficiently large to warrant a diagnosis of large cell lymphoma are associated with a worse prognosis. In these cases, a separate diagnosis of DLBCL should be made. The term *high-grade MALT lymphoma* should be avoided for large B-cell lymphomas in MALT sites, because it may lead to inappropriate treatment with antibiotics instead of aggressive cytotoxic therapy.

IMMUNOPHENOTYPE AND GENETIC FEATURES. The tumor cells express sIg, usually IgM but occasionally IgG or IgA, and lack IgD, and 40% have monotypic cytoplasmic Ig, indicating plasmacytoid differentiation. They express B-cell–associated antigens (CD19, CD20, CD22, CD79a) and are usually negative for CD5 and CD10. Immunophenotyping studies are useful in confirming malignancy (light-chain restriction) and in excluding B-CLL (CD5+), mantle cell (CD5+), and follicle center (CD10+ CD43–, CD11c–, usually cytoplasmic Ig–) lymphomas.

Ig genes are rearranged, and the variable region has a high degree of somatic mutation, as well as intraclonal diversity consistent with a germinal center or post–germinal center stage of B-cell development.[126] Ig heavy-chain variable regions are those often found in autoantibodies, consistent with studies showing that the antibodies produced by the tumor cells have specificity against self-antigens. The bcl-1 and bcl-2 genes are germline; trisomy 3 (60%) and t(11;18)(q21;q21) (25% to 40%) are the most common reported cytogenetic abnormalities.[127] Interestingly, neither of these abnormalities is common in primary large cell lymphomas of the gastrointestinal tract. Translocation t(14;18) involving the Ig heavy-chain locus and the MLT1 gene may occur, more often in nongastric than in gastric MALT lymphoma.[128]

Analysis of the t(11;18) breakpoint has shown fusion of the apoptosis-inhibitor gene API2 to a novel gene at 18q21, named *MLT*, in cases of MALT lymphoma.[129] A gene involved in a breakpoint in MALT lymphomas with t(1;14) has been cloned; named *BCL-10*, it is an apoptosis-promoting gene that in mutated form may cause cellular transformation.[130] API2 and BCL-10 appear to be involved in the NFκB pathway.

Correlation of clinical and genetic features has shown that patients with gastric MALT lymphoma and t(11;18) tend to have more advanced, deeply invasive tumors and do not respond to *H pylori* eradication. t(11;18) is found with varying frequency in MALT lymphomas from various sites: 25% to 40% of gastric cases, 40% to 60% of pulmonary cases, and seldom in thyroid, skin, orbital, and cutaneous cases.[131]

Tumors with t(11;18) tend to have this as their only cytogenetic abnormality, whereas those with trisomy 3 often have complex karyotypes; t(11;18) and trisomy 3 appear to be mutually exclusive.[132] Furthermore, tumors with t(11;18) appear to be less likely to transform to DLBCLs. Thus, there appear to be two pathways of lymphomagenesis in MALT lymphomas: one involving prolonged dependence on *H pylori* infection, with acquisition of multiple cytogenetic abnormalities and risk of progression to DLBCL, and another involving early t(11;18), which confers independence from *H pylori* and has a low risk of other cytogenetic abnormalities or progression.

POSTULATED NORMAL COUNTERPART. The postulated normal counterpart is a post–germinal center memory B cell with capacity to differentiate into marginal zone, monocytoid, and plasma cells.

CLINICAL FEATURES. Extranodal marginal zone B-cell (MALT) lymphoma accounts for the majority of low-grade gastric lymphomas and almost 50% of all gastric lymphomas[133]; in other sites, such as the ocular adnexa, they make up approximately 40% of the cases, and they account for the majority of low-grade pulmonary lymphomas. Patients are usually older adults, although they may be in their 20s and 30s. A slight female predominance has been reported in some series. The majority of patients present with localized stage I or II extranodal disease, involving glandular epithelial tissues of various sites. The stomach is the most frequent site, but most low-grade lymphomas (and former pseudolymphomas) presenting in the lung, thyroid, salivary gland, and orbit are of this type; skin and soft tissues may also be the presenting site. Many patients have a history of autoimmune disease, such as Sjögren's syndrome or Hashimoto's thyroiditis, or of *Helicobacter* gastritis in the case of gastric MALT lymphoma. Acquired MALT secondary to autoimmune disease or infection in these sites is thought to be the substrate for lymphoma development.

Proliferation of the cells of marginal zone lymphoma at certain sites depends on the presence of activated, antigen-driven T cells; in gastric tumors, it has been shown that the T cells are driven by *H pylori* antigens. Therapy directed at the antigen (*H pylori* in gastric lymphoma) results in regression of most early lesions.[134] The long-term prognosis of these patients is not known, however, and patients treated with antibiotic therapy require long and careful follow-up. The disease known as *Mediterranean abdominal lymphoma*, a *heavy-chain disease*, and *immunoproliferative small intestinal disease*, which occurs in young adults in eastern Mediterranean countries, is another example of a MALT-type lymphoma that may respond to antibiotic therapy in its early stages and has been shown to be associated with chronic *C jejuni* infection.[41]

THERAPY OF MUCOSA-ASSOCIATED LYMPHOID TISSUE LYMPHOMAS. The indolent extranodal lymphomas associated with MALT involve the gastrointestinal tract, salivary glands, breast, thyroid, orbit, conjunctiva, skin, lung, and, less commonly, other sites. As these diseases tend to remain localized for long periods of time, local treatment [surgery or radiation therapy (RT)] is effective at long-term control of disease. In particular, low doses of RT (30 Gy) almost always control sites of disease. These doses are somewhat lower than used for patients with localized follicular grade 1 and 2 disease. Retrospective studies provide dose control data for MALT lymphoma.[135,136] Local control rates ranged from 97% to 100%; 5-year PFS and OS were approximately 75% and 95%, respectively.

One-half or more of patients with gastric NHL have the indolent MALT type. The optimal treatment of gastric MALT lymphoma remains to be determined. Gastric MALT lymphoma is frequently associated with chronic gastritis and *H pylori* infection. Because it has been postulated that *H pylori* infection leads to the accumulation of MALT in the stomach and that gastric MALT lymphomas arise within this acquired MALT tissue, promising results have been seen with the use of antibiotics for gastric MALT NHL. In one study from the German MALT Lymphoma Group, 33 patients with low-grade MALT were treated with antibiotics. At 1-year median follow-up more than 70% of patients remained in complete remission. However, in a follow-up study, 22 of 31 patients in continuous complete remission (median follow-up, 16 months) had a monoclonal B-cell population on PCR analysis, leaving open the question of durability of CR after antibiotics.[137] Nonetheless, the standard treatment for patients with gastric MALT who are positive for *H pylori* is antibiotics and follow-up endoscopy 3 and 6 months later. Patients who have a CR should be followed without further treatment. Patients who have a partial response and remain *H pylori* positive should receive a second course of antibiotics before proceeding to more definitive treatment.

Patients who are negative for *H pylori* are unlikely to respond to antibiotics; initial treatment of *H pylori*–negative patients should be RT in most instances. For patients who have persistent disease after antibiotics, local regional irradiation therapy is the treatment of choice. Good results have been obtained with total or partial gastrectomy; however, this approach has been associated with long-term morbidity. Local and regional radiation through the three-field approach (anterior and two lateral fields to minimize radiation to the left kidney) provides local control and relief of symptoms in greater than 90% of patients.

The use of chemotherapy for MALT lymphomas has received limited attention, as this indolent NHL does not routinely require the use of systemic treatment in patients with early-stage disease. In one study of 24 patients with low-grade MALT treated with daily cyclophosphamide or chlorambucil for 12 to 24 months, the CR rate at 1 year was 75%, and approximately 50% continued to be in remission at the time of the study.[138] Although these results are favorable, control of limited disease is superior with RT, and the use of chemotherapy should be limited to patients with advanced or recurrent disease. MALT lymphomas can be disseminated and present at an advanced stage in approximately one-third of cases.[139] Dissemination is usually to lymph nodes but can involve other extranodal sites. Patients with widespread MALT lymphoma should be treated with strategies similar to those described for follicular lymphoma.

Nodal Marginal Zone B-Cell Lymphoma

Nodal marginal zone B-cell lymphoma is a primary nodal lymphoma with features identical to lymph nodes involved by MALT lymphoma, but without evidence of extranodal disease. Monocytoid B cells may be prominent. This diagnosis should not be made in patients with MALT lymphoma at other sites, Sjögren's syndrome, or when another low-grade B-cell lymphoma (follicular, mantle cell) is present in the same node.

MORPHOLOGY. Two morphologic types have been described: cases that resemble MALT lymphoma and cases that more closely resemble splenic marginal zone lymphoma (SMZL). Those that resemble MALT lymphoma show aggregates of monocytoid B cells in a parafollicular, perivascular, and perisinusoidal distribution, with preserved germinal centers and mantle zones. Those that resemble SMZL have infiltrates of marginal zone cells surrounding reactive follicles with germinal centers, but with attenuated mantle zones. Nodal marginal zone lymphoma with features resembling progressively transformed germinal centers has been reported to occur in young males, with localized presentation and good clinical outcome.[140]

IMMUNOPHENOTYPE AND GENETIC FEATURES. The cases that resemble SMZL express IgD and lack CD5, CD23, and cyclin D1. Those that resemble MALT lymphoma are IgD negative and have an immunophenotype identical to that of extranodal marginal zone B-cell lymphoma (MALT).

POSTULATED NORMAL COUNTERPART. The postulated normal counterpart is a post–germinal center marginal zone or monocytoid B cells of nodal type.

CLINICAL FEATURES AND THERAPY. Nodal marginal zone B-cell lymphoma is a rare disorder, accounting for 1% of the cases in the international study of the REAL.[89] The patients presented with isolated or generalized nodal disease; bone marrow was involved in 30%, and, rarely, peripheral blood may be involved. A retrospective survey of 180 patients with pathologically reviewed extragastric MALT lymphomas from 20 institutions revealed that the median age was 59 years (range, 21 to 92 years). Ann Arbor stage I disease was present in 115 patients (64%) and stage II disease in 16 (9%).[141] Most cases were in the low or low-intermediate risk groups according to the IPI.

Patients were treated with a variety of therapeutic strategies, including chemotherapy in 78 cases. The 5-year OS rate was 90%, and the 5-year PFS was 60%. At a median follow-up of 3.4 years, only 6 patients showed histologic transformation. The optimal therapy for patients with monocytoid B-cell lymphoma is not known. Patients are frequently treated with regimens that are used for follicular lymphoma.

Splenic Marginal Zone Lymphoma with or without Villous Lymphocytes

SMZL is a neoplasm of small B lymphocytes that surround and replace splenic white pulp germinal centers, merging with an outer marginal zone of larger cells with pale cytoplasm admixed with large transformed blasts. Small and large cells infiltrate red pulp, often with villous lymphocytes in the peripheral blood.

MORPHOLOGY. In the spleen, the neoplastic cells of SMZL occupy the mantle and marginal zones of the splenic white pulp, usually with a central residual germinal center, which may be either atrophic or hyperplastic. The cells in the mantle zone are small, with slight nuclear irregularity and scant cytoplasm, whereas those in the marginal zone have more dispersed chromatin and abundant, pale cytoplasm and are admixed with centroblasts and immunoblasts. The red pulp is involved with a diffuse and a micronodular pattern and sinus infiltration. Epithelioid histiocytes may be present singly or in clusters and, particularly in the bone marrow, may give rise to the differential diagnosis of an infectious process. Splenic hilar lymph nodes are often involved; the neoplastic cells form vague nodules, often without a central germinal center, and a marginal zone pattern may or may not be present. The marrow usually contains discrete lymphoid aggregates, without a marginal zone pattern, with or without diffuse lymphoid infiltration and often with intrasinusoidal neoplastic cells. When tumor cells are present in the peripheral blood, they often have abundant cytoplasm with small surface "villous" projections (splenic lymphoma with villous lymphocytes) or may appear plasmacytoid.

IMMUNOPHENOTYPE AND GENETIC FEATURES. The tumor cells are IgM+, IgD+, CD5–, CD10–, CD43–, CD23–; express B-cell antigens (CD19, CD20, CD22) and bcl-2; and lack CD11c and CD25. In the majority of cases, lack of CD5 serves to distinguish this disorder from B-CLL, and lack of CD103 and CD25 is useful in distinguishing it from HCL. The cells are cyclin D1 negative by immunoperoxidase staining.

Analysis of the Ig variable region genes indicates a high degree of somatic mutation, consistent with a post–germinal center stage of B-cell development.[142] More recently, ongoing mutations of V region genes, similar to germinal center cells, have been reported. However, a study found somatic mutations in only 50%.[143] BCL-2 is germline. Early reports that t(11;14)(q13;132), BCL-1 rearrangement, and cyclin D1 overexpression were common are now thought to have reflected inclusion of cases of leukemic mantle cell lymphoma. Trisomy 3, found in nodal and extranodal marginal zone lymphoma, is detected in only a small number of cases, and the t(11;18)(q21;q21) has not been reported.[144] Interstitial deletions of 17q31-32 are found in approximately 40%. Studies

suggest that there are two subsets of SMZL: those with and some without somatic mutations; those that lack mutations often have interstitial deletions of 7q and are associated with a worse prognosis.

POSTULATED NORMAL COUNTERPART. The normal counterpart is thought to be a post–germinal center, memory B cell of splenic type (50%) or a naive B cell (50%).

CLINICAL FEATURES AND THERAPY. SMZL accounts for only 1% to 2% of chronic lymphoid leukemia found on bone marrow examination but up to 25% of low-grade B-cell neoplasms in splenectomy specimens.[145] It may make up the majority of chronic B-cell leukemia and low-grade splenic lymphomas that do not fit the defining criteria of B-CLL, lymphoplasmacytic lymphoma, mantle cell lymphoma, follicular lymphoma, or hairy cell leukemia. Patients typically present with weakness, fatigue, or symptoms related to splenomegaly. Physical examination revealed splenomegaly in almost all patients and hepatomegaly in up to 40% of patients, but lymphadenopathy is rare.[145] Lymphocytosis is a uniform finding, but extreme lymphocytosis is unusual. Anemia and thrombocytopenia are present in a minority of patients. In some series more than one-half of the patients have been shown to have a monoclonal Ig. Although most commonly seen in elderly men, the disease can occur in both genders and in young patients. Although SMZL is usually confined to the spleen, bone marrow, and blood, unusual sites of involvement such as leukemic meningitis have been described.

Most patients have an indolent course and require no immediate therapy or respond to splenectomy.[145] For patients in whom splenectomy is inappropriate, splenic radiation can be an alternative. Systemic treatment options include oral alkylating agents or purine analogues, with or without monoclonal antibodies, as for follicular lymphoma.

Follicular Lymphoma

Follicular lymphoma is defined as a lymphoma of follicle center B cells (centrocytes and centroblasts), which has at least a partially follicular pattern

MORPHOLOGY. Follicular lymphoma is composed of a mixture of centrocytes (cleaved follicle center cells) and centroblasts (large noncleaved follicle center cells) and by definition has at least a partially follicular pattern. Rare lymphomas with a follicular growth pattern consist almost entirely of centroblasts. The proportion of centroblasts varies from case to case, and the clinical aggressiveness of the tumor increases with increasing numbers of centroblasts. Numerous criteria have been proposed for grading follicular lymphoma, but reproducibility is poor. The WHO classification uses the cell-counting method of Mann and Berard (Table 41.2-9), which has been shown to have better reproducibility and predictive value than other schemes. The bone marrow is frequently involved by lymphoid aggregates that are generally paratrabecular. Splenic involvement is typically predominantly white pulp.

In addition to typical follicular lymphoma, two variants are recognized, whose relationship to follicular lymphoma remains controversial: cutaneous follicle center lymphoma and diffuse follicle center lymphoma.

TABLE 41.2-9. Follicular and Mantle Cell Lymphomas: Grading and Variants

---

FOLLICULAR LYMPHOMA
Grades
Grade 1: 0–5 centroblasts per high-power field
Grade 2: 6–15 centroblasts per high-power field
Grade 3: >15 centroblasts per high-power field
3a: >15 centroblasts, but centrocytes are still present
3b: Centroblasts form solid sheets with no residual centrocytes
Variants
Cutaneous follicle center lymphoma
Diffuse follicle center lymphoma
Grade 1: 0–5 centroblasts per high-power field
Grade 2: 6–15 centroblasts per high-power field
MANTLE CELL LYMPHOMA
Variant: blastoid

IMMUNOPHENOTYPE AND GENETIC FEATURES. The tumor cells of follicular lymphoma usually express sIg; approximately 60% are IgG and 40% either IgG or, less often, IgA. The tumor cells express pan-B-cell–associated antigens; most are CD10+, and they are CD5–, CD23–/+, and CD43– (most cases). Rare cases of CD5+ follicular lymphoma have been reported. Tightly organized meshworks of FDCs are present in follicular areas. Most cases are bcl-2+, and nuclear bcl-6 is expressed by at least some of the neoplastic cells.[146] The Ki-67+ fraction is lower than that of reactive follicles.

Ig heavy- and light-chain genes are rearranged, with extensive and ongoing somatic mutations, similar to normal germinal center cells. t(14;18)(q32;q21) and *BCL-2* gene rearrangement are present in the majority of the cases.[147] Abnormalities of 3q27 or *BCL6* rearrangement, or both, are found in approximately 15% of follicular lymphomas, whereas 5' mutations of the *BCL6* gene are found in approximately 40%. Translocations involving *BCL6* appear to be associated with an increased risk of transformation to DLBCL.[148]

Most cases have complex karyotypes, and t(14;18) is rarely the sole abnormality.[149] Analysis of cases of the rare grade 3B follicular lymphoma have shown that t(14;18) and 3q27 translocations are mutually exclusive, suggesting that some cases may be more closely related to follicular lymphoma and others to *de novo* DLBCL.

Microarray analysis has shown that follicular lymphomas have a gene expression signature very similar to that of normal germinal center cells, with the exception of overexpression of BCL2 and cell-cycle regulatory genes, and loss of genes associated with cell adhesion.[150] One study suggests that cases with a signature closer to that of normal germinal center cells are less likely to respond to therapy with anti-CD20 antibody.[151] Transformation to DLBCL is associated with p53 mutations and with acquisition of a variety of other genetic abnormalities, some of which may be targets for therapy.[152] The pattern of gene expression in transformed follicular lymphoma differs from that of *de novo* DLBCL, possibly explaining the different clinical behavior.[153]

POSTULATED NORMAL COUNTERPART. The postulated normal counterpart is a germinal center B cell—both centrocytes and centroblasts.

CLINICAL FEATURES. Follicular lymphoma is the second most common lymphoma in the United States and western Europe, accounting for approximately 30% of all NHLs and up to 70% of low-grade lymphomas reported in American and European clinical trials.[89] Thus, our understanding of the clinical features and response to treatment of low-grade lymphoma is essentially that of follicular lymphoma. Follicular lymphoma affects predominantly older adults, with a slight female predominance. Most patients have widespread disease at diagnosis, usually predominantly involving lymph nodes, but also spleen, bone marrow, and occasionally peripheral blood or extranodal sites. Despite the advanced stage, the clinical course is generally indolent, with median survivals in excess of 8 years; however, the disease is not usually curable with available treatment. In the international study of the REAL, the few patients (7%) with IPI scores of 4/5 have a much worse prognosis, with a median survival of only 1 year.[89]

THERAPY OF LOCALIZED FOLLICULAR LYMPHOMA. RT alone is standard treatment for patients with CS I to II follicular grade I to II lymphoma. Nine large series (defined as 50 or more patients per study) reporting results of treatment for follicular grade I to II are shown in Table 41.2-10.[154–162] All but one study contains stage I and stage II patients (in approximately equal frequencies). The 10-year freedom from treatment failure in these studies ranges from 41% to 49%. The 10-year OS (all causes) ranges from 43% to 79%, with a median survival of 11.9 to 15.3 years. Nearly all patients were treated with RT alone except for those in the Foundation Bergonie study, in which the majority of patients received some form of systemic treatment.[160] The freedom from treatment failure and OS in this combined RT and chemotherapy study was no better than in the radiation-alone studies. The majority of patients had follicular lymphoma grade I and grade II histologies; however, follicular lymphoma grade III patients were included in some of the series (noted in Table 41.2-10).

Adverse prognostic factors for freedom from treatment failure are analyzed by multivariate analysis in many of the studies (see Table 41.2-10). Age was the adverse factor most often reported and was seen in five of the nine studies. Follicular grade 3 histology, extensive CS IIA disease, bulky disease (defined as greater than 2 or 3 cm), and extranodal presentations also were reported, but each of these adverse factors were seen in only one or two of the nine studies. No significant difference appears to be present in outcome between follicular grade I versus grade II disease.

No large prospective or randomized studies have evaluated the dose and field size of RT for patients with stage I to II follicular grade I to II lymphoma. The median radiation doses vary from 30 to 40 Gy in eight of the nine series, with the two largest series reporting a median dose of 35 Gy.[156,158] Infield recurrences range from 0% to 11%, with higher percentages occurring in patients with bulky disease or those who receive a radiation dose of less than 30 Gy. Based on these data, the authors recommend 30 to 36 Gy, with a boost to areas of initial involvement to 36 to 40 Gy for early-stage follicular grade I to II lymphoma. Bulky disease should be treated to the upper end of the range; 30 to 36 Gy should suffice for smaller disease. When there is a possibility of significant morbidity from treatment, such as long-term xerostomia from irradiation of the salivary glands in an elderly patient, slightly lower doses should be considered (i.e., 25 to 30 Gy).

TABLE 41.2-10. Radiation Therapy Alone for Early-Stage Low-Grade Follicular Non-Hodgkin's Lymphoma (Selected Trials Containing 50 or More Patients)

Report	Patients(n)/ Med FU/% CT	Stage	10-Y FFTF/OS	Median RT Dose to the Tumor	RT Field Size	Grade Dist	Adverse Prog Factors (FFTF)
Princess Margaret Hospital[158]	573 10.6 y 27%	I (64%) II (36%)	48%/>60%	35 Gy	IF	FG1 (33%) FG2 (32%) FG3 (35%)	Ext CS II >2 cm disease
BNLI[156]	208 NA 0%	I (100%)	47%/64%	35 Gy (suggested)	NA	FG1 (39%) FG2 (35%) FG3 (5%) Other (21%)	Age ≥50
Stanford University[159]	177 7.7 y 5%	I (41%) II (59%)	44%/64%	35–50 Gy	IF/RF/EF (77%) TLI (23%)	FG1 (57%) FG2/3 (43%)	Age >60 Extranodal site RT fields <TLI
Foundation Bergonie[160]	103 8.3 y 70%	I (44%) II (56%)	49%/56%	35–40 Gy	IF (54%) RF (46%)	NA	Age >60
M. D. Anderson[155]	80 19 y 0%	I (41%) II (59%)	41%/43% at 15 y	40 Gy	IF (9%) RF (54%) EF (37%)	FG1 (63%) FG2 (37%)	CS IIA >3 cm disease
Edinburgh[161]	64 5 y 2%	I (58%) II (42%)	49%/78%	30–40 Gy (82%) >40 Gy (18%)	NA	FG1 (78%) FG2 (3%) Other (19%)	NA
University of Florida[154]	72 8.5 y 7%	I (75%) II (25%)	46%/59%	NA	IF (53%) EF (43%) TNI/WA (4%)	NA	NA
NCI[157]	54 9 y 10%	I (50%) II (50%)	48%/69%	36 Gy	IF (38%) EF (48%) TLI/TBI (14%)	—	Age ≥45
Royal Marsden Hospital[162]	58 NA 0%	I (69%) II (31%)	43%/79%	40 Gy	IF (52%) EF (48%)	FG1 (64%) FG2 (21%) Other (15%)	Field size not significant for recurrence

BNLI, British National Lymphoma Investigation; DFS, disease-free survival; EF, extended-field radiation therapy (RT), mantle or whole abdominal (WA) fields (M.D. Anderson), mantle, WA, inverted Y (Stanford, Royal Marsden), mantle, Inv Y (National Cancer Institute); FFTF, freedom from treatment failure; FG, follicular grade; grade/stage dist, grade/stage distribution; IF, involved field; Med FU, median follow-up time; prog, prognostic; NA, not reported; NCI, National Cancer Institute; OS, overall survival (all causes); PFS, progression-free survival; RF, regional field RT, one to three adjacent nodal regions (Wilder); RFS, recurrence/relapse-free survival; TBI, total body irradiation; TLI, total lymphoid irradiation; TNI, total nodal irradiation.

The role of combination chemotherapy in the management of early-stage follicular lymphoma is unclear. Randomized studies conducted in the 1970s failed to demonstrate that non–adriamycin-containing combination chemotherapy regimens plus RT were superior to RT alone.[163,164] A more recent British National Lymphoma Investigation study randomized 148 patients to receive either RT alone or RT plus chlorambucil chemotherapy.[165] No differences were found in freedom from recurrence or survival between the groups. A single-arm study of 91 stage I to II patients treated at the M. D. Anderson Hospital with COP (cyclophosphamide, vincristine, and prednisone) or CHOP-B (cyclophosphamide, doxorubicin, vincristine, prednisone plus bleomycin) chemotherapy in addition to RT demonstrated an improved freedom from recurrence compared to historic controls but no OS differences.[166]

The choice of therapy may lie in the careful assessment of prognostic factors. Most patients with Ann Arbor clinical stage I or II follicular grade I to II lymphoma should have a good prognosis after local-regional RT alone. For patients whose prognosis is less certain, such as those with stage II disease with multiple sites of involvement or bulky nodes, or patients with follicular lymphoma grade III histology, chemotherapy followed by involved-field irradiation may provide more durable remissions.

THERAPY OF DISSEMINATED FOLLICULAR LYMPHOMA. The optimal treatment strategy for patients with advanced-stage follicular lymphoma is controversial. Although many years of clinical investigation have failed to prove that immediate aggressive therapy improves survival compared with conservative therapy, the median survival of only 7 to 8 years from diagnosis in patients with stage III and IV disease has prompted the investigation of novel treatment approaches.[167] Despite the indolent nature of the follicular lymphomas, most patients ultimately die of their disease, and the median OS of patients with follicular NHL has not changed in the past 30 years. The National Cancer Institute initiated a prospective randomized study comparing conservative treatment (no initial therapy) with aggressive combined modality therapy with ProMACE [prednisone, methotrexate-leucovorin, doxorubicin (Adriamycin), cyclophosphamide, etoposide]/MOPP [mechlorethamine (Mustargen), vincristine (Oncovin), procarbazine, prednisone] chemotherapy followed by low-dose (24 Gy) total lymphoid RT.[168] Eighty-nine patients were randomized. The disease-free survival was significantly higher in the combined modality therapy group at 4 years (51%

vs. 12%); however, no differences in OS were seen. Patients with follicular lymphoma who are followed without therapy sometimes have spontaneous regressions that can be complete. Thus, although there is no proof that early aggressive chemotherapy is superior to an initial watch-and-wait approach, improvements in survival depend on the willingness of investigators and patients to participate in clinical trials of new therapeutic approaches.

When a decision is made to treat a patient with disseminated follicular lymphoma using cytotoxic chemotherapeutic agents, a wide variety of choices are available. In general, CRs occur more rapidly with combination chemotherapy regimens, but it is unclear that the ultimate treatment result is superior with combinations.

Chemotherapy. When single alkylating agents (cyclophosphamide or chlorambucil) are directly compared with combinations of three drugs (COP), significant differences in long-term outcome, including survival, are not observed.[169] Moreover, in an analysis conducted by the Southwest Oncology Group of 415 patients treated with a variety of chemotherapy regimens, doxorubicin-containing treatment did not prolong the overall median survival of low-grade lymphoma patients compared with results with less aggressive programs.[170] A Cancer and Leukemia Group B study randomized 228 patients with stage III or IV follicular small cleaved lymphoma or follicular mixed lymphoma to single-agent oral cyclophosphamide or the combination CHOP-B. Treatment was continued in responders for 2 years beyond maximal response. At 10 years with either cyclophosphamide or CHOP-B, respectively, there was no significant difference in overall time to failure (25% failure free vs. 33%) or survival (44% alive vs. 46%).[171] One important advantage to combination chemotherapy programs is speed of response and a possibly prolonged disease-free interval compared with less intense programs.

The subdivision of patients with follicular lymphoma into those with predominantly small cells (follicular small cleaved cell), those with an intermediate number of small and large cells (follicular mixed), and those with more large cells (follicular large cell) is difficult.[89] However, even considering the imprecision of the distinction, patients classified as having follicular large cell lymphoma have a shorter remission duration and OS than patients with the other subtypes. The incorporation of an anthracycline into the initial treatment regimen seems to be more important in patients with follicular large cell lymphoma.[172]

More recent chemotherapy studies have focused on purine analogue–containing regimens. A study from Canada randomized 91 patients to fludarabine or CVP (cyclophosphamide, vincristine, and prednisone).[173] No difference in response rates was seen, with 64% (CR, 9%) for fludarabine versus 52% (CR, 7%) for CVP (*P* =.72). With a median follow-up of 42 months, median PFS (11.0 vs. 9.1 months; *P* =.03) and tumor-free survival (15 vs. 11 months; *P* =.02) were superior in patients receiving fludarabine. No difference in median OS was detected (57 months for fludarabine vs. 44 months for CVP).

Combinations of fludarabine with mitoxantrone have demonstrated very high response rates. The Southwest Oncology Group treated 78 patients with this combination, and complete remission was demonstrated in 34 patients (44%) and partial remission was demonstrated in 39 patients (50%).[174] With a median follow-up time of 5.5 years, the median PFS was 32 months; 88% of all patients are alive at 4 years, which is not sta-

tistically better than historical controls treated with the CHOP regimen.

Autologous Stem Cell Transplantation. Two trials of autologous hematopoietic stem cell transplantation (HSCT) incorporated in the primary therapy of patients with follicular lymphoma have reported high CR rates, but with continued observation it does not appear that this modality is curative for the majority of patients.[175,176] In addition, the incidence of secondary myelodysplasia after these treatments may exceed 15%, tempering the enthusiasm of this approach.[177]

Biologic Therapy. Interferon-α has long been known to be an active drug in the treatment of patients with follicular lymphoma and has an objective response rate of 30% to 55% when used as a single agent with relapsed disease.[178] The value of adding interferon to standard combination chemotherapy regimens has been tested in a number of clinical trials. Several prospective randomized trials have conflicting results, with some suggesting a survival benefit[179] whereas other larger trials failed to demonstrate it.[180] Because of significant toxicity, and the availability of other options, interferon is rarely used in the United States for patients with NHL.

Because of the toxicity of chemotherapy and interferon, investigators have examined the role of monoclonal antibody therapy as initial treatment for patients with follicular NHL. A phase II study treated 50 patients with stage II to IV follicular lymphoma and low tumor burden with single-agent rituximab as first therapy.[181] The overall response rate at 50 days was 73%. Toxicity for both of these studies was minimal.

Hainsworth et al.[182] have also used rituximab (375 mg/m² IV per week for 4 consecutive weeks) as initial therapy in patients with indolent lymphoma. Patients who did not progress received an additional 4-week course of rituximab every 6 months for 2 years. In 62 chemotherapy-naive patients, most of whom had stage III or IV disease, overall response rates at 6 weeks and at maximum response were 47% and 73%, with 7% and 37% complete remissions, respectively. At a median follow-up of 30 months, median PFS was 34 months.

Preliminary results of a study randomizing patients to rituximab maintenance (single infusion every 2 months × 4) versus observation after suggest a significant failure-free survival benefit to the maintenance strategy.[183] However, preliminary results of a study comparing scheduled maintenance to retreatment with rituximab on progression showed no difference in duration of rituximab benefit.[184] Although maintenance therapy with rituximab appears to be safe, additional follow-up of these studies and results from other ongoing clinical trials are necessary to determine optimal timing of maintenance and whether a survival benefit is present with these approaches.

Several approaches of vaccination have been used in clinical trials of patients with follicular NHL. The most frequent target of vaccination approaches is the Id. In phase II clinical trials, anti-Id immune responses occur after vaccination in approximately 50% of patients, and these patients had prolonged PFS compared with historic controls.[188–190] Currently, there are randomized trials evaluating the role of Id vaccination after standard chemotherapy for patients with newly diagnosed follicular NHL.

Chemotherapy-Biologic Combinations. The highest response rates have been observed with the addition of the monoclonal antibody rituximab to chemotherapy combinations as an initial treatment strategy. A small phase II study demonstrated a very high response rate (95%) and a median PFS of approximately 5 years after the combination of CHOP chemotherapy with rituximab,[185] which led to widespread use of this regimen. The Southwest Oncology Group has reported preliminary results of a phase II trial evaluating CHOP chemotherapy followed by rituximab.[186] It did not demonstrate the same magnitude of benefit as the prior trial. Preliminary reports of randomized trials comparing CVP with and without rituximab[187] have demonstrated superior PFS with the addition of rituximab to chemotherapy, with a suggestion of an OS benefit. At the present time, the majority of patients in the United States receive a rituximab-containing regimen as initial therapy.

Radioimmunotherapy. Finally, use of the radiolabeled monoclonal antibody iodine 131 tositumomab in previously untreated patients has also been reported to produce a high CR rate. Between 1996 and 1999, 76 patients with previously untreated follicular NHL received iodine 131 (^{131}I) tositumomab therapy on a phase II, single-center study.[191] Fifty-six patients (74%) had a confirmed CR. Forty-five of these patients remained in CR with a follow-up of 30 to 66 months. The Southwest Oncology Group reported the outcome of a novel chemoimmunotherapeutic approach, combining standard induction chemotherapy (CHOP) followed by consolidation with ^{131}I tositumomab. This phase II trial included 90 patients with previously untreated advanced-stage follicular NHL.[192] The overall response rate to the entire treatment regimen (chemotherapy + ^{131}I tositumomab) was 90%, including 67% complete remissions. The 2-year PFS was estimated to be 81%, which is better than observed historically with CHOP alone[170] or CHOP with rituximab.[185] Longer follow-up and results of an ongoing randomized study are necessary before this approach can be adopted to the majority of patients.

SUMMARY: INITIAL TREATMENT OF FOLLICULAR LYMPHOMA.

Patients with early-stage follicular lymphoma should be considered for treatment with primary RT. Clearly, many treatment options exist for the majority of patients with newly diagnosed, disseminated follicular lymphoma. Whenever possible, the authors strongly encourage participation in clinical trials. Observation is an option for certain asymptomatic patients; however, this approach has no chance at improving survival for these individuals. Monoclonal antibodies, particularly rituximab, are frequently incorporated into chemotherapy regimens and have activity as a single agent for patients with nonbulky disease. For symptomatic patients, or those with bulky disease requiring a rapid response, combination chemotherapy regimens including alkylating agents or purine analogues are appropriate. The role of consolidation or maintenance therapy with rituximab, radioimmunoconjugates, Id vaccination, or more aggressive approaches, including autologous stem cell transplantation (ASCT) as part of initial therapy, remain to be defined.

THERAPY FOR PROGRESSIVE DISEASE.

Almost all patients with follicular lymphoma, despite CR to initial chemotherapy, relapse and are candidates for salvage treatment. In an asymptomatic patient, particularly if the individual is elderly, observation without treatment can be an acceptable option. Local RT can be used in a palliative manner.

A wide variety of second-line chemotherapy regimens have been used in patients with follicular lymphoma. When the initial therapy is repeated, patients with follicular lymphoma often respond. In one series using chlorambucil, the response rate was 68% for the second course of therapy, in contrast to 70% in the initial treatment.[193] Purine analogue–containing chemotherapy regimens are oten used in the relapsed setting. Preliminary results of a cooperative German study, in which patients with relapsed or refractory follicular or mantle cell lymphoma after treatment with CHOP were randomly assigned to receive four cycles of chemotherapy with fludarabine, cyclophosphamide, and mitoxantrone (FCM), with or without rituximab, reveal that overall response rates were 89% with FCM-R and 54% with FCM.[194]

Radiolabeled antibodies directed against CD20 also have high response rates in patients with relapsed follicular lymphoma.[195,196] The first radioimmunoconjugate, yttrium 90 ibritumomab tiuxetan (Zevalin, IDEC Pharmaceuticals, La Jolla, CA), was approved by the Food and Drug Administration in February 2002 for the treatment of patients with relapsed or refractory B-cell low-grade or transformed NHL, including individuals with rituximab-refractory follicular NHL. A phase III randomized study compared yttrium 90 ibritumomab tiuxetan radioimmunotherapy with rituximab in 143 patients with relapsed or refractory low-grade, follicular, or transformed CD20 (+) NHL.[197] The overall response rate was 80% for the yttrium 90 ibritumomab tiuxetan group versus 56% for the rituximab group, which reached statistical significance. However, there was no statistically significant benefit in response duration or survival between the two groups. ^{131}I tositumomab (Bexxar) has also been approved for the treatment of recurrent indolent and transformed B-cell NHL, with results similar to ibritumomab tiuxetan in the rituximab-refractory patient population.[198] Other treatments, such as use of antisense molecules, proteosome inhibitors, and tumor vaccines, have also been shown to produce objective responses.

Autologous[199,200] and allogeneic[201] HSCTs have been used for patients with relapsed follicular lymphoma. Patients transplanted after multiple treatment failures have a poorer outcome.[202] A single randomized study has been published addressing the role of autologous transplantation.[203] Patients with recurrent follicular lymphoma received three cycles of CHOP chemotherapy. Responding patients with limited bone marrow infiltration were eligible for random assignment to three further cycles of chemotherapy (C), unpurged HSCT (U), or purged HSCT (P). Due to poor accrual, the study was closed prematurely, and only 89 patients in total were randomized. With a median follow-up of 69 months, HSCT significantly improved PFS and OS compared with chemotherapy alone; however, the study was underpowered to address the purging question.

An International Bone Marrow Transplantation Registry study retrospectively evaluated 904 patients undergoing transplantation for follicular lymphoma. A total of 176 (19%) received allogeneic, 131 (14%) received purged autologous, and 597 (67%) received unpurged autologous transplants.[202] In multivariate analyses, allotransplantation had higher transplant-related mortality and lower disease recurrence. Purged autotransplantation had a 26% lower recurrence risk than unpurged autotransplantation. Five-year probabilities of survival were 51%, 62%, and 55% after allogeneic, purged autotransplantation, and unpurged autotransplantation, respectively. To decrease the transplant-related mortality associated with allogeneic transplantation and foster a graft-versus-lymphoma effect, there has been great interest in the use of nonmyeloablative conditioning regimens for patients with indolent lymphoma.[204] Studies are under way to define appropriate patients to consider for this approach.

THERAPY OF TRANSFORMED DISEASE. In a patient with follicular lymphoma who progresses with transformation to a DLBCL, treatment is almost always indicated. The clinical manifestations of histologic transformation to DLBCL typically include rapidly progressive lymphadenopathy (i.e., often localized); the development of new symptoms, such as fevers, night sweats, weight loss, and pain; or both. In general, histologic transformation to DLBCL has a poor prognosis and frequently a rapidly fatal outcome. In a series from Stanford, previously untreated patients and patients with limited disease at transformation had improved prognosis.[205] Although the median survival for all patients with transformation was only 22 months, those who achieved a CR to therapy after histologic conversion had an actuarial survival of 75% at 5 years.

Patients who have not previously received an anthracycline-containing regimen should be treated with CHOP. Other chemotherapy regimens used as salvage treatment for DLBCL (see later in Salvage Therapy) are also effective. Young patients who respond to salvage chemotherapy should be considered for consolidation with high-dose therapy and ASCT because selected patients with histologic transformation, particularly those whose transformation occurs early in the course of their disease and who remain chemosensitive, may experience prolonged survival after ASCT.[206] Significant responses, of relatively short duration, have also been observed in patients treated with radioimmunotherapy, particularly ^{131}I tositumomab.[207] Patients who respond to therapy for transformed disease often have recurrences at a later date with indolent, follicular lymphoma.

Mantle Cell Lymphoma

Mantle cell lymphoma is a neoplasm of monomorphous small to medium-sized B cells with irregular nuclei, which resemble the cleaved cells (centrocytes) of germinal centers and overexpress cyclin D1. Neoplastic transformed cells (centroblasts or immunoblasts) are absent.

MORPHOLOGY. Mantle cell lymphoma may have a diffuse, nodular mantle zone or mixed pattern in lymph nodes. Most cases are composed of monomorphous small to medium-sized lymphoid cells, with slightly irregular or "cleaved" nuclei; however, the morphology in different cases can range from lymphocyte-like to large cleaved or lymphoblast-like.

Neither neoplastic centroblasts, immunoblasts, nor pseudo-follicles are seen. Despite the small size and bland appearance of the cells, they often have more mitotic activity than other small cell lymphomas. Bone marrow involvement is typically nodular and may be paratrabecular, and the splenic white pulp may be involved. Gastrointestinal involvement may mimic MALT lymphoma; lymphoepithelial lesions are less common, but immunophenotyping may be required. On smears the cells may resemble small lymphocytes or prolymphocytes.

IMMUNOPHENOTYPE AND GENETIC FEATURES. The tumor cells express strong IgM and IgD, which is often of λ light-chain type, and strongly express B-cell–associated antigens; most coexpress CD5, similar to B-CLL/SLL, and are usually, but not always, CD23 negative. A prominent, irregular meshwork of FDC is found even in diffuse cases. Nuclear cyclin D1 protein is present in all cases and is the gold standard for the diagnosis.

Ig heavy- and light-chain genes are rearranged and lack somatic mutations in 80% or more of the cases, indicating a pregerminal center stage of differentiation. A t(11;14)(q13;q32) in the majority of the cases results in rearrangement of the *BCL1* locus and overexpression of the cyclin D1 gene, which encodes a cell-cycle–associated protein that is not normally expressed in lymphoid cells. Overexpression of this protein may explain the high proliferation fraction and aggressive clinical course of this histologically low-grade lymphoma. The translocation can be detected by fluorescence *in situ* hybridization on touch preparations, bone marrow or blood smears, or nuclei extracted from paraffin sections. More than 90% of cases have genetic abnormalities in addition to the t(11;14), detectable by classic cytogenetics or comparative genomic hybridization (CGH).[208]

Abnormalities in expression of other genes associated with the cell cycle are often present, including mutations of the CDK inhibitors p16 and p17 in blastoid variants and decreased expression of p27, another CDK inhibitor, in the majority of the cases.[209] Cases of the blastoid variant have a high incidence of tetraploidy and p53 gene mutations.[210] Ataxia-telangiectasia mutations are frequent.[211]

Molecular profiling of gene expression in mantle cell lymphoma has shown abnormalities of apoptosis-regulating pathways favoring cellular survival, when compared with normal B lymphocytes.[212] Microarray analysis detects distinct signatures in mantle cell lymphoma compared with SLL and marginal zone lymphoma.[213]

POSTULATED NORMAL COUNTERPART. Mantle cell lymphoma is thought to correspond in most cases to a naive B cell of follicle mantle or germinal center origin that is distinct from the recirculating B cell of B-CLL/SLL and the later centrocyte of follicle center lymphomas.

CLINICAL FEATURES. Mantle cell lymphoma accounts for approximately 7% of adult NHLs in the United States and Europe.[89] In a review of 376 cases of disseminated low-grade lymphoma (Working Formulation categories A through E), mantle cell lymphoma made up 10%.[214] It is a tumor of older adults, with a marked male predominance (75%). The majority (70%) of patients are in stage IV at diagnosis; sites involved include lymph nodes, spleen, Waldeyer's ring, bone marrow (greater than 60%), blood (up to 50%), and extranodal sites, especially the gastrointestinal tract (lymphomatous polyposis).[215] The course is moderately aggressive. The median OS in most series is 3 years, with no plateau in the curve, and failure-free survival is approximately 1 year. The blastoid variant is reported in some studies to be more aggressive.[216]

THERAPY. Because mantle cell lymphoma was widely accepted as an entity only in the last decade, the number of therapeutic trials is not as extensive as for some other types of NHL. Localized mantle cell lymphoma is quite rare, seen in only 13% of unselected patients in one large series.[35] The failure-free survival of patients treated for localized mantle cell lymphoma is quite poor, suggesting that unrecognized dissemination was usually present. The optimal treatment for these patients is not known. Approaches reported in these individuals include involved-field radiation and the combination of CHOP chemotherapy and involved-field irradiation.

Most patients present with disseminated disease. Single-agent chemotherapy has been used less commonly than in other small cell lymphomas, with chlorambucil, fludarabine, and cladribine being the most commonly used agents. The most frequently used combination regimens have been CVP and CHOP. Overall response rates have ranged between 60% and 80% and CR rates between 30% and 60%. A randomized trial comparing CVP and CHOP showed no significant difference in OS (84% vs. 88%) and failure-free survival (41% vs. 58%).[217] A phase II study evaluated the combination of CHOP and rituximab for newly diagnosed mantle cell lymphoma and demonstrated an improved response rate, with no evidence of prolongation of PFS.[218] Other regimens including rituximab and chemotherapy appear very active in short follow-up.[194]

A chemotherapy regimen that was originally used for patients with leukemia, called *hyper-CVAD* (cyclophosphamide, vincristine, doxorubicin, dexamethasone), has been used in mantle cell lymphoma and has a high CR rate.[219] In a historic control study from M. D. Anderson Cancer Center, hyper-CVAD had a superior 3-year event-free survival to CHOP (72% vs. 28%). Sequential phase II studies using this regimen have incorporated consolidation with either high-dose chemotherapy and ASCT or with rituximab, with similar outcomes.

Because of the poor long-term outlook, patients with mantle cell lymphoma who are sufficiently young and healthy often undergo autologous or allogeneic bone marrow transplantation at best response. The long-term benefits of autologous and allogeneic transplantation are still uncertain,[220] although long-term survivors with both approaches are reported. A study from M. D. Anderson Cancer Center evaluating 18 patients who were treated with a nonmyeloablative conditioning regimen and allogeneic stem cell support suggested safety of this approach, with 82% survival median of 26 months' follow-up.[221]

Patients who relapse and are not candidates for transplantation or those who relapse after transplantation can be treated with rituximab or salvage chemotherapy regimens. A preliminary report including 22 patients with relapsed or refractory mantle cell lymphoma has demonstrated a 55% response rate to the proteosome inhibitor bortezomib.[222] Confirmatory studies are ongoing evaluating this agent. Finally, the authors have observed that advanced-stage patients with mantle cell lymphomas are very responsive to low doses of RT (20 to 25 Gy), allowing for large fields to be used for bulky disease not responsive to chemotherapy. CRs are often achieved with these doses that are durable and significantly improve patient quality of life.

Given the relatively poor prognosis of patients with mantle cell lymphoma, the authors strongly advocate participation in clinical trials of novel agents. Young patients should be considered for high-dose therapy and autologous or allogeneic stem cell support. Long-term follow-up of ongoing studies is required to determine the optimal induction chemotherapy regimen.

Diffuse Large B-Cell Lymphoma

DLBCL is a neoplasm of large, transformed B cells with nuclear size equal to or exceeding that of a normal macrophage or more than twice the size of a normal lymphocyte. The cytologic features differ among cases, and morphologic and clinical variants exist. This is a heterogeneous category, likely containing diverse entities. DLBCL as described here is primary, but cases may arise through transformation of small B-cell lymphomas, such as small lymphocytic, lymphoplasmacytic, splenic marginal zone, extranodal marginal zone, and follicular lymphomas.

MORPHOLOGY. DLBCLs are a heterogeneous group of neoplasms. They are typically composed of large cells (3 times the size of normal lymphocytes) that resemble centroblasts or immunoblasts, most often with a mixture of the two. Several morphologic variants can be recognized, but their clinical significance is debated. The centroblastic type (80% of the cases) is composed of cells resembling germinal center centroblasts, with one to three peripheral nucleoli and a narrow rim of basophilic cytoplasm, often with a variable admixture of immunoblasts. Some cases have multilobated centroblasts. The immunoblastic type (10% of the cases) has more than 90% immunoblasts with a prominent central nucleolus and abundant, basophilic cytoplasm, often with plasmacytoid differentiation. These cases are more common in immunosuppressed patients. In nonimmunosuppressed patients, they have been reported in some studies to have a worse prognosis, whereas others have failed to confirm this. In the anaplastic type, the cells are morphologically similar to those of T/null ALCL, with pleomorphic nuclei, abundant cytoplasm and sinusoidal growth pattern, and CD30 expression. Although these have been called *B-ALCL*, they do not have the same distinctive clinical or genetic features of T/null ALCL and are considered a morphologic variant of large B-cell lymphoma. Two other distinctive morphologic and immunophenotypic variants of DLBCL are the plasmablastic type, which often occurs in HIV-positive patients, and a rare ALK-positive variant with a translocation involving the ALK protein.

T-CELL–RICH/HISTIOCYTE-RICH LARGE B-CELL LYMPHOMA. Some cases of large B-cell lymphoma have a prominent background of reactive T cells and, often, histiocytes, so-called T-cell or histiocyte-rich large B-cell lymphoma.[223] They may resemble Hodgkin's lymphoma of either lymphocyte predominance or mixed-cellularity type. In contrast to those with Hodgkin's lymphoma, patients with T-cell/histiocyte-rich large B-cell lymphoma typically present with disseminated disease involving the liver and spleen and have an aggressive clinical course, but with OS similar to that of DLBCL of the usual type.[224] The relationship of this disease to lymphocyte predominance or classic Hodgkin's lymphoma, or both, remains to be elucidated. Genetic analysis using CGH has shown that nodular lymphocyte predominance Hodgkin's lymphoma cells have a greater number of genetic imbalances than T-cell–rich large B-cell lymphoma, suggesting that they are distinct entities.

BONE MARROW INVOLVEMENT IN DIFFUSE LARGE B-CELL LYMPHOMA. Bone marrow involvement in DLBCL may take two forms. In approximately 10% of the cases, large cell lymphoma is present in the marrow. However, approximately 20% may show so-called discordant marrow involvement, aggregates of small atypical lymphoid cells consistent with involvement by low-grade lymphoma, particularly follicular lymphoma.[225] Several studies have shown that discordant marrow involvement is not associated with CNS involvement, in contrast to marrow involvement wit DLBCL, and the OS is similar to that of patients of similar stage with negative bone marrows; however, late relapses are more common.[226]

IMMUNOPHENOTYPE AND GENETIC FEATURES. DLBCLs express one or more B-cell–associated antigens (CD19, CD20, CD22, CD79a), as well as CD45 and often sIg. They may coexpress CD5 or CD10. In various studies, 25% to 80% express bcl-2 protein, and this may be associated with a worse prognosis.[227] Approximately 70% express bcl-6 protein, consistent with a germinal center origin, independent of bcl-6 gene rearrangement.

The only marker clearly associated with prognosis at this time is expression of bcl-2 protein, which is associated with a worse progosis.[228] A number of studies have attempted to define germinal center and non–germinal center phenotypes in DLBCL, using markers such as bcl-6, CD10 (germinal center), and MUM1/IRF4 and CD138 (post–germinal center). In some anatomic sites, a germinal center immunophenotype, particularly bcl-6 expression, has been associated with a better prognosis.[229]

Ig genes are rearranged, and most have somatic mutations in the variable region genes. The *BCL2* gene is rearranged in 15% to 30%; it is associated with disseminated nodal disease but not with either a worse prognosis or with bcl-2 protein expression. The *c-MYC* gene is rearranged in 5% to 15%, and the *BCL6* gene is rearranged in 20% to 40% of cases and shows mutations in the 5' noncoding region in 70%.[230] The 5' noncoding mutations of the bcl-6 gene and the Ig variable region gene mutations are found in normal germinal center cells; their presence in DLBCL is consistent with a germinal center or post–germinal center stage of differentiation. Microarray analysis of gene expression by one group has delineated three categories of DLBCL: one with a germinal center–like signature, one with an activated B-cell signature, and a third, intermediate group.[231] Signatures have been shown to correlate with survival by some but not others.[232]

POSTULATED NORMAL COUNTERPART. Proliferating peripheral B cells include centroblasts or immunoblasts in most cases.

CLINICAL FEATURES. DLBCL was the most common lymphoma in the international study of the REAL, accounting for 31% of the cases.[89] Patients typically present with a rapidly enlarging symptomatic mass, with B symptoms in one-third of the cases. Localized (stage I or II) extranodal disease occurs in up to 30%; bone marrow involvement was seen in only 16%. Up to 40% of DLBCLs are extranodal; common sites include the gastrointestinal tract, bone, and CNS. The prognosis was highly associated with the IPI score. Large B-cell lymphoma may occur as a high-grade transformation of several low-grade B-cell lymphomas (B-CLL, lymphoplasmacytic lymphoma, follicular lymphoma, MALT lymphoma, SMZL). DLBCL of certain extranodal sites, such as the CNS, may be clinically distinctive and may have specific treatment protocols.

THERAPY OF LOCALIZED DIFFUSE LARGE B-CELL LYMPHOMA. Four prospective randomized trials have further evaluated the role of RT in patients with early-stage DLBCL (Table 41.2-11). The Southwest Oncology Group trial randomized 401 stage I and nonbulky stage II patients to receive either three cycles of CHOP and involved-field irradiation (40 to 55 Gy) or eight cycles of CHOP alone.[233] The 5-year PFS (77% vs. 64%, $P = .03$) and OS (82% vs. 72%, $P = .02$) results favored the CHOP and involved-field RT treatment arm, although at 5 to 10 years this survival benefit is less apparent, with late disease recurrences observed in the RT arm. A separate analysis of PFS and OS was performed using a modified IPI. Patients with zero or one risk factor had a higher PFS and OS compared to those with two or three risk factors. As a result of this trial, combination chemotherapy and adjuvant RT have become the standard care for patients with stage I to II DLBCL. Individuals with a higher modified IPI or poor prognostic pretreatment factors have a higher recurrence risk, suggesting that new treatment approaches are needed for these patients.

The Eastern Cooperative Oncology Group randomized 352 patients with bulky stage I (mediastinal or retroperitoneal involvement or masses greater than 10 cm), stage IE, and stage II to IIE disease to eight cycles of CHOP chemotherapy with or without RT. Patients with no response or progression to chemotherapy were removed from the study. Individuals in complete remission were randomized to 30 Gy involved-

TABLE 41.2-11. Chemotherapy versus Combined Modality Therapy for Stage I/II Intermediate- or High-Grade Lymphoma: Prospective Randomized Trials

Study	Patients (n)	Stage	CT	RT Dose (Gy)	% CR or PR	% FFS	% Survival (Y)
ECOG[234]	352	CS I (EN/B) and all CS II, CS I–II	CHOP × 8 (CR)	—	61 (CR)	58	70 (6)
			CHOP × 8 (CR)	30 (IF)	—	73[a]	84 (6)[b]
			CHOP × 8 (PR)	40 (IF)	28 (PR)	60	64 (6)
SWOG[233]	401	CS I/IE (B/NB) and CS II (NB)	CHOP × 8	—	73	64	72 (5)
			CHOP × 3	40–55	75	77[a]	82 (50)[a]
GELA[235]	518	IPI 0, 1	CHOP × 4	—	—	69	78
		CS I–II	CHOP × 4	40	—	64	70
GELA[236]	631	CS I–II	ACVBP	—	—	83[b]	89[b]
		Low risk	CHOP × 3	30–40	—	74	80

B, bulky disease; CR, complete response; CT, chemotherapy; ECOG, Eastern Cooperative Oncology Group; EN, extranodal; FFS, failure-free survival; GELA, Groupe d'Etude des Lymphomes de l'Adulte; IF, involved field; IPI, International Prognostic Index; NB, no bulky disease; PR, partial response; RT, radiation therapy; SWOG, Southwest Oncology Group.
[a]Significant difference between RT and no RT; borderline significant difference between RT and no RT, $P = .06$.
[b]Significantly better result with ACVBP (doxorubicin, cyclophosphamide, vindesine, bleomycin, prednisone).

field RT or no further treatment.[234] Patients in partial remission received 40 Gy to the site(s) of pretreatment involvement plus radiation to contiguous uninvolved region(s). In patients randomized after complete unmission, the 5-year disease-free survival (73% vs. 58%, P = .03), freedom from recurrence (73% vs. 58%, P = .04), and survival (84% vs. 70%, P = .06) all favored the patients who received adjuvant involved-field irradiation.[58] At 10 years, the disease-free survival continues to favor the addition of RT (57% vs. 46%, P = .04), but the survival differences no longer are statistically significant, similar to the aforementioned Southwest Oncology Group trial. In the patients who achieved a partial remission, 28% converted to a complete remission with the addition of 40 Gy RT. To date, the detailed results of this study have not been published.

The results of two European randomized trials were presented as abstracts at the 2002 American Society of Hematology meetings. Fillet and Bonnet[235] compared CHOP × 4 with CHOP × 4 followed by 40 Gy in 518 patients more than 60 years of age who all had an age-adjusted IPI score of zero. The 5-year event-free survival (CHOP 69% vs. CHOP + RT 64%) and OS (CHOP 78% vs. CHOP + RT 70%) did not differ between the two regimens. Additional follow-up of this study is required before definitive conclusions are made. Reyes et al.[236] compared CHOP × 3 followed by 30 to 40 Gy involved-field radiotherapy with the chemotherapy regimen ACVBP (doxorubicin, cyclophosphamide, vindesine, bleomycin, prednisone) followed by consolidation chemotherapy using methotrexate, ifosfamide, etoposide, and cytarabine in 631 patients with low-risk, localized aggressive lymphoma. Event-free survival (CHOP + RT 74% vs. ACVBP 83%) and OS (CHOP + RT 80% vs. ACVBP 89%) was significantly better in the chemotherapy-alone arm. Unfortunately, a significant number of patients in this study had bulky disease, and for these individuals CHOP × 3 + RT would have been predicted to be inadequate.

In summary, abbreviated CHOP chemotherapy plus involved-field RT is excellent therapy for patients with low-risk, nonbulky early-stage DLBCL. Patients with poor prognostic features, such as advanced stage, tumor bulk, or high LDH, may benefit from additional systemic therapy or clinical trials involving novel agents.

THERAPY OF DISSEMINATED DIFFUSE LARGE B-CELL LYMPHOMA. Disseminated DLBCL is a curable disease. More than 40 randomized clinical trials have been reported to identify the best treatment regimen for patients with advanced diffuse aggressive lymphoma. The majority of these trials have not found a significant treatment advantage for any particular regimen. The most widely quoted trial was carried out in the United States comparing CHOP, m-BACOD, ProMACE/CytaBOM, and MACOP-B (Table 41.2-12).[237] This trial was carried out because of enthusiasm generated by single-arm trials showing apparent superiority of m-BACOD, ProMACE/CytaBOM, and MACOP-B over the older CHOP regimen. This study of 899 patients showed no improvement in failure-free survival or OS with the newer regimen but did find increased toxicity with m-BACOD and MACOP-B. The 6-year OS for the four regimens were CHOP, 33%; m-BACOD, 36%; ProMACE/CytaBOM, 34%; and MACOP-B, 32%. The conclusion from the study was that the less complicated and less expensive CHOP regimen should be considered the treatment of choice. This has been widely applied, and today most patients with DLBCL or other aggressive lymphomas receive CHOP-based chemotherapy.

Attempts have been made to improve the response to CHOP by combining it with the monoclonal antibody rituximab. An early study of 33 patients showed a 97% response rate and a 73% CR rate.[238] The Groupe d'Etude des Lymphomes de l'Adulte (GELA) group randomized 399 previously untreated patients with DLBCL, 60 to 80 years old, to receive either eight cycles of CHOP every 3 weeks or eight cycles of CHOP plus rituximab given on day 1 of each cycle.[239] With a median follow-up of 2 years, the addition of rituximab to the CHOP regimen increased the CR rate (76% vs. 63%, P = .005) and prolonged event-free survival and OS in these patients, without a clinically significant increase in toxicity. A larger (n = 632) intergroup United States study randomized a similar population of patients to CHOP versus CHOP with rituximab given on a different schedule,[185] as described in follicular lymphoma.[240] Responding patients then were randomized to receive either rituximab maintenance therapy (4 doses every 6 months for 2 years) or no maintenance. Preliminary results suggest a PFS benefit to the addition of rituximab; however, no OS benefit is yet apparent.

Based largely on the published results from GELA, CHOP with rituximab therapy (all therapy administered on day 1) has emerged to become the standard initial treatment for advanced-stage DLBCL in the United States. An unplanned subgroup analysis of the GELA trial demonstrated that the benefit of rituximab appeared limited to patients with lymphoma that overexpressed bcl-2 on immunohistochemistry.[241]

TABLE 41.2-12. Treatment of Aggressive Non-Hodgkin's Lymphoma (Approximately 80% Diffuse Large B Cell): A Comparison of Four Regimens

Regimen	Complete Remission (%)	Partial Remission (%)[a]	3-Y Failure-Free Survival (%)	Overall Survival (%)
CHOP	44	36	41	54
m-BACOD	48	34	46	52
ProMACE/CytaBOM	56	31	46	50
MACOP-B	51	32	41	50

[a]Some patients who responded partially had only a residual mass on imaging studies and might actually have been in complete remission.

Ongoing research will better define groups of patients with large cell lymphoma who benefit from monoclonal antibody therapy.

Other attempts to improve the response to CHOP involve adjuvant therapy with high-dose therapy and autologous bone marrow transplantation.[242] Several studies have now concluded that all patients with aggressive lymphoma do not benefit when stem cell transplantation is incorporated into their initial treatment strategy compared with patients who are treated with conventional strategy of initial chemotherapy followed by stem cell transplant at first relapse.[243,244] Thus, there seems to be no indication to add ASCT to the initial combination chemotherapy treatment for *all* patients with aggressive lymphoma.

However, when the IPI[88] was retrospectively applied to the GELA LNH-87 study, a failure-free (59% vs. 39%) and OS benefit (65% vs. 52%) was demonstrated for the high-/intermediate-risk and high-risk groups.[245] A retrospective subset analysis of an Italian trial yielded similar results.[246]

All positive trials have incorporated a standard course of induction therapy (rather than an abbreviated course) before consolidative transplantation. An international consensus conference reached the conclusion that autologous high-dose therapy and autotransplantation in patients with high-risk IPI scores seemed to provide benefit,[247] and this is the subject of an ongoing intergroup randomized trial in the United States. At the present time, the authors do not recommend routine use of ASCT as consolidative therapy for newly diagnosed large cell lymphoma outside a clinical trial.

SALVAGE THERAPY. The phrase *salvage therapy* encompasses subsequent treatment administered to patients who failed to achieve an initial remission and the treatment administered to patients who relapse from complete remission. A major prognostic factor for patients receiving any form of salvage therapy relates to the chemotherapy sensitivity of the lymphoma (i.e., those who achieve an initial complete remission and then relapse generally have a better prognosis than patients who are primarily resistant to chemotherapy). Patients with lymphoma that progresses on the previous chemotherapy regimen have a poorer outlook than those who have stable or partially responding disease. Patients who have been in complete remission and then relapse require a rebiopsy before salvage therapy is initiated. Some patients who present with DLBCL are found to have a follicular lymphoma at the time of relapse.

The initial step in planning salvage chemotherapy is to determine the goal of treatment. Some patients who fail to achieve an initial remission or relapse from complete remission can be cured. This is less likely in elderly patients, those with extensive disease, and those with a poor performance status. In such patients less intensive, palliative treatments might be better pursued.

Radiotherapy can frequently be used to alleviate the symptoms at a particular site of involvement in patients with relapsed DLBCL. This can frequently be accomplished with minimal morbidity. However, the chance for cure with salvage radiotherapy is extremely small. Palliative chemotherapy approaches include single-agent treatment with vincristine, cytarabine, alkylating agents, or anthracyclines. Responses to single-agent rituximab occur approximately 30% of the time and are generally of brief duration.[248]

Most patients receive second-line combination chemotherapy regimens. These regimens usually incorporate drugs such as cisplatin, ifosfamide, etoposide, and cytarabine, often in combination with rituximab. For example, Memorial Sloan-Kettering Cancer Center has published results of ICE chemotherapy (ifosfamide, carboplatin, and etoposide), in patients with recurrent aggressive NHL.[249] The overall response rate was 66%, with no treatment-related mortality. This was a very effective cytoreduction and mobilization regimen in patients with NHL and has become a widely used salvage option for those who are eligible for subsequent ASCT. The chances for achieving a complete remission with salvage therapy have varied widely in different studies but generally fall in the 20% to 40% range. A subset of completely responding patients can be long-term survivors, with the overall cure rate for salvage chemotherapy in patients with relapsed DLBCL being approximately 5% to 10%.

An international randomized trial referred to as the *PARMA study* defined the role of bone marrow transplant in relapsed DLBCL.[104] In this trial, 109 patients who had relapsed from complete remission and responded to two cycles of DHAP (dexamethasone, cytarabine, and cisplatin) were randomly allocated to high-dose chemotherapy using the BEAC regimen (carmustine, etoposide, cytarabine, cyclophosphamide) or continued treatment with DHAP. Both groups were to receive involved-field radiotherapy. Bone marrow transplantation was associated with a superior failure-free survival (51% vs. 12% at 5 years) and OS (53% vs. 32% at 5 years). It is important to remember that the trial enrolled only young patients at first relapse who remained chemosensitive. Although this is the only randomized trial in this patient population, a United States cooperative group phase II trial achieved nearly identical results in a similar patient population.[250] Salvage ABMT, as currently used, results in survival of approximately 50% of all patients who actually receive transplants; however, it only adds 10% to the number of newly diagnosed patients with aggressive lymphoma who can be cured with CHOP chemotherapy, because only a minority of all patients meet all the selection criteria for transplantation. For these patients, however, high-dose therapy and autologous bone marrow transplantation are the treatments of choice.

Allogeneic bone marrow transplantation has been used less frequently for patients with DLBCL. Although occasional patients failing autologous transplantation can have prolonged survival with allogeneic transplantation, overall results from the North American Bone Marrow Transplant Registry have favored autologous transplantation. In a report from the European Bone Marrow Transplantation Registry, recurrence rates after allogeneic transplantation were lower than those after autologous transplantation.[251] However, there was no OS advantage due to increased transplant-related mortality after allogeneic transplantation. Ongoing studies in high-risk patients are evaluating "tandem" transplantation (autologous transplant followed by nonmyeloablative allogeneic transplantation), with encouraging preliminary results.

Primary Mediastinal (Thymic) Large B-Cell Lymphoma

Mediastinal (thymic) large B-cell lymphoma is a subtype of DLBCL arising in the mediastinum, of putative thymic B-cell origin, with distinctive clinical, immunophenotypic, and genotypic features.

MORPHOLOGY. Primary mediastinal large B-cell lymphoma usually involves the thymus at presentation. The tumor is composed of large cells with variable nuclear features, resembling centroblasts, large centrocytes, or multilobated cells, often with pale or "clear" cytoplasm. Less often, the tumor cells resemble immunoblasts. Reed-Sternberg–like cells may be present. Many patients have fine, compartmentalizing sclerosis.

IMMUNOPHENOTYPE AND GENETIC FEATURES. The tumor cells are usually Ig negative but express B-cell–associated antigens (CD19, CD20, CD22, CD79a) and CD45.[270] Most cases are bcl-6 positive, and approximately 25% are CD10 positive. Ig heavy- and light-chain genes are rearranged; the bcl-2 gene is usually germline. Bcl-6 gene rearrangements are uncommon. Amplification of the *REL* oncogene has been described in some cases. Expression of the MAL gene associated with T-cell development and the interleukin-4–expressed gene 1 has been demonstrated to be characteristic of primary mediastinal B-cell lymphoma and not other DLBCLs. Analyses of gene expression using microarray technology have shown an expression signature distinct from nodal DLBCL and resembling, in some respects, that of classic Hodgkin's lymphoma, including activation of the JAK-2 and NFκ pathways.[252]

POSTULATED NORMAL COUNTERPART. The postulated normal counterpart is a B cell of the thymic medulla.

DIFFERENTIAL DIAGNOSIS. The major differential diagnoses clinically are thymoma, germ cell tumor, and Hodgkin's disease.

CLINICAL FEATURES AND THERAPY. Primary DLBCL of the mediastinum is a distinct clinicopathologic entity, requiring knowledge of morphology, immunophenotype, and presenting site for the diagnosis.[89] It accounted for 7% of DLBCLs (2.4% of all NHLs) in the international REAL study. It has a female predominance and a median age in the fourth decade; patients present with a locally invasive anterior mediastinal mass originating in the thymus, with frequent airway compromise and superior vena cava syndrome.[253] Relapses tend to be extranodal, including liver, gastrointestinal tract, kidneys, ovaries, and CNS.

Although early studies suggested an unusually aggressive, incurable tumor, others have reported cure rates similar to those for other large cell lymphomas with aggressive therapy, usually combining chemotherapy with mediastinal irradiation. With no evidence to the contrary, the authors recommend treating these patients similarly to other patients with localized diffuse large cell lymphoma (i.e., CHOP ± rituximab and involved-field RT). The prognosis of patients with localized mediastinal large cell NHL is similar to that of other patients with poor-prognosis early-stage disease; approximately 50% of patients are alive without disease at 5 years. Individuals who present with a pleural effusion or who remain gallium positive after CHOP have a worse prognosis. Patients without bulky disease have a better prognosis. Individuals with disseminated disease should be treated like other patients with disseminated DLBCL.

In a study by Zinzani et al.,[254] 50 patients with primary mediastinal large B-cell lymphoma were prospectively treated with MACOP-B followed by RT. CT and gallium 67 citrate single-photon emission (GaSPECT) were obtained at diagnosis, at the end of chemotherapy, and at 3 months after RT. Three patients with progressive disease during chemotherapy were excluded from the analysis. After chemotherapy, 31 of 47 (66%) patients had a positive GaSPECT. Among these 31 patients, 22 became GaSPECT negative after RT. None of the patients with a negative GaSPECT after treatment relapsed at a median follow-up of 39 months.

Intravascular Large B-Cell Lymphoma

Rare cases of large cell lymphoma, usually of B-cell type, present with a disseminated intravascular proliferation of large lymphoid cells, involving small blood vessels, without an obvious extravascular tumor mass or leukemia. This tumor has also been variously known as *intravascular lymphomatosis*, *angiotropic lymphoma*, and *malignant angioendotheliomatosis*. The neoplastic lymphoid cells are mainly lodged in the lumina of small vessels in many organs. The tumor cells may resemble centroblasts or immunoblasts and express B cell–associated antigens. Malignant cells are rarely seen in cerebrospinal fluid, blood, or bone marrow. The organs most commonly involved are CNS, kidneys, lungs, and skin, but virtually any site may be involved. Patients present with a variety of symptoms related to organ dysfunction secondary to vascular occlusion. Because of this, the diagnosis is difficult, and many reported cases were diagnosed at autopsy. If a timely diagnosis is made and combination chemotherapy instituted, many patients achieve complete remission, and long-term survival appears to be possible.[283]

Large B-Cell Lymphoma, Lymphomatoid Granulomatosis Type

The entity described as lymphomatoid granulomatosis has been shown in most cases to be an EBV-positive large B-cell lymphoma with a T-cell–rich background.[255] Patients typically present with extranodal disease, most commonly involving lung, CNS, and/or kidneys. Evidence of past or present immunosuppression may be found. The infiltrates show extensive necrosis, often with only a few atypical large B cells in a background of small T lymphocytes; the infiltrate may be angiocentric as well as angioinvasive. Although the infiltrates may resemble those of nasal-type NK/T-cell lymphoma, there is no biologic and little clinical overlap, because the latter is an NK/T-cell neoplasm that involves the upper airway and midfacial region, skin, and sometimes the gastrointestinal tract, but only rarely the lung or CNS. Lymphomatoid granulomatosis is graded according to the number of large B cells. The lower-grade cases are not typically treated as lymphoma; grade 3 cases fulfill the criteria for large B-cell lymphoma in a T cell–rich background and may be clinically aggressive. The prognosis for this entity is variable and in general is approached like disseminated DLBCL. In addition to combination chemotherapy, responses have been reported using interferon-α and high-dose therapy and autologous stem cell support.[255]

Primary Effusion Lymphoma

Primary effusion lymphoma is a recently recognized disease that occurs most often in immunosuppressed patients, either with HIV or in the posttransplant setting, but occasional cases in nonimmunosuppressed patients have been reported.[30] Patients present with effusions in serous cavities—pleura, pericardium, or peritoneum. Occasionally, infiltration of other tissues may be seen. The clinical course is usually very aggressive. The tumor cells are large, often pleomorphic cells resembling either bizarre plasma cells or the cells of ALCL. They often lack B cell–associated antigens such as CD20 and are bcl-6 negative but may be CD79a positive and CD45 positive, sometimes contain cytoplasmic Ig, and often express CD30 and the plasma cell–associated antigen CD138. Ig genes are clonally rearranged. They typically contain EBV and the Kaposi's sarcoma herpesvirus/HHV-8.[256] The prognosis of this disease is poor.

Burkitt's Lymphoma

Burkitt's lymphoma is a highly aggressive B-cell neoplasm, often presenting in extranodal sites or as an acute leukemia, composed of monomorphic, medium-sized cells with basophilic cytoplasm and a high proliferation fraction. Translocation and deregulation of *C-MYC* on chromosome 8 is a constant feature. EBV is found in a proportion of the cases. The morphology, immunophenotype, and genetics of Burkitt's lymphoma are discussed in detail in Chapter 40.

Burkitt's lymphoma was one of the first malignancies to be shown to be curable with chemotherapy,[257] and the majority of adult patients should be curable today with aggressive combination chemotherapy regimens. High-dose regimens (such as CODOX-M-IVAC) of fairly brief duration are used to treat patients with Burkitt's lymphoma.[258] Importantly, these regimens include higher doses of alkylating agents than CHOP. Patients with localized disease are cured in approximately 90% of the cases with these intensive regimens, and cure rates within excess of 50% have been reported in patients with extensive disease. When treated with similar regimens, adults and children have comparable outcomes.[258] Because of the propensity for CNS metastases, treatment regimens for Burkitt's lymphoma always involve prophylactic therapy to the CNS. Salvage therapy for patients with relapsed Burkitt's lymphoma has generally been unsatisfactory. However, occasional patients can be cured with autologous bone marrow transplantation.[259]

T-CELL AND NATURAL KILLER CELL NEOPLASMS

Precursor T-Lymphoblastic Lymphoma/Leukemia (Precursor T-Cell Acute Lymphoblastic Leukemia/Precursor T-Cell Lymphoblastic Lymphoma)

Precursor T-lymphoblastic lymphoma/leukemia is a neoplasm of lymphoblasts committed to the T-cell lineage, typically composed of small to medium-sized blast cells with scant cytoplasm, moderately condensed to dispersed chromatin and indistinct nucleoli, variably involving bone marrow and blood (precursor T-cell acute lymphoblastic leukemia), thymus, and/or lymph nodes (precursor T-lymphoblastic lymphoma). The morphology, immunophenotype and genetic features, and therapy are discussed in detail in Chapter 42. Clinically, a case is defined as lymphoma if there is a mediastinal or other mass and fewer than 25% blasts in the bone marrow and as leukemia if there are greater than 25% bone marrow blasts, with or without a

mass. Therapy should be similar to regimens used to treat acute lymphocytic leukemia.

Mature T Cell: Mycosis Fungoides

For a discussion of mycosis fungoides, see Chapter 41.3.

Adult T-Cell Lymphoma and Leukemia

Adult T-cell lymphoma and leukemia is a peripheral T-cell neoplasm usually composed of highly pleomorphic cells, caused by the human retrovirus, human T-cell leukemia virus type 1 (HTLV-1).

MORPHOLOGY. In lymph nodes, the infiltrate is diffuse with architectural effacement. Neoplastic cells are usually medium to large sized with nuclear pleomorphism. Reed-Sternberg–like cells and giant cells with convoluted or cerebriform nuclei may be present. Rare cases may be composed of small atypical lymphocytes or may resemble ALCL. Cells with hyperlobated nuclei (flower cells) are common in the peripheral blood in leukemic cases. Bone marrow infiltrates are usually patchy.

IMMUNOPHENOTYPE AND GENETIC FEATURES. Tumor cells express T-cell–associated antigens (CD2, CD3, CD5) but usually lack CD7. Most cases are CD4+, CD8–. Rare cases are CD4–, CD8+ or CD8+, CD4+. CD25 is typically positive. Some cells may be CD30+, but they are ALK negative.

Clonally integrated HTLV-1 genes are found in all cases. The TCR genes are clonally rearranged.[260] Abnormalities of chromosome 14q11, involving the TCRα gene, 14q32 involving the IgH gene, deletions at 6q, trisomy 3, and monosomy X and Y are common.[261] Complex karyotypes may be associated with a worse prognosis. Several viral genes appear to be involved in lymphomagenesis.

POSTULATED NORMAL COUNTERPART. The normal counterparts are peripheral CD4+ T cells in various stages of transformation.

CLINICAL FEATURES. ATL is one manifestation of infection by HTLV-1. Tropical spastic paraparesis and HTLV-1–associated myelopathy appear to be more common manifestations of infection than ATL. The diagnosis is established when a patient with a typical clinical and pathologic syndrome is found to have antibodies to HTLV-1. Most patients are adults, although children are occasionally seen with the disorder when they received transfusions in infancy. The virus can be acquired by vertical transmission from mother to child, sexual transmission, or via blood products. Most cases occur in Japan or the Caribbean, with sporadic cases found elsewhere in the world.

In the United States, the diagnosis is frequently difficult; ATL is not considered because many clinicians are not acquainted with the syndrome. Several variants have been described depending on the clinical features: acute, lymphomatous, chronic, and smoldering. The most common *acute type* presents with neoplastic cells in the blood, skin rashes, generalized lymphadenopathy, hepatosplenomegaly, and hypercalcemia. The *lymphomatous type* is characterized by prominent lymphadenopathy but no blood involvement. The *chronic type* shows skin lesions and an increased white blood cell count with absolute lymphocytosis but no hypercalcemia. The *smoldering type* shows normal blood lymphocyte counts, with 5% circulating neoplastic cells. Patients frequently have skin or pulmonary lesions, but hypercalcemia is not present. Progression from chronic and smoldering to acute types eventually occurs in up to 25% of the cases. Peripheral blood and bone marrow are the most frequent sites of involvement, but any organ can be involved by the disease, including gastrointestinal tract, liver, lung, and CNS.

THERAPY. The treatment of ATL has been unsatisfactory. Patients with the chronic or smoldering syndromes can sometimes be followed without therapy for extended periods of time. When the disease becomes asymptomatic, combination chemotherapy regimens have usually been used. Although patients may respond to the initial combination chemotherapy regimen, the OS remains poor, with fewer than 10% of the patients surviving 5 years after the initiation of therapy. A variety of the new treatment approaches has been studied, including new chemotherapeutic agents, monoclonal antibodies, biologic agents, and allogeneic bone marrow transplantation. In one study, 15 patients with T-cell leukemia/lymphoma, 8 of whom were in partial or complete remission, were treated with interferon-α and zidovudine.[262] Median survival of the nonresponders was 6 months, whereas 55% of the responders were alive at 4 years.

Peripheral T-Cell Lymphoma, Not Otherwise Categorized

Peripheral T-cell lymphoma, not otherwise categorized, comprises a group of predominantly nodal and occasionally extranodal T-cell lymphomas, which do not have consistent immunophenotypic, genetic, or clinical features. Therefore, for the time being, these presumably diverse cases are lumped under the heading peripheral T-cell lymphoma, not otherwise categorized, or unspecified. This category includes heterogeneous diseases that require further definition.

MORPHOLOGY. Peripheral T-cell lymphomas, not otherwise categorized, typically contain a mixture of small and large atypical cells and are classified as diffuse small cleaved, mixed, large cell, and immunoblastic in the Working Formulation. Admixed eosinophils or epithelioid histiocytes may be numerous; the term *lymphoepithelioid cell (Lennert's) lymphoma* has been used for cases rich in epithelioid cells. Because of their relative rarity and heterogeneity, it has been impossible to arrive at a generally useful classification. For the time being, these tumors are simply designated "peripheral T-cell lymphomas, unspecified."

IMMUNOPHENOTYPE AND GENETIC FEATURES. T-cell–associated antigens are variably expressed, and aberrant phenotypes are common (CD3+/– CD2+/– CD5+/– CD7–/+); CD4 is more often expressed than CD8, and tumors may be CD4– CD8–. B-cell–associated antigens are for the most part lacking, although CD20+ cases have been reported. The TCR genes are usually clonally rearranged; Ig genes are germline. Most cases have numeric and structural chromosomal abnormalities; trisomies 3, 5, and 7 are common, as are 6q deletions,

but no specific cytogenetic or oncogene abnormality has been reported. Complex karyotypes are common in cases with larger cells.[263]

POSTULATED NORMAL COUNTERPART. These lymphomas correspond to mature (peripheral) T cells in various stages of transformation.

CLINICAL FEATURES. Peripheral T-cell lymphomas accounted for only 6% of lymphomas in the international study of the REAL, reflecting their rarity in American and European populations.[89] The median age was in the seventh decade, and 65% of the patients had stage IV disease. Blood eosinophilia, pruritus, and hemophagocytic syndromes may occur; lymph nodes, skin, liver, spleen, and other viscera may be involved. The clinical course is aggressive, and relapses may be more common than in large B-cell lymphoma. In the international REAL study, this group had one of the lowest overall and failure-free survival rates.

THERAPY. Treatment regimens used for peripheral T-cell lymphoma are the same as those used for DLBCL, with the omission of rituximab. Because of the poorer OS in peripheral T-cell lymphoma as compared with DLBCL, bone marrow transplantation is more frequently required. Bone marrow transplantation may be as effective in peripheral T-cell lymphoma as in DLBCL.[264] In the setting of recurrent disease, purine analogues and Campath-1H (anti-CD52 monoclonal antibody) may have modest activity.

Angioimmunoblastic T-Cell Lymphoma

Angioimmunoblastic T-cell lymphoma is a peripheral T-cell lymphoma characterized by systemic disease, a polymorphous infiltrate involving lymph nodes, and a prominent proliferation of high endothelial venules and FDCs.

MORPHOLOGY. The nodal architecture is effaced; peripheral sinuses are typically open and even dilated, but the abnormal infiltrate often extends beyond the capsule into the perinodal fat. Prominent arborizing high endothelial venules are present, many of which show thickened or hyalinized periodic acid–Schiff–positive walls. Clusters of epithelioid histiocytes and numerous eosinophils and plasma cells may be present. Expanded aggregates of FDCs, visible on immunostained sections, surround the proliferating blood vessels and may have the appearance of "burnt-out" germinal centers. The lymphoid cells are a mixture of small lymphocytes, immunoblasts, plasma cells, and medium-sized cells with round nuclei and clear cytoplasm. B-immunoblasts may be numerous.

IMMUNOPHENOTYPE AND GENETIC FEATURES. Tumor cells express T-cell–associated antigens (CD2+ CD3+ CD4+ CD5+ CD7–) and usually CD4, but many non-neoplastic CD4+ and CD8+ cells are often present; CD4 may be lost on some or all of the cells. CD10 expression on some of the neoplastic cells has been reported in the majority of the cases. The neoplastic cells have a chemokine receptor profile consistent with Th1 cells. Expanded clusters of CD21+ CD35+ CD23+ FDCs are present in extrafollicular areas and around proliferated venules. The latter feature is useful in distinguishing this disorder from other T-cell lymphomas. Polyclonal plasma cells and B-immunoblasts may be numerous.

The TCR genes are rearranged in 75% and IgH in 10%, corresponding to expanded B-cell clones. EBV genomes are detected in many cases and are usually in large B cells; trisomy 3 or 5, or both, are common.[265]

POSTULATED NORMAL COUNTERPART. The normal counterpart is presumed to be a peripheral CD4+ T cell.

CLINICAL FEATURES. Angioimmunoblastic T-cell lymphoma is one of the more common peripheral T-cell lymphomas encountered in Western countries. In the Kiel Registry, it accounted for 20% of all T-cell lymphomas and approximately 4% of all lymphomas. Angioimmunoblastic T-cell lymphoma is clinically distinctive: Patients typically have generalized lymphadenopathy, fever, weight loss, skin rash, and polyclonal hypergammaglobulinemia and are susceptible to infections. The course is moderately aggressive, with occasional spontaneous remissions, and is not reliably predicted by the histologic appearance.

THERAPY. Approximately 30% of the patients may have initial remission on corticosteroids alone, but most require some form of cytotoxic chemotherapy. Median survivals range from 15 to 24 months, and curability has not been well established. In some patients, a secondary EBV-positive large B-cell lymphoma develops. A prospective but nonrandomized trial compared an anthracycline-based combination chemotherapy regimen with prednisone followed by combination chemotherapy only if the disease progressed. Initial chemotherapy yielded a higher complete remission rate (64% vs. 29%) and median survival (19 vs. 11 months).[266]

Extranodal Natural Killer/T-Cell Lymphoma, Nasal Type (Formerly Angiocentric Lymphoma)

Extranodal NK/T-cell lymphoma, nasal type, is an extranodal lymphoma, usually with an immature NK-cell phenotype and EBV+, with a broad morphologic spectrum and with frequent necrosis and angioinvasion, most commonly presenting in the midfacial region but also in other extranodal sites. It is designated NK/T, because, although most cases appear to be of NK lineage, some have a cytotoxic T-cell phenotype.

MORPHOLOGY. Extranodal NK/T-cell lymphoma is typically characterized by a polymorphous infiltrate composed of a mixture of normal-appearing small lymphocytes and atypical lymphoid cells of varying size, along with plasma cells and occasionally eosinophils and histiocytes. A characteristic feature is invasion of vascular walls and occlusion of lumina by lymphoid cells with varying degrees of cytologic atypia; however, this is not seen in all the cases. Prominent ischemic necrosis of tumor cells and normal tissue is usually present. The term *angiocentric lymphoma* has proven confusing, because angiocentricity is not evident in all cases. Because the most characteristic presentation is midfacial and the cells have T- and NK-cell features, the term *extranodal NK/T-cell lymphoma, nasal-type* has been proposed and is used in the WHO classification.

IMMUNOPHENOTYPE AND GENETIC FEATURES. The atypical cells in most cases are CD2+ CD56+, surface CD3–, and

cytoplasmic CD3+. They are typically CD4– CD8– but may express CD4 or CD7. Most cases express cytotoxic granule proteins such as Granzyme B and TIA-1.

The TCR and Ig genes are usually germline; EBV genomes are generally present and clonal and are detectable in the majority of the cells in most cases by *in situ* hybridization for EBER-1.[267] CGH in nine cases revealed frequent losses at 1p, 17p, and 12q and gains at 2q, 13q, and 10q. *TP53* and *FAS* gene mutations are common.

POSTULATED NORMAL COUNTERPART. The normal counterpart is an activated NK cell in most cases and a cytotoxic T cell in some cases.

CLINICAL FEATURES. Nasal-type T/NK lymphoma is a rare disorder in the United States and Europe but is more common in Asia and in native populations in Peru. It may affect children or adults. Extranodal sites are invariably involved, including nose, palate, upper airway, gastrointestinal tract, and skin. The clinical course is typically aggressive, with relapses in other extranodal sites. Hemophagocytic syndromes may occur. Some cases of the aggressive variant of NK cell leukemia and lymphoma may be related to this disorder.

THERAPY. Patients with localized NK/T-cell lymphoma in the nasal pharynx can be cured with a combination of chemotherapy and local radiotherapy. With radiotherapy alone, treatment failure is frequent. Patients with disseminated NK/T-cell lymphoma have an extremely poor outlook. Occasional long-term survivors are seen using the CHOP regimen. Less aggressive regimens have a uniformly poor outcome.

High-dose chemotherapy and autologous bone marrow transplantation can be curative in some patients after relapse from standard therapy. Because of the poor results with standard chemotherapeutic approaches, incorporation of bone marrow transplantation as a primary management of patients with disseminated NK/T-cell lymphoma in the setting of a clinical trial may be appropriate.

Enteropathy-Type T-Cell Lymphoma

Enteropathy-type T-cell lymphoma is a tumor of intraepithelial T lymphocytes, showing varying degrees of transformation but usually composed of large lymphoid cells.

MORPHOLOGY. Enteropathy was originally termed *malignant histiocytosis of the intestine* but has since been conclusively shown to be a T-cell lymphoma.[268] On gross examination, circumferentially oriented jejunal ulcers are present, often multiple and frequently with perforation. A mass may or may not be present. The tumor may involve liver, spleen, lymph nodes, and other viscera, such as the stomach, gallbladder, and skin.

The tumors contain a variable admixture of small, medium/mixed, large, or anaplastic tumor cells, often with a high content of intraepithelial T cells in adjacent mucosa. Rare cases contain small to medium-sized monomorphic cells. Large numbers of histiocytes and eosinophils are often present and may obscure the tumor cells.

The adjacent mucosa may or may not show villous atrophy; this varies depending on the segment analyzed, because in sprue, villous atrophy is most prominent in the proximal small intestine and may be absent in distal jejunum or ileum. Early lesions may show mucosal ulceration with only scattered atypical cells and numerous reactive histiocytes, without formation of large masses; these lesions are nonetheless clonal. Intraepithelial lymphocytes in adjacent mucosa may also be clonal. Clonal TCR gene rearrangements have been found in cases of celiac disease that is unresponsive to a gluten-free diet (refractory sprue), suggesting that these cases represent early T-cell lymphoma.

IMMUNOPHENOTYPE AND GENETIC FEATURES. The tumor cells express pan-T-antigens (CD3+ CD5– CD7+), are usually CD4– CD8–/+, and express the mucosal lymphoid antigen CD103. CD30 may be positive in some cells. CD56 is expressed in the small cell variant. Expression of cytotoxic T-cell–associated proteins (Granzyme B, TIA-1, perforin) is seen in many of the cases. Detection of a CD3+ CD5– CD8– T-cell population in the mucosa may be a marker for early lymphoma.

The TCRβ gene is clonally rearranged; no specific cytogenetic abnormality has been described. Patients have the HLA DQA1*0501, DQB1*0201 genotype associated with celiac disease. Partial trisomy of chromosome 1q is found in 16% of cases and has been detected in intraepithelial T cells in cases of refractory celiac sprue.[269]

POSTULATED NORMAL COUNTERPART. The normal counterpart is believed to be an intestinal intraepithelial cytotoxic T cell.

CLINICAL FEATURES AND THERAPY. Enteropathy-type T-cell lymphoma occurs in adults, typically with a rather brief history of gluten-sensitive enteropathy, as the initial event in a patient found to have villous atrophy in the resected intestine or without evidence of enteropathy but with either or both antigliadin antibodies or the typical HLA type (DQA1*0501, DQB1*0201) in patients with celiac disease. It is uncommon in most areas of the United States and Europe but is seen with increased frequency in places in which gluten-sensitive enteropathy is common. Treatment of celiac disease with a gluten-free diet effectively prevents the development of lymphoma, so that lymphoma does not usually develop in patients diagnosed with celiac disease early in life and patients with lymphoma rarely have a long history of celiac disease. Patients present with abdominal pain, often associated with jejunal perforation; stomach or colon is affected less often, and other viscera, skin, or soft tissues may be involved. The course is aggressive, and death usually occurs from multifocal intestinal perforation due to refractory malignant ulcers. A poor response to therapy has been reported. It is probably related to the severe nutritional and immunologic abnormalities found in patients with uncontrolled celiac disease.

Hepatosplenic T-Cell Lymphoma

Hepatosplenic T-cell lymphoma is an extranodal, systemic neoplasm of cytotoxic T cells, usually γδ but occasionally αβ, with sinusoidal infiltration of spleen, liver, and bone marrow.

MORPHOLOGY. Hepatosplenic T-cell lymphoma produces a sinusoidal infiltrate in liver and spleen, as well as bone marrow, of medium-sized lymphoid cells with round nuclei, moderately condensed chromatin, and moderately abundant, pale cytoplasm. Mitotic activity is generally low. The white pulp is atrophic. Erythrophagocytosis may be prominent in splenic and bone marrow sinuses.

IMMUNOPHENOTYPE AND GENETIC FEATURES. The tumor cells are CD2+ and CD3+, CD5–, CD4–, CD8–, CD16+, CD56+/–, and most cases lack the αβ TCR protein, expressing instead the γδ complex. However, a number of clinically and histologically similar cases expressing the αβ receptor have been reported. Cytotoxic granule protein TIA-1 is typically expressed, but Granzyme B and perforin are absent, indicating a nonactivated cytotoxic T-cell phenotype.

The TCRγ and TCRδ genes are rearranged; the TCRβ gene may be rearranged or germline. The tumor cells are EBV negative. Isochromosome 7q is characteristic of both types; trisomy 8 is also common in many cases.

POSTULATED NORMAL COUNTERPART. The postulated normal counterpart is an immature cytotoxic T cell, usually γδ but occasionally αβ.

CLINICAL FEATURES AND THERAPY. Hepatosplenic T-cell lymphoma is a rare neoplasm, and diagnosis is often difficult. These patients frequently present as with a multisystem disease, with hepatomegaly, splenomegaly, or both.[270] The absence of lymphadenopathy and the sinusoidal pattern of infiltration of the liver, spleen, and bone marrow make the diagnosis difficult. Frequently, only the demonstration of a T-cell gene rearrangement leads to the correct diagnosis.

A series of 21 patients with hepatosplenic T-cell lymphoma revealed the median age to be 34 years.[270] Patients had splenomegaly (n = 21), hepatomegaly (n = 15), and thrombocytopenia (n = 20). Unusual sites of involvement, such as skin, nasal cavity, gastrointestinal tract, lung, mucosa, and larynx, have also been described. Marrow involvement can be demonstrated by phenotyping in all patients. Isochromosome arm 7q was documented in 9 of 13 patients.

Complete remission can occur with combination chemotherapy, but most patients relapse. In the aforementioned series, prognosis was poor; median survival time was 16 months, and all but two patients ultimately died despite consolidative or salvage high-dose therapy.

Subcutaneous Panniculitis-Like T-Cell Lymphoma

Subcutaneous panniculitis-like T-cell lymphoma is a cytotoxic T-cell lymphoma that infiltrates subcutaneous tissues. It is composed of atypical lymphoid cells of varying size, often with necrosis and karyorrhexis.

MORPHOLOGIC FEATURES. A variable mixture of small, medium, and large atypical cells is present in the subcutis, sparing the dermis, often containing irregular, hyperchromatic nuclei and pale cytoplasm. Apoptosis and karyorrhexis of tumor cells are prominent. Reactive histiocytes with phagocytized nuclear debris or lipid, or both, are numerous. Granulomas may be present. Individual adipocytes are rimmed by neoplastic cells. Cases of the γδ T-cell type may show more infiltration of the deep dermis.

IMMUNOPHENOTYPE AND GENETIC FEATURES. Most cases express pan-T-antigens and usually CD8, although they may be CD4+ and express cytotoxic granule proteins TIA-1 and perforin and, in most cases, the αβ TCR. Occasional cases derive from γδ T cells. TCRs are usually rearranged. No specific cytogenetic abnormalities have been described.

POSTULATED NORMAL COUNTERPART. The normal counterpart is a mature cytotoxic T cell.

CLINICAL FEATURES AND THERAPY. Patients present with one or more subcutaneous nodules and are often misdiagnosed as having panniculitis. Hemophagocytic syndrome is common. The disease may present in an indolent fashion but typically becomes aggressive. Patients may respond to combination chemotherapy regimens, but the responses are usually transient. These lymphomas are generally radiosensitive, and radiotherapy can be used to control symptoms. However, the long-term outlook with this disorder is poor.

Anaplastic Large Cell Lymphoma

Anaplastic large T/null cell lymphoma, primary systemic type, is a T-cell lymphoma consisting of large lymphoid cells with pleomorphic, multiple, or horseshoe-shaped nuclei and abundant cytoplasm, a cohesive growth pattern, and sinusoidal spread in lymph nodes. It expresses CD30 and either T-cell or no lineage-specific antigens, involving lymph nodes or extranodal sites but not limited to the skin.

MORPHOLOGY. The tumor is usually composed of large blastic cells with round or pleomorphic, often horseshoe-shaped or multiple nuclei with multiple or single prominent nucleoli and with abundant cytoplasm, which gives the cells an epithelial or histiocyte-like appearance. The so-called hallmark cell has an eccentric nucleus and a prominent, eosinophilic Golgi region. The tumor cells grow in a cohesive pattern and often preferentially involve the lymph node sinuses or paracortex. In some cases, the tumor cells have a more monomorphous appearance, with round to oval nuclei and no Reed-Sternberg–like cells; these cases have in common with the more anaplastic cases a low nuclear-cytoplasmic ratio, with dense, abundant cytoplasm and a cohesive, often sinusoidal growth pattern. Lymphohistiocytic and small cell variants have been described, more commonly in children. Study of cytogenetic and molecular genetic abnormalities as well as clinical features suggests that these cases belong to the same disease entity as the more anaplastic cases.

IMMUNOPHENOTYPE AND GENETIC FEATURES. The tumor cells are CD30+ and usually express CD25 and epithelial membrane antigen; they are typically CD45+ and CD15–. Approximately 60% express one or more T-cell–associated antigens: CD2 and CD4 are most consistently expressed, as is CD43. CD3, CD5, and CD7 are often negative. Cytotoxic granule proteins are expressed by most cases. The ALK protein is detected in 60% to 85% of the cases using the ALK1 monoclonal antibody, showing nuclear and cytoplasmic staining in cases with the t(2;5), because nucleophosmin is a nuclear protein. Membrane or cytoplasmic staining may be seen in cases with variant translocations. ALK+ cases are more common in children and have a better prognosis than ALK– cases.[271]

The majority of the cases have rearranged TCR genes; 10% have no rearrangement of TCR or Ig genes. Primary systemic ALCL often have a t(2;5)(p23;q35), which results in a fusion of the nucleophosmin gene on chromosome 5 to a novel tyrosine kinase gene on chromosome 2, called *ALK*. Rare cases of B-cell lymphoma with the t(2;5) have been reported. Variant translocations have been described, which also result in overexpression of ALK protein but without the nuclear localization.[272]

Based on current information, t(2;5) and ALK expression are not considered defining features of ALCL; however, the positive cases are clinically homogeneous: young patients with a relatively good prognosis, whereas ALK– cases are often older adults with more aggressive disease. Thus, ALK staining or t(2;5) should be assessed in all cases, and ALK– cases should be specifically designated.

CLINICAL FEATURES. ALCL represents approximately 2% of all lymphomas but approximately 10% of childhood lymphomas and 50% of large cell pediatric lymphomas. Primary systemic ALCL may involve lymph nodes or extranodal sites, including the skin, but is not localized to the skin. Tumors that present with systemic disease (with or without skin involvement) have a bimodal age distribution in children and adults and are associated with the t(2;5), particularly in children, in 20% to 40% of the cases. Patients may present with isolated lymphadenopathy or extranodal disease in any site, including gastrointestinal tract and bone.[3] In adults the tumor is aggressive but potentially curable, similar to other aggressive lymphomas. Cases with the t(2;5) have a significantly better prognosis than cases that lack the t(2;5).

THERAPY. Treatment regimens used for anaplastic cell lymphoma of the primary systemic type are the same as used in DLBCL, without rituximab therapy. Treatment results have been excellent, with better survival in ALK+ patients (71% to 93%) than in ALK– patients (31% to 37%). Excellent results are seen in adults as well as children. In patients with recurrent or refractory disease, preliminary results of two studies have suggested clinical activity of monoclonal antibodies directed against CD30 in patients with anaplastic T-cell lymphoma.[273]

SPECIAL CLINICAL SITUATIONS

CHILDREN

See Chapter 41.1 for a discussion of lymphomas and leukemias in children.

ELDERLY PATIENTS

The incidence of NHL increases with age, and more than 50% of patients are beyond 60 years of age at diagnosis. The IPI demonstrated that NHL patients older than 60 years of age had a significantly lower complete remission rate, greater chance of relapsing from remission (relative risk, 1.8), and higher risk of death (relative risk, 1.96).[88] Several explanations may account for the poorer outcome in elderly adults. Some analyses have shown that older patients were more likely to have mortality from chemotherapy-related toxicity than younger patients, despite similar complete remission rates. Other studies have identified higher relapse rates in elderly patients. Still other analyses have shown inferior survival in elderly patients to be a result of increased deaths from cardiovascular disease and other nonrelapse causes. A Non-Hodgkin's Lymphoma Classification Project demonstrated that elderly patients were more likely to have a high IPI than were younger individuals.[274] Older patients are also more likely to have comorbid conditions. These factors have often led to arbitrary dose reductions or use of less aggressive therapy, which may reduce the possibility of cure. This is exemplified by Southwest Oncology Group studies that revealed a complete remission rate of 37% in patients 65 years of age and above who received initial 50% dose reductions of cyclophosphamide and doxorubicin.[275] Complete remission rates were 52%, a rate similar to those of younger patients, when full-dose chemotherapy was used.

Some analyses have shown that less intensive regimens may be associated with diminished mortality and equivalent outcomes when compared with more aggressive regimens in elderly NHL patients. In general, these regimens have used anthracyclines with less cardiotoxicity than doxorubicin, have substituted mitoxantrone for doxorubicin, or have used short-duration weekly therapy.[276] Although these regimens may be well tolerated, selection bias and lack of appropriate comparisons make it difficult to determine whether these novel regimens are superior to standard regimens, and more recent studies suggest that doxorubicin is superior to mitoxantrone in this population.[277]

Several prospective randomized trials have examined results of NHL treatments in elderly patients. As previously stated in the section Therapy of Disseminated Diffuse Large B-Cell Lymphoma, in two randomized trials, the addition of rituximab to CHOP has demonstrated superior PFS compared with CHOP alone in patients 60 years of age or older.[239,240] Preliminary results of a German randomized trial comparing conventional CHOP, CHOP every 14 days, CHOP with etoposide, and CHOP with etoposide every 14 days in patients older than age 60 demonstrated superior progression-free and OS in the CHOP every-14-day arm compared with standard CHOP.[278] The addition of etoposide was overly toxic. Ongoing randomized trials are addressing whether rituximab adds benefit to the dose-dense regimen.

Elderly patients who participate in clinical trials may be subject to selection bias, although these results suggest that these patients may be able to tolerate aggressive anthracycline-containing regimens. When adverse characteristics such as poor performance status are excluded, elderly NHL patients may have outcomes similar to those of younger patients.[279] The use of colony-stimulating factors (CSFs) may allow elderly patients to receive planned chemotherapy doses, although they may be less effective for the oldest patients and do not entirely prevent neutropenic complications. A randomized trial showed that the routine addition of granulocyte-CSF to CHOP did not improve response rates or survival in elderly patients with aggressive lymphoma and that the rate of hospitalization and infection was not different between the two arms.[280]

The authors initially approach elderly patients with aggressive lymphoma in a similar manner to younger patients, with intent to cure. Supportive care with filgrastim or pegfilgrastim, transfusions, and antibiotic support is often required. These patients may be eligible for ongoing national clincial trials and should be considered for participation whenever possible.

POSTTRANSPLANT LYMPHOPROLIFERATIVE DISORDERS

The risk of developing lymphoma is markedly increased after solid organ transplantation. PTLDs occur in 0.8% to 20.0% of transplanted patients.[281] Although a mortality of 60% to 80% is frequently reported, more favorable outcomes have been described. Identical disorders are seen after allogeneic bone marrow transplantation, especially in recipients of T-cell–depleted marrow. PTLDs are almost always EBV related, although cases unrelated to EBV have been described. The development of PTLD results from proliferation of EBV-transformed B-cell clones when patients receive immunosuppressive therapy after transplantation.[282] Occasional cases of Hodgkin's disease and T-cell NHL have been reported. Most PTLDs after solid organ transplants are host derived.

The histologic appearance of PTLD is highly variable. Classification systems with clinical relevance have been proposed.[283] Lesions may be polymorphic or monomorphic. In some cases the appearance may resemble infectious mononucleosis, and other cases may be indistinguishable from aggressive NHL or plasmacytomas. Lesions may be polyclonal, oligoclonal, or monoclonal.

PTLD after solid organ transplantation has several unique features, which differentiates it from NHL in the immunocompetent host. Most patients present with lymphadenopathy or a mass; however, extranodal involvement, a poor prognostic indicator in large cell lymphoma, is often present. In many series, isolated extranodal disease is the most common presentation of PTLD, and, similar to AIDS-related lymphoma, a minority of patients have disease confined to the lymphatic system. CNS involvement occurred in 22% of PTLDs in a registry experience of more than 1000 patients.[284] Other common extranodal sites include the lung and gastrointestinal tract, which may be associated with a better prognosis. An unusual site of involvement is the allograft, which occurred 22% of the time in a study evaluating heart, lung, and liver transplants. Particularly in lung transplant patients, this phenomenon has been confused with rejection, emphasizing the importance of experienced hematopathology in evaluating questionable biopsies. Diagnosis is made by autopsy in a minority of cases, often when concomitant infection or rejection is present.

The two major risk factors for the development of PTLD after organ transplantation are pretransplant negative recipient EBV serology and the degree of posttransplant immunosuppression. Prophylactic approaches should include elimination, when possible, of these risk factors. Very few prospective trials of PTLD treatment have been performed, and management decisions must be individualized. Initial management should consist of reduction or cessation of immunosuppression. Patients in whom early-onset PTLD develops are most likely to benefit from this approach. Many investigators recommend concurrent administration of acyclovir or ganciclovir, although the value of this approach has been questioned. Surgical excision or RT may be curative for patients with localized PTLD. Surgery should be considered for patients with isolated PTLD in renal transplants. Responses have also been reported with anti–B-cell monoclonal antibodies, including rituximab.[285] This modality is often considered before the use of chemotherapy. Patients who fail to respond to reduction of immunosuppression or antibody therapy can be treated with anthracycline-based combination chemotherapy.[286,287] Durable remissions can be seen, although mortality is higher than in nonimmunosuppressed NHL patients. Interferon can also be considered for patients who are not progressing rapidly.[288] In the setting of PTLD after bone marrow transplantation, donor leukocyte infusion is standard therapy and is highly effective.[289]

HUMAN IMMUNODEFICIENCY VIRUS–ASSOCIATED NON-HODGKIN'S LYMPHOMA

The risk of developing NHL is markedly increased in patients infected with HIV type 1. Large cell lymphomas, small non–cleaved cell NHL, and primary CNS lymphoma are considered AIDS-defining conditions. AIDS-related lymphomas are B-cell neoplasms. Virtually all primary CNS lymphomas and approximately 50% of other AIDS-related NHL are EBV related. Most cases are classified as small non–cleaved cell histology or diffuse large cell lymphoma. The risk of low-grade NHL may also be increased, although these lymphomas are not considered to be diagnostic of AIDS. Small non–cleaved cell lymphomas are associated with c-myc activation in virtually all cases and are frequently associated with p53 mutations. Rearrangements of bcl-6 are detected in approximately 40% of diffuse large cell lymphomas. Primary effusion lymphoma is seen in 1% to 3% of AIDS patients and is associated with HHV-8.

AIDS-associated NHL usually behaves aggressively. Systemic symptoms are common, along with involvement of extranodal sites. Gastrointestinal tract involvement is common, as well as unusual sites such as anus and rectum, skin and soft tissues, and heart. Approximately 15% of cases are primary CNS lymphomas.

Before the highly active antiretroviral therapy era, aggressive chemotherapy regimens were associated with significant toxicity. A randomized trial comparing m-BACOD with reduced-dose m-BACOD demonstrated median survival rates of 31 weeks and 35 weeks, respectively (*P* = .25), with less toxicity in the low-dose arm.[290] More recently, standard CHOP chemotherapy has been combined with antiretroviral therapy and infection prophylaxis with improved results. The AIDS Malignancy Consortium conducted a randomized trial comparing CHOP and rituximab therapy with standard CHOP chemotherapy.[291] Preliminary results from this trial suggest similar CR rates (58% vs. 50%) but a possible increased infection risk associated with rituximab in this setting. Importantly, with a median of 26 weeks of follow-up, median CR duration has not been reached in either group, suggesting significant improvement over historic results with lower-dose chemotherapy regimens.

Other investigators have advocated infusional chemotherapy regimens, such as EPOCH (etoposide, doxorubicin, vincristine, cyclophosphamide, prednisone), for these patients; however, no randomized data exist. In general, the authors recommend standard doses of CHOP, without rituximab, for these patients, in combination with highly active antiretroviral therapy. Antiretroviral therapy and prophylactic antibiotics should be continued during therapy. Opinions differ on the use of CNS prophylaxis, although patients with small non–cleaved cell histology and those with sinus or testicular involvement should receive prophylactic intrathecal therapy. For patients with relapsed or refractory disease, there is an evolving literature suggesting tolerability and clinical benefit to high-dose therapy and ASCT in selected settings.

The prognosis for AIDS patients with primary CNS lymphoma is also poor. Standard therapy has consisted of whole brain irradiation, although median survival is 3 to 4 months. Patients may respond to high-dose methotrexate, and the role of combined modality therapy is being investigated. No standardized approaches have been developed for primary effu-

sion lymphoma, and these patients should probably be treated like other patients with AIDS-related NHL.

EXTRANODAL SITES

Primary Central Nervous System Lymphoma

Primary CNS lymphoma is the subject of Chapter 41.4.

Testicle

Primary testicular NHL accounts for approximately 1% to 9% of all testicular neoplasms and is the most common testicular neoplasm in men over the age of 60. Testicular lymphoma is frequently associated with involvement of Waldeyer's ring, skin and subcutaneous tissue, lung, and CNS.[292] Involvement of the contralateral testis is common at diagnosis or later in the course of disease. Most tumors are classified as diffuse large cell histology or immunoblastic lymphoma, although Burkitt's lymphoma is common in children, and follicular lymphomas and other histologic subtypes have been described.

Most series have reported poor outcomes with relatively few long-term survivors. Orchiectomy is universally recommended as initial therapy for patients with localized disease. Although long-term disease-free survival has been described after orchiectomy alone, the vast majority of patients relapse, and this is not adequate therapy, even for those with stage IE disease. Furthermore, relapse rates exceeding 50% have been observed in the majority of reports in which adjuvant RT was used after orchiectomy. Relapses often occur in extranodal sites, particularly the CNS, and this suggests that testicular NHL is usually a systemic disease, even when clinically localized.[292]

These poor results have led to the use of chemotherapy after orchiectomy for patients with stage IE and IIE disease. The best results in patients with stage IE and IIE disease have been reported by the Vancouver group.[293] Patients were treated with a brief course of doxorubicin-based chemotherapy followed by scrotal radiation for stage IE patients and additional pelvic and paraaortic radiation for patients with stage IIE disease. The 4-year OS and relapse-free survival rates were 93%, as compared with 50% in a historic control group treated with orchiectomy and radiation alone. No relapses in the contralateral testis or CNS were observed, and the routine use of CNS prophylaxis was thought to be unnecessary.

However, other groups have reported CNS relapses and contralateral testis relapse after doxorubicin-based chemotherapy and RT in stage IE patients. High rates of parenchymal CNS relapse after aggressive combination chemotherapy[292] have led the authors to recommend high-dose systemic methotrexate prophylaxis in conjunction with standard CHOP and rituximab therapy. Because of low morbidity and the high rate of contralateral testis recurrence, the authors also recommend prophylactic scrotal radiation after completion of chemotherapy.

Skin

After the gastrointestinal tract, the skin is the second most common extranodal site primarily involved by NHL. As opposed to lymph nodes and most other extranodal sites of presentation of lymphoma, the skin is unusual in that T-cell lymphomas occur more frequently than B-cell lymphomas. The most common cutaneous T-cell lymphoma, mycosis fungoides, is dealt with in Chapter 41.3. The most common presentation is a new or unusual skin lesion.

Skin lymphomas can be classified using the WHO classification. However, the European Organization for Research on the Treatment of Cancer has also developed a classification that specifically deals with primary cutaneous lymphomas.[294] An important feature interpreting any histologic diagnosis of a cutaneous lymphoma is to remember that the clinical behavior may be different than when the same diagnosis is identified in nodal or other extranodal sites. It is also important to realize that full-thickness biopsies usually are required for diagnosis. The diagnosis of cutaneous lymphomas can be extremely difficult, even with immunohistochemical and molecular genetics studies. Repeat biopsies are sometimes required for a definite diagnosis. In addition, the clinical history may be important in making the diagnosis. Lymphomatoid papulosis is histologically quite similar to CD30+, T/null-cell lymphomas in the skin. Often a history of chronic recurring lesions is the key to making the correct diagnosis. The clinical spectrum of cutaneous CD30+ lymphoproliferative disorders ranges from the benign behavior of lymphomatoid papulosis to an aggressive ALCL. Peripheral T-cell lymphomas that are CD30– can involve the skin and typically follow an aggressive clinical course. Tumors with a high proportion of large cells seem to be more aggressive. Angiocentric lymphomas can also have cutaneous presentations and are associated with a highly aggressive course.

Primary B-cell lymphomas in the skin are less common but occur more frequently than previously appreciated. These can include marginal zone lymphoma and DLBCLs. Marginal zone lymphomas of the skin are typically of MALT type. These lymphomas have an excellent survival with local therapy, although local recurrence sometimes occurs. Primary DLBCL occurring on the trunk tends to behave indolently and can be managed with local therapy, in contrast to those that occur on the legs, which tend to follow a more aggressive course.

REFERENCES

1. Seow A, Lee J, Sng I, et al. Non-Hodgkin's lymphoma in an Asian population: 1968–1992 time trends and ethnic differences in Singapore. *Cancer* 1996;77(9):1899.
2. Jemal A, Tiwari RC, Murray T, et al. Cancer statistics, 2004. *CA Cancer J Clin* 2004;54(1):8.
3. Sehn LH, Donaldson J, Chhanabhai M, et al. Introduction of combined CHOP-rituximab therapy dramatically improved outcome of diffuse large B-cell lymphoma in British Columbia. *Blood* 2003;102:29a.
4. Cote TR, Biggar RJ, Rosenberg PS, et al. Non-Hodgkin's lymphoma among people with AIDS: incidence, presentation and public health burden. AIDS/Cancer Study Group. *Int J Cancer* 1997;73(5):645.
5. Corn BW, Marcus SM, Topham A, et al. Will primary central nervous system lymphoma be the most frequent brain tumor diagnosed in the year 2000? *Cancer* 1997;79(12):2409.
6. Ziegler JL. Burkitt's lymphoma. *N Engl J Med* 1981;305(13):735.
7. Doglioni C, Wotherspoon AC, Moschini A, et al. High incidence of primary gastric lymphoma in northeastern Italy. *Lancet* 1992;339(8797):834.
8. Anderson JR, Armitage JO, Weisenburger DD. Epidemiology of the non-Hodgkin's lymphomas: distributions of the major subtypes differ by geographic locations. Non-Hodgkin's Lymphoma Classification Project. *Ann Oncol* 1998;9(7):717.
9. Herrinton LJ, Goldoft M, Schwartz SM, Weiss NS. The incidence of non-Hodgkin's lymphoma and its histologic subtypes in Asian migrants to the United States and their descendants. *Cancer Causes Control* 1996;7(2):224.
10. Chiu BC, Weisenburger DD. An update of the epidemiology of non-Hodgkin's lymphoma. *Clin Lymphoma* 2003;4(3):161.
11. Dinse GE, Umbach DM, Sasco AJ, et al. Unexplained increases in cancer incidence in the United States from 1975 to 1994: possible sentinel health indicators? *Annu Rev Public Health* 1999;20:173.
12. Filipovich AH, Mathur A, Kamat D, Shapiro RS. Primary immunodeficiencies: genetic risk factors for lymphoma. *Cancer Res* 1992;52[19 Suppl]:5465s.
13. Wolfe F, Fries JF. Rate of death due to leukemia/lymphoma in patients with rheumatoid arthritis. *Arthritis Rheum* 2003;48(9):2694.
14. Gelfand JM, Berlin J, Van Voorhees A, Margolis DJ. Lymphoma rates are low but increased in patients with psoriasis: results from a population-based cohort study in the United Kingdom. *Arch Dermatol* 2003;139(11):1425.
15. Voulgarelis M, Moutsopoulos HM. Malignant lymphoma in primary Sjögren's syndrome. *Isr Med Assoc J* 2001;3(10):761.
16. Royer B, Cazals-Hatem D, Sibilia J, et al. Lymphomas in patients with Sjögren's syndrome are marginal zone B-cell neoplasms, arise in diverse extranodal and nodal sites, and are not associated with viruses. *Blood* 1997;90(2):766.
17. Gale J, Simmonds PD, Mead GM, et al. Enteropathy-type intestinal T-cell lymphoma: clinical features and treatment of 31 patients in a single center. *J Clin Oncol* 2000;18(4):795.
18. Young LS, Murray PG. Epstein-Barr virus and oncogenesis: from latent genes to tumours. *Oncogene* 2003;22(33):5108.
19. Kennedy G, Komano J, Sugden B. Epstein-Barr virus provides a survival factor to Burkitt's lymphomas. *Proc Natl Acad Sci USA* 2003;100(24):14269.
20. Gaidano G, Carbone A, Dalla-Favera R. Genetic basis of acquired immunodeficiency syndrome–related lymphomagenesis. *J Natl Cancer Inst Monogr* 1998(23):95.
21. Subar M, Neri A, Inghirami G, et al. Frequent c-myc oncogene activation and infrequent presence of Epstein-Barr virus genome in AIDS-associated lymphoma. *Blood* 1988;72(2):667.
22. Liebowitz D. Epstein-Barr virus and a cellular signaling pathway in lymphomas from immunosuppressed patients. *N Engl J Med* 1998;338(20):1413.
23. Overbaugh J. HTLV-1 sweet-talks its way into cells. *Nat Med* 2004;10(1):20.
24. Arisawa K, Soda M, Endo S, et al. Evaluation of adult T-cell leukemia/lymphoma incidence and its impact on non-Hodgkin lymphoma incidence in southwestern Japan. *Int J Cancer* 2000;85(3):319.
25. Blayney DW, Jaffe ES, Blattner WA, et al. The human T-cell leukemia/lymphoma virus associated with American adult T-cell leukemia/lymphoma. *Blood* 1983;62(2):401.
26. Mori N, Fujii M, Ikeda S, et al. Constitutive activation of NF-kappaB in primary adult T-cell leukemia cells. *Blood* 1999;93(7):2360.
27. Manel N, Kim FJ, Kinet S, et al. The ubiquitous glucose transporter GLUT-1 is a receptor for HTLV. *Cell* 2003;115(4):449.
28. Antman K, Chang Y. Kaposi's sarcoma. *N Engl J Med* 2000;342(14):1027.
29. Cesarman E, Chang Y, Moore PS, et al. Kaposi's sarcoma–associated herpesvirus-like DNA sequences in AIDS-related body-cavity-based lymphomas. *N Engl J Med* 1995;332(18):1186.
30. Nador RG, Cesarman E, Chadburn A, et al. Primary effusion lymphoma: a distinct clinicopathologic entity associated with the Kaposi's sarcoma–associated herpes virus. *Blood* 1996;88(2):645.
31. Sun Q, Matta H, Chaudhary PM. The human herpes virus 8–encoded viral FLICE inhibitory protein protects against growth factor withdrawal–induced apoptosis via NF-kappa B activation. *Blood* 2003;101(5):1956.
32. Mele A, Pulsoni A, Bianco E, et al. Hepatitis C virus and B-cell non-Hodgkin lymphomas: an Italian multicenter case-control study. *Blood* 2003;102(3):996.
33. Musto P. Hepatitis C virus infection and B-cell non-Hodgkin's lymphomas: more than a simple association. *Clin Lymphoma* 2002;3(3):150.
34. Arcaini L, Paulli M, Boveri E, et al. Splenic and nodal marginal zone lymphomas are indolent disorders at high hepatitis C virus seroprevalence with distinct presenting features but similar morphologic and phenotypic profiles. *Cancer* 2004;100(1):107.
35. Nakatsuka S, Liu A, Dong Z, et al. Simian virus 40 sequences in malignant lymphomas in Japan. *Cancer Res* 2003;63(22):7606.
36. Ferber D. Virology. Monkey virus link to cancer grows stronger. *Science* 2002;296(5570):1012.
37. Vilchez RA, Madden CR, Kozinetz CA, et al. Association between simian virus 40 and non-Hodgkin lymphoma. *Lancet* 2002;359(9309):817.
38. Shivapurkar N, Harada K, Reddy J, et al. Presence of simian virus 40 DNA sequences in human lymphomas. *Lancet* 2002;359(9309):851.
39. Parsonnet J, Hansen S, Rodriguez L, et al. *Helicobacter pylori* infection and gastric lymphoma. *N Engl J Med* 1994;330:1267.
40. Zucca E, Bertoni F, Roggero E, et al. Molecular analysis of the progression from *Helicobacter pylori*–associated chronic gastritis to mucosa-associated lymphoid-tissue lymphoma of the stomach. *N Engl J Med* 1998;338(12):804.
41. Lecuit M, Abachin E, Martin A, et al. Immunoproliferative small intestinal disease associated with *Campylobacter jejuni*. *N Engl J Med* 2004;350(3):239.
42. Munksgaard L, Frisch M, Melbye M, Hjalgrim H. Incidence patterns of Lyme disease and cutaneous B-cell non-Hodgkin's lymphoma in the United States. *Dermatology* 2000;201(4):351.
43. Ferreri AJ, Guidoboni M, Ponzoni M, et al. Evidence for association between *Chlamydia psittaci* infection and ocular adnexal lymphoma. *Proc ASCO* 2003;22:565a.
44. Hardell L, Eriksson M, Nordstrom M. Exposure to pesticides as risk factor for non-Hodgkin's lymphoma and hairy cell leukemia: pooled analysis of two Swedish case-control studies. *Leuk Lymphoma* 2002;43(5):1043.
45. Zhang Y, Holford TR, Leaderer B, et al. Hair-coloring product use and risk of non-Hodgkin's lymphoma: a population-based case-control study in Connecticut. *Am J Epidemiol* 2004;159(2):148.
46. Raaschou-Nielsen O, Hansen J, McLaughlin JK, et al. Cancer risk among workers at Danish companies using trichloroethylene: a cohort study. *Am J Epidemiol* 2003;158(12):1182.
47. Ward MH, Mark SD, Cantor KP, et al. Drinking water nitrate and the risk of non-Hodgkin's lymphoma. *Epidemiology* 1996;7(5):465.
48. Morton LM, Holford TR, Leaderer B, et al. Cigarette smoking and risk of non-Hodgkin lymphoma subtypes among women. *Br J Cancer* 2003;89(11):2087.
49. Ng AK, Bernardo MP, Weller E, et al. Long-term survival and competing causes of death in patients with early-stage Hodgkin's disease treated at age 50 or younger. *J Clin Oncol* 2002;20(8):2101.
50. Ng AK, Bernardo MV, Weller E, et al. Second malignancy after Hodgkin disease treated

with radiation therapy with or without chemotherapy: long-term risks and risk factors. *Blood* 2002;100(6):1989.

51. McMichael AJ, Giles GG. Have increases in solar ultraviolet exposure contributed to the rise in incidence of non-Hodgkin's lymphoma? *Br J Cancer* 1996;73(7):945.

52. Alexander FE. Blood transfusion and risk of non-Hodgkin lymphoma. *Lancet* 1997;350 (9089):1414.

53. Korsmeyer SJ, Hieter PA, Ravetch JV, et al. Developmental hierarchy of immunoglobulin gene rearrangements in human leukemic pre-B-cells. *Proc Natl Acad Sci U S A* 1981;78(11):7096.

54. Shipp MA, Richardson NE, Sayre PH, et al. Molecular cloning of the common acute lymphoblastic leukemia antigen (CALLA) identifies a type II integral membrane protein. *Proc Natl Acad Sci U S A* 1988;85(13):4819.

55. Longacre TA, Foucar K, Crago S, et al. Hematogones: a multiparameter analysis of bone marrow precursor cells. *Blood* 1989;73(2):543.

56. Klein U, Kuppers R, Rajewsky K. Human IgM+IgD+ B cells, the major B cell subset in the peripheral blood, express V kappa genes with no or little somatic mutation throughout life. *Eur J Immunol* 1993;23(12):3272.

57. Delves PJ, Roitt IM. The immune system. First of two parts. *N Engl J Med* 2000;343(1):37.

58. Hockenbery DM, Zutter M, Hickey W, et al. BCL2 protein is topographically restricted in tissues characterized by apoptotic cell death. *Proc Natl Acad Sci U S A* 1991;88(16):6961.

59. Inghirami G, Foitl DR, Sabichi A, et al. Autoantibody-associated cross-reactive idiotype-bearing human B lymphocytes: distribution and characterization, including Ig VH gene and CD5 antigen expression. *Blood* 1991;78(6):1503.

60. Zukerberg LR, Medeiros LJ, Ferry JA, Harris NL. Diffuse low-grade B-cell lymphomas. Four clinically distinct subtypes defined by a combination of morphologic and immunophenotypic features. *Am J Clin Pathol* 1993;100(4):373.

61. Liu YJ, Zhang J, Lane PJ, et al. Sites of specific B cell activation in primary and secondary responses to T cell–dependent and T cell–independent antigens. *Eur J Immunol* 1991;21(12):2951.

62. MacLennan IC. Germinal centers. *Annu Rev Immunol* 1994;12:117.

63. Cattoretti G, Chang CC, Cechova K, et al. BCL-6 protein is expressed in germinal-center B cells. *Blood* 1995;86(1):45.

64. French DL, Laskov R, Scharff MD. The role of somatic hypermutation in the generation of antibody diversity. *Science* 1989;244(4909):1152.

65. Peng HZ, Du MQ, Koulis A, et al. Nonimmunoglobulin gene hypermutation in germinal center B cells. *Blood* 1999;93(7):2167.

66. Shen HM, Peters A, Baron B, et al. Mutation of BCL-6 gene in normal B cells by the process of somatic hypermutation of Ig genes. *Science* 1998;280(5370):1750.

67. Liu YJ, Joshua DE, Williams GT, et al. Mechanism of antigen-driven selection in germinal centres. *Nature* 1989;342(6252):929.

68. Wabl MR, Forni L, Loor F. Switch in immunoglobulin class production observed in single clones of committed lymphocytes. *Science* 1978;199(4333):1078.

69. Allman D, Jain A, Dent A, et al. BCL-6 expression during B-cell activation. *Blood* 1996;87(12):5257.

70. Berek C. The development of B cells and the B-cell repertoire in the microenvironment of the germinal center. *Immunol Rev* 1992;126:5.

71. Klein U, Klein G, Ehlin-Henriksson B, et al. Burkitt's lymphoma is a malignancy of mature B cells expressing somatically mutated V region genes. *Mol Med* 1995;1(5):495.

72. Tierens A, Delabie J, Michiels L, et al. Marginal-zone B cells in the human lymph node and spleen show somatic hypermutations and display clonal expansion. *Blood* 1999;93(1):226.

73. Klein U, Kuppers R, Rajewsky K. Evidence for a large compartment of IgM-expressing memory B cells in humans. *Blood* 1997;89(4):1288.

74. Kuppers R, Hajadi M, Plank L, et al. Molecular Ig gene analysis reveals that monocytoid B cell lymphoma is a malignancy of mature B cells carrying somatically mutated V region genes and suggests that rearrangement of the kappa-deleting element (resulting in deletion of the Ig kappa enhancers) abolishes somatic hypermutation in the human. *Eur J Immunol* 1996;26(8):1794.

75. Harris NL, Jaffe ES, Diebold J, et al. World Health Organization Classification of Neoplastic Diseases of the Hematopoietic and Lymphoid Tissues: Report of the Clinical Advisory Committee Meeting—Arlie House, Virginia, November, 1997. *J Clin Oncol* 1999;17(12):3835.

76. Spits H, Lanier LL, Phillips JH. Development of human T and natural killer cells. *Blood* 1995;85(10):2654.

77. Engel P, Gribben JG, Freeman GJ, et al. The B7-2 (B70) costimulatory molecule expressed by monocytes and activated B lymphocytes is the CD86 differentiation antigen. *Blood* 1994;84(5):1402.

78. Meuer SC, Schlossman SF, Reinherz EL. Clonal analysis of human cytotoxic T lymphocytes: T4+ and T8+ effector T cells recognize products of different major histocompatibility complex regions. *Proc Natl Acad Sci U S A* 1982;79(14):4395.

79. Delves PJ, Roitt IM. The immune system. Second of two parts. *N Engl J Med* 2000;343(2):108.

80. Croce CM, Tsujimoto Y, Erikson J, Nowell P. Chromosome translocations and B cell neoplasia. *Lab Invest* 1984;51(3):258.

81. McDonnell TJ, Deane N, Platt FM, et al. bcl-2-immunoglobulin transgenic mice demonstrate extended B cell survival and follicular lymphoproliferation. *Cell* 1989;57(1):79.

82. Rosenberg CL, Wong E, Petty EM, et al. PRAD1, a candidate BCL1 oncogene: mapping and expression in centrocytic lymphoma. *Proc Natl Acad Sci U S A* 1991;88(21):9638.

83. Downing JR, Shurtleff SA, Zielenska M, et al. Molecular detection of the (2;5) translocation of non-Hodgkin's lymphoma by reverse transcriptase–polymerase chain reaction. *Blood* 1995;85(12):3416.

84. Dierlamm J, Baens M, Wlodarska I, et al. The apoptosis inhibitor gene API2 and a novel 18q gene, MLT, are recurrently rearranged in the t(11;18)(q21;q21)p6ssociated with mucosa-associated lymphoid tissue lymphomas. *Blood* 1999;93(11):3601.

85. Lee MS, Chang KS, Cabanillas F, et al. Detection of minimal residual cells carrying the t(14;18) by DNA sequence amplification. *Science* 1987;237(4811):175.

86. Siebert R, Matthiesen P, Harder S, et al. Application of interphase fluorescence in situ hybridization for the detection of the Burkitt translocation t(8;14)(q24;q32) in B-cell lymphomas. *Blood* 1998;91(3):984.

87. Falini B, Mason DY. Proteins encoded by genes involved in chromosomal alterations in lymphoma and leukemia: clinical value of their detection by immunocytochemistry. *Blood* 2002;99(2):409.

88. A predictive model for aggressive non-Hodgkin's lymphoma. The International Non-Hodgkin's Lymphoma Prognostic Factors Project. *N Engl J Med* 1993;329(14):987.

89. Armitage JO, Weisenburger DD. New approach to classifying non-Hodgkin's lymphomas: clinical features of the major histologic subtypes. Non-Hodgkin's Lymphoma Classification Project. *J Clin Oncol* 1998;16(8):2780.

90. A clinical evaluation of the International Lymphoma Study Group classification of non-Hodgkin's lymphoma. The Non-Hodgkin's Lymphoma Classification Project. *Blood* 1997;89(11):3909.

91. Rahmouni A, Montazel JL, Divine M, et al. Bone marrow with diffuse tumor infiltration in patients with lymphoproliferative diseases: dynamic gadolinium-enhanced MR imaging. *Radiology* 2003;229(3):710.

92. Janicek M, Kaplan W, Neuberg D, et al. Early restaging gallium scans predict outcome in poor-prognosis patients with aggressive non-Hodgkin's lymphoma treated with high-dose CHOP chemotherapy. *J Clin Oncol* 1997;15(4):1631.

93. Kostakoglu L, Leonard JP, Kuji I, et al. Comparison of fluorine-18 fluorodeoxyglucose positron emission tomography and Ga-67 scintigraphy in evaluation of lymphoma. *Cancer* 2002;94(4):879.

94. Friedberg JW, Chengazi V. PET scans in the staging of lymphoma: current status. *Oncologist* 2003;8(5):438.

95. Elstrom R, Guan L, Baker G, et al. Utility of FDG-PET scanning in lymphoma by WHO classification. *Blood* 2003;101(10):3875.

96. Hoffmann M, Kletter K, Becherer A, et al. 18F-fluorodeoxyglucose positron emission tomography (18F-FDG-PET) for staging and follow-up of marginal zone B-cell lymphoma. *Oncology* 2003;64(4):336.

97. Romer W, Hanauske AR, Ziegler S, et al. Positron emission tomography in non-Hodgkin's lymphoma: assessment of chemotherapy with fluorodeoxyglucose. *Blood* 1998;91(12):4464.

98. Allal AS, Dulguerov P, Allaoua M, et al. Standardized uptake value of 2-[(18)f] fluoro-2-deoxy-d-glucose in predicting outcome in head and neck carcinomas treated by radiotherapy with or without chemotherapy. *J Clin Oncol* 2002;20(5):1398.

99. Zinzani PL, Magagnoli M, Chierichetti F, et al. The role of positron emission tomography (PET) in the management of lymphoma patients [see comments]. *Ann Oncol* 1999;10 (10):1181.

100. Weihrauch MR, Re D, Scheidhauer K, et al. Thoracic positron emission tomography using 18F-fluorodeoxyglucose for the evaluation of residual mediastinal Hodgkin disease. *Blood* 2001;98(10):2930.

101. Carbone PP, Kaplan HS, Musshoff K, et al. Report of the Committee on Hodgkin's Disease Staging Classification. *Cancer Res* 1971;31:1860.

102. Decaudin D, Lepage E, Brousse N, et al. Low-grade stage III–IV follicular lymphoma: multivariate analysis of prognostic factors in 484 patients—a study of the Groupe d'Etude des Lymphomes de l'Adulte. *J Clin Oncol* 1999;17(8):2499.

103. Federico M, Vitolo U, Zinzani PL, et al. Prognosis of follicular lymphoma: a predictive model based on a retrospective analysis of 987 cases. Intergruppo Italiano Linfomi. *Blood* 2000;95(3):783.

104. Philip T, Guglielmi C, Hagenbeek A, et al. Autologous bone marrow transplantation as compared with salvage chemotherapy in relapses of chemotherapy-sensitive non-Hodgkin's lymphoma. *N Engl J Med* 1995;333:1540.

105. Cheson BD, Horning SJ, Coiffier B, et al. Report of an international workshop to standardize response criteria for non-Hodgkin's lymphomas. NCI Sponsored International Working Group. *J Clin Oncol* 1999;17(4):1244.

106. Dohner H, Stilgenbauer S, Benner A, et al. Genomic aberrations and survival in chronic lymphocytic leukemia. *N Engl J Med* 2000;343(26):1910.

107. Crespo M, Bosch F, Villamor N, et al. ZAP-70 expression as a surrogate for immunoglobulin-variable-region mutations in chronic lymphocytic leukemia. *N Engl J Med* 2003;348(18):1764.

108. Di Raimondo F, Giustolisi R, Cacciola E, et al. Autoimmune hemolytic anemia in chronic lymphocytic leukemia patients treated with fludarabine. *Leuk Lymphoma* 1993;11(1–2):63.

109. Keating MJ, O'Brien S, Lerner S, et al. Long-term follow-up of patients with chronic lymphocytic leukemia (CLL) receiving fludarabine regimens as initial therapy. *Blood* 1998;92(4):1165.

110. Rai KR, Peterson BL, Appelbaum FR, et al. Fludarabine compared with chlorambucil as primary therapy for chronic lymphocytic leukemia. *N Engl J Med* 2000;343(24):1750.

111. Leporrier M, Chevret S, Cazin B, et al. Randomized comparison of fludarabine, CAP, and CHOP in 938 previously untreated stage B and C chronic lymphocytic leukemia patients. *Blood* 2001;98(8):2319.

112. Byrd JC, Peterson BL, Morrison VA, et al. Randomized phase 2 study of fludarabine with concurrent versus sequential treatment with rituximab in symptomatic, untreated patients with B-cell chronic lymphocytic leukemia: results from Cancer and Leukemia Group B 9712 (CALGB 9712). *Blood* 2003;101(1):6.

113. Castagna L, Sarina B, Santoro A. Fludarabine plus rituximab for untreated B-cell chronic lymphocytic leukemia. *Blood* 2003;102(6):2309; author reply, 2309.

114. Byrd JC, Murphy T, Howard RS, et al. Rituximab using a thrice weekly dosing schedule in B-cell chronic lymphocytic leukemia and small lymphocytic lymphoma demonstrates clinical activity and acceptable toxicity. *J Clin Oncol* 2001;19(8):2153.

115. McLaughlin P, Hagemeister FB, Romaguera JE, et al. Fludarabine, mitoxantrone, and dexamethasone: an effective new regimen for indolent lymphoma. *Blood* 1996;14:1262.

116. Khouri IF, Keating MJ, Vriesendorp HM, et al. Autologous and allogeneic bone marrow transplantation for chronic lymphocytic leukemia: preliminary results. *J Clin Oncol* 1994;12(4):748.

117. Sahota SS, Garand R, Bataille R, et al. VH gene analysis of clonally related IgM and IgG from human lymphoplasmacytoid B-cell tumors with chronic lymphocytic leukemia features and high serum monoclonal IgG. *Blood* 1998;91(1):238.

118. Iida S, Rao PH, Nallasivam P, et al. The t(9;14)(p13;q32) chromosomal translocation associated with lymphoplasmacytoid lymphoma involves the PAX-5 gene. *Blood* 1996;88(11):4110.

119. Krenacs L, Himmelmann AW, Quintanilla-Martinez L, et al. Transcription factor B-cell-specific activator protein (BSAP) is differentially expressed in B cells and in subsets of B-cell lymphomas. *Blood* 1998;92(4):1308.

120. Dimopoulos MA, Alexanian R. Waldenström's macroglobulinemia. *Blood* 1994;83(6):1452.

121. Agnello V, Chung RT, Kaplan LM. A role for hepatitis C virus infection in type II cryoglobulinemia. *N Engl J Med* 1992;327(21):1490.

122. Papamichael D, Norton AJ, Foran JM, et al. Immunocytoma: a retrospective analysis from St Bartholomew's Hospital—1972 to 1996. *J Clin Oncol* 1999;17(9):2847.

123. Dimopoulos MA, Weber D, Delasalle KB, et al. Treatment of Waldenström's macroglobulinemia resistant to standard therapy with 2-chlorodeoxyadenosine: identification of prognostic factors. *Ann Oncol* 1995;6(1):49.

124. Dimopoulos MA, Zervas C, Zomas A, et al. Treatment of Waldenström's macroglobulinemia with rituximab. *J Clin Oncol* 2002;20(9):2327.

125. Mitsiades CS, Mitsiades N, Richardson PG, et al. Novel biologically based therapies for Waldenström's macroglobulinemia. *Semin Oncol* 2003;30(2):309.

126. Qin Y, Greiner A, Trunk MJ, et al. Somatic hypermutation in low-grade mucosa-associated lymphoid tissue-type B-cell lymphoma. *Blood* 1995;86(9):3528.

127. Ott G, Katzenberger T, Greiner A, et al. The t(11;18)(q21;q21) chromosome translocation is a frequent and specific aberration in low-grade but not high-grade malignant non-Hodgkin's lymphomas of the mucosa-associated lymphoid tissue (MALT-) type. *Cancer Res* 1997;57(18):3944.

128. Streubel B, Lamprecht A, Dierlamm J, et al. T(14;18)(q32;q21) involving IGH and MALT1 is a frequent chromosomal aberration in MALT lymphoma. *Blood* 2003;101(6):2335.

129. Morgan JA, Yin Y, Borowsky AD, et al. Breakpoints of the t(11;18)(q21;q21) in mucosa-associated lymphoid tissue (MALT) lymphoma lie within or near the previously undescribed gene MALT1 in chromosome 18. *Cancer Res* 1999;59(24):6205.

130. Willis TG, Jadayel DM, Du MQ, et al. Bcl10 is involved in t(1;14)(p22;q32) of MALT B cell lymphoma and mutated in multiple tumor types. *Cell* 1999;96(1):35.

131. Ye H, Liu H, Attygalle A, et al. Variable frequencies of t(11;18)(q21;q21) in MALT lymphomas of different sites: significant association with CagA strains of H pylori in gastric MALT lymphoma. *Blood* 2003;102(3):1012.

132. Schreuder MI, Hoeve MA, Hebeda KM, et al. Mutual exclusion of t(11;18)(q21;q21) and numerical chromosomal aberrations in the development of different types of primary gastric lymphomas. *Br J Haematol* 2003;123(4):590.

133. Bierman PJ. Gastrointestinal lymphoma. *Curr Treat Options Oncol* 2003;4(5):421.

134. Wotherspoon AC, Doglioni C, Diss TC, et al. Regression of primary low-grade B-cell gastric lymphoma of mucosa-associated lymphoid tissue type after eradication of Helicobacter pylori. *Lancet* 1993;342:575.

135. Tsang RW, Gospodarowicz MK, Pintilie M, et al. Stage I and II MALT lymphoma: results of treatment with radiotherapy. *Int J Radiat Oncol Biol Phys* 2001;50(5):1258.

136. Hitchcock S, Ng AK, Fisher DC, et al. Treatment outcome of mucosa-associated lymphoid tissue/marginal zone non-Hodgkin's lymphoma. *Int J Radiat Oncol Biol Phys* 2002;52(4):1058.

137. Neubauer A, Thiede C, Morgner A, et al. Cure of Helicobacter pylori infection and duration of remission of low-grade gastric mucosa–associated lymphoid tissue lymphoma. *J Natl Cancer Inst* 1997;89(18):1350.

138. Hammel P, Haioun C, Chaumette MT, et al. Efficacy of single-agent chemotherapy in low-grade B-cell mucosa-associated lymphoid tissue lymphoma with prominent gastric expression. *J Clin Oncol* 1995;13:2524.

139. Zinzani PL, Magagnoli M, Galieni P, et al. Nongastrointestinal low-grade mucosa–associated lymphoid tissue lymphoma: analysis of 75 patients. *J Clin Oncol* 1999;17(4):1254.

140. Taddesse-Heath L, Pittaluga S, Sorbara L, et al. Marginal zone B-cell lymphoma in children and young adults. *Am J Surg Pathol* 2003;27(4):522.

141. Zucca E, Conconi A, Pedrinis E, et al. Nongastric marginal zone B-cell lymphoma of mucosa-associated lymphoid tissue. *Blood* 2003;101(7):2489.

142. Zhu D, Oscier DG, Stevenson FK. Splenic lymphoma with villous lymphocytes involves B cells with extensively mutated Ig heavy chain variable region genes. *Blood* 1995;85(6):1603.

143. Algara P, Mateo MS, Sanchez-Beato M, et al. Analysis of the IgV(H) somatic mutations in splenic marginal zone lymphoma defines a group of unmutated cases with frequent 7q deletion and adverse clinical course. *Blood* 2002;99(4):1299.

144. Brynes RK, Almaguer PD, Leathery KE, et al. Numerical cytogenetic abnormalities of chromosomes 3, 7, and 12 in marginal zone B-cell lymphomas. *Mod Pathol* 1996;9(10):995.

145. Franco V, Florena AM, Iannitto E. Splenic marginal zone lymphoma. *Blood* 2003;101(7):2464.

146. Harris NL, Nadler LM, Bhan AK. Immunohistologic characterization of two malignant lymphomas of germinal center type (centroblastic/centrocytic and centrocytic) with monoclonal antibodies. Follicular and diffuse lymphomas of small-cleaved-cell type are related but distinct entities. *Am J Pathol* 1984;117(2):262.

147. Levy S, Mendel E, Kon S, et al. Mutational hot spots in Ig V region genes of human follicular lymphomas. *J Exp Med* 1988;168(2):475.

148. Akasaka T, Lossos IS, Levy R. BCL6 gene translocation in follicular lymphoma: a harbinger of eventual transformation to diffuse aggressive lymphoma. *Blood* 2003;102(4):1443.

149. Tilly H, Rossi A, Stamatoullas A, et al. Prognostic value of chromosomal abnormalities in follicular lymphoma. *Blood* 1994;84(4):1043.

150. Husson H, Carideo EG, Neuberg D, et al. Gene expression profiling of follicular lymphoma and normal germinal center B cells using cDNA arrays. *Blood* 2002;99(1):282.

151. Bohen SP, Troyanskaya OG, Alter O, et al. Variation in gene expression patterns in follicular lymphoma and the response to rituximab. *Proc Natl Acad Sci U S A* 2003;100(4):1926.

152. Martinez-Climent JA, Alizadeh AA, Segraves R, et al. Transformation of follicular lymphoma to diffuse large cell lymphoma is associated with a heterogeneous set of DNA copy number and gene expression alterations. *Blood* 2003;101(8):3109.

153. de Vos S, Hofmann WK, Grogan TM, et al. Gene expression profile of serial samples of transformed B-cell lymphomas. *Lab Invest* 2003;83(2):271.

154. Kamath SS, Marcus RB Jr, Lynch JW, et al. The impact of radiotherapy dose and other treatment-related and clinical factors on in-field control in stage I and II non-Hodgkin's lymphoma. *Int J Radiat Oncol Biol Phys* 1999;44(3):563.

155. Wilder RB, Jones D, Tucker SL, et al. Long-term results with radiotherapy for stage I–II follicular lymphoma. *Int J Radiat Oncol Biol Phys* 2001;51:1219.

156. Vaughan Hudson B, Vaughan Hudson G, MacLennan KA, et al. Clinical stage 1 non-Hodgkin's lymphoma: long-term follow-up of patients treated by the British National Lymphoma Investigation with radiotherapy alone as initial therapy. *Br J Cancer* 1994;69(6):1088.

157. Lawrence TS, Urba WJ, Steinberg SM, et al. Retrospective analysis of stage I and II indolent lymphomas at the National Cancer Institute. *Int J Radiat Oncol Biol Phys* 1988;14(3):417.

158. Gospodarowicz M, Lippuner T, Pintilie M, et al. Stage I and II follicular lymphoma: long-term outcome and pattern of failure following treatment with involved field radiation therapy alone. *Int J Radiat Biol Oncol Phys* 1999;45:217a.

159. Mac Manus MP, Hoppe RT. Is radiotherapy curative for stage I and II low-grade follicular lymphoma? Results of a long-term follow-up study of patients treated at Stanford University. *J Clin Oncol* 1996;14:1282.

160. Soubeyran P, Eghbali H, Bonichon F, et al. Localized follicular lymphomas: prognosis and survival of stages I and II in a retrospective series of 103 patients. *Radiother Oncol* 1988;13(2):91.

161. Taylor RE, Allan SG, McIntyre MA, et al. Low grade stage I and II non-Hodgkin's lymphoma: results of treatment and relapse pattern following therapy. *Clin Radiol* 1988;39(3):287.

162. Pendlebury S, Awadi ME, Ashley S, et al. Radiotherapy results in early stage low grade nodal non-Hodgkin's lymphoma. *Radiother Oncol* 1995;36:167.

163. Monfardini S, Banfi A, Bonadonna G, et al. Improved five year survival after combined radiotherapy-chemotherapy for stage I–II non-Hodgkin's lymphoma. *Int J Radiat Oncol Biol Phys* 1980;6(2):125.

164. Landberg TG, Hakansson LG, Moller TR, et al. CVP-remission-maintenance in stage I or II non-Hodgkin's lymphomas: preliminary results of a randomized study. *Cancer* 1979;44(3):831.

165. Kelsey SM, Newland AC, Hudson GV, Jelliffe AM. A British National Lymphoma Investigation randomised trial of single agent chlorambucil plus radiotherapy versus radiotherapy alone in low grade, localised non-Hodgkin's lymphoma. *Med Oncol* 1994;11(1):19.

166. McLaughlin P, Fuller L, Redman J, et al. Stage I–II low-grade lymphomas: a prospective trial of combination chemotherapy and radiotherapy. *Ann Oncol* 1991;2[Suppl 2]:137.

167. Horning SJ, Rosenberg SA. The natural history of initially untreated low-grade non-Hodgkin's lymphoma. *N Engl J Med* 1984;311(23):1471.

168. Young RC, Longo DL, Glatstein E, et al. Watchful-waiting VS aggressive combined modality therapy in the treatment of stage III–IV indolent non-Hodgkin's lymphoma. *Proc Am Soc Clin Oncol* 1987;6:200a.

169. Lister TA, Cullen MH, Beard ME, et al. Comparison of combined and single-agent chemotherapy in non-Hodgkin's lymphoma of favourable histological type. *Br Med J* 1978;1(6112):533.

170. Dana BW, Dahlberg S, Nathwani BN, et al. Long-term follow-up of patients with low-grade malignant lymphomas treated with doxorubicin-based chemotherapy or chemoimmmunotherapy. *J Clin Oncol* 1993;11:644.

171. Peterson BA, Petroni GR, Frizzera G, et al. Prolonged single-agent versus combination chemotherapy in indolent follicular lymphomas: a study of the cancer and leukemia group B. *J Clin Oncol* 2003;21(1):5.

172. Bartlett NL, Rizeq M, Dorfman RF, et al. Follicular large-cell lymphoma: intermediate or low grade? *J Clin Oncol* 1994;12(7):1349.

173. Klasa RJ, Meyer RM, Shustik C, et al. Randomized phase III study of fludarabine phosphate versus cyclophosphamide, vincristine, and prednisone in patients with recurrent low-grade non-Hodgkin's lymphoma previously treated with an alkylating agent or alkylator-containing regimen. *J Clin Oncol* 2002;20(24):4649.

174. Velasquez WS, Lew D, Grogan TM, et al. Combination of fludarabine and mitoxantrone in untreated stages III and IV low-grade lymphoma: S9501. *J Clin Oncol* 2003;21(10):1996.

175. Freedman AS, Neuberg D, Mauch P, et al. Long-term follow-up of autologous bone marrow transplantation in patients with relapsed follicular lymphoma. *Blood* 1999;94(10):3325.

176. Horning SJ, Negrin RS, Hoppe RT, et al. High-dose therapy and autologous bone marrow transplantation for follicular lymphoma in first complete or partial remission: results of a phase II clinical trial. *Blood* 2001;97(2):404.

177. Friedberg JW, Neuberg D, Stone RM, et al. Outcome in patients with myelodysplastic syndrome after autologous bone marrow transplantation for non-Hodgkin's lymphoma. *J Clin Oncol* 1999;17(10):3128.

178. Cheson BD. The curious case of the baffling biological. *J Clin Oncol* 2000;18(10):2007.

179. Hagenbeek A, Carde P, Meerwaldt JH, et al. Maintenance of remission with human recombinant interferon alfa-2a in patients with stage III and IV low-grade malignant non-Hodgkin's lymphoma. *J Clin Oncol* 1998;16(1):41.

180. Fisher RI, Dana B, LeBlanc M, et al. Interferon alpha consolidation after intensive chemotherapy does not prolong the progression-free survival of patients with low grade non-Hodgkin's lymphoma: results of Southwest Oncology Group randomized phase III study 8809. *J Clin Oncol* 2000;18:2010.

181. Colombat P, Salles G, Brousse N, et al. Rituximab (anti-CD20 monoclonal antibody) as single first-line therapy for patients with follicular lymphoma with a low tumor burden: clinical and molecular evaluation. *Blood* 2001;97(1):101.

182. Hainsworth JD, Litchy S, Burris HA, et al. Rituximab as first-line and maintenance therapy for patients with indolent non-Hodgkin's lymphoma. *J Clin Oncol* 2002;20(20):4261.
183. Gielmini M, Schmitz SFH, Cogliatti SB, et al. Maintenance treatment with 2-monthly rituximab after standard weekly × 4 rituximab induction significantly improves event-free survival in patients with follicular lymphoma. *Ann Oncol* 2002;13:112a.
184. Hainsworth JD, Litchy S, Greco FA. Scheduled rituximab maintenance therapy versus rituximab retreatment at progression in patients with indolent non-Hodgkin's lymphoma responding to single-agent rituximab: a randomized trial of the Minnie Pearl Cancer Research Network. *Blood* 2003;102(11):69a.
185. Czuczman MS, Grillo-Lopez AJ, White CA, et al. Treatment of patients with low-grade B-cell lymphoma with the combination of chimeric anti-CD20 monoclonal antibody and CHOP chemotherapy. *J Clin Oncol* 1999;17(1):268.
186. Maloney DG, Press OW, Braziel RM, et al. A phase II trial of CHOP followed by rituximab chimeric monoclonal anti-CD20 antibody for treatment of newly diagnosed follicular non-Hodgkin's lymphoma: SWOG 9800. *Blood* 2001;98.
187. Marcus R, Imrie K, Belch A, et al. An international multi-centre randomized, open-label, phase III trial comparing rituximab added to CVP chemotherapy to CVP alone in untreated stage III/IV follicular non-Hodgkin's lymphoma. *Blood* 2003;102(11):28a.
188. Hsu FJ, Caspar CB, Czerwinski D, et al. Tumor-specific idiotype vaccines in the treatment of patients with B-cell lymphoma—long-term results of a clinical trial. *Blood* 1997;89(9):3129.
189. Kwak LW, Campbell MJ, Czerwinski DK, et al. Induction of immune responses in patients with B-cell lymphoma against the surface-immunoglobulin idiotype expressed by their tumors. *N Engl J Med* 1992;327(17):1209.
190. Timmerman JM, Czerwinski DK, Davis TA, et al. Idiotype-pulsed dendritic cell vaccination for B-cell lymphoma: clinical and immune responses in 35 patients. *Blood* 2002;99(5):1517.
191. Kaminski MS, Tuck M, Regan D, et al. High response rates and durable remissions in patients with previously untreated, advanced-stage, follicular lymphoma treated with tositumomab and iodine I-131 tositumomab (Bexxar). *Blood* 2002;100(11):356a.
192. Press OW, Unger JM, Braziel RM, et al. A phase 2 trial of CHOP chemotherapy followed by tositumomab/iodine I 131 tositumomab for previously untreated follicular non-Hodgkin lymphoma: Southwest Oncology Group Protocol S9911. *Blood* 2003;102(5):1606.
193. Johnson PW, Rohatiner AZ, Whelan JS, et al. Patterns of survival in patients with recurrent follicular lymphoma: a 20-year study from a single center. *J Clin Oncol* 1995;13(1):140.
194. Hiddemann W, Forstpointer R, Fiedler F, et al. The addition of rituximab to combination chemotherapy with fludarabine, cyclophosphamide, mitoxantrone (FCM) results in a significant increase of overall response as compared to FCM alone in patients with relapsed or refractory follicular (FCL) and mantle cell lymphomas (MCL). Results of a prospective randomized comparison of the German Low Grade Study Group (GLSG). *Blood* 2001;98:844a.
195. Dillman RO. Radiolabeled anti-CD20 monoclonal antibodies for the treatment of B-cell lymphoma. *J Clin Oncol* 2002;20(16):3545.
196. Cheson BD. Radioimmunotherapy of non-Hodgkin lymphomas. *Blood* 2003;101(2):391.
197. Witzig TE, Gordon LI, Cabanillas F, et al. Randomized controlled trial of yttrium-90–labeled ibritumomab tiuxetan radioimmunotherapy versus rituximab immunotherapy for patients with relapsed or refractory low-grade, follicular, or transformed B-cell non-Hodgkin's lymphoma. *J Clin Oncol* 2002;20(10):2453.
198. Kaminski MS, Zelenetz AD, Press OW, et al. Pivotal study of iodine I 131 tositumomab for chemotherapy-refractory low-grade or transformed B-cell non-Hodgkin's lymphomas. *J Clin Oncol* 2001;19(19):3918.
199. Apostolidis J, Gupta RK, Grenzelias D, et al. High-dose therapy with autologous bone marrow support as consolidation of remission in follicular lymphoma: long-term clinical and molecular follow-up. *J Clin Oncol* 2000;18(3):527.
200. Freedman AS, Neuberg D, Mauch P, et al. Long-term follow-up of autologous bone marrow transplantation in patients with relapsed follicular lymphoma. *Blood* 1999;94(10):3325.
201. van Besien K, Sobocinski KA, Rowlings PA, et al. Allogeneic bone marrow transplantation for low-grade lymphoma. *Blood* 1998;92(5):1832.
202. van Besien K, Loberiza FR Jr, Bajorunaite R, et al. Comparison of autologous and allogeneic hematopoietic stem cell transplantation for follicular lymphoma. *Blood* 2003;102(10):3521.
203. Schouten HC, Qian W, Kvaloy S, et al. High-dose therapy improves progression-free survival and survival in relapsed follicular non-Hodgkin's lymphoma: results from the randomized European CUP trial. *J Clin Oncol* 2003;21(21):3918.
204. Khouri IF, Keating M, Korbling M, et al. Transplant-lite: induction of graft-versus-malignancy using fludarabine-based nonablative chemotherapy and allogeneic blood progrenitor-cell transplantation as treatment for lymphoid malignancies. *J Clin Oncol* 1998;16(8):2817.
205. Yuen AR, Kamel OW, Halpern J, Horning SJ. Long-term survival after histologic transformation of low-grade follicular lymphoma. *J Clin Oncol* 1995;13(7):1726.
206. Friedberg JW, Neuberg D, Gribben JG, et al. Autologous bone marrow transplantation after histologic transformation of indolent B cell malignancies. *Biol Blood Marrow Transplant* 1999;5(4):262.
207. Zelenetz AD, Saleh M, Vose J, et al. Patients with transformed low grade lymphoma attain durable responses following outpatient radioimmunotherapy with tositumomab and iodine I 131 tositumomab (Bexxar). *Blood* 2002;100(11):357a.
208. Swerdlow SH, Yang WI, Zukerberg LR, et al. Expression of cyclin D1 protein in centrocytic/mantle cell lymphomas with and without rearrangement of the BCL1/cyclin D1 gene. *Hum Pathol* 1995;26(9):999.
209. Onciu M, Schlette E, Medeiros LJ, et al. Cytogenetic findings in mantle cell lymphoma cases with a high level of peripheral blood involvement have a distinct pattern of abnormalities. *Am J Clin Pathol* 2001;116(6):886.
210. Greiner TC, Moynihan MJ, Chan WC, et al. p53 mutations in mantle cell lymphoma are associated with variant cytology and predict a poor prognosis. *Blood* 1996;87(10):4302.
211. Fang NY, Greiner TC, Weisenburger DD, et al. Oligonucleotide microarrays demonstrate the highest frequency of ATM mutations in the mantle cell subtype of lymphoma. *Proc Natl Acad Sci U S A* 2003;100(9):5372.
212. Martinez N, Camacho FI, Algara P, et al. The molecular signature of mantle cell lymphoma reveals multiple signals favoring cell survival. *Cancer Res* 2003;63(23):8226.
213. Thieblemont C, Nasser V, Felman P, et al. Small lymphocytic lymphoma, marginal zone B-cell lymphoma, mantle cell lymphoma exhibit distinct gene-expression profiles allowing molecular diagnosis. *Blood* 2004;103:2727.
214. Fisher RI, Dahlberg S, Nathwani BN, et al. A clinical analysis of two indolent lymphoma entities: mantle cell lymphoma and marginal zone lymphoma (including the mucosa-associated lymphoid tissue and monocytoid B-cell subcategories): a Southwest Oncology Group study. *Blood* 1995;85:1075.
215. Romaguera JE, Medeiros LJ, Hagemeister FB, et al. Frequency of gastrointestinal involvement and its clinical significance in mantle cell lymphoma. *Cancer* 2003;97(3):586.
216. Bosch F, Lopez-Guillermo A, Campo E, et al. Mantle cell lymphoma: presenting features, response to therapy, and prognostic factors. *Cancer* 1998;82(3):567.
217. Meusers P, Englehard M, Bartels H, et al. Multicentre randomized therapeutic trial for advanced centrocytic lymphoma: anthracycline does not improve the prognosis. *Hematol Oncol* 1989;7:365.
218. Howard OM, Gribben JG, Neuberg D, et al. Rituximab and CHOP induction therapy for newly diagnosed mantle cell lymphoma: molecular complete responses are not predictive of progression-free survival. *J Clin Oncol* 2002;20(5):1288.
219. Khouri IF, Romaguera JE, Kantarjian H, et al. Hyper-CVAD and high-dose methotrexate/cytarabine followed by stem-cell transplantation: an active regimen for aggressive mantle-cell lymphoma. *J Clin Oncol* 1998;16(12):3803.
220. Freedman AS, Neuberg D, Gribben JG, et al. High-dose chemoradiotherapy and anti-B-cell monoclonal antibody-purged autologous bone marrow transplantation in mantle-cell lymphoma: no evidence for long-term remission. *J Clin Oncol* 1998;16(1):13.
221. Khouri IF, Lee MS, Saliba RM, et al. Nonablative allogeneic stem-cell transplantation for advanced/recurrent mantle-cell lymphoma. *J Clin Oncol* 2003;21(23):4407.
222. Goy A, Hart S, Pro B, et al. Report of a phase II study of proteasome inhibitor bortezomib in patients with relapsed or refractory indolent or aggressive lymphomas. *Blood* 2003;102(11):180a.
223. Achten R, Verhoef G, Vanuytsel L, et al. T-cell/histiocyte-rich large B-cell lymphoma: a distinct clinicopathologic entity. *J Clin Oncol* 2002;20(5):1269.
224. Bouabdallah R, Mounier N, Guettier C, et al. T-cell/histiocyte-rich large B-cell lymphomas and classical diffuse large B-cell lymphomas have similar outcome after chemotherapy: a matched-control analysis. *J Clin Oncol* 2003;21(7):1271.
225. Fisher DE, Jacobson JO, Ault KA, Harris NL. Diffuse large cell lymphoma with discordant bone marrow histology. Clinical features and biological implications. *Cancer* 1989;64(9):1879.
226. Robertson LE, Redman JR, Butler JJ, et al. Discordant bone marrow involvement in diffuse large-cell lymphoma: a distinct clinical-pathologic entity associated with a continuous risk of relapse. *J Clin Oncol* 1991;9(2):236.
227. Barrans SL, Carter I, Owen RG, et al. Germinal center phenotype and bcl-2 expression combined with the International Prognostic Index improves patient risk stratification in diffuse large B-cell lymphoma. *Blood* 2002;99(4):1136.
228. Gascoyne RD, Adomat SA, Krajewski S, et al. Prognostic significance of Bcl-2 protein expression and Bcl-2 gene rearrangement in diffuse aggressive non-Hodgkin's lymphoma. *Blood* 1997;90(1):244.
229. Lossos IS, Jones CD, Warnke R, et al. Expression of a single gene, BCL-6, strongly predicts survival in patients with diffuse large B-cell lymphoma. *Blood* 2001;98(4):945.
230. Kramer MH, Hermans J, Wijburg E, et al. Clinical relevance of BCL2, BCL6, and MYC rearrangements in diffuse large B-cell lymphoma. *Blood* 1998;92(9):3152.
231. Rosenwald A, Wright G, Chan WC, et al. The use of molecular profiling to predict survival after chemotherapy for diffuse large B-cell lymphoma. *N Engl J Med* 2002;346(25):1937.
232. Shipp MA, Ross KN, Tamayo P, et al. Diffuse large B-cell lymphoma outcome prediction by gene-expression profiling and supervised machine learning. *Nat Med* 2002;8(1):68.
233. Miller TP, Dahlberg S, Cassady JR, et al. Chemotherapy alone compared with chemotherapy plus radiotherapy for localized intermediate- and high-grade non-Hodgkin's lymphoma. *N Engl J Med* 1998;339:21.
234. Horning S, Glick J, et al. Final report of E1484: CHOP v CHOP + radiotherapy for limited stage diffuse aggressive lymphoma. *Blood* 2001;98:724a.
235. Fillet G, Bonnet C. Radiotherapy is unnecessary in elderly patients with localized aggressive non-Hodgkin's lymphoma: results of the GELA LNH 93-4 study. *Blood* 2002;100:92a.
236. Reyes F, Lepage E, et al. Superiority of chemotherapy alone with the ACVBP regimen over treatment with three cycles of CHOP plus radiotherapy in low risk localized aggressive lymphoma: the LNH93-1 GELA study. *Blood* 2002;100:93a.
237. Fisher RI, Gaynor ER, Dahlberg S, et al. A phase III comparison of CHOP vs. m-BACOD vs. ProMACE-CytaBOM vs. MACOP-B in patients with intermediate or high grade non-Hodgkin's lymphoma: results of SWOG-8516 (Intergroup 0067), the National High Priority Lymphoma Study. *Ann Oncol* 1993;5:591.
238. Vose JM, Link BK, Grossbard ML, et al. Phase II study of rituximab in combination with CHOP chemotherapy in patients with previously untreated, aggressive non-Hodgkin's lymphoma. *J Clin Oncol* 2001;19(2):389.
239. Coiffier B, Lepage E, Briere J, et al. CHOP chemotherapy plus rituximab compared with CHOP alone in elderly patients with diffuse large-B-cell lymphoma. *N Engl J Med* 2002;346(4):235.
240. Haberman TM, Weller EA, Morrison VA, et al. Phase III trial of rituximab-CHOP vs. CHOP with a second randomization to maintenance rituximab or observation in patients 60 years of age and older with diffuse large B cell lymphoma. *Blood* 2003;102(11):6a.
241. Mounier N, Briere J, Gisselbrecht C, et al. Rituximab plus CHOP (R-CHOP) overcomes bcl-2–associated resistance to chemotherapy in elderly patients with diffuse large B-cell lymphoma (DLBCL). *Blood* 2003;101(11):4279.
242. Fisher RI. Autologous stem-cell transplantation as a component of initial treatment for poor risk patients with aggressive non-Hodgkin's lymphoma: resolved issues versus remaining opportunities. *J Clin Oncol* 2002;20(22):4411.

243. Haioun C, Lepage E, Gisselbrecht C, et al. Comparison of autologous bone marrow transplantation with sequential chemotherapy for intermediate-grade and high-grade non-Hodgkin's lymphoma in first complete remission: a study of 464 patients. Groupe d'Etude des Lymphomes de l'Adulte. *J Clin Oncol* 1994;12(12):2543.

244. Santini G, Salvagno L, Leoni P, et al. VACOP-B versus VACOP-B plus autologous bone marrow transplantation for advanced diffuse non-Hodgkin's lymphoma: results of a prospective randomized trial by the non-Hodgkin's Lymphoma Cooperative Study Group. *J Clin Oncol* 1998;16(8):2796.

245. Haioun C, Lepage E, Gisselbrecht C, et al. Survival benefit of high-dose therapy in poor-risk aggressive non-Hodgkin's lymphoma: final analysis of the prospective LNH87-2 protocol—a Groupe d'Etude des Lymphomes de l'Adulte study. *J Clin Oncol* 2000;18(16):3025.

246. Santini G, Salvagno L, Leoni P, et al. VACOP-B versus VACOP-B plus autologous bone marrow transplantation for advanced diffuse non-Hodgkin's lymphoma: results of a prospective randomized trial by the non-Hodgkin's Lymphoma Cooperative Study Group. *J Clin Oncol* 1998;16:2796.

247. Shipp MA, Abeloff MD, Antman KH, et al. International consensus conference on high-dose therapy with hematopoietic stem cell transplantation in aggressive non-Hodgkin's lymphomas: report of the jury. *J Clin Oncol* 1999;17:423.

248. Coiffier B, Haioun C, Ketterer N, et al. Rituximab (anti-CD20 monoclonal antibody) for the treatment of patients with relapsing or refractory aggressive lymphoma: a multicenter phase II study. *Blood* 1998;92(6):1927.

249. Moskowitz CH, Bertino JR, Glassman JR, et al. Ifosfamide, carboplatin, and etoposide: a highly effective cytoreduction and peripheral-blood progrenitor-cell mobilization regimen for transplant-eligible patients with non-Hodgkin's lymphoma. *J Clin Oncol* 1999;17(12):3776.

250. Stiff PJ, Dahlberg S, Forman SJ, et al. Autologous bone marrow transplantation for patients with relapsed or refractory diffuse aggressive non-Hodgkin's lymphoma: value of augmented preparative regimens—a Southwest Oncology Group trial. *J Clin Oncol* 1998;16(1):48.

251. Chopra R, Goldstone AH, Pearce R, et al. Autologous versus allogeneic bone marrow transplantation for non-Hodgkin's lymphoma: a case-controlled analysis of the European Bone Marrow Transplant Group Registry data. *J Clin Oncol* 1992;10(11):1690.

252. Savage KJ, Monti S, Kutok JL, et al. The molecular signature of mediastinal large B-cell lymphoma differs from that of other diffuse large B-cell lymphomas and shares features with classical Hodgkin lymphoma. *Blood* 2003;102(13):3871.

253. van Besien K, Kelta M, Bahaguna P. Primary mediastinal B-cell lymphoma: a review of pathology and management. *J Clin Oncol* 2001;19(6):1855.

254. Zinzani PL, Martelli M, Magagnoli M, et al. Treatment and clinical management of primary mediastinal large B-cell lymphoma with sclerosis: MACOP-B regimen and mediastinal radiotherapy monitored by (67)gallium scan in 50 patients. *Blood* 1999;94(10):3289.

255. Wilson WH, Kingma DW, Raffeld M, et al. Association of lymphomatoid granulomatosis with Epstein-Barr viral infection of B lymphocytes and response to interferon-alpha 2b. *Blood* 1996;87(11):4531.

256. Otsuki T, Kumar S, Ensoli B, et al. Detection of HHV-8/KSHV DNA sequences in AIDS-associated extranodal lymphoid malignancies. *Leukemia* 1996;10(8):1358.

257. Ziegler JL, Magrath IT, Olweny CL. Cure of Burkitt's lymphoma. Ten-year follow-up of 157 Ugandan patients. *Lancet* 1979;2(8149):936.

258. Magrath I, Adde M, Shad A, et al. Adults and children with small non-cleaved-cell lymphoma have a similar excellent outcome when treated with the same chemotherapy regimen. *J Clin Oncol* 1996;14(3):925.

259. Philip T, Biron P, Philip I, et al. Massive therapy and autologous bone marrow transplantation in pediatric and young adults Burkitt's lymphoma (30 courses on 28 patients: a 5-year experience). *Eur J Cancer Clin Oncol* 1986;22(8):1015.

260. Poiesz BJ, Ruscetti FW, Gazdar AF, et al. Detection and isolation of type C retrovirus particles from fresh and cultured lymphocytes of a patient with cutaneous T-cell lymphoma. *Proc Natl Acad Sci U S A* 1980;77(12):7415.

261. Itoyama T, Chaganti RS, Yamada Y, et al. Cytogenetic analysis and clinical significance in adult T-cell leukemia/lymphoma: a study of 50 cases from the human T-cell leukemia virus type-1 endemic area, Nagasaki. *Blood* 2001;97(11):3612.

262. Matutes E, Taylor GP, Cavenagh J, et al. Interferon alpha and zidovudine therapy in adult T-cell leukaemia lymphoma: response and outcome in 15 patients. *Br J Haematol* 2001;113(3):779.

263. Lepretre S, Buchonnet G, Stamatoullas A, et al. Chromosome abnormalities in peripheral T-cell lymphoma. *Cancer Genet Cytogenet* 2000;117(1):71.

264. Vose JM, Peterson C, Bierman PJ, et al. Comparison of high-dose therapy and autologous bone marrow transplantation for T-cell and B-cell non-Hodgkin's lymphomas. *Blood* 1990;76(2):424.

265. Anagnostopoulos I, Hummel M, Finn T, et al. Heterogeneous Epstein-Barr virus infection patterns in peripheral T-cell lymphoma of angioimmunoblastic lymphadenopathy type. *Blood* 1992;80(7):1804.

266. Siegert W, Agthe A, Griesser H, et al. Treatment of angioimmunoblastic lymphadenopathy (AILD)-type T-cell lymphoma using prednisone with or without the COPBLAM/IMVP-16 regimen. A multicenter study. Kiel Lymphoma Study Group. *Ann Intern Med* 1992;117(5):364.

267. Elenitoba-Johnson KS, Zarate-Osorno A, Meneses A, et al. Cytotoxic granular protein expression, Epstein-Barr virus strain type, and latent membrane protein-1 oncogene deletions in nasal T-lymphocyte/natural killer cell lymphomas from Mexico. *Mod Pathol* 1998;11(8):754.

268. Isaacson PG, O'Connor NT, Spencer J, et al. Malignant histiocytosis of the intestine: a T-cell lymphoma. *Lancet* 1985;2(8457):688.

269. Verkarre V, Romana SP, Cellier C, et al. Recurrent partial trisomy 1q22-q44 in clonal intraepithelial lymphocytes in refractory celiac sprue. *Gastroenterology* 2003;125(1):40.

270. Belhadj K, Reyes F, Farcet JP, et al. Hepatosplenic gammadelta T-cell lymphoma is a rare clinicopathologic entity with poor outcome: report on a series of 21 patients. *Blood* 2003;102(13):4261.

271. Shiota M, Nakamura S, Ichinohasama R, et al. Anaplastic large cell lymphomas expressing the novel chimeric protein p80NPM/ALK: a distinct clinicopathologic entity. *Blood* 1995;86(5):1954.

272. Benharroch D, Meguerian-Bedoyan Z, Lamant L, et al. ALK-positive lymphoma: a single disease with a broad spectrum of morphology. *Blood* 1998;91(6):2076.

273. Ansell S, Byrd J, Horwitz S, et al. Phase I/II study of a fully human anti CD-30 monoclonal antibody in Hodgkin's disease and anaplastic large cell lymphoma. *Blood* 2003;102(11):181a.

274. Effect of age on the characteristics and clinical behavior of non-Hodgkin's lymphoma patients. The Non-Hodgkin's Lymphoma Classification Project. *Ann Oncol* 1997;8(10):973.

275. Dixon DO, Neilan B, Jones SE, et al. Effect of age on therapeutic outcome in advanced diffuse histiocytic lymphoma: The Southwest Oncology Group experience. *J Clin Oncol* 1986;4:295.

276. Rigacci L, Carpaneto A, Alterini R, et al. Treatment of large cell lymphoma in elderly patients with a mitoxantrone, cyclophosphamide, etoposide, and prednisone regimen: long-term follow-up results. *Cancer* 2003;97(1):97.

277. Osby E, Hagberg H, Kvaloy S, et al. CHOP is superior to CNOP in elderly patients with aggressive lymphoma while outcome is unaffected by filgrastim treatment: results of a Nordic Lymphoma Group randomized trial. *Blood* 2003;101(10):3840.

278. Pfreundschuh M, Truemper L, Kloess M, et al. 2-weekly vs. 3-weekly CHOP with and without etoposide for patients >60 years of age with aggressive non-Hodgkin's lymphoma (NHL): results of the completed NHL-B-2 trial of the DSHNHL. *Ann Oncol* 2002;13[Suppl 2].

279. Gomez H, Hidalgo M, Casanova L, et al. Risk factors for treatment-related death in elderly patients with aggressive non-Hodgkin's lymphoma: results of a multivariate analysis. *J Clin Oncol* 1998;16(6):2065.

280. Doorduijn JK, van der Holt B, van Imhoff GW, et al. CHOP compared with CHOP plus granulocyte colony-stimulating factor in elderly patients with aggressive non-Hodgkin's lymphoma. *J Clin Oncol* 2003;21(16):3041.

281. Opelz G, Henderson R. Incidence of non-Hodgkin lymphoma in kidney and heart transplant recipients [see comments]. *Lancet* 1993;342(8886–8887):1514.

282. Paya CV, Fung JJ, Nalesnik MA, et al. Epstein-Barr virus–induced posttransplant lymphoproliferative disorders. ASTS/ASTP EBV-PTLD Task Force and the Mayo Clinic Organized International Consensus Development Meeting. *Transplantation* 1999;68(10):1517.

283. Hanto DW. Classification of Epstein-Barr virus–associated posttransplant lymphoproliferative diseases: implications for understanding their pathogenesis and developing rational treatment strategies. *Annu Rev Med* 1995;46:381.

284. Penn I, Porat G. Central nervous system lymphomas in organ allograft recipients. *Transplantation* 1995;59(2):240.

285. Milpied N, Vasseur B, Parquet N, et al. Humanized anti-CD20 monoclonal antibody (rituximab) in post transplant B-lymphoproliferative disorder: a retrospective analysis on 32 patients. *Ann Oncol* 2000;11[Suppl 1]:113.

286. Garrett TJ, Chadburn A, Barr ML, et al. Posttransplantation lymphoproliferative disorders treated with cyclophosphamide-doxorubicin-vincristine-prednisone chemotherapy. *Cancer* 1993;72(9):2782.

287. Swinnen LJ, Mullen GM, Carr TJ, et al. Aggressive treatment for postcardiac transplant lymphoproliferation. *Blood* 1995;86(9):3333.

288. O'Brien S, Bernert RA, Logan JL, Lien YH. Remission of posttransplant lymphoproliferative disorder after interferon alfa therapy. *J Am Soc Nephrol* 1997;8(9):1483.

289. Papadopoulos EB, Ladanyi M, Emanuel D, et al. Infusions of donor leukocytes to treat Epstein-Barr virus–associated lymphoproliferative disorders after allogeneic bone marrow transplantation. *N Engl J Med* 1994;330(17):1185.

290. Kaplan LD, Straus DJ, Testa MA, et al. Low-dose compared with standard-dose m-BACOD chemotherapy for non-Hodgkin's lymphoma associated with human immunodeficiency virus infection. National Institute of Allergy and Infectious Diseases AIDS Clinical Trials Group. *N Engl J Med* 1997;336(23):1641.

291. Kaplan LD, Lee J, Scadden DT. No benefit from rituximab in a randomized phase III trial of CHOP with or without rituximab for patients with HIV-associated non-Hodgkin's lymphoma: updated data from AIDS Malignancies Consortium study 010. *Blood* 2003;102(11):409a.

292. Zucca E, Conconi A, Mughal TI, et al. Patterns of outcome and prognostic factors in primary large-cell lymphoma of the testis in a survey by the International Extranodal Lymphoma Study Group. *J Clin Oncol* 2003;21(1):20.

293. Connors JM, Klimo P, Voss N, et al. Testicular lymphoma: improved outcome with early brief chemotherapy. *J Clin Oncol* 1988;6(5):776.

294. Willemze R, Kerl H, Sterry W, et al. EORTC classification for primary cutaneous lymphomas: a proposal from the Cutaneous Lymphoma Study Group of the European Organization for Research and Treatment of Cancer. *Blood* 1997;90(1):354.

LYNN D. WILSON
GLENN W. JONES
MICHAEL GIRARDI
RICHARD L. EDELSON
PETER W. HEALD

SECTION **3**

Cutaneous T-Cell Lymphomas

Cutaneous T-cell lymphoma (CTCL) is a malignancy of T lymphocytes with a propensity to home to the skin and may present with a wide range of potential clinical manifestations. Although previously considered as distinct clinical entities, mycosis fungoides (MF), Sézary syndrome (SS), reticulum cell sarcoma of the skin, and several other cutaneous lymphocytic dyscrasias are now recognized as different clinical presentations of CTCL. The clinical value of the umbrella classification of CTCL is twofold. First, it highlights the relationship between distinct clinical presentations, which can nevertheless evolve into one another (i.e., the patch/plaque MF can develop into the erythrodermic SS) or may coexist. Second, it emphasizes the clinical relevance of advances in understanding the biologic behavior of CTCL cells, including their propensity to home to skin and to the T-cell zones of lymphoid structures. Still, it remains useful for clinicians to attach the subtype of CTCL to the name (e.g., MF-CTCL) because the management scheme and prognosis for subtypes may differ.

PATHOBIOLOGY

MF comprises the vast majority of CTCL, and thus much of what is understood about CTCL pathobiology stems from investigation of MF and its variants. Furthermore, erythrodermic/leukemic MF and SS patients have provided opportunities to isolate and study the malignant CTCL cells directly from the peripheral blood. CTCL is a clonal neoplasm, typically of mature CD4+ helper T (T_H) cells that are capable of stimulating immunoglobulin synthesis by B cells driven by the secretion of interleukin-4 and other cytokines.[1,2] CTCL cells express many of the same surface molecules as their nonmalignant counterparts, including CD45R0, a marker of "activated/memory" T cells. They use surface proteins such as the cutaneous lymphoid antigen (CLA) and chemokine receptors to home to skin.

CLA is the physiologic ligand of endothelial cell E-selectin, a cell adhesion molecule expressed on the surface of endothelial cells of cutaneous venules during chronic inflammation. Interactions between CLA on the surface of CTCL cells and E-selectin on endothelial cells allow CTCL cells to roll along the walls of cutaneous venules. Chemokine receptor CCR4 expressed by the CTCL cells binds chemokine CCL17 that has adhered to the luminal side of the endothelium, facilitating T-cell leukocyte function antigen 1 binding to endothelial cell intracellular adhesion molecule-1 and fostering extravasation into the dermis.[3]

Once MF-CTCL cells emerge within, or enter into the skin, the most striking trait is their profound epidermotropism. Although specimens from early lesions of MF-CTCL have lymphocytes in both the epidermis and dermis, clonality studies on dissected cells demonstrated that virtually all of the lympho-cytes found in the epidermis belong to the malignant clone, whereas the dermis contains a predominance of nonmalignant lymphocytes. Once in the epidermis, CTCL cells appear to become activated, and they have a well-described ability to generate cytokines, predominantly of the T_H2 phenotype. In addition to producing cytokines, MF-CTCL cells are exposed to a complex paracrine environment composed of many growth factors and cytokines elaborated by keratinocytes and stromal fibroblasts, macrophages, endothelial cells, and normal and neoplastic T lymphocytes.

In more advanced stages of disease, MF-CTCL cells appear to lose their dependence on epidermal cell adhesion molecules and cytokines so that epidermotropism is either diminished (to permit the development of tumor nodules that extend deep into the dermis) or lost completely (to permit dissemination of the neoplastic T cells to nodal and visceral sites). At this phase, the clinical presentation of MF-CTCL may become indistinguishable from that of other peripheral T-cell lymphomas, although the broad involvement of the skin usually remains a distinguishing feature. Even in advanced stages, the distinctive tissue distribution of the malignant cells (skin infiltration, preferential localization in interfollicular regions of lymph nodes, variable involvement of the peripheral blood, and avoidance of bone marrow) remains evident.

EPIDEMIOLOGY

CTCL is a relatively rare neoplasm, and the Surveillance, Epidemiology, and End Results program[4] reported that the incidence of MF-CTCL (the most common form of CTCL) had increased 3.2-fold between 1973 and 1984. The overall incidence rate is approximately 4 per 1 million according to Surveillance, Epidemiology, and End Results program data. The actual incidence rate may be an order of magnitude higher, given possible underreporting and the difficulty and confusion in making the diagnosis. The incidence of MF-CTCL rises with age such that the majority of patients are between 40 and 60. The disease is 2.2 times more common in males than in females, and incidence rates are somewhat higher in African Americans than in whites.

ETIOLOGY

Given the inherent immunologic nature of the neoplastic cells responsible for this disorder, it has been proposed that chronic exposure to occupational chemicals, pesticides, or tobacco may predispose to the development of MF-CTCL; however, none of these potential associations has survived scrutiny.[5,6] The observations that the disease is more common in African Americans than whites and that it often presents first in areas normally shielded from the sun (i.e., "bathing trunk" distribution) together suggest that actinic exposure may actually inhibit the evolution of the malignant clone from normal "cutaneous T cells." It is noteworthy that the epidermotropic collections of MF-CTCL cells, referred to histologically as "Pautrier's microabscesses," may represent congregation of malignant T cells around Langerhans cells, the dendritic antigen-presenting cells of the epidermis, and that

Langerhans cells are quite sensitive to ultraviolet (UV) damage. This observation has suggested that epidermotropic CTCL cells may receive growth signals from their contact with Langerhans cells. Therefore, it is possible that UV damage of Langerhans cells may interrupt this growth signal and inhibit the replication of CTCL cells in UV exposed skin sites. It is also intriguing that the often profound response of patch/plaque stage MF-CTCL to UV treatment may reflect this phenomenon as well. The association between human T-cell leukemia virus type 1 infection and adult T-cell leukemia-lymphoma (ATLL) or Epstein-Barr virus in conjunction with nasal natural killer (NK)/T-cell lymphoma is not reflected in the epidemiology of MF-CTCL. There is no clustering and no evidence of maternal transmission of the disease.

CLINICAL PRESENTATION

As more information has been gathered regarding the distinct clinical presentations, natural histories, and basic research associated with the various CTCLs, two classification systems have been developed. These classification schemes now provide the clinician with a basic framework from which to manage the various CTCL disease categories (Table 41.3-1).[7,8]

MYCOSIS FUNGOIDES

The classic MF presentation of CTCL typically progresses through the following four distinct phases:

1. A prediagnostic phase, with an asymptomatic, scaling erythematous macular eruption often in sun-shielded areas (i.e., "bathing trunk" distribution) that lasts for months to years during which the diagnosis may be suspected but cannot be confirmed by standard clinical or histopathologic means.
2. A patch phase, with thin, barely palpable, erythematous and eczematous lesions whose histologic features are at least "consistent with" the diagnosis of MF-CTCL.
3. A plaque phase, with more readily palpable erythematous lesions.
4. A tumor phase, where the neoplastic infiltrate extends below the upper dermis.

Painful and/or pruritic erythroderma may arise *de novo* or during any of the earlier described phases and is not always associated with frank T-cell leukemia (as in SS). Infrequently, MF-CTCL presents with cutaneous tumor nodules in the absence of patches or plaques (as in *tumor d'emblée*). Patients may also present with or progress to involvement of visceral organs.

MYCOSIS FUNGOIDES VARIANTS

Although MF may manifest cutaneous lesions of diverse color, morphology, and distribution (e.g., pink to red to violaceous to brown, eczematous to psoriasiform, nummular to oval to annular to linear) and may variably demonstrate tropisms or other findings histologically (e.g., follicular mucinosis, granulomatous inflammation), several variants of MF have been described in which certain clinicopathologic features predominate. Alopecia mucinosa is characterized by follicular papules with hair loss clinically and infiltrative, perifollicular clonal T cells, admixed with other mononuclear cells histologically. The accumulation of acid mucopolysaccharides in the sebaceous glands and root sheaths of hair follicles results in the histologic pattern termed *follicular mucinosis*. Overall, 15% to 30% of alopecia mucinosa–follicular mucinosis patients either have or will develop CTCL. Rarely, the folliculotropic pattern may be seen, with or without mucinosis, manifesting clinically as acneiform or cystic lesions with a predilection for the head and neck regions. Any follicular variant of MF may prove more difficult to treat by skin-directed therapies [e.g., psoralen and UVA light (PUVA), topical nitrogen mustard (NM)] alone. The use of a systemic retinoid may be of profound benefit in certain patients.

Pagetoid reticulosis, or Woringer-Kolopp disease, typically presents as a solitary cutaneous lesion of long duration, characterized histologically by marked numbers of abnormal CLA+ clonal T cells infiltrating the epidermis. The underlying dermis may be involved with a mixed inflammatory cell infiltrate. Clonal T-cell gene rearrangements have been observed in Woringer-Kolopp disease, which, in all likelihood, represent an indolent, particularly epidermotropic, variant of CTCL. Unilesional disease responds well to local radiotherapy or surgical excision. A disseminated, more aggressive disease that shows a similar histologic pattern of striking epidermal involvement is called the *Ketron-Goodman variant*, which has been characterized by clonal CD8+ cells.

Granulomatous slack skin is a very rare MF variant in which patients develop folds or pendulous bags of lax skin, most commonly in the axillae, neck, breast, or groin areas. Histologically, there is a striking granulomatous inflammation, with multinucleated giant cells admixed with atypical T cells. The lax skin is attributed to a marked destruction of elastin fibers by the granulomatous inflammation. It should be noted that approximately one-third of such cases have been associated with Hodgkin's disease.

TABLE 41.3-1. EORTC and WHO Classifications of Cutaneous Lymphomas

EORTC Classification of Cutaneous Lymphomas	WHO Classification of Cutaneous Lymphomas
INDOLENT	
Mycosis fungoides	Mycosis fungoides
Mycosis fungoides variants	Mycosis fungoides variants
Follicular mycosis fungoides	Follicular mycosis fungoides
Pagetoid reticulosis	Pagetoid reticulosis
CTCL, large cell lymphoma CD30+	Primary cutaneous CD30+ anaplastic large cell lymphoma
Lymphomatoid papulosis	Lymphomatoid papulosis
AGGRESSIVE	
Sézary syndrome	Sézary syndrome
CTCL, large cell CD30– Immunoblastic	Peripheral T-cell lymphoma (unspecified)
Pleomorphic	
PROVISIONAL	
Granulomatous slack skin	Granulomatous slack skin
CTCL, pleomorphic, small/medium-sized	Peripheral T-cell lymphoma (unspecified)
Subcutaneous panniculitis-like T-cell lymphoma	Subcutaneous panniculitis-like T-cell lymphoma

CTCL, cutaneous T-cell lymphoma; EORTC, European Organization for Research and Treatment of Cancer; WHO, World Health Organization.

NON–MYCOSIS FUNGOIDES CUTANEOUS T-CELL LYMPHOMA

Lymphomatoid Papulosis and CD30+ Cutaneous T-Cell Lymphoma

Lesions of lymphomatoid papulosis often appear as groups of erythematous or violaceous papules and/or nodules that can variably develop central necrosis and involution, leaving residual pigment or superficial atrophic scars. Histologically, lesions may show various patterns (referred to as *type A, B,* and *C*) sharing a component of CD30+ atypical T cells often showing clonality by analysis of TCR gene rearrangement status. The natural history is often indolent, and spontaneous remission is possible. Effective control (e.g., PUVA, low-dose methotrexate) resulting in long-lasting remission has been identified. Depending on the clinical series, from 5% to 20% of patients with lymphomatoid papulosis eventually develop a non–B-cell lymphoma, most often CTCL. Regressing atypical histiocytosis is considered a variant of lymphomatoid papulosis.[9]

Lymphomatoid papulosis should be distinguished from primary cutaneous CD30+ large T-cell lymphoma, the latter of which is more often paucilesional, less likely to show involution, and more likely to show dermal sheets of large, anaplastic CD30+ T cells histologically. Patients with CD30+ large T-cell lymphoma may present with tumor-like lesions with central ulceration, which may or may not undergo spontaneous regression. Systemic involvement is unusual, and cutaneous lesions may be treated with radiation therapy alone. However, lesions often relapse, even though the overall clinical course may be indolent.[10–12] Thus, a diagnosis of CD30+ large T-cell lymphoma is ultimately determined by clinical and histologic correlation with an emphasis on disease behavior. Patients with systemic disease, who are age older than 60 years, or whose tumors do not spontaneously regress appear to have a less favorable prognosis. Anaplastic (vs. nonanaplastic) cell histology generally does not imply a poorer prognosis.

Adult T-Cell Leukemia-Lymphoma

ATLL is a disorder that develops in some human T-cell leukemia virus type 1–infected individuals. The clinical presentation of ATLL is often acute, with rapidly growing cutaneous lesions, hypercalcemia, marked lymphadenopathy, and infiltration of visceral organs.[13,14] Patients also present with systemic symptoms such as drenching night sweats and weight loss, and in marked contrast to MF-CTCL, the diagnosis of ATLL is usually made soon after presentation. ATLL patients may present with a leukemic form with extremely high white blood cell counts or a lymphomatous variant. Such patients are often severely immunocompromised and are susceptible to a variety of opportunistic pathogens. In the smoldering form, lesions may be more consistent with patches and plaques, which is more consistent with classic MF. Often, biopsy reveals cells with epidermotropism as in MF with CD4+, CD3+, CD25+, and CD8– expression. Aggressive systemic therapy is often used in managing aggressive presentations.

CD30– Large T-Cell Lymphoma

Typically patients may present with diffuse nodules over the skin surface. Cells are often pleomorphic, but large cells occupy a significant proportion of the infiltrate. Cells may also appear immunoblastic. This entity must be differentiated from other forms of CTCL that may have a similar clinical appearance, as therapeutic management in this case requires more aggressive systemic chemotherapy. MF with subsequent large cell transformation should be given differential diagnostic consideration, as it represents a distinct clinical entity from *de novo* CD30– lymphoma of T cells involving the skin. CD30– disease often presents without prior patch/plaque formation.

Subcutaneous Panniculitis-Like T-Cell Lymphoma

Subcutaneous panniculitis-like T-cell lymphoma, previously termed *cytophagocytic histiocytic panniculitis*, is a rare variant of CD8+ CTCL featuring subcutaneous tumors. The prognosis is particularly poor when the hemophagocytic syndrome is present. In addition to subcutaneous nodules, patients may offer history of more traditional B-cell lymphoma "B-type" symptoms such as fever and weight loss.

CD56+ "Nasal-Type" NK/T-Cell Lymphoma

CD56 is a marker expressed on NK and so-called NK/T cells, the latter of which also express T-cell markers, including CD3. Nasal-type NK/T-cell lymphomas are associated with chronic Epstein-Barr virus infection, tend to be angiocentric histologically, and have a relatively higher incidence in Asia and South America. True nasal NK/T-cell lymphoma, a subtype previously referred to as *lethal midline granuloma*, reflects the capacity for presentation in the nasal cavity ultimately replacing the nasal tissue with a necrotic tumor. Both nasal-type and nasal NK/T-cell lymphoma demonstrate aggressive behavior.

APPROACH TO THE PATIENT WITH MYCOSIS FUNGOIDES

The most important clinical prognostic variables are the type of lesion, the percent of the total skin surface involved, nodal involvement, dissemination to visceral sites, and the presence of CTCL cells in the circulation. These parameters have been codified in the modified TNM staging classification (Table 41.3-2) proposed by the Cutaneous T-Cell Lymphoma Workshop in 1979. Recently, the International Society for Cutaneous Lymphomas has proposed criteria for identification of the SS: (1) absolute Sézary count 1000 cells/μL or more; (2) CD4:CD8 ratio of 10 or more due to increase in CD3+ or CD4+ cells by flow cytometry; (3) aberrant expression of pan-T-cell markers (CD2, CD3, CD4, CD5) by flow cytometry; deficient CD7 expression on T cells (or expanded CD4+, CD7– cells of 40% or more) is a tentative criterion; (4) increased lymphocyte count with T-cell clone in blood identified by Southern blot or polymerase chain reaction; and (5) a chromosomally abnormal T-cell clone.[15]

SKIN LESIONS

Prognosis in MF-CTCL patients depends on both the type of lesions and the extent of cutaneous involvement. All patients should have the number and distribution of each type of lesion and an estimate of the total skin surface involved by CTCL carefully recorded before initiation of therapy. Patients with

TABLE 41.3-2. Staging Classification for Mycosis Fungoides (Tumor, Node, Metastasis)

T1	Patches and/or plaques involving <10% body surface area
T2	Patches and/or plaques involving ≥10% body surface area
T3	One or more cutaneous tumors
T4	Erythroderma
N0	Lymph nodes clinically uninvolved
N1	Lymph nodes clinically enlarged but not histologically involved
N2	Lymph nodes clinically nonpalpable but histologically involved
N3	Lymph nodes clinically enlarged and histologically involved
M0	No visceral disease
M1	Visceral disease present
B0	No circulating atypical cells (Sézary cells)
B1	Circulating atypical cells (Sézary cells)

STAGE GROUPINGS

IA	T1	N0	M0
IB	T2	N0	M0
IIA	T1–2	N1	M0
IIB	T3	N0–1	M0
IIIA	T4	N0	M0
IIIB	T4	N1	M0
IVA	T1–4	N2–3	M0
IVB	T1–4	N0–3	M1

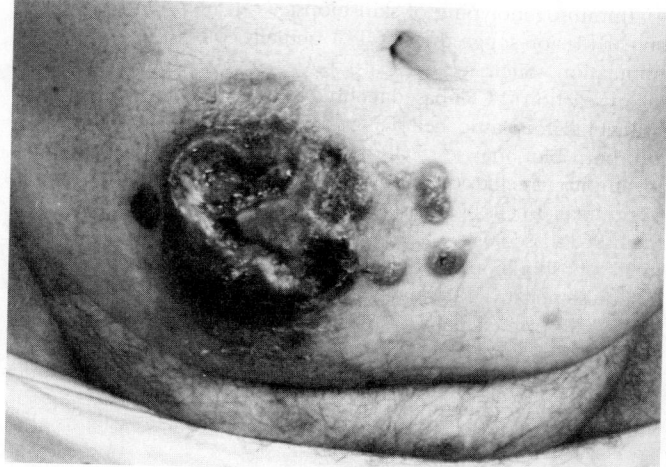

FIGURE 41.3-2. Tumor (T3 disease). (See Color Fig. 41.3-2 in the CD-ROM.)

account when attempting to estimate the prognosis for an individual patient.

Skin biopsies at multiple sites are necessary to establish the diagnosis and to define the T stage because lesion morphology varies even for different lesions from the same patient. The histopathologic criteria for the diagnosis of early CTCL are not firmly established, and there is significant interobserver variability in the pathologic interpretation of the same specimens[17] such that accurate definition of T stage and diagnostic correlation with pathologic material is not simple. Such problems are especially evident for early patch or plaque lesions, where only a small fraction of the infiltrating T lymphocytes (confined exclusively to the epidermis) is actually neoplastic. Most of the cells in the underlying, often much more impressive dermal infiltrate are nonneoplastic reactive CD4+ and CD8+ T lymphocytes, and that in part likely represents the host's immune response to the neoplastic clone. This typical histopathologic pattern can be significantly modified by prior therapy because even topical steroids can significantly alter the intensity and appearance of both the neoplastic and nonneoplastic lymphoid infiltrates.

MF-CTCL biopsy specimens should be reviewed by dermatopathologists with specific experience and interest in the study and diagnosis of CTCL. Specimens that exhibit epidermal collections of lymphocytes (i.e., Pautrier's microabscesses) with characteristic hyperchromatic, irregularly shaped nuclei are interpreted as "diagnostic" for CTCL, and those that exhibit at least two of these features (epidermal collections of lymphocytes, atypical nuclei, or absence of spongiosis) are judged "consistent with" CTCL. Histopathologic features of "transformation" to a high-grade lymphoma such as an enlarged pale nucleus and prominent nucleoli or loss of normal T-cell markers are all associated with a poorer prognosis.

Skin biopsies should also be immunophenotyped to better define the identity of the benign and neoplastic cell populations present in the cutaneous lesions. Several studies have reported correlations between the immunophenotypes of the cells present in the infiltrates and stage of disease. In general, as disease progresses, fewer CD8+ cells are observed, and the relative ratio of CD4+ to CD8+ cells increases, but CD8+ levels have been correlated with prognosis.[18]

patches or plaques that involve less than 10% of the body surface (stage T1) are far more likely to be cured or palliated long term than those with the same types of lesions occupying 10% or greater of the skin surface (stage T2) (Fig. 41.3-1). Prognosis is significantly worse for patients with cutaneous tumors (T3), although it is better for patients with less than 10% of their skin surface involved by tumors than for those with more extensive involvement (Fig. 41.3-2).[16] Prognosis is poorer still for patients with erythroderma, either alone or in combination with patches, plaques, and tumors. Most stage groupings are heterogeneous for survival, and subgroups overlap in survival expectations between stages, a factor that must be taken into

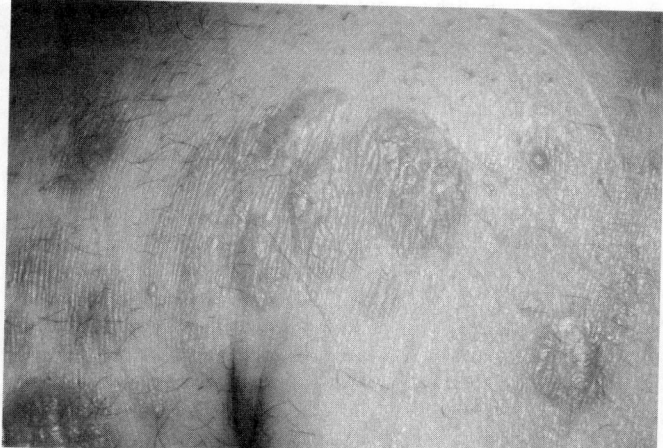

FIGURE 41.3-1. Patch/plaque (T1 to T2 disease). (See Color Fig. 41.3-1 in the CD-ROM.)

Immunogenotyping of skin biopsies can help define whether an early lesion suggestive of CTCL actually contains a clonal T-cell population. Such analyses are best performed by polymerase chain reaction (PCR)-based techniques because one rarely obtains sufficient neoplastic cell DNA from skin biopsies for routine Southern blot analyses. PCR is performed with primers designed to amplify T-cell receptor (TCR) γ chain rearrangements that occur in all T cells before rearrangement of the α and β chain loci. Such PCR-based assays are able to detect clonal T-cell populations in 90% of skin biopsies that show diagnostic CTCL pathology. The 10% false-negative rate may reflect the fact that the currently available PCR primer pairs amplify only 90% of γ chain variable regions. This high degree of sensitivity contrasts with the somewhat lower (79%) sensitivity of standard Southern blot techniques that require significantly more DNA.[19]

LYMPH NODES

The incidence of lymphadenopathy increases with T stage and is associated with a poorer prognosis. Imaging studies (computed tomography scan or magnetic resonance imaging) are recommended at initial evaluation, especially for those with advanced disease, as well as during follow-up, to detect enlargement of thoracic, abdominal, or pelvic nodes. Enlarged lymph nodes are biopsied at initial staging and subsequently if enlargement is detected on physical examination or imaging studies. In clinical practice, biopsy of uninvolved nodal sites is uncommon. Because a proportion of patients with CTCL may have other lymphomas (B or T cell; e.g., Hodgkin's), possibly concurrently, biopsy of clinically significant lymph nodes is recommended.

Flow cytometry, immunophenotyping, and Southern blotting (or PCR-based) genotyping for clonality are recommended for all nodal samples and may detect neoplastic T cells even in so-called reactive, dermatopathic (stage N1) nodes not obviously involved by CTCL. In a study of lymph node samples from 17 patients with stage N1 disease, eight showed evidence of clonal T-cell abnormalities consistent with CTCL on Southern blotting, and these eight patients had a poorer prognosis than those whose nodes were free of CTCL. Another study of lymph nodes in patients with CTCL revealed that specific histologic factors were predictive of outcome. Those patients with small cell infiltrates had a median survival of 40 months, and those with high-grade immunoblastic features had a median survival of only 9 months.[20]

PERIPHERAL BLOOD

The level of circulating neoplastic cells in MF-CTCL patients correlates adversely with prognosis and is an important parameter to document and quantitate both at presentation and during follow-up. In normal individuals, none of the more than 50 available anti-Vβ monoclonal antibodies react with more than 2% to 5% of the circulating peripheral T cells. As shown in Table 41.3-3, it is possible to use these monoclonal antibodies to detect and precisely quantitate the levels of circulating CTCL cells. Such analyses have revealed a remarkable clinical heterogeneity within patients who present with T4 disease. In most, the level of circulating CTCL cells is actually much higher than estimated by less sensitive techniques.[21] In some, the expansion of the neoplastic T-cell clone is accompanied by depression of normal T cells to levels comparable with those observed in advanced acquired immunodeficiency syndrome. Such a *de facto* T-cell

TABLE 41.3-3. Peripheral Blood Values of Six Patients with Advanced Cutaneous T-Cell Lymphoma

Patient	Total Lymphocyte Count[a]	CD4:CD8 Ratio[b]	Sézary Syndrome (%)[c]	Vβ (%)[d]
1	7184	50	32	67
2	794	10	10	32
3	684	13	7	74
4	3276	17	9	78
5	5160	90	13	87
6	3650	14	5	59

[a]Normal range, 1500–3000.
[b]Normal range, 0.5–3.5.
[c]Sézary cells are expressed as a percentage of lymphocytes; normal range, 0–5%.
[d]Percentage of lymphocytes expressing a particular β chain variable region; normal range, 0–5%. In patients in whom there is an identifiable Vβ region, the values in this column represent the percentage of lymphocytes that are malignant.

deficiency may both explain the susceptibility of erythrodermic CTCL patients to infection by bacterial, viral, and fungal pathogens[22] and contribute to the progression of the disease, which is often held in check by host immune mechanisms.

In the absence of specific anti-CTCL monoclonal antibodies, routine flow can accurately detect and quantitate circulating CTCL. Flow cytometry should be performed with antibodies to the CD4, CD8, CD3, CD45R0, and CD20 antigens. The ratio of CD4+ to CD8+ cells is normally 0.5 to 3.5; elevations in this ratio correlate with total leukocyte count and with extent of skin disease in CTCL patients. An elevated ratio of CD4+ to CD8+ cells above 4.5:1.0 strongly suggests significant levels of circulating CTCL cells, and a routine leukocyte count, manual differential, and smear supplemented by a measurement of the CD4:CD8 ratio serve as a good initial screen for circulating CTCL cells. If flow cytometric analysis reveals a marked elevation of the CD4:CD8 ratio or an elevation in the percentage of CD45R0+ cells, it is worthwhile to perform flow cytometry with anti-Vβ monoclonals to determine whether a clonal expansion of T cells is present.

If any of the above studies suggest the presence of circulating CTCL cells, then the more laborious and expensive TCR gene rearrangement studies to confirm their presence are also worthwhile. Even standard Southern blot assay for TCR rearrangement can detect a neoplastic clone, which represents only 1% of the total lymphocyte population, and thus is far more sensitive in detecting circulating CTCL cells than any of the earlier mentioned techniques, including flow cytometry. Nonetheless, in only about 10% of CTCL cases with circulating cells are Southern blots the only laboratory abnormality. In one study of 11 CTCL patients in whom circulating CTCL cells were documented by Southern blotting, 10 also had CD4:CD8 ratios greater than 10:1. Only one patient's CD4:CD8 ratio was less than 2:1.

PATIENT EVALUATION

HISTORY

The duration of the eruption and the evolution of its distribution should be carefully noted. The patient should also be asked about cutaneous integrity, temperature imbalance, fissuring, pruritus, and the use of moisturizers and any medications and infections that may produce rashes that can mimic CTCL.

PHYSICAL EXAMINATION

A complete physical examination should be performed, with particular attention to the skin and lymph nodes. Examination of the skin should record the number of lesions, including their type (patch, plaque, tumor, or erythroderma), distribution, and the percentage of skin surface involved by CTCL lesions. Evaluation of the abdomen may detect hepatosplenomegaly, and the site, size, and number of palpable peripheral lymph nodes should be recorded.

DIAGNOSTIC TESTS

Dermatopathology

At least two skin biopsies should be obtained for routine hematoxylin and eosin histopathology. Frozen specimens should be harvested for immunophenotyping for the CD2, CD3, CD4, CD5, CD7, CD8, CD19, CD20, CD25, CD30, CD45R0, CD56, TCR β, and δ antigens. PCR for γ chain rearrangements and, if available, β chain rearrangements should be performed on either the paraffin or frozen-section tissue.

Peripheral Blood Evaluation

A complete blood cell count with differential and smear examination supplemented by a flow cytometric analysis of peripheral blood lymphocytes to screen for circulating CTCL cells should be performed. Flow cytometric analysis can measure peripheral blood involvement by revealing an elevation of the CD4:CD8 ratio, an increase in CD4+CD7− or CD4+CD26− lymphocytes, or an elevation of CD45R0+ lymphocytes. The interpretation of these findings is facilitated by the demonstration of the malignant clone by PCR testing for gene rearrangement in the peripheral blood. The latter, in turn, is facilitated by similar PCR testing on the patient's skin biopsy. If the clone is detectable in skin, the test is useful in the peripheral blood. If the clone is undetectable by PCR, this method is not interpretable when done on the peripheral blood.

Other Studies

A posteroanterior and lateral chest radiograph should be performed in all patients. Computed tomography or magnetic resonance scans of the chest, abdomen, and pelvis evaluate mediastinal, retroperitoneal, and pelvic nodes as well as supplement physical examination of the axillary and inguinal nodes in patients with T3 and T4 disease.[23] Enlarged nodes should be biopsied (preferably by excision rather than needle sampling) to document both the presence of neoplastic T cells and the histopathologic pattern of involvement (i.e., dermatopathic adenopathy vs. more extensive replacement). The latter can be supplemented by immunophenotypic and TCR rearrangement analyses to document the presence of neoplastic T cells. Bone marrow evaluation is not routinely performed unless abnormalities are noted on complete blood cell count or smear.

PRINCIPLES OF THERAPY

The therapy for CTCLs and specifically MF-CTCL is quite distinct from that of nodal lymphomas. Hence, many of the successful therapeutic strategies for B-cell lymphomas are inappropriate for CTCL. CTCL is first and foremost a disease of *cutaneous* lymphocytes even though they may travel via the blood stream analogous to their nodal counterparts. Hence, early-stage disease that is localized to the skin has an excellent chance of cure or long-term control with therapies directed to the skin alone. In contrast, disease that has established itself in lymph nodes or visceral sites (liver, lung, central nervous system) can be palliated but rarely cured. Thus, the goal of therapy helps dictate the treatment strategies as shown (Table 41.3-4). Two major goals are remission [complete response (CR)] and palliation. The many modalities used are noted (see Table 41.3-4), and the selection of a given treatment is influenced most by the extent of the skin involvement (T status). Success is defined by reducing the tumor burden to zero for the remittive regimens and by limiting the impact of disease (and therapy) on daily activities for palliative agents. Because CTCL is immunosuppressive in various degrees, most of these therapies incorporate features that help target CTCL cells and relatively spare other cells and tissues. Many of these therapies act directly on CTCL cells (e.g., they are directly cytotoxic) but also have indirect effects (e.g., alter the cutaneous environment) that may play a role in disease control.[24]

(LOCALIZED) SKIN-DIRECTED THERAPY

Skin-directed modalities include those for localized disease (radiotherapy, bexarotene, carmustine) and those applicable to total skin therapy (topical chemotherapy with NM, phototherapy, and total skin electron-beam therapy (TSEBT)]. All skin-directed therapies exert their primary effects on disease confined to the skin. Most are capable of destroying CTCL cells directly, probably by triggering T-lymphocyte apoptosis,[25] and many may interfere with the local production of cytokines by epithelial and stromal cells necessary for neoplastic T-cell survival and proliferation.

Localized External-Beam Radiation

MF-CTCL lesions are extremely radioresponsive, and a dose-response relationship has been demonstrated.[26,27] Very-low-energy x-rays as well as electrons can be used to treat localized primary or recurrent patches, plaques, and tumors. Doses between 20 and 36 Gy are effective in fractional sizes of 1 to 2 Gy depending on the size and location of the lesions. Local treatment of isolated lesions is very effective, and the CR rate exceeds 90%, even for tumors. Cotter and coworkers demonstrated that zero of nine patients failed when treated with doses in excess of 30 Gy, with a minimum of 1 year follow-up.[26] Local radiotherapy is rarely first-line, as 96% of patients present with many cutaneous lesions. Local x-ray or electron-beam therapy in similar doses is also quite effective in clearing isolated lesions that fail to respond to PUVA or recur after CR to PUVA or TSEBT.

Approximately 7% of patients with IA disease present with a solitary cutaneous lesion or several in proximity. Wilson et al.[28] found that the rate of clinical remission after local external-beam radiotherapy is very high (approximately 95%). A total of 21 patients were evaluated, with a minimum follow-up of 1

TABLE 41.3-4. Treatment Options by Stage

Stage	Initial Treatment	Treatment for Relapsed or Refractory Disease
Unilesional patch T1N0M0 (stage IA)	Localized, superficial radiotherapy Topical BCNU Topical NM Topical bexarotene PUVA UVB	Same as initial treatment
Limited patch/plaque T1N0–1M0 (stage IA)	Topical NM Topical BCNU PUVA UVB (if only patches) TSEBT ± PUVA or NM	Same as initial treatment TSEBT Topical or oral bexarotene IFN-α alone PUVA + IFN-α Topical corticosteroids
Extensive patch/plaque: symptoms controlled, minimal plaque thickness T2N0–1M0 (stage IA, IIA)	Topical NM Topical BCNU PUVA ± IFN-α UVB (if only patches) TSEBT + adjuvant PUVA or NM	Same as initial treatment TSEBT Topical or oral bexarotene IFN-α alone Topical corticosteroids
Extensive patch/plaque: symptomatic, indurated plaques T2N0–1M0 (stage IB, IIA)	TSEBT + adjuvant PUVA or NM	Topical NM Topical BCNU PUVA + IFN-α Topical or oral bexarotene Topical corticosteroids Repeat TSEBT
Cutaneous tumors T3N0–1M0 (stage IIB)	TSEBT + adjuvant NM or photopheresis Bexarotene Denileukin diftitox	Topical NM and local radiotherapy Oral bexarotene Denileukin diftitox Systemic chemotherapy Repeat TSEBT
Erythroderma T4N0–1M0 (stage III)	TSEBT + adjuvant photopheresis PUVA + IFN-α Photopheresis alone IFN-α	Methotrexate Oral bexarotene Denileukin diftitox Gemcitabine Fludarabine ± IFN-α Pentostatin ± IFN-α 2-Chlorodeoxyadenosine Standard B-cell lymphoma chemotherapy Repeat TSEBT Allogeneic transplant
Nodal or visceral disease (stage IV)	Clinical trial Allogeneic transplant Methotrexate TSEBT Topical NM Topical BCNU PUVA + IFN-α Topical corticosteroids Localized, superficial radiotherapy	Same as initial treatment Systemic chemotherapy as listed above
Transformed to large cell variant	Same as stage IV Consider rituximab if CD20+ Trimetrexate Allogeneic transplant	Same as stage IV

BCNU, carmustine; IFN, interferon; NM, nitrogen mustard; PUVA, psoralen and ultraviolet A light; TSEBT, total skin electron-beam therapy; UVB, ultraviolet B light.

year and treated to a median dose of 20 Gy. Seventeen of the 21 patients received 20 Gy or higher. With a median follow-up of 36 months, the actuarial disease-free survival rates at 5 and 10 years were 75% and 64%, with a local control rate of 83% at 10 years. Acute and chronic toxicities were minor, and such treatment does not preclude TSEBT in the future.

Topical Bexarotene Gel

The approval of bexarotene gel for the topical therapy of CTCL was based on a multicenter trial of 50 patients with refractory disease. Patients were instructed to use the gel once daily and up to twice daily if tolerated. Within 4 to 8 weeks, there was an irritant dermatitis noted. This became the dose-limiting toxicity and could be managed by dose reduction and decreased frequency. The overall response rate was 44%. The impact of the gel can be demonstrated by looking at the body surface area (BSA) assessments. The average involved BSA was 8% (typical of the most common presentation of CTCL), and after 4 to 8 weeks, the BSA increased to 10% because of the irritation. After the gel was decreased after months 3 or 4, the BSA was reduced to 1% on average. The drug is not absorbed to any significant levels. The irritant dermatitis generally limits the use of the gel to patients with BSA of less than 15% due to discomfort. Typically, bexarotene gel is applied to lesions with a frequency dictated by the irritant response, once or twice a day. The involved areas are kept in an irritated state for 12 weeks; the patient holds off therapy for a month and then is evaluated for persistent disease.[29]

Carmustine

Another topical chemotherapeutic agent useful in the treatment of CTCL is carmustine. Ointment-based preparations of carmustine are stable. The selection of a concentration of 10 to 30 mg/dL depends on the size of the lesions being treated. Carmustine is absorbed and leads to bone marrow suppression if too high a concentration is used over too large an area. However, given the marked variability in absorption, it is best to use the 20 mg/dL for up to 10% of BSA and monitor blood counts weekly. An irritant response may occur; however, cutaneous hypersensitivity reactions to topical carmustine are rare, and in one series, such reactions interfered with continuation of therapy in only 10 of 152 patients. However, significant erythema in the treated areas and posttreatment telangiectasia occur in one of three patients.[30] A typical course of topical carmustine would extend for 3 to 4 months to induce a remission. Hyperpigmentation at the sites of application is common.

(EXTENSIVE) SKIN-DIRECTED THERAPY

Nitrogen Mustard

Total skin therapy for T1 and T2 CTCL can be carried out with topical mechlorethamine (NM). Supply issues complicate topical NM therapy, and patients can rarely obtain enough vials for daily aqueous-based NM therapy. Ointment-based NM is less likely to induce allergic reactions, and in its typical formulation of 10 mg/dL, NM in Aquaphor is stable at room temperature. The ointment is applied to the total skin for a minimum of 6 hours a day. No laboratory monitoring is necessary, and allergic

sensitization is what requires periodic examinations. Other side effects of topical NM therapy include induction of second cutaneous malignancies (e.g., squamous cell carcinomas) and hyperpigmentation and hypopigmentation. Between 64% and 90% of NM-treated patients with T1 and T2 CTCL can achieve a CR to therapy. In one series of 243 patients, the response rate was better in those with less extensive disease.[31] Although many patients appear to be cleared by topical NM therapy, seven of eight patients relapse within 3 years unless a maintenance topical NM regimen has been instituted. Maintenance topical NM can also be used to prevent or delay relapse of cutaneous lesions in patients who have achieved a CR to TSEBT or to treat minimal patch or plaque recurrences after such therapy.[32]

Phototherapy

Keratinocytes have mechanisms for managing UV light–induced injuries. Lymphocytes, however, are extremely sensitive to UV light in the form of UVB (290 to 320 nm), narrow-band UVB (311 nm), and photochemotherapy with oral PUVA (320 to 400 nm) light. Thus, a disease such as CTCL, in which lymphocytes are admixed with keratinocytes, is amenable to phototherapy because lymphocytes can be eliminated while keratinocytes survive.

Currently, narrow-band UVB is becoming more popular, and its efficacy in CTCL has been confirmed. Patients typically are treated three to four times per week at a facility for approximately 30 to 40 treatments to achieve a remission. After that, frequency is decreased to a maintenance schedule at weekly intervals. Broad-band UVB has the same treatment schedule.[33]

Photochemotherapy with orally administered PUVA irradiation of the skin (PUVA) therapy is successful in a wide range of CTCLs. Even in patients with thick plaques, PUVA may induce a remission if UVB has failed. In addition, there is more experience in using interferon-α and bexarotene (discussed later) in conjunction with PUVA for partially responding patients. PUVA therapy requires the ingestion of 0.6 mg/kg of 8-methoxypsoralen 1 to 2 hours before the exposure of the skin surface to UVA light (320 to 400 nm). Alternatively, the drug may be dissolved in bath water and applied to the skin, for minimal absorption, before light exposure. To induce remission, treatments should begin three times per week at doses that are minimally phototoxic. After most of the lesions have cleared, the frequency of PUVA can be decreased to twice weekly until the patient has achieved a CR. However, patients should probably not be considered "cured" until they have remained disease-free for at least 5 years after completing therapy. Recent reports suggest that PUVA therapy may result in true "cures," or help slow disease progression, because the mortality rate from early disease was decreased after the adoption of PUVA as the standard therapy for CTCL in Scandinavia.[34] It is recommended that PUVA maintenance be started at once-weekly intervals, eventually extended to once-monthly sessions, subsequent to a CR, and that maintenance be continued for several years to reduce the risk of early relapse of disease.

Total Skin Electron-Beam Therapy

Treatment of the entire cutaneous surface with TSEBT is technically much more challenging than local x-ray therapy and should be attempted only in centers with appropriate equipment and in which a close working relationship has been established between dermatologists and radiation oncologists committed to and experienced in the treatment of patients with CTCL. Several recent publications have detailed the history and evolution of TSEBT, from 1952 through to the present, including consideration of physical dosimetry, radiobiology, and all published clinical results.[35] Electrons ranging in energy between 4 and 7 MeV are used to homogeneously treat the epidermis and dermis. Structures below the deep dermis are relatively spared because most of the dose (80%) is typically administered within the first 10 mm of depth, and less than 5% beyond 20 mm depth. Generally, doses to skin target are in the range of 30 to 36 Gy. Blood and superficial lymph nodes may receive 20% to 40% of the skin surface dose, and this may be clinically important. Many technical factors contribute to a high-quality TSEBT technique, and these are well understood. Technical factors such as completeness of skin treatment, surface dose, and energy or penetration of the electrons are related to clinical outcomes; more intense TSEBT is associated with a greater rate of complete remission and better progression-free experience, and low dose per fraction is associated with reduced acute and chronic side effects. Variations in technique from institution to institution are noted. These arise from local solutions to technical difficulties, specific machine characteristics and beam geometries, potential positioning of patients, and the use of a vertex reflector, for example. Any method of TSEBT should meet the basic requirements of the international consensus method of TSEBT, particularly where TSEBT is administered with curative intent.[35]

TSEBT may be administered as just one in a sequence of treatments for CTCL in a particular patient. For example, TSEBT is excellent treatment for patients with diffuse involvement with thick plaques or cutaneous tumors and is also suitable for patients with symptomatic erythroderma–T4 disease.[36,37] TSEBT is also an excellent alternative for patients with extensive patches or thin plaques refractory to PUVA or other skin-directed therapies. When used in these ways, TSEBT is typically delayed after diagnosis of CTCL until other topical, and even systemic therapies, have been administered and disease has become progressive or refractory. In contrast, TSEBT may be used as an important component of a radiation-based management strategy to control CTCL. This clinical strategy uses radiation whenever and wherever it seems clinically indicated, with the intent to minimize time spent with disease, treatments and related procedures, and toxicities.[36] From this perspective, TSEBT is offered to patients with "early" or stage IA disease at the time of initial diagnosis. Supplemental patch radiotherapy fields to regions of skin that are relatively underdosed are required to reduce isolated failures in those regions, which otherwise occur approximately 19% of the time.[38] Further, for patients at high risk for more generalized relapse in skin subsequent to TSEBT, adjuvant therapies are seriously considered to build on the initial effects of TSEBT. Subsequently, TSEBT may be administered to a patient several times using a variety of dose schedules, as clinically required to help control progressive disease.

RESULTS

Clinical CR rates for patients with T1 or T2 (patch or plaque) disease range from 71% to 98% and are higher in patients with

less extensive disease. Representative data on progression-free and overall survival are presented (Tables 41.3-5 and 41.3-6). Patients with T1 and T2 disease treated with TSEBT have disease-free and overall survivals of 50% to 65% and 80% to 90%, respectively, at 5 years, although patients with antecedent or coexisting lymphomatoid papulosis or alopecia mucinosa–follicular mucinosis appear to have shorter disease-free survival after TSEBT than those who do not. Patients with more advanced T3 and T4 disease fare significantly worse, with 5-year disease-free

TABLE 41.3-5. Progression-Free Survival and Remission Rates for Mycosis Fungoides Patients after Total Skin Electron-Beam Therapy

	No. of Patients	CR (%)	Progression-Free Survival		
			2.5 Y (%)	5.0 Y (%)	7.5 Y (%)
NEWLY DIAGNOSED					
IA	99	95	68	54	51
IB	58	88	41	20	9
IIA	13	85	18	18	—
IIB	12	75	42	31	16
III	8	75	45	45	—
IVA	6	83	42	—	—
IVB	1	100	—	—	—
FAILED PRIOR THERAPY					
IA	22	73	54	27	27
IB	24	83	34	34	34
IIA	13	77	50	17	—
IIB	14	43	0	—	—
III	2	50	—	—	—
IVA	7	71	—	—	—
IVB	3	67	—	—	—

CR, complete response.
Note. Ascertained by stage. Data recorded at Hamilton Regional Cancer Center (282 patients).

TABLE 41.3-6. Overall Survival at 5 and 10 Years for Mycosis Fungoides Patients after Total Skin Electron-Beam Therapy

	No. of Patients	Overall Survival	
		5 Y (%)	10 Y (%)
NEWLY DIAGNOSED			
IA	99	95	92
IB	58	91	81
IIA	13	63	63
IIB	12	55	41
III	8	50	50
IVA	6	100	100
IVB	1	—	—
FAILED PRIOR THERAPY			
IA	22	83	—
IB	24	76	76
IIA	13	42	31
IIB	14	34	26
III	2	—	—
IVA	7	67	—
IVB	3	—	—

Note. Data recorded at Hamilton Regional Cancer Center (282 patients).

and overall survivals of approximately 20% and 50%, respectively. However, those T3 patients with less than 10% of the total skin surface involved by CTCL have significantly better disease-free and overall survival after TSEBT than those with more extensive disease.[16] For patients with erythrodermic MF (T4) who are managed with TSEBT alone (32 to 40 Gy), without concomitant or neoadjuvant therapy, the CR rate is approximately 70%. The 5-year progression-free, cause-specific, and overall survivals are 26%, 52%, and 38%.[37]

Palliation of adenopathy or visceral involvement in patients with N3 disease can be accomplished by the use of appropriate high-energy orthovoltage or megavoltage photons to doses of 20 to 30 Gy. Even 6 to 8 Gy in three fractions are sufficient (e.g., when combined with TSEBT). Combinations of TSEBT with total nodal radiation have been investigated. Although feasible, such combinations do not appear to prolong survival and may be associated with hematologic toxicities not observed with TSEBT alone.

As part of a radiation-based clinical management strategy commencing at the time of diagnosis with MF-CTCL, TSEBT as first-line monotherapy may be followed at the time of progression or relapse, with a judicious use of either local radiation (e.g., for isolated skin relapse) or mechlorethamine or PUVA (for more widespread recurrences).[32,39] Results arising from a limited application of such second-line therapies are impressive, with many patients remaining free of disease at long-term follow-up (e.g., 10 years following a second-line therapy). For example, the median time to a third occurrence of disease with this strategy at Hamilton, Ontario, exceeded 15 years for patients with newly diagnosed stage IA disease who were initially managed with TSEBT monotherapy and then limited second-line therapy as required for their second occurrence of disease. It was 7.5 years for patients with IB disease. With a radiation-based strategy centered on TSEBT as first-line monotherapy, the 15-year actuarial risk of dying from MF was 1% for patients with stage IA disease, and 7% for patients with stage IB disease. Although not formally measured nor compared within a randomized trial between strategies, the dermatologic quality of life seems high when using a radiation-based strategy built around TSEBT as monotherapy.[38]

Toxicity

TSEBT is well tolerated by most patients, and acute sequelae either during or within the initial 6 months after treatment may include pruritus, desquamation, alopecia, epilation, hypohidrosis, xerosis, erythema, lower extremity edema, bullae of the feet, and onychoptosis. Chronic changes can include atrophy of the skin, telangiectasia, alopecia, hypohidrosis, and xerosis. Because of the superficial penetration of the electron beam, patients do not experience gastrointestinal nor hematologic toxicities. Second malignancies such as squamous and basal cell carcinomas, as well as malignant melanomas, have been observed in patients treated with TSEBT, particularly in patients exposed to multiple therapies that are themselves known to be mutagenic, such as PUVA and mechlorethamine. It is interesting that additional x-ray or electron-beam irradiation after TSEBT does not appear to increase the risk of second cutaneous malignancies.[40]

Repeat Treatment

For patients who suffer diffuse cutaneous recurrences after TSEBT not amenable to other skin-directed therapies, a sec-

ond course of TSEBT is both feasible and worthwhile. At Yale, a total of 14 patients have received two, and five patients, three courses of TSEBT. The median total dose after these additional courses was 57 Gy, and 86% of the patients achieved a CR after the second course, with a median disease-free interval of 11.5 months. Median dose was 36 Gy for the first course, 18 Gy for the second, and 12 Gy for the third.[41] A similar experience was reported from Stanford, where 15 patients were identified who had been treated with a second course of TSEBT (median dose of 20 Gy), with a CR rate of 40%.[42] Nine of these patients had a partial response to therapy, and the median total dose for the entire group was 56 Gy. In both series, repeat courses were relatively well tolerated, and sequelae were similar to those observed during and after the first course of therapy. Both studies and unpublished data from Hamilton in a further 39 patients suggest that the palliative benefits of additional courses of TSEBT outweigh their risks in appropriately selected patients. Criteria for retreatment include an extended disease-free interval after the first course of TSEBT, CR to the initial course, diffuse cutaneous involvement, or the failure of other potentially curative skin-directed or palliative systemic modalities.

Combined and Sequential Therapy

Both PUVA and NM are well-established and effective topical therapies for patients with limited skin disease. It is of great interest to combine either of these with TSEBT, and the most logical application would be to use either PUVA or NM as adjuvant therapy subsequent to achieving a CR with TSEBT. At Yale, adjuvant use of PUVA after TSEBT in patients with T1 and T2 disease significantly decreased cutaneous relapse. Patients treated with adjuvant PUVA after TSEBT had a 5-year disease-free survival of 85%, compared with 50% for those not receiving PUVA ($P < .02$). The median disease-free survival for the T1 patients receiving adjuvant PUVA was not reached at 103 months, versus 66 months for the non-PUVA group ($P < .01$). For those with T2 disease, the disease-free survival figures were 60 and 20 months, respectively ($P < .03$).[39] A pilot study in Hamilton confirms these findings, but with a short median follow-up of 1.5 years as of late 2003. There were 23 patients with stages IA to IB disease receiving TSEBT plus PUVA as compared with a nonrandomized control group of 58 patients who received identical TSEBT (both the consensus TSEBT as monotherapy plus supplemental radiation fields to regions of skin that are underdosed in TSEBT, as determined by thermoluminescent dosimeters). The 3-year estimated progression-free experience was 100% with combined therapy and 65% with TSEBT as monotherapy ($P = .04$). Approximately 20% of those receiving PUVA experienced minor adverse effects (nausea or localized skin irritation) during their 20- to 30-week course of 60 applications of PUVA. Adjuvant topical NM also appears able to delay cutaneous recurrence after TSEBT. In 1999, Chinn et al. from Stanford showed that TSEBT with or without NM provided improved response rates compared with mustard alone for those patients with T2 and T3 level disease (76% vs. 39%, $P < .03$ for T2; 44% vs. 8%, $P < .05$ for T3). For those with patch/plaque (T2), adjuvant mustard offered improved freedom from relapse after TSEBT compared with no adjuvant treatment. No significant survival differences were noted between the groups.[32]

Concurrent use of systemic chemotherapy with TSEBT was evaluated in a randomized clinical trial conducted by Kaye and coworkers, where a combination of TSEBT (30 Gy) and combination chemotherapy was compared with a regimen of sequential skin-directed therapies followed by TSEBT if cutaneous lesions progressed.[43] Those patients who received concurrent TSEBT and chemotherapy suffered considerable hematologic toxicity but had a significantly higher CR rate than those who did not. However, there was no statistically significant difference between the two groups with respect to either disease-free (12.9 vs. 21.3 months; $P = .19$) or overall survival at 75 months.

Several nonrandomized studies have suggested that the adjuvant use of single or combination systemic therapy after TSEBT might be of benefit in the treatment of CTCL. In a study of adjuvant doxorubicin-cyclophosphamide after TSEBT, the disease-free survival was longer for those patients who received adjuvant chemotherapy for the first 2 to 3 years of follow-up. However, this early advantage was no longer apparent after 5 years. In contrast, extracorporeal photochemotherapy (ECP) administered during and after TSEBT appears to improve survival ($P<.06$) for patients with T3 or T4 disease who have achieved a CR to TSEBT; however, the group of treated patients was small, and the data are retrospective.[44] Wilson et al. identified a significant improvement in cause-specific survival for erythrodermic patients (blood status both B0 and B1) treated with the combination of TSEBT and ECP compared with those not treated with ECP.[45] The 2-year progression-free, cause-specific, and overall survivals for those receiving TSEBT/ECP were 66%, 100%, and 88%, compared with 36%, 69%, and 63% for those not managed with the combination. The series was nonrandomized/retrospective.

SYSTEMIC THERAPY

Given the intrinsic immunologic nature of the cells responsible for MF-CTCL, it is reasonable that agents that either directly or indirectly modulate T-cell function or other aspects of host immune response should be applied to the therapy of MF-CTCL. Systemic therapies that are successful in managing CTCL are often biologic therapies that tend to spare toxicity to the immune system and targeting toxicity on CTCL cells.

Photopheresis (Extracorporeal Photochemotherapy)

ECP, or photopheresis, involves the removal of a portion of the patient's blood, pheresis of white blood cells away from red blood cells, and exposure of the pheresed white blood cells to UVA in the presence of injected psoralen. The irradiated cells are then reinfused back into the patient. The reinfusion of the killed, irradiated CTCL cells appears to selectively stimulate host immune responses against neoplastic T cells. Evidence that such clone-specific immunization actually occurs has come from several different lines of investigation.

Currently, ECP is frequently used as monotherapy for CTCL, but its combination with other therapies is currently under study. ECP is initially administered on a once-a-month schedule, with therapy continued until maximal clearing is established. An additional 6 months of therapy may be administered to consolidate the clinical response. After the patient's

disease has stabilized, the interval between ECP treatments is gradually prolonged by 1 week per cycle every three cycles. After the interval between treatments has reached 8 weeks for three cycles, therapy can be discontinued.

Patients may experience transient responses 1 to 2 days after photopheresis but begin to show sustained clinical improvement as early as the second month of therapy. However, some do not clear or achieve their maximal response until 12 months after starting therapy. On the average, after 4 to 6 months of therapy, a sustained decrease in erythema, scaling, and pruritus is observed. Patients often notice more subtle changes such as the return of body hair, loss of rigors, and return of the ability to sweat.

Previous reports suggested that conventional systemic therapies are ineffective in prolonging the survival of patients with erythrodermic CTCL. A population-based estimate in one tumor registry survey revealed a 31-month median survival for patients with erythematous skin related to CTCL. A similar analysis of erythrodermic Mycosis Fungoides Cooperative Group patients yielded a 30-month survival. In contrast, patients in the original cohort of ECP patients were found to have a median survival of 60 months, or twice as long as had been obtained with prior conventional systemic therapies.[46-48]

No side effects of ECP that compromise continued administration have been observed in more than 7 years of follow-up. Patients with CTCL in the original cohort treated with ECP have also been carefully studied to determine whether this therapy exerted any adverse effects on host immune response, but none were found. Lymphocyte and leukocyte counts never decreased to low levels. Lymphocyte stimulation studies showed no evidence of immunosuppression, even after years of therapy. Delayed hypersensitivity tests revealed improvement in recall responses after photopheresis; in fact, most of the patients had to experience significant improvement in their erythroderma to allow the skin testing studies to be performed.

Bexarotene (Retinoid Therapy)

Retinoids have found a role in the management of several malignancies, including all-*trans*-retinoic acid therapy of acute promyelocytic leukemia and topical alitretinoin in the treatment of Kaposi's sarcoma. Each retinoid has distinct binding patterns with respect to the major classes of retinoid receptors: RAR and RXR. Initial studies demonstrated that the retinoids approved for acne and psoriasis (binding both RAR and RXR) could produce responses in MF-CTCL. These nonspecific retinoids had also been combined with other therapies such as PUVA, interferon, and TSEBT. Bexarotene is an oral RXR selective retinoid with activity both topically and orally. In a clinical trial of heavily pretreated refractory CTCL, oral monotherapy with bexarotene had a 50% response rate in a group of 94 patients with plaque, tumor, or erythrodermic CTCL. The ideal starting dose is 300 mg/m² as a single dose taken with a meal. The most frequent toxicity is hypertriglyceridemia necessitating antilipemic therapy in the majority of patients. Bexarotene is useful as an oral monotherapy and as a topical gel monotherapy and is now in several combination regimens. In the monotherapy trials, bexarotene was dosed at 300 mg/m² (average dose 450 to 675 mg/d, taken as capsules with the evening meal). Responses were seen at all stages of the disease: 57% at stage IIB, 32% at stage III, 44% at stage IVA, and 40% at stage IVB. Patients were entered at 26 of 43 centers, and at least one response was observed at each of eight centers enrolling more than two patients at 300 mg/m²/d. Responses were paralleled by the secondary end points: decrease in overall BSA involvement, overall tumor aggregate area, and improvement in pruritus. In addition to the 25 primary efficacy end point responders, 20 additional patients clearly benefited by a reduction in BSA involvement by MF-CTCL. There was substantial and progressive improvement in the total BSA involved with CTCL lesions as well as conversion of plaque disease to patch. Pruritus decreased in index lesions in patients regardless of their use of concomitant antipruritic therapy. Notably, there was substantial improvement in the aggregate volume of cutaneous tumors over time. Nine patients in the 300 mg/m²/d group had one or more tumors at baseline. Four of these patients had improvement in size or number, and four tumors resolved completely.[49,50]

A median overall response rate of 50% is unexpectedly high, given the advanced disease stage and the refractory nature of the patients enrolled in the study. These patients had a median duration of disease of 7.3 years, with an expected median survival of only 2.5 to 5.0 years, depending on stage. Response rates in the range of 50% to 60% are reported for oral retinoids administered as single agents. In the previous studies of retinoids, not all required biopsy confirmation nor were they limited to refractory patients.

Bexarotene has a high response rate as a single agent, and the duration of disease control is quite long in responding patients. Although there appeared to be a dose relationship with respect to efficacy, the higher doses were also associated with a higher rate of adverse events and dose-limited toxicities. The most common were hyperlipidemia/hypercholesterolemia and neutropenia. Elevations in the lipids occurred rapidly, within 2 to 4 weeks, and the use of lipid-lowering agents is often necessary for controlling the lipid levels. Dose reductions of bexarotene capsules were also required in some patients. Patients started on bexarotene develop central hypothyroidism with low thyroid-stimulating hormone and free thyroxine levels within weeks of starting the medication. Symptoms of hypothyroidism may be subtle because they include fatigue/asthenia, depression, cold intolerance, constipation, and so forth, and these findings may be attributed to malignancy. Supplementation with levothyroxine while patients were on bexarotene was found to alleviate the symptoms and improve tolerance to treatment. The condition was reversible within 1 to 2 weeks of stopping therapy.

There was a surprisingly low incidence of infections and sepsis seen in this study of advanced patients. Neutropenia, when it occurred, was mainly due to decreases in polymorphonuclear lymphocytes. Use of stem factor support was limited to only a few patients. Patients taking bexarotene were treated as outpatients, with monthly monitoring visits, and tolerated the therapy with high levels of satisfaction. As a palliative agent, oral bexarotene also requires minimal disruption of the patient's life. There are few symptomatic side effects, it can be taken at home, and blood work must be followed monthly.

Denileukin Diftitox

Development of denileukin diftitox followed Waldmann's original investigation of a monoclonal antibody against interleukin-2

receptor (CD25), which had shown efficacy in preliminary studies.[51] Activated T cells may develop avid receptors for this growth factor. By attaching a toxin to a carrier that binds to the interleukin-2 receptor, targeted malignant T cells can then be destroyed, sparing non–interleukin-2 receptor–bearing bystander cells. It is a recombinant protein produced from fusing the gene for diphtheria toxin with the gene for interleukin-2. The drug preferentially binds to activated T cells via the high-affinity interleukin-2 receptor. In patients with CTCL, the population of activated T cells is dominated by the malignant clone. By selectively targeting growing T cells, the drug spares tissues that normally suffer in the cytotoxic therapy of CTCL—bone marrow, mucosa, and hair, for example.

On average, five prior therapies had been exhausted before patients were entered in to the initial denileukin diftitox trial. This is important in understanding the 30% response rate. Of these responders, most were tumor or plaque patients. One of the useful properties of denileukin diftitox is that it is not a skin carcinogen, nor does it compromise the structure of the skin. In the management of a chronic lymphoma such as CTCL, the cumulative effects of cutaneous carcinogenic therapies create a need for an alternative mode for therapy. Thus, potential candidates for this therapy are those who have exhausted several skin-directed therapies and need a nonmutagenic modality.

The second major criterion for entry into the clinical trial was that a skin biopsy or a peripheral blood sample had to demonstrate measurable expression of the high-affinity interleukin-2 receptor (CD25) on the targeted cells. There are three major drawbacks to using this in practice as a way to select patients. The first is that there have been several responders who had no measurable CD25 expression in their skin biopsies. The explanation for this is most likely in the sensitivity of immunoperoxidase testing when compared with fusion toxin toxicity. The level of CD25 expression on a given cell may be well below the level of immunoperoxidase detection (e.g., 500 per cell), yet able to confer toxicity via the fusion toxin. Another drawback to the CD25 testing is the uncertainty over whether the CD25 is expressed on malignant or nonmalignant lymphocytes in the sample being tested. In the absence of large cell transformation, it is extremely difficult to distinguish reactive cutaneous T cells from malignant ones. One advantage to doing a complete immunoperoxidase evaluation on the patient at the time of diagnosis is that there is at least a baseline value for the level of CD25 expression. In the routine staging of patients and characterization of the malignant clone, one may find that the infiltrate is markedly CD25+, suggesting an enhanced sensitivity to denileukin diftitox, but a low level expression of CD25 does not preclude responsiveness.

Patients are given intravenous infusions of the denileukin diftitox over a 30-minute period, 5 days in a row, and repeated every 3 weeks. Using doses of 9 μg/kg/d and 18 μg/kg/d, it was possible to demonstrate the dose responsiveness of the efficacy of interleukin-2 fusion toxin in treating CTCL. The toxicities were also dose-responsive. A vascular leak syndrome occurred at severe levels in 13% of patients. Pretreatment with systemic corticosteroids appears to minimize this complication. Overall, the response rate in heavily treated patients was 30%.[52–55] Almost all responses occurred within the first three infusion cycles and were maximal at eight cycles. Tumor and plaque lesions appeared to be the most responsive. Patient selection for fusion toxin therapy traditionally depends on skin biopsy or flow cytometry demonstration of lymphocytes expressing the high-affinity interleukin-2 receptor (CD25). However, dramatic responses have occurred in CD25– CTCLs. In some patients with remission and subsequent recurrence, retreatment has recaptured a response.

Interferons

Interferon-α at doses of 3 to 6 megaunits can help to clear skin lesions refractory to PUVA alone. Although the systemic side effects of such therapy can be troublesome, some patients experience no significant toxicity. Whereas all three interferons, γ, β, and α, have been studied in CTCL, most clinical studies have been performed with interferon-α. Early studies have reported a CR rate of 10% to 27%, with response duration of less than 6 months with doses ranging from 3 to 12 megaunits/m^2 three times per week (with the lower dose being the best tolerated). As with other therapies, the extent of prior treatment correlated inversely with the clinical response. With interferon-γ, partial responses were attained in one-third of the patients, and improvements in the therapeutic response to PUVA have also been observed, as mentioned earlier. Kuzel reported a series of 39 patients (stages I to IV) treated with interferon-$α_{2a}$ in combination with phototherapy and found a 90% response rate (62% CR), with a median duration of 28 months and survival of 62 months.[56]

All interferons induce similar toxicities. The first week of interferon therapy may be complicated by flu-like syndrome with fever, myalgia, fatigue, and listlessness. After these acute symptoms remit, patients are often left with residual mild, chronic fatigue. Long-term toxicities of concern include neuropathy, dementia, and myelopathy. Interferon therapy can also be complicated by such autoimmune phenomena as proteinuria, thrombocytopenia, and anemia.

Allogeneic Transplant: Stem Cell and Bone Marrow

The initial attempts at bone marrow transplantation used ablative doses of chemotherapy followed by restoration of the marrow precursors. After these initial investigations, the technology shifted toward nonmyeloablative transplantation of allogeneic stem cells from HLA-identical siblings. In one series of three patients with a matching sibling, all patients achieved full donor engraftment and clearance of clonal T cells leading to durable complete remissions but experienced high incidence of infections, which proved fatal in one case. These results suggest that nonmyeloablative transplantation of allogeneic stem cells is a novel and potentially curative therapy for patients with advanced T-cell lymphomas who have a histocompatible sibling.[57]

Systemic Chemotherapy

Chemotherapy has been traditionally associated with increased toxicity in the management of CTCL.[43] Presumably, the immunosuppressive effects of advancing CTCL make patients particularly prone to the suppressive effects of chemotherapy. In addition, central lines in patients with CTCL tend to become infected due to the continuous seeding by bacteria from open skin lesions. Thus, there are two strategies with chemotherapy

in the management of CTCL: traditional intravenous chemotherapy and low-dose oral chemotherapy. There have not been any formal studies comparing these two distinct dosing regimens. The oral agents used in managing CTCL patients are chlorambucil, methotrexate, and etoposide. Methotrexate is probably the most commonly used, at doses at 15 to 50 mg/wk. If chlorambucil or etoposide is used, the peripheral blood count must be carefully monitored. More intense intravenous regimens with cytotoxic chemotherapy are used to offer palliation to patients with CTCL. Single-agent therapy can yield CRs in approximately 30% of patients, but the response durations are relatively short.

Infusional chemotherapy strategies for CTCL use agents that tend to exhibit selectivity for CTCL cells. One of the more unique strategies is to use pegylated doxorubicin. This agent tends to remain intravascular, but in areas such as inflamed lesional skin of CTCL, there is tissue perfusion with the cytotoxic drug. A pilot study of 34 patients with CTCL showed complete response in 15, with only six patients having grade 3 or 4 adverse effects.[58]

Due to the sensitivity of lymphocytes to adenosine toxicity, several studies have reported that the adenine nucleotide derivatives, 2'-deoxycoformycin, 2-chlorodeoxyadenosine, and fludarabine might be useful in the treatment of CTCL. Although these agents are active against T lymphocytes through their inhibition of the enzyme adenosine deaminase, their clinical usefulness in CTCL has been less than initially hoped. In early studies, response rates of approximately 40% were reported for both 2'-deoxycoformycin and 2-chlorodeoxyadenosine, whereas fludarabine was somewhat less effective. However, the duration of these responses was relatively short, and severe myelosuppression was often observed. Combinations of these agents with interferon have been studied, but preliminary results reveal no significant advantages over either modality alone.

Overall, combination systemic therapy yields CR rates of 35% to 50% in MF-CTCL, but there is no significant advantage in the use of drug combinations over single-agent therapy. Chemotherapy may be helpful for patients who are in need of symptomatic palliation when other modalities have proved ineffective or when visceral disease is symptomatic.

OTHER CLINICAL MANAGEMENT ISSUES

Many dimensions of a patient may be affected with a diagnosis of CTCL, and more clinical and research attention should be paid to the complex physical, emotional, mental, and spiritual needs of patients with CTCL. A simple exchange of information about CTCL and providing various treatments for CTCL in and of themselves may not meet important needs of the patients nor guarantee high patient satisfaction. Patients who have CTCL require a lot of time, compassion, and support. Many patients are interested in complementary therapies, and they want to look at their overall health risk as it relates to lifestyle, as approximately half of all patients with MF die from cardiovascular causes or other cancers and not from CTCL. Furthermore, approximately 10% of patients with MF also have anxiety and mood (e.g., depression) disorders. Ideally, patients are approached as whole persons with a combination of patient education, short-term counseling, interdisciplinary teamwork (e.g., full nursing role), appropriate consultations (e.g., psychiatry, infectious diseases), practical support for patients (e.g., a place to stay during TSEBT when from out of town), and, not least, eliciting and clarifying patient values. Further research into these aspects of care and other factors that contribute to the overall CTCL experience is a priority.

REFERENCES

1. Weiss LM, Hu E, Wood GS, et al. Clonal rearrangements of T-cell receptor genes in mycosis fungoides and dermatopathic lymphadenopathy. *N Engl J Med* 1985;313:539.
2. Berger CL, Eisenberg A, Soper L, et al. Dual genotype in cutaneous T cell lymphoma: immunoglobulin gene rearrangement in clonal T cell. *J Invest Dermatol* 1988;90:73.
3. Ferenczi K, Fuhlbrigge RC, Pinkus J, et al. Increased CCR4 expression in cutaneous T cell lymphoma. *J Invest Dermatol* 2002;119:1405.
4. Weinstock MA, Reynes JF. The changing survival of patients with mycosis fungoides. *Cancer* 1999;85:208.
5. Tuyp E, Burgoyne A, Aitchison T, et al. A case-control study of possible causative factors in mycosis fungoides. *Arch Dermatol* 1987;123:196.
6. Whittemore AS, Holly E, Lee IM, et al. Mycosis fungoides in relation to environmental exposures and immune response: a case-control study. *J Natl Cancer Inst* 1989;81:1560.
7. Willemze R, Kerl H, Sterry W, et al. EORTC classification for primary cutaneous lymphomas. A proposal from the Cutaneous Lymphoma Study Group of the European Organization for Research and Treatment of Cancer (EORTC). *Blood* 1997;90:354.
8. Sander CA, Flaig MJ, Jaffe ES. Cutaneous manifestations of lymphoma: a clinical guide based on the WHO classification. *Clin lymphoma* 2001;2:86.
9. Zackheim HS. Lymphomatoid papulosis associated with mycosis fungoides: a study of 21 patients including analyses for clonality. *J Am Acad Dermatol* 2003;49:620.
10. Liu HL, Hoppe RT, Kohler S, et al. Cd30⁺ cutaneous lymphoproliferative disorders: the Stanford experience in lymphomatoid papulosis and primary cutaneous anaplastic large cell lymphoma. *J Am Acad Dermatol* 2003;49:1049.
11. Pauli M, Berti E, Rosso R, et al. CD 30/Ki-1-positive lymphoproliferative disorders of the skin clinicopathologic correlation and statistical analysis of 86 cases: a multicentric study from the European organization for research and treatment of cancer cutaneous lymphoma project group. *J Clin Oncol* 1995;13:1343.
12. Beljaards RC, Kaudewitz P, Berti E, et al. Primary cutaneous CD 30-positive large cell lymphoma: definition of a new type of cutaneous lymphoma with a favorable prognosis. A European Multicenter Study of 47 patients. *Cancer* 1993;71:2097.
13. Hollsberg P, Hafler DA. Pathogenesis of diseases induced by human lymphotropic virus type 1 infection. *N Engl J Med* 1993;328:1173.
14. Bunn PA, Schechter GP, Blayney D, et al. Clinical course of retrovirus-associated adult T-cell lymphoma in the United States. *N Engl J Med* 1983;309:257.
15. Vonderheid EC, Bernengo MG, Burg G, et al. Update on erythrodermic cutaneous T-cell lymphoma: report of the International Society for Cutaneous Lymphomas. *J Am Acad Dermatol* 2002;46:95.
16. Quiros PA, Kacinski BM, Wilson LD. Extent of skin involvement as a prognostic indicator of disease free and overall survival in T3 stage cutaneous T-cell lymphoma patients treated with total skin electron beam radiation therapy. *Cancer* 1996;77:1912.
17. Olerud JE, Kulin PA, Chew DE, et al. Cutaneous T-cell lymphoma: evaluation of pretreatment skin biopsy specimens by a panel of pathologists. *Arch Dermatol* 1992;128:501.
18. Hoppe RT, Medeous LJ, Warnke RA, et al. CD8 positive tumor infiltrating lymphocytes influence the long term survival of patients with mycosis fungoides. *J Am Acad Dermatol* 1995;32:448.
19. Wood GS, Tung RM, Crooks CF, et al. Detection of early cutaneous T-cell lymphoma. *J Invest Dermatol* 1994;103:34.
20. Vonderheid EC, Tan E, Sobel EL, et al. Clinical implications of immunologic phenotyping in cutaneous T cell lymphoma. *J Am Acad Dermatol* 1987;17:40.
21. Heald P, Yan SL, Latkowski J, et al. Profound deficiency in normal circulating T-cells in erythrodermic cutaneous T-cell lymphoma. *Arch Dermatol* 1994;130:198.
22. Axelrod PI, Lorber B, Vonderheid EC. Infections complicating mycosis fungoides and Sézary syndrome. *JAMA* 1992;267:1354.
23. Bass JC, Korobkin MT, Cooper KD, et al. Cutaneous T-cell lymphoma: CT in evaluation and staging. *Radiology* 1993;186:273.
24. Kim YH, Liu HL, Mraz-Gernhard S, et al. Long-term outcome of 525 patients with mycosis fungoides and Sézary syndrome: clinical prognostic factors and risk for disease progression. *Arch Dermatol* 2003;139:926.
25. Dewey WC, Ling CC, Meyn RE. Radiation-induced apoptosis: relevance to radiotherapy. *Int J Radiat Oncol Biol Phys* 1995;33:781.
26. Cotter GW, Baglan RJ, Wasserman TH, et al. Palliative radiation treatment of cutaneous mycosis fungoides: a dose response. *Int J Radiat Oncol Biol Phys* 1983;9:1477.
27. Hoppe RT, Fuks Z, Bagshaw MA. Radiation therapy in the management of cutaneous T-cell lymphomas. *Cancer Treat Rep* 1979;63:625.
28. Wilson LD, Kacinski BM, Jones GW. Local superficial radiotherapy in the management of minimal stage IA cutaneous T-cell lymphoma (mycosis fungoides). *Int J Radiat Oncol Biol Phys* 1998;40:109.
29. Breneman D, Duvic M, Kuzel T, et al. Phase 1 and 2 trial of bexarotene gel for skin-directed treatment of patients with cutaneous T-cell lymphoma. *Arch Dermatol* 2002;138:325.
30. Zackheim HS, Epstein EH, Crain WR. Topical carmustine (BCNU) for cutaneous T cell lymphoma: a 15-year experience in 143 patients. *J Am Acad Dermatol* 1990;22:802.
31. Vonderheid EC, Tan ET, Cantor AF, et al. Long term efficacy, curative potential, and carcinogenicity of topical mechlorethamine chemotherapy and cutaneous T-cell lymphoma. *J Am Acad Dermatol* 1989;20:416.
32. Chinn DM, Chow S, Kim YH, et al. Total skin electron beam therapy with or without topical nitrogen mustard or nitrogen mustard alone as initial treatment of T2 and T3 mycosis fungoides. *Int J Radiat Oncol Biol Phys* 1999;43:951.
33. Cerroni L, Kerl H, Wolf P. Narrowband (311-nm) UV-B therapy for small plaque parapsoriasis and early-stage mycosis fungoides. *Arch Dermatol* 1999;135:1377.
34. Swanbeck G, Roupe G, Sandstrom MH. Indication of a considerable decrease in the death rate in mycosis fungoides by PUVA therapy. *Acta Dermatovener* 1994;74:465.
35. Jones GW, Kacinski BM, Wilson LD, et al. Total skin electron radiation in the management of mycosis fungoides: consensus of the European Organization for Research and Treatment of Cancer (EORTC) Cutaneous Lymphoma Project Group. *J Am Acad Dermatol* 2002;47:364.
36. Jones G, Wilson LD, Fox-Goguen L. Total skin electron beam therapy for patients with mycosis fungoides. *Hematol Oncol Clin North Am* 2003;17:1421.
37. Jones GW, Rosenthal D, Wilson LD. Total skin electron radiation for patients with erythrodermic cutaneous T-cell lymphoma (mycosis fungoides and the Sézary syndrome). *Cancer* 1999;85:1985.
38. Jones GW, Wong R, Sur R, et al. 15-year results of total skin electron beam (TSEBT) radiation as first line management for newly diagnosed stage IA-IB mycosis fungoides. *Int J Radiat Oncol Biol Phys* 2003;57(2 Suppl):S291.
39. Quiros PA, Jones GW, Kacinski BM, et al. Total skin electron beam therapy followed by adjuvant psoralen/ultraviolet A light in the management of patients with T1 and T2 cutaneous T-cell lymphoma (mycosis fungoides). *Int J Radiat Oncol Biol Phys* 1997;38:1027.
40. Licata AG, Wilson LD, Braverman IM, et al. Malignant melanoma and other second cutaneous malignancies in cutaneous T-cell lymphoma (the influence of additional therapy after total skin electron beam radiation). *Arch Dermatol* 1995;131:432.
41. Wilson LD, Quiros PA, Kolenik SA, et al. Additional courses of total skin electron beam therapy in the retreatment of patients with cutaneous T-cell lymphoma. *J Am Acad Dermatol* 1996;35:69.
42. Becker M, Hoppe RT, Knox SJ. Multiple courses of high-dose total skin electron beam therapy in the management of mycosis fungoides. *Int J Radiat Oncol Biol Phys* 1995;32:1445.
43. Kaye FJ, Bunn PA, Steinberg SM, et al. A randomized trial comparing combination electron-beam radiation and chemotherapy with topical therapy in the initial treatment of mycosis fungoides. *N Engl J Med* 1989;321:1784.
44. Wilson LD, Licata AL, Braverman IM, et al. Systemic chemotherapy and extracorporeal photochemotherapy for T3 and T4 cutaneous T-cell lymphoma patients who have achieved a complete response to total skin electron beam therapy. *Int J Radiat Oncol Biol Phys* 1995;32:987.
45. Wilson LD, Jones GW, Kim D, et al. Experience with total skin electron beam in combination with extracorporeal photopheresis in the management of patients with erythrodermic (T4) mycosis fungoides. *J Am Acad Dermatol* 2000;43:54.
46. Edelson RL, Berger CL, Gasparro F, et al. Treatment of cutaneous T cell lymphoma by extracorporeal photochemotherapy: preliminary results. *N Engl J Med* 1987;316:297.
47. Heald PW, Rook A, Perez M, et al. Treatment of erythrodermic cutaneous T-cell lymphoma patients with photopheresis. *J Am Acad Dermatol* 1992;27:427.
48. Heald P, Laroche L, Knobler R. Photoinactivated lymphocyte therapy of cutaneous T-cell lymphoma. *Dermatol Clin* 1994;12:443.
49. Duvic M, Martin AG, Kim Y, et al. The Worldwide Bexarotene Study Group. Phase 2 and 3 clinical trial of oral bexarotene (Targretin capsules) for the treatment of refractory or persistent early-stage cutaneous T-cell lymphoma. *Arch Dermatol* 2001;137:581.
50. Duvic M, Hymes K, Heald P, et al. Worldwide Study Group. Bexarotene is effective and safe for treatment of refractory advanced-stage cutaneous T-cell lymphoma: multinational phase II–III trial results. *J Clin Oncol* 2001;19:2456.
51. Waldmann TA. Anti-IL-2 receptor monoclonal antibody (anti-Tac) treatment of T-cell lymphoma. *Important Advan Oncol* 1994;131.
52. Olsen E, Duvic M, Frankel A, et al. Pivotal phase III trial of two dose levels of denileukin diftitox for the treatment of cutaneous T-cell lymphoma. *J Clin Oncol* 2001;19:376.
53. Kuzel TM. DAB(389)IL-2 (denileukin diftitox, ONTAK): review of clinical trials to date. *Clin Lymphoma* 2000;1[Suppl 1]:S33.
54. Foss FM, Borkowski TA, Gilliom M, et al. Chimeric fusion protein toxin DAB486IL-2 in advanced mycosis fungoides and the Sézary syndrome: correlation of activity and interleukin-2 receptor expression in a phase II study. *Blood* 1994;84:1765.
55. Foss FM, Bacha P, Osann KE, et al. Biological correlates of acute hypersensitivity events with DAB(389)IL-2 (denileukin diftitox, ONTAK) in cutaneous T-cell lymphoma: decreased frequency and severity with steroid premedication. *Clin Lymphoma* 2001;1:298.
56. Kuzel TM, Roenigk HH, Samuelson E, et al. Effectiveness of interferon alpha-2A combined with phototherapy for mycosis fungoides and the Sézary syndrome. *J Clin Oncol* 1995;13:257.
57. Soligo D, Ibatici A, Berti E, et al. Treatment of advanced mycosis fungoides by allogeneic stem-cell transplantation with a nonmyeloablative regimen. *Bone Marrow Transplant* 2003;31:663.
58. Wollina U, Dummer R, Brockmeyer NH, et al. Multicenter study of pegylated liposomal doxorubicin in patients with cutaneous T-cell lymphoma. *Cancer* 2003;98:993.

LISA M. DEANGELIS
JOACHIM YAHALOM

SECTION **4**

Primary Central Nervous System Lymphoma

Primary central nervous system lymphoma (PCNSL) is the term applied to non-Hodgkin's lymphoma (NHL) arising in and confined to the central nervous system (CNS). In the past, this tumor was called *microglioma*, reticulum cell sarcoma or perivascular sarcoma, but its lymphocytic origin, usually the B cell, is now well established. How a lymphoma develops within the CNS, which lacks lymph nodes and lymphatics, remains an unanswered question; however, lymphocytes do traffic in and out of the CNS normally, and these lymphocytes are probably the source of PCNSL.

PCNSL was once a rare tumor, accounting for only 0.5% to 1.2% of intracranial neoplasms, and usually associated with congenital, acquired or iatrogenic immunodeficiency states such as Wiskott-Aldrich syndrome or renal transplantation. The highest incidence (1.9% to 6.0%) was in patients with the acquired immunodeficiency syndrome (AIDS); however, the frequency of AIDS-related PCNSL has dramatically fallen since the institution of highly active antiretroviral therapy (HAART) and improved control of the immune suppression.

A dramatic increase in the incidence of PCNSL has occurred among apparently immunocompetent individuals. A U.S. epidemiologic study using the Surveillance, Epidemiology, and End Results registry revealed a more than three-fold increase in the incidence of PCNSL from the interval between 1973 to 1984 compared with 1985 to 1997.[1] This increase was part of an overall increase in all extranodal NHLs, but proportionately the rise was greatest in the CNS. The increase in PCNSL was seen in all age groups, both genders, and whether one included or excluded never-married men, in an effort to separate the effects of AIDS on the data. However, the rate of increase was slowing after 1985, and this was confirmed in a second study showing a decreased rate after 1995 in patients younger than age 60, whereas the rate remained elevated in patients 60 or older.[1,2] This change cannot be attributed to new diagnostic techniques or the adoption of a uniform nosology,[1] but the reason for this marked rise in PCNSL is unknown.

CLINICAL FEATURES

GENERAL

PCNSL affects all ages. Its peak incidence is in the sixth and seventh decades in immunocompetent patients but younger in immunosuppressed patients.[3] Among apparently immunocompetent individuals, there is a 3:2 male-to-female ratio, but in the AIDS population, more than 90% are men.[4]

By definition, if lymphoma is found outside of the CNS using abdominal, pelvic, and chest computed tomography scans, body positron emission tomography, or bone marrow biopsy in patients suspect for PCNSL, the diagnosis is not PCNSL but rather NHL metastatic to the nervous system. The absence of systemic tumor even at autopsy in virtually all patients confirms the primary nature of this brain tumor even though the cell of origin is not neuroectodermal.

BRAIN

Most PCNSLs present with symptoms of an intracranial mass lesion. The specific presenting symptoms and signs reflect the location of the tumor, with focal cerebral deficits occurring in approximately half of patients.[3] Because the frontal lobe is the most frequently involved region of the brain and multiple lesions are often seen, changes in personality and level of alertness are more common presenting symptoms in PCNSL than in other brain tumors. Headaches and symptoms of increased intracranial pressure are also seen frequently. Because PCNSL affects deep brain structures and not cerebral cortex, seizures are less common than in patients with other brain tumors, occurring in only 10% of patients as a presenting sign. PCNSL also generally grows more rapidly than glioma, and thus, symptoms are usually present for only weeks to a few months before a diagnosis is made.

PCNSL is usually disseminated within the CNS at diagnosis. Brain lesions are multifocal in 40% of immunocompetent patients and almost 100% of AIDS patients. Multiple lesions may cause diagnostic confusion with brain metastases, particularly because 13% of PCNSL patients have a history of a prior systemic malignancy.[5] Furthermore, PCNSL widely infiltrates brain parenchyma, and at autopsy disease is usually seen microscopically in areas where magnetic resonance images were completely normal.[6] Many lesions are periventricular, allowing tumor cells to gain easy access to the cerebrospinal fluid (CSF). At least 42% of patients have demonstrable leptomeningeal seeding on the basis of a positive CSF cytologic examination, leptomeningeal invasion seen pathologically, or unequivocal radiographic evidence of subarachnoid tumor, but patients rarely have symptoms or signs of leptomeningeal lymphoma.[7] At autopsy, many patients have leptomeningeal tumor either from direct invasion into the ventricular system by periventricular tumor or by local involvement of the leptomeninges overlying a cortical lesion.

EYE

The eye, distinct from the orbit, is a direct extension of the brain, and approximately 20% of PCNSL patients have ocular involvement at diagnosis.[8] Conversely, 80% to 90% of patients with ocular lymphoma eventually develop cerebral lymphoma, usually after a several year latency.[9] Ocular lymphoma typically involves the vitreous, retina or choroid, but optic nerve infiltration can also occur.[9,10] Orbital lymphoma is not PCNSL but rather metastasis from systemic NHL. Ocular lymphoma can present with blurred vision or floaters or may be clinically silent; it may begin unilaterally, but most patients eventually develop bilateral but asymmetric disease. A cellular infiltrate of the vitreous can be visualized only by slit-lamp examination; choroidal or retinal lesions often require indirect ophthalmoscopy. Lymphoma can be identified in vitrectomy specimens of patients with cells in the vitreous, obviating the need for brain biopsy[9]; false-negative biopsy may occur when patients have too few vitreal lymphocytes for the pathologist to examine or if the patient has been given corticosteroids to treat a presumed uveitis.[9,10]

LEPTOMENINGES

Primary leptomeningeal lymphoma in the absence of a parenchymal brain mass is rare, accounting for approximately 7% of PCNSLs.[11,12] Patients can present with progressive leg weakness, urinary incontinence or retention, cranial neuropathies, increased intracranial pressure, confusion, or a combination of these symptoms. Symptoms are usually present for only 2 to 3 months before diagnosis, but an occasional patient can have symptoms for 1 to 2 years before the diagnosis is made.[11] Diagnosis is established by demonstration of malignant lymphocytes in the CSF or on meningeal biopsy. The CSF invariably shows an elevated protein concentration, and a lymphocytic pleocytosis often in excess of 100 cells/μL; CSF glucose is low in approximately one-third of patients. Gadolinium magnetic resonance imaging scan of the head or spine reveals meningeal enhancement, hydrocephalus but no brain tumors, or multiple intradural nodules.

SPINAL CORD

Primary spinal cord lymphoma is even less common than primary leptomeningeal lymphoma.[13,14] Lymphoma in the spinal cord parenchyma can occur in isolation or accompany brain lymphoma. Patients present with painless bilateral limb weakness, usually involving the legs; sensory symptoms and signs may initially follow a radicular pattern, but eventually a sensory level may be found. CSF may be normal or have a mildly elevated protein concentration with a few lymphocytes. Prognosis has been poor with patients surviving only a few months from the onset of symptoms, but this is often due to the fact that the diagnosis was not made until autopsy and no appropriate therapy was administered.

DIAGNOSTIC TESTS

CRANIAL IMAGING

Magnetic resonance imaging scan should be the standard imaging technique for any patient with a cerebral neoplasm. The magnetic resonance image of PCNSL is usually quite distinctive, and the diagnosis may be suspected on the basis of the radiographic appearance alone. The tumor has an isointense signal on the pre-gadolinium T1 magnetic resonance image, and after contrast administration, there is dense and diffuse enhancement.[15] The lesions often have indistinct borders, and the amount of surrounding edema is quite variable. Unlike brain metastases or malignant gliomas, ring enhancement is rarely seen.

Prominent contrast enhancement is characteristic of PCNSL, occurring in more than 90% of patients; however, nonenhancing lesions may be seen in approximately 10% of patients, particularly at recurrence. Magnetic resonance spectroscopy may provide additional diagnostic information; PCNSL has marked elevation of lipid and a much higher choline/creatine ratio than all grades of astrocytoma.[16] This magnetic resonance spectroscopy pattern may suggest the diagnosis of PCNSL.

The radiographic features of PCNSL may differ in the immunosuppressed patient from the characteristic image seen in immunocompetent individuals.[17] In the AIDS patient, multiple lesions are seen in more than 70% of patients. Ring enhancement is common, reflecting the higher incidence of necrosis seen pathologically in this group. Spontaneous hemorrhage may occur, and nonenhancing lesions were seen in more than one-fourth of patients in one series.[17] It is impossible to distinguish PCNSL in the AIDS patient from infections, such as toxoplasmosis or from other cerebral processes, on the basis of magnetic resonance imaging alone. Positron emission tomography or single photon emission computed tomography can differentiate between PCNSL and CNS infection with a high degree of reliability.[18,19] PCNSL is hypermetabolic in comparison to infection, which is usually hypometabolic.

LUMBAR PUNCTURE

A lumbar puncture should be part of the diagnostic evaluation of every patient with PCNSL. The protein concentration is elevated in 85% of patients, although rarely above 150 mg/dL. The glucose concentration is usually normal but can be low when florid leptomeningeal tumor is present. A CSF pleocytosis is seen in more than half of patients and always consists of lymphocytes, either reactive or malignant (see later in Pathology). An unequivocally positive CSF cytology eliminates the need for a brain biopsy. This may be particularly important in the immunosuppressed or desperately ill patient at increased risk for a surgical complication. Tumor markers, such a β_2-microglobulin, lactate dehydrogenase isoenzymes, and β-glucuronidase, can, when the level is elevated, provide circumstantial evidence for tumor invasion of the leptomeninges. Occasionally, immunohistochemical stains of CSF demonstrate a monoclonal population of cells establishing the neoplastic nature of the pleocytosis even if the cells appear cytologically benign.[21] Detecting a monoclonal population of lymphocytes in the CSF by polymerase chain reaction of immunoglobulin gene rearrangements may also prove useful.[20]

Systemic lymphomas in immunocompromised patients are often associated with the Epstein-Barr virus (EBV), and using *in situ* hybridization and polymerase chain reaction, EBV has been detected in the tumor tissue of most AIDS-related PCNSLs and some non-AIDS patients with this neoplasm[22]; EBV may play an important role in the development of PCNSL in immunosuppressed patients, comparable to the presumed role it plays in systemic polyclonal and monoclonal lymphoid proliferations seen in the immunocompromised host. Regardless of its role in the genesis of the neoplasm, it may serve a useful diagnostic function. Using polymerase chain reaction, EBV has been detected in the CSF of AIDS patients with PCNSL but not in the CSF of AIDS patients without PCNSL; this approach may offer a simple, noninvasive diagnostic alternative to brain biopsy in the AIDS population.[23] Identification of EBV DNA in the CSF of an AIDS patient, combined with demonstration of hypermetabolic lesions on positron emission tomography or single photon emission computed tomography, can accurately diagnose PCNSL and exclude other CNS processes with a high degree of accuracy.[19] Biopsy can be avoided in such patients and definitive treatment for PCNSL instituted.

PATHOLOGY

Histologically, PCNSL may be any type of NHL but is usually an intermediate- or high-grade malignant subtype. Most are diffuse large cell; large cell, immunoblastic; or lymphoblastic lymphomas. Response to treatment and prognosis are not related to pathologic subtype. However, most series contain so few patients in any given category that it is possible a relationship may have been missed; prospective studies with a large number of patients may reveal differences comparable to that seen for systemic lymphomas. At this time, all PCNSLs are treated in the same manner regardless of subtype or cell of origin.

PCNSL can grow as sheets of cells, but a characteristic vasocentric growth pattern with tumor infiltrating the brain parenchyma between involved blood vessels is found in virtually all cases. In immunocompetent patients, neither necrosis nor hemorrhage is a dominant histologic feature. In autopsy specimens, microscopic tumor is always found in multiple regions of the CNS that appeared normal on neuroimaging studies.[6]

More than 98% of PCNSLs are B-cell lymphomas. Immunohistochemistry to demonstrate monoclonal heavy or light immunoglobulin chain production, or immunoglobulin gene rearrangement, can be useful in some diagnostically difficult cases. Studies of clonality have demonstrated that multifocal PCNSL lesions arise from a single neoplastic clone.[24] A study of adhesion molecules revealed an identical pattern of expression for PCNSL and systemic lymphomas. Bcl-1 and bcl-2 rearrangements have not been detected in PCNSL, and no unique molecular marker has been identified that discriminates PCNSL from its systemic counterparts. However, a recent study suggests that Bcl-6 expression was associated with longer survival in patients treated with high-dose methotrexate.[25] PCNSL from AIDS and non-AIDS patients has been studied for evidence of human herpesvirus 8 as a potential cause of chronic antigenic stimulation leading to tumor formation, but none has been found.[26] The few T-cell PCNSLs must be distinguished from reactive T lymphocytes that may infiltrate the more typical B-cell tumor.[27,28] This is usually straightforward, but in lesions partially treated by corticosteroids, the reactive T cells may be all that is apparent on a biopsy specimen, making accurate diagnosis difficult (see Management and Therapy and Corticostroids).

MANAGEMENT AND THERAPY

The appropriate management of a patient with PCNSL requires a correct diagnosis. This may be difficult because the clinical presentation of PCNSL is not distinctive, and other primary and secondary brain tumors are much more common; however, the method outlined here and in Corticosteroids can aid in the approach to a patient who harbors this tumor (Table 41.4-1).

When a magnetic resonance imaging scan reveals an intracranial mass, the radiographic appearance may strongly suggest the diagnosis of PCNSL (e.g., multiple lesions, a deep or periventricular location, diffuse and dense contrast enhancement, poorly defined borders and relatively little edema surrounding the mass). In addition, the clinical setting may suggest the diagnosis (e.g., an immunocompromised patient). If PCNSL is a reasonable diagnostic consideration, corticosteroids should be withheld unless the patient is in immediate danger of herniation, a rare situation. Corticosteroids may alter or even eliminate the ability to establish the diagnosis pathologically. Histologic confirmation is essential, by stereotactic biopsy, by lumbar puncture demonstrating leptomeningeal lymphoma, or by vitreous biopsy demonstrating lymphomatous cells because inflammatory lesions can mimic PCNSL on mag-

TABLE 41.4-1. Management of Primary Central Nervous System Lymphoma

SURGERY
Avoid corticosteroids before diagnostic biopsy
Biopsy for diagnosis
Resection should be avoided

CHEMOTHERAPY
Should be considered at diagnosis for every patient
Must penetrate the blood–brain barrier
  High-dose with central nervous system penetration (e.g., methotrexate)
  Lipophilic (e.g., procarbazine)
Must have antilymphoma activity
Should be given before radiotherapy

RADIOTHERAPY
Must be whole brain, 3600–4500 cGy if used
Avoid boost
3600 cGy to eyes, if indicated
May be deferred in patients aged 60 y or older who have a complete response to chemotherapy

netic resonance imaging. If the patient requires the immediate use of corticosteroids or if PCNSL was not considered originally and the patient was placed on corticosteroids, a repeat magnetic resonance imaging scan should be done to evaluate for possible resolution or marked shrinkage of the lesion(s). Biopsy should still be attempted if the lesion(s) is reduced in size but still evident; however, nondiagnostic tissue is frequently obtained after corticosteroids. Steroid-induced resolution of an intracranial mass does not establish the diagnosis of PCNSL because other neoplasms and nonneoplastic contrast-enhancing processes such as multiple sclerosis or sarcoidosis can resolve after steroid administration.

Using the clinical staging criteria developed for systemic lymphomas, PCNSL corresponds to stage IE—that is, disease confined to a single extra nodal site. Systemic stage IE disease has a 100% complete response rate and at least a 70% 10-year survival or cure rate with focal radiotherapy (RT). Despite the highly responsive nature of PCNSL to cranial RT, median survival is only 12 to 18 months with a 3% to 4% 5-year survival rate.[8,29] This short survival is due to tumor recurrence. Relapse occurs primarily in the brain, often in regions remote from the original site but within the prior radiation port, and also occurs in the leptomeninges and eye. Systemic lymphoma is found in only 7% to 8% of autopsied patients, and the vast majority of these patients have a single focus of clinically silent disease thought to represent a systemic metastasis from recurrent nervous system tumor.[8]

Regardless of treatment, recent studies clearly indicate the importance of prognostic factors. Age and performance status are the strongest factors, observed in almost all studies. Each can have a profound impact on outcome, particularly in patients aged 60 or older or with a Karnofsky performance status of 70 or less.

Because of its poor prognosis, new treatment approaches have been developed. These therapeutic strategies differ depending on the immunologic status of the patient. Thus, the description of existing and potential treatment regimens for PCNSL are divided into those for the immunologically intact patient and those who have a diminished immune system from a preexisting condition.

IMMUNOLOGICALLY NORMAL PATIENTS

CORTICOSTEROIDS

A unique feature of PCNSL in comparison to other brain tumors is its exquisite sensitivity to corticosteroids. At least 40% of patients have significant shrinkage or disappearance of tumor masses on magnetic resonance imaging scan after administration of corticosteroids.[30] This apparent remission is due to a direct cytotoxic effect by the corticosteroids; biopsy after steroid administration often yields normal, necrotic, or nondiagnostic tissue. Clinically, disappearance of PCNSL lesions is accompanied by improvement that may last long after the corticosteroids have been discontinued. There are isolated reports of patients being cured or having prolonged survival after treatment with steroids alone. However, achievement of clinical improvement after the administration of corticosteroids does not require resolution or diminution of tumor, as many patients have amelioration of symptoms without any detectable change in tumor size on computed tomography scan, a situation similar to glioma and probably related to stabilization of the blood–brain barrier. Regardless of apparent tumor regression, steroid-induced remission is short-lived in most patients and is not definitive treatment.

SURGERY

Surgery is important to confirm the histologic diagnosis but has no therapeutic role. The mean survival of patients with PCNSL with supportive care alone is 1 to 3 months. Surgical resection adds little, prolonging the average survival to only 3 to 5 months. Unlike malignant glioma, where extensive resection is an important component of therapy, surgical extirpation is usually ineffective in PCNSL because of its multifocal and infiltrative nature. Furthermore, the deep location of many PCNSLs leaves the patient susceptible to severe postoperative deficits if a complete resection is attempted. Therefore, stereotactic biopsy is the diagnostic method of choice that also allows for biopsy of deep lesions that cannot be approached safely by conventional surgery. If craniotomy is undertaken because the diagnosis of PCNSL is not considered preoperatively, an intraoperative frozen section can often establish the diagnosis of PCNSL; the procedure should be terminated, as further resection is unnecessary.

RADIOTHERAPY

Whole brain RT (WBRT) combined with corticosteroids has been the conventional treatment for PCNSL, yielding median survivals of 12 to 18 months (Table 41.4-2). There have been no prospective studies to ascertain the optimal dose or fractionation of WBRT in the treatment of this disease, but retrospective data suggest that 4000 to 5000 cGy improved survival over lower doses.[8] The Radiation Therapy Oncology Group (RTOG) conducted a prospective study of PCNSL patients treated with 4000 cGy WBRT plus a 2000 cGy boost to the involved area to assess whether dose intensification improved outcome.[29] Median survival was only 12.2 months, and most recurrences were in the boosted field.

Because of the risk of late neurotoxicity when RT is combined with chemotherapy, attempts have been made to reduce

TABLE 41.4-2. Treatment Regimens for Primary Central Nervous System Lymphoma

Treatment	Median Survival (Mo)	5-Y Survival (%)	Reference(s)
WBRT	12–18	3–4	3
CHOP + WBRT	9.5–16.0	—	34–36
MTX + WBRT + HDAC	42	30	38
MVP + WBRT + HDAC	60	50	37
MVP + WBRT + HDAC	37	32	31
BBBD + IA MTX	40.7	46	44
Single-agent MTX[a]	NR (23)	—	39
MTX + BEAM + ASCR[b]	NR (28)	—	41

ASCR, autologous stem cell rescue; BBBD, blood–brain barrier disruption; BEAM, carmustine (BCNU), etoposide, cytarabine, melphalan; CHOP, cyclophosphamide, doxorubicin, vincristine, and prednisone; HDAC, high-dose cytarabine; IA, intraarterial; MTX, methotrexate; MVP, methotrexate, vincristine, and prednisone; WBRT, whole brain radiotherapy.
[a]NR, not reached, median follow-up was 23 mo.
[b]NR, not reached, median follow-up was 28 mo.

the dose or volume of RT. The RTOG recently reported a study using a high-dose methotrexate-based regimen in combination with 4500 cGy WBRT.[31] During the trial, the protocol was changed such that only 3600 cGy WBRT in a hyperfractionated schedule was given to patients who achieved a complete response with the pre-RT chemotherapy. Survival and disease control were identical regardless of WBRT dose, although the neurotoxicity was not reduced, suggesting that even lower doses of RT are necessary to decrease the risk of leukoencephalopathy. These data are in contrast to those reported by Bessell et al., who used a pre-RT regimen of cyclophosphamide, doxorubicin, and vincristine with dexamethasone plus carmustine, vincristine, and cytarabine to reduce the dose of WBRT from 4500 cGy to 3060 cGy in patients who achieved a complete response.[32] No difference in outcome was observed for older patients, but in patients younger than 60 years, survival was significantly better (3-year overall survival 92% vs. 60%, $P = .04$) if the full dose of WBRT was used.

The need for WBRT has been examined by Shibamoto et al., who reviewed PCNSL patients treated with focal RT only. Patients treated with RT using margins of less than 4 cm had higher out-field recurrences (83%) compared with those treated with 4 cm or more margins.[33] Collectively, these data suggest that the whole brain port remains necessary to achieve optimal benefit from RT in PCNSL, but a boost does not improve local control. Furthermore, a reduced dose of WBRT may provide adequate disease control if combined with effective chemotherapy, but this requires additional study.

The primary treatment of ocular disease is 3500 to 4500 cGy RT over 4 to 5 weeks to the globe.[9] Because ocular lymphoma is predominately a binocular process, both eyes should be irradiated even when only monocular disease can be detected on slit-lamp examination. Most patients experience both symptomatic improvement and resolution of cells in the vitreous after RT; however, some have vitreal clearing without improved vision, and others may not respond to RT. The incidence of ocular toxicity from RT in this disease is unknown but may increase with improved survival because many of the complications are delayed. Conjunctivitis, retinal atrophy, vitreous hemorrhage, and cataract formation have all been reported in PCNSL patients after ocular RT.

Craniospinal irradiation has been proposed as the initial therapy of PCNSL because of the high incidence of clinically evident meningeal tumor at recurrence and the invariable demonstration of leptomeningeal infiltration at autopsy. Little data exist to evaluate this approach, although in the few patients treated with neuraxis RT, there is a suggestion of improved survival over WBRT alone. However, irradiation of such a large portion of the bone marrow compromises the patient's ability to tolerate subsequent systemic chemotherapy, which is likely necessary at relapse. Administration of intrathecal chemotherapy at diagnosis is an effective alternative to neuraxis RT to treat leptomeningeal lymphoma and is associated with less systemic toxicity.

CHEMOTHERAPY

No large prospective trials have compared chemotherapy plus RT with RT alone, but accumulated data from multiple phase II studies clearly document the chemosensitivity of PCNSL to systemic chemotherapy and superior outcomes with combined modality therapy. It is improbable that a phase III trial will ever be mounted to study this issue given the small number of patients with PCNSL and the extended number of years necessary to complete such a protocol.

Most studies have focused on the use of preradiation chemotherapy for two reasons:

1. It permits an assessment of response to treatment. Almost all patients have a complete, albeit short-lived response to RT, and therefore, no measurable disease is present to assess adjuvant chemotherapy. This is particularly important in PCNSL, where investigators are still trying to identify active agents and regimens that are effective against comparable systemic NHLs cannot simply be adopted (see later in Systemic Non-Hodgkin's Lymphoma Regimens).
2. Drugs, particularly methotrexate, before RT may reduce late neurologic toxicity. Opening of the blood–brain barrier by cranial irradiation may persist for weeks to months after completion of RT. This continued breakdown of the blood–brain barrier permits greater drug concentrations to accumulate in normal brain tissue. Completion of chemotherapy before cranial irradiation should minimize normal brain exposure to potentially neurotoxic chemotherapeutic agents. This enhanced neurotoxic potential of multimodality therapy likely applies to other agents in addition to methotrexate.

SYSTEMIC NON-HODGKIN'S LYMPHOMA REGIMENS

Several investigators have used chemotherapeutic regimens successful in the treatment of systemic NHL for use in PCNSL. The combination of preradiation cyclophosphamide, doxorubicin, vincristine, and prednisone (CHOP) or dexamethasone has been studied most extensively. Early reports described responses of brain lesions to CHOP, although patients quickly developed florid leptomeningeal tumor or multifocal brain recurrence in sites distant from the original location of disease before chemotherapy could be completed. In contrast to these data, there are isolated patients reported to have prolonged survival with CHOP plus WBRT, although many of these patients also received intrathecal methotrexate. There have now been two multicenter phase II studies and one prospective randomized phase III trial that definitively establish the poor efficacy and high toxicity of CHOP for PCNSL.[34–36] The RTOG conducted a study in which patients received three cycles of CHOP followed by cranial irradiation.[34] The median survival was only 12.8 months for the 51 patients treated. A separate multi-institutional trial of preradiation CHOP had 46 evaluable patients, with an estimated median survival of approximately 9.5 months.[35] Only 54% of patients completed two cycles of CHOP to begin RT; the others had disease progression or toxicity, with a 15% mortality. The prospective trial was terminated before completion because of poor accrual, but there was no difference in survival or failure-free survival in patients treated with WBRT alone compared with WBRT and CHOP.[36] Therefore, CHOP or similar regimens have no role in the treatment of PCNSL, and they should not be used; these agents should have excellent activity against PCNSL tumor cells, but they are unable to penetrate an intact blood–brain barrier. Adequate drug concentrations are likely achieved only in areas of bulky disease seen on magnetic resonance imaging scan, which accounts for the initial resolution of tumor masses; however, the drugs are unable to reach microscopic disease that persists behind a relatively preserved blood–brain barrier. Although issues of drug delivery may only partially explain the difficulty treating PCNSL, these data strongly argue for the use of drugs that can permeate the blood–brain barrier.

HIGH-DOSE METHOTREXATE

High-dose methotrexate is the single most important agent for the treatment of PCNSL. Originally chosen because of its ability to penetrate the blood–brain barrier and its known activity against lymphoma, methotrexate is now the cornerstone of PCNSL therapy despite the small role it plays in the treatment of comparable systemic lymphomas. Sensitivity to methotrexate may indicate a fundamental biologic difference between PCNSL and NHL.

Methotrexate has been used as a single agent and in combination with other drugs (Table 41.4-3). Doses have ranged from 1 g/m^2 to 8 mg/m^2, without a clear indication that more is necessarily better. However, doses of 3 g/m^2 or more penetrate into the CNS more reliably than lower doses. Several phase II trials using a high-dose methotrexate-based regimen in combination with WBRT have all shown improved survival (median of 33 to 60 months) over WBRT alone. To date, the best results have been achieved combining high-dose methotrexate with vincristine and procarbazine before WBRT, giving a median survival of 60 months (Figs. 41.4-1 and 41.4-2).[37] A large multicenter phase II trial based on this regimen was completed by the RTOG and median survival was 37 months, less than seen in the single institution experience.[31,37] Part of this difference may have been the reduction in methotrexate dose from 3.5 g/m^2 to 2.5 g/m^2, but other factors, such as unfamiliarity in the administration of high-dose methotrexate, undoubtedly contributed to the decreased outcome observed when the regimen was used in the multicenter setting.

All methotrexate-based regimens, when combined with WBRT, carry a significant risk of severe, irreversible neurotoxicity charac-

TABLE 41.4-3.   Active Chemotherapy Regimens

Week	1	2	3	4	5	6[a]	11	16	20
Current Memorial Sloan-Kettering Cancer Center Regimen									
Methotrexate	X		X		X				
Vincristine	X		X		X				
Procarbazine	X →		X		X →				
Intra-Ommaya methotrexate[b]		X		X					
Whole brain radiotherapy[c]						X			
High-dose cytarabine							X	X	X

Days	1	2	3–7	8–16	17–23	24–28
Scheme for Blood–Brain Disruption with Chemotherapy[d]						
Cyclophosphamide	X	X				
Blood–brain barrier disruption[e]	X	X				
Intraarterial methotrexate	X	X				
Leucovorin		X	X			
Procarbazine			X	X		
Dexamethasone			X	X		
Dexamethasone taper					X	

Week	1	3	5[f]
Harvard Regimen			
Methotrexate	X	X	X

[a]Repeat through week 10.
[b]Intra-Ommaya methotrexate given only to patients with a positive cerebrospinal fluid cytology.
[c]Radiotherapy eliminated in all patients 60 y or older and some 45 y or older.
[d]This 28-day course is repeated for 12 cycles.
[e]Two arterial distributions treated per cycle (e.g., left carotid and vertebral). Infusions are rotated each cycle such that each vascular territory is treated eight times over the 1-y course of therapy.
[f]Methotrexate repeated every 2 wk for a complete response plus two cycles or a maximum of eight cycles; this is followed by a maintenance schedule every 28 d for 11 cycles.

terized by dementia, ataxia, and incontinence.[38] Patients aged 60 and older are most vulnerable to this toxicity. This has led to the development of several regimens using chemotherapy alone. The above regimen using methotrexate, vincristine, and procarbazine achieved an identical median survival of 33 months in patients 60 years of age or older whether or not WBRT was included. However, patients who received WBRT died of neurotoxicity, whereas those who did not died of recurrent PCNSL. There has been recent interest using single-agent methotrexate at a dose of 8 g/m^2 as sole therapy over a protracted maintenance period. A recent report on 25 patients achieved a median progression-free survival of 12.8 months, and median overall survival was not reached at 23 months.[39] However, an identical regimen was used in a prospective multicenter trial in Germany that had to be closed early because only 29.7% of patients achieved a complete response and 37.8% progressed on treatment.[40] These data suggest that single-agent methotrexate has limited efficacy and rarely produced sustained disease control. There is a recent report using high-dose methotrexate as an induction regimen followed by high-dose chemotherapy with carmustine (BCNU), etoposide, cytarabine, and melphalan and autologous stem cell rescue without cranial RT.[41] Fourteen of the 28 patients had an objective response to induction and proceeded to transplant. Overall event-free survival was only 5.6 months for all patients and 9.3 for the transplanted patients; however, overall survival was not reached, with a median follow-up of 28 months. Six of the 14 transplanted patients (43%)

remain free of disease at last follow-up. These data suggest that a high-dose chemotherapy approach may be useful in some patients.

The high incidence of leptomeningeal involvement by PCNSL led to the incorporation of intrathecal or intra-Ommaya metho-

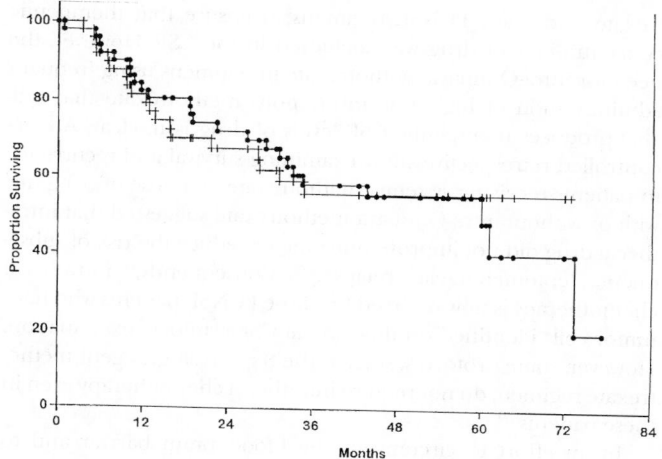

FIGURE 41.4-1.   A Kaplan-Meier curve demonstrating overall (•) and disease-free (*hatch marks*) survival for 52 patients treated with methotrexate, procarbazine, vincristine, cranial irradiation, and high-dose cytarabine. Median survival is 60 months.

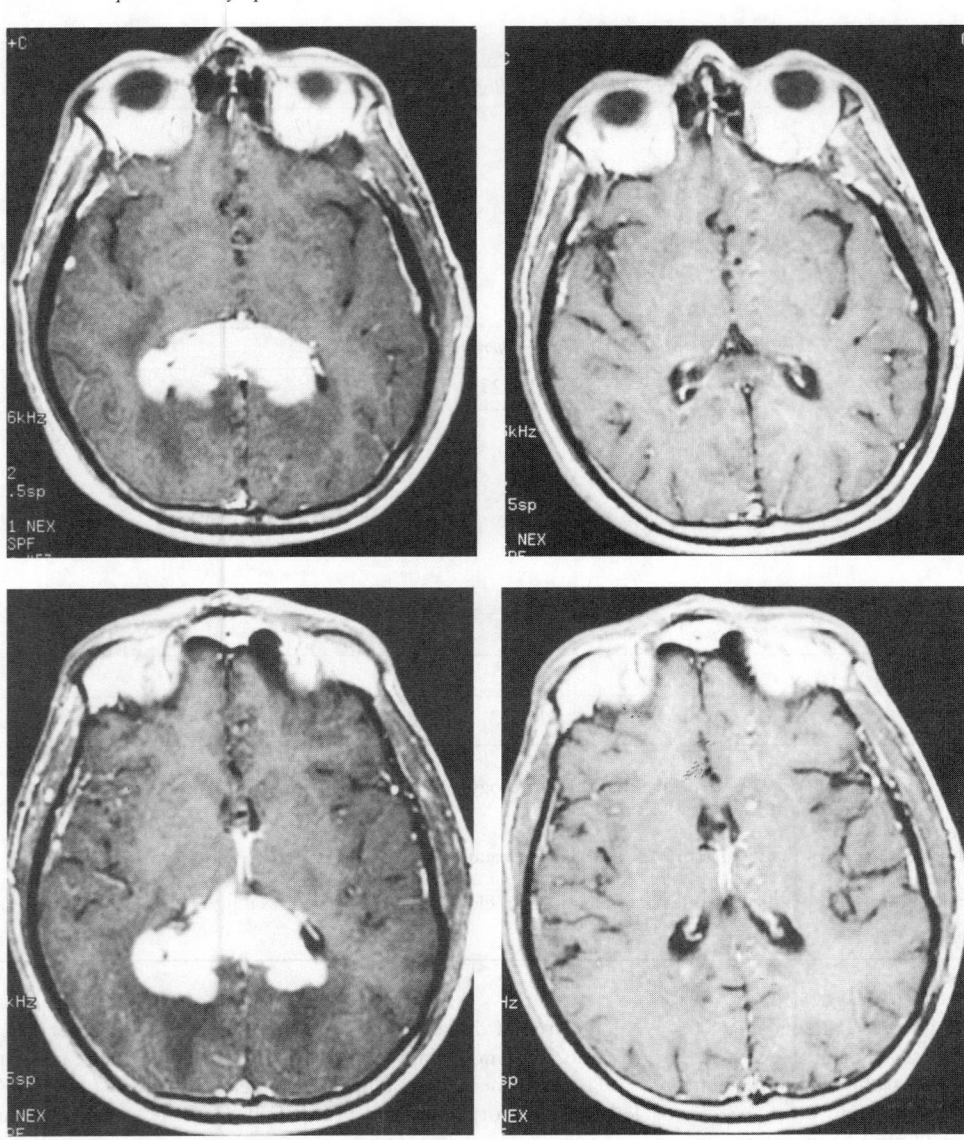

FIGURE 41.4-2. Gadolinium-enhanced magnetic resonance imaging scans demonstrating a complete response of primary central nervous system lymphoma to high-dose methotrexate, procarbazine, and vincristine. Note the prominent and diffuse enhancement pattern and periventricular location so characteristic of primary central nervous system lymphoma.

trexate into many PCNSL regimens to ensure that therapeutic concentrations of drug were achieved in the CSF. However, the need for intra-Ommaya methotrexate in regimens using frequent administration of high-dose intravenous methotrexate that reliably produces therapeutic CSF levels of drug is unclear. A case-controlled retrospective study examining survival and recurrence in patients receiving systemic methotrexate at a dose of 3.5 g/m^2 with or without intra-Ommaya methotrexate suggested that intrathecal drug did not improve outcome or reduce the risk of subsequent leptomeningeal relapse.[42] Consequently, intrathecal chemotherapy is now reserved for those PCNSL patients who have tumor cells identified on their initial CSF cytologic examination. However, some protocols, such as the 8 g/m^2 single-agent methotrexate regimen, do not require intrathecal chemotherapy even in these patients.[39]

In an effort to circumvent the blood–brain barrier and to deliver multiagent treatment, McAllister et al. used blood–brain barrier disruption followed by intraarterial methotrexate in combination with systemic cyclophosphamide, procarbazine, and dexamethasone without cranial irradiation.[44] Their 74

patients had a median survival of 40.7 months; however, 28% received cranial irradiation. These results are superior to WBRT alone but are quite comparable to regimens using systemic high-dose methotrexate without requiring the technically complex and potentially complicated procedure of repeated angiography over the course of 1 year.

Ocular lymphoma may be treated with chemotherapy.[9] The most effective agents are high-dose methotrexate and high-dose cytarabine, both of which can achieve therapeutic concentrations in the vitreous. Clinical responses have been observed. Experience is too limited to know if using systemic chemotherapy to treat isolated ocular lymphoma reduces the risk of subsequent CNS relapse. Recurrent ocular lymphoma can also be treated with intravitreal methotrexate, which can give a sustained remission.

RECURRENT DISEASE

There is no established second-line therapy for patients with recurrent PCNSL. The choice of treatment depends on the site of relapse (e.g., isolated ocular relapse or leptomeningeal lymphoma) and the patient's prior therapy. However, most relapses occur within the first 2 years of diagnosis, and the overwhelming majority occur in the brain. If the patient did not receive WBRT as part of the initial therapy, it is available at relapse. Most patients respond to WBRT, and some can have a durable response that lasts several years. Ocular RT should be used for recurrent ocular lymphoma if not previously administered.

Some investigators recommend using high-dose methotrexate at relapse even if it was used at diagnosis. The authors usually avoid it because drug resistance is easily acquired to methotrexate and cumulative neurotoxicity can be a major problem; however, in patients with a long disease-free interval after initial treatment incorporating methotrexate, the drug is a reasonable option at recurrence. Other drugs that have been reported useful include high-dose cytarabine (3 g/m^2), temozolomide, the PCV regimen (procarbazine, lomustine, and vincristine) and thiotepa. High-dose chemotherapy with thiotepa, busulfan, and cyclophosphamide followed by autologous stem cell rescue showed promising results, with a 3-year survival of 64%, in patients with recurrent or refractory PCNSL.[43] There are isolated promising reports using rituximab, but there is limited penetration of this large molecule into the brain parenchyma and CSF after intravenous administration.[45] There are ongoing studies exploring its use intrathecally.

IMMUNOCOMPROMISED PATIENTS

AIDS-related PCNSL is treated in the same way as in immunocompetent patients, although in general treatment is less effective and more toxic in immunodeficient patients. The initiation of treatment first requires an accurate diagnosis of PCNSL. In the non-AIDS immunocompromised patient, a stereotactic biopsy should be performed when an intracranial mass lesion is first diagnosed. In AIDS patients, this diagnosis may be established if both EBV DNA is identified in the CSF by polymerase chain reaction and a hypermetabolic lesion is seen on positron emission tomography or single photon emission computed tomography imaging.[18,19,22,23] However, if only one of these tests is positive, biopsy is necessary. There is no role for a therapeutic trial with antitoxoplasmosis antibiotics for a cerebral mass lesion in an AIDS patient. This delays accurate diagnosis, usually resulting in clinical deterioration that ultimately compromises outcome.

AIDS-related PCNSL usually occurs in patients with low CD4 counts, often less than 25×10^6 cells/L.[46,47] Age is not an important prognostic factor in AIDS PCNSL because most patients are young; however, performance status is a critical factor that strongly predicts outcome.[46]

The most important component of PCNSL therapy in the immunosuppressed population is treatment of the underlying immune deficiency. In organ transplant recipients, this may necessitate reduction or elimination of immunosuppressive therapy. In AIDS, it means institution or a change in HAART. HAART plays a critical role in the successful treatment of AIDS PCNSL regardless of the nature of the tumor-specific therapy.[47–49] The absolute CD4 count should not be used to determine the choice of PCNSL therapy because coinstitution of HAART improves the underlying immune suppression. There are some reports that institution of HAART plus anti-EBV–directed therapy, such as ganciclovir, may be sufficient to eradicate PCNSL in some AIDS patients without any specific antitumor therapy.[49]

In addition to HAART, corticosteroids and cranial irradiation remain the mainstay of treatment for PCNSL in immunosuppressed patients. Use of corticosteroids should be limited because they can contribute to the underlying immunosuppressive process, but they are still useful for the short-term control of neurologic symptoms and may be necessary during a course of WBRT. AIDS patients with PCNSL respond to cranial irradiation; median survival is 4 to 5 months for those who receive WBRT without HAART, but survival may exceed a few years for those treated with HAART plus WBRT.[47,48]

Chemotherapy for PCNSL has been used infrequently in immunodeficient patients. High-dose methotrexate has been successful for some AIDS patients with PCNSL. Forsyth et al. reported on 10 patients treated with chemotherapy and WBRT.[50] The median survival was only 3.5 months; however, two patients survived more than 1 year, and one is alive more than 7 years after diagnosis. Jacomet et al. treated 15 patients with 3 g/m^2 methotrexate as sole therapy.[51] Median survival was 9.7 months, with some patients surviving more than a year. Recent experience combining HAART with chemotherapy demonstrates that this is well-tolerated and with no increase in toxicity.[52] However, chemotherapy should be avoided in patients with active comorbid conditions. Antinori et al. have shown that monitoring CSF EBV DNA levels can predict response to chemotherapy and may be a useful adjunct to standard neuroimaging.[53] Although experience with chemotherapy in AIDS patients has been relatively limited, patients in good neurologic condition without active opportunistic infections should be considered for a high-dose methotrexate-based regimen combined with HAART because these patients may have prolonged disease control and survival.

REFERENCES

1. Olson JE, Janney CA, Rai RD, et al. The continuing increase in the incidence of primary central nervous system non-Hodgkin lymphoma. A Surveillance, Epidemiology, and End Results analysis. *Cancer* 2002;95:1504.
2. Kadan-Lottick NS, Skluzacek MC, et al. Decreasing incidence rates of primary central nervous system lymphoma. *Cancer* 2002;95:193.
3. DeAngelis LM. Primary central nervous system lymphomas. *Curr Treat Options Oncol* 2001;2:309.
4. So YT, Choucair A, Davis RL, et al. Neoplasms of the central nervous system in acquired immunodeficiency syndrome. In: ML Rosenblum, RM Levy, DE Bredesen, eds. *AIDS and the nervous system.* New York: Raven Press, 1988:285.
5. DeAngelis LM. Primary central nervous system lymphoma as a secondary malignancy. *Cancer* 1991;67:1431.
6. Lai R, Rosenblum MC, DeAngelis LM. Primary CNS lymphoma: a whole brain disease? *Neurology* 2002;59:1557.
7. Balmaceda C, Gaynor JJ, Sun M, et al. Leptomeningeal tumor in primary central nervous systems lymphoma: recognition, significance, and implications. *Ann Neurol* 1995;38:202.
8. DeAngelis LM. Current management of primary central nervous system lymphoma. *Oncology* 1995;9:63.
9. Hormigo AH, DeAngelis LM. Primary ocular lymphoma: clinical features, diagnosis, and treatment. *Clin Lymphoma* 2003;4:22.
10. Peterson K, Gordon KB, Heinemann MH, et al. The clinical spectrum of ocular lymphoma. *Cancer* 1993;72:843.
11. Lachance DH, O'Neill BP, Macdonald DR, et al. Primary leptomeningeal lymphoma: report of 9 cases, diagnosis with immunocytochemical analysis, and review of the literature. *Neurology* 1991;41:95.
12. Kim HJ, Ha CK, Jeon BS. Primary leptomeningeal lymphoma with long-term survival: a case report. *J Neurooncol* 2000;48:47.
13. Nakamizo T, Inoue H, Udaka F, et al. Magnetic resonance imaging of primary spinal intramedullary lymphoma. *J Neuroimaging* 2002;12:183.
14. Herrlinger U, Weller M, Kuker W. Primary CNS lymphoma in the spinal cord: clinical manifestations may precede MRI detectability. *Neuroradiology* 2002;44:239.
15. Gliemroth J, Kehler U, Gaebel C, et al. Neuroradiological findings in primary cerebral lymphomas of non-AIDS patients. *Clin Neurol Neurosurg* 2003;105:78.

16. Harting I, Hartmann M, Jost G, et al. Differentiating primary central nervous system lymphoma from glioma in humans using localized proton magnetic resonance spectroscopy. *Neurosci Lett* 2003;342:163.

17. Thurnher MM, Rieger A, Kleibl-Popov C, et al. Primary central nervous system lymphoma in AIDS: a wider spectrum of CT and MRI findings. *Neuroradiology* 2001;43:29.

18. Hoffman JM, Waskin HA, Schifter T, et al. FDG-PET in differentiating lymphoma from nonmalignant central nervous system lesions in patients with AIDS. *J Nucl Med* 1993;34:567.

19. Antinori A, DeRossi G, Ammassari A, et al. Value of combined approach with thallium-201 single-photon emission computed tomography and Epstein-Barr virus DNA polymerase chain reaction in CSF for the diagnosis of AIDS-related primary CNS lymphoma. *J Clin Oncol* 1999;17:554.

20. Gleissner B, Siehl J, Korfel A, et al. CSF evaluation in primary CNS lymphoma patients by PCR of the CDR III IgH genes. *Neurology* 2002;58:390.

21. Li C-Y, Witzig TE, Phyliky RL, et al. Diagnosis of B-cell non-Hodgkin's lymphoma of the central nervous system by immunocytochemical analysis of cerebrospinal fluid lymphocytes. *Cancer* 1986;57:737.

22. DeAngelis LM, Wong E, Rosenblum F, et al. Epstein-Barr virus in AIDS and non-AIDS primary central nervous system lymphoma. *Cancer* 1992;70:1607.

23. Clinque P, Brytting M, Vago L, et al. Epstein-Barr virus DNA in cerebrospinal fluid from patients with AIDS-related primary lymphoma of the central nervous system. *Lancet* 1993;342:398.

24. Pilozzi E, Talerico C, Uccini S, et al. B cell clonality in multiple localizations of primary central nervous system lymphomas in AIDS patients. *Leuk Lymphoma* 2003;44:963.

25. Braaten KM, Betensky RA, deLeval L, et al. BCL-6 expression predicts improved survival in patients with primary central nervous system lymphoma. *Clin Cancer Res* 2003;9:1063.

26. Montesinos-Rongen M, Hans VH, Eis-Hubinger AM, et al. Human herpes virus-8 is not associated with primary central nervous system lymphoma in HIV-negative patients. *Acta Neuropathol* 2001;102:489.

27. Gijtenbeek JM, Rosenblum MK, DeAngelis LM. Primary central nervous system T-cell lymphoma. *Neurology* 2001;57:716.

28. Ng CS, Chan JKC, Hui PK, et al. Large B-cell lymphomas with a high content of reactive T-cells. *Hum Pathol* 1989;20:1145.

29. Nelson DF, Martz KL, Bonner H, et al. Non-Hodgkin's lymphoma of the brain: can high dose, large volume radiation therapy improve survival? Report on a prospective trial by the radiation therapy oncology group (RTOG): RTOG 8315. *Int J Radiat Oncol Biol Phys* 1992;23:9.

30. Weller M. Glucocorticoid treatment of primary CNS lymphoma. *J Neurooncol* 1999;43:237.

31. DeAngelis LM, Seiferheld W, Schold SC, Radiation Therapy Oncology Group Study 93-10. Combination chemotherapy and radiotherapy for primary central nervous system lymphoma: Radiation Therapy Oncology Group Study 93-10. *J Clin Oncol* 2002;20:4643.

32. Bessell EM, Lopez-Guillermo A, Villa S, et al. Importance of radiotherapy in the outcome of patients with primary CNS lymphoma: an analysis of the CHOD/BVAM regimen followed by two different radiotherapy treatments. *J Clin Oncol* 2002;20:231.

33. Shibamoto Y, Hayabuchi N, Hiratsuka J-I, et al. Is whole-brain irradiation necessary for primary central nervous system lymphoma? Patterns of recurrence after partial-brain irradiation. *Cancer* 2003;97:128.

34. Schultz C, Scott C, Sherman W, et al. Preirradiation chemotherapy with cyclophosphamide, doxorubicin, vincristine, and dexamethasone for primary CNS lymphomas: initial report of Radiation Therapy Oncology Group protocol 88-06. *J Clin Oncol* 1996;14:556.

35. O'Neill BP, O'Fallon JR, Earle JD, et al. Primary central nervous system Non-Hodgkin's lymphoma: survival advantages with combined initial therapy? *Int J Radiat Oncol Biol Phys* 1995;33:663.

36. Mead GM, Bleehen NM, Gregor A, et al. A medical research council randomized trial in patients with primary central non-Hodgkin lymphoma. Cerebral radiotherapy with and without cyclophosphamide, doxorubicin, vincristine, and prednisone chemotherapy. *Cancer* 2000;89:1359.

37. Abrey LE, Yahalom J, DeAngelis LM. Treatment for primary CNS lymphoma: the next step. *J Clin Oncol* 2000;18:3144.

38. Abrey LE, DeAngelis LM, Yahalom J. Long-term survival in primary CNS lymphoma. *J Clin Oncol* 1998;16:859.

39. Batchelor T, Carson K, O'Neill A, et al. Treatment of primary CNS lymphoma with methotrexate and deferred radiotherapy: a report of NABTT 96-07. *J Clin Oncol* 2003;21:1044.

40. Herrlinger U, Schabet M, Brugger W, et al. German Cancer Society Neuro-Oncology Working Group NOA-03 multicenter trial of single-agent high-dose methotrexate for primary central nervous system lymphoma. *Ann. Neurol* 2002;51:247.

41. Abrey LE, Moskowitz CH, Mason WP, et al. Intensive methotrexate and cytarabine followed by high-dose chemotherapy with autologous stem cell rescue in patients with newly diagnosed primary CNS lymphoma: an intent-to-treat analysis. *J Clin Oncol* 2003;21:4151.

42. Khan RB, Shi W, Thaler TH, et al. Is intrathecal methotrexate necessary in the treatment of primary CNS lymphoma? *J Neurooncol* 2002;58:175.

43. Soussain C, Suzan F, Hoang-Xuan K, et al. Results of intensive chemotherapy followed by hematopoietic stem-cell rescue in 22 patients with refractory or recurrent primary CNS lymphoma or intraocular lymphoma. *J Clin Oncol* 2001;19:742.

44. McAllister LD, Doolittle ND, Guastadisegni PE, et al. Cognitive outcomes and long-term follow-up results after enhanced chemotherapy delivery for primary central nervous system lymphoma. *Neurosurgery* 2000;46:51.

45. Pels H, Schulz H, Manzke O, et al. Intraventricular and intravenous treatment of a patient with refractory primary CNS lymphoma using rituximab. *J Neurooncol* 2002;59:213.

46. Raez LE, Patel P, Feun L, et al. Natural history and prognostic factors for survival in patients with acquired immune deficiency syndromes (AIDS)-related primary central nervous system lymphoma (PCNSL). *Crit Rev Oncol* 1998;9:199.

47. Hoffmann C, Tabrizian S, Wolf E, et al. Survival of AIDS patients with primary central nervous system lymphoma is dramatically improved by HAART-induced immune recovery. *AIDS* 2001;15:2119.

48. Skiest DJ, Crosby C. Survival is prolonged by high active antiretroviral therapy in AIDS patients with primary central nervous system lymphoma. *AIDS* 2003;17:1787.

49. Raez L, Cabral L, Cai JP, et al. Treatment of AIDS-related primary central nervous system lymphoma with zidovudine, ganciclovir, and interleukin 2. *AIDS Res Hum Retroviruses* 1999;15:713.

50. Forsyth PA, Yahalom J, DeAngelis LM. Combined-modality therapy in the treatment of primary central nervous system lymphoma in AIDS. *Neurology* 1994;44:1473.

51. Jacomet C, Girard PM, Lebrette MG, et al. Intravenous methotrexate for primary central nervous system non-Hodgkin's lymphoma in AIDS. *AIDS* 1997;11:1725.

52. Gates AE, Kaplan LD. AIDS malignancies in the era of highly active antiretroviral therapy. *Oncology* 2002;16:657.

53. Antinori A, Cingolani A, DeLuca A, et al. Epstein-Barr virus in monitoring the response to therapy of acquired immunodeficiency syndrome-related primary central nervous system lymphoma. *Ann Neurol* 1999;45:259.

VOLKER DIEHL
NANCY LEE HARRIS
PETER M. MAUCH

SECTION 5

Hodgkin's Lymphoma

HISTORY

A great deal has been written about the life and accomplishments of Thomas Hodgkin.[1] In his historic paper entitled "On Some Morbid Appearances of the Absorbent Glands and Spleen" presented to the Medical Chirurgical Society in London on January 10, 1832, Thomas Hodgkin described the clinical history and postmortem findings of the massive enlargement of lymph nodes and spleens of six patients studied at Guy's Hospital in London and of a seventh patient who had been seen by Robert Carswell in 1828.[2] Without a microscope, Hodgkin recognized that these patients had suffered from a disease that started in the lymph nodes located along the major vessels in the neck, chest, or abdomen, rather than from an inflammatory condition.

In 1856, Sir Samuel Wilks, a Guy's Hospital pathologist, described ten postmortem cases that had "a peculiar enlargement of the lymphatic glands frequently associated with disease of the spleen." By 1865, Dr. Wilks had collected 15 cases, which were described in a second paper entitled "Cases of the Enlargement of the Lymphatic Glands and Spleen (or Hodgkin's Disease) with Remarks."[3] This linked Hodgkin's name permanently to this newly identified disease. Wilks's initial descriptions provided some of the earliest understanding of Hodgkin's lymphoma (HL). He described the disease as a cancer that started and remained in the lymph nodes for a long time, perhaps years, before involving the spleen and then spreading to other organs. He also noted anemia, weight loss, and fevers in some of the patients with HL.

Although other physicians had provided descriptions of the characteristic giant cells present in the lymph nodes and spleens of patients with HL, Dr. W. S. Greenfield in 1878 was the first to contribute drawings of them from a low microscopic magnification of a lymph node specimen.[4] Despite Greenfield's findings, Dr. Carl Sternberg in 1898 and Dr. Dorothy Reed in 1902 are credited with the first definitive microscopic descriptions of HL.[5,6]

Both Sternberg and Reed, along with many other physicians, believed that HL was caused by an associated infection rather than by a separate malignant process of the lymph nodes. Proponents of the infection theory cited the frequent association of HL with tuberculosis. Eight of Sternberg's 13 cases of HL had coexistent tuberculosis, and he believed HL to be a variant of tuberculosis. Other physicians believed that HL was a cancer of the lymph nodes. Clinical and pathologic studies that became available in the early twentieth century helped to confirm their view.[7] Despite the very strong evidence for the malignant nature of HL over the last century, it has only recently been shown that Hodgkin's-Reed-Sternberg (H-RS) cells are clonal, which confirms their origin from a single malignant cell.[8]

ETIOLOGY AND EPIDEMIOLOGY

Approximately 7500 new cases of HL are diagnosed each year in the United States. Slightly more men than women develop this malignancy (1.4:1.0). In economically developed countries, HL shows an age-related bimodal incidence. The first peak occurs in the third decade of life and a much smaller peak occurs after the age of 50 years.[9–11] The incidence of HL by age also differs by histologic subtype.[10]

A number of studies have suggested that there is a genetic predisposition for HL. There is an increased incidence in Jews and also among first-degree relatives of individuals with the disease.[12] Siblings appear to have a twofold to fivefold increased risk; in siblings of the same sex there is as much as a ninefold increased risk.[13] There is an increased risk among parent–child pairs but not among spouses, which again suggests a genetic predisposition. Also, HL has been linked with certain HLA antigens.[14,15]

There is less support for most other potential causes of HL. In contrast to other malignancies, HL is rarely seen as a second malignancy, and incidence does not appear to be increased in patients with illness- or treatment-related chronic immunosuppression. Although HL has been noted in patients with acquired immunodeficiency syndrome (AIDS), there remains lack of evidence that there is a direct correlation with the immune suppression associated with AIDS.[16] In fact, in those on the highly active antiretroviral therapy regimen, the incidence of Hodgkin's lymphoma seems to increase with rising numbers of CD4 cells. In contrast, there is increasing evidence to suggest a viral etiology for HL. In economically developed countries, studies report an association between HL in younger patients and higher level of maternal education, decreased numbers of siblings and playmates, early birth order, and residence in single-family dwellings in childhood.[17,18] This association between HL and childhood factors that decrease exposure to infectious agents at an early age has led investigators to propose that the epidemiologic features of HL appear to mimic those of a viral illness that has an age-related host response to infection.

BIOLOGY AND CELL OF ORIGIN

LINEAGE ORIGIN AND CLONALITY OF HODGKIN'S-REED-STERNBERG CELLS

Specific Morphologic Features of Hodgkin's Lymphoma

Lymph nodes affected by HL consist of a heterogeneous mixture of lymphocytes, histiocytes, eosinophils, plasma cells, fibroblasts, and other cells. The mononuclear Hodgkin's cells and their polynucleated counterparts, the Reed-Sternberg cells, which were early considered to represent the malignant substrate of the disease, comprise only 0.1% to 1.0% of the entire cell population in classic HL (CHL), that is, lymphocyte-rich CHL (LRCHL) and the nodular sclerosing (NSHL), mixed-cellularity (MCHL), and lymphocyte-depleted (LDHL) subtypes.[19] Similarly, in nodular lymphocyte-predominant HL (NLPHL, or nodular paragranuloma) the pathognomonic lymphocytic and histiocytic (L&H) cells represent only a small minority of the total cell population. This scarcity of the putative tumor cells was one of the major obstacles in understanding the nature of these cells. Although in the lymphocyte-predominant subtype of HL (LPHL), H-RS cells consistently express B-cell–specific surface antigens (CD19, CD20), in CHL in the majority of cases H-RS cells express the activation markers Ki-1 (CD30), Leu-M1 antigen (CD15), the interleukin-2 (IL-2) receptor (CD25), the transferrin receptor (CD71), and HLA class II molecules (HLA-DR)—not, however, surface antigens, which helped to determine their physiologic counterpart.[20] Until recently, the application of conventional molecular-genetic methods for a more detailed analysis of H-RS cells was not possible due to their scarcity. In addition, these cells could not be enriched from tissue affected by HL, presumably due to their fragility. Thus, over decades, the cell of origin of the H-RS cells remained an enigma.

Cell Lines and Animal Models

The establishment of permanently growing cell lines has permitted the biologic and genetic characterization of the tumor cell population in numerous human neoplasias. In contrast, outgrowth of a cell line is extremely rare in HL. The first two permanent cell lines (designated L428 and L540) were established in 1979 from patients with advanced-stage HL (clinical stage IVB).[21] These cell lines were grown out from a pleural effusion and bone marrow. With few exceptions, all subsequently established cell lines were also obtained from body fluids (bone marrow, pleural effusion, peripheral blood) of patients with advanced-stage disease.[22] This observation may reflect an *in vivo* adaptation of the cells to the conditions of suspension culture as a prerequisite for *in vitro* outgrowth. So far, only 15 cell lines have been established that may be regarded as HL derived. Analysis of immunophenotype, karyotype, immunoglobulin (Ig), or T-cell receptor gene rearrangements of these cell lines revealed heterogeneous results, as in the analysis of primary tissue, so that no conclusion could be drawn regarding the cell of origin of HL. In addition, their derivation from primary H-RS cells could not be determined unequivocally.[22] A novel Epstein-Barr virus (EBV)–negative cell line (L1236) has been established from peripheral blood mononuclear cells of a patient with advanced HL of the MC subtype[23] (Fig. 41.5-1). When single-cell polymerase chain reaction (PCR) was used, it could be shown that the genomic sequences of the Ig gene

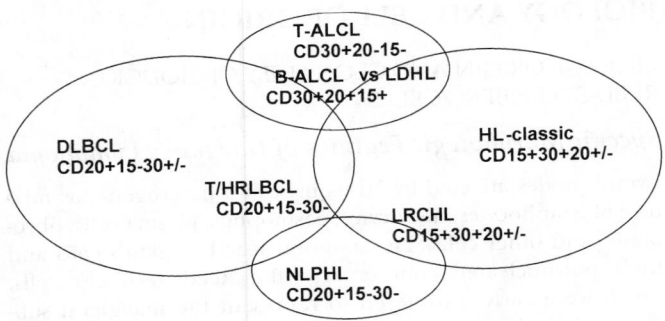

FIGURE 41.5-1. Differential diagnosis of Hodgkin's lymphoma (HL). There is morphologic overlap between classic HL; nodular lymphocyte-predominant HL (NLPHL); T-cell/histiocyte-rich large B-cell lymphoma (T/HRLBCL); large B-cell lymphoma, anaplastic type (B-ALCL); and T-cell anaplastic large cell lymphoma (T-ALCL). Immunophenotyping can be useful in the differential diagnosis. DLBCL, diffuse large B-cell lymphoma; LDHL, lymphocyte-depleted HL; LRCHL, lymphocyte-rich classic HL.

rearrangements of the H-RS cells in the patient's bone marrow were identical to those detected in L1236 cells.[24] Thus, the derivation from the primary H-RS cells could definitely be proved on the molecular level in this cell line.

HL-derived cell lines were successfully used for the discovery of H-RS cell–associated antigens, which include CD30 (Ki-1), CD70, and Ki-27[25,26]; for cloning the CD30 gene[27]; and for studying the CD30 signal transduction pathway. They also enabled the *in vitro* testing of new immunotherapeutic modalities such as ricin A–linked anti-CD30 immunotoxins,[28] saporin-linked anti-CD30 immunotoxins,[29] anti-CD16/CD30 bispecific antibodies,[30] and CD30 anti-idiotype vaccine.

Although none of these HL-derived cell lines could be grown reproducibly in thymus-aplastic T-cell–deficient nude mice, the HL-derived cell lines L540, HL-MyZ, L428, and L1236 have been shown to disseminate intralymphatically after inoculation into T- and B-cell–deficient severe combined immunodeficiency (SCID) mice.[23,31] The SCID mouse model is used for the preclinical *in vivo* testing of new experimental therapeutic approaches.[31] Unfortunately, however, no reproducible growth of primary H-RS cells has been observed after transplantation of biopsy material.[32]

Results of Single-Cell Analysis: Hodgkin's-Reed-Sternberg Cells Are Clonal Lymphoma Cells Derived from B Cells

A methodologic breakthrough in the biologic analysis of H-RS cells was achieved by the establishment of micromanipulation of immunophenotyped single cells from frozen sections, which allowed for the amplification and analysis of genes derived from a single cell. Kuppers et al. amplified rearranged Ig heavy chain (H) genes from single H-RS cells micromanipulated from two cases of CHL and from one case of LPHL.[33] Sequence analysis revealed the clonal B-cell origin of the H-RS cells in all three cases. In 14 of 15 further cases of CHL,[24,34–36] again clonal rearranged Ig genes were detected in the H-RS cells. Clonal Ig gene rearrangements in H-RS cells of CHL were also found by others using micromanipulation and single-cell PCR.[37] Similarly, using the new method, clonally related Ig gene rearrangements were detected in L&H cells isolated from frozen-tissue sections of LPHL.[38] Thus, there is overwhelming

evidence that at least a substantial proportion of cases (if not all) of CHL and LPHL represent monoclonal, B-cell–derived disorders. The view of H-RS cells as clonal lymphoma cells derived from B-cells was further supported by the detection of clonally related H-RS cells in relapsing disease using the rearranged Ig genes as a clone-specific marker gene[39,40] as well as by the detection of clonal EBV genomes[41] and clonal cytogenetic aberrations in H-RS cells[42] obtained from different lymph nodes of the same patient.

Two publications reported on the detection of rare cases of CHL harboring rearranged clonal T-cell receptor genes with lack of Ig gene rearrangements.[43] These findings unequivocally prove the hypothesis that, in some rare instances, CHL is a T-cell–derived lymphoma.

Derivation of Hodgkin's-Reed-Sternberg Cells from Preapoptotic Germinal Center B Cells

The site of physiologic contact between a specific antigen and a B lymphocyte is the germinal center (GC) of a lymph node.[44] This contact results in the accumulation of somatic mutations in the Ig genes leading to the expression of antibodies with higher affinity for the respective antigen due to amino acid exchanges. However, somatic mutations might also result in a lower affinity of the antibody or even in generation of a stop codon. When B cells lose their ability to express an antibody or express an antibody with lower affinity, they subsequently undergo apoptosis within the GC. Induction of apoptotic cell death in GC B cells is mediated through activation of the CD95/Fas cell surface receptor.[45–47] Activation of Fas by its adequate ligand leads to activation of a signaling cascade that results in apoptosis. All other B cells that accumulate favorable mutations are rescued from apoptosis by up-regulation of cellular FLICE (FADD-homologous ICE/CED-3-like protease) inhibitory protein (c-FLIP), a potent and specific inhibitor of the Fas signaling pathway.[46,47] These B cells clonally expand and can accumulate further mutations to improve the affinity of their antibody. After leaving the GC, they differentiate into B memory cells or plasma cells. In a substantial proportion of LPHL cases the clonal L&H cells revealed ongoing mutations, which provides evidence that L&H cells are GC-derived B cells further depending on antigen binding and selection.[38,48] In this context, L&H cells are comparable to follicular lymphoma cells. Although follicular lymphoma cells frequently harbor the chromosomal translocation t(14;18), which results in activation of the bcl-2 gene, the transforming event in L&H cells remains unknown. H-RS cells of CHL differ from those of follicular lymphoma as well as from those of LPHL in that, in a considerable fraction of cases, they accumulate crippling somatic mutations within potentially functional Ig gene rearrangements that prevent further antibody expression.[34] These crippling mutations do not necessarily have to be located within the coding region of Ig genes. One case of MCHL has been described in which a somatic mutation within a regulatory element of the IgH promoter was associated with down-regulation of Ig gene expression.[49] Furthermore, the lack of B-cell–specific transcription factors important for Ig expression and B-cell receptor signaling may centrally be involved in the failure of H-RS cells to express Ig.[50–53] The Ig gene mutation pattern and the detection of crippling mutations rendering potential functional Ig gene rearrangements nonfunctional suggests that H-RS cells as a rule grow independently from antigen selection and even antibody expression. Indeed, no Ig gene expression in H-RS cells could be demonstrated by several groups. In addition, the pattern of Ig gene mutations found in H-RS cells is characteristic of B cells that were not exposed to the full selective pressure of the GC. The mechanisms that prevent negative selection of the H-RS cells in the GC are therefore important issues in understanding the transformation process that leads to clonal growth of these lymphoma cells. Consequently, the hypothesized apoptosis resistance could be demonstrated experimentally.[54,55] Because inherited Fas gene mutations observed in a rare lymphoproliferative syndrome lead to a 51-fold increased risk specifically for development of HL, it was intriguing to see if somatic Fas gene mutations might also underlie the Fas resistance observed in the spontaneous cases of CHL. However, mutations affecting the functionality of the Fas death receptor were observed in only a minute fraction of primary cases of CHL.[56–58] Interestingly, c-FLIP has been shown to be strongly expressed by H-RS cells *in vitro* and in primary biopsy specimens.[55,58] c-FLIP may interrupt transmission of the Fas death signal, thereby preventing negative selection of the preapoptotic GC B-cell precursor.

It is now generally accepted that H-RS cells are in most cases genetically derived from GC B cells; however, the lack of unambiguous phenotypic lineage determination is also characteristic of CHL. In addition to the aforementioned immunohistochemical studies, a report on global gene expression of H-RS cells supports this view because the authors were able to show extensive down-regulation of B-cell receptor–associated signaling molecules and of other important B-cell markers.[53] Importantly, the gene expression signature of H-RS cells was found not to be related to that of GC B cells but to resemble much more the one of *in vitro*–activated peripheral blood B cells and EBV-immortalized B-cell lines.[59] Disappointing the expectations, the possible extinction of the B cellular transcription program by fusion with a non–B cell has now been ruled out.[60,61] Taken together, a general lineage promiscuity is a central feature of CHL. However, few data exist that might help to explain this phenomenon.

GENETIC ALTERATIONS IN HODGKIN'S LYMPHOMA

Chromosomal Instability

Conventional karyotype analyses of Hodgkin's and Reed-Sternberg cells are hampered by the low number of obtainable mitoses from lymph node suspensions and their poor chromosome banding qualities.[62] In addition, karyotypes cannot unequivocally be attributed to the malignant cells, because the cellular compartment with the highest mitotic index in affected tissue is that of nonmalignant lymphocytes in the neighborhood of the H-RS cells. Thus, proliferating cells with a normal karyotype most probably represent reactive lymphoid cells.[63] Depending on the histologic subtype, between 42% (LPHL) and 75% (NSHL) of cases studied yielded evaluable metaphases. In karyotype analyses performed by different groups, the percentage of abnormal karyotypes varied considerably between 22% and 83%. Although numerical and structural cytogenetic abnormalities were observed, a specific chromosomal marker of HL—like, for instance, the Burkitt's lymphoma–specific chromosomal translocations—has not yet been defined.[64] In a study of 60 lymph nodes obtained from untreated patients with HL, in approximately half of the analyzable cases numerical or structural aberrations, or both, were found.[65] Among HL-associated chromosomal abnormalities, aneuploidy (100%) with hyperdiploidy (70%) is the most frequent. Chromosomes 1, 2, 5, 12, and 21 are often triplicated. In a few cases, loss of chromosomes was reported: For example, chromosomal translocations or deletions were found in two-thirds of cases.[65] Fluorescence *in situ* hybridization (FISH) of DNA probes on interphase nuclei has now extended the potential of conventional karyotyping, because numerical chromosomal aberrations can be detected within nonproliferating cells. The FISH method can be combined with immunophenotyping to allow characterization of CD30+ cells within an HL-derived lymph node. FISH revealed numerical chromosomal aberrations in H-RS cells of every case analyzed even if conventional karyotype analysis failed to demonstrate any chromosomal abnormality.[66] These numerical aberrations were either clonal[67] or differed from metaphase to metaphase, which probably points to a chromosomal instability within the H-RS cells. Peripheral blood lymphocytes from patients with HL show a much greater number of abnormal metaphases when incubated with cytostatic drugs than do lymphocytes from normal controls.[62] Studies have focused on the molecular evidence of genetic instability. By the use of comparative genomic hybridization and FISH technology on primary H-RS cells, several studies were able to show that specific gains (and, less prominently, losses) of chromosomal regions are a typical feature of CHL.[68–70] Among the regions affected were loci containing the JAK2 and the REL genes. Both genes are involved in important stimulatory signaling pathways. Therefore, these novel findings provide nice mechanistic explanations of how stimulatory pathways might become dissected from their physiologic regulation. One study aimed at detecting chromosomal regions affected by hemizygotic allelic losses.[71] A region that was recurrently affected by allelic imbalances in more than 90% of primary CHL cases was identified on chromosome band 6q25, a region suspected for a long time to harbor a tumor suppressor gene. The identification of this putative tumor suppressor gene shows great promise for the basic understanding of the biology of CHL.

Taken together, an intrinsic genetic instability, inferable from a broad spectrum of numerical and complex structural chromosomal abnormalities with lack of a typical pattern, is a central feature of CHL. Moreover, molecular studies were able to define the putative target loci of this instability. It is conceivable that this might have considerable pathogenetic relevance by affecting tumor suppressor genes or oncogenes or both. The causes underlying the genetic instability in CHL remain elusive, however.

Molecular Genetic Analyses

Analysis of whole tissue sections for genomic alterations or deregulated expression of the oncogenes MYC, JUN, RAF, and RAS did not reveal any characteristic pattern.[72] Because the t(14;18) translocation results in overexpression of the bcl-2 protein, preventing apoptotic death of follicular lymphoma cells, many attempts were made using PCR to detect breakpoints in the major breakpoint region (mbr) of t(14;18) in H-RS cells. In several studies, the t(14;18) translocation was found in 0% to 39% of HL cases.[73] However, it remained unproven in the positive cases whether the translocation was localized in the H-RS cells, particularly because the detection of the bcl-2 protein by immunohistochemistry *in situ* was not congruent with the detection of the translocation itself in all cases. In a report using micromanipulation of single H-RS cells followed by PCR, the t(14;18) was shown to be localized in non-malignant bystander B cells and not in a single case in the H-RS cells.[74] Similarly, no pathogenetic role could be established for the npm-alk fusion transcript resulting from the chromosomal translocation t(2;5) consistently found in ALCL of T-cell origin.[75,76] The retinoblastoma (RB) tumor suppressor gene that is involved in cell-cycle regulation is mutated or deleted, or both, on both alleles in many malignancies, which results in the absence of RNA and protein. However, in most of the HL cases analyzed, expression of the RB protein was found.[73] Mutations in the p53 tumor suppressor, which are commonly found in most human cancers, are also not a typical feature of H-RS cells as determined by single-cell PCR.[77] In addition, mutations in the BCL10 gene could not be detected in CHL.[56] Thus, although genetic instability is a characteristic feature of H-RS cells, the accumulation of subtle gene alterations in important genes, as they may result from defects in the DNA mismatch repair machinery, are not a typical feature of CHL. Of importance, the functionality of the most important mismatch repair system was demonstrated in H-RS cells.[78]

CONSTITUTIVELY ACTIVE SIGNALING PATHWAYS IN CLASSIC HODGKIN'S LYMPHOMA

Nuclear Factor κB

Dissection of stimulatory signaling pathways from their regulatory circuits is a central feature of human cancers.[79] CHL does not make an exception in this respect, because several important signaling pathways were found to be constitutively activated in H-RS cells. For example, the transcription factor nuclear factor κB (NFκB) was shown to be constitutively active in cultured as well as in primary H-RS cells.[80,81] Moreover, abrogation of NFκB activity in H-RS–derived cell lines leads to induction of massive cell death by down-regulation of a highly antiapoptotic and proproliferative gene expression program.[82,83] Thus, NFκB seems to be a central modulator of survival and proliferation in CHL. Of interest, c-FLIP, the factor that is suspected to contribute essentially to the H-RS cells' evasion of the GC, is an NFκB target and gene, and it was demonstrated to be regulated by this transcription factor in a CHL-derived cell line. NFκB may thereby directly lead to disruption of the principal apoptosis pathway that is needed for negative selection in the GC, which allows the preapoptotic H-RS cell precursor to survive. Several mechanisms were identified that might underlie constitutive activation of NFκB. Good examples are constitutively active CD30 or CD40 signaling, autonomous RANK signaling, and expression of EBV-encoded LMPs (latent membrane proteins) 1 and 2a.[84–89] These findings share an important effector mechanism: They lead to nuclear translocation of NFκB and to induction of transcription of its target genes. It is not clear, however, which of these mechanisms is the dominant one. In normal lymphocytes, NFκB is retained in the cytoplasm by its inhibitors, IκB proteins, and among them the most important seems to be IκBα.[90] Activation of distinct signaling pathways leads to activation of Iκ kinases and subsequent phosphorylation of IκBα, which in turn releases NFκB that translocates to the nucleus and induces the transcription of its target genes. In search for genetic alterations that might underlie malignant transformation of the putative H-RS cells' precursors, deleterious mutations in the IκBα gene were detected in a considerable fraction of EBV-negative cases.[91,91a] In the mutated cases, cytoplasmic retention of NFκB likely is abolished, which thus facilitates its constitutive transcriptional activity. Moreover, Jarrett et al.[91b] demonstrated mutations in the IκBα gene in 15 of 26 primary CHL cases, 11 of which were EBV negative. These findings add substantial weight to the concept that IκBα mutations may represent important transforming events in CHL in the absence of EBV or other viruses. In summary, constitutively active NFκB is a central mediator of survival and proliferation of H-RS cells of CHL. It has therefore become a prominent target for novel therapeutic approaches that aim directly at the transformed cell. Multiple mechanisms were identified that may contribute to its constitutive activation. Among them, mutations of the IκBα gene and expression of EBV-encoded latent gene products appear to give feasible explanations for this phenotype.

Signal Transducer and Activator of Transcription Family and Activator Protein 1

An additional class of transcription factors has been found to be constitutively active in CHL. The signal transducer and activator of transcription (STAT) family includes several members. Among them, STAT3, STAT6, and STAT5a were found to be constitutively active in H-RS cells of CHL.[92,93] STAT3 activity was found to be disrupted from its physiologic regulatory circuits because it did not depend on IL-6 receptor signaling and the subsequent activation of Janus kinases (Jaks). Importantly, the Jak2 genomic locus was shown to be recurrently amplified in CHL, which thus provides a nice mechanistic explanation for this finding.[68] STAT6 was, however, dependent on IL-13 signaling. Because IL-13 and its adequate receptor are expressed by H-RS cells, this may account for the observed STAT6 activation. Activator protein 1 (AP-1) was identified as an additional constitutively active transcription factor in CHL.

Taken together, H-RS cells harbor multiple signaling pathways that are uncoupled from their negative regulatory circuits. This may essentially contribute to their activated phenotype and to their dissection from the physiologic organistic growth control.

EPSTEIN-BARR INFECTION IN HODGKIN'S LYMPHOMA

Individuals who contract infectious mononucleosis have a twofold to threefold increased risk for developing HL. Elevated IgG and IgA titers against the viral capsid antigen in predisease sera were also shown to correlate with an increased risk for HL.[94] Weiss et al. were the first to detect EBV DNA in total lymph nodes affected by HL using Southern blotting.[95] *In situ* hybridization with Epstein-Barr early region–specific RNA probes (EBER-ISH) combines high sensitivity with high specificity in allowing visualization of EBV infection in distinct H-RS cells. EBER 1 and 2 RNAs are small, EBV-encoded, nonpolyadenylated transcripts of high abundance (approximately 10^6 copies per viral genome). When EBER-ISH was used, approximately 50% of the HL cases in industrialized countries were found to harbor the virus in the H-RS cells,[96,97] whereas in several developing countries more than 90% of HL patients carry the virus in their tumor cells.

H-RS cells show a specific expression pattern of viral latent genes with expression of LMP1, LMP2a, and Epstein-Barr nuclear antigen-1 (EBNA-1).[87,89,98,99] This pattern is identical to that found in nasopharyngeal carcinoma endemic in the southwest of China. It differs from that of other EBV-associated neoplasias like endemic Burkitt's lymphoma or immunoblastic B-cell lymphoma in immunocompromised patients. Except for EBNA-1, all latent viral proteins represent targets for cytotoxic T lymphocytes.[77] Thus, EBV-infected cells either express the complete set of latent viral genes in an immunocompromised host [immunoblastic non-Hodgkin's lymphoma (NHL)] or they down-regulate these proteins—except EBNA-1 in Burkitt's lymphoma—possibly to escape the host's immune response. So far, it remains unclear how the specific latent viral gene expression pattern in HL (EBNA-2 negative, LMP positive) and the pronounced T-cell proliferation in affected lymph nodes relate to each other.

The functional relevance of expression of LMPs in H-RS cells is undoubted. LMP1 has transforming potential. Transformation of epithelial cells after transfection of LMP1 has been described.[101] In lymphocytes, apoptosis can be prevented by LMP1 via up-regulation of the bcl-2 gene.[44] LMP1 is also a target for cytotoxic T cells. In addition, it up-regulates (partly in cooperation with EBNA-2) numerous cellular genes, for example, activation-associated antigens (CD23, CD30, CD39) and adhesion molecules [intracellular adhesion molecule-1 (ICAM-1), lymphocyte function–associated antigen-3 (LFA-3)]. Thus it may render a cell indirectly more susceptible to a T-cell response.[37] Knecht et al.[101a] described in some HL cases mutations in the carboxy-terminal part of the LMP1 gene identical to those previously reported in LMP isolates from Chinese nasopharyngeal carcinoma. These authors discussed an association of these mutations with a clinically more aggressive phenotype of CHL. The most important functions of both LMP1 and LMP2a, however, may be represented by the fact that both proteins can activate NFκB, a phenotype that is considered to be one of the most important activational transcription factors that is constitutively active in CHL. LMP1 does so by mimicking a constitutively active CD40 receptor, a pathway that is physiologically activated in antigen-stimulated B cells and that terminates in activation of NFκB.[101] LMP2a, in contrast, shuts down B-cell receptor expression. One would expect such a B cell to rapidly undergo apoptotic cell death, as it no longer fulfills the main criterion for positive selection. The B cell that is latently infected by EBV, however, circumvents this dilemma by up-regulation of the downstream signaling elements of the B-cell receptor—again a process that activates NFκB. Thus, EBV may hide the infected B cell from immune recognition, providing it with the needed prosurvival signals usually assigned by follicular dendritic cells and T cells. In the case of CHL, EBV infection provides a conclusive scenario underlying the transformation of the preapoptotic GC B-cell precursor—lacking Ig expression—that is considered to be the founder of the H-RS cells.

There are, however, some problems with this neat picture. Notably, EBV is present in the H-RS cells in only approximately 50% of CHL cases in the Western world.[99] It was speculated that integration of fragments of the EBV genome into the nuclei of H-RS cells might prevent their detection in the EBV-negative cases. In one study, this mechanism of "hit-and-run" transformation has been ruled out in CHL.[102] It is thus most unlikely that EBV infection accounts for more than the extensively described 50% positive cases. Therefore, other mechanisms have to be taken into account that might underlie HL genesis in the negative cases. Additionally, LMP2a predominantly interacts with Lyn and Syk tyrosine kinases in B cells.[103] These proteins were shown to be absent in H-RS cells.[53] The interaction of LMP2a with the host signaling machinery might therefore be more complicated than previously thought.

There are now much data on what is supposed to be the cellular progeny and on what is thought to govern malignant transformation in CHL. IκBα mutations and EBV infection, among others, provide a good illustration of a possible HL genesis scenario. These and other factors have a common effector mechanism: They may lead to constitutive activation of the transcription factor NFκB. By up-regulation of its antiapoptotic (e.g., c-FLIP) and proproliferative target genes, NFκB might essentially contribute to circumvention of the negative selection by the Fas death pathway. This in turn may allow the transformed preapoptotic GC B cell to proliferate and to give rise to systemic lymphoma disease.

IMMUNOLOGY OF HODGKIN'S LYMPHOMA: CELLULAR IMMUNE DEFICIENCIES

Hodgkin's lymphoma is characterized by the predominance of a reactive infiltrate consisting of T cells, B cells, neutrophils, and eosinophils surrounding few malignant H-RS cells. This morphology suggests a major role in the interplay between the tumor and the host immune system. Although H-RS cells and the H-RS–derived cell lines express several molecules that are necessary for efficient antigen presentation (major histocompatibility complex class I and class II, CD80, CD86, CD54, and CD58),[23,104] an effective immune response is not mounted. The T cells, in the vast majority CD4+ T-cell receptor-αβ positive and only very scarce CD8+ cytotoxic T lymphocytes, are characterized by the expression of activation markers like CD38, CD69, CD71, and major histocompatibility complex class II, but lack CD26 and CD25, the IL-2 receptor. This may be due to the concerted interplay of various chemokines and cytokines secreted by H-RS cells as summarized in Table 41.5-1. Especially, the predominant secretion of Th2 T helper cell–favoring cytokines and chemokines may inhibit an effective cytotoxic Th1 response in favor of a primarily humoral Th2 response.[105] This Th2-biased immune response is further strengthened by the surrounding eosinophils attracted by chemokines like eotaxin.[106] Moreover, secretion of IL-10[107] and transforming growth factor-β[107a] by the H-RS cells, in conjunction with the inability of T cells to secrete IL-2, suppresses an effective immune reaction. On the other hand, H-RS cells seem to be highly dependent on their specific microenvironment, as demonstrated by the difficulty in culturing these cells. All established cell lines are derived from patients with advanced stages of HL, in which the malignant clone lost its dependence on the surrounding cells and spread into the blood system, the pleural cavity, or the bone marrow.[23,108] In summary, H-RS cells effectively escape the host immune system by modulating the immune response in the direction of an impaired Th2 response, which even seems to support the growth of the malignant cells constituting CHL.

TABLE 41.5-1. Cytokines and Chemokines Expressed in H-RS Cells and the Surrounding T Cells

Cytokine/ Chemokine	Expression in H-RS Cell Lines	Expression in H-RS Cells (%)	References
IL-4	2/8	2	Wolf et al., 1996[23]; Klein et al., 1992[427]; Skinnider et al., 2002[420]
IL-13	4/5	93	Skinnider et al., 2002[420]; Kapp et al., 1999[428]; Skinnider et al., 2001[429]; Ohshima et al., 2001[464]
IL-5	2/6	95	Klein et al., 1992[427]; Kapp et al., 1999[428]; Samoszuk and Nansen, 1990[430]
IL-6	5/7	75	Wolf et al., 1996[23]; Klein et al., 1992[427]; Hsu et al., 1992[431]; Jucker et al., 1991[432]
IL-9	0/1	58	Merz et al., 1991[433]
IL-10	2/7	32	Wolf et al., 1996[23]; Herbst et al., 1996[99]; Beck et al., 2001[434]
IL-12	ND	85	Schwaller et al., 1995[435]
IL-2	0/7	22	Merz et al., 1991[433]; Dukers et al., 2000[436]; Hsu et al., 1992[431]
IFN-γ	2/3	47	Wolf et al., 1996[23]; Gerdes et al., 1990[437]; Dukers et al., 2000[436]
TARC	4/4	88	Van den Berg et al., 1999[438]; Peh et al., 2001[465]
MDC	ND	87	Teruya-Feldstein et al., 1999[439]; Hedvat et al., 2001[440]
Eotaxin	1/5	63	Teruya-Feldstein et al., 1999[439]; Jundt et al., 1999[441]
IP-10	ND	100	Teruya-Feldstein et al., 1999[439]; Buri et al., 2000[442]
Mig	ND	100	Teruya-Feldstein et al., 1999[439]; Buri et al., 2000[442]
MIP-1α	ND	100	Teruya-Feldstein et al., 1999[439]; Buri et al., 2000[442]
IL-8	ND	61	Foss et al., 1996[443]
TNF-α	7/7	69	Wolf et al., 1996[23]; Klein et al., 1992[427]; Foss et al., 1993[444]; Hsu et al., 1993[445]; Kretschmer et al., 1990[446]; Sappino et al., 1990[447]
LT-α	5/6	77	Hsu et al., 1993[445]; Kretschmer et al., 1990[446]; Foss et al., 1993[444]
CD40L	0/4	100	Gruss et al., 1994[448]; Carbone et al., 1995[449]; Murray et al., 2001[450]
CD30L	0/3	100	Smith et al., 1993[451]; Gruss et al., 1994[448]; Pinto et al., 1996[452]; Molin et al., 2001[453]
RANKL	2/2	100	Fiumara, 2001[86]
IL-1	3/6	58	Klein et al., 1992[427]; Hsu et al., 1993[445]; Ruco et al., 1990[454]; Xerri et al., 1992[455]; Benharroch et al., 1996[456]; Hsu et al., 1986[457]; Ree et al., 1987[458]
TGF-β	1/1	61	Kadin et al., 1990[459]; Newcom et al., 1988[460]
IL-3	0/6	25	Merz et al., 1991[433]
IL-7	ND	77	Foss et al., 1995[443]
GM-CSF	2/6	0	Klein et al., 1992[427]; Kapp et al., 1999[428]

GM-CSF, granulocyte-macrophage colony-stimulating factor; H-RS, Hodgkin's-Reed-Sternberg; IFN, interferon; IL, interleukin; IP, interferon-inducible protein; LT, lymphotoxin; MDC, macrophage-derived chemokine; Mig, monokine induced by γ-interferon; MIP, macrophage inflammatory protein; ND, no data; RANKL, receptor activator of nuclear factor κB ligand; TARC, thymus and activation-regulated chemokine; TGF, transforming growth factor; TNF, tumor necrosis factor.

PATHOLOGY

DEFINITION OF HODGKIN'S LYMPHOMA

The clinical features and responses to treatment of HL differ dramatically from those of most NHLs, which suggests that a specific immunologic reaction is important not only in the definition but also in the clinical behavior of this disease. Studies in the 1980s showed that in NLPHL, the RS cell variants expressed B-cell–associated antigens,[109] whereas those of most cases of NSHL and MCHL lacked these antigens.[110] This difference in immunophenotype, together with the observation that NLPHL had a more indolent clinical course,[111] led to the suggestion that NLPHL was a low-grade B-cell lymphoma and should be removed from the category of HL and placed with the NHLs. However, both immunophenotypic and, more recently, molecular genetic studies have shown that CHL of NSHL and MCHL types can express B-cell–associated antigens and, like NLPHL, can have rearranged immunoglobulin genes.[34,112] Furthermore, NLPHL and CHL share the feature of having a small number of neoplastic cells in a reactive background, which distinguishes both from most B-cell NHLs. Thus, although it is now known that the neoplastic cells in most cases of both LPHL and CHL are monoclonal B cells, their distinctive pathologic and clinical features still warrant placing them together in a separate category from other lymphoid neoplasms.[100] It is important for both pathologists and oncologists to recognize that HL is two distinct diseases. Therefore, current classifications include two main categories of HL: CHL (NSHL, MCHL, and LDHL) and NLPHL. In summary, the Hodgkin's lymphomas are defined as lymphomas containing one of the characteristic types of RS cells in a background of nonneoplastic cells. Cases are subclassified according to the morphology and immunophenotype of the RS cells and the composition of the cellular background. The differences in the morphology of the RS cells and the composition of the cellular background have formed the basis for the pathologic subclassification of HL (Table 41.5-2).

CLASSIFICATIONS OF HODGKIN'S LYMPHOMA

The early classification of Jackson and Parker[113] recognized three categories: paragranuloma, granuloma, and sarcoma. The distinction between the three categories was based on the ratio of neoplastic to normal cells, which increased from paragranuloma to granuloma to sarcoma, and predicted decreasing survival. In 1966, Lukes and Butler[113a] recognized that the category of granuloma could be subdivided into two categories, NS and MC, that were characterized by distinctive morphology and clinical features. Lukes and Butler also recognized that there were two variants of what they called *lymphocytic or histiocytic predominance type* (replacing paragranuloma)—a nodular and a diffuse variant—which they found differed in prognosis. The Lukes and Butler

TABLE 41.5-2. Classifications of Hodgkin's Lymphoma (HL)

Jackson and Parker[a]	Lukes and Butler[b]	Rye Conference[c]	REAL Classification[d]	WHO Classification[e]
Paragranuloma	Lymphocytic and/or histiocytic, nodular	Lymphocyte predominant	Nodular lymphocyte predominant	Lymphocyte predominant, nodular
	Lymphocytic and/or histiocytic, diffuse		Classic HL	Classic HL
			Lymphocyte-rich classic HL[f]	Lymphocyte-rich classic HL
Granuloma	Nodular sclerosis	Nodular sclerosis	Nodular sclerosis	Nodular sclerosis
	Mixed cellularity[g]	Mixed cellularity[g]	Mixed cellularity	Mixed cellularity
Sarcoma	Diffuse fibrosis	Lymphocytic depleted	Lymphocyte depleted	Lymphocyte depleted
	Reticular			Unclassifiable classic HL

REAL, Revised European-American Lymphoma; WHO, World Health Organization.
[a]Jackson JH, Parker JF. Hodgkin's disease. General considerations. *N Engl J Med* 1944;230:1.
[b]Lukes RJ, Butler JJ. The pathology and nomenclature of Hodgkin's disease. *Cancer Res* 1966;26:1063.
[c]Lukes RJ, Craver LF, Hall TC, et al. Report of the nomenclature committee. *Cancer Res* 1966;26:1311.
[d]Harris NL, Jaffe ES, Stein H, et al. A revised European-American classification of lymphoid neoplasms: a proposal from the International Lymphoma Study Group. *Blood* 1994;84:1361.
[e]Harris NL, Jaffe ES, Diebold J, et al. The World Health Organization classification of hematological malignancies report of the Clinical Advisory Committee Meeting, Airlie House, Virginia, November 1997. *Mod Pathol* 2000;13:193.
[f]Includes some lymphocytic and/or histiocytic nodular cases.
[g]Includes unclassifiable cases.

classification was modified and simplified at the Rye conference in 1966.[114] The Rye classification has remained the standard classification since that time. In 1994, the International Lymphoma Study Group introduced an updated classification, incorporating new immunologic and molecular data, as part of the Revised European-American Lymphoma (REAL) Classification.[115] These concepts have been incorporated into the new World Health Organization (WHO) classification of hematologic malignancies, a joint effort of the Society for Hematopathology and the European Association of Hematopathologists.[419]

There are several major differences between the REAL/WHO classification of HL and older classifications. Most important is the recognition, as stated earlier, that there are two distinct diseases that have been called HL: CHL, which consists predominantly of NSHL and MCHL, and NLPHL (Table 41.5-3). Simply a predominance of lymphocytes in the background is not sufficient to classify a case as NLPHL; cases that have the RS cell morphology and immunophenotype of CHL, even if they contain predominantly lymphocytes, are classified as LRCHL. A second difference is that, in the Lukes-Butler and Rye classifications, MCHL was a heterogeneous category, including both typical cases and all other cases that did not fit into one of the other categories. The authors now recommend that MCHL be restricted to typical cases and that unclassifiable cases be classified as "HL unclassifiable." Finally, it is now clear that immunophenotype is important in the subclassification of HL, both in distinguishing NLPHL from classic types and in distinguishing HL from NHL; thus, the immunophenotype is included in the definitions of HL in the REAL/WHO classification. Typical freedom from treatment failure (FFTF) and survival curves for the main histologic subtypes are illustrated using the German Hodgkin Study Group (GHSG) data in Figure 41.5-2.

NODULAR LYMPHOCYTE-PREDOMINANT HODGKIN'S LYMPHOMA

Morphologic Features

NLPHL is defined as having at least a partially nodular growth pattern. Diffuse areas are present in a minority of the cases,

and it is controversial whether purely diffuse cases exist.[116] The RS cell variants differ from mononuclear and "classic" RS cells: They have vesicular, polylobulated nuclei and distinct but small, usually peripheral nucleoli, without perinucleolar halos; these have been called L&H cells (lymphocytic or histiocytic of Lukes and Butler) or "popcorn" cells, because of the resemblance of their nuclei to an exploded kernel of corn.[114] In fact, they resemble "exploded" centroblasts. Although popcorn cells may be very numerous, usually no classic, diagnostic RS cells

TABLE 41.5-3. Morphologic and Immunophenotypic Features of Nodular Lymphocyte-Predominant and Classic Hodgkin's Lymphoma

	Classic HL	NLPHL
Pattern	Diffuse, interfollicular, nodular	Nodular, at least in part
Tumor cells	Diagnostic RS cells; mononuclear or lacunar cells	L&H or popcorn cells
Background	Lymphocytes, histiocytes, eosinophils, plasma cells	Lymphocytes, histiocytes
Fibrosis	Common	Rare
CD15	+	−
CD30	+	−
CD20	±	+
CD45	−	+
EMA	−	+
EBV (in RS cells)	+ (~50%)	−
Background lymphocytes	T cells > B cells	B cells > T cells
CD57+ T cells	−	+
Ig genes (single-cell PCR)	Rearranged, clonal, mutated, "crippled"	Rearranged, clonal, mutated, ongoing

+, present; −, absent; EBV, Epstein-Barr virus; EMA, epithelial membrane antigen; HL, Hodgkin's lymphoma; Ig, immunoglobulin; L&H, lymphocytes and histiocytes; NLPHL, nodular lymphocyte-predominant Hodgkin's lymphoma; PCR, polymerase chain reaction; RS, Reed-Sternberg.

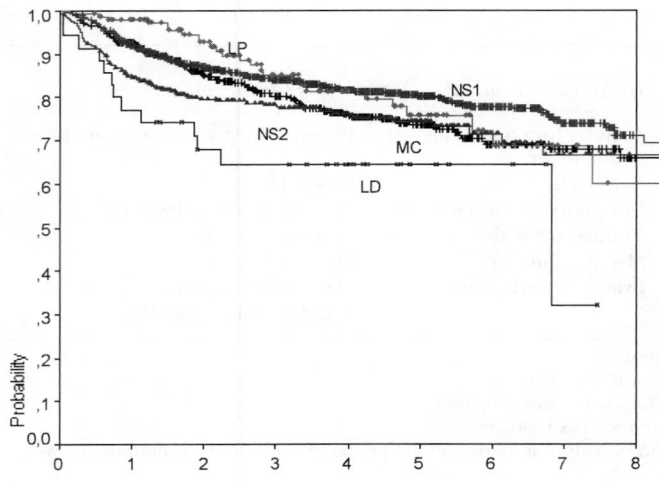

A Freedom from treatment failure (years)

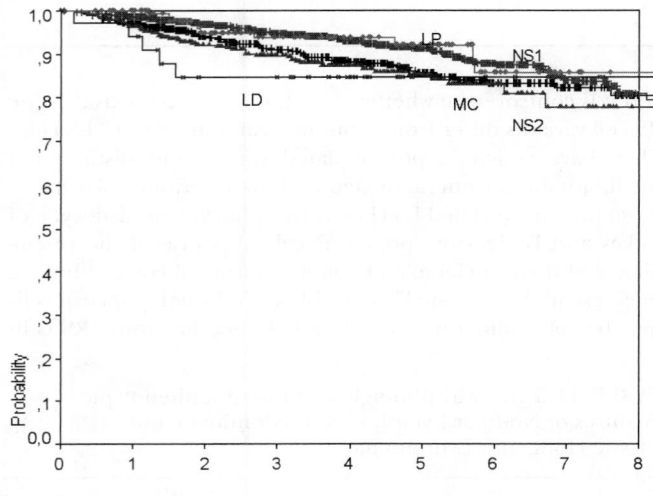

B Survival (years)

FIGURE 41.5-2. **A:** Reviewed histologic subtype: freedom from treatment failure in German Hodgkin Study Group (GHSG) trials, 1988 to 1998, all stages. Lymphocyte depleted (LD), n = 35; lymphocyte predominant (LP), n = 144; mixed cellularity (MC), n = 596; nodular sclerosis grade 1 (NS1), n = 1397; nodular sclerosis grade 2 (NS2), n = 361. Significant (*P* ≤.01) comparisons: NS1 vs. NS2, *P*= .0012; LP vs. LD, *P*= .0088; NS1 vs. LD, *P* = .0017. **B:** Reviewed histologic subtype: survival in GHSG trials, 1988 to 1998. LD, n = 35; LP, n = 144; MC, n = 596; NS1, n = 1397; NS2, n = 361. Significant (*P*≤.01) comparisons: NS1 vs. NS2, *P* = .0021. (See Color Fig. 41.5-2 in the CD-ROM.)

are found. In occasional cases, however, the RS cells may resemble classic or lacunar types; in such cases, immunophenotyping is helpful in establishing the diagnosis. The background is predominantly lymphocytes; clusters of epithelioid histiocytes may be numerous; plasma cells, eosinophils, and neutrophils are rarely seen and, if present, are not numerous.[117] Occasional sclerosis may cause some cases to resemble NSHL.

Progressive Transformation of Germinal Centers

A distinctive type of follicular lymphoid hyperplasia, known as progressive transformation of GCs (PTGC), is seen focally in approximately 20% of lymph nodes involved by NLPHL and may be seen in the absence of HL in other lymph nodes in the same patient.[118] PTGC is characterized by enlarged follicles that contain numerous small B cells of mantle zone type. These follicles may closely resemble the nodules of NLPHL. This phenomenon has given rise to speculation that NLPHL may arise from PTGC. PTGC is usually seen as a single or only a few enlarged follicles in a setting of nonspecific reactive follicular lymphoid hyperplasia; however, on occasion, the enlarged follicles may be numerous and associated with prominent lymph node enlargement, particularly in adolescents and young adults.[119]

Nodular Lymphocyte-Predominant Hodgkin's Lymphoma and Large B-Cell Lymphoma

Patients with NLPHL have a slightly higher risk of developing NHL than patients with other types of HL.[120] Transformation of NLPHL to large B-cell lymphoma, usually with a B-cell phenotype and often monoclonal with respect to immunoglobulin (both phenotype and genotype), is most common. Hansmann et al.[121] reported a 2.6% incidence in a series of 537 cases, and the British National Lymphoma Investigation (BNLI) reported a 2% incidence in 182 cases.[120] The range in more recent reports is from 2.0% to 6.5%.[122] The large B-cell lymphoma does not necessarily consist of typical L&H cells and usually resembles other diffuse large B-cell lymphomas (DLBCLs).[121] Most cases studied have had a B-cell immunophenotype, with B-lineage antigen expression in the majority and monotypic Ig expression in 30% to 50%. In some cases, a clonal relationship between the LPHL and the DBCL has been shown by molecular genetic analysis.[123]

In addition to the cases that progress to DLBCL, cases are found in which NLPHL is composite with DLBCL in the same lymph node, either at the time of diagnosis or at relapse.[124] In the reported cases, the prognosis of these patients appears to be significantly better than that for patients with the usual DLBCL, and patients who respond to treatment may later relapse with only NLPHL.[124]

Immunophenotype

The immunophenotype is an important part of the definition of NLPHL. In contrast to CHL, the atypical cells are CD45+ and express B-cell–associated antigens (CD19, CD20, CD22, CD79a) and epithelial membrane antigen (EMA), but lack CD15 and CD30. In contrast to typical B-cell lymphomas, however, they are usually immunoglobulin-negative by routine techniques. J chain has been demonstrated in many cases.[125] Studies using *in situ* hybridization for light-chain messenger RNA have shown clonal expression in the atypical cells.[126] Popcorn cells also express the nuclear protein encoded by the bcl-6 gene, which is associated with normal GC B-cell development, and the activation-associated molecules CD40 and CD86 (B7/BB1), which are involved in B-cell interaction with T cells.[127]

The nodules of LPHL are actually altered follicles or GCs. The small lymphocytes in the nodules are a mixture of polyclonal B cells with a mantle zone phenotype (IgM and IgD positive), and numerous T cells, many of which are CD57+, similar to the T-cell population in normal and progressively transformed GCs.[128] T cells in NLPHL may show significant nuclear enlargement and irregularity, resembling centrocytes. In contrast to the T cells in reactive or progressively transformed follicles, which are scattered singly and often concentrated in the light zone or at the junction with the mantle zone, the T cells in NLPHL form small aggregates, often giving the follicle a broken-up, moth-eaten, or irregular contour. They typically surround the neoplastic B cells, forming rings, rosettes, or collarettes. Although several reports suggest that the T cells surrounding popcorn cells are mostly CD57+,[129,130] this can be difficult to demonstrate in many cases, and absence of CD57+ cells in the rosettes does not argue against the diagnosis. A prominent concentric meshwork of follicular dendritic cells is present within the nodules. The interfollicular region contains predominantly T cells; when there are diffuse areas, the background lymphocytes are also predominantly T cells, and the follicular dendritic cell meshwork is lost.[131]

Clinical Features

NLPHL accounts for 4% to 5% of cases in most series. The median age of patients is the midthirties, but cases may be seen in both children and the elderly. The male to female ratio is 3:1 or higher. NLPHL usually involves peripheral lymph nodes, with sparing of the mediastinum. Approximately 80% of the patients in most series have stage I or II disease at the time of diagnosis, but rarely patients may present with stage III or IV disease, with a concomitantly worse prognosis. Over 90% of patients have a complete response to therapy, and 90% are alive at 10 years. The cause of death is often NHL, other cancers, or complications of treatment, rather than HL.[122,132]

CLASSIC HODGKIN'S LYMPHOMA

CHL is defined by the presence of classic, diagnostic RS cells in a background of either nodular sclerosis (NS), MC, or lymphocyte depletion, with (when studied) the immunophenotype of CHL (CD15+ CD30+, T- and B-cell–associated antigens usually negative). CHL includes NSHL, MCHL, and LDHL, as well as the proposed new category of LRCHL. Because the immunophenotype, genetic features, and postulated normal counterpart are the same for all of the classic types, these are discussed together at the end of this section.

Nodular Sclerosis Hodgkin's Lymphoma

MORPHOLOGIC FEATURES. NSHL by definition has at least a partially nodular pattern, with fibrous bands separating the nodules in most cases; diffuse areas are common, as is necrosis. The characteristic cell is the lacunar-type RS cell, which may be very numerous. These are cells with characteristically multilobated nuclei and small nucleoli, with abundant, pale cytoplasm that retracts in formalin-fixed sections, producing an empty space, or lacuna. Diagnostic RS cells are also present but may be rare. The background usually contains lymphocytes, histiocytes, plasma cells, eosinophils, and neutrophils.[114]

In some cases with characteristic lacunar cells and a nodular or diffuse pattern, fibrous bands may be absent, and the differential diagnosis with NLPHL may be difficult. These cases have been called the *cellular phase* of NSHL[114]; in one series, the clinical course of these cases was slightly worse than that of typical NSHL.[133] Another morphologic variant, syncytial NSHL, has been described

in which, focally, the NS pattern is lost and there are large sheets of cells resembling lacunar RS cell variants. The prognosis of this variant was not reported to be different from that of typical NSHL. However, other studies have suggested that NSHL with lymphocyte depletion is associated with large mediastinal masses, advanced stage, and poor response to radiation therapy alone.[134]

GRADING OF NODULAR SCLEROSIS HODGKIN'S LYMPHOMA. The BNLI developed a system for grading NSHL (grade 1 and grade 2), based on the number and atypia of the RS cells in the nodules.[135] Cases of grade 2 NSHL overlap with the syncytial and LD variants described earlier in Morphologic Features. Based on this system, 75% to 85% of the cases in most series are grade 1 and 15% to 25% are grade 2. In the BNLI series, grade 2 (NS2) tumors were associated with a worse prognosis than grade 1 (NS1) tumors, with patients with NS2 tumors having an increased rate of relapse, shorter survival, and worse response to initial therapy (see Fig. 41.5-2). The BNLI studies have been criticized because some series included patients whose lymphomas were not pathologically staged and because, compared to some other series, their patients had relatively poor outcomes. A recent study from the GHSG found that four factors—tissue, eosinophilia, bizarre Reed-Sternberg cells, and lymphocyte depletion—were significantly associated with poor outcome in NSHL, with eosinophilia being the most important factor.[135a]

Results from American and European centers have been conflicting, showing either no influence of grade on outcome or a significantly worse outcome for patients with NS2.[136,137] In general, when a center reports either a relatively high rate of relapse or relatively poor survival, patients with NS2 are found to have a significantly worse outcome than patients with NS1; conversely, when overall relapse rates are low and survival high, grade has no impact on outcome.[137] This phenomenon was illustrated most clearly in a study of 195 patients treated in the Netherlands.[138] For patients treated between 1972 and 1980, when overall survival was relatively poor, patients with grade 2 NSHL had a significantly worse outcome (5-year overall survival for those with NS1, 83%; for those with NS2, 43%), whereas for those treated between 1981 and 1992, grade had no impact on outcome (5-year overall survival for patients with NS1, 81%; for those with NS2, 82%).

The impact of NS2 on survival is most evident in patients who experience relapse. Those with NS2 have significantly shorter survival after relapse than those with NS1. Taken together, these results suggest that more aggressive therapy benefits patients with grade 2 disease; they also suggest the possibility that patients with NS1 could be treated less aggressively and still do as well. It could be argued that, in future studies, NSHL should be consistently graded and that trials of less aggressive initial treatment for NS1 might be appropriate.

CLINICAL FEATURES. NSHL is the most common subtype of HL in developed countries (60% to 80% in most series). It is most common in adolescents and young adults but can occur at any age. Incidence in females equals or exceeds that in males. The mediastinum and other supradiaphragmatic sites are commonly involved.

Mixed-Cellularity Hodgkin's Lymphoma

MORPHOLOGIC FEATURES. In MCHL, the infiltrate is usually diffuse or at most vaguely nodular, without band-forming sclerosis, although fine interstitial fibrosis may be present. RS cells are of the classic, diagnostic type and are usually easily identified. Many mononuclear variants are usually also present; rare lacunar cells may be seen. Diagnostic RS cells are large cells with bilobed, double, or multiple nuclei, with a large, eosinophilic, inclusion-like nucleolus in at least two lobes or nuclei. The infiltrate typically contains lymphocytes, epithelioid histiocytes, eosinophils, and plasma cells.[114]

CLINICAL FEATURES. MCHL comprises 15% to 30% of HL cases in most series. It may be seen at any age and lacks the early-adulthood peak of NSHL. Involvement of the mediastinum is less common than in NSHL, and abdominal lymph node and splenic involvement are more common.

Lymphocyte-Depleted Hodgkin's Lymphoma

MORPHOLOGIC FEATURES. The infiltrate in LDHL is diffuse and often appears hypocellular, due to the presence of diffuse fibrosis and necrosis. There are large numbers of RS cells and bizarre "sarcomatous" variants, with a paucity of other inflammatory cells. Confluent sheets of RS cells and variants may occur and rarely predominate (reticular variant or Hodgkin's sarcoma).[114] Before the availability of immunophenotyping studies, many cases diagnosed as LDHL were, in reality, cases of large B-cell lymphoma or T-cell lymphoma, often of the ALCL type. Cases of the reticular variant of LDHL may be difficult to distinguish from ALCL.[139]

CLINICAL FEATURES. LDHL is the least common variant of HL, comprising fewer than 1% of the cases in recent reports. It is most common in older people, in individuals positive for human immunodeficiency virus (HIV),[100] and in nonindustrialized countries. LDHL frequently presents with abdominal lymphadenopathy and spleen, liver, and bone marrow involvement, without peripheral lymphadenopathy.[140] The stage is usually advanced at diagnosis; however, response to treatment is reported not to differ from that of other subtypes of comparable stage.[134]

Immunophenotype of Classic Hodgkin's Lymphoma

In most cases of NSHL, MCHL, and LDHL, the tumor cells are CD15+, CD30+, CD45–. The frequency with which CD15 and CD30 are detected varies in reported series, probably because of technical problems. With microwave antigen retrieval and use of an anti-IgM secondary antibody, the GHSG reported 83% of 1751 cases to be positive for CD15, 96% positive for CD30, and 5% positive for CD20. Expression of B-cell antigens has been reported in a variable number of cases, usually only weakly and in a minority of the cells.[141] Thus, expression of B-cell antigens does not exclude a diagnosis of HL if the morphologic features are typical.

The diagnosis of HL is still made on routine sections, and immunophenotyping studies are an adjunct to the diagnosis. In a morphologically typical case, immunophenotyping studies are not absolutely needed; however, they are becoming more standard practice. Failure to detect CD15 or CD30 or expression of a B-cell–associated antigen does not preclude a diagnosis of HL; however, absence of both CD15 and CD30 and expression of CD20 should prompt reexamination of the slides and consideration of either NLPHL or LRCHL. Expression of

T-cell antigens is distinctly unusual and should prompt both re-review of the slides and molecular genetic analysis of the T-cell receptor gene.

In addition to CD15 and CD30, RS cells express CD25, HLA-DR, ICAM-1, CD95 (apo-1/fas), and both CD40 and CD86 (B7), molecules associated with B-cell activation and interaction with T cells. T cells surrounding the RS cells express both CD40 ligand and CD28, the ligand for CD86. In contrast to NLPHL, the RS cells of CHL lack the nuclear bcl-6 protein associated with follicle center B cells.[142] In EBV-positive cases, the tumor cells express EBV LMP but not EBNA-2.

Immunophenotype and Clinical Behavior of Classic Hodgkin's Lymphoma

Several studies have addressed the impact of immunophenotype on the survival of patients with CHL, with varying results. The GHSG study found that patients whose lymphomas lacked CD15 but expressed CD30 had a significantly worse freedom from relapse and overall survival than patients with CD15+ lymphomas. Coexpression of CD20 with CD15 or CD30, or both, had no impact on outcome, but patients whose lymphomas expressed CD20 alone had poor survival. This result is similar to that reported by McBride and coworkers[143] and raises the question of whether these may represent cases of T-cell–rich large B-cell lymphoma (see Lymphocyte-Rich Classic Hodgkin's Lymphoma).

Lymphocyte-Rich Classic Hodgkin's Lymphoma

MORPHOLOGIC FEATURES. Some cases of HL with RS cells of classic type, both by morphology and immunophenotype, may have a background infiltrate that consists predominantly of lymphocytes, with rare or no eosinophils. The term *lymphocyte-rich classic Hodgkin's lymphoma* was proposed for these cases in the REAL classification. Some cases of LRCHL have a nodular pattern, with remnants of regressed GCs in the nodules, and RS cells and variants located within the mantle zones and interfollicular regions,[144] mimicking NLPHL. This has been termed *follicular Hodgkin's lymphoma*, or nodular LRCHL.[145]

Of 426 cases initially diagnosed as LPHL, review and immunophenotyping by a panel formed by the European Task Force on Lymphoma (ETFL) revealed that only 51% were confirmed as NLPHL, whereas 27% were LRCHL with a nodular pattern, with RS cells in the mantles of reactive follicles and in the interfollicular regions.[145] In a study by the GHSG,[116] a similar rate of misdiagnosis of NLPHL was found; only 44% of 208 cases considered by at least one pathologist as LPHL had the immunophenotype of LPHL, whereas 56% were CHL. When the expert panel reclassified the cases by morphology alone, only 75% of the cases classified as LPHL and 88% of the cases classified as CHL were confirmed by immunophenotyping. Thus, cases of LRCHL may very closely resemble NLPHL and require immunophenotyping for differential diagnosis.

IMMUNOPHENOTYPE. Cases of LRCHL have the immunophenotype of CHL, with expression of CD15 and CD30 by the RS cells. As in other types of CHL, CD20 is coexpressed in 3% to 5% of cases.[145] In nodular areas, the background lymphocytes are predominantly B cells, as in LPHL, and follicular meshworks of follicular dendritic cells are seen with antibodies to CD21 or CD35. Staining for follicular dendritic cells often reveals a small, dense aggregate of these cells consistent with a regressed GC, associated with a broad mantle zone with more loosely spaced follicular dendritic cell processes. The RS cells are found within the mantle area or at the junction of the mantle and interfollicular regions. CD57+ T cells may also be present and may rim the RS cells; thus, it is really the immunophenotype of the RS cells that distinguishes this from NLPHL.

CLINICAL FEATURES. The frequency of LRCHL among cases classified as HL can be roughly calculated from the two GHSG reports.[146] Of 1959 cases of HL with immunophenotyping for CD15, CD30, and CD20, LRCHL comprised 6% (116 cases) and LPHL 5% (92 cases). In the ETFL and GHSG series, the clinical features of LRCHL at presentation seem to be intermediate between those of LPHL and CHL: As in NLPHL, patients had early-stage disease and lacked bulky disease or B symptoms; as in both NLPHL and MCHL and in contrast to NLPHL, they lacked mediastinal disease and a predominance of males was seen; and as in MCHL, patients had an older median age than in either NLPHL or NSHL. In the ETFL series, the overall survival of patients with both LPHL and LRCHL was excellent but was not significantly different from that of patients with other types of HL. However, patients with NLPHL had an increased frequency of multiple relapses and better survival after relapse, compared with patients with LRCHL, NSHL, and MCHL. In the GHSG study, the overall survival of patients with LRCHL was significantly worse than that of patients with NLPHL. These data do not clearly define LRCHL as a distinct entity but are consistent with either an early phase of MCHL or a novel subtype. It is suggested that this category continue to be recognized within the classification of HL, so that additional data can be collected.

Association of Classic Hodgkin's Lymphoma with Other Lymphomas

CHL may be associated with other lymphomas, most often of B-cell type.[147] These lymphomas may occur before, simultaneously with, or after HL. Patients treated for HL are at risk for development of high-grade B-cell lymphomas (DLBCL or Burkitt's or Burkitt's-like lymphoma), which have been presumed to arise in a setting of immune suppression secondary to ther-

apy for HL; the estimated risk ranges from 1% to 5%. However, EBV has not been demonstrated in the secondary lymphomas, in contrast to the situation for most immunosuppression-associated NHLs. Numerous cases of CHL associated with follicular lymphoma or DLBCL have been reported. The HL may precede, follow, or occur simultaneously with the NHL.[147,148] Two cases of HL occurring with NHL (one case of composite HL and follicular lymphoma and one case of DLBCL followed by HL) were studied by single-cell PCR; a common clone was found in the HL and the NHL in both cases.[149] Rare cases of B-cell chronic lymphocytic leukemia may contain cells with the morphology and immunophenotype of classic RS cells, whereas in other cases patients with typical chronic lymphocytic leukemia may go on to develop HL—an HL variant of Richter's syndrome.[150] Several such cases have been studied using single-cell PCR. In the majority of the cases, the RS cells were of the same clone as the chronic lymphocytic leukemia cells, whereas in one case, they were clonally unrelated.[151] Finally, cases of mycosis fungoides or lymphomatoid papulosis associated with HL have been reported.[152] Thus, it is clear that patients with CHL are at some increased risk for development of NHL. In some patients, a single neoplastic B cell can give rise to both HL and NHL, whereas in others, it appears that either immunosuppression or other unknown factors can give rise to two independent malignancies.

Differential Diagnosis of Classic Hodgkin's Lymphoma

Two lymphomas have been described in recent years that have significant morphologic overlap with HL and may cause problems in differential diagnosis (see Fig. 41.5-1): T-cell/histiocyte-rich large B-cell lymphoma (T/HRLBCL) and T-cell ALCL. In addition, DLBCLs with anaplastic cytology may be difficult to distinguish from HL with lymphocyte depletion (Table 41.5-4).

T-CELL/HISTIOCYTE-RICH LARGE B-CELL LYMPHOMA. In the last few years, several groups have reported an unusual type of lymphoma with morphologic features reminiscent of diffuse lymphocyte predominance (LP) or MCHL, with a predominance of small T lymphocytes and scattered large neoplastic cells that express B-cell antigens. Patients typically present with advanced-stage disease and have a poor prognosis.[143] The term *histiocyte-rich* or *T-cell–rich large B-cell lymphoma* has been

TABLE 41.5-4. Differential Diagnosis of Hodgkin's Lymphoma (HL)

Diagnosis	Morphology (Large Cells)	Immunophenotype (Large Cells)	T-Cell Rings	Genetics (Southern Blot)
NLPHL	Popcorn cells	CD20+, EMA+, CD15–, CD30–	+	Ig polyclonal
Classic HL, lymphocyte-rich	Classic RS cells	CD20–, EMA–, CD15+, CD30+	+	Ig polyclonal
PTGC	Centroblasts	CD20+, EMA–, CD15–, CD30–	–	Ig polyclonal
Follicular lymphoma	Centroblasts	CD20+, EMA– (Ig monoclonal)	–	Ig monoclonal
T-cell, histiocyte-rich large B-cell lymphoma	Centroblasts, immunoblasts, popcorn cells	CD20+, EMA+, CD15–, CD30– (Ig monoclonal±)	–	Ig monoclonal
Anaplastic large-cell lymphoma (T-cell)	Horseshoe-shaped nuclei, paranuclear hof	CD20–, EMA±, CD15–, CD30+, T-Ag±	–	TCR monoclonal
Large B-cell lymphoma, anaplastic subtype	Bizarre, large cells, RS-like cells	CD20+, EMA±, CD15–, CD30+	–	Ig monoclonal

Ag, antigen; EMA, epithelial membrane antigen; Ig, immunoglobulin; NLPHL, nodular lymphocyte-predominant Hodgkin's lymphoma; PTGC, progressive transformation of germinal centers; RS, Reed-Sternberg; TCR, T-cell receptor.
Note: EMA may be difficult to detect in formalin-fixed tissues. Classic HL may be CD20+ (15%) or CD15+ (15%).

used for these cases. The cases that resemble HL are different from earlier cases reported as T-cell–rich B-cell lymphoma, many of which are simply B-cell lymphomas of follicle center or large cell type in which T cells comprise 50% or more of the infiltrate. Whether T/HRLBCL constitutes a distinct disease or is simply an aggressive variant of LPHL is not clear. However, it is important to distinguish it from either NLPHL or CHL, because of its aggressive clinical course.

T/HRLBCL is a diffuse lymphoma with a lymphocyte-rich background, with small clusters of epithelioid histiocytes and scattered large mononuclear cells, which suggests either LPHL or CHL. The large cells may resemble popcorn cells, immunoblasts, centroblasts, or all three.

The neoplastic cells express CD20 and other pan-B antigens, may or may not express cytoplasmic light chains, and may or may not have detectable Ig gene rearrangement by Southern blot analysis or whole-section PCR. Like LPHL, they are often EMA positive, but are CD15– and CD30– and EBV negative. The background lymphocytes are T cells that are CD57–, and follicular dendritic cell aggregates are not seen.

The immunophenotype of the large cells is of limited value in the differential diagnosis with LPHL, because it is similar; however, readily detectable Ig light chains would tend to favor a diagnosis of T/HRLBCL. In addition, staining for CD20 may reveal a nodular pattern and a B-cell–rich background, which would favor NLPHL. Follicular aggregates of follicular dendritic cells (anti-CD21) also favor NLPHL, as do large numbers of CD57+ cells. In distinguishing T/HRLBCL from CHL, immunophenotyping is essential and helpful. If the large cells express CD20 and lack CD15 and CD30, the diagnosis of T/HRLBCL is strongly favored, whereas expression of either CD15 or CD30 strongly favors a diagnosis of CHL. Furthermore, in cases diagnosed as CHL that express only CD20, the prognosis appears to be significantly worse than in cases expressing CD15 or CD30, or both, with or without CD20.[143,146]

ANAPLASTIC LARGE CELL LYMPHOMA. ALCL is a T-cell lymphoma characterized by large malignant cells with prominent nucleoli and abundant cytoplasm, which may resemble mononuclear or multinucleated RS cell variants.[153] However, the tumor cells grow in cohesive sheets and frequently involve lymph node sinuses—a pattern that is unusual in HL. In addition, the neoplastic cells are usually smaller than RS cells, have less conspicuous nucleoli without perinucleolar halos, and often have bean-shaped or horseshoe-shaped nuclei, with a prominent paranuclear hof, in contrast to the round nuclei of mononuclear RS cells.[154] ALCL incidence has a bimodal age distribution, with a peak in childhood and another in adulthood.

A subtype of ALCL, called *Hodgkin's-related ALCL*, was described (modified to *Hodgkin's-like* in the REAL classification, a provisional entity).[155] This variant was characterized by cytologic features similar to those of common ALCL—confluent sheets of tumor cells, a cohesive growth pattern, and sinus infiltration—but with architectural features that resemble HL of the NS type, with nodular growth of tumor cells and occasional fibrous bands. The immunophenotype of ALCL-HL was reported to be similar to that of common ALCL, but some cases had CD15 expression and EBV infection. There has been an ongoing debate about whether Hodgkin's-like ALCL is a variant of HL, a variant of ALCL, a heterogeneous mixture of the two, or a distinct disease.

Analysis of the t(2;5) associated with ALCL has helped in resolving this problem. Studies of the translocation have shown that it is absent in cases of typical HL.[76,156] In immunophenotyping studies using antibodies to either the ALK protein or the p80 fusion product of the t(2;5), several groups have found the protein to be present in a subset of ALCL cases but not in HL. Cases diagnosed as ALCL-HL typically lack the ALK protein.[157]

Most hematopathologists now believe that cases reported in the literature as Hodgkin's-like ALCL are heterogeneous. Some represent LD variants of HL, either NSHL type (syncytial, lymphocyte depleted, or NS2) or LDHL (Hodgkin's sarcoma), whereas others are cases of ALCL with a nodular growth pattern. Most cases can be resolved as either HL (CD45–, CD15+, T-cell antigen negative, CD20–/+, t(2;5) negative, ALK1 negative, EMA negative) or ALCL (CD45+, CD15–, T-cell antigen positive, CD20–, t(2;5) positive, ALK1 positive, EMA positive).

In cases that are histologically borderline between HL and T-cell ALCL, immunophenotyping on paraffin sections for CD45, CD15, CD30, CD20, EMA, pan-T antigens, and ALK1, and, if necessary, genetic studies should be undertaken to resolve the differential diagnosis. Expression of CD15 or CD20 tends to exclude a diagnosis of T-cell ALCL (CD20+ cases may be either HL or DLBCL), whereas expression of CD45, T-cell antigens, ALK1, or EMA tends to exclude HL. Southern blot or whole section PCR analysis showing T-cell antigen receptor gene rearrangement would tend to exclude HL and confirm the diagnosis of ALCL. Ig gene rearrangement would not usually be detectable in HL using the aforementioned techniques and this would favor DLBCL, but presence of a weak band would not exclude HL. Cases that cannot be resolved by immunophenotyping or genetic studies should be considered unclassifiable; clinical judgment should be used in deciding whether to perform another biopsy or to treat for either HL or ALCL. The category of *Hodgkin's-like ALCL* will be eliminated from the proposed WHO classification.

In summary, the data currently available suggest that there is no true borderline between HL and ALCL of T-null type as defined in the REAL classification: HL is in most cases a B-cell neoplasm, whereas ALCL is a T-cell neoplasm. There is morphologic but not biologic overlap between HL and ALCL. HL may *resemble* ALCL by having areas of lymphocyte depletion—that is, it may be ALCL-like—but this is a morphologic resemblance only, not a true biologic borderline. Similarly, ALCL may *resemble* HL by having areas of nodularity, sclerosis, or granulocyte infiltration—that is, it may be Hodgkin's-like—but again, this is not a true biologic borderline. In contrast, because HL is a B-cell neoplasm, there may be a *true* biologic borderline between B-cell lymphomas and HL of any type—between DLBCL and NLPHL, between T/HRLBCL and either MCHL or LPHL, and between anaplastic large B-cell lymphoma, CD30+ type, and LD variants of CHL. It is these latter areas that present the currently most challenging differential diagnoses.

DIAGNOSIS AND STAGING

NATURAL HISTORY AND PATTERNS OF SPREAD

The Swiss radiotherapist Rene Gilbert is credited with first reporting that HL spread by contiguity from one lymph node chain to adjacent chains.[19,158] His work was extended by Vera Peters, Henry Kaplan, and others, who evaluated the use of prophylactic radiation therapy to lymph nodes adjacent to those involved with disease.[159,160] The development of new radiographic studies and the routine use of staging laparotomy improved understanding of the presentation and evolution of HL.[160–162] There is considerable evidence that HL begins in a single group of lymph nodes and then spreads to contiguous lymph nodes. Eventually the malignant cells may become more aggressive, invade blood vessels, and spread to organs in a manner similar to that in other malignancies. This is more likely to occur in patients with stage III than with stage I or II HL.

One study of over 700 patients evaluated contiguous nodal involvement as determined by a combination of clinical and surgical staging.[163] Evidence for contiguous spread was most convincing for patients with NS or MC histologic type. The mediastinum, left side of the neck, and right side of the neck were each involved in more than 60% of patients with HL of MC or NS histologic type. These sites were involved four or more times as often as other nodal sites above or below the diaphragm, which suggests that most cases of NSHL or MCHL begin in the chest or neck. Significant associations were found between involvement in the mediastinum and the right or left neck, the neck and the ipsilateral axilla, the mediastinum and the hilum, and the spleen and abdominal nodes. There was a negative association between involvement of the right and left neck if the mediastinum was not involved, which suggests that spread from one neck to the other occurred through the mediastinal nodes. A study evaluating sites of relapse in patients with minimal-stage IIIA HL treated with radiation therapy alone provides additional information.[164] It appears that when the spleen is involved with HL, even minimally, there is a high risk of extranodal involvement. This suggests that HL spreads from above the diaphragm to the spleen, perhaps through the vascular system, and that splenic involvement may herald spread to extranodal sites through a similar process.

Most patients with NSHL or MCHL have a central pattern of lymph node involvement (cervical, mediastinal, paraaortic). In contrast, certain nodal chains (mesenteric, hypogastric, presacral, epitrochlear, popliteal) are seldom involved. The spleen is involved more frequently in patients with adenopathy below the diaphragm, systemic symptoms, and MC histologic type. Involvement of the liver in an untreated patient is rare and almost always occurs with concomitant splenic involvement. Infiltration of the bone marrow is usually focal and almost invariably associated with extensive disease and systemic symptoms. In the great majority of patients, the initial pattern of spread occurs nonrandomly and predictably via lymphatic channels to contiguous lymph node chains. This important observation, first made over 50 years ago, continues to form the basis for determination of treatment strategies in patients with apparently localized HL treated with radiation therapy alone.

STAGING CLASSIFICATIONS

The advent of new imaging modalities and the frequent use of combined modality treatment have made staging procedures simpler and less invasive in recent years. The latest international staging classification was proposed in 1989 during a meeting held in the Cotswolds, England.[165] The Cotswolds clas-

TABLE 41.5-5. Cotswolds Staging Classification for Hodgkin's Lymphoma

STAGE I	Involvement of a single lymph node region or lymphoid structure (e.g., spleen, thymus, Waldeyer's ring) or involvement of a single extralymphatic site (IE).
STAGE II	Involvement of two or more lymph node regions on the same side of the diaphragm (hilar nodes, when involved on both sides, constitute stage II disease); localized contiguous involvement of only one extranodal organ or site and lymph node region(s) on the same side of the diaphragm (IIE). The number of anatomic regions involved should be indicated by a subscript (e.g., II$_3$).
STAGE III	Involvement of lymph node regions on both sides of the diaphragm (III), which may also be accompanied by involvement of the spleen (III$_S$) or by localized contiguous involvement of only one extranodal organ site (IIIE) or both (III SE).
III$_1$	With or without involvement of splenic, hilar, celiac, or portal nodes.
III$_2$	With involvement of paraaortic, iliac, and mesenteric nodes.
STAGE IV	Diffuse or disseminated involvement of one or more extranodal organs or tissues, with or without associated lymph node involvement.
DESIGNATIONS APPLICABLE TO ANY DISEASE STAGE	
A	No symptoms.
B	Fever (temperature, >38°C), drenching night sweats, unexplained loss of >10% body weight within the preceding 6 months.
X	Bulky disease (a widening of the mediastinum by more than one-third or the presence of a nodal mass with a maximal dimension >10 cm).
E	Involvement of a single extranodal site that is contiguous or proximal to the known nodal site.
CS	Clinical stage.
PS	Pathologic stage (as determined by laparotomy).

sification (Table 41.5-5) is a modification of the Ann Arbor classification using information from staging and treatment over the previous 20 years.

Some of the recommended modifications include adding a criteria for clinical involvement of the spleen and liver, which require evidence of focal defects obtained with two imaging techniques; eliminating consideration of abnormalities of liver function; adding the suffix *X* to designate bulky disease (greater than 10 cm maximum dimension); adding a new category of response to therapy (i.e., unconfirmed or uncertain complete remission) to accommodate the difficulty of persistent radiologic abnormalities of uncertain significance after primary therapy; and separately classifying certain cases of localized extranodal disease (e.g., in lung, pleura, chest wall, bone) contiguous to involved nodes as the appropriate lymph node system stage followed by the subscript *E*. The *E* designation excludes multiple extranodal deposits or bilateral lung extension, which constitute stage IV disease. Recommended staging procedures are listed in Table 41.5-6.

An adequate surgical biopsy specimen, possibly from more than one intact lymph node, is required for histopathologic examination.

RADIOGRAPHIC STAGING ABOVE THE DIAPHRAGM

Over 60% of patients with newly diagnosed HL have radiographic evidence of intrathoracic involvement. Frontal and lat-

TABLE 41.5-6. Recommended Staging

Adequate surgical biopsy reviewed by an experienced hemopathologist

Detailed history with attention to the presence or absence of systemic symptoms

Careful physical examination, emphasizing node chains, size of liver and spleen, and Waldeyer's ring inspection

Routine laboratory tests: complete blood cell count, erythrocyte sedimentation rate, and liver function tests

Chest radiograph (posteroanterior and lateral) with measurement of mass-thoracic ratio

Chest and abdominal computed tomography

Radioisotopic evaluation with gallium 67 or positron emission tomography when the results of other conventional diagnostic procedures are not conclusive

Core-needle biopsy of bone marrow from the posterior iliac crest in patients with stage IIB–IV disease

Needle or surgical biopsy of any suspicious extranodal (e.g., hepatic, osseous, pulmonary, cutaneous) lesion(s)

Cytologic examination of any effusion

Staging laparotomy (with splenectomy, needle and wedge biopsy of the liver, and biopsies of paraaortic, mesenteric, portal, and splenic hilar lymph nodes) in rare circumstances in early-stage Hodgkin's lymphoma in which the use of limited radiation therapy alone depends on pathologic staging

---

eral chest radiographs should be routinely ordered and also represent a low-cost method for subsequent surveillance.

Computed (axial) tomography (CT) has become the standard thoracic staging examination for patients with HL, both for determination of sites of initial involvement in the chest and for determination of the extent of the mediastinal adenopathy. CT scanning is especially good at detecting pulmonary disease, pleural or pericardial involvement, apical cardiac nodal enlargement, and extension into the chest wall, and in defining the extent of involved axillary lymph nodes. A slice from a thoracic CT scan can demonstrate extensive axillary and pleural disease that is not apparent on plain chest radiography. Such information has considerable potential to alter clinical management. Identification of the extent of thoracic disease helps define the use of combination chemotherapy and the dose, extent, and need for radiation therapy.

Large mediastinal adenopathy has been defined as a ratio greater than one-third between the largest transverse diameter of the mediastinal mass and the transverse diameter of the thorax at the diaphragm on a standing posteroanterior chest radiograph.[166] Others have defined extensive mediastinal disease as greater than 35% of the thoracic diameter at T-5 or T-6, or as more than 5 to 10 cm in width. Patients with large mediastinal adenopathy have an increased risk of experiencing relapse in nodal and extranodal sites above the diaphragm after radiation therapy alone.[167,168] These patients make up 20% to 25% of those with clinical stage I or II disease, generally present with involvement of multiple supradiaphragmatic nodal chains, and may have extension of tumor into the lung, pericardium, or chest wall.[167] Systemic symptoms are frequently present.

After initial chemotherapy, residual abnormalities often remain on thoracic CT scanning. The use of gallium 67 scanning or positron emission tomography (PET) or both may aid in the management and follow-up of patients in this setting. The gallium scan is a sensitive indicator of disease above the diaphragm, particularly when a dose of 10 mCi and single photon emission CT (SPECT) techniques are used. A negative result on a follow-up gallium scan supports the supposition that there is no active disease after the completion of treatment, even in the presence of a residual abnormality on the CT scan. However, this study is a relative and not absolute indicator of the presence and absence of disease. In the absence of adjuvant involved-field radiation therapy, recurrences may occur in the initially involved site after chemotherapy alone despite a negative result on gallium scan after chemotherapy. In addition, most of the data showing that a negative gallium scan has prognostic importance in patients with early-stage disease has been obtained from patients receiving both chemotherapy and radiation therapy.

Whole body PET measuring [^{18}F]fluorodeoxyglucose activity may be a more sensitive imaging modality than gallium scanning, although more data are needed. Data have reported on the impact of positive and negative PET results in the initial evaluation and treatment of HL.[169,170] However, as with the gallium 67 scan, PET scanning is not an absolute indicator of cure after chemotherapy alone, and at present there is no information supporting the use of these studies to guide whether or not to use adjuvant involved-field radiation in patients with early-stage disease.

RADIOGRAPHIC STAGING BELOW THE DIAPHRAGM

CT, lymphangiography, magnetic resonance imaging, and gallium scanning all have limitations in the radiologic evaluation of the abdominal nodes. No single study is reliable for detecting HL in normal-size nodes, and all studies have a 20% to 25% false-negative rate due to the inability to detect occult HL in the spleen.[162,171] Ninety percent of patients whose disease is up-staged have splenic involvement, either alone or in addition to involvement of other infradiaphragmatic nodal sites.[162] During the past few years, bipedal lymphangiography has given way to CT scanning as the radiologic examination of choice for abdominal staging. In part, this is because lymphangiography is difficult to perform and interpret, and very few departments currently have the expertise to perform the examination. PET and gallium scanning (with SPECT) are complementary studies to CT. With the infrequent use of staging laparotomy and splenectomy in the staging of HL, the risk of over-staging based on a single radiographic test of abdominal involvement (false-positive) has greater potential consequences. Therefore, the authors strongly recommend that two separate studies (i.e., CT and gallium-PET scanning) be used to assess abdominal involvement. Positive findings on both tests should be used to confirm abdominal involvement.

STAGING LAPAROTOMY

Staging laparotomy was extensively used when radiation therapy was the preferred treatment for early-stage HL and when it was mandatory to define the extent of abdominal disease to help determine whether there was an indication for the initial use of chemotherapy. With many groups using prognostic factors to determine treatment for HL, laparotomy has disappeared as a routine staging procedure. Its use should be reserved for patients with limited disease who are to receive radiation therapy alone.

CLINICAL PRESENTATION

In general, HL patients present with peripheral lymphadenopathy. The nodes usually are not tender, and changes in the overlying skin are unusual. Tenderness and skin changes are thought to reflect rapid growth with stretching of nodal capsules. In most cases, the nodes are discrete and freely movable. Occult presentation with central (chest and abdomen) lymphadenopathy, visceral involvement, or systemic symptoms of the disease is more uncommon. The most characteristic clinical presentation of HL is enlarged superficial lymph nodes in young adults, with the most frequent locations being cervical and supraclavicular (60% to 80%), high in the neck or axillary. Less often, enlarged nodes are found in the inguinal-femoral region.

A mediastinal involvement is discovered often by routine staging chest radiography, and even fairly large masses may occur without producing local symptoms. Symptoms of retrosternal chest pain, cough, or shortness of breath may be clinical signs of an intrathoracic disease presentation. A bulky mediastinal mass is not uncommonly associated with small amounts of pericardial and pleural fluid, but malignant effusions, diagnosed by thoracocentesis or pleural biopsy, are rare.

Involvement of the liver in a newly diagnosed patient is uncommon and occurs almost always with concomitant splenic involvement; HL limited to the spleen is rare. Patients may present with abdominal swelling secondary to hepatomegaly or splenomegaly or, rarely, with ascites. Infradiaphragmal lymphadenopathy may give rise to discomfort and pain in the retroperitoneum, the paravertebral region, or the loin region, particularly in the supine position, due to nodular compression of nerves or nerve roots. Advanced intraabdominal disease may be associated with obstruction of the ureters or compression of the renal vein, or ascites, or both.

Bone marrow infiltration is usually focal and in most cases associated with extensive disease including systemic symptoms. Laboratory findings such as leukopenia, anemia, thrombocytopenia, and an elevated alkaline phosphatase level may give indications of bone marrow infiltration.

Involvement of the central nervous system is rare, although invasion of the epidural space can occur by nodular extension from the paraaortic region through the intervertebral foramina, presenting with neurologic symptoms and pain as leading clinical features.[172] Several paraneoplastic neurologic syndromes have been reported in association with HL but all are very rare.

Complaints due to extranodal manifestations of disease may occur, such as cough from pulmonary infiltration, jaundice from hepatic involvement, or abdominal pain from disease adjacent to the bowel. Gastrointestinal involvement is an extremely rare event and might occur as infiltration from mesenteric lymph nodes. Initial symptoms of disease limited to extranodal tissue are much rarer in HL than in NHLs.

A significant proportion of patients with undiagnosed HL present with systemic symptoms before the discovery of enlarged lymph nodes. Typical symptoms are fever, drenching night sweats, and weight loss (B symptoms, relating to the Ann Arbor classification). This characteristic HL-associated fever occurs intermittently and recurs at variable intervals for several days or weeks. Fever and drenching night sweats are found in 25% of all patients at the time of first presentation; the incidence increases to 50% in patients with more advanced disease. Other nonspecific symptoms are pruritus, fatigue, and the development of pain shortly after drinking alcohol. This pain is usually transient at the site of nodal involvement and may be severe. Pruritus, although currently not a defined B

symptom, may be an important systemic symptom of disease but occurs infrequently, in fewer than 20% of patients. It often occurs months or even a year before HL is first diagnosed.[173] The underlying pathophysiologic mechanisms leading to pruritus are unknown, but it may be due to an autoimmune reaction in which a number of cytokines are activated by tumor lysis.

TREATMENT METHODS

RADIOTHERAPY

Principles

The early treatment of HL with crude x-rays in 1901 followed the discoveries by Roentgen, Becquerel, and the Curies at the end of the nineteenth century. The first reports of x-ray treatments that would dramatically shrink enlarged lymph nodes produced great excitement and premature predictions for the successful treatment of HL.[174] During the first two decades of the twentieth century, physicians mainly used two methods to treat HL with radiation. Small doses of radiation were administered to the entire trunk at weekly intervals for many weeks, or radiation was given in a single massive dose just to the tumor. Neither method controlled the HL, and both caused severe side effects.[19] Enlarged nodes usually shrank with both techniques, but recurrence and spread to previously uninvolved nodes invariably followed. After several courses of radiotherapy, the HL became more resistant to treatment, and very few patients survived for 5 years after diagnosis. These multiple recurrences were not attributed to poor radiotherapy techniques but were viewed as inherent to the HL itself. Therefore, most physicians stopped using radiation as a means to cure HL by 1920. For the next 40 years, in most centers, treatment was mainly palliative to shrink large nodes that were painful or interfered with movement, eating, or breathing.

The development of modern radiation therapy techniques for the treatment of HL began with the work of Gilbert, a Swiss radiotherapist, in the 1920s. He began to advocate treatment of apparently uninvolved adjacent lymph node chains that might contain suspected microscopic disease, as well as the evident sites of lymph node involvement. Peters also adapted this technique at the Princess Margaret Hospital in the late 1930s and early 1940s. In her historic paper published in the *American Journal of Roentgenology* in 1950, Peters provided evidence that patients with limited HL could be cured with aggressive radiation therapy that treated involved nodal disease as well as adjacent nodal sites.[159] She did this by identifying a group of patients with limited-stage HL that was cured with high-dose, fractionated radiation therapy. She reported 5-year and 10-year survival rates of 88% and 79%, respectively, for patients with disease limited to a single lymph node region, rates that were notably high for a disease in which virtually no one survived for 10 years. Nevertheless, the concept that early-stage HL might be curable with radiation therapy using higher doses and larger fields was slow to be accepted. Before the 1960s, most patients with limited HL were treated not at all or only with small doses of radiation.

No one deserves more credit than Henry Kaplan for the development of successful modern treatment for HL. His accomplishments are many, and include pioneering work on the development of the linear accelerator,[160] definition of radiation field sizes and doses for a curative approach for early HL,[160] refinement and improvement of diagnostic staging techniques, development of models for translating laboratory findings into clinical practice, and promotion of early randomized clinical trials in the United States.

Techniques

Excellent results in the treatment of early-stage HL have been achieved through careful delineation of disease and meticulous attention to technique.[175] Treatment machine–generated verification films should be used to assure proper alignment. Daily doses of no more than 180 to 200 cGy to the mantle field (unless the treatment field includes the entire heart or entire lung, in which case the dose should be limited to 150 cGy/d or less) reduces risks to both the heart and lungs. Adjusting treatment on the basis of off–central axis dose calculations can reduce dose inhomogeneity from differences in patient separation within the large mantle field. Extended source-to-skin distances of 110 cm or greater rather than a source-to-skin distance of 100 cm also reduces tissue inhomogeneity. Proper use of megavoltage energies ensures that superficial nodes are not underdosed in the build-up region. A 4- to 6-MV linear accelerator should be used for mantle and pelvic fields, whereas higher energies (10 to 15 MV) can be used for treating paraaortic nodes.

The mantle field encompasses the submandibular, cervical, supraclavicular, infraclavicular, axillary, mediastinal, subcarinal, and hilar lymph nodes. A total dose of 3000 cGy to the entire mantle field is sufficient for patients with supradiaphragmatic HL when radiation therapy alone is used. Areas of initial involvement should receive a total dose of 3600 to 4000 cGy through the addition of a cone-down field. Reduction of the radiation dose to 3000 cGy to areas of initial involvement is recommended for patients receiving combined modality therapy, especially when there has been a good response to initial chemotherapy. When at least four cycles of chemotherapy have been given, prophylactic radiation to initially uninvolved sites is probably not needed. Further reduction to 1500 to 2500 cGy may be desirable in prepubertal patients receiving combined modality treatment or occasionally in patients with extensive nodal involvement receiving radiation to large fields after chemotherapy.

There is an increasing use of involved-field irradiation after chemotherapy in the treatment of early-stage HL. Involved-field irradiation should encompass the entire involved lymph node region as defined by the initial definitions described by Stanford University Medical School.[19] For example, the ipsilateral cervical and supraclavicular nodes, and the inguinal and femoral nodes constitute single regions.

Mantle paraaortic-splenic irradiation after a negative finding on laparotomy is occasionally used as a radiotherapy-alone approach for patients with early-stage disease. The paraaortic field encompasses the paraaortic nodes down to the fourth or fifth lumbar vertebral interspace (L-4 or L-5). Without staging laparotomy and splenectomy, the entire spleen must be irradiated. A CT scan should be used to localize the position of the spleen and enable blocking of as much of the left kidney as possible. The dose to the paraaortic lymph nodes should be 3000 cGy when there is no known disease and radiation therapy alone is used. Beam divergence from the mantle and

paraaortic fields creates the potential for an overdose at the spinal cord. A number of different matching techniques have been described.[176]

Prophylactic pelvic irradiation is rarely used in the modern-day treatment of supradiaphragmatic HL. However, pelvic irradiation continues to be used for patients presenting with stage I or II infradiaphragmatic HL. Use of iliac wing blocks to spare bone marrow and a pelvic block to shield the bladder and central pelvic organs should be part of the treatment technique (which includes irradiation of inguinal and femoral nodes). Loss of fertility in both males and females is a risk with the use of pelvic irradiation for subdiaphragmatic HL, and techniques should be used to reduce this risk whenever possible.[177]

CHEMOTHERAPY

The development of chemotherapy programs for HL is a story of success. After the discovery of the cytotoxic effects of nitrogen mustard in the 1940s, a number of different drugs, including chlorambucil, cyclophosphamide, procarbazine, vinblastine, and vincristine were developed and showed efficacy in HL. Response rates were 50% to 60%, with 10% to 30% complete responses. However, relapse was seen in almost all cases, and no cure could be achieved.

Based on work in a murine leukemia cell line, Skipper and colleagues[177a] postulated a model of tumor cell kill based on a logarithmic cell growth and a logarithmic response to cytotoxic agents. From this model, the authors predicted that response to chemotherapy would be dependent on tumor burden, drug dose, and kinetics of residual tumor cells. It was further postulated that the simultaneous use of several drugs with different modes of action might yield superior results. The combination of drugs might be tolerated if the toxicities were nonoverlapping. Initial attempts with two-drug combinations revealed the potential of this approach.

The important role of this model was realized in 1967, when DeVita and colleagues[177b] reported on a four-drug combination chemotherapy program, MOPP [nitrogen mustard, vincristine (Oncovin), procarbazine, and prednisone]. This combination established the curability of over 50% of patients with stage III and IV disease.

The development of MOPP was a milestone in oncology, demonstrating that advanced-stage HL could be cured. The differences in survival between historical controls and MOPP-treated patients were so dramatic that randomized clinical trials were not needed to validate these results. Further information on chemotherapy is given later in the chapter in the section Advanced-Stage Disease.

Combined Modality Chemotherapy

In addition to the many factors that affect either chemotherapy or radiation therapy when used alone, there are several issues that arise specifically because of potential interaction and summing of effects when they are combined. It is important to remember that the purpose of adding a second modality is to overcome resistance to the first, and in the case of adding irradiation to chemotherapy for HL, it seems likely that full-dose irradiation may be needed to overcome primary resistance to chemotherapy. Of particular interest are two German trials,[178] in which patients with stage IA+B, IIA+B, and IIIA disease with extensive mediastinal or splenic involvement or E lesions were treated with two-course cyclophosphamide, vincristine, procarbazine, and prednisone (COPP) and doxorubicin (Adriamycin), bleomycin, vinblastine, and dacarbazine (ABVD) followed by irradiation. In the first trial (HD1), responders to chemotherapy were then given extended-field irradiation with a dose to nonbulky sites assigned randomly to be either 20 Gy or 40 Gy. In the second trial (HD5), a similar group of patients received 30 Gy to the nonbulky sites. Bulky sites received 40 Gy in each trial. Failure-free survival was the same in all groups, which strongly implied that, after optimal chemotherapy, irradiation dose, at least to nonbulky sites, can be reduced without sacrificing efficiency.

Furthermore, the recently closed studies of the GHSG involving patients with early-stage (HD10)[178a] and intermediate-stage (HD11)[178b] Hodgkin's lymphoma showed exactly the same results for FFTF and overall survival whether patients were given 20 Gy or 30 Gy after two (early stage) or four (intermediate stage) courses of ABVD chemotherapy.

The risk of two important late complications of irradiation may be reduced by lowering the dose. Studies of late sequelae of treatment for HL suggest that the risk of second neoplasms, especially breast cancer in women, may be reduced by lowering the radiation dose.[179,180] The other late toxicity possibly associated with radiation dose is cardiovascular toxicity. A Stanford University study found that a higher dose of irradiation to the mediastinum was associated with increased mortality from cardiac disease.[181]

An alternative approach to reduce toxicity from irradiation when used in combined modality treatment is to reduce not the dose but the extent of the field encompassed. Several trials involving patients with limited-stage HL have shown that good results can be achieved when chemotherapy is combined with involved-field irradiation compared to irradiation alone to an extended field.[168,182] The ability to preserve efficacy while limiting toxicity by reducing the size of the treatment fields is one of the most attractive aspects of using combined modality treatment.

The same theoretical considerations that apply to irradiation are also relevant when one considers reduction of the dose of chemotherapy used in combined modality treatment. The section, Early-Stage Favorable Disease, later examines these results in more detail.

In theory, either chemotherapy or radiation therapy could come first in the sequence of combined modality treatment. In practice, it is almost always desirable for chemotherapy to be given first. The reason for this includes early effective treatment of disseminated disease, delay in induction of irreversible loss of bone marrow function, and the opportunity to use smaller, potentially less toxic radiation treatment fields after chemotherapy has induced tumor regression.

HIGH-DOSE CHEMOTHERAPY PLUS STEM CELL SUPPORT

Principles

High-dose chemotherapy (HDCT) has been used extensively to treat patients with relapsed and refractory HL. Implicit in the rationale for this approach is the assumption of a steep dose-response relation for lymphoma patients subjected to che-

moradiotherapy. Although care must be exercised in interpreting clinical results, both animal models and clinical studies support the existence of such a relationship.

The use of autologous bone marrow or peripheral blood stem cells (PBSCs) to support intensification of chemotherapy as salvage treatment has changed the options available for patients experiencing relapse. Autologous transplantation involves the replacement of hematopoietic stem cells that have been irreversibly injured by HDCT or radiotherapy or both. This can be accomplished either with bone marrow cells obtained by multiple aspirations from the posterior iliac crest under anesthesia or with PBSCs collected by apheresis. The use of PBSC has surpassed the use of bone marrow, and PBSCs may be used exclusively in the future. The advantage of using PBSC includes avoidance of general anesthesia and more rapid hematopoietic reconstitution.

Conditioning Regimens

Several conditioning regimens have been used and have been summarized previously.[183] The most commonly used are cyclophosphamide, carmustine (BCNU), and etoposide (CBV), and BCNU, etoposide, cytarabine, and melphalan (BEAM) given in different dose schedules. When BCNU-containing regimens are used, careful clinical monitoring to detect early signs of delayed lung toxicity is important, particularly when BCNU doses of 450 mg/m^2 are given. Mucositis and enterocolitis represent the most significant nonhematologic toxicities associated with high-dose melphalan. Total body irradiation has been used only in a few studies, due to the fact that many HL patients have already received thoracic irradiation by the time they have reached the transplant stage and the treatment-related mortality of patients undergoing preparation with regimens containing total body irradiation is high.[184,185] Although the toxicity profiles differ with these regimens, there is currently no evidence to support the superiority of any particular regimen in HL.

In recent years sequential HDCT is increasingly being used in the treatment of solid tumors and lymphoma. First results from phase II studies show that this kind of therapy offers safe and effective treatment.[186,187] In accordance with the Norton-Simon hypothesis, after initial cytoreduction, a few non–cross-resistant agents are given at short intervals.[188] In general, autologous stem cell transplantation (ASCT) and the use of growth factors allow the application of the most effective drugs in highest doses at intervals of 1 to 3 weeks. Sequential HDCT therapy permits the highest possible dosing in minimum time.

Incorporation of Radiotherapy into High-Dose Chemotherapy Programs

The rationale for incorporation of radiotherapy into HDCT programs stems from the observation that disease progression after HDCT often occurs in sites of prior involvement. Several investigators showed that in 65% to 95% of cases the sites of failure are involved immediately before HDCT.[184,189] Retrospective analysis suggests that radiation therapy may be incorporated as cytoreductive treatment before HDCT or as a consolidative therapy after HDCT.[190,191] However, there is no prospective clinical trial to answer questions regarding the extent of the radiation field, the timing of treatment, and the appropriate dose to use. The complementary role of radiation therapy in salvage HDCT is uncertain and remains to be investigated.

CHOICE OF TREATMENT

PROGNOSTIC FACTORS AND TREATMENT GROUPS

A prognostic factor is a measurement or classification of an individual patient, performed at or soon after diagnosis, that gives information on the likely outcome of the disease. This information is generally phrased in terms of probabilities—for instance, the probability of cure for various values of a prognostic factor. It may be used for informing the patient or, in the context of clinical trials, for defining or describing the study population or adjusting the data analysis; however, for the clinician the most important role of the prognostic factor is to help choose an appropriate treatment strategy.

In HL, patients have been traditionally divided into two or three prognostic groups, chiefly according to stage and B symptoms but also with various other factors taken into consideration. Most basically, stage IIIB or IV, or advanced-stage, disease has been associated with the poorest prognosis, and these patients have been assigned an intensive chemotherapy protocol, sometimes followed by adjuvant radiotherapy. Further prognostic factors were often used to assign patients with stage IIIA or IIB disease to the advanced-stage group. Among the remaining patients with early-stage disease, who had previously continued to receive radiotherapy alone, an "unfavorable" subgroup was often defined to select patients for combined modality therapy. Each group has thus been associated with a typical standard treatment strategy:

- Early stages, favorable: radiation alone (extended field)
- Early stages, unfavorable: moderate amount of chemotherapy (typically four cycles) plus radiation
- Advanced stages: extensive chemotherapy (typically eight cycles) with or without consolidatory (usually local) radiation

These "typical" strategies are not uniformly applied, and the investigation of alternatives, for instance, the use of chemotherapy in patients with favorable early-stage disease, is continuing, as is reported in the following sections. In the aforementioned scheme, two divisions between the three prognostic groups must be defined, each division possibly delineated by a different set of factors. Furthermore, the attempt has been made to identify patients with advanced-stage disease who have a particularly high risk of failure so that they can receive intensified therapy, for example, early HDCT with stem cell support.[192] This approach, however, has not shown any benefit when compared with six to eight courses of conventional chemotherapy such as ABVD.[193]

The selection of factors and the definition of the prognostic groups vary among institutions, as does the choice of treatment.

Prognostic factors are rarely the subject of specific clinical studies but are discovered and evaluated using data from large cohorts of uniformly treated, well-documented, and reliably followed-up patients, usually in large clinical trials.[194,195] The diversity of diagnostic and treatment strategies used for the early stages, as well as statistical problems caused by the low rate of treatment failure events, has led to the reporting and use of different prognostic factors by different institutions and trial groups.

In the following sections, recognized prognostic factors are described for early stages treated with radiotherapy alone, for early stages treated with chemotherapy, and for advanced stages (treated with chemotherapy). Such factors are required to show independent prognostic value in multivariate analyses including data for a large number of patients. This account refers in general to clinically staged patients, because laparotomy is now rarely performed. The use of these factors to define prognostic groups for treatment purposes, as practiced by various institutions and study groups, is described.

Prognostic Factors for Early Stages (Clinical Stage I or II) Treated with Radiotherapy Alone

Recognized adverse factors are as follows:

- Advanced age: correlates with the presence of occult abdominal disease and with poor results of salvage therapy; may also be associated with treatment complications leading to reduced or delayed treatment
- Male gender: small effect only
- Histologic MC subtype: associated with presence of occult abdominal disease
- B symptoms: associated with presence of occult abdominal disease
- Large mediastinal mass: some evidence of increased relapse rate in thorax (little data, because few patients with large mediastinal masses were treated with radiotherapy alone)
- Greater number of involved nodal regions
- Elevated erythrocyte sedimentation rate (ESR)
- Anemia
- Low serum albumin level

These factors are relevant to the decision as to which patients with early-stage disease should be categorized as falling into the "unfavorable" group and receive combined modality therapy because the prognosis with radiotherapy alone is relatively poor. Major study groups have used criteria as described later. Patients in the "favorable" category were generally given radiation only, although the additional application of mild chemotherapy has increased recently.

The European Organization for Research and Treatment of Cancer (EORTC) has, since 1982, defined patients with clinical stage I and II disease (supradiaphragmatic only) as unfavorable if they had *any* of the following factors: age over 50 years, asymptomatic with an ESR more than 50 mm/h, B symptoms with ESR more than 30 mm/h, and large mediastinal mass, based on the results of earlier EORTC trials H1 and H2. In previous trials, stage II disease, MCHL or LDHL histologic type, and number of involved regions had also been counted as adverse factors.[196]

The GHSG has, since 1988, assigned combined modality treatment to patients with clinical stage I or II disease with any of the following adverse factors: large mediastinal mass; three lymph node areas involved, ESR elevated for patients with B symptoms, 30 mm/h or more; ESR elevated for patients without B symptoms, 50 mm/h or more; localized extranodal infiltration (E lesions); and massive splenic involvement.[197] Owing to the rarity of splenectomy, the last-mentioned factor was seldom reported and was abandoned for the present trial generation. It can be difficult to distinguish consistently between E

TABLE 41.5-7. Definition of Treatment Groups by Two Large Cooperative Trials

		GHSG		EORTC/GELA
RISK FACTORS (RF)	A	Large mediastinal mass	A'	Large mediastinal mass
	B	Extranodal disease	B'	Age ≥50 y
	C	Elevated ESR[a]	C'	Elevated ESR[a]
	D	≥3 involved regions	D'	≥4 involved regions
TREATMENT GROUP				
Lymphocyte predominant		NLPHL histology in CS I–II with no RF		NLPHL histology in supradiaphragmatic CS I–II
Early stage favorable		CS I–II with no RF		CS I–II supradiaphragmatic with no RF
Early stage unfavorable		CS I, CS IIA with one or more RF; CS IIB with C/D but without A/B		CS I–II supradiaphragmatic with one or more RF
Advanced stage		CS IIB with A/B; CS III–IV		CS III–IV

CS, clinical stage; EORTC, European Organization for Research and Treatment of Cancer; ESR, erythrocyte sedimentation rate; GELA, Groupe d'Etude des Lymphomes de l'Adulte; GHSG, German Hodgkin Study Group; NLPHL, nodular lymphocyte-predominant Hodgkin's lymphoma.
[a]Erythrocyte sedimentation rate ≥50 mm/h without or ≥30 mm/h with B symptoms.

lesions and stage IV disease, and varying assessments of the prognostic value of this feature have been obtained by different investigators (Table 41.5-7). Stanford began in 1980 to give combined modality treatment to patients with clinical stage I or II disease with large mediastinal masses or multiple E lesions.

The EORTC has investigated the use of localized radiotherapy in a "very favorable" subgroup of patients with early-stage disease. Inclusion criteria were female with stage IA HL younger than 40 years of age, NS or LP histologic type, without elevated ESR or large mediastinal mass. However, a 30% long-term failure rate was observed, and this policy was not continued.

Prognostic Factors for Early Stages (Clinical Stage I or II) Treated with Chemotherapy

Despite the different mode of action of chemotherapy compared with radiotherapy, similar prognostic factors have emerged from analyses of cohorts treated with radiation and with combined modalities. All the factors listed earlier for radiation-treated patients [see Prognostic Factors for Early Stages (Clinical Stage I or II) Treated with Radiotherapy Alone] have also been reliably confirmed in cohorts that also received chemotherapy,[198,199] either in early or advanced stages. This similarity of prognostic effects is supported by the observation from a metaanalysis of radiation therapy versus combined modality treatment in early stages that the size of the difference in failure-free survival between these two treatment strategies was essentially constant for different prognostic groups.[200]

As a consequence, the prognostic factors relevant to the division between unfavorable early-stage and advanced-stage cases, that is, between moderate and extensive chemotherapy, are essentially the same as those listed earlier for the division between favorable and unfavorable [see Prognostic Factors for Early Stages (Clinical Stage I or II) Treated with Radiotherapy Alone]. However, generally only patients with stage IIB or III disease are given advanced-stage treatment due to the presence of these factors.

The EORTC includes in its advanced-stage cohorts those with stage III and IV disease only, without regard to other factors, as did the U.S. National Cancer Institute (NCI) and several U.S. cooperative groups.

In the GHSG, all patients with stage III and IV disease plus patients with stage IIB HL with large mediastinal mass or E

lesions are included in the advanced-stage group. Earlier trials included in the unfavorable early-stage category either all patients with stage IIIA disease or just those without any of the five GHSG factors listed earlier in Prognostic Factors for Early Stages (Clinical Stage I or II) Treated with Radiotherapy Alone. This gradual shift to more use of intensive therapy was based on prognostic factor analyses.

Certain other trial groups include other patients with stage I or II disease in the "advanced" prognostic group, for instance, those with stage IB and IIB or bulky stage II disease.[201]

Prognostic Factors for Advanced Stages

The more uniform treatment modality and the greater frequency of treatment failure events has permitted the determination of more conclusive and generally applicable results for prognostic factor analyses for the advanced stages than for the early stages. The results of the International Prognostic Factors Project on Advanced Hodgkin's Disease,[198] although not necessarily including all possible factors, can be taken as reliable (Table 41.5-8).

All these factors were highly significant in the multivariate analysis of data from 5141 patients treated at 25 centers, and their prognostic power was confirmed in an independent sam-

TABLE 41.5-8. Final Cox Regression Model (International Prognostic Factors Project)

Factor	Log Hazard Ratio	P Value	Relative Risk
Serum albumin <4 g/dL	0.40 ± 0.10	<.001	1.49
Hemoglobin <10.5 g/dL	0.30 ± 0.11	.006	1.35
Male gender	0.30 ± 0.09	.001	1.35
Stage IV disease	0.23 ± 0.09	.011	1.26
Age ≥45 y	0.33 ± 0.10	.001	1.39
White blood cell count ≥15,000/mm³	0.34 ± 0.11	.001	1.41
Lymphocyte count < 600/ mm³ or < 8% of white blood cell count	0.31 ± 0.10	.002	1.38

(From ref. 198, with permission.)

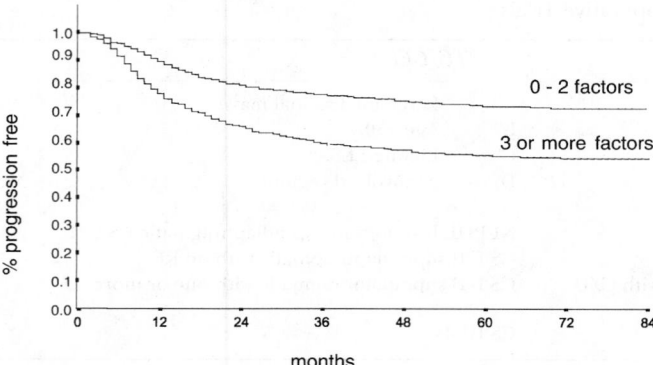

FIGURE 41.5-3. Freedom from treatment failure for patients with fewer than three, or three or more prognostic factors as defined by the International Prognostic Factors Project on Advanced Hodgkin's Disease.

ple. Note that the factors serum albumin level, hemoglobin level, and age 45 years or older are also prognostic for patients with early-stage disease. All seven factors were associated with similar relative risks of between 1.26 and 1.49. Therefore, Hasenclever and Diehl[198] recommended combining these factors into a single score by simply counting the number of adverse factors, to give an integer prognostic score between 0 and 7. However, even patients with five or more factors (7% of cases) had a 5-year failure-free rate of over 40%. The best failure-free rate was close to 80% for those with at most one factor (29% of cases), which suggests that a group of advanced-stage patients with a relatively favorable prognosis could be recognized (1618 patients included in the final analysis for FFTF according to whether the prognostic score was 0 to 2 or 3 or higher) (Fig. 41.5-3).

A number of other factors have been shown to correlate with prognosis in advanced stages, but their independent importance is not proven due to conflicting results or lack of confirmation in a large data set, or both. These include higher pathologic grade in NSHL, tissue eosinophilia, inguinal involvement, and high levels of serum lactate dehydrogenase and β_2-microglobulin.

Factors relevant to advanced-stage patients may be used to identify patients either for treatment intensification or for treatment reduction. Reduction can be achieved by creating a modified protocol or by including these patients in the early-stage group.

Concerning intensification, various investigators have treated a poor-prognosis subset of advanced-stage patients, who had attained a remission by conventional chemotherapy, with HDCT accompanied by hematologic stem cell support.[192,202] Proctor et al.[202] constructed a continuous numerical index for this purpose as a weighted sum of the variables of age, stage, lymphocyte count, hemoglobin level, and presence of bulky disease, and included patients with an index higher than 0.5 in the poor prognosis subset. Carella's group[275] included patients with two or more of the following factors: high lactate dehydrogenase level, very large mediastinal mass, two or more extranodal sites, inguinal involvement, low hematocrit, and bone marrow involvement. However, none of these methods could consistently select a subset with a failure rate of less than 40% with conventional therapy. This

means that the early high-dose approach is unlikely to show a clinically relevant long-term survival benefit compared with conventional treatment.[203]

Concerning treatment reduction, the short-duration, reduced-dose Stanford V chemotherapy regimen (mechlorethamine, doxorubicin, vincristine, vinblastine, etoposide, bleomycin, and prednisone) with or without radiotherapy is currently being tested in patients with bulky stage II or advanced-stage disease who have at most two adverse factors as defined by the International Prognostic Factors Project on Advanced Hodgkin's Disease.[204] Stanford V is, however, not merely a reduction of therapy but rather a rescheduling with lower total doses but greater dose intensities. No data are available on the results of treatment reduction in a favorable subset of those with advanced-stage disease.

In conclusion, the three-level scheme of division into early-stage favorable, early-stage unfavorable, and advanced-stage cases remains valid according to current knowledge (see Table 41.5-7). Separation of very favorable early-stage or poor-risk advanced-stage patients for especially mild or intensive therapy, respectively, does not appear justified. Several prognostic factors, other than clinical stage, are used in making the divisions between favorable, unfavorable, and advanced cases, and no universally valid set of factors has been determined. Nevertheless, the list of reliably confirmed, independent prognostic factors, given earlier in Prognostic Factors for Early Stages (Clinical Stage I or II) Treated with Chemotherapy and Prognostic Factors for Advanced Stages, encompasses most of the factors used by the major institutions and study groups. For patients with early- and advanced-stage disease receiving radiotherapy or chemotherapy or both, the set of relevant factors is fairly similar.

The search for biologically specific factors directly related to tumor activity is now an important research goal, but thus far no reliable and clinically robust factors have been described.

EARLY-STAGE FAVORABLE DISEASE

Reduction of Staging or Treatment: Ongoing and Recently Completed Trials

Increasing concern for the long-term consequences of treatment has prompted many investigators to reexamine the aggressive approaches developed for the staging and treatment of early-stage HL in the 1970s and 1980s. Many of the ongoing and recently completed studies were developed in an attempt to reduce the long-term complications of treatment without increasing mortality from HL. These include studies that

- investigate reduction of radiation dose or reduction of field size in pure radiotherapy
- seek an optimal, short, and less toxic chemotherapy regimen, or an optimal radiation volume in combined radiotherapy
- evaluate chemotherapy alone

Clinical Trials of Radiation Therapy Alone

RADIATION DOSE REDUCTION. Although a few studies have comprehensively reviewed dose-response data for HL, only one prospective randomized study is available.[205] This multicenter trial by the GHSG evaluated the tumoricidal doses for subclinical involvement by HL.[206] A total of 376 patients with laparotomy-staged favorable-prognosis stage IA to IIB HL were enrolled. Only patients without risk factors were included in the trial. Any one of the following risk factors was cause for exclusion: large mediastinal adenopathy, massive splenic involvement, extranodal disease, an ESR of more than 30 mm/h and B symptoms, an ESR of more than 50 mm/h and no B symptoms, or more than three regions of involvement. Patients were randomly assigned to receive either 40-Gy extended-field radiation therapy or 30-Gy extended-field radiation therapy followed by an additional 10 Gy to involved lymph node regions.

The 5-year FFTF results favored the arm receiving the 30-Gy extended field plus 10 Gy over the arm receiving the 40-Gy extended field (81% vs. 70%, respectively; *P* = .026). The 5-year FFTF and survival rates were (nonsignificantly) higher in the reduced-dose arm, which suggests that 30 Gy is sufficient for treating subclinical involvement of HL with radiotherapy alone.[206]

RADIATION FIELD SIZE REDUCTION

Mantle Irradiation Alone in Patients with Clinical Stage IA and IIA Disease. The use of mantle irradiation alone for early-stage HL is attractive because all treatment is completed within 5 weeks, patients avoid the long-term risks of radiation to the upper abdomen, and the potential for salvage with combination chemotherapy is not compromised. Results of prospective and retrospective studies of mantle irradiation alone for unselected clinical stage I or II patients have been disappointing. The EORTC H1 trial, one of the first studies to evaluate the role of chemotherapy in the treatment of early-stage HL, randomly assigned patients with clinical stage I or II disease to receive mantle irradiation alone or irradiation combined with vinblastine chemotherapy. All clinical stage I or II patients were enrolled. Fewer recurrences were seen in patients who received both mantle irradiation and vinblastine chemotherapy. However, relapse rates were high in both groups. The freedom from recurrence was only 38% in the mantle-alone group, and the 15-year survival rate was only 58%. This suggests that mantle irradiation alone is not adequate treatment for unselected patients with clinical stage I or II HL and that vinblastine is only partially effective in eliminating recurrences, many of which occurred below the diaphragm.[207] Similarly, the Toronto series reported that the 10-year rate of freedom from recurrence was only 54%.[208] These high recurrence rates in unselected patients are not surprising, because over 20% of clinical stage I or II patients have occult abdominal involvement, and lack of treatment of potential abdominal disease (with radiation therapy or chemotherapy) will result in higher recurrence rates than achieved with more extensive treatment. When mantle irradiation was restricted to clinically staged, asymptomatic patients with a single involved lymph node region (clinical stage IA), better results were seen, with 10- to 15-year freedom-from-recurrence rates of 58% to 81%.[209] Therefore, most groups have abandoned mantle field irradiation alone.

Mantle Irradiation Alone in Clinically Staged Patients with a Very Low Risk of Abdominal Involvement. Patients with a very low risk of abdominal involvement include female patients with clinical stage IA NSHL, patients with clinical stage IA HL with LP histology, and patients with clinical stage IA interfollicular HL.[162] A similar subgroup of patients was defined by the EORTC

(women younger than 40 years of age with clinical stage IA LP or NS histology, and an ESR of less than 50 mm/h) and was treated with mantle irradiation alone without staging laparotomy in the EORTC trials H7VF (VF for very favorable) and H8VF trials. In the H7VF trial, 40 patients were treated with mantle irradiation alone; complete remission was reached in 95%. However, 23% of patients relapsed, yielding a 6-year event-free survival rate of 66%, a relapse-free survival rate of 73%, and overall and cause-specific survival rates of 96%.[210] The relapse rates were thought to be unacceptably high in this selected subgroup of stage IA patients. The very favorable subgroup is now treated according to the EORTC strategy for the favorable subgroup.

Mantle Irradiation Alone in Patients with Favorable-Prognosis Stage IA and IIA Disease. To determine the role of prophylactic abdominal irradiation in early-stage HL, the EORTC H5 trial (1977 to 1982) compared the use of mantle and paraaortic-splenic pedicle irradiation to mantle irradiation alone in patients with favorable early-stage HL.[196,207] This study included only patients with NS or LP histology, age of 40 years or younger, pathologic stage I or II disease with mediastinal adenopathy, and an ESR of less than 70 mm/h. No differences were seen in disease-free survival or overall survival between the two treatment groups with or without paraaortic irradiation. A 1997 update of this trial showed no statistical difference between the two treatment arms, either for treatment failure probability (*P* = .62) or overall survival (*P* = .69).

In 1989, a single-arm prospective trial was initiated at Harvard University Medical School (Joint Center for Radiation Therapy) investigating mantle irradiation alone in patients with laparotomy-staged IA and IIA HL. The objectives were to identify patients most suitable for mantle irradiation alone, to establish guidelines for follow-up after treatment, to evaluate the requirement for staging laparotomy, and to provide an assessment of risk versus gain for the reduction of treatment in early-stage HL. The eligibility criteria for the study included negative findings on laparotomy, the absence of large mediastinal adenopathy and B symptoms, and NS or LP histology. Thoracic CT scanning and gallium scanning were required to establish the extent of thoracic involvement, and patients with HL in hilar, subcarinal, or cardiophrenic lymph node regions were not eligible for the trial. Eighty-four patients have been enrolled. The 5-year actuarial rate of freedom from recurrence exceeds 80%. These excellent results with mantle irradiation alone also have been seen in other retrospective studies.[211]

Clinical Trials of Combined Chemotherapy and Radiotherapy

Randomized trials of combined modality therapy are based on the premise that this approach results in a very high freedom from recurrence in early-stage HL and that efficacy can be maintained when using less toxic chemotherapy and radiation therapy regimens.

LESS TOXIC CHEMOTHERAPY WITH RADIATION (COMPARISON WITH RADIATION ALONE). Trials of less toxic chemotherapy plus radiotherapy use chemotherapy regimens given for four or six cycles in combination with radiation therapy. The regimens are combined with involved-field or regional (mantle) radiation therapy on the premise that the drugs being tested will be able to provide both prophylactic control at adjacent sites and control of occult abdominal disease in clinically staged patients without upper abdominal and splenic irradiation. Analysis of patterns and frequency of failure will eventually provide better guidelines for designing optimal regimens to control occult HL not appreciated on physical examination or radiographic evaluation. If successful, these regimens should reduce treatment-related morbidity and mortality by reducing both the amount and toxicity of chemotherapy and by using smaller radiation volumes.

With the objective of reducing acute toxicity and chronic morbidity (sterility, increased risk of leukemia), Horning and colleagues developed a "nontoxic" chemotherapy regimen—vinblastine, methotrexate, and bleomycin (VBM)—which was tested in a randomized trial of pathologic stage IA to IIB and IIIA patients. The trial compared subtotal or total nodal irradiation to involved-field irradiation (44 Gy) followed by VBM.[212] The freedom from disease progression at 9 years favored involved-field irradiation and VBM (98%) over subtotal nodal or total nodal irradiation (78%) (*P* = .01). No differences were seen in overall survival (*P* = .09). The BNLI has confirmed the efficacy of VBM with involved-field irradiation, but in their experience this approach produced unacceptable pulmonary and hematologic toxicity.[213] Favorable results with VBM and extended-field radiation therapy in clinical stage IA or IIA HL also have been reported by the Gruppo Italiano per lo Studio Dei Linformi.[214] In that study of 50 patients, the 5-year progression-free survival rate was 82%. Sixteen percent of patients in the trial experienced pulmonary toxicity.

Based on the Stanford trial results reported in Combined Modality Therapy, a follow-up Stanford University trial has been completed.[182] Patients with clinical stage IA or IIA HL (staging laparotomy and splenectomy were eliminated) were treated either with subtotal nodal and splenic irradiation or two cycles of VBM, followed by regional (mantle) irradiation, followed by four additional cycles of VBM (with a reduced bleomycin dose). No differences in 4-year freedom from disease progression or survival were noted between the two arms of the trial.

A regimen of EBVP II (epirubicin, bleomycin, vinblastine, and prednisone, one dose per cycle) and involved-field irradiation (n = 168) versus mantle and paraaortic-splenic irradiation (n = 165) for treatment of patients with favorable-prognosis clinical stage IA or IIA disease was tested in the EORTC H7F trial (1988 to 1993). The EORTC EBVP II regimen was proposed as a regimen that was potentially less toxic but similar in effectiveness to ABVD. In the H7F randomized trial for patients with favorable disease, six cycles of EBVP were combined with involved-field radiation and the results compared with those for subtotal nodal and splenic irradiation in patients with favorable clinical stage I and II disease. At 6 years, the relapse survival rate was significantly higher for patients on the combined chemotherapy and radiation therapy arm than for those on the radiotherapy-alone arm (92% vs. 81%, respectively; *P* = .004). The 6-year survival rate was excellent in both treatment arms (98% vs. 96%, respectively; *P* = .156).[215,216] In contrast, in the H7U trial for patients with unfavorable disease, EBVP and involved-field radiation therapy was inferior to MOPP plus doxorubicin, bleomycin, vinblastine (ABV) and involved-field radiation therapy, which suggests that the use of prognostic factors is crucial in selecting patients for treatment using reduced chemotherapy and radiation therapy regimens.

REDUCED NUMBER OF CHEMOTHERAPY CYCLES. The trials noted here use combination chemotherapy and radiation therapy with fewer than four cycles of chemotherapy. Although the primary goal of these trials is to evaluate the efficacy of short courses of chemotherapy, new regimens are also being tested [i.e., Stanford V; doxorubicin, cyclophosphamide, etoposide, vincristine, bleomycin, prednisone (VAPEC-B)]. The optimal extent of radiation therapy needed is less certain in the short-course trials. For example, there are at least limited data that four to six cycles of chemotherapy are sufficient to control occult abdominal disease in the majority of clinical stage I and II patients.[167,217] With short-course chemotherapy there are very few data on the effectiveness of different regimens in controlling HL outside of the involved regions as defined by physical examination or radiographic evaluation. This uncertainty is reflected in some of the trial designs that use subtotal nodal and splenic radiation rather than involved-field or mantle radiation in combination with chemotherapy. Ongoing and recently completed short-course trials are listed in Table 41.5-9.

The GHSG HD7 trial (1994 to 1998) randomly assigned 643 favorable clinical stage IA to IIB HL patients to subtotal nodal and splenic irradiation alone or to two courses of ABVD and the radiation therapy regimen.[218] The final analysis of the data for 617 patients showed an advantage in FFTF favoring the patients receiving ABVD (91%) over those treated with irradiation alone (75%; *P* <.0001) (see Table 41.5-9). There are several questions raised by this study. First, with an expected long-term FFTF in favorable clinical stage IA and IIA HL of approximately 70% to 75% with radiation therapy alone, is the added benefit in FFTF with two courses of ABVD worth the extra risk from the doxorubicin and bleomycin? Second, is salvage more difficult in patients who experience recurrence after subtotal nodal and splenic irradiation and two courses of ABVD than after subtotal nodal and splenic irradiation alone? These are questions that can be answered only with longer follow-up.

The GHSG HD10 trial (closed January 2003) had essentially the same eligibility criteria as the GHSG HD7 trial. Patients were randomly assigned to four arms, namely, the four combinations of two or four cycles of ABVD followed by 20 or 30 Gy of involved-field radiation therapy. The third interim analysis in August 2003 with 847 patients accrued showed that after a median follow-up of 28 months there was no difference between two and four cycles of ABVD, and, furthermore, no difference between 20 and 30 Gy of involved-field radiation therapy, with an FFTF of 97% and overall survival rate of 99%. This trial demonstrates very clearly that two cycles of ABVD followed by 20 Gy of involved-field radiation therapy are sufficient to control occult HL in the abdomen and to prevent recurrence of HL in apparently uninvolved sites adjacent to known HL (adjacent to the irradiated involved site). A longer follow-up period is necessary, however, to exclude late relapses and toxic side effects.

In a Manchester pilot study and BNLI trial, VAPEC-B chemotherapy for 4 weeks and involved-field irradiation was compared with mantle irradiation alone. Preliminary reports from the Manchester pilot study using the relatively brief 4-week VAPEC-B regimen in early-stage HL provide background data for the ongoing BNLI trial. In the Manchester study, 111 clinical stage IA and IIA patients without mediastinal bulk were randomly, starting in 1989, to receive either limited radiother-

TABLE 41.5-9. Clinical Trials in Favorable-Prognosis Stage I and II Hodgkin's Lymphoma (HL): Trials to Identify the Optimal Number of Chemotherapy Cycles

Trial	Eligibility	Treatment Regimens	No. of Patients	Outcome
GHSG HD7, 1994–1998	CS IA–IIB *without* large mediastinal mass (≥0.33 m/t ratio); massive splenic involvement; localized extranodal involvement; ESR ≥50 mm/h in A, ≥30 mm/h in B; three or more involved areas	A: EFRT 30 Gy (IFRT 40 Gy) B: 2 ABVD + EFRT 30 Gy (IFRT 40 Gy)	305 312	FFTF, 75%; SV (60 mo) 94% FFTF, 91%; SV (60 mo), 94% (FFTF: *P*<.0001; SV: *P*=NS)
GHSG HD10, 1998–2003	CS IA–IIB *without* large mediastinal mass (≥0.33 m/t ratio); localized extranodal involvement; ESR ≥50 mm/h in A, ≥30 mm/h in B; three or more involved areas	A: 2 ABVD + IFRT (30 Gy) B: 2 ABVD + IFRT (20 Gy) C: 4 ABVD + IFRT (30 Gy) D: 4 ABVD + IFRT (20 Gy)	204 210 218 215	Overall FFTF (24 mo), 97% Overall survival (24 mo), 99% After 4 ABVD: FFTF, 96.5%; SV, 98.7% After 2 ABVD: FFTF, 96.7%; SV, 98.2% After 30 Gy: FFTF, 97.3%; SV, 99.0% After 20 Gy: FFTF, 97.9%; SV, 99.3%
BNLI	CS IA–IIA *without* large mediastinal disease	A: 1 VAPEC-B + IFRT (30–40 Gy) B: Mantle RT 30–35 Gy (IFRT 30–40 Gy)	Open	Open
SWOG 9133/ CALGB 9391	CS IA–IIA *without* age <16 y; large mediastinal disease; pericardial involvement	A: 3 (doxorubicin + vinblastine) + STLI (S) (36–40 Gy) B: STLI (S) (36–40 Gy)	166 163	FFTF, 94%; SV (3 y), 98% FFTF, 81%; SV (3 y), 96% (FFTF: *P*<.001; SV: *P*=NS)
EORTC/GELA H8F	CS IA–IIB *without* age ≥50 y; ESR ≥50 mm/h in A, ≥30 mm/h in B; ≥4 sites of disease; large mediastinal disease	A: 3 MOPP/ABV + IFRT (36 Gy) B: STLI (S)	271 272	RFS, 99%; SV (4 y), 99% RFS, 80%; SV (4 y), 95% (RFS: *P*<.0001; SV: *P*<.0816)
GHSG HD13	CS IA–IIB *without* large mediastinal mass (≥0.33 m/t ratio); localized extranodal involvement; ESR ≥50 mm/h in A, ≥30 mm/h in B; three or more involved areas	A: 2 ABVD + 30 Gy IFRT B: 2 ABV + 30 Gy IFRT C: 2 AVD + 30 Gy IFRT D: 2 AV + 30 Gy IFRT	Open; started 01/2003	Open
Stanford V for favorable CS IA–IIA HL	CS I–II *without* B symptoms; age <16 y and >60 y; large mediastinal disease; ≥2 extranodal sites	Stanford V for 8 wk + modified IFRT (30 Gy)	65	Median FU, 16 mo; FFP (3 y), 94.6%; SV, 96.6%

ABV, doxorubicin (Adriamycin), bleomycin, vinblastine; ABVD, doxorubicin, bleomycin, vinblastine, dacarbazine; AV, doxorubicin and vinblastine; AVD, doxorubicin, vinblastine, dacarbazine; BNLI, British National Lymphoma Investigation; CALGB, Cancer and Leukemia Group B; CS, clinical stage; EFRT, extended-field radiotherapy; EORTC, European Organization for Research and Treatment of Cancer; ESR, erythrocyte sedimentation rate; FFP, freedom from progression; FFTF, freedom from treatment failure; FU, follow-up; GELA, Groupe d'Etude des Lymphomes de l'Adulte; GHSG, German Hodgkin Study Group; IFRT, involved-field radiation therapy; MOPP, mechlorethamine, vincristine, procarbazine, prednisone; m/t ratio, mass to thorax ratio; NS, not significant; RFS, relapse-free survival; RT, radiotherapy; Stanford V, mechlorethamine, doxorubicin, vinblastine, prednisone, vincristine, bleomycin, VP-16; STLI (S), subtotal nodal irradiation (splenic irradiation); SV, survival; SWOG, Southwest Oncology Group; VAPEC-B, doxorubicin, cyclophosphamide, etoposide, vincristine, bleomycin, prednisone.

apy alone or VAPEC-B followed by local irradiation only to the involved regions. At a median follow-up of 3.3 years, there were only two recurrences in the arm receiving VAPEC-B plus local irradiation (progression-free survival rate at 3 years was 91%).[219] The current BNLI study has a similar design; however, the radiotherapy-alone arm includes full mantle irradiation rather than irradiation of a more limited field (see Table 41.5-9).

The Southwest Oncology Group (SWOG) and Cancer and Leukemia Group B (CALGB) study of three cycles of adjuvant doxorubicin and vinblastine plus subtotal nodal and splenic irradiation versus subtotal nodal and splenic irradiation alone in patients with clinical stage IA to IIA HL is ongoing (see

Table 41.5-9). For 329 patients who have been enrolled on the study, freedom-from-progression rates at 3 years were 94% for the combined modality arm and 81% for the radiation-only arm.[220] The questions raised by this study are similar to those raised by the GHSG HD7 study (see earlier in Radiotherapy: Reduced Number of Chemotherapy Cycles). These include the potential extra toxicity of the doxorubicin and vinblastine in a group of patients with an expected favorable prognosis after treatment with radiation therapy alone, and the overall strategy in trial design of giving enough chemotherapy to eliminate the need for abdominal irradiation.

The EORTC H8F trial (1993 to 1998), which compared three cycles of MOPP/ABV hybrid and involved-field irradiation with mantle and paraaortic-splenic irradiation for treatment of patients with favorable-prognosis clinical stage IA and IIA HL, was activated in 1993 (see Table 41.5-9). This trial should give answers to the following important questions: Are three cycles of standard chemotherapy sufficient to control subclinical HL in patients with favorable-prognosis clinical stage IA and IIA HL? Can patients who experience relapse after three cycles of MOPP/ABV and involved-field radiation therapy be cured with alternative treatment short of HDCT and stem cell rescue? The one concern of the trial is the use of the hybrid regimen, which confers some risk of sterility and leukemogenesis in these favorable-prognosis HL patients. Use of ABVD and EBVP is proposed for the H9 trials.

The modified Stanford V trial for early-stage favorable-prognosis HL involved a relatively short, but intensive, chemotherapy regimen given for 12 weeks to patients with poor-prognosis stage I and II disease.[221,222] A modification of this trial has been opened for patients with favorable-prognosis clinical stage IA and IIA HL, using 8 weeks of the Stanford V regimen and modified involved-field irradiation to sites of initial involvement (identified radiographically as nodal enlargement of 1.5 cm or greater). The chemotherapy regimen includes mechlorethamine (6 mg/m^2 on weeks 1 and 5), doxorubicin (25 mg/m^2 on weeks 1, 3, 5, and 7), vinblastine (6 mg/m^2 on weeks 1, 3, 5, and 7), prednisone (40 mg/m^2 on days 1 to 36 then tapered off), vincristine (1.4 mg/m^2 on weeks 2, 4, 6, and 8), bleomycin (5 mg/m^2 on weeks 2, 4, 6, and 8), and VP-16 (60 mg/m^2 on days 15 and 16, and days 43 and 44). This study will evaluate the ability of brief but intense chemotherapy to control HL outside of initially involved sites in patients with favorable-prognosis clinical stage I and II HL (see Table 41.5-9).

RADIATION VOLUME AND DOSE. Two trials involving favorable-prognosis early-stage HL evaluated radiation dose to involved sites after chemotherapy. GHSG-initiated trial HD10, comparing 30 Gy with 20 Gy of radiotherapy after two or four courses of ABVD, is described in Combined Modality Chemotherapy (see Table 41.5-9). The EORTC H9F trial is evaluating 36 Gy, 20 Gy, or no radiation to involved sites in patients who have achieved a complete remission after six cycles of EBVP II.

Clinical Trials of Chemotherapy Alone

Probably the first published experience of the use of MOPP chemotherapy alone in early stages of childhood HL comes from Uganda, where no radiation therapy was available.[223] Several small retrospective studies have also reported treatment with MOPP alone.[224] Based on this limited experience, two randomized studies were devised to compare radiation therapy alone to MOPP chemotherapy alone in laparotomy-staged patients. Both studies have median follow-up times of 7.5 to 8.0 years. Although both studies are now dated because of the use of the MOPP regimen and the requirement for staging laparotomy, results from these trials provide valuable information for the design of future protocols.

CHEMOTHERAPY VERSUS RADIATION. The NCI study was initially designed to include patients with intermediate-prognosis HL. Although the trial included patients with favorable-prognosis pathologic stage IIA disease, the most favorable patients (pathologic stage IA patients with peripheral sites) were not included in the trial and were treated with radiation therapy

alone. Patients with an unfavorable prognosis (B symptoms, large mediastinal adenopathy, and limited stage III disease) were included in the trial.[225] Patients were randomly assigned to receive 6 months of MOPP chemotherapy alone or subtotal nodal irradiation alone. After researchers recognized that patients with massive mediastinal involvement and pathologic stage IIIA disease were not optimal candidates for radiation therapy alone, the randomization criteria were changed while the study was ongoing. No difference in disease-free or overall survival was seen at 10 years.

The Italian prospective study randomized patients with pathologic stage I to IIA HL to receive either 6 months of MOPP alone or subtotal nodal irradiation alone.[226] There were no differences in freedom from progression. However, the survival rate was significantly higher in patients treated with radiation therapy alone (93%) than in those treated with chemotherapy alone (56%). The difference in survival was attributed to the failure of salvage in patients experiencing relapse after MOPP chemotherapy. These results are similar to the poor results of salvage ABVD in patients who experienced relapse after MOPP for advanced HL. Both the NCI and the Italian studies found greater acute toxicities in patients who received MOPP chemotherapy. In the Longo et al. study,[225] more than 50% of patients treated with MOPP had at least one hospital admission for fever and neutropenia.

The National Cancer Institute of Canada (NCIC) Clinical Trial Group HD6 study is a modification of the NCI and Italian studies with the randomization of clinically staged, rather than pathologically staged, patients and the use of ABVD as the chemotherapy regimen. Favorable-prognosis patients (NS or LP histology, age younger than 40, ESR less than 50 mm/h, one to three sites of involvement) are randomly assigned to receive either subtotal nodal irradiation and splenic irradiation or four cycles of ABVD alone. This study will test the efficacy of four cycles of ABVD alone in favorable-prognosis early-stage HL. The study is open for accrual.

CHEMOTHERAPY VERSUS COMBINED MODALITY THERAPY. In 1977, the Grupo Argentino de Tratamiento de la Leucemia Aguda (GATLA) and Grupo Latinoamericano de Tratamiento de Hematopatías Malignas (GLATHEM) cooperative groups initiated a randomized study[226a] of chemotherapy with cyclophosphamide, vinblastine, procarbazine, and prednisone (CVPP) alone for six cycles (cyclophosphamide, 600 mg/m^2 and vinblastine, 6 mg/m^2 on day 1; and procarbazine, 100 mg/m^2 and prednisone, 40 mg on days 1 through 14) versus CVPP plus radiation therapy consisting of 30 Gy to involved areas for patients with clinical stage I or II disease. Overall, the 7-year disease-free survival rate was 71% for chemotherapy and radiation therapy compared to 62% for chemotherapy alone ($P = .01$); survival rates were 89% and 81%, respectively ($P = .3$). In a subgroup of patients with favorable-prognosis clinical stage I or II disease, no differences were observed in actuarial rates of disease-free survival (77% vs. 70%), or overall survival (92% vs. 91%), respectively, for CVPP and involved-field irradiation versus CVPP alone. In comparing these results with other adult studies, one should note that in this study and in the subsequent GATLA study nearly 50% of the patients were younger than 16 years of age. It is possible that treatment approaches with chemotherapy alone may be more successful in children than in adult patients.

In the subsequent GATLA study, patients with favorable prognosis were randomized to CVPP for three cycles versus six cycles. At 5 years the actuarial event-free survival rates (80% vs. 84%) and overall survival rates (91% vs. 92%) were not significantly different.[227]

In the ongoing EORTC three-armed H9F trial, patients with favorable-prognosis clinical stage I and II HL who achieve a complete remission after six cycles of EBVP are randomly assigned to receive 36 Gy of involved-field irradiation, 20 Gy of involved-field irradiation, or no radiation therapy.

The Memorial Sloan-Kettering Cancer Center trial randomly assigns clinical stage I to IIIA patients without large mediastinal adenopathy or bulky disease who have achieved a complete remission after six cycles of ABVD to receive either mantle irradiation (35 Gy) or no further treatment. This trial has enrolled approximately 120 patients out of a planned total of 200 patients.

Recommendations and Future Directions

Standard care currently provides a number of treatment options for patients with early-stage favorable-prognosis HL. These include the use of mantle irradiation alone for selected patients with negative laparotomy staging, mantle-paraaortic and splenic irradiation without laparotomy staging, and combination chemotherapy and radiation therapy, often with a reduced number of cycles of chemotherapy and reduction of radiation field sizes and doses, for instance, ABVD for four cycles followed by involved-field irradiation to 20 to 30 Gy.

Current clinical trials are evaluating the use of alternative chemotherapy combinations, shortened courses of chemotherapy, chemotherapy with smaller radiation fields or lower radiation doses, and chemotherapy without radiation therapy. Fortunately, death from HL in favorable-prognosis early-stage patients is unusual, and mortality from other causes occurs many years later. Therefore, survival is not a useful parameter to evaluate midterm results in early-stage HL. Current trials must be judged by rates of freedom from first recurrence, acute morbidity, and new criteria such as quality of life and perhaps cost effectiveness. Trials aiming at high freedom-from-first-recurrence rates may not provide the optimum treatment once long-term (10- to 20-year) data are available. Treatment-related mortality may exceed HL mortality in patients with favorable-prognosis early-stage disease. New methods in decision analysis should also help in the design of trials and in the analysis of retrospective data.

Despite the increasing availability of guidelines for the treatment of HL, there must remain room for individualization of treatment. With different treatment options, some of which may result in a higher recurrence risk at the gain of less toxic initial treatment, patient preferences must be assessed. In addition, treatment should be individualized when a particular treatment approach might result in a higher risk of a serious late complication (e.g., risk of late breast cancer in young female patients treated with large radiation fields). This is an exciting time for the development of new strategies in the treatment of early-stage HL. Many of the ongoing trials ask questions that will allow optimization of treatment for early-stage patients and minimize long-term toxicity.

EARLY-STAGE UNFAVORABLE DISEASE

There were numerous studies analyzing clinical prognostic factors for patients with stage I and II HL in the 1970s and 1980s.[200,207] Based on these studies, clinical investigators have defined favor-

able and unfavorable prognostic groups of patients with stage I and II HL in an effort to refine the design of clinical trials and to tailor treatment in accordance with prognostic factors. Although the definition of favorable and unfavorable-prognosis early-stage HL continues to vary among different cooperative groups and institutions, there are three factors signifying poor prognosis that are used as grouping criteria in most clinical trials: large mediastinal adenopathy or bulky disease, presence of B symptoms, and older age. For each prognostic group, the goal is to define the precise amount of treatment that both minimizes recurrence and mortality from HL and provides the least risk for long-term toxicity. Patients with unfavorable disease require, in general, more aggressive treatment than those with favorable disease. However, the likelihood of cure for patients with unfavorable stage I or II disease is still high, and therefore consideration of long-term toxicity remains an important issue in the treatment of these patients.

A number of clinical trials comparing radiation therapy alone versus combined modality therapy for the treatment of unfavorable-prognosis stage I and II HL were conducted in the 1970s and 1980s. The high recurrence rates with radiation therapy alone led to the development of strategies in current trials that use various combinations of chemotherapy and radiation therapy. To illustrate, one large trial conducted by the EORTC (H5U) randomized patients with unfavorable prognostic factors to total nodal irradiation or to MOPP chemotherapy (six cycles) and mantle irradiation. Although overall survival did not differ (69% in both arms at 15 years), treatment failure rates strongly favored the chemotherapy arm (35% vs. 16%; $P<.001$).

Trials to Identify the Best Chemotherapy Combination

The evolution of studies to identify the best chemotherapy combination for unfavorable early-stage HL paralleled analogous trials for treatment of advanced-stage disease. Early trials compared MOPP with MOPP-like combinations, later trials compared these combinations with ABVD, and finally, the most recent trials compare new intense chemotherapy combinations with ABVD.

The first combined modality trial to test MOPP against ABVD in unfavorable-prognosis patients was the Milan study conducted between 1974 and 1982. This study used split-course treatment (three cycles of chemotherapy preceding and after subtotal nodal irradiation) and showed no significant difference in freedom from progression.[228] However, in the EORTC H6U trial (1982 to 1988) comparing split-course MOPP and ABVD,[229,230] although the 10-year survival was equivalent in both arms, the FFTF rate was significantly higher with ABVD than with MOPP.

The GATLA trial and the EORTC H7U trial (Table 41.5-10) compared the use of modified nonalkylating agent regimens with standard alkylating agent regimens in treatment of patients with unfavorable-prognosis early-stage disease. All patients received combined radiation therapy and chemotherapy. In both trials the arms receiving modified chemotherapy had significantly higher recurrence rates.

In the EORTC trial the recurrence rate was high enough to result in early closure of the trial. Although, in favorable-prognosis stage I and II HL, less toxic and less intense chemotherapy regimens have been effective in combined modality therapy programs, this does not appear to be the case for patients with unfavorable-prognosis disease. In the GATLA trial, the event-free survival rate was 66% for the combination of

TABLE 41.5-10. Randomized Clinical Trials in Unfavorable-Prognosis Stage I and II Hodgkin's Lymphoma: Trials to Identify the Optimal Chemotherapy Combination

Trial	Eligibility	Treatment Regimens	No. of Patients	Outcome
EORTC H6U, 1982–1988	CS I–II *with* large mediastinal mass (≥0.33 m/t ratio) or ESR ≥50 mm/h in A, ≥30 mm/h in B or three or more involved areas	A: 3 MOPP + mantle RT + 3 MOPP B: 3 ABVD + mantle RT + 3 ABVD	165 151	FFP (6 y), 88% (arm B) vs. 76% (arm A); *P* = .01; Not significant for survival [97% (arm B) vs. 85% (arm A); *P* = .22]
Istituto Nazionale Tumori, Milan, 1974–1982	PS IIB	A: 3 MOPP + STLI/TLI + 3 MOPP B: 3 ABVD + STLI/TLI + 3 ABVD	33 36	FFP (5 y), 66% FFP (5 y), 72% (*P* = .2)
GATLA, 1986–1992	Score of age, B symptoms, stage, number of sites, and bulky disease	A: 3 CVPP + IFRT (30 Gy) + 3 CVPP B. 3 AOPE + IFRT (30 Gy) + 3 AOPE	92 84	EFS, 85%; SV (5 y), 95% EFS, 66%; SV (5 y), 87% (EFS: *P* = .009; SV, *P* = .16)
EORTC H7U, 1988–1992	CS IA–IIA *with* age >50 y or ESR ≥50 mm/h in A, ≥30 mm/h in B or large mediastinal mass (≥0.33 m/t ratio)	A: 6 EBVP II + IFRT (36 GY) B: 6 MOPP/ABV + IFRT	160 156	EFS, 68%; SV (6 y), 82% EFS, 90%; SV (6 y), 89% (EFS: *P* <.0001; SV: *P* = .18)
EORTC H9U, 1998	Same as H7U	A: 6 ABVD + IFRT (30 Gy) B: 4 ABVD + IFRT C: 4 BEACOPP + IFRT	Open	Interim analysis: FFP overall, 90%
GHSG HD11, 1998–2003	CS IA–IB, IIA *with* age ≥50 y or ESR ≥50 mm/h or CS IIB and ESR ≥30 mm/h or large mediastinal disease	A: 4 ABVD + IFRT (30 Gy) B: 4 ABVD + IFRT (20 Gy) C: 4 BEACOPP + IFRT (30 Gy) D: 4 BEACOPP + IFRT (20 Gy)	264 257 262 268	Overall FFTF (24 mo), 90% Overall survival (24 mo), 97% After 4 × ABVD: FFTF, 89%; SV, 98% After 4 × BEACOPP: FFTF, 91%; SV, 97% After 30 Gy: FFTF, 93%; SV, 98% After 20 Gy: FFTF, 91%; SV, 99%
GHSG HD14	CS IA–IB, IIA *with* age ≥50 y or ESR ≥50 mm/h or CS IIB and ESR ≥30 mm/h or large mediastinal disease	A: 4 ABVD + IFRT (30 Gy) B: 2 BEACOPP escalated + 2 ABVD + IFRT (30 Gy)	Open, started 01/2003	Open
ECOG 2496, 1998–	Large mediastinal disease	A: 6 ABVD + IFRT (36 Gy) to bulky sites (>5 cm) B: 12 weeks Stanford V + IFRT to bulky sites	Open	Open

ABV, doxorubicin (Adriamycin), bleomycin, vinblastine; ABVD, doxorubicin, bleomycin, vinblastine, dacarbazine; AOPE, doxorubicin, vincristine, prednisone, etoposide; BEACOPP, bleomycin, etoposide, doxorubicin, cyclophosphamide, vincristine, procarbazine, prednisone; CS, clinical stage; CVPP, cyclophosphamide, vinblastine, procarbazine, prednisone; EBVP, epirubicin, bleomycin, vinblastine, prednisone; ECOG, Eastern Cooperative Oncology Group; EFS, event-free survival; EORTC, European Organization for Research and Treatment of Cancer; ESR, erythrocyte sedimentation rate; FFP, freedom from progression; FFTF, freedom from treatment failure; GATLA, Grupo Argentino de Tratamento de la Leucemia Aguda; GHSG, German Hodgkin Study Group; IFRT, involved-field irradiation; MOPP, mechlorethamine, vincristine, procarbazine, prednisone; m/t ratio, mass to thorax ratio; NS, not significant; PS, pathologic stage; Stanford V, mechlorethamine, doxorubicin, vinblastine, prednisone, vincristine, bleomycin, VP-16; RT, radiation therapy; STLI, subtotal nodal irradiation; SV, survival; TLI, total lymphoid irradiation.

doxorubicin, vincristine, prednisone, and etoposide versus 85% (*P* = .009) for CVPP.[227] In the EORTC trial, the event-free survival rate was 68% for EBVP II and involved-field radiotherapy versus 90% (*P* = .0001) for MOPP plus ABV.[215]

Several nonrandomized trials also have evaluated alternative chemotherapy regimens using reduced numbers of cycles of chemotherapy or modified chemotherapy regimens.[231,232] At Stanford, the Stanford V regimen, administered for 3 months, was followed by involved-field irradiation to 36 Gy in 38 patients with large mediastinal disease. No patients had relapsed or died (at a median follow-up of 40 months).[233]

Based mainly on trials in advanced HL, ABVD has become the standard regimen used in patients with clinical stage I and II disease. A number of current trials compare combined modality therapy using ABVD with more intense, novel regimens. Both the EORTC H9U and GHSG HD11 studies of com-

bined modality therapy are comparing four cycles of ABVD with four cycles of BEACOPP baseline (bleomycin, etoposide, doxorubicin, cyclophosphamide, vincristine, procarbazine, and prednisone). At the fourth interim analysis in August 2003, 1051 patients were evaluable, randomized to treatment between May 1998 and July 2002. At a median follow-up of 28 months, there was no difference between the arms receiving four cycles of ABVD and four cycles of BEACOPP baseline, nor between those receiving 20 and 30 Gy of involved-field radiation therapy. The FFTF rate for the total group was 90.0%, and the overall survival rate was 97.4%. There was no significant difference between the four groups in either complete responses, partial responses, progression, relapses, or deaths. In Eastern Cooperative Oncology Group (ECOG) trial 2496 of combined modality therapy, six cycles of ABVD are being compared to 3 months of therapy with the Stanford V regimen.

Trials to Identify the Optimal Number of Cycles of Chemotherapy

Two large, randomized trials are currently evaluating whether four cycles of combination chemotherapy and radiation therapy is sufficient treatment compared to six cycles of chemotherapy and radiation therapy. The closed EORTC H8U study randomized patients to combined modality therapy with four or six cycles of MOPP/ABV. The EORTC H9U trial, opened since 1998, randomizes patients to receive four to six cycles of ABVD.[218] A number of retrospective or prospective single-arm studies have evaluated the role of number of cycles of chemotherapy in patients with large mediastinal disease.[232,234,235] The results vary and the number of patients studied is small; a more definitive answer will need to come from the large randomized trials listed earlier.

Trials to Identify the Appropriate Radiation Therapy Volume

Several randomized trials have addressed the question of radiation therapy volumes in combined modality programs. The French trial reported by Zittoun and colleagues randomized 218 patients with stage I and II unfavorable-prognosis disease to receive six cycles of MOPP sandwiched around involved-field (40-Gy) or extended-field (40-Gy) irradiation.[236] The 6-year disease-free survival rates were 87% and 93%, respectively (*P* = .15). The Milan study reported by Bonfante et al. incorporated only four months of chemotherapy (ABVD), followed by involved-field irradiation (36 Gy) or subtotal nodal irradiation (30 to 36 Gy).[236a] The 5-year freedom-from-progression rates were 96% and 93%, respectively (Table 41.5-11).

The three-arm EORTC and Groupe d'Etude les Lymphomes de l'Adulte H8U trial randomized patients to four cycles of MOPP/ABV plus involved-field radiation or subtotal nodal irradiation. The GHSG HD8 trial, conducted between 1993 and 1998, used two cycles (four months) of COPP/ABVD followed by either involved-field or extended-field irradiation to 30 Gy (see Table 41.5-11). Preliminary evidence from these randomized trials, as well as several nonrandomized studies, suggests that radiation fields may be safely limited to involved regions in most combined modality programs when at least 4 months of chemotherapy is given.[236b,237,238]

Trials of Chemotherapy Alone versus Combined Modality Therapy

Only one prospective trial of chemotherapy alone versus combined modality therapy in treatment of unfavorable-prognosis stage I and II HL has been reported. The GATLA randomly assigned 104 patients with unfavorable disease characteristics to six cycles of CVPP alone or six cycles of CVPP sandwiched around involved-field irradiation (30 Gy). The 7-year survival rates were 66% and 84% and the freedom-from-relapse rates were 34% and 75% (*P* <.001), both favoring combined modality treatment.[239]

The ongoing NCIC HD6 trial evaluates patients with unfavorable disease characteristics but excludes patients with large mediastinal adenopathy or bulky disease. Patients are randomized to receive combined modality therapy with two cycles of ABVD followed by irradiation (an extended mantle plus splenic irradiation or mantle plus paraaortic and splenic irradiation) or four to six cycles of ABVD alone (depending on the rapidity of response).

Recommendations and Future Directions

The outcome of treatment for patients with unfavorable-prognosis stage I or II HL has improved dramatically in the past three decades. Mainly, this is due to the use of combined modality therapy, because historically radiation therapy alone and chemotherapy alone were associated with recurrence rates of approximately 50%. Current clinical trials are exploring new combinations of radiation therapy and chemotherapy to try to

---

TABLE 41.5-11. Randomized Clinical Trials in Unfavorable-Prognosis Stage I and II Hodgkin's Lymphoma: Trials to Identify the Appropriate Radiation Volume

Trial	Eligibility	Treatment Regimens	No. of Patients	Outcome
French Cooperative, 1976–1981	CS I–II *without* age >45 y; ≥3 involved areas; bulky disease	A: 3 MOPP + IFRT (40 Gy) + 3 MOPP B: 3 MOPP + EFRT (40 Gy) + 3 MOPP	82 91	DFS, 87%; SV (6 y), 92% DFS, 93%; SV (6 y), 91% (DFS: *P* = NS; SV: *P* = NS)
Istituto Nazionale Tumori, Milan, 1990–1997	All CS I–II	A: 4 ABVD + STLI B: 4 ABVD + IFRT	65 68	FFP, 96%; SV (5 y), 93% FFP, 94%; SV (5 y), 94% (FFP: *P* = NS; SV: *P* = NS)
EORTC/GELA H8U, 1993–1998	CS IA–IIB *with* age ≥50 y; ESR ≥50 mm/h in A, ≥30 mm/h in B; ≥4 involved sites; large mediastinal disease	A: 6 MOPP/ABV + IFRT (36 Gy) B: 4 MOPP/ABV + IFRT (36 Gy) C: 4 MOPP/ABV + STLI	335 333 327	RFS, 94%; SV (4 y), 90% RFS, 95%; SV (4 y), 95% RFS, 96%; SV (4 y), 93% (RFS: *P* = NS; SV: *P* = NS)
GHSG HD8, 1993–1998	CS IA–IIB *with* ESR ≥50 mm/h in A, ≥30 mm/h in B; ≥3 involved sites; large mediastinal disease	A: 4 COPP/ABVD + EFRT B: 4 COPP/ABVD + IFRT	532 532	FFTF, 86%; SV (5 y), 91% FFTF, 84%; SV (5 y), 92% (FFTF: *P* = NS; SV: *P* = NS)

ABV, doxorubicin (Adriamycin), bleomycin, vinblastine; ABVD, doxorubicin, bleomycin, vinblastine, dacarbazine; COPP, cyclophosphamide, vincristine, procarbazine, prednisone; CS, clinical stage; DFS, disease-free survival; EFRT, extended-field radiotherapy; EORTC, European Organization for Research and Treatment of Cancer; ESR, erythrocyte sedimentation rate; FFP, freedom from progression; FFTF, freedom from treatment failure; GELA, Groupe d'Etude des Lymphomes de l'Adulte; GHSG, German Hodgkin Study Group; IFRT, involved-field radiotherapy; MOPP, mechlorethamine, vincristine, procarbazine, prednisone; NS, not significant; RFS, relapse-free survival; STLI, subtotal nodal irradiation; SV, survival.

reduce late morbidity and mortality while maintaining a high probability of freedom from first recurrence.

A confusing aspect of the literature and current clinical trials is the variable definition of "unfavorable prognosis." Given the common use of combined modality therapy even in favorable-prognosis HL, it is time to reach a consensus on what constitutes "unfavorable." This may require a change in current eligibility criteria of some trials. For example, current combined modality management protocols for favorable-prognosis disease may be sufficient for patients who have three sites of disease or an ESR higher than 50 mm/h, factors considered unfavorable by some clinical trials groups. Detailed analysis of completed clinical trials may permit this redefinition, which would allow some patients to be treated with less aggressive management approaches. In contrast, there are data to suggest that patients with large mediastinal disease are not treated adequately with some of the lower-intensity regimens used for favorable-prognosis patients, and more aggressive management may always be required for this cohort of patients.

ADVANCED-STAGE DISEASE

Basic Regimens

MOPP: THE FIRST GENERATION. Initially, the four-drug MOPP regimen was administered with each drug given at full dose over 2 weeks, with a complete remission rate of 81%. Complete remission rates of 73% to 81%, long-term freedom from progression of 36% to 52%, and long-term overall survival of 50% to 64% were obtained in major trials of MOPP in advanced-stage disease.[240–242]

Despite the good initial results with MOPP therapy, several groups investigated alternative regimens to improve the efficacy or reduce toxicities. The CALGB showed that omission of the alkylating agents nitrogen mustard or procarbazine from the MOPP regimen was associated with inferior complete remission rates.[243] Thus the four-drug principle was considered a standard at that time, to which all alternative combinations had to be compared.

Modifications of the MOPP scheme included the substitution of an alkylating agent like cyclophosphamide or chlorambucil for mechlorethamine or a vinca alkaloid like vinblastine or vincristine as well as alteration of the doses of procarbazine and prednisone.

The ECOG compared a five-drug regimen containing carmustine, cyclophosphamide, vinblastine, procarbazine, and prednisone (BCVPP) with MOPP.[244] Their results showed that BCVPP was associated with a significantly higher freedom-from-progression rate (50% vs. 33%) and overall survival rate (83% vs. 75%) than did MOPP at 5 years. However, the interpretation of these results is complicated by the inclusion of previously treated patients.

In the United Kingdom the mechlorethamine, vinblastine, procarbazine, and prednisone (MVPP) combination was used and showed results comparable to those of MOPP, with complete response rates of 60% to 80% and 5-year overall survival rates of 70% to 80%.[245,246] Also in the United Kingdom, the chlorambucil, vinblastine, procarbazine, and prednisone (ChlVPP) regimen was developed and showed similar efficacy to MOPP with less acute toxicity, although a randomized comparison was not performed (Table 41.5-12). The BNLI performed a randomized trial to com-

pare chlorambucil, vincristine, procarbazine, and prednisone (LOPP) with MOPP. No significant differences were observed in complete response or overall survival rates.[247]

Taken together, several MOPP-like regimens showed similar efficacy with less acute gastrointestinal and neurologic toxicity.

ABVD: THE SECOND GENERATION. MOPP and derivatives had two limitations: (1) still only approximately 50% of patients could be cured, and (2) the alkylating agent–based combination was associated with an increased risk of sterility and acute leukemia.

In an attempt to develop a regimen for patients for whom MOPP treatment had failed, Bonadonna and colleagues introduced the ABVD regimen.[248] Vinblastine had demonstrated high activity as a single agent and lacked cross-resistance with vincristine in human tumors. Both doxorubicin and bleomycin were very active drugs and showed objective responses in approximately 50% of patients. Dacarbazine was added because it was active as a single agent and also showed synergism with doxorubicin.

The Milan group compared three cycles of MOPP or ABVD followed by extended-field irradiation and three additional cycles of the same chemotherapeutic regimen. A significant difference in favor of ABVD was achieved, with freedom-from-progression rates of 63% for MOPP versus 81% for ABVD.[249]

Both MOPP and ABVD were highly active regimens and had nonoverlapping toxicities. It was therefore straightforward to test combinations of MOPP and ABVD to further increase treatment results.

The Milan group randomized patients with stage IV disease to receive MOPP or MOPP/ABVD for up to 12 cycles. The results were emphatically in favor of the alternating program, with a statistically significant difference in freedom from progression at 8 years (36% for MOPP vs. 65% for MOPP/ABVD; $P <.005$). Subsequently, three large cooperative trial groups (ECOG, CALGB, and EORTC) have confirmed these findings and demonstrated superior results for the combination of MOPP/ABVD compared to MOPP or a MOPP derivative. The ECOG compared the MOPP derivative BCVPP with MOPP followed by ABVD. Both complete response and overall survival rates were superior with the MOPP/ABVD combination.[244]

In a three-arm trial, the CALGB compared 6 to 8 cycles of MOPP, 6 to 8 cycles of ABVD, and 12 cycles of MOPP alternating with ABVD. At 10 years, the failure-free survival rates were 38% for MOPP, 55% for ABVD, and 50% for MOPP/ABVD ($P = .02$). Overall survival was not significantly different, although there was a trend in favor of ABVD or MOPP/ABVD compared to MOPP alone.[250]

The EORTC compared two courses of MOPP alternating with two courses of ABVD to a total of eight courses with eight courses of MOPP alone. Radiotherapy was given to initial bulk or residual masses after chemotherapy. MOPP/ABVD was associated with a significantly higher failure-free survival rate at 6 years (43% for MOPP, 60% for MOPP/ABVD).[251]

Thus, ABVD alone and MOPP/ABVD were more effective than MOPP alone. In addition, ABVD alone had the advantage of less acute and long-term toxicities.

DURATION OF THERAPY. In the original NCI studies of MOPP, two additional monthly cycles were given after a complete remission was achieved.[252] Bonadonna et al. initially applied up to 12 cycles of MOPP, and later in the alternating program 8 cycles,

TABLE 41.5-12. Randomized Clinical Trials in Advanced-Stage Hodgkin's Lymphoma: Major Trials for Which Results Have Been Recently Published or Not Yet Published

Trial	Eligibility	Treatment Regimens	No. of Patients	Outcome
Manchester (Radford et al.)	—	A: 6 ChlVPP/EVA ± RT (bulk/resid) B: 11 VAPEC-B ± RT (bulk/resid)	144 138	FFTF, 82%; SV (5 y), 89% FFTF, 62%; SV (5 y), 79% (FFTF: *P* = .006; SV: *P* = .04)
GHSG HD9 (Diehl)	CS IIB with large mediastinal involvement, massive splenic involvement, or E lesions; CS III, IV	A: 8 COPP/ABVD ± RT (bulk/resid) B: 8 BEACOPP baseline ± RT (bulk/resid) C: 8 BEACOPP escalated ± RT (bulk/resid)	260 469 466	FFTF, 69%; SV (5 y), 83% FFTF, 76%; SV (5 y), 88% FFTF, 87%; SV (5 y), 91% (*P* <.0001; A vs. C: *P* <.002)
GHSG HD12 (Diehl)	CS IIB with large mediastinal involvement or E lesions; CS III, IV	A: BEACOPP (escalated × 8) ± RT (bulk/resid) B: BEACOPP (escalated × 8) C: BEACOPP (escalated × 4 + baseline × 4) ± RT (bulk/resid) D: BEACOPP (escalated × 4 + baseline × 4)	Began 01/1998; planned: n = 1200	Final analysis planned for 2006
GHSG HD15 (Diehl)	CS IIB with large mediastinal involvement or E lesions; CS III, IV	A: 8 BEACOPP escalated + EPO/placebo + IFRT (30 Gy for PET-positive PR) B: 6 BEACOPP escalated + EPO/placebo + IFRT (30 Gy for PET-positive PR) C: 8 BEACOPP-14 + EPO/placebo + IFRT (30 Gy for PET-positive PR)	Opened 01/2003	Open
EORTC 20884 (09/1989–03/2000)	CS III and IV	6–8 MOPP/ABV + (if CR after 6 cycles): →A: IFRT (24–30 Gy) →B: No further treatment Not randomized PR	Total: 736 172 161 85 250	 EFS, 79%; SV (5 y), 91% EFS, 84%; SV (5 y), 85% (EFS: *P* = .35; SV: *P* = .10) EFS, 79%; SV, 87%
GELA (Fermé & Diviné)	IPS 0–2	A: 6 ABVD ± RT (bulk) B: Intensified conventional CT ± RT (bulk)	ne	ne
GELA/EBMT H96-1 (Fermé & Diviné)	IPS 3+	A: Brief intensified CT then HDCT + ASCT ± RT (bulk) B: 8 ABVD ± RT (bulk)	83 80	FFS, 75%; SV (5 y), 86% FFS, 82%; SV (5 y), 88% (FFS: *P* = .4; SV: *P* = .6)
UKLG (BNLI) LY09 (Hancock)	Disease requiring systemic therapy: CS I–II with bulk or >3 sites; CS III–IV	A: 6–8 ABVD ± RT (bulk/resid) B: 6–8 ChlVPP/PABlOE ± RT (bulk/resid) *or* 6–8 ChlVPP/EVA ± RT (bulk/resid)	Recruitment: 04/1997–09/2001; n = 807	SV (3 y), 91% SV (3 y), 88%
UKLG (BNLI) phase II study (Hancock)	CS IIB, III, IV with large mediastinal involvement or ≥2 extranodal sites	A: 6–8 ABVD ± RT (bulk) B: Stanford V ± RT (bulk)	Began 03/1998; planned: n = 80	End point: response; phase III trial to follow
SNLG HDIII (Proctor et al.[193])	SNLG index <0.5 (high risk)	3 PVACEBOP ± RT (bulk) + (if response): →A: Melphalan, VP-16 then HDCT + ASCT →B: 2 PVACEBOP	n = 107, randomized n = 65	Median follow-up, 6 y OS, 78% (all patients) TTF (5 y), arms not different TTF, 79 ± 11% TTF, 85 ± 7% (TTF: *P* = .35)
SWOG/ECOG 2496 (Horning & Coltman)	CS II with bulk and III and IV; IPS 0–2	A: 6–8 ABVD ± RT (bulk) B: Stanford V ± RT	Open	Open
Global study, EORTC 20012	CS III and IV	A: 8 ABVD B: 4 BEACOPP escalated + 4 BEACOPP baseline	Opened 01/2003	Open
SWOG/ECOG	CS II with bulk and III and IV; IPS 3+	No radiation A: ABVD B: ABVD then HDCT (BCNU, VP-16, cyclophosphamide) + ASCT	—	—

ABV, doxorubicin (Adriamycin), bleomycin, vinblastine; ABVD, doxorubicin, bleomycin, vinblastine, dacarbazine; ASCT, autologous stem cell transplantation; BEACOPP, bleomycin, etoposide, doxorubicin, cyclophosphamide, vincristine, procarbazine, prednisone; BEACOPP-14, BEACOPP regimen with 14-d interval between courses; ChlVPP, chlorambucil, vinblastine, procarbazine, and prednisone; COPP, cyclophosphamide, vincristine, procarbazine, prednisone; CR, complete response; CS, clinical stage; CT, computed tomography; ECOG, Eastern Cooperative Oncology Group; EFS, event-free survival; EORTC, European Organization for Research and Treatment of Cancer; EPO, erythropoietin; EBMT, European Bone Marrow Transplant Registry; EVA, etoposide, vincristine, and doxorubicin; FFS, failure-free survival; FFTF, freedom from treatment failure; GELA, Groupe d'Etude des Lymphomes de l'Adulte; GHSG, German Hodgkin Study Group; HDCT, high-dose chemotherapy; IFRT, involved-field radiotherapy; IPS, international prognostic score (International Prognostic Factors Project); MOPP, mechlorethamine, vincristine, procarbazine, prednisone; OS, overall survival; PABlOE, prednisolone, doxorubicin, bleomycin, vincristine, etoposide; PET, positron emission tomography; PR, partial response; PVACEBOP, prednisolone, vinblastine, doxorubicin, chlorambucil, etoposide, bleomycin, vincristine, procarbazine; resid, residual; RT, radiotherapy; SNLG, Scotland and Newcastle Lymphoma Group; Stanford V, mechlorethamine, doxorubicin, vinblastine, prednisone, vincristine, bleomycin, VP-16; SV, survival; SWOG, Southwest Oncology Group; TTF, time to treatment failure; UKLG (BNLI), United Kingdom Lymphoma Group (British National Lymphoma Investigation); VAPEC-B, doxorubicin, cyclophosphamide, etoposide, vincristine, bleomycin, prednisolone.

without reduction in efficacy.[242] The CALGB trial demonstrated that 8 cycles of ABVD was comparable to 12 cycles of alternating MOPP/ABVD.[253] A total of 8 to 12 cycles of chemotherapy was given in the more recent phase III trials. Thus, although the optimal duration is not known precisely, eight cycles of MOPP, ABVD, or a combination appears to be sufficient. PET may be useful to differentiate between residual disease or fibrosis in this situation.

There are ongoing studies testing the positive and negative predictability of PET findings after chemotherapy in patients with advanced stages of HL to answer the following questions: How many cycles are needed to control the disease? Is consolidative radiation therapy needed?

The ongoing GHSG HD15 trial delivers radiation therapy only to residual lesions larger than 2.5 cm or rest tumors that have not shrunk by more than 70% of the initial size.

There is no role, however, for maintenance therapy in advanced HL.

Hybrid Regimens: The Third Generation

The theoretic basis for multidrug regimens is the predicted advantage of the early introduction of all active agents to avoid development of resistant tumor cell clones. This idea is based on a model proposed by Goldie and Coldman,[254] who related the drug sensitivity of tumors to their spontaneous mutation rate. This model formed the basis of hybrid schemes that were tested by several groups in treatment of advanced-stage HL.

Groups in Vancouver and Milan independently designed two hybrids of MOPP and ABVD to test the Goldie-Coldman hypothesis prospectively.[254] The NCIC compared the MOPP/ABV hybrid with alternating MOPP and ABVD in patients with stage IIIB or IV HL. At 5 years there was no significant difference between arms in overall survival rates; however, the hybrid regime was associated with higher hematologic and nonhematologic toxicities.[255]

The Milan group compared their MOPP/ABV hybrid with alternating MOPP and ABVD. Freedom-from-progression and overall survival rates at 10 years were not significantly different between the hybrid and alternating arms.[201]

The GHSG compared a new hybrid scheme of COPP, ABV, and ifosfamide, methotrexate, and etoposide (IMEP) with their standard COPP/ABVD regimen. Complete response, FFTF, and overall survival rates showed no statistically significant difference between treatment arms.[256,256a]

A second intergroup trial that compared a MOPP/ABV hybrid with ABVD was conducted in the United States and recruited a total of 856 patients with stage III or IV HL or recurrent disease after radiotherapy. This study was prematurely stopped by the Data and Safety Monitoring Committee because an excess of treatment-related deaths and second malignancies was observed with the hybrid regimen. At 3 years similar failure-free survival rates were observed for ABVD (65%) and MOPP/ABV (67%). From this trial it was concluded that ABVD and MOPP/ABV are equally effective but that ABVD is less toxic and should remain the standard treatment.

The potential relevance of scheduling was exemplified in a BNLI study in which a significant difference was found between a LOPP and etoposide, vincristine, and doxorubicin (EVA) hybrid regimen and a regimen of LOPP alternating with EVA that contained identical total doses. The complete remission rate was significantly lower in the hybrid arm, and the trial was stopped prematurely.[257]

To summarize, the Goldie-Coldman hypothesis could not be proven in treatment of advanced-stage HL, although this could be due to the fact that the optimal hybrid regimen had not been identified. ABVD has emerged as the standard against which newer treatments must be compared. With ABVD therapy, 60% to 70% of patients are free of disease at 5 years. ABVD is much less likely to cause severe myelotoxicity, acute leukemia, or sterility than treatment programs that contain significant doses of alkylating agents.

New Chemotherapy Regimens: The Fourth Generation—Stanford V, ChlVPP/EVA, VAPEC-B

The success of ABVD in the CALGB and intergroup trials indicated that alkylating agents are not essential for curative treatment for advanced HL. However, the pulmonary toxicity of bleomycin, which is especially pronounced in children and in combination with mediastinal irradiation, remains a major concern with ABVD. A number of drugs showing high efficacy in treatment of relapsed HL have become candidates for use in first-line therapy. The topoisomerase inhibitor etoposide has received special interest by several groups, because a 20% to 60% response rate in refractory HL was reported with single-agent etoposide.[258] Based on these considerations, several etoposide-containing drug regimens were developed recently.

At Stanford, the regimen Stanford V was developed.[221] The regimen was given weekly over a total of 12 weeks. Sophisticated consolidative radiotherapy to sites of initial bulky disease was used. In this phase II trial 126 patients were recruited. The estimated 5-year freedom from progression was 89% and the overall survival was 96% at a median observation time of 4.5 years in this single-center study. Reduced long-term toxicities with preserved fertility was a major goal and could be achieved both in men and women. An intergroup trial comparing the Stanford V regimen with ABVD has been initiated in selected patients with low-risk advanced HL. Similarly, the Manchester group developed an abbreviated, 11-week chemotherapy program, VAPEC-B. In a randomized trial, VAPEC-B and the hybrid ChlVPP/EVA regimen were compared with radiotherapy delivered to previous bulk disease or residual disease.[259] This study was stopped after 26 months due to a threefold increase in the rate of progression after VAPEC-B. At a median follow-up of 4.9 years, results showed significant differences in favor of the ChlVPP/EVA regimen in terms of freedom from progression (82% vs. 62% at 5 years), event-free survival (78% vs. 58% at 5 years), and overall survival (89% vs. 79% at 5 years). The Southampton group developed another abbreviated weekly chemotherapy regimen of prednisone, doxorubicin, cyclophosphamide, etoposide, bleomycin, vincristine, methotrexate (PACE-BOM).[260] Radiotherapy was delivered to residual disease. A 64% failure-free survival rate was reported after a median observation time of 5 years.

Caution should be exercised when comparing results across different trials; in particular, the amount of consolidative radiation used can vary widely. Large randomized trials provide the only reliable comparisons between regimens. Table 41.5-13 shows the doses and scheduling of polychemotherapy regimens in HL.

Dose Density and Dose Intensity

In several animal models, a clear relationship between chemotherapy dose and tumor response has been demonstrated. In HL, retrospective analyses of drug delivery with MOPP chemo-

TABLE 41.5-13. Polychemotherapy Regimens Used in Hodgkin's Lymphoma

Drug	Dose (mg/m²)	Route	Schedule (D)	Cycle Length (D)
MOPP				21
Mechlorethamine	6	IV	1, 8	
Oncovin (vincristine)	1.4	IV	1, 8	
Procarbazine	100	PO	1–14	
Prednisone	40	PO	1–14	
COPP				28
Cyclophosphamide	650	IV	1, 8	
Oncovin (vincristine)	1.4	IV	1, 8	
Procarbazine	100	PO	1–14	
Prednisone	40	PO	1–14	
LOPP				28
Leukeran (chlorambucil)	10 total	PO	1–10	
Oncovin (vincristine)	1.4	IV	1, 8	
Procarbazine	100	PO	1–10	
Prednisone	25	PO	1–14	
ABVD				28
Adriamycin (doxorubicin)	25	IV	1, 15	
Bleomycin	10	IV	1, 15	
Vinblastine	6	IV	1, 15	
Dacarbazine	375	IV	1, 15	
MOPP/ABV HYBRID				28
Mechlorethamine	6	IV	1	
Oncovin (vincristine)	1.4[a]	IV	1	
Procarbazine	100	PO	1–7	
Prednisone	40	PO	1–14	
Adriamycin (doxorubicin)	35	IV	8	
Bleomycin	10	IV	8	
Vinblastine	6	IV	8	
BEACOPP (BASELINE)				21
Bleomycin	10	IV	8	
Etoposide	100	IV	1–3	
Adriamycin (doxorubicin)	25	IV	1	
Cyclophosphamide	650	IV	1	
Oncovin (vincristine)	1.4[a]	IV	8	
Procarbazine	100	PO	1–7	
Prednisone	40	PO	1–14	
BEACOPP-14				14
Bleomycin	10	IV	8	
Etoposide	100	IV	1–3	
Adriamycin (doxorubicin)	25	IV	1	
Cyclophosphamide	650	IV	1	
Oncovin (vincristine)	1.4[a]	IV	8	
Procarbazine	100	PO	1–7	
Prednisone	80	PO	1–7	
INCREASED-DOSE BEACOPP				22
Cyclophosphamide	1250	IV	1	
Adriamycin	35	IV	1	
Etoposide	200	IV	1–3	
Procarbazine	100	PO	1–7	
Prednisone	40	PO	1–14	
Oncovin (vincristine)	1.4 (maximum 2 mg)	IV	8	
Bleomycin	10	IV	8	
G-CSF	—	SC	From d 8	
ChlVPP/EVA				28
Chorambucil	6	PO	1–7	
Vinblastine	6	IV	8	
Procarbazine	90	PO	1–7	
Prednisolone	50	PO	1–7	
Etoposide	75–100	PO	1–5	
Vincristine	1.4	IV	1	
Adriamycin (doxorubicin)	50	IV	8	

(continued)

TABLE 41.5-13. *(Continued)*

Drug	Dose (mg/m²)	Route	Schedule (D)	Cycle Length (D)
				50
ChlVPP/PABlOE				
Chorambucil	6	PO	1–14	
Vinblastine	6	IV	1, 8	
Procarbazine	100	PO	1–14, 29–43	
Prednisolone	30	PO	1–14	
Adriamycin (doxorubicin)	40	IV	29	
Bleomycin	10	IV	29, 36	
Oncovin (vincristine)	1.4[a]	IV	29, 36	
Etoposide	200	PO	30–32	
STANFORD V				12 wk
Mechlorethamine	6	IV	Wk 1, 5, 9	
Adriamycin (doxorubicin)	25	IV	Wk 1, 3, 5, 7, 9, 11	
Vinblastine	6	IV	Wk 1, 3, 5, 7, 9, 11	
Vincristine	1.4[a]	IV	Wk 2, 4, 6, 8, 10, 12	
Bleomycin	5	IV	Wk 2, 4, 6, 8, 10, 12	
Etoposide	60 × 2	IV	Wk 3, 7, 11	
Prednisone	40	IV	Wk 1–10 q.o.d.	
G-CSF	—	PO	Dose reduction or delay	
MEC				28
Mechlorethamine	6	IV	1 (courses 1, 3, 5)	
Lomustine (CCNU)	100	PO	1 (courses 2, 4, 6)	
Vindesine	3	IV	1	
Melphalan (Alkeran)	6	PO	1–3	
Prednisone	40	PO	1–14	
Epidoxorubicin	40	IV	8	
Vincristine	1.4	IV	8	
Procarbazine	100	PO	8–14	
Vinblastine	6	IV	1	
Bleomycin	10	IV	15	
VAPEC-B				11 wk
Vincristine	1.4[a]	IV	Wk 2, 4, 6, 8, 10	
Adriamycin (doxorubicin)	35	IV	Wk 1, 3, 5, 7, 9, 11	
Prednisolone	50	PO	Wk 1–6	
Etoposide	75–100 × 5	PO	Wk 3, 7, 11	
Cyclophosphamide	350	IV	Wk 1, 5, 9	
Bleomycin	10	IV	Wk 2, 4, 6, 8, 10	

G-CSF, granulocyte colony-stimulating factor.

[a]Vincristine dose capped at 2 mg.

therapy showed that patients receiving less than the optimal doses had inferior results.[261] Such dose effects were detected independently for mustard, procarbazine, and vincristine.

There are two principal ways to test dose intensity: Doses of cytotoxic drugs can be intensified by increasing individual drug dose, shortening the interval between treatments, or both. The first two strategies increase dose intensity; raising the dose as well as shortening the time schedule increases the dose density. Because there are no or at most very few new drugs on the market for improving treatment of solid tumors and hematologic malignancies, many researchers have started to investigate the impact of dose intensity and dose density. This dose density concept was transferred to clinical trials in 1992 by the GHSG with the time- and dose-intensified BEACOPP regimen.

Until that time, no prospective randomized trials to analyze the role of dose intensity and dose density in the treatment of advanced HL had been conducted. Two German trials testing these questions prospectively were started around 1992. A rather small study was initiated by Gerhartz et al.[262] comparing conventional COPP/ABVD with a dose- and time-escalated COPP/ABVD regimen given with granulocyte-macrophage colony-stimulating factor support. The delivered dose intensity in the dose-intensified arm was 1.22 compared with 0.92 in the standard arm (1.0 = standard intended dose). The GHSG has conducted a series of clinical trials to address the role of dose intensity in treatment of advanced HL in a comprehensive way. A mathematical model of tumor growth and chemotherapy effects was developed and fitted to the data for 705 patients treated by the GHSG.[263] This model predicted that moderate dose escalation would increase tumor control by 10% to 15% at 5 years. The BEACOPP regimen was devised and used as a standard combination for dose escalation.[264] After excellent tolerability and efficacy were established in a pilot trial, a second study of escalated BEACOPP was performed in which doxorubicin was increased to a fixed level and doses of cyclophosphamide and etoposide were increased in a stepwise fashion with granulocyte colony-stimulating factor support.[265] Maximum practicable doses were found to be 190% of cyclophosphamide and 200% of etoposide.

The GHSG then designed a three-arm study comparing COPP/ABVD, standard BEACOPP, and escalated BEACOPP for treatment of patients with advanced HL.[266] Radiotherapy was

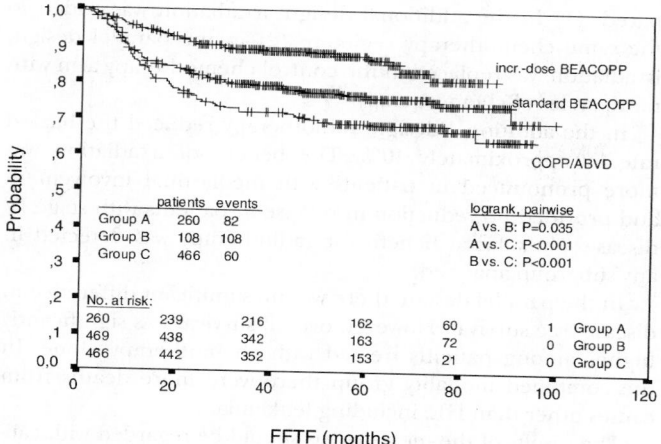

FIGURE 41.5-4. Treatment of advanced-stage Hodgkin's lymphoma (FFTF, HD9 trial of the German Hodgkin Study Group.) BEACOPP, bleomycin, etoposide, doxorubicin, cyclophosphamide, vincristine, procarbazine, and prednisone; COPP/ABVD, cyclophosphamide, vincristine, procarbazine, and prednisone plus doxorubicin, bleomycin, vinblastine, and dacarbazine; FFTF, freedom from treatment failure; incr., increased.

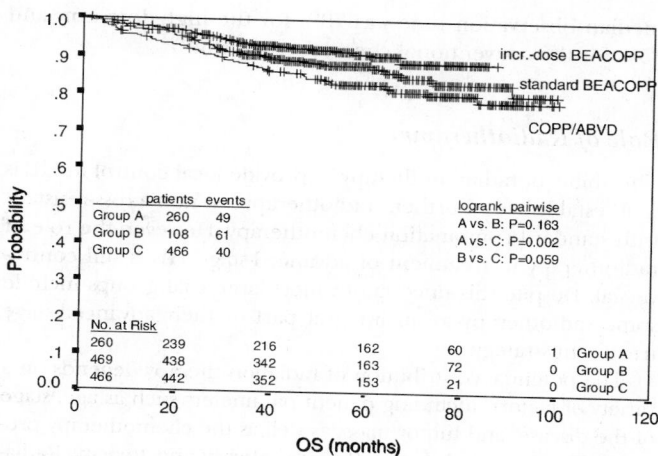

FIGURE 41.5-5. Treatment of advanced-stage Hodgkin's lymphoma (OS, HD9 trial of the German Hodgkin Study Group.) BEACOPP, bleomycin, etoposide, doxorubicin, cyclophosphamide, vincristine, procarbazine, and prednisone; COPP/ABVD, cyclophosphamide, vincristine, procarbazine, and prednisone plus doxorubicin, bleomycin, vinblastine, and dacarbazine; incr., increased; OS, overall survival.

prescribed for bulky disease at diagnosis or for residual disease after eight cycles of chemotherapy, and approximately two-thirds of patients received consolidation radiotherapy. In 1996, at the time of a planned interim analysis, the COPP/ABVD arm of this trial was closed to accrual because of superior outcomes in the combined BEACOPP arms.[266] In the final analysis in July 2001, 1195 of 1201 patients could be evaluated: 260 in the COPP/ABVD group, 469 in the standard BEACOPP group, and 466 in the increased-dose BEACOPP group. At a median observation time of approximately 5 years, the rate of FFTF was 69% for COPP/ABVD, 76% for standard BEACOPP, and 87% for the increased BEACOPP group (P = .004 for the comparison between the COPP/ABVD group and the BEACOPP baseline group, and P <.001 for the comparisons between the increased-dose BEACOPP group and the COPP/ABVD group and the standard BEACOPP group). The 5-year rates for overall survival were 83%, 88%, and 91% for COPP/ABVD, standard BEACOPP, and increased BEACOPP, respectively (P = .002 for the comparison between the COPP/ABVD group and the increased BEACOPP group). Rates of early progression were significantly lower with increased-dose BEACOPP than with COPP/ABVD or with standard BEACOPP (10%, 8%, and 2%, respectively).[267] Although there was a trend in the overall survival rate in favor of BEACOPP, this was only just significant (P = .06) at this point of analysis in 2001. Furthermore, the increased BEACOPP arm overcame the adverse prognostic variables identified by Hasenclever and Diehl.[198]

Figures 41.5-4 and 41.5-5 show the Kaplan-Meier analysis of the probability of FFTF and overall survival, respectively.

As expected, increased BEACOPP was associated with greater hematologic toxicity, including a greater use of both red blood cell and platelet transfusions; there was no difference between COPP/ABVD and standard BEACOPP. There were nine cases of acute myeloid leukemia (AML) and myelodysplastic syndrome (MDS) in the increased BEACOPP group, two in the standard BEACOPP group, and one in the COPP/ABVD group; the total rate of second neoplasias was highest in the COPP/ABVD arm, however.

As an example of a time-intensified chemotherapy regimen, the GHSG evaluated the BEACOPP-14 regimen, in which the

intervals between the BEACOPP treatment courses were shortened to 14 days. The aim was to maintain the high efficacy of the BEACOPP schedule while reducing toxicity, especially the rate of AML and MDS. The regimen was tested in a multicenter pilot study, with the final analysis showing an estimated FFTF of 90% and an overall survival of 97%. Acute hematotoxicity was similar to that of baseline and intensified BEACOPP.[268] Chisesi et al. conducted a randomized trial to test the MEC regimen [mechlorethamine, lomustine (CCNU), vindesine, melphalan, prednisone, epidoxorubicin, vincristine, procarbazine, vinblastine, bleomycin] against the ABVD and Stanford V regimens. Results in terms of FFS and response were superior for both ABVD and MEC.[269]

High-Dose Chemotherapy as Introductory Treatment

HDCT is frequently used in patients with first or later relapses of HL. Numerous phase II trials and two randomized trials from the BNLI and the GHSG have indicated better results with a high-dose program than with conventional treatment.[270–272] For advanced-stage HL, however, limited data concerning the role of HDCT are available. The Genoa group of Carella et al.[273] conducted a phase II trial of myeloablative therapy and autografting in patients with poor risk features described by Straus et al.[274] Subsequently, the European Bone Marrow Transplant Registry (EBMT) initiated a prospective study in poor-risk patients comparing HDCT and autografting (arm A) with additional chemotherapy after four cycles of ABVD-containing chemotherapy (arm B). Results revealed no promising option to improve outcome in advanced-stage disease with first-line HDCT. After a median follow-up of 48 months, the 5-year failure-free survival rates for HDCT with ASCT and additional ABVD were 75% and 82%, respectively.[275] Proctor et al. used their previously published model to identify at-risk patients for participation in a study in which patients were randomized to additional chemotherapy or HDCT and autografting after three cycles of a hybrid regimen and radiotherapy to bulky sites.[202,274] There was no difference between the two groups: The time to treatment failure after 6 years' median observation time was 79% for the high-dose arm and 85% for the conventional chemotherapy arm.[193]

Role of Radiotherapy

The ability of radiation therapy to provide local control in HL is well established. Further, radiotherapy is non–cross-resistant with standard combination chemotherapy. However, the role of radiotherapy in treatment of advanced-stage HL is still controversial. Despite this uncertainty, most large trial groups include some radiotherapy as an integral part of their advanced-stage treatment strategy.

The potential contribution of radiation therapy depends on a variety of factors, including patient parameters such as age, stage of the disease, and tumor mass, as well as the chemotherapy program. The field and dose influence efficacy and toxicity. Radiation therapy for advanced HL can be considered in three clinical settings. First, radiotherapy may be used as an adjuvant after complete remission with standard chemotherapy. Second, radiotherapy may be an integrated component of a combined modality program, possibly with reduced or brief chemotherapy. Finally, radiotherapy can serve as a non–cross-resistant treatment for patients with partial or uncertain response after chemotherapy.

Combined Modality Therapy

The role of radiotherapy in advanced-stage disease in combination with polychemotherapy has not been not fully evaluated and remains highly controversial. Although the contribution of radiotherapy is not clear, most large investigative groups include radiotherapy in their phase III trials.

There have been several reports indicating that patients treated with chemotherapy alone failed to completely respond or progressed, primarily in previously involved nodal sites. In a SWOG study, 80% of relapses after chemotherapy with nitrogen mustard, vincristine, prednisone, bleomycin, doxorubicin, and procarbazine (MOP-BAP) were detected in initially involved sites.[276] A number of authors have reported that approximately 30% of selected patients who experience relapse after chemotherapy can achieve long-term remissions with radiotherapy. However, the benefits of consolidative radiotherapy must be balanced against the risk for serious side effects, particularly second malignancy in the irradiated field.

A number of phase III trials have investigated the role of consolidative radiotherapy after primary chemotherapy with divergent results. After MOP-BAP chemotherapy, 61% of patients who achieved complete remission were randomized to low-dose involved-field radiotherapy or no further treatment in a SWOG study.[276] In this trial no significant differences in remission duration or overall survival were detected.

The GHSG compared the role of low-dose (20-Gy) involved-field radiotherapy versus two cycles of further chemotherapy consolidation in 288 patients who showed a complete response after initial chemotherapy with COPP/ABVD. There was no significant difference in freedom-from-progression or overall survival rates between treatment arms.[277]

To overcome the insufficient power of the randomized studies with too few patients to detect a relevant difference, Loeffler et al.[278] performed a metaanalysis of 14 studies involving more than 1700 patients in total. Two study designs were compared: (1) In the additional design, irradiation was added to the same chemotherapy regimen; (2) in the parallel design, irradiation was replaced in the control chemotherapy arm with more cycles of chemotherapy.

In the additional design, radiotherapy reduced the hazard rate by approximately 40%. The benefit of irradiation was more pronounced in patients with mediastinal involvement and provided no reduction in relapse in patients with stage IV disease. No survival benefit for radiotherapy was detected in any subgroup analyzed.

In the parallel design, there was no significant difference in disease-free survival. However, overall survival was significantly higher among patients treated with chemotherapy alone. In the combined modality group there were more deaths from causes other than HL, including leukemia.

The results of the metaanalysis should be regarded with caution, because the studies were initiated 20 or more years ago and because in most instances MOPP-based chemotherapy regimens were used, which are not regarded as standard therapy today.

The most important issue today relates to the added efficacy of radiotherapy as adjuvant treatment to modern anthracycline-containing chemotherapy regimens and the added late toxicity of this combined modality. Prospective randomized trials, such as the comparison of a MOPP/ABV hybrid regimen with and without consolidative radiotherapy by the EORTC, are needed to address these questions.[279] In the EORTC trial patients in complete remission after MOPP/ABV chemotherapy received two further chemotherapy cycles followed by randomization to involved-field radiotherapy or observation. The final analysis in June 2003 encompassed 421 patients in complete remission who were randomized to receive either additional involved-field radiotherapy or no further treatment. The 5-year event-free survival and 5-year overall survival rates were higher (84% and 91%) in the group receiving no further treatment than in the group receiving additional involved-field radiotherapy (79% and 85%).[280] A study using a similar approach with a potentially more active chemotherapy, BEACOPP, was performed by the GHSG. In this HD12 trial patients with advanced HL (stage IIB with large mediastinal mass, B symptoms, and extranodal disease, and all stage III and IV disease) were randomized to eight cycles of increased BEACOPP or four cycles of increased BEACOPP plus four cycles BEACOPP baseline. Subsequently patients were randomized to receive radiotherapy to initial bulky and residual disease or no further treatment. The third interim analysis of this study performed in March 2003 encompassed 904 evaluable patients for the chemotherapy comparison and 869 evaluable patients for the radiotherapy comparison. At a median observation time of 24 months, the FFTF rate for the total group was 89.2% and the overall survival rate was 94.6%. There was no difference between the arms with and without radiotherapy, when prescribed radiotherapy was considered, in either FFTF or overall survival. The important messages from these two trials are the following:

> Consolidative radiation in treatment of advanced stages of HL after use of an effective, anthracycline-containing chemotherapy regimen [ABVD, M-COPP/ABV(D), BEACOPP, MEC] can be restricted to patients who do not show a complete response or show a partial response and is not needed by patients who experience a complete response or unconfirmed complete response. This cuts down the num-

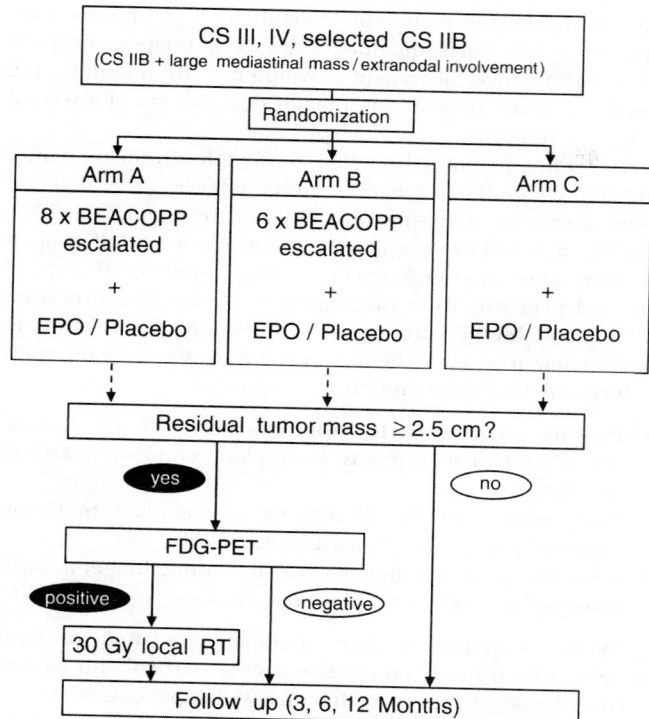

FIGURE 41.5-6. HD15 trial design. CS, clinical stage; BEACOPP, bleomycin, etoposide, doxorubicin, cyclophosphamide, vincristine, procarbazine, and prednisone; EPO, erythropoietin; FDG-PET, [¹⁸F]Fluorodeoxyglucose positron emission tomography; RT, radiotherapy. (See Color Fig. 41.5-6 in the CD-ROM.)

ber of patients receiving consolidative radiation from around 70% in earlier studies to 20% to 30%.

It is mandatory to evaluate further in prospective clinical trials (1) the diagnostic value of PET for the assessment of residual

disease, and (2) the amount of radiation (dose and field size) needed to offer a robust and long-lasting complete response.

The recently begun GHSG HD15 trial involving patients with advanced-stage HL addresses some of these issues. Figure 41.5-6 shows the design of the HD15 trial.

Conclusions

After more than 30 years of clinical research, advanced-stage HL became a curable disease in most instances. Doxorubicin-containing chemotherapy has emerged as the standard against which modern strategies must be compared. With modern chemotherapy, 60% to 70% of patients are alive and free of disease at 5 years (Table 41.5-14). ABVD has a favorable toxicity profile and causes less myelotoxicity, acute leukemia, and sterility relative to many previous treatment programs containing alkylating agents. However, 20% to 30% of patients eventually experience relapse and are then frequently treated with high-dose regimens.

There are two major goals in advanced HL: (1) to improve the cure rate and (2) to reduce acute and late toxicities. The definition of prognostic factors has allowed identification of patients who are at a higher risk for relapse as well as those for whom less toxic approaches might be tested. The optimal approach or program has not yet been identified, although new chemotherapy regimens with increased efficacy such as Stanford V and BEACOPP have been identified. These new drug combinations hold the promise of achieving these goals, but efficacy and toxicity data must mature before their contributions can be assessed with certainty (see Table 41.5-12). Although the addition of radiotherapy improved disease control in some trials, a survival benefit was not identified and the role of radiotherapy remains controversial.

Recommendations for primary treatment of early-stage (favorable and unfavorable) and advanced-stage HL outside clinical trials are given in Table 41.5-15.

TABLE 41.5-14. Results of Polychemotherapy Regimens in Advanced-Stage Disease

Regimen	RT (%)	CR (%)	EFS/FFP/FFTF %	Years	Parameter	Survival %	Years	Reference
ABVD	0	82	61	5	FFP	73	5	250
MOPP/ABVD	0	83	65	5	FFP	75	5	250
MOPP/ABV	0	83	64	8	FFP	79	5	424
ABVD	0	71	65	5	FFS	87	5	425
MOPP/ABV	NS	73	67	5	FFS	85	5	425
MOPP/ABVD	NS	76	67	5	FFP	83	5	426
MOPP/ABV	NS	80	71	5	FFP	81	5	426
ChlVPP/EVA	NS	65	73	5	EFS	83	5	259
COPP/ABVD	63	83	69	3	FFTF	86	3	266
BEACOPP, baseline	72	88	79	3	FFTF	90	3	266
MOPP/ABV	67	95	82	5	EFS	84	5	279
Stanford V	86	99	89	5	FFP	93	5	233
BEACOPP, escalated	72	96	88	3	FFTF	91	3	266
BEACOPP-14	70	94	90	3	FFTF	97	3	268

ABV, doxorubicin (Adriamycin), bleomycin, vinblastine; ABVD, doxorubicin, vinblastine, bleomycin, dacarbazine; BEACOPP, bleomycin, etoposide, doxorubicin, cyclophosphamide, vincristine, procarbazine, prednisone; BEACOPP-14, BEACOPP regimen with 14-d interval between courses; ChlVPP, chlorambucil, vinblastine, procarbazine, and prednisone; COPP, cyclophosphamide, vincristine, procarbazine, prednisone; CR, complete response; EFS, event-free survival; FFP, freedom from progression; FFTF, freedom from treatment failure; MOPP, mechlorethamine, vincristine, procarbazine, prednisone; Stanford V, mechlorethamine, doxorubicin, vinblastine, prednisone, vincristine, bleomycin, VP-16; NS, not specified; RT, radiotherapy.

TABLE 41.5-15. Recommendations for Primary Treatment Outside Clinical Trials

Group	Stage	Recommendation
Early stages (favorable)	CS I–II A/B no RF	EFRT (30–36 Gy) *or* 4–6 cycles CT[a] + IFRT (20–36 Gy)
Early stages (unfavorable)	CS I–II A/B + RF	4–6 cycles CT[b] + IFRT (20–36 Gy)
Advanced stages	CS IIB + RF; CS III A/B; CS IV A/B	6–8 cycles CT[c] + RT (20–36 Gy) to residual lymphoma and bulk

CS, clinical stage; CT, chemotherapy; EFRT, extended-field radiotherapy; IFRT, involved-field radiotherapy; RF, risk factors (see Table 41.5-7); RT, radiotherapy.

[a]ABVD [doxorubicin (Adriamycin), bleomycin, vinblastine, and dacarbazine], EBVP (epirubicin, bleomycin, vinblastine, and prednisone), or VBM (vinblastine, bleomycin, and methotrexate).

[b]ABVD, Stanford V (mechlorethamine, Adriamycin, vinblastine, vincristine, etoposide, bleomycin, and prednisone), or MOPP/ABV [mechlorethamine, vincristine (Oncovin), procarbazine, and prednisone/Adriamycin, bleomycin, vinblastine].

[c]ABVD, MOPP/ABV, ChlVPP/EVA (chlorambucil, vinblastine, procarbazine, and prednisone/etoposide, vincristine, and Adriamycin), or BEACOPP (bleomycin, etoposide, Adriamycin, cyclophosphamide, vincristine, procarbazine, and prednisone) escalated.

PROGRESSIVE AND RELAPSED DISEASE

Diagnosis and Staging at Disease Progression or Relapse

Although late relapses more than 10 years after primary treatment have been reported in HL, relapse generally occurs within 1 to 5 years after primary therapy.[281] At relapse, a new histologic analysis should be performed, because the risk for second tumors—NHL or solid tumors—is increased.[282,283] Moreover, a proportion of patients with NHL are initially misdiagnosed as having HL, or composite lymphomas are not detected during first diagnosis.[284] Therefore, another biopsy at the time of relapse or disease progression is required.

For all patients with relapsed or primary progressive HL, clinical and radiographic restaging is recommended. Because most patients receive salvage treatment, restaging has prognostic and therapeutic importance. Isolated nodal recurrence is associated with a better prognosis than disseminated relapse, and salvage treatment strategies vary depending on prior therapy and time of failure. The issue of how to define complete remission, partial remission, no change, and progressive disease after salvage treatment is vital, because salvage therapies are generally more intense and more toxic than first-line regimens. In salvage therapy studies, the response criteria are usually defined as in first-line therapies. However, in most series reported, a minimum duration of response of 4 weeks after the end of a salvage therapy is required.

Prognostic Factors

The likelihood of successful salvage therapy is determined by biologic features, which may be linked to certain clinical features. Adverse prognostic factors for patients with treatment failure include the treatment modality used in first-line therapy, age, relapse sites, quantity of disease at relapse, and presence or absence of systemic symptoms. In addition, the duration of first remission is a major determinant of a second complete response.

It was first noted in 1979 that the length of remission after first-line chemotherapy had a marked effect on the ability of patients to respond to subsequent salvage treatment.[285] In 1992, the NCI updated its experience with the long-term follow-up of patients who experienced relapse after polychemotherapy.[286] Derived primarily from investigations involving failures after MOPP and MOPP variants, the conclusions are relevant to other chemotherapy programs. On this basis, chemotherapy failures can be divided into three subgroups:

- Primary progressive HL (approximately 10% of all diagnosed HL patients), that is, a complete remission was never achieved
- Early relapse within 12 months of complete remission (approximately 15% of all HL cases)
- Late relapse after complete remission lasting longer than 12 months (approximately 15% of all HL cases)

When conventional chemotherapies are used to treat patients with primary progressive disease, virtually no patient survives longer than 8 years. In contrast, for patients with early relapse or late relapse, the projected 20-year survival rates have been found to be 11% and 22%, respectively.[286]

Patients who experience treatment failure after first-line radiotherapy, combination chemotherapy, or combined modality therapy can be divided into two groups, and their treatment selected accordingly:

- Relapse after irradiation for early-stage disease
- Relapse after primary chemotherapy

Relapse after Irradiation for Early-Stage Disease

Primary radiation therapy alone has been used more extensively in the past than in current practice. The survival of patients treated with conventional chemotherapy after relapse of irradiated early-stage disease is at least equal to that of advanced-stage patients initially treated with chemotherapy. Overall survival and disease-free survival range from 57% to 71%.[200,287,288]

Patients who relapse after radiation therapy alone for localized HL (stage I and II) have satisfactory results with combination chemotherapy and are not considered candidates for HDCT and ASCT.

The relapse rates after radiotherapy vary from 19% to 35%, with the highest rates being in the series that included only clinical rather than laparotomy staging. The majority of patients in these series had salvage treatment based on MOPP or similar regimens. The range of 10-year survival was 57% to 71%, which resembles the results of primary treatment with MOPP in patients with advanced disease. This suggests that prior radiotherapy does not cause drug resistance or a clinically significant compromise of chemotherapy dose intensity.

Stage at relapse is an important prognostic variable in radiation treatment failures. A study from Stanford including more than 100 patients with HL that relapsed after subtotal or total nodal irradiation showed that conventional salvage chemotherapy is sufficient in patients with limited-stage HL having no systemic symptoms on recurrence (stage IA and IIA). After 10 years, 90% of these patients remained disease free.[288] In contrast, the 10-year disease-free survival rates for those with stage IIIA disease and for those with stage IV disease or B symptoms at the time of relapse were 58% and 34%, respectively. An analysis using the International Database on Hodgkin's Disease showed a worse prognosis for patients whose relapse included an extranodal site and stage IV disease at relapse and for those patients older than 40 years of age.[289]

Patients with LPHL or NSHL histology fared better than those with MCHL or LDHL: 10-year freedom from relapse for patients with favorable histologic types was 67% versus 47% (P = .04) for patients with unfavorable histologic types.[287,290,291]

The original experience using systemic therapy for radiation treatment failures was based on the use of MOPP. The likelihood of freedom from second relapse was 57% at 10 years.[292] However, there are sufficient data from doxorubicin-based regimens to indicate that the principles for selecting a salvage regimen for treatment of relapse after radiotherapy are the same as the principles for selecting a primary treatment for advanced disease.

Based on the available evidence, ABVD has superior effects when compared with MOPP for treatment of recurrence after radiation therapy. The Milan Cancer Institute observed a disease-free survival rate of 81% with ABVD variants compared to 54% with MOPP.[293]

Relapse after Primary Chemotherapy

Treating recurrence after primary chemotherapy is a difficult issue. The choice is between the following:

- Salvage radiotherapy
- Conventional salvage chemotherapy
- HDCT followed by ASCT

SALVAGE RADIOTHERAPY. There are relatively few instances in which radiotherapy alone would be considered the standard salvage treatment because the perception is that recurrence indicates disseminated disease. However, salvage radiotherapy offers a potentially curative option with low morbidity for a select subset of patients. Salvage radiotherapy is a valid treatment alternative in patients without B symptoms who have not been given radiation previously or who relapse locally outside the initial radiation field.

This approach has been reported in series of more than 100 patients. Wirth et al. reported the experience of salvage radiotherapy in 51 patients with relapsed or refractory HL.[250] Twenty-three patients (45%) achieved a complete response after irradiation. Five-year failure-free survival and overall survival were 26% and 57%, respectively. Significant prognostic factors influencing failure-free survival were B symptoms at the time of salvage radiotherapy, extranodal involvement, and histologic type. For overall survival, significant factors were B symptoms, age, and number of prior chemotherapy regimens. For patients who relapsed in supradiaphragmatic nodal sites without B symptoms, 5-year failure-free survival and overall survival were 36% and 75%, respectively.

Table 41.5-16 demonstrates that selected patients who experience relapse after chemotherapy in an isolated nodal site without systemic symptoms can undergo salvage by radiother-

TABLE 41.5-16. Salvage Radiotherapy Alone for Relapse after Chemotherapy

No. of Patients	FFP	OS	Prognostic Factor for FFP	Reference
53	26% (5 y)	57% (5 y)	B symptoms, extranodal sites, histology	209
44	38% (5 y)	48% (5 y)	Extranodal sites	421
28	40% (5 y)	63% (5 y)	Duration of response	422
10	38% (5 y)	60% (5 y)	ne	423

FFP, freedom from progression; ne, not evaluated; OS, overall survival.

apy alone. Comparing radiotherapy with other types of salvage treatment is difficult, because the selection criteria for the different forms of treatment vary and no randomized study exists.

CONVENTIONAL SALVAGE CHEMOTHERAPY. Since 1990, a number of new salvage chemotherapy regimens have been tested that incorporate drugs not used in the initial combination. Because most first-line management programs use MOPP, ABVD, or combinations of both, new salvage regimens have been designed anticipating resistance to these drugs in patients who have experienced relapse.[294–297]

Primary progressive disease and early relapse suggest cellular resistance to conventional doses of drugs. Patients with primary refractory HL after treatment with MOPP or alternative regimens usually respond poorly to second or third induction attempts and have a particularly poor prognosis (life expectancy of less than 1.5 years). Fewer than 50% of patients who experience relapse after a short initial remission achieve a second complete remission, even when treated with non–cross-resistant regimens, and median survival of such patients is 2.5 to 4.0 years. For the vast majority of these patients, second-line chemotherapy followed by HDCT is required. In contrast, more than 80% of patients with late relapse achieve a second complete remission with MOPP or alternative regimens and have a median survival of longer than 4 years.[286] The Milan and NCI data suggest that late relapse does not necessarily imply resistance, because retreatment with the initial first-line regimen may result in response. An important goal for any retreatment in late relapse is the achievement of a second complete response, because nearly 50% of second complete responses result in prolonged progression-free survival.[298]

Table 41.5-17 lists the second-line salvage regimens for HL published since 1985. Detailed analysis and interpretation are difficult because in some trials the number of patients is small, the clinical status of patients varied, the duration of first remission is heterogeneous, and a large number of these patients also received subsequent HDCT plus ASCT. No randomized trial exists comparing the effectiveness of different conventional salvage chemotherapy regimens.

HIGH-DOSE CHEMOTHERAPY PLUS STEM CELL SUPPORT. Most clinical results on the use of HDCT with ASCT are derived from transplant centers in which a great deal of selection is used in referral and in the decision to treat with HDCT and ASCT. The encouraging results from numerous phase II studies and analyses using transplant registry data, as well as the

TABLE 41.5-17. Salvage Regimens for Hodgkin's Lymphoma at Conventional Dosages

Regimen	No. of Patients	RR (%)	Plus HDCT (no. of patients)	RFS (%)	Reference
CEP	58	54	—	16	461
CEVD	32	48	—	22	296
Dexa-BEAM	56	56	19	25	294
Mini-BEAM	44	84	26	36	462
MIME	47	63	—	8	295
DHAP	19	68	—	ne	297
ASHAP	56	70	39	40	463
MINE	100	75	72	46	298

ASHAP, doxorubicin (Adriamycin), high-dose arabinoside, and cisplatin (platinum); CEP, CCNU, etoposide, and prednimustine; CEVD, CCNU, etoposide, vindesine, and dexamethasone; Dexa-BEAM, dexamethasone, BCNU, etoposide, arabinoside, and melphalan; DHAP, dexamethasone, high-dose arabinoside, and platinum; HDCT, high-dose chemotherapy; MIME, methyl-GAG, ifosfamide, methotrexate, and etoposide; MINE, methyl-GAG, ifosfamide, vinorelbine, and etoposide; Mini-BEAM, BCNU, etoposide, arabinoside, and melphalan; MOPLACE, methotrexate, vincristine (Oncovin), prednisone, leucovorin, arabinoside, cyclophosphamide, and etoposide; ne, not evaluated; RR, response rate; RFS, relapse-free survival.

TABLE 41.5-18. Randomized Studies in Relapsed Hodgkin's Lymphoma: High-Dose Chemotherapy versus Conventional Salvage Therapy

No. of Patients	Treatment	Outcome	P Value	Follow-Up	Reference
40	2–3 × Mini-BEAM	10% EFS	.025	3 y	301
	BEAM	53% EFS			
142	4 × Dexa-BEAM	39% FFTF	.025	3 y	302
	2 × Dexa-BEAM + BEAM	53% FFTF			

BEAM, BCNU, etoposide, arabinoside, and melphalan; Dexa-BEAM, dexamethasone, BCNU, etoposide, arabinoside, and melphalan; EFS, event-free survival; FFTF, freedom from treatment failure; Mini-BEAM, lower-dose BEAM regimen.

reduction of the early transplant-related mortality to less than 5%, have led to the widespread acceptance of HDCT as an important component in the management of progressive and relapsed HL. HDCT followed by ASCT has been shown to produce 30% to 70% long-term disease-free survival in selected patients with primary progressive and relapsed disease.[296,299,300]

Although results of HDCT have generally been better than those observed after conventional-dose salvage therapy, the validity of this comparison has been questioned because of the lack of randomized trials. The most compelling evidence for the superiority of high-dose therapy in relapsed HL comes from two reports from the BNLI and the GHSG together with the EBMT. In the BNLI trial, patients with relapsed or refractory HL were treated with a combination of BCNU, etoposide, cytarabine, and melphalan at a conventional dose level (mini-BEAM) or a high dose level (BEAM) with autologous bone marrow transplantation. The actuarial 3-year event-free survival was significantly better in patients who received HDCT (53% vs. 10%).[301]

The largest randomized, multicenter trial was performed by the GHSG and EBMT to determine the benefit of HDCT in relapsed HL. Patients with relapse after polychemotherapy were randomized to receive either four cycles of dexa-BEAM (dexamethasone and BEAM) or two cycles of the dexa-BEAM regimen followed by HDCT (BEAM) and ASCT. The interim analysis of data for 142 evaluable patients revealed that, for 115 patients with partial or complete responses after two cycles of chemotherapy, the FFTF was 53% in the HDCT group versus 39% for the patients receiving an additional two cycles of conventional chemotherapy (Table 41.5-18).[302]

High-Dose Chemotherapy in Primary Progressive Hodgkin's Lymphoma

Patients with primary progressive disease, defined as progression during induction treatment or within 90 days after the end of treatment, have a particularly poor prognosis. Treatment of patients with primary progressive HL has consisted of salvage chemotherapy, radiotherapy, and HDCT with ASCT. Conventional salvage regimens have given disappointing results in the vast majority of patients: Response to salvage treatment is low and the duration of response is often short. The 8-year overall survival ranges from 0% to 8%. FFTF in patients in second remission is 0% at 4 to 8 years in small series reported.[286,303] Extensive disease often limits the use of radiotherapy.

In contrast, the data on the use of HDCT and ASCT in these patients are more promising. The EBMT reported their analysis of data for 175 patients with primary progressive disease who received HDCT and ASCT.[304] The 5-year actuarial progression-free and overall survival rates were 32% and 36%, respectively. The Autologous Blood and Marrow Transplant Registry reported a progression-free survival of 38% and an overall survival of 50% at 3 years in 122 patients with primary induction failure.[305] In single-institution series evaluating the efficacy of HDCT exclusively in cases of induction failure, Reece et al. reported a 42% progression-free survival at a median of 3.6 years.[306] Similarly, an updated report from Stanford University showed an event-free survival of 49% at 4 years.[271] Gianni et al. reported an event-free survival of 31% at 4 years.[294] The studies by Yuen et al.[307] and André et al.[308] reported improved outcome after HDCT and ASCT compared with outcomes for historical control groups given conventional chemotherapy for induction failures. Thus, HDCT and ASCT should be considered for HL patients with primary induction failure.

The GHSG retrospectively analyzed data for 206 patients with progressive disease to determine outcome after salvage therapy and identify prognostic factors. The 5-year freedom from second failure and overall survival for all patients were 17% and 26%, respectively. As reported by transplant centers, the 5-year freedom from second failure and overall survival for patients treated with HDCT were 42% and 48%, respectively, but only 33% of all patients received HDCT. A high proportion of those patients rapidly succumb to progressive disease. Life-threatening severe toxicity on salvage treatment occurred in 11% of patients. Insufficient stem cell harvest, poor performance status, and older age also contributed to ineligibility for HDCT. In a multivariate analysis, Karnofsky performance score at disease progression ($P < .0001$), age ($P = .019$), and sensitivity to first-line chemotherapy ($P =$

.0003) were significant prognostic factors for survival. In conclusion, HDCT is an effective treatment for a proportion of patients with primary progressive HL.[309] Due to the poor outcome of HL patients with progressive disease, future trials must aim at identifying patients at very high risk for induction failure and modifying primary treatment in this group to avoid progressive disease.

High-Dose Chemotherapy in Early and Late Relapsed Hodgkin's Lymphoma

Patients undergoing transplantation at first relapse from complete remission can often be cured with HDCT and ASCT.[300,310,311] At present, patients with early relapse are good candidates for HDCT followed by ASCT. A report from Stanford in which historical controls were used found a 4-year event-free survival of 56% for patients with early relapse compared to 19% for patients who received standard-dose salvage chemotherapy.[307] In addition, the HDR-1 study showed better FFTF for patients with early relapse after HDCT than with relapse after conventional chemotherapy.[302] Although the results reported for HDCT in patients with late relapse have been superior to those reported in most series of conventional chemotherapy, the use of HDCT in late relapses has been an area of controversy. Patients with late relapse have high second complete remission rates even with conventional chemotherapies, and overall survival rates range from 40% to 55%. The HDR-1 study of the GHSG showed improved FFTF and overall survival after HDCT compared with conventional chemotherapy in patients with late relapses. Therefore, HDCT should be considered as standard treatment even for patients with late relapses.[302]

PROGNOSTIC FACTORS IN RELAPSED HODGKIN'S LYMPHOMA TREATED WITH HIGH-DOSE CHEMOTHERAPY AND AUTOLOGOUS STEM CELL TRANSPLANTATION. Several published studies have evaluated the importance of prognostic factors for patients with HL undergoing HDCT with subsequent stem cell support.[270,300,312] Adverse prognostic factors identified by multivariate analysis include age, chemoresistance, disease status, poor performance status, extranodal disease, female sex, elevated lactate dehydrogenase level, and failure of more than two prior regimens. An important variable that affects outcome is the ability of conventional salvage chemotherapy to reduce tumor volume before HDCT. Patients who experience relapse after chemotherapy but respond to subsequent conventional salvage therapy make up most of the long-term survivors in transplantation programs. Nevertheless, the role of conventional salvage chemotherapy before HDCT has not clearly been defined. Several studies have confirmed that a subset of patients with disease resistant to conventional salvage therapy clearly benefit from HDCT, with reported long-term survival of 10% to 31%.[270,305,310,313] The answer to the question of how many patients with chemoresistant disease benefit from HDCT and ASCT largely depends on the definition of chemoresistance and the number and intensity of courses of chemotherapy administered to reduce the tumor burden. Accordingly, chemoresistant patients should not routinely be excluded from transplantation programs.

ALLOGENEIC STEM CELL TRANSPLANTATION. Allogeneic stem cell transplantation (alloSCT) has clear advantages compared with autologous transplantation. Donor cells uninvolved by malignancy are used, and this avoids the risk of infusing occult lymphoma cells that, despite purging, may contribute to

TABLE 41.5-19. Recommendations for Treatment of Relapsed and Primary Progressive Hodgkin's Lymphoma

Relapse after first-line radiotherapy	Conventional chemotherapy
Nodal relapse (CS I + II)	Salvage radiotherapy
No B symptoms	
No prior radiotherapy	
Primary progressive disease	HDCT + ASCT
Early relapse	HDCT + ASCT
Late relapse	HDCT + ASCT

ASCT, autologous stem cell transplantation; CS, clinical stage; HDCT, high-dose chemotherapy.

relapse in patients who undergo autologous transplantation. In addition, donor lymphoid cells can potentially mediate a graft-versus-lymphoma effect. As in all allograft studies, issues of donor availability and age constraints have limited the use of alloSCT in treatment of HL. Moreover, in all reports using alloSCT, a high treatment-related mortality rate of up to 75% was observed in patients with HL, which casts doubt on the feasibility of this approach in larger series.[314–316] In most circumstances, allogeneic transplantation from HLA-identical siblings is not recommended for patients with HL. The reduced relapse rate associated with a graft-versus-tumor effect is offset by lethal graft-versus-host toxicity.

Recommendations

In conclusion, patients who experience relapse after radiation therapy alone for localized HL have satisfactory results with combination chemotherapy and are not considered candidates for HDCT with ASCT. The current data support the use of HDCT with ASCT for patients with relapsed and refractory HL after combination chemotherapy (Table 41.5-19).

SPECIAL CASES

LYMPHOCYTE-PREDOMINANT HODGKIN'S LYMPHOMA

The early-stage characteristics, indolent course, and relatively good prognosis of LP variants of HL have been recognized since the 1930s.[317] Earlier studies consistently demonstrated that patients with an LP variant of HL enjoyed a better prognosis than those with other forms.[318] However, the introduction of clinical staging[159] showed that the extent of disease was a more important prognostic factor than histologic type and that the localized nature of LPHL could well account for the good prognosis of this subtype. In addition, modern therapeutic strategies were able to improve survival and cure rates for all types of patients, and prognostic differences due to histologic type were often no longer evident.[133,319] The clinical relevance of the revised REAL[115] and WHO classifications, particularly the distinction between LPHL and LRCHL, has been clarified by the international retrospective study of the ETFL.[320] The many smaller studies of LPHL paint a similar picture.[321–323]

Clinical Features

LPHL patients show an age distribution similar to that of MCHL cases, and are somewhat older on average than NSHL patients

TABLE 41.5-20. Characteristics of 219 Cases Confirmed as LPHL in the European Task Force on Lymphoma Project Compared with Nodular Sclerosis and Mixed-Cellularity Cases in the 1988–1994 Trials of the German Hodgkin Study Group

	LPHL (n = 219)	NSHL (n = 599)	MCHL (n = 174)
Median age (y)	35	30	35
Male gender (%)	74	49	73
Stage I (%)	53	10	21
Stage II (%)	28	47	32
Stage III (%)	14	29	35
Stage IV (%)	6	14	13
B symptoms (%)	10	42	35

LPHL, lymphocyte-predominant Hodgkin's lymphoma; NSHL, nodular sclerosis Hodgkin's lymphoma; MCHL, mixed-cellularity Hodgkin's lymphoma.

(Table 41.5-20). Approximately 75% of patients are male, which is again similar to MCHL and different from NSHL (about 50%). Fifty-three percent of LPHL patients have stage I disease and only 6% have stage IV disease. Thus, the proportion of early-stage cases is consistently high in comparison with CHL, and stage IV cases are consistently rare, although not negligible. B symptoms are present in only 10% of cases, far less than in CHL. LPHL seems to favor the peripheral upper neck and inguinal node sites, and to occur relatively seldom in central sites such as the mediastinum and upper abdomen.[163]

Treatment Results

There is some evidence to support the hypothesis that certain LPHL patients do well without any therapy beyond excision. Of the 51 nodular LPHL cases reported by Miettinen et al.,[324] 31 were given no treatment except possibly surgical removal of the tumor, because malignant disease was not suspected. After 7 years' median follow-up, only seven of the untreated patients died. These results must be cautiously interpreted, because it is likely that especially mild examples would predominate in this retrospective sample. Most LPHL patients have received first-line therapy similar to that prescribed for CHL patients. LPHL appears to relapse just as frequently as other subtypes, but the relapse is less aggressive, which results in frequent multiple relapses and good survival rates (see Fig. 41.5-2).

Transformation to Non-Hodgkin's Lymphoma

The possibility of occurrence of NHL after primary LPHL is clinically important for several reasons. The treatment should be chosen to prevent the development or progression of an NHL; it should avoid inducing a secondary NHL; and a monitoring and diagnostic strategy should be chosen to detect and correctly identify recurrent and secondary tumors. In an analysis of the International Database on Hodgkin's Disease,[325] a significantly higher risk for secondary NHL (increased by a factor of 1.8) was found for LPHL patients than for patients with NSHL and MCHL. Several smaller LPHL studies report incidence of secondary NHL, indicating a rate of 2% to 3% on average. Miettinen et al.[324] reported four secondary NHLs among 31 cases of untreated LPHL, which suggesting that some, if not all, such NHLs develop independently of treatment.

Consequences for Future Treatment

Although the prognosis superiority of LPHL compared with CHL is scarcely discernible with modern treatment programs, the relatively good prognosis of LPHL cases with earlier, less intensive treatment does indicate a potential for treatment reduction. Furthermore, as many patients with LPHL died of fatal treatment-related secondary leukemias and solid tumors as died from HL directly. This suggests that current treatment strategies might be too intensive, particularly when other late effects such as cardiac and pulmonary complications are taken into account. Disadvantages of treatment reduction could include a greater risk of disease progression or of development of an NHL.

Caution is needed in identifying those patients for whom treatment reduction is an option. First, immunostaining is needed for a reliable differential diagnosis between LPHL, CHL, and certain NHL variants. Second, patients with advanced-stage LPHL (20% to 25%) had overall survival and tumor-free survival rates substantially worse than those of patients with early-stage LPHL and similar to those of patients with advanced-stage CHL.[320] This implies that thorough staging and, in the case of advanced-stage disease, aggressive treatment are needed irrespective of histologic subtype.

A watch-and-wait treatment strategy, in which patients are monitored without treatment until the disease shows signs of progression, has been advocated for LPHL and for other indolent lymphomas. However, most authors report only anecdotal untreated cases.[324] A prospective study with explicit inclusion criteria is required to assess the feasibility, risks, and benefits of a watch-and-wait strategy. The EORTC is at present adopting a watch-and-wait approach for patients with stage I supradiaphragmatic LPHL after complete resection of the tumor; the involved field is to be irradiated only if the disease progresses. The GHSG is now treating patients with clinical stage IA LPHL without risk factors with involved-field radiation.

Involved-field radiotherapy has been shown to be inferior to more extensive irradiation in early-stage CHL but might be adequate for the very localized, less aggressive LP subtype. Two study groups, the EORTC and the GHSG, are currently treating certain early-stage LPHL patients with involved-field irradiation.

A new development potentially relevant to LPHL is the use of immunotherapy. The monoclonal antibody rituximab, in particular, is directed against the B-cell restricted CD20 antigen. This antigen is expressed by the L&H cells of LPHL but rarely by the H-RS cells of CHL. First experiences with indolent follicular B-cell lymphomas have shown good results, with approximately 55% overall responses even in heavily pre-treated patients.[326] This therapy is at present being tested in the treatment of relapsed and refractory LPHL by the GHSG.

The International Task Force on Hodgkin's Lymphoma plans a global study to compare 30-Gy involved-field irradiation versus observation versus rituximab therapy in LPHL patients with stage I and II disease.

HODGKIN'S LYMPHOMA IN THE ELDERLY PATIENT

HL treatment results, reflected in complete remission, relapse, and survival rates, tend to worsen with increasing age of the patient at diagnosis. There is no definite threshold age for the onset of this effect, although many authors report changes appearing at around age 60 and older.

HL rarely occurs in patients older than 60 years of age. Two basic problems in the management of elderly patients emerge as a recurrent theme: a high rate of toxicities during treatment and frequent early relapses. Various factors are considered to contribute to this poor prognosis. First, older patients differ from younger patients in disease characteristics: Advanced clinical stage and MC histology[327] are more frequent. Second, the older patient may be more likely to suffer treatment complications, which in turn influence the intensity of delivered therapy.

The patient's physical and mental condition, disease history, and the presence of concurrent disorders influence the treatment strategy. Age in general is not a contraindication for aggressive treatment. Biologically young patients in good physical and mental condition should be treated in a stage-adapted manner, as in conventional treatment protocols. In this subgroup rates of complete remission, relapse-free survival, and overall survival appear to be as good as in younger cohorts.[328] Combined modality treatment with a mild chemotherapy regimen and limited irradiation (i.e., two cycles of ABVD plus involved-field radiotherapy) is increasingly considered the standard therapy in favorable early-stage HL. If no chemotherapy can be administered, mantle or inverted-Y fields should be irradiated, possibly at a reduced dose. For patients with intermediate-stage (unfavorable early-stage) disease, two to four cycles of chemotherapy may be administered before involved-field radiotherapy.

In advanced stages, treatment should also be given with curative intent. The well-established ABVD combination (six to eight cycles) represents a safe regimen, whereas protocols with severe hematologic toxicities should be avoided. The time-intensified BEACOPP regimen, which has proved especially effective in advanced-stage HL patients aged up to 65 years, appears to be too toxic for patients older than 65 years.[329] Support with hematopoietic growth factors (granulocyte colony-stimulating factor) should be given liberally, because infectious complications due to prolonged neutropenia are common. Close monitoring for toxicity (i.e., electrocardiography, echocardiography, pulmonary function testing) and response to treatment are important to adjust treatment at an early time.

Treatment for those patients with impairment of lung, liver, heart, or kidney should be individually adapted. Depending on preexisting impairment of organs, single drugs with organ-specific toxicities (i.e., bleomycin, doxorubicin) may be omitted from the chemotherapy regimen, replaced, or modified in dose. Involved-field radiotherapy, oral combination therapy (CCNU, etoposide, prednimustine), or use of less aggressive drugs such as gemcitabine[330] in the initial treatment as well as the combination of vinblastine, bleomycin, and methotrexate[331] are possible treatment alternatives.

HODGKIN'S LYMPHOMA DURING PREGNANCY

The peak incidence of HL occurs at female reproductive age. Therefore, the association with pregnancy is not uncommon. One case of HL has been reported per 1000 to 6000 deliveries, which makes it the fourth most common cancer diagnosed during pregnancy.[332] Several studies have shown that pregnancy does not worsen the clinical course of the disease and

that the 20-year survival of pregnant women with HL is no different from that of nonpregnant women.[333]

The clinical presentation of HL is not influenced by pregnancy. However, there are significant limitations on staging and treatment of the pregnant patient. CT should be avoided because it exposes the fetus to ionizing radiation. Ultrasonography, which is without known adverse fetal effects, is helpful not only to assess fetal development but also to detect the presence of lymphadenopathy. Magnetic resonance imaging can be used to complete the radiologic staging because it appears to be free from genetic hazards. Decisions about the need for chest radiography should be made on the basis of clinical examination.

If HL is diagnosed in the first trimester, most experts agree that a therapeutic abortion should be encouraged. If the woman wishes to continue her pregnancy, treatment should be deferred until the second trimester at least, because the options for therapy at the beginning of pregnancy are rather limited. If therapy is indicated, a supradiaphragmatic radiation with doses less than 10 Gy or a vinblastine chemotherapy for more advanced disease may be commenced.

In the second or third trimester, stage I or II disease may be closely observed, and treatment should be postponed until an early delivery, usually at 32 to 34 weeks. If there is any sign of rapid disease progression, in supradiaphragmatic lymphadenopathy radiotherapy alone is recommended. Most studies indicate doses of 10 to 44 Gy to the classic mantle field or the involved field with abdominal shielding to protect the fetus. In the second and third trimesters, the risk of adverse sequelae for the fetus from supradiaphragmatic radiation is low. In infradiaphragmatic lymphadenopathy and in stage III or IV disease, combination chemotherapy is the treatment of choice. Because most chemotherapeutic agents freely cross the placenta and enter the fetal circulation, not only the patient but also the fetus must be closely monitored. Chemotherapy administered in the second and third trimesters may increase the risk of intrauterine growth retardation, microcephaly, and mental retardation.[334] Application of cytotoxic drugs shortly before birth may be particularly hazardous, because the placenta is also the primary means of drug elimination, and metabolism and excretion are delayed in the neonatus. The current concept is that antimetabolites, especially methotrexate, carry a high risk of teratogenesis, whereas alkylating agents, doxorubicin, bleomycin, etoposide, and the vinca alkaloids appear acceptable.[334] The ABVD regimen may be used when chemotherapy is indicated beyond the first trimester. Because chemotherapeutic agents reach significant levels in milk, mothers are best advised not to breast feed during treatment.

HODGKIN'S LYMPHOMA IN HUMAN IMMUNODEFICIENCY VIRUS–POSITIVE PATIENTS

Epidemiology and Clinical Presentation

The majority of recent studies demonstrate a slight increase in the incidence of HL in young adult and middle-aged homosexual males. They also suggest that with regard to risk behavior HL associated with HIV infection occurs preferentially in intravenous drug users. An increased incidence of HL among other risk groups such as hemophiliacs or women with an increased risk for AIDS has not been convincingly demonstrated.

Several sets of data support the thesis that EBV infection probably represents a relevant factor in the pathogenesis of HIV-associated HL. First, EBV is found in H-RS cells in 80% to 100% of HL tissue specimens from HIV-infected patients, whereas in the HIV-negative population EBV is found in 50% to 70% of HL specimens.[335] Second, a pathogenetic role of EBV in HIV-associated HL is supported by the fact that tumor cells in virtually all cases of HIV-associated HL express EBV-encoded LMP1.[336]

A characteristic of HL in HIV-infected patients is the predominance of unfavorable histologic subtypes.[337] Most studies in Europe and the United States reported MCHL to be the most frequent histologic subtype among HIV-infected patients (40% to 100%). NSHL was less frequent (0% to 40%) in the HIV population than in HIV-negative persons. The incidence of the LP subtype was rather low (0% to 4%); in contrast, more than 20% of all cases were classified as LDHL.[338]

At the time of diagnosis, 70% to 90% of all patients with HIV-associated HL present with advanced disease. Extranodal involvement is frequent (60%), with the most common sites being bone marrow, liver, and spleen. In contrast to non–HIV-related HL in the general population, in which the involvement of contiguous lymph node groups is typical and dissemination and infiltration of extranodal sites are late occurrences, in HIV-infected patients noncontiguous spread of lymphoma can be observed, such as liver involvement without splenic disease, or lung involvement without mediastinal adenopathy. Bone marrow involvement occurs in 40% to 50% of patients and is the first indicator of the presence of HL in nearly 20% of cases.[339] HL tends to develop as an earlier manifestation of HIV infection, presenting in patients with a median CD4+ count in the range of 275 to 306 cells/μL.[16] At the time of diagnosis, the majority of patients have persistent generalized lymphadenopathy, and in 50% of cases lymphoma may be concurrently present with persistent generalized lymphadenopathy in the same lymph node group.[340] Therefore, it is important to be aware of HIV-associated HL as a differential diagnosis.

Treatment

Treatment is difficult considering the underlying immune deficiency caused by HIV infection itself and may increase the risk for opportunistic infections by inducing further immunosuppression. Survival of patients with HIV-associated HL is short, typically 12 to 18 months, and the incidence of opportunistic infections is increased due to standard therapy regimens. Because most patients suffer from advanced HL they have been treated with combination chemotherapy regimens such as MOPP and ABVD, but the response has been poor in comparison with that of HIV-unrelated HL. Retrospective evaluations[341] show a complete response rate far below that of HIV-negative patients with HL, poor tolerance of chemotherapy, and need for dose reduction or delay of treatment or both. Other prospective studies show that tailored chemotherapy regimens with moderate bone marrow toxicity such as epirubicin, bleomycin, and vinblastine, in combination with antiretroviral treatment with zidovudine, result in a substantial decrease in opportunistic infections, yet overall survival was not significantly improved.[342] Improvement of response rate and median survival could be achieved by full-dose regimens such as

EBVP[343] or ABVD[344] combined with antiretroviral treatment, prophylaxis for the most common opportunistic organism, *Pneumocystis carinii*, and the use of granulocyte colony-stimulating factor.[345] Preliminary data for treatment with the BEACOPP regimen showed promising results with regard to complete remission, toxicity and median survival.[346]

In summary, treatment of HIV-associated HL demands a special approach. Therefore, it will likely be a combination of probably unconventional chemotherapy, antiretroviral agents, prophylaxis for opportunistic infections, and the use of hematopoietic growth factors that will lead to cure of HIV-associated HL. However, the individual components of the recipe are not yet defined.

SEQUELAE

LONG-TERM COMPLICATIONS OF TREATMENT

Long-term complications of mantle irradiation include lung, heart, and thyroid dysfunction, second primary cancers, and Lhermitte's syndrome (Table 41.5-21). Complications such as transverse myelitis and constrictive pericarditis should not occur with the use of modern radiation therapy techniques. Other long-term toxicities are not totally avoidable but can be reduced in severity or frequency.

Pulmonary Complications

Radiation pneumonitis typically occurs 1 to 6 months after completion of mantle irradiation. Once it resolves, there are usually no long-term sequelae. A mild nonproductive cough, low-grade fever, and dyspnea on exertion characterize symptomatic radiation pneumonitis. The overall incidence of symptomatic pneumonitis is less than 5% after mantle irradiation; patients who have large mediastinal adenopathy or who receive combined chemotherapy and radiation therapy have a twofold to threefold greater risk (10% to 15%).[347] Radiographically, pneumonitis is characterized by the formation of infiltrates confined to the original radiation fields. Infection rather than pneumonitis is more likely if the infiltrates extend into areas of

TABLE 41.5-21. Treatment-Related Complications after Curative Therapy for Hodgkin's Lymphoma

---

POTENTIALLY FATAL
Acute myelomonocytic leukemia
Diffuse, high-grade non-Hodgkin's lymphoma
Solid tumors (mostly lung and breast cancer)
Overwhelming bacterial sepsis after splenectomy or spleen irradiation (OPSI)
SERIOUS
Myocardial damage from radiation and anthracyclines
Lung fibrosis from radiation plus bleomycin
Sterility in men and women
Growth abnormalities in children and adolescents
Opportunistic infections
Psychological problems
MINOR
Chemical or clinical hypothyroidism
Long-term alteration of lymphocyte function

the lung initially protected from radiation. Severe pneumonitis may require treatment with steroids.

Cardiac Complications

Various cardiac complications including arrhythmias, myocardial infarction, coronary artery disease, pericarditis, myocarditis, pericardial effusion, and tamponade have been documented after radiation therapy to the mediastinum.[347,348] In many of the earlier studies, these complications were related to treatment techniques that resulted in a high radiobiologic dose to the anterior mediastinum and heart. Current practice, which restricts the dose to the whole heart, blocks the subcarinal region partway into treatment, delivers treatments equally from front and back, and allows less overall radiation dose and smaller treatment volumes due to the use of preradiation chemotherapy has yielded more satisfactory results. Studies have shown a modest increase in cardiac mortality after mantle irradiation. Boivin and colleagues have demonstrated an increased age-adjusted risk of death from myocardial infarction after mediastinal irradiation.[349] When data were analyzed by year of diagnosis of HL, the risk was much greater for patients treated in 1966 or earlier (relative risk, 6.33; 95% confidence interval, 1.73 to 23.16) than for those treated in 1967 or later (relative risk, 1.97; 95% confidence interval, 0.75 to 5.17), which suggests an important role for modern treatment techniques in reducing the risk of complications.

The risk of chronic cardiomyopathy appears to increase as the cumulative dose of doxorubicin exceeds 400 to 450 mg/m^2. It is still unknown whether there is an increased risk for cardiomyopathy at lower cumulative doses (as are commonly given with ABVD) in patients treated with mediastinal radiation before or after chemotherapy. Careful cardiac evaluation of patients treated with combined radiation therapy and chemotherapy is recommended because of concerns that mediastinal irradiation may predispose to accelerated coronary arteriosclerosis and this risk may be further increased by the administration of anthracyclines. Consideration should also be given to using lower doses and blocking the lower portion of the heart whenever possible.

Secondary Neoplasia

The occurrence of second malignancies, including acute leukemia, NHL, and a variety of solid tumors, has in recent years become a well-acknowledged reality that adversely affects survival of some patients cured of HL. Some of these cases may represent chance association. However, physicians should be aware that HL patients are at higher risk of developing a second neoplasm.

A number of reports have stressed the possibility that the occurrence of acute nonlymphocytic leukemia is closely related to the use of drug combinations containing alkylating agents. The use of ABVD in chemotherapy regimens for HL has reduced the risk of leukemia. In most studies the use of radiation therapy in combination with chemotherapy does not increase the risk over that for chemotherapy alone, although there may be an increased risk when chemotherapy is combined with extensive irradiation (i.e., total lymphoid irradiation). There does not appear to be an increased risk for developing acute nonlymphoblastic leukemia after radiation therapy alone.

The total incidence of acute leukemia, which usually occurs within the first 10 years after initial treatment, is reported in most published series to range from 2% to 6%.[350] The classic form of treatment-related leukemia is characterized by a relatively long latency period (3 to 5 years), a preceding myelodysplastic phase, trilineage bone marrow dysplasia, and abnormalities of chromosome 5 or 7 or both. Topoisomerase II inhibitors, primarily the epipodophyllotoxins but also anthracyclines when given in combination with alkylating agents, have been implicated in the development of a clinically and cytogenetically distinct form of secondary acute myeloid leukemia in both adult and pediatric patients.[351]

The update on secondary AML and MDS in the GHSG database involved 5411 patients treated in studies HD1 through HD9 between 1978 and 1998. There was a 1% incidence of secondary AML and MDS after a median observation time of 55 months. Treatment protocols included a variety of treatment options ranging from palliation to alloSCT. No difference in overall survival between patients undergoing alloSCT and those receiving conventional or palliative treatment could be observed. The outcome was very poor: 85% of patients (39 of 46) developing secondary AML or MDS did not survive longer than 1 year after diagnosis. After 24 months, the overall survival rate was 8%.[352]

Nearly all cases of NHL occurring after HL are of intermediate-grade or high-grade histology and are similar to lymphomas seen in patients with immunodeficiency diseases or under chronic immunosuppression for organ transplantation or autoimmune disorders. These lymphomas have a cumulative risk of 1.2% to 2.1% at 15 years.[353,354]

The actual incidence of solid tumors, which have not revealed a particular histopathologic pattern, is not known because the full extent of the expression of the risk of a second neoplasm may not be appreciated for another decade. The solid tumors tend to occur in the second decade after treatment and thus far appear to represent a hazard of both radiotherapy and chemotherapy. The major risk appears to be lung cancer, mostly among smokers, and breast cancer among women when irradiated at a young age.[180,350,355,355a,355b] Other cancers include sarcomas, melanomas, connective tissue and bone tumors, and salivary, stomach, and skin cancers.[354,356]

A major argument against the use of radiation therapy as primary or adjunct therapy in HL has been its potential to induce secondary solid tumors. A large study of the BNLI encompassing 2846 patients included 987 patients who were treated with chemotherapy alone.[357] The BNLI study showed that the relative risk of developing a secondary solid tumor after chemotherapy alone was 5.7. This was not significantly different from the relative risk after radiotherapy alone (4.8) or after combined modality therapy (5.8). Furthermore, a case-control study by a collaborative group of population-based registries and cancer centers that maintains data on 25,665 cases of HL[358] showed that HL patients treated with chemotherapy alone had approximately twice the risk of developing lung cancer of those treated by radiotherapy alone or by both modalities. Most of these data are for MOPP or MOPP-like regimens, and little is known of the relation between the use of ABVD and the risk of second solid tumors.

Gonadal Dysfunction

Many patients who complete successful treatment for HL go on to raise healthy children. However, under some circumstances gonadal dysfunction is an important iatrogenic toxicity that considerably affects the quality of life of patients after HL. Three to six cycles of MOPP or MOPP-like chemotherapy induces azoospermia in 50% to 100% of male patients. This finding is associated with germinal hyperplasia and increased follicle-stimulating hormone levels, with normal levels of luteinizing hormone and testosterone. Only 10% to 20% of patients eventually show recovery of spermatogenesis after a long interval. After MOPP alternated with ABVD, the incidence of permanent azoospermia is approximately 50%. With full-course MOPP chemotherapy, approximately half of women become amenorrheic with occurrence of age-dependent premature ovarian failure (older than 30 years, 75% to 85%; younger than 30 years, approximately 20%).

The Milan Cancer Institute has reported that the administration of ABVD chemotherapy produces only limited and transient germ cell toxicity in men and no drug-induced amenorrhea in women.[359] To circumvent chemotherapy-induced sterility, the use of drug regimens not containing alkylating agents, procarbazine, or nitrosourea derivatives is highly recommended. An alternative for men undergoing MOPP or MOPP/ABVD is sperm storage before chemotherapy. The usefulness of the administration of analogues of gonadotropin-releasing hormone in men or oral contraceptives in premenopausal women remains to be fully defined; however, the limited data available have been discouraging.

OTHER COMPLICATIONS

Minor complications can be summarized as follows. Hypothyroidism is a common event (approximately 30%) after mantle field irradiation, typically picked up by means of an elevated level of thyroid-stimulating hormone.[347] Hormone replacement therapy is required. Herpes zoster is another common complication. It is self-limited and usually occurs in one to two contiguous dermatomes within the first 2 years after treatment. Herpes zoster affects 15% to 20% of patients treated with radiation therapy or chemotherapy alone, but the incidence appears higher in patients treated with combined radiation therapy and chemotherapy. Cutaneous dissemination and visceral involvement from varicella zoster virus infection are rare. Early treatment with antiviral agents may limit the intensity and duration of the infection. Acute transient radiation myelopathy or Lhermitte's sign (paresthesias down the dorsal portion of the extremities when the neck is flexed) occurs in 10% to 15% of patients after mantle irradiation. This particular complication typically occurs 6 weeks to 3 months after radiotherapy and is self-limited, resolving in weeks to months. Xerostomia is a temporary complication of mantle irradiation; salivary secretion returns to normal usually within 6 months of treatment. However, xerostomia may be prolonged if the patient is over 40 years of age at treatment or if Waldeyer's ring is treated. Fluoride supplementation and careful dental care minimize the risks of radiation caries. The risk of postsplenectomy sepsis is present, particularly in children,[360] but can be minimized by immunization with pneumococcal vaccine; in more recent years, vaccines have been developed against *Haemophilus* and *Neisseria*, the other microorganisms associated with a small but finite risk of overwhelming postsplenectomy sepsis.

QUALITY OF LIFE

A review of most randomized clinical trials in HL reveals that quality of life has been neglected as a primary or even a secondary outcome measure. After a review of the literature in pediatric oncology, Bradlyn et al. demonstrated that only 3% of all randomized clinical trial reports reviewed (n = 70) included quality-of-life data.[361] However, mainly retrospective analyses involving long-term survivors of HL have been performed.[362,363] These analyses show that a substantial subgroup of patients still experience serious sequelae of the disease and its treatment many years after the end of treatment. In one study, men earning less than US$15,000 yearly, persons currently unemployed, single individuals, those who experienced serious illness from treatment, and less-educated persons were found to be at high risk for maladaption years after treatment. Furthermore, 22% of the 273 patients studied met the criterion suggested for a psychiatric diagnosis.[362] Currently, it remains unclear at which point in the course of the disease patients with good coping capacity can be distinguished from those without. To characterize phases of readaption and maladaption more precisely, quality-of-life assessment has to be implemented in prospective randomized clinical trials. To ensure completeness of data, quality-of-life investigations should be a mandatory component of the clinical trial design and part of the inclusion criteria.[364]

The assessment of quality of life has become an essential tool in clinical trials in recent years, in particular in the evaluation of therapies given to patients with chronic illnesses such as cancer. Although survival and survival without disease have long been used as the sole end points in clinical trials, this is no longer accepted today, because other characteristics are now considered to be as important as survival by both patients and physicians. Among these, treatment burden, treatment-related toxicity, and their psychological and social impacts are of great importance.

Obviously, this change originates from the dramatic improvement in the efficacy of cancer treatments, particular in HL. Effective therapies, however, have several drawbacks that might limit their use. Chemotherapy and radiation therapy induce severe acute and late toxicities that may diminish the long-term benefit of curative treatment. Several studies with a quality-of-life approach have highlighted the difficulties survivors may experience even long after the treatment, such as general fatigue, poor health, and social problems.

NEW DRUGS FOR TREATMENT OF HODGKIN'S LYMPHOMA

VINORELBINE

Vinorelbine belongs to the family of vinca alkaloids and is a semisynthetic analogue of vinblastine (5' nor-anidro-vinblastine). The main side effect of vinorelbine is myelosuppression. WHO grade 3 or 4 neutropenia occurs in up to 70% of patients but is of very short duration with a low incidence of infectious complications.[365] Vinorelbine used as single-agent therapy in HL was administered in all studies on a weekly schedule at 30 mg/m². Devizzi et al. reported on 22 patients with HL refractory or resistant to at least two chemotherapy regimens, of whom 50% (n = 11) showed an objective response (complete response in 3, partial response in 8) with a median duration of 6 months.[366] Benchekroun et al. evaluated the response to vinorelbine in untreated patients with advanced HL.[367] Thirty-two patients received four weekly doses of vinorelbine before MOPP/ABVD chemotherapy. Ninety percent achieved a partial remission.

IDARUBICIN

Idarubicin is a semisynthetic drug that was first purified in 1976. Idarubicin differs from its parent drug daunorubicin only by the replacement of the C4 methoxyl group in the D ring with a hydrogen atom. This modification has major consequences in terms of the pharmacokinetic characteristics: Idarubicin is much more lipophilic and can be administered orally. Its main metabolite, idarubicinol, is as active as the parent compound. In addition, idarubicin has shown greater cytotoxicity than daunorubicin or doxorubicin *in vitro*. Idarubicin exhibits less cardiotoxicity at equally effective doses compared with other anthracyclines, whereas hematotoxicity and mucositis appear to be more pronounced. The GHSG is currently conducting a clinical phase II study in which idarubicin (8 mg/m² on days 1 and 2) is administered together with etoposide (60 mg/m² on days 1 through 4), ifosfamide (1000 mg/m² on days 1 through 4, continuous infusion), and dexamethasone (20 mg/m² on days 1 through 4) to patients with relapsed or refractory HL.[367a]

GEMCITABINE

Gemcitabine is a new pyrimidine antimetabolite with unique metabolic and mechanistic properties among the nucleoside analogue.[368] It is a derivative of deoxycytidine with fluorine substituted for the two hydrogen atoms in the 2' position of the deoxyribose sugar. Although structurally similar to cytarabine, gemcitabine differs pharmacokinetically and pharmacologically. It acts as a competitive substrate for incorporation into the DNA, where it leads to chain termination. Based on the impressive results against solid tumors like non–small cell lung cancer and pancreatic cancer, gemcitabine was given in a multicenter clinical phase II study to patients with multiple relapsed or refractory HL who had received at least two prior chemotherapy regimens.[330] Gemcitabine was administered on a weekly schedule of 1250 mg/m² on days 1, 8, and 15 of a 28-day cycle. An interim analysis of this trial showed an overall response of 39%, with complete remissions in 2 of 23 patients and partial remissions in 7 of 23. Another ten patients had stable disease. Myelosuppression was the main toxicity.[368a]

IMMUNOTHERAPY

Tumor cells that survive intensive therapy in small quantities are defined as minimal residual disease. These partially dormant chemoresistant lymphoma cells might be eradicated by new immunotherapeutic strategies with a different mechanism of action. Current approaches comprise passive immunotherapy with antibody-based regimens for specific targeting of malignant cells as well as active immunotherapy with modulation of the cellular immune response using cytokines, tumor vaccines, or gene transfer. The combination of immunotherapeutic strategies and standard chemotherapeutic regimens seems to be most promising: Due to their different mechanisms of action, cross-resistance of malignant cells is expected to be rare. Furthermore, the side effects of these two treatment modalities differ, so that toxicity is not usually additive.

PASSIVE IMMUNOTHERAPY

Systemically administered chemotherapeutic agents kill all rapidly dividing cells, whereas monoclonal antibodies can target tumor cells selectively. Normal cells that lack specific tumor antigens are not harmed. HL seems to be an ideal target for antibody-based therapeutic approaches for several reasons. First, H-RS cells express many different cell surface antigens, such as CD15, CD25, CD30, CD40, and CD80 (B7-1) that are present on only a minority of normal human cells.[153] Due to low cross-reactivity with healthy human tissue, side effects should be rare. Second, because many different markers can be detected on the surface of Hodgkin's cells, "cocktails" (combinations of various antibody conjugates targeting different Hodgkin's-specific antigens) might be useful for selective immunotherapy. If one malignant antigen-deficient cell clone is resistant to one antibody, cells might still be targeted by the second or third antibody conjugate administered at the same time. Third, the number of malignant cells that have to be killed is small, because the majority of cells in the involved lymph nodes are reactive bystander cells. Finally, lymphomas are well vascularized,[369] so that intravenously administered antibody conjugates can easily reach their target cells. Therefore, chemotherapy or radiotherapy or both can be used for treatment of bulky disease, whereas immunotherapeutic agents are applied thereafter to eliminate minimal residual disease and thus prevent relapses.

Native Monoclonal Antibodies

Ideally, the therapeutic antibody targets an antigen present only on the tumor cells with high specificity and has no cross-reactivity with normal human tissue. The mechanisms of action of native antibodies include complement activation, antibody-dependent cellular toxicity, phagocytosis of antibody-coated target cells, inhibition of cell-cycle progression, and induction of apoptosis. In early phase I and II trials, use of native antibodies has produced moderate adverse effects, such as chills, fever, dyspnea, nausea, diarrhea, and myalgia. Toxicity was usually related to the number of circulating tumor cells and the development of human antimouse antibodies (HAMA). New chimeric antibodies that consist of human constant and murine variable regions rarely induce HAMA formation.

In the early 1990s, Engert et al. evaluated more than 40 different murine monoclonal antibodies for activity against Hodgkin's-derived cell lines *in vitro* without finding any antitumor activity.[370] Surprisingly, about a decade later two anti-CD30 antibodies were identified with remarkable *in vitro* and *in vivo* activity when used in their native forms. One of them (SGN-30) is derived from the murine AC10 antibody and has been humanized. The other one is a primarily human anti-CD30 antibody (5F11). Both antibodies directly induce apoptosis of CD30+ cell lines as well as antibody dependent cellular cytotoxicity and have shown their activity in mouse models.[371,372] In addition, both antibodies are currently being evaluated in clinical studies. The SGN-30 antibody has shown activity in HL as well as in ALCL, whereas the clinical study of the 5F11 antibody is still ongoing. If the preliminary results showing activity in the phase I trial can be confirmed in phase II studies, these antibodies might become interesting new drugs for combination with established cytotoxic regimens to eliminate quiescent H-RS cells.

The chimeric monoclonal anti-CD20 antibody rituximab (IDEC-C2B8) has now been approved by the U.S. Food and Drug Administration for the treatment of patients with relapsed advanced follicular NHL after a pivotal trial demonstrated response rates of up to 50% in 166 patients.[373] Because the CD20 antigen is expressed on all malignant cells in paragranuloma and LPHL, this entity might be a good target for treatment with rituximab. An international study has shown the safety and efficacy of rituximab therapy in patients with relapsed or refractory LPHL and in others with multiple relapsed CD20+ CHL. Twelve of 14 patients showed a response to rituximab, including 8 with complete and 4 with partial remissions. Thus, rituximab should be incorporated into the treatment of relapsed LPHL.

Immunotoxins

Immunotoxins generally consist of a binding moiety and a toxin moiety, which are either covalently linked via a chemical linker or generated by recombinant fusion technology. The binding domain is usually a monoclonal antibody, a Fab' fragment, a single-chain variable fragment, or a cytokine, whereas the toxin is of bacterial or plant origin. Recombinant toxins are constructed by fusing coding regions of toxins such as diphtheria toxin or *Pseudomonas* exotoxin A to ligand genes.[374] These defined, compact molecules are easy to modify and more economical to produce than their chemically linked counterparts.[375] Immunotoxins can bind selectively to their target cells. After internalization of the construct by endocytosis, the toxin is transferred to the ribosomal subunits, where it interferes with protein synthesis and thus kills the tumor cell.

Another interesting target for selective immunotherapy in HL is the IL-2 receptor (CD25), which is expressed on the majority of H-RS cells.[376] In a phase I study, 15 patients with refractory Hodgkin's lymphoma were treated with the anti-CD25 immunotoxin RFT5.dgA.[377] All patients in this trial were heavily pretreated with a mean of five prior chemotherapeutic regimens, including autologous bone marrow transplantation. Most side effects were related to vascular leak syndrome. Clinical responses included two partial remissions, one minor response, and three cases of disease stabilization. In a subsequent multicenter phase II trial, the overall response rate was 20%. Two new anti-CD25 immunotoxins, DAB486IL-2 and DAB389IL-2, generated by fusing the cytokine IL-2 to a truncated form of the diphtheria toxin, were tested in phase I and II clinical studies for CD25+ hematologic malignancies, including chronic lymphocytic leukemia, Sézary's syndrome, HL, and NHL.[378] One complete remission lasting more than 2 years was reported with DAB486IL-2.[379] However, 27 other patients with refractory disease showed no response. Side effects were hypersensitivity-like symptoms, fatigue, and reversible hepatotoxicity. A correlation between the concentrations of antiimmunotoxin antibody and the incidence of side effects was demonstrated in 50% of all patients presenting with preexisting antibodies after immunization against diphtheria in early childhood.[378] Therefore, repeated application of the immunotoxin was impossible in these patients. Diminishing the immunogenicity of immunotoxins might decrease HAMA formation in humans. Promising approaches include deleting immunodominant epitopes and humanizing the antibody moiety of the immunotoxin.[379,380]

A variety of monoclonal antibodies have been evaluated for their potential clinical use as a ricin A chain immunotoxin against HL.[381,382] The most potent anti-CD30 immunotoxin, Ki-4.dgA, has been investigated in a clinical dose escalation trial.[383] Seventeen patients with refractory or relapsed Hodgkin's lymphoma were treated intravenously with one to three cycles of Ki-4.dgA. All patients receiving 10 mg/m^2 experienced a vascular

leak syndrome of NCI toxicity grade 3. There was only one partial remission in 15 patients evaluable for response. Treatment results were promising in a pilot study with the immunotoxin Ber-H2-Sap6 consisting of the anti-CD30 antibody Ber-H2 chemically linked to the soapwort toxin saporin-S6. Twelve patients with advanced refractory HL were treated with one or two infusions of 0.8 mg/kg Ber-H2-Sap6.[29] Four patients achieved a partial response with a substantial decrease of tumor mass lasting 6 to 10 weeks. Fever, malaise, anorexia, fatigue, mild myalgias, weight gain, and a fourfold to fivefold increase in liver enzyme levels were the main toxicities. Because responses were only short and partial, new anti-CD30 immunotoxins were developed by covalently conjugating murine Ber-H2 to momordin, dianthin, and pokeweed antiviral protein from seeds.[384] In humans, sequential application of anti-CD30 antibodies linked to distinct ribosome-inactivating proteins might prevent formation of human antibodies against the individual toxins.

Radioimmunoconjugates

Radioimmunoconjugates are constructed by linking a monoclonal antibody to radioisotopes without significantly altering the immunologic specificity of the protein. The most important advantage of these constructs compared to all other antibody-based therapeutic strategies is that β-particles emitted by radionuclides can kill adjacent tumor cells through a crossfire effect, regardless of whether cells express the target antigen.[385] In contrast to external-beam radiation therapy, radiolabeled antibodies deliver radiation continuously at a low dose rate to the whole body, including occult micrometastases.[386] Currently, both nonmyeloablative and myeloablative strategies involving radiolabeled antibodies are being investigated for imaging and treatment of HL.

Low-energy radionuclides are coupled to monoclonal antibodies either for diagnostic use (immunoscintigraphy) or low-dose radioimmunotherapy without severe myelosuppression.[387,388] So far, polyclonal antiferritin radioimmunoconjugates have been administered to patients with refractory or relapsed HL. Ferritin is a tumor-associated protein that was first described in Hodgkin's lymphoma.[389] Efficacy was promising, but treatment was limited due to chronic bone marrow toxicity.[390] HRS-1 and HRS-3 were the first anti-CD30 antibodies labeled with radioisotopes (iodine 123, iodine 131) for immunoscintigraphy.[391,392] Twenty out of 25 evaluable patients with HL showed a true-positive result during staging and restaging examinations: Nodal, splenic, bone marrow, and muscle involvement were imaged, and many of these sites had previously been undetected. In this study sensitivity was 87% with an acceptable specificity. Toxicity was mild, with only one patient dropping out because of iodine intolerance. A phase I trial has been initiated investigating the safety of the technetium 99m–labeled anti-CD30 antibody Ber-H2 for immunoscintigraphy and possibly immunotherapy in patients with refractory HL and large cell anaplastic lymphoma. Preliminary results suggest good tolerance of the therapy with no major side effects and satisfactory efficacy for imaging or detecting HL lesions. Thus, a murine anti-CD30 antibody (Ki-4) was linked to iodine and evaluated for activity in relapsed HL in a clinical phase I and II study. Six of 21 patients showed a response, but also approximately one-third of the patients experienced severe bone marrow suppression. Thus, future trials involving modern radioisotopes (indium 111, yttrium 90, rhenium 186) are warranted.[393]

Stem cell support for hematopoietic recovery might be necessary in high-dose radioimmunotherapy. A phase I and II study of treatment with yttrium 90–labeled polyclonal antiferritin antibodies for refractory HL followed by autologous bone marrow transplantation was performed by Vriesendorp et al.[394] Seven of 17 patients achieved complete remissions lasting from 2 months to more than 26 months, and four patients experienced partial remissions (2 to 6 months). Twelve patients received a reduced dose (20 mCi) due to bone marrow involvement or unsuccessful marrow harvest. Complete remissions were observed in two and partial remissions in five of these patients. At all doses, response rates were better in patients with small tumor burden. Based on these encouraging results, radioimmunotherapy appears to be a new promising option, either alone or in combination with other chemotherapy or immunotherapy.

Bispecific Monoclonal Antibodies

Bispecific monoclonal antibodies contain two different recognition sites, one for antigens on tumor cells and another for antigens on immunologic effector cells, such as macrophages, T lymphocytes, or natural killer cells.[395] For treatment of HL with natural killer cell–activating bispecific antibodies, a CD16/CD30 bispecific antibody was constructed using hybridoma technology.[30] Heavily pretreated patients with refractory HL received intravenous infusions of the CD16/CD30 (A9/HRS-3) antibody four times every 3 or 4 days.[396] Fifteen patients with refractory HL were treated with escalating doses. Side effects were rare and consisted of short-lasting fever, pain in involved lymph nodes, and a maculopapulous rash. A total of one complete and one partial remission (lasting 16 months and 3 months, respectively), three minor responses (one lasting more than 11 months), and one mixed response were observed. Another clinical trial investigated a bispecific molecule against CD30 and CD64 (high-affinity receptor for the Fc part of IgG, Fcγ-R1). In this study, ten patients were included and six patients received the maximum dose of 80 mg/m²/cycle. One patient achieved a complete remission and three achieved a partial remission, which shows the potential of antibody-mediated cellular cytotoxicity in treatment of HL.[397]

The development of HAMA in the majority of patients as well as the high incidence of allergic reactions even in HAMA-negative patients who are reexposed to bispecific antibodies are the major problems with therapy using bispecific antibodies. This obstacle might be resolved by the construction of less immunogenic bispecific single-chain antibodies[398] or diabodies. Diabodies are formed by linking the variable regions of the heavy and light chains (V_H and V_L, respectively) of two different antibodies A and B to form two different crossover chains V_HA-V_LB and V_HB-V_LA. Recombinant DNA technology might also reduce the problem of producing bispecific antibodies in sufficient quantity and quality needed for administration in humans.

Prodrugs

The construction of antibodies carrying small enzymes capable of converting relatively nontoxic prodrugs into active anticancer agents allows the destruction of malignant cells that express a certain epitope as well as adjacent antigen-deficient tumor cell variants.[399,400] Alkaline phosphatase is the most frequently used enzyme for converting relatively noncytotoxic prodrugs such as mitomycin phosphate or etoposide phosphate into the active cytostatic drugs mitomycin and etoposide. For experimental use in HL, Sahin et al.[402a] constructed the HRS-3/AP-1 bispecific monoclonal antibody directed against the CD30 antigen and alkaline phosphatase. Bispecific monoclonal antibodies were used to prevent the need for forming antibody-enzyme conjugates chemically. After incubation of HRS-3/AP-1 and alkaline phosphatase with the Hodgkin's-derived cell line L540, mitomycin phosphate was converted into mitomycin alcohol, which was 100 times more toxic to L540 cells than mitomycin phosphate. Antigen-negative bystander cells were also killed once mitomycin phosphate had been activated. It is expected that this approach will lead to less destruction of normal cells than with conventional systemic therapy using the same drugs, because the major portion of the active drug will be released at the target site itself.

Vascular Targeting

Instead of targeting tumor cells directly, immunoconjugates can also be used to selectively occlude tumor vasculature. Because malignant cells are highly dependent on sufficient blood supply, local interruption of the tumor vasculature results in growth inhibition of the majority of dependent cells. Endothelial cells of tumor vessels are in direct contact with the blood stream, whereas tumor cells are often poorly accessible to circulating immunoconjugates. Because tumor endothelial cells are not transformed, it is unlikely that they acquire mutations that render them resistant to therapy. It might even be possible to identify antigens that are universally expressed on the endothelial cells of many different types of tumors.

Endoglin has been identified as a potential antigen for selective vascular targeting in HL.[401] It is part of the transforming growth factor-β receptor and is expressed on proliferating endothelial cells in humans and mice. The antibody MJ7/18, which binds selectively to murine endoglin, has been used for investigating expression of endoglin on vascular endothelia of SCID mice bearing human Hodgkin's lymphoma. After intravenous injection of MJ7/18 into tumor-bearing mice, endoglin was demonstrated to be significantly up-regulated on tumor vessels, whereas vessels in normal organs were not or only weakly stained. These results suggest that endoglin can serve as a target for selective immunotherapy of human HL using MJ7/18, for example, but careful determination of cross-reactivities with normal human tissue will be necessary.

ACTIVE IMMUNOTHERAPY

Therapeutic strategies modulating the cellular immune response have been investigated in lymphoma patients for more than 25 years. Because immunotherapy with bacille Calmette-Guérin had suggested therapeutic effects when combined with chemotherapy in patients with AML and breast cancer,[402] several randomized clinical trials were initiated involving patients with advanced HL as well. Because of a documented lack of therapeutic benefit and a higher frequency of unacceptable toxicity, trials investigating bacille Calmette-Guérin treatment were discontinued.[403]

Cytokines

IL-2 was one of the first immunotherapeutic agents used for anticancer therapy. Several clinical studies were performed to investigate the efficacy of recombinant IL-2 alone or in combination with autologous lymphokine-activated killer cells (adoptive immunotherapy) in patients with refractory HL in the late 1980s and early 1990s.[404–406] Toxicity was mild, mainly consisting of fever, rash, hypotension, and anemia. In these clinical pilot trials, several transient partial remissions were achieved in heavily pretreated patients with relapsed or refractory disease. Although these preliminary results were regarded as promising, no clinical studies have been published since then. IL-2 has been used in combination with a bispecific antibody to enhance the response rates, but with limited success.

Case reports of a few patients who received interferon for treatment of viral infection observed minor responses in HL. Therefore, some pilot studies were conducted to investigate the efficacy of interferon in salvage or maintenance therapy for HL.[407–410] Preliminary results suggest a limited activity of interferon-α in patients with relapsed or refractory HL.

A recombinant fusion protein of an anti-CD30 single-chain variable fragment and IL-12 has been shown to induce efficient lysis of CD30+ tumor cells by natural killer cells. The fusion protein is designed to overcome the H-RS cell–mediated anergy of the infiltrating lymphocytes and to convert the Th2 polarization to a Th1-like response.[411]

Vaccination

Active specific immunotherapy is the main principle behind tumor cell vaccination: Tumor cell antigens or their anti-idiotype vaccine is administered to the patient for stimulation of a specific immune response. Problems of vaccination are the limited availability of purified material and the development of immune tolerance against autogenic tumor antigens.[412,413] One of the earliest strategies investigated for active specific immunotherapy is the replacement of tumor antigen with monoclonal antibodies that carry structures of the tumor antigen as an "internal image." According to the network theory proposed by Nils Jerne,[414] any nominal antigen can induce a cascade of specific antibodies termed Ab1, Ab2, Ab3, etc. The second generation of antibodies (Ab2) raised against the antigen-binding site of the antitumor antibody (Ab1) can mimic the confirmation of the original antigen like an internal image. These internal images can induce specific antitumor responses like the nominal antigen and can thus substitute for tumor antigen as vaccine material. To develop a vaccine for HL, different monoclonal antibodies were evaluated as tumor-specific Ab1 for the induction of internal-image antibodies mimicking structures of the tumor antigen.[415] The most promising internal-image antibody, 9G10, against HRS-4 was used to generate monoclonal anti–anti-idiotypic antibodies (Ab3). Analyses of Ab3 hybridoma (4A4) showed specific binding to the CD30 antigen. 4A4 induced complement-dependent cytotoxicity to CD30+ Hodgkin's cells and prevented subcutaneous growth of solid human Hodgkin's tumors in SCID mice.[416]

GENE THERAPY

Modulation of EBV-directed T-cell activity might be another interesting new immunotherapeutic option. Heslop et al. developed EBV-specific cytotoxic T lymphocytes for treatment of EBV-associated lymphoma after bone marrow transplantation. Donors' blood samples were used for generation of EBV-transformed B-cell lines (lymphoblastoid cell lines) and for production of cytotoxic T lymphocytes.[417] Incubation of activated cytotoxic T cells with lymphoblastoid cell lines of the same probe induced formation of EBV-specific cytotoxic T lymphocytes. In three of ten patients who had elevated levels of EBV DNA after allogeneic transplantation, levels normalized after infusion of the EBV-specific cytotoxic T cells. EBV-specific cytotoxic T lymphocytes were isolated for an adoptive transfer in patients with EBV-positive HL.[418] Nine patients with active relapsed HL and four who were in complete remission after first or subsequent therapy were treated with autologous EBV-specific cytotoxic T lymphocytes. A 100-fold reduction of EBV DNA was observed in all patients; in two of them, B symptoms ceased.

REFERENCES

1. Hellman S. A brief consideration of Thomas Hodgkin and his times. In: Mauch PM, Armitage JO, Diehl V, et al., eds. *Hodgkin's disease*. Philadelphia: Lippincott Williams & Wilkins, 1999:3.
2. Hodgkin T. On some morbid appearances of the absorbent glands and spleen. *Medico-Chirugical Trans* 1832;17:68.
3. Wilks S. Cases of enlargement of the lymphatic glands and spleen (or Hodgkin's disease), with remarks. *Guys Hosp Rep* 1865;11:56.
4. Greenfield W. Specimens illustrative of the pathology of lymphadenoma and leucocythemia. *Trans Pathol Soc Lond* 1878;29:272.
5. Sternberg C. Uber eine eigenartige unter dem Bilde der Pseudoleukamie verlaufende Tuberculose des lymphatischen Apparates. *Zeitschr Heilk* 1898;19:21.
6. Reed D. On the pathological changes in Hodgkin's disease, with special reference to its relation to tuberculosis. *Johns Hopkins Hosp Rep* 1902;10:133.
7. Benda C. Zur Histologie der pseudoleukamischen Geschwulste. *Verhandl deut patholog Gesell* 1904:7.
8. Stein H, Hummel M. Hodgkin's disease: biology and origin of Hodgkin and Reed-Sternberg cells. *Cancer Treat Rev* 1999;25(3):161.
9. MacMahon B. Epidemiological evidence of the nature of Hodgkin's disease. *Cancer* 1957;10:1045.
10. Correa P, O'Conor G, Berard C. International comparability and reproducibility in histologic subclassification of Hodgkin's disease. *J Natl Cancer Inst* 1973;50:1429.
11. Greco R, Acheson R, Foote F. Hodgkin's disease in Connecticut from 1935 to 1962. *Arch Intern Med* 1974;134:1039.
12. Bernard S, et al. Hodgkin's disease: case control epidemiological study in Yorkshire. *Br J Cancer* 1987;55(1):85.
13. Razis DV, Diamond HD, Craver LF. Familial Hodgkin's disease: its significance and implications. *Ann Intern Med* 1959;51:933.
14. Bryden H, et al. Determination of HLA-A*02 antigen status in Hodgkin's disease and analysis of an HLA-A*02-restricted epitope of the Epstein-Barr virus LMP-2 protein. *Int J Cancer* 1997;72(4):614.
15. Poppema S, Visser L. Epstein-Barr virus positivity in Hodgkin's disease does not correlate with an HLA A2-negative phenotype. *Cancer* 1994;73(12):3059.
16. Lowenthal D, et al. AIDS-related lymphoid neoplasia: the Memorial Hospital experience. *Cancer* 1988;61:2325.
17. Mueller N. Hodgkin's disease. In: Schnottenfeld D, Fraumeni J, eds. *Cancer epidemiology and prevention*, vol 2. New York: Oxford University Press, 1992.
18. Gutensohn N. Social class and age at diagnosis of Hodgkin's disease: new epidemiologic evidence for the "two-disease hypothesis." *Cancer Treat Rep* 1982;66(4):689.
19. Kaplan H. *Hodgkin's disease*, vol 2. Cambridge, MA: Harvard University Press, 1980.
20. Haluska FG, et al. The cellular biology of the Reed-Sternberg cell. *Blood* 1994;84:1005.
21. Diehl V, et al. Characteristics of Hodgkin's disease-derived cell lines. *Cancer Treat Rep* 1982;66(4):615.
22. Diehl V, et al. The cell of origin in Hodgkin's disease. *Semin Oncol* 1990;17(6):660.
23. Wolf J, et al. Peripheral blood mononuclear cells of a patient with advanced Hodgkin's lymphoma give rise to permanently growing Hodgkin-Reed Sternberg cells. *Blood* 1996;87(8):3418.
24. Kanzler H, et al. Molecular single cell analysis demonstrates the derivation of a peripheral blood-derived cell line (L1236) from the Hodgkin/Reed-Sternberg cells of a Hodgkin's lymphoma patient. *Blood* 1996;87(8):3429.
25. Stein H, et al. Identification of Hodgkin and Sternberg-Reed cells as a unique cell type derived from a newly detected small-cell population. *Int J Cancer* 1982;30(4):445.
26. Schwab U, et al. Production of a monoclonal antibody specific for Hodgkin and Sternberg-Reed cells of Hodgkin's disease and a subset of normal lymphoid cells. *Nature* 1982;299(5878):65.
27. Durkop H, et al. Molecular cloning and expression of a new member of the nerve growth factor receptor family that is characteristic for Hodgkin's disease. *Cell* 1992;68(3):421.
28. Engert A, et al. Antitumor effects of ricin A chain immunotoxins prepared from intact

antibodies and Fab' fragments on solid human Hodgkin's disease tumors in mice. *Cancer Res* 1990;50(10):2929.

29. Falini B, et al. Response of refractory Hodgkin's disease to monoclonal anti-CD30 immunotoxin. *Lancet* 1992;339(8803):1195.

30. Hombach A, et al. A CD16/CD30 bispecific monoclonal antibody induces lysis of Hodgkin's cells by unstimulated natural killer cells *in vitro* and *in vivo*. *Int J Cancer* 1993;55(5):830.

31. Winkler U, et al. Successful treatment of disseminated human Hodgkin's disease in SCID mice with deglycosylated ricin A-chain immunotoxins. *Blood* 1994;83(2):466.

32. Kapp U, et al. Hodgkin's lymphoma-derived tissue serially transplanted into severe combined immunodeficient mice. *Blood* 1993;82(4):1247.

33. Kuppers R, et al. Hodgkin disease: Hodgkin and Reed-Sternberg cells picked from histological sections show clonal immunoglobulin gene rearrangements and appear to be derived from B cells at various stages of development. *Proc Natl Acad Sci U S A* 1994;91(23):10962.

34. Kanzler H, et al. Hodgkin and Reed-Sternberg cells in Hodgkin's disease represent the outgrowth of a dominant tumor clone derived from (crippled) germinal center B cells. *J Exp Med* 1996;184(4):1495.

35. Irsch J, et al. Isolation of viable Hodgkin and Reed-Sternberg cells from Hodgkin disease tissues. *Proc Natl Acad Sci U S A* 1998;95(17):10117.

36. Vockerodt M, et al. Detection of clonal Hodgkin and Reed-Sternberg cells with identical somatically mutated and rearranged VH genes in different biopsies in relapsed Hodgkin's disease. *Blood* 1998;92(8):2899.

37. Hummel M, et al. Hodgkin's disease with monoclonal and polyclonal populations of Reed-Sternberg cells [see comments]. *N Engl J Med* 1995;333(14):901.

38. Marafioti T, et al. Origin of nodular lymphocyte-predominant Hodgkin's disease from a clonal expansion of highly mutated germinal-center B cells [see comments]. *N Engl J Med* 1997;337(7):453.

39. Jox A, Wolf J, Diehl V. Hodgkin's disease biology: recent advances. *Hematol Oncol* 1997;15(4):165.

40. Jox A, et al. Clonal relapse in Hodgkin's disease [Letter]. *N Engl J Med* 1997;337(7):499.

41. Brousset P, et al. Persistence of the same viral strain in early and late relapses of Epstein-Barr virus–associated Hodgkin's disease. *Blood* 1994;84(8):2447.

42. Inghirami G, et al. The Reed-Sternberg cells of Hodgkin disease are clonal. *Proc Natl Acad Sci U S A* 1994;91(21):9842.

43. Seitz V, et al. Detection of clonal T-cell receptor gamma-chain gene rearrangements in Reed-Sternberg cells of classic Hodgkin disease. *Blood* 2000;95(10):3020.

44. Rajewsky K. Clonal selection and learning in the antibody system. *Nature* 1996;381(6585):751.

45. Silvy A, et al. The differentiation of human memory B cells into specific antibody-secreting cells is CD40 independent. *Eur J Immunol* 1996;26(3):517.

46. Hennino A, et al. FLICE-inhibitory protein is a key regulator of germinal center B cell apoptosis. *J Exp Med* 2001;193(4):447.

47. van Eijk M, et al. Death-receptor contribution to the germinal-center reaction. *Trends Immunol* 2001;22(12):677.

48. Ohno T, et al. Clonality in nodular lymphocyte-predominant Hodgkin's disease [see comments]. *N Engl J Med* 1997;337(7):459.

49. Jox A, et al. Somatic mutations within the untranslated regions of rearranged Ig genes in a case of classical Hodgkin's disease as a potential cause for the absence of Ig in the lymphoma cells. *Blood* 1999;93(11):3964.

50. Stein H, et al. Down-regulation of BOB.1/OBF.1 and Oct2 in classical Hodgkin disease but not in lymphocyte predominant Hodgkin disease correlates with immunoglobulin transcription. *Blood* 2001;97(2):496.

51. Re D, et al. Deregulation of immunoglobulin gene transcription in the Hodgkin-Reed Sternberg cell line L1236. *Br J Haematol* 2001;115(2):326.

52. Hertel CB, et al. Loss of B cell identity correlates with loss of B cell-specific transcription factors in Hodgkin/Reed-Sternberg cells of classical Hodgkin lymphoma. *Oncogene* 2002;21(32):4908.

53. Schwering I, et al. Loss of the B-lineage–specific gene expression program in Hodgkin and Reed-Sternberg cells of Hodgkin lymphoma. *Blood* 2003;101(4):1505.

54. Re D, et al. Cultivated H-RS cells are resistant to CD95L-mediated apoptosis despite expression of wild-type CD95. *Exp Hematol* 2000;28(3):348.

55. Thomas RK, et al. Constitutive expression of c-FLIP in Hodgkin and Reed-Sternberg cells. *Am J Pathol* 2002;160(4):1521.

56. Re D, et al. Lack of BCL10 mutations in Hodgkin's disease-derived cell lines. *Br J Haematol* 2000;109(2):420.

57. Muschen M, et al. Somatic mutations of the CD95 gene in Hodgkin and Reed-Sternberg cells. *Cancer Res* 2000;60(20):5640.

58. Maggio EM, et al. Low frequency of FAS mutations in Reed-Sternberg cells of Hodgkin's lymphoma. *Am J Pathol* 2003;162(1):29.

59. Kuppers R, et al. Identification of Hodgkin and Reed-Sternberg cell–specific genes by gene expression profiling. *J Clin Invest* 2003;111(4):529.

60. Kuppers R, et al. Evidence that Hodgkin and Reed-Sternberg cells in Hodgkin disease do not represent cell fusions. *Blood* 2001;97(3):818.

61. Re D, et al. Cell fusion is not involved in the generation of giant cells in the Hodgkin-Reed Sternberg cell line L1236. *Am J Hematol* 2001;67(1):6.

62. Fonatsch C, et al. Chromosomal in situ hybridization of a Hodgkin's disease–derived cell line (L540) using DNA probes for TCRA, TCRB, MET, and rRNA. *Hum Genet* 1990;84(5):427.

63. Rowley J. Chromosomes in Hodgkin's disease. *Cancer Treat Rep* 1982;66(4):639.

64. Thangavelu M, Le BM. Chromosomal abnormalities in Hodgkin's disease. *Hematol Oncol Clin North Am* 1989;3(2):221.

65. Tilly H, et al. Cytogenetic studies in untreated Hodgkin's disease. *Blood* 1991;77(6):1298.

66. Weber-Matthiesen K, et al. Numerical chromosome aberrations are present within the CD30+ Hodgkin and Reed-Sternberg cells in 100% of analyzed cases of Hodgkin's disease [see comments]. *Blood* 1995;86(4):1464.

67. Inghirami G, Frizzera G. Role of the bcl-2 oncogene in Hodgkin's disease [Editorial]. *Am J Clin Pathol* 1994;101(6):681.

68. Joos S, et al. Genomic imbalances including amplification of the tyrosine kinase gene JAK2 in CD30+ Hodgkin cells. *Cancer Res* 2000;60(3):549.

69. Martin-Subero JI, et al. Recurrent involvement of the REL and BCL11A loci in classical Hodgkin lymphoma. *Blood* 2002;99(4):1474.

70. Barth TF, et al. Gains of 2p involving the REL locus correlate with nuclear c-Rel protein accumulation in neoplastic cells of classical Hodgkin lymphoma. *Blood* 2003;101(9):3681.

71. Re D, et al. Allelic losses on chromosome 6q25 in Hodgkin and Reed Sternberg cells. *Cancer Res* 2003;63(10):2606.

72. Steenvoorden AC, Janssen JW, Drexler HD. Ras mutations in Hodgkin's disease. *Leukemia* 1988;2:325.

73. Weiss L, et al. Absence of the t(2; 5) in Hodgkin's disease [see comments]. *Blood* 1995;85(10):2845.

74. Gravel S, Delsol G, Al Saati T. Single-cell analysis of the t(14; 18)(q32; q21) chromosomal translocation in Hodgkin's disease demonstrates the absence of this translocation in neoplastic Hodgkin and Reed-Sternberg cells. *Blood* 1998;91(8):2866.

75. Herbst H, et al. ALK gene products in anaplastic large cell lymphomas and Hodgkin's disease. *Blood* 1995;86(5):1694.

76. Elmberger P, et al. Transcripts of the npm-alk fusion gene in anaplastic large cell lymphoma, Hodgkin's disease, and reactive lymphoid lesions. *Blood* 1995;86(9):3517.

77. Kuppers R. Identifying the precursors of Hodgkin and Reed-Sternberg cells in Hodgkin's disease: role of the germinal center in B-cell lymphomagenesis. *J Acquir Immune Defic Syndr* 1999;21[Suppl 1]:S74.

78. Re D, et al. Proficient mismatch repair protein expression in Hodgkin and Reed Sternberg cells. *Int J Cancer* 2002;97(2):205.

79. Hanahan D, Weinberg RA. The hallmarks of cancer. *Cell* 2000;100(1):57.

80. Bargou R, et al. High-level nuclear NF-κB and Oct-2 is a common feature of cultured Hodgkin/Reed-Sternberg cells. *Blood* 1996;87(10):4340.

81. Bargou R, et al. Constitutive nuclear factor-κB-RelA activation is required for proliferation and survival of Hodgkin's disease tumor cells. *J Clin Invest* 1997;100(12):2961.

82. Hinz M, et al. Constitutive NF-κB maintains high expression of a characteristic gene network, including CD40, CD86, and a set of antiapoptotic genes in Hodgkin/Reed-Sternberg cells. *Blood* 2001;97(9):2798.

83. Hinz M, et al. Nuclear factor κB-dependent gene expression profiling of Hodgkin's disease tumor cells, pathogenetic significance, and link to constitutive signal transducer and activator of transcription 5a activity. *J Exp Med* 2002;196(5):605.

84. Horie R, et al. Ligand-independent signaling by overexpressed CD30 drives NF-κB activation in Hodgkin-Reed-Sternberg cells. *Oncogene* 2002;21(16):2493.

85. Annunziata CM, et al. Hodgkin disease: pharmacologic intervention of the CD40-NF κB pathway by a protease inhibitor. *Blood* 2000;96(8):2841.

86. Fiumara P, et al. Functional expression of receptor activator of nuclear factor κB in Hodgkin disease cell lines. *Blood* 2001;98(9):2784.

87. Pallesen G, et al. Expression of Epstein-Barr virus latent gene products in tumour cells of Hodgkin's disease [see comments]. *Lancet* 1991;337(8737):320.

88. Herbst H, et al. Expression of latent membrane proteins (LMP) of Epstein-Barr virus in malignant lymphomas [in German]. *Verh Dtsch Ges Pathol* 1991;75:175.

89. Niedobitek G, et al. Immunohistochemical detection of the Epstein-Barr virus-encoded latent membrane protein 2A in Hodgkin's disease and infectious mononucleosis. *Blood* 1997;90(4):1664.

90. Li Q, Verma IM. NF-κB regulation in the immune system. *Nat Rev Immunol* 2002;2(10):725.

91. Emmerich F, et al. Overexpression of IκBα without inhibition of NF-κB activity and mutations in the IκBα gene in Reed-Sternberg cells. *Blood* 1999;94(9):3129.

91a. Cabannes E, Khan G, Aillet F, Jarrett R, Hay R. Mutations in the IkBa gene in Hodgkin's disease suggest a tumour suppressor role for IkappaBalpha. *Oncogene* 1999;18:3063.

91b. Jarrett RF, Lake A, Andrew L, et al. Somatic IkBa mutations are a frequent occurrence in Hodgkin lymphoma. *Blood* 2002;100:4333(abst).

92. Kube D, et al. STAT3 is constitutively activated in Hodgkin cell lines. *Blood* 2001;98(3):762.

93. Skinnider BF, et al. Signal transducer and activator of transcription 6 is frequently activated in Hodgkin and Reed-Sternberg cells of Hodgkin lymphoma. *Blood* 2002;99(2):618.

94. Fang W, Nath KA, Mackey MF. CD40 inhibits B cell apoptosis by upregulating bcl-xL expression and blocking oxidant accumulation. *Am J Physiol* 1997(272):950.

95. Weiss L, et al. Epstein-Barr viral DNA in tissues of Hodgkin's disease. *Am J Pathol* 1987;129(1):86.

96. Cabanillas F, et al. Cytogenetic features of Hodgkin's disease suggest possible origin from a lymphocyte. *Blood* 1988;71(6):1615.

97. Bonecchi R, Bianchi G, Bordignon PP. Differential expression of chemokine receptors and chemotactic responsiveness of type 1 T helper cells (Th1s) and Th2s. *J Exp Med* 1998;187:129.

98. Herbst H, et al. Epstein-Barr virus latent membrane protein expression in Hodgkin and Reed-Sternberg cells. *Proc Natl Acad Sci U S A* 1991;88(11):4766.

99. Herbst H, Raff T, Stein H. Phenotypic modulation of Hodgkin and Reed-Sternberg cells by Epstein-Barr virus. *J Pathol* 1996;179(1):54.

100. Mason D, et al. Nodular lymphocyte predominance Hodgkin's disease. A distinct clinicopathological entity [Editorial]. *Am J Surg Pathol* 1994;18(5):526.

101. Gires O, Zimber-Strobl U, Gonnella R. Latent membrane protein 1 of Epstein-Barr virus mimics a constitutively active receptor molecule. *EMBO J* 1997;16:6131.

101a. Knecht H, Bachmann E, Brousset P, et al. Deletions within the LMP1 oncogene of Epstein-Barr virus are clustered in Hodgkin's disease and identical to those observed in nasopharyngeal carcinoma. *Blood* 1993;82:2937.

102. Staratschek-Jox A, et al. Detection of Epstein-Barr virus in Hodgkin-Reed-Sternberg cells: no evidence for the persistence of integrated viral fragments in latent membrane protein-1 (LMP-1)–negative classical Hodgkin's disease. *Am J Pathol* 2000;156(1):209.

103. Fruehling S, et al. Identification of latent membrane protein 2A (LMP2A) domains essential for the LMP2A dominant-negative effect on B-lymphocyte surface immunoglobulin signal transduction. *J Virol* 1996;70(9):6216.

104. Poppema S, van den Berg A. Interaction between host T cells and Reed-Sternberg cells in Hodgkin lymphomas. *Semin Cancer Biol* 2000;10(5):345.
105. Skinnider BF, Mak TW. The role of cytokines in classical Hodgkin lymphoma. *Blood* 2002;99(12):4283.
106. Maggio E, et al. Chemokines, cytokines and their receptors in Hodgkin's lymphoma cell lines and tissues. *Ann Oncol* 2002;13[Suppl]1:52.
107. Herbst H, et al. Frequent expression of interleukin-10 by Epstein-Barr virus-harboring tumor cells of Hodgkin's disease. *Blood* 1996;87(7):2918.
107a. Hsu S, Hsu P. Autocrine and paracrine functions of cytokines in malignant lymphomas. *Biomed Pharmacother* 1994;48:433.
108. Drexler H. Recent results on the biology of Hodgkin and Reed-Sternberg cells. II. Continuous cell lines. *Leuk Lymphoma* 1993;9(1–2):1.
109. Pinkus G, Said J. Hodgkin's disease, lymphocyte predominance type, nodular—further evidence for a B cell derivation. L & H variants of Reed-Sternberg cells express L26, a pan B cell marker. *Am J Pathol* 1988;133(2):211.
110. Hall P, d'Ardenne A, Stansfeld A. Paraffin section immunohistochemistry. II. Hodgkin's disease and large cell anaplastic (Ki1) lymphoma. *Histopathology* 1988;13(2):161.
111. Regula DJ, Hoppe R, Weiss L. Nodular and diffuse types of lymphocyte predominance Hodgkin's disease. *N Engl J Med* 1988;318(4):214.
112. Brauninger A, Kuppers R, Strickler JG. Hodgkin and Reed-Sternberg cells in lymphocyte predominant Hodgkin disease represent clonal populations of germinal center–derived tumor B cells. *Proc Natl Acad Sci U S A* 1997;94:9337.
113. Jackson HJ, Parker FJ. *Hodgkin's disease and allied disorders*. New York: Oxford University Press, 1947.
113a. Lukes RJ, Butler JJ. The pathology and nomenclature of Hodgkin's disease. *Cancer Res* 1966;26:1063.
114. Lukes R, Butler J, Hicks E. Natural history of Hodgkin's disease as related to its pathological picture. *Cancer* 1966;19:317.
115. Harris NL, Jaffe ES, Stein H. A revised European-American classification of lymphoid neoplasms: a proposal from the International Lymphoma Study Group. *Blood* 1994;84:1361.
116. von Wasielewski R, Werner M, Fischer R. Lymphocyte-predominant Hodgkin's disease: an immunohistochemical analysis of 208 reviewed Hodgkin's disease cases from the German Hodgkin Study Group. *Am J Pathol* 1997;150:793.
117. Burns B, Colby T, Dorfman R. Differential diagnostic features of nodular L & H Hodgkin's disease, including progressive transformation of germinal centers. *Am J Surg Pathol* 1984;8(4):253.
118. Poppema S, Kaiserling E, Lennert K. Nodular paragranuloma and progressively transformed germinal centers: ultrastructural and immunohistochemical findings. *Virchows Arch B Cell Pathol Incl Mol Pathol* 1979;31:211.
119. Ferry J, Zukerberg L, Harris N. Florid progressive transformation of germinal centers. A syndrome affecting young men, without early progression to nodular lymphocyte predominance Hodgkin's disease. *Am J Surg Pathol* 1992;16(3):252.
120. Bennett M, et al. Non-Hodgkin's lymphoma arising in patients treated for Hodgkin's disease in the BNLI: a 20-year experience. British National Lymphoma Investigation. *Ann Oncol* 1991;2[Suppl 2]:83.
121. Hansmann M, Wacker H, Radzun H. Paragranuloma is a variant of Hodgkin's disease with predominance of B-cells. *Virchows Arch A Pathol Anat Histopathol* 1986;409(2):171.
122. Orlandi E, Lazzarino M, Brusamolino E. Nodular lymphocyte predominance Hodgkin's disease (NLPHD): clinical behavior and pattern of progression in 66 patients. Paper presented at: Third International Symposium on Hodgkin's Lymphoma, 1995, Cologne, Germany.
123. Wickert R, et al. Clonal relationship between lymphocytic predominance Hodgkin's disease and concurrent or subsequent large-cell lymphoma of B lineage. *Blood* 1995;86(6):2312.
124. Sundeen J, Cossman J, Jaffe E. Lymphocyte predominant Hodgkin's disease nodular subtype with coexistent "large cell lymphoma." Histological progression or composite malignancy? [see comments]. *Am J Surg Pathol* 1988;12(8):599.
125. Stein H, et al. Reed-Sternberg and Hodgkin cells in lymphocyte-predominant Hodgkin's disease of nodular subtype contain J chain. *Am J Clin Pathol* 1986;86(3):292.
126. Stoler M, et al. Lymphocyte predominance Hodgkin's disease. Evidence for a kappa light chain–restricted monotypic B-cell neoplasm. *Am J Pathol* 1995;146(4):812.
127. Carbone A, et al. Expression of functional CD40 antigen on Reed-Sternberg cells and Hodgkin's disease cell lines. *Blood* 1995;85(3):780.
128. Timens W, Visser L, Poppema S. Nodular lymphocyte predominance type of Hodgkin's disease is a germinal center lymphoma. *Lab Invest* 1986;54(4):457.
129. Poppema S. The nature of the lymphocytes surrounding Reed-Sternberg cells in nodular lymphocyte predominance and in other types of Hodgkin's disease. *Am J Pathol* 1989;135(2):351.
130. Kamel O, et al. Leu 7 (CD57) reactivity distinguishes nodular lymphocyte predominance Hodgkin's disease from nodular sclerosing Hodgkin's disease, T-cell-rich B-cell lymphoma and follicular lymphoma. *Am J Pathol* 1993;142(2):541.
131. Hansmann M, et al. Diffuse lymphocyte-predominant Hodgkin's disease (diffuse paragranuloma). A variant of the B-cell-derived nodular type. *Am J Pathol* 1991;138(1):29.
132. Krayalcin G, Behm F, Geiser P. Lymphocyte predominant Hodgkin disease: clinicopathologic features and results of treatment—the Pediatric Oncology Group experience. *Med Pediatr Oncol* 1997;29:519.
133. Colby T, Hoppe R, Warnke R. Hodgkin's disease: a clinicopathologic study of 659 cases. *Cancer* 1982;49(9):1848.
134. Kant J, et al. The pathologic and clinical heterogeneity of lymphocyte-depleted Hodgkin's disease. *J Clin Oncol* 1986;4(3):284.
135. Bennett M, et al. The prognostic significance of cellular subtypes in nodular sclerosing Hodgkin's disease: an analysis of 271 non-laparotomised cases (BNLI report no. 22). *Clin Radiol* 1983;34(5):497.
135a. Von Wasielewski S, Franklin J, Fischer R, et al. Nodular sclerosing Hodgkin disease: new grading predicts prognosis in intermediate and advanced stages. *Blood* 2003;101(10):4063.
136. Wijlhuizen T, et al. Grades of nodular sclerosis (NSI-NSII) in Hodgkin's disease. Are they of independent prognostic value? *Cancer* 1989;63(6):1150.
137. Hess J, et al. Histopathologic grading of nodular sclerosis Hodgkin's disease. Lack of prognostic significance in 254 surgically staged patients. *Cancer* 1994;74(2):708.
138. van Spronsen D, Vrints L, Erdkamp F. Disappearance of prognostic value of subclassification of nodular sclerosing Hodgkin's disease in south-east Netherlands since 1972. Paper presented at: Third International Symposium on Hodgkin's Lymphoma, 1995, Cologne, Germany.
139. Stein H, et al. The nature of Hodgkin and Reed-Sternberg cells, their association with EBV, and their relationship to anaplastic large-cell lymphoma. *Ann Oncol* 1991;2[Suppl 2]:33.
140. Neiman R, Rosen P, Lukes R. Lymphocyte depletion Hodgkin's disease. A clinicopathological entity. *N Engl J Med* 1973;288:751.
141. Falini B, et al. Expression of lymphoid-associated antigens on Hodgkin's and Reed-Sternberg cells of Hodgkin's disease. An immunocytochemical study on lymph node cytospins using monoclonal antibodies. *Histopathology* 1987;11(12):1229.
142. Falini B, Dalla Favara R, Pileri S. BCL-6 gene rearrangement and expression in Hodgkin's disease. Paper presented at: Third International Symposium on Hodgkin's Lymphoma, 1995, Cologne, Germany.
143. McBride J, et al. T-cell–rich B large-cell lymphoma simulating lymphocyte-rich Hodgkin's disease [see comments]. *Am J Surg Pathol* 1996;20(2):193.
144. Ashton-Key M, et al. Follicular Hodgkin's disease. *Am J Surg Pathol* 1995;19(11):1294.
145. Diehl V, Stein H, Sextro M. Lymphocyte predominant Hodgkin's disease: a European Task Force on Lymphoma project. *Blood* 1996;88:294a.
146. Wasielewski R, Mengel M, Fischer R. Classical Hodgkin's disease: clinical impact of the immunophenotype. *Am J Pathol* 1997;151:1123.
147. Jaffe E, Zarate-Osorno A, Medeiros L. The interrelationship of Hodgkin's disease and non-Hodgkin's lymphomas—lessons learned from composite and sequential malignancies. *Semin Diagn Pathol* 1992;9(4):297.
148. Travis L, et al. Hodgkin's disease following non-Hodgkin's lymphoma. *Cancer* 1992; 69(9):2337.
149. Brauninger A, et al. Identification of common germinal-center B-cell precursors in two patients with both Hodgkin's disease and non-Hodgkin's lymphoma [see comments]. *N Engl J Med* 1999;340(16):1239.
150. Rubin D, et al. Richter's transformation of chronic lymphocytic leukemia with Hodgkin's-like cells is associated with Epstein-Barr virus infection. *Mod Pathol* 1994;7(1):91.
151. Kuppers R, Rajewsky K. The origin of Hodgkin and Reed/Sternberg cells in Hodgkin's disease. *Annu Rev Immunol* 1998;16:471.
152. Brousset P, et al. Hodgkin's disease following mycosis fungoides: phenotypic and molecular evidence for different tumour cell clones. *J Clin Pathol* 1996;49(6):504.
153. Stein H, et al. The expression of the Hodgkin's disease associated antigen Ki-1 in reactive and neoplastic lymphoid tissue: evidence that Reed-Sternberg cells and histiocytic malignancies are derived from activated lymphoid cells. *Blood* 1985;66(4):848.
154. Benharroch D, et al. ALK-positive lymphoma: a single disease with a broad spectrum of morphology. *Blood* 1998;91(6):2076.
155. Zinzani P, et al. Anaplastic large-cell lymphoma: clinical and prognostic evaluation of 90 adult patients [see comments]. *J Clin Oncol* 1996;14(3):955.
156. Sarris A, et al. Long-range amplification of genomic DNA detects the t(2;5)(p23; q35) in anaplastic large-cell lymphoma, but not in other non-Hodgkin's lymphomas, Hodgkin's disease, or lymphomatoid papulosis. *Ann Oncol* 1997;8[Suppl 2]:59.
157. Pulford K, et al. Detection of anaplastic lymphoma kinase (ALK) and nucleolar protein nucleophosmin (NPM)-ALK proteins in normal and neoplastic cells with the monoclonal antibody ALK1. *Blood* 1997;89(4):1394.
158. Gilbert R. Radiotherapy in Hodgkin's disease (malignant granulomatosis): anatomic and clinical foundations, governing principles, results. *AJR Am J Roentgenol* 1939;41:198.
159. Peters M. A study of survivals in Hodgkin's disease treated radiologically. *AJR Am J Roentgenol* 1950;63:299.
160. Kaplan H. The radical radiotherapy of regionally localized Hodgkin's disease. *Radiology* 1962;78:553.
161. Peters M. Prophylactic treatment of adjacent areas in Hodgkin's disease. *Cancer Res* 1966;26:1232.
162. Mauch P, et al. Prognostic factors for positive surgical staging in patients with Hodgkin's disease [see comments]. *J Clin Oncol* 1990;8(2):257.
163. Mauch P, et al. Patterns of presentation of Hodgkin disease. Implications for etiology and pathogenesis [see comments]. *Cancer* 1993;71(6):2062.
164. Marcus K, et al. Improved survival in patients with limited stage IIIA Hodgkin's disease treated with combined radiation therapy and chemotherapy. *J Clin Oncol* 1994;12(12):2567.
165. Lister T, et al. Report of a committee convened to discuss the evaluation and staging of patients with Hodgkin's disease: Cotswolds meeting [published erratum appears in *J Clin Oncol* 1990;8(9):1602] [see comments]. *J Clin Oncol* 1989;7(11):1630.
166. Mauch P, Goodman R, Hellman S. The significance of mediastinal involvement in early stage Hodgkin's disease. *Cancer* 1978;42(3):1039.
167. Hughes-Davies L, et al. Stage IA-IIB Hodgkin's disease: management and outcome of extensive thoracic involvement. *Int J Radiat Oncol Biol Phys* 1997;39(2):361.
168. Hoppe R, et al. The management of stage I–II Hodgkin's disease with irradiation alone or combined modality therapy: the Stanford experience. *Blood* 1982;59(3):455.
169. Spaepen K, et al. Can positron emission tomography with [^{18}F]-fluorodeoxyglucose after first-line treatment distinguish Hodgkin's disease patients who need additional therapy from others in whom additional therapy would mean avoidable toxicity? *Br J Haematol* 2001;115(2):272.
170. Naumann R, et al. Prognostic value of positron emission tomography in the evaluation of post-treatment residual mass in patients with Hodgkin's disease and non-Hodgkin's lymphoma. *Br J Haematol* 2001;115(4):793.
171. Castellino R, et al. Predictive value of lymphography for sites of subdiaphragmatic disease encountered at staging laparotomy in newly diagnosed Hodgkin's disease and non-Hodgkin's lymphoma. *J Clin Oncol* 1983;1(9):532.
172. Sapozink M, Kaplan H. Intracranial Hodgkin's disease. A report of 12 cases and review of the literature. *Cancer* 1983;52(7):1301.

173. Gobbi P, et al. Reevaluation of prognostic significance of symptoms in Hodgkin's disease. *Cancer* 1985;56(12):2874.

174. Pusey W. Cases of sarcoma and of Hodgkin's disease treated by exposures to X-rays: a preliminary report. *JAMA* 1902;38:166.

175. Kinzie J, et al. Patterns of care study: Hodgkin's disease relapse rates and adequacy of portals. *Cancer* 1983;52(12):2223.

176. Lutz W, Larsen R. Technique to match mantle and para-aortic fields. *Int J Radiat Oncol Biol Phys* 1983;9(11):1753.

177. Horning S, et al. Female reproductive potential after treatment for Hodgkin's disease. *N Engl J Med* 1981;304(23):1377.

177a. Skipper HE, Schabel FM Jr. Spontaneous AK leukemia (lymphoma) as a model for human leukemias and lymphomas. *Cancer Chemother Rep* 1972;3(1):3.

177b. De Vita VT, et al. Combination chemotherapy in the treatment of advanced Hodgkin's disease. *Ann Intern Med* 1970;73:881.

178. Loeffler M, et al. Dose-response relationship of complementary radiotherapy following four cycles of combination chemotherapy in intermediate-stage Hodgkin's disease. *J Clin Oncol* 1997;15(6):2275.

178a. Diehl V, Stein H, Hummel M, et al. Optimisation of combined modality treatment intensity in early stage Hodgkin's lymphoma: interim results of the HD10 trial of the GHSG. ASH Educational Book, 2003.

178b. Diehl V, Stein H, Hummel M, et al. Intensification of chemotherapy and concomitant dosis reduction of radiotherapy in intermediate stage Hodgkin's lymphoma: interim results of the HD11 trial of the GHSG. ASH Educational Book, 2003.

179. Bhatia S, et al. Breast cancer and other second neoplasms after childhood Hodgkin's disease [see comments]. *N Engl J Med* 1996;334(12):745.

180. van Leeuwen FE, et al. Roles of radiation dose, chemotherapy, and hormonal factors in breast cancer following Hodgkin's disease. *J Natl Cancer Inst* 2003;95(13):971.

181. Hancock S, Tucker M, Hoppe R. Factors affecting late mortality from heart disease after treatment of Hodgkin's disease. *JAMA* 1993;270(16):1949.

182. Horning S, et al. Stanford-Kaiser Permanente G1 study for clinical stage I to IIA Hodgkin's disease: subtotal lymphoid irradiation versus vinblastine, methotrexate, and bleomycin chemotherapy and regional irradiation. *J Clin Oncol* 1997;15(5):1736.

183. Reece D, Phillips G. Intensive therapy and autotransplantation in Hodgkin's disease. *Stem Cells* 1994;12(5):477.

184. Phillips G, Wolff S, Herzig R. Treatment of progressive Hodgkin's disease with intensive chemoradiotherapy and autologous bone marrow transplantation. *Blood* 1989;73:2086.

185. Jagannath S, et al. High-dose cyclophosphamide, carmustine, and etoposide and autologous bone marrow transplantation for relapsed Hodgkin's disease. *Ann Intern Med* 1986;104(2):163.

186. Josting A, Mapara M, Reiser M. Novel three phase, high-dose sequential chemotherapy with autologous stem cell support for relapsed or refractory Hodgkin's and high-grade non-Hodgkin's lymphoma. *Ann Oncol* 1999;10[Suppl 3]:638.

187. Gianni A, et al. High-dose sequential chemo-radiotherapy with peripheral blood progenitor cell support for relapsed or refractory Hodgkin's disease—a 6-year update. *Ann Oncol* 1993;4(10):889.

188. Norton L, Simon R. The Norton-Simon hypothesis revisited. *Cancer Treat Rep* 1986;70:163.

189. Reece D, et al. Intensive therapy with cyclophosphamide, carmustine, etoposide +/− cisplatin, and autologous bone marrow transplantation for Hodgkin's disease in first relapse after combination chemotherapy [see comments]. *Blood* 1994;83(5):1193.

190. Yahalom J, et al. Accelerated hyperfractionated total-lymphoid irradiation, high-dose chemotherapy, and autologous bone marrow transplantation for refractory and relapsing patients with Hodgkin's disease. *J Clin Oncol* 1993;11(6):1062.

191. Poen J, Hoppe R, Horning S. High-dose therapy and autologous bone marrow transplantation for relapsed/refractory Hodgkin's disease: the impact of involved field radiotherapy on patterns of failure and survival [see comments]. *Int J Radiat Oncol Biol Phys* 1996;36(1):3.

192. Goldstone A. The case for and against high-dose therapy with stem cell rescue for early poor prognosis Hodgkin's disease in first remission. *Ann Oncol* 1998;9[Suppl 5]:S83.

193. Proctor SJ, et al. A population-based study of intensive multi-agent chemotherapy with or without autotransplant for the highest risk Hodgkin's disease patients identified by the Scotland and Newcastle Lymphoma Group (SNLG) prognostic index. A Scotland and Newcastle Lymphoma Group study (SNLG HD III). *Eur J Cancer* 2002;38(6):795.

194. Mauch P, Tarbell N, Weinstein H. Stage IA and IIA supradiaphragmatic Hodgkin's disease: prognostic factors in surgically staged patients treated with mantle and paraaortic irradiation. *J Clin Oncol* 1988;6:1576.

195. Loeffler M, Pfreundschuh M, Hasenclever D. Prognostic risk factors in advanced Hodgkin's disease. Report of the German Hodgkin Study Group. *Blut* 1988;56:273.

196. Carde P, Burger JM, Henry-Amar M. Clinical stages I and II Hodgkin's disease: a specifically tailored therapy according to prognostic factors. *J Clin Oncol* 1988;6:239.

197. Loeffler M, Pfreundschuh M, Rühl U. Risk factor adapted treatment of Hodgkin's lymphoma: strategies and perspectives. *Recent Results Cancer Res* 1989;117:142.

198. Hasenclever D, Diehl V. A prognostic score for advanced Hodgkin's disease. International Prognostic Factors Project on Advanced Hodgkin's Disease [see comments]. *N Engl J Med* 1998;339(21):1506.

199. Lagarde P, et al. Brief chemotherapy associated with extended field radiotherapy in Hodgkin's disease. Long-term results in a series of 102 patients with clinical stages I-IIIA. *Eur J Cancer Clin Oncol* 1988;24(7):1191.

200. Specht LK, Hasenclever D. Prognostic factors of Hodgkin's disease. In: Mauch PM, Armitage JO, Diehl V, et al., eds. *Hodgkin's disease.* Philadelphia: Lippincott Williams & Wilkins, 1999.

201. Viviani S, et al. Alternating versus hybrid MOPP and ABVD combinations in advanced Hodgkin's disease: ten-year results. *J Clin Oncol* 1996;14(5):1421.

202. Proctor S, et al. A numerical prognostic index for clinical use in identification of poor-risk patients with Hodgkin's disease at diagnosis. The Scotland and Newcastle Lymphoma Group (SNLG) Therapy Working Party. *Leuk Lymphoma* 1992;7[Suppl]:17.

203. Hasenclever D, Schmitz N, Diehl V. Is there a rationale for high-dose chemotherapy as first line treatment of advanced Hodgkin's disease? German Hodgkin's Lymphoma Study Group (GHSG). *Leuk Lymphoma* 1995;15[Suppl 1]:47.

204. Horning SJ, Yahalom J, Tesch H. Treatment of stage III-IV Hodgkin's disease. In: Mauch PM, Armitage JO, Diehl V, et al., eds. *Hodgkin's disease.* Philadelphia: Lippincott Williams & Wilkins, 1999:496.

205. Vijayakumar S, Myrianthopoulos L. An updated dose-response analysis in Hodgkin's disease [see comments]. *Radiother Oncol* 1992;24(1):1.

206. Duhmke E, et al. Randomized trial with early-stage Hodgkin's disease testing 30 Gy vs. 40 Gy extended field radiotherapy alone. *Int J Radiat Oncol Biol Phys* 1996;36(2):305.

207. Tubiana M, Henry-Amar M, Carde P. Toward comprehensive management tailored to prognostic factors of patients with clinical stages I and II in Hodgkin's disease. The EORTC Lymphoma Group controlled clinical trials: 1964–1987. *Blood* 1989;73:47.

208. Sutcliffe S, et al. Prognostic groups for management of localized Hodgkin's disease. *J Clin Oncol* 1985;3(3):393.

209. Wirth A, et al. Mantle irradiation alone for clinical stage I-II Hodgkin's disease: long-term follow-up and analysis of prognostic factors in 261 patients. *J Clin Oncol* 1999;17(1):230.

210. Noordijk E, Kluin-Nelemans J. Stage I or II Hodgkin's disease: more chemotherapy and less irradiation [see comments] [in Dutch]. *Ned Tijdschr Geneeskd* 1997;141(26):1281.

211. Ganesan T, et al. Radiotherapy for stage I Hodgkin's disease: 20 years experience at St. Bartholomew's Hospital. *Br J Cancer* 1990;62(2):314.

212. Horning S, Hoppe R, Hancock S. Vinblastine, bleomycin, and methotrexate: an effective adjuvant in favorable Hodgkin's disease. *J Clin Oncol* 1988;6:1822.

213. Bates N, et al. Efficacy and toxicity of vinblastine, bleomycin, and methotrexate with involved-field radiotherapy in clinical stage IA and IIA Hodgkin's disease: a British National Lymphoma Investigation pilot study. *J Clin Oncol* 1994;12(2):288.

214. Gobbi P, et al. Vinblastine, bleomycin, and methotrexate chemotherapy plus extended-field radiotherapy in early, favorably presenting, clinically staged Hodgkin's patients: the Gruppo Italiano per lo Studio dei Linfomi experience. *J Clin Oncol* 1996;14(2):527.

215. Noordijk E, Carde P, Hagenbeek A. Combination of radiotherapy and chemotherapy is advisable in all patients with clinical stage I-II Hodgkin's disease. Six-year results of the EORTC-GPMC controlled clinical trials H7-VF, H7-F and H7-U. *Int J Radiat Oncol Biol Phys* 1997;39:173(abst).

216. Carde P, Noordijk E, Hagenbeek A. Superiority of EBVP chemotherapy in combination with involved field irradiation over subtotal nodal irradiation in favorable clinical stage I-II Hodgkin's disease: The EORTC-GPMC H7F randomized trial. *Proc Am Soc Clin Oncol* 1997;16:13.

217. Andrieu J, et al. Chemotherapy—radiotherapy association in Hodgkin's disease, clinical stages IA, II2A: results of a prospective clinical trial with 166 patients. *Cancer* 1980;46(10):2126.

218. Diehl V, Sieber M, Rüffer U. Treatment of early-stage Hodgkin's disease: considerations in the use of chemotherapy. Paper presented at: Annual Meeting of American Society of Clinical Oncology, 1998, Los Angeles, CA.

219. Radford J, Cowen R, Ryder W. Four weeks of neo-adjuvant chemotherapy significantly reduces the progression rate in patients treated with limited field radiotherapy for clinical stage IA/IIA (CS IA/IIA) Hodgkin's disease. Results of a randomized pilot. *Ann Oncol* 1996;7:66.

220. Press OW, et al. Phase III randomized intergroup trial of subtotal lymphoid irradiation versus doxorubicin, vinblastine, and subtotal lymphoid irradiation for stage IA to IIA Hodgkin's disease. *J Clin Oncol* 2001;19(22):4238.

221. Bartlett N, et al. Brief chemotherapy, Stanford V, and adjuvant radiotherapy for bulky or advanced-stage Hodgkin's disease: a preliminary report. *J Clin Oncol* 1995;13(5):1080.

222. Horning SJ, Bennett JM, Bartlett NL. Twelve weeks of chemotherapy (Stanford V) and involved field radiotherapy (RT) are highly effective for bulky and advanced stage Hodgkin's disease: a limited institution ECOG pilot study. *Blood* 1996;88:2681.

223. Olweny C, Katongole-Mbidde E, Klife C. Childhood Hodgkin's disease in Uganda: a 10-year experience. *Cancer* 1978;42:787.

224. Colonna P, Andrieu J. MOPP chemotherapy alone: a suitable treatment for early stages of Hodgkin's disease? [Letter]. *Lancet* 1985;1(8439):1224.

225. Longo D, et al. Radiation therapy versus combination chemotherapy in the treatment of early-stage Hodgkin's disease: seven-year results of a prospective randomized trial [see comments]. *J Clin Oncol* 1991;9(6):906.

226. Biti G, et al. Extended-field radiotherapy is superior to MOPP chemotherapy for the treatment of pathologic stage I-IIA Hodgkin's disease: eight-year update of an Italian prospective randomized study [see comments]. *J Clin Oncol* 1992;10(3):378.

226a. Duhmke E, Connors JM, Pavlovsky S, Cosset J-M, Hoppe R. Treatment of clinical stage I–II Hodgkin's disease. In: Mauch PM, Armitage JO, Diehl V, Hoppe RT, Weiss LM, eds. *Hodgkin's disease.* Philadelphia: Lippincott Williams & Wilkins, 1999:435.

227. Pavlovsky S, et al. Randomized trial of CVPP for three versus six cycles in favorable-prognosis and CVPP versus AOPE plus radiotherapy in intermediate-prognosis untreated Hodgkin's disease. *J Clin Oncol* 1997;15(7):2652.

228. Santoro A, Viviani S, Zucali R. Comparative results and toxicity of MOPP vs ABVD combined with radiotherapy (RT) in PS IIB, III (A,B) Hodgkin's disease (HD). Paper presented at: Annual Meeting of the American Society of Clinical Oncology, 1983, San Diego, CA.

229. Carde P, Noordijk N, Hagenbeek A. Superiority of MOPP/ABV over EBVP in combination with involved field irradiation in unfavorable clinical stage I-II Hodgkin's disease: The EORTC H7U randomized trial. *Proc Am Soc Clin Oncol* 1993;12:362.

230. Cosset J, Ferme C, Noordijk E. Combined modality therapy for poor prognosis stages I and II Hodgkin's disease. *Semin Radiat Oncol* 1996;6:185.

231. Hagemeister F, et al. Treatment of early stages of Hodgkin's disease with Novantrone, vincristine, vinblastine, prednisone, and radiotherapy. *Semin Hematol* 1994;31(2 Suppl 3):36.

232. Andre M, et al. Results of three courses of Adriamycin, bleomycin, vindesine, and dacarbazine with subtotal nodal irradiation in 189 patients with nodal Hodgkin's disease (stage I, II and IIIA). *Hematol Cell Ther* 1997;39(2):59.

233. Horning S, Rosenberg S, Hoppe R. Brief chemotherapy (Stanford V) and adjuvant radiotherapy for bulky or advanced Hodgkin's disease: an update. *Ann Oncol* 1996;7[Suppl 4]:105.

234. Brusamolino E, et al. Early-stage Hodgkin's disease: long-term results with radiotherapy alone or combined radiotherapy and chemotherapy. *Ann Oncol* 1994;5[Suppl 2]:101.
235. Colonna P, et al. Mediastinal tumor size and response to chemotherapy are the only prognostic factors in supradiaphragmatic Hodgkin's disease treated by ABVD plus radiotherapy: ten-year results of the Paris-Ouest-France 81/12 trial, including 262 patients [see comments]. *J Clin Oncol* 1996;14(6):1928.
236. Zittoun R, Audebert A, Hoerni B, et al. Extended versus involved fields irradiation combined with MOPP chemotherapy in early clinical stages of Hodgkin's disease. *J Clin Oncol* 1985;3:207.
236a. Bonfante V, Vivani S, Devizz IL, et al. Ten-year experience with ABVD plus radiotherapy: subtotal nodal (STNI) versus involved-field (IFRT) in early stage Hodgkin's disease (abstract). *Proc Am Soc Clin Oncol* 2001;20:281a.
236b. Engert A, Schiller P, Josting A, et al. Involved-field radiotherapy is equally effective and less toxic compared with extended-field radiotherapy after four cycles of chemotherapy in patients with early-stage unfavorable Hodgkin's lymphoma: results of the HD8 trial of the German Hodgkin's Lymphoma Study Group. *J Clin Oncol* 2003;21:3601.
237. Andrieu J, Bayle-Weisgerber C, Boiron M. The chemotherapy-radiotherapy sequence in the management of Hodgkin's disease. Results of a clinical trial. *Eur J Cancer* 1979;48:153.
238. Preti A, et al. Hodgkin's disease with a mediastinal mass greater than 10 cm: results of four different treatment approaches. *Ann Oncol* 1994;5[Suppl 2]:97.
239. Pavlovsky S, et al. Randomized trial of chemotherapy versus chemotherapy plus radiotherapy for stage I-II Hodgkin's disease. *J Natl Cancer Inst* 1988;80(18):1466.
240. DeVita VJ, Hubbard SM. Hodgkin's disease. *N Engl J Med* 1993;328:560.
241. Longo D, et al. Twenty years of MOPP therapy for Hodgkin's disease. *J Clin Oncol* 1986;4(9):1295.
242. Bonadonna G, Valagussa P, Santoro A. Alternating non-cross-resistant combination chemotherapy or MOPP in stage IV Hodgkin's disease. A report of 8-year results. *Ann Intern Med* 1986;104(6):739.
243. Nissen NI, Pajak TF, Glidewell O. A comparative study of a BCNU containing 4-drug program versus MOPP versus 3-drug combinations in advanced Hodgkin's disease: a cooperative study by the Cancer and Leukemia Group B. *Cancer* 1979;43:31.
244. Bakemeier R, et al. BCVPP chemotherapy for advanced Hodgkin's disease: evidence for greater duration of complete remission, greater survival, and less toxicity than with a MOPP regimen. Results of the Eastern Cooperative Oncology Group study. *Ann Intern Med* 1984;101(4):447.
245. Nicholson WM, Beard ME, Crowther D. Combination chemotherapy in generalized Hodgkin's disease. *Br Med J* 1970;3:7.
246. Sutcliffe SB, Wrigley PF, Peto J. MVPP chemotherapy regimen for advanced Hodgkin's disease. *Br Med J* 1978;1:679.
247. Hancock B. Randomised study of MOPP (mustine, Oncovin, procarbazine, prednisone) against LOPP (Leukeran substituted for mustine) in advanced Hodgkin's disease. British National Lymphoma Investigation. *Radiother Oncol* 1986;7(3):215.
248. Bonadonna G, et al. Combination chemotherapy of Hodgkin's disease with Adriamycin, bleomycin, vinblastine, and imidazole carboxamide versus MOPP. *Cancer* 1975;36 (1):252.
249. Santoro A, Bonadonna G, Valagussa P. Long-term results of combined chemotherapy-radiotherapy approach in Hodgkin's disease: superiority of ABVD plus radiotherapy versus MOPP plus radiotherapy. *J Clin Oncol* 1987;5:27.
250. Wirth A, Corry J, Laidlaw C, Matthews J, Liew KH. Salvage radiotherapy for Hodgkin's disease following chemotherapy failure *Int J Radiat Oncol Biol Phys* 1997;39:599.
251. Somers R, et al. A randomized study in stage IIIB and IV Hodgkin's disease comparing eight courses of MOPP versus an alteration of MOPP with ABVD: a European Organization for Research and Treatment of Cancer Lymphoma Cooperative Group and Groupe Pierre-et-Marie-Curie controlled clinical trial. *J Clin Oncol* 1994;12(2):279.
252. DeVita VJ, Simon RM, Hubbard SM. Curability of advanced Hodgkin's disease with chemotherapy. Long-term follow-up of MOPP-treated patients at the National Cancer Institute. *Ann Intern Med* 1980;92:587.
253. Canellos GP, Anderson JR, Propert KJ. Chemotherapy of advanced Hodgkin's disease with MOPP, ABVD, or MOPP alternating with ABVD. *N Engl J Med* 1992;327:1478.
254. Goldie JH, Coldman AJ. A mathematic model for relating the drug sensitivity of tumors to their spontaneous mutation rate. *Cancer Treat Rep* 1979;63:1727.
255. Jones S, et al. Comparison of Adriamycin-containing chemotherapy (MOP-BAP) with MOPP-bleomycin in the management of advanced Hodgkin's disease. A Southwest Oncology Group Study. *Cancer* 1983;51(8):1339.
256. Sieber M, Tesch H, Pfistner B, et al. Rapidly alternating COPP/ABV/IMEP is not superior to conventional alternating COPP/ABVD in combination with extended-field radiotherapy in intermediate-stage Hodgkin's lymphoma: final results of the German Hodgkin's Lymphoma Study Group Trial HD5. *J Clin Oncol* 2002;20(2):476.
256a. Sieber M, Tesch H, Pfistner B, et al. Treatment of advanced Hodgkin's disease with COPP/ABV/IMEP versus COPP/ABVD and consolidating radiotherapy: final results of the German Hodgkin's Lymphoma Study Group HD6 trial. *Ann Oncol* 2004;15:276.
257. Hancock BW, Vaughan Hudson G, Vaughan Hudson B, et al. Hybrid LOPP/EVA is not better than LOPP alternating with EVAP: a prematurely terminated British National Lymphoma Investigation randomized trial. *Ann Oncol* 1994;5:117.
258. Schmoll H. Review of etoposide single-agent activity. *Cancer Treat Rev* 1982;9[Suppl]:21.
259. Radford JA, et al. ChlVPP/EVA hybrid versus the weekly VAPEC-B regimen for previously untreated Hodgkin's disease. *J Clin Oncol* 2002;20(13):2988.
260. Simmonds P, et al. PACE BOM chemotherapy: a 12-week regimen for advanced Hodgkin's disease. *Ann Oncol* 1997;8(3):259.
261. Carde P, MacKintosh F, Rosenberg S. A dose and time response analysis of the treatment of Hodgkin's disease with MOPP chemotherapy. *J Clin Oncol* 1983;1(2):146.
262. Gerhartz HH, Schwencke H, Bazarbashi S. Randomized comparison of COPP/ABVD vs. dose and time-escalated COPP/ABVD with GM-CSF support for advanced Hodgkin's disease. *Blood* 1997;90[Suppl 1]:389.
263. Hasenclever D, Loeffler M, Diehl V. Rationale for dose escalation of first line conventional chemotherapy in advanced Hodgkin's disease. German Hodgkin's Lymphoma Study Group. *Ann Oncol* 1996;7[Suppl 4]:95.
264. Diehl V. Dose-escalation study for the treatment of Hodgkin's disease. The German Hodgkin Study Group (GHSG). *Ann Hematol* 1993;66(3):139.
265. Diehl V, et al. BEACOPP: a new regimen for advanced Hodgkin's disease. German Hodgkin's Lymphoma Study Group. *Ann Oncol* 1998;9[Suppl 5]:S67.
266. Diehl V, et al. BEACOPP, a new dose-escalated and accelerated regimen, is at least as effective as COPP/ABVD in patients with advanced-stage Hodgkin's lymphoma: interim report from a trial of the German Hodgkin's Lymphoma Study Group. *J Clin Oncol* 1998;16(12):3810.
267. Diehl V, et al. Standard and increased-dose BEACOPP chemotherapy compared with COPP-ABVD for advanced Hodgkin's disease. *N Engl J Med* 2003;348(24):2386.
268. Sieber M, et al. 14-day variant of the bleomycin, etoposide, doxorubicin, cyclophosphamide, vincristine, procarbazine, and prednisone regimen in advanced-stage Hodgkin's lymphoma: results of a pilot study of the German Hodgkin's Lymphoma Study Group. *J Clin Oncol* 2003;21(9):1734.
269. Chisesi T, et al. ABVD versus Stanford V versus MEC in unfavourable Hodgkin's lymphoma: results of a randomised trial. *Ann Oncol* 2002;13[Suppl 1]:102.
270. Chopra R, et al. The place of high-dose BEAM therapy and autologous bone marrow transplantation in poor-risk Hodgkin's disease. A single-center eight-year study of 155 patients. *Blood* 1993;81(5):1137.
271. Horning S, et al. High-dose therapy and autologous hematopoietic progenitor cell transplantation for recurrent or refractory Hodgkin's disease: analysis of the Stanford University results and prognostic indices. *Blood* 1997;89(3):801.
272. Reece D, Phillips G. Intensive therapy and autologous stem cell transplantation for Hodgkin's disease in first relapse after combination chemotherapy. *Leuk Lymphoma* 1996;21(3–4):245.
273. Carella A, et al. Autologous bone marrow transplantation as adjuvant treatment for high-risk Hodgkin's disease in first complete remission after MOPP/ABVD protocol. *Bone Marrow Transplant* 1991;8(2):99.
274. Straus D, et al. Prognostic factors among 185 adults with newly diagnosed advanced Hodgkin's disease treated with alternating potentially noncross-resistant chemotherapy and intermediate-dose radiation therapy. *J Clin Oncol* 1990;8(7):1173.
275. Federico M, et al. High-dose therapy and autologous stem-cell transplantation versus conventional therapy for patients with advanced Hodgkin's lymphoma responding to front-line therapy. *J Clin Oncol* 2003;21(12):2320.
276. Fabian C, et al. Low-dose involved field radiation after chemotherapy in advanced Hodgkin disease. A Southwest Oncology Group randomized study. *Ann Intern Med* 1994;120(11):903.
277. Diehl V, et al. Further chemotherapy versus low-dose involved-field radiotherapy as consolidation of complete remission after six cycles of alternating chemotherapy in patients with advance Hodgkin's disease. German Hodgkin's Study Group (GHSG). *Ann Oncol* 1995;6(9):901.
278. Loeffler M, et al. Meta-analysis of chemotherapy versus combined modality treatment trials in Hodgkin's disease. International Database on Hodgkin's Disease Overview Study Group [see comments]. *J Clin Oncol* 1998;16(3):818.
279. Raemaekers J, et al. Patients with stage III/IV Hodgkin's disease in partial remission after MOPP/ABV chemotherapy have excellent prognosis after additional involved-field radiotherapy: interim results from the ongoing EORTC-LCG and GPMC phase III trial. The EORTC Lymphoma Cooperative Group and Groupe Pierre-et-Marie-Curie. *Ann Oncol* 1997;8[Suppl 1]:111.
280. Aleman BM, et al. Involved-field radiotherapy for advanced Hodgkin's lymphoma. *N Engl J Med* 2003;348(24):2396.
281. Canellos GP, Horvich A. Management of recurrent Hodgkin's disease. In: Mauch P, Armitage JO, Diehl V, et al., eds. *Hodgkin's disease.* Philadelphia: Lippincott Williams & Wilkins, 1999:507.
282. van Leeuwen FE, Klokman WJ, Hagenbeek A, et al. Second cancer risk following Hodgkin's disease: a 20-year follow-up study. *J Clin Oncol* 1994;12(2):312.
283. Henry-Amar M. Second cancers after treatment of Hodgkin's disease: experience at the International Database on Hodgkin's disease (IDHD) [in French]. *Bull Cancer* 1992;79(4):389.
284. Hansmann M, et al. Morphological and immunohistochemical investigation of non-Hodgkin's lymphoma combined with Hodgkin's disease. *Histopathology* 1989;15(1):35.
285. Fisher R, et al. Prolonged disease-free survival in Hodgkin's disease with MOPP reinduction after first relapse. *Ann Intern Med* 1979;90(5):761.
286. Longo D, et al. Conventional-dose salvage combination chemotherapy in patients relapsing with Hodgkin's disease after combination chemotherapy: the low probability for cure. *J Clin Oncol* 1992;10(2):210.
287. Horwich A, Specht L, Ashley S. Survival analysis of patients with clinical stages I or II Hodgkin's disease who have relapsed after initial treatment with radiotherapy alone. *Eur J Cancer* 1997;33(6):848.
288. Roach M, et al. Prognostic factors for patients relapsing after radiotherapy for early-stage Hodgkin's disease. *J Clin Oncol* 1990;8(4):623.
289. Mauch P, Henry-Amar M. International Database on Hodgkin's Disease: a cooperative effort to determine treatment outcome. *Ann Oncol* 1992;3[Suppl 4]:59.
290. Healey EA, Tarbell NJ, Kalish LA. Prognostic factors for patients with Hodgkin's disease in first relapse. *Cancer* 1993;71:2613.
291. Specht L, Horwich A, Ashley S. Salvage of relapse of patients with Hodgkin's disease in clinical stages I or II who were staged with laparotomy and initially treated with radiotherapy alone. A report from the International Database on Hodgkin's Disease. *Int J Radiat Oncol Biol Phys* 1994;30(4):805.
292. Cannellos G, Young RC, DeVita VD. Combination chemotherapy for advanced Hodgkin's disease in relapse following extensive radiotherapy. *Clin Pharmacol Ther* 1972;13:750.
293. Santoro A, et al. Salvage chemotherapy in Hodgkin's disease irradiation failures: superiority of doxorubicin-containing regimens over MOPP. *Cancer Treat Rep* 1986;70(3):343.
294. Pfreundschuh M, et al. Dexa-BEAM in patients with Hodgkin's disease refractory to

multidrug chemotherapy regimens: a trial of the German Hodgkin's Disease Study Group. *J Clin Oncol* 1994;12(3):580.
295. Hagemeister F, et al. MIME chemotherapy (methyl-GAG, ifosfamide, methotrexate, etoposide) as treatment for recurrent Hodgkin's disease. *J Clin Oncol* 1987;5(4):556.
296. Rodriguet M, Schoppe W, Fuchs R. Lomustine, etoposide, vindesine, and dexamethasone (CEVD) in Hodgkin's disease refractory to cyclophosphamide, vincristine, procarbazine, and prednisone (COPP) and doxorubicin, bleomycin, vinblastine, and dacarbazine (ABVD): a multi-center trial of the German Hodgkin's Study Group. *Cancer Treat Rep* 1987;71:1203.
297. Velasquez WS, Jagannath S, Hagemeister FB. Dexamethasone, high-dose ara-C and cisplatin as salvage treatment for relapsing Hodgkin's disease. *Proc Am Soc Hematol* 1986;68:242.
298. Ferme C, et al. The MINE regimen as intensive salvage chemotherapy for relapsed and refractory Hodgkin's disease [see comments]. *Ann Oncol* 1995;6(6):543.
299. Bierman P, et al. High dose chemotherapy followed by autologous hematopoietic rescue in Hodgkin's disease: long-term follow-up in 128 patients. *Ann Oncol* 1993;4(9):767.
300. Josting A, et al. Favorable outcome of patients with relapsed or refractory Hodgkin's disease treated with high-dose chemotherapy and stem cell rescue at the time of maximal response to conventional salvage therapy (Dex-BEAM). *Ann Oncol* 1998;9(3):289.
301. Linch D, et al. Dose intensification with autologous bone-marrow transplantation in relapsed and resistant Hodgkin's disease: results of a BNLI randomised trial. *Lancet* 1993;341(8852):1051.
302. Schmitz N, Sextro M, Pfistner B. HDR-1: high-dose therapy (HDT) followed by hematopoietic stem cell transplantation (HSCT) for relapsed chemosensitive Hodgkin's disease (HD): final results of a randomized GHSG and EBMT trial (HD-R1). *Proc Am Soc Clin Oncol* 1999;Suppl 5:18.
303. Bonfante V, et al. Outcome of patients with Hodgkin's disease failing after primary MOPP-ABVD [see comments]. *J Clin Oncol* 1997;15(2):528.
304. Sweetenham JW, Carella AM, Taghipour G. High-dose therapy and autologous stem cell transplantation for adult patients with Hodgkin's disease who fail to enter remission after induction chemotherapy: results in 175 patients reported to the EBMT. *J Clin Oncol* 1999;17:3101.
305. Lazarus H, et al. Autotransplants for Hodgkin's disease in patients never achieving remission: a report from the Autologous Blood and Marrow Transplant Registry. *J Clin Oncol* 1999;17(2):534.
306. Reece D, et al. High-dose cyclophosphamide, carmustine (BCNU), and etoposide (VP16-213) with or without cisplatin (CBV +/− P) and autologous transplantation for patients with Hodgkin's disease who fail to enter a complete remission after combination chemotherapy. *Blood* 1995;86(2):451.
307. Yuen A, et al. Comparison between conventional salvage therapy and high-dose therapy with autografting for recurrent or refractory Hodgkin's disease. *Blood* 1997;89(3):814.
308. André M, et al. Comparison of high-dose therapy and autologous stem-cell transplantation with conventional therapy for Hodgkin's disease induction failure: a case-control study. Societé Française de Greffe de Moelle. *J Clin Oncol* 1999;17(1):222.
309. Josting A, et al. Treatment of primary progressive Hodgkin's and aggressive non-Hodgkin's lymphoma: is there a chance for cure? *J Clin Oncol* 2000;18(2):332.
310. Brice P, et al. Prognostic factors for survival after high-dose therapy and autologous stem cell transplantation for patients with relapsing Hodgkin's disease: analysis of 280 patients from the French registry. Societé Française de Greffe de Moelle. *Bone Marrow Transplant* 1997;20(1):21.
311. Sweetenham J, et al. High-dose therapy and autologous stem cell rescue for patients with Hodgkin's disease in first relapse after chemotherapy: results from the EBMT. Lymphoma Working Party of the European Group for Blood and Marrow Transplantation. *Bone Marrow Transplant* 1997;20(9):745.
312. Crump M, et al. High-dose etoposide and melphalan, and autologous bone marrow transplantation for patients with advanced Hodgkin's disease: importance of disease status at transplant. *J Clin Oncol* 1993;11(4):704.
313. Wheeler C, et al. High-dose cyclophosphamide, carmustine, and etoposide with autologous transplantation in Hodgkin's disease: a prognostic model for treatment outcomes. *Biol Blood Marrow Transplant* 1997;3(2):98.
314. Milpied N, et al. Allogeneic bone marrow transplant is not better than autologous transplant for patients with relapsed Hodgkin's disease. European Group for Blood and Bone Marrow Transplantation. *J Clin Oncol* 1996;14(4):1291.
315. Anderson J, et al. Allogeneic, syngeneic, and autologous marrow transplantation for Hodgkin's disease: the 21-year Seattle experience. *J Clin Oncol* 1993;11(12):2342.
316. Gajewski J, et al. Bone marrow transplants from HLA-identical siblings in advanced Hodgkin's disease. *J Clin Oncol* 1996;14(2):572.
317. Rosenthal SR. Significance of tissue lymphocytes in the prognosis of lymphogranulomatosis. *Arch Pathol* 1936;21:628.
318. Westling P. Studies of the prognosis in Hodgkin's disease. *Acta Radiol* 1965;245:5.
319. Culine S, et al. Relationship of histological subtypes to prognosis in early stage Hodgkin's disease: a review of 312 cases in a controlled clinical trial. The Groupe Pierre-et-Marie-Curie. *Eur J Cancer Clin Oncol* 1989;25(3):551.
320. Diehl V, et al. Clinical presentation, course, and prognostic factors in lymphocyte-predominant Hodgkin's disease and lymphocyte-rich classical Hodgkin's disease: report from the European Task Force on Lymphoma Project on Lymphocyte-Predominant Hodgkin's Disease [see comments]. *J Clin Oncol* 1999;17(3):776.
321. Hansmann M, et al. Clinical features of nodular paragranuloma (Hodgkin's disease, lymphocyte predominance type, nodular). *J Cancer Res Clin Oncol* 1984;108(3):321.
322. Orlandi E, et al. Nodular lymphocyte predominance Hodgkin's disease: long-term observation reveals a continuous pattern of recurrence. *Leuk Lymphoma* 1997;26(3–4):359.
323. Pappa V, et al. Nodular type of lymphocyte predominant Hodgkin's disease. A clinical study of 50 cases. *Ann Oncol* 1995;6(6):559.
324. Miettinen M, Franssila K, Saxen E. Hodgkin's disease, lymphocytic predominance nodular. Increased risk for subsequent non-Hodgkin's lymphomas. *Cancer* 1983;51(12): 2293.
325. Henry-Amar M. Second cancer after the treatment for Hodgkin's disease: a report from the International Database on Hodgkin's Disease. *Ann Oncol* 1992;3[Suppl 4]:117.
326. Maloney DG, Grillo-Lopez AJ, Bodkin DJ. IDEC-C2B8: results of a phase I multiple-dose trial in patients with relapsed non-Hodgkin's lymphoma. *J Clin Oncol* 1997;15:3266.
327. Lokich L, Pinkus G, Moloney W. Hodgkin's disease in the elderly. *Oncology* 1974;29:484.
328. Specht L, Nissen N. Hodgkin's disease and age. *Eur J Haematol* 1989;43(2):127.
329. Franklin J, Sieber M, Paulus U. Toxicity and feasibility of the BEACOPP regimen for advanced Hodgkin's disease older than 65 years. *Ann Oncol* 1999;2:157.
330. Tesch H, Santoro A, Fiedler F. Phase II study of gemcitabine in pretreated Hodgkin's disease. Results of a multicenter study. *Blood* 1997;90:339.
331. Gherlinzoni F, Zinziani, PL, Magagnoli M. VBM regimen for Hodgkin's disease in the elderly. *Leuk Lymphoma* 1998;29:72.
332. Sadural E, Smith LG. Haematological malignancies during pregnancy. *Clin Obstet Gynecol* 1995;38:535.
333. Gelb AB, Van de Rijn M, Warnke RA. Pregnancy-associated lymphomas. A clinicopathologic study. *Cancer* 1996;78:304.
334. Fisher P, Hancock B. Hodgkin's disease in the pregnant patient. *Br J Hosp Med* 1996;56(10):529.
335. Tirelli U, et al. Hodgkin's disease and human immunodeficiency virus infection: clinicopathologic and virologic features of 114 patients from the Italian Cooperative Group on AIDS and Tumors. *J Clin Oncol* 1995;13(7):1758.
336. Carbone A, et al. Immunophenotypic and molecular analyses of acquired immune deficiency syndrome–related and Epstein-Barr virus–associated lymphomas: a comparative study. *Hum Pathol* 1996;27(2):133.
337. Tirelli U, et al. Hodgkin disease and infection with the human immunodeficiency virus (HIV) in Italy [Letter]. *Ann Intern Med* 1988;108(2):309.
338. Bellas C, et al. Pathological, immunological, and molecular features of Hodgkin's disease associated with HIV infection. Comparison with ordinary Hodgkin's disease. *Am J Surg Pathol* 1996;20(12):1520.
339. Andrieu J, et al. Hodgkin's disease during HIV1 infection: the French registry experience. French Registry of HIV-Associated Tumors. *Ann Oncol* 1993;4(8):635.
340. Tirelli U, et al. Hodgkin's disease in 92 patients with HIV infection: the Italian experience. GICAT (Italian Cooperative Group on AIDS & Tumors). *Ann Oncol* 1992;3[Suppl 4]:69.
341. Rubio R. Hodgkin's disease associated with human immunodeficiency virus infection. A clinical study of 46 cases. Cooperative Study Group of Malignancies Associated with HIV Infection of Madrid. *Cancer* 1994;73(9):2400.
342. Errante D, et al. Combined antineoplastic and antiretroviral therapy for patients with Hodgkin's disease and human immunodeficiency virus infection. A prospective study of 17 patients. The Italian Cooperative Group on AIDS and Tumors (GICAT). *Cancer* 1994;73(2):437.
343. Tirelli U, Erranta D, Gisselbrecht C. Epirubicin, bleomycin, vinblastine and prednisone (EBVP) chemotherapy in combination with antiretroviral therapy and primary use of G-CSF for patients with Hodgkin's disease and HIV Infection (HD-HIV). *Proc Am Soc Clin Oncol* 1996;15:304.
344. Levine AM, Cheung T, Tulpule A. Preliminary results of AIDS Clinical Trials Group (ACTG) study no. 149: phase II trial of ABVD chemotherapy with G-CSF in HIV-infected patients with Hodgkin's disease (HD). *AIDS* 1997;14:12.
345. Tirelli U, Carbone A, Strau DJ. HIV-related Hodgkin's disease. In: Mauch PM, Armitage JO, Diehl V, et al., eds. *Hodgkin's disease.* Philadelphia: Lippincott Williams & Wilkins, 1999:701.
346. Hartmann P, Winkler U, Franzen C. BEACOPP chemotherapeutic regimen for treatment of HIV-infected patients with Hodgkin's lymphoma. *Blood* 1998;92:540.
347. Tarbell N, Thompson L, Mauch P. Thoracic irradiation in Hodgkin's disease: disease control and long-term complications. *Int J Radiat Oncol Biol Phys* 1990;18(2):275.
348. Hancock S, et al. Intercurrent death after Hodgkin disease therapy in radiotherapy and adjuvant MOPP trials [published erratum appears in *Ann Intern Med* 1991;114(9):810]. *Ann Intern Med* 1988;109(3):183.
349. Boivin J, Hutchison G. Coronary heart disease mortality after irradiation for Hodgkin's disease. *Cancer* 1982;49(12):2470.
350. Van Leeuwen FE, Swerdlow AJ, Valaguss P. Hodgkin's disease. In: Mauch PM, Armitage JO, Diehl V, et al., eds. *Hodgkin's disease.* Philadelphia: Lippincott Williams & Wilkins, 1999:607.
351. Sandoval C, et al. Secondary acute myeloid leukemia in children previously treated with alkylating agents, intercalating topoisomerase II inhibitors, and irradiation. *J Clin Oncol* 1993;11(6):1039.
352. Josting A, et al. Secondary myeloid leukemia and myelodysplastic syndromes in patients treated for Hodgkin's disease: a report from the German Hodgkin's Lymphoma Study Group. *J Clin Oncol* 2003;21(18):3440.
353. Valagussa P. Second neoplasms following treatment of Hodgkin's disease. *Curr Opin Oncol* 1993;5(5):805.
354. Van Leeuwen F, Somers R, Taal B. Increased risk of lung cancer, non-Hodgkin's lymphoma and leukemia following Hodgkin's disease. *J Clin Oncol* 1989;7:1046.
355. Hancock S, Tucker M, Hoppe R. Breast cancer after treatment of Hodgkin's disease. *J Natl Cancer Inst* 1993;85(1):25.
355a. van Leeuwen FE, Klokman WJ, Veer MB, et al. Long-term risk of second malignancy in survivors of Hodgkin's disease treated during adolescence or young adulthood. *J Clin Oncol* 2000;18:487.
355b. Behringer K, Josting A, Schiller P, et al. Solid tumors in patients treated for Hodgkin's disease: a report from the German Hodgkin Lymphoma Study Group. *Ann Oncol* 2004;15:1079.
356. Hancock S, Hoppe R. Long-term complications of treatment and causes of mortality after Hodgkin's disease. *Semin Radiat Oncol* 1996;6:225.
357. Swerdlow A, et al. Risk of second primary cancers after Hodgkin's disease by type of treatment: analysis of 2846 patients in the British National Lymphoma Investigation. *BMJ* 1992;304(6835):1137.
358. Kaldor J, et al. Lung cancer following Hodgkin's disease: a case-control study. *Int J Cancer* 1992;52(5):677.
359. Bonadonna G. Modern treatment of malignant lymphomas: a multidisciplinary approach? The Kaplan Memorial Lecture. *Ann Oncol* 1994;5[Suppl 2]:5.

360. Chilcote R, Baehner R, Hammond D. Septicemia and meningitis in children splenectomized for Hodgkin's disease. *N Engl J Med* 1976;295(15):798.

361. Bradlyn A, Harris C, Spieth L. Quality of life assessment in pediatric oncology: a retrospective review of phase III reports. *Soc Sci Med* 1995;41:1463.

362. Kornblith A, et al. Hodgkin disease survivors at increased risk for problems in psychosocial adaptation. The Cancer and Leukemia Group B. *Cancer* 1992;70(8):2214.

363. Joly F, et al. Late psychosocial sequelae in Hodgkin's disease survivors: a French population-based case-control study. *J Clin Oncol* 1996;14(9):2444.

364. Aaronson NK. Assessing the quality of life of patients in cancer clinical trials: common problems and common sense solution. *Eur J Cancer* 1992;8:1304.

365. Devizzi L, et al. Vinorelbine: a new promising drug in Hodgkin's disease. *Leuk Lymphoma* 1996;22(5–6):409.

366. Devizzi L, et al. Vinorelbine: an active drug for the management of patients with heavily pretreated Hodgkin's disease. *Ann Oncol* 1994;5(9):817.

367. Benchekroun S, Chouffai Z, Harif M. Clinical study of Navelbine activity in Hodgkin's disease. Phase II study. In: Pierre-Fabre Oncologie, ed. *Navelbine (vinorelbine): update and new trends.* Montrouge, France: Libbey Eurotext, 1991:261.

367a. Engert A, Schnell R, Kupper F, et al. A phase-II study with idarubicin, ifosfamide and VP-16 (IIVP-16) in patients with refractory or relapsed aggressive and high grade non-Hodgkin's lymphoma. *Leuk Lymphoma* 1997;24:513.

368. Plunkett W, Huang P, Searcy CE. Gemcitabine: preclinical pharmacology and mechanism of action. *Semin Oncol* 1996;23(5 Suppl 10):3.

368a. Santoro A, Bredenfeld H, Devizzi L, et al. Gemcitabine in the treatment of refractory Hodgkin's disease: results of a multicenter phase II study. *J Clin Oncol* 2000;18:2615.

369. Kaplan H. Hodgkin's disease: unfolding concepts concerning its nature, management and prognosis. *Cancer* 1980;45(10):2439.

370. Engert A, et al. Immunotoxins constructed with anti-CD25 monoclonal antibodies and deglycosylated ricin A-chain have potent anti-tumour effects against human Hodgkin cells in vitro and solid Hodgkin tumours in mice. *Int J Cancer* 1991;49(3):450.

371. Wahl AF, et al. The anti-CD30 monoclonal antibody SGN-30 promotes growth arrest and DNA fragmentation in vitro and affects antitumor activity in models of Hodgkin's disease. *Cancer Res* 2002;62(13):3736.

372. Borchmann P, et al. The human anti-CD30 antibody 5F11 shows in vitro and in vivo activity against malignant lymphoma. *Blood* 2003;102(10):3737.

373. McLaughlin P, Cabanillas F, Grillo-Lopez AJ. IDEC-C2B8 anti-CD20 antibody: final report on a phase III pivotal trial in patients with relapsed low-grade or follicular lymphoma. *Blood* 1996;88:349.

374. Fitzgerald D, Pastan I. Targeted toxin therapy for the treatment of cancer. *J Natl Cancer Inst* 1989;81:1455.

375. Kreitman RJ, Pastan I. Recombinant toxins. *Adv Pharmacol* 1994;28:193.

376. Strauchen JA, Breakstone BA. IL-2 receptor expression in human lymphoid lesions. Immunohistochemical study of 166 cases. *Am J Pathol* 1987;126(3):506.

377. Engert A, et al. A phase-I study of an anti-CD25 ricin A-chain immunotoxin (RFT5-SMPT-dgA) in patients with refractory Hodgkin's lymphoma. *Blood* 1997;89(2):403.

378. LeMaistre CF, Meneghetti C, Rosenblum M. Phase I trial of an interleukin-2 (IL-2) fusion toxins (DAB486IL-2) in hematologic malignancies expressing the IL-2 receptor. *Blood* 1992;79:2547.

379. Tepler I, et al. Phase I trial of an interleukin-2 fusion toxin (DAB486IL-2) in hematologic malignancies: complete response in a patient with Hodgkin's disease refractory to chemotherapy. *Cancer* 1994;73(4):1276.

380. Riechmann L, et al. Reshaping human antibodies for therapy. *Nature* 1988;332(6162):323.

381. Schnell R, et al. Development of new ricin A-chain immunotoxins with potent antitumor effects against human Hodgkin cells in vitro and disseminated Hodgkin tumors in SCID mice using high-affinity monoclonal antibodies directed against the CD30 antigen. *Int J Cancer* 1995;63(2):238.

382. Engert A, et al. Experimental treatment of human Hodgkin's disease with ricin A-chain immunotoxins. *Leuk Lymphoma* 1994;13(5–6):441.

383. Staak J, Schnell R, Schwartz C. Clinical experience with a novel ricin A-chain immunotoxin (Ki-4.dgA) in patients with refractory CD30+ lymphoma. *Onkologie* 1999;22:132.

384. Terenzi A, et al. Anti-CD30 (BER-H2) immunotoxins containing the type-1 ribosome-inactivating proteins momordin and PAP-S (pokeweed antiviral protein from seeds) display powerful antitumour activity against CD30+ tumour cells in vitro and in SCID mice. *Br J Haematol* 1996;92(4):872.

385. Nourigat C, Badger CC, Bernstein ID. Treatment of lymphoma with radiolabeled antibody: elimination of tumor cells lacking target antigen. *J Natl Cancer Inst* 1990;82(1):47.

386. O'Donoghue JA. The impact of tumor cell proliferation in radioimmunotherapy. *Cancer* 1994;73(3[Suppl]):974.

387. Perez P, et al. Specific targeting of cytotoxic T cells by anti-T3 linked to anti-target cell antibody. *Nature* 1985;316(6026):354.

388. Herpst J, et al. Survival of patients with resistant Hodgkin's disease after polyclonal yttrium 90-labeled antiferritin treatment. *J Clin Oncol* 1995;13(9):2394.

389. Order SE, Porter M, Hellmann S. Evidence for a tumor associated antigen. *N Engl J Med* 1971;285:471.

390. Lenhard RJ, et al. Isotopic immunoglobulin: a new systemic therapy for advanced Hodgkin's disease. *J Clin Oncol* 1985;3(10):1296.

391. Carde P, et al. Immunoscintigraphy of Hodgkin's disease: in vivo use of radiolabelled monoclonal antibodies derived from Hodgkin cell lines. *Eur J Cancer* 1990;26(4):474.

392. da Costa L, Carde P, Lumbroso JD, et al. Immunoscintigraphy in Hodgkin's disease and anaplastic large cell lymphomas: results in 18 patients using the iodine radiolabeled monoclonal antibody HRS-3. *Ann Oncol* 1992;3[Suppl 4]:53.

393. Winkler U, Stein H, Scheidhauer K. Radioimmunoconjugates for the therapy of Hodgkin's lymphoma: preliminary data of a clinical study using the anti-CD30 antibody 99mTc-BerH2. Paper presented at: Fourth International Symposium on Hodgkin's Lymphoma; March 28–April 1, 1998; Cologne, Germany.

394. Vriesendorp H, et al. Phase I–II studies of yttrium-labeled antiferritin treatment for end-stage Hodgkin's disease, including Radiation Therapy Oncology Group 87-01 [published erratum appears in *J Clin Oncol* 1991;9(8):1516]. *J Clin Oncol* 1991;9(6):918.

395. Milstein C, Cuello AC. Hybrid hybridomas and their use in immunohistochemistry. *Nature* 1983;305(5934):537.

396. Hartmann F, et al. Treatment of refractory Hodgkin's disease with an anti-CD16/CD30 bispecific antibody [published erratum appears in *Blood* 1998;91(5):1832]. *Blood* 1997;89(6):2042.

397. Borchmann P, et al. Phase 1 trial of the novel bispecific molecule H22xKi-4 in patients with refractory Hodgkin lymphoma. *Blood* 2002;100(9):3101.

398. Mack M, Riethmüller G, Kufer P. A small bispecific antibody construct expressed as a functional single-chain molecule with high tumor cell cytotoxicity. *Proc Natl Acad Sci U S A* 1995;92:7021.

399. Senter PD, Saulnier MG, Schreiber GJ. Anti-tumor effects of antibody alkaline phosphatase conjugates in combination with etoposide phosphate. *Proc Natl Acad Sci U S A* 1988;85:4842.

400. Bagshawe KD, et al. A cytotoxic agent can be generated selectively at cancer sites. *Br J Cancer* 1988;58(6):700.

401. Schiefer D, Huang X, Trieu V. Enhanced expression of endoglin on blood vessels of human Hodgkin's lymphoma xenografted in SCID mice. *Ann Hematol* 1995;73:707.

402. Perloff M, Holland J, Bekesi JG. Chemoimmunotherapy of breast cancer. *Proc Am Assoc Cancer Res* 1976;17:308.

402a. Sahin U, Hartmann F, Senter P, et al. Specific activation of the prodrug mitomycin phosphate by a bispecific anti-CD30/anti-alkaline phosphatase monoclonal antibody. *Cancer Res* 1990;50:6944.

403. Vinciguerra V, et al. MER immunotherapy and combination chemotherapy for advanced, recurrent Hodgkin's disease. Cancer and Leukemia Group B study. *Cancer Clin Trials* 1981;4(2):99.

404. Margolin K, et al. Phase II trial of high-dose interleukin-2 and lymphokine-activated killer cells in Hodgkin's disease and non-Hodgkin's lymphoma. *J Immunother* 1991;10(3):214.

405. Bernstein Z, et al. Interleukin-2 lymphokine-activated killer cell therapy of non-Hodgkin's lymphoma and Hodgkin's disease. *J Immunother* 1991;10(2):141.

406. Tourani J, et al. Interleukin-2 therapy for refractory and relapsing lymphomas. *Eur J Cancer* 1991;27(12):1676.

407. Janssen JT, et al. Phase I study of recombinant human interferon alpha-2C in patients with chemotherapy-refractory malignancies. *Oncology* 1985;42[Suppl 1]:3.

408. Leavitt RD, et al. Alfa-2b interferon in the treatment of Hodgkin's disease and non-Hodgkin's lymphoma. *Semin Oncol* 1987;14(2 Suppl 2):18.

409. Koziner B. Alpha interferon in patients with progressive and/or recurrent Hodgkin's disease. *Eur J Cancer* 1991;27[Suppl 4]:S79.

410. Rybak M, et al. Interferon therapy of relapsed and refractory Hodgkin's disease: Cancer and Leukemia Group B study 8652. *J Biol Response Mod* 1990;9(1):1.

411. Heuser C, et al. Anti-CD30-IL-12 antibody-cytokine fusion protein that induces IFN-gamma secretion of T cells and NK cell-mediated lysis of Hodgkin's lymphoma-derived tumor cells. *Int J Cancer* 2003;106(4):545.

412. Greene MI. Cellular and genetic basis of immune reactivity to tumor cells. *Contemp Top Mol Immunol* 1980;11:81.

413. Howie SM, McBride WH. Tumor-specific T-helper activity can be abrogated by two distinct suppressor-cell mechanisms. *Eur J Immunol* 1982;12:671.

414. Jerne N. Towards a network theory of the immune system. *Ann Immunol* 1974;125:373.

415. Hsu SM, et al. Effect of monoclonal antibodies anti-2H9, anti-IRac, and anti-HeFi-1 on the surface antigens of Reed-Sternberg cells. *J Natl Cancer Inst* 1987;79:1091.

416. Pohl C, et al. CD30-specific AB1-AB2-AB3 internal image antibody network: potential use as anti-idiotype vaccine against Hodgkin's lymphoma. *Int J Cancer* 1993;54(3):418.

417. Heslop HE, Brenner MK, Rooney CM. Long-term restoration of immunity against Epstein-Barr virus infection by adoptive transfer of gene-modified virus specific T-lymphocytes. *Nat Med* 1996;2:551.

418. Roskrow M, et al. Epstein-Barr virus (EBV)-specific cytotoxic T lymphocytes for the treatment of patients with EBV-positive relapsed Hodgkin's disease. *Blood* 1998;91(8):2925.

419. Harris NL. World Health Organization classification of neoplastic diseases of the hematopoietic and lymphoid tissues: report of the Clinical Advisory Committee meeting—Airlie House, Virginia, November 1997. *J Clin Oncol* 1999;17:3835.

420. Skinnider BF, Kapp U, Mak TW. The role of interleukin 13 in classical Hodgkin lymphoma. *Leuk Lymphoma* 2002;43:1203.

421. Brada M, Eeles R, Ashley S, Nichols J, Horwich A. Salvage radiotherapy in recurrent Hodgkin's disease. *Ann Oncol* 1992;3(2):131.

422. Leigh BR, Fox KA, Mack CF, et al. Radiation therapy salvage of Hodgkin's disease following chemotherapy failure. *Int J Radiat Oncol Biol Phys* 1993;27:855.

423. Pezner RD, Lipsett JA, Vora N, Forman SJ. Radical radiotherapy as salvage treatment for relapse of Hodgkin's disease initially treated by chemotherapy alone: prognostic significance of the disease-free interval. *Int J Radiat Oncol Biol Phys* 1994;30:965.

424. Glick JH, Young ML, Harrington D, et al. MOPP/ABV hybrid chemotherapy for advanced Hodgkin's disease significantly improves failure-free and overall survival: the 8-year results of the intergroup trial. *J Clin Oncol* 1998;16:19.

425. Duggan DB, Petroni GR, Johnson JL, et al. Randomized comparison of ABVD and MOPP/ABV hybrid for the treatment of advanced Hodgkin's disease: report of an intergroup trial. *J Clin Oncol* 2003;21:607.

426. Connors JM, Klimo P, Adams G, et al. Treatment of advanced Hodgkin's disease with chemotherapy—comparison of MOPP/ABV hybrid regimen with alternating courses of MOPP and ABVD: a report from the National Cancer Institute of Canada clinical trials group. *J Clin Oncol* 1997;15:1638.

427. Klein S, Jucker M, Diehl V, Tesch H. Production of multiple cytokines by Hodgkin's disease derived cell lines. *Hematol Oncol* 1992;10(6):319.

428. Kapp U, Yeh WC, Patterson B, et al. Interleukin 13 is secreted by and stimulates the growth of Hodgkin and Reed-Sternberg cells. *J Exp Med* 1999;189:1939.

429. Skinnider BF, Elia AJ, Gascoyne RD, et al. Interleukin 13 and interleukin 13 receptor are frequently expressed by Hodgkin and Reed-Sternberg cells of Hodgkin lymphoma. *Blood* 2001;97:250.

430. Samoszuk M, Nansen L. Detection of interleukin-5 messenger RNA in Reed-Sternberg cells of Hodgkin's disease with eosinophilia. *Blood* 1990;75:13.

431. Hsu SM, Xie SS, Hsu PL, Waldron JA Jr. Interleukin-6, but not interleukin-4, is expressed by Reed-Sternberg cells in Hodgkin's disease with or without histologic features of Castleman's disease. *Am J Pathol* 1992;141:129.

432. Jucker M, Abts H, Li W, et al. Expression of interleukin-6 and interleukin-6 receptor in Hodgkin's disease. *Blood* 1991;77:2413.

433. Merz H, Houssiau FA, Orscheschek K, et al. Interleukin-9 expression in human malignant lymphomas: unique association with Hodgkin's disease and large cell anaplastic lymphoma. *Blood* 1991;78:1311.

434. Beck A, Pazolt D, Grabenbauer GG, et al. Expression of cytokine and chemokine genes in Epstein-Barr virus-associated nasopharyngeal carcinoma: comparison with Hodgkin's disease. *J Pathol* 2001;194:145.

435. Schwaller J, Tobler A, Niklaus G, et al. Interleukin-12 expression in human lymphomas and nonneoplastic lymphoid disorders. *Blood* 1995;85:2182.

436. Dukers DF, Jaspars LH, Vos W, et al. Quantitative immunohistochemical analysis of cytokine profiles in Epstein-Barr virus-positive and -negative cases of Hodgkin's disease. *J Pathol* 2000;190:143.

437. Gerdes J, Kretschmer C, Zahn G, et al. Immunoenzymatic assessment of interferon-gamma in Hodgkin and Sternberg-Reed cells. *Cytokine* 1990;2:307.

438. van den Berg A, Visser L, Poppema S. High expression of the CC chemokine TARC in Reed-Sternberg cells. A possible explanation for the characteristic T-cell infiltrate in Hodgkin's lymphoma. *Am J Pathol* 1999;154:1685.

439. Teruya-Feldstein J, Jaffe ES, Burd PR, et al. Differential chemokine expression in tissues involved by Hodgkin's disease: direct correlation of eotaxin expression and tissue eosinophilia. *Blood* 1999;93:2463.

440. Hedvat CV, Jaffe ES, Qin J, et al. Macrophage-derived chemokine expression in classical Hodgkin's lymphoma: application of tissue microarrays. *Mod Pathol* 2001;14:1270.

441. Jundt F, Anagnostopoulos I, Bommert K, et al. Hodgkin/Reed-Sternberg cells induce fibroblasts to secrete eotaxin, a potent chemoattractant for T cells and eosinophils. *Blood* 1999;94:2065.

442. Buri C, Korner M, Scharli P, et al. CC chemokines and the receptors CCR3 and CCR5 are differentially expressed in the nonneoplastic leukocytic infiltrates of Hodgkin disease. *Blood* 2001;97:1543.

443. Foss HD, Herbst H, Gottstein S, et al. Interleukin-8 in Hodgkin's disease. Preferential expression by reactive cells and association with neutrophil density. *Am J Pathol* 1996;148:1229.

444. Foss HD, Herbst H, Oelmann E, et al. Lymphotoxin, tumour necrosis factor and interleukin-6 gene transcripts are present in Hodgkin and Reed-Sternberg cells of most Hodgkin's disease cases. *Br J Haematol* 1993;84:627.

445. Hsu SM, Waldron JW Jr, Hsu PL, Hough AJ Jr. Cytokines in malignant lymphomas: review and prospective evaluation. *Hum Pathol* 1993;24:1040.

446. Kretschmer C, Jones DB, Morrison K, et al. Tumor necrosis factor alpha and lymphotoxin production in Hodgkin's disease. *Am J Pathol* 1990;137:341.

447. Sappino AP, Seelentag W, Pelte MF, Alberto P, Vassalli P. Tumor necrosis factor/cachectin and lymphotoxin gene expression in lymph nodes from lymphoma patients. *Blood* 1990;75:958.

448. Gruss HJ, Herrmann F, Drexler HG. Hodgkin's disease: a cytokine-producing tumor—a review. *Crit Rev Oncog* 1994;5:473.

449. Carbone A, Gloghini A, Gruss HJ, Pinto A. CD40 ligand is constitutively expressed in a subset of T cell lymphomas and on the microenvironmental reactive T cells of follicular lymphomas and Hodgkin's disease. *Am J Pathol* 1995;147:912.

450. Murray PG, Flavell JR, Baumforth KR, et al. Expression of the tumour necrosis factor receptor-associated factors 1 and 2 in Hodgkin's disease. *J Pathol* 2001;194:158.

451. Smith CA, Gruss HJ, Davis T, et al. CD30 antigen, a marker for Hodgkin's lymphoma, is a receptor whose ligand defines an emerging family of cytokines with homology to TNF. *Cell* 1993;73:1349.

452. Pinto A, Aldinucci D, Gloghini A, et al. Human eosinophils express functional CD30 ligand and stimulate proliferation of a Hodgkin's disease cell line. *Blood* 1996;88:3299.

453. Molin D, Glimelius B, Sundstrom C, Venge P, Enblad G. The serum levels of eosinophil cationic protein (ECP) are related to the infiltration of eosinophils in the tumours of patients with Hodgkin's disease. *Leuk Lymphoma* 2001;42:457.

454. Ruco LP, Pomponi D, Pigott R, et al. Cytokine production (IL-1 alpha, IL-1 beta, and TNF alpha) and endothelial cell activation (ELAM-1 and HLA-DR) in reactive lymphadenitis, Hodgkin's disease, and in non-Hodgkin's lymphomas. An immunocytochemical study. *Am J Pathol* 1990;137:1163.

455. Xerri L, Birg F, Guigou V, et al. In situ expression of the IL-1-alpha and TNF-alpha genes by Reed-Sternberg cells in Hodgkin's disease. *Int J Cancer* 1992;50:689.

456. Benharroch D, Prinsloo I, Apte RN, et al. Interleukin-1 and tumor necrosis factor-alpha in the Reed-Sternberg cells of Hodgkin's disease. Correlation with clinical and morphological "inflammatory" features. *Eur Cytokine Net* 1996;7:51.

457. Hsu SM, Zhao X. Expression of interleukin-1 in Reed-Sternberg cells and neoplastic cells from true histiocytic malignancies. *Am J Pathol* 1986;125:221.

458. Ree HJ, Crowley JP, Dinarello CA. Anti-interleukin-1 reactive cells in Hodgkin's disease. *Cancer* 1987;59:1717.

459. Kadin ME, Agnarsson BA, Ellingsworth LR, Newcom SR. Immunohistochemical evidence of a role for transforming growth factor beta in the pathogenesis of nodular sclerosing Hodgkin's disease. *Am J Pathol* 1990;136:1209.

460. Newcom SR, Kadin ME, Ansari AA, Diehl V. L-428 nodular sclerosing Hodgkin's cell secretes a unique transforming growth factor-beta active at physiologic pH. *J Clin Invest* 1988;82:1915.

461. Santoro A, Viviani S, Valagussa P, Bonfante V, Bonadonna G. CCNU, etoposide, and prednimustine (CEP) in refractory Hodgkin's disease. *Semin Oncol* 1986;13(1 Suppl 1):23.

462. Colwill R, Crump M, Couture F, et al. Mini-BEAM as salvage therapy for relapsed or refractory Hodgkin's disease before intensive therapy and autologous bone marrow transplantation. *J Clin Oncol* 1995;13:396

463. Rodriguez J, Rodriguez MA, Fayad L, et al. ASHAP: a regimen for cytoreduction of refractory or recurrent Hodgkin's disease. *Blood* 1999;93:3632.

464. Ohshima K, Akaiwa M, Umeshita R, et al. Interleukin-13 and interleukin-13 receptor in Hodgkin's disease: possible autocrine mechanism and involvement in fibrosis. *Histopathology* 2001;38:368.

465. Peh SC, Kim LH, Poppema S. TARC, a CC chemokine, is frequently expressed in classic Hodgkin's lymphoma but not in NLP Hodgkin's lymphoma, T-cell-rich B-cell lymphoma, and most cases of anaplastic large cell lymphoma. *Am J Surg Pathol* 2001;25:925.

CHAPTER 42

Acute Leukemias

SECTION 1

D. GARY GILLILAND
GLEN DAVID RAFFEL

Molecular Biology of Acute Leukemias

Our understanding of the molecular genetics of acute leukemias has improved dramatically over the past decade. Fueled in part by the availability of the complete sequence of the human genome, more than 100 different mutations have been identified that can be causally implicated in the pathogenesis of acute leukemias. At first glance, the plethora of mutations presents a discouraging prospect for the development of molecular targeted therapies. However, far more mutations are identified than there are phenotypes of acute leukemia, and a theme is developed in this chapter that many of these mutations must target similar signal transduction or transcriptional pathways. Thus, it is plausible to consider therapeutic approaches that target these shared pathways of transformation. Although many mutations remain to be identified, those observed thus far have provided critical insights into the pathophysiology of leukemia and the development of novel therapeutic targets.

LEUKEMIC STEM CELL

An important emerging concept in the pathobiology of leukemia is the existence of a "leukemic stem cell." In normal hematopoietic development, there is a rare population of hematopoietic stem cells that have self-renewal capacity and give rise to multipotent hematopoietic progenitors. These multipotent myeloid or lymphoid progenitors do not have self-renewal capacity but mature into normal terminally differentiated cells in the peripheral blood, including T and B cells, mast cells, eosinophils, erythrocytes, neutrophils, monocytes, and platelets. It is hypothesized that there is a leukemic stem cell that has limitless self-renewal capacity and gives rise to clonogenic leukemic progenitors that do not have self-renewal capacity but are incapable of normal hematopoietic differentiation.

The first convincing evidence in support of the existence of a leukemic stem cell was derived from experiments in which human leukemic cells were injected into immunodeficient NOD-SCID mice (nonobese diabetic mice with severe combined immunodeficiency disease).[1,2] These data show that the resultant leukemias are derived from as few as 1:1000 to 1:10,000 cells, indicating that there is a rare population of human leukemic cells that have self-renewal capacity in this assay. These cells have similar immunophenotypes to normal self-renewing hematopoietic progenitors and suggest that the leukemogenic mutation occurs in a hematopoietic stem cell that has self-renewal capacity. In support of this hypothesis, clonal cytogenetic abnormalities, such as the t(9;22), have been detected in primitive hematopoietic progenitors such as CD34+CD38– cells (reviewed in ref. 3).

Data suggest, however, that it may be the leukemic oncogenes themselves that confer properties of self-renewal. In a murine system, leukemia oncogenes such as *MLL-ENL* (mixed-lineage leukemia 1-eleven nineteen leukemia) can confer properties of self-renewal to purified committed hematopoietic progenitors that have no capacity for self-renewal.[4] These data indicate that certain targets of the *MLL-ENL* gene, and other leukemia oncogenes, confer properties of self-renewal. Further investigation will be required to determine to what extent these findings can be extrapolated to other leukemia oncogenes and to human leukemia. However, these observations may provide some of the tools necessary to understand genes that conspire to confer limitless self-renewal and may be targets for therapeutic intervention. In addition, these transcriptional programs may be commandeered to confer properties of self-renewal to adult somatic tissues for therapeutic purposes such as tissue regeneration.

RECURRING CHROMOSOMAL ABNORMALITIES IN ACUTE LEUKEMIA

Nonrandom chromosomal abnormalities can be detected in the majority of cases of acute leukemia using high-resolution banding techniques. These include balanced reciprocal chromosomal translocations, such as t(8;21)(q22;q22) or t(15;17)(q22;q21); internal deletions of single chromosomes, such as 5q- or 7q-; gain or loss of whole chromosomes (+8 or –7); or chromosome inversions, such as inv(3), inv(16), or inv(8). Complex chromosomal

abnormalities are observed in approximately 15% of *de novo* cases that do not have an antecedent hematologic disorder; this constitutes a clinical group of patients with particularly poor prognoses. Selected recurring cytogenetic abnormalities observed in acute leukemias are annotated in Table 42.1-1.

Initial insights into the pathobiology of acute leukemias were derived from analysis and molecular cloning of recurring chromosomal translocations.[5] First, it appears that certain genomic loci are associated with specific subtypes of leukemia. For example, more than 40 different recurring translocations target the *MLL* gene locus on chromosome 11q23 and are generally associated with a myelomonocytic or monocytic acute myeloid leukemia (AML) phenotype (FAB M4 or M5). As another example, five different translocations target the retinoic acid receptor alpha locus (RAR-α), including the t(15;17)(q22;q21), which is the most common of these, and are all associated with an acute promyelocytic leukemia (APL) phenotype (FAB M3). Other examples, as detailed later, include the translocations that target the T-cell receptor (TCR) or immunoglobulin (Ig) enhancer loci that

TABLE 42.1-1.   Selected Examples of Cytogenetic and Molecular Abnormalities in Leukemia

Cytogenetic Abnormality	Genes Involved	Derivation of Abbreviation	Protein Characterization	Disease
FUSIONS INVOLVING THE CORE-BINDING FACTORS (CBFs)				
t(8;21)(q22;q22)	CBFA2T1/ETO (8q22)	Eight twenty-one	Zinc finger protein	AML
	CBFA2/AML1 (21q22)	Acute myeloid leukemia 1	α subunit of CBF complex	
inv(16)(p13q22)	MYH11 (16p13)	Myosin heavy chain 11	Smooth muscle myosin heavy chain	AML
	CBFB/CBFβ (16q22)	Core-binding factor-β	β subunit of CBF complex	
t(3;21)(q26;q22)	EVI1 (3q26)	Ecotropic virus integration site 1	Multiple zinc fingers	MDS, AML
	CBFA2/AML1 (21q22)	Acute myeloid leukemia 1	α subunit of CBF complex	CML-BC
t(12;21)(p13;q22)	TEL (12p13)	Translocation ETS leukemia	ETS-related transcription factor	ALL
	CBFA2/AML1 (21q22)	Acute myeloid leukemia 1	α subunit of CBF complex	
FUSIONS INVOLVING *MLL*				
t(4;11)(q21;q23)	AF4 (4q21)	*ALL1* fused chromosome 4	Transactivator	ALL, AML
	MLL (11q23)	Mixed-lineage leukemia	*Drosophila* trithorax homologue	
t(11;19)(q23;p13.3)	MLL (11q23)	Mixed-lineage leukemia	*Drosophila* trithorax homologue	AML, ALL
	ENL (19p13.3)	Eleven nineteen leukemia	Transcription factor	
t(9;11)(p22;q23)	AF9 (9p22)	*ALL1* fused chromosome 9	Nuclear protein, ENL homology	AML, ALL
	MLL (11q23)	Mixed-lineage leukemia	*Drosophila* trithorax homologue	
t(11;22)(q23;q13)	MLL (11q23)	Mixed-lineage leukemia	*Drosophila* trithorax homologue	AML
	P300 (22q13)	Protein 300 kD	Adenoviral E1A-associated protein	
t(1;11)(q21;q23)	AF1q (1q21)	*ALL1* fused chromosome 1q	No homology to any known protein	AML
	MLL (11q23)	Mixed-lineage leukemia	*Drosophila* trithorax homologue	
+11 (sole) or normal cytogenetics	MLL (11q23)	Mixed-lineage leukemia	*Drosophila* trithorax homologue MLL partial tandem duplication	AML
FUSIONS INVOLVING *RAR*-α				
t(15;17)(q22;q12-21)	PML (15q21)	Promyelocytic leukemia	Zinc finger protein	APL
	RAR-α (17q21)	Retinoic acid receptor-α	Retinoic acid receptor-α	
t(11;17)(q23;q21)	PLZF (11q23)	Promyelocytic leukemia zinc finger	Zinc finger protein	APL
	RAR-α (17q21)	Retinoic acid receptor-α	Retinoic acid receptor-α	
Fusions involving *E2A*				
t(1;19)(q23;p13.3)	PBX1 (1q23)	Pre-B transformation 1	Homeodomain	ALL
	E2A (19p13.3)	Early region 2A	bHLH transcription factor	
t(17;19)(q22;p13.3)	HLF (17q22)	Hepatic leukemia factor	Leucine zipper	ALL
	E2A (19p13.3)	Early region 2A	bHLH transcription factor	
FUSIONS INVOLVING NUCLEOPORIN GENES AND HOX GENES				
t(6;9)(p23;q34)	DEK (6p23)	Not relevant to molecule	Transcription factor	AML
	CAN/NUP214 (9q34)	Nuclear pore 214	Nucleoporin	
t(7;11)(p15;p15)	HOXA9 (7p15)	Homeobox A9	Homeobox protein	AML/MDS
	NUP98 (11p15)	Nuclear pore 98	Nucleoporin	AML

(continued)

TABLE 42.1-1. *(Continued)*

Cytogenetic Abnormality	Genes Involved	Derivation of Abbreviation	Protein Characterization	Disease
FUSIONS INVOLVING OTT AND MAL				
t(1;22)(p13;q13)	OTT (1p13) MAL (22q13)	One twenty-two megakaryocytic acute leukemia	*Spen* homologue unknown	AML (M7)
TRANSLOCATIONS INVOLVING THE IMMUNOGLOBULIN ENHANCER LOCI				
t(8;14)(q24;q32)	MYC (8q24)	Myelocytomatosis virus	bHLH/bZIP transcription factor	ALL
	IGH (14q32)	Immunoglobulin heavy chain	Ig heavy chain promoter	
t(2;8)(p12;q24)	IGK (2p12)	Immunoglobulin κ-chain	Igκ-chain promoter	ALL
	MYC (8q24)	Myelocytomatosis virus	bHLH/bZIP transcription factor	
t(8;22)(q24;q11)	MYC (8q24)	Myelocytomatosis virus	bHLH/bZIP transcription factor	ALL
	IGL (22q11)	Immunoglobulin λ-chain	Igλ-chain promoter	
TRANSLOCATIONS INVOLVING THE T-CELL RECEPTOR GENES				
t(1;14)(p32;q11)	TAL1/SCL (1p33)	T-cell acute leukemia 1/stem cell leukemia	bHLH transcription factor	ALL
	TCRα/δ (14q11)	T-cell receptor-α/δ	T-cell receptor promoter	
t(1;7)(p32;q34)	TAL1/SCL (1p32)	T-cell acute leukemia 1/stem cell leukemia	bHLH transcription factor	ALL
	TCRβ (7q34)	T-cell receptor-β	T-cell receptor promoter	
t(7;9)(q34;q34)	TCRβ (7q34)	T-cell receptor-β	T-cell receptor promoter	ALL
	TAL2/SCL2 (9q34)	T-cell acute leukemia 2/stem cell leukemia	bHLH transcription factor	
t(7;19)(q34;p13)	TCRβ (7q34)	T-cell receptor-β	T-cell receptor promoter	ALL
	LYL1 (19p13)	Lymphoid leukemia 1	bHLH transcription factor	
t(8;14)(q24;q11)	MYC (8q24)	Myelocytomatosis virus	bHLH/bZIP transcription factor	ALL
	TCRα/δ (14q11)	T-cell receptor-α/δ	T-cell receptor promoter	
t(11;14)(p15;q11)	LMO1 (11p15)	LIM only 1	Zinc finger	ALL
	TCRα/δ (14q11)	T-cell receptor-α/δ	T-cell receptor promoter	
t(11;14)(p13;q11)	LMO2 (11p13)	LIM only 2	Zinc finger	ALL
	TCRα/δ (14q11)	T-cell receptor-α/δ	T-cell receptor promoter	
t(7;10)(q34;q24)	TCRβ (7q34)	T-cell receptor-β	T-cell receptor promoter	ALL
	HOX11 (10q24)	Homeobox 11	Homeobox gene	

ALL, acute lymphoblastic leukemia; AML, acute myeloid leukemia; APL, acute promyelocytic leukemia; bHLH, basic helix-loop-helix; bZIP, basic region/leucine zipper; CBF, core-binding factor; CML, chronic myeloid leukemia; CMML, chronic myelomonocytic leukemia; ENL, eleven nineteen leukemia; ETS, E twenty-six retrovirus; Ig, immunoglobulin; LIM, Lin-11, Isl-2, Mec-3 homeodomain; MDS, myelodysplastic syndrome; MLL, mixed-lineage leukemia; T-PLL, T-cell prolymphocytic leukemia.

are associated with T- and B-cell leukemias, respectively. Second, it appears that most chromosomal translocations associated with AMLs target transcription factors that are important for normal hematopoietic development. For example, more than a dozen translocations target the core-binding factor (CBF). As detailed in Chromosomal Translocations that Target Core-Binding Factor, CBF is a heterodimeric transcription factor comprised of an AML1 (RUNX1) subunit and a CBFβ subunit.[6] Both components of CBF are essential for definitive hematopoiesis. The translocations that target CBF, such as the t(8;21), result in expression of dominant negative inhibitors of normal CBF function, such as the AML1/ETO fusion. Thus, one consequence of many of these chromosomal translocations in acute leukemias is impaired hematopoietic differentiation. A third general observation has been that fusion genes associated with acute leukemias are necessary but not sufficient to cause acute leukemia.

CHROMOSOMAL TRANSLOCATIONS THAT TARGET CORE-BINDING FACTOR

CBF is targeted by more than a dozen different chromosomal translocations in acute leukemias, including the t(8;21) or inv(16), observed in approximately 20% of AMLs, and the t(12;21), present in approximately 25% of patients with pediatric B-cell acute lymphoblastic leukemia (ALL).[6] As discussed in Chapter 42.2, adult patients with CBF leukemias have a favor-

able prognosis when high-dose cytosine arabinoside is incorporated into therapy, and the TEL/AML1 fusion that is expressed as a consequence of t(12;21) in children confers a favorable prognosis among B-cell ALL.[6]

CBF is a heterodimeric hematopoietic transcription factor that is critical for normal hematopoietic development. Loss of function of either subunit results in a complete lack of definitive hematopoiesis.[7,8] The AML1 (RUNX1, CBFA2) subunit of CBF contacts DNA but only weakly transactivates target genes as a monomer. When bound to its heterodimeric partner CBFβ, which does not itself contact DNA, transactivation of CBF target genes is dramatically enhanced.[6] CBF transactivates a spectrum of target genes that are important in normal myeloid development, including cytokines [e.g., granulocyte-macrophage colony-stimulating factor (GM-CSF)] and cytokine receptors (such as M-CSF receptor), as well as in lymphoid development, such as the TCRβ enhancer and the Ig heavy-chain loci. Because CBF targets include cytokines and cytokine receptors that are important for normal hematopoietic development, a mutation or gene rearrangement that resulted in loss of function of either AML1 or CBFβ might be expected to impair hematopoietic differentiation.[6]

Compelling evidence has been shown that translocations that target CBF result in loss of function through dominant negative inhibition. The AML1/ETO fusion associated with t(8;21) and the CBFβ/SMMHC (smooth muscle myosin heavy chain) fusion associated with inv(16) are dominant negative inhibitors of CBF and impair hematopoietic differentiation. Expression of either the AML1/ETO or CBFβ/SMMHCC fusion genes from their endogenous promoter in mice completely inhibits the function of the residual AML1 or CBFβ alleles, resulting in a lack of definitive hematopoiesis and resultant embryonic lethality.[7,8] The phenotype observed is the same as that seen in *AML1–/–* or *CBFβ–/–* mice, indicating that the AML1/ETO or CBFβ/SMMHC fusions, respectively, act as complete dominant negative inhibitors of the native proteins. Repression of CBF target genes by the AML1/ETO or CBFβ/SMMHC fusions is mediated by aberrant recruitment of the nuclear corepressor complex, as it is for the PML/RAR-α fusion (see refs. 9 and 19). Thus, it has been suggested that histone deacetylase, a component of the corepressor complex, may be a therapeutic target for leukemias associated with translocations that target CBF and other leukemogenic transcription factors.[10]

Murine models of leukemia have also provided convincing evidence that expression of the CBF fusions alone is not sufficient to cause acute leukemia. Because AML1/ETO expression during development results in an embryonic lethal phenotype, conditional alleles of AML1/ETO were developed to test the effects of expression in adult bone marrow. Leukemia does not develop in adult animals expressing AML1/ETO in the bone marrow, although AML/ETO confers the ability to serially replate in methylcellulose culture, a measure of self-renewal potential. AML can only be induced in this system using chemical mutagens such as N-ethyl-nitroso-urea. Similarly, expression of CBFβ/SMMHC in adult hematopoietic cells results in leukemia only after a markedly prolonged latency, and the latency can be shortened using mutagenesis strategies.[11,12] Taken together, these data indicate that translocations that target CBF impair hematopoietic differentiation and confer certain properties of leukemic stem cells, such as the ability to serially replate, but are not sufficient to cause leukemia.

CHROMOSOMAL TRANSLOCATIONS THAT TARGET THE RETINOIC ACID RECEPTOR ALPHA GENE

The empiric observation that all-*trans*-retinoic acid (ATRA) induces complete responses in patients with APL drove the subsequent cloning of the t(15;17)(q22;q21) fusion gene involving the RAR-α locus. Several groups demonstrated at approximately the same time that the RAR-α (*RARα*) gene on chromosome 17 was fusion to a novel partner that was eventually identified as the promyelocytic leukemia (PML) gene.[13–15] Two reciprocal fusion RNA species are produced as a consequence of the translocation, *RARα/PML* and *PML/RARα*. The PML/RAR-α fusion protein contains the zinc finger of PML fused to the DNA- and protein-binding domains of RAR-α. Several other chromosomal translocations associated with an APL phenotype have been cloned and characterized. Each of these targets the *RARα* locus, with fusion to various partners (see Table 42.1-1). The best studied of these is the PLZF/RAR-α fusion, which also aberrantly recruits the nuclear corepressor complex (see Table 42.1-1). However, in contrast with the PML/RAR-α fusion, ATRA is not able to relieve corepression mediated by the PLZF/RAR-α fusion and thus is not effective in patients who harbor the t(11;17) associated with this fusion gene.[16]

As with CBF fusions, the PML/RAR-α fusion protein functions as a dominant inhibitory oncogene for RAR-α–interacting proteins, including RXR-α. In addition, the PML/RAR-α fusion interferes with the function of the native PML protein, which is thought to function as a tumor suppressor gene based on analysis of mice that are deficient in PML.[17] Collectively, the dominant interfering activities of the PML/RAR-α fusion protein result in a block in differentiation at the promyelocyte stage of development. The clinical response of these patients to ATRA, as discussed in Chapter 42.2, is explained by the ability of this retinoid to bind to the PML/RAR-α fusion protein and reverse repression of target genes required for normal hematopoietic development. The ability of the PML/RAR-α fusion protein to repress transcription is due in part to the aberrant recruitment of the nuclear corepressor complex, including histone deacetylase,[18–20] suggesting that pharmacologic agents that inhibit histone deacetylases may be useful in therapy of APL.[10,21,22]

The transforming properties of the *PML/RARα* fusion gene have been tested in murine models. Expression of PML/RAR-α in transgenic mice from promoters that direct expression to the promyelocyte compartment, such as cathepsin G or MRP8, result in an APL-like phenotype.[23–25] However, there is approximately a 6-month lag before the development of leukemia, incomplete penetrance of approximately 15% to 30%, and acquired karyotypic abnormalities, all suggesting that second mutations are required for induction of leukemia. Coexpression of the PML/RAR-α and RAR-α/PML under the cathepsin G promoter results in increased penetrance but prolonged latency and acquisition of cytogenetic abnormalities, still supporting the need for additional mutation.[26] In at least some cases, activating mutations in FLT3, as discussed below in the section Activating Mutations in FLT3 and KIT, may be the additional mutation required. ATRA is efficacious, in leukemic animals expressing both PML/RAR-α and activated FLT3, and this model has allowed for preclinical testing of novel agents currently in clinical trials, such as arsenic trioxide.[27]

CHROMOSOMAL TRANSLOCATIONS THAT TARGET HOX FAMILY MEMBERS

The large HOX family of transcription factors is important in patterning in vertebrate development and also plays a critical role in normal hematopoietic development (reviewed in ref. 28). *HOX* genes may also be targeted by chromosomal translocations, with examples including the NUP98/HOXA9 and NUP98/HOXD13 fusions, associated with t(7;11) and t(2;11), respectively (see Table 42.1-1).[29,30] *HOX* gene expression is tightly regulated during hematopoietic development. HOXA9, for example, is expressed in early hematopoietic progenitor cells but is down-regulated during hematopoietic differentiation and is undetectable in terminally differentiated cells. It has been suggested that unregulated overexpression of the HOXA9 moiety from the constitutively active NUP98 promoter may result in aberrant differentiation. Experimental support for this hypothesis includes the observation that the NUP98/HOXA9 fusion protein can transform 3T3 fibroblasts, an activity that requires the HOXA9 DNA-binding domain.[31]

The contribution of the NUP98 moiety to leukemic transformation is not fully understood. NUP98 is normally a component of the nuclear pore complex and is constitutively and ubiquitously expressed. However, several lines of evidence suggest that NUP98 contributes more than a constitutively activated promoter. For example, NUP98 motifs known as *FG repeats* are essential for transformation and may serve to recruit transcriptional coactivators, such as CBP/p300, to HOXA9

DNA-binding sites.[31] In murine models of leukemia, overexpression of HOXA9 alone is not sufficient to cause AML, but coexpression of HOXA9 with transcriptional cofactors, such as MEIS1, results in efficient induction of AML. Thus, the NUP98 moiety in the context of the NUP98/HOXA9 fusion may serve multiple functions, including provision of an active promoter, and recruitment of transcriptional coactivators such as CBP/p300 that subserve the function of other cofactors such as MEIS1. Epidemiologic evidence that the NUP98 contributes to leukemogenesis includes the observation that there are now a spectrum of fusion proteins involving components of the nuclear pore that are targeted by chromosomal translocations in acute leukemias. These include *NUP98* and *NUP214* fused to a diverse group of partners, including *HOX* family members, *HOXA9* and *HOXD13*, and the *DDX10*, *PMX1*, and *DEK* genes, respectively.

It has been hypothesized that dysregulated *HOX* gene expression may be important in leukemias that do not directly target HOX family members. Several proteins that are upstream of HOX expression have been implicated in AML as fusion genes associated with AML. The most frequent of these are *MLL* gene rearrangements (see Chromosomal Translocations That Target the *MLL* Gene and Fig. 42.1-1). More than 40 chromosomal translocations target *MLL* and result in fusions of *MLL* with a broad spectrum of partners. However, a common biologic feature of all of these may be the ability to dysregulate *HOX* gene expression during hematopoietic development in that *HOX* genes have been shown to be direct targets of various *MLL* fusions.[32] For example, t(12;13) associated with AML results in expression of high levels of CDX2 from the *TEL* locus.[33,34] CDX2 is a homeotic protein that regulates expression of HOX family members in the colonic epithelium. As in hematopoietic development, *HOX* gene expression is highest in colonic stem cells in the colonic crypts and is downregulated with maturation to mature epithelial cells. It is thus plausible that high levels of expression of CDX2 dysregulate HOX expression in hematopoietic progenitors and result in leukemia. Evidence to support this includes the ability of CDX2 to induce leukemia in murine retroviral transduction models.[34] Although CDX2 is not normally expressed in hematopoietic cells, a family member, CDX4, has been cloned and appears to play a similar role in hematopoietic development as CDX2 does in the gut. Of note, CDX4 in hematopoietic cells appears to either be downstream or epistatic with MLL in regulation of *HOX* gene expression.[35]

Taken together these data indicate that the NUP98/HOXA9 fusion transforms hematopoietic progenitors in part through dysregulated overexpression and by transactivation mediated through the NUP98 transactivation domain that recruits CBP. Evidence indicates, however, like other gene rearrangements involving hematopoietic transcription factors, expression of NUP98/HOXA9 alone is not sufficient to cause leukemia. In murine bone marrow transplant models, NUP98/HOXA9 induces AML only after markedly prolonged latencies indicative of a requirement for second mutation.

CHROMOSOMAL TRANSLOCATIONS THAT TARGET THE *MLL* GENE

As noted earlier in Recurring Chromosomal Abnormalities in Acute Leukemia, the *MLL* locus is involved in more than 40 different chromosomal translocations with a remarkably diverse group of fusion partners,[36] and are associated with mostly FAB subtype M4 or M5, and fewer with M2 AML. Patients who have received prior chemotherapy for cancer and develop AML [therapy-related myelodysplastic syndrome (MDS)/AML, t-AML] often have abnormalities in 11q23, especially those patients treated with topoisomerase inhibitors such as epipodophyllotoxins or topotecan. Chromosomal translocations involving band 11q23 translocations result in expression of a fusion gene containing amino-terminal *MLL* sequences fused to a wide variety of fusion partners. The function of most of the fusion partners is poorly understood and there has been no common functional motif or activity ascribed to all partners. However, specific fusions may be associated with specific leukemic phenotypes. The MLL/AF4 fusion associated with t(4;11) is frequently observed in infant leukemias and is associated with an ALL phenotype in more than 90% of cases, whereas the MLL/AF9 fusion associated with the t(9;11) is almost exclusively associated with AML. Certain MLL fusion genes also have prognostic significance. For example, patients with t(9;11)(p22;q23) have a better outcome than those with other translocations involving 11q23.

The MLL gene encodes a large, ubiquitously expressed protein. The *Drosophila* protein trithorax, a homologue of *MLL*, regulates patterning and *HOX* gene expression during development. It has been hypothesized, in part based on these observations, that MLL might be required for maintenance of *HOX* gene expression. In support of this hypothesis, mice that lack *Mll* express HoxA7 but are not able to maintain its expression.[37] Mice that have homozygous deficiency for *Mll* have an embryonic lethal phenotype at day postconception 10.5. Even heterozygous animals have developmental anomalies in the axial skeleton and hematopoietic deficits including anemia.[37] Thus, as for other genes targeted by chromosomal translocations, *MLL* is important for normal hematopoietic development.

The function of *MLL* is not fully understood, but cell culture and murine models have provided some insight into transforming activity of the fusion proteins. The MLL protein of the fusion protein retains the amino terminal AT hooks that facilitate binding to DNA, as well as a methyltransferase domain. With the exception of CBP/p300, the function of the remaining broad spectrum of divergent fusion partners is poorly understood. In fact, the remarkable divergence of partners has suggested that alteration in the *MLL* gene itself is a critical required event for transformation. In support of a central role of *MLL* rearrangement in AML, it has been reported that partial tandem duplications (PTDs) of *MLL* are associated with AML, in particular AML associated with +11.[38] Data demonstrating that MLL is a processed polypeptide provide further support for this hypothesis. MLL is processed by proteolytic cleavage into two component parts by a novel protease called *taspase 1*.[39] Cleavage is required for normal regulation of expression of anterior and posterior *HOX* gene paralogs during development. It has thus been suggested that MLL fusion genes, which are not cleavable, may mimic the uncleaved native MLL protein, thereby dysregulating *HOX* gene expression in leukemias.[39]

MLL fusion genes have transforming properties in serial replating assays in retrovirally transduced hematopoietic progenitors[36] as well as in murine models of disease.[40,41] Although various MLL fusions have similar transforming properties *in vitro*, there are distinctive differences in disease penetrance and latency in the murine models, depending on the

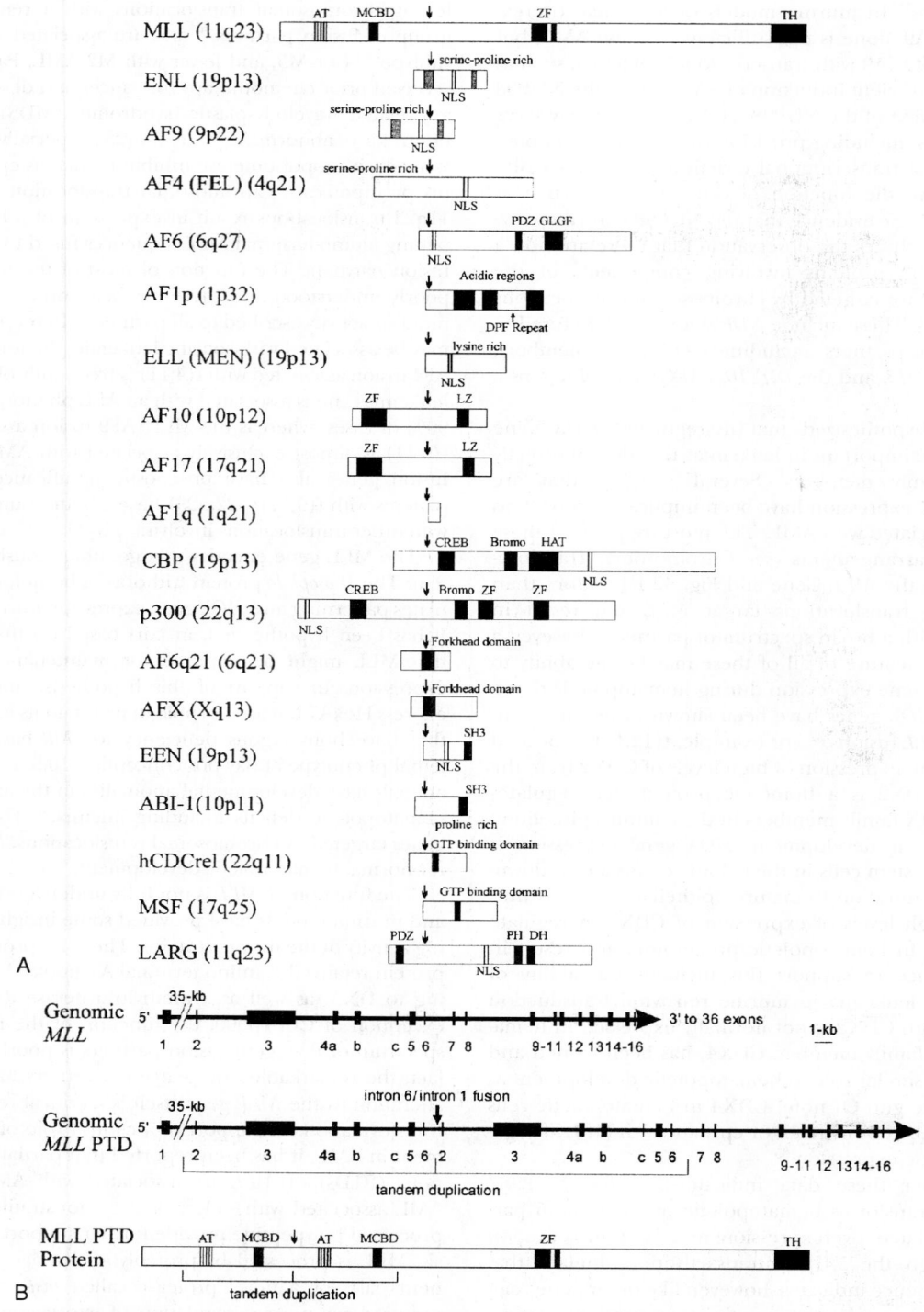

FIGURE 42.1-1. **A:** The MLL protein and several known fusion partners with various motifs identified. Protein motifs are indicated in black. The shaded gray regions in ENL and AF9 indicate known regions of homology. Fusion breakpoints are indicated by arrows. AF1q is unique in that its fusion breakpoint occurs six nucleotides upstream of its open reading frame, resulting in a fusion protein without functional domains. **B:** The genomic structures of *MLL* and *MLL* with an exon 6–exon 2 partial tandem duplication (PTD) are shown. Exons are indicated by *vertical lines and boxes,* and introns are indicated by the *horizontal line* for each structure. The *vertical arrow* indicates point of unique self-fusion that results from the PTD. The predicted protein structure for MLL with the 6-2 PTD is illustrated below and can be compared with the wild-type protein at the top of the figure **(A).** AT, AT hooks; bromo, bromodomain; CREB, cyclic adenosine monophosphate response element–binding protein site; DH, *Dbl* homology domain; DPF, aspartic acid–proline-phenylalanine repeat; GLGF, glycine-leucine-phenylalanine domain; HAT, histone acetyltransferase activity; LZ, leucine zipper; MCBD, methyl CpG–binding domain; NLS, nuclear localization signal; PDZ, PDZ domain; PH, pleckstrin homology domain; SH3, *Src* homology domain 3; TH, trithorax homology (SET domain); ZF, zinc fingers.

fusion partner. It is possible that the MLL gene rearrangement may be critical for transformation, whereas the fusion partners confer properties related to differences in disease phenotype. The long latency of disease in murine knock-in and bone marrow transplant models of leukemia supports the hypothesis that MLL fusions, like the PML/RAR-α and CBF-related fusion proteins, require second mutations to cause leukemia.[40,41]

The t(4;11)(q21;q23) may also be observed in AML, particularly in infants and children. This translocation was originally described in association with ALL, but later studies documented the myeloid or hybrid nature of blasts in some of the patients. New insights into pathogenesis of infant acute leukemia associated with the t(4;11) MLL/AF4 fusion have been gained from analysis of global patterns of gene expression.[42] These analyses indicate that infant leukemia with the MLL/AF4 fusion represents a distinct subclass of leukemia that can be readily delineated from AML or ALL by gene expression profiles. These data, and the target genes that are overexpressed in infant leukemia with the MLL/AF4 fusion such as FLT3,[42] suggest novel approaches to therapy of this subtype of leukemia.

As noted above in the section Leukemic Stem Cell, data indicate that certain *MLL* fusion genes may also confer properties of self-renewal to hematopoietic progenitors. MLL/ENL expression in common myeloid progenitors or granulocyte-monocyte progenitors in a murine system conferred properties of self-renewal, including the ability to serially replate in methylcellulose cultures and to engender a transplantable AML phenotype in recipient animals.[4] These data indicate that leukemogenic mutations may occur in cells that have no intrinsic self-renewal capacity and yet confer these properties by activation of specific transcriptional programs. These exciting observations provide tools for identification of target genes that confer properties of self-renewal and may have value as therapeutic targets for treatment of leukemia and for developing systems for tissue regeneration.

CHROMOSOMAL TRANSLOCATIONS THAT INVOLVE TRANSCRIPTIONAL COACTIVATORS AND CHROMATIN REMODELING PROTEINS

Several translocations associated with leukemia involve transcriptional coactivators and chromatin modifying proteins that have no apparent DNA-binding specificity. These include the MLL/CBP and MOZ/CBP fusions that involve the transcriptional coactivator CBP and the MLL/p300 and MOZ/TIF2 fusions, which involve the coactivators p300 and TIF2, respectively. Although TIF2 itself is not known to have histone acetylase transferase (HAT) activity, a hallmark of the coactivators CBP and p300, it has a well-characterized CBP interaction domain that serves to recruit CBP into a complex with MOZ/TIF2. Thus, recruitment of CBP/p300 is a shared theme among this group of fusion genes.

The transcriptional targets and transformation properties of this class of fusion proteins are not fully understood. Transduction of MLL/CBP into primary murine bone marrow cells followed by transplantation results in a long-latency AML. The activity requires the MLL moiety, and the bromo and HAT domains of CBP, and the long latency in this model suggests a need for second mutations. MOZ/TIF2 also results in leukemia in a similar model system. MOZ is a HAT protein that contains a nucleosome-binding domain and an acetyl–coenzyme A–

binding catalytic domain. Mutational analysis shows that leukemogenic activity requires MOZ nucleosome-binding activity and CBP recruitment activity, but the MOZ HAT activity is dispensable. These data would be consistent with a CBP gain-of-function in which CBP is recruited to MOZ nucleosome-binding sites.[48] However, it has also been hypothesized that the leukemogenic potential of this class of fusions may be related to dominant negative interference with CBP/p300 or that the translocation leads to simple loss of function of CBP expressed from one allele. In support of this hypothesis, loss of a single allele of CBP/p300 in the human Rubinstein-Taybi syndrome increases predisposition to malignancies including colon cancer and mice that are heterozygous for CBP that develop hematopoietic tumors.[49]

T(1;22) TRANSLOCATION ASSOCIATED WITH INFANT ACUTE MEGAKARYOBLASTIC LEUKEMIA

Until recently, little was known about the molecular pathogenesis of acute megakaryoblastic leukemias (AMKLs; FAB M7), due in part to the difficulty in obtaining adequate quantities of material for analysis from densely fibrotic bone marrow. GATA-1 has been shown to be mutant in patients with Down syndrome in whom AMKL develops.[50] In addition, the t(1;22) that is associated with the majority of non-Down AMKL in infants has been cloned. The translocation results in expression of the *OTT/MAL* fusion gene.[51,52] The role of the fusion in transformation of megakaryoblasts is not known, but OTT contains three amino-terminal RNA recognition motifs and a Spen paralog and ortholog C-terminal motif that is conserved in *Drosophila* and may function as a positive regulator of the RAS pathway. The *MAL* gene is ubiquitously expressed and has several functional motifs, including a coiled-coil dimerization motif and a proline-rich transcriptional activation domain and has been shown to be a cofactor for serum response factor (SRF).[52a] However, the function of these genes in leukemogenesis is not known.

DELETIONS AND NUMERIC ABNORMALITIES IN ACUTE LEUKEMIAS

Deletions of all or part of chromosomes 5 and 7 and trisomy 8 are among the most common chromosomal abnormalities associated with gain or loss of genetic material but are not associated with a specific FAB subtype of AML. They are considerably more frequent in older patients, whereas the frequency of the specific translocations and inversions described above decreases with age. These same abnormalities (+8, –7, –5/5q-) are more common in patients with an antecedent MDS, therapy-related AML, or exposure to environmental mutagens. Specific translocations or inversions are relatively less common in these patient groups. An exception to this is AML, which develops in patients who have received high doses of epipodophyllotoxins (VP-16 or VM-26) for treatment of a previous malignancy. As noted in Chromosomal Translocations That Target the *MLL* Gene, translocations involving 11q23 are commonly observed in this setting.

The high frequency of deletions of the long arm of chromosome 5 (5q-) is of interest because the genes encoding several hematopoietic growth factors and their receptors are located on this arm, including *GM/CSF* (5q23-31), *IL-3* (5q23-31), and *IL-4* (5q23-31). The *M-CSF* receptor, c-*fms*, and the *PDGFβR* are also on this chromosome, at 5q33. In some 5q- chromosome defects, one or more of these genes may be deleted. An intensive effort has been made to identify putative tumor suppressor genes in several critically deleted regions of chromosome 5q, as well as 7q and 20q.[53-56] In addition, genomic wide loss of heterozygosity screens have identified a spectrum of other smaller recurrent deletions associated with AML.[57]

However, as yet no gene has been identified that meets the criteria for a classic tumor suppressor in which one allele is deleted and the other allele harbors a loss-of-function mutation in the 5q, 7q, or 20q deleted regions in MDS or AML. Several possible explanations can be made for the difficulty in identification of classic tumor suppressors, despite the availability of complete genomic sequence and detailed annotations of expressed sequences in these regions. The residual allele may be affected by epigenetic mutations that interfere with expression, such as promoter or aberrant methylation, or both, but do not affect coding sequence. These types of mutations are more difficult to detect. Alternatively, it is possible that haploinsufficiency for one or more genes in the critically deleted loci is responsible for the MDS/AML phenotype. Haploinsufficiency for the transcription factor AML1 has been reported in a familial leukemia syndrome, and haploid gene dosage is increasingly being identified as a genetic basis for inherited human diseases.[58,59]

CHROMOSOMAL TRANSLOCATIONS THAT RESULT IN OVEREXPRESSION OF OTHERWISE NORMAL GENES

The chromosomal translocations described thus far result in expression of aberrant fusion genes. Chromosomal translocations may also result in overexpression of otherwise normal genes as a result of juxtaposition of a gene not normally expressed in adult hematopoietic tissues adjacent to an active promoter or enhancer. Most of those identified thus far involve the Ig or TCR enhancer loci, and thus most of these are associated with lymphoid malignancies.

CHROMOSOMAL TRANSLOCATIONS INVOLVING THE IMMUNOGLOBULIN LOCI

The prototypical example of juxtaposition of an Ig enhancer locus to an oncogene resulting in B-cell leukemia and lymphoma is the t(8;14)(q24;q32), resulting in overexpression of the *MYC* bHLH/bZIP transcription factor on chromosome 8 due to juxtaposition to the Ig heavy-chain enhancer on chromosome 14. Similar phenotypes ensue from juxtaposition to other Ig enhancers in the human genome, such as the Igκ locus on chromosome 2 or the Igλ locus on chromosome 22, and are characterized as B-ALL or lymphoma (see Table 42.1-1). Overexpression of MYC from Ig enhancers in murine models results in B-cell leukemias and lymphomas, confirming a central role for MYC overexpression in transformation. However, the mechanism of transformation of *MYC*, and, indeed, a complete understanding of its target genes, is not fully understood. MYC is fully active as a transcription factor when heterodimerized with MAX. MAX is normally a homodimer, or a heterodimer complexed with MAD, which represses transcription. Overexpression of MYC is thought to shift the equilibrium in favor of an MYC-MAX

homodimer that transactivates genes that confer the leukemic phenotype to B cells.

CHROMOSOMAL TRANSLOCATIONS INVOLVING THE T-CELL RECEPTOR

T-cell leukemias are often associated with overexpression of a number of genes due to juxtaposition to the TCR enhancer loci (*TCRβ* at chromosome 7q34 or *TCRα/δ* at chromosome 14q11). Overexpression is thus associated with T-cell phenotypes, including T-cell ALL and lymphoma. For example, T-cell ALL may be associated with overexpression of bHLH family members that include TAL1/SCL, TAL2/SCL2, LYL1, HOX11, LMO2, LMO1, and MYC (see Table 42.1-1; reviewed in ref. 60). In addition to the minority of T-ALL cases with gene rearrangements involving these loci, it has been demonstrated that many patients without evident cytogenetic abnormalities overexpress TAL1, LMO2, or HOX11.[60] Overexpression of HOX11 has been associated with a favorable prognosis.

POINT MUTATIONS IN ACUTE LEUKEMIA

Although intensive effort has focused on chromosomal translocations in leukemia, in part because of their high frequency in various kinds of leukemia, it has become increasingly clear that point mutations play an important role in a spectrum of leukemias (Table 42.1-2). It is likely that more of these will be discovered in the coming years, aided in part by the completion of the human genome sequence and high-throughput sequencing strategies.

ONCOGENIC RAS MUTATIONS

Activating mutations in RAS may be associated with AML and MDS, typically at codons 12, 13, or 61 or N- or K-RAS. The reported incidence varies widely between studies from 25% to 44% (reviewed in ref. 61). One carefully conducted cooperative group trial in which mutant RAS alleles were assessed by direct sequencing reported an 18% incidence of N- or K-RAS mutations and a poor prognosis conferred on RAS mutations.[62] Considerable effort has been devoted to developing small-

TABLE 42.1-2. Point Mutations in Acute Leukemia

Mutation	Frequency in AML (%)
SIGNAL TRANSDUCTION PATHWAYS—ACTIVATING	
FLT3-ITD	~20–25
FLT3 activation loop	~5–10
RAS (N- and K-)	~15–20
KIT (D816V and D816Y)	~5
PTPN11	<5
TRANSCRIPTION FACTORS—LOSS OF FUNCTION	
RUNX1 (AML1; more common in +21 and FAB M0)	<5
C/EBPα (more common in FAB M2)	<5
GATA-1 (more common in FAB M7 in Down syndrome)	<5

AML, acute myeloid leukemia.

molecule inhibitors of RAS activation, with a focus on prenylation inhibitors, including farnesyl transferase and geranyl-geranylation inhibitors that preclude appropriate targeting of activated RAS to the plasma membrane.[63,64] Specifically targeting activated RAS mutants remains an attractive option, and prenyltransferase inhibitors appear to have activity in AML. However, clinical activity is not correlated with the presence of activating mutations in RAS[63,64] or even with inhibition of the target farnesyl transferase itself. Several possible interpretations can be made of these observations, including the possibility that RAS is activated by mechanisms other than intrinsic point mutations (e.g., constitutively activated tyrosine kinases such as FLT3), or that other proteins that are targets of prenylation are important in leukemia pathogenesis, or that farnesyl transferase inhibitors target an as yet unidentified target.

ACTIVATING MUTATIONS IN FLT3 AND KIT

Perhaps the most exciting recent development in pathogenesis of AMLs has been identification and characterization of activating mutations in hematopoietic tyrosine kinases. Substantial evidence has been shown that chromosomal translocations that activate tyrosine kinases can contribute to the pathogenesis of chronic myeloid leukemia (CML) syndromes. The most common of these is the *BCR/ABL* gene rearrangement, but other examples include the TEL/ABL, TEL/PDGFβR, TEL/JAK2, H4/PDGFβR, HIP1/PDGFβR, and rabaptin/PDGFβR fusion proteins. However, these fusion genes are only rarely encountered in AMLs. Approximately 1% to 2% of cases of *de novo* AML have the *BCR/ABL* gene rearrangement. In addition, there are very rare cases of disease progression from CML to AML associated with acquisition of second mutations such as the *NUP98/HOXA9*, *AML1/ETO*, or *AML1/EVI1* rearrangement noted in Table 42.1-1. However, until recently there had been no direct evidence for involvement of activated tyrosine kinases in the majority of cases of AML by cytogenetic, fluorescence *in situ* hybridization, or spectral karyotype analysis. However, point mutations in the tyrosine kinase activation loop and juxtamembrane (JM) mutations that activate *FLT3* and *c-KIT* have been identified in a significant proportion of AML cases. These findings may have important therapeutic implications with the demonstration of the efficacy of molecular targeting of the ABL kinase in BCR/ABL-positive CML and CML blast crisis with imatinib.[65,66]

Activating mutations in *FLT3* have been reported in approximately 30% to 35% of cases of AML.[67,68] In 20% to 25% of cases, ITDs of the JM domain result in constitutive activation of FLT3. These can range in size from a few to more than 50 amino acids and are always in frame. Because of the extensive variability in size and exact position of the repeats within the JM domain, it has been hypothesized that these are loss-of-function domains that impair an autoinhibitory domain, resulting in constitutive kinase activation in the absence of ligand. In support of this hypothesis, the crystallographic structure of FLT3 demonstrates a 7 amino acid extension of the JM domain that intercalates into the catalytic domain, thereby precluding kinase activation.[69] It is likely that ITD mutations in this region would disrupt structure of the autoinhibitory domain, resulting in kinase activation. In an additional 5% to 10% of cases, so-called activating loop mutations occur near position D835 in the tyrosine kinase.[70,71] Several large studies have confirmed the frequency of these mutations in adult and pediatric AML populations and the fact that mutations in *FLT3* appear to confer a poor prognosis.[72–74]

FLT3 mutations may occur in conjunction with known gene rearrangements, such as *AML1/ETO*, *PML/RARα*, CBFβMYH11, or MLL. Analogous activating loop mutations at position D816 have also been reported in *C-KIT* in approximately 5% of cases of AML. These data suggest that constitutive activation of tyrosine kinases may play an important role in the pathogenesis of acute leukemia as well as in CML. Based on these data, it is plausible that additional mutations that activate hematopoietic tyrosine kinases may be discovered.

LOSS-OF-FUNCTION POINT MUTATIONS IN *AML1*, *C/EBPα*, AND *GATA-1*

AML1 (also known as *RUNX1*, *CBFA2*) is a frequent target of translocations in human leukemias. In addition to frequent involvement of AML1 as a consequence of chromosomal translocations, it has been determined that loss-of-function mutations in *AML1* are responsible for the inherited leukemia syndrome FPD/AML (familial platelet disorder with propensity to develop acute myelogenous leukemia).[58,75] In addition, approximately 3% to 5% of sporadic cases of AML harbor loss-of-function mutations in *AML1*,[75,76] with a higher frequency in M0 AML (25%) and in AML or MDS with trisomy 21. It is not known whether loss-of-function mutations in *AML1* confer the favorable prognosis associated with translocations involving the *AML1* gene.

C/EBPα is a hematopoietic transcription factor that is required for normal myeloid lineage development. Because many translocations associated with AML phenotypes result in loss of function of hematopoietic transcription factors, it has been hypothesized that *C/EBPα* may also be a target for loss-of-function mutations in human leukemia. Evidence to support this hypothesis has been reported. Point mutations that result in expression of a mutant C/EBPα protein that has dominant negative activity for wild-type C/EBPα have been reported in a fraction of M2 AML cases.[77] Thus, these mutations would be predicted to impair hematopoietic differentiation. More recent data indicate that *C/EBPα* mutations confer a favorable prognosis.[78]

GATA-1 mutations are associated with a subset of AMKLs (FAB M7), in particular leukemias arising in patients with Down syndrome (constitutional trisomy 21). These mutations appear to result in loss of function or dysregulation of GATA-1 and are thought to contribute to leukemogenesis.[50] The mechanism through which hypomorphic alleles of *GATA-1* contribute to leukemogenesis in the context of +21 is not known. *GATA-1* mutations thus far have only been associated with Down syndrome and have not been observed in other infant AMKLs, including those with the t(1;22) described earlier in t(1;22) Translocation Associated with Infant Acute Megakaryoblastic Leukemia.

MUTATIONAL COMPLEMENTATION GROUPS IN ACUTE LEUKEMIAS

Several lines of evidence indicate that more than one mutation is necessary for the pathogenesis of acute leukemia. First, there

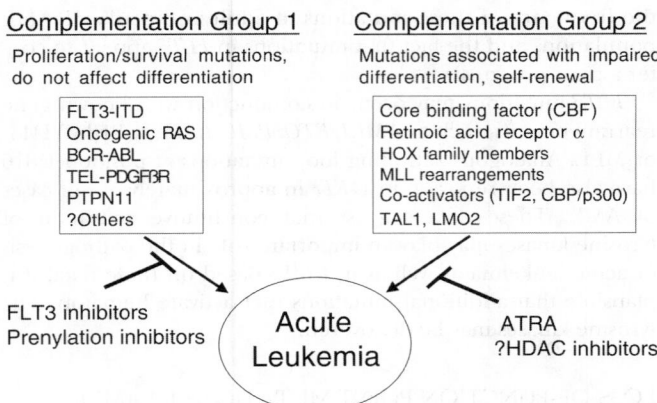

FIGURE 42.1-2. Cooperating mutations in acute leukemia. Leukemia is composed of two broad complementation groups, defined by lack of concurrence of any two mutations in the same complementation group in the same patient. One group is characterized by activating mutations in signal transduction pathways, such as FLT3-ITD or oncogenic N-RAS. When expressed alone, these mutations confer a proliferative or survival advantage, or both, but do not affect differentiation. The second group exemplified by AML1/ETO or PML/RAR-α are associated with impaired differentiation and the ability to confer properties of self-renewal to hematopoietic progenitors. Together, the complementation groups collaborate to engender the acute leukemia phenotype. This model has important therapeutic implications in that each of the complementation groups can be potentially targeted for therapeutic intervention, such as small-molecule inhibitors of FLT3 or RAS, or agents that override the block in differentiation, such as all-*trans*-retinoic acid (ATRA) or possibly histone deacetylase (HDAC) inhibitors.

is evidence for acquisition of additional cytogenetic abnormalities with disease progression from CML to AML (i.e., CML blast crisis). Published examples of progression in BCR/ABL-positive CML include acquisition of t(3;21) *AML1/EVI1*, t(8;21) *AML1/ETO*, or t(7;11) *NUP98/HOXA9* gene rearrangements. Progression of chronic myelomonocytic leukemia to AML in a patient with the *TEL/PDGFβR* gene rearrangement was associated with acquisition of a t(8;21) *AML1/ETO* gene rearrangement.[79] Second, expression of the AML1/ETO or CBFβ/MYH11 fusion proteins in murine models is not sufficient to cause AML.[11,12] Chemical mutagens must be used in these contexts to generate second mutations that cause the AML phenotype. Third, evidence indicates that in some cases the *TEL/AML1* gene rearrangement associated with pediatric ALL may be acquired *in utero*, but ALL does not develop until years later, indicating a requirement for a second mutation.[80] Fourth, AML develops in transgenic mice that express the PML/RAR-α fusion protein only after a long latency of 3 to 6 months, with incomplete penetrance, indicating a need for a second mutation.[23–25]

The genetics epidemiology of AML provides important clues to the nature of the collaborating mutations. One broad complementation group in AML (Fig. 42.1-2) is comprised of mutations that activate signal transduction pathways. These include activating mutations in FLT3, RAS, and KIT and, more rarely, the BCR/ABL and TEL/PDGFβR fusion associated with disease progression in CML. These can be viewed as a complementation group because, although they are collectively present in approximately 50% of cases of AML, they rarely, if ever, occur together in the same patient.

A second complementation group, typified by translocations involving hematopoietic transcription factors, includes

AML1/ETO, CBFβ/SMMHC, PML/RARα, NUP98/HOXA9, MLL gene rearrangements, and *MOZ/TIF2* and they are never observed together in the same leukemia. In general, this second class of mutations impair hematopoietic differentiation and may confer properties of self-renewal to the leukemic stem cell but are not sufficient to cause leukemia when expressed alone (see Recurring Chromosomal Abnormalities in Acute Leukemia). However, one mutation from each of these two complementation groups often coexists in the same leukemia. For example, activating mutations in FLT3 or RAS have been observed in association with virtually all of the fusion genes in the second class described earlier.[81]

Support has also been given for the hypothesis of collaborating classes of leukemia oncogenes derived from analysis of genotypes of CML patients who progress to AML (also called *CML blast crisis*). Some cases of BCR/ABL-positive CML progress to AML associated with acquisition of the t(7;11) translocation associated with expression of the *NUP98/HOXA9* fusion gene discussed above. As another example, TEL/PDGFβR-positive chronic myelomonocytic leukemia may progress to AML associated with acquisition of the t(8;21) translocation related to expression of the AML1/ETO fusion. These cases of disease progressions from CML to AML suggest the hypothesis that constitutively activated tyrosine kinases cooperate with mutations in hematopoietic transcription factors to cause the AML phenotype.

These findings suggest a hypothesis for pathogenesis of AML in which there are two broad classes of cooperating mutations (see Fig. 42.1-2).[81] One class, exemplified by activating mutations in *FLT3* or *RAS*, confer either a proliferative or survival advantage, or both, to hematopoietic progenitors but do not affect differentiation. These mutations do not confer self-renewal capacity as assessed in part by the ability to serially replate in culture or to serially transplant disease in murine models.[82,83] A second class of mutations, exemplified by *AML1/ETO, CBFβ/SMMHC, PML/RARα, NUP98/HOXA9, MLL* gene rearrangements, and *MOZ/TIF2* serve primarily to impair hematopoietic differentiation and confer properties of self-renewal. Together, these cooperating mutations induce the AML phenotype characterized by enhanced proliferative and survival advantage, impaired differentiation, and limitless self-renewal capacity. Experimental evidence supports this model of cooperativity in murine models between BCR/ABL and NUP98/HOXA9,[84] TEL/PDGFβR and AML1/ETO,[85] and FLT3/ITD and PML/RAR-α.[86] These findings have important therapeutic implications in that it may be possible to target both classes of mutations. For example, in APL with activating mutations in FLT3, it may be possible to target FLT3 with small-molecule inhibitors and PML/RAR-α with ATRA (see Chapter 42.2, Fig. 42.1-2, and ref. 87).

CONCLUSION

Identification of a large number of disease alleles associated with acute leukemias over the past decade has provided important insights into the pathophysiology and therapy. Of the more than 100 mutations identified in hematopoietic cells of patients with leukemias, most can be segregated into two broad complementation groups. One group, epitomized by FLT3 and RAS mutations, confer proliferative and survival advantage to cells, whereas a second complementation group, exemplified by AML1/ETO and PML/RAR-α, impair hematopoietic differentiation. Each of these classes of mutations is a potential target for therapeutic intervention with agents such as ATRA or histone deacetylase inhibitors to overcome the block in differentiation and small-molecule inhibitors of FLT3 or RAS to block constitutive activation of signal transduction pathways and may exemplify a mechanism-based approach to future AML treatment.

REFERENCES

1. Bonnet D, Dick JE. Human acute myeloid leukemia is organized as a hierarchy that originates from a primitive hematopoietic cell. *Nat Med* 1997;3:730.
2. Cobaleda C, et al. A primitive hematopoietic cell is the target for the leukemic transformation in human Philadelphia-positive acute lymphoblastic leukemia. *Blood* 2000;95:1007.
3. Deininger MW, Goldman JM, Melo JV. The molecular biology of chronic myeloid leukemia. *Blood* 2000;96:3343.
4. Cozzio A, et al. Similar MLL-associated leukemias arising from self-renewing stem cells and short-lived myeloid progenitors. *Genes Dev* 2003;17:3029.
5. Rowley JD. The role of chromosome translocations in leukemogenesis. *Semin Hematol* 1999;36[4 Suppl 7]:59.
6. Speck NA, Gilliland DG. Core-binding factors in haematopoiesis and leukaemia. *Nat Rev Cancer* 2002;2:502.
7. Wang Q, et al. Disruption of the Cbfa2 gene causes necrosis and hemorrhaging in the central nervous system and blocks definitive hematopoiesis. *Proc Natl Acad Sci U S A* 1996;93:3444.
8. Okuda T, et al. AML1, the target of multiple chromosomal translocations in human leukemia, is essential for normal fetal liver hematopoiesis. *Cell* 1996;84:321.
9. Lutterbach B, et al. ETO, a target of t(8;21) in acute leukemia, interacts with the N-CoR and mSin3 corepressors. *Mol Cell Biol* 1998;18:7176.
10. Pandolfi PP. Histone deacetylases and transcriptional therapy with their inhibitors. *Cancer Chemother Pharmacol* 2001;48[Suppl 1]:S17.
11. Castilla LH, et al. The fusion gene Cbfβ blocks myeloid differentiation and predisposes mice to acute myelomonocytic leukemia. *Nat Genet* 1999;23:144.
12. Higuchi M, et al. Expression of a conditional AML1-ETO oncogene bypasses embryonic lethality and establishes a murine model of human t(8;21) acute myeloid leukemia. *Cancer Cell* 2002;1:63.
13. Goddard AD, et al. Characterization of a zinc finger gene disrupted by the t(15;17) in acute promyelocytic leukemia. *Science* 1991;254:1371.
14. Kakizuka A, et al. Chromosomal translocation t(15;17) in human acute promyelocytic leukemia fuses RAR alpha with a novel putative transcription factor, PML. *Cell* 1991;66:663.
15. de The H, et al. The PML-RAR-alpha fusion mRNA generated by the t(15;17) translocation in acute promyelocytic leukemia encodes a functionally altered RAR. *Cell* 1991;66:675.
16. Zelent A, et al. Translocations of the RARalpha gene in acute promyelocytic leukemia. *Oncogene* 2001;20:203.
17. Salomoni P, Pandolfi PP. The role of PML in tumor suppression. *Cell* 2002;108:165.
18. Grignani F, et al. Fusion proteins of the retinoic acid receptor-alpha recruit histone deacetylase in promyelocytic leukaemia. *Nature* 1998;391:815.
19. He LZ, et al. Distinct interactions of PML-RARalpha and PLZF-RARalpha with co-repressors determine differential responses to RA in APL. *Nat Genet* 1998;18:126.
20. Lin RJ, et al. Role of the histone deacetylase complex in acute promyelocytic leukaemia. *Nature* 1998;391:811.
21. He LZ, et al. Histone deacetylase inhibitors induce remission in transgenic models of therapy-resistant acute promyelocytic leukemia. *J Clin Invest* 2001;108:1321.
22. Pandolfi PP, et al. Transcription therapy for cancer. *Oncogene* 2001;20:3116.
23. Grisolano JL, et al. Altered myeloid development and acute leukemia in transgenic mice expressing PML-RAR alpha under control of cathepsin G regulatory sequences. *Blood* 1997;89:376.
24. He LZ, et al. Acute leukemia with promyelocytic features in PML/RARalpha transgenic mice. *Proc Natl Acad Sci U S A* 1997;94:5302.
25. Brown D, et al. A PMLRARalpha transgene initiates murine acute promyelocytic leukemia. *Proc Natl Acad Sci U S A* 1997;18:2551.
26. Zimonjic DB, et al. Acquired, nonrandom chromosomal abnormalities associated with the development of acute promyelocytic leukemia in transgenic mice. *Proc Natl Acad Sci U S A* 2000;97:13306.
27. Tallman MS, et al. Acute promyelocytic leukemia: evolving therapeutic strategies. *Blood* 2002;99:759.
28. Thorsteinsdottir U, Sauvageau G, Humphries RK. Hox homeobox genes as regulators of normal and leukemic hematopoiesis. *Hematol Oncol Clin North Am* 1997;11:1221.
29. Borrow J, et al. The t(7;11)(p15;p15) translocation in acute myeloid leukaemia fuses the genes for nucleoporin NUP98 and class I homeoprotein HOXA9. *Nat Genet* 1996;12:159.
30. Nakamura T, et al. Fusion of the nucleoporin gene NUP98 to HOXA9 by the chromosome translocation t(7;11)(p15;p15) in human myeloid leukemia. *Nat Genet* 1996;12:154.
31. Kasper LH, et al. CREB binding protein interacts with nucleoporin-specific FG repeats that activate transcription and mediate NUP98-HOXA9 oncogenicity. *Mol Cell Biol* 1999;19:764.
32. Hanson RD, et al. Mammalian Trithorax and polycomb-group homologues are antagonistic regulators of homeotic development. *Proc Natl Acad Sci U S A* 1999;96:14372.
33. Chase A, et al. Fusion of ETV6 to the caudal-related homeobox gene CDX2 in acute myeloid leukemia with the t(12;13)(p13;q12). *Blood* 1999;93:1025.
34. Rawat VP, et al. Ectopic expression of the homeobox gene Cdx2 is the transforming event in a mouse model of t(12;13)(p13;q12) acute myeloid leukemia. *Proc Natl Acad Sci U S A* 2004;101:817.
35. Davidson AJ, et al. cdx4 mutants fail to specify blood progenitors and can be rescued by multiple hox genes. *Nature* 2003;425:300.
36. Ayton PM, Cleary ML. Molecular mechanisms of leukemogenesis mediated by MLL fusion proteins. *Oncogene* 2001;20:5695.
37. Yu BD, et al. MLL, a mammalian trithorax-group gene, functions as a transcriptional maintenance factor in morphogenesis. *Proc Natl Acad Sci U S A* 1998;95:10632.
38. Whitman SP, et al. The partial nontandem duplication of the MLL (ALL1) gene is a novel rearrangement that generates three distinct fusion transcripts in B-cell acute lymphoblastic leukemia. *Cancer Res* 2001;61:59.
39. Hsieh JJ, et al. Proteolytic cleavage of MLL generates a complex of N- and C-terminal fragments that confers protein stability and subnuclear localization. *Mol Cell Biol* 2003;23:186.
40. Dobson CL, et al. The mll-AF9 gene fusion in mice controls myeloproliferation and specifies acute myeloid leukaemogenesis. *EMBO J* 1999;18:3564.
41. Lavau C, et al. Retrovirus-mediated gene transfer of MLL-ELL transforms primary myeloid progenitors and causes acute myeloid leukemias in mice. *Proc Natl Acad Sci U S A* 2000;97:10984.
42. Armstrong SA, et al. MLL translocations specify a distinct gene expression profile that distinguishes a unique leukemia. *Nat Genet* 2002;30:41.
43. Rowley JD, et al. All patients with the t(11;16)(q23;p13.3) that involves MLL and CBP have treatment-related hematologic disorders. *Blood* 1997;90:535.
44. Giles RH, et al. Detection of CBP rearrangements in acute myelogenous leukemia with t(8;16). *Leukemia* 1997;11:2087.
45. Taki T, et al. The t(11;16)(q23;p13.3) translocation in myelodysplastic syndrome fuses the MLL gene to the CBP gene. *Blood* 1997;89:3945.
46. Carapeti M, et al. A novel fusion between MOZ and the nuclear receptor coactivator TIF2 in acute myeloid leukemia. *Blood* 1998;91:3127.
47. Liang J, et al. Acute mixed lineage leukemia with an inv(8)(p11q13) resulting in fusion of the genes for MOZ and TIF2. *Blood* 1998;92:2118.
48. Deguchi K, et al. MOZ-TIF2-induced acute myeloid leukemia requires the MOZ nucleosome binding motif and TIF2-mediated recruitment of CBP. *Cancer Cell* 2003;3:259.
49. Kung AL, et al. Gene dose-dependent control of hematopoiesis and hematologic tumor suppression by CBP. *Genes Dev* 2000;14:272.
50. Wechsler J, et al. Acquired mutations in GATA1 in the megakaryoblastic leukemia of Down syndrome. *Nat Genet* 2002;32:148.
51. Mercher T, et al. Recurrence of OTT-MAL fusion in t(1;22) of infant AML-M7. *Genes Chromosomes Cancer* 2002;33:22.
52. Ma Z, et al. Fusion of two novel genes, RBM15 and MKL1, in the t(1;22)(p13;q13) of acute megakaryoblastic leukemia. *Nat Genet* 2001;28:220.
52a. Miralles F, Posern G, Zaromytidou AI, Treisman R. Actin dynamics control SRF activity by regulation of its coactivator MAL. *Cell* 2003;113:329.
53. Olney HJ, Le Beau MM. The cytogenetics of myelodysplastic syndromes. *Best Pract Res Clin Haematol* 2001;14:479.
54. Lai F, et al. Transcript map and comparative analysis of the 1.5-Mb commonly deleted segment of human 5q31 in malignant myeloid diseases with a del(5q). *Genomics* 2001;71:235.
55. Kratz CP, et al. Genomic structure of the PIK3CG gene on chromosome band 7q22 and evaluation as a candidate myeloid tumor suppressor. *Blood* 2002;99:372.
56. Asimakopoulos FA, Green AR. Deletions of chromosome 20q and the pathogenesis of myeloproliferative disorders. *Br J Haematol* 1996;95:219.
57. Sweetser DA, et al. Loss of heterozygosity in childhood de novo acute myelogenous leukemia. *Blood* 2001;98:1188.
58. Song WJ, et al. Haploinsufficiency of CBFA2 (AML1) causes familial thrombocytopenia with propensity to develop acute myelogenous leukemia (FPD/AML). *Nat Genet* 1999;23:166.
59. Seidman JG, Seidman C. Transcription factor haploinsufficiency: when half a loaf is not enough. *J Clin Invest* 2002;109:451.
60. Ferrando AA, et al. Gene expression signatures define novel oncogenic pathways in T cell acute lymphoblastic leukemia. *Cancer Cell* 2002;1:75.
61. Beaupre DM, Kurzrock R. RAS and leukemia: from basic mechanisms to gene-directed therapy. *J Clin Oncol* 1999;17:1071.
62. Neubauer A, et al. Mutations in the ras proto-oncogenes in patients with myelodysplastic syndromes. *Leukemia* 1994;8:638.
63. Karp JE. Farnesyl protein transferase inhibitors as targeted therapies for hematologic malignancies. *Semin Hematol* 2001;38[3, Suppl 7]:16.
64. Sebti SM, Hamilton AD. Farnesyltransferase and geranylgeranyltransferase I inhibitors in cancer therapy: important mechanistic and bench to bedside issues. *Expert Opin Investig Drugs* 2000;9:2767.
65. Sawyers CL. Molecular studies in chronic myeloid leukemia patients treated with tyrosine kinase inhibitors. *Semin Hematol* 2001;38[3 Suppl 8]:15.
66. Appelbaum FR. Perspectives on the future of chronic myeloid leukemia treatment. *Semin Hematol* 2001;38[3 Suppl 8]:35.
67. Stirewalt DL, Radich JP. The role of FLT3 in haematopoietic malignancies. *Nat Rev Cancer* 2003;3:650.
68. Gilliland DG, Griffin JD. The roles of FLT3 in hematopoiesis and leukemia. *Blood* 2002;100(5):1532.
69. Griffith J, et al. The structural basis for autoinhibition of FLT3 by the juxtamembrane domain. *Mol Cell* 2004;13:169.

70. Yamamoto Y, et al. Activating mutation of D835 within the activation loop of FLT3 in human hematologic malignancies. *Blood* 2001;97:2434.
71. Griffin JD. Point mutations in the FLT3 gene in AML. *Blood* 2001;97:2193A.
72. Abu-Duhier F, et al. FLT3 internal tandem duplication mutations in adult acute myeloid leukaemia define a high-risk group. *Br J Haematol* 2000;111:190.
73. Kiyoi H, et al. Prognostic implication of FLT3 and N-RAS gene mutations in acute myeloid leukemia. *Blood* 1999;93:3074.
74. Meshinchi S, et al. Prevalence and prognostic significance of Flt3 internal tandem duplication in pediatric acute myeloid leukemia. *Blood* 2001;97:89.
75. Michaud J, et al. In vitro analyses of known and novel RUNX1/AML1 mutations in dominant familial platelet disorder with predisposition to acute myelogenous leukemia: implications for mechanisms of pathogenesis. *Blood* 2002;99:1364.
76. Osato M, et al. Biallelic and heterozygous point mutations in the runt domain of the AML1/PEBP2alphaB gene associated with myeloblastic leukemias. *Blood* 1999;93:1817.
77. Pabst T, et al. Dominant-negative mutations of C/EBPalpha, encoding CCAAT/enhancer binding protein-alpha, in acute myeloid leukemia. *Nat Genet* 2001;27:263.
78. Preudhomme C, et al. Favorable prognostic significance of CEBPA mutations in patients with de novo acute myeloid leukemia: a study from the Acute Leukemia French Association (ALFA). *Blood* 2002;100:2717.
79. Golub TR, et al. Fusion of PDGF receptor beta to a novel ets-like gene, tel, in chronic myelomonocytic leukemia with t(5;12) chromosomal translocation. *Cell* 1994;77:307.
80. Wiemels JL, et al. Prenatal origin of acute lymphoblastic leukaemia in children. *Lancet* 1999;354:1499.
81. Gilliland DG. Molecular genetics of human leukemias: new insights into therapy. *Semin Hematol* 2002;39[4 Suppl 3]:6.
82. Kelly LM, et al. FLT3 internal tandem duplication mutations associated with human acute myeloid leukemia induce myeloproliferative disease in a murine bone marrow transplant model. *Blood* 2002;99:310.
83. Chan IT, et al. Conditional expression of oncogenic K-ras from its endogenous promoter induces a myeloproliferative disease. *J Clin Invest* 2004;113:528.
84. Dash AB, et al. A murine model of CML blast crisis induced by cooperation between BCR/ABL and NUP98/HOXA9. *Proc Natl Acad Sci U S A* 2002;99:7622.
85. Grisolano JL, et al. An activated receptor tyrosine kinase, TEL/PDGFbetaR, cooperates with AML1/ETO to induce acute myeloid leukemia in mice. *Proc Natl Acad Sci U S A* 2003;100:9506.
86. Kelly LM, et al. PML/RARalpha and FLT3-ITD induce an APL-like disease in a mouse model. *Proc Natl Acad Sci U S A* 2002;99:8283.
87. Gilliland DG. FLT3-activating mutations in acute promyelocytic leukaemia: a rationale for risk-adapted therapy with FLT3 inhibitors. *Best Pract Res Clin Haematol* 2003;16:409.

DAVID A. SCHEINBERG
PETER G. MASLAK
MARK A. WEISS

SECTION **2**

Management of Acute Leukemias

Acute leukemias are clonal, uncontrolled neoplastic proliferations of immature cells of the hematopoietic system, which are characterized by aberrant or arrested differentiation. Leukemia cells accumulate in the bone marrow, ultimately replacing most of the normal hematopoietic cells and their functions, thus resulting in the signs and symptoms of the disease. These include, most prominently, anemia, hemorrhage, infection, and their consequences. Leukemia cells circulate into the blood and other tissues throughout the body, with patterns characteristic of the particular type of leukemia. The acute leukemias, which can be broadly grouped as either lymphocytic or myelogenous, can be identified phenotypically and genetically and are characterized by a rapid clinical course that usually necessitates immediate treatment. Acute leukemias are derived from and biologically resemble, in many features, primitive hematopoietic progenitor cells; in contrast, chronic leukemias have the phenotype and biologic character of more mature cells. Chronic myeloid leukemia, however, may transform to an acute, blastic phase over time and will thereafter more closely resemble an acute leukemia in its biology, clinical course, and need for therapy.

The acute lymphocytic leukemias (ALLs) are distinguished generally from the lymphomas because the latter resemble more mature lymphoid cells and typically inhabit the lymph nodes, spleen, or other extramedullary sites before spreading to involve the blood or bone marrow. Certain lymphomas, such as lymphoblastic lymphomas and Burkitt's lymphomas, retain features of the leukemias and the lymphomas but are derived from immature cells and require aggressive therapy similar to that used for ALL. Other lymphomas, and sometimes multiple myelomas, however, may spread widely into the blood and bone marrow and, in such a phase, can be described as *leukemic* but are not true leukemias.

Leukemia (meaning *white blood*) was originally described in 1845 by Virchow. Although acute leukemias are relatively rare cancers, they are the most carefully studied, best characterized, and, in some cases, most curable, of the neoplasms. Numerous subtypes have been defined based on morphology, genetics, immunophenotype, and biologic behavior. Oncogenes responsible for leukemogenesis are now identified, and there is an enlarging body of knowledge regarding the molecules and pathways regulating leukemia cell growth and function. Multiple drugs of different classes capable of killing and altering the growth of leukemia cells are now available; the therapeutic strategies that have been developed often result in clinical remissions of adult leukemias and, in a smaller fraction of patients, result in cures. Despite these advances, however, acute leukemia remains, for most adult patients, a fulminant and incurable disease, requiring immediate diagnosis and treatment, whose course is often complicated by the severity of the treatments themselves.[1]

EPIDEMIOLOGY AND ETIOLOGY

INCIDENCE

The acute leukemias are rare diseases but have a disproportionately large impact on cancer survival statistics among children and younger adults. Although the acute leukemias account for fewer than 2% of all cancers, these diseases are the first and second leading causes of death due to cancer in the United States in men and women, respectively, under 40 years of age.[1,2] The incidence rate of acute myelogenous leukemias (AMLs) in the United States is approximately 2.5 per 100,000 persons; for ALL, the rate is approximately 1.3 per 100,000 persons. AML has a slight male predominance (1.3:1.0) and accounts for 25% of acute and chronic leukemias. AML affects approximately 9000 people a year in the United States.[1,2] ALL affects approximately 4000 people, with a similar predominance of males. The incidences of acute leukemias in the United States have not changed substantially over the last 20 years, although there is a slight trend upward among younger patients and a slight fall in the number of diagnoses in those over 65 years of age. Incidence rates for acute leukemia are similar worldwide. In ALL, the incidence rates in African Americans are approximately two-thirds those seen in whites; in AML, rates are more similar

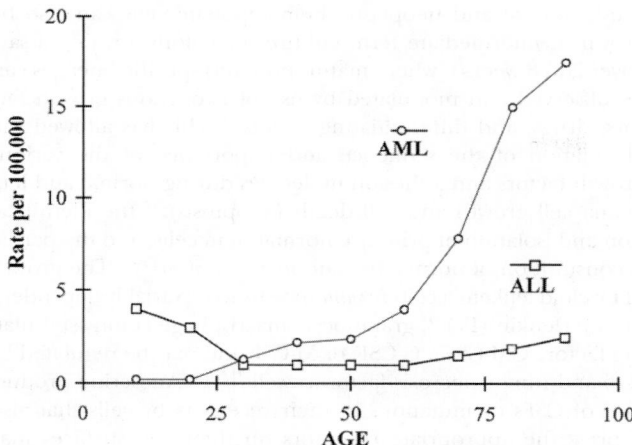

FIGURE 42.2-1. Age-specific incidence of acute myelogenous leukemia (AML) and acute lymphoblastic leukemia (ALL) in the United States. (From ref. 2, with permission.)

between these two groups. Interestingly, age-specific incidences differ dramatically between ALL, which has a median age at diagnosis of 11 years, and AML, which has a median age of 66 years.[1] AML is unusual below the age of 40, but incidence rises progressively with age from approximately 1 per 100,000 at age 40 to more than 15 per 100,000 at age 65 or older. In contrast, ALL has its peak incidence at less than 10 years and has a second smaller rise in persons older than 65 years (Fig. 42.2-1).

SECONDARY LEUKEMIAS

For most patients with acute leukemia, the cause of the disease is unknown. Because leukemias are the result of a genetic alteration in a clonogenic cell, which can often be identified by a chromosomal translocation, deletion, or mutation, known and suspected carcinogens have been explored as causative agents in acute leukemia. A clear cause of leukemia can be found in the minority of patients with a history of prior chemotherapy or radiation therapy. Such secondary leukemias, 90% of which are myeloid, are notoriously difficult to treat. The chromosomal abnormalities often observed in these secondary leukemias are associated with a poor prognosis, even when observed in patients without a history of prior therapy or toxic exposure.

Secondary myeloid leukemias first became apparent in the early survivors of Hodgkin's disease, and it appears that older age at treatment increases the risk.[3,4] Studies initially linked the use of alkylating agents such as nitrogen mustard to the increased risk. Among large cohorts of patients treated with chemotherapy and radiotherapy for Hodgkin's disease, many cases of secondary leukemia were found, mostly AML. Dose-related increases in secondary leukemia occurred. More recent studies have not linked radiotherapy, when used alone, to an increased risk.[5] Mechlorethamine (nitrogen mustard), procarbazine, cyclophosphamide, lomustine, teniposide, and chlorambucil were all implicated in the increased risk. The risk for secondary AML was greatest between 2 and 9 years after therapy, with 85% of cases occurring before the tenth year.[4,5]

Curative therapy for childhood ALL has a risk of inducing secondary AML as well.[6] The increased risk of AML occurred within 6 years and was originally associated with use of an epi-podophyllotoxin (etoposide or teniposide) or alkylating agent. The risk from epipodophyllotoxins was proportional to the dose intensity of the drug rather than the cumulative dose, with the highest risks associated with weekly or twice-weekly administration.[6] In contrast, secondary AML was not increased in pediatric ALL protocols in which epipodophyllotoxins were not used.

Several additional studies in adults and children have now confirmed the association between treatment with epipodophyllotoxins and secondary AML,[7] in particular, monocytic and other leukemias, with abnormalities of chromosome 11q23. Promyelocytic leukemias with t(15;17) have also been associated with etoposide and with other chemotherapeutic agents such as doxorubicin that target topoisomerase II.[8]

Dose-dependent risks for secondary AML have also been observed in adults treated with alkylating agents, including platinum-based drugs, and radiotherapy for breast cancer and ovarian cancer[9] and for a variety of neoplasms treated with an autologous bone marrow transplant after high-dose radiation or low-dose radiation and alkylating agent therapy.[6,10,11] Among the alkylating agents, cyclophosphamide appears to hold less risk; a study of the incidence of secondary leukemia in patients with breast cancer treated with moderate doses of cyclophosphamide confirms this lower level of risk.[11]

OCCUPATIONAL AND ENVIRONMENTAL EXPOSURES

The clear relationship between the atomic bomb radiation[12] or use of carcinogenic therapies and the development of secondary leukemias has led to the exploration of the possible leukemogenic role of other potential carcinogens in the environment, such as low-dose radiation, chemicals, cigarette smoke, high altitude, airline flight, and electromagnetic radiation.[13,14]

Although electromagnetic fields have received considerable attention as a possible carcinogen, the actual risk of leukemia from exposure to commercial and residential power fields remains controversial.[14,15] A large number of conflicting reports have been published, but there is a lack of clear dose-response relationship, and a causal relationship between leukemia and electromagnetic fields, either as a consequence of occupational exposure or residential power use, has little current support.

ALL and AML risks increased as a result of exposure to the atomic bombs.[12] Risks associated with occupational exposure to low-dose radiation are controversial. Early suspicions that paternal exposure at power plants resulted in an increased risk for subsequent children of the exposed workers have been disputed.[16]

Cigarette smoke contains numerous carcinogens and has been linked in a dose-dependent manner to leukemia,[17,18] particularly in patients older than 60 years, and to specific chromosomal alterations known to be associated with chemical mutagens. As much as 20% of AML may be attributable to smoking.[18]

Occupational exposure to benzene has been established as a cause of AML,[19] but low-level exposure in the workplace, for example, less than 10 ppm, has not been clearly established as a risk. Other occupational exposures to solvents, such as to toluene or butadiene in the shoe and rubber industries, or hair dyes, have not been shown conclusively to increase leukemia risk.

OTHER RISK FACTORS

Viruses, and in particular RNA retroviruses, have been found to cause many neoplasms in experimental animals, including leukemia of mice[20] and cats; a human retrovirus, human T-cell leukemia virus type 1, has been identified as the cause of a T-cell lymphoma/leukemia in humans.[21] A clear retroviral cause for acute leukemia in humans has not been identified. Epstein-Barr virus (EBV), a DNA virus, has been associated with oncogenesis in acute B-cell leukemias; Burkitt's lymphomas, especially those of endemic origin; and human immunodeficiency virus–associated lymphomas.[22] EBV may function by increasing lymphoid proliferation in patients; this provides a setting in which a second oncogenic event, possibly myc oncogene activation, can result in the clonal, neoplastic proliferation.[22] It has not been demonstrated, however, that simple infection with either an RNA- or DNA-based virus alone is a cause of acute leukemia.

Although leukemias are acquired disorders, there may be significant genetic and immunologic predispositions that allow their occurrence. Several genetic syndromes are associated with increased risk of leukemias, including Down syndrome, Fanconi's anemia, Bloom's syndrome, and ataxia-telangiectasia.[23,24] Down syndrome is associated with a 20-fold increased risk of leukemia; this is typically a megakaryoblastic leukemia in children younger than 4 years of age and a pre-B ALL in children who are older.[25] These true leukemias must be differentiated from a *transient abnormal myeloproliferative* disorder (TAM).[26] Patients with TAM are neonates with hepatosplenomegaly, modest elevations in blasts, and pancytopenia. Although TAM is a clonal disorder, in two-thirds of cases the disease has a benign course.

An immunologic predisposition for acute leukemia has not been clearly delineated. However, analyses of human leukocyte antigen (HLA) types with specific cytogenetically defined subgroups of AML have pointed to associations between certain HLA-A, -B, -C, and -DR types and common chromosomal translocations or deletions.[27] These correlations may become increasingly important as an understanding of the possible immune response to these breakpoints becomes clear.[28]

BIOLOGY OF ACUTE LEUKEMIAS

More is known about the pathobiology of the acute leukemia cell than about any other neoplasm. This is the consequence of a confluence of recent discoveries regarding hematopoietic growth factors, hematopoietic stem cells and progenitor cells, oncogenes, and transcription factors. These discoveries were made possible by the availability of acute leukemia cell lines capable of immortal growth in culture, reliable assays for hematopoietic cell growth, and sensitive tests for specific gene and protein mutation and expression. The important concepts about leukemia cell growth and function are likely to be useful paradigms that will aid in understanding all cancers.

Cell lines derived from and biologically resembling acute myeloid and acute lymphoid leukemias have been available for 25 years and have allowed careful study of the growth of leukemia cells under controlled conditions and of the effects of antileukemic agents. Mouse models mimicking human leukemias can be prepared by oncogene transfections in transgenic mice.[29,30] In addition, cell lines and fresh acute leukemias have been propagated in immunocompromised nude or SCID (severe combined immunodeficiency) mice, thus also allowing controlled study of new therapies under *in vivo* conditions.

Fresh normal and neoplastic hematopoietic cells can also be grown in intermediate term cultures or colony-forming assays (over 2 to 8 weeks), where maturation into specific lineages can be observed and modulated by use of exogenous growth factors, drugs, and differentiating agents.[31] This has allowed the elucidation of the sequence and importance of the various growth factors and adhesion molecules during normal and leukemia cell growth and cell death (apoptosis),[32] the identification and isolation of primitive normal stem cells, and the partial reconstitution of normal hematopoiesis *ex vivo*.[31–33] The growth of myeloid leukemia cells *in vitro* appears to be variably dependent on interleukin (IL)-3, granulocyte-macrophage colony-stimulating factor (GM-CSF), G-CSF, or M-CSF and may be regulated by IL-6 and tumor necrosis factor as well.[31,34,35] Autocrine production of CSFs or mutations in their receptors by cells that also express the appropriate receptors on their cell surfaces may allow unregulated proliferation in the absence of exogenous factors or as a consequence of added factors.[36,37] Comparable assays *in vivo* using immunosuppressed mice that allow spleen colony formation or complete bone marrow reconstitution have demonstrated that viable hematopoiesis for an entire animal may require as few as 30 hematopoietic stem cells.[38]

Enzyme marker studies using glucose 6-phosphate dehydrogenase have shown that leukemia cells derive from a single clonogenic cell.[39] Depending on the cell of origin, the leukemia clone may involve cells of more than one lineage, for example, erythroid and myeloid, or only one lineage. Unlike normal hematopoiesis, the clonogenic leukemia cell generally retains only a limited ability to differentiate into different lineages.[40] The cells responsible for leukemia colony growth *in vitro* represent a more primitive subset of the entire leukemia cell population.

Considerable aberrancy is seen in the differentiation of leukemia cells, as compared to normal cells, when the cell is examined for surface protein phenotype.[41] Abnormalities in apoptosis, or programmed cell death, may also be present that lead to persistence of the leukemic clone[32] or abnormalities that increase telomerase, which promotes longevity.[42] Apoptotic death may still be induced with appropriate growth factors *in vitro* or, in the case of promyelocytic leukemia, by clinical use of retinoic acid (see Acute Promyelocytic Leukemia). It is likely that many leukemogenic translocations or mutations (see Cytogenetics and Molecular Genetics of Acute Leukemias, later in this chapter, and Chapter 42.1) result in dysregulation of the cell cycle.[43]

Heterogeneity of the cells that comprise the entire leukemic population is frequently seen.[39,44] Although the leukemic clone may involve multiple lineages, typically leukemia blasts are phenotypically of one lineage; within this lineage stages of maturation may vary within the population, suggesting incomplete control of differentiation. The phenotypic heterogeneity of the leukemia colony-forming cell also suggests that leukemias may arise at various stages of differentiation. This concept was surmised based on the morphologic and phenotypic characteristics of different leukemias; evidence supporting the concept has been demonstrated in patients with acute promyelocytic leukemia (APL), in which the leukemia clone can be positively identified by use of sensitive polymerase chain reaction (PCR) techniques for the t(15;17). In most cases, the most primitive hematopoietic cells remained normal, whereas more mature progenitors contained the neoplastic translocation.[45]

Despite the achievement of a complete clinical remission after therapy of acute leukemia, normal hematopoiesis derived from cells originally involved with the leukemic clone is sometimes present.[46] Apparently normal granulocytes have exhibited persistence of chromosomal markers of the original leukemia.[47] The continued presence of clonal hematopoiesis may suggest the existence of a "preleukemic" clone of cells that has a proliferative advantage to other normal cells.[46] In spite of this, hematopoiesis in patients in remission is usually polyclonal or oligoclonal.[48]

DIAGNOSIS AND CLASSIFICATION OF ACUTE LEUKEMIAS

CLINICAL PRESENTATION

Although the signs and symptoms are relatively nonspecific, the diagnosis of acute leukemia is usually made easily with the history of the illness, the physical examination, and an examination of the blood smear and bone marrow aspirate smear. Additional laboratory examinations (complete blood cell counts, coagulation profile, chemistry profile) or diagnostic imaging (chest x-ray; abdominal sonogram) are important in the management of the disease but are not usually necessary for diagnosis. Patients with acute leukemia typically present with a 1- to 4-month history of fatigue or malaise, easy bruisability or frank bleeding, dyspnea, minimal to modest weight loss, fever, bone pain, or abdominal pain (Table 42.2-1). Excessive bleeding after a minor dental procedure or severe epistaxis may bring the patient to the physician's attention. In adults with an antecedent myelodysplastic syndrome, symptoms may date back to up to a year or more.

TABLE 42.2-1. Diagnosis and Evaluation of Acute Leukemia

SYMPTOMS
Fatigue, malaise, dyspnea
Easy bruisability, weight loss
Bone pain or abdominal pain (less common)
Neurologic symptoms (rare)
SIGNS
Anemia and pallor
Thrombocytopenia, hemorrhage, ecchymoses, petechiae, fundal hemorrhage
Fever and infection (pneumonia, sepsis, perirectal abscess)
Adenopathy, hepatosplenomegaly, mediastinal mass
Gum or skin infiltration (rare)
Renal enlargement and insufficiency (rare)
Cranial neuropathy (rare)
IMPORTANT LABORATORY AND DIAGNOSTIC TESTS
Complete blood cell count and differential
Coagulation studies, including fibrinogen
Blood electrolytes and chemistries, including creatinine, uric acid, calcium, phosphorus
Examination of the peripheral blood smear
Examination of the bone marrow aspirate smear and biopsy
Leukemia blast cell surface phenotype, cytogenetics (and molecular genetics if indicated)
Examination of the cerebrospinal fluid (in all patients with acute lymphoblastic leukemias; in patients with acute myelogenous leukemias, only if indicated)
Computed tomography of the chest (in lymphoblastic lymphoma) or of the abdomen (in mature B-cell acute lymphoblastic leukemias)
Human leukocyte antigen typing (for younger patients)

The physical examination typically shows pallor, consistent with anemia, and hemorrhage (in the gums, as epistaxis, in the stool, in the skin as petechiae or ecchymoses, or as fundal hemorrhage). Less commonly, there is hepatic or splenic enlargement and lymphadenopathy. Fever and infection, usually of respiratory origin, are frequent; sepsis may occur. Neurologic signs and symptoms are rare at presentation but may include cranial neuropathies and, occasionally in ALL, nausea, vomiting, and headache.

The laboratory examination is notable for anemia and thrombocytopenia in most patients, with severe thrombocytopenia (platelet count less than $50,000/\mu L$) in more than half of the patients. The white blood cell (WBC) count can be normal, reduced, or elevated; fewer than 20% of patients have greater than $100,000$ cells/μL, and an equal number have fewer than 5000 cells/μL. Acute monocytic leukemias and T-cell leukemias may have the highest WBC counts. Examination of the peripheral blood smear shows blasts in almost all cases. Peripheral blasts may be absent in some patients with lymphoblastic lymphoma. Peripheral blood myeloblast levels in excess of $100,000/\mu L$ represent a medical emergency requiring prompt reduction in the blast level to prevent the signs and symptoms of leukostasis (see later in Principles of Clinical Management of Acute Myelogenous Leukemia). The prothrombin time and partial thromboplastin time may be elevated. In APL, this coagulopathy is often associated with reduced fibrinogen and other evidence of disseminated intravascular coagulation (DIC), another medical emergency that must be treated urgently (see later in Principles of Clinical Management of Acute Myelogenous Leukemia). Subclinical DIC may be present in any form of acute leukemia.

Blood chemistries are typically normal, but in advanced disease, or in infiltrative cases such as with monocytic leukemias, there may be evidence of renal dysfunction (elevated creatinine). Renal infiltration and enlargement can be documented with sonography. In cases of high cell turnover and cell death, such as in patients with mature B-cell ALL (ALL-L3), there may be evidence of "tumor lysis syndrome" at presentation; this syndrome is more commonly seen during the rapid lysis of large numbers of ALL cells, and less often AML cells, during chemotherapy. The laboratory picture of tumor lysis syndrome consists of hypocalcemia, hyperkalemia, hyperphosphatemia, increased lactate dehydrogenase, hyperuricemia, and renal insufficiency; if untreated this syndrome can be fatal (see later in Principles of Clinical Management of Acute Myelogenous Leukemia).

The clinical presentation of AML cannot usually be distinguished from ALL without examination of the blasts for genotype, immunophenotype, and morphology (see later). Particular signs and symptoms, however, are more frequent with certain disease subgroups than with others. Bone pain is more common in ALL, as are signs and symptoms of central nervous system (CNS) infiltration. Lymph node and organ infiltration and enlargement are also more common in ALL and in monocytic subtypes of AML. Gum involvement is seen most frequently in acute monocytic leukemia (AML-M5). Mediastinal masses are found in greater than 50% of patients with T-cell ALL. However, the overlap in symptoms and signs among the leukemia subtypes requires a pathologic diagnosis to be made in all cases. Therefore, a bone marrow aspirate and biopsy, with appropriate cytochemical, immunochemical, and genetic evaluations, must be performed in all cases.

The differential diagnosis of acute leukemia includes other neoplastic hematopoietic disorders, such as lymphomas, myelodysplastic syndromes, multiple myeloma, aplastic anemia, severe megaloblastic anemia due to folate or vitamin B$_{12}$ deficiency, severe lymphocytosis due to infection such as with EBV, severe monocytosis due to tuberculosis, and bone marrow failure with release of early cells such as in myelophthisis due to carcinoma. Examination of the bone marrow nearly always excludes the nonhematopoietic conditions because of the presence of increased numbers of blasts. Careful morphologic examination and immunophenotyping of the cells then excludes virtually all the hematopoietic conditions based on lineage and maturational stage; one exception is the myelodysplastic syndromes, which often differ from the acute leukemias only in the percentage of blasts in the marrow. Up to one-third of AMLs in patients older than 60 years have evolved from a prior myelodysplastic syndrome or hematologic disorder, suggesting that the distinction between refractory anemia with excess blasts or refractory anemia with excess blasts in transformation and true AML after myelodysplasia may be clinically unimportant. These conditions each respond more poorly to chemotherapy then *de novo* AML and progressive leukemia, and bone marrow failure leading to death is the typical outcome.

CLASSIFICATION OF ACUTE LEUKEMIA

Modern classifications of acute leukemia must answer three questions to be diagnostically and prognostically useful:

1. What is the lineage?
2. What is the maturational stage?
3. What is the genotype?

Although traditional classifications relied primarily on morphology and cytochemistry,[49] these limited characterizations are not always adequate for classifying leukemias into groups that assign the most appropriate therapy or predict outcome. Knowledge of the exact immunophenotype and the genotype, either via cytogenetic analysis or molecular analysis, is critically important before one commences the most appropriate definitive treatment, such as high-dose consolidation chemotherapy, bone marrow transplantation, or prolonged maintenance therapy.

MORPHOLOGY AND CYTOCHEMISTRY

The French-American-British (FAB) group has proposed a widely used classification of eight different types of acute myeloid leukemias (M0 to M7) and three types of acute lymphoid leukemias (L1 to L3) based on morphology and cytochemistry; monoclonal antibody–based immunophenotype is also used in undifferentiated cases in which morphology and cytochemistry are inconclusive[49-51] (Table 42.2-2). More recently, the World Health Organization (WHO) has prepared a new classification that expands the number of myeloid leukemia subgroups and better incorporates genotypic data.[52] In addition, the acute lymphoid leukemias are classified primarily based on lineage rather than morphology (Table 42.2-3). Because the treatments of acute lymphoid and acute myeloid leukemias may differ significantly, the most important first step in the diagnostic assignment is to distinguish the lymphoid and myeloid lineages to assign therapy. Among the lymphoid neoplasms, the distinction of Burkitt's-type mature B-cell subtype is a second impor-

tant step, as treatment strategies and prognosis differ with this subgroup. Among the myeloid leukemias, prompt identification of APL is necessary because retinoic acid differentiation therapy is instituted instead of, or concurrently with, chemotherapy. Moreover, a significant risk of highly morbid coagulopathy is associated with APL. Because current therapies for most morphologic subtypes of AML, except for promyelocytic leukemia, are generally similar, and outcomes are generally poor, the usefulness of morphologic classifications is somewhat limited. In addition, morphology and cytochemistry are not diagnostic in 10% to 15% of cases or can be misleading in a small percentage of patients. Moreover, concordance of diagnosis among reviewers may only be 70% to 85%.[53] For these reasons the morphologic classification should always be accompanied by immunophenotypic and genotypic analysis[51-54]; the latter data allow better prediction of outcome and, hence, are a guide to choosing therapeutic options.

Modern classifications of AML are based on morphologic examination for lineage, confirmation of lineage by cytochemical stains, quantitation of the number of blasts, and estimation of the degree of differentiation of the cells (see Table 42.2-3). Myeloid leukemia blasts are typically large with round or irregular, smoothly grained nuclei and with moderate cytoplasm, often containing granules or Auer rods; this latter feature is pathognomonic for myeloblasts (Fig. 42.2-2). In contrast, lymphoid blasts are typically small, with more regular nuclei, clumpier chromatin, and scant, agranular cytoplasm (see Fig. 42.2-2). A cytoplasmic tail, making the cell resemble a "hand mirror," is sometimes seen. B-lineage leukemia blasts are not distinguishable from T-lineage leukemia blasts based on morphology alone, except if they are mature B-cell Burkitt's type (see Fig. 42.2-2) blasts, which have characteristic voluminous, vacuolated, basophilic cytoplasm. Myeloblasts can be graded according to the number and quality of granules; for example, a type 1 blast has no granules, a type II blast has up to 15 delicate granules, and a type III blast has numerous azurophilic granules. The blasts associated with chronic myelogenous leukemia (CML) in "blast crisis" cannot be distinguished on morphologic or phenotypic grounds alone.

The most important stains for determining lineage initially include myeloperoxidase, which can be positive (golden brown) even in the absence of visible primary azurophilic granules, and Sudan black B, which stains primary and secondary granule lipids black. Myeloid differentiation is inferred if either of these stains is positive in 3% or more blasts. AS-D chloroacetate esterase is another stain (red or blue) for maturing myeloid granules; alpha-naphthyl butyrate esterase staining (red/brown) is indicative of monocytic differentiation. Acid phosphatase is generally most useful in T-cell ALL, where it stains as a block or patch.

In the small subset of cases in which lineage cannot be indicated by morphology or cytochemistry, immunophenotyping using specific monoclonal antibodies usually determines lineage to be myeloid. This group is designated as undifferentiated AML. The poorer prognosis of this subgroup makes their distinction from ALL and other AML subtypes important.

Another subgroup that is difficult to classify due to its pleomorphic morphology and unhelpful cytochemistry is acute megakaryoblastic leukemia (AML-M7).[52] The lineage can sometimes be identified by cytoplasmic blebs; electron microscopy for platelet peroxidase is confirmatory, although this is not usu-

TABLE 42.2-2. Classification of Acute Leukemia

Subtype (Incidence)	Bone Marrow Morphology	Typical Immunophenotype	Associated Genotype	Comments
AML-M0, undifferentiated AML (5% of AML)	Type 1 blasts >30%; cytochemistry negative	CD13, 33, 34, HLA-DR	NA	Poorer prognosis
AML-M1, AML with minimal maturation (15% of AML)	Types 1 and II blasts >90%; Sudan black or peroxidase positive; occasional Auer rods present	CD13, 14, 15, 33, 34, HLA-DR	Occasionally inv(3)	Inv(3) associated with thrombocytosis
AML-M2, AML with maturation (25% of AML)	Types I, II, and III blasts >30% and <90%; <20% monocytic cells; strong positive Sudan black, peroxidase, or chloroacetate esterase; many Auer rods possible	CD13, 15, 33, 34, HLA-DR	t(8;21) in one-half of cases	t(8;21) has a favorable prognosis; seen in younger adults; associated with extramedullary involvement and splenomegaly
AML-M3, promyelocytic leukemia (APL; 10% of AML)	>30% blasts and abnormal promyelocytes; multiple Auer rods, sometimes in bundles; heavy granulation; strong positive cytochemistry	CD13, 33, 15, less CD34, HLA-DR negative	t(15;17)	Best prognosis of all acute myeloid leukemias; capable of differentiation with retinoic acid therapy; a high risk of disseminated intravascular coagulation; seen in younger adults
AML-M3v (variant)	Abnormal promyelocytes lack granules or Auer rods; weaker cytochemical stains	As for M3, CD2(+)	As for M3	As for M3, may be mistaken for monocytic leukemia
AML-M4, myelomonocytic leukemia (25% of AML)	As for M2, except that monocytic lineage cells are >20% and <80%; peripheral blood has >5000 monocytes/μL; alpha-naphthol stain is positive	CD13, 14, 15, 33, 34, HLA-DR positive	NA	Evidence of monocytic and granulocytic differentiation; extramedullary involvement can be seen
AML-M4eo, myelomonocytic leukemia with eosinophilia	Abnormal basophilic eosinophils are seen in the marrow, which is similar to that of M4	As for M4	inv(16); other 16 abnormalities	Good prognosis; extramedullary involvement is often seen
AML-M5 A, monocytic leukemia (5% of AML)	Large blasts with >80% of cells of the monocytic lineage; >80% of cells are monoblasts; alpha-naphthol stain is positive	CD13, 14, 33, 34, HLA-DR	Abnormal 11q23	Poorer prognosis; often seen in older adults; extramedullary disease (skin, gingival, and central nervous system involvement) common
AML-M5 B, monocytic leukemia with differentiation (5% of AML)	As for M5 A except that <80% of monocytic lineage are blasts	As for M5 A, CD34(-)	As for M5 A	As for M5 A; t(8,16) associated with erythrophagocytosis
AML-M6, erythroid leukemia (5% of AML)	>50% of nucleated cells are erythroid; often dysmorphic; >30% of nonerythroid cells are blasts; periodic acid–Schiff is block positive	CD13, 33, 41, 71, HLA-DR, glycophorin A	Deletions 5 and 7 are often seen	Poorer prognosis; often preceded by a myelodysplastic syndrome; seen in older patients
AML-M7, megakaryoblastic leukemia (10% of AML)	>30% blasts of megakaryocytic origin with blebs; micromegakaryoblasts often present; megakaryocytic fragments are seen in the blood; peroxidase is usually negative; alpha-naphthol and periodic acid–Schiff may be positive; platelet peroxidase is positive by electron microscopy	CD41, 61	Occasional inv(3); t(3;3) trisomy 21; t(9;22); t(1;22) in infants	Poor prognosis; often a fibrotic bone marrow makes diagnosis difficult; can be seen in Down syndrome children <3 y old but must be distinguished from transient abnormal myeloproliferative disorder; is often associated with prior myelodysplastic syndromes, chronic myeloid leukemia blast crisis, or myeloproliferative disorders
ALL-L1 (30% of adult ALL)	Small cells with minimal cytoplasm and no granules; rare nucleoli; TdT positive	If B-lineage: CD10, 19, 20, 22, 34, HLA-DR, cytoplasmic Ig; if T-lineage: CD2, 5, 7, 10, 34	t(9;22); t(4;11); t(1;9); hyperdiploid	Most common subtype in children
ALL-L2 (65% of adult ALL)	Larger cells with moderate amounts of cytoplasm and prominent nucleoli; TdT positive	As for ALL-L1	As for ALL-L1	Most common subtype in adults
ALL-L3, B-cell or Burkitt's type leukemia (5% of ALL)	Large round cells with deeply basophilic cytoplasm and vacuoles	CD10, 19, 20, 21, 22, surface Ig	t(8;14); t(2;8); t(8;22)	Poor prognosis with standard ALL treatment regimens

ALL, acute lymphoblastic leukemias; AML, acute myelogenous leukemia; HLA, human leukocyte antigen; Ig, immunoglobulin; NA, not available; TdT, terminal deoxynucleotidyl transferase.

TABLE 42.2-3. World Health Organization Classification of Acute Leukemias

ACUTE MYELOID LEUKEMIAS (AML)
AML with recurrent cytogenetic translocations
  AML with t(8;21)(q22;q22) [AML1 (CBF-α)/ETO]
  Acute promyelocytic leukemia [AML with t(15;17)(q22;q11-12)]
    (PML/RAR-α) and variants (PLZF/RAR-α), (NPM/RAR-α),
    (NuMA/RAR-α), (STAT 5b/RAR-α)
  AML with abnormal bone marrow eosinophils [inv(16)(p13q22) or
    t(16;16)(p13;q22); (CBFαβ/MYH11)]
  AML with 11q23 (MLL) abnormalities
AML with multilineage dysplasia
  With prior myelodysplastic or myelodysplastic/myeloproliferative
    syndrome
  Without prior myelodysplastic syndrome
AML and myelodysplastic syndrome, therapy related
  Alkylating agent related
  Topoisomerase II inhibitor related
  Other types
AML not otherwise categorized
  AML minimally differentiated
  AML without maturation
  AML with maturation
  Acute myelomonocytic leukemia
  Acute monoblastic and monocytic leukemia
  Acute erythroid leukemia
    Erythroleukemia (erythroid/myeloid)
    Pure erythroid leukemia
  Acute megakaryoblastic leukemia
    Variant: AML/transient myeloproliferative disorder in Down syn-
      drome
  Acute basophilic leukemia
  Acute panmyelosis with myelofibrosis
  Myeloid sarcoma
Acute leukemia of ambiguous lineage
  Undifferentiated acute leukemia
  Bilineal acute leukemia
  Biphenotypic acute leukemia
PRECURSOR B- AND T-CELL NEOPLASMS
Precursor B-lymphoblastic leukemia/lymphoma (precursor B-cell
  acute lymphoblastic leukemia)
Precursor T-lymphoblastic leukemia/lymphoma
MATURE B-CELL NEOPLASMS
Burkitt's lymphoma/Burkitt's cell leukemia

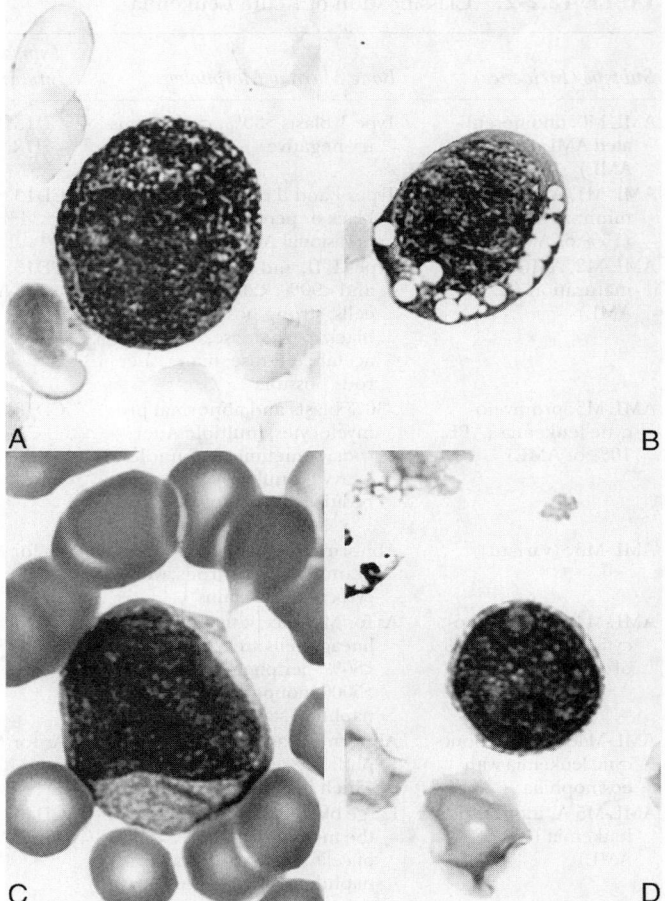

FIGURE 42.2-2. Morphologic appearance of cells typically involved in the various forms of acute leukemia. **A:** Abnormal promyelocyte found in acute promyelocytic leukemia. Numerous cytoplasmic granules tend to obscure the nuclear-cytoplasmic border. **B:** Involved cells in Burkitt's leukemia/lymphoma are relatively large and deeply basophilic and have characteristic vacuoles. **C:** Myeloid blast that characterizes acute myelogenous leukemia is mononuclear with a characteristic cytoplasmic inclusion, the Auer rod. **D:** Lymphoid blast of acute lymphocytic leukemia has a "regular" appearance with a thin rim of cytoplasm. Cells are magnified approximately 100 to 200 ×.

ally a routinely or rapidly available test. Monoclonal antibodies to platelet-specific antigens CD41 and CD61 are usually helpful, but false-positives are seen often. This disease is often associated with bone marrow fibrosis and pancytopenia that obscures the percentage of blasts in aspirates and necessitates the use of a bone marrow biopsy for morphologic diagnosis.

The FAB classification of ALL into L1 and L2 subtypes is based on an examination of blasts for nuclear-cytoplasmic ratio, the number and quality of nucleoli, the regularity of the nuclear membrane outline, and cell size: In general, L1 has a small size in greater than 50% of cells, a high nuclear-cytoplasmic ratio in 75% or more cells, up to one small ill-defined nucleolus in greater than 75% of cells, and a regular nuclear membrane in greater than 75% of cells. L2 generally has the opposite characteristics. L1-type blasts are found more often among children and have denoted a better prognosis. L2 is more common in adults but has little prognostic significance in this population. L3-ALL is easily distinguished by its homogeneous large cells and basophilic cytoplasm with prominent vacuolization. L3-ALL cells usually express cell surface immunoglobulin. The ALLs are usually distinguished cytochemically by the absence of myeloid-specific immunophenotypic markers or cytochemical staining and by the presence of lymphoid immunophenotypic patterns. The WHO classification simplifies these three FAB groups into precursor B-cell or T-cell neoplasms, as the morphologic distinctions do not predict clinical features well.[54]

Additional diagnostic subgroups not classified by the FAB criteria are delineated in the WHO classification. As more information about the importance of specific genotypes is gained, it is likely that additional subdivisions will be suggested.

IMMUNOPHENOTYPING OF ACUTE LEUKEMIAS

Approximately 100 antigen groups, known as *clusters of differentiation* (CDs), have been identified on the surface of hematopoietic cells by monoclonal antibodies. These antigens are predominantly cell surface glycoproteins, and rarely carbohydrates or glycolipids. Although no leukemia-specific antigens have been identified, the CD antigen characterization of hematopoietic cells using a panel of antibodies can establish lineage with reasonable certainty and may suggest maturational stages of cells. Expression on a cell population of antigens not usually found together can also provide strong evidence for neoplasia. Currently, immunophenotyping plays an important role in the understanding of hematopoietic biology and in the diagnosis of leukemia. The immunophenotype is used (1) to confirm the diagnosis in cases in which the classification is clear; (2) to make a diagnosis when morphology and cytochemistry are equivocal, as in undifferentiated AML; (3) to identify biphenotypic leukemias; (4) to characterize aberrant antigen expression that can be used to identify a neoplastic clone, even when found as minimal residual disease, as in clinical remission; and (5) to assist in assigning leukemias into prognostic groups.

The lineage and state of maturation of normal hematopoietic cells can be identified by use of a flow cytometer to determine the cell size, granularity, and presence or absence of a panel of cell surface or cytoplasmic differentiation antigens (designated by their CD numbers). Such analyses, termed *multidimensional* or *multiparameter flow cytometry*, are now available at most cancer centers or at commercial laboratories. Pathways describing the phenotype of normal B, T, and myeloid cells have been constructed[55–58] (Fig. 42.2-3). Acute leukemias can also be characterized by a similar panel of markers, and in general, lineage can be assigned by examination of expression of the same antigens as those found in normal cells.[41]

Acute lymphoid leukemias of T-cell lineage are characterized by expression of the T-cell markers CD2, CD5, CD7, and sometimes CD1 or dual staining of CD4 and CD8. T-cell ALL or lymphoblastic lymphoma may also express the B-lineage markers CD10 and CD21. Acute lymphoid leukemias of B-cell lineage express CD19, CD10, CD22, and, depending on maturational stage, CD20 and surface immunoglobulin. Acute myeloid leukemias express CD13, CD15, CD33, and, more often if monocytoid, CD14. Terminal deoxynucleotidyl transferase (TdT) is expressed by most lymphoid blasts and approximately 20% of myeloid blasts. CD34 can be expressed by blasts of all lineages, especially if the cells are primitive. HLA-DR is found on virtually all B-lineage leukemias, on most myeloid and monocytic leukemias (except promyelocytic leukemia), and on a rare T-cell ALL.

The pathways of antigen expression, with regard to maturational stage, however, are often aberrant in leukemias.[41,58] In some cases there is also abnormal expression of antigens not expected to be found in the lineage.[59–61] Although such "infidelity" of antigen expression may prevent exact assignment of the maturational stage of the leukemia cell, it may distinguish that cell as neoplastic from within a larger population of normal cells. Thus, aberrant antigen expression, which can be an antigen of the wrong lineage, the simultaneous expression of antigens of different stages of maturation, or the lack of an expected antigen, can provide a useful diagnostic marker for the leukemia cells.[59] In addition, such a marker may allow the flow cytometric detection of the leukemia cells at a level of 1 cell in 1000 to 100,000 normal cells, even in patients who have apparently normal bone marrow and blood examination by morphologic criteria (see Table 42.2-4).[62,63] The prognostic sig-

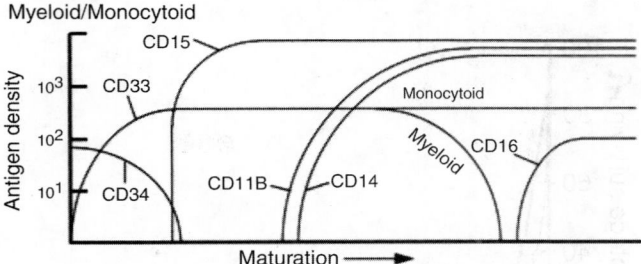

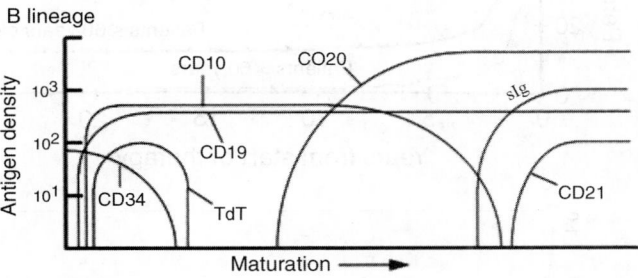

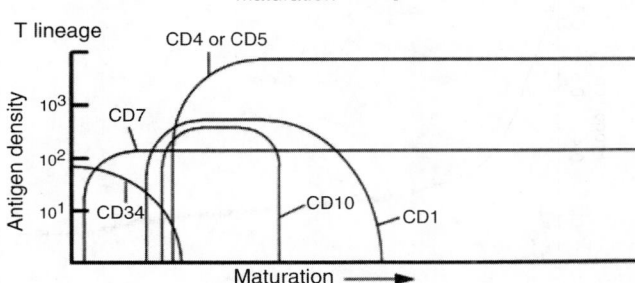

FIGURE 42.2-3. Schematic diagram of selected important antigens expressed on normal hematopoietic cells and acute leukemia cells throughout the differentiation and maturation of the normal cells. Acute leukemia cells may express these antigens aberrantly as described in the text. (From ref. 58, with permission.)

nificance of this detection is not yet clear but is likely to predict relapse.

Mixed-lineage leukemias are being increasingly identified as use of larger numbers of immunophenotypic markers becomes widespread.[54] These leukemias exhibit the phenotype of more than one and sometimes more than two lineages.[61] In most cases, this is the result of blasts that co-express markers of several lineages; in other rare cases, blasts of different lineages coexist in the same patient.[64] In the former, more common, cases, the blasts may be obviously derived from one lineage, based on morphologic, cytochemical, and immunophenotypic criteria; at the same time, the blasts express apparently aberrant markers from another lineage. Myeloid marker–positive ALL and lymphoid marker–positive AML occur frequently. In some cases, assignment of true lineage is more difficult. Scoring systems designed to weigh certain markers have been developed to assign lineage in these difficult cases.[53]

Although several clinical entities of leukemias with aberrant phenotypes have been described, there is considerable overlap in the immunophenotypes, rendering such proposed subgroupings difficult to interpret. In addition, the aberrant markers found on AML blasts are associated with a variety of karyotypes and FAB or WHO subgroups. The prognostic signif-

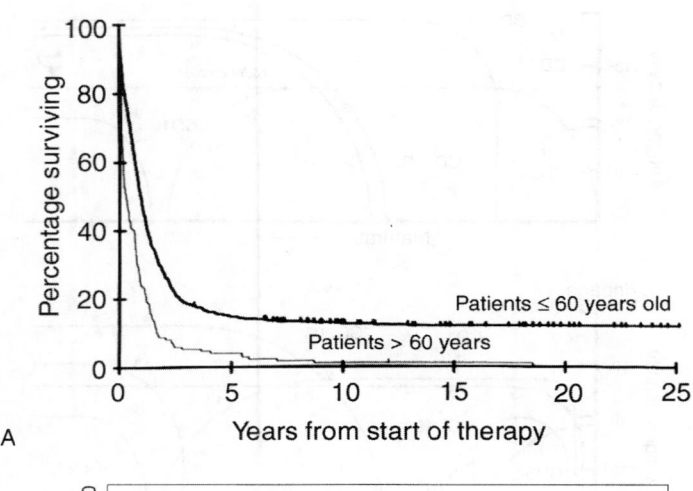

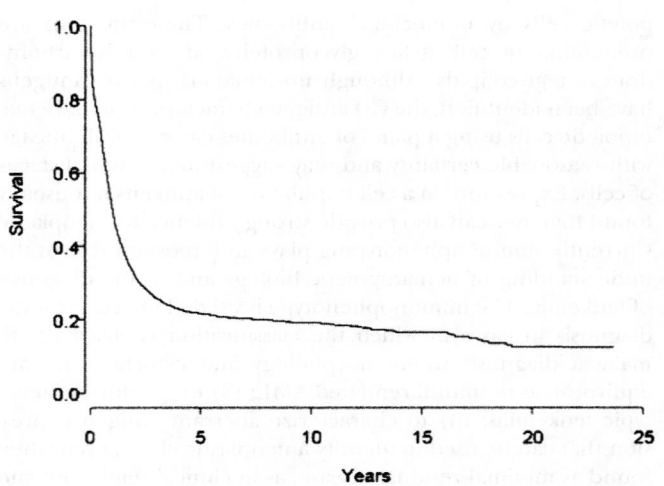

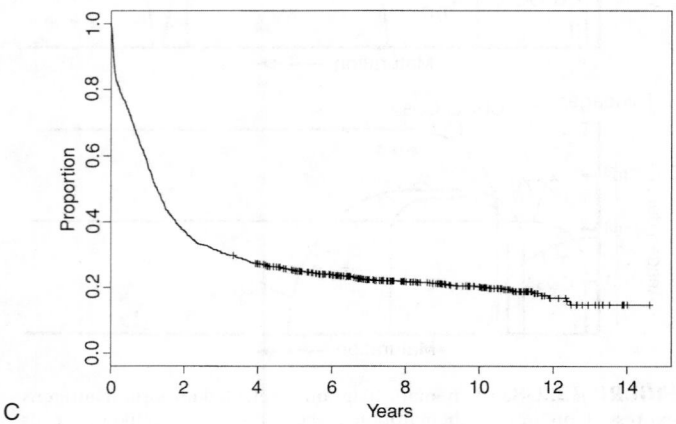

FIGURE 42.2-4. Representative survival curves for acute myelogenous leukemia (AML). **A:** Overall survival for 25 years of follow-up in 687 patients with AML treated on protocols at Memorial Sloan-Kettering Cancer Center, New York. Patients older than 60 years have a substantially worse prognosis. (Data accrued by B. D. Clarkson, C. Little, D. Tyson, L. Megharian, and D. A. Scheinberg.) **B:** Survival of 2985 patients enrolled on Eastern Cooperative Oncology Group protocols for newly diagnosed AML (acute promyelocytic leukemia excluded). Median survival is 12.1 months, and the 5-year survival is 22%. (From ref. 80, with permission.) **C:** Survival for 1213 patients with *de novo* AML treated on five sequential Cancer and Leukemia Group B therapeutic protocols. Patients with t(15;17) and t(9;22) were excluded from the analysis. Median survival is 1.2 years. (From ref. 81, with permission.)

icance of mixed-lineage phenotype or the expression of aberrant markers is unclear.

CYTOGENETICS AND MOLECULAR GENETICS OF ACUTE LEUKEMIAS

The frequent presence of nonrandom chromosomal translocations, oncogene mutations, and tumor suppressor gene abnormalities in leukemia cells has allowed substantial progress to be made in understanding the pathogenesis of acute leukemias,[65–70] in diagnosing and developing prognostic models for subtypes of leukemia,[71–74] and in assessing the effects of therapy or detecting early relapse.[74] The molecular genotype or karyotype is rapidly becoming the gold standard for diagnosis and prognosis in many subtypes of acute leukemia. A detailed discussion of the molecular biology of hematopoietic cancer is found in Chapter 42.1.

In ALL, the presence of t(9;22), found in up to 30% of adults −7 or +8, t(4;11), and t(8;14), diagnostic of mature Burkitt's-type B-cell ALL, is a poor prognostic sign. Abnormal karyotypes are seen in approximately 80% of patients with AML.[73] In AML, t(15;17), t(8;21), and inv (16) or t(16;16) has a favorable prognosis, whereas +8, −5, del (5q), −7, del (9q), del (7q), −20, +11, +13, inv (3), and involvement of 11q23 are unfavorable. Distinct pathologic and clinical syndromes, such as APL, are strongly associated with t(15;17); myeloid leukemia with maturation;

(FAB) AML-M2, with t(8;21); FAB AML-M4EO; myelomonocytic leukemia with abnormal eosinophils with inv (16) or del 16p; and megakaryocytic AML-M7 with t(1;22).[73,75] Chemotherapeutic agents that interfere with DNA–topoisomerase II, such as epipodophyllotoxins or anthracyclines, can result in the balanced translocations described above[76,77] and often appear 1 to 3 years after chemotherapy. In contrast, alkylating agents more typically yield −5, −7 and complex chromosomal abnormalities 2 to 9 years later, frequently initiate as myelodysplastic syndromes, and have a particularly poor prognosis.[78]

PRINCIPLES OF THERAPY OF ACUTE LEUKEMIA

Despite significant advances in understanding the biology of these diseases, clinical progress has lagged behind the experimental data, and the majority of adult patients diagnosed with acute leukemia ultimately die as a result of the disease[79–81] (Fig. 42.2-4). The pattern of response is marked by an initial sensitivity to therapy, resulting in a transient abatement of the disease process. Eventually, however, remnants of the original leukemic clone are able to expand to the point at which they are clinically apparent and once again dominate the bone marrow, compromising many of the vital functions provided by the mature cellular elements of the peripheral blood. Relapse is therefore the rule rather than the exception; even in the modern era, only a relatively small number of patients may be cured.

TABLE 42.2-4.   Current Methods Used Frequently for Detection of Minimal Residual Disease

Technique	Typical No. of Cells Analyzed	Materials Analyzed	Limits of Sensitivity (%)	Example
Morphology	100–200	Intact cells	5	Standard definition of complete response and relapse
Cytogenetics	20–100	Cells capable of dividing in culture	1–5	Inv(16) in remission bone marrow
Fluorescence *in situ* hybridization	100–500	DNA	1–2	PML/RAR-α in acute promyelocytic leukemia, trisomy 17 in acute lymphoblastic leukemias
Southern blot	1,000,000	DNA	1–2	TCR gene rearrangements
Multiparameter flow cytometry	50,000–1,000,000	Intact cells	0.01–0.001	Aberrant immunophenotype: CD34/56
Polymerase chain reaction	1,000,000	RNA; DNA	<.0001	PML/RAR-α in acute promyelocytic leukemia; BCR/ABL in chronic myelogenous leukemia

The goal of therapy in acute leukemia is the eradication of the leukemic clone with the ultimate restoration of the peripheral blood counts. This is generally accomplished by chemotherapy that is able to induce a state of relative aplasia in the bone marrow. Unfortunately, such therapy is not specific for leukemia cells, and any remaining normal precursor hematopoietic cells are also lost. Bone marrow function is affected, and the individual patient needs to be supported through the aplasia by transfusions as well as antimicrobials. Relieved of the suppressive effects of the leukemic blasts, the normal hematopoietic stem cells can proliferate, repopulate the bone marrow, and reestablish polyclonal hematopoiesis. This return to a normal state is only temporary, as residual leukemia cells are present, albeit in relatively small numbers undetectable by conventional means.

The transient nature of the initial clinical response can be best understood in the context of the large number of leukemia cells that are present when the disease is clinically detectable and the limitations of modern chemotherapy to effectively reduce this critical leukemia mass to zero. Animal models have been used to estimate that there are approximately 10^{12} leukemia cells in the body at the time of diagnosis. The standard chemotherapy regimens are able to kill approximately 2 to 3 logs of leukemia cells, resulting in a 99.0% to 99.9% reduction in the total tumor mass.[82] The remaining leukemia cells are present but relatively rare when compared to the overall numbers of hematopoietic cells present in the bone marrow, and they escape detection by conventional means simply by a dilutional effect. Therefore, based on standard morphologic criteria, the patient is said to be in complete remission (CR).

The clinical experience with such a response shows that if patients are not treated with any further therapy, the majority experience a relapse of disease within a relatively brief period of time. The genesis of this recurrence can be traced to leukemia cells, which remain after the initial therapy. Although standard morphologic evaluation shows no evidence of residual leukemia, a state of minimal residual disease exists. Estimates for the number of remaining leukemia cells can be as high as 10 billion. A number of laboratory techniques have been introduced into clinical practice with the intent of increasing the resolution of detecting any remaining leukemia cells (Table 42.2-4).[59,60,62,63,83–88] Although none of the available assays is ideal in discriminating minimal residual disease to the greatest level of sensitivity, current studies are attempting to validate such measures by correlation with clinical data. The ultimate goal is to establish a readily available, specific and sensitive assay that could be used to form the basis for therapeutic decisions in individual patients. The paradigm for such a test has been provided by the reverse transcriptase–based (RT) PCR assay used to detect the PML/RAR-α gene rearrangement in APL (see Acute Promyelocytic Leukemia, later in this chapter) or molecular analysis used to detect BCR/ABL in CML (see Chapter 43.1).

The primary goal of the initial chemotherapy in AML is to achieve CR. Despite the limitations of morphologic evaluation, standards have been adopted to define clinical outcomes and establish reference points from which different therapies can be compared. CR is defined as fewer than 5% blasts in the bone marrow that have regenerated normally.[86] Evidence for normal regeneration includes an acceptable degree of cellularity (greater than 20% as determined in the bone marrow biopsy) and restoration of normal hematopoiesis (as reflected by peripheral blood values of at least 1500 neutrophils/μL and 100,000 platelets/μL). A modification of this definition has been proposed that allows a lower level of recovery for the platelets (CRp).[89] This modification has not been embraced as a standard of defining response, and the application of this definition largely remains confined to a small number of antibody-based studies. Red cell parameters such as hemoglobin or hematocrit are not usually considered in this definition. In addition, the peripheral blood may not contain any evidence of detectable disease, such as circulating blasts or extramedullary collections of leukemia cells. The use of growth factors may complicate such determinations, as a small number of circulating blasts may be present during their continued use. The remission criteria must be sustained for a period of at least 4 weeks or until the next course of therapy is administered.

CR is the only significant form of clinical response in acute leukemia, which is meaningful for the patient. The ability to achieve such a response is directly correlated with survival. Although some clinical trials may report responses with less strict criteria for the recovery of hematopoiesis or allow the presence of residual blasts and define such responses as partial remissions, the inability to decrease leukemia cells below a critical level in the bone marrow is generally a treatment failure and has grave implications for the survival of the patient. Therefore, the determination that a particular drug or combination of drugs is "active" in this disease is very different from the statement that the agent(s) are potentially curative.

Current treatment schemas generally divide therapy into two basic phases: induction and postremission therapy. The purpose of remission therapy is to achieve a CR, ridding the bone marrow of morphologically apparent disease. The goal of postremission therapy is to sustain this response, eradicate minimal residual disease, and effect cure. Different approaches to postremission therapy have evolved based on clinical experience. Definitions to describe these different approaches have been adopted in the lexicon of the clinician.[90] Consolidation therapy is used to describe chemotherapy that is similar to induction therapy and given in the immediate postremission period (usually within 6 months of achieving CR). The doses of the drugs used are either equivalent or slightly attenuated. Intensification is consolidation with the application of higher doses of active agents. *Maintenance* is defined as therapy given over a prolonged period of time (usually greater than 6 months) in which greatly attenuated doses of active agents are used. As such, the toxicity of maintenance is usually considerably less than the other forms of postremission treatment.

Relapse is the clinical recurrence of the disease and is usually heralded by a change in peripheral blood counts, which were previously normal. The reappearance of blasts on examination of the peripheral blood is frequent although not always present. Isolated extramedullary relapse is relatively infrequent in AML. Examination of the bone marrow is mandatory in suspected cases of relapse, as such a diagnosis has grave implications for the patient and will radically affect current management. Relapse is confirmed by the demonstration of greater than 5% blasts in the bone marrow. In situations in which there is only a borderline increase in blasts but the clinical suspicion of relapse is great, it may be necessary to repeat the bone marrow examination in 1 to 2 weeks to confirm the diagnosis.[86]

PRINCIPLES OF CLINICAL MANAGEMENT OF ACUTE MYELOGENOUS LEUKEMIA

The care of the patient with acute leukemia rests on the ability to support the individual through a period of approximately 4 to 6 weeks during which the complications from the myelosuppressive therapy administered to treat the disease are most acute. Successful clinical management requires a detailed understanding of the most frequently encountered complications accompanied by early therapeutic intervention designed to minimize morbidity. With regard to these basic principles, many of the improvements in the overall outcome for leukemia patients can be directly traced to advances in supportive care.

Infection and hemorrhage are the primary causes of death in patients with leukemia.[85] Although many patients with acute leukemia initially present to medical attention with fever and neutropenia, these complications develop in virtually all patients after treatment with chemotherapy. Untreated, infection in the neutropenic patient can be rapidly fatal. Therefore, the early institution of antibiotic therapy is necessary and represents the current standard of care.[91] Initial antibiotic therapy must provide a broad spectrum of antibacterial coverage with an emphasis on gram-negative organisms. The flora indigenous to a particular institution may determine the choice of the antibiotic(s) used as first-line therapy. Common regimens include an antipseudomonal penicillin or cephalosporin coupled with an aminoglycoside. Monotherapy with a third-generation cephalosporin, such as ceftazidime, or a carbapenem, such as imipenem, has also been advocated as an acceptable alternative.

Changes in the initial antibiotic therapy can be made when the organism(s) are isolated from culture and the antibiotic sensitivity is determined or, in cases in which no source is identified, fever persists despite broad-spectrum coverage. Fever that continues without an identifiable source after 3 to 5 days of broad-spectrum antibacterial therapy usually requires empiric antifungal therapy. In the past, amphotericin was the drug of choice for this indication. More recently, liposomal preparations of amphotericin have been introduced and used because of an advantage in the toxicity profile.[92] Cost remains an obstacle to the routine widespread use of these agents. Alternatively, azoles such as fluconazole and itraconazole have been studied and compare favorably with amphotericin as empiric therapy in several randomized studies.[93,94] An important consideration in the use of these agents is the limited activity of fluconazole against *Aspergillus* species and certain non-*albicans Candida* species, organisms that may be clinically significant in the patient undergoing therapy for acute leukemia. Data from several clinical studies have suggested that an echinocandin, caspofungin, alone and in combination, may be active against some resistant fungi.[95] Voriconazole, a second-generation azole, has also been shown to be effective therapy for documented invasive aspergillosis and may represent a better alternative than either fluconazole or itraconazole for use in the leukemia patient.[96] The superiority of voriconazole over amphotericin for empiric use in treating febrile neutropenia remains somewhat controversial.

The algorithm for the treatment of the febrile leukemia patient can be modified according to host or institutional factors. Patients with indwelling central venous catheters or other prosthetic devices may require the early institution of vancomycin. Antimicrobial agents should be continued until the absolute neutrophil count has risen above 500/μL. Patients who have a documented bacterial source of infection should complete at least a 10- to 14-day course of therapy. Those patients with a documented/suspected invasive fungal infection may require a more prolonged course of therapy. The recent availability of an oral form of voriconazole has facilitated continued treatment of such infections, shifting therapy from the hospital to the outpatient setting.

Despite the accepted approach to the empiric therapy of febrile neutropenia in patients with leukemia outlined above, there is considerable controversy regarding infection prophylaxis, use of protected environments and reverse isolation, granulocyte transfusions, or the use of hematopoietic growth factors to accelerate neutrophil recovery.[97,98] Although the duration of neutropenia has consistently been shortened by the use of G-CSF or GM-CSF after chemotherapy in a number of studies, the effect on morbidity and mortality has been variable, and therefore no consensus has been reached.[99–101] The most effective means to prevent infections have generally been the simplest approaches. Frequent hand washing by staff and visitors may be particularly effective at preventing spread of resistant organisms that fester in the modern hospital environment. Careful attention to oral hygiene with regular use of oral rinsing and cleaning with a soft-tipped (sponge) device to prevent gingival trauma may prove useful. Rectal or vaginal examinations are generally avoided.

The ability to sustain the patient through the period of cytopenia is often directly dependent on a fully functional blood bank that can provide immediate access to blood products. Although individual patients may vary with regard to their particular physiologic requirements, the hemoglobin level is generally maintained at or above 8 g/dL. Patients with other medical comorbidities (pulmonary disorders or coronary heart disease) may require more aggressive transfusional support to remain free of symptoms. Hemorrhage and reduction in the platelet count below 5000 to 10,000/µL have a direct relationship. The prophylactic use of platelet transfusions to prevent spontaneous hemorrhage has become the standard of care. The routine use of platelet transfusions has had a significant impact on the incidence of hemorrhagic death. Patients with uncomplicated thrombocytopenia can be transfused when the platelet count falls below 10,000/µL. Patients who are febrile or who have other medical conditions that increase the risk of hemorrhage may require prophylactic platelet transfusions at a higher threshold.[102,103]

The inability to increase the platelet count despite aggressive transfusional support represents a difficult management problem. Some patients become refractory to platelet transfusions as a result of alloimmunization resulting from multiple prior transfusions. Alternatively, persistent fever or DIC may also result in increased platelet destruction. It is difficult to overcome this problem once it develops by simply increasing the amount of random donor platelets infused. Instead, efforts have focused on preventing alloimmunization from occurring. Common strategies include prevention of sensitization through the use of single related donor platelets or HLA-matched platelets or by leukofiltration during the administration of platelet transfusions. Platelets from a potential bone marrow donor are avoided in patients who are eligible for allogeneic stem cell transplantation and reserved only for life-threatening situations.

Coagulopathy may be present in addition to thrombocytopenia. DIC is the most commonly described entity and may result in either hemorrhage or thrombosis. Although this complication is most frequently associated with APL, it may also occur in other forms of leukemia at presentation [i.e., AML M5 t(8;16)] or with the institution of cytotoxic therapy (ALL). Although multiple mechanisms have been proposed, one common hypothesis purports the release of procoagulant substances from the leukemia cells as they lyse or undergo apoptosis as responsible for the clinical syndrome. Alternatively, there has been interest in primary fibrinolysis as a possible explanation for significant hemorrhage in the patient.[104]

Although there is no standard approach for the therapy of leukemia-associated coagulopathy, a number of basic principles can help the clinician manage this difficult problem. Laboratory tests that are often useful as indicators of coagulopathy include the platelet count, prothrombin time, activated partial thromboplastin time, fibrinogen, fibrin split products, and D-dimer. Clinical management relies on frequent monitoring of the patient using these indirect indicators of the ongoing process. Therapeutic intervention is often based on clinical deterioration of the patient or a worsening trend in a laboratory value such as the fibrinogen. Historically, the approach of managing the coagulopathy associated with APL involved the use of continuous infusion of low-dose unfractionated heparin (7 to

10 U/kg/h) titrated to a rising fibrinogen level. The data to support this approach were mostly anecdotal, and it has been replaced by the practice of instituting early treatment with retinoic acid as well as aggressive blood product support.[104,105] Platelet and fresh frozen plasma are transfused to maintain the platelet count above 50,000/µL and the fibrinogen level above 100 mg/dL. The hemostatic abnormalities typically abate after approximately 4 to 8 days or when the leukemia burden has been reduced.

Metabolic abnormalities can exist in the leukemia patient either at presentation secondary to increased cell turnover as a consequence of defective hematopoiesis or with the institution of therapy that results in massive cell death.[106] Patients rarely present with disorders of potassium or calcium but instead such electrolyte abnormalities develop as a result of continuing therapy with aminoglycosides, amphotericin, or other agents that affect renal function. Rapid leukemia cell death in the face of high tumor burden releases large amounts of intracellular metabolites; notably uric acid, potassium, and phosphate, which may cause a life-threatening metabolic condition known as *tumor lysis syndrome*. Uric acid, a product of purine metabolism, may deposit in joints, causing a gout arthropathy or, more importantly, in the renal parenchyma or collecting system, resulting in renal failure. Although dialysis can be instituted to support the patient through the period of renal failure, the primary approach to tumor lysis syndrome lies in the prevention of this disorder. This is accomplished through vigorous hydration, which results in brisk urine output (greater than 150 mL/h) along with the administration of allopurinol coincident to or before the administration of the cytotoxic therapy. The doses of allopurinol administered range from 300 to 900 mg/d. Alkalinization of the urine (by the addition of sodium bicarbonate to the intravenous fluids or by the administration of the carbonic anhydrase inhibitor acetazolamide) to increase the solubility of the uric acid can be undertaken in patients who are refractory to other maneuvers or in those who are allergic to allopurinol.

Life-threatening complications may result as a consequence of uncontrolled electrolyte abnormalities. Cardiac arrhythmias resulting from disturbances in potassium, magnesium, or calcium balance may be particularly difficult to manage in a neutropenic patient with multiple coincident medical problems. Therefore, the best approach is early attention to these metabolic disturbances when they are easily reversible. This is often best accomplished by aggressive hydration during the initial phases of therapy. The resulting diuresis serves to clear toxic by-products as the leukemia cells are rapidly killed. Additional benefit may be gained by using oral phosphate binders (aluminum hydroxide or calcium acetate) to minimize absorption of additional phosphate from dietary sources. In situations in which hyperkalemia is complicated by renal insufficiency, cation exchange resins (Kayexalate) may be indicated. Extreme circumstances may require dialysis to correct multiple abnormalities until normal renal function recovers.

Tumor lysis syndrome most commonly occurs in acute lymphoid leukemias (particularly Burkitt's type) where there is a high cell turnover and rapid tumor growth rate. Management of this disorder is most problematic in the setting of hyperleukocytosis (peripheral blast counts greater than 100,000/µL). Patients with AML have less of a risk for development of tumor lysis than patients with ALL. However, in AML, hyperleukocytosis may result in viscosity changes caused by sludging of the large and "sticky" myeloblasts in the microvasculature (leukostasis). Such changes in blood flow may compromise cerebral or pulmonary function and may be accompanied by hemorrhage that in turn may be fatal. The ability to rapidly decrease a rising circulating blast count is, therefore, an important factor for survival in these patients. Leukapheresis can be used, but this is often a temporizing measure, as the blasts tend to rapidly accumulate. Instead, immediate therapy with cytotoxic chemotherapy should be undertaken, with careful attention to the expected metabolic complications discussed above.

TREATMENT OF NEWLY DIAGNOSED ACUTE MYELOGENOUS LEUKEMIA

Without therapy, AML typically results in the patient's death within a relatively short period of time. Although it is possible to sustain patients briefly with supportive interventions such as transfusions and antimicrobials, they ultimately succumb to the consequences of bone marrow failure: infection or hemorrhage.[85] Most patients typically first seek medical attention for symptoms related to one of these complications, and these individuals require immediate supportive therapeutic intervention to sustain life. Other patients may not present acutely, and the diagnosis is made as part of a methodical workup. Not all patients are candidates for cytotoxic therapy. Some have a poor performance status unrelated to the acute illness, whereas others have active severe medical comorbidities that preclude the administration of chemotherapy. In such instances, a strategy placing an emphasis on supportive care may be more appropriate. The risks, potential benefits, and alternatives of therapy should be carefully considered in each case and discussed with the patient and, when appropriate, the family.

Several prognostic factors have been identified in AML (Table 42.2-5). The difference in treatment results among various regimens using similar chemotherapy may, in part, be caused by the frequency of these negative prognostic characteristics within a study population.[107] Multiple studies have demonstrated the prognostic importance of cytogenetic abnormalities in AML, making this the single most important predictor of response.[81,108,109]

TABLE 42.2-5. Prognostic Features in Adult Acute Leukemia

ACUTE MYELOGENOUS LEUKEMIA (AML)

Age: Older age is associated with a reduced incidence of complete response.

Antecedent hematologic disorder or secondary AML: These subgroups have a lower incidence of complete response and a reduced overall survival.

Cytogenetics: t(15;17), t(8;21), and inv (16) denote good prognostic subgroups. Abnormalities of chromosome 5 or 7, trisomy 8, and 11q23 denote poor prognostic subgroups.

ACUTE LYMPHOCYTIC LEUKEMIA

White blood cell count: High count is associated with a poor prognosis.

Leukemic cell immunophenotype: T cell has a favorable prognosis, pre–B-cell has an intermediate prognosis, whereas mature B-cell disease has a poor prognosis with standard regimens.

Age: Older age is associated with a worse prognosis.

Philadelphia chromosome–positive disease has a worse prognosis.

Time to complete response: Patients requiring more than 4–5 wk to achieve a complete response have a lower likelihood of being cured.

Among the cytogenetic abnormalities that impart a favorable prognosis are t(15;17), t(8;21), t(16;16), or inv(16). Poor prognostic chromosomal abnormalities include abnormalities of chromosome 5 or 7, translocations involving 11q23, trisomy 8, or changes that are defined as complex because they involve multiple chromosomes (greater than 3). Age is inversely associated with the ability to achieve remission.[110,111] In patients older than 60 years of age, standard chemotherapy results in CR in approximately 30% to 50%, compared with the 65% to 80% CR rate reported in younger patient cohorts. AML that occurs as a consequence of prior cytotoxic chemotherapy or that has developed from an antecedent hematologic disorder (e.g., myelodysplastic syndrome) has a particularly poor prognosis with a lower incidence of achieving CR and a shorter duration of survival than patients with *de novo* AML.[112] In 2002, a number of studies have identified an internal tandem duplication in the FLT3 gene as a negative prognostic factor for patients with AML.[113] Such findings underscore the increasingly important role that molecular genetics has come to have in understanding some of the clinical features of AML.

Historically, the diagnosis of acute leukemia has been a "death sentence," as the physician had few therapeutic options. During the 1940s, Sidney Farber ushered in the modern era of chemotherapy by effectively using the first antimetabolites in pediatric patients with ALL. Subsequently, a number of other single agents were demonstrated to have antileukemia activity, at first in the laboratory and later in the clinic. Many of the drugs initially used in adult AML had been pioneered in pediatric ALL. Not surprisingly, because these agents have limited activity in AML, the results from the early clinical trials were disappointing. The introduction of cytarabine (Ara-C) in the early 1960s radically changed the therapy of AML.

Cytarabine is the most important drug currently in use to treat AML. Much of the focus in clinical research in the last 30 years has involved attempts at increasing the drug's efficacy either by combining it with other agents, escalating the dose, or altering the schedule of administration. Despite all the modifications made in treatment in the last few years, cytarabine remains the cornerstone of AML therapy.

INDUCTION

Standard induction therapy is based on the combination of cytarabine with either an anthracycline or anthracenedione. The CR rate in newly diagnosed AML patients younger than 60 years of age ranges from 50% to 82% depending on the distribution of other major prognostic factors within the population studied (Table 42.2-6).[107] Cytarabine was first used as a single agent in the 1960s and was able to induce responses in approximately 20% to 30% of patients. Cytarabine was subsequently used in combination, at first with 6-thioguanine and later with daunorubicin.[114] These combinations increased the CR rate up to approximately 40% to 50%. When the doses of the cytarabine and daunorubicin used were increased, the response rates further improved, establishing a dose-response relationship with these drugs. Cytarabine given for 7 days at 100 mg/m^2/d administered as a continuous infusion with daunorubicin given at 45 mg/m^2/d for 3 days became the standard regimen and is referred as the *3 + 7* or *7 + 3 regimen*. In some instances, patients

TABLE 42.2-6. Representative Treatment Regimens in Newly Diagnosed Acute Myelogenous Leukemia and Acute Promyelocytic Leukemia

Source	Study Group	Induction	Postremission	Complete Response (%)	Outcome	Comments
CALGB[110]	AML: <60 y >60 y	D/A 3 + 7	Cyclic maintenance with A/D/P/ VCR	72/31	12-mo median duration complete response	Standard induction
ECOG[139]	*De novo* AML <65 y	DAT	High-dose Ara-C/AMSA vs. allogeneic bone marrow transplant	68	27% event-free survival (4 y) in high-dose Ara-C/AMSA group	Addition of 6-thioguanine; high-dose Ara-C intensification
ALSG[118]	*De novo* AML <70 y	A/D/VP-16 7-3-7	A/D/VP-16 5-2-5	59	17-mo median survival	Addition of VP-16 to standard 3 + 7
MSKCC[119]	*De novo* AML <60 y	IDR/A 3 + 5	IDR/A 2 + 4 × 5	80	20-mo median survival	Idarubicin substituted as anthracycline
UCLA[126]	AML	D/IDAC	High-dose Ara-C/Mito→Mito/VP-16→high-dose Ara-C/D or allogeneic bone marrow transplant	74	28% DFS (4 y)	Cytarabine dose increased in induction (intermediate dose)
ALSG[127]	*De novo* AML <60 y	D/high-dose Ara-C/VP-16	A/D/VP-16 5-2-5 IDR/A	74	42% actual DFS (4 y)	Cytarabine dose further increased in induction (high dose)
CALGB[141]	*De novo* AML	3 + 7	High-dose Ara-C vs. intermediate-dose Ara-C vs. standard-dose Ara-C × 4 cycles	64	Probability of remaining in CCR greatest in high-dose Ara-C group for patients <60 y old	Establishes high-dose Ara-C as postremission chemotherapy of choice
GIMEMA-AIEOP[197]	APL	ATRA/IDR	IDR/A→Mito/VP-16→IDR/A followed by maintenance	95	79% 2-y event-free survival	Combination retinoid/chemotherapy as induction; chemotherapy or retinoid as maintenance

A, cytarabine; ALSG, Australian Leukemia Study Group; AML, acute myelogenous leukemia; AMSA, amsacrine; APL, acute promyelocytic leukemia; Ara-C, cytarabine; ATRA, all-*trans* retinoic acid; CALGB, Cancer and Leukemia Group B; CCR, continuous complete remission; D, daunorubicin; DFS, disease-free survival; ECOG, Eastern Cooperative Oncology Group; GIMEMA-AIEOP, Gruppo Italiano Malattie Ematologiche Maligne dell Adulto-Associazione Italiana di Ematologia ed Oncologia Pediatrica; IDAC, intermediate-dose cytarabine; IDR, idarubicin; Mito, mitoxantrone; MSKCC, Memorial Sloan-Kettering Cancer Center; P, prednisone; T, 6-thioguanine; UCLA, University of California, Los Angeles; VCR, vincristine; VP-16, etoposide.

who did not achieve a CR with one course of therapy could still achieve CR if they received a second cycle of therapy or an attenuated version of the first course (2 + 4). A randomized trial by the Cancer and Leukemia Group B (CALGB) reported a 59% CR rate using 3 + 7 induction therapy and found this response to be superior to a shorter course of similar therapy.[111,115]

The initial success of increasing the response rate through dose intensification prompted a series of studies that sought to improve on the 3 + 7 combination by either adding agents or further increasing the doses. Because 6-thioguanine was identified as one of the first drugs that could successfully be combined with cytarabine, it was added to daunorubicin/cytarabine to form the DAT or TAD regimen. The CALGB conducted a randomized study comparing 3 + 7 with DAT and found that the addition of 6-thioguanine provided no significant benefit.[116] Modestly increasing the cytarabine dose by extending the infusion to a total of 10 days was also found to be without an advantage. A subsequent study failed to show a statistical advantage to doubling the cytarabine dose during a 7-day infusion, although a greater number of treatment-related deaths were noted in the patients younger than 60 years.[117] Despite this

finding, the 200-mg/m^2 dose has been adopted as a standard in the 3 + 7 regimen.

As new drugs with antileukemia activity became available, new combinations were introduced in an attempt to improve on the standard 3 + 7 induction regimen (see Table 42.2-6). The substitution of doxorubicin for daunorubicin produced no significant benefit but did result in greater gastrointestinal toxicity.[110] In a study conducted by the Australian Leukemia Study Group, the addition of etoposide to the 3 + 7 regimen produced an improved remission duration in a younger cohort of patients but did not affect overall survival.[118] Although mitoxantrone, amsacrine, rubidazone, and aclarubicin have all been substituted for daunorubicin in induction therapy, none of these clinical trials was able to demonstrate unequivocal superiority of any of these second-generation regimens over the previously established standard.

The synthetically modified daunorubicin derivative, idarubicin, has generated the most interest as a potential replacement for the parent compound in AML therapy. Three randomized trials have compared idarubicin with daunorubicin and have demonstrated an increased response rate in patients less than 60 years old who received the idarubicin-containing regimen.[119–121] In addition, more patients treated with idarubicin were able to achieve CR after one course of therapy. The toxicity of the idarubicin-containing regimen was similar to the daunorubicin control arm. In two of the studies, the idarubicin combination demonstrated a survival advantage. An update of these data, however, showed that a survival advantage persisted in only one of the trials with long-term follow-up.[122] In addition, the Eastern Cooperative Oncology Group (ECOG) conducted a trial that randomized elderly patients (older than age 55 years) between induction regimens using daunorubicin, idarubicin, or mitoxantrone and failed to show any advantage to using the newer agents.[123]

The conflicting data from the clinical trials have thus made the choice of anthracycline somewhat controversial and possibly of little clinical importance. Criticism of the randomized idarubicin studies has centered on the issue of dose equivalency when comparing idarubicin at a dose of 12 or 13 mg/m^2 to daunorubicin at a dose of 45 or 50 mg/m^2. The CR rates for the daunorubicin arm (58%, 58%, and 59%, respectively) in each of the three randomized studies were lower than for other studies that reported the results with a standard 3 + 7 regimen. Other nonrandomized trials have used higher doses of daunorubicin (70 to 90 mg/m^2) and have described response rates similar to those of idarubicin, suggesting that the dose of the anthracycline may be more important than the choice of the anthracycline used.[124]

Dose intensification of cytarabine has previously been demonstrated to overcome drug resistance and induce remission in some patients with relapsed disease. Such an approach has been applied to the initial induction regimen in an effort to improve treatment outcomes. Cytarabine doses ranging from 0.5 to 6.0 g/m^2/d for 3 to 8 days have been investigated.[125] The effect of using higher doses of cytarabine as part of the induction regimen has been variable. A University of California, Los Angeles, study randomized patients between 3 + 7 induction and an intermediate-dose cytarabine (500 mg/m^2 q12h × 12 doses) regimen and found that the CR rate and the actuarial 4-year disease-free survival were similar in the two cohorts.[126] Two other randomized studies, however, have shown a benefit to high-dose cytarabine-based inductions.[127,128] This benefit was not achieved by increasing the CR rate but by producing more durable responses with a superior disease-free survival. Toxicity was also increased with the high-dose regimens. This was particularly evident during the subsequent postremission therapy when the infection rate increased and the time to recover peripheral blood counts was delayed.

Hematopoietic growth factors have been used in an attempt to ameliorate the toxicity resulting from dose-intensive approaches. In the elderly, significant toxicity with standard dose regimens had prevented testing dose escalation to improve treatment outcomes. Treatment-related mortality in patients who are older than 60 years of age is higher compared with younger patients treated with similar therapy. As the hematopoietic growth factors were used with increasing frequency throughout the field of oncology to help support patients in the setting of high-dose therapy, this approach was tested in the elderly patient with AML. At first, there was concern over the use of myeloid growth factors in AML, given the potential for increasing leukemia cell growth. A large Japanese study conducted in patients with relapsed disease did not, however, demonstrate stimulation of leukemia cells when G-CSF was used after chemotherapy.[99] Several large randomized trials were subsequently conducted in an attempt to clarify the role of growth factors in AML therapy.[100,101,129–132] Although these studies have demonstrated a decrease in the duration of neutropenia, the clinical impact of this effect has remained controversial. A study from ECOG was able to show a decrease in treatment-related mortality with GM-CSF, whereas another large randomized study from CALGB was not able to demonstrate any significant clinical benefit from this growth factor.[100,129] Different forms of GM-CSF were used in these two studies, which could account for the disparity in outcomes. Moreover, large numbers of patients were removed from both arms of the CALGB study because of toxicity, which could have affected the outcome. Using G-CSF, the French AML Cooperative Study Group demonstrated an increased CR rate but no benefit in survival.[101] The Southwest Oncology Group also investigated G-CSF in older (older than 55 years) patients and found a reduction in the time to neutrophil recovery and a decreased duration of infection but no difference in either CR rate or overall survival.[131] Another European/Australian phase III study showed similar response and survival data in the G-CSF and control groups but a reduction in measures of treatment-related toxicity, such as duration of fever, requirement for antimicrobials, and duration of hospitalization.[130] This study was not confined to an older poor-risk population and included all patients above 16 years old diagnosed with *de novo* AML during the study period. Hence, despite extensive investigation no overwhelming consensus has emerged from the clinical trials advocating the routine use of growth factor support of standard AML therapy. Although using these growth factors is relatively safe and the duration of neutropenia has consistently been reduced, the benefits have been variable across patient populations, and economic data supporting their use have been sparse.[133]

An alternative rationale for growth factor use in AML is based on the ability of the myeloid growth factors to increase leukemia cell proliferation and increase their sensitivity to cell cycle–specific agents. G-CSF and GM-CSF have been used to "prime" patients' leukemia with the intent of modifying sensitivity to cytarabine-based regimens. Unfortunately, the degree of biologic effect needed to significantly alter drug sensitivity and produce the desired clinical effect is unknown and underscores the difficulty with translating *in vitro* phenomena to the practice of medicine. ECOG conducted a study in elderly AML (older than 55 years) in which a subset of patients were randomized and received GM-CSF before cytarabine and either daunorubicin, idarubicin, or mitoxantrone.[123] Although some of the correlative laboratory studies were able to demonstrate an increase in proliferation in some of the patients who received GM-CSF, there was no difference in the clinical outcomes for the patients who received growth factor compared with the placebo group. The Dutch-Belgian Hemato-Oncology Group and the Swiss Group for Clinical Cancer Research investigated the effect of G-CSF on priming before chemotherapy in adult AML patients less than 60 years of age in a large randomized study.[134] Response rates were similar in the growth factor and control groups. Disease-free survival was, however, superior in the G-CSF group, although no effect was seen on overall survival. Despite the results from this single trial, the role of growth factors as a tool for drug sensitization in AML outside the context of a clinical trial remains unclear.

POSTREMISSION THERAPY

In the modern era, postremission therapy can be administered in many forms, including standard-dose chemotherapy, high-dose chemotherapy, and autologous or allogeneic stem cell transplantation. Although the optimal form of postremission therapy is controversial, the need for such treatment is widely accepted. As previously discussed in Induction, current induction therapy is unable to provide adequate cell kill so that residual leukemia cells, although often undetectable by standard means, survive the initial therapy. If left unchecked, these cells proliferate, expand, and eventually result in clinical recrudescence of disease. Postremission therapy is necessary to eradicate minimal residual disease past the point at which it can become clinically meaningful. The benefit of postremission therapy was established by two randomized multicenter trials showing that maintenance therapy was superior to no further treatment in prolonging remission duration.[135,136] This concept of continuing low-dose therapy over a prolonged period of time was further modified by subsequent clinical trials and eventually evolved into schemas that became known as *maintenance therapy*. The CALGB addressed the question regarding the duration of maintenance therapy in a randomized study that compared 36 months versus 8 months of treatment. No benefit was found for the prolonged therapy.[116] Additional studies have suggested that more intensive therapy delivered within a shorter period of time offered clinical benefit, and the concept of modern consolidation therapy was formed.[137,138] One study from ECOG randomized patients less than 65 years of age to receive either one course of intensive consolidation versus 2 years of maintenance therapy and found superior survival in patients receiving the more intensive therapy.[139] These findings have led to the current "state-of-the-art" recommendations for AML therapy, which include induction and intensive postremission therapy (including stem cell transplantation) but no maintenance (Table 42.2-7). This dogma has been challenged by the experience reported in APL, however (see later in Acute Promyelocytic Leukemia).[140]

The logical progression in the evolution of modern postremission therapy was to further intensify the chemotherapy used in this setting. The rationale for dose escalation was based on the efficacy of high-dose Ara-C regimens in overcoming relative drug resistance and successfully treating some patients with relapsed disease. The goal with such therapy is to enhance the degree of cell kill, eliminating greater amounts of leukemia and placing the residual leukemia burden below critical levels. A number of non-randomized trials using cytarabine doses ranging from 1 to 3 g/m^2 (typically given every 12 hours for 6 to 12 doses) have reported disease-free survivals ranging from 30% to 40%.[125] These results were superior compared with the 12% to 20% survival reported with standard dose-attenuated consolidation regimens. The most compelling clinical evidence for intensification therapy was, however, provided by a large randomized study conducted by the CALGB. After achieving remission with a standard 3 + 7 regimen, patients with *de novo* AML were randomized to receive four courses of cytarabine at one of three dose levels: 100 mg/m^2/d for 5 days by continuous infusion (standard-dose arm), 400 mg/m^2/d for 5 days by continuous infusion (intermediate-dose arm), or 3

TABLE 42.2-7. State-of-the-Art Treatment Programs for Adult Acute Leukemia

ACUTE MYELOCYTIC LEUKEMIA

Anthracycline- and cytarabine-based induction regimens.

Intensive postremission therapy; either bone marrow transplant or high-dose cytarabine is required for prolonged remission.

Maintenance therapy and central nervous system (CNS) prophylaxis are not generally indicated.

ACUTE PROMYELOCYTIC LEUKEMIA

Retinoic acid and anthracycline/cytarabine-based treatment.

Management of disseminated intravascular coagulation

    Administration of cryoprecipitate or fresh frozen plasma to maintain fibrinogen greater than 100 mg/dL

    Platelet transfusions to maintain daily platelet count greater than 50,000 μL.

Bone marrow transplantation/high-dose cytarabine therapy reserved for relapsed disease.

ACUTE LYMPHOCYTIC LEUKEMIA

Four or five drug induction regimens using anthracyclines, cyclophosphamide, and/or asparaginase in addition to vincristine and prednisone.

Intensive consolidation therapy based on cytarabine combined with anthracyclines, epipodophyllotoxins, or antimetabolites.

Protracted maintenance therapy (approximately 2 y) based on oral methotrexate combined with mercaptopurine.

Prophylactic intrathecal chemotherapy (with or without cranial radiotherapy) for CNS prophylaxis.

---

g/m^2 twice daily via a 3-hour infusion on days 1, 3, and 5 (high-dose arm). Among the treatment groups, the probability of remaining in continuous CR was greatest in the patients less than 60 years of age who had received the high-dose cytarabine after remission therapy.[141] A subsequent analysis of this trial according to cytogenetic data underscored the importance of this prognostic factor, with prolonged disease-free survival in 84% of the patients with favorable cytogenetics[142] [defined as t(8;21) or inv(16)]. Although the results from this trial have been used to support the use of single-agent high-dose cytarabine intensification as the sole form of postremission therapy, all patients received four courses of maintenance therapy in the form of dose-attenuated cytarabine and daunorubicin in addition to the four courses of high-dose cytarabine. The effect of such therapy on outcomes is uncertain and has caused some speculation as to whether comparable results can be achieved by administering high-dose cytarabine intensification alone, as is the current practice. Still, results from this trial appear similar to those of studies using allogeneic stem cell transplantation as postremission therapy and have essentially shaped the standard of care for AML.

ALLOGENEIC BONE MARROW TRANSPLANTATION

The application of bone marrow or stem cell transplantation as postremission therapy was initially thought to represent the extreme in dose intensification, although subsequently the immunology underlying this treatment modality has increasingly been appreciated as having an important role in its antileukemia effect. High doses of chemotherapy with or without total body radiation are used in an effort to maximize leukemia cell kill. Near or total myeloablation is a consequence of this therapy. Hematopoiesis is restored by the infusion of stem cells harvested from an HLA-compatible donor, thereby rescuing the patient from the lethal consequences of complete bone marrow failure. The donor bone marrow/peripheral blood stem cells (graft) also have a number of immunologic effects on the host. Because of differences in HLA composition, the graft may reject the host, resulting in graft-versus-host disease (GVHD). This complication has systemic consequences, including increasing the risk of infection, and represents a leading source in morbidity and mortality in patients who undergo allogeneic stem cell transplantation.[143] The immunologic effects of the graft may also contain antileukemic activity as evidenced by the lower relapse rate observed in patients with GVHD. This graft-versus-leukemia (GVL) effect may represent a major mechanism in the way allogeneic bone marrow transplantation (alloBMT) cures some patients with AML and may account for the lower relapse rates seen with alloBMT compared with syngeneic (or autologous) transplants where similar conditioning regimens are used.[144] GVL has also come under increasing scrutiny as alternative transplants using nonmyeloablative conditioning regimens are investigated in hosts who were previously unable to undergo stem cell transplantation because of concerns over treatment-related toxicity.[145]

Despite the large number of treatment-related complications and the difficulty in managing these clinical problems, alloBMT is effective antileukemia therapy. Efficacy was first established in a small number of heavily pretreated patients with refractory AML. At that time, such patients had no other treatment options, and the ability to provide some form of therapy that could successfully treat their advanced disease was considered a major breakthrough. The concept that treatment outcomes could be improved and the toxicity lessened if stem cell transplantation was applied earlier in the course of the disease led to a number of nonrandomized clinical trials from large tertiary care centers or cooperative groups. Generally, these trials showed that alloBMT using an HLA-compatible donor for patients in the first CR of AML resulted in a 5-year disease-free survival of approximately 45% to 50%, with relapse rates ranging from 10% to 20%.[146] The fact that the low relapse rate did not translate to prolonged survival in these patients could be explained by the finding that significant numbers of patients succumb to transplant-related complications as GVHD, infection, or interstitial pneumonia. Therefore, alternative mechanisms of failure as represented by the treatment-related toxicity affected the overall survival of this group of patients.

Therefore, although alloBMT is an effective therapy with a relatively low incidence of relapse, major criticisms of this treatment for patients in first remission from AML are that it is quite toxic, very expensive, and, given the results from a number of large randomized studies, not necessarily superior to other forms of dose-intensive therapy. With a conventional graft and standard conditioning, the complication rate increases with increasing age, prompting some centers to restrict this therapy to patients younger than 60 years. As the median age of patients with AML is approximately 65 years, most individuals with this disease are not eligible for this form of therapy. Because of specific entry criteria, BMT trials report results in groups of younger patients who may also do well with other forms of intensive therapy. Such patients represent a good risk population and may not be representative of the majority of patients with AML. The introduction of the nonmyeloablative transplant may further break the age barrier, although the outcomes for such treatments may not be the same as the historic BMT data and require validation by clinical trials.

Only approximately 30% of patients eligible for a conventional BMT have an HLA-compatible donor. Despite meeting minimum eligibility requirements of age and availability of donors, a significant number of patients still fail to proceed with alloBMT for a variety of reasons.[147] Given this rather large attrition rate, it has been estimated that alloBMT (in its current form) is applicable in only 2% to 10% of patients with AML.[79] Strategies using alternative donors, such as unrelated HLA-matched or haplotype-mismatched donors, continue to evolve and may increase the number of patients who are able to proceed with this form of therapy. The results from these alternative transplants have generally been inferior to those of the more conventional grafts.[148] In addition, newer methods of molecular typing are better able to define the HLA type and select truly identical donors, which may result in decreased toxicity and improved overall survival.[149]

AUTOLOGOUS STEM CELL TRANSPLANTATION (AUTO BONE MARROW TRANSPLANTATION)

Despite ongoing efforts to expand the donor pool for alloBMT, the majority of patients do not have an acceptable HLA-matched donor and therefore are unable to undergo alloBMT. In an effort to extend the potential benefits of high-dose therapy to these patients, investigators turned to using bone marrow that was obtained from the patient while in remission as the source of hematopoietic reconstitution.[150] Such an approach was also thought to provide the antileukemic effects associated with high-dose conditioning regimens while avoiding toxic complications, particularly GVHD. One major disadvantage, however, is the potential contamination of the autologous stem cells by residual clonogeneic leukemia cells. Given the present model of tumor cell burden and the effect of currently available chemotherapy on cell kill (see earlier in Postremission Therapy), the ability of the initial chemotherapy to render the individual free of minimal residual disease below a critical mass unable to reproduce the disease is unlikely. The inability of readily available laboratory techniques to reliably detect this minimal residual disease and predict clinical relapse represents a major challenge in the clinical management of acute leukemia. Therefore, concern exists that despite the high-dose conditioning regimens designed to eradicate residual leukemia cells in the patient, relapse will ultimately recur because undetectable residual leukemias are reinfused with the graft. Proof of this hypothesis was offered by an innovative study from St. Jude Children's Hospital.[151] Cells in the autologous bone marrow graft were marked with a neomycin-resistant gene before transplantation into two patients with AML. After clinical relapse of the patients, the neomycin-resistant gene marker was detected in the leukemic blasts of both patients, implying that the "remission" bone marrow graft that had been reinfused contributed to disease recurrence.

Despite such evidence and the compelling rationale for attempting removal of minimal residual disease from the stem cell graft, the clinical benefits of purging the graft remain unclear. Clinical trials using unpurged bone marrow as the source for hematopoietic reconstitution in first remission have reported treatment results comparable to studies using grafts purged through a variety of mechanisms.[150] Results from these trials have generally reported disease-free survival of approximately 40% to 50%. Relapse rates (50% to 60%) are higher than for alloBMT, but, as expected, the transplant-related toxicity is less. In studies that have used either immunologic or pharmacologic methods to purge bone marrow grafts, there has been a profound suppression of normal bone marrow progenitors resulting in a clinically prolonged period of hematologic recovery. Some association has been made, however, between the degree of myelosuppression as evidenced by either the granulocyte-macrophage colony-forming unit or CD34 yields and the relative freedom from relapse.[152-154]

Peripheral blood stem cells represent an alternative to bone marrow as a source of hematopoietic reconstitution, and autologous transplants using this approach have been investigated in AML.[155] Data from such transplants in other malignancies suggested an advantage in terms of enhanced hematologic recovery. In addition, collection of stem cells from the peripheral blood is easier for the patient, as it does not require a surgical procedure with the risk of general anesthesia. A theoretic advantage was also thought to exist because of a difference in recovery rates between the leukemic and normal stem cell compartments. In response to a priming stimulus such as chemotherapy, the normal stem cells are thought to have a temporary growth advantage and appear in the peripheral blood before clonogenic leukemia precursors. Therefore, harvesting early in the recovery process would yield a product relatively free from contamination. Evidence to support this hypothesis is rather scant and replete with the difficulties previously discussed in measuring minimal residual disease. Using standard cytogenetic analysis, however, one study was unable to detect an abnormal karyotype in cells collected early in the recovery process.[156] Further support for this practice has been provided by the experience in harvesting Philadelphia chromosome–negative cells in chronic-phase CML after dose-intensive chemotherapy. Despite the availability of more sensitive laboratory tests, the validation of this hypothesis specifically in AML has remained elusive.

Although some of the clinical trials using peripheral blood stem cells have reported a decrease in the duration of neutropenia and thrombocytopenia, the effect of treatment outcomes has been variable, with most groups reporting relapse rates similar to those seen when unpurged bone marrow has been used for reconstitution.[157] Other studies have shown a superior leukemia-free survival using purged bone marrow as the graft. Few groups have attempted *ex vivo* manipulation of the peripheral blood stem cell product. Instead, a number of studies have intensified the chemotherapy given in the postremission setting before harvesting the potential graft in an effort to maximize cell kill of the residual leukemia cells and effect an *in vivo* purge.[150,158-160] The difficulty with such a strategy is that the cumulative effect of multiple chemotherapy regimens may also decrease the cell yield from the stem cell harvest, impacting engraftment. Despite such concerns this approach has been used with peripheral blood stem cell and bone marrow grafts. The clinical results from these trials have been among the best reported for autologous transplantation in the first remission of AML.

In contrast to efforts to purge the autologous graft before actual transplant, there has been some interest in modifying the graft after infusion to recapitulate the GVL effect seen in alloBMT. Although immunopotentiation may be an intellectually attractive strategy, it is hampered by the relative lack of effective agents that could be used to achieve the desired clinical effect. Some investigators have described an autologous GVL (or graft-versus-tumor) effect with the use of cyclosporin in the posttransplant setting. Several small clinical trials have been reported in breast cancer and in AML, but the effect of the cyclosporin on treatment outcome is unclear.[161] Immunomodulation with IL-2 has the largest experience. Some early studies were marked by toxicity and an inability to administer the IL-2. A study from the City of Hope reported a 2-year disease-free survival of 74% in patients who received an autologous stem cell transplant followed by IL-2.[162] Because this study also used an *in vivo* purge with a high-dose cytarabine-based regimen, it may be difficult to differentiate the contribution that the immunomodulation had on this group of patients. No data regarding immunologic reconstitution or measurements of minimal residual disease were reported with this trial. An ongoing clinical trial conducted by CALGB uses IL-2 after autologous stem cell transplantation in a cohort of young patients.

ASSESSING THE OPTIONS FOR POSTREMISSION THERAPY IN ACUTE MYELOGENOUS LEUKEMIA

At the present time the options for postremission therapy in patients less than 60 years of age with AML involve three forms of dose-intensive treatments: allogeneic or autologous stem cell transplantation or high-dose chemotherapy. The various forms of therapy have been applied either alone or in combination. An ECOG trial suggested little benefit from increasing doses of the postremission chemotherapy before alloBMT.[163] A number of randomized clinical trials have directly compared the different postremission approaches in an effort to establish the optimal therapy.[160,164-166] Although many of the initial comparisons favored alloBMT over chemotherapy with regard to treatment outcomes, the postremission chemotherapy used in these trials consisted of dose-attenuated consolidation regimens. With the current standard of care, these regimens would be considered suboptimal for patients less than 60 years of age. More recently, comparisons have been undertaken with patients who have undergone alloBMT from HLA-compatible donors and those who have received some high-dose chemotherapy regimen (usually some variation of high-dose cytarabine) or autologous BMT (autoBMT). The results from several of these trials are summarized in Table 42.2-8. Generally, these trials have reported a decreased relapse rate in the alloBMT arm accompanied by greater treatment-related morbidity/mortality without a significant benefit in overall survival. In fact, a large U.S. intergroup study showed marginally better overall survival in patients treated with a single course of high-dose cytarabine after a standard cytarabine/idarubicin consolidation. In contrast, the Medical Relapse Center 10 trial reported a decreased relapse rate, with a survival benefit for patients who received autoBMT in addition to three cycles of intensive postremission chemotherapy. Direct comparisons of these studies are complicated, however, by the different amounts of therapy that patients received before the autoBMT (*in vivo* purging) as well as the difference in conditioning regimens used before the autologous transplant.

Despite significant effort and large numbers of patients, the results from these randomized studies have thus failed to provide a clear answer to the question of the best postremission therapy. In the absence of a standard, the approach to AML patients in first remission may vary from center to center. An assessment of risk based on a well-described prognostic factor such as karyotype is part of the decision-making process for individual patients. Patients with good-risk cytogenetics [i.e., t(8;21) or inv(16)] are usually treated with three to four cycles of high-dose postremission chemotherapy. For younger

TABLE 42.2-8. Randomized Comparisons of Dose-Intensive Postmission Regimens

Study	Comparison	Outcomes
Burnett et al.[159]	Autologous BMT (unpurged) vs. observation	Superior DFS and OS at 7 y in autoBMT group
Zittoun et al.[160]	Allogeneic BMT vs. autologous BMT (unpurged) vs. IC	DFS best with allogeneic BMT; equivalent OS
Harousseau et al.[164]	Allogeneic BMT vs. autologous BMT (unpurged) vs. IC	No difference in DFS or OS between arms
Cassileth et al.[165]	Allogeneic BMT vs. autologous BMT (purged) vs. IC	No difference in DFS between arms, marginal advantage in OS for IC
Sucio et al.[166]	Allogeneic stem cell transplant vs. autologous stem cell transplant (unpurged)	Superior DFS for bad/very bad risk cytogenetic group with allogeneic stem cell transplant; similar survival from CR

BMT, bone marrow transplantation; CR, complete remission; DFS, disease-free survival; IC, intensive chemotherapy; OS, overall survival.

patients with poor-risk cytogenetics, many centers recommend alloBMT using alternative donors if a related donor is unavailable. For the standard-risk group, some centers continue to advocate alloBMT for suitable candidates with HLA-compatible donors, whereas other centers reserve BMT for relapse. This strategy is based on the relative equivalence of treatment outcomes. Despite the higher risk of relapse with chemotherapy, BMT can provide effective salvage therapy with equivalent overall survival for some patients who fail chemotherapy-based consolidation. Therefore, holding the BMT in reserve until relapse may avoid unnecessary toxicity in those patients who may be cured by chemotherapy alone. Patients should, however, have either a potential related donor (if available) identified or stem cells (peripheral blood or bone marrow) harvested and cryopreserved during the first remission in the event relapse occurs and a salvage strategy based on stem cell transplantation becomes necessary.[167,168] Standard treatment options are limited for patients who are not candidates for BMT; unfortunately, they represent the largest group of patients.

TREATMENT OF RELAPSED ACUTE MYELOGENOUS LEUKEMIA

The majority of patients with AML relapse and ultimately succumb to the sequelae of resistant disease. Chemotherapy alone is not curative in the relapsed setting. Data from multiple trials suggest that a median survival of only a few months is typical after a second remission is obtained.[169] Allogeneic and autologous stem cell transplantation has been reported to provide prolonged disease-free survival in approximately 30% to 40% of patients treated either early in first relapse or in second remission.[168,170] Therefore, patients who have relapsed and are able to undergo BMT should do so, as this represents their best chance for cure. The ability to proceed with stem cell transplantation, either allogeneic or autologous, is directly dependent on anticipating that such a modality can be used in the future and identifying a potential source of hematopoietic reconstitution relatively early in the patient's clinical course.

The timing of BMT for relapsed disease is somewhat controversial. One strategy relies on the ability of salvage or "second-line" chemotherapy to decrease the leukemia burden below a detectable level and induce a second CR. Unfortunately, most patients who relapse well within a year of completing chemotherapy from AML are unable to achieve a second CR with currently available chemotherapy, and the ability to proceed with alloBMT may be compromised by any additional morbidity incurred with this chemotherapy. Such concerns are particularly relevant, as many of the "high-dose" chemotherapy regimens have been moved to the early phases of treatment, limiting the use of such therapies on relapse. Data from the Fred Hutchinson Cancer Center have suggested that alloBMT performed early in first relapse yields similar results to those transplants performed after a second CR has been obtained.[168] Although a number of centers have adopted this strategy, it requires that patients be able to proceed with alloBMT in a timely manner. The feasibility of this approach may be problematic, as the availability of the donor and the ability of the transplant facility to accommodate the transplant may cause delay and force the patient to receive some form of chemotherapy before alloBMT in an effort to control the underlying disease. Further complicating such a approach is the lack of a uniform definition for "early relapse" and concerns over the maximum allowable amount of residual disease that would allow transplantation to be successful.

A similar strategy has been advocated for patients proceeding to autoBMT.[170] Patients who relapse with disease and previously had stem cells (either peripheral blood or bone marrow) harvested and cryopreserved can proceed directly to autoBMT. Concerns complicating this approach include potential contamination of the graft, particularly if the harvest took place close to the time of relapse, which might suggest residual disease was present in the bone marrow. If no provision has been made for the patient and stem cells have not been collected in first CR, a second remission must be obtained. A number of studies have reported a durable disease-free survival of approximately 30% in patients who have received autoBMT in second CR and approximately 20% in third CR. Results were not dependent on whether purged or unpurged marrow was used as the source of hematopoietic reconstitution.

Most patients however, are not candidates for any type of conventional stem cell transplant. For such individuals, the immediate goal in treating relapse is to induce a second remission. The ability to achieve a second remission is primarily dependent on the duration of the first remission.[169,171] Several groups have found that response rates to salvage therapies are lower in patients with first remission durations of 6 to 12 months. Patients with an exceptionally short remission duration (less than 6 months) are unlikely to respond to any of the standard agents currently available. In such patients, the use of investigational approaches is appropriate.[172] Alternatively, patients who relapse after a year in remission may achieve a second remission by repeating the original induction regimen. Because of the potential cumulative toxicity of the anthracyclines, patients who have received these agents in the past require evaluation of cardiac function before additional retreatment with these agents.

Because most patients with relapsed disease do not respond to repetition of the original induction regimen, investigators have sought to define the underlying basis for clinical drug resistance, with the ultimate goal of identifying new therapies. One mechanism of drug resistance that has been suspected to be clinically relevant is the multidrug-resistant (MDR) phenotype. Initially, this laboratory phenomenon described the observation that cell lines can become cross-resistant to unrelated, structurally diverse chemotherapeutic agents. This mechanism of resistance was eventually linked to a 170- to 180-kD glycoprotein that functions as a drug efflux pump decreasing the intracellular accumulation of drugs, resulting in decreased cytotoxicity of these agents. The MDR phenotype has been observed in cells from approximately 70% of patients with relapsed or refractory disease and also in 25% to 30% of patients with untreated AML.[173] One group reported a particularly high incidence of expression among the elderly. The correlation between clinical response and the expression of the MDR phenotype has varied among studies.[174–176] This underscores the complexity of clinical drug resistance and suggests that alternative mechanisms may play an important role in determining drug resistance of AML cells to current chemotherapy. Other potential mediators of drug resistance such as lung resistance protein have been described, and the relationship of this resistant phenotype to MDR and therapeutic outcomes remains under investigation.[177] The emphasis on the MDR data has led to clinical trials using modulators that alter this phenotype and potentially restore chemotherapy sensitivity. Among the agents tested as clinical MDR modifiers are verapamil, quinine cyclosporin A, and the cyclosporin derivative PSC-833.[178] These studies have been undertaken in relapsed disease and "upfront" as part of a strategy to increase remission rates and improve survival. Although treatment with MDR modifiers has proven to be feasible, toxicity of these agents has been a major problem, and the overall efficacy of such a strategy remains to be established. A major criticism of MDR modification is that resistance to the most important antileukemia agent, cytarabine, is not affected by MDR. Several investigators have attempted to modify cytarabine efficacy in several different ways: increasing the intracellular concentration of the drug by giving high-dose cytarabine or combining cytarabine with fludarabine or attempting to exploit the cytokinetic properties of the myeloid growth factors to recruit leukemia cells into S phase, thereby increasing the sensitivity to the drug.[123,134]

Among the drugs tested in the relapsed setting, high-dose cytarabine, either alone or in combination, has consistently been found to have the greatest antileukemia activity.[125] Although the doses and schedule of cytarabine has varied somewhat between studies, high-dose cytarabine is usually given at 2- to 3-g/m^2 every 12 hours for 8 to 12 doses. Several centers now administer the cytarabine once or twice a day on an every-other-day schedule in an effort to decrease toxicity. Responses to high-dose cytarabine-based regimens have ranged from approximately 30% to 50%. Other active drugs, such as daunorubicin, mitoxantrone, idarubicin, and etoposide, have been combined with high-dose cytarabine, but the advantage of these combinations has not been established in randomized studies. Substantial differences in treatment results between trials containing similar agents may be explained by patient selection and the relatively small numbers of patients treated in these studies.

Patients who fail to achieve remission after receiving either two courses of standard-dose therapy or one course of a high-dose cytarabine-containing regimen can be considered as having primary refractory disease. The prognosis for such patients is exceptionally poor, and the response to salvage regimens using standard agents is rare. Approximately 20% to 40% of these patients who are able to undergo alloBMT can achieve a durable remission.[179] The ability to salvage primary refractory disease with alloBMT underscores the importance of identifying potential donors early in the treatment course of patients who may be eligible for BMT. Patients who are not transplant candidates should be enrolled in investigational studies.

As more patients receive some form of high-dose therapy as the initial treatment, the options at relapse have changed. For some patients who have relapsed after high-dose cytarabine-based postremission therapy, studies suggest that either autoBMT or alloBMT can be curative. Those patients who are not candidates for stem cell transplantation may undergo therapy with alternative salvage regimens. Although the early reports of potentially non–cross-resistant combinations such as mitoxantrone/etoposide or topotecan/cytarabine were encouraging, subsequent studies have shown that these regimens are relatively ineffective. The combination of cyclophosphamide/etoposide given in near myeloablative doses has been shown to induce remission in approximately 30% of patients with disease refractory to high-dose cytarabine-containing regimens in a small phase I/II study.[180] Remissions achieved with these salvage regimens usually have a short duration.

The overwhelming need in leukemia therapy thus is the identification of new effective agents for clinical use. As discussed later in Targeted, Biologic, and Immunologic Therapies of Acute Leukemias, many of the newer agents currently being tested have emerged as the underlying biology of the disease has become better understood and new targets are identified. The promise of these targeted therapies is that they are specific to the leukemia cells and do not have the toxicities associated with conventional chemotherapy. The targeted therapy that has received considerable attention is the drug gemtuzumab ozogamicin, an immunoconjugate composed of an anti-CD33 monoclonal antibody linked to the antitumor antibiotic calicheamicin. CD33 is expressed on most AML cells, and the mechanism underlying the antileukemia properties of this compound is that this agent will target the surface protein and deliver the chemotherapy directly to the leukemia cells. Early studies were promising in that activity was established by the ability of the agent to clear blasts from the peripheral blood.[181] Subsequent phase II studies revealed a CR rate of approximately 15%, although higher response rates have been reported when nonstandard definitions of response are considered.[89] Despite this relatively modest response rate, gemtuzumab ozogamicin was approved by the U.S. Food and Drug Administration for use in patients with relapsed AML older than 60 years whose duration of previous CR was greater than 3 to 6 months because the other options for such patients were virtually nonexistent.[182] Subsequent studies have attempted to broaden the application of this agent but have failed to establish significant efficacy in other patient populations. In addition, some of these studies have reported venoocclusive disease in addition to prolonged myelosuppression as treatment-related toxicities negating any potential benefit of a targeted approach.[183]

Relapse of AML after alloBMT poses a difficult management problem, as patients often have a median survival of only 3 to 4 months.[184] Unfortunately, results are not significantly improved with current therapy, and the toxicity of chemotherapy is often amplified in the posttransplant setting. Treatment options are determined by the performance status of the patient as well as the interval from transplant to relapse. Although a CR rate of approximately 35% has been reported with standard induction regimens, patients who relapse within the first 100 days after BMT are unlikely to respond and have a high treatment-related mortality. Selected young patients who relapse after 1 year may be candidates for a second alloBMT, but their survival at 3 years has been reported to be approximately 10%. Therapeutic approaches, including the use of G-CSF, modulation of the GVL effect by discontinuing immunosuppressive therapy, or infusion of donor leukocytes, have been reported to induce remission in this setting. Although donor leukocyte infusions have received much attention, most of these data have been generated in patients with CML, and the results of such immunologic manipulations as the sole form of therapy in relapsed AML have been routinely disappointing. More recently, investigators have attempted cytoreduction of the leukemia with chemotherapy before donor leukocyte infusion and have reported higher response rates.[185,186] Other investigators have focused efforts on the effects of natural killer cell alloreactivity to propagate a GVL effect, and clinical strategies using such an approach are currently under development.[187]

ACUTE PROMYELOCYTIC LEUKEMIA

APL represents a distinct entity among the myeloid leukemias. The unique biology that characterizes the disease also serves to make it the paradigm for targeted antineoplastic therapy. Historically, the recognition of this disorder separate from the rest of AML has been stressed because of the coagulopathy associated with the disease and the potential for lethal hemorrhage, particularly with the institution of cytotoxic therapy. The incorporation of all-*trans* retinoic acid (ATRA) into upfront therapy further underscores the importance of rapid and accurate diagnosis.

When treatment is with standard cytarabine/anthracycline-based chemotherapy, there is a higher rate of peri-induction mortality in APL than in the other AML subtypes, primarily because of coagulopathy-related complications.[188] A variety of supportive interventions have been introduced in an effort to support the patient through the bleeding diathesis associated with the disease, but these complications remain the most significant source of treatment morbidity, and death resulting from such complications remains a major reason for induction failure. Despite the early hazards associated with the institution of chemotherapy, the long-term survival in APL has been superior to that of the other AML subtypes even before the introduction of ATRA.[189]

The introduction of ATRA as the therapy of choice changed the emphasis from cytotoxic therapy and established differentiation therapy as a feasible and effective modality in the treatment of human cancer. The initial experience with ATRA was reported by Huang et al.[190] and subsequently confirmed by other groups.[191,192] ATRA is not a cytotoxic agent but instead induces a proliferation coincident with maturation of the leukemic clone, which eventually results in terminal differentiation and apoptotic cell death. CR is obtained in 90% to 95% of newly diagnosed cases of APL without inducing aplasia. Instead of worsening APL-related coagulopathy, stabilization and improvement of the coagulation parameters occur within days of the institution of ATRA therapy. The therapeutic effects of ATRA are not restricted to *de novo* disease but are also seen in patients who have relapsed after chemotherapy, as demonstrated by CR rates between 85% and 90% in this patient population.

Despite the many advantages of ATRA therapy, it is not without potential complications. Although there is prompt resolution of the coagulopathy, many trials continue to report 10% to 15% peri-induction mortality as a result of thrombosis/hemorrhage as well as the occurrence of a unique toxicity named the *retinoic acid syndrome* (RAS) or more recently called *APL differentiation syndrome*.[193,194] Approximately 25% of patients develop symptoms consistent with "capillary leak," having features similar to those of acute respiratory distress syndrome or endotoxic shock. RAS is characterized by fever, dyspnea, peripheral edema with weight gain, pleural and pericardial effusions, hypotension, and occasionally renal failure. Untreated, RAS can lead to a rapid clinical deterioration and may result in death.

The pathogenesis of RAS and its relationship to the other biologic effects observed with ATRA remain unclear. The description of a similar symptom complex in patients with APL who have not yet received ATRA has raised the question of whether this syndrome is instead directly related to the underlying disease process.[195] Leukocytosis, which is seen in up to 40% of patients with the institution of ATRA and may be an indicator of a biologic response, has been associated with RAS in some studies.[196] This observation has led investigators to advocate the early administration of chemotherapy along with ATRA. Such an approach has been highly successful in reducing the incidence of RAS in some studies.[197] Because RAS may occur in as many as one-third of the cases regardless of leukocytosis, alternative strategies have been developed. Early therapy with a short course of high-dose steroids (dexamethasone, 10 mg IV twice a day for 3 or more days) at the first onset of symptoms can effectively halt the progression of RAS and has markedly reduced the mortality from this complication.[198–200] Alternatively, the Australian Leukaemia Study Group has used steroid prophylaxis with ATRA therapy to avoid RAS.[201]

Although highly successful in inducing remission, ATRA alone is insufficient therapy for APL. If left on a continuous schedule of ATRA, patients eventually develop resistance to this agent. They are unable to sustain adequate plasma concentrations of the drug and generally relapse within a few months. In addition, most patients have persistent minimal residual disease and remain positive for PML/RAR-α, the molecular marker of APL, after ATRA monotherapy. These observations have led to the incorporation of standard chemotherapeutic agents into the treatment of APL.

Initially, ATRA in conjunction with anthracycline/Ara-C–based postremission treatment regimens was used as sequential therapy in phase II studies and resulted in improved disease-free survival compared to historic controls treated with similar chemotherapy administered without the retinoid. Subsequently, large randomized studies from Europe and North America demonstrated the superiority of ATRA-containing regimens over chemotherapy alone.

In an effort to exploit the sensitivity of APL to anthracycline, the Italian cooperative group GIMEMA-AIEPO moved chemotherapy up to induction by including idarubicin with the ATRA and developed the *AIDA* regimen.[197] Ninety-five percent of patients achieved CR with AIDA induction and, when followed by three courses of postremission chemotherapy, the actuarial event-free survival at 2 years was reported to be 79%. RAS developed in only 2.5% of patients. Sequential ATRA/chemotherapy was subsequently compared with simultaneous administration of these agents during induction in two large randomized studies.[140,202] The Medical Research Center study demonstrated a better CR rate, reduced relapse risk, and superior survival among APL patients who presented with a low peripheral blood cell count and received concomitant ATRA/chemotherapy. In the European APL group trial, patients receiving ATRA plus chemotherapy also had a lower relapse rate. In addition, those who received maintenance in the form of either chemotherapy, intermittent ATRA, or a combination of both had superior overall survival compared with those who received no maintenance. Taken together these trials established the basis for the current standard of care in APL therapy: combined ATRA and chemotherapy induction followed by multiple courses of consolidation therapy, followed by maintenance therapy with either chemotherapy, ATRA, or both.[140] The duration and composition of the optimal maintenance schedule are still under investigation.

The molecular genetics of APL have proven not only to be a useful model in understanding the process of leukemogenesis but have also been shown to have clinical applications. The unique disruption of the RAR-α locus results in novel fusion genes that, given the current level of sophistication in the clinical laboratory, are readily detectable and provide a useful tool for the clinician. The PML/RAR-α fusion product defines sensitivity to ATRA, and the ability of RT-PCR to readily detect PML/RAR-α allows for rapid genetic confirmation of the diagnosis, which, given the variant subtypes, can be difficult even for the experienced morphologist.[74,203] In addition to helping confirm the diagnosis, RT-PCR has facilitated the detection of minimal residual disease, introducing the concept of molecular remission into planning an effective treatment strategy. Therefore, APL has become a paradigm for the use of molecular techniques to monitor therapy.[204,205]

Despite the high remission rate and the prolonged survival, approximately 30% of patients with APL treated in the large randomized studies relapsed. Similar to the experience with other AML subtypes, such patients were incurable with chemotherapy alone, and achieving a second remission in these individuals was often difficult. Many are resistant to rechallenge with the retinoid, particularly if the relapses occur early (within 3 to 6 months). The introduction of arsenic trioxide to the treatment of APL radically changed the therapy for relapsed disease. Initially, the drug was tested in a number of small studies using heavily pretreated patients with few other therapeutic options and produced a high CR rate.[206] These results were subsequently confirmed in a large U.S. multicenter study that showed an 85% CR rate but also a high rate of conversion of the PCR assay from positive to negative in the converters.[207] Despite this result, the ability of arsenic trioxide to sustain remissions and effect cure is unclear. For relapsed patients who are able to achieve remission, allogeneic and autologous stem cell transplantation has, however, been reported to result in long term-survival. Such results with an autologous transplant are dependent on the pretransplant status of minimal residual disease, as 75% of the patients who were PCR negative before undergoing the

autograft were able to remain in clinical and molecular remission with a median follow-up of 28 months.[208]

The therapy of APL in the modern era has been marked by great clinical success accompanied by a new understanding of the fundamental biology of the disease. The promise for future success in APL and, indeed, in all of medical oncology may lie in hypothesis-driven drug design. The observation that arsenic trioxide leads to increased apoptosis of the leukemia cells has prompted investigators to combine this agent with the differentiating effects of ATRA in an attempt to amplify and complement the mechanisms by which each drug exerts a clinical effect. *In vitro*, this combination has been found to be synergistic, and clinical trials exploring various combination schemas have been undertaken. Monoclonal antibodies targeting the CD33 antigen have been used in this disorder and been found to convert the RT-PCR for PML/RAR-α from positive to negative, suggesting activity against minimal residual disease. As models of leukemogenesis based on the interaction of novel transcriptional fusion products such as PML/RAR-α with corepressor binding proteins and histone deacetylases become more refined, the interest in compounds that affect this process at various control points has grown, and efforts to test these agents in clinical trials are currently under way.

GENERAL PRINCIPLES FOR THE TREATMENT OF ADULT ACUTE LYMPHOCYTIC LEUKEMIA

Treatment of adults with ALL has been modeled on therapy developed for childhood ALL. The similarity between the childhood and adult forms of this disease allows for inferences to be drawn from experience in the pediatric population. Adults with ALL, however, have a far poorer outcome when compared to children. A broad review of the St. Jude experience in pediatric ALL demonstrated a dramatic stepwise improvement in treatment results over the last 30 years.[209] Unfortunately, adults with ALL have not shared in this remarkable success story.[210] Some of this difference can be attributed to differences in the incidence of the various cytogenetic subgroups. Those subgroups with an adverse prognosis [particularly t(9;22) and t(4;11)] are more common in adults compared with children, whereas those with a favorable prognosis [such as hyperdiploidy or t(12;21)] are much more common in children than in adults. Another important factor is that adults are less able to tolerate intensive therapy, and intensive therapy may be vitally important for the successful treatment of ALL. Supporting this view are two (nonrandomized) studies indicating that adolescents appear to do better when treated on the typically more aggressive pediatric regimens compared to less intensive adult regimens, which are typically designed to be tolerable for patients up to the age of 60 years (or even older).[211,212]

Treatment of adult ALL can be divided into four broad categories: induction, consolidation (sometimes termed *intensification*), maintenance, and CNS prophylaxis. At presentation, many patients are quite ill with active infection or hemorrhage, or both, and induction regimens for adult ALL have typically emphasized relatively myeloid-sparing cytotoxic agents.

Consolidation therapy is administered at a relatively higher level of intensity to patients already in CR. Before beginning this phase of therapy, patients have normal blood counts and a generally good performance status. They are therefore able to tolerate significant myelosuppression with acceptable toxicity.

Maintenance therapy is administered to patients in remission after the more intensive consolidation therapy. It is given at a low level of intensity, but for a protracted period of time. Current opinion is that 2 years of maintenance therapy is required for optimal results.

The fourth category of treatment is CNS prophylaxis. It is either administered concurrently with systemic chemotherapy or in some programs during a brief interruption in systemic consolidation treatments. CNS prophylaxis is required because, despite aggressive systemic therapy, the CNS remains a sanctuary site, and without specific meningeal-directed therapy, CNS disease will develop in approximately 35% of adult patients.

To understand the natural history of adult ALL and to assign specific therapy, the FAB subclassification (described earlier in Morphology and Cytochemistry) proves less useful than an immunophenotypic subclassification as recognized by the WHO, which classifies three major groups: The most common subtype is pre-B-cell ALL, which comprises approximately 70% of patients. The term pre-B refers to the fact that these cells are committed to the B-cell lineage, as manifested by immunoglobulin gene rearrangement (with detectable cytoplasmic immunoglobulin in most cases) and expression of typical early B-cell markers such as CD19 and TdT but do not express the hallmark of the mature B cell, surface immunoglobulin. In addition to CD19 and TdT, the lymphoblasts of patients with pre-B-cell ALL frequently express CD10 (a neutral endopeptidase), which was previously known as the common ALL antigen.

The second subtype of ALL is T-cell disease. In many cases T-cell ALL and lymphoblastic lymphoma are essentially the same disease. This disease typically affects young adults and has a significant male predominance. The malignant process begins as a rapidly growing mediastinal mass with early dissemination to the bone marrow. Patients present with symptoms related to their mediastinal mass (cough, dyspnea, chest pain) or to bone marrow involvement (infection and bleeding). Patients without evident bone marrow involvement at diagnosis are said to have lymphoblastic lymphoma. Those with scant bone marrow involvement are said to have stage IV lymphoblastic lymphoma, and those with significant (greater than 30% of cells) bone marrow involvement are said to have T-cell ALL. These distinctions are largely semantic and are without important clinical implications. Given the confusion that frequently arises from the "lymphoma versus leukemia" nomenclature, the authors prefer describing this syndrome as *T lymphoblastic disease*. All patients with T lymphoblastic disease require therapy as for ALL.

The third and least common subtype (approximately 5% of adult ALL) is mature B-cell ALL. As the name implies, these leukemic cells are slightly more mature than their pre-B-cell counterparts and express surface immunoglobulin. The typical patient is a young man who presents with a rapidly growing abdominal mass (initial sites are typically the appendix and the ileocecal valve) and early dissemination to the bone marrow. The most common presentation is with symptoms related to the abdominal mass (pain, bloating, and small bowel obstruction) or to bone marrow involvement (infection and bleeding). Patients who present to medical attention without evidence of bone marrow involvement are said to have Bur-

kitt's lymphoma. Once significant bone marrow infiltration occurs, this disease is called mature *B-cell ALL*. In contrast to pre-B-cell ALL and T-cell ALL, mature B-cell ALL requires a distinctly different treatment regimen for optimal results (see the end of this section).

PROGNOSTIC FEATURES IN ADULT ACUTE LYMPHOCYTIC LEUKEMIA

Several evaluations of prognostic features in adult ALL have been made. The two "classic" multivariate analyses were both published in 1988 and were performed by the German multicenter group and the Memorial Sloan-Kettering group.[213,214] Other analyses have in general supported these two studies and have led to five widely accepted prognostic features: WBC count, age, leukemic cell immunophenotype, Philadelphia chromosome–positive (Ph+) disease, and time to achieve CR (see Table 42.2-5).

Multivariate analyses indicate that a high WBC count at diagnosis is associated with poor prognosis. The likelihood of achieving a CR is reduced and the duration of remission (and overall survival) is shorter in those who achieve a CR. An increased WBC count probably has prognostic significance, in part on the basis as a measure of tumor burden but also because of its correlation with adverse cytogenetics [e.g., t(4;11) and t(9;22)]. A high WBC count is probably a continuous variable (the higher the count the worse the prognosis), and different studies have used different levels of elevated WBC count as their cut off for an adverse feature. In the Memorial Hospital study, WBC counts greater than 10,000/μL were associated with a lower frequency of achieving a CR, whereas counts greater than 20,000/μL were associated with a shorter duration of CR. The German study indicated that WBC counts greater than 30,000/μL carry an adverse prognosis. Interestingly, high WBC counts portend a poor prognosis for B-lineage disease; for patients with T-cell disease, this prognostic feature is less important.

Older age is also associated with a worse prognosis. Age is probably a continuous variable (the older the patient the worse the prognosis). In pediatric series adolescent patients typically have the worst prognosis, although in adult series this is almost always the most favorable group. Different studies have defined different ages as being "poor" prognosis, the two most important being age 35 from the German group and age 60 from the Memorial Hospital study.

The immunophenotype of the leukemic cell also carries prognostic implication.[213–215] T-cell disease has a favorable prognosis, pre-B-cell (common) ALL has an intermediate prognosis, and mature B-cell disease has a poor prognosis when treated with standard ALL regimens. Newer regimens have resulted in better survival for this group (see Treatment of Mature B-Cell Acute Lymphocytic Leukemia). Previously, "null" cell ALL was considered to have a poor prognosis. Modern immunophenotyping has essentially eliminated this entity. It is possible that in the past some acute leukemias now classified as AML-M0 would have been considered null cell ALL; not surprisingly, these would fare poorly with vincristine/prednisone-based therapy.

Ph+ disease carries a very poor prognosis. In the pre-imatinib era (it remains unknown what impact imatinib will have) adult patients with this entity were essentially never cured by chemotherapeutic regimens. A minority of patients with this disease may be cured if they undergo allogeneic transplant in first CR.[216] Other cytogenetic abnormalities also have prognostic implications, but their frequency is not sufficient to be noted in multivariate analysis. Most notable of these is the poor prognosis associated with t(4;11).

Time to achieve a complete response during induction therapy carries significant prognostic implications. Patients who require more than 4 or 5 weeks[214] to achieve a complete response have a lower likelihood of being cured. It is not clear if this reflects an "innate" sensitivity to (and curability by) the chemotherapeutic agents used or rather that rapid cytoreduction of the leukemic cell mass minimizes the opportunity for drug resistance to develop and ultimately allows for cure of the patient.

TREATMENT OF NEWLY DIAGNOSED ADULT PATIENTS WITH ACUTE LYMPHOCYTIC LEUKEMIA

A variety of different treatment regimens for adults with ALL have been developed over the last 30 years. These regimens, which borrow heavily from advances made in childhood ALL, have many features in common. Current therapy can induce CR in approximately 65% to 90% of adults. Unfortunately, the majority of these patients subsequently relapse, and overall only 20% to 30% of adults with ALL will prove to be cured of their disease (Fig. 42.2-5).[217–226] The mainstay of induction therapy for ALL has been the combination of vincristine and prednisone. These drugs achieve a complete response in approximately 50% of patients. The addition of an anthracycline to induction therapy was demonstrated in a randomized trial to increase the likelihood of achieving a complete response (83% vs. 47%).[227] Interestingly (and frequently overlooked), this increased incidence of CR did not translate into improved survival for the patients randomized to receive the anthracycline. However, lacking support from randomized clinical trials, further intensification of induction therapy with cyclophosphamide or L-asparaginase is now widely accepted as improving remission induction, and one or both of these drugs are therefore included in essentially all induction regimens. Current induction regimens are therefore labeled as "four-drug" (vincristine, prednisone, anthracycline, and cyclophosphamide or

asparaginase) or "five-drug" (vincristine, prednisone, anthracycline, cyclophosphamide, and asparaginase) regimens. Currently, no data are available to favor one of these induction regimens over another.

Consolidation therapy has evolved over time to include several drugs given in varying sequence. Although there is no "standard" consolidation therapy, some generalizations can be made. The drug most prominently used in consolidation of adult ALL is cytarabine (Ara-C). Consolidation regimens include cytarabine combined with other drugs, most typically anthracyclines, epipodophyllotoxins, alkylators, or antimetabolites (e.g., methotrexate or thioguanine). Multiple studies seem to indicate the value of such consolidations. Most of them are uncontrolled phase II studies or comparisons with historic controls.[218,221,223,224] The experience at M. D. Anderson Cancer Center is typical in this regard, in which implementation of such therapy increased 3-year survival from 15% to 40%.[228] A randomized phase III trial demonstrating the importance of cytarabine-containing consolidations was reported by Fière et al.[217] In this study, after remission induction, patients were randomized to receive consolidation therapy with cytarabine, doxorubicin, and asparaginase or to receive maintenance therapy immediately. Three-year disease-free survival in the consolidation arm was markedly superior at 38% to the no-consolidation arm at 0% (*P* <.005). Although most authors accept that intensive consolidations are beneficial, there is a report by Ellison et al.[229] of a randomized trial that failed to show significant benefit to cytarabine-based consolidation.

Protracted maintenance therapy is a feature unique to treatment strategies for acute lymphoblastic leukemia. All other chemotherapeutically "curable" human malignancies are typically cured with 3 to 6 months of therapy. In pediatric ALL, maintenance therapy is clearly necessary, and most regimens prescribe 2 to 3 years of such treatment. In adults, the necessity of maintenance therapy has been less clearly addressed. Only a few studies have failed to use maintenance therapy, and the low reported disease-free survival seen in the CALGB study (18% at 3 years) and the ECOG study (13% at 4 years) suggests the importance of maintenance therapy in adult ALL.[230,231] A third study that attempted to avoid maintenance therapy by using intensive consolidation also concluded that maintenance therapy is important.[232] The two most important drugs in maintenance chemotherapy are oral methotrexate and mercaptopurine in combination. In pediatric ALL, these two drugs alone can be sufficient for maintenance therapy; in adults, however, most maintenance regimens are typically intensified by incorporating other active agents, such as vincristine, prednisone, anthracyclines, and cyclophosphamide.

The CNS, along with the eye and the testis, is viewed as a "sanctuary" site. These are areas where penetration of systemically administered cytotoxic agents is compromised, leading to the potential of localized relapse. In adults ocular relapse is extremely rare. Testicular disease occurs occasionally in patients with mature B-cell ALL, less frequently in patients with Ph+ ALL, and extremely uncommonly in other adults with ALL. Of the three sanctuary sites, CNS relapse is by far the most common. The incidence of CNS disease at presentation in adult ALL is typically 5% to 10%. Risk factors for development of CNS disease include high WBC count at diagnosis and mature B-cell immunophenotype. Patients who do not receive prophylactic therapy have a cumulative risk of approximately 35% of developing CNS involvement during the course of their disease. Prophylaxis with intrathecal chemotherapy (with or without

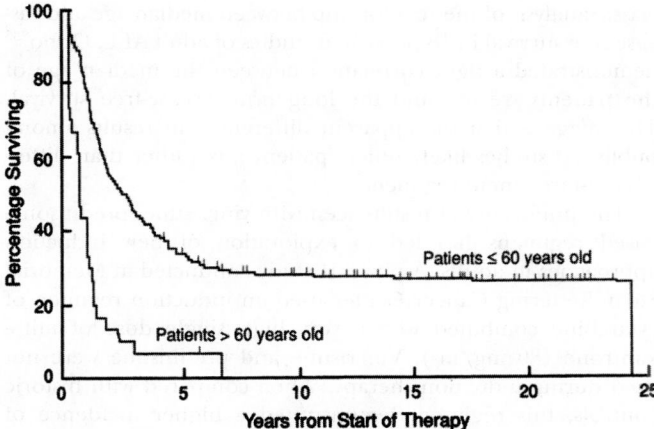

FIGURE 42.2-5. Overall survival with 25-year follow-up for 272 patients with acute lymphocytic leukemia treated on protocols at Memorial Sloan-Kettering Cancer Center, New York. Patients older than 60 years have a substantially worse prognosis. (Data accrued by B. D. Clarkson, C. Little, D. Tyson, L. Megharian, and D. A. Scheinberg.)

TABLE 42.2-9. Representative Chemotherapy Studies in Adult Acute Lymphoblastic Leukemia

Study	Patients (n)	Median Age	Complete Response (%)	Disease-Free Survival	
				Percentage	At Year
Linker et al.[221]	109	25	88	42	5
Hussein et al.[223]	168	28	68	30	5
Kantarjian et al.[225]	204	39	91	39	5
Cuttner et al.[231]	164	32	63	20	5
Ellison et al.[229]	277	33	64	29	5
Fière et al.[217]	218	33	77	40	3
Stewart et al.[222]	68	38	76	18	5

whole brain irradiation) effectively reduces the cumulative incidence to approximately 10%. Intrathecal chemotherapy can be delivered by lumbar puncture or intraventricularly via Ommaya reservoir. If whole brain irradiation is used, intrathecal chemotherapy can be delivered by lumbar puncture (and requires fewer treatments) to achieve acceptable results. Patients not receiving whole brain irradiation as part of their prophylaxis require a greater number of intrathecal treatments and should probably have these treatments administered via an Ommaya reservoir. Patients should achieve a CR of their systemic disease before having an Ommaya reservoir placed to avoid this surgery in the subset of patients who have primary refractory disease or die during induction therapy. Intrathecal chemotherapy does not require adjustments for body surface area, and a typical adult dose is 12 mg methotrexate (or 60 mg cytarabine). A variety of administration schedules have been used, but for patients not receiving brain irradiation, the authors recommend administering six doses during the first 2 to 3 months of treatment, two doses per month during consolidation therapy, and two doses for every 3 to 4 months of maintenance therapy. For patients receiving prophylactic intrathecal therapy via lumbar puncture, it is important to defer such treatments in two circumstances. First, in patients with circulating blasts in the peripheral blood, a traumatic lumbar puncture can "seed" the CNS and actually cause leukemic meningitis.[233] The second setting in which to avoid performing a lumbar puncture is in patients with thrombocytopenia (platelet count less than 50,000/μL) or (more important) coagulopathy, as such patients are at an increased risk for epidural hematomas that can result in lower extremity paralysis.

The addition of whole brain radiotherapy to intrathecal chemotherapy can reduce the amount of intrathecal chemotherapy required for adequate CNS prophylaxis (and obviate the need for an Ommaya reservoir); however, concerns of late toxicity, including loss of cognitive function and leukoencephalopathy,[234] have led many investigators to omit whole brain radiotherapy from prophylactic regimens. CNS prophylaxis, although effective at reducing the incidence of CNS relapse, has no demonstrable effect on systemic relapse or overall survival.[235]

Features common to state-of-the-art treatment programs for adult ALL are summarized in Table 42.2-7. Over the last three decades, treatment regimens that incorporate these features have been developed at many centers. Multiple formulations have been tested that vary the drug dose and schedule during induction, the number and intensity of chemotherapy cycles during consolidation, and the sequencing and duration of maintenance. Despite 30 years of experience

with multiple variations of this treatment strategy, no single formulation appears to be superior to the others. The wide variation in reported outcomes of clinical trials would superficially suggest the superiority of certain regimens (Table 42.2-9). Closer inspection, however, does not support this view. Interpretation of the literature is complicated primarily by differences in patient mix and duration of follow-up. It is easy to understand how duration of follow-up impacts disease-free survival. Figure 42.2-5 indicates overall survival for 272 adult patients with ALL treated at Memorial Sloan-Kettering Cancer Center on several sequential treatment protocols. All of these treatment regimens were designed according to the principles listed in Table 42.2-7. Although 2-year survival is almost 50%, the survival curve continues to fall and a plateau is not reached until 6 years out at approximately 24%. Therefore, studies that report only 2- or 3-year survival markedly overestimate their actual results and can appear superior to regimens that report 5-year survival.

The prognostic features of patients treated on a particular study are as important as duration of follow-up in interpreting the results of clinical trials in adult ALL. Certain patients with adult ALL, such as those with Ph+ disease, have little likelihood of long-term survival. Because these patients may constitute 15% to 30% of unselected adults with ALL, their inclusion onto clinical trials can have a major impact on reported results. Age is another important selection criterion that can vary from study to study, with a major impact on reported survival. In a classic analysis of the relationship between median age and disease-free survival in 18 published studies of adult ALL, Ohno[236] demonstrated a tight correlation between the median age of the patients treated and the long-term disease-free survival. This suggests that the apparent differences in results among published studies likely reflect patient mix rather than differences in treatment regimen.

The uniformity of results seen with vincristine/prednisone-based regimens has led to exploration of new induction approaches in adults. A phase II study conducted at Memorial Sloan-Kettering Cancer Center used an induction regimen of cytarabine combined with a very high single dose of mitoxantrone (80 mg/m²). Vincristine and prednisone were not used during induction therapy. When compared with historic controls, this regimen demonstrated a higher incidence of complete response (P = .056), a lower incidence of failure with resistant disease (P = .028), a significantly reduced time to CR (P = .003), and a trend to improved survival.[237] This regimen appeared to have particularly good activity in patients with Ph+ disease. A prospective multicenter randomized trial comparing this regimen to a standard four-drug induction regimen is currently ongoing and nearing completion.

TREATMENT OF RELAPSED OR REFRACTORY ADULT PATIENTS WITH ACUTE LYMPHOCYTIC LEUKEMIA

Most current induction regimens obtain complete responses in 65% to 90% of newly diagnosed patients. Early deaths account for some of the induction failures, but in most studies 10% to 25% of patients have disease that is resistant to vincristine/prednisone-based regimens. In addition to these primary refractory patients, 60% to 70% of patients who achieve a complete response relapse. Treatment of relapsed and refractory patients is therefore an important and common problem. Numerous regimens have been reported in the setting of relapsed ALL. The most important regimens can be divided into two main groups: those that repeat the regimens used for newly diagnosed patients (this strategy is not used for primary refractory patients) and those that involve high-dose chemotherapy. High-dose regimens appear to obtain a greater incidence of second CRs when compared to re-induction with vincristine/prednisone-based regimens. The high-dose regimens with the greatest likelihood for inducing a second CR are high-dose cytarabine-based regimens.

High-dose cytarabine has been used alone and in combination with a number of different agents. In combination with L-asparaginase,[238–240] doxorubicin,[241] idarubicin,[242,243] or mitoxantrone,[244–247] complete responses as high as 72% have been reported in relapsed patients with ALL. Issues of patient mix make it difficult to assess if a specific regimen is superior to others, but in general a combination of high-dose cytarabine and an anthracycline has the greatest likelihood of achieving a second complete response in relapsed patients (or a first CR in refractory patients). The toxicity of these regimens needs to be balanced against the benefits of achieving a CR.

Unfortunately, second complete responses are very difficult to maintain, and typically each succeeding response is briefer than the preceding one. Patients with a suitable related allogeneic transplant option should probably be referred for such a transplant in second CR.[248] The role of autologous or matched unrelated transplants in relapsed adult ALL have not been clearly established and should be considered investigational.

CENTRAL NERVOUS SYSTEM RELAPSE IN ADULT ACUTE LYMPHOCYTIC LEUKEMIA

CNS relapse occurs in approximately 10% of patients who have received appropriate prophylaxis. In the majority of patients, simultaneous (synchronous) bone marrow relapse can be documented. In occasional patients, CNS relapse may occur without demonstrable systemic relapse (so-called isolated CNS relapse); however, this event almost always predicts subsequent bone marrow relapse, and patients with isolated CNS relapse should first receive CNS-directed therapy and then systemic re-induction chemotherapy. Treatment of established CNS disease requires a combination of radiotherapy and intrathecal chemotherapy. Radiotherapy should consist of 1800 to 2400 cGy (in 150- to 200-cGy fractions) administered to the whole brain. Higher doses should be avoided because of the risk of late toxicity and the fact that some patients may later require total body irradiation as part of a conditioning regimen for an allogeneic transplant. Despite encouraging results in children, spinal radiotherapy should generally be avoided in adults, because the dose of radiotherapy to marrow-bearing areas will subsequently limit the ability to administer necessary systemic chemotherapy. Intrathecal therapy with methotrexate (12 mg) for patients with established CNS disease should preferably be administered intraventricularly via an Ommaya reservoir. Intrathecal chemotherapy can be given as often as two or three times a week (typically at least 48 hours should elapse between doses) until the cerebrospinal fluid is cleared of leukemic blasts, then twice a week for 3 weeks and twice a month for 2 or 3 additional months. Patients in whom CNS disease develops despite prophylaxis with intrathecal methotrexate or those who do not clear the blasts from the cerebrospinal fluid promptly (within 2 treatments) with methotrexate should receive intraventricular therapy with cytarabine at a dose of 60 mg.

BONE MARROW TRANSPLANT FOR ADULT ACUTE LYMPHOCYTIC LEUKEMIA

HLA–identical sibling bone marrow transplants have been used in adults with ALL in a variety of settings. This intense treatment approach has the ability to eradicate leukemia in a subset of patients with disease that is refractory to conventional chemotherapy. Unfortunately, the lack of availability of HLA-matched donors and the toxicity and mortality seen with transplant limit the utility of this approach. Significant controversy exists over the use and timing of allogeneic transplant in adult ALL. Analysis of patterns of failure highlight a fundamental difference in the use of this modality for ALL compared with AML. Patients with AML (in first or second CR) treated with allogeneic transplant tend to fail because of treatment-related mortality (infectious complications, GVHD, etc.). Failure because of relapsed AML after allogeneic transplant (for patients in first or second CR) is relatively uncommon. The results for ALL, however, indicate that even for patients who survive the transplant, there is a significant relapse rate, and overall very few patients are long-term disease-free survivors.

The ability of allogeneic transplants to cure malignant diseases rests in part on the ability of the transplanted (donor) immune system to eliminate residual leukemic cells; this is known as the *GVL effect.* Evidence suggests that this effect may be less important in ALL than in either AML or CML. Data from the International Bone Marrow Transplant Registry compared identical twin (syngeneic) to HLA-identical sibling (allogeneic) transplants.[249] Presumably, GVL should be more pronounced in the allogeneic transplants than in the syngeneic transplants. In this study, there was a significantly higher relapse rate in the identical twin transplants for AML and CML, but not for ALL. This finding implies that GVL is less important in ALL. A second indication that GVL is less active in ALL comes from an analysis of studies of donor T-cell infusions used to treat leukemia that has relapsed after allogeneic bone marrow transplant. In this study donor lymphocyte infusions produced CRs in 73% of patients with CML, 29% of patients with AML, and 0% of patients with ALL.[185] The lack of GVL in ALL may in part explain the high relapse rate and the relatively low incidence of long-term disease-free survival after allogeneic transplant for adult ALL transplanted after first CR.

A review of the published experience of allogeneic bone marrow transplants in adult ALL confirms that only a small fraction of patients are cured by this modality. The results of 192 adults with ALL transplanted at the Fred Hutchinson Cancer Center report a 5-year disease-free survival of only 15% for patients transplanted in second CR or beyond.[248] Another study that suggested more favorable results is difficult to interpret because this study presents combined results for pediatric and adult patients or patients in first CR (who may already be cured) with higher-risk patients.[250]

The ability to cure a small subset of relapsed patients with allogeneic transplant has led investigators to test this modality in first CR. Unfortunately, two large comparisons of allogeneic transplant versus standard chemotherapy for patients in first CR have failed to demonstrate an improved survival for the transplant arm.[251,252] In one of these studies, subset analysis suggests a benefit for certain high-risk patients.[251] This benefit has not been confirmed in the other study.[252] Currently, the only group for whom allogeneic transplant in first CR can be routinely recommended are patients with t(9;22) and t(4;11) disease. For other adult patients, allogeneic transplant should be reserved for second CR.

Autologous transplant for adult ALL is even less effective than allogeneic transplant.[253] The extremely poor results for patients in second CR or beyond has led to this modality being tested in first CR. Unfortunately, a nonrandomized[219] and randomized trial[254] showed no benefit for autotransplant compared with maintenance chemotherapy. This modality should be considered experimental and not be routinely performed in first CR.

TREATMENT OF MATURE B-CELL ACUTE LYMPHOCYTIC LEUKEMIA

Mature B-cell ALL is an uncommon disorder that accounts for approximately 5% of all patients with ALL. This disease has an extremely poor prognosis when treated with traditional ALL regimens such as those described earlier in Treatment of Newly Diagnosed Adult Patients with Acute Lymphocytic Leukemia. Studies have been reported, however, indicating that a majority of patients with mature B-cell ALL can be cured with certain intensive regimens. The important features of regimens for this disease are rapid cycling of drugs, fractionated cyclophosphamide, high-dose methotrexate, and intensive CNS prophylaxis. Maintenance therapy does not appear to be necessary for this subtype and is not used in these regimens. A retrospective review of the French experience with this form of therapy indicates that 12 of 22 (55%) patients over the age of 18 were cured in this "poor-risk" group of patients.[255]

IMATINIB FOR PHILADELPHIA CHROMOSOME–POSITIVE ACUTE LYMPHOCYTIC LEUKEMIA

The uniformity of results seen with vincristine/prednisone-based regimens has led to exploration of new induction approaches in adults. For patients with Philadelphia chromosome/BCR-ABL–positive ALL (Ph+ ALL), the introduction of imatinib, an ABL-specific tyrosine kinase inhibitor, holds significant promise. This agent has profoundly changed the treatment and outcome of patients with CML.[256] The t(9;22) translocation results in the deregulated tyrosine kinase activity of the BCR/ABL fusion protein. As previously noted in Prognostic Features

in Adult Acute Lymphocytic Leukemia, adult patients with Ph+ ALL have a poor prognosis with a very high rate of relapse. Imatinib has been demonstrated to induce a complete response in approximately 30% of patients with relapsed or refractory Ph+ ALL.[257] Unfortunately, the median time to progression in that study was only 66 days, reflecting the rapid development of resistance to imatinib.[258,259] As a consequence imatinib is only one part of the answer, but for some patients it may provide a relatively nontoxic "bridge" to allogeneic transplant. Combining imatinib with other active agents as part of an initial treatment program is an area of active investigation.

GRANULOCYTE SARCOMAS, LEUKEMIA CUTIS, AND OTHER EXTRAMEDULLARY LEUKEMIC INVOLVEMENT

Acute leukemia cells may diffusely infiltrate any organ of the body during the course of disease or may form collections and large masses known as *granulocytic sarcomas*, or as *chloromas*, because of their green hue from the myeloperoxidase. Diffuse involvement of the skin by acute leukemia cells is referred to as *leukemia cutis* and should be distinguished from Sweet's syndrome, which is an infiltration of the skin by neutrophils. The initial presentation of acute leukemia at a primary extramedullary site, with normal marrow and blood findings, is extremely rare.[260] However, if extramedullary leukemia is misdiagnosed as carcinoma or lymphoma and treated without leukemia-specific therapy, the prognosis is poor; overt leukemia usually appears within a year, and death occurs at a median of 3 months later. In contrast, granulocytic sarcomas may occur secondarily in approximately 5% of patients, especially in those with (8;21) or (9;11) translocations or inv(16) chromosome abnormalities, and in patients with other monocytic leukemias.[260,261]

The occurrence of extramedullary disease virtually always heralds systemic relapse and should be treated as such.[260] Specific therapy directed at the extramedullary disease, unless it is located in the CNS, is usually not indicated. Treatment of CNS leukemia is discussed in Central Nervous System Relapse in Adult Acute Lymphocytic Leukemia. The prognostic significance of extramedullary disease is usually negative, even when it is associated with other good prognostic signs [e.g., t(8;21)].[261] Extramedullary disease is treated by systemic therapy of the kind used to consolidate or intensify systemic leukemia (see Postremission Therapy). Leukemia cutis has been treated by external electron-beam therapy, but this treatment has been associated with fatal dermatitis in patients who had also received anthracyclines commonly used to treat AML.[262]

Involvement of the CNS is rare at presentation in AML, in contrast to ALL, in which it occurs frequently; therefore, in the absence of symptoms of neurologic involvement, examination of the cerebrospinal fluid in patients with AML is not indicated at presentation. In patients with ALL, the cerebrospinal fluid should be examined routinely during the initiation of treatment and prophylactic intrathecal chemotherapy should be administered; more aggressive therapy should be initiated if the cerebrospinal fluid is involved. In AML, CNS disease is more common in patients with high blast counts in the blood and with monocytic leukemias, especially the M4EO variant.[263,264] Cranial neuropathies, when present, are most likely to involve the fifth or seventh nerves. Leukemic infiltration of the cranial nerves can occasionally be detected by computed tomography or magnetic resonance, but the diagnosis is usually made by demonstration of leukemia blasts in the cerebrospinal fluid. Some patients may not display positive cerebrospinal fluid findings; emergency treatment with irradiation and intrathecal methotrexate is sometimes indicated even without diagnostic cerebrospinal fluid.

Neurologic symptoms such as headache or confusion may also be the consequence of leukostasis and microemboli in the cerebral microvasculature; this is a rare occurrence except in myeloid leukemias with blood blast counts in excess of 100,000/μL.[265] In these cases, urgent therapy (either by leukapheresis or chemotherapy) to lower the blast count is indicated.

TARGETED, BIOLOGIC, AND IMMUNOLOGIC THERAPIES OF ACUTE LEUKEMIAS

Modern attempts to treat acute leukemias with agents designed to alter the biology and growth of the leukemia cells or to kill the cells via immunologic means have met with variable success.[266–268] Early work focused on nonspecific immunostimulators such as interferon, IL-2, and linomide in the setting of advanced disease; more recently these agents have been proposed for use after induction therapy to eliminate residual leukemia.[269–271] Interferon has demonstrated sporadic and limited success in inducing remissions in acute lymphoblastic leukemia of children but has never achieved the consistent results observed in hairy cell leukemia or CML.[266,269,272] Moreover, the lack of potency and requirement for prolonged use to achieve effects, combined with the marked toxicity of interferons (including fever, malaise, myalgia, neurologic disorders, and cytopenias) make chronic use as a long-term agent for postremission or maintenance therapy difficult. A mechanism of action of interferon in treating acute leukemia has not been demonstrated.

IL-2, which promotes the growth of T cells and natural killer cells and activates natural killer cells to become LAK cells (lymphokine-activated killer cells), has demonstrated potent activity *in vitro* in stimulating autologous effector cells to kill leukemia blasts and to block leukemia cell growth in culture *in vitro* and in mouse models.[270,271,273] Clinical trials of IL-2 have shown significant antileukemia effects in inverse relationship to the leukemic burden[270,274]; therefore, recent studies have focused on the use of IL-2 in patients in remission or after transplantation. Preliminary evidence has shown that relapse rates may be reduced in AML but not in ALL.[271,275] IL-2 has been under investigation as a means to enhance specific therapy with monoclonal antibodies directed to AML cells because of its ability to enhance antibody-dependent cellular cytotoxicity.[276]

Specific monoclonal antibody therapy of acute leukemia has been under investigation since 1981 using passively infused murine monoclonal antibodies, radiolabeled monoclonal antibodies, immunotoxins, and, most recently, genetically engineered humanized monoclonal antibodies.[181,267,268,276–279] Passive serotherapy in relapsed ALL and AML has generally not been effective due to the lack of antibody potency, rapid loss of the target antigen from the leukemia cell surface, and development of human antimurine antibody responses. Attempts to use genetically engineered humanized antibodies, which have greater potency and can be repeatedly infused, have begun to show activity in the setting of residual disease, particularly in APL.[280] The first antibody-drug conjugate, composed of a humanized antibody to CD33 covalently attached to calicheamicin, known as *gemtuzumab ozogamicin*, was approved by the U.S. Food and Drug Administration for older patients with AML.[182] Randomized trials to assess the effectiveness of this approach in combination with other cytotoxic agents and in other patient populations are in progress.

The application of radiolabeled monoclonal antibodies as ablative agents before bone marrow transplantation in patients with acute leukemia is also under study.[281,282] Complete response rates approaching 100% have been achieved using these combined modalities, without detriment to engraftment or significant worsening of toxicity associated with the transplant; the demonstration of a therapeutic advantage of this approach in survival awaits randomized studies.

Antibody therapy can also be used *ex vivo* to purge bone marrow of residual leukemia before autologous reinfusion.[283] Although initial clinical results are encouraging, randomized studies confirming the efficacy of this approach have not been reported. Active specific immunotherapy (vaccine therapy) and passive specific T-cell therapies have been explored for their potential in the treatment of leukemias. In principle, peptide sequences derived from oncogene products, translocated fusion proteins, minor alloantigens, or differentiation antigens may serve as leukemia-specific targets for stimulated cytolytic T cells.[284] These cells can be generated *in vivo* by vaccination,[284,285] *ex vivo* for future donor or autologous cell infusions, or by use of the leukemia cells after their transformation into highly stimulating dendritic cells.[286] Such approaches are most likely to be effective in the setting of minimal disease or transplantation.

The ever-enlarging body of knowledge relating to the molecular pathways involved in leukemia cell pathogenesis is leading to a series of new potential targets for interruption of, or reversal of, leukemogenesis.[67] This effort has been spurred on by the success of imatinib inhibition of bcr-abl kinases in acute and chronic leukemias. This includes the ras oncogene pathway, where inhibitors of the ras farnesyltransferase are showing promise in late-stage clinical trials of AML[287]; the FLT-3 receptor kinase pathway, which is also under attack by several new compounds in trial;[288] and apoptotic pathways, which are currently under study in humans using antisense strategies that down-regulate the antiapoptotic protein bcl-2.[289] Other important molecular targets that will likely soon by addressed in clinical trials of leukemia include the JAK-STAT pathway, the MEK, SRC, abl, PDGFR and kit kinases, telomerase, and proteosomes.[290]

CONCLUSION

Two decades of empiric therapy in leukemia have led to long-term cures in an increasing fraction of adult patients with acute leukemia. Advances in the molecular genetics, immunology, and biology of normal and neoplastic hematopoiesis have produced significant progress in understanding the pathogenesis of acute leukemia. This knowledge is leading to an explosion of new, sensitive molecular assays for minimal disease, new diagnostic and prognostic tests, and more specific and less toxic therapies. Unfortunately, there is still a large gap between the patients who initially achieve remission and those who are ultimately cured. The appropriate care of patients with leukemia requires specialized resources and remains a difficult and complicated task with significant morbidity and mortality. Patients with acute leukemias should continue to be referred to cancer centers and enrolled in investigational treatment protocols until a greater fraction of patients achieves long-term survival.

REFERENCES

1. Xie, Y, Davies, S, Xiang Y, et al. Trends in leukemia incidence and survival in the United States (1973–1998). *Cancer* 2003;97:2229.
2. Jemal, A, Murray, T, Samuels, A, et al. Cancer statistics, 2003. *CA Cancer J Clin* 2003;53:5.
3. Swerdlow A, Barber J, Vaughan Hudson G, et al. Risk of second malignancy after Hodgkin's disease in a collaborative British cohort: the relation to age at treatment. *J Clin Oncol* 2000;18:498.
4. Dores G, Metayer C, Curtis R, et al. Second malignant neoplasms among long-term survivors of Hodgkin's disease: a population-based evaluation over 25 years. *J Clin Oncol* 2002;20:3484.
5. Armitage J, Carbone P, Connors J, et al. Treatment-related myelodysplasia and acute leukemia in non-Hodgkin's lymphoma patients. *J Clin Oncol* 2003;21:897.
6. Pui C-H, Ribeiro R, Hancock M, et al. Acute myeloid leukemia in children treated with epipodophyllotoxins for acute lymphoblastic leukemia. *N Engl J Med* 1991;325:1682.
7. DeVore, R, Whitlock, J, Hainsworth, J, et al. Therapy-related acute nonlymphocytic leukemia with monocytic features and rearrangement of chromosome 11q. *Ann Intern Med* 1989;110:740.
8. Detourmignies L, Castaigne S, Stoppa A, et al. Therapy related acute promyelocytic leukemia: a report on 16 cases. *J Clin Oncol* 1992;10:1430.
9. Travis L, Holowaty E, Bergfeldt K, et al. Risk of leukemia after platinum-chemotherapy for ovarian cancer. *N Engl J Med* 1999;340:351.
10. Pedersen-Bjergaard J, Andersen M, Christiansen D. Therapy-related acute myeloid leukemia and myelodysplasia after high-dose chemotherapy and autologous stem cell transplantation. *Blood* 2000;95:3273.
11. Tallman M, Gray R, Bennett J, et al. Leukemogenic potential of adjuvant chemotherapy for early stage breast cancer: the Eastern Cooperative Oncology Group experience. *J Clin Oncol* 1995;13:1557.
12. Preston D, Kusumi S, Tomonaga M, et al. Cancer incidence in atomic bomb survivors. Part III: Leukemia, lymphoma and multiple myeloma, 1950–1987. *Radiat Res* 1994;137:S68.
13. Gundestrup M, Storm H. Radiation-induced acute myeloid leukaemia and other cancers in commercial jet cockpit crew: a population-based cohort study. *Lancet* 1999;354:2029.
14. Linet M, Hatch E, Kleinerman R, et al. Residential exposure to magnetic fields and acute lymphoblastic leukemia in children. *N Engl J Med* 1997;337:1.
15. Taubes G. Another blow weakens EMF-cancer link. *Science* 1995;269:1816.
16. Doll R, Evans H, Darby S. Paternal exposure not to blame. *Nature* 1994;367:678.
17. Sandler D, Shore D, Anderson J, et al. Cigarette smoking and risk of acute leukemia: associations with morphology and cytogenetic abnormalities in bone marrow. *J Natl Cancer Inst* 1993;85:1994.
18. Siegel M. Smoking and leukemia: evaluation of a causal hypothesis. *Am J Epidemiol* 1993;138:1.
19. Austin A, Delzell E, Cole P. Benzene and leukemia: a review of the literature and risk assessment. *Am J Epidemiol* 1988;127:419.
20. Ben-David Y, Bernstein A. Friend virus-induced erythroleukemia and the multistage nature of cancer. *Cell* 1991;66:831.
21. Poiesz B, Ruscetti F, Gazdar A, et al. Detection and isolation of type C retrovirus particles from fresh and cultured lymphocytes of patient with cutaneous T-cell lymphoma. *Proc Natl Acad Sci U S A* 1980;77:7415.
22. Lombardi L, Newcomb E, Dalla-Favera R. Pathogenesis of Burkitt's lymphoma: expression of an activated c-myc oncogene causes the tumorigenic conversion of EBV-infected human B lymphoblasts. *Cell* 1987;49:161.
23. Pui C-H. Childhood leukemias. *N Engl J Med* 1995;332:1618.
24. Taylor A, Metcalfe J, Thick J, et al. Leukemia and lymphoma in ataxia telangiectasia. *Blood* 1996;82:423.
25. Hasle H, Clemmensen I, Mikkelsen M. Risks of leukaemia and solid tumours in individuals with Down's syndrome. *Lancet* 2000;355:165.
26. Groet J, McElwaine S, Spinelli M, et al. Acquired mutations in GATA1 in neonates with Down's syndrome with transient myeloid disorder. *Lancet* 2003;361:1617.
27. Joventino L, Stock W, Lane N, et al. Certain HLA antigens are associated with specific morphologic and cytogenetic subsets of acute myeloid leukemia. *Leukemia* 1995;9:433.
28. Bocchia M, Korontsvit T, Xu A, et al. Specific human cellular immunity to bcr-abl oncogene-derived peptides. *Blood* 1996;82:3587.
29. Pandolfi P. Knocking in and out genes and trans genes: the use of the engineered mouse to study normal and aberrant hemopoiesis. *Semin Hematol* 1998;35:136.
30. Forster A, Pannell R, Drynan L, et al. Engineering *de novo* reciprocal chromosomal translocations associated with MII to replicate primary events of human cancer. *Cancer Cell* 2003;3:449.
31. Metcalf D. The roles of stem cell self-renewal and autocrine growth factor production in the biology of myeloid leukemia. *Cancer Res* 1989;49:2305.
32. Wickremasinghe R, Hoffbrand A. Biochemical and genetic control of apoptosis: relevance to normal hematopoiesis and hematological malignancies. *Blood* 1999;93:3587.
33. Timens W. Cell adhesion molecule expression and homing of hematologic malignancies. *Crit Rev Oncol Hematol* 1995;19:111.
34. Moore M. Hematopoietic reconstruction: new approaches. *Clin Cancer Res* 1995;1:3.
35. Hoang T, Nara N, Wong G, et al. Effects of recombinant GM-CSF on the blast cells of acute myeloblastic leukemia. *Blood* 1986;68:313.
36. Freedman M, Bonilla M, Fier C, et al. Myelodysplasia syndrome and acute myeloid leukemia in patients with congenital neutropenia receiving G-CSF therapy. *Blood* 2000;96:429.
37. Ward A, van Aesch Y, Schelen A, et al. Defective internalization and sustained activation of truncated granulocyte-colony stimulating factor receptor found in severe congenital neutropenia/acute myeloid leukemia. *Blood* 1999;93:447.
38. Spangrude G, Heimfeld S, Weissman I. Purification and characterization of mouse hematopoietic stem cells. *Science* 1988;241:58.
39. Fialkow P, Singer J, Adamson J, et al. Acute nonlymphocytic leukemia: heterogeneity of stem cell origin. *Blood* 1981;57:1068.
40. Griffin J, Lowenberg B. Clonogeneic cells in acute myeloblastic leukemia. *Blood* 1986;68:1185.
41. Terstappen L, Safford M, Unterhalt M, et al. Flow cytometric characterization of acute myeloid leukemia: IV. Comparison to the differentiation pathway of normal hematopoietic progenitor cells. *Leukemia* 1992;6:993.
42. Norrback K-F, Roos G. Telomeres and telomerase in normal and malignant haematopoietic cells. *Eur J Cancer* 1997;33:774.
43. Hirama T, Koeffler H. Role of the cyclin-dependent kinase inhibitors in the development of cancer. *Blood* 1995;86:841.
44. Sabbath K, Ball E, Larcom P, et al. Heterogeneity of clonogenic cells in acute myeloblastic leukemia. *J Clin Invest* 1985;75:746.
45. Turhan A, Lemoine F, Debert C, et al. Highly purified primitive hematopoietic stem cells are PML/RAR negative and generate nonclonal progenitors in acute promyelocytic leukemia. *Blood* 1995;85:2154.
46. Singer J, Fialkow P. Nature of remission in acute myeloid leukemia: more questions than answers. *Leukemia* 1992;6:60.
47. Fearon E, Burke P, Schiffer C, et al. Differentiation of leukemia cells to polymorphonuclear leukocytes in patients with acute nonlymphocytic leukemia. *N Engl J Med* 1986;315:15.
48. LoCoco F, Pelicci P, D'Adamo F, et al. Polyclonal hematopoietic reconstitution in leukemia patients at remission after suppression of specific gene rearrangements. *Blood* 1993;82:606.
49. Bennett J, Catovsky D, Daniel M, et al. Proposed revised criteria for the classification of acute myeloid leukemia (AML-M0). *Br J Haematol* 1991;78:325.
50. Cheson B, Cassileth P, Head D, et al. Report of the National Cancer Institute sponsored workshop on definitions of diagnosis and response to acute myeloid leukemia. *J Clin Oncol* 1990;8:813.
51. Catovsky, D, Matutes, E, Buccheri, V, et al. A classification of acute leukaemia for the 1990s. *Ann Hematol* 1991;62:16.
52. Jaffe E, Harris N, Stein H, et al. In: Kleihues P, Sobin L, eds. *World Health Organization classification of tumours. Pathology and genetics of tumours of haematopoietic and lymphoid tissues.* Lyons: IARC Press, 2001.
53. Bennett J, Catovsky D, Daniel M, et al. The morphological classification of acute lymphoblastic leukaemia: concordance among observers and clinical correlations. *Br J Haematol* 1981;47:553.
54. Harris N, Jaffe E, Diebold J, et al. World Health Organization classification of neoplastic diseases of the hematopoietic and lymphoid tissues: report of the clinical advisory committee meeting—Airlie House, Virginia, November 1998. *J Clin Oncol* 1999;17:3835.
55. Loken M, Shah V, Datilio K, et al. Flow cytometric analysis of human bone marrow: I. Normal erythroid development. *Blood* 1987;70:1316.
56. Terstappen L, Huang S, Picker L. Flow cytometric assessment of human T-cell differentiation in thymus and bone marrow. *Blood* 1992;79:666.
57. Terstappen L, Safford M, Loken M. Flow cytometric analysis of human bone marrow: III. Neutrophil development. *Leukemia* 1990;4:657.
58. Terstappen L. Cell differentiation and maturation in normal bone marrow and acute leukaemia. In: *Flow cytometry clinical applications.* Oxford: Blackwell Science, 1995:101.
59. Reading C, Estey E, Huh Y, et al. Expression of unusual immunophenotype combinations in acute myelogenous leukemia. *Blood* 1993;81:3083.
60. San Miguel J, Martinez A, Macedo A, et al. Immunophenotyping investigation of minimal residual disease is a useful approach for predicting relapse in acute myeloid leukemia patients. *Blood* 1997;90:2465.
61. Greaves M, Chan L, Furley A, et al. Lineage promiscuity in hematopoietic differentiation and leukemia. *Blood* 1986;67:1.
62. Syrjälä M, Anttila V-J, Ruutu T, Jansson S-E. Flow cytometric detection of residual disease in acute leukemia by assaying blasts co-expressing myeloid tic antigens. *Leukemia* 1994;8:1564.
63. Campana D, Pui C-H. Detection of minimal residual disease in acute leukemia: methodologic advances and clinical significance. *Blood* 1995;8:1416.
64. Ferrara F, Del Vecchio L. Clinical relevance of acute mixed-lineage leukemias. *Leukemia Lymphoma* 1993;12:11.
65. Rowley J. Recurring chromosome abnormalities in leukemia and lymphoma. *Semin Hematol* 1990;27:122.
66. Yoeh E, Ross M, Shurtleff S, et al. Classification subtype discovery, and prediction of outcome in pediatric lymphoblastic leukemia by gene expression profiling. *Cancer Cell* 2002;1:133.
67. Scandura J, Boccuni P, Cammenga J, et al. Transcription factor fusions in acute leukemia: variations on a theme. *Oncogene* 2002;21:3422.
68. Gilliland D. Molecular genetics of human leukemia. *Leukemia* 1998;12:S7.
69. Look A. Oncogenic transcription factors in the human acute leukemias. *Science* 1997;278:1059.
70. Korsmeyer S. Chromosomal translocations in lymphoid malignancies reveal novel protooncogenes. *Annu Rev Immunol* 1992;10:785.
71. Wetzler M, Dodge R, Mrózek K, et al. Prospective karyotype analysis in adult acute lymphoblastic leukemia: the cancer and leukemia group B experience. *Blood* 1999;93:3983.
72. Dabaja B, Faderl S, Thomas D, et al. Deletions and losses in chromosomes 5 or 7 in adult acute lymphocytic leukemia: incidence, associations and implications. *Leukemia* 1999;13:869.

73. Mrózek K, Heinonen K, de la Chapelle A, et al. Clinical significance of cytogenetics in acute myeloid leukemia. *Semin Oncol* 1997;24:17.
74. Miller W Jr, Levine K, DeBlasio A, et al. Detection of minimal residual disease in acute promyelocytic leukemia by reverse transcription polymerase chain reaction assay for the PML/RARα fusion mRNA. *Blood* 1993;82:1689.
75. Koeffler H. Syndromes of acute nonlymphocytic leukemia. *Ann Intern Med* 1987;107:748.
76. Levine E, Bloomfield C. Leukemias and myelodysplastic syndromes secondary to drug, radiation, and environmental exposure. *Semin Oncol* 1992;19:47.
77. Rubin C, Arthur D, Woods W, et al. Therapy-related myelodysplastic syndrome and acute myeloid leukemia in children: correlation between chromosomal abnormalities and prior therapy. *Blood* 1991;78:2982.
78. Pedersen-Bjergaard J, Philip P. Two different classes of therapy related and de-novo acute myeloid leukemia. *Cancer Genet Cytogenet* 1991;55:119.
79. Brinker H. Estimates of overall treatment results in acute non-lymphocytic leukemia based on age-specific rates of incidence and of complete remission. *Cancer Treat Rep* 1985;69:5.
80. Rowe J. Current standard therapy of adult acute myeloid leukemia. In: *American Society of Hematology education book.* American Society of Hematology, 2001:62.
81. Byrd J, Mrózek K, Dodge R, et al. Pretreatment cytogenetic abnormalities are predictive of induction success, cumulative incidence of relapse, and overall survival in adult patients with de novo acute myeloid leukemia: results from Cancer and Leukemia Group B (CAMGB 8461). *Blood* 2002;100:4325.
82. Skipper H, Schabel F, Jay R, et al. Experimental evaluation of potential antitumor agents: on the criteria and kinetics associated with curability of experimental leukemia. *Cancer Treat Rep* 1974;4:137.
83. Anastasi J, Vardiman J, Rudinsky R, et al. Direct correlation of cytogenetic findings with morphology using in situ hybridization: An analysis of suspicious cells in bone marrow specimens of two patients completing therapy for acute lymphoblastic leukemia. *Blood* 1991;77:2456.
84. Ryan D. Detection of minimal residual disease by flow cytometry. In: Bauer DR, Shankey TV, eds. *Clinical flow cytometry. Principles and application.* Baltimore: Williams & Wilkins, 1993:479.
85. Estey E, Keating M, McCredie K, et al. Causes of initial remission failure in acute myelogenous leukemia. *Blood* 1982;60:309.
86. Cheson B, Cassileth P, Head D, et al. Report of the National Cancer Institute sponsored workshop on definitions of diagnosis and response to acute myeloid leukemia. *J Clin Oncol* 1990;8:813.
87. Freireich E, Cork A, Stass S, et al. Cytogenetics for detection of minimal residual disease in acute myeloblastic leukemia. *Leukemia* 1992;6:500.
88. Mortuza F, Papaioannou M, Moreira I, et al. Minimal residual disease tests provide an independent predictor of clinical outcome in adult acute lymphoblastic leukemia. *J Clin Oncol* 2002;20:1094.
89. Sievers E, Larson R, Stadtmauer E, et al. Efficacy and safety of gemtuzumab ozogamicin in patients with CD33-positive acute myeloid leukemia in first relapse. *J Clin Oncol* 2001; 19:3244.
90. Bloomfield C. Post-remission therapy in acute myeloid leukemia. *J Clin Oncol* 1985;3:1470.
91. Hughes W, Armstrong D, Bodey G, et al. 2002 Guidelines for the use of antimicrobial agents in neutropenic patients with cancer. *CID* 2002;34:730.
92. Walsh T, Finberg R, Arndt C, et al. Liposomal amphotericin B for empirical therapy in patients with persistent fever and neutropenia. *N Engl J Med* 1999;340:764.
93. Winston D, Hathom J, Schuster M, et al. A multicenter, randomized trial of fluconazole versus amphotericin B for empiric antifungal therapy of febrile neutropenic patients with cancer. *Am J Med* 2000;108:282.
94. Boogaerts M, Winston D, Bow E, et al. Intravenous and oral itraconazole versus intravenous amphotericin B deoxycholate as empirical antifungal therapy for persistent fever in neutropenic patients with cancer who are receiving broad-spectrum antibacterial therapy. A randomized, controlled trial. *Ann Intern Med* 2001;135:412.
95. Aliff T, Maslak P, Jurcic J, et al. Refractory *Aspergillus* pneumonia in patients with acute leukemia: successful therapy with combination caspofungin and liposomal amphotericin. *Cancer* 2003;97:1025.
96. Walsh T, Pappas P, Winston D, et al. Voriconazole compared with liposomal amphotericin B for empirical antifungal therapy in patients with neutropenia and persistent fever. *N Engl J Med* 2002;346:225.
97. Hathorn J. Critical appraisal of antimicrobials for prevention of infections in immunocompromised hosts. *Hematol Oncol Clin North Am* 1993;7:1051.
98. Strauss R. Therapeutic granulocyte transfusions in 1993. *Blood* 1993;81:1675.
99. Ohno R, Tomonaga M, Kobayashi T, et al. Effect of granulocyte colony-stimulating factor after intensive induction therapy in relapsed or refractory acute leukemia. *N Engl J Med* 1990;323:871.
100. Rowe J, Andersen J, Mazza J, et al. A randomized placebo-controlled phase III study of granulocyte-macrophage colony-stimulating factor in adult patients (>55 to 70 years of age) with acute myelogenous leukemia: a study of the Eastern Cooperative Oncology Group (E1490). *Blood* 1995;86:457.
101. Dombret H, Chastang C, Fenaux P, et al. A controlled study of recombinant human granulocyte colony-stimulating factor in elderly patients after treatment for acute myelogenous leukemia. *N Engl J Med* 1995;332:1678.
102. Gmur J, Burger J, Schanz U, et al. Safety of stringent prophylactic platelet transfusion policy for patients with acute leukemia. *Lancet* 1991;338:1223.
103. Beutler E. Platelet transfusions: the 20,000 μL trigger. *Blood* 1993;81:1411.
104. Tallman M, Kwaan H. Reassessing the hemostatic disorder associated with acute promyelocytic leukemia. *Blood* 1992;79:543.
105. Goldberg M, Ginsburg D, Mayer R, et al. Is heparin administration necessary during induction chemotherapy for patients with acute promyelocytic leukemia? *Blood* 1987;69:187.
106. O'Regan S, Carson S, Chesney R, et al. Electrolyte and acid base disturbances in the management of leukemia. *Blood* 1977;49:345.
107. Keating A, Baker M. Effect of exclusion criteria on interpretation of clinical outcome in AML. In: Gale RP, Ash RC, Champlin RE, et al., eds. *Acute myelogenous leukemia: Progress and controversies.* New York: Wiley-Liss: 1990:235.
108. Keating M, Smith T, Kantarjian H, et al. Cytogenetic pattern in acute myelogenous leukemia: a major reproducible determinant of outcome. *Leukemia* 1988;2:403.
109. Slovak M, Kopecky K, Cassileth P, et al. Karyotypic analysis predicts outcome of preremission and postremission therapy in adult acute myeloid leukemia: a Southwest Oncology Group/Eastern Cooperative Oncology Group study. *Blood* 2000;96:4075.
110. Yates J, Gildewell O, Wiernik P, et al. Cytosine arabinoside with daunorubicin or adriamycin for therapy of acute myelocytic leukemia: A CALGB study. *Blood* 1982;60:454.
111. Rai K, Holland J, Glidewell O, et al. Treatment of acute myelocytic leukemia: a study by Cancer and Leukemia Group B. *Blood* 1981;58:1203.
112. Gajewski J, Ho W, Nimer S, et al. Efficacy of intensive chemotherapy for acute myelogenous leukemia associated with a preleukemic syndrome. *J Clin Oncol* 1989;7:1637.
113. Gilliland D, Griffin J. The roles of FLT3 in hematopoiesis and leukemia. *Blood* 2002;100:1532.
114. Carey R, Ribas-Mundo M, Ellison R, et al. Comparative study of cytosine arabinoside therapy alone and combined with thioguanine, mercaptopurine, or daunorubicin in acute myelocytic leukemia. *Cancer* 1975;36:1560.
115. Yates J, Wallace H Jr, Ellison R, et al. Cytosine arabinoside (NSC 63878) and daunorubicin (NSC 83142) therapy in acute nonlymphocytic leukemia. *Cancer Chemother Rep* 1973;57:485.
116. Preisler H, Davis R, Kirshner J, et al. Comparison of three remission induction regimens and two post-induction strategies for the treatment of acute nonlymphocytic leukemia: a Cancer and Leukemia Group B study. *Blood* 1987;9:1441.
117. Dillman R, David R, Green M, et al. A comparative study of two different doses of cytarabine for acute myeloid leukemia: a phase III trial of cancer and Leukemia Group B. *Blood* 1991;78:2520.
118. Bishop J, Lowenthal R, Joshua D, et al. Etoposide in acute nonlymphocytic leukemia. *Blood* 1990;75:27.
119. Berman E, Heller G, Santorsa J, et al. Results of a randomized trial comparing idarubicin and cytosine arabinoside with daunorubicin and cytosine arabinoside in adult patients with newly diagnosed acute myelogenous leukemia. *Blood* 1991;77:1666.
120. Vogler W, Velez-Garcia E, Weiner R, et al. A phase III trial comparing idarubicin and daunorubicin in combination with cytarabine in acute myelogenous leukemia: a Southeastern cancer study group study. *J Clin Oncol* 1992;10:1103.
121. Wiernik P, Banks P, Case J, et al. Cytarabine plus idarubicin or daunorubicin as induction and consolidation therapy for previously untreated adult patients with acute myeloid leukemia. *Blood* 1992;79:313.
122. Berman E, Wiernick P, Vogler R, et al. Long-term follow-up of three randomized trials comparing idarubicin and daunorubicin as induction therapies for patients with untreated acute myeloid leukemia. *Cancer* 1997;80:2181.
123. Rowe J, Neuberg D, Friedenberg W, et al. A phase III study of three induction regimens and of priming with GM-CSF in older adults with acute myeloid leukemia: a trial by the Eastern Cooperative Oncology Group. *Blood* 2004;103:429.
124. Gale R, Cline M. High remission induction rate in acute myeloid leukaemia. *Lancet* 1977;1:497.
125. Bolwell B, Cassileth P, Gale R. High dose cytarabine: a review. *Leukemia* 1988;2:253.
126. Schiller G, Gajewski J, Nimer S, et al. A randomized study of intermediate versus conventional-dose cytarabine as intensive induction for acute myelogenous leukaemia. *Br J Haematol* 1992;81:170.
127. Bishop J, Matthews J, Young G, et al. High dose cytosine arabinoside (Ara-C) in induction prolongs remission in acute myeloid leukemia (AML): updated results of a randomized phase III trial. *Blood* 1996;87:1710.
128. Weick J, Kopecky K, Appelbaum F, et al. A randomized investigation of high-dose versus standard-dose cytosine arabinoside with daunorubicin in patients with previously untreated acute myeloid leukemia: a Southwest Oncology Group study. *Blood* 1996;88:2841.
129. Stone R, Berg D, George S, et al. Granulocyte-macrophage colony-stimulating factor after initial chemotherapy for elderly patients with primary acute myelogenous leukemia. *N Engl J Med* 1995;332:1671.
130. Heil G, Hoelzer D, Sanz M, et al. A randomized, double-blind, placebo-controlled, phase III study of filgrastim in remission induction and consolidation therapy for adults with de novo acute myeloid leukemia. *Blood* 1997;90:4710.
131. Godwin J, Kopecky K, Head D, et al. A double-blind placebo-controlled trial of granulocyte colony-stimulating factor in elderly patients with previously untreated acute myeloid leukemia: a Southwest Oncology Group study (9031). *Blood* 1998;91:3607.
132. Witz F, Sadoun A, Perrin M, et al. A placebo-controlled study of recombinant human granulocyte-macrophage colony-stimulating factor administered during and after induction treatment for de novo acute myelogenous leukemia in elderly patients. Groupe Ouest Est Leucemies Aigues Myeloblastiques (GOELAM). *Blood* 1998;91:2722.
133. Clavio M, Quintino S, Moasoudi B, et al. Cost of de novo acute myeloid leukemia induction therapy in adults: analysis of EORTC-GIMEMA AML10 and FLANG regimens. *J Exp Clin Cancer Res* 2001;20:165.
134. Lowenberg B, van Putten W, Theobald M, et al. Effect of priming with granulocyte colony-stimulating factor on the outcome of chemotherapy for acute myeloid leukemia. *N Engl J Med* 2003;349:743.
135. Buchner T, Urbanitz D, Hiddemann W, et al. Intensified induction and consolidation with and without maintenance chemotherapy for acute myeloid leukemia: two multicenter studies of the German AML Cooperative Group. *J Clin Oncol* 1985;3:1583.
136. Cassileth P, Harrington D, Hines J, et al. Maintenance chemotherapy prolongs remission duration in adult acute nonlymphocytic leukemia. *J Clin Oncol* 1988;6:583.
137. Cassileth P, Begg C, Bennett J, et al. A randomized study of the efficacy of consolidation therapy in adult acute nonlymphocytic leukemia. *Blood* 1984;63:843.
138. Sauter C, Berchtold W, Foop M, et al. Acute myelogenous leukemia: Maintenance chemotherapy after early consolidation does not prolong survival. *Lancet* 1984:1:379.

139. Cassileth P, Lynch E, Hines J, et al. Varying intensity of postremission therapy in acute myeloid leukemia. *Blood* 1992;79:1924.
140. Fenaux P, Chastang C, Chevret S, et al. A randomized comparison of all trans retinoic acid (ATRA) followed by chemotherapy and ATRA plus chemotherapy and the role of maintenance therapy in newly diagnosed acute promyelocytic leukemia. The European APL Group. *Blood* 1999;94:1192.
141. Mayer R, David R, Schiffer C, et al. Intensive postremission chemotherapy in adults with acute myeloid leukemia. *N Engl J Med* 1994;331:896.
142. Bloomfield C, Lawrence D, Byrd J, et al. Frequency of prolonged remission duration after high-dose cytarabine intensification in acute myeloid leukemia varies by cytogenetic subtype. *Cancer Res* 1998;58:4173.
143. Sullivan K, Weiden P, Storb R, et al. Influence of acute and chronic graft-versus-host disease on relapse and survival after bone marrow transplantation from HLA-identical siblings as treatment of acute and chronic leukemia. *Blood* 1989;73:1720.
144. Horowitz M, Gale R, Sondel P, et al. Graft-versus-leukemia reactions after bone marrow transplantation. *Blood* 1990;75:555.
145. Giralt S, Estey E, Albitar M, et al. Engraftment of allogeneic hematopoietic progenitor cells with purine analog–containing chemotherapy: harnessing graft-versus-leukemia without myeloablative therapy. *Blood* 1997;89:4531.
146. Stockerl-Goldstein K, Blume K. Allogeneic hematopoietic cell transplantation for adult patients with acute myeloid leukemia. In: Thomas E, Blume KG, Forman SJ, eds. *Hematopoietic cell transplantation.* Malden, MA: Blackwell Science, 1999:823.
147. Berman E, Little C, Gee T, et al. Reasons that patients with acute myelogenous leukemia do not undergo allogeneic bone marrow transplantation. *N Engl J Med* 1992;326:156.
148. Sierra J, Storer B, Hansen J, et al. Unrelated donor marrow transplantation for acute myeloid leukemia: an update of the Seattle experience. *Bone Marrow Transplant* 2000;26:397.
149. Petersdorf E, Gooley T, Anasetti C, et al. Optimizing outcome after unrelated marrow transplantation by comprehensive matching of HLA class I and II alleles in the donor and recipient. *Blood* 1998;92:3515.
150. Gorin N-C. Autologous stem cell transplantation for adult acute leukemia. *Curr Opinion Oncol* 2002;14:152.
151. Brenner M, Rill D, Moen R, et al. Gene-marking to trace origin of relapse after autologous bone-marrow transplantation. *Lancet* 1993;341:85.
152. Gorin N-C, Labopin M, Laporte J-P, et al. Importance of marrow dose on posttransplant outcome in acute leukemia: models derived from patients autografted with mafosfamide-purged marrow at a single institution. *Exp Hematol* 1999;27:1822.
153. Keating S, Sucio S, deWitte T, et al. The stem cell mobilizing capacity of patients with acute myeloid leukemia in complete remission correlates with relapse risk: results of the EORTC-GIMEMA AML-10 trial. *Leukemia* 2003;17:60.
154. Feller N, Schuurhuis G, van der Pol M, et al. High percentage of CD34-positive cells in autologous AML peripheral blood stem cell products reflects inadequate in vivo purging and low chemotherapeutic toxicity in a subgroup of patients with poor clinical outcome. *Leukemia* 2003;17:68.
155. To L, Juttner C. Peripheral blood stem cell autografting: a new therapeutic option for AML. *Br J Haematol* 1987;66:285.
156. To L, Russell J, Moore S, et al. Residual leukemia cannot be detected in very early remission peripheral blood stem cell collections in acute non-lymphoblastic leukemia. *Leuk Res* 1987;11:327.
157. Körbling M, Fliedner T, Holle R, et al. Autologous blood stem cell (ABSCT) versus purged bone marrow transplantation (pABMT) in standard risk AML: influence of source and cell composition of the autograft on hemopoietic reconstitution and disease-free survival. *Bone Marrow Transplant* 1991;7:343.
158. Stein A, O'Donnell M, Chai A, et al. In vivo purging with high-dose cytarabine followed by high dose chemoradiotherapy and reinfusion of unpurged bone marrow for adult acute myelogenous leukemia in first complete remission. *J Clin Oncol* 1996;14:2206.
159. Burnett A, Goldstone A, Stevens R, et al. Randomized comparison of addition of autologous bone-marrow transplantation to intensive chemotherapy for acute myeloid leukaemia in first remission: Results of MRC AML 10 trial. *Lancet* 1998;351:700.
160. Zittoun R, Mandelli F, Willemze R, et al. Autologous or allogeneic bone marrow transplantation compared with intensive chemotherapy in acute myelogenous leukemia. *N Engl J Med* 1995;332:217.
161. Baron F, Gothot A, Salmon J-P, et al. Clinical course and predictive factors for cyclosporin-induced autologous graft-versus-host disease after autologous haematopoietic stem cell transplantation. *Br J Haematol* 2000;111:745.
162. Stein A, O'Donnell M, Slovak M, et al. Interleukin-2 after autologous stem-cell transplantation for adult patients with acute myeloid leukemia in first complete remission. *J Clin Oncol* 2003;21:615.
163. Tallman M, Rowlings P, Milone G, et al. Effect of postremission chemotherapy before human leukocyte antigen–identical sibling transplantation for acute myelogenous leukemia in first complete remission. *Blood* 2000;96:1254.
164. Harousseau J-L, Cahn J-Y, Pignon B, et al. Comparison of autologous bone marrow transplantation and intensive chemotherapy as postremission therapy in adult acute myeloid leukemia. *Blood* 1997;90:2978.
165. Cassileth P, Harrington D, Appelbaum F, et al. Chemotherapy compared with autologous or allogeneic bone marrow transplantation in the management of acute myeloid leukemia in first remission. *N Engl J Med* 1998;339:1649.
166. Sucio S, Mandelli F, de Witte T, et al. Allogeneic compared with autologous stem cell transplantation in the treatment of patients younger than 46 years with acute myeloid leukemia (AML) in first complete remission (CR1): an intention-to-treat analysis of the EORTC/GIMEMA AML-10 trial. *Blood* 2003;102:1232.
167. Schiffman K, Clift R, Appelbaum F, et al. Consequences of cryopreserving first remission autologous marrow for use after relapse in patients with acute myeloid leukemia. *Bone Marrow Transplant* 1993;11:227.
168. Clift R, Buckner C, Appelbaum F, et al. Allogeneic marrow transplantation during untreated first relapse of acute myeloid leukemia. *J Clin Oncol* 1992;10:1723.
169. Keating M, Kantarjian H, Smith T, et al. Response to salvage therapy and survival after relapse in acute myelogenous leukemia. *J Clin Oncol* 1989;7:1071.
170. Petersen F, Lynch M, Clift R, et al. Autologous marrow transplantation for patients with acute myeloid leukemia in untreated first relapse or in second complete remission. *J Clin Oncol* 1993;11:1353.
171. Hiddemann W, Martin W, Sauerland C, et al. Definition of refractoriness against conventional chemotherapy in acute myeloid leukemia: a proposal based on the results of retreatment by thioguanine, cytosine arabinoside, and daunorubicin (TAB 9) in 150 patients with relapse after standardized first line therapy. *Leukemia* 1990;4:184.
172. Vey N, Keating M, Giles F, et al. Effect of complete remission on survival in patients with acute myelogenous leukemia receiving first salvage therapy. *Blood* 1999;93:3149.
173. Maslak P, Hegewisch-Becker S, Godfrey L, et al. Flow cytometric determination of the multi-drug resistant phenotype in acute leukemia. *Cytometry* 1994;17:84.
174. Leith C, Kopecky K, Godwin J, et al. Acute myeloid leukemia in the elderly: assessment of multidrug resistance (MDR1) and cytogenetics distinguishes biologic subgroups with remarkably distinct responses to standard chemotherapy. A Southwest Oncology Group study. *Blood* 1997;89:3323.
175. Leith C, Chen I-M, Kopecky K, et al. Correlation of multidrug resistance (MDR1) protein expression with functional dye/drug efflux in acute myeloid leukemia my multiparameter flow cytometry: identification of discordant CD34+/MDR1–/efflux+ and MDR1+/efflux– cases. *Blood* 1995;86:2329.
176. Filipits M, Suchomel R, Zochbauer S, et al. Multidrug resistance associated protein in acute myeloid leukemia: no impact on treatment outcome. *Clin Cancer Res* 1997;3:1419.
177. Filipits M, Pohl G, Stranzl T, et al. Expression of the lung resistance protein predicts poor outcome in de novo acute myeloid leukemia. *Blood* 1998;91:1508.
178. Baer M, George S, Dodge R, et al. Phase 3 study of the multidrug resistance modulator PSC-833 in previously untreated patients 60 years of age and older with acute myeloid leukemia: Cancer and Leukemia Group B study 9720. *Blood* 2002;100:1224.
179. Forman S, Schmidt G, Nademanee A, et al. Allogeneic bone marrow transplantation as therapy for primary induction failure for patients with acute leukemia. *J Clin Oncol* 1991;9:1570.
180. Brown R, Herzig R, Wolff S, et al. High-dose etoposide and cyclophosphamide without bone marrow transplantation for resistant hematologic malignancy. *Blood* 1990;76:473.
181. Sievers E, Appelbaum F, Spielberger R, et al. Selective ablation of acute myeloid leukemia using antibody-targeted chemotherapy: A phase I study of an anti-CD33 calicheamicin immunoconjugate. *Blood* 1999;93:3678.
182. Bross P, Beitz J, Chen G, et al. Approval summary: gemtuzumab ozogamicin in relapsed acute myeloid leukemia. *Clin Cancer Res* 2001;7:1490.
183. Giles F, Kantarjian H, Kornblau S, et al. Mylotarg (gemtuzumab ozogamicin) therapy is associated with hepatic venoocclusive disease in patients who have not received stem cell transplantation. *Cancer* 2001;92:406.
184. Kumar L. Leukemia: management of relapse after allogeneic bone marrow transplantation. *J Clin Oncol* 1994;12:1710.
185. Kolb H-J, Schattenberg A, Goldman J, et al. Graft-versus-leukemia effect of donor lymphocyte transfusions in marrow grafted patients. *Blood* 1995;86:2041.
186. Levine J, Braun T, Penza S, et al. Prospective trial of chemotherapy and donor leukocyte infusions for relapse of advanced myeloid malignancies after allogeneic stem-cell transplantation. *J Clin Oncol* 2002;20:405.
187. Ruggeri L, Capanni M, Urbani E, et al. Effectiveness of donor natural killer cell alloreactivity in mismatched hematopoietic transplants. *Science* 2002;295:2097.
188. Kantarjian H, Keating M, Walters R, et al. Acute promyelocytic leukemia: M. D. Anderson Hospital experience. *Am J Med* 1986;80:789.
189. Head D, Kopecky K, Weick J, et al. Effect of aggressive daunomycin therapy on survival in acute promyelocytic leukemia. *Blood* 1995;86:1717.
190. Huang M, Ye Y, Chen S, et al. Use of all-trans retinoic acid in the treatment of acute promyelocytic leukemia. *Blood* 1988;72:567.
191. Degos L, Dombret H, Chomienne C, et al. All-trans retinoic acid as a differentiating agent in the treatment of acute promyelocytic leukemia. *Blood* 1995;85:2643.
192. Warrell R Jr. Differentiation therapy of acute promyelocytic leukemia with tretinoin (all-trans-retinoic acid). *N Engl J Med* 1991;324:1385.
193. Frankel S, Eardley A, Lauwers G, et al. The "retinoic acid syndrome" in acute promyelocytic leukemia. *Ann Intern Med* 1992;117:292.
194. DiBona E, Avvisati G, Castaman G, et al. Early haemorrhagic morbidity and mortality during remission induction with or without all-trans retinoic acid in acute promyelocytic leukaemia. *Br J Haematol* 2000;108:689.
195. Stadler M, Ganser A, Hoelzer D. Acute promyelocytic leukemia. *N Engl J Med* 1994; 330:140.
196. Castaigne S, Chomienne C, Daniel M, et al. All-trans retinoic acid as a differentiation therapy for acute promyelocytic leukemia. I. Clinical results. *Blood* 1990;76:1704.
197. Mandelli F, Diverio D, Avvisati G, et al. Molecular remission in PML/RARα-positive acute promyelocytic leukemia by combined all-trans retinoic acid and idarubicin (AIDA) therapy. *Blood* 1997;90:1014.
198. Warrell R, Maslak P, Eardley A, et al. Treatment of acute promyelocytic leukemia with all-trans retinoic acid: An update of the New York experience. *Leukemia* 1994;8:929.
199. Vahdat L, Maslak P, Miller W Jr, et al. Early mortality and the retinoic acid syndrome in acute promyelocytic leukemia: impact of leukocytosis, low-dose chemotherapy, PML/RARα isoform, and CD13 expression in patients treated with all-trans retinoic acid. *Blood* 1994;8:3843.
200. Tallman M, Andersen J, Schiffer C, et al. Clinical description of 44 patients with acute promyelocytic leukemia who developed the retinoic acid syndrome. *Blood* 2000;95:90.
201. Wiley I, Firkin F. Reduction of pulmonary toxicity by prednisolone prophylaxis during all-trans retinoic acid treatment of acute promyelocytic leukemia. *Leukemia* 1995;9:774.

202. Burnett A, Grimwade D, Solomon E, et al. Presenting white blood cell count and kinetics of molecular remission predict prognosis in acute promyelocytic leukemia treated with all-trans retinoic acid: result of the randomized MRC trial. *Blood* 1999;93:4131.

203. Miller W Jr, Kakizuka A, Frankel S, et al. Reverse transcription polymerase chain reaction for the rearranged retinoic acid receptor clarifies diagnosis and detects minimal residual disease in acute promyelocytic leukemia. *Proc Natl Acad Sci U S A* 1992;89:2694.

204. Jurcic J, Nimer S, Scheinberg D, et al. Prognostic significance of minimal residual disease detection and PML/RAR-α isoform type: long-term follow-up in acute promyelocytic leukemia. *Blood* 2001;98:2651.

205. LoCoco F, Diverio D, Avvisati G, et al. Therapy of molecular relapse in acute promyelocytic leukemia. *Blood* 1999;94:2225.

206. Soignet S, Maslak P, Wang Z-G, et al. Complete remission after treatment of acute promyelocytic leukemia with arsenic trioxide. *N Engl J Med* 1998;339:1341.

207. Soignet S, Frankel S, Douer D, et al. United States multicenter study of arsenic trioxide in relapsed acute promyelocytic leukemia. *J Clin Oncol* 2001;19:3852.

208. Meloni G, Diverio D, Vignetti M, et al. Autologous bone marrow transplantation for acute promyelocytic leukemia in second remission: prognostic relevance of pretransplant minimal residual disease by reverse-transcription polymerase chain reaction of the PML/RARα fusion gene. *Blood* 1997;90:1321.

209. Rivera G, Pinkel D, Simone J, et al. Treatment of acute lymphoblastic leukemia: 30 years' experience at St. Jude Children's Research Hospital. *N Engl J Med* 1993;329:1289.

210. Hoelzer D, Thiel E, Löffler H, et al. Acute lymphoblastic leukemia—progress in children, less in adults. *N Engl J Med* 1993;329:1343.

211. Boissel N, Auclerc M-F, Lheritier V, et al. Should adolescents with acute lymphoblastic leukemia be treated as old children or young adults? Comparison of the French FRALLE-93 and LALA-94 trials. *J Clin Oncol* 2003;21:774.

212. Stock W, Sather H, Dodge R, et al. Outcome of adolescents and young adults with ALL: a comparison of Children's Cancer Group (CCG) and Cancer and Leukemia Group B (CALGB) regimens. *Blood* 2000;96:467a.

213. Hoelzer D, Thiel E, Löffler H, et al. Prognostic factors in a multicenter study for treatment of acute lymphoblastic leukemia in adults. *Blood* 1988;71:123.

214. Gaynor J, Chapman D, Little C, et al. A cause-specific hazard rate analysis of prognostic factors among 199 adults with acute lymphoblastic leukemia: the Memorial Hospital experience since 1969. *J Clin Oncol* 1988;6:1014.

215. Boucheix C, David B, Sebban C, et al. Immunophenotype of adult acute lymphoblastic leukemia, clinical parameters and outcome: an analysis of a prospective trial including 562 tested patients (LALA87). *Blood* 1994;84:1603.

216. Barrett A, Horowitz M, Ash R, et al. Bone marrow transplantation for Philadelphia chromosome–positive acute lymphoblastic leukemia. *Blood* 1992;79:3067.

217. Fière D, Extra J, David B, et al. Treatment of 218 adult acute lymphoblastic leukemias. *Semin Oncol* 1987;14:64.

218. Hoelzer D, Thiel E, Löffler H, et al. Intensified therapy in acute lymphoblastic and acute undifferentiated leukemia in adults. *Blood* 1984;64:38.

219. Kantarjian H, Walters R, Keating M, et al. Results of the vincristine, doxorubicin, and dexamethasone regimen in adults with standard- and high-risk acute lymphocytic leukemia. *J Clin Oncol* 1990;8:994.

220. Larson R, Dodge R, Burns C, et al. A five-drug remission induction regimen with intensive consolidation for adults with acute lymphoblastic leukemia: Cancer and Leukemia Group B study 8811. *Blood* 1995;85:2025.

221. Linker C, Levitt L, O'Donnell M, et al. Treatment of adult acute lymphoblastic leukemia with intensive cyclical chemotherapy: a follow-up report. *Blood* 1991;78:2814.

222. Stewart K, Keating A, Sutton D, et al. Adult acute lymphoblastic leukaemia: the value of therapy intensification. *Leukemia Lymphoma* 1991;4:103.

223. Hussein K, Dahlberg D, Head D, et al. Treatment of acute lymphoblastic leukemia in adults with intensive induction, consolidation, and maintenance chemotherapy. *Blood* 1989;73:57.

224. Schauer P, Arlin Z, Mertelsmann R, et al. Treatment of acute lymphoblastic leukemia in adults: results of the L-10 and L-10M protocols. *J Clin Oncol* 1983;1:462.

225. Kantarjian H, O'Brien S, Smith T, et al. Results of treatment with hyper-CVAD, a dose-intensive regimen, in adult acute lymphocytic leukemia. *J Clin Oncol* 2000;18:547.

226. Linker C, Damon L, Ries C, et al. Intensified and shortened cyclical chemotherapy for adult acute lymphoblastic leukemia. *J Clin Oncol* 2002;20:2464.

227. Gottlieb A, Weinbert V, Ellison R, et al. Efficacy of daunorubicin in the therapy of adult acute lymphocytic leukemia: a prospective randomized trial by Cancer and Leukemia Group B. *Blood* 1984;64:267.

228. Preti A, Kantarjian H, Management of adult acute lymphocytic leukemia: present issues and key challenges. *J Clin Oncol* 1994;12:1312.

229. Ellison R, Mick R, Cuttner J, et al. The effects of postinduction intensification treatment with cytarabine and daunorubicin in adult acute lymphocytic leukemia: a prospective randomized clinical trial by Cancer and Leukemia Group B. *J Clin Oncol* 1991;9:2002.

230. Cassileth P, Anderson J, Bennett J, et al. Adult acute lymphocytic leukemia: the Eastern Cooperative Oncology Group experience. *Leukemia* 1992;6:178.

231. Cuttner J, Mick R, Budman D, et al. Phase III trial of brief intensive treatment of adult acute lymphoblastic leukemia comparing daunorubicin and mitoxantrone—a CALGB study. *Leukemia* 1991;5:425.

232. Dekker A, van't Veer M, Sizoo W, et al. Intensive postremission chemotherapy without maintenance therapy in adults with acute lymphoblastic leukemia. Dutch Hemato-Oncology Research Group. *J Clin Oncol* 1997;15:476.

233. Burger B, Zimmerman M, Mann G, et al. Diagnostic cerebrospinal fluid examination in children with acute lymphoblastic leukemia: significance of low leukocyte counts with blasts or traumatic lumbar puncture. *J Clin Oncol* 2003;21:184.

234. Inati A, Sallan S, Cassady J, et al. Efficacy and morbidity of central nervous system "prophylaxis" in childhood acute lymphoblastic leukemia: eight years' experience with cranial irradiation and intrathecal methotrexate. *Blood* 1983;61:297.

235. Omura G, Moffitt S, Vogler W, et al. Combination chemotherapy of adult acute lymphoblastic leukemia with randomized central nervous system prophylaxis. *Blood* 1980;55:199.

236. Ohno R. Current progress in the treatment of adult acute leukemia in Japan. *Jpn J Clin Oncol* 1993;22:85.

237. Weiss M, Maslak P, Feldman E, et al. Cytarabine with high dose mitoxantrone induces rapid complete remissions in adult acute lymphoblastic leukemia (ALL) without the use of vincristine or prednisone. *J Clin Oncol* 1996;14:2480.

238. Capizzi R, Poole M, Cooper M, et al. Treatment of poor risk acute leukemia with sequential high-dose Ara-C and asparaginase. *Blood* 1984;63:694.

239. Amadori S, Papa G, Meloni G, et al. Daunorubicin, cytosine arabinoside and 6-thioguanine (DAT) combination therapy for the treatment of acute nonlymphocytic leukemia. *Leuk Res* 1979;3:147.

240. Wells R, Feusner J, Devney R, et al. Sequential high dose cytosine arabinoside–asparaginase treatment in advanced childhood leukemia. *J Clin Oncol* 1985;3:998.

241. Ishii E, Mara T, Ohkubo K, et al. Treatment of childhood acute lymphoblastic leukemia with intermediate-dose cytosine arabinoside and adriamycin. *Med Pediatr Oncol* 1986;14:73.

242. Giona F, Testi A, Amadori G, et al. Idarubicin and high-dose cytarabine in the treatment of refractory and relapsed acute lymphoblastic leukemia. *Ann Oncol* 1990;1:51.

243. Tan C, Steinherz P, Meyers P. Idarubicin in combination with high-dose cytosine arabinoside in patients with acute leukemia in relapse. *Proc Annu Meet Am Assoc Cancer Res* 1990;31:A1133(abst).

244. Feldman E, Alberts D, Arlin Z, et al. Phase I clinical and pharmacokinetic evaluation of high-dose mitoxantrone in combination with cytarabine in patients with acute leukemia. *J Clin Oncol* 1993;11:2002.

245. Hiddemann W, Kreutzman H, Straif K, et al. High-dose cytosine arabinoside in combination with mitoxantrone for the treatment of refractory acute myeloid and lymphoblastic leukemia. *Semin Oncol* 1987;14:73.

246. Kantarjian H, Walters R, Keating M, et al. Mitoxantrone and high dose cytosine arabinoside for the treatment of refractory acute lymphocytic leukemia. *Cancer* 1990;65:5.

247. Leclerc J, Rivard G, Blanch M, et al. The association of once a day high-dose Ara-C followed by mitoxantrone for three days induces a high rate of complete remission in children with poor prognosis acute leukemia. *Blood* 1988;72[Suppl]:210(abst).

248. Doney K, Fisher L, Appelbaum F, et al. Treatment of adult acute lymphoblastic leukemia with allogeneic bone marrow transplantation. Multivariate analysis of factors affecting acute graft-versus-host disease, relapse, and relapse-free survival. *Bone Marrow Transplant* 1991;7:453.

249. Gale R, Horowitz M, Ash R, et al. Identical-twin bone marrow transplants for leukemia. *Ann Intern Med* 1994;120:646.

250. Weisdorf D, Woods W, Nesbit M Jr, et al. Allogeneic bone marrow transplantation for acute lymphoblastic leukaemia: risk factors and clinical outcome. *Br J Haematol* 1994;86:62.

251. Sebban C, Lepage E, Vernant J-P, et al. Allogeneic bone marrow transplantation in adult acute lymphoblastic leukemia in first complete remission: a comparative study. *J Clin Oncol* 1994;12:2580.

252. Zhang M-J, Hoelzer D, Horowitz M, et al. Long-term follow-up of adults with acute lymphoblastic leukemia in first remission treated with chemotherapy or bone marrow transplantation. *Ann Intern Med* 1995;123:428.

253. Attal M, Blaise D, Marit G, et al. Consolidation treatment of adult acute lymphoblastic leukemia: a prospective, randomized trial comparing allogeneic versus autologous bone marrow transplantation and testing the impact of recombinant interleukin-2 after autologous bone marrow transplant. *Blood* 1995;86:1619.

254. Fière D, Lepage E, Sebban C, et al. Adult acute lymphoblastic leukemia: a multicentric randomized trial testing bone marrow transplantation as postremission therapy. *J Clin Oncol* 1993;11:1990.

255. Soussain C, Patte C, Ostronoff M, et al. Small noncleaved cell lymphoma and leukemia in adults. A retrospective study of 65 adults treated with the LMB pediatric protocols. *Blood* 1995;85:664.

256. Druker B, Talpaz M, Resta D, et al. Efficacy and safety of a specific inhibitor of the BCR-ABL tyrosine kinase in chronic myeloid leukemia. *N Engl J Med* 2001;344:1031.

257. Ottmann O, Druker B, Sawyers C, et al. A phase 2 study of imatinib in patients with relapsed or refractory Philadelphia chromosome–positive acute lymphoid leukemias. *Blood* 2002;100:1965.

258. Hoffman W, Jones J, Lemp N, et al. Ph+ acute lymphoblastic leukemia resistant to the tyrosine kinase inhibitor STI571 has a unique BCR-ABL gene mutation. *Blood* 2002;99:1860.

259. Hofman W-K, Komor M, Wassmann B, et al. Presence of the BCR-ABL mutation Glu255Lys prior to STI571 (imatinib) treatment in patients with Ph+ acute lymphoblastic leukemia. *Blood* 2003;102:659.

260. Byrd J, Edenfield W, Shields D, et al. Extramedullary myeloid cell tumors in acute nonlymphocytic leukemia: a clinical review. *J Clin Oncol* 1995;13:1800.

261. Byrd J, Weiss R, Arthur D, et al. Extramedullary leukemia adversely affects hematologic complete remission rate and overall survival in patients with t(8;21) (q22;q22): results from Cancer and Leukemia Group B 8461. *Blood* 1999;93:2143.

262. Baer M, Barcos M, Farrell H, et al. Acute myelogenous leukemia with leukemia cutis. *Cancer* 1989;63:2192.

263. Cassileth P, Sylvester L, Bennett J, et al. High peripheral blast counts in adult acute myelogenous leukemia is a primary risk factor for CNS leukemia. *J Clin Oncol* 1988;6:495.

264. Holmes R, Keating MJ, Cork A. A unique pattern of central nervous system leukemia in acute myelomonocytic leukemia associated with inv(16) (p13q22). *Blood* 1985;65:1071.

265. McKee LJ, Collins R. Intravascular leucocyte thrombi and aggregates as a course of morbidity and mortality in leukemia. *Medicine* 1974;52:463.

266. Schiffer C. Interferon studies in the treatment of patients with leukemia. *Semin Oncol* 1995;18:1.

267. Caron P, Scheinberg D. Immunotherapy for acute leukemias. *Curr Opinion Oncol* 1994;6:715.

268. Jurcic J, Scheinberg D. Recent developments in the radioimmunotherapy of cancer. *Curr Opinion Immunol* 1994;6:715.

269. Meyers J, Flournoy N, Sanders J, et al. Prophylactic use of human leukocyte interferon after allogeneic marrow transplantation. *Ann Intern Med* 1987;107:809.

270. Foa R. Does interleukin-2 have a role in the management of acute leukemia? *J Clin Oncol* 1993;11:1817.

271. Soiffer R, Murray C, Gonin R, et al. Effect of low-dose interleukin-2 on disease relapse after T-cell–depleted allogeneic bone marrow transplantation. *Blood* 1994;84:964.

272. Maslak P, Weiss M, Berman E, et al. Granulocyte colony stimulating factor following chemotherapy in elderly patients with newly diagnosed acute myelogenous leukemia. *Leukemia* 1996;10:32.

273. Lotzová E, Savary C, Herberman R. Induction of NK cell activity against fresh human leukemia in culture with interleukin 2. *J Immunol* 1987;138:2718.

274. Meloni G, Foa R, Vignetti M, et al. Interleukin-2 may induce prolonged remissions in advanced acute myelogenous leukemia. *Blood* 1994;84:2158.

275. Benyunes M, Massumoto A, Higuchi C, et al. Interleukin-2 with or without lymphokine-activated killer cells as consolidative immunotherapy after autologous bone marrow transplantation for acute myelogenous leukemia. *Bone Marrow Transplant* 1993;12:159.

276. Kossman S, Scheinberg D, Jurcic J, et al. A phase I trial of humanized monoclonal antibody HuM195 (anti-CD33) with low dose interleukin-2 (IL-2) in acute myelogenous leukemia. *Clin Cancer Res* 1999;5:2748.

277. Caron P, Dumont L, Scheinberg D. Super-saturating infusional humanized anti-CD33 monoclonal antibody HuM195 in myelogenous leukemia. *Clin Cancer Res* 1998;4:1421.

278. Jurcic J, Larson S, Sgouros G, et al. Targeted α particle immunotherapy for myeloid leukemia. *Blood* 2002;100:1233.

279. Jurcic J, DeBlasio T, Dumont L, et al. Molecular remission induction with retinoic acid and anti-CD33 monoclonal antibody HuM195 in acute promyelocytic leukemia. *Clin Cancer Res* 2000;6:372.

280. Jurcic J, DeBlasio T, Dumont L, et al. Molecular remission induction without relapse and after anti-CD33 antibody in APL. 1998. *Clin Cancer Res* 2000;18:2620.

281. Schwartz MA, Lovett D, Redner A, et al. A dose-escalation trial of M195 labeled with iodine 131 for cytoreduction and marrow ablation in relapsed or refractory myeloid leukemias. *J Clin Oncol* 1993;11:294.

282. Matthews D, Appelbaum F, Eary J, et al. Development of a marrow transplant regimen for acute leukemia using targeted hematopoietic irradiation delivered by 131I-labeled anti-CD45 antibody combined with cyclophosphamide and total body irradiation. *Blood* 1995;85:1122.

283. Selvaggi K, Wilson J, Mills L, et al. Improved outcome for high-risk acute myeloid leukemia patients using autologous bone marrow transplantation and monoclonal antibody–purged bone marrow. *Blood* 1994;83:1698.

284. Pinilla-Ibarz J, Cathcart K, Korontsvit T, et al. Vaccination of patients with chronic myelogenous leukemia with bcr-abl oncogene breakpoint fusion peptides generates specific immune responses. *Blood* 2000;95:1781.

285. Molldrem J, Dermine S, Parker K, et al. Targeted T-cell therapy for human leukemia: cytotoxic T lymphocytes specific for a peptide derived from proteinase 3 peptide preferentially lyse human myeloid leukemia cells. *Blood* 1996;88:2450.

286. Claxton D, McMannis J, Champlin R, et al. Therapeutic potential of leukemia-derived dendritic cells: preclinical and clinical progress. *Crit Rev Immunol* 2001;21:147.

287. Lancet J, Karp J. Farnesyltransferase inhibitors in hematologic malignancies: new horizons in therapy. *Blood* 2003;17:123.

288. Levis M, Small D. FLT3: ITDoes matter in leukemia. *Leukemia* 2003;17:1738.

289. Campos L, Sabido O, Rouault J, Guyotat D. Effects of BCL-2 antisense oligodeoxynucleotides on in vitro proliferation and survival of normal marrow progenitors and leukemic cells. *Blood* 1994;84:595.

290. Ravandi F, Talpaz M, Kantargian H, et al. Cellular signaling pathways: new targets in leukaemia therapy. *Br J Haematol* 2002;116:57.

CHAPTER **43**

Chronic Leukemias

SECTION **1**

BRIAN J. DRUKER
STEPHANIE J. LEE

Chronic Myelogenous Leukemia

Chronic myelogenous leukemia (CML; also called *chronic myeloid leukemia* or *chronic granulocytic leukemia*) is a clonal hematopoietic disorder caused by an acquired genetic defect in a pluripotent stem cell. CML behaves as a bi- or triphasic illness, with most patients diagnosed in a relatively indolent chronic or stable phase that is characterized by excessive numbers of myeloid lineage cells with full maturation. After an average of 4 to 6 years, a more aggressive, advanced phase intervenes, with a malignant clone losing the capacity for terminal differentiation. The advanced phase can be further subdivided into an accelerated phase and a blastic phase, with survival in the blastic phase measured in months.

Treatment options for patients with CML include allogeneic stem cell transplantation (SCT) and a variety of nontransplant therapies. CML has been the leading indication for SCT, which is the only proven curative therapeutic option. However, SCT is associated with substantial morbidity and mortality. Although treatments for CML were, historically, based empirically, this disease has become a paradigm for understanding leukemogenesis and targeted drug development. It is now known that the BCR-ABL protein, which results from a balanced, reciprocal translocation involving chromosomes 9 and 22, functions as a constitutively activated tyrosine kinase and has a central role in the pathogenesis of CML. Knowledge of the molecular pathogenesis led to the development of imatinib mesylate (Gleevec, Glivec, formerly STI 571), a

drug that specifically inhibits the BCR-ABL tyrosine kinase.[1] Imatinib is now the treatment of choice for patients who are not undergoing allogeneic SCT. Integration of the various treatment modalities is a controversial and evolving issue.

EPIDEMIOLOGY

CML accounts for approximately 15% of all leukemias, with 4000 to 5000 new cases diagnosed in the United States annually. The incidence of CML is 1.6 to 2.0 cases per 100,000 persons per year, and the incidence is similar in all countries worldwide.[2] Although CML occurs in all age groups, its incidence increases with each decade of life, making it mainly a disease of adults. According to the Surveillance, Epidemiology, and End Results (SEER) program, the median age at diagnosis is 66 years,[2] which is much higher than reported in single-institutional series. The disease has a slight male predominance (2.2:1.3).[2]

The only known risk factor for development of CML is exposure to radiation in high doses. This is evident from studies of survivors of the atom bomb explosions in Japan in 1945 and from follow-up of patients treated with radiation for ankylosing spondylitis and cervical cancer.[3–5] No known association has been found between CML and infectious agents or chemical exposures, and no familial predisposition has been implicated in CML; thus, patients can be counseled that CML is neither preventable nor heritable.

PATHOGENESIS

The discovery of the Philadelphia (Ph) chromosome in 1960 made CML the first human neoplasm to be characterized by a

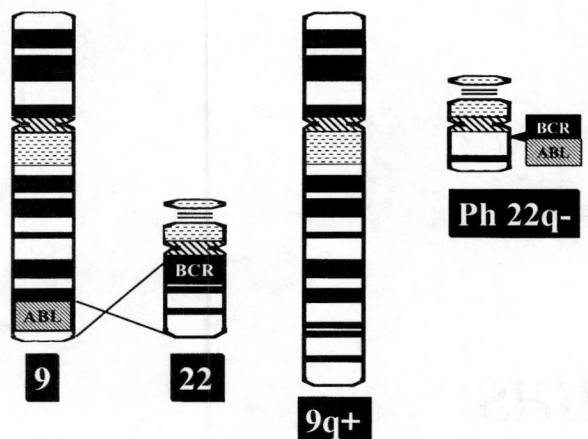

FIGURE 43.1-1. Diagrammatic representation of the formation of the Philadelphia (Ph) chromosome. The normal chromosomes 9 and 22 are shown, along with the derivative chromosomes 9q+ and 22q- (Ph). The approximate positions of the normal *ABL* gene at 9q34 and *BCR* at 22q11, and the *BCR-ABL* fusion gene formed as a result of the translocation, are shown.

consistent cytogenetic marker.[6] In 1973, the Ph chromosome, a shortened chromosome 22 (22q-), was shown to be the result of a balanced, reciprocal translocation between the long arms of chromosomes 9 and 22, t(9;22) (q34;q11) (Fig. 43.1-1).[7] In the 1980s, the *BCR-ABL* chimeric gene and protein formed as a result of the (9;22) translocation, was characterized, and its central role in the pathogenesis of CML was established.[8,9] The Ph chromosome and *BCR-ABL* are found in cells of the myeloid, erythroid, and megakaryocytic lineages; in some B cells; and also in a small proportion of T cells but are absent from other cells of the body, establishing CML as a clonal disorder that originates in a pluripotent hematopoietic stem cell. Despite the presence of *BCR-ABL* in erythroid precursors, expansion of erythroid lineage cells is distinctly uncommon in patients with CML.

The (9;22) translocation transposes the *ABL* (Abelson) protooncogene from chromosome 9 into a relatively small, 5.8-kb genomic region on chromosome 22 named the *breakpoint cluster region* (*bcr*).[10] Although the genomic breakpoints in the *ABL* gene are highly variable, they always occur upstream of the second exon (a2), resulting in translocation of exons 2 to 11 of ABL. Two slightly different chimeric *BCR-ABL* genes are present in patients with CML, depending on the precise location of the breakpoint in the *BCR* gene. Breaks can occur between exons b2 (also known as *e13*) and b3 (e14), yielding a b2a2 fusion messenger RNA (mRNA), whereas a break occurring between exons b3 and b4 produces a b3a2 fusion mRNA (Fig. 43.1-2).[9] Historically, this was referred to as the *major breakpoint cluster region* (*M-BCR*). In the majority of patients, either b2a2 or b3a2 transcripts are present, but, occasionally, patients have both transcripts in their leukemia cells. Although the b3a2 mRNA encodes a BCR-ABL protein that is 25 amino acids larger than that encoded by the b2a2 transcript, both are referred to as *p210BCR-ABL* and have similar prognoses.

The Ph chromosome and the *BCR-ABL* fusion gene are not pathognomonic for CML, being found in 25% to 50% of adult patients with acute lymphoblastic leukemia (ALL) and rare cases of acute myeloid leukemia. In adults with Ph chromosome–positive ALL, one-third have *BCR-ABL* transcripts indistinguishable from those found in CML. In two-thirds, the genomic breakpoint on chromosome 22 occurs in the first intron of the *BCR* gene (between e1 and e2) in an area termed the *minor breakpoint cluster region* (*m-BCR*), resulting in a protein of 190 kD (p190), also referred to as *p185* (see Fig. 43.1-2). Approximately 5% of children with ALL are Ph chromosome positive, and 95% of these patients have the p190 form of BCR-ABL. The p190 transcript is rarely found in patients with CML. An uncommon Ph chromosome–positive chronic neutrophilic leukemia has also been described with an e19a2 *BCR-ABL* mRNA product that encodes a 230-kD protein (p230). The genomic breakpoint of the BCR gene at e19 is also referred to as the *micro-breakpoint cluster region* (*μ-BCR*). Yet, other types of fusions have been observed in isolated cases.

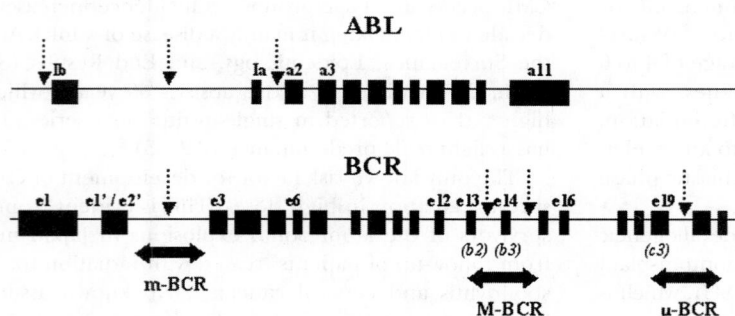

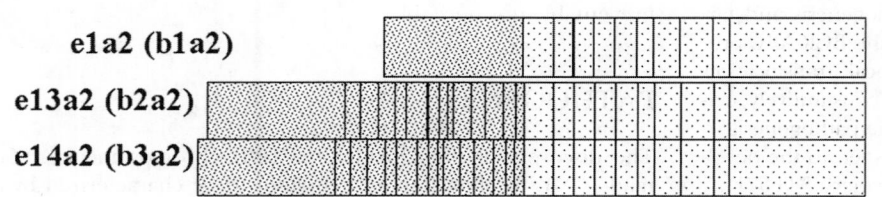

FIGURE 43.1-2. Schematic representation of the genomic structure of the normal *ABL* and *BCR* genes (*top*) and various fusion transcripts generated by the different *BCR-ABL* fusion genes (*bottom*). The b2a2 or the b3a2 transcript is found in the majority of patients with chronic myeloid leukemia. See text for details.

The BCR-ABL fusion protein resides in the cytoplasm and has constitutive tyrosine kinase activity compared to the tightly regulated activity of the normal *ABL* product (p145).[11] The BCR-ABL tyrosine kinase binds to and phosphorylates numerous intracellular proteins, resulting in the activation of various signaling pathways. Current efforts are directed at linking these pathways to the specific pathologic defects that characterize CML.[9] These defects include: increased proliferation or decreased apoptosis of a hematopoietic stem cell or progenitor cell, leading to a massive increase in myeloid cell numbers; premature release of immature myeloid cells into the circulation, postulated to be due to a defect in adherence of myeloid progenitors to marrow stroma; and genetic instability resulting in disease progression. An example of a signaling pathway that is activated by BCR-ABL that links to an increased proliferative rate is the RAS pathway. The antiapoptotic protein BCL_{XL} is up-regulated in BCR-ABL–expressing cells in a STAT-5–dependent pathway, and phosphorylation and inactivation of the proapoptotic molecule BAD occurs as a consequence of AKT activation.[9] Despite the increasing complexity of BCR-ABL signal transduction, all of the transforming functions of BCR-ABL are dependent on its tyrosine kinase activity, making this disease an ideal candidate for a therapy directed against this activity.

DIAGNOSIS AND CLINICAL COURSE

CLINICAL MANIFESTATIONS

Ninety percent of patients with CML are diagnosed in the chronic or stable phase. Ten percent to 20% of patients in older series and as many as 50% in more recent studies present without symptoms and are diagnosed as a result of finding an elevated white blood count on routine blood sampling. The most common presenting symptoms of CML are related to anemia, splenomegaly, and increased cell turnover. Thus, symptoms include fatigue, left upper quadrant pain, abdominal distention or discomfort, early satiety, weight loss, and night sweats. Occasionally, patients may present with a hyperviscosity syndrome with manifestations such as stroke, priapism, stupor, or visual changes caused by retinal hemorrhage and require leukapheresis. The most common physical finding in patients with CML is splenomegaly, with the magnitude of splenomegaly correlating well with the degree of leukocytosis. Ecchymoses are frequently observed, but spontaneous bleeding is uncommon. Lymphadenopathy is not usually seen in the chronic phase.

LABORATORY TESTS

Peripheral Blood and Bone Marrow

The diagnosis of CML is frequently suspected from examination of the peripheral blood and bone marrow. The white blood cell (WBC) count in the chronic phase of CML usually exceeds 50×10^9/L at the time of diagnosis and can range up to 800×10^9/L. During the chronic phase, leukemic cells retain the capacity to differentiate normally, and WBC function is normal. The peripheral blood smear shows a full spectrum of myeloid cells from blasts to neutrophils, with blasts comprising less than 15% and usually less than 5% of the WBC differential. Basophilia is invariably present, and its absence should prompt consideration of other myeloproliferative disorders. Eosino-

philia is also commonly present. The majority of patients have thrombocytosis, and, on occasion, the platelet count may be more than 1000×10^9/L. Most patients with CML have a normochromic, normocytic anemia that is inversely proportional to the degree of leukocytosis.

Blood levels of leukocyte alkaline phosphatase are low or undetectable in most patients with CML. As transcobalamin I is produced by granulocytes, serum B12 levels are increased in proportion to the total WBC count. Uric acid and LDH are also frequently elevated, reflecting the increased WBC mass and turnover.

The bone marrow in patients with chronic-phase CML is markedly hypercellular, with a predominance of myeloid cells with full maturation. As in the peripheral blood, the myeloblast percentage in the marrow is less than 15% and most commonly less than 5%, and basophilia is also present. Megakaryocytes are usually increased in number and may form clusters. Occasional micromegakaryocytes may be present. Erythroid hypoplasia is frequently present and may seem exaggerated because of the increased myeloid-erythroid ratio. Erythroid precursors are otherwise morphologically unremarkable. Reticulin fibrosis is usually absent or mild but may become more prominent with disease progression.

Cytogenetics

Cytogenetic analysis of 20 to 30 bone marrow metaphases has been the standard method to detect the Ph chromosome, which is present in the majority of cells at diagnosis. Cytogenetics can also detect other chromosomal abnormalities that may be an indication of disease progression. Although most patients have a typical t(9;22), approximately 5% have variant translocations. These variant translocations may be simple, involving chromosome 22 and a chromosome other than chromosome 9, or they may be complex, involving one or more other chromosomes in addition to chromosomes 9 and 22.[12]

Molecular Testing

The diagnosis of classic or typical CML is defined by the presence of *BCR-ABL*. In 90% of patients, its presence can be inferred by the detection of the Ph chromosome using standard cytogenetics. In the 10% of patients with a hematologic picture resembling CML who lack a detectable Ph chromosome, at least half have a *BCR-ABL* fusion gene detectable by fluorescence *in situ* hybridization (FISH) or reverse transcription–polymerase chain reaction (RT-PCR). These Ph chromosome–negative, *BCR-ABL*–positive patients have a clinical course that is indistinguishable from that of Ph chromosome–positive, *BCR-ABL*–positive patients.[13] In contrast, the small subset of patients who are Ph chromosome negative and *BCR-ABL* negative may have a more aggressive clinical course.[14]

FISH detects the colocalization of large, fluorescently labeled genomic probes specific to the *BCR* and *ABL* genes. FISH can be performed on metaphase or interphase cells and on peripheral blood. At diagnosis, when typically 90% of cells are *BCR-ABL* positive, FISH is a highly accurate diagnostic test, as false-negative results are uncommon. However, due to the random colocalization of the signals from the *BCR* and *ABL* probes, 8% to 10% of normal cells score positive, making FISH less useful at low disease burdens. A lower false-positive rate can be obtained with D-FISH, for *dual*-FISH, which uses probes that span the breakpoint region.[15]

RT-PCR to amplify the unique sequences created by the fusion of *BCR* and *ABL* is a highly sensitive technique that is ideal for the detection of minimal residual disease.[16,17] PCR testing can either be qualitative, providing information as to the presence or absence of the *BCR-ABL* transcript, or quantitative, assessing the amount of *BCR-ABL* message. False-positive and false-negative results are both possible with RT-PCR, and rigorous controls are required to detect these instances. False-negatives can be due to poor-quality RNA or failure of the reaction, whereas false-positives are usually due to contamination of the sample.

DIFFERENTIAL DIAGNOSIS

Anyone presenting with a WBC count over $50 \times 10^9/L$ with a peripheral blood smear showing a full spectrum of myeloid lineage cells plus basophilia should be suspected of having CML. The diagnosis of chronic-phase CML can be confirmed by the presence of the *BCR-ABL* gene as described in Cytogenetics and Molecular Testing, earlier in this chapter, and by the absence of advanced-phase features as described below in the section Advanced-Phase Disease. The differential diagnosis includes a leukemoid reaction, which is typically seen in patients with underlying infections. In patients with a leukemoid reaction, the WBC count is usually less than $50 \times 10^9/L$ and the peripheral blood smear consists predominantly of segmented neutrophils and bands, often with toxic granulations. Less mature myeloid cells are rarely seen, there is no basophilia, the leukocyte alkaline phosphatase is elevated, and the Ph chromosome and *BCR-ABL* are absent. Approximately 5% of patients with CML present with extreme thrombocytosis and a minimally elevated WBC count, resembling essential thrombocytosis, but are distinguished by the presence of the *BCR-ABL* gene. Although patients with CML may have an increase in monocyte numbers corresponding to the leukocytosis, there is relative monocytopenia, which differentiates CML from chronic myelomonocytic leukemia. In addition, patients with chronic myelomonocytic leukemia and other myeloproliferative disorders frequently lack the basophilia that is seen with CML and lack the *BCR-ABL* gene.

CLINICAL COURSE AND PROGNOSIS

Historically, progression of CML to blast crisis occurred in 5% to 10% of patients in the first 2 years after diagnosis, and thereafter, the annual progression rate increased to 20% to 25%. To guide patient management, various prognostic scales have been developed to predict the probability of disease progression. The best known of these is the Sokal score, which was derived from approximately 800 CML patients treated in the 1960s and 1970s.[18] Input of patient age, platelet count, peripheral blast count, and spleen size at diagnosis into an equation allows separation of the population into three groups: high, intermediate, and low risk of disease progression, with median survivals of 3, 4, and 5 years, respectively. Many of these patients received therapies not currently in use, such as busulfan, splenectomy, and intensive chemotherapy, and the Sokal index is less efficient in discriminating out-

come in interferon (IFN)-α–treated patients. However, a revised score, the Euro score, which also incorporates peripheral blood eosinophils and basophils, can identify risk groups in patients treated with IFN-α.[19] Whether either of these scores will discriminate outcome for patients treated with imatinib is unknown.

Data suggest that genomic deletions in the *ABL* gene on chromosome 9q+ and telomere length may have prognostic significance,[20,21] but these findings need to be validated in larger clinical trials. Clonal cytogenetic abnormalities in addition to the Ph chromosome are present at diagnosis in some patients, with the most common being duplication of the Ph chromosome, trisomy 8, iso-17q, and trisomy 19. Although iso-17q has been associated with a poorer prognosis, the prognostic significance of the other chromosomal abnormalities is less clear.[22]

TREATMENT OF CHRONIC-PHASE DISEASE

Currently available therapies for CML range from relatively nontoxic oral medications to high-dose chemoradiotherapy with allogeneic SCT. Randomized studies have been useful in comparing approaches within a single modality, but no randomized studies have directly compared transplant and nontransplant therapies. Although allogeneic SCT is regarded as the only curative therapy, the inability to identify a suitably matched donor and the risks of the procedure deter many patients from being transplanted. For patients who are candidates for SCT, shared decision making between the patient and physician is essential to acknowledge differing assessments of risk and benefits. Discussion of therapy is divided below into nontransplant and transplant approaches. Table 43.1-1 summarizes criteria for assessment of responses to therapy.

BUSULFAN

Busulfan, an oral alkylating agent, was introduced in 1953 and was used extensively until randomized trials documented that

TABLE 43.1-1. Criteria for Hematologic and Cytogenetic Responses in Chronic Myelogenous Leukemia

Response	*Parameters*
COMPLETE HEMATOLOGIC RESPONSE	Complete normalization of peripheral counts (WBC $<10 \times 10^9/L$, platelets $<450 \times 10^9/L$, no immature cells such as blasts, promyelocytes, or myelocytes); no signs or symptoms of disease, no palpable splenomegaly
CYTOGENETIC RESPONSE (IN PATIENTS WITH COMPLETE HEMATOLOGIC RESPONSE)	
Major	
Complete	No Ph chromosome–positive metaphases
Partial	1–34% Ph chromosome–positive metaphases
Minor	35–90% Ph chromosome–positive metaphases

Ph, Philadelphia; WBC, white blood cells.

hydroxyurea had superior efficacy and fewer side effects.[23] Busulfan therapy is associated with significant toxicity, including severe and prolonged myelosuppression, pulmonary fibrosis, and infertility, but may still be useful for patients who are intolerant of or resistant to other available therapies. Busulfan is used as part of some conditioning regimens in allogeneic SCT, but it should not be used in patients awaiting allogeneic SCT, as its use is associated with an adverse outcome.

HYDROXYUREA

Hydroxyurea is a well-tolerated oral agent that inhibits DNA synthesis by inhibiting ribonucleotide reductase. It can effectively and rapidly control blood counts in the majority of patients with CML. Treatment with hydroxyurea requires close monitoring, as excessive lowering of the WBC count can occur, particularly in the initial stages of therapy. Rare side effects include nausea, skin rashes, and mouth or leg ulcers. Initial daily doses of hydroxyurea range from 1 to 4 g, depending on the WBC count, presence of symptoms, and urgency to lower the WBC count. The maintenance dose usually ranges between 0.5 and 2.0 g/d and is titrated to keep the WBC count between 5 and 20×10^9/L. Although hydroxyurea is effective in controlling the WBC count and reducing splenomegaly, it rarely results in a cytogenetic response and does not prevent disease progression.

INTERFERON-α

IFN-α is a naturally occurring glycoprotein, produced by leukocytes in response to stress, that was first reported to be an effective treatment for CML in the early 1980s.[24] Although the mechanism of action of IFN-α in CML is unknown, it can inhibit cellular proliferation, restore adhesion of hematopoietic cells to marrow stroma, and modulate the immune system. The commercially available recombinant drug is administered as a subcutaneous injection. Multiple studies have confirmed that IFN-α induces complete or partial hematologic remissions in 50% to 80% of previously untreated patients with CML. In contrast to hydroxyurea or busulfan, cytogenetic responses are observed in 40% to 60% of IFN-α–treated patients. This includes 10% to 38% of major cytogenetic responses and 7% to 26% of complete cytogenetic responses.[25] In a metaanalysis of 1554 patients with CML enrolled in seven prospective, randomized trials, IFN-α–treated patients had a statistically significant better survival than patients treated with hydroxyurea ($P = .001$) or busulfan ($P = .00007$) alone.[26] Survival at 5 years was 57% for patients treated with IFN-α versus 42% in the chemotherapy-treated groups ($P < .00001$).[26]

The clinical use of IFN-α is limited by its toxicity profile, with side effects including flu-like symptoms of fevers, chills, myalgias, and fatigue encountered early during treatment. With ongoing therapy, many patients experience chronic fatigue, depression, insomnia, weight loss, peripheral neuropathy, alopecia, stomatitis, diarrhea, loss of recent memory, autoimmune disorders, and abnormalities in liver enzymes.[27] The toxicity of IFN-α increases with increasing dose and patient age, and it should be used with caution in patients with a history of serious depression. Thrombocytopenia, leukopenia, and mild anemia are common with IFN-α therapy, and mild to moderate leukopenia may be necessary to achieve optimal clinical benefits from IFN-α.

The survival benefit in the IFN-α studies is primarily limited to patients who tolerate IFN-α well and have a major cytogenetic response. As the median time to best cytogenetic response is 12 to 24 months, efforts have been directed at identifying patients who are likely to benefit most from IFN-α therapy using pretreatment and early-response parameters. Using the Euro score to segregate patients into different risk categories for response to IFN-α, "low-risk" patients have an expected median survival of 96 to 104 months[19] and an expected major cytogenetic response rate of approximately 50%.[28] In contrast, patients with "high-risk" disease can be expected to have a median survival of 42 months[19] and a major cytogenetic response rate of no more than 20%.[28] Achievement of a complete hematologic response (CHR) after 3 to 6 months of IFN-α therapy is associated with a higher likelihood of attaining a major cytogenetic response and improved survival.[29,30]

Efforts to improve IFN-α response rates or to minimize toxicity have included evaluating optimal dosing, combining IFN-α with other agents, and administering pegylated IFN-α. Although higher doses of IFN-α (5 million units/m^2) are associated with higher rates of major cytogenetic response, tolerance of IFN-α is a major problem with higher dose regimens. The addition of cytosine arabinoside (Ara-C) to IFN-α showed significantly improved hematologic and cytogenetic response rates over IFN-α alone in two randomized studies, but a survival advantage was only demonstrated in one of these studies.[31,32] Not surprisingly, the combination of IFN-α and cytarabine is associated with increased gastrointestinal and marrow toxicity. Attachment of IFN-α to polyethylene glycol (PEG) prolongs the half-life of IFN-α, allowing weekly administration, and may improve the tolerance of IFN-α therapy. Randomized studies comparing various PEG–IFN-α preparations to regular IFN-α are ongoing.

IMATINIB

Imatinib mesylate has rapidly become the treatment of choice for patients with chronic-phase CML who are not candidates for immediate SCT.[33] Imatinib is an orally administered inhibitor of the BCR-ABL tyrosine kinase; thus, it targets the molecular pathogenetic event in CML. Other tyrosine kinases inhibited by imatinib are the platelet-derived growth factor receptors, KIT, and ARG (*ABL*-related gene). Based on remarkable activity in phase I clinical trials,[34] a phase II trial of imatinib was initiated. Four hundred fifty-four patients with confirmed chronic-phase disease who were refractory to or intolerant of IFN-α were treated with an imatinib dose of 400 mg PO daily.[35] With a median follow-up of 29 months, 96% of patients achieved a CHR, with the median time to CHR being less than 1 month. Imatinib induced major cytogenetic responses in 64% of patients, with a complete cytogenetic response rate of 48%. The estimated progression-free survival at 24 months was 87% (Table 43.1-2).

In this phase II study, cytogenetic responses have been durable and correlate with improved progression-free and overall survival. Thus, once a patient achieves a major cytogenetic response, it is estimated that 24 months later, 91% of these patients will not have lost this response. Achievement of a major cytogenetic response at 3, 6, or within 12 months was associated with a statistically significant improvement in overall survival. For example, if a patient achieves a major cytogenetic response within 12 months, the estimated survival at 24 months

TABLE 43.1-2. Phase II Results with Imatinib

	Chronic Phase (IFN Failure)[35] (n = 454)	Accelerated Phase[93] (n = 181)	Blast Crisis[94] (n = 229)
CHR (%)	96	40	9
MCR (%)	64	28	16
CCR (%)	48	20	7
Disease progression at 24 mo (%)	13	50	90

CCR, complete cytogenetic response; CHR, complete hematologic response; IFN, interferon; MCR, major cytogenetic response.

is 99%, as compared to 86% for patients with less than a major cytogenetic response ($P < .001$). Baseline features that independently predicted a high rate of major cytogenetic responses were the absence of blasts in the peripheral blood, a hemoglobin greater than 12 g/dL, fewer than 5% blasts in the marrow, CML disease duration of less than 1 year, and a prior cytogenetic response to IFN-α.[35]

A phase III randomized study (n = 1106) compared imatinib at 400 mg/d to IFN-α plus Ara-C in newly diagnosed patients with chronic-phase CML. Baseline characteristics of patients randomized to each treatment were well balanced for all features evaluated, including age, WBC count, Sokal and Euro scores, and time from diagnosis. With a median follow-up of 19 months, patients randomized to imatinib had significantly better results than patients treated with IFN-α plus Ara-C in all parameters measured (Table 43.1-3), including rates of CHR, major and complete cytogenetic responses, discontinuation of assigned therapy due to intolerance, and progression to accelerated phase or blast crisis.[36] Quality of life was maintained on the imatinib arm and worsened on the IFN-α plus Ara-C arm.

Responses with imatinib are rapid, with noticeable decreases in the WBC count after 1 to 2 weeks and normalization within 4 to 6 weeks. The decline in the platelet count is typically delayed by 1 to 2 weeks. Bone marrow morphologies revert to normal in the majority of patients treated with imatinib, even patients without cytogenetic responses.

TABLE 43.1-3. Phase III Results of Imatinib versus Interferon-α (IFN-α) plus Cytarabine for Patients with Newly Diagnosed Chronic-Phase Chronic Myelogenous Leukemia[a]

	Imatinib, 400 mg/d (n = 553)	IFN-α + Ara-C (n = 553)
CHR (%)	97	69
MCR (%)	87	35
CCR (%)	76	14
Intolerance[b] (%)	3	31
Progressive disease[b] (%)	3	8.5

Ara-C, cytosine arabinoside; CCR, complete cytogenetic response; CHR, complete hematologic response; MCR, major cytogenetic response.
[a]Results are with a median follow-up of 19 months.
[b]Intolerance leading to discontinuation of first-line therapy. Progressive disease to accelerated phase or blast crisis. (All of these differences are highly statistically significant with $P < .001$.)
(From ref. 36, with permission.)

The most common nonhematologic adverse events of imatinib are nausea; muscle cramps; fluid retention, particularly periorbital edema; diarrhea; musculoskeletal pain; fatigue; and skin rashes. Only a minority of patients experienced grade 3/4 toxicity, and most side effects can be managed successfully with supportive measures.[37] Grade 3 or 4 myelosuppression occurs in fewer than 12% of patients and is probably a therapeutic effect, as the majority of hematopoiesis in patients with CML is derived from Ph chromosome–positive stem cells, particularly in patients with advanced disease.[38] As there is minimal suppression of normal hematopoiesis by imatinib, dose reductions below 300 mg/d are unlikely to assist in the recovery of normal hematopoiesis but may allow emergence of imatinib-resistant leukemic clones. Thus, among possible approaches to managing myelosuppression, interruption of treatment, not dose reduction, is the preferred course of action. In general, for chronic-phase patients, treatment should only be interrupted for an absolute neutrophil count of less than 1.0×10^9/L and a platelet count less than 50×10^9/L. These parameters can be modified for patients with more advanced disease. The use of myeloid growth factors while continuing therapy with imatinib is under investigation.

Because of the risk of myelosuppression, patients should have complete blood counts checked weekly to every other week during the first 2 months of imatinib therapy. In the absence of significant myelosuppression, the frequency of hematologic monitoring can then be reduced. Liver function tests should also be monitored regularly during imatinib therapy, as a 1% to 2% incidence of significant abnormalities has occurred in these tests. Evidence is emerging that cytogenetic responses and levels of BCR-ABL transcripts correlate with progression-free survival. Therefore, bone marrow cytogenetics should be monitored every 6 months until a complete cytogenetic response is obtained. Thereafter, quantitative RT-PCR for BCR-ABL, if available, should be monitored every 3 to 6 months on peripheral blood or bone marrow, as this provides a more sensitive assessment of residual disease and may allow earlier detection of relapse. In patients with a complete cytogenetic response, bone marrows should still be monitored yearly, as new cytogenetic abnormalities in Ph chromosome–negative clones have developed in some patients.[39] The significance of these abnormalities is unclear, but there have been reports of some of these patients developing myelodysplasia.

Thus far, relapses in chronic-phase patients treated with imatinib have been uncommon. In contrast, relapses have been a significant problem with single-agent imatinib for advanced-phase disease. The two most common mechanisms mediating relapse are point mutations in the BCR-ABL kinase that render the kinase less sensitive to imatinib and BCR-ABL amplification.[40,41] In some relapsed patients, dose escalation has resulted in transiently improved responses. Whether the same or differing mechanisms mediate cytogenetic resistance (failure to achieve a cytogenetic response) or molecular persistence (failure to eradicate all BCR-ABL–positive cells) remains to be seen.

Despite the fact that 74% of newly diagnosed patients with CML treated with imatinib achieve a complete cytogenetic response, only 5% of patients have undetectable levels of BCR-ABL transcripts when analyzed by RT-PCR.[42] To improve on these response rates, combinations of imatinib with IFN-α or Ara-C or higher doses of imatinib have been investigated in

TABLE 43.1-4.   Summary of Transplant Outcomes

	Related Donor		Unrelated Donor	
	Hematologic Relapse (%)	5- to 15-Y Disease-Free Survival (%)	Hematologic Relapse (%)	5-Y Disease-Free Survival (%)
Chronic phase	5–15	40–80	5–7	40–70
Accelerated phase	10–25	20–40	15	20–40
Blast crisis	25–58	0–25	50	0–5

phase I and II studies. Each of these has slightly improved cytogenetic response rates, as compared to 400 mg/d imatinib, but at the cost of increased toxicity.[43–45] Randomized studies comparing imatinib at 400 mg/d to imatinib at 400 mg/d with PEG–IFN-α to imatinib at 400 mg/d plus Ara-C to imatinib at 800 mg/d are ongoing, with end points of molecular responses at 1 year and survival.

STEM CELL TRANSPLANTATION

Allogeneic hematopoietic SCT remains the only proven therapy that can consistently eradicate all evidence of CML. Extensive experience has illustrated the durability of disease control with SCT and the potential short- and long-term complications. Transplantation is available to fewer than half of patients because older age and significant comorbid disease are clinical contraindications. In North America and Europe, approximately 85% of people have at least one HLA-matched donor available. Given that the chance of matching one full sibling is 25%; approximately 30% of patients have a matched sibling donor, whereas 5% match additional family members. For patients without a matched family member, large international registries offer searchable lists of over 7 million volunteers willing to provide stem cells. This system allows another 50% of patients to find a matched unrelated donor. Historically, CML has been the leading indication for unrelated donor transplantation because the disease was otherwise incurable and its indolence allowed time to find an unrelated donor and arrange the transplant.

If allogeneic SCT is performed while the patient is still in chronic phase using an HLA-matched sibling donor, 5-year survival rates are 60% to 80%, with a 10-year disease-free survival rate of 50% to 60% and a 15-year survival rate of 43%.[46–49] For younger patients without a sibling donor, SCT performed early in the disease course from unrelated donors offers similar results, although the available follow-up is shorter.[50,51] Long-term overall quality of life after allogeneic SCT is quite good, although a subset of patients report some physical limitations and many specific problems.[52,53] Approximately 50% to 60% of patients experience chronic graft-versus-host disease (GVHD), which is the leading cause of nonrelapse mortality more than 2 years after SCT.[49,54,55]

Major Prognostic Features and Methods

The two most frequently used prognostic scoring systems applicable to nontransplant therapy, the Sokal and Euro systems, do not predict outcome after allogeneic SCT. Instead, a variety of disease-, patient-, treatment- and transplant-prognostic factors have been identified. For example, the European Group for Blood and Marrow Transplantation (EBMT) studied 3142 patients to develop a prognostic model specific to allogeneic SCT. Five

major adverse prognostic factors were identified: accelerated or blastic phase, disease duration greater than 12 months, patient age greater than 20 or 40 years, a male patient with a female donor, and transplantation from an unrelated donor. Higher scores, indicating worse prognostic factors, are associated with greater transplant-related mortality.[56] As with all prognostic models, few factors are absolute contraindications and, in aggregate, only offer a rough estimate of expected outcome.

STAGE OF DISEASE AND TIME FROM DIAGNOSIS TO STEM CELL TRANSPLANTATION. Stage of disease before transplantation is one of the most consistent predictors of outcome in related and unrelated donor SCT (Table 43.1-4 and Fig. 43.1-3). Patients in early chronic phase do much better than those who are transplanted while in accelerated phase, blast crisis, or subsequent stable phase after treatment for advanced disease. The poorer outcomes are attributable to higher transplant-related mortality and relapse. For example, whereas first chronic phase is associated with 5-year survival rates of 60% to 80% in sibling SCT, survival estimates roughly halve if the procedure is performed for accelerated phase or second chronic phase (20% to 40%) and halve again if the patient is in blast crisis (5% to 20%). The one exception is patients classified as being in accelerated phase solely on the basis of cytogenetic abnormalities beyond a single Ph chromosome, who have a similar outcome with SCT to those in chronic phase.[57,58]

Increasing time from diagnosis to SCT is associated with worse outcomes in related and unrelated donor transplantation. This effect is observable after a 6-month delay in children and a 1-year delay for adults and is primarily due to higher transplant-related mortality rather than to relapse (Fig. 43.1-4).[50,56,59]

No clear reason for the poorer outcomes associated with a delay in transplantation have been identified. At one time, pro-

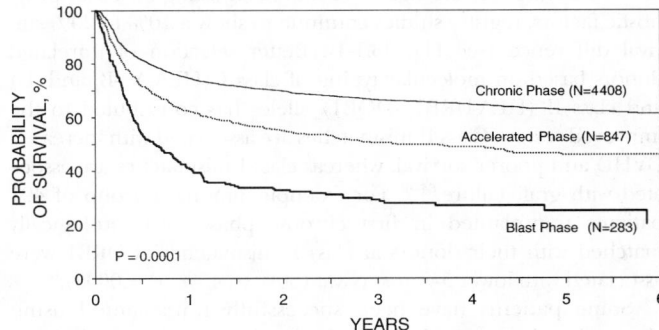

FIGURE 43.1-3.   Probability of survival after HLA-identical sibling stem cell transplantation for chronic myelogenous leukemia by disease status pretransplant, 1991 through 1997. (International Bone Marrow Transplant Registry data, with permission.)

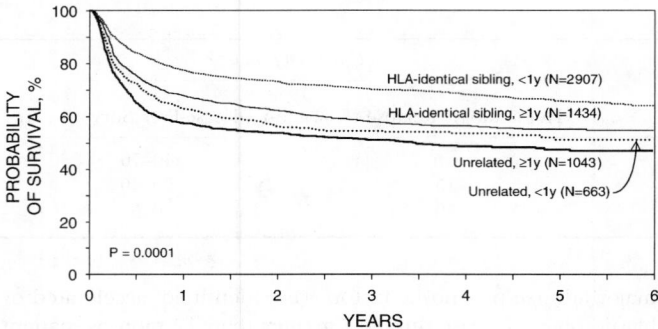

FIGURE 43.1-4. Probability of survival after stem cell transplantation for chronic myelogenous leukemia in chronic phase, by donor type and disease duration, 1995 through 2000. (International Bone Marrow Transplant Registry, with permission.)

longed busulfan exposure was thought to be the culprit. However, busulfan is rarely used now, and the difference is still observable. IFN was then suspected, but the majority of evidence suggests that pretransplant IFN does not adversely affect the outcome of SCT, and, in fact, some intriguing reports found lower relapse rates.[59–61] For now, if a patient is receiving IFN and preparing for transplantation, the literature suggests minimizing the duration of therapy and discontinuing treatment at least 90 days in advance of the procedure.[62,63] The short duration of follow-up and small number of patients treated with imatinib before SCT precludes comment about any effect on transplant outcomes.

AGE AND GENDER. Older age has been identified in most studies as an adverse prognostic factor for allogeneic SCT. The effect seems to be linear, with increasing transplant-related mortality observed above the age of 20 and quite noticeably increasing above the age of 50. CML is rare in childhood, but an analysis reported comparable survival rates to adult patients, with a 3-year survival rate of 65% to 75% in first chronic phase.[59]

Most analyses have found that male patients with female donors have higher transplant-related mortality than all other gender combinations. This may be due to female alloreactivity against antigens encoded on the Y chromosome.[50,56]

DONOR TYPE AND MATCHING. Donor type and degree of HLA matching also predict the success of allogeneic SCT, although in the most recent studies, the outcomes of related and unrelated donor SCT are converging.[50,55] However, adjusting for other prognostic factors, registry studies continue to show a 10% to 20% survival difference (see Fig. 43.1-4). Better selection of unrelated donors based on molecular typing of class I (HLA-A, -B, and -C) and class II (HLA-DRB1, -DQB1) alleles has contributed to the improved results. Class II mismatches are associated with increased GVHD and poorer survival, whereas class I mismatches are associated with graft failure.[64–66] For example, among a group of 491 patients transplanted in first chronic phase and serologically matched with their donors at class I, mismatches at DRB1 were associated with lower 5-year survival (30% vs. 45%, P = .0008).[66]

Some patients have been successfully transplanted using alternative donors such as haploidentical family members or unrelated donor umbilical cord blood. Syngeneic (identical twin) transplantation is associated with low transplant-related mortality but a 60% relapse rate.

PREPARATIVE REGIMEN. The major myeloablative conditioning regimens used for CML are cyclophosphamide and total body irradiation (TBI; 12 to 14 Gy) or busulfan and cyclophosphamide. Randomized studies suggest that the major outcomes are similar with these regimens.[48] Because orally administered busulfan has an unpredictable pharmacokinetic profile, targeting dose to optimize area under the curve may improve results.[67] A randomized trial comparing lower (12 Gy) and higher (15.75 Gy) TBI showed that overall survival was similar because the lower relapse rate in the higher TBI group was offset by greater treatment-related mortality.[68]

Reduced-intensity conditioning regimens, otherwise known as *nonmyeloablative* or *mini* preparative regimens, emphasize immunosuppression rather than myeloablation. The goal of chemoradiotherapy is to allow engraftment, with the hope that subsequent immune reconstitution from the donor, with or without additional lymphocyte infusions, will eradicate residual disease. Given that CML is uniquely sensitive to immunologic approaches, the disease is a prime target for these reduced-intensity conditioning approaches. Common regimens include combinations of fludarabine, busulfan, low-dose TBI, T-cell antibodies, and other immunosuppressive drugs. Many centers have shown that these procedures can be performed in the outpatient setting, avoiding the high early mortality associated with conditioning toxicity and prolonged neutropenia. However, infections and acute and chronic GVHD remain significant problems. In one report of 24 patients conditioned with fludarabine, busulfan, and anti–T-lymphocyte globulin, the projected leukemia-free survival at 5 years was 85%.[69] Further studies with larger numbers of patients and longer follow-up will determine the general applicability of this approach.

STEM CELL SOURCE. Donor stem cells can be obtained either from peripheral blood (PBSC) or marrow. The theoretic advantages of PBSC include earlier engraftment, lower early mortality, better immune reconstitution, and a lower relapse rate, perhaps modulated via increased chronic GVHD. Use of PBSC is associated with higher rates of chronic GVHD,[70] and CML patients are more prone to this complication than people with other diagnoses. In early chronic-phase CML, survival is probably identical with either marrow or PBSC, whereas PBSC may be preferable in advanced disease.

One intriguing option is the use of growth factor–stimulated bone marrow. Two randomized studies suggested a better outcome for CML patients receiving stimulated marrow as compared to stimulated PBSC or unstimulated marrow.[71,72]

GRAFT-VERSUS-HOST DISEASE PROPHYLAXIS AND CLINICAL GRAFT-VERSUS-HOST DISEASE. The major modes of GVHD prophylaxis are immunosuppressive medications and T-cell depletion. Immunosuppressive approaches are more common, usually with a calcineurin inhibitor (cyclosporine or tacrolimus) and methotrexate given on days 1, 3, 6, and 11 after stem cell infusion. With immunosuppressive approaches, relapse rates are minimized, but GVHD is more common. T-cell depletion is associated with lower rates of acute and chronic GVHD but higher rates of relapse, graft failure, and Epstein-Barr virus–associated lymphoproliferative disorders.[73,74] Approaches that combine T-cell depletion with later donor lymphocyte infusion (DLI) have been reported, with promising results.[75] The greater genetic disparity expected with unrelated donor transplantation may mitigate some of the risks of T-cell depletion but also negates some of the benefits. Regardless of the method of GVHD prophylaxis, patients with detectable but minimal (grade I) acute GVHD have the highest overall survival after HLA-matched sibling SCT compared to those with no GVHD (increased relapse rates) or grade II to IV GVHD (higher transplant-related mortality).[50]

Disease Monitoring after Transplantation

Relapses can be considered molecular (PCR positivity), cytogenetic (detection of the Ph chromosome), or clinical (hematologic evidence of CML). The definition of residual or relapsed disease after SCT is controversial and somewhat dependent on the frequency of testing, the sensitivity and specificity of the testing method, the number and type of cells being tested, whether changes over time are considered, the type of donor and method of GVHD prophylaxis, and time since transplant.[76] Complicating the definition of relapse is the observation that molecular evidence of CML clearly remains even after myeloablative conditioning but disappears with time in most patients.[77,78] Approximately 10% to 15% of patients transplanted from sibling donors while in chronic phase relapse hematologically, compared to fewer than 5% for matched, unrelated donor recipients. At the other extreme, approximately 10% of patients remain PCR positive for years after SCT.[67,79]

The definition of relapse post-SCT has important clinical consequences as well. Early intervention after relapse offers the best chance of controlling disease, but overtreatment can result in serious toxicity. Most relapses occur early, with half during the first posttransplant year and fewer than 5% occurring after 5 years.[80] Although careful serial monitoring is necessary to detect imminent relapse, the high sensitivity of molecular testing results in a relatively low positive predictive value for any individual time point. It is hoped that newer, more accurate tests such as quantitative PCR for the BCR-ABL transcript will allow careful monitoring and detection of rising leukemia burden before cytogenetic or clinical relapse.

Management of Relapse after Transplantation

Many options are available for managing relapse after transplantation, but all approaches work best when leukemia burden is minimal. IFN or imatinib can return patients to complete remission with undetectable BCR-ABL transcripts by RT-PCR.[81,82] Other approaches include withdrawal of immunosuppression or DLIs from the original donor. In recognition of the excellent prognosis of CML patients who reenter remission after relapse, the current leukemia-free survival methodology allows them to be included on the disease-free survival curve.[83] Patients may also choose to undergo a second transplant from the same or different donor if sufficient time has elapsed to allow recovery from the first procedure.

CML is uniquely sensitive to the graft-versus-leukemia (GVL) effect and has been a model for eradicating malignant disease through manipulation of the immune system. Of the patients who relapse cytogenetically or hematologically into chronic phase, 60% to 80% can be salvaged by DLIs alone without further cytotoxic chemotherapy, although responses take several months to manifest.[84,85] These remissions are durable, and 5-year disease-free survival rates are approximately 50%. In con-trast, accelerated phase and blast crisis are much less responsive. Risks of DLI are significant and include acute GVHD, pancytopenia with infectious risks, and chronic GVHD resulting in a reported treatment-related mortality of 8% to 20%. Efforts to decrease the toxicity of DLI by selectively infusing subsets of lymphocytes (CD8 depleted), inserting a suicide gene before infusion, minimizing the dose of donor lymphocytes, spreading out the dosing schedule, or expanding specific T-cell clones *ex vivo* before infusion appear to have some success.

The biologic basis for the GVL effect, and whether it can be separated from a generalized GVHD phenomenon, is controversial.[79,86] Because GVL responses can be observed without apparent GVHD, it is likely that leukemia-specific antigens can be recognized by the immune system. Hypothesized antigens include peptides derived from the BCR-ABL fusion protein; tissue-specific peptides, such as those derived from proteinase 3 or the Wilms' tumor protein; or minor histocompatibility peptides.

Autologous Stem Cell Transplantation

Although CML is a stem cell disease, it arises from a somatic mutation, and normal progenitors are detectable in most patients with CML. In theory, these normal stem cells could be used to reconstitute patients after destruction of leukemia cells. However, in practice, autologous procedures with or without attempts to purge the marrow graft have been plagued by high transplant-related toxicity and relapse rates.[87] Estimated disease-free survival rates are approximately 10% even when Ph-negative stem cells can be harvested and transplanted.[88]

TREATMENT DECISIONS

Even before imatinib, it was difficult to recommend a treatment algorithm for CML. No studies have directly compared transplant and nontransplant approaches. Previous quantitative attempts to weigh the tradeoffs between early risks from SCT and late risks of disease progression with nontransplant therapies include decision analysis, cohort studies, and multivariate modeling. These studies conclude that younger patients or those with higher-risk CML do better in the long term with early SCT. Mortality is initially higher with transplant approaches, but overall survival is superior once the curve plateaus.[89,90] A representative analysis is shown in Figure 43.1-5.

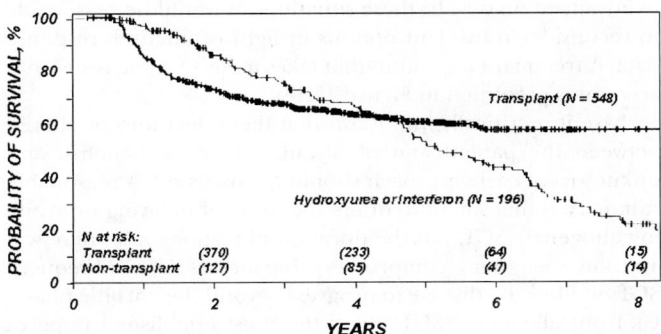

FIGURE 43.1-5. Adjusted probabilities (from COX regression models) of survival after diagnosis of chronic myeloid leukemia in persons receiving HLA-identical sibling bone marrow transplants or nontransplant therapy with hydroxyurea or interferon. (From ref. 89, with permission.)

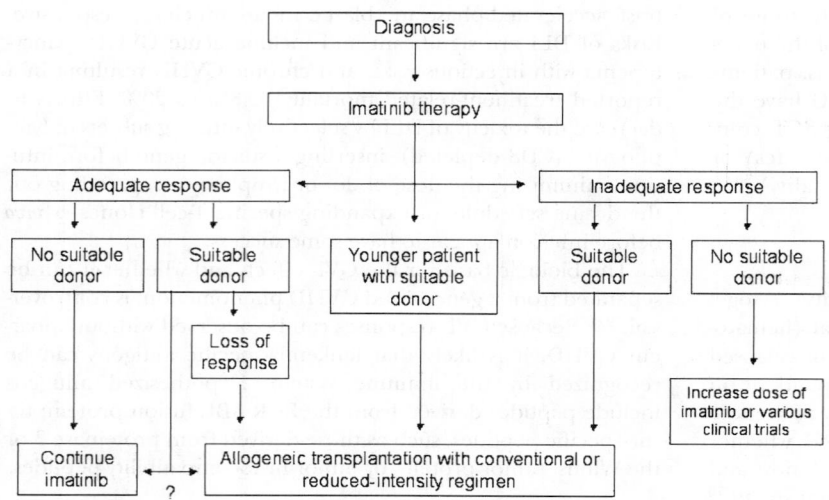

FIGURE 43.1-6.   Clinical decision making in chronic myeloid leukemia (CML). Most newly diagnosed patients with chronic-phase CML are started on therapy with imatinib. For some younger or high-risk patients with suitable donors, an allogeneic stem cell transplant (SCT) can be considered, regardless of response to imatinib. In the remainder of patients, a decision regarding allogeneic SCT transplant might be delayed until it is determined whether an adequate response to imatinib is observed. The difficulty with this is that what constitutes an adequate response to imatinib has not been clearly defined, and it is not evident whether delaying a transplant will have an adverse impact on a subsequent transplant. For patients who do not have an adequate response or lose their response to imatinib, consideration would again be given to allogeneic SCT if a suitable donor can be identified. In the absence of a donor, other treatment options would be explored. (Adapted from ref. 33.)

Imatinib is highly efficacious and well tolerated, with a 99% overall survival rate in the first year of therapy. This fact, plus the lack of long-term follow-up and inability to predict responses before a trial of therapy, have complicated the decision-making process. Other questions include whether patients receiving imatinib can be successfully monitored for loss of response, whether other nontransplant or transplant interventions can salvage people whose disease progresses on imatinib, and whether the data for delaying a transplant beyond 1 to 2 years applies to imatinib-treated patients. Also complicating the decision-making process are efforts to develop less toxic allogeneic transplant procedures that may improve the safety of transplantation and extend the spectrum of patients eligible for transplantation procedures; however, the long-term outcomes of these reduced-intensity procedures are unknown.

It should also be emphasized that treatment decisions are dynamic processes that may be revisited with evolving data. Although fewer patients are undergoing immediate SCT since the introduction of imatinib, this is not an irrevocable decision. For example, of patients who remain greater than 95% Ph chromosome positive after 1 year, approximately 25% will either lose a CHR or progress to advanced-phase disease in the next year, but an equivalent percentage will achieve a major cytogenetic response. Similarly, patients who do not have a CHR within 3 months have a higher rate of disease progression to advanced phases. In these situations, it would be reasonable to reconsider transplant options in light of imatinib response data. A treatment algorithm that takes many of these issues into account is presented in Figure 43.1-6.

Last, it is critically important that these decisions be shared between the patient and physician. The risks, benefits, and unknowns of each approach should be discussed. A reasonable summary is that imatinib offers the hope of delaying or avoiding allogeneic SCT, but the duration of responses is unknown, and any delay may compromise the success of a subsequent SCT or allow the disease to progress beyond the chronic phase. Up-front allogeneic SCT offers the most established hope of cure based on long-term data from thousands of patients, but at the cost of substantial toxicity and risk of death from the procedure itself. Physicians can offer recommendations based on the medical facts of age, health, and available donors, but patients must decide which approach is best based on their personal assessment of the risks and benefits given their own circumstances.

ADVANCED-PHASE DISEASE

In approximately 20% of patients in chronic phase, the disease transforms abruptly into an acute leukemia. This is called *blast crisis* or *blastic transformation*. Morphologically, the bone marrow of blastic-phase CML has greater than 30% blasts. Approximately 65% of patients evolve to blast crisis with myeloid lineage blasts, 30% have blasts of pre–B lymphoid origin, and 5% have undifferentiated or T-cell blasts. On occasion, an isolated blast phase of extramedullary origin may occur while the patient's blood and marrow otherwise meet criteria for chronic-phase disease.

In the majority of patients, the transformation to advanced phase occurs gradually, with the disease becoming more difficult to control with medical therapy. The intermediate period during which the patient is no longer in chronic phase but is not yet clearly in blastic transformation has been termed the *accelerated phase*. The criteria for defining the accelerated phase are highly variable (Table 43.1-5), and only the MD Anderson criteria have been correlated with a median survival of 18 months or less. In some patients, a myelofibrotic picture characterizes the accelerated phase, where there is massive splenomegaly with extensive marrow fibrosis and extramedullary hematopoiesis.

Clonal cytogenetic abnormalities besides a single Ph chromosome may be acquired in patients with CML as their disease progresses, and up to 80% of patients with overt blastic transformation have additional cytogenetic abnormalities.[91] The molecular basis of disease progression is poorly defined, but point mutations or deletions in the *p53* tumor suppressor gene have been observed in up to 25% of patients with myeloid blast crisis, and as many as 50% of patients with lymphoid transformation show homozygous deletion in the *p16* tumor suppressor gene.[92]

Imatinib has single-agent activity in accelerated and blast crisis, with a higher response rate and durability in patients with accelerated-phase disease (see Table 43.1-2).[93,94] Significantly improved outcomes for response and survival were observed for advanced-phase patients treated with 600 mg/d

TABLE 43.1-5. Criteria for Accelerated Phase of Chronic Myeloid Leukemia

International Bone Marrow Transplant Registry	MD Anderson Cancer Center
WBC difficult to control with busulfan or hydroxyurea	Peripheral blood blasts ≥15% but <30%
Rapid WBC doubling time (<5 d)	Peripheral blood blasts and promyelocytes ≥30%
Peripheral blood or marrow blasts ≥10% but <30%	Peripheral blood basophils ≥20%
Peripheral blood or marrow blasts and promyelocytes ≥20%	Platelet count <100 × 10⁹/L unrelated to therapy
Peripheral blood basophils and eosinophils ≥20%	Clonal evolution
Anemia or thrombocytopenia unresponsive to busulfan or hydroxyurea	
Persistent thrombocytosis	
Clonal evolution	
Progressive splenomegaly and myelofibrosis	

WBC, white blood cell count.

imatinib as compared to 400 mg/d. Even though this was a retrospective subgroup analysis, these data are the basis for recommending 600 mg/d imatinib for advanced-phase patients. With combination chemotherapy, 20% of patients in myeloid transformation and 50% of those in lymphoid blast transformation achieve a second chronic phase, which is usually short lived. The results for treatment of myeloid blast crisis with imatinib compare favorably to those of historical controls treated with chemotherapy. However, the high relapse rates suggest that imatinib should be viewed as either a bridge to allogeneic SCT or that patients should be enrolled in clinical trials combining imatinib with other agents. The results of allogeneic SCT in advanced-phase disease are discussed in Stage of Disease and Time from Diagnosis to Stem Cell Transplantation, earlier in this chapter, and are summarized in Table 43.1-4.

FUTURE DIRECTIONS

Other agents in development include second-generation ABL kinase inhibitors that have increased potency or specificity as compared to imatinib or are capable of inhibiting some of the mutant forms of BCR-ABL that are observed in patients who have developed resistance to imatinib.[95,96] A variety of signal transduction inhibitors that impact pathways downstream of imatinib are also under development. These include farnesyl transferase inhibitors, RAF, and MEK inhibitors. Arsenic trioxide, historically the first clinically useful therapy for CML, has seen a resurgence in interest, with *in vitro* data demonstrating that arsenic trioxide can down-regulate BCR-ABL protein expression.[97] Similarly, geldanamycin analogues have been shown to down-regulate BCR-ABL expression.[98] Many of these agents have additive to synergistic effects when combined with imatinib, and combination clinical trials are envisioned. A number of novel chemotherapeutic agents are being developed, including homoharringtonine, decitabine, and troxacitabine, which have shown some activity in patients with CML.[99] Last, vaccine strategies are undergoing investigation. These include vaccinations with BCR-

ABL junction peptides; generation of specific, cytotoxic T cells; or vaccination with autologous proteins, such as heat-shock protein 70.[99] If these immune strategies show promise, they may be most useful in eliminating residual disease after therapy with imatinib. With improvements in the safety of SCT, it is possible that some combination of nontransplant therapy combined with SCT or immunotherapy may eventually offer the greatest benefit for the most patients.

REFERENCES

1. Druker BJ, Lydon NB. Lessons learned from the development of an abl tyrosine kinase inhibitor for chronic myelogenous leukemia. *J Clin Invest* 2000;105:3.
2. Ries LAG, Eisner MP, Kosary CL, et al. *SEER cancer statistics review, 1975–2000.* Bethesda, MD: National Cancer Institute, 2003.
3. Brown WM, Doll R. Mortality from cancer and other causes after radiotherapy for ankylosing spondylitis. *BMJ* 1965;5474:1327.
4. Boice JD Jr, Day NE, Andersen A, et al. Second cancers following radiation treatment for cervical cancer. An international collaboration among cancer registries. *J Natl Cancer Inst* 1985;74:955.
5. Kato H, Schull WJ. Studies of the mortality of A-bomb survivors. 7. Mortality, 1950–1978: part I. Cancer mortality. *Radiat Res* 1982;90:395.
6. Nowell PC, Hungerford DA. A minute chromosome in human chronic granulocytic leukemia. *Science* 1960;132:1497.
7. Rowley JD. A new consistent abnormality in chronic myelogenous leukaemia identified by quinacrine fluorescence and Giemsa staining [Letter]. *Nature* 1973;243:290.
8. de Klein A, van Kessel AG, Grosveld G, et al. A cellular oncogene is translocated to the Philadelphia chromosome in chronic myelocytic leukemia. *Nature* 1982;300:765.
9. Deininger MW, Goldman JM, Melo JV. The molecular biology of chronic myeloid leukemia. *Blood* 2000;96:3343.
10. Groffen J, Stephenson JR, Heisterkamp N, et al. Philadelphia chromosome breakpoints are clustered within a limited region, bcr, on chromosome 22. *Cell* 1984;36:93.
11. Konopka JB, Watanabe SM, Witte ON. An alteration of the human c-abl protein in K562 unmasks associated tyrosine kinase activity. *Cell* 1984;37:1035.
12. Mitelman F. The cytogenetic scenario of chronic myeloid leukemia. *Leuk Lymphoma* 1993;11[Suppl 1]:11.
13. Cortes JE, Talpaz M, Beran M, et al. Philadelphia chromosome-negative chronic myelogenous leukemia with rearrangement of the breakpoint cluster region. Long-term follow-up results. *Cancer* 1995;75:464.
14. Kurzrock R, Bueso-Ramos CE, Kantarjian H, et al. BCR rearrangement-negative chronic myelogenous leukemia revisited. *J Clin Oncol* 2001;19:2915.
15. Dewald GW, Wyatt WA, Juneau AL, et al. Highly sensitive fluorescence in situ hybridization method to detect double BCR/ABL fusion and monitor response to therapy in chronic myeloid leukemia. *Blood* 1998;91:3357.
16. Wang YL, Bagg A, Pear W, et al. Chronic myelogenous leukemia: laboratory diagnosis and monitoring. *Genes Chromosomes Cancer* 2001;32:97.
17. Schoch C, Schnittger S, Bursch S, et al. Comparison of chromosome banding analysis, interphase- and hypermetaphase-FISH, qualitative and quantitative PCR for diagnosis and for follow-up in chronic myeloid leukemia: a study on 350 cases. *Leukemia* 2002;16:53.
18. Sokal JE, Cox EB, Baccarani M, et al. Prognostic discrimination in "good-risk" chronic granulocytic leukemia. *Blood* 1984;63:789.
19. Hasford J, Pfirrmann M, Hehlmann R, et al. A new prognostic score for survival of patients with chronic myeloid leukemia treated with interferon alfa. Writing Committee for the Collaborative CML Prognostic Factors Project Group. *J Natl Cancer Inst* 1998;90:850.
20. Huntly BJ, Bench A, Green AR. Double jeopardy from a single translocation: deletions of the derivative chromosome 9 in chronic myeloid leukemia. *Blood* 2003;102:1160.
21. Brummendorf TH, Holyoake TL, Rufer N, et al. Prognostic implications of differences in telomere length between normal and malignant cells from patients with chronic myeloid leukemia measured by flow cytometry. *Blood* 2000;95:1883.
22. Kantarjian HM, Smith TL, McCredie KB, et al. Chronic myelogenous leukemia: a multivariate analysis of the associations of patient characteristics and therapy with survival. *Blood* 1985;66:1326.
23. Hehlmann R, Heimpel H, Hasford J, et al. Randomized comparison of busulfan and hydroxyurea in chronic myelogenous leukemia: prolongation of survival by hydroxyurea. The German CML Study Group. *Blood* 1993;82:398.
24. Talpaz M, McCredie KB, Mavligit GM, et al. Leukocyte interferon-induced myeloid cytoreduction in chronic myelogenous leukemia. *Blood* 1983;62:689.
25. Silver RT, Woolf SH, Hehlmann R, et al. An evidence-based analysis of the effect of busulfan, hydroxyurea, interferon, and allogeneic bone marrow transplantation in treating the chronic phase of chronic myeloid leukemia: developed for the American Society of Hematology. *Blood* 1999;94:1517.
26. Chronic Myeloid Leukemia Trialists' Collaborative Group. Interferon alfa versus chemotherapy for chronic myeloid leukemia: a meta-analysis of seven randomized trials. *J Natl Cancer Inst* 1997;89:1616.
27. O'Brien S, Kantarjian H, Talpaz M. Practical guidelines for the management of chronic myelogenous leukemia with interferon alpha. *Leuk Lymphoma* 1996;23:247.

28. Kantarjian HM, Smith TL, O'Brien S, et al. Prolonged survival in chronic myelogenous leukemia after cytogenetic response to interferon-alpha therapy. The Leukemia Service. *Ann Intern Med* 1995;122:254.

29. Mahon FX, Faberes C, Pueyo S, et al. Response at three months is a good predictive factor for newly diagnosed chronic myeloid leukemia patients treated by recombinant interferon-alpha. *Blood* 1998;92:4059.

30. Sacchi S, Kantarjian HM, Smith TL, et al. Early treatment decisions with interferon-alfa therapy in early chronic-phase chronic myelogenous leukemia. *J Clin Oncol* 1998;16:882.

31. Guilhot F, Chastang C, Michallet M, et al. Interferon alfa-2B combined with cytarabine versus interferon alone in chronic myelogenous leukemia. French Chronic Myeloid Leukemia Study Group. *N Engl J Med* 1997;337:223.

32. Baccarani M, Rosti G, de Vivo A, et al. A randomized study of interferon-alpha versus interferon-alpha and low-dose arabinosyl cytosine in chronic myeloid leukemia. *Blood* 2002;99:1527.

33. Peggs K, Mackinnon S. Imatinib mesylate—the new gold standard for treatment of chronic myeloid leukemia. *N Engl J Med* 2003;348:1048.

34. Druker BJ, Talpaz M, Resta DJ, et al. Efficacy and safety of a specific inhibitor of the BCR-ABL tyrosine kinase in chronic myeloid leukemia. *N Engl J Med* 2001;344:1031.

35. Kantarjian H, Sawyers C, Hochhaus A, et al. Hematologic and cytogenetic responses to imatinib mesylate in chronic myelogenous leukemia. *N Engl J Med* 2002;346:645.

36. O'Brien SG, Guilhot F, Larson RA, et al. Imatinib compared with interferon and low-dose cytarabine for newly diagnosed chronic-phase chronic myeloid leukemia. *N Engl J Med* 2003;348:994.

37. Deininger MW, O'Brien SG, Ford JM, et al. Practical management of patients with chronic myeloid leukemia receiving imatinib. *J Clin Oncol* 2003;21:1637.

38. Petzer AL, Eaves CJ, Lansdorp PM, et al. Characterization of primitive subpopulations of normal and leukemic cells present in the blood of patients with newly diagnosed as well as established chronic myeloid leukemia. *Blood* 1996;88:2162.

39. Bumm T, Muller C, Al-Ali HK, et al. Emergence of clonal cytogenetic abnormalities in Ph- cells in some CML patients in cytogenetic remission to imatinib but restoration of polyclonal hematopoiesis in the majority. *Blood* 2003;101:1941.

40. Shah NP, Nicoll JM, Nagar B, et al. Multiple BCR-ABL kinase domain mutations confer polyclonal resistance to the tyrosine kinase inhibitor imatinib (STI571) in chronic phase and blast crisis chronic myeloid leukemia. *Cancer Cell* 2002;2:117.

41. Hochhaus A, Kreil S, Corbin AS, et al. Molecular and chromosomal mechanisms of resistance to imatinib (STI571) therapy. *Leukemia* 2002;16:2190.

42. Hughes T, Kaeda J, Branford S, et al. Molecular responses to imatinib (STI571) or interferon + Ara-C as initial therapy for CML: results in the IRIS study. *Blood* 2002;100:93a.

43. Hochhaus A, Fischer T, Brummendorf TH, et al. Imatinib (Glivec) and pegylated interferon α 2a (Pegasys) phase I/II combination study in chronic phase chronic myelogenous leukemia. *Blood* 2002;100:164a.

44. Gardembas M, Rousselot P, Tulliez M, et al. Results of a prospective phase II study combining imatinib mesylate and cytarabine for the treatment of Philadelphia-positive chronic myelogenous leukemia patients in chronic phase. *Blood* 2003;102:4298.

45. Cortes JE, Talpaz M, O'Brien S, et al. High rates of major cytogenetic response in patients with newly diagnosed chronic myeloid leukemia in early chronic phase treated with imatinib at 400 mg or 800 mg daily. *Blood* 2002;100:95a.

46. Clift RA, Storb R. Marrow transplantation for CML: the Seattle experience. *Bone Marrow Transplant* 1996;17:S1.

47. Horowitz MM, Rowlings PA, Passweg JR. Allogeneic bone marrow transplantation for CML: a report from the International Bone Marrow Transplant Registry. *Bone Marrow Transplant* 1996;3[Suppl 17]:S5.

48. Socie G, Clift RA, Blaise D, et al. Busulfan plus cyclophosphamide compared with total-body irradiation plus cyclophosphamide before marrow transplantation for myeloid leukemia: long-term follow-up of 4 randomized studies. *Blood* 2001;98:3569.

49. Gratwohl A, Brand R, Apperley J, et al. Graft-versus-host disease and outcome in HLA-identical sibling transplantations for chronic myeloid leukemia. *Blood* 2002;100:3877.

50. Hansen JA, Gooley TA, Martin PJ, et al. Bone marrow transplants from unrelated donors for patients with chronic myeloid leukemia. *N Engl J Med* 1998;338:962.

51. McGlave PB, Shu XO, Wen W, et al. Unrelated donor marrow transplantation for chronic myelogenous leukemia: 9 years' experience of the national marrow donor program. *Blood* 2000;95:2219.

52. Lee SJ, Fairclough D, Parsons SK, et al. Recovery after stem-cell transplantation for hematologic diseases. *J Clin Oncol* 2001;19:242.

53. Kiss TL, Abdolell M, Jamal N, et al. Long-term medical outcomes and quality-of-life assessment of patients with chronic myeloid leukemia followed at least 10 years after allogeneic bone marrow transplantation. *J Clin Oncol* 2002;20:2334.

54. Socie G, Stone JV, Wingard JR, et al. Long-term survival and late deaths after allogeneic bone marrow transplantation. Late Effects Working Committee of the International Bone Marrow Transplant Registry. *N Engl J Med* 1999;341:14.

55. Weisdorf DJ, Anasetti C, Antin JH, et al. Allogeneic bone marrow transplantation for chronic myelogenous leukemia: comparative analysis of unrelated versus matched sibling donor transplantation. *Blood* 2002;99:1971.

56. Gratwohl A, Hermans J, Goldman JM, et al. Risk assessment for patients with chronic myeloid leukemia before allogeneic blood or marrow transplantation. Chronic Leukemia Working Party of the European Group for Blood and Marrow Transplantation. *Lancet* 1998;352:1087.

57. Clift RA, Buckner CD, Thomas ED, et al. Marrow transplantation for patients in accelerated phase of chronic myeloid leukemia. *Blood* 1994;84:4368.

58. Konstantinidou P, Szydlo RM, Chase A, et al. Cytogenetic status pre-transplant as a predictor of outcome post bone marrow transplantation for chronic myelogenous leukaemia. *Bone Marrow Transplant* 2000;25:143.

59. Cwynarski K, Roberts IA, Iacobelli S, et al. Stem cell transplantation for chronic myeloid leukemia in children. *Blood* 2003;102:1224.

60. Giralt S, Szydlo R, Goldman JM, et al. Effect of short-term interferon therapy on the outcome of subsequent HLA-identical sibling bone marrow transplantation for chronic myelogenous leukemia: an analysis from the international bone marrow transplant registry. *Blood* 2000;95:410.

61. Lee SJ, Klein JP, Anasetti C, et al. The effect of pretransplant interferon therapy on the outcome of unrelated donor hematopoietic stem cell transplantation for patients with chronic myelogenous leukemia in first chronic phase. *Blood* 2001;98:3205.

62. Morton AJ, Gooley T, Hansen JA, et al. Association between pretransplant interferon-α and outcome after unrelated donor marrow transplantation for chronic myelogenous leukemia in chronic phase. *Blood* 1998;92:394.

63. Hehlmann R, Hochhaus A, Kolb HJ, et al. Interferon-alpha before allogeneic bone marrow transplantation in chronic myelogenous leukemia does not affect outcome adversely, provided it is discontinued at least 90 days before the procedure. *Blood* 1999;94:3668.

64. Petersdorf EW, Longton GM, Anasetti C, et al. Association of HLA-C disparity with graft failure after marrow transplantation from unrelated donors. *Blood* 1997;89:1818.

65. Devergie A, Apperley JF, Labopin M, et al. European results of matched unrelated donor bone marrow transplantation for chronic myeloid leukemia. Impact of HLA class II matching. Chronic Leukemia Working Party of the European Group for Blood and Marrow Transplantation. *Bone Marrow Transplant* 1997;20:11.

66. Petersdorf EW, Kollman C, Hurley CK, et al. Effect of HLA class II gene disparity on clinical outcome in unrelated donor hematopoietic cell transplantation for chronic myeloid leukemia: the US National Marrow Donor Program Experience. *Blood* 2001;98:2922.

67. Radich JP, Gooley T, Bensinger W, et al. HLA-matched related hematopoietic cell transplantation for chronic-phase CML using a targeted busulfan and cyclophosphamide preparative regimen. *Blood* 2003;102:31.

68. Clift RA, Buckner CD, Appelbaum FR, et al. Allogeneic marrow transplantation in patients with chronic myeloid leukemia in the chronic phase: a randomized trial of two irradiation regimens. *Blood* 1991;77:1660.

69. Or R, Shapira MY, Resnick I, et al. Nonmyeloablative allogeneic stem cell transplantation for the treatment of chronic myeloid leukemia in first chronic phase. *Blood* 2003;101:441.

70. Cutler C, Giri S, Jeyapalan S, et al. Acute and chronic graft-versus-host disease after allogeneic peripheral-blood stem-cell and bone marrow transplantation: a meta-analysis. *J Clin Oncol* 2001;19:3685.

71. Morton J, Hutchins C, Durrant S. Granulocyte-colony-stimulating factor (G-CSF)-primed allogeneic bone marrow: significantly less graft-versus-host disease and comparable engraftment to G-CSF-mobilized peripheral blood stem cells. *Blood* 2001;98:3186.

72. Ji SQ, Chen HR, Wang HX, et al. Comparison of outcome of allogeneic bone marrow transplantation with and without granulocyte colony-stimulating factor (lenograstim) donor-marrow priming in patients with chronic myelogenous leukemia. *Biol Blood Marrow Transplant* 2002;8:261.

73. Goldman JM, Gale RP, Horowitz MM, et al. Bone marrow transplantation for chronic myelogenous leukemia in chronic phase. Increased risk for relapse associated with T-cell depletion. *Ann Intern Med* 1988;108:806.

74. Devergie A, Reiffers J, Vernant JP, et al. Long-term follow-up after bone marrow transplantation for chronic myelogenous leukemia: factors associated with relapse. *Bone Marrow Transplant* 1990;5:379.

75. Elmaagacli AH, Peceny R, Steckel N, et al. Outcome of transplantation of highly purified peripheral blood CD34+ cells with T-cell add-back compared with unmanipulated bone marrow or peripheral blood stem cells from HLA-identical sibling donors in patients with first chronic phase chronic myeloid leukemia. *Blood* 2003;101:446.

76. Faderl S, Talpaz M, Kantarjian HM, et al. Should polymerase chain reaction analysis to detect minimal residual disease in patients with chronic myelogenous leukemia be used in clinical decision making? *Blood* 1999;93:2755.

77. Radich JP, Gehly G, Gooley T, et al. Polymerase chain reaction detection of the BCR-ABL fusion transcript after allogeneic marrow transplantation for chronic myeloid leukemia: results and implications in 346 patients. *Blood* 1995;85:2632.

78. Lin F, van Rhee F, Goldman JM, et al. Kinetics of increasing BCR-ABL transcript numbers in chronic myeloid leukemia patients who relapse after bone marrow transplantation. *Blood* 1996;87:4473.

79. van Rhee F, Szydlo RM, Hermans J, et al. Long-term results after allogeneic bone marrow transplantation for chronic myelogenous leukemia in chronic phase: a report from the Chronic Leukemia Working Party of the European Group for Blood and Marrow Transplantation. *Bone Marrow Transplant* 1997;20:553.

80. Guglielmi C, Arcese W, Hermans J, et al. Risk assessment in patients with Ph+ chronic myelogenous leukemia at first relapse after allogeneic stem cell transplant: an EBMT retrospective analysis. The Chronic Leukemia Working Party of the European Group for Blood and Marrow Transplantation. *Blood* 2000;95:3328.

81. Higano CS, Chielens D, Raskind W, et al. Use of alpha-2a-interferon to treat cytogenetic relapse of chronic myeloid leukemia after marrow transplantation. *Blood* 1997;90:2549.

82. Olavarria E, Ottmann OG, Deininger M, et al. Response to imatinib in patients who relapse after allogeneic stem cell transplantation for chronic myeloid leukemia. *Leukemia* 2003;17:1707.

83. Klein JP, Keiding N, Shu Y, et al. Summary curves for patients transplanted for chronic myeloid leukaemia salvaged by a donor lymphocyte infusion: the current leukaemia-free survival curve. *Br J Haematol* 2000;109:148.

84. Porter DL, Collins RH Jr, Shpilberg O, et al. Long-term follow-up of patients who achieved complete remission after donor leukocyte infusions. *Biol Blood Marrow Transplant* 1999;5:253.

85. Porter DL, Collins RH, Hardy C, et al. Treatment of relapsed leukemia after unrelated donor marrow transplantation with unrelated donor leukocyte infusions. *Blood* 2000;95:1214.

86. Gratwohl A, Hermans J, Apperley J, et al. Acute graft-versus-host disease: grade and outcome in patients with chronic myelogenous leukemia. Working Party Chronic Leukemia of the European Group for Blood and Marrow Transplantation. *Blood* 1995;86:813.

87. Bhatia R, Verfaillie CM, Miller JS, et al. Autologous transplantation therapy for chronic myelogenous leukemia. *Blood* 1997;89:2623.
88. Koziner B, Dengra C, Lucero G, et al. Autologous stem cell transplantation for patients with chronic myeloid leukemia. The Argentine Group of Bone Marrow Transplantation (GATMO) experience. *Cancer* 2002;95:2339.
89. Gale RP, Hehlmann R, Zhang MJ, et al. Survival with bone marrow transplantation versus hydroxyurea or interferon for chronic myelogenous leukemia. The German CML Study Group. *Blood* 1998;91:1810.
90. Lee SJ, Kuntz KM, Horowitz MM, et al. Unrelated donor bone marrow transplantation for chronic myelogenous leukemia: a decision analysis. *Ann Intern Med* 1997;127:1080.
91. O'Brien S, Thall PF, Siciliano MJ. Cytogenetics of chronic myelogenous leukaemia. *Baillieres Clin Haematol* 1997;10:259.
92. Sill H, Aguiar RC, Schmidt H, et al. Mutational analysis of the p15 and p16 genes in acute leukaemias. *Br J Haematol* 1996;92:681.
93. Talpaz M, Silver RT, Druker BJ, et al. Imatinib induces durable hematologic and cytogenetic responses in patients with accelerated phase chronic myeloid leukemia: results of a phase 2 study. *Blood* 2002;99:1928.
94. Sawyers CL, Hochhaus A, Feldman E, et al. Imatinib induces hematologic and cytogenetic responses in patients with chronic myelogenous leukemia in myeloid blast crisis: results of a phase II study. *Blood* 2002;99:3530.
95. Huron DR, Gorre ME, Kraker AJ, et al. A novel pyridopyrimidine inhibitor of Abl kinase is a picomolar inhibitor of Bcr-abl-driven K562 cells and is effective against STI571-resistant Bcr-abl mutants. *Clin Cancer Res* 2003;9:1267.
96. La Rosee P, Corbin AS, Stoffregen EP, et al. Activity of the Bcr-Abl kinase inhibitor PD180970 against clinically relevant Bcr-Abl isoforms that cause resistance to imatinib mesylate (Gleevec, STI571). *Cancer Res* 2002;62:7149.
97. Perkins C, Kim CN, Fang G, et al. Arsenic induces apoptosis of multidrug-resistant human myeloid leukemia cells that express Bcr-Abl or overexpress MDR, MRP, Bcl-2, or Bcl-x(L). *Blood* 2000;95:1014.
98. Gorre ME, Ellwood-Yen K, Chiosis G, et al. BCR-ABL point mutants isolated from patients with imatinib mesylate-resistant chronic myeloid leukemia remain sensitive to inhibitors of the BCR-ABL chaperone heat shock protein 90. *Blood* 2002;100:3041.
99. Druker BJ, O'Brien SG, Cortes J, et al. Chronic myelogenous leukemia. *Hematology (Am Soc Hematol Educ Program)* 2002;111.

SECTION 2

SUSAN O'BRIEN
MICHAEL J. KEATING

Chronic Lymphoid Leukemias

Chronic lymphocytic leukemia (CLL) is a monoclonal hematopoietic disorder characterized by a progressive expansion of lymphocytes of B-cell lineage. These small, mature-appearing lymphocytes accumulate in the blood, bone marrow, lymph nodes, and spleen. CLL is a common leukemia in the Western world; it accounts for 25% to 30% of all adult leukemias.[1] In Asian countries, CLL represents only 5% of leukemias, with the T-cell phenotype predominating. These geographic and ethnic differences in incidence are most likely the result of genetic factors; Japanese who have settled in Hawaii do not have a higher incidence of CLL than native Japanese.[2] Population studies have not linked the development of CLL to known occupational or environmental risk factors.[3] CLL has a strong familial aggregation, with a two- to sevenfold higher prevalence among family clusters than in the general population.[4] Approximately 7000 to 8000 new cases are diagnosed in the United States annually, with a male-female ratio of 1.6 to 2.0:1.[5] The median age at diagnosis is 65 years.

MOLECULAR BIOLOGY

IMMUNOPHENOTYPING

Clonality of CLL is confirmed by restriction on the cell surface membrane for either kappa or lambda light chains[1] and by the presence of immunoglobulin gene rearrangements.[1] In addition, these cells possess unique idiotypic specificities and often have cytogenetic or molecular abnormalities.[6,7] With the use of sensitive techniques, monoclonal proteins can be detected in the serum of many patients,[8] although only 5% to 10% of patients produce large enough quantities to be detected by serum electrophoresis. CLL cells usually express the B-cell markers CD19, CD20, CD21, CD23, and CD24; most CLL cells are also positive for Ia (DR and DC) and Fc receptors and have receptors for mouse erythrocytes (Table 43.2-1).[9] Some surface markers that are usually found on normal B cells, including CD22, are found infrequently on CLL cells. In addition to B-cell antigens, CLL cells express CD5, an antigen also found on T cells. Although CD5 can be found on normal B cells, these cells are predominantly in the fetal circulation or in the tonsils of normal adults. They usually would not be detected in the peripheral blood using standard immunophenotyping techniques.

SOMATIC MUTATION

Because CD5-positive B cells are found in the fetal spleen and because surface immunoglobulin D is present on cells that have not encountered antigen in the germinal center, it was long presumed that CLL cells are naive B cells. Normal B-cell development involves an antigen-independent phase and an antigen-dependent phase. During the antigen-independent phase, B cells undergo rearrangement of the V, D, and J genes in the bone marrow. Somatic mutation of the heavy- and light-chain genes occurs after encounter with antigen in the germinal center. Somatic mutations have occurred when there is less than 98% sequence homology with the germline gene. The figure of 98% is used because polymorphisms may account for lesser degrees of disparity.[10]

In the 1990s, data emerged that a significant percentage of patients with CLL evidenced somatic mutation in their VH genes. Subsequently, it was confirmed that approximately 50% of patients have mutated VH genes and that this provides significant prognostic information; patients with unmutated VH genes have significantly shorter survival.[11] The characterization of VH gene sequences is labor intensive and has not been readily exportable to clinical laboratories. Thus, correlates with mutation status that may be more easily identified would be useful in clinical care. A correlation between expression of CD38 and lack of somatic mutation has been described.[12] Although the correlation is significant and the presence of CD38, irrespective of mutation status, is associated with inferior survival, a significant minority of patients have mutated VH genes and yet express CD38, and vice versa. These patients may have an intermediate prognosis.[13]

The presence of roughly two equal groups of patients with different prognoses based on VH mutation status suggested that CLL, rather than a disease of naive B cells, might be two separate malignancies, one derived from a naive B cell that expressed unmutated VH genes and the other derived from a memory B cell that had been exposed to antigen and displayed mutated VH

TABLE 43.2-1. Immunophenotyping in Chronic B-Cell Leukemia

Disease	sIg	CD5	CD23	FMC7	CD22	CD79b	CD10
CLL	Weak	++	++	–/+	Weak/–	Weak/–	–
B-PLL	Strong	–/+	–/+	++	+	++	–
HCL	Strong	–	–	++	++	+	–
SLVL	Strong	–/+	–/+	++	++	++	–
FL	Strong	–	–	++	++	++	++
MCL	Strong	++	–/+	++	++	++	–/+

+, present; –, not present; B-PLL, B-cell prolymphocytic leukemia; CLL, chronic lymphocytic leukemia; FL, follicular lymphoma; HCL, hairy cell leukemia; MCL, mantle cell lymphoma; sIg, surface immunoglobulin; SLVL, splenic lymphoma with villous lymphocytes.

genes. This hypothesis has been examined by several groups using gene expression profiling.[14,15] Both groups found that mutated and unmutated CLL show a common pattern of expression that is clearly distinguishable from that of other lymphomas, as well as normal B cells. Nevertheless, although the overall profile was similar, many genes were differentially expressed between the two groups. The gene that was most differentially expressed in one series was ZAP-70, with unmutated cases having significant expression of ZAP-70. Interestingly, this protein is found in T cells, where it transduces signals from the T-cell receptor. It was subsequently shown that ligation of the B-cell receptor in CLL cells that expressed ZAP-70 produced greater tyrosine phosphorylation of cytosolic proteins than did stimulation of CLL cells that did not express ZAP-70. Expression of ZAP-70 was analyzed in 56 patients with CLL. This expression correlated with mutational status, disease progression, and survival (Figs. 43.2-1 and 43.2-2).[16]

MOLECULAR ABNORMALITIES

Conventional chromosome banding has identified cytogenetic abnormalities in 40% to 50% of CLL cases.[6] This technique is hampered by the low mitotic activity of CLL cells. Fluorescence *in situ* hybridization (FISH) using genomic DNA probes has enhanced the ability to detect molecular abnormalities. This technique can detect aberrations in interphase cells. The use of FISH has shown molecular abnormalities in up to 80% of cases of CLL.[7]

13q deletion is the most common genetic aberration found in CLL by FISH (55%), followed by 11q deletion (18%), 12q trisomy (16%), and 17p deletion (7%).[7] Before the use of FISH, trisomy 12 was the most frequently detected chromosomal abnormality in CLL by conventional cytogenetic methods.[6] Structural abnormalities of 13q were often missed by Giemsa banding, presumably because of the small size of the deletion. The prognosis of CLL varies with the chromosomal abnormality. When divided into five prognostic categories—17p deletion, 11q deletion, 12q trisomy, normal karyotype, and 13q deletion (as sole abnormality)—the survival times were 32, 79, 114, 111, and 133 months, respectively. Patients with 17p or 11q deletion had more advanced disease with extensive lymphadenopathy.

The frequency of 13q deletion has led to a search for a potentially new tumor suppressor gene in that location. At least eight genes were identified and screened for alterations at the

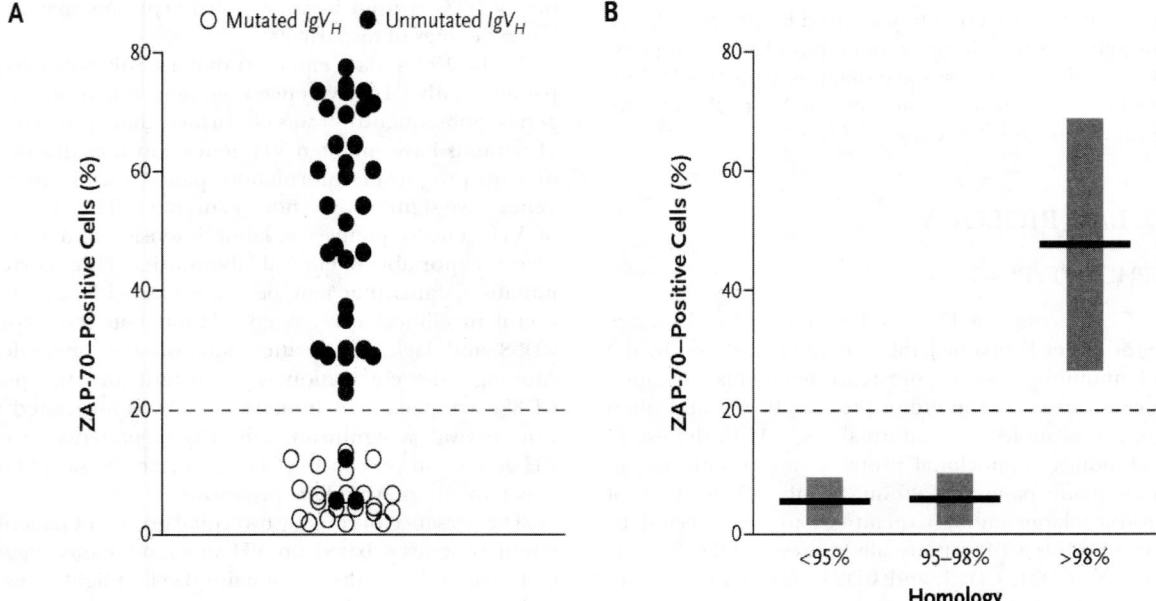

FIGURE 43.2-1. Correlation of the level of expression of ZAP-70 and immunoglobulin heavy-chain variable-region (IgV$_H$) mutational status **(A)** and IgV$_H$ sequence homology **(B)**.

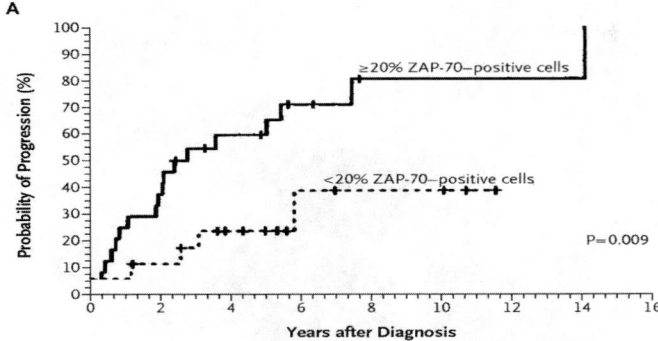

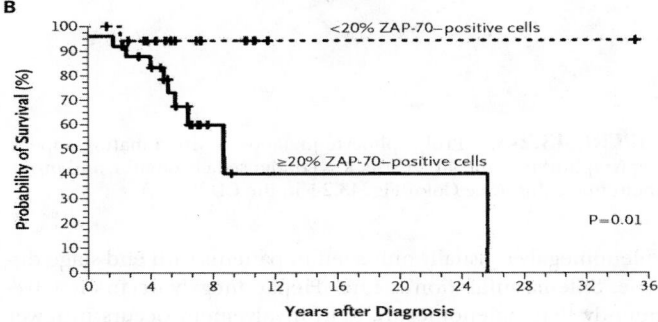

FIGURE 43.2-2. Kaplan-Meier estimates of the actuarial risk of disease progression **(A)** and the likelihood of survival **(B)** among patients with Binet stage A chronic lymphocytic leukemia, according to the level of expression of ZAP-70.

DNA or RNA level, or both, but studies have failed to find consistent involvement of any of those genes. It was found that micro-RNAs (MiR genes) MiR15 and MiR16 are deleted or down-regulated in two of three cases of CLL.[17] The purpose of these noncoding RNAs is uncertain; they may act similarly to small interfering RNAs. Identification of MiR15 and MiR16 target genes may elucidate their mechanism of action.

Another important finding that may significantly aid in identifying factors leading to the development of CLL is a murine model whereby mice accumulate an expanded CD5+ B-cell population, initially in the peritoneal cavity and then in the bone marrow; in addition, older mice develop a CLL-like disorder.[18] This transgenic mouse model was established with the T-cell leukemia-1 gene under the control of a V_H promoter. This model can also be used to test novel anti-CLL therapies in the future.

IMMUNE ABNORMALITIES

Early in the disease, the absolute number of T cells may be increased in untreated B-cell CLL with inversion of the T-helper–T-suppressor cell ratio.[19,20] The CD4-CD8 ratio continues to drop with disease progression or after therapy with nucleoside analogs or alemtuzumab. Assessment of the qualitative function of the T cells has been inconclusive. Normal and decreased CD4 cell function has been reported. Similarly, decreased, normal, or excessive CD8 cell function has been seen. Others have shown that T-cell functions may be impaired by immunosuppressive factors produced by B-CLL cells.[19] The

pathogenesis of the hypogammaglobulinemia in CLL is poorly understood. Impaired B-cell function and regulatory abnormalities of T cells, including the reversal of the normal helper–suppressor cell ratio, may play a role. In addition, CLL-derived natural killer (NK) cells have been shown to suppress immunoglobulin secretion by normal B cells *in vitro*.

DIAGNOSIS

The International Workshop on CLL (IW-CLL) and the National Cancer Institute–sponsored Working Group on CLL (NCI-WG) have outlined diagnostic criteria for CLL.[21,22]

IW-CLL CRITERIA

1. A sustained peripheral blood lymphocyte count greater than $10 \times 10^9/L$
2. A bone marrow aspirate showing greater than 30% lymphocytes
3. Peripheral blood lymphocytes identified as monoclonal B cells

Two of the three criteria are enough to establish a diagnosis.

NCI-WG CRITERIA

1. A peripheral blood lymphocyte count greater than $5 \times 10^9/L$, with less than 55% of the cells being atypical.
2. The lymphocytes should be monoclonal B lymphocytes expressing B-cell surface antigens (CD19, CD20, CD23), low-density surface immunoglobulin (M or D), and CD5 positivity.

A lymphocyte count greater than $5 \times 10^9/L$ was specified by the NCI-WG to distinguish CLL from small lymphocytic lymphoma. However, it is arguable as to whether that distinction is clinically relevant.

Other B-cell malignancies may also present with increased circulating lymphoid cells and should be differentiated from CLL. The diseases that may be confused with CLL are prolymphocytic leukemia (PLL), the leukemic phase of non-Hodgkin's lymphoma (mantle cell lymphoma, follicular lymphoma, or splenic lymphoma with circulating villous lymphocytes), and hairy cell leukemia (HCL). Immunophenotyping is helpful in differentiating these disorders (Figs. 43.2-3 to 43.2-5; see Table 43.2-1).

CLINICAL MANIFESTATIONS

With the use of routine blood testing, the number of CLL patients who are asymptomatic at diagnosis has increased to approximately 40%. Some patients may remain asymptomatic for long periods of time. Approximately 60% of CLL patients present with various symptoms, including constitutional. The most common complaint is fatigue, but this is generally not severe. Sometimes enlarged lymph nodes or the development of an infection is the initial manifestation of disease. Bacterial infections, such as pneumonia, are more common in patients who present with advanced-stage disease. Infections secondary to opportunistic organisms, particularly herpes zoster, may occur. An exaggerated skin reaction to a bee sting or an insect

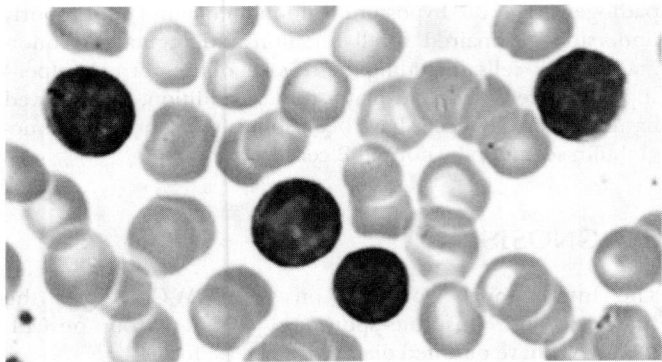

FIGURE 43.2-3. Chronic lymphocytic leukemia. Peripheral smear showing mature-appearing lymphocytes. (See Color Fig. 43.2-3 in the CD-ROM.)

bite is frequent (Well's syndrome). B symptoms are quite uncommon in patients with CLL. In contrast to the situation in lymphoma, fever in the absence of infection is rare in CLL. The lymph nodes, when enlarged, are usually discrete, freely movable, and nontender. Splenomegaly may occur, but massive

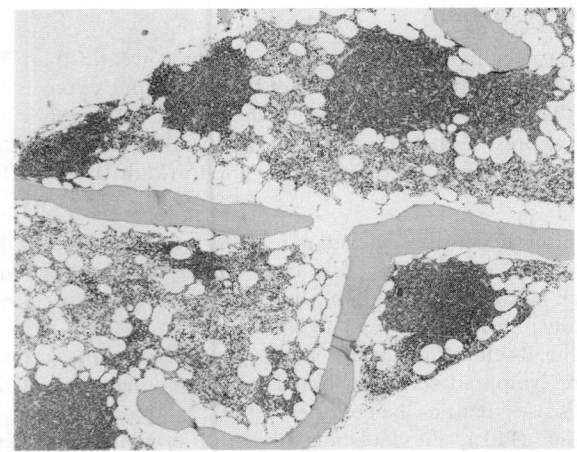

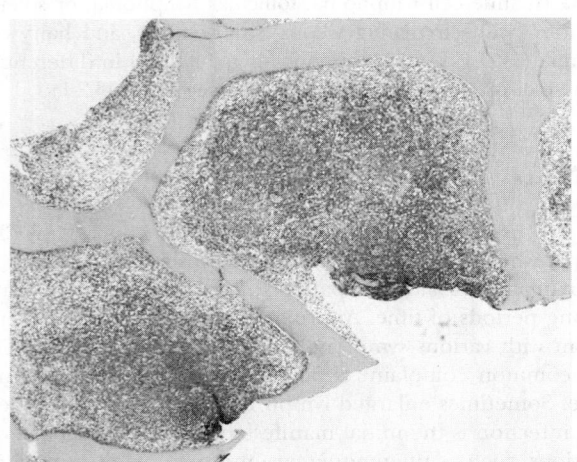

FIGURE 43.2-4. Chronic lymphocytic leukemia. Bone marrow infiltration may range from nodular/focal (**A**) to diffuse (**B**). (See Color Fig. 43.2-4 in the CD-ROM.)

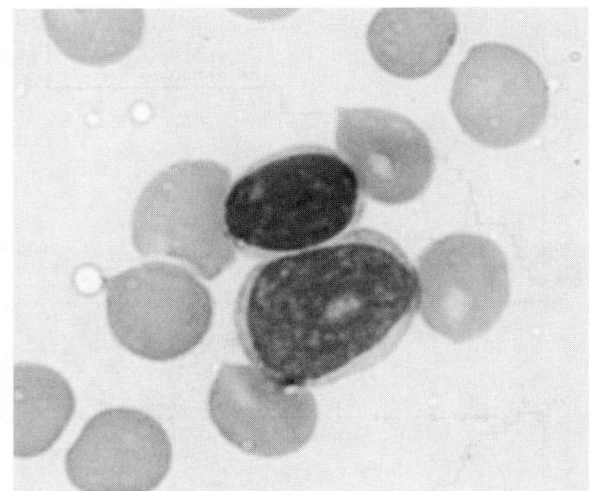

FIGURE 43.2-5. Prolymphocyte juxtaposed with a mature-appearing lymphocyte. Note larger size, less condensed chromatin, and prominent nucleolus. (See Color Fig. 43.2-5 in the CD-ROM.)

splenomegaly is usually only seen in patients with end-stage disease. Splenic infarction is rare. Hepatomegaly occurs less frequently than splenomegaly. Skin involvement occurs in fewer than 5% of cases. Leptomeningeal leukemia is rare and, if present, is usually seen in patients with refractory disease.

LABORATORY FINDINGS

Lymphocytosis, consisting of mature lymphocytes, is almost universal. Absolute lymphocyte counts range from $5 \times 10^9/L$ to $500 \times 10^9/L$. Unlike in acute myeloid leukemia, leukostasis is uncommon in CLL, probably because of the small size and pliable nature of the cells. Rarely, patients with a white blood cell count of less than $5 \times 10^9/L$ may be found to have CLL based on phenotyping of the lymphocytes. The event that prompts such analysis may be the development of hemolytic anemia or autoimmune thrombocytopenia. Marrow infiltration by lymphocytes varies from 30% to 100%, with normal or increased cellularity. The lymphocyte count usually increases over time, but fluctuations in the lymphocyte counts of untreated patients may occur, particularly in the setting of infection. In most cases, the lymphocytes are small and mature appearing, but there may be variations in cell morphology, with some lymphocytes being larger or atypical, whereas others may be plasmacytoid or cleaved or there may be prolymphocytes. The French-American-British (FAB) classification system divides patients into three groups depending on the percentage of abnormal cells.[23] In typical CLL, greater than 90% of the cells are small; in CLL/PLL, 11% to 54% of the cells are prolymphocytes; and in atypical CLL, there is heterogeneous morphology, but 10% or fewer of the cells are prolymphocytes. Ruptured lymphocytes or "smudge" cells are commonly seen in the peripheral smear, reflecting fragility and distortion during preparation of the peripheral smear on the glass slide. Three types of lymphoid infiltration of the marrow can be seen in biopsy specimens: nodular, interstitial, and diffuse. Sometimes, a mixture of the first two patterns is seen. Patients with diffuse infiltration usually have advanced disease and a worse prognosis. Nodular and interstitial patterns may be grouped together as "nondiffuse" and are associated with less advanced disease and better outcome.

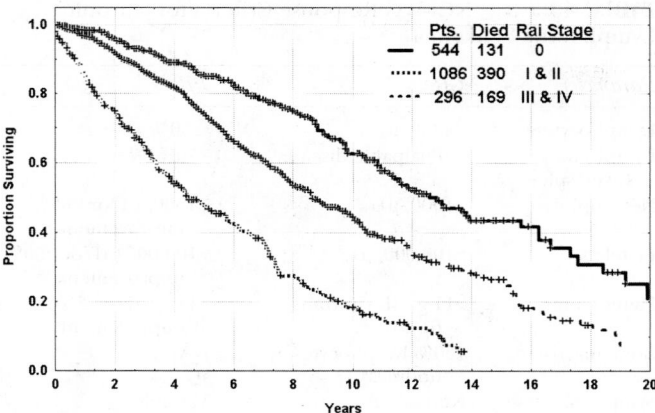

Pts.	Died	Rai Stage
544	131	0
1086	390	I & II
296	169	III & IV

FIGURE 43.2-6. Survival of 1926 previously untreated patients (Pts.) seen at the M. D. Anderson Cancer Center according to Rai stage.

Anemia (hemoglobin less than 11 g/dL) and thrombocytopenia (platelet count less than 100×10^9/L) are frequent with disease progression but occur in only a minority of patients at the time of initial diagnosis. A positive direct antiglobulin test is seen in approximately 25% of cases, but overt autoimmune hemolytic anemia (AIHA) occurs less frequently. The incidence of a positive direct antiglobulin test (Coombs') increases significantly with disease stage.[24] Autoimmune thrombocytopenia is usually diagnosed on the basis of a low platelet count in the presence of adequate numbers of megakaryocytes in the bone marrow. Neutropenia may also be encountered. These cytopenias may be the result of bone marrow failure due to "packed" marrow by CLL or occur as a result of an immune-mediated process or hypersplenism. Hypogammaglobulinemia occurs in approximately 50% of patients with CLL. At diagnosis, it may be noted in fewer than 10% of patients, but its incidence increases significantly with disease progression. Usually, all three immunoglobulin classes (G, A, and M) are decreased, but in some patients only one or two may be low. Significant hypogammaglobulinemia and neutropenia result in increased susceptibility of patients with CLL to bacterial infections.

AUTOIMMUNE COMPLICATIONS

When autoantibodies are present in CLL, they are usually targeted against hematopoietic cells, resulting in AIHA, immune thrombocytopenia, immune-mediated granulocytopenia, and pure red cell aplasia.[25] AIHA is the most frequently occurring of these. Several factors indicate that antibodies against blood cell

antigens are not produced by the leukemic clone. These autoantibodies are polyclonal and are usually immunoglobulin G.[26] The severity of the autoimmune phenomenon does not necessarily correlate with the severity of CLL, and such events may develop in patients whose disease is responding to therapy with fludarabine. Prednisone (P) is the most commonly used treatment for autoimmune complications, with high initial response rates. Relapses are not uncommon. Cyclosporin A is another effective therapy and can produce good results, even in steroid-refractory patients.[27] The monoclonal antibodies rituximab and alemtuzumab have also been used in some patients in whom standard therapy fails and have produced responses.

STAGING

The natural history of CLL is variable, with survival times ranging from 2 to 20 years from diagnosis. In 1975, Rai et al.[28] developed a staging system consisting of five stages (Rai 0 to IV) based on Dameshek's model of orderly disease progression in CLL (Fig. 43.2-6; Table 43.2-2). The Rai staging system was later modified[29] into a three-stage system: low risk (Rai 0), intermediate risk (Rai I, II), and high risk (Rai III, IV). A similar staging system was developed in Europe by Binet et al.[30]; Binet stages A, B, and C generally correspond to low-risk, intermediate-risk, and high-risk disease in Rai staging. Both classifications are based on the extent of marrow compromise (i.e., anemia, thrombocytopenia) in advanced stages and increasing tumor burden in the earlier stages. Both staging systems have been recognized as simple and accurate predictors of survival (see Table 43.2-2), although most patients in the high-risk group (Rai III, IV; Binet C) have a progressive clinical course and short survival. The course of the disease is not uniform in the other risk groups. Patients in the low- and intermediate-risk groups may have an indolent disease course that spans years or even decades, or the course may be progressive and associated with a shortened survival. Thus, it is important to identify prognostic factors that will predict the clinical course of CLL in these risk groups. Several prognostic factors have been found to be associated with shortened survival in CLL. These include a short lymphocyte doubling time (less than 12 months), a diffuse pattern of bone marrow infiltration, advanced age and male gender,[69] abnormal karyotype, high serum levels of β_2-microglobulin and soluble CD23, and a CLL-PLL category (11% to 54% prolymphocytes in the blood).[31] Newer prognostics in CLL include the mutational status of genes, CD38 expression, and ZAP-70 protein, as previously described in Somatic Mutation.

Investigators from Spain have shown that patients presenting with low absolute lymphocyte counts (less than 30×10^9/

TABLE 43.2-2. Staging of Chronic Lymphocytic Leukemia

Rai Stage	Modified Rai Stage	Description	Binet Stage	Description
0	Low risk	Lymphocytosis only	A	Two or fewer lymphoid-bearing areas
1	Intermediate risk	Lymphocytosis and lymphadenopathy	B	Three or more lymphoid-bearing areas
2	Intermediate risk	Lymphocytosis and splenomegaly with/without lymphadenopathy	—	—
3	High risk	Lymphocytosis and anemia (hemoglobin, <11 g/dL)	C	Anemia (hemoglobin, <10 g/dL) or thrombocytopenia (platelets, 100×10^6/dL)
4	High risk	Lymphocytosis and thrombocytopenia (platelets, $<100 \times 10^6$/dL)	—	—

L), a hemoglobin greater than 12 g/dL, and a bone marrow biopsy showing a nondiffuse (interstitial or nodular) pattern of lymphoid infiltration have a survival similar to that of an age-matched population.[32] Similarly, a group in France have found that patients with Binet stage A disease with a hemoglobin greater than 12 g/dL and lymphocytosis less than 30×10^9/L had a survival time equal to that of an age- and sex-matched French population.[33]

TREATMENT AND RESPONSE CRITERIA

An unusual feature of CLL compared to other leukemias is that the diagnosis is not necessarily an indication to initiate treatment. This is true for several reasons. CLL is a disease of the older population, it may be diagnosed in an asymptomatic patient and have a prolonged course, and it is not curable with current treatment approaches. Thus, given that most patients are greater than 60 years old, may have significant comorbid conditions associated with aging, and may have indolent disease, a significant fraction of patients will die of other causes and may never require therapy for CLL.

The NCI-WG indications to initiate treatment for CLL[34] include constitutional symptoms attributable to CLL: weight loss (greater than 10% of baseline weight within the preceding 6 months), extreme fatigue, Eastern Cooperative Oncology Group performance status of 2 or greater, fever (temperature greater than 38°C or 100.5°F for at least 2 weeks), or night sweats without evidence of infection; evidence of progressive bone marrow failure characterized by the development of, or worsening of, anemia or thrombocytopenia, or both; AIHA or autoimmune thrombocytopenia, or both, poorly responsive to corticosteroid therapy; massive (greater than 6 cm below the left costal margin) or progressive splenomegaly; massive (greater than 10 cm in longest diameter) or progressive lymphadenopathy; progressive lymphocytosis defined as an increase in the absolute lymphocyte count by greater than 50% over a 2-month period, or a doubling time predicted to be less than 6 months. Hypogammaglobulinemia or monoclonal gammopathy is not a sufficient criterion to initiate therapy.

Several European groups conducted trials in the 1980s to evaluate whether immediate treatment in patients with early-stage disease could improve survival.[35] These large randomized trials of chlorambucil (CLB) therapy versus a watch-and-wait approach were consistent in showing no benefit to early treatment. Nevertheless, given the significantly better therapies available in the twenty-first century, this question has been raised again. A limitation of randomizing all early-stage patients is that approximately half of them may never require therapy for their disease, thus diluting any potential benefit to an early treatment arm. The discovery of important prognostic factors that can identify early-stage patients with a high likelihood of developing progressive disease may now allow such randomized trials to be conducted.

The response criteria published in 1988 by the NCI-WG on CLL were revised in 1996 (Table 43.2-3).[22] The main change in the criteria was that patients with residual lymphoid nodules on bone marrow biopsy would now be included with patients achieving partial response (PR) and subclassified as having nodular PR (nPR). This was based on data showing that the duration of nPR was significantly shorter than that of complete

TABLE 43.2-3. NCI-WG Response Criteria for Chronic Lymphocytic Leukemia

Parameter	CR	PR
Lymphocytes	≤4000/μL	≥50% ↓
Lymph nodes (liver, spleen)	No palpable disease	≥50% ↓
Neutrophils	≥1500/μL	≥1500/μL or ≥50% improvement
Platelets	>100,000/μL	>100,000/μL or ≥50% improvement
Hemoglobin	>11 g/dL (untransfused)	>11 g/dL or ≥50% improvement
Bone marrow	<30% lymphocytes, no nodules[a]	NA
Symptomatology	None	Variable

↓, decrease; CR, complete response; NA, not applicable; NCI-WG, National Cancer Institute-sponsored Working Group; PR, partial response.
[a]Less than 30% lymphocytes in marrow with residual nodules = nodular PR.

response (CR). Traditionally, flow cytometry studies have shown that in many patients achieving CR or nPR, a population of cells coexpressing CD5 and CD19 persist; in addition, few patients evidence a return to a germline immunoglobulin gene pattern by Southern blot analysis. With the use of two-color flow cytometry, greater than 5% CD5 and CD19 cells reflect minimum residual disease; these patients have a shorter remission duration than those who are MRD negative.

A sensitive four-color flow cytometry assay was developed to differentiate CLL cells from normal B cells on the basis of CD19/CD5/C2D0/CD79b expression.[36] The assay that detects one CLL cell in 10^4 to 10^5 leukocytes was used to assess MRD in 25 patients achieving morphologic CR; MRD was defined as greater than 0.05% CLL cells in the bone marrow. Six patients who were MRD positive had significantly shorter event-free survival and overall survival than did 19 patients who were MRD negative (median survival 39 months for MRD-positive patients vs. all MRD-negative patients alive at a median follow-up of 22 months ($P = .007$).

Polymerase chain reaction (PCR) techniques can also be applied to the assessment of MRD. Consensus primers for rearrangement of IgH gene can be used in 70% to 80% of patients and may detect 1 in 10^4 residual cells. Allele-specific oligonucleotide primers generated for individual patients are more sensitive, detecting 1 in 10^6 CLL cells. Development of quantitative PCR techniques may aid in following patients over time.

CHEMOTHERAPY WITH ALKYLATING AGENTS

For many decades, chemotherapy in CLL consisted of two alkylating agents: CLB and cyclophosphamide (CTX); they could be given with or without corticosteroids. Various doses and schedules of CLB have been used. Commonly used oral schedules include a daily dose of 0.08 mg/kg (4 to 8 mg total dose per day) or an intermittently pulsed schedule of 0.8 mg/kg (30 to 40 mg/m²) given every 2 weeks.[37] CLB is usually administered for several months, and the dose is adjusted to avoid myelosuppression, which is the main toxicity. One study suggested that continuous administration of CLB might be associated with an increased incidence of epithelial cancers in patients with CLL. CTX is usually given at a daily dose of 1 to 2 mg/kg. The overall response rate with either CLB or CTX is approximately 40% to 60%, with 3% to 5% CR.

P has been administered as a single agent, the main indication being treatment of autoimmune phenomena. It is usually given at a dose of 1 mg/kg orally and tapered once a response is noted. An initial increase in the absolute lymphocyte count may be observed due to demargination of lymphocytes. Anemia and thrombocytopenia improve in approximately two-thirds of patients.

Alkylating agents have been combined with steroids in an attempt to improve response rates. One small study compared CLB and P to CLB alone.[37] Although a higher overall response (OR) rate and CR rate were obtained with CLB plus P compared to CLB alone (87% and 20% vs. 45% and 9%, respectively), no difference in median survival was demonstrated. Jaksic et al.[37] compared high-dose daily CLB, 15 mg/d (given until CR or toxicity), to that of CLB, 75 mg given once a week for 6 weeks combined with P. A significantly higher response rate was noted with the continuous CLB arm versus the intermittent CLB plus P arm (70% vs. 31%, respectively). A survival advantage was also noted for patients who received continuous CLB. The cumulative dose for the continuous CLB arm was five to six times that given in the intermittent CLB plus P arm.

Some trials reported good results using CTX, vincristine, and P (CVP or COP) in patients with advanced CLL. Subsequently, the French Cooperative Group on CLL randomized patients with Binet stage B disease to CLB or COP; there was no difference in the rate of disease progression to a more advanced stage or survival between the two groups.[37] Similarly, the Eastern Cooperative Oncology Group conducted a randomized trial comparing CLB and P versus CVP and reported no difference in CR rate, duration of response, or survival. In another trial, the COP regimen was compared to a French CHOP regimen (cyclophosphamide, doxorubicin, vincristine, prednisone) in which doxorubicin at a dose of 25 mg/m² was added to COP. Patients with Binet stage C disease faired better with the CHOP regimen.[37] However, a similarly designed trial demonstrated no difference in survival with CHOP versus CLB and P in Binet stage B patients. CHOP was compared to daily high-dose CLB; there was a higher response rate with high-dose CLB (89% vs. 76%). Thus, CLB used in a traditional palliative mode may not take advantage of the dose response seen with alkylating agents. The use of anthracyclines in CLL is based on only one study (French CHOP).

PURINE ANALOGS

Several purine analogs have demonstrated major clinical activity in indolent lymphoid malignancies. Fludarabine monophosphate (Fludara), 2-chlorodeoxyadenosine (2-CdA), and pentostatin (deoxycoformycin) are all active agents in the treatment of CLL.[37]

In an initial phase II study, 31 patients received fludarabine intravenously at 20 mg/m²/d for 5 days. Four patients achieved PR (3) or CR (1), and 15 patients had clinical improvement. In a larger phase II trial conducted at M. D. Anderson Cancer Center, fludarabine was given at a dosage of 30 mg/m²/d for 5 days; a response rate of 59% was observed in 68 previously treated patients, with 15% achieving CR. Higher response rates

were seen in earlier-stage disease. A subsequent study explored the combination of fludarabine and P. Response rates were identical to those seen with single-agent fludarabine, but the addition of P was associated with an increased incidence of *Pneumocystis carinii* and *Listeria monocytogenes* infections. The major side effects associated with fludarabine were related to myelosuppression and immunosuppression, with low CD4 counts lasting for several months to years after completion of fludarabine treatment.[37]

Single-arm studies have evaluated fludarabine in previously untreated patients. Here response rates are higher at 70% to 80% and CR can be seen in 10% to 25%.[37] An oral formulation of fludarabine has been evaluated in relapsed patients with CLL.[38] Seventy-eight patients received oral fludarabine, 40 mg/m²/d for 5 days every 4 weeks for six to eight cycles. The OR rate was 51%, almost identical to prior trials using the intravenous formulation as a salvage regimen.

2-CdA has also been evaluated in CLL, with comparable efficacy.[37] Like fludarabine, 2-CdA is myelosuppressive and immunosuppressive, with infections being the major toxicity. Although initial data suggested that patients with disease resistant to fludarabine might respond to 2-CdA, this finding was not confirmed. Experience with pentostatin in CLL has been limited, but response rates appear lower than with the other nucleoside analogs.[37]

COMPARATIVE STUDIES

A European randomized trial compared six cycles of fludarabine with six cycles of CAP (CTX, 750 mg/m² on day 1; doxorubicin, 50 mg/m² on day 1; and P, 40 mg/m² on days 1 through 5 every 3 weeks) in 196 patients with Binet stage B or C CLL (Table 43.2-4).[39] In previously treated patients, a significantly higher OR rate of 48% (13% CR) was observed with fludarabine compared to CAP (27% OR, 6% CR). In previously untreated patients the response rates with fludarabine (71% OR, 23% CR) were similar to those with CAP (60% OR, 17% CR), but the duration of response was significantly longer with fludarabine (*P*<.001). In addition there was a trend for longer survival in previously untreated patients receiving fludarabine (*P* = .087). The French Cooperative Group on CLL randomized nearly 1000 previously untreated patients to one of three regimens: fludarabine, CHOP, or CAP.[40] OR rates were 71%, 71%, and 58%, respectively (*P*<.0001). Median survival times were 69, 67, and 70 months. Infection rates were similar, but extramedullary toxicity was less with fludarabine.

Results from an Intergroup trial in previously untreated patients with CLL showed significantly higher OR and CR rates in patients treated with fludarabine versus those given CLB.[41] The study, which enrolled 509 patients, administered standard-dose fludarabine or CLB at a single dose of 40 mg/m² every 4 weeks. A third arm, fludarabine at 20 mg/m²/d for 5 days plus CLB at 20 mg/m² on day one every 4 weeks, was closed early because of toxicity. Crossover was permitted for patients with no response or early relapse. The OR rate with fludarabine was 63% with 20% CR; the OR rate with CLB was 37% with 4% CR rate. Although a longer duration of response and an improved progression-free survival were noted in patients treated with fludarabine, no difference in survival was found between the two groups. Half of the patients who failed to respond to CLB responded to fludarabine, including a 14% CR rate; in contrast

TABLE 43.2-4.   Randomized Trials of Fludarabine versus Alkylating Agent–Based Therapy in Previously Untreated Patients with Chronic Lymphocytic Leukemia

| Trial | Percent Response | | Response Duration (Mo) | Median Survival (Mo) |
	Overall Response	Complete Response		
F vs. CAP (n = 100)	71 vs. 60	23 vs. 17	NR vs. 7[a]	NR vs. 53[b]
F vs. CLB (n = 372)	63 vs. 37[a]	20 vs. 4[a]	25 vs. 14[a]	66 vs. 56[c]
F vs. CHOP vs. CAP (n = 938)	71 vs. 71 vs. 58	40 vs. 30 vs. 15[a]	32 vs. 30 vs. 28[b]	69 vs. 67 vs. 70

CAP, cyclophosphamide, adriamycin, prednisone; CHOP, cyclophosphamide, adriamycin, vincristine, prednisone; CLB, chlorambucil; F, fludarabine; NR, not reached.
[a]$P < .001$.
[b]$P = .087$.
[c]$P = .10$.

only 7% of patients who failed to respond to fludarabine achieved PR with CLB.

Clearly, fludarabine is the most effective single agent in the treatment of CLL and is even as effective as alkylating agent–based combination therapy. It is not surprising that no trial has shown an improvement in survival with fludarabine given that even in previously untreated patients CR occurs in only a minority. It is unlikely that overall survival will be impacted until CR occurs in the majority of patients.

Purine analogs have been demonstrated to interfere with DNA repair mechanisms after exposure of cells to alkylating agents *in vitro*. Such experiments provided a rationale for combining fludarabine and CTX (FC) in patients with CLL. Several studies using this regimen have varied slightly in dose/schedule, but all produced OR rates of 82% to 94% in previously treated patients and 85% to 100% in previously untreated patients.[42–44] CR rates in patients receiving this regimen as initial therapy have ranged from 21% to 47%, higher than that seen with single-agent fludarabine. Two ongoing randomized trials are comparing fludarabine to FC as initial therapy for CLL.

BIOLOGIC THERAPIES

INTERFERON-α

Interferon-α decreases the lymphocyte count and has produced partial remissions in patients with early-stage CLL but is ineffective in advanced disease. Interferon-α has been given as maintenance therapy in patients who responded to fludarabine, but no improvement in response rate or time to progression was observed.[45]

MONOCLONAL ANTIBODIES

Rituximab is a chimeric monoclonal antibody targeted against the CD20 antigen, which is expressed on malignant and on normal B cells.[46] Several trials have evaluated the efficacy of rituximab in the treatment of CLL. Standard-dose rituximab (375 mg/m² weekly × 4) induces responses in up to 30% of previously treated patients; all responses are partial.[46] Higher doses of rituximab have also been studied. A dose-escalation study using doses of 500 mg/m² to 2250 mg/m² in 50 patients with lymphoid malignancies produced an OR rate of 40%; all of the responses were PRs.[47] When the dose levels were grouped into

the lower doses (500 to 825 mg/m²), intermediate doses (1000 to 1500 mg/m²), or highest dose (2250 mg/m²), a significant dose response was observed, ranging from 23% at the lower doses up to 80% at the highest dose ($P = .007$). A different intensification strategy administered standard-dose rituximab, 375 mg/m², three times a week for a total of 12 doses over a 4-week period. The overall response rate was 45%. Only one patient achieved a CR.[48]

This antibody has also been used as initial therapy of patients with CLL. Forty-four with advanced-stage CLL received rituximab at the standard dose for 4 weeks; maintenance rituximab was given weekly × 4 every 6 months for 2 years. The response rate at 6 weeks was 51%, with 4% complete remission. The median progression-free survival was 18.6 months.[49]

The only significant toxicity seen with this antibody is infusion-related side effects such as fever and chills. These are generally mild to moderate and usually only observed with the first dose. Although B cells are targeted by rituximab, trials to date have shown no subsequent decrease in immunoglobulin levels, and infection rates are low.

RITUXIMAB IN COMBINATION

In vitro data suggest that rituximab and fludarabine may potentiate each other. A Cancer and Leukemia Group B (CALGB) trial randomized patients with previously untreated CLL to standard-dose fludarabine for six cycles or a combination of fludarabine and rituximab for six cycles.[50] Patients in both arms of the trial received a 4-week consolidation with rituximab. High overall response rates were seen in both arms, but the concurrent arm had a significantly higher CR rate (33%) compared to patients receiving fludarabine alone (15%). The CR rate increased after consolidation, being 47% in the concurrent arm and 28% in the sequential arm. It was of note that the incidence of grade 3 to 4 neutropenia was increased in patients who received the combination of rituximab and fludarabine (77%) when compared to patients receiving fludarabine alone (41%). No significant difference was seen in the incidence of infection between the two arms. Rituximab has also been combined with fludarabine and CTX (FCR) in previously untreated patients with CLL.[51] Rituximab was given at 375 mg/m² on cycle 1 and at 500 mg/m² for subsequent cycles (total = 6). Fludarabine, 25 mg/m², and CTX, 250 mg/m², were given for 3 days in each cycle. The overall response rate was 95%; the CR rate was 68%. Molecular responses were observed with this combination. Approximately 50% of patients in CR were PCR negative at completion of therapy. The median time to progression has not been reached, with a median follow-up of 2 years.

ALEMTUZUMAB

Alemtuzumab is a humanized monoclonal antibody that binds to the CD52 antigen, which is expressed on more than 95% of human T and B lymphocytes at various stages of differentiation.[52] Data on the activity of alemtuzumab in patients with CLL is rapidly accumulating. The largest study to date enrolled 93 patients with fludarabine-refractory disease. Alemtuzumab was given intravenously at escalating doses up to 30 mg during the first week and subsequently 30 mg three times a week for 12 weeks. Complete remission and partial remission were observed in 2% and 31% of patients, respectively. Fifty-five patients (59%) had stable disease.[52] Alemtuzumab was very effective at eliminating disease in the peripheral blood and bone marrow; bulky lymphadenopathy was less sensitive to therapy, a pattern of response observed on other studies of alemtuzumab. Infusion-related adverse events are seen in the majority of patients with the initial doses. Of more concern is the T-cell suppression that occurs with this agent. As a consequence, a significant incidence of infections (especially cytomegalovirus reactivation) is associated with therapy. Antibacterial and antiviral prophylaxis should always be used with alemtuzumab. Subcutaneous administration of alemtuzumab may be better tolerated. In 41 previously untreated patients with CLL, alemtuzumab subcutaneously thrice weekly was associated with a response rate of 87% (CR, 19%; PR, 68%). Transient skin reactions were seen in 90% of patients, but other side effects were uncommon.[53]

A potentially more optimal use of monoclonal antibodies is in eradication of MRD after debulking with a chemotherapy-based regimen. Two trials have shown that alemtuzumab can be used to improve response rates after a fludarabine-based regimen and that molecular remissions may occur.[54,55]

BONE MARROW TRANSPLANTATION

Allogeneic bone marrow transplantation has not been a viable option in CLL in the past because of the prohibitive toxicity of this approach in a population of older patients. Thus, data are limited. The use of nonmyeloablative transplants has broadened the eligibility to include older patients and may make this approach to treatment more common. The largest series was reported by the European Blood and Marrow Transplant Registry in patients with CLL younger than 60 years from 30 centers worldwide transplanted between 1984 and 1992.[56] Most patients received CTX and total body irradiation followed by HLA-matched marrow from siblings. The 3-year probability of survival was 46%, with a projected survival at 5 years of 30% to 40%. Chronic graft-versus-host disease developed in 16 of 27 evaluable patients. Smaller single-institution studies have shown impressive survival times given that most patients were chemorefractory before transplant.[57] Early data with nonmyeloablative allogeneic transplants indicate almost universal engraftment, although the development of chimerism was slower than with myeloablative transplants. Patients with sensitive disease who were transplanted had a better outcome than those who had resistant disease.[58,59] With the recognition that 60% of CLL patients younger than 55 years eventually develop progressive disease and have a median survival probability of only 5 years after therapy, innovative therapies with curative intent, including the use of stem cell transplantation, will play an increasing role in the future. Auto bone marrow transplantation has also been evaluated.[57,60] The procedure appears to be safe, with a lower relapse rate in patients who transplanted in first remission as an intensification procedure compared to those who received their transplant as a salvage regimen for active disease.

SPLENECTOMY

A number of studies have suggested hematologic and survival benefits from splenectomy in patients with CLL. Splenectomy may be beneficial in individuals with immune-mediated cytopenias such as AIHA and idiopathic thrombocytopenic purpura after failure of corticosteroids or in improving blood counts in patients with hypersplenism. In a study from M. D. Anderson Cancer Center,[61] perioperative mortality among 55 patients was 9%, mostly related to a poor preoperative performance status. Improvements in the platelet count, neutrophil count, and hemoglobin occurred in 81%, 59%, and 33% of patients, respectively. Among Rai stage IV patients, a trend for improved survival was observed using a case-control analysis.

THERAPEUTIC CONSIDERATIONS FOR SPECIFIC PROBLEMS IN PATIENTS WITH CHRONIC LYMPHOCYTIC LEUKEMIA

The most common cause of morbidity in patients with CLL is infection. Because hypogammaglobulinemia is a contributing factor to patients' increased susceptibility to infections, a randomized double-blind study evaluated the use of intravenous immunoglobulin (IVIg), 400 mg/kg, versus placebo given every 3 weeks for 1 year to 84 patients with CLL. A significant reduction in bacterial infections was seen in the group treated with IVIg, but no statistically significant difference was observed in the number of life-threatening infections or nonbacterial infections. Because of the high cost of this therapy, monthly IVIg therapy is best used in hypogammaglobulinemic patients who experience repeated bacterial infections. The autoimmune complications of CLL can be treated with P or cyclosporine. The majority of patients respond to P, but those who are steroid refractory may benefit from IVIg, splenectomy, or danazol.

SECOND MALIGNANCIES AND TRANSFORMATION

Approximately 25% of patients with CLL develop second neoplasms, the most common being skin cancer. The second neoplasm is the cause of death in 7% to 10% of patients. In approximately 2% to 6% of patients, CLL may evolve into a high-grade lymphoma of the diffuse large cell type (Richter's transformation). Usually, Richter's lymphoma arises from the same original CLL clone, and its onset is heralded by fever, weight loss, a rising lactate dehydrogenase, and an asymmetric rapid lymph node enlargement.[62] Because the lymphoma may be patchy, a gallium scan, usually negative in CLL, may aid in identifying a "hot" lymph node–bearing area for biopsy. The prognosis of Richter's lymphoma is poor, with a median survival of only 5 months. PLL develops in approximately 2% to 5% of CLL patients. This transformation is different immunophenotypically and clinically from primary or *de novo* PLL. Secondary PLL is marked by the development of progressive refractory anemia and thrombocytopenia, progressive splenomegaly, and an increase in the percentage of prolymphocytes to greater than 30% of the leukemia cells. As with Richter's lymphoma, PLL transformation portends a poor prognosis despite aggressive therapy.

PROLYMPHOCYTIC LEUKEMIA

PLL is characterized by a high number of circulating prolymphocytes, splenomegaly, minimal lymphadenopathy, and a median survival of less than 3 years. This leukemia can be present at diagnosis or evolve from CLL.[63] When the latter occurs it has the same implication as a Richter's transformation, with a median survival of 6 to 9 months. Prolymphocytes are larger and less homogeneous than CLL cells and have abundant clear cytoplasm, clumped chromatin, and a prominent nucleolus. Prolymphocytes can be of either B- or T-cell type. B-PLL cells usually do not express CD5 but stain strongly for surface immunoglobulin and FMC7 (see Table 43.2-1). In 20% of cases of PLL, T-cell markers are expressed.

Splenectomy and lymphoma-like regimens have been used to treat PLL without much success. Nucleoside analog–based regimens appear to be the most effective, and alemtuzumab (Campath-1H) also has shown promising activity in T-PLL.[64]

LARGE GRANULAR LYMPHOCYTE LEUKEMIA

Large granular lymphocytes (LGLs) are larger than normal lymphocytes and contain azurophilic granules in their cytoplasm. LGLs comprise 10% to 15% of peripheral blood mononuclear cells and are predominantly of NK cell phenotype, a smaller fraction being of T-cell phenotype. The lymphoproliferative disorders of LGL number four: reactive/transient LGL expansion, chronic LGL lymphocytosis, indolent LGL leukemia, and aggressive LGL leukemia.[65] Clonal expansion of LGL can be of NK cell or T-cell phenotype; the T-cell phenotype comprises 80% of LGL leukemias. T-LGL cells have a CD3+/CD57+/CD56– immunophenotype, and NK-LGL express CD3–/CD56+/CD57–. Clonality of T-LGL can be established by T-cell receptor gene rearrangement studies. LGL leukemia is usually indolent. Patients present with cytopenias, including neutropenia with accompanying infections, pure red cell aplasia, thrombocytopenia, and anemia. Serologic abnormalities, such as positive rheumatoid factor or antinuclear antibody, or both; hypergammaglobulinemia; and high β_2-microglobin, are frequent. A small percentage of LGL leukemias present have a more aggressive course, and these cases tend to have an NK cell phenotype. Because lymphocyte counts are usually not elevated, diagnosis requires a high degree of suspicion and a careful examination of the peripheral blood smear and bone marrow. Although the disease is usually indolent, most patients require treatment for cytopenias. Various therapies, including low-dose methotrexate (10 mg/m² PO once weekly), cyclosporine (2 mg/kg PO every 12 hours), or CTX (100 mg PO daily) with or without oral P (1 mg/kg PO daily), have all been effective. Complete remissions may be seen in up to 50% of cases. Lymphoma-type regimens, for example, CHOP, have not been effective for aggressive disease.

HAIRY CELL LEUKEMIA

HCL is a rare B-cell lymphoproliferative disorder that affects adults and represents 2% of all leukemias. It has a marked male preponderance. Most patients have cytopenias; splenomegaly is also frequent.[66] Hairy cells can be seen in the peripheral blood, but at low frequency, and therefore are easily missed. These cells are twice as large as normal lymphocytes, with the nuclei showing a loose chromatin pattern and villi-like cytoplasmic projections (best viewed under phase contrast microscopy). Hairy cells infiltrate the bone marrow in an interstitial or focal pattern, with clear zones in between cells ("fried egg appearance"). Marrow reticulin is increased, and aspirates may result in a dry tap. Immunophenotypic analysis of hairy cells shows the presence of CD19, CD20, CD22, CD25, and CD103, and, in contrast to CLL, hairy cells are negative for CD5 and CD23. Hairy cells also stain strongly for surface immunoglobulin and FMC7. Use of CD103 antibody, which stains tartrate-resistant acid phosphatase, has obviated the need for cytochemical staining for tartrate-resistant acid phosphatase.

HCL has no staging system. For many years the only effective therapy was splenectomy. Pentostatin (2' deoxycoformycin) and cladribine (2-CdA) are the nucleoside analogs that are the mainstay of treatment of HCL.[67] Pentostatin is administered at 4 mg/m² every 2 weeks until maximum response, and 2-CdA is given at 0.1 mg/kg/d as a continuous intravenous infusion for 7 days, or the same total dose can be administered as a 2-hour infusion over 5 days. Because 2-CdA involves a single course of therapy and produces remission rates comparable to those of pentostatin, 2-CdA is used more frequently in the United States for the treatment of HCL. Multiple series have reported high response rates, with patients remaining in remission for many years. The majority of relapsed patients achieve second remission when retreated with pentostatin or 2-CdA. The choice of agent may depend on the duration of the first remission: If less than 3 years, an alternate agent should be used; if greater than 5 years, the same agent should be given. The role of interferon-α is currently limited to patients who are unresponsive to nucleoside analogs.

A certain percentage of patients may relapse with 2-CdA–resistant disease. In addition, 10% to 20% of patients have a variant form of HCL with high numbers of circulating hairy cells and a poor response to nucleoside analogs. Classic and variant hairy cells strongly express CD22, an adhesion molecule found on B cells. Data suggest marked efficacy of a recombinant immunotoxin, BL22, in the treatment of chemotherapy-resistant HCL.[68] This immunotoxin contains the variable domain of the anti-CD22 monoclonal antibody, RFB4, which is fused to a fragment of *Pseudomonas* exotoxin called *PE38*; this fragment lacks the domain necessary for cell binding and contains only the domain responsible for cell death. Between 0.2 and 4.0 mg BL22 was administered intravenously over 30 minutes daily for 3 days. Patients were retreated at intervals of 3 weeks or more and could receive a total of 16 cycles of BL22 or 2 cycles beyond complete remission. Of 16 patients who were resistant to 2-CdA, 11 achieved a complete remission and 2 a partial remission with BL22. After a median follow-up of 16 months (range, 10 to 23), 3 of 11 patients in CR relapsed and were retreated; all 3 patients achieved a second complete remission. Common side effects included transient hypoalbuminemia and elevated aminotransferase levels. In 2 of 16 patients, a reversible hemolytic-uremic syndrome developed. This high complete remission rate in refractory patients has not been described with any other agent.

REFERENCES

1. O'Brien S, delGiglio A, Keating M. Advances in the biology and treatment of B-cell chronic lymphocytic leukemia. *Blood* 1995;85:307.
2. Yanagihara ET, Blaisdell RK, Hayashi T, Lukes RJ. Malignant lymphoma in Hawaii-Japanese: a retrospective morphologic survey. *Hematol Oncol* 1989;7:219.
3. Preston DL, Kusumi S, Tomonoga M, et al. Cancer incidence in atomic bomb survivors. Part III. Leukemia, lymphoma and multiple myeloma. *Radiat Res* 1994;137[Suppl 2]:S68.
4. Houlston RS, Catovsky D, Yuille MR. Genetic susceptibility to chronic lymphocytic leukemia. *Leukemia* 2002;16:1008.
5. Jemal A, Murray T, Samuels A, et al. Cancer statistics, 2003. *CA Cancer J Clin* 2003;53:5.
6. Juliusson G, Oscier DG, Fitchett M, et al. Prognostic subgroups in B-cell chronic lymphocytic leukemia defined by specific chromosome abnormalities. *N Engl J Med* 1990;323:720.
7. Dohner H, Stilgenbauer S, Dohner K, et al. Chromosome aberrations in B-cell chronic lymphocytic leukemia: reassessment based on molecular cytogenetic analysis. *J Mol Med* 1999;77:266.
8. Beaume A, Brizard A, Dreyfus B, et al. High incidence of serum monoclonal Igs detected by a sensitive immunoblotting technique in B-cell lymphocytic leukemia. *Blood* 1994;84:1216.
9. Geisler CH, Larsen JK, Hansen NE, et al. Prognostic importance of flow cytometric immunophenotyping of 540 consecutive patients with B-cell chronic lymphocytic leukemia. *Blood* 1991;78:1795.
10. Naylor M, Capra JD. Mutational status of Ig V_H genes provides clinically valuable information in B-cell chronic lymphocytic leukemia. *Blood* 1999;94(6):1837.
11. Hamblin TJ, Davis Z, Gardiner A, et al. Unmutated Ig V(H) genes are associated with a more aggressive form of chronic lymphocytic leukemia. *Blood* 1999;94:1848.
12. Damle RN, Wasil T, Fais F, et al. Ig V gene mutation status and CD38 expression as novel prognostic indicators in chronic lymphocytic leukemia. *Blood* 1999;94:1840.
13. Hamblin TJ, Orchard JA, Ibbotson RE, et al. CD38 expression and immunoglobulin variable region mutations are independent prognostic variables in chronic lymphocytic leukemia, but CD38 expression may vary during the course of the disease. *Blood* 2002;99:1023.
14. Rosenwald A, Alizadeh AA, Widhopf G, et al. Relation of gene expression phenotype to immunoglobulin mutation genotype in B cell chronic lymphocytic leukemia. *J Exp Med* 2001;194(11):1639.
15. Klein U, Tu Y, Stolovitzky GA, et al. Gene expression profiling of B cell chronic lymphocytic leukemia reveals a homogeneous phenotype related to memory B cells. *J Exp Med* 2001;194(11):1625.
16. Crespo M, Bosch F, Villamor N, et al. ZAP-70 expression as a surrogate for immunoglobulin-variable-region mutations in chronic lymphocytic leukemia. *N Engl J Med* 2003;348:1764.
17. Calin GA, Dumitru CD, Shimizu M, et al. Frequent deletions and down-regulation of micro-RNA genes miR15 and miR16 at 13q14 in chronic lymphocytic leukemia. *Proc Natl Acad Sci U S A* 2002;99(24):15524.
18. Bichi R, Shinton SA, Martin ES, et al. Human chronic lymphocytic leukemia modeled in mouse by targeted TCL1 expression. *Proc Natl Acad Sci U S A* 2002;99(10):6955.
19. Decker T, Flohr T, Trautmann P, et al. Role of accessory cells in cytokine production by T cells in chronic B-cell lymphocytic leukemia. *Blood* 1995;86(3):1115.
20. Scrivener S, Goddard RV, Kaminski ER, et al. Abnormal T-cell function in B-cell chronic lymphocytic leukaemia. *Leuk Lymphoma* 2003;44(3):383.
21. International Workshop on chronic lymphocytic leukemia. Chronic lymphocytic leukemia: recommendations for diagnosis, staging and response criteria. *Ann Intern Med* 1989;110:236.
22. Cheson BD, Bennett JM, Grever M, et al. National Cancer Institute-sponsored Working Group guidelines for chronic lymphocytic leukemia: revised guidelines for diagnosis and treatment. *Blood* 1996;87:4990.
23. Bennet JM, Catovsky D, Daniel MT, et al. Proposals for the classification of chronic (mature) B and T lymphoid leukemias. *J Clin Pathol* 1989;42:567.
24. Mauro FR, Foa R, Cerretti C, et al. Autoimmune hemolytic anemia in chronic lymphocytic leukemia: clinical, therapeutic, and prognostic features. *Blood* 2000;95(9):2786.
25. Diehl LF, Ketchum LH. Autoimmune disease and chronic lymphocytic leukemia: autoimmune hemolytic anemia, pure red cell aplasia, and autoimmune thrombocytopenia. *Semin Oncol* 1998;24:80.
26. Kipps TJ, Carson DA. Autoantibodies in chronic lymphocytic leukemia and related systemic autoimmune disease. *Blood* 1993;81:2475.
27. Cortes J, O'Brien S, Loscertales J, et al. Cyclosporin A for the treatment of cytopenia associated with chronic lymphocytic leukemia. *Cancer* 2001;92:2016.
28. Rai KR, Sawitsky A, Cronkite EP, et al. Clinical staging of chronic lymphocytic leukemia. *Blood* 1975;46:219.
29. Rai KR. A critical analysis of staging in CLL. In: Gale RP, Rai KR, eds. *Chronic lymphocytic leukemia: recent progress and future direction.* UCLA Symposia on Molecular and Cellular Biology, New Series. Vol 59. New York: Liss, 1987:253.
30. Binet J-L, Auquier A, Dighiero G, et al. A new prognostic classification of chronic lymphocytic leukemia derived from a multivariate survival analysis. *Cancer* 1981;48:198.
31. Zwiebel JA, Cheson BD. Chronic lymphocytic leukemia: staging and prognostic factors. *Semin Oncol* 1998;25:42.
32. Montserrat E, Rozman C. Chronic lymphocytic leukemia: prognostic factors and natural history. *Baillieres Clin Haematol* 1993;6:849.
33. Dighiero G, Maloum K, Desablens B, et al. Chlorambucil in indolent chronic lymphocytic leukemia. *N Engl J Med* 1998;338:1506.
34. Cheson BC, Bennett JM, Grever M, et al. National Cancer Institute-sponsored Working Group guidelines for chronic lymphocytic leukemia: revised guidelines for diagnosis and treatment. *Blood* 1996;87:4990.
35. Chemotherapeutic options in chronic lymphocytic leukemia: a meta-analysis of the randomized trials. CLL Trialists' Collaborative Group. *J Natl Cancer Inst* 1999;91:861.
36. Rawstron AC, Kennedy B, Evans PA, et al. Quantitation of minimal disease levels in chronic lymphocytic leukemia using a sensitive flow cytometric assay improves the prediction of outcome and can be used to optimize therapy. *Blood* 2002;99(5):1873.
37. Robak T, Kasznicki M. Alkylating agents and nucleoside analogues in the treatment of B cell chronic lymphocytic leukemia. *Leukemia* 2002;16:1015.
38. Boogaerts MA, Van Hoof A, Catovsky D, et al. Activity of oral fludarabine phosphate in previously treated chronic lymphocytic leukemia. *J Clin Oncol* 2001;19(22):4252.
39. Johnson S, Smith AG, Löffler H, et al. Multicenter prospective randomized trial of fludarabine versus cyclophosphamide, doxorubicin, and prednisone (CAP) for treatment of advanced stage chronic lymphocytic leukemia. *Lancet* 1996;347:1432.
40. Leporrier M, Chevret S, Cazin B, et al. Randomized comparison of fludarabine, CAP, and ChOP in 938 previously untreated stage B and C chronic lymphocytic leukemia patients. *Blood* 2001;98(8):2319.
41. Rai KR, Peterson B, Elias I, et al. A randomized comparison of fludarabine and chlorambucil for patients with previously untreated chronic lymphocytic leukemia: a CALGB, SWOG, CTG/NCI-C and ECOG Intergroup Study. *N Engl J Med* 2000;343:1750.
42. Flinn IW, Byrd JC, Morrison C, et al. Fludarabine and cyclophosphamide with filgrastim support in patients with previously untreated indolent lymphoid malignancies. *Blood* 2000;96:71.
43. O'Brien SM, Kantarjian HM, Cortes J, et al. Results of the fludarabine and cyclophosphamide combination regimen in chronic lymphocytic leukemia. *J Clin Oncol* 2001;19:1414.
44. Hallek M, Schmitt B, Wilhelm M, et al. Fludarabine plus cyclophosphamide is an efficient treatment for advanced chronic lymphocytic leukaemia (CLL): results of a phase II study of the German CLL Study Group. *Br J Haematol* 2001;114:342.
45. O'Brien S, Kantarjian H, Beran M, et al. Interferon maintenance therapy for patients with chronic lymphocytic leukemia in remission after fludarabine therapy. *Blood* 1995;86:1296.
46. Avivi I, Robinson S, Goldstone A. Clinical use of rituximab in haematological malignancies. *Br J Cancer* 2003;89:1389.
47. O'Brien SM, Kantarjian H, Thomas DA, et al. Rituximab dose-escalation trial in chronic lymphocytic leukemia. *J Clin Oncol* 2001;19:2165.
48. Byrd JC, Murphy T, Howard RS, et al. Rituximab using a thrice weekly dosing schedule in B-cell chronic lymphocytic leukemia and small lymphocytic lymphoma demonstrates clinical activity and acceptable toxicity. *J Clin Oncol* 2001;19:2153.
49. Hainsworth JD, Litchy S, Barton JH, et al. Single-agent rituximab as first-line and maintenance treatment for patients with chronic lymphocytic leukemia or small lymphocytic lymphoma: a phase II trial of the Minnie Pearl Cancer Research Network. *J Clin Oncol* 2003;21(9):1746.
50. Byrd JC, Peterson BL, Morrison VA, et al. Randomized phase 2 study of fludarabine with concurrent versus sequential treatment with rituximab in symptomatic, untreated patients with B-cell chronic lymphocytic leukemia: results from Cancer and Leukemia Group B 9712 (CALGB 9712). *Blood* 2003;101:6.
51. Lin TS, Lucas MS, Byrd JC. Rituximab in B-cell chronic lymphocytic leukemia. *Semin Oncol* 2003;30:483.
52. Moreton P, Hillmen P. Alemtuzumab therapy in B-cell lymphoproliferative disorders. *Semin Oncol* 2003;30(4):493.
53. O'Brien S, Giles FJ. Monoclonal antibodies in the treatment of lymphoid leukemia. *Drugs Today* 2003;39(7):541.
54. Montillo M, Cafro AM, Tedeschi A, et al. Safety and efficacy of subcutaneous Campath-1H for treating residual disease in patients with chronic lymphocytic leukemia responding to fludarabine. *Haematologica* 2002;87(7):695.
55. O'Brien SM, Kantarjian HM, Thomas DA, et al. Alemtuzumab as treatment for residual disease after chemotherapy in patients with chronic lymphocytic leukemia. *Cancer* 2003;98(12):2657.
56. Michallet M, Archimbaud E, Bandini G, et al. HLA-identical sibling bone marrow transplantation in younger patients with chronic lymphocytic leukemia. *Ann Intern Med* 1996;124:311.
57. Dreger P, Montserrat E. Autologous and allogeneic stem cell transplantation for chronic lymphocytic leukemia. *Leukemia* 2002;16:985.
58. Khouri IF, Keating M, Korbling M, et al. Transplant-lite: induction of graft-versus-malignancy using fludarabine-based non-ablative chemotherapy and allogeneic blood progenitor-cell transplantation as treatment for lymphoid malignancies. *J Clin Oncol* 1998; 16:2817.
59. Dreger P, Brand R, Hansz J, et al. Treatment-related mortality and graft-versus-leukemia activity after allogeneic stem cell transplantation for chronic lymphocytic leukemia using intensity-reduced conditioning. *Leukemia* 2003;17:841.
60. van Besien K, Keralavarma B, Devine S, et al. Allogeneic and autologous transplantation for chronic lymphocytic leukemia. *Leukemia* 2001;15:1317.
61. Seymour JF, Cusack JD, Lerner SA, et al. Case/control study of the role of splenectomy in chronic lymphocytic leukemia. *J Clin Oncol* 1997;15:52.
62. Giles FJ, O'Brien S, Keating M. Chronic lymphocytic leukemia in (Richter's) transformation. *Semin Oncol* 1998;25:117.
63. Hercher C, Robain M, Davi F, et al. A multicentric study of 41 cases of B-prolymphocytic leukemia: two evolutive forms. *Leuk Lymphoma* 2001;42(5):981.
64. Cao TM, Coutre SE. T-cell prolymphocytic leukemia: update and focus on alemtuzumab (Campath-1H). *Hematology* 2003;1:1.
65. Lamy T, Loughran TP Jr. Clinical features of large granular lymphocyte leukemia. *Semin Hematol* 2003;40:185.
66. Allsup DJ, Cawley JC. The diagnosis and treatment of hairy-cell leukaemia. *Blood Reviews* 2002;16:255.
67. Mey U, Strehl J, Gorschluter M, et al. Advances in the treatment of hairy-cell leukaemia. *Lancet Oncol* 2003;4:86.
68. Kreitman RJ, Wilson WH, Bergeron K, et al. Efficacy of the anti-CD22 recombinant immunotoxin BL22 in chemotherapy-resistant hairy-cell leukemia. *N Engl J Med* 2001;345(4):241.

SECTION **3**

STEFAN FADERL
HAGOP M. KANTARJIAN

Myelodysplastic Syndromes

Myelodysplastic syndromes (MDS) are clonal hematopoietic stem cell disorders whose common denominator is dysplasia in one or more hematopoietic cell lineages (Fig. 43.3-1).[1] Dysplasia reflects accelerated apoptosis, and the combination of apoptosis and excessive cell proliferation results in the paradoxic picture of peripheral blood cytopenias with hypercellular marrows.[2] MDS have been historically referred to as *refractory anemia* (RA), *preleukemia*, or *smoldering leukemia*, terminologies reflecting the proximity of MDS to acute myeloid leukemia (AML) and its capacity to evolve into AML over time. However, restricting the view of MDS to a purely preleukemic condition ignores differences between the two disorders: (1) The clinical picture and prognosis of MDS are more defined by cytopenias, and most patients will not progress to AML, and (2) distinct biologic differences exist that identify MDS as an entity separate from AML.[3]

Assessment of patients with MDS and choice of appropriate therapies remain challenging. Recent years witnessed the development of various classifications that assign patients to risk groups as defined by percent of blasts, karyotype abnormalities, or severity of cytopenias. However valuable they have proved to be, none takes into full account the heterogeneity of MDS. Further exploration of cytogenetic-molecular abnormalities and better insights into the pathophysiology of MDS will help define its pathophysiology, dissect its various subtypes, and provide the scientific rationale for new therapeutic targets.

INCIDENCE AND EPIDEMIOLOGY

MDS is primarily a disease of the elderly. The median age of onset is between 60 and 70 years of age. Although uncommon in children, up to 20% of children with AML may experience a prior myelodysplastic phase. A slight male predominance is typical throughout all age groups. Approximately 5000 to 7000 new cases of MDS are diagnosed each year in the United States.[4] With a median survival of 1 to 3 years, the estimated prevalence is 10,000 to 20,000 cases. The true incidence of MDS may be higher, as: (1) the diagnosis is often overlooked; (2) cases are not always reported; (3) patients do not receive any specific therapy because of old age, the perceived indolent nature of the disease, comorbidities, and lack of effective low-risk treatment modalities; and (4) MDS may be misdiagnosed as aplastic anemia, AML, or myeloproliferative disorders.

ETIOLOGY

The etiology of MDS remains unknown in most cases.[4] MDS is more common in males, in persons with agricultural and industrial occupations, or with exposure to smoking, hair dyes, pesticides, herbicides, organic chemicals, and heavy metals. Other risk factors include benzene, other solvents (e.g., toluene, xylene), chloramphenicol, and marrow-damaging agents including chemotherapeutic agents (e.g., alkylating agents). Occupational exposure to stone and cereal dusts, exhaust gases, nitro-organic explosives, ammonia, diesel fuel, and other petrochemical derivatives has also been associated with MDS. MDS occurs at a higher incidence after exposure to ionizing radiation. A dose-dependent increase of MDS has occurred in atomic bomb survi-

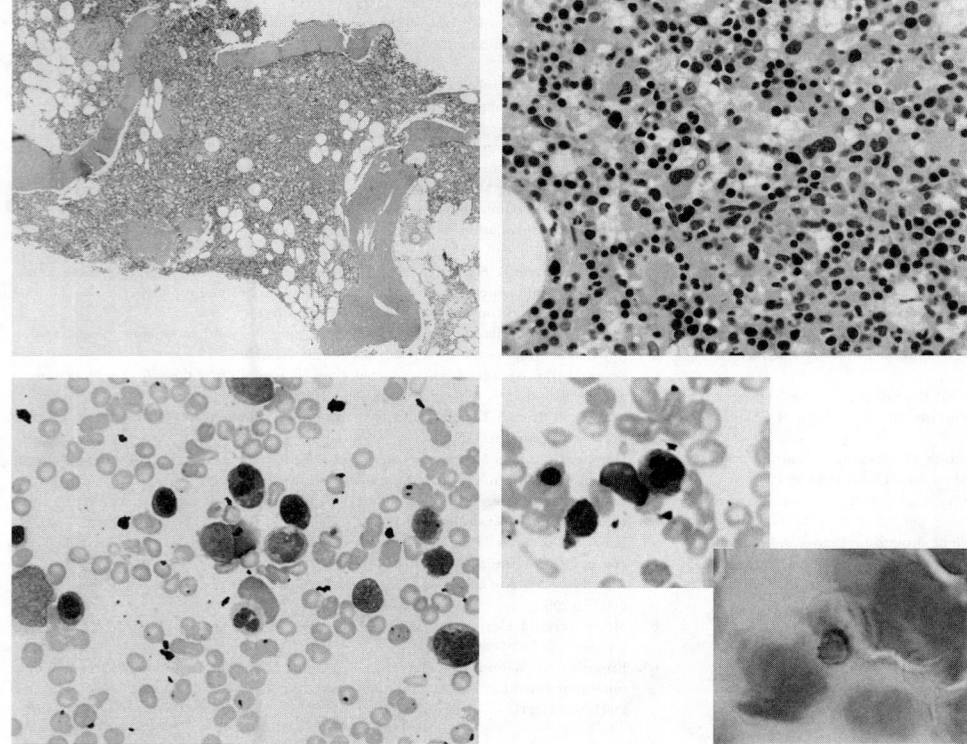

FIGURE 43.3-1. Composite illustrating ineffective hematopoiesis with hypercellular marrow, including dysplastic megakaryocytes, smear with increased blasts (refractory anemia with excess of blasts in transformation), dysgranulopoiesis, dyserythropoiesis, and ringed sideroblasts. (Courtesy of Dr. Carlos Bueso-Ramos, Hematopathology, M. D. Anderson Cancer Center.) (See Color Fig. 43.3-1 in the CD-ROM.)

vors in Japan, even many years after the original exposure. A number of MDS cases have been described in decontamination workers after the Chernobyl nuclear plant accident. Likewise, chronic exposure to low-dose radiation (radiopharmaceuticals) has been found to increase the risk of MDS.[5–7]

A clear association with any of these predisposing factors is found in 20% to 30% of patients [secondary MDS, treatment-related MDS (t-MDS)].[8] The incidence of t-MDS is increasing because of longer survival times currently achieved for tumors that formerly had a rather poor prognosis. The incidence of t-MDS is 10% to 15% at 10 years in patients with Hodgkin's disease and 14% at 4 years in patients aggressively treated for small cell lung cancer.[8] Among patients with Hodgkin's disease or non-Hodgkin's lymphoma undergoing autologous stem cell transplantation (SCT) with high-dose cyclophosphamide and total body irradiation, the estimated cumulative risk of t-MDS at 5 years is 11% to 18%.[9,10] Alkylating agents (cyclophosphamide, melphalan, procarbazine, chlorambucil) are associated with the highest risk of developing t-MDS. A link has been established between exposure to topoisomerase II inhibitors, such as etoposide, and t-MDS; in these t-MDS, rearrangements of the *MLL* gene on chromosome 11q23 are found, and the latency time from exposure to development of t-MDS is shorter (approximately 2 years). Combinations of alkylating agents and radiation therapy may be synergistic, especially in older patients.

Secondary and t-MDS should be distinguished from primary MDS. The age of onset is approximately 10 years earlier than in primary MDS, dysplasia is more prominent, cytopenias are more severe, progression is more rapid, and outcome is worse. Even patients with fewer than 5% marrow blasts may progress more rapidly to AML or die from complications of relentlessly worsening blood cytopenias.[11]

CLASSIFICATION AND PROGNOSTIC FACTORS

FRENCH-AMERICAN-BRITISH CLASSIFICATION

The French-American-British (FAB) classification remains the predominant point of reference by which MDS are grouped together.[12] The FAB classification categorizes patients with MDS based on the percentage of blood and marrow blasts, the presence of marrow ringed sideroblasts, the number of peripheral monocytes, and the presence of Auer rods. Five subtypes of MDS

are defined (Table 43.3-1): RA, RA with ringed sideroblasts (RARS), RA with excess of blasts (RAEB), RAEB in transformation (RAEB-t), and chronic myelomonocytic leukemia (CMML).

The FAB classification distinguishes low-risk from high-risk MDS but has a number of weaknesses.[13] It is based purely on morphology and does not account for additional prognostic markers, particularly the cytogenetic analysis. Some cytogenetic abnormalities, such as the 5q- abnormality, define distinct MDS entities that are not reflected in the FAB scheme. The FAB nomenclature describes progression through different stages of one disease (from RA or RARS to RAEB, RAEB-t, and AML) rather than different disease entities whose commonality need not be defined by percentage of blasts. The term *refractory anemia*, born out of tradition, has become misleading itself. Patients with isolated thrombocytopenia or neutropenia and unambiguous morphologic evidence of MDS fall into the same subtype as those with RA. Patients with trilineage cytopenias usually have a less favorable prognosis than those with cytopenia in one cell lineage, a circumstance that is not considered in the RA category. The rigid structure of the FAB terminology thus either excludes many cases of MDS that defy the current classification (e.g., hypocellular MDS, MDS with extensive fibrosis) or creates problems in which patients fit criteria for more than one subtype (e.g., 1×10^9/L or greater peripheral blood monocytes and 10% blasts in the marrow). The inclusion of CMML as part of the MDS is also problematic.[14] CMML is often a hybrid disease of multilineage dysplasia in the erythroid-megakaryocytic lineages (feature of MDS) and proliferation (more characteristic of myeloproliferative syndromes) with leukocytosis and splenomegaly. Thus, CMML may be a separate disease category. The group of RAEB is also very heterogeneous. A patient with 6% marrow blasts may have a different prognosis than one with 19% blasts. Auer rods have been associated with favorable rather than poor prognosis.[15] Another drawback is the failure to separate t-MDS from *de novo* MDS. This is relevant, as patients with t-MDS often have severe cytopenias and multilineage dysplasia even with low marrow blast counts, evolve more frequently into AML, and have a worse prognosis overall.

WORLD HEALTH ORGANIZATION CLASSIFICATION

To address these concerns, the World Health Organization has suggested a new classification for MDS (Table 43.3-2).[16] The groups of RA and RARS have been divided into those with unilin-

TABLE 43.3-1. French-American-British (FAB) Classification of Myelodysplastic Syndromes

Subtype	Frequency (%)	Blasts (%) Marrow	Blasts (%) Blood	Transformation to AML (%)	Other
RA	10–40	<5	≤1	10–20	—
RARS	10–20	<5	≤1	10	>15% RS
RAEB	25–30	5–20	<5	40–50	—
RAEB-t	10–30	21–29	≥5	50–60	Auer rods
CMML	10–20	≤20	<5	20	>10^9 monocytes

AML, acute myeloid leukemia; CMML, chronic myelomonocytic leukemia; RA, refractory anemia; RAEB, refractory anemia with excess of blasts; RAEB-t, refractory anemia with excess of blasts in transformation; RARS, refractory anemia with ringed sideroblasts; RS, ringed sideroblasts.

TABLE 43.3-2. World Health Organization (WHO) Classification of Myelodysplastic Syndromes

WHO	Abbreviation	FAB Equivalent[a]
Refractory anemia (unilineage)	RA	Refractory anemia (RA)
5q- syndrome	—	—
Refractory cytopenias with multilineage dysplasia	RCMD	—
Refractory anemia with ringed sideroblasts (unilineage)	RARS	Refractory anemia with ringed sideroblasts (RARS)
Refractory cytopenias with multilineage dysplasia	RCMD (with RS)	—
Refractory anemia with excess of blasts-I (<10% blasts)	RAEB-I	RAEB
Refractory anemia with excess of blasts-II (≥10% blasts)	RAEB-II	—

RS, ringed sideroblasts.

[a]The French-American-British (FAB) category of refractory anemia with excess of blasts in transformation (RAEB-t) has been removed. Patients with 20% marrow or greater or blood blasts, or both, are considered to have a diagnosis of acute myeloid leukemia by WHO criteria. (Data from ref. 16.)

eage and multilineage dysplasias. The 5q- syndrome is now defined based on the presence of fewer than 5% marrow blasts, thrombocytosis, and the characteristic morphologic findings of micromegakaryocytes. RAEB consists of two groups, RAEB-I (5% to 10% blasts) and RAEB-II (11% to 19% blasts). RAEB-t has been eliminated, and patients with 20% blasts or greater are considered to have AML based on the equally poor prognosis of high-risk MDS and AML.[17] CMML has been recognized as a separate entity characterized by either myelodysplastic or myeloproliferative features. A category of unclassifiable MDS has been added.

Although an advance over the FAB classification, the World Health Organization nomenclature is still entirely based on morphology and blast count. Its capacity to capture the heterogeneity of the clinical and biologic behavior of MDS is therefore doubtful.

INTERNATIONAL PROGNOSTIC SCORING SYSTEM

The International Prognostic Scoring System (IPSS) has been developed through a multivariate analysis of 816 patients with *de novo* MDS who did not receive any therapy other than supportive care.[18] The IPSS is based on the percent of marrow blasts, the presence of cytogenetic abnormalities, and the degree of cytopenia (Table 43.3-3). It assigns points to each of the factors and divides patients into low, intermediate-1, intermediate-2, and high-risk groups, with corresponding median survival times of 5.7, 3.5, 1.2, and 0.4 years, respectively.

The IPSS was developed in newly diagnosed untreated patients; survival was calculated from diagnosis. It may therefore not apply to other groups of patients, for example, previously treated patients or those referred to tertiary care centers. For example, the median survival of patients with IPSS low and intermediate-1 groups referred to M. D. Anderson Cancer Center were only 2.1 and 1.2 years, respectively.[19] The IPSS criteria do not include a number of important cellular or molecular markers, such as the degree of marrow apoptosis, aberrant intracellular molecular expressions of various genes (e.g., the methylation status of $p15^{INK4b}$; mutations of *Ras*, *Fms*, and *p53*; abnormal expression of *Bcl-2*), marrow stromal derangements, or production of inhibitory cytokines [tumor necrosis factor (TNF)-α, transforming growth factor (TGF)-β].

BIOLOGY AND PATHOPHYSIOLOGY OF MYELODYSPLASTIC SYNDROMES

A plethora of insights into the numerous pathophysiologic processes of MDS have highlighted its biologic complexity. Models of disease biology have emerged that will lead to a better understanding of the highly interconnected biologic processes in MDS and permit a more rational approach to therapy.

Any useful hypothesis for MDS pathogenesis has to reconcile the seemingly paradoxic occurrence of peripheral cytopenias and hypercellular marrows and the gray zones between MDS and marrow failure syndromes such as aplastic anemia on the one hand and between MDS and AML on the other. The reasons for marrow failure in MDS are multifactorial: decreased marrow

TABLE 43.3-3. International Prognostic Scoring System (IPSS) for Myelodysplastic Syndromes

Prognostic Variable	Score Value				
	0	0.5	1	1.5	2.0
Marrow blasts (%)	<5	5–10	—	11–20	21–30
Karyotype[a]	Good	Intermediate	Poor		
Cytopenias[b]	0/1	2/3			

Combined Score	IPSS Risk Group	5-Y Survival (%)	Progression to AML (%)[c]
0	Low	55	15
0.5–1.0	Int-1	35	30
1.5–2.0	Int-2	7	65
>2	High	0	100

AML, acute myeloid leukemia; Int, intermediate.
[a]Good: diploid, -Y, del(5q), del(20q); poor: complex, chromosome 7 abnormalities; intermediate: others.
[b]Hemoglobin less than 10 g/dL, neutrophils less than 1.5×10^9/L, platelets less than 100×10^9/L.
[c]At 5 years.

production of colony-stimulating factors, increased production of hematopoietic inhibitors, changes in the bone marrow microenvironment through elaboration of angiogenic mediators and others, excessive apoptosis in hematopoietic progenitors, and acquisition of additional molecular insults, resulting in uncoupling of proliferation and differentiation of marrow progenitor cells, leading to the acute leukemia phenotype.[20]

The clonality of MDS has been confirmed by X-chromosome inactivation studies, expression patterns of a single isozyme of glucose-6-phosphate dehydrogenase in hematopoietic progenitors, restriction fragment length polymorphisms of several X-chromosome probes as well as highly polymorphic triplet expansion repeat polymorphisms at the human androgen receptor locus on the X chromosome, and the presence of random chromosomal abnormalities in these patients.[21] The clonal process involves mainly myeloid cells but has also been demonstrated in erythroid and B-lymphoid lineages. Some hematopoietic population subsets in MDS are nonclonal, including primitive progenitors (CD34 positive, Thy 1 positive) and T cells. In addition, hematopoietic recovery in remission marrows is frequently nonclonal. Clonality is often difficult to prove and may precede detectable changes such as cytogenetic abnormalities.

Cytogenetic abnormalities occur in 30% to 80% of patients with primary MDS and in 80% to 100% of those with t-MDS.[22] Cytogenetic abnormalities constitute "fingerprints" for the underlying molecular defects, but the exact role of most of the chromosomal changes in MDS remains elusive. Deletions of the long arm of chromosomes 5 (5q-), 7 (7q-), and 20 (20q-) are common deletions in MDS and AML. Chromosome 5 abnormalities are of particular interest, as several genes involved in hematopoiesis have been mapped to this region. These include macrophage colony-stimulating factor (M-CSF), granulocyte-M-CSF (GM-CSF), interleukin (IL)-4 and IL-5, CD14, interferon regulatory factor-1, the receptors for platelet-derived growth factor (PDGF) and M-CSF (c-fms), and others. *Ras* mutations are detected in 20% to 40% of patients with MDS and may be more common in CMML. No clear association has been found between the presence of *Ras* mutations and prognosis in MDS; some investigators have reported increased risk of progression to leukemia and shorter survival times with *Ras* mutations.[23] Mutations of Flt3, a receptor tyrosine kinase, have been described in one-third of patients with AML and 5% to 10% of patients with MDS. Activation of Flt3 may occur through internal tandem duplications or point mutations of the juxtamembrane domain. Mutations in tyrosine kinases such as Flt3 are attractive targets for small-molecule inhibitors, currently tested in clinical trials.[24]

The inciting events in MDS remain undefined. In some patients, normal hematopoiesis may be suppressed by polyclonal, unaffected CD8-positive T cells directed against major histocompatibility complex class I restricted antigens.[25] The anti–granulocyte-macrophage colony-forming unit (GM-CFU) effect may be reversed or prevented by *in vitro* growth of T cell–depleted marrows or incubation of marrow with cyclosporin A. These observations suggested an exaggerated immune response after injury to hematopoietic progenitors and provided the rationale for the use of immunosuppressive therapy in MDS with antithymocyte globulins (ATG), cyclosporin A, or steroids.

The GM-CFUs are decreased in the blood and bone marrow of patients with MDS.[26] Erythroid and megakaryocytic colony formation are also often abnormal. *In vitro* cultures do not always mirror the hematopoietic activity *in vivo*, as patients with low or absent numbers of GM-CFU may still maintain adequate neutrophil counts. Deficiency of growth factors or excessive release of hematopoietic growth factors as an explanation for decreased colony formation has not been consistently proven in most patients. Although the addition of growth factors (erythropoietin, G-CSF, GM-CSF, IL-3) in semisolid cultures may increase colony formation, growth stimulation frequently remains suboptimal.[27]

Dysplasia reflects excessive apoptosis of the hematopoietic progenitors. According to one hypothesis, the primary lesion in MDS is the high cell death rate, which is counterbalanced by a compensatory phase of excessive hematopoiesis. This is supported by studies demonstrating increased apoptosis and proliferation and may explain the apparent paradox of peripheral cytopenias in the presence of hypercellular marrows.[28] The rate of apoptosis in CD34-positive cells in MDS was significantly higher than in AML. On the other hand, apoptosis is lower in the 5q- syndrome.[29] Increased apoptosis has been observed in the cellular elements of the marrow microenvironment, suggesting that the primitive stem cell involved may be a progenitor to hematopoietic and stromal cells.

A number of proapoptotic cytokines may contribute to excessive apoptotic cell death in MDS. High levels of TNF-α and the effect of TNF-α on induction of Fas expression on CD34-positive cells may play a role. A pathophysiologic role of TNF-α in MDS is suggested by the following: (1) TNF-α messenger RNA is overexpressed in marrows from MDS but not in normal marrows or marrows from AML, and (2) increased TNF-α production is restricted to earlier MDS phases (RA, RARS). The source of TNF-α in MDS appears to be marrow monocytes and macrophages, which may be stimulated by elevated M-CSF levels, for example, through point mutations in c-fms, which encodes the M-CSF receptor. That TNF-α production is relevant is suggested by (1) enhanced *in vitro* growth in MDS by incubation with TNF-α neutralizing antibodies, (2) the correlation of TNF-α levels with severity of anemia, (3) poor response to erythropoietin, and (4) the increased rates of apoptosis. This suggests that strategies to suppress TNF-α levels may help therapeutically.[30]

Involvement of the Fas/Fas ligand system in MDS pathophysiology has been proposed. Increased expression of Fas in MDS is correlated with ineffective erythropoiesis and, in some studies, with survival. The Fas ligand–expressing cells are more frequent in MDS than normal control marrows, and Fas ligand is detected on lymphocytes and other cell lines in MDS.[30] Other antiapoptotic signaling pathways, including bcl-2 overexpression, may be important in advanced MDS states.

How can these observations fit into a multistep sequence of pathophysiologic events in MDS? It is possible that an initial injury results in suppression of normal hematopoietic progenitor growth and differentiation, directly or through stimulation of an immunologic response by polyclonal CD8-positive T cells. The cytotoxic suppressor cells induce hematopoietic suppression through production of proapoptotic cytokines, such as TNF-α, the Fas/Fas ligand system, and perhaps TGF-β and c-myc. These processes are more prominent in the early phases of MDS (RA, RARS), resulting in excessive apoptosis and cytopenias, and are more amenable to therapeutic strategies, such as growth factors, antiapoptotic mediators (anti–TNF-α), and immunomodulation (cyclosporin A, ATG, steroids). As proliferation continues, and perhaps through genomic instability, additional molecular hits (bcl-2 overexpression, p53 mutations, Ras mutations and dysfunction, hypermethylation of p15^{INK4b}) may shift the balance from excessive apoptosis toward maturation arrest and unchecked proliferation of hematopoietic progenitor cells, a process that may predominate in more advanced MDS phases (RAEB, RAEB-t). In these later stages of MDS, more appropriate investigations include AML-like strategies to suppress the abnormal clone or ones directed against specific molecular targets.[20]

CLINICAL MANIFESTATIONS

Disease manifestations are due to cytopenia-associated problems, including fatigue, pallor, infections, and bleeding. Lymphadenopathy and hepatosplenomegaly are uncommon, occurring in fewer than 10% to 20% of patients. Patients with CMML present more often with other extramedullary manifestations, such as skin, subcutaneous, and gingival involvement. Central nervous system involvement is rare in MDS and in CMML. Patients with CMML and significant leukocytosis may present with organ infiltration and dysfunction, including pulmonary insufficiency, cardiac decompensation, and renal failure. This may be exacerbated once treatment has started, and bilateral lung infiltrates (leukemic cell necrosis and inflammation) and a picture resembling adult respiratory distress syndrome may develop. Worsening renal dysfunction and tumor lysis complications may also develop. Patients presenting with severe leukocytosis, monocytosis, and organ dysfunction may benefit from leukapheresis, measures to prevent tumor lysis (allopurinol, alkalinization, hydration, oral aluminum hydroxide to bind calcium), steroids, and, at times, early hemodialysis for renal failure.

LABORATORY FEATURES

Anemia is the most common laboratory feature; neutropenia and thrombocytopenia frequently occur. Monocytosis greater than $1 \times 10^9/L$ in the peripheral blood supports the diagnosis of CMML. Smears of the bone marrow and blood show various degrees of dysplasia (mild, moderate, severe) in one or more lineages (myeloid, erythroid, megakaryocytic). Whereas the degree and lineage involvement by dysplasia have been correlated with prognosis, assessment of dysplasia remains subjective. Blasts in MDS are myeloid in origin as determined by histochemistry (myeloperoxidase positive, positive monocytic stains) and by immunophenotyping (CD13, CD14, CD33 positivity), although some cases exhibit B-lineage lymphoid (CD19 or CD10) or mixed-lineage morphologies. Immunophenotypic clustering of blasts by flow cytometry may become a useful tool for diagnosis and determination of response to therapy.[31]

Bone marrow biopsies or aspirates are usually hypercellular but may be normo- or hypocellular. The diagnosis of hypocellular MDS may be important in the context of immune-mediated mechanisms and of immunomodulatory strategies, as, in these cases, a significant overlap to aplastic anemia may exist. Other abnormalities include hypogranulation or hyposegmentation (Pelger-Huët–like) of granulocytes; anisocytosis, poikilocytosis, and macrocytosis of red blood cells; and marrow dyserythro-

poiesis, including ringed sideroblasts, asynchronous maturation, abnormal nuclear shapes, and chromatin clumping. Peripheral platelet dysplasia may be noted, with large, abnormally granular platelets or hypogranular platelets. Marrow micromegakaryocytes are also frequent.

Cytochemical stains of importance in the workup of MDS include stains for (1) iron to assess iron content and to identify ringed sideroblasts, (2) myeloperoxidase to identify abnormal granulation of myeloblasts, (3) periodic acid–Schiff to identify abnormal erythroblasts, (4) reticulin to define the degree of fibrosis, and (5) platelet antibodies to mark micromegakaryocytes. Blood chemistries should include vitamin B_{12} and folic acid levels to exclude vitamin deficiency–induced MDS-like changes. Serum and urinary lysozymes may be increased in CMML; hypokalemia (lysozyme-induced renal tubular loss), renal dysfunction (leukemic involvement), and hyperuricemia may be present. Testing for the human immunodeficiency virus (HIV) excludes MDS-like changes associated with HIV positivity. Additional abnormalities observed in MDS include polyclonal gammopathies in up to one-third of patients, monoclonal gammopathies or hypogammaglobulinemia, the presence of autoimmune antibodies, and B- or T-cell abnormalities.

DIFFERENTIAL DIAGNOSIS

Dysplastic changes in the bone marrow are not pathognomonic for MDS and may occur with other conditions. Therefore, the first concern is to exclude more treatable conditions associated with cytopenias. Such conditions include vitamin B_{12} or folic acid deficiencies; nutritional deficiencies in general (anorexia nervosa); exposure to antibiotics, chemotherapy, ethanol, benzene, or lead; or a regenerating bone marrow after a hypoplastic phase induced by drugs or infections. Patients with HIV-positive disease also present with cytopenias and marrow dysplasia. Other conditions associated with myelodysplasia and cytopenia include chronic inflammation, tuberculosis, liver disorders, hypersplenism, Hodgkin's disease, lymphomas, and metastatic disease to the marrow. In these situations, appropriate tests and an observation period will clarify the diagnosis.

SUBTYPES OF MYELODYSPLASTIC SYNDROMES

5q- SYNDROME

The 5q- syndrome is associated with an interstitial deletion of the long arm of chromosome 5 between bands q12 and q32 as the sole cytogenetic abnormality.[32] The typical characteristics of 5q- include macrocytic anemia, leukopenia, and normal to elevated platelet counts. The bone marrow is variably hypercellular and may contain small, dysplastic, monolobulated megakaryocytes. This constellation of findings was associated with *de novo* MDS and a benign clinical course characterized by prolonged survival and absence of transformation to AML. 5q- syndrome is rare; the median patient age is 65 years, and there is a female predominance. Lower levels of apoptosis in 5q- syndrome (detected by less disruption of mitochondrial membrane potential and decreased annexin V positivity) have been described and may explain the milder clinical course of this MDS subtype. Additional cytogenetic abnormalities, when present, are associated with a worse prognosis. Recent large studies have shown that patients with the 5q- abnormality may present with thrombocytopenia and can progress to AML. 5q- has also been demonstrated in other hematologic diseases (e.g., myeloproliferative disorders, AML). Furthermore, the characteristic monolobulated megakaryocytes are not specific for the 5q- syndrome but have also been demonstrated in patients with a normal chromosome 5.

MYELODYSPLASTIC SYNDROMES WITH MYELOFIBROSIS

Myelofibrosis may predominate in some MDS cases, but severe fibrosis is uncommon. The incidence of MDS with myelofibrosis is difficult to ascertain and may vary according to the MDS subtype. One problem in establishing an accurate diagnosis in these cases is the difficulty of acquiring sufficient marrow aspirate material to determine blast percentage and accompanying dysplasia in fibrotic marrow samples. The prognosis of these patients is difficult to predict, and the disease process should be carefully monitored. In some instances, it is difficult to distinguish MDS with myelofibrosis from acute or chronic myelofibrosis, acute megakaryocytic leukemia (FAB M7), and occasionally hairy cell leukemia.[33]

HYPOPLASTIC MYELODYSPLASTIC SYNDROMES

Some patients with MDS may present with a hypoplastic bone marrow, which is referred to as *hypoplastic MDS*.[34] This may be confused with aplastic anemia. Both conditions may be induced by T-cell suppression of normal hematopoiesis and may benefit from immunomodulatory therapies such as steroids, cyclosporin A, or ATG.

MYELODYSPLASTIC SYNDROMES WITH EOSINOPHILIA OR BASOPHILIA

In up to 15% of patients, marrows from those with MDS contain abnormally high numbers of eosinophils or basophils, or both. These patients have a higher incidence of specific and complex cytogenetic abnormalities, their conditions evolve more frequently into AML, and they have a poor survival.[35]

CHRONIC MYELOMONOCYTIC LEUKEMIA

Although originally included in the FAB classification as a subtype of MDS, CMML is now recognized as a separate disease entity.[16] It is a hybrid disorder characterized by (1) increased myeloid proliferation with a prominent monocytic component (absolute blood monocyte count, 1×10^9/L or greater) and (2) trilineage dysplasia.[36] CMML shares features of MDS and a myeloproliferative disorder. A relatively high incidence of myelofibrosis has been reported in CMML. Immunologic abnormalities (autoantibody production, polyclonal increase of serum immunoglobulins) occur more frequently than in MDS. In contrast to MDS, CMML marrows show excessive growth of GM-CFU colony formation. Patients with CMML are usually older (median age, 65 years) with a male-female ratio of 2:1. Anemia or thrombocytopenia, or both, is common at presentation.

Hepatosplenomegaly is present in 25% to 50% of patients. Extramedullary disease involves the skin and subcutaneous tissues; gingival or central nervous system involvement is rare. Leukocytosis and monocytosis may be associated with leukemic organ infiltration including lungs and kidneys. This may result in pulmonary insufficiency, which may be subtle at presentation but may be exacerbated with therapy (tumor lysis and pulmonary capillary leak). Renal involvement may be manifest by modest rises in creatinine, which worsen with initial therapy, partly because of tumor lysis, but later revert to normal levels. Cytogenetic abnormalities are less frequent than in MDS and, when present, involve monosomy 7, trisomy 8, or other structural changes including 12p.[37] In recent years a number of balanced reciprocal translocations have been cloned that result in abnormal activation of tyrosine kinase domains such as the PDGF-β receptor in fusion proteins resulting from translocation t(5;12) (TEL/PDGF-βR), t(9;12) (either TEL/ABL or TEL/JAK2), and others. Constitutive activation of these kinase domains leads to activation of downstream signaling pathways and to abnormal proliferation and survival of these cells. The significance of these fusion proteins lies in their role as potential targets for therapeutic agents such as imatinib mesylate (STI 571, Gleevec), a potent inhibitor of PDGF-β receptor and BCR-ABL kinases. Reports have indicated activity in a subset of CMML patients harboring recurrent translocations such as t(5;12) that activate tyrosine kinase domains.[38]

Although more is known about the pathophysiology of CMML than of other MDS subtypes, CMML remains a heterogeneous group of disorders with widely differing median survivals ranging from 3 months to more than 60 months (median survival, 18 months). Patients without significant anemia, thrombocytopenia, or excessive marrow blasts (5% or greater) may survive beyond 5 years. Characteristics associated with shorter survival typically include anemia, increased marrow blasts, presence of immature cells in the peripheral blood, and perhaps excessive monocytosis. In a multivariate analysis, a high peripheral blood lymphocyte count (greater than 2.5×10^9/L) has also been identified as an independent poor prognostic indicator of survival.[39] Some survival-associated prognostic factors for CMML appear to differ from those for MDS (e.g., cytogenetic abnormalities).

THERAPY OF MYELODYSPLASTIC SYNDROMES

GENERAL APPROACH

The therapeutic approach to MDS is still largely characterized by a rather passive stance, considering supportive care the generally accepted standard of care. This may be due to (1) the prejudicial attitude of research toward MDS (older patients, incurable disease); (2) the prevailing notion that MDS is an indolent disorder; (3) the older age and the presence of concomitant medical problems of patients with MDS, making aggressive treatment approaches (AML-type chemotherapy, SCT) risky; and (4) the fact that the results of most trials performed to date in MDS are not encouraging, with the resultant view that no current treatment strategy can change the natural history or improve the prognosis of MDS. Undoubtedly, therapeutic decisions in MDS are challenging, but therapeutic nihil-

TABLE 43.3-4. Response Criteria in Myelodysplastic Syndromes: Hematologic Improvement

Category	Response	
	Major	Minor
Erythroid (HI-E)	↑ Hb >2 g/dL if Hb <11 g/dL; transfusion independence	↑ Hb 1–2 g/dL; ↓ transfusion requirements 50%
Platelets (HI-P)	↑ plts ≥30 × 10⁹ if plts <100 × 10⁹; stable platelet count; transfusion independence	↑ plts 50% (net increase >10 × 10⁹/L but ≤30 × 10⁹/L)
Neutrophils (HI-N)	↑ ANC ≥100% or by >0.5 × 10⁹/L if pretreatment ANC <1.5 × 10⁹/L	↑ ANC ≥100%, but net increase <0.5 × 10⁹/L

↑, increased; ↓, decreased; ANC, absolute neutrophil count; Hb, hemoglobin; plts, platelets.
(Data from ref. 40.)

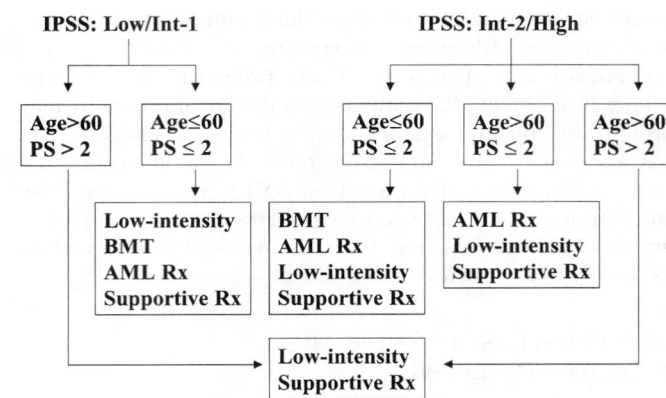

FIGURE 43.3-2. Treatment algorithm. Decision of low- versus high-intensity treatment based on International Prognostic Scoring System (IPSS) score, age, and performance status. AML, acute myeloid leukemia; BMT, bone marrow transplant; Int, intermediate; PS, prognostic score; Rx, treatment.

ism should nevertheless be rebutted. Although effective treatments for MDS are limited, there are several agents that, at least in some patients, hold promise. The belief that MDS is incurable except with allogeneic SCT is now questioned by studies using AML-type chemotherapy that result in long-lasting remissions in some patients.

Among interpretation of clinical trials, there is considerable heterogeneity. Most trials are small in numbers, have short-term follow-ups, and use nonstandardized response criteria, making comparison among different trials difficult. An international working group proposed a set of standardized response criteria for clinical trials in MDS (Table 43.3-4).[40] These may have to be revised, as categories of "minor" response can often be achieved by simple and spontaneous recovery of counts. The treatment goals in MDS differ from those of other hematologic malignancies. MDS is a chronic process that involves a significant amount of morbidity and mortality from the impact of peripheral blood cytopenias and not, for most patients, necessarily from progression to AML. As such, improvement of hematologic indices, quality of life, and disease-related complications are important in the overall evaluation of these patients.

One crucial aspect is to predict which patient will respond to which therapy and when to use it best. This question can be approached by resorting to the IPSS alone or in combination with the FAB classification (Fig. 43.3-2). An indolent course is generally seen only in patients with RA or RARS or with a low IPSS score. High-risk patients include RAEB and RAEB-t (FAB) and the high- and intermediate-2 IPSS group. Patients in the IPSS intermediate-1 group depend on the population under study, being lower risk in community-based studies and higher risk in studies from tertiary care referral centers.[19] Patients with low-risk MDS and minimal findings should be observed. Should they develop significant cytopenias and complications, they may benefit from hematopoietic growth factor support, high doses of vitamins (e.g., B₆) or androgens in some patients, or immunomodulatory strategies (e.g., steroids, cyclosporin A, ATG). Patients should be encouraged to participate in clinical trials. The goal of these low-intensity programs is to produce hematologic improvement. Because of the poor prognosis of high-risk MDS patients,

efforts should be made to enroll them in investigational studies, including targeted therapies [e.g., farnesyltransferase inhibitors (FTIs), monoclonal antibodies], AML-type induction chemotherapy, or SCT. The high-intensity programs are aimed at changing the natural history of MDS.[41]

SUPPORTIVE CARE

Supportive care includes transfusion of packed red blood cells for symptomatic anemia or transfusion of platelets for severe thrombocytopenia or thrombocytopenic bleeding. Blood products should be used diligently: (1) Repeated platelet transfusion may result in refractoriness to such supportive measures, and (2) repeated transfusion of red blood cells, especially in patients who have received more than 20 U of packed cells, leads to iron accumulation. Iron chelation therapy consists of, for example, desferrioxamine, 20 to 40 mg/kg (1.0 to 2.5 g/d) subcutaneously or intravenously (IV) over 9 to 16 hours daily. Patients with neutropenia should be counseled about signs and symptoms of infections and to seek prompt medical attention in these situations. Even in nonneutropenic patients, neutrophils may be dysfunctional, predisposing these patients to infectious episodes. Should these measures fail, trials of vitamins (D, A, retinoids), differentiating agents (hexamethylene bisacetamide, sodium phenylbutyrate), androgens, or steroids may be indicated in occasional patients. The overall success rate of these approaches has, however, been disappointing, and they should not be generally recommended.

LOW-INTENSITY THERAPY

Low-intensity therapy includes hematopoietic growth factors alone or in combination, biologic response modifiers, so-called targeted therapies (e.g., FTIs), differentiating therapy, low-intensity chemotherapy, and epigenetic therapy. Most of these agents are currently evaluated in clinical trials, and limited information is available with regard to their mechanism of action, optimal dose and schedule, toxicities, or appropriate selection of patients.

HEMATOPOIETIC GROWTH FACTORS

Erythropoietin has improved anemia and reduced transfusion requirements in up to 20% to 30% of selected patients, despite elevated endogenous erythropoietin levels in 85% of patients. Responses are most favorable in patients with RA, RARS, or the 5q- syndrome and in individuals who require less than 2 U of packed red cell transfusions per month, with low serum erythropoietin levels (less than 500 mU/mL), and low levels of TNF-α.[42] Patients who do not respond after 4 to 6 weeks can be given erythropoietin in combination with either G-CSF or GM-CSF, which may improve the response rate (to approximately 40%).[43] Combinations of erythropoietin with all-*trans*-retinoic acid have also shown synergistic activity resulting not only in erythroid but also in neutrophil and platelet responses. Combinations of erythropoietic proteins and thalidomide have resulted in a high incidence of thromboembolic complications and should therefore be used with caution.[44] Darbepoietin, a modified form of erythropoietin, has a prolonged serum half-life and increased *in vivo* biologic activity, thus necessitating less frequent dosing. Clinical trials of darbepoetin in patients with MDS are ongoing.

Although G-CSF and GM-CSF have been shown to improve neutropenia in 70% to 80% of patients, no data have shown them to reduce infectious episodes, prolong survival, or influence the rate of transformation to AML. Their use appears reasonable in patients with MDS and recurrent neutropenic febrile episodes but is not recommended for chronic prophylactic use alone in MDS.[1]

IL-11 is a megakaryocytic growth factor that attenuates thrombocytopenia and reduces the need for platelet transfusions after myelosuppressive chemotherapy in patients with nonmyeloid malignancies. A report indicated platelet responses in up to 38% of patients with MDS who received low doses of IL-11 $(10\,\mu g/kg/d)$.[45]

Immunomodulation

Some aspects of the pathophysiology of MDS point toward a role of exaggerated CD8-positive T-cell responses against hematopoietic progenitors, especially during early-stage MDS. Patients with MDS have therefore been assumed to be good candidates for immunosuppressive therapies (ATG or antilymphocyte globulins, cyclosporin A, steroids) similar to patients with aplastic anemia. ATG in unselected MDS patients can result in improvement of hematologic indices, including reduction of transfusion requirements in 15% to 30% of patients. Addition of cyclosporines or steroids, or both, does not appear to improve response rates any further.[46] As these agents are derived from horses, goats, and other animals, problems with serum sickness and other toxicities may be significant, especially in older patients.[47] Reports that patients with MDS and expression of the HLA-DR15 antigen have a higher incidence of responses to immunosuppression need to be investigated further.

Epigenetic Therapy: Role of Hypomethylation

Global and gene-specific DNA methylation is frequent in many solid tumors and hematologic cancers, including MDS, in which the calcitonin gene and the cell-cycle inhibitor p15INK4b are frequently hypermethylated.[48] The association of aberrant DNA methylation with tumor resistance and progression has generated interest in the use of such hypomethylating agents as 5-azacytidine, 5-aza-2'-deoxycytidine (decitabine), or the histone deacetylase and methyltransferase antisense inhibitors.

5-Azacytidine has produced responses in up to half of the patients with MDS and trilineage improvement in approximately one-third. Based on these results, the Cancer and Leukemia Group B (CALGB) compared observation (n = 92) with 5-azacytidine, 75 mg/m² subcutaneously daily for 7 days every 4 weeks (n = 99) in patients with high-risk MDS. Responses occurred in 63% of 5-azacytidine–treated patients [6% complete response (CR), 10% partial response (PR), 47% hematologic improvement] versus 7% in the observation arm. The median times to leukemia transformation (21 vs. 13 months; $P < .01$), median survival (24 months vs. 14 months), and quality of life were superior in patients treated with 5-azacytidine.[49]

Decitabine has a similar structure to 5-azacytidine but has more potent hypomethylating activity. Decitabine has demonstrated activity against a number of myeloid malignancies at higher doses but was associated with severe and prolonged myelosuppression. *In vitro* data suggested that decitabine exerts a dual effect on normal and neoplastic cells. At higher doses, it is cytotoxic; at lower doses cytotoxicity is minimal and the treated cells exhibited marked reduction of DNA methyltransferase activity, reduced overall and gene-specific DNA methylation, and reactivation of silenced genes including tumor suppressor genes.

In a multicenter phase II study, Wijermans et al.[50] treated 66 elderly patients (median age, 66 years) with decitabine, 45 mg/m²/d (15 mg/m² IV over 4 hours every 8 hours), for 3 days every 6 weeks. Twenty-five patients had a high IPSS risk score. Overall, 48% responded (20% CR, 4% PR, 24% hematologic improvement); the response rate was 64% in the high-risk group. The median response duration was 7.4 months; survival from diagnosis was 22 months and, from the start of therapy, 15 months. Myelosuppression was common, and the treatment-related mortality was 7%. Significant platelet responses were observed. Of 53 patients who had received at least one course of decitabine, 35 (66%) experienced increased platelet counts, which exceeded $100 \times 10^9/L$ in 19 (36%). In an update of 169 patients (median age, 70 years; 71 patients in the high-risk group by IPSS) who received decitabine at a dose of 45 to 50 mg/m² daily for 3 days every 6 weeks, the overall response rate was 49% (51% among high-risk patients). The median response duration was 9.5 months, and the median survival 15 months. Responses were independent of age.[51] Hospitalization and quality of life were improved.

Methylation status of p15 and p16 before and after therapy with decitabine was analyzed. Hypermethylation of the p15 gene was detected in 15 of 23 patients (65%), whereas the p16 region was unmethylated in all samples. Among 12 patients with p15 hypermethylation, demethylated epigenotypes and reestablishment of normal p15 protein expression were observed in 9 (75%). However, responses to decitabine also occurred without p15 hypermethylation, suggesting that p15 is only one molecular target for demethylation or that decitabine may induce anti-MDS activity through mechanisms other than hypomethylation.[52]

In a lower dose, prolonged exposure schedule of decitabine (15 mg/m²/d IV over 1 hour daily for 10 days), trying to establish a minimally "biologic" effective dose, responses occurred in four (2 CR, 2 hematologic improvement) of seven patients with MDS with minimal toxicities.[52a] Future trials will expand the low-dose schedule in phase II trials and evaluate combinations of decitabine with histone deacetylase inhibitors and other active agents, such as topoisomerase I inhibitors, retinoids, or interferon-α. A randomized study of decitabine versus supportive care is ongoing.

Arsenicals

Arsenic trioxide has been approved for the treatment of relapsed or refractory acute promyelocytic leukemia, for which it produces high response rates (CR, 80%) and durable remissions (2-year CR rate, 40%). Arsenic trioxide has multiple mechanisms of actions, including induction of apoptosis, tumor cell differentiation, and inhibition of proliferation and angiogenesis. The impact of arsenic trioxide on multiple tumor pathways has led to its investigation in other hematologic malignancies, including MDS. In a phase II trial of patients with low- and high-risk MDS, arsenic trioxide was administered at a dosage of 0.25 mg/kg IV daily for 5 days a week for 2 weeks, followed by 2 weeks off.[53] Hematologic improvement was observed in 6 of 25 patients (24%). Alternative dosing schedules of arsenic trioxide, combinations of arsenic trioxide with other agents (e.g., thalidomide), or novel preparations such as oral tetra arsenic tetrasulfide (As_4S_4) are being explored.

Angiogenesis Inhibitors

Angiogenesis and angiogenic factors play an important role in the pathophysiology of solid tumors and hematologic malignancies. Increased marrow vascularity and increased levels of angiogenic factors [e.g., vascular endothelial growth factor (VEGF), basic fibroblast growth factor, angiogenin, TNF-α, TGF-α, TGF-β, and others] have been demonstrated in MDS.[54] These may also play a role in outcome of patients with MDS and thus provide potential targets for therapy. Antiangiogenesis agents being investigated for MDS include PTK787, an inhibitor of VEGF receptor tyrosine kinases, especially VEGFR-2/KDR; bevacizumab, a novel anti-VEGF monoclonal antibody; and SU5416.

Thalidomide

Thalidomide has a long and colorful history. First introduced in 1953 as a sedative-hypnotic, it was soon associated with disastrous fetal malformations occurring in the offspring of mothers who used thalidomide during pregnancy. Since its abandonment from the prescription drug market in the 1960s, further studies of the activities of thalidomide revealed additional properties that led to a renaissance of thalidomide, especially in cancer therapy: (1) Immunomodulation, in which thalidomide stimulates CD8-positive T lymphocytes, leads to a shift from Th1 to Th2 responses, and inhibits T-cell proliferation; (2) anticytokine effects, in which thalidomide inhibits production of TNF-α and other cytokines; and (3) antiangiogenesis, in which thalidomide has been shown to inhibit basic fibroblast growth factor– and VEGF-induced angiogenesis.[55]

Objective responses with thalidomide at doses of 200 to 800 mg orally daily were reported in only one of nine patients in one study. Another study reported clinical benefits in 16 of 82 (20%) patients.[56] Ten of the patients who were previously trans-

fusion dependent became transfusion independent. A multicenter phase II trial of thalidomide at doses of 200 mg to 1000 mg orally demonstrated limited therapeutic activity.[57] Hematologic improvement occurred in only 1 of 43 (3%) patients with favorable IPSS scores and in 6 of 30 (20%) patients with unfavorable IPSS scores. Frequent adverse events included fatigue, reversible neurotoxicity, constipation, and skin rashes/dryness.

The activity of thalidomide in MDS may be improved by combination with other agents, including topoisomerase inhibitors or hematopoietic growth factors (erythropoietin, darbepoietin). Novel thalidomide analogs with increased immunomodulatory activity and more selective cytokine inhibitory properties are under development.[55] Both groups of analogs inhibit TNF-α, with up to 10,000-fold increased potency compared with the parent compound, and have fewer side effects.

Cytokine Modulation and Antiapoptosis Therapy

Excessive apoptosis and up-regulation of cytokines such as TNF-α and Fas ligand contribute to ineffective hematopoiesis, at least in the early stages of MDS. TNF-α is a pleiotropic cytokine with potent hematopoietic inhibitory activity. It is composed of two subunits, p55 and p75, of which p55 appears to transduce the inhibitory effects of TNF-α on hematopoietic stem cells.[58,59] Macrophages and monocytes are the source for increased levels of TNF-α. Elevated levels of TNF-α are restricted to earlier stages of MDS and were not found in patients with AML.

Several anti–TNF-α strategies have been developed. Pentoxifylline-based combinations (ciprofloxacin, ciprofloxacin-amifostine-dexamethasone) have been ineffective. Blockade of TNF-α by a soluble TNF-receptor fusion protein (etanercept; Enbrel) or a chimeric human-murine monoclonal antibody (Remicade) that neutralizes TNF-α by inhibiting its binding to p55 and p75 receptors has been more successful, with hematologic improvements occurring in 20% of the patients.[60,61] Results are preliminary, however.

Farnesyltransferase Inhibition

Ras proteins couple signals of activated growth factor receptors to downstream mitogenic effectors that result in the activation of transcription factors and expression of protooncogenes. Mutations of Ras have been described in 20% to 40% of patients with MDS. Abnormal activations of Ras can occur in the absence of Ras mutations. Several inhibitors of the Ras–mitogen-activated protein kinase pathway have been developed and are in clinical trials. Most agents act by inhibiting FTIs, enzymes necessary for localization of Ras to the cell membrane. FTIs may also inhibit angiogenesis. Ras activation up-regulates VEGF expression, and suppression of Ras activity through FTIs has been shown to lead to significant decreases in the expression and secretion of VEGF.

R115777 (Zarnestra) is a novel, orally available FTI that has shown activity in phase I studies of patients with solid tumors and leukemias. In a phase II study in patients with MDS at doses of 600 mg orally b.i.d. in cycles of 4 weeks followed by 2 weeks of rest, 3 of 28 patients responded (2 CR and 1 PR).[62] All responders were patients with high-risk MDS. Toxicities included myelosuppression, constitutional symptoms, neurotoxicity, and skin reactions in up to 41% of the patients, suggesting a lower dose of 300 mg orally b.i.d. as more appropriate for future use. Use of other FTIs [lonafarnib (Sarasar)] has demonstrated similar results, with hematologic improvements in up to 20% of patients. Optimization of dose and schedule, identification of MDS patients more likely to respond to inhibition of Ras pathways, and combinations of FTIs with other agents will be of interest.

Other Novel Agents

Given the heterogeneity in the pathophysiology of MDS, numerous other approaches are being investigated. Among additional novel agents undergoing clinical trials in MDS are antisense oligonucleotides to inactivate p53 RNA, the proteasome inhibitor PS-341 [bortezomib (Velcade)], glutathione analogs with myelostimulant activity (TLK199), imatinib mesylate (Gleevec), the FLT3 inhibitors, and homoharringtonine, a plant alkaloid with activity in AML and CML.

HIGH-INTENSITY THERAPY

High-intensity therapy includes AML-type combination regimens and SCT. These approaches are currently the only ones that change the natural course of MDS and produce cures. However, they have an attendant increased risk of treatment-related mortality and morbidity. They are thus usually reserved for patients with high-risk MDS, as the prognosis is as unfavorable as in AML. Age and performance status have to be considered in the treatment decision. High-intensity therapy is most appropriate for patients less than 60 years of age and good performance status (see Fig. 43.3-2).

Acute Myeloid Leukemia–Type Regimens

With intensive chemotherapy in MDS, remission rates ranged from between 40% and 60%.[63,64] With appropriate supportive care measures and prophylactic antibiotics, the mortality was less than 10% to 20%. Factors positively influencing outcome among patients with MDS treated with intensive chemotherapy included age less than 50 years, normal karyotype, and FAB diagnosis of RAEB-t. These studies confirmed that long-term event-free survival was possible with intensive chemotherapy and, in age-comparable groups, was similar to allogeneic SCT. However, CR duration and survival were unsatisfactory.

Beran et al.,[65] in a multivariate analysis, analyzed the outcome of 394 newly diagnosed patients with high-risk MDS treated with chemotherapy combinations (idarubicin/cytarabine; fludarabine/cytarabine; fludarabine/cytarabine/idarubicin; topotecan/cytarabine; cyclophosphamide/cytarabine/topotecan). Overall CR rate was 58% and was significantly associated with karyotype, performance status, age, duration of antecedent hematologic disorder, and treatment in laminar airflow rooms. No difference was found in CR rate based on the regimen used. Topotecan-based regimens had the lowest induction mortality, especially in patients older than 65 years. Overall survival was similar to that of patients treated with idarubicin and cytarabine.

Improvement in outcome may thus not come from more intensified therapy but from innovative postremission strategies (targeted therapies, immunomodulation, anticytokines), new drugs (e.g., novel nucleoside analogs such as clofarabine or troxacitabine; novel topoisomerase I inhibitors such as 9-aminocamptothecin, 9-nitocamptothecin, DX8951F), new formulations of older drugs (liposomal or polyethylene glycol preparations), or different dose schedules.

Stem Cell Transplantation

Allogeneic SCT is applicable to a small subset of MDS patients because of age restrictions, concomitant medical conditions, and donor availability. Results from several large centers indicated disease-free survival rates of 30% to 50%.[66] Results were better in younger patients, with low-risk MDS, and if transplant was applied within 1 year from diagnosis. Failure was primarily due to transplant-associated mortality in low-risk MDS and to disease recurrence in high-risk MDS. With allogeneic SCT in MDS, the long-term follow-up studies showed 3-year survival rates of 23%, similar to intensive chemotherapy. In an update of the International Bone Marrow Transplant Registry, 452 recipients of HLA-identical sibling transplants were reviewed.[67] The median age was 38 years, and most (60%) had high-risk MDS. Overall survival at 3 years was 42%. Survival was more favorable with young age and platelet counts greater than $100 \times 10^9/L$. The incidence of relapse was higher in patients with high percentages of marrow blasts at transplantation, with high IPSS scores, and with T-cell–depleted transplants. When patients were evaluated by the IPSS, the disease-free survival was 60% in the low-risk, 36% in the intermediate-1, and 28% in intermediate-2 risk groups.[66] This compared to 5-year survival rates of 55%, 35%, and 7%, respectively, for unselected patients not receiving SCT. Thus, SCT benefited mostly high-risk MDS patients, but the appropriate timing and optimal marrow ablation regimen remain disputed.

Results from matched unrelated donor programs still lag behind those of matched-related sibling transplants. In an update from the National Marrow Donor Program in MDS, the 2-year survival rate was 29%, the transplant-related mortality 54%, and the relapse probability 14%.[68] Better survival rates (3-year relapse-free survival rate of 59%) have been reported by the Seattle group using conditioning regimens with targeted busulfan and cyclophosphamide.[69]

Although autologous SCT has been advocated as a treatment for MDS, its application is limited to patients who have achieved CR, could be harvested, and were candidates for the procedure. Other transplantation modalities include nonmyeloablative SCT ("mini"-SCT) and transplantation using umbilical cord blood. Few data exist to evaluate the impact of these approaches in MDS.

Improvement in the results of SCT may occur through (1) targeted marrow-ablative approaches, (2) reductions in SCT-related mortality, (3) effective chemotherapy or immunomodulation before and after allogeneic SCT, and (4) broader application of safer procedures in the setting of matched unrelated donor transplants.

CONCLUSION

Progress in MDS remains modest. Although many novel agents have been introduced into clinical trials in MDS in recent years, the major challenge remains a thorough understanding of the pathophysiology of the disease. As the biology of this heterogeneous disorder becomes better understood, further attempts at classification and identification of risk groups will become more relevant clinically. In particular, improved classification may allow more appropriate therapies for low- versus high-risk groups and a better definition of the status of SCT. It is hoped that new targets will be identified and new targeted therapies be developed based on a better knowledge of the pathophysiologic processes in MDS.

REFERENCES

1. Heaney M, Golde D. Myelodysplasia. *N Engl J Med* 1999;340:1649.
2. Shetty V, Hussaini S, Alvi S, et al. Excessive apoptosis, increased phagocytosis, nuclear inclusion and cylindrical confronting cisternae in bone marrow biopsies of myelodysplastic syndrome patients. *Br J Haematol* 2002;116:817.
3. Albitar M, Manshouri T, Shen Y, et al. Myelodysplastic syndrome is not merely "preleukemia." *Blood* 2002;100:791.
4. Aul C, Gatterman N, Schneider W. Epidemiological and etiological aspects of myelodysplastic syndromes. *Leuk Lymphoma* 1995;16:247.
5. Nisse C, Lorthois C, Dorp V, et al. Exposure to occupational and environmental factors in myelodysplastic syndromes: preliminary results of a case-control study. *Leukemia* 1995;9:693.
6. Nagata C, Shimizu H, Hirashima K, et al. Hair dye use and occupational exposure to organic solvents as risk factors for myelodysplastic syndrome. *Leuk Res* 1999;23:57.
7. Kimura A, Takeuchi Y, Tanaka H, et al. Atomic bomb radiation increases the risk of MDS. *Leuk Res* 2001;25:S13.
8. Park DJ, Koeffler HP. Therapy-related myelodysplastic syndromes. *Semin Hematol* 1996;33:256.
9. Stone RM, Neuberg D, Soiffer R, et al. Myelodysplastic syndrome as a late complication following autologous bone marrow transplantation for non-Hodgkin's lymphoma. *J Clin Oncol* 1994;12:2535.
10. Darrington DL, Vose JM, Anderson JR, et al. Incidence and characterization of secondary myelodysplastic syndrome and acute myelogenous leukemia following high-dose chemotherapy and autologous stem cell transplantation for lymphoid malignancies. *J Clin Oncol* 1994;12:2527.
11. Estey EH. Prognosis and therapy of secondary myelodysplastic syndromes. *Haematologica* 1998;83:543.
12. Bennett JM, Catovsky D, Daniel MT, et al. Proposals for the classification of the myelodysplastic syndromes. *Br J Haematol* 1982;51:189.
13. Verhoef GEG, Pittaluga S, Wolfe-Peters CDE, et al. FAB classification of myelodysplastic syndromes: merits and controversies. *Ann Hematol* 1995;71:3.
14. Germing U, Gattermann N, Minning H, et al. Problems in the classification of CMML—dysplastic versus proliferative type. *Leuk Res* 1998;22:871.
15. Seymour J, Estey E. The contribution of Auer rods to the classification and prognosis of myelodysplastic syndromes. *Leuk Lymphoma* 1995;17:79.
16. Harris NJ, Jaffe ES, Diebold J, et al. World Health Organization classification of neoplastic diseases of the hematopoietic and lymphoid tissues: report of the Clinical Advisory Committee meeting, Airlie House, Virginia, November 1997. *J Clin Oncol* 1999;17:3835.
17. Estey E, Thall P, Beran M, et al. Effect of diagnosis (refractory anemia with excess blasts, refractory anemia with excess blasts in transformation, or acute myeloid leukemia [AML]) on outcome of AML-type chemotherapy. *Blood* 1997;90:2969.
18. Greenberg P, Cox C, LeBeau MM, et al. International scoring system for evaluating prognosis in myelodysplastic syndromes. *Blood* 1997;89:2079.
19. Estey E, Keating M, Pierce S, et al. Application of the international scoring system for myelodysplasia to M.D. Anderson patients. *Blood* 1997;90:2843.
20. Rosenfeld C, List A. A hypothesis for the pathogenesis of myelodysplastic syndromes: implications for new therapies. *Leukemia* 2000;14:2.
21. Van Der Lely N, Poddighe P, Wessels J, et al. Clonal analysis of progenitor cells by interphase cytogenetics in patients with acute myeloid leukemia and myelodysplasia. *Leukemia* 1995;9:1167.
22. Schoch C, Schnittger S, Bursch S, et al. Resolving complex aberrant karyotypes in MDS and AML evolving from MDS with 24-color FISH: a study of 40 cases. *Leuk Res* 2001;25:S2.
23. Kurzrock R, Cortes J, Kantarjian H. Clinical development of farnesyltransferase inhibitors in leukemias and myelodysplastic syndromes. *Semin Hematol* 2002;29:20.
24. Gilliland DG, Griffin JD. The roles of Flt3 in hematopoiesis and leukemia. *Blood* 2002;100:1532.
25. Molldrem JJ, Jian YZ, Stetler-Stevenson M, et al. Hematological response of patients with myelodysplastic syndrome to antithymocyte globulin is associated with a loss of lymphocyte-mediated inhibition of CFU-GM and alterations in T-cell receptor Vβ profiles. *Br J Haematol* 1998;102:1314.
26. Greenberg P. In vitro hemopoietic cell culture studies in MDS. *Semin Oncol* 1992;19:34.
27. Stella CC, Cazzola M, Bergamaschi G, et al. Growth of human hematopoietic colonies from patients with myelodysplastic syndromes in response to recombinant human granulocyte-macrophage colony-stimulating factor. *Leukemia* 1989;3:363.
28. Raza A, Mundle S, Shetty V, et al. A paradigm shift in myelodysplastic syndromes. *Leukemia* 1996;10:1648.
29. Washington LT, Jilani I, Estey E, Albitar M. Less apoptosis in patients with 5q- syndrome than in patients with refractory anemia. *Leuk Res* 2002;26:899.
30. Gersuk GM, Beckham C, Loken MR, et al. A role for tumour necrosis factor-alpha, Fas and Fas-ligand in marrow failure associated with myelodysplastic syndrome. *Br J Haematol* 1998;103:176.
31. Ogata K, Nakamura K, Yokose N, et al. Clinical significance of phenotypic features of blasts in patients with myelodysplastic syndrome. *Blood* 2002;100:3887.
32. Nimer SD, Golde DW. The 5q- abnormality. *Blood* 1987;70:1705.
33. Steensma DP, Hanson CA, Letendre L, Tefferi A. Myelodysplasia with fibrosis: a distinct entity? *Leuk Res* 2001;25:829.
34. Wong KF, So CC. Hypoplastic myelodysplastic syndrome—a clinical, morphologic, or genetic diagnosis? *Cancer Genet Cytogenet* 2002;138:85.
35. Matsushima T, Handa H, Yokohama A, et al. Prevalence and clinical characteristics of myelodysplastic syndrome with bone marrow eosinophilia and basophilia. *Blood* 2003;101:3386.
36. Bennett JM, Catovsky D, Daniel MT, et al. The chronic myeloid leukemias: guidelines for distinguishing chronic granulocytic, atypical chronic myeloid and chronic myelomonocytic leukemia. *Br J Haematol* 1994;87:746.
37. Alessandrino EP, Orlandi E, Brusamolino E. Chronic myelomonocytic leukemia: clinical features, cytogenetics, and prognosis in 30 consecutive cases. *Hematol Oncol* 1985;3:147.
38. Magnusson MK, Meade KE, Nakamura R, et al. Activity of STI571 in chronic myelomonocytic leukemia with a platelet-derived growth factor beta receptor fusion oncogene. *Blood* 2002;100:1088.
39. Onida F, Kantarjian HM, Smith TL, et al. Prognostic factors and scoring system in chronic myelomonocytic leukemia: a retrospective analysis of 213 patients. *Blood* 2002;99:840.
40. Cheson BD, Bennett JM, Kantarjian HM, et al. Report of an international working group to standardize response criteria for myelodysplastic syndromes. *Blood* 2000;96:3671.
41. NCCN practice guidelines for the myelodysplastic syndromes. National Comprehensive Cancer Network. *Oncology (Huntington)* 1998;12:53.
42. Hellstrom-Lindberg E. Efficacy of erythropoietin in the myelodysplastic syndromes: a meta-analysis of 205 patients from 17 studies. *Br J Haematol* 1995;89:67.
43. Hellstrom-Lindberg E, Ahlgren T, Beguin Y, et al. Treatment of anemia in myelodysplastic syndromes with granulocyte colony-stimulating factor plus erythropoietin: results from a randomized phase II study and long-term follow-up of 71 patients. *Blood* 1998;92:68.
44. Steurer M, Sudmeier I, Stauder R, Gastl G. Thromboembolic events in patients with myelodysplastic syndrome receiving thalidomide in combination with darbepoietin-alpha. *Br J Haematol* 2003;121:101.
45. Kurzrock R, Cortes J, Thomas DA, et al. Pilot study of low-dose interleukin-11 in patients with bone marrow failure. *J Clin Oncol* 2001;19:4165.
46. Molldrem JJ, Leifer E, Bahceci E, et al. Antithymocyte globulin for treatment of the bone marrow failure associated with myelodysplastic syndromes. *Ann Intern Med* 2002;137:156.
47. Steensma DP, Dispenzieri A, Breanndan S, et al. Antithymocyte globulin has limited efficacy and substantial toxicity in unselected anemic patients with myelodysplastic syndrome. *Blood* 2003;101:2156.
48. Aoki E, Uchida T, Ohashi H, et al. Methylation status of the p15INK4B gene in hematopoietic progenitors and peripheral blood cells in myelodysplastic syndromes. *Leukemia* 2000;14:586.
49. Silverman LR, Demakos EP, Peterson BL, et al. Randomized controlled trial of azacitidine in patients with the myelodysplastic syndrome: a study of the cancer and leukemia group B. *J Clin Oncol* 2002;20:2429.
50. Wijermans P, Luebbert M, Verhoef G, et al. Low-dose 5-aza-2'-deoxycytidine, a DNA hypomethylating agent, for the treatment of high-risk myelodysplastic syndrome: a multicenter phase II study in elderly patients. *J Clin Oncol* 2000;18:956.
51. Wijermans PW, Luebbert M, Verhoef G. Low dose decitabine for elderly high risk MDS patients: who will respond? *Blood* 2002;100:96a.
52. Daskalakis M, Nguyen TT, Nguyen C, et al. Demethylation of a hypermethylated p15/INK4B gene in patients with myelodysplastic syndrome by 5-aza-2'-deoxycitidine (decitabine) treatment. *Blood* 2002;100:2957.
52a. Issa JP, Garcia-Manero G, Giles FJ, et al. Phase 1 study of low-dose prolonged exposure schedules of the hypomethylating agent 5-aza-2'-deoxycytidine (decitabine) in hematopoietic malignancies. *Blood* 2004;103:1635.
53. List AF, Schiller GJ, Mason J, et al. Trisenox® (arsenic trioxide, ATO) in patients (pts) with myelodysplastic syndromes (MDS): preliminary findings in a phase II clinical study. *Blood* 2002;100:790a.
54. Albitar M. Angiogenesis in acute myeloid leukemia and myelodysplastic syndrome. *Acta Haematol* 2001;106:170.
55. Thomas DA, Kantarjian HM. Current role of thalidomide in cancer treatment. *Curr Opin Oncol* 2000;12:564.
56. Raza A, Meyer P, Dutt D, et al. Thalidomide produces transfusion independence in long-standing refractory anemias of patients with myelodysplastic syndromes. *Blood* 2001;98:958.
57. Moreno-Aspitia A, Geyer S, Li C-Y, et al. N998B: multicenter phase II trial of thalidomide (Thal) in adult patients with myelodysplastic syndromes (MDS). *Blood* 2002;100:96a.
58. Selleri S, Anderson S, Young NS, Maciejewski JM. IFN-γ and TNF-α mediates hematopoietic suppression in vitro through apoptosis of hematopoietic progenitors. *J Cell Physiol* 1995;156:538.
59. Tsimberidou AM, Giles FJ. TNF-alpha targeted therapeutic approaches in patients with hematologic malignancies. *Expert Rev Anticancer Ther* 2002;2:277.
60. Deeg HJ, Gotlib J, Beckham C, et al. Soluble TNF receptor fusion protein (etanercept) for the treatment of myelodysplastic syndrome: a pilot study. *Leukemia* 2002;16:162.
61. Raza A, Lisak LA, Tahir S, et al. Hematologic improvement in response to anti-tumor necrosis factor (TNF) therapy with remicade® in patients with myelodysplastic syndromes (MDS). *Blood* 2002;100:795a.
62. Kurzrock R, Kantarjian HM, Cortes JE, et al. Farnesyltransferase inhibitor R115777 in myelodysplastic syndrome: clinical and biological activities in the phase I setting. *Blood* 2003;102:4527.
63. de Witte T, Suciu S, Peetermans M, et al. Intensive chemotherapy for poor prognosis myelodysplasia (MDS) and secondary acute myeloid leukemia (sAML) following MDS of more than 6 months duration. A pilot study by the Leukemia Cooperative Group of the European Organization for Research and Treatment in Cancer (EORTC-LCG). *Leukemia* 1995;9:1805.
64. Estey E. Treatment of acute myelogenous leukemia and myelodysplastic syndromes. *Semin Hematol* 1995;32:132.
65. Beran M, Shen Y, Kantarjian H, et al. High-dose chemotherapy in high-risk myelodysplastic syndrome—covariate-adjusted comparison of five regimens. *Cancer* 2001;92:1999.
66. Appelbaum FR, Anderson A. Allogeneic bone marrow transplantation for myelodysplastic syndrome: outcomes analysis according to IPSS score. *Leukemia* 1998;12[Suppl 1]:S25.
67. Sierra J, Perez WS, Rozman C, et al. Bone marrow transplantation from HLA-identical siblings as treatment for myelodysplasia. *Blood* 2002;200:1997.
68. Castro-Malaspina H, Harris RE, Gajewski J, et al. Unrelated donor marrow transplantation for myelodysplastic syndromes: outcome analysis in 510 transplants facilitated by the National Marrow Donor Program. *Blood* 2002;99:1943.
69. Deeg HJ, Storer B, Slattery JT, et al. Conditioning with targeted busulfan and cyclophosphamide for hemopoietic stem cell transplantation from related and unrelated donors in patients with myelodysplastic syndrome. *Blood* 2002;100:1201.

Nikhil C. Munshi
Kenneth C. Anderson

CHAPTER **44**

Plasma Cell Neoplasms

Plasma cell neoplasms represent a spectrum of diseases characterized by clonal proliferation and accumulation of immunoglobulin (Ig)-producing terminally differentiated B cells. The spectrum includes clinically benign common conditions such as monoclonal gammopathy of unknown significance (MGUS) as well as rare disorders such as Castleman's disease and α heavy-chain disease; indolent conditions such as Waldenström's macroglobulinemia (WM), the more common malignant entity plasma cell myeloma, a disseminated B-cell malignancy; and a more aggressive form, plasma cell leukemia, with circulating malignant plasma cells in the blood. All of these disorders share common features of plasma cell morphology, production of Ig molecules, and immune dysfunction. A plasma cell neoplasm is considered to originate from a single B cell, with resultant monoclonal protein secretion that characterizes its type. Occasional oligoclonal or polyclonal protein abnormalities are observed in conditions such as Castleman's disease. Current laboratory data based on complementarity determining region III confirm the monoclonal origin of this disease.[1]

There are five major classes of Ig synthesized by normal B cells and plasma cells: IgG, IgA, IgM, IgD, and IgE. The dysfunctional plasma cells secrete one of these molecules or, in some instances, produce only κ or λ light-chain molecules.[2,3] Usually, intact Ig molecules are secreted by the plasma cells; however, there may be a discrepancy in the production of the heavy and light chains leading to an imbalance with an excess of free light chain that is excreted in the urine (Bence Jones proteinuria). On occasion, plasma cells do not secrete any paraproteins (nonsecretory-type myeloma); however, they usually have cytoplasmic Ig and produce low levels of Igs undetectable by current methods. Although myeloma can be associated with any of the Ig subtypes, the IgM type is predominantly associated with other malignant conditions such as WM and chronic lymphocytic leukemia (CLL).

The clinical manifestations of plasma cell dyscrasias range from total absence of any symptoms in subjects with MGUS to formation of tumors; paraproteinemia; hypogammaglobulinemia due to decreased levels of the uninvolved Igs; bone disease, especially osteolytic lesions; hematopoietic and immune dysfunction; kidney function abnormalities; and infection problems. These clinical manifestations are the result of a variety of pathogenic mechanisms, including cytokine production by the tumor or by the microenvironment, effect of the tumor mass itself, the deposition of the M protein into various organs, suppression of T- and B-cell functions, and occasionally autoimmune disorders.

HISTORY

The earliest evidence of myeloma has been found in the Egyptian mummies; however, the first published clinical description of the disease was reported in 1850 in England. A patient, Thomas Alexander McBean, presented to Dr. William Macintyre of London in 1845 with symptoms of episodes of fatigue, diffuse bone pain, and urinary frequency. The urinalysis test results detected a urinary protein with the heat properties often observed for urinary light chains, and Macintyre called the disorder "mollities and fragilitas ossium" based on the patient's bony symptoms.[4] Later that year, Dr. Henry Bence Jones also tested urine specimens provided by Macintyre and corroborated the heat properties of urinary light chains. Bence Jones thought that the protein was the "hydrated deuteroxide of albumin" (now called *Bence Jones proteins*) and published his findings several years before Macintyre published his case report.[5] Bence Jones also emphasized the potential importance of looking for this urinary protein in other cases with mollities ossium. After the patient died in 1846, a surgeon, Dr. John Dalrymple, examined several bones and made gross and microscopic observations. His drawings are consistent with the morphology of myeloma cells.

The term *multiple myeloma* (MM) was coined by Rustizky in 1873 after his independent observation in a similar patient with multiple bone lesions. Kahler in 1889 published a review on this condition, and the disease became known, particularly in Europe, as Kahler's disease.[6] Ellinger, in 1899, described the increased serum proteins and sedimentation rate in myeloma. In 1900, Wright described the involvement of plasma cells in this neoplasm, countering the original belief that it originated from the red marrow, and for the first time he described roentgenographic abnormality in myeloma, which to date remains one of the diagnostic tests.

The development of bone marrow aspiration in 1929,[7] electrophoresis to separate serum proteins in 1937,[8] and a later report of a specific spike in the gamma globulin region enhanced the diagnosis and understanding of myeloma. Identification of the heavy and light chains in the monoclonal protein by immunoelectrophoresis was described by Grabar in 1953 and confirmed the monoclonality of Ig in this disease. Other developments in recent times include understanding of the role of the bone marrow microenvironment in myeloma cell growth, survival, and antiapoptosis, and development of drug resistance through cell–cell interaction and activation of cytokine networks. The significance of chromosomal translocation in myeloma pathobiology and, more recently, gene expression profiling and proteomics are providing insights into the molecular pathogenesis of the disease.

No effective systemic therapy existed before 1947, when urethan was reported to show an effect in a few patients. However, a subsequent randomized trial indicated that the survival of patients receiving urethan was inferior to that observed with a placebo.[9] The first successful use of chemotherapeutic agent in myeloma was reported in 1958 by Blokhin and colleagues with the use of a racemic mixture of D- and L-phenylalanine mustards (Sarcolysine). Subsequently, the D- and L-isomers of phenylalanine mustard were tested separately, and the antimyeloma activity was found to reside in the L-isomer, melphalan. In 1962, Bergsagel from the Southwest Oncology Group reported remissions in approximately one-third of myeloma patients treated with melphalan.[10] Administration of high doses of glucocorticoid was first reported to induce remissions in relapsing or refractory myeloma in 1967.[11] The use of melphalan in combination with prednisone was then studied extensively.[12] The role of high-dose therapy was investigated by McElwain and Powles in 1983, and addition of bone marrow and subsequently stem cell transplantation with improved safety and further dose escalation was later evaluated.[13] In the last several years, improved understanding of the role of the bone marrow microenvironment in myeloma biology and development of drug resistance has led to identification of novel agents, such as thalidomide and its analogue immunomodulatory agents, proteasome inhibitors, and bisphosphonates, that target myeloma cells in their microenvironment and can overcome resistance to conventional therapy.

EPIDEMIOLOGY

According to the data from the Surveillance, Epidemiology, and End Results program in 2002, MM is a relatively uncommon malignancy in the United States, representing 1.0% of all malignancies in whites and 2.0% in African Americans. Among hematologic malignancies, it constitutes 10% of the tumors and ranks as the second most frequently occurring hematologic cancer in the United States after non-Hodgkin's lymphoma. At any one time, the prevalence of myeloma is more than 40,000 cases and estimated new cases in 2003 were approximately 14,600; 10,900 patients died from myeloma in 2002. The disease is more common in men and has average annual age-adjusted (1970 U.S. standard) incidence rates per 100,000 of 4.7 in men and 3.2 in women among whites, whereas the incidence is 10.2 in men and 6.7 in women among African Americans. The increased incidence in African Americans is not explained by factors such as social or economic conditions, household size, or family income.[14] The incidence data for other ethnic groups including Native Hawaiians, Hispanics, American Indians from New Mexico, and Alaskan Natives also show higher myeloma rates relative to U.S. whites in the same geographic area; however, the Chinese and Japanese populations have a lower incidence than whites. The incidence of MM has slowly increased in the U.S. white population since 1970; however, the incidence among African Americans has increased more prominently during the 1970s and 1980s and was still increasing in the 1990s.

The incidence of myeloma and other plasma cell disorders increases with advancing age. The median age at diagnosis is 71 years. The mortality pattern also closely follows the incidence curves for age distribution, with a median age at death of 70 years in men and 71 years in women. As seen in Figure 44-1, fewer than 2% of patients are younger than 40 years of age, whereas more than 50% of patients are older than 70 years. A similar age distribution is also observed in other related plasma cell disorders, including MGUS and WM.

ETIOLOGY: ENVIRONMENTAL EXPOSURE

Exposure to ionizing radiation is the strongest single factor linked to an increased risk of MM.[15] This has been documented in atomic bomb survivors with a five times greater incidence than the control group and a latent period of approximately 20 years from exposure.[16] People exposed to low levels of radiation also demonstrate an increased incidence of myeloma, including radiologists, people employed in the nuclear industry, and those handling radioactive materials. An increase in myeloma risk with increasing numbers of diagnostic radiographs was demonstrated without an increased risk of leukemia or lymphoma, which suggests that even a low level of radiation may be a risk factor for myeloma. An association between exposure to various chemicals and the risk of MM remains ill defined. Exposures to metals, especially nickel; agricultural chemicals; benzene and petroleum products; other aromatic hydrocarbons; and silicon have been considered as potential risk factors.[15,17–19] Alcohol and tobacco consumption has not been clearly linked to myeloma. Among medications, only mineral oil used as a laxative has been reported to be associated with an increased risk of MM in some patients.[20,21]

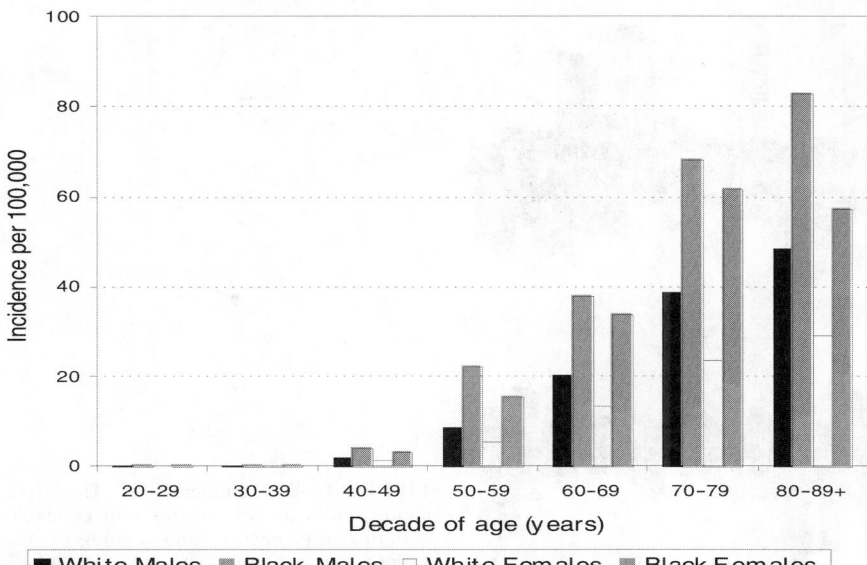

FIGURE 44-1. Multiple myeloma average annual age-, sex-, and race-specific incidence per 100,000 in the United States, 1996 to 2000. Increase in incidence is noted with advancing age, and higher incidence is observed in males than in females and in African Americans than in the white population.

Hereditary and genetic factors may predispose to myeloma development.[22,23] Among 37 families with at least two family members who had myeloma, occurrence among siblings was reported in 25 of the families. However, direct genetic linkage has not been established. Myeloma risk also appears to be enhanced by the presence of HLA-Cw2 in both African American and white populations.

MGUS has been considered a premalignant condition; however, the rate of conversion to myeloma remains extremely low and is often associated with additional genetic changes.[24,25] Repeated infections or antigenic stimulation of the plasma cell compartment has also been proposed as a possible predisposing condition for myeloma. In one interesting case report in the literature, prior therapy with horse antiserum against tetanus led to subsequent development of MGUS, which lasted for three decades before conversion to MM. At the time of myeloma diagnosis, the serum IgG component was found to react specifically against horse α_2-macroglobulin.[26] This report suggests an initial antigen-driven stimulation of monoclonal protein-producing plasma cells, which eventually become malignant after acquiring additional genetic alterations. MGUS has been observed in mice, and in that species it is dependent on strain of mice, aging, preexisting immune status, and antigenic stimulation. MGUS has been associated with immune disorders and infectious diseases. In one report of 57 patients with MGUS who had undergone evaluation for *Helicobacter pylori* infection for various gastrointestinal symptoms, 39 (68%) had evidence of *H pylori* infection and 11 of these 39 patients (28%) had normalization of the serum paraproteins after eradication of *H pylori* infection.[27] Seropravelance of *H pylori*, however, has not been consistently correlated with MGUS.[28] Development of MGUS has also been reported in T-cell deficiency disorders as in acquired immunodeficiency syndrome.[29]

Epidemiologic studies have not been able to conclusively establish an association between MM and infectious or autoimmune diseases. Although an initial report suggested the presence of the human herpesvirus-8 (HHV-8, Kaposi's sarcoma herpesvirus) in the bone marrow dendritic cells of the majority of patients with MM,[30] analogous to its association with other lymphoproliferative diseases such as Castleman's disease,[31] body cavity lymphoma,[32] and Kaposi's sarcoma,[33] other investigators have failed to identify HHV-8 in myeloma cells or dendritic cells from various sources, including mobilized peripheral blood stem cells (PBSCs).[34–37] Because HHV-8 produces unique gene products, including possible growth-promoting factors for myeloma such as analogues of interleukin-6 (IL-6), insulin-like growth factor-1 (IGF-1), and an IL-8, the possible linkage of HHV-8 to myeloma was intriguing. However, even antibodies against HHV-8 have not been observed in MM.[38]

PATHOGENESIS

Myeloma occurs not only in humans but also in mice, canines, and hamsters. In fact, genetic susceptibility to plasma cell tumors has been demonstrated in an inbred strain of mice. A common factor in various species has been considered to be the prevalence of endogenous retroviruses.[39,40] Animal models are now providing a basis for understanding the role of activation of oncogenes, tumor suppressor genes, and cytokines, and the role of the bone marrow microenvironment not only in causing bone destruction but also in sustaining and promoting growth, survival, drug resistance, and genetic instability.

MURINE MODEL

In C57BL/Ka strains of inbred mice, 16% spontaneously develop monoclonal gammopathies without tumor formation by 2 years.[39,41,42] Of interest, however, the C57BL/Ka strain with a high incidence of spontaneous monoclonal gammopathies is relatively resistant to induction of plasmacytoma by mineral oil. In other strains, such as BALB/c, which have a low spontaneous incidence of monoclonal gammopathies, induction of plasmacytoma or myeloma is observed after intraperitoneal injection of mineral oil or its clinically defined component, pristane.[39] Production of such tumors

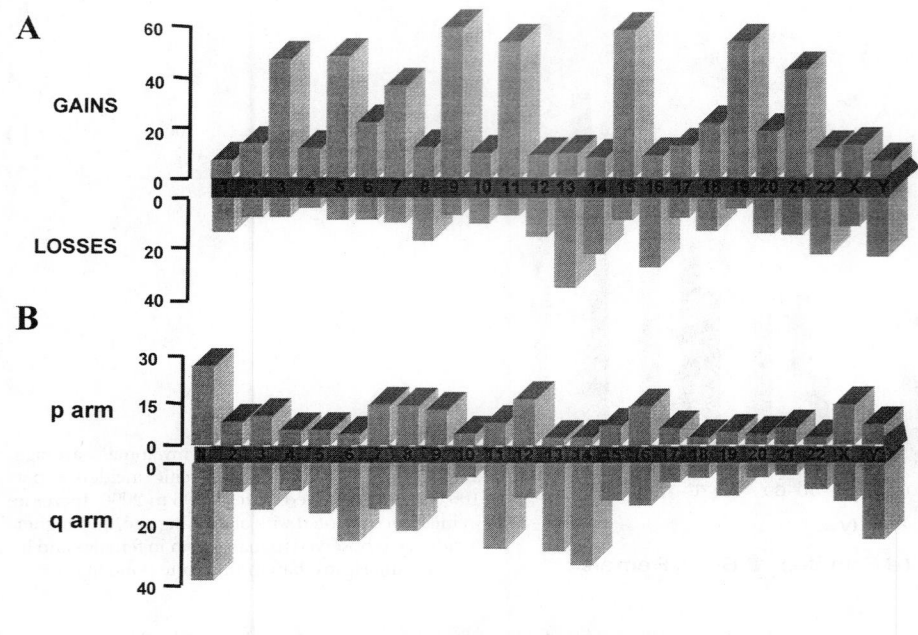

AVG. 11 EVENTS / KARYOTYPE

FIGURE 44-2. Summary of karyotypic abnormalities in 158 patients with evaluable abnormal cytogenetics from a study of 492 patients demonstrating "chromosomal chaos." **A:** Numeric changes with trisomies (gain) and monosomies (loss). **B:** Structural changes involving short (p) and long (q) arm. (Courtesy of Jeffery R. Sawyer.)

can be blocked by administration of indomethacin and accelerated by subsequent infection of the mice with Abelson's virus. Plasmacytomas develop within the oil or other foreign body–mediated granulomas and lymphoplasmacytic infiltration. Plasmacytoma progression is associated with dysregulated expression of *c-myc*, as a result of a translocation analogous to t(8;14) in humans. These plasmacytomas produce IgAs, and a growth factor present in the peritoneal fluid has been confirmed to be IL-6.

An association between antigenic stimulation of normal B cells and development of plasmacytoma has been demonstrated in the pristane oil–treated BALB/c mouse model. When animals are raised in a germ-free environment, incidence of myeloma after mineral oil stimulation is markedly reduced, whereas that of other lymphoid neoplasms increases.[39] These studies suggest an important role of immune stimulation in myeloma development.

Human myeloma cell lines can grow and disseminate in a severe combined immunodeficiency (SCID) mouse model, providing a unique opportunity to study this disease in an *in vivo* setting.[43,44] The introduction of fetal human bone into SCID mice (SCID-hu) has allowed engraftment and proliferation of primary human myeloma cells in more than 80% of mice with human myeloma–specific Ig and light chains detected in murine blood samples.[45,46] In this murine model of primary human disease, the fetal bone undergoes osteoporotic and osteolytic change as a consequence of clonotypic plasma cell proliferation and production of human cytokines.[47] Of interest, the murine bones remain uninvolved, at least in the early stages of the disease.[45] This model provides a unique opportunity to study the importance of stromal cell–myeloma cell interactions, cytokines, and chemokines, as well as genetic and molecular mechanisms critical for myeloma growth and dissemination *in vivo*. This model also can provide clues to the origin of myeloma stem cells, as well as the opportunity to eval-uate new treatment approaches targeting the myeloma cell and its microenvironment.

CYTOGENETIC AND MOLECULAR GENETIC ALTERATIONS

Myeloma karyotypes are complex with an average of 11 numeric and structural abnormalities per cell.[48–50] The relative incidence of gain or loss of various chromosomes with involved p and q arms is shown in Figure 44-2. The inherent problem in the low proliferative activity of the tumor cells and possible clonal evolution have been obstacles to identifying specific chromosomal and molecular changes in myeloma. The frequency and complexity of the chromosomal aberration increase with advanced disease and are uniformly abnormal in plasma cell leukemia. Detection of a complex karyotype predicts poor prognosis. The newer techniques of multicolor fluorescent *in situ* hybridization (FISH) and spectral karyotyping, along with refined G-banding techniques, have identified many nonrandom changes in a large number of patients.[51–53] When these techniques are used, involvement of at least one chromosome is detected in more than 90% of patients.

The Ig heavy-chain gene at 14q32 is involved in translocation in 20% to 40% of cases assessed by conventional cytogenetics; however, by molecular and FISH techniques, it is detectable at a higher frequency, ranging from 50% in MGUS to 90% in advanced myeloma.[48,49,54] The demonstration of this abnormality in MGUS suggests its involvement in the initial step of the transformation.[55–57] Light-chain translocations involving Igλ (22q11) or Igκ (2p12) are less commonly observed and occur in only 20% of cases, even in advanced MM. The most common translocation involving 14q32 results in overexpression of cyclins D1 (on 11q13), and D3 (on 6p21).[54,58] The other biologically important partner chromosome regions are 4p16 (FGFR3 and MMSET), 8q24 (*c-myc*) 16q23 (c-MAF), and 20q11 (MAFB) (Table 44-1).

TABLE 44-1. Nonimmunoglobulin Sites for Illegitimate Switch Recombination in Multiple Myeloma

Chromosome Region	Frequency (% Patients)	Gene(s)	Function
11q13	30	*Cyclin D1*	Induces growth
4p16	25	*FGFR3, MMSET*	Growth factor
8q24	5	*c-myc*	Growth and apoptosis
16q23	1	*c-maf*	Transcription factor
6p25	<1	*IRF4*	Transcription factor

The 4p16 region contains *FGFR3* and *MMSET* genes. *FGFR3* and its activating mutations trigger mitogen-activated protein kinase (MAPK) signaling and growth of myeloma cells.[59] Mutated *FGFR3* also confers resistance to caspase 3–related apoptosis.[60–63] This translocation also activates the *MMSET* gene, a homologue of *MLL1* that is also independently involved in 11q23 translocation. With the enhanced sensitivity of spectral karyotyping, a nonrandom involvement of t(14:16) (q32:q22-23) has been described. Molecular analysis of the locus at chromosome band 16q22 shows fusion of Ig heavy chain with the sequence near the cmaf oncogene, a b-ZIP transcription factor.[64] In addition, translocation partners t(9;14) involving *PAX-5* gene and t(6;14) involving *IRF4* genes have been described.[65,66] In the majority of cases, however, the translocating partner chromosome locus is not yet identified. Although 14q32 is one of the common translocations, its role in myeloma pathogenesis remains unclear due to the variety of partner chromosomes involved and its lack of prognostic significance.

Standard cytogenetic techniques did not identify rearrangements involving 8q24, which contains c-*myc* oncogene and is commonly involved in murine plasmacytoma. However, FISH analyses in one study identified karyotypic abnormalities that involve c-*myc* in 45% cases of advanced myeloma.[67] A study with interphase FISH confirmed c-*myc* rearrangement in 15% of MM cases, with increasing frequency correlated with severity of disease. Interestingly, c-*myc* involvement was heterogeneous, which suggests evolution of disease.[68] Changes in c-myc in the form of either abnormal size transcript or high level of expression have also been reported.[69,70]

Partial or complete deletion of chromosome arm 13q confers a poor prognosis, even after high-dose therapy.[71] When the *Rb1* gene is used as a probe, FISH analysis reveals Rb1 deletion in more than 40% of these patients.[72] In a detailed analysis of chromosome arm 13q with an 11-probe FISH panel, more than 80% of 50 patients showed molecular deletions, with 13q14 representing a critical region most frequently involved.[73] In addition, constitutive phosphorylation of pRB in myeloma cells can be further enhanced by IL-6.[74] Cyclin D, cyclin-dependent kinases, and cyclin-dependent kinase inhibitors p15 and p16 (ink), p21 and p27 (cip), and p57 (kip) have also been investigated in myeloma due to their effect on pRb phosphorylation. Abnormalities in p16 and p15 have been reported in 75% and 67% of myeloma patients, respectively, which suggests an important defect in the pRb regulatory pathway.[75–77]

One of the commonly altered genes in many malignancies is p53. In myeloma, abnormalities in p53 are detected in fewer than 10% of patients with early-stage disease.[78,79] However, p53 abnormalities represent an important late event associated with progression to an aggressive form of the disease. A study of p53 gene mutations in 52 patients with myeloma showed 7 of 52 patients to have p53 abnormalities, all with advanced clinically aggressive acute or leukemic stage of MM.[78] One study showed poor prognosis in patients with p53 gene deletion, as assessed by FISH, after standard-dose therapy.[80] In contrast to samples from primary patient, mutations in p53 are more commonly detected in myeloma cell lines, which are usually derived from patients with aggressive myeloma. MDM2, an important inhibitor of p53 function, is overexpressed in the majority of myeloma cell lines; however, increased MDM2 expression is infrequently observed in primary myeloma cells.[81]

An important antiapoptotic gene, *BCL-2*, is uniformly overexpressed in low-grade non-Hodgkin's lymphoma. In this family of genes, *BCL-2* and *BCL-XL* are antiapoptotic genes, whereas *BAX*, *BAD*, and *BCL$_{XS}$* are proapoptotic genes. A balance between these genes determines cell survival. The t(14:18) translocation involving the *BCL-2* gene is quite rare in myeloma (2% to 3% of cases). However, numerous myeloma cells lines as well as primary cells express high levels of BCL-2.[82,83] Its relationship to development of drug resistance, as well as radiation resistance, in myeloma cells is also well described.[84–86] However, one study involving 63 patients showed a significant correlation between BCL-2 expression and resistance to therapy with interferon (IFN) but not with melphalan and prednisone.[87] The association of BCL-2 expression with prognosis remains controversial, because one small study failed to show a correlation with short survival. BCL-XL is up-regulated in myeloma cells as a consequence of IL-6–induced activation of signal transducer and activator of transcription 3 (STAT3).[88] It confers a drug-resistant phenotype and, in conjunction with bcl-2, leads to increased genetic instability. These molecular changes, coupled with abnormalities of gp130, nuclear factor κB (NFκB), and STATs, promote progression of myeloma.[89]

High telomerase activity has also been demonstrated in myeloma cells, relative to normal cells and other malignant cell lines.[90] Although the clinical implication of this activity remains under investigation, telomerase activity confers growth and survival and is therefore an additional target for therapeutic intervention.

DISEASE EVOLUTION

MM is a germinal center–derived tumor with mainly post-switch B-cell phenotype characterized by extensive Ig gene hypermutation in a pattern suggesting antigen selection. This is reflected in the exceedingly rare occurrence of IgM myeloma. Somatic mutations of other loci, such as BCL-6, have also been reported in myeloma B cells, along with characteristic Ig gene rearrangement.[91] Similar mechanisms may be affecting other cell-cycle control genes whose products regulate cell proliferation and malignant transformation.

As in most malignancies, pathogenesis of MM appears to be associated with dysregulated expression and function of multiple key cellular genes controlling apoptosis, cell growth, and proliferation. Understanding the evolution of myeloma from MGUS has provided a background for defining a multistep process involving alterations in various oncogenes and tumor suppressor genes. One report suggests the presence of 14q32 abnormalities in patients with MGUS, with the addition of chromosome 13 change associated with a transformation to overt MM.[55] This has led to a theory

TABLE 44-2. Adhesion Molecule Expression on Normal Plasma Cells, Multiple Myeloma Cells, and Plasma Cell Leukemia Cells

	Normal Plasma Cell	MM Cell	PCL Cell
ADHESION MOLECULES			
CD11a	+	−	−
CD11b	−	−	+
CD44	+	+	+
CD54	+	+	+
CD56	−	+	−
CD58	−	+	ND
LFA-1	−	−/+	+
VLA-4	+	+	ND
VLA-5	+	+	−
MPC-1	+	+	−
RHAMM	−	+	±
Syndecan-1	+	+	−
SURFACE MOLECULES			
CD19	+	−	−
CD28	−	−	+
CD38	+	+	+
CD40	+	+	+[a]
CD45	+	−[b]	

MM, multiple myeloma; ND, not determined; PCL, plasma cell leukemia.
[a]CD40 expression is enhanced on PCL cells relative to normal plasma cells and MM cells.
[b]CD45 on immature myeloma cells.

that one subset of myelomas may derive from prior MGUS with a high incidence of monosomy 13, whereas in a second group of *de novo* myelomas other genetic abnormalities may be involved.[55]

MICROENVIRONMENT

Myeloma cells express adhesion molecules that mediate interaction with the microenvironment, including both bone marrow stromal cell (BMSC) elements and extracellular matrix proteins (Table 44-2). These adhesion molecules mediate both homotypic and heterotypic adhesion. Adhesion not only plays a role in migration and localization of myeloma cells in the bone marrow but also induces tumor cell growth and survival. For example, syndecan-1, a cell surface transmembrane heparan sulfate proteoglycan

present on MM cells, interacts with type I collagen and regulates growth of MM cells; it also mediates increased osteoclast activity.[92–94] Elevated levels of syndecan-1 shed into serum correlates with increased tumor mass, decreased matrix metalloproteinase-9 activity in serum, and poor prognosis.[92] Besides the adhesion-induced signaling mediating growth, survival, and antiapoptosis, binding of myeloma cells to BMSCs also induces transcription and secretion of cytokines IL-6, IGF-1, vascular endothelial growth factor (VEGF), stromal cell–derived factor-1 (SDF-1), and tumor necrosis factor-α (TNF-α),[95–99] which mediate tumor cell growth, survival, drug resistance, and migration[125] (Figs. 44-3 and 44-4).

The biologic and clinical relevance of increased angiogenesis, although established in solid tumors, has only recently been appreciated in hematologic malignancies. Higher bone marrow microvessel density has been reported in MM patients than in individuals with MGUS.[100–102] Moreover, in patients with myeloma the degree of microvessel density has been correlated with prognosis.[103,104] Immunohistochemical studies show that the angiogenic factor VEGF is expressed by MM cells.[105] Levels of hepatocyte growth factor, which also promotes angiogenesis, are increased in the serum of myeloma patients and predict for poor outcome, especially in patients with increased β_2-microglobulin (β_2M) levels.[106] Finally, novel agents such as thalidomide inhibit angiogenesis and can also overcome drug resistance in myeloma.

ROLE OF CYTOKINES

Myeloma cells and BMSCs produce cytokines, including IL-6,[95] IGF-1,[99] VEGF,[97] SDF-1,[98] TNF-α,[96] TGF-β,[107] IL-21,[108] and others that mediate tumor cell growth, survival, antiapoptosis, migration, and development of drug resistance.

Interleukin-6

IL-6 is an essential growth and survival factor for myeloma. The IL-6 receptor (IL-6R) expressed by myeloma cells is composed of two polypeptide components: the α chain (gp80, IL-6Rα) and the signal-transducing element, the β chain (gp130). The gp130 component is shared by a family of cytokines, including oncostatin M and leukemia inhibitory factor. Interaction of IL-6 with its receptor activates RAS/RAF/MEK/ERK, Janus kinase (JAK)/STAT, and phosphatidylinositol 3 kinase (PI3K)/AKT signaling pathways, mediating growth, survival, and drug resistance (see Fig. 44-4). IL-

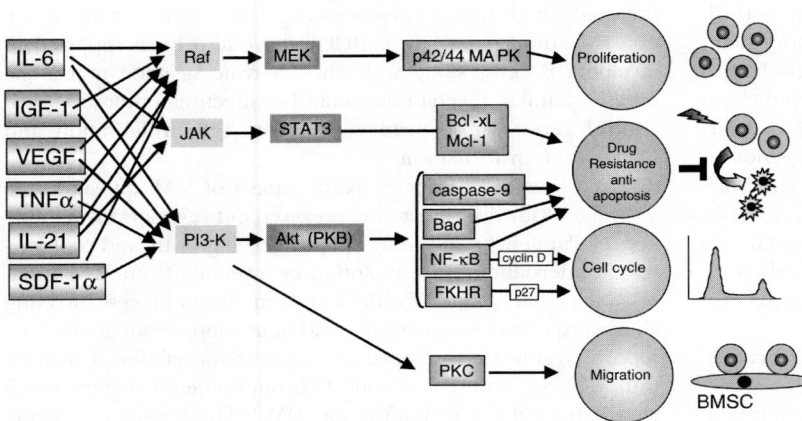

FIGURE 44-3. The RAS/Raf/mitogen-activated protein kinase (MAPK) kinase (MEK) pathway mediates proliferation of multiple myeloma (MM). Janus kinase (JAK)/signal transducer and activator of transcription 3 (STAT3), along with up-regulation of Bcl-xL and Mcl-1, mediate survival. Phosphatidylinositol 3 kinase (PI3-K)/Akt, through downstream activation of Bad and nuclear factor κB (NF-κB) or inactivation of caspase-9, or both, mediates antiapoptosis. NF-κB and forkhead in rhabdomyosarcoma (FKHR) modulate cyclin D and KIP1, thereby regulating cell-cycle progression. Signaling through PI3-K induces downstream protein kinase C (PKC) activity and MM cell migration. BMSC, bone marrow stromal cells; IGF-1, insulin-like growth factor-1; IL, interleukin; SDF-1α, stromal cell–derived factor-1α; TNFα, tumor-necrosis factorα; VEGF, vascular endothelial growth factor. (Adapted from ref. 125.) (See Color Fig. 44-3 in the CD-ROM.)

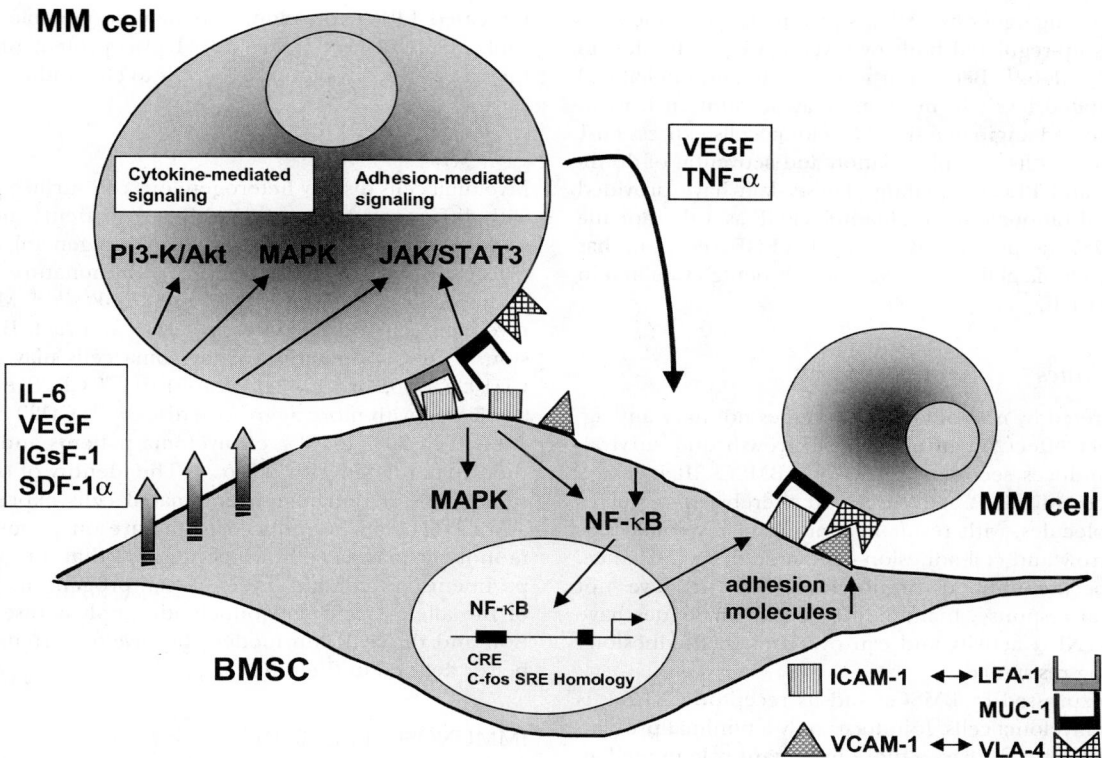

FIGURE 44-4. Multiple myeloma (MM) cells' interaction with and adhesion to the bone marrow stromal cells (BMSCs) lead to adhesion- and cytokine-mediated signaling. MM cell binding to BMSCs induces the activation of p42/44 mitogen-activated protein kinase (MAPK) and nuclear factor κB (NF-κB) in BMSCs. The activation of NF-κB up-regulates adhesion molecules on BMSCs. Cytokines secreted through this interaction include interleukin-6 (IL-6), tumor necrosis factor-α (TNF-α), and vascular endothelial growth factor (VEGF), which activate the main signaling pathways [p42/44 MAPK, Janus kinase (JAK)/signal transducer and activator of transcription 3 (STAT3), and phosphatidylinositol 3 kinase (PI3-K)/AKT] and their downstream targets, which triggers MM cell growth, survival, and migration. ICAM1, intercellular adhesion molecule-1; LFA1, lymphocyte function–associated antigen-1; MUC1, mucin 1; SDF-1α, stromal cell–derived factor-1α; VCAM1, vascular cell adhesion molecule-1; VLA4, very late antigen 4. (Adapted from ref. 125.) (See Color Fig. 44-4 in the CD-ROM.)

6 is mainly produced by stromal cells after binding to myeloma cells and is also triggered by other cytokines, including TNF-α,[96] IL-1β, and VEGF in the bone marrow milieu.[97] IL-6 mediates both autocrine and paracrine growth of myeloma cells. It increases the proportion of cells in S phase, prevents apoptosis of malignant plasma cells, and confers resistance to antitumor agents such as dexamethasone. Dexamethasone-induced apoptosis is mediated by cytochrome *c*, but not Smac (second mitochondria-derived activator of caspases) release from mitochondria into the cytosol, followed by caspase 9 and caspase 3 activation[109]; IL-6 blocks caspase 9 activation, thereby protecting cells against dexamethasone-induced apoptosis.[110] Soluble IL-6Rα, shed by myeloma cells into serum, can amplify the response of myeloma cells to IL-6; both high serum IL-6Rα levels and high serum IL-6 levels portend poor prognosis. IL-6 and soluble IL-6Rα also mediate enhanced bone resorption by osteoclasts. To date IL-6 has been targeted therapeutically using antibodies specific for IL-6 or its receptor, as well as using IL-6 superantagonist (SANT-7), which binds IL-6R but does not trigger downstream signaling. These treatment approaches have produced only transient responses in a small number of patients. Neutralizing anti–IL-6 murine monoclonal antibodies have been administered either locally (malignant pleural effu-

sions) or intravenously in patients with advanced MM. Although clinical responses were not seen, therapy led to reduced survival and proliferation of malignant plasma cells, which confirms a role for IL-6 in mediating myeloma growth *in vivo*.

Insulin-Like Growth Factor-1

IGF-1 is a growth and survival factor in human MM that activates PI3K and MAPK signaling pathways mediating proliferation and antiapoptosis.[111,112] It induces more potent protection against dexamethasone than does IL-6. IGF-1 also up-regulates FLIP, XIAP, and A1/Bfl1[111] and increases telomerase, thereby further enhancing tumor cell growth and survival.[113] IGF-1 mediates adhesion and migration of myeloma cells via β$_1$ integrin.[99] These studies have identified IGF-1 as a novel therapeutic target; both antibodies and small molecule inhibitors against IGF-1 show promise in preclinical studies.

Vascular Endothelial Growth Factor

VEGF has only modest proliferative effects on myeloma cells; however, it plays a more important role in triggering tumor cell migration and angiogenesis.[114,115] Its production in bone marrow milieu is up-regulated both by myeloma cell adhesion to BMSCs and by IL-6.[116] Because it is a specific endothelial cell mitogen, elevated levels in myeloma may account, at least in part, for increased angiogenesis.[105] Myeloma cells express Flt-1 and VEGF triggers its phosphorylation and activation of downstream MEK and PKCα signaling. These data have provided the preclinical rationale for evaluating VEGF as a therapeutic target. PTK787, a potent inhibitor of VEGF receptor, has shown antimyeloma activity *in vitro*[117] and is being evaluated in early clinical trials.

Other Cytokines

TNF-α is secreted by myeloma cells and does not have any significant direct effect on myeloma cell growth and survival; however, it induces secretion of IL-6 by BMSCs. It is also a strong inducer of NFκB activation and thereby up-regulates adhesion molecules, with resultant binding of myeloma cells to bone marrow and cell adhesion–mediated drug resistance. Although specific antibody inhibitors of TNF-α have not shown clinical response, thalidomide and its analogues have potent anti–TNF-α activity and can overcome cell adhesion–mediated drug resistance.

SDF-1 is expressed by BMSCs, and its receptor, CXCR4, is expressed by myeloma cells. It induces only a minimal proliferative effect; however, it plays a more important role in mediating migration.

IL-21 induces proliferation and inhibits apoptosis independent of IL-6 signaling. It triggers phosphorylation of JAK, STAT3, and ERK1/2 (p44/42 MAPK). TNF-α up-regulates expression of both IL-21 and the IL-21 receptor.

TGF-β is produced by MM cells and induces secretion of IL-6 by BMSCs; it also contributes to the immunosuppressive characteristic of myeloma.

Drug Resistance

Intrinsic and acquired resistance of plasma cells to conventional chemotherapy is common, and as a result only 50% of patients achieve a partial response, with few complete responses. Drug resistance is mediated by several mechanisms.[118] First, altered intracellular drug concentration may be due to overexpression of the MDR1 gene, encoding for P-glycoprotein, an integral membrane protein that functions as an adenosine triphosphate–dependent drug efflux pump. Cyclosporine A and verapamil inhibit P-glycoprotein function and have been tested as chemosensitizers but achieved only modest short-term benefit in clinical studies.[119] PSC 833, a nonimmunosuppressive and nonnephrotoxic derivative of cyclosporine D, has also been evaluated in a phase II trial, with limited success.[120] Second, the multidrug resistance–associated protein (MRP), a member of the adenosine triphosphate–binding cassette transporter gene superfamily, may also confer clinical drug resistance.[121] Third, expression of lung resistance–related protein (LRP) a member of the class of major vault proteins, is associated with poor response and shortened survival.[122] Vault proteins are multisubunit proteins localized to the nuclear membrane that are implicated in transport of substances such as alkylating agents to the nucleus. Dose intensification of melphalan has been shown to overcome the resistance due to

increased LRP expression.[123] It may be possible to combine vault protein inhibitors with P-glycoprotein inhibitors to increase sensitivity of myeloma cells to chemotherapy.

PHENOTYPE

Myeloma cells display heterogeneous cell surface phenotypes, with differences both among different patients and within the same patient at different disease stages. In general, all myeloma cells express high levels of CD38, with immature plasma cells additionally expressing CD45 and IL-6R.[124,126] More mature myeloma cells do not express CD45 and lack IL-6R expression.[127] A subpopulation of myeloma cells may also express CD10, CD56, or CD49e (VLA-5).[127–129] CD28 expression is associated with more aggressive disease[130]; CD20 expression is present in 20% to 30% of myeloma patients and can be further up-regulated with IFN-α.[131] The identity of the myeloma stem cell still remains an enigma. B cells expressing CD19 and CD11b can be induced to mature on stromal cells into monotypic plasma cells, which suggests that this cellular compartment may contain myeloma cell progenitors.[132] With use of the allele-specific oligonucleotide polymerase chain reaction and the SCID-hu model, the myeloma stem cell will be better defined in the future.

IMMUNOSUPPRESSION

Myeloma patients present with suppressed immune function due to a variety of factors. Most significant is suppression of uninvolved Igs; for example, in patients with IgG myeloma, there is suppression of serum IgA and IgM levels.[133] The factors causing this suppression include a direct effect of monoclonal Ig, increased soluble Fc receptor or Fc-expressing cells, suppression of helper cell functions, and macrophage-related factors that affect B-cell maturation to plasma cells.[134] Recovery of uninvolved Igs to normal levels after effective therapy has been associated with both improved survival and protection from infectious complications.

The total T-cell count may be decreased; however, in a substantial number of patients it may be normal, with no significant changes in CD8 cells.[136,137] A stage-dependent suppression of natural killer cells has been observed.[138] Deficiency of CD4 helper cells is also pronounced. In one study the proliferation and frequency of Epstein-Barr virus– and influenza A–specific T cells were significantly reduced in a cohort of 24 newly diagnosed or conventionally treated MM patients compared with 19 healthy individuals, suggest an impaired CD8+ T-cell response in MM patients.[140] A defect in natural killer T-cell function has also been detected in patients with progressive myeloma when compared to patients with MGUS or nonprogressive disease.[141]

Anti-idiotype T-cell response has been demonstrated in the majority of patients, with higher idiotype-specific T-cell frequency in MGUS and early stage of myeloma compared to advanced disease.[142] This observation has lead to a provocative hypothesis that immunologic response plays an important role in controlling proliferation of the malignant clone in the early stages of the disease, whereas loss of immune regulation is associated with evolution to an overt or more aggressive form of the disease. These data also provide the scientific basis for the development of idiotype-specific T-cell responses for therapeutic purposes, through either vaccination *in vivo* or production of idiotype- or myeloma-specific cytotoxic T lymphocytes *in vitro.*[143]

CLINICAL MANIFESTATIONS

Patients with MM may be entirely asymptomatic and diagnosed on routine blood testing or may present with a myriad of symptoms: hematologic manifestations, bone-related problems, infections, various organ dysfunctions, neurologic complaints, or bleeding tendencies (Table 44-3). These signs and symptoms result from direct tumor involvement in bone marrow or extramedullary plasmacytomas, the effect of the protein produced by the tumor cells deposited in various organs, production of cytokines by the tumor cells or by the bone marrow microenvironment, and effects on the immune system.

ANEMIA

A normochromic normocytic anemia is usually observed in myeloma patients due to tumor cell involvement of the marrow as well as inadequate erythropoietin responsiveness. The suppressive effects of various cytokines on erythropoiesis and the effect of renal dysfunction on erythropoietin production are also contributing factors. High Ig levels exacerbate the anemia due to dilutional effects. Anemia gives rise to fatigue, weakness, and occasionally shortness of breath. In the Durie-Salmon staging system, the level of anemia is considered to be one of the criteria reflective of the tumor mass load. Erythropoietin administration is therefore an important supportive care therapy for patients with symptomatic anemia. In one study, improvement in hemoglobin by more than 2 g/dL was observed in 60% of treated patients, and responses were more frequent in patients with low erythropoietin levels than in patients with normal or high levels (72% vs. 20%).

RENAL FAILURE

Nephropathy is one of the serious adverse complications that can be observed at the time of clinical presentation. The etiology of renal failure can be multifactorial. The most common cause is development of light-chain tubular casts leading to interstitial nephritis (myeloma kidney).[144] Another common cause of renal

TABLE 44-3. Clinical Features of Multiple Myeloma

Symptoms	*Common Cause*
Bone pain	Pathologic fracture
Easy fatigability	Anemia
Polyuria	Hypercalcemia
Nausea and vomiting	Renal failure, hypercalcemia
Recurrent infections	Low uninvolved immunoglobulin, low CD4 count
Paraplegia	Cord compression
Confusion, central nervous system symptoms	Hyperviscosity or hypercalcemia
Neurologic symptoms	Nerve compression, amyloidosis, POEMS syndrome

POEMS, polyneuropathy, organomegaly, endocrinopathy, monoclonal gammopathy, and skin changes.

dysfunction is hypercalcemia and hypercalciuria leading to osmotic diuresis, volume depletion, and prerenal azotemia. Other modes of kidney involvement in myeloma include light-chain deposition disease, which is more commonly associated with κ light-chain proteins and impaired glomerular filtration; AL amyloidosis, which is more frequently associated with λ light chain (especially λ light-chain subtype VI) and may have an initial presentation as nephrotic range proteinuria; and renal calcium deposition, leading to interstitial nephritis.[145–147] The presence of λ light chains in the urine is also more commonly associated with myeloma kidney. Bence Jones proteins bind to a common peptide segment of Tamm-Horsfall glycoprotein to promote heterotypic aggregation.[148] Tamm-Horsfall protein deposition in the kidney and its measurement in the urine may therefore be a sensitive test to predict renal dysfunction.[149] Additional factors exacerbating renal failure in myeloma patients include use of nonsteroidal antiinflammatory drugs for pain control, hyperuricemia, use of nephrotoxic chemotherapeutic agents, use of intravenous contrast for radiographic studies, and use of bisphosphonates as well as calcium deposition and stones in the kidney. The proteinuria observed in patients with amyloidosis is more often nonspecific, which can help to differentiate it from typical myeloma-related kidney disease characterized by excessive light-chain excretion.[150] Pathologic renal changes similar to human myeloma-related nephropathy develop in IL-6 transgenic mice expressing IL-6 under metallothionein-1 promoter, which indicates a relationship between constitutive high IL-6 expression in the liver, dysproteinemia and long acute-phase response, and renal changes.[151]

HYPERCALCEMIA AND BONE DISEASE

The mechanism of bone abnormalities in myeloma, especially destruction, is an unbalanced process of increased osteoclast activity and suppressed osteoblast activity. These changes are due to an increase in osteoclast-activating factors produced predominantly by the bone marrow microenvironment but also by myeloma cells.[152,153] These factors include IL-1β, TNF-β (lymphotoxin), and IL-6.[154,156] The receptor activator of NFκB ligand (RANKL) plays an important role in osteoclast differentiation via its receptor RANK located on the osteoclast membrane. A member of the TNF family, it was originally described as a factor secreted by T cells that induces maturation of dendritic cells. RANKL is also secreted by stromal cells and osteoblasts and induces differentiation and maturation of osteoclast progenitors. Moreover, its production is elicited by factors such as parathyroid hormone, parathyroid hormone-related peptide, and osteoclast-activating factors.[153,157] Osteoprotegerin acts as a decoy receptor for RANKL and has been implicated in the development of bone changes in myeloma. In addition, a soluble factor produced by myeloma cells, dickoppf-1 DKK1, inhibits osteoblast activity (Fig. 44-5).[158,159] All of these factors contribute to the development of osteoporosis and lytic bone lesions. Radiographic findings of such destruction are shown in Figure 44-8. These bone changes frequently involve the vertebral column and result in compression fractures, lytic bone lesions, and related pain.

A new onset of back pain or other bone pain is a frequent presenting symptom in myeloma patients. Changes in the cytokine milieu and bone destruction may also lead to development of hypercalcemia, which is observed in approximately 25% of patients at some stage of the disease. Symptoms of high

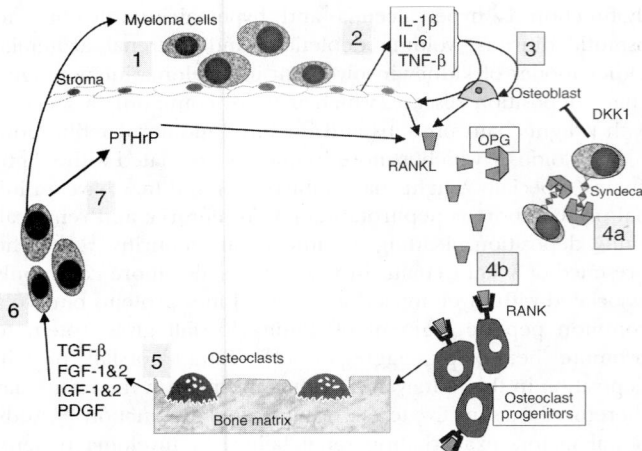

FIGURE 44-5. Biology of bone destruction in multiple myeloma (MM). 1: MM cells adhere to stroma. 2: Stromal cells secrete osteoclast-activating factors (OAFs). 3: OAFs stimulate stroma and osteoblasts to secrete receptor activator of nuclear factor κB ligand (RANKL). 4a: DKK1 produced by myeloma cells blocks osteoblast activity. 4b: RANKL is blocked by osteoprotegerin (OPG). OPG levels are reduced in MM due to syndecan trapping of OPG. 5: Increased osteoclastic activity leads to increased cytokine release from the bone matrix. 6: These cytokines stimulate MM cell growth, which increases process no. 1. 7: These cytokines also cause release of parathyroid hormone–related peptide (PTHrP) from MM cells, which activates stromal cells to secrete additional RANKL. FGF-1&2, fibroblast growth factors 1 and 2; IGF-1&2, insulin-like growth factors 1 and 2; IL-1β, interleukin-1β; IL-6, interleukin-6; PDGF, platelet-derived growth factor; TGF-β, transforming growth factor-β; TNF-β, tumor necrosis factor-β.

calcium levels include mental status changes, lethargy, constipation, and vomiting. High paraprotein levels, low albumin levels, or both, commonly observed in patients with myeloma, calls for measurement of ionized calcium. Hypercalcemia may also contribute to renal failure and should therefore be considered an oncologic emergency requiring prompt intervention.

INFECTIONS

Myeloma patients are at risk for developing recurrent bacterial infections due to deficiencies in both humoral and cellular immunity.[134,161,162] Various factors including high monoclonal Ig levels, soluble Fc receptor in serum, and transforming growth factor-β (TGF-β) lead to suppression of B-cell function, which in turn leads to depressed level of uninvolved Igs.[107,163] This impairment in the patients' ability to mount humoral responses predisposes patients to infections with bacteria that are ordinarily opsonized by specific antibodies against bacterial antigens. Patients also have profound T-cell dysfunction due to various immunosuppressive cytokines such as TGF-β secreted by the microenvironment and Fas ligand present on the membrane of the myeloma cells. The therapy for myeloma, which frequently includes high-dose corticosteroids, also increases the infection-related risks in these patients.

NEUROLOGIC SYMPTOMS

The most common cause of neurologic abnormalities is a tumor mass effect, especially compression of the spinal cord or cranial or spinal nerves. This may present as motor or, less frequently, sensory problems. Depositions of amyloid in the paraneural vessels or vasa nervorum may lead to polyneuropathies. An interesting constellation of symptoms described as POEMS syndrome (polyneuropathy, organomegaly, endocrinopathy, monoclonal gammopathy, and skin changes) is observed in osteosclerotic myeloma with prominent sensory neuropathy.[164–166] The biologic and cellular basis of these manifestations is not yet well understood. Leptomeningeal involvement in myeloma has been described, usually in the late phase of the disease and with manifestations involving the central nervous system (CNS).[168] Paraneoplastic CNS syndromes have also been described, possibly related to an immune mechanism directed at proteins present in the CNS, including the cerebellum. In addition, neurologic symptoms may occur as a consequence of hypercalcemia or hyperviscosity.

HYPERVISCOSITY

The M components in myeloma can cause hyperviscosity and compromise circulation when the serum Ig levels exceed certain levels. The incidence is highest in WM with IgM, followed by IgA myeloma (25% patients), and is least common in IgG myeloma (fewer than 10% of patients).[169–171] It can also be observed when Igs have a self-aggregating property that leads to increased viscosity: For example, the IgG3 subclass is more commonly associated with hyperviscosity. The syndrome is usually observed when serum viscosity exceeds 4.0 CP relative to normal serum and manifests with circulatory compromise involving the CNS, kidneys, and lungs; it may also be associated with bleeding complications. Due to varying characteristics of idiotypes, the same level of increased viscosity may produce different severity of symptoms in individual patients. Maintaining a high level of suspicion for this syndrome is important in treating any patient with paraproteinemia and either mental changes or pulmonary distress, because prompt plasmapheresis can alleviate symptoms and avoid irreversible organ damage.

COAGULOPATHY

Myeloma patients may acquire coagulation abnormalities related to the high level of paraprotein, which interferes with the normal coagulation cascade, or may exhibit specific antibody activity that leads to a clinical syndrome similar to acquired deficiency of factor VIII.[173,174] Additional factors, such as thrombosis in capillary circulation associated with hyperviscosity and anoxia, leads to coagulation-related complications in 15% of patients with IgG myeloma and in more than 33% of patients with IgA myeloma. Although platelet counts are not suppressed in the early stages of myeloma, functional abnormalities of platelets have been described and may also contribute to bleeding.

Patients may also present in a hypercoagulable state related to acquired deficiencies in protein C, protein S, or lupus anticoagulants that lead to thromboembolic complications.[175] The Fab fragment of the myeloma protein binds to fibrin and may prevent its aggregation.[176] In addition, factor X deficiency is reported in patients with systemic AL amyloidosis[177]; however, an inhibitor has not been demonstrated *in vitro* to account for this manifestation.

Therapy may also increase the hypercoagulable state in myeloma. An increased incidence of deep venous thrombosis (12% to 24%) is observed in patients taking thalidomide, especially along with dexamethasone or other combination chemotherapies. In one study 12 of 50 patients (24%) receiving thalidomide developed deep venous thrombosis, compared to 2 of 50 (4%) patients receiving identical therapy without thalidomide.[178] Activated protein C resistance in the absence of factor V Leiden mutation and high serum homocysteine levels are associated with an increased risk of thrombotic complications.[179]

EXTRAMEDULLARY DISEASE

Extramedullary disease manifestations are uncommon in patients with myeloma at presentation. However, such manifestations have been observed in the setting of advanced-stage disease or relapse after allogeneic transplantation. Solitary or multiple extramedullary plasmacytomas have been described in the liver, spleen, lymph nodes, kidneys, subcutaneous tissues, and brain parenchyma. Extramedullary involvement may be suspected in patients who have more aggressive features of myeloma, including high lactate dehydrogenase levels, immunoblastic morphology, high tumor cell labeling index, and complex karyotypic features.[180]

DIAGNOSIS

Because myeloma patients present with a variety of symptoms not specific to the disease, the diagnosis of myeloma is quite often delayed. An older patient with a new onset of unexplained back pain or bone pain, recurrent infection, anemia, or renal insufficiency should be screened for myeloma. Additional findings such as hyperproteinemia or proteinuria, anemia, hypoalbuminemia, low Ig levels, or marked elevation of erythrocyte sedimentation rate should prompt a further complete evaluation for diagnosis of plasma cell myeloma.

The initial evaluation includes a hemogram, complete skeletal radiographic survey, serum and urine protein electrophoresis and immunofixation, quantitative Ig levels, urinary protein excretion in 24 hours, and bone marrow aspiration and biopsy (Table 44-4). The diagnostic criteria for MGUS, smoldering and indolent myeloma, and MM are shown in Table 44-5.

STAGING AND RISK ASSESSMENT

After preliminary investigation, more detailed cellular and molecular studies are required to stage myeloma and evaluate other prognostic variables that determine the patient's probable outcome.

PROTEIN ELECTROPHORESIS

Among patients with myeloma, 70% have IgG subtype whereas 20% have IgA subtype, with an additional 5% to 10% having production of monoclonal light chains only. A small proportion of patients, fewer than 1%, produce monoclonal IgD, IgE, or IgM or have nonsecretory myeloma. Suppression of uninvolved Igs (e.g., IgM and IgA in IgG myeloma) is present in the

TABLE 44-4. Patient Evaluation

PRESENCE AND CHARACTERIZATION OF MONOCLONAL PROTEIN
Serum protein electrophoresis
Quantitative immunoglobulin
24-H urine: total protein and Bence Jones protein immunofixation of urine and serum, serum-free light chains
RADIOLOGIC EVALUATION
Skeletal survey
Magnetic resonance imaging with short time inversion recovery images
Bone densitometry
LABORATORY EVALUATION
Complete blood cell count with reticulocyte and differential count
Chemistry panel (renal, calcium, albumin, uric acid, lactate dehydrogenase)
β_2-Microglobulin, C-reactive protein
BONE MARROW
Aspirate and biopsy
  Cytogenetics
  Flow cytometry (DNA-cIg)
  Plasma cell labeling index
SPECIALIZED STUDIES FOR SELECTED PATIENTS
Abdominal fat pad or rectal biopsy for amyloid
Solitary lytic lesion biopsy
Serum viscosity if IgM component or high IgA levels or serum M component >7 g/dL

cIg, cytoplasmic immunoglobulin; Ig, immunoglobulin.

majority of the patients at diagnosis. Suppression of all of the three major classes of Ig should raise the possibility that the patient may have light-chain-only disease or nonsecretory disease. When multiple Ig class suppression is associated with a small M peak on serum protein electrophoresis, a less common variety of myeloma involving IgD or IgE may be suspected. Patients producing intact Ig can also have excess light-chain production and excretion in the urine (Fig. 44-6). The distribution of κ and λ light chains in the majority of myeloma cases is similar, except in IgD myeloma in which λ light chain is more common. Currently there is no difference in therapeutic approach to the different types of myeloma; however, patients with IgA myeloma, despite a higher initial response rate, have inferior survival.

Myeloma plasma cells usually produce a single, abnormal, unique, monoclonal antibody with a constant isotype and light-chain restriction. Rare occurrences of biclonal and triclonal cases have been reported at the time of diagnosis.[181] Occurrence of isotype switch and appearance of abnormal protein bands have, however, been reported in myeloma patients after therapy, especially high-dose therapy.[182] This appears to be related to recovery of normal Ig production rather than alteration in disease biology. This change is also associated with improved survival. Occasionally, patients with initially intact Ig production relapse with only Bence Jones proteinuria (light-chain escape), nonsecretory disease, or high lactate dehydrogenase disease, and this change has been correlated with more aggressive disease.[183]

Further analysis of a unique variable region in the myeloma-related idiotype (e.g., complementarity determining region III) provides information on the monoclonal nature of the protein and also provides a tool to investigate minimal residual disease by polymerase chain reaction using allele-specific oligo-

TABLE 44-5. Diagnostic Criteria for Multiple Myeloma, Myeloma Variants, and Monoclonal Gammopathy of Unknown Significance

MULTIPLE MYELOMA

Major criteria
  I. Plasmacytoma on tissue biopsy
  II. Bone marrow plasmacytosis with >30% plasma cells
  III. Monoclonal globulin spike on serum electrophoresis exceeding 3.5 g/dL for IgG or 2 g/dL for IgA, ≥1 g/24 h of κ or λ light-chain excretion on urine electrophoresis in the presence of amyloidosis

Minor criteria
  a. Bone marrow plasmacytosis 10% to 30%
  b. Monoclonal globulin spike present but less than the level defined above
  c. Lytic bone lesions
  d. Suppressed uninvolved immunoglobulins; IgM <50 mg/dL, IgA <100 mg/dL, or IgG <600 mg/dL

Diagnosis is confirmed when any of the following features are documented in symptomatic patients with clearly progressive disease. The criterion of three minor criteria that must include a + b—that is,

  I + b, I + c, I + d (I + a not sufficient)
  II + b, II + c, II + d
  III + a, III + c, III + d
  a + b + c, a + b + d

INDOLENT MYELOMA (SAME AS MYELOMA EXCEPT)

No bone lesions or only limited bone lesion (≤3 lytic lesions); no compression fractures
M component levels: (a) IgG <7 g/dL; (b) IgA <5/dL
No symptoms or associated disease features, that is,
  Performance status >70%
  Hemoglobin >10 g/dL
  Serum calcium normal
  Serum creatinine <2 mg/dL
  No infections

SMOLDERING MYELOMA (SAME AS INDOLENT MYELOMA EXCEPT)

No bone lesions
Bone marrow plasma cells ≤30%

MONOCLONAL GAMMOPATHY OF UNKNOWN SIGNIFICANCE

Monoclonal gammopathy
M component level
  IgG ≤3.5 g/dL
  IgA ≤2 g/dL
  Bence Jones protein ≤1 g/24 h
Bone marrow plasma cells <10%
No bone lesions
No symptoms

Ig, immunoglobulin.

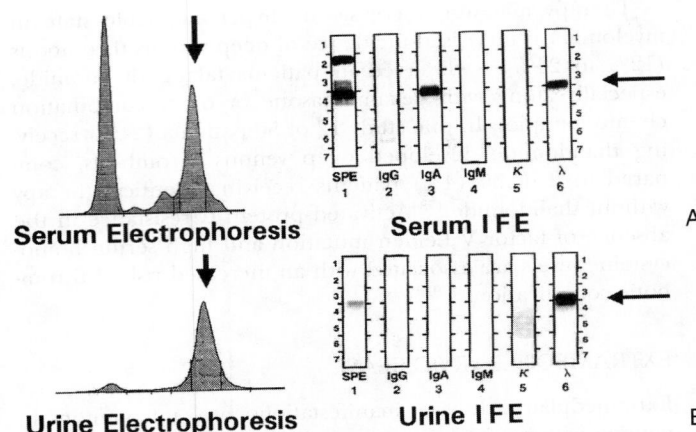

FIGURE 44-6. **A:** Serum and urine protein electrophoresis showing abnormal monoclonal protein bands (*arrow*). Quantitation of the M protein is performed by nephelometric measurement of the band. **B:** Identification of serum and urine M component by immunofixation electrophoresis (IFE). The labels indicate the specificity of the antiserum used in developing the immunofixation pattern. The top is immunoglobulin A (IgA)-γ in serum and the bottom is free γ light chain in urine. SPE, serum protein electrophoresis.

nucleotide, which thus allows determination of molecular complete remissions.[184]

BONE MARROW EXAMINATION

Various degrees of bone marrow infiltration are observed in myeloma, with the majority of patients having an excess number of plasma cells (more than 5%). The pattern of bone marrow involvement (diffuse vs. nodular) is important, because patients with nodular disease seem to have poorer outcomes (in contrast to CLL).[185] The morphology of the plasma cell seems to be an important factor determining severity of the disease. This is based on histologic examination (Bartl grade)

in which grade I suggests a slow-growing disease, whereas grade III represents plasmablastic disease with an aggressive course.[186] There is also an increased incidence of cytogenetic abnormalities in patients with higher-grade disease. Plasma cells contain cytoplasmic Igs with a constant heavy and light chain, which can be evaluated by flow cytometric analysis or immunohistochemical staining of plasma cells.[187] When coupled with DNA staining using propidium iodide, two-parameter analysis can detect changes in DNA content in myeloma cells (Fig. 44-7). DNA aneuploidy is observed in the bone marrow of more than 80% of patients, which suggests the existence of chromosomal abnormalities in the majority of patients.[187] This analysis also provides an objective marker to evaluate response to therapy and to distinguish reactive from clonal plasmacytosis, especially in nonsecretory disease. A hypodiploid tumor cell has also been associated with refractoriness to standard-dose therapy.

CYTOGENETICS

Because the myeloma cell represents a mature differentiated cell with low proliferative activity, cytogenetic abnormalities are not frequently found. Abnormalities are detected in only one-third of patients at the time of diagnosis; however, repeated analysis improves the yield to almost one-half of patients. The normal karyotypic pattern observed in the remaining half most likely originates from dividing normal hematopoietic cells.[48]

As described previously in Cytogenetic and Molecular Genetic Alterations, a complex karyotypic pattern is frequently observed, and its distribution is shown in Figure 44-2. Although a predominant constant cytogenetic abnormality has not been described, certain recurrent changes have been noticed. These include the common B-cell tumor-related changes in the 14q32 region involving the IgH region, chromosome arm 1q, and chromosome 13–related changes.[188–190] A longitudinal analysis in patients undergoing high-dose che-

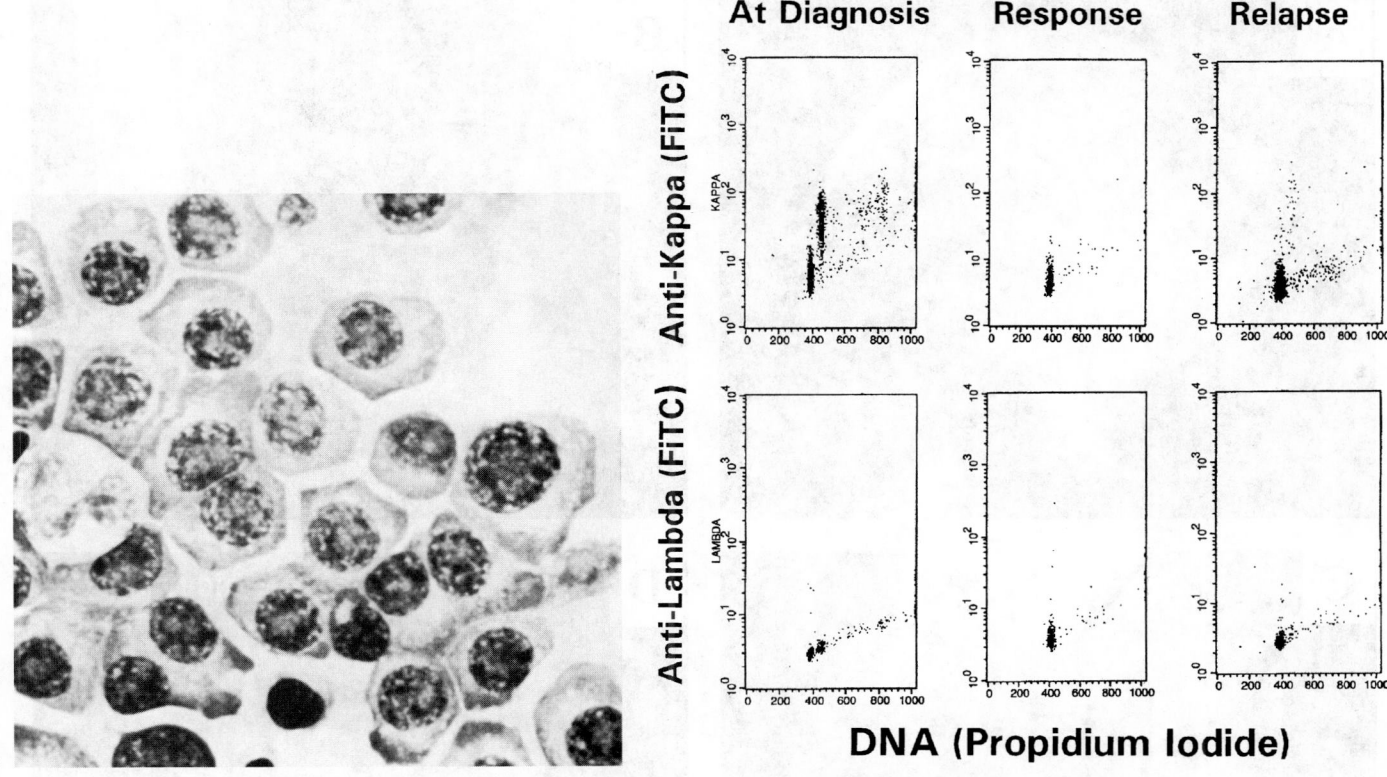

FIGURE 44-7. **A:** Bone marrow plasma cells in a patient with immunoglobulin G myeloma showing neoplastic plasma cells at various stages of differentiation. **B:** Two-parameter flow cytometry of DNA content of bone marrow cells (abscissa, propidium iodide) and cytoplasmic immunoglobulin [ordinate, anti-κ or anti-γ fluorescein isothiocyanate (FiTC)]. At diagnosis, approximately 45% hyperdiploid tumor cells with κ light-chain restriction are seen (**left panel**); at the time of maximal response no hyperdiploid light-chain–restricted cells are noted (**middle panel**); at the time of early relapse, reappearance of a small hyperdiploid and κ light-chain–restricted population (fewer than 1%) is indicative of reemergence of a small number of clonal cells, which may not yet be apparent on cytologic examination of the bone marrow (**right panel**). A population of κ restricted but diploid cells may represent a second clone.

motherapy has shown cytogenetic evolution, which portends poor prognosis.[191] Detection of chromosome 13 deletion abnormalities at diagnosis, as well as after high-dose chemotherapy, has now been reported to carry a poor prognosis. The application of FISH technology has improved the ability to detect genetic changes by using interphase cells. The Rb-1 probe detects an abnormality on the 13q14 region, and its deletion has been reported in more than 40% of patients as detected by interphase FISH, which also predicts poor outcome after standard-dose therapy.[192] Interphase FISH analysis for numeric chromosomal aberrations has identified trisomies of chromosomes 6, 9, and 17, which predict favorable outcomes.[52] Plasma cell leukemia has been reported to frequently contain a t(11:14); however, this translocation has also been detected in patients with MGUS, without any prognostic relevance.[193]

LABELING INDEX

The proportion of cycling myeloma cells is small early in the disease; bromodeoxyuridine or tritiated thymidine methods show a median of 1% cycling cells at diagnosis. The labeling index has important prognostic significance, because patients with more than 1% cells in S phase in bone marrow have worse outcomes.[187,194,195]

RADIOGRAPHIC EVALUATION

The radiographic survey of bone is a standard diagnostic evaluation. It shows osteopenia in an early phase of the disease and, with increasing tumor burden, lytic punched-out lesions (Fig. 44-8). Osteosclerotic lesions are observed in POEMS syndrome.[164,166] Due to the predominant osteolytic activity with osteoblastic inactivity, bone scans seldom give positive results unless a recent fracture has occurred and are therefore not useful in the diagnosis of MM.

Because demineralization of bone (osteoporosis) is one of the common manifestations of myeloma, measurement of bone mineral density (BMD) by dual-energy X-ray absorptiometry is an important evaluation at diagnosis.[196] In a study of 66 patients at diagnosis, the majority of patients had decreased BMD with a lumbar mean BMD value (Z score) of −1.24 ± 1.45. After standard-dose therapy, lumbar BMD increased by 0.7%, whereas in a group treated with high-dose therapy BMD improved by 4.6% ($P = .02$).[197] Similar improvements in BMD have also been noted in patients undergoing high-dose therapy with addition

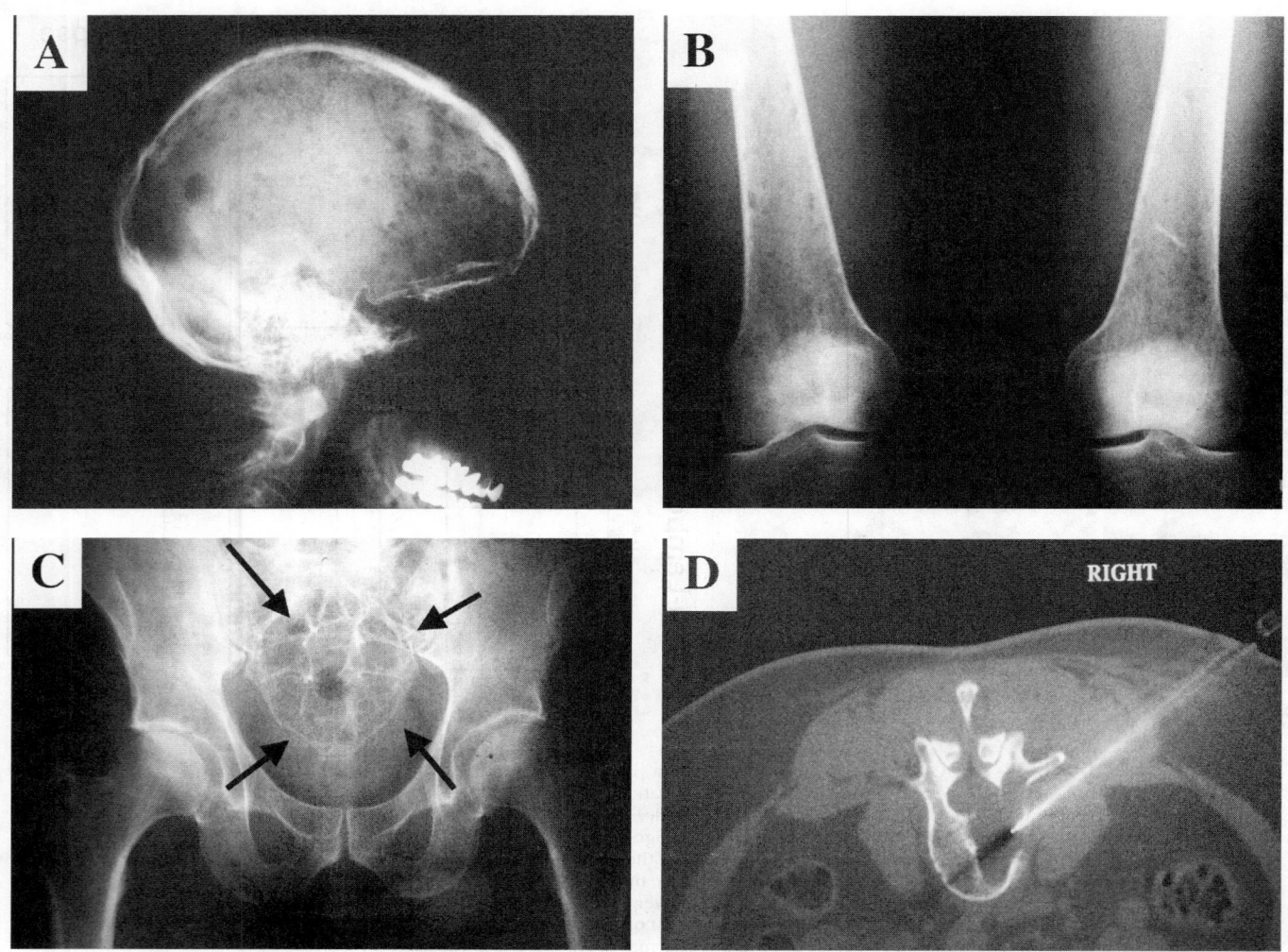

FIGURE 44-8.   Typical skeletal changes on radiograph. **A:** Example of punched-out lytic lesions in skull. **B:** Small lytic lesions in the left femur. **C:** Large lytic lesion (*arrows*) in the sacrum. **D:** Fine-needle aspiration biopsy of the vertebral lesion. (Courtesy of Hemendra Shah.)

of bisphosphonates.[198] Differential effects of pamidronate on cortical and cancellous bone have been described in patients with myeloma undergoing autotransplantation.[197,198]

Magnetic resonance imaging (MRI) of bone marrow provides a better assessment of tumor burden and is essential in the workup of patients with solitary plasmacytomas of bone.[199] More than 95% of myeloma patients have abnormalities on MRI: One-third have diffuse involvement of the bone marrow, one-third have focal lesions, and the remaining third have heterogeneous focal and diffused marrow involvement (Fig. 44-9*A*). Because myeloma is a macrofocal disease, random bone marrow sampling may not be diagnostic or predictive of disease status. MRI short tau inversion recovery (STIR) images provide a better assessment of tumor burden in myeloma.[200,203] A focal marrow plasmacytoma can be further analyzed through computed tomography (CT)–guided fine-needle aspiration, which allows cytologic diagnosis and further risk assessment based on evaluation of the results of cytogenetic and FISH analysis, as well as labeling index. As therapies become more effective, the MRI pattern may change (see Fig. 44-9*B*); diffuse involvement of the marrow may evolve into focal disease. Nor-

malization of MRI abnormalities may provide a better definition of complete responses. Positron emission tomography has also been evaluated in a small number of studies and may provide a better functional definition of lesions observed on MRI or CT, as well as allowing selection of lesions for biopsy.[204]

DIFFERENTIAL DIAGNOSIS

In the presence of lytic bone lesions and greater than 30% marrow plasmacytosis, the diagnosis of myeloma can be readily established. However, in the absence of lytic bone lesions or diffuse osteoporosis, other criteria are required to differentiate overt myeloma from MGUS.[205] These include anemia, high levels of monoclonal protein in serum and urine, and marrow plasmacytosis (see Table 44-5).[206,207] Distinguishing smoldering myeloma and MGUS may be difficult, because this distinction is based on levels of serum monoclonal proteins and marrow plasmacytosis.[208] As shown in Table 44-6, anemia, bone lesions, and MRI abnormalities are absent in the majority of the

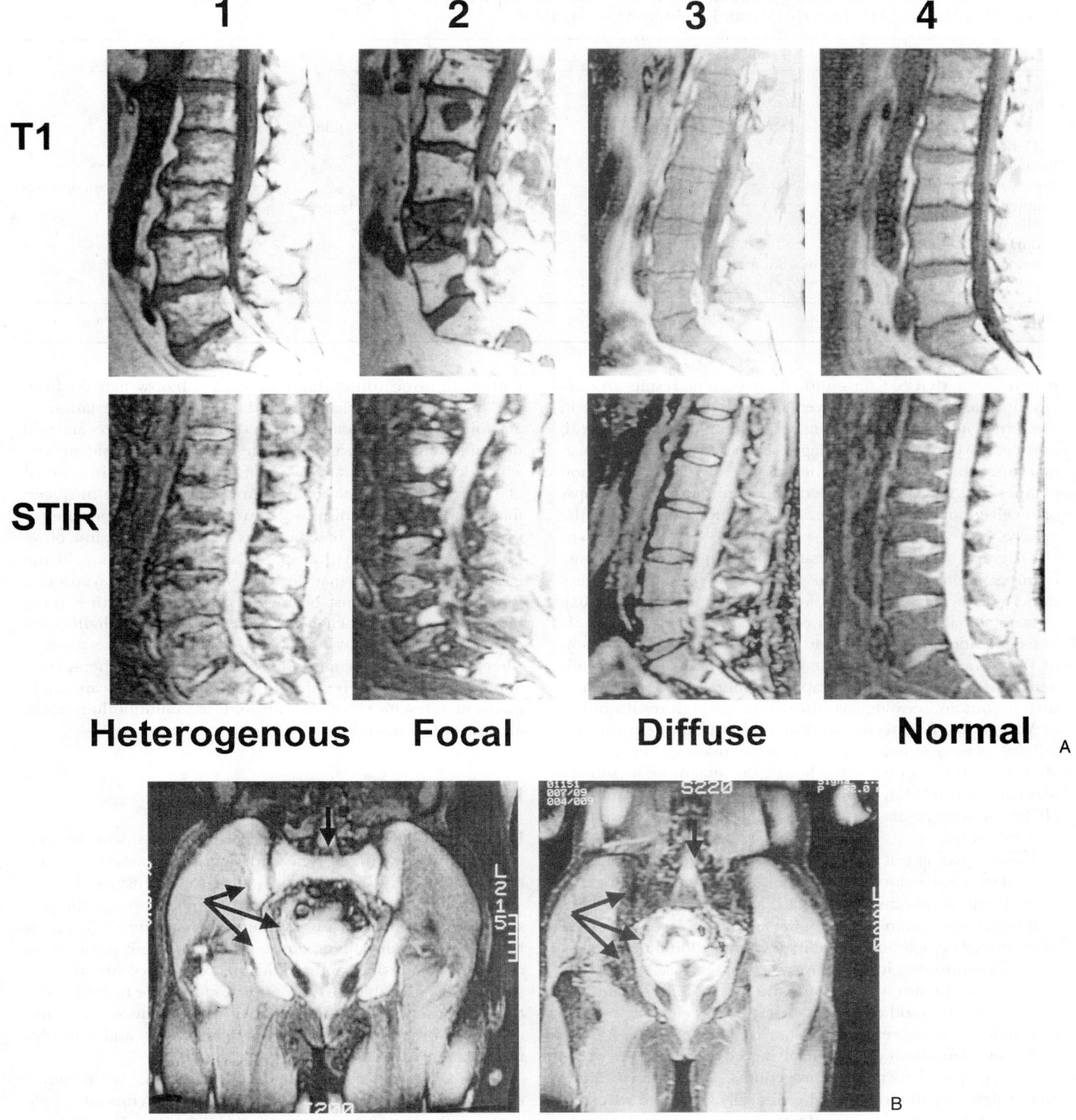

1   **2**   **3**   **4**

T1

STIR

Heterogenous   Focal   Diffuse   Normal

A

B

FIGURE 44-9.   A: Magnetic resonance imaging (MRI) pattern in multiple myeloma at diagnosis. T1-weighted and short tau inversion recovery (STIR) imaging shows that approximately one-third of patients present with a heterogeneous pattern (1), focal plasmacytoma lesions (2), or diffuse homogeneous hyperintense marrow pattern (3). Hyperintensity of marrow on STIR image is suggestive of uniform marrow involvement by myeloma. A few patients have the hypointense and homogenous pattern also seen in healthy individuals (4). **B:** The hyperintense marrow pattern suggestive of extensive marrow involvement before therapy (*left; arrows*) changes to a hypointense pattern after complete response and normalization of marrow (*right; arrows*). Fine-needle aspiration examination in 72 patients with MRI-detected focal disease showed tumor in 92%, which indicates that MRI-detected focal lesions in myeloma represent tumor.

TABLE 44-6. Major Diagnostic Criteria among Monoclonal Gammopathy of Unknown Significance (MGUS), Smoldering Multiple Myeloma (SMM), and Multiple Myeloma (MM)

	MGUS	SMM	MM
M component			
IgG	<3 g/dL	>3 g/dL, stable	>3 g/dL
IgA	<1 g/dL	>1 and <2 g/dL, stable	>2 g/dL
Light chain/urine	<1 g/24 h	>1 g/24 h	>1 g/24 h
Plasma cells on marrow biopsy	<10%	>10% but <20%	>10%
Bone lesions on skeletal survey	No lesions	No lytic lesions	Lytic lesions or osteoporosis
Magnetic resonance imaging	No focal lesions	Focal lesions can be present	—
β_2-Microglobulin levels	Normal	Normal	High or normal
Plasma cell labeling index	<1%	<1%	Can be >1%
Renal failure, hypercalcemia, anemia, bone pain, extramedullary disease	Absent	Absent	Present

Ig, immunoglobulin.

patients with MGUS. Conventional cytogenetic results are usually normal in MGUS; however, monoclonal plasma cells in some individuals with MGUS may be aneuploid. Patients with nonsecretory myeloma are diagnosed based on marrow plasmacytosis and presence of bone lesions. MRI to detect abnormalities and CT- or MRI-guided fine-needle aspiration biopsy of involved anatomic sites are important for follow-up of the disease.

Diagnosis of solitary plasmacytoma of bone or soft tissue requires intense investigation to rule out systemic disease. Bone marrow examination in a true solitary lesion is normal, with no clonal cell population evidenced on DNA cytoplasmic Ig examination. MRI evaluation for myelomatous involvement of the bone marrow helps detect early lesions, before their detection by standard radiographic examination. Detection of such lesions and cytologic confirmation through results of CT- or MRI-guided fine-needle aspiration biopsy may help confirm solitary plasmacytoma and its genetic makeup. In case of MGUS, such detection may change the diagnosis to solitary plasmacytoma or MM. It is important to note that patients with MGUS or solitary plasmacytoma seldom have suppression of uninvolved Igs.

Besides plasma cell neoplasms, various other conditions can present with monoclonal Ig secretion. These conditions include other B-cell neoplasms such as CLL and B-cell non-Hodgkin's lymphoma; autoimmune conditions such as cold agglutinin diseases, mixed cryoglobulinemia, hypergammaglobulinemia, and Sjögren's syndrome; inflammatory or storage diseases such as lichen myxedematosus, Gaucher's disease, sarcoidosis, and cirrhosis, and, rarely, other malignancies such as chronic myeloid leukemia or colon, breast, or prostate cancer.

Protein deposition disease involving various organs requires additional special diagnostic procedures. Deposition of amyloid protein (amyloidosis) can be clinically suspected based on macroglossia, vascular fragility (raccoon's eyes, periorbital subcutaneous hemorrhages), carpal tunnel syndrome, organomegaly, nephropathy, and cardiomegaly with arrhythmia. Detection of Congo red–positive amyloid in perivascular areas and subcutaneous fat, bone marrow, or rectal biopsy specimens with classic apple-green birefringence when visualized under polarized light are diagnostic of AL amyloid. Electrocardiography may reveal low voltage, and echocardiographic evaluation shows thickening of the interventricular septum or classic speckled

pattern in myocardium. Endomyocardial biopsy may establish the diagnosis of cardiac amyloid. Another manifestation of amyloid deposition is autonomic dysfunction due to amyloid deposition in the vasa nervorum of the autonomic nerves, which leads to orthostatic hypotension. Deposition in adrenal glands leads to hypoadrenalism. Amyloid deposition in spleen may lead to hyposplenism with thrombocytosis. Deposition in liver may be suspected based on elevated levels of alkaline phosphatase and γ-glutamyl transpeptidase, and deposition in the gastrointestinal tract may lead to malabsorption syndrome. Renal dysfunction must be further investigated with a renal biopsy, because light-chain cast nephropathy or light-chain deposition disease may be reversible after aggressive therapy, whereas deposition of amyloid requires a different therapeutic approach. Because deposition of Ig and light chain can mimic many manifestations of AL amyloidosis, immunofluorescent analysis of unfixed tissue is important for diagnosis.

PROGNOSTIC VARIABLES

Patients with MM have variable disease courses, with survival ranging from less than 1 year with aggressive disease to more than 10 years with indolent presentation or sensitive disease. Various characteristics have been identified to predict the possible course of the disease. Evaluation of prognostic factors is important to define therapeutic strategies, permit comparison of clinical trial results, and predict life expectancy after diagnosis. As shown in Table 44-7, prognostic factors are related to the tumor burden, intrinsic properties of the tumor, host and microenvironmental influences, and treatment- and intervention-related factors.

Studies measuring *in vitro* Ig production by patients' myeloma cells have led to the development of clinically applicable methods to estimate tumor mass. A clinical staging system for MM using standard laboratory measurement, developed by Durie and Salmon, has been applied to predict clinical outcomes after standard-dose chemotherapy.[209] As shown in Table 44-8, this system is based on monoclonal protein or Ig levels in serum, light-chain excretion in a 24-hour urine sample, hypercalcemia, anemia, extent of bone lesions, and renal failure. In a study by the National Cancer Institute of Canada, overall survival after standard-dose therapy was 49

TABLE 44-7. Prognostic Variables

TUMOR BURDEN–RELATED FACTORS
β_2-Microglobulin level
Serum immunoglobulin level
Number of lytic bone lesions
Hemoglobin level
Serum calcium level
Percentage of bone marrow plasmacytosis
Albumin level

TUMOR BIOLOGY–RELATED FACTORS
Monosomy 13 or 13q–
Plasma cell labeling index
Bartl grade
Mitotic activity
Immunoglobulin A myeloma
C-reactive protein level
Lactate dehydrogenase level
Soluble interleukin-6 receptor level
Renal failure

TUMOR MICROENVIRONMENT–RELATED FACTORS
Bone marrow microvessel density
Serum syndecan-1 level
Matrix metalloproteinase 9 level
Soluble CD16 level

TREATMENT-RELATED FACTORS
≤12 mo of prior therapy
Tandem transplantation
Second transplant within 6 mo
Achievement of complete response

PATIENT-RELATED FACTORS
Albumin level
Performance status
Presence of other organ problems not related to myeloma

TABLE 44-8. Myeloma Staging System

Criteria	Measured Myeloma Cell Mass (Cells × $10^{12}/m^2$)
STAGE I	
All of the following	<0.6 (low)
Hemoglobulin >10 g/dL	
Normal serum calcium (<12 mg/dL)	
Skeletal survey normal bone structure (Scale 0) or solitary bone plasmacytoma or osteoporosis only	
Low M component production rates	
IgG value <5 g/dL	
IgA value <3 g/dL	
Urine light-chain M component on electrophoresis <4 g/24 h	
STAGE II	
Overall data not as minimally abnormal as shown for stage I and no single value abnormal as defined for stage III	0.6–1.2 (intermediate)
STAGE III	
One or more of the following	>1.2 (high)
Hemoglobin value <8.5 g/dL	
Serum calcium value >12 mg/dL	
Advanced lytic bone lesions, three or more	
High M component production rates	
IgG value >7 g/dL	
IgA value >5 g/dL	
Urine light-chain M component on electrophoresis >12 g/24 h	
Subclassification	
A = relatively normal renal function (serum creatinine value >2 mg/dL)	
B = abnormal renal function (serum creatinine value ≥2 mg/dL)	

Ig, immunoglobulin.
(From Alexanian R, Balcerzak S, Bonnet JD, et al. Prognostic factors in multiple myeloma. *Cancer* 1975;36:1192, with permission.)

---

months for patients with low disease burden (stage I) and 25 months for those with high tumor burden (stage III). When renal failure was included in the staging system, patients with stage IIIA disease had a median survival of 30 versus 15 months for those with stage IIIB disease.[210] The accuracy and predictive value of the Durie-Salmon system are less pronounced in patients undergoing high-dose chemotherapy. The high-dose chemotherapy is probably able to reduce the disease burden to a greater extent, with patient outcome depending on tumor biology–related factors. Because the Durie-Salmon system considers tumor burden–related variables and depends on subjective interpretation of lytic bone lesions, additional variables have been investigated to better assess patient prognosis.

β_2M has been identified as one of the most consistent predictors of survival in plasma cell myeloma. β_2M is the light-chain gene of the class I histocompatibility antigens expressed on the surface of all nucleated cells and is shed into the blood. Its renal excretion explains its elevation in renal failure. In MM, β_2M level therefore reflects both tumor burden and renal function.[211,212] High β_2M levels (more than 2.5 mg/L) carry a poor prognosis for treatment with both standard-dose and high-dose therapy.[213] Other independent factors associated with poor prognosis include elevated levels of C-reactive protein (CRP), serum IL-6, serum soluble IL-6R, and IgA isotype.[214] Because CRP levels reflect IL-6 activity and elevated CRP levels can be associated with acute-phase reactions, including inflammation and infections, the predictive value of elevated CRP in myeloma is important only when other possible causes for its elevation are ruled out.

The bone marrow plasmacytosis reflects tumor burden but does not predict survival. Peripheral blood monoclonal plasma cells predict for survival in myeloma: in a study of 254 patients, a blood monoclonal plasma cell count of 4% or higher in 57% of patients was associated with a median survival of 2.4 years compared with 4.4 years in patients with less than 4% circulating plasma cells.[215]

Among the various other disease biology–related variables, Bartl grading of tumor cells correlates with survival in patients undergoing high-dose chemotherapy. Flow cytometric measurement of DNA content in monoclonal cells identified by cytoplasmic Ig can identify hypodiploid tumor cells, which are associated with resistance to standard-dose chemotherapy.[216] Plasma cell proliferation rate, as measured by the labeling index, is a valuable prognostic factor: a labeling index higher than 2% predicts inferior survival. One study combining β_2M and labeling index identified a low-risk group (both parameters low), an intermediate-risk group (one parameter high), and a high-risk group (both parameters high) to have median survival times of 71 months, 40 months, and 15 months, respectively.[195]

Cytogenetic abnormalities have been identified as a major prognostic factor in plasma cell myeloma. Abnormalities involving chromosome 13 carry a poor prognosis, with short survival even after high-dose chemotherapy. In a study of 1000 patients receiving high-dose chemotherapy with melphalan 200 mg/m^2, the three most significant adverse variables associated with a shorter survival were the presence of chromosome 13 abnormality, β_2M level of more than 2.5 mg/L at the time of transplantation, and more than 12 months of prior conventional-dose therapy. Additional tumor-related factors predictive of inferior survival include increased soluble IL-6R level, elevated serum lactate dehydrogenase level with extramedullary disease, and increased tumor cell mitotic activity (more than one per high-power field).

Among the microenvironment-related factors, bone marrow microvessel density has been identified as an important prognosticator. High microvessel density in bone marrow (four or more per high-power field) at diagnosis confers shorter event-free survival (2.7 vs. 4.3 years; P = .03) and overall survival (7.9+ vs. 4.3 years; P = .006) after high-dose chemotherapy.[217] This may be reflective of increased VEGF expression by myeloma cells or other microenvironmental factors.[105] An increased level of serum syndecan-1 has been described to portend poor prognosis. Soluble CD16 levels have been correlated with disease activity: significantly lower levels of soluble CD16 are found in sera from patients with MM than in sera from MGUS patients and normal controls; moreover, within myeloma, a stage-dependent decrease in soluble CD16 has been observed.[218]

Among therapy- and intervention-related prognostic factors, having received more than 12 months of prior standard-dose therapy affects survival, especially in patients undergoing high-dose chemotherapy. Age older than 65 years is associated with inferior survival after standard-dose therapy; however, age does not appear to predict poor survival after high-dose therapy.[219]

Because high-dose therapy and the newer biologically based therapies such as thalidomide and bortezomib (Velcade) are able to overcome drug resistance, some traditional prognostic factors such as Durie Salmon staging are no longer predictive of survival. Additional molecular studies with FISH analysis,[220] expression of proteins of the bcl family and p53, activation of STAT and NFκB pathways, and gene microarray analysis may identify additional prognostic factors.

TREATMENT

The diagnosis of a monoclonal gammopathy does not always require immediate treatment of the patient. Although MM is generally a disseminated disease, patients may present with solitary plasmacytomas that can be treated with local therapy only or with indolent asymptomatic myeloma, which can smolder for a long period before becoming symptomatic and requiring treatment.

SOLITARY PLASMACYTOMA

Solitary plasmacytoma requires specialized techniques for accurate staging, including a CT scan and MRI to exclude more disseminated disease. Solitary plasmacytomas of bone involve vertebral bodies in one-third of patients and frequently affect

men (70%) at a younger age (median, 56 years).[221] A monoclonal protein in the serum is observed in 24% to 54% of patients, but in the remaining cases no detectable monoclonal protein is seen, even on immunofixation. Extramedullary plasmacytomas are diagnosed less frequently and require a workup, including MRI and positron emission tomography to rule out additional sites or disseminated disease. The optimal therapy for true solitary plasmacytoma is curative-dose radiotherapy at 4000 to 5000 cGy.[222,223] With this dose, local tumor recurrence rate has been less than 10%; 30% of patients with solitary bone lesions, compared to more than 70% of patients with solitary extramedullary plasmacytomas, achieve long-term disease-free survival.[224,225] Monoclonal protein disappears after radiotherapy in 25% to 50% of patients, which suggests possible eradication of disease; conversely, reappearance of monoclonal protein predicts for recurrence of disease. With better staging using MRI, true solitary plasmacytoma of the bone can be cured in a high proportion of patients.

INDOLENT MYELOMA

Myeloma patents with a low tumor mass and slowly progressive disease may present without specific symptoms. Such patients generally have less than 20% bone marrow plasmacytosis and low monoclonal protein levels, as shown in Table 44-5.[208,226] They have no lytic bone lesions, no hypercalcemia or renal disease, and hemoglobin levels higher than 10 g/dL. In patients with indolent light-chain disease, Bence Jones proteinuria does not exceed 10 g/d. These patients do not present with cytogenetic abnormalities when conventional karyotyping is used and often have a low labeling index and low serum β_2M levels. Features predictive of early progression to symptomatic myeloma include presence of lytic bone lesions, high serum myeloma protein levels (more than 3 g/dL IgG or more than 2 g/dL IgA), and focal MRI abnormalities.[227] Median time to progression is 26 months for all patients, 10 months for patients with bone lesions and high monoclonal protein level, and 61 months for those without these features. Patients with indolent myeloma are not treated with chemotherapy until disease progression, onset of symptoms, or development of new lytic bone lesions; however, pamidronate therapy has been used to delay onset of bone-related complications. An evaluation of thalidomide treatment in 31 patients with indolent myeloma showed responses in 66% of patients, with the potential to delay progression to symptomatic disease.[228] In the future, gene expression profiling of tumor cells from these patients may provide important prognostic information and define the need for early chemotherapeutic intervention in selected patients.

SYMPTOMATIC MULTIPLE MYELOMA

Standard-Dose Therapy

Oral melphalan and prednisone were the first successful combination chemotherapy for myeloma. Subsequently various other single agents and combination chemotherapy regimens have been investigated and reported to have significant antimyeloma activity.

MELPHALAN AND PREDNISONE. Treatment with oral melphalan and prednisone was introduced 35 years ago and has remained the standard of therapy, providing symptomatic relief as well as tumor mass reduction.[229] A partial response, defined as a greater than 50% reduction in monoclonal protein, has been observed in 50% to 60% of patients, with 3% to 5% of patients achieving a complete response. The absorption of oral melphalan is unpredictable, which requires its ingestion on an empty stomach and an increase in dose if the patient does not develop cytopenia.[230] With the availability of an intravenous formulation, dose and pharmacokinetics are now predictable. In patients receiving melphalan and prednisone, a prompt response is associated with poor survival, reflecting a highly proliferative tumor. The median response duration is 18 months and overall survival is 24 to 36 months. Frequent complications after melphalan and prednisone therapy include the development of cytopenia and, with chronic administration, myelodysplastic changes in the marrow. Melphalan and prednisone should not be used as induction therapy in patients eligible for high-dose therapy and stem cell transplantation, because the ability to mobilize adequate numbers of stem cells decreases with prolonged use of this combination.

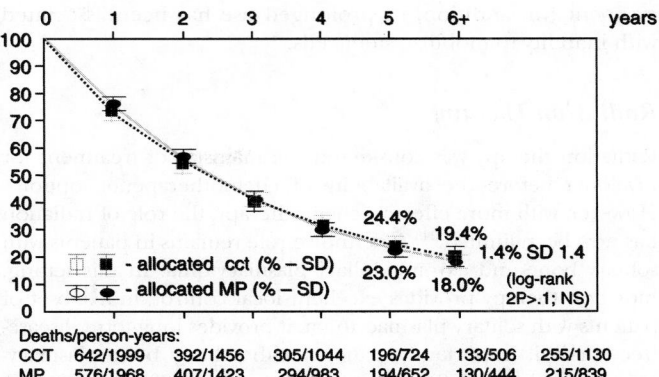

FIGURE 44-10. Results of a metaanalysis of randomized trials comparing combination chemotherapies (CCTs) with melphalan and prednisone (MP). No significant survival differences were noted between results for patients randomized to receive CCT and those randomized to receive MP. NS, not significant; SD, standard deviation. (See Color Fig. 44-10 in the CD-ROM.)

OTHER ALKYLATING AGENT–BASED COMBINATIONS.

Various chemotherapeutic combinations have been investigated in myeloma, including combinations of vincristine, cyclophosphamide, carmustine (BCNU), melphalan, doxorubicin (Adriamycin), and prednisone. Commonly used regimens include vincristine, BCNU, melphalan, cyclophosphamide, and prednisone (VBMCP) and vincristine, melphalan, cyclophosphamide, and prednisone/vincristine, BCNU, doxorubicin, and prednisone (VMCP/VBAP).[231-234,237] In randomized studies these combinations achieved response rates, as well as event-free and overall survival rates, similar to those for melphalan and prednisone. A metaanalysis of 18 published studies involving 3814 patients randomized to receive either melphalan and prednisone or various other chemotherapeutic combinations showed that outcome after melphalan and prednisone and outcome after other chemotherapeutic combinations are equivalent (Fig. 44-10).

VINCRISTINE, DOXORUBICIN, AND DEXAMETHASONE AND HIGH-DOSE DEXAMETHASONE.

The role of high-dose corticosteroids was initially investigated in the late 1960s, and therapeutic benefit was seen in small numbers of patients. Glucocorticoids down-regulate IL-6 production and induce apoptosis *in vitro*. The molecular mechanism of steroid-induced apoptosis in myeloma involves a decrease in NFκB activity through inhibitor of κB (IκB) activation. Interestingly, myeloma cells can be rescued from glucocorticoid-mediated killing by addition of IL-6 to *in vitro* cultures or by co-culturing them with stromal cells, which are a source of IL-6 *in vivo*. High-dose dexamethasone was evaluated in combination with vincristine and doxorubicin (VAD): vincristine at 0.25 mg/m² and doxorubicin 9 mg/m² given by continuous infusion over 24 hours for 4 days along with dexamethasone 40 mg orally on days 1 to 4, 9 to 12, and 17 to 20, with cycles repeated every 5 weeks.[238,239] More than 50% of patients with refractory myeloma showed rapid and marked responses, defined as more than 75% cytoreduction; efficacy was better in patients responsive to prior therapy. Response to VAD was much faster than response to other combination therapies, with a median tumor halving time of 21 days versus more than 6 weeks. The advantages of this combination include quick response, effec-

tiveness in treating hypercalcemia, quick relief of bone pain, applicability in patients with renal failure, and lack of cumulative bone marrow stem cell damage, which allows for subsequent successful mobilization and collection of stem cells. Studies of high-dose dexamethasone alone given in doses similar to that used in the VAD regimen have shown response rates similar to those observed with VAD in primary resistant myeloma, which indicates that dexamethasone is clearly an important agent in VAD. In a study evaluating corticosteroid dose intensity, chemotherapy regimens with higher corticosteroid doses yielded higher response rates and improved survival ($P = .02$).[240] VAD is associated with minimal bone marrow toxicity, and continuous infusion of doxorubicin prevents cardiac toxicity. Randomized comparisons of VAD and other chemotherapeutic combinations have failed to show any survival benefit for VAD. Addition of cyclophosphamide to VAD (CVAD) has been shown to achieve responses in up to 40% of patients with VAD-refractory disease.

INTERFERON.

The role and efficacy of IFN in the management of myeloma remain controversial. It has been shown to achieve up to 20% responses in patients with relapsed myeloma. Its mode of action remains multifactorial: direct growth inhibition, as well as antiangiogenic and immunomodulatory activity, may contribute to its overall action. However, in combination with other chemotherapeutic regimens, it has failed to demonstrate beneficial effect.[241] In a metaanalysis of 16 trials involving 2286 patients, response rate was 45.9% for patients treated with chemotherapy versus 54.4% for those receiving chemotherapy with IFN. The difference in overall survival was 5 months. The role of IFN in maintenance therapy after standard-dose therapy has been evaluated, with some studies showing significant prolongation of survival.[241,243] A metaanalysis of eight trials involving 929 patients showed prolongation of relapse-free survival by 7 months and of overall survival by 5 months in patients receiving IFN. In younger patients and those with lower tumor burden, IFN maybe more effective. To date, however, IFN has not achieved benefit after high-dose therapy.[244] It is associated with flu-like symptoms, weight loss, impotence, depression, mental status changes, and cytopenia; in addition, its prolonged use has been associated with inability to mobilize stem cells.

Radiation Therapy

Radiation therapy was considered the mainstay of treatment for myeloma before the availability of chemotherapeutic options. However, with more effective chemotherapy, the role of radiation has now been limited.[245] A definitive role remains in patients with solitary bone and extramedullary plasmacytoma. In this setting, radiation therapy provides excellent local control; in a subset of patients with solitary plasmacytoma, it provides long-term disease-free survival. Importantly, patients with solitary bone plasmacytoma treated with definitive radiation therapy (4000 to 5000 cGy) have a progression-free survival rate of 30%, compared to 70% for those with extramedullary plasmacytomas.[222–225,246] The indication for radiation therapy in MM remains palliation, in cases of impending pathologic fracture and for treatment of spinal cord compression. In patients with bone pain or symptomatic soft tissue masses, radiation is only considered when chemotherapeutic options have failed.[247,248] Radiation to bone marrow–containing areas, such as the pelvic bone, should be used judiciously if there is need for collection of stem cells. The dose of palliative radiation therapy ranges from 1500 to 2500 cGy. Studies to date have failed to show any benefit of hemibody radiation in MM. However, total body radiation has been used before allogeneic and autologous transplantation. More recent studies have demonstrated that total body radiation does not provide additional cytoreductive potential. High-dose melphalan and total body radiation conditioning before transplant increases treatment-related morbidity and mortality and delays immune recovery compared to high-dose melphalan alone. Studies using nonmyeloablative regimens followed by allogeneic stem cell transplantation use low-dose radiation and achieve adequate engraftment without myeloablation and associated toxicity of total body irradiation.

High-Dose Therapy with Peripheral Blood Stem Cell Support

The low incidence of complete responses with standard-dose induction chemotherapy, even in newly diagnosed patients, suggests a marked drug resistance acquired during a prolonged subclinical course of the disease, evidenced by the presence of complex karyotypic aberrations and multiple molecular changes. This observation led to a pilot study by the late Tim McElwain and his colleagues at the Royal Marsden Hospital evaluating the role of melphalan dose escalation (140 mg/m^2). They reported complete remissions in refractory patients[13]; however, treatment-related mortality was high due to bone marrow toxicity. Bone marrow support in subsequent studies improved the treatment-related mortality; further dose escalation of melphalan to 200 mg/m^2 and addition of total body irradiation provided further improvement in response.[249]

NEWLY DIAGNOSED PATIENTS. Initial demonstration of the activity of high-dose melphalan therapy led to a series of evaluations of the role of high-dose therapy with stem cell support in myeloma. These studies reported complete remissions in up to 50% of patients, with extension of event-free survival and overall survival to more than 3 years and more than 5 to 6 years, respectively.[250–254]

The superiority of high-dose chemotherapy with autologous bone marrow support was confirmed in a randomized trial conducted by Intergroupe Français du Myélome. The response rate (50% or greater reduction in myeloma protein) in 100 patients receiving high-dose therapy (melphalan, 140 mg/m^2, plus total body irradiation) was 81% (22% complete remission) compared with 57% (5% complete remission) ($P < .001$) in a similar number of patients receiving standard-dose chemotherapy consisting of VMCP alternating with BVAP (BCNU, vincristine, doxorubicin, and prednisone). Significantly longer event-free survival (median, 28 vs. 18 months) and overall survival (median, 57 vs. 42 months) were reported after high-dose therapy (Fig. 44-11). The projected 5-year event-free and overall survival rates were 28% and 52% after high-dose therapy compared to 10% and 12% after standard-dose therapy, respectively.[255]

A similar response and survival benefit has been reported more recently from the Medical Research Council trial VII, which randomly assigned 407 patients to receive either standard-dose chemotherapy or high-dose chemotherapy with transplantation.[256] A Spanish trial involving 164 patients treated with either high-dose chemotherapy or conventional therapy also showed a superior complete response rate in the

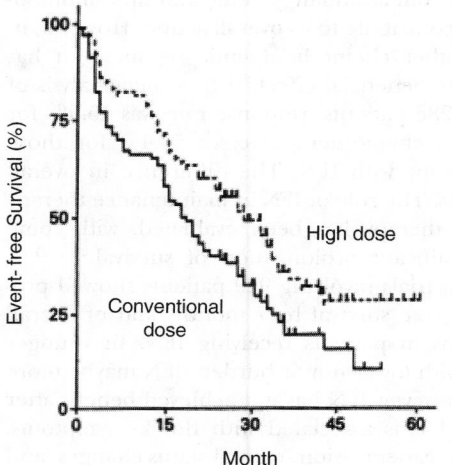
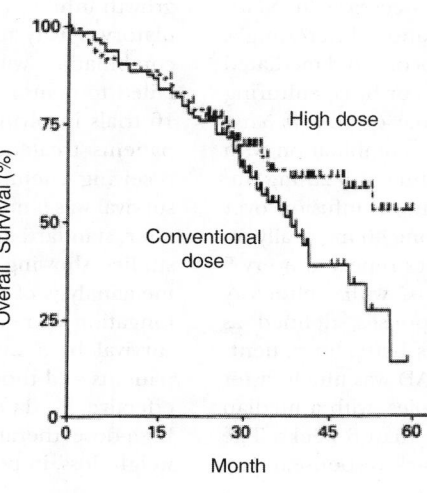

FIGURE 44-11. Comparative trials of high-dose chemotherapy (HDCT) versus standard-dose chemotherapy (SDCT). IFM-90 (Intergroupe Français de Myélome) randomized trial with 100 patients accrued to each arm comparing SDCT using vincristine, melphalan, cyclophosphamide, and prednisone (VMCP) and BCNU, vincristine, doxorubicin, and prednisone (VBAP) with high-dose chemotherapy using melphalan, 140 mg/m^2, plus total body irradiation (800 cGy). Higher complete response rates and significantly longer event-free and overall survival were noted with high-dose chemotherapy.

TABLE 44-9.   Results of Large Randomized Studies Comparing Standard-Dose Therapy with High-Dose Chemotherapy (HDCT)

Study	Regimen	No. of Patients	CR (%)	EFS (Median, Mo)	OS (Median, Mo)
Attal et al.[255]	Conventional	100	5[a]	18[a]	37[a]
	HDCT	100	22	27	52% at 60
Fermand et al.[252]	Conventional	96	—	18.7[b]	50.4[b]
	HDCT	94	—	24.3	55.3
Blade et al.[257]	Conventional	83	11[a]	34.3[b]	66.9[b]
	HDCT	81	30	42.5	67.4
Child et al.[256]	Conventional	200	8.5[a]	19.6[a]	42.3[a]
	HDCT	201	44	31.6	54.8
Barlogie et al.[244]	Conventional	252	15[b]	21[a]	53[b]
	HDCT	258	17	25	58

CR, complete response; EFS, event-free survival; OS, overall survival.
[a]Significant difference.
[b]No significant difference.

high-dose chemotherapy arm, with a trend for prolonged event-free and overall survival in the high-dose chemotherapy arm (Table 44-9).[257] In contrast, the Myélome Autogreffe group trial reported by Fermand et al. involving 190 newly diagnosed MM patients failed to show superiority of high-dose chemotherapy.[258] More recently, a U.S. intergroup study randomizing patients between high-dose chemotherapy and conventional therapy followed by delayed high-dose chemotherapy at relapse failed to show superiority of high-dose chemotherapy for either achievement of complete response or lengthening of overall survival; event-free survival benefit was modest (4 months) in the high-dose therapy group.

TANDEM TRANSPLANTS. Attempts to further improve the results of autotransplantation have included intensification with tandem transplants. Harousseau et al. were the first to report the feasibility of tandem autologous bone marrow trans-plantation, with a 69% complete response rate in a small, select group of patients.[259] Barlogie et al. investigated use of a sequential non–cross-resistant remission induction regimen followed by tandem autologous transplantations ("total therapy") in 231 newly diagnosed patients.[260] Forty-one percent of patients achieved complete response after two transplanta-tions, and the median event-free and overall survival times were 43 months and 68 months, respectively.

Attal et al. of the Intergroupe Francophone du Myélome (IFM-94) reported a randomized comparison of single high-dose chemotherapy (melphalan, 140 mg/m², and total body irradiation to 8 Gy) and double high-dose chemotherapy (melphalan, 200 mg/m², followed by melphalan, 140 mg/m², and total body irradiation to 8 Gy)[213] in 399 newly diagnosed patients. This study reports no significant differences in rates of complete response or very good partial response between the two arms (42% vs. 50%, respectively, $P = 0.10$); however,

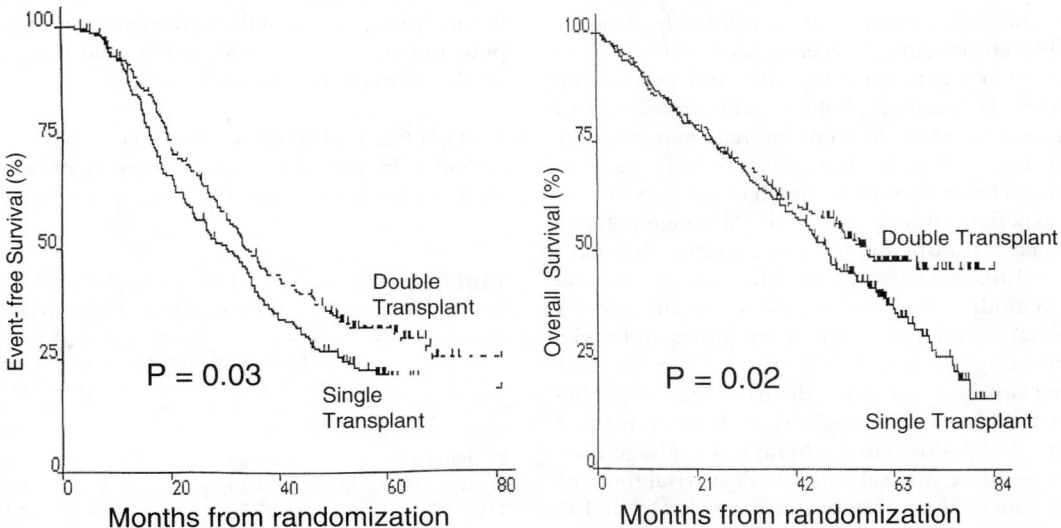

FIGURE 44-12.   Comparative trial of single versus double high-dose chemotherapy (HDCT). IFM-94 (Intergroupe Francophone du Myélome) trial with 399 patients randomized to receive single HDCT with melphalan, 140 mg/m², plus total body irradiation (800 cGy) or first HDCT with melphalan, 140 mg/m², and subsequent second HDCT with melphalan, 140 mg/m², plus total body irradiation (800 cGy). Superior event-free and overall survival were noted with double HDCT.

TABLE 44-10.   Single versus Double Intensive Therapy: Preliminary Results of Randomized Trials

Study	No. of Patients	Median Follow-Up (Mo)	Results
Dutch-Belgian Hemato-Oncology Cooperative Group[a]	261	33	Higher CR rate (28% vs. 11%)
Bologna	178	30	No difference in EFS and OS
Myélome Autogreffe group trial 95	228	40	No difference in EFS and OS
Intergroupe Francophone du Myélome trial 94[213]	399	60	Better EFS and OS with double intensive therapy

CR, complete response; EFS, event-free survival; OS, overall survival.
[a]2×70 mg/m^2 melphalan ± chemotherapy + total body irradiation + peripheral blood stem cell transplantation.

there was a significant improvement in the double high-dose chemotherapy arm in probability of event-free survival at 7 years (10% vs. 20%; $P = .03$) and estimated overall survival at 7 years (21% vs. 42%; $P = .01$) (Fig. 44-12). The Myélome Autogreffe group (n = 193), Dutch-Belgian Hemato-Oncology Cooperative Group (n = 255), and Bologna (n = 178) trials, with a median follow-up of 27 to 30 months, have not yet shown a significant benefit for tandem transplantation (Table 44-10).

Various factors need special consideration in the management of myeloma with high-dose chemotherapy. These factors include source of stem cells, conditioning regimen, timing of transplantation, and tumor cell purging.

TIMING OF HIGH-DOSE THERAPY. To obtain high-quality hematopoietic stem cells, ideal timing for stem cell collection is early in the course of the induction treatment. Ability to collect adequate stem cells (2×10^6 CD34+ cells/kg or more) in patients with less than 12 months of prior therapy is 86% compared to 48% in patients with more than 24 months of prior therapy.[261]

Multi-institutional trials demonstrating that high-dose therapy prolongs remission duration and survival but is not curative have led to the exploration question of whether high-dose chemotherapy should be used early after diagnosis rather than delayed to treat relapsed myeloma. To evaluate this important question, Fermand et al. randomly assigned 185 newly diagnosed patients to receive three or four cycles of vinblastine, doxorubicin, methotrexate, and prednisone (VAMP) followed by early high-dose chemotherapy and autotransplantation (n = 91), or conventional chemotherapy with VMCP for 1 year.[258] The latter group of patients were offered high-dose chemotherapy if they had primary refractory disease or experienced relapse (n = 94). Although patients who underwent early transplantation had significantly longer event-free survival times (39 vs. 13 months), overall survival was identical in both arms (median, 64.6 months and 64 months). Importantly, the time without symptoms and toxicity analysis reflecting quality of life (mean, 27.8 vs. 22.3 months) showed superior results for the early high-dose chemotherapy arm (Table 44-11). Vesole et al. have confirmed the effectiveness of high-dose chemotherapy as a salvage therapy, recording event-free survival and overall survival times of 21 months and longer than 43 months, respectively, in 135 patients with advanced refractory MM.[262] In this study, patients with primary unresponsive disease had better outcomes than patients with resistant relapse (progression on last salvage chemotherapy), with event-free survival of 37 versus 17 months, respectively ($P = .0004$), and overall survival of

greater than or equal to 43 versus 21 months, respectively ($P = .0003$). Gertz et al. of the Mayo Clinic have reported a similar experience for 64 patients undergoing elective delayed transplantation at the time of progression after standard therapy.[263]

The intergroup trial in the United States, which randomly assigned patients to up-front high-dose therapy or standard-dose therapy with high-dose therapy as a salvage treatment showed only modest event-free survival benefit for early transplantation.

HIGH-DOSE REGIMEN. High-dose melphalan (140 to 200 mg/m^2), with or without total body irradiation, is the most common conditioning regimen used in myeloma treatment.[214,249,262,264,265] Melphalan's predominant myelotoxicity and metabolism independent of renal function are ideal for MM patients, who commonly have renal function abnormalities. Melphalan seems to be superior to thiotepa when given with total body irradiation, with patients achieving longer relapse-free and overall survival times.[265] A combination regimen containing high-dose carboplatin with etoposide and cyclophosphamide, or a combination with cyclophosphamide, BCNU and VP-16 (CBV), has achieved only occasional responses in patients with resistant disease.[266,267] No regimen has shown marked superiority over others. The addition of total body irradiation has not been shown to improve cytoreduction and in fact increases morbidity and treatment-related mortality. A poor outcome in one study using total body irradiation was attributed to delayed immune recovery.

STEM CELL PURGING. Myeloma cell contamination as evaluated by polymerase chain reaction or sensitive immuno-fluorescence is universally observed in stem cell products. Purg-

TABLE 44-11.   Stem Cell Transplantation as Up-Front versus Rescue Treatment: Results of Randomized Trial[258]

	Early Transplantation (n = 91)	Late Transplantation (n = 94)
CR	19%	5%[a]
Median EFS	39 mo	13 mo[a]
Median OS	64.6 mo	64 mo
TWISTT	27.8 mo	22.3 mo

CR, complete response; EFS, event-free survival; OS, overall survival; TWISTT, time without symptoms, treatment, and treatment toxicity.
Note: Median follow-up, 58 mo.
[a]Significant difference.

ing of tumor cells by positive selection of CD34+ cells leads to a 3 to 5 log unit reduction in contamination.[268,269] Negative selection using the monoclonal antibody cocktail containing CD10 (common acute lymphoblastic leukemia antigen), CD20 (a pan B-cell antigen), and plasma cell–associated antigen-1 or peanut agglutinin and anti-CD19 antibodies results in undetectable levels of myeloma cells by conventional flow cytometry.[253] The early follow-up results from these studies have not revealed any significant advantage in responses or survival, but they consistently show a delay in engraftment after transplantation. A multicenter, randomized study comparing CD34-selected PBSCs versus unselected PBSCs in 131 patients failed to show any significant difference in event-free survival or overall survival time.[270] Even when cells were purged using fluorescence-activated cell sorting of very early hematopoietic stem cells (CD34+,Thy1+, Lin–), relapses were frequent and patients had delayed hematopoietic engraftment and suppressed immune status for prolonged periods of time.[271,272] Because of these data, emphasis is now on strategies to improve responses to high-dose chemotherapy, rather than on purging of autografts.

HEMATOPOIETIC STEM CELL SOURCE. Mobilized PBSCs provide more rapid engraftment than bone marrow stem cells. Myeloma patients with less than 1 year of prior therapy had faster granulocyte and platelet recovery after PBSC transplantation than after bone marrow autografting.[273] The duration of prior chemotherapy, especially with stem cell–damaging agents (melphalan, BCNU, and high doses of cyclophosphamide), along with radiation to bone marrow–containing areas, significantly affects the ability to procure adequate quantities of PBSCs as well as engraftment kinetics after transplantation.[274] After treatment with cyclophosphamide and granulocyte-macrophage colony-stimulating factor, normal PBSCs are mobilized during the first 3 days of leukapheresis, whereas peak levels of contaminating myeloma cells are present on subsequent days. These myeloma cells show a higher labeling index and a more immature phenotype (CD19+).[275]

Management of Older Patients

Because the incidence of myeloma increases with age, the role of high-dose chemotherapy has been evaluated in patients older than 65 years of age. Older age does not impact stem cell mobilization or engraftment.[219] The feasibility and efficacy of high-dose chemotherapy with PBSC transplantation have been evaluated in 70 patients, 70 years or older (median age, 72 years; range, 70 to 83 years) treated with melphalan (200 mg/m² or 140 mg/m²).[276] Of note, treatment-related mortality was higher (16%) among the initial 25 patients receiving melphalan at 200 mg/m². Complete response was achieved in 27% of patients, but median complete response duration was only 1.5 years, with 3-year event-free survival and overall survival rates projected at 20% and 31%, respectively. Although this study confirms the feasibility of high-dose chemotherapy in older patients with MM, it also indicates a higher risk in this patient population, highlighting the need for strict patient selection based on clinical status.

Management of Patients with Renal Dysfunction

One-third of patients with overt MM present with renal insufficiency. With hydration, control of hypercalcemia, and effective therapy, it is reversible in 50% of cases. Renal dysfunction of less than 6 months' duration and rapid initiation of therapy with reduction in monoclonal protein levels are associated with higher likelihood of improvement in renal function. Improved renal function is observed mainly in patients with light-chain cast nephropathy and light-chain deposition disease; therefore, renal biopsy is used to identify these reversible conditions and the need for aggressive treatment. Because the pharmacokinetics of melphalan are unaltered by renal failure, such patients are potentially candidates for high-dose therapy.[277] Based on this observation, high-dose melphalan and PBSC transplantation were used to treat 81 patients with MM and renal dysfunction (creatinine level higher than 2 mg/dL).[278] In this setting, renal failure had no impact on the quality of stem cell collection and engraftment. However, treatment-related mortality rates were 6% and 13% after the first and second autologous stem cell transplantations, respectively, and melphalan at 200 mg/m² caused excessive toxicity. Complete remission was achieved in 31 patients (38%) after tandem stem cell transplantations, and the probabilities of event-free survival and overall survival to 3 years were 48% and 55%, respectively. Dose reduction and close monitoring are therefore needed to ensure the safety of the procedure, and the role of transplantation in the setting of renal failure remains investigational.

Importantly, novel therapies have provided alternative strategies for treatment of myeloma in the setting of renal failure. Thalidomide, bortezomib, and arsenic trioxide all have been evaluated in this setting. Ease of administration, limited toxicity, and effectiveness make these the primary modes of therapy for myeloma patients with renal failure.

Maintenance Therapy

Despite improvements in remission rates, there is no clear plateau in the survival curves after conventional or high-dose chemotherapy. Although the proportion of patients achieving complete response has increased, all patients eventually experience relapse. Various maintenance therapies have been evaluated in MM in an effort to sustain remission. IFN-α is the most widely evaluated agent as maintenance therapy; however, randomized studies have demonstrated only modest improvements in event-free survival and overall survival times (5 to 12 months) in patients achieving remission with standard-dose therapy, and its role after high-dose chemotherapy has not been confirmed.[279] Low-dose prednisone administered on alternate days prolonged remission duration after standard-dose therapy in a single randomized study.[280] Thalidomide and its analogue immunomodulatory drug 3 (IMiD3), with and without added dexamethasone; bisphosphonates; and immune manipulations such as idiotype vaccination and protein-pulsed dendritic cell-based vaccination are all strategies under evaluation as maintenance treatments to prolong event-free survival and overall survival in myeloma.

Allogeneic Transplantation

SYNGENEIC TRANSPLANTATION. Bensinger et al. have reported their experience with 11 patients receiving syngeneic transplants: 5 patients achieved complete response and three achieved partial response. The 1996 update showed one patient from each group alive 9 and 15 years after transplantation,

TABLE 44-12. Studies of Allogeneic Transplantation for Newly Diagnosed Myeloma

Study	No. of Patients	TRM (%)	CR (%)	OS (Actuarial)	EFS (Actuarial)
Gahrton et al.[135]	162	41	44	28% at 84 mo	45% at 60 mo
Bensinger et al.[139]	80	44	36	20% at 54 mo	24% at 54 mo
Alyea et al.[284]	61[a]	5	28	40% at 36 mo	20% at 38 mo

CR, complete response; EFS, event-free survival; OS, overall survival; TRM, treatment-related mortality.
[a]T-cell depleted.

respectively.[281] A larger experience from the European Bone Marrow Transplant Registry was reviewed by Gahrton et al. Twenty-five patients undergoing syngeneic transplants were compared with 125 case-matched patients undergoing autotransplantation or allogeneic transplantation.[282] The complete remission rate was not significantly different between the three graft groups (twin, 68%; autologous, 48%; allogeneic, 58%). However, patients undergoing syngeneic transplantation had significantly superior median survival time compared with those receiving autologous transplants (72 vs. 25 months; P = .009) and allogeneic transplants (72 vs. 16 months; P = .008).

ALLOGENEIC TRANSPLANTATION. Allogeneic transplantation has remained a difficult procedure in myeloma. An older population with limited donor availability, coupled with frequent renal impairment, has restricted the use of matched-sibling transplantation in MM. In addition, the almost 50% 1-year mortality has limited the use of this procedure to only a high-risk patient population. Importantly, the allogeneic graft–versus–myeloma effect may result in a favorable long-term outcome after allogeneic transplantation. Results of three large studies are listed in Table 44-12. A retrospective analysis of case-matched European Bone Marrow Transplant Registry data compared outcomes for 189 patients receiving allografts and an equal number of patients from the same time period receiving autotransplants. This study showed a superior median survival for patients undergoing autotransplantation compared to those undergoing allogeneic transplantation (34 vs. 18 months, respectively).[283] The 1-year treatment-related mortality was significantly higher after allogeneic transplantation (41% for allotransplantation and 13% for autotransplantation). However, patients undergoing allogeneic transplantation and surviving the first year showed a tendency toward better progression-free survival and overall survival.

A very low transplant-related mortality of 10% has been reported in a single-center study at the Dana-Farber Cancer Institute in which selective depletion of CD6+ T cells was the sole form of prophylaxis for graft-versus-host disease (GVHD).[284] However, the median progression-free survival time was 12 months, and the median overall survival time was 22 months, a result inferior to that institute's previous experience in autologous transplantation. Case-matched comparative studies at other single institutions have also failed to show a survival advantage for allotransplantation.[285]

DONOR LYMPHOCYTE INFUSIONS. A graft-versus-myeloma effect has been demonstrated by the induction of complete response with donor lymphocyte infusion (DLI) at relapse after allogeneic transplantation.[286] In a large study, Lokhorst et al. reported six complete response and eight partial response after

DLI in 27 patients after allotransplantation.[287] Five of these patients remained disease free more than 30 months after DLI. However, DLI was associated with acute GVHD in 55% of patients and chronic GVHD in 26% of patients. Five patients experienced bone marrow aplasia, which was fatal in two cases. A similar DLI experience has been reported by Salama et al.[288] Several strategies have been explored to reduce GVHD after DLI,[289,290] including lowering the number of T cells infused, selectively depleting CD8+ T cells, and using herpes simplex virus thymidine kinase gene transduction of DLI to allow for administration of ganciclovir to deplete T cells if significant GVHD develops. Immunizing donors with idiotype vaccine may allow selective transfer of T cells specific for graft-versus-myeloma without increasing the incidence of GVHD.

NONMYELOABLATIVE TRANSPLANTATION. Studies in a canine model showed that a nonmyeloablative dose of total body irradiation could lead to successful engraftment when used in conjunction with a combination of cyclosporine and mycophenolate mofetil.[291] This animal experience, coupled with reduced day 100 transplant-related mortality in pilot studies in patients, has allowed for matched-sibling allogeneic transplantation in patients who were otherwise considered poor risks for the standard allogeneic preparative regimen. Results from three large studies are listed in Table 44-13. Badros et al. first reported on 31 patients undergoing allogeneic transplantation after nonmyeloablative conditioning with melphalan (100 mg/m²). Transplant-related mortality in the first 120 days was low (10%). Nineteen patients (61%) achieved complete response or near-complete response; however, acute GVHD developed in 18 patients (58%) and chronic GVHD was seen in 10 patients (35%).[292] Giralt et al. used reduced-intensity conditioning with fludarabine and melphalan in 16 patients. Successful engraftment was observed in all patients; however, the 100-day mortality rate was 20% and the 1-year mortality rate was 40%, with only six patients alive after a median follow-up period of 15 months.[293]

Maloney et al. have evaluated the combination of initial autotransplantation for tumor cytoreduction followed by nonmyeloablative matched-sibling allogeneic transplantation in 54 patients.[294] The treatment was performed in an outpatient setting with a low 100-day mortality (2%). The overall response rate was 83%, with 53% complete responses. At a median follow-up of 552 days after allografting, overall survival was 78%. However, GVHD continued to be a problem; 38% of patients developed acute GVHD and 46% developed chronic GVHD requiring therapy.

Although the early clinical results with nonmyeloablative transplantation are encouraging, this strategy is associated with significant morbidity due to acute and chronic GVHD and a

TABLE 44-13.   Representative Studies of Mini-Allogeneic Transplantation in Myeloma

Study	Conditioning	No of Patients	TRM (%)	Response (%)	Acute GVHD (%)	Chronic GVHD (%)	PFS	OS
Badros et al.[292]	Mel or Mel/TBI/Flu	31	10 (early) 20 (late)	CR 61 PR 10	58	32	1 y: 86%	1 y: 86%
Kroger et al.[155]	PBSCT + Mel/Flu/ATG	17	18	CR 73 PR 20	63	40	2 y: 56%	2 y: 74%
Maloney et al.[294]	PBSCT + TBI/MMF/cyc	31	16	CR 43 PR 31	45	55	—	1 y: 81%

ATG, antithymocyte globulin; CR, complete response; cyc, cyclosporin; EFS, event-free survival; Flu, fludarabine; GVHD, graft-versus-host disease; Mel, melphalan; MMF, mycophenolic acetate; OS, overall survival; PBSCT, peripheral blood stem cell transplantation; PFS, progression-free survival; PR, partial response; TBI, total body irradiation; TRM, treatment-related mortality.

mortality rate of 20% at 1 year. It should therefore be used only in the context of clinical trials attempting to improve patient outcome by both enhancing efficacy and reducing toxicity.

Novel Biologically Based Agents

Despite improvements in complete responses and prolongation of overall and event-free survival, myeloma remains an incurable disease in the majority of patients. Novel treatment approaches specifically targeting the mechanisms whereby myeloma cells grow and survive in the bone marrow can overcome resistance to standard-dose and high-dose therapies and thereby offer great potential to improve patient outcomes.

Myeloma cells adhere to the extracellular matrix and to BMSCs, which promotes proliferation, survival, drug resistance, and migration. These effects are partially mediated through various cytokines, including IL-6, VEGF, TNF-α, and IGF-1. The growth, survival, drug resistance, and migration are mediated via the RAS/RAF MAPK, JAK/STAT, PI3K/AKT, and protein kinase C signaling cascades, respectively. Novel therapies not only directly target myeloma cells but also target the bone marrow microenvironment.

THALIDOMIDE. The rationale for the use of thalidomide in myeloma was its known antiangiogenic activity, coupled with reports of increased angiogenesis in MM bone marrow. Studies during the last several years have confirmed the efficacy of thalidomide in refractory relapsed MM. A phase II study involving 169 such patients investigated the use of thalidomide in incremental doses of 200 to 800 mg. In this group of patients with advanced posttransplantation-relapsed myeloma, a partial response was attained in 26% patients, with an overall response rate of 34%.[295,296] Subsequently, the efficacy of thalidomide has been confirmed in several phase II studies (Table 44-14).[160,167,172,235] The major toxicities of thalidomide are somnolence, constipation, neurologic symptoms, fatigue, and deep venous thrombosis. Based on *in vitro* results showing synergism as well as reversal of resistance, thalidomide has been combined with dexamethasone. This combination has achieved response rates of more than 50% in relapsed patients and 70% in newly diagnosed patients (Table 44-15).[236,242,296a,296b] Studies confirm that thalidomide and its more potent IMiD analogues not only act to inhibit angiogenesis but also act directly on MM cells. In addition, they abrogate the adhesion of MM cells to BMSCs and block the secretion of MM growth and survival factors such as IL-

6, TNF-α, VEGF, and fibroblast growth factor, which are triggered by the binding of MM cells to BMSCs (Fig. 44-13). These agents also induce immune responses by expanding the number and function of natural killer cells and provide T-cell costimulatory signals through the B7-CD28 pathway.[297] A derived phase I clinical trial of IMiD3 (CC 5013) has shown at least a 25% reduction in paraprotein levels (minimal response) in 15 of 24 patients (63%), including 11 patients who had received prior thalidomide therapy. Stable disease (less than 25% reduction in paraprotein) was observed in an additional 2 patients (8%).[297a] Therefore, 17 of 24 patients (71%) demonstrated benefit from treatment. Importantly, no significant somnolence, constipation, or neuropathy was seen in this study. However, myelosuppression was the dose-limiting toxicity observed at the highest dose level. These results therefore provide the basis for the evaluation of CC 5013, either alone or in combination, to treat patients with MM at earlier stages of disease. A phase II trial of CC 5013 in patients with relapsed or refractory MM achieved a 10% complete response rate, 25% partial response rate, and 40% stable disease rate, without attendant somnolence, constipation, or neuropathy. Formal evaluation of thalidomide or CC 5013, alone or with dexamethasone, for treatment of newly diagnosed patients and as maintenance therapy is ongoing.

BORTEZOMIB. Bortezomib is the prototype proteasome inhibitor. MM cell adhesion to BMSCs triggers the transcription and secretion of IL-6 in BMSCs via an NFκB-dependent mechanism, and bortezomib was originally used in MM due to its blockade of NFκB activation and related paracrine IL-6 production in BMSCs. Bortezomib also acts directly on MM

TABLE 44-14.   Thalidomide Salvage Therapy for Multiple Myeloma

Study	No. of Patients	Dose (mg/d)	Response Rate (%)
Barlogie et al.[295]	169	200–800	32[a]
Yakoub-Agha et al.[160]	83	50–800	46
Kumar et al.[167]	32	200–800	31
Durie et al.[172]	33	50–400	24

[a]Two-year event-free survival and overall survival rates of 20% and 48%, respectively.

TABLE 44-15. Results of Combination Chemotherapy with Thalidomide Plus Dexamethasone in Relapsed and Newly Diagnosed Multiple Myeloma

Study	Patient Population	No. of Patients	Therapy and Dosing	Response Rate (%)
Palumbo et al.[236]	Relapsed	120	100 mg/d T + 40 mg D	52
Dimopoulos et al.[242]	Refractory	44	200–400 mg/d T + 20 mg/m² D	55
Weber et al.[296a]	Newly diagnosed	40	200–800 mg/d T + 20 mg D	72
Rajkumar et al.[296b]	Newly diagnosed	50	200–400 mg/d T + 40 mg D	64

D, dexamethasone; T, thalidomide.

cells to induce apoptosis, even of tumor cells resistant to known conventional therapeutic agents.[297b] It overcomes the protective effects of IL-6 and adds to the anti-MM effects of dexamethasone. Importantly, it acts in the microenvironment to inhibit the binding of MM cells to BMSCs, the transcription and secretion of IL-6 and other cytokines triggered by MM to BMSC adhesion, and bone marrow angiogenesis.[297c] Based on exciting results in an animal model and a confirmed safety profile in a phase I study that in fact showed responses in myeloma patients, a multicenter phase II trial of bortezomib in MM was completed in 2002. Two hundred and two patients with refractory relapsed MM were treated with 1.3 mg/m² of bortezomib twice weekly for 2 weeks, followed by 1 week without treatment, for up to eight cycles (24 weeks). Dexamethasone (20 mg by mouth daily) was added to the regimen in patients with a suboptimal response.[297d] Of 193 heavily pretreated evaluable patients, 35% showed a response, including 7 patients in whom myeloma protein became undetectable and 12 patients in whom myeloma protein was detectable only by immunofixation. The median duration of response was 12 months, and the median overall survival was 16 months. Grade 3 adverse events included thrombocytopenia (28%), fatigue (12%), peripheral neuropathy (12%), and neutropenia (11%). Based on this study confirming bortezomib as an active agent in patients with relapsed and refractory MM, the U.S. Food and Drug Administration approved the drug for clinical use. Addition of dexamethasone in this study improved responses in 19% patients, which confirmed synergism between these two agents. A randomized study comparing bortezomib with dexamethasone in treatment of relapsed myeloma was prematurely closed due to superior results with bortezomib. Evaluation of this agent in treatment of newly diagnosed patients and in combination with other agents is under way.[297e]

ARSENIC TRIOXIDE. Arsenic trioxide is another commercially available agent that targets both the MM cell and its microenvironment.[297f] At a clinically achievable level, it induces apoptosis of drug-resistant MM cell lines and patient cells via activation of caspase 9. Arsenic trioxide also decreases binding of MM cells to BMSCs and inhibits secretion of IL-6 and VEGF induced by adhesion of MM to BMSCs. It also inhibits telomerase and induces immune effects. A phase I clinical study of arsenic trioxide showed at least a minimal response in 3 of 14 patients with refractory relapsed disease.[297g] An additive effect of arsenic trioxide with dexamethasone and ascorbic acid has been observed *in vitro*.[297h] Based on these results, an on-going phase I and II study is evaluating the safety and efficacy of arsenic trioxide in combination with

dexamethasone and ascorbic acid in patients with relapsed MM. The most common toxicities include myelosuppression, neuropathy, and Q-T prolongation.

BISPHOSPHONATES. The second- and third-generation bisphosphonates pamidronate and zoledronate reduce skeletal complications and bone pain in myeloma (Table 44-16).[298,299] Their mechanism of action includes down-regulation of osteoclast activity, decreased IL-6 production, activation of γ/δ T cells with antimyeloma activity, and induction of apoptosis of osteoclasts through inhibition of farnesyl and geranyl-geranyl transferase activity.[300,301] In addition to reducing bone-related problems, continued administration of pamidronate over 21 months conferred some survival advantage to patients receiving salvage chemotherapy and pamidronate compared with those receiving chemotherapy alone (21 vs. 14 months; $P = .041$).[298,302] *In vitro* cytotoxic effects of bisphosphonates have been observed in myeloma cell lines,[303,304] patient cells *in vitro*, and tumor specimens in the SCID-hu *in vivo* model. Preliminary reports of frequent administration of pamidronate alone (every 2 weeks) have shown response or delay in disease progression in occasional patients.[305] Pamidronate, 90 mg, and zoledronic acid, 4 mg, are equipotent in reducing bone-related problems in myeloma. Infusion time for zoledronic acid is 15

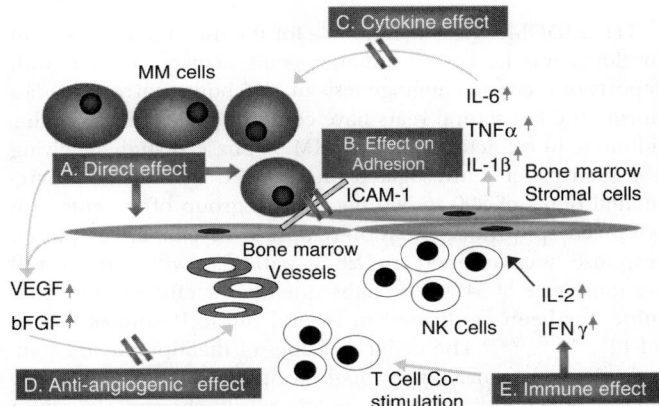

FIGURE 44-13. Potential mechanisms of action of thalidomide and its analogues. **A:** Direct effect on the multiple myeloma (MM) cells. **B:** Inhibition of MM cell–blood marrow stromal cell (BMSC) adhesion. **C:** Inhibition of cytokine production in the microenvironment. **D:** Antiangiogenic effects through inhibition of the proangiogenic cytokines. **E:** Modulation of immune function, especially natural killer (NK) cells and T cells. bFGF, basic fibroblast growth factor; ICAM, intracellular adhesion molecule; IFN, interferon; IL, interleukin; TNFα, tumor necrosis factor-α; VEGF, vascular endothelial growth factor. (See Color Fig. 44-13 in the CD-ROM.)

TABLE 44-16. Summary of Published Placebo-Controlled Trials of Bisphosphonates in Patients with Multiple Myeloma

	Belch et al.[a]	*Lahtinen et al.*[b]	*Berenson et al.*[298]
Number of evaluable patients	166	336	377
Bisphosphonate therapy	Etidronate, 5 mg/kg daily (oral)	Clodronate, 2.4 g/d (oral) for 24 mo	Pamidronate, 90 mg (IV q4wk × 9 cycles)
Lytic bone lesions	0	+	0
Pathologic fractures	0	0	+
Radiation therapy	NA	NA	+
Bone pain	0	0	+
Hypercalcemia	0	0	+
Survival	–	0	+

0, no effect; +, beneficial effect; –, harmful effect; NA, not assessed.
[a]Belch A, Shelley W, Bergsagel Q, et al. A randomized trial of maintenance versus no maintenance melphalan and prednisone in responding multiple myeloma patients. *Br J Cancer* 1988;57:94.
[b]Lahtinen R, Laakso M, Palva I, Virkkunen P, Elomaa I. Randomized, placebo-controlled multicentre trial of clodronate in multiple myeloma. Finnish Leukaemia Group [published erratum appears in *Lancet* 1992;340:1420]. *Lancet* 1992;340:1049.

minutes compared to 1 to 2 hours for pamidronate. Patients on long-term bisphosphonate therapy should be monitored for development of renal toxicity.

OTHER POTENTIAL AGENTS AND FUTURE DIRECTIONS. Both *in vitro* systems and *in vivo* animal models have been developed to characterize mechanisms of MM cell homing to bone marrow, as well as factors such as MM cell–BMSC interactions, cytokines, and angiogenesis that promote MM cell growth, survival, drug resistance, and migration in the bone marrow milieu. These model systems have allowed the development of several promising biologically based therapies that can target the MM cell and the bone marrow microenvironment, including thalidomide and revlimid, bortezomib, VEGF receptor tyrosine kinase inhibitor PTK787, histone deacetylase (HDAC) inhibitors suberoylanilide hydroxamic acid (SAHA) and LAQ 824, 2 methoxyestradiol, arsenic trioxide, and lysophosphatidic acid acyltransferase-beta (LPAAT) inhibitor; that can target MM cells directly, including telomerase inhibitor GRN 163, heat-shock protein 90 inhibitor 17 AAG, TNF-related apoptosis-inducing ligand, statins, IGF-1 receptor inhibitor; and that can target only the bone marrow microenvironment, including IκB kinase inhibitors and P38MAPK inhibitors (Fig. 44-14). It is the authors' hypothesis that drugs in these classes will need to be combined to achieve complete eradication of MM cells, and the authors are presently studying their mechanisms of action at the gene and protein level to provide the framework for their rational combination in clinical trials to overcome drug resistance and improve patient outcome.

Proteomic and genomic studies are now providing the preclinical rationale for molecularly based combination therapy. For example, these studies have defined the preclinical rationale for combining bortezomib with conventional DNA-damaging agents and with stress response (heat-shock protein-90) inhibitors. Ultimately it may be possible to carry out gene and protein profiling, both to select cocktails of targeted therapies for specific patients and to define targets of sensitivity and resistance to develop next-generation, more potent, and less toxic therapies.

WALDENSTRÖM'S MACROGLOBULINEMIA

Dr. Jan Waldenström first described a condition in two patients characterized by bleeding tendencies in mucosa, anemia, lymphadenopathy, and high serum viscosity with high-molecular-mass M component.[306] WM is characterized by excess lymphoplasmacytic cells and differs from myeloma in various aspects, including absence of lytic bone disease and presence of hepatosplenomegaly or lymphadenopathy or both.

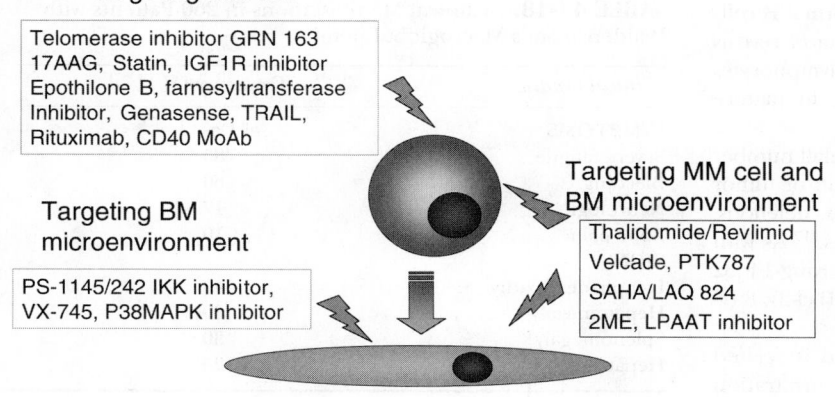

Targeting MM cell

Telomerase inhibitor GRN 163
17AAG, Statin, IGF1R inhibitor
Epothilone B, farnesyltransferase
Inhibitor, Genasense, TRAIL,
Rituximab, CD40 MoAb

Targeting BM microenvironment

PS-1145/242 IKK inhibitor,
VX-745, P38MAPK inhibitor

Targeting MM cell and BM microenvironment

Thalidomide/Revlimid
Velcade, PTK787
SAHA/LAQ 824
2ME, LPAAT inhibitor

FIGURE 44-14. Novel therapies in preclinical or clinical development targeting the multiple myeloma (MM) cells or their microenvironment, or both. BM, bone marrow; IGF1R, insulin-like growth factor-1 receptor; IKK, IκB kinase; LPAAT, lysophosphatidic acid acyltransferase-beta; SAHA, suberoylanilide hydroxamic acid; TRAIL, tumor necrosis factor–related apoptosis-inducing ligand. (See Color Fig. 44-14 in the CD-ROM.)

TABLE 44-17. Immunophenotype of Waldenström's Cells

Surface Molecule	Peripheral Blood B Cells	Chronic Lymphocytic Leukemia	Waldenström's Macroglobulinemia	Multiple Myeloma
sIg	++	+	+	0
cIg	0	0	+	++
CD5	0	++	±	0
CD10	0	0	±	+
CD19	++	++	+	0/+
CD20	++	+	++	0/+
CD21	++	++	+	0
CD22	++	+	++	0
CD23	++	++	0	0
CD38	0	0	+	++
PCA1	0	0	+	++

cIg, cytoplasmic immunoglobulin; sIg, surface immunoglobulin; +, positive; ++, strongly positive; ±, variable; 0, negative.

Macroglobulinemia is less frequent than myeloma, with approximately 1500 new cases annually in the United States. Its incidence is higher in males and in whites than in African Americans. The median age at diagnosis is 63 years.[307] Familial occurrence and a case of WM in monozygotic twins have been reported.[308,309] Interestingly, a patient working with canaries developed macroglobulinemia, and the monoclonal serum IgM reacted with an antigen in canary droppings, which suggests a role for constant antigenic stimulation in the pathogenesis.[310] The low prevalence of the disease has limited detailed epidemiologic and pathogenetic studies. Like myeloma, WM cells are postantigen selected memory B cells, with somatic hypermutation and rearrangement in the variable region and unique complimetarity determining region. In contrast to normal B cells, which produce IgM as a primary immune response and with further antigenic stimulation and selection undergo class switching to produce IgG, WM cells are arrested before class switching and produce IgM. No clonal diversity is observed and no isotype switching is reported.

Viral infections with hepatitis C virus appear to be a significant risk factor for development of cryoglobulinemia, which is often associated with WM. The role of infection with Kaposi's sarcoma–associated herpesvirus, identified in bone marrow dendritic cells from patients with WM, and of hepatitis G virus infection in pathogenesis is undefined.[311–313] Phenotypically the malignant cells are surface and cytoplasmic Ig-positive cells expressing pan B-cell markers, including CD19, CD20, and CD22. CD5 and CD23 are expressed in small number of cases. The immunophenotypic differences among cells in MM, WM, and CLL and normal B cells are shown in Table 44-17.[314] Bone marrow examination reveals monotypic cells ranging from small lymphocytes, to lymphocytes with varying levels of plasmacytoid differentiation, to mature plasma cells with mast cells and Dutcher bodies.

Chromosomal changes have been reported in a small number of patients with WM, mainly due to low proliferation of tumor cells. Complex karyotypic changes include trisomies, deletions, and structural abnormalities of various chromosomes.[315] As with myeloma and other B-cell tumors, translocations involving 14q32 are reported with various partners: chromosomes 18 (bcl-2), 8 (c-myc), 11 (PRAD-1), and 9 (PAX-5).[316,317]

The clinical presentation of WM is variable and is related both to high IgM levels and lymphoplasmacytic cell infiltration of various organs.[318] Manifestations related to tissue infiltration include cough and dyspnea, diarrhea and gastrointestinal bleeding, skin plaques, periorbital exophthalmos, and nerve palsies. The large molecular size of IgM leads to higher serum viscosity than is observed with comparable levels of IgG or IgA. Hyperviscosity is rarely seen with IgG or IgA levels of less than 5 g/dL, whereas IgM levels above 3 g/dL lead to clinical manifestations. Relative plasma viscosity above 5 cP is usually associated with symptoms. Hyperviscosity may present with fatigue, blurred vision, headache, shortness of breath, mucosal bleeding, and mental status changes or coma. Type I cryoglobulinemia due to physicochemical interactions with the paraprotein is observed in a small number of patients, who present with purpura, urticaria, Raynaud's phenomenon, acrocyanosis, malleolar ulcers, or necrosis.[319] Cryoglobulinemia type II due to antibody reactivity causes arthralgias, proteinuria, renal failure, polyneuropathy, and mononeuritis.[314,320] Additional presenting features may be related to the presence of cold agglutinins, which leads to a mild hemolytic anemia or exacerbation of Raynaud's phenomenon. Severe demyelinating sensorimotor neuropathies are observed in 10% of patients, one-half of whom have detectable antibodies against myelin-associated glycoprotein (anti-MAG antibodies).[321–323] Sensory or ataxic neuropathy is observed more commonly in patients with anti-MAG antibodies. The frequencies of common presenting features are listed in Table 44-18.

TABLE 44-18. Clinical Manifestations in 260 Patients with Waldenström's Macroglobulinemia

Clinical Findings	Frequency (%)
SYMPTOMS	
Severe fatigue	85
Bleeding	60
Neurologic	17
Bone pain	10
SIGNS	
Lymphadenopathy	40
Hepatomegaly	30
Splenomegaly	30
Hepatosplenomegaly	25

TABLE 44-19. Waldenström's Macroglobulinemia: Proposed Diagnostic Criteria

- Immunoglobulin M monoclonal gammopathy of any concentration
- Bone marrow infiltration by small lymphocytes showing plasmacytoid and plasma cell differentiation
- Intertrabecular pattern of bone marrow infiltration
- Immunophenotype of surface immunoglobulin M+ CD5± CD10– CD19+ CD20+ CD22+ CD23– CD25+ CD27+ FMC7+ CD103– CD138–[a]

[a]Variations from this immunophenotypic profile can occur. In these instances, however, care should be taken to satisfactorily exclude other lymphoproliferative disorders. This is most relevant in CD5+ cases, in which chronic lymphocytic leukemia and mantle cell lymphoma require specific exclusion before a diagnosis of Waldenström's macroglobulinemia can be made.

Laboratory evaluation usually shows anemia; however, leukopenia and thrombocytopenia are uncommon in untreated patients. Elevated erythrocyte sedimentation rate, monoclonal IgM protein in serum with occasional light chains in the urine, and elevated β_2M levels may be present. Bone marrow shows typical lymphoplasmacytic infiltration, with the presence of mast cells. CT evaluation of chest, abdomen, and pelvis may show lymphadenopathy, with enlargement of liver or spleen or both. A skeletal survey is performed to rule out IgM myeloma; bone lesions are not seen in WM. Specialized testing may be required, depending on clinical findings or involvement of other organs. For example, tissue infiltration may require confirmation with biopsy. The diagnostic criteria proposed by a consensus panel are listed in Table 44-19.

Patients who are asymptomatic may not require immediate cytoreductive therapy, because early therapy does not alter the outcome. Patients with preserved hemoglobin and low β_2M levels are ideal candidates for observation. Clear criteria were proposed by the consensus panel at the second international workshop on WM to distinguish patients with symptomatic WM who require therapy from those with asymptomatic WM and IgM MGUS (Table 44-20). Patients with high IgM-related symptoms due to hyperviscosity, hemolytic anemia, neuropathy, and cryoglobulinemia may benefit from plasmapheresis without conventional chemotherapy.[324–326]

Patients who are symptomatic from the disease or have marked hepatosplenomegaly, cytopenia, or progressive disease require treatment. Chlorambucil alone or combined with steroids achieves response, defined as a greater than 50% decrease in paraprotein levels and tumor mass, in 60% to 75% of previously untreated patients; however, complete responses are observed in fewer than 5% of patients.[327] Responses are gradual, and peak response may not occur for 12 to 18 months. Treatment is continued until maximal reduction is observed. Median survival after diagnosis is more than 10 years. More aggressive combination therapy with multiple agents has achieved response rates of more than 80%; however, there is no associated improvement in overall survival. Importantly, prolonged therapy with alkylating agent has lead to development of myelodysplastic syndrome or acute myeloid leukemia in up to 10% of patients.

The purine analogues fludarabine at a dose of 25 mg/m² intravenously for 5 days every 4 weeks and cladribine at a dose of 0.1 mg/kg by continuous infusion for 7 days have produced responses in up to 80% of previously untreated patients, with complete responses in 10% of patients. The effectiveness of purine analogue therapy in previously treated patients has been in the range of 30%, with higher responses in patients relapsing after cessation of prior therapy and less frequent responses in patients with resistant relapse.[328–331] Patients experiencing relapse after receiving one purine analogue do not usually respond to another purine analogue. In a large prospective multicenter study of the Southwest Oncology Group involving newly diagnosed patients, however, fludarabine showed a response rate of only 39%.[332] Younger patients are found to respond better than older patient populations. Anemia, β_2M level above 2.5 mg/dL, and IgM level above 4 g/dL were predicative of poor outcome in that study. The major side effects of purine analogues are prolonged cumulative cytopenia and immunosuppression leading to infection with opportunistic organisms. Nonchemotherapeutic treatment options include rituxan (anti-CD20 monoclonal antibody), which achieved a

TABLE 44-20. Classification of Waldenström's Macroglobulinemia and Related Disorders

	IgM monoclonal protein[a]	BM infiltration[b]	Symptoms Attributable to IgM	Symptoms Attributable to Tumor Infiltration[c]
WM symptomatic	+	+	+	+
WM asymptomatic	+	+	–	–
IgM-related disorders[d]	+	–	+	–
MGUS	+	–	–	–

BM, bone marrow; IgM, immunoglobulin M; MGUS, monoclonal gammopathy of unknown significance; WM, Waldenström's macroglobulinemia; +, positive; –, negative.
[a]The consensus panel considered it to be inappropriate to define an IgM concentration to distinguish MGUS from WM. However, it is important to note that the IgM concentration rarely if ever exceeds 3 g/dL in MGUS.
[b]Patients with unequivocal bone marrow infiltration by lymphoplasmacytic lymphoma are considered to have WM, whereas patients without evidence of infiltration are considered to have MGUS. However, it is acknowledged that in some patients equivocal evidence of bone marrow infiltration is demonstrable. This may be manifest in a number of ways and includes the detection of clonal B cells by flow cytometry or polymerase chain reaction in the absence of morphologic evidence of bone marrow infiltration. Alternatively, patients may have equivocal bone marrow infiltrates without confirmatory phenotypic studies. It is considered that these patients should be classified as having MGUS until further data become available.
[c]Symptoms attributable to tumor infiltration include any of the following: constitutional symptoms, cytopenia(s), and organomegaly.
[d]It is well recognized that a population of patients exists who have symptoms attributable to the IgM monoclonal protein but no overt evidence of lymphoma. Such patients may present with symptomatic cryoglobulinemia, amyloidosis, or autoimmune phenomena such as peripheral neuropathy and cold agglutinin disease. It is appropriate to consider these patients as a clinically distinct group, and the term *IgM-related disorders* is proposed.

20% to 30% response rate in small studies,[314] and IFN-α, which showed a 30% response rate.[333,334] High-dose dexamethasone pulsing has produced some responses in patients with refractory disease.[335,336] There have been reports of occasional responses after splenectomy.[337,338] The role of high-dose chemotherapy has been evaluated in six patients who received extensive prior therapy. Five patients achieved a partial response and one patient achieved a complete response.[339] However, because prolonged prior therapy affects stem cell mobilization with purine analogues and chlorambucil, mobilization at an earlier stage of the treatment is necessary. The role of thalidomide in management of this disease remains under investigation.

REFERENCES

1. Bakkus MH. Ig gene sequences in the study of clonality. *Pathol Biol (Paris)* 1999;47:128.
2. Macro M, Andre I, Comby E, et al. IgE multiple myeloma. *Leuk Lymphoma* 1999;32:597.
3. Blade J, Kyle RA. Nonsecretory myeloma, immunoglobulin D myeloma, and plasma cell leukemia. *Hematol Oncol Clin North Am* 1999;13:1259.
4. Macintyre W. Case of mollities and fragilitas ossium, accompanied with urine strongly charged with animal matter. *Med Chir Trans Lond* 1859;33:211.
5. Bence Jones H. On a new substance occurring in the urine of a patient with mollities and fragilitas ossium. *Philos Trans R Soc Lond* 1848;55:673.
6. Kahler O. Zur Symptomatologie des multiplen Myeloma: beobachtung von Albumosurie. *Prog Med Wochenschr* 1889;14:33.
7. Arinkin M. Die intravitale Untersuchungs-Methodik des Knochenmarks. *Folia Haematol (Lepiz)* 1929;38:233.
8. Tiselius A. Electrophoresis of serum globulin. II. Electrophoretic analysis of normal and immune sera. *Biochem J* 1937;31:1464.
9. Holland JR, Hosley H, Scharlau C, et al. A controlled trial of urethane treatment in multiple myeloma. *Blood* 1966;27:328.
10. Bergsagel D. Evaluation of new chemotherapeutic agents in the treatment of multiple myeloma. IV. L-Phenylalanine mustard (NSC-8806). *Cancer Chemother Rep* 1962;21:87.
11. Salmon SE, Shadduck RK, Schilling A. Intermittent high-dose prednisone (NSC-10023) therapy for multiple myeloma. *Cancer Chemother Rep* 1967;51(1):179.
12. Alexanian R, Bonnet J, Gehan E, et al. Combination chemotherapy for multiple myeloma. *Cancer* 1972;30:382.
13. McElwain T, Powles R. High-dose intravenous melphalan for plasma-cell leukemia and myeloma. *Lancet* 1983;1:822.
14. Cohen HJ, Crawford J, Rao MK, Pieper CF, Currie MS. Racial differences in the prevalence of monoclonal gammopathy in a community-based sample of the elderly [published erratum appears in *Am J Med* 1998;105(4):362]. *Am J Med* 1998;104:439.
15. Riedel DA, Pottern LM. The epidemiology of multiple myeloma. *Hematol Oncol Clin North Am* 1992;6:225.
16. Ichimaru M, Ishimaru T, Mikami M, Matsunaga M. Multiple myeloma among atomic bomb survivors in Hiroshima and Nagasaki, 1950–76: relationship to radiation dose absorbed by marrow. *J Natl Cancer Inst* 1982;69:323.
17. Bergsagel DE, Wong O, Bergsagel PL, et al. Benzene and multiple myeloma: appraisal of the scientific evidence. *Blood* 1999;94:1174.
18. Lundberg I, Milatou-Smith R. Mortality and cancer incidence among Swedish paint industry workers with long-term exposure to organic solvents. *Scand J Work Environ Health* 1998;24:270.
19. Salmon SE, Kyle RA. Silicone gels, induction of plasma cell tumors, and genetic susceptibility in mice: a call for epidemiologic investigation of women with silicone breast implants [Editorial; Comment]. *J Natl Cancer Inst* 1994;86:1040.
20. Doody MM, Linet MS, Glass AG, et al. Risks of non-Hodgkin's lymphoma, multiple myeloma, and leukemia associated with common medications. *Epidemiology* 1996;7:131.
21. Linet MS, Harlow SD, McLaughlin JK. A case-control study of multiple myeloma in whites: chronic antigenic stimulation, occupation, and drug use. *Cancer Res* 1987;47:2978.
22. Brown LM, Linet MS, Greenberg RS, et al. Multiple myeloma and family history of cancer among blacks and whites in the U.S. *Cancer* 1999;85:2385.
23. Grosbois B, Jego P, Attal M, et al. Familial multiple myeloma: report of fifteen families. *Br J Haematol* 1999;105:768.
24. Kyle RA, Therneau TM, Rajkumar SV, et al. A long-term study of prognosis in monoclonal gammopathy of undetermined significance. *N Engl J Med* 2002;346:564.
25. Avet-Loiseau H, Facon T, Daviet A, et al. 14q32 translocations and monosomy 13 observed in monoclonal gammopathy of undetermined significance delineate a multistep process for the oncogenesis of multiple myeloma. Intergroupe Francophone du Myélome. *Cancer Res* 1999;59:4546.
26. Seligmann M, Sassy C, Chevalier A. A human IgG myeloma protein with anti-2 macroglobulin antibody activity. *J Immunol* 1973;110:85.
27. Malik AA, Ganti AK, Potti A, Levitt R, Hanley JF. Role of *Helicobacter pylori* infection in the incidence and clinical course of monoclonal gammopathy of undetermined significance. *Am J Gastroenterol* 2002;97:1371.
28. Rajkumar SV, Kyle RA, Plevak MF, Murray JA, Therneau TM. *Helicobacter pylori* infection and monoclonal gammopathy of undetermined significance. *Br J Haematol* 2002;119:706.
29. Konrad RJ, Kricka LJ, Goodman DB, Goldman J, Silberstein LE. Brief report: myeloma-associated paraprotein directed against the HIV-1 p24 antigen in an HIV-1-seropositive patient. *N Engl J Med* 1993;328:1817.
30. Rettig MB, Ma HJ, Vescio RA, et al. Kaposi's sarcoma–associated herpesvirus infection of bone marrow dendritic cells from multiple myeloma patients [see comments]. *Science* 1997;276:1851.
31. Soulier J, Grollet L, Oksenhendler E, et al. Kaposi's sarcoma–associated herpesvirus-like DNA sequences in multicentric Castleman's disease [see comments]. *Blood* 1995;86:1276.
32. Said W, Chien K, Takeuchi S, et al. Kaposi's sarcoma–associated herpesvirus (KSHV or HHV8) in primary effusion lymphoma: ultrastructural demonstration of herpesvirus in lymphoma cells. *Blood* 1996;87:4937.
33. Schalling M, Ekman M, Kaaya EE, Linde A, Biberfeld P. A role for a new herpes virus (KSHV) in different forms of Kaposi's sarcoma. *Nat Med* 1995;1:707.
34. Cull GM, Carter GI, Timms JM, et al. Low incidence of human herpesvirus 8 in stem cell collections from myeloma patients. *Bone Marrow Transplant* 1999;23:759.
35. Tarte K, Chang Y, Klein B. Kaposi's sarcoma-associated herpesvirus and multiple myeloma: lack of criteria for causality. *Blood* 1999;93:3159; discussion, 3163.
36. Yi Q, Ekman M, Anton D, et al. Blood dendritic cells from myeloma patients are not infected with Kaposi's sarcoma–associated herpesvirus (KSHV/HHV-8). *Blood* 1998;92:402.
37. Tarte K, Olsen SJ, Yang Lu Z, et al. Clinical-grade functional dendritic cells from patients with multiple myeloma are not infected with Kaposi's sarcoma–associated herpesvirus. *Blood* 1998;91:1852.
38. Brander C, Raje N, O'Connor PG, et al. Absence of biologically important Kaposi sarcoma–associated herpesvirus gene products and virus-specific cellular immune responses in multiple myeloma. *Blood* 2002;100:698.
39. Potter M. Experimental plasmacytomagenesis in mice. *Hematol Oncol Clin North Am* 1997;11:323.
40. Radl J. Multiple myeloma and related disorders. Lessons from an animal model. *Pathol Biol (Paris)* 1999;47:109.
41. Radl J. Animal model of human disease. Benign monoclonal gammopathy (idiopathic paraproteinemia). *Am J Pathol* 1981;105:91.
42. Radl J, Croese JW, Zurcher C, Van den Enden-Vieveen MH, de Leeuw AM. Animal model of human disease. Multiple myeloma. *Am J Pathol* 1988;132:593.
43. Huang YW, Richardson JA, Vitetta ES. Anti-CD54 (ICAM-1) has antitumor activity in SCID mice with human myeloma cells. *Cancer Res* 1995;55:610.
44. Feo-Zuppardi FJ, Taylor CW, Iwato K, et al. Long-term engraftment of fresh human myeloma cells in SCID mice. *Blood* 1992;80:2843.
45. Urashima M, Chen BP, Chen S, et al. The development of a model for the homing of multiple myeloma cells to human bone marrow. *Blood* 1997;90:754.
46. Yaccoby S, Barlogie B, Epstein J. Primary myeloma cells growing in SCID-hu mice: a model for studying the biology and treatment of myeloma and its manifestations. *Blood* 1998;92:2908.
47. Yaccoby S, Pearse RN, Johnson CL, et al. Myeloma interacts with the bone marrow microenvironment to induce osteoclastogenesis and is dependent on osteoclast activity. *Br J Haematol* 2002;116:278.
48. Sawyer J, Waldron J, Jagannath S, Barlogie B. Cytogenetics findings in 200 patients with multiple myeloma. *Cancer Genet Cytogenet* 1995;82:41.
49. Dewald GW, Kyle RA, Hicks GA, Greipp PR. The clinical significance of cytogenetic studies in 100 patients with multiple myeloma, plasma cell leukemia, or amyloidosis. *Blood* 1985;66:380.
50. Gould J, Alexanian R, Goodacre A, et al. Plasma cell karyotype in multiple myeloma. *Blood* 1988;71:453.
51. Sawyer JR, Lukacs JL, Thomas EL, et al. Multicolour spectral karyotyping identifies new translocations and a recurring pathway for chromosome loss in multiple myeloma. *Br J Haematol* 2001;112:167.
52. Perez-Simon JA, Garcia-Sanz R, Tabernero MD, et al. Prognostic value of numerical chromosome aberrations in multiple myeloma: a FISH analysis of 15 different chromosomes. *Blood* 1998;91:3366.
53. Rasillo A, Tabernero MD, Sanchez ML, et al. Fluorescence in situ hybridization analysis of aneuploidization patterns in monoclonal gammopathy of undetermined significance versus multiple myeloma and plasma cell leukemia. *Cancer* 2003;97:601.
54. Hallek M, Bergsagel LP, Anderson KD. Multiple myeloma: increasing evidence for a multistep transformation process. *Blood* 1998;91:3.
55. Avet-Loiseau H, Li JY, Morineau N, et al. Monosomy 13 is associated with the transition of monoclonal gammopathy of undetermined significance to multiple myeloma. Intergroupe Francophone du Myélome. *Blood* 1999;94:2583.
56. Drach J, Angerler J, Schuster J, et al. Interphase fluorescence in situ hybridization identifies chromosomal abnormalities in plasma cells from patients with monoclonal gammopathy of undetermined significance. *Blood* 1995;86:3915.
57. Hayman SR, Bailey RJ, Jalal SM, et al. Translocations involving the immunoglobulin heavy-chain locus are possible early genetic events in patients with primary systemic amyloidosis. *Blood* 2001;98:2266.
58. Chesi M, Bergsagel PL, Brents LA, et al. Dysregulation of cyclin D1 by translocation into an IgH gamma switch region in two multiple myeloma cell lines [see comments]. *Blood* 1996;88:674.
59. Hart KC, Robertson SC, Kanemitsu MY, et al. Transformation and Stat activation by derivatives of FGFR1, FGFR3, and FGFR4. *Oncogene* 2000;19:3309.
60. Chesi M, Nardini E, Brents LA, et al. Frequent translocation t(4;14)(p16.3;q32.3) in multiple myeloma is associated with increased expression and activating mutations of fibroblast growth factor receptor 3. *Nat Genet* 1997;16:260.
61. Li Z, Zhu YX, Plowright EE, et al. The myeloma-associated oncogene fibroblast growth factor receptor 3 is transforming in hematopoietic cells. *Blood* 2001;97:2413.
62. Chesi M, Brents LA, Ely SA, et al. Activated fibroblast growth factor receptor 3 is an oncogene that contributes to tumor progression in multiple myeloma. *Blood* 2001;97:729.

63. Plowright EE, Li Z, Bergsagel PL, et al. Ectopic expression of fibroblast growth factor receptor 3 promotes myeloma cell proliferation and prevents apoptosis. *Blood* 2000;95:992.
64. Chesi M, Bergsagel PL, Shonukan OO, et al. Frequent dysregulation of the c-maf proto-oncogene at 16q23 by translocation to an Ig locus in multiple myeloma. *Blood* 1998;91: 4457.
65. Iida S, Rao PH, Butler M, et al. Deregulation of MUM1/IRF4 by chromosomal translocation in multiple myeloma. *Nat Genet* 1997;17:226.
66. Mahmoud MS, Huang N, Nobuyoshi M, et al. Altered expression of Pax-5 gene in human myeloma cells. *Blood* 1996;87:4311.
67. Shou Y, Martelli ML, Gabrea A, et al. Diverse karyotypic abnormalities of the c-myc locus associated with c-myc dysregulation and tumor progression in multiple myeloma. *Proc Natl Acad Sci U S A* 2000;97:228.
68. Avet-Loiseau H, Gerson F, Magrangeas F, et al. Rearrangements of the c-myc oncogene are present in 15% of primary human multiple myeloma tumors. *Blood* 2001;98:3082.
69. Selvanayagam P, Blick M, Narni F, et al. Alteration and abnormal expression of the *c-myc* oncogene in human multiple myeloma. *Blood* 1988;71.
70. Greil R, Fasching B, Loidl P, Huber H. Expression of the c-myc proto-oncogene in multiple myeloma and chronic lymphocytic leukemia: an in situ analysis. *Blood* 1991;78:180.
71. Tricot G, Sawyer J, Jagannath S, et al. Poor prognosis in multiple myeloma is associated only with partial or complete deletion of chromosome 13 or abnormalities involving 11q and not with other karyotype abnormalities. *Blood* 1995;86:4250.
72. Dao DD, Sawyer JR, Epstein J, et al. Deletion of the retinoblastoma gene in multiple myeloma. *Leukemia* 1994;8:1280.
73. Shaughnessy J, Barlogie B. Chromosome 13 deletion in myeloma. *Curr Topics Microbiol Immunol* 1999;246:199.
74. Urashima M, Ogata A, Chauhan D, et al. Interleukin-6 promotes multiple myeloma cell growth via phosphorylation of retinoblastoma protein. *Blood* 1996;88:2219.
75. Ng MH, Chung YF, Lo KW, et al. Frequent hypermethylation of p16 and p15 genes in multiple myeloma. *Blood* 1997;89:2500.
76. Urashima M, Teoh G, Ogata A, et al. Characterization of p16(INK4A) expression in multiple myeloma and plasma cell leukemia. *Clin Cancer Res* 1997;3:2173.
77. Kawano MM, Mahmoud MS, Ishikawa H. Cyclin D1 and p16INK4A are preferentially expressed in immature and mature myeloma cells, respectively. *Br J Haematol* 1997;99:131.
78. Neri A, Baldini L, Trecca D, et al. p53 gene mutations in multiple myeloma are associated with advanced forms of malignancy. *Blood* 1993;81:128.
79. Portier M, Moles JP, Mazars GR, et al. p53 and RAS gene mutations in multiple myeloma. *Oncogene* 1992;7:2539.
80. Drach J, Ackermann J, Fritz E, et al. Presence of a p53 gene deletion in patients with multiple myeloma predicts for short survival after conventional-dose chemotherapy. *Blood* 1998;92:802.
81. Teoh G, Urashima M, Ogata A, et al. MDM2 protein overexpression promotes proliferation and survival of multiple myeloma cells. *Blood* 1997;90:1982.
82. Pettersson M, Jernberg-Wiklund H, Larsson LG, et al. Expression of the Bcl-2 gene in human multiple myeloma cell lines and normal plasma cells. *Blood* 1992;79:495.
83. Puthier D, Pellat-Deceunynck C, Barille S, et al. Differential expression of Bcl-2 in human plasma cell disorders according to proliferation status and malignancy. *Leukemia* 1999;13:289.
84. Gazitt Y, Fey V, Thomas C, Alvarez R. Bcl-2 overexpression is associated with resistance to dexamethasone, but not melphalan, in multiple myeloma cells. *Int J Oncol* 1998;13:397.
85. Tu Y, Renner S, Xu F, et al. BCL-X expression in multiple myeloma: possible indicator of chemoresistance. *Cancer Res* 1998;58:256.
86. Iyer R, Ding L, Batchu RB, et al. Antisense p53 transduction leads to overexpression of bcl-2 and dexamethasone resistance in multiple myeloma. *Leuk Res* 2003;27:73.
87. Sangfelt O, Osterborg A, Grander D, et al. Response to interferon therapy in patients with multiple myeloma correlates with expression of the Bcl-2 oncoprotein. *Int J Cancer* 1995;63:190.
88. Catlett-Falcone R, Landowski TH, Oshiro MM, et al. Constitutive activation of Stat3 signaling confers resistance to apoptosis in human U266 myeloma cells. *Immunity* 1999;10:105.
89. Feinman R, Koury J, Thames M, et al. Role of NF-κB in the rescue of multiple myeloma cells from glucocorticoid-induced apoptosis by bcl-2. *Blood* 1999;93:3044.
90. Shammas MA, Shmookler Reis RJ, Akiyama M, et al. Telomerase inhibition and cell growth arrest by G-quadruplex interactive agent in multiple myeloma. *Mol Cancer Ther* 2003;2:825.
91. Sahota SS, Davis Z, Hamblin T, et al. Discordant somatic mutation of immunoglobulin variable region genes and bcl-6 genes in chronic lymphocytic leukemia. *Blood* 1999;94:662a.
92. Dhodapkar MV, Kelly T, Theus A, et al. Elevated levels of shed syndecan-1 correlate with tumour mass and decreased matrix metalloproteinase-9 activity in the serum of patients with multiple myeloma [published erratum appears in *Br J Haematol* 1998;101(2):398]. *Br J Haematol* 1997;99:368.
93. Dhodapkar MV, Weinstein R, Tricot G, et al. Biologic and therapeutic determinants of bone mineral density in multiple myeloma. *Leuk Lymphoma* 1998;32:121.
94. Yang Y, Yaccoby S, Liu W, et al. Soluble syndecan-1 promotes growth of myeloma tumors in vivo. *Blood* 2002;100:610.
95. Chauhan D, Uchiyama H, Urashima M, Yamamoto K, Anderson KC. Regulation of interleukin-6 in multiple myeloma and bone marrow stromal cells. *Stem Cells* 1995;15:35.
96. Hideshima T, Chauhan D, Schlossman R, Richardson P, Anderson KC. The role of tumor necrosis factor α in the pathophysiology of human multiple myeloma: therapeutic applications. *Oncogene* 2001;20:4519.
97. Dankar B, Padro T, Leo R, et al. Vascular endothelial growth factor and interleukin-6 in paracrine tumor-stromal cell interactions in multiple myeloma. *Blood* 2000;95:2630.
98. Hideshima T, Chauhan D, Hayashi T, et al. The biological sequelae of stromal cell-derived factor-1α in multiple myeloma. *Mol Cancer Ther* 2002;1:539.
99. Tai YT, Podar K, Catley L, et al. Insulin-like growth factor-1 induces adhesion and migration in human multiple myeloma cells via activation of β_1-integrin and phosphatidylinositol 3'-kinase/AKT signaling. *Cancer Res* 2003;63:5850.
100. Vacca A, Ribatti D, Roncali L, et al. Bone marrow angiogenesis and progression in multiple myeloma. *Br J Haematol* 1994;87:503.
101. Rajkumar SV, Fonseca R, Witzig TE, Gertz MA, Greipp PR. Bone marrow angiogenesis in patients achieving complete response after stem cell transplantation for multiple myeloma. *Leukemia* 1999;13:469.
102. Rajkumar SV, Mesa RA, Fonseca R, et al. Bone marrow angiogenesis in 400 patients with monoclonal gammopathy of undetermined significance, multiple myeloma, and primary amyloidosis. *Clin Cancer Res* 2002;8:2210.
103. Munshi NC, Wilson C. Increased bone marrow microvessel density in newly diagnosed multiple myeloma carries a poor prognosis. *Semin Oncol* 2001;28:565.
104. Kumar S, Fonseca R, Dispenzieri A, et al. Bone marrow angiogenesis in multiple myeloma: effect of therapy. *Br J Haematol* 2002;119:665.
105. Bellamy WT, Richter L, Frutiger Y, Grogan TM. Expression of vascular endothelial growth factor and its receptors in hematopoietic malignancies. *Cancer Res* 1999;59:728.
106. Seidel C, Borset M, Turesson I, et al. Elevated serum concentrations of hepatocyte growth factor in patients with multiple myeloma. The Nordic Myeloma Study Group. *Blood* 1998;91:806.
107. Urashima M, Ogata A, Chauhan D, et al. Transforming growth factor-β1: differential effects on multiple myeloma versus normal B cells. *Blood* 1996;87:1928.
108. Brenne AT, Baade Ro T, Waage A, et al. Interleukin-21 is a growth and survival factor for human myeloma cells. *Blood* 2002;99:3756.
109. Chauhan D, Hideshima T, Rosen S, et al. Apaf-1/Cytochrome c-independent and Smac-dependent induction of apoptosis in multiple myeloma cells. *J Biol Chem* 2001;276:24453.
110. Chauhan D, Pandey P, Hideshima T, et al. SHP2 mediates the protective effect of interleukin-6 against dexamethasone-induced apoptosis in multiple myeloma cells. *J Biol Chem* 2000;275:27845.
111. Mitsiades CS, Mitsiades N, Poulaki V, et al. Activation of NF-κB and up-regulation of intracellular anti-apoptotic proteins via the IGF-1/Akt signaling in human multiple myeloma cells: therapeutic implications. *Oncogene* 2002;21:5673.
112. Qiang YW, Kopantzev E, Rudikoff S. Insulinlike growth factor-I signaling in multiple myeloma: downstream elements, functional correlates, and pathway cross-talk. *Blood* 2002;99:4138.
113. Akiyama M, Hideshima T, Hayashi T, et al. Cytokines modulate telomerase activity in a human multiple myeloma cell line. *Cancer Res* 2002;62:3876.
114. Podar K, Tai YT, Davies FE, et al. Vascular endothelial growth factor triggers signaling cascades mediating multiple myeloma cell growth and migration. *Blood* 2001;98:428.
115. Podar K, Tai YT, Lin BK, et al. Vascular endothelial growth factor-induced migration of multiple myeloma cells is associated with β_1 integrin- and phosphatidylinositol 3-kinase-dependent PKC alpha activation. *J Biol Chem* 2002;277:7875.
116. Gupta D, Treon SP, Shima Y, et al. Adherence of multiple myeloma cells to bone marrow stromal cells upregulates vascular endothelial growth factor secretion: therapeutic applications. *Leukemia* 2001;15:1950.
117. Lin B, Podar K, Gupta D, et al. The vascular endothelial growth factor receptor tyrosine kinase inhibitor PTK787/ZK222584 inhibits growth and migration of multiple myeloma cells in the bone marrow microenvironment. *Cancer Res* 2002;62:5019.
118. Gieseler F, Nussler V. Cellular resistance mechanisms with impact on the therapy of multiple myeloma [Editorial]. *Leukemia* 1998;12:1009.
119. Pilarski LM, Yatscoff RW, Murphy GF, Belch AR. Drug resistance in multiple myeloma: cyclosporin A analogues and their metabolites as potential chemosensitizers. *Leukemia* 1998;12:505.
120. Sonneveld P, Marie JP, Huisman C, et al. Reversal of multidrug resistance by SDZ PSC 833, combined with VAD (vincristine, doxorubicin, dexamethasone) in refractory multiple myeloma. A phase I study. *Leukemia* 1996;10:1741.
121. Abbaszadegan MR, Futscher BW, Klimecki WT, List A, Dalton WS. Analysis of multidrug resistance-associated protein (MRP) messenger RNA in normal and malignant hematopoietic cells. *Cancer Res* 1994;54:4676.
122. Filipits M, Drach J, Pohl G, et al. Expression of the lung resistance protein predicts poor outcome in patients with multiple myeloma. *Clin Cancer Res* 1999;5:2426.
123. Raaijmakers HG, Izquierdo MA, Lokhorst HM, et al. Lung-resistance–related protein expression is a negative predictive factor for response to conventional low but not to intensified dose alkylating chemotherapy in multiple myeloma. *Blood* 1998;91:1029.
124. Pilarski LM, Jensen GS. Monoclonal circulating B cells in multiple myeloma. A continuously differentiating, possibly invasive, population as defined by expression of CD45 isoforms and adhesion molecules. *Hematol Oncol Clin North Am* 1992;6:297.
125. Hideshima T, Anderson KC. Molecular mechanisms of novel therapeutic approaches for multiple myeloma. *Nat Rev Cancer* 2002;2:927.
126. Hata H, Xiao HQ, Petrucci MT, et al. Interleukin-6 gene expression in multiple myeloma: a characteristic of immature myeloma cells. *Blood* 1993;81:3357.
127. Kawano MM, Huang N, Harada H, et al. Identification of immature and mature myeloma cells in the bone marrow of human myelomas. *Blood* 1993;82:564.
128. Epstein J, Barlogie B, Katzmann J, Alexanian R. Phenotypic heterogeneity in aneuploid multiple myeloma indicates pre-B cell involvement. *Blood* 1988;71:861.
129. Kawano MM, Mahmoud MS, Huang N, et al. High proportions of VLA-5- immature myeloma cells correlated well with poor response to treatment in multiple myeloma. *Br J Haematol* 1995;91:860.
130. Robillard N, Jego G, Pellat-Deceunynck C, et al. CD28, a marker associated with tumoral expansion in multiple myeloma. *Clin Cancer Res* 1998;4:1521.
131. Treon SP, Shima Y, Preffer FI, et al. Treatment of plasma cell dyscrasias by antibody-mediated immunotherapy. *Semin Oncol* 1999;26:97.
132. Thomas X, Xiao HQ, Chang R, Epstein J. Circulating B lymphocytes in multiple myeloma patients contain an autocrine IL-6 driven pre-myeloma cell population. *Curr Topics Microbiol Immunol* 1992;182:201.
133. Pilarski LM, Andrews EJ, Mant MJ, Ruether BA. Humoral immune deficiency in multiple myeloma patients due to compromised B-cell function. *J Clin Immunol* 1986;6: 491.

134. Munshi NC. Immunoregulatory mechanisms in multiple myeloma. *Hematol Oncol Clin North Am* 1997;11:51.

135. Gahrton G, Tura S, Ljungman P, et al. Prognostic factors in allogeneic bone marrow transplantation for multiple myeloma. *J Clin Oncol* 1995;13:1312.

136. Mellstedt H, Holm G, Pettersson D, et al. T cells in monoclonal gammopathies. *Scand J Haematol* 1982;29:57.

137. Mills KH, Cawley JC. Abnormal monoclonal antibody–defined helper/suppressor T-cell subpopulations in multiple myeloma: relationship to treatment and clinical stage. *Br J Haematol* 1983;53:271.

138. Osterborg A, Nilsson B, Bjorkholm M, Holm G, Mellstedt H. Natural killer cell activity in monoclonal gammopathies: relation to disease activity. *Eur J Haematol* 1990;45:153.

139. Bensinger WI, Buckner CD, Anasetti C, et al. Allogeneic marrow transplantation for multiple myeloma: an analysis of risk factors on outcome. *Blood* 1996;88:2787.

140. Maecker B, Anderson KS, von Bergwelt-Baildon MS, et al. Viral antigen-specific CD8+ T-cell responses are impaired in multiple myeloma. *Br J Haematol* 2003;121:842.

141. Dhodapkar MV, Geller MD, Chang DH, et al. A reversible defect in natural killer T cell function characterizes the progression of premalignant to malignant multiple myeloma. *J Exp Med* 2003;197:1667.

142. Yi Q, Osterborg A, Bergenbrant S, et al. Idiotype-reactive T-cell subsets and tumor load in monoclonal gammopathies. *Blood* 1995;86:3043.

143. Yi Q, Osterborg A. Idiotype-specific T cells in multiple myeloma: targets for an immunotherapeutic intervention? *Med Oncol* 1996;13:1.

144. Solomon A, Weiss DT, Kattine AA. Nephrotoxic potential of Bence Jones proteins [see comments]. *N Engl J Med* 1991;324:1845.

145. Khamlichi AA, Rocca A, Touchard G, et al. Role of light chain variable region in myeloma with light chain deposition disease: evidence from an experimental model. *Blood* 1995;86:3655.

146. Pozzi C, Fogazzi GB, Banfi G, et al. Renal disease and patient survival in light chain deposition disease. *Clin Nephrol* 1995;43:281.

147. Clark AD, Shetty A, Soutar R. Renal failure and multiple myeloma: pathogenesis and treatment of renal failure and management of underlying myeloma. *Blood Rev* 1999;13:79.

148. Huang ZQ, Sanders PW. Localization of a single binding site for immunoglobulin light chains on human Tamm-Horsfall glycoprotein. *J Clin Invest* 1997;99:732.

149. Huang ZQ, Kirk KA, Connelly KG, Sanders PW. Bence Jones proteins bind to a common peptide segment of Tamm-Horsfall glycoprotein to promote heterotypic aggregation. *J Clin Invest* 1993;92:2975.

150. Kyle RA, Greipp PR. Amyloidosis (AL): clinical and laboratory features in 229 cases. *Mayo Clin Proc* 1983;58:665.

151. Fattori E, Della Rocca C, Costa P, et al. Development of progressive kidney damage and myeloma kidney in interleukin-6 transgenic mice. *Blood* 1994;83:2570.

152. Mundy GR, Raisz LG, Cooper RA, Schechter GP, Salmon SE. Evidence for the secretion of an osteoclast stimulating factor in myeloma. *N Engl J Med* 1974;291:1041.

153. Roodman GD. Mechanisms of bone lesions in multiple myeloma and lymphoma. *Cancer* 1997;80:1557.

154. Bataille R, Manolagas SC, Berenson JR. Pathogenesis and management of bone lesions in multiple myeloma. *Hematol Oncol Clin North Am* 1997;11:349.

155. Kroger N, Schwerdtfeger R, Kiehl M, et al. Autologous stem cell transplantation followed by a dose-reduced allograft induces high complete remission rate in multiple myeloma. *Blood* 2002;100:755.

156. Garrett R, Durie B, Nedwin G, et al. Production of lymphotoxin, a bone resorbing cytokine, by cultured human myeloma cells. *N Engl J Med* 1987;317:526.

157. Tricot G. New insights into the role of microenvironment in multiple myeloma. *Lancet* 2000;355:248.

158. Tian E, Zhan F, Walker R, et al. The role of the Wnt-signaling antagonist DKK1 in the development of osteolytic lesions in multiple myeloma. *N Engl J Med* 2003;349:2483.

159. Lacey DL, Timms E, Tan HL, et al. Osteoprotegerin ligand is a cytokine that regulates osteoclast differentiation and activation. *Cell* 1998;93:165.

160. Yakoub-Agha I, Attal M, Dumontet C, et al. Thalidomide in patients with advanced multiple myeloma: a study of 83 patients—report of the Intergroupe Francophone du Myelome (IFM). *Hematol J* 2002;3:185.

161. Broder S, Humphrey R, Durm M, et al. Impaired synthesis of polyclonal (non-paraprotein) immunoglobulins by circulating lymphocytes from patients with multiple myeloma: role of suppressor cells. *N Engl J Med* 1975;293:887.

162. Jacobson DR, Zolla-Pazner S. Immunosuppression and infection in multiple myeloma. *Semin Oncol* 1986;13:282.

163. Cook G, Campbell JD, Carr CE, Boyd KS, Franklin IM. Transforming growth factor beta from multiple myeloma cells inhibits proliferation and IL-2 responsiveness in T lymphocytes. *J Leukoc Biol* 1999;66:981.

164. Soubrier MJ, Dubost JJ, Sauvezie BJM. POEMS syndrome: a study of 25 cases and a review of the literature. *Am J Med* 1994;97:543.

165. Lacy MQ, Gertz MA, Hanson CA, Inwards DJ, Kyle RA. Multiple myeloma associated with diffuse osteosclerotic bone lesions: a clinical entity distinct from osteosclerotic myeloma (POEMS syndrome). *Am J Hematol* 1997;56:288.

166. Miralles GD, O'Fallon JR, Talley NJ. Plasma-cell dyscrasia with polyneuropathy. The spectrum of POEMS syndrome. *N Engl J Med* 1992;327:1919.

167. Kumar S, Gertz MA, Dispenzieri A, et al. Response rate, durability of response, and survival after thalidomide therapy for relapsed multiple myeloma. *Mayo Clin Proc* 2003;78:34.

168. Leifer D, Grabowski T, Simonian N, Demirjian ZN. Leptomeningeal myelomatosis presenting with mental status changes and other neurologic findings. *Cancer* 1992;70:1899.

169. Pruzanski W, Watt JG. Serum viscosity and hyperviscosity syndrome in IgG multiple myeloma. Report on 10 patients and a review of the literature. *Ann Intern Med* 1972;77:853.

170. Preston FE, Cooke KB, Foster ME, Winfield DA, Lee D. Myelomatosis and the hyperviscosity syndrome. *Br J Haematol* 1978;38:517.

171. Chandy KG, Stockley RA, Leonard RC, et al. Relationship between serum viscosity and intravascular IgA polymer concentration in IgA myeloma. *Clin Exp Immunol* 1981;46:653.

172. Durie BG. Low-dose thalidomide in myeloma: efficacy and biologic significance. *Semin Oncol* 2002;29:34.

173. Perkins HA, MacKenzie MR, Fudenberg HH. Hemostatic defects in dysproteinemias. *Blood* 1970;35:695.

174. Lackner H. Hemostatic abnormalities associated with dysproteinemias. *Semin Hematol* 1973;10:125.

175. Deitcher SR, Erban JK, Limentani SA. Acquired free protein S deficiency associated with multiple myeloma: a case report. *Am J Hematol* 1996;51:319.

176. Coleman M, Vigliano EM, Weksler ME, Nachman RL. Inhibition of fibrin monomer polymerization by lambda myeloma globulins. *Blood* 1972;39:210.

177. Furie B, Greene E, Furie BC. Syndrome of acquired factor X deficiency and systemic amyloidosis in vivo studies of the metabolic fate of factor X. *N Engl J Med* 1977;297:81.

178. Zangari M, Anaissie E, Barlogie B, et al. Increased risk of deep-vein thrombosis in patients with multiple myeloma receiving thalidomide and chemotherapy. *Blood* 2001;98:1614.

179. Zangari M, Saghafifar F, Anaissie E, et al. Activated protein C resistance in the absence of factor V Leiden mutation is a common finding in multiple myeloma and is associated with an increased risk of thrombotic complications. *Blood Coagul Fibrinolysis* 2002;13:187.

180. Barlogie B, Smallwood L, Smith T, Alexanian R. High serum levels of lactic dehydrogenase identify a high-grade lymphoma-like myeloma. *Ann Intern Med* 1989;110:521.

181. Pizzolato M, Bragantini G, Bresciani P, et al. IgG1-kappa biclonal gammopathy associated with multiple myeloma suggests a regulatory mechanism. *Br J Haematol* 1998;102:503.

182. Zent CS, Wilson CS, Tricot G, et al. Oligoclonal protein bands and Ig isotype switching in multiple myeloma treated with high-dose therapy and hematopoietic cell transplantation. *Blood* 1998;91:3518.

183. Kozuru M, Uike N, Takahira H, et al. Immunoglobulin class switch from IgA1 to IgG2 and simultaneous association with Bence Jones proteinuria in the escape phase in a myeloma patient treated with interferon alpha. *Br J Haematol* 1997;98:114.

184. Billadeau D, Quam L, Thomas W, et al. Detection and quantitation of malignant cells in the peripheral blood of multiple myeloma patients. *Blood* 1992;80:1818.

185. Barlogie B, Gale RP. Multiple myeloma and chronic lymphocytic leukemia: commonalities and differences in biology and therapy. *Leuk Lymphoma* 1991;27.

186. Bartl R, Frisch B. Clinical significance of bone marrow biopsy and plasma cell morphology in MM and MGUS. *Pathol Biol (Paris)* 1999;47:158.

187. Barlogie B, Alexanian R, Pershouse M, Smallwood L, Smith L. Cytoplasmic immunoglobulin content in multiple myeloma. *J Clin Invest* 1985;76:765.

188. Bergsagel PL, Nardini E, Brents L, Chesi M, Kuehl WM. IgH translocations in multiple myeloma: a nearly universal event that rarely involves c-myc. *Curr Topics Microbiol Immunol* 1997;224:283.

189. Tricot G, Sawyer JR, Jagannath S, et al. Unique role of cytogenetics in the prognosis of patients with myeloma receiving high-dose therapy and autotransplants. *J Clin Oncol* 1997;15:2659.

190. Sawyer JR, Tricot G, Mattox S, Jagannath S, Barlogie B. Jumping translocations of chromosome 1q in multiple myeloma: evidence for a mechanism involving decondensation of pericentromeric heterochromatin. *Blood* 1998;91:1732.

191. Govindarajan R, Jagannath S, Flick J, et al. Preceding standard therapy is the likely cause of MDS after autotransplants for multiple myeloma. *Br J Haematol* 1996;95:349.

192. Dao DD, Sawyer JR, Epstein J, et al. Deletion of the retinoblastoma gene in multiple myeloma. *Leukemia* 1994;8:1280.

193. Avet-Loiseau H, Li JY, Facon T, et al. High incidence of translocations t(11;14)(q13;q32) and t(4;14)(p16;q32) in patients with plasma cell malignancies. *Cancer Res* 1998;58:5640.

194. Witzig TE, Gonchoroff NJ, Katzmann JA, et al. Peripheral blood B cell labeling indices are a measure of disease activity in patients with monoclonal gammopathies. *J Clin Oncol* 1988;6:1041.

195. Greipp PR, Lust JA, et al. Plasma cell labeling index and beta 2-microglobulin predict survival independent of thymidine kinase and C-reactive protein in multiple myeloma [see comments]. *Blood* 1993;81:3382.

196. Mariette X, Khalifa P, Ravaud P, et al. Bone densitometry in patients with multiple myeloma [see comments]. *Am J Med* 1992;93:595.

197. Mariette X, Bergot C, Ravaud P, et al. Evolution of bone densitometry in patients with myeloma treated with conventional or intensive therapy. *Cancer* 1995;76:1559.

198. Chodimella U, Dhodapkar M, Weinstein R, et al. Differential effects of pamidronate (PAM) on cortical and cancellous bone in patients with myeloma (MM) undergoing autotransplants (AT). *Proc Am Soc Clin Oncol* 1998;10.

199. Moulopoulos LA, Dimopoulos MA, Weber D, et al. Magnetic resonance imaging in the staging of solitary plasmacytoma of bone. *J Clin Oncol* 1993;11:1311.

200. Moulopoulos LA, Dimopoulos MA, Smith T, et al. Prognostic significance of magnetic resonance imaging in patients with asymptomatic multiple myeloma. *J Clin Oncol* 1995;13:251.

201. Moulopoulos LA, Dimopoulos MA. Magnetic resonance imaging of the bone marrow in hematologic malignancies. *Blood* 1997;90:2127.

202. Vande Berg BC, Lecouvet FE, Michaux L, et al. Magnetic resonance imaging of the bone marrow in hematological malignancies. *Eur Radiol* 1998;8:1335.

203. Kusumoto S, Jinnai I, Itoh K, et al. Magnetic resonance imaging patterns in patients with multiple myeloma. *Br J Haematol* 1997;99:649.

204. el-Shirbiny AM, Yeung H, Imbriaco M, et al. Technetium-99m-MIBI versus fluorine-18-FDG in diffuse multiple myeloma. *J Nucl Med* 1997;38:1208.

205. Kyle RA. Monoclonal gammopathy of undetermined significance. *Am J Med* 1978;64:814.

206. Merlini G, Waldenström JG, Jayakar SD. A new improved clinical staging system for multiple myeloma based on analysis of 123 treated patients. *Blood* 1980;55:1011.

207. Woodruff RK, Wadsworth J, Malpas JS, Tobias JS. Clinical staging in multiple myeloma. *Br J Haematol* 1979;42:199.

208. Kyle RA, Greipp PR. Smoldering multiple myeloma. *N Engl J Med* 1980;302:1347.

209. Durie B, Salmon S. Clinical staging system for myeloma: correlation of measured myeloma cell mass with presenting clinical features, response to treatment, and survival. *Cancer* 1975;36:842.

210. Bergsagel DE, Bailey AJ, Langley GR, et al. The chemotherapy on plasma-cell myeloma and the incidence of acute leukemia. *N Engl J Med* 1979;301:743.

211. Child JA, Norfolk DR, Cooper EH. Serum beta 2-microglobulin in myelomatosis [Letter]. *Br J Haematol* 1986;63:406.

212. Garewal H, Durie BG, Kyle RA, et al. Serum beta 2-microglobulin in the initial staging and subsequent monitoring of monoclonal plasma cell disorders. *J Clin Oncol* 1984;2:51.

213. Attal M, Harousseau JL, Facon T, et al. Single versus double autologous stem-cell transplantation for multiple myeloma. *N Engl J Med* 2003;349:2495.

214. Vesole DH, Tricot G, Jagannath S, et al. Autotransplants in multiple myeloma: what have we learned? *Blood* 1996;88:838.

215. Witzig TE, Gertz MA, Lust JA, et al. Peripheral blood monoclonal plasma cells as a predictor of survival in patients with multiple myeloma [see comments]. *Blood* 1996;88:1780.

216. Barlogie B, Alexanian R, Dicke KA, et al. High-dose chemoradiotherapy and autologous bone marrow transplantation for resistant multiple myeloma. *Blood* 1987;70:869.

217. Munshi N, Wilson C, Penn J, et al. Angiogenesis in newly diagnosed multiple myeloma (MM): poor prognosis with increased microvessel density (MVD) in bone marrow biopsies (BMBX). *Blood* 1998;92:98a.

218. Mathiot C, Galon J, Tartour E, et al. Soluble CD16 in plasma cell dyscrasias. *Leuk Lymphoma* 1999;32:467.

219. Siegel DS, Desikan KR, Mehta J, et al. Age is not a prognostic variable with autotransplants for multiple myeloma. *Blood* 1999;93:51.

220. Facon T, Avet-Loiseau H, Guillerm G, et al. Chromosome 13 abnormalities identified by FISH analysis and serum beta2-microglobulin produce a powerful myeloma staging system for patients receiving high-dose therapy. *Blood* 2001;97:1566.

221. Dimopoulos MA, Moulopoulos A, Delasalle K, Alexanian R. Solitary plasmacytoma of bone and asymptomatic multiple myeloma. *Hematol Oncol Clin North Am* 1992;6:359.

222. Mill WB, Griffith R. The role of radiation therapy in the management of plasma cell tumors. *Cancer* 1980;45:647.

223. Liebross RH, Ha CS, Cox JD, et al. Solitary bone plasmacytoma: outcome and prognostic factors following radiotherapy. *Int J Radiat Oncol Biol Phys* 1998;41:1063.

224. Corwin J, Lindberg RD. Solitary plasmacytoma of bone vs. extramedullary plasmacytoma. *Cancer* 1979;43:1007.

225. Woodruff RK, Malpas JS, White FE. Solitary plasmacytoma. II: Solitary plasmacytoma of bone. *Cancer* 1979;43:2344.

226. Alexanian R. Localized and indolent myeloma. *Blood* 1980;56:521.

227. Dimopoulos MA, Moulopoulos A, Smith T, Delasalle KB, Alexanian R. Risk of disease progression in asymptomatic multiple myeloma. *Am J Med* 1993;94:57.

228. Rajkumar SV, Gertz MA, Lacy MQ, et al. Thalidomide as initial therapy for early-stage myeloma. *Leukemia* 2003;17:775.

229. Bergsagel DE, Sprague CC, Austin C, Griffith KM. Evaluation of new chemotherapeutic agents in the treatment of myeloma IV: phenylalanine mustard. *Cancer Chemother Rep* 1962;21:87.

230. Alexanian R, Haut A, Khan AU, et al. Treatment for multiple myeloma. Combination chemotherapy with different melphalan dose regimens. *JAMA* 1969;208:1680.

231. Boccadoro M, Marmont F, Tribalto M, et al. Multiple myeloma: VMCP/VBAP alternating combination chemotherapy is not superior to melphalan and prednisone even in high-risk patients. *J Clin Oncol* 1991;9:444.

232. Gregory WM, Richards MA, Malpas JS. Combination chemotherapy versus melphalan and prednisolone in the treatment of multiple myeloma: an overview of published trials [see comments]. *J Clin Oncol* 1992;10:334.

233. Salmon SE, Haut A, Bonnet JD, et al. Alternating combination chemotherapy and levamisole improves survival in multiple myeloma: a Southwest Oncology Group study. *J Clin Oncol* 1983;1:453.

234. MacLennan IC, Chapman C, Dunn J, Kelly K. Combined chemotherapy with ABCM versus melphalan for treatment of myelomatosis. The Medical Research Council Working Party for Leukaemia in Adults [see comments]. *Lancet* 1992;339:200.

235. Neben K, Moehler T, Benner A, et al. Dose-dependent effect of thalidomide on overall survival in relapsed multiple myeloma. *Clin Cancer Res* 2002;8:3377.

236. Palumbo A, Bertola A, Falco P, et al. Efficacy of low-dose thalidomide and dexamethasone as first salvage regimen in multiple myeloma. *Hematol J* 2004;5:318.

237. Cohen HJ, Silberman HR, Tornyos K, Bartolucci AA. Comparison of two long-term chemotherapy regimens, with or without agents to modify skeletal repair, in multiple myeloma. *Blood* 1984;63:639.

238. Barlogie B, Smith L, Alexanian R. Effective treatment of advanced multiple myeloma refractory to alkylating agents. *N Engl J Med* 1984;310:1353.

239. Alexanian R, Barlogie B, Dixon D. High-dose glucocorticoid treatment of resistant myeloma. *Ann Intern Med* 1986;105:8.

240. Salmon SE, Crowley JJ, Grogan TM, et al. Combination chemotherapy, glucocorticoids, and interferon alfa in the treatment of multiple myeloma: a Southwest Oncology Group study [see comments]. *J Clin Oncol* 1994;12:2405.

241. Mandelli F, Avvisati F, Amadori S, et al. Maintenance treatment with recombinant interferon alfa-2b in patients with multiple myeloma responding to conventional induction chemotherapy. *N Engl J Med* 1990;322:1430.

242. Dimopoulos MA, Zervas K, Kouvatseas G, et al. Thalidomide and dexamethasone combination for refractory multiple myeloma. *Ann Oncol* 2001;12:991.

243. Ludwig H, Cohen AM, Polliack A, et al. Interferon-alpha for induction and maintenance in multiple myeloma: results of two multicenter randomized trials and summary of other studies. *Ann Oncol* 1995;6:467.

244. Barlogie B, Kyle RA, Anderson KC, et al. Comparable survival in multiple myeloma (MM) with high dose therapy (HDT) employing mel 140 mg/m² + TBI 12 Gy autotransplants versus standard dose therapy VBMCP and no benefit from interferon (IFN) maintenance: results of intergroup trial S9321. *Blood* 2003;102:42a.

245. Hu K, Yahalom J. Radiotherapy in the management of plasma cell tumors. *Oncology* 2000;14:101.

246. Woodruff RK, Whittle JM, Malpas JS. Solitary plasmacytoma. I: Extramedullary soft tissue plasmacytoma. *Cancer* 1979;43:2340.

247. Wallington M, Mendis S, Premawardhana U, Sanders P, Shahsavar-Haghighi K. Local control and survival in spinal cord compression from lymphoma and myeloma. *Radiother Oncol* 1997;42:43.

248. Rowell NP, Tobias JS. The role of radiotherapy in the management of multiple myeloma. *Blood Rev* 1991;5:84.

249. Barlogie B, Dicke KA, Alexanian R. High dose melphalan for refractory myeloma—the M. D. Anderson experience. *Hematol Oncol* 1988;6:167.

250. Cunningham D, Paz-Ares L, Milan S, et al. High-dose melphalan and autologous bone marrow transplantation as consolidation in previously untreated myeloma. *J Clin Oncol* 1994;12:759.

251. Bensinger WI, Rowley SD, Demirer T, et al. High-dose therapy followed by autologous hematopoietic stem-cell infusion for patients with multiple myeloma. *J Clin Oncol* 1996;14:1447.

252. Fermand JP, Ravaud P, Chevret S, et al. High-dose therapy and autologous blood stem cell transplantation in multiple myeloma: preliminary results of a randomized trial involving 167 patients. *Stem Cells* 1995;13:156.

253. Anderson KC, Andersen J, Soiffer R, et al. Monoclonal antibody-purged bone marrow transplantation therapy for multiple myeloma. *Blood* 1993;82:2568.

254. Harousseau JL, Attal M, Divine M, et al. Autologous stem cell transplantation after first remission induction treatment in multiple myeloma. A report of the French Registry on Autologous Transplantation in Multiple Myeloma. *Stem Cells* 1995;13:132.

255. Attal M, Harousseau JL, Stoppa AM, et al. A prospective, randomized trial of autologous bone marrow transplantation and chemotherapy in multiple myeloma. Intergroupe Français du Myélome. *N Engl J Med* 1996;335:91.

256. Child JA, Morgan GJ, Davies FE, et al. High-dose chemotherapy with hematopoietic stem-cell rescue for multiple myeloma. *N Engl J Med* 2003;348:1875.

257. Blade J, Surenda A, et al. High-dose therapy autotransplantation/intensification vs. continued conventional chemotherapy in multiple myeloma patients responding to initial treatment chemotherapy. Results of a prospective randomized trial from the Spanish Cooperative group PETHEMA. *Blood* 2001;98:815a.

258. Fermand JP, Ravaud P, Chevret S, et al. High-dose therapy and autologous peripheral blood stem cell transplantation in multiple myeloma: up-front or rescue treatment? Results of a multicenter sequential randomized clinical trial. *Blood* 1998;92:3131.

259. Harousseau JL, Milpied N, Laporte JP, et al. Double-intensive therapy in high-risk multiple myeloma. *Blood* 1992;79:2827.

260. Barlogie B, Jagannath S, Desikan KR, et al. Total therapy with tandem transplants for newly diagnosed multiple myeloma. *Blood* 1999;93:55.

261. Tricot G, Jagannath S, Vesole D, et al. Peripheral blood stem cell transplant for multiple myeloma: identification of favorable variables for rapid engraftment in 225 patients. *Blood* 1995;85:588.

262. Vesole DH, Barlogie B, Jagannath S, et al. High-dose therapy for refractory multiple myeloma: improved prognosis with better supportive care and double transplants. *Blood* 1994;84:950.

263. Gertz MA, Lacy MQ, Inwards DJ, et al. Early harvest and late transplantation as an effective therapeutic strategy in multiple myeloma. *Bone Marrow Transplant* 1999;23:221.

264. Desikan KR, Fassas A, Siegel D, et al. Superior outcome with melphalan 200 mg/m² (MEL 200) for scheduled second autotransplant compared to MEL+TBI or CTX for myeloma (MM) in pre-tx-2 PR. *Blood* 1997;90:231a.

265. Jagannath S, Barlogie B. Autologous bone marrow transplantation for multiple myeloma. *Hematol Oncol Clin North Am* 1992;6:437.

266. Fermand JP, Levy Y, Gerota J, et al. Treatment of aggressive multiple myeloma by high-dose chemotherapy and total body irradiation followed by blood stem cells autologous graft. *Blood* 1989;73:20.

267. Ventura GJ, Barlogie B, Hester JP, et al. High dose cyclophosphamide, BCNU and VP-16 with autologous blood stem cell support for refractory multiple myeloma. *Bone Marrow Transplant* 1990;5:265.

268. Vescio RA, Hong CH, Cao J, et al. The hematopoietic stem cell antigen, CD34, is not expressed on the malignant cells in multiple myeloma. *Blood* 1994;84:3283.

269. Schiller G, Vescio R, Freytes C, et al. Transplantation of CD34+ peripheral blood progenitor cells after high-dose chemotherapy for patients with advanced multiple myeloma. *Blood* 1995;86:390.

270. Stewart AK, Vescio R, Schiller G, et al. Purging of autologous peripheral-blood stem cells using CD34 selection does not improve overall or progression-free survival after high-dose chemotherapy for multiple myeloma: results of a multicenter randomized controlled trial. *J Clin Oncol* 2001;19:3771.

271. Gazitt Y, Reading CC, Hoffman R, et al. Purified CD34+ Lin– Thy+ stem cells do not contain clonal myeloma cells. *Blood* 1995;86:381.

272. Tricot G, Gazitt Y, Leemhuis T, et al. Collection, tumor contamination, and engraftment kinetics of highly purified hematopoietic progenitor cells to support high dose therapy in multiple myeloma. *Blood* 1998;91:4489.

273. Harousseau JL, Attal M, Divine M, et al. Comparison of autologous bone marrow transplantation and peripheral blood stem cell transplantation after first remission induction treatment in multiple myeloma. *Bone Marrow Transplant* 1995;15:963.

274. Tricot G, Jagannath S, Vesole D, et al. Peripheral blood stem cell transplants for multiple myeloma: identification of favorable variables for rapid engraftment in 225 patients. *Blood* 1995;85:588.

275. Gazitt Y, Tian E, Barlogie B, et al. Differential mobilization of myeloma cells and normal hematopoietic stem cells in multiple myeloma after treatment with cyclophosphamide and granulocyte-macrophage colony-stimulating factor. *Blood* 1996;87:805.

276. Badros A, Barlogie B, Siegel E, et al. Autologous stem cell transplantation in elderly multiple myeloma patients over the age of 70 years. *Br J Haematol* 2001;114:600.

277. Tricot G, Alberts DS, Johnson C, et al. Safety of autotransplants with high-dose melphalan in renal failure: a pharmacokinetic and toxicity study. *Clin Cancer Res* 1996;2:947.

278. Badros A, Barlogie B, Siegel E, et al. Results of autologous stem cell transplant in multiple myeloma patients with renal failure. *Br J Haematol* 2001;114:822.
279. Browman G, Bergsagel D, Sicheri D, et al. Randomized trial of interferon maintenance in multiple myeloma: a study of the National Cancer Institute of Canada Clinical Trials Group. *J Clin Oncol* 1995;13:2354.
280. Berenson JR, Crowley JJ, Grogan TM, et al. Maintenance therapy with alternate-day prednisone improves survival in multiple myeloma patients. *Blood* 2002;99:3163.
281. Bensinger WI, Demirer T, Buckner CD, et al. Syngeneic marrow transplantation in patients with multiple myeloma. *Bone Marrow Transplant* 1996;18:527.
282. Gahrton G, Svensson H, Bjorkstrand B, et al. Syngeneic transplantation in multiple myeloma—a case matched comparison with autologous and allogeneic transplantation. *Bone Marrow Transplant* 1999;24:741.
283. Bjorkstrand B, Ljungman P, Svensson H, et al. Allogenic bone marrow transplantation versus autologous stem cell transplantation in multiple myeloma: a retrospective case-matched study from the European Group for Blood and Marrow Transplantation. *Blood* 1996;88:4711.
284. Alyea EP, Anderson KC. Allotransplantation for multiple myeloma. *Cancer J* 2001;7:166.
285. Mehta J, Tricot G, Jagannath S, et al. Salvage autologous or allogeneic transplantation for multiple myeloma refractory to or relapsing after a first-line autograft? *Bone Marrow Transplant* 1998;21:887.
286. Tricot G, Vesole DH, Jagannath S, et al. Graft-versus-myeloma effect: proof of principle. *Blood* 1996;87:1196.
287. Lokhorst HM, Schattenberg A, Cornelissen JJ, et al. Donor lymphocyte infusions for relapsed multiple myeloma after allogeneic stem-cell transplantation: predictive factors for response and long-term outcome. *Blood* 2000;18:3031.
288. Salama M, Nevill T, Marcellus D, et al. Donor leukocyte infusions for multiple myeloma. *Bone Marrow Transplant* 2000;26:1179.
289. Munshi NC, Govindarajan R, Drake R, et al. Thymidine kinase (TK) gene-transduced human lymphocytes can be highly purified, remain fully functional and are killed efficiently with ganciclovir. *Blood* 1997;89:1334.
290. Soiffer RJ, Alyea EP, Hochberg E, et al. Randomized trial of CD8+ T-cell depletion in the prevention of graft-versus-host disease associated with donor lymphocyte infusion. *Biol Blood Marrow Transplant* 2002;8:625.
291. Storb R, Yu C, Zaucha JM, et al. Stable mixed hematopoietic chimerism in dogs given donor antigen, CTLA4Ig, and 100 cGy total body irradiation before and pharmacologic immunosuppression after marrow transplant. *Blood* 1999;94:2523.
292. Badros A, Barlogie B, Siegel E, et al. Improved outcome of allogeneic transplantation in high-risk multiple myeloma patients after nonmyeloablative conditioning. *J Clin Oncol* 2002;20:1295.
293. Giralt S, Aleman A, Anagnostopoulos A, et al. Fludarabine/melphalan conditioning for allogeneic transplantation in patients with multiple myeloma. *Bone Marrow Transplant* 2002;30:367.
294. Maloney DG, Molina AJ, Sahebi F, et al. Allografting with nonmyeloablative conditioning following cytoreductive autografts for the treatment of patients with multiple myeloma. *Blood* 2003;102:3447.
295. Barlogie B, Desikan R, Eddlemon P, et al. Extended survival in advanced and refractory multiple myeloma after single-agent thalidomide: identification of prognostic factors in a phase 2 study of 169 patients. *Blood* 2001;98:492.
296. Singhal S, Mehta J, Desikan R, et al. Antitumor activity of thalidomide in refractory multiple myeloma [see comments]. *N Engl J Med* 1999;341:1565.
296a. Weber D, Rankin K, Gavino M, Delasalle K, Alexanian R. Thalidomide alone or with dexamethasone for previously untreated multiple myeloma. *J Clin Oncol* 2003;21:16.
296b. Rajkumar SV, Hayman S, Gertz MA, et al. Combination therapy with thalidomide plus dexamethasone for newly diagnosed myeloma. *J Clin Oncol* 2002;20:4319.
297. Raje N, Anderson K. Thalidomide—a revival story [Editorial; Comment]. *N Engl J Med* 1999;341:1606.
297a. Richardson PG, Schlossman RL, Weller E, et al. Immunomodulatory drug CC-5013 overcomes drug resistance and is well tolerated in patients with relapsed multiple myeloma. *Blood.* 2002;100:3063.
297b. Hideshima T, Richardson P, Chauhan D, et al. The proteasome inhibitor PS-341 inhibits growth, induces apoptosis, and overcomes drug resistance in human multiple myeloma cells. *Cancer Res* 2001;61:3071.
297c. Mitsiades N, Mitsiades CS, Poulaki V, et al. Molecular sequelae of proteasome inhibition in human multiple myeloma cells. *Proc Natl Acad Sci U S A* 2002;99:14374.
297d. Richardson PG, Barlogie B, Berenson J, et al. A phase 2 study of bortezomib in relapsed, refractory myeloma. *N Engl J Med* 2003;348:2609.
297e. Mitsiades N, Mitsiades CS, Richardson PG, et al. The proteasome inhibitor PS-341 potentiates sensitivity of multiple myeloma cells to conventional chemotherapeutic agents: therapeutic applications. *Blood* 2003;101:2377.
297f. Hayashi T, Hideshima T, Akiyama M, et al. Arsenic trioxide inhibits growth of human multiple myeloma cells in the bone marrow microenvironment. *Mol Cancer Ther* 2002;1:851.
297g. Munshi NC, Tricot G, Desikan R, et al. Clinical activity of arsenic trioxide for the treatment of multiple myeloma. *Leukemia* 2002;16:1835.
297h. Bahlis NJ, McCafferty-Grad J, Jordan-McMurry I, et al. Feasibility and correlates of arsenic trioxide combined with ascorbic acid-mediated depletion of intracellular glutathione for the treatment of relapsed/refractory multiple myeloma. *Clin Cancer Res* 2002;8:3658.
298. Berenson JR, Lichtenstein A, Porter L, et al. Efficacy of pamidronate in reducing skeletal events in patients with advanced multiple myeloma. *N Engl J Med* 1996;334:488.
299. Apperley JF, Croucher PI. Bisphosphonates in multiple myeloma. *Pathol Biol (Paris)* 1999;47:178.
300. Berenson JR, Lipton A. Bisphosphonates in the treatment of malignant bone disease. *Ann Rev Med* 1999;50:237.
301. Shipman CM, Croucher PI, Russell RG, Helfrich MH, Rogers MJ. The bisphosphonate incadronate (YM175) causes apoptosis of human myeloma cells in vitro by inhibiting the mevalonate pathway. *Cancer Res* 1998;58:5294.
302. Berenson JR, Lichtenstein A, Porter L, et al. Long-term pamidronate treatment of advanced multiple myeloma patients reduces skeletal events. Myeloma Aredia Study Group. *J Clin Oncol* 1998;16:593.
303. Aparicio A, Gardner A, Tu Y, et al. In vitro cytoreductive effects on multiple myeloma cells induced by bisphosphonates. *Leukemia* 1998;12:220.
304. Shipman CM, Rogers MJ, Apperley JF, et al. Anti-tumour activity of bisphosphonates in human myeloma cells. *Leuk Lymphoma* 1998;32:129.
305. Dhodapkar MV, Singh J, Mehta J, et al. Anti-myeloma activity of pamidronate in vivo. *Br J Haematol* 1998;103:530.
306. Waldenström J. Incipient myelomatosis or essential hyperglobulinemia with fibrinogenopenia: a new syndrome? *Acta Med Scand* 1944;117:216.
307. Groves FD, Travis LB, Devesa SS, Ries LA, Fraumeni JF Jr. Waldenström's macroglobulinemia: incidence patterns in the United States, 1988–1994. *Cancer* 1998;82:1078.
308. Fine JM, Muller JY, Rochu D, et al. Waldenström's macroglobulinemia in monozygotic twins. *Acta Med Scand* 1986;220:369.
309. Renier G, Ifrah N, Chevailler A, et al. Four brothers with Waldenström's macroglobulinemia. *Cancer* 1989;64:1554.
310. James JM, Brouet JC, Orvoenfrija E, et al. Waldenström's macroglobulinaemia in a bird breeder: a case history with pulmonary involvement and antibody activity of the monoclonal IgM to canary's droppings. *Clin Exp Immunol* 1987;68:397.
311. Izumi T, Sasaki R, Shimizu R, et al. Hepatitis C virus infection in Waldenström's macroglobulinemia [Letter]. *Am J Hematol* 1996;52:238.
312. Izumi T, Sasaki R, Tsunoda S, et al. B cell malignancy and hepatitis C virus infection. *Leukemia* 1997;11:516.
313. Silvestri F, Barillari G, Fanin R, et al. Risk of hepatitis C virus infection, Waldenström's macroglobulinemia, and monoclonal gammopathies [Letter; Comment]. *Blood* 1996;88:1125.
314. Dimopoulos MA, Panayiotidis P, Moulopoulos LA, Sfikakis P, Dalakas M. Waldenström's macroglobulinemia: clinical features, complications, and management. *J Clin Oncol* 2000;18:214.
315. Calasanz MJ, Cigudosa JC, Odero MD, et al. Cytogenetic analysis of 280 patients with multiple myeloma and related disorders: primary breakpoints and clinical correlations. *Genes Chromosomes Cancer* 1997;18:84.
316. van den Akker TW, Radl J, Franken-Postma E, Hagemeijer A. Cytogenetic findings in mouse multiple myeloma and Waldenström's macroglobulinemia. *Cancer Genet Cytogenet* 1996;86:156.
317. Nishida K, Taniwaki M, Misawa S, Abe T. Nonrandom rearrangement of chromosome 14 at band q32.33 in human lymphoid malignancies with mature B-cell phenotype. *Cancer Res* 1989;49:1275.
318. Waldenström JG. Macroglobulinemia—a review. *Haematologica* 1986;71:437.
319. Andriko JA, Aguilera NS, Chu WS, Nandedkar MA, Cotelingam JD. Waldenström's macroglobulinemia: a clinicopathologic study of 22 cases. *Cancer* 1997;80:1926.
320. Pruzanski W, Chu R, Damji NF, Galler S, Norman CS. Anemia, splenomegaly and hyperviscosity syndrome. *Can Med Assoc J* 1980;123:731.
321. Dalakas MC, Flaum MA, Rick M, Engel WK, Gralnick HR. Treatment of polyneuropathy in Waldenström's macroglobulinemia: role of paraproteinemia and immunologic studies. *Neurology* 1983;33:1406.
322. Meier C, Roberts K, Steck A, et al. Polyneuropathy in Waldenström's macroglobulinaemia: reduction of endoneurial IgM-deposits after treatment with chlorambucil and plasmapheresis. *Acta Neuropathol* 1984;64:297.
323. Virella G, Lopes-Virella MF. Effects of therapeutically useful thiols (DL-penicillamine and alpha-mercaptopropionylglycine) on immunoglobulins. *Clin Exp Immunol* 1970;7:85.
324. Waldenström JG. Plasmapheresis—bloodletting revived and refined. *Acta Med Scand* 1980;208:1.
325. Waldenström JG. Plasmapheresis and cold sensitivity of immunoglobulin molecules. II. A study of macroglobulinemia polyclonalis spuria and immune complex disease. *Acta Med Scand* 1984;216:467.
326. Buskard NA, Galton DA, Goldman JM, et al. Plasma exchange in the long-term management of Waldenström's macroglobulinemia. *Can Med Assoc J* 1977;117:135.
327. Petrucci MT, Avvisati G, Tribalto M, Giovangrossi P, Mandelli F. Waldenström's macroglobulinaemia: results of a combined oral treatment in 34 newly diagnosed patients. *J Intern Med* 1989;226:443.
328. Kantarjian HM, Alexanian R, Koller CA, Kurzrock R, Keating MJ. Fludarabine therapy in macroglobulinemic lymphoma. *Blood* 1990;75:1928.
329. Dimopoulos MA, O'Brien S, Kantarjian H, et al. Fludarabine therapy in Waldenström's macroglobulinemia. *Am J Med* 1993;95:49.
330. Dimopoulos MA, Kantarjian H, Weber D, et al. Primary therapy of Waldenström's macroglobulinemia with 2-chlorodeoxyadenosine. *J Clin Oncol* 1994;12:2694.
331. Zinzani PL, Gherlinzoni F, Bendandi M, et al. Fludarabine treatment in resistant Waldenström's macroglobulinemia. *Eur J Haematol* 1995;54:120.
332. Dhodapkar M, Jacobson J, Gertz M, et al. Phase II intergroup trial of fludarabine in Waldenström's macroglobulinemia: results of Southwest Oncology Group trial (SWOG 9003) in 220 patients. *Blood* 1997;90:577a.
333. Rotoli B, De Renzo A, Frigeri F, et al. A phase II trial on alpha-interferon (alpha IFN) effect in patients with monoclonal IgM gammopathy. *Leuk Lymphoma* 1994;13:463.
334. Legouffe E, Rossi JF, Laporte JP, et al. Treatment of Waldenström's macroglobulinemia with very low doses of alpha interferon. *Leuk Lymphoma* 1995;19:337.
335. Clamon GH, Corder MP, Burns CP. Successful doxorubicin therapy of primary macroglobulinemia resistant to alkylating agents. *Am J Hematol* 1980;9:221.
336. Jane SM, Salem HH. Treatment of resistant Waldenström's macroglobulinemia with high dose glucocorticosteroids. *Aust N Z J Med* 1988;18:77.
337. Humphrey JS, Conley CL. Durable complete remission of macroglobulinemia after splenectomy: a report of two cases and review of the literature. *Am J Hematol* 1995;48:262.
338. Takemori N, Hirai K, Onodera R, Kimura S, Katagiri M. Durable remission after splenectomy for Waldenström's macroglobulinemia with massive splenomegaly in leukemic phase. *Leuk Lymphoma* 1997;26:387.
339. Desikan KR, Dhodapkar M, Siegel D, et al. High-dose therapy with autologous peripheral blood stem cell support for Waldenström's macroglobulinemia: a pilot study. *Br J Hematol* 1999;105:993.

Susanne M. Arnold
Frank S. Lieberman
Kenneth A. Foon

CHAPTER **45**

Paraneoplastic Syndromes

Tumors may produce signs and symptoms distant from the primary site or its metastases, and these are referred to as *paraneoplastic syndromes*. The syndromes may be due to (1) tumor production of substances that directly or indirectly cause distant symptoms, (2) depletion of normal substances that leads to a paraneoplastic manifestation, or (3) host response to the tumor that results in the syndrome. Perhaps the best-characterized paraneoplastic syndromes are those producing polypeptide hormones, such as adrenocorticotropic hormone (ACTH) or parathyroid hormones, that affect organ function at remote sites. Such paraneoplastic syndromes parallel the underlying malignancy, and successful treatment of the tumor leads to disappearance of the syndrome (hormone). Additional tumor-derived proteins responsible for paraneoplastic syndromes have been identified, including various growth factors and cytokines such as interleukin-1 (IL-1) and tumor necrosis factor (TNF). Malignancies may produce antibodies that lead to neurologic paraneoplastic syndromes such as the Eaton-Lambert syndrome. Many paraneoplastic syndromes, especially those of an immune or neurologic etiology, do not predictably resolve with treatment of the underlying malignancy.

The paraneoplastic syndrome may be the first sign of a malignancy, and its recognition may be critical for early cancer detection. Proteins secreted in paraneoplastic syndromes may be used as tumor markers. In some situations, the underlying disease cannot be treated, but the symptoms and complications of the paraneoplastic syndrome can be successfully managed. This chapter reviews the wide range of paraneoplastic syndromes, including endocrine, hematologic, gastrointestinal (GI), renal, cutaneous, and neurologic paraneoplastic syndromes.

ENDOCRINOLOGIC MANIFESTATIONS OF CANCER

Cancers can produce endocrine syndromes or "ectopic" hormone syndromes through the production of cytokines, protein hormones, or hormone precursors by the tumor. Rarely cancers can metabolize steroids to biologically active forms, which results in paraneoplastic syndromes. In general, treatment of the underlying malignancy results in resolution of the endocrinologic paraneoplastic syndrome.

ECTOPIC ADRENOCORTICOTROPIC HORMONE SYNDROME

First described by Brown in 1928, the syndrome of ectopic ACTH was further characterized in 1965 in 88 patients with Cushing's syndrome and cancer.[1] This report was the first to suggest that tumors produced ACTH or an ACTH-like substance that led to adrenal hyperplasia and hypercortisolism, and thus the term *ectopic ACTH production* was coined. Subsequently, the gene responsible, the proopiomelanocortin (POMC) gene, was cloned. POMC contains not only ACTH, but melanocyte-stimulating hormone, β-lipotropin, endorphins, and enkephalins.[2] Tumors process POMC in different ways—small cell lung cancers (SCLCs), for example, release a higher level of ACTH precursors in the circulation, whereas carcinoid tumors produce intact ACTH in large amounts.[1,3] Ectopic ACTH production is commonly associated with SCLC but can also be found in a variety of neoplasms (Table 45-1). Although 3% to 7% of patients with SCLC develop Cushing's syndrome, many patients with SCLC secrete ACTH precursors without developing the syndrome.[4]

TABLE 45-1.   Tumors Associated with Ectopic Adrenocorticotropic Hormone

Tumor Type	Liddle, Island, Ney, et al.[1]	Crapo[4]	Howlett, Drury, Perry, et al.[a]	Wajchenberg, Mendonca, Liberman, et al.[2]	Odell[b]
Small cell lung carcinoma	50	49	19	8	50
Bronchial carcinoid	8	8	37	17	2
Thymic carcinomas	10	12	12	25	10
Pancreas	10	6	12	25	10
Pheochromocytoma	3	2	6	25	5
Medullary cancer of the thyroid	2	6	—	—	5
Gastrointestinal carcinoid	6	—	—	—	—
Adenocarcinoma	7	2	—	—	—
Miscellaneous	10	10	12	—	18

[a]Howlett TA, Drury PL, Perry L, et al. Diagnosis and management of ACTH-dependent Cushing's syndrome: comparison of the features in ectopic and pituitary ACTH production. *Clin Endocrinol* 1986;24:699.
[b]Odell W. Endocrine/metabolic syndromes of cancer. *Semin Oncol* 1997;214:299.

Clinical Presentation

The differential diagnosis of a patient with hypercortisolism includes Cushing's disease, adrenal dysfunction, ectopic ACTH production, and corticotropin-releasing hormone (CRH) overproduction. Pituitary overproduction (Cushing's disease) is the cause in over 55% of patients, followed in frequency by adrenal dysfunction, ectopic ACTH production (occurring in 11% to 25%), and CRH overproduction, which is quite rare.[5,6] Cushing's disease is more common in young women than in young men (3:1), whereas older individuals of both genders (at higher risk for lung cancer) typically have ectopic ACTH production. Signs and symptoms of classic hypercortisolism include truncal obesity, purple striae, hypertension, fatigue, moon facies, buffalo hump, weakness, depression, amenorrhea, hirsutism, and edema. In contrast, ectopic ACTH production from SCLC causes myopathy with weakness, muscle wasting, weight loss, hyperpigmentation, and hypokalemia. Carcinoid tumors that secrete ectopic ACTH may cause signs and symptoms that overlap those of pituitary-dependent Cushing's disease and paraneoplastic ACTH overproduction.

Diagnosis

Distinguishing between pituitary adenoma, ectopic ACTH production, and primary adrenal disorders is the primary focus of the diagnostic workup (Fig. 45-1). The two most common screening tests for cortisol overproduction are measurement of the 24-hour urinary free cortisol level and the low-dose dexamethasone suppression test. In healthy subjects cortisol production should be suppressed by a relatively low dose of dexamethasone, whereas patients with Cushing's disease or ectopic ACTH production are not affected.

With reliable radioassays of ACTH, plasma levels can be determined early in the diagnostic workup. In primary adrenal disease, ACTH levels are low, whereas in ACTH-dependent Cushing's syndrome the ACTH level is elevated. Classically, plasma ACTH and ACTH precursor levels in ectopic ACTH production are much higher than in Cushing's disease (pituitary adenoma); however, there is a great deal of overlap, particularly in the case of slow-growing malignancies such as carcinoids. If normal or elevated ACTH levels are present (which thus eliminates primary adrenal disease), a high-dose

dexamethasone suppression test is indicated. High-dose dexamethasone suppresses cortisol production in patients with Cushing's disease but in those with ectopic ACTH production or primary adrenal disorders.[6] False-positive results are seen when dexamethasone is metabolized more rapidly than normal through drug–drug interactions (such as with diphenylhydantoin or phenobarbital) or in disease states such as thyrotoxicosis. Furthermore, bronchial carcinoids can show ACTH and cortisol suppression with high-dose dexamethasone testing in 40% to 50% of cases.[7]

The metyrapone and CRH stimulation tests have been developed because of the limitations of the dexamethasone suppression test. In both tests the sensitivity of pituitary adenoma to stimulation by either cortisol deprivation (metyrapone) or directly by CRH is exploited. Metyrapone blocks the production of cortisol in the adrenal by inhibiting the conversion of 11-deoxycortisol to cortisol, which leads to an increased ACTH

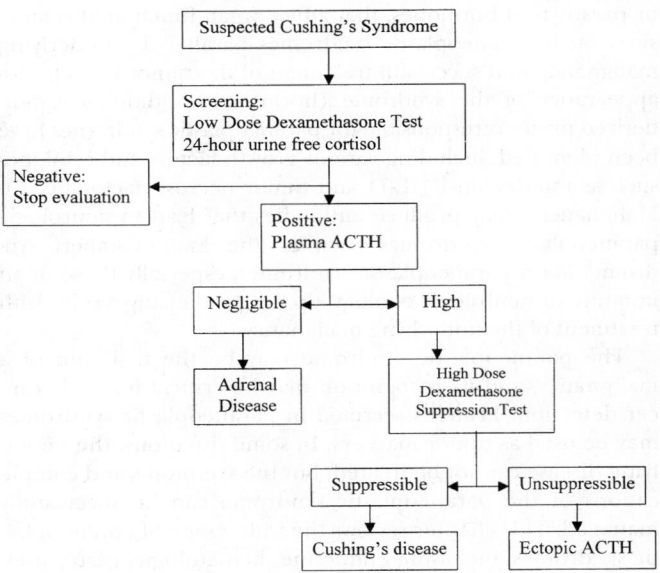

FIGURE 45-1.   Diagnostic algorithm for the evaluation of patients with suspected Cushing's syndrome. See text for details of various tests. ACTH, adrenocorticotropic hormone.

secretion in normal patients; it thus tests the integrity of the adrenal-cortisol-pituitary feedback loop. Patients with Cushing's disease show stimulated ACTH production, whereas ectopic ACTH production is unaffected. In the largest reported study, the metyrapone test correctly predicted Cushing's in 71% of patients with ACTH-dependent Cushing's syndrome. Combining the dexamethasone suppression test and the metyrapone test improved the predictive accuracy to 82%.[8] CRH stimulation causes increased ACTH levels in pituitary adenomas but not in ectopic ACTH-producing tumors. In one report of 41 patients with ACTH-dependent hypercortisolism, 29 of 33 patients with pituitary adenomas showed stimulation when given ovine CRH, whereas none of the 8 patients with ectopic ACTH production showed stimulation.[9] This led to a sensitivity of 88%, a specificity of 100%, and a diagnostic accuracy of 90%, which compared favorably with the standard dexamethasone suppression test. Again, the combination of CRH stimulation and dexamethasone suppression led to a superior diagnostic accuracy of 98%.

Once the diagnosis of ectopic ACTH production has been established, localization is the most important aspect of therapy. Because a major portion of patients with ectopic ACTH secretion have lung cancer, plain radiography followed by computed tomography (CT) detects more than 90% of the lung tumors associated with ACTH production.[7] The exception is bronchial carcinoid tumors, which are visualized on 36% of initial radiographs but are localized by CT scan in approximately 85% of cases.[10] Octreotide receptor scintigraphy has been promoted for localizing ACTH-producing tumors, because many such tumors have octreotide receptors.[11] An additional advantage of localizing tumors with octreotide receptor scintigraphy is the suggestion of possible therapy with either somatostatin analogues or radiolabeled octreotide.

Treatment

Surgery is the treatment of choice in patients with early-stage tumors producing Cushing's syndrome because it can completely alleviate symptoms. In one series of 41 patients with ectopic ACTH production and absence of SCLC, 16 of 21 patients (76%) with localized tumors were cured of Cushing's syndrome through surgery. Specifically, 81% of bronchial carcinoid tumors were cured by resection, and 9 of 12 patients (75%) with occult ACTH production experienced palliation with bilateral adrenalectomy.[12] Although bilateral adrenal removal is effective in treating Cushing's syndrome, the patient must have lifelong glucocorticoid and mineralocorticoid replacement. Patients with severe muscle weakness and uncontrolled hypertension are candidates for this approach. The use of laparoscopic adrenalectomy has been reported to provide effective palliation in patients with Cushing's syndrome, with minimal morbidity and no mortality reported.[13]

The majority of patients do not have surgically resectable disease and may have ongoing symptoms related to Cushing's syndrome. Medical therapy for ectopic ACTH production centers on inhibiting cortisol production with mitotane, aminoglutethimide, metyrapone, or ketoconazole (Table 45-2).[14-16] Mitotane is effective in lowering cortisol levels; however, it is rarely used because of its severe toxicity and slow onset of action. Aminoglutethimide used alone has limited success, but when combined with metyrapone is an effective treatment. Because of its rapid onset of action and favorable toxicity profile, ketocona-

TABLE 45-2. Drugs Used for Treating Ectopic Adrenocorticotropic Hormone Production

Drug	Dose
Ketoconazole	400–1200 mg/d
Metyrapone	500–4000 mg/d
Aminoglutethimide	500–2000 mg/d
Mitotane	4–12 g/d
Sandostatin	300–1500 µg/d

zole has evolved as the therapy of choice for ectopic ACTH. In one small study,[16] 66% of patients with ectopic ACTH production had a hormonal response and symptomatic improvement with ketoconazole at a dosage of 400 to 1200 mg/d. A minority developed symptomatic hypoadrenalism.

Primary suppression of ACTH production can be accomplished by cytotoxic chemotherapy for the primary malignancy or octreotide suppression of ACTH release. In general, chemotherapy alone is not associated with control of Cushing's syndrome but is combined with adrenal suppression in most cases. If patients show significant localization with octreotide receptor scintigraphy, a trial of octreotide may be in order. Use of the combination of ketoconazole and octreotide has also been reported.[17]

SYNDROME OF INAPPROPRIATE ANTIDIURETIC HORMONE PRODUCTION

Recognition of the syndrome of inappropriate antidiuretic hormone production (SIADH) as a paraneoplastic syndrome was first reported in 1957,[18] with confirmation of this hypothesis in 1968, when arginine vasopressin was extracted from cancers associated with the syndrome.[19] Although the majority of SCLC specimens test positive for arginine vasopressin by radioimmune assay, only 3% to 15% of patients with SCLC have the syndrome.[20]

The pathophysiology of SIADH is well described. After vasopressin is released, it binds to specific receptors in the renal collecting ducts and ascending limb of the loop of Henle. Excess water is reabsorbed and increased sodium is delivered to the distal nephron. This increases intravascular volume, which in turn increases renal perfusion and decreases proximal tubular resorption of sodium. Antidiuretic hormone secretion continues in SIADH despite the decrease in plasma osmolality, causing eventual hyponatremia.[21]

Clinical Features and Diagnosis

The cardinal features of SIADH are water intoxication and hyponatremia, including the following principal findings: decreased serum osmolarity, inappropriate elevation of urine osmolarity with urine sodium levels higher than 20 mEq/L, euvolemia (absence of hypovolemia), normal renal function, normal adrenal function, and normal thyroid function. Most patients are asymptomatic, but when symptoms develop they generally reflect central nervous system toxicity. In the early stages, patients complain of fatigue, anorexia, headaches, and mildly altered mental status. As the syndrome progresses, patients may experience continued delirium, confusion, and seizures. Ultimately, patients develop refractory seizures, coma, and, in rare cases, death. Most patients, however, experience minimal symptoms and are discovered to have hyponatremia on routine laboratory evaluation.

In evaluating a patient with hyponatremia and cancer, other causes of hyponatremia need to be considered. In general, the first step in evaluating patients with hyponatremia is to assess volume status. SIADH is one of the euvolemic hyponatremic states. Therefore, it is necessary to rule out states associated with volume overload such as congestive heart failure, nephrotic syndrome, malignant ascites, and significant liver disease. It is also essential to exclude extrarenal volume depletion and renal sodium wasting. Once the patient is determined to be euvolemic, other causes of euvolemic hyponatremia must be ruled out, including hypothyroidism, renal dysfunction, and Addison's disease. A careful review of medications is also essential.

Once the diagnosis of SIADH is made, a wide variety of causes must be considered, including central nervous system diseases, pulmonary diseases, and drug effects. Tumor-associated SIADH is a diagnosis of exclusion. For the purposes of treatment, however, differentiating tumor-related SIADH from other causes of SIADH is not necessary. It is rarely necessary to perform a water-loading test to make the diagnosis of SIADH. Because these patients are often unable to excrete free water, they can develop significant water intoxication, which leads to serious morbidity in this setting. The principal malignancy associated with SIADH is SCLC (75% of cases), although others have been described (non–small cell lung cancer, head and neck cancer, and others).

Treatment

As with any syndrome associated with ectopic hormone production, treating the underlying disease is the most effective means of controlling SIADH. Chemotherapy treatment of the associated SCLC is generally associated with improvement in the syndrome. SIADH has not been shown to be a negative prognostic factor in terms of response to chemotherapy. In situations in which brain metastases are present, the addition of radiation therapy is important.

Supportive measures such as fluid restriction and pharmacologic therapy can be undertaken to treat SIADH. Patients with sodium levels under 130 mmol/L are placed on free water restriction (500 mL/d), in addition to being treated for the primary malignancy.[22] In the event that the serum sodium level does not normalize, pharmacologic agents such as demeclocycline that inhibit the effect of arginine vasopressin on the kidneys are indicated. The recommended dosage of demeclocycline is 600 to 1200 mg/d in divided doses. Other less common medications that have reported efficacy include fludrocortisone, urea, and lithium. Finally, in severe cases in which patients have life-threatening convulsions or coma, patients can be treated with hypertonic saline solution with intravenous furosemide. It is important not to raise the serum sodium level too rapidly (the recommendation is 1 mEq/L/h) due to the risk of central pontine myelinolysis.[23] It is generally thought that hypertonic saline and furosemide treatment should be carried out in the intensive care unit setting.

HYPOCALCEMIA

Although most of the discussion regarding disturbance of calcium balance and malignancy revolves around hypercalcemia,

hypocalcemia is actually more common in patients with bone metastases. Tumors associated with lytic bone metastases such as breast, prostate, and lung cancers can lead to hypocalcemia.[24] Hypocalcemia can also occur in patients whose tumors secrete calcitonin (i.e., medullary carcinoma of the thyroid and, rarely, breast cancer, colorectal cancer, SCLC, and carcinoid). Patients are rarely symptomatic but occasionally develop tetany and neuromuscular irritability. Asymptomatic patients can show mild neuromuscular dysfunction by electromyography. Therapy, consisting of calcium infusion, is reserved for those patients with findings of neuromuscular irritability or symptoms such as tetany and seizures. Signs of neuromuscular irritability including Chvostek's sign and Trousseau's sign (carpal spasm with decreased blood flow) indicate the need for calcium infusion. For a discussion of hypercalcemia, please refer to Chapter 49.4.

ONCOGENOUS OSTEOMALACIA

Rickets is a well-recognized inborn error of metabolism, whereas the adult counterpart, osteomalacia, is usually secondary to intestinal malabsorption syndrome, renal tubular acidosis, and chronic renal insufficiency. Oncogenous osteomalacia is a rare syndrome characterized by osteomalacia, hypophosphatemia, hyperphosphaturia, and decreased vitamin D levels. Mean age at diagnosis is approximately 35 years. Patients typically present with bone pain, phosphaturia, renal glycosuria, hypophosphatemia, normocalcemia with normal parathyroid hormone function, low levels of 1,25-dihydroxyvitamin D_3, and increased alkaline phosphatase levels. The proposed mechanisms include inhibition of the conversion of 1,25-dihydroxyvitamin D_3 and a tumor-secreted *phosphaturic substance*. It is usually associated with benign mesenchymal tumors including hemangiomas and hemangiopericytomas but rarely is seen with multiple myeloma and prostate cancer.[25,26] The typical tumor involves prominent giant cells, spindle cells, and a high degree of vascularity. Approximately one-half of the tumors are in the lower extremities, and the remaining tumors are divided between the head and neck and upper extremities, with some patients having tumors at multiple sites. The definitive therapy is removal of the tumor, if possible. Otherwise, treatment requires large doses of vitamin D and phosphate.

GONADOTROPIN SECRETION

The human hormones with gonadotropic properties are follicle-stimulating hormone (FSH), luteinizing hormone (LH), and human chorionic gonadotropin (HCG).[27] These three hormones are composed of two polypeptide chains: α and β subunits. The α subunit is common to all of the hormones and the β subunit determines biologic and immunologic specificity. The pituitary produces fluctuating levels of FSH and LH, whereas biologically active HCG is produced by the placenta and is normally found only in pregnant women. Although many studies have shown elevations of HCG in nonmalignant chronic diseases, values for the α and β subunits of HCG are significantly higher in cancer patients than in patients with nonmalignant disease.[27]

Gonadotropin secretion may occur in pituitary tumors, gestational trophoblastic tumors, germ cell tumors, hepatoblastomas in children, bronchogenic carcinomas, and GI cancers.[28,29]

Gonadotropins measured in tumors arising in gestational tissue, testes, ovaries, and endocrine organs are valuable tumor markers and are discussed in Chapters 31, and 32, and 34.

The frequency of symptoms associated with tumor-produced gonadotropin is unknown. The most common problem is that of a male patient presenting with unexplained gynecomastia. In this situation, β-HCG level should be determined, and a careful examination of the testes and radiographic examination of the chest and mediastinum should be performed. Germ cell tumors of the testes or extragonadal sites and lung cancers are the most frequent causes of the combination of gynecomastia and HCG elevation, whereas adrenal carcinoma, hepatoma, GI tract tumors, and tumors of the genitourinary tract are less common causes.[30–32] Histologic specimens have revealed that all of these tumors contain syncytial giant cells or choriocarcinomatous elements similar to trophoblastic germ cell tumors. Treatment of the underlying malignancy can resolve gynecomastia. Because the α subunit of HCG is identical to that of thyroid-stimulating hormone, rare cases of hyperthyroidism in the setting of excess HCG due to testis cancer have been reported.[33] Other cases of hyperthyroidism have been noted in choriocarcinoma due to the same mechanism.[34] In these cases thyrotoxicosis is rare, and treatment with antithyroidal drugs (e.g., propylthiouracil or methimazole) or chemotherapy resolves the hyperthyroidism.[33]

TUMOR-PRODUCED HUMAN PLACENTAL LACTOGEN, GROWTH HORMONE–RELEASING HORMONE, AND PROLACTIN

Human placental lactogen has been detected in a small percentage of patients with nontrophoblastic nongonadal tumors. This may be associated with elevated levels of estrogen, HCG, and gynecomastia. The detection of human placental lactogen in nonpregnant women is diagnostic of malignancy.[35]

Elevated growth hormone levels have been reported in rare patients with gastric and lung cancer.[36] Whether this is due to ectopic production or overproduction by cells that retain the ability to secrete growth hormone from primordial origin remains controversial. Growth hormone–releasing hormone production has also been reported in nonpituitary tumors and, as in pituitary tumors, results in acromegaly.[37] This 44–amino acid peptide has been isolated from pancreatic tumors as well as bronchial and foregut carcinoids. Secretion of growth hormone–releasing hormone can be controlled by administration of long-acting somatostatin analogues. The definitive therapy is removal of the tumor, whenever possible.

Patients with cancers of the lung, colon, breast, ovary, and cervix, and with renal adenocarcinoma have been reported who have elevated prolactin levels and, rarely, galactorrhea.[38] Symptoms can be subtle. Male patients may only exhibit decreased libido, whereas postmenopausal women may have no symptoms. Treatment of the tumor decreases prolactin levels. Because these cases are extremely rare, it is important to exclude the presence of a pituitary lesion in patients with elevated prolactin levels.

HYPOGLYCEMIA

Insulinomas frequently produce hypoglycemia; however, hypoglycemia associated with non–islet cell tumors is an unusual paraneoplastic syndrome. Mesenchymal tumors, including a variety of sarcomas and mesotheliomas, are the most common cause of non–islet cell–induced hypoglycemia. Rarely, adrenal carcinomas, GI cancers, and varied other tumors have been associated with hypoglycemia.[38,39] These tumors are typically large, often invade the liver, and have a protracted course. The patient may present with typical signs and symptoms of hypoglycemia, including generalized neurologic abnormalities.

The causes of paraneoplastic hypoglycemia are varied: production of nonsuppressible insulin-like growth factor-1 (IGF-1) and IGF-2, hypermetabolism of glucose, production of substances stimulating ectopic insulin release, production of hepatic glucose inhibitor, insulin binding by a monoclonal protein, insulin receptor proliferation, or rarely ectopic insulin production.[40–43] The most likely mechanism is tumor production of IGFs (also called *somatomedins*), a family of peptide hormones normally produced by the liver under growth hormone regulation.[44,45] Several reports have specifically identified excess production of pro–IGF-2, which binds to insulin and IGF receptors in malignancy. This down-regulates growth hormone secretion and decreases hepatic production of IGF-binding proteins with eventual hypoglycemia.[46]

The treatment of paraneoplastic hypoglycemia initially involves glucose infusion. After this, tumor debulking should be carried out, although the long-term effect of debulking is poorly understood. If treatment of the tumor is not possible, then the use of subcutaneous and long-acting intramuscular glucagons, high-dose corticosteroids, or somatostatin analogues may be considered.

HEMATOLOGIC MANIFESTATIONS OF CANCER

Paraneoplastic syndromes that involve hematopoietic cells and clotting factors are extremely common. Although the etiologies of most of these paraneoplastic abnormalities remain unexplained, advances in the understanding of hormones and growth factors that regulate hematopoiesis has led to a better understanding of some of these disorders.

ERYTHROCYTOSIS

The most common solid tumor leading to erythrocytosis is renal cell carcinoma, which is often associated with elevated serum erythropoietin levels. The next most common malignancy leading to erythrocytosis is hepatoma, in which erythrocytosis is also secondary to erythropoietin production. Other tumors leading to erythrocytosis include Wilms' tumor, hemangiomas, cerebellar hemangioblastoma, uterine fibroids, adrenal tumors, and pheochromocytomas.[47] In adrenal cortical tumors and virilizing ovarian tumors, it is hypothesized that the production of androgenic hormones and prostaglandins[48] can enhance the effect of erythropoietin and lead to erythrocytosis.

It is important to rule out other causes of erythrocytosis, even in the presence of a tumor. Polycythemia rubra vera is typically associated with elevated white cell and platelet counts as well as splenomegaly. There are obvious causes of polycythemia secondary to arterial desaturation associated with hemoglobinopathies, carboxyhemoglobinemia, and chronic hypoxic states.

Erythropoietin can be measured in the blood when it is suspected that it is overproduced secondary to a tumor. Erythrocytosis secondary to tumors is usually not high enough to require treatment, but if the hematocrit is extremely high (i.e., higher than 55% in a man or higher than 50% in a woman) phlebotomy can be used. Control of the tumor usually controls the erythrocytosis, as well.

ANEMIA

The most common anemias in cancer patients are normocytic normochromic anemia of chronic disease, anemia secondary to bone marrow invasion (often associated with leukoerythroblastosis), and anemia secondary to chemotherapy and radiation treatment. Normochromic, normocytic anemia of cancer is a common paraneoplastic syndrome, characterized by low serum iron levels, normal or increased ferritin levels, normal iron stores, and a low serum erythropoietin level. It is thought that IL-1, TNF, and transforming growth factor-β are produced by tumors and effect a decreased erythropoietin response.[49,50]

A rare cause of anemia in cancer patients is pure red cell aplasia. One well-described paraneoplastic syndrome is that of thymoma and pure red cell aplasia with associated hypogammaglobulinemia.[51] Pure red cell aplasia may also be associated with a variety of lymphoid malignancies, including chronic lymphocytic leukemia (CLL) and large granular lymphocytic lymphoma and leukemia.[52] Rarely, pure red cell aplasia is associated with solid tumors.

Autoimmune hemolytic anemias are typically associated with B-cell malignancies, including CLL and lymphomas, and arise secondary to immunoregulatory abnormalities in these diseases, rather than to a direct secretion of tumor-derived substances. Hallmarks of the disease are a positive direct antiglobulin test result, elevated reticulocyte count, decreased haptoglobin level, and elevated lactate dehydrogenase level. Warm antibody hemolytic anemia is most commonly associated with lymphomas, CLL, and mucin-producing adenocarcinomas. Cold agglutinin disease is most common in Waldenström's macroglobulinemia and lymphomas.[52] Autoimmune hemolytic anemia is rarely associated with solid tumors; however, an association with ovarian, GI, lung, breast, and renal cell cancers has been reported.[52] Corticosteroid treatment appears to be less effective in autoimmune hemolytic anemia associated with carcinomas than in those that are idiopathic or associated with lymphoid malignancies. The Coombs' test result may revert to negative with control of the tumor.

Microangiopathic hemolytic anemia is characterized by fragmentation of red cells, and although often observed in thrombotic thrombocytopenic purpura and the hemolytic-uremic syndrome, it has also been reported in association with malignancy.[50,53] Such patients may have intimal proliferation of arterioles, intravascular tumor growth, or intravascular fibrin precipitation, with or without thrombocytopenia. Disseminated intravascular coagulation (DIC) may contribute to microangiopathic hemolytic anemia in metastatic carcinomas by inducing the red cell fragmentation from fibrin strands. Patients typically have pronounced schistocytosis with *microspherocytes*, spherocyte-shaped erythrocytes smaller than 5 μm in diameter. The reticulocyte count is typically increased, and a leukoerythroblastic blood picture may predominate. Microangiopathic hemolytic anemia is typically associated with adenocarcinoma of the GI tract, heart, lung, and prostate. The mechanism remains unknown. The microangiopathic hemolytic anemia syndrome may respond to effective anticancer therapy.

GRANULOCYTOSIS

Granulocytosis with elevation of the white blood cell count above $15 \times 10^9/L$ without infection or leukemia is common in neoplasms.[54] Neoplasms most commonly associated with granulocytosis include Hodgkin's disease, lymphoma, and a variety of solid tumors, including gastric, lung, pancreatic, and brain cancer, and malignant melanoma. Paraneoplastic granulocytosis consists of mature neutrophils, in contrast to chronic myelogenous leukemia, in which more immature forms are seen, along with basophils and eosinophils, a decreased leukocyte alkaline phosphatase level, elevated vitamin B_{12} level and vitamin B_{12}–binding capacity, and the presence of the Philadelphia chromosome. The common mechanism associated with tumor-associated granulocytosis is tumor production of growth factors, including granulocyte colony-stimulating factor, granulocyte-macrophage colony-stimulating factor, IL-3, IL-1, and a variety of others.[55,56]

GRANULOCYTOPENIA

Granulocytopenia is typically secondary to chemotherapy, radiation therapy, or tumor infiltration of bone marrow. Rarely, tumors may produce a factor that suppresses granulopoiesis by interfering with any number of growth factors. As well, there are rare reports of antibodies against granulocytes in patients with Hodgkin's disease and non–chemotherapy-induced neutropenia.[57] Neutropenia associated with large granular lymphocytic leukemia and lymphoma may be caused by immune dysregulation of T cells. The preferred therapy for severe granulocytopenia is direct stimulation with growth factors, including granulocyte colony-stimulating factor or granulocyte-macrophage colony-stimulating factor.

EOSINOPHILIA AND BASOPHILIA

Eosinophilia is commonly associated with Hodgkin's disease and mycosis fungoides and is rarely associated with other lymphomas and solid tumors. The tumor cells may be producing a factor that specifically stimulates eosinophil production, such as granulocyte-macrophage colony-stimulating factor, IL-3, or IL-5.[58] Extremely high eosinophil counts can cause symptoms similar to those of Löffler's syndrome, which is associated with nodular pulmonary infiltrates with cough and fever in rare cases. Basophilia is associated with chronic myelogenous leukemia and a variety of other myeloproliferative disorders but does not typically give rise to symptoms.

THROMBOCYTOSIS

Thrombocytosis is quite common in cancer patients and may be associated with Hodgkin's disease, lymphomas, and a variety of carcinomas and leukemias.[59] Thrombocytosis is expected early in the course of a variety of myeloproliferative diseases, including polycythemia rubra vera and chronic myelogenous leukemia. In patients with cancer and thrombocytosis it is important to exclude underlying secondary causes such as inflammatory disorders, hemorrhage, iron deficiency, hemolytic anemia, and splenectomy. The thrombocytosis secondary to malignancies may be caused by overproduction of thrombopoietin.[60] Thrombosis and hemorrhage are rarely associated with this paraneoplastic syndrome, and treatment is not generally indicated.

THROMBOCYTOPENIA

Thrombocytopenia in cancer patients is typically secondary to therapy, DIC, or tumor infiltration of bone marrow. A syndrome similar to idiopathic thrombocytopenic purpura is commonly seen in lymphoid malignancies including CLL and lymphomas, as well as Hodgkin's disease. Rarely, solid tumors such as lung, breast, and GI cancers have been associated with a similar syndrome.[61,62] These patients may have bleeding, petechiae, and purpura and may respond to high-dose prednisone, splenectomy, or both. Other common causes of thrombocytopenia, such as use of heparin, thiazide diuretics, and a variety of other drugs, should be ruled out. As is typical of nonparaneoplastic idiopathic thrombocytopenic purpura, patients have adequate or increased megakaryocytes in the bone marrow and do not respond to transfusion of platelets.

THROMBOPHLEBITIS

The association of cancer and thrombophlebitis was first observed by Trousseau.[63] Recurrent deep venous thrombosis, warfarin resistance, and thrombosis at unusual sites should increase suspicion of occult malignancy in a patient without a known cancer diagnosis. The greatest risk of migratory thrombophlebitis is with pancreatic cancer; however, it may be seen in a variety of adenocarcinomas, including breast, ovarian, and prostate cancer. The activation of coagulation factors V, VII, IX, and XI as well as fibrinogen and fibrin degradation products occurs. Increased secretion of plasminogen activators and decrease in their inhibitors, activation of platelets, and increased platelet aggregation all assist in increasing thrombosis risk.[64] Clearly, cancer-related thrombosis represents a complex imbalance of coagulation and fibrinolysis: increased fibrinogen and platelet catabolism; decreased levels of protein C, protein S, and antithrombin; direct generation of thrombin; and thrombocytosis all represent abnormalities associated with malignancy.[65]

There have been several advances in the diagnostic accuracy of testing for venous thromboembolism (VTE) in the past few years, including a standardized clinical model to determine pretest probability of VTE, the measurement of plasma D-dimer, compression ultrasonography, and impedance plethysmography.[64] Studies in cancer patients suspected of having VTE have confirmed that normal results on the D-dimer test, compression ultrasonography, or impedance plethysmography and a low pretest probability of VTE can reliably exclude VTE.[64,66] The treatment may include unfractionated heparin, low-molecular-weight heparin, and warfarin. Studies conducted over the past 15 years have proven that low-molecular-weight heparin is as effective and safe as unfractionated heparin,[64,67] and several metaanalyses indicate that use of low-molecular-weight heparin may decrease mortality in cancer patients with thrombosis.[68,69] Treatment of the underlying malignancy is the most definitive therapy, but is usually unsuccessful in these particular diseases.

DISSEMINATED INTRAVASCULAR COAGULATION AND COAGULOPATHIES

As stated previously in Thrombophlebitis, cancer patients often have elevated levels of fibrin or fibrinogen degradation products, thrombocytosis, and hyperfibrinogenemia, representing overcompensated DIC with fibrinolysis.[64] Overt DIC occurs in 7% of patients with solid tumors (primarily adenocarcinomas). Older age, breast cancer, male gender, advanced stage, and the presence of necrosis in the tumor specimen are independent risk factors for DIC.[70] Thrombocytopenia, prolonged prothrombin time and partial thromboplastin time, decreased fibrinogen levels, and increased levels of fibrin degradation products and D-dimer are the hallmarks of DIC in cancer patients.[70] Acute promyelocytic leukemia (APL) often has associated DIC,[71] due to an increase in the phospholipid binding protein annexin II on APL cells. Annexin II causes increased production of plasmin and a cascade of unopposed fibrinolysis that triggers bleeding.[72] In patients with APL all-*trans*-retinoic acid rapidly reverses DIC,[72] whereas among patients with solid tumors, only 33% had resolution of their DIC with cancer therapy in one study.[70] The presence of DIC also is prognostic of poorer survival in early-stage and advanced malignancies.[70] Plasma and platelet transfusions can be used for patients with DIC and serious bleeding, whereas heparin should be reserved for patients with DIC who develop thrombosis (in the absence of severe thrombocytopenia). A variety of other therapies including antiplatelet drugs and fibrinolytic inhibitors and activators has been suggested, but these have no proven efficacy. Use of ε-aminocaproic acid is contraindicated except in the rare case of DIC caused by primary fibrinolysis, in which it may be used with caution.

Several other paraneoplastic coagulopathies have been reported. Acquired von Willebrand factor (vWF) is seen in plasma cell dyscrasias, gastric and adrenal carcinomas, leukemias, and lymphomas. Spontaneous mucosal bleeding may be present, and laboratory tests reveal prolonged partial thromboplastin time and bleeding time, as well as decreased vWF antigen levels, vWF ristocetin cofactor activity, and ristocetin platelet aggregation. Desmopressin acetate, vWF concentrates, and intravenous immunoglobulin are indicated in severe cases, as is treatment of the underlying malignancy.[73] Acquired hemophilia (factor VIII autoantibodies) has been reported in patients with solid tumors, paraproteinemias, and lymphoproliferative disorders. Spontaneous mucosal or intramuscular bleeding is characteristic, and increased partial thromboplastin time and normal prothrombin time are seen. In addition to treatment of the underlying cancer, plasmapheresis and administration of factor VIII concentrates, corticosteroids, and cyclophosphamide have been used as treatment.[64,74]

NONBACTERIAL THROMBOTIC ENDOCARDITIS

Nonbacterial thrombotic endocarditis may lead to thrombotic or hemorrhagic complications and may occur with or without DIC. It is characterized by sterile, verrucous fibrin-platelet lesions on the left-sided heart valves. Nonbacterial endocarditis should be suspected in cancer patients who present with ischemic embolic events and is most commonly seen with adenocarcinomas of the lung and pancreas.[75] Although some patients may have heart murmurs, the majority do not, and echocardiography is diagnostic. Treatment of the underlying malignancy is the primary therapy. Anticoagulants are contra-indicated because of the high risk of bleeding.

GASTROINTESTINAL MANIFESTATIONS OF CANCER

PROTEIN-LOSING ENTEROPATHY

Paraneoplastic protein-losing enteropathy was initially thought to be due to impaired protein synthesis. However, it has been shown that synthesis of proteins in these patients is normal or slightly increased, whereas the serum half-life of protein is dramatically decreased.[76] Protein-losing enteropathy results from increased mucosal permeability to serum proteins due to abnormal cellular structure, mucosal erosion or ulceration, or lymphatic obstruction. Hypoalbuminemia can be seen with virtually any cancer of the GI tract, including esophageal, gastric, and colonic cancer, carcinoid syndrome,[77] and Kaposi's sarcoma. Intestinal involvement of lymphoid malignancies, including Hodgkin's disease and non-Hodgkin's lymphoma, can lead to protein-losing enteropathy.

In contrast to renal protein loss, the protein loss in GI disorders is independent of the protein's size; therefore, proteins of various sizes such as albumin, immunoglobulins, and ceruloplasmin all are lost equivalently. In hypoproteinemia caused by both GI and non-GI disorders, proteins of long serum half-life (i.e., albumin) tend to be affected more than proteins of shorter serum half-life (i.e., retinol-binding protein). Levels of other serum constituents that depend on carrier proteins, such as iron, copper, and calcium, may be depressed when patients develop hypoproteinemic states.

The diagnosis of protein-losing enteropathy is generally identified on routine blood chemistry evaluation. Patients show variable rates of peripheral edema and debilitation. Other sources of hypoproteinemia such as malnutrition and liver disease must be excluded. Measurement of levels of α_1-antitrypsin, a protein that is excreted unchanged in the stool, is used to confirm the diagnosis and quantitate the degree of protein loss.[78] Diarrhea and the presence of fecal occult blood can lead to abnormal test results.

Aside from treatment of the primary malignancy, many patients require dietary therapy. For example, patients with lymphatic obstruction need a low-fat diet and may require the use of medium-chain triglycerides, which do not require intestinal lymphatic transport. With appropriate treatment of the cancer and dietary therapy, approximately 50% of patients show improvement.[76]

ANOREXIA AND CACHEXIA IN THE CANCER PATIENT

Cancer anorexia-cachexia syndrome (CACS), as it is now known, is the most common paraneoplastic syndrome. Hallmarks of this syndrome include anorexia, weight loss (specifically of lean body mass), muscle atrophy, anemia, asthenia, and alteration in the metabolism of all energy substrates. Cancer cachexia indicates a poor prognosis.[79] CACS affects over 50% of all cancer patients to a mild degree, but 15% experience loss of greater than 10% of baseline body weight.[80]

In the past decade, significant advances have been made in understanding the molecular mechanism underlying this dis-order, and both humoral and tumor-derived factors have been implicated. TNF-α is important for the induction of cachexia and, along with other mediators, such as IL-6, interferon-γ, leukemia inhibitory factor, transforming growth factor-β, and IL-1, is important for the maintenance of the cachectic state.[81] A wasting syndrome results when these factors dominate the body's anticachectic pathways, which include IL-4, IL-10, IL-13, and others.

Cachectic patients demonstrate a decrease in efficiency of energy expenditure compared to noncachectic patients. Uncoupling proteins affect this efficiency at the level of the mitochondria by altering the protein gradient generated during respiration, and this appears to be mediated by TNF.[81] Muscle protein loss is a result of increased degradation, decreased protein synthesis, and increased apoptosis secondary to increased activity of the adenosine triphosphate–ubiquitin–proteasome complex.[81,82] Aside from endogenous mediators, tumor-derived proteolysis-inducing factor has been implicated in increased muscle protein degradation, decreased protein synthesis, direct muscle proteolysis, and inhibition of glucose utilization by muscle cells.[83] Tumors also produce factors that change the patient's perception of food, particularly taste and smell, which leads to a lack of enjoyment in eating. The central nervous system's control of appetite can be altered by tumor factors, such as serotonin, and by anatomic and psychologic factors, which causes secondary anorexia that complicates the paraneoplastic syndrome and makes a pharmacologic solution to cachexia difficult. Although treatment with individual anticytokine antibodies reverses specific features of CACS *in vitro*, no single antibody eradicates all aspects of the syndrome.[84]

When clinically evaluating a cancer patient for CACS, appetite, intake over prior weeks, weight, and weight loss are all critical. Plasma proteins such as albumin have limited value in evaluating CACS, because they are affected by factors other than nutrient status. Treating patients with malnutrition and cancer is similar to treating other forms of severe stress such as that associated with burns, trauma, and sepsis; the primary objective is adequate caloric intake excluding calories from protein sources. Whenever possible, the GI tract should be used for nutritional support. Although total parenteral nutrition is an option, numerous studies have found no survival benefit to its use in cancer patients, with an increase in infectious and mechanical complications.[85] The Harris-Benedict equation is useful for determining basal caloric needs. Generally, stress factors of cancer (estimated at 20% to 30% of the basal metabolic rate) are added to the patient's caloric needs. If other forms of stress are present, such as infection, these factors should be added. In addition to meeting the caloric needs, 1.0 to 1.5 g of protein per kg of body weight is also given, and 25% to 40% of nonprotein calories should be in the form of lipids. In complex cases, a 24-hour urine collection to test for nitrogen loss should be undertaken at least 24 hours after nutritional support begins. A positive nitrogen balance indicates that the patient is receiving adequate caloric intake.

Pharmacologic approaches to improving nutritional status in the cancer patient include use of appetite stimulants, corticosteroids and progestational agents, prokinetics, antidepressants, analgesics, and antiemetics. Unfortunately, most of these medications are of marginal benefit. Several studies have examined the usefulness of corticosteroids and found that they can increase appetite and elevate mood but do not cause significant weight gain and are limited because of progressive muscle weakness.[86,87] Progestational agents, including megestrol acetate and medroxyprogesterone acetate, have been found to improve appetite and caloric intake, and reduce loss of fat tissue in patients with cancer or acquired immunodeficiency syndrome in more than a dozen randomized trials reviewed.[88] The dose range for megestrol acetate is 160 to 1600 mg, but 300 to 480 mg/d is adequate for most patients. The major risk of progestational agents is an increased likelihood of thromboembolic events. Prokinetic drugs such as metoclopramide reduce nausea and early satiety but do not lead to increase in body mass.[87] Cannabinoids such as dronabinol, thalidomide, melatonin, and anabolic steroids have all been used, but without definitive evidence of improvement in cancer patients.

Unfortunately, the current therapy for CACS remains largely ineffective. Nutritional support, counseling, and the use of progestational or prokinetic agents continue to play the predominant role in management. Novel agents such as cytokine inhibitors have yet to be tested in humans, but animal testing is under way. Future strategies that move beyond nutritional improvement to counteracting the metabolic disarray in cancer cachexia is essential.

RENAL MANIFESTATIONS OF NONRENAL CANCER

Patients with nonrenal carcinoma may develop treatment-related nephropathies, tubular interstitial defects, glomerular abnormalities, and fluid and electrolyte disorders. Radiation nephritis and drug-induced toxicities from antineoplastic drugs (e.g., cisplatin), antibiotics, analgesics, and radiographic contrast agents all induce various forms of renal failure. Infiltrative disorders from leukemias and lymphomas, tubular precipitation abnormalities such as protein cast nephropathy, uric acid nephropathy, hypercalcemic nephropathy, and obstructive nephropathy lead to tubular interstitial diseases. Membranous glomerulopathy, minimal-change disease, amyloidosis, and consumptive coagulopathy all lead to glomerular abnormalities. Finally, hypercalcemia, hypocalcemia, hyponatremia, and tumor lysis syndrome, covered in other chapters of this book, lead to fluid and electrolyte disorders. Although renal manifestations of systemic cancer and its therapy are common, several classes of renal insult are specifically paraneoplastic in nature.

GLOMERULAR DISORDERS

Most cases of membranous nephropathy are idiopathic, but in an early report of 101 patients with idiopathic nephrotic syndrome, 11% had cancer and 8% had membranous nephropathy.[89] In 80% of cases of paraneoplastic nephrotic syndrome, the diagnosis is made concurrently or after that of the malignant disease. Nephrosis-range proteinuria, hypertension, and microscopic hematuria characterize the syndrome. Immune complexes are thought to play a role in malignancy-associated glomerular disease. The responsible antigens include fetal antigens, autologous nontumor antigens, tumor-associated antigens, and viral antigens.[90] Nephrotic syndrome may resolve with successful treatment of the underlying malignancy. Other standard therapies include loop diuretics to symptomatically treat the peripheral edema associated with the syndrome. As

well, careful monitoring for the development of thrombosis, especially renal vein thrombosis, is warranted in severe protein wasting.

Other glomerular diseases include membranoproliferative glomerulonephritis[91] and minimal-change disease. Hodgkin's disease is the cause of most cases of minimal-change disease, with lymphoproliferative disorders, pancreatic carcinoma, and mesothelioma also reported. There is a parallel relationship between the activity of the lymphoma and the degree of proteinuria. Other cancer-associated glomerulopathies include focal and segmental glomerulosclerosis with CLL, T-cell lymphomas, and acute myelogenous leukemia; immunoglobulin A (IgA) nephropathy with lung, head and neck, and pancreatic cancers, mycosis fungoides, and liposarcoma; and membranoproliferative glomerulonephritis with CLL, Burkitt's and other lymphomas, hairy cell leukemia, and malignant melanoma. Rarely, rapidly progressive glomerulonephritis has been associated with lymphoma and monoclonal gammopathies.[91]

MICROVASCULAR LESIONS

Hemolytic-uremic syndrome is most often seen after use of chemotherapeutic agents such as mitomycin C but has also been reported in malignancy. Giant hemangiomas and hemangioendotheliomas[92] and specific malignancies such as APL and prostate, gastric, and pancreatic cancers are the most common culprits. A renal vasculitis secondary to Henoch-Schönlein purpura has also been reported in a patient with lung cancer, but this is an extremely rare complication of malignancy. More frequent is the association of renal vasculitis secondary to a process such as cryoglobulinemia, a known complication of hepatocellular carcinoma and concomitant hepatitis C disease.[91]

TUMOR INFILTRATION

Autopsy series show that the kidney is commonly affected by infiltrative and metastatic processes[93]; 40% to 60% of patients with leukemia have tumor infiltration of the kidney. There is a strong association between bone marrow involvement by tumor and renal infiltration. In both non-Hodgkin's lymphoma as well as Hodgkin's disease the involvement tends to be nodular and bilateral, whereas in leukemia the involvement is infiltrative.[93] Treatment of the underlying malignancy often results in resolution of the renal lesions. Other tubular abnormalities, such as protein cast precipitation syndrome, paraprotein disease, uric acid nephropathy, hypercalcemia, and obstructive uropathy, are discussed in Chapters 44 and 49.4.

CUTANEOUS MANIFESTATIONS OF CANCER

A wide variety of cutaneous syndromes is associated with malignancies and may precede, be concurrent with, or follow the discovery of the underlying malignancy. It is critical that, once a potential cutaneous paraneoplastic syndrome has been diagnosed, an appropriate systemic evaluation for a neoplasm be undertaken. The initial workup includes detailed medical history, physical examination, and routine screening laboratory tests. This is followed by studies directed by the abnormalities

TABLE 45-3.   Pigmented Lesions and Keratoses

Disease	Description	Malignancy	Cause	Comments
Acanthosis nigricans[a]	Gray-brown symmetric velvety plaques on the neck, axilla, flexor areas, and anogenital region	Adenocarcinomas; predominantly gastric	Unknown	Benign form present from birth and associated with various syndromes
Tripe palms[a]	Hyperpigmented velvety thickened palms with hyperkeratotic ridges	Gastric, lung	Unknown	Often associated with acanthosis nigricans
Generalized melanosis	Diffuse gray-brown skin pigmentation	Melanoma, adrenocorticotrophic hormone–producing tumors	Melanin deposits in dermis	May be seen in benign conditions
Leser-Trélat sign[a]	Sudden appearance of seborrheic keratoses	Gastric, lymphoma, breast	Unknown	Differentiate from benign seborrheic keratoses
Acrokeratosis paraneoplastica or Bazex's disease[a]	Symmetric, psoriasiform acral hyperkeratosis	Squamous cell carcinoma of the esophagus, head and neck, lung	Unknown	Predominantly male disorder
Paget's disease	Erythematous keratotic patch over areola/nipple, urogenital, or perianal area	Breast, uterine, ovarian, prostate, anal	Paget cells are either cancerous or Langerhans' cells	Occurs in fewer than 3% of breast cancers; extramammary Paget's overlies the area of cancer
Sweet's syndrome[a]	Erythematous painful raised cutaneous plaques	Hematologic malignancies, various carcinomas	Unknown	May respond to steroids; 10% to 15% associated with cancer
Pyoderma gangrenosum[a]	Painful papules, ulcers, violaceous borders and purulent exudates	Basal, squamous skin cancers; cutaneous T-cell non-Hodgkin's lymphoma	Unknown	Neutrophilic infiltrate

[a]True paraneoplastic syndrome.

PIGMENTED LESIONS AND KERATOSES

Acanthosis nigricans is characterized by gray-brown hyperpigmented, velvety plaques that often affect the neck, axilla, flexor areas, and anogenital region (Table 45-3). The malignant and benign forms are very similar in appearance, but the malignant form progresses rapidly, and pruritus is common. The malignant variety may precede the tumor, occur simultaneously, or even follow the appearance of the tumor. It is typically associated with adenocarcinomas of the GI tract, predominantly gastric cancer, but has also been associated with a variety of other adenocarcinomas, including lung, breast, ovarian, and even hematologic malignancies.[94] The pathogenesis remains uncertain.

Tripe palms are often associated with acanthosis nigricans. Patients show thickened palms with exaggerated hyperkeratotic ridges, a velvety texture, and brown hyperpigmentation.[95] Tripe palms usually occur in patients with lung and gastric cancer.

Melanosis is caused by abnormal deposition of melanin, which results in diffuse gray-brown pigmentation in the skin.[96] Melanosis may appear before or after the primary melanoma is detected, and it is often accentuated in light-exposed areas of the upper body. Histopathologic examination demonstrates melanin granules in perivascular or interstitial melanophages; free granules may be seen in the dermis. Melanosis can also be caused by ACTH-producing tumors.[97]

The Leser-Trélat sign refers to the sudden appearance (or increase in the number and size) of seborrheic keratoses secondary to an occult malignancy. These can appear 5 months before or up to 10 months after the diagnosis of malignancy,[98] and adenocarcinoma of the stomach is the most common cause. Association with lymphoma, breast and colon cancers, and squamous cell carcinoma is also reported.[99] Treatment of the malignancy results in involution of the seborrheic keratoses.

Acrokeratosis paraneoplastica or Bazex's syndrome is characterized by symmetric psoriasiform acral hyperkeratosis. It is predominantly associated with male gender and squamous cell carcinoma of the esophagus, head and neck, or lungs.[100] The skin lesions precede the detection of the tumor in 60% of cases. Cross-reaction between the basement membrane and tumor antigens as well as secretion of growth factors such as IGF-1 or transforming growth factor-α are postulated to cause this syndrome.[101]

Paget's disease of the breast is characterized by erythematous keratotic patches over the areola, nipple, or accessory breast tissue and is associated with breast cancer.[102] Extramammary Paget's disease is an erythematous exudative dermatitis located on the vulva in women, the genitals in men, and the perianal area in both sexes. Histopathologically, Paget's disease demonstrates large pale cells within the epidermis and often in the cutaneous appendages. Extramammary Paget's disease is associated with an internal malignancy in 50% of cases, usually carcinoma of the uterus, rectum, bladder, vagina, or prostate gland. Most of these cancers are usually related to the site of the dermatosis.

NEUTROPHILIC DERMATOSES

Sweet's syndrome is associated with fever, neutrophilia, and the appearance of erythematous painful raised cutaneous plaques on the face, neck, and upper extremities. Histopathologic

TABLE 45-4. Erythemas

Disease	Description	Malignancy	Cause	Comments
Erythema gyratum repens[a]	Advancing concentric rings of erythema with trailing scales	Lung, breast, uterus, gastrointestinal cancers	Unknown	80% Associated with malignancies
Necrolytic migratory erythema[a]	Macules and papules progressing to epidermal necrolysis	Glucagonoma	Glucagon or metabolic product	Somatostatin beneficial
Flushing[a]	Episodic reddening of face and neck	Carcinoids, medullary thyroid carcinoma	Serotonin or other vasoactive peptides	—
Exfoliative dermatitis	Progressive erythema followed by scaling	Cutaneous T-cell and other lymphomas, Hodgkin's disease	Unknown	Accounts for 10–20% of all exfoliative dermatitis

[a]True paraneoplastic syndrome.

examination demonstrates a dermal infiltration of well-differentiated neutrophils, unlike leukemia cutis, which contains immature myeloid blasts. Association with malignancy occurs in 20% of cases. Acute myelogenous leukemia is the most common malignancy, although association with myeloproliferative and lymphoproliferative disorders, myelodysplastic syndromes, and carcinomas has also been reported.[103] Sweet's syndrome may precede the detection of malignancy by many years or occur concomitantly. The cause is thought to be hypersensitivity, and response to corticosteroids is usually prompt.

The lesions of pyoderma gangrenosum appear as painful papules that subsequently ulcerate with violaceous irregular borders and a purulent, hemorrhagic exudate with a necrotic base. Histopathologic examination demonstrates a lymphocytic vasculitis or neutrophilic infiltrate. Pyoderma gangrenosum is associated with basal and squamous cell carcinomas as well as with cutaneous T-cell lymphomas.[104]

ERYTHEMAS

Erythema gyratum repens presents as rapidly advancing concentric rings of erythema with trailing scales on the trunk and proximal extremities and precedes malignancy more than 80% of the time (Table 45-4).[105] It is associated with lung, breast, uterine, and GI tract malignancies.

Necrolytic migratory erythema is solely associated with glucagonoma and is characterized by erythematous macules and papules that progress to blistering and epidermal necrosis on the central face, lower abdomen, perineum, and buttocks.[106] The eruption clears after resection of the tumor, but in metastatic glucagonoma may wax and wane. Somatostatin is beneficial due to its suppression of glucagon secretion.[98]

Flushing is an episodic reddening of the face and neck, lasting a few minutes, typically associated with the carcinoid syndrome but also seen with leukemia, medullary carcinoma of the thyroid, renal cell carcinoma, and other malignancies.[107,108] Vasoactive peptides such as serotonin are thought to mediate this syndrome.[108]

Exfoliative dermatitis is a progressive erythema followed by scaling that is classically associated with cutaneous T-cell lymphoma but may be seen in other lymphomas.[109]

Multicentric reticulohistiocytosis is a disease that manifests as violaceous papules overlying joints with associated arthritis mutilans in 50% of patients. Twenty-eight percent of patients develop malignancies, including pancreatic and squamous cell lung car-

cinomas and metastatic melanoma. The disease results from the destructive effects of proteinases,[110] and treatments including corticosteroids, nonsteroidal antiinflammatory medications, and immunosuppressive agents have been ineffective.[110]

ENDOCRINE AND METABOLIC LESIONS

A variety of metabolic disorders cause paraneoplastic manifestations in the skin. Systemic nodular panniculitis or subcutaneous fat necrosis is characterized by violaceous nodules, is associated with adenocarcinoma of the pancreas, and may be accompanied by polyarthralgia, fever, and eosinophilia.[111] Cushing's syndrome is associated with broad purple striae, hyperpigmentation, telangiectasia, atrophy of the skin, facial plethora, acne vulgaris, ecchymosis, and mild hirsutism. Addison's syndrome can occur with adrenocortical carcinoma and is characterized by generalized hyperpigmentation, especially in scars, pressure points, and points of friction. Hirsutism is associated with virilism and is caused by increased levels of glucocorticoids and testosterone, typically from adrenal and ovarian tumors. Carcinoid syndrome may cause telangiectasias and scleroderma-like and pellagra-like skin changes. Many of these lesions resolve with treatment of the underlying malignancy.

BULLOUS LESIONS

Paraneoplastic pemphigus (PNP) is most frequently seen in B-cell lymphoproliferative disorders, including lymphomas and CLL as well as Castleman's disease, thymoma, Waldenström's macroglobulinemia, and spindle cell neoplasms.[112] It occurs after the malignancy in two-thirds of cases. Patients develop painful Castleman's ulcers and intraepidermal and lichenoid skin lesions, as well as stomatitis. Internal organ involvement is common, and respiratory failure causes death in 30% of patients with this disorder.[113] In contrast to other types of pemphigus, microscopic evidence of inflammation is a hallmark of PNP. Patients with PNP demonstrate autoantibodies to desmosomal plakins, lectin, desmogleins 1 and 3, and bullous pemphigoid antigen 1, which cause acantholytic blistering,[98,113,114] although the pathogenesis is incompletely understood. The course of the disease is progressive and independent of the underlying malignancy, particularly the stomatitis. Corticosteroids and cyclosporine are beneficial.[112] Mycophenolate mofetil is added in patients with refractory disease.[115]

TABLE 45-5. Miscellaneous Lesions

Disease	Description	Malignancy	Cause	Comments
Acquired ichthyosis[a]	Generalized dry, crackling skin, hyperkeratosis, rhomboidal scales	Hodgkin's disease, other lymphomas, multiple myeloma, Kaposi's sarcoma	Unknown	Should be differentiated from hereditary ichthyosis, which occurs before age 20 y
Dermatomyositis[a]	Erythema or telangiectasias of the knuckles, chest, periorbital region	Miscellaneous	Unknown	Malignant disease reported in up to 50%, precedes carcinoma by days to years
Pachydermoperiostosis[a]	Thickening of skin, lips, ears, lids; forehead; scalp; clubbing; excessive sweating	Lung	Unknown	May be seen in lung cancer, and lung abscess and benign tumors
Hypertrichosis lanuginosa acquisita (malignant down)[a]	Rapid development of fine, long, silky hair, especially on ears and forehead	Lung, colon, bladder, uterus, gallbladder	Unknown	High association with cancer
Amyloid	Waxy yellow plaques and nodules	Multiple myeloma, Waldenström's macroglobulinemia	Unknown	Also associated with primary systemic amyloidosis
Muir-Torre syndrome[a]	Sebaceous gland neoplasm	Colon cancer, lymphoma	Unknown	
Pruritus[a]		Lymphomas, leukemias, multiple myeloma, central nervous system tumors, abdominal tumors	Unknown	Failure to determine a cutaneous cause of generalized pruritus necessitates an evaluation for an underlying systemic disease

[a]True paraneoplastic syndrome.

MISCELLANEOUS LESIONS

Acquired ichthyosis is characterized by generalized dry, crackling skin, hyperkeratosis and rhomboidal scales of the extensor surfaces (Table 45-5). It is most commonly associated with Hodgkin's disease but may be seen with lymphomas, multiple myeloma, Kaposi's sarcoma,[116] and other malignancies. It tends to develop after the malignancy and runs a parallel course. Topical lubricants and keratolytics are helpful for symptomatic relief.

Dermatomyositis may be idiopathic or paraneoplastic, and has been linked to malignancy in over 25% of cases. It is characterized by a heliotrope rash of the periorbital skin and Gottron's papules (erythematous papules on the extensor surfaces of joints, which may also show telangiectasias).[117] Patients also exhibit proximal muscle weakness, scalp pruritus, poikiloderma, periungual telangiectasias, and erythema. The most common cancers associated with dermatomyositis are those of the genital organs in women and respiratory tract in both sexes.[98] Malignancy can precede, follow, or occur simultaneously with dermatomyositis; the most frequent pattern is onset of cancer within 1 year of the diagnosis of dermatomyositis.

Pachydermoperiostosis is characterized by thickening of the skin and creation of new folds; thickened lips, ears, and lids; macroglossia; clubbing; thickening of the forehead and scalp; and excessive sweating.[118] The cause of this syndrome is unknown, but it is most often associated with bronchogenic carcinoma.

Hypertrichosis lanuginosa acquisita (malignant down) is the sudden appearance of downy hair on the entire body. Lung cancer is the most commonly associated malignancy, followed by colon, bladder, ovarian, uterine, and pancreatic cancers.[119]

Pruritus may be the initial feature of an occult malignancy or the clinical manifestation of a previously diagnosed tumor. It is most frequently associated with Hodgkin's disease but may be seen with polycythemia vera, cutaneous T-cell lymphomas, and a variety of other diseases.[120] Severe pruritus localized in the nostrils has been reported in some patients with advanced brain tumors.

Amyloid deposits, which may manifest as macroglossia, superficial waxy yellow and pink elevated nodules on the skin, may be associated with multiple myeloma or Waldenström's macroglobulinemia. They may also be associated with benign disorders such as primary systemic amyloidosis.

Muir-Torre syndrome is a sebaceous gland neoplasm that may precede, follow, or coexist with visceral cancers.[121] It is most often associated with GI tract adenocarcinoma of the colon or genitourinary tract, or lymphoma.

Numerous additional hereditary disorders associated with cutaneous manifestations of malignancy are described in Table 45-6.

NEUROLOGIC MANIFESTATIONS OF CANCER

Neurologic diseases are defined as paraneoplastic when they occur in increased frequency in patients with cancer and are not related to a direct effect of tumor, infection, metabolic abnormalities, or toxicity of therapy (Table 45-7).[122,123] Autoantibodies and evidence for cellular autoimmunity directed against neuronal, glial, or muscle cell antigens have been identified in a number of paraneoplastic neurologic disorders (Table 45-8).[124,125] Over the past four decades, different investigators identified and reported these disorders using a variety of names. This review follows the nosology used by Posner.[123]

Paraneoplastic disorders are rare, but accurate diagnosis is important. For patients without a known malignancy, correct diagnosis may lead to discovery and early treatment of the underlying malignancy. Effective treatment of the neurologic disorder may improve neurologic dysfunction and improve quality of life. Equally important, proper diagnosis of a paraneoplastic disorder spares the patient an extensive and expensive search for alternative causes of the neurologic dysfunction.

Paraneoplastic disorders are diagnosed by the identification of stereotypic clinical syndromes and, when appropriate, confirmatory laboratory studies to demonstrate evidence of autoimmunity. Autoantibodies against specific neural antigens characterize sev-

TABLE 45-6. Hereditary Disorders

Disease	Description	Malignancy	Heredity	Comments
Cowden's disease (multiple hamartoma syndrome)	Fibromas of oral mucosa with "cobblestoning" of the tongue, facial trichilemmomas	Thyroid, breast carcinomas	Autosomal dominant	Associated with multiple hamartomas, lipomas, neuromas, hemangiomas, thyroid adenomas
Gardner's syndrome	Bony exostoses, epidermal cysts, sebaceous cysts, dermoid tumors, lipomas, fibromas	Adenocarcinoma of large or small bowel	Autosomal dominant	Hallmark is polyposis of the colon
Peutz-Jeghers syndrome	Hamartomatous polyps of the GI tract and mucocutaneous pigmentation of the lips, face, and oral mucosa	GI adenocarcinomas	Autosomal dominant	Associated with benign or malignant neoplasm
Keratosis palmaris et plantaris (tylosis)	Hyperkeratosis of palms and soles after age 10 y	Esophageal carcinoma	Autosomal dominant	95% Incidence of carcinoma by age 65 y
Neurofibromatosis (von Recklinghausen)	Neurofibromas, café au lait spots	Pheochromocytoma	Autosomal dominant	Malignancies develop in a minority of patients
Nevoid basal cell carcinoma syndrome	Multiple basal cell carcinomas, pits on soles and palms, jaw cysts, skeletal abnormalities	Medulloblastoma, fibrosarcoma (jaw)	Autosomal dominant	Infrequent association with internal malignancy
Tuberous sclerosis (Bourneville)	Pigmented macules, adenomas, fibromas	Neurologic malignancies	Autosomal dominant	Malignancies develop in a minority of patients
Cerebelloretinal hemangioblastoma (von Hippel-Lindau)	Retinal malformation, papilledema	Neurologic malignancies	Autosomal dominant	Malignancies develop in a minority of patients
Encephalotrigeminal syndrome (Sturge-Weber)	Capillary or cavernous hemangiomas within the cutaneous distribution of the trigeminal nerve	Neurologic malignancies	Autosomal dominant	Malignancies develop in a minority of patients
Ataxia-telangiectasia	Telangiectasias	Lymphomas, leukemias	Autosomal recessive	IgA ± IgE deficiency; sinopulmonary infections, tumors in <10%
Bloom's syndrome	Photosensitivity, telangiectasias, erythema of face	Leukemias	Autosomal recessive	Stunted growth, high incidence
Fanconi's anemia	Patchy hyperpigmentation	Leukemias	Autosomal recessive	High incidence
Chédiak-Higashi syndrome	Recurrent pyoderma, giant melanosomes, dilution of skin and hair color	Lymphomas	Autosomal recessive	High incidence
Werner's syndrome (adult progeria)	Scleroderma-like changes, premature aging, leg ulcers, short stature	Sarcomas, meningiomas, others	Autosomal recessive	Cancers in approximately 10%
Wiskott-Aldrich syndrome	Eczematous dermatitis, pyoderma	Lymphomas	Sex linked (male)	>10% Incidence
Bruton's sex-linked agammaglobulinemia	Recurrent infections	Lymphomas, leukemias	Sex linked	>5% Incidence

GI, gastrointestinal; IgA, immunoglobulin A; IgG, immunoglobulin G.

eral neurologic disorders.[124] In some disorders—for instance, Lambert-Eaton myasthenic syndrome (LES) associated with SCLC[126] or myasthenia gravis associated with thymoma[127]—the antibodies are clearly important to the pathogenesis of the disease and immunosuppression is clearly effective therapeutically.[128,129] For other disorders, such as encephalomyeloneuritis associated with SCLC, the role of the antibody response in producing neurologic dysfunction is less clear.[130,131]

SUBACUTE SENSORY NEURONOPATHY AND ENCEPHALOMYELONEURITIS

Most frequently associated with SCLC, subacute sensory neuronopathy and encephalomyeloneuritis (SSN-EMN) may affect multiple sites within the central and peripheral nervous sys-

TABLE 45-7. Estimated Incidence of Neurologic Disorders That Are Paraneoplastic Syndromes

Syndrome	% Paraneoplastic
Lambert-Eaton myasthenic syndrome	60
Subacute cerebellar degeneration	50
Subacute sensory neuronopathy	20
Opsoclonus-myoclonus (children)	50
Opsoclonus-myoclonus (adults)	20
Sensory motor peripheral neuropathy	10
Encephalomyelitis	10
Dermatomyositis	10

(From Posner JB. Paraneoplastic syndromes. *Neurol Clin* 1991;9:919, with permission.)

TABLE 45-8. Antineuronal Antibodies and Associated Paraneoplastic Syndromes and Cancers

Antibody	Site of Activity	Genes	Cellular Function	Clinical Syndrome	Cancers
Anti-Hu (ANNA-1)	Panneuronal	HuD, HuC, Hel-N1/N2	RNA binding	Paraneoplastic encephalo-myelitis, paraneoplastic sensory neuronopathy, PCD, autonomic dysfunction	SCLC, sarcoma, neuroblastoma
Anti-Ri (ANNA-2)	Central nervous system neurons	Nova-1	RNA binding	Paraneoplastic opsoclonus-myoclonus, PCD	Breast, gynecologic, SCLC, bladder
Anti-Yo (APCA)	Purkinje cell	CDR34/62/3, PCD-17	Leucine zipper	PCD	Ovary, uterus, breast, SCLC
Anti-Tr	Purkinje cell	MAZ	Leucine zipper Interacts with DCC gene product	PCD	Hodgkin's, non-Hodgkin's lymphoma
Anti-VGCC	Presynaptic neuromuscular junction	MysB, Synaptotagmin	Ach release	Lambert-Eaton myasthenic syndrome	SCLC, Hodgkin's disease
Anti-CAR	Photoreceptors	Recoverin	Calcium binding	Cancer-associated retinopathy	SCLC, melanoma
Antiamphiphysin	Synapse, central nervous system neurons	Amphiphysin	Synaptic vesicle protein	Stiff-person syndrome, encephalitis	Breast, SCLC
Anti-AchR	Postsynaptic neuromuscular junction	?MHC	Ach receptor	Myasthenia	Thymoma
Anti-CV2, anti–CRMP-5	Oligodendrocyte	CRMP-5	Axonal growth factor	Neuropathy, uveitis, chorea, ataxia	SCLC, renal cell, breast, lymphoma
Anti-AchR (nicotinic)	Postsynaptic, ganglionic	Nicotinic AchR	AchR, nicotinic	Dysautonomia	SCLC, thymoma
Anti-Ta	Nucleus	Ma1, Ma2	?	Limbic encephalitis	Testis

Ach, acetylcholine; AchR, acetylcholine receptor; ANNA, antineuronal nuclear antibody; APCA, antiparietal cell antibody; CAR, carcinoma-associated retinal; CRMP, collapsin response mediator protein-2; MHC, major histocompatibility complex; PCD, paraneoplastic cerebellar degeneration; SCLC, small cell carcinoma of the lung; VGCC, voltage-gated calcium channel.

tem.[132] When SSN-EMN occurs in patients with SCLC, antibodies called anti-Hu antibodies are usually present in the serum, and high titers of antibodies to the Hu antigen are almost never seen in patients without SCLC.[132] Diagnosis of SSN-EMN and documentation of anti-Hu antibody should lead to the search for an SCLC, which is often localized at the time of diagnosis of the neurologic disorder. Low-titer anti-Hu antibodies have been documented in patients with SCLC and no neurologic disease,[133] and the association with localized SCLC suggests that anti-Hu antibodies are a marker for systemic immune suppression of tumor progression.

The range of presentations and extent of neurologic involvement in patients with paraneoplastic disorders associated with anti-Hu antibodies are quite broad. One presentation is a pure sensory neuropathy.[134,135] The disorder progresses relentlessly over days to weeks, and sensory nerve action potentials are lost.[135] The cerebrospinal fluid (CSF) usually demonstrates increased protein concentration and a lymphocytic pleocytosis, and in SSN associated with anti-Hu antibody, the dorsal root ganglia show lymphocytic infiltration and loss of neurons.[136] At postmortem examination, inflammatory changes in other regions of the nervous system have been seen in approximately half of SSN patients studied. Most cases of SSN are associated with other autoimmune disorders rather than with cancer, and anti-Hu antibodies are absent. The association of anti-Hu antibodies with Sjögren's syndrome is probably spurious.[137] Immunosuppression is usually ineffective,[138] but spontaneous remission may occur. Treatment of the underlying SCLC may ameliorate signs of neu-

rologic dysfunction,[138] and treatment of Hodgkin's disease with chemotherapy was followed by clinical improvement in one patient.[139]

LIMBIC ENCEPHALITIS

The clinical, radiologic, and immunobiologic features of limbic encephalitis (LE) have been described in two analyses encompassing 250 patients.[140,141] LE may be mistaken for herpes simplex encephalitis, because it presents with memory disturbance, agitation, and seizures. Magnetic resonance imaging (MRI) may show mesial temporal contrast enhancement or T2 signal hyperintensities.[142] The CSF shows increased protein concentration and a lymphocytic pleocytosis. Symptoms of SSN or involvement of brainstem or spinal cord may be present. Biopsy of temporal lobe may show perivascular lymphocytic infiltrates. In autopsy specimens, neuronal loss and gliosis are most prominent in limbic and insular cortex.[140,141]

Molecular characterization of target antigens divides this syndrome into distinguishable diseases. Most cases of LE are associated with SCLC, and anti-Hu antibodies are present in serum and CSF.[140,141] Patients with testicular cancer and LE harbor a different antibody[143] than those with SCLC. In a series of 13 patients with testicular cancer and LE, 10 harbored antibodies against a novel onconeural antigen named *Ma2*. Ma2 is a 40-kD protein not found in normal testis, but it is widely expressed in the normal human CNS as well as dorsal root ganglia. A related onconeural antigen, Ma1, normally found in the testis, is associated with cerebellar or brainstem dysfunction in patients with lung, breast, parotid gland, or colon cancer.[144] Breast cancer is the underlying malignancy in perhaps 5% of cases; anti-Ri antibodies have been reported in this setting.[145] A patient with thymoma and a novel autoantibody directed against synaptic vesicles has been reported.[146] LE has also been reported with Hodgkin's disease and non-Hodgkin's lymphoma.[147,148]

LE may be one of the more treatable forms of CNS paraneoplastic disorder.[140,141] More than 40% of patients followed for longer than 8 months in one series had some neurologic improvement. Treatment of the underlying tumor seems more effective than immunosuppression. This experience adds to earlier reports of improvement after successful treatment of an underlying lung cancer.[149] The distinction between anti-Ma2– and anti-Hu–associated LE is important clinically, because anti-Ma2–associated LE appears to have a better prognosis. Orchiectomy and aggressive treatment of residual disease appear to be the most effective treatment for anti-Ma2–associated LE.[144] Immunosuppression has been less successful, but one patient improved after treatment with corticosteroids and intravenous IgG.

Patients with LE should be tested for anti-Hu antibody; male patients should undergo examination of the testes and should be tested for anti-Ma2 antibodies. Detection of anti-Hu or anti-Ma antibodies indicates the likelihood of SCLC or testicular cancer, respectively. Rarely, small cell cancers of other organs, including poorly differentiated small cell carcinoma of the prostate, have been found as the only systemic cancer in patients with LE and anti-Hu antibodies.[150,151]

Brainstem encephalitis and myelitis usually occur together and in association with LE.[152] MRI scanning must exclude metastatic tumor. Most cases are associated with anti-Hu antibodies but other autoantibodies may be present. Brainstem encephalitis and myelitis are usually rapidly and relentlessly progressive.

AUTONOMIC NEUROPATHY

A pure paraneoplastic autonomic neuropathy is rare, but approximately 25% of patients with anti-Hu syndrome and SSN-EMN have autonomic dysfunction.[132] Progressive paraneoplastic autonomic failure may rarely be the first manifestation of an occult malignancy. Bladder dysfunction, bowel immotility and obstipation, and postural hypotension may be disabling.[153] The disorder is usually associated with SCLC and autoantibodies that react with neurons in the myenteric plexus.[153] In a series reported by the Mayo Clinic, 42% of patients with subacute autonomic neuropathy demonstrated antibodies directed against the nicotinic acetylcholine receptor.[154,155] Autonomic dysfunction may occur in patients with myasthenia gravis; in some, gastroparesis was the only manifestation, but severe pandysautonomia has been reported.[156] In some, antibodies against the ganglionic nicotinic acetylcholine receptor were identified.[155,156] The intestinal dysmotility may respond to anticholinesterase inhibitors. In rabbits, immunization with the recombinant α_3 subunit of the nicotinic neuronal acetylcholine receptor produces profound dysautonomia.[157]

PROGRESSIVE CEREBELLAR DEGENERATION

Subacute cerebellar degeneration in an adult without a family history of cerebellar disease demands investigation to exclude underlying tumor.[123] Posner has classified progressive cerebellar degeneration (PCD) into subcategories based on the underlying tumor, associated clinical features, and presence of specific associated autoantibodies.[123]

Patients usually complain first of difficulty with walking, which progresses over weeks to months. Diplopia and vertigo may be early symptoms. Loss of dexterity, dysarthria, and oscillopsia associated with nystagmus appear. The disorder usually leaves patients incapacitated.[158] Subtle motor system or cognitive dysfunction may be present.[159] Imaging may show diffuse cerebellar atrophy,[159,160] but contrast-enhancing lesions or lesions with mass effect are not part of PCD. CSF testing usually shows a lymphocytic pleocytosis and mildly elevated protein concentration during the early phase of the disorder, and oligoclonal bands have been reported.[158] The most common pathologic finding is diffuse, extensive loss of cerebellar Purkinje cells.[158] Inflammatory changes are frequently minimal in the Purkinje cell layer and more prominent in the surrounding white matter, leptomeninges, or in the region of the dentate nucleus.

Anti-Yo PCD is most commonly associated with ovarian or breast carcinoma, and patients are almost exclusively women. Frequently, the neurologic disorder antedates discovery of the tumor. The Yo antigen is one of a family of three cerebellar degeneration–related (cdr) antigens identified by expression cloning.[158,161–163] Only Yo, or CDR2, is transcribed in human tumors. The disorder is subacute in onset and usually progressive. Most patients develop downbeating nystagmus, oscillopsia, and diplopia. The PCD renders patients unable to walk, and dysarthria is frequently severe. Once the disorder reaches this stage, treatment with immunosuppression or effective treatment of the underlying malignancy rarely produces significant improvement. Early recognition of the syndrome may allow more effective attempts at immunosuppressive therapy.

Patients with PCD and Hodgkin's disease are predominantly male and younger than the females with anti-Yo PCD.[164] The disorder frequently develops in patients already treated for Hodgkin's disease. This type of PCD also seems to be molecularly heterogeneous. Antibodies against a novel onconeural antigen named Tr have been found in patients with Hodgkin's disease and PCD.[165,166] PCD associated with Hodgkin's disease appears to have a better prognosis for recovery than the anti-Yo–associated syndrome.[164] Spontaneous improvement was seen in 15% of cases in one series, and one patient improved significantly with effective treatment of Hodgkin's disease.[165] As the patient responded to treatment, the anti-Tr antibody declined tenfold in serum and disappeared from the CSF.[165] The target antigen for anti-Tr is a zinc finger protein (MAZ) identified by screening a human cerebellar expression library.[167] This protein interacts with DCC protein in neurons, the receptor for a neuronal survival factor, netrin-1.[167] Other patients with Hodgkin's disease demonstrate antibodies against metabotropic glutamate receptor type 1. Anti–metabotropic glutamate receptor type 1 antibodies appear to be directly pathophysiologically related to cerebellar dysfunction in a mouse model of passive adoptive transfer of disease.[168]

A study of 50 patients with PCD suggests that molecular characterization has prognostic significance.[169] Patients with anti-Ri had better functional outcomes and longer survival than patients seropositive for anti-Yo and anti-Hu antibody. Effective antitumor treatment was the most important determinant of outcome and duration of survival. All seven patients in this series who improved had complete remission of the under-lying tumor after systemic therapy.[169]

Antibody-negative PCD may occur in conjunction with LES. Approximately 30 patients have been reported; in some no tumor has been identified.[170] The most common associated tumor is SCLC. The PCD may not remit, even as the myas-thenic syndrome responds to immunosuppression.

Approximately 15% of patients with anti-Hu antibodies develop PCD as the first manifestation of disease. In these patients, signs suggesting multisystem involvement are often present. Identification of the anti-Hu antibody directs the search for SCLC.

PCD has been associated with a variety of other solid tumors and with myelogenous leukemia and monoclonal gammopa-thy.[123] It is unclear whether these cases are causally related to the associated tumors.

PARANEOPLASTIC VISION LOSS

Paraneoplastic disorders are a rare cause of vision loss in can-cer patients. Paraneoplastic visual syndromes may be identified by the clinical history, ophthalmologic examination, retinal electrophysiologic studies, and the presence or absence of autoantibodies.[171] Retinal disorders are the most common. Within this class, the photoreceptor degenerations are the best characterized.[172]

Patients with photoreceptor degeneration commonly note night blindness, photopsias, and blurred vision. If cones are involved, loss of color perception may occur. Electroretino-grams are abnormal, and ophthalmoscopic examination may show retinal arteriolar attenuation.[172]

A number of different autoantibodies have been described in association with photoreceptor degeneration, but the most common is the anti-CAR (carcinoma-associated retinal antigen) antibody. The target antigen is recoverin, a calcium-binding mol-ecule involved in the transduction of light signaling in verte-brate photoreceptors.[173] The majority of patients with anti-CAR have cancer, usually SCLC, but a similar syndrome has been reported in patients with no detectable cancer.[174] Usually the vision loss is relentlessly progressive and blindness is the ulti-mate result, but occasional patients have responded to high-dose corticosteroids, plasmapheresis, or intravenous IgG.[174]

Antibodies directed against a variety of retinal antigens, including neurofilaments,[175] have been reported in patients with photoreceptor degeneration in addition to CAR. Most patients suffered from SCLC, non–small cell lung cancer, or breast cancer. Antibody against a photoreceptor antigen impli-cated in autosomal recessive retinitis pigmentosa, TLUP-1, has been reported in a patient with cancer-associated retinopathy and endometrial cancer.[176] Some patients with anti-Hu syn-drome develop retinal photoreceptor degeneration. Treatment of the underlying tumor usually does not modify the course of the visual syndrome. Three cases of isolated cone dystrophy have been reported.[177]

Progressive vision loss with retinal pigmentary abnormalities has been separated into several syndromes. Most commonly associated with melanoma or adenocarcinomas of the gut,[177] these disorders have distinctive ophthalmoscopic appearances. Melanoma-associated retinopathy (MAR) most commonly appears at the stage of metastatic melanoma and is more com-mon in men than in women.[177] Only rods are affected, and progressive blindness is unusual. Autoantibodies against rod bipolar cells may be recognizing a lipid antigen.[178] Intravitreal injection of human MAR IgG into monkeys produces the elec-troretinal abnormalities of the syndrome.[179] Acquired night blindness has been reported in association with melanoma.[177]

A small number of patients with paraneoplastic optic neu-ropathies have been reported.[180-183] Primary cancers include SCLC, lymphoma, neuroblastoma, glucagonoma, nasopharyn-geal carcinoma, non–small cell lung cancer, thymoma, and myeloma.[177] Ophthalmoscopic examination may reveal optic disk pallor but not retinal pigmentary changes or vascular attenuation. Optic neuropathy may be associated with anti-CV2 antibodies; these patients frequently have concomitant cerebel-lar dysfunction and sensorimotor neuropathy.[181] Electroretino-grams are normal, but visual evoked potentials are delayed. Patients do not complain of photopsia; instead, progressive scotomas related to optic nerve dysfunction develop. The autoimmune optic neuropathies seem to have a better visual prognosis as a class than the melanoma-associated and other cancer-associated retinopathies.[177] Patients with paraneoplastic optic neuropathy improve with immunosuppression, but, as with other paraneoplastic disorders, most reports of visual recovery have been associated with treatment of the cancer.[177] Steroids have been the most frequently used immunosuppres-sive treatment. For MAR patients, aggressive multimodality antimelanoma therapy with surgery, radiation, and immuno-therapy improve aspects of visual function.[184] A patient with multiple myeloma and an antibody directed against an antigen in retinal ganglion cells recovered completely after high-dose chemotherapy and stem cell transplantation obliterated the autoantibody.[183]

Patients with overlap syndromes combining retinopathy and optic neuropathy have been reported. Autoantibodies to recov-erin may be seen in other autoimmune retinal disorders, such as retinitis pigmentosa.[177]

OPSOCLONUS-MYOCLONUS

Opsoclonus-myoclonus (OM), a disorder of ocular motility and multifocal myoclonus, was first described in children with neuro-blastoma. Although earlier reports suggested that half of pediat-ric cases were paraneoplastic, probably only 5% are associated with cancer. Because the OM antedates the discovery of neuro-blastoma in many children, search for underlying neuroblas-toma is necessary in any child who develops OM. The peak age of onset for the disorder is 18 months, and girls are preferentially affected. Significant neurologic dysfunction frequently persists in children with OM and neuroblastoma.[185] Favorable disease stage at the time of diagnosis of the neuroblastoma correlates with a higher risk of neurologic sequelae in pediatric patients with OM, but the presence of antineuronal antibodies does not.[186] Success-ful treatment of the neuroblastoma may be associated with a bet-ter neurologic outcome.[185] Although antineuronal antibodies are frequently detected in children with OM and neuroblastoma, no one antigen seems to be the common target. Antineurofila-ment antibodies were implicated in one pediatric case,[187] and anti-Hu antibodies in another patient.[188]

A novel antibody, anti-Ri, has been reported in several adult patients with opsoclonus and truncal ataxia or other cerebellar signs. These cases were associated with breast or gynecologic cancers.[189] Anti-Ri antibodies recognize 55- and 80-kD bands on denaturing Western blots of cortical neurons. It is unclear whether the neurologic prognosis is different for antibody-negative and anti-Ri–associated OM. The target antigen is Nova, an RNA-binding protein, and antibodies derived from patients recognize a region of the protein necessary for RNA interaction,[190] which suggests a mechanism for antibody-mediated toxicity.

In a series of 24 adult patients with OM, 12 of 14 patients with paraneoplastic OM had no detectable autoantibodies. The ten idiopathic cases were monophasic, with good recovery in most patients. The paraneoplastic cases were relentlessly progressive despite administration of immunosuppressive therapy in five patients with refractory tumors, but at least partial recovery occurred in patients whose tumors were successfully treated.[191] Paraneoplastic OM has also been associated with Hodgkin's disease; these patients do not have anti-Ri antibodies.[192] In a study of 21 patients with OM, including idiopathic OM as well as SLSC- and neuroblastoma-related cases, 25 putative targets were identified by probing a brainstem complementary DNA library. The target proteins included members of postsynaptic density protein families, or proteins restricted to neurons, including RNA- and DNA-binding and zinc finger proteins.[193]

PARANEOPLASTIC MOTOR NEURON DISORDERS

Most cases of motor neuron disorders in patients with cancer probably represent the concomitant occurrence of two common disorders in the same patient. However, paraneoplastic motor neuron disorders (PMNDs) do occur, and diagnosis is important, because patients may improve after tumor removal or immunosuppression.[194] Experienced neuromuscular clinicians believe that PMND can be differentiated from amyotrophic lateral sclerosis (ALS) using clinical and electrophysiologic criteria and discourage an extensive search for occult malignancy in patients with typical ALS. However, PMND with a variable mixture of upper and lower motor neuron signs has been reported in association with both lymphoproliferative malignancies and solid tumors.[194–199]

Patients with PMND were separated into three different groups[196] in a series reported by Memorial Sloan-Kettering Cancer Center. One group harbored anti-Hu antibodies.[196,197] In these patients, progressive motor neuron dysfunction is part of a more complex syndrome incorporating features of the anti-Hu syndrome. A second group of five women with primary lateral sclerosis and breast cancer were identified; none had anti-Hu antibodies or other autoantibodies. A third group of patients developed a syndrome resembling ALS and had a variety of underlying solid tumors.

Patients with Hodgkin's disease or non-Hodgkin's lymphoma, paraproteinemia, and a mixed upper and lower motor neuron syndrome have been reported. Lower motor neuron syndromes, as well as a mixture of lower and upper motor neuron signs, have been reported in association with myeloproliferative disorders and paraproteinemias.[194] A rapidly progressive, painless lower motor neuron syndrome occurred in a patient with angiocentric lymphoma.[198]

Case reports suggest that patients may improve substantially after effective treatment of the underlying malignancy or, less clearly, with immunosuppressive therapy.[129] Remission of the motor neuron syndrome has been reported after nephrectomy in a patient with renal cell carcinoma[195] and after successful treatment of lung cancer.[199] A case of breast cancer associated with lower motor neuron syndrome and autoantibodies directed against isoforms of beta-IV spectrin and other undefined nodal antigens has also been reported.[200]

Posner has suggested that the predominantly lower motor neuron disorder termed *subacute motor neuronopathy* or *spinal muscular atrophy* is an opportunistic viral syndrome.[123] This syndrome has been reported with Hodgkin's disease and non-Hodgkin's lymphoma. Patients present with multifocal motor weakness. Sensory complaints may be present. The CSF is usually acellular with mildly elevated protein levels. These patients often spontaneously stabilize neurologically. A subacute motor axonal neuropathy and ophthalmoplegia in a patient with melanoma treated with a MAGE vaccine was associated with anti-GQ1b antibodies.[201]

One of the authors treated a patient who survived 15 years after diagnosis of metastatic adenocarcinoma of the colon and then developed a rapidly progressive motor neuron disorder and dementia (F. Lieberman, *unpublished observation*, 1998). An antibody reactive with anterior horn cells in spinal cord and pyramidal cells in cortex was identified in the patient's serum. Treatment with intravenous IgG produced a transient improvement in leg strength and ambulation, but the patient died of neurogenic respiratory failure despite a subsequent trial of high-dose methylprednisolone.

PARANEOPLASTIC PERIPHERAL NEUROPATHIES

Subacute sensorimotor neuropathy usually presents with progressive distal, symmetric sensory loss and weakness, more severe in the legs.[202] Lung cancer is the most commonly associated malignancy. In approximately two-thirds of patients, the neuropathy precedes the diagnosis of cancer or is noted at the time of diagnosis. CSF is usually acellular, and protein concentration may be mildly elevated. Neurophysiologic studies usually indicate an axonal process and nerve biopsy specimens show a mixture of axonal injury and demyelination. This disorder is usually relentlessly progressive, but some patients stabilize after tumor removal and some patients appear to benefit from corticosteroid therapy.[123] Women with breast cancer may develop a slowly progressive sensorimotor neuropathy with proximal weakness and upper motor neuron signs.[194–202] This disorder is frequently indolent.

A novel antigen, CV2, has been reported as the target antigen in a group of patients presenting with sensorimotor neuropathy, cerebellar degeneration, and uveitis.[203] Optic neuropathy may also occur. The CV2 antigen is a member of the Ulip/CRMP family of proteins, involved in axonal growth and guidance. Anti-Hu antibodies were simultaneously present in 20% of the patients. Limited pathologic studies suggest that Schwann cells may be the site of injury in the peripheral nervous system and oligodendrocytes in the central nervous system.

Acute polyradiculoneuropathy (APN) appears to occur in increased frequency in patients with Hodgkin's disease. The clinical features of APN in Hodgkin's disease are similar to those of idiopathic Guillain-Barré syndrome.[204] Treatment of the Hodgkin's disease does not clearly modify the course of the neuropathy. No specific autoantibodies have been identified in these patients. APN associated with Hodgkin's disease may respond to plasmapheresis or intravenous gamma globulin.[205] APN has also been reported in association with leukemias, non-Hodgkin's lymphoma, and multiple myeloma.[204,205] Leukemic or lymphomatous infiltration of the peripheral nerves may be clinically indistinguishable from APN.[206] Relapsing and remitting forms of APN have also been reported in association with a variety of solid tumors, leukemia, and lymphoma,[205] but it is possible that these cases represent coincidence of idiopathic inflammatory polyneuropathy in a patient with cancer. A patient with hepatocellular carcinoma and APN demonstrated antineutrophil cytoplasmic antibodies.[207] Several cases of chronic inflammatory demyelinating polyneuropathy have been associated with melanoma.[208] Concomitant vitiligo suggests an autoimmune disorder, perhaps directed against shared cell surface ganglioside antigens.[209]

A number of different syndromes are associated with plasma cell dyscrasias.[210,211] Typical osteolytic multiple myeloma is only rarely associated with clinically significant peripheral neuropathy. Most commonly, the neuropathy is a sensorimotor neuropathy and is relatively mild. Pure sensory neuropathy has also been reported. Patients with osteolytic myeloma also develop more severe neuropathies that clinically resemble Guillain-Barré syndrome or chronic inflammatory demyelinating polyneuropathy.[210] Secondary amyloidosis may also cause a relentless, often painful, sensorimotor neuropathy in patients. Unfortunately, the progressive neuropathies rarely respond to immunosuppressive therapy of any form.[210,211]

Although osteosclerotic myeloma represents only 2% of cases of multiple myeloma, 50% of patients with osteosclerotic myeloma develop peripheral neuropathy.[210] The association with progressive sensorimotor neuropathy is crucial to recognize, because this neuropathy frequently improves after radiation therapy or chemotherapy. Bone scanning is insensitive, and a metastatic bone survey is necessary to identify the sclerotic bone lesion. M protein (IgG or IgA) may be missed unless immunoelectrophoresis or immunofixation is performed on the serum specimen and urine. Nonmalignant plasma cell dyscrasias may also be associated with neuropathy, and the response to treatment is quite variable.[210]

A distinctive syndrome combining polyneuropathy, hepatosplenomegaly, endocrinopathy, skin changes, and paraproteinemia, known as the POEMS syndrome, is associated with osteosclerotic myeloma. The natural history and features of the neuropathy are the same as those for patients with osteosclerotic myeloma who do not meet all the diagnostic criteria for POEMS.[210] Chemotherapy may be beneficial for patients with POEMS and disseminated plasmacytoma.

Painful mononeuritis multiplex due to small vessel vasculitis has been linked to underlying malignancy in a small number of patients. SCLC, prostate cancer, endometrial cancer, lymphoma, and renal cell carcinoma have been implicated.[194] In some patients, the mononeuritis multiplex is part of a more generalized vasculitis, with muscle involvement and elevated sedimentation rate. In other patients, the vasculitis appears limited to the peripheral nerves. Nerve biopsy is necessary for diagnosis. Mononeuritis multiplex may be a presentation of the anti-Hu syndrome; the cases of prostate carcinoma associated with the vasculitic syndrome have been small cell, undifferentiated carcinomas. In one case, the prostate cancer was associated with anti-Hu antibodies. Immunosuppression or plasmapheresis may be beneficial, and removal of a resectable associated cancer has been followed by improvement as well.

Inflammatory brachial neuritis is usually not linked with malignancy, but when paraneoplastic, is most frequently associated with Hodgkin's disease.[123] Because metastatic plexopathy is far more common than the paraneoplastic disorder, imaging studies should be performed to identify tumor infiltration of the plexus when paraneoplastic neuritis is considered. Unlike radiation-induced plexopathy, the inflammatory disorder is frequently painful at onset.

NEUROMUSCULAR JUNCTION DISORDERS

Typical myasthenia gravis (MG) is associated with thymoma in approximately 15% of cases, and autoantibodies against contractile proteins of striated muscle are associated with increased probability of underlying thymoma.[194] All patients with MG should undergo CT scanning of the chest to identify thymic neoplasms. In patients with thymoma, the MG may remit after thymectomy.[194] In most cases, the thymoma is not invasive and can be definitively treated by thymectomy.

LES is one paraneoplastic neurologic disorder for which the immunobiology is clinically relevant, and the molecular understanding of the disease is applicable to the clinic.[212] In approximately 60% of patients with LES, the disorder is associated with an underlying cancer, usually SCLC.[194,213] Proximal weakness is a common presenting complaint, but bulbar symptoms are uncommon. In most patients, LES is not a pure motor syndrome. Paresthesias are frequently reported. The abnormality of autonomic function has been termed *cholinergic dysautonomia*[214]; patients may report dry mouth or erectile dysfunction. Characteristic electrophysiologic abnormalities include augmentation of the compound motor action potential with repetitive stimulation.[213]

Antibodies directed against protein epitopes in the voltage-gated calcium channel of presynaptic neurons are present in most patients with LES.[215] Passive transfer of antibody reproduces the characteristic electrophysiologic abnormality in animal models of LES.[216] Immunization with a component of the P/Q-type calcium channel, synaptotagmin, produces autoantibodies and clinical disease in an animal model of LES.[217]

Most patients with LES benefit from plasmapheresis and immunosuppressive therapy.[213] Drugs that increase presynaptic acetylcholine release may also decrease symptoms; 3,4-diaminopyridine is one such agent that has relatively minimal side effects.

PARANEOPLASTIC SYNDROMES WITH MUSCLE RIGIDITY

Stiff-person syndrome presents with muscle stiffness and rigidity, predominately in the paraspinal and abdominal muscles, and muscle spasms.[194] Stiff-person syndrome has been reported in association with breast cancer, Hodgkin's disease, and colon cancer. Paraneoplastic stiff-person syndrome is associated with antibodies against amphiphysin, a synaptic protein involved in vesicle endocytosis. Antibodies against glutamic acid decarboxylase have also been reported, and some patients have antibodies to both amphiphysin and glutamic acid decarboxylase.[194] Patients frequently improve with effective treatment for the underlying tumor, and steroids may also be beneficial.

Paraneoplastic neuromyotonia is a syndrome of spontaneous and continuous muscle fiber activity of peripheral origin.[194] Unlike stiff-person syndrome this abnormal activity persists during sleep and electromyographs show high-frequency burst discharges. The disorder frequently develops in association with MG in thymoma. Hodgkin's disease, plasma cell dyscrasias, and SCLC have been associated with neuromyotonia.[194] Autoantibodies against voltage-gated potassium channels have been found in some patients with paraneoplastic neuromyotonia. The disorder may improve spontaneously or with plasmapheresis. Whether antineoplastic treatment benefits these patients in general is unclear.

DERMATOMYOSITIS

Although most patients with dermatomyositis do not have cancer, patients with the disorder do seem to be at higher risk for discovery of a cancer.[194] Breast cancer is the most commonly associated cancer in women, and lung and GI cancer in men. Association with tumors of the pancreas, melanoma, germ cell tumors, nasopharyngeal carcinoma, and lymphoma has also been reported.

An immune-mediated intramuscular angiopathy leads to ischemia and muscle fiber necrosis. Deposits of IgG, IgM, and complement are found in small blood vessels. Cellular inflammatory infiltrates include B cells, macrophages, and CD4+ T cells.

Immunosuppression has not been tested specifically in patients with underlying cancer, but the modalities that are effective in idiopathic dermatomyositis seem effective in the paraneoplastic disorder. It is unclear if antineoplastic therapy leads to improvement in the muscle disease in the absence of concomitant immunosuppression.

MOVEMENT DISORDERS

If one excludes cerebellar syndromes and paraneoplastic encephalomyelitis, paraneoplastic movement disorders are rare. Usually the movement disorder accompanies other signs of brainstem dysfunction. Disorders of excess movement predominate. Chorea has been reported in association with brainstem signs in patients with SCLC,[218–220] acute lymphocytic leukemia,[221] renal cell carcinoma,[222] and Hodgkin's disease.[223] A normal MRI scan does not exclude paraneoplastic chorea.[224] Patients with chorea in association with CRMP-5 neuronal antibody may also manifest sensorimotor neuropathy, autonomic dysfunction, and visual symptoms.[225] Another similar patient improved clinically and radiologically after successful systemic chemotherapy.[226] Antibody immunoreactivity with optic nerve, retina, or choroid was not demonstrated, so the relationship of the visual syndrome to the paraneoplastic choreiform disorder is unclear. Rubral tremor in extremity has been described as a paraneoplastic syndrome.[227]

Paraneoplastic parkinsonian syndromes are extremely rare.[228] Rapidly progressive parkinsonism and autonomic failure have been reported in a man with multiple myeloma. At necropsy, no inflammatory changes were detected in the basal ganglia or elsewhere in the brain.[229] The relationship between the myeloma and the movement disorder is unclear.

In summary, for most of the paraneoplastic neurologic syndromes, treatment is currently unsatisfactory. A recurring observation regarding outcome is that effective tumor ablation, either with surgery or systemic therapies, is more effective than immunosuppression in producing clinical neurologic improvement. However, recovery after effective tumor therapy is variable and frequently incomplete, perhaps because the burden of

neuronal cell loss is great by the time the diagnosis of paraneoplastic neurologic disorder is established. Immunosuppression with corticosteroids, plasma exchange, intravenous IgG, and immunoadsorption is variably effective.[230] In a small and heterogeneous series of patients treated with extracorporeal immunoadsorption, there was a 75% response rate.[231] For many of the paraneoplastic syndromes, there is no evidence-based rationale for choosing the type or sequence of immunotherapy. The ease and safety of intravenous IgG lead to its frequent choice as the first-line therapy for antibody-mediated or antibody-associated disorders.[232]

MISCELLANEOUS PARANEOPLASTIC SYNDROMES

HYPERTROPHIC OSTEOARTHROPATHY

A clinical syndrome that is presumably hypertrophic osteoarthropathy (HOA) has been described in the medical literature since the age of Hippocrates. In 1992, an international workshop on HOA met in Florence, Italy, and established a consensus for the diagnosis, classification, and assessment of this syndrome.[233] To fulfill the diagnostic criteria for this disease, both digital clubbing and periostosis must be present. Digital clubbing can be defined as paronychial soft tissue expansion associated with the loss of the curved linear lucency normally present at the junction between the nail and the skin. This may progress to a prominent bulbus enlargement of the distal end of the digit, representing an underlying increase in vascular and connective tissues. Periostosis is represented by periosteal proliferation in tubular bones, particularly the tibia and femur. Incomplete forms of HOA include clubbing alone, isolated periostosis, and pachydermia associated with any of the minor manifestations of the syndrome (synovial effusions, seborrhea, folliculitis, hyperhidrosis, hypertrophic gastropathy, and acroosteolysis).[234]

HOA can be characterized as primary or secondary, generalized or localized. The localized forms are seen in patients with hemiplegia, aneurysm, infectious arthritis, and patent ductus arteriosis. The generalized syndromes are associated with a variety of pulmonary, cardiac, liver, intestinal, and mediastinal diseases, as well as miscellaneous problems. Malignancy-related HOA is most commonly caused by non–small cell lung cancer and metastasis to the lungs. The mediastinal cancers associated with HOA are esophageal carcinoma, thymoma, primary mediastinal germ cell tumor, and metastasis to the mediastinum.

As with many paraneoplastic syndromes, successful treatment of the underlying disease is associated with a rapid resolution of the problem. However, in most cases of lung cancer, the disease is generally in an advanced state, and therefore successful treatment is difficult. Patients with severe pain have been successfully treated with nonsteroidal antiinflammatory drugs.[235] Surgery and other arthritic treatments such as colchicine have been less successful.[236] Many times the symptoms can be quite debilitating and do not respond to therapy.

FEVER

Thirty percent of patients with cancer develop fever at some point during the course of their malignancy,[237] with the majority having an underlying infection. Other causes of fever in cancer patients include tumor, drug fever, reaction to blood products, and autoimmune disease. The major differential point in determining whether the fever is due to infection is the presence or absence of neutropenia. In patients with low white blood cell counts, infection causes more than two-thirds of all fevers, whereas patients with normal white blood cell counts are infected far less frequently. Twenty percent of fevers in non-neutropenic patients are secondary to infection, whereas 45% remain unexplained after complete evaluation.[238]

In the absence of infection, it is thought that cancer cells can produce cytokines, which cause fever. Renal cell carcinoma is the most common cancer associated with fever, with fever occurring in up to one-half of patients.[239] Hepatoma patients develop fever one-third of the time.[240] Pel-Ebstein fever is seen in patients with Hodgkin's disease and is an important prognostic feature of this disease. Fever is also seen in patients with non-Hodgkin's lymphoma.[241] Acute leukemia, osteosarcoma, atrial myxoma, adrenal carcinoma, pheochromocytoma, and hypothalamic tumors are also rarely associated with the development of fever.

The endogenous pyrogens have been well described over the past 20 years. IL-1 has replaced the term *endogenous pyrogen*, which was initially used to describe this cytokine associated with Hodgkin's disease.[242] Subsequently, IL-1 has been shown to increase circulating neutrophils and cortisol and to be intimately involved in the acute-phase response. TNF (α and β subtypes) has also been shown to cause fever, although it does not use the same receptors as IL-1 and appears to induce IL-1.[243] Many other cytokines have been implicated in paraneoplastic fever, including interferon and IL-6.

The most important point in the management of fever in patients with cancer is evaluating for infection, which can be life threatening in neutropenic patients. If infection is excluded, nonsteroidal antiinflammatory drugs are a reasonable means to manage patients with fever. Nonsteroidal drugs inhibit cyclooxygenase, reducing prostaglandin E_2 synthesis. Some investigators use the response to nonsteroidal antiinflammatory drugs to differentiate fever caused by infection from that caused by a tumor. In two separate studies, response to indomethacin and naproxen was associated with a high incidence of tumor-related fever compared with infectious causes.[244,245] Corticosteroids are also effective antipyretics, both by inhibiting prostaglandin E_2 and blocking transcription of messenger RNA for pyrogenic cytokines.[246]

REFERENCES

1. Liddle GW, Island DP, Ney RL, et al. Non-pituitary neoplasms and Cushing's syndrome. *Arch Intern Med* 1963;11:471.
2. Wajchenberg BL, Mendonca BB, Liberman B, et al. Ectopic adrenal corticotropic hormone syndrome. *Endocr Rev* 1994;15:752.
3. Terzolo M, Reimondo G, Ali A, et al. Ectopic ACTH syndrome: molecular basis and clinical heterogeneity. *Ann Oncol* 2001;12[Suppl 2]:S83.
4. Crapo L. Cushing's syndrome: a review of diagnostic tests. *Metabolism* 1979;28:955.
5. Wajchenberg BL, Mendonca BB, Liberman B, et al. Ectopic ACTH syndrome. *J Steroid Biochem Mol Biol* 1995;53:139.
6. Oldfield EH, Doppman JL, Nieman LK, et al. Petrosal sinus sampling with and without corticotropin-releasing hormone for the differential diagnosis of Cushing's syndrome. *N Engl J Med* 1991;325:897.
7. Pass HI, Doppman J, Nieman L, et al. Management of the ectopic ACTH-syndrome due to thoracic carcinoids: the HIH experience and review of the world literature. *Ann Thorac Surg* 1990;50:52.
8. Avgerinos PC, Wanovski JA, Oldfield EH, et al. The metyrapone and dexamethasone suppression tests for the differential diagnosis of the adrenocorticotropin-dependent Cushing syndrome: a comparison. *Ann Intern Med* 1994;121:318.
9. Nieman LK, Chrousos GP, Oldfield EH, et al. The ovine corticotropin-releasing hormone stimulation test and the dexamethasone suppression test in the differential diagnosis of Cushing's syndrome. *Ann Intern Med* 1986;105:862.
10. Leinung MC, Young WF Jr, Whitaker MD, et al. Diagnosis of corticotropin-producing bronchial carcinoid tumors causing Cushing's syndrome. *Mayo Clin Proc* 1990;65:1315.
11. de Herder WW, Krenning EP, Malchoff CD, et al. Somatostatin receptor scintigraphy: its value in tumor localization in patients with Cushing's syndrome caused by ectopic corticotropin or corticotropin-releasing hormone secretion. *Am J Med* 1994;96:305.
12. Zeiger MA, Pass HI, Doppman JD, et al. Surgical strategy in the management of non-small cell ectopic adrenal corticotropic hormone syndrome. *Surgery* 1992;112:994.
13. Pujol J, Viladrich M, Rafecas A, et al. Laparoscopic adrenalectomy. A review of 30 initial cases. *Surg Endosc* 1999;13:488.
14. Misbin RI, Canary J, Willard D. Aminoglutethimide in the treatment of Cushing's syndrome. *J Clin Pharmacol* 1976;16:645.
15. Jeffcoate WJ, Rees LH, Tomlin S, et al. Metyrapone in the long-term management of Cushing's disease. *BMJ* 1977;2:215.
16. Winquist EW, Laskey J, Crump M, et al. Ketoconazole in the management of paraneoplastic Cushing's syndrome secondary to ectopic adrenal corticotropin production. *J Clin Oncol* 1995;13:157.
17. Vignati F, Loli P. Additive effect of ketoconazole and octreotide in the treatment of severe adrenocorticotropin-dependent hypercortisolism. *J Clin Endocrinol Metab* 1996;81:2885.
18. Schwartz WB, Bennet W, Curelop S, et al. A syndrome of renal sodium loss in hyponatremia probably resulting from inappropriate secretion of anti-diuretic hormone. *Am J Med* 1957;23:529.
19. Vorherr H, Massry S, Utiger R, et al. Anti-diuretic principle in malignant tumor extracts from patients with inappropriate ADH syndrome. *J Clin Endocrinol Metab* 1968;28:162.
20. Lokich JJ. The frequency in clinical biology of ectopic hormone syndromes of small cell carcinoma. *Cancer* 1982;50:2111.
21. Hays R. Alteration in luminal membrane structure by antidiuretic hormone. *Am J Physiol* 1983;245:289.
22. Glover D, Glick J. Metabolic oncologic emergencies. *CA Cancer J Clin* 1987;37:302.
23. Ayus J, Krothapali R, Arieff A. Treatment of symptomatic hyponatremia and its relation to brain damage. *N Engl J Med* 1987;317:1190.
24. Raskin P, McClain CJ, Medsger TA. Hypocalcemia associated with metastatic bone disease. *Arch Intern Med* 1973;132:539.
25. Ryan EA, Reiss E. Oncogenous osteomalacia. Review of the world literature of 42 cases and report of two new cases. *Am J Med* 1984;77:501.
26. Siris ES, Clemens TL, Dempster DW, et al. Tumor-induced osteomalacia. Kinetics of calcium, phosphorus, and vitamin D metabolism and characteristics of bone histomorphometry. *Am J Med* 1987;82:307.
27. Blackman MR, Weintraub BD, Rosen SW, et al. Human placental and pituitary glycoprotein hormones and their subunits as tumor markers: a quantitative assessment. *J Natl Cancer Inst* 1980;65:81.
28. Kenimer JG, Hershman JM, Higgins HP. The thyrotropin in hydatidiform moles is human chorionic gonadotropin. *J Clin Endocrinol Metab* 1975;40:481.
29. Anderson T, Waldmann TA, Javadpour N, et al. Testicular germ-cell neoplasms: recent advances in diagnosis and therapy. *Ann Intern Med* 1979;90:373.
30. Kahn CR, Rosen SW, Weintraub BD, et al. Ectopic production of chorionic gonadotropin and its subunits by islet cell tumors: a specific marker for malignancy. *N Engl J Med* 1977;197:565.
31. Bender RA, Weintraub BD, Rosen SW. Prospective evaluation of two tumor-associated proteins in pancreatic adenocarcinoma. *Cancer* 1979;45:591.
32. Broder LE, Weintraub BD, Rosen SW, et al. Placental proteins and their subunits as tumor markers in prostatic carcinoma. *Cancer* 1977;40:211.
33. Kellner O, Voigt W, Schneyer U, et al. HCG induced hyperthyreosis in germ cell cancer. *Anticancer Res* 2000;20:5135.
34. Cave WT Jr, Dunn JT. Choriocarcinoma with hyperthyroidism: probable identity of the thyrotropin with human chorionic gonadotropin. *Ann Intern Med* 1976;85:60.
35. Rosen SW, Weintraub BD, Vaitukaitis JL, et al. Placental proteins and their subunits as tumor markers. *Ann Intern Med* 1975;82:71.
36. Steiner H, Dahlback O, Waldenstrom J. Ectopic growth-hormone production and osteoarthropathy in carcinoma of the bronchus. *Lancet* 1968;1:783.
37. Boizel R, Labat F, Bachelot I, et al. Acromegaly due to a growth hormone releasing hormone secreting bronchial carcinoid tumor. Further information on the abnormal responsiveness of the somatotroph cells and their recovery after successful treatment. *J Clin Endocrinol Metab* 1987;64:304.
38. Blackman MR, Rosen SW, Weintraub BD. Ectopic hormones. *Adv Intern Med* 1978;23:85.
39. Odell WD, Wolfsen AR. Humoral syndromes associated with cancer. *Ann Rev Med* 1978;29:379.
40. Sluiter WJ, Marrink J, Houwen B. Monoclonal gammopathy with an insulin binding IgG(k) M-component associated with severe hypoglycemia. *Br J Haematol* 1986;62:679.
41. Stuart CA, Prince MJ, Peters EJ, et al. Insulin receptor proliferation: a mechanism for tumor-associated hypoglycemia. *J Clin Endocrinol Metab* 1986;63:879.
42. Kiang DT, Bauer GE, Kennedy BJ. Immunoassayable insulin in carcinoma of the cervix associated with hypoglycemia. *Cancer* 1973;31:801.
43. Silvert CK, Rossini AA, Ghazvinian S, et al. Tumor hypoglycemia: deficient splanchnic glucose output and deficient glucagon secretion. *Diabetes* 1976;25:202.
44. Zapf J, Walter H, Froesch ER. Radioimmunological determination of insulin-like growth factors I and II in normal subjects and in patients with growth disorders and extrapancreatic tumor hypoglycemia. *J Clin Invest* 1981;68:3121.
45. Gorden P, Hendricks CM, Kahn CR, et al. Hypoglycemia associated with non-islet cell tumor and insulin like growth factors. *N Engl J Med* 1981;305:1452.
46. Ron D, Powers A, Pandian M, et al. Increased IGF-II production and consequent suppression of GH secretion: a dual mechanism for tumor-induced hypoglycemia. *J Clin Endocrinol Metab* 1989;68:701.

47. Hammond D, Winnick S. Paraneoplastic erythrocytosis and ectopic erythropoietins. *Ann N Y Acad Sci* 1974;230:219.

48. Lees LH. The biosynthesis of hormones by nonendocrine tumors—a review. *J Endocrinol* 1975;67:143.

49. Spivak J. Cancer-related anemia: its cause and characteristics. *Semin Oncol* 1994;21[Suppl 3]:3.

50. Frenkel E, Bick R, Rutherford C. Anemia of malignancy. *Hematol Oncol Clin North Am* 1997;10:861.

51. Vasavada PJ, Bournigal LJ, Reynolds RW. Thymoma associated with pure red cell aplasia and hypogammaglobulinemias. *Postgrad Med* 1973;54:93.

52. Akard LP, Brandt J, Lee L, et al. Chronic T cell lymphoproliferative disorder and pure red cell aplasia. *Am J Med* 1987;83:1069.

53. Antman KH, Skarin AT, Mayer RJ, et al. Microangiopathic hemolytic anemia and cancer: a review. *Medicine (Baltimore)* 1979;58:377.

54. Robinson WA. Granulocytosis in neoplasia. *Ann N Y Acad Sci* 1974;230:212.

55. Hocking W, Goodman J, Golde E. Granulocytosis associated with tumor production of colony stimulating factor. *Blood* 1983;61:600.

56. Sato K, Fujii Y, Kakiuchi T, et al. Paraneoplastic syndrome of hypercalcemia and leukocytosis caused by squamous carcinoma cells (T3M-1) producing parathyroid hormone-related protein, interleukin 2, and granulocyte colony stimulating factor. *Cancer Res* 1989;49:4740.

57. Heyman M, Walsh T. Autoimmune neutropenia and Hodgkin's disease. *Cancer* 1987;59:1903.

58. Weller P. The immunobiology of eosinophils. *N Engl J Med* 1991;324:1110.

59. Levin J, Conley CL. Thrombocytosis associated with malignant disease. *Arch Intern Med* 1964;114:497.

60. Estrov Z, Talpaz M, Maligit G, et al. Elevated plasma thrombopoietin activity in patients with cancer related thrombocytosis. *Am J Med* 1995;98:551.

61. Doan C, Bouroncle BA, Wiseman BK. Idiopathic and secondary thrombocytopenic purpura. Clinical study and evaluation of 381 cases over a period of 28 years. *Ann Intern Med* 1960;53:861.

62. Bellone JD, Kunicki TS, Aster RH. Immune thrombocytopenia associated with carcinoma. *Ann Intern Med* 1983;99:470.

63. Trousseau A. Phlegmasia alba dolens. Clinique medicale de l'Hotel-Dieu de Paris, London. *N Sydenham Soc* 1865;3:94.

64. DeSancho MT, Rand JH. Bleeding and thrombotic complications in critically ill patients with cancer. *Crit Care Clin* 2001;17:559.

65. Bick R, Struass J, Frenkel E. Thrombosis and hemorrhage in oncology patients. *Hematol Oncol Clin North Am* 1997;10:875.

66. Ginsberg JS, Kearon C, Douketis J, et al. The use of D-dimer testing and impedance plethysmographic examination in patients with clinical indication of deep venous thrombosis. *Arch Intern Med* 1997;157:1077.

67. Levine M, Gent M, Hirsch J, et al. A comparison of low molecular weight heparin administered primarily at home with unfractionated heparin administered in the hospital for proximal deep venous thrombosis. *N Engl J Med* 1996;334:667.

68. Green D, Hull RD, Brant R, et al. Lower mortality in cancer patients treated with low-molecular weight heparin versus standard heparin. *Lancet* 1992;339:1476.

69. Siragusa S, Cosmi B, Piovella F, et al. Low-molecular-weight heparins and unfractionated heparin in the treatment of patients with acute venous thromboembolism: results of a meta-analysis. *Am J Med* 1996;100:269.

70. Sallah S, Wan JH, Nguyen NP, et al. Disseminated intravascular hemolysis in solid tumors: clinical and pathologic studies. *Thomb Haemost* 2001;86:828.

71. Grainick HR, Abrell E. Studies of the procoagulant and fibrinolytic activity of promyelocytes in acute promyelocytic leukemia. *Br J Haematol* 1973;24:59.

72. Menell JS, Cesarman GM, Jacovina AT, et al. Annexin II and bleeding in acute promyelocytic leukemia. *N Engl J Med* 1999;340:994.

73. Veyradier A, Jenkins CS, Fressinaud E, et al. Acquired von Willebrand's syndrome: from pathophysiology to management. *Thromb Haemost* 2000;84:175.

74. Sallah S, Singh P, Hanrakan LP. Antibodies against Factor VIII in patients with solid tumors: successful treatment of cancer may suppress inhibitor formation. *Haemostasis* 1998;28:244.

75. Gonzales Quintela A, Candela M, et al. Non-bacterial thrombotic endocarditis in cancer patients. *Acta Cardiol* 1991;46:1.

76. Waldmann TA. Protein losing enteropathy. *Gastroenterology* 1966;50:422.

77. Schwartz M, Jarnum S. Protein losing gastroenteropathy: hypoproteinemia due to gastrointestinal protein loss of varying aetiology, diagnosed by means of 131I-albumin. *Dan Med Bull* 1961;8:1.

78. Strygler B, Nicor MJ, Santangelo WC, et al. Alpha1-anti-trypsin excretion in stool in normal subjects and in patients with gastrointestinal disorders. *Gastroenterology* 1990;99:1380.

79. Harvey KB, Bothe A, Blackburn GL. Nutritional assessment and patient outcome during oncologic therapy. *Cancer* 1979;43:2065.

80. DeWys WD, Begg D, Lavin PT, et al. Prognostic effect of weight loss prior to chemotherapy in cancer patients. *Am J Med* 1980;69:491.

81. Argiles JM, Moore-Carrasco R, Fuster G, et al. Cancer cachexia: molecular mechanisms. *Int J Biochem Cell Biol* 2003;35:405.

82. Carbo N, Busquets S, Van Royen M, et al. TNF-α is involved in activating DNA fragmentation in skeletal muscle. *Br J Cancer* 2002;86:1012.

83. Todorove P, Carink J, MeDevitt B, et al. Characterization of cancer cachectic factor. *Nature* 1999;22:739.

84. Moldawer LL, Copeland EM. Proinflammatory cytokines, nutritional support, and the cachexia syndrome: interactions and therapeutic options. *Cancer* 1997;79:1828.

85. Body JJ. The syndrome of anorexia-cachexia. *Curr Opin Oncol* 1999;11:255.

86. Della G, Cuna R, Pelligini A, et al. Effect of methylprednisolone sodium succinate on quality of life in preterminal cancer patients: a placebo-controlled, multicenter study. *Eur J Cancer Clin Oncol* 1989;25:1817.

87. Strasser F, Bruera ED. Update on anorexia and cancer. *Hematol Oncol Clin North Am* 2002;16:589.

88. Maltoni M, Nanni O, Scarpi E, et al. High-dose progestins for the treatment of cancer anorexia-cachexia syndrome: a systematic review of randomised clinical trials. *Ann Oncol* 2001;12:289.

89. Lee JC, Yamauchi H, Hopper J. The association of cancer and nephrotic syndrome. *Ann Intern Med* 1966;64:41.

90. Eagen JW, Lewis EJ. Glomerulopathies of neoplasia. *Kidney Int* 1977;11:297.

91. Maesaka J, Mittel S, Fishbane S. Paraneoplastic syndromes of the kidney. *Semin Oncol* 1997;24:373.

92. Lesesne J, Rothschild N, Erickson B. Cancer-associated hemolytic-uremic syndrome: analysis of 85 cases from a national registry. *J Clin Oncol* 1989;7:781.

93. Shapiro JH, Ramsay CG, Jacobson HG, et al. Renal involvement in lymphomas and leukemias in adults. *AJR Am J Roentgenol* 1962;88:928.

94. Brown J, Winkelmann RK. Acanthosis nigricans, a study of 90 cases. *Medicine* 1968;47:33.

95. Cohen RP, Grossman ME, Almeida L, et al. Tripe palms and cancer. *Clin Dermatol* 1993;11:165.

96. Sexton M, Snyder CR. Generalized melanosis in occult primary melanoma. *J Am Acad Dermatol* 1989;20:261.

97. Nelson DH, Meakin JW, Thorn GW, et al. ACTH-producing pituitary tumors following adrenalectomy for Cushing's syndrome. *Ann Intern Med* 1960;52:560.

98. Boyce S, Harper J. Paraneoplastic dermatoses. *Dermatol Clin* 2002;20:523.

99. Holdiness MR. The sign of Leser-Trélat. *Int J Dermatol* 1986;25:564.

100. Richard M, Giroux JM. Acrokeratosis paraneoplastica (Bazex's syndrome). *J Am Acad Dermatol* 1987;16:178.

101. Bolognia JL. Bazex's syndrome. *Clin Dermatol* 1993;11:37.

102. Ashikari R, Park K, Huvos AG, et al. Paget's disease of the breast. *Cancer* 1970;26:680.

103. Cohen PR, Talpaz M, Kurzrock R. Malignancy-associated Sweet's syndrome. *J Clin Oncol* 1988;6:1887.

104. Cohen P, Kurzrock R. Mucocutaneous paraneoplastic syndromes. *Semin Oncol* 1997;24:334.

105. Solomon H. Erythema gyratum repens. *Arch Dermatol* 1969;100:639.

106. Hashizume T, Kiryu H, Noda K, et al. Glucagonoma syndrome. *J Am Acad Dermatol* 1988;19:377.

107. Murray JS, Paton RR, Pope CE. Pancreatic tumor associated with flushing and diarrhea. *N Engl J Med* 1961;264:436.

108. Wilkin JK. Flushing reactions: consequences and mechanisms. *Ann Intern Med* 1981;95:468.

109. Nicolis GD, Helwig EB. Exfoliative dermatitis: a clinicopathologic study of 135 cases. *Arch Dermatol* 1973;108:788.

110. Rapini R. Multicentric reticulohistiocytosis. *Clin Dermatol* 1993;11:107.

111. MacMahon HE, Brown PA, Shen EM. Acinar cell carcinoma of the pancreas with subcutaneous fat necrosis. *Gastroenterology* 1965;49:555.

112. Anhalt GJ. Paraneoplastic pemphigus. *Adv Dermatol* 1997;12:77.

113. Nousari H, Anhalt G. Pemphigus and bullous pemphigoid. *Lancet* 1999;354:667.

114. Amagai M, Nishikawa T, Nousari HC, et al. Antibodies against desmoglein 3 (pemphigus vulgaris antigen) are present in sera from patients with paraneoplastic pemphigus and cause acantholysis in vivo in neonatal mice. *J Clin Invest* 1998;102:775.

115. Williams JV, Marks JG, Billingsley EM. Use of mycophenolate mofetil in the treatment of paraneoplastic pemphigus. *Br J Dermatol* 2000;142:506.

116. Young L, Steinman HK. Acquired ichthyosis in a patient with acquired immunodeficiency syndrome and Kaposi's sarcoma. *J Am Acad Dermatol* 1987;16:395.

117. Sigurgeirsson B, Lindelöf B, Edhag O, et al. Risk of cancer in patients with dermatomyositis or polymyositis. *N Engl J Med* 1992;326:363.

118. Vogl A, Goldfischer S. Pachydermoperiostosis. Primary or idiopathic hypertrophic osteoarthropathy. *Am J Med* 1962;33:166.

119. Hegedus SI, Schorr WF. Acquired hypertrichosis lanuginosa and malignancy. *Arch Dermatol* 1972;106:84.

120. Lober CW. Should the patient with generalized pruritus be evaluated for malignancy? *J Am Acad Dermatol* 1988;19:350.

121. Finan MC, Connolly SM. Sebaceous gland tumors and systemic disease: a clinicopathologic analysis. *Medicine* 1984;63:232.

122. Clouston, PD, De Angelis LM, Posner JB. The spectrum of neurologic disease in patients with systemic cancer. *Ann Neurol* 1992;31:268.

123. Paraneoplastic syndromes. In: Posner JB, ed. *Neurologic complications of cancer*. Philadelphia: FA Davis,1995:353.

124. Dalmau J, Posner JB. Neurologic paraneoplastic antibodies (anti-Yo, anti-Hu, anti-Ri): the case for a nomenclature based on antibody and antigen specificity. *Neurology* 1994;44:2241.

125. Posner JB, Furneaux HM. Paraneoplastic syndromes. In: Waksman BH, ed. *Immunologic mechanisms in neurologic and psychiatric disease*. New York: Raven Press, 1990:187.

126. Leys K, Lang G, Johnston I, et al. Calcium channel autoantibodies in Lambert-Eaton myasthenic syndrome. *Ann Neurol* 1991;29:307.

127. Williams CL, Hay JE, Huiatt TW, et al. Paraneoplastic IgG striational autoantibodies produced by clonal thymic B cells and in serum of patients with myasthenia gravis and thymoma react with titin. *Lab Invest* 1992;66:331.

128. Verma P, Oger J. Treatment of acquired autoimmune myasthenia gravis: a topic review. *Can J Neurol Sci* 1992;19:360.

129. Das A, Hochberg FH, McNelis S. A review of the therapy of paraneoplastic neurologic syndromes. *J Neurooncol* 1999;41:181.

130. Hormigo A, Lieberman F. Nuclear localization of anti-Hu antibody is not associated with in vitro cytotoxicity. *J Neuroimmunol* 1994;55:205.

131. Smitt PAE, Manley G, Posner JB. High titer antibodies but no disease in mice immunized with the paraneoplastic antigen HuD. *Neurology* 1994;44:[Suppl 2]376.

132. Dalmau J, Graus F, Rosenblum MK, et al. Anti-Hu associated paraneoplastic encephalomyelitis/sensory neuronopathy. A clinical study of 71 patients. *Medicine (Baltimore)* 1972;71:59.

133. Dalmau J, Furneaux HM, Gralla RJ, et al. Detection of the anti-Hu antibody in the serum of patients with small cell lung cancer—a quantitative Western blot analysis. *Ann Neurol* 1990;27:544.

134. Horwich MS, Cho L, Porro RS, et al. Subacute sensory neuropathy: a remote effect of carcinoma. *Ann Neurol* 1979;2:7.

135. Donofrio PD, Alessi AG, Alberts JW, et al. Electrodiagnostic evaluation of carcinomatous sensory neuronopathy. *Muscle Nerve* 1989;12:508.

136. Henson RA, Russell DS, Wilkinson M. Carcinomatous neuropathy and myopathy: a clinical and pathological study. *Brain* 1954;77:82.

137. Sillevis-Smitt P, Manley G, Moll JW, et al. Pitfalls in the diagnosis of autoantibodies associated with paraneoplastic neurologic disease. *Neurology* 1996;46:1739.

138. Graus F, Vega F, Delattre J-Y, et al. Plasmapheresis and antineoplastic treatment in CNS paraneoplastic syndromes with antineuronal autoantibodies. *Neurology* 1992;42:536.

139. Sagar HJ, Read DJ. Subacute sensory neuropathy with remission: an association with lymphoma. *J Neurol Neurosurg Psychiatry* 1982;45:83.

140. Graus F, Keime-Guibert F, Rene R, et al. Anti-Hu associated paraneoplastic encephalomyelitis: analysis of 200 patients. *Brain* 2001;124:1138.

141. Gultekin S, Rosenfeld MR, Voltz R, et al. Paraneoplastic limbic encephalitis: neurological symptoms, immunological findings, and tumour association in 50 patients. *Brain* 2000;123:1481.

142. Dirr LY, Elster AD, Donofrio PD, et al. Evolution of brain MRI abnormalities in limbic encephalitis. *Neurology* 1990;40;1300.

143. Voltz R, Guletkin SH, Rosenfeld MR, et al. A serologic marker of paraneoplastic limbic and brain-stem encephalitis in patients with testicular cancer. *N Engl J Med* 1999;340:1788.

144. Dalmau J, Guletkin SH, Voltz R, et al. Ma1, a novel neuron and testis-specific protein is recognized by the serum of patients with paraneoplastic neurological disorders. *Brain* 1999;122:27.

145. Rojas-Marcos I, Rousseau A, Keime-Guibert F, et al. Spectrum of paraneoplastic neurologic disorders in women with breast and gynecologic cancer. *Medicine (Baltimore)* 2003;82:216.

146. Knudsen A, Storstein A, Oltedal L, et al. Pyramidal cell antibodies associated with limbic encephalitis and thymoma. *Acta Neurol Scand* 2003;107:431.

147. Kung S, Mueller PS, Geda YE, et al. Delirium resulting from paraneoplastic limbic encephalitis caused by Hodgkin's disease. *Psychosomatics* 2002;43:498.

148. Thuerl C, Muller K, Laubenberger J, et al. MR imaging of autopsy-proved paraneoplastic limbic encephalitis in non-Hodgkin's lymphoma. *AJNR Am J Neuroradiol* 2003;24:507.

149. Brennan LV, Craddock PR. Limbic encephalopathy as a nonmetastatic complication of oat cell lung cancer: its reversal after treatment of the primary lung lesion. *Am J Med* 1983;75:518.

150. Modrego PJ, Cay A, Pina MA, et al. Paraneoplastic subacute encephalitis caused by adenocarcinoma of the prostate; a clinicopathologic report. *Acta Neurol Scand* 2002;105:351.

151. Stern RC, Hulette CM. Paraneoplastic limbic encephalitis associated with small cell carcinoma of the prostate. *Mod Pathol* 1999;12:818.

152. Babikian VL, Stefansson K, Dieperink MF, et al. Paraneoplastic myelopathy: antibodies against protein in normal spinal cord and underlying neoplasm. *Lancet* 1985;2:49.

153. Veilleux M, Bernier JP, Lamarche JB. Paraneoplastic encephalomyelitis and subacute dysautonomia due to an occult atypical carcinoid tumour of the lung. *Can J Neurol Sci* 1990;17:324.

154. Lennon VA, Sas DF, Busk MF, et al. Enteric neuronal autoantibodies in pseudoobstruction with small-cell lung carcinoma. *Gastroenterology* 1991;100:137.

155. Vernino S, Low PA, Fealey RD, et al. Autoantibodies to ganglionic acetylcholine receptors in autoimmune autonomic dysfunction. *N Engl J Med* 2000;343:847.

156. Vernino S, Cheshire WP, Lennon VA. Myasthenia gravis with autoimmune autonomic neuropathy. *Auton Neurosci* 2001;88:187.

157. Lennon VA, Ermilov LG, Szurszewski JH, et al. Immunization with neuronal nicotinic acetylcholine receptor induces neurologic autoimmune disease. *J Clin Invest* 2003;111:907.

158. Peterson K, Rosenblum MK, Kotanides H, et al. Paraneoplastic cerebellar degeneration. I. A clinical analysis of 55 anti-Yo positive patients. *Neurology* 1992;42:1931.

159. Posner JB. Paraneoplastic cerebellar degeneration. *Prin Pract Oncol Update* 1991;5:1.

160. Greenberg HS. Paraneoplastic cerebellar degeneration: a clinical and CT study. *J Neurooncol* 1984;2:377.

161. Dropcho E, Chen Y, Posner J, et al. Cloning of a brain protein identified by autoantibodies from a patient with paraneoplastic cerebellar degeneration. *Proc Natl Acad Sci U S A* 1987;84:4552.

162. Fathallah-Shaykh H, Wolf S, Wong E, et al. Cloning of leucine-zipper protein recognized by the sera of patients with antibody-associated paraneoplastic cerebellar degeneration. *Proc Natl Acad Sci U S A* 1991;88:3451.

163. Sakai K, Mitchell DJ, Tsukamoto T, et al. Isolation of a complementary DNA clone encoding an autoantigen recognized by an anti-neuronal antibody from a patient with paraneoplastic cerebellar degeneration. *Ann Neurol* 1990;28:692.

164. Hammack J, Kotanides H, Rosenblum MK, et al. Paraneoplastic cerebellar degeneration II. Clinical and immunologic findings in 21 patients with Hodgkin's disease. *Neurology* 1990;42:1938.

165. Peltola J, Hietaharju A, Rantala I, et al. A reversible neuronal antibody (anti-Tr) associated paraneoplastic cerebellar degeneration in Hodgkin's disease. *Acta Neurol Scand* 1998;98:360.

166. Graus F, Dalmau J, Valldeoriola F, et al. Immunological characterization of a neuronal antibody (anti-Tr) associated with paraneoplastic cerebellar degeneration and Hodgkin's disease. *J Neuroimmunol* 1998;74:55.

167. Bataller L, Wade DF, Graus F, et al. The MAZ protein is an autoantigen of Hodgkin's disease and paraneoplastic cerebellar dysfunction. *Ann Neurol* 2003;53:123.

168. Coesmans M, Sillevis Smitt PA, Linden DJ, et al. Mechanisms underlying cerebellar motor deficits due to mGluR1-autoantibodies. *Ann Neurol* 2003;53;325.

169. Shams'ili S, Grefkens J, de Leeuw B, et al. Paraneoplastic cerebellar degeneration associated with antineuronal antibodies: analysis of 50 patients. *Brain* 2003;126:1409.

170. Clouston PD, Saper CB, Arbizu T, et al. Paraneoplastic cerebellar degeneration III: cerebellar degeneration, cancer and the Lambert-Eaton syndrome. *Neurology* 1992;42:1944.

171. Tang RA, Kellaway J, Young SE. Ophthalmic complications of systemic cancer. *Oncology* 1991;3:59.

172. Thirkill CE, FitzGerald P, Sorgott RC, et al. Cancer associated retinopathy (CAR syndrome) with antibodies reactive with retinal, optic nerve, and cancer cells. *N Engl J Med* 1989;321:1589.

173. Thirkill CB, Taft RC, Tyler NK, et al. The cancer associated retinopathy antigen is a recoverin-like protein. *Invest Ophthalmol Vis Sci* 1992;33:2768.

174. Kiltner JL, Thirkill CE. The 22Kda antigen in optic nerve and retinal diseases. *J Neuroophthalmol* 1999;19:71.

175. Kornguth SE, Kalinke T, Grunwald GV, et al. Anti-neurofilament antibodies in the sera of patients with small cell carcinoma of the lung and with visual paraneoplastic syndrome. *Cancer Res* 1986;462:2588.

176. Kikuchi T, Arai J, Shibuki H, et al. Tubby-like protein 1 as an autoantigen in cancer associated retinopathy. *J Neuroimmunol* 2000;103:26.

177. Chan JW. Paraneoplastic retinopathies and optic neuropathies. *Surv Ophthalmol* 2003;48:12.

178. Nudelman E, Hakomori S, Kannagi R, et al. Characterization of a human melanoma associated ganglioside antigen defined by a monoclonal antibody, 4.2. *J Biol Chem* 1982;257:12752.

179. Lei B, Bush RA, Milam AH, et al. Human melanoma-associated retinopathy(MAR) antibodies alter the retinal ON response of the monkey ERG in vivo. *Invest Ophthalmol Vis Sci* 2000;41:262.

180. Malik S, Furlan AJ, Sweeney PJ, et al. Optic neuropathy: a rare paraneoplastic syndrome. *J Clin Ophthalmol* 1992;12:137.

181. De la Sayette V, Bertran F, Honnorat J, et al. Paraneoplastic cerebellar syndrome and optic neuritis with anti-CV2 antibodies: clinical response to excision of the primary tumor. *Arch Neurol* 1998;55:405.

182. Luiz JE, Lee AG, Keltener JL, et al. Paraneoplastic optic neuropathy and autoantibody production in small cell carcinoma of the lung. *J Neuroophthalmol* 1998;18:178.

183. Lieberman FS, Odel J, et al. Bilateral optic neuropathy with IgG multiple myeloma improved after myeloablative chemotherapy. *Neurology* 1999;57:414.

184. Keltner JL, Thirkill CE, Yip PT. Clinical and immunologic characteristics of melanoma associated retinopathy syndrome: eleven new cases and a review of 51 previously published cases. *J Neuroophthalmol* 2001;21:173.

185. Russo C, Cohn SL, Petruzzi MJ, et al. Long-term neurologic outcome in children with opsoclonus-myoclonus associated with neuroblastoma: a report from the Pediatric Oncology Group. *Pediatr Med Oncol* 1997;28:284.

186. Rudnick E, Khakoo Y, Antunes NL, et al. Opsoclonus-myoclonus-ataxia syndrome in neuroblastoma: clinical outcome and antineuronal antibodies—a report from the Children's Cancer Study Group Study. *Med Pediatr Oncol* 2001;36:612.

187. Noetzel MJ, Cawley LP, James VL, et al. Antineurofilament protein antibodies in opsoclonus/myoclonus. *J Neuroimmunol* 1987;15:137.

188. Fisher PG, Wechsler SD, Singer HS. Anti-Hu antineuronal antibody in neuroblastoma-associated paraneoplastic syndrome. *Pediatr Neurol* 1994;10:309.

189. Budde-Steffen C, Anderson NE, Rosenblum MK. An antineuronal autoantibody in paraneoplastic opsoclonus. *Ann Neurol* 1988;23:528.

190. Buckanovich RJ, Yang YY, Darnell RB. The onconeural antigen Nova-I is a neuron-specific RNA-binding protein, the activity of which is inhibited by paraneoplastic antibodies. *J Neurosci* 1996;16:1114.

191. Bataller L, Graus F, Saiz A, et al. Clinical outcome in adult onset idiopathic or paraneoplastic opsoclonus myoclonus. *Brain* 2001;124:437.

192. Kay CL, Davie-Jones GAB, Singal R, et al. Paraneoplastic opsoclonus-myoclonus in Hodgkin's disease. *J Neurol Neurosurg Psychiatry* 1993;56:831.

193. Bataller L, Rosenfeld MR, Graus F, et al. Autoantigen diversity in the opsoclonus myoclonus syndrome. *Ann Neurol* 2003;53:347.

194. Rudnicki SA, Dalmau J. Paraneoplastic syndromes of the spinal cord, nerve, and muscle. *Muscle Nerve* 2000;23:1800.

195. Evans BK, Fagan MD, Arnold T, et al. Paraneoplastic motor neuron disease and renal cell carcinoma: improvement after nephrectomy. *Neurology* 1990;40:960.

196. Forsyth PA, Dalmau J, Graus F, et al. Motor neuron syndromes in cancer patients. *Ann Neurol* 1997;47:722.

197. Verna A, Berger JR, Snodgrass S, et al. Motor neuron disease: a paraneoplastic process associated with anti-Hu antibody and small cell lung carcinoma. *Ann Neurol* 1996;40:112.

198. Rubio A, Poole RM, Bara HS, et al. Motor neuron disease and angiotropic lymphoma. *Arch Neurol* 1997;54:92.

199. Mitchell DM, Olezak SA. Remission of a syndrome indistinguishable from motor neuron disease after resection of bronchial carcinoma. *Br Med J* 1979;2:176.

200. Berghs S, Ferracci F, Maksimova E, et al. Autoimmunity to BIV spectrum in paraneoplastic lower motor neuron syndrome. *Proc Natl Acad Sci U S A* 2001;12:6945.

201. Klooss L, Sillevis Smitt P, Ang CW, et al. Paraneoplastic ophthalmoplegia and subacute motor axonal neuropathy associated with anti-GQ1b antibodies in a patient with malignant melanoma. *J Neurol Neurosurg Psychiatry* 2003;74:507.

202. Antoine JC, Mosnier J-F, Absi L, et al. Carcinoma associated paraneoplastic peripheral neuropathies in patients with and without anti-onconeural antibodies. *J Neurol Neurosurg Psychiatry* 1999;67:7.

203. Yu Z, Kryzer TJ, Griesmann GE, et al. CRMP-5 neuronal autoantibody: marker of lung cancer and thymoma related autoimmunity. *Ann Neurol* 2001;49:146.

204. Lisak RP, Mitchell M, Zweiman B, et al. Guillain-Barré syndrome and Hodgkin's disease: three cases with immunological studies. *Ann Neurol* 1977;1:72.

205. Smitt PS, Posner JB. Paraneoplastic peripheral neuropathy. In: Latov N, Wokke JH, Kelly JJ Jr, eds. *Immunological infectious disease of the peripheral nerves.* Cambridge: Cambridge University Press, 1998:225.

206. Baron KD, Rowland LP, Zimmerman HM. Neuropathy with malignant tumor-metastases. *Neur Ment Dis* 1962;56:10.

207. Walcher J, Witter T, Rupprecht HD. Hepatocellular carcinoma presenting with paraneoplastic demyelinating polyneuropathy and PR-3 antineutrophil cytoplasmic antibody. *J Clin Gastroenterol* 2002;35:364.

208. Bird SDI, Brown MD, Shy ME, et al. Chronic inflammatory demyelinating polyneuropathy associated with malignant melanoma. *Neurology* 1996;46:822.

209. Weiss MD, Luciano CA, Semino-Mora C, et al. Molecular mimicry in chronic inflammatory demyelinating polyneuropathy and melanoma. *Neurology* 1998;51:1738.

210. Kelly JJ Jr. Polyneuropathies associated with myeloma, POEMs, and non-malignant IgG and IgA monoclonal gammopathies. In: Latov N, Wokke JH, Kelly JJ Jr, eds. *Immunological infectious disease of the peripheral nerves.* Cambridge: Cambridge University Press, 1998:225.

211. Ropper AH, Gorson KC. Neuropathies associated with paraproteinemia. *N Engl J Med* 1998;338:1601.

212. Takamori M. An autoimmune channelopathy associated with cancer: Lambert-Eaton myasthenic syndrome. *Intern Med* 1999;38:86.

213. Tim RW, Massey JM, Sanders DB. Lambert-Eaton myasthenic syndrome (LEMS). Clinical and electrodiagnostic features and response to therapy in 59 patients. *Ann N Y Acad Sci* 1998;841:823.

214. Khurana RK, Koski CL, Mayer RF. Autonomic dysfunction in Lambert-Eaton myasthenic syndrome. *J Neurol Sci* 1988;85:77.

215. Voltz R, Carpentier AF, Rosenfeld MR, et al. P/Q-type voltage-gated calcium channel antibodies in paraneoplastic disorders of the central nervous system. *Muscle Nerve* 1999;22:119.

216. Flink MT, Atchison WD. Passive transfer of Lambert-Eaton syndrome to mice induces dihydropyridine sensitivity of neuromuscular transmission. *J Physiol* 2002;543:567.

217. Takamori M, Komai K, Iwasa K. Antibodies to calcium channel and synaptotagmin in Lambert-Eaton myasthenic syndrome. *Am J Med Sci* 2000;319:204.

218. Albin RL, Bromberg MB, Penney JB, et al. Chorea and dystonia: a remote effect of carcinoma. *Mov Disord* 1988;3:162.

219. Dieti HW, Pulst SM, Engelhardt P, et al. Paraneoplastic brainstem encephalitis with acute dystonia and central hypoventilation. *J Neurol* 1982;227:22.

220. Heckman JG, Lang CI, Druschky A, et al. Chorea resulting from paraneoplastic encephalitis. *Mov Disord* 1997;12:464.

221. Schiff DE, Ortega JA. Chorea, eosinophilia, and lupus anticoagulant associated with acute lymphoblastic leukemia. *Pediatr Neurol* 1992;8:466.

222. Kujawa LA, Niemi VR, Tomasi MA, et al. Ballistic-choreic movements as the presenting feature of renal cancer. *Arch Neurol* 2001;58:1133.

223. Batchelor TT, Pletten M, Palmer-Toy DE, et al. Chorea as a paraneoplastic complication of Hodgkin's disease. *J Neurooncol* 1998;36:185.

224. Tremont-Lukats IW, Fuller GNM, Ribalta T, et al. Paraneoplastic chorea: case study with autopsy confirmation. *J Neurooncol* 2002;4:192.

225. Vernino S, Tuite P, Alder CH, et al. Paraneoplastic chorea associated with CRMP-5 neuronal antibody and lung carcinoma. *Ann Neurol* 2002;51:625.

226. Croteau D, Oainati A, Dalmau J, et al. Response to cancer therapy in a patient with a paraneoplastic choreiform disorder. *Neurology* 2001;57:719.

227. Simonetti F, Peergami P, Aktipi KM, et al. Paraneoplastic "rubral" tremor—a case report. *Mov Disord* 1998;13:12.

228. Golbe LI, Miller DC, Duvoisin RC. Paraneoplastic degeneration of the substantia nigra with dystonia and Parkinsonism. *Mov Disord* 1989;4:147.

229. Fahn S, Brin MR, Dwork AF, et al. Case 1: rapidly progressive Parkinsonism, incontinence, impotency, and a levodopa-induced moaning in a patient with multiple myeloma. *Mov Disord* 1996;11:298.

230. Giometto B, Taraloto B, Graus F. Autoimmunity in paraneoplastic neurological syndromes. *Brain Pathol* 1999;9:261.

231. Batchelor TT, Platten M, Hochberg FH. Immunoadsorption therapy for paraneoplastic syndromes. *J Neurooncol* 1998;40:131.

232. Blaes F, Strittmatter M, Merkelbach S. Intravenous immunoglobulins in the therapy of paraneoplastic disorders. *J Neurol* 1992;246:299.

233. Martinez-Lavin M, Matucci-Cerinic M, Jajic I, et al. Hypertrophic osteoarthropathy: consensus on its definition, classification, assessment and diagnostic criteria. *J Rheumatol* 1993;20:1386.

234. Matucci-Cerinic M, Lotti T, Jajic I, et al. The clinical spectrum of pachydermoperiostosis (primary hypertrophic osteoarthropathy). *Medicine* 1991;70:208.

235. Martinez-Lavin M, Weisman MH, Pineda CJ. Hypertrophic osteoarthropathy. In: Schumacher HR Jr, ed. *Primer on rheumatic diseases,* 9th ed. Atlanta: Arthritis Foundation, 1988:240.

236. Matucci-Cerinic M, Ceruso M, Lotti T, et al. The medical and surgical treatment of finger clubbing and hypertrophic osteoarthropathy. A blind study with colchicine and a surgical approach to finger clubbing resection. *Clin Exp Rheumatol* 1992;10[Suppl 7]:67.

237. Greenberg SB, Taber L. Fever of unknown origin. In: Mackowiak PA, ed. *Fever: basic mechanisms in management.* New York: Raven Press, 1991:183.

238. Pizzo PA, Robichaud KJ, Wesley R, et al. Fever in the pediatric and young adult patient with cancer. *Medicine* 1982;61:153.

239. Friocourt L, Jouquan J, Khoury S, et al. Fever in adult renal cancer. In: *Renal tumors: proceedings of the first international symposium on kidney tumors.* New York: Alan R. Liss, 1982:283.

240. Ashraf SJ, Arya SC, El-Sayed M, et al. A profile of primary hepatocellular carcinoma patients in the Gizan area of Saudi Arabia. *Cancer* 1986;58:2163.

241. Larson EB, Featherstone HJ, Petersdorf RG. Fever of undetermined origin: diagnosis and follow-up of 105 cases, 1970–1980. *Medicine* 1982;61:269.

242. Bodel P, Ralph P, Wenc K, et al. Endogenous pyrogen production by Hodgkin's disease and human histiocytic lymphoma cell lines in vivo. *J Clin Invest* 1980;65:514.

243. Dinarello C, Cannon J, Wolff S, et al. Tumor necrosis factor (cachectin) is an endogenous pyrogen and induces production of interleukin 1. *J Exp Med* 1986;163:1433.

244. Warshaw AL, Carey RW, Robinson DR. Control of fever associated with visceral cancers by indomethacin. *Surgery* 1981;89:414.

245. Chang JC, Gross HM. Utility of naproxen in the differential diagnosis of fever of undetermined origin in patients with cancer. *Am J Med* 1983;76:597.

246. Dinarello C, Bunn P. Fever. *Semin Oncol* 1997;24:288.

F. Anthony Greco
John D. Hainsworth

CHAPTER **46**

Cancer of Unknown Primary Site

Patients with cancer of unknown primary site are common. The exact incidence is unknown because many of these patients are "assigned" other diagnoses and are therefore not accurately represented in tumor registries (discussed later in Carcinoma of Unknown Primary Site As a Distinct Clinicopathologic Entity). Nonetheless, in the United States, unknown primary cancers accounted for approximately 2% of all cancer diagnoses reported by Surveillance, Epidemiology, and End Results (SEER) registries between 1973 and 1987.[1] International registries from seven other countries have listed the frequencies from 2.3% to 7.8%.[2] The authors believe a more realistic estimate of the incidence of these patients is 5% of all invasive cancers in the United States per year (approximately 80,000 to 90,000 patients). Within this heterogenous patient group, there are several clinical presentations and histologic tumor types. The largest group of patients has metastatic carcinoma of unknown primary site. Others have equivocal histologic diagnoses and tumors that are difficult to classify using the time-honored method of light microscopic examination. Specialized pathologic studies are essential in delineating the type of neoplasm present in many of these patients and at times may suggest the site of origin. Extreme heterogeneity in clinical presentations, histologic appearances, and natural histories has made systematic evaluation of these patients difficult, and an established base of knowledge has developed slowly. Only a few investigators have been interested in detailed studies of these patients. Therefore, past information often suffers from many generalizations and is not representative of the entire patient population. Much of these data are derived from grouping all patients and deal primarily with results of various chemotherapeutic regimens.

Over the past few decades, several important issues have changed in oncology. Combination chemotherapy, often used with surgery or radiation therapy, has proven to be potentially curative for selected patients with several metastatic tumors. In addition, palliation and prolongation of survival have been demonstrated for patients with many other tumor types after systemic therapy. Furthermore, treatment continues to evolve and improve, as illustrated by the introduction in the past few years of several new and useful biologic targeted agents, such as rituximab, trastuzumab, imatinib, and gefitinib. These therapeutic improvements have relevance for patients with cancers of unknown primary site because some of these neoplasms are likely to be responsive to these therapies.

Diagnostic pathology has improved remarkably. The more routine use of electron microscopy and immunohistochemistry and the emerging field of molecular genetics are contributing to the more precise diagnosis of neoplasms. It is possible to define more reliably the histology and, at least in selected patients, the origin and biology of their neoplasms. In concert with the evolving diagnostic techniques, several clinical syndromes and features are being recognized and are helping physicians to better understand and manage these patients. Oncologists are continually rethinking the issues with respect to patients with cancers of unknown primary site.

Appropriate patient management requires an understanding of several clinicopathologic features that help to identify several subsets of patients with more responsive tumors. A patient with cancer of unknown primary site typically develops symptoms or signs at a metastatic site, and the diagnosis is made by biopsy of a metastatic lesion. History, physical examination, and other appropriate evaluation of the patient fail to identify the primary site. The initial biopsy should be generous because many studies may be required. Routine light microscopic histology establishes the neoplastic process and provides a practical classification sys-

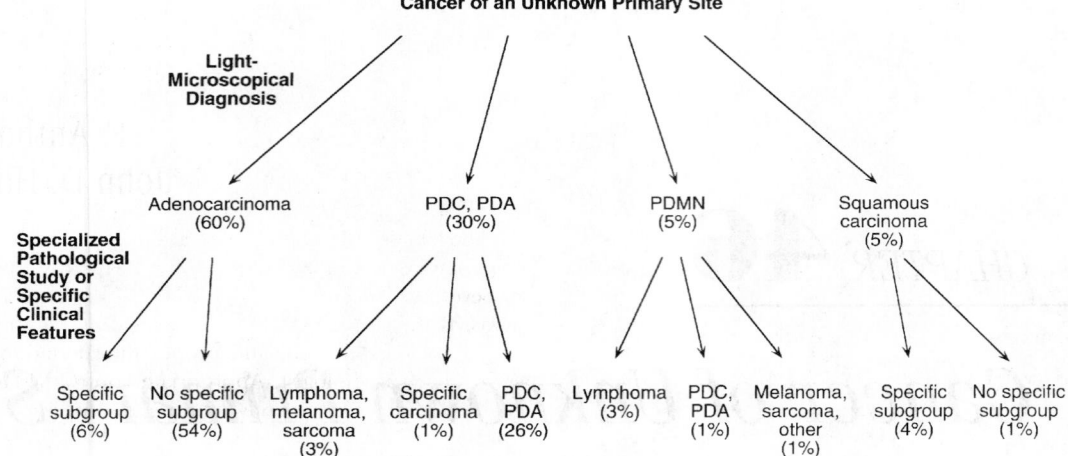

FIGURE 46-1.   Relative size of various clinical and histologic subgroups of patients as determined by optimal clinical and pathologic evaluation. PDA, poorly differentiated adenocarcinoma; PDC, poorly differentiated carcinoma; PDMN, poorly differentiated malignant neoplasm. (From Hainsworth JD, Greco FA. Treatment of patients with cancer of an unknown primary site. *N Engl J Med* 1993;329:257, with permission.)

tem on which the patient can be subsequently evaluated and managed. In the broad category of cancers of unknown primary site, there are four major light microscopic diagnoses: (1) poorly differentiated neoplasm, (2) poorly differentiated carcinoma (with or without features of adenocarcinoma), (3) well-differentiated and moderately well-differentiated adenocarcinoma, and (4) squamous cell carcinoma.

These diagnoses vary to some extent with respect to clinical characteristics, recommended diagnostic evaluation, treatment, and prognosis. After appropriate clinical and pathologic evaluation, the approximate size of the various groups and subsets of patients are illustrated in Figure 46-1.

POORLY DIFFERENTIATED NEOPLASMS OF UNKNOWN PRIMARY SITE

If the pathologist is confident of a cancer but cannot differentiate a general category of neoplasm (e.g., carcinoma, lymphoma, melanoma, sarcoma), this tumor is designated a *poorly differentiated neoplasm*. A more precise diagnosis is essential in this group of patients because many have responsive tumors. Approximately 5% of all patients with cancers of unknown primary site (approximately 4000 patients annually in the United States) present with this diagnosis by initial light microscopic appearance, but few remain without a defined lineage after specialized pathologic study. The most frequent tumor for which effective therapy is available is non-Hodgkin's lymphoma. In reported series, 35% to 65% of poorly differentiated neoplasms were found to be lymphomas after further pathologic study.[3–6] Most of the remaining tumors in this group are carcinomas. Melanoma and sarcoma together account for less than 15% of all patients.

The evaluation of poorly differentiated tumors requires specialized pathologic studies. Immunoperoxidase tumor staining, electron microscopy, and genetic analysis can be helpful in the differential diagnosis. The most common cause of a nonspecific light microscopic diagnosis is an inadequate or poorly handled biopsy specimen. If possible, fine-needle aspiration biopsy should not be

performed in these patients as an *initial* diagnostic procedure because the histologic pattern is not preserved and the ability to perform special studies is limited. The authors have documented several instances where a fine-needle aspiration has suggested a specific diagnosis, proven later to be incorrect by an incisional biopsy. Frequently, a more definitive diagnosis can be made by obtaining a larger biopsy. Communication with the pathologist is important because special tissue processing may be necessary for some pathologic studies. In addition, all the clinical information may also help the pathologist narrow down or be more certain of the diagnosis. Some neoplasms remain unclassifiable by light microscopy, even with an adequate biopsy specimen. Additional pathologic study is always indicated in these tumors.

IMMUNOPEROXIDASE TUMOR STAINING

Immunoperoxidase staining is the most widely available specialized technique for the classification of neoplasms. Immunoperoxidase staining often can be done on formalin-fixed, paraffinized tissue, which broadens its applicability, making repeat biopsy unnecessary in some patients. Immunoperoxidase antibodies are either monoclonal or polyclonal and are directed at cell components or products, which can include enzymes [e.g., prostatic acid phosphate, neuron-specific enolase (NSE)], normal tissue components [e.g., keratin, desmin, vimentin, neurofilaments, common leukocyte antigen (CLA)], hormones and hormone receptors (e.g., estrogen receptor), oncofetal antigens [e.g., α-fetoprotein (AFP)], carcinoembryonic antigen (CEA), and other substances (e.g., S-100 protein, chromogranin). Many new antibodies are being developed, making this area of diagnostic pathology a dynamic and evolving field. Specific diagnoses usually cannot be made on the basis of immunoperoxidase staining alone because none of these reagents is directed at tumor-specific antigens. Although cytokeratin stains, particularly cytokeratins 7 and 20, may suggest (at least statistically) various primary sites[7–12] by their presence or absence, the authors have not found this to be accurate enough to rely on routinely. Staining can also be extremely

TABLE 46-1. Immunoperoxidase Tumor Staining Patterns Useful in the Differential Diagnosis of Poorly Differentiated Neoplasms

Tumor Type	Immunoperoxidase Staining
CARCINOMA	Epithelial stains (e.g., CK 7, 20 variable)
	EMA (+) CLA, S-100, vimentin (−)
Colorectal carcinoma	CK 7 (−); CK 20 (+)
Lung carcinoma	
Adenocarcinoma	TTF-1 (+)
Other	
Non–small cell carcinoma	CK 7 (+), CK 20 (−)
	TTF-1 (−)
Small cell carcinoma	TTF-1 (+), chromogranin (+)
	NSE (+)
Neuroendocrine carcinoma	NSE, chromogranin, synaptophysin (+)
	Epithelial stains (+)
Germ cell tumor	HCG, AFP (+)
	Placental alkaline phosphatase (+)
	Epithelial stains (+)
Prostate carcinoma	PSA (+), rare false (−) and (+)
	Epithelial stains (+)
	CK 7 (−), CK 20 (−)
Breast carcinoma	ER, PR (+)
	Her-2-neu (+)
	CK 7 (+), CK 20 (−)
	Gross cystic fluid protein 15 (+)
	Epithelial stains (+)
Thyroid carcinoma	
Follicular/papillary	Thyroglobulin (+), TTF-1 (+)
Medullary	Calcitonin (+)
LYMPHOMA	CLA (+), rare false (−)
	EMA occasionally (+)
	All other stains (−)
SARCOMA	
Mesenchymal	Vimentin (+)
	Epithelial stains usually (−)
Rhabdomyosarcoma	Desmin (+)
Angiosarcoma	Factor VIII antigen (+)
Gastrointestinal stromal tumor	CD117 (c-kit) (+)
MELANOMA	S-100, vimentin, HMB45 (+)
	NSE often (+)
	Synaptophysin (−)
	Epithelial stains (−)

+, positive result; −, negative result; AFP, α-fetoprotein; CK, cytokeratin; CLA, common leukocyte antigen; EMA, epithelial membrane antigen; ER, estrogen receptor; HCG, human chorionic gonadotropin; NSE, neuron-specific enolase; PR, progesterone receptor; PSA, prostate-specific antigen; TTF-1, thyroid transcription factor-1.

variable, and a particular stain may be negative, yet other data may nonetheless support a particular tumor type. For example, a neuroendocrine carcinoma does not invariably stain with all neuroendocrine reagents. Therefore, results must be interpreted in conjunction with the light microscopic appearance and the clinical picture. Some immunoperoxidase staining patterns that are useful in the differential diagnosis of neoplasms are outlined in Table 46-1.

Several important questions can usually be answered by immunoperoxidase staining. The CLA stain usually can be used to make the important distinction between lymphoma and carcinoma.[13,14] Staining for NSE, chromogranin, and synaptophysin can suggest a neuroendocrine carcinoma (e.g., small cell carcinoma, carcinoid, islet cell tumor).[15–17] Staining for prostate-specific antigen (PSA) strongly suggests prostate carcinoma in a male with metastatic adenocarcinoma.[17,18] Certain staining characteristics can suggest breast carcinoma (e.g., estrogen or progesterone receptors, gross cystic fluid protein 15), amelanotic melanoma (e.g., positive staining for S-100 protein, vimentin, HMB45), or sarcoma (e.g., positive staining for desmin, vimentin, factor VIII antigen, c-kit-CD117 stain).[19–24] Staining for human chorionic gonadotropin (HCG) or AFP can suggest the diagnosis of a germ cell tumor in an appropriate clinical situation.[25,26]

Several problems are associated with immunoperoxidase stains. Technical expertise is required to perform these tests accurately and reproducibly, and proper interpretation requires an experienced pathologist. Appropriate control slides are stained and examined concurrently because nonspecific staining occasionally is a problem. Care must be taken to avoid overinterpretation because no staining pattern is entirely specific. Certain stains, particularly CLA and PSA, are relatively specific; however, false-positive and false-negative results can occur with any of these stains. For example, some carcinomas stain with vimentin, some sarcomas stain with keratin, and a wide variety of carcinomas (other than neuroendocrine and germ cell tumors) stain with NSE and HCG.

In some circumstances, diagnoses based on immunoperoxidase staining in patients with poorly differentiated neoplasms of unknown primary site can be used to plan therapy and predict outcome. Undifferentiated neoplasms identified as lymphoma on the basis of positive CLA staining respond well to the combination chemotherapy used for non-Hodgkin's lymphoma.[3] In 35 patients with equivocal routine light microscopic histology and positive CLA staining, treatment with a variety of standard lymphoma regimens resulted in an actuarial disease-free survival of 45% at 30 months. Their outcome was similar to a group of concurrently treated patients who had non-Hodgkin's lymphomas with typical light microscopic histology. In patients diagnosed on the basis of immunoperoxidase staining with tumors other than lymphoma, only limited data exist concerning treatment outcome.

ELECTRON MICROSCOPY

A diagnosis can be made by electron microscopy in some poorly differentiated neoplasms. Electron microscopy is not widely available, requires special tissue fixation, is relatively expensive, and should be reserved for the study of neoplasms whose lineage is unclear after routine light microscopy and immunoperoxidase staining. Like immunoperoxidase staining, electron microscopy is reliable in differentiating lymphoma from carcinoma. It may be superior to immunoperoxidase staining for the identification of poorly differentiated sarcoma. Other structures such as neurosecretory granules (neuroendocrine tumors) or premelanosomes (melanoma) can suggest a particular tumor. Undifferentiated tumors often have nonspecific ultrastructural features; therefore, the absence of a particular ultrastructural finding cannot be used to rule out a specific diagnosis. Some neoplasms defy further classification despite specialized pathologic study.

In some instances, electron microscopy provides evidence for adenocarcinoma or squamous cell carcinoma. Features of adenocarcinoma include intercellular and intracellular lumina and surface microvilli. Squamous carcinomas are characterized by frequent and prominent desmosomes and by prominent bundles of prekeratin filaments in the adjacent cytoplasm. It usually is not possible to determine the origin of poorly differentiated adenocarcinoma or squamous carcinoma by electron microscopic features. Treatment implications for adenocarcinoma and squamous carcinoma recognized only by ultrastructural features are unclear.

GENETIC ANALYSIS

The identification of chromosomal abnormalities and genetic changes associated with neoplasms is becoming increasingly important. The use of tumor-specific chromosomal abnormalities in diagnosis is still limited, but it is likely that future research will identify many additional specific genetic abnormalities.

Chromosomal abnormalities have been well characterized in several hematopoietic neoplasms. Most B-cell non-Hodgkin's lymphomas are associated with tumor-specific immunoglobulin gene rearrangements, and typical chromosomal changes have been identified in some B-cell and T-cell lymphomas and in Hodgkin's disease.[27,28] In the rare instance when the diagnosis of lymphoma cannot be definitively established with either immunoperoxidase staining or electron microscopy, detection of chromosomal translocations t(14:18); t(8:14); t(11:14) and others or the presence of an immunoglobulin gene rearrangement provides definitive diagnostic information.

A few other nonrandom chromosomal rearrangements associated with nonlymphoid tumors have been identified. A chromosomal translocation, t(11:22), has been found in peripheral neuroepitheliomas, in desmoplastic small round cell tumors, and frequently in Ewing's tumor.[29–31] An isochromosome of the short arm of chromosome 12 (i12p) and other chromosome 12 abnormalities are found in a large percentage of germ cell tumors.[32,33] A genomic hybridization technique has been developed that can detect extra 12p material in paraffin-embedded tissue specimens.[34] This technique will likely improve the applicability of testing because tissue culture is not necessary. Other hybridization procedures are under development to detect a number of genetic abnormalities characteristic of several neoplasms and should be helpful diagnostically in several selected tumors. Many other nonrandom cytogenetic abnormalities found in other tumors include t(2:13) in alveolar rhabdomyosarcoma; 3p deletion in small cell lung cancer; 1p deletion in neuroblastoma; t(X:18) in synovial sarcoma; and 11p deletion in Wilms' tumor. Epstein-Barr viral genomes have been identified in the tumor cells of patients with cervical lymph node metastases of unknown primary site, highly suggesting nasopharyngeal primaries.[35,36] Among head and neck tumors, Epstein-Barr virus has been associated only with nasopharyngeal carcinoma. Because some of these tumor types are poorly differentiated and are often metastatic at the time of diagnosis, identification of these genetic changes may provide a specific diagnosis. Genetic diagnosis has been applied successfully to a subset of patients with carcinoma of unknown primary site suspected of having germ cell tumors [discussed later in Poorly Differentiated Carcinoma (with or without Features of Adenocarcinoma) of Unknown Primary Site].

DNA microarrays have been studied in several neoplasms,[37] and this technique holds promise as a method to classify neoplasms based on gene expression profiling, perhaps identifying specific genetic patterns or fingerprints independent of previous histologic and biologic knowledge. In the future, this and other techniques may identify more specific tumor lineages or primary tumor types subject to specific therapies in patients with unknown primary cancers. The technology is now available to classify unknown primary carcinoma by gene expression, which also has the potential to identify their primary origin and provide prognostic information as well as clues to more specific targeted therapy by pharmacogenomic evaluation. As more precise and specific genetic lesions are identified in primary neoplasms and their metastases (e.g., lung, breast, ovary, germ cell), these data can be expected to provide more useful diagnostic and therapeutic information for unknown primary cancers. The identification of germ cell tumors has already met this expectation, [discussed in Poorly Differentiated Carcinoma (with or without Features of Adenocarcinoma) of Unknown Primary Site.]

POORLY DIFFERENTIATED CARCINOMA (WITH OR WITHOUT FEATURES OF ADENOCARCINOMA) OF UNKNOWN PRIMARY SITE

The understanding of the various subsets of patients with poorly differentiated carcinoma has improved considerably in the last 15 years. In concert with identification of several important clinical features, specialized pathology has continued to improve, and consequently several "favorable subsets" of patients have been identified within this large group with specific therapeutic implications. When considering the group as a whole, the demographic features have not changed; however, when excluding these more "favorable subsets," the clinical characteristics of the remaining patients with poorly differentiated carcinoma are more similar to those with well-differentiated adenocarcinoma. Patients with poorly differentiated carcinoma account for approximately 30% of carcinoma of unknown primary sites (approximately 25,000 patients annually in the United States), and approximately one-third of these patients' tumors have some features of adenocarcinomatous differentiation (poorly differentiated adenocarcinoma). Some of the patients in this group have extremely responsive neoplasms, and therefore careful clinical and pathologic evaluation is crucial in patients with poorly differentiated carcinoma.

CLINICAL CHARACTERISTICS

The clinical characteristics in this diverse group of patients appear to differ, albeit with a considerable overlap, from the characteristics of patients with well-differentiated adenocarcinoma. As mentioned, when the now recognizable more treatable subsets of patients are excluded, the demographic features are more like those with well-differentiated adenocarcinoma. When considering the whole group as compared with well-differentiated adenocarcinoma, the median age is younger and there is often a history of rapid progression of symptoms (often less than 30 days) and/or objective evidence of rapid tumor growth. The location of metastasis also differs, with the predominant sites of involvement more often involving peripheral lymph nodes, mediastinum, and retroperitoneum. Some of these relatively distinctive clinical features are useful in identifying chemotherapy responsive subsets of patients.

PATHOLOGIC EVALUATION

Light microscopic features that can differentiate chemotherapy-responsive tumors from nonresponsive tumors have not been identified.[38] Even with careful retrospective review of these tumors, responsive tumors of well-defined types (e.g., germ cell tumor, lymphoma) are only rarely identified.

These tumors should routinely undergo additional pathologic study with immunoperoxidase staining; in selected tumors, electron microscopy and genetic analysis are also appropriate. The use of routine light microscopy alone is not adequate to assess these tumors. The information provided by these additional pathologic studies has been summarized (discussed earlier in Poorly Differentiated Neoplasms of Unknown Primary Site). The frequency of more specific diagnoses, particularly lymphoma, is much lower in the carcinoma group than in the group initially diagnosed by routine light microscopy as poorly differentiated neoplasm. This is not surprising because carcinoma is a more specific diagnosis. Other diagnoses may still be suggested. To assess the clinical usefulness of immunoperoxidase tumor-cell staining in patients with poorly differentiated carcinoma of unknown primary site, the authors retrospectively performed a battery of stains on archival tumors, from patients treated prospectively.[39] Poorly differentiated carcinoma or poorly differentiated adenocarcinoma was diagnosed on the basis of routine light microscopic examination, and all patients were treated before the technology of immunoperoxidase staining was routinely used (1978 to 1983). Therefore, results of immunoperoxidase staining could be correlated with clinical outcome in this group of similarly treated patients with a long follow-up. Immunoperoxidase staining confirmed the diagnoses of poorly differentiated carcinoma in 49 patients (56%) and yielded other diagnoses in 16 patients (18%): melanoma (eight), lymphoma (four), prostatic carcinoma (one), and neuroendocrine tumor (three). In 24 patients (28%), the immunoperoxidase-staining pattern was inconclusive; electron microscopy was occasionally helpful in clarifying the diagnosis in these patients. Seventy-five patients (86%) received combination chemotherapy with a cisplatin-based regimen, and 24 patients (28%) had a complete response. Nine of these patients were later given specific diagnoses by immunoperoxidase staining; lymphoma was diagnosed in four patients, melanoma in four patients, and yolk sac tumor in one patient. All patients with an immunoperoxidase diagnosis of lymphoma had clinical features compatible with lymphoma and are long-term survivors. Patients with immunoperoxidase features suggesting melanoma were surprisingly responsive to chemotherapy, with three of seven complete responses and two long-term survivors. Patients with melanoma diagnosed by immunoperoxidase staining alone should not be excluded from a trial of chemotherapy. Immunoperoxidase staining is useful in the routine evaluation of metastatic poorly differentiated carcinoma of unknown primary site, as it can occasionally suggest the lineage of the tumor and have specific therapeutic implications. Others have reported similar findings in patients treated with cisplatin-containing chemotherapy.[40]

Electron microscopy can be useful for a small minority of these carcinomas. In general, electron microscopy should be reserved for those tumors not diagnosed by immunoperoxidase stains. Lymphoma can be diagnosed reliably in most instances in those tumors mistakenly believed to be carcinoma. In addition, sarcoma, melanoma, mesothelioma, and neuroendocrine tumors occasionally are defined by subcellular features. Neuroendocrine differentiation is particularly important and is discussed later in Neuroendocrine Carcinoma of Unknown Primary Site.

Chromosomal or genetic analysis is becoming an increasingly important method of diagnosis. Specific abnormalities have been identified in several neoplasms (discussed earlier in Genetic Analysis). Evaluation for these abnormalities may be useful in patients with poorly differentiated carcinoma of unknown primary site. In reference to germ cell tumors, Motzer and colleagues performed genetic analysis on tumors in 40 patients with the "extragonadal germ cell syndrome" or "midline carcinomas of uncertain histogenesis."[41] In 12 of the 40 patients with poorly differentiated carcinoma, abnormalities of chromosome 12 (e.g., i[12p]; del [12p]; multiple copies of 12 p) were diagnostic of germ cell tumor. Other specific abnormalities were diagnostic of melanoma (two patients), lymphoma (one patient), peripheral neuroepithelioma (one patient), and desmoplastic small cell tumor (one patient). Of the germ cell tumors diagnosed on basis of genetic analysis, five achieved a complete response to cisplatin-based chemotherapy. This confirms the authors' previously formulated hypothesis that some of these patients have histologically atypical germ cell tumors.[42,43] These genetic findings can be diagnostic in these patients. Additional specific genetic abnormalities or gene expression profiling in solid tumors will likely further improve the ability to establish tumor lineage or biology, and, it is hoped, also identify specific targets to improve therapy. Preliminary results using polymerase chain reaction and *in situ* hybridization to identify Epstein-Barr viral genomes in neck nodes have established an occult nasopharyngeal primary in some patients (discussed earlier in Genetic Analysis).

Autopsy data looking specifically at patients with poorly differentiated carcinoma of unknown primary site are limited. The number of postmortem examinations in medicine in general is declining. Based on the limited necropsy data the authors have accumulated, it appears that primary sites are found in only a minority of these patients (40%). These findings are contrary to those for well-differentiated adenocarcinoma of unknown primary site, in which the primary site is found in most patients (more than 75%) at autopsy.[44,45]

DIAGNOSTIC EVALUATION

A history, physical examination, routine laboratory testing, and chest radiograph should be obtained in each patient. Any clues are followed with appropriate diagnostic testing. Computed tomography (CT) scans of the chest and abdomen should be performed in all patients in this group because of the frequency of mediastinal and retroperitoneal involvement. Serum levels of HCG and AFP should be measured because substantial elevations of these markers suggest the diagnosis of germ cell tumor. Serum tumor markers such as CEA, CA 125, CA 19-9, and CA 15-3 can be helpful in monitoring response to chemotherapy but are too nonspecific to be useful in diagnosis. Positron emission tomography (PET) scanning appears to have a role in locating the primary cancer and metastatic sites when all other tests are inconclusive. Several series of patients with unknown primary patients,[46-49] including head and neck presentations,[50-54] have demonstrated that PET can detect the primary tumor in approximately 30% of these patients (20% to 60%), and in the authors' view, PET is now an indicated procedure.

TREATMENT

When additional pathologic studies identify a specific neoplasm (e.g., lymphoma, sarcoma), appropriate therapy can be administered. Patients with elevated serum levels of HCG or AFP and clinical features highly suggestive of extragonadal germ cell tumor (e.g., mediastinal or retroperitoneal mass) should be treated with chemotherapy effective for germ cell tumors, even when pathologic examination is not diagnostic.

Most patients have multiple metastases and only the nonspecific diagnoses of poorly differentiated carcinoma or poorly differentiated adenocarcinoma despite additional pathologic study. The first reports showing that some of these patients (a small subset) have highly responsive tumors appeared in the late 1970s.[43,55-57] Most of these patients were young men with mediastinal tumors; serum levels of HCG or AFP were frequently elevated. Although the histology was not diagnostic, these patients were thought to have histologically atypical extragonadal germ cell tumors. Several other tumor lineages have subsequently been identified in some of these patients (i.e., thymoma, neuroendocrine tumors, sarcomas, lymphomas), but many others still defy precise classification.

Further evidence for the responsiveness of many other tumors in patients with poorly differentiated carcinoma of unknown primary site has accumulated since 1978. Based on the encouraging results in a few patients treated from 1976 to 1978, the authors prospectively studied the role of cisplatin-based therapy in patients with poorly differentiated carcinoma of unknown primary site. In a series of reports, the authors documented a high overall response rate and long-term disease-free survival in a minority of these patients.[38,39,42,58-60] The patient characteristics of 220 such patients, accumulated between 1978 and 1989, are summarized in Table 46-2. Most of the patients in this group did not have clinical characteristics strongly suggestive of extragonadal germ cell tumor. However, involvement of the mediastinum, retroperitoneum, and peripheral lymph node groups was relatively common, clinical features now known to be associated with a more favorable prognosis. In the early years of this study, most patients received treatment with cisplatin, vinblastine, and bleomycin with or without doxorubicin, then the most commonly used regimen for the treatment of advanced testicular cancer. Later, as etoposide replaced vinblastine, these patients received cisplatin and etoposide with or without bleomycin. All patients received an initial treatment trial of two courses of therapy, and responding patients received a total of four treatment courses. Major tumor responses were seen in 138 of 220 patients (62%), and 58 patients (26%) had complete response to treatment.

The authors' most recent update of this initial group of patients shows the following: 12% (26 patients) of the entire group have remained alive and free of tumor at a minimum follow-up of 6 years, with a range of 6 to 17 years (median of 11 years). Fourteen patients who were relapse-free at a minimum of 11 months at the time of the authors' original report[60] can-

TABLE 46-2. Clinical Characteristics of 220 Patients with Poorly Differentiated Carcinoma of Unknown Primary Site

Characteristics	Number of Patients (%)
GENDER	
Female	54
Male	166
RACE	
White	209
African American	9
Asian American	2
PERFORMANCE STATUS	
ECOG 0, 1	188
ECOG 2, 3	32
DOMINANT METASTATIC SITE	
Mediastinum	43 (20)
Retroperitoneum	42 (19)
Lung	29 (13)
Lymph nodes (cervical, axillary, inguinal)	20 (9)
Liver	11 (5)
Pleura-peritoneum	6
Bone	5
Pelvic mass	4
Pancreas	3
Soft tissue	2
Brain	2
Other (one each)	3
Multiple sites (no dominant site)	50 (23)
SERUM TUMOR MARKERS	
HCG (N = 206)	
Normal	174
Elevated	32 (16)
AFP (N = 201)	
Normal	190
Elevated	11 (5)
LDH (N = 199)[a]	
Normal	103
Elevated	96 (48)
CEA (N = 127)	
Normal	80
Elevated	47 (37)
NUMBER OF METASTATIC SITES	
1	57 (26)
2	67 (31)
3	60 (27)
>3	36 (16)

AFP, α-fetoprotein; CEA, carcinoembryonic antigen; ECOG, Eastern Cooperative Oncology Group; HCG, human chorionic gonadotropin; LDH, lactate dehydrogenase.
[a]Thirty-two of 96 patients had liver metastases as possible source for elevated LDH.

not be documented now as alive and free of the original tumor. Six patients are lost to follow-up, and each was known to be alive and relapse-free at 1.0, 2.5, 3.0, 3.5, 4.0, and 7.0 years, respectively. Four patients died with progressive carcinoma of unknown primary site 1, 1, 7, and 7 years after initial chemotherapy. Three patients developed new cancers (one brain tumor, one pancreatic carcinoma, one lymphoma) 9, 9, and 17 years, respectively, after the initial therapy. One patient died of an unrelated cause (4 years after therapy).

The survival curves for the entire group of 220 patients and for the subset of 58 (26%) who had a complete response to

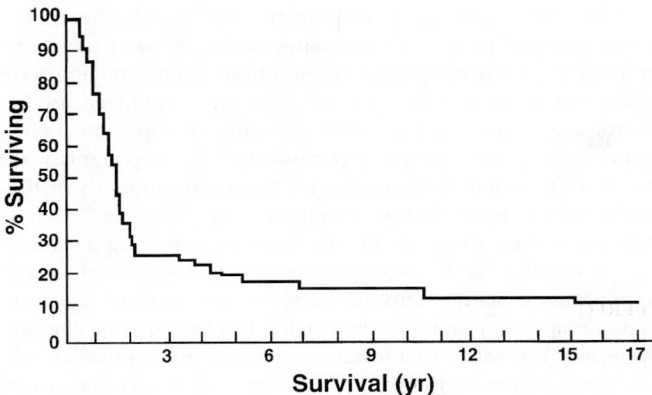

FIGURE 46-2. Survival curve for all 220 patients with poorly differentiated carcinoma (12% at 17 years).

chemotherapy are shown in Figures 46-2 and 46-3. The median survival of complete responders was approximately 3 years. Median survival for all patients was 20 months. Of the 58 complete responders, 22 patients remain alive and relapse-free (38%), representing 10% of the entire group of 220. These long-term survival statistics are not censored. Patients who are lost to follow-up (six), died of second unrelated cancers (three), or died of other causes (one) are all are included as deaths on the curves. It is of note that 50 of the 220 patients were treated by oncologists outside the authors' center, and their long-term results are equivalent. These results in this large series of patients is historically important and supported, at that time, the notion that some of these poorly differentiated histologic types represent more sensitive tumors than well-differentiated adenocarcinoma, and substantial prolongation of life was possible for some of these patients with the expectation of cure for a small minority.

In those relatively rare patients with features highly suggestive of an extragonadal germ cell tumor (two or more features of the extragonadal germ cell syndrome), the authors continue to recommend a classic accepted regimen for the treatment of testicular or extragonadal germ cell tumors.

The authors now are certain that their original prospective clinical trial of the 220 patients with poorly differentiated carci-

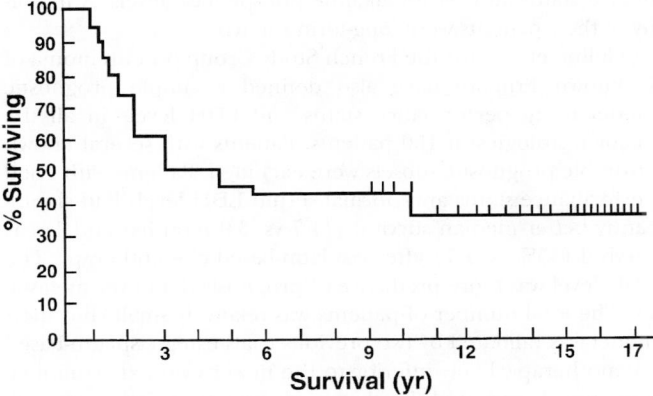

FIGURE 46-3. Survival curve of complete responders (38% at 17 years).

noma was heavily weighted with patients now known to represent "favorable subsets," each with a relatively good prognosis. These subsets included (1) patients with two or more features of the extragonadal germ cell syndrome; (2) patients with poorly differentiated neoplasms otherwise not specified; (3) patients with anaplastic lymphoma diagnosed as carcinoma in years past but routinely diagnosed today by specialized pathology; (4) patients with primary peritoneal carcinoma; (5) patients with poorly differentiated neuroendocrine carcinoma; and (6) patients with predominant sites of tumor involving the retroperitoneum, mediastinum, and peripheral lymph nodes. Although the nature of many of these carcinomas remains obscure even today, a number of these patients were subsequently proven to have lymphoma, neuroendocrine tumors, thymic carcinomas, or germ cell tumors. In the authors' original series,[60] 58 patients (26%) had a complete response to cisplatin-based chemotherapy, 45 of these 58 had predominant sites of tumor in the retroperitoneum, mediastinum, and peripheral lymph nodes, and 20 remain alive (unpublished observation). Many of these patients had highly responsive neoplasms, identified more readily today by specialized pathology. Other investigators also demonstrated the responsiveness of selected poorly differentiated carcinomas.[61–66] Complete remissions were seen in a minority (10% to 20%) of these patients, and a small cohort (5% to 10%) were long-term disease-free survivors. These results were usually seen with platinum-based chemotherapy, often with etoposide with or without bleomycin.

The authors' more recent or modern experience has excluded or stratified these more favorable subsets of patients in their clinical trials, with the remaining patients having more unfavorable features. Once all the more favorable subsets of patients are excluded, the remaining patients have a similar prognosis to the large majority of the well-differentiated adenocarcinoma group, and thus the authors now include all these patients in new clinical trials.

Since 1989, the authors have either seen or collected clinical and pathologic data from other physicians on 900 additional patients with carcinomas of unknown primary site. These data, along with more recent data from prospective clinical trials in 396 patients performed by the Minnie Pearl Cancer Research Network, have formed the basis of the authors' current grouping of the patients with unfavorable prognoses, regardless of histology, in recent clinical trials.

Since 1995, the Minnie Pearl Cancer Research Network has treated 396 patients in five sequential prospective clinical trials incorporating several newer cytotoxic agents (paclitaxel, docetaxel, gemcitabine, irinotecan). Most of the patients with favorable prognostic features were excluded from these trials (discussed later in Chemotherapy for Metastatic Carcinoma of Unknown Primary Site). These results suggest a major improvement in clinical benefit and survival with these newer therapies.

PROGNOSTIC FACTORS

Patients have been analyzed for clinical and pathologic features predictive of treatment responsiveness and long-term survival. Prognostic features evaluated included age, sex, smoking history, serum tumor marker status (HCG, AFP), serum lactate dehydrogenase (LDH) and CEA, number of metastatic sites, predominant site of tumor involvement, and light microscopic histology (poorly differentiated carcinoma vs. poorly differentiated adenocarcinoma). Several features were independently predictive of favorable treatment outcome, including tumor location in the retroperitoneum or peripheral lymph nodes, tumor limited to one or two metastatic sites, younger age (younger than 35 years), negative smoking history, and normal LDH and CEA. In recent years, specialized pathology became available to diagnose some of the more responsive tumors, but clinical features also remain important to help identify subsets of patients with varying prognoses. Some of the highly responsive tumors cannot be otherwise identified despite extensive pathologic evaluation.

More than two decades ago, the authors hypothesized that the highly responsive carcinomas probably were unrecognized or histologically atypical extragonadal germ cell tumors. The authors still believe that some of the highly responsive tumors are germ cell tumors that are marker-negative and are not identifiable using all available pathologic methods. Patients with clinical features highly suggestive of extragonadal germ cell tumors were analyzed for response to therapy and long-term survival. This group included 34 men younger than age 45 years who had predominant disease in the mediastinum or retroperitoneum. Six of these men had elevated serum levels of AFP, HCG, or both. The histologic features of all tumors in this group were re-reviewed, and only one had typical features of a germ cell tumor (yolk sac tumor).[38] In this group, 29 of 34 patients (85%) responded to therapy, with 17 patients (50%) having complete response. Seven patients in this group (20%) remain disease-free. Therefore, selection of patients with *clinical features* highly suggestive of extragonadal germ cell tumor, despite the nondiagnostic histology, defines a subgroup with a higher complete response rate and long-term survival than the group as a whole (see also later in Special Issues in Carcinoma of Unknown Primary Site). Strong support for the hypothesis that some of these patients have extragonadal germ cell tumors has been provided by Motzer and colleagues, as previously discussed, who demonstrated chromosome 12 abnormalities diagnostic of germ cell tumors in several young men with poorly differentiated midline carcinomas of unknown primary site.[41] The excellent response to treatment and survival (50% complete responders, 20% disease-free survival) for patients in the authors' initial series with clinical features highly suggestive of extragonadal germ cell tumor suggests that these are germ cell tumors, albeit histologically atypical. These treatment results do not differ greatly from those in patients with known extragonadal germ cell tumors treated with standard cisplatin-based therapy.[67,68] If feasible, genetic analysis on tumor tissue should be done as a diagnostic test for selected patients with carcinoma of unknown primary site.

Responsive tumors are heterogeneous in their origin, and only a small subset of patients has histologically atypical germ cell tumors. A few of the patients have non-Hodgkin's lymphoma. Certain lymphomas may be confused with anaplastic carcinomas; some lymphomas, notably the Ki-1 lymphomas, also can stain positively with epithelial membrane antigen, further complicating their differentiation from carcinoma.[69] It is hoped that this confusion will be minimized or eliminated with the routine use of immunoperoxidase staining for CLA. Another group of highly responsive tumors are poorly differentiated neuroendocrine carcinomas (discussed later in Neuroendocrine Carcinoma of Unknown Primary Site).

The nature of the other responsive tumors in this heterogeneous group of patients remains speculative, but over time, several other specific neoplasms are now more readily recognized. Malignant thymoma is a tumor recently recognized to be responsive to cisplatin-based therapy, with some patients experiencing long-term complete remissions.[70] Some patients with poorly differentiated carcinoma located predominantly in the mediastinum have thymic carcinoma or thymoma. A few patients in the authors' original series who were long-term survivors were identified as having melanoma on the basis of immunoperoxidase stains. This diagnosis seems unusual because melanoma is a tumor that is usually unresponsive to chemotherapy. It is possible that unknown primary melanomas identifiable only by immunoperoxidase staining or electron microscopy represent a uniquely chemotherapy-sensitive subset or in fact are occasionally misdiagnosed and represent an entirely different tumor. It is possible that some responsive tumors represent a heretofore undefined tumor type. Alternatively, some may represent highly undifferentiated, and therefore perhaps chemotherapy-sensitive, epithelial tumors from occult primary sites, which are usually much less responsive to systemic therapy. It is likely that future knowledge and refinements in genetic diagnosis (DNA profiling) will establish the identity of many of these tumors.

Prognostic factors have also been evaluated by others[71–74] in patient groups containing all the histologic types of unknown primary cancer. At M. D. Anderson Hospital, a heterogeneous group of patients with various histologic subtypes was analyzed retrospectively. Those with clinical features of extragonadal germ cell tumors were excluded, and only a minority of patients with poorly differentiated carcinoma received cisplatin-based treatment as used in the treatment of germ cell tumors. Some of the same clinical features as the authors previously identified were found to be important prognostic features, including limited number of metastatic sites involved, tumor location in lymph nodes (including mediastinum and retroperitoneum) other than the supraclavicular lymph nodes, and female sex (also seen in the authors' recent series). In addition, the relatively poor outcome of patients with adenocarcinoma (as compared with other histologies) and liver metastasis was confirmed.

Van der Gaast et al.[73] evaluated 79 patients with poorly differentiated carcinoma and found three groups with median survivals of 4 years, 10 months, and 4 months based on performance status and serum alkaline phosphatase levels. A minority of their patients were long-term survivors.

Culine et al.[74] for the French Study Group on Carcinoma of Unknown Primary have also defined a simple prognostic model using performance status and LDH levels in all the major histologies in 150 patients. Patients with several known favorable prognostic subsets were excluded. Patients with good performance status and normal serum LDH levels had significantly better median survival (11.7 vs. 3.9 months) and 1-year survival (45% vs. 1%) after cisplatin-based chemotherapy. The LDH level was more predictive of prognosis than liver metastasis. The total number of patients was relatively small, and their model was validated by two previous trials using cisplatin-based chemotherapy, likely inferior to the newer cytotoxic combinations now being used. Furthermore, long-term follow-up at 2, 3, and 5 years is now necessary rather than making conclusions about the effectiveness of therapy based primarily on median survival. Others have also reported liver metastases,[60,71,72] poor performance status,[60,71,72] and heavy smoking history[60] as poor prognostic factors. Further validation of prognostic models in larger numbers of patients receiving the new cytotoxic combination therapies and with end points of survivals at 1 year and beyond are required. An accurate prognostic model will be helpful to better design and interpret clinical studies.

Although prognostic features are useful, occasional excellent responses are seen even in patient subgroups with unfavorable features. At present, even these patients should be considered for a trial of chemotherapy.

NEUROENDOCRINE CARCINOMA OF UNKNOWN PRIMARY SITE

Improved pathologic methods for diagnosing neuroendocrine tumors have resulted in the recent recognition of a wider spectrum of these neoplasms. The incidence of unknown primary neuroendocrine tumors is not known, but an estimate is approximately 4000 patients a year in the United States. Most of the well-described adult neuroendocrine tumors have distinctive histology and a known primary site of origin (Table 46-3). The well-differentiated or low-grade neuroendocrine tumors (typical carcinoid, islet cell tumors, and others) occasionally present with metastases, without a recognizable primary site, and usually possess an indolent biologic behavior. Carcinoid tumors of unknown primary site appear to be increasing.[1] A second group of neuroendocrine tumors is poorly differentiated by light microscopy but has neuroendocrine histologic features (typical small cell, atypical carcinoid, or poorly differentiated neuroendocrine carcinoma) and acts aggressively. A third group of neuroendocrine tumors, recently recognized, has high-grade biology and no distinctive neuroendocrine features by light microscopy. The initial diagnosis in this group is usually poorly differentiated carcinoma, and neuroendocrine features are recognized only when immunoperoxidase staining or, more definitively, electron microscopy is performed. Neuroendocrine carcinomas of unknown primary site occur in each of these three categories.

LOW-GRADE NEUROENDOCRINE CARCINOMA

Metastatic neuroendocrine tumors with histologic features typical of low-grade well-differentiated carcinoid or islet cell tumor are occasionally found without obvious primary site.

TABLE 46-3. Adult Neuroendocrine Tumors with Known Primary Sites

Indolent Biology	Aggressive Biology
Carcinoid tumor (many primary sites)	Small cell lung cancer, atypical or poorly differentiated carcinoids (many primary sites)
Islet cell tumor, pancreas	Extrapulmonary small cell carcinoma (many primary sites)
Pheochromocytoma, adrenal	Peripheral neuroepithelioma (usually in adolescents)
Medullary carcinoma, thyroid	Merkel cell tumor, skin
Paraganglioma-neurons	Neuroblastoma, adrenal

The incidence of unknown primary low-grade neuroendocrine carcinoma appears to be increasing.[1] Metastatic tumor usually involves the liver and/or bone and is sometimes associated with clinical syndromes produced by the secretion of bioactive substances (e.g., carcinoid syndrome, glucagonoma syndrome, VIPomas, Zollinger-Ellison syndrome). In some of these patients, further evaluation reveals primary sites in the small intestine, rectum, pancreas, or bronchus.

As predicted by the histologic appearance, these tumors usually exhibit an indolent biology, and slow progression over years is likely. Management should follow guidelines established for metastatic carcinoid or islet cell tumors from obvious known primary sites. These neoplasms are usually refractory to intensive systemic chemotherapy, and cisplatin-based chemotherapy produces low response rates.[75] Depending on the clinical situation, appropriate management may include local therapy (resection of isolated metastasis, hepatic artery ligation/embolization, cryotherapy, radiofrequency ablation), treatment with somatostatin analogues, streptozocin, doxorubicin, 5-fluorouracil (5-FU)–based systemic therapy, or symptomatic management.

SMALL CELL CARCINOMA

Patients with a history of cigarette smoking and small cell undifferentiated carcinoma at a metastatic site usually have a lung primary. A positive stain for thyroid transcription factor-1 is highly suggestive of a lung primary. CT of the chest and fiberoptic bronchoscopy should be performed. Perhaps PET scanning may be useful in this setting, but data are limited. If a pulmonary lesion is identified, the patient should be treated according to recommendations for small cell lung cancer. Small cell carcinoma can also arise from a variety of extrapulmonary primary sites. Patients with localizing symptoms or signs should have appropriate diagnostic studies performed.

When no primary site is identified, patients with small cell carcinoma should be treated with combination chemotherapy as recommended for small cell lung cancer. The authors have found that a regimen of paclitaxel, carboplatin, and oral etoposide is a very active therapy for these patients and have continued to evaluate this regimen. These tumors are initially chemotherapy-sensitive, and major palliative benefit can be derived from treatment. An occasional patient enjoys long-term benefit. In the rare instance when the tumor appears at a single metastatic site, the addition of radiation therapy or resection to combination chemotherapy, or both, should be considered.

POORLY DIFFERENTIATED NEUROENDOCRINE CARCINOMA

In approximately 10% of poorly differentiated carcinomas, electron microscopy reveals neurosecretory granules, a finding diagnostic of neuroendocrine carcinoma. These tumors have been called "poorly differentiated neuroendocrine tumors," "atypical carcinoids," or "primitive neuroectodermal tumors." In some of these tumors, neuroendocrine features are recognizable by light microscopy; in others the diagnosis is simply "poorly differentiated carcinoma." Although electron microscopy is the most accurate means of pathologic diagnosis, most of the tumors also have typical immunoperoxidase-staining patterns, with positive staining for NSE, chromogranin, and/or synaptophysin.

TABLE 46-4. Poorly Differentiated Neuroendocrine Tumors of Unknown Primary Site in 51 Patients

Features	Number of Patients
CLINICAL CHARACTERISTICS	
Male	34
Female	17
Smoking (>10 pack-years)	25
DOMINANT TUMOR SITE	
Retroperitoneum	13
Peripheral lymph nodes	7
Mediastinum	6
Bone	6
Liver	6
Other	8
Multiple sites (no dominant site)	6
TREATMENT	
Cisplatin-based combinations	38
Cyclophosphamide, doxorubicin, vincristine with or without etoposide	8
Surgical excision only	3
Radiation therapy only	2
RESPONSE TO CHEMOTHERAPY	
Complete response	13 (26%)
Partial response	20
No response or nonevaluable	10
Continuously disease-free	8 (15%)

The authors previously reported a group of 29 patients with poorly differentiated neuroendocrine tumors,[58] and later updated their experience to include 51 patients, 46 treated with combination chemotherapy (Table 46-4). Most of these patients had clinical evidence of high-grade tumor, and most had metastases in multiple sites. Thirty-three of 43 evaluable patients (77%) responded to chemotherapy with a cisplatin-based combination regimen. Thirteen patients (26%) had complete responses, and eight remained continuously disease-free more than 2 years after completion of therapy.

The authors are currently evaluating the combination of paclitaxel, carboplatin, and oral etoposide in patients with poorly differentiated neuroendocrine tumors of unknown primary site. Thirty-two patients have been treated since 2000.[76] There have been 16 men and 16 women, and 27 of the 32 were initially called poorly differentiated carcinoma but later defined as neuroendocrine tumors by immunoperoxidase staining (25 patients) or electron microscopy (2 patients). Most of these patients had several sites of metastasis, with predominant tumor in the liver (18 patients), nodes (6 patients), and mediastinum (2 patients). Twenty-four of the 32 patients received four courses of chemotherapy with paclitaxel, carboplatin, and oral etoposide. Of the 28 evaluable patients, there have been 4 complete responders, 12 partial responders, 11 stable responders, and 1 progressive tumor. Preliminary results showed that ten patients remained alive from 12 to 35 months, and four remained progression-free.

The origin of these poorly differentiated neuroendocrine carcinomas remains unclear. In four of the authors' patients, specific diagnoses were made either subsequently in their clinical course or at autopsy. Two patients had carcinoid tumors with undifferentiated growth pattern (both presented with abdominal carcinomatosis), one had small cell lung cancer, and one had extragonadal germ cell tumor with predominant neuroendocrine differentiation. It is likely that some additional patients, with small cell histology, had small cell lung cancer with occult primary tumor; however, more than half of these patients had no smoking history, and the absence of overt pulmonary involvement makes this diagnosis unlikely in most patients. It is probable that some of these tumors are undifferentiated variants of well-recognized neuroendocrine tumors (e.g., carcinoid tumor), without a recognizable primary site. In the undifferentiated form, the clinical and pathologic characteristics no longer resemble the characteristics of the more differentiated counterpart. Anaplastic or atypical carcinoid tumors arising in the gastrointestinal tract are responsive to platinum-based chemotherapy, whereas carcinoid tumors with typical histology are usually resistant.[75] A few reports of patients with "extrapulmonary small cell carcinoma of unknown primary site" have also documented chemotherapy responsiveness and occasional long-term survival after systemic therapy.[77,78] However, the term "extrapulmonary small cell carcinoma" implies the existence of a known primary site (e.g., head and neck, salivary gland, prostate, cervix, esophagus, bladder); these tumors, described by the authors, are therefore more aptly described as "neuroendocrine carcinoma of unknown primary site," unless an obvious primary site is present.

Although the origin(s) of these poorly differentiated neuroendocrine tumors remains undefined, the presence of neurosecretory granules in the tumors of patients with poorly differentiated carcinoma identifies a highly treatable subgroup. Molecular genetic studies may be helpful if an 11:22 translocation (peripheral neuroepithelioma, soft tissue Ewing's sarcoma, or desmoplastic small round cell tumor) or i(12p) abnormality (germ cell tumor) is identified. All patients otherwise not specifically diagnosed should be treated with a trial of combination chemotherapy. As in small cell neuroendocrine carcinomas, these tumors are very sensitive to combination chemotherapy. Some patients with a single site of tumor involvement may be curable with local treatment modalities alone; however, adjuvant chemotherapy should also be administered in these patients if clinically feasible.

ADENOCARCINOMA OF UNKNOWN PRIMARY SITE

CLINICAL CHARACTERISTICS

Well-differentiated and moderately well-differentiated adenocarcinoma are the most frequent light microscopic diagnoses in patients with carcinoma of unknown primary site, accounting for approximately 60% of patients (approximately 50,000 patients annually in the United States). These are the patients that many physicians associate with the entity of unknown primary cancer. Typically, patients with this diagnosis are elderly and have metastatic tumors at multiple sites. The sites of tumor involvement frequently determine the clinical presentation; common metastatic sites include lymph nodes, liver, lung, and bone.

The clinical course is often dominated by symptoms and signs related to the metastases. The primary site becomes obvious in only 15% to 20% of patients during life.[79] At autopsy, however, 70% to 80% of patients have a primary site detected. The most common primaries identified at autopsy are the lung and pancreas, accounting for approximately 40%.[44] Other gastrointestinal sites (e.g., stomach, colon, liver) are frequent, although adenocarcinomas from a wide variety of other primary sites are encountered occasionally. Adenocarcinomas of the breast, prostate, and ovary are rare in this group of patients. There also seems to be an unexpected metastatic pattern observed for several of these tumors; for example, occult pancreatic primaries more frequently involve bone rather than liver and occult prostate and lung cancer less often involving bone. The authors are not at all certain that the clinical course or response to various therapies of occult primary cancers is similar to the known primaries.

Historically as a group, patients with metastatic adenocarcinoma of unknown primary site have a very poor prognosis, with inexorable progression and a median survival of only 3 to 4 months. This is not surprising, considering the fact that many of these patients appear to harbor lung or gastrointestinal neoplasms. Many patients in this group have widespread metastases and poor performance status at the time of diagnosis. However, it is an error to stereotype *all* patients with adenocarcinoma of unknown primary site because within this large group are subsets of patients with more favorable prognoses, as discussed later in Pathologic Evaluation. In addition, chemotherapy has improved considerably in the past several years, and many patients now are candidates for chemotherapy with a reasonable expectation of clinical benefit and improved survival.

PATHOLOGIC EVALUATION

The diagnosis of well-differentiated or moderately well-differentiated adenocarcinoma is based on light microscopic features, particularly the formation of glandular structures by neoplastic cells. The authors have considered patients with well-differentiated or moderately well-differentiated adenocarcinoma as one group. These histologic features are shared by adenocarcinomas, and the site of the primary tumor usually cannot be determined by histologic examination. Certain histologic features typically are associated with a particular tumor type (e.g., papillary features with ovarian cancer and signet ring cells with gastric cancer). However, these characteristics are not specific enough to be used as definitive evidence of the primary site. Immunoperoxidase stains and electron microscopy are of limited value in identifying the site of origin of most well-differentiated or moderately well-differentiated adenocarcinomas. The stain for PSA is an exception because it is relatively specific for prostate cancer, and it should be used in men with suggestive clinical findings. Positive immunoperoxidase staining for estrogen or progesterone receptors, gross cystic fluid protein 15, or the Her2-neu suggests metastatic breast cancer in women with metastatic adenocarcinoma. Neuroendocrine stains (e.g., NSE, chromogranin, synaptophysin) can occasionally identify an unsuspected neuroendocrine neoplasm. Several other stains or batteries of stains have been evaluated,[7–12] but none are truly tumor-specific and, if used, should be in connection with all the other clinical data.

The diagnosis of poorly differentiated adenocarcinoma should be viewed differently, as stressed earlier in Clinical Characteristics, because some of these patients are representative of subsets with distinctive tumor biology and responsiveness to systemic therapy. This diagnosis is usually made when only minimal or questionable glandular formation is seen on histologic examination or, on occasion, when tumors exhibit positive staining for mucin but have no glandular features. Well-differentiated adenocarcinoma, poorly differentiated adenocarcinoma, and poorly differentiated carcinoma are diagnoses that probably represent parts of a spectrum of tumor differentiation rather than specific, sharply demarcated entities. These histologies represent a heterogeneous group of tumors with various biologic and clinical properties. Different pathologists may use slightly different criteria for making each of these three diagnoses. It is therefore appropriate to perform additional study with immunoperoxidase staining, electron microscopy, and genetic studies in poorly differentiated adenocarcinomas. Guidelines for the evaluation and treatment of patients with poorly differentiated adenocarcinoma are provided earlier in Poorly Differentiated Carcinoma (with or without Features of Adenocarcinoma) of Unknown Primary Site.

DIAGNOSTIC EVALUATION

The clinical evaluation of these patients is similar to that described for patients with poorly differentiated carcinoma of unknown primary site. An exhaustive search for the primary site is not indicated because it rarely can be found. Therefore, the clinical evaluation should be performed to evaluate any suspicious clinical symptoms or signs and to determine the extent of metastatic disease. Initial evaluation should include a thorough history and physical examination, standard laboratory screening tests (i.e., complete blood count, liver function tests, serum creatinine, urinalysis), and chest radiography. All men should have a serum PSA determination, and all women should undergo mammography. CT scans of the abdomen can identify a primary site in 10% to 35% of patients and frequently are useful in identifying additional sites of metastatic disease.[80,81] Additional symptoms, signs, or abnormal physical and laboratory findings should be evaluated with appropriate diagnostic studies. Extensive imaging evaluation of asymptomatic areas is rarely useful in identifying a primary site, is expensive, and often results in confusing or false-positive results. However, an argument can be made to consider gastrointestinal endoscopy because several of these tumors are now more treatable than previously.

PET is an important addition for the evaluation of potential primary sites, as discussed earlier in Diagnostic Evaluation in Poorly Differentiated Carcinoma (with or without Features of Adenocarcinoma) of Unknown Primary Site. The availability of various tumor markers (CEA, CA 15-3, CA 19-9, CA 125, β-HCG, AFP) has not proven, in general, to be useful for diagnosis or prognosis but can be used to follow the response to therapy.[82,83]

TREATMENT

The group of patients with adenocarcinoma of unknown primary site contains several clinically defined subgroups for which useful rather specific therapy can be given. Although most tumors within these clinically defined subgroups are well- or moderately differentiated adenocarcinomas, it should be kept in mind that some tumors are poorly differentiated carcinomas. Chemotherapy can also be useful for some patients who do not

TABLE 46-5. Therapy for Women with Peritoneal Adenocarcinomatosis of Unknown Primary Site

Study	Number of Patients	Therapy	Complete Response Rate (%)	Long-Term Survival (%)	Median Survival (Mo)
Lele et al., 1988[90]	23	Surgical cytoreduction and cisplatin-based chemotherapy	22	26	19
Strnad et al., 1989[92]	18	Surgical cytoreduction and cisplatin-based chemotherapy	39	17	23
Dalrymple et al., 1989[91]	31	Surgical cytoreduction and cisplatin-based or chlorambucil chemotherapy	10	6	11
Ransom et al., 1990[93]	33	Surgical cytoreduction and cisplatin-based chemotherapy	13	9	17
Fromm et al., 1990[94]	74	Surgical cytoreduction, cisplatin alone, or in combination or melphalan alone	20	25	24
Bloss et al., 1993[95]	33	Surgical cytoreduction, cisplatin-based chemotherapy	35	15	20
Piver et al., 1997[96]	46	Surgical cytoreduction, cisplatin-based chemotherapy: paclitaxel-based chemotherapy	40	Not reported	19

fit into any of these subgroups (discussed later in Chemotherapy for Metastatic Carcinoma of Unknown Primary Site).

Peritoneal Carcinomatosis in Women

Adenocarcinoma causing diffuse peritoneal involvement is typical of ovarian carcinoma, although carcinomas from the gastrointestinal tract, lung, or breast can occasionally produce this clinical syndrome. Several women have been described with diffuse peritoneal carcinomatosis who had no primary site found in the ovaries or elsewhere in the abdomen at the time of laparotomy.[84–89] These patients frequently had histologic features typical of ovarian carcinoma, such as papillary configuration or psammoma bodies. This syndrome has been termed "multifocal extraovarian serous carcinoma" or "peritoneal papillary serous carcinoma." It is now clear that many of these patients have a primary peritoneal carcinoma. In the early 1980s, several anecdotal case reports documented excellent responses to cisplatin-based chemotherapy in women with this syndrome.[84–87] This tumor is more common in women with a family history of ovarian cancer, and prophylactic oophorectomy, as expected, does not protect them from this tumor.[88] Like ovarian carcinoma, the incidence of primary peritoneal carcinoma is increased in women with BRCA1 mutations.[89]

Table 46-5 summarizes the results of seven series including a total of 258 women with this syndrome.[90–96] The clinical features are similar to ovarian carcinoma or abdominal carcinomatosis. Many patients have elevated serum levels of CA 125 antigen. An occasional patient presents with pleural effusion only, but metastases outside the peritoneal cavity are unusual. The histologic features are similar to ovarian carcinoma (usually papillary configurations but also other histologies, including poorly differentiated carcinoma). The initial treatment plan for most patients included laparotomy with surgical cytoreduction; most received cisplatin-based combination chemotherapy. A few patients received cisplatin, chlorambucil, or melphalan alone. Other investigations documented the activity of paclitaxel.[96] A summary of the historical results in 258 women are as follows: Twenty-two percent (range of 10% to 40%) of all patients had a complete response to chemotherapy, the median survival was 18

months (range of 11 to 24 months), and the long-term survival (more than 2 years) was 16% (range of 6% to 26%). These results from several trials confirm the chemosensitivity of these tumors in some women with this syndrome.

The site of origin of these carcinomas is likely from the peritoneal surface (primary peritoneal carcinoma). Because ovarian epithelium is in part an extension of the mesothelial surface, some carcinomas arising from the peritoneal (mesothelial) surface may share a similar lineage (müllerian derivation) and biology with ovarian carcinoma. Support for this hypothesis has been strengthened by the demonstration of gene expression profiles nearly identical to ovarian carcinoma (B. I. Sikic, *personal communication*, 2003). Therefore, optimal management of these patients should follow guidelines for the management of advanced ovarian cancer, including aggressive surgical cytoreduction followed by postoperative chemotherapy. Carboplatin plus paclitaxel or similar regimens considered optimal for the treatment of advanced ovarian cancer would seem a reasonable choice for initial chemotherapy, and the results are likely to be similar to those of ovarian carcinoma. Several other confirmatory results have been reported since 1997, this clinical pathologic entity is now generally accepted, and the patients are now usually included in therapeutic trials with ovarian cancer.

Papillary peritoneal carcinomatosis has also been reported in men[97]; however, it is difficult to confirm the precise biology, and some of these tumors may be metastatic from an occult primary from elsewhere. The study of gene expression patterns in these patients may be very revealing, particularly if they match those seen in women. A trial of chemotherapy should be administered to good performance status patients.

Women with Axillary Lymph Node Metastases

Breast cancer should be suspected in women who have axillary lymph node involvement with adenocarcinoma. Occasionally, the histology is poorly differentiated carcinoma. Men with occult breast cancer can present in this fashion but are rare. The initial lymph node biopsy should include estrogen and progesterone receptors. Elevated levels provide strong evidence for the diagnosis of breast cancer.[98] If no other metastases are identified, these patients may have stage II breast cancer with an occult primary, which is potentially curable with appropriate therapy. PET and magnetic resonance imaging have identified occult breast cancer even with normal mammography.[99–101] Modified radical mastectomy has been recommended in such patients, even when physical examination and mammography are normal. An occult breast primary has been identified after mastectomy in 44% to 80% of patients.[102–104] Primary tumors are usually less than 2 cm in diameter; in occasional patients, only noninvasive tumor is identified in the breast.[105] Prognosis after primary therapy is similar to that of other patients with stage II breast cancer.[102–106] Radiation therapy to the breast after axillary lymph node dissection represents a reasonable alternative primary therapy. Either neoadjuvant or adjuvant systemic chemotherapy is indicated in this setting, similar to standard therapy for stage II breast cancer.

Women with metastatic sites in addition to the axillary lymph nodes may have metastatic breast cancer with an occult primary. These women should be managed as if they have metastatic breast cancer. Elevated serum levels of CA 15-3 or CA 27-29 suggest the possibility of breast cancer. Estrogen and progesterone receptor and Her-2-neu status is of particular importance in these patients because they may derive major palliative benefit from hormonal therapy, chemotherapy, and trastuzumab.

Men with Possible Prostate Carcinoma

PSA concentrations should be measured in men with adenocarcinoma of unknown primary site. These tumors can also be stained for PSA. Even when clinical features (i.e., metastatic pattern) do not suggest prostate cancer, a positive PSA (serum or tumor stain) is reason for a trial of hormonal therapy.[107,108] Osteoblastic bone metastases are also an indication for an empiric hormone trial, regardless of the PSA findings.

SQUAMOUS CARCINOMA OF UNKNOWN PRIMARY SITE

Squamous carcinoma at a metastatic site represents approximately 5% of all patients with unknown primary carcinomas (approximately 4000 patients annually in the United States). Effective treatment is available for patients with certain clinical syndromes (approximately 90% of patients), and appropriate evaluation is important.

SQUAMOUS CARCINOMA INVOLVING CERVICAL AND SUPRACLAVICULAR LYMPH NODES

The cervical lymph nodes are the most common metastatic site. Patients are usually middle-aged or elderly, and frequently they have abused tobacco or alcohol. When the upper or middle cervical lymph nodes are involved, a primary tumor in the head and neck region should be suspected. Clinical evaluation should include an examination of the oropharynx, hypopharynx, nasopharynx, larynx, and upper esophagus by direct endoscopy, with biopsy of any suspicious areas. CT of the neck better defines the disease in the neck and occasionally identifies a primary site. PET scanning is indicated, as it may also

identify primary sites.[50–54,109] Detection of Epstein-Barr virus genome in the tumor tissue is highly suggestive of a nasopharyngeal primary site[35,36] (discussed earlier in Genetic Analysis), particularly in poorly differentiated carcinomas. Other genetic studies of squamous cell carcinoma of the head and neck region have shown genetic alterations in "normal tissue" as a precursor of invasive carcinoma.[110] Further study is indicated, as these findings do not yet have a practical application. When the lower cervical or supraclavicular lymph nodes are involved, a primary lung cancer should be suspected. Fiberoptic bronchoscopy should be performed if the chest radiograph and head and neck examinations are normal, as this has a high yield, frequently identifying a lung primary.[111]

When no primary site is identified, local treatment should be given to the involved neck. The reported results in more than 1400 patients are primarily retrospective single-institution experiences, often using a variety of treatment modalities.[112–134] In many of these series, a large minority of patients had poorly differentiated carcinoma and adenocarcinoma. A substantial percentage, usually 30% to 40%, of patients achieved long-term disease-free survival after local treatment modalities. The results obtained using radical neck dissection, high-dose radiation therapy, or a combination of these modalities have been similar. The volume of tumor in the involved neck influences outcome, with N1 or N2 disease having a significantly higher cure rate than N3 or massive neck involvement.[132,134] Poorly differentiated carcinoma also represents a poor prognostic factor in these patients. When resection alone is used as the primary treatment modality, a primary tumor in the head and neck subsequently becomes apparent in 20% to 40% of patients. Primary tumors surface less commonly when radiation therapy is used, presumably due to the eradication of occult head and neck primary sites within the radiation field. Radiation therapy dosages and techniques should be similar to those used in patients with primary head and neck cancer,[123] and the nasopharynx, oropharynx, and hypopharynx may be included in the irradiated field. Patients with low cervical and supraclavicular nodes do not do as well because lung cancer is a frequent site of occult primary tumors. Patients with no detectable disease below the clavicle should be treated with aggressive local therapy because 10% to 15% of these patients have long-term disease-free survival. Chemotherapy should also be considered for these patients.

The role of chemotherapy for metastatic squamous carcinoma in cervical lymph nodes is controversial. A nonrandomized comparison of patients treated with local modalities alone or with local modalities combined with chemotherapy (cisplatin and 5-FU) showed a higher complete response rate (81% vs. 60%) and longer median survival time (more than 37 vs. 24 months) in patients also receiving chemotherapy.[126] Combined modality treatment with concurrent chemotherapy and radiotherapy in locally advanced head and neck carcinoma is now standard and accepted, and it is also reasonable for these unknown primary patients. In those who receive local therapy first, adjuvant platinum-based or paclitaxel-based chemotherapy should be considered.

SQUAMOUS CARCINOMA INVOLVING INGUINAL LYMPH NODES

Most patients with a tumor in inguinal lymph nodes have a detectable primary site in the genital or anorectal areas. Careful examination of vulva, vagina, cervix, penis, and scrotum is important, with biopsy of any suspicious areas. Digital examination and anoscopy should be performed to exclude lesions in the anorectal area. Identification of a primary site in these patients is important because curative therapy is available for carcinomas of the vulva, vagina, cervix, and anus, even after spread to regional lymph nodes. Nearly 50% of these patients with inguinal presentations have poorly differentiated carcinoma. For the patient in whom no primary site is identified, surgical resection with or without radiation therapy to the inguinal area sometimes results in long-term survival. These patients, regardless of histology, should also be considered for neoadjuvant or adjuvant chemotherapy.

SQUAMOUS CARCINOMA METASTATIC TO OTHER SITES

Metastatic squamous carcinoma in areas other than the cervical or inguinal lymph nodes usually represents metastasis from an occult primary lung cancer. CT scans of the chest and fiberoptic bronchoscopy should be considered. Chemotherapy with regimens used in the treatment of non–small cell lung cancer may be considered in patients with good performance status. Other rare presentations include primaries from the head and neck, esophagus, anus, and skin.

Patients with the diagnosis of poorly differentiated squamous carcinoma should be evaluated carefully, particularly if other clinical features are atypical for lung cancer (i.e., young patient, non-smoker, unusual metastatic sites). Occasionally, adenocarcinomas, particularly in the breast, undergo squamous differentiation at metastatic sites. As with the diagnosis of poorly differentiated adenocarcinoma, this histologic diagnosis (squamous cell) is sometimes based on minimal histologic findings. Additional pathologic evaluation with immunoperoxidase stains, electron microscopy, and molecular studies should be considered. When the diagnosis remains unclear, such patients should be considered for a trial of therapy for poorly differentiated carcinoma.

CHEMOTHERAPY FOR METASTATIC CARCINOMA OF UNKNOWN PRIMARY SITE

Approximately 90% of patients with well-differentiated or moderately differentiated adenocarcinoma of unknown primary site are not represented in one of the several favorable prognostic clinical subgroups. Furthermore, approximately 80% of patients with poorly differentiated carcinoma do not conform to a known favorable prognostic subgroup. In the past, chemotherapy of various types has produced low response rates, very few complete responses, and even fewer long-term survivals.[2,135,136] The results of chemotherapy in several reported series of 10 or more patients from 1964 to 2002 are briefly summarized as follows: A total of 1515 patients were reported in 45 trials.[2,136] The only single agent studied adequately in previously untreated patients was 5-FU, with response rates ranging from 0% to 16%. Cisplatin has been reported as a single drug in only one series,[137] with a response rate of 19%. Other single agents, including methotrexate, doxorubicin, mitomycin C, vincristine, and semustine, have been reported with response rates from 6% to 16%.[138] The FAM regimen (5-FU, doxorubicin, mitomycin C) and various modifications have been used often, based on the demonstrated activity of these combina-

tion regimens in some gastrointestinal cancers.[139–150] The combination of 5-FU and leucovorin has not been evaluated adequately but does not appear active in patients with liver metastasis with an unknown primary,[151] a group most likely to have gastrointestinal primaries. The overall response rates from all these prospective clinical trials varied from 8% to 39% (mean of 20%), complete responders less than 1%, median survival of 4 to 15 months (mean of 6 months), survival beyond 2 years rare (rarely reported), and disease-free survival beyond 3 years nonexistent (none reported).

Since 1991, many cisplatin-based combination chemotherapy regimens have been reported.[2,136,137] In two small, randomized comparisons[139,142] (subject to many confounding factors) of doxorubicin with or without cisplatin, no difference in median survival was observed, but there was more toxicity in the cisplatin-containing arms. A third, more recent, small, randomized trial[61] did show the superiority of cisplatin, epirubicin, and mitomycin C compared with mitomycin C alone (median survival of 9.4 vs. 5.4 months). The authors have also seen some useful clinical responses to cisplatin- or carboplatin-based chemotherapy, as well as 5-FU plus leucovorin.

These data need to be viewed with several factors in mind. Some of the series are small and large randomized comparisons are lacking. In addition to adenocarcinomas, some patients with poorly differentiated carcinoma of unknown primary site were included in many of these series. The patients were not standardly evaluated or compared in reference to sites of metastasis (nodal vs. visceral), performance status, sex, age, as well as other known prognostic factors.

Recently, the chemotherapy has improved considerably for patients with adenocarcinoma and poorly differentiated carcinoma who do not fit or conform to a specific "treatable" or favorable subset. The introduction of several new drugs with rather broad-spectrum antineoplastic activity is changing the standard treatment for patients with several common epithelial cancers. These drugs include the taxanes, gemcitabine, vinorelbine, irinotecan, and topotecan.

Since 1995, the Minnie Pearl Cancer Research Network has completed five sequential prospective phase II trials incorporating paclitaxel,[152,153] docetaxel,[153,154] gemcitabine,[155] and irinotecan[156] into the first-line therapy for 396 patients with carcinoma of unknown primary site. Only patients with carcinoma of unknown primary site (any histology) who were not defined in a "treatable" or favorable subset were eligible for these trials (with the exception of eight patients with poorly differentiated neuroendocrine carcinoma on the first two trials). The chemotherapy regimens, patient characteristics, response rates, and survivals are summarized in Tables 46-6 and 46-7. The total response rate for all patients treated in the five clinical trials was 30% (107 of 353 evaluable patients), with 85 (94%) partial responders and 22 (6%) complete responders. With a minimum follow-up of 1 year and maximum follow-up of 8 years, the median survival was 9.1 months, and the 1-, 2-, 3-, 5-, and 8-year survivals were 38%, 19%, 12%, 8%, and 6%, respectively (Fig. 46-4). The median progression-free survival is 5 months, and the 1-, 2-, 3-, 5-, and 8-year progression-free survivals are 17%, 7%, 5%, 4%, and 3%, respectively (Fig. 46-5). The toxicity of all these regimens was generally moderate, primarily myelosuppression, with a total of eight (2%) treatment-related deaths.

Long-term follow-up on the 144 patients in the first three trials is of interest; the minimum follow-up was 4.8 years

TABLE 46-6. Chemotherapy Regimens and Patient Characteristics of Five Consecutive Prospective Phase II Studies in 396 Patients from 1995 to 2002 by the Minnie Pearl Cancer Research Network

Characteristics	Study 1[152] Paclitaxel, Carboplatin, Etoposide	Study 2[154] Docetaxel, Cisplatin	Study 3[154] Docetaxel, Carboplatin	Study 4[155] Paclitaxel, Carboplatin, Gemcitabine	Study 5[156] Paclitaxel, Carboplatin, Etoposide, followed by Gemcitabine, Irinotecan	Total
NUMBER OF PATIENTS	71	26	47	120	132	396
AGE (Y)						
Median	72	60	56	58	59	62
Range	31–82	34–74	23–76	21–85	29–83	21–85
MALE/FEMALE	35/36	13/13	25/22	64/56	67/65	203/193
HISTOLOGY						
Adenocarcinoma (well differentiated)	34 (48%)	13 (50%)	18 (38%)	63 (53%)	59 (44%)	187 (47%)
PDC or PDA	30 (42%)	11 (43%)	28 (60%)	56 (46%)	72 (55%)	197 (50%)
Neuroendocrine carcinoma (poorly differentiated)	6 (9%)	2 (7%)	0 (0%)	0 (0%)	0 (0%)	8 (2%)
Squamous carcinoma	1 (1%)	0 (0%)	1 (2%)	1 (1%)	1 (1%)	4 (1%)
ECOG PERFORMANCE STATUS						
0	9 (13%)	10 (38%)	9 (19%)	27 (27%)	24 (18%)	79 (20%)
1	50 (70%)	10 (38%)	26 (55%)	77 (64%)	97 (73%)	260 (66%)
2	12 (17%)	6 (24%)	12 (26%)	16 (14%)	11 (9%)	57 (14%)
NUMBER OF ORGAN SITES INVOLVED						
1	28 (39%)	7 (27%)	15 (32%)	42 (35%)	41 (31%)	133 (34%)
2 or more	43 (61%)	19 (73%)	32 (68%)	78 (65%)	91 (69%)	263 (66%)

ECOG, Eastern Cooperative Oncology Group; PDC, poorly differentiated carcinoma; PDA, poorly differentiated adenocarcinoma.

TABLE 46-7. Response to Therapy and Survival

	Study 1	Study 2	Study 3	Study 4	Study 5	Total
Number of patients	71	26	47	120	132	396
Partial response/complete response	48%/15%	22%/4%	22%/0%	21%/4%	23%/6%	30%/6%
1-Y survival	48%	40%	33%	42%	35%	38%
2-Y survival	20%	28%	28%	23%	16%	19%
3-Y survival	14%	16%	15%	14%	Too early	12%
5-Y survival	12%	13%	10%	Too early	Too early	10%
8-Y survival	8%	Too early	Too early	Too early	Too early	8%
Minimum follow-up (y)	6.7	6	4.8	3	1	1
Range of follow-up (y)	6.7–8.0	6.0–6.7	4.8–5.8	3.0–4.6	1–2	1–8

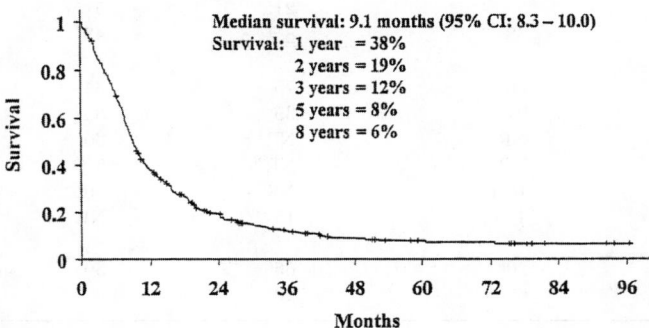

FIGURE 46-4. Unknown primary carcinoma trials: combined overall survival. Survival curve for 396 patients treated on five sequential prospective phase II trials by the Minnie Pearl Cancer Research Network. CI, confidence interval.

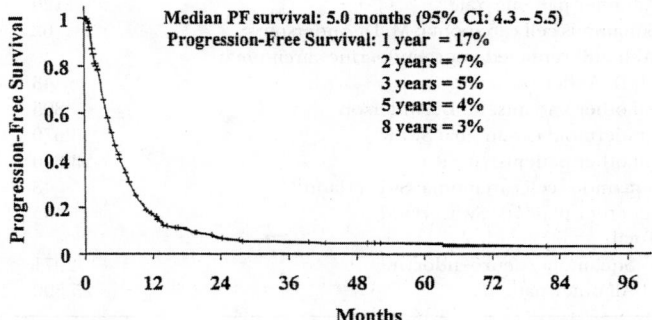

FIGURE 46-5. Unknown primary carcinoma trials: progression-free (PF) survival curve for 396 patients treated on five sequential prospective phase II trials by the Minnie Pearl Cancer Research Network. CI, confidence interval.

TABLE 46-8.   Unknown Primary Cancer: Survival of All Patients[a]

Study	Number of Patients	Median Survival (Mo)	1-Y Survival (%)	5-Y Survival (%)
Yale University[161]	1268	5	23	6
M. D. Anderson[162]	1000	11	43	11
University of Kansas[163]	686	6	21.5	5.1
Charity Hospital[164]	453	4	13.9	3.3
Johns Hopkins[165]	245	3	18	2
Mayo Clinic[166]	150	4	12	0.7
SEER[1]	26,050	NR	NR	5
Southeast Netherlands[167]	1024	2.75	15	NR
Switzerland[168]	543	4	15	NR
Total	31,419	5	22	5

NR, not reported; SEER, Surveillance, Epidemiology, and End Results registries.
[a]Includes treated and untreated patient groups, all histologies and clinical presentations.

(range of 4.8 to 8.0 years); the median survival was 10 months; and the 1-, 2-, 3-, 5-, and 8-year survivals were 42%, 22%, 18%, 12%, and 10%, respectively. The actuarial survival curves look very similar for the 252 additional patients treated in studies 4 and 5. There have been no significant differences in survival when comparing the survival curves of all five phase II studies. When evaluating the effectiveness of new therapy, survival and progression-free survival at 1 year and beyond are more important milestones than median survival.

There was no difference in survival for adenocarcinoma versus the poorly differentiated carcinomas. Women survived significantly longer than men, and those with performance status 0 or 1 (Eastern Cooperative Oncology Group scale) lived longer than those with performance status 2. Subsequent trials recently reported by others[2,62,157–160] have confirmed the activity of the newer cytotoxic agents; however, long-term follow-up has not been reported.

In the absence of randomized prospective clinical trials proving that any form of chemotherapy improves the survival of these patients versus best supportive care alone, one might reasonably question if survival is indeed improved. The authors rely largely on historical control data, which are associated with several difficulties, particularly the heterogeneous patient population, with so many variables representing multiple subsets of patients. Nonetheless, if one concentrates on prospective clinical trial survival data[2,136] nearly all the results are reported as median survivals. In some of these trials, the 1-year survivals were 10% to 20%, and 2-, 3-, and 5-year survivals were not reported, likely because of either early reporting or all the patients had died. Retrospective reviews of patient survival are useful but suffer from even greater variability than prospective results.

The authors have reviewed several reports of survival for patients with unknown primary cancer[1,161–168] in an attempt to better define the natural history of this syndrome (Table 46-8). Most of these reports were retrospective; therefore, treatments were not uniform, and some patients received no systemic therapy. In addition, these series usually contained patients now known to fit into specific treatable or favorable subsets. These historical series represent 31,419 reported patients (see Table 46-8). The median survival was 5 months, with a 1-year survival of 22% and 5-year survival of 5%. It is very likely that survival at 1 year and beyond is largely represented by subsets of patients with a more favorable prognosis who received local therapy (surgery or radiotherapy) or those with very indolent tumors (e.g., carcinoids). This is supported by data illustrated in Table 46-9. Squamous or epidermoid carcinoma and well-differentiated neuroendocrine carcinoma (carcinoid, islet cell–type histology) reported from some series (total of 2971 patients) had median, 1-year, and 5-year survivals of 20 months, 66% and 30%, respectively. All the remaining patients in these series (total of 25,890 patients) had median, 1-year, and 5-year survivals of 6 months, 20%, and 5%, respectively.

The aggregate information from these historical data makes a very compelling argument that the newer chemotherapy regi-

TABLE 46-9.   Survival of Patients with Squamous Cell Carcinoma and Well-Differentiated Neuroendocrine Carcinoma[a]

Study	Number (N)	Median Survival (Mo)	1-Y Survival (%)	5-Y Survival (%)
Squamous cell carcinoma: Yale[161]	148	9	39	15
All other patients: Yale	1120	5	21	5
Squamous cell carcinoma: M. D. Anderson[162]	62	38	85	43
Well-differentiated neuroendocrine carcinoma:				
M. D. Anderson	43	26	75	34
All other patients: M. D. Anderson	895	9	35	8
Epidermoid carcinoma: SEER[1]	2670	NR	NR	30
All other patients: SEER	23,380	NR	NR	5
Squamous cell carcinoma: Switzerland[168]	48	10.1	NR	NR
All other patients: Switzerland	495	4	15	NR
Total				
Squamous/neuroendocrine	2971	20[b]	66[b,c]	30[c]
All other patients	25,890	6[b]	20[b]	5[c]

NR, not reported; SEER, Surveillance, Epidemiology, and End Results registries.
[a]Includes treated and untreated patients.
[b]SEER data not included in calculation (not reported).
[c]Switzerland data not included in calculation (not reported).

mens as administered in prospective clinical studies by the community-based Minnie Pearl Research Network to 396 patients with relatively poor prognostic features produces a meaningful prolongation of survival for these patients. The long-term survivals of these 396 patients at 1, 2, 3, 5, and 8 years are 38%, 19%, 12%, 8%, and 6%, respectively. These survival results at 2 years are comparable to the 1-year survival of the historical control patients.

Several other groups have reported early follow-up data with the newer cytotoxic drugs, including paclitaxel-, docetaxel-, gemcitabine-, and irinotecan-based regimens,[157–160] and the median survivals are similar to the 396 patients reported here; however, long-term follow-up has not yet been reported. The improvements in these therapies are best seen and documented at 1-, 2-, 3-, and 5-year survival end points. Far less than 50% of the patients are long-term survivors; consequently, major differences may not be appreciated by comparing only median survival data. It may be erroneous to believe a new therapy is improved or not based on small changes in median survival alone. The standard therapy for good-performance-status patients with carcinoma of unknown primary site is with one of the newer cytotoxic combinations as reported in the 396 patients in this chapter, or as reported by others.[157–160]

These new survival data are encouraging. Many of the more common patients with unknown primary adenocarcinoma or poorly differentiated carcinoma who do not fit or conform to any previously defined "treatable" or favorable subset can now attain substantial clinical benefit from the new cytotoxic drug combinations. Despite the fact that randomized trials of treatment versus no treatment are still lacking, the median survival as well as 1-, 2-, 3-, and 5-year survival results are superior to the survivals recorded from the past. The authors are not aware of other progression-free survival data reported in the literature. The survival for patients with unknown primary carcinoma now compares favorably to the survivals of several other groups of advanced carcinoma patients receiving various types of chemotherapy, including, for example, extensive-stage small cell lung cancer and advanced non–small cell lung cancer. Certainly, there is vast room for improvement, and basic and clinical research remains a priority to further enhance the therapy for these patients.

SPECIAL ISSUES IN CARCINOMA OF UNKNOWN PRIMARY SITE

BIOLOGY OF THE PRIMARY TUMOR

The biology of the primary tumor in patients with unknown primary neoplasms remains an enigma. The authors believe the clinical and biologic information available highly suggest that many of these patients represent a distinct entity. However, there are other patients with tumors that conform or behave like known primary cancers. Although it is accepted that at least some of these patients have occult primaries found occasionally during the course of their disease, and more commonly at autopsy, there are several other potential explanations for the apparent absence of a primary cancer. First, some of these primary cancers may inexplicably regress or involute entirely despite the fact that metastasis already occurred. This theory is supported by the scarring seen occasionally in the testicle of patients with metastatic germ cell neoplasms (i.e.,

"burned-out primary"). Second, some of these tumors may have arisen from embryonic epithelial "rest cells" that did not complete their appropriate migration *in utero* to their designated tissue/organ. Extragonadal germ cell tumors with primaries in the mediastinum, retroperitoneum, or undescended testicular cancer are known examples of this phenomenon. Third, some of these patients have an unrecognized primary neoplasm (not an unknown primary cancer) such as an extragonadal germ cell tumor, lymphoma, melanoma, or sarcoma, which, of course, has arisen from these lineages virtually anywhere in the body. Fourth, the pathogenesis of some of these carcinomas may arise or result from a specific genetic lesion present in all cells, and these tumors might be expected to have a similar gene expression distinct from specific carcinomas of recognized primary sites, as is suggested by the unusual occurrence of metastatic adenocarcinoma of unknown primary site in monozygotic twin brothers with primary immunodeficiency disorder (X-linked hyper-immunoglobulin M syndrome).[169] Finally, some of these neoplasms may arise from adult stem cells exhibiting plasticity.[170,171] Hematopoietic stem cells appear to be able to give rise or transform into liver cells as well as muscle, gastrointestinal, skin, and brain cells.[170] Therefore, some unknown primary tumors might continue to reflect the differentiation or transformation of adult stem cells and may be "tumors of adult stem cells." For example, seemingly metastatic adenocarcinoma in bone, liver, lymph node, or elsewhere may, in fact, arise from an adult stem cell with the capacity to become any type of cell and to develop as a "primary" neoplasm in any of these tissues.[171] All unknown primary tumors certainly possess a metastatic phenotype; however, when a primary is clinically occult, the natural history may in some patients vary from known primary cancers.

Karyotypic analysis of metastatic carcinoma of unknown primary site often demonstrates diverse multiple complex abnormalities and is not yet helpful in most instances for diagnosis or classification (see earlier in Genetic Analysis) but is more representative of advanced neoplasms of many types (e.g., various chromosomal 1p abnormalities).[172] Thus far, there is no direct evidence to support a common/nonrandom genetic profile for even a portion of unknown primary tumors. However, recently gene expression profiles of known primary tumors suggest that the metastatic potential of tumors is encoded in the bulk of a primary tumor, rather than rare cells within the primary tumor with an ability to metastasize.[173] Overexpression of p53, bcl-2, C-myc, Ras and Her-2-neu have been observed in unknown primary carcinomas.[174–177] However, there is controversy about the frequency of expression and the clinical relevance of these observations. Tumors that strongly express p53 and bcl-2 may be more responsive to platinum-based chemotherapy.[175] The authors have shown that 10% of poorly differentiated carcinomas are strongly positive for Her-2 staining,[177] and obviously these patients may be reasonable candidates for a trial of anti-Her-2-neu antibody therapy (trastuzumab). Furthermore, the vascular endothelial growth factor[178,179] and the epidermal growth factor receptor are commonly expressed in epithelial neoplasms of many types including unknown primary carcinoma (unpublished observations) and therapy with epidermal growth factor receptor and vascular endothelial growth factor inhibitors are being explored.

A better understanding of the biology of unknown primary cancer is likely to be forthcoming, particularly with the development and study of gene expression profiling of these and other neoplasms.

CARCINOMA OF UNKNOWN PRIMARY SITE AS A DISTINCT CLINICOPATHOLOGIC ENTITY

The authors have been struck over the past two decades by the number of times patients and their referring physicians (often oncologists) are very frustrated by unknown primary cancer. They are often somewhat obsessed with finding the primary site or at least giving the patient a more specific diagnosis. There are many reasons underlying these feelings. Some patients think their oncologist is not clever enough as a diagnostician and seek the advice of others. Some oncologists feel relatively inadequate and wonder what other test(s) they might order; some have been relatively tentative, not feeling confident in recommending any therapy. Certainly a reasonable clinical and pathologic evaluation of these patients and their tumors is indicated, being aware of possible primary sites and the relevance in particular patients. However, once these considerations and evaluation are complete and there is no additional helpful information, as often is the case, one should stop, discuss the issue with the patient/family, and accept the clinicopathologic diagnosis as an unknown primary. Patients are better served, and physicians eventually feel more comfortable and therefore manage these patients more effectively once their patients accept and understand this diagnosis as a distinct clinicopathologic entity.

A second practical issue in the United States is the determination of reimbursement for chemotherapy by Medicare for cancer diagnoses. Other than Federal Drug Administration approval for a specific tumor type, reimbursement is most typically determined by Medicare (and several other third-party insurers) by consulting the two compendia—*American Hospital Formulary Drug Information* and *United States Pharmacopeia Drug Information*. Their listing is by an indication index of tumor types (International Classification of Disease 9 codes) and a generic drug index. The list is based on published literature showing "effectiveness" or clinical benefit in a specific tumor type. This is a particularly arbitrary system. The diagnosis code for unknown primary cancer previously not included in the compendia has been recently listed by *American Hospital Formulary Drug Information* and *United States Pharmacopeia Drug Information*. For the first time ever, three drugs are listed as indicated for patients with unknown primary cancer (paclitaxel, carboplatin, etoposide). Other drugs more recently studied (docetaxel, gemcitabine, and irinotecan) are also being considered by the compendia.

Medicare usually does not pay for any drug not listed as an indication. Many patients with unknown primary cancer are coded as another diagnosis by oncologists. At times this is a "good guess" or statistical probability of the possible primary tumor. For example, patients with lung lesions or mediastinal node involvement are often coded as having non–small cell lung cancer; patients with liver metastases are coded as colon or pancreatic cancer. Furthermore, patients are at times assigned a diagnosis based on the pathology report alone (e.g., adenocarcinoma consistent with pancreatic or colon primary, or by cytokeratin-staining results). This activity, in turn, causes the true incidence of unknown primary cancer to be underestimated but does allow for reimbursement for some drug costs

by a system that otherwise has not "approved" therapies for patients with unknown primary cancer. The authors consider it a minor victory for unknown primary patients to now be recognized by the compendia with a diagnostic code and to have a few drugs listed as indicated for their therapy.

There are now more than enough clinical and pathologic data to classify patients confidently as having an unknown primary cancer, and global acceptance of this entity will help these patients establish an identity, stimulate more interest by physician investigators, and eventually improve the general understanding of these patients and their tumors.

EXTRAGONADAL GERM CELL CANCER SYNDROME

Selected patients with poorly differentiated carcinoma almost certainly have germ cell tumors, although the histologic features are atypical, even when generous pathologic specimens are available for study. Chromosomal analysis (see earlier in Genetic Analysis in Poorly Differentiated Neoplasms of Unknown Primary Site) may provide a definitive diagnosis in some of these patients, particularly if their tumor cells contain specific chromosome 12 abnormalities. Even if not found or in the absence of a genetic study, young people who have mediastinal or retroperitoneal masses or multiple lung nodules with or without elevated serum levels of HCG or AFP should be suspected of harboring a germ cell tumor. Lymphomas, neuroendocrine tumors, and other tumors (i.e., sarcoma, melanoma, thymic carcinoma) should be ruled out by immunoperoxidase stains, electron microscopy, or, if necessary, cytogenetic studies. The "extragonadal germ cell cancer syndrome" was described in 1979.[55,56] The full syndrome has the following features: (1) It occurs in young men (younger than 50 years); (2) tumors are predominantly located in the midline (mediastinum, retroperitoneum) or multiple pulmonary nodules; (3) the symptom interval is short (less than 3 months), and there is a history of rapid tumor growth; (4) serum levels of HCG, AFP, or both are elevated; and (5) there is a good response to previously administered radiation therapy or chemotherapy.

Few patients have all elements of this syndrome [see earlier in Prognostic Factors in Poorly Differentiated Carcinoma (with or without Features of Adenocarcinoma) of Unknown Primary Site]. These clinical features are those of extragonadal germ cell tumors, but without a definitive histology or molecular marker, the diagnosis is equivocal. In rare cases, women can have these tumors, and the other features are also not absolute. Any two features suggest the possibility of a germ cell tumor. Since 1979, the authors have documented the correct diagnosis in some of these patients by repeat biopsies, by review and study of previous pathologic material, and at autopsy. Lymphoma, neuroendocrine carcinoma, thymic carcinoma, sarcoma, melanoma, and metastatic carcinoma can simulate the syndrome. However, the majority of these tumors are poorly differentiated carcinoma, not otherwise specified. Because these patients may have atypical germ cell tumors, treatment with cisplatin-based chemotherapy as used in advanced testicular cancer is recommended.

SINGLE SITE OF NEOPLASM

In the situation in which only one site of neoplasm is identified (e.g., one node group, one mass), the possibility of an unusual primary tumor mimicking metastatic disease should be considered. Several unusual tumors could present in this fashion, including Merkel-cell tumors; skin adnexal tumors (e.g., apocrine, eccrine, and sebaceous carcinomas); and even sarcomas, melanomas, or lymphomas that are mistakenly interpreted as metastatic carcinoma (pathologically and clinically). Patients with one site of involvement (brain, liver, subcutaneous tissue, bone, intestine, lymph node, or other sites) usually have metastatic carcinoma, and many other sites are present but are not detectable. In the absence of any other documented metastatic disease, these patients should be treated with aggressive local therapy (i.e., resection, radiation therapy, or both) because a minority enjoy long-term disease-free survival. Isolated axillary carcinoma in women often arises from an occult breast cancer, and in general, these patients should be treated like stage II breast carcinoma (see earlier in Women with Axillary Lymph Node Metastases). Patients who present with isolated cervical, supraclavicular, and inguinal adenopathy often have squamous cell carcinoma (see earlier in Squamous Carcinoma of Unknown Primary Site), but a minority harbor poorly differentiated carcinoma and adenocarcinoma. In addition to definitive local therapy, the authors believe these patients should also receive either neoadjuvant or adjuvant chemotherapy with one of the newer regimens, but it is difficult to know if this treatment is superior to local therapy alone.

UNSUSPECTED GESTATIONAL CHORIOCARCINOMA

In young women with poorly differentiated carcinoma or anaplastic neoplasms, particularly with lung nodules, be aware of the possibility of metastatic gestational choriocarcinoma. The history of recent pregnancy, spontaneous abortion, or missed menstrual periods should suggest the possibility. In this group of patients, serum HCG levels are invariably elevated. On occasion, biopsy specimens do not show the classic appearance of choriocarcinoma but simply that of metastatic carcinoma, usually poorly differentiated. Ultrasound or CT scan of the abdomen may show an enlarged uterus, and a dilation and curettage may be indicated in these patients. Most of these patients are curable with single-agent methotrexate.

UNSUSPECTED GASTROINTESTINAL STROMAL TUMOR

Patients with predominant abdominal masses and a diagnosis of carcinoma or sarcoma (particularly leiomyosarcoma) of unknown primary site should have their biopsy specimen stained for c-kit (CD117). In some circumstances, a repeat biopsy is indicated to be sure the patient does not have a gastrointestinal stromal tumor. The authors have seen a few patients with unsuspected gastrointestinal stromal tumor, later proven by biopsy review or repeat biopsy, who responded favorably to imatinib. It is reasonable to do a CD117 stain on all sarcomas of unknown primary site, but data are still lacking as to the effectiveness of imatinib in this setting.

ISOLATED PLEURAL EFFUSION

An isolated pleural effusion containing carcinoma occasionally represents metastatic disease from occult ovarian carcinoma or primary peritoneal carcinoma. Even when the patient has no symptoms or signs and an abdominopelvic CT scan and PET scan are normal, the primary may reside in the abdomen or pelvis. These occult abdominal neoplasms may arise from the ovary or the peritoneal surface (see earlier in Peritoneal Carcinomatosis in Women) and most characteristically cause a pleural effusion. Should there be no clue of neoplasm in the abdomen, an elevated serum CA 125 level suggests the possibility of this phenomenon. In the absence of clinical findings in the abdomen, laparoscopy or exploratory laparotomy might be diagnostic, but these procedures are not therapeutic in this setting. Some of these tumors are particularly responsive to chemotherapy with a taxane/platinum regimen.

An isolated pleural effusion can be a manifestation of a peripheral lung carcinoma (usually adenocarcinoma), a mesothelioma, or, rarely, a metastatic tumor from other sites. In a series of 42 patients, a primary lung cancer was eventually found in 15 patients (36%).[180] Diagnosis may be difficult; at times, the primary is not apparent even after chest tube drainage. Cytology usually shows adenocarcinoma. Electron microscopy may reveal ultrastructural features diagnostic of mesothelioma. The therapy of these patients is difficult. In those with poor performance status or advanced age, a trial of tamoxifen or megestrol acetate is reasonable. In fit patients, a trial of chemotherapy for unknown primary carcinoma should be considered. In one small series of patients,[180] chemotherapy produced symptomatic improvement in 78% of patients (29 of 37 patients). Thirty of 37 patients had their pleural effusion reduced by chemotherapy, and their median survival was 12 months (3 to 60+ months).

GERM CELL TUMORS WITH METASTASES OF OTHER HISTOLOGIES

On occasion, patients with germ cell tumors, particularly extragonadal primaries, may have a metastatic lesion that consists of only somatic tumor cells. This is particularly true for neuroendocrine or sarcomatous differentiation but can include any histologies. Patients therefore may be diagnosed as having a neuroendocrine tumor or sarcoma. In these rare instances, a primary germ cell tumor (usually extragonadal) is present elsewhere and subsequently is clinically apparent. It is difficult to make the diagnosis initially. An elevated plasma AFP or HCG level is suggestive. The presence of a mediastinal, retroperitoneal, or testicular mass supports this possibility. Chromosomal analysis of tumor tissue may be diagnostic if a specific chromosome 12 abnormality is found. If the patient has metastatic germ cell tumor with metastases of other histologies, the treatment of choice is cisplatin-based chemotherapy. These patients appear to have a worse prognosis than those with typical germ cell tumors, probably because the somatic cell tumors are less sensitive to chemotherapy.

MELANOMA AND AMELANOTIC MELANOMA

Approximately 10% to 15% of all melanomas presenting with an unknown primary site are believed to be amelanotic. The authors have viewed this diagnosis with considerable skepticism. At times, the only reason for the pathologic diagnosis is the similarity of the histologic pattern to melanoma, even though no pigment is demonstrated. In the authors' experience, detailed pathologic and molecular study has occasionally revealed a group of other specific diagnoses, including lymphomas, neuroendocrine tumors, germ cell tumors, sarcomas, and poorly differentiated carcinoma (not otherwise specified).

Melanosomes or premelanosomes seen on electron micrographs have been considered diagnostic of melanoma, but on rare occasion these structures are seen in other tumors. Some believe amelanotic melanomas do not always form premelanosomes, raising the question as to whether they are really melanomas. Immunoperoxidase panels are also useful in suggesting the diagnosis of melanoma (see Table 46-1). It is of interest that in the authors' original series[60] of 220 patients with poorly differentiated carcinoma, nine were later believed to perhaps be amelanotic melanoma on the basis of immunoperoxidase stains and/or electron microscopy. These particular patients generally responded well to cisplatin-based chemotherapy, and several had long-term survival, an unexpected result for melanoma.

The history of a resected, abraded, or frozen pigmented skin lesion would certainly favor a metastatic melanoma in an individual. In addition, the rare primary visceral melanoma should be considered (e.g., eye, adrenal, bowel) as the source of the disease in questionable cases. For patients with the pathologic diagnosis of amelanotic melanoma and no history or clinical features to support this diagnosis, treatment based on guidelines for unknown primary cancer should be considered. Patients with multiple metastases should be considered for empiric chemotherapy (discussed earlier in Chemotherapy for Metastatic Carcinoma of Unknown Primary Site). If only one site is involved (particularly a single nodal site), definitive local treatment with resection plus/minus radiation therapy is indicated.

UNKNOWN PRIMARY CANCER IN CHILDREN

There are scant data in children, and, as expected, many of the unknown primary neoplasms represent embryonal malignancies[181] (i.e., rhabdomyosarcoma, neuroblastoma, Ewing's sarcoma, Wilms' tumor, hepatoblastoma, germ cell tumors, lymphomas, and poorly differentiated neuroendocrine tumors). The authors have seen a few examples of some of these tumors in children and adolescents when the initial diagnosis or primary site was uncertain. In addition, well-differentiated adenocarcinoma and poorly differentiated carcinoma of unknown primary site occur in children, but they are exceedingly rare. Because most of these neoplasms in children can be diagnosed by specialized pathology, the therapy is usually not an issue, but in those rare patients with carcinoma, not otherwise specified, the authors favor following the same management plan as for adults.

EVOLVING ROLE OF PROGNOSTIC FACTORS: THERAPEUTIC IMPLICATIONS

The prognoses of the subgroups of patients with squamous cell carcinoma, poorly differentiated neoplasm (otherwise not classified), and neuroendocrine carcinoma and those with a single small site of metastasis are relatively good. Some other patients with poorly differentiated carcinoma have chemotherapy-responsive tumors, and complete responses and long-term survival have been documented for a minority of patients. On the other hand, the larger group of patients with well-differentiated adenocarcinoma has had relatively resistant tumors, with virtually no complete responses to chemotherapy and no long-term survivals. In the past several years, subsets of patients with a more favorable prognosis or other "favorable" prognostic factors have

TABLE 46-10. Favorable Prognostic Factors in Cancer of Unknown Primary Site

DEFINITE

Poorly differentiated malignant neoplasm (not otherwise classified) (60% = lymphomas)

Extragonadal germ cell syndrome (PDA or PDC)

Retroperitoneal, mediastinal, and/or peripheral lymph node involvement (PDA, PDC, WDA)

Squamous cell carcinomas (head/neck or inguinal area)

Isolated axillary adenopathy—women, rare in men (WDA, PDC, PDA)

Peritoneal carcinoma—women, rare in men (WDA, PDC, PDA)

Blastic bone mets or increased PSA in serum or tumor—men (WDA, PDA, PDC)

Neuroendocrine carcinoma—high-grade or poorly differentiated (small cell and others)

Neuroendocrine carcinoma—low-grade or well-differentiated (carcinoid/islet cell type)

Single site of metastasis (WDA, PDC, PDA)

Performance status 0, 1 (with otherwise favorable features)

Normal serum LDH (with otherwise favorable features)

PROBABLE

Women

Nonsmoker

Two sites of metastasis

Estrogen and/or progesterone receptor–positive tumor

Normal serum CEA

CEA, carcinoembryonic antigen; LDH, lactate dehydrogenase; PDA, poorly differentiated adenocarcinoma; PDC, poorly differentiated carcinoma; PSA, prostate-specific antigen; WDA, well-differentiated adenocarcinoma.

been recognized. These subsets of patients, many managed with specific therapies, have a better prognosis than the group as a whole. The authors have stressed that both pathologic and clinical factors can now define several patients with a better prognosis (Table 46-10) (also see earlier in Prognostic Factors).

Although there are undoubtedly other unrecognized favorable features, it appears that most patients who do not fit into a favorable subset have a poor prognosis, regardless of their initial light microscopic diagnosis (well-differentiated adenocarcinoma or poorly differentiated carcinoma). These patients have recently been treated with several of the newer cytotoxic combinations (taxanes, gemcitabine, and irinotecan), with modest improvements in the response rate (with some complete responses) and survival (see earlier in Chemotherapy for Metastatic Carcinoma of Unknown Primary Site). Furthermore, the newer cytotoxic combinations appear more effective with less toxicity than cisplatin-based chemotherapy, even for those patients within favorable prognostic subsets who otherwise require chemotherapy. The one exception is patients with at least two features of the extragonadal germ cell syndrome, where cisplatin-based therapy remains the treatment of choice. Further study of the patients with poor prognoses is necessary to continue to build on the progress seen with newer cytotoxic agent–based combination chemotherapies.

CONCLUSION

The recognition of subsets of responsive tumors in patients within the large heterogeneous population of cancers of

TABLE 46-11. Carcinoma of Unknown Primary Site: Summary of Evaluation and Therapy of Responsive Subsets

	Clinical Evaluation[a]	*Special Pathologic Studies*	*Subsets*	*Therapy*	*Prognosis*
Adenocarcinoma (well-differentiated or moderately differentiated)	Chest, abdominal CT scan; PET scan Men: Serum PSA Women: Mammogram Serum CA 15-3 Serum CA 125 Additional studies to evaluate symptoms, signs	Men: PSA stain Women: ER, PR	1. Women, axillary node involvement[b] 2. Women, peritoneal carcinomatosis[b] 3. Men, blastic bone metastases, high serum PSA, or PSA tumor staining 4. Single metastatic site[b] 5. Other groups (see text)	1. Treat as primary breast cancer 2. Surgical cytoreduction plus chemotherapy 3. Hormonal therapy for prostate cancer 4. Lymph node dissection, radiotherapy 5. Newer chemotherapy	Survival improved with specific therapy Survival improved
Squamous carcinoma	Cervical node presentation[b] Panendoscopy PET scan Supraclavicular presentation[b] Bronchoscopy PET scan Inguinal presentation[b] Pelvic, rectal exams, anoscopy PET scan	Genetic analysis	1. Cervical adenopathy Nasopharyngeal cancer (identified by PCR for Epstein-Barr viral genes) 2. Supraclavicular 3. Inguinal adenopathy	1. Radiation therapy, neck dissection, chemotherapy 2. Radiation therapy, chemotherapy 3. Inguinal node dissection, radiation therapy, chemotherapy	25–50% 5-y survival 5–15% 5-y survival 15–20% 5-y survival
Poorly differentiated carcinoma, poorly differentiated adenocarcinoma	Chest, abdominal CT scans, serum HCG, AFP; PET scan; additional studies to evaluate symptoms, signs	Immunoperoxidase staining Electron microscopy Genetic analysis	1. Atypical germ cell tumors (identified by chromosome 12 abnormalities) 2. Extragonadal germ cell syndrome (two features) 3. Lymph node predominant tumors (mediastinum, retroperitoneum, peripheral nodes) 4. Gastrointestinal stromal tumors (identified by CD117 stain) 5. Other groups (see text)	1. Treatment for germ cell tumor 2. Cisplatin/etoposide 3. Newer chemotherapy 4. Imatinib 5. Newer chemotherapy	40–50% cure rate Survival improved (10–20% cured) Survival improved Survival improved Survival improved
Neuroendocrine carcinoma	Chest, abdominal CT	Immunoperoxidase staining Electron microscopy	1. Low-grade 2. Small cell carcinoma 3. Poorly differentiated	1. Treat as advanced carcinoid 2,3. Paclitaxel/carboplatin/etoposide or platinum/etoposide	Indolent biology/long survival High response rate survival improved; rarely cured

AFP, α-fetoprotein; CT, computed tomography; ER, estrogen receptor; HCG, human chorionic gonadotropin; PCR, polymerase chain reaction; PET, positron emission tomography; PR, progesterone receptor; PSA, prostate-specific antigen.
[a]In addition to history, physical examination, routine laboratory tests, and chest x-ray films.
[b]May also present with poorly differentiated carcinoma, and management and outcome are similar.

unknown primary site represents an improvement in the management of these patients. Approximately 40% of all patients fall within a defined subset with important treatment implications (see Fig. 46-1). These patients with more responsive tumors can often be defined with appropriate clinical and pathologic evaluation. A summary of treatable subsets and an outline of the evaluation necessary for their identification are given in Table 46-11. As the therapy for various neoplasms improves, the outcomes for patients with cancers of unknown primary site are likely to improve. Recently, several combination chemotherapy regimens using newer agents have been useful in previously unresponsive subgroups of patients. A therapeutic trial is the only absolute method to determine if a patient has a responsive tumor. Even for responsive carcinomas, the tumor origin, biology, and precise lineage often continue to be an enigma. However, groups of patients with insensitive tumors remain. Improved therapy for these patients will probably follow advances in the understanding of the biology and treatment of non–small cell lung cancer, pancreatic cancer, and the other gastrointestinal cancers because many insensitive carcinomas either arise from these occult primary sites or share a common biology.

The authors have established a registry, a repository for pathologic material, and are collecting and cataloging patient data from other physicians around the country. Pathologic material, clinical summaries, and follow-up data on all such patients are being requested. A bank of unstained slides is maintained, so that special stains developed in the future may be evaluated rapidly. The authors have also established a frozen tissue bank for genetic studies, particularly DNA profiling. These data eventually may provide a better assessment of the frequency and spectrum of these neoplasms and improve knowledge of their lineage, biology, and, subsequently, successful therapy for these patients.

REFERENCES

1. Muir C. Cancer of unknown primary site. *Cancer* 1995;75:353.
2. Pavlidis N, Briasoulis E, Hainsworth J, Greco FA. Diagnostic and therapeutic management of cancer of an unknown primary. *Eur J Cancer* 2003;39:1990.
3. Horning SJ, Carrier EK, Rouse RV, et al. Lymphomas presenting as histologically unclassified neoplasms: characteristics and response to treatment. *J Clin Oncol* 1989;17:1281.
4. Hales SA, Gatter KC, Heryet A, Mason DY. The value of immunocytochemistry in differentiating high-grade lymphoma from other anaplastic tumours: a study of anaplastic tumours from 1940 to 1960. *Leuk Lymphoma* 1989;1:59.
5. Gatter KC, Alcock C, Heryet A, Mason DY. Clinical importance of analysing malignant tumours of uncertain origin with immunohistochemical techniques. *Lancet* 1985;1:1302.
6. Azar HA, Espinoza CG, Richman AV, et al. Undifferentiated large cell malignancies: an ultrastructural and immunocytochemical study. *Hum Pathol* 1982;13:323.
7. Wong NP, Zee S, Zarbo RJ, et al. Coordinate expression of cytokeratins 7 and 20 defines unique subsets of carcinoma. *Appl Immunohistochem* 1995;3:99.
8. Tot T. Cytokeratins 20 and 7 as biomarkers: usefulness in discriminating primary from metastatic adenocarcinoma. *Eur J Cancer* 2002;38:758.
9. Brown RW, Campagna LB, Dunn JK, Cagle PT. Immunohistochemical identification of tumor markers in metastatic adenocarcinoma. A diagnostic adjunct in the determination of primary site. *Am J Clin Pathol* 1997;107:12.
10. Kaufman O, Deidesheimer T, Muehlenberg M, Deicke P, Dietel M. Immunohistochemical differentiation of metastatic breast carcinomas from metastatic adenocarcinomas of other common primary sites. *Histopathology* 1996;29:233.
11. Lagendijk JH, Mullink H, VanDiest PJ, Meijer GA, Meijer CJ. Tracing the origin of adenocarcinomas with unknown primary using immunohistochemistry: differential diagnosis between colonic and ovarian carcinomas as primary sites. *Hum Pathol* 1998;29:491.
12. Tot T. Adenocarcinomas metastatic to the liver: the value of cytokeratins 20 and 7 in the search for unknown primary tumors. *Cancer* 1999;85:171.
13. Warnke RA, Gatter KC, Falini B, et al. Diagnosis of human lymphoma with monoclonal antileukocyte antibodies. *N Engl J Med* 1983;109:1275.
14. Battifora H, Trowbridge IS. A monoclonal antibody useful for the differential diagnosis between malignant lymphoma and nonhematopoietic neoplasms. *Cancer* 1983;51:816.
15. Tapra FJ, Polak JM, Barbosa AJA, et al. Neuron-specific enolase is produced by neuroendocrine tumors. *Lancet* 1981;1:808.
16. O'Connor DT, Burton D, Deftos LJ. Immunoreactive human chromogranin A in diverse polypeptide hormone producing human tumors and normal endocrine tissues. *J Clin Endocrinol Metab* 1983;57:1084.
17. Mackey B, Ordonez NG. Pathological evaluation of neoplasms with unknown primary tumor site. *Semin Oncol* 1993;20:206.
18. Allhof EP, Proppe KH, Chapman CM. Evaluation of prostate-specific acid phosphatase and prostate-specific antigen. *J Urol* 1983;57:1084.
19. Denk H, Knepler R, Artlieb U, et al. Proteins of intermediate filaments: an immunohistochemical and biochemical approach to the classification of soft tissue tumors. *Am J Pathol* 1983;110:193.
20. Osborn M, Weber K. Biology of disease: tumor diagnosis by intermediate filament type—a novel tool for surgical pathology. *Lab Invest* 1983;48:372.
21. Kahn HJ, Marks A, Thom H, et al. Role of antibody to S-100 protein in diagnostic pathology. *Am J Clin Pathol* 1983;79:341.
22. Gown AM, Vogel AM, Hoak D, et al. Monoclonal antibodies specific for melanocytic tumors distinguish subpopulations of melanocytes. *Am J Pathol* 1986;123:195.
23. Kaufmann O, Deidesteimer T, Muehlenberg M, et al. Immunohistochemical differentiation of metastatic breast carcinomas from metastatic adenocarcinomas of other primary sites. *Histopathology* 1996;29:233.
24. Miettinen M, Lasota J. Gastrointestinal stromal tumors—definition, clinical, histological, immunohistochemical, and molecular genetic features and differential diagnosis. *Virchows Arch* 2001;438:1.
25. Bosman FT, Giard RWM, Nieuwenhuijen-Kruseman AC, et al. Human chorionic gonadotrophin and alpha fetoprotein in testicular germ cell tumors: a retrospective immunohistochemical study. *Histopathology* 1980;4:673.
26. Kurman KJ, Scardino PT, McIntire KR, et al. Cellular localization of alpha fetoprotein and human chorionic gonadotropin in germ cell tumors of the testis using an indirect immunoperoxidase technique: a new approach to classification utilizing tumor markers. *Cancer* 1977;40:2136.
27. Arnold A, Cossman J, Bakhshi A, et al. Immunoglobulin-gene rearrangements as unique clonal markers in human lymphoid neoplasms. *N Engl J Med* 1983;309:1593.
28. Rowley JD. Recurring chromosome abnormalities in leukemia and lymphoma. *Semin Hematol* 1990;27:122.
29. Turc-Carel C, Philip I, Berger MP, et al. Chromosomal translocation in Ewing's carcoma. *N Engl J Med* 1983;309:497.
30. Whang-Peng J, Triche TJ, Knutsen T, et al. Chromosome translocation in peripheral neuroepithelioma. *N Engl J Med* 1984;311:584.
31. Gerald WL, Ladanyi M, de Alava E, et al. Clinical, pathologic and molecular spectrum of tumors associated with t(11;22) (p13;q12): desmoplastic small round-cell tumors and its variants. *J Clin Oncol* 1998;16:3028.
32. Atkin NB, Baker MC. Specific chromosome change, i(12p), in testicular tumors. *Lancet* 1982;2:1349.
33. Ilson DH, Motzer RJ, Rodriguez E, et al. Genetic analysis in the diagnosis of neoplasms of unknown primary tumor site. *Semin Oncol* 1993;20:229.
34. Summersgill B, Goker H, Osin P, et al. Establishing germ cell origin of undifferentiated tumors by identifying gain of 12p material using comparative genomic hybridization analysis of paraffin-embedded samples. *Diagn Mol Pathol* 1998;7:260.
35. Yuge NK, Mochiki M, Nibu K, et al. Detection of Epstein-Barr virus in metastatic lymph nodes of patients with nasopharyngeal carcinoma and a primary unknown cancer. *Arch Otolaryngol Head Neck Surg* 2003;129:338.
36. Feinmesser R, Miyazaki I, Chenng R, et al. Diagnosis of nasopharyngeal carcinoma by DNA amplification of tissue obtained by fine-needle aspiration. *N Engl J Med* 1992;326:17.
37. Ramaswamy S, Golub TR. DNA microarrays in clinical oncology. *J Clin Oncol* 2002;20:1932.
38. Hainsworth JD, Wrigth EP, Gray GF Jr, Greco FA. Poorly differentiated carcinoma of unknown primary site: Correlation of light microscopic findings with response to cisplatin-based combination chemotherapy. *J Clin Oncol* 1987;5:1272.
39. Hainsworth JD, Wright EP, Johnson DH, Davis BW, Greco FA. Poorly differentiated carcinoma of unknown primary site; clinical usefulness of immunoperoxidase staining. *J Clin Oncol* 1991;9:1931.
40. Van der Gaast A, Verweij J, Planting AS, et al. The value of immunohistochemistry in patients with poorly differentiated adenocarcinoma and undifferentiated carcinoma of unknown primary site. *J Cancer Res Clin Oncol* 1996;122:181.
41. Motzer RJ, Rodriguez E, Reuter VE, et al. Molecular and cytogenic studies in the diagnosis of patients with midline carcinoma of unknown primary site. *J Clin Oncol* 1995;13:274.
42. Greco FA, Vaughn WK, Hainsworth JD. Advanced poorly differentiated carcinoma of unknown primary site: recognition of a treatable syndrome. *Ann Intern Med* 1986;104:547.
43. Richardson RL, Schoumacher RA, Fer MF, et al. The unrecognized extragonadal germ cell cancer syndrome. *Ann Intern Med* 1981;94:181.
44. Nystrom JS, Weiner JM, et al. Metastatic and histologic presentations in unknown primary cancer. *Semin Oncol* 1977;4:53.
45. Mayordomo JI, Guerra JM, Guijarro C, et al. Neoplasms of unknown primary site: a clinicopathological study of autopsied patients. *Tumori* 1993;79:321.
46. Kole AC, Nieweg OE, Prium J, et al. Detection of unknown occult primary tumors using positron emission tomography. *Cancer* 1998;82:1160.
47. Lassen U, Daugaard G, Eigtved A, Damgaard K, Friberg L. 18F-FDG whole body positron emission tomography (PET) in patients with unknown primary tumors (UPT). *Eur J Cancer* 1999;35:1076.
48. Bohuslavizki KH, Klutmann S, Kroger S, Sonnemann U, et al. FDG PET detection of unknown primary tumors. *J Nucl Med* 2000;41:816.
49. Rades D, Kuhnel G, Wildfang I, et al. Localized disease in cancer of unknown primary (CUP): the value of positron emission tomography (PET) for individual therapeutic management. *Ann Oncol* 2001;12:1605.
50. Stokkel MP, Terhaard CH, Hordijk GJ, van Rijk PP. The detection of unknown primary tumors in patients with cervical metastases by dual-head positron emission tomography. *Oral Oncol* 1999;35:390.
51. Aassar OS, Fischbein NJ, Caputo GR, et al. Metastatic head and neck cancer: role and usefulness of FDG PET in locating occult primary tumors. *Radiology* 1999;210:177.
52. Jungehulsing M, Scheidhauer K, Damm M, et al. 2(F)-fluoro-2-deoxy-D-glucose positron emission tomography is a sensitive tool for detection of occult primary cancer (carcinoma of unknown primary syndrome) with head and neck lymph node manifestation. *Otolaryngol Head Neck Surg* 2000;123:294.
53. Dede F, Ajoedi ND, Ansari SM, et al. Metastatic thyroid cancer occurring as an unknown primary lesion: the role of F-18 FDG positron emission tomography. *Clin Nucl Med* 2001;26:396.
54. Nieder C, Gregoire V, Ang KK. Cervical lymph node metastases from occult squamous cell carcinoma: cut down a tree to get an apple? *Int J Radiat Oncol Biol Phys* 2000;50:727.
55. Richardson RL, Greco FA, Wolff S, et al. Extragonadal germ cell malignancy: value of tumor markers in metastatic carcinoma of young males. *Proc Am Assoc Cancer Res* 1979;20:204(abst).
56. Hainsworth JD, Greco FA. Poorly differentiated carcinoma of unknown primary site. In: Fer MF, Greco FA, Oldham R, eds. *Poorly differentiated neoplasms and tumors of unknown origin.* Orlando, FL: Grune & Stratton, 1986:189.
57. Fox RM, Woods RL, Tattersall MHN. Undifferentiated carcinoma in young men: the atypical teratoma syndrome. *Lancet* 1979;1:1316.

58. Hainsworth JD, Johnson DH, Greco FA. Poorly differentiated neuroendocrine carcinoma of unknown primary site: a newly recognized clinicopathologic entity. *Ann Intern Med* 1988;109:364.
59. Hainsworth JD, Greco FA. Treatment of patients with cancer of an unknown primary site. *N Engl J Med* 1995;329:257.
60. Hainsworth JD, Johnson DH, Greco FA. Cisplatin-based combination chemotherapy in the treatment of poorly differentiated carcinoma and poorly differentiated adenocarcinoma of unknown primary site: results of a 12 year experience at a single institution. *J Clin Oncol* 1992;10:912.
61. Falkson CI, Cohen GL. Mitomycin C, epirubicin and cisplatin versus mitomycin C alone as therapy for carcinoma of unknown primary origin. *Oncology* 1998;55:116.
62. Pavlidis N, Kalofonos H, Bafaloukos D, et al. Cisplatin/Taxol combination chemotherapy in 72 patients with metastatic cancer of unknown primary site: a phase II trial of the Hellenic Cooperative Oncology Group. *Proc Am Soc Clin Oncol* 1999;18:195a(abst).
63. Raber MN, Faintuch J, Abbruzzese J, et al. Continuous infusion 5-fluorouracil, etoposide and cis-diamminedichloroplatinum in patients with metastatic carcinoma of unknown primary site. *Ann Oncol* 1991;2:519.
64. Pavlidis N, Kosmidis P, Skaros D, et al. Subsets of tumors responsive to cisplatin or combinations in patients with carcinoma of unknown primary site. *Ann Oncol* 1992;3:631.
65. van der Gaast A, Verweij J, Henzen-Logmans SC, Rodenburg CJ, Stoter G. Carcinoma of unknown primary; identification of a treatable subset. *Ann Oncol* 1990;1:119.
66. Briasoulis E, Txavaris N, Fountzilas G, et al. Combination regimen with carboplatin, epirubicin and etoposide in metastatic carcinomas of unknown primary site: a Hellenic Cooperative Oncology Group phase II trial. *Oncology* 1998;55:426.
67. Hainsworth JD, Einhorn LH, Williams SD, et al. Advanced extragonadal germ-cell tumors: successful treatment with combination chemotherapy. *Ann Intern Med* 1982;97:7.
68. Israel A, Bosl GJ, Golbey RB, et al. The results of chemotherapy for extragonadal germ-cell tumors in the cisplatin era: the Memorial Sloan-Kettering Cancer Center experience (1975–1982). *J Clin Oncol* 1985;3:1073.
69. Agnarsson BA, Kadin ME. Ki-1 positive large cell lymphoma: a morphologic and immunologic study of 19 cases. *Am J Surg Pathol* 1988;12:264.
70. Loehrer PJ, Jiroutek M, Aisner J, et al. Combined etoposide, ifosfamide, and cisplatin in the treatment of patients with advanced thymoma and thymic carcinoma: an intergroup trial. *Cancer* 2001;1:2010.
71. Abbruzzese JL, Abbruzzese MC, Hess KR, et al. Unknown primary carcinoma: natural history and prognostic factors in 657 consecutive patients. *J Clin Oncol* 1994;12:1272.
72. Lenzi R, Hess KR, Abbruzzese MC, et al. Poorly differentiated carcinoma and poorly differentiated adenocarcinoma of unknown primary origin: favorable subsets of patients with unknown primary cancer? *J Clin Oncol* 1997;15:2056.
73. van der Gaast A, Verweij J, Planting AST, et al. Simple prognostic model to predict survival in patients with undifferentiated carcinoma of unknown primary site. *J Clin Oncol* 1995;13:1720.
74. Culine S, Kramar A, Saghatchian M, et al. Development and validation of a prognostic model to predict the length of survival in patients with carcinoma of unknown primary site. *J Clin Oncol* 2002;20:4679.
75. Moertel CG, Kovals LK, O'Connell MJ, et al. Treatment of neuroendocrine carcinomas with combined etoposide and cisplatin: Evidence of major therapeutic activity in the anaplastic variants of these neoplasms. *Cancer* 1991;68:227.
76. McKay CE, Hainsworth JD, Burris AA, et al. Treatment of metastatic poorly differentiated neuroendocrine carcinoma with paclitaxel/carboplatin/etoposide: a Minnie Pearl Cancer Research Network phase II trial. *Proc Am Soc Clin Oncol* 2002;21:158a.
77. van der Gaast A, Verwey J, Prins E, Splinter TAW. Chemotherapy as treatment of choice in extrapulmonary undifferentiated small cell carcinoma. *Cancer* 1990;65:422.
78. Kasimis BS, Wuerker RB, Malefatto JP, Moran EM. Prolonged survival of patients with extrapulmonary small cell carcinoma arising in the neck. *Med Pediatr Oncol* 1983;11:27.
79. Schildt RA, Kennedy PS, Chen TT, et al. Management of patients with metastatic adenocarcinoma of unknown origin: a Southwest Oncology Group study. *Cancer Treat Rep* 1983;67:77.
80. McMillan JH, Levine E, Stephens RH. Computed tomography in the evaluation of metastatic adenocarcinoma from an unknown primary site. *Radiology* 1982;143:143.
81. Karsell PR, Sheedy PF, O'Connell MJ. Computerized tomography in search of cancer of unknown origin. *JAMA* 1982;248:340.
82. Currow DC, Findlay M, Cox K, Harnett PR. Elevated germ cell markers in carcinoma of unknown primary site do not predict response to platinum-based chemotherapy. *Eur J Cancer* 1996;32A:2357.
83. Pavlidis N, Kalef-Ezra J, Briasoulis E, et al. Evaluation of six tumor markers in patients with carcinoma of unknown primary. *Med Ped Oncol* 1994;22:162.
84. Hochstere H, Wernz JC, Muggia FM. Intra-abdominal carcinomatosis with histologically normal ovaries. *Cancer Treat Rep (Lett)* 1984;68:931.
85. Gooneratne S, Sassone M, Blaustein A, Talerman A. Serous surface papillary carcinoma of the ovary: a clinicopathologic study of 26 cases. *Int J Gynecol Pathol* 1982;1:258.
86. Chen KT, Flam MS. Peritoneal papillary serous carcinoma with long-term survival. *Cancer* 1986;58:1371.
87. August CZ, Murad TM, Newton M. Multiple focal extraovarian serous carcinoma. *Int J Gynecol Pathol* 1985;4:11.
88. Tobacman JK, Greene MH, Tucker MA, et al. Intra-abdominal carcinomatosis after prophylactic oophorectomy in ovarian cancer-prone families. *Lancet* 1982;2:795.
89. Schorge JO, Muto MG, Welch WR, et al. Molecular evidence for multifocal papillary serous carcinoma of the peritoneum in patients with germ-line BRCA1 mutations. *J Natl Cancer Inst* 1998;90:841.
90. Lele SB, Piver MJ, Mathara J, et al. Peritoneal papillary carcinoma. *Gynecol Oncol* 1988;31:315.
91. Dalrymple JC, Bannatyne P, Russell P, et al. Extraovarian peritoneal serous papillary carcinoma: a clinicopathologic study of 31 cases. *Cancer* 1989;64:110.
92. Strnad CM, Grosh WW, Baxter J, et al. Peritoneal carcinomatosis of unknown primary site in women. *Ann Intern Med* 1989;111:213.
93. Ransom DT, Patel SR, Keeney GL, et al. Papillary serous carcinoma of the peritoneum: a review of 33 cases treated with cisplatin-based chemotherapy. *Cancer* 1990;66:1091.
94. Fromm GL, Gershenson DM, Silva EG. Papillary serous carcinoma of the peritoneum. *Obstet Gynecol* 1990;75:89.
95. Bloss JD, Liao SY, Buller RE, et al. Extraovarian peritoneal serous papillary carcinoma: a case-control retrospective comparison to papillary adenocarcinoma of the ovary. *Gynecol Oncol* 1993;50:347.
96. Piver MS, Eltabbakh GH, Hempling RE, et al. Two sequential studies for primary peritoneal carcinoma: induction with weekly cisplatin followed by either cisplatin/doxorubicin/cyclophosphamide or paclitaxel/cisplatin. *Gynecol Oncol* 1997;67:141.
97. Shah IA, Jayram L, Gani OJ, et al. Papillary serous carcinoma of the peritoneum in a man. *Cancer* 1998;82:860.
98. Bhatia SK, Saclarides TJ, Witt TR, et al. Hormone receptor studies in axillary metastases from occult breast cancer. *Cancer* 1987;59:1170.
99. Block EF, Meyer MA. Positron emission tomography in diagnosis of occult adenocarcinoma of the breast. *Am Surg* 1998;64:906.
100. Schorn C, Fischer U, Luftner-Nagel S, Westerhof JP, Grabbe E. MRI of the breast in patients with metastatic disease of unknown primary. *Eur Radiol* 1999;9:470.
101. Henry-Tillman RS, Fischer U, Luftner-Nagel S, et al. MRI of the breast in patients with metastatic disease of unknown primary. *Eur Radiol* 1999;9:470.
102. Ashikari R, Rosen PP, Urban JA, Senoo T. Breast cancer presenting as an axillary mass. *Ann Surg* 1976;183:415.
103. Patel J, Nemoto T, Rosner D, et al. Axillary lymph node metastases from an occult breast cancer. *Cancer* 1981;47:2923.
104. Merson M, Andreola S, Galimberti V, et al. Breast carcinoma presenting as axillary metastases without evidence of a primary tumor. *Cancer* 1992;70:504.
105. Rosen PP. Axillary lymph node metastases in patients with occult noninvasive breast carcinoma. *Cancer* 1980;46:1298.
106. Ellerbroek N, Holmes F, Singletary E, et al. Treatment of patients with isolated axillary nodal metastases from an occult primary carcinoma consistent with breast origin. *Cancer* 1990;66:1461.
107. Tell DT, Khoury JM, Taylor HG, et al. Atypical metastasis from prostate cancer: clinical utility of the immunoperoxidase technique for prostate-specific antigen. *JAMA* 1985; 253:3574.
108. Gentile PS, Carloss HW, Huang T-Y, et al. Disseminated prostate carcinoma simulating primary lung cancer. *Cancer* 1988;62:711.
109. Braams JW, Pruim J, Kole AC, et al. Detection of unknown primary head and neck tumor by positron emission tomograph. *Int J Oral Maxillofac Surg* 1997;26:112.
110. Califano J, Westra WH, Koch W, et al. Unknown primary head and neck squamous carcinoma: molecular indemnification of the site of origin. *J Natl Cancer Inst* 1999;91:599.
111. Jones AS, Cook JA, Phillips DE, et al. Squamous carcinoma presenting as an enlarged cervical lymph node. *Cancer* 1993;72:1756.
112. Barrie JR, Knapper WH, Strong EW. Cervical nodal metastases of unknown origin. *Am J Surg* 1970;120:466.
113. Jesse RH, Perez CA, Fletcher GH. Cervical lymph node metastasis: unknown primary cancer. *Cancer* 1973;31:854.
114. Coker DD, Casterline PF. Chambers RG, Jacques DA. Metastases to lymph nodes of the head and neck from an unknown primary site. *Am J Surg* 1977;134:517.
115. Jose B, Bosch A, Caldwell WL, Frias Z. Metastasis to neck from unknown primary tumor. *Acta Radiol Oncol* 1979;18:161.
116. Nordstrom DG, Tewfik HH, Latourette HB. Cervical lymph node metastases from an unknown primary. *Int J Radiat Oncol Biol Phys* 1979;5:73.
117. Fermont AC. Malignant cervical lymphadenopathy due to an unknown primary. *Clin Radiol* 1980;31:355.
118. Leipzig B, Winter ML, Hokanson JA. Cervical nodal metastases of unknown origin. *Laryngoscope* 1981;91:593.
119. Pacini P, Olmi P, Cellai E, Chiavacci A. Cervical lymph node metastases from an unknown primary tumour. *Acta Radiol Oncol* 1981;20:311.
120. Spiro RH, DeRose G, Strong EW. Cervical node metastasis of occult origin. *Am J Surg* 1983;146:441.
121. Mobit-Tabatabasi MA, Dasmaphapatra KS, Rush BF Jr, Ohanian M. Management of squamous cell carcinoma of unknown origin in cervical lymph nodes. *Am Surg* 1986;52:152.
122. Yang ZY, Hu YH, Yan JH, et al. Lymph node metastases in the neck from an unknown primary: report on 113 patients. *Acta Radiol Oncol* 1983;22:17.
123. Carlson LS, Fletcher GH, Oswald MJ. Guidelines for the radiotherapeutic techniques for cervical metastases from an unknown primary. *Int J Radiat Oncol Biol Phys* 1986;12:2101.
124. McCunniff AJ, Raber M. Metastatic carcinoma of the neck from an unknown primary. *Int J Radiat Oncol Biol Phys* 1986;12:1849.
125. Bataini JP, Rodriguez J, Jaulerry C, et al. Treatment of metastatic neck nodes secondary to an occult epidermoid carcinoma of the head and neck. *Laryngoscope* 1987;97:1080.
126. De Braud F, Heilbrun LK, Ahmed K, et al. Metastatic squamous cell carcinoma of an unknown primary localized to the neck: advantages of an aggressive treatment. *Cancer* 1989;64:510.
127. Marcial-Vega VA, Cardenes H, Perez CA, et al: Cervical metastasis from unknown primaries: radiotherapeutic management and appearance of subsequent primaries. *Int J Rad Oncol Biol Phys* 1990;19:919.
128. LeFebvre JL, Coche-Dequeant D, Van JT, et al. Cervical lymph nodes from unknown primary tumor in 190 patients. *Am J Surg* 1990;160:443.
129. Weir L, Keane T, Cummings B, et al. Radiation treatment of cervical lymph node metastasis from an unknown primary: an analysis of outcome by treatment volume and other prognostic factors. *Radiother Oncol* 1995;35:206.

130. Brizel DM, Albers ME, Fisher SR, et al. Hyperfractionated irradiation with or without concurrent chemotherapy for locally advanced head and neck cancer. *N Engl J Med* 1998;338:1798.

131. Wendt TG, Grabenbauer GG, Rodel CM, et al. Simultaneous radiochemotherapy versus radiotherapy alone in advanced head and neck cancer: a randomized multicenter study. *J Clin Oncol* 1998;16:1318.

132. Coletier PJ, Garden AS, Morrison WH, et al. Postoperative radiation for squamous cell carcinoma metastatic to cervical lymph nodes from an unknown primary site: outcomes and patterns of failure. *Head Neck* 1998;20:674.

133. Fernandez JA, Suarez C, Martinez JA, et al. Metastatic squamous cell carcinoma in cervical lymph nodes from an unknown primary tumor: prognostic factors. *Clin Otolaryncol* 1998;23:158.

134. Medini E, Medini AM, Lee CK, Gapany M, Levitt SR. The management of metastatic squamous cell carcinoma in cervical lymph nodes from an unknown primary. *Am J Clin Oncol* 1998;21:121.

135. Sporn JR, Greenberg BR. Empirical chemotherapy for adenocarcinoma of unknown primary tumor site. *Semin Oncol* 1993;20:261.

136. Greco FA, Hainsworth JD. Cancer of unknown primary site. In: Devita VT, Hellman S, Rosenberg SA, eds. *Cancer principles and practice of oncology*, 6th ed. Philadelphia: Lippincott Williams & Wilkins, 2001:2537.

137. Wagener DJT, de Muelder PHM, Burghouts JT, et al. Phase II trial of cisplatin for adenocarcinoma of unknown primary site. *Eur J Cancer*, 1991;27:755.

138. Casciato DA. Metastasis of unknown origin. In: Haskell E, ed. *Cancer treatment*, 4th ed. Philadelphia: W. B. Saunders Company, 1995:1128.

139. Milliken ST, Tattersall MHN, Woods RL, et al. Metastatic adenocarcinoma of unknown primary site: a randomized study of two combination chemotherapy regimens. *Eur J Cancer Clin Oncol* 1987;23:1645.

140. McKeen E, Smith F, Haidak D, et al. Fluorouracil, adriamycin and mitomycin-C for adenocarcinoma of unknown origin. *Proc Am Assoc Cancer Res* 1980;21:358(abst).

141. Woods RL, Fox RM, Tattersall MHN, et al. Metastatic adenocarcinoma of unknown primary: a randomized study of two combination-chemotherapy regimens. *N Engl J Med* 1980;303:87.

142. Eagan RT, Thermean TM, Rubin J, et al. Lack of value for cisplatin added to mitomycin-doxorubicin combination chemotherapy for carcinoma of unknown primary site. *Am Clin Oncol* 1987;10:82.

143. Goldberg RM, Smith FP, Ueno W, et al. Fluorouracil, adriamycin and mitomycin in the treatment of adenocarcinoma of unknown primary. *J Clin Oncol* 1986;4:395.

144. Kambhu I, Kelsen D, Niedzwiecki D, et al. Phase II trial of mitomycin-C, vindesine, and adriamycin and predictive variables in the treatment of patients with adenocarcinoma of unknown primary site. *Proc Am Assoc Cancer Res* 1986;27:734(abst).

145. Flore JJ, Kelsen DP, Gralla RJ, et al. Adenocarcinoma of unknown primary origin. Treatment with vindesine and doxorubicin. *Cancer Treat Rep* 1985;69:591.

146. Valentine J, Rosenthal S, Arseneau JC. Combination chemotherapy for adenocarcinoma of unknown primary origin. *Cancer Clin Trial* 1979;2:265.

147. Rudnick S, Tremont S, Staab E, et al. Evaluation and therapy of adenocarcinoma of unknown primary. *Proc Am Soc Clin Oncol* 1981;1:379(Abst).

148. Sulkes A, Uziely B, Isacson R, et al. Combination chemotherapy in metastatic tumors of unknown origin. *Ist J Med Sci* 1988;24:604.

149. van der Gaast A, Verweij J, Planting AST, et al. 5-Fluorouracil, doxorubicin, and mitomycin C (FAM) combination chemotherapy for metastatic adenocarcinoma of unknown primary. *Eur J Cancer Clin Oncol* 1988;24:765.

150. Treat J, Falchuk SC, Tremblay C, et al. Phase II trial of methotrexate-FAM in adenocarcinoma of unknown primary. *Eur J Cancer Clin Oncol* 1989;25:1053.

151. Nole F, Colleoni M, Buzzoni R, et al. Fluorouracil plus folinic acid in metastatic adenocarcinoma of unknown primary site suggestive of a gastrointestinal primary. *Tumori* 1993;79:116.

152. Hainsworth JD, Erland JB, Kalman CA, et al. Carcinoma of unknown primary site: treatment with one-hour paclitaxel, carboplatin and extended schedule etoposide. *J Clin Oncol* 1997;15:2385.

153. Greco FA, Gray J, Burris HA, et al. Taxane-based chemotherapy with carcinoma of unknown primary site. *Cancer J* 2001;7:203.

154. Greco FA, Erland JB, Morrissey LH, et al. Phase II trials with docetaxel plus cisplatin or carboplatin. *Ann Oncol* 2000;11:211.

155. Greco FA, Burris HA, Litchy S, et al. Gemcitabine, carboplatin, and paclitaxel for patients with unknown primary site: a Minnie Pearl Cancer Research Network study. *J Clin Oncol* 2002;20:1651.

156. Greco FA, Hainsworth JD, Yardley DA, et al. Sequential paclitaxel/carboplatin/etoposide followed by irinotecan/gemcitabine for patients with carcinoma of unknown primary site: a Minnie Pearl Cancer Research Network phase II trial. *Proc Am Soc Clin Oncol* 2002;21:161a.

157. Briasoulis E, Kalofonos H, Bafaloukos D, et al. Carboplatin plus paclitaxel in unknown primary carcinoma: a phase II Hellenic Cooperative Oncology Group study. *J Clin Oncol* 2000;18:3101.

158. Lastra E, Munoz A, Rubio I, et al. Paclitaxel, carboplatin, and oral etoposide in the treatment of patients with carcinoma of unknown primary site. *Proc Am Soc Clin Oncol* 2000;19:579a.

159. Mukai H, Watanabe T, Ando M, et al. A safety and efficacy trial of docetaxel and cisplatin in patients with cancer of unknown primary. *Proc Am Soc Clin Oncol* 2003;22:646.

160. Culine S, Lortholary A, Voigt JJ, et al. Cisplatin in combination with either gemcitabine or irinotecan in carcinomas of unknown primary site: results of a randomized phase II study trial for the French Study Group on Carcinomas of Unknown Primary. *J Clin Oncol* 2003;21:3479.

161. Altman E, Cadman E. An analysis of 1,539 patients with cancer of unknown primary site. *Cancer* 1986;57:120.

162. Hess KR, Abbruzzese MC, Lenzi R, et al. Classification and regression free analysis of 1000 consecutive patients with unknown primary carcinoma. *Clin Cancer Res* 1999;5:3403.

163. Holmes FT, Fouts TL. Metastatic cancer of unknown primary site. *Cancer* 1970;26:816.

164. Krementz ET, Cerise EJ, Foster DC, et al. Metastases of undetermined source. *Curr Probl Cancer* 1979;4:1.

165. Markman M. Metastatic adenocarcinoma of unknown primary site: analysis of 245 patients seen at the Johns Hopkins Hospital from 1965–1979. *Med Ped Oncol* 1982;10:569.

166. Moertel CG, Reitmeier RJ, Schutt AJ, et al. Treatment of the patient with adenocarcinoma of unknown primary site. *Cancer* 1972;30:1469.

167. Van de Wouw AJ, Janssen-Heijnen MLC, Coebergh JWW, et al. Epidemiology of unknown primary tumors; incidence and population-based survival of 1285 patients in Southeast Netherlands 1984–1992. *Eur J Cancer* 2002;38:409.

168. Levi F, Te VC, Erler G, et al. Epidemiology of unknown primary tumors. *Eur J Cancer* 2002;38:1810.

169. Wood LA, Venner PM, Pabst HF. Monozygotic twin brothers with primary immunodeficiency presenting with metastatic adenocarcinoma of unknown primary. *Acta Oncologica* 1998;37:771.

170. Korbling M, Katz RL, Khanna A, et al. Hepatocytes and epithelial cells of donor origin in recipients of peripheral blood stem cells. *N Engl J Med* 2002;346:738.

171. McCulloch EA. Stem cells and diversity. *Leukemia* 2003;17:1042.

172. Abbruzzese JL, Lenzi R, Raber MN, et al. The biology of unknown primary tumors. *Semin Oncol* 1993;20:238.

173. Ramaswamy S, Ross KN, Lander ES, Golab TR. A molecular signature of metastasis in primary solid tumors. *Nat Genet* 2003;33:49.

174. Bar-Eli M, Abbruzzese JL, Lee-Jackson D, et al. P53 gene mutation spectrum in human unknown primary tumors. *Anticancer Res* 1993;13:1619.

175. Briasoulis E, Tsakos M, Fountzilas G, et al. Bc12 and p53 protein expression in metastatic carcinoma of unknown primary origin; biological and clinical implications. A Hellenic Cooperative Oncology Group study. *Anticancer Res* 1998;18:1907.

176. Pavlidis N, Briasoulis E, Baj M, et al. Overexpression of C-myc, Ras and C-erb-2 oncoproteins in carcinoma of unknown primary origin. *Anticancer Res* 1995;15:2563.

177. Hainsworth JD, Lennington WJ, Greco FA. Overexpression of Her-2 in patients with poorly differentiated carcinoma or poorly differentiated adenocarcinoma of unknown primary site. *J Clin Oncol* 2000;18:632.

178. Karavasilis V, Tsanou E, Malamon-Mitsi V, et al. Microvessel density and vascular endothelial growth factor in cancer of unknown primary. An immunohistochemical study. *Proc ESMO* 2002;51.

179. Hillen HF, Hak LE, Joosten-Achjanie SR, et al. Microvessel density in unknown primary tumors. *Int J Cancer* 1997;74:81.

180. Bonnefoi H, Smith IE. How should cancer presenting as a malignant pleural effusion be managed? *Br J Cancer* 1996;74:832.

181. Kuttesch JF, Parham DM, Kaste SC, et al. Embryonal malignancies of unknown primary origin in children. *Cancer* 1995;75:115.

James F. Pingpank, Jr.

CHAPTER **47**

Peritoneal Carcinomatosis

Peritoneal carcinomatosis is the dissemination and implantation of tumor cells throughout the peritoneal cavity and often results in significant morbidity without systemic metastases. Tumors may originate from a local or distant site. Frequently, a diagnosis is not established until after the vague signs and symptoms of early disease have given way to debilitating effects of extensive local and regional disease. The traditional assumption that such advanced tumor burden represents an incurable and untreatable condition is no longer valid. Mounting evidence suggests that aggressive management of local disease through novel regional combination therapies can have significant impact on the quality of a patient's life through symptom control, while also effectively mitigating tumor progression. Although it is possible to draw parallels across all types of peritoneal carcinomatosis, the primary tumor histologic type dictates the clinical management of the regional disease as well as the pattern of potential disease recurrence after therapy. Unlike in the majority of other advanced malignancies, attempts at symptom palliation and disease control often significantly overlap, such as in the control of ascites or the relief of a bowel obstruction. For these reasons, there is benefit to be realized from treating peritoneal carcinomatosis as a distinct regional disease entity. This chapter provides an overview of the biologic basis of this regional pattern of tumor spread. Included is a discussion of concepts regarding the classification and diagnostic evaluation of peritoneal tumors, followed by a review of the local, regional, and systemic treatment approaches to this protean group of diseases.

PATHOPHYSIOLOGY

The peritoneal cavity is a potential space with a lining of mesothelial cells overlying an extensive vascular and lymphatic capillary network. The underlying basement membrane serves as a barrier to the easy efflux of molecular and cellular material. The cavity is filled with a small volume of fluid, with a characteristic pattern of production, circulation, and absorption.[1] Several pathologic states, including the presence of infection or malignancy, may lead to increased fluid absorption or decreased resorption or both.[2] Fluid is filtered into and out of the peritoneal cavity through the peritoneum, with the net flow of fluid based on intraperitoneal hydrostatic pressure. Fluid absorption is thought to occur throughout the peritoneum, with 80% returned via the portal circulation. Proteins and cellular material cannot penetrate the peritoneal basement membrane and are absorbed through lymphatic channels and pores located primarily on the undersurface of the diaphragm and throughout the omentum. The presence of peritoneal carcinomatosis results in the blockage of these channels with tumor cells, which prohibits the efflux of protein and peritoneal fluid.[3] Watters and Buck demonstrated the presence of mesothelial cell–lined channels extending directly from the peritoneal cavity into adjacent lymphatics concentrated in the diaphragm.[4] Intraperitoneal iodine 125–labeled albumin has been used to verify the role of these channels in the absorption of macromolecules along the diaphragmatic and nonvisceral peritoneum.[5] The flow of fluid and cellular material throughout the abdomen is governed by gravity along with diaphragmatic and intestinal movement. The patterns of peritoneal fluid flow determine the flow of particulate material throughout the peritoneal cavity and give clues to the patterns of tumor dissemination in patients with peritoneal carcinomatosis. The most common sites of disease are in the right lower quadrant (local spread of primary appendiceal tumors), the right diaphragm and hepatoduodenal ligament, the omentum, and the pelvic visceral and nonvisceral peritoneum.[6]

Hagiwara and colleagues detailed the presence of immunologic filters called *milky spots* concentrated in the omentum, hepatoduodenal ligament, base of the mesentery, pouch of Douglas, and the appendiceal epiploicae. These appear to function as lymphatic and immunologic filters, similar to nodal tissue in solid organs, and have been proposed to serve as a trapping area for clumps of tumor cells.[7] The location of milky spots and lymphatic channels, the constant movement of abdominal viscera, the ebb and flow of ascites, and gravity all contribute to the pattern of tumor dissemination.

Peritoneal carcinomatosis may arise from primary tumors of the peritoneal lining (mesothelioma, primary peritoneal carcinoma), extension from intraabdominal viscera with low risk (mucinous adenocarcinoma of the appendix, ovarian cancer) or high risk (adenocarcinoma of the colon, stomach, or pancreas) of concurrent systemic metastases, or spread from extraabdominal malignancies (melanoma, breast cancer). Each of these subtypes exhibits distinct patterns of disease spread and is addressed individually.

Intraperitoneal viscera, including the ovary and appendix, are the most common source of tumors presenting with isolated peritoneal carcinomatosis. Primary gastrointestinal malignancies access the peritoneal cavity via two distinct mechanisms, correlating with the phenotype of the primary tumor. High-grade, poorly differentiated tumors spread through primary organ invasion with subsequent cell shedding and distant organ attachment, often with concurrent lymphatic or hematologic metastases. Low-grade, well-differentiated tumors disseminate via a pressure-burst phenomenon, common to slow-growing tumors such as mucinous tumors of the appendix and ovary, in which the slow tumor growth permits the sheer volume of tumor cells to rupture through viscera and contaminate the peritoneum with tumor cells.[8] Traditionally, this is a pattern seen in tumors of low or absent malignant potential. Other less common sources of peritoneal carcinomatosis include hematogenous spread from distant sites, including melanoma and breast cancer, or iatrogenic seeding from tumor manipulation during biopsy or surgical procedures, seen with hepatocellular carcinoma and adenocarcinoma of the gallbladder, respectively.

The mere presence of free-floating tumor cells within the peritoneal cavity does not universally correlate with peritoneal carcinomatosis. Attachment, implantation, and proliferation are all necessary steps in the establishment and growth of intraperitoneal disease.[9] Characteristics favoring the establishment of lymphatic or hematogenous metastases, or both, do not always favor intraperitoneal tumor seeding. Up-regulation of adhesion molecules correlates with a "sticky" tumor phenotype, and low immunogenicity of these tumor cells may allow escape from immune surveillance. For established tumors to grow once successful implantation has occurred, induction of new vessel growth must be possible, or tumors must be capable of obtaining nutrients from ascitic fluid. Traditionally, these characteristics are present in slow-growing, low-grade tumors.

DIAGNOSTIC EVALUATION

In the absence of signs or symptoms of disease, the majority of patients with peritoneal carcinomatosis are diagnosed at laparotomy for a known primary gastrointestinal malignancy. Those with more advanced tumor burdens often present with massive ascites and signs of partial bowel obstruction and generalized inanition. Although regular follow-up and serial imaging is the rule in patients with resected gastrointestinal malignancies, early diagnosis of small-volume peritoneal carcinomatosis is rarely possible. The difficulties in obtaining accurate staging information frustrate attempts at disease staging and frequently lead to unnecessary surgical interventions. Generally, peritoneal disease identified at the time of laparotomy for high-grade bowel obstruction or hepatic metastases is beyond the scope of effective regional therapy.

The preoperative staging of peritoneal disease is limited by the insensitivity of traditional imaging modalities such as computed tomography (CT), ultrasonography, and magnetic resonance imaging (MRI). For both CT and ultrasonography, detection of peritoneal implants 1 cm or less approximates 25%.[10] These studies are most sensitive for the detection of omental metastases or indirect evidence of tumor such as the presence of ascites or extracellular mucin, mesenteric thickening, or matting of loops of bowel. Several authors have examined the usefulness of MRI in this setting with mixed results. Low and colleagues reported that MRI was superior to helical CT in the assessment of bowel and mesenteric thickening,[11] whereas Balestreri et al. demonstrated sensitivity and specificity of 84% and 100%, respectively, for the detection of peritoneal recurrence in ovarian carcinoma.[12] The author does not routinely use MRI in the assessment of these patients, because CT is easier to obtain, preferred by patients, and does not sacrifice image quality.

The use of metabolic imaging such has positron emission tomography (PET) for assessing metastatic disease has gained favor in recent years. Overall, PET has not shown efficacy in the evaluation of lesions smaller than 1 cm in diameter. Fong et al. reported that extrahepatic peritoneal nodules smaller than 1 cm were not detected when fluorine F 18 fluorodeoxyglucose PET was used in the preoperative evaluation of patients undergoing resection of hepatic metastases from colorectal cancer.[13] A more recent report describes detection of peritoneal disease in 14 of 24 patients with peritoneal metastases, including 4 patients without CT detection of tumor implants.[14]

Peritoneal cytologic analysis has been used to identify or exclude a malignancy in patients with new-onset ascites, with or without a history of cancer, as well as to investigate patients with apparently resectable tumors for the presence of free-floating intraperitoneal malignant cells. Cytologic analysis of several primary gastrointestinal malignancies, including those of the colon, pancreas, stomach, and appendix, has been performed in an attempt to identify patients with increased risk for developing local versus systemic recurrence.[15,16] The presence of tumor cells in peritoneal washings obtained at the time of surgical resection correlates with increased local recurrence and decreased survival, even in the absence of nodal or systemic metastases. The existence of this subset of tumors in which local, intraperitoneal recurrence has the potential to affect overall survival has fueled interest in exploring local therapies as potential adjuvants to surgical resection.

HISTOLOGIC SUBTYPES

PSEUDOMYXOMA PERITONEI

Much confusion surrounds the diagnosis of *pseudomyxoma peritonei*. Werth first used the term to describe the pathologic findings in a patient with a ruptured ovarian cystadenoma and copious gelatinous intraperitoneal material.[17] Subsequently, the term has been used to include the presence of extracellular mucin arising from the benign and malignant tumors of the appendix and large bowel as well as primary peritoneal tumors, which has led to confusion among both patients and clinicians regarding the clinical and prognostic significance of this pathologic finding. Simply put, although the intraperitoneal mucin is frequently the source of symptoms at presentation, disease classification is based on the origin and pathologic characteristics of the primary tumor. Pseudomyxoma peritonei should never be used as a diagnosis, but rather to describe the clinical picture associated with the release of extracellular mucin into the peritoneal cavity with or without the presence of malignant cells. Once mucin has gained access to the peritoneal cavity, attachment to other viscera is common and is associated with abdominal distention but relatively few, if any, symptoms. The most important prognostic factor associated with pseudomyxoma peritonei is the presence (or absence) of malignancy. The diagnosis of malignancy may not be excluded until thorough pathologic examination of the primary tumor has been completed. A continuum of appendiceal tumors producing mucinous ascites extends from benign adenomas of the appendix to low-grade, mucinous adenocarcinomas to, less commonly, poorly differentiated adenocarcinomas. Ronnet et al. have divided these tumors into three groups based on pathologic and prognostic information.[18] Disseminated peritoneal adenomucinosis (DPAM) includes peritoneal tumors with scant cellularity in the presence of abundant extracellular mucin. Endothelial cells present are histologically bland with low-grade adenomatous features, minimal cytologic atypia, and low mitotic activity. Lesions comprising peritoneal mucinous carcinomatosis display abundant glandular formation, hyperchromatic nuclei, and overall cytologic atypia consistent with low-grade malignancies. Tumors classified as peritoneal mucinous carcinomatosis with intermediate or discordant features represent an intermediate group of tumors having features consistent with DPAM but with focal areas of well-differentiated mucinous adenocarcinoma. Significantly improved disease-free and overall survival is associated with the absence of malignant cells in DPAM.[19] Grossly, the diagnosis of malignancy includes the presence of lymph node metastases, or an invasive phenotype, or both, noted at laparotomy. Histologic evaluation should include examination of the primary tumor, peritoneal implants, and extracellular mucin and demonstrates moderate to abundant cellularity, pleomorphic nuclear changes with or without cellular atypia, or the presence of invasion in malignant tumors. The determination of the location of the primary tumor may be difficult in cases of extensive tumor spread throughout the peritoneal cavity. This is especially true in women, in whom ovarian involvement is frequent at early stages of tumor dissemination.

Benign tumors of the appendix may present with copious amounts of extracellular mucin with minimal cellularity and without evidence of invasion or cellular atypia. Benign tumors grow slowly, occlude the appendiceal lumen, and eventually rupture via a pressure-burst phenomenon, which leads to the release of nonmalignant cells throughout the peritoneum along with ever-increasing amounts of extracellular mucin. These cells may become adherent to structures throughout the peritoneal cavity, including the omentum and ovaries, but lack the ability to initiate

lymphatic or hematogenous metastases or tissue invasion. For both men and women, the appendix is almost universally the source of diffuse intraperitoneal tumor spread of benign histologic type in the presence of extensive mucin. Benign or borderline tumors, or tumors of low malignant potential of ovarian origin are common but rarely produce the pseudomyxoma peritonei seen with their malignant counterparts. The series of Ronnet et al.[8] is one of the few series to look at these tumors separately from those with malignant characteristics. Sixty-five patients with DPAM were treated with maximal tumor debulking and cytoreduction followed by intraperitoneal mitomycin C and 5-fluorouracil (5-FU) in the immediately postoperative period. All patients were also treated with an additional three courses of adjuvant systemic therapy using the same two drugs. Median survival had not been achieved in over 6 years (median) of follow-up. These findings are supported by a report from van Ruth and colleagues, in a review of data for 62 patients presenting with pseudomyxoma peritonei, all of whom were treated with aggressive operative cytoreduction followed by direct application of hyperthermic intraperitoneal mitomycin C.[20] Additional systemic chemotherapy was reserved for patients with pathologic evidence of malignancy using the Ronnet criteria. With such prolonged survivals, aggressive surgical management of symptomatic lesions is warranted, which often necessitates multiple laparotomies over many years. Operative principles include organ preservation, especially regarding gastrointestinal tract length, in light of the potential for multiple surgical interventions over a patient's lifetime. In this group of patients, morbidity and mortality are frequently due to the nutritional and physiologic effects of multiple surgical interventions over a prolonged period. At present, there is no clear role for intraperitoneal or systemic chemotherapy over isolated surgical cytoreduction in this patient population.

MUCINOUS ADENOCARCINOMA OF THE APPENDIX AND COLON

Adenocarcinoma of the appendix presents in two distinct forms, malignant mucinous adenocarcinoma, often with associated pseudomyxoma peritonei, and adenocarcinoma of the appendix with histologic characteristics similar to those of primary tumors of the colon and rectum. The pathologic criteria separating low-grade, mucinous adenocarcinoma (also mucinous cystadenocarcinoma) from the more aggressive histologic type are vague and vary among institutions. In general, these low-grade tumors display patterns of intraperitoneal spread similar to those of benign adenomucinosis, but with histologic examination of the primary tumor and mucinous implants demonstrates malignant characteristics. Several series detailing institutional experiences with all patients presenting with pseudomyxoma peritonei report that approximately half of patients display frankly malignant tumors.[20–23] Although the vast majority of low-grade mucin-producing tumors are appendiceal in origin, a small percentage of such tumors originate in the large bowel.[24] Histologic characteristics of these tumors include moderate to extensive cellularity within the peritoneal implants, with cytologic atypia and increased mitotic activity present in cells of the primary tumor and surface implants. The significance of lymph node metastases or intraperitoneal organ invasion is controversial. When present, these pathologic criteria are associated with a poorer prognosis and are considered to be representative of high-grade tumors by several investigators. The largest series of patients with mucinous adeno-

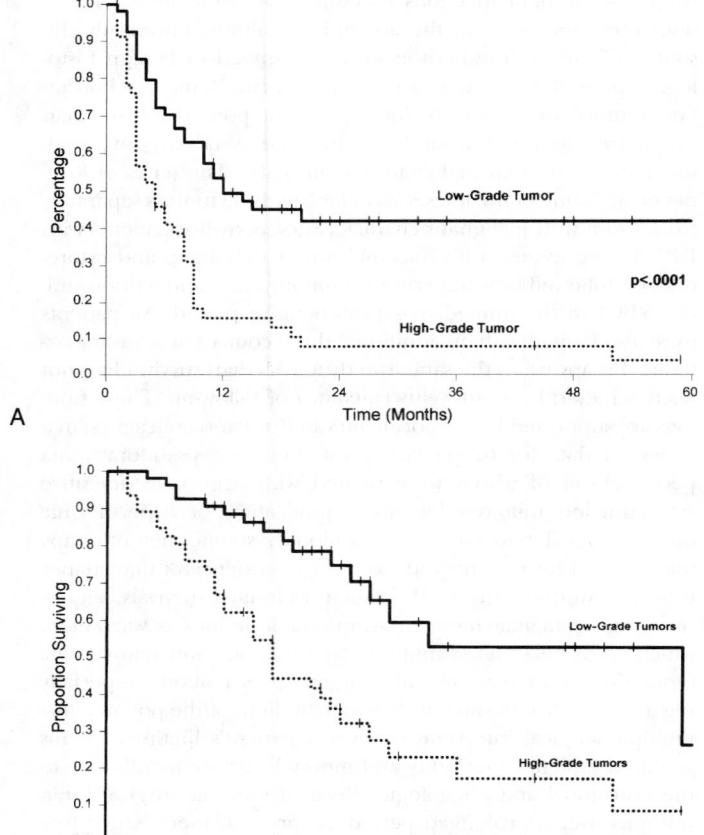

A

B

FIGURE 47-1. Impact of tumor grade on progression-free (**A**) and overall survival (**B**). Patients with low-grade, well-differentiated tumors of gastrointestinal origin exhibited statistically significant improvements in disease-free and overall survival compared to patients with poorly differentiated tumors who underwent the same degree of surgical debulking and intraperitoneal hyperthermic chemotherapy.

carcinoma of the appendix was reported by Sugarbaker and Chang and describes 385 patients.[22] On multivariate analysis, the histopathologic characteristics of the tumor and the completeness of cytoreduction influenced outcome. Several reports have verified these findings, including two supporting the use of these pathologic criteria to define separate prognostic groups. In a series of 94 consecutively treated patients with all classes of adenocarcinoma of the appendix, Sarr and coworkers at the Mayo Clinic reported the presence of high-grade, "colonic-type" tumors in 45% of patients.[25] This finding was associated with higher-grade tumors and higher stage and, ultimately, poorer prognosis to mucinous tumors. The series of the author and colleagues at the Surgery Branch of the National Cancer Institute revealed similar results (Fig. 47-1), and this group now classifies higher-grade, non–mucin-producing tumors of the appendix with other colonic neoplasms, not with low-grade mucinous tumors.[26]

PRIMARY GASTROINTESTINAL MALIGNANCIES

Peritoneal carcinomatosis, alone or in combination with systemic metastases, is a frequent mode of spread from primary adenocarcinoma of the pancreas, stomach, gallbladder, and large and small bowel. In patients with transmural invasion of primary tumors, the entire peritoneal cavity is at risk for seeding with metastatic disease. The presence of peritoneal disease is a sign of the aggressive nature of these tumors and is frequently associated with unresectable primary tumors or the presence of systemic metastases. Great variability exists in the range of biologic behavior and aggressiveness of these tumors, with prognosis dependent on the source of the primary tumor. In the author's and colleagues' series of 101 patients with primary gastrointestinal adenocarcinoma presenting with peritoneal metastases, 47 primary tumors were classified high grade. In patients in whom complete resection of all peritoneal carcinomatosis was attained, the disease-free and overall survivals (24 vs. 12 months; $P = .0025$) were significantly improved over those of patients in whom complete resection was not possible. In this series, all patients received intraoperative hyperthermic chemotherapy (cisplatin, 250 mg/m^2) during a 90-minute perfusion after tumor resection was completed.[6] Culliford et al. reported on 64 patients with peritoneal carcinomatosis from primary colonic adenocarcinoma treated with cytoreduction followed by intraperitoneal 5-FU and leucovorin. The majority of patients presented with synchronous metastases. Median survival was 34 months, and the ability to resect all disease was associated with increased survival on multivariate analysis.[27] The positive impact of complete resection on survival has been supported in other series for appendiceal,[28] colorectal,[29] and gastric cancer,[30] but when complete resection of the primary tumor along with all peritoneal metastases is not possible, surgical intervention merely delays the inevitable need for intravenous therapy. Operative intervention should be reserved for clinical trials or circumstances of very limited disease in which complete resection is possible or to provide palliation to patients with bowel obstruction or gastrointestinal bleeding. The role of regional chemotherapy after complete cytoreduction in this group of patients remains undefined.

The poor prognosis associated with the progression to peritoneal carcinomatosis has led to attempts at adjuvant treatment of tumors at high risk for the development of peritoneal spread but without visible carcinomatosis. Due to the low likelihood of successful complete surgical resection of peritoneal carcinomatosis from high-grade tumors and the poor intraperitoneal penetration of intravenous chemotherapy, the greatest potential benefit for regional therapy lies in the adjuvant treatment of patients with completely resected primary tumors with a high likelihood of local or regional recurrence. Studies performing cytologic examination of ascites or peritoneal washings or determining the presence of transmural invasion after potentially curative resection of pancreatic, gastric, or colonic malignancies have demonstrated an increase in local or intraperitoneal recurrence rate associated with the presence of malignant cells.[30–33] Data regarding adjuvant intraperitoneal therapy for high-risk tumors have been mixed. Yu et al. randomized 248 patients with stage II or III gastric cancer to surgical resection alone or to resection plus postoperative intraperitoneal mitomycin C and 5-FU, but an increase in survival with adjuvant therapy was seen only in the subset of patients with stage III cancer.[34] Other series involving similar patients using intraperitoneal cisplatin or mitomycin C did not show statistically significant improvements in local control or survival, except in patients with serosal invasion by tumors.[35,36]

PRIMARY PERITONEAL MESOTHELIOMA

Primary peritoneal mesothelioma arises from the mesothelial cells lining the peritoneal cavity. Like pleural mesothelioma, peritoneal mesothelioma is a rare malignancy (2 cases per million) of increasing incidence. Traditional pathologic classification has divided peritoneal mesothelioma into three separate groups based on microscopic appearance and prognosis. Kass described benign, borderline, and malignant subsets of tumors.[37] Benign tumors include adenomatoid and localized fibrous mesothelioma, are the least common of the three subtypes, and tend to be the most localized. The intermediate, or borderline, group includes multicystic and well-differentiated papillary peritoneal mesotheliomas. For tumors in either of these two groups, the natural history of disease is characterized by tumor recurrences necessitating repeated surgical resection for control of the tumor. Associated intraabdominal complications such as ascites and obstruction are infrequent and, when present, may indicate the presence of malignant histology. In a retrospective series of 22 patients with well-differentiated papillary mesothelioma, surgical resection was performed with or without additional therapy.[38] Long-term follow-up was available for the majority of patients, and no patient death was attributable to recurrent or progressive disease. Complications associated with adjuvant radiation therapy or chemotherapy appeared to have a greater impact on morbidity and mortality than that of disease progression. Careful pathologic evaluation is required to confirm the presence of a well-developed papillary pattern of mesothelioma cells with bland appearance and cuboidal epithelium, which is characteristic of well-differentiated papillary mesothelioma, and to exclude the presence of isolated foci of more aggressive histology, consistent with diffuse malignant mesothelioma.

Three histologic subtypes of malignant peritoneal mesothelioma have been described—epithelial, sarcomatoid, and mixed (elements of both epithelial and sarcomatoid)[39]—all of which are associated with exposure to asbestos. Reported associations between asbestos exposure and malignant mesothelioma range from 50% to 83%, but the link appears to be less than that seen with pleural mesothelioma.[40] Other potentially causative agents include abdominal radiation and simian virus 40 exposure. The epithelial type is the most common and carries the best prognosis, although significant variability in extent of disease at presentation is common. Great variability in disease stage exists within the subtype of epithelial mesothelioma, with some patients presenting with small-volume, superficial disease, and others with a more invasive form of epithelial mesothelioma. The volume of ascites is not associated with overall tumor volume or invasiveness. The sarcomatoid and mixed tumors are more rapidly growing tumors associated with an invasive phenotype and often present with large numbers of tumor implants along the majority of visceral and nonvisceral peritoneal surfaces with an accompanying desmoplastic reaction. Complete resection of these tumors is often not possible. With all three types of malignant mesothelioma, progression of disease is predominantly within the peritoneal cavity, occasionally with local mesenteric lymphatic spread, but with infrequent distant metastases. Local extension through the diaphragm is seen in a minority of patients. The most frequent cause of death is the overall debilitation associated with the metabolic effects of the tumor volume, decreased nutritional intake, and the protein loss and dehydration associated with the massive ascites and frequent paracentesis.

The natural history of peritoneal mesothelioma is poorly characterized because of the rarity of the disease and the lack of a uniform clinical and pathologic staging system. Presenting symptoms are often vague and longstanding, with late presentation being associated with massive ascites, diffuse omental replacement with tumor, and thick carpeting of tumor along diaphragmatic and mesenteric surfaces.[41] Symptoms are related to the volume of ascites and the impact of mesenteric or serosal tumor implants on bowel function. In rare, very advanced tumors, massive tumor volume leads to diffuse compression of abdominal viscera with early satiety and overall inanition. Malnutrition is a frequent complicating factor, secondary to poor intake from early satiety, the catabolic effects of the large tumor volume, and protein loss caused by frequent paracentesis for control of ascites. Median survival in untreated patients is less than 1 year. The presence of malnutrition significantly impairs any patient's ability to tolerate therapeutic interventions. This is especially pronounced with regard to intravenous chemotherapy, in which the therapeutic impact is slow and continued paracentesis is needed.

Diagnosis of malignant mesothelioma may be established with minimal cellular material. In patients presenting with progressive ascites, CT frequently demonstrates a greatly thickened omentum secondary to complete replacement with tumor. In the author's experience, diagnosis can be universally established via paracentesis or percutaneous fine-needle aspiration or core biopsy in patients presenting with such advanced disease, with laparotomy reserved for therapeutic measures. In a smaller subset of patients, diagnosis is established at laparotomy or laparoscopy for other conditions, such as appendicitis or cholecystitis, or as part of an infertility workup. This group tends to have significantly less disease at presentation than do symptomatic individuals.

Treatment of malignant mesothelioma has evolved over the past two decades, with growing enthusiasm for combination therapies, often involving aggressive surgical debulking in combination with a chemotherapeutic regimen. Early series established the futility of simple surgical debulking, because complete removal of all gross tumor is rarely possible. Median survival was less than 1 year.[42] Multiple regimens of single-agent or combination systemic chemotherapy have been examined, including those using gemcitabine, doxorubicin (Adriamycin), pemetrexed, and platinum compounds. Most series included both peritoneal and pleural mesothelioma. Results have been disappointing, with overall response rates of less than 30% and of limited duration.[43] In an attempt to overcome the problem of drug delivery to intraperitoneal tumors, direct intraperitoneal administration was performed with encouraging results. Markman and Kelsen reported median survival of 9 months in 19 patients treated with intraperitoneal cisplatin and mitomycin C.[44] Although the observed median survival did not differ greatly from that of historic controls, 47% of patients experienced palliation of ascites and four patients (21%) survived longer than 3 years. Langer and colleagues at the Fox Chase Cancer Center reported a median survival of 22 months with the combination of intraperitoneal cisplatin and etoposide after aggressive surgical debulking.[45] Trimodality therapy using surgical resection followed by combination chemotherapy and whole abdomen irradiation was reported by Lederman et al.[46] Six of ten treated patients remained disease-free 6 years after therapy, but this approach has not been widely accepted due to significant gastrointestinal toxicity. All of these trials were plagued by small numbers of patients and the absence of control groups but gave credibility to the strategy of combination surgical resection and regional chemotherapy.

Several groups have reported encouraging results in larger series incorporating surgical resection with a 90-minute continuous hyperthermic peritoneal perfusion with chemotherapy. Loggie et al. reported on a series of 12 patients treated with operative debulking and hyperthermic intraperitoneal mitomycin C, with permanent control of ascites in 86% of patients and median survival of 34 months at publication.[47] Additional series from the national cancer institutes of Italy[48] and the United States[49] describe similar long-term control of ascites along with 3-year overall survival of 66% and 59%, respectively, using platinum-based hyperthermic perfusions. In the 49 patients treated in the series reported by Feldman et al., the presence of previous debulking surgery, absence of deep tissue invasion, and minimal residual disease after resection were associated with improved progression-free and overall survival (Fig. 47-2).[49] The role of additional postoperative systemic chemotherapy in patients with residual disease has yet to be adequately addressed.

PRIMARY PERITONEAL MALIGNANCIES

A small group of infrequently occurring tumors of unclear origin arising in the peritoneal cavity have been termed *primary peritoneal carcinoma*.[50,51] Patients are almost exclusively women, although isolated reports have described the presence of such tumors in male patients.[52] Presenting symptoms are nonspecific, including abdominal distention and early satiety secondary to massive ascites. These tumors diffusely involve the peritoneal surface and have a histologic appearance similar to that of ovarian carcinoma and must be differentiated from mesothelioma by immunohistochemistry. Unlike with primary ovarian tumors, ovarian involvement, when present, is superficial, not invasive. Chu et al. established the following criteria to confirm the diagnosis of primary peritoneal carcinoma over ovarian carcinoma: both ovaries must be normal in size; the amount of extraovarian involvement must be greater than the involvement on the surface of the ovary; the ovarian component must be smaller than 5 mm × 5 mm within the ovary and otherwise confined to the surface of the ovary; and the cytologic characteristics must be of the serous type.[50]

Treatment of primary peritoneal carcinoma follows programs established for ovarian carcinoma, with operative tumor debulking and adjuvant chemotherapy, because these tumors display a sensitivity to platinum-based chemotherapy which mimics that of ovarian tumors. Regimens of platinum combined with paclitaxel have led to median survivals of 40 months compared to 24 months with platinum alone.[39]

GYNECOLOGIC TUMORS

Peritoneal extension from ovarian, endometrial, and cervical carcinomas is not uncommon. In a significant number of patients, local or diffuse peritoneal involvement may represent the clinically significant aspect of the disease. Ovarian malignancies tend to spread throughout the peritoneal cavity, with frequent omental replacement in concert with multiple implants on bowel mesentery and serosa. Correct staging of ovarian malignancies includes thorough assessment of peritoneal surfaces. In distinction to gastrointestinal malignancies, ample evidence suggests a benefit to less than complete cytoreduction as part of a multimodality approach, including intravenous or intraperitoneal chemotherapy. Therapy has been shown to significantly impact the ascites frequently seen with this disease. The use of abdominal external-beam radiation therapy has been more widely accepted in the treatment of extrauterine spread of uterine endometrial cancer, with 70% 10-year survival seen in high-risk patients.[53]

TREATMENT

TECHNIQUE OF SURGICAL RESECTION

Surgical resection is the treatment of choice for patients with significant peritoneal carcinomatosis secondary to benign and low-grade appendiceal tumors, mesothelioma, and ovarian cancer. Maximal tumor debulking is desired but frequently is not possible due to the diffuse nature of the disease. The goal of surgical therapy is to relieve symptoms caused by tumor bulk and malignant ascites, effectively "resetting the clock" with regard to tumor progression. In patients with benign conditions, this is completed with surgical resection alone. The goal for patients with malignancies is to control symptoms and debulk tumor with an eye toward additional therapy. In multiple series examining the effect of combination therapy for peritoneal malignancies, the degree of tumor debulking achieved remains the most important prognostic factor across multiple tumor types.[51,54,55]

Experimental therapies now center on the delivery of intraperitoneal chemotherapy via continuous infusion after tumor debulking has been performed. In these circumstances, tumor penetration by chemotherapy is enhanced by cytoreduction to lesions of 5 mm or smaller.[56] For patients with malignant tumors, even after complete removal of all gross tumor, most investigators would advocate additional therapy, because residual microscopic disease surely exists.

Careful preoperative assessment of disease and treatment planning are important to maximize tumor debulking and potential effectiveness of chemotherapy, while limiting toxicity and potential postoperative complications. As described earlier in Pathophysiology, a characteristic pattern of spread exists and dictates the extent of surgical resection. The most common sites of disease include the greater and lesser omentum, the falciform ligament, and the splenic hilum. The peritoneum overlying both hemidiaphragms (right more than left), pelvic viscera, and small bowel mesentery is also frequently involved. Complete removal of the greater and lesser omentum is possible and is routinely performed at the author's institution. When involved, the peritoneum may be stripped off the entirety of both hemidiaphragms, the right and left paracolic gutters, and the majority of the pelvis. When the spleen or splenic hilum is involved with tumor, splenectomy is performed. The presence of significant tumor volume in the pelvis

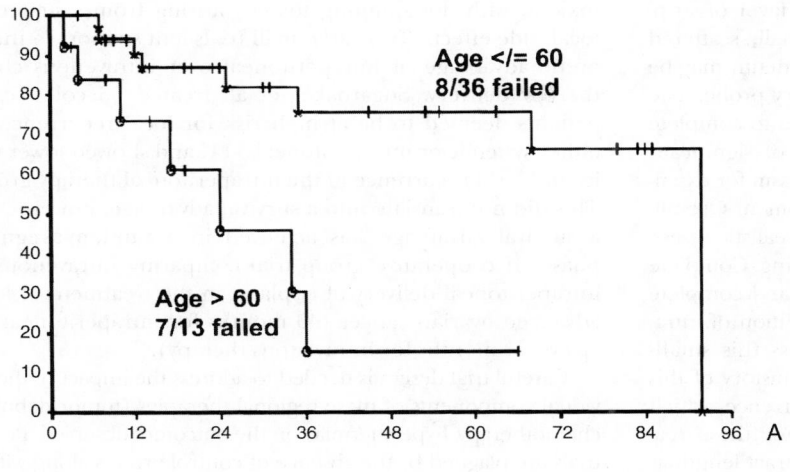

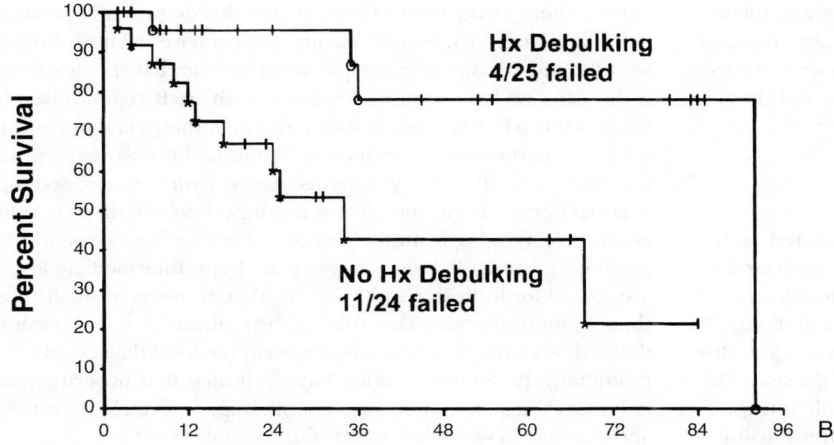

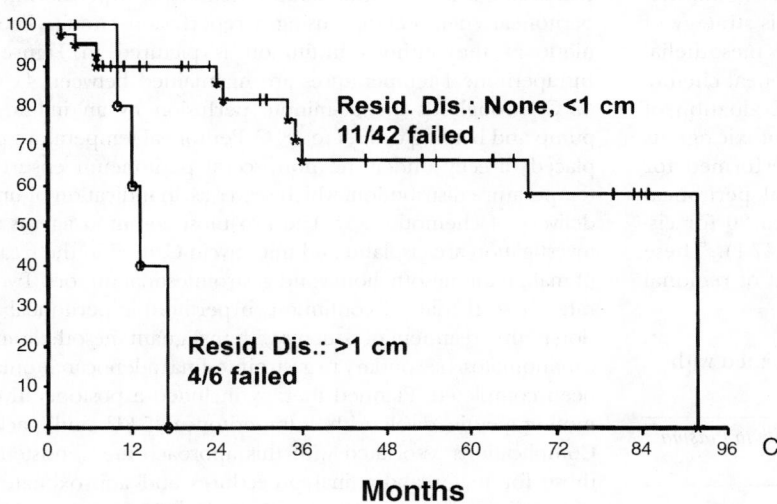

FIGURE 47-2. Factors impacting survival in patients with malignant mesothelioma undergoing surgical debulking and hyperthermic chemotherapeutic perfusion. Multivariate analysis of data for a series of 49 patients successfully treated with aggressive surgical resection and intraoperative chemotherapy revealed that age younger than 60 years (**A**), a history (Hx) of prior surgical debulking (**B**), and the ability to resect all disease to a volume of less than 1 cm (**C**) correlated with increased survival. Resid. Dis., residual disease.

and along the hepatoduodenal ligament and small bowel mesentery requires tailored operative approaches. In the pelvis, a complete peritonectomy of the nonvisceral peritoneum may be completed along with a total abdominal hysterectomy and bilateral salpingo-oophorectomy. If a low anterior resection is performed, it is protected with a loop ileostomy, because

the author's experience reveals an increased anastomotic leak rate after a colocolostomy is performed in the setting of hyperthermic intraperitoneal chemotherapy. A low anterior resection is reserved for those patients in whom complete tumor debulking is possible. Isolated areas of dense small bowel involvement may be treated with resection, but all attempts should be made to minimize bowel resections in favor of stripping of tumor from the peritoneal surface. Small, scattered implants along the visceral and mesenteric peritoneum may be controlled with fulguration, using a ball-tip cautery probe. The hepatoduodenal ligament is the most resistant area to complete removal of advanced disease, and the presence of significant tumor in this location should temper one's enthusiasm for extensive surgical debulking in other areas of the abdomen. Overall, the extent of resection should be governed by a realistic assessment of the potential for successful surgical debulking. Complete removal of all microscopic tumor is not possible, and complete peritonectomy is not generally endorsed. The addition of intraperitoneal chemotherapy is designed to address this small-volume residual disease. In addition, the natural history of this group of diseases is one of continued local recurrence, which necessitates multiple therapeutic interventions. For these reasons, the maintenance of as much gastrointestinal tract length as possible remains a key component of therapy. Sugarbaker advocates a more aggressive approach toward involved areas, including (1) omentectomy and splenectomy, (2) left upper quadrant stripping, (3) right upper quadrant stripping, (4) lesser omentectomy and cholecystectomy, (5) pelvic peritonectomy with hysterectomy and sigmoid colectomy, and (6) antrectomy.[57]

INTRAPERITONEAL CHEMOTHERAPY

These aggressive cytoreduction strategies have gained wider acceptance over the last decade but have yet to be subjected to objective assessment. Multiple studies have demonstrated improved prognosis when complete surgical debulking is achieved. This most likely represents favorable patterns of disease growth or intervention at an earlier stage of disease. The majority of recent series have included hyperthermic intraperitoneal chemotherapy delivered via continuous infusion using a roller pump and a heating element. Preclinical models have demonstrated effective delivery of locally applied chemotherapy to lesions of 10 mm or less.[58] In addition, this strategy of local delivery exploits the barrier created by the mesothelial lining, allowing high concentrations of intraperitoneal chemotherapy with minimal systemic drug exposure. Evaluation of peritoneal cavity and plasma concentration of cytotoxic agents delivered into the peritoneal cavity has been performed for multiple agents. Local drug delivery achieves a peak peritoneal cavity to plasma concentration ratio ranging from 20 for cisplatin to more than 1000 for paclitaxel (Table 47-1). These agents have been delivered with a limited amount of regional

TABLE 47-1. Pharmacokinetic Advantages Associated with Intraperitoneal Antineoplastic Drug Delivery

Agent	Peak Peritoneal Cavity to Plasma Concentration Ratio
Carboplatin	18
Cisplatin	20
Mitomycin C	72
Methotrexate	92
5-Fluorouracil	298
Doxorubicin	474
Mitoxantrone	620
Paclitaxel	>1000

toxicity, with dose-limiting toxicity arising from systemic, not local, side effects. Two early small trials lent support to the theoretic advantage of intraperitoneal over intravenous chemotherapy delivery. Sugarbaker et al. treated 66 colon cancer patients deemed to be at high risk for local recurrence with either systemic or intraperitoneal 5-FU and showed lower toxicity and local recurrence in the intraperitoneal therapy group.[59] This did not translate into a survival advantage, however. Such a survival advantage was achieved in a random-assignment phase III cooperative group trial comparing intravenous and intraperitoneal delivery of cisplatin in the treatment of locally advanced ovarian cancer (49 months for intraperitoneal therapy vs. 41 months for intravenous therapy).[60]

Careful trial design is needed to address the impact of the individual components of these regional therapies (tumor debulking, chemotherapy, hyperthermia) on the outcomes observed. Previous trials are plagued by the absence of control groups along with the lack of a standard system of tumor staging. In addition, as discussed earlier, there is no clear consensus on the degree of operative debulking necessary. Several staging systems have been proposed, with the most comprehensive put forth by Sugarbaker. His system divides the abdomen into 12 regions, with each region given a score of 0 (no tumor seen) to 3 (tumor larger than 5 cm, or confluent). The peritoneal cancer index is the sum of the scores in all 12 regions.[61] Several other groups use more basic systems, scoring residual disease at the completion of surgical debulking on a four-point scale, ranging from the absence of any visible disease to the presence of multiple lesions larger than 1 cm. Intermediate levels are scored for individuals with low or high numbers of small (less than 5 mm) lesions. The role of hyperthermia is not clearly defined, yet it has theoretic advantages in the local delivery of chemotherapy. Preliminary studies have indicated that hyperthermia enhances the penetration of chemotherapy into malignant cells and may have a synergistic effect with chemotherapy.[62]

One area in which a large degree of standardization has been established is in the intraoperative delivery of hyperthermic intraperitoneal chemotherapy using a reperfusion circuit. The technique at the author's institution is pictured in Figure 47-3. Intraperitoneal temperatures are maintained between 41°C and 42°C throughout the 90-minute perfusion by an in-line roller pump and heating coil set to 48°C. Peritoneal temperature probes placed directly under the nonvisceral peritoneum ensure even temperature distribution, which serves as an indication of uniform delivery of chemotherapy. The two most common agents under investigation are cisplatin and mitomycin C, used in the treatment of malignant mesothelioma and gastrointestinal tumors. Two separate phase II trials of continuous hyperthermic peritoneal perfusion in the treatment of patients with malignant mesothelioma and carcinomatosis secondary to gastrointestinal adenocarcinoma have been completed. Planned therapy included a postoperative chemotherapeutic dwell with intraperitoneal 5-FU and paclitaxel. Complications associated with this approach are consistent with those for major abdominal procedures and approximate 25%, with perioperative mortality less than 5%.[26] At present, a phase III, random-assignment trial has been initiated involving patients with low-grade, mucinous tumors of the gastrointestinal tract that compares surgical debulking alone to debulking with continuous hyperthermic peritoneal perfusion with cisplatin. Randomization occurs intraoperatively, once all disease has been maximally debulked. Patients in whom debulking down to residual disease of less than 1 cm in any area is not possible are removed from the

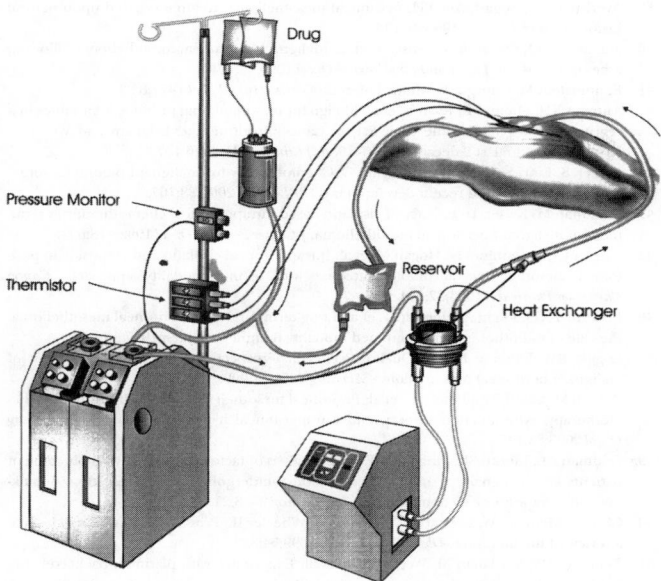

FIGURE 47-3. National Cancer Institute's peritoneal perfusion technique. Chemotherapy solution is circulated through a roller pump and heat exchanger and into the abdominal cavity. A single inflow catheter is placed in the area of greatest tumor location, with outflow taken from the opposite end of the abdomen. Indirect assurance of uniform chemotherapy distribution is established using three intraperitoneal temperature probes.

study before randomization. All patients receive four courses of postoperative intravenous chemotherapy (5-FU, leucovorin, oxaliplatin). The primary end point of the study is disease-free survival, with overall survival as a secondary end point.

OTHER INTRAPERITONEAL THERAPIES

The ability to limit systemic exposure of anticancer agents through regional delivery systems is especially attractive for novel therapies. Photodynamic therapy uses intravenous delivery of a sensitizing agent such as photofrin, a derivative of hematoporphyrin, which has preferential affinity for malignant cells. After time is allowed for clearance of the dye from normal cells, the peritoneum is exposed to laser light, which results in the formation of intracellular free radical compounds. Early results in the treatment of peritoneal carcinomatosis and sarcomatosis are encouraging but are tempered by the occurrence of significant local and systemic toxicity.[63] Other approaches under investigation include intraperitoneal delivery of gene therapy, in which it is thought that direct application of vector onto tumor deposits may improve transduction efficiency.[64] Fujiyama et al. reported animal studies of intraperitoneal delivery of cisplatin-impregnated microspheres designed for slow-release delivery of drug over 14 days.[65] Although these animal experiments did not reveal increased therapeutic effect over an equal dose of aqueous cisplatin, less toxicity was observed, which allows for dose escalation.

PALLIATION

Complications of peritoneal carcinomatosis, including obstruction and ascites, can be among the most vexing problems facing medical and surgical oncologists. Tumor progression can lead to partial or complete bowel obstruction, resulting in severe abdominal pain and cramping along with intractable nausea and vomiting. Before surgical intervention is undertaken to relieve obstruction, a thorough evaluation, including CT scan and upper gastrointestinal series, should be performed to assess the location and degree of obstruction in addition to the overall tumor volume. Evaluation of the entire bowel is mandatory, often with the use of a rectal contrast agent, to assure the absence of a second obstruction distal to the clinically apparent lesion. The decision between bypass and resection should be based on the overall health of the patient, the amount of intraperitoneal and extraperitoneal disease, and the presence or absence of gastrointestinal bleeding. In patients with unresectable obstructing or near-obstructing lesions of the pelvis, an end colostomy may be necessary. Diffuse carcinomatosis often results in functional, not anatomic, obstruction, which may be effectively palliated only through placement of a gastrostomy tube. Blair and coworkers at City of Hope National Medical Center reported on a series of 63 patients undergoing operative palliation of malignant bowel obstruction secondary to nongynecologic malignancies.[66] Median survival was 90 days, with 45% of patients tolerating a regular diet on hospital discharge a mean of 12 days after surgery. On univariate analysis, poorer prognosis was associated with malignant obstruction as the initial presentation of malignancy, the presence of ascites, and noncolorectal primary tumors. In a series of 69 patients undergoing resection of melanoma metastatic to the gastrointestinal tract, curative resection was associated with 49-month survival compared with 5.4 months for palliative procedures.[67]

Refractory malignant ascites can significantly impact both the patient's quality of life and duration of survival in peritoneal carcinomatosis. Ten percent to 15% of patients with gastrointestinal tract cancer develop malignant ascites.[68] Conservative management through diuretic therapy is effective in up to 47% of patients, although randomized trials have not been performed.[69] Spironolactone therapy, starting at 150 mg/d, may be necessary for prolonged periods to establish and maintain control of the ascites. Direct drainage of ascitic fluid through paracentesis and surgically placed peritoneovenous shunts provides immediate relief, but with increased complications compared with diuretic therapy. Repeated paracenteses increase the rate of infectious complications and hypoalbuminemia, which makes this an impractical long-term solution. Peritoneal shunts (Denver and LeVeen shunts) remove ascitic fluid and return it to the systemic circulation. Successful, prolonged control of ascites is possible in up to 70% of patients. Complications include disseminated intravascular coagulation, pulmonary emboli, pulmonary edema, and the rare tumor embolus.[70] Other therapies under investigation include the use of inhibitors of vascular endothelial growth factor and matrix metalloproteinase, two cytokines shown to be present in elevated amounts in malignant ascites.[71,72]

REFERENCES

1. Henriksen JH, Winkler K. Peritoneum and ascites formation. In: Bengmark S, ed. *The peritoneum and peritoneal access.* London: Wright Publishers, 1989:94.
2. Feldman GB, Knapp RC, Order SE, Hellman S. The role of lymphatic obstruction in the formation of ascites in a murine ovarian carcinoma. *Cancer Res* 1972;32:1663.
3. Garrison RN, Galloway RH, Heuser LS. Mechanisms of malignant ascites production. *J Surg Res* 1987;42:126.
4. Watters WB, Buck RC. Scanning electron microscopy of mesothelial regeneration in the rat. *Lab Invest* 1972;26(5):604.

5. Flessner MF, Fenstermachner JD, Blasberg RG, Dedrick RL. Peritoneal absorption of macromolecules studied by quantitative autoradiography. *Am J Physiol* 1985;248:H26.
6. Sugarbaker P. Observations concerning cancer spread within the peritoneal cavity and concepts supporting an ordered pathophysiology. In: Sugarbaker P, ed. *Peritoneal carcinomatosis: principles of management.* Boston: Kluwer Academic Publishers, 1996:79.
7. Hagiwara A, Rakanhashi T, Sawai K, et al. Milky spots at the implantation site for malignant cells in peritoneal dissemination in mice. *Cancer Res* 1993;53:687.
8. Ronnet BM, Shmookler BM, Sugarbaker PH, Kurman RJ. Pseudomyxoma peritonei: new concepts in diagnosis, origin, nomenclature, and relationship to mucinous borderline (low malignant potential) tumors of the ovary. *Anat Pathol* 1997;2:197.
9. Weiss L. Metastatic inefficiency: intravascular and intraperitoneal implantation of cancer cells. *Cancer Treat Res* 1996;82:1.
10. Archer AG, Sugarbaker PH, Jelinek JS. Radiology of peritoneal carcinomatosis. *Cancer Treat Res* 1996;82:263.
11. Low RN, Semelka RC, Worawattarakul S, Alzate GD, Sigeti JS. Extrahepatic abdominal imaging in patients with malignancy: comparison of MR imaging and helical CT, with subsequent surgical correlation. *Radiology* 1999;21:625.
12. Balestreri L, Bison L, Sorio R, et al. Abdominal recurrence of ovarian cancer: value of abdominal MR in patients with positive CA125 and negative CT. *Radiol Med* 2002;104(5–6):426.
13. Fong Y, Saldinger PF, Akhurst T, et al. Utility of 18F-FDG positron emission tomography scanning on selection of patients for resection of hepatic colorectal metastases. *Am J Surg* 1999;178:282.
14. Turlakow A, Yeung HW, Salmon AS, Macapinlac HA, Larson SM. Peritoneal carcinomatosis: role of 18F-FDG PET. *J Nucl Med* 2003;44:1407.
15. Kanellos I, Demetriades H, Zintzaras E, et al. Incidence and prognostic value of positive peritoneal cytology in colorectal cancer. *Dis Colon Rectum* 2003;46:535.
16. Nakatsuka A, Yamaguchi K, Shimizu S, et al. Positive washing cytology in patients with pancreatic cancer indicates a contraindication of pancreatectomy. *Int J Surg Invest* 1999;1:311.
17. Werth H. Klinische und anatomische untersuchungen zue lehre von deh bauchgeschwuelsten und der laparotomie. *Arch Gynakol* 1884;24:100.
18. Ronnet BM, Zahn CM, Kurman RJ, et al. Disseminated peritoneal adenomucinosis and peritoneal mucinous carcinomatosis. *Am J Surg Pathol* 1995;19(12):1390.
19. Ronnet BM, Yan H, Kurman RJ, et al. Patients with pseudomyxoma peritonei associated with disseminated peritoneal adenomucinosis have a significantly more favorable prognosis than patients with peritoneal mucinous carcinomatosis. *Cancer* 2001;92:85.
20. van Ruth S, Acherman YIZ, van de Vijvert MJ, et al. Pseudomyxoma peritonei: a review of 62 cases. *Eur J Surg Oncol* 2003;29:682.
21. Gough DB, Donohue JH, Schutt JA, et al. Pseudomyxoma peritonei: long-term patient survival with an aggressive regional approach. *Ann Surg* 1994;219:112.
22. Sugarbaker PH, Chang D. Results of treatment of 385 patients with peritoneal surface spread of appendiceal malignancy. *Ann Surg Oncol* 1999;6:727.
23. Harshen R, Jyothirmayi R, Mithal N. Pseudomyxoma peritonei. *Clin Oncol* 2003;15:73.
24. Green JB, Timmcke AE, Mitchell WT, et al. Mucinous carcinoma—just another colon cancer? *Dis Colon Rectum* 1993;36:49.
25. Nitecki SS, Wolff BG, Schlinkert R, Sarr MG. The natural history of surgically treated primary adenocarcinoma of the appendix. *Ann Surg* 1994;219:51.
26. Pingpank JF, Libutti SK, Bartlett DL, et al. Aggressive surgical resection/debulking and continuous hyperthermic peritoneal perfusion (CHPP) with cisplatin (CDDP) for patients with peritoneal carcinomatosis from primary gastrointestinal adenocarcinoma. *Proc Am Assoc Cancer Res* 2003:R4487.
27. Culliford AT, Brooks AD, Sharma S, et al. Surgical debulking and intraperitoneal chemotherapy for established peritoneal metastases from colon and appendix cancer. *Ann Surg Oncol* 2001;8:787.
28. Sugarbaker PH, Jablonski KA. Prognostic features of 51 colorectal and 130 appendiceal cancer patients with peritoneal carcinomatosis treated by cytoreductive surgery and intraperitoneal chemotherapy. *Ann Surg* 1995;221:124.
29. Elias D, Blot F, El Otmany A, et al. Curative treatment of peritoneal carcinomatosis arising from colorectal cancer by complete resection and intraperitoneal chemotherapy. *Cancer* 2001;92:71.
30. Roviello F, Marrelli D, de Manzoni G, et al. Prospective study of peritoneal recurrence after curative surgery for gastric cancer. *Br J Surg* 2003;90:1113.
31. Lennon AM, Mulcahy HE, Hyland JMP, et al. Peritoneal involvement in stage II colon cancer. *Am J Clin Pathol* 2003;119:108.
32. Ishikawa O, Wada H, Ohigashi H, et al. Postoperative cytology for drained fluid from the pancreatic bed after "curative" resection of pancreatic cancers: does it predict both the patient's prognosis and the site of cancer recurrence? *Ann Surg* 2003;238:103.
33. Leach SD, Rose JA, Lowy AM, et al. Significance of peritoneal cytology in patients with potentially resectable adenocarcinoma of the pancreatic head. *Surgery* 1995;118:472.
34. Yu W, Whang I, Averbach A, Chang D, Sugarbaker PH. Morbidity and mortality of early postoperative intraperitoneal chemotherapy as adjuvant therapy for gastric cancer. *Am Surg* 1998;64:1104.
35. Sautner T, Hofbauer F, Depisch D, Schiessel R, Jakesz R. Adjuvant intraperitoneal cisplatin chemotherapy does not improve long-term survival after surgery for advanced gastric cancer. *J Clin Oncol* 1994;12:970.
36. Ikeguchi M, Kondou A, Oka A, et al. Effects of continuous hyperthermic peritoneal perfusion on prognosis of gastric cancer with serosal invasion. *Eur J Surg* 1995;161:581.
37. Kass ME. Pathology of peritoneal mesothelioma. In: Sugarbaker PH, ed. *Peritoneal carcinomatosis: drugs and diseases.* Boston: Kluwer Academic Publishers, 1996:213.
38. Daya D, McCaughey WTE. Well-differentiated papillary mesothelioma of the peritoneum: a clinicopathologic study of 22 cases. *Cancer* 1990;65:292.
39. Averbach AM, Sugarbaker PH. Peritoneal mesothelioma: treatment based upon natural history. *Cancer Treat Res* 1996;81:193.
40. Manavoglu O, Orhan B, Evrensel T, et al. Malignant peritoneal mesothelioma following asbestos exposure. *J Environ Pathol Toxicol Oncol* 1996;15:191.
41. Kannerstein M, Churg J. Peritoneal mesothelioma. *Hum Pathol* 1977;8:83.
42. Antman KH, Shemin R, Ryan L, et al. Malignant mesothelioma; prognostic variables in a registry of 180 patients, the Dana-Farber Cancer Institute and Brigham and Women's Hospital over the last 2 decades, 1965–1985. *J Clin Oncol* 1988;6:147.
43. Tomek S, Emri S, Krejcy K, Manegold C. Chemotherapy for malignant pleural mesothelioma: past results and recent developments. *Br J Cancer* 2003;88:167.
44. Markman M, Kelsen D. Efficacy of cisplatin-based intraperitoneal chemotherapy as treatment of malignant peritoneal mesothelioma. *J Cancer Res Clin Oncol* 1992;118:547.
45. Langer CJ, Rosenblum N, Hogan M, et al. Intraperitoneal cisplatin and etoposide in peritoneal mesothelioma: favorable outcome with a multimodality approach. *Cancer Chemother Pharmacol* 1993;32:204.
46. Lederman GS, Recht A, Herman T, et al. Long-term survival in peritoneal mesothelioma: the role of radiotherapy and combined modality treatment. *Cancer* 1987;59:1882.
47. Loggie BW, Fleming RA, McQuellon RP, et al. Prospective trial for the treatment of malignant peritoneal mesothelioma. *Am Surg* 2001;67:999.
48. Deraco M, Casali P, Inglese MG, et al. Peritoneal mesothelioma treated by induction chemotherapy, cytoreduction surgery, and intraperitoneal hyperthermic perfusion. *J Surg Oncol* 2003;83:147.
49. Feldman AL, Libutti SK, Pingpank JF, et al. Analysis of factors associated with outcome in patients with malignant peritoneal mesothelioma undergoing surgical resection/debulking and intraperitoneal chemotherapy. *J Clin Oncol* 2003;21(24):4560.
50. Chu CS, Menzin AW, Leonard DG, Rubin SC, Wheeler JE. Primary peritoneal carcinoma: a review of the literature. *Obstet Gynecol Surv* 1999;54:323.
51. Kennedy AW, Markman M, Webster KD, et al. Experience with platinum-paclitaxel chemotherapy in the initial management of papillary serous carcinoma of the peritoneum. *Gynecol Oncol* 1998;71:288.
52. Jermann M, Vogt P, Pestalozzi BC. Peritoneal carcinoma in a male patient. *Oncology* 2003;64:468.
53. Stewart KD, Martinez AA, Weiner S, et al. Ten-year outcome including patterns of failure and toxicity for adjuvant whole abdominopelvic irradiation in high-risk and poor histologic feature patients with endometrial carcinoma. *Int J Rad Oncol Biol Phys* 2002;54:527.
54. Portilla AG, Sugarbaker PH, Chang D. Second-look surgery after cytoreduction and intraperitoneal chemotherapy for peritoneal carcinomatosis from colorectal cancer: analysis of prognostic features. *World J Surg* 1999;23:23.
55. Bristow RE, Montz FJ, Lagasse LD, Leuchter RS, Karlan BY. Survival impact of surgical cytoreduction in stage IV epithelial ovarian cancer. *Gynecol Oncol* 1999;72:278.
56. Alexander HR, Bartlett DL, Libutti SK. National Cancer Institute experience with regional therapy for unresectable primary and metastatic cancer of the liver or peritoneal cavity. In: Markman M, ed. *Regional chemotherapy; clinical research and practice . Current Clinical Oncology series.* Totowa, NJ: Humana Press, 2000:127.
57. Sugarbaker PH. Peritonectomy procedures. *Ann Surg* 1995;221:29.
58. Los G, Mutsaers PH, van der Vijgh WJ, et al. Direct diffusion of cis-diamminedichloroplatinum(II) in intraperitoneal rat tumors after intraperitoneal chemotherapy: a comparison with systemic chemotherapy. *Cancer Res* 1989;49:3380.
59. Sugarbaker PH, Gianola FJ, Speyer JC, et al. Prospective, randomized trial of intravenous versus intraperitoneal 5-fluorouracil in patients with advanced primary colon or rectal cancer. *Surgery* 1985;98:414.
60. Alberts DS, Liu PY, Hannigan EV, et al. Intraperitoneal cisplatin plus intravenous cyclophosphamide versus intravenous cisplatin plus cyclophosphamide for stage III ovarian cancer. *N Engl J Med* 1996;335:1950.
61. Sugarbaker PH. Successful management of microscopic residual disease in large bowel cancer. *Cancer Chemother Pharmacol* 1999;43:S15.
62. Benoit L, Duvillard C, Rat P, Chauffert B. The effect of intra-abdominal temperature on the tissue and tumor diffusion of intraperitoneal cisplatin in a model of peritoneal carcinomatosis in rats. *Chirurgie* 1999;124:375.
63. Menon C, Kutney SN, Lehr SC, et al. Vascularity and uptake of photosensitizer in small human tumor nodules: implications for intraperitoneal photodynamic therapy. *Clin Can Res* 2001;7:3904.
64. Lechanteur C, Pricen F, Lo Bue S, et al. HSV-1 thymidine kinase gene therapy for peritoneal carcinomatosis. *Adv Exp Med Biol* 1998;341:119.
65. Fujiyama J, Nakase Y, Osaki K, et al. Cisplatin incorporated microspheres: development and fundamental studies for its clinical application. *J Control Release* 2003;89:397.
66. Blair SL, Chu DZJ, Schwarz RE. Outcome of palliative operations for malignant bowel obstruction in patients with peritoneal carcinomatosis for nongynecological cancer. *Ann Surg Oncol* 2001;8:632.
67. Ollila DW, Essner R, Wanek LA, Morton DL. Surgical resection for melanoma metastatic to the gastrointestinal tract. *Arch Surg* 1996;131:975.
68. Ringenberg QS, Doll DC, Loy TS, Yarbro JW. Malignant ascites of unknown origin. *Cancer* 1989;64:753.
69. Gough IR, Balderson GA. Malignant ascites: a comparison of peritoneovenous shunting and nonoperative management. *Cancer* 1993;71:2377.
70. Schumacher DL, Saclarides TJ, Staren ED. Peritoneovenous shunts for palliation in patients with malignant ascites. *Ann Surg Oncol* 1994;1:378.
71. Luo JC, Toyoda M, Shibuya M. Differential inhibition of fluid accumulation and tumor growth in two mouse ascites tumors by an antivascular endothelial growth factor/permeability factor neutralizing antibody. *Cancer Res* 1998;58:2594.
72. Talbot DC, Brown PD. Experimental and clinical studies on the use of matrix metalloproteinase inhibitors for the treatment of cancer. *Eur J Cancer* 1996;32A:2528.

CHAPTER 48

Immunosuppression-Related Malignancies

SECTION **1**

ROBERT YARCHOAN
RICHARD F. LITTLE

AIDS-Related Malignancies

Patients with human immunodeficiency virus (HIV) infection have a substantially increased incidence of certain tumors, including some that are rarely seen in patients without underlying HIV infection. Three malignant conditions are now considered as AIDS defining when they occur in HIV-infected individuals: Kaposi's sarcoma (KS), certain aggressive non-Hodgkin's lymphomas (NHLs), and invasive cervical cancer.[1] Over the past decade, it has become increasingly evident that most tumors highly associated with HIV are caused by oncogenic viruses.[2,3] In addition to these AIDS-defining tumors, individuals with HIV infection are at substantially increased risk of developing a number of other neoplasms[4,5] (Table 48.1-1). However, it is worth noting that many common cancers do not appear with greater frequency in AIDS patients than in the general population. This fact would suggest that immunosurveillance may not be important in keeping such tumors in check during their early pathogenesis.

Since the advent of highly active antiretroviral therapy (HAART) in 1995, there has been a decrease in the incidence of most AIDS-related malignancies. This has led many to assume that the epidemic of these malignancies is no longer a major public health problem. However, no person has yet been cured of HIV infection, and since the introduction of life-

extending HAART, the total number of persons living with AIDS in the United States has increased by more than 50%.[6] Thus, the denominator of those at risk for AIDS-related malignancies has increased. It is difficult to predict what the future of this dynamic epidemic will hold, but it is not unreasonable to hypothesize that as AIDS patients live longer, their cumulative risk of developing AIDS-related malignancies will increase.[7] Thus, in absence of curative therapy for AIDS, oncologists can expect to see more such cases in coming years.

KAPOSI'S SARCOMA

EPIDEMIOLOGY

In 1872, Moritz Kaposi[8] first described several cases of a multicentric purplish tumor appearing predominantly on the lower extremity of elderly men. This form of KS, now called *classic KS*, is found predominantly in individuals living near the Mediterranean Sea or in Ashkenazi Jews. A more aggressive form of KS, now called *endemic KS*, was subsequently recognized in Africa. This form generally occurs earlier in life, often in the third or fourth decades, frequently involves the lymph nodes, and occurs in a higher percentage of females than does classic KS. Also, it can develop in children, causing severe morbidity in this setting.

In 1982, a cluster of cases of KS among young homosexual men in New York City was one of the first epidemiologic signs of the AIDS epidemic.[9,10] This was a striking epidemiologic finding given that only three cases had been reported in the period 1961 to 1979 for the same age group in two major New York

TABLE 48.1-1. Post–Acquired Immunodeficiency Syndrome Relative Risks of Various Malignant Conditions in Patients with Acquired Immunodeficiency Syndrome

Tumor	Relative Risk	95% Confidence Interval
Kaposi's sarcoma	310.2	291.6–329.5
Non-Hodgkin's lymphoma	112.9	103.6–123.4
Invasive cervical cancer	2.9	0.7–16.0
Anal cancer	31.7	11.6–69.2
Non–acquired immunodeficiency syndrome–related cancers	1.9	1.5–2.3
Angiosarcoma	36.7	4.4–132.5
Soft tissue sarcoma	7.2	1.5–21.0
Hodgkin's disease	7.6	4.1–13.1
Leukemia	11.0	3.0–28.3
Multiple myeloma	4.5	0.9–13.2
Brain	3.5	1.4–7.2
Seminoma or germinoma	2.9	1.1–6.3
Squamous cell carcinoma, unusual sites	6.8	1.4–19.8
Lung, adenocarcinoma	2.5	1.0–5.0

Note. Relative risk calculations based on comparisons of the cancer experiences of people with acquired immunodeficiency syndrome and those of the general population younger than 70 years by matching population-based cancer and acquired immunodeficiency syndrome registries in the United States and Puerto Rico.
(Data from ref. 4.)

City hospitals. KS is now the most common tumor seen in HIV-infected patients. In developed Western nations, it was found that those HIV-infected patients at highest risk for development of KS were men who had sex with other men[11] or women whose male sexual partners had sex with other men. It was relatively uncommon in individuals whose risk for HIV was injection drug use, blood transfusion, or use of factor VIII. These observations suggested that KS was not caused solely by HIV but rather involved the presence of another infectious agent.[12] Further support for this hypothesis came from the observation that KS periodically developed in transplant recipients and in gay men who were HIV seronegative.

In 1994, Drs. Chang, Moore, and colleagues discovered a new herpesvirus, called the *Kaposi's sarcoma–associated herpesvirus* (KSHV) or *human herpesvirus-8*, and subsequent studies showed that this was an essential causative agent for all forms of KS.[13,14] A number of epidemiologic studies showed that the seroprevalence of KSHV generally paralleled the incidence of KS.[15,16] For example, in Africa, the majority of individuals are infected with KSHV, and KS prevalence exceeds that of most other tumors in some populations. KSHV infection is also relatively common in southern Italy and other countries in which classic KS is frequently observed. In other countries, such as those in northern Europe, KSHV infection is relatively rare. Thus, varying prevalence of KSHV infection appears to be a principal cause of variations in the incidence of KS.

Retrospective analyses of HIV and KSHV exposure patterns show that the epidemic of KSHV infection in gay men in the United States emerged almost simultaneously with that of HIV.[17] Since the mid-1990s, a decreasing incidence of KS has occurred among homosexuals in the United States and other Western industrialized countries.[18] Before 1985, KS was reported

as the initial manifestation of AIDS in approximately 30% of cases,[19] but in the period from 1992 to 1997 it was the initial manifestation in 12.5%.[1] The decrease in KS as the index disease for AIDS in recent years has occurred in part because the Centers for Disease Control and Prevention (CDC) revised its definition of AIDS in 1992 to include a CD4 cell count under $200/mm^3$, and thus cases of KS that occur at lower CD4 cell counts are excluded from the index-case count. However, a further decline in incident cases from 60 to 20 per 1000 person-years occurred between 1992 and 1997,[1] suggesting that this was more than just the result of a change in the case definition of AIDS. This decrease in KS incidence appears to be in part due to a decrease in the seroincidence of KSHV after 1983, in concert with efforts to encourage safer sex practices among gay men at risk for HIV infection. Also, as discussed later in Treatment, improved treatments for the underlying HIV infection have contributed to the decline in KS incidence.[20] At the same time, it should be noted that KS is a much more common cause of morbidity and mortality in some parts of the world than it is in the United States. In certain parts of sub-Saharan Africa, KS represents almost half of all cancer cases in males and is the second most frequent tumor in females.[21]

A number of unresolved questions remain regarding the transmission of KSHV infection. Sexual as well as nonsexual transmission can occur.[22] Blood-borne transmission can occur, but appears to be relatively inefficient.[23] KSHV infection from donor to solid-organ transplant recipients and subsequent development of KS have been documented.[24] It appears that there is relatively little KSHV in semen, but frequent shedding into saliva of infected individuals.[25] KSHV transmission from mother to child may be relatively frequent, possibly due to premastication of food by the mother in feeding younger children or through child-to-child salivary contact. Recent evidence suggests that the frequent spread of KSHV infection among men having sex with other men may be related to the use of saliva as a lubricant. If this is borne out, it may provide an opportunity to reduce the spread of KSHV (and the incidence of KS) through education aimed at reducing salivary transmission of KSHV.

Although KSHV appears to be an essential factor for the development of KS, it is usually not sufficient. Co-infection with KSHV and HIV increases the risk of developing KS by as much as 500- to 10,000-fold as compared with KSHV infection alone. Individuals infected with KSHV but not HIV can develop KS, but it is rare and usually occurs after their fifth decade of life. However, the 10-year probability of developing KS after co-infection with HIV and KSHV approaches 50%.[26] Also, there is evidence that the risk of KS is higher for those who acquire KSHV subsequent to HIV infection,[27] suggesting that there is an important role for immune surveillance of KSHV and the risk of KS. The majority of cases occur when the CD4 cell count is below $200/mm^3$, and the risk increases substantially as the CD4 cell count falls below $100/mm^3$.[20] Since the advent of HAART, the incidence of KS has dropped markedly, partly due to immune protection.

PATHOGENESIS

KS is a multicentric tumor that arises simultaneously in multiple nonmetastatic sites (Fig. 48.1-1). The lesions are character-

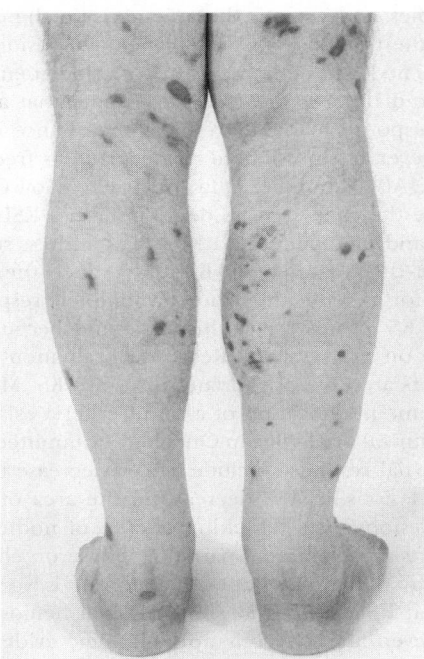

FIGURE 48.1-1. Cutaneous manifestations of Kaposi's sarcoma. (See Color Fig. 48.1-1 in the CD-ROM.)

TABLE 48.1-2. Mimics of Human Genes in the Kaposi's Sarcoma–Associated Herpesvirus Genome

Viral Gene	Human Analog	Function, Comment
ORF K6/ vMIP1	MIP	T helper type 2 chemoattractant; angiogenic activity
ORF K4/ vMIP2	MIP	T helper type 2 chemoattractant; angiogenic activity
ORF K4.1/ vMIP3	MIP	T helper type 2 chemoattractant; angiogenic activity
ORF K2/vIL-6	IL-6	B-cell growth factor; angiogenic factor
ORF74/ vGPCR	IL-8 receptor	Constitutively active GPCR; induces proliferation and angiogenic activity
ORF K9/ vIRF-1	IRF	Inhibits interferon signaling in infected cells
ORF K11.5/ vIRF-2	IRF	Inhibits interferon signaling in infected cells
ORF16/vBcl-2	Bcl-2	Inhibits apoptosis
ORF72/vCYC	D-type cyclins	Cell-cycle control
ORF K13/ vFLIP	FLIP	Inhibits Fas-mediated apoptosis; latent gene

FLIP, FLICE-inhibitory protein; GPCR, G protein–coupled receptor; IL, interleukin; IRF, interferon regulatory factors; MIP, macrophage inflammatory protein.

ized by vascular slits filled with blood, and this accounts for their purplish hue. Microscopically, the tumors are heterogeneous but characterized by a predominance of KSHV-infected spindle-shaped cells that are thought to be derived from lymphatic endothelial cells.[28,29] Thus, the lesions can be viewed as representing an abnormal angiogenic state that is directly and indirectly caused by KSHV infection. Some evidence has been shown that advanced KS may involve monoclonal proliferation,[30] although this is not universally accepted. However, a substantial body of evidence indicates that hyperproliferation of endothelial-derived spindle cells induced by angiogenic and other factors is important at all stages of the disease.[29,31–34] Most of this hyperproliferation appears to be directly or indirectly induced by KSHV.

A study of the genome of KSHV showed that it encodes for a number of mimics of human genes, including several with direct angiogenesis activity (Table 48.1-2). For example, it encodes for viral homologues to human interleukin-6 (IL-6) and three homologues of macrophage inhibitory protein that have been shown to have angiogenic activity.[29,32] It also induces other cellular angiogenic factors, which have the potential for stimulating spindle cells as well as angiogenesis, and can upregulate cell surface expression for these angiogenic cytokines, providing for autocrine and paracrine effects in tumorigenesis. For example, ORF74 of KSHV encodes for a constitutively active G protein–coupled receptor (KSHV-GPCR) that induces production of vascular endothelial growth factor and other angiogenic factors, in part by activating hypoxia-inducible factor.[33,34] Evidence has also shown that the proangiogenic effects induced by KSHV are enhanced by factors that activate the KSHV-GPCR over constitutive levels.[35,36] This can occur in response to a variety of chemokines. Also, the HIV protein, Tat, can collaborate with KSHV-GPCR in activating KSHV-infected cells. Such observations suggest a role for endogenous factor

dysregulation and a multifactorial role of HIV in KS pathogenesis. These mechanisms may partly explain why HAART can be of therapeutic benefit in AIDS-KS.

Nearly all the spindle cells in KS lesions are infected with KSHV.[2,37] Most are latently infected and express KSHV latency-associated nuclear antigen. Indeed, detection of this antigen in lesions by immunohistochemistry can be useful in making the pathologic diagnosis of KS. Evidence for lytic KSHV replication is found in a minority of these cells, and paracrine angiogenesis and endothelial cell proliferation by certain KSHV lytic gene products (including viral IL-6 and ORF74) is believed to be important in the development of KS lesions. Evidence has shown that KSHV can be induced to undergo lytic replication by hypoxia,[38] and it is possible that the tendency of KS to arise in the feet, which are relatively hypoxic, is in part the result of hypoxia-induced KSHV reactivation.

STAGING AND PROGNOSIS

The unique clinical presentation of KS requires a departure from standard tumor staging. Because lesions arise simultaneously at multiple sites without an obvious primary site (see Fig. 48.1-1), almost all KS patients would be classified as having metastatic disease using the standard oncology staging. However, multiple areas of skin involvement may not necessarily imply a worse prognosis relative to more focal involvement. Indeed, it is not at all clear how to use the term *metastatic* in relation to KS.

Uniform staging is central to response assessment and is necessary to help compare results among trials and with historic controls. The most widely used staging system for KS, devised before the widespread use of HAART, is the AIDS Clinical Trials Group Oncology Committee TIS staging system. Evaluation suggests that this system requires some refinement since the advent of

TABLE 48.1-3. Revised and Proposed AIDS Clinical Trials Group Staging Classification for Kaposi's Sarcoma[a]

	Good Risk (0; All of the Following)	Poor Risk (1; Any of the Following)
Tumor (T)	Confined to skin and/or lymph nodes and/or non-nodular oral disease confined to the palate	Tumor-associated edema or ulceration; extensive oral KS; gastrointestinal KS; KS in other non-nodal viscera
Immune system (I; not included if HIV sensitive to HAART)[39]	CD4 cells ≥150/μL	CD4 cells <150/μL
Systemic illness (S)	No history of opportunistic infection or thrush; no "B" symptoms (unexplained fever, night sweats, >10% involuntary weight loss, or diarrhea) persisting more than 2 wk; performance status ≥70 (Karnofsky)	History of opportunistic infections and/or thrush; "B" symptoms present; performance status <70; other HIV-related illness (e.g., neurologic disease, lymphoma)

HAART, highly active antiretroviral therapy; HIV, human immunodeficiency virus; KS, Kaposi's sarcoma.
[a]Based on refs. 39 and 40. The revised CD4 cutoff of 150 cells/μL[40] is lower than the original proposal of 200 cells/μL. However, in the HAART era, CD4 cells do not appear to confer prognostic information. Examples of staging: In the pre-HAART era, a patient with KS restricted to the skin, CD4 count of 10 cells/μL, and a history of *Pneumocystis carinii* pneumonia would be $T_0I_1S_1$ and would be considered poor risk.[40] Suggested revision since HAART would be staged as T_0S_1 and would be considered good risk.[39]

HAART[39] (Table 48.1-3). The original AIDS Clinical Trials Group TIS system scores patients based on the extent of tumor involvement (T), the immune status of the patient (I), and other AIDS-related systemic illness (S) in an attempt to stratify risk of poor prognosis.[40] Risk is assigned as overall either good or poor, depending on the presence or absence of localized tumor versus more extensive tumor with associated edema, ulceration, visceral disease, or extensive oral KS; CD4 cells over or below 150/mm³; and the presence or absence of antecedent opportunistic infections (OIs), thrush, constitutional symptoms, other HIV-related illness, and Karnofsky performance status. Good risk is designated with a subscript 0 and poor risk by the subscript 1, the summary taking the form T_0 or $_1I_0$ or $_1S_0$ or $_1$. Pre-HAART, a patient who is poor risk in any single category is considered poor risk overall. In the era of HAART, CD4 level does not seem to provide prognostic information.[39] Two different risk categories have been identified: a good risk (T_0S_0, T_1S_0, T_0S_1) and a poor risk (T_1S_1). This latter approach most likely is dependent on the ability to respond to HAART. It is possible that the original TIS may be more applicable for patients with multidrug-resistant HIV infection.

TREATMENT

A number of therapeutic modalities are available, each with advantages and disadvantages that must be weighed in the overall clinical context that can be considered in any given case. Broadly, these include HAART (for HIV-associated KS),

local therapies, and systemic therapies. It is worth noting at the onset that the treatment of KS is generally considered palliative; there is no known treatment that can rid patients of KSHV infection, and there is no evidence to date that achieving a complete response markedly reduces the chance of a recurrence. However, it is possible to render patients free of detectable disease. Also, a number of factors (such as low CD4 count) can increase the chance of KS developing in a KSHV-infected individual, and therapeutic strategies that address such factors can help in the treatment of KS and reduce the chance of recurrence for patients who achieve a complete response.

Because KS lesions are multicentric and because of their appearance on the skin, the Response Evaluation Criteria in Solid Tumors are not appropriate for use in KS. Most clinical trials use some modification of a set of criteria established by the AIDS Clinical Trials Group Oncology Committee.[41,42] Criteria for a partial response include a 50% decrease in the total number of lesions, a 50% decrease in the area of measured cutaneous lesions, or a flattening of 50% of nodular lesions. Most patients who achieve a partial response on clinical trials do so through flattening of nodular lesions. It is worth keeping in mind that KS lesions may show residual hemosiderin pigmentation even after there is no pathologic evidence of disease, and biopsy of such a residual pigmented lesion may be useful in establishing that such a patient has achieved a pathologic complete response.

Highly Active Antiretroviral Therapy

It is now clear that HAART should be considered fundamental to the oncologic therapy for AIDS-KS.[20,43] Whether additional therapy is required is dependent on a number of factors that must be individually assessed for each patient. In considering a rational treatment plan, it is important to assess the likelihood of inducing a satisfactory response with HAART alone and whether the addition of other therapies is indicated for a given individual. HAART can induce responses in up to 74% of patients and is most likely to have a beneficial effect in previously untreated patients with relatively little KS who are naive to antiretroviral therapy, in whom the viral load can be suppressed, and in whom an increment of 150 or more CD4 cells/mm³ is realized with HAART initiation.[43] However, if such a patient has severe morbidity associated with the KS or is psychologically distressed by the visible lesions, additional therapy should be considered, so that a meaningful therapeutic benefit can be realized more quickly. In such patients, however, HAART should also be administered whenever possible. Laboratory evidence has shown that protease inhibitor antiretroviral drugs may have some direct antiangiogenic therapy and may promote regression of KS by that mechanism.[44] However, one clinical study has failed to find a difference between HAART regimens containing a protease inhibitor and those without one.[20] Clinicians should be on the lookout for additional clinical studies addressing this question.

Local Therapy

Local therapies may be useful for limited mucocutaneous disease and include such modalities as cryotherapy, photodynamic therapy, intralesional injections, radiation therapy (RT), and topical application of various drugs. Surgical biopsy is important for making a definitive diagnosis of KS before potentially toxic therapies are used. However, it is the authors' opinion that, except under unusual circumstances, surgical excision is not the best choice for the management of local lesions. Indeed, there is evidence that KS can first develop in surgical wounds,[45] perhaps because of tissue hypoxia at the edge of the wound,[38] and the authors have observed KS reappear in wound tissue after wide excisions.

Radiotherapy is useful for localized disease but does not control disease outside of the treatment area. In addition, there are reports of a decreased tolerance to radiation among AIDS-KS patients, particularly on the mucosal surfaces, where severe mucositis can occur.[46] Often the outcome is not completely satisfactory because of chronic residual lymphedema, postirradiation telangiectasias, permanent woody skin changes, and reappearance of KS in the area of previous irradiation. The use of carbon dioxide laser therapy to remove tumors of the mouth, oropharynx, and larynx has been reported to result in immediate improved oral intake with less toxicity than is sometimes seen with radiation to the oral cavity.[47] Photodynamic therapy has been reported to be effective in KS, yielding high response rates, and has the advantage over other local therapies in that 40 to 50 lesions can be treated during a single session.[48] It is frequently associated with moderate pain and then photosensitivity for a number of weeks after the treatment.

Cryotherapy is easy to administer and, unlike surgical excision, it can be accomplished without local anesthesia. However, the cosmetic outcome from cryotherapy can be imperfect, particularly in dark-skinned individuals, due to permanent destruction of melanocytes. Topical 9-*cis*-retinoic acid (Panretin Gel) is U.S. Food and Drug Administration approved for use in KS and may result in responses in more than 45% of lesions, but can cause local inflammation and lightening of the skin, yielding inadequate cosmesis in some cases. Intralesional injection or iontophoresis of low-dose vinblastine (0.1 mL of 0.1 mg/mL) or 3% sodium tetradodecyl sulfate injection (0.1 to 0.3 mL) causes a nonspecific necrosis or sclerosis of mucocutaneous tissue with sometimes reasonable cosmetic outcome for small lesions but can be quite painful when administered.

Systemic Therapy

Systemic therapy in addition to HAART should be considered in AIDS-KS if HAART alone is thought to be insufficient therapy and if the tumor burden is not amenable to treatment by local modalities (Table 48.1-4). It is impossible to give a hard and fast rule to determine which patients should be treated with systemic therapies. In considering such approaches, it is worth remembering that the treatment is palliative and often must be continued for a prolonged period. The risk of cumulative toxicity of a given therapy must be weighed against the anticipated benefit. The tumor response to cytotoxic chemotherapy is generally more rapid than antiretroviral therapy alone and occurs in a higher percentage of patients. Cytotoxic chemotherapy is thus often appropriate for patients with KS in whom either a rapid response is desired (and worth the drug toxicity) or who would not be able to tolerate worsening of their disease. Cytotoxic chemotherapy is often indicated for those with extensive cutaneous KS, life-threatening KS, symptomatic visceral KS, substantial pulmonary KS, ulcerating KS, or tumor-related pain. Social withdrawal due to the presence of

TABLE 48.1-4. Therapies for Patients with Advanced Kaposi's Sarcoma

Therapy	Response Rates
COMMONLY USED STANDARD THERAPIES	
HAART	Variable; should be optimized whenever possible in combination with other therapies
Liposomal anthracyclines	
Doxorubicin	59%[52]
Daunorubicin	25%[50]
Paclitaxel	59–71%[53,54]
ALTERNATIVE THERAPIES	
Interferon-α	Variable, CD4 cell dependent
Adriamycin/bleomycin/vinca alkaloids (ABV)	24–88% (Higher response rates with higher doxorubicin doses, but greater toxicity)
Vincristine/vinblastine	45%
Bleomycin/vinca alkaloids	23%

HAART, highly active antiretroviral therapy.

KS is also an important indication for the use of systemic chemotherapy in KS.

Immunotherapy with interferon-α was identified as being active in KS in the early 1980s, particularly in patients with greater than 200 CD4 cells/mm^3 and disease limited to the skin.[49] Interferon should be used in combination with HAART, and there is some evidence that it is effective in patients with lower CD4 counts when so combined. The use of interferon-α is associated with a decreased white blood cell count, flu-like symptoms, and sometimes depression. Interferon-α is most appropriate for disease that is associated with relatively minor morbidity.

During the first decade of the AIDS epidemic, several cytotoxic chemotherapeutic agents were shown to have activity against KS, including the vinca alkaloids, bleomycin, etoposide, and doxorubicin. For some time, the standard of care was to treat milder disease requiring cytotoxic chemotherapy with the vinca alkaloids and more severe disease with a combination of vinca alkaloids, bleomycin, and doxorubicin (ABV).[50]

In the past several years, newly developed monotherapeutic approaches have largely supplanted earlier, more toxic, combination therapies. Approved monotherapy regimens include the liposomal anthracyclines or paclitaxel, used in combination with HAART, for patients requiring cytotoxic chemotherapy.[51] Liposomal formulations of anthracyclines were developed because such formulations have a smaller volume of distribution than the unencapsulated drugs. They also remain in the circulation for a relatively longer time. A related advantage is that they have greater relative uptake in the KS tissue than other tissues as compared to the unencapsulated drugs, in part because of the sequestering of blood that occurs in the lesions. These features all lead such liposomal formulations to have greater tumor specificity and relatively less toxicity than the parent unencapsulated drugs. Two such agents, liposomal daunorubicin (DaunoXome) and pegylated liposomal doxorubicin (Doxil) are now approved by the U.S. Food and Drug Administration for the treatment of KS. In randomized trials, both preparations were found to have equal or better efficacy with less toxicity than the previous standard of care,

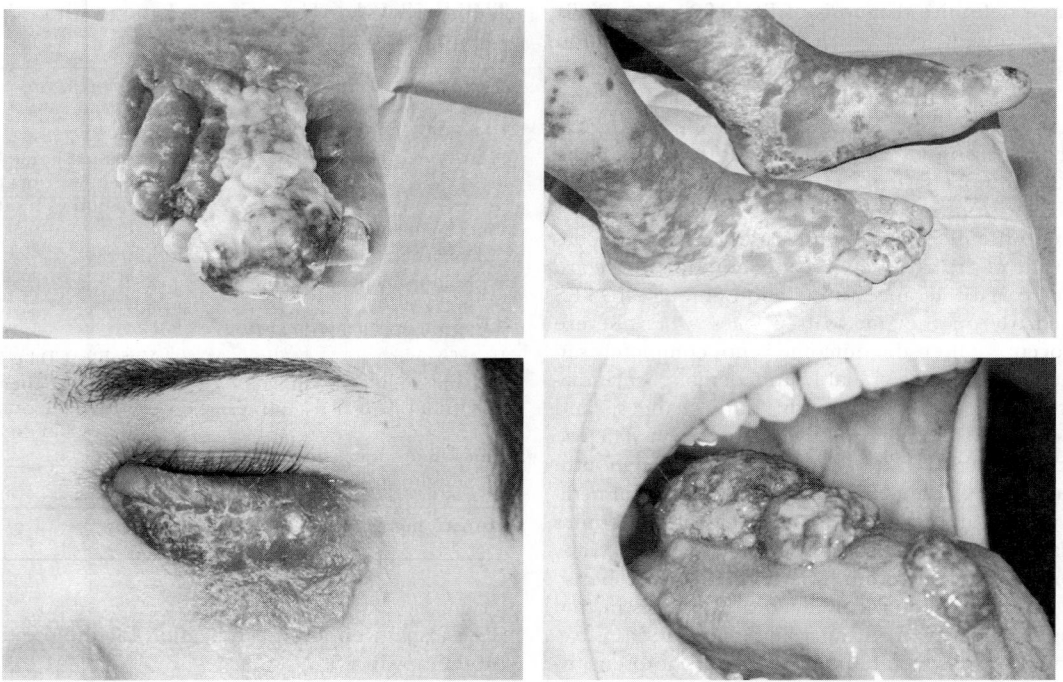

FIGURE 48.1-2. Mucocutaneous manifestations of Kaposi's sarcoma in the era of highly active antiretroviral therapy. (See Color Fig. 48.1-2 in the CD-ROM.)

which was a combination of doxorubicin, vinca alkaloids, and bleomycin.[50,52] Pre-HAART, response rates of nearly 50% were anticipated, and this is improved with concomitant HAART administration.

Paclitaxel was also developed for use in KS based on observations that it targets cellular microtubules (such as vinca alkaloids, shown to be active in KS, albeit causing the opposite effect) and its *in vitro* inhibition of a KS-derived spindle cell line.[53] Responses ranging from 59% to 71% were demonstrated in two phase II trials.[53,54] Largely based on these findings, the U.S. Food and Drug Administration approved paclitaxel as second-line therapy for KS in 1997, although some oncologists recommend it as first-line therapy for life-threatening KS. The principal toxicities in patients with AIDS are neutropenia, alopecia, and neuropathy; doses can be titrated in individual patients to identify a dose that provides an antitumor response with acceptable toxicity. Hypersensitivity due to the cremophor in the preparation requires premedication when using paclitaxel, and 10 mg dexamethasone is generally adequate. In this regard, it is worth remembering that corticosteroids can induce dramatic acceleration of KS growth, and except in such cases in which it is needed (such as for premedication of paclitaxel), pharmacologic doses of systemic steroids should be avoided in patients with KS whenever possible.

The number of cycles of chemotherapy required varies among patients. A general strategy is to treat patients until a reasonable response plateau or remission is attained and then to either stop or increase the time between the doses to maintain the response. Patients with substantial benefit from HAART are most likely to be able to suspend chemotherapy after an early response and maintain or even improve on the tumor response with HAART continuation. However, even with substantial HAART benefit, some patients require ongoing antitumor therapy in addition to HAART, and this is sometimes an indefinite requirement, especially in patients with resistant HIV or aggressive KS. Chronic chemotherapy can be associated with cumulative treatment-related toxicities that can limit the ability to continue therapy. Such considerations serve to emphasize the ongoing considerable challenge remaining in developing better therapy for this condition and serve as a reminder that, although extraordinarily useful in AIDS-KS, HAART is no panacea for this life-threatening tumor[55] (Fig. 48.1-2).

Experimental Approaches to the Treatment of Kaposi's Sarcoma

Development of nontoxic pathogenesis-based therapies would represent a further advance in treatment of AIDS-KS, and a number of approaches, as outlined below, are under active development.

ANTIANGIOGENESIS APPROACHES. KS is a highly vascular tumor, and for this reason, there is currently an interest in exploring the use of angiogenesis inhibitors in patients with KS. Compounds with antiangiogenic activity that have shown evidence of meaningful benefit include thalidomide,[42,56] Col-3,[57] and IL-12.[55] IL-12 has been shown to be a potent inhibitor of angiogenesis, possibly through induction of inducible protein 10, a potent inhibitor of angiogenesis.[58] However, it has other activities, such as induction of type 1 (cytotoxic) T-cell immunity and production of interferon-γ, and it is quite possible that these effects may contribute to its activity in KS. Other possible antiangiogenic compounds, such as antivascular endothelial growth factor antibody or other inhibitors of steps involved in angiogenesis, may be useful in KS.

ANTI–KAPOSI'S SARCOMA–ASSOCIATED HERPESVI-RUS AND MOLECULAR TARGETED APPROACHES. A randomized clinical trial of oral ganciclovir demonstrated that administration of this agent was associated with a lower rate of KS development.[59] This result indicates that an antiherpes drug can reduce the incidence of KS, although it still remains unclear as to how it can affect established lesions. In a small trial of cidofovir in KS, seven of seven patients had disease progression, possibly because of its lack of effect on the early genes in KSHV replication, such as K2/vIL-6 or ORF74/vGPCR, which appear to be most important in the pathogenesis of KS.[60] However, it may be possible to develop other antiviral approaches with therapeutic benefit.

Based on KSHV expression of c-kit receptors, imatinab mesylate (Gleevec) was administered to five patients, four of whom had pathologically confirmed tumor response.[61] Immunohistochemistry showed strong immunoreactivity in the endothelial and spindle cells for phosphorylated and nonphosphorylated c-kit in tumors before treatment, providing compelling justification for further study of this novel targeted approach.

AIDS-ASSOCIATED LYMPHOMAS

EPIDEMIOLOGY AND OVERVIEW

Aggressive non-Hodgkin's B-cell lymphoma was included in the case definition of AIDS in 1985 owing to the increased incidence of these tumors in people with AIDS. Compared to the general population, the risk of developing lymphoma is up to 250-fold higher and, unlike the case with KS, is independent of the particular risk group for HIV acquisition.[62] Additionally, in HIV-infected patients, more than 80% of lymphomas that occur are high-grade B-cell lymphomas,[63] whereas only 10% to 15% of lymphomas among HIV not-infected patients are of this type.[64] NHL is now the second most common AIDS-associated malignancy and is the AIDS-defining diagnosis in roughly 3% of HIV-positive patients, although it is uncertain what percentage of patients already diagnosed with AIDS develop lymphoma. The risk of AIDS-related lymphoma (ARL) increases with the degree and duration of immunosuppression. Since the advent of HAART, the incidence of ARL has decreased by approximately 50%, owing to a decrease in the number of individuals with highly depleted CD4 cells.[62] Importantly, however, the incidence of ARL in patients with any given CD4 count has not been affected by HAART, and as mentioned above, the number of ARL cases is likely to increase as the population of longer-surviving HIV-infected individuals increases with HAART. Also, it is quite possible that the cumulative risk of a given patient developing ARL will increase as patients live longer with a given CD4 count.

Tumor histology and prognosis are related to immune status in ARL[65] (Table 48.1-5). Poor-prognosis immunoblastic tumors tend to occur more frequently with highly advanced immune depletion, and since the advent of HAART, the incidence of these tumors has decreased substantially (most notably the primary brain lymphomas), resulting in a greater relative proportion of the incident cases of better-prognosis diffuse large B-cell centroblastic tumors and Burkitt's lymphomas.[62] Thus, HAART has affected the biology and the epidemiology of ARL, and this changing bioepidemiology is a substantial contributor to the increase in overall survival from approximately 6 to 18 months to 20 months since HAART was introduced as standard therapy for HIV infection.[62,66]

PATHOPHYSIOLOGY

The lymphoproliferative disorders of immune-dysfunction syndromes can serve as a model for ARL pathophysiology. A common theme is that the tumors are often associated with oncogenic viruses and that the specific tumor types vary according to the immune defect.[3] Similarly, ARL histogenesis is influenced by the degree of immune depletion, in part explaining why ARL histologic subtypes track with the CD4 cell count.[66–68] It

TABLE 48.1-5. Comparison of HIV-Associated Lymphomas

Histogenetic Origin	Histology	Viral Associations (%)		Histogenetic Markers (%)		Pathobiologic Markers (%)				CD4 Cells	Prospects for Chemosensitivity
		EBV	KSHV	MUM1	Syn-1	BCL-2	BCL-6	P53	c-MYC		
Germinal center	Burkitt's	<50	0	<15	0	0	100	60	100	May be relatively well preserved	Favorable
	DLBCL centroblastic	<30	0	<30	0	0	>75	Rare	0–50	May be relatively well preserved	Favorable
	Primary brain DLBCL	100	0	>50	<60	90	<50	0	0	<50/mm³	Responds to radiation
Postgerminal center	DLBCL immunoblastic	>80	Rare	100	>50	30	0	0	0–20	Usually low	Poor
	Primary effusion lymphoma	>90	100	100	>90	0	0	0	0	Usually low	Poor
	Plasmablastic (oral cavity associated)	>70	Rare	100	100	0	0	Rare	0	Usually low	Poor

DLBCL, diffuse large B-cell lymphoma (centroblastic, immunoblastic are morphologic variants in the World Health Organization classification system of lymphoid malignancies)[75]; EBV, Epstein-Barr virus; KSHV, Kaposi's sarcoma–associated herpesvirus.
(Adapted from refs. 66–68, 98, and 138.)

is not entirely clear what the relative contribution of immune dysregulation and immune depletion is in lymphomagenesis. For example, chronic stimulation by HIV or other factors may play a role. Aberrant somatic hypermutation of the immunoglobulin V genes appears to be a frequent event in ARL of germinal center (GC) or post-GC B-cell histogenic origin,[69] and the finding that the V_H4 family of immunoglobulin variable genes are frequently hypermutated in ARL[70] supports a role of immune stimulation in ARL development. In some cases, there are intraclonal variants of aberrant hypermutations, suggesting that this can be an ongoing event during lymphomagenesis.[69]

Further highlighting the combined role of immune dysfunction and stimulation is the finding that fewer regional DNA–copy number alterations are seen in diffuse large B-cell lymphomas (DLBCLs) in HIV-infected compared to not-infected patients, suggesting that fewer somatic genomic changes are needed for progression to lymphoma in HIV-immunocompromised hosts.[71] Elevated cytokine levels, including IL-6, IL-10, and tumor necrosis factor-β, are often seen in ARL, suggesting a role for immune dysregulation in lymphomagenesis.[65,72] Consistent with this concept is the finding that chemokine receptor mutations affect the risk of lymphoma. For example, the 3'A variant of stromal cell–derived factor 1 (SDF1) chemokine appears to double and quadruple the NHL risk in heterozygotes and homozygotes for this variant, respectively.[73] Of interest, the SDF1-3'A chemokine variant is carried by 37% of whites and 11% of blacks and may contribute to the lower risk of ARL in blacks compared with whites. The HIV co-receptor CCR5 deletion variant CCR5-Δ32 appears to confer an approximately threefold protection against NHL, independently of its HIV protective effect.[74] The CCR5-Δ32 mutation may be protective against NHL through a mechanism involving a decreased response of B cells to the mitogenic activity of the chemokine RANTES (regulated on activation, normally T cell expressed and secreted). It is possible that such factors may provide a means of assessing the risk of NHL in HIV-infected persons and provide insights for the development of preventive and treatment approaches.

CLASSIFICATION AND TUMOR BIOLOGY

ARL are histologically heterogeneous and are almost invariably derived from monoclonal B-cell populations.[65] The World Health Organization recognizes three major categories of HIV-associated B-cell lymphomas: (1) Burkitt's, (2) DLBCL, and (3) the rarely occurring primary effusion lymphomas (PELs), also termed *body cavity lymphomas*.[75] The HIV-associated DLBCL are mainly comprised of the centroblastic and immunoblastic histologic subtypes. As mentioned earlier in Epidemiology and Overview, the relative proportion of the various tumor types has shifted since the advent of HAART.

It has been long established that distinct clinical and biologic characteristics of ARL track with the immune status.[65] These observations have been confirmed through histogenetic markers and microarray assays of gene expression that have reinforced the correlation between the immune environment and tumor histogenesis (see Table 48.1-5). The heterogeneity of genetic lesions involved in ARL pathogenesis includes chromosomal translocations that deregulate the expression of various protooncogenes and appears to some extent to be influenced by the immune status.[65–67,76] The resulting tumor biology is a major determinant of treatment sensitivity, as confirmed by

gene expression patterns that predict treatment outcome in HIV-unrelated DLBCL.[77] A closer examination of this follows.

Immunoblastic tumors that arise in the setting of advanced immune depletion are more likely to be of post-GC B-cell origin, expressing the histogenic markers syndecan-1 and MUM-1 and the antiapoptotic protein bcl-2. It has been found that bcl-2 expression and activation of the NF-κB signaling pathway confer resistance to apoptosis in the post-GC B-cell tumors, and this could partially explain the poor prognosis of these tumors.[78] Also, 70% to 90% of these tumors are Epstein-Barr virus (EBV) associated, whereas only 30% to 50% of Burkitt's and centroblastic DLBCL are EBV associated. The immunoblastic tumors often exhibit EBV latency type 3 expression and in particular express EBNA-2 and LMP-1, which are EBV-specific antigenic targets.[79] It has been hypothesized that as immune injury advances, EBV-specific cytotoxic T-cell responses become impaired, thus allowing immune escape of the emerging lymphomatous clone. The EBV gene LMP-1 may be involved in lymphomagenesis by increasing the threshold for cells to undergo programmed cell death,[80] at least through up-regulation of the cellular antiapoptotic oncogene, bcl-2,[81] which may be densely expressed in immunoblastic cases.[82] EBNA-2 expression has been reported to be associated with extranodal disease,[83] which is a prominent feature of the immunoblastic HIV-related DLBCL. If EBV is found in centroblastic and Burkitt's cases, EBNA-2 and LMP-1 are not typically expressed, underscoring the importance of other genetic lesions in these tumors.[68]

HIV-related centroblastic DLBCL and Burkitt's lymphoma have a tendency to occur when the immune system has not yet suffered extensive injury from HIV, and these tumors are more likely to express bcl-6, lacking the aforementioned histogenic markers associated with post-GC B-cell immunoblastic tumors. Pathobiologic and microarray analysis confirm their GC B-cell origin.[65,67,76] Microarray analysis has confirmed superior survival in GC B-cell–derived DLBCL compared to DLBCL having activated B-like expression patterns in the HIV not-related setting,[77] a finding that appears to also describe bcl-2–negative DLBCL in ARL.[66] Such data reinforce the idea that the improved survival of patients with ARL in the HAART era is most likely due to the relative shift in the greater proportionate incidence of tumors with GC B-cell histogenic origin rather than any putative specific treatment effect of HAART during lymphoma therapy.[66]

Other pathobiologic markers of tumor resistance such as p53 mutation and c-myc expression also are correlated with histogenetic origin and histology. Those tumors derived from GC B cells are more likely to show c-myc activation; this occurs in essentially 100% of Burkitt's cases and up to 50% of centroblastic DLBCL, but rarely in immunoblastic lymphomas.[65] Burkitt-like lymphomas may be a morphologic variant in a continuum from Burkitt's to DLBCL in the context of the range of immunodepletion that occurs in HIV-infected patients. The frequency of EBV infection in AIDS–Burkitt-like lymphoma (80%) is similar to that in diffuse large cell lymphoma, but the pattern of viral latency is similar to that seen in Burkitt's lymphoma (i.e., no LMP-1 or EBNA-2 expression) in approximately 60% of the cases. Also, patients with AIDS–Burkitt-like lymphoma usually have a relatively low CD4 count, similar to that seen in the diffuse large-cell immunoblastic lymphomas. The clinical manifestations can also vary from Burkitt's lymphoma. For example, these tumors do not seem to share the predilection for central nervous system (CNS) involvement associated with Burkitt's lymphoma. p53 mutations are seen in

40% to 60% of ARL but appear to be unrelated to prognosis, a distinction that may suggest a different pathobiology for this marker compared to non-AIDS–related NHL.[66]

The precise histogenetic derivation and the molecular pathogenesis of AIDS–primary CNS lymphoma (AIDS-PCNSL) are poorly understood. Essentially all of these tumors are EBV associated. Evidence suggests that they may be segregated into two major biologic categories based on the expression pattern of bcl-6, LMP-1, and bcl-2.[84] A substantial proportion of these tumors appear to be derived from GC B cells, although they show immunoblastic histology.[85] This finding may have therapeutic implications.

The rarely occurring tumor PEL, also of post-GC B-cell origin,[86] exhibits distinctive clinical and biologic features, including immunoblastic morphology and indeterminate immunophenotype. Monoclonality can be established by the finding of clonal immunoglobulin gene rearrangements, indicating late B-cell genotype derivation that may have undergone antigenic selection.[87] These tumors are universally associated with KSHV and appear to follow the same epidemiologic pattern as KS.[88] The majority of PEL are also EBV positive.

It is unclear why PEL develop in the pleural spaces, although study of the KSHV genome may provide insights into this predilection. Hypoxia can activate lytic KSHV replication,[89] and there is some evidence that KSHV-encoded vBcl-2 is up-regulated by hypoxia.[90] Activation of vBcl-2 and other KSHV genes may contribute to the development of lymphoma in the relatively hypoxic environment of the pleural spaces and may also help to explain why these tumors are poorly responsive to chemotherapy. These observations may provide insights toward developing novel therapeutic strategies for this rare tumor.

Other lymphomas that are seen with increased frequency in the setting of HIV include Hodgkin's disease (HD), polymorphic lymphoproliferative disorders resembling posttransplant-associated lymphoproliferative disease, and lymphomatoid granulomatosis, but these are non–AIDS defining. Multicentric Castleman's disease (MCD) is sporadically reported in HIV-infected patients and is of interest because of its association with KSHV and other similarities with lymphomagenesis.[75] Affected patients may have a 15-fold increased risk of lymphoma compared to the general HIV-infected population.

KSHV-associated MCD is likely to be a unique entity from other forms of MCD. Almost all MCD in HIV infection are KSHV related, whereas approximately 50% of MCD occurring in non–HIV-infected individuals are KSHV related. Although poorly described, the disease has a short median survival of less than 2 years and is probably a cytokine-driven syndrome related to the highly lytic state of the KSHV found in the tumors.[91,92] Many of the symptoms of MCD appear to derive from hyperproduction of viral or cellular IL-6. No standard therapy is recognized for KSHV-MCD, but case reports have suggested possible roles of interferon-α, rituximab,[93] and antiviral therapy.[94]

CLINICAL PRESENTATION AND STAGING OF PERIPHERAL LYMPHOMAS

ARL frequently present as advanced stage III or IV disease and behave aggressively, with unusual patterns of organ involvement.[95,96] The majority of patients present with either a rapidly growing mass lesion or the development of systemic "B" symptoms (unexplained fever, drenching night sweats, or unexplained weight loss in excess of 10% of the normal body weight). Extranodal involvement is common, including the bone marrow (25% to 40%), gastrointestinal tract (26%), and CNS (17% to 32%).

In addition to the standard NHL staging for patients not HIV infected, the CD4 cell count, HIV viral load, and CNS assessment should be performed in all ARL cases. Computed tomography of the brain with contrast is adequate to assess for large parenchymal brain lesions, but magnetic resonance imaging with gadolinium has the potential advantage of revealing evidence of leptomeningeal involvement by lymphoma. Cytologic examination of the cerebrospinal fluid should be performed in all cases.

The surrogate factor most correlated with prognosis is the CD4 cell count. With standard therapy, in the pre-HAART era, patients with fewer than 100 CD4 cells/mm^3 have a median survival of approximately 4 months, whereas those with 100 or greater CD4 cells/mm^3 have a median survival of 11 months.[97] Since the advent of HAART, there has been a modest improvement in survival to 20 months.[62] Although this improvement has been attributed to concurrent administration of HAART with chemotherapy, there are thus far no data that specifically confirm this impression, and high response rates and long-term disease-free survival equivalent to those seen in HIV-unrelated DLBCL can be achieved without concurrent antiretroviral therapy[66] (Fig. 48.1-3). An explanation that fits the available data is that the principal basis for the improved survival is a bioepidemiologic shift in ARL linked to the immunologic effects of HAART during lymphomagenesis.[98] The international prognostic index for lymphoma may be of some utility in AIDS-lymphomas, although its use is not widely reported and may need reassessment in the HAART era. In any case, such clinical criteria are nonspecific, and the available evidence suggests that these markers are of limited utility. More specific disease diagnosis based on tumor biology using methods such as gene expression analysis have better prognostic value and have already been developed, although they are not yet widely applied.[77]

TREATMENT OF PERIPHERAL AIDS-RELATED LYMPHOMAS

Treatment of ARL must take into consideration the fact that two interrelated life-threatening diseases characterize the diag-

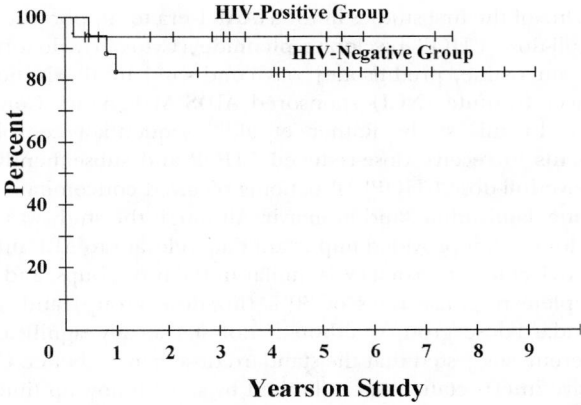

FIGURE 48.1-3. Progression-free survival in human immunodeficiency virus (HIV)-related and unrelated bcl-2–negative diffuse large B-cell lymphoma treated with dose-adjusted etopside, prednisone, vincristine, cyclophosphamide, and doxorubicin (EPOCH). (From ref. 66, with permission.)

TABLE 48.1-6. Selected Regimens and Outcomes for AIDS-Associated Non-Hodgkin's Lymphoma

Regimen	Evaluable Patients (n)	Median Baseline CD4 Cells/mm³	Complete Response Rate (%)	Median Overall/Disease-Free Survival (Mo)	Author
Low- or standard-dose m-BACOD	175	100 (low), 107 (standard)	41 (low), 52 (standard)	8/8	Kaplan et al.[99]
Low- or standard-dose CHOP plus HAART	53	119	35 (low), 37 (standard)	Not available (limited follow-up)	Ratner et al.[100]
Infusional CDE	48	70	46	8/15	Sparano et al.[139]
Infusional CDE + rituximab + HAART	29	132	86	Not available (limited follow-up)	Tirelli et al.[106]
Various chemotherapy + HAART (retrospective)	44	144	52 (71% in long-term HAART responders)	12/not available	Antinori et al.[105]
Dose-adjusted EPOCH (HAART deferment until chemotherapy completion)	39	198	74	Not yet reached (at 53 mo, OS is 60% and DFS is 92%)	Little et al.[66]

CDE, cyclophosphamide, doxorubicin, VP-16; CHOP, cyclophosphamide, doxorubicin, vincristine, prednisone; DFS, disease-free survival; EPOCH, etoposide, prednisone, vincristine, cyclophosphamide, doxorubicin; HAART, highly active antiretroviral therapy; m-BACOP, moderate-dose methotrexate, bleomycin, doxorubicin (Adriamycin), cyclophosphamide, vincristine (Oncovin), dexamethasone; OS, overall survival.

nosis. This fact has underscored the approach to treatment of this disease (Table 48.1-6). Optimal care of ARL requires that the care team has substantial expertise in lymphoma and in the management of patients with HIV infection.

Issues that predominated and constrained therapeutic approaches early in the epidemic have been modified somewhat by advances in HIV therapy. Before HAART, chemotherapy-associated toxicity, such as febrile neutropenia, that would generally be tolerated in HIV not-infected patients, was often poorly tolerated, and reduction of such toxicity was the guiding principle that led to the development of low-dose chemotherapy for ARL.[99] However, the development of HAART has resulted in better tolerance of chemotherapy in the majority of patients with ARL, and this has led to a new standard of care that recognizes the presumed therapeutic advantage of standard-dose chemotherapy for most patients. No standard of care has been defined that dictates a specific chemotherapy regimen in ARL, and identifying the best chemotherapeutic regimen for various subsets of patients is one focus of clinical research. Other important unresolved areas are the potential role of rituximab and how to coordinate treatment of the ARL with AIDS care and HAART.

One of the first studies in the HAART era to support the use of full-dose CHOP [cyclophosphamide (Cytoxan), doxorubicin, vincristine, prednisone] was conducted by the National Cancer Institute (NCI)–sponsored AIDS Malignancy Consortium. In this study, Ratner et al.[100] sequentially enrolled patients to receive dose-reduced CHOP and subsequently to receive full-dose CHOP. All patients received concomitant stavudine, lamivudine, and indinavir. Although the study was not randomized, it provided important data relevant to ARL in the HAART era. The toxicity was similar in the two groups, and the complete response rates of 30% (low-dose group) and 47% (standard-dose group), although not statistically significantly different, suggested that the standard dose may be better. Conclusive interpretations were limited by short follow-up time in the study.

This was also one of the first studies to document the complicated pharmacokinetic interactions that occur with coadministration of HAART and chemotherapy. Pharmacokinetic data were collected and compared to those of historic controls

who received CHOP without HAART. Elimination of cyclophosphamide was decreased from 70 mL/min/m² in historic controls to 39 mL/min/m² in the study patients. Doxorubicin elimination and the area under the time concentration curve of indinavir were similar to those in previous studies of these agents. The study supports the feasibility of such an approach, because there were no obvious clinical complications. However, in an uncontrolled study such as this, subtle toxicity effects could be difficult to demonstrate. In another trial that assessed pharmacokinetics of chemotherapy and antiretroviral therapy, plasma etoposide levels were reported to be decreased by 11% to 38% on chemotherapy cycles given with didanosine compared to cycles without didanosine administration.[101] These results serve as a reminder that there may be complex and unexpected drug interactions when one attempts to combine chemotherapy with complicated anti-HIV regimens, that these interactions are dependent on the specific drugs and administration schedules, and that these interactions may affect the outcome of either therapy. Rigorous study of the myriad interactions between antiretroviral drugs and drugs used to treat lymphoma has become somewhat impractical as the number of anti-HIV drugs continues to expand.[102]

These studies, as well as several epidemiologic and retrospective studies reported during the last several years, have given rise to the notion that improvements in ARL overall survival are due to coadministration of HAART with antineoplastic therapy. However, there are no controlled data that specifically address this issue, and the potential confounding factors that are inherent in such studies[103] introduce some uncertainty into this view. Also, as noted earlier in Clinical Presentation and Staging of Peripheral Lymphomas, there is an alternative interpretation that fits the available data. Most of the data include patients who were already receiving HAART at the time the lymphoma was diagnosed, and it is thus difficult to differentiate whether the improved outcome is due to the effect of HAART during lymphomagenesis or to its coadministration with the antineoplastic chemotherapy. Central to this, one must consider the complicated interrelationship of HAART, immune status, and tumor histogenesis. With this in mind, it is worthwhile to critically examine some of the studies.

Vaccher et al.[104] retrospectively compared a group of 24 patients with HIV-NHL who were treated with CHOP chemotherapy plus HAART with a group of 80 earlier patients who were treated with either CHOP or a CHOP-like regimen before the introduction of HAART. Substantially greater World Health Organization grade 3 to 4 myelotoxicity and neurotoxicity occurred in the patients who received CHOP-HAART compared with those who received chemotherapy alone, but the OI rates and mortality were significantly higher in the no-HAART group. Although the concurrent HAART may have resulted in the decreased OI rate, an alternative explanation may be that standards of care for OI prophylaxis and CD4 cell status at lymphoma diagnosis explain the difference, as HAART-induced immune reconstitution has decreased the size of the at-risk population with extremely advanced immune suppression. In another retrospective study, Antinori et al.[105] reported that those who had long-term virologic responses to HAART had improved lymphoma outcome. The overall complete response rate was 52%, but the subset analysis yielded differential responses between groups defined as HAART responders or HAART failures/HAART naive. Although the former group had a complete response rate of 71% compared to the latter group's response rate of 30%, the groups were different by virtue of the criteria on which they were defined and selected, and this uncontrolled bias precludes the ability to assign attribution to concurrent HAART as the factor causing the different outcome. Again, an alternative explanation may be that the immunologic milieu in those responding to HAART was sufficiently different from the others that tumor histogenesis was differentially affected, giving rise to biologically distinct tumors more responsive to therapy. Thus, there may or may not be a specific therapeutic role for HAART, but the retrospective data in question do not resolve the issue. In any case, these data do not support the notion that concurrent HAART decreases the efficacy of a bolus chemotherapy regimen.

Another important issue in ARL is whether the use of rituximab will confer benefit when added to combination chemotherapy in a manner similar to that for non–HIV-related NHL. Preliminary analysis of concomitant HAART (no specific regimen) and CDE (cyclophosphamide, doxorubicin, VP-16) plus rituximab appears favorable, as shown by a high complete response rate of 86%.[106] Although encouraging, full scrutiny of these data is limited by a short follow-up time of 9 months, and, therefore, whether an improvement occurs in progression-free and disease-free survival cannot yet be assessed.

The most definitive examination of rituximab in ARL to date was a randomized trial conducted by investigators of the NCI-sponsored AIDS Malignancy Consortium. Standard-dose CHOP with HAART (no specific regimen) was given to all patients randomized to receive rituximab or no rituximab.[107] Complete responses were seen in 58% of those randomized to receive rituximab and in 50% of those who did not. Although there was no statistical difference in the efficacy, the rituximab arm had more treatment-related deaths (15% vs. 2%). Some evidence in HIV-unrelated NHL suggests that rituximab confers a benefit only in DLBCL expressing bcl-2.[108] Because ARL rarely express bcl-2, rituximab may have a limited role in this disease[66] and yet may have contributed to toxicity. Longer-term follow-up for this study is not available.

A study conducted at the NCI has provided information about the potential for satisfactory therapeutic results with ARL in the era of HAART.[66] This was a phase II study of 39 patients with a median potential follow-up of 53 months. The

Drug	Total Dose (mg/m²/d)	Route	Day 1 2 3 4 5 6 14 22
Etoposide	50	CIV	x---x---x---x---
Vincristine	0.4	CIV	x---x---x---x---
Doxorubicin	10	CIV	x---x---x---x---
**Cyclophosphamide			
CD4 < 100	187	IV	x
CD4 ≥ 100	375	IV	x
Prednisone	60	PO	x x x x x
Filgrastim			xxxxx
New Cycle Begins			x

FIGURE 48.1-4. Dose-adjusted EPOCH [etoposide, prednisone, vincristine (Oncovin), cyclophosphamide, and doxorubicin] for AIDS-related lymphoma. **First cycle only. Subsequent cycles adjusted down by 187 mg/m² if absolute neutrophil count <500/mm³; otherwise, increase by 187 mg/m² to a maximum of 750 mg/m².

study used a dose-adjusted modification of etoposide, prednisone, vincristine, cyclophosphamide, and doxorubicin (DA-EPOCH) (Fig. 48.1-4). Antiretroviral therapy was deferred until completion of chemotherapy (maximum of six cycles), and then HAART was optimized. The basis of this dose-adjusted strategy was to balance the chemotherapy-related immune injury with optimal dose intensity for best curative potential of the regimen using myelotoxicity as a surrogate marker for individual patient tolerance to chemotherapy. The decision by the research team to suspend antiretroviral therapy during the period of chemotherapy was based on a number of considerations. One was that cytotoxic chemotherapy for lymphoma is expected to deplete the CD4 cell compartment by 800 or more cells/mm³ in HIV not-infected patients.[109] By contrast, fewer than 20 CD4 cells/mm³ would be predicted lost due to HIV alone, even at high viral loads, during the 16 weeks of DA-EPOCH.[110] Thus, an important therapeutic goal of HAART (e.g., maintenance or increase, or both, in the CD4 cell compartment) would not be realized during chemotherapy, but the potential risks of such therapy would remain. Such risks include overlapping toxicities, unpredictable pharmacokinetic interactions that could change the therapeutic effects of the antilymphoma and the anti-HIV drugs, and an increase in the likelihood that patients would not adhere to the HAART regimen because of toxicities from the ARL therapy. These risks could adversely affect the curative potential of the lymphoma treatment (e.g., dose delays or reductions, or both) and the long-term control of HIV (e.g., poor absorption or adherence leading to resistant HIV). Also, any theoretic benefit that HAART may have in protecting the normal lymphocytes during chemotherapy could also have the undesirable effect of protecting the malignant lymphocytes from the effects of the cytotoxic drugs. Moreover, HAART deferment on the basis of these considerations appeared consistent with guidelines for the use of antiretroviral agents in HIV-1 infected adults and adolescents set forth by the Panel on Clinical Practices for Treatment of HIV Infection convened by the Department of Health and Human Services.[111]

Although the study was not designed to address whether antiretroviral drug suspension is better, equivalent, or inferior to concomitant HAART, it did demonstrate that for bcl-2–negative tumors, ARL outcome is equivalent to that in HIV-unrelated DLBCL selected for equivalent clinical indices, and it established ARL as a highly curable tumor[66] (see Fig. 48.1-3). Moreover, HIV viral loads were controlled as expected for uncomplicated HIV infection, and CD4 counts recovered to baseline within 12 months after HAART reinstitution, a similar pattern seen in HIV not-infected patients receiving similar therapy.[112] Although selection bias is always a concern in single-institution studies such as this, no known disease elements in aggressive NHL predict a disease-free survival of 92% at 53 months with standard CHOP, which thus argues against selection bias as accounting for the results. Consideration of the tumor biology, however, may help explain the results: ARL tend to densely express markers associated with high tumor proliferation, an adverse pathobiologic marker with standard bolus CHOP[113] but not with EPOCH[114]; ARL tend to be associated with multidrug-resistance proteins that would confer resistance to CHOP but might be overcome with infusional therapy[115]; and a greater proportion of ARL since HAART express pathobiologic markers of GC B-cell histogenesis than the HIV not-infected series. A multi-institutional trial conducted by investigators of the NCI extramural AIDS Malignancy Consortium is under way to further investigate the approach.

A high percentage (15% to 20%) of HIV-associated lymphomas have involvement of the CNS at presentation.[97] Therefore, in HIV-associated lymphomas, routine CNS prophylaxis with intrathecal methotrexate or cytosine arabinoside should be considered standard practice. Markers of increased risk of CNS involvement include sites of extranodal involvement and EBV detection by polymerase chain reaction (PCR) analysis of the CSF,[116] but these data cannot yet be incorporated into standard-of-care decision making to identify those for whom intrathecal prophylaxis is unnecessary. CNS involvement by lymphoma confers an extremely poor prognosis, and combination intrathecal chemotherapy and whole brain radiotherapy are often required, but the toxic effects may defeat the goals of this approach.[66]

PRIMARY CENTRAL NERVOUS SYSTEM LYMPHOMA IN AIDS

OVERVIEW AND PATHOLOGY

In the pre-HAART era, PCNSL comprised approximately 19% of ARL, which is substantially higher than its representation in non–AIDS-NHL (approximately 1%). PCNSL occurs most frequently in patients with a CD4 cell count of less than $50/mm^3$ and can occur in the setting of other CNS pathology such as toxoplasmosis. Computed tomography or magnetic resonance scans usually demonstrate single or multiple contrast-enhancing masses that are not reliably distinguishable from toxoplasmosis or other CNS processes. HAART has profoundly reduced the incidence of these tumors.[62]

Definitive diagnosis of focal brain lesions in AIDS patients requires biopsy and yields a greater than 92% diagnostic rate. However, there is often some reluctance to do this procedure. Although stereotactic biopsy is generally safe, the location of some lesions poses technical challenge and can introduce potential morbidity to the patient as well as risk to the surgical team. Therefore, in many medical centers it has become standard practice to treat AIDS patients who have focal brain lesions and antitoxoplasmosis antibodies empirically with antitoxoplasmosis therapy, reserving biopsy for those patients who are seronegative for antitoxoplasma antibodies or fail to respond to

treatment. However, delay in diagnosis can adversely affect survival in AIDS-PCNSL. Such factors necessitate consideration of alternative, less invasive diagnostic modalities. If a brain biopsy is performed, it is important to remember that corticosteroids administered to control intracerebral swilling can have a rapid antitumor response and cause false-negative biopsies even in the face of lymphoma. In such a situation, it is important to perform the biopsy as soon after the first dose of steroid as possible or even, if deemed safe, before the steroid therapy.

A major advance in the field based on a study by Antinori et al.[117] is the relatively noninvasive diagnostic capability using CSF EBV-DNA detection by PCR and thallium 201 single photon emission computed tomography. The basis for this approach is the observation that nearly all HIV-related PCNSLs are associated with EBV infection and that detection of CSF EBV-DNA by PCR in HIV-infected patients with brain lesions is reliably associated with PCNSLs.[118] The presence of increased uptake and positive EBV-DNA had 100% sensitivity and 100% positive predictive value. Because PCNSL likelihood is extremely high in patients with hyperactive lesions and positive EBV-DNA, brain biopsy may be avoided, and patients could promptly undergo definitive therapy. These results suggest that if both tests are positive, radiotherapy for PCNSL can commence without delay, whereas if both tests are negative, there is 100% negative predictive value against lymphoma. This is one of the very rare situations in oncology in which it may be acceptable medical practice to administer RT (or chemotherapy) without a tissue diagnosis of cancer. Readers should be alert, however, for future studies that may affect the recommendations for management of such patients. Discordance between the two tests requires biopsy for prompt diagnosis or, if this cannot be obtained, presumptive therapy for toxoplasmosis and then lymphoma therapy if no response is observed.

TREATMENT

PCNSL is highly responsive to whole brain irradiation, and a substantial proportion of patients can be expected to have complete tumor eradication; however, they have a high likelihood of subsequently succumbing to OI or recurrent PCNSL, even within the radiation field. In a study of 55 AIDS patients with biopsy-proven primary CNS lymphomas, all tumors responded clinically and radiologically to whole brain RT consisting of 4000 rads in 267-rad fractions over 3 weeks or an equivalent dose.[119] The mean duration of survival from the appearance of symptoms consistent with the mass lesion was significantly greater in patients who received RT than in those who did not (134 vs. 42 days). Autopsy findings showed that patients who did not receive RT generally died from tumor progression, whereas those who completed RT often died of OIs. Such observations emphasize the need for early diagnosis and treatment and for effective treatment of OIs and HAART optimization.[119] Because these tumors nearly universally develop only after the CD4 cells have fallen below $50 \text{ cells}/mm^3$, the therapeutic approach may best be to include HAART to achieve rapid immune reconstitution. Most patients do not benefit with high-dose chemotherapy, in part because of excessive toxicity in AIDS patients.[120] Also, if immune reconstitution in fact is useful as part of the treatment for this condition, use of immunosuppressive high-dose chemotherapy could be counterproductive, but clinical data are inadequate to define this. Surgery has no therapeutic role in PCNSL because microscopic tumor infiltration into brain parenchyma extends from the site of primary involvement.

HODGKIN'S DISEASE

EPIDEMIOLOGY AND PATHOGENESIS

Although HD is not an AIDS-defining condition, it has a clear association with HIV disease: It presents in HIV-infected patients with distinct clinical and biologic characteristics that distinguish it from its HIV-negative counterpart ("primary" HD), and it occurs with somewhat increased frequency among HIV-infected patients.[4] Among HIV-infected patients, the most common histologic HD subtype is mixed cellularity, followed by lymphocyte depletion.[121] EBV infection appears to be more predominant among cases of HIV-associated HD (78% to 100% of cases) than in cases of primary HD (15% to 58% of cases).

CLINICAL PRESENTATION, TREATMENT, AND PROGNOSIS

Patients with HIV-associated HD generally present at a younger age, with higher-stage disease, less frequent mediastinal involvement, more frequent involvement of extranodal sites of disease, and more frequent occurrence of B symptoms compared to their HIV not-infected counterparts[121] (Table 48.1-7). Immune status is often relatively good, with more than 275 CD4 cells/mm^3 in patients diagnosed with HIV-associated HD.

Prognosis is generally poorer for HIV-HD than for primary HD. HIV-HD patients frequently have a number of features that have been associated with poor prognosis in primary non-HIV–associated HD, including male sex, large number of sites involved, and mixed cellularity or lymphocyte-depleted histology. In general, complete response rates are relatively high with systemic chemotherapy (50% to greater than 80%), but relapse of HD is common. For patients successfully treated for HD, long-term control of HIV may improve survival compared to the pre-HAART era.

No real separate standard of care is available for HIV-HD, but conventional chemotherapy regimens such as ABVD (doxorubicin, bleomycin, vinblastine, and dacarbazine) or combined modality therapy are used.[122] Because of the occurrence of multiple poor prognostic factors in HIV-HD, most oncologists advocate use of systemic chemotherapy in all clinically staged patients. CNS evaluation and prophylaxis are not indicated because the CNS is distinctly uncommonly involved.

ANOGENITAL CANCERS IN HUMAN IMMUNODEFICIENCY VIRUS INFECTION

Cervical cancer was added to the CDC list of AIDS-defining conditions in 1993.[123] Anal cancer, although not an AIDS-defining condition, is also relatively prevalent among HIV-infected women and homosexual and bisexual men with HIV infection.[124] These cancers are associated with human papillomavirus (HPV) infection and appear to be more aggressive in HIV-infected than in non–HIV-infected individuals. It is thus recommended that HIV-infected women undergo regular periodic cervical Papanicolaou (Pap) testing. The CDC has recommended cytologic screening as part of the initial evaluation when HIV seropositivity is diagnosed. The CDC recommends that if the initial Pap smear is normal, at least one additional evaluation should be repeated within 6 months.[125] If the repeat is normal, reevaluation should be done at least annually. If the initial or follow-up Pap smear shows severe inflammation with reactive squamous cellular changes, another Pap smear should be collected within 3 months. If the initial or follow-up Pap smear shows squamous intraepithelial lesions or atypical squamous cells of undetermined significance, the woman should be referred for a colposcopic examination of the lower genital tract and, if indicated, undergo colposcopically directed biopsies. HIV infection is not an indication for colposcopy among women with normal Pap smears. Because of the common occurrence of HPV-associated cytologic abnormalities in the anal mucosa of HIV-infected women and homosexual men, some experts have suggested that routine periodic cytologic examination of the anal mucosa should also be considered in

TABLE 48.1-7. Comparison of Human Immunodeficiency Virus–Associated Hodgkin's Disease and Primary Hodgkin's Disease

Feature	Reference[121]		Reference[140]		Reference[141]
	HIV+ (n = 114)	HIV– (n = 104)	HIV+ (n = 45)	HIV– (n = 407)	HIV+ (n = 46)
Age (median)	29	38	30	31	27
CD4 (median)	275	N/A	306	N/A	—
Histology (%)					
MC	45	29	49	20	41
LD	21	—	4	—	22
NS	30	59	40	—	22
Mediastinal disease (%)					
NS	27	80	10	71	—
MC	23	21	3	—	—
Stage III–IV (%)	81	44	75	—	89
Extranodal disease (%)	63	29	33	—	>41
Epstein-Barr virus–positive tumor (%)	78	25	—	—	—
B symptoms (%)	77	35	80	—	83
Prior acquired immunodeficiency syndrome diagnosis (%)	17	N/A	11	N/A	6

HIV, human immunodeficiency virus; LD, lymphocyte depleted; MC, mixed cellularity; NS, nodular sclerosing.

high-risk individuals. A model to estimate the clinical benefits and cost effectiveness of screening HIV-positive homosexual and bisexual men for anal squamous intraepithelial lesions and anal squamous cell cancer indicates that Pap screening every 1 to 2 years beginning in early HIV disease would result in an incremental cost-effectiveness ratio of $13,000 to $16,000 per quality-adjusted life year saved and thus offers quality-adjusted life expectancy benefits at a cost comparable with that of other accepted clinical preventive interventions.[126] HPV vaccines have not been evaluated in this setting, but strategies to prevent HPV-related tumors might include this approach.

CERVICAL CANCER

Epidemiology

Squamous intraepithelial lesions, vulvovaginal condyloma acuminatum, and anal intraepithelial neoplasia are seen with approximately fivefold increase in HIV-infected women compared to HIV not-infected women.[127] Among sexually active women, HIV-infected women have a substantially higher rate of persistent HPV infections of the types most strongly associated with intraepithelial lesions and invasive cervical cancer, that is, HPV-16 or HPV-18.[128,129] The increased prevalence of HPV infection among HIV-infected women may explain the increased incidence of squamous intraepithelial lesions in this population.

Greater immune suppression is associated with increased incidence of high-grade cervical intraepithelial neoplasia in HIV-infected women who may also present with invasive cervical cancer at a younger age and with more aggressive advanced-stage disease compared to HIV-seronegative women. This suggests that progression of HPV-associated dysplasia to frank invasive anogenital cancers may be more rapid in this population. In addition, women with a CD4 cell count less than 500/mm^3 appear to be at greater risk for poor outcome.[130] The incidence of invasive cervical cancer appears unchanged since the advent of HAART,[131] but it is unclear whether this is due to reduced usage of these medications among the women at highest risk for HIV and HPV, or some other factor. Likewise, the effect of HAART on the incidence of anal squamous intraepithelial lesions is as yet unclear, but the data suggest that HAART may not result in regression of these lesions.[132] However, progressive immunodeficiency may increase the risk of persistent oncogenic HPV infection, and the amount of HPV-16 DNA in cervicovaginal lavage is significantly increased in those who are HIV infected.[133] Thus, it is plausible that HIV may be a cofactor for the oncogenic effects of HPV.

Therapy

Standard therapy for preinvasive cervical neoplasia, including cryotherapy, laser therapy, cone biopsy, and loop excision, appears to be somewhat less effective in women with HIV infection because of the twofold higher frequency of recurrence even among those with high CD4 cell count.[134] The lower the CD4 count, the higher the risk for recurrence.

Invasive cervical cancer should be approached with the same principles of oncologic management that guide treatment of cervical cancer in HIV-negative patients. Patients with well-controlled HIV infection and relative immune preservation can be expected to have outcomes similar to those of HIV-

negative women, and thus HAART should be included as part of the overall treatment plan when feasible. Also, because advanced HIV disease may be more intolerant of the myelosuppressive effects of RT and combination chemotherapy, HAART can be expected to be of benefit. When such therapy is administered concomitantly with antiretroviral therapy, potential for overlapping toxicity of the various agents should be considered in the therapeutic plan.

ANAL CANCER

Evidence of HPV infection of the anal canal and anal cancer and the immediate precursor lesions, high-grade anal intraepithelial neoplasia, are common among HIV-infected women[127] and among men who have sex with men, especially those with HIV or immunosuppression.[135] A history of recent anal warts predicted for HPV DNA in all men. Anal squamous intraepithelial lesions do not appear to regress in patients receiving HAART, but among those with high CD4 cell counts the effect appears to be variable.

For invasive anal cancer, standard combined chemotherapy and radiation appear to effectively control disease in most patients.[136] Patients with CD4 counts less than 200/mm^3 appear more likely to experience treatment-related toxicity, including cytopenias, intractable diarrhea, or moist desquamation requiring hospitalization or a colostomy either for a therapy-related complication or for salvage. Patients with CD4 of 200/mm^3 or greater appear to have better disease control with acceptable morbidity. Novel regimens such as those using infusional cisplatin and 5-fluorouracil with radiotherapy that appear to have good tolerance among HIV not-infected individuals may be appropriate to consider in HIV-infected individuals, but the specific data are not available.[137]

FUTURE DIRECTIONS

Most AIDS-associated cancers are virally mediated neoplastic processes. In this regard, HIV can play a varied role. It can induce an immunosuppressed host in which oncogenic viral infection and opportunistic neoplasia can develop relatively unchecked, and it can serve to stimulate the immune system to secrete cytokines that promote cellular proliferation and oligoclonal expansions of cells infected with a variety of known oncogenic viruses. Molecular interactions between HIV-related proteins (or factors induced by HIV) and genomic sequences in some of these viruses may modulate their oncogenic potential. Many AIDS-associated cancers thus appear to be preventable. However, as with many other cancers, it is unlikely that behavioral prevention alone can eliminate these epidemic neoplasms. Great strides in the treatment of HIV infection have recently been made, although it is too soon to determine the ultimate effect of these advances on opportunistic neoplastic disease. The greater understanding of the virologic and molecular basis of these cancers may provide opportunities for advancement in prevention and treatment through antiangiogenesis approaches and antiviral, vaccine, and immune-based therapies. Research in AIDS malignancies has the potential to impact on a number of other important fields in oncology, including general tumor angiogenesis, viral oncogenesis, immunologic control of tumors, and molecular pathogenesis of tumors. This should prove to be a fruitful area of research over the next decade.

REFERENCES

1. CDC. *MMWR Surveillance summaries for AIDS-defining opportunistic illnesses, 1992–1997*. Atlanta: Centers for Disease Control and Prevention, 1999:1.
2. Boshoff C, Weiss R. AIDS-related malignancies. *Nat Rev Cancer* 2002;2:373.
3. Little RF, Yarchoan R. Treatment of gammaherpesvirus-related neoplastic disorders in the immunosuppressed host. *Semin Hematol* 2003;40:163.
4. Goedert JJ, Cote TR, Virgo P, et al. Spectrum of AIDS-associated malignant disorders. *Lancet* 1998;351:1833.
5. Grulich AE, Wan X, Law MG, et al. Risk of cancer in people with AIDS. *AIDS* 1999;13:839.
6. CDC. *HIV/AIDS surveillance report*. Atlanta: Centers for Disease Control and Prevention, 2001:13 (No.2).
7. Pluda JM, Venzon DJ, Tosato G, et al. Parameters affecting the development of non-Hodgkin's lymphoma in patients with severe human immunodeficiency virus infection receiving antiretroviral therapy. *J Clin Oncol* 1993;11:1099.
8. Kaposi M. Idiopathisches multiples Pigmensarkom der Haut. *Arch Derm Syph* 1872;4:265.
9. Hymes KB, Cheung T, Greene FB, et al. Kaposi's sarcoma in homosexual men—a report of eight cases. *Lancet* 1981;2:598.
10. MMWR. *Kaposi's sarcoma and Pneumocystis pneumonia among homosexual men—New York City and California*. Atlanta: Centers for Disease Control and Prevention, 1981.
11. Gottlieb MS, Schroff R, Schanker HM, et al. *Pneumocystis carinii* pneumonia and mucosal candidiasis in previously healthy homosexual men: evidence of a new acquired cellular immunodeficiency. *N Engl J Med* 1981;305:1425.
12. Beral V, Peterman TA, Berkelman RL, Jaffe HW. Kaposi's sarcoma among persons with AIDS: a sexually transmitted infection? *Lancet* 1990;335:123.
13. Moore PS, Chang Y. Detection of herpesvirus-like DNA sequences in Kaposi's sarcoma in patients with and without HIV infection. *N Engl J Med* 1995;332:1181.
14. Chang Y, Cesarman E, Pessin M, et al. Identification of herpesvirus-like DNA sequences in AIDS-associated Kaposi's sarcoma. *Science* 1994;266:1865.
15. Gao SJ, Kingsley L, Li M, et al. KSHV antibodies among Americans, Italians and Ugandans with and without Kaposi's sarcoma. *Nat Med* 1996;2:925.
16. Olsen SJ, Chang Y, Moore PS, et al. Increasing Kaposi's sarcoma–associated herpesvirus seroprevalence with age in a highly Kaposi's sarcoma endemic region, Zambia in 1985. *AIDS* 1998;12:1921.
17. O'Brien TR, Kedes D, Ganem D, et al. Evidence for concurrent epidemics of human herpesvirus 8 and human immunodeficiency virus type 1 in US homosexual men: rates, risk factors, and relationship to Kaposi's sarcoma. *J Infect Dis* 1999;180:1010.
18. Eltom MA, Jemal A, Mbulaiteye SM, et al. Trends in Kaposi's sarcoma and non-Hodgkin's lymphoma incidence in the United States from 1973 through 1998. *J Natl Cancer Inst* 2002;94:1204.
19. Safai B, Johnson KG, Myskowski PL, et al. The natural history of Kaposi's sarcoma in the acquired immunodeficiency syndrome. *Ann Intern Med* 1985;103:744.
20. Portsmouth S, Stebbing J, Gill J, et al. A comparison of regimens based on non-nucleoside reverse transcriptase inhibitors or protease inhibitors in preventing Kaposi's sarcoma. *AIDS* 2003;17:F17.
21. Parkin DM, Wabinga H, Nambooze S, Wabwire-Mangen F. AIDS-related cancers in Africa: maturation of the epidemic in Uganda. *AIDS* 1999;13:2563.
22. Mbulaiteye SM, Pfeiffer RM, Whitby D, et al. Human herpesvirus 8 infection within families in rural Tanzania. *J Infect Dis* 2003;187:1780.
23. Atkinson J, Edlin BR, Engels EA, et al. Seroprevalence of human herpesvirus 8 among injection drug users in San Francisco. *J Infect Dis* 2003;187:974.
24. Moore PS. Transplanting cancer: donor-cell transmission of Kaposi sarcoma. *Nat Med* 2003;9:506.
25. Pauk J, Huang ML, Brodie SJ, et al. Mucosal shedding of human herpesvirus 8 in men. *N Engl J Med* 2000;343:1369.
26. Martin JN, Ganem DE, Osmond DH, et al. Sexual transmission and the natural history of human herpesvirus 8 infection. *N Engl J Med* 1998;338:948.
27. Renwick N, Halaby T, Weverling GJ, et al. Seroconversion for human herpesvirus 8 during HIV infection is highly predictive of Kaposi's sarcoma. *AIDS* 1998;12:2481.
28. Skobe M, Brown LF, Tognazzi K, et al. Vascular endothelial growth factor-C (VEGF-C) and its receptors KDR and flt-4 are expressed in AIDS-associated Kaposi's sarcoma. *J Invest Dermatol* 1999;113:1047.
29. Moore PS, Boshoff C, Weiss RA, Chang Y. Molecular mimicry of human cytokine and cytokine response pathway genes by KSHV. *Science* 1996;274:1739.
30. Rabkin CS, Janz S, Lash A, et al. Monoclonal origin of multicentric Kaposi's sarcoma lesions. *N Engl J Med* 1997;336:988.
31. Ensoli B, Nakamura S, Salahuddin SZ, et al. AIDS-Kaposi's sarcoma–derived cells express cytokines with autocrine and paracrine growth effects. *Science* 1989;243:223.
32. Boshoff C, Endo Y, Collins PD, et al. Angiogenic and HIV-inhibitory functions of KSHV-encoded chemokines. *Science* 1997;278:290.
33. Bais C, Santomasso B, Coso O, et al. G-protein–coupled receptor of Kaposi's sarcoma–associated herpesvirus is a viral oncogene and angiogenesis activator. *Nature* 1998;391:86.
34. Sodhi A, Montaner S, Patel V, et al. The Kaposi's sarcoma–associated herpes virus G protein-coupled receptor up-regulates vascular endothelial growth factor expression and secretion through mitogen-activated protein kinase and p38 pathways acting on hypoxia-inducible factor 1alpha. *Cancer Res* 2000;60:4873.
35. Gershengorn MC, Geras-Raaka E, Varma A, Clark-Lewis I. Chemokines activate Kaposi's sarcoma–associated herpesvirus G protein–coupled receptor in mammalian cells in culture. *J Clin Invest* 1998;102:1469.
36. Pati S, Foulke JS Jr, Barabitskaya O, et al. Human herpesvirus 8–encoded vGPCR activates nuclear factor of activated T cells and collaborates with human immunodeficiency virus type 1 Tat. *J Virol* 2003;77:5759.
37. Antman K, Chang Y. Kaposi's sarcoma. *N Engl J Med* 2000;342:1027.
38. Haque M, Davis DA, Wang V, et al. Kaposi's sarcoma–associated herpesvirus (human herpesvirus 8) contains hypoxia response elements: relevance to lytic induction by hypoxia. *J Virol* 2003;77:6761.
39. Nasti G, Talamini R, Antinori A, et al. AIDS-related Kaposi's sarcoma: evaluation of potential new prognostic factors and assessment of the AIDS Clinical Trial Group staging system in the HAART era—the Italian Cooperative Group on AIDS and Tumors and the Italian Cohort of Patients Naive from Antiretrovirals. *J Clin Oncol* 2003;21:2876.
40. Krown SE, Testa MA, Huang J. AIDS-related Kaposi's sarcoma: prospective validation of the AIDS Clinical Trials Group staging classification. AIDS Clinical Trials Group Oncology Committee. *J Clin Oncol* 1997;15:3085.
41. Krown SE, Metroka C, Wernz JC. Kaposi's sarcoma in the acquired immunodeficiency syndrome: a proposal for uniform evaluation, response, and staging criteria. *J Clin Oncol* 1989;7:1201.
42. Little RF, Wyvill KM, Pluda JM, et al. Activity of thalidomide in AIDS-related Kaposi's sarcoma. *J Clin Oncol* 2000;18:2593.
43. Dupont C, Vasseur E, Beauchet A, et al. Long-term efficacy on Kaposi's sarcoma of highly active antiretroviral therapy in a cohort of HIV-positive patients. CISIH 92. Centre d'information et de soins de l'immunodeficience humaine. *AIDS* 2000;14:987.
44. Sgadari C, Barillari G, Toschi E, et al. HIV protease inhibitors are potent anti-angiogenic molecules and promote regression of Kaposi sarcoma. *Nat Med* 2002;8:225.
45. Webster-Cyriaque J. Development of Kaposi's sarcoma in a surgical wound. *N Engl J Med* 2002;346:1207.
46. Kirova YM, Belembaogo E, Frikha H, et al. Radiotherapy in the management of epidemic Kaposi's sarcoma: a retrospective study of 643 cases. *Radiother Oncol* 1998;46:19.
47. Hadderingh RJ, van der Meulen FW. Carbon dioxide laser treatment of oral Kaposi's sarcoma, *Int Conf AIDS* 1989; Vol 5.
48. Bernstein ZP, Wilson BD, Oseroff AR, et al. Photofrin photodynamic therapy for treatment of AIDS-related cutaneous Kaposi's sarcoma. *AIDS* 1999;13:1697.
49. Krown SE, Real FX, Cunningham-Rundles S, et al. Preliminary observations on the effect of recombinant leukocyte A interferon in homosexual men with Kaposi's sarcoma. *N Engl J Med* 1983;308:1071.
50. Gill PS, Wernz J, Scadden DT, et al. Randomized phase III trial of liposomal daunorubicin versus doxorubicin, bleomycin, and vincristine in AIDS-related Kaposi's sarcoma. *J Clin Oncol* 1996;14:2353.
51. Kumar PP, Little RF, Yarchoan R. Update on Kaposi's sarcoma: a gammaherpesvirus-induced malignancy. *Curr Infect Dis Rep* 2003;5:85.
52. Stewart S, Jablonowski H, Goebel FD, et al. Randomized comparative trial of pegylated liposomal doxorubicin versus bleomycin and vincristine in the treatment of AIDS-related Kaposi's sarcoma. International Pegylated Liposomal Doxorubicin Study Group. *J Clin Oncol* 1998;16:683.
53. Saville MW, Lietzau J, Pluda JM, et al. Treatment of HIV-associated Kaposi's sarcoma with paclitaxel. *Lancet* 1995;346:26.
54. Gill P, Scadden D, Groopman J, et al. Low dose paclitaxel (Taxol) is highly effective in the treatment of patients with advanced AIDS-related Kaposi's sarcoma. In: *J AIDS & HR*, 1st National AIDS Malignancy Conference, Bethesda, MD, April 1, 1997, Vol 14(4). Philadelphia: Lippincott–Raven, 1997.
55. Little RF, Aleman K, Merced L, et al. *Preliminary results of combination liposomal doxorubicin and interleukin-12 followed by chronic IL-12 maintenance therapy in advanced AIDS-related Kaposi's sarcoma*, 10th Conference on Retroviruses and Opportunistic Infections, Boston, February 10–14, 2003.
56. Bower M, Howard M, Gracie F, et al. *A phase II study of thalidomide for Kaposi's sarcoma: activity and correlation with KSHV DNA load*, 1st National AIDS Malignancy Conference, Bethesda, MD, April 1, 1997, Vol 14(4). Philadelphia: Lippincott–Raven, 1997.
57. Cianfrocca M, Cooley TP, Lee JY, et al. Matrix metalloproteinase inhibitor COL-3 in the treatment of AIDS-related Kaposi's sarcoma: a phase I AIDS malignancy consortium study. *J Clin Oncol* 2002;20:153.
58. Sgadari C, Angiolillo AL, Tosato G. Inhibition of angiogenesis by interleukin-12 is mediated by the interferon-inducible protein 10. *Blood* 1996;87:3877.
59. Martin DF, Kuppermann BD, Wolitz RA, et al. Oral ganciclovir for patients with cytomegalovirus retinitis treated with a ganciclovir implant. Roche Ganciclovir Study Group. *N Engl J Med* 1999;340:1063.
60. Little RF, Merced-Galindez F, Staskus K, et al. A pilot study of cidofovir in patients with Kaposi sarcoma. *J Infect Dis* 2003;187:149.
61. Koon H, Bubley G, Pantanowitz L, et al. *AIDS-related Kaposi's sarcoma: imatinab mesylate–induced regression in C-KIT positive disease*, 7th International Conference on Malignancies in AIDS and Other Immunodeficiencies, Bethesda, MD, April 28–29, 2003.
62. Besson C, Goubar A, Gabarre J, et al. Changes in AIDS-related lymphoma since the era of highly active antiretroviral therapy. *Blood* 2001;98:2339.
63. Levine AM. Lymphoma complicating immunodeficiency disorders. *Ann Oncol* 1994;5[Suppl 2]:29.
64. National Cancer Institute sponsored study of classifications of non-Hodgkin's lymphomas: summary and description of a working formulation for clinical usage. The non-Hodgkin's Lymphoma Pathologic Classification Project. *Cancer* 1982;49:2112.
65. Gaidano G, Carbone A. AIDS-related lymphomas: from pathogenesis to pathology. *Br J Haematol* 1995;90:235.
66. Little RF, Pittaluga S, Grant N, et al. Highly effective treatment of acquired immunodefi-

ciency syndrome–related lymphoma with dose-adjusted EPOCH: impact of antiretroviral therapy suspension and tumor biology. *Blood* 2003;101:4653.

67. Dalla-Favera R. *Mechanisms of genetic lesions in AIDS–associated lymphoma*, 7th International Conference on Malignancies in AIDS and other Immunodeficiencies, Bethesda, MD, 2003.
68. Carbone A. Emerging pathways in the development of AIDS-related lymphomas. *Lancet Oncol* 2003;4:22.
69. Gaidano G, Pasqualucci L, Capello D, et al. Aberrant somatic hypermutation in multiple subtypes of AIDS-associated non-Hodgkin lymphoma. *Blood* 2003;102:1833.
70. Ng VL, Hurt MH, Herndier BG, et al. VH gene use by HIV type 1–associated lymphoproliferations. *AIDS Res Hum Retroviruses* 1997;13:135.
71. Tiirikainen MI, Mullaney BP, Holly EA, et al. DNA copy number alterations in HIV-positive and HIV-negative patients with diffuse large-cell lymphomas. *J Acquir Immune Defic Syndr* 2001;27:272.
72. Martinez-Maza O, Breen EC. B-cell activation and lymphoma in patients with HIV. *Curr Opin Oncol* 2002;14:528.
73. Rabkin CS, Yang Q, Goedert JJ, et al. Chemokine and chemokine receptor gene variants and risk of non-Hodgkin's lymphoma in human immunodeficiency virus-1–infected individuals. *Blood* 1999;93:1838.
74. Dean M, Jacobson LP, McFarlane G, et al. Reduced risk of AIDS lymphoma in individuals heterozygous for the CCR5-delta32 mutation. *Cancer Res* 1999;59:3561.
75. Jaffe ES, Harris NL, Stein H, Vardiman JW. *World Health Organization classification of tumors: pathology & genetics: tumors of haematopoietic and lymphoid tissues.* Lyons: IARC Press, 2001:351.
76. Gaidano G, Capello D, Carbone A. The molecular basis of acquired immunodeficiency syndrome–related lymphomagenesis. *Semin Oncol* 2000;27:431.
77. Rosenwald A, Wright G, Chan WC, et al. The use of molecular profiling to predict survival after chemotherapy for diffuse large-B-cell lymphoma. *N Engl J Med* 2002;346:1937.
78. Kirshenbaum LA. Bcl-2 intersects the NFkappaB signalling pathway and suppresses apoptosis in ventricular myocytes. *Clin Invest Med* 2000;23:322.
79. Redchenko IV, Rickinson AB. Accessing Epstein-Barr virus–specific T-cell memory with peptide-loaded dendritic cells. *J Virol* 1999;73:334.
80. Wang D, Liebowitz D, Kieff E. An EBV membrane protein expressed in immortalized lymphocytes transforms established rodent cells. *Cell* 1985;43:831.
81. Finke J, Lange W, Mertelsmann R, Dolken G. BCL-2 induction is part of the strategy of Epstein-Barr virus. *Leuk Lymphoma* 1994;12:413.
82. Schlaifer D, Brousset P, Attal M, et al. bcl-2 proto-oncogene and Epstein-Barr virus latent membrane protein-1 expression in AIDS-related lymphoma. *Histopathology* 1994;25:77.
83. Hamilton-Dutoit SJ, Rea D, Raphael M, et al. Epstein-Barr virus–latent gene expression and tumor cell phenotype in acquired immunodeficiency syndrome–related non-Hodgkin's lymphoma. Correlation of lymphoma phenotype with three distinct patterns of viral latency. *Am J Pathol* 1993;143:1072.
84. Larocca LM, Capello D, Rinelli A, et al. The molecular and phenotypic profile of primary central nervous system lymphoma identifies distinct categories of the disease and is consistent with histogenetic derivation from germinal center–related B cells. *Blood* 1998;92:1011.
85. Sekita T, Tamaru JI, Kaito K, et al. Primary central nervous system lymphomas express Vh genes with intermediate to high somatic mutations. *Leuk Lymphoma* 2001;41:377.
86. Klein U, Gloghini A, Gaidano G, et al. Gene expression profile analysis of AIDS-related primary effusion lymphoma (PEL) suggests a plasmablastic derivation and identifies PEL-specific transcripts. *Blood* 2003;101:4115.
87. Stamatopoulos K, Kosmas C, Stavroyianni N, et al. Selection of immunoglobulin diversity gene reading frames in B cell lymphoproliferative disorders. *Leukemia* 1999;13:601.
88. Nador RG, Cesarman E, Chadburn A, et al. Primary effusion lymphoma: a distinct clinicopathologic entity associated with the Kaposi's sarcoma–associated herpes virus. *Blood* 1996;88:645.
89. Davis DA, Rinderknecht AS, Zoeteweij JP, et al. Hypoxia induces lytic replication of Kaposi sarcoma–associated herpesvirus. *Blood* 2001;97:3244.
90. Widmer I, Davis D, Haque M, et al. *KSHV viral Bcl-2 (ORF16) promoter region is activated by hypoxia*, 7th International Conference on Malignancies in AIDS and Other Immunodeficiencies: Basic, Epidemiologic, and Clinical Research, National Cancer Institute, Bethesda, MD, April 28–29, 2003.
91. Oksenhendler E, Carcelain G, Aoki Y, et al. High levels of human herpesvirus 8 viral load, human interleukin-6, interleukin-10, and C reactive protein correlate with exacerbation of multicentric Castleman disease in HIV-infected patients. *Blood* 2000;96:2069.
92. Aoki Y, Yarchoan R, Wyvill K, et al. Detection of viral interleukin-6 in Kaposi sarcoma–associated herpesvirus-linked disorders. *Blood* 2001;97:2173.
93. Corbellino M, Bestetti G, Scalamogna C, et al. Long-term remission of Kaposi sarcoma–associated herpesvirus-related multicentric Castleman disease with anti-CD20 monoclonal antibody therapy. *Blood* 2001;98:3473.
94. Casper C, Nichols WG, Huang M-L, et al. *Remission of HHV-8 and HIV-associated multicentric Castleman's disease with ganciclovir treatment*, International Conference on Malignancies in AIDS and Other Immunodeficiencies, Bethesda, MD, April 28–29, 2003.
95. Levine AM, Gill PS, Muggia F. Malignancies in the acquired immunodeficiency syndrome. *Curr Probl Cancer* 1987;11:209.
96. Pluda JM, Yarchoan R, Jaffe ES, et al. Development of non-Hodgkin lymphoma in a cohort of patients with severe HIV infection on long-term antiretroviral therapy. *Ann Intern Med* 1990;113:276.
97. Levine AM. AIDS-associated malignant lymphoma. *Med Clin North Am* 1992;76:253.
98. Little RF, Wilson WH. Update on the pathogenesis, diagnosis, and therapy of AIDS-related lymphoma. *Curr Infect Dis Rep* 2003;5:176.
99. Kaplan LD, Straus DJ, Testa MA, et al. Low-dose compared with standard-dose m-BACOD chemotherapy for non-Hodgkin's lymphoma associated with human immunodeficiency virus infection. National Institute of Allergy and Infectious Diseases AIDS Clinical Trials Group. *N Engl J Med* 1997;336:1641.
100. Ratner L, Lee J, Tang S, et al. Chemotherapy for human immunodeficiency virus–associated non-Hodgkin's lymphoma in combination with highly active antiretroviral therapy. *J Clin Oncol* 2001;19:2171.
101. Sparano J, Wiernik P, Hu X, et al. Pilot trial of infusional cyclophosphamide, doxorubicin, and etoposide plus didanosine and filgrastim in patients with human immunodeficiency virus–associated non-Hodgkin's lymphoma. *J Clin Oncol* 1996;14:3026.
102. Scadden DT. AIDS lymphomas: beginning of an EPOCH? *Blood* 2003;101:4647.
103. Feinstein AR. Clinical biostatistics. XI. Sources of 'chronology bias' in cohort statistics. *Clin Pharmacol Ther* 1971;12:864.
104. Vaccher E, Spina M, di Gennaro G, et al. Concomitant cyclophosphamide, doxorubicin, vincristine, and prednisone chemotherapy plus highly active antiretroviral therapy in patients with human immunodeficiency virus–related, non-Hodgkin lymphoma. *Cancer* 2001;91:155.
105. Antinori A, Cingolani A, Alba L, et al. Better response to chemotherapy and prolonged survival in AIDS-related lymphomas responding to highly active antiretroviral therapy. *AIDS* 2001;15:1483.
106. Tirelli U, Spina M, Jaeger U, et al. Infusional CDE with rituximab for the treatment of human immunodeficiency virus–associated non-Hodgkin's lymphoma: preliminary results of a phase I/II study. *Recent Results Cancer Res* 2002;159:149.
107. Kaplan L. *No benefit from rituximab in a randomized phase III trial of CHOP with or without rituximab for patients with HIV-associated non-Hodgkin's lymphoma*: AIDS Malignancies Consortium Study 010, 7th International Conference on Malignancies in AIDS and Other Immunodeficiencies, Bethesda, MD, April 28–29, 2003.
108. Mounier N, Briere J, Gisselbrecht C, et al. Rituximab plus CHOP (R-CHOP) overcomes bcl-2–associated resistance to chemotherapy in elderly patients with diffuse large B-cell lymphoma (DLBCL). *Blood* 2003;101:4279.
109. Mackall CL, Fleisher TA, Brown MR, et al. Lymphocyte depletion during treatment with intensive chemotherapy for cancer. *Blood* 1994;84:2221.
110. Mellors JW, Rinaldo CR Jr, Gupta P, et al. Prognosis in HIV-1 infection predicted by the quantity of virus in plasma. *Science* 1996;272:1167.
111. *Guidelines for the use of antiretroviral agents in HIV-1 infected adults and adolescents*: The Panel on Clinical Practices for Treatment of HIV Infection convened by the Department of Health and Human Services (DHHS). World Wide Web URL: http://www.aidsinfo.nih.gov, 2004.
112. Mackall CL, Fleisher TA, Brown MR, et al. Age, thymopoiesis, and CD4+ T-lymphocyte regeneration after intensive chemotherapy. *N Engl J Med* 1995;332:143.
113. Miller TP, Grogan TM, Dahlberg S, et al. Prognostic significance of the Ki-67–associated proliferative antigen in aggressive non-Hodgkin's lymphomas: a prospective Southwest Oncology Group trial. *Blood* 1994;83:1460.
114. Wilson WH, Teruya-Feldstein J, Fest T, et al. Relationship of p53, bcl-2, and tumor proliferation to clinical drug resistance in non-Hodgkin's lymphomas. *Blood* 1997;89:601.
115. Tulpule A, Sherrod A, Dharmapala D, et al. Multidrug resistance (MDR-1) expression in AIDS-related lymphomas. *Leuk Res* 2002;26:121.
116. Cingolani A, Gastaldi R, Fassone L, et al. Epstein-Barr virus infection is predictive of CNS involvement in systemic AIDS-related non-Hodgkin's lymphomas. *J Clin Oncol* 2000;18: 3325.
117. Antinori A, De Rossi G, Ammassari A, et al. Value of combined approach with thallium-201 single-photon emission computed tomography and Epstein-Barr virus DNA polymerase chain reaction in CSF for the diagnosis of AIDS-related primary CNS lymphoma. *J Clin Oncol* 1999;17:554.
118. Cingolani A, De Luca A, Larocca LM, et al. Minimally invasive diagnosis of acquired immunodeficiency syndrome–related primary central nervous system lymphoma. *J Natl Cancer Inst* 1998;90:364.
119. Baumgartner JE, Rachlin JR, Beckstead JH, et al. Primary central nervous system lymphomas: natural history and response to radiation therapy in 55 patients with acquired immunodeficiency syndrome. *J Neurosurg* 1990;73:206.
120. Forsyth PA, Yahalom J, DeAngelis LM. Combined-modality therapy in the treatment of primary central nervous system lymphoma in AIDS. *Neurology* 1994;44:1473.
121. Tirelli U, Errante D, Dolcetti R, et al. Hodgkin's disease and human immunodeficiency virus infection: clinicopathologic and virologic features of 114 patients from the Italian Cooperative Group on AIDS and Tumors. *J Clin Oncol* 1995;13:1758.
122. Levine AM, Cheung T, Huang J, Testa M. Prospective, multicenter phase II trial of ABVD chemotherapy with G-CSF in HIV-infected patients with Hodgkin's disease (HD): AIDS Clinical Trials Group (ACTG) study 149. *Proc Am Soc Clin Oncol* 1997;16(meeting abst).
123. MMWR. *1993 revised classification system for HIV infection and expanded surveillance case definition for AIDS among adolescents and adults*, Vol 41(RR-17). Atlanta: Centers for Disease Control and Prevention, 1992.
124. Palefsky JM. Human papillomavirus infection and anogenital neoplasia in human immunodeficiency virus–positive men and women. *J Natl Cancer Inst Monogr* 1998:15.
125. MMWR. *1993 sexually transmitted diseases treatment guidelines*. Atlanta: Centers for Disease Control and Prevention, 1993.
126. Goldie SJ, Kuntz KM, Weinstein MC, et al. The clinical effectiveness and cost-effectiveness of screening for anal squamous intraepithelial lesions in homosexual and bisexual HIV-positive men. *JAMA* 1999;281:1822.
127. Williams AB, Darragh TM, Vranizan K, et al. Anal and cervical human papillomavirus infection and risk of anal and cervical epithelial abnormalities in human immunodeficiency virus–infected women. *Obstet Gynecol* 1994;83:205.
128. Motti PG, Dallabetta GA, Daniel RW, et al. Cervical abnormalities, human papillomavirus, and human immunodeficiency virus infections in women in Malawi. *J Infect Dis* 1996;173:714.
129. Biggar RJ, Melbye M. Marital status in relation to Kaposi's sarcoma, non-Hodgkin's lymphoma, and anal cancer in the pre-AIDS era. *J Acquir Immune Defic Syndr Hum Retrovirol* 1996;11:178.
130. Maiman M, Fruchter RG, Guy L, et al. Human immunodeficiency virus infection and invasive cervical carcinoma. *Cancer* 1993;71:402.

131. Jones J, Hanson D, Ward J. *Effect of antiretroviral therapy on recent trends in cancers among HIV-infected persons,* 2nd National AIDS Malignancy Conference, Bethesda, MD, April 6–8, 1998.
132. Palefsky JM. Anal squamous intraepithelial lesions: relation to HIV and human papillomavirus infection. *J Acquir Immune Defic Syndr* 1999;21[Suppl 1]:S42.
133. Wright T, Sun XW, Ellerbrock TV, Chiasson MA. *Comparison of the amount of HPV 16 DNA in cervicovaginal secretions of HIV-infected and -uninfected women, using quantitative competitive–polymerase chain reaction (QC-PCR),* Vol 12. International Conference on AIDS, Geneva, 1998.
134. Maiman M, Fruchter RG, Serur E, et al. Recurrent cervical intraepithelial neoplasia in human immunodeficiency virus–seropositive women. *Obstet Gynecol* 1993;82:170.
135. Palefsky JM, Holly EA, Ralston ML, Jay N. Prevalence and risk factors for human papillomavirus infection of the anal canal in human immunodeficiency virus (HIV)-positive and HIV-negative homosexual men. *J Infect Dis* 1998;177:361.
136. Hoffman R, Welton ML, Klencke B, et al. The significance of pretreatment CD4 count on the outcome and treatment tolerance of HIV-positive patients with anal cancer. *Int J Radiat Oncol Biol Phys* 1999;44:127.
137. Hung A, Crane C, Delclos M, et al. Cisplatin-based combined modality therapy for anal carcinoma: a wider therapeutic index. *Cancer* 2003;97:1195.
138. Carbone A, Gloghini A, Larocca LM, et al. Expression profile of MUM1/IRF4, BCL-6, and CD138/syndecan-1 defines novel histogenetic subsets of human immunodeficiency virus–related lymphomas. *Blood* 2001;97:744.
139. Sparano J, Lee S, Chen M, et al. *Phase II Trial of Infusional Cyclophosphamide, Doxorubicin, and Etoposide (CDE) in HIV-Associated Non-Hodgkin's Lymphoma (NHL): an Eastern Cooperative Oncology Group (ECOG) trial (E1494).* 3rd Annual AIDS Malignancy Conference, Bethesda, MD, May 26–27, 1999.
140. Levy R, Colonna P, Tourani JM, et al. Human immunodeficiency virus associated Hodgkin's disease: report of 45 cases from the French Registry of HIV-Associated Tumors. *Leuk Lymphoma* 1995;16:451.
141. Rubio R. Hodgkin's disease associated with human immunodeficiency virus infection. A clinical study of 46 cases. Cooperative Study Group of Malignancies Associated with HIV Infection of Madrid. *Cancer* 1994;73:2400.

SECTION 2

STANLEY R. RIDDELL

Transplantation-Related Malignancies

Hematopoietic stem cell transplantation (HSCT) to treat malignant and nonmalignant diseases and transplantation of an allogeneic solid organ to restore organ function are increasingly used therapeutic modalities. Improved management of infections and refined immunosuppressive therapy have significantly improved the survival of transplant recipients. As larger numbers of patients are cured with transplantation, late complications, including the development of malignancy, have become increasingly important in medical management.

IMMUNE SURVEILLANCE AND TUMOR DEVELOPMENT

Burnet hypothesized that a function of the host immune system was to protect against the development of cancer.[1] However, experimental studies in mice with genetic or iatrogenic immunodeficiency initially failed to provide convincing evidence of an increased rate of tumor development, and the immune surveillance hypothesis was nearly abandoned.[2] More recent analysis of mice with genetically characterized defects in the production of natural killer, T, and B lymphocytes or in interferon-γ signaling have identified an increased susceptibility to spontaneous and chemically induced tumors.[3] Thus, prolonged treatment with immunosuppressive drugs could predispose transplant recipients to late tumor development, particularly those with prior exposure to mutagenic chemotherapy or radiation.

Data collected by registries of HSCT or solid organ transplant patients have been invaluable in evaluating the risk of late malignancies.[4,5] The method most commonly used for analysis is computation of the standardized incidence ratio, which compares the incidence of the malignancy observed in patients who have undergone transplantation with the expected incidence in a general population of the same age and gender. HSCT and organ transplant patients exhibit an increased incidence of several malignancies, including those caused by ultraviolet light or by oncogenic viruses, such as Epstein-Barr virus (EBV) and human herpesvirus-8 (HHV-8). Virus-associated malignancies may undergo complete regression with withdrawal of immunosuppressive drugs or restoration of functional T-cell responses to viral antigens by adoptive immunotherapy, which provides direct evidence for the contribution of defects in host immunity in the genesis of these tumors. An increased risk of tumors involving the breast, genitourinary tract, gastrointestinal tract, and lung has not been observed consistently in transplant recipients. This might imply that immune surveillance is less important for these malignancies, although it is possible that the duration of follow-up remains insufficient to detect an increased risk for tumors with a long latency.

HEMATOPOIETIC STEM CELL TRANSPLANT RECIPIENTS

Approximately 12,000 allogeneic and 18,000 autologous stem cell transplantations are performed worldwide each year, primarily for hematologic diseases.[6] Such patients have typically received mutagenic chemotherapy as primary therapy for their disease and receive additional intensive chemotherapy or radiotherapy or both as conditioning for transplantation. Allogeneic HSCT recipients often require prolonged immunosuppressive drug therapy after transplantation and have an increased risk of developing lymphoproliferative disorders and solid tumors, whereas autologous HSCT recipients are at increased risk for secondary acute myeloid leukemia (AML), myelodysplastic syndrome (MDS), and solid tumors. The peak time for the occurrence of these malignancies after transplantation suggests that distinct factors contribute to pathogenesis. Lymphoproliferative disorders associated with EBV infection occur during the first year at the height of the immunodeficiency; AML and MDS primarily occur in the first 3 years after transplantation; and solid tumor occurrence shows a steady increase with time from transplantation (Fig. 48.2-1).

SOLID TUMORS AFTER HEMATOPOIETIC STEM CELL TRANSPLANTATION

Epidemiology

The first large study to examine the development of solid tumors in HSCT recipients evaluated 2145 patients who underwent allogeneic or syngeneic HSCT between 1970 and 1987 as treatment for leukemia or aplastic anemia. In this study, 13 solid tumors

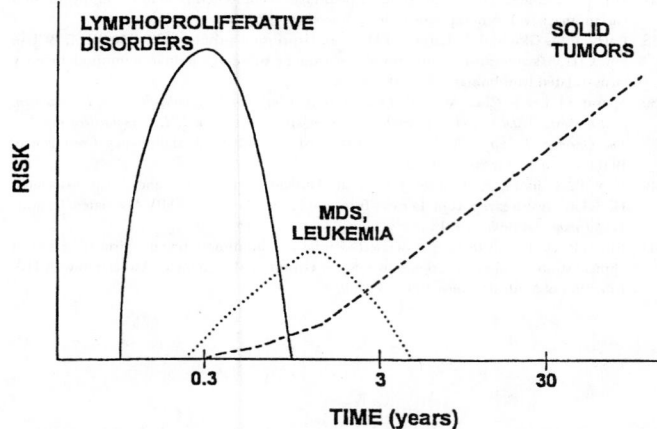

FIGURE 48.2-1. Time course and relative risk of the major categories of malignancies that develop after hematopoietic stem cell transplantation. MDS, myelodysplastic syndrome. (From Deeg HJ, Socie G. Malignancies after hematopoietic stem cell transplantation: many questions, many answers. *Blood* 1998;91:1833, with permission.)

developed a median of 56 months (range, 2.5 to 163.0 months) after transplantation.[7] The histologic types of second malignancies included glioblastoma, melanoma, squamous cell carcinoma of the skin or oral cavity, basal cell carcinoma of the skin, adenocarcinoma of the gastrointestinal tract and lung, and hepatoma.

Subsequent studies of large numbers of patients have confirmed the late development of solid tumors after HSCT and have provided insight into the risk factors for and pathogenesis of these malignancies.[8–11] The largest study of solid tumors in HSCT recipients analyzed 19,220 patients who received allogeneic or syngeneic HSCT between 1964 and 1992.[8] Overall, the ratio of observed to expected (O/E) cases of new solid tumors was 2.7, with a cumulative incidence rate of 2.2% at 10 years and 6.7% at 15 years.[8] The incidence of solid tumors continued to increase even 20 years after HSCT.[9] Cancers that occur with significantly increased frequency in HSCT recipients include melanoma (O/E, 5.0) and cancers of the buccal cavity or oropharynx (O/E, 11.1), liver (O/E, 7.5), brain (O/E, 7.6), thyroid (O/E, 6.6), bone (O/E, 13.4), and connective tissues (O/E, 8.0). The incidence of breast, lung, gastrointestinal, and genitourinary tumors, which represent the most common malignancies in the general population, are not found to be increased in most studies of HSCT recipients.

Several factors increase the risk for the development of solid tumors in HSCT recipients (Table 48.2-1). The risk of developing a tumor after transplantation is 36 times higher than expected for children who are younger than the age of 10 years at the time of transplantation, 4.6 times higher for patients

TABLE 48.2-1. Risk Factors for the Development of Solid Tumors after Hematopoietic Stem Cell Transplantation

MAJOR RISK FACTORS
Young age at the time of transplantation
Pretransplantation cranial irradiation
Total body irradiation in the conditioning regimen
MINOR RISK FACTORS
Chronic graft-versus-host disease
T-cell depletion of the stem cell graft

aged 10 to 29 years, and nearly normal for patients aged 30 years and older. The excess risk in children younger than age 10 years is primarily due to the development of brain and thyroid tumors in patients who have received pretransplantation cranial irradiation.[8,11] Total body irradiation as part of myeloablative therapy was associated with squamous cell carcinoma of the oral cavity, melanoma, thyroid cancer, central nervous system (CNS) tumors, and liver cancer.[8,10]

T-cell depletion of the stem cell graft, acute and chronic graft-versus-host disease (GVHD), and immunosuppressive drug therapy are not associated with an increased risk of most solid tumors.[12] However, immune deficiency or dysregulation may be involved in the development of melanoma and squamous cell carcinoma of the oral cavity. Transplantation of stem cells that are depleted donor T cells to prevent GVHD confers an increased risk for melanoma.[8] In addition, patients who develop chronic GVHD and require longer than 1 year of immunosuppressive therapy exhibit a significantly increased risk of squamous cell carcinoma of the buccal cavity and skin.[8]

Solid tumors also develop with increased frequency in recipients of autologous HSCT, although the available data are derived from analysis of smaller numbers of patients and are not sufficient to accurately define the risk for specific tumors.[13] The solid tumors reported after autologous HSCT are similar to those seen after allogeneic HSCT and include squamous and basal cell carcinoma of the skin, melanoma, CNS tumors, sarcoma, and thyroid carcinoma. Autologous HSCT recipients have delayed immune recovery but do not develop GVHD or receive posttransplantation immunosuppressive drug therapy. Therefore, comparison of the incidence and types of malignancies that occur in autologous and allogeneic HSCT recipients may assist in elucidating distinct contributions of GVHD and immunosuppressive drug therapy to the pathogenesis of tumor development.

Pathogenesis

Second malignancies are a complication of cancer chemotherapy or irradiation in the nontransplantation setting,[14,15] but HSCT appears to contribute further to tumor development. The use of total body irradiation in the conditioning regimen for transplantation is consistently associated with an increased risk of late solid tumor development. Chronic GVHD is a risk factor for squamous cell cancer of the oral cavity, which suggests that chronic inflammation or prolonged treatment with immunosuppressive drugs, or both, may be involved in the development of these tumors.[8,16] The association of T-cell–depleted transplants with an increased risk of melanoma suggests a potential role for defective T-cell function in the pathogenesis of melanoma after HSCT. T cells reactive with melanocyte differentiation antigens such as Melan-A, gp100, and tyrosinase, which are expressed in both normal melanocytes and melanomas, have been identified in normal individuals.[17] A role in immune surveillance has not been proven, but such T cells are expanded in the blood and tumor infiltrates of some patients with melanoma, recognize and kill tumor cells *in vitro*, and can mediate tumor regression after *in vitro* expansion and adoptive transfer to tumor-bearing hosts.[18,19]

Clinical Features, Diagnosis, and Management

The clinical features of solid tumors in HSCT recipients have not been distinguishable from those of tumors of the same histologic type developing in the general population, and diagnosis and management should be performed in accordance with standard practice for tumors of the same stage. All HSCT recipients should be counseled before transplantation regarding the increased risk of solid tumor development and monitored after transplantation for symptoms or signs indicative of a malignancy to ensure early diagnosis and therapy.

Second malignancies are beginning to influence long-term survival of HSCT recipients. New cancers accounted for 6% of the deaths in patients free of their original disease 2 years after allogeneic HSCT.[20] The median follow-up of patients in this study was only 80 months, and tumors that exhibit a longer latency are likely to emerge. Newer approaches to allogeneic HSCT have been developed using less intensive conditioning regimens that do not include total body irradiation or use lower doses of irradiation.[21] The reduced intensity of the conditioning regimens may decrease secondary malignancies resulting from cytotoxic therapy. However, these nonmyeloablative regimens rely on an allogeneic graft-versus-tumor effect to eradicate the underlying malignancy, which is frequently associated with GVHD.[22] Thus, immunosuppressive drug therapy is often required for prolonged periods of time to treat GVHD and may interfere with immune surveillance mechanisms.

LYMPHOPROLIFERATIVE DISORDERS ASSOCIATED WITH EPSTEIN-BARR VIRUS IN HEMATOPOIETIC STEM CELL TRANSPLANT RECIPIENTS

Epidemiology

Posttransplantation lymphoproliferative disorder (PTLD) arising from donor B cells infected with EBV is a life-threatening complication of allogeneic HSCT but rarely occurs after autologous HSCT.[23] In a large multicenter study involving 18,014 patients who received allogeneic HSCT between 1969 and 1992, the cumulative incidence of PTLD was 1.0% at 10 years.[23] PTLD is the most frequent new malignancy in the first 5 years after transplantation, with more than 80% of the cases occurring in the first year and the peak incidence in the third month after transplantation.

The risk of developing a PTLD differs dramatically depending on the type of allogeneic HSCT. The use of major histocompatibility complex–mismatched donors, the administration of anti–T-cell antibodies to the recipient as part of the preparative regimen or for GVHD therapy, and the depletion of T cells from the stem cell graft are associated with an increased risk of PTLD.[23] Recipients of transplants from unrelated donors or donors mismatched at two or more major histocompatibility complex alleles with the recipient have a 3.7-fold greater risk of PTLD than recipients of transplants from matched, related donors. Patients who receive a stem cell transplant that is depleted of T cells to prevent GVHD are at a ninefold higher risk for developing PTLD than those who receive unmodified bone marrow or peripheral blood stem cells.[23] The risk of PTLD is highest when monoclonal antibodies specific only for T cells or for both T cells and natural killer cells, or sheep red blood cell E-rosetting techniques are used for T-cell depletion. In contrast, techniques that eliminate both T and B cells, such as those using the Campath-1 antibody or agglutination with soybean lectin, do not increase the risk of PTLD compared with unmodified HSCT.[23,24] The

low incidence of PTLD with these methods of T-cell depletion is presumably due to the removal of EBV-infected B cells from the stem cell inoculum.

Pathogenesis

EBV, which causes a persistent infection in more than 90% of immunocompetent adults, is directly implicated in the development of PTLD. During primary EBV infection in normal hosts, the virus enters B lymphocytes by an interaction between the viral envelope glycoprotein gp350/220 and the B-cell surface molecule CD21, which normally serves as the receptor for the C3d complement fragment. Some EBV-infected B cells express the entire array of viral genes and undergo lytic infection. Others may enter various forms of latency in which only EBV nuclear antigen-1 (EBNA-1) is expressed or in which a more extensive set of genes (latency III program) that includes EBNA-1, EBNA-2, EBNA-3A, EBNA-3B, EBNA-3C, EBNA-LP, and the latent membrane proteins (LMP) 1, 2A, and 2B are expressed.[25] The *latency III program* induces B-cell proliferation as a result of the coordinated action of EBNA-1, which is required for maintenance of the viral episome; EBNA-2, which functions as a transcriptional activator of viral and cellular genes that regulate cell growth; and LMP-1, which acts to mimic constitutively active CD40 signaling in B cells.[26]

The immunocompetent host mounts a cellular immune response to EBV that is characterized by major expansions of CD3+ CD8+ cytotoxic T lymphocytes (CTLs), which eliminate EBV-infected B cells that express the lytic or latency III program of viral genes.[27] The elimination of proliferating EBV-infected B cells by CTLs assists in terminating acute infection, but the virus persists in the subset of resting memory B cells that express only the EBNA-1 viral gene. The presence of glycine/alanine repeat sequences in EBNA-1 inhibits its translation and proteolytic processing; this limits the presentation to CTLs and allows latently infected B cells to escape immune elimination and provide a reservoir for reactivation.[28,29] Because of this persistent reservoir of virus, memory CTL responses to EBV must be maintained for the life of the host to prevent the outgrowth of EBV-infected B cells.

The balance between host T-cell immunity and persistent EBV in immunocompetent hosts is perturbed in the early stages after allogeneic HSCT. The administration of cytotoxic therapy before HSCT destroys the host T cells required to maintain EBV in a latent state but also eliminates the reservoir of host EBV-infected B cells. The infusion of an unmanipulated allogeneic stem cell graft from an EBV-seropositive donor provides a new source of EBV-infected B cells and replaces the host EBV strain with the EBV strain of the donor.[30] However, reconstitution of EBV-specific T-cell immunity is essential to reestablish control of EBV infection, and a quantitative deficiency of EBV-specific CTLs is common in the first 6 months after allogeneic transplantation.[31] T-cell recovery may be further impaired by T-cell depletion of the stem cell graft, which reduces the number of EBV-specific T cells administered to the recipient, or the use of monoclonal anti–T-cell antibodies for GVHD prophylaxis or therapy, which eliminates EBV-specific T cells *in vivo*. This severe deficiency of EBV-specific CTLs allows the unimpeded activation of lytic infection in memory B cells that can spread to a broad range of target B cells, some of which may activate the latency III program leading to B-cell proliferation.[32]

Clinical Features and Diagnosis

PTLD in HSCT recipients commonly presents with fever, progressive lymphadenopathy, or involvement of pharyngeal lymphoid tissue.[33] PTLD may present with extranodal disease involving the spleen, liver, lungs, gastrointestinal tract, kidneys, and CNS. New approaches that use quantitative polymerase chain reaction to measure the levels of EBV DNA in posttransplantation blood samples have been developed for monitoring of EBV reactivation and diagnosis of PTLD in high-risk patients.[34,35] Additional study is required to standardize the monitoring methodology, define cutoff values for instituting early therapy, and determining the frequency of false-negative results.[36]

The diagnosis of PTLD is usually established by biopsy of involved tissue, which demonstrates proliferating B cells containing EBV. Tumors developing after HSCT almost always consist of oligoclonal or monoclonal populations of donor B cells and most commonly exhibit a monomorphic diffuse large cell morphology, although plasmacytoid variants are also seen.[33] The presence of EBV in the tumor can be established by Southern blot testing of DNA extracted from tumor tissue or by analysis of EBV gene expression in tissue sections. Two EBV-encoded RNAs are abundantly expressed in PTLD and can be detected by *in situ* hybridization.[37] Immunohistochemical staining with antibodies against EBV proteins can also be used to confirm the presence of EBV in the tumor.

Treatment and Prevention

The development of PTLD in HSCT recipients is an ominous sign due to the propensity for these tumors to grow rapidly, and urgent therapy is usually necessary. Reduction in immunosuppression should be considered in all patients, but may be difficult in those with GVHD. Surgical resection or irradiation may be useful as a temporary measure to control localized disease in anatomically critical sites. Efforts to treat PTLD in HSCT recipients with chemotherapy regimens similar to those used to treat non-Hodgkin's lymphoma are rarely successful due to the toxicity of chemotherapy in post-HSCT patients.

The association of deficient EBV-specific T-cell immunity with the development of PTLD has led to efforts to restore T-cell responses to EBV by the adoptive transfer of T cells obtained from the EBV-seropositive stem cell donor. Sixteen of 19 patients with PTLD treated with unirradiated donor lymphocytes achieved complete pathologic and clinical resolution of their disease.[33] Rapid amplification of EBV-specific CTL to levels equivalent to those in normal donors was observed after donor lymphocyte infusion. However, due to the presence of alloreactive T cells in the donor lymphocytes used for therapy, GVHD developed in 50% of treated patients.[33] An approach to cellular treatment of PTLD that alleviates the problem of GVHD uses donor T cells that are enriched for EBV-specific reactivity and depleted for alloreactivity by *in vitro* culture. The infusion of such EBV-specific T-cell lines was effective for treatment of established PTLD in HSCT recipients, and transferred T cells persisted in the blood for longer than 18 months after infusion.[38,39] Limitations of this approach include the emer-

gence of antigen-loss variants if the cell lines infused target only one or a few EBV epitopes and the time required to expand donor EBV-specific T cells *in vitro* for therapy.[40] The safety and efficacy of T-cell therapy for EBV have encouraged the use of EBV-specific T-cell lines as prophylaxis for high-risk patients undergoing T-cell–depleted HSCT. Prophylactic T-cell infusions were highly effective, and the only major impediment to the broader application of T-cell therapy for prevention of PTLD is the technical expertise and resources required.[41]

An alternative therapy for PTLD is to target the proliferating B cells with monoclonal antibodies directed at cell surface molecules. The infusion of monoclonal antibodies directed at CD21 and CD24 induced regression of PTLD in approximately 50% of patients. However, this approach is less effective for patients with oligoclonal or monoclonal disease, and these antibodies are not commercially available.[42] The administration of the anti-CD20 monoclonal antibody rituximab (Rituxan) has been reported to induce remission of PTLD after HSCT, and further studies are in progress to define the response rate and long-term outcome.[43,44] The use of anti-CD20 is also promising as a prophylactic approach for patients with increasing EBV DNA levels.[45]

Antiviral drugs and interferon-α have been used as adjuncts to other modalities. Acyclovir and ganciclovir target the viral thymidine kinase, which is expressed in the replicative phase of EBV infection and not in proliferating EBV-infected B cells. These agents do not inhibit the growth of EBV-transformed B cells *in vitro* and would not be expected to be beneficial for PTLD. Pharmacologic induction of the viral thymidine kinase gene in EBV-infected cells by administration of arginine butyrate has been reported to render EBV-associated PTLD susceptible to ganciclovir therapy and induce a complete regression in four of six patients.[46]

HODGKIN'S DISEASE AND LATE-ONSET NON-HODGKIN'S LYMPHOMAS IN HEMATOPOIETIC STEM CELL TRANSPLANT RECIPIENTS

Epidemiology

In a study of 18,531 allogeneic HSCT recipients, the incidence of Hodgkin's disease was significantly more than expected in the age- and sex-matched general population (O/E, 6.2).[47] There was a trend toward a significantly increased risk in patients who developed grade 3 or 4 GVHD. The majority of cases were of mixed-cellularity histology and contained the EBV genome; however, in contrast to EBV-associated PTLD, which typically occurs in the first 6 months after transplantation, the onset of Hodgkin's disease occurred at a median of 4.2 years after transplantation.[47] Cases of late-onset non-Hodgkin's lymphoma have also been reported in HSCT recipients, but the majority of these are T cell in origin, and an association with lymphotropic viruses, such as EBV or human T-cell lymphotropic virus, has not been demonstrated.[48]

Clinical Manifestations and Management

Hodgkin's disease in HSCT recipients is usually characterized by an aggressive histology, with 75% being mixed-cellularity or lymphocyte-depleted types. Treatment with conventional chemotherapy or radiotherapy is effective, with six of the eight patients in the largest series alive 2.7 to 9.6 years after diagnosis of Hodgkin's disease.[47]

ACUTE MYELOID LEUKEMIA AND MYELODYSPLASTIC SYNDROME AFTER HEMATOPOIETIC STEM CELL TRANSPLANTATION

Epidemiology

AML and MDS are well-recognized complications of conventional chemotherapy and radiotherapy for Hodgkin's disease, non-Hodgkin's lymphoma, breast cancer, and other malignancies.[49–51] Patients who receive high-dose chemotherapy and autologous HSCT for non-Hodgkin's lymphoma and Hodgkin's disease have also been reported to have an increased risk of secondary AML or MDS compared with the general population. In three series, the cumulative incidence of AML and MDS in recipients of autologous HSCT for non-Hodgkin's lymphoma or Hodgkin's disease was 5% at 5 years,[52] 18% at 6 years,[53] and 12% at 6 years,[54] respectively. Risk factors for the development of AML and MDS were age older than 40 years at the time of transplantation, pretransplantation irradiation, pretransplantation alkylating agent therapy, mobilization of stem cells with VP-16, and a low pretransplantation platelet count.[55,56] The use of total body irradiation in doses of more than 12 Gy in the conditioning regimen has been identified as a risk factor for the development of AML and MDS after transplantation in some studies.[56]

Rare cases of the development of leukemia in donor cells after allogeneic HSCT have also been reported.[57] In these cases, the donor reportedly remained healthy and the mechanism of leukemogenesis in the recipient remained unexplained. Inadvertent transplantation of marrow from a donor with AML has also been reported.[58]

Pathogenesis

Secondary AML and MDS in patients who receive conventional chemotherapy or combined chemoradiotherapy results from DNA damage in hematopoietic stem cells caused by alkylating agents, epipodophyllotoxins, or ionizing radiation. It is unclear whether the risk of AML and MDS after HSCT is entirely due to damage to stem cells from prior therapy or if transplantation conditioning or other transplantation factors add further risk. Cytogenetic abnormalities are occasionally found in the marrow of patients being evaluated for autologous HSCT. In a few cases in which the marrow was morphologically normal and was used for transplantation despite the presence of a cytogenetic abnormality, the patients developed MDS or AML in the first 12 months after transplantation.[59] Thus, cytogenetic analysis of the bone marrow should be performed in patients with extensive prior therapy who are being evaluated for HSCT.

Clinical Features and Management

The clinical features of AML and MDS after autologous HSCT are the same as those seen in cases of secondary AML and MDS that develop after conventional chemotherapy or low-dose irradiation. These include abnormalities of chromosomes 5 and 7 and a poor response to therapy. A small number of patients who have developed AML and MDS after autologous HSCT have subsequently been treated with a second high-dose cytotoxic regimen followed by allogeneic HSCT. This approach is complicated by significant regimen-related toxicity but can be curative.

ORGAN TRANSPLANT RECIPIENTS

Recipients of organ allografts generally require lifelong therapy with immunosuppressive drugs to prevent graft rejection and, as a consequence, are at increased risk for the development of a malignancy. The overwhelming majority of tumors arising in solid organ transplant recipients occur in recipient tissues. However, a malignancy of donor cells may occasionally arise in the transplanted organ or be inadvertently transmitted to the recipient via the transplanted organ.[60] Polymorphic DNA markers can be used to determine the origin of the malignancy and should be considered in suspicious cases, because withdrawal of immunosuppression may result in regression of donor-derived malignancies.[61,62] The overall incidence of cancer in organ allograft recipients is increased threefold to fourfold compared with the general population and increases with the length of observation after transplantation.[5,63] The incidence of cancers of the skin and lip, B-cell lymphoproliferative diseases, and Kaposi's sarcoma (KS) are significantly increased in organ allograft recipients. Malignancies that are common in the general population, such as cancers of the breast, lung, prostate, colon, and cervix, are not increased in organ transplant recipients.[5,63]

CANCER OF THE SKIN AND LIP IN ORGAN TRANSPLANT RECIPIENTS

Epidemiology and Risk Factors

The most common neoplasms developing in organ allograft recipients are cancers of the skin or lip.[64] The most dramatic increase is in squamous cell carcinoma, but the risk of developing basal cell carcinoma, melanoma, and Merkel-cell carcinoma is also significantly increased (Table 48.2-2). The incidence of skin cancer in renal transplant recipients was 82% after more than 20 years in a study in Australia, where sun exposure is high,[65] and 40% in a study in the Netherlands.[66] In two studies of heart transplant recipients, the incidence of skin cancer was 44% at 7 years.[67] In the general population, basal cell carcinoma of the skin occurs five times more frequently than squa-

TABLE 48.2-2. Incidence of Nonmelanoma Skin Cancer in Organ Transplant Recipients

Study	Transplant Type	Follow-Up (Y)	Incidence of Nonmelanoma Skin Cancer (%)
Ramsay et al.[65]	Renal	5	29
		10	52
		20	82
Hartevelt et al.[66]	Renal	10	10
		20	40
Lampros et al.[67]	Heart	5	21
		10	35

TABLE 48.2-3.   Risk Factors for Skin Cancer after Organ Transplantation

Sun exposure
Length of time after transplantation
Intensive immunosuppression
Duration of pretransplantation dialysis
Fair skin
HLA mismatching between donor and recipient

mous cell carcinoma, whereas in organ transplant recipients, squamous cell carcinoma occurs four times more frequently than basal cell carcinoma.[64] In addition to an increased incidence of malignant lesions, transplant recipients have a higher incidence of leukoplakia and dysplastic lesions of the lip.[68]

Risk factors for the development of skin cancer in organ transplant recipients have been identified (Table 48.2-3). Features prevalent in patients with skin cancer in the general population, including light skin and blonde or red hair, are also prevalent in transplant recipients with skin cancer. Sun exposure and cigarette smoking are risk factors for the development of cancer of the lip in organ transplant recipients. The length of time from transplantation is an important risk factor and presumably reflects the contributions of immunosuppressive drug therapy to tumorigenesis. Use of more intense immunosuppressive regimens appears to increase the risk for the development of skin cancer, which suggests that newer approaches that do not rely on prolonged immunosuppression to induce tolerance to transplanted organs will be beneficial in reducing risk.[69,70]

Pathogenesis

The pathogenesis of skin and lip cancer in organ transplant recipients is multifactorial and may include underlying genetic predisposition, environmental factors, immunologic alterations induced by the transplant, immunosuppressive drugs, and viral infection.[64] The precise mechanism by which immunosuppressive drug therapy potentiates the development of skin cancer remains elusive. In murine models, tumors induced by ultraviolet light are often highly antigenic when transplanted into syngeneic mice, which suggests that defects in the host immune response contribute to tumor formation.[71] Ultraviolet light induces local immunosuppressive effects that facilitate the establishment of tumors, and immunosuppressive drugs may potentiate this local impairment in host immunity.[72–74] A potential role for cyclosporine in tumorigenesis that is distinct from its immunosuppressive properties has also been suggested. Cyclosporine increases the production of transforming growth factor-β by tumor cells and results in increased tumor cell motility and invasiveness *in vitro* and enhanced tumor growth and metastasis *in vivo*.[75]

Human papilloma virus DNA is detected in a significant fraction of squamous cell carcinomas in organ transplant recipients and may contribute to tumor development, although a causal role has not been established.[76]

Clinical Features, Management, and Prevention

Skin cancers in organ transplant recipients are generally considered to be more aggressive than tumors that develop in the general population. Fifty percent to 80% of patients have multiple lesions, and individual lesions characteristically exhibit greater local invasiveness.[77] Squamous cell carcinomas in organ transplant patients are also more likely to metastasize to lymph nodes and distant sites. Skin cancers in these patients are treated using the same modalities used for tumors in the general population, including surgical excision, cryosurgery, electrocautery, and radiotherapy.

Given the frequency of skin cancers in organ allograft recipients, it is essential to educate patients about the hazards associated with sun exposure, provide strategies for protecting the skin from sunlight, promote awareness of the importance of early detection and treatment, and institute regular dermatologic monitoring.[64] Skin disorders that resemble malignancies, such as warts, hyperkeratoses, and keratoacanthomas, are frequently observed in transplant patients, and a biopsy of suspicious lesions should be performed for accurate diagnosis. Premalignant lesions have been successfully treated with topical tretinoin or a combination of low-dose etretinate and topical tretinoin.[64]

EPSTEIN-BARR VIRUS–ASSOCIATED LYMPHOPROLIFERATIVE DISORDERS IN ORGAN TRANSPLANT RECIPIENTS

Epidemiology

PTLD associated with EBV infection is the second most frequent malignancy in solid organ transplant recipients. The incidence of PTLD during the first year after transplantation is 0.2% for kidney transplant recipients and 1.2% for heart transplant recipients.[78] The incidence of PTLD is highest in the first year after transplantation, but these tumors may develop with increased frequency for more than 6 years after transplantation. PTLD develops in host B cells, although the EBV strain may be derived from reactivation of latent virus in the host or virus transmitted with the donor organ. Transplant recipients who are EBV seronegative and receive an organ from an EBV-seropositive donor are more likely to develop a PTLD than EBV-seropositive recipients.[79]

The drug regimen used to prevent or treat graft rejection influences the risk of PTLD, with the highest risk of PTLD observed in patients who receive cyclosporine, FK-506, or anti-CD3 monoclonal antibodies.[78] Patients receiving heart, lung, or combined heart and lung transplants have a higher incidence of PTLD than patients receiving kidney or liver transplants because intensive immunosuppression must be maintained in these patients to prevent life-threatening graft rejection.

Pathogenesis

The pathogenesis of PTLD occurring in solid organ transplant recipients is similar to that of PTLD in HSCT recipients and reflects defective control of EBV by the host immune response. The immunosuppressive drugs administered to organ transplant patients potently suppress EBV-specific CTL activity *in vitro* and *in vivo*. A study of 30 cardiothoracic transplant recipients who received cyclosporin A and azathioprine as rejection prophylaxis showed that EBV-specific CTL activity in the peripheral blood was suppressed or undetectable in all patients during the first 6 months after transplantation.[80] Recovery of EBV-specific T-cell responses is further impaired in patients who require additional immunosuppressive therapy to treat rejection episodes. PTLD in organ allograft recipients frequently involves the transplanted organ, the CNS, and the gastrointestinal tract, which suggests that immunoregulatory factors in the microenvironment may act in concert with a deficiency of EBV-specific CTL to predispose to tumor development. The organ allograft is a site of chronic antigenic stimulation, and local cytokines produced by alloreactive T cells have been suggested to promote the activation and growth of EBV-infected B cells.[81]

Clinical Features, Diagnosis, and Management

Patients developing PTLD may present with an infectious mononucleosis syndrome, including fever, peripheral lymphadenopathy, and tonsillar enlargement. On occasion, the disease presents with a fulminant course characterized by rapidly progressive diffuse multiorgan involvement and severe systemic symptoms. More commonly, PTLD presents with localized lesions in lymph nodes; in extranodal sites such as the gastrointestinal tract, CNS, lung, and the transplanted organ; or in both nodal and extranodal sites. The diagnosis of PTLD is made by analysis of EBV gene expression in biopsy samples of involved tissue, as described earlier for HSCT recipients (see Lymphoproliferative Disorders Associated with Epstein-Barr Virus in Hematopoietic Stem Cell Transplant Recipients).

A standard approach to the management of PTLD in organ allograft recipients has not been established. Therapy may depend on the site of tumor involvement, the rate of tumor growth, and the necessity to maintain intense immunosuppression. A reduction or withdrawal of immunosuppressive drug therapy can result in expansion of endogenous EBV-specific T cells and complete regression of the tumor.[82] However, this strategy may lead to rejection of the organ allograft, which, except in the case of renal transplant recipients, who can return to dialysis therapy, can have disastrous consequences. Anatomically localized lesions may be amenable to surgical resection or limited-field irradiation, but tumor recurrence is common.

Systemic therapy is usually necessary to control PTLD that fails to regress after a reduction in immunosuppressive therapy. Chemotherapy has been used in patients who fail to respond to a reduction in immunosuppression or who have rapidly progressive disease. In small studies, standard regimens used for non-Hodgkin's lymphoma, such as cyclophosphamide, hydroxydaunorubicin [doxorubicin (Adriamycin)], vincristine (Oncovin), and prednisone or ProMACE-CytaBOM (prednisone, doxorubicin, cyclophosphamide, etoposide, cytarabine, bleomycin, vincristine, methotrexate, leucovorin, and trimethoprim/sulfamethoxazole) have induced durable complete remissions in the majority of patients.[83] However, other studies have reported significantly less promising results due to both a high incidence of infectious complications related to neutropenia and refractory disease. Encouraging results have been obtained for therapy with anti-CD20 antibody (rituximab) alone or in combination with chemotherapy, with response rates of more than 65% reported in small trials.[84,85]

Cellular immunotherapy has also been used to restore EBV-specific T-cell immunity in solid organ transplant recipients with PTLD. Unlike in the case of allogeneic HSCT recipients, who have an immunocompetent stem cell donor who can be used as a source of T cells for therapy, in organ transplant recipients EBV-specific T cells must be generated from the recipient's blood or the blood of partially HLA-matched healthy donors.[86–88] The transfer of EBV-specific T cells has resulted in an increased frequency of EBV-specific CTL in the blood and regression of established PTLD.[86,88]

LATE-ONSET LYMPHOMAS AND HODGKIN'S DISEASE IN ORGAN TRANSPLANT RECIPIENTS

The overwhelming majority of PTLDs are EBV associated and of B-cell origin, but T-cell lymphoproliferative disorders have also been described in organ transplant recipients. The T-cell lymphoproliferations typically occur several years after transplantation, involve the bone marrow and peripheral blood at presentation, and are not related to EBV, human T-cell lymphotropic virus, or HHV-8 infection. The prognosis for these patients is poor even with the administration of chemotherapy and reduction of immunosuppression.[89]

Hodgkin's disease has also been reported in organ allograft recipients, and the tumors are usually EBV positive. The clinical presentation and response to therapy is typical of Hodgkin's disease in the general population.

KAPOSI'S SARCOMA IN ORGAN TRANSPLANT RECIPIENTS

Epidemiology

KS is a slow-growing endothelial cell tumor caused by HHV-8 and occurs up to 500 times more frequently in organ transplant recipients than in the general population.[90] Risk factors for the development of KS in organ transplant recipients include African or Middle Eastern origin and the use of antilymphocyte serum for immunosuppression.[90]

The role of HHV-8 in KS in organ transplant recipients was initially suggested by analysis of the serostatus of recipients and donors. The presence of HHV-8 antibodies before or after transplantation is highly predictive of the development of posttransplantation KS, which supports a role for reactivation of endogenous HHV-8 or transmission of HHV-8 in the pathogenesis of KS.[91] The transmission of HHV-8 by the organ allograft has also been demonstrated, and the endothelial tumors in some organ recipients have been found to be of donor cell origin.[92,93] This remarkable finding suggests that transferred donor KS tumor cells or progenitor cells are able to proliferate as a consequence of immunosuppressive therapy.

Pathogenesis

HHV-8 infection is central to the pathogenesis of KS, and molecular studies of the biology of HHV-8 continue to provide insights into the mechanisms of transformation.[94] The spontaneous regression of KS lesions observed with withdrawal of immunosuppression in organ transplant recipients suggests that cellular immune responses directed against HHV-8 antigens or donor alloantigens may be capable of eliminating KS and implicates T-cell defects in the pathogenesis of these tumors.

Clinical Features and Management

Sixty percent of organ allograft recipients with KS present with localized skin or mucosal lesions, and the remainder present with visceral disease involving the gastrointestinal tract, lungs, and lymph nodes.[90] The diagnosis of KS, which can be difficult in cases of visceral disease, is made by biopsy and histologic analysis. The mainstay of therapy for KS that develops after solid organ transplantation is reduction in immunosuppressive therapy. This intervention alone induces a complete response in approximately 25% of patients.[95] However, reintroduction of intensive immunosuppression to treat episodes of graft rejection has been associated with recurrence of the tumor. Due to the inability to maintain reduced levels of immunosuppression in many organ allograft recipients, chemotherapy using regimens described for KS in human immunodeficiency virus (HIV) infection is frequently required to control KS.[95] Novel, less toxic approaches to treat KS are likely to emerge as the biology of these tumors is better understood and may include antiangiogenesis therapy, treatment with antiviral drugs, or T-cell therapy targeting HHV-8 antigens.[96]

OTHER HUMAN HERPESVIRUS-8–ASSOCIATED MALIGNANCIES IN ORGAN TRANSPLANT RECIPIENTS

HHV-8 has been associated with other malignancies, including primary effusion lymphoma in HIV-infected patients and multicentric Castleman's diseases in both HIV-positive and HIV-negative patients.[94,96] Primary effusion lymphoma with integrated HHV-8 DNA has been reported to occur rarely in solid organ transplant recipients and usually can be distinguished from the more common PTLD by the presence of malignant pleural, peritoneal, or pericardial effusions without tumor mass, or adenopathy. Knowledge of both donor and recipient HHV-8 status before transplantation can help identify patients who are at risk for HHV-8–associated malignancies and are suitable for enrollment in clinical trials of candidate prophylactic agents.

REFERENCES

1. Burnet FM. The concept of immunological surveillance. *Prog Exp Tumor Res* 1970;13:1.
2. Rygaard J, Povlsen CO. Is immunological surveillance not a cell-mediated immune function? *Transplantation* 1974;17:135.
3. Dunn GP, Bruce AT, Ikeda H, Old LJ, Schreiber RD. Cancer immunoediting: from immunosurveillance to tumor escape. *Nat Immunol* 2002;3:991.
4. Horowitz MM, Rowlings PA. An update from the International Bone Marrow Transplant Registry and the Autologous Blood and Marrow Transplant Registry on current activity in hematopoietic stem cell transplantation. *Curr Opin Hematol* 1997;4:395.
5. Penn I. Occurrence of cancers in immunosuppressed organ transplant recipients. *Clin Transpl* 1998;147.
6. Horowitz MM. In: Thomas E, Blume K, Forman S, eds. *Hematopoietic cell transplantation*, 2nd ed. Malden, MA: Blackwell, 1999.
7. Witherspoon RP, et al. Secondary cancers after bone marrow transplantation for leukemia or aplastic anemia. *N Engl J Med* 1989;321:784.
8. Curtis RE, et al. Solid cancers after bone marrow transplantation. *N Engl J Med* 1997;336:897.
9. Baker KS, et al. New malignancies after blood or marrow stem-cell transplantation in children and adults: incidence and risk factors. *J Clin Oncol* 2003;21:1352.
10. Bhatia S, et al. Solid cancers after bone marrow transplantation. *J Clin Oncol* 2001;19:464.
11. Socie G, et al. New malignant diseases after allogeneic marrow transplantation for childhood acute leukemia. *J Clin Oncol* 2000;18:348.
12. Kolb HJ, et al. Malignant neoplasms in long-term survivors of bone marrow transplantation. Late Effects Working Party of the European Cooperative Group for Blood and Marrow Transplantation and the European Late Effect Project Group. *Ann Intern Med* 1999;131:738.
13. Bhatia S, et al. Malignant neoplasms following bone marrow transplantation. *Blood* 1996;87:3633.
14. Andre MP, et al. Second cancers and late toxicities after treatment of aggressive non-Hodgkin lymphoma with the ACVBP regimen. A GELA cohort study on 2837 patients. *Blood* 2004;103:1222.
15. Bhatia S, et al. Breast cancer and other second neoplasms after childhood Hodgkin's disease. *N Engl J Med* 1996;334:745.
16. Ades L, Guardiola P, Socie G. Second malignancies after allogeneic hematopoietic stem cell transplantation: new insight and current problems. *Blood Rev* 2002;16:135.
17. Pittet MJ, et al. High frequencies of naive Melan-A/MART-1-specific CD8(+) T cells in a large proportion of human histocompatibility leukocyte antigen (HLA)-A2 individuals. *J Exp Med* 1999;190:705.
18. Dudley ME, et al. Cancer regression and autoimmunity in patients after clonal repopulation with antitumor lymphocytes. *Science* 2002;298:850.
19. Yee C, et al. Adoptive T cell therapy using antigen-specific CD8+ T cell clones for the treatment of patients with metastatic melanoma: in vivo persistence, migration, and antitumor effect of transferred T cells. *Proc Natl Acad Sci U S A* 2002;99:16168.
20. Socie G, et al. Long-term survival and late deaths after allogeneic bone marrow transplantation. Late Effects Working Committee of the International Bone Marrow Transplant Registry. *N Engl J Med* 1999;341:14.
21. Maris M, Storb R. The transplantation of hematopoietic stem cells after non-myeloablative conditioning: a cellular therapeutic approach to hematologic and genetic diseases. *Immunol Res* 2003;28:13.
22. Mielcarek M, et al. Graft-versus-host disease after nonmyeloablative versus conventional hematopoietic stem cell transplantation. *Blood* 2003;102:756.
23. Curtis RE, et al. Risk of lymphoproliferative disorders after bone marrow transplantation: a multi-institutional study. *Blood* 1999;94:2208.
24. Gross TG, Loechelt BJ. Epstein-Barr virus associated disease following blood or marrow transplant. *Pediatr Transplant* 2003(7 Suppl 3):44.
25. Kieff E. In: Fields B, Knipe D, Howley P, eds. *Fields virology*. Philadelphia: Lippincott–Raven Publishers, 1996:2343.
26. Liebowitz D. Epstein-Barr virus and a cellular signaling pathway in lymphomas from immunosuppressed patients. *N Engl J Med* 1998;338:1413.
27. Callan MF, et al. Large clonal expansions of CD8+ T cells in acute infectious mononucleosis. *Nat Med* 1996;2:906.
28. Levitskaya J, et al. Inhibition of antigen processing by the internal repeat region of the Epstein-Barr virus nuclear antigen-1. *Nature* 1995;375:685.
29. Yin Y, Manoury B, Fahraeus R. Self-inhibition of synthesis and antigen presentation by Epstein-Barr virus-encoded EBNA1. *Science* 2003;301:1371.
30. Gratama JW, et al. Eradication of Epstein-Barr virus by allogeneic bone marrow transplantation: implications for sites of viral latency. *Proc Natl Acad Sci U S A* 1988;85:8693.
31. Lucas KG, Small TN, Heller G, Dupont B, O'Reilly RJ. The development of cellular immunity to Epstein-Barr virus after allogeneic bone marrow transplantation. *Blood* 1996;87:2594.
32. Timms JM, et al. Target cells of Epstein-Barr-virus (EBV)-positive post-transplant lymphoproliferative disease: similarities to EBV-positive Hodgkin's lymphoma. *Lancet* 2003; 361:217.
33. O'Reilly RJ, et al. Biology and adoptive cell therapy of Epstein-Barr virus-associated lymphoproliferative disorders in recipients of marrow allografts. *Immunol Rev* 1997;157:195.
34. Gartner BC, et al. Evaluation of use of Epstein-Barr viral load in patients after allogeneic stem cell transplantation to diagnose and monitor posttransplant lymphoproliferative disease. *J Clin Microbiol* 2002;40:351.
35. Sirvent-Von Bueltzingsloewen A, et al. A prospective study of Epstein-Barr virus load in 85 hematopoietic stem cell transplants. *Bone Marrow Transplant* 2002;29:21.
36. Stevens SJ, et al. Role of Epstein-Barr virus DNA load monitoring in prevention and early detection of post-transplant lymphoproliferative disease. *Leuk Lymphoma* 2002;43:831.
37. Gulley ML, et al. Guidelines for interpreting EBER in situ hybridization and LMP1 immunohistochemical tests for detecting Epstein-Barr virus in Hodgkin lymphoma. *Am J Clin Pathol* 2002;117:259.
38. Rooney CM, et al. Use of gene-modified virus-specific T lymphocytes to control Epstein-Barr-virus-related lymphoproliferation. *Lancet* 1995;345:9.
39. Heslop HE, et al. Long-term restoration of immunity against Epstein-Barr virus infection by adoptive transfer of gene-modified virus-specific T lymphocytes. *Nat Med* 1996;2:551.
40. Gottschalk S, et al. An Epstein-Barr virus deletion mutant associated with fatal lymphoproliferative disease unresponsive to therapy with virus-specific CTLs. *Blood* 2001;97:835.
41. Rooney CM, et al. Infusion of cytotoxic T cells for the prevention and treatment of Epstein-Barr virus-induced lymphoma in allogeneic transplant recipients. *Blood* 1998;92:1549.
42. Benkerrou M, et al. Anti-B-cell monoclonal antibody treatment of severe posttransplant B-lymphoproliferative disorder: prognostic factors and long-term outcome. *Blood* 1998;92:3137.
43. Kuehnle I, et al. CD20 monoclonal antibody (rituximab) for therapy of Epstein-Barr virus lymphoma after hemopoietic stem-cell transplantation. *Blood* 2000;95:1502.
44. Faye A, et al. Chimaeric anti-CD20 monoclonal antibody (rituximab) in post-transplant B-lymphoproliferative disorder following stem cell transplantation in children. *Br J Haematol* 2001;115:112.
45. van Esser JW, et al. Prevention of Epstein-Barr virus-lymphoproliferative disease by molecular monitoring and preemptive rituximab in high-risk patients after allogeneic stem cell transplantation. *Blood* 2002;99:4364.
46. Mentzer SJ, Perrine SP, Faller DV. Epstein-Barr virus post-transplant lymphoproliferative disease and virus-specific therapy: pharmacological re-activation of viral target genes with arginine butyrate. *Transpl Infect Dis* 2001;3:177.
47. Rowlings PA, et al. Increased incidence of Hodgkin's disease after allogeneic bone marrow transplantation. *J Clin Oncol* 1999;17:3122.
48. Zutter MM, et al. Secondary T-cell lymphoproliferation after marrow transplantation. *Am J Clin Pathol* 1990;94:714.
49. Smith RE. Risk for the development of treatment-related acute myelocytic leukemia and myelodysplastic syndrome among patients with breast cancer: review of the literature and the National Surgical Adjuvant Breast and Bowel Project experience. *Clin Breast Cancer* 2003;4:273.

50. van Leeuwen FE, et al. Long-term risk of second malignancy in survivors of Hodgkin's disease treated during adolescence or young adulthood. *J Clin Oncol* 2000;18:487.

51. Ng AK, et al. Second malignancy after Hodgkin disease treated with radiation therapy with or without chemotherapy: long-term risks and risk factors. *Blood* 2002;100:1989.

52. Darrington DL, et al. Incidence and characterization of secondary myelodysplastic syndrome and acute myelogenous leukemia following high-dose chemoradiotherapy and autologous stem-cell transplantation for lymphoid malignancies. *J Clin Oncol* 1994;12:2527.

53. Stone RM, et al. Myelodysplastic syndrome as a late complication following autologous bone marrow transplantation for non-Hodgkin's lymphoma. *J Clin Oncol* 1994;12:2535.

54. Micallef IN, et al. Therapy-related myelodysplasia and secondary acute myelogenous leukemia after high-dose therapy with autologous hematopoietic progenitor-cell support for lymphoid malignancies. *J Clin Oncol* 2000;18:947.

55. Krishnan A, et al. Predictors of therapy-related leukemia and myelodysplasia following autologous transplantation for lymphoma: an assessment of risk factors. *Blood* 2000;95:1588.

56. Miller JS, et al. Myelodysplastic syndrome after autologous bone marrow transplantation: an additional late complication of curative cancer therapy. *Blood* 1994;83:3780.

57. Newburger PE, et al. Leukemia relapse in donor cells after allogeneic bone-marrow transplantation. *N Engl J Med* 1981;304:712.

58. Niederwieser DW, et al. Inadvertent transmission of a donor's acute myeloid leukemia in bone marrow transplantation for chronic myelocytic leukemia. *N Engl J Med* 1990;322:1794.

59. Chao NJ, et al. Importance of bone marrow cytogenetic evaluation before autologous bone marrow transplantation for Hodgkin's disease. *J Clin Oncol* 1991;9:1575.

60. Birkeland SA, Storm HH. Risk for tumor and other disease transmission by transplantation: a population-based study of unrecognized malignancies and other diseases in organ donors. *Transplantation* 2002;74:1409.

61. Conlon PJ, Smith SR. Transmission of cancer with cadaveric donor organs. *J Am Soc Nephrol* 1995;6:54.

62. Herzig KA, et al. Novel surveillance and cure of a donor-transmitted lymphoma in a renal allograft recipient. *Transplantation* 2000;70:149.

63. Sheil AG. Cancer in immune-suppressed organ transplant recipients: aetiology and evolution. *Transplant Proc* 1998;30:2055.

64. Euvrard S, Kanitakis J, Claudy A. Skin cancers after organ transplantation. *N Engl J Med* 2003;348:1681.

65. Ramsay HM, Fryer AA, Hawley CM, Smith AG, Harden PN. Non-melanoma skin cancer risk in the Queensland renal transplant population. *Br J Dermatol* 2002;147:950.

66. Hartevelt MM, Bavinck JN, Kootte AM, Vermeer BJ, Vandenbroucke JP. Incidence of skin cancer after renal transplantation in the Netherlands. *Transplantation* 1990;49:506.

67. Lampros TD, et al. Squamous and basal cell carcinoma in heart transplant recipients. *J Heart Lung Transplant* 1998;17:586.

68. King GN, et al. Increased prevalence of dysplastic and malignant lip lesions in renal-transplant recipients. *N Engl J Med* 1995;332:1052.

69. Jensen P, Moller B, Hansen S. Skin cancer in kidney and heart transplant recipients and different long-term immunosuppressive therapy regimens. *J Am Acad Dermatol* 2000;42:307.

70. Starzl TE, et al. Tolerogenic immunosuppression for organ transplantation. *Lancet* 2003;361:1502.

71. Kripke ML. Immunoregulation of carcinogenesis: past, present, and future. *J Natl Cancer Inst* 1988;80:722.

72. Hill LL, Shreedhar VK, Kripke ML, Owen-Schaub LB. A critical role for Fas ligand in the active suppression of systemic immune responses by ultraviolet radiation. *J Exp Med* 1999;189:1285.

73. Seite S, et al. Alterations in human epidermal Langerhans cells by ultraviolet radiation: quantitative and morphological study. *Br J Dermatol* 2003;148:291.

74. Moodycliffe AM, Nghiem D, Clydesdale G, Ullrich SE. Immune suppression and skin cancer development: regulation by NKT cells. *Nat Immunol* 2000;1:521.

75. Hojo M, et al. Cyclosporine induces cancer progression by a cell-autonomous mechanism. *Nature* 1999;397:530.

76. Harwood CA, et al. Human papillomavirus infection and non-melanoma skin cancer in immunosuppressed and immunocompetent individuals. *J Med Virol* 2000;61:289.

77. Barrett WL, First MR, Aron BS, Penn I. Clinical course of malignancies in renal transplant recipients. *Cancer* 1993;72:2186.

78. Opelz G, Henderson R. Incidence of non-Hodgkin lymphoma in kidney and heart transplant recipients. *Lancet* 1993;342:1514.

79. Shahinian VB, et al. Epstein-Barr virus seronegativity is a risk factor for late-onset post-transplant lymphoproliferative disorder in adult renal allograft recipients. *Transplantation* 2003;75:851.

80. Haque T, et al. A prospective study in heart and lung transplant recipients correlating persistent Epstein-Barr virus infection with clinical events. *Transplantation* 1997;64:1028.

81. Haque T, Crawford DH. The role of adoptive immunotherapy in the prevention and treatment of lymphoproliferative disease following transplantation. *Br J Haematol* 1999;106:309.

82. Khatri VP, et al. Endogenous CD8+ T cell expansion during regression of monoclonal EBV-associated posttransplant lymphoproliferative disorder. *J Immunol* 1999;163:500.

83. Swinnen LJ, Mullen GM, Carr TJ, Costanzo MR, Fisher RI. Aggressive treatment for post-cardiac transplant lymphoproliferation. *Blood* 1995;86:3333.

84. Milpied N, et al. Humanized anti-CD20 monoclonal antibody (rituximab) in post transplant B-lymphoproliferative disorder: a retrospective analysis on 32 patients. *Ann Oncol* 2000;11[Suppl 1]:113.

85. Orjuela M, et al. A pilot study of chemoimmunotherapy (cyclophosphamide, prednisone, and rituximab) in patients with post-transplant lymphoproliferative disease following solid organ transplantation. *Clin Cancer Res* 2003;9:3945S.

86. Khanna R, et al. Activation and adoptive transfer of Epstein-Barr virus-specific cytotoxic T cells in solid organ transplant patients with posttransplant lymphoproliferative disease. *Proc Natl Acad Sci U S A* 1999;96:10391.

87. Comoli P, et al. Infusion of autologous Epstein-Barr virus (EBV)-specific cytotoxic T cells for prevention of EBV-related lymphoproliferative disorder in solid organ transplant recipients with evidence of active virus replication. *Blood* 2002;99:2592.

88. Haque T, et al. Treatment of Epstein-Barr-virus-positive post-transplantation lymphoproliferative disease with partly HLA-matched allogeneic cytotoxic T cells. *Lancet* 2002;360:436.

89. Hanson MN, et al. Posttransplant T-cell lymphoproliferative disorders—an aggressive, late complication of solid-organ transplantation. *Blood* 1996;88:3626.

90. Mendez JC, Paya CV. Kaposi's sarcoma and transplantation. *Herpes* 2000;7:18.

91. Farge D, et al. Human herpes virus-8 and other risk factors for Kaposi's sarcoma in kidney transplant recipients. Groupe Cooperatif de Transplantation d'Ile de France (GCIF). *Transplantation* 1999;67:1236.

92. Regamey N, et al. Transmission of human herpesvirus 8 infection from renal-transplant donors to recipients. *N Engl J Med* 1998;339:1358.

93. Barozzi P, et al. Post-transplant Kaposi sarcoma originates from the seeding of donor-derived progenitors. *Nat Med* 2003;9:554.

94. Aoki Y, Tosato G. Pathogenesis and manifestations of human herpesvirus-8-associated disorders. *Semin Hematol* 2003;40:143.

95. Shepherd FA, et al. Treatment of Kaposi's sarcoma after solid organ transplantation. *J Clin Oncol* 1997;15:2371.

96. Little RF, Yarchoan R. Treatment of gammaherpesvirus-related neoplastic disorders in the immunosuppressed host. *Semin Hematol* 2003;40:163.

CHAPTER 49

Oncologic Emergencies

SECTION 1
JOACHIM YAHALOM

Superior Vena Cava Syndrome

Superior vena cava syndrome (SVCS) is the clinical expression of obstruction of blood flow through the SVC. Characteristic symptoms and signs may develop quickly or gradually when this thin-walled vessel is compressed, invaded, or thrombosed by processes in the superior mediastinum. The first pathologic description of SVC obstruction, in a patient with syphilitic aortic aneurysm, appeared in 1757.[1] In 1954, Schechter[2] reviewed 274 well-documented cases of SVCS reported in the literature; 40% of them were due to syphilitic aneurysms or tuberculosis mediastinitis. These entities have since virtually disappeared, and cancer of the lung is now the underlying process in approximately 70% of patients with SVCS. It is estimated that, in the United States, SVCS develops in 15,000 people each year.[3]

ANATOMY AND PATHOPHYSIOLOGY

The SVC is the major vessel for drainage of venous blood from the head, neck, upper extremities, and upper thorax. It is located in the middle mediastinum and is surrounded by relatively rigid structures, such as the sternum, trachea, right bronchus, aorta, pulmonary artery, and perihilar and paratracheal lymph nodes. The SVC extends from the junction of the right and left innominate veins to the right atrium, for a distance of 6 to 8 cm. The distal 2 cm of the SVC is within the pericardial sac, with a point of relative fixation of the vena cava at the pericardial reflection. The azygos vein, the main auxiliary vessel, enters the SVC posteriorly, just above the pericardial reflection. The width of the SVC is 1.5 to 2.0 cm, and it maintains blood at a low pressure. The SVC is thin walled, compliant, and easily compressible and is vulnerable to any space-occupying process in its vicinity. The SVC is completely encircled by chains of lymph nodes that drain all the structures of the right thoracic cavity and the lower part of the left thorax. The auxiliary azygos vein is also threatened by enlargement of paratracheal nodes. Other critical structures in the mediastinum, such as the main bronchi, esophagus, and spinal cord, may be involved by the same process that led to obstruction of the SVC.[4–6]

When the SVC is fully or partially obstructed, an extensive venous collateral circulation may develop. The azygos venous system is the most important alternative pathway. Carlson[7] found that dogs could not survive sudden ligation of the SVC below the level of the azygos vein, but they tolerated well ligation of the SVC above it. He could, however, successfully obstruct the SVC and the azygos vein in operations performed in two stages, presumably by allowing time for collaterals to form. Other collateral systems are the internal mammary veins, lateral thoracic veins, paraspinous veins, and esophageal venous network. The subcutaneous veins are important pathways, and their engorgement in the neck and thorax is a typical physical finding in SVCS. Despite these collateral pathways, venous pressure is almost always elevated in the upper compartment if the SVC is obstructed. Venous pressures have been recorded as high as 200 to 500 cm H_2O in severe SVCS.[8]

ETIOLOGY AND NATURAL HISTORY

SVCS usually has an insidious onset and progresses to typical symptoms and signs. Review of the data from three series[9–11]

TABLE 49.1-1.   Common Symptoms and Physical Findings of Superior Vena Cava Syndrome

Symptoms	Patients Affected[a] (%)	Physical Findings	Patients Affected[a] (%)
Dyspnea	63	Venous distention of neck	66
Facial swelling and head fullness	50	Venous distention of chest wall	54
Cough	24	Facial edema	46
Arm swelling	18	Cyanosis	20
Chest pain	15	Plethora of face	19
Dysphagia	9	Edema of arms	14

[a]Analysis based on data from 370 patients.[9–11]

(Table 49.1-1) shows dyspnea to be the most common symptom. Dyspnea occurred in 63% of patients with SVCS. A sensation of fullness in the head and facial swelling were reported by 50% of the patients. Other complaints were cough (24%), arm swelling (18%), chest pain (15%), and dysphagia (9%). The characteristic physical findings were venous distention of the neck (66%) and chest wall (54%), facial edema (46%), plethora (19%), and cyanosis (19%). These symptoms and signs may be aggravated by bending forward, stooping, or lying down. Malignant disease is the most common cause of SVCS. The percentage of patients in different series with a confirmed diagnosis of malignancy varies from 78% to 86% (Table 49.1-2). Lung cancer was diagnosed in 65% of 415 patients analyzed in these series.[14,10–12] Armstrong et al.[9] did a retrospective review of 4100 cases treated for bronchogenic carcinoma between 1965 and 1984, and they identified 99 patients (2.4%) with SVCS. Salsali and Cliffton[13] observed SVCS in 4.2% of 4960 patients with lung cancer; 80% of the tumors inducing SVCS were of the right lung. Small cell lung cancer (SCLC) is the most common histologic subtype (Table 49.1-3), and it was found in 38% of the patients who had lung cancer and SVCS. In six large series of SCLC, 9% to 19% of patients demonstrated SVCS.[14–19] The second most common histologic subtype is squamous cell carcinoma, found in 26% of lung cancer patients with SVCS. Lymphoma involving the mediastinum was the cause of SVCS in 8% of patients reported in the series (see Table 49.1-2). Armstrong et al.[9] found SVCS in 1.9% of 952 patients with lymphoma. Perez-Soler et al.[20] identified 36 cases (4%) of SVCS among 915 patients with non-Hodgkin's lymphoma (NHL) treated at the M. D. Anderson Cancer Center. Twenty-

three patients (64%) had diffuse large cell lymphoma, 12 (33%) had lymphoblastic lymphoma, and 1 patient had follicular large cell lymphoma. Of their patients with diffuse large cell lymphoma and lymphoblastic lymphoma, 7% and 21% had SVCS, respectively. In a series of patients with primary mediastinal B-cell lymphoma with sclerosis, SVCS was present in 57% of patients.[21] Hodgkin's lymphoma commonly involves the mediastinum, but it rarely causes SVCS. Other primary mediastinal malignancies that cause SVCS are thymoma and germ cell tumors. Breast cancer is the most common metastatic disease that causes SVCS.[4,10,12] In one report, breast cancer was the cause of SVCS in 11% of cases.[22]

Nonmalignant conditions causing SVCS are not as rare as previously reported.[9,23] When the data were collected from general hospitals, as many as 22% of patients had noncancerous causes of SVCS.[4,10,12] Parish et al.[10] reported 19 patients with benign causes of SVCS, and Schraufnagel et al.[4] included 16 such patients in their series. Fifty percent of the patients in both reports had a diagnosis of mediastinal fibrosis, which was probably due to histoplasmosis. Parish et al.[10] reported six patients with thrombosis of SVC, and in five, the thrombosis developed in the presence of central vein catheters or pacemakers. Sculier and Feld[24] reviewed 24 cases of central venous catheter–induced SVC. Of these, 18 were caused by pacemaker catheters. LeVeen peritoneovenous shunts, Swan-Ganz catheters, and hyperalimentation catheters were also involved. The increasing use of these devices for the delivery of chemotherapy agents or for hyperalimentation contributes to the development of SVCS in the cancer patient.[25] Obstruction of SVC in the pediatric age group is rare and has a different etiologic spectrum. The causative factors are mainly iatrogenic[26] secondary to cardiovascular surgery for congenital heart disease, ventriculoatrial shunt for hydrocephalus, and SVC catheterization for parenteral nutrition. In a report of 175 children with SVCS, 70% were iatrogenic. Of the remaining 53 cases, 37 (70%) were caused by mediastinal tumors, 8 (15%) were caused by benign granuloma, and 4 (7.5%) by congenital anomalies of the cardiovascular system. Two-thirds of the tumors causing SVCS in childhood are lymphomas.[26,27] Of 16 children reported from St. Jude Children's Research Hospital with SVCS at presentation, eight were diagnosed with NHL, four had acute lymphoblastic leukemia, two had Hodgkin's disease, one had neuroblastoma, and one had a yolk sac tumor.[22] Most children in whom SVCS developed late in the course of their malignancy had recurrent solid tumors.[28] Issa et al.[27] reported that mediastinal fibrosis secondary to histoplasmosis caused SVCS in 7 (5%) of the 150 patients reviewed.

TABLE 49.1-2.   Primary Pathologic Diagnoses for Superior Vena Cava Syndrome

Histologic Diagnosis	Bell et al.,[11] 159 Patients (%)	Schraufnagel et al.,[4] 107 Patients (%)	Parish et al.,[10] 86 Patients (%)	Yellin et al.,[12] 63 Patients (%)	Total, 415 Patients (%)
Lung cancer	129 (81)	67 (63)	45 (52)	30 (48)	271 (65)
Lymphoma	3 (2)	10 (9)	8 (9)	13 (21)	34 (8)
Other malignancies (primary or metastatic)	4 (3)	14 (13)	14 (16)	8 (13)	40 (10)
Nonneoplastic	2 (1)	16 (15)	19 (22)	11 (18)	50 (12)
Undiagnosed	21 (13)	—	—	—	21 (5)

TABLE 49.1-3. Lung Cancer Subtypes Associated with Superior Vena Cava Syndrome

Histology	No. of Patients	Percentage of Patients
Small cell	142	38
Squamous cell	97	26
Adenocarcinoma	52	14
Large cell	43	12
Unclassified	34	9
Total	370	100

TABLE 49.1-5. Positive Yield of Diagnostic Procedures for Patients with Superior Vena Cava Syndrome

Procedure	No. of Procedures	No. Positive	Percentage Positive
Sputum cytology	59	29	49
Thoracocentesis	14	10	71
Bone marrow biopsy	13	3	23
Lymph node biopsy	95	64	67
Bronchoscopy	124	65	52
Mediastinoscopy	105	95	90
Thoracotomy	49	48	98

DIAGNOSTIC PROCEDURES

SVCS has long been considered to be a potentially life-threatening medical emergency.[5,23,29] It was common practice to immediately apply radiation therapy with initial high-dose fractions, sometimes even before the histologic diagnosis of the primary lesion was established.[23,29,30] Diagnostic procedures, such as bronchoscopy, mediastinoscopy, thoracotomy, or supraclavicular lymph node biopsy, were often avoided because they were considered to be hazardous in the presence of SVCS.[5,23] However, the safety of these invasive procedures in patients with SVCS has markedly improved, and the modern treatment of SVCS has become disease specific from the outset.[4,31,32,82] Temporizing emergency mediastinal irradiation before biopsy is rarely used because it may preclude proper interpretation of the specimen in almost one-half of patients.[33] The clinical identification of SVCS is simple because the symptoms and signs are typical and unmistakable. The chest film shows a mass in most patients. Only 16% of the patients studied by Parish et al.[10] had normal chest films. The most common radiographic abnormalities are superior mediastinal widening and pleural effusion (Table 49.1-4).

Computed tomography (CT) provides more detailed information about the SVC, its tributaries, and other critical structures, such as the bronchi and the cord.[34] The additional information is necessary because the involvement of these structures requires prompt action for relief of pressure.

CT phlebography provides excellent imaging information on the site and extent of obstruction and the status of collaterals.[35] Helical CT phlebography replaced the combination of CT and digital phlebography that was advocated in the past.[36] The role of magnetic resonance imaging has been insufficiently investigated but appears promising, especially because this modality is noninvasive.[37]

Contrast venography provides important information for determining if the vena cava is completely obstructed or remains patent and extrinsically compressed.[31,38] Dyet and Moghissi[39] demonstrated by venography that 41% of patients with SVCS have a patent SVC that is displaced or involved but not obstructed by a tumor. Another 19% have SVC obstruction below the azygos vein, for which collateral venous compression should be adequate. Venography is valuable if surgical bypass is considered for the obstructed vena cava.[40] Lokich and Goodman[23] stated that venograms are relatively contraindicated because the interruption of the integrity of the vessel wall, in the presence of increased intraluminal pressures, may result in excessive bleeding from the puncture site. However, no evidence of this complication has been reported. Although a venography can confirm the clinical diagnosis and outline the anatomy, priority should still be given to procedures that help establish the histologic diagnosis. Radionuclide technetium 99m venography is an alternative, minimally invasive method of imaging the venous system.[41–43] Although images that are obtained by this method are not as well defined as those achieved with contrast venography, they demonstrate patency and flow patterns. Collateral circulation can be evaluated in a general manner and quantified to some degree by radionuclide venography. Gallium single-photon emission CT may be of value in selected cases.[44]

In 58% of 107 patients reported by Schraufnagel et al.,[4] the SVCS developed before the primary diagnosis was established. The diagnostic procedures used in different studies are summarized in Table 49.1-5. Sputum cytology established the diagnosis for almost one-half of patients. Cytologic diagnosis is as accurate as tissue diagnosis in small cell carcinoma.[45] Bronchoscopy supplies the malignant cells for cytologic evaluation in most cases of small cell disease.[46] In the presence of pleural effusion, thoracocentesis established the diagnosis of malignancy in 71% of patients. Biopsy of a supraclavicular node, especially if there was a suspicious palpatory finding, was rewarding in two-thirds of the reported attempts. SCLC and NHL often involve the bone marrow. A biopsy of the bone marrow may provide the diagnosis and stage for these patients. Mediastinoscopy has a very high success rate for providing a diagnosis, and a complication rate of approximately 5%.[47] Reports by several authors on using mediastinoscopy for patients with SVCS whose histologic diagnosis could not be established with less invasive techniques confirmed the safety and high diagnostic yield of mediastinoscopy.[47,48,82] No periop-

TABLE 49.1-4. Chest Radiographic Findings for 86 Patients with Superior Vena Cava Syndrome

Finding	No. of Patients	Percentage of Patients
Superior mediastinal widening	55	64
Pleural effusion	22	26
Right hilar mass	10	12
Bilateral diffuse infiltrates	6	7
Cardiomegaly	5	6
Calcified paratracheal nodes	4	5
Mediastinal (anterior) mass	3	3
Normal	14	16

(From ref. 10, with permission.)

erative mortality was recorded, and the diagnosis yield was excellent.

Percutaneous transthoracic CT-guided fine-needle biopsy is emerging as an effective and safe alternative to an open biopsy or mediastinoscopy, with a sensitivity rate of 75%.[40,50,82] Successful diagnostic transluminal atherectomy also has been reported.[51] A thoracoscopic biopsy or thoracotomy is diagnostic if all other procedures have failed. Ahmann[31] examined the traditional opinion that diagnostic procedures carry with them significant hazard, primarily excessive bleeding.[23,29] He reviewed 843 invasive and semiinvasive diagnostic procedures and found that only 10 reported complications, none of them fatal. Ahmann[31] and others[12,32] found minimal evidence to suggest that diagnostic procedures such as venographies, thoracotomies, bronchoscopies, mediastinoscopies, and lymph node biopsies carry an excessive risk in patients with SVCS. In 163 patients treated at Memorial Sloan-Kettering Cancer Center for anterior mediastinal mass, 44 underwent general anesthesia. No deaths occurred, and only four patients had prolonged intubation, demonstrating the low risk of modern anesthesia in thoracic patients.[52]

MANAGEMENT

The goals of treatment of SVCS are to relieve symptoms and to attempt the cure of the primary malignant process. SCLC, NHL, and germ cell tumors constitute almost one-half of the malignant causes of SVCS. These disorders are potentially curable, even in the presence of SVCS. The treatment of SVCS should be selected according to the histologic disorder and stage of the primary process. The prognosis of patients with SVCS strongly correlates with the prognosis of the underlying disease.

When the therapeutic goal is only palliation of SVCS, or when urgent treatment of the venous obstruction is required, direct opening of the occlusion should be considered. The newer techniques of endovascular stenting and angioplasty with possible thrombolysis should provide prompt relief of symptoms before more specific cancer therapy.[3,83–85]

SMALL CELL LUNG CANCER

Chemotherapy alone or in combination with thoracic irradiation therapy is the standard treatment for SCLC.[53] Chemotherapy and radiotherapy as initial treatments are effective in rapidly improving the symptoms of SVCS.[19] In an analysis of 50 patients with SCLC who presented with SVCS, investigators from Ontario, Canada recorded a response rate to chemotherapy of 93% and a similar response to mediastinal irradiation of 94%.[19] In this series, 70% of patients remained SVCS free before death. A review of the literature indicated a response rate of 77% and relapse-free rate of 60%.[83] It is of interest that, when the total treatment of SCLC included chemotherapy and radiation, the risk of SVCS recurrence was significantly lower than when the treatment was chemotherapy alone.[19] A small randomized trial, however, could not show that the addition of mediastinal radiation after chemotherapy in patients with SCLC and SVCS increased the protection from local recurrence or improved the survival rate.[16]

Among 643 patients with SCLC, Sculier et al.[15] identified 55 patients (8.5%) with SVCS. In one-half of patients, the manifes-

tations of SVCS developed before the histologic diagnosis was established. In the other patients, the syndrome developed after the pathologic diagnosis of SCLC was made, but before a specific treatment was started. Symptomatic relief of SVCS was obtained in 35 of 48 patients (73%) initially treated with chemotherapy and in 3 of 7 patients (43%) who were initially treated with radiation. Relief of SVCS occurred within 7 to 10 days after initiation of therapy. In SCLC patients with recurrent or persistent SVCS after initial chemotherapy, the obstruction responded in 5 of 7 patients (71%) who received additional chemotherapy and in 25 of 32 patients (78%) who received radiotherapy.[19] These data support retreatment of SVCS for palliation of symptoms.

In some series of SCLC, SVCS was a favorable prognostic sign,[15,16,18] whereas its presence did not affect survival in other reports.[14,17] A study of 408 patients with SCLC by Wurschmidt et al.[18] showed that the presence of SVCS independently predicted for better survival. Other independent predictors for better survival were stage and performance status.[18] The reason for the possible association of SVCS with better prognosis remains obscure. It is of interest to note that some researchers found a higher incidence of brain metastases at the time of diagnosis in SCLC patients with SVCS compared to patients without SVCS.[17,18,53] Although randomized trials of the contribution of thoracic irradiation to chemotherapy have not consistently demonstrated an advantage to the combined modality approach, metaanalysis of these studies showed a small but significant improvement in local control and survival of patients with limited disease with the addition of radiotherapy.[54,55] The optimal sequence of the two modalities, and the dose and fractionation of radiotherapy, have not yet been fully established.[56] However, the use of combination chemotherapy as the initial modality, with subsequent rapid shrinkage of the tumor, may eliminate the necessity of irradiating a large volume of lung tissue. When chemotherapy is administered, the arm veins should be avoided. Veins of the lower extremities provide an alternative simple venous access.

NON–SMALL CELL LUNG CANCER

A review of SVCS in lung cancer by Rowell and Gleeson[83] indicated that chemotherapy relieved SVCS in 59% of patients with non-SCLC; radiotherapy relieved the obstruction in 63% of non-SCLC patients. Nevertheless, in almost 20% of the patients the obstruction has recurred. Response to radiotherapy was higher in patients who had received prior therapy (94% vs. 70%).[83] Another review indicated that the median survival of patients with non-SCLC was shorter in the presence of SVCS (only 6 months) than without SVCS (9 months).[86]

NON-HODGKIN'S LYMPHOMA

The most extensive experience in treating SVCS secondary to NHL is reported from the M. D. Anderson Cancer Center.[20] Twenty-two patients with diffuse large cell lymphoma and eight patients with lymphoblastic lymphoma were evaluated for results of treatment. The patients were treated with chemotherapy alone, chemotherapy combined with irradiation, or radiotherapy alone. All patients achieved complete relief of SVCS symptoms within 2 weeks of the onset of any type of treatment. No treatment modality appeared to be superior in achieving clinical improvement. The presence of dysphagia, hoarseness, or stridor was a major adverse prognostic factor for patients with lymphoma who presented with SVCS. Eighteen of 22 patients (81%) with large cell lymphoma achieved complete response. Relapse occurred in all six patients treated with irradiation alone, in four of seven patients treated with chemotherapy alone, and in five of nine patients treated with chemotherapy and radiotherapy. The median survival rate was 21 months. All eight patients with lymphoblastic lymphoma achieved complete response. Six relapses occurred in this group, and all were in sites that were not initially involved. Median survival was 19 months.

From these results, the researchers concluded that SVCS secondary to lymphoma is rarely an emergency that requires treatment before a histologic diagnosis is made. They recommended that the choice of treatment should be based on the histologic diagnosis and that the patients should undergo, if possible, a complete staging workup before therapy. They advocated chemotherapy as the treatment of choice, because it provides local and systemic therapeutic activity. They suggested that local consolidation with radiation therapy may be beneficial in patients with large cell lymphoma with mediastinal masses larger than 10 cm. A similarly favorable experience in children with T-cell lymphoma or leukemia (nine patients) and Hodgkin's disease (two patients) presenting with SVCS was reported from Israel.[57] Tissue diagnosis was obtained before specific therapy in all children; SVCS responded to chemotherapy within 2 to 10 days, and the overall 3-year disease-free survival rate was 78%.

NONMALIGNANT CAUSES

Patients with nonmalignant causes of SVCS differ significantly from patients with malignant disease. If the cause is not malignant, the patients often have symptoms long before they seek medical advice, it takes more time to establish the diagnosis, and their survival is markedly longer.[4] Schraufnagel et al.[4] reported that the average survival rate was 9 years if the primary process was benign, compared with an average survival of 5 months for patients with lung cancer. Mahajan et al.[58] reviewed the literature of benign SVCS and reported 16 new cases. Twelve (75%) of these 16 patients had a mediastinal granuloma that was attributed to histoplasmosis. Most patients had an insidious onset of SVCS and were relatively young. Ten patients who were available for a follow-up of 1 to 11 years were all doing well at the time of the report. It was suggested that the good prognosis of patients with benign SVCS caused by fibrosing mediastinitis does not provide a role for SVC bypass surgery.[58,59] However, Nieto and Doty[38] advocated surgery for SVCS caused by benign disorders if the syndrome develops suddenly, progresses, or persists after 6 to 12 months of observation for possible collateral development.[38] In patients whose histoplasmosis complement fixation titers suggest active disease, ketoconazole treatment may prevent recurrent SVCS.[60]

CATHETER-INDUCED OBSTRUCTION

In catheter-induced SVCS, the mechanism of obstruction is usually thrombosis. Streptokinase, urokinase, or recombinant tissue-type plasminogen activator may cause lysis of the thrombus early in its formation.[24,61–64] Heparin and oral anticoagulants may reduce the extent of the thrombus and prevent its progression. Removal of the catheter, if possible, is another option and should be combined with anticoagulation to avoid embolization. In patients for whom electrodes of a pacemaker must be changed, the broken wire should be removed to prevent the risk of developing SVCS.[24,61,65] Percutaneous transluminal angioplasty, with or without thrombolytic therapy, and stent insertion have been successfully used to open catheter-induced SVC obstructions.[62,66–69]

TREATMENT

RADIATION THERAPY

In patients with SVCS as a result of non-SCLC, radiotherapy has long been the primary treatment. The likelihood of relieving the symptoms and signs of SVCS is high,[5,9] but the overall prognosis for these patients is poor.[4,5,9,25] In the series of Armstrong et al.,[9] the 1-year survival for these patients was 17%, and the survival at 2 years declined to 2%. More recently, the use of percutaneous metal stent insertion to improve blood flow through the SVC has been introduced as an alternative to palliative radiation therapy in malignant SVCS.[3,70,84,85] Radiotherapy is an optional treatment for most patients with SVCS.[23,29,30] It is also used as an effective initial treatment if a histologic diagnosis cannot be established and the clinical status of the patient is deteriorating. However, some reviews suggest that SVC obstruction alone rarely represents an absolute emergency that requires radiotherapy without a specific diagnosis, and endovascular stenting can be used as an alternative to radiotherapy for obtaining immediate relief of the obstruction.[3,12,31,32,70,84,85] Yet, SVCS may be the earliest manifestation of invasive involvement of additional critical structures in the thorax (Table 49.1-6), such as the bronchi. Under such circumstances, prompt treatment with irradiation may be required without any delay.

The fractionation schedule of radiation that has been recommended includes two to four large initial fractions of 3 to 4 cGy, followed by conventional fractionation to a total dose of 30 to 50 cGy.[5,23,29] However, no data clearly support a particular

TABLE 49.1-6. Complications of Malignant Invasion Associated with Superior Vena Cava Syndrome

Complication	No. of Patients[a] (%)
ESOPHAGUS	
Symptoms of dysphagia or esophageal dysfunction	26 (24)
Anatomic evidence of esophageal invasion	6 (6)
TRACHEA	
Displaced on examination or roentgenogram	7 (7)
Compressed or invaded by lesion	14 (13)
VOCAL CORD PARALYSIS	
Unilateral	6 (6)
Bilateral	3 (3)
PERICARDIUM	
Tamponade	3 (3)
Neoplastic invasion at necropsy	6 (6)

[a]Some patients may have had more than one complication.
(From ref. 4, with permission.)

fractionation scheme.[19] In one study, patients treated with initial high-dose fractions showed a slightly faster symptomatic improvement than patients receiving conventional-dose radiation.[9] Improvement within 2 weeks or less was observed in 70% of those treated with initial high-dose fractions and in 56% of patients receiving conventional-dose therapy. This difference was not statistically significant.

A radiotherapy study evaluated the efficacy of treating patients with SVCS with a short course of hypofractionated irradiation.[71] The study compared a regimen of 8 Gy per fraction once a week to a total dose of 24 Gy to a program of delivering only two fractions of 8 Gy (total of 16 Gy) within 1 week. Transient dysphagia was the main side effect in almost one-half of patients in both programs. The 24-Gy regimen resulted in a complete resolution of symptoms in 56% of patients and a partial response in another 40%. The 16-Gy regimen yielded a complete response in only 28% of patients. The mean time for SVCS recurrence and the median overall survival rate were longer in the higher-dose regimen (6 months and 9 months, respectively) compared to the low-dose regimen (3 months and 3 months, respectively). A more recent study reported on the experience of using only two fractions, 6 Gy each, 1 week apart in 23 elderly (more than 71 years) patients with malignancy-related SVCS.[87] Overall response was 87% with relatively minimal toxicity.

Serial venograms and autopsies[31] suggest that the symptomatic improvement achieved by radiotherapy is not always due to improvement of flow through the SVC. It is probably also a result of the development of collaterals after the pressure in the mediastinum is eased.

The field of radiation for SVCS induced by lung cancer should encompass the gross tumors with appropriate margins and mediastinal, hilar, and supraclavicular lymph nodes. In the series of Armstrong et al.,[9] supraclavicular failures occurred in 8 of 91 patients (9%) receiving radiation therapy to the supraclavicular fossae and in 2 of 6 patients (33%) not receiving therapy to these lymph nodes.[9]

ENDOVASCULAR STENTING AND ANGIOPLASTY

Percutaneous transluminal angioplasty using the balloon technique, insertion of expandable wire stents, or both, have been successfully used to open and maintain the patency of SVC obstruction resulting from malignant and benign causes.[3,69,70,72,83–85] Thrombolysis is often an integral part of the endovascular management of SVCS because thrombosis is frequently a critical component of the obstruction and lysis is necessary to allow the passage of the wire. Balloon dilatation (angioplasty) can also be used before stenting. Most reports have emphasized the use of combination endovascular therapy: thrombolysis, angioplasty, and stent therapy.[3,85] The experience with stenting has been growing rapidly. Most experience has been with three stents: the Gianturco Z-stent, the Wallstent, and the Palmaz stent. The Wallstent is the most commonly used device.[3] It is self-expanding and built of woven stainless steel wire. Its tight weave deters tumor ingrowth. Total occlusion of the SVC is not a contraindication to stent therapy, and a success rate of 85% in total occlusion situations has been reported.[73] The largest experience in using stents to open malignant obstruction of the SVC was reported by Nicholson et al. in Great Britain.[70] The British team used Wallstents in 75 patients and obtained improvement of obstruction in all patients; 90% remained free of symptoms until death. This study retrospectively compared stent therapy with radiation therapy and found that only 12% of patients treated with radiation remained free of SVCS until death. However, long-term experience in maintaining patency after stent therapy in patients with SVCS from benign causes who are expected to have long survival is still limited.[69] Complication rates for endovascular therapy have ranged from 0% to 50% and include bleeding, stent migration, stent occlusion, and pulmonary embolus.[3] Most complications can be successfully treated with percutaneous methods.

SURGERY

The experience with successful direct bypass graft for SVC obstruction is limited. It was recommended that autologous grafts of almost the same size as the SVC should be used.[74] Doty et al.[75] used a composite spiral graft, which was constructed from the patient's saphenous vein. They reported 23 years of experience with this procedure in 16 patients with benign obstruction of SVC; 14 patients maintained patency, and 15 were relieved of symptoms of SVCS. Avashti and Moghissi[76] reported successful bypasses of obstructed SVCs using Dacron prostheses. Magnan et al.[77] used an expanded polytetrafluoroethylene prosthesis to reconstruct the SVC in nine patients with malignancy-induced SVCS and in one patient with chronic mediastinitis. In all, patients' symptoms disappeared promptly after the operation, the grafts remained open, and survival rates at 1, 2, and 5 years were 70%, 25%, and 12.5%, respectively.[77] The preferred bypass route is between an innominate or jugular vein on the left side and the right atrial appendage, using an end-to-end anastomosis.[45] Piccione et al.[78] used the autologous pericardium to reconstruct the SVC after resection for malignant obstruction. In patients with malignancy-induced SVCS, surgical intervention should be considered only after other therapeutic maneuvers with irradiation, chemotherapy, and stenting have been exhausted. Most patients with SVCS of benign origin have long survivals without surgical intervention.[58,59] However, if the process progresses rapidly or if there is a retrosternal goiter or aortic aneurysm, surgical intervention may relieve the obstruction.

THROMBOLYTIC THERAPY

Thrombolysis is an important component of comprehensive endovascular therapy.[3] Successful experience with thrombolytic agents was also obtained in the treatment of catheter-induced SVCS.[24,64,79] A review from the Cleveland Clinic[64,80] of the response of SVCS to thrombolytic therapy showed that 8 of 11 patients (73%) with a central venous catheter lysed after thrombolytic therapy compared with only 1 of 5 patients who responded to thrombolytic therapy in the absence of a central catheter. The higher yield of thrombolytic therapy in patients with catheters is probably related to the mechanism of obstruction, the ability to deliver the agent directly to the thrombus, and earlier recognition of SVCS in patients with malfunctioning catheters. In the Cleveland Clinic experience,[64] urokinase was more effective than streptokinase, and a delay in administering therapy beyond 5 days of symptom onset was associated with a treatment failure. Favorable experience with recombinant tissue-type plasminogen activator as a thrombolytic agent for catheter-induced SVCS has been reported.[62,63]

Many patients who undergo stenting for SVCS receive thrombolytic therapy during or during and after the procedure. The indications, protocol, and risks have not been well studied as of yet.[83]

GENERAL MEASURES

Medical measures other than specific chemotherapy may be beneficial in temporarily relieving the symptoms of SVCS. Bed rest with the head elevated and oxygen administration can reduce the cardiac output and venous pressure. Diuretic therapy and a reduced-salt diet to reduce edema may have an immediate palliative effect, but the risk of thrombosis enhanced by dehydration should not be ignored. Steroids are commonly used, but their effectiveness has never been properly evaluated. They may improve obstruction by decreasing a possible inflammatory reaction associated with tumor or with irradiation. However, Green et al.[81] demonstrated the lack of inflammatory reaction and edema after radiotherapy for experimental SVCS, although documentation in a controlled fashion is lacking. Thrombolytic therapy with urokinase, streptokinase, and recombinant tissue-type plasminogen activator was effective in SVCS induced by indwelling catheters.[62,64,79,80]

RECOMMENDATIONS

In patients without a clear cause of SVCS, an efficient diagnostic effort should be attempted before any oncologic treatment is given. However, percutaneous endovascular intervention should be considered, because it relieves symptoms rapidly without masking the diagnosis. Three deep-cough sputum specimens should be obtained for cytologic analysis. A positive cytologic evaluation provides reliable pathologic information, particularly in the diagnosis of SCLC.[45] If pleural effusion is present, thoracocentesis should be performed and the centrifuge-prepared specimen examined for the presence of malignant cells. If a suspicious lymph node is palpable, particularly in the supraclavicular area, a needle or open biopsy should be the next diagnostic step. In the absence of positive sputum results, pleural effusion, or accessible suspicious lymph node analysis, a bronchoscopy should be performed, and brushing, washing, and biopsy samples should be obtained for cytologic and histologic analysis. If these efforts do not provide the histologic diagnosis of the primary process, percutaneous transthoracic fine-needle biopsy under CT or fluoroscopic guidance is safe and highly effective.[49,51,82] In the rare patient for whom less-invasive procedures have failed to establish the diagnosis, the location of the suspicious lesion in the chest and the experience of the surgical team should determine whether mediastinoscopy or thoracotomy is performed.

During the diagnostic process, the patient can benefit from bed rest with the head elevated and with oxygen administration. Some clinicians advocate the use of diuretics and steroids (6 to 10 mg dexamethasone given orally or intravenously every 6 hours) as a temporary palliative measure if the patient is uncomfortably symptomatic. Anticoagulation is of no proven benefit and may interfere with diagnostic procedures. After the cause of SVCS has been established, treatment of the primary process should promptly follow. Combination chemotherapy with an appropriate regimen is the treatment of choice for SCLC and NHL. Radiation therapy of the lesion and adjacent nodal areas may enhance control after initial response to chemotherapy. Non-SCLC causing SVCS is best treated with radiation therapy or endovascular stent insertion, or both. The incorporation of CT scan information into a carefully designed treatment plan may enable the administration of a total radiation dose of more than 5000 cGy, which may provide long-term local control for some patients. Most patients with nonmalignant causes for SVCS have an indolent course and a good prognosis. Percutaneous transluminal angioplasty or stent insertion should be considered an effective alternative to surgery. However, the long-term maintenance of patency with stent insertion is still unknown. Surgery is indicated only when the process is rapidly progressing or caused by a retrosternal goiter or an aortic aneurysm. If SVCS is induced by a catheter, the catheter should be removed if possible. Heparin should be administered during the removal of the catheter to prevent embolization. In catheter-induced SVCS, urokinase, streptokinase, or recombinant tissue-type plasminogen activator is of value if used early in the thrombotic process.[60–62,80] The clinical course of SVCS rarely represents an absolute emergency. In these situations, the bronchus is likely to be obstructed by the same basic process, and irradiation may have to be started immediately, even before the histologic diagnosis is established.

REFERENCES

1. Hunter W. The history of an aneurysm of the aorta, with some remarks on aneurysms in general. *Med Observ Inq* 1757;1:3.
2. Schechter MM. The superior vena cava syndrome. *Am J Med Sci* 1954;227:46.
3. Schindler N, Vogelzang RL. Superior vena cava syndrome. Experience with endovascular stents and surgical therapy. *Surg Clin North Am* 1999;79:683.
4. Schraufnagel DE, Hill R, Leech JA, Pare JAP. Superior vena caval obstruction. Is it an emergency? *Am J Med* 1981;70:1169.
5. Davenport D, Ferree C, Blake D, Raben M. Radiation therapy in the treatment of superior vena caval obstruction. *Cancer* 1978;42:2600.
6. Rubin P, Hicks GL. Biassociation of superior vena caval obstruction and spinal-cord compression. *N Y State J Med* 1973;73:2176.
7. Carlson HA. Obstruction of the superior vena cava: an experimental study. *Arch Surg* 1934;29:669.
8. Roswit B, Kaplan G, Jacobson HG. The superior vena cava syndrome in bronchogenic carcinoma. *Radiology* 1953;61:722.
9. Armstrong BA, Perez CA, Simpson JR, Hederman MA. Role of irradiation in the management of superior vena cava syndrome. *Int J Radiat Oncol Biol Phys* 1987;13:531.
10. Parish JM, Marschke RF, Dines DE, Lee RE. Etiologic considerations in superior vena cava syndrome. *Mayo Clin Proc* 1981;56:407.
11. Bell DR, Woods RL, Levi JA. Superior vena caval obstruction: a 10-year experience. *Med J Aust* 1986;145:566.
12. Yellin A, Rosen A, Reichert N, Lieberman Y. Superior vena cava syndrome. The myth—the facts. *Am Rev Respir Dis* 1990;141:1114.
13. Salsali M, Cliffton EE. Superior vena caval obstruction in carcinoma of lung. *N Y State J Med* 1969;69:2875.
14. Dombernowsky P, Hansen HH. Combination chemotherapy in the management of superior vena caval obstruction in small-cell anaplastic of the lung. *Acta Med Scand* 1978;204:513.
15. Sculier JP, Evans WK, Feld R, et al. Superior vena caval obstruction in small cell lung cancer. *Cancer* 1986;57:847.
16. Spiro SG, Shah S, Harper PG, et al. Treatment of obstruction of the superior vena cava by combination chemotherapy with and without irradiation in small-cell carcinoma of the bronchus. *Thorax* 1983;38:501.
17. Urban T, Lebeau B, Chastang C, et al. Superior vena cava syndrome in small-cell lung cancer. *Arch Intern Med* 1993;153:384.
18. Wurschmidt F, Bunemann H, Heilmann HP. Small cell lung cancer with and without superior vena cava syndrome: a multivariate analysis of prognostic factors in 408 cases. *Int J Radiat Oncol Biol Phys* 1995;33:77.
19. Chan RH, Dar AR, Yu E, et al. Superior vena cava obstruction in small-cell lung cancer. *Int J Radiat Oncol Biol Phys* 1997;38:513.
20. Perez-Soler R, McLaughlin P, Velasquez WS, et al. Clinical features and results of management of superior vena cava syndrome secondary to lymphoma. *J Clin Oncol* 1984;2:260.
21. Lazzarino M, Orlandi E, Paulli M, et al. Primary mediastinal B-cell lymphoma with sclerosis: an aggressive tumor with distinctive clinical and pathologic features. *J Clin Oncol* 1993;11:2306.

22. Chen JC, Bongard F, Klein SR. A contemporary perspective on superior vena cava syndrome. *Am J Surg* 1990;97:1005.

23. Lokich JJ, Goodman R. Superior vena cava syndrome: clinical management. *JAMA* 1975;231:58.

24. Sculier JP, Feld R. Superior vena cava obstruction system: recommendation for management. *Cancer Treat Rev* 1985;12:209.

25. Bertrand M, Presant CA, Klein L, Scott E. Iatrogenic superior vena cava syndrome. A new entity. *Cancer* 1984;54:376.

26. Janin Y, Becker J, Wise L, et al. Superior vena cava syndrome in childhood and adolescence: a review of the literature and report of three cases. *J Pediatr Surg* 1982;17:290.

27. Issa PY, Brihi ER, Janin Y, Slim MS. Superior vena cava syndrome in childhood: report of ten cases and review of the literature. *Pediatrics* 1983;71:337.

28. Ingram L, Rivera GK, Shapiro DN. Superior vena cava syndrome associated with childhood malignancy: analysis of 24 cases. *Med Pediatr Oncol* 1990;18:476.

29. Perez CA, Present CA, Van Amburg AL III. Management of superior vena cava syndrome. *Semin Oncol* 1978;5:123.

30. Scarantino C, Salazar OM, Rubin R, et al. The optimum radiation schedule in the treatment of superior vena caval obstruction: importance of ^{99m}Tc scintiangiograms. *Int J Radiat Oncol Biol Phys* 1979;5:1987.

31. Ahmann FR. A reassessment of the clinical implications of the superior vena cava syndrome. *J Clin Oncol* 1984;2:961.

32. Shimm DS, Lugue GL, Tigsby LC. Evaluating the superior vena cava syndrome. *JAMA* 1981;245:951.

33. Loeffler JS, Leopold KA, Recht A, et al. Emergency prebiopsy radiation for mediastinal masses: impact on subsequent pathologic diagnosis and outcome. *J Clin Oncol* 1986;4:716.

34. Yedlicka JW, Schultz K, Moncada R, Flisak M. CT findings in superior vena cava obstruction. *Semin Roentgenol* 1989;24:84.

35. Qanadli SD, El Hajjam M, Bruckert F, et al. Helical CT phlebography of the superior vena cava: diagnosis and evaluation of venous obstruction. *AJR Am J Roentgenol* 1999;172:1327.

36. Moncada R, Cardella R, Demos TC, et al. Evaluation of superior vena cava syndrome by axial CT and CT phlebography. *AJR Am J Roentgenol* 1984;143:731.

37. Hansen ME, Spritzer CE, Sostman HD. Assessing the patency of mediastinal and thoracic inlet veins: value of MR imaging. *AJR Am J Roentgenol* 1990;155:1177.

38. Nieto AF, Doty DB. Superior vena cava obstruction: clinical syndrome, etiology and treatment. *Curr Probl Cancer* 1986;10:442.

39. Dyet JF, Moghissi K. Role of venography in assessing patients with superior vena cava obstruction caused by bronchial carcinoma for bypass operations. *Thorax* 1980;35:628.

40. Stanford W, Jolles H, Ell S, Chiu LC. Superior vena cava obstruction: a venographic classification. *AJR Am J Roentgenol* 1987;148:259.

41. Son YH, Wetzel RA, Wilson WA. ^{99m}Tc pertechnetate scintiphotography as diagnostic and followup aids in major vascular obstruction due to malignant neoplasm. *Radiology* 1968;91:349.

42. Van Houtte P, Fruhling J. Radionuclide venography in the evaluation of superior vena cava syndrome. *Clin Nucl Med* 1981;6:177.

43. Conte FA, Orzel JA. Superior vena cava syndrome and bilateral subclavian vein thrombosis: CT and radionuclide venography correlation. *Clin Nucl Med* 1986;11:698.

44. Swayne LC, Kaplan IL. Gallium SPECT detection of neoplastic intravascular obstruction of superior vena cava. *Clin Nucl Med* 1989;14:823.

45. Yesner R, Gersti B, Auerbach O. Application of the World Health Organization classification of lung carcinoma to biopsy material. *Ann Thorac Surg* 1965;1:33.

46. Ihde DC, Cohen MH, Bernath AM, et al. Serial fiberoptic bronchoscopy during chemotherapy of small cell carcinoma of the lung. *Chest* 1978;74:531.

47. Mineo TC, Ambrogi V, Nofroni I, et al. Mediastinoscopy in superior vena cava obstruction: analysis of 80 consecutive patients. *Ann Thorac Surg* 1999;68:223.

48. Jahangiri M, Goldstraw P. The role of mediastinoscopy in superior vena caval obstruction. *Ann Thorac Surg* 1995;59:453.

49. Cosmos L, Haponik EF, Dariak JJ, Summer WR. Neoplastic superior vena caval obstruction: diagnosis with percutaneous needle aspiration. *Am J Med Sci* 1987;293:99.

50. Reyes CV, Thompson KS, Massarani-Wafai R, et al. Utilization of fine-needle aspiration cytology in the diagnosis of neoplastic superior vena caval syndrome. *Diagn Cytopathol* 1998;19:84.

51. Dake MD, Zemel G, Dolmatch BL, Katzen BT. The cause of superior vena cava syndrome diagnosis with percutaneous atherectomy. *Radiology* 1990;174:957.

52. Ferrari LR, Bedford RF. General anesthesia prior to the treatment of anterior mediastinal masses in pediatric cancer patients. *Anesthesiology* 1990;72:991.

53. Seifter EJ, Ihde DC. Therapy of small cell lung cancer: a perspective on two decades of clinical research. *Semin Oncol* 1988;15:278.

54. Warde P, Payne D. Does thoracic irradiation improve survival and local control in limited stage small cell carcinoma of the lung? A meta-analysis. *J Clin Oncol* 1992;10:890.

55. Pignon JP, Arriagada R, Ihde DC, et al. A meta-analysis of thoracic radiotherapy for small-cell lung cancer. *N Engl J Med* 1992;327:1618.

56. Murray N, Coy P, Pater JL, et al. Importance of timing for thoracic irradiation in the combined modality treatment of limited-stage small-cell lung cancer. *J Clin Oncol* 1993;11:336.

57. Yellin A, Mandel M, Rechavi G, et al. Superior vena cava syndrome associated with lymphoma. *Am J Dis Child* 1992;146:1060.

58. Mahajan V, Strimlan V, Van Ordstrand HS, Loop FD. Benign superior cava syndrome. *Chest* 1975;68:32.

59. Effler DB, Groves LK. Superior vena caval obstruction. *J Thorac Cardiovasc Surg* 1962;43:574.

60. Urshel HC Jr, Razzuk MA, Netto GJ, Disiere J, Chung SY. Sclerosing mediastinitis: improved management with histoplasmosis titer and ketoconazole. *Ann Thorac Surg* 1990;50:215.

61. Goudevonos JA, Reid PG, Adams PC, Holden MP, Williams DO. Pacemaker-induced superior vena cava syndrome: report of four cases and review of the literature. *Pacing Clin Electrophysiol* 1989;12:1890.

62. Fine DG, Shepherd RF, Welch TJ. Thrombolytic therapy for superior vena cava syndrome [Letter]. *Lancet* 1989;1:1200.

63. Greenberg S, Kosinski R, Daniels J. Treatment of superior vena cava thrombosis with recombinant tissue type plasminogen activator. *Chest* 1991;99:1298.

64. Gray BH, Olin JW, Grador RA, et al. Safety and efficacy of thrombolytic therapy for superior vena cava syndrome. *Chest* 1991;99:54.

65. Blackburn T, Dunn M. Pacemaker-induced superior vena cava syndrome: consideration of management. *Am Heart J* 1988;116:893.

66. Grace AA, Sutters M, Schofield PM. Balloon dilation of pacemaker-induced stenosis of the superior vena cava. *Br Heart J* 1991;65:225.

67. Montgomery JH, D'Souza VJ, Dyer RB, et al. Non-surgical treatment of the superior vena cava syndrome. *Am J Cardiol* 1985;56:829.

68. Sunder SK, Ekong EA, Sivalingam K, Kumar A. Superior vena cava thrombosis due to pacing electrodes: successful treatment with combined thrombolysis and angioplasty. *Am Heart J* 1992;123:790.

69. Kee ST, Kinoshita L, Razavi MK, et al. Superior vena cava syndrome: treatment with catheter-directed thrombolysis and endovascular stent placement. *Radiology* 1998;206:187.

70. Nicholson AA, Ettles DF, Arnold A, et al. Treatment of malignant superior vena cava obstruction: metal stents or radiation therapy. *J Vasc Interv Radiol* 1997;8:781.

71. Rodrigues CI, Njo KH, Karim ABMF. Hypofractionated radiation therapy in the treatment of superior vena cava syndrome. *Lung Cancer* 1993;10:221.

72. Shah R, Sabanathan S, Lowe RA, et al. Stenting in malignant obstruction of superior vena cava. *J Thorac Cardiovasc Surg* 1996;112:335.

73. Crowe MT, Davies CH, Gaines PA, et al. Percutaneous management of superior vena cava occlusions. *Cardiovasc Intervent Radiol* 1995;18:367.

74. Scherck JP, Kerstein MD, Stansel HC. The current status of vena caval replacement. *Surgery* 1974;76:209.

75. Doty JR, Flores JH, Doty DB. Superior vena cava obstruction: bypass using spiral vein graft. *Ann Thorac Surg* 1999;67:1111.

76. Avashti RB, Moghissi K. Malignant obstruction of the superior vena cava and its palliation. *J Thorac Cardiovasc Surg* 1977;74:244.

77. Magnan PE, Thomas P, Giudicelli R, Fuentes P, Branchereau A. Surgical reconstruction of the superior vena cava. *Cardiovasc Surg* 1994;2:598.

78. Piccione W Jr, Faber LP, Warren WH. Superior vena caval reconstruction using autologous pericardium. *Ann Thorac Surg* 1990;50:417.

79. Meister FL, McLaughlin TF, Tenney RD, Sholkoff SD. Urokinase. A cost-effective alternative treatment of superior vena cava thrombosis and obstruction. *Arch Intern Med* 1989;149:1209.

80. Comerota AJ. Safety and efficacy of thrombolytic therapy for superior vena caval syndrome. *Chest* 1991;99:3.

81. Green J, Rubin P, Holzwasser G. The experimental production of superior vena cava obstruction. *Radiology* 1963;81:406.

82. Porte H, Metois D, Finzi L, et al. Superior vena cava syndrome of malignant origin. Which surgical procedure for which diagnosis? *Eur J Cardiothorac Surg* 2000;17:384.

83. Rowell NP, Gleeson FV. Steroids, radiotherapy, chemotherapy and stents for superior vena caval obstruction in carcinoma of the bronchus: a systematic review. *Clin Oncol* 2002;14:338.

84. Lazarou S, Koutoulidis V, Ladopoulos CH, Vlachos L. Stent therapy for malignant superior vena cava syndrome: should be first line therapy or simple adjunct to radiotherapy. *Eur J Radiol* 2002;47:247.

85. Garcia Monaco R, Bertoni H, Pallota G, et al. Use of self-expanding vascular endoprostheses in superior vena cava syndrome. *Eur J Cardiothorac Surg* 2003;24:208.

86. Chen Y-M, Yang S, Perng R-P, Tsai C-M. Superior vena cava syndrome revisited. *Jpn J Clin Oncol* 1995;25:32.

87. Lonardi F, Gioga G, Agus G, et al. Double-flash, large-fraction radiation therapy as palliative treatment of malignant superior vena cava syndrome in the elderly. *Support Care Cancer* 2002;10:156.

JOACHIM M. BAEHRING

SECTION 2

Increased Intracranial Pressure

Increase in intracranial pressure (ICP) is a common neurologic complication of patients with cancer involving the nervous system. Various mechanisms have to be considered. Large cerebral metastases are the most common cause and can give rise to intracranial hemorrhage. Coagulopathies predispose to subdural hemorrhage. The immunocompromised host is at risk for infections of the nervous system, such as fungal or bacterial meningitis or a bacterial abscess resulting in increased ICP. Subependymal or leptomeningeal masses located at "bottlenecks" of spinal fluid pathways, such as the foramen of Monro or the aqueduct of Sylvius, raise pressure by obstructing spinal fluid flow. Communicating hydrocephalus reflects decreased reabsorption of spinal fluid in leptomeningeal carcinomatosis. Dural sinus stenosis from dural metastases causes a syndrome resembling idiopathic intracranial hypertension (IIH). A cancer-related hypercoagulable state can lead to dural sinus thrombosis or extracranial venous outflow obstruction.

This chapter provides an overview of the various mechanisms of increased ICP, the clinical manifestations, diagnosis, and treatment options.

PATHOPHYSIOLOGIC CONSIDERATIONS

Intracranial volume is not expandable in an adult due to its containment by the skull and the dura. The brain itself has an average volume of 1400 mL, spinal fluid of 52 to 160 mL, and blood of 150 mL.[1] Increase in the volume of one compartment is at the expense of the other two (Monro-Kellie hypothesis). If brain volume increases as a result of a brain tumor, spinal fluid volume decreases as a compensatory mechanism. Up to an ICP of 200 to 250 mm cerebrospinal fluid (CSF) compartmental volume increase results in only minor increases in ICP as long as CSF flow is not obstructed, the rate between CSF production and reabsorption remains constant, and the dural venous sinuses remain open. The intracranial compliance decreases with rising ICP; that is, with rising pressure, increase in volume leads to a disproportionate increase in pressure. This is reflected in the occurrence of plateau waves in patients with increased ICP. Plateau waves are acute elevations of ICP up to 1300 mm CSF lasting 5 to 20 minutes. They are of pathogenetic significance because they further compromise cerebral perfusion in patients with increased ICP.[2] Plateau waves have been suspected to cause intermittent symptoms of increased ICP with orthostasis in patients with brain tumors.[3]

Volume changes within the brain parenchyma leading to increased ICP in cancer patients are caused by primary or secondary brain tumors, vasogenic edema, or indirect neurologic complications of cancer (Fig. 42.2-1*B*). Vasogenic edema results from an increased leakage of a plasma filtrate into brain tissue through leaky capillaries within a brain tumor or surrounding a brain abscess or cerebral hemorrhage. Cytotoxic edema is induced by ischemic injury, cytotoxic chemotherapy agents, or toxic metabolites in liver failure. Breakdown of the adenosine triphosphate-dependent transmembranous ion transport system leads to intracellular entrapment of water. Extraaxial mass lesions arise from neoplastic growth (dural tumors such as metastases, meningioma, or lymphoma), infection (subdural empyema), or hemorrhage (subdural hematoma in the coagulopathic or thrombocytopenic patient).

Increased ICP can also be the consequence of an imbalance between CSF production and reabsorption. Spinal fluid is produced at an average rate of 21 to 22 mL/h. CSF represents a plasma filtrate passively diffusing through the choroid plexus of the lateral, third, and fourth ventricles. It is reabsorbed within the arachnoid granulations overlying the cerebral hemispheres. Mass lesions in proximity to bottlenecks of CSF flow (foramen of Monro, cerebral aqueduct, medullary foramina, basilar subarachnoid cisterns) cause obstructive or "noncommunicating" hydrocephalus. Carcinomatosis or meningitis interferes with CSF reabsorption. With chronic obstruction of the arachnoid granulations, spinal fluid pressure reaches a new equilibrium within the high normal range, giving rise to a condition called *normal-pressure hydrocephalus* (NPH) characterized by ventricular enlargement out of proportion to age-related cortical atrophy. Increased production of CSF is a rare cause of raised ICP.

IIH (pseudotumor cerebri) denotes a syndrome characterized by signs of increased ICP in the absence of mass lesions or hydrocephalus. Pathologically poorly defined, an increasing number of patients are found to have partial obstruction of dural venous sinuses. Iatrogenic causes of IIH include isotretinoin, tetracycline antibiotics, and sulfonamides.

Acute increases in arterial and venous pressure result in an increase in ICP. Cerebral perfusion is kept constant over a wide arterial pressure range (50 to 160 mm Hg). Once this autoregulatory mechanism fails, further increase in arterial blood pressure results in a passive increase of ICP. Venous obstruction can be reproduced with the Queckenstedt maneuver (manual compression of both internal jugular veins). Dural venous sinus pressure fluctuates with intrathoracic pressure changes. Thus, coughing, sneezing, and straining (Valsalva maneuver) are accompanied by an increase in ICP. In a patient with increased ICP and decreased intracranial compliance, gagging or coughing can lead to transient decompensation and acute onset of symptoms (syncope in patients with colloid cyst of the third ventricle; plateau waves).

Depending on etiology and location of an increase in cerebral parenchymal or extraaxial volume, patients may have relatively few symptoms until herniation ensues. The faster the pathologic process evolves, the more likely is the patient to have symptoms. Cingulate or transfalcian herniation denotes lateral shift of a hemisphere underneath the falx cerebri. Vascular structures (ipsilateral anterior cerebral artery, internal cerebral vein, vein of Galen) can be compromised. In transtentorial herniation, the diencephalon is forced through the tentorial notch as a consequence of a supratentorial mass lesion. Infratentorial masses can result in an upward herniation of posterior fossa structures. Uncal herniation, most often encountered in temporal lobe mass lesions, leads to compression of the midbrain at the level of the tentorial notch. When ICP exceeds 40 to 50 mm Hg, cerebral blood flow is diminished, irreversibly damaging the brain.

EPIDEMIOLOGY AND PATHOGENESIS

Brain metastases are the most common cause of increased ICP in a cancer patient. In adults, lung cancer and melanoma are particularly prone to seeding to the brain.[4] Cerebral metastasis can be further complicated by intratumoral hemorrhage. Although lung cancer is the most common primary tumor leading to hemorrhagic brain seeding, the relative incidence of hemorrhagic transformation of a cerebral metastasis is highest in melanoma, choriocarcinoma, renal cell carcinoma, and papillary thyroid cancer.[5] In children, the brain metastases most commonly associated with intracranial hemorrhage are Ewing's sarcoma, rhabdomyosarcoma, and melanoma.[6] Secondary cerebral volume increase in cancer patients results from hemorrhage, ischemia, infection, or autoimmune inflammatory processes. Cerebral hemorrhage from coagulopathies typically occurs in patients with hematologic malignancies such as acute lymphocytic or myelocytic leukemia.[7] Diffuse cerebral edema and increased ICP in patients with leukemia can be the mere result of leukostasis and occurs at blast counts exceeding $4 \times 10^5/\mu L$. Higher counts are usually required in lymphoblastic leukemia, because the cells are smaller and less adherent than myeloid blasts.[8] Increase in ICP can also be the consequence of diffuse cerebral hemorrhages in disseminated intravascular coagulopathy.

Herpes simplex encephalitis gives rise to extensive vasogenic edema affecting the medial temporal and inferior frontal lobe. Depending on disease burden, patients with cerebral toxoplasmosis, aspergillosis, or candidiasis can present with signs of increased ICP as well. Autoimmune inflammatory encephalomyelitis has been described as a rare entity in patients after bone marrow transplantation. Brain abscess complicates neurosurgical interventions for resection of metastases, drainage of cerebral hemorrhage, or placement of ventricular catheters.

Primary brain tumors with a predilection for subependymal or intraventricular location, such as subependymal giant cell astrocytoma, lymphoma, subependymoma, choroid plexus papilloma, ependymoma, meningioma, colloid cyst, central neurocytoma, chordoid glioma of the third ventricle, or thalamic tumors, can cause spinal fluid obstruction early in their course. A syndrome resembling NPH has been observed in long-term survivors of whole brain or, less commonly, partial brain irradiation. Fibrosis of arachnoid granulations has been suspected to play a role in the pathogenesis of this entity that is also characterized by extensive white matter demyelination and frank necrosis. Selected patients seem to respond favorably to ventriculoperitoneal shunting.[9–11] An acute imbalance between CSF production and reabsorption occurs in opportunistic meningeal infections in the immunocompromised cancer patient. *Cryptococcus neoformans* meningitis is almost invariably associated with elevation of ICP. After splenectomy patients are susceptible to meningitis with encapsulated bacteria. The pathogenesis of communicating hydrocephalus in patients with spinal cord tumors or nonobstructive masses of the cerebellopontine angle is not well understood. Most commonly ependymomas, but also schwannoma, meningioma, neurofibroma, and glioma, might release protein degradation products or cells into CSF that obstruct the arachnoid granulations.[12,13] However, the protein level is rarely elevated in these patients. Others have suspected blockage of the lumbar CSF reservoir,[14–16] arachnoiditis, or increased fibrinogen levels[17] as the cause of this syndrome. Retinoic acid, a differentiating agent used for the treatment of promyelocytic leukemia, has been associated with episodes of communicating hydrocephalus, likely as a consequence of decreased CSF reabsorption.[18] Rarely is increased ICP caused by CSF overproduction. Patients with choroid plexus papillomas, especially if they are multifocal, are at risk.[19]

The hypercoagulable state in cancer patients can manifest itself as dural venous sinus thrombosis. The incidence is increased in patients receiving L-asparaginase therapy. Increased ICP is the only manifestation of cerebral venous thrombosis in more than one-third of patients.[20] Nonthrombotic causes of dural sinus stenosis or occlusion are dural mass lesions such as meningioma or diffuse meningiomatosis of the convexity, metastases from breast or prostate cancer, non-Hodgkin's lymphoma, Ewing's sarcoma, plasmocytoma, or neuroblastoma that either compress or invade the sinus.[21–23] Venous hypertension can also arise from metastases at the base of the skull causing obstruction of the internal jugular vein or from compression of the superior vena cava by mediastinal masses. Lesions giving rise to the syndrome of IIH compromise the distal superior sagittal sinus or the torcula Herophili.[24]

CLINICAL PRESENTATION

Headache is the most common complaint of patients with increased ICP. In its classic form it is severe, relentless, and resistant to common analgesics and reaches maximum intensity on awakening in the morning.[25] Decreased venous drainage in the supine position likely accounts for this observation. Frequently, patients report immediate relief from their headache by vomiting. However, the majority of patients have nonspecific tension-type or migraine-like headaches. If ICP continues to rise, nausea and vomiting ensue. Cognitive complaints such as slowness to respond and inattentiveness reflect frontal lobe dysfunction. The patient becomes increasingly somnolent and ultimately falls into a coma.

Funduscopic examination reveals papilledema in approximately half of patients with increased ICP. Absence of venous pulsations within the center of the optic disc is an early finding, whereas papilledema with blurring of the disc margins or small hemorrhages characterizes later stages. The Foster-Kennedy syndrome—optic nerve atrophy as a result of a sphenoid wing meningioma and contralateral papilledema from increased ICP—is rarely seen in the days of improved neuroimaging methods and earlier diagnosis. Focal neurologic deficits can help localize the mass that accounts for the pressure increase. Gaze paresis to the side opposite the lesion indicates involvement of the frontal center for horizontal gaze. Posterior frontal masses cause contralateral hemiparesis. Hemianesthesia or complex neglect syndromes reflect parietal lobe pathology. Temporal and occipital lobe disease causes visual field deficits. An upward gaze paresis occurs in patients with tumors of the tectal region such as pineal neoplasms or metastases. Paresis of extraocular muscles results from stretch injury of the fourth or sixth nerve or uncal herniation with compression of the third nerve. However, the clinician must be aware of "false" localizing signs. Temporal lobe tumors can cause compression of the cerebral peduncle at the tentorial notch on the opposite side, resulting in a hemiparesis on the same side as the mass lesion (Kernohan's syndrome). The patient falls easily, particularly backward.

Symptoms are aggravated by vasogenic edema surrounding intraparenchymal masses and partially or completely resolve with medical management. Hyponatremia as a result of inappropriate secretion of antidiuretic hormone is observed as a metabolic complication of increased ICP. Sphincter incontinence occurs in chronic increased ICP. Patients with acute meningitis present with classic signs of meningeal irritation, including photophobia, phonophobia, and a Kernig or Brudzinski sign. In meningeal carcinomatosis, these signs are frequently absent.

Increased ICP in infants results in an increased head circumference. Chronic hydrocephalus can be recognized on plain radiographs of the skull as focal thinning of the tabula interna of the skull ("Lückenschädel"). This is accompanied by personality changes and loss of previously acquired motor skills. Herniation of one cerebellar tonsil causes a head tilt and neck stiffness.[26] Tectal masses result in upgaze inhibition, light-near dissociation of pupillary response, and convergence-retraction nystagmus (Parinaud's syndrome). Pressure on the mesencephalic tegmentum leads to pathologic lid retraction and an upward gaze palsy (setting-sun sign).

Slowly progressive, static ICP changes are accompanied by few or no symptoms. Clinical deterioration is profound when dynamic pressure changes such as plateau waves or abnormal intracranial compartmentation or herniation occur.[27] Signs and symptoms of increased ICP manifest earlier in patients with lesions of the posterior fossa because of the small size of this compartment. In uncal herniation from temporal lobe masses or herpes encephalitis, ipsilateral compression of the third nerve leads to pupillary dilatation before extraocular dysmotility. With progression of shift of brain substance, a complete third nerve palsy ensues and signs of midbrain dysfunction appear. Patients develop contralateral hemiparesis from pressure on the cerebral peduncle and ultimately become stuporous. Increasing pressure from hemispheric or diencephalic mass lesions results in central (transtentorial) herniation. Central herniation leads to a progressive syndrome reflecting sequential damage to brainstem structures in a rostrocaudal fashion. At the early "diencephalic" stage, mild changes in the patient's alertness are accompanied by periodic breathing, yawning, or hiccuping. Pupils are small but remain reactive to light. With further progression of central herniation, the patient becomes obtunded or stuporous. Roving eye movements reflect diffuse cortical dysfunction and preservation of lower brainstem gaze centers. Noxious stimuli elicit flexion of upper extremities and extension of lower extremities (decorticate posturing). Midsize pupils that are unresponsive to light indicate midbrain dysfunction. Damage to the mesencephalic reticular activating system produces coma. Central neurogenic hyperventilation denotes a fast and regular breathing pattern. The triad of changes in breathing pattern, arterial hypertension, and bradycardia is known as the *Kocher-Cushing reflex*.[28] Noxious stimulation elicits extension of all limbs (decerebrate posturing). Absence of oculocephalic reflex (doll's head maneuver) and horizontal eye movements to caloric stimulation of the vestibular system indicate damage to pontine structures. Breathing becomes apneustic. Further progression leads to herniation of the cerebellar tonsils through the foramen magnum. At the preterminal stage, breathing is ataxic and the blood pressure drops.

The syndrome of raised ICP and cerebral herniation can evolve slowly over days to weeks or acutely over hours. Rapid progression usually indicates hemorrhage. Subdural hematomas in patients with coagulopathies can evolve so rapidly that signs of cerebral herniation are present before an imaging study can be obtained. Hemorrhage into a metastatic focus is typically characterized by the sudden onset of focal neurologic signs including seizures. Intraparenchymal hemorrhage as a result of coagulopathy leads to slowly progressive neurologic deterioration.[7]

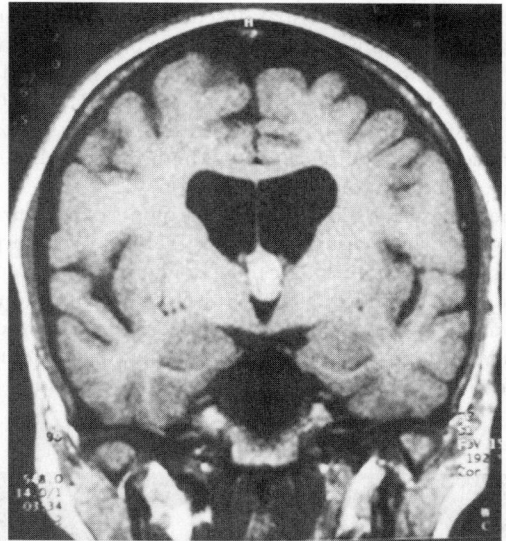

A

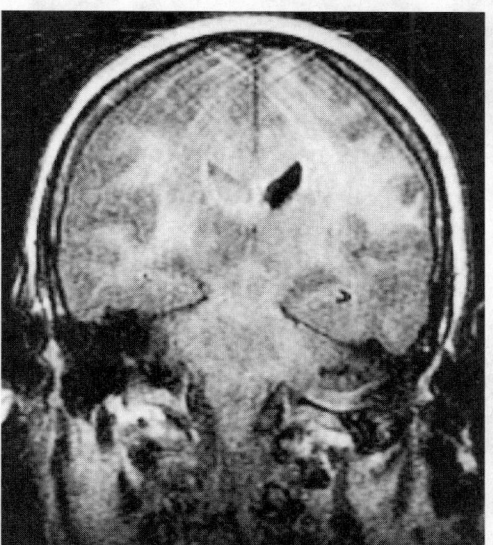

B

FIGURE 49.2-1. **A:** Mechanisms of increased intracranial pressure. Intermittent obstructive hydrocephalus caused by the "pressure valve" effect of a colloid cyst of the foramen of Monro. This 38-year-old patient had experienced several presyncopal episodes and was experiencing positional headaches. The lateral ventricles are dilated [unenhanced T1-weighted magnetic resonance imaging (MRI), coronal section (**A**)]. **B:** A 78-year-old woman with gliomatosis cerebri. Hyperintense signal on this coronal fluid attenuated inversion recovery MRI demarcates the extent of cerebral infiltration by neoplastic cells and vasogenic edema. Extensive effacement of the sulcal pattern and early transtentorial herniation are present (**B**).

A peculiar syndrome is associated with tumors causing a pressure valve effect, such as a colloid cyst of the foramen of Monro (Fig. 49.2-1). Patients, typically in their late childhood or early adulthood, report sudden onset of severe imbalance, headache, and nausea that is frequently brought on by positional changes (bending down) or Valsalva maneuvers. Sudden deaths have occurred, and these patients require close observation until appropriate therapy can be provided.[29,30]

IIH (pseudotumor cerebri) is mostly characterized by nocturnal or hypnopompic headaches aggravated by Valsalva maneuver. Nonspecific visual changes, diplopia due to sixth nerve palsy, and transient visual obscuration are less frequent manifestations. On physical examination, papilledema is the most striking abnormality.[31] The blind spot is enlarged. It is presumed that the disorder is due to decreased CSF absorption. Dural sinus thrombosis or nonthrombotic stenosis of dural sinuses not complicated by hemorrhagic infarction results in a pseudotumor-like presentation.

Another characteristic clinical syndrome is recognized in patients with chronic disturbance of spinal fluid reabsorption. These patients or, more likely, their family members report a combination of cognitive decline, precipitate micturition, and gait apraxia.[32,33] Dementia is usually of the subcortical type. Precipitate micturition reflects dysfunction of the cortical center for bladder control (paracentral lobule). Minimal bladder filling

results in the uncontrollable urge to urinate. The gait disturbance is characterized by difficulty initiating ambulation and postural instability with retropulsion. Strength is preserved.

DIAGNOSIS

The history and clinical examination detect the presence of increased ICP. Imaging studies are helpful in determining its cause and confirming the clinical impression. The most readily available imaging study is unenhanced computed tomography. The study is adequate to determine the presence of intraventricular and subarachnoid CSF flow obstruction (Fig. 49.2-2), as well as uncal, transfalcian, and transtentorial herniation

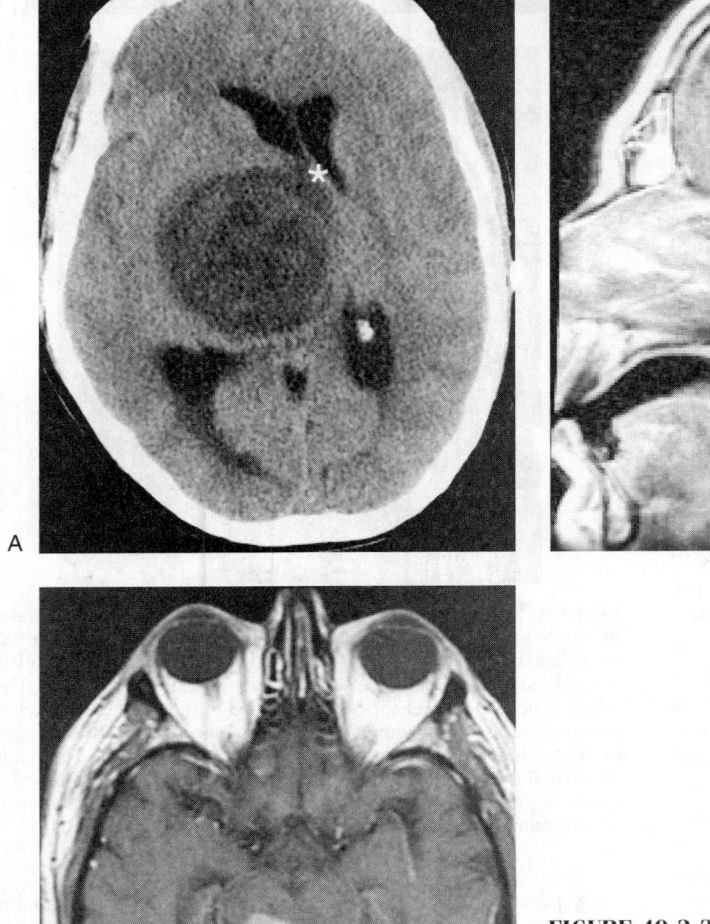

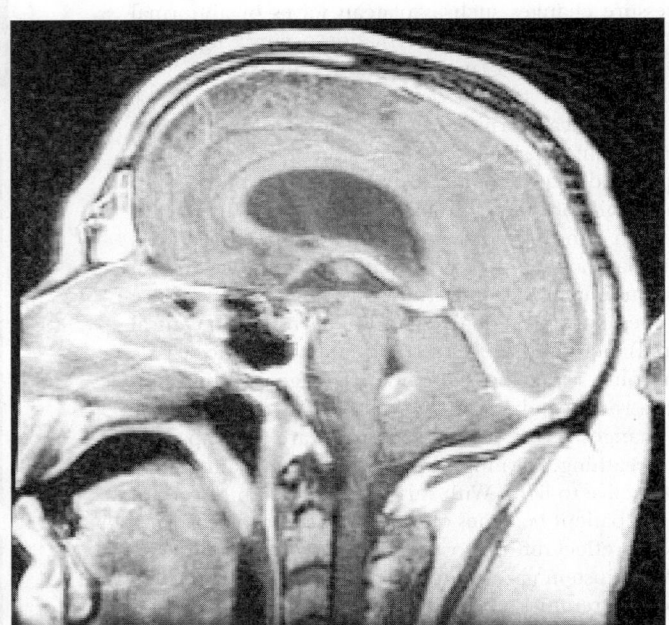

FIGURE 49.2-2.   Obstructive hydrocephalus. **A:** A 45-year-old patient with an anaplastic astrocytoma of the right thalamus. Computed tomography revealed obstruction at the level of the foramen of Monro (*asterisk*). **B:** A 55-year-old patient with a midbrain metastasis from an adenocarcinoma of the lung. Partial obstruction is present at the level of the cerebral aqueduct. The temporal horns of the lateral ventricles are dilated [T1-weighted magnetic resonance imaging (MRI) with gadolinium]. **C:** A 38-year-old patient with seeding of non–small cell lung cancer to the floor of the fourth ventricle. He presented with intractable headaches, nausea, vomiting, and severe back pain indicative of obstructive hydrocephalus and leptomeningeal spread to the spinal canal (T1-weighted MRI with gadolinium, sagittal view).

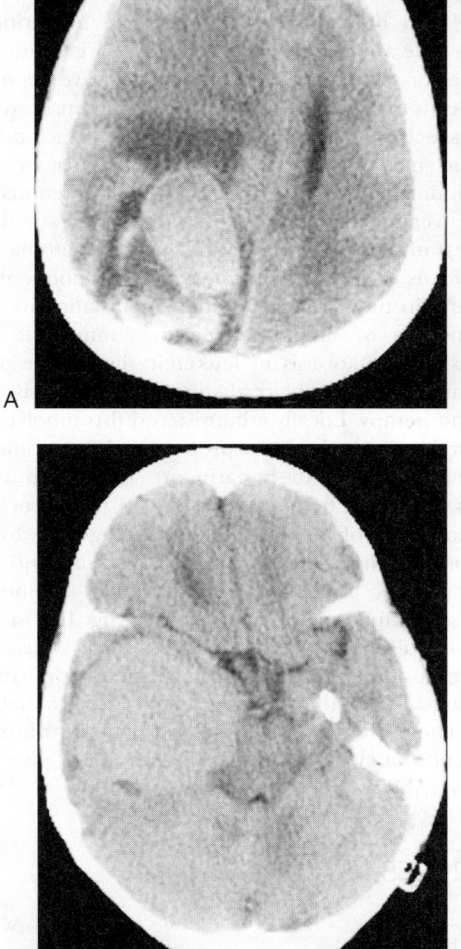

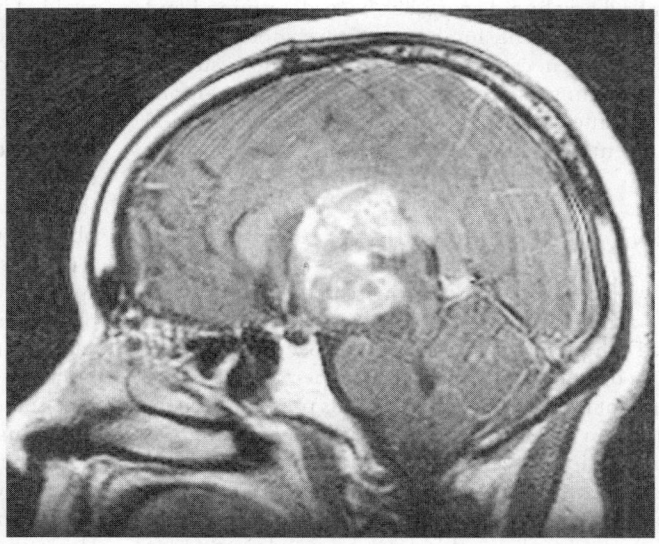

FIGURE 49.2-3. Cerebral herniation. **A:** Unenhanced computed tomography scan of the head shows a hemorrhagic brain metastasis in a 42-year-old woman with malignant melanoma. The metastasis exerts mass effect on the right lateral ventricle. Transfalcian herniation of the right hemisphere is present. **B:** A 37-year-old woman with an anaplastic astrocytoma of the diencephalon. Imminent transtentorial herniation is present (T1-weighted magnetic resonance imaging with gadolinium, sagittal view). **C:** A 25-year-old woman in whom a large right temporal meningioma developed years after whole brain radiation therapy for acute lymphoblastic leukemia in early childhood. The tumor compresses the cerebral peduncle and displaces the midbrain (unenhanced computed tomography).

(Fig. 49.2-3). The presence of intracranial hemorrhage or a neoplastic or infectious mass lesion can be identified and emergency treatment initiated. Transependymal edema is seen as periventricular hypodensity and indicates CSF flow obstruction.

More detailed neuroanatomic imaging and the distinction between a neoplastic, infectious, inflammatory, or ischemic process require magnetic resonance imaging (MRI) and magnetic resonance spectroscopy. The use of intravenous gadolinium is advised because most conditions associated with increased ICP in cancer patients cause breakdown of the blood–brain barrier and thus can be better visualized with contrast dye. CSF flow studies (cine–MRI) are helpful to evaluate the functional significance of minute structural lesions within or surrounding the cerebral aqueduct. Slit-like ventricles in the correct clinical setting are indicative of IIH. Coronal images through the orbit may reveal dilatation of the optic nerve sheaths in this condition. *Ex vacuo* ventricular dilatation out of proportion to cortical atrophy is characteristic for NPH. MRI of the spine should be considered in patients with unexplained communicating hydrocephalus. Obstruction or infiltration of dural venous sinuses is best visualized with magnetic resonance venography.[34]

Scintigraphic cisternography can document spinal fluid circulation abnormalities such as NPH. Early ventricular filling with tracer substance after lumbar injection and delayed or absent demarcation of subarachnoid space overlying the cerebral hemispheres is indicative of decreased reabsorption of CSF through the arachnoid granulations.

CSF pressure can be measured directly through a lumbar puncture performed in the lateral decubitus position. Puncture of the subarachnoid space below the level of spinal fluid obstruction bears the risk of initiating or aggravating cerebral herniation. The risk is considerable in mass lesions of the posterior fossa. Computed tomography should be obtained before lumbar puncture in patients with signs of increased ICP. Compartmentation (obstructive hydrocephalus at the foramen of Monro or cerebral aqueduct; obliteration of basal cisterns as a result of transtentorial or transforaminal herniation) prohibits puncture of the subarachnoid space below the level of obstruction. When unperturbed communication between the intraventricular and subarachnoid space has been determined and the basal cisterns are patent, lumbar puncture should not be delayed if it is deemed necessary for accurate diagnosis such as in cryptococcal meningitis. Transcranial Doppler sonography is helpful in the intensive care unit for monitoring cerebral perfusion in patients with increased ICP.

TREATMENT

In the majority of cases, the onset of increased ICP in cancer patients is protracted over days to weeks. After increased ICP is recognized and symptomatic measures have been initiated to lower pressure, a diagnostic procedure can be performed before definitive treatment is provided. Fewer patients present an emergency and require an immediate neurosurgical intervention.

The patient with increased ICP is best positioned with head and upper trunk slightly elevated. Body temperature elevation is treated with antipyretics. Serum osmolality is kept in the high normal range. Isotonic saline solutions are recommended for intravenous hydration.

Corticosteroids are effective agents for the initial management of increased ICP caused by vasogenic edema. No benefit has been convincingly shown for cytotoxic edema of an acute ischemic stroke, intracranial hemorrhage secondary to remote effects of cancer, or spinal fluid obstruction. Moderate (6 to 10 mg dexamethasone every 6 hours) to high doses (up to 100 mg/d dexamethasone) are used. A superior therapeutic effect has not been shown for high doses, and the risk of adverse reactions, in particular gastroduodenal ulceration, is considerable. Corticosteroids should be avoided if central nervous system lymphoma is considered in the differential diagnosis and a tissue diagnosis has not yet been established. Dexamethasone and related drugs induce lymphocytic apoptosis and may obscure morphologic diagnosis.

Osmotic diuresis through infusion of hyperosmolar agents such as mannitol or glycerol is an alternative or additional treatment option. Most commonly used are intravenous infusions of 20% to 25% mannitol solutions given at an initial dose of 0.75 to 1.0 g/kg body weight followed by 0.25 to 0.50 g/kg body weight every 3 to 6 hours. Monitoring of serum osmolality is required. The effect is transient, and treatment should be stopped if the target serum osmolality is exceeded (300 mOsm/L).

Monitoring in the neurologic intensive care unit is required in patients with depressed mental status secondary to ICP elevation. Careful blood pressure adjustment needs to avoid blood pressure peaks without decreasing cerebral perfusion. The most rapid method to decrease ICP is intubation with mechanical hyperventilation. The pCO_2 should be decreased to 25 to 30 mm Hg. Lower pCO_2 levels are avoided because cerebral perfusion is decreased. The effect of hyperventilation is transient, and, thus, other measures such as corticosteroid use and osmotic diuresis need to be instituted expeditiously.

Obstructive hydrocephalus constitutes a neurosurgical emergency. Rapid neurologic deterioration with signs of cerebral herniation mandate the immediate placement of an external ventriculostomy. Permanent drainage of CSF through a ventriculoperitoneal shunt or endoscopic placement of a third ventriculostomy may be necessary when the cause of spinal fluid flow obstruction cannot be definitively treated. Although filter systems are available, ventriculoperitoneal shunting is avoided in patients with leptomeningeal tumor to prevent peritoneal seeding.

NPH responds favorably to ventriculoperitoneal shunting. It is the task of the clinician to carefully select patients who may benefit from this procedure. Individuals with a short history of the classic clinical triad of gait apraxia, precipitate micturition, and cognitive decline are most likely to respond. Large-volume spinal fluid releases or scintigraphic cisternography have been used as objective means to predict outcome of a shunting procedure.

Disease-specific treatment of increased ICP in addition to symptomatic management with corticosteroids or osmotic diuresis is indicated in the majority of cases. Infectious complications are treated with antimicrobial therapy. Patients with a brain abscess undergo surgical drainage. A hematoma within a metastatic focus is resected if located in a noneloquent area of the brain and in the absence of widely metastatic disease. Subdural hematoma or empyema requires immediate surgical decompression. Leukostasis in leukemic diseases responds to hydration and whole brain irradiation, leukapheresis, and systemic chemotherapy. Locally administered thrombolytic agents (tissue plasminogen activator or urokinase) or systemic intravenous anticoagulation with heparin are used in dural sinus thrombosis. Petechial hemorrhages due to thrombocytopenia require transfusion of blood platelets. A coagulopathy can be corrected using transfusion of fresh frozen plasma and substitution of vitamin K. Increased ICP secondary to medication requires discontinuation of the causative drug. IIH in the cancer patient is typically caused by malignant dural sinus compression and responds to local surgical treatment or irradiation. Leptomeningeal carcinomatosis is treated with irradiation and intrathecal chemotherapy. CSF flow obstruction prohibits intrathecal injection of cytotoxic agents because it can give rise to a severe, irreversible toxic encephalomyelopathy.

REFERENCES

1. Fishman RA. *Cerebrospinal fluid in diseases of the nervous system.* Philadelphia: W.B. Saunders Company, 1992.
2. Lundberg N. Continuous recording and control of ventricular fluid pressure in neurosurgical practice. *Acta Psychiatrica Scand* 1960;36[Suppl 149]:1960.
3. Watling CJ, Cairncross JG. Acetazolamide therapy for symptomatic plateau waves in patients with brain tumors. Report of three cases. *J Neurosurg* 2002;97:224.
4. Lassman AB, DeAngelis LM. Brain metastases. *Neurol Clin* 2003;21:1.
5. Posner JB. *Neurologic complications of cancer.* Philadelphia: FA Davis Company, 1995.
6. Kaste SC, Rodriguez-Galindo C, Furman WL, Langston J, Thompson SJ. Imaging aspects of neurologic emergencies in children treated for non-CNS malignancies. *Pediatr Radiol* 2000;30:558.
7. Quinn JA, DeAngelis LM. Neurologic emergencies in the cancer patient. *Semin Oncol* 2000;27:311.
8. Choo-Kang LR, Jones DM, Fehr JJ, Eskenazi AE, Toretsky JA. Cerebral edema and priapism in an adolescent with acute lymphoblastic leukemia. *Pediatr Emerg Care* 1999;15:110.
9. DeAngelis LM, Delattre JY, Posner JB. Radiation-induced dementia in patients cured of brain metastases. *Neurology* 1989;39:789.
10. Thiessen B, DeAngelis LM. Hydrocephalus in radiation leukoencephalopathy: results of ventriculoperitoneal shunting. *Arch Neurol* 1998;55:705.
11. Perrini P, Scollato A, Cioffi F, et al. Radiation leukoencephalopathy associated with moderate hydrocephalus: intracranial pressure monitoring and results of ventriculoperitoneal shunting. *Neurol Sci* 2002;23:237.
12. Caviness JA, Tucker MH, Pia SK, Tam DA. Hydrocephalus as a possible early symptom in a child with a spinal cord tumor. *Pediatr Neurol* 1998;18:169.
13. Rifkinson-Mann S, Wisoff JH, Epstein F. The association of hydrocephalus with intramedullary spinal cord tumors: a series of 25 patients. *Neurosurgery* 1990;27:749.
14. Phan TG, Krauss WE, Fealey RD. Recurrent lumbar ependymoma presenting as headache and communicating hydrocephalus. *Mayo Clin Proc* 2000;75:850.
15. Costello F, Kardon RH, Wall M, et al. Papilledema as the presenting manifestation of spinal schwannoma. *J Neuroophthalmol* 2002;22:199.
16. Kordas M, Czirjak S, Doczi T. The spinal tumour related hydrocephalus. *Acta Neurochir (Wien)* 1997;139:1049.

17. Pirouzmand F, Tator CH, Rutka J. Management of hydrocephalus associated with vestibular schwannoma and other cerebellopontine angle tumors. *Neurosurgery* 2001;48:1246.

18. Colucciello M. Pseudotumor cerebri induced by all-trans retinoic acid treatment of acute promyelocytic leukemia. *Arch Ophthalmol* 2003;121:1064.

19. Di Rocco C, Iannelli A. Poor outcome of bilateral congenital choroid plexus papillomas with extreme hydrocephalus. *Eur Neurol* 1997;37:33.

20. Biousse V, Ameri A, Bousser MG. Isolated intracranial hypertension as the only sign of cerebral venous thrombosis. *Neurology* 1999;53:1537.

21. Gironell A, Marti-Fabregas J, Bello J, Avila A. Non-Hodgkin's lymphoma as a new cause of non-thrombotic superior sagittal sinus occlusion. *J Neurol Neurosurg Psychiatry* 1997;63:121.

22. Kim AW, Trobe JD. Syndrome simulating pseudotumor cerebri caused by partial transverse venous sinus obstruction in metastatic prostate cancer. *Am J Ophthalmol* 2000;129:254.

23. Thomas DA, Trobe JD, Cornblath WT. Visual loss secondary to increased intracranial pressure in neurofibromatosis type 2. *Arch Ophthalmol* 1999;117:1650.

24. Goldsmith P, Burn DJ, Coulthard A, Jenkins A. Extrinsic cerebral venous sinus obstruction resulting in intracranial hypertension. *Postgrad Med J* 1999;75:550.

25. Forsyth PA, Posner JB. Headaches in patients with brain tumors: a study of 111 patients. *Neurology* 1993;43:1678.

26. Kelly KM, Lange B. Oncologic emergencies. *Pediatr Clin North Am* 1997;44:809.

27. Plum F, Posner JB. *The diagnosis of stupor and coma.* Philadelphia: FA Davis, 1980.

28. Cushing HW. Some experimental and clinical observations concerning states of increased intracranial tension. *Am J Med Sci* 1902;124:375.

29. Aronica PA, Ahdab-Barmada M, Rozin L, Wecht CH. Sudden death in an adolescent boy due to a colloid cyst of the third ventricle. *Am J Forensic Med Pathol* 1998;19:119.

30. Jeffree RL, Besser M. Colloid cyst of the third ventricle: a clinical review of 39 cases. *J Clin Neurosci* 2001;8:328.

31. Foley J. Benign forms of intracranial hypertension—"toxic" and "otitic" hydrocephalus. *Brain* 1955;78:1.

32. Hakim S, Adams RD. The special clinical problem of symptomatic hydrocephalus with normal cerebrospinal fluid pressure. *J Neurol Sci* 1965;2:307.

33. Fisher CM. Hydrocephalus as a cause of disturbance of gait in the elderly. *Neurology* 1982;32:1358.

34. Chaudhuri R, Tarnawski M, Graves MJ, Graves PE, Cox TC. Dural sinus occlusion due to calvarial metastases: a CT blind spot. *J Comput Assist Tomogr* 1992;16:30.

SECTION 3

JOACHIM M. BAEHRING

Spinal Cord Compression

Compression of the spinal cord is one of the most devastating neurologic complications of cancer, affecting 5% to 10% of cancer patients.[1] The majority of cases result from spinal metastases with extension into the epidural space. Pain is the most common initial clinical manifestation of metastases to the axial skeleton. Within weeks, neurologic impairment ensues and is irreversible if treatment is not initiated promptly. Malignant spinal cord compression (MSCC) is a diagnostic challenge, especially in patients without a history of cancer. Back pain is one of the most common ailments in the general population and, in the vast majority of cases, results from degenerative changes of the spine. Early identification of patients at risk of MSCC is essential, because limited workup, symptomatic management, and bed rest—a common practice in patients with "benign" back pain—almost invariably leads to profound neurologic morbidity.

This chapter describes the clinical syndromes, diagnosis, and treatment of epidural cancer metastases. Metastases below the conus medullaris—corresponding to the level of the first lumbar vertebra in adults—giving rise to isolated radiculopathies or a cauda equina syndrome are included.

EPIDEMIOLOGY

Epidemiologic data must be interpreted with respect to possible selection bias. Population-based studies frequently underestimate the incidence of a disease because they primarily rely on administrative data. Important clinical information is frequently missing, and the completeness and accuracy of available data are unknown. Data from referral centers for cancer treatment are expected to overestimate the incidence of cancer-related cord compression because patients are more likely to be referred to such an institution if they develop a complication requiring emergent and multimodality care.[2]

The majority of patients with MSCC are older than 50 years of age. The lifetime incidence in cancer patients is 1% to 6%, although autopsy series have revealed higher numbers (5% to 10%).[2–5] The most common types of cancer associated with spinal cord compression are breast, prostate, and lung cancer and lymphoma.[1,2–4,6–9] The cumulative incidence of MSCC is disease specific and is highest in multiple myeloma (8%), prostate cancer (7%), nasopharyngeal cancer (6.5%), and breast cancer (5.5%).[2] The median interval between cancer diagnosis and manifestation of MSCC ranges from 6.0 to 12.5 months. Late axial bone metastases causing cord compression are more common in breast cancer (43 months).[3] In only 1 in 500 cancer patients is spinal cord compression part of the presenting oncologic syndrome.[2] However, 20% of MSCC cases lack a history of cancer.[4,10] MSCC as the primary manifestation of a malignancy is more common in non-Hodgkin's lymphoma, myeloma, and lung cancer, especially the small cell variant; it is almost unheard of in breast cancer.[11,12] Two-thirds of MSCC cases affect the thoracic spine. The lumbar spine is involved in 20%. MSCC at the level of the cervical and sacral spine is rare.[1,7,9,13,14] Colon and prostate cancer metastases seem to have a predilection for the lumbosacral spine. Multiple epidural metastases are detected on initial presentation in up to one-third of patients in whom the whole axial skeleton is investigated.[15] Local recurrence after irradiation is rare, but one in ten patients develops a second metastatic deposit causing cord compression at a different spine level within 5 months of the first event.[1,7]

The tumor spectrum causing cord compression is quite different in the pediatric population. The majority of cases of cord compression in children are caused by neuroblastoma and Ewing's sarcoma. Primary vertebral osteosarcoma and lymphoma are less common. Cord compression at initial manifestation of the tumor occurs more frequently than in the adult population.[16]

PATHOPHYSIOLOGY

The most common mechanisms of spinal cord compression are the direct extension of tumor from a hematogenous metastasis to a vertebral body into the epidural space and the pathologic fracture of a vertebral body infiltrated by a metastatic deposit that results in cord injury by a bone fragment or spinal instability (Fig. 49.3-1). Involvement of posterior spinal

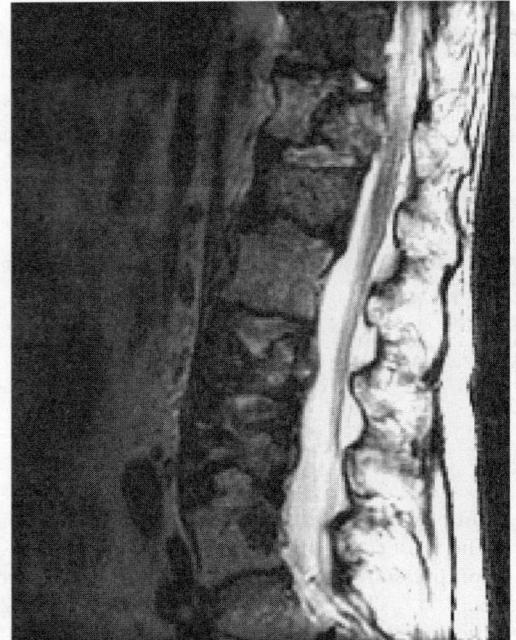
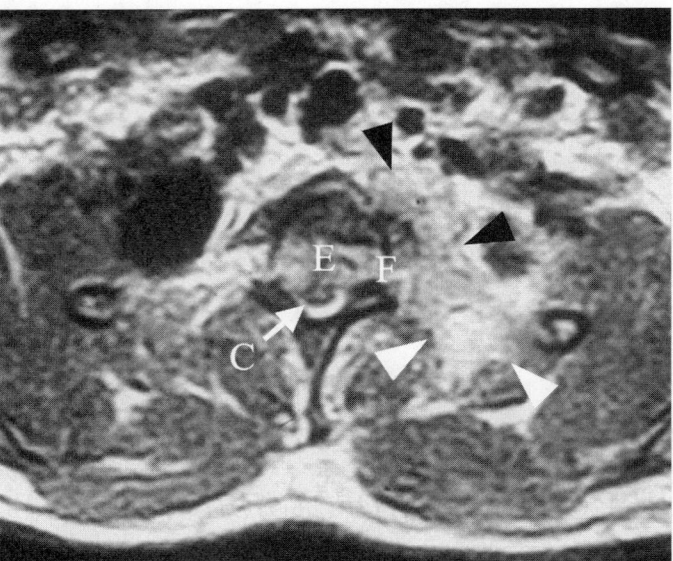

FIGURE 49.3-1. **A:** T2-weighted magnetic resonance imaging (MRI; sagittal view) of the lumbosacral spine of a 53-year-old patient with metastatic renal cell cancer shows a pathologic fracture of the T-12 vertebral body, posterior dislocation of a bone fragment, and compression of the spinal cord. **B:** T1-weighted MRI with gadolinium (axial view) of a 19-year-old patient with Ewing's sarcoma of the T-2 vertebral body. The tumor has extended into the epidural space (E) and compresses the spinal cord (C, *arrow*). The mass has grown through the intervertebral foramen (F) into the paravertebral space (*black* and *white arrowheads*). The patient had noticed that his left pupil had become smaller (Horner's syndrome). He then started having intermittent upper back pain aggravated by coughing and of difficulty walking upstairs and initiating urination.

elements with nerve root impingement is less common.[17] Transforaminal progression of paravertebral tumor is encountered in lymphoma and neuroblastoma. Other paravertebral tumors such as the Pancoast's tumor of the lung apex infiltrate the epidural space after destruction of a vertebral body. Primary hematogenous seeding to the epidural space is a rare cause of MSCC.[6] Spinal cord compression can also result from intradural mass lesions (meningioma, nerve sheath tumors, large leptomeningeal metastases; Fig. 49.3-2) or intraneural spread of neurogenic tumors. Nonmetastatic causes are epidural hematoma in patients with coagulopathy or abscess in an immunocompromised host.

The mechanism of cord injury is not entirely understood. The early myelopathy associated with MSCC may be due to impairment of venous drainage leading to intramedullary vasogenic edema. Irreversible cord necrosis results from ischemia. Pathologic fracture of a vertebral body and posterior displacement of bone fragments leads to mechanical cord destruction. On histopathologic examination, demyelination or necrosis of white matter is the predominant finding at the level of cord compression, whereas gray matter is relatively well preserved.[8]

Bone, particularly the axial skeleton, is one of the most common organ systems involved by metastatic spread. Up to one-third of patients dying of cancer develop metastases to the spine at some point during their illness.[18] Release of bone-derived growth factors and cytokines, capillary structure, and peculiar blood flow phenomena may facilitate deposition and growth of metastases.[19,20] Venous blood from intraabdominal and intrathoracic organs is drained not only through the vena cava but also through the vertebral and epidural venous plexus (Batson's plexus). This low-pressure circulation without valves and with frequent flow reversal depending on intrathoracic and intraabdominal pressure appears to be an ideal transportation system for cancer cells.

The complex syndrome of back pain is comprised of local, radicular, and referred components. Pain-sensitive structures of the spine are the vertebral periosteum, the posterior longitudinal ligament, and the synovia of the facet joints. They are innervated by branches of the segmental spinal nerve. Pain from metastatic tumor spread to the spine ensues when the cancer infiltrates the periosteum. Radicular pain results from compression or infiltration of a nerve root. Pain can also be the consequence of irritation of long tracts of the spinal cord (funicular pain) or paravertebral muscle spasm.

Micturition is frequently impaired in patients with MSCC. A brief review of the anatomy of bladder control helps to explain the patient's symptoms. Excitatory input to the detrusor muscle promoting bladder emptying is parasympathetic and involves sacral spinal cord segments. Relaxation of the internal sphincter is transmitted through the sympathetic nervous system. Preganglionic neurons originate from thoracic and upper lumbar cord segments. The external sphincter muscle is innervated by anterior horn motor neurons of the sacral cord (nucleus of Onufrowicz). Voluntary bladder control requires sensory input from stretch receptors within the bladder wall. This signal is transmitted to the pontine micturition center, which also receives descending input from the paracentral lobule of the frontal lobe. The coordinated inhibition of internal

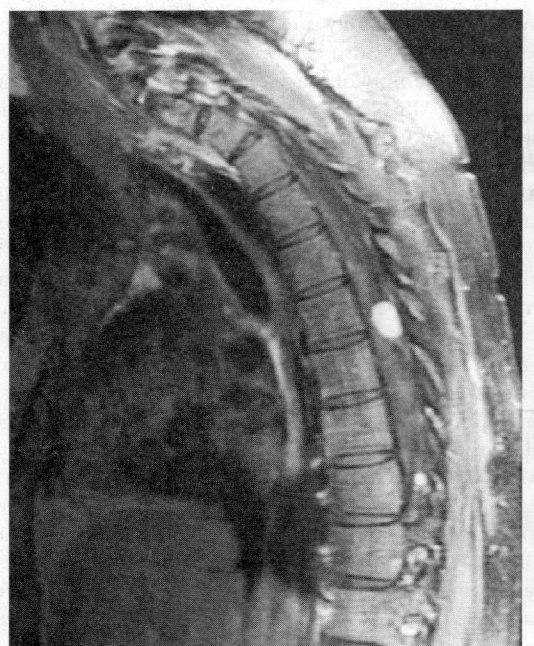 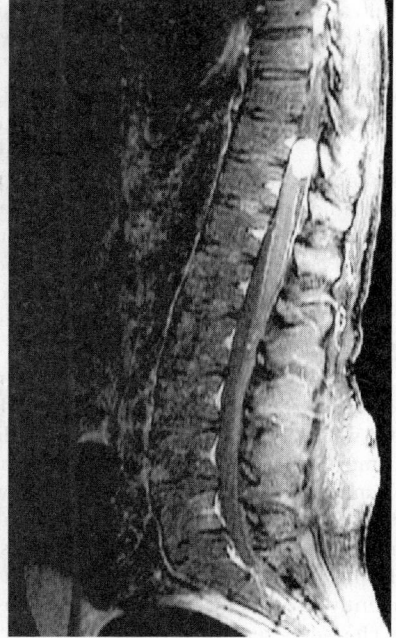

FIGURE 49.3-2. Topical differential diagnosis of cord compression. **A:** This T1-weighted magnetic resonance image (MRI) with gadolinium and fat suppression (thoracic spine, sagittal view) demonstrates an intradural, extramedullary mass lesion with cord compression in a 32-year-old woman with neurofibromatosis type 2 and a meningioma of the spinal canal. **B:** Leptomeningeal metastasis with cord infiltration and compression at the level of the T-10 vertebral body in a 27-year-old patient with leptomeningeal spread of a diencephalic yolk sac tumor. The tumor infiltrated the thoracic spinal cord, giving rise to Brown-Séquard syndrome below the level of infiltration [T1-weighted MRI with gadolinium and fat suppression, lower spine, sagittal view (**B**)].

A,B

and external sphincter is mediated through the pontine micturition center. Spinal cord compression above the conus results in lack of voluntary control of micturition. Reflex emptying is possible but incomplete. Destruction of the sacral spinal cord leads to external sphincter insufficiency, unawareness of bladder fullness, and overflow incontinence. The mechanisms for control of defecation are similar.

CLINICAL PRESENTATION

Pain is the most common presenting symptom in patients with metastases involving the axial skeleton.[3,4,13,14] Any back pain in a patient with a cancer known to frequently seed to spine or epidural space should be considered of metastatic origin until proven otherwise. In its early stage, the pain may be localized to the affected spinal segment. Pain likely ensues when the richly innervated periosteum is involved. The vertebral body affected by metastatic spread is tender to percussion. The pain resulting from an epidural mass effect is typically exacerbated by sneezing, coughing, or the Valsalva maneuver. Because the recumbent position aggravates the pain, many patients experience maximum pain intensity on awakening in the morning or even have to sleep in a sitting position. Compression of a nerve root is associated with excruciating pain in the corresponding radicular distribution. It has a lancinating character and is likewise aggravated by the Valsalva maneuver. Radicular pain in the thoracic region is usually bilateral, whereas cervical and lumbar radiculopathies are unilateral.[21] Paravertebral muscle spasm caused by nerve root irritation from a metastasis results in straightening of the physiologic cervical or lumbar lordosis. Straight leg raising (Lasègue maneuver) or, more specifically, crossed straight leg raising (passive elevation of the contralateral, pain-free leg) exacerbates a radiculopathy. Referred pain may mimic a radiculopathy. Especially with intraneural tumor spread, neuropathic features (allodynia, hyperpathia, hyperalgesia) may predominate.

Neurologic symptoms typically evolve within weeks to months of the onset of back pain.[10,14] Hyperacute presentation with the evolution of paraplegia within hours to days of onset of neurologic symptoms is not uncommon in bronchogenic carcinoma. A much slower course is typical for metastases from breast cancer.[8] Motor dysfunction (paraparesis or quadriparesis, spasticity) is the earliest sign and occurs before sensory disturbance. Only one-third of patients report lower extremity weakness as an initial symptom. However, at diagnosis, fewer than one-third of patients are ambulatory.[3,4,13] Typical early complaints are leg "heaviness" and difficulty climbing stairs or getting up from a chair. Because the majority of malignancy-related cord compressions occur at the level of the thoracic spinal cord, most patients present with a paraparesis. The rare patient with a cervical spinal cord metastasis is expected to have a quadriparesis, which varies in degree, and, if the high cervical cord is compromised, respiratory insufficiency. Epidural progression of metastases to the upper lumbar spine results in a conus medullaris syndrome with distal lower extremity weakness, saddle paraesthesias, and overflow leakage from bladder and bowel.

Ataxia in a patient with MSCC reflects compression of spinocerebellar pathways.

Only a few patients report diminished sensation to all sensory qualities below the level of compression at initial presentation. The level of hypesthesia is usually two to three segments below the metastatic lesion. Discrepancy of up to ten levels above or below the lesion has been described.[13] Tingling paresthesias radiating down the spine into the extremities on brisk flexion of the neck (Lhermitte's sign) indicates an intrinsic or extrinsic spinal cord process.

Symptoms of neurogenic bladder dysfunction are less common at symptom onset but are frequently overlooked or rationalized by the patient. A detailed micturition history is indispensable, because patients are unlikely to report their symptoms until their compensatory mechanisms fail. New onset of nocturia or pollakiuria in the correct clinical setting should alarm the physician, and a common explanation by the patient that "I've been drinking a lot" should be disregarded. Alarming symptoms of bladder dysfunction are hesitancy and urinary retention. At diagnosis, almost half of patients with MSCC are incontinent or require catheterization.[4]

The presence of Horner's syndrome (the combination of miosis, ptosis, and enophthalmos) indicates transforaminal progression of tumors located at the level of the cervicothoracic junction and infiltration of the stellate ganglion.

DIFFERENTIAL DIAGNOSIS

Infiltration of the lumbosacral plexus or peripheral nerves originating from it (femoral, sciatic nerve) has to be distinguished from malignant epidural compression of a root or the cauda equina. With unilateral involvement, bladder and bowel symptoms are absent; however, bilateral infiltration of plexus or nerve has been seen in neurolymphomatosis and perineural spread from pelvic malignancies. Herpes zoster is encountered at spinal levels previously or concurrently affected by cancer.[8,22]

The cauda equina syndrome is characterized by an asymmetric painful lumbosacral polyradiculopathy, a patchy sensory deficit corresponding to multiple lumbar and sacral nerve roots, and bladder and bowel incontinence. In a cancer patient, this syndrome raises suspicion of leptomeningeal carcinomatosis. The presence of signs and symptoms referable to intracranial disease (headache, asymmetric cranial neuropathies) facilitates the diagnosis.

Intraparenchymal spinal cord metastases and primary cord tumors are rare but may resemble epidural disease. Metastatic cord tumors predominantly arise from small cell lung cancer and breast cancer.[23] Infectious myelitis (caused by herpes simplex or human T-lymphotropic virus) and autoimmune myelitis are examples of myelopathies not directly related to cancer that have to be distinguished from MSCC. Predominance of transverse myelopathic features in the absence of pain is indicative of an intraparenchymal process.

Spinal cord hemisyndromes indicate intrinsic spinal cord disease. A classical Brown-Séquard syndrome characterized by leg weakness and loss of proprioception on the side of cord infiltration and loss of pain and temperature sensation on the opposite side is rarely seen, but incomplete variants exist. Leptomeningeal spread of highly aggressive tumors can lead to spinal cord infiltration causing an overlap syndrome of extrinsic and intrinsic cord disease.

DIAGNOSIS

The mere complaint of back pain in a cancer patient frequently does not lead to an immediate workup for vertebral metastases. Only the occurrence of more severe symptoms such as sphincter dysfunction or paraparesis sets off a comprehensive diagnostic procedure.[3] In spite of the availability of sensitive diagnostic tests, the average time between onset of symptoms and definitive diagnosis is still 3 months (range, 37 to 205 days). Two-thirds of this time passes after the patient reports the symptoms to a health professional.[13] An interesting pattern was observed in a Scottish study. The rate of cord compression diagnosis steadily increased throughout the course of the week and reached its peak on Friday.[13]

With the availability of magnetic resonance imaging (MRI), the diagnosis of MSCC has been simplified. The decision to use this tool is dependent on the clinical evaluation. New onset or change in character of preexisting back pain in a cancer patient or atypical back pain in the absence of a cancer history warrants measures beyond plain radiography and symptomatic therapy. Degenerative spine disease mostly affects the lower cervical and lower lumbar spine, the segments of largest motion. The pain waxes and wanes and responds to bed rest and symptomatic treatment with nonsteroidal antiinflammatory agents. Pain located in the thoracic spine, pain that progresses in spite of conservative measures, or pain aggravated by supine position should raise the suspicion for MSCC.

MRI of the whole spine is the most sensitive diagnostic test when MSCC is suspected in a cancer patient. The study can accurately identify the level of the metastatic lesion and guide the radiation oncologist in planning the treatment field. Multiple levels of involvement present in up to one-third of patients with metastatic spinal cord compression are recognized.[15,24] Vertebral metastases without protrusion into the epidural space are detected before a potentially irreversible cord syndrome ensues. Metastases can be distinguished from other pathologic processes involving the axial skeleton, epidural and intradural space, and spinal cord. Bacterial abscesses typically cause end plate destruction and invasion of the disc space, whereas metastatic deposits leave the latter intact. Leptomeningeal carcinomatosis appears as nodular or linear tumor deposits in the medullary pia and along intradural nerve roots. Intradural extramedullary tumors such as meningioma or nerve sheath tumors can be easily diagnosed by their characteristic appearance and enhancement with contrast dye. Intramedullary metastases or primary tumors cause enlargement of the cord and thus can be distinguished from infectious or inflammatory myelitis, which does not expand the transverse diameter of the cord.

Plain films of the spine lack sufficient sensitivity. Series of the pre-MRI era found signs of vertebral metastasis at the level of the cord compression on plain x-ray films in 80% of patients.[14] Multiple levels of involvement are missed. The local extent of metastatic disease is frequently underestimated, and paraspinal tumors with transforaminal extension may be entirely missed.

Myelography after intrathecal injection of water-soluble contrast dye with or without computed tomography (myelography, computed tomographic myelography) was the diagnostic procedure of choice in the pre-MRI era. The study requires a lumbar puncture with a large-bore needle and injection of contrast dye. Epidural lesions resulting in complete block of the subarachnoid space obscure the extent of disease. Characterization of metastatic deposits rostral to the block requires a second procedure with cervical and suboccipital injection of dye. The study remains an option for patients in whom MRI is contraindicated.

Scintigraphic examination of the skeletal system is most useful as a screening procedure for bone metastases. Its resolution, specificity, and sensitivity are inadequate to evaluate a patient with signs or symptoms of epidural metastasis and to predict the level of cord compromise.[13] Myeloma may completely evade scintigraphic detection.

Positron emission tomography is likewise most useful as a staging procedure and cannot substitute for more detailed anatomic imaging procedures.

Accurate treatment planning requires a tissue diagnosis. If cancer initially presents with MSCC, a biopsy is mandatory before initiation of therapy. This can be done by excisional biopsy of the mass or by computed tomography–guided needle biopsy.

A lumbar puncture is of no diagnostic value in epidural cancer. However, the procedure might be considered in a patient presenting with transverse myelopathy or cauda equina syndrome before the results of imaging studies are known. Complete obliteration of the subarachnoid space by an epidural metastasis results in compartmentation of the spinal canal with the possibility of herniation ("coning") after pressure reduction in the compartment below the level of obstruction by a lumbar puncture. Although cord herniation is a rare event, an MRI scan of the spine is advisable whenever MSCC is suspected before a lumbar puncture is performed. Thrombocytopenic cancer patients are at risk of developing a spinal epidural hematoma at the site of a lumbar puncture. A platelet transfusion may be required before the procedure can be safely performed.

TREATMENT

Treatment with corticosteroids should be initiated immediately when MSCC is suspected. Corticosteroids not only facilitate pain management but also reduce vasogenic cord edema and may prevent additional damage to the spinal cord from decreased perfusion. After an initial intravenous bolus, dosages of up to 10 mg every 6 hours are most commonly used. Oral bioavailability is excellent, and intravenous application is only required in patients who cannot swallow. Protocols using higher dosages (initial bolus of 100 mg followed by 96 mg divided in four doses for 3 days and a subsequent rapid taper) may achieve better pain control, but it remains unclear if their use leads to an improvement in recovery or preservation of motor function and sphincter control.[14,25,26] Complications of steroid use (gastroduodenal ulceration, hallucinations, euphoria, insomnia, generalized burning sensation) are more likely with use of higher dosages.[27]

At the time of diagnosis, two-thirds of patients are treated with initial radiotherapy and one in five or six patients is treated with initial surgical decompression. One-fourth of patients with MSCC are provided comfort care only due to widespread disease and poor quality of life.[2]

Conventional external-beam radiation therapy is the most commonly used treatment modality. Various treatment schedules have been applied with comparable results. Most protocols consist of five to ten applications of 3 to 4 Gy. Others have provided higher daily doses (5 Gy) during a 3-day induction phase followed by daily fractions of 3 Gy over 5 days for consolidation.[14] In the palliative situation, single fractions of 8 Gy may be preferable. Response to treatment depends on histologic features of the tumor. As one would anticipate, patients with relatively radiosensitive tumors (breast cancer, lymphoma) have a higher chance of regaining or preserving motor function than patients with less radiosensitive tumors (non–small cell lung cancer, melanoma, renal cell carcinoma).[14] Stereotactic radiosurgery of spinal metastases is feasible, but it remains to be shown if patients benefit from this approach.[28]

Strontium 89 therapy is used as palliative treatment for widely disseminated bone metastases from prostate cancer. It provides pain control but cannot reverse the neurologic syndrome from epidural cord compression.

The role of surgical decompression in patients with MSCC is still subject to controversial discussion. For the majority of patients, a benefit from surgical intervention has not been convincingly shown.[29] Commonly accepted indications are the lack of a recent history of cancer, involvement of a previously irradiated segment, progressive painful radiculopathy in spite of irradiation, cord compression resulting from pathologic fracture, spinal instability, and metastatic deposits from relatively radioresistant tumors.[3,17,24] Younger patients are more likely to undergo surgical debulking.[2] Posterior exposure with laminectomy at the level of cord compression has been a common approach. The metastatic focus, usually located within the vertebral body, cannot be completely visualized and thus at best can be only partially removed. Laminectomy may increase the degree of instability in kyphotic deformities as a result of pathologic fracture. Thus an anterior approach for surgical decompression is favored in selected patients. This procedure, reserved for patients with the possibility of long-term survival, includes resection of the affected vertebral body and implantation of stabilizing instrumentation. Frequently, two surgical sessions are required.[17,30] Surgical morbidity is considerable. A posterolateral transpedicular approach with stabilizing instrumentation is a feasible alternative.[17]

Treatment guidelines are similar in the pediatric population. Surgical intervention is recommended for patients with rapid neurologic deterioration or a severe transverse myelopathy at initial presentation. As in adults, neurologic improvement after surgery is the exception.[16]

Systemic chemotherapy is an appropriate treatment only for patients with MSCC caused by highly chemosensitive tumors such as non-Hodgkin's lymphoma. Radiation or surgical intervention may not be necessary.[11,31]

It is unclear if asymptomatic patients benefit from incidental detection of epidural metastases. The treatment decision is dependent on tumor type and the patient's condition. Observation and serial MRI scans may be appropriate until pain ensues.

Bisphosphonates are now widely used, particularly in the treatment of breast cancer and multiple myeloma. Monthly provision of intravenous pamidronate at a dose of 90 mg in combination with other treatment modalities for the underlying cancer significantly reduces skeletal morbidity.[19]

PROGNOSIS

Naturally, the prognosis for the patient with epidural metastasis and cord compression is dependent on the type and extent of the underlying malignancy. Untreated, patients with MSCC succumb within a month of diagnosis. The median overall survival of patients with MSCC ranges from 3 to 16 months.[1–4,7,30,32] Patients with therapy-sensitive tumors such as lymphoma or myeloma live longer (for lymphoma, 6 to 14 months) than patients with solid tumors.[2,3,7,33] Most patients die of systemic tumor progression.

The most important determinant of functional outcome is the severity of neurologic damage at the time treatment is initiated. Eighty percent of patients who are treated when a significant neurologic deficit is absent and 50% of those with mild transverse myelopathy at initiation of treatment, but only 5% of patients who are paraplegic when definitive treatment is begun, remain ambulatory or regain the ability to walk after treatment.[1,4,6,7,9] Late return of function within 6 to 20 months of treatment has been observed in long-term survivors of MSCC with non-Hodgkin's lymphoma.[9,11] The faster the neurologic deficit evolves, the lower is the chance for recovery of motor function after treatment.[33]

CONCLUSION

Malignant epidural spinal cord compression is a devastating complication affecting 5% to 10% of cancer patients. In the majority of cases it carries a grim prognosis, but there are a substantial number of patients, especially those with lymphoma, myeloma, or prostate cancer, who have the potential for long-term survival. The major determinant of outcome is the patient's functional status at initiation of therapy. Accurate diagnosis in a timely fashion is paramount and requires MRI of the whole spine. Radiation therapy in combination with corticosteroids is the adequate treatment for most patients. Selected patients benefit from surgical intervention.

REFERENCES

1. Helweg-Larsen S, Sorensen PS, Kreiner S. Prognostic factors in metastatic spinal cord compression: a prospective study using multivariate analysis of variables influencing survival and gait function in 153 patients. *Int J Radiat Oncol Biol Phys* 2000;46:1163.
2. Loblaw DA, Laperriere NJ, Mackillop WJ. A population-based study of malignant spinal cord compression in Ontario. *Clin Oncol (R Coll Radiol)* 2003;15:211.
3. Kovner F, Spigel S, Rider I, et al. Radiation therapy of metastatic spinal cord compression. Multidisciplinary team diagnosis and treatment. *J Neurooncol* 1999;42:85.
4. Bach F, Larsen BH, Rohde K, et al. Metastatic spinal cord compression. Occurrence, symptoms, clinical presentations and prognosis in 398 patients with spinal cord compression. *Acta Neurochir (Wien)* 1990;107:37.
5. Loblaw DA, Laperriere NJ. Emergency treatment of malignant extradural spinal cord compression: an evidence-based guideline. *J Clin Oncol* 1998;16:1613.
6. Posner JB. Back pain and epidural spinal cord compression. *Med Clin North Am* 1987;71:185.
7. Maranzano E, Latini P. Effectiveness of radiation therapy without surgery in metastatic spinal cord compression: final results from a prospective trial. *Int J Radiat Oncol Biol Phys* 1995;32:959.
8. Barron KD, Hirano A, Araki S, Terry RD. Experiences with metastatic neoplasms involving the spinal cord. *Neurology* 1959;9:91.
9. Helweg-Larsen S. Clinical outcome in metastatic spinal cord compression. A prospective study of 153 patients. *Acta Neurol Scand* 1996;94:269.
10. Schiff D, O'Neill BP, Suman VJ. Spinal epidural metastasis as the initial manifestation of malignancy. *Neurology* 1997;49:452.
11. McDonald AC, Nicoll JA, Rampling RP. Non-Hodgkin's lymphoma presenting with spinal cord compression; a clinicopathological review of 25 cases. *Eur J Cancer* 2000;36:207.
12. Bach F, Agerlin N, Sorensen JB, et al. Metastatic spinal cord compression secondary to lung cancer. *J Clin Oncol* 1992;10:1781.
13. Levack P, Graham J, Collie D, et al. Don't wait for a sensory level—listen to the symptoms: a prospective audit of the delays in diagnosis of malignant cord compression. *Clin Oncol (R Coll Radiol)* 2002;14:472.
14. Greenberg HS, Kim JH, Posner JB. Epidural spinal cord compression from metastatic tumor: results with a new treatment protocol. *Ann Neurol* 1980;8:361.
15. Schiff D, O'Neill BP, Wang CH, O'Fallon JR. Neuroimaging and treatment implications of patients with multiple epidural spinal metastases. *Cancer* 1998;83:1593.
16. Bouffet E, Marec-Berard P, Thiesse P, et al. Spinal cord compression by secondary epi- and intradural metastases in childhood. *Childs Nerv Syst* 1997;13:383.
17. Healey JH, Brown HK. Complications of bone metastases: surgical management. *Cancer* 2000;88[Suppl 12]:2940.
18. Abrams HL, Spiro R, Goldstein N. Metastases in carcinoma. *Cancer* 1950;3:74.
19. Coleman RE. Metastatic bone disease: clinical features, pathophysiology and treatment strategies. *Cancer Treat Rev* 2001;27:165.
20. Coleman RE. Skeletal complications of malignancy. *Cancer* 1997;80[Suppl 8]:1588.
21. Posner JB. Neurological complications of systemic cancer. *Med Clin North Am* 1971;55:625.
22. Mullins GM, Flynn JP, el Mahdi AM, McQueen JD, Owens AH, Jr. Malignant lymphoma of the spinal epidural space. *Ann Intern Med* 1971;74:416.
23. Schiff D, O'Neill BP. Intramedullary spinal cord metastases. *Neurology* 1996;47:906.
24. Hardy JR, Huddart R. Spinal cord compression—what are the treatment standards? *Clin Oncol (R Coll Radiol)* 2002;14:132.
25. Sorensen S, Helweg-Larsen S, Mouridsen H, Hansen HH. Effect of high-dose dexamethasone in carcinomatous metastatic spinal cord compression treated with radiotherapy: a randomized trial. *Eur J Cancer* 1994;30A:22.
26. Delattre JY, Arbit E, Rosenblum MK, et al. High dose versus low dose dexamethasone in experimental epidural spinal cord compression. *Neurosurgery* 1988;22:1005.
27. Heimdal K, Hirschberg H, Slettebo H, Watne K, Nome O. High incidence of serious side effects of high-dose dexamethasone treatment in patients with epidural spinal cord compression. *J Neurooncol* 1992;12:141.
28. Ryu S, Fang YF, Rock J, et al. Image-guided and intensity-modulated radiosurgery for patients with spinal metastasis. *Cancer* 2003;97:2013.
29. Young RF, Post EM, King GA. Treatment of spinal epidural metastases. Randomized prospective comparison of laminectomy and radiotherapy. *J Neurosurg* 1980;53:741.
30. Sundaresan N, Sachdev VP, Holland JF, et al. Surgical treatment of spinal cord compression from epidural metastasis. *J Clin Oncol* 1995;13:2330.
31. Wong ET, Portlock CS, O'Brien JP, DeAngelis LM. Chemosensitive epidural spinal cord disease in non-Hodgkin's lymphoma. *Neurology* 1996;46:1543.
32. Maranzano E, Latini P, Checcaglini F, et al. Radiation therapy in metastatic spinal cord compression. A prospective analysis of 105 consecutive patients. *Cancer* 1991;67:1311.
33. Rades D, Blach M, Nerreter V, Bremer M, Karstens JH. Metastatic spinal cord compression. Influence of time between onset of motoric deficits and start of irradiation on therapeutic effect. *Strahlenther Onkol* 1999;175:378.

SECTION 4

ANTONIO TITO FOJO

Metabolic Emergencies

Metabolic emergencies in cancer patients continue to present challenges to the practicing oncologist. Because they are often encountered in patients with advanced cancer, prompt recognition and the institution of adequate therapy are essential. However, the availability of better therapies has made these difficult problems increasingly manageable.

TUMOR LYSIS SYNDROME

GENERAL

Spontaneous or treatment-induced cell death leads to a constellation of metabolic abnormalities that together comprise tumor lysis syndrome (TLS). Although it can occur as a result of ongoing cell death in a rapidly growing tumor, it occurs most frequently after the administration of cytotoxic chemotherapy to patients with hematologic malignancies, in which a large percentage of cells are proliferating and drug-sensitive. In these patients, TLS occurs a few hours to a few days after the initiation of therapy. Cell death leads to the release of potassium, phosphate, uric acid, and other purine metabolites, overwhelming the kidney's capacity for clearance, with resultant hyperkalemia, hyperphosphatemia and secondary hypocalcemia, and hyperuricemia (discussed later in Hyperuricemia). Significant increases in serum lactate dehydrogenase (LDH) occur frequently. Unchecked, TLS can progress to lactic acidosis and acute renal failure. Although established TLS is associated with a high morbidity and mortality, judicious prophylaxis can lead to successful treatment or even prevention. A higher mortality among patients with solid tumors who developed TLS is likely a consequence of less preemptive prophylaxis and reduced awareness of the occurrence of this problem in solid tumors.

Although TLS has been reported in association with a wide variety of tumors, it occurs most frequently in rapidly growing, chemosensitive myelolymphoproliferative malignancies. In these patients, TLS is most likely to occur in those presenting with either large, bulky adenopathy or high white blood cell counts. The highest incidence of TLS occurs in patients with myeloproliferative diseases, acute leukemias, and high-grade non-Hodgkin's lymphomas, especially Burkitt's lymphoma.[1-4] In high-grade non-Hodgkin's lymphoma, an incidence as high as 42% has been reported, although clinically significant TLS occurred in only 6% of patients.[5] The latter percent is more in agreement with a pan-European retrospective chart review that identified TLS in 3.4%, 5.2%, and 6.1% of patients with acute myeloid leukemia, acute lymphocytic leukemia, and non-Hodgkin's lymphoma, respectively, with an overall mortality of 0.9% for all patients and 17.5% for patients who developed TLS.[6] By comparison, TLS occurs infrequently in solid tumors, most likely due to the longer doubling time, low growth fraction, and slow response to treatment compared with lymphoproliferative malignancies.[7] When it occurs in solid tumors, it usually occurs with tumors that are sensitive to chemotherapy, although less sensitive tumors may lead to TLS if bulky, metastatic disease is present, as evidenced by a high serum LDH.

Although the onset can be spontaneous, it occurs most frequently within days of the institution of chemotherapy but has also been reported after ionizing radiation, including total body irradiation in the transplant setting, embolization, radiofrequency ablation, monoclonal antibody therapy, glucocorticoids, and interferon and in the setting of hematopoietic stem cell transplantation.[8]

Risk factors include (1) the presence of bulky disease, bulky adenopathy, hepatosplenomegaly or a high leukocyte count, or both, often evidenced by elevated pretreatment LDH; (2) elevated pretreatment uric acid; (3) compromised renal function, as evidenced by biochemical abnormalities or decreased urine output; and (4) the use of potentially nephrotoxic drugs.

The clinical presentation can range from asymptomatic laboratory abnormalities to clinical changes secondary to the electrolyte disturbances, including cardiac arrhythmias and cardiac arrest (hyperkalemia), neuromuscular irritability, tetany, seizures and mental status changes (hypocalcemia), acute renal failure (hyperuricemia and hyperphosphatemia), and metabolic acidosis (acute renal failure and lactic acidosis).

PATHOGENESIS

Cell lysis with the release of intracellular contents at a rate that exceeds the kidney's capacity to clear them is the most important etiologic factor in TLS. Rapidly dividing cells have a high nucleic acid turnover, and some cancer cells, particularly lymphoid cells, contain higher levels of phosphate than their normal counterparts.[9]

Hyperkalemia poses the greatest immediate threat. Although release of intracellular potassium from dying cells is the principal cause of hyperkalemia, it has been suggested that falling adenosine triphosphate levels before cell lysis can lead to leakage of potassium, accounting for the fact that a rise in serum potassium is often the first sign of TLS. Electrocardiographic abnormalities can be trivial or can include malignant arrhythmias, sinus node dysfunction, and conduction disturbances. Common changes include peaked T waves and QRS widening.

Other manifestations of hyperkalemia include neuromuscular symptoms manifested as muscle cramps, weakness, and paresthesias and constitutional symptoms such as nausea, vomiting, and diarrhea.

Hyperuricemia, although not posing an immediate threat, is the most common finding. Uric acid elevation occurs as the purine nucleotides, guanosine, and adenosine are catabolized in the liver, first to inosine, then to hypoxanthine and xanthine, before oxidation to uric acid. The real culprit is not the hyperuricemia but the increased renal uric acid excretion that occurs as a result of this. With a pKa of 5.4, uric acid is soluble at physiologic pH but poorly soluble in acidic urine, and when present in high concentrations crystallizes in the renal parenchyma, distal tubules, and collecting ducts, where luminal pH is 5, leading to intraluminal tubular obstruction and oliguria.

Hyperphosphatemia, like hyperkalemia and hyperuricemia, follows cell lysis, resulting in hyperphosphaturia and hypocalcemia. The latter occurs directly as a result of tissue precipitation of calcium phosphate and secondarily to inappropriately low levels of plasma 1,25-dihydroxyvitamin D_3 (calcitriol).[10] Hypocalcemia leads to increased levels of parathyroid hormone, with a resultant decrease in phosphate reabsorption in the proximal tubule, accentuating the hyperphosphaturia and enhancing the risk of nephrocalcinosis and tubular obstruction. Clinically, hypocalcemia may manifest as muscle twitches, cramps, carpopedal spasm, paresthesia, or tetany, with more severe symptoms, including mental status changes, confusion, delirium, hallucinations, and seizures, seen only rarely. Severe hypocalcemia can complicate hyperkalemia and its associated electrocardiographic changes as well as lead to hypotension.

Acute renal failure occurring in the setting of tumor lysis is usually multifactorial. Contributing factors include intravascular volume depletion, precipitation of nucleic acid metabolites, most notably uric acid and calcium phosphate crystals in the renal tubules (acute nephrocalcinosis).

THERAPY

In approaching a patient with potential TLS, the physician should remember that it is "easier to stay out of trouble than get out of trouble." In the modern era, all patients are likely to have serum blood urea nitrogen, creatinine, electrolytes, calcium, phosphate, and uric acid measured on presentation, and these can alert the physician and guide preventive management. Preventive measures include foremost the institution of adequate/vigorous hydration, the start of allopurinol therapy, and treatment with oral phosphate binders, beginning preferably 24 hours before the administration of chemotherapy. Together these measures seek to achieve a high urine flow while reducing the uric acid burden, thus increasing the elimination of potassium and minimizing the likelihood that uric acid and/or calcium phosphate will precipitate in renal tissue and tubules.

Aggressive hydration is the single most important intervention, and this should begin as soon as possible, administering intravenous fluids at a rate of 3000 mL/m²/d so as to maintain a high urine output. When possible, tumor therapy should be delayed so that hydration can be administered. Alkalinization of the urine remains controversial. Although alkalinization is recommended to avoid crystallization of uric acid, it favors precipitation of calcium/phosphate complexes in renal tubules, a concern in patients with concomitant hyperphosphatemia. Furthermore, the metabolic alkalemia that may result from the administration of bicarbonate to achieve alkalinization can worsen the neurologic manifestations of hypocalcemia. Thus, alkalinization of the urine is not uniformly recommended and in the majority of cases should be avoided. Administration of 100 mEq intravenous sodium bicarbonate maintains urine pH above 7.5, a pH value that is needed not because of uric acid, which has a pKa of 5.4, but because of xanthine, which as a pKa of approximately 7.4.

Hyperkalemia should be treated aggressively. Cation exchange resins that bind potassium and promote bowel elimination should be used, recognizing their value will be delayed. Calcium gluconate antagonizes the cardiac effects of hyperkalemia and can be especially helpful in patients with concomitant hypocalcemia. Ten to 30 mL of a 10% solution provides immediate but transient benefit. Sodium bicarbonate can be used to correct acidemia, thus shifting potassium back into cells; administering hypertonic dextrose and insulin can augment the latter. Loop diuretics can be used to eliminate excess potassium in patients without renal failure; hemodialysis is indicated in those with renal impairment.

Hyperphosphatemia and its resultant hypocalcemia should be managed with oral phosphate binders such as aluminum hydroxide, 30 mL four times a day. Administration of hypertonic dextrose and insulin can be used but are rarely needed. Because calcium administration can promote metastatic calcifications, it should be avoided except as needed in the management of hyperkalemia.

Hyperuricemia should also be managed aggressively, given its central role in the development of acute renal failure. Allopurinol, an analogue of the natural purine base hypoxanthine, lowers uric acid by inhibiting xanthine oxidase, the enzyme responsible for converting hypoxanthine to xanthine and in turn xanthine to uric acid. Its active metabolite, oxypurinol, also inhibits xanthine oxidase. Because both allopurinol and oxypurinol inhibit the synthesis of uric acid but have no effect on preexisting uric acid, uric acid levels usually do not fall until after 48 to 72 hours of treatment. Furthermore, inhibition of xanthine oxidase leads to increased plasma levels of hypoxanthine and xanthine, with increased renal excretion of both metabolic products. Like uric acid, hypoxanthine and especially xanthine (pKa = 7.4) may precipitate, leading to the formation of stones and contributing to acute renal failure. Allopurinol is available as both an oral and an intravenous preparation. Oral allopurinol, the formulation familiar to most physicians, has a bioavailability of 50% and is usually administered at a dose of 300 mg/d, either as a single 300-mg tablet or 100 mg three times a day. In the management of patients with TLS, doses as high as 400 mg/m^2/d may be used. Alternately, allopurinol may be administered intravenously to adult patients at a dose of 200 to 400 mg/m^2/d and to children at a starting dose of 200 mg/m^2/d, titrating the dose to achieve the desired level of serum uric acid.[11] Intravenous allopurinol was approved as Aloprim in 1999 by the U.S. Food and Drug Administration for "the management of patients with leukemia, lymphoma, and solid tumor malignancies receiving cancer therapy which causes elevations of serum and urinary uric acid levels and who cannot tolerate oral therapy." Because the cost of intravenous allopurinol can be as much as $400 to $1000 a day, its use should be reserved for critically ill patients or where oral administration is medically precluded, not possible because of emesis/bowel obstruction, or uncertain to result in sufficient absorption. In patients receiving intravenous allopurinol, a switch to oral administration should occur as soon as possible. Allopurinol should be discontinued if allergic reactions such as skin rashes and urticaria are noted. The incidence of allergic reactions is increased in patients receiving amoxicillin, ampicillin, or thiazide diuretics. Finally, the doses of allopurinol should be adjusted for creatinine clearance as follows: 300 mg/d for a clearance greater than 20 mL/min; 200 mg/d for a clearance of 10 to 20 mL/min; 100 mg/d for a clearance of 3 to 10 mL/min; and 100 mg every 36 to 48 hours for a clearance less than 3 mL/min. An alternate approach to the treatment of hyperuricemia involves the use of the enzyme urate oxidase, an even more expensive option. This is discussed later in greater detail in Hyperuricemia.

If acute renal failure develops, conventional hemodialysis is the preferred mode of dialysis because it is far more effective in eliminating uric acid and phosphate than peritoneal dialysis. Immediate hemodialysis is recommended. Indeed, in patients presenting with TLS hemodialysis should be started before cytotoxic therapy is administered.

HYPERURICEMIA

GENERAL

Although hyperuricemia can occur in the setting of TLS, it is frequently noted in patients with cancer as an isolated finding. For example, a pan-European retrospective chart review performed in 17 centers in four countries that examined the charts of 755 patients with acute lymphocytic leukemia, acute myeloid leukemia, or non-Hodgkin's lymphoma identified hyperuricemia without TLS in 13.6% of cases, with TLS in an additional 5.3%.[6]

PATHOGENESIS

Allopurinol, the standard of treatment of hyperuricemia for decades, has been used successfully in patients with and without a diagnosis of cancer. Together with increased physician awareness, it has been a major contributor to the reduced occurrence of severe TLS characterized by acute renal failure. Allopurinol and its metabolite, oxypurinol, inhibit xanthine oxidase, the enzyme responsible for converting hypoxanthine to xanthine and in turn to uric acid. Thus, both allopurinol and oxypurinol inhibit the formation of uric acid; however, neither has an effect on preexisting uric acid. Detractors point out that allopurinol has no effect on preexisting uric acid and therefore has a slow onset of action, is ineffective in as many as 43% of patients, is known to elicit allergic reactions, and can interfere with the metabolism of some chemotherapeutic agents. Supporters note that it has been administered to millions of patients with few severe adverse events, with an incidence of allergic reactions not too dissimilar to that of many drugs, is easy to use, and is inexpensive.

Urate oxidase catalyzes the oxidation of uric acid to allantoin, a catabolite that is five- to tenfold more soluble than uric acid in urine and is rapidly excreted by the kidneys.[12] Urate oxidase is found in most mammals but is not expressed in humans, a result of a nonsense mutation in the coding region during evolution.[13] Thus, uric acid is the end product of purine metabolism in humans, whereas allantoin is the final metabolite produced in other mammals. Uricozyme, a nonrecombinant urate oxidase extracted from *Aspergillus flavus*, has been available in France and Italy for more than two decades for the treatment of hyperuricemia.[14] Because of encouraging results and a 4.5% incidence of hypersensitivity reactions, recombinant urate oxidase, rasburicase (Fasturtec/Elitek) was developed. Rasburicase is produced in *Saccharomyces cerevisiae* using a urate oxidase complementary DNA from *A flavus*.

THERAPY

Because urate oxidase degrades uric acid rather than prevents its synthesis as does allopurinol, rapid reduction in uric acid occurs after its administration without a buildup of precursors. Studies in both adults and children have shown that in the overwhelming majority of patients uric acid levels are normalized within 4 hours of rasburicase injection, usually falling to a level of 0.5 to 1.0 mg/dL; these levels are maintained throughout the treatment course. Although the majority of patients treated with rasburicase have not required hemodialysis, a small percentage have required dialysis despite normalization of uric acid levels. This latter observation is not unexpected, given the multifactorial nature of acute renal failure in TLS and the fact that rasburicase affects only one component, albeit the most significant one.

A rasburicase dose of 0.15 to 0.20 mg/kg has been recommended, with an interval of 12 hours in the first few days and 24 hours thereafter for a total of 5 days. However, with a rare exception (patients with very high serum levels of uric acid), 0.15 mg/kg is usually sufficient, and given a half-life of 16 to 21 hours, a dose of 0.15 mg/kg every 24 hours is likely to be adequate in the overwhelming majority of patients.[15] Side effects include skin rash, mild nausea and vomiting, and rarely a hypersensitivity reaction including anaphylaxis. Antibodies against rasburicase or its epitopes occur in approximately 10% to 20% of patients, and subsequent retreatment appears to be associated with a higher incidence of allergic reactions, without affecting efficacy because to date the antibodies do not appear to be blocking activity.[16] Note that rasburicase should not be given to patients with glucose-6-phosphate dehydrogenase deficiency because hydrogen peroxide, a by-product of the urate oxidase reaction, presents a burden to these patients that can lead to hemolysis.

Although the efficacy of rasburicase over allopurinol in preventing acute renal failure secondary to hyperuricemia is less clear, its rapid onset of action and ability to lower preexisting elevated uric acid levels are distinct advantages that rasburicase possesses over allopurinol. This may allow one to begin chemotherapy treatment without delay, a desirable course of action in a patient with a rapidly proliferating chemosensitive tumor and hyperuricemia. However, one must remember that rasburicase has no effect on the other manifestations of TLS, and these must continue to be addressed. Because at the present time a 5-day course of therapy with rasburicase is approximately 2000 to 3000 times more expensive than a 5-day course of allopurinol and three to six times more than intravenous allopurinol, cost needs to be factored into decision making.[6,15] Furthermore, although the price of rasburicase may fall, it is likely to remain substantially higher than allopurinol and continue to influence decision making. Rasburicase can be justified only if it would prevent severe tumor lysis from occurring, and increasing

awareness of this complication, combined with aggressive prevention, made enormous impact on the therapy of TLS before the availability of rasburicase. Although some studies suggest that rasburicase can reduce the need for dialysis, no differences or only clinically insignificant differences in serum creatinine have been reported in other studies, and at the present time the data do not definitively prove that less dialysis is required in rasburicase-treated patients.[16,17] Given this, a reasonable strategy to consider pending studies that define alternate rasburicase administration strategies might be the following:

1. Continue to rely on the triad of aggressive hydration, management of electrolyte disturbances, and institution of allopurinol. These should begin immediately on presentation.
2. Evaluate patients for their TLS risk, and administer rasburicase at the time therapy must be started to high-risk patients with the potential for hyperuricemia. A conservative approach can be adapted with administration of rasburicase to adults with a uric acid greater than 7.5 mg/dL and children with a level above 5.5 mg/dL. In these patients, administer a single 0.15 mg/kg dose of rasburicase (0.2 mg/kg for those with higher serum levels of uric acid), and follow the levels of uric acid. Administer additional doses of rasburicase only to patients with uric acid levels above an arbitrary number, such as 5 mg/dL; remember that a few additional uric acid measurements are far less expensive than a dose of rasburicase.
3. Finally, be certain that serum samples obtained for uric acid are immediately cooled to 0°C to 4°C to prevent *ex vivo* enzymatic degradation of uric acid because this will result in a falsely low level.

CANCER AND HYPONATREMIA

GENERAL

Water and sodium homeostasis is frequently disordered in patients with cancer.

Optimal homeostasis requires a delicate balance between renal free water clearance and renal sodium metabolism. The hormone arginine vasopressin (AVP) is charged with renal free water clearance; atrial natriuretic peptide together with the renin-angiotensin-aldosterone system regulates renal sodium metabolism.

Hyponatremia, commonly defined as serum sodium lower than 130 mEq/L, occurs commonly, with a reported incidence of 3.7% in medical cancer patients.[18] Clinical manifestations of hyponatremia range from none to impaired consciousness progressing to coma and generalized hypotonia, or seizure activity all secondary to cerebral edema. Less dramatic symptoms, including anorexia, nausea, and asthenia, are often difficult to ascribe to a single cause in cancer patients. Electroencephalographic changes showing diffuse slowing or epileptic activity in a patient having seizures can also be observed. The differential diagnosis is extensive and includes, among others, head injuries, pulmonary infections, space-occupying intracranial lesions, recent surgical intervention or radiation therapy, gastrointestinal losses, cardiac failure, diabetes, hypothyroidism, and iatrogenic causes secondary to the administration of hypotonic fluids or one of many drugs, including diuretics. Among medical cancer patients, inappropriate secretion of AVP [syndrome of inappropriate antidiuretic hormone (SIADH)] and sodium depletion each account for approximately one-third of cases. The most common causes of sodium depletion include gastrointestinal or renal losses or reduced intake. Other etiologies more likely to occur in cancer patients than the general patient population include hyponatremia associated with third spacing of fluids such as might occur with ascites and pseudohyponatremia as might occur in a patient with multiple myeloma and hyperproteinemia.

PATHOGENESIS

SIADH occurs as a result of ectopic production of antidiuretic hormone also known as *arginine vasopressin*, or *AVP*.[19] *SIADH* is defined as a hypoosmolar hyponatremia with excessive natriuresis (20 mEq/L or more). The latter results in a urine osmolarity that is "abnormally high relative" to plasma osmolarity. Hypouremia and hypouricemia with a high urine output of both urea and uric acid are observed. Renal, adrenal, and thyroid function must be normal, and edema must not be present on clinical examination.[20] Distinguishing SIADH from other causes of hyponatremia can be difficult but is supported by a low plasma urea and uric acid; a high urinary Na^+ and Cl^-; and high fractional excretion of Na^+, Cl^-, urea, and uric acid, because all four are eliminated at a higher rate in SIADH compared with depletional causes of hyponatremia. Fractional excretions performed on random urine samples are also useful.[21] If plasma vasopressin levels are measured, they are found to be elevated despite the low plasma osmolality.

In cancer patients, hyponatremia secondary to inappropriate secretion of AVP (SIADH) occurs as a paraneoplastic syndrome or as a complication of therapy. The inappropriate secretion of AVP can originate from its normal source, the hypothalamus, as a consequence of dysregulation, or can be ectopic in origin, arising from the cancer cells themselves. Hypothalamic dysregulation can result from damage to afferent nerves from peripheral baroreceptors, with inappropriate hypothalamic stimulation leading to AVP release. In cases of ectopic production, AVP is detectable in plasma and correlates with detectable AVP mRNA or immunoreactive peptides in tumor cells. Although inappropriate AVP secretion can occur with any cancer, it is most frequently reported with small cell lung cancer, head and neck carcinomas, hematologic malignancies, and non–small cell lung cancer.[18] Drugs reported to cause SIADH include cyclophosphamide, and its isomeric analogue, ifosfamide; the vinca alkaloids, including vincristine, vinblastine and vinorelbine; carboplatin; and cisplatin, although the latter more frequently causes renal salt wasting.

Besides SIADH, there is increasing awareness of an alternate mechanism of cerebral mediated salt losses referred to as *cerebral salt wasting syndrome* (CSWS). Two major criteria must be met for a diagnosis of CSWS: (1) a cerebral lesion and (2) high urinary excretion of Na^+ and Cl^-, in a patient with contraction of the extracellular fluid volume. Although the frequency of CSWS is far less than SIADH or sodium depletion, it is important to make the correct diagnosis because the management is different.

THERAPY

The first step in the treatment of hyponatremia in the cancer patient is to identify the cause. If the diagnosis is SIADH, the aim of therapy is to restore serum sodium and osmolality to normal, with the rapidity of correction guided by the severity of the clinical presentation and the pace with which the hyponatremia developed. If the evidence suggests that hyponatremia developed slowly over a prolonged period of time, it is likely that some equilibration has occurred and that correction can and should proceed over several days. Patients in whom hyponatremia develops rapidly are more likely to present with severe clinical symptoms but can tolerate more rapid correction. If the hyponatremia is thought to be drug-induced, the offending agent(s) should be discontinued. Fortunately, most cases present with mild hyponatremia and can be managed with judicious water restriction and intravenous or even oral salt administration. In asymptomatic patients with serum sodium levels below 125 mmol/L, intravenous saline is indicated; in symptomatic patients or those with a very low serum sodium (consider values below 115 mmol/L), more aggressive measures must be taken, including the administration of (1) hypertonic (3%) saline at a rate of 50 to 100 mL per hour, followed by intravenous saline at a rate of 100 to 250 mL per hour as tolerated by the patient's cardiovascular status, to correct any volume deficits that may have developed; (2) oral or intravenous furosemide at a dose of 20 to 40 mg or at a dose appropriate for the patient's preexisting renal function, but only if the patient is deemed to be euvolemic or once the patient's volume status has been corrected; and (3) if these measures prove inadequate or in more severe cases, demeclocycline, at a dose of 300 to 600 mg twice daily. If the diagnosis is CSWS, aggressive fluid and electrolyte replacement, with mineralocorticoid supplementation (fludrocortisone 100 to 400 µg/d), is indicated.

Strategies to prevent hyponatremia from occurring include (1) curtailing free water intake and encouraging salt consumption; (2) avoiding the offending agent or instituting careful in-hospital metabolic monitoring with appropriate therapy if the drug must be used again; and (3) ideally effecting a reduction in tumor burden.

LACTIC ACIDOSIS AND CANCER

GENERAL

Lactic acidosis is occasionally reported in cancer patients as a cause of metabolic acidosis. Among cancer patients, spontaneous lactic acidosis can occur in patients with hematologic and lymphoid malignancies as well as solid tumors, having been described in patients with breast, colon, ovarian, and small cell lung cancer, among others. In some patients with TLS, the occurrence of a metabolic acidosis that cannot be accounted by the degree of renal insufficiency can be caused by lactic acidosis. Not surprisingly, the occurrence of metabolic acidosis in cancer patients is a poor prognostic sign.

PATHOGENESIS

Although most patients with lactic acidosis present or evolve to a more severe acidosis, lactic acidosis is defined as a pH of 7.35 or less, with a plasma lactate concentration of 5 mEq/L or more.[22] Lactic acid production normally occurs under conditions of hypoxia in all peripheral tissues, and after its release into the circulation, 90% of lactic acid is metabolized in the liver, where it is converted to pyruvate, with the remaining 10% metabolized or excreted by the kidney. Extensive evidence indicates that tumor cells rely on anaerobic glycolysis disproportionately, unlike normal cells. Because of this, they produce large quantities of lactate, and this can lead to an imbalance between lactate production by tumor cells and its use by the liver. The essential role of liver metabolism to avert lactic acid accumulation explains the common clinical observation that patients with compromised liver function are more likely to develop severe lactic acidosis. In patients with cancer, compromise of liver function can occur when extensive hepatic metastases replace a substantial portion of the liver parenchyma. In these patients, once established, lactic acidosis can progress inexorably.

Among patients with leukemias and lymphomas, lactic acidosis usually occurs in adults and has an extremely poor prognosis.[22] Liver involvement is frequently present and in a substantial proportion of patients contributes to hypoglycemia. Some have suggested that the loss of mitochondrial membrane potential ($\Delta\psi$m) during programmed cell death, or apoptosis, results in compensatory glycolysis with accumulation of lactic acid and acidosis.[23] Although this thesis has to be more extensively tested, it could account for the fact that lactic acidosis is more frequently observed in patients with leukemia and lymphoma, two diseases in which cancer cell death by apoptosis is more likely to occur.

THERAPY

Lactic acidosis usually develops in patients with extensive disease and frequently progresses rapidly. Even with maximal supportive therapy, mortality rates of 60% to 90% are common.[24] The developing acidosis can lead to cardiac arrhythmias and hypotension with the potential for cardiovascular collapse. Consequently, an aggressive therapeutic approach is indicated and includes the following:

1. Aggressively support blood pressure with fluids and vasopressors as indicated. The goal in doing this is to preclude generalized hypoperfusion that leads to further accumulation of lactic acid.
2. The use of sodium bicarbonate is controversial because no controlled study has shown improvement in outcome. However, in a patient with acidosis severe enough to impact hemodynamic function and the response to catecholamines, judicious use of sodium bicarbonate can be supported.
3. Hemodialysis and hemofiltration with a bicarbonate-based replacement fluid have been used successfully in patients with lactic acidosis not associated with malignancy.
4. Attempts to correct the underlying cause are essential but often very difficult if not impossible. If the lactic acidosis is a complication of the patient's cancer, it does not resolve unless chemotherapy brings about a significant and sustained cytoreduction.

HYPERCALCEMIA AND CANCER

GENERAL

Hypercalcemia is the most common paraneoplastic syndrome, occurring in approximately 10% to 20% of patients with advanced cancer. Although it has been reported with nearly every tumor type, it occurs most frequently in patients with multiple myeloma and those with cancer of the breast, kidney, lung, and head and neck.

Symptoms of hypercalcemia include nausea, vomiting, constipation, polyuria, and disorientation. Clinical evidence of volume contraction may be apparent. Severe hypercalcemia is a poor prognostic sign. Since the mid-1990s, the early and widespread use of bisphosphonates has resulted in a decrease in the frequency and severity of hypercalcemia in cancer patients.

PATHOGENESIS

Hypercalcemia can occur as result of focal bone destruction (osteolytic) or more frequently as a humoral paraneoplastic syndrome. Focal bone destruction can be mediated by local (paracrine) factors secreted by tumor cells infiltrating bone, including a variety of cytokines and growth factors that increase bone resorption by directly stimulating osteoclasts or more likely by interacting with osteoblasts, which, in turn, up-regulate osteoclast-activating factors. Alternately, hypercalcemia can occur as a paraneoplastic syndrome caused by tumor-produced factors that affect bone resorption and/or tubular calcium reabsorption. The systemic factor most commonly secreted by tumor cells, parathyroid hormone–related protein (PTHrP), mediates a humoral form of malignant hypercalcemia, often referred to as *humoral hypercalcemia of malignancy*. Circulating PTHrP is found in approximately 80% of hypercalcemic cancer patients. PTHrP stimulates an increase in bone resorption together with an increase in renal tubular calcium reabsorption, leading to hypercalcemia. In addition, PTHrP can synergize local (paracrine) factors, including interleukin-1, interleukin-6 and tumor necrosis factor-α, further contributing to hypercalcemia. Evidence also suggests that PTHrP may promote tumor progression and skeletal metastases, underscoring the complex nature of this syndrome.[25] With both focal bone destruction and humoral hypercalcemia of malignancy, inhibition of osteoblast activity and stimulation of osteoclast-mediated resorption lead to an uncoupling of bone resorption and formation. As a result, the deoxypyridinoline to osteocalcin ratio increases markedly, distinguishing this hypercalcemia from that associated with primary hyperparathyroidism, in which bone coupling is maintained.[26] Hypercalcemia induces an osmotic diuresis while inhibiting antidiuretic hormone. The resultant polyuria together with nausea and vomiting leads to progressive dehydration, reduced glomerular filtration, and increased calcium resorption, further worsening the hypercalcemia. Although hypercalcemia has been reported with most tumors, humoral hypercalcemia is most frequently encountered in patients with carcinomas of the breast, lung, kidney, and head and neck, whereas hypercalcemia with skeletal metastases is seen most often in patients with multiple myeloma.

THERAPY

The therapeutic interventions used depend on the presentation. Asymptomatic patients with a serum calcium level of 3.25 mmol/L or less can be managed conservatively, whereas symptomatic patients or those with a serum calcium level above 3.25 mmol/L require immediate aggressive measures.

Although hydration results at most in only a mild 0.5 mmol/L (approximately 2 mg/dL) decrease in serum calcium levels, it is a simple, rapid, and effective intervention that can also preclude continued renal calcium reabsorption. Therefore, the first intervention should be intravenous hydration with isotonic saline. Outpatient hydration can be used for nonurgent cases, whereas inpatient hydration is mandatory for those requiring immediate therapy. Infusion of 1 to 2 L of isotonic saline over 2 hours expands the intravascular volume and when combined with 20 to 40 mg of intravenous furosemide can enhance calcium excretion by increasing delivery to and blocking transport of calcium and sodium from the loop of Henle.

Together with hydration, the bisphosphonates are currently the cornerstone of therapy for malignancy-associated hypercalcemia. Bisphosphonates are simple chemical compounds based on a phosphorus-carbon-phosphorus backbone, similar to pyrophosphate but with a carbon replacing the central oxygen. The carbon renders the molecules resistant to hydrolysis but allows the retention of pyrophosphate-like inhibition of bone resorption. Although their mechanism of action is complex and not fully understood, they inhibit both normal and pathologic bone resorption via direct and indirect effects on osteoclasts. The affinity of bisphosphonates for hydroxyapatite leads to their concentration in bone at the interface between active osteoclasts and the bone resorption surface. From here, they are subsequently released and internalized by osteoclasts at the time of bone resorption. Evidence indicates that non–nitrogen-containing bisphosphonates such as clodronate resemble pyrophosphate and are metabolized intracellularly to nonhydrolyzable analogues of adenosine triphosphate that inhibit adenosine triphosphate–dependent intracellular enzymes and are thus cytotoxic, whereas nitrogen-containing bisphosphonates (aminobisphosphonates), including pamidronate, ibandronate, and zoledronate, inhibit protein prenylation and bone resorption by osteoclasts by inhibiting the mevalonate pathway.[27–29] Because of poor oral absorption, they must be administered intravenously. Several bisphosphonates have been used in the treatment of hypercalcemia of malignancy, including the following:

1. Clodronate is a second-generation bisphosphonate of intermediate potency. Usually given by mouth, the recommended intravenous dose is 300 to 500 mg/d for 3 to 5 days or a single 900- to 1500-mg dose administered over 4 to 30 hours. The latter regimen achieved normocalcemia in 80% of cases but was associated with an increase in creatinine in one-fifth of those treated.[30] In the palliative setting, clodronate can be given by subcutaneous infusion, with mild local reaction in one third as the principal side effect.[31]

2. Pamidronate, a nitrogen-containing bisphosphonate, has been shown to be more effective than clodronate, achieving normocalcemia in as many as 90% of patients, for a longer period of time than clodronate. The usual dose is 90 mg administered as a single intravenous infusion over 1 to 2 hours; a 60-mg dose can be used in patients with lower serum calcium levels, although the higher dose is preferable in patients with a humoral component.[32,33]

3. Ibandronate, like pamidronate, contains a single nitrogen atom in an aliphatic side chain. A 6-mg dose administered as a 2-hour infusion normalizes serum calcium in more than 75% of patients.[34]

4. Zoledronate, a third-generation bisphosphonate containing a heterocyclic nitrogen, is more potent than pamidronate and the current best choice, with a success rate exceeding 90%.[35] A 4- to 8-mg dose can be administered intravenously over only 5 to 15 minutes, an attractive advantage over pamidronate in the outpatient setting. Normalization of serum calcium occurs in 4 to 10 days and lasts 4 to 6 weeks.

As a group, the bisphosphonates are well tolerated, with a small incidence of fever, the most frequently reported adverse event for pamidronate, zoledronate, and ibandronate. Management of the fever includes the use of antipyretics, decreasing the rate of the intravenous infusion, and switching to another agent because having a fever with one does not mean it will happen with the other. Transient hypocalcemia and hypophosphatemia and a reversible increase in serum creatinine can also occur.

Bisphosphonates are most effective in the therapy of hypercalcemia associated with multiple myeloma but are also efficacious in the setting of solid tumors with skeletal metastases. However, they may be less effective in the treatment of patients with humoral-mediated hypercalcemia because, although they are potent inhibitors of bone resorption, they have no effect on tubular calcium reabsorption mediated by humoral factors, including PTHrP. Although one study has shown a correlation between pretreatment levels of PTHrP and the time to reach normocalcemia after pamidronate administration, zoledronate was equally effective regardless of serum PTHrP.[35,36] Where diminished responsiveness is ascribed to elevated PTHrP, gallium nitrate should be considered the therapy of choice.

Gallium nitrate was originally developed as an anticancer agent and accumulates in skeletal tissues, where it inhibits bone resorption, possibly by reducing the solubilization of hydroxyapatite crystals, and inhibits the activity of osteoclasts.[37,38] In addition, gallium nitrate appears to inhibit tubular calcium resorption and PTH secretion, making it very effective in patients with parathyroid carcinomas. Gallium nitrate administered as a 5-day 200 mg/m^2/d continuous infusion results in a gradual reduction of serum calcium over the 5-day infusion. Side effects include nausea, vomiting, and renal impairment in approximately 10% of patients. Although randomized, double-blind studies have shown gallium nitrate to be more effective than the bisphosphonates, the 5-day schedule of administration is more cumbersome than the 1-day administration of the bisphosphonates, often limiting its use to the acute setting. However, it should be tried in patients with hypercalcemia refractory to the bisphosphonates.

Two other agents available for the treatment of hypercalcemia are plicamycin and calcitonin. Plicamycin (mithramycin) is a cytotoxic antibiotic that acts by blocking RNA synthesis in osteoclasts. At a dose of 25 µg/kg intravenously over 3 to 6 hours, plicamycin lowers serum calcium levels within 12 hours, with a maximum effect at approximately 48 hours. However, because the effect lasts only several days, repeated doses must be administered at 3- to 7-day intervals. Although widely used in the past, the occurrence of side effects, including thrombocytopenia and transient elevation in serum transaminases and creatinine as well as the availability of other agents, currently limits its use to patients with severe symptoms or those refractory to other therapies. Calcitonin, a polypeptide hormone secreted by the parafollicular cells of the thyroid, inhibits osteoclast-mediated bone resorption while promoting urinary calcium and sodium excretion. It is safe and nontoxic, and a 4 to 8 IU/kg intramuscular or subcutaneous injection every 6 to 8 hours can bring about a rapid decline of serum calcium within 2 to 6 hours of administration. The need for frequent administration and the occurrence of tachyphylaxis within a few days of instituting therapy limit its use to the acute setting, where it should be used in combination with longer-acting agents.

Agents in development include osteoprotegerin (OPG), a naturally occurring soluble receptor that inhibits bone resorption by inhibiting osteoclast differentiation. OPG is part of a cytokine system that belongs to the tumor necrosis factor superfamily.[39] The components include the ligand RANKL (receptor activator of nuclear factor κB ligand), its specific receptor RANK (receptor activator of nuclear factor κB), and OPG, a soluble "decoy" receptor. In bone marrow, RANKL is found in both a membrane-bound and a soluble form. The receptor, RANK, is expressed on chondrocytes, mature osteoclasts, and their hematopoietic precursors. By binding to RANK, RANKL can increase bone resorption by increasing osteoclast formation from hematopoietic precursors (regulating proliferation, differentiation, fusion, and activation of osteoclast precursor cells) and by increasing osteoclast activity and inhibiting osteoclast apoptosis. The activity of RANKL, also known as *osteoclast differentiation factor* or *OPG ligand*, is counterbalanced physiologically by circulating OPG, with the net effect dependent on the local ratio of osteoclast differentiation factor to OPG. By acting as a decoy, intravenous administration of OPG has potent hypocalcemic effects in murine models of humoral hypercalcemia.[40] It should be noted that RANKL is also important for T-cell dendritic cell interactions, promoting dendritic cell survival, and that OPG inhibits dendritic cell survival by inducing apoptosis. This may become an important consideration in its use as an antihypercalcemic agent and even more important if used chronically.

The activity of both the bisphosphonates and gallium nitrate is thought to be mediated in part by inhibiting the adhesion of tumor cells to the bone matrix. Because of this, the bisphosphonates and gallium nitrate have been used to prevent the development and progression of bone metastases. Several clinical trials have documented their effectiveness in this setting, and they are widely and increasingly being used in prophylaxis, an approach that will likely reduce the incidence of acute hypercalcemia. It is likely that the bisphosphonate(s) that eventually achieve wide use in prophylaxis will also be used in the acute setting as physicians become increasingly comfortable with their administration. Furthermore, although animal studies suggest OPG may be somewhat better than the bisphosphonates, its future use or that of any other new agent depends on achieving superiority over agents that are very effective. Obviously the best therapy is the development of more effective anticancer agents.

CANCER-RELATED HEMOLYTIC-UREMIC SYNDROME

GENERAL

Hemolytic-uremic syndrome (HUS) is a microvascular disorder characterized histopathologically by disseminated microthrombi occluding the microvasculature. HUS is often associated with the presence of large von Willebrand's factor multimers capable of agglutinating circulating platelets. The hallmark of this syndrome, a Coombs'-negative hemolytic anemia with an elevated schistocyte count, results from the fragmentation of erythrocytes as they pass through clogged arterioles. The disseminated microthrombi lead to ischemic organ damage, most commonly of the kidneys and brain, with resultant renal insufficiency a well as a range of neurologic symptoms. Although TTP and HUS represent a spectrum with considerable overlap of symptoms, renal insufficiency invariably occurs in HUS but is often milder in TTP, in which neurologic symptoms often predominate.

PATHOGENESIS

In cancer patients, HUS has been reported (1) as a manifestation of the cancer itself; (2) as a complication of chemotherapy; (3) in the setting of bone marrow transplantation; and (4) more recently as a problem in patients receiving antibodies and immunotoxins. In untreated patients, HUS has been described primarily in those with disseminated cancer, although a few reports have described HUS as a manifestation of occult or early cancers.[41] Although it has been reported more frequently with adenocarcinomas of the breast, lung, pancreas, prostate, and stomach it has also been reported in patients with lymphomas as well as other malignancies.[42] In treated patients, a diverse group of chemotherapeutic agents have been implicated in the etiology of HUS. A 1986 review that identified 39 patients with chemotherapy-related HUS implicated mitomycin C and 5-fluorouracil as the most frequent culprits.[43] More recently, numerous reports of gemcitabine-associated HUS have appeared, reflecting the widespread use of this agent.[44] Other agents that have been implicated in the etiology of this syndrome include bleomycin, cisplatin, cytosine arabinoside, daunomycin, deoxycoformycin, estramustine, and semustine.[45] Although some have reported HUS in a high percentage of patients undergoing bone marrow transplant the incidence may be overestimated, given the difficulty in establishing a diagnosis.[45,46] Finally, it appears that the use of targeted therapies does not reduce the occurrence of this complication, as evidenced by reports describing HUS in patients receiving immunotoxins.

The clinical manifestations of fulminant HUS include the classic pentad of microangiopathic hemolytic anemia, thrombocytopenia, fever, rapidly progressive renal failure, and neurologic deficits. Acute respiratory distress syndrome can also develop in some patients. In this setting, a high mortality rate has been reported because the therapy of this difficult-to-treat syndrome is made even more difficult in a patient with a severe underlying disease. In other patients, a subacute presentation with microangiopathic changes, mild thrombocytopenia, and gradual deterioration of renal function has been described. The main differential is disseminated intravascular coagulopathy.

THERAPY

Although a definitive treatment approach for cancer-associated HUS remains to be established, a consensus is beginning to emerge. When a given therapy is implicated as causative, this should be discontinued. Blood pressure should be controlled. The value of steroids is uncertain precluding a recommendation for their routine use. Hemodialysis is indicated in patients with renal failure. Although the efficacies of therapeutic plasma exchange using fresh frozen plasma as the substitution fluid and of immunoadsorption chromatography are arguable, either or both should be initiated promptly at diagnosis in all patients.[45,47,48] Because of more widespread availability, therapeutic plasma exchange with fresh frozen plasma is usually started first. Initially, an exchange volume of 1.0 to 1.5 times the calculated plasma volume (45 to 80 mL/kg) must be used daily. The frequency can be adjusted only after sustained improvement is noticed (LDH of more than 300 U/L and platelet count of more than 150×10^9/L for several days). This therapy may need to be continued for months. Cryosupernatant plasma has been reported to be at least as effective as fresh frozen plasma. Greater success can be expected in patients with smaller tumor burdens or those in whom anticancer therapy is effective and in cases where vigilance has led to an early diagnosis. Some have also suggested that treatment may be more efficacious when HUS occurs as a manifestation of the underlying cancer than as a complication of therapy.[41]

REFERENCES

1. Cohen LF, Balow JE, Magrath IT, Poplack DG, Ziegler JL. Acute tumor lysis syndrome. A review of 37 patients with Burkitt's lymphoma. *Am J Med* 1980;68:486.
2. Altman A. Acute tumor lysis syndrome. *Semin Oncol* 2001;28(2 Suppl 5):3.
3. Sallan S. Management of acute tumor lysis syndrome. *Semin Oncol* 2001;28(2 Suppl 5):9.
4. Fleming DR, Doukas MA. Acute tumor lysis syndrome in hematologic malignancies. *Leuk Lymphoma* 1992;8:315.
5. Hande KR, Garrow GC. Acute tumor lysis syndrome in patients with high-grade non-Hodgkin's lymphoma. *Am J Med* 1993;94:133.
6. Annemans L, Moeremans K, Lamotte M, et al. Pan-European multicentre economic evaluation of recombinant urate oxidase (rasburicase) in prevention and treatment of hyperuricaemia and tumour lysis syndrome in haematological cancer patients. *Support Care Cancer* 2003;11:249.
7. Baeksgaard L, Sorensen JB. Acute tumor lysis syndrome in solid tumors—a case report and review of the literature. *Cancer Chemother Pharmacol* 2003;51:187.
8. Abou Mourad Y, Taher A, Shamseddine A. Acute tumor lysis syndrome in large B-cell non-Hodgkin lymphoma induced by steroids and anti-CD 20. *Hematol J* 2003;4:222.
9. Ettinger DS, Harker WG, Gerry HW, Sanders RC, Saral R. Hyperphosphatemia, hypocalcemia, and transient renal failure. Results of cytotoxic treatment of acute lymphoblastic leukemia. *JAMA* 1978;239:2472.
10. Dunlay RW, Camp MA, Allon M, et al. Calcitriol in prolonged hypocalcemia due to the tumor lysis syndrome. *Ann Intern Med* 1989;110:162.
11. Feusner J, Farber JE. Role of intravenous allopurinol in the management of acute tumor lysis syndrome. *Semin Oncol* 2001;28(2 Suppl 5):13.
12. Brogard JM, Coumaros D, Franckhauser J, Stahl A, Stahl J. Enzymatic uricolysis: a study of the effect of a fungal urate-oxydase. *Rev Eur Etud Clin Biol* 1972;17:890.
13. Yeldandi AV, Yeldandi V, Kumar S, et al. Molecular evolution of the urate oxidase-encoding gene in hominoid primates: nonsense mutations. *Gene* 1991;109:281.
14. Patte C, Sakiroglu C, Ansoborlo S, et al. Urate-oxidase in the prevention and treatment of metabolic complications in patients with B-cell lymphoma and leukemia, treated in the Societe Francaise d'Oncologie Pediatrique LMB89 protocol. *Ann Oncol* 2002;13:789.
15. Yim BT, Sims-McCallum RP, Chong PH. Rasburicase for the treatment and prevention of hyperuricemia. *Ann Pharmacother* 2003;37:1047.
16. Navolanic PM, Pui CH, Larson RA, et al. Elitek-rasburicase: an effective means to prevent and treat hyperuricemia associated with tumor lysis syndrome, a meeting report, Dallas, Texas, January 2002. *Leukemia* 2003;17:499.
17. Goldman SC, Holcenberg JS, Finklestein JZ, et al. A randomized comparison between rasburicase and allopurinol in children with lymphoma or leukemia at high risk for tumor lysis. *Blood* 2001;97:2998.
18. Berghmans T, Paesmans M, Body JJ. A prospective study on hyponatraemia in medical cancer patients: epidemiology, aetiology and differential diagnosis. *Support Care Cancer* 2000;8:192.
19. Johnson BE, Chute JP, Rushin J, et al. A prospective study of patients with lung cancer and hyponatremia of malignancy. *Am J Respir Crit Care Med* 1997;156:1669.
20. Rossi NF, Schrier RW. Hyponatremic states. In: Maxwell MH, Kleeman CR, Narins RG, eds. *Clinical disorders of fluid and electrolyte metabolism*, 4th ed. New York: McGraw-Hill, 1987:461.
21. Musch W, Thimpont J, Vandervelde D, et al. Combined fractional excretion of sodium and urea better predicts response to saline in hyponatremia than do usual clinical and biochemical parameters. *Am J Med* 1995;99:348.
22. Sillos EM, Shenep JL, Burghen GA, et al. Lactic acidosis: a metabolic complication of hematologic malignancies: case report and review of the literature. *Cancer* 2001;92:2237.
23. Tiefenthaler M, Amberger A, Bacher N, et al. Increased lactate production follows loss of mitochondrial membrane potential during apoptosis of human leukaemia cells. *Br J Haematol* 2001;114:574.
24. van der Beek A, de Meijer PH, Meinders AE. Lactic acidosis: pathophysiology, diagnosis and treatment. *Neth J Med* 2001;58:128.
25. Esbrit P. Hypercalcemia of malignancy—new insights into an old syndrome. *Clin Lab* 2001;47:67.
26. Nakayama K, Fukumoto S, Takeda S, et al. Differences in bone and vitamin D metabolism between primary hyperparathyroidism and malignancy-associated hypercalcemia. *J Clin Endocrinol Metab* 1996;81:607.
27. Benford HL, Frith JC, Auriola S, Monkkonen J, Rogers MJ. Farnesol and geranylgeraniol prevent activation of caspases by aminobisphosphonates: biochemical evidence for two distinct pharmacological classes of bisphosphonate drugs. *Mol Pharmacol* 1999;56:131.
28. Russell RG, Rogers MJ. Bisphosphonates: from the laboratory to the clinic and back again. *Bone* 1999;25:97.
29. Luckman SP, Hughes DE, Coxon FP, et al. Nitrogen-containing bisphosphonates inhibit the mevalonate pathway and prevent post-translational prenylation of GTP-binding proteins, including Ras. *J Bone Miner Res* 1998;13:581.
30. Purohit OP, Radstone CR, Anthony C, Kanis JA, Coleman RE. A randomised double-blind comparison of intravenous pamidronate and clodronate in the hypercalcaemia of malignancy. *Br J Cancer* 1995;72:1289.
31. Walker P, Watanabe S, Lawlor P, et al. Subcutaneous clodronate: a study evaluating efficacy in hypercalcemia of malignancy and local toxicity. *Ann Oncol* 1997;8:915.
32. Nussbaum SR, Younger J, Vandepol CJ, et al. Single-dose intravenous therapy with pamidronate for the treatment of hypercalcemia of malignancy: comparison of 30-, 60-, and 90-mg dosages. *Am J Med* 1993;95:297.
33. Vinholes J, Guo CY, Purohit OP, Eastell R, Coleman RE. Evaluation of new bone resorption markers in a randomized comparison of pamidronate or clodronate for hypercalcemia of malignancy. *J Clin Oncol* 1997;15:131.
34. Pecherstorfer M, Herrmann Z, Body JJ, et al. Randomized phase II trial comparing different doses of the bisphosphonate ibandronate in the treatment of hypercalcemia of malignancy. *J Clin Oncol* 1996;14:268.
35. Major P, Lortholary A, Hon J, et al. Zoledronic acid is superior to pamidronate in the treatment of hypercalcemia of malignancy: a pooled analysis of two randomized, controlled clinical trials. *J Clin Oncol* 2001;19:558.
36. Walls J, Ratcliffe WA, Howell A, Bundred NJ. Response to intravenous bisphosphonate therapy in hypercalcaemic patients with and without bone metastases: the role of parathyroid hormone-related protein. *Br J Cancer* 1994;70:169.
37. Warrell RP Jr, Bockman RS, Coonley CJ, Isaacs M, Staszewski H. Gallium nitrate inhibits calcium resorption from bone and is effective treatment for cancer-related hypercalcemia. *J Clin Invest* 1984;73:1487.
38. Warrell RP Jr. Gallium nitrate for the treatment of bone metastases. *Cancer* 1997;80(8 Suppl):1680.
39. Hofbauer LC, Neubauer A, Heufelder AE. Receptor activator of nuclear factor-kappaB ligand and osteoprotegerin: potential implications for the pathogenesis and treatment of malignant bone diseases. *Cancer* 2001;92:460.
40. Capparelli C, Kostenuik PJ, Morony S, et al. Osteoprotegerin prevents and reverses hypercalcemia in a murine model of humoral hypercalcemia of malignancy. *Cancer Res* 2000;60:783.
41. Mungall S, Mathieson P. Hemolytic uremic syndrome in metastatic adenocarcinoma of the prostate. *Am J Kidney Dis* 2002;40:1334.
42. Gordon LI, Kwaan HC. Cancer- and drug-associated thrombotic thrombocytopenic purpura and hemolytic uremic syndrome. *Semin Hematol* 1997;34:140.
43. Sheldon R, Slaughter D. A syndrome of microangiopathic hemolytic anemia, renal impairment, and pulmonary edema in chemotherapy-treated patients with adenocarcinoma. *Cancer* 1986;58:1428.
44. Walter RB, Joerger M, Pestalozzi BC. Gemcitabine-associated hemolytic-uremic syndrome. *Am J Kidney Dis* 2002;40:E16.
45. Kaplan AA. Therapeutic apheresis for cancer related hemolytic uremic syndrome. *Ther Apher* 2000;4:201.
46. Verburgh CA, Vermeij CG, Zijlmans JM, van Veen S, van Es LA. Haemolytic uraemic syndrome following bone marrow transplantation. Case report and review of the literature. *Nephrol Dial Transplant* 1996;11:1332.
47. Snyder HW Jr, Mittelman A, Oral A, et al. Treatment of cancer chemotherapy-associated thrombotic thrombocytopenic purpura/hemolytic uremic syndrome by protein A immunoadsorption of plasma. *Cancer* 1993;71:1882.
48. von Baeyer H. Plasmapheresis in thrombotic microangiopathy-associated syndromes: review of outcome data derived from clinical trials and open studies. *Ther Apher* 2002;6:320.

JONATHAN A. COLEMAN
MCCLELLAN M. WALTHER

SECTION 5

Urologic Emergencies

In the course and management of many malignancies, it is not uncommon to see involvement of the genitourinary system. Extrinsic compression or direct invasion of the urinary tract by locally advanced tumors as well as sequelae from treatment such as surgical, radiation, chemotherapeutic interventions or unrelated medical conditions can impact the urinary system. Initial evaluation of symptoms of sepsis, hematuria, urinary obstruction, priapism, and voiding dysfunction leads to diagnosis and appropriate early treatment. Although many of these problems can be conservatively managed, urologic emergencies can occur that require immediate attention and treatment to avoid significant morbidity.

URINARY TRACT INFECTION

URINARY SEPSIS

Neutropenic sepsis occurs in 1.1% to 14.0% of patients after each cycle of chemotherapy. These episodes are most frequently associated with malignancies that impair granulocyte function or with more intensive bone marrow suppression regimens such as CHOP-M [cyclophosphamide, doxorubicin (Adriamycin), vincristine, prednisone, with methotrexate] or similar agents. As many as 8.9% of sepsis cases in this setting are caused by uropathogens. Urinary tract infections are most frequently associated with urethral catheterization and require surveillance in immunocompromised patients.

Treatment includes broad-spectrum antibiotic coverage until sensitivity results are available (see Chapter 53). The initiation of broad-spectrum intravenous antibiotics is appropriate empiric antibiotic treatment and associated with improved survival and shorter hospital stays compared with inappropriate empiric antibiotic coverage.[1,2] Use of antibiotics before hospital admission, advanced patient age, and male gender are risk factors for resistant uropathogens.[3]

Signs and symptoms of urinary obstruction in the setting of infection, including altered renal function, decreased urine output, flank pain, urinary retention, rectal pain, or tender prostate or urethra on examination, require immediate evaluation of the genitourinary system in addition to the use of systemic antibiotics. When the diagnosis of obstruction is made, urgent steps must be made to relieve it. Percutaneous nephrostomy provides direct drainage to the renal pelvis, which is critical in the case of ureteral obstruction and urosepsis. Percutaneous nephrostomy access has a greater placement success rate than retrograde ureteral catheterization and allows a means for irrigation of viscous purulent fluid if drainage is not adequate.

PERIURETHRAL ABSCESS

Periurethral abscess is a life-threatening infection of the male urethra and periurethral tissues.[4] Patients present with sepsis and perineal or scrotal abscess or phlegmon. Urethral strictures, found in 60% to 85% of these patients, cause a high urethral voiding pressure and lead to periurethral extravasation of infected urine, particularly after urethral instrumentation.[4,5] The infection can range from a small abscess confined by Buck's fascia, to an extensive necrotizing fasciitis of the penis, scrotum, and perineum.

The differential diagnosis includes tissue edema, follicular abscess, perirectal abscess, Fournier's gangrene, and penile or urethral cancer. Physical examination identifies urethral involvement, extent of phlegmon, and crepitance caused by gas-forming organisms. Urinalysis and culture usually isolate gram-negative and anaerobic bacteria. Retrograde urethrogram demonstrates diagnostic extravasation of contrast into the periurethral tissues.

Treatment of periurethral abscess consists of emergent débridement and suprapubic drainage of urine. In the presulfonamide era, mortality was at least 50%.[5] Broad-spectrum antibiotic coverage for gram-negative organisms and anaerobes, using aminoglycoside and cephalosporins, has been associated with a 1.6% mortality.[4] Additional débridement and skin grafts or secondary wound closure can be required with extensive tissue necrosis.

As many as 20% of patients develop recurrent periurethral abscess during follow-up, apparently due to extensive urethral stricture disease. Evaluation after resolution of sepsis should exclude contributory factors, such as an unstable bladder, urethral diverticula, or perineal fistula. Construction of a perineal urethrostomy may prevent abscess recurrence and should be considered if significant urethral disease is present.[4,5]

CYSTITIS

Cystitis, defined symptomatically as an irritation of the bladder, presents with suprapubic discomfort, frequency, dysuria, and urgency. Severe manifestations include urge incontinence and hematuria. Patients may present with acute exsanguinating hematuria but more commonly develop milder symptoms and pathologic disease. The etiology may be related to a toxic chemical agent, radiation, thrombocytopenia with subsequent bleeding, or myelosuppression with associated infection.

General measures taken in the initial evaluation of patients with symptomatic cystitis should exclude urinary infection and the presence of malignancy involving the bladder or its associated innervation. Symptomatic relief of discomfort on voiding can be obtained with urinary analgesics such as phenazopyridine hydrochloride (Pyridium). Suprapubic discomfort, frequency, urgency, and urge incontinence require antispasmodics to obtain relief; oxybutynin chloride (Ditropan), tolterodine tartrate (Detrol), propantheline bromide (Pro-Banthine), hyoscyamine sulfate (Cystospaz, Levsin), and flavoxate hydrochloride (Urispas) are used for this purpose. Combinations of drugs, sometimes including antiseptics, are often helpful. These include Urised (methenamine, methylene blue, phenyl salicylate, benzoic acid, atropine sulfate, and hyoscyamine), and Pyridium Plus (phenazopyridine, hyoscyamine, and butabarbital). Severe symptoms may require belladonna and opium rectal suppositories. Patients with mild voiding dysfunction associated with chronic bladder pain may benefit from a trial of tricyclic antidepressants.[6] Treatment measures unique to each etiology are included below.

CHEMICAL CYSTITIS

Oxazaphosphorines

Cyclophosphamide (Cytoxan), the most commonly used oxazaphosphorine, is an alkylating agent first used in the treatment of malignant tumors in Europe in 1957. Currently, cyclophosphamide (Cytoxan) has a role in the treatment of solid tumors and lymphomas, as well as benign inflammatory states, Wegener's granulomatosis and rheumatoid arthritis being the most common. Other oxazaphosphorines—ifosfamide, trophosphamide, and sufosfamide—have been used since the 1970s for the treatment of solid malignancies and lymphomas. Dose-limiting toxicity with these compounds is usually urinary tract toxicity.

Urinary symptoms, including frequency, urgency, dysuria, and nocturia, develop in as many as 24% of patients treated with oral cyclophosphamide. In patients, microhematuria occurs in 7% to 53% and gross hematuria in 0.6% to 15.0%.[7] Gross hematuria can range from lightly stained urine to exsanguinating hemorrhage. Symptoms usually occur soon after cyclophosphamide is given but may occur years later. Malignant lesions, usually transitional cell carcinoma, occur in 2.0% to 5.5% of patients who receive oral cyclophosphamide for nonmalignant disease.[7] The entire urothelium can be affected, but the bladder is the most frequently involved area.

Bladder pathology has been attributed to toxic metabolites of these compounds. Hepatic microsomal cells break down cyclophosphamide to hydroxycyclophosphamide, then by target cells to aldophosphamide, and then to phosphoramide mustard, the active antineoplastic metabolite, and acrolein, which has no significant antitumor activity.[8] Similarly, ifosfamide is metabolized to iphosphoramide mustard and acrolein. Urinary excretion of acrolein is believed to be the major source of urothelial toxicity. Most normal cells are able to break down the toxic metabolites and diminish their effect. Glutathione is a naturally occurring thiol that can confer such protection in most cells but is present in low levels in urine. Oxazaphosphorine toxicity has been demonstrated in several animal models with their systemic administration and by instillation of their normal metabolic products directly into the bladder.

Bladder damage from these compounds is cumulative and generally dose-related. *Cytoxan cystitis* occurs frequently and early after intravenous therapy, especially dose-intensive regimens. Fibrosis has been found in as many as 25% of children receiving high-dose cyclophosphamide.[9] Severe hematuria and telangiectasia are more common in these patients.[9] Cystitis usually takes weeks to develop after oral treatment but has been seen after as little as one dose. Oxazaphosphorine cystitis is potentiated by prior pelvic radiation.[10]

Laboratory values reveal normal coagulation profiles, a normal platelet count, and negative urine culture. Because these patients are at risk for developing urothelial malignancies, episodes of cystitis and hematuria must be evaluated, including urinalysis and urine cytology. Patients receiving cyclophosphamide develop markedly abnormal urine sediment cytologies, including marked atypia, increased nuclear size, and bizarrely shaped cytoplasm, which frequently resolve with cessation of

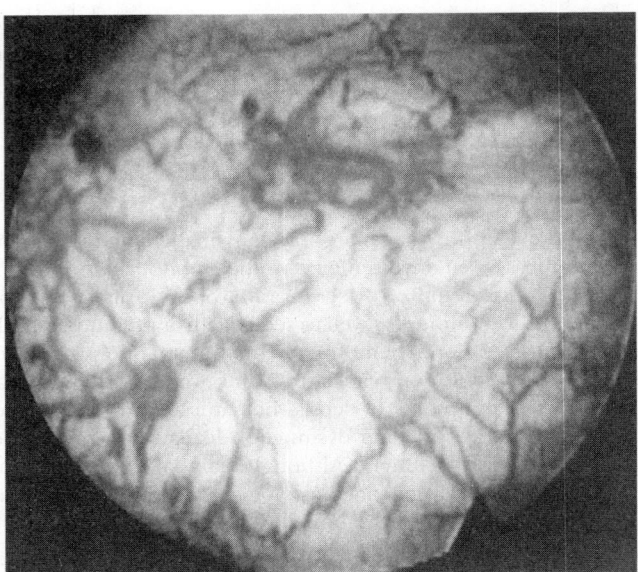

FIGURE 49.5-1. Cyclophosphamide (Cytoxan) cystitis. Microscopic hematuria is found in approximately one-half of patients receiving oral cyclophosphamide. Increased vascularity with fragile "corkscrew" vessels is seen at cystoscopy here. Submucosal hemorrhage adjacent to larger vessels occurred after bladder distension. Fulguration of these small vessels temporarily alleviates bleeding. Radiation cystitis appears similar at cystoscopy.

the drug.[11] These findings can be suggestive of malignancy and need to be interpreted with caution.[12] Patients with abnormal urine cytologies that have not been investigated previously should undergo a thorough urologic evaluation. Cystoscopy may reveal a tumor or changes compatible with cyclophosphamide cystitis (Fig. 49.5-1). Acutely diffuse inflammation is seen. Chronic changes include a pale bladder mucosa with telangiectasia. Areas of edema can be present with patchy hemorrhagic areas that stain with methylene blue, an indicator of mucosal injury. Biopsies reveal hyperemia, hemorrhage, edema, mucosal thinning, and ulceration of the urothelium. Necrosis of mucosa, muscle, and small arterioles and telangiectasia can be present. Atypia can be prominent, and abundant mitoses often occur. These finding are similar to those seen after radiation therapy. Mucosal lesions of cyclophosphamide-induced cystitis may be identified early, before the appearance of microscopic hematuria.[13]

Hemorrhagic cystitis is managed by stopping or reducing the drug. Substituting a different medication, usually azathioprine, is necessary in as many as one-third of patients who develop severe cystitis after chronic oral administration.[14] Hydration and diuresis are routinely used to dilute the metabolites in the urine and minimize their toxicity after intravenous administration.[8] The cystitis usually improves within several days after cessation of the drug but can occasionally persist for months. Patients receiving high doses of oxazaphosphorines require additional measures to counter their effects. Bladder irrigation is helpful in many of these patients taking cyclophosphamide.

Sodium 2-mercaptoethane sulfonate (mesna) was designed to function in the urinary tract to detoxify azophosphorine metabolites with urothelial toxicity. Mesna is a sulfhydryl compound that is administered intravenously and rapidly excreted by the urinary tract. After intravenous administration, mesna undergoes oxidation, forming disulfide bonds and making an unreactive dimer (dimesna). One concern regarding this drug class is that it might affect the antineoplastic properties of oxazaphosphorines. Mesna and dimesna are very hydrophilic and do not normally penetrate cells, explaining its antineoplastic sparing effect.[8] The unreactive form, dimesna, is filtered by the kidneys and undergoes tubular reabsorption, where one-third of it is reduced to its active form, mesna, by glutathione reductase.[8] In the urinary tract, the sulfhydryl group of mesna complexes with the terminal methyl group of acrolein, joining the compound to the double bond of acrolein and forming a nontoxic thioether.[8] The presence of mesna also inhibits spontaneous breakdown of cyclophosphamide to acrolein in the urine. In addition to decreasing chemical cystitis, the risk of bladder cancer is significantly reduced when mesna is used in the Sprague-Dawley rat model.

Oral mesna is well absorbed but slow to achieve adequate urinary concentrations. It has an unpleasant taste that may affect patient compliance, particularly when there is concomitant administration of a chemotherapy that induces nausea. Mesna is best given intravenously and commonly administered in three doses. A loading dose equivalent to 20% [weight per weight (w/w)] of the ifosfamide dose, given 15 minutes before the ifosfamide, is followed by two similar doses 4 and 8 hours after the ifosfamide.[8] Doses as high as 60% to 120% (w/w) have been used with cyclophosphamide, with the same schedule. The timing of dosages of mesna is important, as the half-life of mesna is 35 minutes, whereas that of cyclophosphamide is 4 hours.[8,15] Mesna toxicity is minimal, the major side effects being diarrhea, headaches, and limb pain.

Another thiol compound, N-acetylcysteine, has been used less extensively to ameliorate the effects of oxazaphosphorines. Animal data demonstrate the bladder is protected when given at a dose of 1:1 (w/w) with cyclophosphamide in a similar schedule as mesna. Problems with N-acetylcysteine include a wide distribution in the body, with low urinary levels. High intravenous doses or intravesical administration are required to reach effective concentrations. Conflicting data concerning impairment of antitumor activity have not been resolved.

Bone Marrow Transplantation

Hemorrhagic cystitis occurs in approximately 2% of conditioning regimens not containing cyclophosphamide and is frequently related to thrombocytopenia.[10] The incidence of hemorrhagic cystitis in regimens with cyclophosphamide is 5% to 15%.[10,16,17] Allogeneic bone marrow and unrelated transplantation appear to have a higher risk than autologous bone marrow transplantation.[16,18] Prior cyclophosphamide, radiation, urethral catheterization, infection (bacterial or previous viral), concurrent medication, or coagulation disorders (thrombocytopenia) can all contribute to the development of hemorrhagic cystitis in these patients. Prior administration of busulfan, an alkyl sulfonate, increases the risk of hemorrhagic cystitis to as high as 36%, compared with 4% in patients receiving the same regimen without prior exposure.[19] Concomitant use of these agents is associated with hemorrhagic cystitis in 0.5% to 50.0% of patients.[10,17,20] Patients with acute bleeding have decreased survival compared with patients without bleeding.[16]

Several viruses have been implicated in the etiology of hemorrhagic cystitis in patients undergoing bone marrow transplantation, either as viral reactivation or a new infection. These include polyoma (BK) virus, adenovirus, especially adenovirus 11, papovavirus, influenza A, and cytomegalovirus. Transplantation patients with hematuria in whom viral particles are detected have a longer latency to the onset of hematuria than patients with so-called idiopathic hemorrhagic cystitis (mean onset of 55 vs. 25 to 27 days, respectively).[10] The viral type also has a longer duration than idiopathic cystitis. Viral culture from the urine of affected individuals remains the gold standard of diagnosis; however, the use of polymerase chain reaction and enzyme immunoassay techniques may also be used with reasonable sensitivity and have the ability to obtain a more timely result.[21,22]

It has been recommended patients receiving the combination of cyclophosphamide and busulfan should receive continuous bladder irrigation during treatment. Prophylactic treatment with mesna seems equally efficacious[23–25] and does not appear to affect engraftment.[26] Mesna 60% (w/w) has been an adequate dose in children, but adults appear to require a higher dose [120% to 160% (w/w)].[26] Treatment in these patients is symptomatic.

Intravesical Chemotherapy

Intravesical treatment of superficial bladder tumors with chemotherapeutic agents or biologic modifiers may cause a chemical cystitis or inflammatory response with marked symptoms. Several agents are commonly used. Thiotepa is well tolerated, although 2% to 49% experience cystitis, and approximately one-third develop hematuria. A third of patients receiving epodyl and 26% to 50% of patients receiving Adriamycin develop cystitis. Mitomycin C is best tolerated, with 6% to 33% of patients developing cystitis, and a third develop hematuria. Intravesical gemcitabine is associated with a 17% incidence of hematuria. Most hematuria is microscopic. Significant hemorrhagic cystitis is uncommon with any of these agents. Bladder contractures have rarely been reported in patients receiving thiotepa or mitomycin. Most patients receiving intravesical bacille Calmette-Guérin commonly develop irritative voiding symptoms. Biopsies in patients after bacille Calmette-Guérin treatment reveal acute and chronic inflammatory changes and granuloma formation. Urinary analgesics and antispasmodics are particularly helpful in this group. If symptoms are severe or prolonged, isoniazid and acetaminophen or ibuprofen are given until symptoms resolve. It is uncommon for treatment regimens to be stopped because of toxicity. Bladder symptoms occur with more frequency and severity when using combined intravesical therapy with bacille Calmette-Guérin and interferon-α.

Other

Oral 9-nitrocamptothecin, a water-insoluble topoisomerase I inhibitor, and other camptothecins are associated with dose-related hematuria in up to 25% of patients. Hematuria may be a chemical cystitis related to the significant urinary elimination of the drug, although it can also be associated with profound thrombocytopenia. Increasing fluid intake to 3 L/d has been associated with decreased cystitis and ability to finish treatment.

Busulfan, an alkyl sulfonate used in the treatment of chronic granulocytic leukemia, has also been reported as a cause of hemorrhagic cystitis. As many as 16% of patients in regimens with intravenous busulfan, and without cyclophosphamide, develop hemorrhagic cystitis.[10] Cystoscopy in these patients reveals generalized inflammation and edema. Biopsies demonstrate metaplastic changes in the urothelium, submucosal inflammation, and telangiectasia. Both cystoscopic and histologic findings are similar to radiation or oxazaphosphorine cystitis. Bladder malignancies have not been associated with its use. Given orally, a cumulative dose of 2 to 5 kg appears necessary to induce these changes. Stopping the drug and alleviation of irritative symptoms are the primary treatment.

Other chemotherapeutic regimens that do not include agents with known bladder toxicity appear to be able to induce a cystitis and hematuria without associated thrombocytopenia. The mechanism in these patients is not clear, although bleomycin has been suggested to be the culprit.

INTRAVESICAL PHOTOTHERAPY

Kelly and Snell[27] first performed treatment of superficial bladder tumors with "phototherapy" in 1975. Treatment involves administering an intravenous photosensitizer (usually a hematoporphyrin derivative), waiting 2 days, and then activating the compound with light. The time lag allows preferential uptake of sensitizer by tumor, with normal tissue levels decreasing, thus increasing the therapeutic index. An optical fiber placed in the bladder through a cystoscope transmits light to activate the sensitizer. Patients whose entire bladder mucosa is illuminated develop marked bladder irritation, with suprapubic discomfort, urgency, and urge incontinence. Symptoms can be surprisingly mild the first day after activation but peak in the second and third day. Symptoms improve quickly and usually resolve by 4 to 6 weeks. Cystoscopy initially reveals exuberant local reaction and edema.[27] Biopsies initially reveal coagulative necrosis and hemorrhage. Later, acute and chronic inflammation and atypia are present. The acute response can resolve with little residual effect visually apparent. Bladder fibrosis and reflux are unpredictable side effects of this therapy and have limited the use of this technology. Treatment of the acute symptoms includes Foley drainage to put the bladder to rest and belladonna and opium suppositories for control of bladder discomfort.

RADIATION

Patients undergoing primary radiotherapy of malignant pelvic tumors, most commonly cervical, bladder, and prostate neoplasms, can suffer deliberate or incidental damage to the bladder. The risk is increased when urinary infection is present, when repeated or high-dose radiation is given, or when surgery has been performed in the area. Cyclophosphamide, given systemically in combination with pelvic radiotherapy, greatly increases the risk of radiation cystitis.[28]

In the first 4 to 6 weeks after treatment, an acute inflammatory response with resultant irritative symptoms and/or hematuria develops. Mild symptoms occur in as many as 50% to 82% of patients and generally do not require medication. Hemorrhagic cystitis can occur later, even years after successful treatment, and is frequently associated with tumor recurrence. The time between treatment and development of delayed symptoms (frequency, dysuria, and hematuria), is proportional to the dose received.[29] Patients with late cystitis may also have concomitant bladder ulcers, bladder fibrosis, and ureteral strictures. They require thorough evaluation, as these patients are at increased risk for transi-

tional cell carcinoma of the bladder. Bladder biopsies should be done sparingly, as the bladder mucosa heals poorly.

Cystitis has been reported to develop in 3.7% of patients receiving intravaginal intracavitary radiation alone (3200 cGy) for stage I endometrial carcinoma after radical hysterectomy.[30] When external-beam radiation (4000 to 5400 cGy) is added, 4.0% to 6.5% of patients develop cystitis.[30] Patients undergoing definitive radiation treatment of cervical carcinoma have a risk of cystitis that is dose-related.[31] At doses less than 6000 cGy, the development of cystitis has been strongly linked to recurrent tumor.[31] The incidence of cystitis in this group is 2.8% to 8.0%.[29] Of patients receiving external-beam radiation (3000 to 8500 cGy) for bladder cancer, 1.2% to 18% developed cystitis,[31] 8% hematuria,[31] and 5% a contracted bladder.[31a] Chronic cystitis developed in 15% of patients.[31b]

Radiation to the prostate (5000 to 7200 cGy) and draining lymph nodes (5000 cGy) for cure of prostate cancer elicits dysuria and mild to moderate hematuria in 18% to 40% of patients. Severe dysuria or hematuria develops in 0.8% to 8.3%, and 3.4% to 9% develop strictures or urethral obstruction as a delayed presentation.

During the acute phase, cystoscopy reveals edema, erythema, and increased vascularity, which can be associated with a mild decrease in bladder capacity. Later, the bladder is pale, and telangiectasia is present. Focal areas of hyperemia and bullous edema may be present. Often, there is no focal area of bleeding. With extensive damage, necrosis and calcification can occur. Biopsy findings are dose- and time-dependent. In the first 24 hours, there is erythema due to hyperemia. This develops into a diffuse inflammatory response, with hyperemia, edema, lymphocytic infiltration, and degeneration of the urothelium with atypia.[29] Shallow ulcers are occasionally seen but usually occur as a late response. This response lasts up to 4 months after therapy. Later, sclerosing endarteritis, fibrosis, and atrophy occur. There may be edema and an inflammatory infiltrate. There can be ulceration, and healing is poor. Treatment is symptomatic.

ANTIBIOTICS

Although most cystitis seen in the setting of oncologic care is related to antineoplastic agents, penicillins used in the treatment of chemotherapy-related infections represent another source. Methicillin, nafcillin, ticarcillin, piperacillin, carbenicillin, and penicillin G have all been implicated. The incidence of cystitis associated with the use of these agents is small, occurring in 4% to 8% of patients. Symptoms are typical of cystitis. Laboratory investigation reveals eosinophilia, pyuria, hematuria, proteinuria, and negative urine cultures. The submucosal deposition of C3, immunoglobulins G and M, and dimethoxyphenylpenicilloyl, a methicillin antigen, supports a hypersensitivity etiology. A diffuse hemorrhagic cystitis is seen at cystoscopy. Biopsies show an intense inflammatory reaction with erosion.[32] With repeated use, the time to development of symptoms shortens. Symptoms usually resolve promptly on cessation of the drug or substitution with an unrelated drug.

BLADDER HEMORRHAGE

Severe inflammatory cystitis can result in significant intravesical bleeding and, when left untreated, leads to large clot formation,

TABLE 49.5-1. Management of Bladder Hemorrhage

MEDICAL MANAGEMENT
Maintain platelet count >50,000/μL^3.
Correct prothrombin time, partial thromboplastin time with necessary factors, fresh frozen plasma.
Stop medications that adversely affect clotting.
Minimize constipation, straining to eliminate.
Transfuse with blood as needed.
Sedate as needed.
BEDSIDE MANAGEMENT
Place large-bore Foley and evacuate clots with piston syringe.
If irrigation is clear and bladder is emptied, replace Foley with three-way catheter for continuous irrigation.
OPERATIVE MANAGEMENT
Conservative measures
  Perform cystoscopic evacuation of clots and fulgaration after bleeding parameters are normalized.
  Use three-way continuous bladder irrigation after cystoscopy.
Intravesical instillation for hematuria
  Perform cystoscopic evacuation of clots and fulgaration after bleeding parameters are normalized.
  Obtain cystogram; if no reflux, start continuous bladder irrigation in operating room, choosing less toxic agent (silver nitrate, alum, etc.) first.
  If life-threatening bleeding persists, reevaluate medical management, cystoscopy, fulgarate, exclude reflux, and consider formalin instillation in operating room. Irrigate bladder with saline afterward to remove residual formalin.

causing bladder outlet obstruction and urinary retention. Initial intervention should include patient stabilization, bedside bladder lavage through a large-caliber urethral catheter with sterile water or saline to evacuate clots, and initiation of a continuous bladder irrigation system with sterile isotonic saline solution via a three-way large-caliber catheter. Correction of hematologic abnormalities should be performed if present. When bedside bladder clot evacuation and continuous irrigation are not successful, cystoscopic evacuation of clots with fulguration of bleeding sites cures most patients (Table 49.5-1). Correction of thrombocytopenia before cystoscopy frequently stops bleeding and is necessary for fulguration to be effective and prevent further bleeding episodes. Patients who do not respond to conservative therapy have been successfully treated with intravesical instillation of chemical astringents or fixatives. These treatments should be initiated only after cystogram has excluded vesicoureteral reflux to prevent upper tract damage or systemic absorption. Cystoscopic clot evacuation and fulguration should be performed just before starting these agents.[33] Bladder instillation is performed using gravity drainage, with minimal hydrostatic head required for filling.

Silver nitrate is a cauterizing agent that results in cellular protein coagulation and eschar formation. A 0.5% to 1.0% water solution as continuous bladder irrigation has been used in the management of radiation and chemical cystitis.[34] Chloride salts in solution or from ulcerated mucosal lesions are avoided, as they can result in precipitation of silver chloride. When effective, bleeding usually stops within 24 to 72 hours.

Continuous irrigation with 1% alum is used in a similar manner as silver nitrate.[35] Specific toxicities are related to aluminum absorption and include renal dysfunction, altered mental status, and encephalopathy.[36]

Formalin is a tissue fixative and embalming agent. Because of its potential toxicity, formalin is used only in the management of

patients with life-threatening hematuria unresponsive to other measures. After cystoscopic examination, a 1% to 5% solution of formalin is instilled for 3 to 10 minutes in the operating room.[37,38] Complications and response are directly related to concentration and duration of exposure. Complications include bladder rupture, vesicorectal or vesicovaginal fistula, renal failure, acidosis, altered mental status, and chemical skin burns.[39,40] Formalin toxicity may be abrogated by dialysis to decrease blood levels and correct the metabolic acidosis.

Formaldehyde exists as a gas and has a maximum solubility of 37% in aqueous solution. A 37% aqueous solution of formaldehyde is equivalent to a 100% solution of formalin. Dilution of formaldehyde to formalin in treatment concentrations is best performed in the pharmacy.

Bladder irrigation with any chemical agent can be irritating, with local pain and bladder spasms requiring medical treatment. Complications related to intravesical instillation of chemical agents include ureteral stricture, bladder fibrosis with loss of volume, and death.[37] With signs of toxicity, the bladder irrigation is changed to water or saline to wash out any residual drug. As bladder healing occurs, hematuria can frequently recur if the underlying pathology still exists.

Other less tried regimens have been shown to have activity in the treatment of radiation or cyclophosphamide-induced hemorrhagic cystitis. These include intravesical instillation of prostaglandins,[41] oral pentosanpolysulphate[42] or conjugated estrogens,[41] or hyperbaric oxygen.[43] Endovascular techniques such as selective vesicle artery thrombosis has occasionally been effective for cases of severe bladder hemorrhage that is refractory to first line therapies. Open cystotomy with bladder packing has rarely been used.

URINARY OBSTRUCTION

Urinary obstruction associated with loss of renal function can lead to accumulation of water, urea, and electrolytes, as well as loss of renal concentrating ability. Immediately after release of obstruction, these can lead to brisk postobstruction diuresis, hypovolemia, electrolyte losses, and shock. Most fluid losses in this setting represent a physiologic diuresis of free water and filtered solutes that can be compensated for by oral fluid intake in the mentally competent patient. A pathologic diuresis can result when excessive fluid exchange produces a washout of the concentration gradient at the level of the thin loop of Henle, creating an inability for urine concentration. Patients are monitored hourly for elevated urine output over 200 mL/hr with frequent serum electrolyte studies and, if unable to compensate with oral fluid intake, require intravenous supplementation.[44,45] Rarely, patients with severe fluid and electrolyte disturbances may require dialysis.

UPPER TRACTS

Malignancy

Malignant ureteral obstruction occurs in as many as 4.4% of patients with advanced cancer. Although outcomes are generally dependent on the primary tumor, obstruction of the genitourinary tract by active malignancy is a poor prognostic sign, with less than 60% of patients surviving 6 months. The most common associated malignancies are prostate, bladder, cervical, colon, and lymphoid cancers. Definitive radiation treatment of cervical cancer has been reported to have a continuous increasing risk of recurrence 0.15% per year over 25 years.[46] Ureteral obstruction may be an incidental finding on computed tomography and associated with altered renal function. Radionuclide imaging may be helpful if the clinical picture is not diagnostic of obstruction.[47]

Cystoscopic placement of ureteral stents maintains quality of life better than percutaneous nephrostomy.[48] Stent placement may be difficult when the ureteral orifices are obscured by local tumor invasion. Ureteral stents placed for obstruction at the bladder level are more predisposed to bleeding and obstruction than those placed for retroperitoneal metastases causing extrinsic ureteral obstruction. As many as 49% to 63% of patients with bladder malignancies may end up with percutaneous nephrostomy.

Patients undergoing percutaneous nephrostomy placement can usually undergo antegrade placement of a ureteral stent. These stents can be changed cystoscopically, at which time care should be taken to maintain access to the ureteral orifice. Ureteral stents are generally changed every 3 to 4 months to prevent encrustation and obstruction. Minor hematuria and bladder spasms are often associated with ureteral stent placement and treated symptomatically. As many as 5% of patients have significant bleeding, usually associated with tumor invasion in the bladder.

Patients with ureteral obstruction and urinary conduits may require initial percutaneous nephrostomy, followed by internalization of the ureteral stent. Percutaneous management with ureteroscopic incision of a benign stricture has been effective in up to 57% of patients.[49] Residual ureteral stricture requiring definitive surgical treatment is uncommon, as most responses to treatment are short-lived. Late strictures after radiation therapy have had limited success with excision and ureteral reimplantation.[46]

Untreated patients with bilateral ureteral obstruction succumb to renal failure within a month. Recovery of renal function after relief of obstruction depends on duration of obstruction and initial renal function.[50] Preservation of renal parenchyma and renal function has been reported as long as 5 months after complete unilateral ureteral obstruction. When there is partial ureteral obstruction, return-to-normal function has been reported in 68% of patients, with marked improvement in 24%. Patients with ureteral obstruction from hormone-sensitive prostate cancer have had longer survival than those with gastric, pancreatic, or colon cancer.

LOWER TRACT

Prostate

Urinary voiding symptoms may occur in debilitated patients after surgery, chemotherapy, or significant medical events. Symptoms may range from urinary frequency with decreased force of stream and nocturia to urinary retention.

Urinary retention may be obstructive, pharmacologic, neurogenic, or psychogenic in nature. Patient medical and voiding history are examined, with these factors in mind. Urinary tract infection or prostatitis should be detected early and treated appropriately. Manipulation of the urinary tract or prostate in these patients is kept to a minimum to prevent sepsis.

Relief of urinary obstruction with catheter drainage offers immediate relief. Patients with urethral stricture disease, benign prostatic hypertrophy, prostate cancer, meatal stenosis, or phimosis can be challenging to catheterize. Urethral dilation or use of a specialized angulated (Coudé) catheter to pass an enlarged prostate median lobe may be necessary. Placement of suprapubic trocar drainage is performed when urethral catheterization is not possible or there are concerns about promoting sepsis. Individuals especially trained in their use best perform these procedures. Minor surgical procedures can be performed to relieve phimosis or meatal stenosis.

Permanent effects on ability to void can occur after abdominoperineal resection, radical hysterectomy, or extensive pelvic operations that interrupt normal pelvic parasympathetic innervation to the bladder. Temporary loss of voiding may occur secondary to anticholinergic agents that block detrusor activity, pain that results in increased sympathetic bladder neck tone, and narcotics that inhibit the urge to void. Of patients with urinary retention as a presenting complaint, as many as 18% to 23% reestablish normal voiding if given a voiding trial. Of patients with urinary retention after nonurologic surgery, as many as 69% reestablish normal voiding patterns if placed on intermittent self-catheterization, generally within 3 months.

Evaluation of urinary retention associated with nonsurgical medical disorders is less well defined. Assessment of prehospital admission American Urological Association voiding symptom score in all these patients is helpful in identifying patients who may require treatment of prostate obstruction.[51] Urodynamics may be indicated to distinguish bladder outlet obstruction from impaired detrusor contractility. Transurethral resection of the prostate remains the standard against which other treatment regimens for urinary retention due to benign prostate hypertrophy are measured. Use of alternative methods such as holmium laser resection, urethral stent, or chronic indwelling catheter drainage may be dictated by available technology or patient health.

Patients with urinary retention due to prostate cancer had good relief of obstruction 1 month after bilateral orchiectomy. Similar results have been observed using luteinizing hormone–releasing hormone antagonists, although improvement may take longer. Urethral stents have been used to hasten spontaneous voiding.

Urethral

Patients in whom a catheter cannot be passed may have benign prostatic hypertrophy or urethral stricture disease. A Coudé catheter more easily follows the natural angulation of the urethra into the bladder. A small catheter may pass through a stricture that is not severe. Urethral dilation by trained personnel may be required. Forceful advancement of the catheter is to be avoided, as the integrity of the urethra can be violated, contributing to bleeding, urinary extravasation, local cellulitis, and stricture formation, all of which contribute to making cystoscopic access more difficult.[52] Cystoscopic placement of a Foley catheter may be required in complicated cases or when the etiology of the obstruction is unknown. Urethral bleeding after traumatic catheter placement or inflation of a balloon in the urethra stops when the Foley is in place if coagulation parameters are normal. Urine should be checked for infection and treated appropriately.

Catheter Problems

A Foley catheter balloon may not deflate, preventing its removal. Scissors removal of the valve allows drainage if that is the location of the obstruction. Obstruction at a distal level can be relieved by balloon rupture with a spinal needle under ultrasound guidance.[53] Suprapubic or transvaginal routes are preferred, although transrectal is technically feasible. Retrograde filling of the balloon with mineral oil can also facilitate its spontaneous rupture by degradation of the latex in the balloon. However, any procedure that ruptures the balloon should be followed by cystoscopic examination to look for retained balloon fragments.

PRIAPISM

Priapism is the emergent condition defined as sustained painful erection of the corpora cavernosal tissue not associated with sexual stimulation. Two types of priapism have been described, ischemic (low-flow) and nonischemic (high-flow), with different treatment and prognosis.

Ischemic priapism is associated with decreased penile venous outflow and stasis of blood resulting in intracavernosal blood acidosis and low oxygen tension. Ischemic priapism is treated emergently, as irreversible cellular damage and corporal fibrosis, which can result in erectile dysfunction, occur within 24 to 48 hours. Ischemic priapism may be caused by sickle cell disorders, oral or injected medications, or tumor infiltrate.[54,55] Nonischemic priapism usually results from perineal trauma with injury to the internal pudendal artery with arteriovenous fistula formation. Nonischemic priapism is painless, is not ischemic, can increase in tumescence after sexual stimuli, and can be managed electively.

Patient history may reveal drug use, sickle cell anemia, perineal trauma, or malignancy. Priapism is usually found in men but has been reported rarely in women. On physical examination, the corpora cavernosa are rigid. The glans, an extension of the corpora spongiosa, is usually soft. Voiding symptoms may occur in as many as 25% of patients when tumor involves the corpora spongiosa or urethra. Pseudo-priapism is characterized by rigidity and edema associated with metastases rather than venous stasis. Pain is thought to be due to tissue anoxia. In malignant priapism, tumor infiltration of the cavernosa or invasion of venous drainage is thought to lead to stasis and thrombosis.

As many as 10% of patients develop priapism related to malignancy.[56] Penile metastases are most often symptom-free, with associated priapism in 20% to 53% of patients.[57] Prostate, bladder, and kidney cancer are most commonly involved in adults.[57] Leukemia is the most common malignant cause in children.[56] Needle biopsy or aspiration of the firm corpora cavernosa can confirm the diagnosis. The management of priapism varies according to cause.[58]

Treatment of malignant priapism is initially aimed at relief of pain and anxiety, with hydration, analgesia, and rest.[58] Treatment of the underlying malignancy can be associated with relief.[57] Hormonal therapy of prostate cancer and chemotherapy of leukemia have higher expectations of response. Radiation is palliative if more emergent relief is needed or therapeutic options are limited. Intracavernosal injection of pharmacologic agents has had anecdotal success. Without systemic treatment, survival in malignant priapism is poor, as most patients have metastatic disease at presentation.[57] Sixty percent of patients died a median of 4 months (range of 0.2 to 60.0 months) after developing priapism.[57]

Surgical treatment of priapism involves creation of a vascular shunt between the glans penis and the corpora cavernosa.[59] Under anesthesia, a Tru-cut needle placed through the glans into each corpora cavernosa achieves this. Anoxia occurring during priapism or shunting performed as treatment can result in impotence. A penile prosthesis may be required if the corpora cavernosa become fibrosed and unable to distend in normal fashion.

PARAPHIMOSIS

Paraphimosis is the pathologic state occurring after retraction of the foreskin proximal to the glans penis characterized by local swelling and difficulty in returning the foreskin to its normal position. Retention of the preputial ring proximal to the coronal sulcus is associated with tissue tension greater than lymphatic pressure and results in edema of the prepuce and glans. If not reduced, the edema can become massive, associated with pain and skin breakdown. Manual reduction is usually performed, using anesthetic jelly and pressure to remove edema. The penis is grasped with both hands, placing the last three fingers along the shaft. The index fingers are used to pull the foreskin over the glans, while the thumbs push the glans back through the constricting ring of the prepuce.[52] When this is not possible, a local anesthetic block may be required to release the trapped foreskin.[53] A dorsal slit procedure allows relief of an acute constricting paraphimosis or phimosis if conservative measures fail.

REFERENCES

1. Leibovici L, Shraga I, Drucker M, et al. The benefit of appropriate empirical antibiotic treatment in patients with bloodstream infection. *J Intern Med* 1998;244:379.
2. Leibovici L, Drucker M, Konigsberger H, et al. Septic shock in bacteremic patients: risk factors, features and prognosis. *Scand J Infect Dis* 1997;29:71.
3. Leibovici L, Greenshtain S, Cohen O, Wysenbeek AJ. Toward improved empiric management of moderate to severe urinary tract infections. *Arch Intern Med* 1992;152:2481.
4. Walther MM, Mann BB, Finnerty DP. Periurethral abscess. *J Urol* 1987;138:1167.
5. Baker WJ, Wilkey JL, Barson LJ. An evaluation of the management of peri-urethral phlegmon in 272 consecutive cases at the Cook County Hospital. *J Urol* 1949;61:943.
6. Pranikoff K, Constantino G. The use of amitriptyline in patients with urinary frequency and pain. *Urology* 1998;51:179.
7. Talar-Williams C, Hijazi YM, Walther MM, et al. Cyclophosphamide-induced cystitis and bladder cancer in patients with Wegener's granulomatosis. *Ann Intern Med* 1996;124:477.
8. Schoenike SE, Dana WJ. Ifosfamide and mesna. *Clin Pharm* 1990;9:179.
9. Johnson WW, Meadows DC. Urinary-bladder fibrosis and telangiectasia associated with long-term cyclophosphamide therapy. *N Engl J Med* 1971;284:290.
10. Brugieres L, Hartmann O, Travagli JP, et al. Hemorrhagic cystitis following high-dose chemotherapy and bone marrow transplantation in children with malignancies: incidence, clinical course, and outcome. *J Clin Oncol* 1989;7:194.
11. Forni AM, Koss LG, Geller W. Cytological study of the effect of cyclophosphamide on the epithelium of the urinary bladder in man. *Cancer* 1964;17:1348.
12. Liedberg CF, Rausing A, Langeland P. Cyclophosphamide hemorrhagic cystitis. *Scand J Urol Nephrol* 1970;4:183.
13. Kimura M, Tomita Y, Morishita H, Takahashi K. Presence of mucosal change in the urinary bladder in nonhematuric patients with long-term exposure and/or accumulating high-dose cyclophosphamide. Possible significance of follow-up cystoscopy on preventing development of cyclophosphamide-induced hemorrhagic cystitis. *Urol Int* 1998;61:8.
14. Fauci AS, Haynes BF, Katz P, Wolff SM. Wegener's granulomatosis: prospective clinical and therapeutic experience with 85 patients for 21 years. *Ann Intern Med* 1983;98:76.
15. Anonymous. Cytoxan. In: Schumacher MM, Dowd AL, eds. *Physicians' desk reference*, 45th ed. Oradell, NJ: Medical Economics, 1991:723.

16. Nevo S, Swan V, Enger C, et al. Acute bleeding after bone marrow transplantation (BMT)—incidence and effect on survival. A quantitative analysis in 1,402 patients. *Blood* 1998;91:1469.

17. Seber A, Shu XO, Defor T, Sencer S, Ramsay N. Risk factors for severe hemorrhagic cystitis following BMT. *Bone Marrow Transplant* 1999;23:35.

18. Sencer SF, Haake RJ, Weisdorf DJ. Hemorrhagic cystitis after bone marrow transplantation. Risk factors and complications. *Transplantation* 1993;56:875.

19. Thomas AE, Patterson J, Prentice HG, et al. Haemorrhagic cystitis in bone marrow transplantation patients: possible increased risk associated with prior busulphan therapy. *Bone Marrow Transplant* 1987;1:347.

20. Nevill TJ, Barnett MJ, Klingemann HG, et al. Regimen-related toxicity of a busulfan-cyclophosphamide conditioning regimen in 70 patients undergoing allogeneic bone marrow transplantation. *J Clin Oncol* 1991;9:1224.

21. Raboni SM, Siqueira MM, Portes SR, Pasquini R. Comparison of PCR, enzyme immunoassay and conventional culture for adenovirus detection in bone marrow transplant patients with hemorrhagic cystitis. *J Clin Virol* 2003;27:270.

22. Echavarria MS, Ray SC, Ambinder R, Dumler JS, Charache P. PCR detection of adenovirus in a bone marrow transplant recipient: hemorrhagic cystitis as a presenting manifestation of disseminated disease. *J Clin Microbiol* 1999;37:686.

23. Turkeri LN, Lum LG, Uberti JP, et al. Prevention of hemorrhagic cystitis following allogeneic bone marrow transplant preparative regimens with cyclophosphamide and busulfan: role of continuous bladder irrigation. *J Urol* 1995;153:637.

24. Meisenberg B, Lassiter M, Hussein A, et al. Prevention of hemorrhagic cystitis after high-dose alkylating agent chemotherapy and autologous bone marrow support. *Bone Marrow Transplant* 1994;14:287.

25. Vose JM, Reed EC, Pippert GC, et al. Mesna compared with continuous bladder irrigation as uroprotection during high-dose chemotherapy and transplantation: a randomized trial. *J Clin Oncol* 1993;11:1306.

26. Blacklock H, Ball L, Knight C, Schey S, Prentice G. Experience with mesna in patients receiving allogeneic bone marrow transplants for poor prognostic leukaemia. *Cancer Treat Rev* 1983;10:45.

27. Benson RC, Kinsey JH, Cortese DA, Farrow GM, Utz DC. Treatment of transitional cell carcinoma of the bladder with hematoporphyrin derivative phototherapy. *J Urol* 1983;130:1090.

28. Jayalakshmamma B, Pinkel D. Urinary-bladder toxicity following pelvic irradiation and simultaneous cyclophosphamide therapy. *Cancer* 1976;38:701.

29. Oration JP. Complications following radiation therapy in carcinoma of the cervix and their treatment. *Am J Obstet Gynecol* 1964;88:854.

30. Kucera H, Vavra N, Weghaupt K. Benefit of external irradiation in pathologic stage I endometrial carcinoma: a prospective clinical trial of 605 patients who received postoperative vaginal irradiation and additional pelvic irradiation in the presence of unfavorable prognostic factors. *Gynecol Oncol* 1990;38:99.

31. Dean RJ, Lytton B. Urologic complications of pelvic irradiation. *J Urol* 1978;119:64.

31a. Shiels RA, Nissenbaum MM, Mark SR, Browde S. Late radiation cystitis after treatment for carcinoma of the bladder. *S Afr Med J* 1986;70:727.

31b. Ram MD. Visceral complications of supervoltage radiotherapy for carcinoma of the bladder. *Br J Surg* 1970;57:409.

32. Cook FV, Farrar WE Jr, Kreutner A. Hemorrhagic cystitis and ureteritis, and interstitial nephritis associated with administration of penicillin G. *J Urol* 1979;122:110.

33. West NJ. Prevention and treatment of hemorrhagic cystitis. *Pharmacotherapy* 1997;17:696.

34. Kumar AP, Wrenn ELJ, Jayalakshmamma B, et al. Silver nitrate irrigation to control bladder hemorrhage in children receiving cancer therapy. *J Urol* 1976;116:85.

35. Goel AK, Rao MS, Bhagwat AG, et al. Intravesical irrigation with alum for the control of massive bladder hemorrhage. *J Urol* 1985;133:956.

36. Murphy CP, Cox RL, Harden EA, et al. Encephalopathy and seizures induced by intravesical alum irrigations. *Bone Marrow Transplant* 1992;10:383.

37. Donahue LA, Frank IN. Intravesical formalin for hemorrhagic cystitis: analysis of therapy. *J Urol* 1989;141:809.

38. Dewan AK, Mohan GM, Ravi R. Intravesical formalin for hemorrhagic cystitis following irradiation of cancer of the cervix. *Int J Gynaecol Obstet* 1993;42:131.

39. Vicente J, Rios G, Caffaratti J. Intravesical formalin for the treatment of massive hemorrhagic cystitis: retrospective review of 25 cases. *Eur Urol* 1990;18:204.

40. Sarnak MJ, Long J, King AJ. Intravesicular formaldehyde instillation and renal complications. *Clin Nephrol* 1999;51:122.

41. Miller LJ, Chandler SW, Ippoliti CM. Treatment of cyclophosphamide-induced hemorrhagic cystitis with prostaglandins. *Ann Pharmacother* 1994;28:590.

42. Hampson SJ, Woodhouse CR. Sodium pentosanpolysulphate in the management of haemorrhagic cystitis: experience with 14 patients. *Eur Urol* 1994;25:40.

43. Mathews R, Rajan N, Josefson L, Camporesi E, Makhuli Z. Hyperbaric oxygen therapy for radiation induced hemorrhagic cystitis. *J Urol* 1999;161:435.

44. O'Reilly PH, Brooman PJ, Farah NB, Mason GC. High pressure chronic retention. Incidence, aetiology and sinister implications. *Br J Urol* 1986;58:644.

45. Howards SS. Post-obstructive diuresis: a misunderstood phenomenon. *J Urol* 1973;110:537.

46. McIntyre JF, Eifel PJ, Levenback C, Oswald MJ. Ureteral stricture as a late complication of radiotherapy for stage IB carcinoma of the uterine cervix. *Cancer* 1995;75:836.

47. Dubovsky EV, Russell CD. Advances in radionuclide evaluation of urinary tract obstruction. *Abdom Imaging* 1998;23:17.

48. Yachia D. Overview: role of stents in urology. *J Endourol* 1997;11:379.

49. Meretyk S, Clayman RV, Kavoussi LR, Kramolowsky EV, Picus DD. Endourological treatment of ureteroenteric anastomotic strictures: long-term followup. *J Urol* 1991;145:723.

50. Shokeir AA, Provoost AP, Nijman RJ. Recoverability of renal function after relief of chronic partial upper urinary tract obstruction. *BJU Int* 1999;83:11.

51. Kaplan SA, Olsson CA, Te AE. The American Urological Association symptom score in the evaluation of men with lower urinary tract symptoms: at 2 years of followup, does it work? *J Urol* 1996;155:1971.

52. Neuwirth H, Frasier B, Cochran ST. Genitourinary imaging and procedures by the emergency physician. *Emerg Med Clin North Am* 1989;7:1.

53. Stine RJ, Avila JA, Lemons MF, Sickorez GJ. Diagnostic and therapeutic urologic procedures. *Emerg Med Clin North Am* 1988;6:547.

54. Hamre MR, Harmon EP, Kirkpatrick DV, Stern MJ, Humbert JR. Priapism as a complication of sickle cell disease. *J Urol* 1991;145:1.

55. Banos JE, Bosch F, Farre M. Drug-induced priapism. Its aetiology, incidence and treatment. *Med Toxicol Adverse Drug Exp* 1989;4:46.

56. Winter CC, McDowell G. Experience with 105 patients with priapism: update review of all aspects. *J Urol* 1988;140:980.

57. Chan PT, Begin LR, Arnold D, et al. Priapism secondary to penile metastasis: a report of two cases and a review of the literature. *J Surg Oncol* 1998;68:51.

58. Powars DR, Johnson CS. Priapism. *Hematol Oncol Clin North Am* 1996;10:1363.

59. Kulmala R. Treatment of priapism: primary results and complications in 207 patients. *Ann Chir Gynaecol* 1994;83:309.

CHAPTER 50

Specialized Techniques in Cancer Management

SECTION **1**

JAMES F. PINGPANK, JR.

Vascular Access and Specialized Techniques of Drug Delivery

The development of increasingly complex treatment regimens for patients with advanced malignancies has led to a greater reliance on a variety of intraarterial and intravenous delivery systems. Long-term access may be required for chemotherapy, total parenteral nutrition, or analgesics, or all. Since the introduction of indwelling catheters and infusion systems in 1973, changes and improvements in design have resulted in the development of a diverse group of products to meet specific treatment goals.[1,2] A basic understanding of the selection and maintenance of these devices is important for all clinicians caring for cancer patients. This chapter reviews the issues surrounding catheter selection, insertion techniques, maintenance, and management of frequent catheter-related complications.

CATHETER TYPES

A diverse group of catheters is available, each with their own strengths and weaknesses. Issues critical to the selection of a specific catheter include the number and type of agents to be infused, the length and frequency of the proposed treatment, the use of bolus versus continuous-infusion administration schedules, the potential need for frequent blood draws or the administration of blood products, along with patient and physician preference. The vast majority of catheters are venous, all designed for access to the central venous system. The most useful division of catheter systems is between those with an external component and completely implanted devices, which are accessed percutaneously (Table 50.1-1). Intraarterial delivery systems are considered separately.

EXTERNAL CATHETERS

Catheters with external components are the most frequently used in hospitalized patients and acute care. They are the simplest to insert, exchange, and remove and may be safely used for all aspects of patient care. The most basic of these is the single or multilumen 16-gauge catheter positioned via the internal jugular, subclavian, or femoral vein, and it may be used for intraoperative and acute care as well as longer-term administration of chemotherapy or supportive care. Although these catheters are not tunneled, when inserted under sterile conditions, they may be safely used for 7 to 14 days but are not appropriate for long-term or outpatient use. In addition, these catheters are considered to have the highest risk for migration and infection due to the minimal subcutaneous catheter length and the absence of a subcutaneous cuff.

External catheters designed for more long-term use include Hickman, Groshong, and Broviac (Bard Access Systems, Salt Lake City, UT) catheters, each of which possesses subtle differ-

TABLE 50.1-1. Catheter-Specific Advantages and Disadvantages

Catheter Type	Advantages	Disadvantages
Central indwelling catheter	Low device profile Durable Low routine maintenance	Operating room with sedation for insertion Increased insertion-associated risks (pneumothorax, arterial injury)
Central externalized catheter	Large catheter lumen for cellular therapy and transfusion Durable, low catheter thrombosis rate	Shorter catheter life vs. indwelling ? Increased rate of catheter infections Increased insertion-associated risks (pneumothorax, arterial injury) Ongoing, routine care required
Peripheral port	Local anesthesia for insertion Decreased insertion-associated risks (pneumothorax, arterial injury) Low device profile	? Decreased durability ? Increased rate of catheter infections Increased rates of catheter-associated thrombosis
PICC line	Local anesthesia for insertion Decreased insertion-associated risks (pneumothorax, arterial injury) Easily exchanged for new catheter Ease of use	? Decreased durability ? Increased rate of catheter infections Increased rates of catheter-associated thrombosis Ongoing, routine care required

PICC line, peripherally inserted central catheter.

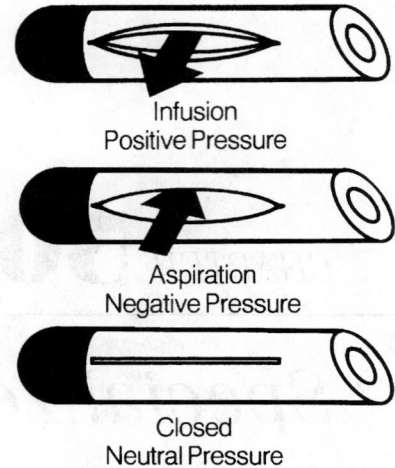

FIGURE 50.1-1. The slit valve along the side of the Groshong catheter tip is designed to prevent passive reflux of blood into the lumen.

ences in design. These catheters are available in single- and double-lumen systems and in a variety of sizes for adult and pediatric patients and are designed to be inserted in an operating room or interventional radiology suite. The longer length of these devices allows for the creation of a subcutaneous tunnel between the skin insertion site and the central vein, which aids in catheter fixation and infection control. In addition, a Dacron cuff is affixed to the catheter, designed to be positioned in the subcutaneous tissue near the skin insertion site. The cuff is intended to promote tissue ingrowth and scarring and serve as an additional protection against catheter infection and migration. Several modifications to the basic design of these Silastic catheters have been marketed in an attempt to improve the function and durability of the catheter. Early data suggested that the use of antibiotic- or silver ion–impregnated cuffs could decrease the incidence of catheter-associated infections,[3] but this was not demonstrated in larger, random-assignment trials.[4] Among different catheters, the most significant design modification is the slit valve design to the Groshong catheter tip (Fig. 50.1-1). This slit valve is designed to stay in a closed position, except in the presence of positive or negative pressure, to prohibit passive blood reflux and subsequent catheter infection or thrombosis, decreasing catheter maintenance, and avoid frequent heparin-containing flushes. However, the frequent loss of valve competence does not obviate the need for regular heparin flushes to prevent device-associated clot.[5]

More recently, an increasing number of central access devices are being placed through more peripheral access sites. These peripherally inserted central catheters (PICC lines) are inserted through a peripheral vein using a Seldinger technique, with the catheter tip positioned in the subclavian, or more central, vein.[6,7] PICC lines offer the potential for long-term access, with a decrease in insertion-associated complications, such as pneumothorax or arterial injury. Catheters may be inserted and maintained by a committed, skilled nursing team, bypassing the need for surgical or interventional radiology–directed line placement, decreasing cost and resource use. Several studies demonstrate safety and durability of these systems for outpatient antibiotic and nutritional therapy when managed by experienced nursing teams.[6,8] Additional studies examining the utility of peripherally placed lines in the acute setting have revealed a greater rate of thrombophlebitis and venous thrombosis over standard centrally placed lines in hospitalized patients as well as in those undergoing hemodialysis.[9]

IMPLANTED DEVICES

The development of completely implantable infusion catheters has greatly simplified the management of patients requiring long-term chemotherapy or nutritional support. The catheter itself is unchanged (Fig. 50.1-2) but is connected to a subcutaneously implanted reservoir, or port, constructed from titanium or, more recently, plastic. These ports contain 1 to 3 mL of heparinized saline and incorporate a compressed, self-sealing silicone diaphragm just below the patient's skin. The diaphragm allows repeated puncture with a noncoring Huber needle, designed with a hole along the side of the needle shaft. When not in use, the entire system is contained below the skin. Single- and double-lumen devices are available. The majority of these ports are placed in the operating room with local anesthesia and intravenous sedation, often with fluoroscopic guidance. The hub of the port is placed along the chest wall, often directly inferior and medial to the deltopectoral groove, where it may be easily palpated and accessed while preserving patient modesty. It is important to fix the port to the underlying pectoralis fascia with interrupted sutures to avoid flipping or migration, which may

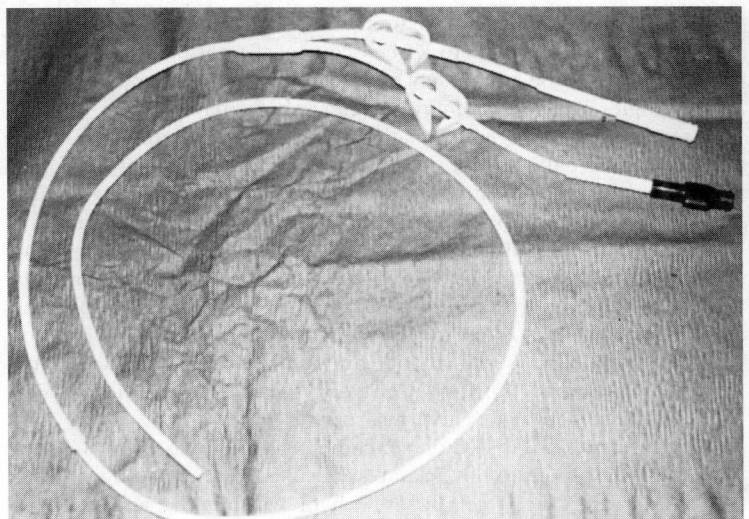 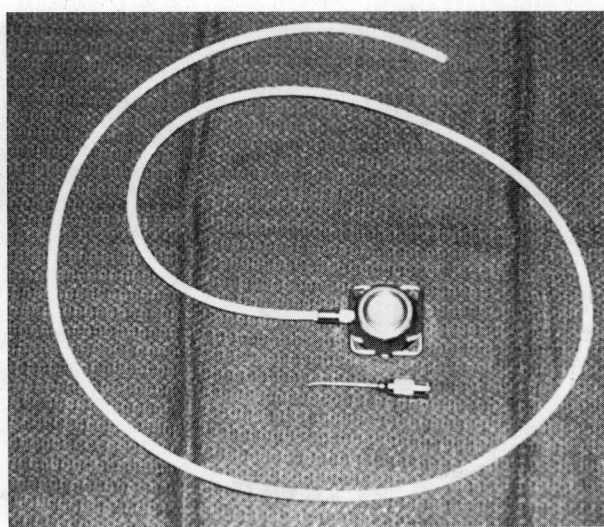

A

B

FIGURE 50.1-2. A: Dual-lumen 10-Fr. Hickman catheter showing the Dacron cuff. **B:** Implantable venous device. A noncoring Huber needle is also shown. The housing of the port can be made of titanium (pictured) or plastic.

kink the catheter. Creation of the subcutaneous port pocket should be accomplished with a minimum of dissection to reduce the risk for seroma formation and subsequent port site infection. Unlike external devices, malfunction or infection of an implanted device requires operative revision or removal, respectively. Management of catheter infections are discussed later in Infections, but infections of the port pocket or overlying skin require device removal, with the skin being allowed to heal by secondary intention. Modern ports are low-profile devices, with expected life span of well over a year when properly cared for. They are compatible with both magnetic resonance imaging and computed tomography scan. Most recently, the development of Passports by Sims Deltec (St. Paul, MN) has permitted the placement of upper extremity ports in the interventional radiology suite. Similar to PICC line insertion, this may be accomplished with local anesthesia.

Several studies have compared complication rates and overall performance of implantable ports and external catheters. Overall, there has been little consistent difference between the two systems with respect to infection rate, catheter-associated thrombosis, and catheter patency, although the implantable devices tend to be more durable.[10,11] Overwhelming studies point to the positive impact of a well-trained, diligent catheter-care staff in preserving long-term function.[12] As noted in External Catheters, recent data suggest increased rates of thrombotic complications in peripherally placed central lines, most certainly related to the relative size of extremity veins. Careful patient selection, including lifestyle, body habitus, and planned therapeutic regimen, remains a central component of catheter durability.

IMPLANTABLE INFUSION PUMPS

Implantable ports offer the advantage of a completely contained system between medication doses. For patients undergoing continuous-infusion therapy, an external pump was necessary. The development of completely implantable subcu-

taneous infusion pumps has helped patients break the reliance on external pumps. Initially developed for the long-term delivery of heparin to patients with venous thrombosis,[13] these pump/catheter systems are now used for a variety of conditions in which continuous drug administration is desired. Infusion pumps are manufactured by Codman/Johnson & Johnson (Raynham, MA) and Medtronic (Minneapolis, MN) and are available for intravenous or intraarterial drug delivery. Modern pumps are constructed from titanium and weigh between 98 and 173 g when empty. Reservoir volumes range from 16 to 60 mL, with available constant infusion rates of 0.3 to 4.0 mL/d. Pumps are surgically implanted in the subcutaneous tissue, usually on the anterior abdominal wall, and accessed percutaneously using noncoring needles. Bolus or sustained administration of a given agent for therapeutic or diagnostic intervention is possible with both pumps, albeit through different mechanisms (Fig. 50.1-3). The main pump chamber contains a reservoir surrounded by a chamber of gas-phase fluorocarbon, which is compressed into a fluid phase on filling of the drug reservoir. Over time, the fluid expands at a constant rate at body temperature, serving as a propellant. These systems may be used for intravenous administration of medications such as insulin, intrathecal administration of narcotics, or intraarterial administration of regional chemotherapy.[14-17] In the care of cancer patients, the administration of systemic and intrathecal narcotics, and intrahepatic chemotherapy via the gastroduodenal artery have been the most common uses of these devices.

Implantable systems capable of delivery of medication at variable rates are under investigation. Early reports regarding these programmable implantable medication systems reported successful euglycemic control in dogs using a battery-powered solenoid pump capable of pulsatile administration of intraperitoneal administration of insulin. Bidirectional communication between the pump and an external transmitter allows for monitoring and regulation of drug delivery.[18] Studies in small numbers of human subjects report reductions in hemoglobin A_{1C},

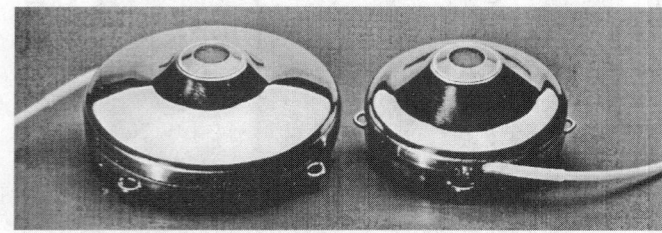

Pump refill

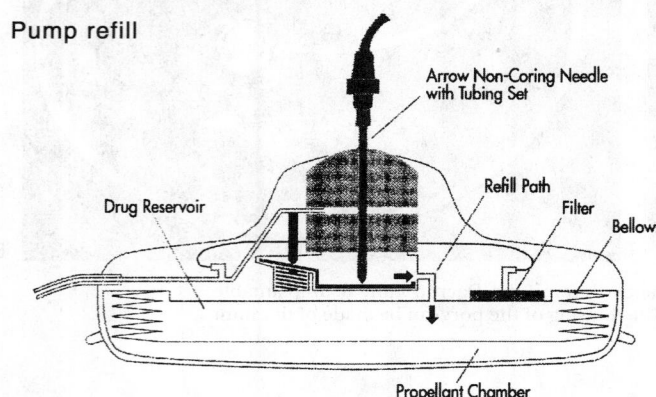

Bolus injection

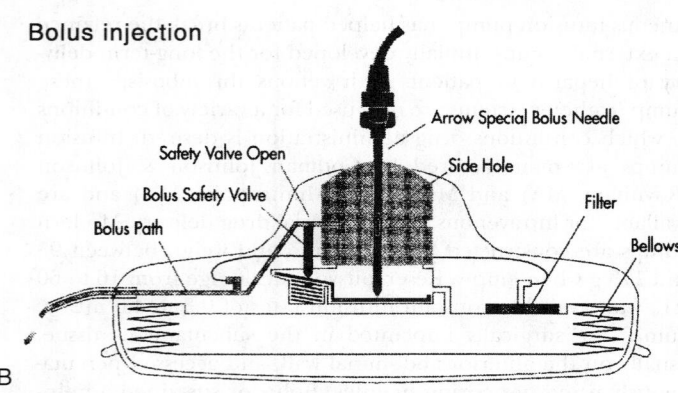

FIGURE 50.1-3. **A:** The implantable infusion pump (Arrow International, Reading, PA), which comes in various sizes. The smaller pump is used for the infusion of narcotic analgesics either intravenously or via an intraspinal route. **B:** A schematic representation of how the pump system works. Body heat causes the propellant to shift from a liquid to a gaseous phase, which compresses the bellows and allows for the drug to be dispensed. When the drug reservoir is refilled, the propellant is compressed and shifts back into a liquid phase.

no episodes of insulin over-delivery, and good patient quality of life.[19] At present, all subcutaneously placed pumps are hampered by the increased cost associated with operative placement and the absence of available data supporting a benefit over conventional therapy.

CATHETER SELECTION

Careful matching of patients with appropriate vascular access systems is essential to avoid patient exposure to unnecessary risks and financial expense. The selection of the proper catheter must take into account numerous factors, including the proposed length of treatment, the number of agents to be used, the need for frequent blood draws or transfusions, and the patient's vascular anatomy. For example, a patient scheduled for a short, 1- to 2-week course of total parenteral nutrition could be adequately treated with a percutaneously placed single- or double-lumen catheter, which may be inserted and removed more easily. Patients with the potential for more aggressive transfusion support or in need of cell transplants are best served by larger external catheters, which are easily accessed and enable infusion of blood products, chemotherapy, and nutritional support. Although these catheters need to be inserted in the operating room, removal is easier than with implanted ports, and more rapid infusion is possible. By contrast, patients requiring prolonged administration of chemotherapy with serial blood draws are ideal candidates for implanted ports, which are low-profile and require little maintenance between treatments.

At present, the choice of catheter is often based on the specialization of the physician responsible for line insertion. PICC lines are placed by nurses with or without the assistance of interventional radiologists, whereas peripheral implanted ports are the responsibility of interventional radiologists. Central catheters, with the exception of single-lumen percutaneous lines, are inserted in the operating room by surgeons, often with fluoroscopic assistance. In the highest-volume centers, the establishment of a vascular access team responsible for catheter selection, insertion, and long-term care has resulted in prolongation of catheter life, a decreased infection rate, and improved efficiency.[20] This team approach aids in hospital-wide standardization as well as accurate assessment of catheter-related complications. Additional factors to consider before selecting a specific access device include a history of previous indwelling catheter, central vein patency, patient age and size, patient immune status, and the need for frequent blood draws. In those patients with a history of multiple previous catheters or catheter-related complications, or both, duplex Doppler examination may be needed to assure vein patency. Other patient factors such as the potential for superior vena cava narrowing or obstruction from mediastinal tumors or the increased risk of thrombosis and cellulitis in postmastectomy and postaxillary dissection patients may limit access sites. Recent data would suggest that establishing central venous access ipsilateral to a breast cancer may be performed safely and effectively.[21]

INSERTION TECHNIQUES

The preferred arena for the insertion of long-term venous access is either the operating room or the interventional radiology suite, where sterility can be ensured. Adequate lighting, analgesia, and staffing are essential to ensure proper catheter placement and maximize catheter life. Although local anesthesia is all that is required for catheter placement, the use of intravenous sedation provides better patient comfort, especially in difficult insertions. Sedation is mandatory in pediatric patients, and general anesthesia is often preferred. Real-time fluoroscopy is helpful in directing guidewires in difficult cases and should be used to confirm catheter tip placement at the junction of the superior vena cava and the right atrium before fixing the catheter to the skin or chest wall.

The most commonly used insertion technique is that initially described by Seldinger, in which a catheter is placed over a percutaneously placed wire.[22] This technique may be used to access any deep or central vein, but in patients with long-term access needs, the internal jugular and subclavian veins are preferred. In difficult cases, access to the central venous system can be obtained via a femoral vein approach, with the port or the catheter exit site placed on the abdominal wall at the level of the umbilicus.

Accessing the subclavian vein demonstrates general technical points. A rolled towel is placed longitudinally between the patient's shoulders to increase the distance between the clavicle and the chest wall. A wide sterile prep and drape are mandatory to allow access to the ipsilateral internal jugular vein if cannulation of the subclavian vein is unsuccessful. It is the author's practice to consent the patient for both sides, in the event of unanticipated difficulty accessing either vein on a given side. Before attempting access on the contralateral side, a chest radiograph is mandatory to confirm the absence of a pneumothorax. Comfortable patient positioning and liberal infiltration with local anesthesia, including along the periosteum of the clavicle, ensure a minimum of patient movement and discomfort. Trendelenburg's position aids in vein access. A finder needle attached to a 5-mL syringe is advanced, bevel up, under the clavicle in the direction of the sternal notch. A constant gentle aspiration is applied until blood freely enters the syringe, indicating venous access. If bright red blood or pulsatile flow is noted, the syringe is withdrawn, and pressure is held. Once the vein has been located, an introducer needle is placed in the same fashion as the finder needle. On access to the vein, the needle hub is rotated 90 degrees, and a flexible guidewire is advanced through the needle into the superior vena cava. If the wire is placed too far, cardiac irritation develops, usually a supraventricular tachycardia, and the wire should be pulled back. If resistance to threading the wire is encountered immediately the needle is likely not in the vein, and the syringe should be used to ensure proper position. Resistance after several centimeters of wire has been threaded may indicate entrance into a smaller vein or central vein stenosis. Fluoroscopy should be used with or without contrast to thread the wire and examine potential venous narrowing. A wire should never be advanced against resistance.

Once the wire has been successfully inserted, fluoroscopy should confirm its location in the vena cava and not in the contralateral subclavian vein or other feeding vessel. Subsequently, a catheter exit site or port placement site should be selected on the anterior chest wall. The skin and subcutaneous tissue surrounding the proposed catheter exit site or port site should be infiltrated with local anesthesia, and a skin incision performed. If a single- or double-lumen external catheter is to be inserted, the incision should be made in a location cosmetically favorable that also allows for easy catheter care. In this circumstance, a second 5-mm incision is made at the site where the guidewire exits the skin. A subcutaneous tunnel is then fashioned between the two incisions, and the catheter is advanced from the exit site to the wire exit site. The catheter should be advanced until the cuff is 1 cm past the skin incision and then measured for proper placement. It is the author's practice to confirm proper catheter length by tracing the path of the catheter along the external chest wall using fluoroscopy before trimming the catheter length. After establishing the proper catheter length, attention is turned toward accessing the subclavian vein. A peel-away sheath and dilator are advanced over

the guidewire into the vein with care. Once the dilator/sheath combination is inside the vein, the sheath should be advanced over the dilator the remainder of its length. This is done to minimize the risk of significant venous injury by the rigid dilator. Once the sheath is completely inside the vein, the dilator is withdrawn and blood return confirmed, and only then is the wire completely removed. If blood return is not observed after removal of the dilator, fluoroscopy should confirm sheath placement and kinking checked for. For this reason, it is best to maintain the wire inside the vein until blood return is ensured.

Once the sheath is in place, the catheter is inserted into the vein through the lumen and the sheath is split and peeled away. To avoid losing access to the vein, the entire length of the catheter should be advanced into position, with placement confirmed via fluoroscopy before removal of the sheath, rather than pulling the sheath back as the catheter is advanced. During sheath removal, the catheter is steadied at the skin with a pair of forceps. Improper placement of the catheter tip increases the rate of associated complications, including cardiac arrhythmias from cardiac irritation and catheter failure associated with thrombosis.[23] The ideal catheter tip position is just inside the right atrium or at the junction of the superior vena cava and the right atrium, keeping in mind that the tip migrates up 1 to 3 cm when the patient is upright. Catheter placement in the subclavian vein is associated with a higher rate of venous thrombosis and catheter failure versus placement in the right atrium or vena cava. The author's technique for using external bony landmarks to estimate proper catheter length is described in Figure 50.1-4. The usual location of the junction of the right atrium and the superior vena cava is 4 to 6 cm below the angle of Louis,

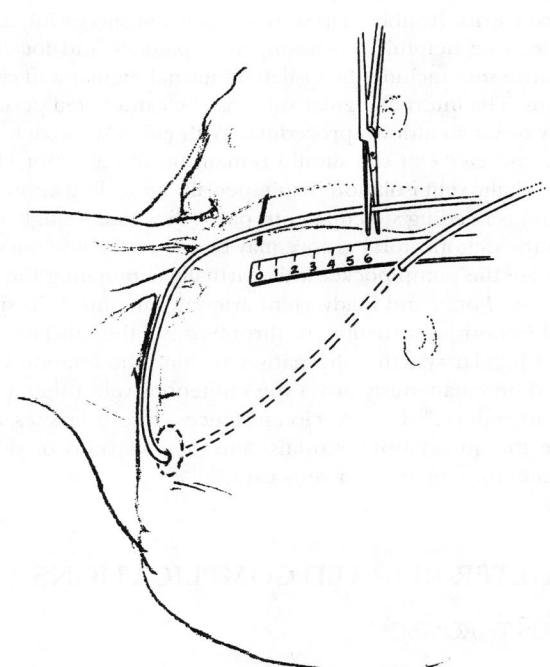

FIGURE 50.1-4.   The length of the catheter can be estimated by simulating its course through the subclavian vein and superior vena cava along the clavicle and right border of the sternum. If the catheter is cut 6 cm inferior to the angle of Louis, it approximates a final position at the superior vena caval and atrial junction. Tip position should be confirmed using fluoroscopy.

but fluoroscopic confirmation of location is essential. An upright chest x-ray should be obtained at the completion of the procedure to document catheter placement and confirm the absence of a pneumothorax, a complication of less than 1% of catheters placed by the subclavian or jugular approach.[24] If an implanted pump is being placed, similar technique is used, except the second incision is placed higher on the chest, just medial to the deltopectoral groove, in a vertical orientation. A subcutaneous pocket is fashioned to accommodate the port after it is attached to the catheter. Care should be taken to ensure the orientation of the port does not kink the catheter at the port hub before placing the anchoring sutures.

Increasingly, real-time ultrasound guidance has been used to aid in catheter insertion, predominantly via a cervical approach. Several recent randomized series have noted decreased rates of arterial puncture and cervical hematoma, shorter procedure times, and increased rates of successful catheter insertion when ultrasound guidance is used versus a more traditional technique based solely on anatomic landmarks.[25,26] In a large nonrandomized series of 493 patients, the overall success rate of ultrasound-guided internal jugular vein cannulation was 94.5%, with cervical hematoma and arterial puncture rates of 4.3% and 1.4%, respectively.[27] Such a benefit does not appear to extend to subclavian vein catheter insertion, where surface landmarks are more consistent and ultrasonic venous examination is more difficult.[28] Although routine use of real-time ultrasonography may not be necessary in experienced hands, its use in patients with poorly defined surface landmarks, thrombocytopenia or coagulation abnormalities, or a history of multiple indwelling central catheters should be encouraged.

Alternatives to subclavian vein access are available when catheter insertion is not possible secondary to anatomic or safety concerns. If subclavian vein access is not successful, ultrasound can be helpful in assessing vein patency and location. Alternative sites include the ipsilated internal jugular and cephalic veins. The internal jugular vein may be cannulated percutaneously or via a cutdown procedure. With either approach, the port or catheter exit site should remain on the anterior chest wall. Cephalic vein isolation is an especially appealing approach for patients needing subcutaneous ports, in whom a single incision in the deltopectoral groove may be used to isolate the vein and create the pump pocket while virtually eliminating the risk of pneumothorax and inadvertent arterial puncture.[29] In situations of stenosis, obstruction, or thrombosis of the subclavian or internal jugular systems, alternatives include the femoral vein, accessed percutaneously or via the saphenous vein using a cutdown procedure.[30] In rare circumstances, insertion sites may include the gonadal, intercostals, and azygous veins or direct placement into the inferior vena cava.[26,31-33]

CATHETER-RELATED COMPLICATIONS

VENOUS THROMBOSIS

Catheter-associated thrombosis is the most common complication associated with long-term indwelling catheters, reported in 30% of 70% of patients, the majority of which are asymptomatic. Symptomatic thrombosis is reported in 5% to 10% of patients with central catheters.[34,35] When present, thrombi remain a source of catheter infection as well as pulmonary emboli and

permanent venous obstruction.[36] The latter complication must always be considered when planning to attempt venous access at or distal to sites previously used. Chronic irritation of the venous endothelium, at the catheter tip, the area of venous entry, or another area of sustained contact, is thought to be the inciting event in the development of catheter-associated thrombi. Recent data suggest that thrombi develop early in the life of the catheter and do not become clinically apparent unless collateral veins do not compensate for the progressive decrease in venous flow.[31]

Management of catheter-associated thrombosis is geared toward catheter preservation and prevention of secondary complications. Immediate catheter removal before attempted salvage is rare, and completion of therapy is often possible. Prompt relief of symptoms through elevation of the affected extremity and decreasing the risk of pulmonary emboli and clot propagation with therapeutic anticoagulation are the most pressing interventions. Traditional strategies based on therapeutic heparinization followed by oral warfarin therapy proved effective in catheter preservation and prevention of clot extension.[33] The true risk of pulmonary emboli from catheter-associated thrombi is unknown, but reviews of upper extremity deep venous thrombosis report an incidence of pulmonary emboli in 10% to 15% of affected patients, some of which were fatal.[37,38] The significance of asymptomatic catheter-associated thrombi is not clear, as few complications of catheter removal were noted in patients with small, asymptomatic clots. Furthermore, modern silicone and polyurethane catheters appear to be less likely associated with severe pulmonary emboli. These risks, and those of chronic venous insufficiency secondary to thrombotic complications, must be weighed in light of the life-threatening malignancy necessitating therapy.

Treatment of clinically significant catheter-associated thrombus is similar to that for other deep venous thrombosis and is centered around long-term anticoagulation. Initial trials were performed using bolus and continuous-infusion intravenous heparin for 24 to 48 hours before initiation of warfarin therapy.[37,38] Presently, initial therapy with low-molecular-weight heparin therapy followed by warfarin allows complete management in the outpatient setting and allows prolonged catheter preservation. Recommendations regarding the length of therapy are based on small, nonrandomized trials and include continuation of therapy for the length of the remaining catheter life and possibly for several weeks after catheter removal.[39] Thrombolytic therapy has been reported as a salvage strategy for maintaining a vital catheter and/or vein. Low-dose recombinant tissue plasminogen activator injected directly into the catheter and clot has been shown effective when used in combination with long-term anticoagulation after catheter removal.[40]

Prophylaxis against catheter-associated thrombosis has been examined using low-molecular-weight heparin or low-dose warfarin. Both strategies appeared effective when compared in randomized, controlled trials of high-risk patients.[41,42] Both trials were conducted in small groups of high-risk patients, leaving questions as to the benefit of such therapy on the majority of cancer patients with indwelling catheter. At present, the author's practice is to individualize therapy based on the patient's risk for thrombosis, the length of therapy, and a history of catheter-related complications.

INFECTIONS

Although subclinical thrombosis is a frequent complication of long-term indwelling catheter, infection is the greatest cause of catheter loss.[43] Risk factors for infectious complications include the type of catheter used, the absence of a skilled team caring for catheters, the lack of of antibiotic-coated catheters, and the length and frequency of catheter use.[44,45] Percutaneously placed short-term catheters are associated with the highest rate of infectious complications but are also accessed more often and for greater periods of time than other types of catheters. The establishment of dedicated care teams/protocols and the use of antibiotic-coated catheters have proven beneficial. Among those catheters designed for long-term use, tunneled catheters with externalized hubs are more likely to develop infections (40%) than implanted subcutaneous devices (5% to 10%).[40,41] Infectious complications decrease in frequency over time. This is thought to be due to the restoration of the skin integrity after insertion.

Skin flora, either the patient's own or transferred from a caregiver, are the most common contaminating organisms.[46] In the period immediately after catheter insertion, infections have the pattern of standard postoperative infections, most commonly presenting as cellulitis or deeper infections in the port pocket or along the catheter. These complications may be treated conservatively with antibiotics if discovered early in their course. The presence of a postoperative abscess mandates catheter removal. Inability to clear acute or chronic infections may indicate the presence of a bacterial biofilm surrounding the catheter, secreted by the infecting organism. Such a film makes delivery of antibiotics difficult, often necessitating catheter removal.[47]

Infectious complications of established venous access devices include those at the catheter exit or access site, infections of the catheter subcutaneous tunnel, and catheter-associated bacteremia. Tenderness and/or erythema at the catheter skin exit site or the port access site is frequently due to *Staphylococcus epidermidis* and may be associated with localized purulent discharge. Signs of systemic infection or sepsis are rare. Catheter preservation is the rule, and local treatment with antibiotic ointment usually is indicated. Cultures of any purulent discharge should be obtained before initiation of therapy. In cases of infection with *Pseudomonas* or atypical mycobacterium species or when blood cultures reveal the offending organism, catheter removal is indicated.[48,49] In the presence of systemic symptoms but negative blood cultures, oral or intravenous antibiotics are usually effective. More deep-seated infections manifest by erythema, tenderness, and fluctuance overlying the port pocket or subcutaneous catheter tunnel. These infections are more difficult to control, even with intravenous antibiotics. Catheter salvage is possible with several weeks of antibiotics, but in the absence of prompt clinical improvement, catheter removal is inevitable.[50]

The presence of a catheter-related source of bacteremia must be documented by blood cultures obtained through the line as well as from a peripheral site. The most common pathogen in catheter-related bacteremia is a coagulase-negative staphylococci and is usually readily treated with vancomycin administered via all lumens of the infected line.[42,46] After 2 to 3 days of antibiotic therapy, peripheral and catheter cultures should be repeated to ensure adequate treatment. After a total of 14 days of therapy, antibiotics should be discontinued and cultures repeated after 48 to 72 hours.[46] Indications for catheter removal include the inability to clear the infection after antimicrobial therapy, continued signs and symptoms of bacteremia, or recurrent infection after completion of a full course

of therapy. Before catheter removal, patients with persistent or recurrent catheter infections may benefit from a short course of low-dose recombinant tissue plasminogen activator designed at treating infections associated with catheter tip fibrin sheath or thrombus. Adequate delivery of antibiotics to the septic focus is not possible without destruction of the associated sheath or thrombus.[51] At the National Institutes of Health, the presence of such a sheath or thrombus is confirmed with a catheter venogram before initiating therapy.

REFERENCES

1. Broviac JW, Cole JJ, Scribner BH. A silicone rubber atrial catheter for prolonged parenteral alimentation. *Surg Gynecol Obstet* 1973;136:602.
2. Hickman RO, Buckner CD, Clift RA. A modified right atrial catheter for access to the venous system in marrow transplant recipients. *Surg Gynecol Obstet* 1979;148:791.
3. Flowers RH, Schwenzer KJ, Koper RF, et al. Efficacy of an attachable subcutaneous cuff for the prevention of intravascular catheter-related infection. A randomized, controlled trial. *JAMA* 1989;261:878.
4. Groeger JS, Lucas AB, Coit D, et al. A prospective, randomized evaluation of the effect of silver impregnated subcutaneous cuffs for preventing tunneled chronic venous access infections in cancer patients. *Ann Surg* 1993;218:206.
5. Mayo DJ, Horne MK, Summers BL, et al. The effects of heparin flush on patency of the Groshong catheter: a pilot study. *Oncol Nurs Forum* 1996;23:1401.
6. Cardella JF, Cardella K, Bacci N, Fox PS, Post JH. Cumulative experience with 1,273 peripherally inserted central catheters at a single institution. *J Vasc Interv Radiol* 1996;7:5.
7. Banton J. Using midlines and PICC lines for chemotherapy regimens. *Oncol Nurs Forum* 1999;26:514.
8. Alhimyary A, Fernandez C, Picard M, et al. Safety and efficacy of total parenteral nutrition delivered via a peripherally inserted central venous catheter. *Nutr Clin Pract* 1996;11:199.
9. Allen AW, Megargell JL, Brown DB, et al. Venous thrombosis associated with the placement of peripherally inserted central catheters. *J Vasc Interv Radiol* 2000;11:1309.
10. May GS, Davis C. Percutaneous catheters and totally implantable access systems: a review of reported infection rates. *J Intraven Nurs* 1988;11:97.
11. Ross MN, Hasse GM, Poole MA, et al. Comparison of totally implanted reservoirs with external catheters as venous access devices in pediatric oncology patients. *Surg Gynecol Obstet* 1988;167:141.
12. Viale PH. Complications associated with implantable vascular access devices in the patient with cancer. *J Infus Nurs* 2003;26:97.
13. Rohde TD, Blackshear PJ, Varco RL, Buchwald H. One year of heparin anticoagulation. An ambulatory subject using a totally implantable infusion pump. *Minn Med* 1977;60:719.
14. Kemeny N, Jarnagin W, Gonen M, et al. Phase I/II study of hepatic arterial therapy with floxuridine and dexamethasone in combination with intravenous irinotecan as adjuvant treatment after resection of hepatic metastases from colorectal cancer. *J Clin Oncol* 2003;21:3303.
15. Rougier P, Laplanche A, Huguier M, et al. Hepatic arterial infusion of floxuridine in patients with liver metastases from colorectal carcinoma: long-term results of a prospective randomized trial. *J Clin Oncol* 1992;10:1112.
16. Hassenbusch SJ, Pillay PK, Magdinec M, et al. Constant infusion of morphine for intractable cancer pain using an implantable pump. *J Neurosurg* 1990;73:405.
17. Hunger-Dathe W, Braun A, Muller UA, et al. Insulin pump therapy in patients with type 1 diabetes mellitus: results of the Nationwide Quality Circle in Germany (ASD) 1999–2000. *Exp Clin Endocrinol Diabetes* 2003;111:428.
18. Saudek CD, Fischell RE, Swindle MM. The programmable implantable medication system (PIMS): design features and pre-clinical trials. *Horm Metab Res* 1990;22:201.
19. Udelsman R, Chen H, Loman K, et al. Implanted programmable insulin pumps: one hundred and fifty-three patient years of surgical experience. *Surgery* 1997;122:1005.
20. Hunter MR. Development of a vascular access team in an acute care setting. *J Infus Nurs* 2003;26:86.
21. Gandhi RT, Getrajdman GI, Brown KT, et al. Placement of subcutaneous chest wall ports ipsilateral to axillary node dissection. *J Vasc Interv Radiol* 2003;14:1063.
22. Jansen RF, Wiggers T, van Geel BN, et al. Assessment of insertion techniques and complication rates of dual-lumen central venous catheters in patients with hematological malignancies. *World J Surg* 1990;14:100.
23. Petersen J, Delaney JH, Brakstad MT, et al. Silicone venous access devices positioned with their tips high in the vena cava are more likely to malfunction. *Am J Surg* 1999;178:38.
24. Miller JA, Singireddy S, Maldjian P, Baker SR. A reevaluation of the radiographically detectable complications of percutaneous venous access lines inserted by four subcutaneous approaches. *Am Surg* 1999;65:125.
25. Slama M, Novara A, Safavian A, et al. Improvement of internal jugular vein cannulation using an ultrasound-guided technique. *Intensive Care Med* 1997;23:916.
26. Teichgraber UK, Benter T, Gebel M, Manns MP. A sonographically guided technique for central venous access. *AJR Am J Roentgenol* 1997;169:731.
27. Mey U, Glasmacher A, Hahn C, et al. Evaluation of an ultrasound-guided technique for central venous access via the internal jugular vein in 493 patients. *Support Care Cancer* 2003;11:148.

28. Bold RJ, Winchester DJ, Madary AR, et al. Prospective, randomized trial of Doppler-assisted subclavian vein catheterization. *Arch Surg* 1998;133:1089.

29. Povoski SP. A prospective analysis of the cephalic vein cutdown approach for chronic indwelling central venous access in 100 consecutive cancer patients. *Ann Surg Oncol* 2000;7:496.

30. Willard W, Coit D, Lucas A, Groeger JS. Long-term vascular access via the inferior vena cava. *J Surg Oncol* 1991;46:162.

31. Torosian MT, Meranze S, McLean G, Mullen JL. Central venous access with occlusive superior central venous thrombosis. *Ann Surg* 1986;203:30.

32. Pokorny WJ, McGill CW, Harberg FJ. Use of azygous vein for central catheter insertion. *Surgery* 1985;97:362.

33. Knox MF, Holton JC, Morris WD, Flippin TA. Translumbar inferior vena cava Groshong catheter placement in a patient with superior vena cava occlusion. *J Ark Med Soc* 1989;85:325.

34. Horne MK, May DJ, Alexander HR, et al. Venographic surveillance of tunneled venous access devices in adult oncology patients. *Ann Surg Oncol* 1995;2:174.

35. De Cicco M, Matovic M, Balestreri L, et al. Central venous thrombosis: an early and frequent complication in cancer patients bearing long-term Silastic catheter. A prospective study. *Thromb Res* 1997;86:101.

36. Raad I, Luna M, Khalil SA, et al. The relationship between the thrombotic and infectious complications of central venous catheters. *JAMA* 1994;271:1014.

37. Becker DM, Philbrick JT, Walker RB. Axillary and subclavian venous thrombosis. Prognosis and treatment. *Arch Intern Med* 1991;151:1934.

38. Hicken GJ, Ameli FM. Management of subclavian-axillary vein thrombosis: a review. *Can J Surg* 1998;41:13.

39. Gould JR, Carloss HW, Skinner WL. Groshong catheter-associated subclavian venous thrombosis. *Am J Med* 1993;95:419.

40. Horne MK, Mayo DJ, Cannon RO, et al. Intra-clot recombinant tissue plasminogen activator in the treatment of deep venous thrombosis of the lower and upper extremities. *Am J Med* 2000;108:251.

41. Monreal M, Alastrue A, Rull M, et al. Upper extremity deep venous thrombosis in cancer patients with venous access devices- prophylaxis with low molecular weight heparin (Fragmin). *Thromb Haemost* 1996;75:251.

42. Bern MM, Lokich JJ, Wallach SR, et al. Very low doses of warfarin can prevent thrombosis in central venous catheters. A randomized prospective trial. *Ann Intern Med* 1990;112:423.

43. Groeger JS, Lucas AB, Thaler HT, et al. Infectious morbidity associated with long-term use of venous access devices in patients with cancer. *Ann Intern Med* 1993;119:1168.

44. Mirro J, Rao BN, Kumar M, et al. A comparison of placement techniques and complications of externalized catheters and implantable port use in children with cancer. *J Pediatr Surg* 1990;25:120.

45. Darouiche RO, Raad II, Heard SO, et al. A comparison of two antimicrobial-impregnated central venous catheters. Catheter Study Group. *N Engl J Med* 1999;340:1.

46. Raad II, Bodey GP. Infectious complications of indwelling vascular catheters. *Clin Infect Dis* 1992;15:197.

47. Costerton JW, Stewart PS, Greenberg EP. Bacterial biofilms: a common cause of persistent infections. *Science* 1999;284:1318.

48. Benezra D, Kiehn TE, Gold JW, et al. Prospective study of infections in indwelling central venous catheters using quantitative blood cultures. *Am J Med* 1988;85:495.

49. Raad II, Vartivarian S, Khan A, Bodey GP. Catheter-related infections caused by the Mycobacterium fortuitum complex: 15 cases and a review. *Rev Infect Dis* 1991;12:1120.

50. Jones GR. A practical guide to evaluation and treatment of infections in patients with indwelling central venous catheters. *J Intraven Nurs* 1998;21:S134.

51. Jones GR, Konsler GK, Dunaway RP. Urokinase in the treatment of bacteremia and candidemia in patients with right atrial catheters. *Am J Infect Control* 1996;24:160.

SECTION 2

H. RICHARD ALEXANDER, JR.

Isolation Perfusion

Vascular isolation and perfusion of a cancer-bearing organ or region of the body (i.e., extremity) using a recirculating extracorporeal perfusion circuit has been in clinical use for almost 50 years. It was originally applied to the limb by Creech et al. in the 1950s for patients with high-grade unresectable extremity sarcoma or in-transit melanoma.[1] In the early 1960s, additional experience with isolated perfusion of the limb or liver was reported by a small number of centers.[2,3] More recently, the technique has been under clinical evaluation for patients with these conditions and has also been used in isolation perfusion of the lung.[4]

Isolation perfusion was initially applied under normothermic conditions using chemotherapeutics alone, and subsequently mild to moderate hyperthermia (38.5° to 42.0°C) became a routine component of treatment.[5] Since 1992, there has been considerable interest in the use of tumor necrosis factor (TNF) used in combination with melphalan and hyperthermia in isolation perfusion.[6–8] This chapter reviews the principles and technique of isolation perfusion and the current status of this treatment modality in clinical practice. The role of the various components of therapy that are routinely used on efficacy and toxicity are reviewed.

PRINCIPLES OF ISOLATION PERFUSION

Isolation perfusion is a specialized surgical technique administered under a general anesthetic and usually for an interval of 60 to 90 minutes. Initially, the vascular supply of a cancer-bearing organ or region such as liver or extremity is isolated, and all collateral blood flow to the area is controlled to avoid any leak of perfusate into the systemic circulation or leak of systemic blood into the perfusion circuit. Once the vessels are cannulated, they are connected to inflow and outflow lines of an extracorporeal bypass circuit that consists of an oxygenator, reservoir, heat exchanger, and roller pump. The heat exchanger, which warms the perfusate, is connected to a closed water-recirculating circuit (Fig. 50.2-1). It has become routine practice during isolated limb perfusion (ILP) to confirm that complete vascular isolation has been achieved using a continuous intraoperative leak-monitoring technique with either radiolabeled iodine 131 human serum albumin or technetium 99–labeled red blood cells.[9,10] Once the perfusion is complete, the vascular bed of the treated region is flushed with several liters of saline and colloid solution to remove any residual intravascular therapeutic agents. Finally, the native vascular blood flow is reestablished to the site, and therapy is completed. Because of the need to place indwelling vascular catheters during treatment, the patient must be systemically anticoagulated, usually using heparin during perfusion. However, the anticoagulation effects can be effectively reversed with protamine sulfate and thawed fresh frozen plasma.

There are several advantages of isolation perfusion as a treatment technique. In practice, complete separation of the regional and systemic circulation can be achieved in most circumstances. This is particularly true for isolation perfusion of the liver.[11] For patients undergoing ILP for in-transit melanoma for high-grade unresectable sarcoma of the extremity, small, less than 1% leaks of perfusate into the systemic circulation can be detected using a leak-monitoring system. Klaase and coworkers[9] reported the frequency of perfusate leak in 383 patients who underwent 438 ILPs using a standardized technique. The cumulative overall leak rate was 0.9%. A leak rate of greater than 5% was encountered in 6.2% of ILPs, and a leak rate of greater than 10% was observed in only 1.4%. During ILP, leak of perfusate can usually be controlled with various maneuvers such as adjustments in flow rate or tightening of the extremity tourniquet.[12] Because treatment is confined to an

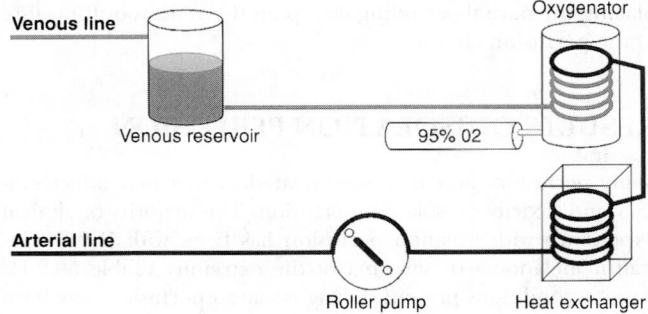

FIGURE 50.2-1. General components of isolated organ perfusion circuit showing the venous reservoir, oxygenator, heat exchanger, and roller pump. Blood flow from the perfused site is collected in a venous reservoir by passage drainage. The roller pump on the arterial side of the circuit can be adjusted to increase or decrease flow rates as appropriate. The oxygenator and heat exchanger are in-line components of this circuit, and the latter can effectively heat the perfusate so that tissue hyperthermia can be routinely achieved.

organ or region of the body, systemic exposure and toxicity secondary to the therapeutic agents can be eliminated or significantly limited.[13] In addition, dose escalation of the therapeutic agents is limited largely by the tissue tolerance of the perfused organ or the extremity.[14] Finally, isolation perfusion allows one to deliver clinically significant levels of hyperthermia, which has direct cytotoxic and synergistic antitumor effects with various chemotherapeutic and biologic agents.[15,16]

ISOLATED LIMB PERFUSION

ILP of the lower extremity is most commonly performed via cannulation of the external iliac vessels and in the arm via the axillary vessels. However, in the lower extremity, ILP can be performed via the femoral or popliteal vessels and in the arm via the brachial vessels under appropriate clinical situations. For the approach to the iliac vessels, a lower abdominal "transplant" incision and a retroperitoneal approach are made. The external iliac artery and vein are dissected from their origin down to the inguinal ligament and small arterial branches and venous tributaries and ligated and divided. This is particularly important in the region of the inguinal ligament to prevent leak of perfusate into the systemic circulation. The hypogastric vein is ligated *in situ*, and the hypogastric artery is temporarily occluded with a vascular occluding clamp. If possible, some of the branches of the hypogastric artery in the pelvis should be identified and ligated to prevent collateral flow across the pelvis. A Steinmann pin is anchored into the anterior superior iliac spine, and the external iliac vessels are cannulated, with the catheter tips in each vessel positioned just below the inguinal ligament. An Esmarch tourniquet is snugly wrapped at the root of the extremity, held in place by the Steinmann pin, and the cannulas are connected to the extracorporeal bypass circuit.

ISOLATED HEPATIC PERFUSION

Isolated hepatic perfusion (IHP) is a more complex treatment to administer and has not gained as widespread or consistent clinical evaluation because of the major nature of the operative procedure, the associated morbidity associated with the treat-

ment, and the fact that initial clinical studies did not clearly document efficacy of the therapy. The unique vascular anatomy of the liver, however, does make it an ideally suitable organ for isolated perfusion. The procedure starts with a right subcostal incision. Once it has been determined that there are no contraindications to proceeding with IHP, the incision is extended, and the liver is extensively mobilized. This includes division of the diaphragmatic attachments of the left and right hepatic lobes and complete dissection of the retrohepatic vena cava from the level of the renal veins to the diaphragm to prevent any leak of perfusate from the retrohepatic inferior vena cava (IVC). A cholecystectomy is performed, and the porta hepatis structures are completely dissected and isolated. Cannulation for inflow to the liver is typically via the gastroduodenal artery alone or the gastroduodenal artery and portal vein.[6] Splanchnic venous flow is shunted to the right atrium using a second veno–veno bypass circuit similar to that used in hepatic transplantation procedures with an inflow cannula positioned in the axillary vein. The venous effluent of the liver is collected from a cannula positioned in an isolated segment of retrohepatic IVC, and therefore during treatment, the IVC flow must also be shunted (Fig. 50.2-2). The external veno–veno bypass circuit results in flow rates of approximately 2 L/min and stable cardiac parameters during treatment.[17]

PERFUSION PARAMETERS

The extracorporeal perfusion circuit typically contains 1 L of perfusate that consists of 700 mL of a balanced salt solution, one unit of type-matched packed red blood cells, and 1500 U of heparin. The resultant hematocrit of approximately 25% provides adequate tissue oxygen retention, and perfusate containing higher hematocrits confers no additional benefit in preventing regional toxicity.[18] Generally, flow rates in the range of 400 to 800 mL/min are achievable and adjusted depending on line pressure, changes in reservoir volume, or the presence of a systemic perfusate leak based on intraoperative monitoring.

Continuous intraoperative leak monitoring to assess for the presence of perfusate leak into the systemic circulation is being used more routinely and is an important component of isolation perfusion therapy when one considers that the perfusate often contains doses of therapeutic agents that are at least 10-fold greater than maximally tolerated systemic doses. Careful monitoring of leak can reduce the severity of systemic complications and may improve response rates.[10,13] A gamma detection camera is positioned either over the precordium of the heart for patients undergoing ILP or over the pump housing of the veno–venous bypass circuit for patients undergoing IHP, both of which serve as a stable reservoir of blood to measure radioactivity. Once the gamma detection camera has been positioned, a small dose of radionuclide is given systemically, and a baseline level of radioactive counts is measured on a strip chart recorder. Then a tenfold higher dose is administered into the perfusion circuit. Therefore, if a 10% leak of perfusate into the systemic circulation occurs, there is a doubling of the amount of radioactivity compared with baseline. Leak rates using this system have been shown to correlate with measured leak rates with TNF or melphalan from the perfusate into the systemic circulation.[9,13]

Despite very careful preoperative preparation, during ILP, the surgeon may encounter several situations that require

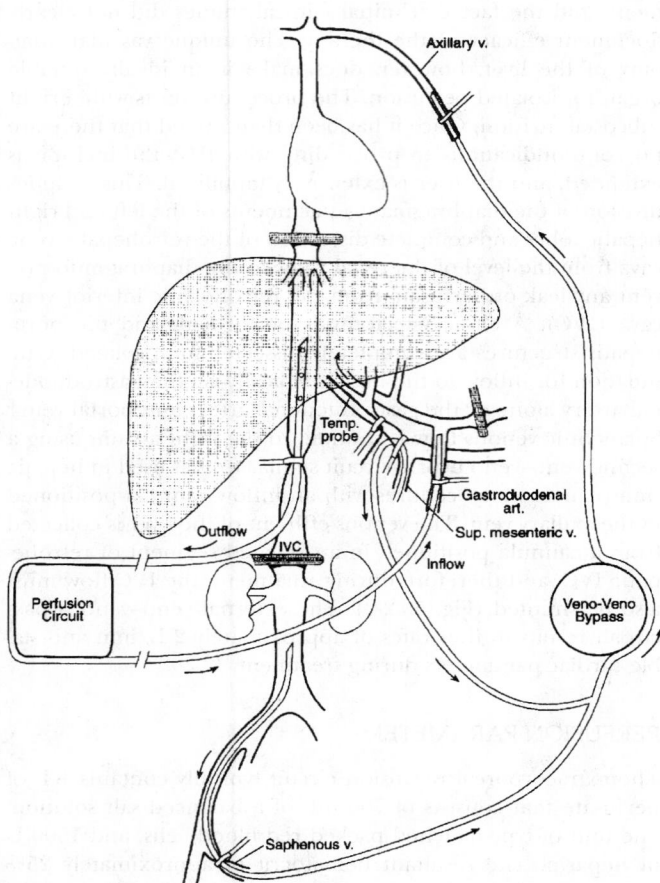

FIGURE 50.2-2. Schematic illustration of the isolated hepatic perfusion circuit. The arterial inflow is via the gastroduodenal artery, and venous outflow is collected from a cannula positioned in an isolated segment of retrohepatic vena cava. The inflow and outflow cannula are connected to a perfusion circuit, as shown in Figure 50.2-1. On the patient's left is the veno–veno bypass circuit, which shunts portal splanchnic and inferior venal caval (IVC) blood flow back to the systemic circulation during therapy.

adjustment in perfusion parameters to minimize a leak of perfusate or blood out of or into the perfusion circuit. Flow rates that indirectly affect arterial line pressure, reservoir volume, and leak of perfusate are continuously monitored. If there is leak of systemic blood into the perfusion circuit, this is reflected by an increase in the reservoir volume in the circuit and can be remedied by increasing flow rates to increase line pressure, tightening the extremity tourniquet, or increasing venous pressure in the circuit by placing a partial-occluding clamp on the venous outflow line. If there is a perfusate leak into the systemic circulation, this is manifested by an increase in radioactive counts detected by the gamma camera and the strip chart recorder, or one may see a decrease in reservoir volume in the perfusion circuit. Under these circumstances, one may decrease flow rates to lower the line pressure or tighten the tourniquet. Rarely, a two-way leak occurs, evidenced by changes in reservoir volume (generally a gain) as well as an increase in radioactivity on the strip chart recorder. This can be a particular difficult and tricky condition to adequately control, and typical steps include decreasing flow rates to stop any systemic leak of perfusate, tightening the tourniquet, and then placing the partial-occluding clamp on the venous outflow line of the perfusion circuit.

RESULTS OF ISOLATION PERFUSION

Many perfusion- and treatment-related factors may affect efficacy and toxicity of isolation perfusion. The majority of clinical experience with isolation perfusion has been with ILP for in-transit melanoma or sarcoma of the extremity (Table 50.2-1). Various conditions present during isolation perfusion may have substantial effects on outcome such as hyperthermia and biologic agents, most notably TNF, and these are discussed here.

HYPERTHERMIA

Hyperthermia has been used in isolation perfusion alone or in combination with chemotherapeutics and TNF. In experimental models, it has direct cytotoxicity against tumor lines and has established synergy with various chemotherapeutics and TNF.[16,19] This latter feature is presumed to be the main contribution of hyperthermia in isolation perfusion. Under hyperthermic conditions, tumor neovasculature responds differently than native blood vessels. At temperatures up to 46°C, normal microvessels dilate, and blood flow increases up to sixfold as a compensatory mechanism to diffuse local heat accumulation.[20] In contrast, tumor-associated microvessels have a diminished capacity to vasodilate, and at comparable temperatures there is stasis and diminution of blood flow, indicating a differential sensitivity between tumor-associated and normal microvasculature.[20]

After the original report of normothermic ILP using chemotherapeutics in 1957 by Creech et al.,[1] most investigators subsequently incorporated some degree of hyperthermia as closed-circuit water-recirculating heat exchangers became available to replace the use of inefficient warm moist towels and infrared lamps to warm perfusate fluid.[21] Stehlin et al. reported results of ILP in 165 patients with extremity sarcoma or melanoma in whom significant hyperthermia was delivered to the perfused limb. They observed that when the perfusate was warmed to 46°C and average tissue temperature was 42°C, there was severe regional toxicity, including pain, edema, blistering, and weakness observed in 70% of patients.[2] When tissue temperatures were reduced to 40°C or less, regional complications were minimal. Compared with historical controls treated identically at that institution, the addition of hyperthermia during ILP with melphalan in patients with extremity melanoma resulted in an increase in response rates from 35% to 80%.[2] Klaase and coworkers reported an analysis of factors associated with toxicity after ILP for melanoma in 425 patients.[22] Tissue temperature of higher than 40°C was the most significant factor associated with increased regional toxicity. In addition, female gender and a decrease in perfusate pH were also associated with worse regional toxicity.

Skibba et al. have reported data on eight patients with unresectable cancer confined to liver treated with a 4 hour IHP using hyperthermia alone to 42.5°C.[23] Toxicity associated with this therapy was substantial; all patients had marked elevation in post-IHP hepatic transaminases and bilirubin and two of eight died in the early postoperative period. There was some transient antitumor activity evidenced by central tumor necrosis on follow-up computed tomography scans. Hyperthermia appears to improve the efficacy chemotherapeutics or biologic agents

TABLE 50.2-1.   Selected Series of Isolation Perfusion Using Tumor Necrosis Factor and Melphalan

Study	Trial Type	Agents	n	CR (%)	PR (%)	Comments
Lienard et al.[25]	Phase II ILP Melanoma/sarcoma	Regimen A: melphalan, 10–13 mg/L TNF, 3–4 mg IFN, 0.2 mg	29	90	10	First report with TNF in ILP
Lienard et al.[48]	Phase III ILP Melanoma	Regimen A vs. melphalan, 10–13 mg/L TNF, 3–4 mg	31 33	78 69	22 22	IFN not necessary
Fraker et al.[49]	Phase III ILP Melanoma	Regimen A vs. Melphalan, 10–13 mg/L	20 23	80 61	10 39	Small trial, inconclusive
Eggermont et al.[38]	Phase II ILP Sarcoma	Melphalan, 10–13 mg/L TNF, 3–4 mg	186	29	53	Limb salvage >80
Vaglini et al.[33]	Phase II ILP Melanoma	Melphalan, 10–13 mg/L TNF, 0.5–4.0 mg IFN, 0.2 mg	10	70	—	Low-dose TNF works
Alexander and Feldman[24]	Phase II IHP Multiple histologies	Melphalan, 1.5 mg/kg TNF, 1.0 mg	50	2	73	TNF used safely in IHP
Posner et al.[29]	Phase I/II ILP Melanoma	TNF alone, 1–4 mg	6	16	34[a]	TNF alone minimal efficacy
Klaase et al.[35]	Phase II ILP Melanoma	Melphalan with or without hyperthermia	120	55	30	30% 10-y survival
Vahrmeijer et al.[41]	Phase I IHP Hyperthermia	Melphalan, 0.5–4.0 mg/kg	24	6	23	Toxicity was leukopenia

CR, complete response; IFN, interferon; IHP, isolated hepatic perfusion; ILP, isolated limb perfusion; PR, partial response; TNF, tumor necrosis factor.
[a]All responses short-lived (one 7-mo CR; two 1-mo PRs).

given via isolation perfusion of the limb or liver. It has marginal, if any, independent antitumor effects, and temperatures higher than 40° to 41°C are associated with unacceptable toxicity.

TUMOR NECROSIS FACTOR

Recombinant TNF became available in the mid-1980s and was evaluated in multiple clinical trials using various methods of administration.[24] However, it was found that humans are very sensitive to the toxic effects of TNF, and at the maximum tolerated doses administered it had very little antitumor activity. Although interest in TNF as a systemically administered antitumor agent waned, enthusiasm for its administration via isolation perfusion grew remarkably in the early 1990s, when Lienard et al. reported initial results in 29 patients treated with a combination of TNF, melphalan, and hyperthermia for in-transit melanoma or high-grade sarcoma of the extremity.[25] The overall response rate in that initial trial was 100%, with 90% of patients having a complete response to treatment (see Table 50.2-1).

TNF is ideally suited for administration via isolation perfusion and is thought to exert its antitumor activity via effects on the tumor-associated neovasculature. TNF has known significant procoagulant activity and increases vascular permeability.[26] There are data showing selective obliteration of tumor neovasculature after ILP with TNF, hyperthermia, and melphalan correlates, with efficacy for patients with high-grade unresectable extremity sarcoma (Fig. 50.2-3).[27] However, there are limited clinical data available using TNF alone via isolation perfusion. Three patients with high-grade extremity sarcoma were treated at the author's institution with hyperthermic ILP and TNF alone, without evidence of significant antitumor activity.[28] One patient had angiographically documented obliteration of tumor-associated neovasculature after ILP; however, he experienced clinical and radiographic tumor progression within 6 weeks, suggesting that the vascular obliteration

observed after TNF may not be sufficient for subsequent tumor regression. Posner and coworkers[29] reported results of ILP with TNF alone in six patients with in-transit melanoma. One had a complete response of 7 months' durations, and two others had brief, less-than-1-month, partial responses. TNF administered alone via IHP has very little antitumor activity.

However, when TNF is used in ILP with melphalan, it is associated with a rapid time course of response in tumors compared with ILP with melphalan alone, and large tumors form eschar reminiscent of the findings in murine models (Fig. 50.2-4). Because TNF causes increased endothelial permeability and has selective procoagulant effects on tumor-associated vasculature, it has been postulated that during isolation perfusion TNF may augment delivery of chemotherapeutics to the tumor by selectively increasing tumor neovascular permeability.[26]

Leak of TNF into the systemic circulation during ILP is associated with transient proinflammatory cytokine production, most notably interleukin-6 and interleukin-8.[30] During IHP with TNF, transient high plasma levels of interleukin-6 and interleukin-8 levels are routinely measured due to hepatic synthesis of these proteins when TNF is in the perfusate.[31] When leak of TNF is kept minimal during ILP and during IHP even when no leak is observed, there are transient and manageable metabolic and hemodynamic alterations that occur from secondary cytokine production.

CURRENT STATUS OF ISOLATED LIMB PERFUSION

The role of TNF in isolation perfusion is still under clinical evaluation and has not conclusively demonstrated in properly designed and conducted prospective random assignment trials. In the initial report from Lienard et al., results from 29 patients

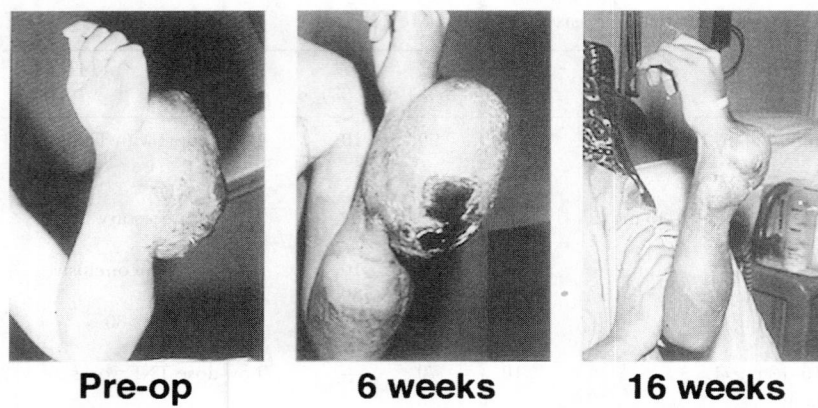

Pre-op   **6 weeks**   **16 weeks**

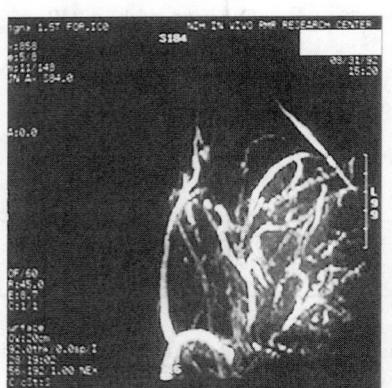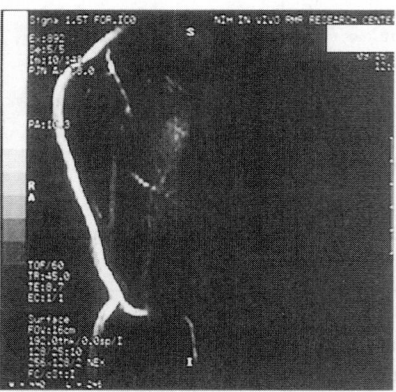

Pre- and Post-ILP MRA

FIGURE 50.2-3. Preperfusion and postperfusion magnetic resonance angiograms (MRAs) showing neovascularity in a large multiply recurrent Ewing's sarcoma arising on the dorsum of a forearm. The patient had small volume pulmonary metastases and was treated with a palliative 90-minute hyperthermic isolated limb perfusion (ILP) using tumor necrosis factor and melphalan. He had a significant regression (*top panel*) that lasted for 2 years until death from systemic disease progression. Three days posttherapy, complete obliteration of the tumor neovasculature was observed with no effect of perfusion on the native blood vessels in the extremity (*bottom panel*).

treated with ILP using a combination of TNF, melphalan, and hyperthermia for in-transit melanoma or high-grade sarcoma of the extremity were presented.[25] In subsequent reports from various institutions, including a follow-up report from Lienard et al. of a larger series of patients, the complete response rates were lower (see Table 50.2-1).[13,32,33] A small prospective random-assignment trial comparing melphalan, TNF, and IFN with melphalan alone showed no difference in overall or complete response rates between the groups.[49] It is also noteworthy that in several trials of ILP using melphalan alone, complete response rates between 55% and 82% have been reported.[34,35] A prospective random-assignment trial comparing melphalan and TNF with melphalan alone administered via ILP for in-transit melanoma of the extremity was closed in Europe because of low accrual, suggesting a bias that TNF for most patients with this histology does not substantially contribute to efficacy compared with melphalan alone. A large multicenter trial of prophylactic ILP after excision of primary lesions

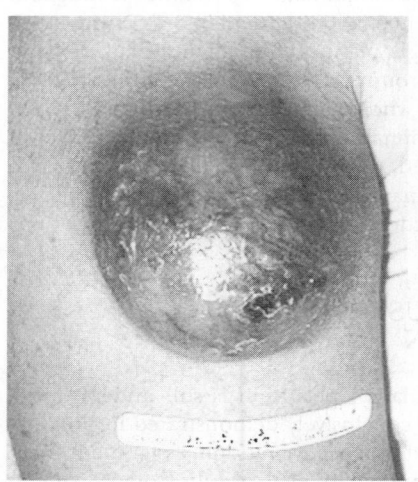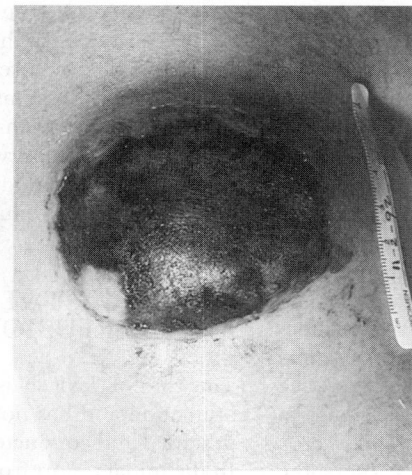

FIGURE 50.2-4. Photographs of a patient treated with isolated limb perfusion using tumor necrosis factor and melphalan for in-transit extremity melanoma. The top panel shows an in-transit site of disease before and 5 days after isolated limb perfusion. Note the rapid eschar formation over the tumor, with sparing of overlying and adjacent normal skin, which is characteristic of a tumor necrosis factor effect.

greater than 1.5 mm in depth showed a decrease in local recurrence with ILP from 6.6% to 3.3% compared with excision alone, with no benefit in survival.[36] Based on these results, prophylactic ILP has been largely abandoned.

ILP has been used for patients with unresectable high-grade extremity sarcoma for palliation, for potential cure in cases of multifocal disease, and as a neoadjuvant therapy to convert an unresectable lesion to a resectable one. Early data reported with ILP using chemotherapeutics alone indicated limited antitumor activity against this histology.[37] A multi-institutional trial using this regimen for patients with high-grade unresectable extremity sarcoma was conducted in Europe, and the results reported in by Eggermont and coworkers.[38] An overall clinical and pathologic response rate of more than 80% and a limb salvage rate of more than 80% using this regimen for patients with unresectable high-grade extremity sarcoma has been confirmed by others, and it is now licensed for use in Europe.[39]

CURRENT STATUS OF ISOLATED HEPATIC PERFUSION

After the initial experience with TNF and melphalan in ILP, several centers have reported results with this regimen used in IHP for patients with unresectable primary or metastatic cancers confined to the liver (see Table 50.2-1).[17,40,41] de Vries and coworkers reported results in eight patients treated with melphalan and TNF and one patient treated with TNF alone for 1 hour at 41°C.[42] IHP was associated with a 33% mortality in the series, but five of six evaluable patients treated with melphalan and TNF had radiographic evidence of antitumor efficacy. Lindner and colleagues also reported considerable toxicity and limited efficacy in 11 patients treated with IHP using TNF and melphalan.[40] The largest series reported using TNF and melphalan via IHP comes from the National Cancer Institute; 34 patients underwent IHP with doses of melphalan and TNF that were derived from previously conducted phase I studies and were higher than those used at other institutions.[17] The treatment-related mortality was 4%, and the investigators observed an overall radiographic response rate of 75%. The group presented follow-up data on 50 patients with metastatic unresectable colorectal cancer to the liver.[43] The cohort was patients who had advanced and largely refractory disease, and treatment mortality in this series was only 2%. In the 32 patients treated with IHP using TNF and melphalan, there was a 74% radiographic partial response rate, with a median time to liver progression of 8.5 months and median survival of 16.5 months. In a second cohort of 19 patients, IHP with melphalan alone was administered followed by hepatic artery infusion therapy using floxuridine and leucovorin. The radiographic partial response rate was 74%, with a median duration of 14.5 months.

The morbidity and treatment mortality with IHP are highest in those reports that represent initial institutional experience with a highly technical procedure using agents that have known regional and systemic toxicity. With continued refinement and experience, the morbidity and mortality associated with the therapy should decrease. With refinements in the technique of IHP and when combined with additional treatments, it may become a more widely offered option for patients with unresectable hepatic malignancies from a variety of histologies (see Chapter 51.3).

STATUS OF ISOLATION PERFUSION OF OTHER SITES

There are very limited data regarding the application of isolation perfusion to other organs. Pass and coworkers from the National Cancer Institute reported results of a phase I isolation lung perfusion with escalating dose TNF for patients with unresectable pulmonary metastases.[44] Twenty patients were treated with unilateral isolated lung perfusion with TNF doses ranging from 0.3 to 6.0 mg. An oxygenated circuit was used analogous to that in either isolation perfusion settings and tissue hyperthermia between 38° and 39.5°C was used. There were no deaths in the study, and short-term regression of metastatic nodules was noted in three patients. Burt et al. reported no observable efficacy in eight patients with unresectable lung metastases who underwent isolated lung perfusion using doxorubicin.[4]

VARIATIONS OF ISOLATION PERFUSION TECHNIQUES

Isolated limb infusion is a new method of regional drug delivery to an extremity that uses percutaneously positioned intravascular occlusion balloons or more simply an extremity tourniquet to confine infused chemotherapy to the affected limb.[45,46] Percutaneous liver perfusion has also been described in which melphalan is infused into the hepatic artery and hepatic venous effluent is captured and filtered using a special double balloon catheter in the retrohepatic IVC.[47] The advantages of these modifications in isolation perfusion are that they avoid the morbidity of an operative procedure, and multiple retreatments can be delivered. On the other hand, because complete vascular isolation is not routinely achieved and the perfusate is infused slowly over a brief 20- to 30-minute interval, hyperthermia cannot be consistently applied, and systemic leak of perfusate may limit the use of biologic agents in this setting.

CONCLUSION

Isolated perfusion of various organs or the extremity using hyperthermia and chemotherapeutics with or without TNF has been shown to have substantial antitumor activity against a variety of histologies. After the initial studies using TNF, there was considerable enthusiasm for its routine use in organ perfusion for the treatment of in-transit melanoma in high-grade extremity sarcoma. Although the data support its use in treatment of high-grade extremity sarcoma, the benefit of TNF in combination with melphalan against in-transit melanoma has not been conclusively demonstrated. Because of the potential toxicity with TNF, its routine use outside of a clinical research trial cannot be advocated. IHP is a promising regional modality for unresectable malignancies confined to the liver, but continued investigation in a clinical research setting is clearly necessary to determine the optimum clinical setting in which to offer this form of therapy. Hyperthermia appears to be an important component of treatment and appears to act primarily by enhancing the tumoricidal effects of melphalan. TNF has no substantial antitumor activity when administered via isolated organ perfusion alone but may enhance the antitumor effects of melphalan against both the extremity tumors such as sarcoma.

REFERENCES

1. Creech O, Krementz ET, Ryan RF, Winblad JN. Chemotherapy of cancer: regional perfusion utilizing an extracorporeal circuit. *Ann Surg* 1958;148:616.
2. Stehlin JS, Giovanella BC, de Ipolyi PD, Muenz LR, Anderson RF. Results of hyperthermic perfusion for melanoma of the extremities. *Surg Gynecol Obstet* 1975;140:339.
3. Ausman RK. Development of a technic for isolated perfusion of the liver. *N Y State J Med* 1961;61:3393.
4. Burt ME, Liu D, Abolhoda A, et al. Isolated lung perfusion for patients with unresectable metastases from sarcoma: a phase I trial. *Ann Thorac Surg* 2000;69:1542.
5. Alexander HR, Fraker DL, Bartlett DL. Isolated limb perfusion for malignant melanoma. *Semin Surg Oncol* 1996;12:416.
6. Alexander HR, Bartlett DL, Libutti SK. Isolated hepatic perfusion: a potentially effective treatment for patients with metastatic or primary cancers confined to the liver. *Cancer J Sci Am* 1998;4:2.
7. Lienard D, Eggermont AM, Kroon BBR, Koops HW, Lejeune FJ. Isolated limb perfusion in primary and recurrent melanoma: indications and results. *Semin Surg Oncol* 1998;14:202.
8. Eggermont AM, Schraffordt KH, Klausner JM, et al. Isolation limb perfusion with tumor necrosis factor alpha and chemotherapy for advanced extremity soft tissue sarcomas. *Semin Oncol* 1997;24:547.
9. Klaase JM, Kroon BBR, van Geel AN, Eggermont AMM, Franklin HR. Systemic leakage during isolated limb perfusion for melanoma. *Br J Surg* 1993;80:1124.
10. Barker WC, Andrich MP, Alexander HR, Fraker DL. Continuous intraoperative external monitoring of perfusate leak using I-131 human serum albumin during isolated perfusion of the liver and limbs. *Eur J Nucl Med* 1995;22:1242.
11. Libutti SK, Bartlett DL, Fraker DL, Alexander HR. Technique and results of hyperthermic isolated hepatic perfusion with tumor necrosis factor and melphalan for the treatment of unresectable hepatic malignancies. *J Am Coll Surg* 2000;191:519.
12. Sorkin P, Abu-Abid S, Lev D, et al. Systemic leakage and side effects of tumor necrosis factor alpha administered via isolated limb perfusion can be manipulated by flow rate adjustment. *Arch Surg* 1995;130:1079.
13. Thom AK, Alexander HR, Andrich MP, et al. Cytokine levels and systemic toxicity in patients undergoing isolated limb perfusion (ILP) with high-dose TNF, interferon-gamma and melphalan. *J Clin Oncol* 1995;13:264.
14. Wieberdink J, Benckhuysen C, Braat RP, van Slooten EA, Olthuis GAA. Dosimetry in isolation perfusion of the limbs by assessment of perfused tissue volume and grading of toxic tissue reactions. *Eur J Cancer Clin Oncol* 1982;18:905.
15. Sakaguchi Y, Makino M, Kaneko T, et al. Therapeutic efficacy of long duration-low temperature whole body hyperthermia when combined with tumor necrosis factor and carboplatin in rats. *Cancer Res* 1994;54:2223.
16. Klostergaard J, Leroux E, Siddik ZH, Khodadadian M, Tomasovic SP. Enhanced sensitivity of human colon tumor cell lines in vitro in response to thermochemoimmunotherapy. *Cancer Res* 1992;52:5271.
17. Alexander HR Jr, Bartlett DL, Libutti SK, et al. Isolated hepatic perfusion with tumor necrosis factor and melphalan for unresectable cancers confined to the liver. *J Clin Oncol* 1998;16:1479.
18. Klaase JM, Kroon BBR, van Slooten GW, van Dongen JA. Comparison between the use of whole blood versus a diluted perfusate in regional isolated perfusion by continuous monitoring of transcutaneous oxygen tension: a pilot study. *J Invest Surg* 1994;7:249.
19. Miller RC, Richards M, Baird C, Martin S, Hall EJ. Interaction of hyperthermia and chemotherapy agents; cell lethality and oncogenic potential. *Int J Hyperthermia* 1994;10:89.
20. Dudar TE, Jain RK. Differential response of normal and tumor microcirculation to hyperthermia. *Cancer Res* 1984;44:605.
21. Stehlin JS. Hyperthermic perfusion with chemotherapy for cancers of the extremities. *Surg Gynecol Obstet* 1969;129:305.
22. Klaase JM, Kroon BBR, van Geel BN, et al. Patient- and treatment-related factors associated with acute regional toxicity after isolated perfusion for melanoma of the extremities. *Am J Surg* 1994;167:618.
23. Skibba JL, Quebbeman EJ, Komorowski RA, Thorsen KM. Clinical results of hyperthermic liver perfusion for cancer in the liver. *Contr Oncol* 1988;29:222.
24. Alexander HR, Feldman AL. Tumor necrosis factor: basic principles and clinical application in systemic and regional cancer treatment. In: Rosenberg SA, ed. *Biologic therapy of cancer*, 3rd ed. Philadelphia: Lippincott Williams & Wilkins, 2000:174.
25. Lienard D, Ewalenko P, Delmotti JJ, Renard N, Lejeune FJ. High-dose recombinant tumor necrosis factor alpha in combination with interferon gamma and melphalan in isolation perfusion of the limbs for melanoma and sarcoma. *J Clin Oncol* 1992;10:52.
26. Friedl J, Puhlmann M, Bartlett DL, et al. Induction of permeability across endothelial cell monolayers by tumor necrosis factor (TNF) occurs via a tissue factor-dependent mechanism: relationship between the procoagulant and permeability effects of TNF. *Blood* 2002;100:1334.
27. Olieman AFT, van Ginkel RJ, Hoekstra HJ, et al. Angiographic response of locally advanced soft-tissue sarcoma following hyperthermic isolated limb perfusion with tumor necrosis factor. *Ann Surg Oncol* 1997;4:64.
28. Fraker D, Alexander HR, Ross M, et al. A phase II trial of isolated limb perfusion with high dose tumor necrosis factor and melphalan for unresectable extremity sarcomas. *Soc Surg Oncol* 1999;53:22.
29. Posner MC, Lienard D, Lejeune FJ, Rosenfelder D, Kirkwood J. Hyperthermic isolated limb perfusion with tumor necrosis factor alone for melanoma. *Cancer J Sci Am* 1995;1:274.
30. Ferroni P, di Filippo F, Martini F, et al. Effects of isolated limb perfusion with tumor necrosis factor-alpha on circulating levels of proinflammatory cytokines. *J Immunother* 2001;24:354.
31. Lans TE, Bartlett DL, Libutti SK, et al. Role of tumor necrosis factor (TNF) on toxicity and cytokine production following isolated hepatic perfusion (IHP). *Clin Cancer Res* 2001;7:784.
32. Lienard D, Lejeune F, Ewalenko I. In transit metastases of malignant melanoma treated by high dose rTNFα in combination with interferon-gamma and melphalan in isolation perfusion. *World J Surg* 1992;16:234.
33. Vaglini M, Santinami M, Manzi R, et al. Treatment of in-transit metastases from cutaneous melanoma by isolation perfusion with tumour necrosis factor-alpha (TNF-α), melphalan and interferon-gamma (IFN-γ). Dose-finding experience at the National Cancer Institute of Milan. *Melanoma Res* 1994;4:35.
34. Minor DR, Allen RE, Alberts D, et al. A clinical and pharmacokinetic study of isolated limb perfusion with heat and melphalan for melanoma. *Cancer* 1985;55:2638.
35. Klaase JM, Kroon BBR, van Geel AN, et al. Prognostic factors for tumor response and limb recurrence-free interval in patients with advanced melanoma of the limbs treated with regional isolated perfusion using melphalan. *Surgery* 1994;115:39.
36. Koops HS, Vaglini M, Suciu S, et al. Prophylactic isolated limb perfusion for localized, high-risk limb melanoma: results of a multicenter randomized Phase III trial. *J Clin Oncol* 1998;16:2906.
37. Klaase JM, Kroon BBR, Benckhuijsen C, et al. Results of regional isolation perfusion with cytostatics in patients with soft tissue tumors of the extremities. *Cancer* 1989;64:616.
38. Eggermont AMM, Koops HS, Klausner JM, et al. Isolated limb perfusion with tumor necrosis factor and melphalan for limb salvage in 186 patients with locally advanced soft tissue extremity sarcomas. *Ann Surg* 1996;224:756.
39. Rossi CR, Foletto M, di Filippo F, et al. Soft tissue limb sarcomas: Italian clinical trials with hyperthermic antiblastic perfusion. *Cancer* 1999;86:1742.
40. Lindner P, Fjalling M, Hafstrom L, Nielsen H, Mattson H. Isolated hepatic perfusion with extracorporeal oxygenation using hyperthermia tumour necrosis factor alpha and melphalan. *Eur J Surg Oncol* 1999;25:179.
41. Vahrmeijer AL, Van Dierendonck JH, Keizer HJ, et al. Increased local cytostatic drug exposure by isolated hepatic perfusion: a phase I clinical and pharmacologic evaluation of treatment with high dose melphalan in patients with colorectal cancer confined to the liver. *Br J Cancer* 2000;82:1539.
42. de Vries MR, Borel Rinkes IH, van de Velder CJH, et al. Isolated hepatic perfusion with tumor necrosis factor a and melphalan: experimental studies in pigs and phase I data from humans. *Recent Results Cancer Res* 1998;147:107.
43. Bartlett DL, Libutti SK, Figg WD, Fraker DL, Alexander HR. Isolated hepatic perfusion for unresectable hepatic metastases from colorectal cancer. *Surgery* 2001;129:176.
44. Pass HI, Mew DJY, Kranda KC, et al. Isolated lung perfusion with tumor necrosis factor for pulmonary metastases. *Ann Thorac Surg* 1996;61:1609.
45. Thompson JF, Siebert GA, Anissimov YG, et al. Microdialysis and response during regional chemotherapy by isolated limb infusion of melphalan for limb malignancies. *Br J Cancer* 2001;85:157.
46. Guadagni S, Russo F, Rossi CR, et al. Deliberate hypoxic pelvic and limb chemoperfusion in the treatment of recurrent melanoma. *Am J Surg* 2002;183:28.
47. Pingpank JF, Libutti SK, Chang R, et al. A phase I feasibility study of hepatic arterial melphalan infusion with hepatic arterial melphalan infusion with hepatic venous hemofiltration using percutaneously placed catheters in patients with unresectable hepatic malignancies. *Am Soc Clin Oncol Proc* 2003;22:282.
48. Lienard D, Eggermont AMM, Schraffordt-Koops H, et al. Isolated limb perfusion with tumour necrosis factor-alpha and melphalan with or without interferon-gamma for the treatment of in-transit melanoma metastases: a multicentre randomized phase II study. *Melanoma Res* 1999;9:491.
49. Fraker DL, Alexander HR, Bartlett DL, Rosenberg SA. A prospective randomized trial of therapeutic isolated limb perfusion (ILP) comparing melphalan (M) versus melphalan, tumor necrosis factor (TNF) and interferon-gamma (IFN): an initial report. *Soc Surg Oncol* 1996;49:6.

CHAPTER 51

Treatment of Metastatic Cancer

DAVID A. LARSON
JAMES L. RUBENSTEIN
MICHAEL W. MCDERMOTT

SECTION **1**

Metastatic Brain Cancer

BRAIN METASTASES

Parenchymal brain metastases are a common manifestation of systemic cancer, far outnumbering primary brain tumors, and are a significant cause of neurologic problems. The incidence is thought to be increasing, because of improved imaging and more frequent screening studies in cancer patients. Current outcome information for different treatment modalities indicates that local control and good neurologic quality of life are commonly achieved. Future studies of standard and novel therapies will no doubt better define patient subsets in which survival is increased.

For decades, whole brain radiotherapy (WBRT) was considered the standard of care in patients with brain metastases. Beginning in the 1970s, WBRT fractionation schemes were studied extensively in large phase III trials. More recently, beginning in the 1990s, focal therapy (surgery or radiosurgery) and combinations of focal and WBRT have been studied in phase III trials, and information gained in those studies can be used to support the use of WBRT, surgery, radiosurgery, or combinations of those as initial therapy. In this chapter the results of phase III trials are emphasized more than are the hundreds of retrospective reports that motivated activation of formal trials. Published outcomes are reported mainly in terms of survival, local control of known brain metastases, and freedom from new brain metastases. Randomized trial outcome data are helpful in determining "best" initial brain therapy, particularly if future salvage therapy, in the event of failure, is not considered. Realistically, however, most patients who are initially candidates for focal therapy remain candidates for and actually receive salvage therapy of some form, unless lost to follow-up. Many investigators have not subjected outcome of initial plus salvage therapy to actuarial analysis, but those who have conclude that in some cases initial choice of therapy may be less important than previously thought.[1] Future studies will undoubtedly investigate the relationship between initial therapy, salvage therapy, outcome, and cost.

Rapid progress in imaging technology must influence current interpretation of previous studies. With the improved sensitivity of today's imaging, some patients who earlier were found to have either a single brain metastasis or no extracranial metastases, or both, might now be found to have multiple intracranial or extracranial metastases, or both, which would confer a less favorable prognosis and might require different therapy. In addition, the use of today's sensitive imaging, together with the more frequent use of high-dose contrast, may increase the apparent size of metastases and delineated radiosurgery target volumes. A small increase in radiosurgery margins has been shown to markedly increase local control.[2]

EPIDEMIOLOGY

The exact incidence of brain metastases is not known. Historical data, based on surgeries performed in patients with clinically favorable cancer, suggested that brain metastases were relatively infrequent, accounting for only one in ten intracranial tumors. Although subsequent estimates vary, they indicate the opposite—that brain metastases actually occur up to ten times more frequently than primary brain tumors. In a Memorial Sloan-Kettering Cancer Center autopsy series, 15% of cancer patients had brain metastases.[3] A Roswell Park Memorial Institute autopsy study found that 55% of melanoma patients had brain metastases.[4] A population-based study in the Netherlands found that brain metastases developed in 8.5% of cancer patients.[5] This latter study showed the 5-year cumulative incidence of brain metastases to be approximately 16%, 10%, 7%, 5%, and 1% for patients with lung cancer, renal cell cancer, melanoma, breast cancer, and colorectal carcinoma, respectively. These incidence estimates for specific pathologies can be applied to estimates of new cancer cases in the United States for 2003 to yield an estimate of approximately 60,000 cases of brain metastases.[6] However, if autopsy-based incidence figures are used, the expected number of cases of brain metastases may be as high as 170,000.[7]

Numerous authors hypothesize that the incidence of brain metastases is expected to increase as a result of several factors: improved cancer treatments, which lead in turn to longer survival; earlier brain screening for those specific cancers that have a predilection for brain metastases; and increased capability of modern imaging to detect early brain metastases. Although this hypothesis seems reasonable, Schouten et al.[5] found no evidence for an increasing incidence of brain metastases, at least over the period 1986 to 1995.

Certain primary cancers have a predilection for spread to the central nervous system (CNS). However, the reported percentage of cases of each primary type that metastasizes to the brain varies considerably, possibly because of methodologic differences between studies. Lassman and De Angelis[8] reviewed nine studies and found the following variation in reported percentages of patients developing brain metastases for specific primary histologies: 18% to 64% (lung cancer), 2% to 21% (breast cancer), 2% to 12% (colorectal cancer), 4% to 16% (melanoma), 1% to 8% (kidney), 1% to 10% (thyroid), and 1% to 18% (unknown primary). The overall rate of brain metastases was 6% to 24% in five cited studies. Some tumors, such as prostate, oropharyngeal, and skin carcinoma, rarely metastasize to the brain. In children the incidence of brain metastases is approximately 6% to 10%, and the most common associated solid primary tumors are sarcoma, Wilms' tumor, neuroblastoma, and germ cell tumor.[9,10]

Considerable variability is found at time of diagnosis of brain metastases. The median interval from diagnosis of cancer to that of brain metastasis is 12 months.[11] For some primary cancers, such as melanoma, breast cancer, renal cell carcinoma, or gynecologic cancer, the median interval is 2 to 3 years.[11] In up to one-third of patients, brain metastases are diagnosed within 1 month of the primary cancer diagnosis[5]; such are referred to as *synchronous metastases*. In rare instances, brain metastases are first diagnosed more than 10 years after the diagnosis of primary cancer.

METASTATIC SPREAD

The metastatic process involves a series of complex, sequential events involving subpopulations of tumor cells. Metastatic cells that successfully colonize the brain must (1) escape from the primary tumor via local invasion; (2) enter the lymphatic or vascular system, which has numerous interconnections; (3) circulate to and exit from the brain microvasculature; (4) evade immune and nonimmune responses; and (5) grow in response to the local brain microenvironment.

Access to the brain by tumor cells is governed by the blood–brain barrier, a physiologic/anatomic structure defined by tight junctions between brain and endothelial cells, a thick basement membrane, and underlying astrocytes that regulate the flow of nutrients, ions, and cells into the brain. For brain metastases to develop, malignant cells must adhere to the luminal surface of brain microvessel luminal cells and then invade the blood–brain barrier. This process involves the expression of various cell surface receptors and degradative enzymes. It is assumed that a series of genetic, biochemical, and biologic properties is responsible for the growth of brain metastases, possibly reflected in as yet poorly understood quantitative changes in the expression of several genes. Successful metastatic growth in the brain likely requires unique tumor cell characteristics that may not be necessary for successful growth at other organ sites.

Brain metastases may occur on the surface of the brain (leptomeninges and meninges) or within the parenchyma (cerebrum, cerebellum, brainstem). The vast majority of brain metastases from solid tumors result from hematogenous spread rather than from dissemination via cerebral spinal fluid or from direct brain invasion by head and neck cancer. Thus, the distribution of brain metastases mainly reflects blood flow, with approximately 80% of lesions found in the cerebrum, 15% in the cerebellum, and 5% in the brainstem.[11,12] Posterior fossa metastases appear to arise disproportionately from pelvic or abdominal primary tumors.[12] It has been hypothesized that cells originating from pelvic or abdominal primary cancers may gain access to the posterior fossa or leptomeninges through Batson's vertebral venous plexus without passing through the lungs.

Within the brain parenchyma, single malignant cells or metastatic emboli with a typical diameter of 100 to 200 μm may lodge in regions where there is a sudden reduction of vascular caliber, such as in the gray/white matter junction. In this area and in the most distal vascular fields, called *border or watershed zones*, blood vessels narrow to a diameter of approximately 50 μm. Hwang et al.[13] examined computed tomography (CT) and magnetic resonance imaging (MRI) studies in 100 patients with 302 evaluable metastatic lesions and found that the major vascular border zones were the sites of growth in 62% of lesions, even though the border zones constituted only 29% of the area. Likewise, the gray/white matter junction was the preferred site for 64% of lesions.

Brain metastases tend to be well circumscribed, without infiltration into surrounding brain tissue, sometimes with associated edema. Some metastases may have associated hemorrhage, particularly from renal cell carcinoma, melanoma, or choriocarcinoma primaries.

CLINICAL PRESENTATION

Brain metastases should be included in the differential diagnosis in any cancer patient in whom new neurologic symptoms or signs develop. Common clinical presentations, in descending order, include headache (24% to 53%), focal weakness (16% to 40%), altered mental status (24% to 31%), seizures (15% to 16%), and ataxia (9% to 20%).[11,14] Occasionally, hemorrhage within a brain metastasis may cause acute onset of neurologic symptoms. More often, neurologic symptoms develop over days or weeks. Data acquired during 1973 to 1993 indicate that only 10% of patients diagnosed with brain metastases by CT or MRI were symptomatic.[11] However, it is possible that a smaller percentage of today's patients are symptomatic, because screening imaging is more frequently performed and imaging modalities are more sensitive.

IMAGING AND DIAGNOSIS

Brain CT is often performed on patients suspected of having brain metastasis. However, MRI is the more sensitive study and is performed if CT is nondiagnostic or if additional information, such as number of lesions, is needed to determine therapy. Recommended pre-gadolinium studies include T2-weighted and T1-weighted sequences. Recommended postgadolinium studies include T1-weighted and fluid-attenuated inversion-recovery sequences. Contiguous thin axial slices without skips are necessary to ensure that the smallest lesions are detected. If the diagnosis of brain metastasis remains in doubt, biopsy should be considered. Patchell et al.[15] reported that, of 54 patients with a single brain lesion who were enrolled on a formal study in which biopsy was required before therapy, 11% had nonmetastatic lesions, including glial tumor, abscess, and inflammatory process.

Two studies have evaluated the role of MRI in patients found to have a single metastasis on CT. Kuhn et al.[16] compared triple-dose gadoteridol MRI with contrast-enhanced CT and conventional-dose gadopentetate dimeglumine MRI studies in four patients with a single intracranial metastasis demonstrated on contrast-enhanced CT. Eighteen total brain metastases, and more than one in all four patients, were demonstrated on gadoteridol MRI, compared to the four seen on CT. In 1999, Schellinger et al.[14] investigated 55 patients with single brain metastasis according to CT and found that 31% had multiple brain metastases on MRI. The two main characteristics for brain metastases missed by CT were smaller diameter and frontotemporal location.

Several studies have demonstrated that the dose of intravenous contrast used for MRI is important in determining the number of brain metastases detected and is without increased toxicity.[16–20] Most recently, Schneider et al.[20] studied 74 patients with one to eight proven intraaxial metastatic lesions to the brain using 0.1-mmol/kg bolus injections of gadobenate dimeglumine at 10-minute intervals over a 20-minute period. Cumulative dosing produced significant dose-related increases in lesion-to-brain ratio and lesion signal intensity enhancement. Significantly more lesions were noted after the second injection compared to the first. In patients with one lesion observed after the first injection, additional lesions were noted in approximately 20% of patients after a second injection. Nevertheless, the use of high-dose contrast is not yet widespread. Whether or not the use of high-dose contrast is more cost effective than standard-dose contrast MRI is unknown, likely because of difficulty in understanding the cost effectiveness of subsequent interventions.

High-dose contrast MRI is potentially most valuable in patients thought to have a single brain metastasis, because the therapeutic approach may be different than if multiple metastases are found. During the CT era, as many as 50% of patients with tumor metastatic to the brain were found to have a single metastasis.[12] However, it is almost certain that the current percentage is lower, given the increased sensitivity of modern imaging. Current patient data acquired with modern CT and MRI technology indicate that approximately 20% of patients thought to have a single brain metastasis based on CT actually have multiple lesions on MRI.[14]

PROGNOSIS

Numerous pre-CT-era studies have shown that survival time in patients with symptomatic brain metastases is approximately 1 to 2 months without therapy, 2 to 3 months with corticosteroid therapy, and 3 to 6 months with WBRT. These survival data are consistent with current outcome data in patients who do not meet selection criteria for focal brain therapy. Retrospective recursive partitioning analysis (RPA) of prognostic factors was performed by Gaspar et al.,[21] who studied more than 1100 patients receiving external-beam radiotherapy after enrolling in various Radiation Therapy Oncology Group (RTOG) brain metastasis trials during 1979 to 1993. The radiotherapy fractionation and dose schedules varied over a broad range. By today's standards some of these individuals would have been candidates for focal therapy. Patients were found to fall into three well-defined prognostic groups, with significantly different median survivals. For RPA class 1 patients [those younger than 65 years, with a Karnofsky performance score (KPS) of 70 or greater, controlled primary tumor, and no extracranial metastases], median survival was 7.1 months. For RPA class 3 patients (those with KPS of less than 70), median survival was 2.3 months. For the remaining patients, those in RPA class 2, median survival was 4.2 months (Fig. 51.1-1).

Today, many diagnoses of brain metastases are made relatively early, while patients are asymptomatic and when aggressive focal therapy, such as surgery or radiosurgery, can be offered. Patients who satisfy selection criteria for focal therapy appear to have a more favorable prognosis. Sneed et al.[22] found that sur-

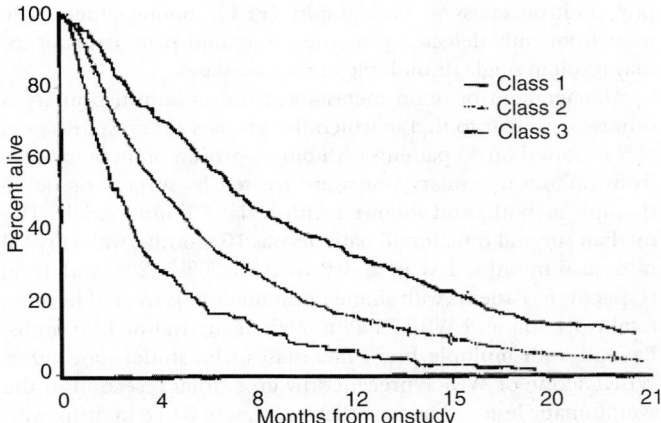

FIGURE 51.1-1. Median survival according to recursive partitioning analysis (RPA) class, based on analysis of 1200 patients treated on three consecutive Radiation Therapy Oncology Group trials conducted between 1979 and 1993, testing several different fractionation schemes and radiation sensitizers. RPA class 1 is comprised of patients less than 65 years old, Karnofsky performance score (KPS) of 70 or greater, controlled primary tumor, and no extracranial metastases. RPA class 3 is comprised of patients with KPS less than 70. RPA class 2 is comprised of all other patients. (From ref. 23, with permission.)

TABLE 51.1-1.   Median Survival According to Recursive Partitioning Analysis Class and Selected Initial Brain Therapy[a]

Initial Treatment	Patients (n)	Median Survival (Mo) by RPA Class		
		Class 1	Class 2	Class 3
WBRT (RTOG phase III trials)[21]	1176	7.1	4.2	2.3
Radiosurgery[22]	265	14.0	8.2	5.3
WBRT + radiosurgery[22]	295	15.2	7.0	5.5
Surgery + WBRT[23]	125	14.8	9.9	6.0

RPA, recursive partitioning analysis; RTOG, Radiation Therapy Oncology Group; WBRT, whole brain radiotherapy.
[a]Patients who satisfied selection criteria for and received focal therapy according to various institutional policies appear to have better median survival than RTOG WBRT trial patients treated during 1977 to 1993. It is not known how many of the RTOG WBRT patients might have met current selection criteria for radiosurgery. RPA class 1 is comprised of patients <65 years old, Karnofsky performance score (KPS) of ≥70, controlled primary tumor, and no extracranial metastases. RPA class 3 is comprised of patients with KPS <70. RPA class 2 is comprised of all other patients.

vival was substantially greater in patients receiving radiosurgery, with or without WBRT, than that found in patients in the RTOG WBRT trials, for each of the three RPA classes. Agboola et al.[23] found improved survival in all three RPA classes for patients undergoing surgical resection and WBRT. These RPA prognostic data are summarized in Table 51.1-1.

UNKNOWN PRIMARY TUMOR

Pavlidis et al.[24] reviewed the management of cancer of unknown primary tumor, which accounts for up to 3% of malignant neoplasms. It represents a heterogeneous group of malignancies that share unique clinical and biologic behavior. In most patients the primary site remains unknown despite extensive workup, including immunohistochemistry, electron microscopy, CT, mammography, positron emission tomography (PET), among others. The most frequently detected primaries, lung and pancreas cancers, may result in single or multiple brain metastases.

Management of brain metastases from unknown primary is otherwise similar to that in which the primary is known. Ruda et al.[25] reported on 33 patients with biopsy-proven brain metastases from unknown primary who were treated by surgery or radiotherapy, or both, and followed with serial CT until death. The median survival time for all patients was 10 months, with survival rates at 6 months, 1 year, and 2 years of 76%, 42%, and 15%, respectively. Patients with single brain metastasis treated by gross total resection and WBRT had a median survival of 13 months. Patients with multiple brain metastases who underwent either WBRT alone or WBRT preceded by gross total resection of the symptomatic lesions had a median survival of 6 to 8 months, with none alive at 2 years. In 85% of patients with a single brain metastasis, a significant improvement in neurologic functions was observed after surgical resection; among patients with multiple brain metastases, a neurologic improvement was observed in all those who had a resection of symptomatic lesions and only in one-half of the patients who had WBRT alone. The number of brain metastases was the only significant factor affecting survival according to univariate and multivariate analysis. Whether this

series is representative of typical unknown primary patients is uncertain, because the primary tumor was eventually found in 82% of patients during the follow-up period, a much larger percentage than that otherwise reported in the literature.

SYMPTOM MANAGEMENT

Corticosteroids

Corticosteroids are generally indicated in brain metastasis patients with symptomatic peritumoral edema. The antiedema effect of corticosteroids is usually attributed to a reduction in the permeability of abnormal tumor capillaries. Dexamethasone is typically used, given its low mineralocorticoid activity and relatively low risk of cognitive impairment and infection. Typical dosing consists of a 10-mg loading dose followed by 16 mg/d in divided doses, although lower doses are often used. Steroids should be tapered as clinically indicated, with taper based primarily on clinical rather than imaging evaluation.

Although clinical experience has established the effectiveness of dexamethasone in reducing symptoms and MRI evidence of peritumoral edema, often within days of symptom onset, the need for corticosteroids in all patients with brain metastases remains uncertain. Few contemporary studies have analyzed the risks and benefits of dexamethasone in patients with brain metastases. Hempen et al.[26] studied 138 patients with primary or metastatic brain tumors treated with radiotherapy. Those with brain metastases (n = 91) were given standard-fraction WBRT over 2 to 3 weeks, and most received dexamethasone with tapering doses, for a mean duration of 6.9 weeks. Clinical improvements possibly attributable to dexamethasone were observed in 33% of patients shortly after it was initiated, in 44% during radiotherapy, and in 11% after radiotherapy. However, side effects possibly attributable to dexamethasone were frequently observed, including hyperglycemia (47%), peripheral edema (11%), psychiatric disorder (10%), oropharyngeal candidiasis (7%), Cushing's syndrome (4%), muscular weakness (4%), and pulmonary embolism (2%). Among 13 patients who received radiotherapy without dexamethasone, treatment was well tolerated, except in 1 patient with brainstem symptoms. Together these limited data suggest that dexamethasone need not be initiated in asymptomatic patients.

Some early studies used radiation dose/fractionation regimens that are currently considered nonstandard. In particular, Harwood and Simson[27] found that 27% of patients treated with rapid fractionation (1000-cGy single fraction) experienced acute signs or symptoms of increased intracranial pressure, now thought to be caused by dose-dependent, radiation-induced permeability of the blood–brain barrier.[28] These data lend support to the widely accepted view that patients receiving high-dose radiosurgery for brain metastases should receive a single loading dose of corticosteroids at the time of radiosurgery. However, there is little evidence suggesting that steroids have a role in standard WBRT for brain metastases absent clinical symptoms related to blood–brain barrier breakdown.

Antiseizure Medication

Approximately 15% of patients with brain metastasis present with seizures, and most such patients are found to have supratentorial lesions. Patients who present with seizures or in whom seizures develop during therapy should be started on antiseizure medications. In the absence of seizures, prophylactic antiseizure medications are generally not started. Forsyth et al.[29] conducted a clinical trial to determine if prophylactic antiseizure medications in brain tumor patients without prior seizures reduced seizure frequency. One hundred newly diagnosed brain tumor patients received antiseizure medications or not in a prospective, randomized, unblinded study. Sixty patients had metastatic tumors, and 40 had primary brain tumors. Subsequent seizures occurred in 26 (26%) of patients. However, seizure-free survivals were similar. At 3 months, 87% of the medicated group and 90% of the nonmedicated group were seizure free. It was concluded that prophylactic antiseizure medications are unnecessary in brain tumor patients who have not had a seizure. These data and conclusions confirm the earlier results of other investigators.[30] A possible exception is the patient with brain metastases in highly epileptogenic areas or the patient with tumors that frequently involve the cortex, such as melanomas. A retrospective study by Byrne et al.[31] found that prophylactic antiepileptic medications in patients with metastatic melanoma reduced the subsequent seizure frequency from 37% to 17%.

Side effects of antiseizure medications include morbilliform rashes, Stevens-Johnson syndrome, shoulder-hand syndrome, or other side effects that would warrant changing or discontinuing therapy. Some antiseizure medications interact with dexamethasone or chemotherapeutic agents, and some stimulate the cytochrome P-450 enzyme system to accelerate the metabolism of chemotherapeutic agents.

Venous Thromboembolism

Venous thromboembolism occurs commonly in cancer patients, resulting in significant morbidity and mortality. Sorensen at al.[32] found the 1-year survival rate for cancer patients with thrombosis to be only 12%, compared to 36% in cancer patients without thrombosis, possibly reflecting thromboembolism and a more aggressive course of cancers associated with it. Patients with brain tumors and thrombosis are thought to be at increased risk for intracranial hemorrhage with anticoagulation. Whether such patients are best managed with inferior vena cava (IVC) filters remains controversial. Levin et al.[33] found a 62% complication rate in 42 patients with intracranial malignancy and venous thrombosis treated with IVC filters. Schiff and DeAngelis[34] reviewed similar patients treated instead with anticoagulation and found that only 3 of 42 (7%) experienced cerebral hemorrhage. They also found that recurrent venous thromboembolism requiring anticoagulation developed in four of ten (40%) patients who received an IVC filter. This may suggest that anticoagulation is safe for patients with those metastatic cancer pathologies that are thought to be less prone to hemorrhage.

TREATMENT

In this section, the results of important randomized trials involving brain metastases are emphasized, when possible, and less emphasis is placed on retrospective studies. On the surface, the randomized trial results tend to make a good case for more treatment rather than less: WBRT *plus* radiosensitizers, WBRT *plus* surgery, WBRT *plus* radiosurgery. Although the few studies defining long-term risks of WBRT indicate relatively low risk of serious side effects in 1-year survivors, provided extended fractionation schemes are used, concern for those risks motivates some practitioners to avoid initial WBRT and instead use focal therapy alone (radiosurgery or surgery). Whether such patients are less than optimally treated is not immediately obvious. Most patients who qualify for focal therapy are likely to be carefully followed, and most are likely to have salvage therapy at the time of brain recurrence. The randomized trials do not report actuarial outcome analysis of initial plus salvage therapy. Sneed et al.,[1] in a retrospective study, found that omission of WBRT in patients receiving initial radiosurgery for up to four brain metastases did not compromise intracranial control, provided salvage therapy information was included in the actuarial outcome analysis.

Whole Brain Radiotherapy

The outcome of WBRT for brain metastasis was first described 50 years ago. Symptomatic improvement was observed in approximately 60% of patients, and median survival times were 3 to 6 months,[35–37] compared to 1 to 2 months without treatment.[38–40] Beginning in 1970, numerous WBRT randomized trials were conducted by the RTOG.[41–45] These trials examined a wide variety of fractionation schemes and drew numerous conclusions. For example, RTOG 6901 and RTOG 7361, involving greater than 1800 patients, found complete or partial clinical responses in 60% to 90% of symptomatic patients, with median duration of improvement in 10 to 12 weeks, and with 75% to 80% of remaining survival time spent in an improved or stable neurologic state. Brain metastases were reported to be the cause of death in 30% to 50% of patients. These trials did not show significant differences with respect to survival times, symptomatic response rates, or duration of symptomatic response.

Studies of ultra-rapid fractionated WBRT (10 Gy in one fraction, 12 Gy in two fractions, 15 Gy in two fractions over 3 days), as carried out by RTOG and other investigators,[41–47] showed a possible increased risk of herniation and death within a few days of treatment and are not recommended. Likewise, no advantage was seen in giving either 50 Gy in 20 fractions or 54.4 Gy at 1.6 Gy twice daily over the more commonly prescribed 30 Gy in 10 fractions.[44,45] As a result, the most common fractionation schemes include 30 Gy in 10 fractions, 37.5 Gy in 15 fractions, and 40 Gy in 20 fractions. Regimens using ten or fewer fractions, which are thought to have increased toxicity, are used in patients with poor prognosis, because they are not expected to live long enough to experience serious side effects. The longer, less toxic regimens, which use smaller daily fractions, are most often used in patients expected to live longer than 6 months.

The most thorough imaging analysis of response rates to WBRT was performed by Nieder et al.,[48] who studied CT responses in 108 patients with 336 measurable lesions after WBRT (30 Gy in ten fractions). They found an overall response rate of 59%, by lesion (complete response rate of 24%, partial response rate of 35%). Complete response rates by tumor type were 37% for small cell carcinoma, 35% for breast cancer, 25% for squamous cell carcinoma, 14% for nonbreast adenocarcinoma, 0% for renal cell carcinoma, and 0% for melanoma. Improved complete response rates were associated with smaller tumor volume and absence of necrosis. Complete response rates were 39% for solid metastases, 15% if less than 50% necrosis, and 11% if 50%

or greater necrosis. Complete response rates were inversely related to volume, ranging stepwise from 52% for lesion volumes of 0.5 mL or less to 0% for lesions greater than 10 mL.[48] In a separate study, Nieder et al.[49] calculated biologically effective dose to compare the effect of various fractionation schemes and found that partial remission rates increased with increasing biologically effective dose but complete remission rates failed to do so, unexpectedly. Other analyses quantify outcome in terms of local control rather than local response. Randomized trials reported by Kondziolka et al.[50] and Patchell et al.[15] indicate that 1-year actuarial local control after WBRT alone is in the range of 0% to 14%. Taken together, these data indicate that long-term control of gross brain metastases after WBRT is unlikely.

Side effects occurring during or shortly after WBRT include hair loss, mild skin reaction, fatigue, and, in some patients, ototoxicity. Hair regrows in 6 to 12 months, skin reactions resolve after several weeks, and fatigue improves after a few months. In occasional patients outpatient myringotomy may be required to relieve radiation-induced fluid buildup behind the tympanic membrane.

The frequency of long-term side effects of WBRT is unclear. The most frequently referenced study is that of DeAngelis et al.,[51] who reported a 1-year rate of dementia of 11% in patients with nonrecurrent brain metastases initially treated with WBRT. This rate must be viewed within the context of the study, which involved 47 patients, with 5 developing dementia. Each of the five received either daily dose fractions greater than 3 Gy or radiation-sensitizing agents. Of 15 patients treated with "safe" radiation fractionation (less than 3 Gy per fraction), none had dementia at 1 year. More recently, Penitzka et al.[52] assessed intelligence, attention, and memory in 29 patients with brain metastases before and after WBRT. They determined that neuropsychological capacity in small cell lung cancer patients was impaired even before prophylactic cranial irradiation, possibly caused by previous chemotherapy. More important, they concluded that therapeutic WBRT delivered in patients with brain metastases other than from small cell lung cancer did not induce a significant decline in cognitive function. Although these two studies are small, they lend support to the notion that risk of brain radiation toxicity is dose and fractionation dependent, but relatively low provided today's standard fractionation schemes are used.

Nieder et al.[53] related use of carbamapazine to risks of symptomatic late toxicity in WBRT patients and found an actuarial rate of 50% among those who had taken carbamapazine during and after radiotherapy, compared to 18% among patients who had not. Some of the side effects of drug treatment may be indistinguishable from those of WBRT, however.

In patients undergoing surgical resection of a single metastasis followed by WBRT (30 Gy in 10 fractions or 40 Gy in 20 fractions), Nieder et al.[54] reported a 42% 2-year actuarial probability of symptomatic mild, moderate, or severe late radiation toxicity, although details regarding the nature of the toxicity were not included. Whether surgery predisposes to increased risk of radiation toxicity is unclear.

Whole Brain Radiotherapy ± Radiation Sensitizers

Radiosensitizers are pharmacologic agents that enhance the lethal effects of radiotherapy when administered together with it. For a radiosensitizer to be practical, its enhanced effects must be greater in tumor tissue than in normal tissue. Two phase III studies have evaluated radiosensitizers in patients with brain metastases.

Mehta et al.[55] reported on survival and neurologic outcomes in a randomized trial of WBRT (30 Gy/ten fractions) with or without daily injections of motexafin gadolinium (MGd). MGd is a redox mediator that selectively targets tumor cells, decreases local oxygen consumption, and is detectable by MRI. A total of 401 patients were enrolled. No significant differences were seen in median survival (5.2 months in the sensitizer arm compared to 4.9 months in the control arm) or median time to neurologic progression (9.5 months compared to 8.3 months). However, among 251 non–small cell lung cancer patients, MGd was found to improve median time to neurologic progression (not reached compared to 7.4 months; $P = .48$). An ongoing phase III study will more definitively determine if patients with brain metastases from non–small cell lung cancer treated with MGd and WBRT retain neurologic function and mentation longer than patients receiving WBRT alone. Kumar et al.[56] examined the impact of anemia in the entire group of 401 patients and found that, although anemia adversely affected survival, the adverse prognostic effect of anemia was overcome by treatment with MGd.

Suh et al.[57] reported results of a randomized trial comparing WBRT (30 Gy/ten fractions) and supplemental oxygen with WBRT after daily injections of RSR13 and supplemental oxygen. RSR13 is an allosteric modifier of hemoglobin that reduces hemoglobin oxygen-binding affinity, facilitates oxygen release, and increases tissue PO_2. A total of 538 patients were enrolled. Patients in the RSR13 arm experienced greater median survival than those in the control arm (5.3 months compared to 4.5 months). Among individuals with breast cancer primaries, median survival was 8.7 months in the RSR arm compared to 4.6 months in the control arm. In addition, an RSR13 dose–response relationship was demonstrated.

Surgery

Surgery is useful to confirm the diagnosis, relieve mass effect, improve local control and survival, and salvage failures after prior therapy. Numerous reports indicate the most important predictor of survival after resection of a single metastasis is favorable status of systemic disease (i.e., "absent" or "controlled"). Reported unfavorable survival factors include poor general medical condition, poor neurologic status, infratentorial tumor location, advanced age, male gender, and short interval from diagnosis of primary cancer to diagnosis of brain metastasis. Surgical advances, such as intraoperative localization and functional mapping, now allow excision of some metastases previously considered unresectable. Nevertheless, thalamic, basal ganglia, and brainstem metastases are not usually considered for resection because of excessive risks of morbidity. Patients with single metastasis in most other sites may be good candidates for surgery. Lang and Sawaya[58] summarized median survivals after surgical resection of brain metastasis, according to primary tumor type, based on 46 published reports. They found the following average median survivals by tumor type: melanoma (7 months), lung cancer (12 months), renal cell cancer (10 months), breast cancer (12 months), and colon cancer (9 months).

Patients with multiple metastases may be candidates for surgery provided each lesion is considered resectable. If all lesions are not

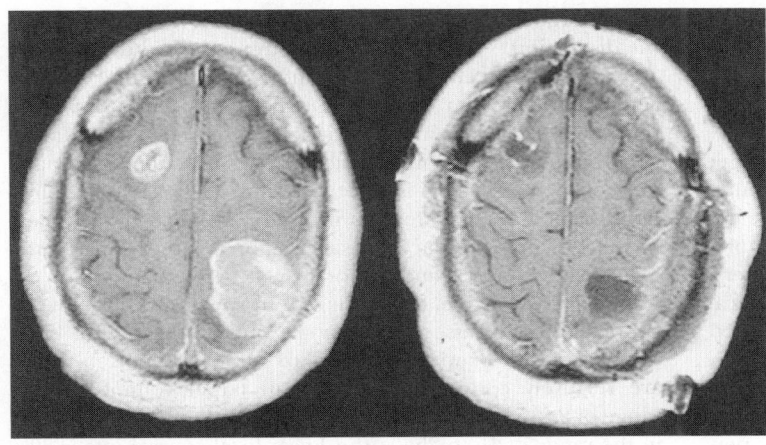

FIGURE 51.1-2. Example of resectable multiple cerebral metastases. Preoperative (**left**) and postoperative (**right**) gadolinium-enhanced T1-weighted axial MRI of bilateral brain metastases. The lesions were resected by two separate craniotomies performed at the same sitting. (From ref. 58, with permission of Wiley-Liss, Inc., a subsidiary of John Wiley & Sons, Inc.)

considered resectable, operation can be considered for those symptomatic lesions that are resectable. The most complete analysis of outcome after surgical resection of multiple lesions is that of Bindal et al.,[59] who reviewed 56 patients undergoing resection for multiple brain metastases. Patients were retrospectively placed in one of two groups: 30 patients who had at least one unresected lesion (group A) and 26 who had all lesions resected (group B). A third group, for comparison purposes, consisted of 26 matched controls with single surgically resected metastasis (group C). Median survivals were 6, 14, and 14 months for groups A, B, and C, respectively. Surgical mortality was 3%, 4%, and 0%; surgical morbidity was 8%, 9%, and 8%, respectively. Among group B patients, 83% of symptomatic patients improved, 11% remained stable, and 6% worsened. These data imply that in patients with multiple brain metastases who are otherwise good surgical candidates surgical resection of all lesions is as effective as surgical resection in patients with a single metastasis. An example of resection of multiple cerebral metastases is shown in Figure 51.1-2.

Modern 30-day surgical mortality after surgical resection of a single metastasis is approximately 0% to 10%.[58] Surgical morbidity includes neurologic deficits (0% to 13%) and nonneurologic complications (0% to 20%), including embolism, thrombosis, and wound infections.[58]

Whole Brain Radiotherapy ± Surgery

Three prospective, randomized trials have evaluated the role of preradiation surgery in patients who receive WBRT. Two of the three provide support for the use of surgery plus WBRT rather than WBRT alone in selected patients with good performance status, controlled extracranial disease, and a single brain metastasis.

In the first trial, Patchell et al.[15] studied 48 patients with a single brain metastasis who were randomized to surgical resection and WBRT versus needle biopsy and WBRT (36 Gy in 12 fractions). Patients in the resection arm had significantly improved local control (80%) compared to those randomized to biopsy and WBRT (48%). Patients in the resection arm also had significantly increased median duration of functional independence (38 vs. 8 weeks), and median survival (40 vs. 15 weeks). Factors found to be associated with longer survival included younger age, no extracranial disease, surgical resection, and longer interval from primary diagnosis to diagnosis of brain metastasis.

In the second trial, Noordijk et al.[60] studied 63 patients with a single brain metastasis who were randomized to surgical resec-

tion and WBRT versus WBRT (40 Gy in 20 fractions). Patients in the resection arm had significantly longer functionally independent median survival (7.5 vs. 3.5 months) and longer median survival (10 vs. 6 months). However, there was no survival benefit for patients with active extracranial disease (5 months in each arm). For patients without active extracranial disease, the median survival time was significantly improved in the resection arm (12 vs. 7 months).

In the third study, Mintz and Cairncross[61] performed a similar trial on 84 patients but failed to find a benefit for surgical resection and WBRT (30 Gy in ten fractions) compared to WBRT alone. The median survival times were 6.3 months in the WBRT-alone arm and 5.6 months in the resection arm. The presence of extracranial metastases was found to be an important predictor of mortality. No significant differences were found in the 30-day mortality, morbidity, or causes of death. The presence of extracranial metastases was an important predictor of mortality (relative risk, 2.3). The mean proportion of days that the Karnofsky performance status was 70% or greater did not differ between the two groups.

Surgery ± Whole Brain Radiotherapy

The benefit of WBRT after surgical resection was addressed in a separate randomized study by Patchell et al.[62] Ninety-five adults who had single metastases to the brain were treated with complete surgical resections and randomly assigned to observation versus postoperative WBRT (50.4 Gy in 28 fractions). The WBRT arm was found to have a significantly decreased risk of local failure (10% vs. 46% for observation), distant brain failure (14% vs. 37%), and any brain failure (18% vs. 70%); longer median time to local failure (greater than 52 vs. 27 weeks); and longer median time to any brain failure (greater than 70 vs. 26 weeks). Patients randomized to WBRT were significantly less likely to die neurologic deaths (14% vs. 44%), although they had similar median survival and length of functional independence.

Radiosurgery

Radiosurgery refers to the delivery of accurately targeted, highly conformal radiation to one or more intracranial targets in a single treatment session using multiple beams. High doses are prescribed and are highly effective at producing cell death.

To minimize damage to normal tissue, it is necessary to prescribe lower doses to larger tumors.

Radiosurgery is most commonly performed with either a cobalt 60 gamma knife using 201 static, radially directed beams or with one of several different linear accelerator (LINAC) radiosurgery systems. Dose distributions in and near the target are similar for the two technologies, and clinical reports generally show similar treatment outcomes. Gamma knife system treatment of brain metastases requires (1) invasive fixation of a stereotactic headframe to the skull on the day of radiosurgery, (2) MRI or CT scans with the headframe in place, (3) identification of target and normal anatomic structures on the acquired images, (4) dose planning, (5) placement of the patient with attached headframe in the gamma knife in mechanical relationship to the 201 gamma knife beam collimators, (6) treatment delivery, and (7) removal of the headframe. Treatments performed with LINAC radiosurgery systems generally follow similar steps, with the obvious difference that a single beam is used to treat the target from many different angles and with additional possible system-dependent differences. Although some LINAC systems use a headframe analogous to that used with the gamma knife, others use a system of implanted screws to which the headframe can be fixed and removed; still others use implanted fiducials that are tracked in real time by a camera in the treatment area. Some noninvasive LINAC systems are based on infrared-detectable diode arrays attached to a bite block and use accurate real-time array tracking. Less accurate systems may rely solely on a simple thermoplastic mask. The Cyberknife (Accuray, Sunnyvale, CA) system deserves separate mention; it uses a small LINAC attached to a robotic arm to treat the target from multiple angles. During treatment, serial orthogonal x-rays are periodically acquired and compared with an extensive library of digitally reconstructed radiographs of the patient's skull to determine updated patient position and to redirect the robotic arm to compensate for any motion. One attraction of noninvasive and removable systems is that treatments need not be carried out on the same day that some of the other steps in the procedure are performed. Another attraction is that multiple fraction radiosurgery is easily performed, although its role is yet to be defined.

Brain metastases considered for radiosurgery typically range from a few millimeters up to several centimeters in maximum dimension. Shaw et al.[63,64] studied the relationship between maximum tolerated radiosurgery dose and volume in an RTOG dose-escalation trial involving patients with recurrent brain tumors. Flickinger et al.[65] calculated logistic dose-response curves fit to the RTOG data to demonstrate the relationship between target size and dose likely to produce a 10% risk of late toxicity: less than 2 cm (21.0 Gy), 2 to 3 cm (16.0 Gy), and 3 to 4 cm (13.5 Gy). Most radiosurgery practitioners use the RTOG data as an approximate, volume-dependent, dose prescription guideline. However, for any given tumor size clinical reports vary considerably regarding dose actually prescribed, ratio of maximum to prescription dose, degree of dose conformity, and so forth. Reported rates of radiation necrosis lie in a low to modest range: 0% (Kondziolka et al.[50]), 2% (Breneman et al.[66]), 4% 2-year actuarial (Flickinger et al.[67]), 10% (Alexander et al.[68]), and 17% (Joseph et al.[69]). Symptoms are usually treated with steroids, but surgery may be necessary to avoid a prolonged course of steroids or to differentiate between progressive tumor and radiation necrosis. In cases in which MRI shows progression,

[^{18}F]fluorodeoxyglucose (FDG)-PET may be useful in making the distinction.[70] Reported rates of chronic steroid dependence are 7% (Mehta et al.[71]), 8% (Alexander et al.[68]), and 11% 2-year actuarial (Flickinger et al.[67]). On the other hand, dramatic postradiosurgery resolution of individual cases of preradiosurgery peritumoral edema is occasionally described, although rates of such resolution are not yet well known. Early complications of radiosurgery are seen in up to 10% of patients. These include seizures, headaches, exacerbation of preexisting neurologic deficits, nausea, and hemorrhage.

In the past decade, hundreds of retrospective clinical investigations have addressed the outcome of radiosurgery for brain metastasis, with or without WBRT or surgery. Reported results are relatively consistent: For median target volumes in the range of 2 to 7 cc and for median prescribed radiosurgery doses in the range of 15 to 25 Gy, the 1-year local control rate is 80% to 90% and does not appear to depend strongly on the number of brain metastases treated, and median survival rates are in the range of 6 to 12 months. Specific actuarial rates of freedom from progression depend on dose, volume, histology, and pattern of MRI or CT enhancement at the time of radiosurgery.[72,73]

Concerns of potential late WBRT toxicity have motivated some investigators to treat initially with radiosurgery alone. Sneed et al.[1] found that omission of WBRT in patients receiving initial radiosurgery for up to four brain metastases did not compromise intracranial control provided salvage therapy information was included in the actuarial outcome analysis, an analysis that is not usually reported. The main argument against initial omission of WBRT is that neurologic deficits may develop in patients who have recurrences. This is supported by Regine et al.,[74] who reported recurrence anywhere in the brain after radiosurgery alone in 17 of 36 patients, with new neurologic deficits seen in 12 of the 17 patients with recurrences. However, whether the specific neurologic deficits were associated with complications at the initial radiosurgery site, recurrences at the initial site, or separate brain sites of microscopic disease that might have been addressed with initial WBRT is not known. In addition, whether omission of initial WBRT is more or less costly is not known, given that omission of WBRT may be more likely to result in future salvage therapies. An ongoing American College of Surgical Oncology Group phase III trial comparing radiosurgery alone to radiosurgery plus WBRT should eventually provide important information.

An issue faced by those who perform radiosurgery has to do with number of brain metastases: How many is too many to treat? In the absence of definitive data, many institutions individualize treatments. At others, institutional policy may allow any number to be treated by extending treatment to several days. In any case, Yan et al.[75] analyzed 183 patients treated with radiosurgery with or without WBRT for newly diagnosed brain metastases. Multivariate analysis was performed to evaluate number of brain metastases as a prognostic factor for survival, adjusting for well-accepted variables, and it was found that number of brain metastases was not significant. Median survival was 14 months for patients with one brain metastasis and did not differ significantly for patients with any number, including eight or greater. Selection factors play an important role, and whether equivalent survival would have been obtained instead with WBRT and follow-up radiosurgery as needed is unknown. Nevertheless, these data imply that some large number may reasonably be treated, even if the maximum number is not precisely known. At the University of California, San Francisco, the percentage of brain metastasis patients treated for three or more brain metastases has increased from 25% (1992) to 50% (2001).

A related issue is one of overall brain dose when multiple lesions are treated. Yamamoto et al.[76] analyzed dose distributions in 80 patients who were each treated with radiosurgery for more than 10 lesions (median, 17; range, 10 to 43). The median brain volumes receiving various doses were 1105 cc received greater than 2 Gy, 309 cc received greater than 5 Gy, 64 cc received greater than 10 Gy, 24 cc received greater than 15 Gy, and 8 cc received greater than 20 Gy. The authors concluded that cumulative brain doses did not exceed the threshold level for necrosis in normal brain.

Radiosurgery or Surgery

To date there have been no formal trials comparing radiosurgery and surgery in patients with brain metastasis, and three retrospective studies have differing results. Auchter et al.[77] reported 122 patients treated with radiosurgery and WBRT who met selection criteria similar to those used in randomized trials of WBRT ± surgical resection. Local control, functional independence, and median survival were comparable to those of the surgery plus WBRT arms of the reported randomized trials.[15,60] Bindal et al.[78] reported 61% versus 87% crude local control rates for radiosurgery with or without WBRT versus surgery with or without WBRT and median survival times of 7.5 versus 16.4 months, respectively. O'Neill et al.[79] compared patients with single metastases who were candidates for either radiosurgery or surgery, most of whom received WBRT in addition. One-year survival probabilities were not significantly different (56% for radiosurgery vs. 62% for surgery). It must be assumed that the differing results have to do with differences in selection factors or surgical or radiosurgical technique, or both.

Whole Brain Radiotherapy ± Radiosurgery

Kondziolka et al.[50] performed the first randomized trial of WBRT with or without radiosurgery boost. Inclusion criteria included KPS of 70 or greater, two to four brain metastases of diameter of 2.5 cm or less, and target greater than 5 mm from the optic chiasm. WBRT consisted of 30 Gy delivered in 12 fractions. Radiosurgery was delivered at any time within 1 month before or after WBRT and consisted of a single dose of 16 Gy. Only 27 patients were enrolled based on early stopping rules. The two arms were well balanced with respect to age, KPS, and presence of extracranial disease. The radiosurgery arm was found to have significantly improved time to local failure (median, 36 vs. 6 months; P = .0005) and time to any brain failure (median, 34 vs. 5 months; P = .002). Nevertheless, survival was not found to differ significantly in the two arms (median 7.5 months for WBRT vs. 11 months for WBRT plus radiosurgery; P = .22), although several patients who failed WBRT alone underwent salvage radiosurgery.

In 1996, the RTOG activated a phase III trial to study WBRT with or without radiosurgery boost (RTOG 9508).[80] Three hundred thirty-three patients with one to three newly diagnosed brain metastases were enrolled between January 1996 and June 2001, with balanced accrual in both arms. Single metastases

had to be considered unresectable (based on location in deep gray matter or in eloquent cortex). Exclusions included patients with metastases to the brainstem or metastases located within 1 cm of the optic apparatus, RPA class 3 patients, and individuals who had received systemic treatment within 1 month of enrollment. WBRT consisted of 37.5 Gy delivered in 3 weeks (15 fractions), and radiosurgery doses were based on tumor size according to RTOG 9005 toxicity information.[63] No survival benefit was seen in patients with multiple metastases. Univariate analysis demonstrated a significant survival advantage in the WBRT plus radiosurgery group for the following patients: those with single brain metastases (median survival, 6.5 vs. 4.9 months; P = .039), patients with tumor size greater than 2 cm (median survival, 6.5 vs. 5.3 months; P = .045), and RPA class 1 patients (median survival, 11.6 vs. 9.6 months; P = .045). Patients in the radiosurgery arm were more likely to have stable or improved KPS through 6 months (43% vs. 27%; P = .03). Multivariate analysis showed radiosurgery improved survival only in patients with single metastases (P < .0001) or RPA 1 (P < .0001). No differences were noted between treatment groups when assessing time to intracranial tumor progression, although the risk of developing a local recurrence was 43% greater in the nonradiosurgery arm. Likewise, the neurologic death rate was similar in the two arms (approximately 34%). Patients in the radiosurgery arm had significantly improved KPS and decreased steroid use at 6 months, although no differences were seen when assessing mental status. No survival advantage was noted based on type of radiosurgery unit used (LINAC vs. gamma knife). The authors concluded that WBRT plus radiosurgery improved performance for all patients with one to three metastases and survival for patients with a single unresectable brain metastasis.

Radiosurgery ± Whole Brain Radiotherapy

The American College of Surgical Oncology Group recently activated a phase III trial to compare radiosurgery alone to radiosurgery plus WBRT for patients with one to three brain metastases and histologically confirmed primary tumor. Exclusions include patients with lesions near the optic apparatus or in the brainstem or with primary germ cell tumor, small cell carcinoma, or lymphoma. The accrual goal is 480 patients over 5 years. Information from this trial is expected to add substantially to our knowledge base.

Brachytherapy

Brachytherapy for brain metastases involves the placement of radioactive sources directly inside a tumor or on the surfaces of a resection cavity to deliver a high dose of radiation locally while minimizing dose to surrounding normal tissue. The isotope most frequently used is iodine 125, either as a permanent or temporary implant, and in most cases without WBRT. Only small numbers of patients have been reported, with selection based on local institutional criteria and with widely varying survival rates, local control, and necrosis rates.[81–85] It is possible to draw only the most general conclusions: Crude local control rates are in the range of 80% to 95%, and median survivals are in the range of 6 to 14 months, for the most part.

Many of the nonbrachytherapy phase III data previously discussed demonstrate specific benefits for patients with a favor-

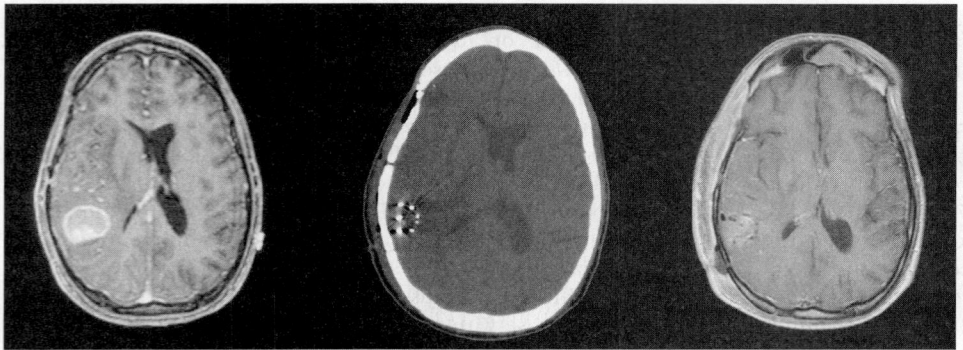

FIGURE 51.1-3.   Example of metastatic melanoma to right parietal lobe, locally recurrent after prior WBRT and radiosurgery, salvaged with surgical resection and brachytherapy. **Left:** Preresection T1-weighted postgadolinium MRI showing recurrent melanoma. **Middle:** Postresection noncontrast CT showing iodine 125 brachytherapy seeds. **Right:** Postresection T1-weighted postgadolinium MRI showing iodine 125 brachytherapy seeds.

able prognosis who initially receive two therapies (either WBRT plus surgery or WBRT plus radiosurgery) rather than one. Absent formal phase I or II studies, and given several reasonable approaches supported by phase III results, brachytherapy must be considered more investigational than other approaches, at least at the time of initial presentation of brain metastases. In patients with recurrent brain metastases, brachytherapy with surgical resection may be a reasonable alternative to surgery alone or radiosurgery (Fig. 51.1-3).

Chemotherapy

Many chemotherapeutic agents do not penetrate the intact blood–brain barrier. This fact, together with that of the known efficacy of radiation treatments, has led to the widespread belief that chemotherapy need not be considered for patients with brain metastases. Micrometastases, small aggregates of metastatic cells, may indeed be protected by an intact blood–brain barrier. However, as micrometastases grow, up-regulation of angiogenic factors leads to the development of new blood vessels. These vessels, which lack the physiologic and anatomic characteristics of vessels constituting the normal blood–brain barrier, contribute to the development of a disrupted barrier, with increased vessel permeability. Disrupted barriers are readily observed on CT or MRI examinations as edema or contrast enhancement, even with tumors as small as a few millimeters. Some studies have demonstrated that the penetration into brain metastases of chemotherapy agents that have limited ability to cross an intact blood–brain barrier does not differ from the penetration into systemic, non-CNS metastases.[86] In addition, some clinical studies report objective response rates to systemic chemotherapy that are similar for systemic and brain metastases. van den Bent[86] has summarized outcome reports of patients with brain metastasis treated with a variety of systemic agents. For specific tumor types and for various chemotherapy regimens, reported brain metastasis response rates are as follows: non–small cell lung cancer (27% to 45%), small cell lung cancer (21% to 40%), breast cancer (47% to 55%), and melanoma (12%). Likewise, approximate median survivals are as follows: non–small cell lung cancer (7 to 8 months), small cell lung cancer (3 to 6 months), breast cancer (6 to 13 months), and melanoma (4.5 months).

Results of a few phase III studies comparing chemotherapy alone with combined chemotherapy and WBRT do not allow firm conclusions,[86] and studies comparing chemotherapy alone to WBRT alone are lacking. Nevertheless, it appears reasonable to consider chemotherapy for brain metastases in specific situations, such as chemosensitive primary tumor, no prior chemotherapy, or systemic metastases requiring chemotherapy.[86] An example of response to chemotherapy is shown in Figure 51.1-4.

Salvage Therapy

Patients who have recurrences in the brain may be candidates for salvage therapy, particularly those in whom nonbrain systemic metastases are either currently of lesser clinical significance or are absent. No matter what the initial therapy, patients who may benefit from possible future salvage therapy are followed at 3-month intervals with repeat brain MRI. Possible tumor enhancement seen after surgery must be distinguished from postsurgical changes, and any seen after WBRT, radiosurgery, or brachytherapy must be distinguished from radiation necrosis. PET scan may be useful to make the latter distinction.[70] An example of positive MRI and negative PET studies after radiosurgery for renal cell metastasis is shown in Figure 51.1-5.

In general, the same array of therapeutic options available for initial treatment can be considered for salvage therapy, including chemotherapy. No reliable data are available that accurately describe the relative frequency of various combinations of first and second therapies. However, in patients who initially receive either WBRT or focal therapy salvage is often performed focally, particularly in those whose primary tumor remains controlled and who otherwise do not have extensive extracranial disease (see Fig. 51.1-3). WBRT is not usually repeated in patients who are expected to live more than 6 months because of concerns of radiation injury. However, in poor-prognosis patients it can be repeated, usually by delivering lower doses and smaller fraction sizes, such as 20 to 25 Gy in 10 fractions or 30 Gy in 30 fractions (1 Gy b.i.d.). Treatment outcomes are similar to those obtained after initial WBRT for RPA class II or III patients, with symptomatic improvement in up to 75% of patients and mean or median survival times of 3 to 5 months.[87–89] The risk of serious radiation toxicity after repeat WBRT is considered low in patients who are unlikely to survive 6 months.

Surgery is not often repeated, although it certainly can be. The largest reported reoperation series is that of Bindal et al.,[90] who reported neurologic improvement in 75% of 48 patients, median survival after reoperation of 11.5 months, and no operative mortality or morbidity. Others have also reported favorable reoperation results, reflecting the positive role for surgery and careful patient selection.

Radiosurgery, on the other hand, is often repeated, although few reports document its efficacy. Chen et al.[91] reviewed 45 patients with five or fewer lesions (176 total lesions) beyond the previously

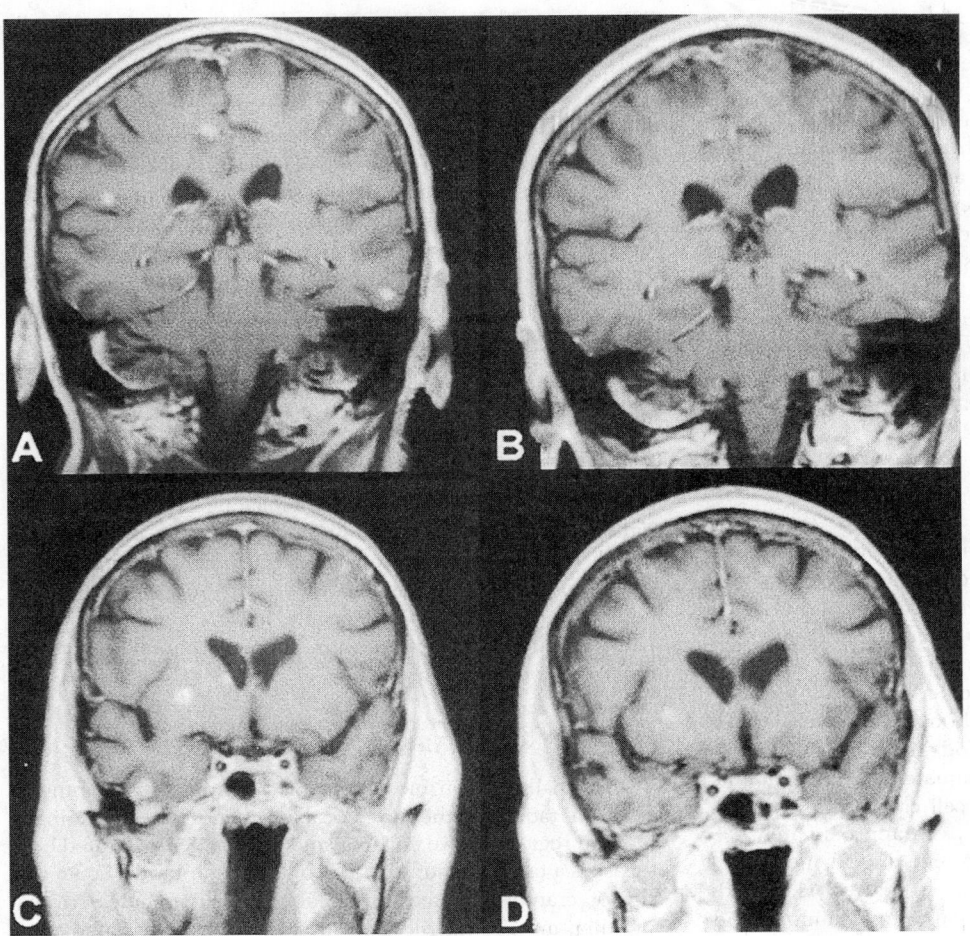

FIGURE 51.1-4. Example of response to chemotherapy, showing magnetic resonance images (MRIs) before and after treatment with temozolomide and gemcitabine for non–small cell lung cancer. Coronal MRIs of the brain after gadolinium administration compare the disease before and after treatment. **A:** Coronal image at the level of the brainstem before treatment showing at least four enhancing lesions consistent with metastases, at the gray-white junction. **B:** Coronal image at the same level as **A** after treatment. **C:** Coronal image at the level of the third ventricle before treatment showing additional enhancing lesions. **D:** Coronal image at the same level as **C** after treatment, showing resolution of most lesions and a greater than 50% decrease in diameter of the remaining lesion. (From Ebert BL, Niemierko E, Shafer K, Salgia R. Use of temozolomide with other cytotoxic chemotherapy in the treatment of patients with recurrent brain metastases from lung cancer. *Oncologist* 2003;8:69, with permission.)

treated radiosurgery volume treated with repeat radiosurgery. Median time between first and second procedures was 17 weeks; median survival after the second procedure was 28 weeks. Ten of the 28 patients underwent two salvage radiotherapies, and 1 underwent a third. The 1-year actuarial freedom from progression of treated tumors was 92%. Hillard et al.[92] studied ten patients who received two or more radiosurgeries to at least three isocenters and who were followed for toxicity for at least 6 months. Seizures developed in one patient in association with radiation necrosis, but no other significant focal or global neurotoxicities were seen.

CARCINOMATOUS MENINGITIS

Dissemination and growth of cancer cells within the leptomeningeal space are among the most serious complications faced by the cancer patient. Early diagnosis of this complication is often elusive, and management represents a significant challenge. The median survival for patients diagnosed with carcinomatous meningitis is 3 to 6 months.

Because carcinomatous meningitis from solid tumors is often associated with an advanced stage of systemic disease and frequently occurs with concomitant parenchymal brain metastases, therapeutic goals may be limited to the palliation of symptoms and to the prevention of further neurologic deterioration. The goals in treating leukemic and lymphomatous meningitis are more optimistic and include significant prolongation of survival and cure. In all cases, early aggressive intervention is critical to preserve neurologic function. Therapeutic intervention relies on traditional approaches with radiation or chemotherapy, or both, with the goal of treating the entire neuraxis.

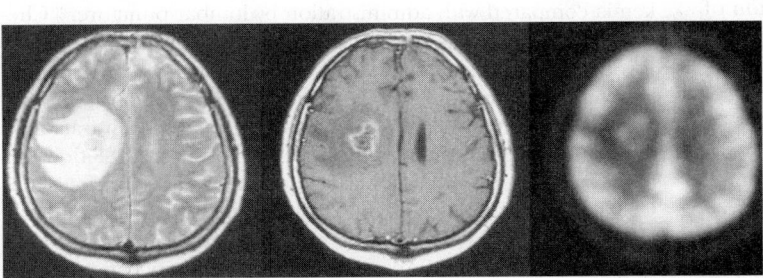

FIGURE 51.1-5. Example of renal cell metastasis treated with radiosurgery, with follow-up magnetic resonance imaging (MRI) and positron emission tomography (PET) studies at 15 weeks. From left to right, the images are T2-weighted MRI, T1-weighted postgadolinium MRI, and [18F]fluorodeoxyglucose(FDG)-PET. MRI was consistent with recurrence. PET was considered negative because only slight FDG accumulation was seen in the margin around the irradiated lesion, a common pattern after radiosurgery. At 41 weeks, the patient showed clinical and radiologic signs of regression. (From ref. 70, with permission.)

PATHOPHYSIOLOGY

Cancer cells may disseminate and seed the leptomeninges by several distinct mechanical pathways: (1) leptomeningeal contamination after resection of metastatic foci within the brain, in particular posterior fossa tumors; (2) hematogenous dissemination resulting in infiltration through arachnoid vessels or the choroid plexus; (3) tumor cell extension along peripheral nerves to the subarachnoid space; and (4) vascular dissemination from the bone marrow within the skull. Once inside the leptomeningeal compartment, tumor cells may spread throughout the neuraxis by bulk cerebrospinal fluid (CSF) flow. Disseminated leptomeningeal deposits may continue to manifest invasiveness by spreading into parenchyma as well as cranial or spinal nerve roots. The molecular features that underlie this pathophysiology have not been defined.

EPIDEMIOLOGY

Approximately 5% of cancer patients are affected by neoplastic meningitis. Although the vast majority of tumor histologies have been associated with this phenotype, this complication occurs most commonly in particular subsets of hematologic and solid tumor patients. Neoplastic meningitis is relatively common in patients with acute lymphoblastic leukemia and with intermediate or high-grade non-Hodgkin's lymphoma. This complication is extremely rare in patients with Hodgkin's disease. Leptomeningeal disease develops in approximately 25% of patients with metastatic melanoma and small cell carcinoma. In addition, carcinomatous meningitis develops in approximately 2% to 5% of breast cancer patients. Leptomeningeal metastases have also been described in less common solid tumors, including germ cell tumors, sarcomas, gastrointestinal tumors, and squamous cell carcinoma. In addition, primary tumors of the CNS such as medulloblastoma or ependymoma often disseminate within the leptomeningeal space throughout the craniospinal axis. Overt leptomeningeal dissemination in patients with astrocytic neoplasms is relatively rare.

CLINICAL PRESENTATION

Leptomeningeal tumor dissemination disrupts neurologic function by at least three distinct processes. Leptomeningeal tumor cell infiltration may result in altered mentation, incontinence, lower motor neuron weakness, back or radicular pain, cranial nerve deficits resulting in diplopia, hearing loss, hoarseness, alterations in taste, dysphagia, meningismus, and headache. Leptomeningeal tumor cell growth may also cause regional disturbances in blood flow in the affected nervous tissue resulting in metabolic dysfunction that produces seizures, stroke-like symptoms, and generalized encephalopathy. Finally, bulky leptomeningeal deposits may result in the obstruction of normal CSF flow pathways, leading to increased intracranial pressure and hydrocephalus.

DIAGNOSTIC STUDIES

A detailed examination of the CSF is usually required to make a diagnosis of neoplastic meningitis. Cytologic evaluation of the CSF, the gold standard, is an extremely insensitive test; 40% to 50% of patients with neoplastic meningitis have negative CSF cytology.[93] Repetitive CSF cytologic evaluations usually result in increased diagnostic sensitivity. Unfortunately, conversion to positive cytology is generally a manifestation of tumor progression and resultant neurologic deterioration. Given the importance of early diagnosis and intervention in treating leptomeningeal disease, there has been significant effort to identify biomarkers for this complication. For example, in the 1980s, it was demonstrated that the tumor antigen carcinoembryonic antigen as well as the enzymatic activity of beta-glucuronidase could be detected in the CSF in patients with brain and leptomeningeal metastases.[94] These biomarkers could facilitate clinical detection of neoplastic meningitis and were shown to rise and fall in parallel with the clinical course. Unfortunately, to date no biomarker has emerged with adequate sensitivity and specificity, and the diagnosis of leptomeningeal cancer relies heavily on cytology and clinical impression.

Approximately 50% of patients with neoplastic meningitis and spinal symptoms have abnormal imaging studies using gadolinium-enhanced MRI.[93] Common radiographic presentations include hydrocephalus without an identifiable mass lesion as well as leptomeningeal contrast enhancement. Abnormal enhancement of the meninges is not specific, however, and may also be seen after lumbar puncture, with infection, trauma, inflammation, or after craniotomy.

RADIATION THERAPY

Effective palliation in most cases of carcinomatous meningitis relies on radiation therapy. Focal irradiation of symptomatic sites and regions where imaging studies have demonstrated bulk disease is a favorable strategy. It avoids the substantial acute toxicity of craniospinal axis irradiation, which includes nausea, vomiting, marked fatigue, and myelosuppression. Craniospinal axis irradiation has a negative impact on bone marrow function, which may significantly compromise the ability to administer subsequent myelosuppressive chemotherapy for the treatment of systemic disease. One strategy, therefore, is to selectively use external-beam irradiation to treat symptomatic sites of disease and to rely on intrathecal chemotherapy to suppress the remainder of the disease in the neuraxis. Examples include external-beam irradiation to the base of the skull in patients with cranial nerve deficits or external-beam irradiation to the lumbosacral plexus in patients with cauda equina syndrome.[95–98]

INTRATHECAL CHEMOTHERAPY

The most reliable means of administering chemotherapy within the leptomeningeal space is through an implanted subcutaneous reservoir and ventricular catheter (Ommaya reservoir). Retrospective analysis suggests that intraventricular administration may result in prolonged remission in patients with leptomeningeal leukemia compared with administration by lumbar puncture.[99] Chemotherapeutic agents administered into the ventricle disseminate through the neuraxis by bulk CSF flow. CSF flow abnormalities are common in patients with leptomeningeal metastases, who frequently present with hydrocephalus and increased intracranial pressure as a result of bulky disease, which obstructs CSF flow. Up to 70% of patients with neoplastic meningitis have obstruction in CSF pathways as detected by radionuclide ventriculography.[100] Obstruction in CSF flow may be reversed with local irradiation. A CSF flow study is therefore recommended for every patient beginning intrathecal chemotherapy via a ventricular catheter because of the potential risk of irreversible neurotoxicity from high sustained concentrations of intrathecal chemotherapy.[97,98]

Cytarabine and methotrexate are the most widely used agents for intrathecal administration in the prophylaxis and treatment of leptomeningeal cancer. Intraventricular administration of methotrexate achieves therapeutic concentrations (more than 1 µmol/L) that persist for up to 48 hours. One approach to the treatment of active neoplastic meningitis is to use twice-weekly intrathecal therapy until CSF clears, followed by weekly and then monthly maintenance therapy until disease progression. Intrathecal methotrexate can cause myelosuppression as well as mucositis, toxicities that can be attenuated by oral leucovorin administration.

Cytarabine is also commonly used in the treatment of neoplastic meningitis. Cytarabine is metabolized by cytidine deaminase. Because of low CNS levels of cytidine deaminase, metabolism of cytarabine occurs relatively slowly in the CSF, resulting in an extended half-life of this drug in the leptomeningeal compartment.[95]

TREATMENT-RELATED TOXICITY

Placement of an intraventricular catheter is associated with an approximate 1% risk of perioperative hemorrhage. Extended use of the device is associated with at least a 5% risk of infection, usually with gram-positive organisms. Ultimately, the development of a necrotizing leukoencephalopathy is the most significant toxicity associated with the treatment of leptomeningeal carcinomatosis. This appears to occur most commonly in patients who receive intrathecal methotrexate after cranial irradiation. The clinical manifestations are initially radiographic, usually bilaterally symmetric abnormalities in white matter. Subsequently, progressive dementia may develop that can progress to substantial debility and to death.[95]

SYSTEMIC CHEMOTHERAPY AND NEW APPROACHES

Most water-soluble chemotherapy drugs are limited by the intact blood–brain barrier, and thus systemic therapy often fails to effectively treat microscopic, nonenhancing disease in brain parenchyma and in the subarachnoid space. An important exception is the high-dose systemic administration of methotrexate, which results in therapeutic drug levels in the CSF; this therapeutic approach has been shown to be active in neoplastic meningitis in lymphoma and in some solid tumors. Moreover, high-dose intravenous methotrexate administration overcomes problems associated with obstruction of CSF flow, which may compromise the subarachnoid administration of drugs. However, an important limitation of this approach is that high-dose methotrexate administration requires detailed inpatient monitoring of fluid status, renal function, urine alkalinization, and leucovorin rescue. Therefore, systemic administration of methotrexate at high doses is not appropriate or practical for all patients.[101]

Finally, there is increasing interest in the administration of targeted, biologic therapies into the leptomeningeal compartment to treat brain and leptomeningeal tumors. Mounting evidence is being compiled that most water-soluble small molecules or monoclonal antibodies exhibit inefficient penetration into the brain or leptomeninges. For example, systemic administration of monoclonal antibodies that target CD20 in B-cell lymphomas or of small molecules that inhibit the bcr-abl tyrosine kinase results in low levels in the CSF.[102,103] The direct administration of biologic therapies within the leptomeningeal compartment to treat brain tumors or neoplastic meningitis, or both, is an area of current early-phase clinical investigation.[102,104]

REFERENCES

1. Sneed PK, Lamborn KR, Forsther JM, et al. Radiosurgery for brain metastases: is whole brain radiotherapy necessary? *Int J Radiat Oncol Biol Phys* 1999;43(3):549.
2. Noel G, Simon JM, Valery CA, et al. Radiosurgery for brain metastasis: impact of CTV on local control. *Radiother Oncol* 2003;68(1):15.
3. Posner JB, Chernik NL. Intracranial metastases from systemic cancer. *Adv Neurol* 1978;19:579.
4. Patel JK, Didolkar MS, Pickren JW, et al. Metastatic pattern of malignant melanoma. A study of 216 autopsy cases. *Am J Surg* 1978;135(6):807.
5. Schouten LJ, Rutten J, Huveneers HA, et al. Incidence of brain metastases in a cohort of patients with carcinoma of the breast, colon, kidney, and lung and melanoma. *Cancer* 2002;94(10):2698.
6. Jemal A, Murray T, Samuels A, et al. Cancer statistics, 2003. *CA Cancer J Clin* 2003;53(1):5.
7. Johnson JD, Young B. Demographics of brain metastasis. *Neurosurg Clin North Am* 1996;7(3):337.
8. Lassman AB, DeAngelis LM. Brain metastases. *Neurol Clin* 2003;21(1):1, vii.
9. Vannucci RC, Baten M. Cerebral metastatic disease in childhood. *Neurology* 1974;24(10):981.
10. Graus F, Walker RW, Allen JC. Brain metastases in children. *J Pediatr* 1983;103(4):558.
11. Nussbaum ES, Djalilian HR, Cho KH, et al. Brain metastases. Histology, multiplicity, surgery, and survival. *Cancer* 1996;78(8):1781.
12. Delattre JY, Krol G, Thaler HT, et al. Distribution of brain metastases. *Arch Neurol* 1988;45(7):741.
13. Hwang TL, Close TP, Grego JM, et al. Predilection of brain metastasis in gray and white matter junction and vascular border zones. *Cancer* 1996;77(8):1551.
14. Schellinger PD, Meinck HM, Thron A. Diagnostic accuracy of MRI compared to CCT in patients with brain metastases. *J Neurooncol* 1999;44(3):275.
15. Patchell RA, Tibbs PA, Walsh JW, et al. A randomized trial of surgery in the treatment of single metastases to the brain. *N Engl J Med* 1990;322(8):494.
16. Kuhn MJ, Hammer GM, Swenson LC, et al. MRI evaluation of "solitary" brain metastases with triple-dose gadoteridol: comparison with contrast-enhanced CT and conventional-dose gadopentetate dimeglumine MRI studies in the same patients. *Comput Med Imaging Graph* 1994;18(5):391.
17. Runge VM, Wells JW, Nelson KL, et al. MR imaging detection of cerebral metastases with a single injection of high-dose gadoteridol. *J Magn Reson Imaging* 1994;4(5):669.
18. Akeson P, Larsson EM, Kristoffersen DT, et al. Brain metastases—comparison of gadodiamide injection-enhanced MR imaging at standard and high dose, contrast-enhanced CT and non–contrast-enhanced MR imaging. *Acta Radiol* 1995;36(3):300.
19. Yuh WT, Fisher DJ, Runge VM, et al. Phase III multicenter trial of high-dose gadoteridol in MR evaluation of brain metastases. *AJNR Am J Neuroradiol* 1994;15(6):1037.
20. Schneider G, Kirchin MA, Pirovano G, et al. Gadobenate dimeglumine-enhanced magnetic resonance imaging of intracranial metastases: effect of dose on lesion detection and delineation. *J Magn Reson Imaging* 2001;14(5):525.
21. Gaspar L, Scott C, Rotman M, et al. Recursive partitioning analysis (RPA) of prognostic factors in three Radiation Therapy Oncology Group (RTOG) brain metastases trials. *Int J Radiat Oncol Biol Phys* 1997;37(4):745.
22. Sneed PK, Suh JH, Goetsch SJ, et al. A multi-institutional review of radiosurgery alone vs. radiosurgery with whole brain radiotherapy as the initial management of brain metastases. *Int J Radiat Oncol Biol Phys* 2002;53(3):519.
23. Agboola O, Benoit B, Cross P, et al. Prognostic factors derived from recursive partition analysis (RPA) of Radiation Therapy Oncology Group (RTOG) brain metastases trials applied to surgically resected and irradiated brain metastatic cases. *Int J Radiat Oncol Biol Phys* 1998;42(1):155.
24. Pavlidis N, Briasoulis E, Hainsworth J, et al. Diagnostic and therapeutic management of cancer of an unknown primary. *Eur J Cancer* 2003;39(14):1990.
25. Ruda R, Borgognone M, Benech F, et al. Brain metastases from unknown primary tumour: a prospective study. *J Neurol* 2001;248(5):394.
26. Hempen C, Weiss E, Hess CF. Dexamethasone treatment in patients with brain metastases and primary brain tumors: do the benefits outweigh the side-effects? *Support Care Cancer* 2002;10(4):322.
27. Harwood AR, Simson WJ. Radiation therapy of cerebral metastases: a randomized prospective clinical trial. *Int J Radiat Oncol Biol Phys* 1977;2(11–12):1091.
28. van Vulpen M, Kal HB, Taphoorn MJ, et al. Changes in blood–brain barrier permeability induced by radiotherapy: implications for timing of chemotherapy (review). *Oncol Rep* 2002;9(4):683.
29. Forsyth PA, Weaver S, Fulton D, et al. Prophylactic anticonvulsants in patients with brain tumour. *Can J Neurol Sci* 2003;30(2):106.
30. Glantz MJ, Cole BF, Friedberg MH, et al. A randomized, blinded, placebo-controlled trial of divalproex sodium prophylaxis in adults with newly diagnosed brain tumors. *Neurology* 1996;46(4):985.
31. Byrne TN, Cascino TL, Posner JB. Brain metastasis from melanoma. *J Neurooncol* 1983;1(4):313.
32. Sorensen HT, Johnsen SP, Norgard B, et al. Cancer and venous thromboembolism: a multidisciplinary approach. *Clin Lab* 2003;49(11–12):615.
33. Levin JM, Schiff D, Loeffler JS, et al. Complications of therapy for venous thromboembolic disease in patients with brain tumors. *Neurology* 1993;43(6):1111.

34. Schiff D, DeAngelis LM. Therapy of venous thromboembolism in patients with brain metastases. *Cancer* 1994;73(2):493.
35. Chao JH, Phillips RH, Nickerson JJ. Roentgen-ray therapy of cerebral metastases. *Cancer* 1954;7:682.
36. Chu FCH, Hilaris BB. Value of radiation therapy in the management of intracranial metastases. *Cancer* 1961;14:577.
37. Order SE, Hellman S, von Essen CF, et al. Improvement in quality of survival following whole-brain irradiation for brain metastasis. *Radiology* 1968;91:149.
38. Lang EF, Slater J. Metastatic brain tumors. Results of surgical and nonsurgical treatment. *Surg Clin North Am* 1964;44:865.
39. Markesbery WR, Brooks WH, Gupta GD, et al. Treatment for patients with cerebral metastases. *Arch Neurol* 1978;35:754.
40. Richards P, McKissock W. Intracranial metastases. *BMJ* 1963;1:15.
41. Borgelt B, Gelber R, Kramer S, et al. The palliation of brain metastases: final results of the first two studies by the Radiation Therapy Oncology Group. *Int J Radiat Oncol Biol Phys* 1980;6(1):1.
42. Borgelt B, Gelber R, Larson M, et al. Ultra-rapid high dose irradiation schedules for the palliation of brain metastases: final results of the first two studies by the Radiation Therapy Oncology Group. *Int J Radiat Oncol Biol Phys* 1981;7(12):1633.
43. Coia LR. The role of radiation therapy in the treatment of brain metastases. *Int J Radiat Oncol Biol Phys* 1992;23(1):229.
44. Kurtz JM, Gelber R, Brady LW, et al. The palliation of brain metastases in a favorable patient population: a randomized clinical trial by the Radiation Therapy Oncology Group. *Int J Radiat Oncol Biol Phys* 1981;7(7):891.
45. Murray KJ, Scott C, Greenberg HM, et al. A randomized phase III study of accelerated hyperfractionation versus standard in patients with unresected brain metastases: a report of the Radiation Therapy Oncology Group (RTOG) 9104. *Int J Radiat Oncol Biol Phys* 1997;39(3):571.
46. Hindo WA, DeTrana FA 3rd, Lee MS, et al. Large dose increment irradiation in treatment of cerebral metastases. *Cancer* 1970;26(1):138.
47. Young DF, Posner JB, Chu F, et al. Rapid-course radiation therapy of cerebral metastases: results and complications. *Cancer* 1974;34(4):1069.
48. Nieder C, Berberich W, Schnabel K. Tumor-related prognostic factors for remission of brain metastases after radiotherapy. *Int J Radiat Oncol Biol Phys* 1997;39(1):25.
49. Nieder C, Nestle U, Walter K, et al. Dose/effect relationships for brain metastases. *J Cancer Res Clin Oncol* 1998;124(6):346.
50. Kondziolka D, Patel A, Lunsford LD, et al. Stereotactic radiosurgery plus whole brain radiotherapy versus radiotherapy alone for patients with multiple brain metastases. *Int J Radiat Oncol Biol Phys* 1999;45(2):427.
51. DeAngelis LM, Delattre JY, Posner JB. Radiation-induced dementia in patients cured of brain metastases. *Neurology* 1989;39(6):789.
52. Penitzka S, Steinvorth S, Sehlleier S, et al. [Assessment of cognitive function after preventive and therapeutic whole brain irradiation using neuropsychological testing.] *Strahlenther Onkol* 2002;178(5):252.
53. Nieder C, Leicht A, Motaref B, et al. Late radiation toxicity after whole brain radiotherapy: the influence of antiepileptic drugs. *Am J Clin Oncol* 1999;22(6):573.
54. Nieder C, Schwerdtfeger K, Steudel WI, et al. Patterns of relapse and late toxicity after resection and whole-brain radiotherapy for solitary brain metastases. *Strahlenther Onkol* 1998;174(5):275.
55. Mehta MP, Rodrigus P, Terhaard CH, et al. Survival and neurologic outcomes in a randomized trial of motexafin gadolinium and whole-brain radiation therapy in brain metastases. *J Clin Oncol* 2003;21(13):2529.
56. Kumar P, Mehta MP, Rodrigus P, et al. Motexafin gadolinium (MGd) overcomes adverse survival effect of anemia in brain metastases (BM) patients treated with whole brain radiation therapy (WBRT): analysis of a phase III randomized trial. *Int J Radiat Oncol Biol Phys* 2003; 57[2 Suppl]: S133.
57. Suh JH, Stea BD, Kresl JJ, et al. A phase 3, randomized, open-label, comparative study of standard whole brain radiation therapy (WBRT) with supplemental oxygen (O_2), with or without RSR13, in patients with brain metastases. *Neuro-oncology* 2003;5(4):345.
58. Lang FF, Sawaya R. Surgical treatment of metastatic brain tumors. *Semin Surg Oncol* 1998;14(1):53.
59. Bindal RK, Sawaya R, Leavens ME, et al. Surgical treatment of multiple brain metastases. *J Neurosurg* 1993;79(2):210.
60. Noordijk EM, Vecht CJ, Haaxma-Reiche H, et al. The choice of treatment of single brain metastasis should be based on extracranial tumor activity and age. *Int J Radiat Oncol Biol Phys* 1994;29(4):711.
61. Mintz AP, Cairncross JG. Treatment of a single brain metastasis: the role of radiation following surgical resection. *JAMA* 1998;280(17):1527.
62. Patchell RA, Tibbs PA, Regine WF, et al. Postoperative radiotherapy in the treatment of single metastases to the brain: a randomized trial. *JAMA* 1998;280(17):1485.
63. Shaw E, Scott C, Souhami L, et al. Single dose radiosurgical treatment of recurrent previously irradiated primary brain tumors and brain metastases: final report of RTOG protocol 90-05. *Int J Radiat Oncol Biol Phys* 2000;47(2):291.
64. Shaw E, Scott C, Souhami L, et al. Radiosurgery for the treatment of previously irradiated recurrent primary brain tumors and brain metastases: initial report of radiation therapy oncology group protocol (90-05). *Int J Radiat Oncol Biol Phys* 1996;34(3):647.
65. Flickinger JC, Kondziolka D, Lunsford LD. Radiobiological analysis of tissue responses following radiosurgery. *Technol Cancer Res Treat* 2003;2(2):87.
66. Breneman JC, Warnick RE, Albright RE Jr, et al. Stereotactic radiosurgery for the treatment of brain metastases. Results of a single institution series. *Cancer* 1997;79(3):551.
67. Flickinger JC, Kondziolka D, Lunsford LD, et al. A multi-institutional experience with stereotactic radiosurgery for solitary brain metastasis. *Int J Radiat Oncol Biol Phys* 1994;28(4):797.
68. Alexander E 3rd, Moriarty TM, Davis RB, et al. Stereotactic radiosurgery for the definitive, noninvasive treatment of brain metastases. *J Natl Cancer Inst* 1995;87(1):34.
69. Joseph J, Adler JR, Cox RS, et al. Linear accelerator-based stereotaxic radiosurgery for brain metastases: the influence of number of lesions on survival. *J Clin Oncol* 1996;14(4):1085.
70. Belohlavek O, Simonova G, Kantorova I, et al. Brain metastases after stereotactic radiosurgery using the Leksell gamma knife: can FDG PET help to differentiate radionecrosis from tumour progression? *Eur J Nucl Med Mol Imaging* 2003;30(1):96.
71. Mehta MP, Rozental JM, Levin AB, et al. Defining the role of radiosurgery in the management of brain metastases. *Int J Radiat Oncol Biol Phys* 1992;24(4):619.
72. Goodman KA, Sneed PK, McDermott MW, et al. Relationship between pattern of enhancement and local control of brain metastases after radiosurgery. *Int J Radiat Oncol Biol Phys* 2001;50(1):139.
73. Shiau CY, Sneed PK, Shu HK, et al. Radiosurgery for brain metastases: relationship of dose and pattern of enhancement to local control. *Int J Radiat Oncol Biol Phys* 1997; 37(2):375.
74. Regine WF, Scott C, Murray K, et al. Neurocognitive outcome in brain metastases patients treated with accelerated-fractionation vs. accelerated-hyperfractionated radiotherapy: an analysis from Radiation Therapy Oncology Group Study 91-04. *Int J Radiat Oncol Biol Phys* 2001;51(3):711.
75. Yan ES, Sneed PK, McDermott MW, et al. Number of brain metastases is not an important prognostic factor for survival following radiosurgery for newly-diagnosed nonmelanoma brain metastases. *Int J Radiat Oncol Biol Phys* 2003;57[2 Suppl]:S131.
76. Yamamoto M, Ide M, Nishio S, et al. Gamma knife radiosurgery for numerous brain metastases: is this a safe treatment? *Int J Radiat Oncol Biol Phys* 2002;53(5):1279.
77. Auchter RM, Lamond JP, Alexander E, et al. A multiinstitutional outcome and prognostic factor analysis of radiosurgery for resectable single brain metastasis. *Int J Radiat Oncol Biol Phys* 1996;35(1):27.
78. Bindal AK, Bindal RK, Hess KR, et al. Surgery versus radiosurgery in the treatment of brain metastasis. *J Neurosurg* 1996;84(5):748.
79. O'Neill BP, Iturria NJ, Link MJ, et al. A comparison of surgical resection and stereotactic radiosurgery in the treatment of solitary brain metastases. *Int J Radiat Oncol Biol Phys* 2003;55(5):1169.
80. Andrews DW, Scott C, Sperduto PW, et al. Whole brain radiation therapy with or without stereotactic radiosurgery boost for patients with one to three brain metastases: phase II results of the RTOG 9508 randomized trial. *Lancet* 2004;363:1665.
81. Bernstein M, Cabantog A, Laperriere N, et al. Brachytherapy for recurrent single brain metastasis. *Can J Neurol Sci* 1995;22(1):13.
82. Bogart JA, Ungureanu C, Shihadeh E, et al. Resection and permanent I-125 brachytherapy without whole brain irradiation for solitary brain metastasis from non–small cell lung carcinoma. *J Neurooncol* 1999;44(1):53.
83. Ostertag CB, Kreth FW. Interstitial iodine-125 radiosurgery for cerebral metastases. *Br J Neurosurg* 1995;9(5):593.
84. McDermott MW, Cosgrove GR, Larson DA, et al. Interstitial brachytherapy for intracranial metastases. *Neurosurg Clin North Am* 1996;7(3):485.
85. Schulder M, Black PM, Shrieve DC, et al. Permanent low-activity iodine-125 implants for cerebral metastases. *J Neurooncol* 1997;33(3):213.
86. van den Bent MJ. The role of chemotherapy in brain metastases. *Eur J Cancer* 2003; 39(15):2114.
87. Wong WW, Schild SE, Sawyer TE, et al. Analysis of outcome in patients reirradiated for brain metastases. *Int J Radiat Oncol Biol Phys* 1996;34(3):585.
88. Cooper JS, Steinfeld AD, Lerch IA. Cerebral metastases: value of reirradiation in selected patients. *Radiology* 1990;174(3 Pt 1):883.
89. Abdel-Wahab MM, Wolfson AH, Raub W, et al. The role of hyperfractionated re-irradiation in metastatic brain disease: a single institutional trial. *Am J Clin Oncol* 1997;20(2):158.
90. Bindal RK, Sawaya R, Leavens ME, et al. Reoperation for recurrent metastatic brain tumors. *J Neurosurg* 1995;83(4):600.
91. Chen JC, Petrovich Z, Giannotta SL, et al. Radiosurgical salvage therapy for patients presenting with recurrence of metastatic disease to the brain. *Neurosurgery* 2000;46(4):860; discussion, 866.
92. Hillard VH, Shih LL, Chin S, et al. Safety of multiple stereotactic radiosurgery treatments for multiple brain lesions. *J Neurooncol* 2003;63(3):271.
93. Chamberlain MC. Neoplastic meningitis: a guide to diagnosis and treatment. *Curr Opin Neurol* 2000;13(6):641.
94. Schold SC, Wasserstrom WR, Fleisher M, et al. Cerebrospinal fluid biochemical markers of central nervous system metastases. *Ann Neurol* 1980;8(6):597.
95. Posner JB. *Neurologic complications of cancer.* Philadelphia: FA Davis Co, 1995.
96. Jayson GC, Howell A. Carcinomatous meningitis in solid tumours. *Ann Oncol* 1996;7(8):773.
97. Grossman SA, Krabak MJ. Leptomeningeal carcinomatosis. *Cancer Treat Rev* 1999;25(2):103.
98. Grossman SA, Krabak MJ. *NCCN clinical practice guidelines for carcinomatous/lymphomatous meningitis.* 1999;13:144.
99. Bleyer WA, Poplack DG. Intraventricular versus intralumbar methotrexate for central-nervous-system leukemia: prolonged remission with the Ommaya reservoir. *Med Pediatr Oncol* 1979;6(3):207.
100. Grossman SA, Trump DL, Chen DC, et al. Cerebrospinal fluid flow abnormalities in patients with neoplastic meningitis. An evaluation using 111indium-DTPA ventriculography. *Am J Med* 1982;73(5):641.
101. Glantz MJ, Cole BF, Recht L, et al. High-dose intravenous methotrexate for patients with nonleukemic leptomeningeal cancer: is intrathecal chemotherapy necessary? *J Clin Oncol* 1998;16(4):1561.
102. Rubenstein JL, Combs D, Rosenberg J, et al. Rituximab therapy for CNS lymphomas: targeting the leptomeningeal compartment. *Blood* 2003;101(2):466.
103. Petzer AL, Gunsilius E, Hayes M, et al. Low concentrations of STI571 in the cerebrospinal fluid: a case report. *Br J Haematol* 2002;117(3):623.
104. Laske DW, Muraszko KM, Oldfield EH, et al. Intraventricular immunotoxin therapy for leptomeningeal neoplasia. *Neurosurgery* 1997;41(5):1039; discussion 1049.

MICHAEL R. JOHNSTON
MARC DE PERROT

SECTION 2

Metastatic Cancer to the Lung

BIOLOGY

The metastatic cascade is a complex process that involves a series of events. Growth and angiogenesis are followed by invasion into surrounding tissue and intravasation into the bloodstream. Circulating tumor cells can then arrest and attach to endothelial cells. Attachment is followed by extravasation, invasion, and growth into the metastatic site. Each of these steps continues to be the subject of intense research.

Tumors can spread to the lung through hematogenous or lymphangitic routes. Lymphangitic metastasis to the lung occurs by retrograde spread from involved lymph nodes through lymphatic channels in the pleura and diaphragm and the thoracic duct to mediastinal and hilar lymph nodes. Widespread dissemination in the lung then occurs through pulmonary lymphatics, leading to the characteristic picture of lymphangitis carcinomatosis (Fig. 51.2-1).

Hematogenous spread arises from deposition of tumor cells and invasion of thin-walled capillaries. Only 0.1% of circulating tumor cells will eventually produce pulmonary metastasis. The large majority of tumor cells are destroyed by blood turbulence, natural killer cells, macrophages, and platelets. Infrequently, hematogenous tumor emboli can cause acute pulmonary hypertension that may be indistinguishable from acute pulmonary thromboembolism. Macroscopic tumor emboli usually arise from primary tumors with direct access to the inferior vena cava or its tributaries. These tumors include sarcomas, germ cell tumors, renal cell carcinomas, and hepatocellular carcinomas. Microscopic tumor emboli with thrombotic microangiopathy characterized by fibrocellular intimal proliferation of small pulmonary arteries have also been described in patients with a history of carcinoma originating in particular from breast or stomach.[1,2]

Large series of autopsies have shown the lung to be the second most common site for the occurrence of metastasis. Weiss and Gilbert[3] showed that in 20% of autopsied patients, the lung was the sole site of metastasis. The clinical incidence of isolated pulmonary metastasis varies with the primary tumor site. Metastasis to the lung is the main cause of treatment failure in 50% to 80% of patients with osteogenic sarcomas and in 30% to 50% of patients with soft tissue sarcomas. Isolated lung metastases, however, are found in only a small proportion of patients (1% to 2%) with carcinomas.

DIAGNOSIS

SIGNS AND SYMPTOMS

Typically, patients with pulmonary metastasis present with a new finding on a radiologic image, either chest radiograph or computed tomography (CT) scan, and no associated symptoms. The patient has most likely been treated for another malignancy with the propensity for spread to the lung. Because previous imaging has probably been performed, this new finding is all the more indicative of metastatic disease. If the tumor is bulky or close to the hilum, symptoms, including shortness of breath, cough, and hemoptysis, may be present. Endobronchial metastasis may obstruct an airway, causing stridor, atelectasis, or pneumonia, depending on the site and degree of obstruction. Tumors most prone to spread to the bronchus include colon carcinoma, renal cell carcinoma, breast carcinoma, and, less frequently, sarcoma and melanoma (Fig. 51.2-2). Invasion of tumor into parietal pleura or chest wall usually results in pain. A spontaneous pneumothorax or hemothorax in a patient with a history of sarcoma is highly suggestive of lung metastasis.

RADIOLOGY

Chest Radiography

Although not as sensitive as other imaging techniques, the chest radiograph is still probably the most specific in the diagnosis of lung metastasis.[4,5] As the most common surveillance tool, the

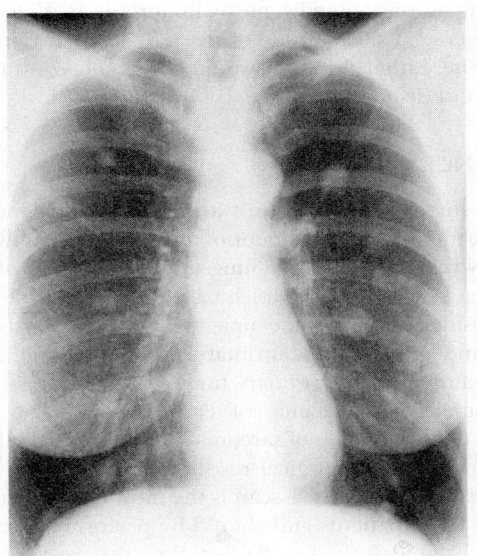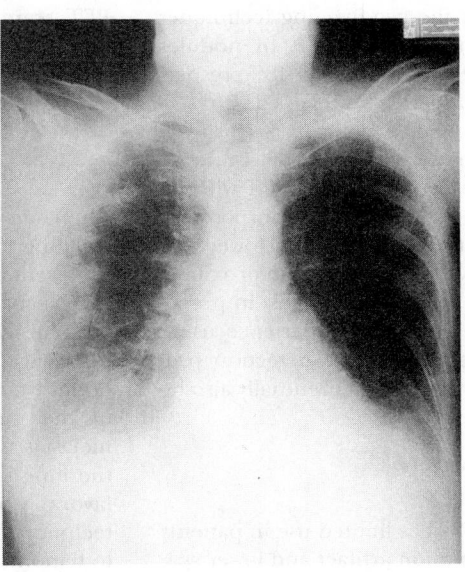

A,B

FIGURE 51.2-1. Chest radiographs of patients with lung metastasis (**A,** Hematogenous metastasis; **B,** lymphangitic metastasis).

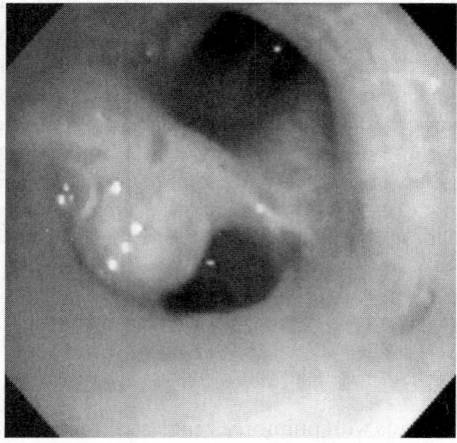

FIGURE 51.2-2. Endobronchial metastasis from chondrosarcoma. The patient also had lung parenchymal metastasis from a previously treated primary tumor in the hand.

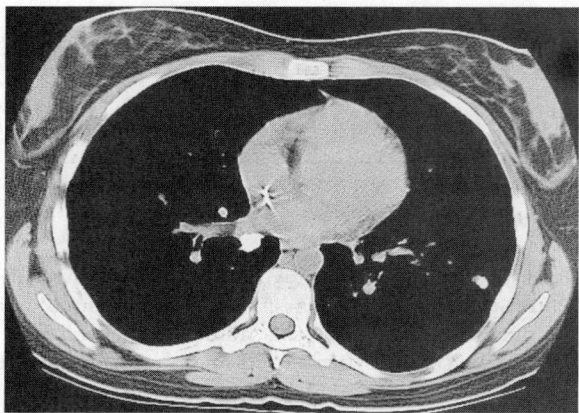

FIGURE 51.2-3. Calcified osteosarcoma metastasis bordering the inferior pulmonary vein in the right lower lobe and another in the left lower lobe. This scan was performed after chemotherapy and shows decreases in the soft tissue component of the nodules, but viable tumor was found in both resected specimens.

chest radiograph is often the first indication of lung metastasis. In addition to demonstrating lung nodules, it may show lobar or segmental collapse indicating endobronchial metastasis, hilar or mediastinal nodal disease, lymphangitic spread, or pleural effusions. A rapidly growing sarcoma metastasis may appear as a cavitating mass, and, in addition, osteosarcoma, chondrosarcoma, and synovial sarcoma may show calcifications within the metastasis (Fig. 51.2-3).

Computed Tomography

With its enhanced contrast resolution and the spatial clarity gained by eliminating overlapping structures, CT is the most effective method of imaging lung metastasis. It is also superior to chest radiography for imaging hilar, mediastinal, and pleural structures.[6] Helical CT with a single breath-hold technique has proven more sensitive than conventional CT and can consistently detect nodules smaller than 5 mm.[7] However, helical CT and high-resolution CT underestimate the actual number of tumor nodules found at surgery. A sensitivity of 82% and 75%, respectively, were found for the two imaging techniques in a retrospective study by Margaritora et al.[8] In nodules smaller than 6 mm, the sensitivity fell to 61% and 48%, respectively. In a prospective study of 13 patients subjected to resection of lung metastasis, Diederich et al.[9] found a 95% sensitivity of helical CT in detecting pulmonary nodules of 6 mm or greater but only 69% with nodules less than 6 mm. CT without intravenous contrast is sufficient for surveillance purposes or for following small, indeterminate lung nodules. However, a contrast-enhanced CT is imperative when tumor is in proximity to hilar or mediastinal structures and preoperatively in preparation for metastasectomy. With increasing experience using low-dose spiral CT scans in lung cancer early-detection programs, it seems likely that this technique may eventually also be applied to surveillance of lung metastasis.

Magnetic Resonance Imaging

Magnetic resonance imaging (MRI) has limited use in patients with lung metastasis. Because of motion artifact and lower spa-

tial resolution, its sensitivity is inferior to that of CT. When compared with helical CT in 23 patients with lung metastasis, MRI found 36% of those nodules seen on CT to be less than 5 mm, 83% of nodules 5 to 10 mm, and 92% of nodules 10 to 15 mm.[10] However, as in primary lung cancer, MRI is very useful in determining tumor invasion into mediastinal and chest wall structures, especially in the superior sulcus. This is particularly important in planning extended surgical resections.

Positron Emission Tomography

The experience with positron emission tomography (PET) in lung metastasis is still quite limited. Lucas et al.[11] found an 87% sensitivity and 100% specificity in a series of patients with soft tissue sarcomas. Thirteen true positives and two false-negatives were found, but histologic confirmation was not obtained on all lesions. If the experience with PET detection of primary lung cancers can be extrapolated to lung metastasis, the downfall will again be the failure to detect small, subcentimeter nodules. Rather than defining the extent of disease in the lung, PET scanning is undoubtedly more important in detecting metastatic disease at sites outside of the lung or recurrence at the primary site. Either discovery would potentially contraindicate lung metastasectomy.

SURVEILLANCE

The issue of surveillance takes on two aspects: surveillance of the lung in patients after treatment of a malignancy known to preferentially metastasize to the lung and surveillance of the lung in patients after resection of lung metastasis. In the first instance considerations include imaging modality; histology, site, stage, and grade of the primary tumor; interval since definitive treatment of the primary tumor; and an assessment of the therapeutic importance of early detection of lung metastasis.[12] More than 80% of sarcomas metastasize initially to the lung, and aggressive surgical resection appears to impact favorably on survival. Chest CT scan is the most useful imaging technique in these patients and should be performed every 3 to 6 months for at least the first 2 years, then progressively less frequently thereafter. Surveillance should continue after 5 years, with chest radiographs every 6 months to 1 year, because metastasis can still present many years after treatment of the original tumor.

Appropriate lung surveillance for patients with extrathoracic carcinomas is more difficult to specify. CT scanning has been suggested for high-grade renal cell carcinomas, testis tumors with intraabdominal disease, and head and neck cancers with which occult primary lung and esophageal cancers may also be detected. For other carcinomas, including breast and colon, chest radiographs or CT scans should be considered at 6- or 12-month intervals, especially in patients with higher-stage primary tumors.

Patients who have had complete resection of lung metastasis require close surveillance. Most cancer centers perform chest CT scans every 3 months for 2 years, then every 6 months for another 3 years. After 5 years, chest radiographs are performed at regular intervals between 6 and 12 months.

TISSUE DIAGNOSIS

In most situations the diagnosis of lung metastasis is all too obvious from the clinical scenario, and obtaining confirmatory tissue is unnecessary. Thus, the young patient with a previously treated osteosarcoma who now has multiple lung nodules generally needs no biopsy before treatment. However, the middle-aged patient with a history of colon or renal cell carcinoma that presents with a new solitary pulmonary nodule should have a tissue diagnosis. Depending on location within the lung and expertise in the local medical community, diagnostic tissue can be obtained by transthoracic needle aspiration or bronchoscopic transbronchial biopsy. In situations in which the extrathoracic malignancy is a carcinoma and biopsy of the lung nodule reveals the same cell type, it is best to consider the lung tumor as a new primary lung cancer rather than a metastatic lesion. At surgery a wedge resection of the lesion and frozen-section diagnosis may reveal the true origin of the lesion. If not, an anatomic lung cancer resection and appropriate lymph node staging should be performed.

TREATMENT

RADIATION

Whole lung irradiation for the treatment of micrometastatic disease within the lung dates back more than 30 years. A low dose, usually less than 20 Gy in divided fractions, is given to patients with known nonpulmonary malignancies that have a high incidence of lung metastasis. It has also been used in patients with cancer and synchronous lung metastasis as either definitive therapy or as a prelude to metastasectomy. Occasionally, the technique is used as an adjuvant to metastasectomy in an effort to prevent further recurrence.

Most of the experience with whole lung irradiation has been with primary tumors of bone, either osteosarcoma or Ewing's sarcoma.[13] In the 1970s and 1980s, a number of studies were done in patients with osteosarcoma, comparing prophylactic lung irradiation with chemotherapy after treatment of the primary tumor. The largest of these studies was a randomized trial in 203 patients performed by the EORTC (European

Organization for Research and Treatment of Cancer). After definitive treatment of the primary tumor, patients were randomized in a three-arm study to 9 months of a modified Rosen chemotherapy protocol, 20 Gy whole lung radiation, or 3 months of chemotherapy and radiation. No difference was found between any of the three arms in either disease-free survival or overall survival at 4 years.[14] The only positive aspects of the radiation were that it did as well as the chemotherapy regimen, at less toxicity, and that more patients were amenable to surgical resection of their lung metastasis.

A similar experience was found in Ewing's sarcoma. In the first Intergroup Ewing's Sarcoma Study, all patients were treated with radiation to the primary tumor and VAC chemotherapy (vincristine, actinomycin D, cyclophosphamide) alone or the addition of doxorubicin to the chemotherapy regimen (VACA) or whole lung radiation.[15] The incidence of lung metastasis decreased from 38% with VAC to 20% with radiation and 10% with VACA. No significant difference was found between radiation and VACA. At 5 years, however, the disease-free survival significantly favored the VACA group (65% vs. 53%; $P < .001$).

Presently, whole lung radiation is not a proven treatment for micrometastatic disease in the lung. It is not without risk. Radiation pneumonitis has been reported in doses as low as 15 Gy, especially when combined with actinomycin D.[16] Pulmonary function studies have shown a decrease in lung volumes and diffusing capacity of the lung for carbon monoxide that usually return to normal within 5 years.[17]

CHEMOTHERAPY

Lung metastases are preferentially treated with chemotherapy for tumors with a high degree of chemosensitivity and for those tumors that typically do not metastasize solely to the lung. Breast cancer metastasis, for example, may respond to hormonal suppression, cytotoxic agents, and molecular targeted therapies. Also, the lung metastasis is usually coincidental to the discovery of widespread metastatic disease. Other primary malignancies for which chemotherapy should strongly be considered as first-line therapy for lung metastasis include germ cell tumors, gynecologic malignancies, and the Ewing's sarcoma family of tumors (ESFT).

SURGERY

History

Surgery specifically for the resection of lung metastasis has been practiced for at least 75 years.[18] In 1927, Divis from Prague reported the removal of a lung metastasis as a separate, planned procedure. Other case reports appeared in the literature, including an often-quoted paper by Barney and Churchill in 1939. They resected a solitary renal cell carcinoma metastasis in a woman who survived for 23 years after the resection. Alexander and Haight[19] published the first series of cases in 1947. These cases were collected from surgeons throughout the United States and included six from the University of Michigan. Twenty-four patients with a solitary lung metastasis, 16 with carcinoma and 8 with sarcoma, underwent resection. One postoperative death occurred, 11 had recurrences, and 12 were disease free from 1 to 12 years later.[19] Other larger series were reported in the 1950s and 1960s in which indications were further expanded to include resection of multiple metastases and re-resection of recurrent disease.

Indications and Strategy

Alexander and Haight[19] were also the first to specify criteria for resection of lung metastasis. They include the following: (1) Metastatic disease is limited to the lung, (2) the primary neoplasm has been treated definitively and is presently controlled, and (3) the patient must be capable of tolerating complete resection of all metastases. These criteria remain applicable today, although sometimes with modifications and provisions.

The rationale for resecting lung metastasis is based on the premise that, before definitive treatment of the primary tumor, viable tumor cells spread hematogenously to the lung. Most of these cells perish, as described earlier in Biology, but some possess the cellular mechanisms needed for invasion and growth. Although the growth pattern of these tumor nodules may vary, the total number within the lung is fixed. Either because of the filtering properties of the pulmonary microcirculation or biologic limitations of the tumor cells, active tumor growth is confined only to the lung. Therefore, resection of these metastatic tumor nodules may potentially render the patient disease free. Because the nodules grow at different rates, detection and localization of small nodules become problematic. CT can image nodules less than 5 mm in size, and careful palpation of the lung may detect nodules as small as 3 mm. Smaller nodules, or those located deep within lung parenchyma, are missed, however. Follow-up imaging studies may again show nodules. These are not new nodules; rather, they are newly discovered nodules that now have reached a detectable size. Reexcision is warranted as long as the patient meets the original criteria for resection. Depending on growth patterns and other influences, such as adjuvant chemotherapy, multiple procedures over months and years may be necessary to keep the patient disease free. Therefore, resection of lung metastasis should never be considered as a one-time surgical therapy.

Two factors have influenced extending indications for metastasectomy beyond the basic criteria initially proposed by Alexander and Haight. The first has to do with improved treatment regimens for the primary neoplasms. These therapies may change our approach to such chemosensitive tumors as breast carcinoma, germ cell tumors, and some bone sarcomas. The second factor is our ability to perform metastasectomies, either first time or redos, with exceptionally low morbidity and mortality. Basic criteria for resection of lung metastasis and examples of some extended indications are listed in Table 51.2-1.

The nonseminomatous germ cell tumors often metastasize to the lung and mediastinal lymph nodes. The tumors may consist of multiple cell types, including benign teratomatous elements.

TABLE 51.2-1.   Basic Criteria and Extended Indications for Metastasectomy

Basic Criteria	Extended Indications
The primary tumor is controlled	Germ cell tumors
The lung is the only site of metastasis	Assessing chemotherapy response
All disease within the lung is resectable	Sarcoma with synchronous lung metastasis

The malignant components are highly responsive to multidrug chemotherapy regimens, but the benign teratomas are not. If lung or mediastinal masses remain after chemotherapy and tumor markers were not, or never were, elevated, resection of residual disease is indicated. Benign teratomas should be removed because they will continue to grow and eventually cause compressive or obstructive symptoms. The resected specimens may also reveal whether active, malignant elements remain that will require consideration of further chemotherapy. Assessing a response to chemotherapy applies to other tumors as well. Any chemosensitive tumor with lung metastasis can be considered for resection of residual lung lesions, even if the patient was originally considered unresectable because of the extent of lung involvement. Resecting the more prominent, or suspicious, of the remaining lesions removes chemoresistant sites and gives pathologic confirmation of disease status.

The diagnosis of a primary sarcoma with synchronous lung metastasis has an ominous prognosis. If a major amputation or ablative surgery is required for control of the primary tumor, the decision to proceed may hinge on resectability of the lung metastasis. Because metastasectomy has far less morbidity and functional disability, it is reasonable to perform the lung resection first. Less than a complete resection of the lung disease would render the patient incurable and obviate aggressive resection of the primary tumor.

Staging

Appropriate staging of a patient for lung metastasectomy begins with a careful assessment of the primary tumor site. This usually entails radiologic imaging, such as MRI for extremity sarcomas, but may also require endoscopy for gastrointestinal tumors. When radiation changes make assessment difficult, needle biopsy may be indicated. Assessing for possible recurrence is usually best accomplished by the physicians who treated the patient for the primary tumor.

Staging for metastatic disease in sites other than the lung depends on the type and origin of the primary tumor. In addition, any history or physical findings that suggest a metastatic focus should be thoroughly investigated. At the very least a bone scan is indicated with all sarcomas of bone and a CT of the abdomen with specific liver imaging for all colon carcinomas. Melanoma, renal cell carcinoma, and breast cancer all deserve a full metastatic workup that includes imaging of the head, chest, abdomen, and bones. Soft tissue sarcomas of the extremities usually metastasize only to the lung initially. However, truncal sarcomas, especially those located in the retroperitoneum, may spread to nodes or intraabdominal sites, including liver and spleen.

Disease within the chest is best staged with a contrast-enhanced spiral CT scan. This technique gives the best definition of parenchymal lung involvement, along with most areas of the mediastinum and chest wall (Fig. 51.2-4). Tumors abutting the pericardium and great vessels or with suspected intra-atrial extension through the pulmonary vein are better assessed for possible invasion with a cardiac-gated MRI. Similarly, tumors with potential invasion into the thoracic inlet require MRI for visualization of the brachial plexus, vertebrae, and subclavian vessels.

The role of PET scanning is still to be determined. In high-grade tumors with high uptake of [^{18}F]fluorodeoxyglucose,

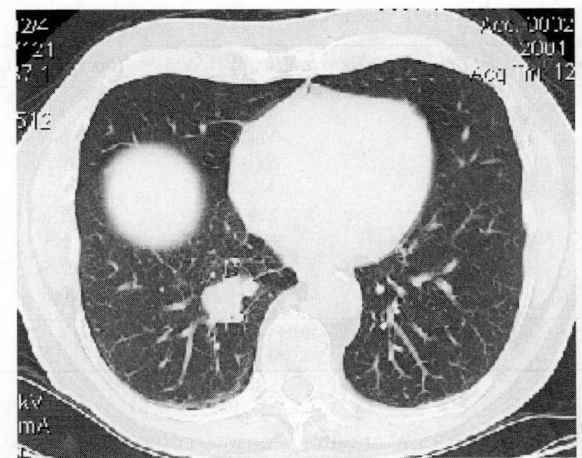 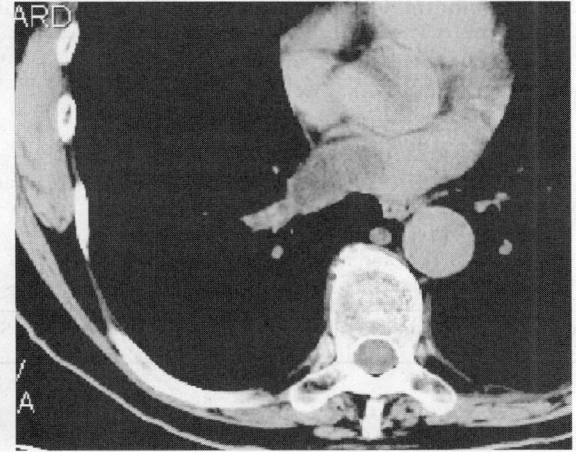

FIGURE 51.2-4. Synovial cell sarcoma metastasis in the right lower lobe (**A**) with extension through the inferior pulmonary vein into the left atrium (**B**).

PET may supplant all other imaging studies for residual disease at the primary site and at metastatic sites other than the lung. The superior spatial definition of the CT scan still makes it necessary for lung imaging. If fusion CT-PET scanning can deliver similar clarity, it may play an important role in staging and patient selection in the future.

Physiologic Assessment

Unlike lung cancer patients, most individuals being considered for resection of lung metastasis have reasonably normal pulmonary and cardiovascular systems. This is especially true for most sarcoma patients, who tend to be young and otherwise healthy. Some notable exceptions can be found, however, in whom careful, directed physiologic assessments are mandatory. In distinction to the sarcoma patient, those with colon, breast, and head and neck primary carcinomas are usually older and may have concurrent lung and heart disease that may need investigating. Patients who received certain chemotherapy agents during treatment of their primary tumor deserve special scrutiny. Bleomycin is used extensively in the treatment of germ cell tumors and can cause interstitial pulmonary fibrosis. Lung volumes and diffusion capacity should be determined preoperatively. Doxorubicin is a commonly used drug for bone and soft tissue sarcomas. It may cause cardiotoxicity, especially at cumulative doses greater than 450 mg/m². A MUGA (multiple gated acquisition) scan or other determination of cardiac ejection fraction is warranted.

Functional evaluation of the patient with recurrent lung metastasis becomes more challenging with each recurrence. Previous nonanatomic lung resections throughout both lungs make an estimation of lung reserve difficult to quantify. Ventilation-perfusion scans are of little help because their quantification is based on relative comparisons between lung zones. Evidence of carbon dioxide retention or pulmonary hypertension is indicative of markedly diminished pulmonary reserve and should mitigate against further extensive lung resections. Spirometry and measurements of maximal oxygen consumption may give some measure of lung function, but absolute values relate to risk only when major anatomic resections are contemplated. The two studies the authors have found most useful in assigning risk are the 6-minute walk and a global quality-of-life instrument.[20] In reality,

patients who have been through multiple lung resection procedures have impressive insight into the degree of their respiratory disability. They often become the final arbiter of whether or not more lung resections can be tolerated.

Prognostic Indicators

A large volume of the literature on lung metastasectomy is focused on the selection of patients for surgery based on clinical factors that may impact on survival. It is hoped that these prognostic indicators can identify those patients who would benefit the most from an aggressive surgical approach to their metastatic lung disease. This could also save certain groups of patients the risk and discomfort of a major procedure that has little chance of impacting on their survival. Over the years a long list of potential indicators has been appraised (Table 51.2-2). In most recent studies three indicators—histology, disease-free interval, and number of tumor nodules—have shown some prognostic validity. However, complete resection stands out as the only prognostic indicator that consistently predicts survival. The classic study by Marcove et al.[21] initially pointed this out. In 145 patients with osteosarcoma lung metastasis, 31% 5-year survival was realized in those treated with complete resection, versus 2% survival for unresectable patients. The International Registry of Lung Metastases study is a more recent example.[22] In this report, 5206 patients resected for lung metastasis of various histologies from 18 institutions in

TABLE 51.2-2. Potential Prognostic Indicators

Age
Disease-free interval
Gender
Histology or grade of the primary tumor
Number of metastases resected
Number of nodules on preoperative imaging study
Resectability
Synchronous versus metachronous
Tumor doubling time
Unilateral versus bilateral
Mediastinal or hilar lymph node metastasis

TABLE 51.2-3.   Significant Survival Advantages of Prognostic Indicators in Selected Studies

Study	Tumor	Subgroup(s) with Improved Survival	DFI (Y)	Resectability (Yes/No)	Resected Nodules (n)
Pastorino et al.[22]	All	Germ cell	3	Yes	1 vs. >1
Billingsley et al.[23]	STS	Gynecologic sarcoma	1	Yes	No
Pfannschmidt et al.[61]	Renal cell	Node negative	2	Yes	≤7 vs. >7
Saito et al.[94]	Colon	CEA <10 ng/mL, node negative	NS	NS	1 vs. >1
Saeter et al.[45]	Osteosarcoma	Response to chemo	NS	Yes	1 vs. >1
Seki et al.[64]	Uterine cervix	Tumor <3 cm	NS	Yes	NS
Liu et al.[62]	Head and neck	Glandular tumors	2	Yes	NS
Friedel et al.[59]	Breast		3	Yes	NS

CEA, carcinoembryonic antigen; DFI, disease-free interval; NS, not stated; STS, soft tissue sarcoma.

Europe and North America were retrospectively reviewed. A median survival of 35 months for completely resected patients, compared to 15 months for those incompletely resected, was highly significant. In a series of 719 patients with lung metastasis from soft tissue sarcoma of the extremities, the median survival of 33 months for fully resected patients was significantly better than the 11-month survival for those receiving nonoperative treatments (Table 51.2-3).[23] Thus, in terms of categorically excluding patients from undergoing metastasectomy, the inability to resect all of the metastatic disease is the only prognostic factor contraindicating surgery. Translating this into practical terms is often difficult. For instance, in a patient with multiple metastases, how many is too many? Numbers alone are not always helpful. Girard et al.[24] report a series of 44 patients who underwent resection of 8 to 110 metastases. Number of nodules resected was not a significant prognostic factor, but complete resectability was. Other issues then become important considerations, including age, intercurrent disease, operative risk factors, and position of the nodules in the lung. In certain situations, such as the young, otherwise healthy sarcoma patient, chest exploration is warranted. Preferably, this is done through an incision in which both lungs can be assessed simultaneously. The number and position of the nodules within the lung are accurately determined and the amount of lung to be removed for complete resection estimated. Unfortunately, video-assisted thoracoscopic surgery (VATS) is not an adequate approach to make this judgment, because it is often the deep-seated nodule close to the hilum and beyond the view of VATS that is the limiting factor for complete removal.

Techniques

ANESTHESIA. Standard thoracic anesthesia techniques are commonly used in all metastasectomy procedures regardless of the particular incision used. These include: continuous arterial blood pressure monitoring, usually with a radial artery line; continuous oxygen saturation and electrocardiographic monitoring; and split-lung ventilation with either a double-lumen endotracheal tube or a bronchial blocker. Prior chemotherapy exposure is an important consideration in intraoperative patient management. Bleomycin and mitomycin are known pulmonary toxins that can cause further lung injury if high fractions of inspired oxygen (FiO_2) concentrations are used. Ideally, the FiO_2 in these patients should be maintained at 40% or lower. Doxorubicin cardiomyopathy may lead to unexplained hypotension and arrhythmias that require inotropic agents or antiarrhythmic drugs. Postoperative pain control measures vary with the surgical inci-

sion. Whereas local anesthetic or intercostal nerve blocks at the incision sites may suffice for VATS, pain control after a lateral thoracotomy or clamshell incision is better managed with a thoracic epidural catheter. Intravenous and oral narcotics may be sufficient for discomfort from a median sternotomy incision because of the stability of its closure and the absence of divided muscles.

INCISIONS. The appropriate incision for metastasectomy depends on the individual patient circumstances and the experience of the surgeon. The overriding consideration is resection of all metastatic disease, not how one chooses to enter the chest. At least in terms of open procedures, there seems to be no difference in ultimate survival between a thoracotomy approach and median sternotomy.[25] Each incision has its own attractions as well as limitations (Table 51.2-4).

Certain circumstances may dictate the choice of surgical approach. For instance, in a patient with a single peripheral nodule and a long disease-free interval, VATS resection followed by careful follow-up seems reasonable. Likewise, the patient with bilateral metastasis, possibly invading the posterior mediastinum, is best approached through a clamshell incision. However, in most situations either sternotomy or lateral thoracotomy (or thoracotomies for bilateral disease) is preferred.[101]

RESECTIONS. Once the chest is entered, the lung is fully mobilized and each lobe is carefully palpated. This is best accomplished with a deflated, nonventilated lung and traction on the lung with an atraumatic lung clamp (Fig. 51.2-5). When bilateral resections are performed at the same setting, the lesser involved lung is resected first so that adequate single lung ventilation can be maintained during resection of the more involved lung. Nodules close to the lung surface are resected using an automatic stapling device, whereas those close to the hilum usually require anatomic segmentectomy or lobectomy. Pneumonectomy is rarely required but is justified if necessary for complete resection.[26,27] Every effort should be made to conserve lung tissue as long as a margin of normal tissue (at least 1 cm) is maintained around the nodule. Lung-sparing procedures, such as sleeve lobectomy and deep precision cautery excision (Perelman technique),[28] should be used whenever possible. Because small nodules can easily be missed, the surgeon and first assistant should independently palpate the lung.

Lung metastasis may spread to hilar and mediastinal lymph nodes; however, the frequency of these secondary metastases is unknown (Fig. 51.2-6). In one series, 9 of 63 patients (14%)

TABLE 51.2-4. Summary of Surgical Incisions

	Lateral Thoracotomy	*Median Sternotomy*	*Clamshell*	*VATS*
Advantages	Familiar approach; optimum exposure to hemithorax	One operation accesses and treats bilateral disease; good exposure to anterior mediastinum	Good exposure to hemithoraces and to entire mediastinum	Low morbidity; good exposure to lung surface and pleural space
Disadvantages	Bilateral disease requires 2 procedures	Limited exposure to left lower lobe	Higher morbidity; longer operating time	Lesions below lung surface difficult to locate; no palpation of lung
Relative patient discomfort	+++	++	++++	+
Special considerations	A lung without evidence of disease on imaging will not be explored	Use with caution in patients who may not tolerate traction on the heart	Problem with malunion of sternum	Reserve for patients with minimal, easily accessible disease and long DFI

DFI, disease-free interval; VATS; video-assisted thoracoscopic surgery.

subjected to ipsilateral mediastinal lymph node dissection (except for subcarinal nodes) had tumor involvement. The primary tumor in eight of these patients was a carcinoma, and the other had a Ewing's sarcoma.[29] Presently, an extensive lymph node dissection cannot be recommended, but resection of enlarged or suspicious nodes should be performed. This is especially pertinent in colon, renal, breast, melanoma, and germ cell tumors, in which mediastinal nodal metastases are not uncommon and may have prognostic implications.

The relative safety of lung metastasectomy, especially when compared with resections for primary lung cancer, is a major factor in promoting its widespread usage (Fig. 51.2-7). Operative morbidity and mortality are substantially lower than in patients with lung cancer. Patients undergoing metastasectomy are, on average, younger, have better cardiopulmonary function, and require less formidable lung resections. Even after multiple previous lung resections, metastasectomy can be accomplished with surprisingly low mortality.[30]

PALLIATIVE PROCEDURES

Most patients with lung metastasis die of progressive disease. Disease within the chest can cause disabling symptoms that may progress to become life threatening. Procedures aimed specifically at palliation can often alleviate symptoms and prolong life. Parenchymal metastases not amenable to complete resection are rarely resected for palliation alone. However, those involving major airways and pericardium or accompanying malignant effusions in the pleural or pericardial spaces often respond well to palliative measures.

Airway

Lung metastasis most commonly involves major airways either by direct extension from a parenchymal lesion or from invasion of tumor in hilar and mediastinal lymph nodes. Of all lung metastases, 2% to 5% directly involve the tracheobronchial tree primarily.[31] Most commonly, these originate from carcinomas of the kidney, colon, and breast, with melanoma and sarcoma being less frequent.[32] These are often unresectable because of their position within the airway or because of the extent of accompanying disease. They present initially as a cough, often with hemoptysis, then progress to severe dyspnea

and stridor if the mainstem bronchi or trachea are involved. Treatment is predicated on the severity of the symptoms. In the patient with life-threatening airway obstruction, immediate rigid bronchoscopic resection is indicated. The Nd:YAG (neodymium:yttrium aluminum garnet) laser is a helpful adjunct in the removal of endobronchial tumor and in controlling bleeding. Tumor regrowth with recurrent obstruction occurs unless more durable methods of control are initiated. If the tumor is chemotherapy resistant, external-beam radiation offers good local control with low morbidity. Other options include endobronchial brachytherapy, photodynamic therapy, and the use of endobronchial stents.[33] These procedures require highly specialized equipment and personnel. All are associated with a

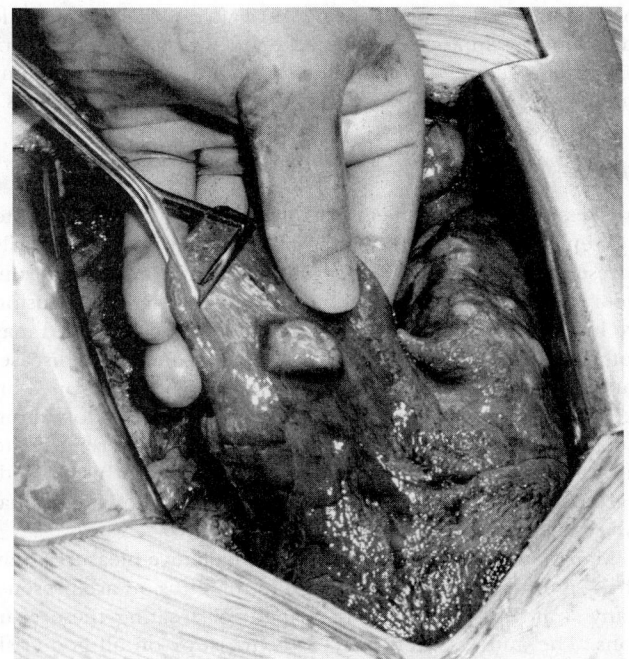

FIGURE 51.2-5. Intraoperative photograph showing palpation of a collapsed lung. The atraumatic clamp on the lung provides traction for precise palpation of the lung parenchyma. A metastatic nodule is clearly visible.

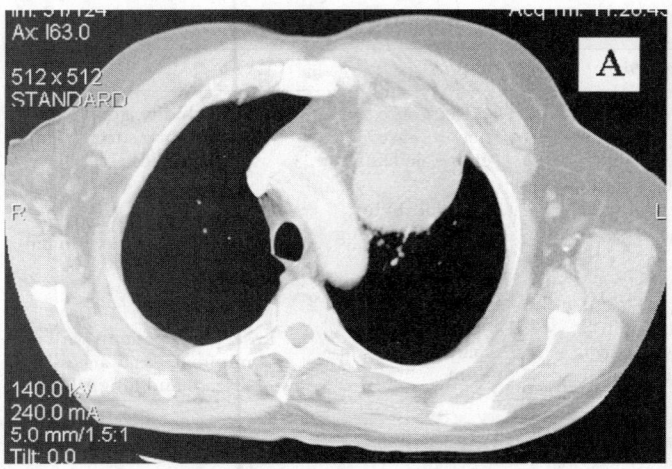
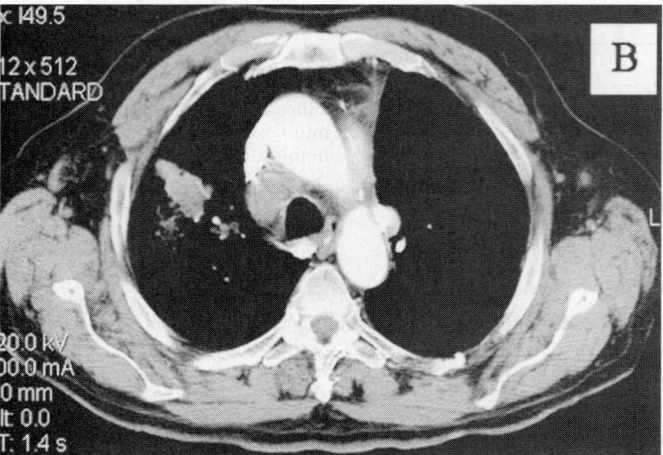

FIGURE 51.2-6.   Chest computed tomography scans of a 72-year-old man with metastatic colon cancer. **A:** The large left upper lobe metastasis was the only site of disease and was resected with a left upper lobectomy. Resected lymph nodes had no metastasis. **B:** Sixteen months later, the patient presents with a right upper lobe mass and bulky mediastinal adenopathy. A primary lung cancer was initially considered, but biopsy showed adenocarcinoma identical to colon primary. No resection was performed.

significant morbidity, which is often justified in an effort to maintain airway patency.

Pericardium

Extension of a lung metastasis onto the pericardium can result in hemodynamically significant pericardial constriction. This is most common with metastatic breast cancer but can occur with other malignancies as well. Patients present with symptoms of low cardiac output but may also have peripheral edema and ascites. If any effusion is present, it should be drained and the pericardium sclerosed.[34] In those patients with pericardial constriction, dramatic palliation of symptoms can be achieved with an anterior pericardiectomy. This is accomplished through a median sternotomy and the resection of all pericardium between the phrenic nerves.

Pleura

Progression of a lung metastasis through the pleura and into adjacent structures signifies aggressive, but not necessarily unresectable, disease.[27] However, when tumor involves the pleural space, diffuse dissemination and a malignant effusion are invariably present. This occurs with all histologies and may not be related to the amount of lung parenchymal disease. Patients usually present with the insidious onset of dyspnea on exertion and cough. Occasionally, a large sarcomatous lung metastasis may rupture into the pleural space, causing acute respiratory symptoms and hemodynamic instability from bleeding into the pleural space. Emergent thoracotomy and palliative resection may be necessary.

Malignant pleural effusions call for palliative measures only when significant symptoms related to the effusion are present. Many strategies have been described for treating these effusions. The authors prefer VATS pleuroscopy on all good-risk patients for complete evacuation of all fluid and direct assessment of lung expansion under anesthesia. If the lung fully expands, talc insufflation poudrage is performed. When the lung fails to expand enough to fill the pleural space, a cuffed

Silastic pleural catheter is placed to facilitate drainage of the effusion on an outpatient basis.[33]

EXPERIMENTAL THERAPIES

Radiofrequency Ablation

Radiofrequency ablation (RFA) has become commonplace in the treatment of metastatic disease to liver and kidney. A small but emerging experience has accrued in the treatment of lung metastasis. Most reports are anecdotal, and there are no controlled trials to date. RFA is confined to patients who are not operative candidates or for the palliation of unresectable lesions (Fig. 51.2-8). In one series of 18 patients with inoperable lung tumors, 13 of which were lung metastases, 10 of the patients had complete or partial responses as scored by a complex radiographic scheme. With a mean follow-up of only 4 months, long-term control cannot be assessed.[35] The authors note that tumors often increase in size after treatment, and therefore size alone may not be a valid indicator of response. Complications have generally been confined to

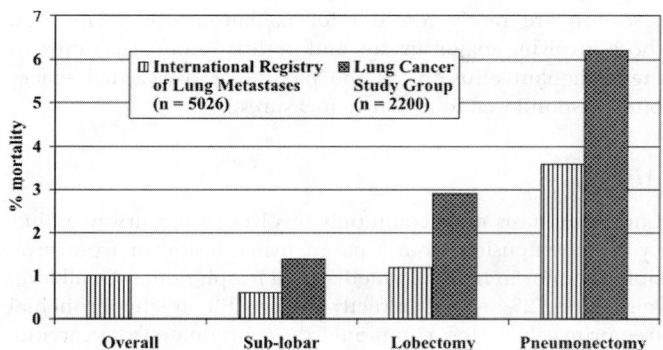

FIGURE 51.2-7.   Comparison of mortality for three different surgical procedures. Rates are taken from two large surgical series of lung resections for lung metastasis[22] and lung cancer.[100] The higher mortality in lung cancer patients is presumably due to their older age and higher incidence of comorbidities.

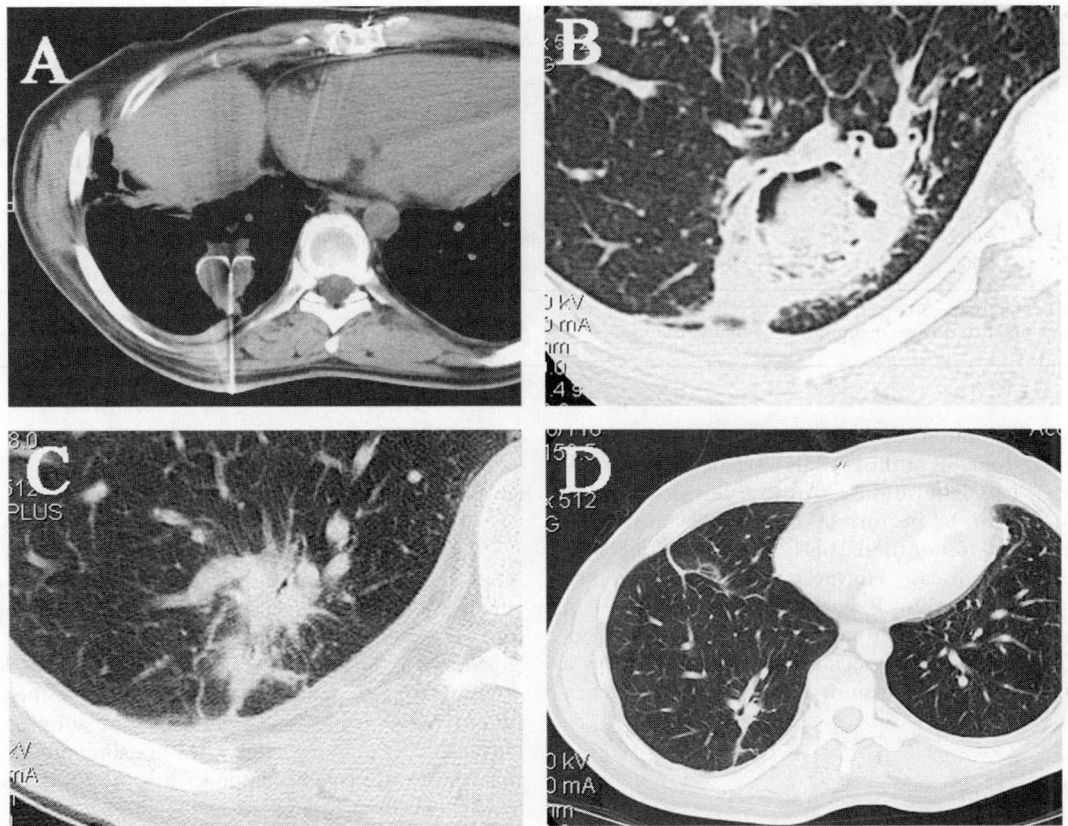

FIGURE 51.2-8. Radiofrequency ablation (RFA) of a neurofibrosarcoma lung metastasis in a 38-year-old man who had undergone four previous metastasectomies. **A:** Umbrella-tined needle is deployed within the metastasis. **B:** One week after RFA, the mass has cavitated. **C:** One month after RFA shows contracture of the mass and obliteration of the cavity. **D:** One year after RFA, only a linear scar remains, and there is no evidence of recurrence.

pneumothorax, pleural effusion, and pneumonitis, although one patient in the study died of massive hemoptysis. However, a prospective pilot study in the authors' institution suggests a cautious approach. Three patients with multiple lung metastases (two from colon and one from a soft tissue sarcoma) underwent technically successful RFA of one metastasis each (mean, 1.9 cm; range, 1.2 to 2.5) followed by complete resection of all lesions 2 to 4 weeks later. Of the three lesions subjected to RFA, 50% to 75% still showed viability as assessed by hematoxylin and eosin staining and immunohistochemistry for the proliferative marker, MIB-1. Further studies of cell viability are under way, but similar findings have been reported in kidney tumors.[36]

Lung Perfusion

Dose-limiting toxicity often preempts the administration of effective systemic chemotherapy for cancer. Isolated perfusion of organs or anatomic regions, such as limbs, has generated mixed results and enthusiasm for many years. Theoretically, lung metastasis is an ideal disease to treat with lung perfusion. Initial tumor seeding in the lung is through the pulmonary circulation, which continues to be a nutrient source for the tumors. In addition, perfusate is dispersed throughout the lung parenchyma, thus exposing multiple nodules and micrometastatic disease simultaneously. Attempts at isolating and perfusing the lung with high-dose chemotherapy date back to the late 1950s. More recently, Johnston[37] described methods of isolating and perfusing one or both lungs for the administration of high-dose chemotherapy. Perfusate is infused through a cannula placed in the pulmonary artery and recovered via a venous cannula positioned in the left atrium. Single-lung perfusion is accomplished by perfusing one lung while ventilating the other. Total lung perfusion requires cardiopulmonary bypass. The perfusion circuit includes a roller pump, heat exchanger, and reservoir. An oxygenator is included in the circuit if control of oxygen and carbon dioxide tension is desired.

Initial research was confined mostly to large, non–tumor-bearing animals. Weksler et al.[38] subsequently described a method of single-lung perfusion in rats. Therapeutic studies in rats with sarcoma or carcinoma lung metastases have now been carried out with a variety of anticancer agents, including doxorubicin, cisplatin, tumor necrosis factor-α, melphalan, FUdR (5-fluoro-2'-deoxyuridine), and gemcitabine.[39] These studies invariably show higher tumor drug levels than those achieved with intravenous drug. Most also show a decrease in the number or size of tumor nodules compared to the untreated lung.

Unfortunately, these encouraging animal data have not been duplicated in clinical trials to date (Table 51.2-5). Despite

TABLE 51.2-5. Phase I Clinical Trials of Lung Perfusion for Pulmonary Metastasis

Study	Year	Patients (n)	Chemotherapy	Toxicity	Response
Johnston et al.[95]	1995	8[a]	Doxorubicin or cisplatin	Two pulmonary complications; 1 death	None
Ratto et al.[40]	1996	6	Cisplatin	Two pulmonary edema	Metastases resected
Pass et al.[96]	1996	16	TNF-α	One systemic TNF toxicity	Three minor responses
Burt et al.[97]	2000	8	Doxorubicin	Major lung injury with 80 mg/m^2	One stable disease
Putnam[98]	2002	16	Doxorubicin	19% Mortality; 23% morbidity	One partial response
Schroder et al.[99]	2002	4	Cisplatin + hyperthermia	Four pulmonary edema	Metastases resected
Van Putte et al.[39]	2003	11	Melphalan	None	Metastases resected

TNF, tumor necrosis factor.
[a]Includes four patients with diffuse bronchioloalveolar carcinoma.

significant lung and tumor drug levels, objective responses were minimal. However, all of these trials were designed as feasibility and phase I toxicity studies. In those terms it is clear that lung perfusion can be performed consistently and with a high degree of safety. Most of these trials enrolled patients with otherwise unresectable disease. However, the study reported by Ratto et al.[40] and the ongoing Belgian/Dutch trial[39] differ in that they use lung perfusion as an immediate adjuvant to surgical resection of patients with resectable disease. If there is a therapeutic future for lung perfusion, this is the most attractive context for its use.

Lung Transplantation

The ideal solution for treating patients with unresectable metastatic cancer to the lung is to entirely remove the diseased organ and replace it with healthy lung. The patient must not have tumor elsewhere, either at the primary tumor site or other metastatic sites. Although this can never be determined with certainty, a long disease-free interval at all sites except the lung and a thorough metastatic workup are encouraging. In this context the indication for lung transplantation would be oncologic rather than respiratory. Thus, it would be potentially curative treatment for localized disease, not replacement of a failed organ.

Solid-organ transplantation for cancer therapy is a proven concept. In patients with hepatocellular carcinoma who have either one tumor mass less than 5 cm in diameter or up to three nodules smaller than 3 cm, the survival at 5 years after liver transplantation is 70% and the recurrence rate is approximately 15%.[41] The experience with lung transplantation for cancer is small and not nearly so promising. de Perrot et al.[42] summarized the world experience with transplantation for bronchioloalveolar carcinoma. Of 26 reported transplants, 13 have recurred, 11 of which were in the transplanted lung.[42]

Lung transplantation for the treatment of metastatic pulmonary disease is anecdotal. In Toronto, the authors performed a bilateral lung transplant for a patient with end-stage lung disease secondary to diffuse bilateral metastatic leiomyoma of the uterus (Fig. 51.2-9). The patient is doing well without evidence of recurrent disease 3 years after transplantation.[43] With survival after lung transplantation for all indications now greater than 50% at 5 years, this treatment strategy may become a viable alternative for highly selected patients with lung metastasis.

RESULTS

SARCOMA

Osteosarcoma

Osteosarcoma metastasizes primarily to the lung and has one of the more favorable histologies in terms of outcome after pulmonary resection. Before effective chemotherapy, the 5-year survival for osteosarcoma was only approximately 10% to 20%, and up to 80% of patients treated by radical resection of the primary tumor died from lung metastasis. An aggressive surgical approach was advocated by Marcove et al.,[21] who documented that the natural history of unresected pulmonary metastasis was associated with a 50% mortality at 1 year, 88% at 2 years, 95% at 3 years, and no survivors at 5 years. Following on this aggressive approach, Martini et al.[44] in 1970 reported the first series of 22 patients with metastatic osteogenic sarcoma who underwent resection of multiple lung metastases. When resection was coupled with induction or adjuvant therapy, a significant increase in survival was achieved. Currently, aggressive medical and surgical treatment attains 5-year survival rates ranging between 30% and 40% in patients with metachronous pulmonary metastasis (Table 51.2-6). Chemotherapy associated with aggressive resection of pulmonary metastasis has transformed a uniformly fatal condition into one with reasonable expectation of long-term outcome. The 5-year survival can achieve 50% in patients undergoing complete resection of metachronous pulmonary metastasis.[45]

The presence of synchronous pulmonary metastasis at the time of diagnosis of the primary tumor is associated with poorer outcome (see Table 51.2-6). However, histologic response to preoperative chemotherapy and complete resection of all sites of tumor correlate with improved long-term survival.[46]

Soft Tissue Sarcoma

Soft tissue sarcomas comprise a family of nonossifying malignant neoplasms arising from mesenchymal connective tissues. They may arise from any site, but extremities are most common. Although metastasis from soft tissue sarcoma, like those from osteogenic sarcoma, is usually confined to the lung, the results of resection are less favorable. In general these tumors are less sensitive to chemotherapy than osteosarcoma, which renders metastasectomy even more compelling. No data have suggested that neoadjuvant therapy improves resectability or survival. Hence, patients who meet standard criteria for resectability should undergo metastasectomy.

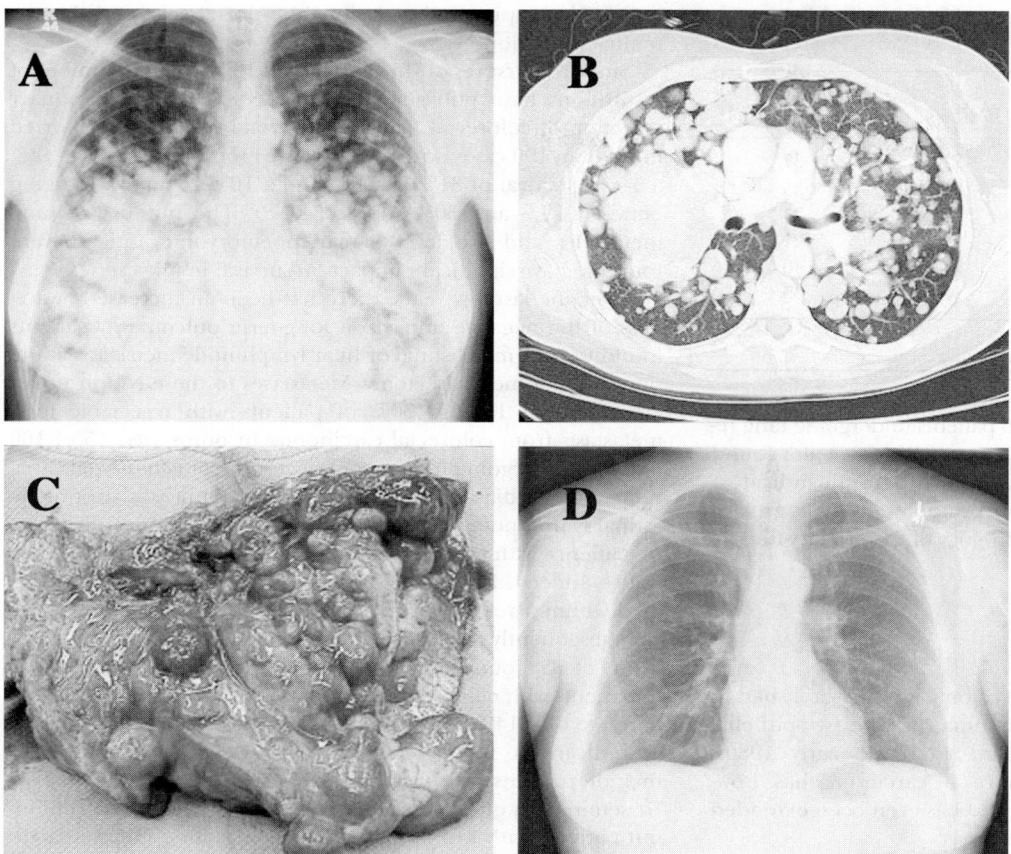

FIGURE 51.2-9. Lung transplantation for innumerable lung metastases from a leiomyoma of the uterus in a young woman. **A,B:** Chest radiograph and computed tomography scan pretransplant. **C:** Recipient lung clearly showing metastatic nodules. **D:** Chest radiograph 3 years after double-lung transplant. No evidence of recurrence is found.

In a review of 3149 patients with soft tissue sarcoma treated at the Memorial Sloan-Kettering Cancer Center between 1982 and 1997, 719 patients either developed or presented with lung metastasis. The likelihood of metastatic disease could be predicted according to the site, grade, and histopathology of the primary soft tissue sarcoma. The most common tumors to develop metastases to the lung were, by order of frequency, leiomyosarcoma, 21%; malignant fibrous histiocytoma, 18%; liposarcoma, 12%; and synovial sarcoma, 14%. Extremity soft tissue sarcomas were also more likely to metastasize to the lung than were visceral sarcomas. Complete resection, disease-free interval greater than 12 months, and low-grade histology were significant favorable prognostic factors, whereas an age older than 50 years at the time of metastases and a diagnosis of liposarcoma or malignant peripheral nerve tumor were unfavorable prognostic factors. Of 213 patients undergoing metastasectomy, 161 patients had a complete resection and achieved a 3-year survival of 46% and 5-year survival

of 37%.[23] These results were significantly better than for patients who had an incomplete resection or who did not undergo surgery. A metaanalysis by the EORTC based on 255 patients reported similar survival rates after complete resection, with 54% at 3 years and 38% at 5 years[47] (Table 51.2-7).

Recurrence in the lung develops in approximately half of the patients who have complete pulmonary resection of soft tissue sarcoma metastases. Median disease-free interval between metastasectomy and lung recurrence is 4 to 6 months. Experience with repeated thoracotomies remains limited, with only a few reports in the literature. The National Cancer Institute and M. D. Anderson Cancer Center reported their experiences with 43 and 39 patients, respectively, and found a median survival of 25 and 28 months after the second thoracotomy if complete resection is achieved.[48,49] Complete resection, a single lung metastasis, and a disease-free interval greater than 18 months were associated with improved survival when compared to patients with incomplete resection or with-

TABLE 51.2-6.   Outcome after Treatment for Lung Metastasis from Osteogenic Sarcoma

Study	Years	Patients (n)	Synchronous/ Metachronous	Cumulative 5-Y Survival (%)
Carter et al.[77]	1977–1983	25	0/25	20
Skinner et al.[78]	1971–1991	114	0/114	37
Meyer et al.[79]	1968–1987	59	0/59	38
Goorin et al.[80]	1972–1981	32	0/32	32
Meyers et al.[46]	1975–1984	62	62/0	11
Bacci et al.[81]	1993–1995	44	44/0	14

TABLE 51.2-7. Surgical Treatment of Pulmonary Metastasis from Soft Tissue Sarcoma

Study	Years	Patients (n)	Cumulative 5-Y Survival (%)
Billingsley et al.[23]	1982–1997	719	37
van Geel et al.[47]	NS	255	35
Casson et al.[49]	1981–1985	68	25
Verazin et al.[82]	1970–1986	78	21
Choong et al.[83]	1976–1992	214	40
Robert et al.[84]	1980–1993	126	35

NS, not stated.

out surgical options. In a series of 86 patients undergoing lung re-resection for metastatic soft tissue sarcoma, Weiser et al.[50] found an estimated 5-year survival of 36%. Poor prognostic indicators included more than three pulmonary nodules, nodules greater than 2 cm, and high-grade histopathology of the primary tumor.

CARCINOMA

Colon

Although the role of lung metastasectomy is well established in the treatment of patients with sarcoma, its role in epithelial cancers (carcinomas) is less clear. Since the early 1980s, metastasectomy for metastatic colorectal carcinoma has, however, become more commonplace and has even been extended to patients with lung and liver metastasis.

Metastatic spread of colorectal carcinoma typically involves regional lymph nodes, liver, and lung. Lung metastasis in the absence of other hematogenous metastasis occurs in only a minority of patients. A report of 1578 patients undergoing curative surgery for colorectal carcinoma found that 137 (8.7%) developed lung metastasis, and only 16 (1%) were candidates for metastasectomy. Although the incidence of liver metastasis was similar between colon and rectal carcinoma, lung metastasis appeared significantly higher (11.5%) after resection of rectal carcinoma than after resection of right (3.8%) or left (3.4%) colon carcinoma.[51] This is likely due to the usually more aggressive nature of rectal tumors

and to their spread directly into the portal vein and the systemic circulation.

Since the first report by Blalock[52] in 1944, a large number of institutions have published their experience with pulmonary resection of colorectal metastasis. Several series have reported more than 100 cases, with an operative mortality of 0% to 1.9%, a 5-year survival of 31% to 44%, and a 10-year survival ranging between 19% and 30% (Table 51.2-8). The number of lung metastases and the level of carcinoembryonic antigen were found to have significant impact on survival in most series.

Over the last few years, there has been an increased awareness of the negative impact on long-term outcome in patients found to have mediastinal or hilar lymph node metastasis at the time of lung metastasectomy. Metastases to these lymph nodes are found in 15% to 30% of patients with resectable lung metastasis from colorectal carcinoma. In one series, 15 of 100 patients undergoing lung metastasectomy from colorectal carcinoma with mediastinal lymph node sampling had hilar or mediastinal lymph node metastasis.[53] Survival was significantly worse in patients with nodal metastasis than in those with normal nodes. Indeed, 14 of the 15 patients with positive lymph nodes died within 5 years after metastasectomy; the lone 5-year survivor subsequently underwent chemotherapy for bone metastasis. Inoue et al.[54] found similar results, with a 5-year survival of 50% in patients with negative mediastinal or hilar lymph nodes, compared to only 14% in those with nodal metastasis.

Indications for resection are now being extended to include patients with liver and lung metastasis (Table 51.2-9). Dissemination of colorectal carcinoma to the liver is common, but patients with resectable liver as well as lung metastasis are rare. The most likely scenario is that of a patient who undergoes curative resection of liver metastasis, only to develop lung lesions later on. Resection of synchronous liver and lung metastasis is even less common and, despite complete surgical resection, is associated with a worse prognosis.[55–57] Resection of liver metastasis after a previous lung metastasectomy has also been reported.[55]

A review of prognostic factors in a series of 86 patients undergoing lung resection for metastasis from colorectal carcinoma found that a previous liver metastasectomy in 13 of these individuals had no impact on long-term outcome. Only complete resection and low preoperative carcinoembryonic antigen level were

TABLE 51.2-8. Survival after Metastasectomy by Primary Site of Carcinoma

Primary Site	Study	Year	Patients (n)	Cumulative 5-Y Survival (%)
Head and neck	Liu et al.[62]	1966–1995	83	50
	Wedman et al.[85]	1978–1994	21	59
Breast	Friedel et al.[59]	NS	467	38
Colorectal	Okumura et al.[53]	1967–1995	159	41
	McCormack et al.[86]	1965–1988	144	40
	McAfee et al.[87]	1960–1988	139	31
	Zink et al.[88]	1988–1999	110	33
Kidney	Pfannschmidt et al.[61]	1985–1999	185	37
	Piltz et al.[89]	1980–2000	105	40
Gynecologic	Fuller et al.[63]	1943–1982	15	36
	Seki et al.[64]	1959–1986	32	52

NS, not stated.

TABLE 51.2-9.   Resection of Lung and Liver Metastases from Colorectal Carcinoma

Study	Year	Patients (n)	Sequence of Metastases (n)	Cumulative 5-Y Survival (%)
Headrick et al.[55]	1980–1998	58	Liver-lung (45) Lung-liver (7) Synchronous (6)	30
Kobayashi et al.[90]	1988–1996	47	Liver-lung (25) Lung-liver (1) Synchronous (21)	31
Regnard et al.[91]	1970–1995	43	Liver-lung (43)	11
Mineo et al.[92]	1987–1998	29	Liver-lung (10) Lung-liver (7) Synchronous (12)	51
Nagakura et al.[57]	1982–2000	27	Liver-lung (17) Synchronous (10)	27
Robinson et al.[56]	1979–1998	25	Liver-lung (12) Lung-liver (5) Synchronous (8)	43
Lehnert et al.[93]	1981–1996	17	Liver-lung (16) Lung-liver (1)	25

statistically significant indicators of a good prognosis in multivariate analysis.[58]

Breast

Lung metastasis from breast carcinoma is more likely to occur through lymphatic channels via internal mammary or mediastinal lymph nodes, or both, than by hematogenous spread. Bone, pleura, and liver metastasis is often present also. Solitary lesions can be resected with good results, but this represents fewer than 1% of all patients with metastatic breast cancer. An analysis of 467 patients from the International Registry reported survival rates of 38% after 5 years, 22% after 10 years, and 20% after 15 years.[59] Most had only one metastasis that was completely resected through a lateral thoracotomy. Significant prognostic factors were a complete resection and a disease-free interval of at least 36 months. Incomplete resection was usually due to metastatic lymph nodes or chest wall and/or diaphragmatic invasion. Patients with a solitary lung metastasis had a survival rate of 44% at 5 years and 23% at 10 and 15 years, but this did not significantly differ from those with multiple metastases. In 19 patients undergoing repeated thoracotomies for recurrent lung metastasis, there was no difference in survival when compared to patients who underwent only one procedure. The 5-year survival was 37% after the first procedure and remained as high as 40% at 5 years after repeated thoracotomies.

Kidney

Metastatic disease develops in approximately 33% of patients with renal cell carcinoma. Common sites include the lung, liver, bone, brain, and adrenal. In a report of 278 patients with renal cell carcinoma, approximately half of those presenting with metastatic disease underwent a potentially curative metastasectomy.[60] The overall survival was 44% at 5 years, compared to 14% with noncurative surgery and 11% in those treated nonsurgically. Predictors of survival included a single site of first recurrence, complete resection, and a disease-free interval greater than 12 months. Other reports have shown the efficacy of lung resection for metastatic renal cell carcinoma. The 5-year survival ranges between 40% and 50% after complete resection in most recent series. The presence of metastasis in mediastinal or hilar lymph nodes is usually associated with significantly worse survival. Pfannschmidt et al.[61] performed systematic hilar and mediastinal lymph node dissection at the time of lung metastasectomy in 191 patients and found a significant drop in 5-year survival from 42% to 24% with positive nodes. Positive mediastinal or hilar lymph nodes remained significant in a multivariate analysis, along with the number of lung metastases and the disease-free interval.[61]

Head and Neck

Head and neck cancers, except for cancers of the lip, tonsil, and adenoid, metastasize initially to the lung. The difficulty is to differentiate between a metastatic lesion and a primary lung carcinoma, because most of these patients are smokers and are at high risk of developing multiple aerodigestive tract malignancies. If the pulmonary nodule is solitary, and if both lung and head and neck tumors are squamous carcinomas, it may be difficult to differentiate between a metastasis and a primary lung cancer. In such cases, if the lesion is resectable, it should be treated as a primary lung carcinoma with curative intent. When multiple lung lesions are detected, metastatic disease can be confirmed histologically with fine-needle aspiration biopsy or surgical biopsy. The efficacy of metastasectomy for head and neck carcinoma is unclear. An analysis of 83 patients operated on between 1966 and 1995 showed an operative mortality of 2%, with complete resection achieved in 86% of the patients and an overall survival of 50% at 5 years.[62] Patients with glandular tumors fared better than those with squamous cell cancer (5-year survival of 64% vs. 34%, respectively). When patients with glandular tumors were analyzed separately according to their histology, those with adenoid cystic carcinoma had a 5-year survival of 84%. Patients with thyroid cancers also have excellent overall survival, regardless of whether they are treated medically or surgically.

Gynecologic Cancers

Isolated lung metastasis from uterine and cervical carcinoma is relatively rare. Fuller et al.[63] reported 15 patients presenting with pulmonary metastasis from gynecologic cancers between 1943 and 1982. Six women had primary tumors involving the cervix, three from the endometrium and two each from ovary, uterine sarcoma, and choriocarcinoma. The 2- and 5-year survivals were 71% and 36%, respectively.

Seki et al.[64] reported 32 patients undergoing metastasectomy for lung metastasis from squamous cell carcinoma of the uterine cervix. More than half of the patients with lesions larger than 3 cm had secondary lymph node involvement and microscopic satellite lesions around the main metastatic nodule. The authors concluded that wedge resection of the metastasis is appropriate for metastatic lesions smaller than 3 cm but suggested that lobectomy with lymph node dissection is necessary for lesions 3 cm in diameter or larger.

Chemotherapy is the primary treatment for metastatic choriocarcinoma. However, on rare occasions pulmonary resection may be necessary to remove lung metastases that persistently secrete human chorionic gonadotropin (HCG) despite chemotherapy. In a series of 43 patients who underwent resection of lung metastasis from chemotherapy-resistant choriocarcinoma, an observed 5-year survival rate of 50% was achieved.[65]

MELANOMA

Although the clinical behavior of melanoma is often unpredictable, in general, resection of pulmonary metastasis has been disappointing. Chemotherapy and immunotherapy are still being used with mixed results. The 5-year survival is usually close to 10%. A report by Mathisen et al.[66] of 49 patients with pulmonary metastasis from melanoma between 1970 and 1986 found a median survival for all patients of 13 months and observed no significant difference in median survival between those undergoing resection of metastatic melanoma (12 months) and those who did not (10.5 months).

Harpole et al.[67] reviewed 945 patients presenting with melanoma lung metastasis. A total of 112 patients underwent pulmonary resection from this group. The 5-year survival in 98 patients with complete resection was 20%, whereas the overall survival of patients managed nonoperatively was 4%.[67] In a review of 328 metastatic melanoma patients from the International Registry of Lung Metastases, a similar survival of 22% at 5 years was found.[68] Factors that predicted better survival by multivariate analysis included complete resection, longer disease-free interval, treatment with chemotherapy, one or two lung metastases only, and the absence of metastatic lymph nodes. Although prognostic factors varied with the studies, most authors found that a disease-free interval greater than 12 months was associated with better prognosis. Ollila et al.[69] observed that a tumor doubling time of less than 60 days was associated with a mean survival of 16 months and no 5-year survivors, whereas the mean survival was 29 months and the 5-year survival was 21% in patients who had a tumor doubling time greater than 60 days.

GERM CELL TUMORS

Nonseminomatous germ cell tumors are characterized by wide dissemination, including lung metastasis, and high sensitivity to

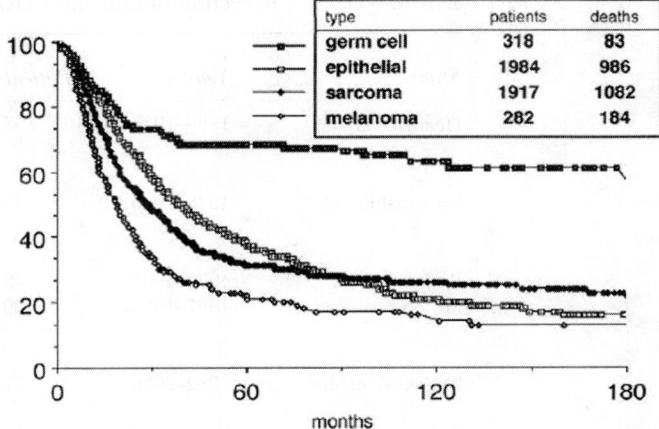

type	patients	deaths
germ cell	318	83
epithelial	1984	986
sarcoma	1917	1082
melanoma	282	184

FIGURE 51.2-10.   Overall survival curves for various tumor histologies from the International Registry of Lung Metastases. Note the significantly better survival in patients with germ cell tumors as compared to carcinomas (epithelial), sarcomas, and melanomas. (From ref. 29, with permission.)

chemotherapy. A cisplatin-based regimen has greatly improved the cure rate from 30% or less in the early 1960s to almost 90% over the past 10 to 20 years.[70] Resection of lung metastasis for germ cell tumors achieved the best long-term survival in the International Registry of Lung Metastases when compared to epithelial tumors (carcinomas), sarcomas, and melanoma (Fig. 51.2-10).

Current indications for resection in these patients are (1) absence of response to chemotherapy, (2) partial response followed by recurrence while on chemotherapy, (3) recurrence after standard and second-line chemotherapy, (4) to determine whether residual viable tumor is present, and (5) to resect enlarging benign teratomatous elements of the tumor. Surgical resection after chemotherapy serves to assess response, remove chemoresistant disease, and direct additional chemotherapy. Hence, resection of all residual disease seen on CT after chemotherapy is important. Often, only benign teratoma is found, because this element of the tumor is resistant to chemotherapy.

Kesler et al.[71] reviewed 268 patients who underwent cisplatin-based chemotherapy followed by at least one surgical procedure to remove residual mediastinal disease from nonseminomatous germ cell tumors of testicular origin. All patients demonstrated metastasis to the middle mediastinum, whereas only 16% of them also presented tumor in the paravertebral sulcus and 7% in the anterior mediastinum. Resected residual disease was necrotic in 15% of the patients, teratomatous in 59%, persistent nonseminomatous germ cell tumor in 15%, and non–germ cell carcinomatous degeneration in 11%. Overall 5- and 10-year survivals were 86% and 74%, respectively. Survival was negatively influenced by an elevated preoperative β-HCG and by the presence of residual mediastinal disease. Steyerberg et al.[72] observed that, in addition to the negative impact of elevated levels of β-HCG and incomplete resection, the number and size of lung metastases, as well as their persistence after chemotherapy, were adverse prognostic factors after multivariate analysis.

Because resection of residual masses containing only necrosis is unnecessary, Steyerberg et al.[73] estimated preoperatively the probability of necrosis, mature teratoma, and cancer in residual pulmonary masses. They found that, if the retroperitoneal lymph node dissection demonstrated only necrotic tissue, the probability of finding necrotic tissue at thoracotomy was high and thoracotomy may not be necessary.[73] Brenner et al.,[74] however, reported discordant histology between the chest and abdomen in 6 of 24 patients undergoing a combined approach, with viable tumor present in the chest, but not in the abdomen, in 1 patient.

EWING'S SARCOMA FAMILY OF TUMORS

The last decade has been marked by key advances in understanding the chromosomal rearrangements that link Ewing's sarcoma, peripheral neuroectodermal tumor, Askin's tumor, and neuroepithelioma. These tumors are currently defined as the ESFT.

ESFT are the second most common primary osseous malignancy in childhood and adolescence. Multimodality therapy has been most successful in these young age groups. Metastatic disease occurs in 20% to 25% of patients with Ewing's tumors and represents the most significant risk factor of poor prognosis. Approximately one-third of primary metastases are limited to the lung and pleura, and these patients seem to fare better than those with bone or bone marrow metastasis.

Strategies to improve outcome of patients with metastatic ESFT include whole lung radiation, dose-intensified chemotherapy, and high-dose therapy followed by autologous bone marrow or peripheral blood stem cell transplantation. The outcome of patients with ESFT and synchronous pulmonary or pleural metastasis, or both, is influenced by the response of the primary tumor to chemotherapy, the presence of metastatic lesions in one or both lungs, and the use of whole lung irradiation.[75] Surgical resection of pulmonary metastasis does not appear to improve survival and should be limited to patients with pulmonary relapse only.[76]

REFERENCES

1. von Herbay A, Illes A, Waldherr R, et al. Pulmonary tumor thrombotic microangiopathy with pulmonary hypertension. *Cancer* 1990;66:587.
2. Roberts KE, Hamele-Bena D, Saqi A, et al. Pulmonary tumor embolism: a review of the literature. *Am J Med* 2003;115:228.
3. Weiss L, Gilbert HA. Pulmonary metastasis. In: Weiss L, Gilbert HA, eds. *Pulmonary metastasis*. Boston: GK Hall, 1978:142.
4. Chang AE, Schaner EG, Conkle DM, et al. Evaluation of computed tomography in the detection of pulmonary metastases: a prospective study. *Cancer* 1979;43:913.
5. Gross BH, Glazer GM, Bookstein FL. Multiple pulmonary nodules detected by computed tomography: diagnostic implications. *J Comput Assist Tomogr* 1985;9:880.
6. Snyder BJ, Pugatch RD. Imaging characteristics of metastatic disease to the chest. *Chest Surg Clin North Am* 1998;8:29.
7. Remy-Jardin M, Remy J, Giraud F, Marquette CH. Pulmonary nodules: detection with thick-section spiral CT versus conventional CT. *Radiology* 1993;187:513.
8. Margaritora S, Porziella V, D'Andrilli A, et al. Pulmonary metastases: can accurate radiological evaluation avoid thoracotomic approach? *Eur J Cardiothorac Surg* 2002;21:1111.
9. Diederich S, Semik M, Lentschig MG, et al. Helical CT of pulmonary nodules in patients with extrathoracic malignancy: CT-surgical correlation. *AJR Am J Roentgenol* 1999;172:353.
10. Kersjes W, Mayer E, Buchenroth M, et al. Diagnosis of pulmonary metastases with turbo-SE MR imaging. *Eur Radiol* 1997;7:1190.
11. Lucas JD, O'Doherty MJ, Wong JC, et al. Evaluation of fluorodeoxyglucose positron emission tomography in the management of soft-tissue sarcomas. *J Bone Joint Surg Br* 1998;80:441.
12. Expert Panel on Musculoskeletal Imaging. ACR Appropriateness Criteria: follow-up examinations for bone tumors, soft-tissue tumors, and suspected metastasis post therapy. American College of Radiology. World Wide Web URL: http://www.acr.org/dyna/?doc=departments/appropriateness_criteria/toc.html, 2002.
13. Whelan JS, Burcombe RJ, Janinis J, et al. A systematic review of the role of pulmonary irradiation in the management of primary bone tumours. *Ann Oncol* 2002;13:23.
14. Burgers JM, van Glabbeke M, Busson A, et al. Osteosarcoma of the limbs. Report of the EORTC-SIOP 03 trial 20781 investigating the value of adjuvant treatment with chemotherapy and/or prophylactic lung irradiation. *Cancer* 1988;1;61:1024.
15. Razek A, Perez CA, Tefft M, et al. Intergroup Ewing's Sarcoma Study: local control related to radiation dose, volume, and site of primary lesion in Ewing's sarcoma. *Cancer* 1980;1;46:516.
16. Baeza MR, Barkley HT Jr, Fernandez CH. Total-lung irradiation in the treatment of pulmonary metastases. *Radiology* 1975;116:151.
17. Ellis ER, Marcus RB Jr, Cicale MJ, et al. Pulmonary function tests after whole-lung irradiation and doxorubicin in patients with osteogenic sarcoma. *J Clin Oncol* 1992;10:459.
18. Martini N, McCormack PM. Evolution of the surgical management of pulmonary metastases. *Chest Surg Clin North Am* 1998;8:13.
19. Alexander J, Haight C. Pulmonary resection for solitary metastatic sarcoma and carcinoma. *Surg Gynecol Obstet* 1947;85:129.
20. Parsons JA, Johnston MR, Slutsky AS. Predicting length of stay out of hospital following lung resection using preoperative health status measures. *Quality of Life Res* 2003;12:645.
21. Marcove R, Martini N, Rosen G. The treatment of pulmonary metastasis in osteogenic sarcoma. *Clin Orthop* 1975;111:65.
22. Pastorino U, Buyse M, Friedel G, et al. Long-term results of lung metastasectomy: prognostic analyses based on 5206 cases. *J Thorac Cardiovasc Surg* 1997;113:37.
23. Billingsley KG, Burt ME, Jara E, et al. Pulmonary metastases from soft tissue sarcoma: analysis of patterns of diseases and postmetastasis survival. *Ann Surg* 1999;229:602.
24. Girard P, Baldeyrou P, Le Chevalier T, et al. Surgical resection of pulmonary metastases. up to what number? *Am J Respir Crit Care Med.* 1994;149:469.
25. Roth JA, Pass HI, Wesley MN, et al. Comparison of median sternotomy and thoracotomy for resection of pulmonary metastases in patients with adult soft-tissue sarcomas. *Ann Thorac Surg* 1986;42:134.
26. Koong HN, Pastorino U, Ginsberg RJ. Is there a role for pneumonectomy in pulmonary metastases? International Registry of Lung Metastases. *Ann Thorac Surg* 1999;68:2039.
27. Putnam JB Jr, Suell DM, Natarajam G, Roth JA. Extended resection of pulmonary metastases: is the risk justified? *Ann Thorac Surg* 1993;55:1440.
28. Cooper JD, Perelman M, Todd TR, et al. Precision cautery excision of pulmonary lesions. *Ann Thorac Surg* 1986;41:51.
29. Loehe F, Kobinger S, Hatz RA, et al. Value of systemic mediastinal lymph node dissection during pulmonary metastasectomy. *Ann Thorac Surg* 2001;72:225.
30. Jaklitsch MT, Mery CM, Lukanich JM, et al. Sequential thoracic metastasectomy prolongs survival by re-establishing local control within the chest. *J Thorac Cardiovasc Surg* 2001;121:657.
31. Baumgartner WA, Mark JB. Metastatic malignancies from distant sites to the tracheobronchial tree. *J Thorac Cardiovasc Surg* 1980;79:499.
32. Heitmiller RF, Marasco WJ, Hruban RH, et al. Endobronchial metastasis. *J Thorac Cardiovasc Surg* 1993;106:537.
33. Johnston MR, Grondin S. The role of endoscopy in the staging and management of lung metastases. *Chest Surg Clin North Am* 1998;8:49.
34. Maher EA, Shepherd FA, Todd TJ. Pericardial sclerosis as the primary management of malignant pericardial effusion and cardiac tamponade. *J Thorac Cardiovasc Surg* 1996;112:637.
35. Herrera LJ, Fernando HC, Perry Y, et al. Radiofrequency ablation of pulmonary malignant tumors in nonsurgical candidates. *J Thorac Cardiovasc Surg* 2003;125:929.
36. Michaels MJ, Rhee HK, Mourtzinos AP, et al. Incomplete renal tumor destruction using radio frequency interstitial ablation. *J Urol* 2002;168:2406.
37. Johnston MR. Lung perfusion and other methods of targeting therapy to lung tumors. *Chest Surg Clin North Am* 1995;5:139.
38. Weksler B, Schneide A, Ng B, et al. Isolated single lung perfusion in the rat: an experimental model. *J Appl Physiol* 1993;74:2736.
39. Van Putte BP, Hendriks JMH, Romijn S, et al. Isolated lung perfusion for the treatment of pulmonary metastases: current mini-review of work in progress. *Surg Oncol* 2003;12:187.
40. Ratto GB, Toma S, Civalleri D, et al. Isolated lung perfusion with platinum in the treatment of pulmonary metastases from soft tissue sarcomas. *J Thorac Cardiovasc Surg* 1996;112:614.
41. Llovet JM, Burroughs A, Bruix J. Hepatocellular carcinoma. *Lancet* 2003;362:1907.
42. de Perrot M, Chernenko S, Waddell TK, et al. Impact of bronchogenic carcinoma in patients undergoing lung transplantation. Results of an international survey. *J Heart Lung Transplant* 2003;22:S161.
43. Shargall Y, Pakhale S, Chamberlain D, et al. Bilateral lung transplantation for metastatic leiomyosarcoma. *J Heart Lung Transplant* 2004;23:912.
44. Martini N, Huvos AG, Mike V, et al. Multiple pulmonary resections in the treatment of osteogenic sarcoma. *Ann Thorac Surg* 1971;12:271.
45. Saeter G, Hoie J, Stenwig AE, et al. Systemic relapse of patients with osteogenic sarcoma. Prognostic factors for long term survival. *Cancer* 1995;75:1084.
46. Meyers PA, Heller G, Healey JH, et al. Osteogenic sarcoma with clinically detectable metastasis at initial presentation. *J Clin Oncol* 1993;11:449.
47. van Geel AN, Pastorino U, Jauch KW, et al. Surgical treatment of lung metastases: the European Organization for Research and Treatment of Cancer–Soft Tissue and Bone Sarcoma Group study of 255 patients. *Cancer* 1996;77:675.
48. Pogrebniak HW, Roth JA, Steinberg SM, et al. Reoperative pulmonary resection in patients with metastatic soft tissue sarcoma. *Ann Thorac Surg* 1991;52:197.
49. Casson AG, Putnam JB, Natarajan G, et al. Efficacy of pulmonary metastasectomy for recurrent soft tissue sarcoma. *J Surg Oncol* 1991;47:1.
50. Weiser MR, Downey RJ, Leung DH, et al. Repeat resection of pulmonary metastases in patients with soft-tissue sarcoma. *J Am Coll Surg* 2000;191:184.
51. Pihl E, Hughes ES, McDermott FT, et al. Lung recurrence after curative surgery for colorectal cancer. *Dis Colon Rectum* 1987;30:417.
52. Blalock A. Recent advances in surgery. *N Engl J Med* 1944;231:261.
53. Okumura S, Kondo H, Tsuboi M, et al. Pulmonary resection for metastatic colorectal cancer: experiences with 159 patients. *J Thorac Cardiovasc Surg* 1996;112:867.
54. Inoue M, Kotake Y, Nakagawa K, et al. Surgery for pulmonary metastases from colorectal carcinoma. *Ann Thorac Surg* 2000;70:380.

55. Headrick JR, Miller DL, Nagorney DM, et al. Surgical treatment of hepatic and pulmonary metastases from colon cancer. *Ann Thorac Surg* 2001;71:975.

56. Robinson BJ, Rice TW, Strong SA, et al. Is resection of pulmonary and hepatic metastases warranted in patients with colorectal cancer? *J Thorac Cardiovasc Surg* 1999;117:66.

57. Nagakura S, Shirai Y, Yamato Y, et al. Simultaneous detection of colorectal carcinoma liver and lung metastases does not warrant resection. *J Am Coll Surg* 2001;193:153.

58. Girard P, Ducreux M, Baldeyrou P, et al. Surgery for lung metastases from colorectal cancer: analysis of prognostic factors. *J Clin Oncol* 1996;14:2047.

59. Friedel G, Pastorino U, Ginsberg RJ, et al. Results of lung metastasectomy from breast cancer: prognostic criteria on the basis of 467 cases of the International Registry of Lung Metastases. *Eur J Cardiothorac Surg* 2002;22:335.

60. Kavolius JP, Mastorakos DP, Pavlovich C, et al. Resection of metastatic renal cell carcinoma. *J Clin Oncol* 1998;16:2261.

61. Pfannschmidt J, Hoffmann H, Muley T, et al. Prognostic factors for survival after pulmonary resection of metastatic renal cell carcinoma. *Ann Thorac Surg* 2002;74:1653.

62. Liu D, Labow DM, Dang N, et al. Pulmonary metastasectomy for head and neck cancers. *Ann Surg Oncol* 1999;6:572.

63. Fuller AF Jr, Scannell JG, Wilkins EW Jr. Pulmonary resection for metastases from gynecologic cancers: Massachusetts General Hospital experience, 1943–1982. *Gynecol Oncol* 1985;22:174.

64. Seki M, Nakagawa K, Tsuchiya S, et al. Surgical treatment of pulmonary metastases from uterine cervical cancer. Operation method by lung tumor size. *J Thorac Cardiovasc Surg* 1992;104:876.

65. Xu LT, Sun CF, Wang YE, et al. Resection of pulmonary metastatic choriocarcinoma in 43 drug-resistant patients. *Ann Thorac Surg* 1985;39:257.

66. Mathisen DJ, Flye MW, Peabody J. The role of thoracotomy in the management of pulmonary metastases from malignant melanoma. *Ann Thorac Surg* 1979;27:295.

67. Harpole DH Jr, Johnson CM, Wolfe WG, et al. Analysis of 945 cases of pulmonary metastatic melanoma. *J Thorac Cardiovasc Surg* 1992;103:743.

68. Leo F, Cagini L, Rocmans P, et al. Lung metastases from melanoma: when is surgical treatment warranted? *Br J Cancer* 2000;83:569.

69. Ollila DW, Stern SL, Morton DL. Tumor doubling time: a selection factor for pulmonary resection of metastatic melanoma. *J Surg Oncol* 1998;69:206.

70. Liu D, Abolhoda A, Burt ME, et al. Pulmonary metastasectomy for testicular germ cell tumors: a 28-year experience. *Ann Thorac Surg* 1998;66:1709.

71. Kesler KA, Brooks JA, Rieger KM, et al. Mediastinal metastasis from testicular nonseminomatous germ cell tumors: patterns of dissemination and predictors of long-term survival with surgery. *J Thorac Cardiovasc Surg* 2003;125:913.

72. Steyerberg EW, Keizer HJ, Zwartendijk J, et al. Prognosis after resection of residual masses following chemotherapy for metastatic nonseminomatous testicular cancer: a multivariate analysis. *Br J Cancer* 1993;68:195.

73. Steyerberg EW, Keizer HJ, Messemer JE, et al. Residual pulmonary masses after chemotherapy for metastatic nonseminomatous germ cell tumor. Prediction of histology. ReHiT Study Group. *Cancer* 1997;79:345.

74. Brenner PC, Herr HW, Morse MJ, et al. Simultaneous retroperitoneal, thoracic, and cervical resection of postchemotherapy residual masses in patients with metastatic nonseminomatous germ cell tumors of the testis. *J Clin Oncol* 1996;14:1765.

75. Paulussen M, Ahrens S, Craft AW, et al. Ewing's tumors with primary lung metastases: survival analysis of 114 (European Intergroup) Cooperative Ewing's Sarcoma Studies patients. *J Clin Oncol* 1998;16:3044.

76. Heij HA, Vos A, de Kraker J, et al. Prognostic factors in surgery for pulmonary metastases in children. *Surgery* 1994;115:687.

77. Carter SR, Grimer RJ, Sneath RS, et al. Results of thoracotomy in osteogenic sarcoma with pulmonary metastases. *Thorax* 1991;46:727.

78. Skinner KA, Eilber FR, Holmes EC, et al. Surgical treatment and chemotherapy for pulmonary metastases from osteosarcoma. *Arch Surg* 1992;127:1065.

79. Meyer WH, Schell MJ, Kumar AP, et al. Thoracotomy for pulmonary metastatic osteosarcoma. An analysis of prognostic indicators of survival. *Cancer* 1987;59:374.

80. Goorin AM, Shuster JJ, Baker A, et al. Changing pattern of pulmonary metastases with adjuvant chemotherapy in patients with osteosarcoma: results from the multiinstitutional osteosarcoma study. *J Clin Oncol* 1991;9:600.

81. Bacci G, Briccoli A, Mercuri M, et al. Osteosarcoma of the extremities with synchronous lung metastases: long-term results in 44 patients treated with neoadjuvant chemotherapy. *J Chemother* 1998;10:69.

82. Verazin GT, Warneke JA, Driscoll DL, et al. Resection of lung metastases from soft-tissue sarcomas. A multivariate analysis. *Arch Surg* 1992;127:1407.

83. Choong PF, Pritchard DJ, Rock MG, et al. Survival after pulmonary metastasectomy in soft tissue sarcoma. Prognostic factors in 214 patients. *Acta Orthop Scand* 1995;66:561.

84. Robert JH, Ambrogi V, Mermillod B, et al. Factors influencing long-term survival after lung metastasectomy. *Ann Thorac Surg* 1997;63:777.

85. Wedman J, Balm AJ, Hart AA, et al. Value of resection of pulmonary metastases in head and neck cancer patients. *Head Neck* 1996;18:311.

86. McCormack PM, Burt ME, Bains MS, et al. Lung resection for colorectal metastases. 10-year results. *Arch Surg* 1992;127:1403.

87. McAfee MK, Allen MS, Trastek VF, et al. Colorectal lung metastases: results of surgical excision. *Ann Thorac Surg* 1992;53:780.

88. Zink S, Kayser G, Gabius HJ, et al. Survival, disease-free interval, and associated tumor features in patients with colon/rectal carcinomas and their resected intra-pulmonary metastases. *Eur J Cardiothorac Surg* 2001;19:908.

89. Piltz S, Meimarakis G, Wichmann MW, et al. Long-term results after pulmonary resection of renal cell carcinoma metastases. *Ann Thorac Surg* 2002;73:1082.

90. Kobayashi K, Kawamura M, Ishihara T. Surgical treatment for both pulmonary and hepatic metastases from colorectal cancer. *J Thorac Cardiovasc Surg* 1999;118:1090.

91. Regnard JF, Grunenwald D, Spaggiari L, et al. Surgical treatment of hepatic and pulmonary metastases from colorectal cancers. *Ann Thorac Surg* 1998;66:214.

92. Mineo TC, Ambrogi V, Tonini G, et al. Long-term results after resection of simultaneous and sequential lung and liver metastases from colorectal carcinoma. *J Am Coll Surg* 2003;197:386.

93. Lehnert T, Knaebel HP, Duck M, et al. Sequential hepatic and pulmonary resections for metastatic colorectal cancer. *Br J Surg* 1999;86:241.

94. Saito Y, Omiya H, Kohno K, et al. Pulmonary metastasectomy for 165 patients with colorectal carcinoma: a prognostic assessment. *J Thorac Cardiovasc Surg* 2002;124:1007.

95. Johnston MR, Minchin R, Dawson CA. Lung perfusion with chemotherapy in patients with unresectable metastatic sarcoma to the lung or diffuse bronchioloalveolar carcinoma. *J Thorac Cardiovasc Surg* 1995;110:368.

96. Pass HI, Mew DJY, Kranda KC, et al. Isolated lung perfusion with tumor necrosis factor for pulmonary metastases. *Ann Thorac Surg* 1996;61:1609.

97. Burt ME, Liu D, Abolhoda A, et al. Isolated lung perfusion for patients with unresectable metastases from sarcoma: a phase I trial. *Ann Thorac Surg* 2000;69:1542.

98. Putnam JB. New and evolving treatment methods for pulmonary metastases. *Semin Thorac Cardiovasc Surg* 2002;14:49.

99. Schroder C, Fisher S, Pieck AC, et al. Technique and results of hyperthermic (41 degrees C) isolated lung perfusion with high doses of cisplatin for the treatment of surgically relapsing or unresectable lung sarcoma metastasis. *Eur J Cardiothorac Surg* 2002;22:41.

100. Ginsberg RJ, Hill LD, Eagan RT, et al. Modern thirty-day operative mortality for surgical resections in lung cancer. *J Thorac Cardiovasc Surg* 1983;86:654.

101. Johnston MR. Median sternotomy for resection of pulmonary metastases. *J Thorac Cardiovasc Surg* 1983;85:516.

SECTION 3

H. RICHARD ALEXANDER, JR.
NANCY E. KEMENY
THEODORE S. LAWRENCE

Metastatic Cancer to the Liver

Metastases to the liver represent the sole or life-limiting component of disease for many patients with a variety of cancers, including colorectal cancer, ocular melanoma, neuroendocrine tumors, and other histologies. The liver is a common site of hematogenous metastases for tumors arising in the gastrointestinal tract, presumably because of the unique venous drainage through the portal venous system to the liver. On the other hand, factors that predispose ocular melanoma to metastasize predominantly to the liver are unknown but must occur through hematogenous spread

via the arterial system. Once metastases to the liver are diagnosed, the prognosis is generally poor. Even with aggressive therapy, the median survival for patients with ocular melanoma in the liver is between 2 and 7 months[1] and 12 to 24 months for patients with colorectal cancer.[2] Because of the unique vascular anatomy of the liver, a number of regional therapies designed to maximize efficacy while minimizing systemic toxicity have been under clinical evaluation. For patients with colorectal cancer, the ability to resect disease is associated with 5-year disease-free survival in 20% to 50% of patients,[3,4] and patients with liver metastases from functional neuroendocrine tumors can derive substantial palliative benefit from resection.[5] Infusional therapy is administered into the hepatic artery using intermittent percutaneous catheterization, usually with particle embolization of the tumor neovasculature (chemoembolization) or via continuous hepatic artery infusion (HAI) therapy with indwelling implantable pumps. Local ablative therapy is administered via laparotomy or percutaneously

TABLE 51.3-1. Various Regional Treatments under Clinical Evaluation for Cancers Confined to the Liver

Treatment	Advantages	Disadvantages
Resection	5-Y survival: 20–50% for colorectal cancer patients	Disease-free survival is low Limited number of patients suitable
Infusional therapy		
Chemoembolization	Can palliate large symptomatic tumor deposits Effects are prompt	May require repeated percutaneous catheterizations Staged treatments are usually necessary
Hepatic artery infusion	Allows significant dose escalation, has high response rates FUDR has high hepatic extraction, minimizing systemic toxicity	Implantable pump is expensive, requires laparotomy
Hepatic perfusion	Allows regional delivery of novel agents	Technically complex to administer
Selective internal radiation	Novel method of delivering radiation with minimal hepatic injury	Inhomogeneous radiation distribution Systemic leak
Local ablative therapy (cryotherapy, RF ablation, local injection)	Can obliterate established hepatic metastases Minimal injury to normal hepatic tissue	Often requires operative procedure to apply treatment Does not treat microscopic disease; limitations on size and number of lesions that can be treated

FUDR, floxuridine; RF, radiofrequency.

placed probes or needles to deliver cryo- or radiofrequency ablation (RFA) of tumors or direct injection of cytotoxic agents such as ethanol. Combined approaches have been used, such as adjuvant HAI after resection or local ablation, in an attempt to prolong disease control in the liver. Newer regional therapies, such as isolated hepatic perfusion (IHP) or selective internal radiation, are being evaluated.

Many of the data regarding regional therapy for hepatic metastases relate to colorectal cancer because of its high incidence. Approximately 150,000 new cases of colorectal carcinoma occur annually in the United States, and 75,000 deaths will occur.[6] Synchronous hepatic metastases are identified in 10% to 20% of patients with colorectal cancer and are the sole or life-limiting component of disease in up to 60% of patients.[7] Only a small proportion of patients have resectable disease,[8] and therefore the vast majority are best suited for a regional therapy, as mentioned above. This section reviews the natural history of patients with hepatic metastases and the recent advances in imaging modalities. The results of resection alone or with adjuvant therapy for patients with resectable disease are presented, as well as results with other regional therapies, such as local ablative techniques, HAI therapies, and newer approaches (Table 51.3-1).

NATURAL HISTORY OF LIVER METASTASES

The natural history of hepatic metastases from different histologies has been largely derived from retrospective studies and

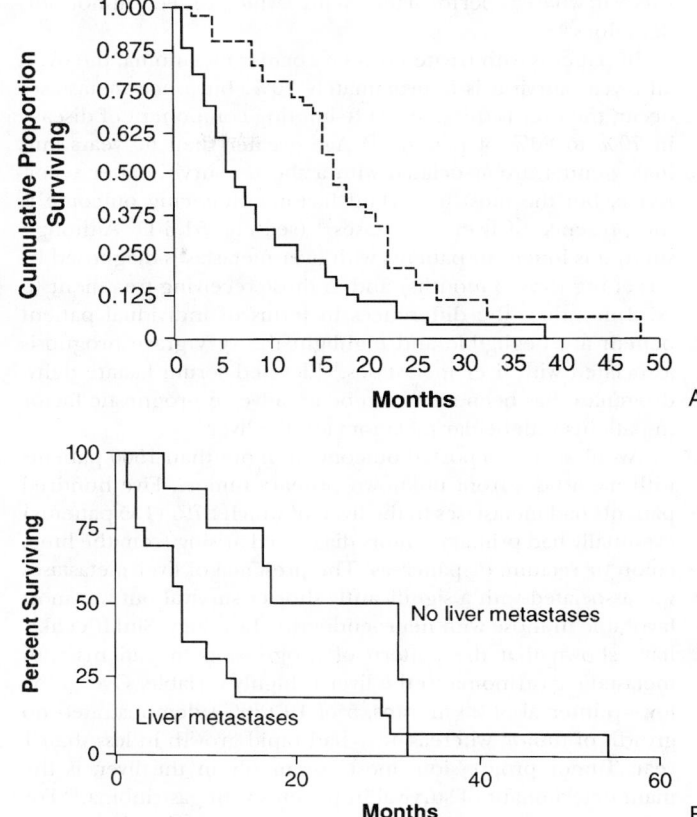

FIGURE 51.3-1. **A:** Survival in patients with untreated colorectal cancer with metastases confined to the liver based on percent hepatic replacement of 20 or less (*dotted line*) or greater than 20 (*solid line*). **B:** Survival in patients with metastatic ocular melanoma with or without hepatic metastases. (Modified from refs. 11 and 13.)

without the benefit of newer imaging modalities. Outcome of patients who are staged using computed tomography (CT), magnetic resonance imaging (MRI), or, for patients with neuroendocrine tumors, somatostatin receptor scintigraphy (SRS), survival may appear better than that of historic controls, for whom the number and extent of hepatic metastases were not easily quantified (Fig. 51.3-1). In addition, there is variability in the rate of progression of disease in the liver. In patients with colorectal cancer metastatic to the liver, for example, there are occasional long-term survivors and considerable disparity between median and mean survival (see Fig. 51.3-1). In one series from Roswell Park Cancer Institute of 30 patients with untreated colorectal cancer metastatic to the liver, the mean survival was 16 months, with a range of 2 to 58 months.[9] Heterogeneity in tumor progression has also been demonstrated in patients with neuroendocrine tumors metastatic to the liver.[10]

In a series of 544 patients with unresectable colorectal liver metastases documented by laparotomy, CT, or ultrasound (US), the factors that independently predicted outcome on multivariate analysis were performance status, extent of liver disease (number of involved segments), abnormal liver tests (prothrombin time and alkaline phosphatase), and site of primary tumor.[8] Those with no adverse factors (i.e., normal performance status and liver tests) had a 1-year survival of 46%. In general, patient factors such as gender or age do not influence survival, whereas performance status, which reflects tumor burden, does.[8,11]

In patients with treated primary ocular melanoma, the overall 5-year survival is approximately 70%, but once metastases occur, the liver is the sole or life-limiting component of disease in 70% to 80% of patients.[12] Age greater than 50 years and male gender are associated with a shorter survival after recurrence, but the most important factor influencing outcome is the presence of liver metastases[13] (see Fig. 51.3-1). Although survival is longer in patients with liver metastases diagnosed by screening (5 vs. 3 months) and in those receiving treatment (5 vs. 2 months), the differences in terms of individual patient benefit are negligible and highlight the very grave prognosis associated with liver metastases.[1] Elevated serum lactate dehydrogenase has been shown to be an adverse prognostic factor in patients with ocular melanoma to the liver.[14]

Ayoub et al.[15] reported outcome in more than 1500 patients with metastases from unknown primary tumors. Five hundred patients had metastases to the liver, of which 27% (135 patients) eventually had primary tumors diagnosed arising from the lung, colon or rectum, or pancreas. The presence of liver metastases was associated with a significantly shorter survival but was most favorable in those with neuroendocrine histology. Sutliff et al.[10] have shown that the pattern of progression in patients with metastatic gastrinoma to the liver is highly variable. Over a follow-up interval of 29 months, 5 of 19 (26%) demonstrated no growth of tumor, whereas 42% had rapid growth in less than 1 year. Tumor progression, most commonly in the liver, is the main determinant of survival in patients with gastrinoma.[16] For individuals with liver metastases from other functional neuroendocrine tumors, the sequelae from uncontrolled hormone production are the main cause of death.

IMAGING OF HEPATIC METASTASES

Currently, several imaging options are available for assessment of liver metastases. Considerable advancements in imaging technology have made it possible to accurately detect the number, size, and distribution of hepatic lesions and frequently distinguish between malignant or benign lesions. The most commonly used tests include CT scan, MRI, US, and, more recently, positron emission tomography (PET), usually using the glucose analogue FDG ([^{18}F]fluorodeoxyglucose). US is commonly used for screening because of its availability, and it is relatively inexpensive, but its most important application is as an intraoperative modality to assess suitably for resection and to gauge the adequacy of treatment when using local ablative therapy. In general, intraoperative US identifies 20% more occult lesions in the liver than does CT scan and therefore should be used with any contemplated resection.[17]

CT scan is used most commonly to assess a patient with possible hepatic metastases. It has the advantages of being widely available and, by using new-generation rapid-acquisition scanners, the entire chest, abdomen, and pelvis can be evaluated in a single breath-hold, eliminating the problem of respiratory misregistration. The overall detection rate of helical CT in detecting colorectal liver metastases is approximately 85%, and the positive predictive value is 96%.[18] Because liver tumors have a variable degree of vascularity and derive their

perfusion from the arterial tree, CT arterioportography has been used to enhance the sensitivity of the test, particularly for hypovascular lesions, but involves placement of a catheter and injection of contrast into the superior mesenteric artery with capture of images during the arterial and the portal venous phase of hepatic perfusion. Dual arterial and venous phase CT scans after intravenous injection of contrast agent using high-speed helical CT scanners are now commonly used in place of CT arterioportography but may have limited additional sensitivity for detection of hypovascular tumors compared to portal phase CT alone. On the other hand, because hypervascular lesions are frequently isoattenuating in relation to normal liver parenchyma, arterial phase helical CT can detect more liver metastases than conventional portal venous phase CT in this setting.

MRI scanning is also used routinely and has particular advantages for imaging of focal liver lesions. The most common contrast agents used with MRI are gadolinium chelates.[19] The optimum MR imaging protocols for evaluation of liver lesions vary depending on the available equipment and contrast agents being used. Although MRI has disadvantages because of motion artifact from the heart or aorta, it can distinguish benign cysts or hemangiomas from malignant lesions based on characteristic findings on T1 versus T2 spin–weighted sequences.

In patients with colorectal liver metastases who have been staged using conventional diagnostic methods, PET scanning identifies additional disease or excludes metastases in 20% of patients.[20] It has a slightly lower detection rate for liver metastases compared to CT, but outcome after liver resection in individuals staged with PET preoperatively may be improved because of better patient selection.[21] SRS has been used with increasing regularity and is extremely accurate in imaging neuroendocrine tumors except insulinoma. In addition, because hemangiomas do not image on SRS, the study can be used to distinguish benign versus malignant lesions when there are equivocal findings on CT or MRI.[22]

RESECTION: TECHNICAL CONSIDERATIONS

The benefit of resection in selected patients with hepatic metastases from colorectal cancer and other histologies such as neuroendocrine tumors has been fairly well established in the literature. The technique of hepatic resection is detailed elsewhere,[23] and several significant advances have been made over the last 10 years that make liver resection a more routine procedure with minimal patient morbidity. At exploration an evaluation to exclude the presence of extrahepatic disease should be done. In patients who have a high risk of harboring unresectable disease, staging laparoscopy can be used to avoid an unnecessary laparotomy.[24] Intraoperative US should be routinely used to screen for the presence of deep-seated or occult metastases and guide the nature of the resection. Segment-oriented resection (vs. nonanatomic wedge excision) using portal pedicle ligation and extrahepatic ligation of the hepatic vein, both of which can be performed using stapling devices, and maintenance of low central venous pressure and the use of intermittent vascular inflow occlusion during parenchyma dissection are all being used more commonly (Fig. 51.3-2).[23] Extensive resection involving contiguous vena cava or reim-

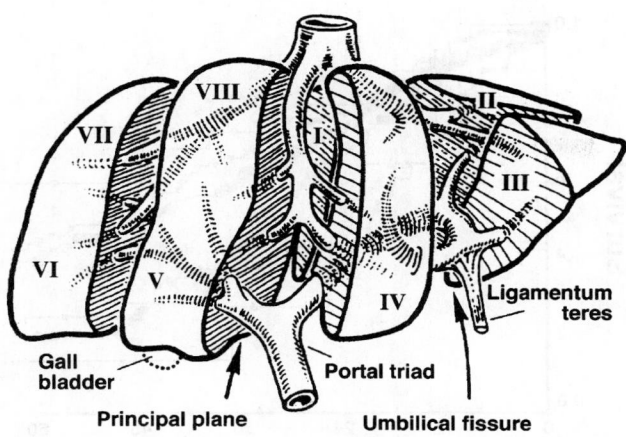

FIGURE 51.3-2. Segments of the liver used in planning hepatic resection. The principal plane divides the right and left lobes of the liver. Extent of hepatic resection planned on the basis of an understanding of the segmental anatomy of the liver has resulted in minimal morbidity and mortality associated with the procedure. (Modified from ref. 4.)

plantation of the hepatic veins is rarely indicated. A prospective random assignment trial of 120 patients undergoing elective hepatic resection and assigned to receive or not receive operative closed suction drains demonstrated no difference in outcome between groups.[25] Selective percutaneous drainage of postoperative fluid collections is necessary in fewer than 10% of patients.

In an analysis of more than 1800 consecutive cases reported from the Memorial Sloan-Kettering Cancer Center, the mortality associated with major hepatic resection was less than 4%, and the extent of surgery as reflected in a greater number of hepatic segments resected and increased blood loss were independently associated with greater morbidity and mortality.[26,27] Diabetes has also been reported as a risk factor for increased morbidity and mortality.[28] Other complications from hepatic resection include hepatic insufficiency, biliary leak, perihepatic abscess, pleural effusion, ileus, or wound infection.[26]

RESULTS OF HEPATIC RESECTION FOR COLORECTAL CANCER

The overall 5-year survival after resection of hepatic metastases in patients with colorectal cancer ranges from 26% to almost 40% in recent series (Table 51.3-2). Factors associated with improved outcome after resection in most series include tumor- and treatment-related variables. Patient characteristics such as age or gender have not been identified as significant prognostic variables, but elevation in preoperative serum carcinoembryonic antigen levels is associated with poorer outcome.[29–31]

Tumor-related factors associated with poor outcome after resection include positive lymph node status of the primary tumor, a disease-free interval between resection of the primary tumor and liver metastases of less than 1 year, and the presence of extrahepatic disease, including regional periportal lymph nodes. With respect to the liver metastases, factors that generally reflect advanced tumor burden, such as increasing number of lesions, size of largest lesion greater than 5 or 10 cm, bilobar distribution of disease, percent hepatic replacement, or weight of resected specimen, have been shown to predict shorter survival compared to those without these parameters (Fig. 51.3-3).[29,32] Technical factors predictive of poor outcome include a positive or close resection margin.[32,33] A series of patients undergoing repeat hepatic resection reported a 5-year survival rate of 34%,[34] and long-term survival after simultaneous or sequential resection of liver and lung metastases in selected patients with colorectal cancer has also been reported.[35]

A clinical scoring system including five widely used and available clinical and pathologic parameters has been proposed to predict outcome after resection of colorectal liver metastases[31] (Table 51.3-3). Based on outcome of 1001 patients undergoing resection with curative intent, increasing clinical risk score was associated with decreased survival (Fig. 51.3-4). Of note, patients with a clinical risk score of 5 had an actuarial 5-year survival of only 14%, and no patient had survived 5 years at the time of the report. These data form a basis for stratification of patients at high risk of recurrence after hepatic resection and may provide a useful method of selecting those suitable for adjuvant treatments postoperatively.

RESULTS OF RESECTION FOR NONCOLORECTAL CANCERS

Series of hepatic resection for tumor histologies other than colorectal cancer have been reported, but the benefit of this approach has not been conclusively demonstrated. Table 51.3-4 summarizes outcomes of selected series of patients with different histologies. Anecdotal reports have been published of long-term survivors after hepatic resection for noncolorectal gastrointestinal primary tumors such as gastric or pancreatic cancer[36]; however, this is not considered standard treatment, as most patients with advanced upper intestinal adenocarcinomas have recurrences at multiple sites in addition to the liver. Five-year survival in patients undergoing resection of neuroendocrine hepatic metastases ranges from 10% to 54%.[5,37] Chen et al.[37] reported that outcome was significantly improved in patients undergoing resection compared to a retrospectively matched cohort who did not undergo resection. Actuarial 5-year survival after resection of clinically isolated hepatic metastases in breast cancer patients is reported between 9%

TABLE 51.3-2. Results of Resection of Colorectal Liver Metastases from Selected Series

Study	Year	n	5-Y Survival (%)	Disease-Free Survival (%)	Median Survival (Mo)	Operative Mortality (%)
Bakalakos et al.[32]	1998	238	29	—	23	1.1
Cady et al.[29]	1998	244	—	30 (5 y)	—	3.6
Fong et al.[31]	1999	1001	37	—	42	2.8
Ambiru et al.[33]	1999	168	26	11 mo (median)	—	3.5

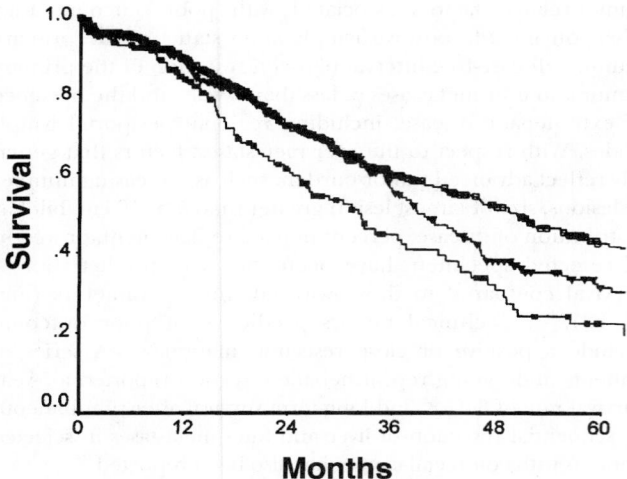

FIGURE 51.3-3.   Five-year overall survival in patients undergoing resection of hepatic metastases from colorectal cancer based on number of lesions. Survival is better in patients with one lesion (*open square*) compared to those with two or three (*filled triangles*) or four or greater (*filled boxes*) lesions. (From ref. 31, with permission.)

and 18%.[38] Based on the typical systemic pattern of recurrence in patients with advanced breast cancer, this approach must be considered palliative in nature with little expectation of long-term disease control. Other histologies for which hepatic resection has been reported include metastatic soft tissue sarcoma[39] and melanoma.[40] Actuarial 5-year survival of 60% has been reported for patients undergoing resection for tumors arising from the genitourinary tract, including testicular, adrenal, ovarian, renal, uterine, and cervical.[41] Presumably, patients with noncolorectal cancers and hepatic metastases were selected for operation based on factors thought to be favorable, such as a long interval of radiographically isolated and resectable liver metastases and good operative risk.

HEPATIC ARTERIAL CHEMOTHERAPY

Until recently, the treatment of hepatic metastases from colorectal cancer had a dismal prognosis, with a median survival of 6 months. With the use of new agents such as irinotecan[42] or

TABLE 51.3-3.   Clinical Risk Score for Tumor Recurrence in Patients Undergoing Resection for Colorectal Metastases to Liver

	Survival (%)			
Score	1-Y	3-Y	5-Y	Median (Mo)
0	93	72	60	74
1	91	66	44	51
2	89	60	40	47
3	86	42	20	33
4	70	38	25	20
5	71	27	14	22

Note: Each risk factor is one point: node-positive primary, disease-free interval less than 12 months, greater than one tumor, size greater than 5 cm, carcinoembryonic antigen greater than 200 ng/mL. (Modified from ref. 31.)

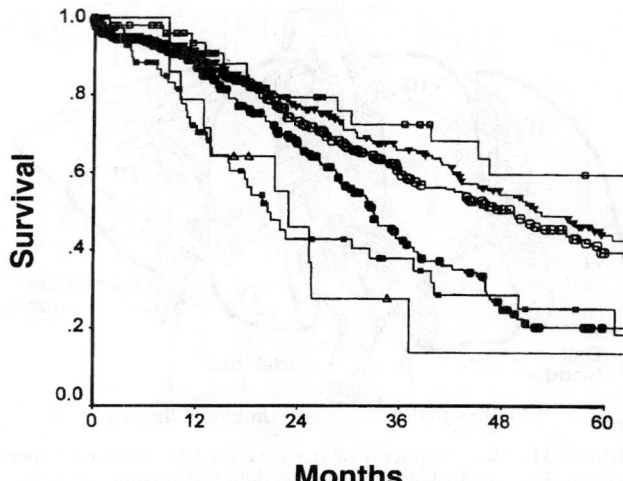

FIGURE 51.3-4.   Five-year overall survival in 1001 patients with metastatic colorectal cancer to the liver undergoing resection with curative intent. Outcome was analyzed based on the absence or presence of various prognostic factors, as outlined in Table 51.3-3. Patients with zero or one prognostic factor had improved survival compared with those with increasing numbers of adverse prognostic variables (*P* <.0001). (*Open box* is score = 0; *filled triangle* score = 1; *open circle* score = 2; *filled circle* score = 3; *filled box* score = 4; *open triangle* score = 5.) (From ref. 31, with permission.)

oxaliplatin[43] in combination with 5-fluorouracil (5-FU) and leucovorin (LV), the median survival has increased to 14 and 19 months, respectively. However, 2-year survival for patients with unresectable disease continues to be approximately 20% to 30%.

The rationale for HAI chemotherapy is that liver metastases are perfused almost exclusively by the hepatic artery, whereas normal hepatocytes derive their blood supply from the portal vein as well as the hepatic artery. The injection of floxuridine (FUDR) into either the hepatic artery or portal vein demonstrates that mean tumor FUDR levels are significantly increased (15-fold) when the drug is injected via the hepatic artery.

The use of drugs that are largely extracted by the liver during the first pass results in high local concentrations of drug

TABLE 51.3-4.   Results of Resection of Noncolorectal Cancers: Selected Series

Study	Histology	n	5-Y Survival (%)	Actuarial Median Survival (Mo)
Chen et al.[37]	Neuroendocrine	15	73	NR
Yao et al.[5]	Neuroendocrine	16	70[a]	NR
Harrison et al.[41]	Genitourinary[b]	34	60	NR
DeMatteo et al.[39]	Sarcoma	56	30	39
Harrison et al.[41]	Breast/melanoma sarcoma	41	26	32
Raab et al.[38]	Breast	34	18	27

NR, not reached.
[a]Four-year actuarial survival.
[b]Includes renal (5), testicular (9), adrenal (7), ovary (7), uterine (4), cervical (2).
(Modified from ref. 112.)

TABLE 51.3-5. Drugs for Hepatic Arterial Infusion

Drug	Half-Life (Min)	Estimated Increased Exposure by HAI
Fluorouracil (FU)	10	5–10-fold
Floxuridine (FUDR)	<10	100–400-fold
Carmustine (BCNU)	<5	6–7-fold
Mitomycin C	<10	6–8-fold
Cisplatin	20–30	4–7-fold
Adriamycin (doxorubicin hydrochloride)	60	2-fold

HAI, hepatic arterial infusion.

with minimal systemic toxicity. FUDR is the best drug to use for regional therapy because 94% to 99% of FUDR is extracted during the first pass, compared to 19% to 55% of 5-FU.[44] The pharmacologic advantage of various chemotherapeutic agents for hepatic arterial infusion is summarized in Table 51.3-5. Drugs with a steep dose-response curve are more useful when given by HAI, because small increases in the concentration of drug result in a large improvement in response. Drugs with a high total body clearance are also more useful for hepatic infusion. The area under the concentration-time curve is a function not only of drug clearance but also of hepatic arterial flow. Because hepatic arterial blood flow has a high regional exchange rate (100 to 1500 mL/min), drugs with a high clearance rate are needed. If a drug is not rapidly cleared, recirculation through the systemic circulation mitigates the advantage of HAI over systemic therapy.

The original HAI trials were performed with percutaneously placed hepatic arterial lines. The inconvenience of the procedures and complications with bleeding and thrombosis led investigators away from the technique, although the response rates were approximately 50%. The development of a totally implantable infusion pump allowed for a more convenient administration of HAI chemotherapy. A number of randomized studies have now been conducted to answer the question of whether HAI therapy is a more effective treatment for metastatic colorectal cancer (Table 51.3-6). Many of the major trials conducted had problems in design, which are outlined below. To determine whether HAI therapy is more effective than systemic therapy for liver metastases before randomization, patients need to be stratified by the percent of liver involvement and the baseline lactate dehydrogenase levels. At Memorial Sloan-Kettering Cancer Center, a randomized trial[45] compared HAI to systemic infusion using the same chemotherapeutic agent (FUDR), same drug schedule (a 14-day continuous infusion), and the same method of administration (pump) in both groups. Patients were stratified for percent of liver involvement and baseline lactate dehydrogenase levels. Individuals with extrahepatic disease or resectable hepatic lesions were considered ineligible for the protocol. The study design allowed for a crossover from systemic therapy to hepatic arterial therapy in the event of tumor progression on systemic therapy. Of the 99 evaluable patients, there were 2 complete and 23 partial responses (53%) in the group receiving HAI and 10 partial responses (21%) in the systemic group. The median survivals for the HAI and systemic groups were 17 and 12 months, respectively. The interpretation of survival results is difficult in this study because 60% of the patients in the systemic group crossed over and received intrahepatic therapy after tumor progression on systemic therapy. Those who did not cross over for technical reasons had a median survival of 8 months, compared to 18 months for those patients who crossed over to hepatic infusion.

A similar randomized study conducted by the Northern California Oncology Group[46] also used FUDR infusion in the HAI and systemic groups. Although 143 patients were entered, only 117 were eligible. A 42% response rate was reported in the HAI group and 10% in the systemic group. The median time to progression was 401 and 201 days (P = .009), and the median survivals were 503 and 484 days, respectively. Although a crossover design was not built into the study, 43% of patients in the systemic group crossed over to intrahepatic therapy, possibly obscuring any difference in survival. Another factor that makes interpretation of survival results difficult in this study is that patients with metastases to hepatic lymph nodes were included in both study groups.

A National Cancer Institute (NCI) study[47] compared HAI to systemic infusion of FUDR in 64 patients. HAI had a signifi-

TABLE 51.3-6. Randomized Studies of Hepatic Arterial Infusion versus Systemic Chemotherapy for Patients with Hepatic Metastases from Colorectal Cancer

Group	Patients (n)	Response (%) HAI	Response (%) SYS	Response (%) P Value	Survival (Mo) HAI	Survival (Mo) SYS	Survival (Mo) P Value
MSKCC[45]	162	53	21	.001	17[a]	12	—
NCOG[46]	143	42	10	.0001	16.6	16	—
NCI[47]	64	62	17	.003	47[b]	13	—
City of Hope[113]	41	56	0	NS	—	NS	—
Mayo Clinic[48]	69	48	21	.02	12.6	10.5	—
French[49]	163	49	14	NS	22[b]	10	.02
English[50]	100	50	0	.01	13	6.3	.03
German[114]	168	43	20	—	12.7	17.6	—
CALGB[53]	135	48	25	.009	22.7	19.8	.027

CALGB, Cancer and Leukemia Group B; HAI, hepatic arterial infusion; MSKCC, Memorial Sloan-Kettering Cancer Center; NCI, National Cancer Institute; NCOG, Northern California Oncology Group; NS, not stated; SYS, systemic chemotherapy.
[a]Sixty-eight percent treated.
[b]Two-year survival.

cantly improved response rate compared with systemic therapy: 62% versus 17%, respectively. Interpretation of survival data is difficult, because 34% of the HAI group never received chemotherapy and 38% of the HAI group had positive portal lymph nodes. Despite these limitations, in the subset of patients without extrahepatic disease, 2-year survival was 47% in the HAI group and 13% in the systemic group ($P = .03$).

Another small study conducted by the Mayo Clinic[48] compared HAI FUDR with systemic bolus FU for 5 days. The trial did not allow a crossover to HAI. Objective tumor responses were observed in 48% of patients receiving HAI FUDR and 21% of patients receiving systemic FU. Time to hepatic progression was significantly longer in the HAI group versus the systemic group (15.7 vs. 6.0 months, respectively). Despite the increase in response rate and time to hepatic progression, survival was similar in the two groups (see Table 51.3-6). In this study the power to detect a survival advantage is very low because of the small number of patients. Of the 36 patients in the HAI group, 14% never received treatment, 19% had extrahepatic disease, 9% had hepatic artery thrombosis, and 6% had pump malfunction.

In a multicenter French trial,[49] 163 patients were randomized to either HAI FUDR or systemic bolus FU. The response rate was 49% in the HAI group and 14% in the systemic group. Median times to hepatic progression for the HAI and systemic groups were 15 and 6 months, respectively (see Table 51.3-6). The 2-year survival was 22% in the HAI group and 10% in the systemic group ($P < .02$). Not all patients in the systemic group received chemotherapy, and some only received therapy when they became symptomatic.

Another study, conducted in England,[50] similar to the French study, had no crossover and a reasonable number of patients in the systemic group. This study addressed quality of life and did demonstrate a significantly longer time with better quality of life in the hepatic arterial group. An increase in survival also occurred: Median survival was 405 and 198 days for the HAI and systemic groups, respectively.

A German multicenter study[51] randomized 168 patients to (1) HAI FUDR, (2) HAI FU/LV, or (3) intravenous FU/LV. The median time to progression was 5.9, 9.2, and 6.6 months; median survival was 12.7, 18.7, and 17.6 months; and tumor response was 43.2%, 45.0%, and 19.7%, respectively. Two-thirds of patients treated with HAI FU/LV experienced severe toxicity, compared to one-third treated with FUDR. It should be pointed out that, although an intention-to-treat analysis was used, only 68.5% of patients randomized to HAI FUDR were treated (see Table 51.3-6). An English study[52] randomized 290 patients to intravenous FU/LV or HAI FU/LV. Median survivals were 13.4 and 14.7 months in the intravenous and HAI arms, respectively. However, 37% of patients allocated to the HAI arm never received treatment. In a metaanalysis[2] combining the results of the seven earliest trials, the use of HAI FUDR in the treatment of nonresectable liver metastases from colorectal cancer produced a significantly better response rate of 41% with HAI, a 14% response rate with systemic FU, and median survival time of 16 versus 13 months, respectively (Fig. 51.3-5).

The Cancer and Leukemia Group B completed a trial[53] in which 135 patients were randomized to systemic FU/LV using a 5-day regimen or HAI FUDR, LV, and dexamethasone. No crossover was permitted. Seventy percent of the patients had greater than 30% liver involvement, 78% had synchronous metastases, and 97% were chemotherapy naive. Response rates

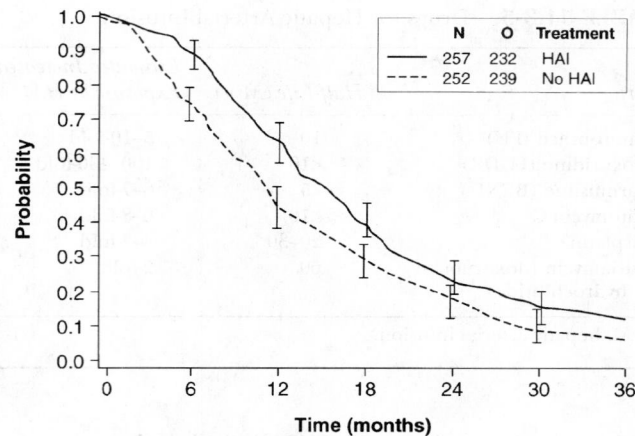

FIGURE 51.3-5. Overall survival in patients with metastatic colorectal cancer to the liver treated with hepatic arterial infusion (HAI) therapy using a fluorodeoxyuridine-based regimen compared to systemic therapy (no HAI). Survival curves based on a metaanalysis of the published literature of phase III random assignment trials compared these two treatment strategies. The number of patients (N) and the observed number of deaths (O) are shown in the legend. HAI therapy has a significantly improved survival compared to those treated with no HAI therapy (log rank test, $P = .0009$). (From ref. 2, with permission.)

were higher in the HAI group (48% vs. 25%). Median survival was significantly better in the HAI arm (22.7 vs. 19.8 months). Quality-of-life measurements, especially at month three and six, were significantly better in the HAI arm.

TOXICITY OF HEPATIC ARTERIAL INFUSION THERAPY WITH FLOXURIDINE

The most common problems with HAI are hepatic toxicity and ulceration of the stomach and duodenum. Myelosuppression, nausea, vomiting, and diarrhea rarely occur with HAI using FUDR. If diarrhea does occur, shunting to the bowel should be suspected. Clinically, biliary toxicity is manifested as elevations of aspartate transaminase (AST), alkaline phosphatase, and bilirubin. In the early stages of toxicity, hepatic enzyme elevations return to normal when the drug is withdrawn and the patient is given a rest period, whereas in more advanced cases, it does not resolve. The bile ducts derive their blood supply almost exclusively from the hepatic artery and thus are undoubtedly perfused with high doses of chemotherapy.

In patients in whom jaundice develops, an endoscopic retrograde cholangiopancreatogram may demonstrate lesions resembling idiopathic sclerosing cholangitis in 5% to 29% of individuals treated by experienced clinicians. Because the ducts are sclerotic and nondilated, sonograms usually do not show dilation. The strictures may be focal and present at the hepatic duct bifurcation, and therefore drainage procedures either by endoscopic retrograde cholangiopancreatogram or by transhepatic cholangiogram may be helpful. Duct obstruction from metastases should first be excluded by CT of the liver.

Close monitoring with liver function tests is necessary to avoid biliary complications. If the serum bilirubin is elevated to 3 mg/dL, no further treatment should be given until the bilirubin returns to normal, and then only after a long rest period, to prevent the development of sclerosing cholangitis. Ulcer disease results from inadvertent perfusion of the stomach and duodenum with drug via the small collateral branches from the hepatic artery and can be prevented by careful dissection of these collaterals at the time of pump placement.[54]

Three approaches have been tried to decrease hepatic toxicity: (1) HAI dexamethasone (D), (2) circadian modification, and (3) HAI FU alternating with FUDR. The hepatic toxicity induced by hepatic arterial infusion of FUDR may be related to portal triad inflammation, which could lead to ischemia of the bile ducts. Hepatic arterial administration of dexamethasone may decrease inflammation and thereby decrease biliary toxicity. In patients with established hepatobiliary toxicity from HAI, dexamethasone promotes resolution of the liver function abnormalities. In a randomized study of FUDR with D versus FUDR alone, there was a trend toward decreased bilirubin elevation in patients receiving FUDR + D compared to the group receiving FUDR alone (9% vs. 30%; $P = .07$).[55] Although the addition of dexamethasone was not associated with the ability to administer a significant increase in the amount of FUDR, the response rate with FUDR + D was 71% versus 40% for FUDR alone ($P = .03$). Survival was also improved: 23 months for FUDR + D versus 15 months for FUDR alone.

Although the dose of FUDR fits into an implanted pump, the dose of FU requires an external pump for infusion or bolus weekly side port injections. Van Riel et al., using a Medi-Port to administer FU infusion, 1000 mg/m^2 for 5 days, reported a 34% response rate in 145 patients, with a 14.3-month median survival.[55a] Arterial thrombosis was seen in 48% and catheter dislocation in 22%. Giving a higher dose of FU (2200 mg/m^2) over 24 hours weekly with LV, objective responses were seen in 28 of 50 (56%) patients, with a median survival of 23 months.[56]

OTHER AGENTS USED WITH HEPATIC ARTERIAL INFUSION

On the basis of the success of systemic FU/LV regimens as well as laboratory studies suggesting that LV may be a better modifier of FUDR than of FU, 63 patients were treated with FUDR and LV by HAI. The overall response rate was 62%, with an improvement in survival: 75% of the patients were alive at 1 year, 66% at 2 years, and 14% at 5 years.[44] However, biliary sclerosis was increased. The addition of other drugs to FUDR, such as carmustine, mitomycin C, and dexamethasone, has produced higher response rates. In patients who have progressed on systemic therapy, new HAI protocols with combined systemic agents have increased response rates. Systemic CPT-11 plus HAI FUDR + dexamethasone produced a 74% response rate in 35 previously treated patients.[57] Thirteen of 15 patients who received previous systemic chemotherapy including CPT-11 responded to this treatment. The addition of systemic oxaliplatin to HAI FUDR and dexamethasone produced an 83% response rate in 30 previously treated patients.[58]

ADJUVANT THERAPY AFTER RESECTION OF COLORECTAL LIVER METASTASES

Approximately 75% of patients who undergo hepatic resection experience recurrent metastases within 2 years, and approxi-

TABLE 51.3-7. Survival after Adjuvant Therapy Subsequent to Liver Resection with Hepatic Arterial Infusion and Systemic Therapy versus Systemic Therapy Alone

Survival Rate Comparisons	HAI + SYS (n = 74)	SYS (n = 82)	P Value
2-Y survival	85%	69%	.02
2-Y hepatic DFS	89%	57%	.00001
2-Y DFS	57%	41%	.07

DFS, disease-free survival; HAI, hepatic arterial infusion; SYS, systemic therapy.
(Modified from ref. 59.)

mately one-half recur in the liver.[31] The utility of systemic chemotherapy in the adjuvant setting after hepatic resection of metastatic colorectal cancer has never been subjected to a randomized trial. Thus, the role of this modality remains unclear. Three large, randomized trials address the question of whether adjuvant therapy with HAI is useful after liver resection. At Memorial Sloan-Kettering Cancer Center,[59] patients were randomized to HAI FUDR + D and systemic 5-FU with or without LV or systemic chemotherapy alone after the resection of hepatic metastases. The end points were 2-year survival and 2-year recurrence-free survival. Patients were stratified according to the number of liver metastases (one, two to four, greater than four) and type of chemotherapy (none, 5-FU ± levamisole, or 5-FU + LV). Numerous other parameters were comparable. Actuarial survival at 2 years was significantly increased with HAI + systemic therapy (SYS) compared to SYS alone (Table 51.3-7). Comparing the HAI + SYS arm with the SYS alone, the rate of hepatic recurrence-free survival at 2 years was 90% and 60%, respectively. Overall progression-free survival was also better with the HAI + SYS arm (see Table 51.3-7).

Five deaths were reported before initiation of therapy, two in the HAI + SYS group and three in the SYS-alone group. During treatment, three deaths occurred: one in the HAI + SYS group and two in the SYS-alone group during treatment. More patients in the HAI + systemic therapy group experienced diarrhea compared to the systemic therapy group, 29% versus 14%, respectively, and nausea, 10% and 5%, respectively. Hepatic enzyme elevations occurred in the following: 29% had a doubling of the serum alkaline phosphatase, 65% had a tripling of the AST, and 18% had increases in their serum bilirubin to greater than 3.0 mg/dL. Biliary abnormalities returned to normal in all but four patients who required biliary stents.

The Eastern Cooperative Oncology Group and Southwest Oncology Group[60] conducted a prospective, randomized, multicenter trial of hepatic resection alone (group A) versus resection followed by 4 cycles of HAI with FUDR and 12 cycles of systemic infusional 5-FU (group B). Only patients with three or fewer hepatic metastases from colorectal cancer were enrolled. Preoperatively, 110 patients were randomized, 56 in A and 54 in B; 11 (19.6%) patients in group A and 21 (38.8%) in group B (treated group) ultimately were withdrawn from the study due to operative findings of either greater than three liver metastases, extrahepatic disease, or no evidence of liver metastases. The 4-year recurrence-free rate was significantly greater with combined modality therapy versus resection alone, 58% and 34%, respectively ($P = .039$). In addition, less involvement of the liver with hepatic recurrence was noted in group B (8) versus group A (24) (P= .035). Overall median survival presently is 47.5 months in the treated group and 34.2 months in the group that had resection only. The authors concluded that, although no overall survival benefit was demonstrated in the interim analysis, a trend toward increased survival was already apparent in the chemotherapy-treated patients.

In a German study,[61] a multicenter randomized trial (26 centers) of hepatic resection versus hepatic resection and adjuvant HAI with 5-FU and LV (HAI 5-FU/LV), patients were stratified according to number of liver metastases (one to two, three to six) and the site of the primary tumor (colon or upper rectum, mid or lower rectum). One hundred thirteen patients were assigned to each group. Despite initial randomization, 24 (21%) in the HAI arm and 18 (16%) patients in the control group did not receive the assigned treatment. In the group randomized to adjuvant treatment, it was not performed for the following reasons: anatomic variants, documentation of extrahepatic disease at time of surgery, technical complications with port placement, patient refusal after randomization, and others. In the control group randomized to resection alone, reasons for not following the randomized assignment were unresectable disease, microscopic residual disease, and extrahepatic disease. Therefore, at the start of the trial, 87 (77%) were actually treated in the HAI + SYS group. At the 18-month interim analysis, the percent relapsing was 33.0% in patients receiving adjuvant therapy and 36.7% in patients treated with resection alone. No survival advantage was seen, and median survival time was reported as 34.5 months in the HAI group versus 40.8 months in the control group (P= .15). In the secondary analysis comparing the "as treated" arm (n = 87) to the group receiving no adjuvant therapy (n = 114), median survival was 44.8 months versus 39.7 months, respectively. Median survival time to liver progression doubled in the group receiving HAI 5-FU/LV as opposed to the control group: 44.8 versus 23.3 months. Finally, median time to progression of disease or death was increased in the group receiving adjuvant HAI 5-FU/LV: 20.0 versus 12.6 months.

The results of this randomized trial must be interpreted with caution. Of the 113 patients randomized, 73 (64.6%) had chemotherapy data available, and only 34 (30%) patients completed the assigned protocol. This suggests that the power to detect a difference, even with an intention-to-treat analysis, was not adequate, given that the majority of patients did not receive their assigned treatment.

NEOADJUVANT CHEMOTHERAPY

Neoadjuvant chemotherapy has been evaluated as a way to decrease hepatic tumor burden to proceed with hepatic resection. Although no randomized prospective trial has been completed regarding this as a treatment strategy, the results of a retrospective analysis have been presented, and they appear promising.

Giacchetti et al.[62] conducted a retrospective review of 151 patients with unresectable liver-only metastases from colorectal cancer who were treated with FU/LV and oxaliplatin followed by attempted liver resection. The criteria used to define unresectability were (1) fewer than four liver metastases, (2) a single tumor greater than 5 cm, (3) tumor in both hepatic lobes,

(4) invasion of the intrahepatic vascular structures, and (5) a high percentage of liver involvement (greater than 25%). These authors' analyses revealed that, of this group, 77 (51%) became resectable after neoadjuvant therapy and 58 of 77 (75%) were able to undergo complete resections. The 5-year survival rate for the 77 patients who underwent hepatic resection was 50%, and progression-free survival was 17 months. For the completely resected patients, median overall survival was not reached, but 72% had relapsed within a median of 12 months.

A prospective trial is under way at the Mayo Clinic enrolling patients considered unresectable due to (1) involvement of all three major hepatic veins, the portal vein bifurcation, or the retrohepatic vena cava; (2) involvement of the main right or main left portal vein and the main hepatic vein of the opposite lobe; (3) disease requiring more than a right or left trisegmentectomy; or (4) six or more metastatic lesions distributed diffusely in both lobes of the liver. In the presence of any of the above, patients are treated with FU, LV, and oxaliplatin. Thus far, Alberts et al.[63] reported on 42 patients with nonoptimally resectable disease treated with FOLFOX. Fourteen had a resection, but 59% had recurrences. Median survival was 31 months. In a retrospective review of unresectable patients at M. D. Anderson Hospital who had HAI therapy followed by surgery, 4 of 26 patients with hepatocellular carcinoma[64] and 22 of 383 with colorectal carcinoma were able to undergo resection or ablative techniques. The four patients with hepatocellular carcinoma have not had re-recurrence, whereas recurrent disease developed in 83% of the patients with colorectal carcinoma.

OTHER LIVER TUMORS

The use of HAI for other metastatic tumors has not been studied as extensively. A response has been demonstrated in patients with breast cancer, even those who progressed on systemic therapy. Neuroendocrine tumors, metastatic melanomas, and gastric leiomyosarcoma also respond to regional therapy. Leyvraz et al.[65] reported an overall response rate of 40% in 31 patients with ocular melanoma metastatic to the liver who were treated with intraarterial fotemustine.

HEPATIC ARTERY INFUSION WITH HEPATIC VENOUS FILTRATION

Another approach to enable the use of high doses of chemotherapy while limiting systemic toxicities involves the use of venous hemofiltration wherein high doses of cytotoxins can be administered into the arterial supply of the liver. Hepatic venous blood is collected via a double-balloon catheter positioned in the retrohepatic vena cava and the balloons are inflated above and below the hepatic veins to isolate and collect hepatic venous effluent. The collected blood is passed through a charcoal filtration device and returned to the systemic circulation. This technique was originally developed at Yale University School of Medicine.[66] It was applied to 23 patients with primary or metastatic hepatic cancers using either high doses of 5-FU (1000 to 5000 mg/m²) in 12 patients or doxorubicin (50 to 120 mg/m²) in 9 patients. The extraction efficiency of the system was 64% to 91% and accompanied

TABLE 51.3-8. Summary of Isolated Hepatic Perfusion Trial Using Tumor Necrosis Factor and Chemotherapeutics

Study	n	Agent(s)	Dose	Results
Hafström and Naredi, 1998[70]	11	Melphalan TNF	0.5 mg/kg 30–200 µg	Mortality 18% Morbidity 45% 3/11 PR
Oldhafer et al., 1998[69]	6	Melphalan TNF	60–140 mg 200–300 µg	Mortality 0% 1/6 CR, 2/6 PR
Alexander et al., 1998[71]	34	Melphalan TNF	1.5 mg/kg 1.0 mg	Mortality 3% 1 CR, 25 PR (75%)

CR, complete response; PR, partial response; TNF, tumor necrosis factor.

by acceptable toxicity. The most common toxicity was neutropenia and transient hypotension due to the catecholamine-depleting effects of the charcoal filters and diminished cardiac return during the procedure. Dose-limiting myelotoxicity was observed at 5000 mg/m² 5-FU and 120 mg/m² doxorubicin.

Investigators at the NCI's Center for Cancer Research have reported results of a phase I trial of escalating doses of melphalan administered via a 30-minute hepatic arterial infusion with hepatic venous hemofiltration using percutaneously placed catheters as previously evaluated at Yale. The average filtration efficiency was 83%, and radiographic evidence of response was observed in 5 of 12 evaluable patients with advanced unresectable metastases from ocular melanoma, colorectal cancer, sarcoma, or biliary neoplasms.[67] At the maximum safe tolerated dose of 3.0 mg/kg melphalan, transient grade 3/4 toxicity was observed in 57% of patients.

ISOLATED HEPATIC PERFUSION

IHP is a regional treatment that has been used at a limited number of centers since its original clinical application 40 years ago and is similar to isolated limb perfusion, used for extremity melanoma or sarcoma, in which the cancer-bearing region is perfused with a recirculating closed circuit containing a reservoir, heat exchanger for delivery of hyperthermia, and roller pump (see Chapter 50.2).[68] IHP is administered via an operative procedure, during which time the liver is extensively prepared to prevent leak of systemic perfusate during treatment. Venous outflow is from a cannula positioned in an isolated segment of the retrohepatic inferior vena cava, and arterial inflow is through a cannula placed in the gastroduodenal artery.

Because of the procedure's technical complexity, the morbidity reported to be associated with it in older series, and the lack of documented efficacy using chemotherapeutics alone,[68] it has not gained widespread or consistent clinical evaluation. However, in the early 1990s, several centers initiated trials of IHP using tumor necrosis factor (TNF) and melphalan, with the benefit of continuous intraoperative leak monitoring using radiolabeled erythrocytes or albumin to ensure minimal or no leak of perfusate during treatment. Data from three centers in Europe and the NCI in Bethesda, Maryland, report results with IHP using TNF and melphalan (Table 51.3-8). Oldhafer et al.[69] reported a series of 12 patients, of whom 6 received TNF and melphalan. Tumor biopsies obtained on posttreatment day one showed tumor necrosis in most patients, and there was an over-

all radiographic response rate of 50% and a median survival of 11 months. A Swedish group treated 11 patients and had an operative mortality of 18%. Antitumor activity was observed in three of six patients with ocular melanoma to the liver and in none of five patients with colorectal cancer. The modest antitumor activity may be secondary to the very low doses of agents used, only 0.2 to 0.3 mg TNF and 0.5 mg/kg melphalan, which are considerably lower than the maximum safe tolerated doses determined in phase I trials at the NCI.[68,70]

Investigators and coworkers from the NCI reported results in 34 patients with metastatic unresectable cancers confined to the liver using 1 mg TNF and 1.5 mg/kg melphalan.[71] Treatment mortality was 3%, and despite the fact that most had received previous therapy and many had very advanced tumor burden in the liver, the overall radiographic response rate was 75%. Responses were consistent across all histologies treated, including ocular melanoma and colorectal cancer, and observed in those with very advanced disease. In 2001, results in 51 patients with isolated unresectable colorectal cancer confined to the liver who were treated with IHP using TNF and melphalan or melphalan alone followed by HAI therapy using FUDR and LV have been presented by the group.[72] Seventy-three percent of patients had failed previous systemic therapy with a 5-FU–based regimen. One treatment-related mortality (2%) occurred. Of note, the overall responses remained similar to their initial report, 77% for patients treated with TNF and melphalan IHP and 74% for patients treated with IHP using melphalan alone, but median time to progression in the liver was significantly prolonged with the addition of HAI therapy (10.0 vs. 14.5 months, respectively). The same group has reported results of hyperthermic IHP with melphalan alone in 29 patients with metastatic ocular melanoma to the liver.[14] Three (10%) radiographic complete responses and 15 partial responses (52%) occurred. Median actuarial overall survival was 12.1 months.

CHEMOEMBOLIZATION FOR METASTATIC CANCER TO THE LIVER

Chemoembolization therapy administers intraarterial chemotherapy followed by infusion of one of a number of embolic agents, such as degradable starch microspheres, gelatin powders, polyvinyl chloride, or pledgets. Responding patients usually undergo multiple procedures over time as tumors and vasculature regrow. This approach has been widely applied in the treatment of primary hepatocellular carcinoma (see Chapter 29.4). For patients

TABLE 51.3-9. Outcome in Patients with Neuroendocrine Tumors Metastatic to the Liver after Chemoembolization

Reference	Histology	Treatment	Patients (n)	Response Rate Objective	Response Rate Hormonal[a]	Median Survival
Ruszniewski et al.[115]	Carcinoid	Embolization only, islet cell	24	6/14	8/14	ND
Kim et al.[116]	Carcinoid	CDDP (150 mg), Dox (50 mg)	30	11/30	16/21	15
	Islet cell	5-FU (350 mg), STP (150–200 mg)				

CDDP, cisplatin; Dox, doxorubicin; 5-FU, 5-fluorouracil; ND, not determined; STP, streptozotocin.
[a]Defined as 50% decrease; expressed as fraction of patients evaluable.

with metastatic cancer, the best accepted use is for patients with unresectable metastases from carcinoid or islet cell tumors, most of which are highly vascular (Table 51.3-9). In addition, the indolent course of disease in many patients presents a setting in which even a partial response can provide long-term palliation. Even patients who do not achieve an objective response have improvements in symptoms resulting from a decrease in tumor-related hormonal secretion. The overall objective response rates are between 30% and 50%, and the great majority of patients show reduced hormone secretion and improvement of symptoms. Median survivals range from 1.5 to 3.0 years and are clearly influenced by patient selection.[73,74] Although there has been a shift in practice from embolization alone to chemoembolization with a variety of agents, there is no clear evidence that the use of chemotherapy improves response or patient outcome.

Chemoembolization has also been attempted for patients with colorectal cancer metastatic to the liver (Table 51.3-10). In contrast to neuroendocrine tumors, most metastatic colorectal cancers demonstrate a more aggressive course within the liver and systemically. Although objective response rates in the range of 30% are obtained, it is not clear that patient survival is prolonged. A small randomized phase II trial suggests no statistically significant benefit of chemoembolization with 5-FU and interferon-α over embolization only.[75] It is important to integrate chemoembolization with the newer systemic chemotherapeutic agents, such as oxaliplatin and irinotecan, for colorectal cancer.

Two groups have investigated the potential value of adjuvant chemotherapy after chemoembolization in patients with gastrointestinal malignancies metastatic to the liver. The Puget Sound Oncology Consortium performed an investigation of alternating systemic continuous-infusion 5-FU (250 mg/m²/d for 28 days) interspersed with two or three transcatheter arterial chemoembolization treatments using foam particles with cis-

platin in 32 patients. Although this group believed that toxicity was acceptable with this regimen, they did have grade 3 toxicities occur in 81% of patients and grade 4 in 31%. Furthermore, the overall 40% response rate, median duration of response of 4.2 months, and overall median survival of 14.3 months are similar to what one might anticipate with systemic chemotherapy alone.[76] A similar experience was published by the Southwest Oncology Group, which combined chemoembolization (collagen mixed with cisplatin, mitomycin C, and doxorubicin) with systemic continuous-infusion 5-FU/LV in 31 patients. This group found an overall response rate of 29%, with a median survival of 14 months.[77] Thus, the value of combining hepatic chemoembolization with adjuvant chemotherapy using agents currently available does not appear promising.

Embolization procedures cause significant pain (requiring narcotic analgesics), fever, nausea, and malaise lasting 2 to 7 days in nearly all patients. Portal venous thrombosis, although rarely seen (in contrast to hepatocellular carcinoma), is an absolute contraindication to hepatic arterial embolization.

LOCAL ABLATIVE THERAPY

Several techniques are being used for local ablation of hepatic metastases, including cryotherapy, percutaneous injection of toxic agents, hyperthermic coagulative necrosis, and newer experimental techniques. The goal of local ablative therapy is to achieve complete necrosis of the tumor with minimal injury to surrounding normal hepatic parenchyma. Currently, its use is indicated in patients who are not surgical candidates, for those whose tumors are not amenable to resection because of multiple tumors involving both lobes, for tumors arising in cirrhotic livers for which preservation of parenchyma is impera-

TABLE 51.3-10. Outcome in Patients with Colorectal Cancer Metastatic to the Liver after Chemoembolization

Study	Treatment	Previously Treated	Patients (n)	Response Rate Objective	Response Rate Carcinoembryonic Antigen[a]	Median Survival (Mo)
Sanz-Altamira et al.[117]	1000 mg 5-FU 10 mg MMC	Yes	40	8/35	18/29	10
Tellez et al.[118]	CDDP, MMC, Dox	Yes	30	17/27	19/20	8.6
McGinn et al.[107]	Radiation, FUDR, MMC	Yes	26	3/25	—	5

CDDP, cisplatin; Dox, doxorubicin; E, embolization; 5-FU, 5-fluorouracil; FUDR, floxuridine; MMC, mitomycin C.
[a]Defined as 50% decrease; expressed as fraction of patients evaluable.

tive, for tumors straddling the interlobar plane that would otherwise require an extended resection, for recurrent tumors after previous resection where re-resection might be unsafe or anatomically impossible, and as an adjunct to surgical resection by treating microscopically positive margins.

Limitations of local ablation therapies include the inability to treat subclinical or occult tumor deposits, inability to treat tumors greater than several centimeters in diameter, inability to treat tumors abutting major vascular structures, and difficulty in assessing the adequacy of tissue destruction during therapy. Real-time US and MRI scanning are routinely used during treatment, but further refinement in technique and imaging is required.

CRYOTHERAPY

Cryotherapy is a term representing the *in situ* destruction of tissue by the freeze-thaw process. The process of freezing tissue can cause direct cellular destruction that is dependent on the magnitude of tissue cooling, and this can be variable during cryosurgery. Microcirculatory failure secondary to freezing within the vasculature and subsequent vascular damage may be additional tumoricidal mechanisms.

Two main technical advances have made cryotherapy applicable to liver tumors on a broad scale. The first is the development of vacuum-insulated cryoprobes that allow controlled freezing of tumors deep within the liver, and the second is the use of intraoperative US to allow precise probe placement into the center of tumors and to monitor the progression of the freeze margin in real time. The most commonly used probes range from 6 to 12 mm in diameter, and a disk-shaped probe can be used for freezing thin surface lesions or a positive or close resection margin. Liquid nitrogen is circulated through the tip of the probes at a temperature of $-196°C$, which results in a probe-tip temperature between $-160°$ and $-180°C$. The probe is placed into the center of the lesion under US guidance directions to assure that uniform freezing will extend symmetrically in all directions from the tip of the probe. Repeated freeze-thaw cycles can improve tumor cell killing, and vascular inflow occlusion to the liver (Pringle maneuver) can improve the cooling rate and may allow successful freezing of larger tumors with smaller probes.

The 8-mm probe can reliably create a spherical ice ball of 3 cm and the 12-mm probe an ice ball of 5 cm in nonischemic liver. Newer cryosurgical systems are designed to allow simultaneous circulation of liquid nitrogen through multiple probes. Smaller 3.6- to 6.3-mm probes can be inserted through laparoscopic ports or percutaneously.[78] The advancing interface between frozen tissue and normal tissue can be monitored by US as a distinct hyperechoic ring. The advancement of this ring is monitored until it extends at least 1 cm beyond the tumor in all directions. The ice ball creates an acoustic shadow, making it impossible to monitor the advancement of all edges simultaneously.

In a review of the published literature results, more than 900 patients treated with the technique were reported,[79] with patient, treatment, and tumor parameters associated with successful outcome detailed.[80,81] Seifert and Morris[81] reported that 116 patients with colorectal cancer treated with cryotherapy had an overall morbidity of 28%. A single mortality occurred

TABLE 51.3-11. Factors with Independent Prognostic Significance in Colorectal Patients Undergoing Cryotherapy of Hepatic Metastases

Low pretreatment carcinoembryonic antigen value
Diameter largest lesion <3 cm
No extrahepatic disease
Node-negative involvement of primary tumor
Metachronous (vs. synchronous) liver metastases
Successful cryotherapy of all hepatic lesions

(Data from ref. 81.)

secondary to treatment (0.9%). Factors found to be independently correlated with favorable outcome after therapy are listed in Table 51.3-11. Weaver et al.[80] reported a median survival of 34 months and an 82% hepatic recurrence rate in 136 patients undergoing 158 cryotherapy procedures. Repeat[82] and laparoscopic treatments[83] have been reported.

A single prospective random assignment trial evaluating cryosurgery versus conventional resection in patients with liver metastases from a variety of histologies has been reported.[84] Liver recurrences and overall survival were similar in the two groups, and the authors concluded that cryotherapy is as effective as surgical resection for liver metastases. However, the heterogeneous nature of the patients treated and the unconventional treatment administered routinely to patients postoperatively make interpretation of the data difficult. Others have reported results in patients with neuroendocrine tumors of the liver, noting good palliation and a greater than 90% reduction in circulating tumor-related functional proteins (i.e., gastrin or 5-hydroxyindoleacetic acid) in more than 90% of patients, for a median of 10 to 13 months after cryotherapy.[85]

In general, cryotherapy is considered a safe and effective means for treating hepatic tumors of all histologies with low morbidity. Cryotherapy has also been used in conjunction with hepatic resection to assist in resection of a deep-seated lesion, to treat an inadequate margin after resection, and, in addition to resection, to preserve hepatic tissue.[86,87] Complications related specifically to cryotherapy include pleural effusions, hepatic cracking with associated intraoperative hemorrhage, biliary fistula, abscess, and myoglobinuria with renal failure.

Bilchik et al.[88] have reported large-scale results with the combination of cryosurgery with or without posttherapy systemic irinotecan or intraarterial FUDR in 153 patients with 5-FU–resistant colorectal liver metastases. Median survival after cryosurgery alone was 13 months, compared to 23.6 and 21.2 months for those treated with adjuvant irinotecan or FUDR, respectively. In this study, tumor size, number, and location were not associated with outcome; only preoperative and posttherapy carcinoembryonic antigen were predictors of outcome.

RADIOFREQUENCY ABLATION

Another form of local ablative therapy for liver tumors is open or percutaneous hyperthermic coagulation. A probe inserted into the middle of a tumor emits radiowaves from its tip, which heats the surrounding tissue. Energy penetrates a few centimeters into the surrounding tissue, causes molecular vibration of dipoles (particularly of water), and is converted to heat, resulting in tissue coagulative necrosis. The success of RFA in successful ablation of primary or metastatic tumor deposits within the liver is influenced by the expertise and diligence of the treating physician to ensure that an adequate zone of thermal necrosis has been delivered to the entire tumor. For large tumors this requires multiple consecutive probe placements. The zone of thermal necrosis can be imaged with intraoperative US, but adequacy of treatment is primarily based on maintaining target temperatures for a set interval of time. Nagata et al.[89] reported results of RFA treatment in 173 patients with primary or hepatic cancers. Additional therapy, including arterial embolization, radiotherapy, immunotherapy, and systemic chemotherapy, was also combined with RFA treatment in this series. Treatments were administered percutaneously, and greater than 80% of patients underwent more than four sessions of RFA. In 45 patients treated with metastatic tumor deposits, there was no response or disease progression in 53%. Curley et al.[90] from the M. D. Anderson Cancer Center treated 123 patients with RFA either using the percutaneous or open operative technique with US guidance. A total of 169 tumors ranging in size from 0.5 to 12 cm (median diameter, 3.4 cm) were ablated. Three-fourths of patients underwent open operative RFA, and no treatment-related deaths occurred in the study. The authors report three tumor recurrences in 169 treated lesions (1.8%) at a median follow-up of 15 months. The low recurrence rate may be due to the fact that many patients were treated operatively to facilitate probe placement and more reliably assess adequacy of therapy. In addition, the authors used inflow occlusion via the Pringle maneuver, which may have enhanced the effectiveness of the thermal ablation. In practice, the technologies behind the various local ablative therapies are evolving, and as smaller probe sizes are developed and techniques for monitoring adequacy of tissue destruction are refined the advantages of one form of ablative therapy over another may become increasingly obscure.

A group of investigators from Japan studied the feasibility of combining intrahepatic artery 5-FU (750 to 1250 mg) administered as a weekly 5-hour infusion with RFA therapy in nine patients with hepatic metastases from colorectal carcinoma.[91] These investigators found the combination to be feasible and safe, with three of nine patients surviving for more than 2 years. More recently, Kesmodel et al.[92] reported results in 51 patients with unresectable colorectal liver metastases who were treated with RFA and HAI using an FUDR-based regimen. Despite this aggressive regional strategy, disease progression in the liver was observed in more than 60%. Overall median survival was 24 months, suggesting that combination therapy may be superior to HAI alone.

OTHER ABLATIVE TECHNIQUES

Percutaneous ethanol injections into malignant deposits in the liver have most broadly been applied to the treatment of patients with hepatocellular carcinomas. The density of tumors associated with hepatocellular carcinoma and the common occurrence of this malignancy in the setting of severe underlying hepatic disease lend themselves to this form of local therapy as opposed to surgical resection, which is often not possible in patients with severe underlying hepatic cirrhosis. Currently, there are no randomized studies comparing the value of percu-

taneous ethanol injection with any of the other local modalities for the treatment of patients with hepatic malignancy. Thus, its value relative to other local techniques is uncertain. Outcome after ethanol treatment is adversely affected by underlying hepatic disease.[93] Patients classified as having Child's A have a 2-year survival, approximately twofold greater than those classified as Child's C (approximately 90% vs. less than 40%, respectively). Although the technique is generally restricted to patients with tumors less than approximately 3 to 5 cm in size, Livraghi et al.[94] published their experience with percutaneous ethanol injection in 108 patients with hepatocellular carcinoma with tumors greater than 5 cm in size performed in a single session under general anesthesia. Despite the size of the lesions treated, this group found a 3-year survival of 57% for those in patients with single lesions measuring 5.0 to 8.5 cm and 42% for those with multiple lesions measuring 5 to 10 cm.[94] The overall rate of major complications in this study was less than 5%, thus suggesting that percutaneous ethanol injections may be a useful modality even in the setting of lesions up to 10 cm in size.

Although no randomized comparisons between percutaneous ethanol injection and hepatectomy have been performed, several studies address this issue through retrospective comparisons or the use of contemporary patient cohorts. In a large retrospective analysis of 391 patients, Livraghi et al.[95] found no difference in 3-year survival for 120 patients treated by surgical resection (79% Child's A; 40% Child's B) versus 155 treated by percutaneous ethanol injection (71% Child's A; 41% Child's B); however, they noted a significantly inferior (threefold lower) survival for those patients who were not treated with either percutaneous ethanol injection or hepatectomy. Similarly, Orlando et al.[96] used a matched historic comparison group to compare the outcome of this untreated group (65 patients) with small hepatocellular carcinomas (less than 4 cm) with 35 patients treated by percutaneous ethanol injection and found that the 3-year survival of those treated with percutaneous ethanol injections was superior to that of the historic comparison group (33% vs. 14%, respectively) but that the primary difference in survival outcome was restricted to those patients with Child's A disease (71% vs. 21%, respectively); those with Child's B had a similar, but poor, 3-year survival outcome regardless of whether they were treated with percutaneous ethanol injections or left untreated (9% for both groups). These results suggest that percutaneous ethanol injections may be associated with a more favorable outcome compared with that of patients who are treated with best supportive care only and that clinical outcome with this form of local therapy may be similar to that of hepatectomy.

Given the potential value of percutaneous ethanol injections and transcatheter arterial embolization, several groups have combined these two approaches. In 86 patients with Child's class A or B cirrhosis and large hepatocellular carcinomas (3.1 to 8.0 cm), Lencioni et al.[97] found 69% and 47% 3- and 5-year survivals with 56% and 82% recurrence rates at 3 and 5 years in patients treated with transcatheter arterial chemoembolization (gelatin sponge with epirubicin emulsified in iodized oil) followed by percutaneous ethanol injection. Investigators in Germany compared the survival of 132 patients with inoperable hepatocellular carcinoma nonrandomly treated with best supportive care (45 patients) or percutaneous ethanol infusion (15 patients), transcatheter arterial chemoembolization (33 patients), or the combination of both local therapies (39 patients).[98] These investigators found that patients treated with a combination of percutaneous ethanol infusion and transarterial chemoembolization had an improved survival when compared to those patients treated with either chemoembolization alone or best supportive care only. However, those treated with chemoembolization alone had larger and more advanced hepatic disease compared to those treated with ethanol alone or the combination of local therapies, because ethanol injections (either alone or combined with chemoembolization) were reserved for those patients with fewer than three lesions with none greater than 5 cm in size. Those assigned to supportive care had disease too advanced to be treated by either chemoembolization or alcohol injections. Given these caveats, the supportive care group had the worst median survival compared with any of the treatment groups (2 vs. 25 months in the combination group). Although these data support the use and feasibility of combining transarterial chemoembolization with percutaneous ethanol injection, the true value of this combined approach versus either approach used individually requires further investigations using a randomized prospective trial design.

RESULTS OF WHOLE LIVER IRRADIATION ± CHEMOTHERAPY

Early studies demonstrated that whole liver radiation produces temporary palliation of pain for patients with cancer that is metastatic to the liver. However, it was soon discovered that doses greater than 30 to 35 Gy could produce a condition that has become known as *radiation hepatitis*.[99] Radiation hepatitis is better described as *radiation-induced liver disease* (RILD), as the pathologic evaluation shows no evidence of hepatitis. Patients in whom RILD develops present 2 weeks to 2 months after the completion of radiation therapy with weight gain and bloating and, in severe cases, confusion. Jaundice as a presenting symptom is uncommon (and suggests that impending liver failure has already developed). Physical examination reveals anicteric ascites and painful hepatomegaly. Laboratory evaluation shows a marked elevation of alkaline phosphatase out of proportion to the typically modest increases in alanine aminotransferase, AST, and bilirubin (which tends to be unconjugated); elevations in prothrombin time and partial thromboplastin time; and thrombocytopenia. Paracentesis and radiologic studies (CT or MRI, or both) fail to show progressive disease. Liver biopsy reveals venoocclusive disease pathologically identical to that resulting from a variety of insults. Although most patients recover in 1 to 2 months, overt liver failure and death develop in 10% to 20%.[100]

Unfortunately, a tolerable whole liver dose produces only short-term palliation and patient survival.[101] This is true regardless of whether the radiation is given daily or twice daily in 1.5-Gy fractions. To attempt to improve on these results, whole liver radiation has been combined with systemic and hepatic arterial chemotherapy. The most widely used drugs have been the fluoropyrimidines, 5-FU and FUDR, as both are cytotoxic and radiosensitizing agents. The objective response rates and survival after combination chemoradiotherapy appear to be somewhat superior to those obtained by radiation alone. Whole liver radiation tolerance does not seem to be affected by the concurrent use of fluoropyrimidines, in contrast with other chemotherapeutic agents such as alkylating agents or mitomycin C, which appear to increase RILD risk.[100] Tolerable courses (5% chance of RILD) for whole liver radiation in patients who have not received alkylator therapy appear to be 21 Gy in 3-Gy fractions, 25 Gy in 2.5-Gy fractions, and 30 Gy in 2-Gy fractions (Table 51.3-12).

Two major techniques are now being explored to increase focal radiation dose: yttrium 90 microspheres and conformal external-beam radiation. A randomized trial demonstrated that the combination of microspheres and hepatic arterial FUDR was superior to hepatic arterial FUDR alone in the treatment of colorectal cancer confined to the liver. Seventy-four patients with unresectable colorectal metastases undergoing implantation of a hepatic arterial infusion pump were randomly assigned to receive a single dose of microspheres (2 to 3 GBq) through the hepatic artery within 4 weeks of surgery. Patients then went on to receive chronic FUDR treatment. The overall response rate and median time to progression were increased in the group receiving microspheres (44% vs. 18%, P <.01, and 16 vs. 10 months, P<.001, respectively), and there was a trend toward an improvement in overall survival.[102] It should be noted that the efficacy of FUDR alone in this study was markedly less than is typically reported in the United States, which leaves open the question of whether the results of this study can be generalized.

Although these initial clinical results using microspheres are interesting, their wider use has been hampered by a lack of

TABLE 51.3-12.   Results of Treatment of Metastatic Cancer to the Liver Treated with Whole Liver Irradiation with Chemotherapy: Selected Series

Study	*Dose (Gy/Fractions)*	*Chemotherapy*	*Route*	*Patients (n)*	*Response (% Total)*	*Median Survival (Mo)*	*Hepatic Toxicity[a]*
Lawrence et al.[119]	33/22	FUDR	HA	19	39[b]	7	0
	36/24	—	—	13	ND	ND	—
Rotman et al.[120]	22.5–32.3/15	5-FU	IV	27	83[c]	6	0
Wiley et al.[121]	25.5/17	5-FU	HA	19	37[b]	6	0

5-FU, 5-fluorouracil; FUDR, floxuridine; HA, intraarterial hepatic infusion; IV, intravenous infusion; ND, not determined.
[a]Number of patients with grade 3 radiation hepatitis.
[b]Objective response (computed tomography or radionuclide scan documenting 50% decrease in bidimensional product).
[c]Subjective response (e.g., decrease in pain).

understanding of dosimetry and by technical factors. Radiation dose has been calculated by assuming that the microspheres are uniformly distributed throughout the liver. This assumption is clearly false, as CT scans and biopsies show selective microsphere deposition in the tumor.[103] Significant strides have been made to better quantify the dosimetry of this technique by using methods similar to those of brachytherapy (placement of radioactive sources inside the tumor).[104] A better understanding of dosimetry and of technical factors, such as the potential for pulmonary shunting (which can lead to radiation pneumonitis),[105] is required before the safe use of microspheres can become routine.

External-beam irradiation can be used to treat patients with localized unresectable metastatic cancer to the liver. These efforts have been based on the hypothesis that, just as substantial fractions of the liver can be resected if the remaining fraction can support liver function, focal high-dose liver radiation can be safely administered if sufficient normal liver is spared. As summarized in the Chapter 29.4, conformal planning can use beams not confined to the axial plane to reduce normal liver irradiation. Furthermore, three-dimensional planned treatment has allowed the development of a quantitative understanding of the relationships among dose, volume, and risk of complication.[106,107]

Phase I/II trials for patients with unresectable intrahepatic cancer using either standard two-dimensional techniques[108] or three-dimensional conformal fractionated external-beam irradiation combined with hepatic arterial FUDR have demonstrated that high-dose focal radiation can produce a greater than 50% response rate in previously treated patients.[109] These results support the hypothesis that the dose delivered is an important prognostic factor in local control and survival for patients with metastatic colorectal cancer. Patients who received greater than 70 Gy had a median survival in excess of 17 months. Importantly, dose was an independent prognostic factor and was not correlated with tumor size. Attempts are under way to give higher radiation doses through technical improvements in dose delivery that treat less normal liver while encompassing the tumor.[110] Another technique for giving high-dose radiation that is applicable to small tumors (median, 2.5 cm in diameter) is to use a single large fraction of 14 to 26 Gy, which has produced up to an 80% rate of control at 18 months.[111]

CONCLUSION

Despite the fact that isolated hepatic metastases are a significant clinical problem frequently associated with a very poor prognosis, there are evolving systemic regional treatment strategies that increasingly expand the options available for patients with this condition. For individuals with resectable hepatic deposits primarily of colorectal, neuroendocrine, or genitourinary origin, the benefit in terms of overall survival or palliation appears to be well established. For patients undergoing resection for colorectal cancer, various patient, tumor, and treatment variables have been identified as important prognostic factors and can be used to select patients for adjuvant therapy. For those with unresectable colorectal cancers confined to the liver, HAI therapy using FUDR-based regimens have high response rates, but the benefit in terms of overall

survival when compared to newer systemic agents has not been conclusively demonstrated. Local ablative therapies have the advantage of being able to ablate local tumor deposits, but their influence on overall survival has not been demonstrated. As the technology behind local ablative treatments advances, they will no doubt become more widely used options in combination with postablation HAI or systemic therapy, or both. Chemoembolization has been used in patients with advanced cancers of the liver and can result in palliation in a significant percentage of those treated. Newer therapies including percutaneous perfusion or IHP and selective internal radiation are under active clinical evaluation and may gain more widespread acceptance with further refinement of treatment in the future. The range of therapies highlight the acknowledged importance and difficulty in treating hepatic metastases and provide an expectation that durable complete disease control within the liver with an associated improvement in quality of life and overall survival can be routinely achieved.

REFERENCES

1. Gragoudas ES, Egan KM, Seddon JM, et al. Survival of patients with metastases from uveal melanoma. *Ophthalmology* 1991;98:383.
2. Meta-Analysis Group in Cancer reappraisal of hepatic arterial infusion in the treatment of nonresectable liver metastases from colorectal cancer. *J Natl Cancer Inst* 1996;88:252.
3. Fong Y, Salo J. Surgical therapy of hepatic colorectal metastasis. *Semin Oncol* 1999;26:514.
4. Yoon SS, Tanabe KK. Surgical treatment and other regional treatments for colorectal cancer liver metastases. *Oncologist* 1999;4:197.
5. Yao KA, Talamonti MS, Nemcek A, et al. Indications and results of liver resection and hepatic chemoembolization for metastatic gastrointestinal neuroendocrine tumors. *Surgery* 2001;130:677.
6. Jemal A, Murray T, Samuels A, et al. Cancer statistics, 2003. *CA Cancer J Clin* 2003;53:5.
7. Görög D, Toth A, Weltner J. Prognosis of untreated liver metastasis from rectal cancer. *Acta Chir Hung* 1997;36:106.
8. Rougier P, Milan C, Lazorthes F, et al. Prospective study of prognostic factors in patients with unresected hepatic metastases from colorectal cancer. *Br J Surg* 1995;82:1397.
9. Palmer M, Petrelli NJ, Herrera L. No treatment option for liver metastases from colorectal adenocarcinoma. *Dis Colon Rectum* 1989;32:698.
10. Sutliff VE, Doppman JL, Gibril F, Venzon DJ, et al. Growth of newly diagnosed, untreated metastatic gastrinomas and predictors of growth patterns. *J Clin Oncol* 1997;15:2420.
11. Finan PJ, Marshall RJ, Cooper EH, Giles GR. Factors affecting survival in patients presenting with synchronous hepatic metastases from colorectal cancer: a clinical and computer analysis. *Br J Surg* 1985;72:373.
12. Seregard S, Kock E. Prognostic indicators following enucleation for posterior uveal melanoma. *Acta Ophthalmol Scand* 1995;73:340.
13. Kath R, Hayungs J, Bornfeld N, et al. Prognosis and treatment of disseminated uveal melanoma. *Cancer* 1993;72:2219.
14. Alexander HR, Libutti SK, Pingpank JF, et al. Hyperthermic isolated hepatic perfusion (IHP) using melphalan for patients with ocular melanoma metastatic to liver. *Clin Cancer Res* 2003;9:6343.
15. Ayoub J-P, Hess KR, Abbruzzese MC, Lenzi R, et al. Unknown primary tumors metastatic to liver. *J Clin Oncol* 1998;16:2105.
16. Yu F, Venzon DJ, Serrano J, et al. Prospective study of the clinical course, prognostic factors, causes of death, and survival in patients with long-standing Zollinger-Ellison syndrome. *J Clin Oncol* 1999;17:615.
17. Jarnagin WR, Bach AM, Winston CB, et al. What is the yield of intraoperative ultrasonography during partial hepatectomy for malignant disease? *J Am Coll Surg* 2001;192:577.
18. Valls C, Andia E, Sanchez A, et al. Hepatic metastases from colorectal cancer: preoperative detection and assessment of resectability with helical CT. *Radiology* 2001;218:55.
19. Awaya H, Ito K, Jonjo K, et al. Differential diagnosis of hepatic tumors with delayed enhancement at gadolinium-enhanced MRI: a pictorial essay. *Clin Imaging* 1998;22:180.
20. Ruers TJ, Langenhoff BS, Neeleman N, et al. Value of positron emission tomography with [F-18]fluorodeoxyglucose in patients with colorectal liver metastases: a prospective study. *J Clin Oncol* 2002;20:388.
21. Strasberg SM, Dehdashti F, Siegel BA, et al. Survival of patients evaluated by FDG-PET before hepatic resection for metastatic colorectal carcinoma: a prospective database study. *Ann Surg* 2001;233:293.
22. Termanini B, Gibril F, Doppman JL, et al. Distinguishing small hepatic hemangiomas from vascular liver metastases in gastrinoma: use of a somatostatin-receptor scintigraphic agent. *Radiology* 1997;202:151.
23. DeMatteo RP, Fong Y, Jarnagin WR, Blumgart LH. Recent advances in hepatic resection. *Semin Surg Oncol* 2000;19:200.
24. Jarnagin WR, Conlon K, Bodniewicz J, et al. A clinical scoring system predicts the yield of diagnostic laparoscopy in patients with potentially resectable hepatic colorectal metastases. *Cancer* 2001;91:1121.

25. Fong Y, Brennan MF, Brown K, et al. Drainage is unnecessary after elective liver resection. *Am J Surg* 1996;171:158.
26. Jarnagin WR, Gonen M, Fong Y, et al. Improvement in perioperative outcome after hepatic resection: analysis of 1,803 consecutive cases over the past decade. *Ann Surg* 2002;236:397.
27. Kooby DA, Stockman J, Ben Porat L, et al. Influence of transfusions on perioperative and long-term outcome in patients following hepatic resection for colorectal metastases. *Ann Surg* 2003;237:860.
28. Little SA, Jarnagin WR, DeMatteo RP, et al. Diabetes is associated with increased perioperative mortality but equivalent long-term outcome after hepatic resection for colorectal cancer. *J Gastrointest Surg* 2002;6:88.
29. Cady B, Jenkins RL, Steele GD Jr, et al. Surgical margin in hepatic resection for colorectal metastasis. A critical and improveable determinant of outcome. *Ann Surg* 1998;227:566.
30. Ohlsson B, Stenram U, Tranberg K-G. Resection of colorectal liver metastases: 25-year experience. *World J Surg* 1998;22:268.
31. Fong Y, Fortner J, Sun RL, et al. Clinical score for predicting recurrence after hepatic resection for metastatic colorectal cancer. *Ann Surg* 1999;230:309.
32. Bakalakos EA, Kim JA, Young DC, Martin EW Jr. Determinants of survival following hepatic resection for metastatic colorectal cancer. *World J Surg* 1998;22:399.
33. Ambiru S, Miyazaki M, Isono T, et al. Hepatic resection for colorectal metastases. *Dis Colon Rectum* 1999;42:632.
34. Petrowsky H, Gonen M, Jarnagin W, et al. Second liver resections are safe and effective treatment for recurrent hepatic metastases from colorectal cancer: a bi-institutional analysis. *Ann Surg* 2002;235:863.
35. Mineo TC, Ambrogi V, Tonini G, et al. Long-term results after resection of simultaneous and sequential lung and liver metastases from colorectal carcinoma. *J Am Coll Surg* 2003;197:386.
36. Bines SD, England G, Deziel DJ, et al. Synchronous, metachronous and multiple hepatic resections of liver tumors originating from primary gastric tumors. *Surgery* 1993;114:799.
37. Chen H, Hardacre JM, Uzra A, et al. Isolated liver metastases from neuroendocrine tumors: does resection prolong survival? *J Am Coll Surg* 1998;187:88.
38. Raab R, Nussbaum KT, Behrend M, Weimann A. Liver metastases of breast cancer: results of liver resection. *Anticancer Res* 1998;18:2231.
39. DeMatteo RP, Shah A, Fong Y, et al. Results of hepatic resection for sarcoma metastatic to liver. *Ann Surg* 2001;234:540.
40. Schwartz SI. Hepatic resection for noncolorectal nonneuroendocrine metastases. *World J Surg* 1995;19:72.
41. Harrison LE, Brennan MF, Newman E, et al. Hepatic resection for noncolorectal, nonneuroendocrine metastases: a fifteen-year experience with ninety-six patients. *Surgery* 1997;121:625.
42. Saltz LB, Cox JV, Blanke C, et al. Irinotecan plus fluorouracil and leucovorin for metastatic colorectal cancer. Irinotecan Study Group. *N Engl J Med* 2000;343:905.
43. Goldberg R, Morton R, Sargent D, et al. N9741: oxaliplatin (Oxal) or CPT-11 + 5-fluorouracil (5-FU)/leucovorin (LV) or Oxal + CPT-11 in advanced colorectal cancer (CRC). Initial toxicity and response data from a GI intergroup study. *Proc Am Soc Clin Oncol* 2002.
44. Kemeny N, Fata F. Hepatic-arterial chemotherapy. *Lancet Oncol* 2001;2:418.
45. Kemeny N, Daly J, Reichman B, et al. Intrahepatic or systemic infusion of fluorodeoxyuridine in patients with liver metastases from colorectal carcinoma. *Ann Intern Med* 1987;107:459.
46. Hohn DC, Stagg RJ, Friedman MA, et al. A randomized trial of continuous intravenous versus hepatic intraarterial floxuridine in patients with colorectal cancer metastatic to the liver: The Northern California Oncology Group trial. *J Clin Oncol* 1989;7:1646.
47. Chang AE, Schneider PD, Sugarbaker PH, et al. A prospective randomized trial of regional versus systemic continuous fluorodeoxyuridine chemotherapy in the treatment of colorectal liver metastases. *Ann Surg* 1987;206:685.
48. Martin JK, O'Connel MJ, Wieand HS, et al. Intra-arterial floxuridine vs systemic fluorouracil for hepatic metastases from colorectal cancer. *Arch Surg* 1990;125:1022.
49. Rougier P, LaPlanche A, Huguier M, et al. Hepatic arterial infusion of floxuridine in patients with liver metastases from colorectal carcinoma: long-term results of a prospective randomized trial. *J Clin Oncol* 1992;10:1112.
50. Allen-Mersh TG, Earlam S, Fordy C, et al. Quality of life and survival with continuous hepatic-artery floxuridine infusion for colorectal liver metastases. *Lancet* 1994;344:1255.
51. Lorenz M, Muller HH. Randomized, multicenter trial of fluorouracil plus leucovorin administered either via hepatic arterial or intravenous infusion versus fluorodeoxyuridine administered via hepatic arterial infusion in patients with nonresectable liver metastases from colorectal carcinoma. *J Clin Oncol* 2000;18:243.
52. Kerr DJ, McArdle CS, Ledermann J, et al. Intrahepatic arterial versus intravenous fluorouracil and folinic acid for colorectal cancer liver metastases: a multicentre randomised trial. *Lancet* 2003;361:368.
53. Kemeny NE, Niedzwiecki D, Hollis DR, et al. Hepatic arterial infusion (HAI) versus systemic therapy for hepatic metastases from colorectal cancer; a CALGB randomized trial of efficacy, quality of life (QOL), cost effectiveness, and molecular markers. *Soc Clin Oncol Proc* 2003;22:252(abst).
54. Ellis LM, Chase JL, Patt YZ, Curley SA. Hepatic arterial infusion chemotherapy for colorectal cancer metastasis to the liver. In: Curley SA, ed. *Liver cancer.* New York: Springer-Verlag, 2000:150.
55. Kemeny N, Seiter K, Niedzwiecki D, et al. A randomized trial of intrahepatic infusion of fluorodeoxyuridine with dexamethasone versus fluorodeoxyuridine alone in the treatment of metastatic colorectal cancer. *Cancer* 1992;69:327.
55a. van Riel JMG, van Groeningen CJ, Albers SHM, et al. Hepatic arterial 5-fluorouracil in patients with liver metastases of colorectal cancer: single-centre experience in 145 patients. *Ann Oncol* 2000;11:1563.
56. Lorenz M, Mueller HH, Mattes E, et al. Phase II study of weekly 24-hour intra-arterial high-dose infusion of 5-fluorouracil and folinic acid for liver metastases from colorectal carcinomas. *Ann Oncol* 2001;12:321.
57. Kemeny N, Gonen M, Sullivan D, et al. Phase I study of hepatic arterial infusion of floxuridine and dexamethasone with systemic irinotecan for unresectable hepatic metastases from colorectal cancer. *J Clin Oncol* 2001;19:2687.
58. Paty P, Fong Y, Harris R, et al. Update of phase I studies of hepatic arterial infusion (HAI) of floxuridine (FUDR) and dexamethasone (DEX) plus: systemic oxaliplatin (Oxal) and irinotecan (CPT-11) or systemic Oxal and fluorouracil (FU) and leucovorin (LV) for unresectable hepatic metastases from colorectal cancer. *Am Soc Clin Oncol Proc* 2003;22:289(abst).
59. Kemeny N, Huang Y, Cohen AM, et al. Hepatic arterial infusion of chemotherapy after resection of hepatic metastases from colorectal cancer. *N Engl J Med* 1999;341:2039.
60. Kemeny MM, Adak S, Gray B, et al. Combined-modality treatment for resectable metastatic colorectal carcinoma to the liver: surgical resection of hepatic metastases in combination with continuous infusion of chemotherapy—an intergroup study. *J Clin Oncol* 2002;20:1499.
61. Lorenz M, Müller H-H, Schramm H, et al. Randomized trial of surgery versus surgery followed by adjuvant hepatic arterial infusion with 5-fluorouracil and folinic acid for liver metastases of colorectal cancer. *Ann Surg* 1998;228:756.
62. Giacchetti S, Itzhaki M, Gruia G, et al. Long-term survival of patients with unresectable colorectal cancer liver metastases following infusional chemotherapy with 5-fluorouracil, leucovorin, oxaliplatin and surgery. *Ann Oncol* 1999;10:663.
63. Alberts S, Donohue J, Mahoney M. Liver resection after 5-fluorouracil and oxaliplatin for patients with metastatic colorectal cancer (MCRC) limited to the liver: a North Center Cancer Treatment Group (NCCTG) phase II study. American Society for Clinical Oncology Conference Proceeding. 2003;22:263..
64. Meric F, Patt YZ, Curley SA, et al. Surgery after downstaging of unresectable hepatic tumors with intra-arterial chemotherapy. *Ann Surg Oncol* 2000;7:490.
65. Leyvraz S, Spataro V, Bauer J, et al. Treatment of ocular melanoma metastatic to the liver by hepatic arterial chemotherapy. *J Clin Oncol* 1997;15:2589.
66. Ravikumar TS, Pizzorno G, Bodden W, et al. Percutaneous hepatic vein isolation and high-dose hepatic arterial infusion chemotherapy for unresectable liver tumors. *J Clin Oncol* 1994;12:2723.
67. Pingpank JF, Libutti SK, Chang R, et al. A phase I feasibility study of hepatic arterial melphalan infusion with hepatic arterial melphalan infusion with hepatic venous hemofiltration using percutaneously placed catheters in patients with unresectable hepatic malignancies. *Am Soc Clin Oncol Proc* 2003;22:282(abst).
68. Alexander HR, Bartlett DL, Libutti SK. Isolated hepatic perfusion: a potentially effective treatment for patients with metastatic or primary cancers confined to the liver. *Cancer J Sci Am* 1998;4:2.
69. Oldhafer KJ, Lang H, Frerker M, et al. First experience and technical aspects of isolated liver perfusion for extensive liver metastasis. Surgery 1998;123:622.
70. Hafström L, Naredi P. Isolated hepatic perfusion with extracorporeal oxygenation using hyperthermia TNFα and melphalan: Swedish experience. Recent Results Cancer Res 1998;147:120.
71. Alexander HR, Bartlett DL, Libutti SK, et al. Isolated hepatic perfusion with tumor necrosis factor and melphalan for unresectable cancers confined to the liver. *J Clin Oncol* 1998;16:1479.
72. Bartlett DL, Libutti SK, Figg WD, et al. Isolated hepatic perfusion for unresectable hepatic metastases from colorectal cancer. *Surgery* 2001;129:176.
73. Schell SR, Camp ER, Caridi JG, Hawkins IF Jr. Hepatic artery embolization for control of symptoms, octreotide requirements, and tumor progression in metastatic carcinoid tumors. *J Gastrointest Surg* 2002;6:664.
74. Gupta S, Yao JC, Ahrar K, et al. Hepatic artery embolization and chemoembolization for treatment of patients with metastatic carcinoid tumors: the M. D. Anderson experience. *Cancer J* 2003;9:261.
75. Salman HS, Cynamon J, Jagust M, et al. Randomized phase II trial of embolization therapy versus chemoembolization therapy in previously treated patients with colorectal carcinoma metastatic to the liver. *Clin Colorectal Cancer* 2002;2:173.
76. Bavisotto LM, Patel NH, Althaus SJ, et al. Hepatic transcatheter arterial chemoembolization alternating with systemic protracted continuous infusion 5-fluorouracil for gastrointestinal malignancies metastatic to liver: a phase II trial of the Puget Sound Oncology Consortium (PSOC 1104). *Clin Cancer Res* 1999;5:95.
77 Leichman CG, Jacobson JR, Modiano M. Hepatic chemoembolization combined with systemic infusion of 5-fluorouracil and bolus leucovorin for patients with metastatic colorectal carcinoma: a Southwest Oncology Group pilot trial. *Cancer* 1999;86:775.
78. Huang A, McCall JM, Weston MD, et al. Phase I study of percutaneous cryotherapy for colorectal liver metastasis. *Br J Surg* 2002;89:303.
79. Seifert JK, Junginger T, Morris DL. A collective review of the world literature on hepatic cryotherapy. *J R Coll Surg Edinb* 1998;43:141.
80. Weaver ML, Ashton JG, Zemel R. Treatment of colorectal liver metastases by cryotherapy. *Semin Surg Oncol* 1998;14:163.
81. Seifert JK, Morris DL. Prognostic factors after cryotherapy for hepatic metastases from colorectal cancer. *Ann Surg* 1998;228:201.
82. Seifert JK, Morris DL. Repeat hepatic cryotherapy for recurrent metastases from colorectal cancer. *Surgery* 1999;125:233.
83. Iannitti DA, Heniford T, Hale J, et al. Laparoscopic cryoablation of hepatic metastases. *Arch Surg* 1998;133:1011.
84. Korpan NN. Hepatic cryosurgery for liver metastases. Long-term follow-up. *Ann Surg* 1997;225:193.
85. Seifert JK, Cozzi PJ, Morris DL. Cryotherapy for neuroendocrine liver metastases. *Semin Surg Oncol* 1998;14:175.
86. Dwerryhouse SJ, Seifert JK, McCall JL, et al. Hepatic resection with cryotherapy to involved or inadequate resection margin (edge freeze) for metastases from colorectal cancer. *Br J Surg* 1998;85:185.
87. Wallace JR, Christians KK, Pitt HA, Quebbeman EJ. Cryotherapy extends the indications for treatment of colorectal liver metastases. *Surgery* 1999;126:766.

88. Bilchik AJ, Wood TF, Chawla SP, et al. Systemic irinotecan or regional floxuridine chemotherapy prolongs survival after hepatic cryosurgery in patients with metastatic colon cancer refractory to 5-fluorouracil. *Clin Colorectal Cancer* 2001;1:36.

89. Nagata Y, Hiraoka M, Nishimura Y, et al. Clinical results of radiofrequency hyperthermia for malignant liver tumors. *Int J Radiat Oncol Biol Phys* 1997;38:359.

90. Curley SA, Izzo F, Delrio P, et al. Radiofrequency ablation of unresectable primary and metastatic hepatic malignancies: results in 123 patients. *Ann Surg* 1999;230:9.

91. Kainuma O, Asano T, Aoyama H. Combined therapy with radiofrequency thermal ablation and intra-arterial infusion chemotherapy for hepatic metastases from colorectal cancer. *Hepato-gastroenterology* 1999;46:1071.

92. Kesmodel SB, Canter RJ, Spitz FR, Fraker DL. Phase II trial of combination radiofrequency ablation (RFA) and hepatic artery infusion (HAI) therapy for colorectal liver metastases. 22 (General Poster Session). Meeting Proceedings; American Society of Clinical Oncology; 39th Annual Meeting, Chicago, IL. 2003;29:5.

93. Giorgio A, Tarantino L, Mariniello N. Percutaneous ethanol injection under general anesthesia for hepatocellular carcinoma: 3 year survival in 112 patients. *Eur J Ultrasound* 1998;8:201.

94. Livraghi T, Benedini V, Lazzaroni S. Long term results of single session percutaneous ethanol injection in patients with large hepatocellular carcinoma. *Cancer* 1998;83:48.

95. Livraghi T, Bolondi L, Buscarini L. No treatment, resection and ethanol injection in hepatocellular carcinoma: a retrospective analysis of survival in 391 patients with cirrhosis. *J Hepatol* 1995;22:522.

96. Orlando A, Cottone M, Virdone R. Treatment of small hepatocellular carcinoma associated with cirrhosis by percutaneous ethanol injection. A trial with a comparison group. *Scand J Gastroenterol* 1997;32:598.

97. Lencioni R, Paolicchi A, Moretti M. Combined transcatheter arterial chemoembolization and percutaneous ethanol injection for the treatment of large hepatocellular carcinoma: local therapeutic effect and long-term survival rate. *Eur Radiol* 1998;8:439.

98. Allgaier HP, Deibert P, Olschewski M. Survival benefit of patients with inoperable hepatocellular carcinoma treated by a combination of transarterial chemoembolization and percutaneous ethanol injection—a single-center analysis including 132 patients. *Int J Cancer* 1998;79:601.

99. Reed GB, Cos AJ. The human liver after radiation injury. A form of veno-occlusive disease. *Am J Pathol* 1966;48:597.

100. Lawrence TS, Robertson JM, Anscher MS, et al. Hepatic toxicity resulting from cancer treatment. *Int J Radiat Oncol Biol Phys* 1995;31:1237.

101. Russell AH, Clyde C, Wasserman TH, et al. Accelerated hyperfractionated hepatic irradiation in the management of patients with liver metastases: results of the RTOG dose escalating protocol. *Int J Radiat Oncol Biol Phys* 1993;27:117.

102. Gray B, van Hazel G, Hope M, et al. Randomised trial of SIR-spheres plus chemotherapy vs. chemotherapy alone for treating patients with liver metastases from primary large bowel cancer. *Ann Oncol* 2001;12:1711.

103. Sarfaraz M, Kennedy AS, Cao ZJ, et al. Physical aspects of yttrium-90 microsphere therapy for nonresectable hepatic tumors. *Med Phys* 2003;30:199.

104. Campbell AM, Bailey IH, Burton MA. Tumour dosimetry in human liver following hepatic yttrium-90 microsphere therapy. *Phys Med Biol* 2001;46:487.

105. Leung TW, Lau WY, Ho SK, et al. Radiation pneumonitis after selective internal radiation treatment with intraarterial 90 yttrium-microspheres for inoperable hepatic tumors. *Int J Radiat Oncol Biol Phys* 1995;33:919.

106. Dawson LA, Normolle D, Balter JM, et al. Analysis of radiation-induced liver disease using the Lyman NTCP model. *Int J Radiat Oncol Biol Phys* 2002;53:810.

107. McGinn CJ, Robertson JM, Lawrence TS, et al. A phase I/II trial of chemoembolization with mitomycin C following hepatic arterial fluorodeoxyuridine/leucovorin and whole liver radiotherapy for patients with intrahepatic malignancies. *Cancer Ther* 1998;1:88.

108. Malik U, Mohiuddin M. External-beam radiotherapy in the management of liver metastases. *Semin Oncol* 2002;29:196.

109. McGinn CJ, Ten Haken RK, Ensminger WD, et al. Treatment of intrahepatic cancers with radiation doses based on a normal tissue complication probability model. *J Clin Oncol* 1998;16:2246.

110. Kitamura K, Shirato H, Seppenwoolde Y, et al. Tumor location, cirrhosis, and surgical history contribute to tumor movement in the liver, as measured during stereotactic irradiation using a real-time tumor-tracking radiotherapy system. *Int J Radiat Oncol Biol Phys* 2003;56:221.

111. Herfarth KK, Debus J, Lohr F, et al. Stereotactic single-dose radiation therapy of liver tumors: results of a phase I/II trial. *J Clin Oncol* 2001;19:164.

112. Bartlett DL, Fong Y. Solitary mall hepatic metastases: when and how? In: Blumgart L, Poston G, eds. *Clinical challenges in hepatobiliary and pancreatic surgery.* Oxford: Isis Medical Media, 1999.

113. Wagman LD, Kemeny MM, Leong L, et al. A prospective, randomized evaluation of the treatment of colorectal cancer metastatic to the liver. *J Clin Oncol* 1990;8:1885.

114. Lorenz M, Muller HH. Randomized, multicenter trial of fluorouracil plus leucovorin administered either via hepatic arterial or intravenous infusion versus fluorodeoxyuridine administered via hepatic arterial infusion in patients with nonresectable liver metastases from colorectal carcinoma. *J Clin Oncol* 2000;18:243.

115. Ruszniewski P, Rougier P, Legmann P. Hepatic arterial chemoembolization in patients with liver metastases of endocrine tumors. *Cancer* 1993;71:2624.

116. Kim YH, Ajani JA, Carrasco CH, et al. Selective hepatic arterial chemoembolization for liver metastases in patients with carcinoid tumor or islet cell carcinoma. *Cancer Invest* 1999;17:474.

117. Sanz-Altamira PM, Spence LD, Huberman MS. Selective chemoembolization in the management of hepatic metastases in refractory colorectal carcinoma. *Dis Colon Rectum* 1997;40:770.

118. Tellez C, Benson IAB, Lyster MT. Phase II trial of chemoembolization for the treatment of metastatic colorectal carcinoma to the liver and review of the literature. *Cancer* 1998;82:1250.

119. Lawrence TS, Dworzanin LM, Walker-Andrews SC. Treatment of cancers involving the liver and porta hepatis with external beam irradiation and intraarterial hepatic fluorodeoxyuridine. *Int J Radiat Oncol Biol Phys* 1990;20:555.

120. Rotman M, Kuruvilla AM, Choi K. Response of colo-rectal hepatic metastases to concomitant radiotherapy and hyperfractionated external radiation therapy. *Int J Radiat Oncol Biol Phys* 1986;12:2179.

121. Wiley AL, Wirtanen GW, Stephenson JA, et al. Combined hepatic artery 5-fluorouracil and irradiation of liver metastases. A randomized study. *Cancer* 1989;64:1783.

SECTION **4**

MARK W. MANOSO
JOHN H. HEALEY

Metastatic Cancer to the Bone

The development of metastatic bone disease is the source of significant morbidity in the cancer population. In the United States, half of the 556,000 individuals who die of cancer each year have metastatic disease.[1] Breast and prostate carcinomas are the most common to develop metastases to bone, with an incidence of 65% to 75% and 68%, respectively.[2,3] In addition, lung, thyroid, and renal carcinoma metastasize to bone in approximately 30% to 40% of cases.[2,3] The decline in the mortality rate over the last few years translates into more people living with cancer and bone metastases. Metastatic bone disease has become an increasingly important quality-of-life issue. Currently, mean survival after metastasis to bone varies greatly depending on tumor type and sites of involvement. Mean survival ranges from a low of 3 months with lung carcinoma to a high of 19 months with thyroid and breast carcinoma.[4] When

patients have only skeletal metastases, their average survival is 12 months, compared to 3 months for both pulmonary and bone metastasis.[5] With prolongation in survival, the challenge is to improve the quality of the patient's remaining life.

The treatment of metastatic disease requires a multidisciplinary approach that addresses systemic and focal disease. The complex nature of metastatic disease requires the combined efforts of a team of medical, surgical, radiation, and orthopedic oncologists. Systemic disease necessitates a combination of chemotherapy, hormonal therapy, immunotherapy, and bisphosphonate therapy. Focal complications are best addressed with surgery or radiotherapy, or both. With metastatic disease to bone, prevention of skeletal complications requires early detection and aggressive management. All members of the team must keep a vigilant eye for the early signs of disease progression and skeletal manifestations.

PRESENTATION

The morbidity associated with metastatic bone disease includes pain, hypercalcemia, pathologic fractures, spinal instability and cord compression, and immobility. Knowledge of the presentation of metastatic bone disease is important in the prevention and treatment of the most severe complications.

The most common symptom of metastatic disease to the skeletal system is pain. Pain may initially be a well-localized or diffuse ache that is worse at night and is unimproved with recumbency. Extremity lesions tend to be well defined and easily identified, in contrast to spine and pelvic sites, which produce vague, diffuse symptoms. With progression the pain worsens with weight-bearing activity. The initial biologic pain comes from the tumor's presence in the bone. The release of inflammatory mediators, neuropeptides, and cytokines, as well as elevation of the intraosseous pressure due to tumor mass effect, irritates intraosseous and periosteal nerve endings. The functional pain is caused by the mechanical weakness of the bone, which can no longer support the normal stresses of daily activities. Mechanical pain usually is associated with bone loss in lytic lesions; however, blastic lesions may weaken the bone sufficiently through the loss of structural integrity to cause functional pain. The development of functional pain is a marker for a bone at risk for fracture.

Another common complication, hypercalcemia of malignancy, occurs most commonly in squamous cell lung cancer, breast cancer, multiple myeloma, and renal cell carcinoma. In breast carcinoma, the historic incidence has ranged from 19.0% to 49.5%.[6,7] The hypercalcemia is mediated by one of two mechanisms in metastatic bone disease. Advanced metastatic disease with severe bone destruction at multiple sites is the more frequent cause of this complication. In addition, tumors such as squamous cell carcinoma may secrete parathyroid hormone–related protein and produce the equivalent of secondary hyperparathyroidism. With decrease in activity because of pain, disuse osteolysis can exacerbate the hypercalcemia. With mild disease, patients are often asymptomatic. With severe disease, patients may develop fatigue, lethargy, nausea, vomiting, anorexia, and disorientation. Early initiation of bisphosphonate therapy may prevent hypercalcemia.

Pathologic fractures may be the first sign of metastatic disease in the skeletal system. In breast carcinoma, as many as 35% of patients with bone disease experience fracture.[7] In one review, an 8% cumulative incidence of long bone pathologic fracture occurred in 1800 cancer patients.[8] Breast, lung, renal, and thyroid cancer have been the most common cause of pathologic fracture.[8]

The spine is the most common site of skeletal metastases, so spinal instability and neurologic abnormalities are common. In one study of 131 patients with spinal metastases, 106 had signs of myelopathy, of whom 52 had additional radicular symptoms.[9] Spinal cord compression, if diagnosed late, leads to loss of ambulation and independence and significantly impacts the quality of remaining life. Loss of proprioception, sphincter control, or motor or sensory function reflects spinal cord compression that needs treatment. Knowledge of the neurologic signs of spinal cord compression can prevent these devastating complications.

PATHOPHYSIOLOGY

Significant strides have been made in characterization of the pathogenesis of metastatic bone disease. Historically, the initial studies of Batson identified the importance of blood flow. He described the high flow, low-pressure, valveless plexus of veins that connects the visceral organs to the spine and pelvis.[10] Batson demonstrated the mechanism of prostate cancer metastasis to the spine. Multiple authors have highlighted the importance of the arterial transportation of microemboli in the development of metastatic bone lesions. Intracardiac[11] and intraaortic[12] injection of tumor cells in rodent models have created patterns of metastatic disease that are identical to clinical distributions. With arterial metastasis, tumor cells are trapped in the terminal ends of the major capillaries running into the bone.

Recent research has focused on the multistep cellular process of metastasis. Initially the cancer cell must disengage from its primary site. The loss of expression of E-cadherin, a cell surface adhesion molecule, has been demonstrated in breast, prostate, colorectal, and pancreatic carcinoma as an early step in cellular disengagement. After invasion of the vascular or lymphatic system, the cancer cell must survive the immune system and then arrest at its final destination. At the distant site, the malignant cell must adhere to the basement membrane, invade the surrounding tissue, induce angiogenesis, and develop into a secondary mass. Cell adhesion molecules from the integrin family, immunoglobulin superfamily (intracellular adhesion molecule, vascular cell adhesion molecule, and platelet endothelial cell adhesion molecule), and selectin family of receptors have been implicated in adhesion to basement membrane proteins such as laminin at the target site.[13] To leave the vascular system, the tumor cell releases matrix metalloproteinases, a diverse family of zinc-dependent endopeptidases, to break down the host tissue and allow invasion.[14] After tissue invasion, angiogenesis is required for continued tumor growth. Microarray analysis of metastatic breast cancer specimens has suggested a metastatic profile of interleukin-11, connective tissue growth factor, and transforming growth factor-β gene overexpression.[15]

Once the metastatic lesion is established in bone, the cytokine expression of the tumor cells and their interaction with osteoclasts and osteoblasts determine the nature of the lesion. Osteoclastic activity has been shown to be increased by tumor expression of interleukin-6[16] and parathyroid hormone–related protein.[17] The inhibition of osteoclastic recruitment and osteoclast function is the basis for bisphosphonate therapy in osteolytic metastatic lesions and Paget's disease. Osteoblastic lesions have been associated with endothelin-1[17] and insulin-like growth factor[18] stimulation of osteoblasts.

DIAGNOSTIC EVALUATION

In a patient with musculoskeletal pain, a thorough history and physical examination is the first step in the evaluation. An assessment of carcinogenic exposure, family history taking, extensive review of systems, and special attention to examination of the thyroid, breast, and prostate gland must be included in the complete evaluation for metastatic bone disease. Skeletal disease presents in one of three scenarios. The first is the presentation of multiple bone lesions in widely metastatic disease. No diagnostic dilemma is present, and the patient can be treated clinically if the treatment would be the same regardless of the disease process, without a tissue diagnosis. In the second scenario, the patient presents with a history of cancer and a new solitary bone lesion. The new bone lesion cannot be assumed to be the first sign of metastatic disease. Solitary foci are frequently the presentation of renal and thyroid carcinoma metastases and plasmacytoma. In the third scenario, the patient has a solitary lesion and no history of cancer. The origin of disease in the third situation is most commonly lung or renal cell carcinoma. In the latter two situations, the patient must be evaluated for a primary lesion of bone as well as for metastatic disease.

After a thorough history taking and physical examination, a skeletal lesion should first be evaluated with plain radiography. Plain radiographs are the most specific but least sensitive for diagnostic purposes. Plain radiographs significantly aid in determining nonoperative versus operative management. Next, the entire skeletal system is evaluated; bone scintigraphy is a quick and highly sensitive means of assessing all the bones of the body for destructive lesions. Because of the low specificity of this modality, all scintigraphic abnormalities should be investigated using plain radiography. The radiographic assessment to evaluate for an unknown primary is completed with a chest radiograph and a computed tomography (CT) scan of the chest, abdomen, and pelvis. The CT scan is particularly useful for lung and intraabdominal carcinomas.[19]

In addition to radiographic studies, the diagnostic workup includes a combination of laboratory tests to identify the primary sites and evaluate for common complications of skeletal metastatic disease. The initial screening laboratory examination includes a complete blood cell count to evaluate for anemia, thrombocytopenia, and myelosuppression; measurement of electrolytes, including calcium, phosphorus, and alkaline phosphatase, to evaluate for hypercalcemia and bone turnover; renal and liver function tests; and erythrocyte sedimentation rate to assess for systemic illness. Additional tests to evaluate for specific diseases should include serum and urine protein electrophoresis for myeloma, parathyroid hormone level for hyperparathyroidism and brown tumors, β_2-microglobulin level for lymphoma and myeloma, prostate-specific antigen level for prostate cancer, and cancer antigen 125 level for breast carcinoma.[19] The combination of laboratory and radiographic evaluations is successful in identifying at least 85% of primary lesions.[19]

After the preliminary workup is completed, a biopsy must be performed to verify the diagnosis before initiation of treatment. Biopsy on its own, however, is poor at identifying a primary metastatic source.[19] With solitary lesions, a primary sarcoma must be ruled out. The differential diagnosis of primary tumors can include malignant fibrous histiocytoma and dedifferentiated chondrosarcoma. For patients with the appropriate history, secondary sarcomas of Paget's disease and postradiation sarcomas should be considered. In addition to malignant lesions, benign mimics are also in the differential diagnosis. Multiple lytic bone lesions can occur with hyperparathyroidism and with the presence of multiple brown tumors. Paget's disease may present as a lytic lesion or as a sclerotic lesion depending on its phase of progression. Multiple scintigraphic hot spots can be caused by multiple fractures associated with osteomalacia and osteoporosis. Multiple osteoporotic compression fractures of the spine are often a diagnostic dilemma and can frequently be distinguished from metastatic disease by magnetic resonance imaging (MRI).

When a site is chosen for biopsy, a non–weight-bearing bone is preferred. With the creation of a biopsy hole in the bone, the risk for fracture is elevated. Scintigraphy can aid in finding an accessible safer site when multiple lesions exist. The method of biopsy can be open or CT-guided needle aspiration. Needle aspiration can be used if a hole exists in the bone or a soft tissue mass is present. Accuracy of needle biopsy findings has been reported to be as high as 89%.[20] If the needle biopsy findings are nondiagnostic or the lesion is confined to the bone, an open biopsy is required. The area should be protected from weight bearing for at least 6 weeks to allow the bone to heal or until surgery is performed to stabilize the bone.

IMAGING OF BONE LESIONS

PLAIN RADIOGRAPHY

Although plain radiographs are relatively insensitive for the detection of metastatic disease, they provide the basis for the initial evaluation, surgical planning, and follow-up evaluation of metastatic bone disease. They are inexpensive and easily obtained, compared to other types of images. The pattern of disease on the plain radiographs can be diagnostic of some primary bone lesions in the evaluation of bone pain. Plain radiographs evaluate the structural integrity of bone and the risk of impending pathologic fracture. This analysis determines if prophylactic surgery is needed. Due to its importance in decision making, plain radiography should be the first test ordered to evaluate bone pain.

The reaction of bone to the metastatic deposits creates one of three characteristic radiographic patterns: osteolytic, osteoblastic, and mixed.[21] The balance between osteoclastic and osteoblastic activity determines which pattern predominates. When bone destruction predominates and the host bone fails to react, an osteolytic pattern is produced. When bone formation predominates, then an osteoblastic pattern is generated. Osteolytic patterns of bone destruction are geographic, moth eaten, or permeative. More aggressive lesions are permeative to moth eaten, whereas slow-growing lesions may be geographic in appearance. No radiographic pattern is diagnostic for a particular type of carcinoma. However, prostate carcinoma tends to have a blastic appearance, whereas breast carcinoma is predominantly mixed or lytic. Lung, thyroid, and renal carcinoma usually appear purely lytic. Location in the bone is occasionally relevant. Lung cancers often produce cortical lytic lesions.

Finally, serial radiographs are required after treatment of metastatic bone lesions. After radiotherapy, serial imaging should be used to monitor for treatment response and resolution of the lesion. In addition, progression of disease after surgical stabilization or palliative radiotherapy can be inexpensively assessed with plain radiography. In the case of multiple myeloma, which may be cold on bone scintigraphy, a plain radiographic bone survey is the most accurate imaging test to assess for new lesions.

BONE SCINTIGRAPHY

Bone scintigraphy is integral in the evaluation of a patient with bone pain because it can detect occult bone lesions. Technetium bone scans rely on the incorporation of tagged diphosphonate into the hydroxyapatite during bone mineralization. Scintigraphy has been reported to be 72%[22] to 84%[23] sensitive in detecting occult bone lesions. Nevertheless, bone scans are not specific, nor do they provide structural detail of the bone.

The imaging highlights regions of bone turnover with areas of new bone deposition. Plain radiography is required to evaluate for diagnostic benign and malignant lesions, which must be differentiated from metastatic disease. Second, very aggressive lesions as are typical of lung carcinoma and melanoma or myeloma, which may not elicit new bone formation, appear cold on scintigraphy.

COMPUTED TOMOGRAPHY

CT scans are not a primary tool for evaluating metastatic bone disease, but they are a useful adjunctive study. CT is especially helpful for the three-dimensional evaluation of bone integrity for preoperative planning in shoulder and pelvic[5] lesions. CT is superior to plain radiography in determining the extent of cortical destruction and the presence of a soft tissue component. In this role, it can identify a target for needle biopsy. Although it depicts bony anatomy well in the spine, MRI is more valuable for assessment of epidural extension and neural compression. MRI is also a better test for evaluating the extent of medullary involvement and the presence of a soft tissue component.

MAGNETIC RESONANCE IMAGING

Because MRI is able to achieve a high contrast between metastatic tumor disease and normal marrow, it is excellently suited for examining the skeletal system.[24] The sensitivity of MRI depends on the varying water content of different tissues. The high fat content of normal bone marrow provides the contrast for the high water content of the tumor mass. On T1-weighted images, the fatty yellow marrow appears bright next to the dark-appearing tumor, but on T2-weighted images the yellow marrow content is dark next to the bright metastatic lesion. Although highly sensitive, MRI has difficulty differentiating infection, inflammation, and metastatic disease of bone. Visualization is impaired in the very young, who have red marrow that lacks the relatively high fat content. In younger patients with red marrow, gadolinium aids in amplification of the metastatic focus.

MRI is a valuable tool in differentiating pathologic compression fractures from osteoporotic compression fractures of the spine. Full-body MRI is currently under investigation as a screening tool for metastatic disease; current studies show it to be equal to or slightly more sensitive than bone scintigraphy.[25] Although MRI provides an excellent anatomic map of the metastatic bone lesion, it is unable to provide information on structural integrity of the skeletal system. MRI is not a stand-alone study and images require correlation with plain radiographs.

POSITRON EMISSION TOMOGRAPHY

Positron emission tomography (PET) is a nuclear medicine technique that uses radioactive [^{18}F]fluorodeoxyglucose as a tracer to highlight metabolically active cells. This nonspecific study can be used to locate an unknown primary or to evaluate for multiple sites of metastatic disease. In a study of patients with metastatic disease and an unknown primary, 27 of 53 primary sites were identified after failure of conventional methods.[26]

In a comparison between PET and technetium bone scan in 110 patients, 19 of 21 osseous lesions were identified by both forms of imaging. However, bone scanning had a false-positive rate of 35 of 54. The accuracy of PET was 98%, whereas the bone scan accuracy was 61%.[27] Although the PET imaging modality shows promise, it is currently only an investigational tool for most cancers. As with bone scanning and MRI, correlation with structural imaging is required for treatment planning.

THERAPEUTIC GOALS

Current management of metastatic bone disease focuses on improvement in the quality of remaining life. Palliative treatment aims at pain relief, maintenance and restoration of function, and reduction in local tumor burden. To maximize function and limit morbidity, close surveillance for the development of metastatic bone disease and its complications is required.

Treatment planning requires an understanding of both systemic and local therapeutic modalities. Symptomatic pain relief frequently requires a combination of medical and radiation therapy. To this end, the use of bisphosphonates in breast, prostate, and renal carcinoma has been shown to delay the onset of skeletal complications. Surgery is indicated when fracture is impending or frank fracture has occurred. Due to the poor healing rates of pathologic fractures, surgical stabilization with methyl methacrylate augmentation or arthroplasty is the only method that can restore function in a timely manner. Reconstruction to manage an impending fracture is both less painful for the patient and more easily performed by the surgeon. However, surgery should not be performed alone. Adjuvant radiotherapy is necessary to prevent local progression of disease. If radiotherapy is left out, the surgical correction will fail as more bone is destroyed. After surgical stabilization and wound healing, the goal of surgery is for the patient to immediately bear weight and resume normal activities.

The intensity of treatment should be tailored to the patient's prognosis and life expectancy. The pretreatment functional status should be measured and followed. Pain relief and maintenance of function are the priorities to optimize the patient's quality of life. Outcome measurement and quality-of-life assessment tools have been developed to evaluate the disease and treatment effects. The Functional Assessment of Cancer Therapy Scale, Short Form 36, International Society of Limb Salvage–Musculoskeletal Tumor Society assessment, Karnofsky Performance Scale, Eastern Cooperative Oncology Group scale, and the Toronto Extremity Salvage Score are all currently used instruments. As new therapeutic modalities are developed, these tools will aid in determining the appropriate therapeutic choice.

THERAPEUTIC MODALITIES

Currently, three main modalities exist for the treatment of metastatic bone disease: medical treatment, radiation therapy, and surgery. These treatments are combined, depending on the severity of bone destruction and the life expectancy of the patient.

MEDICAL THERAPY

Medical management takes aim at systemic disease. Medical oncologists direct this treatment arm. Based on the type of cancer present, therapy may include chemotherapeutic agents, bisphosphonates, hormone therapy, immune therapy, and stem cell or bone marrow transplantation.

Bisphosphonates

Bisphosphonates are analogues of pyrophosphate (P-O-P) in which carbon has replaced the bridging oxygen molecule. Because no enzyme exists that cleaves a C-P bond, bisphosphonates cannot be metabolized by the body. The pharmacologic properties are controlled by the side chains attached to the central carbon. Side chain moieties in the first-generation compounds clodronate and etidronate do not contain nitrogen. The mechanism of action is substitution in the production of adenosine triphosphate, and the product then becomes a toxic adenosine triphosphate analogue that poisons the osteoclast.[28] Second-generation tiludronate and pamidronate have nitrogen-containing chains, and the third-generation risedronate and zoledronate have nitrogen ring side chains. Each succeeding generation is more potent, and toxicities vary. Nitrogen-containing bisphosphonates disrupt the cholesterol synthesis in osteoclasts, which leads to the disruption of the ruffled border and reduced osteoclast recruitment.[29] *In vitro*, all bisphosphonates can induce osteoclast apoptosis. Zoledronic acid is claimed to increase osteoblast function, at least in the short term, although this claim is controversial.

Bisphosphonates are considered safe drugs, with the most common side effects being dyspepsia for oral agents and a combination of bone pain and nausea for intravenous agents. Due to the highly charged phosphate moieties, approximately 1% of the orally ingested drug is absorbed. The drug is readily cleared from the blood, with half binding to the bone surface and the rest rapidly excreted from the kidneys. The tissue selectivity maintains a high dose in the bone where it is needed to decrease osteoclastic activity.[30]

Bisphosphonate therapy is currently indicated for osteoporosis, hypercalcemia of malignancy, active Paget's disease, metastatic bone disease of breast and prostate cancer, and multiple myeloma. For metastatic bone disease, zoledronate, 4 mg, and pamidronate, 90 mg, every 3 to 4 weeks are the approved dosing regimens. Higher doses may cause renal dysfunction in prostate cancer patients. Pamidronate has been shown in several studies to be effective in treating osteolytic disease, and zoledronate has proven efficacy in treating osteoblastic and osteolytic metastatic bone disease.

Two large, randomized, double-blind studies evaluated the effectiveness of pamidronate for treating breast carcinoma metastases. Three hundred seventy-two patients were enrolled in a trial comparing pamidronate with placebo given every 4 weeks for 24 cycles. The pamidronate arm had a significant decrease in skeletal morbidity and a delay in onset of the first skeletal event.[31] The effect was seen after 6 months of therapy. Hortobagyi and associates[32] randomly assigned 382 women receiving chemotherapy for microscopic metastatic breast carcinoma also to receive either pamidronate or placebo. Again, a statistically significant decrease was seen in skeletal morbidity, and the onset of the first skeletal complication was delayed by 7 months.

Lipton et al.[33] first compared zoledronate to pamidronate in a double-blind, randomized study involving 1648 patients with breast carcinoma or multiple myeloma. The two drugs were found to be equally effective in decreasing skeletal complications. Then, among 422 men with metastatic prostate carcinoma, zoledronate significantly improved the rate of skeletal complications, and its effect was seen at 3 months.

Lipton et al.[34] performed a retrospective review of data for 74 renal cell carcinoma patients who were entered into a multicenter, randomized, double-blind study. Again, a statistically significant decrease in the rate of skeletal events occurred, along with a significant delay in the median time to onset of the first event. Although this study was not large, its results suggested that bisphosphonates may be useful for patients with lytic metastases of all histologic types.

Due to the delay in benefit of 3 to 6 months, bisphosphonate therapy should be started early in the disease process. If treatment of osteolytic lesions cannot wait 6 months, then a combination of radiation and surgical treatment may be necessary.

Chemotherapy

In deciding whether to use systemic therapy (chemotherapy, hormonal therapy, or immunotherapy) for the treatment of metastatic bone disease, one must first know the histologic type of tumor. Second, the bone involved must be stable with no risk of pathologic fracture. Tumors that are considered very sensitive to chemotherapeutic agents are small cell lung cancer, Hodgkin's and non-Hodgkin's lymphoma, testicular carcinoma, and all small round blue cell tumors.[35] A second tier of tumors is moderately sensitive to systemic treatments. These are breast carcinoma, ovarian carcinoma, and germ cell cancers.[35] This group has a slower, less complete response to systemic therapy.

For breast carcinoma, treatment options are determined by estrogen and progesterone receptor status. In the literature, significant tumor shrinkage with endocrine therapy is 30% to 65%.[36] In one study among patients with only bone metastases who were treated with a multiagent regimen (5-fluorouracil, doxorubicin, and cyclophosphamide), complete response rate was 7% and partial response rate was 52%, and an additional 32% experienced stabilization of disease.[36] Another large multicenter study evaluated the use of various endocrine agents (megestrol acetate, tamoxifen, aminoglutethimide, dexamethasone, hydrocortisone, and fluoxymesterone) in a placebo arm against pamidronate. A partial response was seen in 21% and a stabilization of disease was seen in an additional 32%.[37]

For prostate cancer, a significant degree of responsiveness to hormonal therapy is seen in up to 80% of tumors. Surgical or chemical castration is the mainstay of treatment. Even in patients with hormone-refractory disease who had skeletal metastases, the use of oral dexamethasone significantly improved pain in 61% of patients in one study.[38] In the same study, bone scan intensity improved in 19% and remained stable in another 38% of patients.[38]

RADIATION THERAPY

External-Beam Radiotherapy

External-beam radiotherapy has become a mainstay in the palliative treatment of metastatic bone disease. The indications for radiotherapy in metastatic bone disease are the relief of pain and the control of localized disease. Suppression of tumor growth is critical for both nonoperatively and operatively treated skeletal disease. The effects of radiotherapy may be seen quickly in lymphoma and myeloma, but the full extent of relief may not be achieved for 3 to 4 weeks. Optimization of pain medication is a necessity, and adjustment is required after treatment.

The use and timing of radiation therapy must be coordinated among specialists. The complication of marrow suppression in irradiated long bones may prevent or delay the use of certain chemotherapeutic options. Equally important is the cooperation of the surgical and radiation oncologists in the treatment of impending and pathologic fractures. Before palliative radiotherapy, the bone must be assessed for risk of fracture and the need for surgery. In one study, 13% of long bone and 6% of spinal sites fractured after radiotherapy.[39] For all carcinoma types combined, pathologic fractures heal in 35% of patients treated with radiotherapy and nonoperative management.[40] Surgery through a previously irradiated field carries increased perioperative risks, especially the risk of infection. Finally, palliative radiotherapy is given typically to a small field to minimize complications; however, the entire bone requires radiation therapy after surgical stabilization. The full length of the bone must be irradiated due to the spread of tumor during the surgical procedure. The whole treatment plan must be understood by all concerned before any part of it is commenced.

Palliative radiotherapy has been shown to provide some relief in 80% to 90% of patients and complete relief in 50% to 85% of patients with localized skeletal disease.[39,41] Multiple authors have found no difference associated with histologic type or total dose in the tumor response to radiotherapy.[39,41] A reanalysis of data from the Radiation Therapy Oncology Group study of the palliation of metastases to bone found a significant improvement in pain relief with protracted dose-fractionation schedules.[42] A nonrandomized study by Arcangeli et al. found a statistically better outcome in breast and prostate carcinoma than in lung carcinoma.[43] In addition, a significant difference in pain relief was seen with higher doses (4050 cGy) delivered over a protracted course than with low-dose short-course regimens.[43] More complete responses are seen with doses of 30 Gy or higher. With the ultimate goal of relieving pain and improving the quality of remaining life, the dose and fractionation pattern are tailored to the area of disease, assessment of toxicity, functional status, life expectancy, and accessibility and availability of the facility to the patient.

Postoperative radiotherapy is used after fixation of impending and pathologic fractures and after decompression and stabilization of the spine. When surgery is planned, radiation should be delivered postoperatively to the entire surgical area. In a retrospective study, 15% of patients treated with surgery alone developed loosening of prostheses or hardware requiring revision surgery, compared to 3% treated with surgery and radiotherapy.[44] In addition, return to a higher level of function was seen in the combined modality group.[44]

In spinal metastatic disease, the earlier the diagnosis is made and treatment is initiated, the better the outcome.[45] Radiotherapy should be the first-line therapy when no surgical indication is present. Indications for surgery include spinal instability, pathologic fracture with structural canal compromise, circumferential epidural tumor, occult primary tumor, and radioresistant tumors. Among those with spinal metastatic disease, 94% of patients who have the ability to walk maintain their ambulatory status after radiotherapy, whereas ambulation is restored in 60% with motor weakness and 11% with paraplegia at presentation.[45]

Patients with the favorable tumor types of breast and prostate carcinoma, myeloma, and lymphoma have an improved outcome when presenting with paresis or paraplegia.[45] After the initiation of treatment, bracing should be considered to prevent peritreatment fractures.

Typically, chemotherapy or hormonal therapy is the mainstay of treatment for widespread systemic disease. With the failure of or the inability to use medical management, another experimental option is the use of hemibody radiotherapy. With hemibody radiation, either the upper or lower one-half of the body receives treatment. Advantages include the treatment of multiple lesions at once and the theoretical prevention of progression in asymptomatic sites. Seventy percent to 90% of patients have some relief of pain and up to 45% have complete relief.[46] Pain relief is reported to start within 3 days. In a randomized phase III trial, breast and prostate carcinomas were found to respond better than other primary histologic types.[46] In addition, 12 Gy delivered over 2 days was equivalent to 15 Gy given over 3 days in terms of posttreatment performance status, narcotic scores, degree of pain relief, and pain-free interval.[46] Severe and life-threatening complications occurred, temporarily, in 12% of patients, and no statistical differences were seen between upper body and lower body treatment.

Complications of external-beam radiotherapy are classified into acute and late events. Acute events are seen early and are often transient. The most common acute events are fatigue and skin irritation. Nausea is common with upper abdominal treatment fields. Esophagitis is common with thoracic spine treatment. Bone marrow suppression with leukopenia, anemia, and thrombocytopenia occurs with significant tumor infiltration of the marrow and wide treatment fields. Patients who are heavily pretreated with chemotherapy are more prone to myelosuppression.

Late complications of palliative radiotherapy are uncommon due to the limited survival and lower doses delivered. After treatment of skeletal disease, the bone should be protected during the posttreatment hyperemia secondary to the healing response. The hyperemia can temporarily further weaken the bone and increase the risk of fracture. Tong et al. reported fracture rates of 4% to 18% depending on total radiation dose.[39] Posttreatment stress fractures may be seen within 3 months after treatment in the pelvis.[47] Careful monitoring for these events helps to limit the increased morbidity of these complications.

Radionuclide Therapy

Systemic radionuclide therapy with strontium 85 and strontium 89 (^{89}Sr), samarium 153 ([153]Sm), or rhenium 188 ([188]Re) is an alternative to the use of hemibody radiation for the treatment of widespread bone metastasis. When attached to bone-seeking carriers, the radioisotope can be delivered in a focused manner to areas of bone turnover. The toxic side affects of external-beam radiotherapy are reduced. The most common adverse reaction is myelosuppression; therefore, systemic radionuclides should not be used in patients undergoing chemotherapy or after hemibody radiotherapy.

[89]Sr has been the most widely studied of the radionuclides. Most trials have shown efficacy against prostate and breast carcinoma. One phase III randomized study of 126 prostate carcinoma patients treated with external-beam radiotherapy plus either ^{89}Sr or placebo showed a significant decrease in narcotic use and progression of pain over 6 months, and decreased levels

of prostate-specific antigen and bone turnover markers in the group receiving ^{89}Sr treatment.[48] One major complication was the need for platelet transfusion, which occurred in 7.5% of patients in the treatment group. Over 80% of patients with prostate or breast cancer who were treated with radionuclide therapy had partial to complete relief of pain at 6 months.[48] A more recent randomized trial with the same treatment arms found no improvement in the ^{89}Sr group; however, this study included multiple histologic types of metastatic carcinoma.[49] The efficacy of ^{89}Sr therapy may be limited to more osteoblastic lesions that allow incorporation of the carrier into bone. Aggressive osteolytic lesions may not respond well to this form of therapy, with poor accumulation at the site of disease.

[153]Sm and [188]Re are less well studied. One double-blind, randomized study of [153]Sm compared treatment at 0.5 and 1.0 mCi/kg and showed a benefit in 72% of the patients who received the higher dose. Because no difference in toxicity was seen, the higher dose was recommended.[50] A similar study of [188]Re treatment in 64 patients with hormone-resistant prostate carcinoma randomly assigned to receive one of to two dosage levels found a lower pain level in 92% of patients in the higher-dose group at 6 months.[51] Neither study found any permanent adverse affects of the radionuclide treatment.

Isotope therapy is promising and should be considered in patients with widespread metastatic bone disease from prostate and breast carcinoma. If radionuclides are used, careful monitoring of renal function and complete blood counts should be performed. [89]Sr has been shown to be safe and effective as an adjunct to external-beam radiotherapy and as a stand-alone agent; failure of one modality of radiation therapy does not preclude the use of the other.

SURGICAL CONSIDERATIONS

Bone Biomechanics and Biology

The overall strength of bone depends on the material properties of collagen and mineral composition as well as the structural properties of bone. Its tensile yield strength and compressive strength are determined by its mineral content.[52] The collagen content has the greatest impact on tensile properties after the yield point has been reached.[53] Chemotherapy and radiotherapy alter bone strength by decreasing its reparative abilities.[54] The second determinant of bone strength, its structural properties, is determined by the shape and distribution of trabecular and cortical bone. Hipp et al. evaluated the mechanical properties of blastic and lytic metastatic lesions; both types of lesions weakened the bone, but lytic ones had a greater effect.[55] Lytic lesions remove both the mineral and organic structure in bone, leading to losses in strength and stiffness, but blastic lesions disrupt only the normal trabecular framework, causing a loss of stiffness and fatigue properties, not loss of strength.

In metastatic bone disease, abnormally weak bone breaks under normal stresses. Osteolytic metastatic disease disrupts the normal trabecular and cortical structure of bone. Disruptions in the cortex can cause stress risers with small holes and create an open section effect with larger lesions. Stress risers are sites within the remaining cortical bone where stress is concentrated around a hole. Small defects with a lesion diameter to bone diameter ratio of 0.2 reduce bending strength to 60%.[56] In an open section defect, the lesion creates a hole that is greater in size than the diameter of the bone; the strength is reduced by 90%.[57] Torsional strength is affected more by smaller lesions than is compression or bending strength.[56] Torsional loads occur with daily activities of pivoting in stance or getting up from a chair during transfer. The pathologic bone tends to fracture in a transverse pattern, unlike normal bone, which breaks in oblique or spiral patterns.

The presence of metastatic disease not only weakens bone but also significantly affects healing. Factors that influence the healing potential of pathologic fractures are histologic diagnosis, expected length of survival, surgical repair, chemotherapy, and postoperative irradiation. A classic study of bone healing in metastatic bone disease showed a 35% union rate after pathologic fractures when all histologic tumor types are grouped together.[40] The best response was seen in multiple myeloma, with a 67% healing rate, followed by renal cell carcinoma with 44% and breast carcinoma with 37%. Lung carcinoma metastatic lesions never healed. Patients living longer than 6 months treated with a cast and less than 30 Gy of radiation had a 65% healing rate. Internal fixation combined with irradiation produced a 90% union rate.[40] Chemotherapy has been shown to slow the healing process.[54] Other systemic factors that may contribute to healing are nutritional status, presence of osteoporosis, and hormone manipulation.

Impending Pathologic Fractures

Numerous studies have focused on predictive factors for impending pathologic fracture; however, no consensus has been reached. In 1964, Snell and Beals studied 19 pathologic femur fractures due to breast carcinoma. By adopting a criterion size of 2.5 cm for a lytic lesion in the femoral cortex or in any bone if painful, they were able to predict 58% of the fractures.[58] After evaluating 104 pathologic fractures, Parrish and Murray recommended prophylactic fixation for femoral shaft fractures in which at least 50% of the diameter of the cortex was destroyed and there was accompanying pain.[59] Murray et al. later revised these criteria to include the presence of pain, destruction of 30% of the cortex, and failure of radiotherapy.[60] Zickel and Mouradian proposed a system based on a retrospective review of data for 34 patients.[61] Criteria for high risk included pure lytic lesions, subtrochanteric lesions, cortical involvement, and increasing pain. They could find no correlation between lesion size and fracture risk. One of largest series evaluated data for 203 patients with 516 metastatic breast carcinoma lesions in the femur.[62] No correlation could be found between lesion size, pain, or lesion pattern and the risk for fracture. Hipp et al. compared three orthopedic oncologists' prediction of strength after viewing plain radiographs and CT scans with actual mechanical testing to failure of handmade defects.[63] Only modest agreement was found between the surgeons' opinion of lesion size and the actual size, and no correlation existed between predicted and actual load-bearing capacity. These results demonstrated the inaccuracy of a pure radiographic assessment of fracture risk.

The first proposed scoring system for predicting pathologic fractures was put forth by Mirels in 1989.[64] Four factors—site, size, pain, and radiographic appearance—are graded on a scale of 1 to 3 (Table 51.4-1). The system was based on a retrospective evaluation of data for 78 patients who developed 27 fractures over a 6-month period. The fracture group had a

TABLE 51.4-1. Mirels's Scoring System to Predict Pathologic Fracture

Variable	Score		
	1	2	3
Site	Upper limb	Lower limb	Peritrochanteric
Pain	Mild	Moderate	Functional
Radiograph	Blastic	Mixed	Lytic
Size (proportion of shaft)	$<\frac{1}{3}$	$\frac{1}{3} - \frac{2}{3}$	$>\frac{2}{3}$

Score	No. of Patients	Fracture Rate (%)
0–6	22	0
7	19	5
8	12	33
9	7	57
10–12	18	100

(Data from ref. 64.)

mean score of 10, and the nonfracture group had a mean score of 7. The two groups overlap, however, in scores of 8 and 9. One-third of the fractures occurred in patients with a score of less than 10. Key points from Mirels's study are the importance of clinical and radiographic parameters.[64] He makes a distinction between biologic and mechanical pain in the assessment of risk for fracture. Mechanical pain, as previously discussed in Presentation, is due to weakness of bone and its inability to support the required load. All patients with functional pain went on to experience fracture. Large lesions, twice the diameter of the bone, were associated with functional pain. Lesions larger than two-thirds the diameter of bone were associated with a significantly increased risk for fracture. Of note, no blastic lesion fractured, and only 48% of lytic lesions fractured. The author recommended radiation therapy for patients with scores of less than 7 and surgery for patients with higher scores.

Finite-element analysis from computer modeling of CT scans has led to a better understanding of bone destruction.[65] Hipp et al. have shown computer models to be accurate in predicting strength for bending and torsional loads in canine femurs.[65] The site of fracture is the area of minimum cortical wall thickness. Variations in cortical destruction are not as important as the site with the thinnest remaining cortex.

At Memorial Sloan-Kettering Cancer Center, a combination of clinical and radiographic parameters has been used for determining the need for prophylactic fixation. Surgery is performed when pain is functional after radiotherapy or is accompanied by endosteal cortical destruction of more than 50% or a cortical defect larger than the diameter of the bone or larger than 2.5 cm. When effective systemic treatment options exist, as for early breast cancer, a trial of systemic therapy can obviate the need for surgery. Conversely, late-stage breast cancer behaves like lung cancer that will not heal, and surgery is indicated.

SURGICAL TREATMENT

Tumor Excision

With metastatic disease of the bone, cure is rarely the intent of surgery. Indications for surgery are need for biopsy, treatment of impending or pathologic fractures of long bones, spinal instabil-

ity, neurologic deficit, and failure of radiation. Treatment options include intralesional or extralesional excision of the tumor before reconstruction. Embolization and cryotherapy are effective surgical adjuvants in the management of metastatic disease.

Intralesional excision is the most common form of tumor removal. Ideally, biopsy can be followed by intralesional curettage and stabilization or reconstruction in the same surgical setting. Combining diagnosis and treatment provides pain relief and the quickest return to function. If definitive surgery is delayed, the bone weakened further by biopsy is at a high risk for fracture. The goal of intralesional curettage is the debulking of all gross tumor, which removes a significant source of pain and an impediment to fracture healing and fixation. Debulking of the tumor aids postoperative radiotherapy in preventing local progression of disease and failure of fixation.[44]

Marginal and wide excision of metastatic disease has a selective role. Marginal resection completely removes the biologic tumor stimulus for pain and allows for segmental joint reconstruction. Microscopic disease is more readily treated with radiotherapy than is gross disease after surgery. Wide excision has been recommended for solitary renal cell carcinoma metastases as a means of possible cure.

Preoperative embolization and cryotherapy have a selective role in the treatment of metastatic disease. Due to the vascularity of thyroid and renal cell carcinoma, preoperative embolization is recommended to greatly reduce intraoperative blood loss. Cryotherapy has been shown to be a useful surgical adjuvant for the removal of microscopic disease after curettage. Adjuvants such as cryotherapy become even more important for local control after failure of radiotherapy or chemotherapy to control tumor growth.

Fracture Treatment

Because conservatively treated pathologic fractures heal poorly, prosthetic replacement and internal fixation are the most efficient manner of relieving pain and restoring function. Surgical management should restore bone strength and allow immediate weight bearing. Stabilization of a fracture requires control of the proximal and distal fracture fragments. Fracture location is an important consideration, and management strategies are different for epiphyseal, metaphyseal, and diaphyseal locations.

EPIPHYSEAL FRACTURES. Epiphyseal fractures are the easiest lesions to manage. Fracture healing occurs rarely and makes operative reduction and internal fixation a poor treatment choice. Cemented prosthetic joint implants provide a reliable means to provide a painless weight-bearing joint surface. All disease at the site should be resected to improve pain control and aid in the effectiveness of postoperative radiation therapy. Stem length should be chosen to treat existing or potential lesions within the same bone.

METAPHYSEAL FRACTURES. Metaphyseal fractures are more complex. Based on the variation in geometry, quality of residual bone, and histologic subtypes, a choice must be made between prosthetic joint replacement and internal fixation. If the patient has an extended life expectancy, systemic therapies are available, and the tumor is radiosensitive, then internal fixation can support the bone while healing occurs. Myeloma, breast cancer, and lymphoma are the more favorable histologic types for fracture healing.

Internal fixation techniques include the use of load-bearing devices (plates) and load-sharing devices (intramedullary nails). Plate fixation is best used in bones that cannot accommodate an intramedullary device or in sclerotic bone that prevents insertion of a nail. Plate and screw fixation does not protect the entire bone and leaves the patient susceptible to a future fracture proximal or distal to the fixation. The increased susceptibility of the remaining bone causes plating to be more prone to failure than is intramedullary nailing. Dijstra et al.[66] evaluated 167 pathologic fractures and found that plate fixation was associated with an 11% failure rate within 7 weeks and a 40% cumulative 5-year failure rate. Although the failure rate of plating is high, most metaphyseal fractures cannot be stabilized with intramedullary fixation.

Prosthetic replacement of metaphyseal lesions can be very difficult. Generally, the bone in the surrounding apophyseal areas should be saved because it helps to retain soft tissue attachments. Examples of these areas are the greater and lesser trochanters of the hip and the greater and lesser tuberosities of the humerus. Securing these attachments to a hemiarthroplasty device in a dependable fashion is difficult. When necessary, supplemental fixation methods with mesh, tension bands, wires, or cable systems can be used, but the constructs are usually unsatisfactory and result in persistent muscle weakness and pain. In addition, it is difficult to assess bone alignment and length accurately when treating metaphyseal fractures with prosthetic replacement. In these instances, the significant bone loss resulting from the metastatic lesion that requires prosthetic replacement also eliminates or distorts the typical bony landmarks needed to orient the reconstruction. Problems with limb length inequality, joint instability, and limb weakness typically follow such surgical attempts.

DIAPHYSEAL FRACTURES. Diaphyseal lesions are treated successfully by intramedullary fixation. Closed and open insertion techniques can be used to stabilize the bone. Interlocked medullary rods restore flexion and bending strength to the weakened bone. Compression strength depends on the magnitude and extent of the bone deficiency. The open insertion technique allows the use of methyl methacrylate cement to fill the void and restore compression strength to the bone. Torsional strength is restored with the use of locking screws or cement fixation.[67]

When multiple lesions are present in the diaphysis, metaphysis, and epiphysis, intramedullary devices may not sufficiently stabilize all of the affected areas. Prosthetic replacement with a long-stemmed device can remove the periarticular disease and provide support for the entire bone. Removal of tumor at the diaphyseal site may aid in pain control and improve the effectiveness of postoperative radiotherapy.

Closed nailing techniques should be reserved for two groups of patients. The first group is preterminal patients with minimal survival expectations in whom local progression of disease and fixation failure is not likely to occur. The second group includes patients with exquisitely radiosensitive tumors that can be controlled by postoperative irradiation. The failure or success of intramedullary nailing is determined by the survival of the patient and tumor type. Nail failure will occur with breakage of the device if the fracture fails to unite.

OTHER MANAGEMENT OPTIONS. Although internal fixation and arthroplasty are the most reliable means of treating pathologic fractures, other treatment options are available. These include cast or brace immobilization, external fixation, and amputation.

External fixation or cast or brace immobilization can be considered for (1) patients with extensive localized disease that cannot be immobilized by internal means; (2) patients who are preterminal and in whom analgesic modalities can control symptoms; and (3) patients in whom sepsis, pneumonia, or other medical problems prevent surgery. These measures can be initiated at the hospital and continued in the outpatient, home, or hospice care setting.

Amputation has a limited role in the treatment of metastatic bone disease. Current indications for amputation include unreconstructable distal extremity lesions, complications of disease such as a fungating tumor, complications of treatment such as recurrent infection, and intractable pain.

Amputation may be the treatment of choice in many acrometastases (metastases that occur in the distal extremity).[68] These are rare, occurring in 0.007% to 0.30% of patients with osseous metastasis, and usually represent a preterminal event. Lung, renal, and esophageal cancer accounted for 48% of the primary lesions in the 31 cases of acrometastases reviewed by Healey et al.[69] Thirty-six percent of the patients required palliative amputations for pain relief. Amputation is suitable for other expendable bones and bones of the distal extremities.[70] In cases of solitary metastasis of renal carcinoma, amputation may extend the disease-free period or be curative. Rehabilitation of the hand is often difficult and time consuming, and amputation can quickly relieve pain and restore function.[68] Major proximal amputations of the lower extremity can be considered when complex reconstruction would be required or after failure of previous surgery.[71] The aggressive treatment methods developed for limb salvage in primary bone tumors are an inappropriate use of time and resources in cases of skeletal metastases. Alternatives to amputation for intractable pain are rhizotomy and chordotomy, which allow retention of the extremity and control of the pain.

A minimally invasive approach to the treatment of metastatic bone lesions has been the radiographically guided percutaneous injection of low-viscosity polymethyl methacrylate for select indications. The injection of cement into fractured vertebral bodies eliminates mechanical instability and improves the compression strength of the vertebral body. In the spine, cement is injected into the pathologic fracture of the vertebral body. If kyphosis of greater than 20 degrees exists, kyphoplasty can be performed in addition to restore height.[72] Fourney et al. retrospectively evaluated 65 vertebroplasties and 32 kyphoplasties performed for pathologic compression fractures in cancer patients.[72] Eighty-four percent of the patients had significant pain relief. Six patients sustained cement leaks, but all were asymptomatic. Reported major complications of vertebroplasty are the extravasation of cement into adjacent nerve foramen, venous emboli, and even spinal cord compression requiring decompression.[73] A similar technique has been described for pelvic lytic lesions in a few small series.[74,75] Moderate to complete pain relief has been reported to occur in 75% to 83% of cases. Major complications are rare, but include intraarticular extension of cement into the hip joint causing chondrolysis and extravasation around the sciatic nerve, worsening the pretreatment level of pain.[75] Because of the complications associated with percutaneous injection of polymethyl methacrylate, it is important to coordinate the procedure to allow for emergent surgical backup to address acute extravasation issues.

Surgical Reconstruction

SPINE. The spine is the most common site of metastatic bone disease, and the most common forms of carcinoma to metastasize to the spine are lung, breast, and prostate.[76] In one autopsy study, patients with a terminal malignancy had an incidence of spinal metastasis of 90% for prostate carcinoma, 75% for breast carcinoma, and 45% for lung carcinoma. Twenty-six percent of these autopsy-proven metastases were not visible on plain radiographs.[76]

Pain is the presenting symptom in 85% of patients with spinal metastases. The pain may be difficult to distinguish from benign spinal disease. Pain from metastatic disease is often unrelenting and not improved with recumbence. Causes of pain may be biologic factors, mechanical instability, pathologic fracture, epidural compression, or nerve root impingement. Neurologic compromise can present as a radiculopathy or myelopathy, or as cauda equina syndrome. An appreciation of these symptoms is critical to prevention of unnecessary suffering or development of a permanent deficit. After treatment of cord compression, bowel and bladder control had the poorest rate of return if they were absent at presentation.[77]

Multiple staging systems have been devised for the determination of treatment and the prediction of outcomes. Tomita's system is an informative approach for treatment planning that combines a description of the affected anatomical areas and the extent of disease. The anatomic sites are divided into the vertebral body, pedicle, lamina and spinous process, epidural space, and paravertebral region as distinct components.[78] Prognosis for spinal metastasis depends on general condition, ambulatory status and pretreatment neurologic function, the primary tumor type, and sites of other metastasis (brain and viscera). Of note, 70% to 90% of patients who are ambulatory at presentation remain ambulatory, whereas 33% to 70% of those who have paraparesis and 11% of those who have paraplegia on presentation regain an ambulatory status.[45,77,79]

The natural history of spinal metastasis is variable. Influential factors are anatomic location of metastases, functional status, treatment, and primary tumor histologic type. Tokuhashi et al. developed a scoring system for the assessment of survival after spinal metastasis.[80] The system used six parameters: general condition, number of extraspinal bone metastases, number of spinal metastases, major internal organ metastases, primary site, and severity of cord paralysis. The total score was found to correlate with postoperative survival. A population-based study in Ontario evaluated survival and complication rates after surgery for metastatic spinal disease and found increasing age, male gender, and primary lung cancer to be the most significant risk factors for mortality within 30 days.[4] Melanoma, lung carcinoma, and upper gastrointestinal tumors had the worst survival, with more than 50% mortality within 90 days of surgery.[4] Tomita et al. reported on 78 patients with epidural metastases who were treated with irradiation and high-dose steroids.[78] They noted a significant difference in mortality when ambulation could be restored. Ambulatory patients had a 53-week survival in contrast to less than 5 weeks for nonambulatory patients.

Radiotherapy, the mainstay treatment for metastatic spine disease, provides control of pain and restoration of function. Maranzano and Latini, in a prospective study involving 275 patients with spinal cord compression, demonstrated the continued effectiveness of radiotherapy and steroids as a means of treatment when no surgical indications were present.[45] Overall, ambulation was maintained or improved in 76% and sphincter control in 44%. Regardless of lesion radiosensitivity, the key factor in outcome was preoperative level of function. Ninety-four percent of ambulatory patients maintained function, whereas 60% of patients who were nonambulatory on presentation experienced return of function.

Surgery is reserved for diagnosis, decompression of neural elements, restoration of mechanical stability, and failure of radiotherapy. Multiple approaches for decompression and stabilization of the spine have been described. Of note, laminectomy alone with radiation has been shown to have a poor outcome.[81] Laminectomy provides inadequate decompression, except in rare cases of posterior element disease only, and without instrumentation frequently leads to progressive deformity and increased neurologic compression. Improved surgical outcomes have occurred with more aggressive tumor removal than with laminectomy alone.

Resection approaches vary from anterior only, to posterolateral with transpedicular decompression, to a combined anterior and posterior approach. The choice of surgical approach is determined by extent and location of disease, the type of reconstruction, and patient comorbidities. The anterior approach alone has been recommended for disease limited to one or two segments with neural compression without posterior extension.[77,79,82] The anterior approach allows direct access for decompression and correction of deformity. Harrington[82] initially reported on 14 patients who underwent anterior resection with cement and pin reconstruction. Twelve patients had a major neurologic deficit preoperatively. Nine experienced complete recovery, two had partial improvement and the condition of one remained unchanged. Weigel et al. evaluated 76 patients treated with a combination of surgical approaches based on the site of disease.[79] Improvement in neurologic function occurred in 62% after anterior surgery, 50% after posterolateral surgery, and 45% after combined procedures. Seventy percent of patients who were nonambulatory at presentation regained the ability to ambulate. Due to local recurrence and new spinal metastases, paraplegia developed in 18% of the patients within 8.4 months on average.

A posterolateral approach allows circumferential decompression with anterior and posterior reconstruction.[83] Bauer evaluated 67 patients with epidural compression treated via a posterior approach with excision of all gross disease and reconstruction. Forty-four of 58 patients had complete or partial neurologic recovery. Thirty-eight of the 44 patients who were alive at 6 months retained their ambulatory ability.[84] Bilsky et al. treated 25 patients with a posterolateral, transpedicular corpectomy with anterior cement and pin reconstruction and posterior instrumentation.[83] Twenty-one had high-grade spinal cord compression preoperatively. All patients experienced significant pain relief. All nine ambulatory patients remained ambulatory. Fifty percent of nonambulatory patients became ambulatory after surgery. The posterolateral approach is particularly suitable for patients with extensive epidural disease and those who have had thoracic radiotherapy or previous thoracotomy, or have significant pulmonary disease, which is a relative contraindication for thoracotomy (Fig. 51.4-1).

En bloc spondylectomy and extralesion resection have been advocated by some for improved palliation and possible cura-

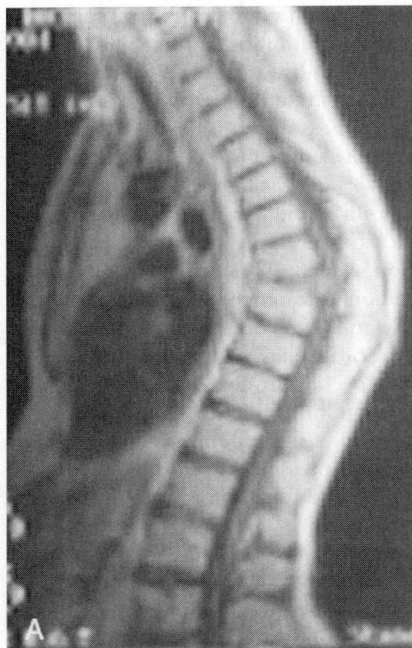

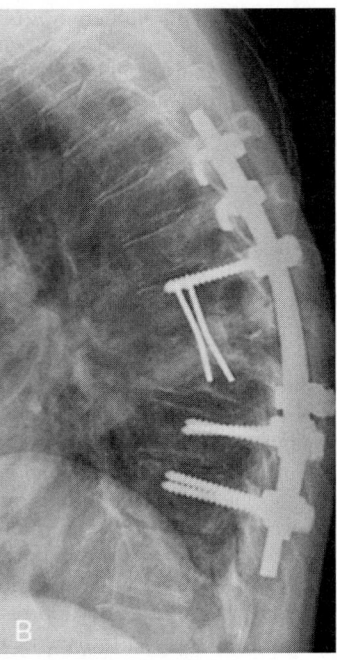

FIGURE 51.4-1.　Metastatic disease of the spine with fracture and nerve root compression. **A:** T1-weighted sagittal magnetic resonance image of T-9 metastatic lesion with pathologic fracture and spinal cord compression. **B:** Postoperative radiograph after decompression, vertebral body reconstruction with cement and pins, and segmental posterior instrumentation using a single-stage posterolateral, transpedicular approach.

tive resection.[78] Tomita et al. described a method for *en bloc* spondylectomy used in 24 patients with metastatic and primary disease.[78] Oncologically sound, this method attempts to remove the posterior elements as one element and the vertebral body as a second element. No local recurrences were seen in 12 survivors at 14 months. In contrast, intralesional excisions are prone to local failure rates as high as 49%.[77]

LOWER EXTREMITY. The femur is the third most common site of skeletal metastases and the most common to require surgical intervention. Sixty-six percent of pathologic

long bone fractures involve the femur. The proximal end and the shaft account for 87% of femoral lesions.[85] Indications for surgery are impending fracture and frank pathologic fracture in patients with a life expectancy of longer than 1 month. The goal of treatment is to provide pain relief and to restore or maintain ambulatory function and mobility. Surgical methods are determined by location of disease.

Lesions of the femoral head and neck are best treated with arthroplasty. Historically, internal fixation has been associated with a high failure rate due to progression of disease and loss of fixation. Advantages of arthroplasty include the fact that all dis-

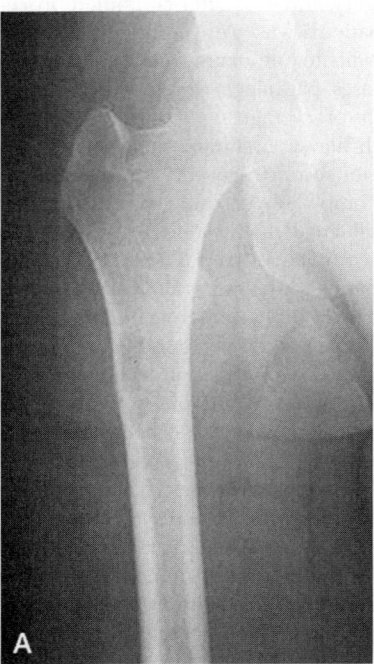

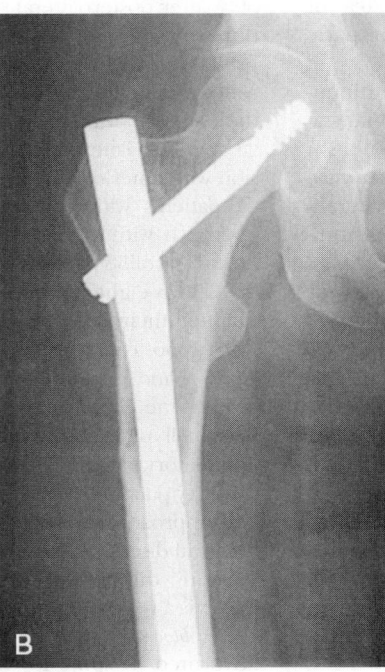

FIGURE 51.4-2.　Impending subtrochanteric pathologic fracture. **A:** Plain radiograph of a subtrochanteric lytic lesion with incomplete fracture. **B:** Postoperative image after curettage and intramedullary nail fixation of subtrochanteric lesion.

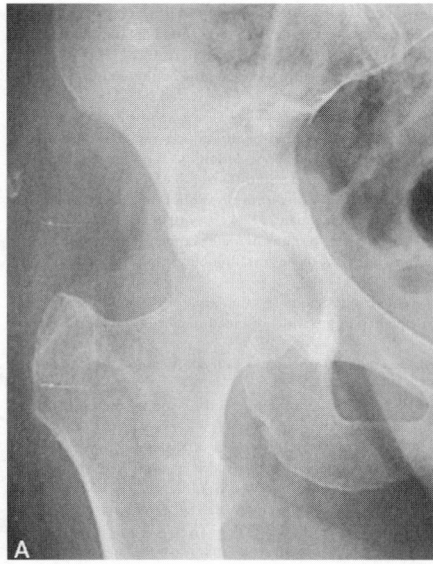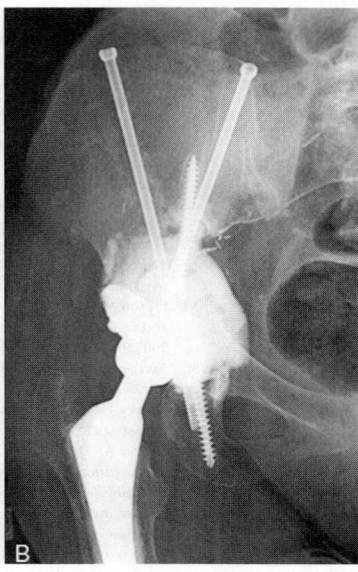

FIGURE 51.4-3.   Acetabular metastatic disease. **A:** Pre-operative plain radiograph of a lytic metastatic lesion of the dome, medial wall, and posterior column of the acetabu-lum. **B:** Plain radiograph after a modified Harrington reconstruction of the acetabulum[5] using antegrade cannu-lated screws, protrusio ring acetabular component, and fix-ation screws and cement.

eased bone can be removed, immediate weight bearing is allowed, and stability does not rely on fracture healing. Technical consider-ations are the use of long stem components for femoral shaft pro-tection and the use of total arthroplasty versus hemiarthroplasty. Long stem components can treat concurrent shaft fractures and protect against future lesions. Risks of embolization and sudden cardiac arrest have been reported with these prostheses.[86] With regard to the second technical point, Habermann and associates reported on the presence of biopsy-proven acetabular disease in 19 of 23 patients with no previously recognized involvement at the time of hip arthroplasty.[85] The disadvantages of total hip arthro-plasty are increased blood loss, operative time, and dislocation rate. Because of the increased complications, hemiarthroplasty is recommended as the routine treatment.

Peritrochanteric lesions (intertrochanteric and subtrochan-teric) can be treated with internal fixation or arthroplasty depend-ing on the remaining bone stock (Fig. 51.4-2). Multiple authors have reported on the use of third-generation cephalomedullary long nails for the treatment of impending and pathologic frac-tures. The largest series evaluated 110 total impending[27] and pathologic[83] peritrochanteric fractures with a mean follow-up of 1.5 years or until death.[87] Mean survival in the series was best for renal and breast carcinoma at 18 and 13 months, respectively. Ninety-two percent of patients became mobile, and complete to moderate pain relief occurred in 93%. Complications included a hardware failure rate of 4% and fatty emboli syndrome in three patients. For intertrochanteric lesions, arthroplasty has been sup-ported as the treatment of choice by some authors.[85,88] The advan-tages of arthroplasty are the same as previously mentioned. The disadvantages are the increased operative time and blood loss. For subtrochanteric and shaft fractures, the treatment of choice has been intramedullary nail fixation.

No matter what method of reconstruction is performed, all fractures require supplemental radiation therapy to treat under-lying disease. Treatment of the fracture frequently exposes new areas to tumor spread. This newly contaminated region must be treated with radiation to avoid tumor proliferation and a new fracture distal to the implant. Only patients with failure of previ-ous radiation therapy should be treated with surgery alone.

PELVIS AND ACETABULUM.   Most patients with pelvic and acetabular metastases have pain; however, it does not always arise directly from the hip joint. Avulsion fractures of the iliac crest or anterior-inferior iliac spine are common and should be treated nonoperatively. However, mechanical insufficiency of the acetabu-lum can be managed only surgically. The indications for surgical treatment of acetabular disease are the failure of nonoperative measures (protected weight bearing, antineoplastic treatment, analgesics, and radiation therapy) to control pain, a pathologic fracture of the acetabulum, or an impending fracture in the ipsi-lateral femur requiring surgery.

Preoperative evaluation, including Judet radiography, must be performed carefully, to define disease in the anterior and posterior acetabular columns. CT scanning is indispensable to evaluate the medial acetabulum and acetabular dome and to define any associ-ated soft tissue mass. It is the best study for assessing overall bone integrity. Pathologic anatomy is better described by a four-part sys-tem that assesses the anterior column, posterior column, acetabu-lar dome, and medial wall as separate components. Bone in each region can then be graded as sufficient or insufficient, where suffi-cient bone provides adequate support for the acetabular compo-nent and insufficient bone does not. Thus, the classification system combines both anatomic and reconstructive considerations.

Marco and associates, using the four-part system, analyzed data for a series of 55 patients who required surgical reconstruction of the acetabulum for metastatic disease.[5] In this series, 10 patients (18%) had insufficiency of both anterior and posterior columns, whereas 36 patients (65%) had single-column insufficiency. Forty-two of 55 patients (76%) had an insufficient medial wall com-bined with either an insufficient column or an insufficient dome, and 47 patients (85%) had an acetabular fracture. In all 55 patients, the reconstruction was reinforced with pins or cannu-lated screws incorporated into cement, using a modified Har-rington technique. This allows for bypass of major acetabular defects with proximal fixation of the socket into the remaining iliac bone. A protrusio ring "revision" hip socket can be used to transfer load to the remaining intact cortical bone when medial wall defects are present (Fig. 51.4-3). A 3-month evaluation of the surviving 41 of the 55 patients (75%) demonstrated a significant reduction in pain in 83% of the patients. Ambulation was restored in 9 of 18 nonambulatory patients, and 14 of 17 patients maintained their ability to ambulate in the community. Of the 21 patients (38%) who had more than 1 year of follow-up, 14 (67%) continued to experience improved pain relief and 12 (57%) remained ambulatory in the community or household. In this series, despite the fact that patients with significant acetabular metastasis had a short life expectancy, the positive effect on both pain relief and functional improvement validated the role of surgery in managing this group. Acetabular reconstruction using the outlined techniques showed a low incidence of fixation failure, supporting the biomechanical stability of the construct, and providing sufficient durability in these patients.

Finally, massive pelvic involvement can be treated by acetabular resection and reconstruction using a saddle prosthesis (Waldemar Link, Hamburg, Germany), as reported by Aboulafia and associates[89] or with a pelvic endoprosthesis. Such aggressive surgical approaches may help select patients with intermediate-term life expectancies.

REFERENCES

1. Jemal A, Murray T, Samuels A, et al. Cancer statistics, 2003. *CA Cancer J Clin* 2003;53:5.
2. Plunkett T, Rubens R. The biology and management of bone metastases. *Crit Rev Oncol Hematol* 1999;31:89.
3. Galasko C. Skeletal metastases. *Clin Orthop* 1985;210:18.
4. Finkelstein J, Zaveri G, Wai E, et al. A population-based study of surgery for spinal metastasis: survival rates and complications. *J Bone Joint Surg Br* 2003;85:1045.
5. Marco R, Sheth D, Boland P, et al. Functional and oncological outcome of acetabular reconstruction for the treatment of metastatic disease. *J Bone Joint Surg Am* 2000;82:642.
6. Galasko C, Burn J. Hypercalcemia in patients with advanced mammary cancer. *BMJ* 1971;3:573.
7. Plunkett T, Smith P, Rubens R. Risk of complications from bone metastases in breast cancer: implications for management. *Eur J Cancer* 2000;36:476.
8. Higinbotham N, Marcove R. Management of pathologic fractures. *J Trauma* 1965;5:792.
9. Stark R, Henson R, Evans S. Spinal metastases: a retrospective survey from a general hospital. *Brain* 1982;105:189.
10. Batson O. The function of the vertebral veins and their role in the spread of metastases. *Ann Surg* 1940;112:138.
11. Arguello F, Baggs R, Frantz C. A murine model of experimental metastasis to bone and bone marrow. *Cancer Res* 1988;48:6876.
12. Powles T, Clark S, Easty D, et al. The inhibition by aspirin and indomethacin of osteolytic tumor deposits and hypercalcemia in rats with Walker tumour, and its possible application to human breast cancer. *Br J Cancer* 1973;28:316.
13. Meyer T, Hart I. Mechanism of tumour metastasis. *Eur J Cancer* 1998;34:214.
14. Cockett M, Murphy G, Birch M, et al. Matrix metalloproteinases and metastatic cancer. *Biochem Soc Symp* 1998;63:295.
15. Kang Y, Siegel P, Shu W, et al. A multigenic program mediating breast cancer metastasis to bone. *Cancer Cell* 2003;3:537.
16. Clohisy D, Perkins S, Ramnaraine M. Review of cellular mechanisms of tumor osteolysis. *Clin Orthop* 2000;373:104.
17. Guise T, Yin J, Mohammad K. Role of endothelin-1 in osteoblastic bone metastasis. *Cancer* 2003;97:779.
18. Roodman G. Role of stromal-derived cytokines and growth factors in bone metastasis. *Cancer* 2002;97:733.
19. Rougraff B, Kneisl J, Simon M. Skeletal metastases of unknown origin. *J Bone Joint Surg Am* 1993;75:276.
20. Agarwal S, Agarwal T, Agarwal R, et al. Fine needle aspiration of bone tumors. *Cancer Detect Prev* 2000;24:602.
21. Dorfman H, Czerniak B. *Metastatic tumors in bone.* St. Louis: Mosby, 1998.
22. Eustace S, Tello R, DeCarvalho V, et al. A comparison of whole-body turboSTIR MR imaging and planar 99mTc-methylene diphosphonate scintigraphy in the examination of patients with suspected skeletal metastases. *AJR Am J Roentgenol* 1997;169:1655.
23. Galasko C. The detection of skeletal metastases from mammary cancer by gamma camera scintigraphy. *Br J Surg* 1969;56.
24. Vanel D, Bittoun J, Tardivon A. MRI of bone metastases. *Eur Radiol* 1998;8:1345.
25. Lauenstein T, Freudenberg L, Goehde S, et al. Whole-body MRI using a rolling table platform for the detection of bone metastases. *Eur Radiol* 2002;12:2091.
26. Bohuslavizki K, Klutmann S, Kroger S, et al. FDG PET detection of unknown primary tumors. *J Nucl Med* 2000;41:816.
27. Bury T, Barreto A, Daenen F, et al. Fluorine-18 deoxyglucose positron emission tomography for the detection of bone metastases in patients with non–small cell lung cancer. *Eur J Nucl Med* 1998;25:1244.
28. Frith J, Monkkonen J, Auriola S, et al. Clodronate and liposome-encapsulated clodronate are metabolized to a toxic ATP analog, adenosine 5'-(beta, gamma-dichloromethylene) triphosphate, by mammalian cells in vitro. *J Bone Miner Res* 1997;12:1358.
29. Rodan G. The development and function of the skeleton and bone metastases. *Cancer* 2003;97:726.
30. Rodan G, Reszka A. Osteoporosis and bisphosphonates. *J Bone Joint Surg Am* 2003;85:8.
31. Theriault R, Lipton A, Hortobagyi G, et al. Pamidronate reduces skeletal morbidity in women with advanced breast cancer and lytic bone lesions: a randomized, placebo-controlled trial. Protocol 18 Aredia Breast Cancer Study Group. *J Clin Oncol* 1999;17:846.
32. Hortobagyi G, Theriault R, Lipton A, et al. Long-term prevention of skeletal complications of metastatic breast cancer with pamidronate. *J Clin Oncol* 1998;16:2038.
33. Lipton A, Small E, Saad F, et al. The new bisphosphonate, Zometa (zoledronic acid), decreases skeletal complications in both osteolytic and osteoblastic lesions: a comparison to pamidronate. *Cancer Invest* 2002;20:45.
34. Lipton A, Zheng M, Seaman J. Zoledronic acid delays the onset of skeletal-related events and progression of skeletal disease in patients with advanced renal cell carcinoma. *Cancer* 2003;98:962.
35. Savage P, Ward W. Medical management of metastatic skeletal disease. *Orthop Clin North Am* 2000;31:545.
36. Harvey H. Issues concerning the role of chemotherapy and hormonal therapy of bone metastases from breast carcinoma. *Cancer* 1997;80:1646.
37. Lipton A, Theriault R, Leff R, et al. Long-term reduction of skeletal complications in breast cancer patients with osteolytic bone metastases receiving hormone therapy, by monthly 90 mg pamidronate (Aredia) infusions. *Proc Am Soc Clin Oncol* 1997:531.
38. Nishimura K, Nonomura N, Yasunaga Y, et al. Low doses of oral dexamethasone for hormone-refractory prostate carcinoma. *Cancer* 2000;89:2570.
39. Tong D, Gillick L, Hendrickson F. The palliation of symptomatic osseous metastases: final results of the study by the Radiation Therapy Oncology Group. *Cancer* 1982;50:893.
40. Gainor B, Buchert P. Fracture healing in metastatic bone disease. *Clin Orthop* 1983;178:297.
41. Vargha Z, Glicksman A, Boland J. Single-dose radiation therapy in the palliation of metastatic disease. *Radiology* 1969;93:1181.
42. Blitzer P. Reanalysis of the RTOG study of the palliation of symptomatic osseous metastasis. *Cancer* 1985;55:1468.
43. Arcangeli G, Giovinazzo G, Saracino B, et al. Radiation therapy in the management of symptomatic bone metastases: the effect of total dose and histology on pain relief and response duration. *Int J Radiat Oncol Biol Phys* 1998;42:1119.
44. Townsend P, Rosenthal H, Smalley S, et al. Impact of postoperative radiation therapy and other perioperative factors on outcome after orthopedic stabilization of impending or pathologic fractures due to metastatic disease. *J Clin Oncol* 1994;12:2345.
45. Maranzano E, Latini P. Effectiveness of radiation therapy without surgery in metastatic spinal cord compression: final results from a prospective trial. *Int J Radiat Oncol Biol Phys* 1995;32:959.
46. Salazar O, Sandhu T, Da Motta N, et al. Fractionated half-body irradiation (HBI) for the rapid palliation of widespread, symptomatic, metastatic bone disease: a randomized phase III trial of the International Atomic Energy Agency (IAEA). *Int J Radiat Oncol Biol Phys* 2001;50:765.
47. Frassica D. Radiation therapy. *Orthop Clin North Am* 2000;31:557.
48. Porter A, McEwan A, Powe J, et al. Results of a randomized phase-III trial to evaluate the efficacy of strontium-89 adjuvant to local field external beam irradiation in the management of endocrine resistant metastatic prostate cancer. *Int J Radiat Oncol Biol Phys* 1993;25:805.
49. Smeland S, Erikstein B, Aas M, et al. Role of strontium-89 as adjuvant to palliative external beam radiotherapy is questionable: results of a double-blind randomized study. *Int J Radiat Oncol Biol Phys* 2003;56:1397.
50. Serafini A, Houston S, Resche I, et al. Palliation of pain associated with metastatic bone cancer using samarium-153 lexidronam: a double-blind placebo-controlled clinical trial. *J Clin Oncol* 1998;16:1574.
51. Palmedo H, Manka-Waluch A, Albers P, et al. Repeated bone-targeted therapy for hormone-refractory prostate carcinoma: randomized phase II trial with the new, high-energy radiopharmaceutical rhenium-188 hydroxyethylidenediphosphonate. *J Clin Oncol* 2003;21:2869.
52. Reilly D, Burstein A, Frankel V, et al. The elastic modulus for bone. *J Biomech* 1974;7:271.
53. Burstein A, Zika J, Heiple K, et al. Contribution of collagen and mineral to the elastic-plastic properties of bone. *J Bone Joint Surg Am* 1975;57:956.
54. Pelker R, Friedlaender G, Panjabi M, et al. Chemotherapy-induced alterations in the biomechanics of rat bone. *J Orthop Res* 1985;3:91.
55. Hipp J, Rosenberg A, Hayes W. Mechanical properties of trabecular bone within and adjacent to osseous metastases. *J Bone Miner Res* 1992;7:1165.
56. McBroom R, Cheal E, Hayes W. Strength reductions from metastatic cortical defects in long bones. *J Orthop Res* 1988;6:369.
57. Pugh J, Sherry H, Futterman B, et al. Biomechanics of pathologic fractures. *Clin Orthop* 1982;169.
58. Snell W, Beals R. Femoral metastases and fractures from breast cancer. *Surg Gynecol Obstet* 1964;119:22.
59. Parrish F, Murray J. Surgical treatment for secondary neoplastic fractures. *J Bone Joint Surg Am* 1970;52:665.
60. Murray J, Bruels M, Lindberg R. Irradiation of polymethylmethacrylate. In vitro gamma radiation effect. *J Bone Joint Surg Am* 1974;56:311.
61. Zickel R, Mouradian W. Intramedullary fixation of pathological fractures and lesions of the subtrochanteric region of the femur. *J Bone Joint Surg Am* 1976;58:1061.
62. Keene J, Sellinger D, McBeath A, et al. Metastatic breast cancer in the femur: a search for the lesion at risk of fracture. *Clin Orthop* 1986;203:282.
63. Hipp J, Springfield D, Hayes W. Predicting pathologic fracture risk in the management of metastatic bone defects. *Clin Orthop* 1995;312:120.

64. Mirels H. Metastatic disease in long bones: a proposed scoring system for diagnosing impending pathologic fractures. *Clin Orthop* 1989;249:256.

65. Hipp J, McBroom R, Cheal E, et al. Structural consequences of endosteal metastatic lesions in long bones. *J Orthop Res* 1989;7:828.

66. Dijstra S, Wiggers T, Van Geel B, et al. Impending and actual pathological fractures in patients with bone metastases of the long bones: a retrospective study of 233 surgically treated fractures. *Eur J Surg* 1994;160:535.

67. Assal M, Zanone X, Peter R. Osteosynthesis of metastatic lesions of the proximal femur with a solid femoral nail and interlocking spiral blade inserted without reaming. *J Orthop Trauma* 2000;14:394.

68. Morris D, House H. The significance of metastasis to the bones and soft tissues of the hand. *J Surg Oncol* 1985;28:146.

69. Healey J, Tumbull A, Miedema B, et al. Acrometastases: a study of twenty-nine patients with osseous involvement of the hands and feet. *J Bone Joint Surg Am* 1986;68:743.

70. Esther R, Bos G. Management of metastatic disease of other bones. *Orthop Clin North Am* 2000;31:647.

71. Malawer M, Buch R, Thompson W, et al. Major amputations done with palliative intent in the treatment of local bony complications associated with advanced cancer. *J Surg Oncol* 1991;47.

72. Fourney D, Schomer D, Nader R, et al. Percutaneous vertebroplasty and kyphoplasty for painful vertebral body fractures in cancer patients. *J Neurosurg* 2003;98:21.

73. Cotten A, Demondion X, Boutry N, et al. Therapeutic percutaneous injections in the treatment of malignant acetabular osteolysis. *Radiographics* 1999;19.

74. Hierholzer J, Anselmetti G, Fuchs H, et al. Percutaneous osteoplasty as a treatment for painful malignant bone lesions of the pelvis and femur. *J Vasc Interv Radiol* 2003;14.

75. Weill A, Kobaiter H, Chiras J. Acetabulum malignancies: technique and impact on pain of percutaneous injection of acrylic surgical cement. *Eur Radiol* 1998;8:123.

76. Wong D, Fornasier V, MacNab I. Spinal metastases: the obvious, the occult, and the impostors. Spine 1990;15:1.

77. King G, Kostuik J, McBroom R, et al. Surgical management of metastatic renal carcinoma of the spine. *Spine* 1991;16:265.

78. Tomita K, Toribatake Y, Kawahara N, et al. Total en bloc spondylectomy and circumspinal decompression for solitary spinal metastasis. *Paraplegia* 1994;32:36.

79. Weigel B, Maghsudi M, Neumann C, et al. Surgical management of symptomatic spinal metastases: postoperative outcome and quality of life. *Spine* 1999;24:2240.

80. Tokuhashi Y, Matsuzaki H, Toriyama S, et al. Scoring system for the preoperative evaluation of metastatic spine tumor prognosis. *Spine* 1990;15:1110.

81. Rao S, Badani K, Schildhauer T, et al. Metastatic malignancy of the cervical spine: a nonoperative history. *Spine* 1992;17:S407.

82. Harrington K. The use of methylmethacrylate for vertebral-body replacement and anterior stabilization of pathological fracture-dislocations of the spine due to metastatic malignant disease. *J Bone Joint Surg Am* 1981;63:36.

83. Bilsky M, Boland P, Lis E, et al. Single stage posterolateral transpedicle approach for spondylectomy, epidural decompression, and circumferential fusion of spinal metastases. *Spine* 2000;25:2240.

84. Bauer H. Posterior decompression and stabilization for spinal metastases. Analysis of sixty-seven consecutive patients. *J Bone Joint Surg Am* 1997;79:514.

85. Habermann E, Sachs R, Stern R, et al. The pathology and treatment of metastatic disease of the femur. *Clin Orthop* 1982;169:70.

86. Patterson B, Healey J, Cornell C, et al. Cardiac arrest during hip arthroplasty with a cemented long-stem component: a report of seven cases. *J Bone Joint Surg Am* 1991;73:271.

87. Van Doorn R, Stapert J. Treatment of impending and actual pathological femoral fractures with the long gamma nail in the Netherlands. *Eur J Surg* 2000;166:247.

88. Damron T, Sim F. Surgical treatment for metastatic disease of the pelvis and the proximal end of the femur. *Instr Course Lect* 2000;49:461.

89. Aboulafia A, Buch R, Mathews J, et al. Reconstruction using the saddle prosthesis following excision of primary and metastatic periacetabular tumors. *Clin Orthop* 1995;314:203.

SECTION **5**

DAO M. NGUYEN
DAVID S. SCHRUMP

Malignant Pleural and Pericardial Effusions

MALIGNANT PLEURAL EFFUSION

Approximately 100,000 cases of malignant pleural effusion (MPE) occur annually in the United States, and MPE is the initial manifestation in 10% to 50% of cancer patients.[1] Two-thirds of MPEs are attributable to lung (35%) or breast (23%) carcinoma and lymphoma (10%). Carcinomas of unknown primary account for an additional 12% of MPE cases. Presence of MPE frequently indicates advanced and incurable disease. Although the overall prognosis of patients with MPE depends on the histologic characteristics and extent of their primary disease, significant palliation can be achieved in these individuals by accurate and timely diagnosis and interventions associated with minimal morbidity.

MPEs typically arise as the result of altered microvascular permeability and diffuse metastatic involvement of mediastinal or subpleural lymphatics. Pulmonary parenchymal tumors (primary or metastatic) may erode the visceral pleura, spilling cells and disrupting the normal resorption of fluid by the visceral pleura. Alternatively, the parietal and visceral pleura themselves are common sites of deposits, which results in increased capillary permeability due to inflammation, overt endothelial disruption, or obstruction of efferent flow with elevated lymphatic hydrostatic pressure (Fig. 51.5-1). Primary or metastatic involvement of hilar or mediastinal lymph nodes obstructs normal visceral and parietal lymphatic drainage, which results in pleural effusion. Typically, involvement of the mesothelial surface results in exfoliation of tumor cells into the pleural fluid; however, few malignant cells are found in the pleural fluid in the setting of submesothelial involvement.

CLINICAL PRESENTATION

MPE can be an initial manifestation of cancer, and up to 50% of individuals presenting with MPE have no history of malignancy.[1] Most patients with MPE are symptomatic, with dyspnea of varying severity being the predominate symptom. Cough and chest discomfort ranging from dull ache (often characterized as heaviness or pressure) to sharp pleuritic pain may also

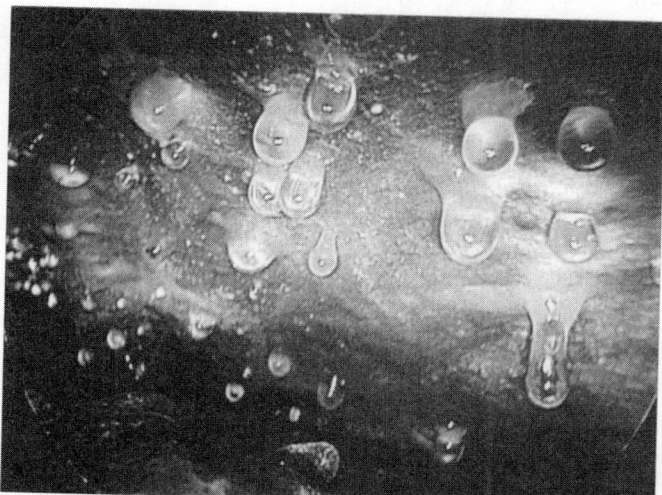

FIGURE 51.5-1. Exudation of pleural fluid from the parietal pleura as viewed through the thoracoscope during video-assisted thoracoscopic talc poudrage of a patient with malignant pleural effusion due to metastatic melanoma. The biopsy specimen from the parietal pleura was positive for melanoma cells. (See Color Fig. 51.5-1 in the CD-ROM.)

be present. Physical examination usually reveals decreased breath sounds with dullness to percussion and diminished tactile fremitus. Tracheal deviation and low cardiac output related to mediastinal compression occasionally may be seen with large effusions.

DIAGNOSIS AND EVALUATION

Radiographic Examinations

Upright posteroanterior, lateral, and lateral decubitus chest radiographs that allow assessment of "free-flowing" pleural effusion should be performed as initial investigations. Particularly in the setting of a newly diagnosed effusion, computed tomography (CT) of the chest should be performed to define fluid loculations, mediastinal or hilar lymphadenopathy, pleural masses, and parenchymal disease. Complete opacification of the hemithorax occurs in approximately 15% of MPE cases. An opacified hemithorax with mediastinal shift toward the contralateral side indicates massive effusion, whereas opacification without a shift may be due to a combination of pleural fluid and lung collapse resulting from proximal airway obstruction, effusion with mediastinal fixation by malignant lymphadenopathy, or malignant mesothelioma.

Invasive Diagnostic Maneuvers

After appropriate radiographic assessment, thoracentesis should be performed to obtain fluid for biochemical and cytopathologic analysis, to relieve symptoms, and to determine the extent of lung expansion after pleural fluid drainage. In the presence of free-flowing effusion, thoracentesis can be safely performed at the level of the posterior sixth or seventh intercostal space, with 1000 to 1500 mL of fluid (or up to 20 mL of pleural fluid per kg of body weight) removed.[2,3] In the presence of a large pleural effusion occupying more than 50% of the pleural cavity, gradual drainage of the fluid is prudent to avoid postexpansion pulmonary edema.[4] If the pleural collection is loculated, ultrasonography- or CT-guided drainage is recommended. A small sample of pleural fluid should be sent for biochemical analysis; the remaining fluid should be processed for cytopathologic examination.

The initial cytologic finding is positive in approximately 50% of patients who are ultimately found to have MPE. If initial cytologic results are negative, one should either consider repeat thoracentesis or proceed directly to thoracoscopy and pleural biopsy. Thoracoscopy, performed either by direct pleuroscopy under local anesthesia with intravenous sedation or with video assistance under general anesthesia, has a diagnostic yield of nearly 100% for malignant disease involving the pleura.[5]

Biochemical and Pathologic Analysis

Pleural fluid obtained by diagnostic thoracentesis should be routinely sent for analysis of protein, glucose, and lactic dehydrogenase (LDH) as well as cell counts, cultures, and pathologic examination. MPE is most commonly exudative (LDH level of more than 200 U/mL, fluid to serum LDH ratio higher than 0.6, fluid to serum protein ratio higher than 0.5).[6] Frequently, fluid is blood-tinged or grossly hemorrhagic due to disruption of capillaries or venules by direct tumor invasion or cytokine-mediated vasodilation. Typically, the pleural fluid is hypercellular with leukocyte counts of 1000 to 10,000 cells/mm^3 (predominantly lymphocytes and monocytes), reactive mesothelial cells, and exfoliated tumor cells. Approximately one-third of MPEs are acidic (pH less than 7.3) with a glucose to serum ratio of less than 0.5. These biochemical parameters correlate with advanced disease, poor response to palliative pleurodesis maneuvers, and diminished survival in patients with MPE.[7,8] Only cytopathologic or histopathologic identification of malignant cells by standard light-microscopical examination of the cellular component of the pleural fluid (either as smears or cell blocks and with or without special cytoimmunohistochemical stainings) or a pleural biopsy specimen is diagnostic of the malignant nature of the pleural effusion.

TREATMENT

Thoracentesis

Thoracentesis may be an appropriate treatment for MPE in patients with limited life expectancy who cannot tolerate any surgical procedure. Recurrent effusions are observed in 97% of individuals within 30 days after thoracentesis. In general, pleurodesis performed immediately after thoracentesis is not effective because residual pleural fluid dilutes the sclerosing agent, diminishing its irritant effects on the pleura. Loculations may form after such treatment, which makes definitive treatment of the pleural effusion more complicated. In patients presenting with MPE as the initial manifestation of breast cancer, small cell lung cancer, germ cell tumors, or lymphoma, thoracentesis followed by systemic chemotherapy may successfully treat the pleural space. However, most patients with MPE require more aggressive intervention to prevent recurrence. Multiloculated MPEs may pose a therapeutic challenge because they are frequently refractory to complete drainage by thoracentesis or tube thoracostomy and thus unsuitable for pleurodesis. Multiple small observational studies have demonstrated that intrapleural instillation of fibrinolytics such as streptokinase or urokinase for loculated MPE is very effective in promoting lysis of fibrinous septations and facilitating complete pleural drainage and successful pleurodesis.[9,10]

Tube Thoracostomy with or without Pleurodesis

After thoracentesis and reexpansion of the lung, pleural fluid should be completely evacuated with a tube thoracostomy to allow apposition of the visceral and parietal pleura. Recurrent effusions are noted in 60% to 100% of patients after tube thoracostomy drainage alone; in general, obliteration of the pleural space either by parietal pleurectomy or instillation of sclerosants causing inflammation and subsequent pleural symphysis is required to ensure durable relief. Chemical pleurodesis is the preferred treatment for patients with MPE, and the efficacy of this intervention depends on (1) complete drainage of the pleural space and reexpansion of the lung to ensure apposition of the pleural surfaces, and (2) instillation of an effective sclerosing agent into the pleural space and retention of this agent in the chest for several hours to induce an inflammatory fibrosis and obliteration of the pleural space by symphysis of the parietal and visceral pleurae.

It has been a common practice to insert a chest tube (28 to 32 Fr.) at the level of the sixth or seventh intercostal space laterally and to direct it posteriorly to the most dependent portion of the pleural cavity. Once complete drainage is achieved (as confirmed by chest radiograph and daily drainage of less than 150 mL), the sclerosing agent (suspended or dissolved in 100 to 150 mL of normal saline) is instilled into the pleural space via the chest tube. The tube is then clamped for 1 to 2 hours to allow retention of sclerosing agent in the pleural space. It is subsequently unclamped and connected to suction and eventually removed when the daily drainage is less than 150 mL. It is also a common clinical practice to rotate the patient by periodically changing the patient's position in bed (lateral decubitus, supine, and prone) to enhance distribution of the sclerosant, as frequently described in most pleurodesis studies. There is little evidence, however, that such maneuvers, which frequently cause some degree of discomfort to patients, are necessary for successful pleurodesis. Moreover, concurrent intrapleural administration of lidocaine (Xylocaine, 3 mg/kg or up to 250 mg) and the sclerosing agent of choice is recommended, because significant pleuritic chest pain occurs in 7% and 40% of patients undergoing chemical pleurodesis using talc and doxycycline, respectively.[11] Pain, discomfort, and anxiety associated with pleurodesis performed at bedside may be alleviated with liberal use of intravenous sedatives and narcotics. This method of treatment typically requires hospitalization and placement of a large-bore chest tube for complete evacuation of the exudative effusion before chemical pleurodesis. However, more recent randomized and nonrandomized studies involving small numbers of patients have indicated that pigtail catheter drainage and sclerosis may be as successful as more traditional chest tube pleurodesis procedures and may be associated with less discomfort. Outpatient management of MPE with a small-bore (10.3-Fr.) all-purpose drainage catheter and bleomycin pleurodesis has been described.[12] Pleural fluid was drained by a catheter connected to a collection bag until drainage was less than 100 mL/d. Bleomycin (60 U in 50 mL of dextrose 5% in water) was then instilled to the chest via the drainage catheter. The tube was removed 24 hours after pleurodesis. Fifty-three percent of patients treated in this manner experienced complete responses, and an additional 25% had partial responses. In another study, MPE was drained by a 12-Fr. van Sonnenberg pigtail catheter inserted under ultrasonographic guidance in 15 patients, 11 of whom had loculated pleural effusions (which necessitated this method of drainage).[13] Talc (5 g suspended in 100 mL of injectable normal saline) was instilled into the pleural cavity once pleural fluid drainage was less than 100 mL/d. Control of MPE was achieved in 80% of these cases. Additional talc instillation was required in two patients to treat residual pockets of effusion and produced good results. These data suggest that outpatient management of MPE may be appropriate in patients with MPE, who typically have limited life expectancy.

Thoracoscopy

Thoracoscopy performed under general anesthesia with or without single lung ventilation provides opportunity for complete drainage of pleural fluid, breakdown of fibrin septation, evaluation of visceral pleura for lung expandability, biopsy of parietal pleura, and pleurodesis by talc insufflation or instillation of other sclerosing agents such as doxycycline or bleomycin. A small incision is made at the level of the seventh intercostal space along the midaxillary line for introduction of the thoracoscope. Pleural biopsy and instillation of the sclerosing agent can be accomplished via the in-line working channel of the thoracoscope. As indicated in selected cases, pleural abrasion or even parietal pleurectomy can be performed with thoracoscopic technique. Large pleural effusions should be partially drained before thoracoscopy to minimize the risk of reexpansion pulmonary edema.

Complications of medical or surgical intervention for MPE include pleuritic pain, low-grade fever, soft tissue hematoma or hemothorax, empyema, expansion pulmonary edema, and talc-induced adult respiratory distress syndrome. Moreover, a high frequency of chest wall tumor recurrence due to seeding of cancer cells (up to 40% of cases) has been observed in association with pleural procedures (needle thoracentesis or pleural biopsy, tube thoracostomy, or thoracoscopy trocar site) performed for pleural effusion due to malignant pleural mesothelioma.[2]

Pleurodesis Agents

Various agents have been used in the last 50 years to induce adhesive obliteration of the pleural space. Intrapleural instillation of nitrogen mustard, thiotepa, 5-fluorouracil, bacille Calmette-Guérin, radioactive zinc, gold, chromium, and phosphorus has been used to treat MPE, but these agents were found to have limited efficacy and unacceptable toxicity. Other pharmacologic and biologic agents (quinacrine, *Corynebacterium parvum*, interferons, interleukin-2, OK432) have also been used in multiple small, uncontrolled trials to treat MPE with varying and frequently disappointing efficacy rates and significant side effects. These agents are no longer in clinical use and are mentioned here only because of historical and academic interest.

Several chemicals have been extensively evaluated in both randomized and nonrandomized clinical studies for their efficacy as pleurodesic agents (Table 51.5-1). None of them except bleomycin is known to possess antitumor activity. They induce intense pleural inflammation and subsequently adhesive fibrosis of the parietal and visceral pleurae.

TETRACYCLINE AND DOXYCYCLINE. Tetracycline was extensively used as a sclerosing agent to treat pleural effusions of benign and malignant origin because of its efficacy, low cost, and safety. The overall efficacy of tetracycline in controlling MPE was 70%.[14,15] The usual dose was 500 to 1000 mg diluted in 100 mL of normal saline. The main side effects were pleuritic pain at the time of drug instillation (20% to 70% of cases) and low-grade fever (33% of patients). Lidocaine (20 mL of

TABLE 51.5-1. Efficiency of Sclerosing Agents Used in Treating Patients with Malignant Pleural Effusion

Agents	Response (%)	
	Mean	Range
Talc	98	72–100
Bleomycin	64	31–85
Tetracycline	72	25–100
Doxycycline	73	68–88

(Adapted from ref. 42.)

1% or 2% solution) could be mixed with tetracycline before administration to decrease pleuritic pain. Injectable tetracycline has not been available in the United States since 1991 because the drug preparations did not meet U.S. Food and Drug Administration purity standards. Because of this, the tetracycline derivatives doxycycline and minocycline have been used for pleurodesis. Three small, uncontrolled clinical trials have reported response rates of 67% to 88% after doxycycline pleurodesis.[16–18] The side effects are similar to those observed with tetracycline. Most patients require repeated doxycycline instillations for successful pleurodesis. In these reported series, only 15% of patients responded to a single treatment, and 9% required more than four instillations. Intrapleural minocycline (300 mg with 20 mL of 1% lidocaine) was given to seven patients with MPE, six of whom responded (86%).[19] The small number of patients studied, unspecified criteria for success, and duration of treatment response make it difficult to compare minocycline with other agents.

BLEOMYCIN. Intrapleural administration of bleomycin (60 to 120 U) achieves pleurodesis in 65% of patients with MPE (range, 62% to 81%).[20–22] Intrapleural bleomycin is well tolerated and associated with few side effects.[23] In a multicenter randomized trial,[14] bleomycin was superior to tetracycline for pleurodesis; 70% of patients treated with bleomycin had successful control of MPE compared to only 47% of patients treated with tetracycline. Unfortunately, bleomycin is expensive; typically each treatment dose ranges from $1100 to $1300. Bleomycin pleurodesis has been compared with less expensive talc pleurodesis in a prospective randomized study of 29 women with MPE secondary to breast cancer. Of 22 evaluable patients (3 of whom had bilateral pleurodesis), all 10 patients (100%) treated with talc experienced complete control of MPE compared to 10 of 15 patients (67%) receiving bleomycin.[22]

TALC. Talc produces an intense chemical pleuritis that effectively obliterates the pleural space. Asbestos-free, gas-sterilized or heat-sterilized talc USP may be administered via chest tube as a slurry (5 g in 100 mL of normal saline) or insufflated as a powder during thoracoscopy or thoracotomy.[24] Talc pleurodesis is highly effective with overall response rates ranging from 80% to 100%.[25–35] Viallat and colleagues reviewed their experience with thoracoscopic talc poudrage pleurodesis for MPE in 360 cases, including 88 mesothelioma patients and 272 individuals with effusions secondary to a variety of malignancies.[32] Approximately 3.0 to 4.5 g of heat-sterilized asbestos-free talc was insufflated via atomizer during thoracoscopy. Pleurodesis was successful in 90% of 327 evaluable patients at 1 month, and 82% of individuals had lifelong pleurodesis. Talc has consistently been shown to be superior to other commonly used sclerosing agents (tetracycline or doxycycline and bleomycin). In a randomized controlled trial, Fentiman and colleagues compared the efficacy of talc poudrage versus tetracycline in 33 breast cancer patients with MPE.[25] Ninety-two percent of patients receiving talc had successful pleurodesis compared to only 42% of patients receiving tetracycline. In another study, successful pleurodesis was observed in 97% of patients undergoing intrapleural talc insufflation by thoracoscopy compared to 70% and 47% of patients receiving bleomycin and tetracycline, respectively.[31] Thoracoscopic talc poudrage was also very effective in producing durable pleurodesis in patients with recalcitrant MPE for

TABLE 51.5-2. Efficacy of Talc Pleurodesis by Thoracoscopic Talc Poudrage or Talc Slurry by Tube Thoracostomy for Malignant Pleural Effusion

	No. of Patients	% Successful Pleurodesis[a]
THORACOSCOPIC TALC POUDRAGE		
Fentiman et al.[25]	12	92
Boniface et al.[26]	270	93
Canto et al.[29]	33	90
Yim et al.[72]	28	96
Ladjimi et al.[27]	218	78
Weissberg et al.[28]	169	92
Canto et al.[29]	128	86
Sanchez-Armengol and Rodriguez-Panadero[30]	119	87
Aelony et al.[35]	42	92
CALBG 9334[3,b]	131	79
Total	1150	89
TALC SLURRY		
Yim et al.[72]	29	90
Webb et al.[34]	28	100
Kennedy et al.[33]	40	78
Zimmer et al.[73]	19	90
CALGB 9334[3,b]	117	70
Total	233	86

CALGB, Cancer and Leukemia Group B.
[a]As defined by parameters delineated in each separate study.
[b]Multi-institution random-assignment clinical trial.

whom prior treatment with tetracycline failed.[35] Many single-institution studies demonstrated the effectiveness of talc pleurodesis either by thoracoscopic insufflation of dry talc into the pleural cavity or by intrapleural instillation of talc slurry via chest tubes, but controversies exist with respect to the cost effectiveness and clinical efficacy of each method (Table 51.5-2). To definitively answer the question regarding the most effective method of performing talc pleurodesis, a random-assignment phase III intergroup clinical trial lead by Cancer and Leukemia Group B (CALGB 9334) was initiated in 1993. A total of 501 patients were accrued to participate in this study, which compared efficacy, cost-effectiveness, and quality of life for talc pleurodesis in MPE using either talc slurry administered via chest tube or talc insufflation by thoracoscopy.[3,36] Despite multiple confounding factors (death rate before 30 days of 13% in the chest tube group and 9% in the thoracoscopy group; talc not administered, lung not expanded more than 90%, lack of follow-up data) that limited the number of patients in each group available for outcome analysis, the rate of recurrent effusion-free survival at 30 days was the same in both groups (chest tube, 70% or 82 of 117; thoracoscopy, 79% or 103 of 131). The 30-day survival rates were similar in both groups. Respiratory complications were greater in the thoracoscopy group ($P = .004$). Based on patients' reports, patients undergoing thoracoscopic talc pleurodesis felt safer, were more comfortable, had better pain control, and experienced less fatigue than those undergoing bedside talc pleurodesis via a chest tube. This quality-of-life advantage should be balanced against the risk of a slight increase in respiratory morbidity after thoracoscopic pleurodesis.[36]

The most commonly reported adverse effects of talc pleurodesis are fever (16% of cases) and pain (7% of cases). Less common complications include empyema, pneumonitis (similar to acute respiratory distress syndrome), and respiratory failure.[37,38] Pulmonary complications noted in earlier series have not been observed as frequently in more recent trials and tend to occur in patients who receive 10 to 12 g of talc or undergo either bilateral pleurodesis or unilateral pleurodesis in conjunction with pleural biopsy (which raised the possibility of talc emboli).

Intrapleural Chemotherapy

Few clinical studies have been conducted to investigate the efficacy of intrapleural chemotherapy for MPE. Regional chemotherapy in the form of intrapleural chemotherapy for malignant mesothelioma is discussed in Chapter 36. The overall response rates for intrapleural chemotherapy are low, and the treatments, even though regional, are associated with significant systemic side effects. Unless studied within the context of a clinical trial, intrapleural chemotherapy has no role in the management of MPE.

Intrapleural treatment with combinations of cisplatin (100 mg/m^2) and cytarabine (600 to 1200 mg/m^2) has been used to treat MPE in two studies.[39] This combination produced a complete response in only 27% of the patients, and adverse effects including pain (66%), cardiopulmonary symptoms (54%), bone marrow suppression (52%), and renal toxicity (34%) were noted in 76% of patients, which suggests that significant systemic absorption of the chemotherapeutic agents occurred in these individuals. Intrapleural doxorubicin at doses ranging from 10 to 40 mg produced complete responses in 12 of 55 evaluable patients (24%).[40] Adverse effects included pain (29%), fever (15%), nausea and vomiting (29%), and anorexia (24%). Repeated escalating doses of etoposide (100 to 225 mg/m^2) were administered intrapleurally to nine patients with MPE,[41] none of whom experienced a clinical response.

Cost Effectiveness of Pleurodesis for Malignant Pleural Effusion

The most effective and economic method for the treatment of MPE is still a matter of debate. It is important for physicians who manage patients with MPE to be knowledgeable regarding the efficacies, toxicities, and costs of available treatment modalities. The estimated costs for commonly used pleurodesis agents, indexed for effectiveness as cost per symptom-free day, are listed in Table 51.5-3. Even though talc itself is not expensive ($0.15 to $0.50 for a 2.5- to 10-g dose), the cost of talc pleurodesis performed by thoracoscopy is high because of operating room and professional fees. The total cost of treatment has been determined to be $20,996 (1992 U.S. dollars). The high success rate may justify the expense of talc pleurodesis. The 6-month cost of talc pleurodesis, estimated to be $149 per symptom-free day, should drop significantly if the procedure is performed by pleuroscopy under intravenous sedation and local anesthesia or by instillation of talc slurry via chest tube. Both of these techniques are as effective as talc poudrage performed by video-assisted thoracoscopic surgery under general anesthesia. Bleomycin is the most expensive pleurodesis agent, with the cost per dose averaging $1140; however, the total cost of treatment is relatively low, because of the high efficiency of achieving pleurodesis with a single administration of this drug. The 6-month cost per symptom-free day was approximately $132 in an analysis reported by Belani and colleagues.[42] Tetracycline and its currently available substitute doxycycline are costly ($159 and $218 per symptom-free day, respectively), given the fact that repeated administrations of these agents are required to achieve successful pleurodesis, which prolongs hospitalization and increases the risk of treatment-related complications.

Pleurectomy

Stripping of the parietal pleura is 100% effective in controlling MPE. Although it may have a role in the treatment of malignant pleural mesothelioma,[43] pleurectomy via thoracotomy is not routinely performed because the morbidity (23%), and mortality (10%) cannot be justified in debilitated patients for whom less invasive and equally successful treatment options may be available. However, several studies have indicated that parietal pleurectomy can be performed via video-assisted thoracoscopic surgery (VATS) with acceptable risk in patients. Waller et al.[44] performed VATS parietal pleurectomy in 19 patients with MPE secondary to mesothelioma or metastatic adenocarcinoma. Symptomatic recurrent effusion occurred in three patients (15.7%). Tumor seeding at the thoracoscopic trocar sites occurred in 5 of 13 mesothelioma patients. More recently, Harvey and colleagues[45] performed VATS pleurectomy in 11 patients (five with non–small cell lung cancer, four with breast cancer, one with mesothelioma, one with cancer of unknown primary) with no recurrences and one death (9%) due to sepsis from a necrotic tumor involving the liver. Other complications included prolonged air leak (one patient) and bleeding requir-

TABLE 51.5-3. Cost of Therapy for Malignant Pleural Effusion by Treatment Type

Treatment Type	Agent Cost	Total Cost of Treatment	Cost per Symptom-Free Day	Cost Drivers
Talc	$0.15–0.50	$20,996	$149	OR facilities
Bleomycin	$1140 (60 U)	$8657	$132	High agent cost
Tetracycline^a	$1977 (500 mg)	$8066	$159	—
Doxycycline	$258 (3 × 500 mg)	$8061	$218	Need for repeated instillation

OR, operating room.
^{a}Not available.
(Adapted from ref. 42.)

ing reoperation and transfusion (one patient). The results of these two small series should not be viewed as justifications for more liberal application of VATS parietal pleurectomy as the first line of treatment for MPE. Instead, parietal pleurectomy should be reserved for malignant effusions that are refractory to less invasive and less expensive interventions.

Pleuroperitoneal Shunt

The pleuroperitoneal shunt, introduced in 1982, has been evaluated as a therapeutic option for the treatment of MPE. It may be used for recurrent effusions that are refractory to tube thoracostomy and pleurodesis or MPE associated with trapped lung.[46] The most commonly used device is the Denver pleuroperitoneal shunt (Denver Biomaterials, Inc., Golden, CO). The shunt is a silicone rubber conduit consisting of a unidirectional valved pump chamber connecting to pleural and peritoneal catheters. The pumping chamber can be implanted into a subcutaneous pocket or exteriorized as an external pumping chamber. Because of the negative pressure differential between the pleural and peritoneal cavities, manual compression of the pumping chamber is required for fluid drainage from the chest. Each compression transports 1.5 mL of fluid, and patients are frequently asked to compress the pump for 5 to 10 minutes four times a day. Implantation of the shunt can be performed under local or general anesthesia. Petrou and colleagues used pleuroperitoneal shunt in 63 patients with recurrent MPE and trapped lung.[46] There were no operative deaths, and complications were noted in five patients (8%). Effective palliation was achieved in more than 95% of cases. Catheter occlusion was noted in eight patients (12%) at 1 week to 4 months after insertion, with five patients requiring replacement or revision of the shunt and three patients requiring shunt removal and treatment of empyema. Contraindications include pleural infection, multiple loculations, inability of the patient to press the chamber, short life expectancy, and obliterated peritoneal space.[47] The need for active pumping of the chamber a minimum of 400 times a day limits its usefulness to patients with excellent performance status. In addition, the shunt may malfunction over time, which further limits its usefulness. Because of this, the pleuroperitoneal shunt should be considered as one of the last alternatives for patients with refractory effusions.

Indwelling Pleural Catheter

Malignant pleural fluid can be drained for prolonged periods of time by a small-caliber biocompatible silicone rubber indwelling catheter such as the Pleurx catheter (Surgimedics, Denver Biomaterials, Inc., Golden, CO). The catheter is inserted under local anesthesia and mild intravenous sedation in the operating room as an inpatient or outpatient procedure. The pleural cavity is accessed at the anterior axillary line around the sixth or seventh intercostal space by a needle through which a guidewire is passed to maintain the tract. A small incision is then made over the wire and a 5- to 8-cm chest wall subcutaneous tunnel is created with a counterincision. The catheter is pulled through the tunnel and out next to the wire. The catheter is then inserted into the pleural cavity using the Seldinger technique and a tear-away plastic sheath. Up to 1500 mL of pleural fluid can be drained immediately after catheter insertion. Residual fluid can be gradually drained at subse-

quent times. The patients and their caretakers are given clear verbal and written instructions on proper techniques to drain the pleural fluid. The pleural fluid is drained completely every second day or more often as dictated by symptoms. The advantages of pleural catheter placement are the ease of insertion and minimal discomfort caused by the catheter, rapid drainage of recurrent symptomatic effusion, and the need for minimal or no hospitalization for catheter insertion and care.

A prospective multi-institutional random-assignment clinical trial comparing the efficacy of the Pleurx pleural catheter versus chest tube and doxycycline sclerotherapy for recurrent symptomatic MPE in 144 patients was reported (randomization ratio of 2:1, with 99 patients having an indwelling catheter and 45 patients undergoing doxycycline pleurodesis).[48] There was no difference between the two groups in performance status or initial dyspnea scores. After treatment, both groups showed similar improvements in respiratory symptoms and had similar morbidity. Initial treatment success was achieved in 68% of patients receiving chest tube and doxycycline pleurodesis versus 92% of patients with the Pleurx catheters. There was no difference between treatment groups in the rate of late failure as defined by recurrence of MPE (13% for the pleural catheter group and 21% for the doxycycline group; $\chi^2 = 0.23$; $P = .631$). Spontaneous pleurodesis was observed in 46% of patients receiving the Pleurx catheter as treatment for their effusions, with a median time to pleurodesis of 29 days (range, 8 to 223 days). The authors concluded that the Pleurx catheter was as effective as doxycycline pleurodesis in relieving symptoms related to MPE. More importantly, the chronic indwelling pleural catheter had a safety and efficacy equivalent to those of the chest tube and sclerosis while requiring less hospitalization (mean, 1.83 days) than the common treatment strategy of chest tube and pleurodesis (mean, 6.83 days). Outpatient management of patients with MPE with Pleurx catheters was evaluated by Putnam and colleagues at the M. D. Anderson Cancer Center.[49] One hundred consecutively treated patients given Pleurx catheters (60 outpatients and 40 inpatients) were compared to 68 patients treated with chest tubes and pleurodesis (all inpatients) with respect to treatment outcome (control of MPE and its symptoms), duration of hospitalization, treatment-related morbidity and mortality, and early hospital charges. This study revealed that outpatient treatment of MPE with a chronic indwelling catheter was safe and effective and was associated with a 19% rate of complications (device malfunction requiring removal, loculation of pleural effusion requiring intervention, and pleural space infection requiring further therapy in the form of percutaneous drainage, antibiotics or other operations). Median durations of hospital stay were 7 days and 0 days for inpatient treatments (Pleurx catheter placement or chest tube placement with pleurodesis) and outpatient Pleurx catheter placement, respectively. The economic impact was significant: for patients treated in hospital, mean charges ranged from $7000 to $11,000, whereas mean charge was $3400 for outpatient treatments. A chronic indwelling pleural catheter is particularly useful for recurrent MPE refractory to pleurodesis or MPE associated with trapped lung.

SUMMARY

The prognosis of patients with MPE varies with the histologic type of the primary tumor. In general, 65% of patients with MPE

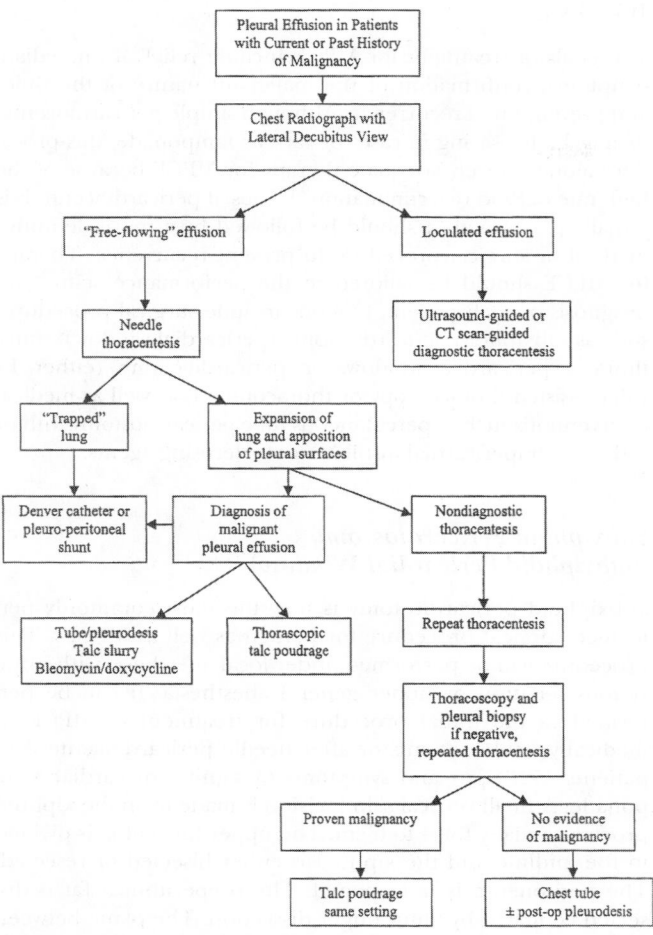

FIGURE 51.5-2. Treatment algorithm for malignant pleural effusion. CT, computed tomography.

are dead within 3 months and 80% are dead within 6 months. Because of this, treatment of MPE should focus on expeditious and cost-efficient palliation. The authors' approach to patients with MPE who have good performance status is talc pleurodesis. Indwelling pleural catheters have been used frequently for intermittent drainage of effusions in patients with trapped lung or limited life expectancy, as well as individuals on protocols requiring sequential analysis of molecular end points in tumor cells readily obtained from malignant effusions. The algorithm for the diagnosis and treatment of malignant pleural is outlined in Figure 51.5-2.

MALIGNANT PERICARDIAL EFFUSION

Patients with malignant pericardial disease may be asymptomatic or may present with a number of manifestations, with pericardial effusion being the most common. Pericardial tamponade due to malignant pericardial effusion (MPCE) accounts for at least 50% of all reported cases of pericardial fluid collection that require intervention. As with cancerous pleural effusions, MPCEs are frequently indicative of advanced incurable malignancy. Overall median survival of patients with MPCE is less than 6 months.

CLINICAL PRESENTATION

In most cases MPCE is observed in patients with a previous diagnosis of cancer, typically at late stages of their disease. MPCE is rarely seen as the initial manifestation of extracardiac malignancy; only 90 cases were reported in the English literature over a 55-year period.[50] The most common symptoms attributed to pericardial effusion are dyspnea, cough, chest pain, fever, and edema. Nonspecific complaints are also frequent, and because of this, pericardial effusion may remain unsuspected in patients in whom nonspecific symptoms are attributed to disease progression. The frequency of cardiac tamponade as the initial manifestation of malignant effusion is highly variable and depends on the rate of fluid accumulation, volume of fluid, and underlying cardiac function. The pericardium may distend over a period of time to accommodate a large volume of fluid before the clinical appearance of tamponade. Impedance of right atrial and ventricular filling by pericardial fluid results in cardiac tamponade. Signs and symptoms of cardiac tamponade include dyspnea, orthopnea, low output (peripheral vasoconstriction; cold, clammy extremities; poor capillary refill; and diaphoresis), jugular venous distention, distant heart sounds, pulsus paradoxus, and narrowed pulse pressure. Electrocardiogram may show low-voltage complexes in all leads and electrical alternans.

DIAGNOSTIC MODALITIES

Radiographic and Echocardiographic Studies

Pericardial effusion in asymptomatic patients is most frequently detected by plain posteroanterior and lateral chest radiographs. The typical finding on chest radiograph is an enlarged globular water-bottle pericardial silhouette. Moreover, when pericardial effusion and tamponade are caused by malignancy, concomitant parenchymal involvement and/or pleural effusion are observed in 30% to 50% of cases.[51] Once pericardial effusion is suspected, echocardiography should be performed to confirm its presence and hemodynamic significance (Fig. 51.5-3). Two-dimensional echocardiography can define the location and amount of effusion, as well as the pres-

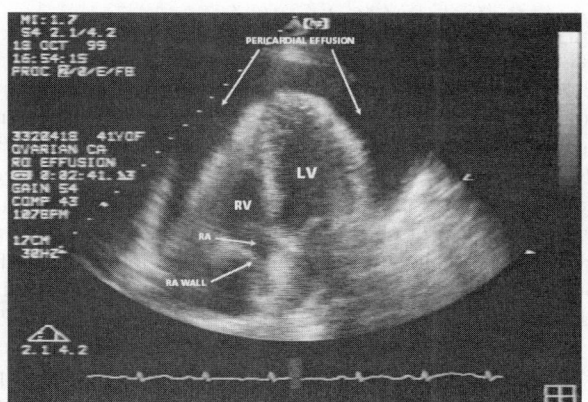

FIGURE 51.5-3. Two-dimensional echocardiography demonstrates a large pericardial effusion with circumferential fluid collection that resulted in a 1.5-cm separation of the visceral and parietal pericardium. Characteristic M-mode finding of ventricular collapse is indicative of early cardiac tamponade. LV, left ventricle; RA, right atrium; RV, right ventricle. (Courtesy of E. E. Tucker, MD, Clinical Center, National Institutes of Health, Bethesda, MD.)

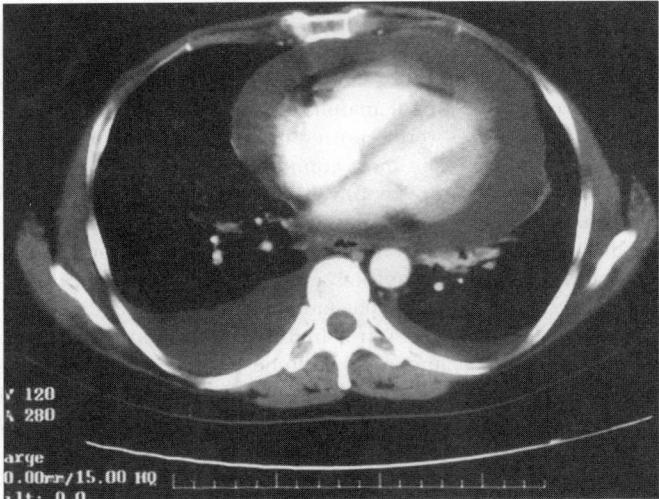

FIGURE 51.5-4. Chest computed tomography scan of a patient with metastatic ovarian cancer shows a large pericardial effusion and bilateral pleural effusion (both effusions were proven to be malignant by cytologic and histopathologic examination of tissue obtained by subxiphoid pericardiostomy and tube thoracostomy).

ence of pericardial or intracardiac masses. Right atrial and ventricular collapse are the most common echocardiographic signs of cardiac tamponade and are identified with a sensitivity ranging from 38% to 60% and a specificity ranging from 50% to 100%.[52] Echocardiography is frequently used to provide guidance for safe and accurate pericardiocentesis. Pericardial effusion can be also be diagnosed by CT scan, which can detect as little as 50 mL of pericardial fluid (Fig. 51.5-4). This is not the diagnostic method of choice for pericardial effusion because it is time-consuming to perform and is no more accurate than echocardiography. CT may be helpful in evaluating intrapericardial masses as well as in defining the nature of the pericardial fluid, because the attenuation coefficients for exudates, chyle, serous fluid, and blood may differ.[53]

Cytopathology and Histopathology

Imaging techniques mentioned earlier in Radiographic and Echocardiographic Studies provide information regarding the amount and hemodynamic significance of pericardial effusion but not regarding its benign or malignant nature. Only 50% to 60% of pericardial effusions in cancer patients are confirmed by cytologic examination to be malignant.[54] Weiner and colleagues[54] reviewed 95 cases of pericardial effusion treated initially by pericardiocentesis. Malignant cells were identified in pericardial fluid from two-thirds of cancer patients; cytologic results correlated with histologic diagnosis of the underlying malignancy in 100% of these individuals. Press and Livingston[55] reviewed 190 cases of MPCE diagnosed by pericardiocentesis. Pericardial fluid was positive for malignant cells in 151 patients with documented neoplastic pericarditis (specificity, 79%); hence, cytologic examination of pericardial fluid remains valuable in the diagnosis of MPCE, especially when results are positive. In contrast, parietal pericardial biopsy results are frequently nondiagnostic because the principal site of malignant infiltration is the visceral pericardium and its subepicardial lymphatics.

TREATMENT

The goals of treatment for MPCE include relief of immediate symptoms, confirmation of the malignant nature of the fluid, and prevention of recurrence. Although simple pericardiocentesis may be life-saving in cases of cardiac tamponade, this procedure alone is rarely adequate therapy for MPCE because of the high rate of fluid reaccumulation.[51] Thus, if pericardiocentesis is initially performed, it should be followed by a more definitive medical or surgical procedure to prevent recurrence. Therapy for MPCE should be tailored to the performance status and prognosis of each patient. Options include surgical procedures such as subxiphoid pericardiostomy (pericardial window), transthoracic pericardial window, or pericardiectomy (either by video-assisted thoracoscopy or thoracotomy), as well as medical interventions such as percutaneous tube pericardiostomy with or without intrapericardial instillation of sclerosing agents.

Subxiphoid Pericardiostomy (Subxiphoid Pericardial Window)

Subxiphoid pericardiostomy is now the most commonly performed surgical procedure for benign as well as MPCEs. This procedure can be performed under local anesthesia with intravenous sedation or under general anesthesia. It can be performed as the initial procedure for treatment of MPCE in medically stable patients or after needle pericardiocentesis in patients with signs and symptoms of significant cardiac tamponade. A small vertical skin incision is made from the xiphoid process caudally for 4 to 6 cm. The upper linea alba is divided in the midline and the xiphoid is either bisected or resected. The peritoneum is not opened. The preperitoneal fat is dissected cephalad by blunt finger dissection. The plane between the posterior sternum and the anterior pericardium is then developed to allow insertion of a retractor to elevate the lower end of the sternum. The pericardium is identified as the bulging grayish white fibrous membrane. The anterior pericardium is then incised, fluid is drained, and samples are collected for cytologic and microbiologic analyses. The pericardium is then digitally explored to identify adhesions and tumor masses. A piece of pericardium (2 to 4 cm²) is excised and submitted for microbiologic as well as pathologic studies. Through a separate stab wound in the upper abdomen, a 28-Fr. curved chest tube is placed in the pericardial space through the pericardial window for postoperative drainage. Some authors advocate leaving the tube in place for 4 to 5 days regardless of the drainage amount to promote local inflammation and fusion of the visceral and parietal pericardium. No attempts are made to create a communication between the pericardial space and either the pleural or peritoneal space. Allen and colleagues noted that autopsies of six patients who had undergone the subxiphoid procedure revealed complete pericardial symphysis with extensive adhesions.[56] A comprehensive review of the clinical experience pertaining to more than 800 patients with effusions of different causes who underwent subxiphoid pericardiostomy has indicated an overall mortality rate of approximately 0.46% (range, 0% to 5%), an overall morbidity rate of approximately 1.53% (range, 0% to 10%), and a recurrence rate of approximately 3.5% (range, 0% to 9.1%). These low mortality, morbidity, and recurrence rates compare very favorably with those obtainable with percutaneous pericardiocentesis and pericar-

TABLE 51.5-4.　Subxiphoid Pericardiostomy and Percutaneous Catheter Drainage for Pericardial Effusions

Subxiphoid Pericardiostomy		*Date*	*No. of Patients*	*Mortality Rate (%)*	*Morbidity Rate (%)*	*Recurrence Rate (%)*
McDonald et al.[74]		2003	150	0	0.7	4.7
Allen et al.[56]		1999	94	0	1.1	1.1
Moores et al.[75]		1995	155	0	0	2.5
Okamoto et al.[76]		1993	51	0	0	3.9
Chan et al.[77]		1991	22	0	0	9.1
Park et al.[59]		1991	10	0	10	0
Sugimoto et al.[78]		1990	28	0	0	7.1
Reitknecht et al.[79]		1985	46	0	0	4.5
Ghosh et al.[80]		1985	108	2	5.5	4.6
Levin and Aaron[81]		1982	28	0	7.0	7.0
Prager et al.[82]		1982	25	1	0	0
Santos and Frater[83]		1977	46	0	0	0
Total/mean			**763**	**0.25**	**2.02**	**3.71**
Percutaneous Catheter Drainage	*Technique*	*Date*	*No. of Patients*	*Mortality Rate (%)*	*Morbidity Rate (%)*	*Recurrence Rate (%)*
McDonald et al.[74]	Catheter	2003	96	0	3.1	15.6
Allen et al.[56]	Catheter	1999	23	4.3	17.4	33.3
Di Segni et al.[84]	Balloon/pericardiostomy	1995	8	0	12.5	0
Ziskind et al.[71]	Balloon/pericardiostomy	1993	50	2.0	20.0	4.0
Celermajer et al.[67]	Catheter	1991	36	3.0	5.6	19.4
Shepherd[51]	Catheter/sclerosis	1987	58	0	10.3	17.0
Kopecky et al.[85]	Catheter	1986	42	0	2.4	24.0
Total/mean			**313**	**1.33**	**10.2**	**16.2**

(Adapted from ref. 56.)

diostomy with or without sclerosis (0.7% mortality, 3.0% morbidity, and 13.0% recurrence) (Table 51.5-4).

Partial Pericardiectomy or Pericardial Window via Thoracotomy

Before the recent resurrection of subxiphoid pericardial window as the preferred surgical treatment for pericardial effusion, pericardial window or even pericardiectomy via a thoracotomy incision was advocated. Piehler and associates[57] reviewed their experience with surgical management of pericardial effusions in 145 patients and suggested that the extent of pericardial resection influenced the incidence of recurrent effusions. However, several series indicated no difference in recurrence rates for patients treated by subxiphoid pericardiostomy and by transthoracic drainage.[58,59] More importantly, postoperative complications (pneumonia, pleural effusion, respiratory failure, cardiac arrhythmia, deep venous thrombosis, and pulmonary embolism) are much less frequent after subxiphoid pericardial drainage than after transthoracic pericardial resection (10% vs. 50%, respectively). Thus, transthoracic pericardial resection is not a suitable initial procedure for drainage of MPCE.

If possible, VATS[60–62] should be used if transthoracic pericardial resection is required for recurrent effusion after subxiphoid pericardiostomy or for diagnosis and treatment of simultaneous pleural and parenchymal pathology. Compared to thoracotomy, minimally invasive approaches are more suitable interventions in debilitated cancer patients. The potential limitation of VATS pericardectomy is the need for general anesthesia and single-lung ventilation. Pericardial resection via laparoscopy or video-assisted subxiphoid pericardial window procedure have been reported[63]; however, there is no added benefit for these expensive minimally invasive techniques compared to standard subxiphoid pericardiostomy. Pericardial-peritoneal shunt, using a Denver pleuroperitoneal catheter with pumping chamber, has been used to treat MPCE in a limited number of patients.[64] Experience with this technique is too limited to allow adequate assessment of its clinical usefulness, although it may be suitable for pericardial effusions that are refractory to repeated pericardiostomy procedures.

Pericardiocentesis

Pericardiocentesis can be life saving when performed on patients with hemodynamically significant cardiac tamponade. Removal of as little as 50 mL of pericardial fluid can significantly improve signs and symptoms of acute tamponade. Traditionally, after subcutaneous infiltration of 1% lidocaine local anesthetic solution, the needle is inserted at the right side of the xiphoid process and directed 45 degrees dorsally aiming toward the tip of the left scapula. In cancer patients with symptomatic pericardial effusion, pericardiocentesis may be used to stabilize the patient before performance of more definitive drainage procedures such as percutaneous tube pericardiostomy or subxiphoid pericardial window.

As the sole treatment for MPCE, pericardiocentesis is associated with recurrence requiring further treatment in up to 70% of cases.[65] This procedure has been associated with a significant incidence of complications, some of which are fatal, even when performed by experienced physicians. Allen et al.[56] observed clinically significant complications in 5 of 23 patients (22%) undergoing percutaneous pericardiocentesis, including three right ventricular perforations (with one fatality) requiring surgical intervention, one ventricular arrhythmia requiring cardioversion, and one pneumothorax. The complication rate observed by Allen et al. exceeds that reported by Vaitkus et al.,[66] who summarized their experience with pericardiocentesis in 139 patients with MPCEs.[67] Percutaneous pericardiocentesis successfully alleviated symptoms in 97% of cases. Morbidity and mortality in this series were 3.0% and 0.7%, respectively.

Echocardiography may reduce complications and improve the success of the pericardiocentesis by delineating the size and location of the effusion relative to cardiac structures. Overall rates of complication and success are approximately 2.4% and 100% after ultrasonographically guided pericardial drainage[68] compared to 4.8% and 90.0% after unassisted pericardiocentesis.[69]

Percutaneous Tube Pericardiostomy and Pericardial Sclerotherapy

The rates of fluid reaccumulation have been reported to range from as low as 44% to as high as 70% after pericardiocentesis.[65] It is now a common practice to place a 9-Fr. pigtail draining catheter into the pericardial space after successful needle pericardiocentesis using the Seldinger technique to enable more complete evacuation of the effusion and provide access for sclerotherapy. Although several agents have been used in the past, tetracycline and its currently available derivative doxycycline have been most extensively evaluated as sclerosing agents for pericardial effusion. Maher and colleagues reported their experience with 93 patients with MPCE treated by percutaneous pericardial drainage followed by tetracycline or doxycycline sclerosis.[65] Successful placement of the pericardiostomy tube was achieved in 85 patients (92%). Pericardial effusion was controlled in 75 patients (88%); 10 patients (12%) did not respond to sclerosis, and 8 of these subsequently underwent surgical pericardiostomy. Sclerotherapy required one to eight instillations of tetracycline or doxycycline (median, three); 50 patients required three or more instillations to control their effusions. Treatment-related complications included (in decreasing order of frequency) pain, catheter occlusion, fever, and atrial arrhythmias. The apparently favorable results of this minimally invasive treatment strategy are offset by the need for repeated instillations of the sclerosing agent to achieve pericardial symphysis. Liu and colleagues conducted a prospective study to evaluate the efficacy and toxicity of bleomycin versus doxycycline as the sclerosing agents for MPCE.[70] Bleomycin was found to be as effective as doxycycline in achieving satisfactory control of MPCE, yet produced much less retrosternal pain. As a result, these authors recommend that bleomycin be considered the first-line chemical sclerosing agent for MPCE.

Percutaneous Balloon Tube Pericardiostomy

Percutaneous balloon tube pericardiostomy, initially advocated by Ziskind and subsequently studied by others, appears to be an extension of the more commonly performed percutaneous tube pericardiostomy. After successful pericardiocentesis, dilatation of the needle tract is performed under fluoroscopy using a balloon catheter. Ziskind and colleagues[71] reported

that this technique was effective in relieving pericardial effusion in 46 of 50 patients (92%). Procedure-related complications included fever (six patients), pleural effusion requiring chest tube placement or thoracentesis (eight patients), small pneumothorax (two patients), and right ventricular injury requiring surgery (one patient), for an overall clinically significant complication rate of 18%. Even though this is an effective minimally invasive technique for pericardial drainage, its widespread application may be limited by the need for specialized equipment as well as interventional cardiologists or radiologists. The high incidence of inadvertent pleural effusions requiring drainage makes this technique less attractive than the others discussed previously.

Local or Systemic Therapies for Malignant Pericardial Effusion

Radiotherapy is generally reserved for MPCE associated with lymphoma or breast carcinoma. Vaitkus and colleagues reviewed the experience of 54 patients treated with radiotherapy as the primary mode of therapy for MPCE.[66] Of these patients, 39 (72%) underwent initial pericardiocentesis. The majority received neither systemic nor other direct pericardial intervention. Radiation therapy was successful in controlling MPCE in 36 patients (66.7%). The highest success rates were noted in leukemia and lymphoma patients and breast cancer patients (93% and 71%, respectively). Surprisingly, 45% of patients with other solid tumors had adequate control of their effusions. Although radiotherapy is noninvasive, it requires repeated visits or even prolonged hospitalization and may theoretically cause acute pericarditis or myocarditis. These potential complications may not be relevant for many patients due to their limited survival.

Patients with MPCE secondary to lymphoma or breast carcinoma may have effusions controlled with systemic chemotherapy. Vaitkus et al.[66] reported their experience with 46 patients with breast cancer (38 patients), lymphoma (2 patients), or other solid tumors (6 patients) treated with systemic chemotherapy. Thirty-six patients (78%) underwent initial therapeutic pericardiocentesis. Systemic chemotherapy prevented recurrence of effusion in 31 patients (67%); successful control of effusion was achieved in over two-thirds of these individuals irrespective of whether or not pericardiocentesis preceded systemic therapy.

SUMMARY

MPCE is frequently an indication of advanced, incurable malignancy. Hence, the goals of intervention include relief of symptoms and prevention of recurrence. The treatment of MPCE should proceed in a stepwise fashion as outlined in Figure 51.5-5. Surgical (subxiphoid pericardiostomy) or medical (ultrasonographically guided percutaneous tube pericardiostomy and sclerotherapy) interventions have acceptable risks and provide excellent results. The authors favor surgical drainage as the primary approach for patients with MPCE because of its simplicity and extremely high success rate without the need for intrapericardial instillation of sclerosing agents and tube manipulations, which may be associated with patient discomfort. Recurrent MPCE can be managed either by repeat pericardiostomy or insertion of a shunt. Patients responding to treatment with complete control of the effusion should have a meaningful survival, with

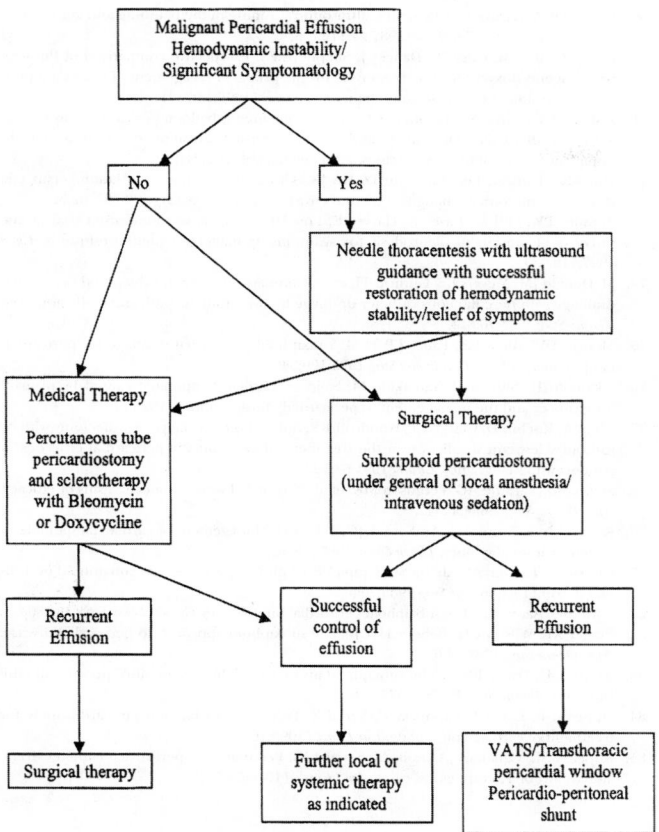

FIGURE 51.5-5.   Treatment algorithm for malignant pericardial effusion. VATS, video-assisted thoracic surgery.

life expectancy (average, 9 months) contingent on the histologic characteristics of the underlying malignancy.

REFERENCES

1. Fenton KN, Richardson JD. Diagnosis and management of malignant pleural effusions. *Am J Surg* 1995;170:69.
2. Antunes G, Neville E, Duffy J, Ali N. BTS guidelines for the management of malignant pleural effusions. *Thorax* 2003;58:ii29.
3. Putnam JB Jr. Malignant pleural effusions. *Surg Clin North Am* 2002;82:867.
4. Ratliff JL, Chavez CM, Jamchuk A, Forestner JE, Conn JH. Re-expansion pulmonary edema. *Chest* 1973;64:654.
5. DeCamp MM Jr, Jaklitsch MT, Mentzer SJ, Harpole DH Jr, Sugarbaker DJ. The safety and versatility of video-thoracoscopy: a prospective analysis of 895 consecutive cases. *J Am Coll Surg* 1995;181:113.
6. Assi Z, Caruso JL, Herndon J, Patz EF Jr. Cytologically proved malignant pleural effusions: distribution of transudates and exudates. *Chest* 1998;113:1302.
7. Sahn SA, Good JT Jr. Pleural fluid pH in malignant effusions. Diagnostic, prognostic, and therapeutic implications. *Ann Intern Med* 1988;108:345.
8. Rodriguez-Panadero F, Lopez MJ. Low glucose and pH levels in malignant pleural effusions. Diagnostic significance and prognostic value in respect to pleurodesis. *Am Rev Respir Dis* 1989;139:663.
9. Davies CW, Traill ZC, Gleeson FV, Davies RJ. Intrapleural streptokinase in the management of malignant multiloculated pleural effusions. *Chest* 1999;115:729.
10. Gilkeson RC, Silverman P, Haaga JR. Using urokinase to treat malignant pleural effusions. *AJR Am J Roentgenol* 1999;173:781.
11. Robinson LA, Fleming WH, Galbraith TA. Intrapleural doxycycline control of malignant pleural effusions. *Ann Thorac Surg* 1993;55:1115.
12. Patz EF Jr. Malignant pleural effusions: recent advances and ambulatory sclerotherapy. *Chest* 1998;113:74S.
13. Thompson RL, Yau JC, Donnelly RF, Gowan DJ, Matzinger FR. Pleurodesis with iodized talc for malignant effusions using pigtail catheters. *Ann Pharmacother* 1998;32:739.
14. Ruckdeschel JC, Moores D, Lee JY, et al. Intrapleural therapy for malignant pleural effusions. A randomized comparison of bleomycin and tetracycline. *Chest* 1991;100:1528.
15. Gravelyn TR, Michelson MK, Gross BH, Sitrin RG. Tetracycline pleurodesis for malignant pleural effusions. A 10-year retrospective study. *Cancer* 1987;59:1973.
16. Heffner JE, Standerfer RJ, Torstveit J, Unruh L. Clinical efficacy of doxycycline for pleurodesis. *Chest* 1994;105:1743.
17. Mansson T. Treatment of malignant pleural effusion with doxycycline. *Scand J Infect Dis Suppl* 1988;53:29.
18. Kitamura S, Sugiyama Y, Izumi T. Intrapleural doxycycline for control of malignant pleural effusion. *Curr Ther Res* 1981;30:515.
19. Hatta T, Tsubota N, Yoshimura M, Yanagawa M. Intrapleural minocycline for postoperative air leakage and control of malignant pleural effusion [in Japanese]. *Kyobu Geka* 1990;43:283.
20. Ostrowski MJ. An assessment of the long-term results of controlling the reaccumulation of malignant effusions using intracavity bleomycin. *Cancer* 1986;57:721.
21. Kessinger A, Wigton RS. Intracavitary bleomycin and tetracycline in the management of malignant pleural effusions: a randomized study. *J Surg Oncol* 1987;36:81.
22. Hamed H, Fentiman IS, Chaudary MA, Rubens RD. Comparison of intracavitary bleomycin and talc for control of pleural effusions secondary to carcinoma of the breast. *Br J Surg* 1989;76:1266.
23. Ostrowski MJ, Halsall GM. Intracavitary bleomycin in the management of malignant effusions: a multicenter study. *Cancer Treat Rep* 1982;66:1903.
24. Colt HG, Russack V, Chiu Y, et al. A comparison of thoracoscopic talc insufflation, slurry, and mechanical abrasion pleurodesis. *Chest* 1997;111:442.
25. Fentiman IS, Rubens RD, Hayward JL. A comparison of intracavitary talc and tetracycline for the control of pleural effusions secondary to breast cancer. *Eur J Cancer Clin Oncol* 1986;22:1079.
26. Boniface E, Guerin JC. Value of talc administration using thoracoscopy in the symptomatic treatment of recurrent pleurisy. Apropos of 302 cases [in French]. *Rev Mal Respir* 1989;6:133.
27. Ladjimi S, M'Raihi L, Djemel A, et al. Results of talc administration using thoracoscopy in neoplastic pleurisies. Apropos of 218 cases [in French]. *Rev Mal Respir* 1989;6:147.
28. Weissberg D, Ben Zeev I. Talc pleurodesis. Experience with 360 patients. *J Thorac Cardiovasc Surg* 1993;106:689.
29. Canto A, Rivas J, Moya J, et al. Pleural effusion of malignant etiology. Thoracoscopic use of talc as an effective method of pleurodesis [in Spanish]. *Med Clin(Barc)* 1985;84:806.
30. Sanchez-Armengol A, Rodriguez-Panadero F. Survival and talc pleurodesis in metastatic pleural carcinoma, revisited. Report of 125 cases. *Chest* 1993;104:1482.
31. Hartman DL, Gaither JM, Kesler KA, et al. Comparison of insufflated talc under thoracoscopic guidance with standard tetracycline and bleomycin pleurodesis for control of malignant pleural effusions. *J Thorac Cardiovasc Surg* 1993;105:743.
32. Viallat JR, Rey F, Astoul P, Boutin C. Thoracoscopic talc poudrage pleurodesis for malignant effusions. A review of 360 cases. *Chest* 1996;110:1387.
33. Kennedy L, Rusch VW, Strange C, Ginsberg RJ, Sahn SA. Pleurodesis using talc slurry. *Chest* 1994;106:342.
34. Webb WR, Ozmen V, Moulder PV, Shabahang B, Breaux J. Iodized talc pleurodesis for the treatment of pleural effusions. *J Thorac Cardiovasc Surg* 1992;103:881.
35. Aelony Y, King RR, Boutin C. Thoracoscopic talc poudrage in malignant pleural effusions: effective pleurodesis despite low pleural pH. *Chest* 1998;113:1007.
36. Fleishman S, Dresler C, Herndon JE, et al. Quality of life (QOL) advantage of sclerosis for malignant pleural effusion (MPE) via talc thoracoscopy over chest tube infusion of talc slurry: a Cancer and Leukemia Group B study. *Proc Am Soc Clin Oncol* 2002;21:355a.
37. Rinaldo JE, Owens GR, Rogers RM. Adult respiratory distress syndrome following intrapleural instillation of talc. *J Thorac Cardiovasc Surg* 1983;85:523.
38. Bouchama A, Chastre J, Gaudichet A, Soler P, Gibert C. Acute pneumonitis with bilateral pleural effusion after talc pleurodesis. *Chest* 1984;86:795.
39. Rusch VW, Figlin R, Godwin D, Piantadosi S. Intrapleural cisplatin and cytarabine in the management of malignant pleural effusions: a Lung Cancer Study Group trial. *J Clin Oncol* 1991;9:313.
40. Masuno T, Kishimoto S, Ogura T, et al. A comparative trial of LC9018 plus doxorubicin and doxorubicin alone for the treatment of malignant pleural effusion secondary to lung cancer. *Cancer* 1991;68:1495.
41. Holoye PY, Jeffries DG, Dhingra HM, et al. Intrapleural etoposide for malignant effusion. *Cancer Chemother Pharmacol* 1990;26:147.
42. Belani CP, Pajeau TS, Bennett CL. Treating malignant pleural effusions cost consciously. *Chest* 1998;113:78S.
43. Soysal O, Karaoglanoglu N, Demiracan S, et al. Pleurectomy/decortication for palliation in malignant pleural mesothelioma: results of surgery. *Eur J Cardiothorac Surg* 1997;11:210.
44. Waller DA, Morritt GN, Forty J. Video-assisted thoracoscopic pleurectomy in the management of malignant pleural effusion. *Chest* 1995;107:1454.
45. Harvey JC, Erdman CB, Beattie EJ. Early experience with videothoracoscopic hydrodissection pleurectomy in the treatment of malignant pleural effusion. *J Surg Oncol* 1995;59:243.
46. Petrou M, Kaplan D, Goldstraw P. Management of recurrent malignant pleural effusions. The complementary role of talc pleurodesis and pleuroperitoneal shunting. *Cancer* 1995;75:801.
47. Ponn RB, Blancafor J, D'Agostino RS, et al. Pleuroperitoneal shunting for intractable pleural effusions. *Ann Thorac Surg* 1991;51:605.
48. Putnam JB Jr, Light RW, Rodriguez RM, et al. A randomized comparison of indwelling pleural catheter and doxycycline pleurodesis in the management of malignant pleural effusions. *Cancer* 1999;86:1992.
49. Putnam JB Jr, Walsh GL, Swisher SG, et al. Outpatient management of malignant pleural effusion by a chronic indwelling pleural catheter. *Ann Thorac Surg* 2000;69:369.
50. Fincher RM. Case report: malignant pericardial effusion as the initial manifestation of malignancy. *Am J Med Sci* 1993;305:106.

51. Shepherd FA, Morgan C, Evans WK, et al. Medical management of malignant pericardial effusion by tetracycline sclerosis. *Am J Cardiol* 1987;60:1161.

52. Chong HH, Plotnick GD. Pericardial effusion and tamponade: evaluation, imaging modalities, and management. *Compr Ther* 1995;21:378.

53. Johnson FE, Wolverson MK, Sundaram M, Heiberg E. Unsuspected malignant pericardial effusion causing cardiac tamponade. Rapid diagnosis by computed tomography. *Chest* 1982;82:501.

54. Wiener HG, Kristensen IB, Haubek A, Kristensen B, Baandrup U. The diagnostic value of pericardial cytology. An analysis of 95 cases. *Acta Cytol* 1991;35:149.

55. Press OW, Livingston R. Management of malignant pericardial effusion and tamponade. *JAMA* 1987;257:1088.

56. Allen KB, Faber LP, Warren WH, Shaar CJ. Pericardial effusion: subxiphoid pericardiostomy versus percutaneous catheter drainage. *Ann Thorac Surg* 1999;67:437.

57. Piehler JM, Pluth JR, Schaff HV, et al. Surgical management of effusive pericardial disease. Influence of extent of pericardial resection on clinical course. *J Thorac Cardiovasc Surg* 1985;90:506.

58. Naunheim KS, Kesler KA, Fiore AC, et al. Pericardial drainage: subxiphoid vs. transthoracic approach. *Eur J Cardiothorac Surg* 1991;5:99.

59. Park JS, Rentschler R, Wilbur D. Surgical management of pericardial effusion in patients with malignancies. Comparison of subxiphoid window versus pericardiectomy. *Cancer* 1991;67:76.

60. Liu HP, Chang CH, Lin PJ, et al. Thoracoscopic management of effusive pericardial disease: indications and technique. *Ann Thorac Surg* 1994;58:1695.

61. Mack MJ, Landreneau RJ, Hazelrigg SR, Acuff TE. Videothoracoscopic management of benign and malignant pericardial effusion. *Chest* 1993;103:390.

62. Hazelrigg SR, Mack MJ, Landreneau RJ, et al. Thoracoscopic pericardiectomy for effusive pericardial disease. *Ann Thorac Surg* 1993;56:792.

63. Yim AP, Ho JK. Video-assisted subxiphoid pericardiectomy. *J Laparoendosc Surg* 1995;5:193.

64. Wang N, Feikes JR, Mogensen T, Vyhmeister EE, Bailey LL. Pericardioperitoneal shunt: an alternative treatment for malignant pericardial effusion. *Ann Thorac Surg* 1994;57:289.

65. Maher EA, Shepherd FA, Todd TJ. Pericardial sclerosis as the primary management of malignant pericardial effusion and cardiac tamponade. *J Thorac Cardiovasc Surg* 1996;112:637.

66. Vaitkus PT, Herrmann HC, LeWinter MM. Treatment of malignant pericardial effusion. *JAMA* 1994;272:59.

67. Celermajer DS, Boyer MJ, Bailey BP, Tattersall MH. Pericardiocentesis for symptomatic malignant pericardial effusion: a study of 36 patients. *Med J Aust* 1991;154:19.

68. Callahan JA, Seward JB, Nishimura RA, et al. Two-dimensional echocardiographically guided pericardiocentesis: experience in 117 consecutive patients. *Am J Cardiol* 1985;55:476.

69. Clarke DP, Cosgrove DO. Real-time ultrasound scanning in the planning and guidance of pericardiocentesis. *Clin Radiol* 1987;38:119.

70. Liu G, Crump M, Goss PE, Dancey J, Shepherd FA. Prospective comparison of the sclerosing agents doxycycline and bleomycin for the primary management of malignant pericardial effusion and cardiac tamponade. *J Clin Oncol* 1996;14:3141.

71. Ziskind AA, Pearce AC, Lemmon CC, et al. Percutaneous balloon pericardiotomy for the treatment of cardiac tamponade and large pericardial effusions: description of technique and report of the first 50 cases. *J Am Coll Cardiol* 1993;21:1.

72. Yim AP, Chan AT, Lee TW, Wan IY, Ho JK. Thoracoscopic talc insufflation versus talc slurry for symptomatic malignant pleural effusion. *Ann Thorac Surg* 1996;62:1655.

73. Zimmer PW, Hill M, Casey K, Harvey E, Low DE. Prospective randomized trial of talc slurry vs bleomycin in pleurodesis for symptomatic malignant pleural effusions. *Chest* 1997;112:430.

74. McDonald JM, Meyers BF, Guthrie TJ, et al. Comparison of open subxiphoid pericardial drainage with percutaneous catheter drainage for symptomatic pericardial effusion. *Ann Thorac Surg* 2003;76:811.

75. Moores DW, Allen KB, Faber LP, et al. Subxiphoid pericardial drainage for pericardial tamponade. *J Thorac Cardiovasc Surg* 1995;109:546.

76. Okamoto H, Shinkai T, Yamakido M, Saijo N. Cardiac tamponade caused by primary lung cancer and the management of pericardial effusion. *Cancer* 1993;71:93.

77. Chan A, Rischin D, Clarke CP, Woodruff RK. Subxiphoid partial pericardiectomy with or without sclerosant instillation in the treatment of symptomatic pericardial effusions in patients with malignancy. *Cancer* 1991;68:1021.

78. Sugimoto JT, Little AG, Ferguson MK, et al. Pericardial window: mechanisms of efficacy. *Ann Thorac Surg* 1990;50:442.

79. Reitknecht F, Regal AM, Antkowiak JG, Takita H. Management of cardiac tamponade in patients with malignancy. *J Surg Oncol* 1985;30:19.

80. Ghosh SC, Larrieu AJ, Ablaza SG, Grana VP. Clinical experience with subxiphoid pericardial decompression. *Int Surg* 1985;70:5.

81. Levin BH, Aaron BL. The subxiphoid pericardial window. *Surg Gynecol Obstet* 1982;155:804.

82. Prager RL, Wilson CH, Bender HW Jr. The subxiphoid approach to pericardial disease. *Ann Thorac Surg* 1982;34:6.

83. Santos GH, Frater RWN. The subxiphoid approach in the treatment of pericardial effusion. *Ann Thorac Surg* 1977;23:477.

84. Di Segni E, Lavee J, Kaplinsky E, Vered Z. Percutaneous balloon pericardiostomy for treatment of cardiac tamponade. *Eur Heart J* 1995;16:184.

85. Kopecky SL, Callahan JA, Tajik AJ, Seward JB. Percutaneous pericardial catheter drainage: report of 42 consecutive cases. *Am J Cardiol* 1986;58:633.

RICHARD B. HOSTETTER
FRANCESCO M. MARINCOLA
DOUGLAS J. SCHWARTZENTRUBER

SECTION 6

Malignant Ascites

The development of intraperitoneal fluid in a patient with known cancer is most likely due to intraperitoneal spread of the disease. If neoplastic cells are identified in the fluid, the term *malignant ascites* is used. This finding has multiple implications:

1. The recognition of small quantities of intraperitoneal fluid may have staging and prognostic significance and alter a planned surgical intervention.

2. If the ascites is giving rise to clinical symptoms, palliative options should be considered even though this may reflect end-stage disease.

3. The presence of malignant ascites does not always imply shortened survival and may be part of a clinical picture amenable to curative efforts.

In such cases as lymphoma and ovarian cancer, strategies aimed at obtaining regression of tumor and prolongation of survival should be considered.

The therapeutic approaches used to treat patients with malignant ascites include extensive surgical debulking in preparation for local or systemic chemotherapy,[1,2] intracavitary chemotherapy with or without hyperthermia,[2–9] phototherapy,[10] instillation of biologic response modifiers,[11–18] and intracavitary particle irradiation.[19] Although prolongation of survival has been attributed to some of these therapies, no definitive study has ever demonstrated effectiveness or superiority of one strategy over the other.[20] It is possible that the lack of randomized clinical trials reflects the skepticism of many investigators about the therapeutic effectiveness of available options and the desire to explore new treatment modalities in the context of phase I or phase II studies.

DIAGNOSIS AND WORKUP

Abdominal distention and changes in abdominal girth are classic symptoms of ascites (Table 51.6-1). Signs of ascites include dullness to percussion, shifting dullness, and fluid wave. These signs may be totally absent in smaller effusions (100 mL or less) diagnosed incidentally during workup for malignancy. Ultrasonography, computerized tomography, or endoscopic ultrasonography[21] may be useful to guide probes into small fluid collections for diagnostic purposes. The widespread availability of laparoscopy in staging of abdominal cancers has increased the accuracy of determining malignant ascites and peritoneal disease.[22]

Nonneoplastic causes of ascites include congestive heart failure, liver failure, renal or pancreatic disease, hypoproteinemia, chylous ascites from trauma or surgery, infectious processes, and benign gynecologic conditions, such as endometriosis. Malignant

TABLE 51.6-1. Assessment of the Patient with Ascites: Diagnosis and Workup

HISTORY
Increasing abdominal girth—"clothes don't fit"
Ingestion and early satiety
Ankle swelling
Easy fatigability
Shortness of breath
PHYSICAL EXAMINATION
Fluid wave
Shifting dullness
RADIOGRAPHIC STUDIES
Abdominal flat plate: generalized ground-glass appearance; air-filled small bowel loops occupy central position and are separated by fluid between loops; and psoas shadows obscured
Ultrasonography, abdominal computed tomography: both are sensitive tests that definitively diagnose small amounts of ascites
PARACENTESIS
Gross character on inspection: bloody, serous, milky, and turbid
Cell count and differential
Chemistries: total protein, lactic dehydrogenase, carcinoembryonic antigen, CA-125, amylase, and bilirubin
Cytologic analysis
Microbiologic analysis: Gram stain and culture
LAPAROSCOPY
When cytologic results are negative yet a high suspicion of malignancy
To gain access to minimal fluid collections
To evaluate for staging and curative intent of therapy

ascites represents approximately 10% of all cases of ascites.[23] In children, rarely is malignancy the cause of ascitic fluid.[23] Approximately one-third of patients with known malignancy have nonmalignant causes of ascites.[24] In a patient with advanced cancer, however, the ascites is most likely malignant. A peritoneal tap is indicated when a definitive diagnosis of malignant ascites is necessary for staging purposes or when surgical resection is planned based on the stage of the disease. Other indications may include determining the presence of malignant ascites in cancer patients with no known intraperitoneal disease or in cryptogenic ascites. This applies particularly to female patients because of the high likelihood of a gynecologic primary that may benefit from tumor debulking followed by systemic or locoregional therapy.[25]

The ascitic fluid should be evaluated by performing a cell count, various chemical analyses, and measurement of tumor and cytologic markers (see Table 51.6-1; Table 51.6-2). Fifty milli-

TABLE 51.6-2. Tools for the Evaluation of Malignant Serous Effusions

Standard biochemical and cytologic determinations
    Ascites/serum ratio for protein, lactic dehydrogenase, fibronectin, cholesterol, erythrocyte and leukocyte count, cultures, Papanicolaou stain of pelleted ascites[26,28,87,88]
Immunochemical stains
    Carcinoembryonic antigen, CA-125, urokinase receptor, human chorionic gonadotropin, vascular endothelial growth factor, estrogen and progesterone receptors[29,30,89–92]
Endoscopic ultrasonographically guided fine-needle aspiration of ascitic fluid
    Small effusions noted during endoscopic ultrasonography[21]
Laparoscopic evaluation and biopsy
    Most sensitive test for ascites of unknown origin[33]

liters of fluid is generally sufficient to collect enough cells for cytologic evaluation; if no cancer cells are found in this amount of fluid, additional volume will generally not be more informative. A serous (rather than bloody) character of the fluid suggests a hydraulic cause such as portal hypertension, cardiac failure, nephrotic syndrome, reduced oncotic pressure, or pancreatic ascites. Infection is generally associated with other systemic symptoms. Tubercular and malignant ascites may be particularly difficult to differentiate because several markers express similar patterns, with the notable exception of the presence of cholesterol.[24,26] The presence of chylous fluid can be related to obstruction or injury of large retroperitoneal lymphatic channels such as is seen with extensive intraabdominal lymphomas, after external-beam radiotherapy,[27] or after surgery.

Peritoneal fluid cytologic examination yields a diagnosis in a large proportion of cases.[24] The presence of elevated ascitic fluid to serum ratios of protein or lactic dehydrogenase, carcinoembryonic antigen, CA-125, fibronectin, cholesterol, human chorionic gonadotropin, or vascular endothelial growth factor favors neoplasm.[26,28–30]

Approximately 20% of patients with malignant ascites present without an identified primary cause.[31] In these patients, particularly in women, attempts to identify the tumor of origin should be undertaken, because the identification of the primary histologic type may influence the treatment strategy.[25] Approximately 75% of women presenting with malignant ascites of unknown origin have a gynecologic source (ovary, uterus, or cervix) and another 10% have a gastrointestinal origin, whereas in men gastrointestinal primaries predominate.[25,31,32] Laparoscopy and biopsy have been useful in identifying the cause of ascites when results of cytologic analysis are negative.[22] In 129 patients with an unknown primary laparoscopy identified carcinomatosis in 60%[33] and laparoscopy with peritoneal biopsy was able to establish the cause of ascites in 86% of these cases. Laparoscopy has been rarely associated with prolonged leak from the port site[33] or port site recurrence and is considered a safe tool for the evaluation of ascites.

TREATMENT OF MALIGNANT ASCITES

Because the pathogenesis of malignant ascites differs from the pathogenesis of most benign ascites, the treatment is often different in many respects.[25] Hormonal changes in the renin-angiotensin-aldosterone system,[34] changes in cytokines giving rise to vascular permeability,[34,35] and obstruction of lymphatic channels[36,37] are believed to be the most relevant factors inducing malignant ascites. Because most of the time there is no underlying venous obstruction or portal hypertension, vascular shunting procedures are not indicated. Many strategies have been used to achieve palliation, because the presence of malignant ascites is perceived as a sign of incurable disease. Paracentesis can effectively palliate the symptoms of malignant ascites.[38] A survey of practicing physicians suggested that the most common means of managing malignant ascites was paracentesis, and it was also felt to be the most effective.[20] After paracentesis, diuretics and peritoneovenous shunting were most commonly used. In particular cases, radical surgical procedures or aggressive intracavitary therapies have been advocated; however, to date few prospective randomized trials have been performed to compare alternative treatments. The encouraging results reported by many phase I or II studies involving intracavitary instillation of chemotherapeutic agents have generally not matured into randomized phase III trials.

The median survival of patients with symptomatic malignant ascites is approximately 2 months.[25] In general, for nonovarian malignant ascites, the focus is on palliation of symptoms.[39] Patients with malignant ascites secondary to ovarian cancer represent an exception because they have a significantly better survival.[40] Patients with large-volume nonovarian malignant ascites have a high mortality (41%) after major abdominal surgery. For these patients, Yazdi et al.[41] have suggested intraperitoneal chemotherapy or peritoneovenous shunt placement at the time of the abdominal operation.

According to Souter et al.,[42] a patient with malignant ascites whose only considered therapeutic goal is palliation should first undergo repeated paracentesis and medical management with diuretics. If the rate of reaccumulation of fluid is rapid, the fluid is not viscous or bloody, there is no evidence of intracavitary loculation,[43] and the expected survival time is longer than 3 months, shunting should be considered. Contraindications for placement of a shunt are the presence of intraperitoneal infection and cardiac or renal insufficiency. Cairns and Malone,[44] in a case report of three patients, noted that the subcutaneous administration of octreotide at dosages of 200 to 600 μg/d reduced pain and ascites formation in a palliative setting.

DIURESIS AND RESTRICTION OF SALT AND FLUID INTAKE

The use of diuretics and restriction of salt and fluid intake are generally the initial therapy for malignant ascites. Oral diuretics are effective in approximately one-third of patients but often at much higher than usual dosages.[34] Pockros et al.[45] noted that cancer patients with portal hypertension–related ascites caused by massive hepatic metastases were most likely to experience palliation when treated with diuretics.

REPEATED PARACENTESIS AND EXTERNAL DRAINS

Repeated abdominal drainage may palliate symptoms of malignant ascites. Gough et al.[46] reported no difference in survival and quality of life between patients treated with repeated abdominal paracentesis and patients treated with peritoneovenous shunts. It is possible to remove up to 5 L of fluid at a time and allow drainage for up to 6 hours at a time with minimal adverse events.[47] However, several concerns are raised by this approach, including the risk of infection, electrolyte and fluid imbalances secondary to the sudden depletion of body fluids, and the risk of intraperitoneal visceral injury. For this reason and for convenience, many catheters and techniques have been developed to provide long-term percutaneous access for repeated drainage of ascites.[48–54] Although good palliation can be achieved in this fashion, the life span of these drains is limited by the need for removal due to malfunction or infection. Lorentzen et al.[55] have reported the use of ultrasonographically guided insertion of peritoneogastric shunts in patients with malignant ascites using a Denver shunt connected to a gastrostomy tube. This technique allows intermittent removal of fluid, which, on pumping, is shunted through the gastrostomy tube to the stomach. Others have advocated peritoneal-urinary drainage for the treatment of refractory

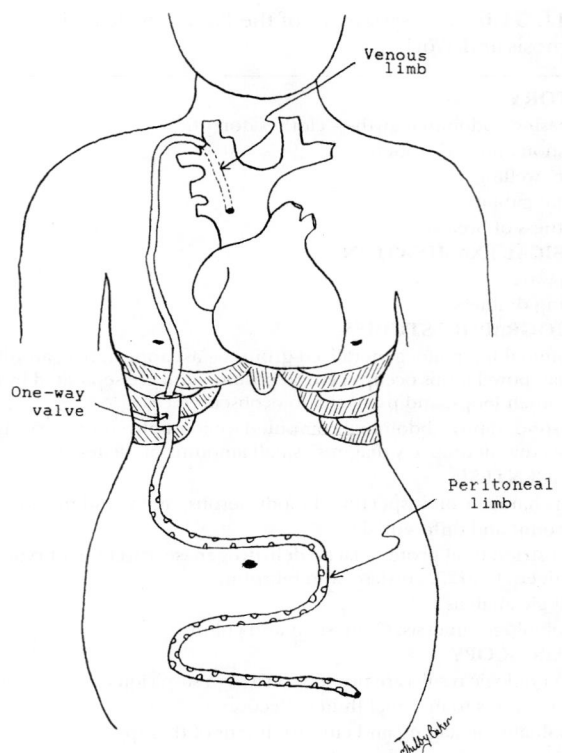

FIGURE 51.6-1.   The peritoneovenous shunt *in situ.*

ascites.[56] These methods have been used less frequently than external drains (in which the ascitic fluid is totally removed from the body) and peritoneovenous shunts (returning the drained fluid from the peritoneal cavity directly to the intravascular space).

PERITONEOVENOUS SHUNTING

The application of shunting procedures to the treatment of malignant ascites has been reported by many authors in many countries.[34,39,57–65] Patients with symptomatic malignant ascites may gain significant benefit from internal peritoneovenous shunting. The devices consist of (1) a length of multiply perforated tubing to be inserted into the free peritoneal cavity, (2) a length of tubing to be inserted into the superior vena cava (or other large venous vessel), and (3) a unidirectional flow valve connecting the two limbs (Fig. 51.6-1). The two most popular devices are the LeVeen shunt and the Denver shunt. The latter has a one-way pump that can be pumped manually by the patient or physician to clear debris. Briefly, the functioning of the shunt takes advantage of the pressure gradient (5 to 15 cm H_2O) existing between the abdominal and thoracic cavities. On inspiration, the further increase in pressure gradient (due to increased negative pressure within the thorax) drains fluid from the abdominal cavity by allowing the unidirectional valve to open. The surgical procedure for the placement of the shunt can be performed under local or general anesthesia. Prophylactic antibiotic coverage is recommended as with the placement of any prosthetic material. In the traditional approach, a muscle-splitting subcostal incision is made and the intraperitoneal portion of the shunt is placed using a nonabsorbable purse-

TABLE 51.6-3.   Patient Survival after Peritoneovenous Shunting

	Underlying Malignancy			Patient Survival	
	Ovarian	GI	Other	Median (Wk)	% Alive at 1 Y
Summary for studies published before 1985	85	52	99	5–16	0–12
Recent investigations (published since 1985)					
Kostroff et al., 1985[62]	11	8	12	8	0
Campioni et al., 1986[93]	8	14	20	7	7
Sonnenfeld and Tyden, 1986[63]	—	16	11	8	0
Roussel et al., 1986[94]	12	10	14	13	0
Soderlund, 1986[64]	7	15	2	7	4
Shepherd and Miller, 1988[95]	2	8	4	6	7
Edney et al., 1989[96]	8	24	13	33	13
Smith et al., 1989[97]	3	23	24	22	4
Holm et al., 1989[68]	1	7	5	NA	0
Gough and Balderson, 1993[46]	9	13	20	20	NA
Schumacher et al., 1994[65]	17	34	38	10	NA
Faught et al., 1995[98]	21	—	4	11	NA
Wickremesekera and Stubbs, 1997[99]	—	21	—	22	NA
Bieligk et al, 2001[39]	0	16	35	7	NA
Zanon et al., 2002[58]	13	29	—	19	NA
Total	197	290	301	5–33	0–13

GI, gastrointestinal (colon, stomach, pancreas, hepatobiliary); NA, not available.

string suture to secure the limb in a watertight fashion. Current product guidelines describe the percutaneous insertion of the peritoneal catheter using a peel-away introducer if allowed by the patient's anatomy. A second incision is made in the neck or groin to expose the internal jugular vein or femoral vein, respectively, in which the venous portion of the shunt will be introduced. Alternatively, the venous catheter may be inserted percutaneously into the subclavian vein. A subcutaneous pocket is fashioned for the pump (over the lower rib cage in the case of a Denver shunt) and a subcutaneous tunnel is developed linking the abdominal and venous incisions. The venous limb is passed through the tunnel and introduced into the central venous system according to the chosen technique. Before placement of the intravenous portion of the shunt, the flow of ascitic fluid through the device needs to be demonstrated to exclude malpositioning or kinking within the abdominal cavity. It is recommended that a portion of the ascites be discarded before placing the venous limb to avoid the dangers of volume overload and early disseminated intravascular coagulation.

The median survival of 788 patients with refractory malignant ascites (gastrointestinal primary in 37%, ovarian primary in 25%, and other malignancies in 38%) undergoing placement of a peritoneovenous shunt was 5 to 33 weeks with 0% to 13% of patients alive at 1 year (Table 51.6-3). Variables such as protein content and number of neoplastic cells in the ascitic fluid[43] have accounted for differences in shunt function and patient survival. The most common limitation of the shunt is in bloody ascites, because the limbs of the shunt frequently become occluded and malfunction early. Immediate postinsertion complications related to placement of the peritoneovenous shunt include shunt malfunction due to technical reasons and pulmonary congestion due to sudden flow of ascitic fluid within the intravascular space.[62,66] Checking the position of the device radiographically before ending the surgical procedure can prevent malfunction; fluid overload can be prevented by discarding a significant portion of ascitic fluid at the time of placement of the shunt.[67,68] Careful preoperative

patient selection and postoperative monitoring of fluid and electrolyte balance are important to minimize this complication. Disseminated intravascular coagulation after shunt placement is a rare event in malignant ascites compared to cirrhotic ascites.[69] However, the coexistence of liver malfunction (e.g., liver metastases) may enhance the risk of coagulopathy.[70] The development of a coagulopathy after placement of a shunt needs to be managed according to standard treatment for this condition. A common postoperative symptom associated with placement of a peritoneovenous shunt is fever, and it should not be considered by itself as a sign of sepsis.[60,62,71] Finally, a rare complication of placement of a peritoneovenous shunt is the development of pulmonary tumor embolization with a possibly fatal outcome.[72]

A significant proportion of shunts stop functioning before the patient's demise because of occlusion, which is independent of the type of device used.[46,61–63,66,68] Although the Denver shunt provides a pump that allows manual flushing at periodic intervals, the literature has failed to demonstrate the functional superiority of this device. It has been reported, however, that flushing of the Denver shunt combined with the administration of thrombolytic agents can occasionally restore shunt function.[66] Relocation of the catheter is usually necessary to establish patency, because thrombolytic agents are infrequently successful in this situation. The goal in reestablishing flow in the system is to correct the source of the problem and avoid replacement of the entire shunt. Shunt malfunction is usually manifested by recurrence of ascites and can be confirmed by failure to visualize technetium 99m macroaggregate albumin in the lungs after intraperitoneal injection of the nucleotide.[73] A shuntogram recorded after percutaneous injection of radiographic contrast agent into the venous limb of the shunt (into the pump reservoir if a Denver shunt) helps determine the site of obstruction. The authors previously described shunt occlusion by thrombofibrinous encasement of the venous limb, which manifests as a characteristic contrast outline of the tubing on shuntogram.[74]

Another complication of peritoneovenous shunt placement is infection in the peritoneal cavity. The development of spontaneous bacterial peritonitis unrelated to operative infection or to perforation of a viscous due to the malignant process is, for unknown reasons, less likely in patients with malignant ascites than in patients with cirrhotic ascites. Evidence of hematologic dissemination of tumor cells from the ascitic fluid and tumor growth along the shunt tract has been reported and is likely to occur relatively often.[61,72,75,76] However, this theoretical risk has not been a clinical problem, most likely because of the limited survival of these patients.

To avoid the massive fluid shifts associated with drainage of refractory ascites, Daimon et al. proposed the use of extracorporeal ultrafiltration of the ascites followed by intravenous reinjection of the ultrafiltered fluid.[77] Among the patients treated in this fashion, two had malignant ascites. This approach was well tolerated, and both patients died of their primary disease free of symptoms related to ascites. The added cost, equipment, and time necessary to perform this procedure, however, make it impractical.

INTRACAVITARY THERAPY

Intracavitary therapies have attempted to target the source of ascites production. Platinum-based drugs used alone or in combination with other agents have been some of the more commonly used chemotherapeutic agents for the treatment of peritoneal carcinomatosis. Hyperthermia has been used to enhance the local effectiveness of intraperitoneally administered chemotherapy. Some have added intravenous thiosulfate and other vasoactive drugs to diminish the side effects related to systemic absorption of the chemotherapy. Park et al.[2] reported their experience in treating 18 patients with primary peritoneal mesothelioma with continuous hyperthermic peritoneal perfusion and cisplatin. Nine of ten patients with ascites had resolution of their ascites postoperatively. The median progression-free survival in this study was 26 months and the overall 2-year survival was 80%, superior to the survival reported in historical controls. Gilly et al. reported resolution of malignant ascites in 11 of 12 patients with ovarian or digestive cancer treated with intraperitoneal chemotherapy and hyperthermia consisting of either cisplatin or mitomycin C after surgical resection of bulk disease.[5] Patients had a median survival of 11.2 months. Loggie et al. reported a median survival of 7.6 months in 39 patients with malignant ascites of gastrointestinal origin treated with cytoreductive surgery and intraperitoneal hyperthermic chemotherapy with mitomycin C.[9] Patients undergoing the same therapy in this study but without ascites (n = 45) had a significantly higher median survival of 27.7 months. The operative mortality in this study was low (6%), and 79% of 39 patients with malignant ascites did not have recurrence of their ascites postoperatively. Complete resolution of massive malignant ascites from various causes was reported by Ben Ari et al. in 38 of 41 patients undergoing continuous hyperthermic peritoneal perfusion and cisplatinum-based chemotherapy.[8] The mean duration of response was 10 months. Other authors have addressed the use of hyperthermia in combination with local chemotherapy for the treatment of peritoneal malignancies and control of ascites with similar results.[6,7]

Biologic response modifiers have been used as an alternative to chemotherapeutic agents for the treatment of intraperitoneal carcinomatosis. Therapy with single-agent interferon-α,[11,13,16] interferon-β,[78] OK-432 streptococcal preparation,[18] bispecific antibody HEA125xOKT3,[14] tumor necrosis factor,[79] and interleukin-2 with or without adoptive administration of lymphokine-activated killer cells[12,15,78] has been reported with variable success. A randomized trial has compared the effectiveness of interleukin-2, interferon-α, or interferon-β for the control of malignant effusions. Results suggested a higher efficacy for interleukin-2, particularly in patients with mesothelioma.[78] Others have reported effectiveness of the combined intraperitoneal administration of interleukin-2 and OK-432 in patients with ascites secondary to gastric malignancy.[80] The authors reported cytologic disappearance of cancer and decrease of ascites in 81% of 22 evaluable patients. Phase I studies of adoptive cellular immunotherapy with intraperitoneal injection of activated human blood monocytes have shown the feasibility of this approach.[81] Triamcinolone hexacetonide, a slowly metabolized corticosteroid, was prospectively used in 12 patients and produced a delay in repeat paracentesis.[17] Ng et al.[82] report a successful case of intraperitoneal rituximab therapy for refractory ascites in low-grade small cell lymphoma with a response duration of 8 months. Radioiodinated monoclonal antibodies directed against tumor markers have also been used.[83]

RADICAL SURGERY

Peritonectomy is an extensive surgical debulking procedure in preparation for intraperitoneal chemotherapy advocated by Sugarbaker et al.[1] The authors reported good long-term results in selected patients affected with peritoneal carcinomatosis, sarcomatosis, and mesothelioma.[84–86] A pilot study by Sindelar et al.[10] describing the use of photodynamic therapy as adjuvant treatment after aggressive debulking of disseminated intraperitoneal malignancies has shown a 26% disease-free survival rate at 18 months. These approaches have been used in selected patients and have not been commonly applied for the treatment of malignant ascites.

CONCLUSION

In summary, malignant ascites represents in most instances a debilitating symptom of end-stage cancer. Purely palliative measures on one extreme and aggressive therapeutic intervention on the other represent the wide range of treatment options. Reported survival of patients treated with curative intent, in general, is better than that of patients undergoing palliative procedures but clearly reflects differences in patient selection (differences in disease stage, histologic type, extent of disease, etc.). Few definitive studies have been performed to evaluate the treatment of malignant ascites. Many questions remain unanswered, such as the value of a peritoneovenous shunt insertion compared to medical management or intermittent drainage, the role of external versus internal drains, and the effectiveness of locoregional curative efforts. The best treatment approach remains one that is individualized to each patient, is multidisciplinary, and is palliative.

REFERENCES

1. Sugarbaker PH. Peritonectomy procedures. *Ann Surg* 1995;221:29.
2. Park BJ, Alexander HR, Libutti SK, et al. Treatment of primary peritoneal mesothelioma by continuous hyperthermic peritoneal perfusion (CHPP). *Ann Surg Oncol* 1999;6:582.
3. Markman M, Howell SB, Lucas WE, Pfeifle CE, Green MR. Combination intraperitoneal chemotherapy with cisplatin, cytarabine, and doxorubicin for refractory ovarian carci-

noma and other malignancies principally confined to the peritoneal cavity. *J Clin Oncol* 1984;2:1321.

4. McClay EF, Howell SB. Intraperitoneal therapy in the management of patients with ovarian cancer. *Hematol Oncol Clin North Am* 1992;6:915.

5. Gilly FN, Carry PY, Brachet A, et al Treatment of malignant peritoneal effusion in digestive and ovarian cancer. *Med Oncol Tumor Pharmacother* 1992;9:177.

6. Sayag AC, Gilly FN, Carry PY, et al. Intraoperative chemohyperthermia in the management of digestive cancers. A general review of literature. *Oncology* 1993;50:333.

7. Fujimoto S, Shrestha RD, Kokubun M, et al. Positive results of combined therapy of surgery and intraperitoneal hyperthermic perfusion for far-advanced gastric cancer. *Ann Surg* 1990;212:592.

8. Ben Ari G, Scott D, Zippel D, et al. Continuous hyperthermic peritoneal perfusion (CHPP) for malignant ascites and irresectable intra-abdominal cancer. *Gan To Kagaku Ryoho* 2000;27[Suppl 2]:436.

9. Loggie BW, Fleming RA, McQuellon RP, Russell GB, Geisinger KR. Cytoreductive surgery with intraperitoneal hyperthermic chemotherapy for disseminated peritoneal cancer of gastrointestinal origin. *Am Surg* 2000;66:561.

10. Sindelar WF, DeLaney TF, Tochner Z, et al. Technique of photodynamic therapy for disseminated intraperitoneal malignant neoplasms. Phase I study. *Arch Surg* 1991;126:318.

11. Bezwoda WR, Seymour L, Dansey R. Intraperitoneal recombinant interferon-alpha 2b for recurrent malignant ascites due to ovarian cancer. *Cancer* 1989;64:1029.

12. Steis RG, Urba WJ, VanderMolen LA, et al. Intraperitoneal lymphokine-activated killer-cell and interleukin-2 therapy for malignancies limited to the peritoneal cavity. *J Clin Oncol* 1990;8:1618.

13. Stuart GC, Nation JG, Snider DD, Thunberg P. Intraperitoneal interferon in the management of malignant ascites. *Cancer* 1993;71:2027.

14. Marme A, Strauss G, Bastert G, Grischke EM, Moldenhauer G. Intraperitoneal bispecific antibody (HEA125xOKT3) therapy inhibits malignant ascites production in advanced ovarian carcinoma. *Int J Cancer* 2002;101:183.

15. Lissoni P, Mandala M, Curigliano G, et al. Progress report on the palliative therapy of 100 patients with neoplastic effusions by intracavitary low-dose interleukin-2. *Oncology* 2001;60:308.

16. Sartori S, Nielsen I, Tassinari D, et al. Evaluation of a standardized protocol of intracavitary recombinant interferon alpha-2b in the palliative treatment of malignant peritoneal effusions. A prospective pilot study. *Oncology* 2001;61:192.

17. Mackey JR, Wood L, Nabholtz J, Jensen J, Venner P. A phase II trial of triamcinolone hexacetonide for symptomatic recurrent malignant ascites. *J Pain Symptom Manage* 2000;19:193.

18. Kageyama Y, Sakai Y, Arai G, et al. Intracavitary administration of OK-432 with subcutaneous priming for malignant ascites in a case of advanced renal cell carcinoma. *Int J Urol* 2002;9:57.

19. Jackson GL, Blosser NM. Intracavitary chromic phosphate (32-P) colloidal suspension therapy. *Cancer* 1981;48:2596.

20. Lee CW, Bociek G, Faught W. A survey of practice in management of malignant ascites. *J Pain Symptom Manage* 1998;16:96.

21. Chang KJ, Albers CG, Nguyen P. Endoscopic ultrasound-guided fine needle aspiration of pleural and ascitic fluid. *Am J Gastroenterol* 1995;90:148.

22. Roskos M, Popp MB. Laparoscopic diagnosis and management of malignant ascites. *Surg Laparosc Endosc Percutan Tech* 1999;9:365.

23. Runyon BA. Care of patients with ascites. *N Engl J Med* 1994;330:337.

24. Runyon BA. Malignancy-related ascites and ascitic fluid humoral tests of malignancy [Editorial]. *J Clin Gastroenterol* 1994;18:94.

25. Parsons SL, Watson SA, Steele RJC. Malignant ascites. *Br J Surg* 1996;83:6.

26. Sood A, Garg R, Kumar R, et al. Ascitic fluid cholesterol in malignant and tubercular ascites. *J Assoc Physicians India* 1995;43:745.

27. Lentz SS, Schray MF, Wilson TO. Chylous ascites after whole-abdomen irradiation for gynecologic malignancy. *Int J Radiat Oncol Biol Phys* 1990;19:435.

28. Bansai S, Kaur K, Bansai AK. Diagnosing ascitic etiology on a biochemical basis. *Hepatogastroenterology* 1998;45:1673.

29. Grossmann M, Hoermann R, Gocze PM, et al. Measurement of human chorionic gonadotropin–related immunoreactivity in serum, ascites and tumour cysts of patients with gynaecologic malignancies. *Eur J Clin Invest* 1995;25:867.

30. Zebrowski BK, Liu W, Ramirez K, et al. Markedly elevated levels of vascular endothelial growth factor in malignant ascites. *Ann Surg Oncol* 1999;6:373.

31. Ringenberg QS, Doll DC, Loy TS, Yarbro JW. Malignant ascites of unknown origin. *Cancer* 1989;64:753.

32. Wilailak S, Linasmita V, Srivannaboon S. Malignant ascites in female patients: a seven year review. *J Med Assoc Thai* 1999;82:15.

33. Chu CM, Lin SM, Peng SM, Wu CS, Liaw YF. The role of laparoscopy in the evaluation of ascites of unknown origin. *Gastrointest Endosc* 1994;40:285.

34. Smith EM, Jayson GC. The current and future management of malignant ascites. *Clin Oncol (R Coll Radiol)* 2003;15:59.

35. Aslam N, Marino CR. Malignant ascites: new concepts in pathophysiology, diagnosis, and management. *Arch Intern Med* 2001;161:2733.

36. Feldman GB, Knapp RC. Lymphatic drainage of the peritoneal cavity and its significance in ovarian cancer. *Am J Obstet Gynecol* 1974;119:991.

37. Coates G, Bush RS, Aspin N. A study of ascites using lymphoscintigraphy with 99m Tc-sulfur colloid. *Radiology* 1973;107:577.

38. McNamara P. Paracentesis—an effective method of symptom control in the palliative care setting? *Palliat Med* 2000;14:62.

39. Bieligk SC, Calvo BF, Coit DG. Peritoneovenous shunting for nongynecologic malignant ascites. *Cancer* 2001;91:1247.

40. Loggie BW, Perini M, Fleming RA, Russell GB, Geisenger K. Treatment and prevention of malignant ascites associated with disseminated intraperitoneal malignancies by aggressive combined-modality therapy. *Am Surg* 1997;63:137.

41. Yazdi GP, Miedema BW, Humphrey LJ. High mortality after abdominal operation in patients with large-volume malignant ascites. *J Surg Oncol* 1996;62:93.

42. Souter RG, Tarin D, Kettlewell MG. Peritoneovenous shunts in the management of malignant ascites. *Br J Surg* 1983;70:478.

43. Qazi R, Savlov ED. Peritoneovenous shunt for palliation of malignant ascites. *Cancer* 1982;49:600.

44. Cairns W, Malone R. Octreotide as an agent for the relief of malignant ascites in palliative care patients. *Palliat Med* 1999;13:429.

45. Pockros PJ, Esrason KT, Nguyen C, Duque J, Woods S. Mobilization of malignant ascites with diuretics is dependent on ascitic fluid characteristics. *Gastroenterology* 1992;103:1302.

46. Gough IR, Balderson GA. Malignant ascites. A comparison of peritoneovenous shunting and nonoperative management. *Cancer* 1993;71:2377.

47. Stephenson J, Gilbert J. The development of clinical guidelines on paracentesis for ascites related to malignancy. *Palliat Med* 2002;16:213.

48. Lomas DA, Wallis PJ, Stockley RA. Palliation of malignant ascites with a Tenckhoff catheter. *Thorax* 1989;44:828.

49. Richard HM III, Coldwell DM, Boyd-Kranis RL, et al. Pleurx tunneled catheter in the management of malignant ascites. *J Vasc Interv Radiol* 2001;12:373.

50. O'Neill MJ, Weissleder R, Gervais DA, Hahn PF, Mueller PR. Tunneled peritoneal catheter placement under sonographic and fluoroscopic guidance in the palliative treatment of malignant ascites. *AJR Am J Roentgenol* 2001;177:615.

51. Kouraklis G. Postoperative drainage in patients with malignant ascites: a safe method. *J Surg Oncol* 2002;79:124.

52. Barnett TD, Rubins J. Placement of a permanent tunneled peritoneal drainage catheter for palliation of malignant ascites: a simplified percutaneous approach. *J Vasc Interv Radiol* 2002;13:379.

53. Iyengar TD, Herzog TJ. Management of symptomatic ascites in recurrent ovarian cancer patients using an intra-abdominal semi-permanent catheter. *Am J Hosp Palliat Care* 2002;19:35.

54. Lee A, Lau TN, Yeong KY. Indwelling catheters for the management of malignant ascites. *Support Care Cancer* 2000;8:493.

55. Lorentzen T, Sengelov L, Nolsoe CP, et al. Ultrasonically guided insertion of a peritoneogastric shunt in patients with malignant ascites. *Acta Radiol* 1995;36:481.

56. Rozenblit GN, Del Guercio LR, Rundback JH, Poplausky MR, Lebovics E. Peritoneal-urinary drainage for treatment of refractory ascites: a pilot study. *J Vasc Interv Radiol* 1998;9:998.

57. Alexander HR, Fraker DL. Shunting procedures for malignant ascites and pleural effusions. In: Lotze MT, Rubin JB, eds. *Regional therapy for malignant ascites and pleural effusions*, 1st ed. Philadelphia: Lippincott–Raven Publishers, 1997:271.

58. Zanon C, Grosso M, Apra F, et al. Palliative treatment of malignant refractory ascites by positioning of Denver peritoneovenous shunt. *Tumori* 2002;88:123.

59. Tueche SG, Pector JC. Peritoneovenous shunt in malignant ascites. The Bordet Institute experience from 1975–1998. *Hepatogastroenterology* 2000;47:1322.

60. Holman JM Jr, Albo D Jr. Peritoneovenous shunting in patients with malignant ascites. *Am J Surg* 1981;142:774.

61. Souter RG, Wells C, Tarin D, Kettlewell MG. Surgical and pathologic complications associated with peritoneovenous shunts in management of malignant ascites. *Cancer* 1985;55:1973.

62. Kostroff KM, Ross DW, Davis JM. Peritoneovenous shunting for cirrhotic versus malignant ascites. *Surg Gynecol Obstet* 1985;161:204.

63. Sonnenfeld T, Tyden G. Peritoneovenous shunts for malignant ascites. *Acta Chir Scand* 1986;152:117.

64. Soderlund C. Denver peritoneovenous shunting for malignant or cirrhotic ascites. A prospective consecutive series. *Scand J Gastroenterol* 1986;21:1161.

65. Schumacher DL, Saclarides TJ, Staren ED. Peritoneovenous shunts for palliation of the patient with malignant ascites. *Ann Surg Oncol* 1994;1:378.

66. Lund RH, Moritz MW. Complications of Denver peritoneovenous shunting. *Arch Surg* 1982;117:924.

67. Reinhold RB, Lokich JJ, Tomashefski J, Costello P. Management of malignant ascites with peritoneovenous shunting. *Am J Surg* 1983;145:455.

68. Holm A, Halpern NB, Aldrete JS. Peritoneovenous shunt for intractable ascites of hepatic, nephrogenic, and malignant causes. *Am J Surg* 1989;158:162.

69. Ragni MV, Lewis JH, Spero JA. Ascites-induced LeVeen shunt coagulopathy. *Ann Surg* 1983;198:91.

70. Tempero MA, Davis RB, Reed E, Edney J. Thrombocytopenia and laboratory evidence of disseminated intravascular coagulation after shunts for ascites in malignant disease. *Cancer* 1985;55:2718.

71. Greig PD, Langer B, Blendis LM, Taylor BR, Glynn MF. Complications after peritoneovenous shunting for ascites. *Am J Surg* 1980;139:125.

72. Smith RR, Sternberg SS, Paglia MA, Golbey RB. Fatal pulmonary tumor embolization following peritoneovenous shunting for malignant ascites. *J Surg Oncol* 1981;16:27.

73. Singh A, McAfee JG, Thomas FD, Grossman ZD. Radionuclide assessment of peritoneovenous shunt patency. *Clin Nucl Med* 1979;4:447.

74. Schwartzentruber DJ, Leapman SB, Filo RS, Madura JA. Thrombofibrinous sheath occlusion of peritoneovenous shunts. *Surgery* 1987;102:534.

75. Maat B, Oosterlee J, Spaas JA, White H, Lammes FB. Dissemination of tumour cells via LeVeen shunt [Letter]. *Lancet* 1979;1:988.

76. Tarin D, Price JE, Kettlewell MG, et al. Mechanisms of human tumor metastasis studied in patients with peritoneovenous shunts. *Cancer Res* 1984;44:3584.

77. Daimon S, Yasuhara S, Saga T, et al. Efficacy of extracorporeal ultrafiltration of ascitic fluid as a treatment of refractory ascites. *Nephrol Dial Transplant* 1998;13:2617.

78. Lissoni P, Barni S, Tancini G, et al. Intracavitary therapy of neoplastic effusions with cytokines: comparison among interferon alpha, beta and interleukin-2. *Support Care Cancer* 1995;3:78.

79. del Mastro L, Venturini M, Giannessi PG, et al. Intraperitoneal infusion of recombinant human tumor necrosis factor and mitoxantrone in neoplastic ascites: a feasibility study. *Anticancer Res* 1995;15:2207.

80. Yamaguchi Y, Satoh Y, Miyahara E, et al. Locoregional immunotherapy of malignant ascites by intraperitoneal administration of OK-432 plus IL-2 in gastric cancer patients. *Anticancer Res* 1995;15:2201.

81. Wiesel ML, Faradji A, Grunebaum L, et al. Hemostatic changes in human adoptive immunotherapy with activated blood monocytes or derived macrophages. *Ann Hematol* 1992;65:75.

82. Ng T, Pagliuca A, Mufti GJ. Intraperitoneal rituximab: an effective measure to control recurrent abdominal ascites due to non-Hodgkin's lymphoma. *Ann Hematol* 2002;81:405.

83. Buckman R, De Angelis C, Shaw P, et al. Intraperitoneal therapy of malignant ascites associated with carcinoma of ovary and breast using radioiodinated monoclonal antibody 2G3. *Gynecol Oncol* 1992;47:102.

84. Sugarbaker PH, Jablonski KA. Prognostic features of 51 colorectal and 130 appendiceal cancer patients with peritoneal carcinomatosis treated by cytoreductive surgery and intraperitoneal chemotherapy. *Ann Surg* 1995;221:124.

85. Sugarbaker PH. Intraperitoneal chemotherapy for treatment and prevention of peritoneal carcinomatosis and sarcomatosis. *Dis Colon Rectum* 1994;37:S115.

86. Sugarbaker PH, Welch LS, Mohamed F, Glehen O. A review of peritoneal mesothelioma at the Washington Cancer Institute. *Surg Oncol Clin North Am* 2003;12:605.

87. Chen SJ, Wang SS, Lu CW, et al. Clinical value of tumour markers and serum-ascites albumin gradient in the diagnosis of malignancy-related ascites. *J Gastroenterol Hepatol* 1994;9:396.

88. Lee CM, Changchien CS, Shyu WC, Liaw YF. Serum-ascites albumin concentration gradient and ascites fibronectin in the diagnosis of malignant ascites. *Cancer* 1992;70:2057.

89. Nystrom JS, Dyce B, Wada J, Bateman JR, Haverback B. Carcinoembryonic antigen titers on effusion fluid. A diagnostic tool? *Arch Intern Med* 1977;137:875.

90. Pedersen N, Schmitt M, Ronne E, et al. A ligand-free, soluble urokinase receptor is present in the ascitic fluid from patients with ovarian cancer. *J Clin Invest* 1993;92:2160.

91. Vergote IB, Onsrud M, Bormer OP, Sert BM, Moen M. CA125 in peritoneal fluid of ovarian cancer patients. *Gynecol Oncol* 1992;44:161.

92. Kraft A, Weindel K, Ochs A, et al. Vascular endothelial growth factor in the sera and effusions of patients with malignant ascites. *Cancer* 1999;85:178.

93. Campioni N, Pasquali Lasagni R, Vitucci C, et al. Peritoneovenous shunt and neoplastic ascites: a 5-year experience report. *J Surg Oncol* 1986;33:31.

94. Roussel JG, Kroon BB, Hart GA. The Denver type for peritoneovenous shunting of malignant ascites. *Surg Gynecol Obstet* 1986;162:235.

95. Shepherd KE, Miller BJ. Peritoneovenous shunts—devices of last resort. *Can J Surg* 1988;31:444.

96. Edney JA, Hill A, Armstrong D. Peritoneovenous shunts palliate malignant ascites. *Am J Surg* 1989;158:598.

97. Smith DA, Weaver DW, Bouwman DL. Peritoneovenous shunt (PVS) for malignant ascites. An analysis of outcome. *Am Surg* 1989;55:445.

98. Faught W, Kirkpatrick JR, Krepart GV, Heywood MS, Lotocki RJ. Peritoneovenous shunt for palliation of gynecologic malignant ascites. *J Am Coll Surg* 1995;180:472.

99. Wickremesekera SK, Stubbs RS. Peritoneovenous shunting for malignant ascites. *N Z Med J* 1997;110:33.

CHAPTER 52

Hematopoietic Therapy

YANYUN WU
PETER L. PERROTTA
EDWARD L. SNYDER

SECTION **1**

Transfusion Therapy

Despite the increasing use of hematopoietic growth factors, transfusion therapy continues to play an important role in the care of oncology patients. In fact, transfusion therapy has become increasingly critical as improved therapeutic regimens prolong the survival of patients with malignant disease. These patients often require frequent blood transfusions when they develop severe anemia, hemorrhage, thrombocytopenia, and coagulation disorders caused by their disease, treatment, or both.

The development of sterile, disposable, and flexible plastic containers has resulted in the concept of *blood component therapy*.[1] Whole blood is first separated into cellular and noncellular components, including red blood cells, platelets, and plasma. Individual blood components are then stored under optimal conditions and only that portion of blood required by the patient is transfused (Table 52.1-1). Thus, blood resources that often reach critically low inventory levels in the blood bank are more efficiently used.[2] Anticoagulants and additives currently used in blood collection containers allow storage of liquid red cells for up to 42 days. These advances have essentially eliminated the use of whole blood for allogeneic blood transfusion. Cancer patients may also require coagulation factor concentrates, albumin, or immunoglobulin, all of which can be prepared by fractionating human plasma. Cell separators capable of collecting platelets, plasma, granulocytes, peripheral blood stem cells, mononuclear cells, and, more recently, red blood cells[3] are playing an increasingly important role in transfusion medicine.

Routine blood bank procedures including ABO and Rhesus (Rh) typing, antibody screening, and compatibility testing identify most patients at risk for serious immune-mediated red cell transfusion reactions. Furthermore, a better understanding of red cell, platelet, and leukocyte antigen structure, as well as the immune responses to these antigens, has vastly improved transfusion therapy. Changes in recruiting and screening blood donors, as well as advances in the testing of donor blood, have drastically reduced the risk of viral transmission in the United States and Europe. All units of blood collected in the United States are tested for hepatitis B, hepatitis C, human immunodeficiency virus (HIV) types 1 and 2, human T-cell lymphotropic virus (HTLV) types 1 and 2, and syphilis. West Nile virus testing was implemented under a U.S. Food and Drug Administration (FDA) investigational new drug (IND) in 2003. Nucleotide amplification testing (NAT) for hepatitis C and HIV is now performed in most European countries and the United States. Nevertheless, there remain significant risks of transfusion therapy. Complications that are not unique to oncology patients include acute and delayed hemolytic, febrile nonhemolytic, allergic, transfusion-related acute lung injury (TRALI), and septic reactions. Of concern in patients who receive large numbers of allogeneic transfusions is the development of HLA alloimmunization and transfusion-associated graft-versus-host disease (GVHD). The presence of numerous recipient red cell alloantibodies can also severely limit the number of compatible units available for a patient. Development of platelet alloantibodies can result in a refractory state to platelet transfusion. Fortunately, routine precautions taken in oncology patients including leukoreduction and irradiation of all cellular blood

TABLE 52.1-1. Use of Blood Transfusion Components in Oncology Patients

Component	Typical Indications for Oncology Patients
Red blood cells	Symptomatic acute and chronic anemias
Red blood cells frozen and deglycerolized	Symptomatic anemia in patient who has developed alloantibodies to common red cell antigens
Leukocyte reduced components	Symptomatic anemia, reduce febrile reactions from leukocyte antibodies, alternative to cytomegalovirus-seronegative components, prevent HLA alloimmunization
Washed components	Remove potentially harmful plasma antibodies, may decrease severe febrile reactions if leukoreduction is not effective
Platelet components	Thrombocytopenia with bleeding or as a prophylactic measure
HLA matched/selected platelets and cross-match–compatible platelets	HLA-alloimmunized thrombocytopenic patients with decreased platelet survival by immune mechanisms
Fresh frozen plasma	Replacement of labile and stable plasma coagulation factors for which specific factor concentrates are not available, liver dysfunction, disseminated intravascular coagulation, hypofibrinogenemia
Cryoprecipitate	Fibrinogen replacement
Granulocytes by apheresis	Neutropenic patient with documented infection unresponsive to antibiotics

products have reduced the incidence of alloimmunization and transfusion-associated GVHD.

Although the hazards of blood transfusion are relatively small, the expected benefit of a transfusion must still outweigh any risk to the patient. Therefore, practitioners of hematology and oncology need to clearly understand the indications for and complications of blood transfusion therapy to minimize the exposure of patients to unnecessary allogeneic blood products and to prevent wasting of limited blood resources.

BLOOD COMPONENT THERAPY

RED BLOOD CELLS

Preparation and Storage

Red blood cells, formerly called *packed cells*, are prepared by first centrifuging whole blood and then removing most of the plasma. A standard whole blood collection involves removing 450 to 500 mL of whole blood[4] into sterile containers containing an anticoagulant and preservative solution. Solutions composed of citrate, phosphate buffers, and dextrose (CPD) originally allowed storage of red cells for 21 days at 1° to 6°C. It was later found that red cell shelf life could be increased to 35 days by adding adenine to the preservative solution (CPDA-1). Adenine improves cell viability by increasing intracellular adenosine triphosphate levels, whereas dextrose provides a substrate for red cell metabolism. Shelf life is further extended to 42 days by using an additive solution that contains a higher concentration of adenine than is present in CPDA-1 units.[5] The hematocrit of red cell units varies from 70% (CPDA-1) to 55% to 60% (additive solutions containing approximately 100 mL of crystalloid). Citrate contained in blood preservatives inhibits clotting by binding calcium. Symptomatic

hypocalcemia and alkalosis related to citrate toxicity are rare complications of red cell therapy limited to patients undergoing massive transfusion. Red blood cells with rare antigen profiles can be frozen within 6 days of collection if processed without a rejuvenation solution or frozen before the expiration date if processed with a rejuvenation solution, and stored for up to 10 years. They are frozen in approximately 40% glycerol to avoid cell dehydration and damage during the freezing process. Frozen red cells are indicated for oncology patients who have an alloantibody to a high-incidence antigen or who have multiple alloantibodies.

Indications for Red Cell Transfusion

The decision to transfuse red cells is no longer based solely on a patient's hematocrit.[6] The patient's overall clinical status and laboratory parameters are both considered when deciding to transfuse a patient. Symptoms and signs of anemia include excessive fatigue, malaise, headache, tachycardia, and hypotension. Acute blood loss of more than 30% total blood volume leads to hypotensive shock. Oncology patients typically have more slowly developing chronic anemias that are tolerated better than rapid-onset anemia due to the ability of the body's fluid compensatory mechanisms. Red cell transfusion is rarely indicated when the hemoglobin level is higher than 10 g/dL and is often not considered until the hemoglobin is less than 7 g/dL.[7] Younger patients usually tolerate a given degree of anemia better than older patients, who may have underlying coronary, myocardial, or pulmonary disease. Patients with unstable angina or acute myocardial infarction may benefit from red cells when their hemoglobin level is less than 10 g/dL.[8] Thus, red cell transfusion should be based on clinical criteria rather than broadly applied threshold hemoglobin values. Transfusing a single red cell unit typically increases the hemoglobin level by 1 g/dL (and increases the hematocrit by 3%) in the absence of active red cell destruction.

Antibody Screening, Antibody Identification, and Cross-Matching

In all but the most emergent situations, a properly labeled sample must be sent to the blood bank before a red cell unit is issued. This sample is used to type patients' red cells for ABO and Rh status. *Front typing* involves reacting patient red cells with commercial antibodies directed against the A, B, and D antigens. Blood grouping is confirmed during *back typing*, in which patient serum is tested for anti-A and anti-B antibodies using commercial type A and B cells. After blood grouping, recipient serum or plasma is screened for atypical red cell antibodies. Antibody screening is performed by incubating a patient's serum or plasma with two to four commercial group O red screening cells that together express most clinically significant red cell antigens on their membrane surface. If an antibody is present in the patient sample, it reacts with the screening cell(s) and causes red cell agglutination. Antibody screening is often referred to as the *indirect antiglobulin test* (Fig. 52.1-1). Antigen-antibody reactions can be enhanced by adding various substances such as polyethylene glycol, low-ionic strength saline, and albumin. In the past, most blood banks perform *tube testing* in which red cell agglutinates are identified in standard test tubes, but there are a number of newer techniques that are being used to detect antigen-antibody reactions. These include gel systems based on the differential mobility of red cell

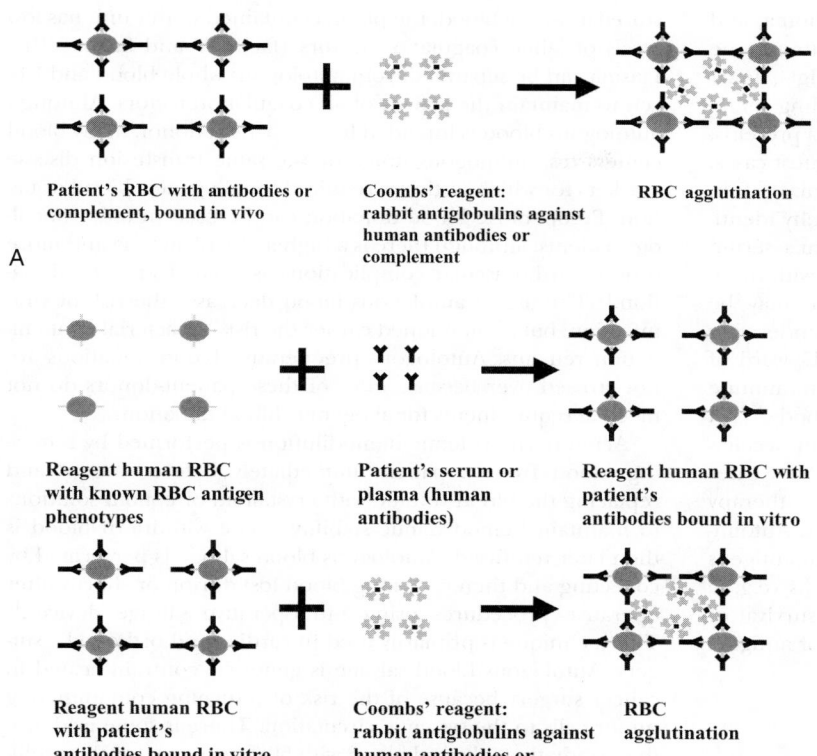

Patient's RBC with antibodies or complement, bound in vivo

Coombs' reagent: rabbit antiglobulins against human antibodies or complement

RBC agglutination

A

Reagent human RBC with known RBC antigen phenotypes

Patient's serum or plasma (human antibodies)

Reagent human RBC with patient's antibodies bound in vitro

Reagent human RBC with patient's antibodies bound in vitro

Coombs' reagent: rabbit antiglobulins against human antibodies or complement

RBC agglutination

B

FIGURE 52.1-1. **A:** Direct anti–human globulin test or direct Coombs' test. **B:** Indirect anti–human globulin test or antibody screen. RBC, red blood cell. (See Color Fig. 52.1-1 in the CD-ROM.)

agglutinates through gel columns, and capture systems in which test red cells are immobilized on microtiter plates. Some of these systems are automated and semiautomated and will likely replace tube testing for the majority of ABO grouping, Rh typing, and antibody screening in the future.

Antibody identification is performed by testing a patient's serum against a *panel* of 8 to 12 commercial group O red cells of known antigen phenotype. The antibody can usually be identified based on the reactivity pattern. A number of techniques are used to facilitate red cell antibody identification. Most use substances that either enhance or suppress the reactivity of a specific antibody. Some patients' sera contain antibodies that react with all panel cells, a situation termed *panreactivity* or *panagglutinins*. Panagglutinins can be caused by (1) a single antibody directed against a high-incidence antigen present on all panel test red cells, (2) multiple antibodies that in total react with all test cells, or (3) an autoantibody. Autoantibodies are often found in warm autoimmune hemolytic anemias, in which case the patient's serum also reacts with his or her own red cells (positive auto control).

The direct antiglobulin test (DAT), or direct Coombs' test (see Fig. 52.1-1), is performed to identify *in vivo* coating of red cells with globulins, immunoglobulin (Ig) G and C3d in particular. It is performed by incubating a suspension of the patient's red cells with antihuman antibodies directed against IgG, IgA, IgM, C3, or C4. A positive DAT result implies that the patient's red cells are coated with the corresponding globulin. DATs are no longer performed on blood from volunteer donors because results are positive for as few as 1 per 7000 blood donors and, more importantly, have no clinical significance.[9] In addition, DATs are not routinely performed at most large medical centers as part of routine pretransfusion testing; the test must be

specifically requested. Positive DAT results are also seen in patients with delayed hemolytic transfusion reactions, autoimmune hemolytic anemia, autoimmune disorders (systemic lupus erythematosus), and malignancy (especially B-cell malignancies such as chronic lymphocytic leukemia).

Cross-matching is performed by reacting patient serum with donor red cells from the unit selected for transfusion. If no reaction is observed, the unit is released as *compatible*. Cross-matching is omitted only in emergent life-threatening situations, in which there is truly insufficient time to perform compatibility testing. Many hospitals supply group O Rh-negative red cells in the emergency or operating rooms until a properly labeled patient sample is received in the blood bank. Transfusion of type-specific un–cross-matched blood (e.g., A-positive unit transfused to A-positive recipient) is permitted only when the recipient's ABO Rh status is known with certainty. Use of type-specific blood is particularly helpful when supplies of O-negative red cells are severely limited during blood shortages. More recently, *computer cross-matches* have been instituted at several hospitals in North America.[10] Patients for whom ABO and Rh types are known and who have a negative antibody screen are provided computer-selected ABO-compatible blood and the cross-matching step described previously is omitted. Although a true serologic cross-match is not performed, the computer cross-match is safe in the vast majority of transfusions if appropriate safeguards are in place to prevent typing errors and to ensure proper patient identification.

Red Cell Autoantibodies

Oncology patients may develop autoimmune hemolytic anemia as a direct result of their disease. In particular, patients with chronic lymphocytic leukemia, non-Hodgkin's lymphoma, and plasma cell disorders frequently develop warm autoimmune hemolytic anemias. Autoantibodies consist of Igs (IgG, IgM) that react with a wide range of self-antigens, including membrane and intracellular components, adsorbed plasma proteins, and nuclear antigens. The DAT result is positive in most cases. Patients with warm autoimmune hemolytic anemias often require transfusion. The blood bank may have difficulty identifying compatible red cell units, because the patient's serum reacts not only with his or her own red cells but also with those of all donor red cells. Therefore, additional time may be required to exclude the presence of a significant underlying alloantibody that is obscured by the autoantibody. Upward of 25% of previously transfused patients with autoimmune hemolytic anemia may have an underlying alloantibody.[11] An underlying alloantibody, if undetected, may result in accelerated red cell destruction of a transfused red cell unit that carries the corresponding antigen. Therefore, transfusion therapy must be carefully planned and used in these patients. Autoimmune antibodies can appear to have specificity for Rh antigens (e.g., anti-e), but transfusing antigen-negative red cells (e.g., e negative) is not indicated because *in vivo* red cell survival of antigen-negative cells is usually no better than that of antigen-positive cells.

BLOOD DONATIONS

Blood donations can be divided into several categories as follows: (1) *autologous* donation is self-donation of blood for one's own use, (2) *allogeneic* or homologous donation is donation of blood for use by others, and (3) *directed* donation is allogeneic donation of blood for use by a specific recipient. Directed donations are useful for some cancer patients. A friend or family member of a potential recipient typically donates a directed donor unit. In fact, blood supplies can be greatly supplemented by relatives and friends of oncology patients during critical periods of their treatment. Depending on institutional guidelines, directed units not needed by the intended recipient may be *crossed over* to the general blood bank supply and distributed to other patients, provided the donor meets all requirements for allogeneic donation.

Autologous Transfusions

The most commonly used forms of autologous transfusion include preoperative blood donation, acute normovolemic hemodilution, and autologous blood salvage. Each type of autologous transfusion may be useful in certain oncology patients.[12] Many blood centers provide autologous preoperative blood donation services in which a patient's blood is drawn and stored for later use, usually during a surgical procedure.[13] Although the criteria for autologous donations are less stringent than those for allogeneic donations, oncology patients are often too anemic to donate their own blood. Patients must feel well on the day of donation and cannot be hypotensive, febrile, or septic. Because of the risk of bacterial contamination of the donated units, the donor cannot have open wounds, such as from a recent biopsy, or have an indwelling vascular or urinary catheter. Platelets and granulocytes contained in an autologous blood unit rapidly degrade with storage and are essentially nonfunctional by the time the unit is transfused. If the autologous unit is stored as whole blood, the plasma contained in this unit has low levels of labile coagulation factors (factor V and factor VIII). Plasma can be separated from autologous whole blood and frozen to maintain the activity of all coagulation factors. Although autologous blood is intended for the patient-donor, many blood centers test autologous units for the same transfusion disease markers for which testing is required for allogeneic blood donation. Preoperative blood donation can be used in older oncology patients, although there is a higher risk of anemia and more serious cardiovascular complications associated with the donation.[14] The use of autologous blood decreases the risk of viral infection, but as mentioned earlier the risk of bacterial contamination remains. Autologous preoperative blood donations are not crossed over because most of these patient-donors do not meet all requirements for allogeneic blood donation.

Acute normovolemic hemodilution is performed by removing blood from a patient immediately before surgery and replacing the blood volume with crystalloid or colloid solutions to maintain hemodynamic stability.[15] The withdrawn blood is then later reinfused. Autologous blood salvage is performed by collecting and then returning blood lost during or shortly after operative procedures using intraoperative salvage devices.[16] This technique is primarily used in cardiac and orthopedic surgery. Autologous blood salvage is generally contraindicated in cancer surgery because of the risk of returning contaminating tumor cells to the systemic circulation. There is some evidence that irradiating salvaged blood with 50 Gy can destroy the proliferative ability of malignant cells, but more studies are needed before this technique can be safely applied in cancer surgery.[17]

Autologous Platelet Donation

Although oncology patients can bank their own red cells through autologous donation, it is not usually feasible for these patients to donate autologous platelets. Platelets stored in the liquid phase at room temperature have a shelf life of only 5 days. Platelets collected by apheresis and preserved frozen in dimethyl sulfoxide (DMSO) can be stored at −80°C.[18] They are then thawed, washed, and resuspended in autologous plasma or other solutions before transfusion. Platelets prepared by this technique do undergo a number of structural and metabolic changes that decrease their recovery and survival compared with liquid-stored platelet concentrates.[19] Furthermore, most patients cannot donate enough platelets to support a full course of induction chemotherapy. It is possible, however, to store significant numbers of frozen autologous platelets for patients who are refractory to platelet transfusion provided the blood bank is technically capable of preparing and storing these specialized products.[20]

The discovery and clinical use of thrombopoietin[21] potentially may increase interest in the concept of autologous platelet donation. Thrombopoietin, like erythropoietin, is an essential regulatory factor for megakaryopoiesis and can stimulate the production of platelets. Oncology patients with anticipated future chemotherapy can receive thrombopoietin and then undergo multiple apheresis collection of platelets. The platelets collected can then be frozen and thawed at the time of transfusion. Early clinical trial data have showed promising safety and efficacy for this attractive approach.[22] Similarly, this strategy may become an important option for oncology patients who are refractory to platelet transfusions. This approach may also be used with normal volunteer platelet apheresis donors, although more safety and efficacy studies need to be done. Concerns have been raised regarding the development of antibodies to neoantigens present on recombinant thrombopoietin.[23]

Directed Blood Donation and Dedicated Donor Units

Directed blood donations are those donations made for a specific patient. These units, most frequently obtained from family members or friends, can greatly augment the blood supply. Donors wishing to make directed donations must meet the same criteria for blood donation as other allogeneic donors. These units undergo all required testing for transmissible diseases, and unexpected positive test results are possible. Thus, it is important that the donor understand that his or her blood will be tested for viral diseases such as HIV and hepatitis C. In fact, directed blood donors are more likely to be positive for some infectious disease markers than other allogeneic blood donors.[24] This increased frequency of positive infectious disease markers in part reflects the higher percentage of first-time donors in the directed donor group.

The cytomegalovirus (CMV) status of the blood donor and the needs of the oncology patient also affect the use of directed blood donation. CMV-seronegative blood products are often required by oncology patients, in particular by those patients who are marrow transplant candidates or recipients. As in the allogeneic donor pool, many directed donor units are seropositive for CMV. Thus, units from some directed donors may not be appropriate for the intended recipient. The patient's oncologist must decide if a CMV-seropositive directed unit can be transfused into a given patient.

Dedicated donor blood units are used primarily for pediatric oncology patients to reduce their exposure to blood from different donors. A dedicated unit is simply a unit of allogeneic red cells that is specifically set aside by the blood bank for use by a single patient. The unit is obtained from the general blood bank stock or from a directed donor. When necessary, small aliquots are removed from the units for transfusion. This approach is not feasible in adult oncology patients because of the larger blood volume requirements. However, a single dedicated unit could supply as many as ten separate transfusions to a pediatric patient and thus dramatically reduce exposure to multiple donors.

Directed platelet donation is possible, although in most cases it is not practical. As stated earlier in Autologous Platelet Donation, platelets have a shelf life of only 5 days, and it usually takes 2 to 3 days to finish all of the required allogeneic donor testing. In addition, to use the direct donation approach, the oncologist has to be able to predict the exact days of platelet transfusion to arrange the direct donation and not to waste the products collected. Also, multiple arrangements for the directed donations have to be made within a short period of time, because patients may require multiple platelet transfusions during a specific time period. The oncologist should consult the blood bank medical director to develop a plan of action for the patient.

PLATELET TRANSFUSION THERAPY

Preparation and Storage

Plastic primary collection bags with attached satellite containers allow harvesting of platelets as a by-product of red cell separation.

In the United States, platelets are usually prepared by the platelet-rich plasma method, whereas the buffy coat method is used in Europe.[25] Each *random-donor* platelet (RDP) unit prepared by differential centrifugation of a single whole blood collection contains at least 5.5×10^{10} platelets suspended in 50 mL of plasma. The FDA-mandated shelf life of all platelet preparations is 5 days when stored at 20° to 24°C under constant agitation in plastic containers that allow adequate oxygen diffusion. Storage longer than 5 days is precluded by the increased risk of bacterial growth and the development of platelet function abnormalities. RDP units are typically administered in four- to six-unit *pools*. In the absence of conditions associated with decreased platelet survival, each RDP unit should increase a recipient's platelet count by 5000 to 10,000/μL. Single-donor platelets (SDPs) prepared by apheresis are often transfused to oncology patients to minimize their exposure to multiple donors. SDP units contain more than 3×10^{11} platelets suspended in approximately 200 mL of plasma. Thus, one SDP unit is equivalent to five to six average RDP units.

ABO type–specific platelets are provided whenever possible. This is because transfusing out-of-type platelets may result in a posttransfusion platelet increment 10% to 20% less than that expected for ABO type–specific platelets.[26,27] In addition, Rh antigens found on the small number of contaminating red cells present in platelet concentrates can be sufficient to immunize a number of Rh-negative recipients. If Rh-negative platelet concentrates are not available for an Rh-negative patient, Rh-positive platelets can be transfused followed by administration of Rh immunoglobulin within 72 hours of transfusion. Intramuscular and intravenous Rh immunoglobulin preparations are available and prevent Rh immunization.[28]

Indications for Platelet Transfusion

Platelets are transfused to thrombocytopenic patients who are actively bleeding or undergoing invasive procedures, or to severely thrombocytopenic patients as a prophylactic precautionary measure.[29] Spontaneous bleeding is rarely encountered when a patient's platelet count is higher than 20,000/μL. In fact, studies suggest that oncology patients receiving chemotherapy can tolerate platelet counts as low as 5000 to 10,000/μL.[30–32] Postsurgical patients with platelet counts higher than 50,000/μL may require platelet transfusions to control or prevent postoperative bleeding. Overall coagulation status should also be considered, because patients with plasma coagulation factor disorders are more likely to bleed at marginal platelet counts. Actively bleeding patients taking aspirin, an irreversible inhibitor of platelet function, may require transfusions at higher platelet counts. Obviously, transfused platelets are similarly inhibited if the patient continues to take aspirin. Platelet transfusions may also be used in patients with congenital or acquired platelet dysfunction to control bleeding or to prevent bleeding in high-risk patients.

Platelet Refractory State

Platelet refractoriness is a major problem for cancer patients who are dependent on platelet transfusions. There are many causes of an apparent lack of response to platelet transfusions, involving either immune or nonimmune mechanisms (Table 52.1-2). In most cases, platelet refractoriness is attributed to nonimmune causes, including sepsis, splenomegaly, and dis-

TABLE 52.1-2. Potential Causes of Platelet Refractoriness in Cancer Patients

Nonimmune	Immune
Hypersplenism	HLA antibodies
Disseminated intravascular coagulation	Platelet-specific antibodies
	Circulating immune complexes
Sepsis	Autoantibodies (autoimmune thrombocytopenia)
Drugs (amphotericin)	
Viremia	
Bleeding	
Radiotherapy, chemotherapy	
Vasculitis	

TABLE 52.1-3. General Guidelines for Granulocyte Transfusions

Absolute neutrophil count <500/μL
Reversible myeloid hypoplasia caused by chemotherapy or disease
Documented infection that has not responded to appropriate antibiotics for a minimum of 24–48 h
Fever of unknown origin unresponsive to broad-spectrum antibiotics

seminated intravascular coagulation.[33] The corrected count increment (CCI) is used to identify patients who are refractory to platelet transfusions through either HLA or platelet alloimmunization. The CCI is calculated as follows:

$$(Post - Pre) \times BSA/(number\ of\ platelets\ transfused \times 10^{-11})$$

where Pre is pretransfusion platelet count, Post is posttransfusion platelet count drawn 1 to 4 hours after completion of the transfusion, number of platelets transfused is calculated at 1 RDP unit = approximately 0.5×10^{11} platelets and 1 SDP unit = approximately 3.0×10^{11} platelets, and BSA is body surface area in square meters. Patients with a low CCI (less than 5000) may benefit from the use of cross-match–compatible platelets or HLA-matched SDPs.

Platelet cross-matching is performed by adding recipient serum to wells coated with donor platelets. After appropriate antibodies and an indicator reagent are added, the compatibility of the patient's serum and the donor's platelets is determined based on reactivity patterns. An incompatible cross-match predicts a poor CCI more than 90% of the time, whereas a cross-match negative for incompatibility is only 50% predictive of a successful transfusion.[34] Depending on a particular hospital's blood supplier, cross-match–compatible platelets or HLA-selected platelets may be more readily available.[35] Some centers use a combination of the two techniques: that is, platelet units are selected for cross-matching based first on the HLA type of the donor and recipient.

Cross-match–compatible and HLA-selected platelets are not readily available in all blood banks. Increasing the dose of standard platelet concentrates can be considered until these products are obtained. For example, a dose of eight to ten RDP units is transfused instead of the more typical four- to six-unit pools. In fact, investigators have suggested that higher platelet doses (approximately 4 to 6×10^{11} platelets per dose) given prophylactically to patients with hematologic malignancies reduce the overall number of platelet transfusions and thus the number of donor exposures.[36] Ideally, the platelets are ABO identical, because ABO incompatibility may decrease posttransfusion platelet increments by 10% to 20%.[37] Some medical centers provide *platelet drips* to bleeding refractory patients. Three-unit RDP pools are continuously infused through an electromechanical pump every 4 hours, which provides a total of 18 RDP units over 24 hours. Use of some electromechanical pumps does not appear to harm platelets or red cells.[38] Platelet drips could theoretically maintain a lower platelet count, but this has not been proven. There are no studies that have fully compared the efficacy of intermittent

platelet boluses and platelet drips in refractory patients. Corticosteroids, chemotherapy, splenectomy, and intravenous Ig, effective treatments for many autoimmune thrombocytopenias, are not useful in platelet-refractory patients.

The use of leukocyte-reduction filters as well as ultraviolet B irradiation decreases the rate of HLA alloimmunization to platelets.[39,40] Therefore, leukocyte-reduced filtered blood products should be provided to oncology patients who require many platelet transfusions (see Leukoreduction later in this chapter). Presumably, leukoreduction removes donor antigen-presenting cells, which may play a key role in initiating HLA alloimmunization.

GRANULOCYTES

Granulocytes continue to play a small role in the supportive care of neutropenic oncology patients with serious infections, primarily allogeneic peripheral blood stem cell and marrow transplant recipients. Improvements in apheresis collection techniques now allow collection of larger numbers of granulocytes (6 to 8×10^{10}) from volunteer donors than was previously possible.[41] These changes include the administration of corticosteroids or growth factors, or both, to white cell donors before apheresis.[42,43] Granulocytes are typically transfused to neutropenic oncology patients who have developed gram-positive or gram-negative bacterial sepsis unresponsive to antibiotic therapy for a minimum of 24 to 48 hours (Table 52.1-3).[44] Granulocyte transfusions have also been used in cases of fungal infection, but with somewhat lower success rate. Granulocytes collected from nonstimulated (no administration of corticosteroids or growth factors) healthy donors contain at least 1×10^{10} neutrophils per unit. These units can be stored for only 24 hours at 20° to 24°C without agitation. Granulocyte units contain 20 to 25 mL of red cells and thus should be ABO compatible and must be cross-matched with the recipient's serum. Donated granulocytes are rarely HLA matched for the recipient, even for those patients with known HLA antibodies, because there are few data suggesting that HLA-matched granulocytes have improved survival and recovery. Granulocytes should be irradiated (2500 cGy) to inactivate the large number of lymphocytes found in the product. Their use is considered for patients who have an absolute neutrophil count of less than 500/μL and a reasonable chance of marrow recovery.

Because of their short half-life, granulocytes are typically provided daily until the patient can maintain an absolute neutrophil count higher than 500/μL without transfusion or until the infection resolves. Infusion of larger numbers of granulocytes (on the order of 6 to 8×10^{10} granulocytes) produces measurable increases in adult recipient neutrophil counts, but the optimal dose and frequency remain undefined. Febrile reactions to granulocytes are common. The reactions seem to be more severe when amphotericin is infused near the time of granulocyte transfusion. Overall, the additional benefit of granulocyte transfusions for these neutropenic patients compared with antibiotic treatment alone is unclear because there are no well-controlled clinical trials. In addition, the clinical benefit of transfusing larger numbers of granulocytes collected from donors stimulated by corticosteroids or growth factors seems probable but has not been proven convincingly. The collection of granulocytes, or any blood component, by apheresis is not an entirely innocuous process. The donor is at risk for uncommon but potentially serious adverse reactions, including hydroxyethyl starch–related fluid retention, hypotension, anaphylaxis, and citrate-induced hypocalcemia. Hydroxyethyl starch is used as a sedimenting agent to maximize granulocyte yields. Minor but typically tolerable side effects of pretreating granulocyte donors with dexamethasone (insomnia, flushing), granulocyte colony-stimulating factor, or both (bone pain, headaches, insomnia) occur in a substantial number of donors.[45] The long-term effects of granulocyte colony-stimulating factor on volunteer donors are unknown.[43]

Adverse recipient reactions to granulocytes are common because of the activity of transfused white cells as well as their degradation products. These reactions are typical of the febrile nonhemolytic transfusion reactions (FNTRs) seen after administration of other blood products. Pulmonary infiltration after granulocyte infusion should be observed carefully. Granulocytes should be transfused slowly, 1 to 2 mL/min through a standard microaggregate filter. Obviously, a leukocyte-reduction filter should *never* be used to administer granulocytes. In addition, the recipient should be premedicated with acetaminophen or some other antiinflammatory agent before the granulocyte transfusion.

PLASMA

Plasma is prepared by centrifuging whole blood and then freezing the removed plasma within 8 hours of collection. Rapid freezing maintains the activity of labile coagulation factors such as factors V and VIII. The most commonly available form of plasma, fresh frozen plasma (FFP), contains all coagulation factors, other plasma proteins, and complement. FFP should not be used only for volume expansion because there is a risk of transfusion-transmitted disease (TTD) and transfusion reactions. Other safer nonplasma substitutes are available. A unit of FFP contains from 180 to 270 mL of plasma. The primary indications for FFP transfusion in oncology patients include deficiencies of multiple coagulation factors as seen in liver disease, disseminated intravascular coagulation, and hypofibrinogenemia.[46] FPP is often used for urgent reversal of warfarin therapy in bleeding patients and before invasive procedures. FFP is not the treatment of choice for replacing most individual clotting factors because of the large volumes that would be required to obtain adequate factor levels. The patient's cardiovascular and fluid status may preclude the use of large amounts of plasma. In fact, large transfusions of FFP can produce fluid overload and subsequent heart failure in some patients. FFP is not the treatment of choice for coagulopathies in cases in which virally inactivated or recombinant products exist, such as for deficiencies of factor VIII (hemophilia A) or factor IX (hemophilia B).

CRYOPRECIPITATE

Cryoprecipitate is prepared by thawing FFP between 1° and 6°C. A single 10- to 15-mL unit of cryoprecipitate contains fibrinogen (100 to 350 mg/bag), factor VIII (at least 80 IU/bag), and some von Willebrand factor, factor XIII, and fibronectin. Thus, a similar dose of fibrinogen can be provided in a much smaller volume compared with FFP. Use of cryoprecipitate is generally limited to patients with severe hypofibrinogenemia (less than 100 mg/dL). Because of the availability of factor concentrates containing von Willebrand factor, such as Humate-P, cryoprecipitate is rarely used for treatment of von Willebrand's disease. Cryoprecipitate should *not* be used *alone* in treating disseminated intravascular coagulation because it contains no factor V. Cryoprecipitate may also be used in patients with uremia and liver failure to control or prevent bleeding, due to the fact that it contains von Willebrand factor. Cryoprecipitate, thrombin, and calcium are combined to make fibrin glue.[47] This biologic sealant is most often used to limit surgical bleeding. Because blood products are used in its manufacture, it may expose the recipient to the risks of TTD.

PLASMA DERIVATIVES

Albumin

Solutions containing 5% human albumin in saline are primarily used to replace intravascular volume and, more rarely, to treat hypoalbuminemia. Their use as a volume expander has decreased because other nonplasma colloidal solutions such as dextran and hydroxyethyl starch are readily available. Albumin is also used to replace plasma removed during apheresis. Albumin prepared in the United States is virally inactivated by heat treatment. Properly prepared albumin has not been reported to transmit viruses, including hepatitis B virus (HBV), hepatitis C virus (HCV), and HIV types 1 and 2. Albumin is not a viable nutritional source for patients with chronic protein deficiency states seen in oncology patients.[48]

Immunoglobulins

Immunoglobulin products include intravenously administered immunoglobulin, intramuscularly administered immunoglobulin, and several specialized products such as Rh(D) immunoglobulin and hepatitis B immunoglobulin. In the United States, immunoglobulin products are prepared from donor plasma screened for TTDs. Individual plasma units are then pooled and separated by alcohol fractionation or by anion exchange chromatography, which results in a product that is considered safe from virus transmission.[49] The clinical indications for intravenous immunoglobulin are still expanding, and currently the use of polyspecific intravenous immunoglobulin includes, but is not limited to, treatment of immune-mediated thrombocytopenias, autoimmune hemolytic anemias, and demyelinating polyneuropathies such as Guillain-Barré syndrome.[50] It is also provided to patients with primary and secondary immune deficiencies. Patients who are IgA-deficient are at risk of anaphylaxis due to production of anti-IgA (often IgG). For these patients, IgA-deficient preparations should be used. Some Ig preparations are manufactured with a chemical inactivation step using solvent and detergent processing to reduce infectivity of lipid-enveloped viruses, including HIV and hepatitis C. Specific immunoglobulin preparations are made from donors with hyperimmune serum and can be used prophylactically or after exposure to prevent infections from viruses such as HBV.

Clotting Factors

Antihemophilic factor (factor VIII), factor IX, and antithrombin III are commercially available derivatives prepared from large pools of human plasma. These products originally were associated with a high risk of transmitting viruses until virus-inactivation methods were developed that did not damage the product's coagulant activity. These methods include heat inactivation and solvent and detergent exposure. Individual coagulation factors of extremely high purity are produced using antibody-affinity purification procedures. Recombinant factors VIII, IX, and VIIa are currently available. Recombinant factors VIII and IX should be used if available for patients with a specific factor deficiency. Currently, the FDA-labeled use for recombinant factor VIIa is treatment of patients with factor VIII or IX inhibitors. It is a very potent agent with potential thrombogenic effects. It may be very useful in many settings, but currently there is no available clinical laboratory testing to monitor its efficacy, and studies are lacking regarding its efficacy and dosing for off-label use. The use of these products in cancer patients is generally limited to replacement of individual clotting factors or to the treatment of patients with specific factor inhibitors. Antithrombin III may be useful in patients with venoocclusive disease with antithrombin III deficiency.

TRANSFUSION REACTIONS AND COMPLICATIONS

Oncology patients, like other transfusion recipients, experience adverse reactions to blood component therapy. Although cancer patients per se are not at an increased risk for the more common febrile and allergic transfusion reactions, they are likely to experience one of these reactions if they are receiving or have received multiple transfusions during their treatment. Most reactions occur during or shortly after a blood transfusion, but reactions may present several hours to days later. In general, transfusion reactions are broadly categorized as immune or nonimmune based on their presumed mechanism (Table 52.1-4). Of particular concern to cancer patients are (1) the development of alloimmunization, or antibodies to red cell or platelet membrane components, through repeated allogeneic blood exposure, and (2) transfusion-associated GVHD, a potentially fatal but uncommon complication. Chronic iron overload and secondary hemochromatosis, long-term complications of red cell transfusion

therapy, also occur in patients with hematologic malignancies who experience long-term survival.[51]

ACUTE INTRAVASCULAR HEMOLYTIC REACTIONS

Acute intravascular hemolytic transfusion reactions (AIHTRs) are serious complications that are usually avoided by carefully adhering to standard protocols for administering blood products. These reactions occur in blood recipients who have preexisting antibodies directed against antigens present on the transfused red cells. ABO incompatibility remains the most common cause of immediate intravascular hemolytic reactions, but they are also caused by incompatibility within other blood group systems such as Duffy (Fy^a, Fy^b) and Kidd (Jk^a, Jk^b). Transfusion of ABO-incompatible blood is typically due to clerical errors involving misidentification of the patient.[52] Proper labeling of clots used by the blood bank for compatibility testing and careful identification of patients are the best ways to prevent potentially fatal ABO-incompatibility reactions. Donor erythrocytes carrying either A or B antigens or both avidly bind to the recipient's naturally occurring anti-A and anti-B antibodies. This binding results in complement fixation, formation of the C5b-9 membrane attack complex, and, finally, hemolysis. It is now clear that biologic response modifiers such as proinflammatory cytokines [interleukin-1 (IL-1), tumor necrosis factor-α], chemokines (IL-8), and complement fragments (C3a, C5a) play a major role in the pathophysiology of AIHTRs.[53]

AIHTRs present as fever, chills, sudden onset of back pain, hypotension, tachycardia, diaphoresis, and dyspnea. The symptoms are usually evident in recipients shortly after the transfusion is begun. Laboratory studies reveal an increase in unconjugated bilirubin up to 2 to 3 mg/dL and marked elevation of lactate dehydrogenase. The classic signs of intravascular hemolysis include acute-onset hemoglobinuria and hemoglobinemia. Results of the DAT or direct Coombs' test become reactive due to the coating of the *donor's* red cells with the *recipient's* antibodies. AIHTRs are medical emergencies. Treatment consists of immediate cessation of the transfusion, close monitoring of vital signs, and use of intravenous fluids to maintain urine output at more than 100 mL/h with or without a loop diuretic (Table 52.1-5). Blood pressure and airway support, administration of pressors, and mechanical ventilation may be necessary. Dialysis should be considered in patients who develop renal failure as a result of acute red cell hemolysis and subsequent acute tubular necrosis.

DELAYED EXTRAVASCULAR HEMOLYTIC REACTIONS

Delayed extravascular hemolytic transfusion reactions (DHTRs) typically occur in patients who initially have a negative antibody screen result on pretransfusion testing but who then experience accelerated destruction of transfused red cells 7 to 14 days after transfusion. In most cases, red cell destruction is caused by an antibody that is of low titer, below the detection limits of most routine screening techniques. On reexposure to the offending antigen, the antibody rapidly forms and binds to the transfused red cells. DHTRs are also caused by primary sensitization in which a patient synthesizes a new antibody. Antibodies implicated in DHTRs usually fix complement only to the C3 level and thus cause extravascular as opposed to intravascular hemolysis. Antibodies most commonly identified in DHTRs include those

TABLE 52.1-4. Complications of Blood Transfusion Therapy in Cancer Patients

Immune Mediated	Nonimmune Mediated
Acute hemolytic transfusion reaction	Transfusion-associated bacterial sepsis
Delayed extravascular hemolytic reaction	Circulatory overload and cardiac failure
Febrile transfusion reaction	Viral transmission
Allergic transfusion reaction	Iron overload
Alloimmunization	Hypocalcemia
Transfusion-associated graft-versus-host disease	Hypothermia
Transfusion-related acute lung injury (TRALI)	Dilutional factor depletion and thrombocytopenia

TABLE 52.1-5.   Identification and Initial Management of Transfusion Reactions in Oncology Patients

Reaction	Symptoms and Signs	Management
Acute intravascular hemolytic reaction	Back pain, fever, hypotension, shock, dyspnea, hemoglobinuria, hemoglobinemia, positive direct Coombs' test result	Stop transfusion, IV fluids, vasopressor support, maintain diuresis, corticosteroids, dialysis if indicated
Delayed extravascular hemolytic reaction	Anemia, jaundice, fever, positive direct Coombs' test result	Stop transfusion, fluid support, follow laboratory results (hematocrit, lactate dehydrogenase, bilirubin)
Febrile reaction	Fever, chills, rigors, mild dyspnea	Stop transfusion, antipyretics, consider leukoreduced product for subsequent transfusions
Allergic (mild)	Pruritus and urticaria *only*	Antihistamines, may continue transfusion if symptoms improve in <30 min, otherwise stop transfusion
Allergic (anaphylactic)	Urticaria, bronchospasm, dyspnea, nausea, hypotension	Stop transfusion, antihistamines, vasopressor support, corticosteroids, consider premedication or washed red blood cells for subsequent transfusions
Septic reaction	Rapid onset of chills, fever, hypotension	Stop transfusion, culture product and patient, vasopressor support, IV fluids, broad-spectrum antibiotics

directed against Rh(E, c), Duffy, Kidd, and Kell blood group antigens. DHTRs are often diagnosed after an unexpected posttransfusion drop in hematocrit, an elevation of unconjugated bilirubin, and the appearance of a new positive DAT result. There is usually a delay of 3 days to 2 weeks between transfusion and the onset of extravascular hemolysis. Only rarely do delayed reactions cause intravascular hemolysis with associated hemoglobinemia and hemoglobinuria. Regardless, these patients should be followed until the hemolysis resolves. Signs and symptoms of DHTRs should be recognized to avoid unnecessary diagnostic procedures used to evaluate an unexpected, unexplained decrease in hematocrit. These patients typically do not develop cytokine storm and are for the most part asymptomatic.

FEBRILE NONHEMOLYTIC REACTIONS

FNTRs after red cell and platelet transfusion are common in cancer patients. They are presumably caused by antibodies (leukoagglutinins) in the recipient that are directed against HLA-specific or leukocyte-specific antigens, or both, on donor white blood cells and platelets. Reactions between leukoagglutinins present in the transfused donor product and recipient leukocyte antigens may also play a role. Formation of leukocyte antigen-antibody complexes then results in complement binding and release of endogenous pyrogens such as IL-1, IL-6, and tumor necrosis factor-α. Cytokines generated by leukocytes during platelet and red cell storage may also contribute to FNTRs.[54] Symptoms typically occur during or several hours after the transfusion and include low-grade (more than 1°C increase) and high-grade fevers accompanied by shaking chills. Rarely, vomiting, dyspnea, hypotension, and decreased oxygen saturation ensue. The severity of symptoms is often directly related to the number of leukocytes contained in the product or the rate of transfusion. Leukoreduction of blood components decreases, but does not eliminate, the frequency of FNTRs,[55,56] and therefore white cell–reduced products should be considered in patients who have experienced febrile reactions. Premedication with an antipyretic such as acetaminophen may minimize mild FNTRs but is not entirely effective. Antihistamines do not prevent or treat FNTRs. Corticosteroids can minimize FNTRs if they are administered several hours before the transfusion and should be considered for patients who have had several severe reactions. Intravenous or intramuscular meperidine can resolve severe rig-

ors in a matter of minutes.[57] If symptoms do not resolve in less than 4 hours or are especially severe, other complications such as sepsis caused by contaminated blood products or a hemolytic reaction should be seriously considered. Under some circumstances, it may be difficult to distinguish between FNTRs and other causes of fever in immunocompromised cancer patients. Specific conditions that can mimic benign FNTRs include preexisting or impending sepsis, infusion of a contaminated unit of blood or platelets, and a hemolytic transfusion reaction.

ALLERGIC REACTIONS

Allergic reactions to plasma, platelets, and red cells are relatively common in cancer patients. They present as pruritus, urticaria, or both, usually in the absence of fever. Allergic reactions are classically IgE mediated, and most symptoms are attributed to histamine release. At times it is difficult to distinguish between allergic and febrile transfusion reactions when urticarial symptoms are accompanied by low-grade fever. Other common symptoms and signs include pruritus, erythema, papular rashes, and wheals. Severe anaphylaxis resulting in bronchospasm and hypotension occur rarely, but can be life threatening. As in other allergic processes, symptoms are not dose related, and severe manifestations can occur after small exposures. Treatment of mild allergic reactions consists of stopping the transfusion and administering diphenhydramine or other antihistamines. For mild allergic reactions (e.g., pruritus and hives only without fever or vasomotor instability), it is reasonable to resume transfusing the same unit provided the symptoms promptly resolve. If the symptoms recur after the transfusion is restarted, a new unit should then be obtained. Severe anaphylactic reactions with bronchospasm and cardiovascular collapse are fortunately rare and should be treated like any other anaphylactic reaction with corticosteroids, vasopressors, and airway support. Washed red cells in which the residual donor plasma has been removed and replaced by saline may benefit patients with repeated or severe allergic reactions.[58] Patient can be premedicated with an H_1 blocker, or a combination of H_1 and H_2 blockers, and steroids if not contraindicated, depending on the severity of previous allergic transfusion reactions. Leukocyte-reduction filters are not helpful because they do not remove the implicated soluble mediators.

SEPTIC REACTIONS

Blood products are rarely contaminated by bacteria during the collection process. This may occur if the donor is transiently bacteremic at the time of collection or if the arm is improperly cleansed before venipuncture.[59] Transfusing blood products that are contaminated by bacteria is potentially dangerous and can result in profound hypotension, shock, and death. Other than blood cultures, there are no laboratory tests to screen for bacterial contamination of red cells. Refrigeration of red cells markedly diminishes the growth of most bacteria, with a bacterial contamination rate of 1 in 30,000 units. The risk of septic transfusion reactions (STRs) is higher for platelet transfusions than for other blood components because platelets are stored at room temperature, with a bacterial contamination rate of 1 in 2000 to 3000 units.[60] Therefore, the American Association of Blood Banks began requiring pretransfusion bacterial testing of platelets starting in March 2004. There are a few testing systems in development for detecting bacteria in platelets.[61,62] Common organisms that cause STRs include gram-positive bacteria (*Staphylococcus* species) and gram-negative bacteria (*Enterobacter, Yersinia, Pseudomonas* species).[63] *Yersinia enterocolitica* has been a common cause of red cell STRs because it grows at a cold temperature and multiplies during refrigerated storage of red blood cell products, and free hemoglobin is a growth factor for this organism.[64] Blood cultures should be obtained for patients who develop high fevers during or shortly after transfusion, especially if they become hypotensive. A Gram stain or acridine orange stain of the suspected contaminated product is helpful when organisms are seen, but this test is not highly sensitive. Both the patient's blood and the implicated blood unit should be cultured whenever an STR is suspected. Other symptoms associated with STRs are attributed to preformed endotoxin and cytokines and include skin flushing, severe rigors, and cardiovascular collapse. These symptoms may occur during transfusion or minutes to hours after the transfusion is completed. Treatment includes administration of fluids and cardiovascular support. Broad-spectrum antibiotics should be started *immediately*, even before culture results can guide further therapy. Severe febrile reactions can mimic STRs, but febrile reactions are self-limited and are generally not associated with profound hypotension.

TRANSFUSION-RELATED ACUTE LUNG INJURY

TRALI was thought to be a rare transfusion complication in the past, but it is now believed to occur as often as 1 in 500 to 1 in 5000 transfusions and with a variety of presentations ranging from mild dyspnea, chills, fever, and hypotension, to severe noncardiogenic pulmonary edema.[65–69] It typically occurs within 6 hours of transfusion and is clinically identical to adult respiratory distress syndrome. The most common clinical findings include the rapid onset of dyspnea, tachypnea, cyanosis, fever, and hypotension.[67] Lung auscultation reveals diffuse crackling and decreased breath sounds. Invasive cardiac monitoring shows normal cardiac pressures and function with hypoxemia and decreased pulmonary compliance. Radiographic findings include diffuse, fluffy infiltrates consistent with pulmonary edema. The presumed cause is immune-mediated reaction of HLA antibodies or other leukoagglutinins with white cells, which subsequently leads to leukocyte activation.[70] Granulocytes are first activated in the peripheral circulation by HLA or other antigen-antibody complexes. The activated leukocytes then migrate to the lungs, where they bind to the pulmonary capillary bed via integrins and other cell adhesion molecules. Proteolytic enzymes are then released that destroy tissue, which results in a capillary leak syndrome and pulmonary edema. More recently, reactive lipid products released from donor cell membranes have been associated with the development of TRALI.[71] TRALI should be suspected in patients with rapid-onset respiratory distress after transfusion therapy or with pulmonary edema without hypervolemia and congestive heart failure. Definitive diagnosis requires identification of HLA, granulocyte antibodies, or both in either the donor's or recipient's serum. The corresponding antigens should also be found on the recipient's or donor's leukocytes. This extensive testing is performed in a few specialized laboratories. Approximately 80% to 90% of patients with TRALI survive with supportive care consisting of aggressive respiratory support, supplemental oxygen delivery, and mechanical ventilation when necessary. Based on the presumed pathogenesis of TRALI, use of leukoreduced blood products could potentially decrease the incidence of TRALI. Corticosteroids may be useful in treating TRALI, but there are no controlled studies demonstrating its efficacy. Use of diuretics is generally contradicted in treatment of TRALI. For unclear reasons, TRALI rarely recurs.

TRANSFUSION-ASSOCIATED GRAFT-VERSUS-HOST DISEASE

Transfusion-associated GVHD is a rare complication of blood transfusion that is fatal in approximately 90% of patients.[72] Transfusion-associated GVHD occurs when donor immunocompetent T and natural killer cells attack recipient cells because these recipient cells appear foreign due to differences in major or minor histocompatibility antigens.[73] GVHD is commonly seen after allogeneic bone marrow transplantation but may also rarely occur in immunodeficient or immunosuppressed patients after blood transfusion. Removing T cells from donor grafts can minimize the occurrence of acute GVHD in oncology patients but is associated with increased graft failure and a decrease in a beneficial graft-versus-leukemia or graft-versus-tumor effect. The risk of transfusion-associated GVHD is related to the number of viable T lymphocytes transfused, the recipient's immune status, and the HLA disparity between donor and recipient. Therefore, patients undergoing multiple transfusions who receive cells from donors who share HLA haplotypes with the recipient (haploidentical) are at greatest risk. Clinically, transfusion-associated GVHD is characterized by the acute onset of rash, abdominal pain, diarrhea, liver function abnormalities, and bone marrow suppression beginning 2 to 30 days after transfusion. The maculopapular rash seen is similar to that observed in acute GVHD after bone marrow transplantation. Biopsy of the skin can confirm the diagnosis. Pancytopenia may be severe in transfusion-associated GVHD and is attributed to destruction of recipient marrow stem cells by donor lymphocytes. Immunosuppressive therapy with prednisone and cyclosporine has not been reported to be effective in transfusion-associated GVHD. There is no known effective treatment for transfusion-associated GVHD other than stem cell transplantation if the donor can be identified promptly, but therapeutic strategies have been proposed based on the presumed mechanism of its onset.[74] Fortunately, transfusion-associated GVHD can be prevented by irradiating products before transfusion. Specifically, irradiating cellular blood products with 2500 cGy inactivates donor lympho-

Transfusion-Transmitted Disease **2409**

cytes and is the most effective method for preventing transfusion-associated GVHD.[75]

POSTTRANSFUSION PURPURA

Posttransfusion purpura is a rare complication of transfusion. It typically presents as a sudden onset of severe thrombocytopenia with a platelet count below 15,000 occurring 5 to 10 days after transfusion. Patients are usually PLA1 negative[76] and have developed anti-PLA1 antibody due to prior transfusions or pregnancies. These strong anti-PLA1 antibodies destroy not only the transfused platelets but also the patient's own platelets through a bystander reaction. Patients are often refractory to platelet transfusions, but the course of the disease is frequently self-limited and may recur. Treatments including administration of intravenous immunoglobulin, steroid therapy, and plasma exchange may be useful.

TRANSFUSION COMPLICATIONS DUE TO THE INFUSION OF HEMATOPOIETIC STEM CELLS

For patients receiving hematopoietic stem cells, transfusion reactions can occur as with transfusion of regular blood components. However, there are certain reactions unique to the transfusion of hematopoietic stem cells. The most common are the acute reactions associated with infusion of DMSO, a cryopreservative used for freezing hematopoietic stem cells. Signs and symptoms of DMSO toxicity include, but are not limited to, an unpleasant taste or smell, nausea, vomiting, diarrhea, chills, hypertension, flushing, hypotension, bronchospasm, pulmonary edema, cardiac arrhythmias, and neurologic symptoms. DMSO toxicity is often dose related; thus, reaction to DMSO might be prevented by slowing the infusion and by washing the components before transfusion.

In patients undergoing allogeneic bone marrow transplantation, mismatch in blood group antigens between donor and recipient may pose additional risks for the recipient. Major mismatch is defined as when the recipient has antibody against donor red blood antigen; minor mismatch is defined as when the donor has antibody against recipient red blood cell antigen. Although mismatch in other blood group antigens such as Rh or Kidd may complicate transplantation as well, ABO mismatch is the most common transfusion-related complication in allogeneic bone marrow transplantation. In major and minor ABO mismatches, stem cell infusion can be complicated by immediate hemolytic transfusion reactions, although these can be generally prevented by red blood cell depletion or plasma depletion, respectively. Delayed hemolysis may occur after bone marrow transplantation. It may be quite severe and is often seen in cases of minor ABO mismatch. Delayed red blood cell engraftment or even pure red blood cell aplasia is a complication in major ABO mismatch. Due to the coexistence of donor and recipient red blood cell and ABO antibodies, it is important to provide blood components compatible with both donor and recipient in cases in which the recipient needs transfusion. Patients should be monitored for hemolysis and delayed red blood cell engraftment if applicable.

TRANSFUSION-TRANSMITTED DISEASE

The risk of transfusion-transmitted disease (TTD), primarily viral transmission, has dramatically decreased over the past 25 years. Bacterial contamination of units is not usually considered a TTD but actually is far more common than viral or fungal transmission. The use of volunteer donors and predonation screening questionnaires were the earliest effective steps taken to reduce the risk of transfusion-related hepatitis and HIV infection. These risks continue to drive government-mandated pretransfusion testing requirements. The development of enzyme immunoassays in the 1970s and nucleotide testing in the late 1990s has further decreased the risk of TTD[77] (Table 52.1-6). Transfusion-associated HIV infection and hepatitis are a persistent problem in parts of the world that do not have access to such screening tests.

Pretransfusion TTD testing in the United States includes screening for syphilis, hepatitis B (hepatitis B surface antigen, anti–hepatitis B core antigen), hepatitis C (anti-HCV, HCV NAT), HIV (anti–HIV-1/HIV-2, HIV NAT), HTLV (anti–HTLV-1/HTLV-2), and West Nile virus (NAT). Assessment of serum alanine aminotransferase, measured in most European countries as a nonspecific surrogate marker of hepatitis, is no longer required by American Association of Blood Banks standards.[5] Positive screening test results are confirmed by supplemental or confirmatory testing. Current estimates of the risk of transfusion-related HIV infection are 1 in 2,135,000 units transfused.[77] After NAT testing for HIV, the *window period* in which HIV could be transmitted by a donor who is infected but who tests negative for HIV was lowered to 11 days.[77] Due to the

TABLE 52.1-6. Risks of Transfusion-Transmitted Disease

Organism	Estimated Risk per Unit Transfused in the United States per Transfusion	Pretransfusion Testing
Hepatitis B virus	1:205,000	HBsAg, anti-HBc
Hepatitis C virus (HCV)	1:1,935,000 (postnucleotide testing)	Anti-HCV, nucleotide testing
Human immunodeficiency virus (HIV) types 1 and 2	1:2,135,000 (postnucleotide testing)	Anti-HIV-1/2, (p24 antigen), nucleotide testing
Human T-cell lymphotropic virus (HTLV) I and II	1:2,993,000	Anti-HTLV-1/2
Cytomegalovirus (CMV)	1:10 to 1:20 (see text)	Some units tested for anti-CMV antibodies
Parvovirus B19	Unknown	None
Bacterial contamination	1:1500 to 1:2500	None
Treponema pallidum	Rare	Rapid plasma reagin
Parasites (*Plasmodium* sp., *Ehrlichia* sp., *Babesia microti*)	Rare	None
vCJD prion	Rare (see text)	Deferral based on history

HBsAg, hepatitis B surface antigen; anti-HBc, hepatitis B core antibody; vCJD, variant Creutzfeldt-Jacob disease.

introduction of NAT testing, there is no added benefit of P24 HIV antigen testing; thus, after the FDA's licensure of an HIV-NAT assay, the American Association of Blood Banks no longer requires testing of donated blood for HIV by P24 antigen.

Routine vaccination of infants and young children with hepatitis B vaccine should also decrease the risk of transfusion-transmitted hepatitis B as these children enter the blood donor pool. Chronic carriers of HBV (positive for hepatitis B surface antigen, positive for anti–hepatitis B core antigen IgG, positive or negative for hepatitis B e antigen, positive or negative for anti–hepatitis B e antigen) can transmit the disease through blood donation or by other blood-borne exposures. Those carriers with measurable hepatitis B e antigen are probably more infectious and, accordingly, more likely to transmit disease through blood exposure or by vertical transmission. The chances of a health care worker's contracting hepatitis B from a single contaminated needle stick are estimated to be between 2% and 40%. By contrast, the chances of acquiring HIV from a single contaminated needle stick are less than 1%. These differences may be at least in part related to the higher number of viral particles present in the blood of carriers of HBV. The rate of transmitting hepatitis C through needle stick is probably on the order of 5%.[78] Health care workers must strictly adhere to universal precautions to protect themselves and their patients.

Genomic testing for HCV RNA was implemented in the United States and Europe to detect seronegative yet infectious units. Nucleotide testing for HCV and HIV is typically performed on samples pooled from multiple donors.[77] The importance of HCV transmission in blood therapy has been confirmed in many countries by retrospective review. During these reviews, recipients of blood components from donors later found to be positive by anti-HCV screening (instituted in 1991) are examined. A large percentage of these recipients, up to 75%, are found to be anti-HCV positive.[79,80] Unlike with HBV, the majority of those recipients who become HCV seropositive develop chronic liver disease. Therefore, these patients must be offered counseling that addresses the complications of hepatitis C, as well as the risk to close contacts and family members.[81] NAT decreases the incidence of transfusion-related hepatitis C by narrowing the window period from approximately 70 to 10 days; the risk of transfusion-transmitted HCV infection is now estimated to be 1 in 1,935,000. Hepatitis G virus has been transferred by blood transfusion, but its significance is unclear, because transfusion-acquired infection has not been associated with acute or chronic hepatitis.[82]

Several techniques have been developed to inactivate viruses in plasma, including solvent and detergent treatment and photochemical inactivation using psoralens and long-wavelength ultraviolet A light.[83] Methods used to inactivate infectious pathogens in cellular blood components as well as FFP are currently under clinical development. Albumin, immunoglobulin, factor concentrates, and other plasma derivatives are also virally attenuated by standard treatment protocols.

Other pathogens such as CMV and parvovirus B19 are common in the general donor population and may pose a serious threat in immunocompromised and splenectomized patients.[84] Approximately 40% to 60% of blood donors have been exposed to CMV during their lifetimes and thus have developed antibodies directed against CMV. However, only approximately 2% of CMV-seropositive donors are actively infected, and in these cases transfusion of their blood to an immuno-

compromised recipient could cause potentially serious disease. The actual risk of posttransfusion seroconversion of a CMV-negative recipient who receives CMV-untested blood depends on the prevalence of CMV seropositivity in the donor population. This prevalence varies widely in different parts of the United States and other countries.

A number of other infectious diseases are known or are suspected to be transmitted by blood transfusion. These include malaria, Chagas' disease, leishmaniasis, and toxoplasmosis.[85] Parvovirus B19 infection, malaria, and babesiosis are of particular risk to immunocompromised patients. The risk of acquiring babesiosis by blood transfusion is unknown because the disorder is endemic in many areas and often results in asymptomatic infection. Small clusters of cases of blood transfusion–associated babesiosis have been described attributed to single asymptomatic blood donors.[86] Thus, oncologists should recognize that babesiosis can cause febrile hemolytic disorders because it is a potentially fatal, yet treatable disease. Transmission of *Borrelia burgdorferi* by transfusion has not yet been documented. The risk of transfusion-transmitted variant Creutzfeldt-Jakob disease, first described in 1996, is unknown.[87] As of this writing, two cases of variant Creutzfeldt-Jakob disease transmission by blood transfusion have been reported from the United Kingdom. Fears of transmitting variant Creutzfeldt-Jakob disease have resulted in implementation of a universal white blood cell reduction policy in the United Kingdom.[88] In the United States, donations are now deferred *indefinitely* from individuals who spent 6 months or more, cumulatively, in the United Kingdom from 1980 through 1996. This policy will likely have a negative effect on blood supplies. Further restrictions are likely to follow as and if more transfusion-transmitted variant Creutzfeldt-Jacob disease cases are reported.

USE OF SPECIAL BLOOD PRODUCTS IN ONCOLOGY PATIENTS

Cancer patients are often immunosuppressed as a result of their disease, treatment, or both. Accordingly, they are prone to a wide variety of viral and bacterial infections and to harmful cell-mediated immune responses. By virtue of their frequent exposure to transfusions, they are highly susceptible to developing HLA alloantibodies that can adversely affect their therapy if appropriate precautions are not taken. Specifically, HLA antibodies are implicated in common febrile transfusion reactions and in the development of refractoriness to platelet transfusions. Thus, oncology patients should receive blood products that have been specially processed to prevent these and other complications.[89] Currently available special blood products include those that are leukoreduced, irradiated, and CMV seronegative or CMV-safe. Patients should be individually considered for each of these products, and the patient's needs must be periodically reevaluated.

LEUKOREDUCTION

Leukocytes contained in blood components can provoke febrile nonhemolytic reactions, induce HLA alloimmunization, and transmit CMV to both immunocompetent and immunosuppressed recipients. Leukocytes are effectively removed from red cell and platelet concentrates by leukocyte-reduction filters. Currently used third-generation leukocyte-reduction filters remove

3 to 4 $\log_{10}$ of the total intact leukocytes found in red cell and platelet concentrates. American Association of Blood Banks standards require that units labeled leukoreduced contain fewer than 5×10^6 residual white cells. Red cells are leukoreduced shortly after blood collection (prestorage leukodepletion), after refrigerated storage (poststorage leukodepletion), or at the bedside during transfusion. Filters are used similarly to leukoreduce platelet concentrates. Platelets collected by modern apheresis devices are designed to directly collect leukoreduced platelets. Many physicians believe that these apheresis products do not require further leukoreduction. White cell reduction by each of these techniques requires quality control measures [using current good manufacturing practices (CGMP)] that verify adequate leukoreduction of cellular blood products.

Leukoreduction decreases the incidence and severity of febrile transfusion reactions and reduces the risk of HLA alloimmunization.[39] Specifically, leukoreduced products are less likely to stimulate the HLA alloantibodies implicated in both febrile transfusion reactions and antibody-mediated platelet reactions. Other generally accepted benefits of white cell reduction include delaying platelet refractoriness and decreasing the risk of transmitting white cell–related infectious agents including CMV and HTLV-1/HTLV-2.[90] Thus, leukodepleted products are recommended for all autologous and allogeneic bone marrow and peripheral blood stem cell transplant recipients and candidates. They are also indicated for patients with leukemia, lymphoma, and aplastic anemia. Patients with solid tumors who are not transplant patients but who have large anticipated cellular blood product needs should also receive leukoreduced products, as should any patient with chronic transfusion needs (i.e., patients with chronic malignancies, thalassemia, or sickle cell disease).

Prestorage leukoreduced products are preferable because they also have minimal cytokines and other biologic response modifiers that play a role in transfusion complications. Many of these proteins are not efficiently removed by leukocyte-reduction filters.[91] This is particularly true for platelet concentrates stored at room temperature, because there is continued elaboration of biologically active substances such as tumor necrosis factor-α, IL-1, and IL-6.[54,92] With the dramatic decrease in the risk of viral transmission, investigators are focusing on the immunomodulatory effects of blood transfusion.[93] These effects involve associations between allogeneic transfusion and bacterial infection, tumor progression, and tumor recurrence.[94,95] Universal leukoreduction of all units of red cells and platelets is required in a number of countries, including the United Kingdom, and is under continuous debate in the United States.

IRRADIATION

Blood components are irradiated to prevent potentially lethal transfusion-associated GVHD by interfering with the ability of lymphocytes to proliferate. Irradiation of blood components is indicated for bone marrow or peripheral blood stem cell transplant recipients, patients with congenital immunodeficiency states, neonates, and premature infants, and for intrauterine exchange transfusion.[96] Directed blood donations made by relatives should also be irradiated. Patients with acquired immunodeficiency syndrome commonly receive irradiated components, although there is no clear increased risk of transfusion-associated GVHD in this population. Standard guidelines recommend irradiating red blood cells, platelets, and granulocytes with a minimum dose of 2500 cGy.[97] Platelets are not adversely affected by this exposure. Irradiated red cell units have a shortened maximum shelf life of 28 days. It is not believed necessary to irradiate FFP or cryoprecipitate because these preparations do not contain viable leukocytes. Leukoreduction is *not* a substitute for irradiation because transfusion-associated GVHD has been described after transfusion of leukoreduced, nonirradiated blood.[98] Bone marrow or peripheral blood stem cells must never be irradiated before transplantation.

There is preliminary evidence from a murine transfusion model that photochemical treatment with psoralen S-59 and long-wavelength ultraviolet light can prevent transfusion-associated GVHD.[99] In a murine transfusion model, clinical and histologic evidence of GVHD could be prevented by both gamma-irradiating or photochemically treating splenic leukocytes. Photochemical treatment was originally developed to inactivate contaminating viruses, bacteria, and leukocytes in blood components. This technology is currently under investigation in the United States and Europe.

CYTOMEGALOVIRUS-SERONEGATIVE AND CYTOMEGALOVIRUS-SAFE COMPONENTS

CMV infection is a leading cause of morbidity and mortality in marrow and solid organ transplant patients. Most serious CMV infections develop in these populations as a result of latent reactivation of recipient CMV, but nevertheless, CMV can be transmitted by blood transfusion. Therefore, blood banks supply products that have a low potential for transmitting CMV. These products include CMV-seronegative units prepared from donors who are CMV IgG antibody negative and leukodepleted components. The latter are blood components leukoreduced in a blood center or laboratory using current good manufacturing techniques and strict quality control measures. Depending on the donor population, as many as 80% to 90% of blood donors may be CMV seropositive. In this situation, the demand for CMV-seronegative products can easily exceed supply. In addition, CMV-seronegative products are capable of transmitting CMV disease; CMV seronegativity does not guarantee that the product is incapable of causing acute CMV disease. Research has suggested that CMV-seronegative and leukodepleted filtered products are equivalent in preventing CMV transmission.[90] In this study, however, all five deaths attributed to CMV pneumonitis occurred in patients who received leukoreduced products. Results of another study argue against the complete equivalence of seronegative and leukodepleted filtered products.[100]

Many transfusion specialists, however, consider quality-assured leukodepleted units to be CMV "safe" in that they are unlikely to transmit CMV disease. In addition to CMV-seronegative marrow and solid organ transplant recipients, CMV-seronegative or CMV-safe components are generally indicated for premature infants, those undergoing intrauterine transfusions, patients with congenital immunodeficiencies, CMV-seronegative pregnant women, and seronegative patients with HIV. The British Committee for Standards in Hematology concluded that leukoreduced components are an "effective alternative" to seronegative products for preventing transfusion-related CMV transmission.

APHERESIS

Apheresis, derived from the Greek word meaning "to take away," is the process of selectively removing one component of whole blood and returning the remainder to the donor or patient. Today, sophisticated and highly automated blood cell separators are available for processing large volumes of donor or patient blood to remove the desired blood component. There are two broad applications of apheresis: apheresis for blood component collection and therapeutic apheresis. Apheresis is currently used in blood centers to collect plasma, platelets, granulocytes, lymphocytes, and peripheral blood stem cells. In the United States, most plasma used by the fractionation industry to produce coagulation factor concentrates, albumin, and immunoglobulin is obtained by *plasmapheresis*. *Plateletpheresis* provides many of the SDPs used by oncology patients. Collecting large numbers of platelets from specific donors is important to many patients who respond poorly to platelet transfusion as a result of alloimmunization to HLA- or platelet-specific antibodies. *Leukapheresis* is used to describe the removal of granulocytes (used for granulocyte transfusions in neutropenic cancer patients), peripheral blood stem cells (autologous or allogeneic), and other mononuclear cells. Red cell units are also collected using automated cell separators.[37]

Therapeutic apheresis is a procedure commonly performed for a variety of conditions.[101] Generally recognized indications for *plasma* exchange include thrombotic thrombocytopenic purpura, Waldenström's macroglobulinemia, myasthenia gravis, chronic inflammatory demyelinating polyneuropathy, Guillain-Barré syndrome, and anti–glomerular basement membrane disease. Plasma exchange may help prevent the initiation or continuation of dialysis in patients with rapidly progressive renal failure secondary to multiple myeloma.[102] Therapeutic plasmapheresis has been used in cancer patients who develop a wide array of paraneoplastic syndromes, but its efficacy has not been confirmed by clinical trials.[103] Simple removal of red cells from patients with polycythemia is performed by simple phlebotomy and does not require a cell separator. On the other hand, automated separators very efficiently exchange red cells in patients in sickle cell crisis and patients with *Babesia* infection. Oncology patients with myeloid leukemias and hyperleukocytosis may require cellular apheresis to prevent hyperviscosity and reduce tumor burden before receiving chemotherapy.

Leukapheresis is typically performed in acute or chronic myeloid leukemia in blast crisis when the white blood cell count exceeds $100,000/\mu L$. Patients may or may not have symptoms of leukostasis or hyperviscosity at these levels. Lymphoid leukemias are less likely to produce leukostatic symptoms but are also treated by leukapheresis in certain situations or when the blast count is rapidly increasing. As blood viscosity increases, flow in cerebral and myocardial circulations slows, which results in tissue hypoperfusion and organ hypoxia. The presence of central nervous system or pulmonary symptoms may be an indication for more urgent care. A single leukapheresis procedure can reduce the leukocyte count by 20% to 50% and reduce hyperviscosity symptoms. On occasion, the cell count may actually rise after leukapheresis as malignant cells are released from the spleen and lymphoid organs. Leukapheresis is rarely needed for chronic myelogenous leukemia in chronic phase. *Thrombocytapheresis* is used for patients with myeloproliferative disease who have platelet counts over $1,000,000/\mu L$. These patients with significant thrombocytosis may be actively hemorrhaging or show signs of thrombosis. The platelet count invariably rebounds after the procedure unless chemotherapy is initiated. Prophylactic plateletpheresis is rarely indicated for such patients. Its use may further decrease with administration of the new drug anagrelide (Agrylin) to decrease platelet count.

EFFECT OF GROWTH FACTORS ON TRANSFUSION MEDICINE

Hematopoietic growth factors as applied to oncologic transfusion therapy are designed to limit the exposure of patients to allogeneic blood.[51,104] The isolation, characterization, and subsequent synthesis of erythropoietin by recombinant technology (rHuEPO) were the most important advances in decreasing red cell transfusions. Use of rHuEPO has dramatically reduced the transfusion needs of patients with various anemias.[105] rHuEPO has also been used to increase the yield of autologous donations and to stimulate erythropoiesis after surgery. Administration of granulocyte colony-stimulating factor has been shown to decrease infection rates in neutropenic patients undergoing chemotherapy, replacing marginally effective granulocyte transfusions. The limitations and risks of platelet transfusion therapy continue to drive the development of agents that stimulate platelet production in oncology patients. There is a rapid increase in the use of growth factors, including FLT-3 ligand, c-MPL ligand (thrombopoietin),[106] and various combinations of growth factors. IL-11, in particular, has been approved by the FDA for prevention of severe thrombocytopenia in patients receiving myelosuppressive chemotherapy. Thrombopoietic growth factors also have the potential to stimulate platelet apheresis donors, increase stem cell harvest yields, and expand progenitor cells *ex vivo*.[107,108] Development of neutralizing antibodies against endogenous thrombopoietin has plagued clinical testing of thrombopoietic growth factors.

BLOOD SUBSTITUTES

Red cell substitutes currently in development include hemoglobin-based oxygen carriers (HBOCs), perfluorocarbon emulsions, and liposome-encapsulated hemoglobin. The two major types of blood substitutes, HBOCs and perfluorocarbon emulsions, are in phase II and III clinical trials. None are currently approved for clinical use in the United States.[109] HBOCs are artificially derived products with oxygen-carrying properties. They are structurally similar to hemoglobin but do not contain red cell stroma, transfusion of which is toxic and leads to renal damage. Development of HBOCs has been hampered by the relatively short half-life of these oxygen carriers in the circulation. Perfluorocarbons are synthetic hydrocarbons that have the ability to carry dissolved oxygen. The particles circulate for only a few hours until they are removed by the reticuloendothelial system. Research efforts to modify or remove red blood cell antigens from donor units are proceeding slowly, but a truly universally compatible red cell unit may one day be achieved.

REFERENCES

1. Simon TL, Dzik WH, Snyder EL, et al. *Rossi's principles of transfusion medicine*, 3rd ed. Philadelphia: Lippincott Williams & Wilkins, 2002.
2. Sullivan MT, McCullough J, Schreiber GB, et al. Blood collection and transfusion in the United States in 1997. *Transfusion* 2002;42(10):1253.

3. Snyder EL, Elfath MD, Taylor H, et al. Collection of two units of leukoreduced RBCs from a single donation with a portable multiple-component collection system. *Transfusion* 2003;43:1695.
4. Brecher ME. *Technical manual,* 14th ed. Bethesda, MD: American Association of Blood Banks, 2002.
5. Menitove J. *Standards for blood banks and transfusion services,* 22nd ed. Bethesda, MD: American Association of Blood Banks, 2003.
6. Goodnough LT. Indications for red cell transfusion. *Vox Sang* 2002;83[Suppl 1]:7.
7. Hasley PB, Lave JR, Kapoor WN. The necessary and the unnecessary transfusion: a critical review of reported appropriateness rates and criteria for red cell transfusions. *Transfusion* 1994;34:110.
8. Hebert PC, Wells G, Blajchman MA, et al. A multicenter, randomized, controlled clinical trial of transfusion requirements in critical care. Transfusion requirements in critical care investigators, Canadian critical care trials group [Comment] [erratum appears in *N Engl J Med* 1999;340(13):1056]. *N Engl J Med* 1999;340(6):409.
9. McCullough J. In: McCullough J, ed. *Transfusion medicine.* New York: McGraw-Hill, 1998.
10. Judd WJ. Requirements for the electronic crossmatch. *Vox Sang* 1998;74:409.
11. Leger R, Garratty G. Evaluation of methods for detecting alloantibodies underlying warm autoantibodies. *Transfusion* 1999;39:11.
12. Toy PT, Menozzi D, Strauss RG. Efficacy of preoperative donation of blood for autologous use in radical prostatectomy. *Transfusion* 1993;33:721.
13. Goodnough LT, Brecher ME, Kanter MH, et al. Transfusion medicine. Second of two parts-blood conservation. *N Engl J Med* 1999;340:525.
14. Gandini G, Franchini M, Bertuzzo D, et al. Preoperative autologous blood donation by 1073 elderly patients undergoing elective surgery: a safe and effective practice. *Transfusion* 1999;39:174.
15. Kreimeier U, Messmer K. Perioperative hemodilution. *Transfus Apheresis Sci* 2002;27(1):59.
16. Rosenblatt MA. Strategies for minimizing the use of allogeneic blood during orthopedic surgery. *Mt Sinai J Med* 2002;69(1–2):83.
17. Hansen E, Knuechel R, Altmeppen J, et al. Blood irradiation for intraoperative autotransfusion in cancer surgery: demonstration of efficient elimination of contaminating tumor cells. *Transfusion* 1999;39:608.
18. Bock M, Schleuning M, Heim MU, et al. Cryopreservation of human platelets with dimethyl sulfoxide: changes in biochemistry and cell function. *Transfusion* 1995;35:921.
19. Funke I, Wiesneth M, Koerner K, et al. Autologous platelet transfusion in alloimmunized patients with acute leukemia. *Ann Hematol* 1995;71(4):169.
20. Torretta L, Perotti C, Pedrazzoli P, et al. Autologous platelet collection and storage to support thrombocytopenia in patients undergoing high-dose chemotherapy and circulating progenitor cell transplantation for high-risk breast cancer. *Vox Sang* 1998;75:224.
21. Kaushansky K, Lok S, Holly RD, et al. Promotion of megakaryocyte progenitor expansion and differentiation by the c-MPL ligand thrombopoietin.[Comment]. *Nature* 1994;369 (6481):568.
22. Vadhan-Raj S, Kavanagh JJ, Freedman RS, et al. Safety and efficacy of transfusions of autologous cryopreserved platelets derived from recombinant human thrombopoietin to support chemotherapy-associated severe thrombocytopenia: a randomised cross-over study. *Lancet* 2002;359(9324):2145.
23. Kuter DJ, Begley CG. Recombinant human thrombopoietin: basic biology and evaluation of clinical studies. *Blood* 2002;100(10):3457.
24. Wallace EL, Churchill WH, Surgenor DM, et al. Collection and transfusion of blood and blood components in the United States, 1992. *Transfusion* 1995;35:802.
25. Murphy S, Heaton WA, Rebulla P. Platelet production in the old world—and the new. *Transfusion* 1996;36:751.
26. Duguesnoy RJ, Anderson AJ, Tomasulo PA, et al. ABO compatibility and platelet transfusions of alloimmunized thrombocytopenic patients. *Blood* 1979;54(3):595.
27. Lozano M, Cid J. The clinical implications of platelet transfusions associated with ABO or Rh(D) incompatibility. *Transfus Med Rev* 2003;17(1):57.
28. Anderson B, Shad AT, Gootenberg JE, et al. Successful prevention of post-transfusion Rh alloimmunization by intravenous Rho (D) immune globulin (WinRho SD). *Am J Hematol* 1999;60:245.
29. Contreras M. Consensus conference on platelet transfusion. Final statement. *Blood Rev* 1998;12:239.
30. British Committee for Standards in Haematology, Blood Transfusion Task Force. Guidelines for the use of platelet transfusions. *Br J Haematol* 2003;122(1):10.
31. Zumberg MS, del Rosario ML, Nejame CF, et al. A prospective randomized trial of prophylactic platelet transfusion and bleeding incidence in hematopoietic stem cell transplant recipients: 10,000/l versus 20,000/microL trigger. *Biol Blood Marrow Transplant* 2002;8(10):569.
32. Corash L. How much do we know about the platelet transfusion threshold?[Comment]. *Transfusion* 2003;43(6):691.
33. Contreras M. Diagnosis and treatment of patients refractory to platelet transfusions. *Blood Rev* 1998;12:215.
34. Friedberg RC, Donnelly SF, Mintz PD. Independent roles for platelet crossmatching and HLA in the selection of platelets for alloimmunized patients. *Transfusion* 1994;34:215.
35. Kekomaki S, Volin L, Koistinen P, et al. Successful treatment of platelet transfusion refractoriness: the use of platelet transfusions matched for both human leucocyte antigens (HLA) and human platelet alloantigens (HPA) in alloimmunized patients with leukaemia. *Eur J Haematol* 1998;60:112.
36. Norol F, Bierling P, Roudot-Thoraval F, et al. Platelet transfusion: a dose-response study. *Blood* 1998;92:1448.
37. Linden JV, Snyder EL, Kalish RI, Napychank PA. In vitro and in vivo evaluation of an electromechanical blood infusion pump. *Lab Med* 1988;19:574.
38. Snyder EL, Rinder HM, Napychank P. In vitro and in vivo evaluation of platelet transfusions administered through an electromechanical infusion pump. *Am J Clin Pathol* 1990;94(1):77.
39. Leukocyte reduction and ultraviolet B irradiation of platelets to prevent alloimmunization and refractoriness to platelet transfusions. The Trial to Reduce Alloimmunization to Platelets Study Group. *N Engl J Med* 1997;337:1861.
40. Novotny VM. Prevention and management of platelet transfusion refractoriness. *Vox Sang* 1999;76:1.
41. Stroncek DF, Jaszcz W, Herr GP, et al. Expression of neutrophil antigens after 10 days of granulocyte-colony-stimulating factor. *Transfusion* 1998;38:663.
42. Heuft HG, Goudeva L, Sel S, et al. Equivalent mobilization and collection of granulocytes for transfusion after administration of glycosylated G-CSF (3 microg/kg) plus dexamethasone versus glycosylated G-CSF (12 microg/kg) alone. *Transfusion* 2002;42(7):928.
43. Stroncek DF, Matthews CL, Follmann D, et al. Kinetics of G-CSF–induced granulocyte mobilization in healthy subjects: effects of route of administration and addition of dexamethasone. *Transfusion* 2002;42(5):597.
44. Klein HG, Strauss RG, Schiffer CA. Granulocyte transfusion therapy. *Semin Hematol* 1996;33:359.
45. McCullough J, Clay M, Herr G, et al. Effects of granulocyte-colony-stimulating factor on potential normal granulocyte donors. *Transfusion* 1999;39:1136.
46. Lundberg G. Practice parameter for the use of fresh-frozen plasma, cryoprecipitate, and platelets. Fresh-Frozen Plasma, Cryoprecipitate, and Platelets Administration Practice Guidelines Development Task Force of the College of American Pathologists. *JAMA* 1994;271:777.
47. Jackson MR, MacPhee MJ, Drohan WN, et al. Fibrin sealant: current and potential clinical applications. *Blood Coagul Fibrinolysis* 1996;7:737.
48. Erstad BL, Gales BJ, Rappaport WD. The use of albumin in clinical practice. *Arch Intern Med* 1991;151:901.
49. Tabor E. The epidemiology of virus transmission by plasma derivatives: clinical studies verifying the lack of transmission of hepatitis B and C viruses and HIV type 1. *Transfusion* 1999;39:1160.
50. Knezevic-Maramica I, Kruskall MS. Intravenous immune globulins: an update for clinicians. *Transfusion* 2003;43(10):1460.
51. Dunphy FR, Harrison BR, Dunleavy TL, et al. Erythropoietin reduces anemia and transfusions: a randomized trial with or without erythropoietin during chemotherapy. *Cancer* 1999;86:1362.
52. Linden JV, Paul B, Dressler KP. A report of 104 transfusion errors in New York State. *Transfusion* 1992;32:601.
53. Capon SM, Goldfinger D. Acute hemolytic transfusion reaction. A paradigm of the systemic inflammatory response: new insights into pathophysiology and treatment [erratum appears in *Transfusion* 1995;35(9):794]. *Transfusion* 1995;35(6):513.
54. Snyder EL. The role of cytokines and adhesive molecules in febrile non-hemolytic transfusion reactions. *Immunol Invest* 1995;24(1–2):333.
55. Snyder EL, Dodd RY. Reducing the risk of blood transfusion. In: *American Society of Hematology Education Program Book.* Washington, DC: American Society of Hematology, 2001:433.
56. Paglino JC, Pomper GJ, Fisch G, et al. Reduction of febrile but not allergic reactions to red cells and platelets following conversion to universal prestorage leukoreduction. *Transfusion* 2004;44(1):16.
57. Burks LC, Aisner J, Fortner CL, et al. Meperidine for the treatment of shaking chills and fever. *Arch Intern Med* 1980;140:483.
58. Heddle NM, Klama L, Meyer R, et al. A randomized controlled trial comparing plasma removal with white cell reduction to prevent reactions to platelets. *Transfusion* 1999;39(3):231.
59. Goldman M, Blajchman MA. Blood product–associated bacterial sepsis. *Transfus Med Rev* 1991;5(1):73.
60. Kuehnert MJ, Roth VR, Haley NR, et al. Transfusion-transmitted bacterial infection in the United States, 1998 through 2000. *Transfusion* 2001;41(12):1493.
61. Werch JB, Mhawech P, Stager CE, et al. Detecting bacteria in platelet concentrates by use of reagent strips. *Transfusion* 2002;42(8):1027.
62. Ortolano GA, Freundlich LF, Holme S, et al. Detection of bacteria in WBC-reduced PLT concentrates using percent oxygen as a marker for bacteria growth. *Transfusion* 2003;43(9):1276.
63. Krishnan LA, Brecher ME. Transfusion-transmitted bacterial infection. *Hematol Oncol Clin North Am* 1995;9:167.
64. Stubbs JR, Reddy RL, Elg SA, et al. Fatal *Yersinia enterocolitica* (serotype 0:5,27) sepsis after blood transfusion. *Vox Sang* 1991;61:18.
65. Kopko PM, Marshall CS, MacKenzie MR, et al. Transfusion-related acute lung injury: report of a clinical look-back investigation. *JAMA* 2002;287:1968.
66. Sazama K. 355 reports of transfusion-associated deaths. *Transfusion* 1990;30:583.
67. Kopko PM, Paglieroni TG, Popovsky MA, et al. TRALI: correlation of antigen-antibody and monocyte activation in donor-recipient pairs. *Transfusion* 2003;43:177.
68. Kao GS, Wood IG, Dorfman DM, et al. Investigations into the role of anti-HLA class II antibodies in TRALI. *Transfusion* 2003;43:185.
69. Silliman CC, Boshkov LK, Mehdizadehkashi Z, et al. Transfusion-related acute lung injury: Epidemiology and a prospective analysis of etiologic factors. *Blood* 2003;101:454.
70. Silliman CC. Transfusion-related acute lung injury. *Transfus Med Rev* 1999;13:177.
71. Silliman CC, Voelkel NF, Allard JD, et al. Plasma and lipids from stored packed red blood cells cause acute lung injury in an animal model. *J Clin Invest* 1998;101(7):1458.
72. Schroeder ML. Transfusion-associated graft-versus-host disease. *Br J Haematol* 2002;117 (2):275.
73. Vogelsang GB, Hess AD. Graft-versus-host disease: new directions for a persistent problem. *Blood* 1994;84:2061.
74. Saigo K, Ryo R. Therapeutic strategy for post-transfusion graft-vs.-host disease. *Int J Hematol* 1999;69:147.
75. Williamson LM, Warwick RM. Transfusion-associated graft-versus-host disease and its prevention. *Blood Rev* 1995;9(4):251.
76. McFarland JG. Posttransfusion purpura. In: Popovsky MA, ed. *Transfusion reactions.* Bethesda, MD: American Association of Blood Banks, 2001:187.

77. Dodd RY, Notari EPT, Stramer SL. Current prevalence and incidence of infectious disease markers and estimated window-period risk in the American Red Cross blood donor population [Comment]. *Transfusion* 2002;42(8):975.

78. Hamid SS, Farooqui B, Rizvi Q, et al. Risk of transmission and features of hepatitis C after needlestick injuries. *Infect Control Hosp Epidemiol* 1999;20:63.

79. Long A, Spurll G, Demers H, et al. Targeted hepatitis C lookback: Quebec, Canada [comment]. *Transfusion* 1999;39(2):194.

80. Dike AE, Christie JM, Kurtz JB, et al. Hepatitis C in blood transfusion recipients identified at the Oxford Blood Centre in the national HCV look-back programme. *Transfus Med* 1998;8(2):87.

81. Zarski JP, Leroy V. Counselling patients with hepatitis C. *J Hepatol* 1999;31:136.

82. Heuft HG, Berg T, Schreier E, et al. Epidemiological and clinical aspects of hepatitis G virus infection in blood donors and immunocompromised recipients of HGV-contaminated blood. *Vox Sang* 1998;74(3):161.

83. Hambleton J, Wages D, Radu-Radulescu L, et al. Pharmacokinetic study of FFP photochemically treated with amotosalen (s-59) and UV light compared to FFP in healthy volunteers anticoagulated with warfarin. *Transfusion* 2002;42(42):1302.

84. Moor AC, Dubbelman TM, VanSteveninck J. Transfusion-transmitted diseases: risks, prevention and perspectives. *Eur J Haematol* 1999;62:1.

85. Dodd RY. Transmission of parasites by blood transfusion. *Vox Sang* 1998;74:161.

86. Dobroszycki J, Herwaldt BL, Boctor F, et al. A cluster of transfusion-associated babesiosis cases traced to a single asymptomatic donor. *JAMA* 1999;281:927.

87. Turner ML, Ironside JW. New-variant Creutzfeldt-Jakob disease: the risk of transmission by blood transfusion. *Blood Rev* 1998;12:255.

88. Murphy MF. New variant Creutzfeldt-Jakob disease (NVCJD): the risk of transmission by blood transfusion and the potential benefit of leukocyte-reduction of blood components. *Transfus Med Rev* 1999;13(2):75.

89. CDC, Infectious Disease Society of America, and the American Society of Blood and Marrow Transplantation. Guidelines for preventing opportunistic infections among hematopoietic stem cell transplant recipients. *Biol Blood Marrow Transplant* 2000;6:665.

90. Bowden RA, Slichter SJ, Sayers M, et al. A comparison of filtered leukocyte-reduced and cytomegalovirus (CMV) seronegative blood products for the prevention of transfusion-associated CMV infection after marrow transplant. *Blood* 1995;86:3598.

91. Geiger TL, Perrotta PL, Davenport R, et al. Removal of anaphylatoxins C3a and C5a and chemokines interleukin 8 and RANTES by polyester white cell-reduction and plasma filters. *Transfusion* 1997;37(11–12):1156.

92. Muylle L, Wouters E, Peetermans ME. Febrile reactions to platelet transfusion: the effect of increased interleukin 6 levels in concentrates prepared by the platelet-rich plasma method. *Transfusion* 1996;36(10):886.

93. Blajchman MA. Transfusion-associated immunomodulation and universal white cell reduction: are we putting the cart before the horse? [Comment]. *Transfusion* 1999;39(7):665.

94. McAlister FA, Clark HD, Wells PS, et al. Perioperative allogeneic blood transfusion does not cause adverse sequelae in patients with cancer: a meta-analysis of unconfounded studies. *Br J Surg* 1998;85:171.

95. Amato AC, Pescatori M. Effect of perioperative blood transfusions on recurrence of colorectal cancer: meta-analysis stratified on risk factors. *Dis Colon Rectum* 1998;41:570.

96. Przepiorka D, LeParc GF, Stovall MA, et al. Use of irradiated blood components: practice parameter [Comment]. *Am J Clin Pathol* 1996;106(1):6.

97. Guidelines on gamma irradiation of blood components for the prevention of transfusion-associated graft-versus-host disease. BCSH Blood Transfusion Task Force. *Transfus Med Rev* 1996;6:261.

98. Akahoshi M, Takanashi M, Masuda M, et al. A case of transfusion-associated graft-versus-host disease not prevented by white-cell reduction filters. *Transfusion* 1992;32:169.

99. Grass JA, Wafa T, Reames A, et al. Prevention of transfusion-associated graft-versus-host disease by photochemical treatment. *Blood* 1999;93(9):3140.

100. Nichols WG, Price TH, Gooley T, et al. Transfusion-transmitted cytomegalovirus infection after receipt of leukoreduced blood products. *Blood* 2003;101(10):4195.

101. Smith JW, Weinstein R, for the AABB Hemapheresis Committee KLH. Therapeutic apheresis: a summary of current indication categories endorsed by the AABB and the American Society for Apheresis. *Transfusion* 2003;43(6):820.

102. Moist L, Nesrallah G, Kortas C, et al. Plasma exchange in rapidly progressive renal failure due to multiple myeloma. A retrospective case series. *Am J Nephrol* 1999;19:45.

103. Graus F, Vega F, Delattre JY, et al. Plasmapheresis and antineoplastic treatment in CNS paraneoplastic syndromes with antineuronal autoantibodies. *Neurology* 1992;42:536.

104. Thatcher N, De Campos ES, Bell DR, et al. Epoetin alpha prevents anaemia and reduces transfusion requirements in patients undergoing primarily platinum-based chemotherapy for small cell lung cancer. *Br J Cancer* 1999;80:396.

105. Goldberg MA. Erythropoiesis, erythropoietin, and iron metabolism in elective surgery: preoperative strategies for avoiding allogeneic blood exposure. *Am J Surg* 1995;170:37S.

106. Kaushansky K, Drachman JG. The molecular and cellular biology of thrombopoietin: the primary regulator of platelet production. *Oncogene* 2002;21(21):3359.

107. Kuter DJ. Thrombopoietins and thrombopoiesis: a clinical perspective. *Vox Sang* 1998;74:75.

108. Kuter DJ, Goodnough LT. Thrombopoietin in healthy donors. *Blood* 2002;99(10):3867; discussion, 3867.

109. Winslow RM. New transfusion strategies: red cell substitutes. *Annu Rev Med* 1999;50:337.

SECTION 2

DENNIS L. COOPER
STUART SEROPIAN

Autologous Stem Cell Transplantation

The use of peripheral blood progenitor cells (PBPCs) in combination with hematopoietic growth factors has removed prolonged myelosuppression as a major barrier to high-dose chemotherapy (HDCT). After HDCT with PBPC rescue, the duration of neutropenia and thrombocytopenia is now only moderately longer than in patients given aggressive standard therapy. The improved therapeutic index of HDCT has resulted in a significant change in practice. For example, advanced age has become less important than comorbidity as a criterion for patient selection. Second, a growing number of patients receive a significant portion of their care as outpatients, which improves the cost effectiveness of treatment. In addition, because treatment-related mortality is now considerably lower than 5% at most centers, exploratory studies have begun of the use of HDCT in treatment of nonmalignant diseases such as refractory autoimmune disorders, including lupus erythematosus, scleroderma, rheumatoid arthritis, and multiple sclerosis.[1] Finally, the standard use of HDCT in the initial management of multiple myeloma is an acknowledg-

ment that HDCT can improve duration and quality of life even when there is little chance of achieving a cure.[2]

Although a substantial percentage of patients are not cured by HDCT, an exciting development in the past few years is the use of HDCT as a platform for the subsequent treatment of minimal residual disease. Adjuvant treatment with rituximab has yielded good preliminary results in patients with B-cell lymphoma but with a surprising incidence of neutropenia.[3] Another strategy that appears promising is that of tandem transplants with HDCT and autologous transplant followed by reduced-intensity allogeneic transplant.[4] By separating the toxicity of ablative treatment from the complications accompanying allogeneic engraftment, maximum cytoreduction and a graft-versus-tumor effect can be achieved sequentially and more safely, particularly in older patients. Alternatively, results suggest that an "allogeneic effect" can be mimicked by the use of posttransplantation interleukin-2, at least in patients with acute myelogenous leukemia.[5] The ability of the host immune system to eradicate minimal residual disease will also be explored by posttransplant vaccination, perhaps augmented by strategies that accelerate immune reconstitution.

Despite the safety and ease with which HDCT can now be performed, there are still several questions and limitations surrounding its use. First, HDCT has not overcome significant drug resistance and to date its role in nonhematolymphoid malignancies has not been confirmed. Second, it seems likely that in many cases in which the bone marrow is involved, tumor cells are mobilized concomitantly with progenitor cells.

Contamination of the stem cell product will assume greater importance when better preparative regimens are developed. Third, a small percentage of patients still cannot achieve acceptable PBPC collections, a finding that highlights persistent gaps in the knowledge of progenitor cell mobilization as well as the fact that there has been little progress in the ability to expand progenitor cells *in vitro*. Finally, late complications, including myelodysplastic syndrome (MDS) and acute myelogenous leukemia, represent a stiff price of success, particularly for patients whose disease is not likely to be soon fatal.

HISTORY

The goal of rebuilding a bone marrow destroyed by radiation was born in the aftermath of the devastation that ended World War II and the subsequent nuclear arms race. In a landmark study published in 1949, Jacobson showed that lead shielding of the spleen in mice protected against death from marrow aplasia after total body irradiation (TBI). However it was another several years before it was determined that cells (rather than a humoral factor) from the spleen had repopulated the bone marrow and restored hematopoiesis. Subsequent experiments confirmed the presence of circulating stem cells in mammals, and in 1975, the presence of pluripotential progenitor cells in the blood of humans was unequivocally demonstrated.

Despite proof of the existence of circulating progenitor cells, it remained questionable whether there were enough of them to safely reconstitute hematopoiesis in patients who had received marrow-ablative therapy. In fact, two patients with Ewing's sarcoma and paroxysmal nocturnal hemoglobinuria failed to engraft with blood progenitor cells from healthy identical twin siblings. In both cases, hematopoiesis was restored by bone marrow infusions from the same donors. The effectiveness of syngeneic bone marrow but not PBPCs was in agreement with laboratory studies that showed important differences in the capacity for self-renewal between blood and marrow progenitor cells.

The first semisuccessful PBPC autografts were reported in 1985 by Juttner et al.[6] Based on earlier experiments showing a marked rebound in granulocyte-macrophage colony-forming units (GM-CFUs) after chemotherapy, they timed apheresis to begin with neutrophil recovery after intensively myelosuppressive chemotherapy. Although this work was replicated in several centers, the broader use of PBPCs was limited by the inability to enumerate progenitor cells and thereby determine the number required for engraftment. In addition, because many patients succumbed to their underlying disease, the durability of these grafts remained indeterminate. In view of the known effectiveness of autologous bone marrow transplantation, PBPC transplantation was reserved for patients who were not eligible for marrow harvest. Potential candidates included those with marrow tumor involvement, prior pelvic irradiation, or bone marrow hypocellularity.

The transition toward the use of PBPCs, now complete for patients undergoing autologous rescue and moving steadily in that direction for patients receiving allogeneic transplants, has been facilitated by technology that allows same-day quantification of progenitor cells and by mobilization strategies that permit a considerably greater number of progenitor cells to be collected from the blood than from the bone marrow.

STEM CELL MOBILIZATION

Hematopoietic growth factors given to enhance neutrophil recovery after chemotherapy have been shown to mimic as well as potentiate the effect of chemotherapy in mobilizing progenitor cells. In addition to neutrophil precursors, megakaryocyte progenitors are also increased; however, in the absence of assays that measured the capacity for self-renewal and pluripotentiality, the ability of circulating "mobilized" progenitor cells to establish permanent trilineage engraftment remained speculative. Accordingly, in most early clinical trials, PBPCs were used in addition to autologous bone marrow. These studies confirmed that neutrophil recovery was more rapid in patients given PBPCs but also surprisingly showed an improvement in platelet and red blood cell recovery.[7] The latter findings provided the rationale for using mobilized PBPCs alone, initially with bone marrow held in reserve and, more recently, without the need to harvest backup bone marrow. Approximately 10 years ago the use of PBPCs surpassed the use of bone marrow for autologous rescue.

The discovery of the CD34 antigen as a progenitor cell marker represents a landmark in the development of strategies to maximize the mobilization and collection of blood progenitor cells. The CD34 antigen was initially described in 1984 on tissue culture cells derived from a patient with acute nonlymphocytic leukemia (ANLL) and was subsequently found to be present on nearly all colony-forming progenitor cells detected by *in vitro* assays.[8] The "stemness" of CD34+ cells was established by successfully engrafting lethally irradiated baboons and later humans with CD34+-selected cells. These studies suggested that both pluripotential and more committed progenitor cells are contained within the small fraction of bone marrow (1% to 2%) and peripheral blood mononuclear cells that are CD34+.

In 1991, the description of a flow cytometric assay for CD34+ cells provided a rapid quantitative analysis of circulating progenitor cells and soon replaced time-consuming *in vitro* assays in which the adequacy of progenitor cell collection was inferred from the number of progenitor colonies formed in agar after 2 weeks of growth.[9] With the availability of same-day results of the CD34+ cell count, apheresis could be timed to coincide with an increasing progenitor cell number rather than with a surrogate marker such as neutrophil recovery. Similarly, because the collected number of CD34+ cells could also be quickly counted, apheresis procedures could be limited to the number required to reach the target number of CD34+ cells. In fact, well-mobilized patients often require only one procedure to achieve an adequate collection.

The CD34+ cell count of the infused product is generally considered the most reliable marker for predicting the rapidity of engraftment after HDCT. The administration of 5×10^6 CD34+ cells/kg or more results in neutrophil and platelet recovery within 14 days in the majority of patients and 95% have recovery within 21 days.[10] With an intermediate CD34+ cell dose (between 2.5 and 5.0×10^6 CD34+ cells/kg), neutrophil recovery may be as rapid as at higher CD34+ cell numbers but a detectable incidence of delayed platelet recovery is reported, particularly in more heavily pretreated patients and in those given myeloid growth factors after transplantation.[11] The minimum number of CD34+ cells/kg that is required for engraftment has not been defined, in part because many regimens are not truly myeloablative. In a study of 48 patients who received 1.0 to 2.5 × 10⁶ CD34+ cells/kg, neutrophil engraftment occurred at a median of day 11, but 19% had delayed platelet engraftment beyond 21 days and 9% had a delay longer than 100 days.[12] The clinical significance of lower CD34+ cell doses is that there is a longer duration of hospitalization, greater use of antibiotics, and an increased and more prolonged need for transfusions. Taken together, these results suggest that the use of 5 × 10⁶ CD34+ cells/kg or more is optimal; the use of 2.5 × 10⁶ CD34+ cells/kg or more is acceptable; and in patients who only achieve between 1.0 and 2.5 × 10⁶ CD34+ cells/kg, the decision to proceed to HDCT must be individualized.

At present, PBPCs are mobilized in most patients with the use of chemotherapy followed by growth factors or with growth factors alone. The combination of myelosuppressive chemotherapy plus growth factors is considered the most productive strategy for mobilizing progenitor cells[13] and, in comparison with the use of growth factors alone, offers the advantage of providing additional treatment against the underlying disorder. In fact, with the robust mobilization produced by this approach, often only a single apheresis is required and the costs and toxicities associated with multiple apheresis can be reduced.

Although much of the earlier stem cell mobilization literature was dominated by the use of intensively myelosuppressive regimens, in most patients standard disease-specific chemotherapy followed by granulocyte colony-stimulating factor (G-CSF) is generally sufficient to collect an adequate number of progenitor cells. For example, in a study involving a group of patients with non-Hodgkin's lymphoma (NHL) in whom HDCT and PBPC treatment were planned as part of initial therapy, Pettengell et al.[14] required only a single apheresis to collect more than 2.5 × 10⁶ CD34+ cells/kg after treatment with standard doses of vincristine, doxorubicin, prednisone, etoposide, cyclophosphamide, and bleomycin (VAPEC-B) plus G-CSF. In more heavily pretreated NHL patients the well-tolerated regimen of ifosfamide, carboplatin, and etoposide (ICE) plus G-CSF resulted in successful mobilization in 86% of patients, and 61% had more than 6 × 10⁶ CD34+ cells/kg collected.[15] Similarly, the outpatient regimen of cyclophosphamide 1.5 g/m² followed by G-CSF 10 μg/kg is a reliable and safe mobilization program for patients with NHL[16] and multiple myeloma[17] that can be timed to avoid the need for weekend apheresis.

An alternative to the use of chemotherapy plus growth factors for stem cell mobilization is the use of growth factors alone. With growth factor mobilization, apheresis can be scheduled and morbidity is reduced because of the absence of chemotherapy. Although the yield of progenitor cells is lower, engraftment is comparable to that observed after mobilization of cells with chemotherapy plus growth factor.[13] The lack of significant acute or known long-term complications from growth factors makes them acceptable for stem cell mobilization in healthy donors.

Disadvantages of growth factor mobilization include need for a greater number of aphereses (and need for a central catheter) and lower progenitor cell collection. The long-term

impact of infusion of a lower number of CD34+ cells on the outcome of treatment is uncertain. Galimberti et al.[18] found a statistically better survival in multiple myeloma patients who received 5 × 10⁶ CD34+ cells/kg or more. Gordan et al.[19] also found a statistically significant improvement in progression-free survival and overall survival in patients with Hodgkin's disease and NHL given a higher number of CD34+ cells and speculated that higher infused doses of CD34+ cells may promote faster immune reconstitution.

G-CSF is the most commonly used cytokine when growth factors are used alone. In normal donors it is superior to granulocyte-macrophage CSF (GM-CSF) and is associated with fewer side effects. It also appears to be the most productive agent when used in combination with aggressive chemotherapy, in which its advantage is enhanced by an earlier neutrophil recovery.[20] Although the combination of GM-CSF and G-CSF may mobilize a higher number of early progenitor cells than either cytokine alone, there is no evidence that this is clinically advantageous. As a result, G-CSF is usually used alone.

INADEQUATE MOBILIZATION OF STEM CELLS

Poor mobilization has been inconsistently linked to a variety of patient characteristics, including age, diagnosis, sex, and degree of marrow infiltration by tumor. Nevertheless, the failure to mobilize enough stem cells to proceed to HDCT (fewer than 1.0 × 10⁶ CD34+ cells/kg) is most strongly associated with the type and number of previous treatments. Thus, in a population of patients with Hodgkin's disease and NHL there was an average decrease of 0.2 × 10⁶ CD34+ cells/kg for every cycle of previous chemotherapy.[21] Although this study did not specifically examine the type of chemotherapy, it is known that some drugs are more toxic to progenitor cells than others. Because of their association with MDS and leukemia, it is not surprising that melphalan, nitrosourea agents, nitrogen mustard, and procarbazine are potent stem cell toxins. Less well known for causing stem cell toxicity are fludarabine, particularly in combination with cyclophosphamide in patients with chronic lymphocytic leukemia,[22] and high cumulative doses (7.5 g/m² or more) of cytosine arabinoside. The latter drug may partially account for the difficulty in mobilizing progenitor cells in patients with acute myelogenous leukemia. The use of wide-field radiation has also been correlated with impaired progenitor cell mobilization. Interestingly, mediastinal radiation was as toxic as pelvic radiation.[21]

When stem cell mobilization is inadequate after treatment with growth factors or chemotherapy plus growth factors, there is no approach that has consistently been effective. In patients who do not show mobilization with G-CSF alone, the use of disease-specific chemotherapy plus G-CSF is reasonable but unproven. In patients who do not have effective mobilization with chemotherapy plus G-CSF, there are no data to suggest that the benefits of more myelosuppressive regimens outweigh the risks associated with prolonged neutropenia. In patients who experience poor mobilization either with G-CSF alone or with chemotherapy plus G-CSF, it appears that a majority of patients can achieve an acceptable (but rarely optimal) number of stem cells using higher doses of G-CSF. Fraipont et al.[23] retrospectively studied 27 patients who required a second mobilization because of an inadequate collection (fewer than 2 × 10⁶ CD34+ cells/kg or fewer than 5 × 10⁴ GM-CFUs) after chemotherapy plus G-CSF. In seven patients who underwent remobilization with chemotherapy plus G-CSF, the yield of the second collection was similar to the first. In 20 patients who underwent remobilization with 10 µg/kg of G-CSF alone, the peripheral blood CD34+ cell count and the number of CD34+ cells collected per apheresis was statistically increased.

Weaver et al.[24] showed that, in patients from whom fewer than 2.5 × 10⁶ CD34+ cells/kg were obtained with the first mobilization, the yield of a second attempt was significantly increased regardless of whether chemotherapy plus G-CSF or G-CSF alone was used. These results suggest that the first attempt had a priming effect on the second or that other factors may have compromised the first mobilization. G-CSF was as effective as the combination of chemotherapy plus G-CSF with a suggestion of an advantage for the use of higher doses of G-CSF. Importantly, the collection from the second mobilization was significantly greater in patients whose initial harvest was better. For example, in fewer than half of the patients with a collection of fewer than 1.5 × 10⁶ CD34+ cells/kg after the first collection were enough cells subsequently collected to proceed with HDCT. Watts et al.[25] used a stricter definition of mobilization failure (fewer than 1 × 10⁶ CD34+ cells/kg and fewer than 1 × 10⁵ GM-CFU/kg) and remobilized 20 patients with similar chemotherapy and higher doses of G-CSF. Only 2 patients achieved more than 2.0 × 10⁶ CD34+ cells/kg with the second collection, but 9 of 20 patients achieved more than 1.0 × 10⁶ CD34+ cells/kg and 14 of 20 patients had enough progenitor cells combined from the first and second collections to proceed to transplantation.

Gazitt et al.[26] used a different strategy and treated mobilization failures (fewer than 0.2 × 10⁶ CD34+ cells/kg after 2 to 3 days of apheresis) with immediate high-dose G-CSF, 32 µg/kg/d, with apheresis beginning approximately 5 days later. An adequate number of progenitor cells to proceed to HDCT was collected in 15 of 17 patients.

Taken together, these studies suggest that in patients who achieve suboptimal collections (1.0 to 2.4 × 10⁶ CD34+ cells/kg), one-half or more may achieve an acceptable (2.5 × 10⁶ CD34+ cells/kg) cumulative stem cell collection after a second mobilization with chemotherapy plus G-CSF or G-CSF alone. Higher doses of G-CSF are generally recommended, although it is controversial whether there is a mobilization dose-response for G-CSF when used in combination with chemotherapy. However, in evaluating these studies, one must consider that there may be a significant biologic difference between suboptimal mobilizers (1.0 to 2.4 × 10⁶ CD34+ cells/kg) and poor mobilizers who achieve fewer than 1.0 × 10⁶ CD34+ cells/kg. Indeed, engraftment data suggest that the former group may not really need or significantly benefit from a second collection, whereas the latter group has a high incidence of transplantation-related mortality despite the supplemental use of backup bone marrow.[27]

In poor mobilizers or nonmobilizers, more effective strategies are clearly required. Combinations of hematopoietic growth factors including GM-CSF plus G-CSF or erythropoietin plus G-CSF have not consistently increased progenitor cell mobilization beyond that achieved with higher doses of G-CSF. Although stem cell factor has been shown to augment the action of G-CSF in progenitor cell mobilization, the impact appears incremental, and there have been no published studies in which a poorly mobilizing group was specifically tested. In addition, the study by Stiff et al.[28] suggested that stem cell factor may be toxic, with mast cell–mediated reactions observed in a small percentage of patients.

There are conflicting data on the use of autologous bone marrow in poor mobilizers. Watts et al.[27] described 12 patients in whom fewer than 1 × 10⁶ CD34+ cells/kg and 1 × 10⁵ GM-CFU/kg could be collected. A subsequent bone marrow harvest was done and both progenitor products were given after HDCT. Five of 12 patients experienced treatment-related mortality; 4 of 11 evaluable patients experienced a delay of neutrophil recovery beyond 21 days and 8 patients experienced delayed platelet recovery. In contrast to these dismal results are those of a study by Rick et al.,[29] who identified 13 patients as poor mobilizers on the basis of a peripheral blood CD34+ cell count of fewer than 10/µL after chemotherapy plus G-CSF mobilization. This group underwent bone marrow harvest at a median of 46 days after failed stem cell mobilization. Ten patients underwent HDCT with autologous bone marrow rescue. Platelet engraftment was delayed but neutrophil engraftment, supportive care, febrile days, and duration of hospitalization were similar to those of historical controls.

Lemoli et al.[30] harvested mobilized bone marrow in a much larger group of 86 poor mobilizers by administering G-CSF 7.5 µg/kg twice daily for 3 days before bone marrow collection. Interestingly, engraftment was surprisingly good despite a median infusion dose of only 0.7 × 10⁶ CD34+ cells/kg. The observation of moderately rapid engraftment without a clear relationship to CD34+ cell dose suggests a qualitative difference between bone marrow and blood progenitor cells. The authors concluded that failure to mobilize is not always due to poor marrow quality and that some patients may acquire a specific defect in mobilization due to chemotherapy. Nevertheless, it should be noted that the definition of a poor mobilizer in the successful bone marrow studies was different and less stringent than that used by Watts et al.[27] For example, 75% of the patients in the Lemoli et al.[30] study were labeled *poor mobilizers* after failing to achieve a peripheral blood CD34 count of more than 10/µL after mobilization with G-CSF alone, a strategy that is less productive than chemotherapy plus G-CSF mobilization. In addition, a major limitation of using bone marrow is the potential for tumor cell contamination, particularly with diseases such as leukemia, myeloma, and lymphoma. Furthermore, the median time between failed mobilization and subsequent HDCT was 2 months, a period that is impractical for patients with aggressive disease. As a result, although mobilized autologous marrow rescue can be considered for selected patients, it should probably not be recommended until other strategies have been attempted.

If it is true that failed mobilization reflects an acquired defect in mobilization rather than poor marrow quality, it seems likely that more effective strategies will be developed as the biology of mobilization is better understood. AMD-3100 is a failed anti–acquired immunodeficiency syndrome therapy that was initially studied because it blocked attachment of the human immunodeficiency virus to the chemokine receptor CXCR4. CXCR4 and its ligand, stromal cell–derived factor-1 (SDF-1), are thought to play a central role in G-CSF–induced progenitor cell mobilization,[31] and a preliminary report of a study involving normal volunteers showed that the combination of AMD-3100 and G-CSF mobilized three times as many CD34+ cells as either drug alone.[32] Ongoing clinical trials, including studies involving poor mobilizers, are in progress.

Exciting preliminary results have been reported with the use of recombinant human growth hormone in combination with G-CSF.[33] Thirteen patients who had previously failed to experience mobilization with chemotherapy plus G-CSF were treated with consecutive cycles of identical chemotherapy followed by G-CSF 5 µg/kg/d for the first mobilization and then with G-CSF 5 µg/kg/d plus growth hormone 100 µg/kg/d for the second mobilization. As a result, each patient served as his or her own control. The results were strikingly better after treatment with the combination of G-CSF and growth hormone, with 13 of 13 patients yielding enough cells to proceed with HDCT (mean, 7×10^6 CD34+ cells/kg) compared with none of the patients given G-CSF alone. After HDCT and rescue with the G-CSF/growth hormone–mobilized stem cells, neutrophil and platelet engraftment were seen at 9 and 13 days, respectively, which indicated that the progenitor cells were functional.

TUMOR CONTAMINATION

One of the early indications for the use of PBPCs rather than bone marrow was known involvement of the marrow by tumor. Implicit in this recommendation was that the blood was likely to be less contaminated with tumor cells than the bone marrow. Several studies conducted during steady-state hematopoiesis in patients with breast cancer, neuroblastoma, and lymphoma confirmed this hypothesis. After mobilization, the advantage of blood over marrow has been reduced in some studies, whereas in others it has been enhanced. For example, Leonard et al. found that in lymphoma patients the decrease in tumor cell contamination of blood compared with marrow in the steady state was negated by mobilization with cyclophosphamide and G-CSF.[34] In contrast, Ladetto et al. found that in multiple myeloma patients mobilized with 5.0 g/m² cyclophosphamide plus G-CSF there were a median of 2.68 log units fewer myeloma cells in blood than in marrow sampled immediately after mobilization.[35] A second course of high-dose cyclophosphamide did not result in a further decrease in tumor cell contamination, which suggests the limits of *in vivo* purging in this patient population. In the latter study and in that by Galimberti et al.[18] tumor cell contamination appeared to remain consistent from one apheresis procedure to another. These studies and that by Knudsen et al.[36] have not confirmed an earlier theory suggesting that tumor cells were mobilized later than progenitor cells after a mobilization procedure.

The clinical significance of administering tumor-contaminated progenitor cells is unclear. Although gene marking studies show that infused tumor cells can contribute to relapse, there are fewer data to suggest that they are the sole or even principal cause of recurrence. In patients with breast cancer two studies have shown comparable outcomes in patients whose stem cell products did and did not show occult tumor cells.[37,38] Similarly, in patients with multiple myeloma, a higher number of circulating tumor cells was associated with a shorter time to recurrence and a decrease in overall survival but was not significant in a multivariable analysis that included β_2-microglobulin level and plasma cell labeling index.[39] These results suggest that a higher level of tumor contamination was a sign of more aggressive disease rather than a direct cause of treatment failure. Galimberti et al.[18] used a highly sensitive

polymerase chain reaction (PCR) assay for detecting contaminating myeloma cells and did not find a relationship between reinfused tumor cells and outcome. They concluded that residual disease rather than contaminated reinfused stem cells was the major source of relapse.

Purging by CD34 cell selection has also been tested in a randomized study involving multiple myeloma patients. Despite a reduction in tumor cell contamination by over 3 log units, there was no benefit in disease-free or overall survival.[40]

Breast cancer and multiple myeloma may not be the ideal diseases to study the impact of reinfused tumor cells because the routine failure to eradicate residual disease may diminish the apparent impact of contaminating tumor cells. In patients with NHL, there is increasing indirect evidence that reinfused tumor cells play a significant role in recurrence. Investigators from the Dana-Farber Cancer Institute showed that, of 48 patients with PCR-negative marrows after purging, only 6 patients experienced relapse.[41] In contrast, 49 of 65 patients whose PCR results remained positive after purging, experienced relapse after transplantation. Despite the impressive outcome after successful purging, an alternative explanation for their findings is that a persistently positive stem cell product is a marker for residual resistant disease, a theory that is supported by the predominant pattern of recurrence in previously involved sites of disease.

Bierman et al.[42] retrospectively reviewed data for over 3000 lymphoma patients from three large databases and compared the outcome after transplantation with syngeneic, allogeneic (T-cell replete vs. depleted), autologous purged and autologous unpurged stem cells. The autologous unpurged group accounted for 60% of the patients, which reflected the prevailing standard of care. Purging was done with a variety of methods, including 4-hydroxyperoxycyclophosphamide, mafosfamide, "other pharmacologic agents," positive selection techniques, and monoclonal antibodies. Relapse rates and overall survival were significantly better after purged autologous and syngeneic transplantation in patients with low-grade lymphoma, which suggests that contaminating lymphoma cells are a significant cause of treatment failure. Transplantation of purged autologous cells was associated with a threefold higher risk of relapse than transplantation of syngeneic cells, which indicates either incomplete purging in many of the patients or the existence of other advantages to receiving syngeneic cells, such as improved immune reconstitution and surveillance. There were no significant differences in relapse rate or outcome in patients with intermediate- or high-grade lymphoma. Interestingly, relapse rates were not significantly lower after allogeneic compared with syngeneic transplants. In addition, neither the absence of the development of chronic graft-versus-host-disease nor the use of T-cell depletion was associated with a higher relapse rate compared with T-cell–replete allogeneic or syngeneic transplantation. These data suggest that the major advantage of donor transplants is that they are tumor free rather than that they produce a graft-versus-lymphoma effect.

Despite the findings of the retrospective study discussed earlier, the time and expense required and the lack of a standardized process have diminished enthusiasm for purging, as has the lack of confirmatory randomized data showing benefit. Nevertheless, the routine use of rituximab in patients with B-cell lymphoma has for the most part made these considerations moot. Rituximab is now used in combination with chemotherapy in most patients with B-cell lymphoma and causes a profound B-cell depletion and the achievement of PCR-negative stem cell products in the vast majority of patients with follicular and mantle cell lymphomas.[43,44] It seems likely that these data in combination with encouraging published clinical trials will stimulate further investigation of transplantation in these patient populations.[45,46]

PRACTICAL CONSIDERATIONS FOR THE POTENTIAL AUTOLOGOUS STEM CELL PATIENT

Because of the potential deleterious effect of prior therapy on stem cell mobilization, the possibility that a patient may be a candidate for HDCT and stem cell rescue should be considered from the time of diagnosis. For example, dexamethasone-based programs have replaced melphalan in the initial treatment of multiple myeloma because of alkylating agent–induced stem cell toxicity. Similarly, fludarabine, which has played an increasingly important role in the treatment of low-grade B-cell disorders, has been identified as a stem cell toxin.[22] These results suggest that for potential HDCT candidates stem cells should be collected before initiation of fludarabine therapy when feasible or at least before extensive treatment.

Progenitor cell mobilization can generally be accomplished with disease-specific chemotherapy plus G-CSF or with G-CSF alone. In general the former strategy is favored by most clinicians because of the additional antineoplastic effect afforded by chemotherapy as well as the higher stem cell yields.[13] In heavily pretreated patients it has been suggested that chemotherapy-induced mobilization is more impaired than cytokine mobilization alone. However, in a retrospective study of multiple myeloma patients the inferiority of G-CSF alone as a mobilizing agent extended to heavily pretreated patients except those with premobilization platelet counts of fewer than $200,000/\mu L$, for whom the advantage of chemotherapy plus G-CSF disappeared.[47]

Despite evidence of a dose-response effect when G-CSF is used alone for mobilization,[48] the data are conflicting regarding the role of higher doses of G-CSF when used in conjunction with chemotherapy. Currently, in most patients, G-CSF 10 $\mu g/kg$ is started 1 to 4 days after chemotherapy to hasten hematopoietic recovery and to increase the yield of progenitor cells. Lower doses of G-CSF can be considered in non–heavily pretreated patients, particularly after intensively myelosuppressive chemotherapy.

The timing of apheresis can be optimized (lower number of procedures) by measuring the blood CD34+ cell count during the period of brisk neutrophil recovery. If collection is started when the CD34+ cell count exceeds $20/\mu L$, more than 2×10^6 CD34+ cells/kg can be collected in one or two procedures in the majority of patients. However, because patients who show less evidence of mobilization (5 to 15 CD34+ cells/μL) may also yield a potentially adequate progenitor cell collection (more than 1×10^6 CD34+ cells/kg) with three or more aphereses, the use of a cutoff of 20 CD34+ cells/μL should be limited to patients who can be anticipated to be good mobilizers (non–heavily pretreated). In settings in which the blood CD34+ cell count is unavailable, it would appear that the best time to begin collection is when the white blood cell count has increased to more than 3000 to 6000/μL *and* the patient has a rising platelet count.[49]

The target number of stem cells is generally at least 2.5×10^6 CD34+ cells/kg, but with more than 5.0×10^6 CD34+ cells/kg, most patients have white blood cell recovery and become independent of platelet transfusions within 2 weeks.[10] Particularly if CD34+ cell selection or tandem transplantations are considered, a higher collection target is desirable. In addition, in one study of multiple myeloma patients, a better disease outcome was independently associated with CD34+ cell dose, although the mechanism of this effect was not studied.[18] In a second study of patients with Hodgkin's disease and NHL, infused CD34+ cell dose was positively associated with progression-free and overall survival.[50] Because the infused dose of CD34+ cells was also correlated with more rapid lymphocyte recovery, the authors speculated that immune reconstitution was faster at higher CD34+ cell doses.

Although, as noted earlier in Stem Cell Mobilization, more than 1×10^6 CD34+ cells/kg is considered sufficient for most patients, 10% to 20% have slowed or incomplete platelet recovery. In addition, because a substantial percentage of patients (including all myeloma patients) eventually require additional treatment, it is unclear whether marrow reserve in such patients will be adequate to sustain aggressive therapy.

There is considerable controversy regarding the usefulness of administering hematopoietic growth factors after progenitor cell infusion. Although most studies show a favorable impact of G-CSF in shortening the period of neutropenia, it is much less certain that this is of clinical benefit. For example, shorter periods of hospitalization after posttransplantation G-CSF may reflect a tendency to discharge patients once they reach a certain white blood cell count rather than a true clinical advantage. It also seems possible that patients who are most likely to benefit from the addition of G-CSF are those who have received fewer progenitor cells; however, the use of G-CSF in this group is also associated with delays in platelet engraftment, which suggests that G-CSF may drive a limited number of progenitor cells toward neutrophil differentiation.[11]

If G-CSF is used after transplantation, most but not all studies suggest that there is little advantage to beginning G-CSF immediately compared to delaying administration 5 to 7 days after stem cell infusion. Demirer et al.[51] found no difference between patients randomly assigned to receive G-CSF either at day 0 or at day 5 but found that both groups had a statistically shorter period of hospitalization, duration of fever, and length of antibiotic use compared to patients who did not receive G-CSF. There does not appear to be any advantage in using higher doses of G-CSF in the posttransplantation period. In one study G-CSF 16 $\mu g/kg/d$ was no more effective than G-CSF 5 $\mu g/kg/d$ in accelerating neutrophil engraftment.[52]

HIGH-DOSE THERAPY REGIMENS: NEW DIRECTIONS

In contrast to allogeneic transplantation for which there is increasing evidence that cure can be achieved by an immunologic effect of the graft,[53,54] cure after autologous rescue requires complete eradication of tumor cells by the high-dose regimen. As a result, allogeneic programs have moved toward immunosuppressive, less toxic programs to facilitate donor engraftment. In contrast, improvement for patients undergoing autologous rescue will require programs with greater antineoplastic activity.

Alkylating agents have provided the nucleus of most preparative programs, primarily because they demonstrate a disproportionate ratio of marrow to nonmarrow toxicity. The relative lack of nonmarrow toxicity provides an opportunity for dose escalation without excessive toxicity. *In vitro* studies also show that alkylating agents have a steep dose-response curve against tumor cell lines and that there is minimal cross-resistance among alkylating agents. In fact, in contrast to drugs such as anthracyclines, vinca alkaloids, and topoisomerase inhibitors, it is extremely difficult even under tissue culture conditions to make tumor cells more than a few-fold resistant to alkylating agents. As a result, minor drug resistance can theoretically be overcome by dose escalation or by the addition of other alkylating agents. Finally, as with other curative regimens, the combination of alkylating agents with nonoverlapping extramyeloid toxicity is theoretically possible with maintenance of near the maximum tolerated dosages of each agent. Thus, most currently used high-dose programs, with the exception of those for multiple myeloma,[55] administer two or more alkylating agents in combination. External-beam radiation, which shares many of the same advantageous biologic features as alkylating agents, cannot be dose-escalated except to very limited fields; thus, the use of TBI has been limited to highly radiation-sensitive neoplasms such as leukemia and lymphoma. However, it is not certain that even in the latter two diseases radiation is superior to chemotherapy.

In clinical practice, dose escalation of alkylating agent–based regimens has been limited by excessive nonmarrow toxicities, including mucositis, pneumonitis, and venoocclusive disease. In fact, new toxicities not predicted by single-agent studies have emerged when high doses of alkylating agents have been used in combination. As a result, the initial promise of many of the currently used programs has not been realized; significant drug resistance has not been overcome by the modest dose escalation permitted by progenitor cells and growth factors. In fact, with the exception of a small percentage of cases in patients with refractory Hodgkin's disease, the vast majority of cures after HDCT and autologous progenitor cell rescue have been observed in patients with chemosensitive lymphoid malignancies.

Several strategies are being explored to improve the results of HDCT. First, as morbidity, mortality, and cost are reduced, HDCT will increasingly be explored earlier in treatment when there is less likelihood of significant drug resistance. High-dose therapy is now considered the standard of care as part of the initial treatment of patients with multiple myeloma,[2,56] and a large retrospective study suggests a survival benefit in patients with high-risk NHL.[57]

A second approach has been to increase the intensity of preparative regimens. Based on favorable reports from single-institution studies, the Southwestern Oncology Group tested the addition of high-dose etoposide to cyclophosphamide and TBI in patients with either relapsed or refractory NHL.[58] Patients who were not candidates for TBI (because of prior irradiation) received BCNU (carmustine) at a dose of 15 mg/kg (adjusted for obese patients) along with the same doses of cyclophosphamide and etoposide used in the TBI regimen. The investigators concluded that the augmented regimens were more effective than previous preparative programs for chemoresistant patients, particularly for those patients who experienced induction failure. However, half of the latter group had a partial or

better response to salvage therapy before transplantation, which indicates that they were not truly resistant. In fact, only 1 of 15 patients with disease larger than 1 cm going into transplantation remained alive and disease free at the time of analysis, which suggests that the more intensive regimen was not able to overcome bulky resistant disease. Further, this program did not appear to be superior in chemosensitive relapsed patients when compared with results in the group's earlier studies. Thus, it remains unclear whether these more intensive and toxic programs represent a significant advance.

In view of the toxicity inherent in increasing the dosages or numbers of drugs included in high-dose regimens, an alternative approach is to give HDCT for two or more cycles. Sequential or tandem transplantations, facilitated by the ability to collect a large number of progenitor cells, have been most intensively compared with single transplantations in patients with multiple myeloma. A report of the French Intergroupe Francophone du Myélome showed a survival advantage in the group that received two courses of HDCT.[59] Nevertheless, enthusiasm for this approach has been tempered by the lack of confirmatory data showing survival advantage from other randomized studies,[60,61] the absence of curative potential even with this highly aggressive treatment, and the emergence of newer drugs that are showing surprising disease activity even in heavily pretreated patients.[62] Moreover, improvement in survival with tandem transplantations appears to be limited to the best-prognosis patients. Patients with chromosome 13 deletion, high β_2-microglobulin levels, or a high plasma cell labeling index have not shown durable responses with this approach.[63]

One of the more promising strategies for intensifying high-dose therapy without concomitantly increasing toxicity is to administer targeted therapy either alone or in combination with chemotherapy. Delivery of radiation in the form of labeled monoclonal antibodies allows higher doses of radiation to be administered to tumor-bearing areas without delivery of similar doses to the lungs and liver.[64,65] Gopal et al.[66] performed a retrospective analysis of 125 consecutively treated patients with follicular lymphoma given either high-dose radioimmunotherapy alone or conventional HDCT with or without TBI. Patients treated with high-dose radioimmunotherapy had a statistically better progression-free and overall survival with no increase in early or late toxicity. The same group has also done a phase I and II study involving patients with relapsed mantle cell lymphoma in which tositumomab was given along with escalating doses of cyclophosphamide and etoposide. Progression-free survival was estimated at 61% in this poor-prognosis group.[65] In a preliminary report, Nademanee et al.[67] treated 18 high-risk patients with B-cell lymphoma with high-dose ibritumomab tiuxetan plus high-dose cyclophosphamide and etoposide. After a median follow-up of 8 months, 17 of 18 patients were alive in remission, and 7 patients with active disease at transplantation had achieved remission. These results suggest that targeted radiation may be a more effective and less toxic alternative to TBI in CD20+ lymphomas.

When HDCT is unlikely to be curative, there is increasing interest in using the achievement of minimal residual disease as a platform for additional posttransplantation therapy. These strategies include the induction of an autologous graft-versus-tumor–like response,[5,68] posttransplantation vaccination,[69] and adjuvant therapy with monoclonal antibodies such as rituximab.[3] Interest in the use of posttransplantation rituximab for

B-cell lymphoma patients is particularly intense because of its lack of severe toxicity and the occurrence of occasional dramatic durable responses in patients who have experienced relapse after autologous transplant.[70,71] A phase II trial in patients with predominately large cell lymphoma has shown encouraging results, with an 83% event-free survival at 2 years.[3] However, a preliminary report of a randomized study comparing adjuvant rituximab with observation after transplantation for aggressive B-cell lymphoma did not show a benefit in event-free survival.[72] Adjuvant rituximab therapy after progenitor cell transplantation also may not be benign. Horwitz et al. described a 54% incidence of grade 3 or 4 neutropenia, with many of the affected patients experiencing multiple episodes up to 1 year after transplantation. The mechanism of the neutropenia was unclear, but it appeared responsive to G-CSF and was not associated with infection.[3] Rose et al.[73] described a patient who received rituximab before and after transplantation who developed agranulocytosis that was resistant to G-CSF but responded to cyclosporine. Attempts at withdrawal of cyclosporine resulted in recurrence of neutropenia 14 months after transplantation. In view of the potential toxicity in this setting and probable reduced benefit of adjuvant rituximab for the increasing number of patients treated previously with rituximab, the use of adjuvant rituximab after transplantation remains investigational.

An innovative new approach for the treatment of minimal residual disease after autologous transplantation is to perform a reduced-intensity allogeneic transplantation in patients with matched donors. The use of reduced-intensity conditioning rather than standard preparative regimens lowers transplant-related mortality and extends the opportunity for allogeneic transplantation to older patients.[54,74] In addition, by performing a standard autologous transplantation first, maximum cytoreduction can be achieved without the morbidity or mortality that may accompany allogeneic engraftment.[4] The standard preparative regimen used during autologous transplantation also provides enough immunosuppression so that a subsequent reduced-intensity program is sufficient to permit engraftment.[4] To date, this approach has been most intensively studied in multiple myeloma because the mortality after standard allogeneic transplantation has been excessive, even in younger patients. Maloney et al.[4] treated 54 patients with this approach and reported a complete response rate of 57% after a median follow-up of 552 days. Most encouraging has been the observation of ongoing reduction in paraprotein levels well after treatment, which suggests a graft-versus-myeloma response. A "biologic randomization" study comparing tandem autologous transplantations with autologous transplantation followed by reduced-intensity allogeneic transplantation in poor-prognosis patients is in progress.

LATE TOXICITY: MYELODYSPLASIA AND SECONDARY LEUKEMIA

The most important factors resulting in myelodysplasia (MDS) and secondary leukemia (ANLL) after autologous transplantation are the type and extent of treatment *before* HDCT. For example, in one study there were no cases of MDS or ANLL in 71 patients with multiple myeloma treated with a brief course of vincristine, doxorubicin, and dexamethasone (VAD) followed

by tandem autologous transplants.[75] In contrast, cytogenetic abnormalities suggestive of MDS and ANLL were observed in 7 of 111 patients who had received an average of 2 years of chemotherapy before autologous transplantation.[75] Similarly, Harrison et al. implicated the use of alkylating agents during initial and salvage treatment rather than HDCT in the development of MDS and ANLL in patients with Hodgkin's disease treated with BCNU, etoposide, cytarabine, and melphalan (BEAM) and autologous transplantation.[76] These findings are supported by laboratory observations showing the presence of clonal hematopoiesis or cytogenetic abnormalities before transplantation in most patients who eventually developed MDS or ANLL after HDCT and autologous transplantation.[77] Given the "multiple-hit" hypothesis regarding most malignancies, it is still likely that HDCT is contributory to the development of MDS and ANLL; however, these data do argue for a dominant role of the treatment before transplantation.

Because patients have been treated heterogeneously before HDCT, it has been difficult to weigh the relative leukemogenic impact of different conditioning regimens. A case-control study does not support the hypothesis that TBI-based regimens are more leukemogenic than chemotherapy-only preparative regimens.[78] Nevertheless, in the absence of data showing that TBI-based programs are superior to HDCT, it seems likely that standard TBI will be used less often in future preparative regimens except as targeted therapy given in the form of radioactive monoclonal antibody.[66]

FUTURE DIRECTIONS

Potential major advances in high-dose therapy include the availability of targeted radioactive monoclonal antibodies and routine *in vivo* purging of B-cell lymphoma patients with rituximab. It seems likely that these two strategies will have their greatest impact in patients with follicular lymphoma. For these patients, one study has shown a survival advantage for high-dose therapy in patients with relapsed disease,[46] and there is increasing evidence that reinfused tumor cells are an important cause of relapse.[42] *In vivo* purging with rituximab before progenitor cell collection and HDCT has also led to greater enthusiasm for the use of HDCT in mantle cell lymphoma, and one study showed that most patients treated using this approach were alive and free of disease after more than 3 years of follow-up.[45] It remains unclear whether posttransplantation rituximab therapy will enhance survival, particularly in patients previously treated with rituximab during induction or salvage therapy or both. Posttransplantation vaccination may further improve disease-free and overall survival with minimal risk for toxicity.[69]

As allogeneic transplantation emerges as a promising treatment for myeloma,[4] low-grade lymphoma,[79] and mantle cell lymphoma,[80,81] prognostic factors will assume greater importance in selecting the most appropriate treatment for individual patients. In myeloma patients, for example, even tandem autologous transplantations have not been very effective for patients with unfavorable pretreatment variables such as chromosome 13 deletion and high levels of β_2-microglobulin. Among patients with lymphoma, a persistently positive result on positron emission tomography after salvage treatment may highlight a group of patients who have chemoresistant disease and for whom autologous transplantation is likely to fail.[82]

Alternatively, because of the morbidity and mortality associated with graft-versus-host-disease, allografts may be reserved for those for whom autologous transplantation fails. A small study has suggested the potential for cure in patients with relapsed NHL.[80]

REFERENCES

1. Openshaw H, Nash RA, McSweeney PA. High-dose immunosuppression and hematopoietic stem cell transplantation in autoimmune disease: clinical review. *Biol Blood Marrow Transplant* 2002;8:233.
2. Attal M, Harousseau JL, Stoppa AM, et al. A prospective, randomized trial of autologous bone marrow transplantation and chemotherapy in multiple myeloma. Intergroupe Français du Myélome. *N Engl J Med* 1996;335:91.
3. Horwitz SM, Negrin RS, Blume K, et al. Rituximab as adjuvant to high dose therapy and autologous hematopoietic cell transplantation for aggressive non-Hodgkin's lymphoma. *Blood* 2004;103(3):777.
4. Maloney DG, Molina AJ, Sahebi F, et al. Allografting with nonmyeloablative conditioning following cytoreductive autografts for the treatment of patients with multiple myeloma. *Blood* 2003;102:3447.
5. Stein AS, O'Donnell MR, Slovak ML, et al. Interleukin-2 after autologous stem-cell transplantation for adult patients with acute myeloid leukemia in first complete remission. *J Clin Oncol* 2003;21:615.
6. Juttner CA, To LB, Haylock DN, et al. Circulating autologous stem cells collected in very early remission from acute non-lymphoblastic leukaemia produce prompt but incomplete haemopoietic reconstitution after high dose melphalan or supralethal chemoradiotherapy. *Br J Haematology* 1985;61:739.
7. Gianni AM, Bregni M, Siena S, et al. Rapid and complete hemopoietic reconstitution following combined transplantation of autologous blood and bone marrow cells. A changing role for high dose chemo-radiotherapy? *Hematol Oncol* 1989;7:139.
8. Civin CI, Strauss LC, Brovall C, et al. Antigenic analysis of hematopoiesis III. A hematopoietic progenitor cell surface antigen defined by a monoclonal antibody raised against KG-1a cells. *J Immunol* 1984;133:157.
9. Siena S, Bregni M, Brando B, et al. Flow cytometry for clinical estimation of circulating hematopoietic progenitors for autologous transplantation in cancer patients. *Blood* 1991;77:400.
10. Weaver CH, Hazelton B, Birch R, et al. An analysis of engraftment kinetics as a function of the CD34 content of peripheral blood progenitor cell collections in 692 patients after the administration of myeloablative chemotherapy. *Blood* 1995;86:3961.
11. Bensinger W, Appelbaum F, Rowley S, et al. Factors that influence collection and engraftment of autologous peripheral-blood stem cells. *J Clin Oncol* 1995;13:2547.
12. Weaver CH, Potz J, Redmond J, et al. Engraftment and outcomes of patients receiving myeloablative therapy followed by autologous peripheral blood stem cells with a low CD34+ cell content. *Bone Marrow Transplant* 1997;19:1103.
13. Narayanasami U, Kanteti R, Morelli J, et al. Randomized trial of filgrastim versus chemotherapy and filgrastim mobilization of hematopoietic progenitor cells for rescue in autologous transplantation. *Blood* 2001;98:2059.
14. Pettengell R, Morgenstern GR, Woll PJ, et al. Peripheral blood progenitor cell transplantation in lymphoma and leukemia using a single apheresis. *Blood* 1993;82:3770.
15. Moskowitz CH, Bertino JR, Glassman JR, et al. Ifosfamide, carboplatin, and etoposide: a highly effective cytoreduction and peripheral blood progenitor-cell mobilization regimen for transplant-eligible patients with non-Hodgkin's lymphoma. *J Clin Oncol* 1999;17:3776.
16. Jones HM, Jones SA, Watts MJ, et al. Development of a simplified single-apheresis approach for peripheral-blood progenitor-cell transplantation in previously treated patients with lymphoma. *J Clin Oncol* 1994;12:1693.
17. Lerro KA, Medoff E, Wu Y, et al. A simplified approach to stem cell mobilization in multiple myeloma patients not previously treated with alkylating agents. *Bone Marrow Transplant* 2003;32:1113.
18. Galimberti S, Morabito F, Guerrini F, et al. Peripheral blood stem cell contamination evaluated by a highly sensitive molecular method fails to predict outcome of autotransplanted multiple myeloma patients. *Br J Haematol* 2003;120:405.
19. Gordan LN, Sugrue MW, Lynch JW, et al. Correlation of early lymphocyte recovery and progression-free survival after autologous stem cell transplant in patients with Hodgkin's and non-Hodgkin's lymphoma. *Bone Marrow Transplant* 2003;31:1009.
20. Weaver CH, Schulman KA, Buckner CD. Mobilization of peripheral blood stem cells following myelosuppressive chemotherapy: a randomized comparison of filgrastim, sargramostim, or sequential sargramostim and filgrastim. *Bone Marrow Transplant* 2001;27: S23.
21. Haas R, Mohle R, Fruhauf S, et al. Patient characteristics associated with successful mobilizing and autografting of peripheral blood progenitor cells in malignant lymphoma. *Blood* 1994;83:3787.
22. Tournilhac O, Cazin B, Lepretre S, et al. Impact of frontline fludarabine and cyclophosphamide combined treatment on peripheral blood stem cell mobilization in B-cell chronic lymphocytic leukemia. *Blood* 2004;103(1):363.
23. Fraipont V, Sautois B, Baudoux E, et al. Successful mobilization of peripheral blood HPCs with G-CSF alone in patients failing to achieve sufficient numbers of CD34+ cells and/or CFU-GM with chemotherapy and G-CSF. *Transfusion* 2000;40:339.
24. Weaver CH, Tauer K, Zhen B, et al. Second attempts at mobilization of peripheral blood stem cells in patients with initial low CD34+ cell yields. *J Hematother* 1998;7:241.
25. Watts MJ, Ings SJ, Flynn M, et al. Remobilization of patients who fail to achieve minimal progenitor thresholds at the first attempt is clinically worthwhile. *Br J Haematol* 2000;111:287.
26. Gazitt Y, Freytes CO, Callander N, et al. Successful PBSC mobilization with high-dose G-CSF for patients failing a first round of mobilization. *J Hematother* 1999;8:173.
27. Watts MJ, Sullivan AM, Leverett D, et al. Back-up bone marrow is frequently ineffective in patients with poor peripheral-blood stem-cell mobilization. *J Clin Oncol* 1998;16:1554.
28. Stiff P, Gingrich R, Luger S, et al. A randomized phase 2 study of PBPC mobilization by stem cell factor and filgrastim in heavily pretreated patients with Hodgkin's disease or non-Hodgkin's lymphoma. *Bone Marrow Transplant* 2000;26:471.
29. Rick O, Beyer J, Kingreen D, et al. Successful autologous bone marrow rescue in patients who failed peripheral blood stem cell mobilization. *Ann Hematol* 2000;79:681.
30. Lemoli RM, de Vivo A, Damiani D, et al. Autologous transplantation of granulocyte colony-stimulating factor-primed bone marrow is effective in supporting myeloablative chemotherapy in patients with hematologic malignancies and poor peripheral blood stem cell mobilization. *Blood* 2003;102:1595.
31. Petit I, Szyper-Kravitz M, Nagler A, et al. G-CSF induces stem cell mobilization by decreasing bone marrow SDF-1 and up-regulating CXCR4. *Nat Immunol* 2002;3:687.
32. Liles WC, Rodger E, Broxmeyer HE, et al. Mobilization and collection of CD34+ progenitor cells from normal human volunteers with AMD-3100, a CXCR4 antagonist, and G-CSF. *Am Soc Hematol* 2002(abst 404).
33. Carlo-Stella C, Di Nicola M, Guidetti A, et al. Use of recombinant human growth hormone plus recombinant human granulocyte colony-stimulating factor for the collection of CD34+ cells in poor mobilizers. *Am Soc Hematol* 2002(abst 401).
34. Leonard BM, Hetu F, Busque L, et al. Lymphoma cell burden in progenitor cell grafts measured by competitive polymerase chain reaction: less than one log difference between bone marrow and peripheral blood sources. *Blood* 1998;91:331.
35. Ladetto M, Omede P, Sametti S, et al. Real-time polymerase chain reaction in multiple myeloma: quantitative analysis of tumor contamination of stem cell harvests. *Exp Hematol* 2002;30:529.
36. Knudsen LM, Rasmussen T, Nikolaisen K, et al. Mobilisation of tumour cells along with CD34+ cells to peripheral blood in multiple myeloma. *Eur J Haematol* 2001;67:289.
37. Cooper BW, Moss TJ, Ross AA, et al. Occult tumor contamination of hematopoietic stem-cell products does not affect clinical outcome of autologous transplantation in patients with metastatic breast cancer. *J Clin Oncol* 1998;16:3509.
38. Weaver CH, Moss T, Schwartzberg LS, et al. High-dose chemotherapy in patients with breast cancer: evaluation of infusing peripheral blood stem cells containing occult tumor cells. *Bone Marrow Transplant* 1998;21:1117.
39. Gertz MA, Witzig TE, Pineda AA, et al. Monoclonal plasma cells in the blood stem cell harvest from patients with multiple myeloma are associated with shortened relapse-free survival after transplantation. *Bone Marrow Transplant* 1997;19:337.
40. Stewart AK, Vescio R, Schiller G, et al. Purging of autologous peripheral-blood stem cells using CD34 selection does not improve overall or progression-free survival after high-dose chemotherapy for multiple myeloma: results of a multicenter randomized controlled trial. *J Clin Oncol* 2001;19:3771.
41. Freedman AS, Neuberg D, Mauch P, et al. Long-term follow-up of autologous bone marrow transplantation in patients with relapsed follicular lymphoma. *Blood* 1999;94:3325.
42. Bierman PJ, Sweetenham JW, Loberiza FR Jr, et al. Syngeneic hematopoietic stem-cell transplantation for non-Hodgkin's lymphoma: a comparison with allogeneic and autologous transplantation—the Lymphoma Working Committee of the International Bone Marrow Transplant Registry and the European Group for Blood and Marrow Transplantation. *J Clin Oncol* 2003;21:3744.
43. Magni M, Di Nicola M, Devizzi L, et al. Successful in vivo purging of CD34-containing peripheral blood harvests in mantle cell and indolent lymphoma: evidence for a role of both chemotherapy and rituximab infusion. *Blood* 2000;96:864.
44. Galimberti S, Guerrini F, Morabito F, et al. Quantitative molecular evaluation in autotransplant programs for follicular lymphoma: efficacy of in vivo purging by rituximab. *Bone Marrow Transplant* 2003;32:57.
45. Gianni AM, Magni M, Martelli M, et al. Long-term remission in mantle cell lymphoma following high-dose sequential chemotherapy and in vivo rituximab-purged stem cell autografting (R-HDS regimen). *Blood* 2003;102:749.
46. Schouten HC, Qian W, Kvaloy S, et al. High-dose therapy improves progression-free survival and survival in relapsed follicular non-Hodgkin's lymphoma: results from the randomized European CUP trial. *J Clin Oncol* 2003;21:3918.
47. Morris CL, Siegel E, Barlogie B, et al. Mobilization of CD34+ cells in elderly patients (≥70 years) with multiple myeloma: influence of age, prior therapy, platelet count and mobilization regimen. *Br J Haematol* 2003;120:413.
48. Weaver CH, Birch R, Greco FA, et al. Mobilization and harvesting of peripheral blood stem cells: randomized evaluations of different doses of filgrastim. *Br J Haematol* 1998;100:338.
49. Zimmerman TM, Michelson GC, Mick R, et al. Timing of platelet recovery is associated with adequacy of leukapheresis product yield after cyclophosphamide and G-CSF in patients with lymphoma. *J Clin Apheresis* 1999;14:31.
50. Gordan LN, Sugrue MW, Lynch JW, et al. Correlation of early lymphocyte recovery and progression-free survival after autologous transplant in patients with Hodgkin's and non-Hodgkin's lymphoma. *Bone Marrow Transplant* 2003;31:1009.
51. Demirer T, Ayli M, Dagli M, et al. Influence of post-transplant recombinant human granulocyte colony-stimulating factor administration on peritransplant morbidity in patients undergoing autologous stem cell transplantation. *Br J Haematol* 2002;118:1104.
52. Bolwell B, Goormastic M, Dannley R, et al. G-CSF post-autologous progenitor cell transplantation: a randomized study of 5, 10, and 16 micrograms/kg/day. *Bone Marrow Transplant* 1997;19:215.

53. Khouri IF, Keating M, Korbling M, et al. Transplant-lite: induction of graft-versus-malignancy using fludarabine-based nonablative chemotherapy and allogeneic blood progenitor-cell transplantation as treatment for lymphoid malignancies. *J Clin Oncol* 1998;16:2817.

54. Slavin S, Nagler A, Naparstek E, et al. Nonmyeloablative stem cell transplantation and cell therapy as an alternative to conventional bone marrow transplantation with lethal cytoreduction for the treatment of malignant and nonmalignant hematologic diseases. *Blood* 1998;91:756.

55. Lahuerta JJ, Grande C, Blade J, et al. Myeloablative treatments for multiple myeloma: update of a comparative study of different regimens used in patients from the Spanish registry for transplantation in multiple myeloma. *Leuk Lymphoma* 2002;43:67.

56. Child JA, Morgan GJ, Davies FE, et al. High-dose chemotherapy with hematopoietic stem-cell rescue for multiple myeloma. *N Engl J Med* 2003;348:1875.

57. Haioun C, Lepage E, Gisselbrecht C, et al. Survival benefit of high-dose therapy in poor-risk aggressive non-Hodgkin's lymphoma: final analysis of the prospective LNH87-2 protocol—a Groupe d'Etude des Lymphomes de l'Adulte study [Comment]. *J Clin Oncol* 2000;18:3025.

58. Stiff PJ, Dahlberg S, Forman SJ, et al. Autologous bone marrow transplantation for patients with relapsed or refractory diffuse aggressive non-Hodgkin's lymphoma: value of augmented preparative regimens—a Southwest Oncology Group trial. *J Clin Oncol* 1998;16:48.

59. Attal M, Harousseau J-L, Facon T, et al. Single versus double autologous stem-cell transplantation for multiple myeloma. *N Engl J Med* 2003;349:2495.

60. Fermand J-P, Marolleau J-P, Alberti C, et al. Single versus tandem high dose therapy supported with autologous blood stem cell transplantation (ABSC) using unselected or CD34 enriched ABSC: preliminary results of a two by two designed randomized trial in 230 young patients with multiple myeloma. *Blood* 2001;98:815a(abst).

61. Cavo M, Tosi P, Zamagni E, et al. The "Bologna 96" clinical trial of single vs double autotransplants for previously untreated multiple myeloma patients. *Blood* 2002;100:179(abst).

62. Richardson PG, Barlogie B, Berenson J, et al. A phase 2 study of bortezomib in relapsed, refractory myeloma. *N Engl J Med* 2003;348:2609.

63. Barlogie B, Jagannath S, Desikan KR, et al. Total therapy with tandem transplants for newly diagnosed multiple myeloma. *Blood* 1999;93:55.

64. Press OW, Eary JF, Gooley T, et al. A phase I/II trial of iodine-131-tositumomab (anti-CD20), etoposide, cyclophosphamide, and autologous stem cell transplantation for relapsed B-cell lymphomas. *Blood* 2000;96:2934.

65. Gopal AK, Rajendran JG, Petersdorf SH, et al. High-dose chemo-radioimmunotherapy with autologous stem cell support for relapsed mantle cell lymphoma. *Blood* 2002;99:3158.

66. Gopal AK, Gooley TA, Maloney DG, et al. High-dose radioimmunotherapy versus conventional high-dose therapy and autologous hematopoietic stem cell transplantation for relapsed follicular non-Hodgkin lymphoma: a multivariable cohort analysis. *Blood* 2003;102:2351.

67. Nademanee A, Molina A, Forman S, et al. A phase I/II study of high-dose radioimmuno-therapy with Zevalin in combination with high-dose etoposide and cyclophosphamide followed by autologous stem cell transplant in patients with poor risk or relapsed B cell non-Hodgkin's lymphoma. *Blood* 2002;100(abst).

68. Park J, Lee MH, Lee HR, et al. Autologous peripheral blood stem cell transplantation with induction of autologous graft-versus-host disease in acute myeloid leukemia. *Bone Marrow Transplant* 2003;32:889.

69. Holman P, Medina B, Corringham R, et al. Early and robust immune responses to idiotype vaccination occur in mantle cell lymphoma and indolent lymphoma patients following autologous stem cell transplantation. *Blood* 2003;102:899a(abst).

70. Tsai D, Moore H, Hardy C, et al. Rituximab (anti-CD20 monoclonal antibody) therapy for progressive intermediate-grade non-Hodgkin's lymphoma after high-dose therapy and autologous peripheral stem cell transplantation. *Bone Marrow Transplant* 1999;24:521.

71. Pan D, Moskowitz CH, Zelenetz AD, et al. Rituximab for aggressive non-Hodgkin's lymphomas relapsing after or refractory to autologous stem cell transplantation. *Cancer J* 2002;8:371.

72. Haioun C, Mounier N, Emile JF, et al. Rituximab vs nothing after high-dose consolidative first line chemotherapy with autologous stem cell transplantation in poor risk diffuse large cell lymphoma. Results of the first interim analysis of the randomized LNH98 GELA study. *Blood* 2003;102:399a(abst).

73. Rose AL, Forsythe AM, Maloney DG. Agranulocytosis unresponsive to growth factors following rituximab in vivo purging [Letter]. *Blood* 2003;101:4225.

74. McSweeney PA, Niederwieser D, Shizuru JA, et al. Hematopoietic cell transplantation in older patients with hematologic malignancies: replacing high-dose cytotoxic therapy with graft-versus-tumor effects. *Blood* 2001;97:3390.

75. Govindarajan R, Jagannath S, Flick JT, et al. Preceding standard therapy is the likely cause of MDS after autotransplants for multiple myeloma. *Br J Haematol* 1996;95:349.

76. Harrison CN, Gregory W, Hudson GV, et al. High-dose BEAM chemotherapy with autologous haemopoietic stem cell transplantation for Hodgkin's disease is unlikely to be associated with a major increased risk of secondary MDS/AML. *Br J Cancer* 1999;81:476.

77. Lillington DM, Micallef IN, Carpenter E, et al. Detection of chromosome abnormalities pre-high-dose treatment in patients developing therapy-related myelodysplasia and secondary acute myelogenous leukemia after treatment for non-Hodgkin's lymphoma. *J Clin Oncol* 2001;19:2472.

78. Metayer C, Curtis RE, Vose J, et al. Myelodysplastic syndrome and acute myeloid leukemia after autotransplantation for lymphoma: a multicenter case-control study. *Blood* 2003;101:2015.

79. Van Besien K, Loberiza FR Jr, Bajorunaite R, et al. Comparison of autologous and allogeneic hematopoietic stem cell transplantation for follicular lymphoma. *Blood* 2003;102:3521.

80. Seropian S, Bahceci E, Cooper DL. Allogeneic peripheral blood stem cell transplantation for high-risk non-Hodgkin's lymphoma. *Bone Marrow Transplant* 2003;32:763.

81. Khouri IF, Lee M-S, Saliba RM, et al. Nonablative allogeneic stem-cell transplantation for advanced/recurrent mantle cell lymphoma. *J Clin Oncol* 2003;21:4407.

82. Spaepen K, Stroobants S, Dupont P, et al. Prognostic value of pretransplantation positron emission tomography using fluorine 18-fluorodeoxyglucose in patients with aggressive lymphoma treated with high-dose chemotherapy and stem cell transplantation. *Blood* 2003;102:53.

SECTION 3

RICHARD W. CHILDS

Allogeneic Hematopoietic Stem Cell Transplantation

For more than 35 years, allogeneic hematopoietic cell transplantation (HCT) has been used successfully to treat patients with advanced hematologic malignancies.[1] Despite its inherent risks, allogeneic transplantation offers many patients with treatment-resistant leukemias the only chance of a cure. The concept that cancer might be cured should high enough doses of cytotoxic agents be deliverable was based on the observation that some malignancies exhibit a steep dose-response effect to radiation and cytotoxic drugs. The permanent eradication of recipient bone marrow (BM) was quickly identified as the major obstacle to dose intensification. With the availability of hematopoietic progenitor cells to rescue BM function, high-dose chemotherapy regimens for a variety of "incurable" cancers became a popular area of investigation. Myeloablative doses of chemoradiotherapy are intended to completely eradicate the malignancy, followed by the infusion of hematopoietic progenitor cells [either BM cells or progenitors mobilized into the blood by granulocyte colony-stimulating factor (G-CSF)] to rescue the patient from ensuing BM aplasia. However, most dose-intensification strategies have failed to cure patients with advanced malignancies. Indeed, in some animal models, exceedingly high doses of total body irradiation (TBI), far more than could be used clinically, are needed to kill all leukemia cells.[2] Furthermore, autologous BM transplants (BMTs) are limited by the risk that cancer cells residing in the autograft might be reinfused into the patient. The use of hematopoietic progenitor cells from a healthy donor to restore marrow function would avoid this risk. This concept was most appropriately applied to malignancies, such as leukemia, which originate in the BM itself. However, several lines of evidence reveal that even the most intense of conditioning regimens often fail to completely eradicate leukemic clones. Rather, a powerful immune reaction generated from transplanted donor T cells against residual leukemia [called *graft-versus-leukemia* (GVL)] occurs in those who achieve durable disease-free survival. Indeed, in murine studies dating back as far as the 1950s, it was observed that leukemia-bearing recipients undergoing an allogeneic transplant have a greater proportion of leukemic cure compared with mice receiving syngeneic transplants.[3] It is through the combination of these two components, dose-intensive tumor killing followed by the GVL effect, that allogeneic HCT has its curative potential.

CONDITIONING REGIMENS

CONVENTIONAL MYELOABLATIVE CONDITIONING

For conventional myeloablative transplantation of hematologic malignancies, the preparative regimen serves two purposes: (1) to provide sufficient immunosuppression to prevent rejection and allow engraftment of donor hematopoietic/immune cells and (2) to eradicate malignant cells. Decisions regarding the choice of a specific preparative regimen are guided by following: the sensitivity of the underlying malignancy to the drugs contained within that regimen; the age and performance status of the patient; the specific toxicities inherent to individual conditioning agents; and the HLA compatibility between the recipient and donor. For many hematologic malignancies, cytoreduction through dose-intensive conditioning is required to optimize the induction of curative GVL effects. Therefore, the conditioning regimen plays a major role in transplant outcome. In general, myeloablative conditioning strategies can be divided into two categories: TBI-based or chemotherapy-based (Table 52.3-1).

Most TBI-based regimens are composed of high-dose cyclophosphamide given as 60 mg/kg intravenously (IV) on 2 consecutive days followed by varying doses of fractionated TBI to a cumulative dose of 1200 to 1500 cGy. Although evidence exists that the higher doses of TBI may have superior efficacy in preventing disease relapse, a concomitant increase in toxicity appears to negate a survival benefit.

Although a number of chemotherapy-based regimens without radiation have been used, the combination of cyclophosphamide (60 mg/kg IV on 2 consecutive days, total dose 120 mg/kg) and busulfan (4 mg/kg orally on 4 consecutive days, total dose 16 mg/kg) has remained a popular conditioning strategy since its initial use in the early 1980s. Similar to the experience with TBI, dose intensification of chemotherapy-based regimens usually results in a reduction in disease relapse. However, such a benefit is typically offset by an increase in toxicity and transplant-related mortality.

The decision guiding preparative regimen choice is often based on the disease-specific activity of the agents contained within the regimen. In general, radiation- and chemotherapy-based regimens have shown equivalence in disease-free survival in acute and chronic myelogenous leukemias. Two randomized trials evaluating cyclophosphamide and busulfan versus TBI and cyclophosphamide in patients with chronic-phase chronic myelogenous leukemia (CML) revealed equal efficacy between both regimens.[4] However, in acute lymphocytic leukemia (ALL), TBI-based regimens may be the treatment of choice, as two randomized trials reported a significantly increased risk of relapse in patients with ALL who received conditioning with chemotherapy alone (busulfan and etoposide or busulfan and cyclophosphamide) compared with regimens containing TBI (TBI and etoposide or TBI and cyclophosphamide).[5,6] The toxicity profile of preparative regimens vary considerably, a factor that often guides the selection of a regimen for an individual patient. In general, TBI-based regimens are associated with a higher risk of secondary malignancies, cataracts, hypothyroidism, and growth retardation, whereas chemotherapy-based regimens, particularly those containing busulfan, are associated with a higher risk of severe mucositis and

TABLE 52.3-1. Toxicity Profiles of Various Myeloablative and Nonmyeloablative Transplant Conditioning Regimens

Reference(s)	Conditioning Agents	Mixed Chimerism	Graft Rejection	VOD	Mucositis
MYELOABLATIVE CONDITIONING					
1,6	Busulfan, 16 mg/kg PO	−	+	++	++
	Cyclophosphamide, 120 mg/kg IV				
1,6	TBI, 1200–1400 cGy	−	+	+	+++
	Cyclophosphamide, 120 mg/kg IV				
NONMYELOABLATIVE CONDITIONING					
109	Busulfan, 8 mg/kg PO	+	+/−	++	+/−
	Fludarabine, 180 mg/m² IV				
	ATG, 40 mg/kg IV				
131	Busulfan, 6.3 mg/kg IV	++	+/−	−	+/−
	Fludarabine, 150 mg/m² IV				
124	TBI, 200 cGy	+++	++	−	−
129	TBI, 200 cGy	+++	+	−	−
	Fludarabine, 90 mg/m² IV				
130	Alemtuzumab (Campath), 100 mg IV	++	−	−	+/−
	Fludarabine, 150 mg/m²				
	Melphalan, 140 mg/m² IV				
123	Cyclophosphamide, 120 mg/kg	+++	−	−	−
	Fludarabine, 125 mg/m² IV				
108	Melphalan, 180 or 140 mg/m²	+	+/−	+/−	+/−
	Fludarabine, 125 mg/m² IV				
107	Fludarabine, 125 or 90 mg/m² IV	++	+/−	−	−
	Cyclophosphamide, 2 g/m² IV				
	Rituximab pre/posttransplant				

−, does not occur; +, rarely occurs; ++, occurs commonly; +++, frequently occurs; ATG, antithymocyte globulin; TBI, total body irradiation, VOD, vasoocclusive disease.

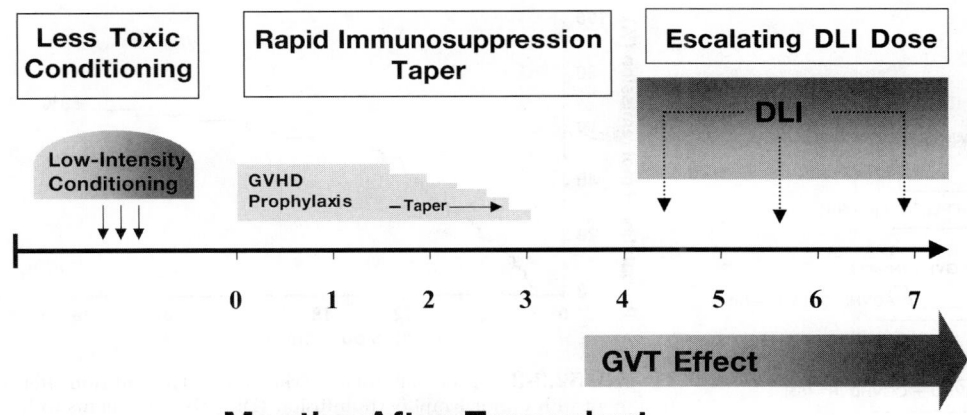

FIGURE 52.3-1. Nonmyeloablative transplant strategy. DLI, donor lymphocyte infusion; GVHD, graft-versus-host disease; GVT, graft-versus-tumor.

venoocclusive disease (VOD), with fewer effects on growth and development. A recent study from the Nordic Transplantation Group reported busulfan-treated patients to have a significantly higher incidence of VOD (12%) and death from graft-versus-host disease (GVHD) (22%) compared with patients receiving conditioning with TBI and cyclophosphamide [1% (*P* = .01) and 3% (*P* <.001), respectively].[6a] Data exist showing patients with high busulfan area under the concentration-time curve levels are at greatest risk for the development of VOD and death. The significant interpatient and intrapatient variability in the absorption of oral busulfan may in part be responsible for the significant variations observed in busulfan pharmacokinetics.[6b] The advent of IV busulfan now allows for more accurate dosing and could potentially lead to a reduction in the toxicities associated with this agent.

NONMYELOABLATIVE CONDITIONING REGIMENS

In recent years, investigators have increasingly explored the use of reduced-intensity preparative regimens in an effort to decrease the risk of regimen-related toxicity and mortality that occur as a consequence of myeloablative conditioning. Nonmyeloablative preparative regimens are given primarily to induce immunosuppression to allow for the engraftment of donor hematopoietic progenitor cells and immune cells, which mediate subsequent GVL effects. Such low-intensity transplants rely primarily on the GVL effect to eradicate the underlying malignancy (Fig. 52.3-1). Furthermore, because host BM cells are not completely destroyed, autologous hematopoiesis may occur, which shortens the time interval of neutropenia compared with patients undergoing a myeloablative transplant.

Although regimens vary considerably between institutions, results have been promising, showing high degrees of donor engraftment with a lower incidence of toxicities such as severe mucositis, pneumonitis, and VOD compared with those receiving conventional high-dose myeloablative regimens. Furthermore, they have proven to be safe in older patients (e.g., older than 55 years) and in those with underlying medical comorbidities who would not be candidates for a myeloablative transplant due to an exceedingly high risk of transplant-related mortality. Remarkably, some regimens do not cause neutropenia, significantly reducing the risk of opportunistic infection and allowing for transplantation to occur in the out-

patient setting. Furthermore, sustained remissions of more than 5 years suggest the procedure may be curative for a number of different malignant and nonmalignant hematologic diseases. The improved safety profile of nonmyeloablative conditioning has made this transplant approach the procedure of choice for patients at high risk for complications associated with dose-intensive regimens. Although long-term follow-up data are not yet available, it is reasonable to anticipate that younger patients may further benefit from a reduction in growth retardation, sterility, and the risk of secondary malignancy that occur with allogeneic HCT. The toxicity profiles of different nonmyeloablative transplant conditioning regimens are shown in Table 52.3-1.

GRAFT-VERSUS-LEUKEMIA EFFECT

The concept that donor immune cells might make an important contribution to the antileukemic effect of allogeneic BMT was based on observations in animal models in the 1950s. Mice with leukemia given syngeneic BMTs died of leukemia, whereas mice given allogeneic BMTs were rescued from leukemia but instead died from acute GVHD.[7] Sentinel observations supporting the existence of a GVL effect in humans included the following: Leukemia relapse occurred less often in patients who developed GVHD after BMT compared with those who never developed GVHD; the incidence of leukemic relapse was increased in identical twin transplants; and the incidence of leukemic relapse was increased and in those receiving T cell–depleted marrow (to prevent acute GVHD). Subsequently, a retrospective study of more than 2000 recipients of HLA-matched sibling BMTs confirmed acute GVHD and chronic GVHD (CGVHD) were both associated with a significant reduction in the risk of disease relapse, whereas T-cell depletion increased the risk of relapse.[8] Results from this study showing the relationship of GVHD, T-cell depletion, and the source of donor cells with relapse are shown in Figure 52.3-2. Data from this registry showed GVL effects vary according to the type of leukemia but were most evident in patients with chronic-phase CML undergoing transplant in early chronic phase. Further indirect evidence for a donor immune-mediated antileukemic effect included the observation that up to 50% of patients who are ultimately cured after allogeneic trans-

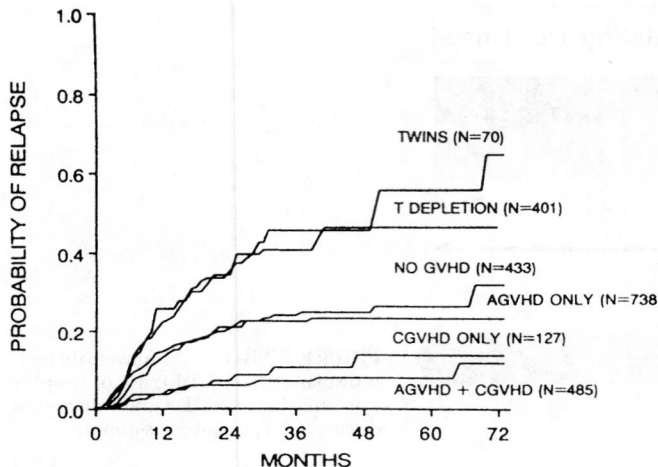

FIGURE 52.3-2.   Actuarial probability of relapse after bone marrow transplantation for early leukemia according to type of graft and development of graft-versus-host disease (GVHD). AGVHD, acute GVHD; CGVHD, chronic GVHD. (From Horowitz MM, Gale RP, Sondel PM, et al. Graft-versus-leukemia reactions after bone marrow transplantation. *Blood* 1990;75:555, with permission.)

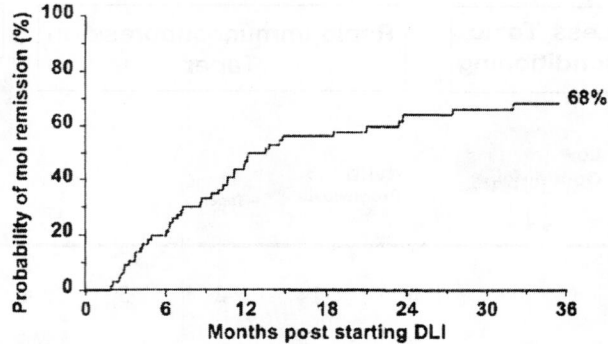

FIGURE 52.3-3.   Probability of achieving molecular remission after treatment with donor lymphocyte infusion (DLI) for 66 patients with chronic myelogenous leukemia in relapse after allogeneic stem cell transplantation. (From ref. 12, with permission.)

plantation have detectable CML bcr/abl transcripts or small numbers of Philadelphia-positive chromosomes for months after allogeneic BMT; their delayed clearance is consistent with an active GVL effect.[9] In addition, abrupt discontinuation of cyclosporine after CML relapse has been associated with reinduction of cytogenetic remissions.[10]

Finally, the most compelling evidence supporting the curative nature of the GVL effect is the observation that durable molecular remissions can be induced in patients with CML in relapse after marrow transplant by the transfusion of donor lymphocytes in the absence of chemotherapy.[11] The efficacy of donor lymphocyte infusions (DLIs) for the treatment of relapsed leukemia is disease-dependent, with remission induction occurring in a substantially higher percentage of patients with chronic-phase CML than patients with advanced CML or other acute leukemias. In general, 70% to 80% of patients with cytogenetic or hematologic relapse of CML can be expected to achieve a molecular remission after DLI. Remissions are usually not observed until months after DLI, consistent with the time required to expand antileukemic T-cell clones (Fig. 52.3-3). The vast majority of patients achieving a molecular remission achieve long-term disease-free survival. The durability of disease response is dependent on stage of disease at relapse; patients with CML with a cytogenetic relapse have a higher probability of achieving long-term disease-free survival after DLI compared with those having a hematologic relapse or relapse in accelerated phase or blast crisis.[12]

In contrast to the relatively high efficacy of DLI in relapsed chronic-phase CML, only a minority of patients with acute leukemias who relapse after allogeneic transplant achieve a durable remission after the infusion of donor lymphocytes. In a report from the European Group for Blood and Marrow Transplant, only 29% of patients with relapsed acute myelogenous leukemia (AML) and none with relapsed ALL (0 of 11) achieved remission after DLI.[13] Furthermore, unlike chronic-phase CML, remissions after DLI for accelerated/blast crisis CML and acute leukemia appear to be of limited duration, with a significant proportion of patients relapsing within a year

of treatment. Disease regression after DLI has also been described in patients with relapsed multiple myeloma, chronic lymphocytic leukemia (CLL), and non-Hodgkin's lymphoma, although too few have been treated to define the efficacy of this approach in these diseases.

The major complication associated with DLI is acute GVHD and CGVHD; up to 70% of patients develop acute GVHD after DLI that may be life-threatening (i.e., grade 3 to 4) in 15% to 20% of cases. The propensity for GVHD after DLI is likely impacted on by the following two factors: (1) Relatively large doses of T lymphocytes have traditionally have been infused (1 to 10×10^7 CD3 cells/kg), and (2) these cells are usually given without GVHD prophylaxis. Two approaches to reduce the incidence of GVHD after DLI have been developed. One approach is to selectively infuse lymphocytes depleted of CD8+ T cells. This approach was investigated based on the experience that CD8+-depleted allografts were associated with a low incidence of GVHD without an increased risk of relapse.[14] Several nonrandomized trials have shown that CD8+-depleted DLI can reinduce remission, with a rate of GVHD that was lower than that observed with unmanipulated DLI.[14] A recent trial that randomized patients to unselected versus CD8-depleted DLI as prophylaxis for disease relapse reported a significantly higher incidence of acute GVHD in the unselected cohort [six of nine patients (67%)] compared with recipients of CD8-depleted DLI [zero of nine patients (0%); $P = .009$]. Importantly, both groups converted from mixed chimerism to full donor chimeras after DLI, suggesting that CD8 depletion reduces the incidence of GVHD without adversely affecting its ability to eradicate recipient hematopoietic cells.[15] An alternative strategy involves the infusion of donor lymphocytes in multiple aliquots, starting at low cell numbers and escalating the dosage at variable intervals until a GVL effect is achieved. A recent trial comparing these two different lymphocyte infusion approaches in patients with relapsed chronic-phase CML revealed a significantly lower incidence of GVHD in the group that received dose-escalating lymphocyte infusions compared with the group receiving traditional single "bulk-dose" regimens (10% vs. 44%). Importantly, although acute GVHD was extremely low in the escalating-dose group, the GVL effect was preserved, with 91% of patients achieving a complete remission (CR) by 2 years.[16]

The other potentially life-threatening complication of DLI is marrow aplasia. Approximately 30% to 40% of patients who receive DLI for relapsed CML develop pancytopenia, which typically occurs at the time of the GVL response. Although most patients still have mixed or complete T-cell chimerism at the time of DLI, myeloid chimerism may be predominantly recipient in origin, originating from the leukemic clone, thus leaving the marrow aplastic after a GVH hematopoietic effect. The duration of aplasia is variable and is directly dependent on the number of residual donor hematopoietic cells. Although in most cases, spontaneous reconstitution of marrow by donor cells usually occurs, some patients have persistent aplasia and may require additional donor stem cell infusions to rescue marrow function. Reconditioning before such stem cell infusions is not required, as most patients have predominantly donor immunity and are therefore tolerant of donor hematopoietic progenitor cells. Although the infusion of donor lymphocytes with stem cells has been used successfully to treat relapsed leukemia, it is unclear if the incidence and severity of BM aplasia are mitigated. A recent nonrandomized study found no significant difference in the incidence (31% vs. 22%), time of onset (41 vs. 48 days), or duration (15 vs. 14 days) of hematologic cytopenias that occurred in two different cohorts of patients receiving either donor lymphocytes alone versus a G-CSF–mobilized (T cell–rich) apheresis product containing a 550-fold higher CD34+ cell dose.[17]

MECHANISMS OF GRAFT-VERSUS-LEUKEMIA EFFECT

Although evidence supporting the GVL effect is overwhelming, the target antigens on leukemic cells as well as the effector cells mediating these antileukemic effects are not fully understood.[18] The high incidence of leukemic relapse in syngeneic transplants suggests that a significant component of the GVL effect is the consequence of donor immune cells targeting allogeneic antigens. Minor histocompatibility antigens [major histocompatibility complex (MHC)-bound peptides derived from the degradation of cellular proteins with amino acid polymorphisms between the patient and donor] can lead to differential recognition by T cells and are likely the dominant targets for both GVHD and the GVL effect. The tissue-restricted pattern of minor histocompatibility antigens likely explains why some patients respond to DLI without the development of GVHD; T-cell populations mediating an antileukemia reaction against minor histocompatibility antigens restricted to hematopoietic cells would not be expected to cause GVHD, in contrast to T cells targeting such antigens expressed broadly on both normal tissue and leukemic cells, where both GVHD and a GVL effect would occur. Indeed, T-cell clones have been generated *in vitro* that specifically recognize minor histocompatibility antigens restricted to leukemic cells and normal hematopoietic cells.[19] Minor histocompatibility antigens may be either MHC class I– or class II–restricted, thus evoking CD8+ and CD4+ alloreactive T-cell responses, respectively. Recently, investigators have shown that CD8+ clones recognizing HA-1 and HA-2, two minor histocompatibility antigens restricted to hematopoietic cells, emerge in the blood of some patients at the time of a GVL effect, further confirming minor antigens to be the dominant target of T cells mediating GVL effects.[20]

Donor T cells targeting tumor antigens restricted or overexpressed on malignant cells might also serve as targets for GVL. T cells specific for peptides derived from several different normal proteins overexpressed on leukemia cells (e.g., proteinase

3, myeloperoxidase, Wilms' tumor protein) can be isolated from some donors and patients who have antileukemic effects *in vitro*. Furthermore, the degradation of proteins restricted to tumor cells might result in the MHC binding and presentation of unique peptides from the region of fusion gene or mutated gene sequence. Although leukemia-restricted peptides would appear to be an attractive target for donor immune cells, as of yet there is no convincing evidence to implicate a specific antileukemic effect in GVL. However, patients with relapsed leukemia who achieve remission after DLI without GVHD lend credence to the notion that GVL may occasionally be a targeted antileukemic process.

Although the full nature of the effector cells mediating GVL are not entirely known, both CD4+ helper T cells and CD8+ cytotoxic T cells with direct antileukemic activity have been isolated from patients after allogeneic BMT.[20] Recent data suggest natural killer (NK) cells may play a particularly important role in the GVL effect against myelogenous leukemia in the setting of haploidentical or partially mismatched allogeneic transplantation when killer immunoglobulin-like receptor (KIR) incompatibility exists in the direction of GVHD (defined as the absence of an MHC class I KIR ligand in the recipient that is present in the donor).[21] However, in the HLA-matched setting, the contribution that NK cells make to GVL is not known.

COMPLICATIONS OF ALLOGENEIC HEMATOPOIETIC STEM CELL TRANSPLANTATION

Allogeneic HCT is associated with a number of complications, many unique to this type of therapy, that can be divided into two general categories: (1) toxicities related to conditioning and (2) toxicities that occur as the consequence of transplanting allogeneic immune cells/tissue into the recipient, namely graft rejection, GVHD, and infectious complications associated with immunosuppression.

The complications associated with myeloablative doses of chemoradiotherapy vary in terms of incidence and severity depending on the intensity and type of agents used in conditioning. These complications may occur as an immediate side effect, at or shortly after the preparative regimen, or in a delayed fashion years after transplantation. Commonly observed immediate toxicities include nausea and vomiting; mucositis; and pancytopenia, including neutropenia associated with associated fever and/or opportunistic bacterial or invasive fungal infection.

High-dose cyclophosphamide may be associated with hemorrhagic cystitis or, more rarely, rapidly progressive heart failure. The routine use of mesna, hydration, and forced diuresis has largely eliminated early hemorrhagic cystitis. In contrast, late hemorrhagic cystitis (occurring beyond 72 hours of cyclophosphamide) remains a continuing problem in allogeneic BMT and is usually viral in etiology (polyomavirus BK or adenovirus), occurring more frequently in profoundly immunosuppressed patients such as recipients of T cell–depleted transplants.[22] High-dose busulfan is associated with grand mal seizures; many busulfan-containing regimens use seizure prophylaxis with phenytoin (Dilantin) or phenobarbital.

Opportunistic infections as a consequence of preparative regimen-induced neutropenia remain a significant complication associated with allogeneic BMT. Most fungal and bacterial infections originate from microorganisms colonizing the skin, oral cavity, perianal area, or gastrointestinal (GI) or respiratory tract. The most common life-threatening bacterial infections occurring during the neutropenic period include gram-negative and aerobic gram-positive bacteria. These pathogens gain entry into the host through indwelling vascular catheters or as a consequence of the breakdown of GI mucosa related to high-dose chemoradiotherapy. Decontamination of the gut with nonabsorbable antibiotics such as neomycin or vancomycin has met with mixed success, with poor patient compliance being a major drawback to this approach. Prophylactic oral quinolones such as ciprofloxacin or norfloxacin appear to decrease the incidence of febrile neutropenia and gram-negative infections, although possibly at the expense of more episodes of gram-positive bacteremia. *Candida* and *Aspergillus* species are the most common fungal pathogens, commonly causing infection during periods of neutropenia or systemic corticosteroid use for GVHD. Oral triazoles, such as fluconazole, have been shown in randomized trials to decrease the incidence of opportunistic candidal infections but have no impact on the incidence of infections with resistant species such as *Aspergillus* or *Candida krusei.* One placebo-controlled randomized study showed patients who received prophylactic fluconazole for 75 days after the transplant not only had a lower incidence of invasive candidiasis (30 of 148 patients vs. 4 of 152 patients, $P < .001$) but also a significantly lower incidence of severe GVHD of the GI tract (20 of 143 patients vs. 8 of 145 patients, $P = .02$), resulting in an overall survival benefit.[23] Although prophylactic itraconazole appears superior to fluconazole in terms of preventing invasive mold infections, the toxicities and poor tolerability of this drug limit its success as a prophylactic antifungal agent. Finally, voriconazole (an orally available broad-spectrum triazole with high activity against *Aspergillus* species) has recently been shown to be at least as effective as amphotericin B in the treatment of acute invasive *Aspergillus* in immunocompromised patients; studies comparing prophylactic voriconazole with fluconazole are currently under way, with the hope this new agent will significantly reduce the risk of invasive *Aspergillus* infections associated with allogeneic transplantation.[24]

VENOOCCLUSIVE DISEASE

One of the most serious life-threatening complications of dose-intensive chemoradiotherapy is VOD of the liver. VOD produces a clinical syndrome of jaundice, tender hepatomegaly, and unexplained weight gain or ascites.[25] Clinically evident VOD occurs in approximately 30% of allogeneic BMT patients conditioned with oral busulfan-containing regimens, with approximately 25% of those affected having severe life-threatening disease leading to progressive liver failure, hepatic encephalopathy, and/or hepatorenal syndrome. The exact pathogenesis of VOD is unknown, although the earliest event is believed to be endothelial damage due to BMT conditioning, leading to fibrinogen and collagen deposition in vessel walls at the interface of hepatic sinusoids and terminal venules, which ultimately become obstructed; histologically, damage to zone 3 hepatocytes is present. Predisposing factors for VOD include a history of liver disease, advanced age, elevated liver enzymes before transplant, short interval from prior treatment with gemtuzumab ozogamicin (Mylotarg) to transplant conditioning (e.g., less than 4 months), use of busulfan in the conditioning regimen, dose intensity of the conditioning regimen, presence of acute GVHD, and transplants from

alternative donors such as matched unrelated or haploidentical donors.[26] The diagnosis of VOD is based on the presence of clinical criteria (jaundice, tender hepatomegaly, and unexplained weight gain or ascites), in which there is a 90% correlation between the presence of all three criteria and a histologic confirmation by liver biopsy. Symptoms of VOD usually occur shortly after the conditioning regimen (e.g., less than 20 days), although late-onset VOD (symptoms developing 24 to 42 days after conditioning) has rarely been described in some patients.[27] Therapy for established VOD is unsatisfactory and consists mostly of measures to support renal function, fluid balance, and coagulation status. Recombinant tissue plasminogen activator and prostaglandin E_1 have had mixed success, making it unclear what, if any, role these agents should play in the treatment of established disease. Defibrotide, a polydeoxyribonucleotide with activity in several vascular disorders, has recently been used with success to treat patients with severe VOD after HCT. A study of 88 patients who developed severe, life-threatening VOD after allogeneic or autologous transplantation provided evidence to support the safety and activity of this agent; 36% of patients had complete resolution of VOD, with 35% of patients surviving more than 100 days after the transplant.[28] The therapeutic drug monitoring of oral busulfan, with appropriate dose adjustments, appears to be useful in reducing the incidence of VOD associated with this agent. Data regarding whether pharmacologic prophylaxis against VOD is effective are currently inconclusive. Two randomized clinical trials have shown a significant reduction in the incidence of VOD in patients taking ursodiol prophylaxis versus those taking placebo (15% vs. 50% and 3% vs. 18.5%, respectively, in each study).[29,30] Because this agent is generally well tolerated, it has increasingly been used as prophylaxis in patients thought to be at high risk for VOD.

PULMONARY COMPLICATIONS

Pulmonary complications occur frequently after allogeneic BMT and may be related to infectious agents, diffuse alveolar hemorrhage (DAH), or pulmonary edema or may have an idiopathic origin. Common life-threatening infectious etiologies include *Aspergillus* or other fungal organisms, respiratory syncytial virus and cytomegalovirus (CMV). Late pneumonia from *Pneumocystis carinii* may occur more than a year after transplantation and is usually related to prolonged CD4+ lymphopenia associated with T-cell depletion of the allograft or acute or CGVHD. Interstitial pneumonitis (IP) syndrome is an inflammatory lung disease that is characterized by diffuse IP and alveolitis sometimes leading to interstitial fibrosis. Clinically, it is characterized by fever, hypoxia, and diffuse pulmonary infiltrates. Animal models have shown that lung irradiation appears to play an important role in the development of IP syndrome after allogeneic BMT. The syndrome occurs in up to 10% to 20% of patients receiving myeloablative conditioning, usually within the first 3 months of transplantation, and is lethal in up to half the cases.[31] Approximately 90% of the cases of IP are related to either CMV infection or have an idiopathic origin (idiopathic IP). The incidence of CMV pneumonitis appears to have decreased significantly over the past 10 years, primarily as the consequence of more sensitive methods to detect early CMV reactivation [e.g., polymerase chain reaction (PCR) for CMV or CMV antigenemia testing] before clinical disease develops. Patient-specific risk factors for IP include older age, prior history of exposure to pulmonary toxic drugs such as bleomycin, history of acute or CGVHD, dose intensity of the conditioning regimen, or the use of TBI.[32] Regimens that use a lower dose rate or total dose of TBI, lung shielding, as well as hyperfractionated TBI may be associated with a lower risk of IP.[33]

Bronchoscopy with bronchoalveolar lavage should be used in all patients with IP to differentiate idiopathic IP from infectious causes or DAH. Empiric use of anti-CMV agents such as ganciclovir or foscarnet should be considered when bronchoalveolar lavage is not feasible. The prognosis of patients developing DAH is extremely poor, with mortality rates in the range of 48% to 80%; survival appears to be worse in those with DAH after allogeneic transplantation (vs. autologous transplants) and in patients who develop this complication more than 30 days after transplant conditioning.[34] Although evidence exists supporting the efficacy of high-dose corticosteroids in patients with DAH, the effectiveness of these agents in the treatment of idiopathic IP remains equivocal.

LATE COMPLICATIONS

The delayed complications associated with allogeneic HCT depend on patient age at transplantation and are primarily the consequence of the effects of long-term damage to normal tissues by either the preparative regimen or CGVHD. These effects include growth retardation, infertility, endocrine failure, avascular joint necrosis, osteopenia, cataracts, renal insufficiency, restrictive pulmonary defects, neurocognitive defects, and secondary malignancies.[35] The use of TBI in the conditioning regimen seems to be the factor associated with the greatest risk for secondary malignancies.[36] A long-term follow-up study of 1036 patients undergoing BMT for a wide range of malignant and nonmalignant conditions reported a 12.6% incidence of secondary neoplasms at 15 years, a rate that was 3.8 times higher than an age-matched control population.[37] The most frequently observed secondary neoplasms are lymphomas, leukemias, and solid tumors (particularly oral cavity and skin). The characteristic time course of secondary malignancies is shown in Figure 52.3-4. The median time from trans-

plant to secondary lymphoma [primarily Epstein-Barr virus (EBV) virus–related], leukemia, and solid tumor is 2.5 months, 6.7 months, and 5 to 6 years, respectively.[36] Increased solid tumor risk appears to be associated with younger patient age at transplantation and the use of radiation in the conditioning regimen. CGVHD and/or treatment for CGVHD are strongly associated with an increased risk of squamous cell carcinoma of the skin.

EPSTEIN-BARR VIRUS LYMPHOPROLIFERATIVE DISORDER

Posttransplant EBV-associated lymphoproliferative disorder (LPD) represents an aggressive and potentially fatal B-cell lymphoid proliferation that occurs after 5% to 30% of allogeneic transplants. This lymphoma originates from EBV-infected B cells, typically of donor origin, and usually stems from a deficiency of EBV-specific cytotoxic T cells associated with the use of immunosuppressive drugs or T-cell depletion of the allograft. EBV LPD can be successfully treated by infusing unmanipulated leukocytes from the donor or donor lymphocytes that have been sensitized *in vitro* to irradiated EBV-transformed B cell lines.[38] Prophylactic infusion of *ex vivo*–generated EBV-specific T cells have been shown to prevent EBV LPD without causing acute GVHD in children receiving T cell–depleted transplants from HLA-mismatched donors.[39] B-cell depletion of the allograft is another strategy that has been used successfully to prevent this disorder. The use of rituximab, a monoclonal antibody to the B-cell antigen CD20, has been shown to be an effective strategy to treat established LPD. Quantitative real-time PCR monitoring for EBV DNA can be used to identify patients at high risk for the development of posttransplant LPD. Furthermore, preemptive therapy with rituximab in patients reactivating EBV by PCR may significantly reduce the risk of development of LPD. One study reported a dramatic reduction in LPD mortality in those with EBV reactivation who received preemptive rituximab (0%) compared with untreated historical controls with viral reactivation (26%; $P = .04$).[40]

GRAFT-VERSUS-HOST DISEASE

GVHD is the consequence of immunocompetent donor T cells targeting recipient tissues that possess antigens absent from the donor.[41] GVHD may manifest as either acute or chronic disease, each with characteristic clinical findings and a distinct pathophysiology. The major target tissues of GVHD are the skin, liver, and GI tract, although other tissues may be involved. The diagnosis of acute GVHD may be based on one or a myriad of characteristic clinical and laboratory findings.[42] Skin manifestations include a "sunburn-like" erythematous maculopapular rash that often involves the palms and soles, and under severe circumstances, may be associated with desquamation. Hepatic involvement is characterized by a rise in alkaline phosphatase and total bilirubin, often in association with a mild to moderate increase in hepatic transaminases. GI GVHD predominantly involves the distal small bowel and colon and clinically is associated with crampy abdominal pain and watery diarrhea, which may be voluminous and bloody under severe circumstances. Endoscopic findings are variable and may range from a grossly normal-appearing bowel, to bowel edema and

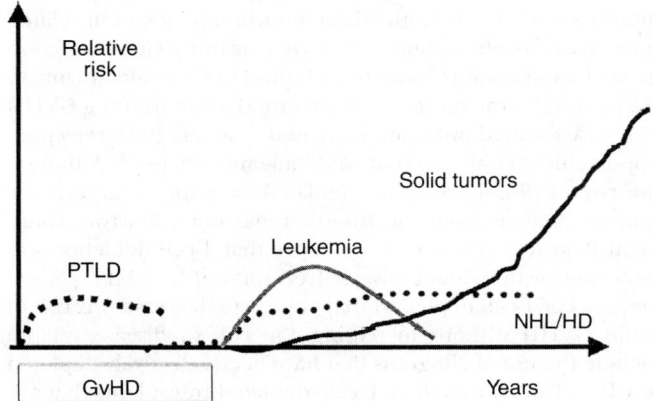

FIGURE 52.3-4. Scheme of time course and relative risk of second malignancies after allogeneic stem cell transplantation. GvHD, graft-versus-host disease; HD, Hodgkin's disease; NHL, non-Hodgkin's lymphoma; PTLD, posttransplant lymphoproliferative disorder. (From ref. 36, with permission.)

TABLE 52.3-2. Glucksberg Clinical Stage and Grade of Acute Graft-Versus-Host Disease

Stage	Skin	Liver	Intestinal Tract
1	Maculopapular rash <25% of body surface	Bilirubin, 34–50 μmol/L	>500 mL diarrhea/d
2	Maculopapular rash 25–50% of body surface	Bilirubin, 51–102 μmol/L	>1000 mL diarrhea/d
3	Generalized erythroderma	Bilirubin, 103–225 μmol/L	>1500 mL diarrhea/d
4	Generalized erythroderma with bullous formation and desquamation	Bilirubin >255 μmol/L	Severe abdominal pain with or without ileus

Grade	Degree of Organ Involvement
I	Stage 1–2 skin rash; no gastrointestinal tract involvement; no liver involvement; no decrease in clinical performance
II	Stage 1–3 skin rash; stage 1 gastrointestinal tract involvement or stage 1 liver involvement (or both); mild decrease in clinical performance
III	Stage 2–3 skin rash; stage 2–3 gastrointestinal tract involvement or stage 2–4 liver involvement (or both); marked decrease in clinical performance
IV	Similar to grade III with stage 2–4 organ involvement; extreme decrease in clinical performance

(From refs. 42 and 43, with permission.)

total denuding of intestinal mucosa in severe cases; colonic biopsy usually reveals pathopneumonic features of crypt cell loss/necrosis with apoptotic bodies and lymphocytic infiltrates, although disease involvement is frequently patchy and can be missed on random biopsy. Upper GI involvement, although more rare, may be associated with recurrent nausea, vomiting, and dyspepsia. Traditionally, acute GVHD has been divided into severity grades I to IV, depending on the extent of skin involvement, volume of diarrhea, or level of bilirubin elevation (Table 52.3-2).[43]

Donor T cells are the principal mediators of GVHD. Antigens that are disparate between patient and donor that serve as targets for GVHD in the HLA-identical transplant setting are referred to as *minor histocompatibility antigens*.[18] Although few *minor histocompatibility antigens* have been characterized to date, increasing evidence suggests the degree of disparity between recipient and donor *minor histocompatibility antigens* is a major determinant for the development of both acute GVHD and CGVHD.[44] The development of GVHD is a multistep process, in which recipient tissues are recognized as foreign by the donor immune system; antigen-presenting cells present recipient alloantigens to donor T cells, resulting in the activation and expansion of GVHD effector populations, ultimately leading to T cell–mediated cytotoxic damage of target tissues. Host antigen-presenting cells were recently shown in a murine model to be the driving force behind the activation of donor CD8+ T cells that mediate acute GVHD.[45]

GVHD remains a significant contributor to transplant-related morbidity and mortality. The incidence and severity of GVHD are determined by a number of variables, including degrees of HLA disparity between patient and donor, use of a T cell–replete versus T cell–depleted allograft, patient age, intensity of the conditioning regimen (e.g., myeloablative versus nonmyeloablative), and the agents used as prophylaxis for GVHD.[46] Furthermore, acute GVHD after allogeneic BMT is often most severe within the first month after transplantation and appears to be exacerbated by conditioning-induced cytokine release from damaged recipient tissues that mature and activate host antigen-presenting cells.

In general, the incidence of clinically significant acute GVHD (grades II to IV) in patients undergoing T cell–replete allogeneic HCT (from an HLA-identical sibling), in which con-

ventional GVHD prophylaxis is used [cyclosporin A (CSA) and methotrexate], is on the order of 30% to 40%, with approximately 15% of patients developing severe grade 3 to 4 disease.[46] The incidence of acute GVHD after unrelated allogeneic transplantation is directly proportional to degree of HLA matching; several recent studies have shown the incidence of acute GVHD after unrelated transplantation to be similar to HLA-identical sibling transplants when using high-resolution HLA-matched donors.[47] However, in recipients of partially matched related donor or partially matched unrelated donor transplants, acute GVHD occurs more frequently, affecting more than 70% of patients.

The two most common methods to prevent acute GVHD include the use of prophylactic immunosuppressive agents and/or the use of allografts in which donor T cells have been partially or completely depleted.[48] Although the combined use of CSA and methotrexate has been found to be superior to either agent alone in the prevention of GVHD, the addition of prednisone to these agents does not appear to offer any additional benefit.[49] Furthermore, prolonging the time course that patients receive CSA (i.e., 24 months) as GVHD prophylaxis does not appear to significantly reduce the incidence of CGVHD compared with those receiving a shorter coarse (i.e., 6 months) of CSA.[50] In both HLA-identical sibling and unrelated transplants, T-cell depletion [both *in vitro* using CD34 selection or *in vivo* using antithymocyte globulin (ATG) or alemtuzumab (Campath)] is the most effective method for preventing GVHD but is associated with an increased risk of graft rejection, opportunistic viral infection, and leukemic relapse.[51] Although the risk of disease relapse is leukemia specific, a large retrospective analysis from the International Bone Marrow Transplant Registry showed clear evidence that T-cell depletion was associated with a lower disease-free survival in CML.[52] Novel methods of T-cell depletion that appear to decrease this risk of acute GVHD without increasing the risk of disease relapse include the use of allografts that have been selectively depleted of CD8+ T cells, as well as T cell–depleted transplants that are followed by delayed scheduled infusions of donor lymphocytes months from the time of the original transplant.[14,15,53]

The mainstay of therapy for the treatment of acute GVHD is corticosteroid therapy, usually in association with CSA or tacrolimus (FK506). Approximately 40% to 60% of patients with grade 2 to 4 GVHD can be expected to respond to these agents. A randomized trial of low-dose (2 mg/kg) versus high-dose (10 mg/kg) methylprednisolone for acute GVHD showed no difference in response rates with either regimen.[54] Response to steroids appears to predict survival. In particular, steroid refractory patients have a dismal prognosis, with 60% to 80% dying from GVHD-related causes; unmitigated GVHD and infectious complications related to prolonged immunosuppression contribute to the high mortality rate observed in these patients. Despite decades of clinical research, no effective standard first-line therapy exists for patients developing steroid-refractory disease. ATG has been used with minimal success (20% to 40% response rate), with no evidence that it improves survival in this setting.[55] Extracorporeal photopheresis and drugs such as continuous IV infusions of CSA or tacrolimus, IV or oral mycophenolate mofetil, and immunosuppressive monoclonal antibodies that target a variety of different T-cell antigens have been used with variable success.[56,57] At the National Heart, Lung, and Blood Institute, a comprehensive strategy to treat patients developing steroid-refractory acute GVHD was developed that consisted of the following: (1) the use of the monoclonal antibody daclizumab (anti-CD25) alone or in combination with infliximab (anti–tumor necrosis factor); (2) tapering of corticosteroids once steroid resistance was diagnosed to decrease the risk of invasive fungal infections; and (3) the routine use of prophylactic broad-spectrum antibiotics in combination with lipid formulations of amphotericin B to prevent opportunistic *Aspergillus* infections. The authors observed a dramatic improvement in the complete response rate and survival of steroid-refractory GVHD in patients receiving infection prophylaxis and monoclonal antibody therapy (100% response; median survival of 453 days) compared with the authors' historical cohort of patients who were treated with ATG alone (17% response; median survival of 42 days; *P* <.001 for survival). These findings strongly suggest that vigorous prophylaxis against opportunistic infectious pathogens combined with immunosuppressive monoclonal antibody therapy can be used successfully to salvage patients developing this usually fatal complication.[57a]

CGVHD occurs in 15% to 50% of long-term survivors of allogeneic BMT and typically manifests with symptoms 3 months to 2 years after transplantation. The etiology of CGVHD appears to be related to alloreactive T cells that infiltrate and damage tissues as well as cause abnormalities in immune regulation.[58] Risk factors for CGVHD include a prior history of acute GVHD, older patient age, use of mismatched or unrelated donors, and a history of DLI for relapsed malignancy. Furthermore, the use of peripheral blood (PB) stem allografts (in contrast to marrow), particularly those containing very high doses of CD34+ cells, also appear to increase this risk. A recently published trial that randomized patients to PB versus BM allografts reported a significantly higher incidence of CGVHD in the recipients of PB transplants (65%) compared with those in the BM group (36%; *P* = .004).[59] However, the higher probability of long-term disease-free survival in patients developing CGVHD appears to offset the deleterious effects of this complication on survival.

Patients with CGVHD are often severely immunocompromised, either as a consequence of the immunosuppressive therapy used to treat the disorder or from the underlying immune deregulation associated with the disease process. CGVHD is lethal in up to 20% of cases, with death predominantly being related to infectious causes.[58] Patients with a particularly poor prognosis include those with hepatic involvement (bilirubin of more than 1.2) and/or thrombocytopenia. CGVHD is traditionally classified as either limited or extensive, limited disease being defined as localized skin involvement with or without mild hepatic involvement and extensive as generalized skin involvement with or without other target organ involvement. The characteristic clinical manifestations are numerous and include lichenoid or sclerodermatous skin involvement, hepatic cholestasis, friable nails, dry eyes (Sjögren's syndrome), fasciitis, xerostomia, lichenoid buccal changes, bronchiolitis obliterans, vaginal dryness, serositis, malabsorption, diarrhea, GI dysmotility, and pancytopenia. Treatment depends on the extent of disease. Systemic disease is typically treated with alternate-day CSA or FK506 and low-dose corticosteroids. Patients not responding to standard therapy often benefit from alternative therapies, including mycophenolate mofetil, psoralen and ultraviolet A light (for skin involvement), oral thalidomide, total lymphoid irradiation, and more recently extracorporeal photopheresis or monoclonal antibodies targeting tumor necrosis factor or activation antigens on T cells.[60] As infections are the main cause of death, prophylaxis for organisms such as *P carinii* and encapsulated bacteria is usually warranted, particularly in those taking systemic immunosuppressive therapy.

GRAFT FAILURE

Failure to achieve or maintain sustained donor hematopoietic engraftment after allotransplantation is referred to as *graft failure*. Graft failure may manifest as persistent neutropenia, without evidence of engraftment (primary graft failure), or as initial engraftment followed by a delayed fall in blood counts (late or secondary graft failure). *Graft rejection* is the term used to describe graft failure that occurs as a consequence of the active rejection of donor hematopoietic cells by immunocompetent host cells that survived the conditioning regimen. Graft rejection manifests as transient donor engraftment followed by a lymphocytosis of recipient origin, which ultimately leads to the rejection of donor hematopoietic cells and pancytopenia, or in some cases (e.g., nonmyeloablative transplants), autologous hematopoietic recovery. The mediators of graft rejection include NK cells or residual recipient T cells recognizing donor mismatched MHC molecules, or in an HLA-matched setting, minor histocompatibility antigens.[61]

Primary graft failure is associated with a significant risk of death from hemorrhage or infection and should be suspected in all transplant patients who remain pancytopenic for more than 3 to 4 weeks. Although graft failure occurs in less than 2% of patients undergoing myeloablative allogeneic HCT from an HLA-identical sibling, the incidence increases for recipients of T cell–depleted transplants, particularly those from HLA-mismatched or unrelated donors. Other risk factors for graft rejection include the infusion of low stem cell numbers (i.e., less than 1×10^6 CD34+ cells/kg), history of multiple blood transfusions, HLA disparity between the patient and donor, use of low-intensity or dose-reduced conditioning regimens, and transplantation for severe aplastic anemia.[62]

It is important to differentiate graft failure from pancytopenia related to other causes, including marrow suppression from infection, medications, or CGVHD. Furthermore, it is important to give early consideration for a second donor stem cell infusion, given the high-risk of opportunistic infection associated with prolonged periods of neutropenia and the difficult logistics of collecting more donor cells. Nonimmunologically mediated graft failure has been successfully treated with hematopoietic growth factors such as granulocyte-macrophage colony-stimulating factor or G-CSF, followed by a second infusion of donor stem cells in those who fail to manifest hematopoietic recovery. Graft rejection, in which donor hematopoietic cells are no longer detectable by cytogenetic or molecular methods, usually requires repeat conditioning to eradicate the host's "rejection" cells, followed by the infusion of a second donor allograft. Although the outcome in those requiring a second donor marrow infusion for graft failure is poor, successful and sustained donor engraftment has been reported in 57% of primary and 37% of secondary graft failure patients.[63]

CYTOMEGALOVIRUS INFECTION

CMV is a member of the herpes virus family that may cause serious and life-threatening pathology after allogeneic BMT. CMV disease occurs most commonly as the consequence of viral reactivation in patients who have a history of prior CMV infection. The cellular immune system plays an important role in the suppression of CMV viral reactivation. Disruption of cellular immunity associated with T-cell depletion (both *in vitro* and *in vivo*), GVHD, or immunosuppressive therapy can lead to CMV reactivation and subsequent disease. The clinical features of CMV disease may include pneumonitis, hepatitis, marrow suppression, upper GI involvement, and colitis. Reactivation tends to occur most commonly 3 weeks to 100 days after transplantation and is most strongly associated with acute GVHD and the pretransplant CMV serologic status of the recipient. Although 40% to 60% of patients who are serologically positive for CMV reactivate this virus after conventional allogeneic transplantation, the risk of reactivation in patients who are serologically negative before transplantation is extremely rare. *In vivo* T-cell depletion with alemtuzumab (anti-CD52) is associated with an increased incidence of CMV reactivation, as high as 85% in some studies.[64] Effective prevention can be achieved through the use of CMV-negative or leukocyte-filtered blood products (in seronegative patient–donor pairs), and prophylactic IV ganciclovir or foscarnet therapy.[65] In addition, a recent randomized trial showed high-dose oral valacyclovir was as effective as IV ganciclovir as posttransplant prophylaxis of CMV.[66] Because up to 60% of patients who are pretransplant seropositive for CMV (defined as "at risk for CMV") never reactivate CMV, an alternative and probably more effective approach is to reserve ganciclovir or foscarnet use for patients with detectable viral reactivation, either by PCR methods or by immunofluorescent techniques designed to detect viral antigen on the surface of neutrophils (CMV antigenemia).[64,66] Both techniques allow for early detection and treatment of CMV reactivation long before symptoms develop.[67] Several studies have shown that immunity to CMV after transplantation is mediated through donor CMV-specific T cells that are transplanted with the allograft. Therefore, for patients at risk for CMV reactivation (i.e., pretransplant CMV serologically positive), a donor who is serologically positive for CMV is actually desirable, as transference of donor immunity against this virus may result in a reduction of CMV-associated morbidity.

SOURCES OF ALLOGENEIC HEMATOPOIETIC STEM CELLS

ALLOGENEIC PERIPHERAL BLOOD STEM CELL TRANSPLANTS

Based on the success of autologous PB stem cell (PBSC) transplants, allogeneic transplant regimens that use PB-derived stem cells as apposed to marrow cells have been used with increasing frequency over the past decade.[68] The recombinant growth factor G-CSF is usually given to donors for 4 to 6 consecutive days (10 to 15 µg/kg/d) to mobilize hematopoietic progenitors into the circulation, followed by one or two leukapheresis procedures. G-CSF-mobilized PBSC transplants contain higher numbers of progenitor cells than marrow grafts, usually in the range of 5 to 10×10^6 CD34+ cells/kg. Allograft CD34+ cell yields after G-CSF mobilization correlate strongly with preapheresis circulating CD34 counts.[69] A recent study of allogeneic stem cell donors demonstrated that a single 25-L apheresis procedure was well tolerated and resulted in similar CD34+ cell yields, with less donor thrombocytopenia and inconvenience compared with two consecutive daily 15-L procedures.[70]

The recovery of both neutrophils and platelets is faster with peripheral blood cells than with marrow. Initial concerns that the 10- to 20-fold higher T-cell dose in PB allografts might be associated with a greater risk of acute GVHD have been dispelled. Indeed, several trials comparing allogeneic BM with PBSC transplantation have shown that PBSCs are associated with a shorter period of neutropenia and red blood cell and platelet transfusion dependence, with an equal probability of acute GVHD.[71–75]

A recently completed phase III trial of allotransplantation in 138 patients with hematologic malignancies found that PBSC grafts were associated with more rapid engraftment and better disease-free and overall survival than marrow grafts, without a greater risk of acute GVHD.[76] Neutrophil engraftment occurred 6 days earlier (day 15 vs. 21), and platelet recovery occurred 8 days earlier (day 13 vs. 21) among those receiving PBSC transplants. The incidence of acute grade 2 to 4 GVHD was equal between groups, occurring in 64% of PBSC and 57% of BM recipients (P = not significant). The cumulative incidence of CGVHD was also similar, occurring in 46% of PBSC and 35% of marrow recipients. This study provided the first evidence that PBSC transplantation may be associated with a survival advantage over conventional marrow transplants. Two-year survival in the PBSC group was 66% versus 54% in the marrow group (P = .06), a finding that led to the early termination of this trial. These, as well as the previously mentioned benefits, have made PBSCs the preferred source of donor hematopoietic progenitors for allogeneic transplantation.

UNRELATED DONORS

Although allogeneic transplantation is potentially curative for a number of hematologic malignancies, two-thirds of patients who would otherwise be candidates for the procedure lack an HLA-identical sibling to serve as a donor. The knowledge that the HLA system played a critical role in transplantation outcomes led to the successful use of HLA-matched unrelated donors and subsequent establishment of volunteer donor registries. As of 2002, more than 7 million typed volunteer donors have been registered worldwide, including 4 million in the National Marrow Donor Program, the single largest registry.[77] It is estimated that approximately 50% to 70% of white patients have an HLA-A–, HLA-B–, and HLA-DR–matched unrelated donor.[78] Because of the growing availability of volunteer unrelated donors, an increasing number of matched unrelated transplants are being performed annually. Nonetheless, a number of factors associated with unrelated transplantation limit the practical application of this transplant approach. Delays of 4 months or longer from the time of the donor search to transplantation frequently result in patients succumbing to their malignancy before the procedure can be performed.[78] The relative rarity of certain HLA haplotypes in ethnic/racial minorities makes finding a suitably matched unrelated donor particularly difficult for these patients.

The results of extensive published data on unrelated donor transplants reveal engraftment rates of 85% to 100%, grade 2 or more acute GVHD in 21% to 98%, CGVHD in 50% to 74%, and disease-free survival rates of 1% to 74%.[79,80] This wide range in outcome is explained mostly by variations in patient populations, transplantation methods, and HLA-typing techniques. The recent use of molecular-based typing has been associated with a significant improvement in transplant outcome, including a decrease in life-threatening acute GVHD and CGVHD.[81] Furthermore, typing beyond HLA-A, -B, and -DR loci may be of further benefit, as other MHC antigens appear to have a significant impact on transplant outcome. HLA class I antigen mismatches that are serologically detectable (including HLA-C) result in a significant increase in the risk of graft failure.[82] T-cell depletion of HLA-matched unrelated donor allografts is associated with a decrease in severe acute GVHD and CGVHD, although relapse may be higher and no net benefit on survival has been observed. Future trials that optimize donor selection, conditioning regimens, and GVHD prophylaxis are required to improve the outcome of HLA-matched unrelated donor transplants.

MISMATCHED RELATED TRANSPLANTS

Because the majority of patients in need of a hematopoietic stem cell transplant have a full-haplotype mismatched relative, haploidentical ("half-matched") or mismatched related donors have increasingly been used as an alternative source of stem cells for patients lacking an HLA-identical sibling. These donors may actually have a closer histocompatibility profile than matched unrelated donors, as the shared donor haplotype is genetically identical to the patient, which may be associated with better matching of minor histocompatibility antigens. Furthermore, potential family donors can usually be identified quickly and are usually more readily available than matched unrelated donors.

Graft rejection, GVHD, and ineffective immunity leading to fatal opportunistic infection are the major immune-mediated complications associated with HLA disparity; the greater the HLA disparity, the higher these risks. Early as well as recent trials comparing outcome in patients receiving partially mismatched related versus matched sibling donor allografts showed that engraftment, GVHD, and survival were inferior in the recipients of partially mismatched transplants.[79] Recently, through the use of modified conditioning regimens and more effective T cell–depletion methods, several groups have begun

to report improved outcome using mismatched family donors, with long-term disease-free survivals in the range of 20% to 40%.[83–85] These results are significant, as most the patients treated on these trials had advanced, "high-risk" hematologic malignancies associated with poor transplant outcome, even in a matched sibling setting. One recent analysis from Italy of 112 patients with hematologic malignancies undergoing haploidentical transplantation showed the risk of disease relapse to be significantly higher in patients with ALL compared with AML.[86] Investigators from this group subsequently observed that that donor-versus-recipient NK cell alloreactivity could eliminate AML relapse and graft rejection and protect patients against GVHD after such haploidentical transplants. Through *in vitro* studies and clinical observations, they demonstrated that when MHC class I killer immunoglobulin G–like receptor (KIR) inhibitory ligands were absent in the recipient that were resent in the donor (KIR incompatibility in the GVH direction), NK cells expand that are not inhibited by ligands expressed on recipient AML, substantially reducing the risk of disease relapse compared with those who receive KIR-compatible transplants.[21] Interestingly, this beneficial NK cell effect was not observed against ALL, perhaps the consequence of these populations lacking activating ligands required to trigger NK cytolytic activity. In murine haploidentical transplant studies, Ruggeri and colleagues[21] demonstrated that such KIR-incompatible, alloreactive NK cells can obviate the need for high-intensity conditioning and reduce the incidence of GVHD. Based on these findings, trials evaluating the impact of the adoptive infusion of alloreactive NK cells in humans undergoing KIR-incompatible mismatched transplantation will likely be evaluated in the future. The impact of KIR incompatibility when using partially mismatched unrelated donors has not yet been defined. One study reported disease-free survival in AML patients was superior in those receiving unrelated allografts with KIR incompatibility in contrast to another retrospective analysis, where KIR ligand incompatibility did not appear to improve the risk of disease relapse or GVHD.[87,88]

Although opportunistic infections and disease relapse remain problematic, recent modifications in transplants using mismatched related donors including the use of reduced-intensity conditioning regimens and high doses of donor CD34+ cells have improved transplant outcome. A recent nonrandomized study comparing transplantation outcomes in patients with hematologic malignancies who received marrow grafts from matched unrelated, one-antigen-mismatched unrelated, or two or more HLA-disparate family donors showed a significantly higher probability of overall survival for matched unrelated patients (58%) versus either mismatched unrelated (34%; $P = .01$) or haploidentical (21%; $P = .002$) patients.[89] Therefore, if available to patients who lack a closely matched family donor, phenotypically matched unrelated donors would seem the most desirable alternative allograft source at this time.

UMBILICAL CORD BLOOD TRANSPLANTATION

Umbilical cord blood is a new and promising source of hematopoietic progenitor cells for transplantation in both malignant and nonmalignant disorders. The realization that cord blood, obtained from the placenta after delivery, contained long-term repopulating progenitor cells, led to its investigational use as a source of stem cells for allogeneic transplantation.[90] Cord blood has been shown to contain primitive hematopoietic stem cells with remarkable proliferative potential, which may overcome the limitation of relatively low absolute cell numbers. Also, the immature lymphocytes in cord blood appear to decrease the risk and severity of acute GVHD and CGVHD, potentially permitting greater HLA disparity and expanding donor availability. Currently, more than 70,000 cryopreserved cord blood units are estimated to be available for use in unrelated transplantation.[77] One major advantage of cord blood transplants over unrelated marrow is the speed with which cord blood units can be made available for transplantation (a median of only 13.5 days in one study). In a trial evaluating umbilical cord transplants in 44 children with malignant and nonmalignant hematologic diseases receiving grafts from an HLA-identical or single-antigen-mismatched donor, 85% engrafted, with only 3% developing grade 2 or higher acute GVHD.[91] A subsequent multi-institutional study from Europe reported similar engraftment rates in 78 recipients of cord blood from related donors, with acute GVHD occurring in 9% of the recipients of HLA-matched cord blood and 50% of the recipients of HLA-mismatched cord blood.[92] Recently, a dose of 1.5×10^7 nucleated cells/kg (recipient weight) has been defined as the minimum acceptable dose of cells required for acceptable engraftment rates and transplant-related mortality after cord blood transplantation. The early success of cord blood transplants has led to the creation of an increasing number of umbilical cord blood banks worldwide. However, graft failure, which is most closely associated with patient size, age, and low cord stem cell doses, remains a significant problem that limits the applicability of this approach in adults. A number of approaches are being developed to overcome the obstacle of low-cell doses in adults, including *ex vivo* expansion of umbilical cord progenitor cells and multiple-unit transplantation using several different cord donors.

RESULTS OF CONVENTIONAL ALLOGENEIC TRANSPLANTATION FOR HEMATOLOGIC MALIGNANCIES

Allogeneic HCT is potentially curative for a number of different hematologic malignancies, including acute and chronic leukemias, myelodysplastic syndromes, myeloproliferative disorders, Hodgkin's and non-Hodgkin's lymphoma, and multiple myeloma. The indications for allogeneic HCT vary according to disease categories and are influenced by variables such as disease-specific prognostic factors (e.g., cytogenetic abnormalities), response to prior therapy, patient age and performance status, disease status (e.g., in remission vs. relapsed refractory disease), and most important, availability of a suitable allogeneic donor to serve as a source for hematopoietic stem cells. The decision whether to proceed with allogeneic transplantation is often difficult and controversial and is ultimately guided by the potential benefits and risks of such therapy. Diseases such as CML, curable only by allotransplantation, are associated with an excellent posttransplant outcome and high probability of long-term disease-free survival, justifying the risks of regimen-related toxicity. Conversely, diseases such as multiple myeloma are associated with a high risk of treatment-related mortality and disease relapse, making the decision to proceed with transplantation more difficult. Nevertheless, for the major-

ity who undergo this approach, allogeneic HCT remains the only therapy with established curative potential.

CHRONIC MYELOGENOUS LEUKEMIA

CML is a clonal myeloproliferative disease of hematopoietic stem cell origin that is characterized by an early chronic phase of 3 to 5 years' duration, followed by an accelerated phase of 3 to 6 months, which ultimately terminates in a fatal blastic phase. Treatment with interferon-α prolongs survival, but only a minority of patients have a sustained cytogenetic remission of the Philadelphia chromosome [reciprocal translocation, t(9;22)(q34;q11)]. Imatinib mesylate (Gleevec) is a tyrosine kinase inhibitor that blocks BCR-ABL kinase activity, resulting in an inhibition of proliferation in Philadelphia-positive hematopoietic progenitor cells. Remarkably, the drug is extremely well tolerated, results in a complete cytogenetic response rate of more than 70%, and was recently shown to have superior efficacy to interferon-α plus cytarabine in a randomized trial.[93] Based on the above, many institutes have begun to use imatinib as first-line treatment for patients with chronic-phase CML, reserving allogeneic transplant for those who fail to achieve a cytogenetic remission. The first-line use of imatinib mesylate in patients with chronic-phase CML has already significantly reduced the number of allogeneic transplantations performed for this leukemia. Nevertheless, allogeneic HCT remains the only treatment approach with proven curative potential in this leukemia. Patient age, disease status (chronic phase vs. accelerated or blastic phase), and the time interval from diagnosis to transplant (i.e., less than 1 year vs. more than 1 year) are the best predictors for long-term disease-free survival. In general, 65% to 80% of patients transplanted with chronic-phase CML can expect to be cured, in contrast to a minority (10% to 20%) who undergo transplantation in accelerated or blastic phase. Patients with chronic-phase CML transplanted within a year from the time of diagnosis have the best outcome, with long-term disease-free survivals of 75% to 80%. A study from the Fred Hutchinson Cancer Center of 196 patients undergoing allogeneic HCT from matched unrelated donors reported a 5-year survival of 75%, a rate that compared favorably to that institution's results using HLA-matched sibling donors.[80] Among hematologic malignancies, CML appears most susceptible to the GVL effect. The majority of CML patients who relapse after an allogeneic HCT can be induced back into remission after treatment with a DLI.[11,12] The sensitivity of this leukemia to the GVL effect was a primary motivation for studies investigating the use of low-intensity nonmyeloablative transplantation (discussed later in Nonmyeloablative Allogeneic Hematopoietic Cell Transplantation) as a less toxic approach for patients with chronic-phase CML. Early results using nonmyeloablative stem cell transplantation (NST) have been promising, with durable molecular remissions reported in a number of different transplant centers.[94] Notably, patients older than age 60 have been successfully treated with minimal conditioning associated toxicity, an important finding given the median age of CML patients at diagnosis is 65 years.[95] As with myeloablative transplants, patients with more advanced disease (accelerated phase/blast crisis) are significantly less likely to achieve long-term disease-free survival after NST compared with patients with earlier-stage disease. Recently, oral imatinib mesylate was reported to induce cytogenetic and molecular remissions in some patients with CML relapsing after allogeneic transplant, including patients who failed DLIs.[96]

ACUTE MYELOGENOUS LEUKEMIA

With the exception of those with favorable or low-risk cytogenetic abnormalities [e.g., t(8;21), t(15;17), inv or del(16)], most patients with AML have a high risk of relapse after chemotherapy-induced remission.[97] Compared with those who receive chemotherapy alone, patients undergoing an allogeneic HCT after first CR (CR1) have a lower probability of relapse, with 5-year disease-free survivals in the range of 46% to 62%.[98,99] AML patients with cytogenetic abnormalities associated with a poor prognosis in CR1 who are unlikely to be cured with chemotherapy alone may be cured after an allogeneic transplant.[100] Furthermore, patients in CR2 or those with untreated relapsed AML can be cured only by allogeneic HCT, albeit they are less likely to achieve long-term disease-free survival (22% to 30%). Therefore, the decision to perform transplant after CR1 is influenced by the predicted increase in disease-free survival versus the risk of regimen-related mortality. Based on these observations, it is reasonable to proceed to transplant in CR1 in patients who are at intermediate or high risk of relapse [e.g., normal karyotype, abnormal chromosome 5 or 7, 3q rearrangements, t(6;9), complex karyotype abnormalities, FLT3 length mutation], withholding the procedure until first relapse or CR2 in low-risk patients. Patients with primary chemotherapy-refractory AML, associated with the worst prognosis, can still be salvaged by an allogeneic HCT in 10% to 15% of cases.

ACUTE LYMPHOBLASTIC LEUKEMIA

Although 65% to 85% of adults with ALL achieve remission with primary chemotherapy, 60% to 70% eventually experience relapse that is rarely curable with salvage chemotherapy. Factors associated with a poor outcome ("high-risk") include age older than 60 years; leukocyte count of more than 30,000 on presentation; and chromosomal translocations involving t(4;11), t(1;19), t(8;14) or the Philadelphia chromosome t(9;22) (found in approximately 15% to 30% of adult ALL cases).[101] In adults, allogeneic HCT in first CR1 is usually reserved for patients with high-risk features, where cure with chemotherapy is unlikely.[102,103] Several studies of allogeneic HCT in high-risk patients transplanted in CR1 have reported long-term disease-free survival in the range of 40% to 61%, rates considerably higher than those observed with chemotherapy alone. Because some patients in CR1 (without high-risk features) are cured with chemotherapy alone, allogeneic HCT is usually reserved for patients who have relapsed disease who achieve a remission with reinduction chemotherapy (e.g., CR2). Furthermore, long-term disease-free survival with allogeneic transplantation in CR2 is in the range of 35% to 40%, which is comparable to disease-free survival of patients undergoing transplantation in CR1. As chemotherapy is considerably more effective in achieving durable remissions in children, allogeneic HCT is usually reserved for those who fail to be cured with primary therapy or have Philadelphia-positive ALL.

MYELODYSPLASTIC SYNDROME

Allogeneic HCT is the only curative therapy available for patients with myelodysplastic syndrome. In general, 30% to 50% of patients with myelodysplastic syndrome can be expected to achieve long-term disease-free survival. Factors associated with improved outcome include younger age, lower pretransplant marrow blast percentage, shorter disease duration, and favorable cytogenetics. A retrospective trial of 131 patients with myelodysplastic syndrome undergoing allogeneic BMT reported disease-free and overall survival rates of 34% and 41%, respectively.[104] Disease-free survival was dependent on pretransplant BM blast percentages with refractory anemia/refractory anemia with ringed sideroblasts (RA/RARS), refractory anemia with excessive blasts (RAEB), RAEB in transformation (RAEB-T), and secondary AML patients having disease-free survivals of 52%, 34%, 19%, and 26%, respectively. A retrospective analysis of transplant events in relation to the International Prognostic Scoring System cytogenetic categories showed that cytogenetic abnormalities alone were highly predictive of posttransplant outcome.[105] The event-free survival for good-, intermediate-, and poor-risk cytogenetic subgroups were 51%, 40%, and 6%, respectively, with corresponding relapse rates of 19%, 12%, and 82%. International Prognostic Scoring System cytogenetic categories were defined as good-risk if patients had normal karyotype, –Y alone, del(5q) alone, or del(20q) alone; poor-risk if patients had anomalies of chromosome 7 or complex cytogenetics (three or more anomalies): and intermediate-risk if other karyotypic anomalies were present that did not meet the criteria for good or poor risk.

OTHER HEMATOLOGIC MALIGNANCIES

The role of allogeneic HCT in multiple myeloma, CLL, Hodgkin's and non-Hodgkin's lymphoma, and myeloproliferative disorders is less well defined than with acute leukemias or chronic-phase CML. Most studies published to date have consisted of relatively small retrospective analyses or anecdotal case reports. Nevertheless, reports of durable remissions in patients with relapsed or chemotherapy-refractory disease, often in association with GVHD or after DLI, provide strong evidence that these diseases are susceptible to a potentially curative GVL effect. Several trials of allogeneic transplantation in CLL have reported long-term disease-free survival rates in the range of 49% to 70%,[106] although mortality associated with myeloablative procedures can be significant (range of 25% to 46%). Nevertheless, there now exist compelling data in the literature that CLL can be cured with an allogeneic transplant.[107] As with other hematologic malignancies, CLL patients with chemotherapy-sensitive disease are significantly more likely to achieve long-term disease-free survival compared with those with more advanced, chemotherapy-resistant disease. Although a number of patients with multiple myeloma have achieved long-term disease-free survival after allogeneic HCT, transplant-related mortality may be as high as 50%, thus limiting the full therapeutic potential of this approach.[106] Regimens with reduced transplant-related toxicities, such as nonmyeloablative hematopoietic transplantation, avoid many transplant-related complications and may ultimately improve disease-free survival compared with myeloablative approaches in a variety of hematologic malignancies (discussed later in Nonmyeloablative Allogeneic Hematopoietic Cell Transplantation).

NONMYELOABLATIVE ALLOGENEIC HEMATOPOIETIC CELL TRANSPLANTATION

Although allogeneic HCT using myeloablative chemoradiotherapy can be curative for patients with hematologic malignancies, its use is marred by a high incidence of treatment-related complications and a 20% to 35% risk of transplant-related mortality. The desirable antitumor effects of dose-intensive conditioning are often offset by its substantial and potentially life-threatening toxicities. Debilitated or older patients with hematologic malignancies are at particularly high risk, thus limiting the applicability of this potentially curative treatment modality to relatively younger patients with a good performance status. Recognition that transplanted donor immune cells can cure patients with leukemia led to the notion that GVL alone, without intensive cytoreductive therapy, might be sufficient to obtain long-term control of hematologic malignancies. Subsequently, investigators began to explore the concept of low-intensity or nonmyeloablative conditioning regimens, immunosuppressive enough to permit engraftment of the donor immune system for the generation of GVL effects while sparing patients the toxicities associated with myeloablative therapy.[108–110] Nonmyeloablative transplantation was first pursued in humans in the late 1990s. Since then, a growing list of transplant centers have reported success using this approach in a number of different hematologic malignancies as well as in patients with nonmalignant hematologic disorders and select solid tumors. Despite the use of low-intensity conditioning, engraftment rates have been high, and long-term remissions, induced purely through a donor immune-mediated antitumor effect have been observed in a variety of malignant diseases. Importantly, regimen-related toxicity and mortality appear to be significantly decreased, thus expanding eligibility for allotransplantation to include older or debilitated patients, as well as allowing for exploration of graft-versus-tumor (GVT) effects in other treatment refractory or incurable malignancies.

NONMYELOABLATIVE CONDITIONING REGIMENS

A variety of low-intensity conditioning strategies have been explored over the past 8 years. These regimens use powerful immunosuppressants to allow engraftment of the donor immune system while reducing overall toxicity associated with myeloablative agents (see Table 52.3-1). Although regimens vary, most incorporate the nucleoside analogue fludarabine because of its profound immunosuppressive effects and low-toxicity profile. By definition, a nonmyeloablative regimen allows for some degree of autologous hematopoietic recovery as a consequence of recipient hematopoietic stem cells surviving the conditioning regimen (e.g., fludarabine plus cyclophosphamide, fludarabine plus low-dose TBI). However, despite a substantial reduction in the dose of conditioning agents, the term "nonmyeloablative" is a misnomer for some reduced-intensity transplant approaches, as the conditioning agents may actually fully eradicate the host's hematopoietic cells. Indeed, this may be the case in heavily pretreated patients receiving conditioning with "dose-reduced" melphalan (i.e., 140 mg/m^2) or busulfan (8 mg/kg).[110] Furthermore, recipient hematopoietic stem cells that survive transplant conditioning are in most cases immunologically eradicated by donor T cells weeks to months after transplantation, a process referred to as *GVH hematopoiesis.*

Although direct comparisons of myeloablative versus nonmyeloablative regimens have not yet been made, preliminary data on the safety of this new approach have been encouraging. Several centers testing different low-intensity transplant regimens in a variety of hematologic and nonhematologic

malignancies have reported regimen-related mortality rates of less than 20%. This mortality risk is remarkably low, given most patients in these trials were precluded from a myeloablative transplant because of a high risk (i.e., 40% or more) of regimen-related mortality related to heavy pretreatment, debilitation, or advanced patient age.[111]

Because nonmyeloablative conditioning does eradicate recipient hematopoietic progenitors, a mixture of both donor and patient myeloid and lymphoid cells is usually detectable at the time of neutrophil recovery. This state, called *mixed chimerism,* has both beneficial and negative effects on transplant outcome. Mixed chimerism can induce donor immune tolerance recipient antigens, leading to a reduction in the incidence of acute GVHD.[112] However, mixed chimerism is also associated with an increased risk of graft failure, and the tolerance it induces may inhibit beneficial GVT effects, leading to a higher risk of disease relapse.[113] These negative aspects of mixed chimerism can be overcome by donor lymphocytes, which induce GVH hematopoietic effects that shift chimerism from mixed to complete donor, thus breaking tolerance and enhancing a GVT effect.[114] Indeed, many nonmyeloablative transplant approaches incorporate a strategy in which low-intensity conditioning achieves a platform of mixed chimerism so that subsequent donor leukocyte infusions or cytokines can be given to induce a donor immune-mediated antitumor effect (see Fig. 52.3-1).

NONMYELOABLATIVE TRANSPLANT TOXICITY

Compared with myeloablative approaches, conditioning-induced toxicity is relatively mild with nonmyeloablative regimens. In general, most patients tolerate the preparative regimen well, without the occurrence of mucositis or the requirement for total parenteral nutrition. VOD occurs infrequently, is usually mild in severity, and is observed predominantly in regimens that contain busulfan (see Table 52.3-1).[110] Most trials have reported transplant-related mortality rates in the range of 7% to 20%, which is remarkably low, given the advanced age and poor performance status of the majority of these patients. A single-institution analysis reported a significant reduction in 6-month transplant-related mortality in patients receiving low-intensity fludarabine-based conditioning (7%) with those receiving a T cell–depleted myeloablative transplant (30%).[115] A nonmyeloablative regimen developed at the Fred Hutchinson Cancer Center that uses low-dose TBI (200 cGy) based conditioning is associated with minimal conditioning-related toxicity, can be given in the outpatient setting, and appears ideally suited for older patients.[116] With the exception of low-dose TBI-based strategies, pancytopenia associated with the conditioning regimen is common. However, the occurrence of partial autologous hematopoietic recovery shortens the overall depth and duration of neutropenia and reduces platelet and red blood cell transfusion requirements. A study comparing transfusions after conditioning with 2 Gy of TBI (with or without fludarabine) versus conventional myeloablative therapy revealed a significant reduction in the percentage of patients requiring red blood cell (63% vs. 96%) and platelet transfusions (23% vs. 100%) after nonmyeloablative versus myeloablative conditioning, respectively.[117]

The decreased mucositis and shortening in neutropenia time associated with reduced-intensity conditioning appear to translate into a reduction in opportunistic bacterial and fungal infections.[118] Nevertheless, 10% to 15% of patients still develop invasive fungal infections that may have lethal consequences. Profound immunosuppression as a consequence of high-dose corticosteroid therapy for GVHD appears to be the major factor putting patients at risk for these opportunistic pathogens.[57a,119] Interventions that affect engrafting donor T cells are the major determinants influencing the risk of CMV reactivation and disease after transplantation. The cumulative incidence of CMV reactivation after T cell–replete NST is similar to patients receiving T cell–replete myeloablative transplants. However, the addition of alemtuzumab to the conditioning regimen (for *in vivo* T-cell depletion) causes a delay in donor immune recovery and substantially increases the risk of viral reactivation in this setting.[120] Importantly, CMV reactivation after NST may be delayed in onset relative to conventional transplants. Therefore, CMV surveillance past transplant day 100, previously defined to be the window of viral risk in recipients of myeloablative procedures, may be necessary.[118]

NST is too new to make any conclusions regarding long-term complications, although it is hoped that the many late side effects attributable to myeloablative conditioning, including growth retardation, sterility, endocrine abnormalities, cataracts, and secondary malignancies, will be observed with reduced frequency compared with conventional myeloablative transplants.

ENGRAFTMENT

The ability to establish engraftment of donor hematopoietic and lymphoid cells is directly related to the degree of host immunosuppression induced by the preparative regimen. Although graft rejection occurs with a higher frequency compared with myeloablative approaches, in general, more than 90% of patients can be expected to have durable donor engraftment. As with myeloablative transplants, *ex vivo* T-cell depletion of the allograft is associated with lower degrees of donor T-cell chimerism and a higher risk of graft rejection.[113] In contrast, *in vivo* T-cell depletion with alemtuzumab is less commonly associated with graft rejection, particularly when DLIs are given after transplantation to patients with mixed chimerism.[121] Regimens that use low-dose TBI alone have a higher incidence of graft rejection (up to 20% in patients with chronic-phase CML), although the addition of fludarabine appears to decrease this risk. Furthermore, the use of BM allografts after low-dose TBI appears to be associated with a greater risk of graft rejection compared with PBSCs.[111]

The kinetics of donor engraftment after NST show considerable variation depending on the type and intensity of agents used for conditioning. At the National Heart, Lung, and Blood Institute, the authors systematically studied lineage specific chimerism in patients with hematologic and nonhematologic malignancies who received an NST from an HLA-identical or single-locus mismatched family after cyclophosphamide (60 mg/kg × 2 days) and fludarabine (25 mg/m² × 5 days) based conditioning.[122,123] Graft rejection was exceedingly rare, with 98% (177 out of 180) of patients achieving sustained donor engraftment; the three patients who rejected their transplant had full autologous hematopoietic recovery in the absence of any cytopenias. In contrast with myeloablative regimens, in which lymphohematopoietic recovery is completely donor, cyclophosphamide/fludarabine-based conditioning resulted in a unique pattern of donor engraftment where significant dif-

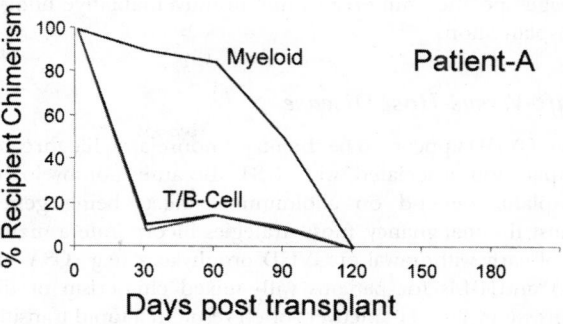

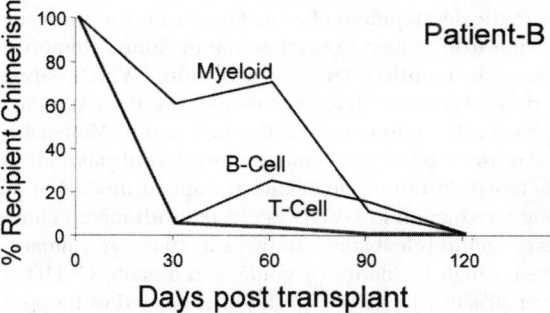

FIGURE 52.3-5. Patients receiving nonmyeloablative conditioning with cyclophosphamide and fludarabine have initial autologous recovery of lymphoid and hematopoietic cells. Recipient cells are gradually immunologically "ablated" as the consequence of a donor immune-mediated graft-versus-host hematopoietic effect.

ferences in chimerism were observed between T cells and myeloid cells (Fig. 52.3-5). After the withdrawal of posttransplant immunosuppression (either CSA alone or in combination with mycophenolate mofetil), and in some cases after a DLI, chimerism transitioned to complete donor in all cellular lineages in the majority of cases. The median time to 100% donor T-cell and myeloid chimerism was 30 (range of 14 to 164) and 88 (range of 21 to 220) days, respectively. BM erythroid (CD71+ cells) and CD34+ progenitor cell chimerism closely approximated myeloid chimerism, whereas NK cells tended to parallel T-cell chimerism.[123] These engraftment profiles contrast NST regimens using low-dose TBI (2 Gy) or "dose-reduced" busulfan or melphalan, where the engraftment of donor myeloid typically occurs quicker compared with donor T cells.[124,125] Furthermore, engraftment profiles may vary significantly among patients receiving the same low-intensity–conditioning regimen. Higher doses of allograft CD34+ cells and, in particular, prior exposure to immunosuppressive chemotherapy, may significantly facilitate and expedite the engraftment of donor lymphohematopoietic cells.

T-cell chimerism appears to be an important determinant of multiple posttransplant events, including the risk of graft rejection, acute GVHD, and the ability to generate a GVL/GVT effect.[113,123,126,127] In general, patients with low degrees of donor T-cell chimerism are at higher risk for graft rejection and disease relapse, in contrast with patients with high degrees of donor T-cell chimerism, where graft rejection and disease relapse occur less frequently. Furthermore, patients with more rapid donor T-cell engraftment may be at an increased risk of developing acute GVHD. These findings highlight the importance of assessing lineage specific chimerism after nonmyeloablative allogeneic transplantation.

Graft-Versus-Host Disease

Acute GVHD appears to be the major nonrelapse life-threatening complication associated with NST. Because nonmyeloablative transplants depend on alloimmune effects being generated against the malignancy, most strategies incorporate a methodology of early withdrawal of GVHD prophylaxis (e.g., CSA/tacrolimus) and DLIs for patients with mixed chimerism or disease progression. These maneuvers often result in a rapid transition of chimerism in the direction of the donor that sometimes is associated with the development of acute GVHD. Furthermore, because conversion from mixed to predominantly donor chimerism may be delayed by months after transplantation, GVHD is also sometimes delayed in onset (i.e., occurring more than 100 days posttransplant) relative to myeloablative transplants. Many early NST regimens used CSA or tacrolimus alone as prophylaxis for GVHD, largely based on nonmyeloablative transplant models in animals showing a reduction in GVHD associated with mixed chimerism. However, nonmyeloablative transplant trials in humans have reported a high incidence of grade 2 to 4 acute GVHD (in the range of 30% to 70%), a complication associated with opportunistic infections and other lethal consequences in up to 15% of patients. Older patient age, prior history of chemotherapy, and rapid T-cell engraftment appear to be associated with an increased risk of GVHD.[122,128] The high incidence of this complication has led to the use of additional immunosuppressive agents (e.g., mycophenolate mofetil, methotrexate) in combination with CSA/tacrolimus as prophylaxis for GVHD. *Ex vivo* T-cell depletion of the allograft decreases the risk of GVHD but may significantly increase the risk of graft rejection. A more promising strategy involves *in vivo* T-cell depletion through the use of alemtuzumab (CAMPATH).[129,130] A study of 129 patients undergoing fludarabine/melphalan-based conditioning reported a significant reduction in acute grade 2 to 4 GVHD in patients who received alemtuzumab plus CSA as GVHD prophylaxis (22%) compared with those receiving CSA plus methotrexate (45%; $P = .006$). Disease-free survival was similar between cohorts, although patients receiving alemtuzumab had a significantly higher incidence of CMV reactivation (85% vs. 24%; $P < .001$) and required a higher number of DLIs to achieve similar control of the malignancy.

The use of matched unrelated donors after nonmyeloablative conditioning has recently been explored at a number of transplant centers.[131] As with myeloablative transplants, the risk of acute GVHD and CGVHD appears directly related to the degree of HLA compatibility between the patient and donor. A study of patients with advanced age (median age, 53 years) receiving a low-dose TBI-based regimen followed by an unrelated donor transplant reported a 44% incidence of grade 2 to 4 acute GVHD and a transplant-related mortality rate of only 16% at 1 year.[111]

Graft-Versus-Leukemia Effect

GVL effects after NST have been observed in a heterogeneous group of hematologic malignancies.[110,131] Durable remissions lasting more than 5 years in patients transplanted with acute and chronic leukemias, myelodysplastic syndromes, multiple myeloma, lymphoid malignancies (e.g., Hodgkin's disease and

non-Hodgkin's lymphoma), and myeloproliferative disorders now exist in the literature. In general, diseases previously defined to be susceptible to GVL/GVT effects after myeloablative procedures appear likewise to be susceptible to the same effect after nonmyeloablative transplantation. Because autologous hematopoietic recovery may occur and because the GVL effect is typically delayed from the time of transplant conditioning, recurrent and sometimes progressive disease may be observed initially after the transplant. Remission of disease may not occur until months after transplantation, often in association with the withdrawal of posttransplant immunosuppression or after the infusion of donor lymphocytes.[110,123]

A number of trials have shown that the GVT effects that follow nonmyeloablative transplantation are most effective against malignancies with slow growth kinetics, in particular chronic leukemias and indolent lymphomas. Indeed several studies have reported durable remissions of CML (see earlier in Chronic Myelogenous Leukemia), low-grade NHL, CLL, mantle cell lymphoma, and multiple myeloma after reduced-intensity allogeneic transplantation.[110,131] In contrast, uncontrolled hematologic malignancies associated with more rapid kinetics typically do not benefit from this approach unless pretransplant cytoreduction is first achieved.[132] Therefore, in diseases such as AML, ALL, myelodysplastic syndrome in transformation to leukemia, and lymphomas, induction of a remission before nonmyeloablative conditioning appears to optimize the chance of long-term disease-free survival.[133] The use of autografting followed by nonmyeloablative allografting has recently been investigated as a method to maximize disease control before allogeneic transplantation[129]; long-term disease-free survival has been observed in patients with Hodgkin's and non-Hodgkin's lymphoma as well multiple myeloma after this approach. The results of these early trials have been encouraging and will likely lead to prospective randomized trials comparing NST with more conventional myeloablative procedures.

Graft-Versus-Solid Tumor

Without evidence to support efficacy, many considered the 25% to 35% risk of regimen-related mortality with myeloablative allogeneic transplantation too high to justify transplant studies in patients with nonhematologic malignancies. However, the ability of DLIs to induce remissions of leukemia provided indisputable evidence of the curative potential of GVL and ultimately the impetus to study for similar beneficial allogeneic immune effects in metastatic solid tumors. The reduced risk of transplant-related mortality associated with nonmyeloablative conditioning provided a safer platform to conduct such trials. Case reports of disease regression in association with GVHD in a few patients with metastatic breast carcinoma undergoing myeloablative allogeneic transplantation led credence to the concept that donor immune cells might have activity against tumors of epithelial origin. However, efforts to systematically investigate for GVT effects in solid tumors have only recently been pursued.[134] At the National Heart, Lung, and Blood Institute, the authors initiated trials of nonmyeloablative HCT in patients with metastatic solid tumors in late 1997, shortly after the successful preliminary results of nonmyeloablative HCT in hematologic malignancies. Although these trials are ongoing, definitive evidence to support the existence of a graft-versus-solid tumor effect in renal cell carcinoma was quickly demonstrated. Ten of

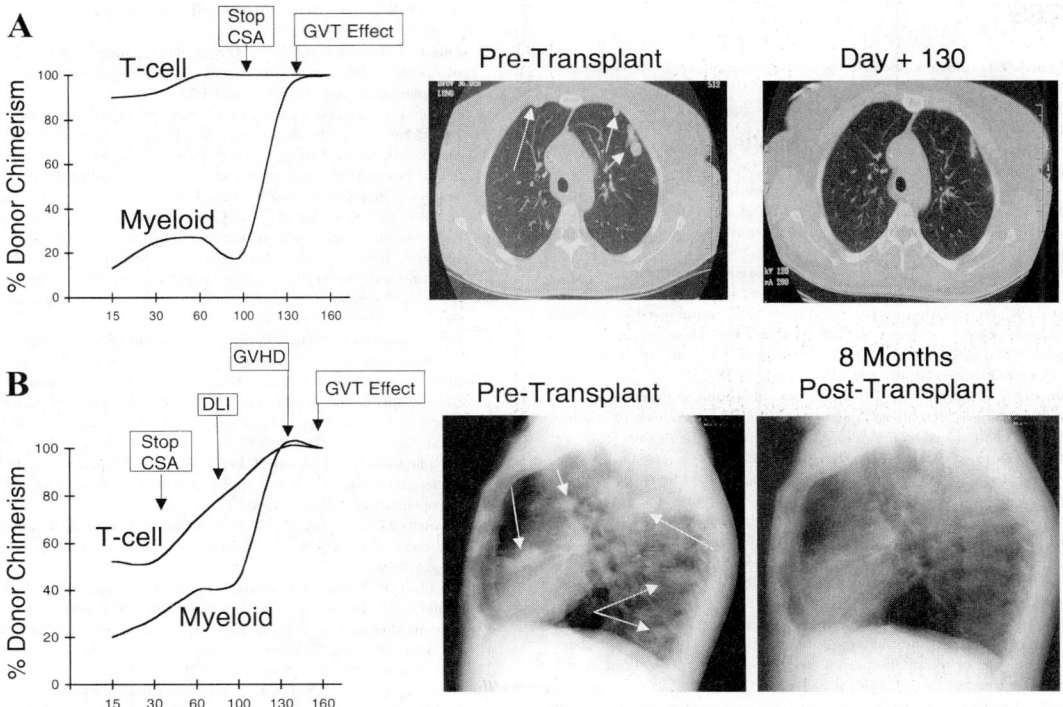

FIGURE 52.3-6.   Relationship of lineage-specific donor engraftment, cyclosporin A (CSA) withdrawal **(A)**, and graft-versus-host disease (GVHD) to a graft-versus-tumor (GVT) effect **(B)** in two patients with metastatic renal cell carcinoma after nonmyeloablative allogeneic hematopoietic cell transplantation. DLI, donor lymphocyte infusion. (From ref. 134, with permission.)

the first 19 patients treated with cyclophosphamide/fludarabine-based conditioning followed by transplantation with HLA-matched PBSCs had regression of their metastatic kidney cancer, typically delayed by 4 to 6 months, consistent with a donor immune-mediated antitumor effect.[135] Furthermore, the observation that disease regression was associated with acute GVHD, the withdrawal of immunosuppression, DLIs, and predominantly complete donor T-cell chimerism provided compelling evidence that these disease responses occurred as a consequence of a GVT effect (Fig. 52.3-6). The first patient treated on study with metastatic renal cell carcinoma remains in remission now more than 6 years after treatment. A number of investigators have recently confirmed that GVT effects can be induced against renal cell carcinoma using a variety of different low-intensity transplant strategies.[134] Of note, patients with stable or slowly growing disease appear much more likely to benefit from this approach compared with patients with rapidly growing tumors, where early death from disease progression may preclude a beneficial GVT effect.

GVT effects after NST have recently been described (mostly case reports) against a number of solid tumors, including metastatic breast, pancreatic, ovarian, and colon cancer.[134] However, longer follow-up and larger case series are needed before the sensitivity of a specific solid tumor to GVT effects and the impact of this approach on survival can be determined. Despite melanoma's reputation as being immunoresponsive, little to no efficacy of nonmyeloablative transplantation in this metastatic tumor has been observed, perhaps the consequence of the rapid kinetics associated with this tumor.[134]

Although proof of concept has been established showing GVT effects are inducible against select solid tumors, the overall response rate of most malignancies to this approach has been relatively low, with most responses only being partial. Although indubitably safer than conventional myeloablative transplantation, a 10% to 15% chance of transplant-related mortality further limits this approach. Therefore, "second-generation" transplant trials focusing on methods to target the alloimmune response specifically to the tumor through adoptive T/NK cell infusion or posttransplant tumor vaccination strategies are needed. Although allogeneic HCT for solid tumors is still in its infancy, developments such as these could lead to more effect transplant trials in the future.

FUTURE PROSPECTS

Allogeneic HCT remains the only curative treatment modality for a large number of patients with hematologic malignancies. Exciting advances in the field over the past decade have made allogeneic transplantation an essential component to the treatment of an increasing number of malignant diseases. Furthermore, an expanded understanding of the requirements for the engraftment of donor cells, as well as the basic immunologic mechanisms involved in GVHD and GVL reactions, has greatly improved both the safety and efficacy of the procedure. The eventual identification of leukemia and tumor-specific antigens will likely lead to more targeted allogeneic immunotherapy approaches that avoid the morbidity associated with GVHD.

REFERENCES

1. Thomas ED, Blume KG. Historical markers in the development of allogeneic hematopoietic cell transplantation. *Biol Blood Marrow Transplant* 1999;5:341.

2. Burchenal JH, Oettgen HF, Holmberg EA, Hemphill SC, Reppert JA. Effect of total-body irradiation on the transplantability of mouse leukemias. *Cancer Res* 1960;20:425.

3. Barnes DW, Loutit JF. Treatment of murine leukaemia with x-rays and homologous bone marrow. II. *Br J Haematol* 1957;3:241.

4. Devergie A, Blaise D, Attal M, et al. Allogeneic bone marrow transplantation for chronic myeloid leukemia in first chronic phase: a randomized trial of busulfan-cytoxan versus cytoxan-total body irradiation as preparative regimen: a report from the French Society of Bone Marrow Graft (SFGM). *Blood* 1995;85:2263.

5. Davies SM, Ramsay NK, Klein JP, et al. Comparison of preparative regimens in transplants for children with acute lymphoblastic leukemia. *J Clin Oncol* 2000;18:340.

6. Blume KG, Kopecky KJ, Henslee-Downey JP, et al. A prospective randomized comparison of total body irradiation-etoposide versus busulfan-cyclophosphamide as preparatory regimens for bone marrow transplantation in patients with leukemia who were not in first remission: a Southwest Oncology Group study. *Blood* 1993;81:2187.

6a. Ringden O, Remberger M, Ruutu T, et al Increased risk of chronic graft-versus-host disease, obstructive bronchiolitis, and alopecia with busulfan versus total body irradiation: long-term results of a randomized trial in allogeneic marrow recipients with leukemia. Nordic Bone Marrow Transplantation Group. *Blood* 1999;93:2196.

6b. Hassan M. The role of busulfan in bone marrow transplantation. *Med Oncol* 1999;16:166.

7. Mathe G, Amiel JL, Schwarzenberg L, Cattan A, Schneider M. Adoptive immunotherapy of acute leukemia: experimental and clinical results. *Cancer Res* 1965;25:1525.

8. Filipovitch A, Shapiro R, Ramsay N, et al. Unrelated donor bone marrow transplantation for correction of lethal congenital immunodeficiencies. *Blood* 1992;80:270.

9. Lenarsky C, Weinberg K, Kohn DB, Parkman R. Unrelated donor BMT for Wiskott-Aldrich syndrome. *Bone Marrow Transplant* 1993;12:145.

10. Higano CS, Brixey M, Bryant EM, et al. Durable complete remission of acute nonlymphocytic leukemia associated with discontinuation of immunosuppression following relapse after allogeneic bone marrow transplantation. A case report of a probable graft-versus-leukemia effect. *Transplantation* 1990;50:175.

11. Kolb HJ, Beisser K, Holler E, et al. Donor buffy coat transfusions for adoptive immunotherapy in human and canine chimeras. *Periodicum Biologorum* 1991;93:81.

12. Dazzi F, Szydlo RM, Cross NC, et al. Durability of responses following donor lymphocyte infusions for patients who relapse after allogeneic stem cell transplantation for chronic myeloid leukemia. *Blood* 2000;96:2712.

13. Kolb HJ, Schattenberg A, Goldman JM, et al. Graft-versus-leukemia effect of donor lymphocyte transfusions in marrow grafted patients. European Group for Blood and Marrow Transplantation Working Party Chronic Leukemia. *Blood* 1995;86:2041.

14. Champlin R, Jansen J, Ho W, et al. Retention of graft-versus-leukemia using selective depletion of CD8-positive T lymphocytes for prevention of graft-versus-host disease following bone marrow transplantation for chronic myelogenous leukemia. *Transplant Proc* 1991;23:1695.

15. Soiffer RJ, Alyea EP, Hochberg E, et al. Randomized trial of CD8+ T-cell depletion in the prevention of graft-versus-host disease associated with donor lymphocyte infusion. *Biol Blood Marrow Transplant* 2002;8:625.

16. Dazzi F, Szydlo RM, Craddock C, et al. Comparison of single-dose and escalating-dose regimens of donor lymphocyte infusion for relapse after allografting for chronic myeloid leukemia. *Blood* 2000;95:67.

17. Flowers ME, Leisenring W, Beach K, et al. Granulocyte colony-stimulating factor given to donors before apheresis does not prevent aplasia in patients treated with donor leukocyte infusion for recurrent chronic myeloid leukemia after bone marrow transplantation. *Biol Blood Marrow Transplant* 2000;6:321.

18. Riddell SR, Berger C, Murata M, Randolph S, Warren EH. The graft versus leukemia response after allogeneic hematopoietic stem cell transplantation. *Blood Rev* 2003;17:153.

19. Falkenburg JH, van de Corput L, Marijt EW, Willemze R. Minor histocompatibility antigens in human stem cell transplantation. *Exp Hematol* 2003;31:743.

20. Marijt WA, Heemskerk MH, Kloosterboer FM, et al. Hematopoiesis-restricted minor histocompatibility antigens HA-1- or HA-2-specific T cells can induce complete remissions of relapsed leukemia. *Proc Natl Acad Sci U S A* 2003;100:2742.

21. Ruggeri L, Capanni M, Urbani E, et al. Effectiveness of donor natural killer cell alloreactivity in mismatched hematopoietic transplants. *Science* 2002;295:2097.

22. Childs R, Sanchez C, Engler H, et al. High incidence of adeno- and polyomavirus-induced hemorrhagic cystitis in bone marrow allotransplantation for hematological malignancy following T cell depletion and cyclosporine. *Bone Marrow Transplant* 1998;22:889.

23. Marr KA, Seidel K, Slavin MA, et al. Prolonged fluconazole prophylaxis is associated with persistent protection against candidiasis-related death in allogeneic marrow transplant recipients: long-term follow-up of a randomized, placebo-controlled trial. *Blood* 2000;96:2055.

24. Herbrecht R, Denning DW, Patterson TF, et al. Voriconazole versus amphotericin B for primary therapy of invasive aspergillosis. *N Engl J Med* 2002;347:408.

25. Bearman SI. The syndrome of hepatic veno-occlusive disease after marrow transplantation. *Blood* 1995;85:3005.

26. Wadleigh M, Richardson PG, Zahrieh D, et al. Prior gemtuzumab ozogamicin exposure significantly increases the risk of veno-occlusive disease in patients who undergo myeloablative allogeneic stem cell transplantation. *Blood* 2003;102:1578.

27. Toh HC, McAfee SL, Sackstein R, et al. Late onset veno-occlusive disease following high-dose chemotherapy and stem cell transplantation. *Bone Marrow Transplant* 1999;24:891.

28. Richardson PG, Murakami C, Jin Z, et al. Multi-institutional use of defibrotide in 88 patients after stem cell transplantation with severe veno-occlusive disease and multisystem organ failure: response without significant toxicity in a high-risk population and factors predictive of outcome. *Blood* 2002;100:4337.

29. Essel J, Schroeder M, Harman G, et al. Ursodiol prophylaxis against hepatic complications of allogeneic BMT: a randomized, double-blind placebo-controlled trial. *Ann Intern Med* 1988;128:975.

30. Ohashi K, Tanabe J, Watanabe R, et al. The Japanese multicenter open randomized trial of ursodeoxycholic acid prophylaxis for hepatic veno-occlusive disease after stem cell transplantation. *Am J Hematol* 2000;64:32.

31. Granena A, Carreras E, Rozman C, et al. Interstitial pneumonitis after BMT: 15 years experience in a single institution. *Bone Marrow Transplant* 1993;11:453.

32. Shanker G, Scott Bryson J, Jennings D, et al. Idiopathic pneumonia syndrome after allogeneic bone marrow transplantation in mice. Role of pretransplant radiation conditioning. *Am J Respir Cell Mol Biol* 1999;20:1116.

33. Gopal R, Ha CS, Tucker SL, et al. Comparison of two total body irradiation fractionation regimens with respect to acute and late pulmonary toxicity. *Cancer* 2001;92:1949.

34. Afessa B, Tefferi A, Litzow MR, Peters SG. Outcome of diffuse alveolar hemorrhage in hematopoietic stem cell transplant recipients. *Am J Respir Crit Care Med* 2002;166:1364.

35. Kolb HJ, Poetscher C. Late effects after allogeneic bone marrow transplantation. *Curr Opin Hematol* 1997;4:401.

36. Ades L, Guardiola P, Socie G. Second malignancies after allogeneic hematopoietic stem cell transplantation: new insight and current problems. *Blood Rev* 2002;16:135.

37. Kolb HJ, Socie G, Duell T, et al. Malignant neoplasms in long-term survivors of bone marrow transplantation. Late Effects Working Party of the European Cooperative Group for Blood and Marrow Transplantation and the European Late Effect Project Group. *Ann Intern Med* 1999;131:738.

38. Papadopoulos EB, Ladanyi M, Emanuel D, et al. Infusions of donor leukocytes to treat Epstein-Barr virus-associated lymphoproliferative disorders after allogeneic bone marrow transplantation. *N Engl J Med* 1994;330:1185.

39. Rooney CM, Smith CA, Ng CY, et al. Infusion of cytotoxic T cells for the prevention and treatment of Epstein-Barr virus-induced lymphoma in allogeneic transplant recipients. *Blood* 1998;92:1549.

40. van Esser JW, Niesters HG, van der Holt B, et al. Prevention of Epstein-Barr virus-lymphoproliferative disease by molecular monitoring and preemptive rituximab in high-risk patients after allogeneic stem cell transplantation. *Blood* 2002;99:4364.

41. Teshima T, Ferrara JL. Understanding the alloresponse: new approaches to graft-versus-host disease prevention. *Semin Hematol* 2002;39:15.

42. Glucksberg H, Storb R, Fefer A, et al. Clinical manifestations of graft-versus-host disease in human recipients of marrow from HL-A-matched sibling donors. *Transplantation* 1974;18:295.

43. Thomas ED, Storb R, Clift RA, et al. Bone-marrow transplantation (second of two parts). *N Engl J Med* 1975;292:895.

44. Goulmy E, Schipper R, Pool J, et al. Mismatches of minor histocompatibility antigens between HLA-identical donors and recipients and the development of graft-versus-host disease after bone marrow transplantation. *N Engl J Med* 1996;334:281.

45. Shlomchik WD, Couzens MS, Tang CB, et al. Prevention of graft versus host disease by inactivation of host antigen-presenting cells. *Science* 1999;285:412.

46. Nash RA, Pepe MS, Storb R, et al. Acute graft-versus-host disease: analysis of risk factors after allogeneic marrow transplantation and prophylaxis with cyclosporine and methotrexate. *Blood* 1992;80:1838.

47. Weisdorf DJ, Anasetti C, Antin JH, et al. Allogeneic bone marrow transplantation for chronic myelogenous leukemia: comparative analysis of unrelated versus matched sibling donor transplantation. *Blood* 2002;99:1971.

48. Chakrabarti S, MacDonald D, Hale G, et al. T-cell depletion with CAMPATH-1H "in the bag" for matched related allogeneic peripheral blood stem cell transplantation is associated with reduced graft-versus-host disease, rapid immune constitution and improved survival. *Br J Haematol* 2003;121:109.

49. Storb R, Pepe M, Anasetti C, et al. What role for prednisone in prevention of acute graft-versus-host disease in patients undergoing marrow transplants? *Blood* 1990;76:1037.

50. Kansu E, Gooley T, Flowers ME, et al. Administration of cyclosporine for 24 months compared with 6 months for prevention of chronic graft-versus-host disease: a prospective randomized clinical trial. *Blood* 2001;98:3868.

51. Perez-Simon JA, Kottaridis PD, Martino R, et al. Nonmyeloablative transplantation with or without alemtuzumab: comparison between 2 prospective studies in patients with lymphoproliferative disorders. *Blood* 2002;100:3121.

52. Marmont AM, Horowitz MM, Gale RP, et al. T-cell depletion of HLA-identical transplants in leukemia. *Blood* 1991;78:2120.

53. Elmaagacli AH, Peceny R, Steckel N, et al. Outcome of transplantation of highly purified peripheral blood CD34+ cells with T-cell add-back compared with unmanipulated bone marrow or peripheral blood stem cells from HLA-identical sibling donors in patients with first chronic phase chronic myeloid leukemia. *Blood* 2003;101:446.

54. Van Lint MT, Uderzo C, Locasciulli A, et al. Early treatment of acute graft-versus-host disease with high- or low-dose 6-methylprednisolone: a multicenter randomized trial from the Italian Group for Bone Marrow Transplantation. *Blood* 1998;92:2288.

55. Arai S, Margolis J, Zahurak M, Anders V, Vogelsang GB. Poor outcome in steroid-refractory graft-versus-host disease with antithymocyte globulin treatment. *Biol Blood Marrow Transplant* 2002;8:155.

56. Bruner RJ, Farag SS. Monoclonal antibodies for the prevention and treatment of graft-versus-host disease. *Semin Oncol* 2003;30:509.

57. Przepiorka D, Kernan NA, Ippoliti C, et al. Daclizumab, a humanized anti-interleukin-2 receptor alpha chain antibody, for treatment of acute graft-versus-host disease. *Blood* 2000;95:83.

57a. Srinivasan R, Chakrabarti S, Walsh T, et al. Improved survival in steroid-refractory acute graft versus host disease after non-myeloablative allogeneic transplantation using a daclizumab-based strategy with comprehensive infection prophylaxis. *Br J Haematol* 2004;124:777.

58. Atkinson K. Chronic graft-versus-host disease. *Bone Marrow Transplant* 1990;5:69.

59. Mohty M, Kuentz M, Michallet M, et al. Chronic graft-versus-host disease after allogeneic blood stem cell transplantation: long-term results of a randomized study. *Blood* 2002;100:3128.

60. Vogelsang GB. How I treat chronic graft-versus-host disease. *Blood* 2001;97:1196.

61. Voogt PJ, Fibbe WE, Marijt WA, et al. Rejection of bone-marrow graft by recipient-derived cytotoxic T lymphocytes against minor histocompatibility antigens. *Lancet* 1990;335:131.

62. Anasetti C, Amos D, Beatty PG, et al. Effect of HLA compatibility on engraftment of bone marrow transplants in patients with leukemia or lymphoma. *N Engl J Med* 1989;320:197.

63. Davies SM, Weisdorf DJ, Haake RJ, et al. Second infusion of bone marrow for treatment of graft failure after allogeneic bone marrow transplantation. *Bone Marrow Transplant* 1994;14:73.

64. Chakrabarti S, Mackinnon S, Chopra R, et al. High incidence of cytomegalovirus infection after nonmyeloablative stem cell transplantation: potential role of Campath-1H in delaying immune reconstitution. *Blood* 2002;99:4357.

65. Atkinson K, Downs K, Golenia M, et al. Prophylactic use of ganciclovir in allogeneic bone marrow transplantation: absence of clinical cytomegalovirus infection. *Br J Haematol* 1991;79:57.

66. Ljungman P, Lore K, Aschan J, et al. Use of a semi-quantitative PCR for cytomegalovirus DNA as a basis for preemptive antiviral therapy in allogeneic bone marrow transplant patients. *Bone Marrow Transplant* 1996;17:583.

67. Cortez KJ, Fischer SH, Fahle GA, et al. Clinical trial of quantitative real-time polymerase chain reaction for detection of cytomegalovirus in peripheral blood of allogeneic hematopoietic stem-cell transplant recipients. *J Infect Dis* 2003;188:967.

68. Korbling M, Przepiorka D, Huh YO, et al. Allogeneic blood stem cell transplantation for refractory leukemia and lymphoma: potential advantage of blood over marrow allografts. *Blood* 1995;85:1659.

69. Moncada V, Bolan C, Yau YY, Leitman SF. Analysis of PBPC cell yields during large-volume leukapheresis of subjects with a poor mobilization response to filgrastim. *Transfusion* 2003;43:495.

70. Bolan CD, Carter CS, Wesley RA, et al. Prospective evaluation of cell kinetics, yields and donor experiences during a single large-volume apheresis versus two smaller volume consecutive day collections of allogeneic peripheral blood stem cells. *Br J Haematol* 2003;120:801.

71. Powles R, Mehta J, Kulkarni S, et al. Allogeneic blood and bone-marrow stem-cell transplantation in haematological malignant diseases: a randomised trial. *Lancet* 2000;355:1231.

72. Schmitz N, Bacigalupo A, Hasenclever D, et al. Allogeneic bone marrow transplantation vs filgrastim-mobilised peripheral blood progenitor cell transplantation in patients with early leukaemia: first results of a randomised multicentre trial of the European Group for Blood and Marrow Transplantation. *Bone Marrow Transplant* 1998;21:995.

73. Bensinger WI, Clift R, Martin P, et al. Allogeneic peripheral blood stem cell transplantation in patients with advanced hematologic malignancies: a retrospective comparison with marrow transplantation. *Blood* 1996;88:2794.

74. Del Canizo MC, Martinez C, Conde E, et al. Peripheral blood is safer than bone marrow as a source of hematopoietic progenitors in patients with myelodysplastic syndromes who receive an allogeneic transplantation. Results from the Spanish registry. *Bone Marrow Transplant* 2003;32:987.

75. Blaise D, Kuentz M, Fortanier C, et al. Randomized trial of bone marrow versus lenograstim-primed blood cell allogeneic transplantation in patients with early-stage leukemia: a report from the Societe Francaise de Greffe de Moelle. *J Clin Oncol* 2000;18:537.

76. Bensinger WI, Martin PJ, Storer B, et al. Transplantation of bone marrow as compared with peripheral-blood cells from HLA-identical relatives in patients with hematologic cancers. *N Engl J Med* 2001;344:175.

77. Grewal SS, Barker JN, Davies SM, Wagner JE. Unrelated donor hematopoietic cell transplantation: marrow or umbilical cord blood? *Blood* 2003;101:4233.

78. McGlave PB, Shu XO, Wen W, et al. Unrelated donor marrow transplantation for chronic myelogenous leukemia: 9 years' experience of the national marrow donor program. *Blood* 2000;95:2219.

79. Szydlo R, Goldman JM, Klein JP, et al. Results of allogeneic bone marrow transplants for leukemia using donors other than HLA-identical siblings. *J Clin Oncol* 1997;15:1767.

80. Hansen JA, Gooley TA, Martin PJ, et al. Bone marrow transplants from unrelated donors for patients with chronic myeloid leukemia. *N Engl J Med* 1998;338:962.

81. Speiser DE, Tiercy JM, Rufer N, et al. High resolution HLA matching associated with decreased mortality after unrelated bone marrow transplantation. *Blood* 1996;87:4455.

82. Petersdorf EW, Hansen JA, Martin PJ, et al. Major-histocompatibility-complex class I alleles and antigens in hematopoietic-cell transplantation. *N Engl J Med* 2001;345:1794.

83. Aversa F, Tabilio A, Velardi A, et al. Treatment of high-risk acute leukemia with T-cell-depleted stem cells from related donors with one fully mismatched HLA haplotype. *N Engl J Med* 1998;339:1186.

84. Veys P, Amrolia P, Rao K. The role of haploidentical stem cell transplantation in the management of children with haematological disorders. *Br J Haematol* 2003;123:193.

85. Tamaki H, Ikegame K, Kawakami M, et al. Successful engraftment of HLA-haploidentical related transplants using nonmyeloablative conditioning with fludarabine, busulfan and anti-T-lymphocyte globulin. *Leukemia* 2003;17:2052.

86. Aversa F, Terenzi A, Felicini R, et al. Haploidentical stem cell transplantation for acute leukemia. *Int J Hematol* 2002;76(Suppl 1):165.

87. Giebel S, Locatelli F, Lamparelli T, et al. Survival advantage with KIR ligand incompatibility in hematopoietic stem cell transplantation from unrelated donors. *Blood* 2003;102:814.

88. Davies SM, Ruggieri L, DeFor T, et al. Evaluation of KIR ligand incompatibility in mismatched unrelated donor hematopoietic transplants. Killer immunoglobulin-like receptor. *Blood* 2002;100:3825.

89. Drobyski WR, Klein J, Flomenberg N, et al. Superior survival associated with transplantation of matched unrelated versus one-antigen-mismatched unrelated or highly human leukocyte antigen-disparate haploidentical family donor marrow grafts for the treatment of hematologic malignancies: establishing a treatment algorithm for recipients of alternative donor grafts. *Blood* 2002;99:806.

90. Gluckman E. Hematopoietic stem-cell transplants using umbilical-cord blood. *N Engl J Med* 2001;344:1860.

91. Wagner JE, Kernan NA, Steinbuch M, Broxmeyer HE, Gluckman E. Allogeneic sibling umbilical-cord-blood transplantation in children with malignant and non-malignant disease. *Lancet* 1995;346:214.

92. Gluckman E, Rocha V, Boyer-Chammard A, et al. Outcome of cord-blood transplantation from related and unrelated donors. Eurocord Transplant Group and the European Blood and Marrow Transplantation Group. *N Engl J Med* 1997;337:373.

93. O'Brien SG, Guilhot F, Larson RA, et al. Imatinib compared with interferon and low-dose cytarabine for newly diagnosed chronic-phase chronic myeloid leukemia. *N Engl J Med* 2003;348:994.

94. Or R, Shapira MY, Resnick I, et al. Nonmyeloablative allogeneic stem cell transplantation for the treatment of chronic myeloid leukemia in first chronic phase. *Blood* 2003;101:441.

95. Goldman JM. Therapeutic strategies for chronic myeloid leukemia in the chronic (stable) phase. *Semin Hematol* 2003;40:10.

96. McCann SR, Gately K, Conneally E, Lawler M. Molecular response to imatinib mesylate following relapse after allogeneic SCT for CML.. *Blood* 2003;101:1200.

97. Grimwade D, Walker H, Oliver F, et al. The importance of diagnostic cytogenetics on outcome in AML: analysis of 1,612 patients entered into the MRC AML 10 trial. The Medical Research Council Adult and Children's Leukaemia Working Parties. *Blood* 1998;92:2322.

98. Bostrom B, Brunning RD, McGlave P, et al. Bone marrow transplantation for acute nonlymphocytic leukemia in first remission: analysis of prognostic factors. *Blood* 1985;65:1191.

99. McGlave PB, Haake RJ, Bostrom BC, et al. Allogeneic bone marrow transplantation for acute nonlymphocytic leukemia in first remission. *Blood* 1988;72:1512.

100. Chalandon Y, Barnett MJ, Horsman DE, et al. Influence of cytogenetic abnormalities on outcome after allogeneic bone marrow transplantation for acute myeloid leukemia in first complete remission. *Biol Blood Marrow Transplant* 2002;8:435.

101. Hoelzer D, Ludwig WD, Thiel E, et al. Improved outcome in adult B-cell acute lymphoblastic leukemia. *Blood* 1996;87:495.

102. Barrett AJ, Horowitz MM, Ash RC, et al. Bone marrow transplantation for Philadelphia chromosome-positive acute lymphoblastic leukemia. *Blood* 1992;79:3067.

103. Chao NJ, Forman SJ, Schmidt GM, et al. Allogeneic bone marrow transplantation for high-risk acute lymphoblastic leukemia during first complete remission. *Blood* 1991;78:1923.

104. Runde V, de Witte T, Arnold R, et al. Bone marrow transplantation from HLA-identical siblings as first-line treatment in patients with myelodysplastic syndromes: early transplantation is associated with improved outcome. Chronic Leukemia Working Party of the European Group for Blood and Marrow Transplantation. *Bone Marrow Transplant* 1998;21:255.

105. Nevill TJ, Fung HC, Shepherd JD, et al. Cytogenetic abnormalities in primary myelodysplastic syndrome are highly predictive of outcome after allogeneic bone marrow transplantation. *Blood* 1998;92:1910.

106. van Besien K, Keralavarma B, Devine S, Stock W. Allogeneic and autologous transplantation for chronic lymphocytic leukemia. *Leukemia* 2001;15:1317.

107. Khouri IF, Keating MJ, Saliba RM, Champlin RE. Long-term follow-up of patients with CLL treated with allogeneic hematopoietic transplantation. *Cytotherapy* 2002;4:217.

108. Giralt S, Estey E, Albitar M, et al. Engraftment of allogeneic hematopoietic progenitor cells with purine analog-containing chemotherapy: harnessing graft-versus-leukemia without myeloablative therapy. *Blood* 1997;89:4531.

109. Slavin S, Nagler A, Naparstek E, et al. Nonmyeloablative stem cell transplantation and cell therapy as an alternative to conventional bone marrow transplantation with lethal cytoreduction for the treatment of malignant and nonmalignant hematologic diseases. *Blood* 1998;91:756.

110. Chakrabarti S, Childs R. Allogeneic immune replacement as cancer immunotherapy. *Expert Opin Biol Ther* 2003;3:1051.

111. Maris MB, Niederwieser D, Sandmaier BM, et al. HLA-matched unrelated donor hematopoietic cell transplantation after nonmyeloablative conditioning for patients with hematologic malignancies. *Blood* 2003;102:2021.

112. Sykes M, Spitzer TR. Non-myeloablative induction of mixed hematopoietic chimerism: application to transplantation tolerance and hematologic malignancies in experimental and clinical studies. *Cancer Treat Res* 2002;110:79.

113. Antin JH, Childs R, Filipovich AH, et al. Establishment of complete and mixed donor chimerism after allogeneic lymphohematopoietic transplantation: recommendations from a workshop at the 2001 Tandem Meetings of the International Bone Marrow Transplant Registry and the American Society of Blood and Marrow Transplantation. *Biol Blood Marrow Transplant* 2001;7:473.

114. Mapara MY, Kim YM, Marx J, Sykes M. Donor lymphocyte infusion-mediated graft-versus-leukemia effects in mixed chimeras established with a nonmyeloablative conditioning regimen: extinction of graft-versus-leukemia effects after conversion to full donor chimerism. *Transplantation* 2003;76:297.

115. Canals C, Martino R, Sureda A, et al. Strategies to reduce transplant-related mortality after allogeneic stem cell transplantation in elderly patients: comparison of reduced-intensity conditioning and unmanipulated peripheral blood stem cells vs a myeloablative regimen and CD34(+) cell selection. *Exp Hematol* 2003;31:1039.

116. Storb R, Yu C, Sandmaier BM, et al. Mixed hematopoietic chimerism after marrow allografts. Transplantation in the ambulatory care setting. *Ann N Y Acad Sci* 1999;872:372;discussion 375.

117. Weissinger F, Sandmaier BM, Maloney DG, et al. Decreased transfusion requirements for patients receiving nonmyeloablative compared with conventional peripheral blood stem cell transplants from HLA-identical siblings. *Blood* 2001;98:3584.

118. Junghanss C, Marr KA, Carter RA, et al. Incidence and outcome of bacterial and fungal infections following nonmyeloablative compared with myeloablative allogeneic hematopoietic stem cell transplantation: a matched control study. *Biol Blood Marrow Transplant* 2002;8:512.

119. Fukuda T, Boeckh M, Carter RA, et al. Risks and outcomes of invasive fungal infections in recipients of allogeneic hematopoietic stem cell transplants after nonmyeloablative conditioning. *Blood* 2003;102:827.

120. Chakrabarti S, Milligan DW, Pillay D, et al. Reconstitution of the Epstein-Barr virus-specific cytotoxic T-lymphocyte response following T-cell-depleted myeloablative and nonmyeloablative allogeneic stem cell transplantation. *Blood* 2003;102:839.

121. Chakrabarti S, McDonald D, Milligan DW. T cell-depleted nonmyeloablative stem cell transplantation: what is the optimum balance between the intensity of host conditioning and the degree of T cell depletion of the graft? *Bone Marrow Transplant* 2001;28:313.

122. Carvallo C, Geller N, Kurlander R, et al. Prior chemotherapy and allograft CD34+ dose impact donor engraftment following nonmyeloablative allogeneic stem cell transplantation in solid tumor patients. *Blood* 2003;103:1560.

123. Childs R, Clave E, Contentin N, et al. Engraftment kinetics after nonmyeloablative allogeneic peripheral blood stem cell transplantation: full donor T-cell chimerism precedes alloimmune responses. *Blood* 1999;94:3234.

124. McSweeney PA, Niederwieser D, Shizuru JA, et al. Hematopoietic cell transplantation in older patients with hematologic malignancies: replacing high-dose cytotoxic therapy with graft-versus-tumor effects. *Blood* 2001;97:3390.

125. Storb RF, Champlin R, Riddell SR, et al. Non-myeloablative transplants for malignant disease. *Hematology (Am Soc Hematol Educ Program)* 2001;375.

126. Keil F, Prinz E, Moser K, et al. Rapid establishment of long-term culture-initiating cells of donor origin after nonmyeloablative allogeneic hematopoietic stem-cell transplantation, and significant prognostic impact of donor T-cell chimerism on stable engraftment and progression-free survival. *Transplantation* 2003;76:230.

127. Ritchie DS, Morton J, Szer J, et al. Graft-versus-host disease, donor chimerism, and organ toxicity in stem cell transplantation after conditioning with fludarabine and melphalan. *Biol Blood Marrow Transplant* 2003;9:435.

128. Antin JH. Stem cell transplantation-harnessing of graft-versus-malignancy. *Curr Opin Hematol* 2003;10:440.

129. Maloney DG, Sandmaier BM, Mackinnon S, Shizuru JA. Non-myeloablative transplantation. *Hematology (Am Soc Hematol Educ Program)* 2002;392.

130. Kottaridis PD, Milligan DW, Chopra R, et al. In vivo CAMPATH-1H prevents graft-versus-host disease following nonmyeloablative stem cell transplantation. *Blood* 2000; 96:2419.

131. Anagnostopoulos A, Giralt S. Critical review on non-myeloablative stem cell transplantation (NST). *Crit Rev Oncol Hematol* 2002;44:175.

132. Fernandez-Aviles F, Urbano-Ispizua A, Aymerich M, et al. Low-dose total-body irradiation and fludarabine followed by hematopoietic cell transplantation from HLA-identical sibling donors do not induce complete T-cell donor engraftment in most patients with progressive hematologic diseases. *Exp Hematol* 2003;31:934.

133. Arnold R, Massenkeil G, Bornhauser M, et al. Nonmyeloablative stem cell transplantation in adults with high-risk ALL may be effective in early but not in advanced disease. *Leukemia* 2002;16:2423.

134. Storb RF, Lucarelli G, McSweeney PA, Childs RW. Hematopoietic cell transplantation for benign hematological disorders and solid tumors. *Hematology (Am Soc Hematol Educ Program)* 2003;372.

135. Childs R, Chernoff A, Contentin N, et al. Regression of metastatic renal-cell carcinoma after nonmyeloablative allogeneic peripheral-blood stem-cell transplantation. *N Engl J Med* 2000;343:750.

SECTION **4**

JENNIFER L. HOLTER
HOWARD OZER

Hematopoietic Growth Factors

The term *hematopoietic growth factors* (HGFs) refers to cytokines that govern hematopoiesis by regulating the proliferation, differentiation, maturation, and viability of the cellular components of blood and their progenitor cells. Cytokines by definition are proteins released by cells that act as intercellular mediators. For the purposes of hematopoiesis, HGFs are primarily produced by cells of the bone marrow, with the exception of erythropoietin (EPO), which is produced by cells of the kidney. However, many other nonmarrow cells can produce HGFs. Table 52.4-1 describes the endogenous cellular sources, inducers, and hematopoietic role of the four major HGFs of importance in cancer therapy: EPO, granulocyte colony-stimulating factor (G-CSF), granulocyte-macrophage colony-stimulating factor (GM-CSF), and interleukin-11 (IL-11).

Recombinant human (rHu) HGFs are commonly used in oncology practice for a variety of purposes, including attenuation of chemotherapy-induced myelosuppression, treatment of hematopoietic malignancies, and management of depressed HGF production in malignancy. Six rHu HGFs are approved for use in the United States; these products are listed in Table 52.4-2. These agents are used in practice to support depressed hematopoiesis; rHu EPO to stimulate erythropoiesis, rHu G-CSF and GM-CSF to stimulate growth of neutrophils; and rHu IL-11 to stimulate thrombopoiesis.

The role of rHu HGFs in cancer therapy is a field of study that is continually evolving. Key areas of research with current growth factors seek to identify the cost-effective application of these agents and to elucidate the true benefits of growth factors in terms of outcomes such as reductions in infection and mortality, improvements in quality of life (QOL), and improved overall progression-free survival. This chapter focuses on reviewing the appropriate use of recombinant HGFs for hematopoiesis in the oncology setting based on evidence from current literature and introduces new HGFs under development.

OVERVIEW OF HEMATOPOIESIS AND HEMATOPOIETIC GROWTH FACTORS

All of the cellular components in blood (erythrocytes, leukocytes, and platelets) are derived from multipotent stem cells located primarily in the bone marrow. As stem cells mature and differentiate, they become progressively committed to specific blood cell lineages with distinct functions. Throughout the maturation process, a number of cells in varying stages of commitment are created; these actively proliferating cells are termed *progenitor cells*. HGFs regulate the proliferation, differentiation, and maturation of the stem cells and progenitor cells. Some HGFs (e.g., Steel factor or Flt3 ligand) regulate stem and early progenitor cells; others (e.g., EPO or G-CSF) regulate more committed progenitors and mature cells (Fig. 52.4-1).

The effects of HGFs are mediated through receptors located on both hematopoietic and nonhematopoietic cells. As such, the physiologic effects of HGFs are numerous and not confined to hematopoiesis. Table 52.4-3 lists the various receptor locations and illustrates the pleiotropic effects of these proteins. An area of both concern and interest is the fact that receptors for all currently applied HGFs are found on various tumor cell lines. Theoretically, HGFs may stimulate proliferation of these tumor cells via signaling through these receptors. Although tumor cell proliferation may be detrimental, HGFs have also been used therapeutically to induce active division of tumor cells to increase sensitivity to conventional chemotherapy. Other research is ongoing to investigate exploitation of these receptor locations by using the HGF as a targeted carrier for anticancer modalities.

The receptors for EPO, G-CSF, and GM-CSF belong to the HGF receptor superfamily sharing homology with receptors for IL-2, thrombopoietin, and other cytokines.[1,2] The IL-11 receptor is a member of a cytokine receptor family that includes IL-6 and leukemia inhibitor factor, among others, that all use the signal transducing receptor subunit gp130 after ligand binding.[3] Important new research has identified the suppressor of cytokine signaling (SOCS) family of proteins. A family of eight compounds (SOCS-1 to SOCS-7 and cytokine-inducible SH2-containing protein), these proteins are implicated in the negative regulation of several cytokine pathways, particularly the receptor-associated tyrosine kinase/signal trans-

TABLE 52.4-1. Endogenous Sources, Inducers, and Roles of Major Hematopoietic Growth Factors

Hematopoietic Growth Factor	Endogenous Sources	Physiologic States That Induce Production	Endogenous Substances That Induce Production	Endogenous Hematopoietic Role
EPO	Kidney Brain Uterus	Hypoxia	Estradiol (uterus)	Stimulates erythropoiesis
G-CSF	Marrow stromal cells Neutrophils Monocytes/macrophages T cells Endothelial cells Fibroblasts Mesothelial cells Epithelial cells Various tumor cell lines	Infection Inflammation Tissue damage	Endotoxin Lipopolysaccharide TNF IL-1β IFN-γ GM-CSF M-CSF IL-3 IL-4	Regulates production, maturation, and function of neutrophil lineage
GM-CSF	Monocytes/macrophages T cells Endothelial cells Fibroblasts Mesothelial cells Epithelial cells Various tumor cell lines	Infection Inflammation Tissue damage	IL-1 IL-6 TNF Endotoxin	Regulates production, maturation, and function of myeloid lineage
IL-11	Bone marrow stromal cells Fibroblasts Chondrocytes Synoviocytes Osteoblasts Trophoblasts Epithelial cells	Thrombocytopenia Respiratory viruses	TGF-β IL-1 TNF Parathyroid hormone Calcium ionophores Phorbol esters	Regulates production and maturation of megakaryocytes Induces platelet production Stimulates erythropoiesis Regulates macrophage proliferation and differentiation

EPO, erythropoietin; G-CSF, granulocyte colony-stimulating factor; GM-CSF, granulocyte-macrophage colony-stimulating factor; IFN, interferon; IL, interleukin; M-CSF, macrophage colony-stimulating factor; TGF, transforming growth factor; TNF, tumor necrosis factor.

ducer and activator of transcription (Jak/STAT) pathways of transcriptional activation. Of particular interest is SOCS-3, identified as a regulator in hematopoiesis. The cytokine G-CSF activates the Jak/STAT pathway, and new data suggest that G-CSF also induces expression of SOCS-3 in neutrophils and a myeloid precursor cell line, suggesting the presence of a negative feedback circuit.[4,5] The SOCS-3 protein also acts as a negative regulator in fetal erythropoiesis.[6]

TABLE 52.4-2. Hematopoietic Growth Factors Approved for Use by the U.S. Food and Drug Administration with Applications in Cancer Therapy

Hematopoietic Growth Factor	Generic Name	Brand Names	Molecular Description	Hematopoietic Effects	Applications in Cancer
EPO	Epoetin alfa	Epogen, Procrit	rHu EPO	Red cell lineage	Anemia associated with chemotherapy, cancer, or myeloproliferative disorders
	Darbepoetin	Aranesp	rHu EPO with altered glycosylation	Red cell lineage	Anemia associated with chemotherapy, cancer, or myeloproliferative disorders
G-CSF	Filgrastim	Neupogen	rHu G-CSF	Neutrophil lineage	Reduce febrile neutropenia in patients receiving myelosuppressive chemotherapy, reduce duration of neutropenia after bone marrow transplantation, mobilize progenitor cells
	Pegfilgrastim	Neulasta	Pegylated rHu G-CSF	Neutrophil lineage	Reduce febrile neutropenia in patients receiving myelosuppressive chemotherapy
GM-CSF	Sargramostim	Leukine	rHu GM-CSF	Myeloid lineage	Reduce duration of neutropenia after bone marrow transplantation, mobilize progenitor cells
IL-11	Oprelvekin	Neumega	rHu IL-11	Megakaryocytes	Treatment of chemotherapy-associated thrombocytopenia

EPO, erythropoietin; G-CSF, granulocyte colony-stimulating factor; GM-CSF, granulocyte-macrophage colony-stimulating factor; IL-11, interleukin-11; rHu, recombinant human.

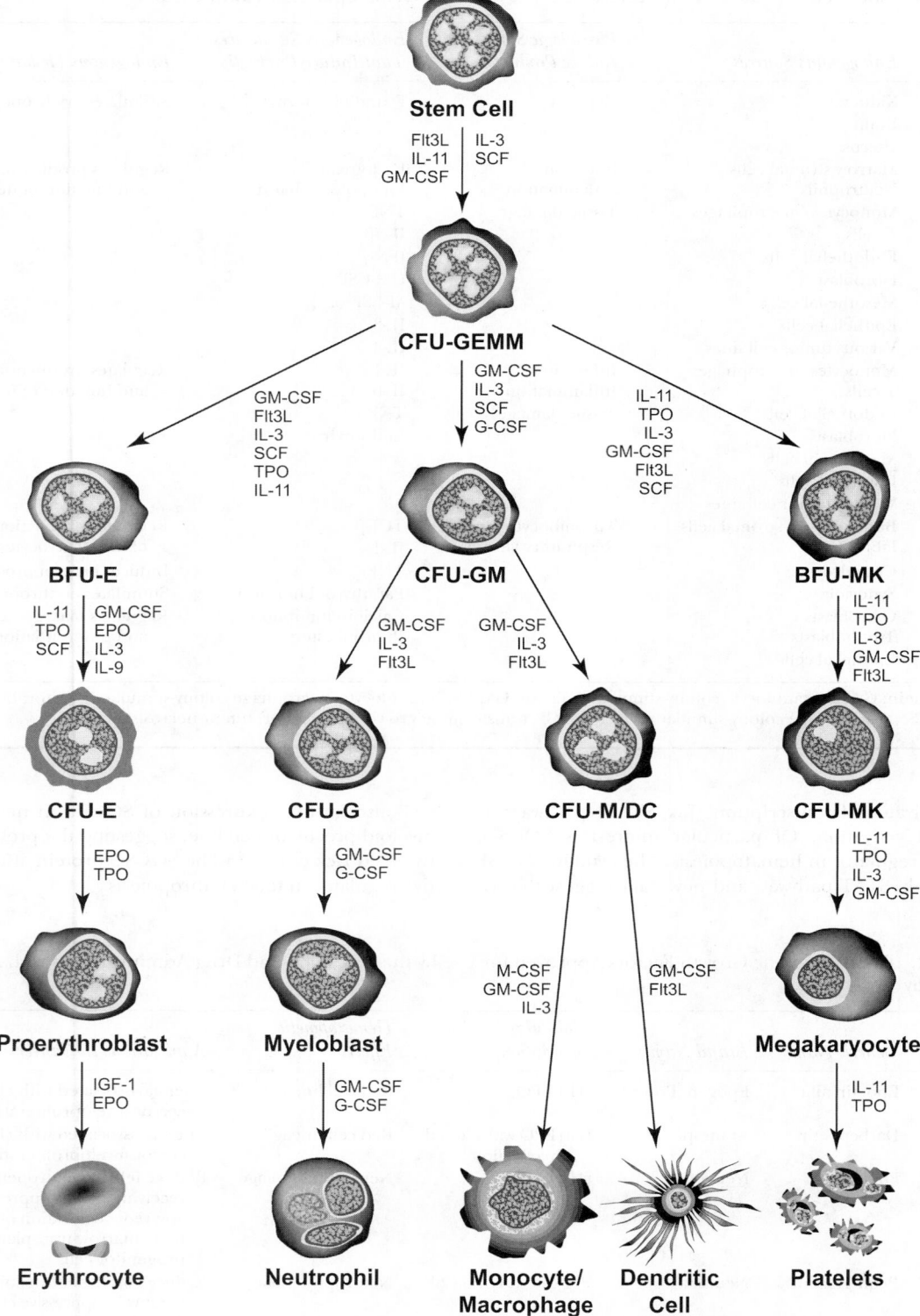

FIGURE 52.4-1. This schematic depiction of the hematopoietic cascade identifies the role of key hematopoietic growth factors and the maturation of blood cells in the process of hematopoiesis. BFU, blast-forming unit; CFU, colony-forming unit; EPO, erythropoietin; Flt3L, flt3 ligand; G-CSF, granulocyte colony-stimulating factor; GM-CSF, granulocyte-macrophage colony-stimulating factor; IGF, insulin-like growth factor; IL, interleukin; M-CSF, macrophage colony-stimulating factor; MK, megakaryocyte; SCF, stem cell factor; TPO, thrombopoietin.

TABLE 52.4-3. Receptor Locations and Pleiotropic Effects of Major Hematopoietic Growth Factors

Hematopoietic Growth Factor	Receptor Locations	Potential Nonhematopoietic Effects
EPO	Breast tumor vasculature	Neuroprotection
	Neurons	Angiogenesis
	Astrocytes	Testosterone production
	Endothelial cells	Mucosal protection
	Leydig cells	Hypertension
	Gastric mucosal cells	
	Vascular smooth muscle cells	
	Cardiomyocytes	
	Myeloid cells	
	Lymphocytes	
	Megakaryocytes	
	Mesangial cells	
	Cancer cell lines	
	Colon adenocarcinoma	
	Pancreatic carcinoma	
	Prostate carcinoma	
	Bladder carcinoma	
	Hepatoma	
	Promyelocytic leukemia	
	Erythroleukemia	
	AML	
	Renal carcinoma	
	Breast carcinoma	
	Neuroblastoma	
	Sarcoma	
	Melanoma	
G-CSF	Neutrophils and their progenitor cells	Antiinflammatory activity
	Monocytes	Sensitization of malignant myeloid tumor cells to chemotherapy
	Platelets	
	Endothelial cells	
	Placenta	
	Endometrium	
	Cancer cell lines	
	Myeloid leukemic cells	
	Epithelial cells	
	Small cell lung carcinoma	
	Ovarian carcinoma	
	Gastric adenocarcinoma	
	Acute promyelocytic leukemia cells	
	Acute lymphoblastic leukemia cells	
	Bladder cancer	
	B-cell lymphoma	
GM-CSF	Myeloid cells	Vaccine adjuvancy
	Dendritic cells	Mucosal protection
	Endothelial cells	Crohn's disease
	Cancer cell lines	Wound healing
	Myeloid leukemias	
	ALL	
	Endometrial carcinoma	
	Renal cell carcinoma	
	Skin carcinoma	
	Glioma	
	Non–small cell lung cancer	
	Malignant plasma cells	
	Prostate cancer	
	Colon carcinoma	
	Melanoma	
	Gastric carcinoma	
	Osteosarcoma	

(continued)

TABLE 52.4-3. (*Continued*)

Hematopoietic Growth Factor	Receptor Locations	Potential Nonhematopoietic Effects

IL-11	Megakaryocyte progenitors
	Myeloid cells
	Lymphocytes
	Osteoclasts/osteoblasts
	Endometrial cells
	Ovarian epithelial cells
	Gastric mucosal cells
	Nerve cells
	Anterior pituitary cells
	Cancer cell lines
	    B-cell chronic lymphocytic leukemia
	    Ovarian, prostate cancer epithelial cells
	    AML
		Mucosal protection and repair
		Antiinflammatory activity
		Increased bone resorption through osteoclast activation
		Inhibition of adipogenesis
		Regulation of neuronal differentiation
		Active in human reproduction

ALL, acute lymphoblastic leukemia; AML, acute myeloid leukemia; EPO, erythropoietin; G-CSF, granulocyte colony-stimulating factor; GM-CSF, granulocyte-macrophage colony-stimulating factor; IL-11, interleukin-11.

ERYTHROPOIETIN

Endogenous EPO is the primary regulator of red blood cell production, and both humans and mice deficient in EPO develop severe anemia. EPO is primarily produced in the kidney, likely by interstitial fibroblasts and proximal tubular cells,[7] in response to hypoxia or decreased red cell oxygen-carrying capacity (see Table 52.4-1). Endogenous serum concentrations vary inversely with red cell oxygen-carrying capacity. Normal serum EPO levels range from approximately 4 to 30 U/L. Serum EPO levels rise as the hematocrit drops below approximately 35% and can rise 100- to 1000-fold with severe anemia. Endogenous EPO levels are often depressed in cancer patients with chronic anemias.[8] Conversely, excess EPO production can lead to secondary polycythemia as a result of renal tumors causing local hypoxia or occasionally direct tumor secretion of EPO.

A recombinant form of human EPO first became available in 1989, and currently three different forms are commercially available. In the United States, epoetin alfa and darbepoetin alfa are approved. Epoetin alfa contains the identical amino acid sequence to endogenous human EPO and has a half-life of approximately 3 to 10 hours in healthy volunteers after intravenous (IV) administration. Darbepoetin alfa is an rHu EPO modified by the addition of two N-glycosylation sites to produce a molecule with a longer half-life of approximately threefold greater than epoetin alfa.[9] Outside of the United States, epoetin beta is available, a protein with an identical amino acid sequence to endogenous human EPO but with a different glycosylation pattern than epoetin alfa. The difference in glycosylation does not appear to significantly alter efficacy compared with epoetin alfa.

Like their endogenous counterparts, rHu EPOs stimulate the proliferation, differentiation, and maturation of committed erythroid progenitors to mature erythrocytes. After administration of rHu EPOs, a rise in the red cell count does not begin to occur until 2 weeks of continuous dosing and may take up to 8 weeks.

The toxicity and side effects of epoetin alfa or darbepoetin alfa are generally minimal. Some patients experience edema on epoetin alfa or darbepoetin alfa therapy. An increase in thrombotic events has been reported with recombinant EPO therapies; however, these appear to be more common in patients with chronic renal failure, particularly those with ischemic heart disease or congestive heart failure. Hypertension can also occur but is similarly more common in patients with chronic renal failure.[10] Patients' hematocrit should be monitored while on therapy to avoid erythrocytosis. As noted in Table 52.4-3, EPO receptors have been identified on cells of breast tumor vasculature[11]; however, no current evidence exists that exogenously administered rHu EPO leads to tumor cell proliferation.[12]

GRANULOCYTE COLONY-STIMULATING FACTOR

Endogenous G-CSF regulates the production, maturation, and function of the neutrophil lineage. Mice and dogs deficient in G-CSF develop severe neutropenia.[13,14] Data from G-CSF-deficient mice suggest that endogenous G-CSF reduces apoptosis and is critical for granulocyte survival; however, G-CSF is not essential for trafficking of granulocytes from the bone marrow to circulation.[15] Endogenous G-CSF is produced by many different cell types, both myeloid and nonmyeloid (see Table 52.4-1). Serum concentrations vary inversely with blood neutrophil concentrations. Normal serum G-CSF levels range from 20 to 100 pg/mL; however, G-CSF levels can exceed 2000 pg/mL in states of bacteremia or neutropenia.

rHu G-CSF is currently available commercially in four forms, of which filgrastim and pegfilgrastim are approved in the United States. Filgrastim is a recombinant protein that has an amino acid sequence identical to endogenous G-CSF, except for the addition of an N-terminal methionine and lack of glycosylation found on human G-CSF. The protein is expressed in *Escherichia coli*.[16] The half-life of rHu G-CSF is approximately 3.5 hours in both cancer patients and healthy subjects after either IV or subcutaneous (SC) dosing; however, clearance appears to increase with blood neutrophil concentration increases.[17,18] Pegfilgrastim is a pegylated version of filgrastim designed for longer residence time, thus necessitating fewer injections. In a study of ten cancer patients, the median half-life of pegfilgrastim was approximately 33 hours.[19] Serum clearance is directly related to blood neutrophil concentrations.[19,20] Outside of the United States, rHu G-CSF is available as lenograstim, a glycosylated recombinant G-CSF expressed in a mammalian cell system (Chinese hamster ovaries), and Nartograstim, an N-terminal–mutated recombinant G-CSF expressed in *E coli*.

When exogenously administered, rHu G-CSF increases the level of circulating neutrophils by accelerating production through reducing transit time from stem cell to mature neutrophil and by inhibiting neutrophil apoptosis.[21] These effects are associated with an increase in the number of neutrophil progenitors in marrow and an increase in the percent of myeloid progenitors in S phase. Evidence suggests that rHu G-CSF may stimulate the entry of quiescent stem and progenitor cells into cell cycle.[22] This activity of G-CSF on acute myeloid leukemia (AML) cell lines has been used therapeutically to stimulate active division of leukemic cell progenitors, thus sensitizing these cells to cytotoxic modalities to improve malignant cell kill.[23]

The neutrophils produced show morphologic changes consistent with activation, including Döhle's inclusion bodies, toxic granulation, and an increase in band forms. At a minimum, these neutrophils are functionally normal as tested with standard assays of phagocytosis and respiratory burst. However, data suggest that G-CSF enhances chemotaxis, phagocytosis, and the oxidative burst of mature neutrophils *in vitro* and increases antibody-dependent cellular cytotoxicity *in vivo*.[21]

Marrow aspirates show a left shift in patients receiving G-CSF or other myeloid growth factors, and after IV administration, neutrophil counts may transiently drop. On discontinuation of recombinant G-CSF, peripheral neutrophil counts decrease by approximately 50% per day and return to baseline in 4 to 6 days.[24] Lymphocytes and monocytes are also marginally increased with rHu G-CSF administration; however, the clinical significance of these changes is not established.

In addition to stimulating neutrophil production, G-CSF mobilizes hematopoietic progenitor cells (HPCs) into the peripheral circulation. The mechanism by which G-CSF stimulates mobilization is not fully understood. However, it has been demonstrated that the presence of G-CSF receptors on HPCs is not required for mobilization by G-CSF.[25] These data suggest that G-CSF may first activate a mature hematopoietic cell via a G-CSF receptor, and this activated cell in turn generates secondary signals leading to HPC mobilization. The nature of these secondary signals is unknown but may involve release of proteases that interact with cellular adhesion molecules or modulation of stromal-derived factor-1 expression in the marrow.[26]

The most common side effect from rHu G-CSF administration is mild to moderate bone pain.[27] Regular white blood cell monitoring should be conducted during therapy to prevent leukocytosis; typically treatment is discontinued when the neutrophil count reaches 10,000 cells/μL in the setting of chemotherapy-induced neutropenia. Rare, serious adverse events include allergic-type reactions (particularly with the first dose), splenic rupture in persons receiving recombinant G-CSF for peripheral blood stem cell (PBSC) mobilization (including healthy donors), and adult respiratory distress syndrome in neutropenic patients with infection.[28,29]

GRANULOCYTE-MACROPHAGE COLONY-STIMULATING FACTOR

Endogenous GM-CSF promotes the growth and differentiation of cells in the neutrophil and monocyte lineages as well as dendritic cells, eosinophils, and, in the presence of EPO, erythrocytes. Mice deficient in GM-CSF do not develop hematopoietic abnormalities but instead develop a syndrome similar to pulmonary alveolar proteinosis.[30] Endogenous GM-CSF is produced by myeloid and nonmyeloid cells, and production is induced by inflammatory stimuli (see Table 52.4-1) Normal endogenous serum concentrations fall below 100 pg/mL and increase with the presence of infection.[31]

rHu GM-CSF is expressed in three different systems, yielding sargramostim, molgramostim, and regramostim. Sargramostim, the only form available in the United States, is an rHu GM-CSF that has an amino acid sequence identical to endogenous GM-CSF, except for a substitution of leucine at position 23. The carbohydrate moiety may also differ from endogenous human GM-CSF. Sargramostim is expressed in yeast (*Saccharomyces cerevisiae*) and is O-glycosylated. After SC administration in healthy subjects, the mean terminal half-life is approximately 2.7 hours. Outside of the United States, rHu GM-CSF is available as molgramostim, a nonglycosylated rHu GM-CSF expressed in *E coli*, and regramostim, a fully glycosylated rHu GM-CSF expressed in Chinese hamster ovary cells. The different formulations appear to have similar pharmacologic activity.

Administration of rHu GM-CSF increases levels of circulating neutrophils, eosinophils, and, to a lesser extent, macrophages and lymphocytes. In addition, rHu GM-CSF exerts immunomodulatory activity on cells of the granulocyte and macrophage lineages. Although endogenous GM-CSF is involved in erythropoiesis and megakaryocyte development, other growth factors are required for final maturation of these cell lines, and rHu GM-CSF has no significant clinical effect on erythrocyte or platelet levels.

The effects of rHu GM-CSF on neutrophils is similar to G-CSF in that it stimulates neutrophil progenitor proliferation; reduces neutrophil apoptosis; and enhances chemotaxis, phagocytosis, and respiratory burst.[32,33] Beyond these effects, rHu GM-CSF stimulates neutrophils and primes them to respond more vigorously to other stimuli.[34] Neutrophils exposed to rHu GM-CSF exhibit enhanced superoxide anion generation and expression of class II major histocompatibility complex molecules. As with rHu G-CSF administration, marrow aspirates show a left shift, and neutrophil counts may transiently drop after IV administration.

The effects of GM-CSF on other cell lineages have led to significant research surrounding the immunomodulatory effects of rHu GM-CSF. On a cellular level, GM-CSF enhances macrophage chemotaxis and phagocytosis and stimulates cytokine release from monocytes that enhance the function of natural killer cells. Further, GM-CSF expands and activates dendritic cells and increases their migration to lymph nodes, stimulates naive T cells, and activates eosinophils.[32] For these reasons, the immunomodulatory properties of rHu GM-CSF are under investigation for various applications, including use as an antitumor vaccine adjuvant.

Typical side effects of sargramostim therapy include injection site reactions, low-grade fever, and myalgias.[35–37] Occasionally, patients experience dyspnea, likely resulting from sequestration of granulocytes in the pulmonary vasculature.[38] As with G-CSF, patients can experience bone pain, and regular white blood cell monitoring should be conducted during therapy to prevent leukocytosis. Typically treatment is discontinued when the neutrophil count reaches 10,000 cells/μL. Rare adverse events include allergic-type reactions with the first dose and fluid retention.

Some data suggest that sargramostim may be associated with a lower risk of serious adverse events compared with molgramostim; however, controlled trials are lacking.[37]

INTERLEUKIN-11

Endogenous IL-11 stimulates proliferation of megakaryocyte progenitor cells and induces megakaryocyte maturation, leading to increased platelet production.[39]

Mice deficient in IL-11 demonstrate normal megakaryocyte development and platelet production, demonstrating that IL-11 alone does not regulate thrombopoiesis.[40,41] *In vitro* murine studies suggest that megakaryocytopoiesis is stimulated at very early developmental stages and that IL-11 is synergistic with Steel factor and IL-3.[42] Like other cytokines, endogenous IL-11 has various sources and inducers (see Table 52.4-1). Serum concentrations of IL-11 are typically undetectable or very low but are elevated in states of thrombocytopenia.[43,44]

Oprelvekin is an rHu IL-11 that has an amino acid sequence identical to endogenous IL-11, except for lacking the amino-terminal proline residue, resulting in a protein with one less amino acid than endogenous IL-11. The molecule is expressed in bacteria (*E coli*) and is nonglycosylated. After SC administration in healthy subjects, the mean terminal half-life is approximately 7 hours.

Oprelvekin stimulates megakaryocytopoiesis and thrombopoiesis through direct action on megakaryocytes and increases megakaryocyte ploidy.[45,46] The platelets produced are morphologically and functionally normal, with no change in platelet reactivity and a normal life span. Platelet counts begin to rise 5 to 9 days after the start of dosing, and after stopping therapy, platelet counts continue to rise for up to 7 days then fall and return to normal in 14 days.

At doses indicated for thrombopoiesis, oprelvekin use is associated with several serious toxicities, including allergic reactions and anaphylaxis. Approximately two-thirds of patients receiving oprelvekin in clinical trials experienced edema, and nearly half experienced dyspnea. Fluid retention has also resulted in exacerbation of existing pleural effusions and atrial arrhythmias. Many patients also become mildly anemic, primarily due to dilutional anemia.[47,48] Rarer adverse events include papilledema. Preliminary data suggest that lower doses may be better tolerated with milder and less frequent toxicity.[49] As noted in Table 52.4-3, IL-11 receptors are located on cancer cell lines, including AML cells. *In vitro* studies with AML cells isolated from patients found IL-11 alone to have little effect on the cell cycle or AML blast apoptosis; however, IL-11 synergistically increased leukemic progenitor cell formation in combination with G-CSF.[50] However, the clinical significance of these findings and other tumor cell receptor locations are not established.

CLINICAL USE OF RECOMBINANT ERYTHROPOIETIN IN CANCER THERAPY

Anemia secondary to malignancy or chemotherapy is a common and important clinical problem that may cause fatigue, tachycardia, and dyspnea and negatively impact a patient's QOL. The presence of anemia is of particular concern in patients who have preexisting cardiovascular morbidity that impairs their ability to compensate for the decreased oxygen-carrying capacity of the

blood.[51] Anemia in the cancer patient can have a multitude of causes, including toxic effects to bone marrow by chemotherapy and radiation; tumor encroachment of the marrow; decreased red cell survival with hemolysis; hypersplenism and blood loss; or poor production secondary to iron, vitamin, or EPO deficiency. Alternatively, anemia can occur without any other underlying known cause other than the cancer itself. This phenomenon is termed "anemia of cancer" and is likely related to anemia of chronic disease. Anemia of chronic disease is typified by a hyporegenerative, normocytic, normochromic anemia associated with reduced serum iron and transferrin saturation but elevated (or normal) ferritin levels. Probable mechanisms for cancer-related anemia include impaired iron use, suppressed erythroid progenitor cell differentiation, insufficient EPO production, and shortened red blood cell survival.[52] Increased use of chemotherapy regimens with higher dose intensities contributes to stem cell damage as a cause of anemia. Other evidence suggests that cisplatin may cause direct tubular injury, leading to reduced EPO synthesis.[12] Radiation of the pelvis and spine is particularly damaging due to the high percentage of marrow in these sites. Studies have demonstrated that endogenous EPO levels are inappropriately low both in patients with anemia of cancer and chemotherapy-induced anemia, suggesting an additional underlying mechanism.[53] Last, marrow progenitor cells may exhibit an impaired response to EPO.

Until the 1990s, transfusions were the only treatment option for anemia. Transfusions, although necessary in acute situations, are a limited resource and carry the increased risk of transfusion-related infection. Over the last decade, clinical trials with rHu EPO products have been conducted in a variety of settings in oncology. These settings include chemotherapy/radiotherapy-induced anemia, anemia associated with myeloid and lymphoproliferative disorders, anemia of cancer, bone marrow transplantation (BMT), and perioperative management of anemia associated with oncologic surgery. Trials have been progressively refined to more accurately identify the true benefits of these products and the factors necessary for optimal outcomes. Such prognostic/outcome-related factors currently evaluated include the appropriate baseline hemoglobin (Hb), the need for concurrent iron repletion, and identification of appropriate dosing and schedule. Recently, the American Society of Clinical Oncology and the American Society of Hematology collaborated to form a panel that produced guidelines for the appropriate use of recombinant EPO products.[54] These guidelines focus on chemotherapy/radiotherapy-induced anemia and anemia associated with myeloid and lymphoproliferative disorders (Table 52.4-4). The following sections discuss results of this collaboration as well as additional data that have been published since the guidelines were created. Also, data on the use of rHu EPO in anemia of cancer, BMT, and surgical oncology are reviewed.

CHEMOTHERAPY- AND RADIATION THERAPY–INDUCED ANEMIA

Epoetin therapy improves clinical measures of efficacy, including Hb and the need for transfusions. Based on evidence from well-controlled trials, epoetin therapy produces significant increases compared with placebo when the baseline Hb concentration is 10 g/dL or less. In these trials, those receiving epoetin showed mean Hb increases of approximately 2 to 3 g/

TABLE 52.4-4. American Society of Clinical Oncology and American Society of Hematology 2002 Guidelines for the Use of Epoetin Therapy[a]: Summary of Recommendations for Epoetin Therapy

Chemotherapy- or radiation-associated anemia	
Baseline Hb <10 g/dL	Epoetin is a recommended treatment option. Transfusion remains an additional option.
Baseline Hb >10 but <12 g/dL	Clinical circumstances should govern whether to use epoetin. Transfusion remains an additional option for severe clinical conditions.
Dosing	Efficacy data are from trials of epoetin dosed thrice weekly starting at 150 U/kg, with consideration of dose escalation to 300 U/kg after 4 wk. A weekly regimen of 40,000 U/wk can be considered based on common clinical practice.
Duration of therapy—nonresponders	It is not beneficial to continue epoetin therapy beyond 6–8 wk in the absence of a response (1–2 g/dL rise in Hb).
Duration of therapy—responders	Insufficient evidence to support "normalization" of Hb levels above 12 g/dL. Epoetin should be dose-titrated or discontinued once the Hb rises to (or near) 12 g/dL.
Iron repletion	Baseline and periodic monitoring of measures of iron deficiency and instituting iron repletion when indicated may be valuable; however, inadequate data exist to specify the optimal guidelines for such monitoring.
Anemia associated with low-risk myelodysplasia	One well-designed trial supports the use of epoetin in this circumstance.
Anemia associated with myeloma, NHL, CLL	There is no sufficient evidence to support the use of epoetin in these patients outside of chemotherapy-related anemia. Tumor reduction should be attempted first; if a rise in Hb does not occur, epoetin may be used according to the guidelines for chemotherapy-associated anemia if clinically indicated. Transfusion remains an additional option.

CLL, chronic lymphocytic leukemia; Hb, hemoglobin; NHL, non-Hodgkin's lymphoma.
[a]These guidelines do not include data published after 2002 or recommendations for the use of darbepoetin alfa.
(From ref. 54, with permission.)

dL. Trials of patients with baseline Hb of more than 10 g/dL showed mixed results. The only well-controlled trial found no significant difference in Hb change. A metaanalysis of all randomized trials found that the use of epoetin decreased the relative odds of receiving a red blood cell transfusion by an average of 62% [odds ratio, 0.38 (95% confidence interval, 0.28 to 0.51)]. The metaanalysis did not test for effect stratified by baseline Hb (Rizzo[54] and Seindenfeld et al.[54a]), The American Society of Hematology/American Society of Clinical Oncology collaboration recommended epoetin therapy for chemotherapy- and radiation therapy–induced anemia if the Hb has declined to 10 g/dL or less; however, epoetin use in patients with less severe anemia is not clearly justified in all patients by the current evidence (Fig. 52.4-2). Clinical judgment should be

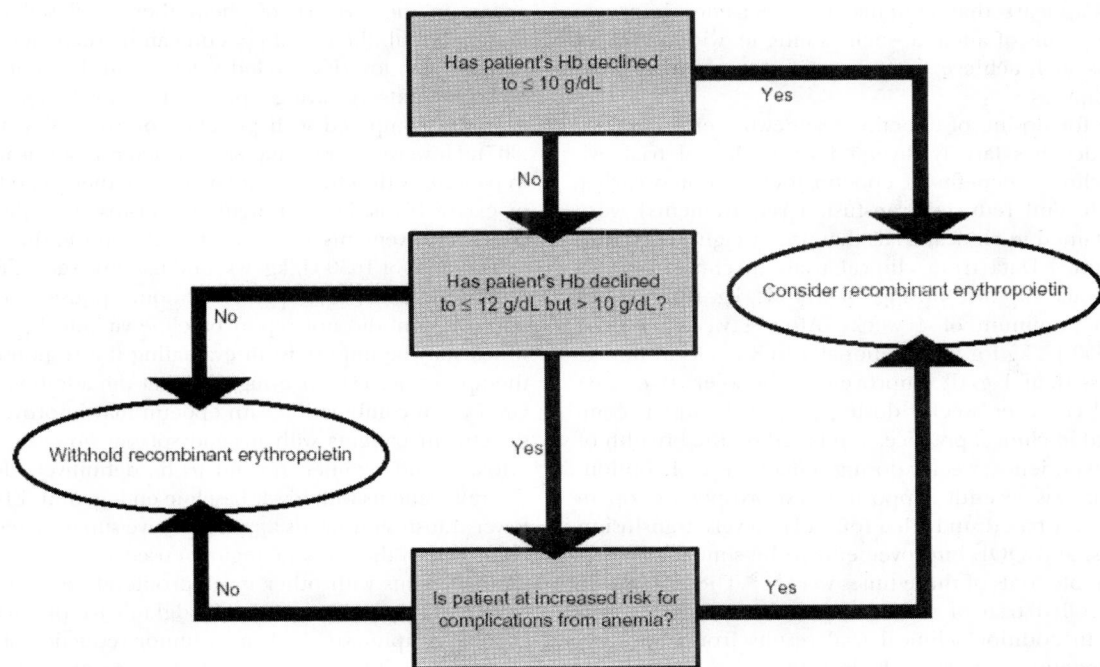

FIGURE 52.4-2. An algorithm for the use of epoetin in chemotherapy-associated anemia according to guidelines proposed by the American Society of Clinical Oncology and the American Society of Hematology. Hb, hemoglobin. (Data from ref. 54.)

used to evaluate epoetin therapy in less severe anemia, with consideration being given to patients at risk for worse outcomes from anemia such as those with preexisting cardiovascular morbidity. Transfusion remains an additional treatment option in severe clinical cases.[54]

Data on the effect of epoetin on QOL appear positive; however, instruments are still under development, and this research is ongoing. Some trials of epoetin therapy, including a recent large randomized controlled trial conducted by Littlewood et al., demonstrated significant improvements in QOL measures, such as fatigue and ability to perform daily activities.[54,55] However, several factors potentially detract from the validity of these trials. First, the nature of conducting these types of trials requires patients to complete surveys at distant time points; thus, dropout rates have been high. Second, the instruments used have been recently developed, and the definition of a clinically meaningful change is still being determined. Despite these difficulties, a multivariate analysis of the Littlewood et al. study maintained the benefits of epoetin therapy as measured by three cancer-specific scales: the Functional Assessment of Cancer Therapy—Fatigue subscale, the Functional Assessment of Cancer Therapy-General, and the Cancer Linear Analog Scale.[56] These improvements correlated with improvements in Hb. Furthermore, data from this analysis demonstrated that prolonged anemia in the placebo group was associated with progressively worsening QOL scores despite small improvements in Hb with time. Still a different analysis of the data from the Littlewood et al. study sought to determine the minimally important clinical difference (MID) in scores measuring QOL. The analysis correlated the minimally important clinical difference in QOL scores with a change of Hb of 1 g/dL. Using this criterion, epoetin therapy was associated with clinically important differences in all of the QOL measures evaluated.[57] Although QOL research is still maturing, it appears that patients do experience improvements in symptoms of anemia, such as fatigue, with increases in Hb and as such achieve those benefits more quickly with epoetin therapy.

Guidance for dosing of epoetin is somewhat enigmatic, as clinical practice has largely diverged from clinical trial evidence. The clinical benefits of epoetin therapy noted earlier (improved Hb and reduced transfusion requirements) were primarily obtained in clinical trials that used weight-based dosing of epoetin.[54] Data from clinical trials in chemotherapy-induced anemia support dosing of 150 U/kg three times weekly for a minimum of 4 weeks. After 4 weeks, a dose increase to 300 U/kg for an additional 4 to 8 weeks in nonresponders (less than 1 g/dL improvement by week 4) can be considered.[54] However, weekly dosing (40,000 U/wk) is commonly applied in clinical practice, and based on the breadth of this clinical experience, weekly dosing remains a viable option. Weekly dosing was recently supported in a prospective, open-label, community-based study that found Hb levels, transfusion requirements, and QOL improvements to be similar to those from comparable trials of three times weekly.[58] The results of a placebo-controlled trial of weekly dosing have not yet been published.[59] In addition, clinical trial results from the long-acting darbepoetin are now available.[60] In a phase 3 randomized, double-blind trial of once-weekly dosing, darbepoetin use resulted in significantly fewer patients requiring transfusions (27% vs. 52%; P <.01) and a significantly higher Hb response

rate (66% vs. 24%; P <.001) compared with placebo in patients with chemotherapy-induced anemia. Further trials will need to confirm these findings and identify the appropriate dosing of darbepoetin.[61,62]

The optimal duration of therapy in patients responding to epoetin therapy is not defined; however, it is recommended that Hb levels should be raised to or near 12 g/dL.[54] No evidence exists for "normalization" of Hb above 12 g/dL. Once the Hb level approaches 12 g/dL, epoetin therapy should be dose-titrated down or discontinued and subsequently reinitiated if indicated. In nonresponders (defined as patients achieving a less than 1 to 2 g/dL rise in Hb), dosing beyond 6 to 8 weeks does not appear to be beneficial.[54]

No controlled trials are available regarding the benefits of iron status monitoring and iron repletion in the setting of cancer. In patients with chronic renal failure, controlled trials were conducted and have demonstrated a role for iron repletion concurrent with epoetin in this setting. These trials have found either improved Hb responses with iron therapy or a decreased requirement in epoetin doses needed to maintain Hb responses compared with patients not receiving iron. IV iron repletion appears superior to oral therapy in this setting; however, the optimal regimen is not yet defined.[63–65] Therefore, baseline and periodic monitoring of iron, total iron-binding capacity, transferrin saturation, or ferritin levels and the institution of iron repletion may be valuable; however, guidelines for specific practices cannot be provided.[54]

ANEMIA RELATED TO MYELOPROLIFERATIVE DISORDERS

Currently, little evidence is available to support the use of epoetin in patients with anemia secondary to myeloproliferative disorders in the absence of chemotherapy. Based on one well-designed trial, the use of epoetin can be recommended only in patients with low-risk myelodysplasia.[66] In this trial, significantly more patients receiving epoetin therapy had a hematologic response compared with placebo controls (37% vs. 11%; P = .007). However, subset analysis revealed no significant difference in patients with refractory anemia and either ringed sideroblasts or excess blasts. Further, neither transfusion requirements nor QOL improvements were reported. Patients in this trial received a fixed dose of 1050 U/kg/wk, and baseline serum EPO levels of more than 200 mU/L predicted nonresponse to epoetin therapy. The trial did not report baseline vitamin B_{12} or iron data, which may be important in evaluating the response to epoetin therapy. Other evidence suggests that the addition of G-CSF or GM-CSF in combination with epoetin may improve response to epoetin in patients with myelodysplasia; however, the optimal cytokine and regimen remain to be definitively determined.[67] Overall, patients with lower baseline endogenous EPO levels and lower transfusion needs appear to have superior response rates, regardless of the cytokine regimen used.

In patients with other myeloproliferative disorders, specifically multiple myeloma, non-Hodgkin's lymphoma (NHL), or chronic lymphocytic leukemia, tumor reduction should generally be applied first due to the lack of strong evidence supporting epoetin therapy for anemia in the absence of chemotherapy in these conditions. Although overall more patients receiving epoetin therapy in trials experienced a hematologic response compared with controls, results were confounded by inadequate reporting.[54] However, it should be noted that in patients with these disorders and anemia associated with chemotherapy, epoetin therapy may be instituted under the guidelines outlined for chemotherapy-induced anemia.

ANEMIA OF CANCER

Some data are available in patients with solid tumors experiencing anemia of cancer; however, the results are not conclusive. A double-blind, randomized, placebo-controlled trial found that epoetin 100 U/kg SC three times weekly significantly increased hematocrit compared with placebo but did not affect transfusion requirements.[68] A second randomized, controlled trial demonstrated significantly increased Hb and exercise capacity in cachectic patients with solid tumors receiving epoetin 4000 to 10,000 U SC three times weekly and indomethacin compared with indomethacin alone.[69] Preliminary data with darbepoetin in this setting suggest benefits in terms of Hb increases and transfusion requirement decreases.[70] However, no firm recommendations are available for use of epoetin therapy in anemia of cancer outside of that associated with chemotherapy or myeloproliferative disorders.[54]

ANEMIA AFTER BONE MARROW TRANSPLANT

Trials in this setting have not demonstrated a reduced need for transfusions in patients receiving autologous transplant; however, epoetin therapy may be useful in allogeneic transplant. Patients receiving epoetin after allogeneic transplant have experienced accelerated erythroid engraftment, increases in Hb, fewer transfusions, and a reduced time to transfusion independence; however, benefits have varied by trial.[71] Recent preliminary evidence suggests timing may play a role. A small, historically controlled study found improvements in transfusions with administration of epoetin on days 35 and 56 after allogeneic transplant but not day 1.[72] As data are limited, however, recommendations for use of epoetin therapy in anemia after BMT are not available.[54]

ANEMIA ASSOCIATED WITH ONCOLOGIC SURGERY

Data in the setting of oncologic surgery are conflicting. Kosmadakis et al. conducted a randomized, double-blind, placebo-controlled trial of perioperative epoetin 300 U/kg and iron 100 mg IV daily for 14 days beginning 7 days preoperatively in patients undergoing surgery for gastrointestinal malignancy.[73] Patients receiving epoetin required fewer intraoperative transfusions (29% vs. 59.3%; P = .023) and fewer postoperative transfusions (3.2% vs. 28%; P = .001). Interestingly, significantly fewer patients receiving epoetin had complications compared with placebo, and a multivariate analysis found epoetin use to be independently associated with increased 1-year survival.[73] In contrast, a second randomized, placebo-controlled trial of epoetin 20,000 U/d for 10 days did not result in a transfusion benefit. Iron repletion was not performed in this trial, which may have affected the outcomes.[74] A randomized, double-blind, placebo-controlled trial of preoperative epoetin in patients undergoing surgery for head and neck cancer demonstrated a trend toward reduced transfusions with epoetin, but the difference did not reach statistical significance. In this trial, patients received three doses of epoetin 600 U/kg before surgery with twice-daily oral iron sulfate 150 mg. Of patients receiving epoetin, 34.5% did not require transfusion compared with 17.2% of those receiving placebo.[75] Thus, future study is needed to best identify the appropriate candidates and epoetin regimen for perioperative use of epoetin in the surgical oncology setting.

PREDICTORS OF RECOMBINANT ERYTHROPOIETIN THERAPY RESPONSE

Despite the demonstrated efficacy of epoetin in several settings, a fair number of patients fail to respond to treatment. In trials of patients with chemotherapy-induced anemia and baseline Hb of 10 g/dL or less, the difference in percentage of patients responding to epoetin compared with controls ranged from approximately 30% to 80%.[54] As such, methods to predict response to epoetin therapy would be both clinically relevant and cost-effective. Work has been done to identify baseline or early predictors of response to epoetin therapy. Preliminary evidence suggests that valuable tools for predicting response to epoetin therapy include baseline serum EPO in patients with lymphoma or myeloma, a 2-week marrow response as measured by the change in Hb and the soluble transferrin receptor increment, and baseline iron status. However, these models require further refinement and validation.[76]

FUTURE AREAS OF RESEARCH IN RECOMBINANT ERYTHROPOIETIN THERAPY

The field of study involving appropriate management of anemia in patients with cancer continues to evolve. Areas requiring additional research to clarify the optimal usage of recombinant EPO therapies are many. Recent advances in health care practitioner awareness of patient QOL issues have fostered research in this field, but much is still to be learned in terms of identifying the appropriate instruments, clinically important differences, and effective trial strategies. Specific to guidelines for use of recombinant EPO therapy, several questions remain unanswered in the oncology setting, including the optimal clinical end points for therapy (maximum target Hb or different end points such as respiratory function); the maximum dosing interval that will provide convenience, safety, and efficacy; the role for and appropriate use of iron supplementation; appropriate use in the pediatric population; and identification of useful baseline efficacy predictors. In concert with the latter, a need for research on the cost-effectiveness of epoetin therapy is warranted.

The question of rHu EPO support and its role in affecting survival and antitumor activity also remains unclear and warrants further study. There are preliminary data suggesting that rHu EPO may have either a positive impact[55] or negative impact on survival.[77] With respect to antitumor activity, preclinical and clinical data have suggested that rHu EPO therapy may improve tumor control and efficacy of chemotherapy and radiation.[78–80] However, a randomized, multicenter, placebo-controlled study was conducted in 351 patients with head and neck cancer and mild anemia (baseline Hb less than 12 to 13 g/dL) that challenges those data.[81] In this trial, patients who received rHu EPO before and during radiation therapy had a higher risk of locoregional tumor progression [relative risk of 1.69 (95% confidence interval, 1.16 to 2.47); $P = .007$]. Various factors may have contributed to these results, including differences in baseline characteristics and a differential effect of rHu EPO in certain subgroups. Overall, the safety and efficacy of rHu EPO therapy for tumor control require further study.

CLINICAL USE OF RECOMBINANT GRANULOCYTE COLONY-STIMULATING FACTORS IN CANCER THERAPY

The G-CSFs, rHu G-CSF and rHu GM-CSF, have been applied in a variety of oncology settings, including the management of chemotherapy-induced neutropenia, hematopoietic reconstitution after stem cell transplant, mobilization and *ex vivo* expansion of HPCs, and as a priming agent in AML. However, research continues to identify the appropriate application of these growth factors within each setting. Key issues include optimizing outcomes and cost-effective use. The American Society of Clinical Oncology recently created updated recommendations for the use of CSFs; these guidelines are summarized in Table 52.4-5 and discussed in the following sections.[82]

NEUTROPENIA ASSOCIATED WITH STANDARD-DOSE CHEMOTHERAPY

Neutropenia and the associated complication of infection often manifest as febrile neutropenia (FN), lead to significant morbidity and mortality in patients receiving cancer chemotherapy, and are often dose-limiting. The incidence of infection directly correlates with the depth and duration of neutropenia. FN typically results in hospitalization for evaluation and initiation of IV broad-spectrum antibiotics, leading to reduced QOL, increased risk for iatrogenic complications, and increased health care utilization costs. Options for reducing the incidence of FN include use of CSFs, chemotherapy dose reduction or delay, and prophylactic antibiotic use. The latter option is used under limited circumstances due to the risk of promoting growth of resistant organisms. Thus, CSFs and reduction of chemotherapy dose intensity remain the two most frequently exercised alternatives.

Prophylactic Colony-Stimulating Factor Use

The decision on whether to administer a CSF as primary prophylaxis (i.e., immediately after the first cycle of chemotherapy before any occurrence of neutropenia), secondary prophylaxis (i.e., immediately after subsequent cycles to reduce the risk of FN after the prior occurrence of FN), or therapeutically (i.e., treating severe neutropenia or FN once it is established) remains a challenge. In particular, the clinical benefit and economic value of routine primary prophylaxis have been extensively debated.

Current evidence indicates that primary prophylaxis with a CSF results in a relative risk reduction of FN by approximately 50%.[82] Significant reductions in documented infections have also been demonstrated. An analysis of five trials that have reported infection-related mortality failed to find a significant reduction with CSF support [summary odds ratio, 0.60 (0.30, 1.22); $P = .16$]; however, the power of the combined analysis was insufficient to determine this outcome. An additional outcome

TABLE 52.4-5. Summary of American Society of Clinical Oncology Guidelines for Administration of Granulocyte Colony-Stimulating Factor and Granulocyte-Macrophage Colony-Stimulating Factor

Indication	Recommendation
Primary prophylactic CSF administration (administration of a CSF beginning with the first cycle of a treatment regimen)	Recommended if: 1. The chemotherapy regimen has an expected 22% or more incidence of FN. 2. A decrease in dose intensity would compromise long-term outcomes (survival/cure). 3. The patient is at increased risk for serious complications or death from FN (e.g., advanced age, prior treatment, low performance status, infection).
Secondary prophylactic CSF administration (administration of a CSF in all subsequent cycles after an episode of FN)	Use if a decrease in dose intensity would compromise long-term outcomes (survival/cure).
Treatment of established FN	Use with antibiotics in patients predicted to have a poor outcome (e.g., organ or intravenous site infection, hypotension, bacteremia, serious comorbidities).
Treatment of established neutropenia in afebrile patients	Not recommended.
Use of CSF to increase dose intensity	Not recommended.
Use of CSF to enable delivery of dose-dense chemotherapy regimens	Use with dose-dense ACT for lymph node–positive breast cancer; results inconclusive with other regimens.
Adjuncts to stem cell transplantation	Use of CSF is warranted for PBSC mobilization and following PBSC or BM transplantation.
Delayed engraftment-graft failure	Use of a CSF is warranted.
Acute myeloid leukemia	Use after induction in patients older than 55 y if determined to be cost-effective based on shortened hospitalization secondary to shortened duration of neutropenia. Routine use in younger patients, postconsolidation, in relapsed disease, or for priming of leukemic cells is not recommended.
Acute lymphoblastic leukemia	Routine use not recommended due to lack of clear benefit and risk for secondary myeloid leukemia in pediatric patients.
Myelodysplastic syndromes	Routine use not recommended.
Concurrent administration of CSFs with chemotherapy and radiation therapy	Avoid.

ACT, doxorubin (Adriamycin), cyclophosphamide, paclitaxel; BM, bone marrow; CSF, colony-stimulating factor; FN, febrile neutropenia; PBSC, peripheral blood stem cell.

demonstrated in these trials was the maintenance of dose intensity of the chemotherapeutic regimen through avoidance of dose reduction or delay secondary to neutropenia. Evidence for long-term clinical benefit from maintaining dose intensity has varied. In patients receiving cyclophosphamide, methotrexate, and 5-fluorouracil as adjuvant therapy for breast cancer, it was determined that those receiving 85% or more of the planned

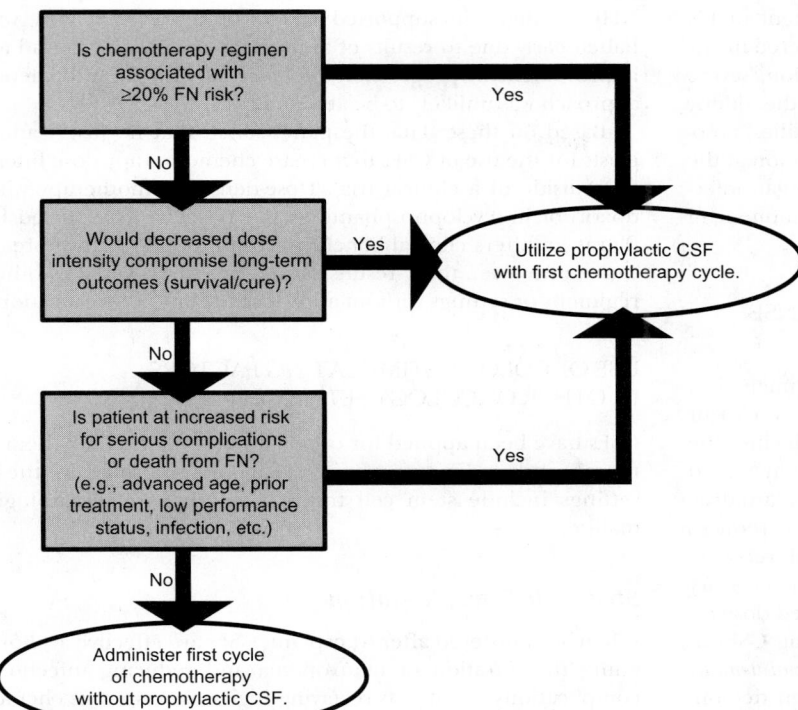

FIGURE 52.4-3. An algorithm for the primary prophylactic use of colony-stimulating factors in chemotherapy-induced neutropenia according to guidelines proposed by the American Society of Clinical Oncology. CSF, colony-stimulating factor; FN, febrile neutropenia. (Data from ref. 82.)

total dose had improved relapse-free survival compared with the control group, which received no chemotherapy. However, those who received 65% or less experienced no improvement compared with controls.[83] Other data in NHL demonstrate reduced complete response rates and/or survival with dose reductions of 20% to 30%.[84] Therefore, in these settings or in those of other responsive and potentially curable malignancies (e.g., germ cell tumors), the use of CSFs to maintain dose intensity may be reasonable. However, this practice is not associated with universal benefit across all regimens and tumor types.

Because primary prophylaxis dictates that all patients receive a CSF, the economic impact of this practice has been extensively studied. Early economic analyses found CSFs to be cost-effective when the risk of FN with a particular regimen exceeded 40%. However, recent analyses have taken a more comprehensive approach to identifying direct costs associated with FN, including total hospitalization costs. These studies suggest that primary prophylactic CSF use is associated with a cost savings when the risk of FN is 20% or higher.[85,86] Special circumstances in patients receiving regimens with a risk of FN below 20% may, however, warrant prophylactic CSF use. These circumstances are any condition that would increase the risk of serious complications or death from FN and include but are not limited to advanced age, prior cancer treatment, low performance status, active infections, and advanced cancer.

The elderly represent an important special population in whom primary prophylaxis is recommended for all patients aged 65 and older receiving moderately toxic chemotherapy. This guideline is also endorsed by the European Organisation for Research and Treatment of Cancer, which based its recommendation on data from trials in NHL, small cell lung cancer, and urothelial tumors that found primary prophylactic rHu G-CSF reduced the incidence of FN and/or infections.[84] Other sup-

porting evidence for this recommendation include the fact that the risk of neutropenic infections increases with age and that some studies suggest mortality from neutropenic infection may be elevated in the elderly.[87–89] In addition, the duration of hospitalization and resulting cost of hospitalization are increased in patients older than 65 years of age.[85]

Together these data led the panel to provide the following recommendations with regard to primary prophylactic use of CSFs: Primary prophylaxis with the CSFs should be considered in any patient (1) receiving a chemotherapy regimen associated with an incidence of FN of 20% or more, (2) in whom a reduction in treatment intensity may compromise disease-free or overall survival, or (3) who is aged 65 and older or is at an increased risk for serious consequences from FN due to other factors (Fig. 52.4-3).

Alternatives to Primary Prophylaxis

Alternatives to primary prophylaxis include secondary prophylaxis, dose reduction or delay, or therapeutic use of CSFs. The panel recommended that secondary prophylaxis with CSFs should be considered in any patient experiencing a prior neutropenic complication that a recurrence of would likely result in treatment delays or dose reductions leading to reduced dose intensity that may compromise disease-free or overall survival or patient QOL. In settings such as palliative chemotherapy or others in which a reduction in dose intensity is not expected to compromise long-term outcomes, dose reduction or delay is considered the preferred option to CSF use.[82]

Therapeutic application of growth factors does not afford the benefit of reducing the incidence of hospitalization due to FN; however, treatment of FN with a CSF may reduce the risk of prolonged hospitalization, which accounts for a significant portion of hospitalization costs.[90,91] As such, routine treatment of FN with a CSF is not recommended but should be considered in any patient at increased risk for prolonged hospitalization, severe complications, or death. These populations include the elderly or those with uncontrolled cancer, serious comorbidities, absolute neutrophil count of less than $100/\mu L$, hospitalization at the time of fever development, hypotension, sepsis, or organ infection.[92,93] Current evidence does not support the treatment of afebrile neutropenia with a CSF.[94,95]

NEUTROPENIA ASSOCIATED WITH DOSE-INTENSE OR DOSE-DENSE CHEMOTHERAPY

Increasing the dose intensity of a chemotherapy regimen (i.e., increasing the total dose of one or more agents per cycle) or administering dose-dense chemotherapy (i.e., reducing the interval between chemotherapy cycles, resulting in an increased dose delivered per unit of time compared with standard-dose therapy) leads to an increased risk of neutropenia or reduces the amount of time a patient has for neutrophil recovery between cycles. As such, the use of CSFs is considered necessary to be able to administer these regimens at the planned dose on schedule. However, the long-term benefits from using CSFs in this manner are still under investigation. Although *maintenance* of dose intensity of standard-dose regimens has been demonstrated to be necessary for optimal outcomes in the certain settings, *increases* in dose intensity with or without CSF support have not been associated with improved outcomes.

Improvements in survival have been demonstrated using CSF support of the dose-dense approach, but a definitive benefit has been found to date only in the setting of dose-dense adjuvant chemotherapy for lymph node–positive breast cancer. The Cancer and Leukemia Group B Trial 9741 evaluated four adjuvant chemotherapy regimens in 2005 women with axillary node–positive breast cancer.[96] Patients received either sequential doxorubicin 60 mg/m^2, paclitaxel 175 mg/m^2, and cyclophosphamide 600 mg/m^2, or concurrent doxorubicin and cyclophosphamide followed by paclitaxel. Each of these regimens was administered either every 3 weeks without CSF support or every 2 weeks with filgrastim support (dose-dense). The primary and secondary end points of the trial were disease-free survival and overall survival. Both disease-free survival (relative risk of 0.74; $P = .010$) and overall survival (relative risk of 0.69; $P = .013$) were improved with the dose-dense regimens.

CSF support of the dose-dense approach has been applied in other settings, with variable results. Two trials in small cell lung cancer found improved survival with dose-dense regimens of either doxorubicin, cyclophosphamide, and etoposide or ifosfamide, carboplatin, etoposide, and vincristine.[97,98] Lenograstim support enabled increased overall dose intensity in the dose-dense arm of doxorubicin, cyclophosphamide, and etoposide. Randomization to rHu GM-CSF or placebo was used in the trial of ifosfamide, carboplatin, etoposide, and vincristine; however, no benefit to therapy with rHu GM-CSF was demonstrated. Conflicting data have been presented in the setting of NHL. Although a survival advantage was found with 14-day cycles of cyclophosphamide, doxorubicin, vincristine, and prednisone (CHOP-14) compared with 21-day cycles in older patients with aggressive NHL, no such benefit was demonstrated in a trial enrolling a lower-risk group of younger patients with aggressive NHL.[99,100] In addition, a Japanese study in advanced, aggressive

NHL of filgrastim-supported CHOP-14 versus CHOP-21 was halted early due to results of an interim analysis that found an improvement in progression-free survival with the dose-dense approach was unlikely to be attained.[101]

Based on these data, the panel stated that no justification exists for the use of CSFs to increase chemotherapy dose intensity outside of a clinical trial. Dose-dense chemotherapy with doxorubicin, cyclophosphamide, and paclitaxel supported by filgrastim offers clinical benefit in lymph node–positive breast cancer; however, these results cannot be extrapolated to other regimens or settings without appropriate clinical investigation.

USE OF COLONY-STIMULATING FACTORS IN OTHER ONCOLOGY SETTINGS

CSFs have been applied for other purposes outside of chemotherapy-induced neutropenia in oncology. Primarily, these settings include stem cell transplantation and hematologic malignancies.

Stem Cell Transplantation

When administered after transplant, CSFs are effective at shortening the duration of neutropenia and reducing infectious complications in patients receiving high-dose cytotoxic chemotherapy with autologous or allogeneic bone marrow or PBSC transplantation. These benefits are also afforded to patients experiencing engraftment failure or delay.

CSFs, alone or in combination with chemotherapy or other cytokines, are effective at mobilizing PBSCs into the circulation for both autologous and allogeneic transplant. Over the last decade, autologous PBSC transplantation has largely replaced autologous BMT due to earlier hematopoietic recovery. Increasingly, PBSC mobilized with CSFs from healthy donors are being used in certain settings for allogeneic PBSC transplant, leading to faster hematopoietic recovery compared with allogeneic BMT. A significant concern with this practice was the theoretical potential for increased incidence and/or severity of graft-versus-host disease due to an increase in the number of lymphocytes found in the PBSC allograft compared with the bone marrow. To date, evidence suggests that, in general, an increase in graft-versus-host disease does not occur, and, in fact, the increase in lymphocytes may result in reduced infection rates in patients receiving allogeneic PBSC transplant compared with BMT.[102,103] However, these data must be confirmed in each setting. For example, a recent retrospective review found that compared with allogeneic BMT, PBSC transplant resulted in an increased incidence of acute graft-versus-host disease (74% vs. 54%, $P = .05$) and reduced leukemia-free and overall survival (21% vs. 32%; $P = .04$ and 24% vs. 34%; $P = .04$, respectively) in patients with acute lymphoblastic leukemia (ALL).[104]

The optimal timing and protocols for CSF administration in either mobilization or posttransplant hematopoietic reconstitution remain under investigation. Other investigations include the use of CSF donor-primed bone marrow for allogeneic BMT, which may result in more rapid engraftment with lower rates of graft-versus-host disease,[105,106] and HGF use for *ex vivo* expansion of HPCs. Although to date, *ex vivo* expansion products of adult progenitor cells have not resulted in increased numbers of stem cells with repopulating potential, expansion of cord blood has. A recent clinical trial suggests that transplant of *ex vivo* expanded cord blood may provide an additional transplant option, with further investigation.[107]

Acute Myeloid Leukemia

CSFs have been used in patients with AML after both induction and consolidation therapy for chemotherapy-induced neutropenia and as priming agents to sensitize leukemic cells to chemotherapy. Generally, primary prophylactic postinduction CSF use has resulted in a decreased time to neutrophil recovery (500 cells/μL) by 2 to 6 days, with resultant reductions in the duration of hospitalization and antibiotic use.[108–116] No consistent effects on complete response rates or patient survival have been demonstrated, nor evidence of leukemia growth stimulation or enhanced drug resistance. The economic benefits of primary CSF use in this setting remain under debate. Similarly, postconsolidation CSF use has resulted in a decreased duration of severe neutropenia with reduced infection rates but no effect on complete response rates or survival.[111,117] Current evidence does not support use of CSFs in the setting of relapsed AML; little data are available to confirm benefits in infection-related morbidity or the lack of leukemic stimulation.

Based on *in vitro* data suggesting that CSFs can sensitize leukemic cells to cell cycle–specific cytotoxic agents, such as cytarabine, several clinical trials were conducted to evaluate this theory. Most trials demonstrated no benefits in terms of response rate, response duration, or survival.[113–115,118–120] However, a recent European multicenter, randomized trial of 640 previously untreated, nonelderly adults with AML found an improvement in disease-free survival.[23] Patients received induction with idarubicin and cytarabine in cycle one and idarubicin and amsacrine in cycle two, each with or without concurrent lenograstim. Although patients with favorable-risk AML and unfavorable-risk AML received no benefits from lenograstim priming, those with standard-risk AML (72% of patients in the trial) experienced significantly reduced event- and disease-free survival and improved overall survival at 4 years (overall survival, 35% vs. 45%; *P* = .02). As such, further investigation to identify the appropriate patient population and regimen for priming is warranted.

Acute Lymphoblastic Leukemia

Data supporting the clinical benefits of postinduction CSFs in both pediatric and adult ALL are variable. Although typically CSFs do result in shortened durations of neutropenia, the impact on other clinical outcomes such as the incidence of infection or FN and the duration of hospitalization is variable.[121–124] No improvements in disease-free survival or overall survival have been demonstrated. Of significant concern is the risk of therapy-related myeloid malignancy associated with CSF use in patients with ALL. A recent analysis of two consecutive pediatric ALL protocols evaluated this risk and found that the rate of therapy-related myeloid malignancy was higher among children receiving postinduction rHu G-CSF compared with those who did not receive rHu G-CSF (11.0% ± 3.5% vs. 2.7% ± 1.3%; *P* = .019).[125] Thus, routine use of CSFs in ALL cannot be recommended.

Myelodysplastic Syndromes

Although CSFs can increase neutrophil counts in patients with myelodysplastic syndromes, these counts decline on discontin-

uation of the CSF. A randomized trial compared rHu G-CSF with best supportive care and found overall survival to be shorter in patients with refractory anemia and excess blasts who received rHu G-CSF.[126] Thus, use of CSFs in this setting cannot be recommended.

DOSING AND TIMING OF COLONY-STIMULATING FACTORS

The recommended dose of filgrastim is 5 μg/kg, and that of sargramostim is 250 μg/m², each administered SC daily. With the exception of PBSC mobilization, doses higher than those recommended do not provide additional clinical benefit.[127,128] For PBSC mobilization, a dose of 10 μg/kg/d for filgrastim may provide an improved stem cell yield.[129,130] Although each can be administered IV, pharmacokinetic data support SC as the preferred route.[131–133]

The benefits documented in clinical trials were achieved with initiation of CSFs within 24 to 72 hours after chemotherapy, although after stem cell infusion, administration within 5 days has been demonstrated to maintain efficacy. For chemotherapy-induced neutropenia, daily injections of filgrastim are typically continued until an absolute neutrophil count of 10,000 cells/μL. After stem cell transplantation, daily CSFs may be discontinued after 3 days of an absolute neutrophil count of 1000 cells/μL with filgrastim or 1500 cells/μL with sargramostim.[82]

Recently introduced was the long-acting pegfilgrastim. Currently approved to reduce the incidence of FN in patients with nonmyeloid malignancies receiving myelosuppressive chemotherapy, pegfilgrastim can be administered once during each chemotherapy cycle. Clinical trials have demonstrated equivalent efficacy to filgrastim in this setting. Of interest is the use of pegfilgrastim to support dose-dense regimens. Preliminary data with dose-dense regimens for lymphoma suggest that pegfilgrastim may have a role in this setting.[134,135] However, concern has been raised due to the lengthened duration of activity of pegfilgrastim. Pegfilgrastim should not be administered in the period between 14 days before and 24 hours after administration of cytotoxic chemotherapy. As such, this use remains investigational.

The concern of administering CSFs in either close proximity to or concurrent with cytotoxic chemotherapy or radiation therapy first arose with a trial of sargramostim in patients receiving cisplatin, etoposide, and thoracic irradiation for small cell lung cancer.[136] Patients receiving sargramostim experienced an increase in thrombocytopenia. Since then, other trials have demonstrated worsened myelosuppression with concurrent filgrastim and chemotherapy.[137,138] Conversely, other regimens have administered concurrent radiation and/or chemotherapy safely concurrent with CSFs.[139] At present, concurrent administration should be applied only in the setting of appropriately designed clinical trials.

CLINICAL USE OF RECOMBINANT INTERLEUKIN-11 IN CANCER THERAPY

At present, platelet transfusion remains the primary therapeutic modality for prevention and treatment of thrombocytopenia in the oncology setting. However, rHu IL-11 (oprelvekin) is a treatment option. Although limited by a high incidence of

TABLE 52.4-6.   Selected Hematopoietic Growth Factors in Clinical Development for Applications in Cancer Therapy

Factor	Other Names	Cellular Targets[a]	Potential Hematopoietic Applications in Cancer[b]
Thrombopoietin	TPO, MGDF	Megakaryocytes	Chemotherapy-associated thrombocytopenia
		Platelets	Generation of megakaryocytes and platelets *in vitro*
Interleukin-3	Interleukin-3, multi-CSF	Multilineage	Accelerate hematopoietic reconstitution
			Mobilize progenitor cells
			Expand progenitor cells *ex vivo*
Flt3 ligand	Flt3L	Multilineage	Mobilize progenitor cells
Leridistim (formerly myelopoietin)	Interleukin-3/G-CSF receptor agonist	Multilineage	Chemotherapy-induced neutropenia and thrombocytopenia
Promegapoietin	Interleukin-3/TPO receptor agonist	Multilineage	Chemotherapy-induced neutropenia and thrombocytopenia
Progenipoietin	Flt3/G-CSF receptor agonist; ProGP-1	Multilineage	Mobilize progenitor cells
Melatonin		CD4/CD8 T cells	Chemotherapy- or radiation therapy–induced myelosuppression

CSF, colony-stimulating factor; Flt3L, flt3 ligand; G-CSF, granulocyte colony-stimulating factor; MGDF, megakaryocyte growth and development factor; TPO, thrombopoietin.
[a]Multilineage includes red cell, neutrophil, monocyte, and megakaryocyte lineages.
[b]Applications are based on preclinical or *in vitro* studies and clinical trials in humans.

edema, oprelvekin is used in profound thrombocytopenia to maintain transfusion requirements. A decreasing supply of platelets and the risk for infection with platelet transfusions may foster increasing use of oprelvekin.

CHEMOTHERAPY-INDUCED THROMBOCYTOPENIA

Randomized placebo-controlled trials have demonstrated reduced platelet transfusion requirements in patients receiving oprelvekin after intensive chemotherapy. In a study of patients with advanced breast cancer receiving cyclophosphamide (3200 mg/m^2) and doxorubicin (75 mg/m^2), fewer patients who received oprelvekin required platelet transfusions (32% vs. 59%; $P = .04$).[140] Similarly, in a trial that evaluated oprelvekin in patients who had required a platelet transfusion in the previous chemotherapy cycle, 70% of oprelvekin patients required transfusions compared with 96% of placebo-treated patients ($P <.05$).[141] In the treatment of chemotherapy-induced thrombocytopenia, the approved dose of oprelvekin is 50 µg/kg daily. Lower doses have been studied in other settings, but such use remains investigational.[49]

THROMBOCYTOPENIA AFTER BONE MARROW TRANSPLANT

No clinical evidence exists for the efficacy of oprelvekin in platelet reconstitution after BMT. In a placebo-controlled trial of oprelvekin in patients with breast cancer who were undergoing autologous BMT with peripheral blood progenitor cell support, the platelet transfusion requirement was not reduced with oprelvekin [12.4 (±10.2) mean platelet transfusions per patient with placebo vs. 9.9 (±3.5) with oprelvekin; $P = 0.34$].[142]

THROMBOCYTOPENIA ASSOCIATED WITH BONE MARROW FAILURE

A pilot study of low-dose oprelvekin 10 µg/kg/d was conducted in patients with bone marrow failure secondary to myelodysplastic syndrome, aplastic anemia, or graft failure.[49] Patients received oprelvekin for two 14-day courses with a 14-day rest period in between courses. Six of 16 patients (38%) had platelet responses with only grade 1 toxicities. These preliminary results are promising; however, further study is required to assess the role of oprelvekin in the setting of bone marrow failure.

HEMATOPOIETIC GROWTH FACTORS IN DEVELOPMENT

A multitude of cytokines and other proteins is involved in the regulation of hematopoiesis. However, to date, only four proteins are available for use in practice. Research is ongoing to identify other regulators of hematopoiesis and to use those already identified for clinical purposes. New compounds are in development and are listed in Table 52.4-6. Key areas of compound development include immunomodulation and targeting early-acting or multiple cytokines for multilineage responses.

CONCLUSION

Clearly, the HGFs play an integral role in the modern management of cancer. Advantages include the ability to reduce the use of red cell and platelet transfusions and the incidence of FN. CSFs have also become integral therapies in stem cell transplant support. Still, questions remain regarding the appropriate specific application of these expensive agents and what benefits are afforded in terms of outcomes such as survival and QOL. Ongoing research is directed at answering these questions and developing new growth factors to further improve management of the hematologic complications of cancer and its treatment.

REFERENCES

1. D'Andrea AD, Fasman GD, Lodish HF. A new hematopoietic growth factor receptor superfamily: structural features and implications for signal transduction. *Curr Opin Cell Biol* 1990;2:648.
2. Fukunaga R, Ishizaka-Ikeda E, Nagata S. Growth and differentiation signals mediated by different regions in the cytoplasmic domain of granulocyte colony-stimulating factor receptor. *Cell* 1993;74:1079.
3. Neben S, Turner K. The biology of interleukin 11. *Stem Cells* 1993;11(Suppl 2):156.

4. Krebs DL, Hilton DJ. SOCS proteins: negative regulators of cytokine signaling. *Stem Cells* 2001;19:378.

5. Hortner M, Nielsch U, Mayr LM, et al. Suppressor of cytokine signaling-3 is recruited to the activated granulocyte-colony stimulating factor receptor and modulates its signal transduction. *J Immunol* 2002;169:1219.

6. Sasaki A, Yasukawa H, Shouda T, et al. CIS3/SOCS-3 suppresses erythropoietin (EPO) signaling by binding the EPO receptor and JAK2. *J Biol Chem* 2000;275:29338.

7. Buemi M, Cavallaro E, Floccari F, et al. The pleiotropic effects of erythropoietin in the central nervous system. *J Neuropathol Exp Neurol* 2003;62:228.

8. Spivak JL. Cancer-related anemia: its causes and characteristics. *Semin Oncol* 1994;21:3.

9. Heatherington AC, Schuller J, Mercer AJ. Pharmacokinetics of novel erythropoiesis stimulating protein (NESP) in cancer patients: preliminary report. *Br J Cancer* 2001;84(Suppl 1):11.

10. Markham A, Bryson HM. Epoetin alfa. A review of its pharmacodynamic and pharmacokinetic properties and therapeutic use in nonrenal applications. *Drugs* 1995;49:232.

11. Acs G, Acs P, Beckwith SM, et al. Erythropoietin and erythropoietin receptor expression in human cancer. *Cancer Res* 2001;61:3561.

12. Lappin TR, Maxwell AP, Johnston PG. EPO's alter ego: erythropoietin has multiple actions. *Stem Cells* 2002;20:485.

13. Lieschke GJ, Grail D, Hodgson G, et al. Mice lacking granulocyte colony-stimulating factor have chronic neutropenia, granulocyte and macrophage progenitor cell deficiency, and impaired neutrophil mobilization. *Blood* 1994;84:1737.

14. Hammond WP, Csiba E, Canin A, et al. Chronic neutropenia. A new canine model induced by human granulocyte colony-stimulating factor. *J Clin Invest* 1991;87:704.

15. Basu S, Hodgson G, Katz M, et al. Evaluation of role of G-CSF in the production, survival, and release of neutrophils from bone marrow into circulation. *Blood* 2002;100:854.

16. Hoglund M. Glycosylated and non-glycosylated recombinant human granulocyte colony-stimulating factor (rhG-CSF)—what is the difference? *Med Oncol* 1998;15:229.

17. Layton JE, Hockman H, Sheridan WP, et al. Evidence for a novel in vivo control mechanism of granulopoiesis: mature cell-related control of a regulatory growth factor. *Blood* 1989;74:1303.

18. Terashi K, Oka M, Ohdo S, et al. Close association between clearance of recombinant human granulocyte colony-stimulating factor (G-CSF) and G-CSF receptor on neutrophils in cancer patients. *Antimicrob Agents Chemother* 1999;43:21.

19. Johnston E, Crawford J, Blackwell S, et al. Randomized dose-escalation study of SD/01 compared with daily filgrastim in patients receiving chemotherapy. *J Clin Oncol* 2000;18:2522.

20. Yowell SL, Crawford J, Holmes FA, et al. Sustained-duration, once-per-chemotherapy-cycle pegfilgrastim demonstrates highly efficient, self-regulating, neutrophil-dependent elimination. *Pharmacotherapy* 2001;21:1281(abst).

21. Boneberg EM, Hartung T. Molecular aspects of anti-inflammatory action of G-CSF. *Inflamm Res* 2002;51:119.

22. Mahmud N, Devine SM, Weller KP, et al. The relative quiescence of hematopoietic stem cells in nonhuman primates. *Blood* 2001;97:3061.

23. Lowenberg B, Van Putten W, Theobald M, et al. Effect of priming with granulocyte colony-stimulating factor on the outcome of chemotherapy for acute myeloid leukemia. *N Engl J Med* 2003;349:743.

24. Stroncek DF, Clay ME, Smith J, et al. Changes in blood counts after the administration of granulocyte colony-stimulating factor and the collection of peripheral blood stem cells from healthy donors. *Transfusion* 1996;36:596.

25. Liu F, Poursine-Laurent J, Link DC. Expression of the G-CSF receptor on hematopoietic progenitor cells is not required for their mobilization by G-CSF. *Blood* 2000;95:3025.

26. Thomas J, Liu F, Link DC. Mechanisms of mobilization of hematopoietic progenitors with granulocyte colony-stimulating factor. *Curr Opin Hematol* 2002;9:183.

27. Stroncek DF, Clay ME, Petzoldt ML, et al. Treatment of normal individuals with granulocyte-colony-stimulating factor: donor experiences and the effects on peripheral blood CD34+ cell counts and on the collection of peripheral blood stem cells. *Transfusion* 1996;36:601.

28. Kroger N, Zander AR. Dose and schedule effect of G-GSF for stem cell mobilization in healthy donors for allogeneic transplantation. *Leuk Lymphoma* 2002;43:1391.

29. Takatsuka H, Takemoto Y, Mori A, et al. Common features in the onset of ARDS after administration of granulocyte colony-stimulating factor. *Chest* 2002;121:1716.

30. Dranoff G, Crawford AD, Sadelain M, et al. Involvement of granulocyte-macrophage colony-stimulating factor in pulmonary homeostasis. *Science* 1994;264:713.

31. Omori F, Okamura S, Shimoda K, et al. Levels of human serum granulocyte colony-stimulating factor and granulocyte-macrophage colony-stimulating factor under pathological conditions. *Biotherapy* 1992;4:147.

32. Mellstedt H, Fagerberg J, Frodin J-E, et al. Augmentation of the immune response with granulocyte-macrophage colony-stimulating factor and other hematopoietic growth factors. *Curr Opin Hematol* 1999;6:169.

33. Sakamoto C, Suzuki K, Hato F, et al. Antiapoptotic effect of granulocyte colony-stimulating factor, granulocyte-macrophage colony-stimulating factor, and cyclic AMP on human neutrophils: protein synthesis-dependent and protein synthesis-independent mechanisms and the role of the Janus kinase-STAT pathway. *Int J Hematol* 2003;77:60.

34. Kaplan SS, Basford RE, Wing EJ, et al. The effect of recombinant human granulocyte macrophage colony-stimulating factor on neutrophil activation in patients with refractory carcinoma. *Blood* 1989;73:636.

35. Jones SE, Schottstaedt MW, Duncan LA, et al. Randomized double-blind prospective trial to evaluate the effects of sargramostim versus placebo in a moderate-dose fluorouracil, doxorubicin, and cyclophosphamide adjuvant chemotherapy program for stage II and III breast cancer. *J Clin Oncol* 1996;14:2976.

36. Beveridge RA, Miller JA, Kales AN, et al. Randomized trial comparing the tolerability of sargramostim (yeast-derived RhuGM-CSF) and filgrastim (bacteria-derived RhuG-CSF) in cancer patients receiving myelosuppressive chemotherapy. *Support Care Cancer* 1997;5:289.

37. Dorr RT. Clinical properties of yeast-derived versus *Escherichia coli*-derived granulocyte-macrophage colony-stimulating factor. *Clin Ther* 1993;15:19.

38. Hovgaard D, Schifter S, Rabol A, et al. In vivo kinetics of 111indium-labelled autologous granulocytes following I.V. administration of granulocyte-macrophage colony-stimulating factor (GM-CSF). *J Haematol* 1992;48:202.

39. Saitoh M, Taguchi K, Momose K, et al. Kinetic analysis of megakaryopoiesis induced by recombinant human interleukin 11 in myelosuppressed mice. *Cytokine* 2001;13:287.

40. Gainsford T, Nandurkar H, Metcalf D, et al. The residual megakaryocyte and platelet production in c-mpl-deficient mice is not dependent on the actions of interleukin-6, interleukin-11, or leukemia inhibitory factor. *Blood* 2000;95:528.

41. Nandurkar HH, Robb L, Begley CG. The role of IL-II in hematopoiesis as revealed by a targeted mutation of its receptor. *Stem Cells* 1998;16 Suppl 2:53.

42. Weich NS, Fitzgerald M, Wang A, et al. Recombinant human interleukin-11 synergizes with steel factor and interleukin-3 to promote directly the early stages of murine megakaryocyte development in vitro. *Blood* 2000;95:503.

43. Chang M, Suen Y, Meng G, et al. Differential mechanisms in the regulation of endogenous levels of thrombopoietin and interleukin-11 during thrombocytopenia: insight into the regulation of platelet production. *Blood* 1996;88:3354.

44. Schwertschlag US, Trepicchio WL, Dykstra KH, et al. Hematopoietic, immunomodulatory and epithelial effects of interleukin-11. *Leukemia* 1999;13:1307.

45. Weich NS, Wang A, Fitzgerald M, et al. Recombinant human interleukin-11 directly promotes megakaryocytopoiesis in vitro. *Blood* 1997;90:3893.

46. Orazi A, Cooper RJ, Tong J, et al. Effects of recombinant human interleukin-11 (Neumega rhIL-11 growth factor) on megakaryocytopoiesis in human bone marrow. *Exp Hematol* 1996; 24:1289.

47. Gordon MS, McCaskill-Stevens WJ, Battiato LA, et al. A phase I trial of recombinant human interleukin-11 (Neumega rhIL-11 growth factor) in women with breast cancer receiving chemotherapy. *Blood* 1996;87:3615.

48. Smith JW. Tolerability and side-effect profile of rhIL-11. *Oncology (Huntingt)* 2000;14(9 Suppl 8):41.

49. Kurzrock R, Cortes J, Thomas DA, et al. Pilot study of low-dose interleukin-11 in patients with bone marrow failure. *J Clin Oncol* 2001;19:4165.

50. Tafuri A, Lemoli RM, Petrucci MT, et al. Thrombopoietin and interleukin 11 have different modulatory effects on cell cycle and programmed cell death in primary acute myeloid leukemia cells. *Exp Hematol* 1999;27:1255.

51. Wintrobe MM, Lukens JN, Lee GR. The approach to the patient with anemia. In: Lee GR, Bithell TC, Foerster J, et al., eds. *Wintrobe's clinical hematology*, 9th ed. Philadelphia: Lea & Febiger, 1993:718.

52. Bron D, Meuleman N, Mascaux C. Biological basis of anemia. *Semin Oncol* 2001;28:1.

53. Miller CB, Jones RJ, Piantadosi S, et al. Decreased erythropoietin response in patients with the anemia of cancer. *N Engl J Med* 1990;322:1689.

54. Rizzo J, Lichtin AE, Woolf SH, et al. Use of epoetin in patients with cancer: evidence-based clinical practice guidelines of the American Society of Clinical Oncology and the American Society of Hematology. *J Clin Oncol* 2002;20:4083.

54a. Seindenfeld J, Aronson N, Piper MA, et al. Use of epoetin for anemia in oncology. Evidence Report/Technology Assessment No. 30, AHRQ Publication No. 1-E009. Rockville, MD: Agency for Healthcare Research and Quality, June 2001.

55. Littlewood TJ, Bajetta E, Nortier JWR, et al. Effects of epoetin alfa on hematologic parameters and quality of life in cancer patients receiving nonplatinum chemotherapy: results of a randomized, double-blind, placebo-controlled trial. *J Clin Oncol* 2001;19: 2865.

56. Fallowfield L, Gagnon D, Zagari M, et al. Multivariate regression analyses of data from a randomised, double-blind, placebo-controlled study confirm quality of life benefit of epoetin alfa in patients receiving non-platinum chemotherapy. *Br J Cancer* 2002;87:1341.

57. Patrick DL, Gagnon DD, Zagari MJ, et al. Assessing the clinical significance of health-related quality of life (HrQOL) improvements in anaemic cancer patients receiving epoetin alfa. *Eur J Cancer* 2003;39:335.

58. Gabrilove JL, Cleeland CS, Livingston RB, et al. Clinical evaluation of once-weekly dosing of epoetin alfa in chemotherapy patients: improvements in hemoglobin and quality of life are similar to three-times-weekly dosing. *J Clin Oncol* 2001;19:2875.

59. Silberstein PT, Witzig TE, Sloan JA, et al. Weekly erythropoietin for patients with chemotherapy induced anemia: a randomized, placebo-controlled trial in the North Central Cancer Treatment Group. *Proc Am Soc Clin Oncol* 2002;21:356a(abst).

60. Vansteenkiste J, Pirker R, Massuti B, et al. Double-blind, placebo-controlled, randomized phase III trial of darbepoetin alfa in lung cancer patients receiving chemotherapy. *J Natl Cancer Inst* 2002;94:1211.

61. Glaspy JA, Jadeja JS, Justice G, et al. Darbepoetin alfa given every 1 or 2 weeks alleviates anaemia associated with cancer chemotherapy. *Br J Cancer* 2002;87:268.

62. Glaspy JA, Jadeja JS, Justice G, et al. A randomized, active-control, pilot trial of front-loaded dosing regimens of darbepoetin-alfa for the treatment of patients with anemia during chemotherapy for malignant disease. *Cancer* 2003;97:1312.

63. Aggarwal HK, Nand N, Singh S, et al. Comparison of oral versus intravenous iron therapy in predialysis patients of chronic renal failure receiving recombinant human erythropoietin. *J Assoc Physicians India* 2003;51:170.

64. Besarab A, Amin N, Ahsan M, et al. Optimization of epoetin therapy with intravenous iron therapy in hemodialysis patients. *J Am Soc Nephrol* 2000;11:530.

65. Macdougall IC, Tucker B, Thompson J, et al. A randomized controlled study of iron supplementation in patients treated with erythropoietin. *Kidney Int* 1996;50:1694.

66. Anonymous. A randomized double-blind placebo-controlled study with subcutaneous recombinant human erythropoietin in patients with low-risk myelodysplastic syndromes. Italian Cooperative Study Group for rHuEpo in Myelodysplastic Syndromes. *Br J Haematol* 1998;103:1070.

67. Kasper C, Zahner J, Sayer HG. Recombinant human erythropoietin in combined treatment with granulocyte- or granulocyte-macrophage colony-stimulating factor in patients with myelodysplastic syndromes. *J Cancer Res Clin Oncol* 2002;128:497.

68. Henry DH, Abels RI. Recombinant human erythropoietin in the treatment of cancer and chemotherapy-induced anemia: results of double-blind and open-label follow-up studies. *Semin Oncol* 1994;21:21.

69. Daneryd P. Epoetin alfa for protection of metabolic and exercise capacity in cancer patients. *Semin Oncol* 2002;29:69.

70. Smith R. Applications of darbepoietin-[alpha], a novel erythropoiesis-stimulating protein, in oncology. *Curr Opin Hematol* 2002;9:228.

71. Klaesson S. Clinical use of rHuEPO in bone marrow transplantation. *Med Oncol* 1999; 16:2.

72. Baron F, Sautois B, Baudoux E, et al. Optimization of recombinant human erythropoietin therapy after allogeneic hematopoietic stem cell transplantation. *Exp Hematol* 2002;30:546.

73. Kosmadakis N, Messaris E, Maris A, et al. Perioperative erythropoietin administration in patients with gastrointestinal tract cancer: prospective randomized double-blind study. *Ann Surg* 2003;237:417.

74. Kettelhack C, Hones C, Messinger D, et al. Randomized multicentre trial of the influence of recombinant human erythropoietin on intraoperative and postoperative transfusion need in anaemic patients undergoing right hemicolectomy for carcinoma. *Br J Surg* 1998; 85:63.

75. Scott SN, Boeve TJ, McCulloch TM, et al. The effects of epoetin alfa on transfusion requirements in head and neck cancer patients: a prospective, randomized, placebo-controlled study. *Laryngoscope* 2002;112:1121.

76. Beguin Y. Prediction of response and other improvements on the limitations of recombinant human erythropoietin therapy in anemic cancer patients. *Haematologica* 2002;87: 1209.

77. Leyland-Jones B. Breast cancer trial with erythropoietin terminated unexpectedly. *Lancet Oncol* 2003;4:459.

78. Silver DF, Piver MS. Effects of recombinant human erythropoietin on the antitumor effect of cisplatin in SCID mice bearing human ovarian cancer: a possible oxygen effect. *Gynecol Oncol* 1999;73:280.

79. Thews O, Koenig R, Kelleher DK, et al. Enhanced radiosensitivity in experimental tumours following erythropoietin treatment of chemotherapy-induced anaemia. *Br J Cancer* 1998;78:752.

80. Glaser CM, Millesi W, Kornek GV, et al. Impact of hemoglobin level and use of recombinant erythropoietin on efficacy of preoperative chemoradiation therapy for squamous cell carcinoma of the oral cavity and oropharynx. *Int J Radiat Oncol Biol Phys* 2001;50:705.

81. Henke M, Laszig R, Rube C, et al. Erythropoietin to treat head and neck cancer patients with anaemia undergoing radiotherapy: randomised, double-blind, placebo-controlled trial. *Lancet* 2003;362:1255.

82. Ozer H, et al. 2003 update of recommendations for the use of hematopoietic colony-stimulating factors: evidence-based clinical practice guidelines. *J Clin Oncol* 2004 (in press).

83. Bonadonna G, Valagussa P. Dose-response effect of adjuvant chemotherapy in breast cancer. *N Engl J Med* 1981;304:10.

84. Repetto L, Biganzoli L, Koehne CH, et al. EORTC Cancer in the Elderly Task Force guidelines for the use of colony-stimulating factors in elderly patients with cancer. *Eur J Cancer* 2003;39:2264.

85. Lyman GH, Kuderer N, Greene J, et al. The economics of febrile neutropenia: implications for the use of colony-stimulating factors. *Eur J Cancer* 1998;34:1857.

86. Lyman GH, Kuderer NM, Djulbegovic B. Prophylactic granulocyte colony-stimulating factor in patients receiving dose-intensive cancer chemotherapy: a meta-analysis. *Am J Med* 2002;112:406.

87. Chrischilles E, Delgado DJ, Stolshek BS, et al. Impact of age and colony-stimulating factor use on hospital length of stay for febrile neutropenia in CHOP-treated non-Hodgkin's lymphoma. *Cancer Control* 2002;9:203.

88. Morrison VA, Picozzi V, Scott S, et al. The impact of age on delivered dose-intensity and hospitalizations for febrile neutropenia in patients with intermediate grade non-Hodgkin's lymphoma receiving initial CHOP chemotherapy: a risk factor analysis. *Clin Lymphoma* 2001;2:47.

89. Armitage JO, Potter JF. Aggressive chemotherapy for diffuse histiocytic lymphoma in the elderly: increased complications with advancing age. *J Am Geriatr Soc* 1984;32:269.

90. Garcia-Carbonero R, Mayordomo JI, Tornamira MV, et al. Granulocyte colony-stimulating factor in the treatment of high-risk febrile neutropenia: a multicenter randomized trial. *J Natl Cancer Inst* 2001;93:31.

91. Aviles A, Guzman R, Garcia EL, Talavera A, Diaz-Maqueo JC. Results of a randomized trial of granulocyte colony-stimulating factor in patients with infection and severe granulocytopenia. *Anticancer Drugs* 1996;7:392.

92. Klastersky J, et al. The Multinational Association for Supportive Care in Cancer Risk Index: a multinational scoring system for the identifying low-risk febrile neutropenic cancer patients. *J Clin Oncol* 2000;18:3083.

93. Talcott JA, Siegel RD, Finberg R, Goldman L. Risk assessment in cancer patients with fever and neutropenia: a prospective, two-center validation of a prediction rule. *J Clin Oncol* 1992;10:316.

94. Gerhartz HH, Stern AC, Wolf-Hornung B, et al. Intervention treatment of established neutropenia with human recombinant granulocyte-macrophage colony-stimulating factor (rhGM-CSF) in patients undergoing cancer chemotherapy. *Leuk Res* 1993;17:175.

95. Hartmann LC, Tschetter LK, Habermann TM, et al. Granulocyte colony-stimulating factor in severe chemotherapy-induced afebrile neutropenia. *N Engl J Med* 1997;336:1776.

96. Citron ML, Berry DA, Cirrincione C, et al. Randomized trial of dose-dense versus conventionally scheduled and sequential versus concurrent combination chemotherapy as postoperative adjuvant treatment of node-positive primary breast cancer: first report of Intergroup trial C9741/Cancer and Leukemia Group B trial 9741. *J Clin Oncol* 2003;21:1.

97. Thatcher N, Girling DJ, Hopwood P, et al. Improving survival without reducing quality of life in small-cell lung cancer patients by increasing the dose-intensity of chemotherapy with granulocyte colony-stimulating factor support: results of a British Medical Research Council Multicenter Randomized Trial. Medical Research Council Lung Cancer Working Party. *J Clin Oncol* 2000;18:395.

98. Steward WP, von Pawel J, Gatzemeier U, et al. Effects of granulocyte-macrophage colony-stimulating factor and dose intensification of V-ICE chemotherapy in small-cell lung cancer: a prospective randomized study of 300 patients. *J Clin Oncol* 1998;16:642.

99. Pfreundschuh M, Truemper L, Kloess M, et al. 2-weekly vs. 3-weekly CHOP with and without etoposide for patients >60 years of age with aggressive non-Hodgkin's lymphoma (NHL): results of the completed NHL-B-2 trial of the DSHNHL. *Blood* 2002;100:774a(abst).

100. Pfreundschuh M, Truemper L, Schmits R, et al. 2-weekly vs. 3-weekly CHOP with and without etoposide in young patients with low-risk (low LDH) aggressive non-Hodgkin's lymphoma: results of the completed NHL-B-1 trial of the DSHNHL. *Blood* 2002;100:(abst).

101. Hotta T, Shimakura Y, Ishizuka N, et al. Randomized phase III study of standard CHOP (S-CHOP) versus biweekly CHOP (Bi-CHOP) in aggressive non-Hodgkin's lymphoma (NHL): Japan Clinical Oncology Group study, JCOG9809. *Proc Am Soc Clin Onc* 2003;22:565(abst).

102. Bensinger WI, Martin PJ, Storer B, et al. Transplantation of bone marrow as compared with peripheral-blood cells from HLA-identical relatives in patients with hematologic cancers. *N Engl J Med* 2001;344:175.

103. Storek J, Dawson MA, Storer B, et al. Immune reconstitution after allogeneic marrow transplantation compared with blood stem cell transplantation. *Blood* 2001;97:3380.

104. Garderet L, Labopin M, Gorin NC, et al. Patients with acute lymphoblastic leukaemia allografted with a matched unrelated donor may have a lower survival with a peripheral blood stem cell graft compared to bone marrow. *Bone Marrow Transplant* 2003;31:23.

105. Ji SQ, Chen HR, Wang HX, et al. Comparison of outcome of allogeneic bone marrow transplantation with and without granulocyte colony-stimulating factor (lenograstim) donor-marrow priming in patients with chronic myelogenous leukemia. *Biol Blood Marrow Transplant* 2002;8:261.

106. Morton J, Hutchins C, Durrant S. Granulocyte-colony-stimulating factor (G-CSF)-primed allogeneic bone marrow: significantly less graft-versus-host disease and comparable engraftment to G-CSF-mobilized peripheral blood stem cells. *Blood* 2001;98:3186.

107. Shpall EJ, Quinones R, Giller R, et al. Transplantation of ex vivo expanded cord blood. *Biol Blood Marrow Transplant* 2002;8:368.

108. Dombret H, Chastang C, Fenaux P, et al. A controlled study of recombinant human granulocyte colony-stimulating factor in elderly patients after treatment for acute myeloid leukemia: AML Cooperative Study Group. *N Engl J Med* 1995;332:1678.

109. Rowe JM, Andersen JW, Mazza JJ, et al. A randomized placebo-controlled phase III study of granulocyte-macrophage colony-stimulating factor in adult patients (>55 to 70 years of age) with acute myelogenous leukemia: a study of the Eastern Cooperative Oncology Group (E1490). *Blood* 1995;86.

110. Stone RM, Berg DT, George SL, et al. Granulocyte-macrophage colony-stimulating factor after initial chemotherapy for elderly patients with primary acute myelogenous leukemia: Cancer and Leukemia Group B. *N Engl J Med* 1995;332:1671.

111. Heil G, Hoelzer D, Sanz MA, et al. The International Acute Myeloid Leukemia Study Group: a randomized, double-blind, placebo-controlled, phase III study of filgrastim in remission induction and consolidation therapy for adults with de novo acute myeloid leukemia. *Blood* 1997;90:4710.

112. Godwin JE, Kopecky KJ, Head DR, et al. A double-blind placebo-controlled trial of granulocyte colony-stimulating factor in elderly patients with previously untreated acute myeloid leukemia: a Southwest Oncology Group study (9031). *Blood* 1998;91:3607.

113. Lowenberg B, Boogaerts MA, Daenen SM, et al. Value of different modalities of granulocyte-macrophage colony-stimulating factor applied during or after induction therapy of acute myeloid leukemia. *J Clin Oncol* 1997;15:3496.

114. Lowenberg B, Suciu S, Archimbaud E, et al. Use of recombinant GM-CSF during and after remission induction chemotherapy in patients aged 61 years and older with acute myeloid leukemia: final report of AML-111, a phase III randomized study of the Leukemia Cooperative Group of European Organisation for the Research and Treatment of Cancer and the Dutch-Belgian Hemato-Oncology Cooperative Group. *Blood* 1997;90:2952.

115. Zittoun R, Suciu S, Mandelli F, et al. Granulocyte-macrophage colony-stimulating factor associated with induction treatment of acute myelogenous leukemia: a randomized trial by the European Organization for Research and Treatment of Cancer Leukemia Cooperative Group. *J Clin Oncol* 1996;14:2150.

116. Witz F, Sadoun A, Perrin M-C, et al. A placebo-controlled study of recombinant human granulocyte-macrophage colony-stimulating factor administered during and after induction treatment for de novo acute myelogenous leukemia in elderly patients. *Blood* 1998;91:2722.

117. Harousseau JL, Witz B, Lioure B, et al. G-CSF after intensive consolidation chemotherapy in acute myeloid leukemia: results of a randomized trial of the Groupe Ouest-Est Leucémies Aigues Myeloblastiques. *J Clin Oncol* 2000;18:780.

118. Bhalla K, Birkhofer M, Arlin A, et al. Effect of recombinant GM-CSF on the metabolism of cytosine arabinoside in normal and leukemic human bone marrow cells. *Leukemia* 1988;2:810.

119. Peterson BA, George SL, Bhalla K, et al. A phase III trial with or without GM-CSF administered before and during high dose cytarabine in patients with relapsed or refractory acute myelogenous leukemia: CALGB 9021. *Proc Am Soc Clin Onc* 1996;14:1749(abst).

120. Ohno R, Naoe T, Kanamaru A, et al. A double-blind controlled study of granulocyte colony-stimulating factor started two days before induction chemotherapy in refractory acute myeloid leukemia. *Blood* 1994;83:2086.

121. Larson RA, Dodge RK, Linker CA, et al. A randomized controlled trial of filgrastim during remission induction and consolidation chemotherapy for adults with acute lymphoblastic leukemia. *Blood* 1998;92:1556.

122. Pui C, Boyett JM, Hughes WT, et al. Human granulocyte colony-stimulating factor after induction chemotherapy in children with acute lymphoblastic leukemia. *N Engl J Med* 1997;336:1781.

123. Laver J, Amylon M, Desai S, et al. Effects of r-metHu granulocyte colony-stimulating factor in an intensive treatment for T-cell leukemia and advanced stage lymphoblastic lymphoma of childhood: a Pediatric Oncology Group pilot study. *J Clin Oncol* 1998;16:522.

124. Heath JA, Steinherz PG, Altman A, et al. Human granulocyte colony-stimulating factor in children with high-risk acute lymphoblastic leukemia: a Children's Cancer Group study. *J Clin Oncol* 2003;21:1612.

125. Relling MV, Boyett JM, Blanco JG, et al. Granulocyte colony-stimulating factor and the risk of secondary myeloid malignancy after etoposide treatment. *Blood* 2003;101:3862.

126. Greenberg P, Taylor K, Larson R, et al. Phase III randomized multicenter trial of G-CSF vs. observation for myelodysplastic syndromes (MDS). *Proc Am Soc Hematol* 1993;82:196a(abst).

127. Hamm J, Schiller JH, Cuffie C, et al. Dose-ranging study of recombinant human granulocyte-macrophage colony-stimulating factor in small-cell lung carcinoma. *J Clin Oncol* 1994;12:2667.

128. Stahel RA, Jost LM, Honegger H, et al. Randomized trial showing equivalent efficacy of filgrastim 5 mg/kg/d and 10 mg/kg/d following high-dose chemotherapy and autologous bone marrow transplantation in high-risk lymphomas. *J Clin Oncol* 1997;15:1730.

129. Grigg AP, Roberts AW, Raunow H, et al. Optimizing dose and scheduling of filgrastim (granulocyte colony-stimulating factor) for mobilization and collection of peripheral blood progenitor cells in normal volunteers. *Blood* 1995;86:4437.

130. Weaver CH, Birch R, Greco FA, et al. Mobilization and harvesting of peripheral blood stem cells: randomized evaluations of different doses of filgrastim. *Br J Haematol* 1998;100:338.

131. Stute N, Furman WL, Schell M, et al. Pharmacokinetics of recombinant human granulocyte-macrophage colony-stimulating factor in children after intravenous and subcutaneous administration. *J Pharm Sci* 1995;84:824.

132. Honkoop AH, Hoekman K, Wagstaff J, et al. Continuous infusion or subcutaneous injection of granulocyte-macrophage colony-stimulating factor: increased efficacy and reduced toxicity when given subcutaneously. *Br J Cancer* 1996;74:1132.

133. Roskos LK, Cheung EN, Vincent M, et al. Pharmacology of filgrastim (r-metHuG-CSF). In: Morstyn G, Dexter TM, Foote MA, eds. *Filgrastim (r-metHuG-CSF) in clinical practice*, 2nd ed. New York: Marcel Dekker, 1998:51.

134. Moore TD, Patel T, Segal ML, et al. *A single pegfilgrastim dose per cycle supports dose-dense (Q14D) CHOP-R in patients with NHL.* Poster presented at American Society of Hematology, 2002.

135. Younes A, Fayad L, Pro B, et al. *Safety and efficacy of prophylactic pegfilgrastim in patients with Hodgkin's disease receiving ABVD chemotherapy.* Poster presentation at the annual meeting of the American Society of Hematology, 2002.

136. Bunn PAJ, Crowley J, Kelly K, et al. Chemoradiotherapy with or without granulocyte-macrophage colony-stimulating factor in the treatment of limited-stage small-cell lung cancer: a prospective phase III randomized study of the Southwest Oncology Group. *J Clin Oncol* 1995;13:1632.

137. Meropol N, Miller L, Korn E, et al. Severe myelosuppression resulting from concurrent administration of granulocyte colony-stimulating factor and cytotoxic chemotherapy. *J Natl Cancer Inst* 1992;84:1201.

138. Rowinsky E, Grochow L, Sartorius S, et al. Phase I and pharmacologic study of high doses of the topoisomerase I inhibitor topotecan with granulocyte colony-stimulating factor in patients with solid tumors. *J Clin Oncol* 1996;14:1224.

139. Livingston R, Ellis G, Gralow J, et al. Dose intensive vinorelbine with concurrent granulocyte colony-stimulating factor support in paclitaxel-refractory metastatic breast cancer. *J Clin Oncol* 1997;15:1395.

140. Isaacs C, Robert NJ, Bailey FA, et al. Randomized placebo-controlled study of recombinant human interleukin-11 to prevent chemotherapy-induced thrombocytopenia in patients with breast cancer receiving dose-intensive cyclophosphamide and doxorubicin. *J Clin Oncol* 1997;15:3368.

141. Tepler I, Elias L, Smith JW, et al. A randomized placebo-controlled trial of recombinant human interleukin-11 in cancer patients with severe thrombocytopenia due to chemotherapy. *Blood* 1996;87:3607.

142. Vredenburgh JJ, Hussein A, Fisher D, et al. A randomized trial of recombinant human interleukin-11 following autologous bone marrow transplantation with peripheral blood progenitor cell support in patients with breast cancer. *Biol Blood Marrow Transplant* 1998;4:134.

Brahm H. Segal
Thomas J. Walsh
Juan C. Gea-Banacloche
Steven M. Holland

CHAPTER **53**

Infections in the Cancer Patient

Infections are major causes of morbidity and mortality in patients with cancer, principally related to the intensity and duration of immunosuppressive chemotherapy. It is essential to know the patient's quantitative and qualitative immune defects and to stratify the risk for specific pathogens in the context of the history, physical examination, radiologic findings, and laboratory data.

Patients with cancer vary both in terms of underlying malignancy and in terms of the level of immunosuppression. Multiple predisposing factors may exist in a single patient, which thus increases the spectrum of likely pathogens. This chapter characterizes the major categories of immunologic deficits in persons with cancer (Tables 53-1 through 53-3), the pathogens to which they are susceptible, and the clinical manifestations and treatment of the major pathogens encountered, and discusses novel approaches to prevention, early diagnosis of infections, and immune augmentation strategies.

FACTORS PREDISPOSING CANCER PATIENTS TO INFECTION

ABSOLUTE NEUTROPHIL COUNT MORE THAN 500/μL AND NO IMMUNOSUPPRESSIVE THERAPY

Certain malignancies are inherently associated with immune deficits. Patients with chronic lymphocytic leukemia (CLL) frequently have hypogammaglobulinemia leading to increased susceptibility to infection with encapsulated bacteria, principally *Streptococcus pneumoniae*.[1] Such patients may have recurrent sinopulmonary infections and septicemia. Although routine administration of immunoglobulin to patients with CLL and hypogammaglobulinemia reduces the frequency of bacterial infections, such therapy is not cost effective.[2]

Patients with multiple myeloma are often functionally hypogammaglobulinemic; the total level of immunoglobulin produced may be elevated, but the repertoire of antibody production is restricted. Savage et al.[3] noted a biphasic pattern of infection among patients with multiple myeloma. Infections by *pneumoniae* and *Haemophilus influenzae* occurred early in the disease and in patients responding to chemotherapy, whereas infections by *Staphylococcus aureus* and gram-negative pathogens occurred more commonly in advanced disease and during neutropenia. One randomized study showed that prophylactic intravenous immunoglobulin protected against serious infections in patients with multiple myeloma.[4] The patients who benefited most from immunoglobulin therapy were those with poor immunoglobulin G antibody responses to pneumococcal vaccination.

Patients with hairy cell leukemia are predisposed to opportunistic atypical mycobacterial infections. Patients with untreated Hodgkin's disease have significant abnormalities in T-cell number and function, which persist in the majority of long-term survivors.[5] However, most opportunistic infections occur during poorly controlled malignancy in the setting of cytotoxic and immunosuppressive therapy. Human T-cell leukemia virus type 1, which is associated with adult T-cell leukemia and lymphoma, may itself be immunosuppressive, predisposing to other infections, including strongyloidiasis and mycobacterial infection. This may in part account for the high rate of infectious complications in adult T-cell leukemia and lymphoma.

Adrenal corticosteroid–producing tumors and ectopic adrenocorticotropic hormone–secreting tumors are associated with an increased risk of bacterial and opportunistic infections. In patients

TABLE 53-1. Factors Predisposing Patients with Cancer to Infection

PHAGOCYTIC CELLS (NEUTROPHILS, MONOCYTES, AND MACROPHAGES)
Quantitative defects: neutropenia
  Cytotoxic chemotherapy
  Radiation therapy
  Leukemic infiltration of marrow
  Tumor-associated autoimmune neutropenia
Qualitative defects
  Corticosteroids
  Antibodies inhibiting cytokine signaling (e.g., infliximab)
T LYMPHOCYTES
Quantitative defects
  Cytotoxic chemotherapy
  Nucleoside analogues (e.g., fludarabine, 2-chlorodeoxyadenosine, and 2-deoxycoformycin)
  Radiation therapy
  Corticosteroids
  Monoclonal antibody preparations targeting lymphocyte subsets (see text)
  Human immunodeficiency virus (HIV) infection
Qualitative defects
  Corticosteroids
  Calcineurin inhibitors
  HIV infection
  Alkylating agents
  Hodgkin's disease
  Human T-cell leukemia virus type 1 infection
  Antibodies inhibiting cytokine signaling (see text)
B LYMPHOCYTES: HYPOGAMMAGLOBULINEMIA OR DYSGAMMAGLOBULINEMIA
Chronic lymphocytic leukemia
B-cell lymphomas
Splenectomy
Corticosteroids
HIV infection
Rituximab
DISRUPTION OF MUCOCUTANEOUS INTEGRITY
Vascular catheters
Peritoneal catheters
Ommaya reservoirs
Urinary stents
Cytotoxic chemotherapy (e.g., cytarabine arabinoside, etoposide, alkylating agents)
Radiation therapy
Herpesvirus infection
OBSTRUCTION OF LUMINAL PASSAGES
Endobronchial tumors
Gastrointestinal and hepatobiliary tumors
Genitourinary tumors
Head and neck tumors

with endogenous Cushing's disease, Graham and Tucker[6] noted the predominance of cryptococcosis, aspergillosis, nocardiosis, and *Pneumocystis jiroveci* (formerly *Pneumocystis carinii*) infection.

Solid tumors may predispose to infection because of anatomic factors. Tumors that overgrow their blood supply become necrotic, thus forming a nidus for infection. Head and neck tumors may erode into the mouth and through fascial planes of the neck, predisposing to serious infections by oral flora. Lemierre syndrome, a septic thrombophlebitis of the neck that may lead to endocarditis and septic embolization, is usually caused by oral *Fusobacterium* species. Head and neck cancers also increase the risk

of aspiration pneumonia. Endobronchial tumors may cause recurrent postobstructive pneumonias. Abdominal tumors may obstruct the genitourinary or hepatobiliary tracts, predisposing to pyelonephritis and cholangitis, respectively. Direct invasion through the colonic mucosa is associated with local abscess formation and sepsis by enteric flora. *Streptococcus bovis* bacteremia is highly associated with colon cancer. Breast tumors increase the risk of mastitis and abscess formation, usually by *S aureus*. Patients with advanced malignancy also commonly suffer from malnutrition, which further increases the risk of infection.

NEUTROPENIA

Neutropenia may develop independently of chemotherapy in certain patients with cancer. In acute leukemia, the marrow may be replaced with malignant cells so that virtually no normal circulating neutrophils exist. Similarly, patients with premalignant hematologic disease, such as myelodysplastic syndrome, may have associated bone marrow failure. However, persons rendered neutropenic by cytotoxic chemotherapy are likely to be at greater risk for life-threatening infections due to the concomitant disruption of epithelial mucosal barriers by such agents.

The relationship between circulating leukocytes and risk of infection was established by Bodey et al.[7] in a classic study of patients receiving treatment for acute leukemia. The frequency of severe infections was highest when the absolute neutrophil count was less than $100/\mu L$ and proportionately less frequent at 100 to $500/\mu L$ and 500 to $1000/\mu L$. This relationship was sustained whether the patient was in relapse or remission, although the overall risk of infection was greater during relapse. In addition to the depth of neutropenia, the risk of infection was strongly related to the duration of neutropenia. The likelihood of survival after severe infections was related to both what the initial neutrophil count was and whether a rise occurred within the first week of onset of infection.

The risk of invasive aspergillosis is directly related to the duration of neutropenia. Gerson et al.[8] showed that aspergillosis was uncommon in patients with leukemia when neutropenia lasted for less than 14 days. However, after 14 days, the risk of aspergillosis increased in direct proportion to the length of neutropenia. Invasive aspergillosis is also a major cause of mortality in patients with persistent neutropenia secondary to aplastic anemia.[9]

LYMPHOPENIA

Relatively little attention has been paid to the absolute lymphocyte count and levels of lymphocyte subsets in relation to infection risk in cancer patients. Fludarabine is a fluorinated analogue of adenine that is a lymphotoxic compound primarily affecting CD4+ lymphocytes. The combination of fludarabine and corticosteroids is more immunosuppressive than either agent alone.[10] Fludarabine plus prednisone results in a uniform depression of CD4+ cells that may persist for several months after completion of therapy. O'Brien et al.[11] found that 14 of 264 patients (5%) with CLL developed either *P jiroveci* pneumonia or listeriosis, and three cases occurred more than a year after therapy in patients who were in remission. In advanced CLL, particularly in patients treated with fludarabine, neutropenia and defects in cell-mediated immunity predispose to infection with an expanded spectrum of pathogens, including opportunistic fungi, *P jiroveci*,

TABLE 53-2. Predominant Immunologic Defects and Associated Pathogens in Patients with Cancer

Abnormality	Bacteria	Fungi	Protozoa	Viruses

Qualitative defect of phagocytic function or neutropenia	Gram positive
	  Staphylococcus aureus
	  Streptococcus sp.
	  Nocardia sp.
	Gram negative
	  Escherichia coli
	  Klebsiella sp.
	  Enterobacter sp.
	  Proteus sp.
	  Other enterobacteriaceae
	  Pseudomonas aeruginosa
	  Stenotrophomonas maltophilia
	  Acinetobacter sp.
		Candida sp.
		Aspergillus sp.
		Fusarium sp.
		Dark-walled molds
		Trichosporon sp.
		Zygomycetes
		Other filamentous fungi		

Defective cell-mediated immunity	*Mycobacterium* sp. *Nocardia* sp. *Listeria monocytogenes* *Salmonella* sp.	*Pneumocystis jiroveci* (*carinii*) *Histoplasma capsulatum* *Coccidioides immitis* *Penicillium marneffei* *Cryptococcus neoformans*	*Toxoplasma gondii* *Strongyloides stercoralis*	Cytomegalovirus Epstein-Barr virus Varicella zoster virus
Defective humoral immunity	*Streptococcus pneumoniae* *Haemophilus influenzae* *Neisseria meningitides*	*Cryptococcus neoformans*		

Listeria monocytogenes, mycobacteria, and herpesviruses.[12] Lymphopenia and T-cell depletion are risk factors for opportunistic viral and fungal infections after allogeneic hematopoietic stem cell transplantation (HSCT).

MUCOSAL IMMUNITY

The mucosal linings of the gastrointestinal, sinopulmonary, and genitourinary tracts constitute the first line of host defense against a variety of pathogens. Chemotherapy and radiation therapy impair mucosal immunity at several different levels. When the physical protective barrier conferred by the epithelial lining is compromised, local flora may invade. Chronic graft-versus-host disease (GVHD) may further compromise mucosal immunity, including by causing defective salivary immunoglobulin secretion. Corticosteroids also profoundly compromise mucosa-associated lymphoid tissue by inducing apoptosis of M cells and depleting lymphoid follicles of T and B cells.[13]

Mucosal epithelial cells secrete a variety of antimicrobial peptides, including lactoferrin (iron sequestration), lysozyme (hydrolysis of peptidoglycan of gram-positive bacteria), and phospholipase A2 (cleavage of structural phospholipids of bacteria). Defensins are small cysteine-rich antibacterial peptides (molecular weight of approximately 4 kD) located in the primary (azurophilic) granules of neutrophils and in a variety of

TABLE 53-3. Time Line of Principal Immune Defects and Infectious Complications in Allogeneic Hematopoietic Stem Cell Transplant Recipients

	Months after Transplantation		
	<1	1–6	>6[a]
Principal immune defect	Neutropenia	T cell, humoral Phagocytic (qualitative)	Humoral

Pathogens	Bacteria
	  Staphylococcus sp.
	  Streptococcus sp.
	  Enterobacteriaceae
	  Pseudomonas aeruginosa
	Fungi
	  Candida sp.
	  Aspergillus sp.
	  Other filamentous fungi
	Viruses
	  Herpes simplex virus
	  Respiratory viruses
		Fungi
		  Aspergillus sp.
		  Candida sp.
		  Cryptococcus neoformans
		  Dimorphic fungi
		  Pneumocystis jiroveci (*carinii*)
		Viruses
		  Cytomegalovirus
		  Epstein-Barr virus
		  Varicella zoster virus
		  Respiratory viruses
			Respiratory viruses
			Varicella zoster virus
			Encapsulated bacteria

[a]Graft-versus-host disease necessitating intensive immunosuppressive therapy leads to lack of reconstitution of phagocytic (qualitative) and cell-mediated immunity, thus prolonging the period of risk for infection with both common bacteria and opportunistic pathogens (see text).

mucosal epithelial cells, including bronchial epithelium and Paneth's cells within small intestinal crypts. Neutropenia and loss of the epithelial cell anatomic barrier and local production of antimicrobial proteins may predispose to typhlitis (neutropenic enterocolitis). Keratinocyte growth factor may protect against mucosal toxicity and attenuate the early phase of GVHD.[14]

CORTICOSTEROIDS

High-dose corticosteroids have profound effects on the distribution and function of neutrophils, monocytes, and lymphocytes. In patients with cancer, corticosteroids are seldom the only immunosuppressive agents being administered, and it is therefore difficult to delineate the degree of impairment in host defense elicited by the corticosteroid regimen alone. Infections in patients with collagen vascular diseases treated with corticosteroids are associated with both impaired phagocytic function (e.g., *S aureus* and enterobacteriaceae infections) and cell-mediated immunity (e.g., herpes zoster and *P jiroveci* infections).[15] In this population, the incidence of infectious complications increases when the adult equivalent of prednisone 20 to 40 mg/d is administered for longer than 4 to 6 weeks.[16]

In patients with cancer, the risk of infections is a function of the dose and duration of corticosteroid therapy as well as other coexisting immunodeficiencies, such as neutropenia, and use of other immunosuppressive agents. Corticosteroids blunt fever and local signs of infection such as peritonitis. In allogeneic HSCT recipients, corticosteroid therapy for GVHD is a major risk factor for invasive filamentous fungal infections, and fever may not be present.[17] Corticosteroids disable neutrophil-mediated killing of *Aspergillus fumigatus* hyphae[18] and directly stimulate hyphal growth[19] *in vitro*, possibly via sterol-binding proteins in the fungus.

INTERLEUKIN-2

Patients receiving high-dose interleukin-2 (IL-2) for malignancy have an increased risk of bacterial infections. Inteleukin-2 causes a profound but reversible defect in neutrophil chemotaxis that may account for the increased frequency of infections.[20] Among 345 patients enrolled in a multicenter study of IL-2, the incidence of bacteremia ranged from 19% to 38%. *S aureus* followed by coagulase-negative staphylococci were the most common pathogens, accounting for 90% of septic episodes. The frequency of sepsis in IL-2 recipients was several-fold greater than in nonneutropenic patients with indwelling central catheters.

SPLENECTOMY AND FUNCTIONAL ASPLENIA

In the spleen, rapid antigen presentation occurs, leading to the production of opsonizing antibodies by B cells. The removal of nonopsonized bacteria protects against encapsulated bacteria to which the patient is not yet immune. Splenic irradiation results in functional asplenia, which predisposes to pneumococcal sepsis. Functional asplenia is also a late complication of severe GVHD.[21] Thus, in allogeneic HSCT recipients, fever in the late transplantation period must be evaluated promptly (as in patients with asplenia) because of the risk of overwhelming infection by encapsulated pathogens (see Tables 53-2 and 53-3).

Asplenic patients are principally at risk for overwhelming sepsis by encapsulated bacteria. The most common pathogen is *S pneumoniae*, but other pathogens include *H influenzae* and *Neisseria meningitidis*. It is best to immunize individuals against encapsulated bacteria at least 2 weeks in advance of splenectomy. If this is not feasible, immunization is still advisable after splenectomy, because such patients remain capable of mounting a protective antibody response. Molrine et al.[22] suggest reimmunization of asplenic persons every 5 years with the pneumococcal polysaccharide vaccine.

Although most cases of pneumococcal sepsis occur within the first 2 years after splenectomy, one-third may occur up to 5 years after splenectomy, and cases of fulminant sepsis have been reported more than 20 years after splenectomy. The Working Party of the British Committee for Standards in Haematology recommends lifelong prophylactic antibiotics in patients who have had a splenectomy, and particularly in the first 2 years after splenectomy; in children up to age 16 years; and in patients with other immune impairment.[23]

Asplenic patients should be advised to seek medical attention rapidly when fever occurs. Prophylaxis with penicillin has been traditionally used after splenectomy. However, the growing frequency of antibiotic resistance among *S pneumoniae* isolates raises concern. Newer-generation quinolones have reliable activity against most penicillin-resistant pneumococci, although quinolone-resistant pneumococcal isolates have become more frequent in association with increased use of these agents. Empirical therapy with ceftriaxone or a newer-generation quinolone is warranted in asplenic patients with fever while culture results are awaited. In areas in which penicillin-resistant *S pneumoniae* is frequent, vancomycin may be added. Some physicians prescribe a personal supply of oral antibiotics for asplenic patients to use if fever occurs and the patients do not have easy access to a medical facility.

Other pathogens of concern in asplenic individuals include *Capnocytophaga canimorsus*, *Babesia*, *Plasmodium*, and *Salmonella* species. Infection with *C canimorsus* (previously DF-2) is typically associated with dog bites and can lead to sepsis with or without evidence of cellulitis. *Babesia microti* is transmitted by the *Ixodes scapularis* tick, which is also the vector for Lyme disease. When in Lyme-endemic regions in the spring to autumn periods, patients should follow basic precautions to avoid tick bites (wear long-sleeved clothing, use tick repellants). Babesiosis is diagnosed by a peripheral blood smear showing characteristic intraerythrocytic inclusions.

HEMATOPOIETIC STEM CELL TRANSPLANTATION

The spectrum of pathogens to which HSCT recipients are most susceptible follows a time line corresponding to the predominant immune defects. In the first month of HSCT, neutropenia is the principal host defense defect, predisposing to bacterial, fungal, and viral infections (see Table 53-3). After myeloid engraftment, qualitative dysfunction of phagocytes persists due to use of corticosteroids and other immunosuppressive agents. The risk of infection by opportunistic viruses and filamentous fungi during this period is strongly associated with the severity of GVHD and the requirement for potent immunosuppressive regimens. Impairment in neutrophil chemotaxis has been noted in some patients and may increase the risk of infection. Alveolar macrophage function was impaired in patients studied within 4 months of allogeneic HSCT.[24]

Defects in cell-mediated immunity persist for several months, even in uncomplicated allogeneic HSCT recipients, predisposing to opportunistic infections, including candidiasis, infection with *P jiroveci*, cytomegalovirus (CMV), and herpes zoster (see Table 53-3). Repopulation of specific T-cell subsets occurs at different rates, which results in a lower than normal CD4+ (T helper cell) to CD8+ (suppressor-cytotoxic T cell) ratio for the first 6 months after engraftment.[25] In addition to low T-cell number, T-cell receptor diversity is reduced.[26] Whereas mature and cooperative T- and B-cell functions are usually reconstituted by 1 to 2 years after engraftment, chronic GVHD is associated with persistently depressed cell-mediated and humoral immunity.

Defective reconstitution of humoral immunity is a major factor contributing to increased infection susceptibility in the late transplantation period. Winston et al.[27] noted a high frequency of pneumococcal infections between 7 and 36 months after transplantation, associated with serum opsonic deficiency for *S pneumoniae*. Kulkarni et al.[28] reported that pneumococcal sepsis occurred a median of 10 months after transplantation (range, 3 to 187 months) and was significantly more frequent in patients with chronic GVHD. Eight of 31 patients (26%) with pneumococcal sepsis were receiving penicillin prophylaxis. Breakthrough infections by penicillin-resistant pneumococci may occur on penicillin prophylaxis. Knowledge about the local patterns of pneumococcal antibiotic sensitivity is key in selecting prophylactic agents.

Pneumococcal vaccination in pediatric allogeneic HSCT recipients produced inconsistent antibody responses when administered within the first 2 years after transplantation, especially in patients with chronic GVHD. Children immunized more than 2 years after transplantation had normal antibody responses.[29] Neither the 23-valent nor 7-valent pneumococcal vaccines covers all pneumococcal strains. Therefore, although pneumococcal vaccination is recommended, it does not obviate the need for antibiotic prophylaxis in high-risk patients. Storek et al.[30] showed that serum antibody levels against poliovirus, *Clostridium tetani*, *H influenzae*, and *S pneumoniae* in allogeneic HSCT recipients correlated more with pretransplantation antibody levels in the recipient than levels in the donor, which suggests that immunization of recipients before transplantation, when feasible, may lead to better antibody levels within the first year after transplantation. The Centers for Disease Control and Prevention (CDC) has published guidelines on vaccination of HSCT recipients and household members.[31]

Allografts from HLA-matched unrelated donors, partially mismatched related donors, and cord blood are associated with a higher risk of GVHD. T-cell depletion delays immune reconstitution and, consequently, carries a greater risk of infectious complications, most notably from opportunistic viral[32] and fungal[33] pathogens. Cord blood transplant recipients have a higher risk of infections than other allograft recipients during the early transplantation period because of slower myeloid engraftment. A high rate of opportunistic infections has been noted after day 100 in cord blood transplant recipients, including invasive aspergillosis, candidemia, pulmonary nontuberculous mycobacterial infection, CMV infection, and respiratory syncytial virus (RSV) infection.[34] Invasive aspergillosis occurred more than 3 years after cord blood transplantation in 2 of the 15 long-term survivors, in association with corticosteroid therapy for GVHD.

Autologous transplants are associated with fewer infectious complications than allogeneic transplants. However, CD34 enrichment of autografts leads to a significant reduction in T cells, natural killer cells, and monocytes, compared with unmanipulated autografts and delaying immune reconstitution. Recipients of CD34-enriched autografts appear to be at a level of risk similar to that of allogeneic HSCT recipients for infection with CMV and other opportunistic organisms.[35]

IMMUNOSUPPRESSIVE AGENTS TO PREVENT AND TREAT GRAFT-VERSUS-HOST DISEASE

Cyclosporin A, tacrolimus, and sirolimus (rapamycin) are used to disrupt T-cell activation and are associated with an increased risk of common bacterial and opportunistic infections. They are often paired with methotrexate, corticosteroids, or other immunosuppressive agents.

Alemtuzumab (Campath-1H) is a humanized monoclonal antibody that targets CD52, which is expressed on normal and most malignant T lymphocytes. This agent has been used in a variety of hematologic malignancies and for T-cell depletion to reduce GVHD in allogeneic HSCT. Alemtuzumab treatment is associated with severe lymphopenia and a high incidence of opportunistic infections. Chakrabarti et al.[36] reported a 50% incidence of CMV infection after nonmyeloablative transplant conditioning with alemtuzumab, 46% of which cases occurred after day 100 of HSCT. In the setting of screening for CMV and preemptive antiviral therapy, CMV disease occurred in only 6% of patients at risk. The median time to CD4+ T-cell count higher than 200/µL was 9 months, which reflected a delay in immune reconstitution. Surveillance for CMV reactivation and preemptive therapy should be considered in alemtuzumab recipients in the early and late transplantation period. CMV surveillance is also recommended for nontransplant recipients treated with alemtuzumab, given the significant frequency of CMV reactivation.[37] Alemtuzumab is associated with other opportunistic infections, including respiratory virus infections, herpes simplex, parvovirus B19–related pure red cell aplasia, invasive aspergillosis, and mycobacterial infection.[37,38]

CTLA-4 and anti-CD40 ligand monoclonal antibodies inhibit costimulatory pathways required for T-cell activation and are thus expected to induce antigen-specific tolerance and disable T-cell activation in response to new pathogens. Anticytokine antibodies include the IL-2 receptor antagonist daclizumab and the tumor necrosis factor-α–inhibiting agents infliximab, etanercept, and adalimumab. Daclizumab is associated with an increased risk of wound infections. Tumor necrosis factor-α is a principal mediator of neutrophil and monocyte activation and inflammation. Use of infliximab in HSCT recipients with severe GVHD was associated with an increased risk of invasive filamentous fungal infections.[39] Visilizumab is a humanized anti-CD3 monoclonal antibody that induces apoptosis selectively in activated T cells. In a pilot study of the use of visilizumab in patients with corticosteroid-refractory GVHD, Epstein-Barr virus (EBV) posttransplantation lymphoproliferative disease (PTLD) developed in two of seven patients but was controlled with rituximab[40] (see Epstein-Barr Virus, later in this chapter).

BACTERIAL INFECTIONS IN CANCER PATIENTS

A shift in the normal respiratory flora toward colonization with aerobic gram-negative bacilli occurs in sick hospitalized patients. Changes in the fibronectin content of cell surfaces in debilitated persons lead to reduced adherence by the normal anaerobic flora, which favors colonization by aerobic gram-negative rods. In immunocompromised patients with cancer, alterations in bowel flora lead to acquisition of more virulent bacteria.[41] These changes are exacerbated by the use of broad-spectrum antibiotics that may suppress the normal anaerobic bowel flora.

Whereas in the 1960s and 1970s gram-negative bacterial pathogens (Enterobacteriaceae and *Pseudomonas aeruginosa*) were the principal causes of bacteremia, gram-positive bacterial infections have since become predominant. They account for approximately two-thirds of nosocomial blood stream infections in patients with hematologic malignancies.[42] In both neutropenic and nonneutropenic patients, coagulase-negative staphylococci account for approximately 30% of infections.[42] This shift toward infection by gram-positive organisms likely reflects the widespread use of implantable venous catheters, quinolone prophylaxis, and availability of more effective agents against gram-negative pathogens. Infection with antibiotic-resistant organisms is a growing problem of particular relevance to patients with cancer (Table 53-4) (see Infection with Resistant Bacterial Pathogens, later in this chapter).

STAPHYLOCOCCUS SPECIES

Coagulase-negative staphylococci are organisms of low intrinsic virulence, and their isolation from blood is frequently dismissed as skin contamination. In patients with cancer, coagulase-negative staphylococci most frequently cause a localized catheter-associated infection and bacteremia. Most nosocomial coagulase-negative staphylococci are resistant to β-lactams, which makes vancomycin the initial drug of choice for such infections. However, given the increased prevalence of vancomycin-resistant enterococci (VRE), an antistaphylococcal β-lactam should be used for sensitive staphylococci.

S aureus is the most common cause of surgical wound infections and can cause both local and systemic disease. In some instances a toxic shock syndrome occurs, manifesting as fever, hypotension, gastrointestinal toxicity, rash, and skin exfoliation. Prompt initiation of antibiotic therapy, fluid resuscitation, removal of surgical packing, and wound débridement are required. Disruptions of the skin barrier from indwelling intravenous catheters or biopsy sites are additional portals of entry.

Serious methicillin-sensitive *S aureus* infections should be treated with an antistaphylococcal penicillin (nafcillin or oxacillin). A transesophageal echocardiogram to evaluate for endocarditis should be considered in cases of *S aureus* bacteremia, including intravascular catheter–associated blood stream infections.[43] Nafcillin is superior to vancomycin in preventing persistent *S aureus* bacteremia and relapse.[44] The authors therefore advise that vancomycin be reserved for patients with methicillin-resistant *S aureus* (MRSA) infections or patients with significant β-lactam allergies (see Infections with Resistant Bacterial Pathogens, later in this chapter).

ENTEROCOCCUS SPECIES

The portal of entry in enterococcal bacteremia may be an indwelling central catheter or defects in the gut mucosa from chemotherapy or radiation toxicity. Tumor invasion of the gut may predispose to bacteremia caused by *Enterococcus* species as well as *Streptococcus bovis*. Ampicillin is the drug of choice for sensitive *Enterococcus* isolates. For serious infections (e.g., bacteremia), addition of an aminoglycoside for synergy is reason-

able, because even sensitive strains are intrinsically tolerant to the bactericidal activity of penicillins and vancomycin.

VIRIDANS GROUP STREPTOCOCCI

Viridans streptococci are α-hemolytic streptococci that are oral commensals. Cytosine arabinoside (Ara-C), a highly mucotoxic agent, and prophylaxis with ciprofloxacin or trimethoprim-sulfamethoxazole (presumably by selecting for resistant streptococci) are the major risk factors for bacteremia caused by viridans streptococci.[45]

Bacteremia in patients previously enrolled in trials studying neutropenic fever was caused by viridans streptococci in 13% of cases.[46] Neutropenic patients with viridans streptococcal bacteremia may have a 24- to 48-hour prodrome of low-grade fever and facial flushing, followed by high fever and chills. In as many as 25% of cases, bacteremia is complicated by a toxic shock–like syndrome characterized by hypotension, respiratory distress, renal failure, and a centrifugal maculopapular rash usually starting on the trunk with subsequent desquamation of the palms and soles. Whereas bacteremia due to viridans streptococci is commonly associated with native valve endocarditis in the general population, endocarditis is rare in neutropenic patients with hematologic malignancies.[47] Septic shock may be more common in children than in adults.[45]

Resistance of viridans streptococci to β-lactams has been increasingly recognized, and penicillin susceptibility should not be presumed.[45] The authors advise using vancomycin as initial therapy for blood stream infections by viridans streptococci pending susceptibility testing.

OTHER GRAM-POSITIVE BACTERIA

There is an emerging spectrum of gram-positive bacterial infections in patients with cancer. *Corynebacterium jeikeium* is a common cutaneous commensal organism that infects prosthetic devices, such as vascular catheters, peritoneal dialysis catheters, prosthetic valves, and ventricular shunts. Blood stream infections in patients with hematologic malignancies are associated with skin lesions in half of cases, pulmonary lesions in approximately one-third, and death in one-third.[48] In neutropenic patients, survival is strongly associated with resolution of neutropenia. *C jeikeium* is resistant to the β-lactams, and vancomycin is the drug of choice. In a series of HSCT recipients with *C jeikeium* bacteremia, all eight patients who received appropriate antibiotic therapy and whose central intravenous catheters were removed survived, regardless of persistence of neutropenia; mortality was more than 50% in patients who received no antibiotics and in those who received antibiotics without removal of the central venous catheter.[49]

Bacillus cereus may be associated with a primary cutaneous infection involving vesicular and pustular lesions, particularly in neutropenic children.[50] *Bacillus subtilis* is often a blood culture contaminant. However, isolation of *B subtilis* from more than one blood culture bottle suggests true bacteremia, and the patient should be treated with vancomycin or clindamycin in addition to catheter removal.[51] *Stomatococcus mucilaginosus* infection maybe particularly virulent in neutropenic patients and has been associated with septic shock, respiratory distress syndrome, and meningitis. *Leuconostoc, Lactobacillus,* and *Pediococcus* species are often vancomycin resistant, but most isolates are susceptible to penicillin.

TABLE 53-4. Antibacterial Agents Commonly Used to Treat Patients with Cancer

Antibiotic	Spectrum	Usual Daily Dose[a]	Comments
Ceftazidime	Enterobacteriaceae *Pseudomonas aeruginosa* Less reliable activity against gram-positive bacteria (e.g., viridans streptococci) Poor activity against anaerobes	2 g q8h	Inactivated by extended-spectrum β-lactamases (ESBLs) and cephalosporinases.
Cefepime	Enterobacteriaceae *P aeruginosa* Most gram-positive bacteria Poor activity against anaerobes	2 g q8h to q12h	Active against most ESBL- and cephalosporinase-producing gram-negative bacteria; active against most streptococci, except *Enterococcus* sp.
Piperacillin-tazobactam	Enterobacteriaceae *P aeruginosa* Most gram-positive bacteria (excluding MRSA) Anaerobes	4.5 g q6h	Broad spectrum of activity.
Carbapenems	Enterobacteriaceae *P aeruginosa* Most gram-positive bacteria (excluding MRSA) Anaerobes	Imipenem: 500 mg q6h Meropenem: 1–2 g q8h Ertapenem: 1 g q.d.	Broad spectrum of activity, including ESBL-producers; inactive against *Stenotrophomonas maltophilia*. Ertapenem is not active against *P aeruginosa*.
Aztreonam	Enterobacteriaceae *P aeruginosa*	2 g q8h	Limited spectrum requires pairing with an agent with gram-positive activity for neutropenic fever; useful for persons with β-lactam allergies.
Vancomycin	Exclusively gram-positive bacteria	1 g q12h	Growing frequency of resistance among *Enterococcus* sp.; rare cases of *Staphylococcus aureus* intermediately sensitive or resistant to vancomycin; *Leuconostoc*, *Pediococcus*, and *Lactobacillus* sp. are intrinsically resistant.
Quinolones	Enterobacteriaceae *P aeruginosa* Newer-generation agents have increased activity against gram-positive bacteria	—	Effective prophylaxis against aerobic gram-negative rods during neutropenia; resistance is an important concern (see text).
Trimethoprim-sulfamethoxazole	Enterobacteriaceae (growing resistance) No activity against *P aeruginosa* Active against *S maltophilia, Burkholderia cepacia, Listeria monocytogenes, P jiroveci, Nocardia* sp.	For serious infections (e.g., PCP or bacteremia) is 5mg/kg IV q8h or PO 2 DS (160-mg) tablets 3 times daily. For prophylaxis against PCP, 1 single strength (80-mg) or 1 DS tablet daily or 1 DS tablet 3d/wk.	Effective prophylaxis against *Pneumocystis jiroveci* (*carinii*); potential hypersensitivity and bone marrow toxicity.
Aminoglycosides	Enterobacteriaceae *P aeruginosa* Synergistic activity against sensitive gram-positive organisms (e.g., *Enterococcus* sp.)	—	Should be paired with an antipseudomonal β-lactam agent if used for neutropenic fever or gram-negative bacteremia. Once-daily dosing less nephrotoxic.
Metronidazole	Exclusively anaerobic activity	500 mg q6–8h	First-choice agent against *Clostridium difficile* (PO).
Linezolid	Exclusively gram-positive activity, including MRSA and VRE	600 mg q12h	Excellent oral bioavailability; reversible marrow suppression and peripheral and optic neuropathy with long-term use; should not be used with adrenergic or serotonergic agents (see text).
Quinupristin-dalfopristin	Similar spectrum as linezolid, but inactive against *Enterococcus faecalis*	7.5 mg/kg q8h	Toxicities include myalgias, reversible liver enzyme abnormalities (see text).
Daptomycin	Member of new class of cyclic lipopeptide antibiotics active against gram-positive bacteria	4 mg/kg daily	FDA-approved for complicated skin infections by susceptible gram-positive bacteria.

DS, double strength; FDA, U.S. Food and Drug Administration; MRSA, methicillin-resistant *Staphylococcus aureus*; PCP, *Pneumocystis carinii* pneumonia; VRE, vancomycin-resistant enterococci.
[a]Doses apply to adults with normal renal function.

ENTEROBACTERIACEAE AND *PSEUDOMONAS AERUGINOSA*

The enterobacteriaceae include several pathogenic species, among them *Escherichia coli* and *Klebsiella, Proteus, Enterobacter,* *Serratia,* and *Citrobacter* species. Patients with neutropenia are at highest risk for bacteremia and life-threatening infections by these pathogens. The principal portal of entry appears to be the alimentary tract, although intravenous catheters may also be a source.

In clinical trials and epidemiologic studies of infections in cancer patients, the incidence of *P aeruginosa* infections was 1% to 2.5% among all patients at the onset of neutropenic fever, and 5% to 12% among patients with microbiologically documented infections.[52] Chatzinikolaou et al.[53] compared 245 cases of *P aeruginosa* bacteremia between 1991 and 1995 at M. D. Anderson Cancer Center to the database from the 1970s and early 1980s. The frequency of *P aeruginosa* bacteremia decreased in patients with solid tumors but was unchanged in patients with acute leukemia (55 cases per 1000 admissions). Approximately half of the cases of *P aeruginosa* bacteremia occurred in outpatients, which underscores the need for regimens for neutropenic fever with activity against *P aeruginosa.*

The site of disease often reflects where colonization has occurred. Colonization of the upper airway may lead to pneumonia after aspiration of infected droplets. Typhlitis (neutropenic enterocolitis) and perineal cellulitis may occur because of colonization of the gut by *P aeruginosa.* Pathologically, *P aeruginosa* invades small arteries and veins, leading to thrombosis, hemorrhage, and infarction. This angioinvasion is most evident in cases of ecthyma gangrenosum: *P aeruginosa* invades cutaneous blood vessels and perivascular connective tissue, which leads to coagulative necrosis. The lesions of ecthyma gangrenosum usually evolve from erythematous macules to papules and ultimately to necrotic nodules and bullae. The lesions may present in any stage with minimal or absent inflammatory infiltrate.

Initial optimal antibiotic therapy for *P aeruginosa* bacteremia consists of an antipseudomonal β-lactam antibiotic and an aminoglycoside. It is reasonable to continue aminoglycoside therapy until clinical stability and sterilization of blood have been achieved.

LEGIONELLA

Patients with compromised cellular immunity are at increased risk for legionellosis. In the cancer population, patients at highest risk include those receiving high-dose corticosteroids and fludarabine, and allogeneic HSCT recipients. The typical presentation is acute pneumonia with either a focal or diffuse infiltrate. Gastrointestinal symptoms and myalgias are common. Culture of sputum or bronchoalveolar lavage (BAL) samples in patients who have not received prior antibiotics is usually diagnostic. The laboratory should be alerted when *Legionella* infection is considered, because this organism grows optimally on buffered charcoal yeast agar. The urine *Legionella* antigen assay is sensitive and specific for *Legionella pneumophila* serogroup 1, the most common *Legionella* isolate; however, it does not detect other *Legionella* species. Sputum culture and a urinary antigen test are the optimal combination in most situations.[54] Direct fluorescent antibody testing on respiratory samples is labor intensive and has variable sensitivity. Acute and convalescent serologic testing is also useful in establishing the diagnosis but entails a delay of at least 4 weeks if the acute titer is negative or intermediate. Polymerase chain reaction (PCR) testing of respiratory secretions is both sensitive and specific for *Legionella* detection, but standardized assays are not commercially available.[54] The two most potent classes of antibiotics against *Legionella* species are the fluoroquinolones (ciprofloxacin, levofloxacin, moxifloxacin, gemifloxacin) and the macrolides (azithromycin).

Infection by *Legionella* species most commonly occurs after inhalation of contaminated droplets from water distribution systems. Nosocomial legionellosis has been linked to contamination of hospital water. A single case of nosocomial legionellosis should be regarded as a sentinel event. Some experts advocate routine testing of hospital water sources for colonization by *Legionella* species and appropriate disinfection, particularly in centers that treat highly immunocompromised patients (for detailed guidelines, see http://www.cdc.gov/ncidod/hip/enviro/Enviro_guide_03.pdf).

CLOSTRIDIUM SPECIES

Clostridium species include highly virulent toxin-producing species as well as relatively nonvirulent saprophytes. Toxin-producing species can cause invasive disease such as myonecrosis (gas gangrene), emphysematous cholecystitis and pyelonephritis, necrotizing enterocolitis (typhlitis), and septic shock (see Intraabdominal Infections later in this chapter). Acute hemolysis may result from toxin-producing *Clostridium perfringens.* Most cases of clostridial sepsis in oncology occur in patients with leukemia or gastrointestinal or genitourinary malignancies.[55] Polymicrobial sepsis with enteric flora is commonly observed with clostridial blood stream infection and is more likely to result in septic shock and death. *C perfringens* and *Clostridium septicum* are the most common causes of clostridial blood stream infections in patients with cancer. *Clostridium tertium* sepsis is less common, but the organism is highly virulent. Infections due to other clostridial species are usually associated with fever without evidence of organ involvement and have a lower mortality rate.

Clostridial myonecrosis is characterized by a rapidly progressive, necrotizing soft tissue infection and systemic toxicity, and requires rapid surgical débridement. A needle aspiration or biopsy specimen of the infected tissue showing large, thick gram-positive rods suggests the diagnosis. However, staining of the organism in clinical material may be variable or appear to show a gram-negative result.

The initial antibiotic regimen for invasive clostridial infection should have broad activity against enteric flora, because deep soft tissue infections are often polymicrobial. In neutropenic patients, metronidazole or clindamycin plus an antipseudomonal cephalosporin (such as ceftazidime or cefepime) or single-agent therapy with imipenem, meropenem, or piperacillin-tazobactam is a reasonable regimen. Clindamycin, in addition to showing antianaerobic activity, has the theoretical benefit of reducing toxin production by targeting the bacterial ribosome.

MYCOBACTERIA

Host defense against *Mycobacterium* species relies principally on cellular immunity. In two large HSCT centers in the United States, *Mycobacterium tuberculosis* infection occurred in approximately 0.1% of patients.[56,57] In Hong Kong, an area highly endemic for *M tuberculosis,* the incidence was 5.5%.[58] Therefore, vigilance for *M tuberculosis* infection is necessary among patients who have resided in countries where the organism is endemic.

In the immunocompromised, the clinical manifestations of infection due to *M tuberculosis* may be atypical, and disseminated disease is more common than in immunocompetent patients. The chest radiographic appearance is highly variable and may include an isolated nodule, an infiltrate, or a diffuse reticulonodular pattern. The chest radiograph may be negative in patients with disseminated or extrapulmonary tuberculosis. Cavitary lung disease is less commonly observed in immunocompromised hosts. Extrapulmonary manifestations may include meningitis, brain abscess, vertebral or paravertebral abscess, septic joint, hepatic and splenic disease, and bone marrow involvement. Patients from countries in which the organism is endemic who consume unpasteurized dairy products are at increased risk of gastrointestinal tuberculosis caused by *Mycobacterium bovis*. In addition, systemic *M bovis* infection may rarely occur after intravesicular therapy with bacille Calmette-Guérin for bladder cancer. Detection of mycobacterial DNA in clinical specimens by PCR may facilitate a more rapid diagnosis, although cultures are required for drug susceptibility testing.

Prevention of infection relies on compliance with established infection control measures, including respiratory isolation of persons with presumed or known active tuberculosis in negative-pressure rooms. Given the low prevalence of tuberculosis in cancer centers in the United States, skin testing should be reserved for patients with some additional risk factor for tuberculosis (such as residence in a country where the disease is endemic).

Infection with nontuberculous mycobacteria (atypical mycobacteria) is well described among patients with cancer, particularly in patients with hematologic malignancies. Clinical manifestations include pneumonia, soft tissue or wound infections, and central catheter infections that may require surgical excision of the infected tunnel site (see Intravascular Catheter–Associated Infections, later in this chapter). Pulmonary *Mycobacterium kansasii* infection is associated with significant chest radiographic findings but relatively indolent symptoms, and responds well to rifampin-containing regimens.[59] *Mycobacterium haemophilum* most commonly causes erythematous papular skin lesions through hematogenous dissemination; pneumonia, arthritis, and osteomyelitis are also observed.[60] This organism has a unique requirement for iron supplementation for growth, and therefore the microbiology laboratory should be alerted that this diagnosis is being considered. Speciation of mycobacterial isolates is essential, because nontuberculous mycobacteria are typically resistant to regimens for *M tuberculosis*. The American Thoracic Society has published guidelines for the diagnosis and treatment of tuberculous[61] and nontuberculous[62] mycobacterial infections.

NOCARDIA

Nocardiosis is an uncommon infection in patients with cancer, but infection is associated with significant morbidity and mortality. Those with a hematologic malignancy, allogeneic HSCT recipients, patients with lymphopenia, and those receiving corticosteroids are at highest risk.[63] Nocardiosis is relatively uncommon in HSCT recipients, with an incidence of less than 1%, and may occur in either the early or late transplantation period.[64]

Bronchopneumonia, lobar pneumonia, nodules, or necrotizing abscesses with cavitation are observed. Empyema and extension to the chest wall may occur. Brain abscess, meningitis, osteomyelitis, soft tissue mass, cutaneous abscess, catheter exit-site infection, liver abscess, bacteremia, and disseminated disease may occur in the presence or absence of pulmonary disease. *Nocardia* species are slender, filamentous, beaded, branching gram-positive rods that are variably acid fast and slow growing. It is important to alert the microbiology laboratory when nocardiosis is suspected so that appropriate stains (a modified acid stain should be included) and culture conditions are used.

High-dose trimethoprim-sulfamethoxazole (trimethoprim, 15 mg/kg daily in three divided doses) is the mainstay of therapy for pneumonia or disseminated infection. Other agents to use in combination include the carbapenems (imipenem or meropenem), minocycline, ceftriaxone, amikacin, and linezolid.[65,66] Surgical drainage or resection should be considered in cases refractory to medical therapy. Resolution of lesions is slow, and therapy must be continued for months.

FUNGAL INFECTIONS

The opportunistic yeasts produce a spectrum of clinical disease that ranges from superficial and mucosal infections to disseminated disease. *Candida* species are endogenous flora that gain access to the blood stream through breeches in anatomical barriers. The bowel is the principal portal of entry in patients with acute leukemia receiving highly mucotoxic regimens.[67]

Filamentous fungi (molds) are ubiquitous soil inhabitants whose conidia (spores) are inhaled on a regular basis. The sinopulmonary tract is the most common portal of entry. The respiratory mucosa and alveolar macrophages constitute the first line of host defense against conidia. At the hyphal stage, circulating neutrophils are most important in controlling infection. Thus, prolonged neutropenia is a critical risk factor for invasive aspergillosis.[8] Repeated cycles of prolonged neutropenia and concomitant corticosteroid therapy further increase the risk of filamentous fungal infection. Most filamentous fungal infections are caused by *Aspergillus* species. In addition, the frequency of rare but emerging pathogenic fungi commonly resistant to amphotericin B has significantly increased over the past 20 years among patients with hematologic malignancies. Table 53-5 summarizes antifungal agents commonly used in patients with cancer.

CANDIDIASIS

Oropharyngeal and Esophageal Candidiasis

Oral mucosal candidiasis (thrush) is common with T-cell immunodeficiency. In patients with cancer, conditions that predispose to oral candidiasis include cytotoxic chemotherapy, corticosteroid therapy, and antibiotic use. Oral candidiasis is usually diagnosed visually. White adherent plaques develop on the palate, buccal mucosa, tongue, or gingiva. The differential diagnosis includes chemotherapy-induced mucositis, bacterial infections, and herpes simplex virus (HSV) infection. A wet mount or Gram stain preparation showing pseudohyphae establishes the diagnosis. A culture of the oral mucosa that grows *Candida* species is not by itself diagnostic, because these species commonly colonize the mouth. Therapy for oropharyngeal candidiasis includes local treatments such as clotrimazole troches or oral fluconazole.

Esophageal candidiasis is more severe and typically causes odynophagia. The differential diagnosis of infectious causes includes HSV, CMV (principally in HSCT recipients), and bacteria. Initial therapy with fluconazole is advised for esophageal candidiasis. Amphotericin B, caspofungin,[68] and voriconazole[69] are options in refractory cases. Most fluconazole-resistant *Candida* isolates are susceptible to voriconazole and to other second-generation azoles, but cross-resistance may occur.

Candidemia

Candida species are the fourth most common cause of nosocomial blood stream infections in the United States.[70] The crude

TABLE 53-5. Antifungal Agents

Antifungal Agent	Comments
AZOLES	
Fluconazole	Acceptable alternative to amphotericin B for candidemia at dosage of 400–800 mg/d; broad range of MICs to *Candida glabrata*; *Candid krusei* is resistant; prophylactic use in high-risk patients (e.g., acute leukemia during neutropenia, hematopoietic transplantation); maintenance therapy for cryptococcal meningitis; inactive against filamentous fungi.
Itraconazole	Active against *Candida* sp., *Aspergillus* sp., dimorphic fungi, dark-walled molds. Cyclodextrin formulation has ↑ bioavailability compared with capsules and can be administered parenterally. Itraconazole solution approved for empirical therapy for neutropenic fever.
SECOND-GENERATION AZOLES	Second-generation antifungal triazoles (voriconazole, posaconazole, and ravuconazole) have broad spectrum of activity, including *Candida* sp. (including most, but not all, fluconazole-resistant isolates), *Aspergillus* sp., dimorphic fungi, *Cryptococcus neoformans*, *Trichosporon* sp., *Fusarium* sp., *Pseudallescheria boydii*, and dark-walled molds.
Voriconazole	New standard of care as initial therapy for invasive aspergillosis; treatment of other filamentous fungi resistant to amphotericin B (*Fusarium* sp., *P boydii*, and dark-walled molds); poor activity against zygomycetes; acceptable alternative to amphotericin B formulations as empirical therapy for neutropenic fever (see text).
Posaconazole[a]	Similar spectrum of activity to voriconazole but active against zygomycetes; growing clinical database from compassionate-use protocols for treatment of *Aspergillus* sp. and other refractory filamentous fungi (*Fusarium* sp., *P boydii*, and dark-walled molds).
Ravuconazole[a]	Phase II studies ongoing.
POLYENES	
Nystatin	Topical agent useful for mucosal candidiasis; parenteral liposomal nystatin is experimental.
Amphotericin B desoxycholate (AMB-D)	Broad spectrum of antifungal activity but with significant infusion-related toxicity and nephrotoxicity.
Lipid formulations of amphotericin B	Equal or superior efficacy and ↓ toxicity compared with AMB-D; ↑↑ pharmacy acquisition cost.
Liposomal amphotericin B	↓ Proven breakthrough fungal infections and ↓ infusion-related toxicity and nephrotoxicity than AMB-D as empirical therapy for persistent neutropenic fever; ↓ infusion-related toxicity and nephrotoxicity than amphotericin B lipid complex as empirical therapy.
Amphotericin B lipid complex	Extensive compassionate-use database for patients with refractory invasive fungal infections or intolerance of AMB-D; successfully used in hepatosplenic candidiasis in pediatric patients; ↑↑ levels in reticuloendothelial system.
Amphotericin B colloidal dispersion	Similar efficacy, ↓ nephrotoxicity, but ↑ infusion toxicity vs. AMB-D in a randomized study of primary therapy for invasive aspergillosis and in a randomized study of empirical therapy for persistent neutropenic fever.
5-FLUCYTOSINE	Randomized studies support combination AMB-D and 5-flucytosine for cryptococcal meningitis; pyrimidine analogue with dose- and duration-dependent myelotoxicity and gastrointestinal toxicity; monitoring of serum levels and adjustment of dosing for azotemia required.
ECHINOCANDINS	Class of antifungal peptides that inhibit synthesis of glucan, a fungal cell wall constituent; potently fungicidal against *Candida* sp., including fluconazole-resistant strains; fungistatic against *Aspergillus* sp., principally acting at growing hyphal tips; infrequent infusion-related events and no nephrotoxicity.
Caspofungin	Compassionate-use study of patients with refractory invasive aspergillosis or intolerance to licensed antifungal agents showing 41% successful responses (superior to those of carefully matched historical controls) led to approval for this indication; favorable rate of successful outcome and ↓ toxicity compared to AMB-D for invasive candidiasis; comparable efficacy and ↓ toxicity compared to liposomal amphotericin B as empirical therapy for neutropenic fever.
Micafungin[a]	Trend toward ↓ invasive aspergillosis and ↓ frequency of empirical antifungal therapy compared with fluconazole in HSCT recipients.
Anidulafungin[a]	Similar efficacy to fluconazole in AIDS-associated *Candida* esophagitis; phase III candidemia trial in progress.

↑, increased; ↑↑, greatly increased; ↓, decreased; AIDS, acquired immunodeficiency syndrome; HSCT, hematopoietic stem cell transplant; MICs, minimal inhibitory concentrations.
[a]Nonlicensed compounds.

mortality of candidemia is 30% to 60%. This high mortality rate reflects the presence of serious comorbidities, such as malignancy, neutropenia, and illness requiring prolonged periods in the intensive care unit. In a European surveillance study of candidemia in cancer patients, the overall 30-day mortality was 39%. Higher mortality rates occurred in older patients, in those with poorly controlled malignancy, and in those infected with *Candida* (*Torulopsis*) *glabrata*.[71] In a retrospective study of 476 cases of candidemia, the mortality rate was 52%. Neutropenia, high APACHE (acute physiology and chronic health evaluation) score, and disseminated disease were associated with poorer outcomes.[72]

C albicans is the most common *Candida* species isolated from the blood. The proportion of non-*albicans Candida* species varies among different centers, but they account for approximately one-half of blood stream isolates. *Candida krusei* is always resistant to fluconazole, and *C glabrata* has a broad range of minimum inhibitory concentrations. *Candida tropicalis* blood stream infection often has a severe course with cutaneous dissemination, arthralgias, myalgias, and renal failure. *Candida parapsilosis* infection is mostly associated with vascular catheters and lipid formulations used for total parenteral nutrition. A minority of *Candida lusitaniae* and *Candida guillermondii* isolates are resistant to amphotericin B.

The sensitivity for detection of candidemia has been significantly improved by the lysis centrifugation system and the BacT/Alert system. However, in single-organ infection and in early disseminated candidiasis, even lysis centrifugation culture has limited sensitivity. Nonculture methods, such as PCR, antigen detection, and detection of metabolites, are investigational.

Early catheter removal may reduce the likelihood of late complications of candidemia.[73] Removal reduced the time to sterilization of the blood in nonneutropenic patients in whom the catheter was the likely portal of entry.[74] The Infectious Diseases Society of America (IDSA) has advised removal of all intravascular catheters in patients with candidemia but noted that this recommendation was stronger for nonneutropenic patients in whom the catheter is the most likely primary source of infection.[75] In patients who have received cytotoxic chemotherapy, candidemia is likely to arise from defects in the gut mucosa rather than from the catheter.[67,76] Nucci and Anaissie[77] noted a lack of association between early central venous catheter removal and improved survival and questioned the routine practice of catheter removal in all candidemic patients. If a multilumen catheter is not immediately removed, the authors advise rotating antifungal infusions through all ports. The authors suggest replacement of all intravenous catheters in the setting of clinical instability, lack of resolution of fever within 2 to 3 days, or persistent candidemia after 1 to 2 days of appropriate antifungal therapy. Ophthalmologic examination to evaluate for retinitis is also advised in patients with candidemia.[78]

Chronic Disseminated Candidiasis

Chronic disseminated candidiasis (also called *hepatosplenic candidiasis*) is a complication of highly mucotoxic chemotherapy regimens, such as those used as induction therapy for acute leukemia. Anttila et al.[79] reported a frequency of chronic disseminated candidiasis of 7% in 562 adult patients receiving treatment for acute leukemia. Survival was highly correlated with whether the leukemia was in remission. The use of azole prophylaxis has likely reduced the frequency of chronic disseminated candidiasis.

The only symptom may be persistent fever after neutrophil recovery. Elevation in levels of liver-associated enzymes is common. After resolution of neutropenia, numerous target lesions in the liver and spleen become apparent by radiologic imaging, such as computed tomography (CT) scan, ultrasonography, or magnetic resonance imaging (MRI). Serial ultrasonographic analyses in patients in whom a high clinical suspicion exists may further enhance the likelihood of detecting new or evolving lesions.[80]

A liver biopsy is required for a definitive diagnosis, but because the lesions are discrete, results of a blind percutaneous biopsy may be falsely negative. If the findings of percutaneous biopsy are nondiagnostic, it is reasonable to initiate antifungal therapy with fluconazole or caspofungin if the clinical setting and radiographic appearance are compatible (Fig. 53-1). If fever does not abate after 5 to 7 days of therapy, an open or laparoscopically guided liver biopsy is recommended.

Chronic disseminated candidiasis is not a contraindication for subsequent chemotherapy or HSCT. Patients in whom fever and lesions have resolved with antifungal therapy can undergo further episodes of neutropenia without progression of the fungal infection if antifungal therapy is reinitiated during the neutropenic periods.[81]

Choi et al.[82] noted an association between chronic disseminated candidiasis in adult patients with acute leukemia and common IL-4 promoter haplotypes. Although preliminary, this study highlights a relatively novel approach to genetics in which polymorphisms of relevant host defense genes in humans are correlated with the risk and pathogenesis of opportunistic infections.

Therapy for Invasive Candidiasis

A large randomized study comparing intravenous fluconazole (400 mg daily) with amphotericin B as therapy for candidemia in nonneutropenic patients found both regimens equally effective, but fluconazole had less toxicity.[83] In a subsequent study of nonneutropenic patients with candidemia, duotherapy with a higher dose of fluconazole (800 mg daily) and amphotericin B led to better clearance of candidemia than fluconazole alone but was associated with significantly more nephrotoxicity and no survival benefit.[84] A randomized trial comparing voriconazole with amphotericin B followed by fluconazole for invasive candidiasis has completed enrollment, and the data are being analyzed.

When caspofungin was compared with conventional amphotericin B in a randomized, double-blinded study in adult patients with invasive candidiasis, there was a trend toward a higher favorable response rate in the caspofungin arm (73% vs. 62%, respectively) in the modified intent-to-treat analysis.[85] Among patients who received the study drug for at least 5 days, caspofungin was statistically superior to amphotericin B (81% vs. 65% successful outcomes, respectively). Caspofungin recipients had significantly fewer clinical adverse experiences, less nephrotoxicity, and less premature discontinuation due to drug-related toxicity. Survival and the rate of sterilization of blood in candidemic patients were similar in the two arms. This study strongly supports the use of caspofungin as initial therapy for invasive candidiasis in adults.

ASPERGILLOSIS

Risk Factors and Clinical Manifestations

Prolonged and persistent neutropenia is a critical risk factor for aspergillosis.[8] More recent studies have reported that the predominance of aspergillosis cases occur in the postengraftment rather than the neutropenic period of allogeneic HSCT, with immunosuppressive therapy for GVHD being a principal risk factor. There are three likely reasons for the increased proportion of invasive filamentous fungal infections in the postengraftment period: (1) shortening of the duration of neutropenia as a result of infusion of larger numbers of myeloid progenitors and treatment with colony-stimulating factors; (2) increased proportion of unrelated donors and HLA-mismatched transplants, which predispose to GVHD; and (3) increased proportion of patients who survive beyond the early transplantation period.

Marr et al.[33] retrospectively evaluated risk factors for invasive aspergillosis in HSCT recipients. Receipt of T-cell–depleted or CD34-selected stem cell products, use of corticosteroids, and presence of neutropenia, lymphopenia, GVHD, CMV disease, and respiratory virus infections were associated with an increased risk of aspergillosis after neutrophil recovery. Invasive aspergillosis more than 6 months after transplantation was associated with chronic GVHD and CMV disease. Late-onset invasive aspergillosis is also a major cause of mortality in recipients of nonmyeloablative allogeneic HSCT, with acute and chronic GVHD and CMV disease being the principal risk factors.[86,87] Marr et al.[88] noted an increase in the frequency of nonfumigatus *Aspergillus* species, zygomycetes, and *Fusarium* and *Scedosporium* species in allogeneic

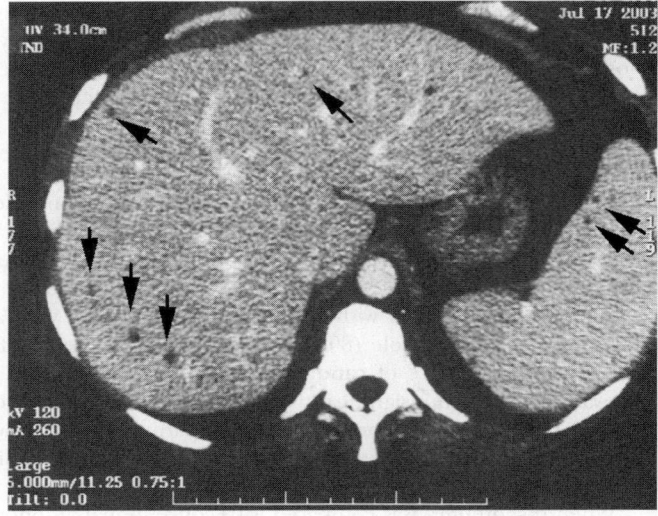

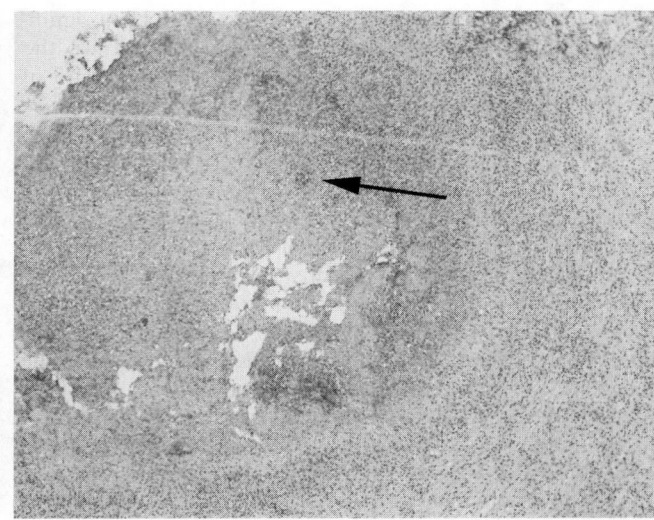

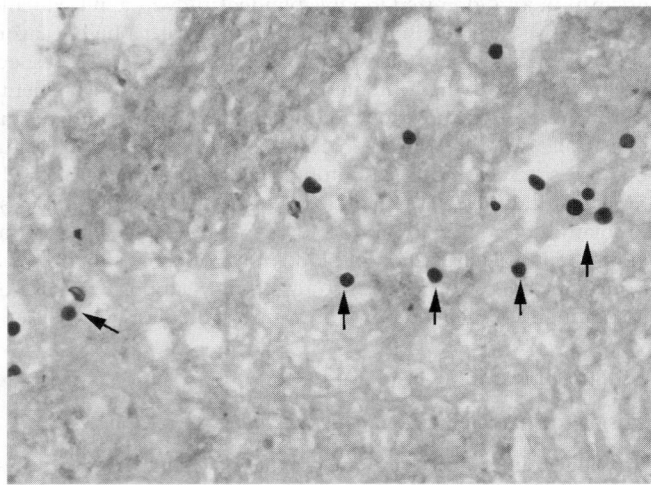

FIGURE 53-1. Hepatosplenic candidiasis. **A:** Abdominal computed tomographic scan to evaluate persistent fever after neutrophil recovery in a patient who underwent induction chemotherapy for acute myelogenous leukemia showed multiple hypodense lesions in the liver and spleen (*arrows*). **B:** Liver biopsy specimen showed discrete abscesses (*arrow*) (hematoxylin and eosin, 40×). **C:** Numerous yeast are evident (*arrows*) after Gomori methenamine silver staining (400×). (See Color Fig. 53-1*B,C* in the CD-ROM.)

HSCT recipients. Patients with relapse of malignancy treated with multiple transplants were at particular risk for infection with these pathogens.

Aspergillosis can involve virtually any organ in the immunocompromised host, but sinopulmonary disease is the most common. In addition to air, hospital water systems may be a source of nosocomial aspergillosis.[89] Invasive aspergillosis in the neutropenic host may present as fever, sinus pain or congestion, cough, pleuritic chest pain, and hemoptysis. Erosion through a large central blood vessel wall can lead to massive pulmonary hemorrhage. The radiographic appearance of pulmonary aspergillosis includes bronchopneumonia, lobar consolidation, segmental pneumonia, nodular lesions resembling septic emboli, and cavitary lesions (Fig. 53-2). The central nervous system is a common target for hematogenous aspergillosis (see Central Nervous System Infection, later in this chapter). Gastrointestinal aspergillosis usually coexists with pulmonary disease, but in rare instances, the gastrointestinal tract is the sole organ involved. Other sites of disseminated aspergillosis include the skin, heart, eye, bone, kidney, liver, and thyroid.

Diagnosis of Invasive Aspergillosis

Early diagnosis of aspergillosis in highly immunocompromised patients remains difficult. Blood culture results are rarely posi-

tive, sputum and BAL cultures have approximately 50% sensitivity in focal pulmonary lesions, and definitive diagnosis often requires an invasive procedure and is usually made only when the disease is advanced. Isolation of an *Aspergillus* species from a sputum or BAL specimen should be presumed to represent invasive disease in neutropenic patients.

Chest CT scans facilitate detection of pulmonary aspergillosis in patients with persistent neutropenic fever; this leads to earlier initiation of therapy, which, in turn, may be associated with an improved outcome.[90] A CT scan may show peripheral or subpleural nodules not apparent on plain chest radiographs (see Fig. 53-2). The "halo sign" is a characteristic chest CT feature of angioinvasive organisms.[91] The hazy alveolar infiltrates appear to correspond to regions of ischemia and are highly suggestive of invasive aspergillosis.[91]

A sensitive double-sandwich enzyme-linked immunosorbent assay for detection of the fungal cell wall constituent galactomannan has been developed. Maertens and colleagues[92,93] reported a high sensitivity and specificity of this assay in detecting early aspergillosis in high-risk patients. With serial sampling of serum, the galactomannan assay generally became positive several days before the onset of clinical symptoms or radiographic findings. Herbrecht et al.[94] reported an overall sensitivity of only 65% in patients with definite invasive aspergillosis and a specificity of 95%.

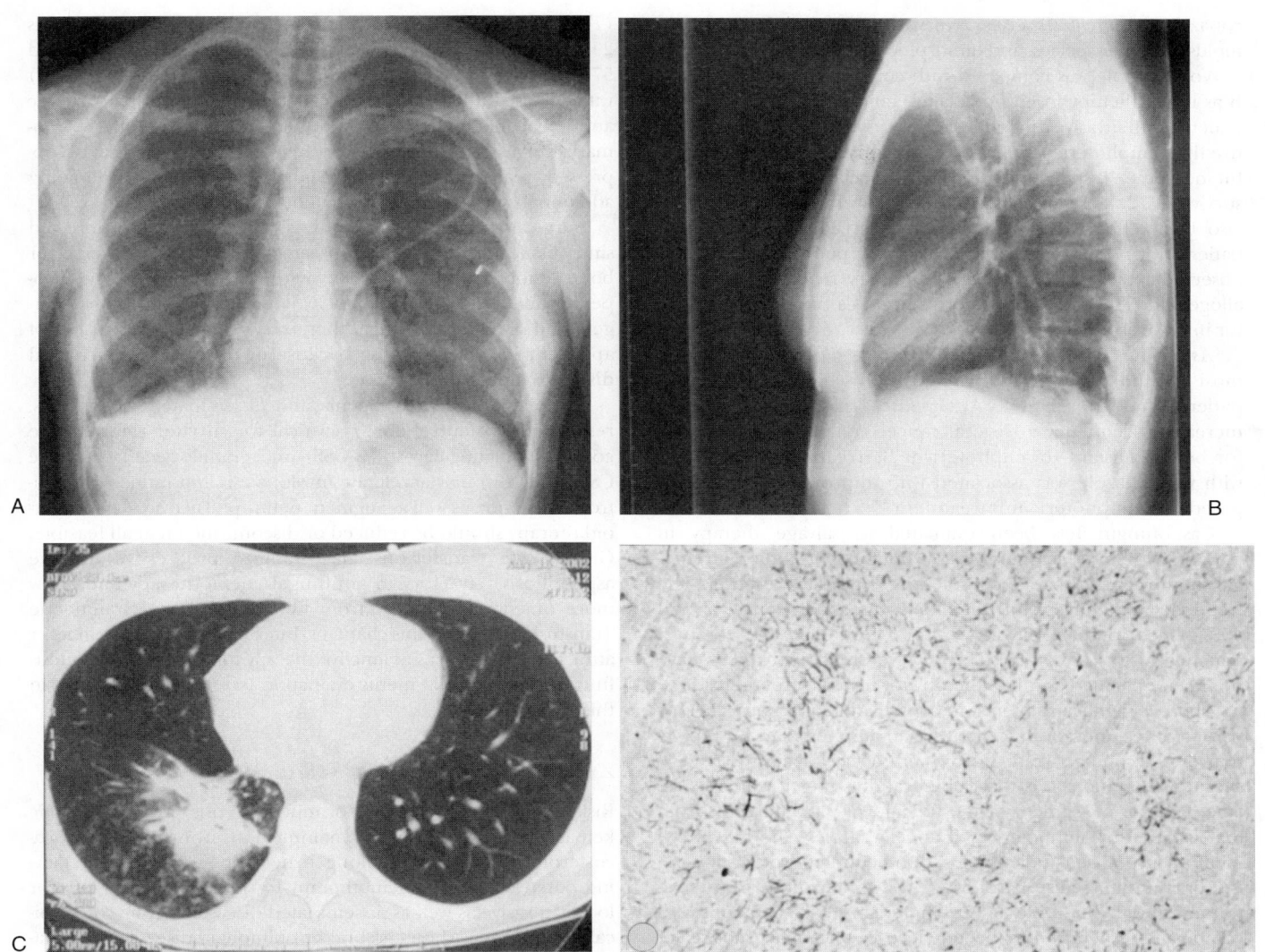

FIGURE 53-2. Aspergillosis. **A,B:** Chest radiographs to evaluate persistent neutropenic fever in a patient with relapsed leukemia showed subtle increased markings in the right lower lung. **C:** Chest computed tomography (CT) scan obtained the same day showed a significant area of consolidation not apparent on the chest radiograph. Bronchoalveolar lavage specimen grew *Aspergillus fumigatus*. This case illustrates the appropriate use of a chest CT scan in patients with persistent neutropenic fever at high risk for invasive mold infection. **D:** Invasive pulmonary aspergillosis in another patient showing necrosis and invasive hyphae (Gomori methenamine silver stain). (From Segal B, Walsh T. Opportunistic fungal infections. In: Cohen J, Powderly WG, eds. *Infectious diseases*, 2nd ed. St. Louis: Mosby, 2004, with permission.)

In a study of 170 patients at high risk for invasive aspergillosis at three North American cancer centers, the galactomannan assay identified 25 of 31 patients with invasive aspergillosis (81% sensitivity) with serial sampling and there was a specificity of 89% (http://www.fda.gov/bbs/topics/NEWS/2003/NEW00907.html). Concomitant antifungal agents with mold activity can reduce the sensitivity of the galactomannan assay, and piperacillin/tazobactam may cause a false positive result. Serial quantitation of galactomannan antigenemia levels has also been used to predict response to antifungal therapy in animal models[95] and in patients.[96] In allogeneic HSCT recipients, a rising galactomannan antigen level was associated with failure of therapy, whereas a stable or decreasing level was predictive of a positive response.[96] The U.S. Food and Drug Administration approved the Platelia *Aspergillus* enzyme immunoassay (Bio-Rad Laboratories, Redmond, WA).

PCR-based detection of aspergillosis is also promising. β-Glucan, a ubiquitous fungal cell wall constituent, is also being evaluated as a diagnostic marker for invasive fungal infection. Additional prospective studies are required to define which diagnostic method, or combination of methods, confers optimal sensitivity and specificity in detecting early *Aspergillus* infection.

Treatment of Invasive Aspergillosis

Lipid formulations of amphotericin B have allowed for greater drug delivery with reduced toxicity. Voriconazole, posaconazole (SCH 56592), and ravuconazole (BMS 207147) are second-generation triazoles that are highly active against filamentous fungi. Currently, only voriconazole is licensed. These agents are active against *Candida* species (including most isolates resistant to fluconazole), *Aspergillus* species, *Scedosporium* species, dematiaceous molds, *Fusarium* species, and dimorphic fungi.

Voriconazole was compared with conventional amphotericin B as initial therapy in an open-label, randomized trial involving patients with invasive aspergillosis.[97] Voriconazole was more effective than amphotericin B (51% vs. 32% of subjects had a successful outcome, respectively) and was associated with improved survival at 12 weeks (71% vs. 58%, respectively). Voriconazole has also been effective as salvage therapy in adult and pediatric patients with invasive aspergillosis.[98,99] The poorest outcome was observed in patients with extrapulmonary aspergillosis and in allogeneic HSCT recipients. Voriconazole is the drug of choice for invasive aspergillosis.

Aspergillus fumigatus followed by *Aspergillus flavus* are the most common species causing invasive disease in neutropenic patients and after HSCT. *Aspergillus terreus* is observed with increasing frequency at several cancer centers and is notable for being resistant to amphotericin B. Treatment of *A terreus* with voriconazole was associated with improved survival compared with amphotericin B treatment.[100]

Caspofungin has been evaluated as salvage therapy in patients with invasive aspergillosis refractory to standard antifungal therapy and in patients intolerant of standard therapy. The frequency of a successful outcome ranged between 40% and 45%, which compares favorably with the outcomes for carefully matched historical controls.[101,102] However, echinocandins have not been evaluated as initial therapy for invasive aspergillosis.

There is significant interest in combination antifungal therapy pairing an echinocandin with either an amphotericin B preparation or a second-generation azole with activity against *Aspergillus* species. The rationale is that echinocandins target a unique site (the β-glucan constituent of the fungal cell wall) different from that targeted by amphotericin B and the azoles (the fungal cell membrane). *In vitro* studies have shown neutral to synergistic activity (but no antagonism) involving the combination of an echinocandin with an azole or amphotericin B preparation, and combination therapy has been effective in animal models of aspergillosis. The published clinical experience involving combination regimens is limited to small series at single centers.[103,104] Randomized studies are required to define the role of combination therapy as primary therapy for invasive aspergillosis.

Several centers reasonably use combination regimens as salvage therapy for refractory aspergillosis. The combination of caspofungin and liposomal amphotericin B (LAMB) as salvage therapy led to a favorable outcome in approximately 40% to 60% of patients with invasive aspergillosis.[104,105] In 47 patients with invasive aspergillosis refractory to amphotericin B preparations, the combination of voriconazole and caspofungin was associated with increased survival compared with voriconazole alone (K. Marr, *personal communication*, 2003). Although their results are encouraging when compared with the historical success rate of salvage regimens for invasive aspergillosis, these studies are retrospective, and therefore other host- and infection-related factors may have influenced the outcome. In cases of invasive aspergillosis refractory to voriconazole, salvage therapy with caspofungin plus a lipid formulation of amphotericin B (5 mg/kg/d or more) is reasonable.

Patients who recover from an episode of invasive aspergillosis are at risk for relapse of infection during subsequent periods of immunosuppression. In a multicenter European series involving 48 patients with aspergillosis who later were treated with HSCT (77% allogeneic), the overall incidence of relapsed infection was 29% among patients who received secondary prophylaxis and 57% among those who did not.[106] Fourteen of 16 patients (88%) with relapsed infection died. Smaller series showed that systemic antifungal therapy (with or without surgical resection) for primary fungal infection followed by secondary prophylaxis suppressed reactivation in the majority of patients undergoing additional cycles of cytotoxic chemotherapy or HSCT.

Surgical excision of locally invasive disease, such as infected sinus tissue, primary cutaneous lesions, intravitreal disease, or bone lesions, should be performed when feasible. In neutropenic patients and in allogeneic HSCT recipients, combined surgery and systemic antifungal therapy should be used in cases of apparent localized disease because of the risk of subclinical dissemination.

In patients with neutropenia and disseminated aspergillosis, resolution of neutropenia is critical for survival. Granulocyte colony-stimulating factor (G-CSF) and granulocyte-macrophage CSF (GM-CSF) may accelerate myelopoiesis and reduce the neutropenic period as well as augment neutrophil activity. Corticosteroid therapy should be reduced or discontinued if at all feasible. Granulocyte transfusions may stabilize progressive invasive aspergillosis refractory to antifungal chemotherapy and allow more time until recovery from neutropenia (see Granulocyte Transfusions, later in this chapter). Interferon-γ (IFN-γ) is another attractive candidate as adjunctive therapy for invasive filamentous fungal infections that merits evaluation (see Interferon-γ, later in this chapter).

ZYGOMYCOSIS

Risk factors for zygomycosis (or mucormycosis) include diabetic ketoacidosis, protein-calorie malnutrition, iron overload, corticosteroid therapy, and prolonged neutropenia. Patients receiving potent cytotoxic chemotherapy for leukemia are at risk for locally invasive as well as disseminated disease. Zygomycosis typically manifests as rhinocerebral or pulmonary disease after inhalation of spores. In rhinocerebral disease, fever, facial pain, and headache are common findings. Contiguous extension may lead to orbital involvement with proptosis and extraocular muscle paresis, involvement of hard palate, and spread to the brain. An eschar over the palate or nasal turbinates is suggestive of zygomycosis, but other filamentous fungi can produce similar findings. Occasionally, isolated primary cutaneous disease may follow minor trauma. Injection drug users may inject contaminating spores directly into the blood stream, which leads to space-occupying lesions of the brain or other organs.

Therapy for zygomycosis involves high-dose amphotericin B (conventional or lipid formulations) plus early and aggressive surgical débridement. Itraconazole and voriconazole are not active against zygomycetes species, and breakthrough zygomycosis has been reported in allogeneic HSCT recipients receiving voriconazole as prophylaxis or empirical antifungal therapy.[107] Posaconazole, a second-generation antifungal azole, led to a successful outcome in 16 of 23 patients (70%) with refractory zygomycosis or intolerance to standard antifungal therapy.[108]

CRYPTOCOCCUS NEOFORMANS INFECTION

Host defense against cryptococcal infection is principally dependent on cellular immunity. Isolated neutropenia is rarely associated with cryptococcal infection. Immunoglobulins directed against capsular epitopes and complement facilitate phagocytosis of the organism and likely play a role in host defense. Among patients with cancer, those with hematologic malignancies, those receiving high-dose corticosteroids, and allogeneic HSCT recipients are at highest risk for cryptococcosis. The principal portal of entry of this organism is likely via inhalation. Spread to the blood and then to the central nervous system is a prerequisite for subsequent development of cryptococcal meningitis.

Meningitis is the most common presentation of cryptococcal infection. Other manifestations include primary pneumonia, fungemia, and cutaneous and visceral dissemination. In the pre–acquired immunodeficiency syndrome (AIDS) era, patients who died early during therapy were more likely to have rapidly progressive infection, cerebrospinal fluid with high opening pressure, a low glucose level, fewer than 20 leukocytes/μL, positive findings on India ink preparation, culture of cryptococci from extraneural sites, and high titers of cryptococcal antigen in serum and cerebrospinal fluid.[109] A more recent study of non–AIDS-associated cryptococcal disease showed that mortality was highest among persons with malignancy.[110] Additional central nervous system complications include development of a mass lesion, obstructive hydrocephalus requiring shunting, and visual loss. Visual loss may be a consequence of endophthalmitis, a space-occupying lesion in the visual pathway, direct invasion of the optic nerve (which may cause visual loss over several hours), or elevated intracranial pressure.

In AIDS-associated cryptococcal meningitis, the optimal regimen currently is amphotericin B (0.7 mg/kg daily) plus 5-flucytosine (100 mg/kg daily) for the first 2 weeks, followed by maintenance fluconazole therapy (400 mg daily).[111] This is an appropriate regimen to use in non–AIDS-associated cryptococcal infection in the absence of modern randomized trials. In neutropenic patients, reduction of the dosage of 5-flucytosine may be considered to avoid delay in myeloid recovery. Because fluconazole is well tolerated, continuing therapy with this agent for several months (or longer if intensive immunosuppressive therapy is continued) is reasonable.

LESS COMMON OPPORTUNISTIC FUNGAL PATHOGENS

Trichosporon *Species*

Trichosporonosis typically occurs in profoundly neutropenic patients and those receiving corticosteroid therapy, and typically manifests with refractory fungemia, funguria, cutaneous lesions, renal failure, pulmonary lesions, and chorioretinitis.[112] Disseminated trichosporonosis may yield a false-positive result on a cryptococcal latex antigen test because of cross-reactivity with the polysaccharide capsule of *Cryptococcus neoformans*. This cross-reactivity may be clinically important, because patients treated with high-dose corticosteroid therapy are at risk for both infections, and *C neoformans* typically responds to amphotericin B therapy, whereas *Trichosporon* species are usually resistant.

Study of *in vitro* and experimental infections indicates that most *Trichosporon* species are inhibited, but not killed, by achievable serum levels of conventional amphotericin B.[113] Fluconazole has superior activity in experimental infections and is the preferred antifungal agent. Combination therapy with high-dose amphotericin B (1.0 to 1.5 mg/kg daily) and fluconazole (800 mg

daily or 12 mg/kg daily in children) may have synergy against some strains based on murine models of trichosporonosis.[114]

Infection with *Blastoschizomyces capitatus* (formerly *Trichosporon capitatus*) usually presents as a chronic disseminated infection, resembling chronic candidiasis.[115] A CT scan may show lesions suggestive of hepatosplenic candidiasis; definitive diagnosis requires positive results on either blood culture or biopsy. Central nervous system involvement is also observed. *B capitatus* does not cross-react with the cryptococcal latex agglutination test.

Malassezia *Species*

Malassezia furfur infection is often associated with lipid-containing parenteral nutrition administered through a central venous catheter in immunocompromised patients or premature infants. Clinical manifestations include persistent fungemia and pulmonary infiltrates. Thrombocytopenia occurs in premature infants but generally not in adults. Blood culture recovery is enhanced by addition of olive oil or other long-chain fatty acids to the culture plates. *M furfur* is often refractory to amphotericin B therapy. Fluconazole is probably the drug of choice, but discontinuation of lipid infusions and removal of the central catheter are also important. In neutropenic patients and patients treated with corticosteroids, a folliculitis resembling disseminated candidiasis may occur. This localized process does not imply disseminated infection. *Malassezia pachydermatis* is a less common cause of infection than *M furfur* and has similar clinical manifestations.

Fusarium *Species*

Fusarium species are soil saprophytes that have been associated with soft tissue infection, onychomycosis, and keratitis in immunocompetent hosts. With the widespread use of intensive antineoplastic therapy for acute leukemia and HSCT, invasive and disseminated fusariosis has become more common.[116] The likelihood of infection by a *Fusarium* species is substantially increased by the presence of disseminated cutaneous lesions and isolation of a mold from blood culture. Skin is an important portal of entry for *Fusarium*.[116] Initial localized manifestations included onychomycosis, paronychia, and cellulitis. Early identification of localized skin disease and débridement may be life-saving. Inhalation of spores is another major portal of entry, leading to fungal sinusitis and pneumonia. *Fusarium* infection may be associated with colonization of hospital water systems,[117] although the outside environment is likely to be the principal reservoir.[118]

Survival of disseminated fusariosis is critically dependent on resolution of neutropenia.[116] *Fusarium* species have variable *in vitro* sensitivity to amphotericin B, and the clinical response has been poor. Use of voriconazole as salvage therapy for fusariosis was associated with a 46% success rate,[119] which compared favorably with the response to amphotericin B.

Scedosporium *Species*

Scedosporium apiospermum (*Pseudallescheria boydii*) and *Scedosporium prolificans* are the principal pathogenic species of *Scedosporium*. In neutropenic patients, *S apiospermum* is a virulent pathogen, infection with which clinically and histologically resembles aspergillosis. Invasion of blood vessels leading to infarction is common. *S apiospermum* causes sinopulmonary disease, endophthalmitis, and dissemination to the central nervous system. The infection can also spread directly from the skin to bone and joint. Establishing a culture-based diagnosis of *S apiospermum* is important because of its frequent resistance to amphotericin B.

The authors advise using voriconazole as first-line therapy for scedosporiosis. Voriconazole led to a successful response in 17 of 27 cases (63%) of *S apiospermum* infection, and the rate of successful outcome was 30% to 40% in disseminated and central nervous system infection.[120] Surgical resection of localized lesions is advised when feasible. *S prolificans* causes a similar spectrum of disease as *S apiospermum* but is generally resistant to all antifungal agents.

Dematiaceous (Dark-Walled) Molds

Dark-walled molds (Phaeohyphomycetes) contain melanin in their cell walls, which imparts a brown or olive-green color in culture. In immunocompromised patients, soft tissue infection, sinusitis, central nervous system infection, pneumonia, fungemia, and disseminated disease are observed. Subcutaneous infection is most frequently caused by *Alternaria* species. *Bipolaris, Cladophialophora* (*Xylohypha* or *Cladosporium*) *bantianum, Wangiella,* and *Dactylaria* species have a strong predisposition to cause central nervous system disease.

Therapy in immunocompromised patients involves surgical excision of localized disease when feasible and systemic antifungal therapy. Sensitivity to amphotericin B is variable, and clinical failures have been reported. Itraconazole has been the preferred agent for phaeohyphomycosis.[121] Voriconazole has *in vitro* activity against dark-walled molds and is also a viable option.

Endemic Dimorphic Fungi

Endemic dimorphic fungi are so named because of their characteristic geographic distribution. These organisms include *Histoplasma capsulatum, Coccidioides immitis, Blastomyces dermatitidis, Paracoccidioides brasiliensis* (endemic in Latin America), and *Penicillium marneffei* (endemic in Southeast Asia). These fungi are dimorphic, existing in nature in the fruiting mycelial stage and converting to the yeast stage at body temperature. Because some of these pathogens may be quiescent during the initial infection and only manifest clinically during depression of cell-mediated immunity, a detailed travel history is essential.

Endemic mycoses in the central United States (e.g., Ohio River valley) include histoplasmosis and blastomycosis. In the immunocompetent host, inhalation of *Histoplasma* microconidia is typically asymptomatic but may manifest with acute fever, pulmonary infiltrates, and hypoxia. Immunocompromised patients have a higher risk of disseminated histoplasmosis involving the liver, spleen, lymph nodes, bone marrow, adrenal glands, mucocutaneous tissues, gastrointestinal tract, and central nervous system. The chest radiograph may show a miliary reticulonodular appearance suggestive of tuberculosis. An acute sepsis syndrome with hypotension and disseminated intravascular coagulation, adrenal crisis, and meningitis are potential lethal complications.

A rapid diagnosis of histoplasmosis can be made by Giemsa staining of a peripheral blood smear of bone marrow aspirate demonstrating characteristic intracellular yeast forms. Lysis centrifugation is the preferred blood culture system. Antigen detection in blood and urine is a sensitive and specific method

in disseminated disease. Antibody detection may also be useful, but false-negative results may occur in immunocompromised patients. Biopsy specimens may show small intracellular or narrow budding yeasts suggestive of the diagnosis, which should be confirmed by culture. Severe pulmonary or disseminated histoplasmosis should be treated with an amphotericin B formulation. Prolonged therapy with itraconazole may be initiated after stabilization of disease and should probably be continued for the duration of immunosuppression.

Infection with *Coccidioides immitis* is endemic in the southwestern United States. In normal persons, infection is usually symptomatic or self-limited. In patients with compromised cell-mediated immunity, *C immitis* is likely to be more virulent. In an early review of *C immitis* infection in immunocompromised patients, disseminated disease occurred in almost half of the cases and was associated with a high mortality rate.[122] Progression of infection was often fulminant, and pulmonary disease frequently manifested after signs of dissemination.[122] Diagnosis is most easily established by serology or demonstration of pathognomonic spherules in sputum or tissue samples. Coccidioidomycosis can involve virtually any organ in disseminated disease but has a particular trophism for bone and the central nervous system. Treatment of disseminated disease generally requires amphotericin B followed by maintenance fluconazole. Intracisternal amphotericin B should be considered in cases of meningitis.

Pneumocystis jiroveci (carinii)

P jiroveci (formerly *P carinii*) is more appropriately classified as a fungus than as a protozoan based on gene sequence data and cell wall constituents. Defective T-cell immunity is the principal risk factor for *P jiroveci* pneumonia (PCP). Sepkowitz et al.[123] reported that corticosteroid use was associated with 204 of 227 cases of PCP (90%) in patients without AIDS at Memorial Sloan-Kettering Cancer Center. The median time that patients received corticosteroids was 2 months, although a minority of patients had received corticosteroids for less than 1 month. Approximately 60% of patients had hematologic malignancies, 25% had solid tumors, 10% were HSCT recipients, and 5% were receiving relatively mild immunosuppressive regimens.

P jiroveci infection can have a more fulminant course in non-AIDS than in AIDS patients, with more rapid progression to respiratory failure.[124] Patients treated with corticosteroids may develop initial clinical manifestations of PCP only during steroid taper. Bilateral interstitial infiltrates are most common in PCP, although unilateral or patchy infiltrates are also observed. Nodules, cavitary lesions, and pleural effusions are less common. In a minority of patients, the chest radiograph is normal. Extrapulmonary *P jiroveci* infection is very rare in patients with cancer and has for the most part been reported only in patients with AIDS.

Diagnosis of PCP relies on visualization of the organism microscopically. Immunofluorescent staining using monoclonal antibodies is more sensitive than cell wall staining methods, such as silver staining or Wright-Giemsa staining.[125] Spontaneously expectorated sputum is generally unsatisfactory for diagnosis, but sputum induction using 3% sodium chloride solution in an ultrasonic nebulizer may yield a satisfactory sample. In a small study of human immunodeficiency virus (HIV)–negative patients with PCP, the diagnostic sensitivity using this method was approximately 60%.[126] BAL is the standard diagnostic modality for PCP. BAL findings may be less sensitive in patients with cancer than in those with HIV infection because of reduced organism burden in HIV-negative patients. Quantitative PCR-based detection of *P jiroveci* in oral washes had acceptable sensitivity and specificity in HIV-infected patients and merits evaluation in other immunocompromised populations.[127]

Trimethoprim-sulfamethoxazole (trimethoprim: 15 mg/kg/d in three divided doses) is the treatment of choice for *P jiroveci* infection. In patients intolerant of this regimen, intravenous pentamidine, dapsone-trimethoprim, and clindamycin-primaquine are acceptable alternatives. Atovaquone may be used for mild to moderate PCP. In patients with moderate or severe PCP (room air PaO$_2$ of 75 torr or less), corticosteroids should be added based on studies of patients with AIDS-associated PCP.[128] In patients who are not responding to therapy, repeat bronchoscopy should be considered to exclude additional pathogens.

Trimethoprim-sulfamethoxazole is highly effective as prophylaxis against PCP. In children with cancer at high risk for PCP, trimethoprim-sulfamethoxazole administered daily or on 3 consecutive days weekly was fully protective, whereas an approximately 20% incidence of PCP was seen in placebo recipients.[129] Defining which patients with cancer will benefit from prophylaxis against *P jiroveci* is often empirical given the absence of controlled studies in several high-risk groups. Children with acute lymphoblastic leukemia and allogeneic HSCT recipients are known high-risk groups that should be offered prophylaxis. In HSCT recipients, the peak risk of PCP is between 1 and 4 months after transplantation, corresponding to the period of most profound T-cell immunodeficiency. Prophylaxis is generally administered shortly after engraftment until at least 6 months after HSCT but should be reinitiated at later periods in the setting of GVHD requiring use of immunosuppressive agents. Adults with acute lymphoblastic leukemia, patients with central nervous system tumors receiving high-dose corticosteroid therapy, and patients receiving corticosteroid therapy combined with either myelotoxic agents or fludarabine are also at high risk for PCP.

VIRAL INFECTIONS

The herpesviruses are the most important viral pathogens in patients with cancer. Pathogens include HSV-1 and HSV-2, varicella zoster virus (VZV), CMV, EBV, and human herpesvirus-6 (HHV-6). These DNA viruses establish a latent phase after primary infection, in which the viral genome resides in target cells for life with the potential to reactivate. Host defense against these viruses is dependent on viral-specific helper and cytotoxic T lymphocytes (CTLs), and thus both the likelihood of reactivation and the severity of disease are augmented during profound T-cell immunosuppression. Table 53-6 summarizes common antiviral agents used in persons with cancer. Detailed reviews and guidelines on prevention of opportunistic viral infections in HSCT recipients have been published.[31,130]

HERPES SIMPLEX VIRUS

HSV predominantly affects patients during profound neutropenia. Among seropositive patients, the incidence of HSV reactivation is approximately 70% after chemotherapy for leukemia[131] or conditioning for HSCT.[132] Among HSCT recipients, HSV disease is most likely to occur within the first month but may occur in later stages during intense immunosuppression.

Oropharyngeal HSV (mostly caused by HSV-1) during neutropenia may be severe, causing gingival disease, stomatitis, and cheilitis, clinically indistinguishable from mucositis after cytotoxic chemotherapy. An oral swab culture for HSV detects viral shedding, which suggests that HSV is contributing to mucosal disease. Local spread of HSV may cause esophagitis, tracheitis, or pneumonia. Documentation of pulmonary involvement requires a biopsy, because respiratory secretions may be contaminated by oral mucosal HSV. Disseminated HSV disease may involve the skin, liver (causing a necrotizing hepatitis), and brain. HSV-2 infection is more likely to cause genital and anal disease. HSV-1 seropositive allogeneic HSCT recipients with HSV-1–negative donors had more frequent and longer episodes of HSV reactivation than those with HSV-1–positive donors, which suggests that HSV-specific cellular immunity may be transferred.[133]

HSV is usually diagnosed by culture. Biopsy specimens show characteristic inclusions with positive results on immunohistochemistry. In patients with significant mucosal disease, it is safest to treat with intravenous acyclovir (5 mg/kg every 8 hours), switching to an oral regimen when the disease has become quiescent. Disseminated HSV disease should be treated with intravenous acyclovir (10 mg/kg every 8 hours).

In all HSV-seropositive patients receiving chemotherapy for acute leukemia[13] and in allogeneic HSCT recipients and in some autologous HSCT recipients at high risk for mucositis during the neutropenic period.[31] A longer period of prophylaxis should be considered in allogeneic HSCT recipients with GVHD or with frequent HSV reactivations before transplantation.[31] Acyclovir-resistant HSV is observed in HSCT recipients and appears to be more common in recipients of allografts from unrelated and HLA-mismatched donors.[130] When clinical acyclovir resistance is suspected, antiviral susceptibility testing of the isolate at a reference laboratory may be useful. Foscarnet is recommended as therapy for acyclovir-resistant HSV; acyclovir cross-resistance is expected with antiviral agents (e.g., famciclovir, ganciclovir) that target the viral thymidine kinase enzyme.

CYTOMEGALOVIRUS

Risk Factors, Clinical Manifestations, and Treatment

CMV is the most serious of the viral pathogens in HSCT recipients, with seropositive recipients at the greatest risk of developing CMV disease. Before the widespread adoption of prophylaxis against CMV, approximately 30% of seropositive transplant recipients developed CMV disease. Seronegative recipients may acquire primary CMV infection from a seropositive donor or from infected blood products. CMV pneumonia is observed in nontransplant patients with leukemia but is uncommon. Risk factors include potent immunosuppressive therapy and granulocyte transfusions from unscreened donors.[134]

CMV-specific T-cell–mediated immunity after allogeneic HSCT is key for protection against CMV disease. Seropositive patients who receive T-cell–depleted allografts or who are treated with agents that deplete T cells (e.g., antithymocyte immunoglobulin, OKT3, alemtuzumab) to prevent or treat GVHD are at increased

TABLE 53-6. Antiviral Agents Commonly Used to Treat Immunocompromised Patients with Cancer

Disease	Antiviral Therapy[a]	Comments
Mucocutaneous herpes	Acyclovir, 5 mg/kg q8h (IV)	—
Acyclovir resistant	Foscarnet, 40 mg/kg q8h (IV)	Antiviral testing available at reference laboratories.
Prophylaxis	Acyclovir, 400 mg t.i.d. (PO)	—
Herpes (disseminated or visceral organ involvement)	Acyclovir, 10 mg/kg q8h (IV)	—
Herpes encephalitis	Acyclovir, 10–12 mg/kg q8h (IV)	PCR of spinal fluid diagnostic method of choice.
Chickenpox	Acyclovir, 10 mg/kg q8h (IV)	—
Herpes zoster		
Single dermatome	Acyclovir, 800 mg 5 times daily or Valacyclovir, 1 g t.i.d (PO) or Famciclovir, 500 mg t.i.d. (PO)	—
>1 Dermatome or disseminated	Acyclovir, 10 mg/kg q8h (IV)	—
Cytomegalovirus (CMV) disease	Ganciclovir, 5 mg/kg q12h (IV) or	Add IV immunoglobulin in cases of pneumonia.
	Foscarnet, 60 mg/kg q8h (IV)	Use foscarnet for ganciclovir-resistant infection and consider in patients with borderline ANC (e.g., <1500/μL).
Prophylaxis (HSCT recipients)	Ganciclovir, 5 mg/kg q12h for 5 d then daily (IV) or	Prophylaxis is typically administered until at least d 100 of HSCT; ganciclovir is started after ANC recovery.
	Acyclovir, 500 mg/m² q8h (IV) for first month, then 800 mg q.i.d. (PO) or	Valganciclovir (prodrug of ganciclovir) merits further evaluation as CMV prophylaxis.
	Valacyclovir, 2 g q.i.d. (PO)	—
Preemptive therapy	Ganciclovir, 5 mg/kg q12h (IV) for 2 wk followed by 5 mg/kg daily 5 d/wk × 2 wk or to d 100 of HSCT or	—
	Foscarnet, 60 mg/kg q12h (IV) for 2 wk followed by 90 mg/kg daily 5 d/wk for 2 wk	—
Influenza	Oseltamivir, 75 mg b.i.d. (PO)	—
	Rimantadine, 200 mg q.d. (PO) or	—
	Amantadine, 100 mg q.d. (PO)	—
Respiratory syncytial virus infection	Ribavirin, 6 g/300 mL water, by aerosol 18 h/d	Some investigators add pooled intravenous immunoglobulin or palivizumab (see text).
Parainfluenza virus infection	Supportive care	—
Adenovirus infection	Cidofovir, 3–5 mg/kg weekly × 2, then every other week	Requires probenecid and hydration; gastroenteritis and cystitis are generally self-limiting and do not require therapy; consider for pneumonia or disseminated disease, although benefit not established.
Chronic hepatitis B	Lamivudine, 100 mg q.d. (PO)	Add or switch to adefovir in cases of resistance.
Chronic hepatitis C	Pegylated interferon-α weekly (SC) and ribavirin b.i.d. (PO)	See http://www.va.gov/hepatitisc for dosing.
Parvovirus B19 infection	Intravenous immunoglobulin (see text)	—

ANC, absolute neutrophil count; HSCT, hematopoietic stem cell transplant; PCR, polymerase chain reaction.
[a]Dosages are for adults with normal renal function.

risk for CMV disease. Hakki et al.[135] showed that CD4+ and CD8+ counts of fewer than 100×10^9/L and 50×10^9/L, respectively; bone marrow as the source of stem cells (peripheral stem cell allografts contain approximately ten times more lymphocytes than bone marrow allografts); and high-dose corticosteroids predicted reduced reconstitution of CMV-specific T-cell immunity at 3 months after allogeneic HSCT.

Among partially T-cell–depleted allogeneic HSCT recipients receiving either preemptive or prophylactic ganciclovir, recipient CMV seropositivity was an adverse risk factor for overall and transplant-related mortality when allografts were from HLA-matched unrelated, but not matched related, donors.[32] Use of a lower dose of antithymocyte immunoglobulin for T-cell depletion appeared to be associated with a better outcome among CMV-seropositive recipients receiving allografts from matched unrelated donors.[136]

Nichols et al.[137] evaluated the effect of CMV serostatus of donors and recipients on mortality among 1750 non–T-cell–depleted allogeneic HSCT recipients in the era of preemptive antiviral therapy. Allografts from CMV-seropositive donors into CMV-seronegative recipients were associated with the highest mortality. This was principally connected with increased bacterial and fungal infections, which suggests an adverse immunomodulatory effect of primary CMV infection.

Ljungman et al.[138] evaluated the effect of CMV donor serostatus on transplant outcome in 7018 CMV-seropositive allogeneic HSCT recipients enrolled in the European Group for Blood and Marrow Transplantation program. Patients receiving allografts from unrelated CMV-seropositive donors had increased overall survival and reduced transplant-related mortality compared to recipient of allografts from unrelated seronegative donors, which suggests that transfer of CMV-specific immunity from donor to recipient may be of benefit.

CMV disease is far less frequent in autologous HSCT recipients, but no less severe. CD34-selected autologous stem cell transplantation is associated with a greater risk of CMV disease than conventional nonselected peripheral stem cell transplantation.[139] The period of risk in autologous transplantation is generally confined to the first 3 months, corresponding to the period of reconstitution of T-cell immunity.

CMV infection, either primary or reactivated, can have protean manifestations. These range from asymptomatic viral shedding, to a self-limited mononucleosis-like syndrome, to life-threatening organ disease. Pulmonary disease typically manifests as an interstitial pneumonitis resembling PCP with hypoxia and progression to respiratory failure. A definitive diagnosis of CMV pneumonitis requires a compatible clinical syndrome plus the histologic documentation of either characteristic CMV inclusions within parenchymal tissue or intracellular inclusions within epithelial cells obtained by BAL. Because CMV can be shed from pulmonary secretions without causing invasive disease, CMV cultured from pulmonary secretions does not definitively indicate CMV disease. However, in an allogeneic HSCT recipient with a compatible chest radiograph, such documentation of CMV infection in the absence of cytologic or histologic evidence of disease should prompt anti-CMV therapy, given the high likelihood of CMV disease.

Both infectious and noninfectious processes may masquerade as, or occur in addition to, pulmonary CMV disease. In one study of late CMV pneumonia (occurring after day 100 of transplantation), approximately half of the cases were associated with concurrent pulmonary infections, including infection with *P aeruginosa*, *Legionella*, *Aspergillus*, *Mycobacteria*, *Nocardia*, *Toxoplasma*, or respiratory viruses.[140] Therefore, diffuse interstitial disease in an HSCT recipient should be evaluated early with BAL and, if feasible, transbronchial biopsy (see Pulmonary Infiltrates, later in this chapter).

Treatment of CMV pneumonia consists of ganciclovir or foscarnet plus immunoglobulin. The expected mortality rate when immunoglobulin therapy is added is between 30% and 50%, which is significantly improved compared with prior series in which ganciclovir alone was used.[141] The addition of immunoglobulin in cases of CMV gastrointestinal disease does not appear to affect outcome.[142] Combination ganciclovir and foscarnet therapy has been used principally in AIDS-associated CMV retinitis, but a limited database exists in allogeneic HSCT recipients. The combination appears to be well tolerated and should be considered in refractory cases. Cidofovir may be considered in cases of CMV disease after failure of or intolerance to ganciclovir or foscarnet.[143] Cidofovir is associated with significant nephrotoxicity, and additional studies are needed before it can be considered for use as initial therapy or in preemptive strategies.

CMV disease can occur at any location within the gastrointestinal tract. In the esophagus, ulcerations resembling HSV or candidal esophagitis occur. Definitive identification of CMV in these cases relies on biopsy or cytologic analysis. CMV colitis is associated with abdominal pain and diarrhea. CMV involvement of enteric vessels may result in hemorrhage and infarction. Treatment of CMV gastroenteritis with ganciclovir suppressed viral replication but produced no clinical benefit or endoscopic improvement compared with placebo.[144] CMV hepatitis should be considered in the setting of fever and elevations of liver enzymes. Other potential viral causes include HSV-1 and HSV-2, hepatitis viruses, and EBV. Analysis of a liver biopsy specimen documenting CMV inclusions is diagnostic. Less common sites of CMV disease in HSCT recipients include the pancreas, brain, spinal cord (transverse myelitis), and adrenals. CMV retinitis, the most common complication in patients with AIDS, is uncommon in transplant recipients. A CMV syndrome associated with fever, pancytopenia, and CMV viremia may precede the development of organ disease.

Prevention of Cytomegalovirus Disease

Because of the high mortality associated with CMV disease, much effort has been focused on prevention. In CMV-seronegative allogeneic HSCT recipients, primary CMV infection may be transmitted from the allograft if the donor is CMV seropositive or from transfusion products. CMV-seronegative HSCT recipients receiving allografts from CMV-seronegative donors should receive only transfusion products from CMV-negative donors or leukocyte-depleted products to avoid primary CMV infection. Use of filtered red blood cell transfusions from CMV-seropositive donors is associated with a small but significant increase in CMV transmission compared with restricting the transfusion product donor pool to CMV-seronegative persons.[145] Therefore, in centers that use filtered red cell products in CMV-seronegative allogeneic HSCT recipients, CMV surveillance appears to be warranted.

The following preventative approaches have been evaluated in allogeneic HSCT recipients at risk for CMV reactivation[141]: (1) prophylaxis: antiviral agents are administered to all CMV-seropositive HSCT recipients (CMV-seronegative recipients receiving seropositive bone marrow were also candidates for antiviral prophylaxis in some studies); and (2) preemptive therapy: initiation of antiviral agents after detection of asymptomatic CMV infection by screening cultures or by molecular testing.

Prophylaxis

In two randomized studies, acyclovir prophylaxis was associated with increased survival, but the rates of CMV reactivation and disease were fairly high.[146,147] Ljungman et al.[148] compared oral valacyclovir (a valine esterified analogue of acyclovir with high oral bioavailability) with acyclovir for prophylaxis in allogeneic HSCT recipients in whom the donor or recipient was CMV seropositive. All patients received initial intravenous acyclovir until day 28 after transplantation or until discharge, and then either oral valacyclovir (2 g four times daily) or acyclovir (800 mg four times daily) until week 18 after transplantation. Oral valacyclovir was more effective than oral acyclovir in preventing asymptomatic CMV reactivation (28% vs. 40%, respectively); there was no difference in CMV disease, adverse events, or overall survival. Thus, valacyclovir and high-dose oral acyclovir are each acceptable agents for CMV prophylaxis, but neither agent obviates the need for surveillance and preemptive therapy with ganciclovir or foscarnet. Winston et al. showed that oral valacyclovir (2 g four times daily) had similar efficacy compared to standard intravenous ganciclovir as prophylaxis in allogeneic HSCT recipients after neutrophil recovery.[148a]

In vitro, ganciclovir, an acyclic nucleoside analogue of guanosine, is approximately 50 times more active against CMV than acyclovir. Two randomized placebo-controlled studies of ganciclovir prophylaxis in CMV-seropositive allogeneic transplant recipients produced similar results.[149,150] Ganciclovir prophylaxis was highly effective at suppressing CMV during the early transplantation period but was associated with higher rates of neutropenia, bacterial and opportunistic infections, and late CMV disease. Ganciclovir prophylaxis did not lead to an improvement in survival.

Nguyen et al.[140] retrospectively reviewed 541 adult allogeneic HSCT patients who had received ganciclovir prophylaxis.

Thirty-five episodes of CMV pneumonia were documented, 26 (74%) of which occurred after day 100. The mortality rate was approximately 75%. Almost all cases of late CMV pneumonia occurred in patients who had GVHD or who had received T-cell–depleted transplants. Reconstitution of CMV-specific T-cell responses was delayed in allogeneic HSCT recipients who received ganciclovir prophylaxis, which conceivably predisposed such patients to late CMV disease.

Preemptive Therapy

Highly sensitive methods for early diagnosis of CMV include detection of the CMV pp65 antigen in peripheral blood leukocytes and detection of CMV DNA by PCR. A single positive finding of CMV antigenemia or two consecutive positive PCR results are triggers for preemptive antiviral therapy. Preemptive ganciclovir therapy based on detection of CMV antigenemia is associated with a similar rate of CMV disease and similar long-term survival rate as for ganciclovir prophylaxis initiated at engraftment.[151]

Einsele et al.[152] randomly assigned allogeneic HSCT recipients to receive preemptive ganciclovir therapy based on PCR detection of CMV in blood or a positive CMV culture (of blood, urine, or throat washings). PCR screening led to earlier detection of subclinical CMV infection than did culture. The PCR screening group had a lower rate of CMV disease, shorter duration of ganciclovir therapy, and lower rates of neutropenia and nonviral infections than the culture group, and overall survival was superior. Discontinuing preemptive ganciclovir therapy in patients whose blood PCR test results became negative appeared to be safe.

Foscarnet and ganciclovir had similar efficacy as preemptive CMV therapy in allogeneic HSCT recipients, but ganciclovir was associated significantly more often with premature discontinuation due to either neutropenia or thrombocytopenia.[153] Renal impairment was observed in only 5% of foscarnet recipients. The frequency of antiviral drug resistance has remained low. However, in the setting of intense immunosuppression for GVHD and prolonged ganciclovir use, the incidence of ganciclovir resistance may be as high as 8%.[154] A rising level of CMV antigenemia early after initiation of preemptive ganciclovir therapy is frequently observed, particularly in patients receiving high-dose corticosteroids, and does not per se indicate resistance to ganciclovir. Continuing or reinitiating ganciclovir induction therapy (5 mg/kg twice daily) appears to be warranted.[155]

Late CMV disease remains a persistent problem in the era of preemptive therapy. In a prospective cohort study, high CMV viral load, lymphopenia, and CMV-specific T-cell immunodeficiency were predictors of late CMV disease and death in seropositive allogeneic HSCT recipients.[156] In a case-control study, CMV disease was significantly delayed after nonmyeloablative compared with standard ablative allogeneic transplantation (median time, 132 vs. 52 days, respectively); interestingly, the overall 1-year incidence was similar in the two groups.[157] The CDC recommends continued CMV surveillance until 1 year after transplantation in high-risk allogeneic HSCT recipients, which include those with chronic GVHD, low CD4+ count (fewer than 50/µL), and CMV infection before day 100 after HSCT.[31]

VARICELLA ZOSTER VIRUS

HSCT recipients and patients receiving intensive steroid therapy are at risk for life-threatening disseminated primary and reacti-

vated VZV infection. Reactivated VZV disease is typically a late complication of allogeneic HSCT, usually occurring 3 months to a year after transplantation. The major risk factor for developing reactivated VZV in allogeneic HSCT recipients is acute and chronic GVHD requiring intensive immunosuppressive therapy.

In immunocompromised patients, VZV infection may manifest with a multidermatomal or disseminated vesicular exanthem associated with hemorrhage and necrosis. Secondary bacterial infections, usually with *Streptococcus pyogenes*, may occur. Infection of viscera can cause hemorrhagic pneumonia, encephalitis, retinal necrosis, hepatitis, and small bowel disease. The diagnosis of cutaneous herpes zoster can usually be made by visual inspection alone. Immunofluorescent staining of material from an unroofed skin lesion or from a skin biopsy can establish the diagnosis within hours. A Tzanck preparation can confirm infection by a herpesvirus but is not specific for VZV.

Intravenous acyclovir (10 mg/kg every 8 hours) is the established treatment for primary varicella (chickenpox) or disseminated herpes zoster. Early initiation of acyclovir therapy reduces progression of disease and usually eliminates mortality. For localized dermatomal herpes zoster, an oral regimen consisting of acyclovir (800 mg five times per day), valacyclovir (1 g three times per day), or famciclovir (500 mg three times daily) is advised. Such patients must be monitored closely for signs of progressive herpes zoster and for streptococcal superinfection. Salicylates should not be used because of the risk of Reye's syndrome.

Lack of a clinical response to therapy should prompt reconsideration of the initial diagnosis and suggest the possibility of a secondary infection or VZV resistance to acyclovir. Resistance of VZV to acyclovir may be increased in HSCT recipients who have received prolonged courses of acyclovir or ganciclovir as prophylaxis for CMV infection. However, in one study of acyclovir prophylaxis against CMV, the small proportion of patients who developed VZV disease were successfully treated with high-dose acyclovir, which indicates that either antiviral resistance did not occur or could be overcome by intensification of the acyclovir regimen.[146]

Prolonged antiviral prophylaxis after allogeneic HSCT to prevent VZV reactivation is controversial. Long-term prophylaxis with higher-dose acyclovir (800 mg twice daily) for 1 year after allogeneic HSCT appeared to prevent VZV reactivation.[158] In a randomized study of acyclovir prophylaxis for CMV, the rate of VZV at day 210 after transplantation was only 3% in patients receiving prolonged high-dose acyclovir.[146] Valacyclovir (500 mg twice daily for prophylaxis) is being used increasingly because of its improved bioavailability. Thrombotic thrombocytopenic purpura observed in patients with AIDS treated with valacyclovir has not been observed in trials of valacyclovir therapy in HSCT recipients.[31]

Nosocomial transmission of VZV is well documented. Patients with chickenpox, those with disseminated herpes zoster, and immunocompromised patients with dermatomal herpes zoster should be placed in contact and respiratory isolation (private negative-pressure room, air exhausted to outside, six or more air exchanges per hour). Varicella zoster immune globulin (VZIG) should be offered to immunosuppressed VZV-seronegative patients after exposures such as prolonged face-to-face contact, a household or playmate contact, or exposure to an infected roommate in a shared hospital room. VZIG should be administered within 96 hours after exposure. The role for chemoprophylaxis after exposure is undefined, but it appears reasonable.

The current varicella vaccine uses the live attenuated Oka strain (Merck). Although the varicella vaccine has been shown to be safe in children with leukemia, its use is contraindicated in immuncompromised persons except in a research protocol. Household contacts and health care workers who have no history of chickenpox and are seronegative for VZV should receive the vaccine to prevent infection by wild-type VZV.[31] If a rash occurs after vaccination, direct contact with immunocompromised persons should be avoided. If inadvertent contact occurs, the use of VZIG is not recommended because of the low transmission rate and the expectation that disease will be mild if it occurs. An outbreak of chickenpox was reported at a day-care center despite vaccination, which indicates that vaccination conferred poor protection in an outbreak setting in healthy children and that breakthrough chickenpox in children remained highly infectious.[159]

An inactivated varicella vaccine was safe and effective in reducing the frequency of herpes zoster in patients with lymphoma undergoing autologous HSCT, and protection correlated with reconstitution of VZV-specific CD4+ T-cell immunity.[160]

EPSTEIN-BARR VIRUS

In the United States, most adults have been infected by EBV. Primary infection is usually asymptomatic but may cause a mononucleosis syndrome. Latent infection persists in B cells and produces no disease in the vast majority of people. EBV-specific CTLs are the principal controllers of the replication of EBV-infected B cells. EBV lymphoproliferative disorders are encountered in patients with severely impaired T-cell immunity, such as those who have AIDS or undergo intensive and prolonged immunosuppressive therapy. EBV-induced PTLD is defined as an abnormal proliferation of B-lymphoid cells in a transplant recipient. The lesions may be composed of polyclonal or monoclonal populations of transformed B cells. PTLD is most common between 1 and 6 months after allogeneic HSCT. Immunosuppressive therapy for GVHD and use of T-cell–depleted allografts increase the risk of PTLD.

Clinical manifestations of PTLD are varied, and a high index of suspicion is required. Patients may have a mononucleosis-like syndrome with fever and localized adenopathy. Disseminated disease may manifest with generalized adenopathy and extranodal organ involvement, including the bowel, liver, bone marrow, and central nervous system. A CT scan of the head, chest, abdomen, and pelvis is useful in a high-risk patient with unexplained fever. Diagnosis of PTLD requires a biopsy specimen showing the characteristic histology and evidence of EBV infection by immunohistochemistry or EBV DNA detection.

Whereas PTLD in organ transplant recipients typically responds to a reduction in the intensity of immunosuppression, PTLD in HSCT recipients may not respond to such conservative measures. Antiviral therapy for PTLD has generally been disappointing. Although antiviral agents may attenuate the lytic cycle of EBV and reduce the frequency of new B-cell clones, they do not affect the replication of EBV-transformed PTLD B cells. Thus, serum EBV DNA levels may paradoxically increase during antiviral therapy. Other strategies include intravenous immunoglobulin, low-dose chemotherapy, anti–IL-6, rituximab (a monoclonal antibody therapy targeted to the B-cell epitope CD20), and donor lymphocyte infusions. Adoptive immunotherapy using donor-derived EBV-specific cytotoxic T-lymphocyte clones is another promising strategy (see Immune Augmentation Strategies, later in this chapter).

HUMAN HERPESVIRUS-6

HHV-6 was first isolated from peripheral blood of patients with lymphoproliferative disorders.[161] This virus was initially called *human B-lymphotrophic virus*, but it was later discovered that the virus is predominantly T-cell trophic. HHV-6 has been recognized as an opportunistic pathogen in solid organ and HSCT recipients. In HSCT recipients, HHV-6 has been associated with a variety of syndromes: fever and rash clinically resembling cutaneous GVHD, bone marrow suppression, encephalitis, and pneumonitis. However, establishing a causal relationship between HHV-6 and these syndromes is made difficult by the fact that HHV-6 is present in the saliva and whole blood of approximately 50% of HSCT recipients—usually between 2 and 4 weeks after transplantation. The evidence supporting a link between HHV-6 infection and encephalitis[162] and interstitial pneumonitis[163] is the most persuasive, based on the *in situ* documentation of HHV-6 in the respective organs using immunohistochemistry, molecular detection methods, and culture. Central nervous system infection may occur in the early and later transplantation periods and is associated with mental status changes, fever, headaches, seizures, focal neurologic deficits, and low-attenuation lesions in the posterior cerebral lobes on MRI. Hippocampal involvement with confusion and memory impairment may occur.

HHV-6 inhibits marrow progenitors *in vitro* and likely has a marrow-suppressive effect *in vivo*. HHV-6 viral load was significantly correlated with delayed platelet engraftment and with the number of platelet transfusions required in allogeneic HSCT recipients.[164] Among allogeneic HSCT recipients, peripheral HHV-6 levels are higher in recipients of allografts from unrelated donors[164] and cord blood,[165] which supports a role for cellular immunity in control of infection.

Singh and Carrigan[166] proposed the following two criteria for the diagnosis of HHV-6 disease: (1) presence of bone marrow suppression, encephalitis, or pneumonitis; and (2) documentation of active infection by culture, PCR testing of an acellular specimen (a positive PCR result from blood cannot distinguish active from latent infection), or immunohistochemistry.

Comparative studies evaluating therapy for HHV-6 have not been performed, and it is therefore not possible to make definitive recommendations about treatment. HHV-6 is sensitive *in vitro* to ganciclovir and foscarnet, and it is reasonable to initiate therapy with either of these agents when HHV-6 disease is proven or strongly suspected. The role of screening for asymptomatic HHV-6 infection and prophylaxis with antiviral agents is unknown.

COMMUNITY RESPIRATORY VIRUSES

Community respiratory viruses include members of the families Orthomyxoviridae (influenza A, B, and C) and Paramyxoviridae (parainfluenza 1 to 4, RSV, and measles), as well as adenoviruses and rhinoviruses. These viruses are important causes of morbidity and mortality in immunocompromised patients. In the era of prophylactic and preemptive therapy for CMV, the proportion of pulmonary infections caused by community respiratory viruses is likely to increase. These viruses are seasonal and are rapidly transmitted from one person to another by respiratory secretions, so the potential exists for nosocomial outbreaks.

Respiratory viruses may account for a significant proportion of undiagnosed or "idiopathic" pneumonias in HSCT recipients in older series. Their importance as pathogens in this population has been documented more recently by centers that routinely screen for community viral pathogens in patients with respiratory illnesses. Immuncompromised persons with symptoms of respiratory infection should be evaluated for respiratory viruses, among other causes, and contact precautions should be considered. Rapid immunodiagnostic methods for common respiratory viruses are widely used and effective. Such rapid methods also have additional potential benefits for early initiation of antiviral agents and implementation of appropriate infection control precautions. Cell culture is generally more sensitive than antigen-detection methods, with the exception of RSV in children, for which antigen detection is highly sensitive. Rapid antigen-detection methods and cell culture are therefore complementary. The CDC has issued guidelines on prevention of community respiratory viral infections.[31]

Respiratory Syncytial Virus

RSV infection is most virulent in patients with leukemia and in HSCT recipients. In patients with leukemia, progression to pneumonia and mortality are more common in the setting of neutropenia.[167] RSV infection can occur throughout the transplantation period—from the preengraftment stage to more than a year after transplantation—although RSV infection in the late transplantation period may have a less aggressive course.[168]

Upper respiratory tract symptoms (sinusitis, coryza, rhinorrhea) usually precede lower respiratory tract involvement (dyspnea, wheezing) and pneumonia but may be absent. The historic mortality from RSV pneumonia in HSCT recipients is approximately 80%.[169] In a preliminary study, patients who received aerosolized ribavirin and intravenous immune globulin containing high RSV-neutralizing titers at least 24 hours before respiratory failure had a 22% mortality rate compared with 100% mortality in patients who either did not receive therapy or in whom treatment was initiated after respiratory failure had occurred.[170]

Rapid diagnosis of RSV is possible by antigen-detection methods. Englund et al.[171] showed that, compared with culture, antigen detection had a sensitivity of 89% in BAL specimens, 15% in nasal-throat washings, and 71% in endotracheal aspirates in symptomatic adult leukemia or HSCT patients. The specificity was 97% to 100% for testing of specimens from these sources. The lower sensitivity of antigen detection in specimens from the upper airway of adults is attributed to a lower viral burden. The low yield of upper airway specimen cultures limits the value of these noninvasive tests in adults with respiratory disease.

In a preliminary study, intravenous ribavirin for treatment of RSV pneumonia in HSCT recipients who at enrollment did not require mechanical ventilation was associated with an eventual 80% mortality rate.[172] In a second strategy, aerosolized ribavirin was administered to patients in whom RSV was isolated from nasopharyngeal washes who had no signs of lower respiratory tract involvement. Pneumonia developed in 8 of 25 patients (32%), and the mortality rate was 29%.[169] These studies suggest that early diagnosis and treatment of RSV in this population may be life-saving. The RSV-specific monoclonal antibody palivizumab appeared to be safe and well tolerated in HSCT recipients with RSV infection in phase I studies[173] and may be considered as adjunctive therapy. There are insufficient data to recommend palivizumab as prophylaxis.

Parainfluenza Viruses

Parainfluenza viruses are important community respiratory viruses in leukemia and HSCT patients. In a review of 45 cases of parainfluenza virus infection in HSCT recipients, 26 patients (58%) had pneumonia, of whom 39% died.[174] Nichols et al.[175] reported parainfluenza virus infections in 7% of HSCT recipients. Approximately 80% of these infections were community acquired, and receipt of a transplant from an unrelated donor was the only independent risk factor. Coexistent pulmonary pathogens were isolated in approximately half of the cases. Treatment with aerosolized ribavirin with or without immunoglobulin did not appear to affect clinical outcome.

Influenza Virus

Influenza virus is the most important respiratory virus globally and the most common cause of excess seasonal mortality in North America (approximately 20,000 deaths in the United States annually). During a winter outbreak period, influenza was diagnosed in approximately 30% of adult patients hospitalized for a respiratory illness at the M. D. Anderson Cancer Center.[174] Pneumonia occurred in 12 of 15 patients (80%) with influenza, and 4 of these patients died. In other centers, the incidence of pneumonia and mortality associated with influenza virus infection was substantially lower.[169]

Amantadine and rimantadine are active against influenza A but not influenza B. In one center, resistance to these agents rapidly developed during therapy for influenza A among patients with leukemia and HSCT recipients.[176] The neuraminidase inhibitors zanamivir and oseltamivir are active against both influenza A and B. They are effective in reducing the duration of influenza illness if started early after onset of symptoms and have a prophylactic benefit during community outbreaks.[177,178] In one series, oseltamivir was found to be safe and appeared to be effective against influenza infection in HSCT recipients.[179] The role of these agents as treatment or prophylaxis in immunocompromised patients with cancer merits further evaluation.

The CDC advises annual administration of the inactivated influenza vaccine to immunocompromised persons and their close contacts (e.g., health care workers and household members). Immunocompromised persons are less likely to mount an adequate antibody response to immunization. Immunization should be provided ideally 2 weeks before chemotherapy. If given during chemotherapy, immunization is preferably administered between cycles. Use of the inhaled live attenuated influenza vaccine FluMist is contraindicated in the immunocompromised patient. Use of the injected inactivated vaccine is preferred for close contacts of immuncompromised patients, including health care workers (http://www.cdc.gov/nip/flu).

Adenovirus

The clinical manifestations of adenovirus infection in HSCT recipients include pneumonia, bronchiolitis, upper respiratory tract infection, renal parenchymal disease, hemorrhagic cystitis, hepatitis, small and large bowel disease, encephalitis, and disseminated infection. Viral shedding in throat secretions, urine, and stool is common, occurring in 5% to 20% of HSCT recipients, and should not be equated with disease. Gastroenteritis and hemorrhagic cystitis are usually self-limited, whereas pneumonia and disseminated disease are associated with a high mortality rate. In a prospective cohort study, adenovirus infection occurred in 41 of 437 allogeneic HSCT recipients (9%).[180] Patients with adenovirus infection were younger and were more likely to have received a transplant from an unrelated donor and to have GVHD. Ribavirin[174] and cidofovir[180,181] have been used for severe adenoviral infections in HSCT recipients, but the database is too small to make conclusions about benefit.

Rhinoviruses

Rhinoviruses are frequent causes of the common cold in immunocompetent persons. The published database on rhinoviral infections in the severely immunocompromised is very limited. In patients with prolonged myelosuppression and in HSCT recipients, rhinoviruses can cause pneumonia with significant morbidity and mortality.[182] Rhinoviral infections often coexist with bacterial and opportunistic infections, which makes the mortality attributable to rhinoviruses difficult to estimate.

Measles Virus

Kaplan et al.[183] conducted an extensive review of measles in immunocompromised patients. Of 40 patients with malignancy (aged 3 months to 22 years), 16 (40%) had no rash, whereas the remainder had either typical or atypical exanthems. Twenty-three (58%) had pneumonitis, 8 (20%) had encephalitis, 6 (20%) had both, and 6 (20%) had no complications. A finding of giant cell pneumonia on histopathologic analysis should raise the concern for measles. The overall fatality rate was 55%. The benefit of ribavirin therapy could not be assessed.

In the developed world, the risk of measles among the immunocompromised is highest during local community outbreaks and potentially after travel to countries where measles is endemic. The measles-mumps-rubella vaccine contains live attenuated viruses and should not be administered to severely immunocompromised persons; if these persons are exposed to measles, immunoglobulin should be administered regardless of prior vaccination status. There is no contraindication to measles-mumps-rubella immunization of healthy household members. Guidelines on administration of measles-mumps-rubella vaccine to HSCT recipients have been published by the CDC.[31]

PARVOVIRUS B19

Parvovirus B19 is a DNA virus that is transmitted via respiratory secretions and blood products, and vertically from mother to fetus. It is the cause of erythema infectiosum (fifth disease), a common, self-limiting febrile exanthem. Infection in immunocompromised persons unable to mount a protective antibody response may cause chronic pure red cell aplasia. Isolated anemia, thrombocytopenia, or pancytopenia may occur. Predisposing conditions include acute and chronic leukemias, myelodysplastic syndrome, lymphoma, HSCT, potent antineoplastic chemotherapy, and systemic steroids.[184] Particularly among children with acute lymphoblastic leukemia, parvovirus B19 infection may mimic leukemic relapse or chemotherapy-induced cytopenia, leading to persistent abnormalities of hematopoiesis.[184] Parvovirus B19 may also cause a virus-associated hemophagocytic syndrome, characterized by fever, histiocytic hyperplasia, and cytopenia.

Diagnosis of parvovirus B19 infection in the immuncompromised patient relies on PCR detection of viral DNA in serum; antibody responses may be disabled in these patients. Treatment consists of intravenous immunoglobulin.

HEPATITIS VIRUSES

Hepatitis B Virus

Abnormalities in liver test results are common in patients with cancer. Among HSCT recipients, the differential diagnosis is broad and includes drug toxicity, GVHD, venoocclusive disease, recurrent malignancy, and infectious hepatitis. Patients who receive multiple transfusions of blood and pooled plasma products may be at a higher risk for transfusion-associated viral hepatitis, despite the highly effective screening methods currently used to test blood products.

Reactivation of latent hepatitis B virus (HBV) is a well-recognized complication in patients with chronic HBV infection receiving cytotoxic or immunosuppressive therapy. In a prospective study of 100 Chinese patients who received induction chemotherapy for lymphoma, hepatitis developed in 67% of patients positive for the hepatitis B surface antigen (HB_sAg) compared to 14% of HB_sAg-negative patients.[185] Reactivation of HBV (as determined by serum levels of HBV DNA and hepatitis B e antigen) was associated with icteric hepatitis, but infrequently with liver failure and mortality. In a prospective study of 305 patients with lymphoma, the prevalence of hepatitis C virus (HCV) and HBV infection was 16% and 3.2%, respectively. No reactivation in HCV-positive patients occurred during chemotherapy. In contrast, HBV reactivation occurred in approximately 80% of HBV-infected patients and was associated with a 37% mortality rate. Thus, HBV should be considered to be an opportunistic pathogen in heavily immunosuppressed persons with hematologic malignancies.

Symptomatic hepatitis may manifest after withdrawal of immunosuppressive agents or between cycles of chemotherapy when recovery of immune responses occurs.[186] This reactivation is most likely due to an increase in HBV synthesis during immunosuppressive therapy followed by a rebound in host immune responses to HBV infection when therapy is stopped.

Although the HB_sAg carrier state is not a contraindication to HSCT, such patients may be at a higher risk for fulminant hepatitis as a result of reactivation. HBV reactivation manifesting as an elevation in liver-associated enzyme levels is common in both allogeneic and autologous HSCT recipients. In one series, significant liver disease was more severe and occurred earlier after transplantation in autologous HSCT recipients than in allogeneic HSCT recipients, but only 1 of 33 patients (3%) died of liver failure.[187] Among HB_sAg-positive autologous HSCT recipients, the pretransplantation HBV DNA viral load was the most important risk factor for posttransplantation HBV reactivation.[188] Lowering the HBV viral load with antiviral agents in patients with chronic HBV infection undergoing transplantation should be considered. In a small randomized study, lamivudine (100 mg daily) starting 1 week before until 52 weeks after allogeneic HSCT significantly reduced HBV exacerbation.[189]

Chronic HBV hepatitis has been reported in patients with negative results on serologic studies. Vergani et al.[190] reported 23 cases of histologically proven HBV infection in children with leukemia and liver disease, none of whom had detectable HBV serum antigens or antibodies. In eight of the children, HBV markers subsequently appeared in the serum within 15 months of cessation of chemotherapy. Bréchot et al.[191] documented HBV DNA in 59% of liver samples but in only 10% of serum samples in patients with chronic liver disease and negative test results for HB$_s$Ag. The process of "reverse seroconversion" in which HBV reactivation occurs in patients with prior HBV immunity (hepatitis B surface antibody and core antibody positive) is uncommon but well described in allogeneic HSCT recipients.[192]

Vaccination against HBV should be considered in seronegative patients with cancer. However, among HSCT recipients, active immunization in the immediately pretransplantation and posttransplantation periods is often ineffective as a result of defective T-cell and B-cell function. Adoptive transfer of T-cell immunity specific to HBV can be achieved after allogeneic HSCT from immune donors and was associated with resolution of HBV infection in HSCT recipients with pretransplantation chronic HBV infection.[193] This suggests that HBV immunization of non–HBV-infected allogeneic HSCT donors may confer protection in recipients with preexisting chronic HBV infection.

Hepatitis C Virus

Before routine blood screening began in 1991, HSCT recipients were at significant risk for HCV infection. HCV infection can cause both early and late complications in HSCT recipients. In a longitudinal cohort study, pretransplantation HCV infection plus an elevated serum aspartate transaminase level predicted severe venoocclusive disease (relative risk, 9.6),[194] whereas HCV infection without elevated transaminase levels did not. An acute flare of hepatitis occurred in approximately one-third of HCV-positive patients 4 to 5 months after transplantation and was usually self-limited.[194] Frickhofen et al.[195] also noted an association between pretransplantation HCV infection and severe venoocclusive disease in the early transplantation period.

Approximately one-half of HCV-positive transplant recipients continue to have mild to moderate elevations in liver enzyme levels 5 to 10 years after transplantation.[194] Cirrhosis was identified in approximately 1% of all HSCT recipients surviving 1 year or longer.[196] Of cases of cirrhosis manifesting more than 10 years after transplantation, 93% were attributed to HCV.[196] To try to avoid cirrhosis, therapy should be considered in transplant recipients with chronic HCV infection who have not taken immunosuppressive agents for at least 6 months, have normal marrow recovery, and have no GVHD.[197] Randomized studies have shown the superiority of pegylated IFN-α plus ribavirin over standard IFN-α plus ribavirin or pegylated IFN alone (see http://www.va.gov/hepatitisc).

HCV is universally transmitted from HCV RNA–positive donors to their recipients.[197] If an HCV-positive donor is the best available match, treatment of the donor with anti-HCV therapy before stem cell harvest may be considered to try to eliminate detectable viral replication and reduce the likelihood of HCV transmission. IFN-α should be stopped at least 1 week before har-

vest to avoid problems with engraftment.[197] Significant hepatic dysfunction is uncommon in nontransplanted HCV-positive patients receiving chemotherapy for hematologic malignancies.

Other Transfusion-Associated Hepatitis Viruses

Hepatitis G virus is a newly discovered transfusion-associated virus that can establish persistent asymptomatic infection. Surveillance studies have not established a role for this virus in non–A-E acute transfusion-related hepatitis or chronic liver disease.[198] TT is another virus capable of establishing persistent infection whose pathogenicity remains questionable.[199] In a Japanese study, TT viral DNA was detected with far greater frequency in HSCT recipients than in blood donors and in one patient was temporally associated with elevated serum hepatic enzyme levels.[200] Conceivably, these and other transfusion-associated viruses yet to be discovered may be agents of non–A-E hepatitis in heavily transfused persons with cancer and in hepatitis-associated aplastic anemia.

WEST NILE VIRUS

In 2002, there were 4156 reported cases of West Nile virus infection in the United States involving 44 states. Most human cases of West Nile virus infection are acquired from infected mosquitos. Blood products and stem cell and organ allografts are other potential modes of transmission. Immunosuppression may increase the risk of central nervous system disease after West Nile virus infection. Allogeneic HSCT recipients are likely at higher risk for more severe West Nile virus infection based on their prolonged immunocompromised state.[201] As of July 2003, all blood donations collected in the United States are being screened for West Nile virus by nucleic acid amplification detection, but rare cases of donors with low-level viremia may be missed The CDC has also issued guidelines for avoiding mosquito bites to prevent infection by West Nile virus (http://www.cdc.gov/ncidod/dvbid/westnile/index.htm).

SMALLPOX VACCINE

Since the terrorist events of September 2001, new emphasis has been focused on bioterrorism preparedness, including smallpox vaccination. Because live vaccinia virus is used in the vaccine preparation, smallpox vaccination is contraindicated in persons deemed to be at higher risk for vaccinia complications, including patients with cancer receiving chemotherapy or radiation therapy, transplant recipients, and persons with household contacts that fall into these categories (see http://www.cdc.gov/smallpox for a complete description of contraindication criteria). The CDC considers that appropriate infection control practices and site care should prevent transmission of vaccinia virus from vaccinated health care workers to patients. Thus, administrative leave is not routinely required for newly vaccinated health care workers.

PARASITIC INFECTIONS

TOXOPLASMOSIS

Reactivation of *Toxoplasma gondii* may cause life-threatening disease in patients with profound deficits in T-cell immunity. In a review of 128 reported cases of toxoplasmosis in patients with neoplastic disorders, 59 patients had Hodgkin's disease, 12 had non-Hodgkin's lymphoma, and 36 had acute or chronic leukemia.[202] Risk factors include therapy with corticosteroids, cytotoxic agents, or radiation, and poorly controlled malignancy.

Toxoplasmosis is an uncommon complication of HSCT, occurring in fewer than 1% of patients. In the largest series of toxoplasmosis in allogeneic HSCT recipients, almost all patients were seropositive before transplantation, and 73% had acute moderate to severe GVHD.[203] The median day of onset of disease was 64 days after HSCT. Sixty-three percent of patients died, and 22% were first diagnosed at autopsy.

Central nervous system disease with altered mental status, coma, seizures, cranial nerve abnormalities, and motor weakness are the most common findings.[202] Cerebrospinal fluid is usually normal; however, a mononuclear pleocytosis and elevated protein level may be seen. Heart, lungs, liver, spleen, lymph nodes, bone marrow, pancreas, spleen, and skeletal muscle may also be involved.

Definitive diagnosis of toxoplasmosis relies on demonstration of tachyzoites and cysts in histopathologic sections. Use of electron microscopy and immunostaining may facilitate diagnosis. Visualization of the organism in cerebrospinal fluid using Giemsa staining is diagnostic of disease, but the sensitivity of this method is low. PCR applied to serum and tissue samples has become widely used and may facilitate earlier diagnosis of toxoplasmosis and complement histopathologic methods.[203,204]

The treatment of choice for toxoplasmosis is oral sulfadiazine (4 to 6 g/d in four divided doses) plus pyrimethamine (loading dose of 200 mg, followed by 50 to 75 mg/d). Folinic acid should be administered to reduce myeloid toxicity. Whether maintenance therapy is required after quiescence of disease is unknown. It is reasonable to continue a maintenance regimen (sulfadiazine 2 g/d plus pyrimethamine 50 mg/d) during periods of immunosuppressive therapy. In patients intolerant of sulfonamides, clindamycin and primaquine may be used instead.

STRONGYLOIDIASIS

Strongyloides stercoralis is an intestinal nematode that typically causes localized infection but can cause disseminated disease, or hyperinfection syndrome, in immunocompromised patients. *S stercoralis* is endemic in tropical and subtropical regions, but the parasite is also observed in Europe and rural areas in the southeastern United States. Cross-infection between humans through fecal contact appears most likely.[205] *S stercoralis* can establish an asymptomatic chronic gastrointestinal infection through autoinfection. The hyperinfection syndrome can occur years after the initial infection in the setting of immunosuppression. It results from penetration of filariform larvae through the intestinal mucosa, followed by dissemination. Secondary bacterial infection results from passage of enteric bacteria through the bowel as a consequence of gastrointestinal strongyloidiasis and may result in peritonitis, bacteremia, and meningitis. This underscores the need to obtain a thorough history about prior residence in endemic areas. Among reported cases of hyperinfection syndrome associated with cancer, approximately 90% of patients had a hematologic malignancy.[205]

Patients from endemic areas or with unexplained peripheral eosinophilia should be screened for *S stercoralis* infection by serologic testing before receiving immunosuppressive agents. The CDC advises that potential HSCT recipients with a positive serologic test result or unexplained eosinophilia despite a negative serologic result receive prophylaxis with ivermectin.[31] This recommendation can reasonably be applied to other patients receiving potent immunosuppressive regimens as well. All infected patients should have at least three negative stool test results after completion of treatment before beginning chemotherapy.

FOOD- AND WATER-BORNE INFECTIONS

Immunocompromised persons are at increased risk for serious infections by food- and water-borne pathogens. *Salmonella* and *Campylobacter* species can cause dysentery and sepsis. In patients with cancer, the risk of *Salmonella* sepsis may be increased by splenectomy, gastrectomy, and hypochlorhydria, as well as by significantly impaired cellular immunity such as in those receiving corticosteroids or allogeneic HSCT recipients. Undercooked fish and seafood from marine, estuarine, and brackish water (particularly in the region of the Gulf states and Mexico) may harbor *Aeromonas* and *Vibrio* species. Underlying hepatic or neoplastic disease (especially leukemia) predisposes to sepsis and severe soft tissue infections by these organisms (see Skin Lesions and Soft Tissue Infections, later in this chapter).

Listeria monocytogenes is a gram-positive rod that principally infects neonates, the elderly, and persons with compromised cellular immunity. Bacteremia and meningitis are the most common manifestations. Infection is acquired by ingestion of contaminated food products, and outbreaks are well described. Safdar et al.[206] reported an incidence of listeriosis of 0.47% in allogeneic HSCT recipients. T-cell–depleted allografts and CMV viremia appeared to be associated with an increased risk of listeriosis. Nontransplant patients with hematologic malignancies receiving corticosteroids and fludarabine are also at increased risk for listeriosis. Systemic listeriosis should be treated with parenteral ampicillin with or without gentamicin or with trimethoprim-sulfamethoxazole in penicillin allergic patients.

Cryptosporidium parvum can cause a protracted and disabling diarrhea in immunocompromised patients, particularly those with AIDS. Water-borne outbreaks have occurred in the United States, and immunocompromised persons and their health care providers must be aware of local outbreaks and take appropriate precautions. Diagnosis is made by visualization of the organism in stool using a modified acid-fast stain, enzyme immunoassay, or PCR. Paromomycin, azithromycin, and nitazoxanide are most commonly used for cryptosporidiosis, but therapy is generally unsatisfactory.

Isospora and *Cyclospora* species are other enteric coccidians that may cause prolonged diarrhea. Microsporidiosis typically manifests as a protracted diarrhea but may cause disseminated disease, including central nervous system involvement, sinusitis, pneumonitis, keratitis, and renal failure in severely compromised persons. Diagnosis is made by visualization using light or electron microscopy or DNA detection.

Acanthamoeba species may cause an insidious granulomatous encephalitis in immunocompromised patients, such as those receiving high-dose corticosteroid therapy, transplant recipients, and patients with AIDS. Skin manifestations include persistent ulcers, nodules, or subcutaneous abscesses. HSCT recipients may have a more fulminant course characterized by obtundation, coma, and seizures, associated with a necrotizing meningoencephalitis and hydrocephalus. A diagnosis may be established by analysis of cerebrospinal fluid or biopsy specimen showing characteristic amoebic trophozoites. The treatment of choice is parenteral pentamidine.

The CDC has issued guidelines on travel (http://www.cdc.gov/travel) and food- and water-related precautions for HIV-infected persons[207] that are generally applicable to immuncompromised patients with cancer.

NEUTROPENIC FEVER

INITIAL EVALUATION

Patients with cancer and neutropenic fever often have infection, and bacteremia is documented in approximately 20% of cases.[208] Because of the high likelihood of occult infection in a patient with febrile neutropenia without localizing symptoms or signs, and the potential for rapid progression to severe sepsis, prompt initiation of empirical antibiotic therapy is essential. The likelihood of bacteremia is related to the intensity of neutropenia (with an absolute neutrophil count of fewer than $100/\mu L$ carrying the greatest risk) and the duration of neutropenia. A rapid fall in the neutrophil count may also be a risk factor for infection, whereas evidence of marrow recovery, even if the neutrophil count is still fewer than $500/\mu L$, is a positive prognostic factor. Concomitant use of corticosteroid therapy raises the likelihood of infection with opportunistic pathogens such as *P jiroveci* that characteristically affect patients with defects in cell-mediated immunity. This chapter uses the following established criteria for neutropenic fever: (1) a single oral temperature measurement of higher than $38.3°C$ ($101°F$) or a temperature of $38°C$ ($100.4°F$) or higher for longer than 1 hour and (2) neutropenia with an absolute neutrophil count of fewer than $500/\mu L$ or fewer than $1000/\mu L$ with predicted rapid decline to fewer than $500/\mu L$.

Fever is a sensitive but nonspecific sign of infection in neutropenic patients, and other findings of infection are often lacking.[209] Sputum production in cases of pneumonia and drainage from an infected wound may be absent. The lack of reliable physical examination findings to identify patients with infection constitutes the rationale for initiating empirical antibacterial therapy in patients with neutropenic fever.

A meticulous physical examination is necessary. Mucositis is commonly observed after chemotherapy and may be difficult to distinguish from gingivostomatitis caused by reactivation of HSV infection. In patients with prolonged neutropenia or those who receive concomitant high-dose corticosteroid therapy, fungal infection of the palate, typically by *Aspergillus* species or zygomycetes, constitutes a surgical emergency. A black necrotic eschar is the most common sign of such infections. Palpation over the anterior sinuses and an ophthalmologic examination should be performed. A detailed inspection of the skin, including the nails, may disclose a lesion suggestive of systemic infection or a possible portal of entry. Examples include ecthyma gangrenosum caused by *P aeruginosa*, or erythematous papules caused by disseminated candidiasis. Catheter sites and sites of prior skin penetration (e.g., surgical wounds and biopsy sites) should be palpated. The perineum

and perianal region are easily missed sources of infection that need careful inspection and palpation.

The initial evaluation should include the following: complete blood count and differential, serum chemistry including liver-associated enzyme levels, at least two sets of cultures of blood from different sites, and a urine culture. An initial chest radiograph in the absence of clinical signs of pulmonary infection is of low yield in ambulatory adult patients with neutropenic fever.[210] The authors advise chest radiography as part of the initial evaluation of neutropenic fever in patients requiring hospitalization and in patients at higher risk for infections (e.g., those with hematologic malignancies, anticipated prolonged neutropenia, use of systemic corticosteroids).

The volume of blood collected for culture should be in accordance with the blood culture system used. In adults at least 20 mL of blood is required for optimal sensitivity for detecting blood stream infection. A metaanalysis showed little benefit to culturing blood from two sites in patients with central venous catheters.[211] In the authors' opinion, collecting blood culture specimens from at least two ports of a central catheter without venipuncture is acceptable. Specimens from potential sites of infection, such as skin lesions or sputum, should be obtained before instituting antibiotics. However, febrile neutropenia should be considered a medical emergency, and prompt initiation of empirical antibiotics should not be delayed if culture material is not immediately available.

There are numerous potential causes of fever in this patient group, including drugs, transfusion reactions, colony growth factors, thrombophlebitis, and tumor per se. Serum levels of inflammatory markers such as reactive protein and procalcitonin have been evaluated as correlates of infection in patients with neutropenic fever, but there are currently no validated criteria against which to interpret them. Therefore, prompt initiation of appropriate antibiotic therapy is still required in all febrile neutropenic patients.

ANTIBIOTIC REGIMENS

Empirical antibiotic therapy at the outset of neutropenic fever became standard of care more than 30 years ago, largely based on improved survival in patients with sepsis due to *P aeruginosa* and other aerobic gram-negative rods.[212] Numerous studies of monotherapy and combination therapy have been conducted that further delineate the advantages and disadvantages of various empirical regimens for neutropenic fever. The IDSA has published evidence-based guidelines on antibiotic therapy for neutropenic fever without a documented source.[213] Initial antibiotic regimens are divided into three categories: (1) monotherapy, (2) duotherapy without vancomycin, and (3) vancomycin plus one or two drugs.

Monotherapy

Since the mid-1980s, the development of broad-spectrum antipseudomonal antibiotics has led to a reevaluation of the need for combination antibiotic therapy. Obviating the need for an aminoglycoside would be expected to reduce nephrotoxicity in a patient population frequently treated with nephrotoxic drugs. Pizzo et al.[214] showed that ceftazidime monotherapy was as safe and effective as a combination regimen in patients with neutropenic fever. De Pauw et al.[215] subsequently compared ceftazidime with piperacillin plus tobramycin in treatment of approximately 800 episodes of neutropenic fever in patients with leukemia or HSCT. The mean duration of neutropenia was 18 days. The two regimens were similar with regard to control of infections and infection-related mortality, but fewer adverse reactions occurred in the ceftazidime arm. Therefore, ceftazidime monotherapy is effective empirical therapy in high-risk patients with febrile neutropenia.

The IDSA considered the following four antibiotics to be appropriate as empirical monotherapy for neutropenic fever: ceftazidime, cefepime, imipenem, and meropenem.[213] A disadvantage of ceftazidime monotherapy is the modest or absent activity against certain gram-positive pathogens (e.g., viridans streptococci, enterococci) and gram-negative pathogens with extended-spectrum β-lactamases and chromosomally mediated inducible β-lactamases (see Infection with Resistant Bacterial Pathogens, later in this chapter).

Cefepime is a fourth-generation cephalosporin active against aerobic gram-negative rods and most gram-positive organisms observed in patients with cancer. The carbapenems (imipenem and meropenem) and piperacillin-tazobactam are active against these pathogens and anaerobes. Ertapenem is a carbapenem that is poorly active against *P aeruginosa* and is therefore not appropriate empirical therapy for neutropenic fever.

In a randomized study of 399 episodes of neutropenic fever comparing ceftazidime with imipenem as initial therapy, the survival rate was approximately 98% for both regimens.[216] Imipenem treatment was linked with more *Clostridium difficile*–associated diarrhea, nausea, and vomiting. In another randomized study, imipenem with or without amikacin was compared to ceftazidime with or without amikacin as initial therapy in 750 episodes of neutropenic fever.[217] The success rate (resolution of clinical and laboratory signs of infection without modification of the initial regimen) was poorest in the ceftazidime monotherapy arm (59%) but was similar in the other three arms (71% to 76%). The majority of failures were due to coagulase-negative staphylococci and viridans streptococci. Nevertheless, overall mortality was less than 1%.

In a multicenter French study involving 400 patients with neutropenic fever, empirical therapy with cefepime yielded survival similar to that with imipenem (95% vs. 98%, respectively) but caused less gastrointestinal toxicity.[218] Another randomized trial compared cefepime with imipenem in treatment of 251 patients with neutropenic fever requiring hospitalization.[219] Sixty-seven percent of patients had leukemia, and 55% had an absolute neutrophil count of fewer than 100/μL at study entry. The response to therapy was similar (68% for imipenem and 75% for cefepime), and both drugs were well tolerated.

Meropenem is a carbapenem with a spectrum similar to that of imipenem, except for enhanced activity against gram-negative bacteria and less activity against gram-positive bacteria. In a large multicenter study involving 958 patients with febrile neutropenia, meropenem monotherapy was as effective as ceftazidime plus amikacin as initial empirical therapy.[220] In another randomized study, meropenem was more effective than ceftazidime as empirical therapy for neutropenic fever, with the greatest benefit occurring in severely neutropenic patients, HSCT recipients, and patients given antibiotic prophylaxis before study entry.[221] Both regimens were well tolerated, with rash and gastrointestinal symptoms being the most common adverse events.

Piperacillin-tazobactam, a broad-spectrum antipseudomonal penicillin, was compared with cefepime in an open-label, randomized study of empirical therapy in 528 patients with hematologic malignancies and neutropenic fever.[222] The end-of-treatment success rate was 45% in piperacillin-tazobactam recipients and 36% in cefepime recipients (*P* = .04). Adverse events were similar. Therefore, piperacillin-tazobactam (4.5 g every 6 hours) is an acceptable monotherapy regimen for empirical therapy of neutropenic fever.

A metaanalysis of 29 randomized clinical trials pooled data from 4795 febrile episodes and a subset of 1029 bacteremic episodes. Similar efficacy was found for empirical monotherapy and aminoglycoside-containing combination regimens.[223] With highly effective monotherapy regimens for neutropenic fever, initial empirical combination regimens may be most appropriate for patients in unstable condition and at institutions at which multidrug-resistant pathogens are frequently encountered. To facilitate comparisons between studies and standardization of trials, the Immuncompromised Host Society and the Multinational Association for Supportive Care in Cancer (MASCC) proposed specific guidelines on the methodology for conducting clinical trials involving patients with cancer and neutropenic fever.[224]

Duotherapy without Vancomycin

The standard duotherapy regimen for empirical therapy of neutropenic fever is an antipseudomonal β-lactam plus an aminoglycoside. The β-lactam–aminoglycoside synergy was thought to be important in effecting a rapid resolution of bacteremia. This hypothesis was supported by clinical data when applied to the early carboxy- and acylureido-penicillins. Pairing an antipseudomonal β-lactam with a quinolone may provide broad-spectrum activity against resistant gram-negative pathogens and avoid aminoglycoside-related nephrotoxicity. In a large randomized study of 471 febrile episodes, ciprofloxacin plus piperacillin was as effective as tobramycin plus piperacillin as empirical therapy for neutropenic fever.[225] However, with the advent of broader-spectrum cephalosporins and carbapenems, combination regimens are usually not required for primary empirical management of neutropenic fever.

Use of an aminoglycoside alone for treatment of infection with gram-negative bacteria is not recommended because of the high failure rate. Ceftriaxone plus an aminoglycoside, which has the potential for single daily dosing, was effective in some studies.[226] A metaanalysis of randomized trials showed equivalence between ceftriaxone-containing combination regimens and regimens with a β-lactam with antipseudomonal activity as empirical therapy for neutropenic fever.[227] However, ceftriaxone does not have reliable activity against *P aeruginosa*. Therefore, in patients at significant risk for *P aeruginosa* infection, ceftriaxone plus an aminoglycoside may be suboptimal.

When to Add Vancomycin

The rationale for adding vancomycin to an empirical regimen for neutropenic fever stems from the increased proportion of infections caused by gram-positive bacteria. This change in the proportion of infections in neutropenic patients from predominantly those caused by gram-negative bacteria to those caused by gram-positive bacteria is associated with the widespread use of tunneled catheters. Infection by coagulase-negative staphylococci, which are usually resistant to β-lactams, has become the most common cause of bacteremia in patients with cancer. In addition, MRSA is resistant to β-lactams and *Enterococcus* species are resistant to cephalosporins. Although ceftazidime has *in vitro* activity against most viridans streptococci, serious infection by these pathogens has occurred in neutropenic patients receiving ceftazidime alone.[46]

Randomized studies have shown no benefit of routine addition of vancomycin to standard antibacterial regimens as initial empirical therapy for neutropenic fever.[228,229] Because of the emergence of VRE in association with vancomycin use, the IDSA[213] and the National Comprehensive Cancer Network (NCCN)[230] appropriately advise against the routine use of vancomycin as initial empirical therapy for neutropenic fever.

Cometta et al.[231] evaluated the need for the addition of vancomycin in patients with hematologic malignancies and HSCT recipients who had persistent neutropenic fever. There was no difference between the addition of vancomycin and the addition of placebo with regard to defervescence, episodes of grampositive bacteremia, or use of empirical amphotericin B. One limitation was the addition of vancomycin or teicoplanin in approximately 40% of patients after on-study vancomycin (or placebo) was stopped.

The authors suggest that addition of vancomycin be reserved for specific settings, which include (1) clinically apparent, catheter-related infection; (2) positive blood culture for a grampositive bacterium before identification and susceptibility testing; (3) known colonization with MRSA or penicillin- and cephalosporin-resistant pneumococci; and (4) hypotension or septic shock without an identified pathogen (Fig. 53-3). Some experts add vancomycin in treatment of patients with neutropenic fever at high risk for viridans group streptococci (e.g., prior quinolone prophylaxis, severe mucositis associated with cytarabine-containing regimens); this must be weighed against the significant downside of selection for vancomycin-resistant pathogens.[45] Empirical vancomycin should be discontinued after 2 to 3 days if the initial culture results are negative or show a pathogen such as methicillin-sensitive *S aureus* for which other antibiotics can be used.

In neutropenic febrile patients with allergies to β-lactams, vancomycin plus aztreonam is an acceptable regimen[232] (see Table 53-4). Aztreonam monotherapy is not advised because it has no activity against gram-positive bacteria. To avoid excessive use of vancomycin, the authors advise that patients be questioned carefully about the nature and severity of a prior β-lactam allergy. In patients with a history of an uncomplicated rash to a penicillin (absence of urticaria, anaphylaxis, respiratory symptoms, or other significant complications), ceftazidime and cefepime may be safely used without the need for skin testing.[233]

MODIFICATIONS IN THERAPY FOR NEUTROPENIC FEVER

Resolution of Fever within First 3 to 5 Days of Treatment and Persistent Neutropenia

If the fever rapidly abates after initiation of empirical therapy in a patient with an unremarkable physical examination and negative culture results, one should assume that an occult infection existed that has responded to antibiotics. Pizzo et al.[234] randomly assigned patients with prolonged neutropenia and an undiffer-

entiated fever to either discontinuation of empirical antibiotics on day 7 of therapy or continuation of therapy until resolution of neutropenia. Of patients who had become afebrile, 40% had recurrent fever after antibiotics were stopped, which leads to the conclusion that day 7 of therapy was too early to stop antibiotics in the setting of persistent neutropenia. In a subsequent study, discontinuation of antibiotics on day 14 of therapy was shown to be safe in patients who remained afebrile during therapy but who were still neutropenic.[235]

Since these early studies, attempts have been made to identify lower-risk patients in whom early discharge from an oral regimen could be safely done while the patients were still neutropenic (see Lower-Risk Patients with Neutropenic Fever, later in this chapter). The IDSA recommends that, in lower-risk adults with undifferentiated neutropenic fever who responded to empirical intravenous antibiotics, the regimen may be changed to ciprofloxacin plus amoxicillin-clavulanate.[213] In higher-risk patients, intravenous antibiotic therapy should be continued.

Persistent or Recurrent Neutropenic Fever

After selection of an initial empirical regimen for neutropenic fever, close observation of the patient is necessary. Modifications of the initial antibiotic regimen should be made on the basis of new physical examination findings pointing to a previously inapparent focus of infection, signs of clinical instability, and radiographic and culture data. The initial empirical antibacterial regimen need not be changed solely on the basis of persistent or recurrent neutropenic fever in a clinically stable patient.

Recurrent neutropenic fever after response to the initial antibiotic regimen raises the possibility of a breakthrough infection. A careful physical examination for a new focus of infection, repeat blood cultures, and chest radiography or CT scanning are warranted. Changes suggestive of sepsis, such as declining blood pressure, reduction in urine output, rigors, or tachypnea, warrant an empirical modification of the initial regimen. Sepsis due to aerobic gram-negative rods is typically not accompanied by localizing symptoms or physical examination findings. A suitable salvage regimen must be tailored to the common nosocomial pathogens at a given center. Vancomycin, a carbapenem, and an aminoglycoside are an example of a broad-spectrum regimen appropriate for neutropenic fever in the unstable patient (see Septic Shock, later in this chapter).

New symptoms and signs of infection in neutropenic patients may be subtle and need to be aggressively investigated. A new erythematous papular lesion may provide initial evidence for isolated cutaneous or disseminated infection by bacterial or fungal pathogens, and biopsy and culture are necessary. Ecthyma gangrenosum resulting from *P aeruginosa* infection may initially manifest as an erythematous papule and later progress to a necrotic ulcerative lesion (see Skin Lesions and Soft Tissue Infections, later in this chapter). Catheter exit sites, surgical wounds, and biopsy sites should be meticulously inspected and palpated for signs of infection. In the neutropenic patient, fever and local tenderness may be the only signs of infection. A diffuse maculopapular rash is suggestive of a drug reaction, but a culture should be performed to rule out an infectious cause. Blurred vision may represent keratitis or endophthalmitis caused by bacterial, viral, or candidal species, or a central nervous system process. Sinopulmonary symptoms in a patient with persistent neutropenia (10 days or longer) or in a patient receiv-

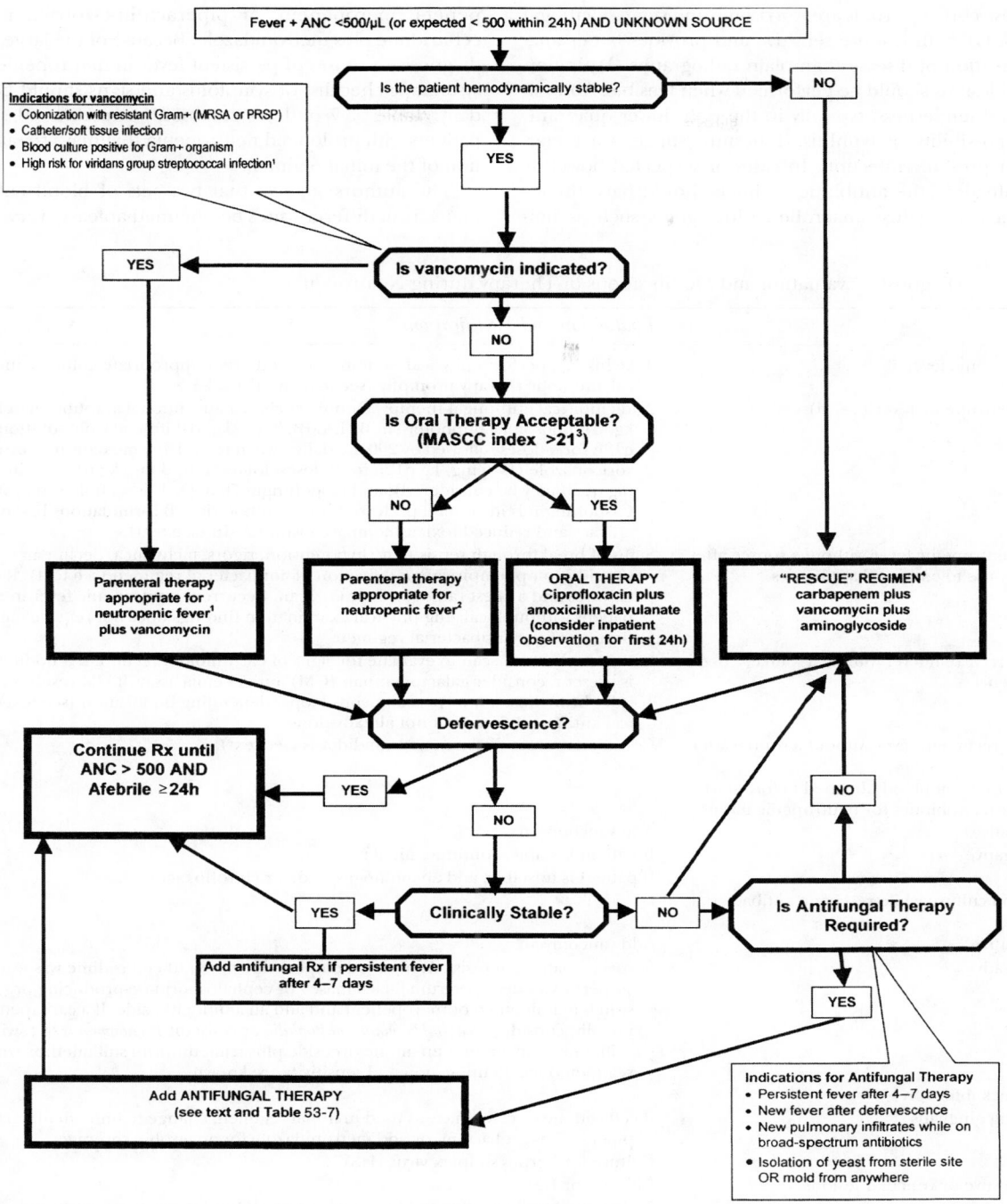

FIGURE 53-3. Algorithm for initial mangement and modifications in therapy of patients with neutropenic fever. See text and Tables 53-5 and 53-7 for more detailed descriptions. ANC, absolute neutrophil count; MASCC, Multinational Association for Supportive Care in Cancer; MRSA, methicillin-resistant *Staphylococcus aureus*; PRSP, penicillin-resistant *Streptococcus pneumoniae*; Rx, treatment. [1]Some experts add vancomycin in patients with neutropenic fever at high risk for viridans group streptococcal infection (e.g., prior quinolone prophylaxis, severe mucositis associated with cytarabine-containing regimens); this must be weighed against the significant downside of selection for vancomycin-resistant pathogens. [2]In a stable patient with undifferentiated neutropenic fever who does not require vancomycin, appropriate parenteral monotherapy consists of ceftazidime, cefepime, imipenem, meropenem, or piperacillin/tazobactam. [3]MASCC index: Burden of illness: no or mild symptoms, +5; moderate symptom, +3; no hypotension, +5; no chronic obstructive pulmonary disease, +4; solid tumor or no previous fungal infection in patients with hematologic malignancies, +4; no dehydration, +3; outpatient status, +3; and age younger than 60 years, +2. A MASCC index of 21 or more has been associated with a relatively low frequency of severe complications. See text for a detailed discussion. [4]This "rescue" antibacterial regimen will vary between institutions depending on the local patterns of antibiotic resistance. Carbapenem + aminoglycoside (or fluoroquinolone) + vancomycin is an acceptable initial regimen that should be tailored once culture results are know.

ing high-dose corticosteroids are worrisome and suggest a fungal infection. A CT scan is more sensitive and provides better anatomic delineation of disease than plain radiographs. Aspiration or biopsy of lesions should be performed when feasible. Abdominal pain and tenderness, typically in the right lower quadrant, raises the possibility of typhlitis. Tenesmus suggests a rectal, perineal, or prostatic infection. In cases of suspected bowel or perianal infection, the antibiotic regimen should have broad-spectrum activity against anaerobes, with agents such as imipenem, meropenem, or piperacillin-tazobactam alone, or ceftazidime plus metronidazole. Because of the large differential diagnosis of causes of persistent fever in neutropenic patients, a systematic checklist of symptoms and signs should be evaluated daily. Table 53-7 outlines commonly encountered scenarios in patients with prolonged neutropenia that may warrant modification of the initial regimen.

The authors suggest that two sets of blood culture specimens from different sites be obtained at least every 48 hours in

TABLE 53-7.   Diagnostic Evaluation and Modifications of Therapy during Neutropenia

Findings	*Evaluation and Modifications*
Initial neutropenic fever	Take history, perform physical examination, and order appropriate cultures; initiate empirical antibiotic therapy promptly (see text and Fig. 53-3).
Persistent neutropenic fever (4–7 d)	Add empirical antifungal therapy. Options include conventional amphotericin B (0.7 mg/kg/d), liposomal amphotericin B (LAMB; 3 mg/kg/d); itraconazole solution (IV 200 mg q12h for 4 doses followed by 200 mg daily; switch to oral 400 mg daily may be considered); voriconazole (IV 6 mg/kg q12h for 2 doses, followed by 3 mg/kg q12h; switch to oral 200 mg q12h may be considered); and caspofungin 70 mg × 1 dose, followed by 50 mg daily). Caspofungin is in general preferred over amphotericin B formulations based on equal efficacy and reduced toxicity compared with LAMB (see text).
Recurrent neutropenic fever without a source after initial response to empirical antibiotics	Signs of breakthrough sepsis (e.g., hypotension, rigors, tachypnea, decline in urine output) should prompt empirical modification of antibacterial regimen (see text). Repeat blood cultures and a chest radiograph or CT scan. Recurrent neutropenic fever in a stable patient without localizing physical examination findings does not require empirical modification of the antibacterial regimen.
Persistent or recurrent fever without a source, ≥10 d of neutropenia	Consider chest CT scan to evaluate for signs of early mold infection. If a nodule or infiltrate is present, consider galactomannan (GM) antigenemia assay. If GM result is negative, consider bronchoscopy or percutaneous biopsy depending on location (see text). Add empirical antifungal therapy if not already done.
Persistent or recurrent fever without a source after ANC recovery	Consider chronic disseminated candidiasis (see text).
Positive culture from blood obtained before starting empirical antibiotics for neutropenic fever	
Gram positive	Add vancomycin.
Gram negative	If patient is stable, continue initial regimen.
	If patient is unstable, add an aminoglycoside or ciprofloxacin.
Positive blood culture while receiving antibacterial therapy	
Gram positive	Add vancomycin.
Gram negative	Suspect a pathogen resistant to initial empirical regimen. If ceftazidime was used initially, suspect extended-spectrum β-lactamase– or cephalosporinase-producing organisms; switch to imipenem or meropenem and add an aminoglycoside. If a carbapenem was used initially, consider *Stenotrophomonas maltophilia* or resistant *Pseudomonas* sp.; switch to piperacillin-tazobactam plus an aminoglycoside plus trimethoprim-sulfamethoxazole. Modify regimen once identification and sensitivity are known.
Head and neck infection	
Necrotizing gingivitis	If ceftazidime or cefepime was used in initial regimen, change to imipenem, meropenem, or piperacillin-tazobactam, or add metronidazole for anaerobic coverage.
	Culture for herpes simplex virus (HSV).
Oral ulcerative or vesicular lesions	Culture for HSV.
	For documented or suspected mucocutaneous HSV infection, give acyclovir 5 mg/kg q8h.
Sinus tenderness	Suspect aerobic gram-negative rod (Enterobacteriaceae or *Pseudomonas aeruginosa*). Perform sinus CT scan if no improvement after 2–3 d of empirical antibiotics. With prolonged neutropenia (≥10 d) or concomitant high-dose corticosteroids, invasive mold infections become more likely and initiation of empirical voriconazole is advised. In cases of confirmed or suspected zygomycosis, a lipid formulation of amphotericin B (5 mg/kg/d) should be used instead of voriconazole (see text). Examine palate and nasal mucosa for signs of invasive infection. Perform sinus CT scan to evaluate extent of disease and to guide diagnostic and therapeutic drainage.
Respiratory tract	
Upper respiratory tract symptoms	Screen for community respiratory viruses.
New infiltrate after resolution of neutropenia	May be inflammatory response to old infection.
	If the patient is asymptomatic, observe; if symptomatic and not responding to antibacterial agents, consider BAL.[a]

(*continued*)

TABLE 53-7. *(Continued)*

Findings	Evaluation and Modifications
New infiltrate while neutropenic	Suspect resistant bacteria or mold infection.
	Perform chest CT scan to evaluate extent of disease and to detect other lesions. perform sputum cultures and GM antigenemia assay; if GM assay nondiagnostic, bronchoscopy or percutaneous biopsy is warranted based on location of lesion. If pneumonia developed in hospital, broaden antibiotic regimen to cover nosocomial pathogens. Consider MRSA, resistant, and gram-negative pathogens, and nosocomial legionellosis (see text). Consider empirical addition of voriconazole (IV 6 mg/kg q12h for 2 doses followed by 4 mg/kg q12h). Diffuse infiltrates raise concern for community respiratory viruses (particularly during winter), *Pneumocystis jiroveci* (*carinii*) (in setting of concomitant corticosteroid therapy), bacterial pneumonia, CMV (in acute leukemia, may be associated with neutropenia), and noninfectious causes (e.g., aspiration hemorrhage, aspiration, drug toxicity, respiratory distress syndrome, congestive heart failure). BAL recommended.
Gastrointestinal tract	
Retrosternal burning, odynophagia	Consider esophagitis. Suspect *Candida* or herpes simplex virus esophagitis. Bacterial esophagitis and CMV (primarily in allogeneic HSCT recipients) also possible. Add fluconazole (400 mg PO or IV) and acyclovir (5 mg/kg q8h IV) empirically. If no response in 3 d, consider endoscopy.
Acute abdominal pain	Differential diagnosis includes same causes as in nonneutropenic patient (e.g., cholecystitis, appendicitis) plus typhlitis (neutropenic colitis).
	Ensure that antibiotic regimen has adequate anaerobic activity (e.g., imipenem, meropenem or piperacillin-tazobactam). Provide bowel rest.
	Abdominal and pelvic CT scan. Monitor for need for surgical intervention (see text).
Perianal cellulitis	Broaden antibiotic regimen to include anaerobic activity. Provide local care. Consider pelvic CT scan to evaluate extent of disease. Monitor need for surgical drainage (see text).
Central venous catheter (surgically implanted)	
Exit-site cellulitis	Add vancomycin.
Tunnel infection	Add vancomycin; remove catheter.
Collection around catheter	Incise and drain; if infected, add appropriate antibiotics and remove catheter.
Local infection	Remove catheter. Perform local débridement.
Aspergillus sp.	May require excision of tunnel tract.
Mycobacterium sp.	Add appropriate antimicrobial agents (see text).
Catheter-associated bacteremia	Add appropriate antibiotics.
	Remove catheter for infection by a highly resistant bacterial pathogen (e.g., *Bacillus* sp., *Corynebacterium* jeikeium JK, *Mycobacterium* sp., and possibly *Candida* sp. (see text).

ANC, absolute neutrophil count; BAL, bronchoalveolar lavage; CT, computed tomography; CMV, cytomegalovirus; HSCT, hematopoietic stem cell transplant; MRSA, methicillin-resistant *Staphylococcus aureus*.
*The differential diagnosis of pneumonia in immunocompromised patients is broad, and the authors advise early BAL or percutaneous biopsy (depending on location of the lesion). Studies must be tailored to the individual patient. In highly immunocompromised patients perform gram staining; culture for bacteria, mycobacteria, fungi, *Nocardia* sp., *Legionella* sp., herpesviruses, CMV, and community respiratory viruses (particularly during winter); and cytologic analysis for *P jiroveci*.

patients with persistent neutropenic fever to avoid delay in making appropriate modifications to the antibiotic regimen in cases of breakthrough infection during neutropenia. For pathogens that are not reliably isolated from the blood (e.g., fungal species), frequent collection of blood culture specimens may increase the likelihood of making an earlier diagnosis. In addition, the common use of deep central catheters makes line infection an ever-present and easily detected cause of fever.

In patients with persistent neutropenic fever, the authors advise continuation of antibiotics for the duration of neutropenia. With regard to the minority of patients with prolonged neutropenia in whom neutrophil recovery is not expected to occur, expert opinion is divided. These patients generally have a hematologic malignancy or are HSCT recipients who would be categorized as "higher risk." The database is inadequate to make a definitive recommendation on managing these patients. Some experts consider stopping antibiotics after 2 weeks if no source of infection was identified and the patient is carefully observed.[213] Others suggest using an oral quinolone-based regimen. Indefinite continued intravenous therapy is the most con-

servative option, but this may not be acceptable to the patient because of quality-of-life issues. Ciprofloxacin plus amoxicillin-clavulanate and an oral azole with activity against molds (itraconazole or voriconazole) may be an acceptable long-term option for oral therapy.

Although infection is presumed to be the cause in most cases of neutropenic fever, infections identified by physical examination (e.g., cellulitis) or microbiologically account for 30% to 50% of cases.[236] Cell wall–deficient bacteria are induced *in vitro* and *in vivo* by antibiotics that act on the cell wall (e.g., β-lactams and vancomycin). Because of the fragile cell wall, these bacteria are typically not recovered in standard blood culture systems.[236]

Empirical Antifungal Therapy

The rationale for empirical antifungal therapy for persistent febrile neutropenia is that meticulous clinical examination and collection of culture specimens are not sufficiently sensitive for early detection of fungal infections. Before standard implementation of empirical antifungal therapy, there was a correlation between prolonged neutropenic fever and mortality in patients with cancer, and fungal infection was frequently found at autopsy.[237] Two randomized prospective studies showed that empirical amphotericin B therapy was associated with a trend toward fewer serious fungal infections in antibiotic-treated neutropenic patients with persistent fever.[237,238] Because fungal infections are uncommonly encountered in the first 7 days of neutropenic fever, empirical antifungal therapy is typically begun between days 4 and 7 of neutropenic fever. Empirical antifungal therapy should be continued for the duration of neutropenia.

In a large randomized study of patients with neutropenic fever unresponsive to standard antibacterial agents, LAMB therapy was associated with fewer proven breakthrough fungal infections and less infusion-related and renal toxicity compared with conventional desoxycholate amphotericin B.[239] In a secondary pharmacoeconomic analysis, use of LAMB significantly increased the overall cost of hospitalization from the time of the first dose of study drug until discharge.[240]

In an open randomized study, intravenous followed by oral itraconazole solution (cyclodextrin formulation) was as effective as, but less toxic than, conventional amphotericin B as empirical therapy for neutropenic fever,[241] which leads to the approval of itraconazole solution for this indication. Prior use of prophylactic fluconazole was similar in both groups, an important consideration given the potential for cross-resistance of fungal pathogens to different classes of azoles. Fluconazole has shown similar efficacy and improved tolerance compared with amphotericin B as empirical therapy for neutropenic fever in two randomized studies.[242,243] However, given its lack of activity against filamentous fungi, the authors suggest that fluconazole is more suitable as prophylaxis during neutropenia rather than as empirical therapy in patients at high risk for invasive filamentous fungal infection (e.g., acute leukemia and allogeneic HSCT patients).

Newer-generation azoles and echinocandins are attractive candidates for antifungal prophylaxis and empirical therapy for neutropenic fever. Voriconazole was compared with LAMB in a nonblinded, randomized study of empirical antifungal therapy in patients with persistent neutropenic fever (n = 837 patients, 72% with hematologic malignancies) unresponsive to antibacterial agents.[244] Treatment success was stringently defined and required fulfillment of all criteria grouped into a composite outcome. The overall success rates were 26% with voriconazole and 31% with LAMB. Empirical voriconazole was associated with fewer breakthrough fungal infections (1.9% vs. 5.0%), with the greatest protective benefit occurring in the protocol-defined high-risk patients (those with relapsed acute leukemia and allogeneic HSCT patients). Infusion-related toxicity and nephrotoxicity were more common in the LAMB arm, whereas transient visual changes and visual hallucinations were more common in the voriconazole arm. Because of the lack of proof of noninferiority of voriconazole compared to LAMB based on prespecified end points for a successful outcome, voriconazole was not approved by the U.S. Food and Drug Administration for use as empirical antifungal therapy. In the authors' opinion, the results of this trial support voriconazole as a reasonable alternative to amphotericin B formulations as empiric therapy, despite the lack of U.S. Food and Drug Administration approval for this indication.

Caspofungin was compared with LAMB as empirical therapy for persistent neutropenic fever in a randomized double-blind study.[245] The overall success rate as defined by a prespecified composite analysis was 34% in both arms. Response to baseline fungal infections (mostly candidiasis and aspergillosis) was superior in caspofungin recipients. Drug-related toxicities and premature withdrawals due to drug-related adverse events were significantly lower in caspofungin recipients. There was a trend toward improved 7-day posttherapy survival in caspofungin recipients compared to LAMB recipients (92.6% vs. 89.2%, respectively; *P* = .051), and in patients with a baseline fungal infection, mortality was 44.4% in LAMB recipients and 11.1% in caspofungin recipients (*P*<.01). The results of this study strongly supports the use of caspofungin as an option for empirical antifungal therapy.

The selection of an empirical antifungal agent should be tailored to the individual patient and should broadly consider risk of breakthrough fungal infection, toxicity, and pharmacoeconomic factors as opposed to solely the pharmaceutical acquisition costs.

Persistent Fever after Resolution of Neutropenia

In most cases, an undifferentiated fever that has persisted during neutropenia resolves around the time of myeloid recovery. In a minority of patients, a "fever of unknown origin" persists for several days after myeloid recovery. As in the neutropenic period, evaluation of fever after myeloid recovery begins with a methodical assessment of both noninfectious causes such as drug fever (e.g., due to recombinant growth factors, β-lactam antibiotics), transfusion reactions, and deep venous thrombosis, as well as infectious causes.

A careful physical examination may show a site of infection that was inapparent during neutropenia, such as a perirectal process. A chest radiograph should be obtained, because pulmonary infection may not be apparent radiographically during neutropenia. Blood and urine cultures, complete blood cell count, serum chemistry tests, and measurement of liver enzyme levels should be performed. An elevated alkaline phosphatase level should prompt consideration of hepatosplenic candidiasis, even if blood cultures were negative for *Candida* species. CT, MRI, and ultrasonography are complementary imaging modalities and may show discrete bull's-eye lesions (see Candidiasis, earlier in this chapter).

Unlike in the neutropenic period, empirical antibiotics can be discontinued after resolution of neutropenia in patients who are stable with an undifferentiated fever and negative culture data. If a source of infection is known, then antibiotic therapy targeted to the specific pathogen(s), rather than broad-spectrum empirical regimens used for neutropenic fever, is advised.

OUTPATIENT MANAGEMENT OF NEUTROPENIC FEVER

Lower-Risk Patients with Neutropenic Fever

Over the past decade, studies have shown that patients with febrile neutropenia can be stratified according to their risk of developing major or life-threatening infectious complications. Prospective randomized studies have shown that patients in the lowest-risk group are appropriate candidates for carefully monitored empirical outpatient antibiotic therapy.

Rubin et al.[246] evaluated the association between response to initial empirical antibacterial therapy and duration of neutropenia in patients with undifferentiated neutropenic fever. Patients with neutropenia of 7 days' duration or less had response rates of 95%, patients with neutropenia of intermediate duration had response rates of 79%, and those with neutropenia of longer than 14 days' duration had only a 32% response rate. In patients who had experienced defervescence after initiation of empirical antibiotic therapy, the risk for recurrent fever was directly related to the duration of neutropenia. Therefore, patients with long-duration neutropenia are less able to contain ongoing infections or are more likely to develop new infections (or both) after initiation of appropriate empirical antibiotic treatment.

Talcott et al.[247,248] developed a model for prediction of risk for serious complications and mortality in patients with febrile neutropenia that was based on a retrospective analysis of data for 261 patients and was validated prospectively in 444 patients with cancer and febrile neutropenia. The model identified the following groups with a high risk of substantial morbidity (25% to 40%) and mortality (12% to 18%): (1) individuals who are inpatients at the time of fever and neutropenia (primarily patients with hematologic malignancy or HSCT recipients); (2) outpatients with concurrent comorbidity (hypotension, organ dysfunction, altered mentation, uncontrolled bleeding, etc.); and (3) outpatients with uncontrolled progressive malignancy. In contrast, outpatients without significant comorbidity and with controlled malignancy (referred to as Talcott group IV) had a low rate of morbidity (2% to 5%) and no infection-related mortality.

Klastersky et al.[249] further refined risk stratification for complications in patients with neutropenic fever. Febrile neutropenic cancer patients were observed prospectively in a study of the MASCC. Independent factors assessable at fever onset predicting low risk of complications were identified in 756 patients. When logistic regression modeling was used, the following factors were found to be associated with low risk: (1) burden of illness characterized by low or moderate symptoms, (2) bureden of illness characterized by moderate symptoms, (3) absence of hypotension, (4) absence of chronic obstructive pulmonary disease, (5) presence of solid tumor or absence of previous fungal infection in patients with hematologic malignancies, (6) outpatient status, (7) absence of dehydration, and (8) age younger than 60 years. These variables predicting low risk were assigned an integer weight, and a risk index score consisting of the sum of these integers was derived. In the validation set of 383 patients, the risk index accurately identified patients at low risk for complications. A score of 21 or higher identified low-risk patients with a positive predictive value of 91%, a specificity of 68%, and a sensitivity of 71%.

The Talcott and MASCC risk index models are based on clinical criteria assessed at the time of initial evaluation of neutropenic fever. Neither risk stratification considers the duration or degree of neutropenic fever, both of which predict the risk of complications of neutropenic fever and the likelihood that the initial antibiotic regimen will require modification. At the time of initial evaluation of neutropenic fever, the physician may not be able to accurately estimate the duration of neutropenia, unless there is already evidence of neutrophil recovery. Both the IDSA[213] and the NCCN[230] appropriately include short duration of neutropenia (less than 7 days) as a factor predictive of low risk in febrile neutropenic patients.

Adult Patients

There are obvious benefits to outpatient management of patients with neutropenic fever in terms of improved quality of life, avoidance of exposure to nosocomial pathogens, and cost savings. The greatest concern about outpatient management of neutropenic fever relates to the possibility of occurrence of life-threatening complications that may be reversible if detected and treated early (e.g., with intravenous fluid, vasopressors, broadening of antibiotic coverage). Deriving and prospectively validating a risk stratification model that accurately identifies lower-risk patients is key in selecting patients for outpatient management of neutropenic fever. The second requirement is demonstration of the safety and efficacy of outpatient regimens in well-designed prospective studies. Three strategies have been evaluated for outpatient management of febrile neutropenia: (1) initial inpatient therapy followed by outpatient management, (2) initial outpatient management with intravenous antibiotics, and (3) initial outpatient management with oral antibiotics.

Two randomized studies showed that oral ciprofloxacin plus amoxicillin-clavulanate was as safe and effective as parenteral regimens in hospitalized patients with neutropenic fever.[226,250] Both studies evaluated lower-risk patients, but the inclusion of patients with hematologic malignancies and patients with an expected duration of neutropenia of as long as 10 days after the onset of fever reflects more liberal criteria for risk stratification. Patients with comorbidities predictive of a higher risk of complications (e.g., hemodynamic instability; neurologic, hepatic, respiratory, or renal impairment; catheter infections; inability to take oral medications) were excluded. These studies were conducted in hospitalized patients, and therefore extrapolations should not be made about the feasibility of this oral regimen in the outpatient setting.

Talcott's group studied 30 low-risk patients with primarily hematologic malignancies and febrile neutropenia.[251] Standard intravenous antibiotics were administered for the initial 2 days in the hospital, followed by home antibiotic therapy with gentamicin plus either mezlocillin or ceftazidime. No patient died, but the incidence of serious complications and the high hospital admission rate in this pilot study suggested that criteria for selecting patients for outpatient therapy required further refinement.

Rubenstein et al.[252] compared outpatient oral ciprofloxacin (750 mg three times per day) plus clindamycin with parenteral clindamycin and aztreonam in 83 low-risk febrile neutropenic patients with solid tumors or leukemia. Patients were observed for 2 hours, then both oral and parenteral groups were sent home to complete therapy. No mortality or severe complications occurred in either group. The oral arm had additional renal toxicity, perhaps related to dehydration. The authors considered the parenteral regimen to have greater safety than the oral one. Subsequently, the oral regimen was changed to ciprofloxacin (500 mg) plus amoxicillin-clavulanate (500 mg) every 8 hours, and the parenteral regimen was unchanged in a study of 179 patients with mostly solid tumors. Outcomes were similar, with 90% and 87% response rates in the oral and parenteral arms, respectively. Patients with solid tumors had higher response rates than those with hematologic malignancies. All patients survived without major infectious complications or antibiotic-related toxicity.

Malik et al.[253] conducted a prospective, randomized study comparing the use of oral ofloxacin with the use of combination parenteral antibiotics (amikacin plus carbenicillin, cloxacillin, or piperacillin) in 122 hospitalized febrile neutropenic patients in Pakistan. This study was not confined to low-risk patients. The overall response to antibiotics was 77% in the oral therapy arm and 73% in the parenteral therapy arm. Mortality rates in the oral therapy group and parenteral therapy group were similar (7% and 10%, respectively). These researchers subsequently compared oral ofloxacin administered in the outpatient and in the inpatient setting in the treatment of 169 patients with febrile neutropenia.[254] Only low-risk patients as generally defined by the Talcott criteria were enrolled. Successful treatment with ofloxacin was more likely in cases in which no source of fever was documented by cultures or physical examination. Mortality was 4% in the group initially treated as outpatients versus 2% in the group initially treated as inpatients.

Klastersky and colleagues applied the MASCC risk index to identify lower-risk patients (those with a score of 21 or higher) with neutropenic fever for treatment as outpatients with ciprofloxacin plus amoxicillin-clavulanate after an initial 24-hour period of hospitalization (cited in ref. 230). This pilot study suggested that a 24-hour period of inpatient observation may provide important data relevant to selecting patients for outpatient antibiotic therapy from among those who, on initial presentation with febrile neutropenia, meet the criteria for lower risk as defined by the MASCC model.

These and other studies have supported the safety of outpatient antibiotic therapy for low-risk patients with neutropenic fever.[255] However, the ability to draw broad conclusions is limited. The prospective, randomized studies described earlier each enrolled fewer than 200 patients and therefore lacked sufficient power to detect small differences between treatment groups. Pooling data from different studies for a metaanalysis is made difficult by the differences in eligibility criteria, choice of antibiotics, criteria for hospital admission, and criteria for a successful outcome.

Both the IDSA[213] and the NCCN[230] support the use of outpatient oral antibiotic therapy in carefully selected lower-risk patients with febrile neutropenia. In adults, the use of ciprofloxacin plus amoxicillin-clavulanate is recommended. In patients allergic to penicillins, the NCCN guidelines recommend replacing amoxicillin-clavulanate with clindamycin; however, the database on the use of ciprofloxacin plus amoxicillin-clavulanate is more extensive, and the latter should be considered the regimen of choice. In the authors' opinion, there is an insufficient database to recommend quinolone monotherapy in patients with neutropenic fever.

A key component of outpatient management of neutropenic fever is ensuring adequate observation by staff experienced in the management of this patient population. Patients must live in close proximity to a facility that can provide emergency care (e.g., fluid resuscitation, intravenous antibiotics) should the need arise. Only centers with the required infrastructure, including the accessibility of trained staff 24 hours per day, should treat lower-risk febrile neutropenic patients in the outpatient setting.

Pediatric Patients

The Talcott and MASCC models apply to adults with neutropenic fever and should not be extrapolated to pediatric patients. Klaassen et al.[256] prospectively derived a risk stratification model for pediatric patients with neutropenic fever. Patients were excluded if they had another medical condition requiring inpatient observation or an abnormal chest radiograph. Prespecified exclusion comorbidity criteria included hypotension, hypoxia requiring supplemental oxygen, respiratory distress, pain requir-

ing intravenous narcotics, and vomiting or diarrhea requiring fluid resuscitation. Significant bacterial infection or unexpected death from infection occurred in 43 of the 227 episodes. Children with an absolute monocyte count of 100/μL or higher were at the lowest risk for significant bacterial infections. The prognostic value of the monocyte count was validated prospectively in a separate group of pediatric patients. In a retrospective series involving 509 pediatric patients with neutropenic fever, lack of signs of sepsis on admission (chills, hypotension, requirement for intravenous hydration), absolute neutrophil count higher than 100/μL, and resolution of fever within 48 hours of initiation of therapy accurately distinguished patients who could be discharged on oral agents.[257] Santolaya et al. derived and prospectively validated a risk prediction model for invasive bacterial infections in children with neutropenic fever consisting of the following variables: serum C-reactive protein greater than 90 mg/L, hypotension, relapsed leukemia, platelet count less than 50,000/μL, and recent receipt of chemotherapy. [257a]

Oral cefixime, a third-generation cephalosporin, has been successfully used in randomized trials involving pediatric patients with neutropenic fever.[258] Quinolones are the only class of oral antibiotics with activity against *P aeruginosa* and therefore fill an important niche in the outpatient management of febrile neutropenic in adults. Quinolone use in pediatric patients with neutropenic fever is controversial because of the possible increased risk of arthropathy. Studies of the outpatient treatment of lower-risk pediatric patients with neutropenic fever using ciprofloxacin-containing regimens have shown encouraging results. However, the number of patients studied is limited.[259–262]

There are insufficient data to recommend initial outpatient oral therapy for pediatric patients with neutropenic fever.[213] Lower-risk pediatric patients have been given early discharge on cefixime therapy after at least 48 hours of intravenous antibiotics and inpatient observation. However, the withdrawal of cefixime from the United States and other markets creates an important need for additional studies. Quinolone use in pediatric patients with neutropenic fever merits further evaluation in randomized trials.

ANTIBACTERIAL PROPHYLAXIS IN AFEBRILE NEUTROPENIC PATIENTS

Despite improvements in the antibacterial agents used in febrile neutropenia, persistent and profound neutropenia remains the most important predictor of life-threatening infections. Administration of prophylactic agents at the onset of neutropenia therefore has potential appeal as a means of reducing the incidence of infections during this high-risk period. However, concern for the emergence of antibiotic-resistant bacteria plus the lack of a survival benefit associated with antibacterial prophylaxis has led to a reasonable recommendation by the IDSA against routine prophylaxis in neutropenic patients.[213]

Today, antibacterial prophylaxis for neutropenia is largely restricted to quinolones and trimethoprim-sulfamethoxazole. These agents have activity against enterobacteriaceae without significant activity against commensal intestinal anaerobes and thus provide "selective decontamination" of the gut. A metaanalysis of trials of fluoroquinolone prophylaxis in neutropenic patients showed a clear benefit in reducing aerobic gram-negative rod infections.[263] Engels et al.[263] evaluated 18 trials encompassing 1408 patients in whom quinolones were compared to either placebo or trimethoprim-sulfamethoxazole. Patients who received quinolones had approximately 80% fewer gram-negative infections than those not given prophylaxis, which led to an overall reduction in total infections. The reduction in fever was small and, in blinded trials, was not significant. Prophylaxis did not affect mortality.

The frequency of infections with quinolone-resistant gram-negative isolates, gram-positive infections, and fungal infections was not significantly affected by quinolone prophylaxis in the metaanalysis.[263] However, although quinolones have remained effective in preventing gram-negative bacterial infections, infection with quinolone-resistant gram-negative organisms has developed during prophylaxis at several centers. Gomez et al.[264] evaluated the clinical and microbiologic outcomes of patients with leukemia and febrile neutropenia during a period in which ciprofloxacin prophylaxis was used and a subsequent period in which quinolone prophylaxis was abandoned due to a high prevalence of quinolone-resistant enterobacteriaceae. There were no differences between the two cohorts with respect to rates of bacteremia or significant complications, but incidence of quinolone-resistant *E coli* was higher in the group that received prophylaxis.

To try to overcome the inadequate activity of quinolones against gram-positive bacteria, combination prophylactic regimens have been used that pair a quinolone with an agent with activity against gram-positive agents (e.g., a penicillin or rifampin). A metaanalysis showed that addition of gram-positive prophylaxis reduced total bacteremic episodes as a result of a decrease in streptococcal and coagulase-negative staphylococcal infections.[265] However, combination regimens were associated with increased side effects and did not affect the frequency of undifferentiated neutropenic fever, total documented infections, or infectious mortality. Newer-generation quinolones with enhanced activity against streptococci are potential candidates for prophylactic use and warrant further study.

In comparative studies, trimethoprim-sulfamethoxazole has, in general, been less effective than quinolones with regard to protection against gram-negative infections.[263] The authors suggest that in neutropenic patients trimethoprim-sulfamethoxazole prophylaxis be reserved for specific groups at high risk for *P jiroveci* infection [see *Pneumocystis Jiroveci (Carinii)*]. Trimethoprim-sulfamethoxazole prophylaxis may also reduce the frequency of nocardiosis, listeriosis, and toxoplasmosis in persons with compromised T-cell immunity.

ANTIFUNGAL PROPHYLAXIS IN NEUTROPENIC AND ALLOGENEIC HEMATOPOIETIC STEM CELL TRANSPLANT RECIPIENTS

Two double-blinded, placebo-controlled trials have shown that prophylactic fluconazole controlled yeast colonization and reduced the rate of mucosal candidiasis and invasive *Candida* infections in HSCT recipients.[266,267] The use of empirical amphotericin B to treat prolonged neutropenic fever also was delayed. A reduction in mortality was noted in the study by Slavin et al.,[267] in which most of the patients were allograft recipients. This effect of fluconazole was found to confer significant long-term improvement in survival, possibly by reducing *Candida* antigen–induced gut GVHD.[268] Lower-dose fluconazole (200 mg daily) appears to be as effective as the standard dose (400 mg daily).[269] Fluconazole prophylaxis in this population was associated with colonization by azole-resistant *Candida* strains.[270]

In a metaanalysis, antifungal prophylaxis with either azoles or low-dose amphotericin B reduced the frequency of superficial and invasive fungal infection and fungal infection–related mortality in HSCT recipients and in nontransplant patients with acute leukemia and prolonged neutropenia.[271] Viscoli et al.[272] noted an association between antifungal prophylaxis and an increased risk of bacteremia based on a retrospective analysis of clinical trials. This possible association merits evaluation in a prospective study. In a randomized trial, fluconazole prophylaxis reduced fungal colonization, invasive infection, and fungal infection–related mortality in nontransplant patients with leukemia and in autologous transplant recipients.[273] The benefit of fluconazole prophylaxis was greatest in autologous transplant recipients not receiving colony growth factor support and in patients receiving mucotoxic regimens consisting of cytarabine plus anthracyclines—a finding that is consistent with the bowel's being a principal portal of entry for *Candida* blood stream infections. Other studies of nontransplant patients with acute leukemia showed no significant benefit of fluconazole prophylaxis.[274,275] The major concerns with prophylactic fluconazole are the emergence of resistant *Candida* species and the lack of activity against filamentous fungi.

The erratic bioavailability of itraconazole in capsule form argues against its use in highly immunocompromised neutropenic patients. The cyclodextrin formulation of itraconazole is an attractive candidate for prophylactic use in patients with prolonged neutropenia because intravenous administration leads to therapeutic levels by 3 days[276] and oral absorption is significantly improved over that for the capsule form. Itraconazole solution has been safe and effective as prophylaxis during prolonged neutropenia in several studies.[277,278] The oral solution may cause significant gastrointestinal symptoms. Itraconazole may also cause myocardial depression and should not be used in persons with a significantly reduced ejection fraction.

Winston et al.[279] compared itraconazole with fluconazole as prophylaxis in allogeneic HSCT recipients in an open-label, multicenter, randomized trial. Antifungal prophylaxis was administered from day 1 until day 100 after transplantation. The frequency of invasive fungal infections (mostly due to *Candida* and *Aspergillus* species) was significantly lower in itraconazole recipients. Although there was a trend toward reduction in fungal infection–related mortality in itraconazole recipients, the overall 180-day mortality was similar in the groups receiving itraconazole and fluconazole.

In another randomized study, itraconazole or fluconazole prophylaxis was administered to allogeneic HSCT recipients for the first 180 days after transplantation and until 4 weeks after therapy for GVHD was stopped.[280] There were fewer invasive mold infections in itraconazole recipients (5%) than in fluconazole recipients (12%); the rates of invasive candidiasis were similar. Hepatic toxicity and discontinuation due to gastrointestinal intolerance were more common in itraconazole recipients. No difference in survival or in fungal infection–free survival occurred. Itraconazole use led to an increase in cyclophosphamide metabolites, which in turn correlated with hyperbilirubinemia and nephrotoxicity during the early transplantation period.[281] This reinforces the fact that itraconazole and the newer-second generation triazoles, which are potent inhibitors of cytochrome P-450 isoenzymes, have high potential for drug–drug interactions. A multicenter randomized trial comparing fluconazole with voriconazole as prophylaxis in allogeneic HSCT recipients has begun.

The echinocandin micafungin was compared with fluconazole as prophylaxis in 882 HSCT recipients in a randomized, double-blind study.[282] The frequency of breakthrough candidiasis was less than 1% in both arms. One micafungin recipient (0.2%) and seven fluconazole recipients (1.5%) developed invasive aspergillosis (*P* = .07). Significantly fewer micafungin recipients than fluconazole recipients required empirical antifungal therapy for persistent neutropenic fever.

PROTECTIVE ENVIRONMENTS

The rationale for protective environments for neutropenic and other highly immunocompromised patients (e.g., allogeneic HSCT recipients) is derived from the same principle as selective decontamination by prophylactic antibiotics. By reducing the frequency of colonization by virulent bacteria, a "germ-free" environment was considered to be important in protecting neutropenic patients from infection.

Such stringent measures, however, are not necessary for the majority of neutropenic patients. The availability of more effective antibacterial agents, the shift in predominance of infectious organisms from gram-negative to gram-positive pathogens in neutropenic patients, and the lack of evidence supporting the benefit of protective isolation have led to the adoption of less restrictive methods of isolation at most centers. The cost and excess labor required to maintain stringent isolation and the additional emotional burden that patients and families must endure further argue against the routine use of such measures.

Isolation of aerobic gram-negative bacteria from food in hospitals is well known. Uncooked vegetables often contain relatively large burdens of *E coli*, *Klebsiella* species, and *P aeruginosa*.[283] Thus, although not validated by controlled studies, it is reasonable to omit such foods from the diets of neutropenic patients. Careful hand washing before and after patient contact remains the most effective method for preventing nosocomial infection.

Although well-designed clinical trials have not validated the use of high-efficiency particulate air (HEPA) filtration, the CDC recommends that allogeneic HSCT recipients be placed in rooms with HEPA filters.[31] The principal benefit of HEPA filtration is likely to be prevention of mold infections. In a retrospective analysis, HEPA filters provided protection to highly immunocompromised patients with hematologic malignancies in the setting of an outbreak of aspergillosis.[284] It is reasonable to use HEPA filtration for nontransplant patients with prolonged neutropenia.

SYNDROMES

BACTEREMIA IN NEUTROPENIC AND IMMUNOCOMPROMISED PATIENTS

Bacteremia is a common complication of antineoplastic cytotoxic chemotherapy. The dominant risk factor for bacteremia is the duration of neutropenia. In an analysis of neutropenic fever trials, Hann et al.[208] showed that neutropenia lasting 1 to 5 days before trial entry was associated with a relative risk of bacteremia of 5.2 compared to no neutropenia; neutropenia of 6 to 15 days had a relative risk of 7.35. Patients with a hematologic disease or HSCT recipients were more likely to have bacteremia than patients with solid tumors. Shock predicted bacteremia with a relative risk of 5.6.

A positive blood culture result may dictate modification of the initial antibiotic regimen (see Table 53-7). Although coagulase-negative *Staphylococcus* species and *Corynebacterium* (diphtheroid) species are common blood culture contaminants, patients with cancer often have indwelling intravenous catheters, which can be portals of entry for these bacteria. The likelihood of blood stream infection is increased if these organisms are isolated from more than one blood culture. The authors therefore advise obtaining at least two sets of blood culture specimens from separate sites. *C jeikeium* is a virulent pathogen that causes catheter-associated bacteremia and disseminated organ infection. Isolation of this organism from a single blood culture requires prompt initiation of vancomycin therapy. Similarly, isolation of *S aureus* from a single blood culture (or from the urine of a febrile patient) should be considered to represent hematogenous infection.

If a gram-negative organism is isolated from blood collected before the initiation of antibiotic treatment, an appropriate parenteral regimen used empirically at the onset of neutropenic fever can be maintained while awaiting drug sensitivity data as long as the patient is clinically stable.[285] The standard empirical antibiotic regimens for neutropenic fever and the specific regimen adopted at a given institution are selected to provide reliable coverage against likely gram-negative pathogens. If the patient is unstable or if the gram-negative organism is isolated after initiation of antibiotics (i.e., breakthrough bacteremia), change to a new regimen is warranted (see Table 53-7 for specific suggestions). Once antibiotic susceptibilities are known, therapy should be tailored appropriately.

SEPTIC SHOCK

Shock and multiple-organ dysfunction are dreaded complications of sepsis. In patients with neutropenia, prompt initiation of broad-spectrum antibiotic therapy directed against commonly encountered blood-borne pathogens is essential (e.g., *S aureus*, viridans group streptococci, enterobacteriaceae, and *P aeruginosa*). Unlike in the stable patient with neutropenic fever, there is likely not to be an opportunity to modify antibiotic therapy based on culture data if the initial regimen does not provide adequate coverage. The initial selection should be tailored to the antibiotic susceptibility of the predominant pathogens at a given center. A combination regimen consisting of vancomycin, a carbapenem (imipenem or meropenem), and an aminoglycoside is a reasonable initial regimen. A quinolone may be considered instead of an aminoglycoside in patients with significant renal impairment. At centers in which *Stenotrophomonas maltophilia* infection is common, addition of trimethoprim-sulfamethoxazole should be considered. Modifications should be made once culture and sensitivity data are known.

In septic shock, several interventions need to be made rapidly. If a nidus of infection is identified, surgical débridement should be performed emergently, and material sent for culture and staining for bacteria and fungi. Fluid resuscitation, oxygen delivery, invasive hemodynamic monitoring, and vasopressor agents may be required. A randomized study showed that use of hydrocortisone (intravenously 50 mg every 6 hours) plus fludrocortisone (orally 50 μg daily) reduced mortality in patients with septic shock and insufficient adrenal reserve (as defined by an adrenocorticotropic hormone stimulation test) without increasing adverse events.[286] Activated protein C is an important regulator of coagulation and inflammatory responses during sepsis, and low levels of activated protein C in sepsis correlate with a poor outcome.

Administration of drotrecogin alfa (Xigris), or recombinant human activated protein C, significantly reduced mortality compared with placebo (24.7% vs. 30.8% mortality, respectively) in patients with severe sepsis.[287] Use of drotrecogin alfa may be associated with an increased risk of bleeding. Because this trial of activated protein C involved a general patient population with sepsis, the results cannot be extrapolated to highly immunocompromised patients, who are likely to have additional comorbidities, including thrombocytopenia.

INFECTION WITH RESISTANT BACTERIAL PATHOGENS

Gram-Positive Bacteria

The incidence of nosocomial MRSA blood stream infections in the United States is increasing. In a 3-year surveillance study of over 10,000 cases of nosocomial bacteremia, almost 30% of *S aureus* isolates were methicillin resistant.[70] MRSA isolates are resistant to all β-lactam antibiotics and often are cross-resistant to multiple classes of antibiotics. Preventing emergence and spread of these organisms requires careful attention to infection control guidelines and judicious use of antibiotics.[288]

Clinical infections caused by *S aureus* strains with intermediate vancomycin resistance have been reported sporadically, generally in patients receiving prolonged courses of vancomycin.[289,290] There have been reports of two clinical infections by vancomycin-resistant *S aureus* occurring as a result of transfer of the *vanA* gene from *Enterococcus*.[291,292] Given the intrinsic virulence of *S aureus* and its propensity to cause serious nosocomial infections, the acquisition of vancomycin resistance is of particular concern for the future.

Approximately 50% of *Enterococcus faecium* and the minority of *Enterococcus faecalis* isolates are resistant to vancomycin[70] and are typically multiply resistant to penicillin, ampicillin, and aminoglycosides. VRE blood stream infection is an important cause of morbidity in patients with cancer. Outbreaks of VRE occur by contact transmission and have been documented in cancer centers.[293] Hospitalized patients with cancer may be particularly prone to VRE colonization and blood stream infection based on multiple coexisting risk factors: use of cephalosporins, vancomycin, and agents with anaerobic activity[294]; prolonged hospitalization; neutropenia; and chemotherapy-induced mucositis. Prevention and infection control methods, including prudent use of antibiotics (restriction of vancomycin usage), isolation of colonized and infected patients, surveillance, hand washing, and use of appropriate barrier protections are key for reducing rates of VRE infection.[288]

Linezolid and quinupristin-dalfopristin meet an important unmet need based on their activity against clinically relevant gram-positive pathogens, including MRSA, penicillin-resistant pneumococci, and VRE.[295] Linezolid is the first of a new class of synthetic antimicrobial agents, the oxazolidinones, to be approved for use in patients. It is active against both *E faecalis* and *E faecium*. Linezolid had similar efficacy to vancomycin in a randomized study of patients with MRSA infections[296] and in patients with nosocomial pneumonia in which linezolid and vancomycin were each paired with aztreonam.[297] In a secondary analysis, linezolid was associated with improved survival and clinical cure rates compared with vancomycin in the subset of patients with nonsocomial MRSA pneumonia.[297a]

There have been case reports of reversible thrombocytopenia, anemia, and neutropenia associated with linezolid therapy. In an open-label compassionate-use study of linezolid for resistant gram-positive infections, linezolid was shown to be safe and effective in treating resistant gram-positive infections in neutropenic cancer patients.[298] The potential marrow-suppressive effects of prolonged linezolid therapy in patients receiving cytotoxic chemotherapy merits additional evaluation. Linezolid is a weak, reversible monoamine oxidase inhibitor and may interact with adrenergic or serotonergic agents. Peripheral and optic neuropathy may complicate long-term linezolid use and are not always reversible.

Quinupristin-dalfopristin is a 30:70 mixture of quinupristin and dalfopristin, which are semisynthetic streptogramin antibiotics. This combination is safe and effective in serious vancomycin-resistant *E faecium* infections, but is not active against *E faecalis*. It had activity similar to that in comparator arms in randomized studies involving hospitalized patients with complicated soft tissue infections[299] and nosocomial pneumonia.[300] Quinupristin-dalfopristin inhibits the metabolism of agents cleared through cytochrome P-4503A4. The most common adverse effects are arthralgias, myalgias, and conjugated hyperbilirubinemia.

Daptomycin is a novel cyclic lipopeptide antibiotic that is potently cidal against common gram-positive bacterial pathogens, including *Staphylococcus* and *Streptococcus* species. It is U.S. Food and Drug Administration approved for complicated soft tissue infections caused by susceptible gram-positive pathogens. Daptomycin should not be used for pneumonia because it is inactivated by surfactant.

Resistance to linezolid and quinupristin-dalfopristin among *S aureus* and enterococcal isolates has so far been rare. However, isolation of resistant pathogens at individual centers highlights the need for judicious use of these agents. Additional antibacterial agents with activity against gram-positive pathogens that have been approved or are in clinical trials include the ketolides and ramoplanin, an oral nonabsorbed antimicrobial with activity against VRE and *C difficile*.

Gram-Negative Bacteria

Infections due to enterobacteriaceae and other gram-negative bacteria (such as *S maltophilia* and *Acinetobacter* species) that are highly resistant to antibiotics due to production of β-lactamases are increasing. Bush et al.[301] grouped β-lactamases according to their substrates and inhibition by the β-lactamase inhibitor clavulanic acid as follows: group 1 cephalosporinases are not well inhibited by clavulanic acid (also referred to as Bush group 1 β-lactamases); group 2 penicillinases, cephalosporinases, and extended-spectrum β-lactamases are generally inhibited by β-lactamase inhibitors; and group 3 metallo-β-lactamases hydrolyze penicillins, cephalosporins, and carbapenems, and confer broad resistance to almost all β-lactam antibiotics. Table 53-4 lists antibacterial agents commonly used in patients with cancer.

E coli and *Klebsiella* isolates should be screened for production of extended-spectrum β-lactamases.[302] The carbapenems (imipenem, meropenem, and ertapenem) have consistent bactericidal activity against strains producing extended-spectrum β-lactamases and are the drugs of choice in serious infections by these pathogens. The chromosomally mediated β-lactamases (Bush group 1) may not be expressed initially (repressed) but are induced (de-repressed) after exposure to broad-spectrum cephalosporins and confer resistance to multiple classes of antibiotics. Thus, resistance may develop during therapy. This group of β-lactamases is characteristic of *Enterobacter* species but is also observed in *Citrobacter, Serratia,* and indole-positive *Proteus* species. In an observational study of bacteremia by *Enterobacter* species, selection of hyperproducer mutants was associated with prior use of third-generation cephalosporins, and blood stream infection by these mutants was associated with a higher mortality rate.[303] In the setting of sepsis or other serious infections by *Enterobacter* species, use of a carbapenem is advised.

The proportion of infections caused by multidrug-resistant *P aeruginosa* has increased in the United States.[304] Emergence of resistance to cephalosporins and carbapenems during therapy may occur. In a case-control study of nosocomial *P aeruginosa* infection, receipt of imipenem, piperacillin-tazobactam, vancomycin, or aminoglycosides was each associated with isolation of imipenem-resistant *P aeruginosa,* which illustrates the complex relationship between antibiotic use and selection for resistant pathogens.[305] Quinolone-resistant *P aeruginosa* is being observed with increasing frequency, a finding that reinforces the need for judicious use of these agents. Serious infections due to strains of *P aeruginosa* resistant to all common antipseudomonal agents are an increasingly serious problem. Colistin administered parenterally[306] or in aerosol form (in infections limited to the lung)[307] may be considered as salvage therapy. Consultation with an infectious diseases specialist is advised.

S maltophilia colonizes hospital environments and establishes carriage in patients who have been treated with broad-spectrum antimicrobial agents. This organism has become an increasingly important cause of nosocomial infections in patients with cancer.[308] Clinical manifestations include catheter-associated cellulitis, bacteremia, pneumonia, endocarditis, mastoiditis, meningitis, and disseminated nodular soft tissue infection.[309] *S maltophilia* is resistant to carbapenems and is often broadly resistant to other agents. It elaborates a metallo-β-lactamase that hydrolyzes carbapenems. The majority of strains are susceptible to trimethoprim-sulfamethoxazole, which is the preferred initial antibiotic for this organism.

Acinetobacter species are gram-negative coccobacilli that colonize hospital environments and have caused nosocomial outbreaks. The risk of infection has been associated with use of quinolones.[310] Many blood stream infections have been catheter related and have responded to catheter removal and antimicrobial therapy.[311] Infection was polymicrobial in 25% of cases.[311] *Acinetobacter* species are often resistant to multiple classes of antibiotics, including carbapenems, and therapy must be tailored to individual antibiotic susceptibility.

INTRAVASCULAR CATHETER–ASSOCIATED INFECTIONS

Tunneled, cuffed vascular catheters have been used extensively in patients with cancer to provide long-term central venous access for blood drawing and infusions. Catheter infections have been divided into several categories. Greene[312] distinguished exit-site from tunnel infections based on whether inflammation extended more than 2 cm from the exit site. Purulent discharge from the exit site may be present; however, in neutropenic patients, local erythema and tenderness may be the only signs of infection, which makes it difficult to distinguish infection from sterile inflammation associated with mild trauma. Tunnel infections manifest with inflammation extending along the subcutaneous tract through which the catheter was inserted. The third major category is catheter-related bacteremia or fungemia, which may occur with or without signs of

localized infection. A fivefold to tenfold greater organism recovery from cultures of blood drawn from the catheter compared with peripheral blood cultures is highly suggestive of catheter infection. The differential time to positivity of cultures of blood drawn from the catheter and blood drawn from the vein is also useful in identifying catheter-associated blood stream infection.[313] The fourth category is a septic thrombophlebitis in which a catheter-associated venous thrombus is documented in association with positive blood cultures.

Most bacterial exit-site infections can be cured with antibiotics alone without catheter removal. Newman et al.[314] identified 160 exit-site infections in association with 690 Hickman catheters placed, most caused by *Staphylococcus epidermidis* or *S aureus.* Treatment was usually with vancomycin, and only 6% of infections resulted in catheter removal. In another study, 55 of 65 exit-site infections were successfully treated with antibiotics and local care alone.[315]

In contrast to exit-site infections, tunnel infections generally require catheter removal because of failure of antibiotic therapy alone. Persistently positive blood cultures for longer than 3 days or recurrences of bacteremia due to the same pathogen despite adequate antibiotic therapy suggest antibiotic failure and require catheter removal. Certain pathogens (e.g., fungi, *Mycobacterium fortuitum* complex, *Bacillus* species, and antibiotic-resistant bacteria) are unlikely to clear or are prone to cause relapse without catheter removal. In cases of tunnel infection caused by *M fortuitum* or *Mycobacterium chelonae,* surgical excision of the tissue surrounding the tunnel may be required as well.[316]

In cases of septic thrombophlebitis, prompt catheter removal and initiation of antimicrobial therapy are essential. Anticoagulation is generally used, although its value has not been clearly established. Septic phlebitis of a central vein usually does not require surgical drainage if the catheter is removed. When a focus of infection exists in the soft tissue around the vein, surgical drainage may be necessary.

For nonsurgically implanted catheters, use of chlorhexidine and silver sulfadiazine–coated catheters reduces the risk of catheter-related blood stream infections compared with use of standard noncoated catheters and is cost effective in patients at high risk for catheter-related blood stream infections.[317] Use of central catheters coated on both the internal and external surfaces with minocycline and rifampin was associated with lower rates of catheter-related blood stream infections compared with use of first-generation chlorhexidine and silver sulfadiazine–coated catheters in which only the external surface was coated.[318] Detailed guidelines for the prevention of catheter-related infections have been proposed by the CDC.[317]

SKIN LESIONS AND SOFT TISSUE INFECTIONS

In the heavily immunocompromised patient with cancer, the differential diagnosis of skin lesions is often broad.[319] Drug reactions are probably the most common noninfectious cause of cutaneous lesions. β-lactams, sulfa antibiotics, and cytosine arabinoside are common offenders. Cutaneous lesions may be manifestations of the underlying malignancy. Mixed cryoglobulinemia may produce cutaneous vasculitis. Sweet's syndrome is characterized by fever and skin lesions, which may be papular, nodular, or ulcerative and may be misdiagnosed as cellulitis. Histologically, a dense neutrophilic infiltrate located mostly in the mid and upper dermis is diagnostic. Sweet's syndrome is associated with hematologic malignancies and may occur during the neutropenic period. GVHD typically presents as a diffuse maculopapular rash, and involvement of the gut and liver is common. Biopsy of skin lesions for histologic analysis and culture is prudent to rule out infection.

Infections of the skin either can be localized or can be manifestations of systemic infection. Ecthyma gangrenosum–like lesions can be caused by *S aureus*, enteric gram-negative rods, and filamentous fungi, including *Aspergillus*, zygomycetes, and *Fusarium* species. Ecthyma gangrenosum begins as a raised erythematous papule or nodule that progresses to a bluish black necrotic lesion within 12 to 24 hours. A central area of necrosis surrounded by erythema is typical. Hemorrhagic bullae may occur. Pathologically, ecthyma gangrenosum is a necrotizing process in which masses of bacteria are often observed within the vessel wall. In neutropenic patients, infiltrating white cells may be absent. Ecthyma gangrenosum is the most characteristic skin lesion associated with systemic *P aeruginosa* infection, but it is not pathognomonic.

Local soft tissue infection by *P aeruginosa* and other aerobic gram-negative rods can rapidly spread through fascial planes in the neutropenic patient, causing extensive necrosis and fulminant sepsis. The initial signs at the site of entry may be mild, pain and tenderness may be out of proportion to erythema, and purulence is likely to be absent. A specimen from needle aspiration of the lesion showing gram-negative bacilli establishes the diagnosis of invasive infection; however, a negative finding on aspiration does not rule out the diagnosis. Prompt surgical débridement and parenteral antibiotics (e.g., an antipseudomonal penicillin and an aminoglycoside) may be life saving.

S maltophilia can cause a variety of dermatologic infections, including mucocutaneous ulcerations, primary cellulitis, a metastatic nodular cellulitis, and ecthyma gangrenosum (see Infection with Resistant Bacterial Pathogens: Gram-Negative Bacteria, earlier in this chapter). *Aeromonas hydrophila* is a gram-negative rod that grows in fresh and brackish waters. However, among immunocompromised patients with cancer, *Aeromonas* sepsis may occur without recent water or fish exposure.[320] *Vibrio vulnificus* can cause disease in those who eat contaminated seafood or have an open wound that is exposed to seawater. In the immunocompromised, particularly in persons with liver disease, *V vulnificus* can cause life-threatening sepsis and blistering skin lesions. *Aeromonas* species and *V vulnificus* are generally sensitive to third-generation cephalosporins (e.g., ceftazidime).

Septicemia caused by viridans streptococci is associated with facial flushing and rash. The rash is usually maculopapular, starting on the trunk and extending to the face and extremities. Skin exfoliation of the palms and soles may occur in 25% of patients 2 weeks after the onset of the rash, likely the result of acquisition of a plasmid producing a toxic shock syndrome toxin.

Bacteremia caused by *C jeikeium* is commonly associated with skin lesions in neutropenic patients. The skin lesions often occur at catheter sites and at sites of trauma, such as bone marrow aspiration, and may only become apparent after resolution of neutropenia.[48] The lesions may be cellulitic, ulcerative, or pustular. If diphtheroids are isolated from a skin lesion, the microbiology laboratory should specifically be asked to evaluate for *C jeikeium*. *Bacillus* species are rare causes of skin infection but can be associated with impetiginous, ulcerative, and necrotic skin lesions. *C jeikeium* and *Bacillus* species are sensitive to vancomycin.

Clostridium species are gram-positive anaerobes that may cause deep soft tissue infection involving the fascia and muscle (see *Clostridium* Species, earlier in this chapter). Typically, a small dusky or purplish lesion on the leg or abdominal wall rapidly expands, and as infection progresses, the lesions become necrotic, bullous, and hemorrhagic. Systemic toxicity including fever, malaise, and mental status changes occurs early. Because the infection occurs in the deep soft tissue, tenderness and evidence of vascular compromise typically precede the development of cellulitis. A rapidly progressive deep soft tissue infection with gas formation suggests clostridial myonecrosis (or polymicrobial necrotizing fasciitis). Needle aspiration specimens characteristically show the organism in the setting of a mild or absent inflammatory response. Extensive surgical débridement may be life saving if initiated early, but the mortality rate is high.[55]

The characteristic skin lesions of disseminated candidiasis are raised erythematous discrete papules, measuring approximately 0.5 to 1.0 cm in diameter. The lesions are usually not tender. Concurrent myalgias raise the possibility of *Candida* myositis. The yeast is cultured from skin lesion specimens in approximately half the cases. Therefore, a negative culture result does not rule out the diagnosis. Biopsy and fungal staining of cutaneous lesions can provide an immediate clue to the diagnosis, prompting the early addition of antifungal therapy. Blood cultures are typically positive.

Trichosporonosis may manifest as sepsis and disseminated infection in neutropenic patients.[321] Skin lesions occur in 30% of disseminated infections and are characterized by nontender erythematous nodules, which may become necrotic. Histologically, budding yeast are present in the dermis, as distinguished from *Candida* species, which produce pseudohyphae. High-dose azole therapy is the treatment of choice.

Cutaneous infection by filamentous fungi may be primary or may result from systemic infection. Primary cutaneous infection with molds can occur in immunocompetent patients by traumatic inoculation. However, progression to angioinvasion, infarction, extension to the deep soft tissue fascia and muscle, and dissemination may occur in the highly immunocompromised. Walmsley et al.[322] described 16 cases of primary cutaneous aspergillosis in children, most of whom had leukemia or lymphoma or had undergone HSCT. Eleven cases were related to use of intravenous arm boards, and five cases were attributed to hematogenous dissemination. Clinically, these lesions resemble ecthyma gangrenosum associated with disseminated *P aeruginosa* infection. Histologically, hyphal elements are present and may cause angioinvasion and infarction. Primary cutaneous fusariosis has a varied appearance, including cellulitis, paronychia, onychomycosis resembling dermatophyte infection, papular and nodular lesions, and subcutaneous nodules[116] (see *Fusarium* Species, earlier in this chapter). Primary localized cutaneous infection with a mold requires surgical resection and has an excellent prognosis.[323] In the neutropenic patient, the likelihood of subclinical systemic infection is high, and therefore systemic antifungal therapy is warranted.

SINUSITIS

In immunocompetent patients, sinusitis results principally from inadequate drainage of mucous secretions from the sinus cavities. Respiratory bacterial pathogens, including *S pneumoniae*, *H influenzae*, and *Moraxella catarrhalis* predominate. In patients with neutropenia or other highly immunocompromised patients, infections by *P aeruginosa*, enterobacteriaceae, and molds are more common.

Treatment of sinusitis in immunocompetent patients with cancer involves a standard antibiotic regimen, such as amoxicillin-clavulanate, azithromycin, clarithromycin, or a cephalosporin with activity against respiratory pathogens. In cases in which an obstructing tumor interferes with drainage from the maxillary sinuses, surgical creation of an antral window may be required to facilitate drainage.

In neutropenic patients with symptoms or signs of sinusitis, a regimen with activity against gram-negative bacteria (such as ceftazidime) should be administered. If no improvement occurs within 3 days, a CT scan of the sinuses with diagnostic aspiration of fluid collections is recommended. A sinus endoscopy may also be useful to visualize the upper airways and to obtain diagnostic material.

Infections by community respiratory viruses may initially manifest with sinus congestion or nonspecific upper airway symptoms. A high index of suspicion for such viruses is necessary for early therapy and prevention of nosocomial outbreaks. Examination of a nasopharyngeal wash sample may rapidly establish the diagnosis (see Community Respiratory Viruses, earlier in this chapter).

Invasive fungal sinusitis in immunocompromised patients often has devastating results. Infection by *Aspergillus* species is most common in patients with persistent neutropenia (e.g., aplastic anemia) and in HSCT recipients. Zygomycetes are classically associated with rhinocerebral disease, which leads to necrosis of the palate and extension to surrounding structures. Sinusitis by emerging fungal pathogens, including *Fusarium* species, dark-walled molds, and *Scedosporium* species are being recognized more. Symptoms and signs suggestive of fungal sinusitis include fever, nasal congestion, headache, maxillary tenderness, and periorbital swelling. Sinus endoscopy may show necrotic material or ulceration. Hyphal invasion into blood vessels leads to tissue infarction and hemorrhage. Extension to the brain and disseminated infection may occur.

Invasive fungal sinusitis in patients with hematologic malignancies and HSCT recipients is principally caused by *Aspergillus* species (*A flavus* and *A fumigatus*). Less common infection-causing mold include zygomycetes, *Fusarium* species, *Scedosporium* species, and dark-walled molds. Therapy for invasive mold infections involves a combined medical and surgical approach. Voriconazole is the drug of choice for invasive aspergillosis. Because voriconazole has poor activity against zygomycetes, a lipid formulation of amphotericin B (5 mg/kg/d) should be used for suspected or confirmed zygomycosis. When feasible, surgical resection of involved tissue should be performed, because medical therapy alone is unlikely to contain infection in the setting of neutropenia or severe immunosuppression. Antifungal therapy should be continued even if all of the visualized necrotic tissue is fully débrided, because of the likelihood of inapparent local and disseminated disease.

PULMONARY INFILTRATES

Immunocompent Patients

In patients with cancer, pulmonary infiltrates pose a difficult diagnostic challenge. Numerous noninfectious causes of pulmonary infiltrates include congestive heart failure, pulmonary hemorrhage, infarction, drug-induced pneumonitis, radiation injury, tumor, bronchiolitis obliterans, and acute respiratory distress syndrome. In addition, common processes can have atypical radiographic appearances, and two or more pulmonary processes can exist simultaneously in this patient population. Careful history taking should solicit information on the time course of respiratory symptoms, sick contacts (e.g., to identify community respiratory viral infections, tuberculosis), recent hospitalization, travel, animal exposures, and exposure to droplets from water distribution systems (suggestive of *Legionella*). Severe acute respiratory syndrome should be considered in patients with compatible symptoms and recent travel in endemic areas (http://www.cdc.gov/ncidod/sars).

In patients with cancer who do not have neutropenia and are not undergoing immunosuppressive therapy, initial empirical treatment for suspected bacterial community-acquired pneumonia should be according to IDSA guidelines.[324] Sputum culture specimens should be collected before therapy is started if feasible. In patients who do not require hospital admission based on a validated pneumonia severity index[324] and who have not received antibiotics recently, administration of a macrolide (azithromycin or clarithromycin) or a newer-generation quinolone (moxifloxacin, gatifloxacin, levofloxacin, or gemifloxacin) is advised. Such a regimen can treat most of the common community-acquired pathogens, including "atypical" pneumonia (due to *Chlamydia*, *Mycoplasma*, and *Legionella* species). For patients requiring hospital admission, the authors advise therapy pairing a macrolide with either ceftriaxone or cefotaxime, or monotherapy with a newer-generation quinolone. For patients with severe community-acquired pneumonia (e.g., those requiring admission to an intensive care unit), the authors advise broad-spectrum coverage with an antipseudomonal β-lactam plus a newer-generation quinolone. A parapneumonic effusion should be aspirated and the sample submitted for Gram staining, bacterial culture, and measurement of protein, lactate dehydrogenase, and pH.

Neutropenic Patients

In patients who have had neutropenia for less than 1 week, pulmonary infections are likely to be caused by enterobacteriaceae, *P aeruginosa*, or *S aureus*. Because of neutropenia, physical findings of consolidation and sputum production may be absent. Blood cultures, a chest radiograph, and, if possible, a sputum specimen for Gram staining and culture should be obtained. In suspected acute bacterial pneumonia, it is essential to initiate appropriate empirical antibiotic therapy promptly and to closely monitor the response in an inpatient setting. The precise selection depends on several variables, including recent use of antibiotics, presence of community-acquired versus nosocomial pneumonia, and the local antibiotic sensitivity data.

For nosocomial pneumonia, therapy with an antipseudomonal β-lactam is advised. Some experts advise adding an aminoglycoside or quinolone, but the value of combination regimens over monotherapy has not been established. If the pneumonia is community acquired (i.e., present before admission or developing within 4 days of hospitalization), addition of a macrolide or quinolone is warranted to treat atypical pathogens. Empirical addition of a macrolide or quinolone is also warranted in cases of nosocomial pneumonia in which hospital-acquired legionellosis is suspected (see *Legionella*, earlier in this chapter). Vancomycin or linezolid should be added for pneumonia in patients colonized with MRSA and for nosocomial pneumonia at centers in which MRSA is common. Particularly during winter months, community-acquired respiratory viruses should also be considered. RSV and parainfluenza are significant pathogens during neutropenia in patients receiving chemotherapy for acute leukemia and in HSCT recipients.

If clinical improvement occurs within 48 to 72 hours, no further diagnostic measures are necessary, and antibiotic therapy should be continued until neutropenia resolves and for at least 10 to 14 days. Once neutropenia resolves, an appropriate oral antibiotic regimen could be administered for the remainder of the course.

In cases of refractory pneumonia, bacterial infection resistant to the initial antibiotic regimen and nonbacterial pathogens, particularly filamentous fungi, must be considered. A CT scan of the chest is useful in defining the location and morphology of the lesions and in guiding diagnostic procedures. Presence of the halo sign in a persistently febrile neutropenic patient is highly suggestive of invasive aspergillosis; however, angioinvasive infections by other organisms, including other filamentous fungi and *P aeruginosa*, may produce similar findings.

Development of a new or progressive infiltrate while the patient is taking broad-spectrum antibacterial agents in patients with prolonged neutropenia (10 days or longer) is most worrisome and suggests invasive aspergillosis. Addition of voriconazole should be considered while diagnostic results are awaited (see Table 53-7). Empirical modification of the antibacterial regimen in keeping with the predominant local hospital pathogens (e.g., MRSA, *S maltophilia*) is also warranted in the setting of a rapidly progressive pneumonia. A positive galactomannan assay result in a patient with prolonged neutropenia, fever, and a compatible pulmonary infiltrate is sufficient evidence of invasive aspergillosis.[325] If results of the galactomannan assay and routine cultures (blood, sputum) are negative, an invasive diagnostic procedure is warranted (see Diagnostic Evaluation, later).

Patients with Defects in Cellular Immunity

Patients with impaired cellular immunity (see Tables 53-1 through 53-3) are at increased risk for infection with common bacteria and opportunistic organisms, including fungi (*Aspergillus* and other filamentous fungi, *C neoformans*, dimorphic fungi), *Legionella*, *P jiroveci*, *M tuberculosis*, nontuberculous mycobacteria, *Nocardia* species, and viral pathogens. CMV and community respiratory viruses can cause severe pulmonary infection in HSCT recipients and in nontransplant patients with hematologic malignancies. Influenza may cause severe disease in these and less immunocompromised persons (e.g., the elderly and persons with preexisting comorbidities). In winter months, upper respiratory tract symptoms and bronchospasm favor the diagnosis of RSV infection. Diffuse necrotizing pneumonia caused by VZV and HSV are also encountered in transplant recipients. Patients receiving concomitant steroid therapy in addition to cytotoxic therapy are at particular risk for *P jiroveci* infection and, to a lesser degree, for histoplasmosis, coccidioidomycosis, cryptococcosis, strongyloidiasis, and reactivation of tuberculosis.

Diagnostic Evaluation

For patients who either are not responding to antibacterial therapy or whose clinical course is not suggestive of an acute bacterial process, an expeditious approach to establishing the diagnosis is indicated. Examination of a sample obtained by sputum induction with hypertonic saline is diagnostic of *P jiroveci* pneumonia in non–HIV-infected patients in approximately 60% of cases.[126] Sputum, either spontaneously expectorated or induced, is also of value in diagnosing tuberculosis. BAL has a high diagnostic sample yield when alveolar infiltrates are present as in pneumonia caused by *P jiroveci*, *M tuberculosis*, and respiratory viruses. The sensitivity of BAL testing for focal lesions such as nodules is variable. For lesions larger than 2 cm, the sensitivity of BAL testing ranges from 50% to 80%, but for smaller lesions, the diagnostic yield is usually less than 15%.[326] Quantitative cultures of specimens obtained by BAL or a protected brush catheter may increase the specificity in the diagnosis of bacterial pneumonia and aid in distinguishing it from upper airway colonization in ventilated patients.

BAL testing is relatively insensitive for diagnosis of aspergillosis and detects only approximately 50% of cases.[327] Percutaneous biopsy may increase the diagnostic yield, but in thrombocytopenic patients, the risk of bleeding may be unacceptably high. Video-assisted thoracic surgery has been used successfully to diagnose interstitial lung disease with significantly less morbidity than open lung biopsy. Open lung biopsy is the definitive diagnostic method and also allows for easier visualization and control of bleeding. False-negative results occur in approximately 5% of open lung biopsy procedures as a result of sampling error in the case of patchy lesions. In a small series, open lung biopsy had a poor diagnostic yield in allogeneic HSCT recipients with diffuse infiltrates.[328] The galactomannan antigen assay may be particularly useful in establishing a probable diagnosis of invasive aspergillosis without the need for an invasive procedure in high-risk patients who have compatible clinical and radiographic findings (see Diagnosis of Invasive Aspergillosis, earlier in this chapter).

The microbiologic evaluation should be tailored to the clinical manifestations and nature of immunocompromise. In highly immunocompromised patients (e.g., those receiving chemotherapy for acute leukemia, HSCT recipients), the following studies of BAL and lung biopsy specimens should be considered: culture and stains for bacteria, fungi, *Legionella*, mycobacteria, *Nocardia*, HSV, CMV, and community respiratory viruses (both rapid antigen methods and shell vial culture), and cytologic or immunofluorescent studies for *P jiroveci*.

CARDIAC INFECTIONS

Cardiac infections are relatively uncommon in patients with cancer. Infection can occur as a complication of thoracic surgery, such as a pneumonectomy, in which dehiscence of the bronchial stump can lead to a bronchopleural fistula and infection of the pleural space with extension to the pericardium. Meticulous and repeated débridements of infected tissue and repair of fistulas are necessary.

Endocarditis can occur as a complication of catheter-associated bacteremia or a septic thrombophlebitis of the neck. In neutropenic patients, dental procedures should be avoided, but if they are necessary, antibiotic prophylaxis (amoxicillin) is recommended to avoid secondary bacteremia. Echocardiography is warranted in patients with bacteremia and signs suggestive of endocarditis, such as a new murmur or embolic phenomena. Fungal endocarditis (due principally to *Candida* species) may result from cardiac surgery or illicit drug use and generally requires removal of the infected valve because of the poor penetration of antifungal agents into the vegetation and the propensity for large vessel embolization. Rarely, filamentous fungi may also cause myocardial abscesses with direct extension to and destruction of the contiguous valve in profoundly immunosuppressed patients. Pericardial aspergillosis is a rare but highly lethal complication in profoundly immunosuppressed patients. It usually results from contiguous spread from the lungs or myocardium.[329] Clinical manifestations include chest pain, a pericardial friction rub, and pericardial constriction and tamponade.

Other pathogens associated with myopericarditis or endocarditis include *T gondii, C neoformans, H capsulatum, Mycobacterium* species, *Nocardia* species, *Bartonella* species, and viruses (e.g., HSV, CMV, influenza).

OROPHARYNGEAL INFECTIONS

Oropharyngeal infections in patients with cancer usually result from the combination of neutropenia and mucositis (see Mucosal Immunity, earlier in this chapter). The differentiation of chemotherapy-induced mucosal erosions and mucositis with superimposed bacterial infection is difficult. HSV is commonly shed in oral secretions and may produce mucosal ulcerations resembling chemotherapy-induced mucositis and necrotizing gingivitis. Oral mucosal candidiasis is most common in patients with profound T-cell deficiencies, such as those receiving high-dose steroid therapy. Diagnosis is usually made by visual inspection alone, although in cases of uncertainty, a wet-mount preparation showing pseudohyphal forms is confirmatory. A swab culture is not of diagnostic value because *Candida* species are commensals in the oral cavity. Filamentous fungi (e.g., *Aspergillus* species and zygomycetes) can cause invasive disease of the hard palate and other oral cavity structures, principally in patients with prolonged neutropenia. The involved mucosa may initially have a dusky or violaceous appearance followed by necrosis, eschar formation, and ulceration. Urgent surgical débridement plus systemic antifungal therapy may be life-saving.

Patients with oral mucosal disease may have difficulty eating because of pain. Malnourishment and dehydration may be severe if parenteral nutrition and fluid replacement are not initiated. Severe local infection with spread to adjacent tissue structures may occur, including paranasal sinusitis and septic thrombophlebitis. Disrupted oral mucosa may be a portal of entry for bacterial pathogens, leading to systemic infection.

Dental disease should ideally be treated in advance of initiating chemotherapy and radiation therapy to allow for an adequate healing time. Plaque should be removed by scaling and curettage, and severely decayed or periapically infected teeth should be removed. A dentist experienced in the care of cancer patients should perform the initial clinical and radiographic evaluation and provide regular follow-up examinations.

Chemical plaque control agents such as chlorhexidine mouth rinses are used routinely in patients with cancer, and different cancer centers use various rinsing protocols to enhance oral hygiene. Use of such rinses has lead to a reduction in microbial counts, but their value with regard to reducing oral disease and systemic infection remains unproven.[330]

EPIGLOTTITIS

Epiglottitis should be considered in patients with fever and pain in the throat, odynophagia, difficulty handling upper airway secretions, and signs of upper airway compromise. The combination of neutropenia and mucotoxic chemotherapy and radiation therapy predisposes patients to epiglottitis. Pathogens in this setting include common respiratory pathogens such as *S pneumoniae* and *H influenzae*, gram-negative rods, and fungi. *Candida* epiglottitis, an unusual complication of neutropenia, may represent localized disease or disseminated infection.[331] Antifungal therapy with fluconazole or caspofungin is warranted.

If epiglottitis is suspected, care should be taken to avoid unnecessary manipulations of the upper airway (e.g., probing of the oral cavity with tongue depressors). Urgent consultation with an otolaryngologist should be obtained, and evaluation of the upper airway and procurement of a specimen for culture may be performed in the operating room. Tracheal intubation may be required.

ESOPHAGITIS

Esophagitis is encountered commonly in patients with cancer. A gradual onset of retrosternal chest pain or burning and odynophagia are the most common symptoms. The differential diagnosis includes candidiasis, HSV infection, CMV infection (principally in HSCT recipients), bacterial infections, and aspergillosis. Radiation therapy to the chest may produce an erosive esophagitis clinically indistinguishable from infection.

The evaluation of esophagitis requires consideration of the patient's immune status. Patients with prolonged neutropenia and HSCT recipients are more likely to have an infection. *Candida* infection is probably the most common cause. However, more than one infection may be present. Oral mucosal candidiasis increases the likelihood of *Candida* esophagitis. However, the use of prophylactic oral topical antifungal agents may protect against thrush while leaving the patient susceptible to esophageal candidiasis.

In highly immunocompromised patients with symptoms suggestive of esophagitis, two general strategies have been used. In the first, an endoscopy is performed initially. Whitish plaques are suggestive of candidiasis, whereas ulcers suggest viral infection. Brushings and biopsy specimens have the highest diagnostic yield. A brushing may suffice instead of a biopsy, which may carry the risk of bleeding, particularly in patients with thrombocytopenia.

In the second approach, empirical therapy is administered initially. Fluconazole, with or without high-dose acyclovir (10 mg/kg every 8 hours), is administered for *Candida* or HSV, respectively. Alternatively, fluconazole may be administered initially, followed by acyclovir if no clinical response has occurred within 2 days. A history of oral HSV infections or presence of anti-HSV antibodies should prompt early initiation of acyclovir therapy. In the setting of concurrent neutropenic fever, appropriate broad-spectrum antibacterial agents with activity against oral flora (e.g., imipenem, meropenem, or piperacillin-tazobactam) should be added empirically. If symptoms do not rapidly abate, endoscopy should be performed.

Diagnosis of bacterial esophagitis relies on demonstration of bacterial invasion of the esophageal wall. Bacteria causing local disease include gram-positive cocci, gram-negative rods, and mixed organisms.[332] Esophagitis may be complicated by bacteremia due predominantly to gram-positive pathogens (viridans streptococci, *S aureus, Bacillus* species). Erosive esophagitis may rarely lead to esophageal rupture or life-threatening bleeding.

INTRAABDOMINAL INFECTION

Common causes of an acute abdomen in the general population (such as cholecystitis, pancreatitis, appendicitis, and diverticulitis) also occur in patients with malignancy. Intraabdominal tumors, depending on their location, may lead to an obstructive cholangitis (e.g., pancreatic and hepatobiliary tumors) or erosion through a viscus. In some instances, tumor may replace most of the bowel wall, with perforation after initiation of cytoreductive chemotherapy.

Patients with prolonged neutropenia are at risk for typhlitis, which results from a combination of neutropenia and defects in the bowel mucosa related to cytotoxic chemotherapy. It is most common in patients with leukemia who have undergone intensive cytotoxic chemotherapy. Very rarely, typhlitis has been reported in patients with leukemia who have not received chemotherapy. Typhlitis is also observed in patients with solid tumors receiving taxanes.[333,334] Pediatric patients appear to be at greater risk for typhlitis than adults. *P aeruginosa* is the principal pathogen, although enterobacteriaceae, clostridia, and *Candida* species may also cause typhlitis. Pathologically, typhlitis is characterized by ulceration and necrosis of the bowel wall, hemorrhage, and masses of organisms. In the setting of neutropenia, inflammation may be sparse.

Typhlitis has a wide range of severity. Presumptive diagnostic criteria for typhlitis include fever, abdominal pain and tenderness, and radiologic evidence of right colonic inflammation in patients with neutropenia.[335] Nausea, vomiting, and diarrhea (sometimes bloody) are the most common associated symptoms. Abdominal distention, tenderness, and a right lower quadrant fullness or mass reflect thickened bowel. Pericecal collections may occur. Tenderness is usually localized to the right lower quadrant but may become diffuse. Septicemia by *P aeruginosa* and enterobacteriaceae is common; prostration and hypotension may be presenting signs.[335] Septicemia may be caused by multiple organisms, including anaerobes. Clostridial species are the most common anaerobic pathogens and may cause a devastating myonecrosis (see *Clostridium* Species, earlier in this chapter).

A CT scan should be obtained for patients with suspected typhlitis or undiagnosed abdominal pain in the setting of neutropenia fever. Positive CT scan findings are present in approximately 80% of cases of typhlitis[335] and include a right lower quadrant inflammatory mass, pericecal fluid, soft tissue inflammatory changes, localized bowel wall thickening and mucosal edema, and a paralytic ileus. Usually, disease is limited to the cecum, but more extensive involvement of the large bowel and disease of the terminal ileum may occur. Typhlitis was the most common finding in a review of cases of gastrointestinal abnormalities identified by CT scan in neutropenic patients; other abnormalities in descending order included *C difficile* colitis, GVHD of the bowel, CMV-related colitis, and bowel ischemia.[336]

Treatment of typhlitis requires broad-spectrum antibiotics with activity against aerobic gram-negative rods and anaerobes (e.g., imipenem, meropenem, or piperacillin-tazobactam), and supportive care, including administration of intravenous fluids, bowel rest, and nasogastric decompression, should be instituted. The indications for surgery are derived from clinical experience rather than trials. Shamberger et al.[337] proposed the following criteria for surgical intervention: (1) persistent gastrointestinal bleeding after resolution of neutropenia, thrombocytopenia, and clotting abnormalities; (2) free intraperitoneal perforation; (3) uncontrolled sepsis despite fluid and vasopressor support; and (4) an intraabdominal process (such as appendicitis) that would require surgery in the absence of neutropenia. When these criteria were used, 20 of 25 pediatric patients with typhlitis were managed without surgery, and only 1 patient died of typhlitis. In cases of a localized peritonitis, a pericecal collection, or a suspected sealed-off cecal perforation in a clinically stable neutropenic patient, surgical intervention may be delayed until resolution of neutropenia, given the increased surgical mortality during neutropenia. Surgical intervention involves resection of necrotic bowel, usually entailing a right hemicolectomy, ileostomy, and mucous fistula.

Patients with cancer are at high risk for *C difficile* colitis due to prolonged stays in the hospital, where environmental transmission is likely to occur, and receipt of broad-spectrum antibiotics. Clinical manifestations include asymptomatic carriage, colitis without pseudomembrane formation, pseudomembranous colitis, and fulminant colitis. In severe *C difficile* disease, paralytic ileus, toxic dilatation of the colon, and bowel perforation may occur. An abdominal film typically shows a dilated colon with mucosal edema (thumbprinting).

Oral metronidazole is the standard therapy for *C difficile* colitis. Because of the risk of selection for VRE, oral vancomycin should be reserved for refractory cases and for patients intolerant of metronidazole. Patients to whom oral agents cannot be administered should receive parenteral metronidazole, because biliary excretion of the drug and exudation from inflamed colon generally result in adequate luminal concentrations of the drug. Intravenous vancomycin is of no value in this setting because of inadequate luminal levels. In cases involving toxic dilatation of the colon or perforation, subtotal colectomy, diverting ileostomy, or colostomy may be required.

Endoscopic diagnosis of pseudomembranous colitis relies on visualization of characteristic raised, adherent, yellow plaques on the colonic mucosa. The mainstay of diagnosis is detection of *C difficile* toxin A, toxin B, or both with a cytotoxin test or enzyme immunoassay. Enzyme immunoassays that detect both toxins are preferred because of higher sensitivity. Approximately 20% of patients experience reinfection or relapse after initial therapy. Retreatment with metronidazole and limitation of the use of broad-spectrum antibiotics are advised.

ANORECTAL INFECTIONS

Anorectal infections in patients with malignancy may be life-threatening. Infection may follow the development of an anal fissure. Tiny abrasions may be a portal of entry or infection may originate in the anal crypts. Once anorectal infection is established, fascial extension to the external genitalia, pelvic floor, retroperitoneum, and peritoneal cavity may occur. Anorectal infections, with or without extensive regional spread, may lead to septicemia.

Patients with leukemia receiving intensive cytotoxic chemotherapy are at greatest risk for anorectal infections, with an incidence of approximately 5% in older series. The incidence may have decreased with the advent of colony-stimulating factors. The most common pathogens are enterobacteriaceae, anaerobes, enterococci, and *P aeruginosa*.[338,339] In most cases, the infection is polymicrobial. Recovery from neutropenia is the most important prognostic indicator for a positive outcome.[338]

Fever often precedes symptoms and signs suggestive of anorectal infection, and perirectal pain, often exacerbated by defecation, may initially occur in the absence of physical examination findings.[339] Therefore, serial examinations of the perianal region are necessary. In one series, point tenderness and poorly demarcated induration were the most consistent signs of perianal infection.[339] Advanced disease was heralded by soft tissue breakdown and necrosis and progressive extension to the adjacent perineal and pelvic structures.

In a patient with neutropenic fever, the presence of perirectal pain or local tenderness should prompt early administration of antibiotics with activity against anaerobes (e.g., imipenem, meropenem, or piperacillin-tazobactam). The authors advise against a digital rectal examination in the setting of neutropenia or thrombocytopenia to avoid traumatizing the friable mucosa. A CT scan may be useful to show the extent of perirectal involvement and drainable collections. Stool softeners, sitz baths, warm compresses, and analgesics should be provided.

Most cases of anorectal infection can be managed with appropriate broad-spectrum antibiotics and supportive measures without surgical intervention.[340] Indications for surgery include progression of disease locally or continued sepsis despite adequate antibiotic therapy, obvious tissue necrosis, or fluctuance. With adequate surgical drainage, pain typically resolves within 2 days.[339] At surgery, perirectal lesions usually are found to consist of necrotic cavities filled with tissue debris.[339]

CENTRAL NERVOUS SYSTEM INFECTION

Central nervous system infections in patients with cancer can be divided into surgical and nonsurgical complications. Common related surgical procedures include resection of tumor, insertion of a shunt for hydrocephalus, and insertion of a reservoir to facilitate delivery of chemotherapeutic agents and easy sampling of cerebrospinal fluid. Patients with cancer involving the brain typically receive high-dose steroids and local radiation therapy, which may further increase the risk of infections.

Infections related to implanted hardware may manifest in a variety of ways. Infection of a shunt or an Ommaya reservoir may manifest with malfunction of the device. Overt signs of meningitis, such as meningismus and photophobia, do not usually occur, but most patients have fever. Change in mental status may be the only sign of infection. A CT scan may suggest meningitis, ventriculitis, or a brain abscess if the device is infected at the proximal end. Evaluation of the cerebrospinal fluid is required for a diagnosis. Infection may occur in the more distal region of the device manifesting as a soft tissue infection. In cases of ventriculoatrial shunts, a distal site of infection may cause persistently positive blood cultures, thrombophlebitis, right-sided endocarditis, or septic pulmonary emboli. Distal ventriculoperitoneal shunt infections are associated with peritonitis and intraabdominal collections.

Coagulase-negative staphylococci, *S aureus,* and *Propionibacterium acnes* are the most common organisms infecting intraventricular devices. Enterobacteriaceae and *P aeruginosa* account for approximately 10% of infections. Coagulase-negative staphylococci and *P acnes* usually cause indolent late postoperative infections.

Removal of the entire device plus systemic antibiotic therapy is the most effective approach to eradicate infection. Parenteral and intraventricular instillation of antibiotics without hardware removal has met with variable success; however, recrudescence of infection is common. Antibiotic therapy should be tailored to the specific pathogen isolated. In an acutely ill patient with suspected meningitis related to prior neurosurgery, empirical therapy with parenteral vancomycin should be administered to cover *Staphylococcus, Streptococcus,* and *Propionibacterium* species in combination with an agent with activity against enterobacteriaceae and *P aeruginosa* (e.g., ceftazidime).

Central nervous system infections unrelated to neurosurgery are relatively uncommon in patients with cancer. In two series, the incidence of central nervous system infections in HSCT recipients was approximately 2%.[341,342] In a review of 58 cases of brain abscess after HSCT, 92% were caused by fungi.[343] *Aspergillus* species accounted for approximately 60% of isolates and one-third were caused by *Candida* species. Approximately 90% of cases of central nervous system aspergillosis were associated with a pulmonary focus, whereas most cases of *Candida* brain abscess were associated with candidemia or neutropenia. Only 4 of 58 patients had a bacterial brain abscess and 1 patient had cerebral toxoplasmosis. The mortality rate in this series was 97%.

Manifestations of CNS aspergillosis include focal seizures, hemiparesis, cranial nerve palsies, and hemorrhagic infarcts due to vascular invasion. In most cases, concurrent pneumonia is present and may require chest CT scan for detection. *Aspergillus* brain abscesses are typically multiple, hypodense, and nonenhancing with little mass effect. CT scans with contrast enhancement initially may reveal no focal lesions but usually evolve to focal ring-enhancing or hemorrhagic lesions. MRI may further facilitate early detection. Intermediate T2 signal surrounded by a rim of higher signal may be observed. A retrospective analysis of data for 86 patients with CNS aspergillosis treated with voriconazole either as primary or salvage therapy showed that 34% experienced a complete or partial response.[344] This success rate compares very favorably to that in previous series in which the frequency of successful responses to amphotericin B was almost nil.

Other less common causes of central nervous system infection in patients with cancer include herpesviruses (HSV, VZV, CMV, EBV, and HHV-6), adenovirus, *L monocytogenes, Acanthamoeba, Nocardia* species, *Mycobacterium* species, and *T gondii.*

DEMENTIAS

Patients with cancer may develop a chronic dementia related to leukoencephalopathy, a debilitating complication of therapy for their malignancy. The combination of cranial radiation therapy and intrathecal or systemic methotrexate has been most closely linked with leukoencephalopathy, although other intrathecal regimens may produce similar findings.

Progressive multifocal encephalopathy (PML) is a demyelinating disease associated with lytic infection of oligodendrocytes by the human polyomavirus JC virus. Patients may develop rapidly progressive dementia as well as focal motor or cerebellar findings. Today, this disease is most commonly seen in patients with advanced AIDS, which reflects the critical role of cell-mediated immunity in controlling this infection. Occasionally, PML is seen in heavily immunocompromised persons with hematologic malignancies and in HSCT recipients. MRI typically shows unilateral or bilateral white matter disease without mass effect or enhancement. Diagnosis is established either by examination of brain biopsy specimen or by detection of the JC virus in spinal fluid by PCR. There is no established therapy for PML. In patients with AIDS who have PML, highly active antiretroviral therapy has produced mixed results. By extrapolation, it is logical to try to reduce immunosuppressive therapy in persons with cancer and PML as a means of augmenting cell-mediated immunity.

GENITOURINARY INFECTIONS

Patients with cancer may be at increased risk for serious urinary tract infections as a result of breeches of the normal anatomy of the genitourinary system, colonization by pathogenic organisms, and defects in host defenses. The most common mechanism of seeding of the bladder is via the ascending route. Barriers to entry and proliferation of pathogens include the presence of normal perineal flora, urination, mucosal epithelial lining, phagocytes, and possibly immunoglobulin secretion (immunoglobulin A and immunoglobulin G).

A bladder catheter greatly facilitates colonization of the normally sterile bladder. A strong correlation exists between pre-catheterization rectal and periurethral isolates and organisms subsequently isolated from the urinary tract after bladder catheterization. Obstruction to urine flow permits colonization and multiplication of bacteria. In patients with cancer, obstruction of urine flow may result from tumors either within or impinging on the genitourinary tract. Tumors associated with hypercalcemia or hyperuricemia predispose to urinary stones. Impaired bladder emptying resulting in urine stasis may result from tumors involving the spinal cord. Urinary intestinal diversions are associated with a high incidence of bacteriuria and may predispose to clinically significant infections after myeloablative chemotherapy.

The epithelial lining of the bladder and a layer of mucopolysaccharide form a protective barrier against bacterial colonization and invasion. Injury to the bladder mucosa by cytotoxic agents likely increases the risk of infection. During neutropenia, the genitourinary tract may be an important portal of entry for systemic infections. Alternatively, the kidney may be secondarily seeded as a consequence of hematogenous infection. Neutropenic patients with a urinary tract infection are less likely to have dysuria and pyuria and are far more likely to become bacteremic than are nonneutropenic patients.[209]

Infection of the prostate, seminal vesicles, epididymis, and testes may represent localized disease or hematogenous seeding. Common causative bacteria include enterobacteriaceae, *P aeruginosa*, *S aureus*, and enterococci. Less common pathogens include *Salmonella* species, *M tuberculosis* (more likely to involve the kidneys and ureters), *Nocardia* species, *Candida* species *Blastomyces dermatitidis*, and *C neoformans*.

Asymptomatic candiduria is common in patients with bladder catheters. Management of candiduria is limited by lack of knowledge about the natural history of this infection, specifically with regard to predicting in which patients systemic infection will occur. Fluconazole is effective in eradicating candiduria in the short term, but recurrent infection is likely.[345] Removal of indwelling bladder catheters and cessation of antibacterial

agents frequently lead to clearing of candiduria. Therefore, routine treatment of asymptomatic candiduria is not warranted. Because of the risk of candidemia after genitourinary tract manipulations, candiduria should be treated before such procedures are performed. The authors suggest that patients with neutropenic fever and candiduria receive systemic antifungal therapy because of the potential for occult candidemia.

Hemorrhagic cystitis is a common consequence of cytotoxic regimens, which cause direct bladder mucosal injury and thrombocytopenia. In HSCT recipients with unexplained hematuria occurring beyond the early period (during which it is an expected toxicity of the preparative regimen), a viral cause should be considered. Adenovirus, the polyomavirus BK virus, and, rarely, CMV have been associated with hemorrhagic cystitis. Adenovirus and BK virus hemorrhagic cystitis are usually self-limiting, and the value of antiviral therapy is unclear. BK virus is associated with nephropathy in renal transplant recipients.[346] It is unclear whether BK virus causes renal disease in other immuncompromised groups.

INFECTIONS IN SURGICAL ONCOLOGY

Patients undergoing surgery for malignancies are at risk for infections as a result of anatomic factors and impaired host defense. Colonization is a prerequisite to clinically significant infection. Thus, patients undergoing head and neck surgery are at risk for infections by skin and oral mucosal flora. Patients undergoing resection of hepatobiliary or gastrointestinal tumors are at risk for infections by gastrointestinal flora. Superimposed on these anatomic factors are risk factors specific to the oncology patient. These include tumor obstruction of hollow viscera, infection of the tumor itself (e.g., a tumor abscess), extensive debulking that may be required for gynecologic and other malignancies, intraperitoneal instillation of chemotherapy (such as in gynecologic malignancies), and prolonged use of surgical drains. Prior radiation therapy interferes with wound healing and predisposes to more serious or protracted infection. Nodal dissection impairs lymphatic drainage and increases the likelihood of infection. Surgical oncology patients are also prone to serious infections that are not contiguous with the surgical site, such as catheter-related sepsis and ventilator-associated pneumonia. Such patients benefit from care by a multidisciplinary team, including intensivists and infectious disease specialists. The authors agree with the evidence-based guidelines of the American Society of Health-System Pharmacists on antimicrobial prophylaxis for surgery.[347]

Patients with head and neck cancers who undergo procedures that breach the upper aerodigestive tract mucosa are at significant risk for infection. Penel et al.[348] prospectively evaluated 165 consecutive surgical procedures for head and neck cancer involving the aerodigestive tract at Oscar Lambret Cancer Center over 2 years. The overall rate of wound infection was 42%. Tumor stage, previous chemotherapy, duration of preoperative hospital stay, presence of a permanent tracheostomy, and hypopharyngeal and laryngeal cancers were associated with an increased risk of infection. In a prospective randomized trial, a 3-day course of prophylactic antibiotics was no more effective than the standard 1-day regimen in treatment of patients undergoing head and neck surgery.[349] Preoperative radiotherapy was associated with more severe infections and late wound complications. Similarly, no benefit of prolonged perioperative prophylaxis was identified either in clean (n = 201) or clean-contaminated (n = 207) surgeries for head and neck cancer in a retrospective analysis.[350] Among clean-contaminated procedures, factors affecting postoperative wound infection rates were performance of bilateral neck dissections, disease stage, type of laryngectomy, and prior tracheotomy.[350] Among clean procedures, radical neck dissection was associated with a higher rate of infections.

Surgeries for gastrointestinal, esophageal, gastric, and pancreatic malignancies were associated with the highest frequency of postoperative infections.[351] In addition to increasing morbidity and mortality, such surgery-related infections significantly increase the duration of hospitalization and cost.[351]

Surgical procedures involving hepatobiliary tumors may be associated with severe and protracted infections. The biliary tract is usually sterile. However, patients with obstructive malignancies are usually treated with stents or diverting procedures that enable colonization of the biliary tract with intestinal flora. Bacterial colonization of the biliary tract at the time of surgery increases the risk of postoperative infection. In a retrospective analysis of 170 therapeutic biliary drainage procedures in 90 patients with cancer, the overall infection rate was 61%, despite the fact that most patients received prophylactic antibiotics.[352] Cholangitis and bacteremia were the most common manifestations and enterobacteriaceae, *Enterococcus* species, and *Candida* species were the most frequent pathogens.

Chemoembolization and radiofrequency ablation of hepatic tumors are effective in reducing tumor bulk but also create a necrotic bed that may be seeded by intestinal bacteria, which predisposes to infection. The incidence of infection after these procedures is approximately 1%. Kim et al.[353] identified prior biliary enteric anastomosis as the primary determinant in development of a liver abscess after subsequent chemoembolization. Seven of 157 cases (4.5%) were complicated by a liver abscess, and 6 of these cases occurred in patients who had undergone a Whipple procedure before chemoembolization. Indeed, a liver abscess occurred in six of seven patients who had undergone a Whipple procedure before embolization. In the absence of a randomized study, administration of prophylactic antibiotics active against enteric flora should be considered in patients undergoing hepatic chemoembolization or radiofrequency ablation with a history of prior biliary stenting or reconstruction. Bacterial hepatic abscesses in patients with cancer require percutaneous or open drainage and a prolonged course of appropriate antibiotics until all clinical and radiographic signs of infection have resolved.

Patients with cancer undergoing major abdominal surgery are also at risk for nosocomial candidiasis, which reflects the fact that *Candida* species colonize gastrointestinal and vaginal mucosa. Other risk factors for candidemia relevant to this patient group include use of triple-lumen catheters and need for parenteral nutrition.[354] In patients with gastrointestinal perforations or anastomotic leaks, prophylaxis with fluconazole reduced the frequency of peritoneal candidiasis and may be warranted in this high-risk group.[355]

Malnutrition is an important and often overlooked condition predisposing to postoperative infections and morbidity. Randomized studies have shown the value of perioperative enteral nutrition in reducing serious postoperative infections and hospitalization days in patients with cancer.[356,357]

IMMUNE AUGMENTATION STRATEGIES

COLONY GROWTH FACTORS

Normal myelopoiesis requires myeloid stem cells. Under the influence of stem cell factor, IL-3, and GM-CSF, these give rise to the colony-forming unit–granulocyte-macrophage. G-CSF acts at a later stage in concert with other growth factors to specifically drive granulopoiesis. Primary administration of CSFs has reduced the incidence of febrile neutropenia by approximately 50% in randomized trials in adults in whom the incidence of neutropenic fever was higher than 40% in the control group. In patients with acute myelogenous leukemia, CSFs produce a modest decrease in the duration of neutropenia, which in some studies has translated into a reduction in the duration of fever, use of antibiotics, and hospitalization.[358,359] This benefit has mainly been demonstrated in patients 55 years of age or older and after consolidation chemotherapy. With the exception of one placebo-controlled study in which GM-CSF administration was associated with a lower frequency of fatal fungal infections and early mortality in patients with acute myelogenous leukemia,[360] CSFs have not produced a survival advantage.

The American Society of Clinical Oncology has recommended that prophylactic CSFs (G-CSF and GM-CSF) be used only in populations in whom the frequency of febrile neutropenia is likely to exceed 40%.[361] The society's guidelines also considered that certain patients receiving a relatively nonmyelosuppressive regimen may benefit from CSFs if they are at high risk for infectious complications. Examples of such risk factors include preexisting neutropenia, extensive prior chemotherapy or pelvic irradiation leading to a reduction in myeloid reserves, a history of recurrent febrile neutropenia with chemotherapy of similar or lower dose intensity, an open wound, and poor performance status. In the authors' opinion, patients with prior serious or life-threatening infection such as typhlitis or an invasive fungal infection should also be considered for CSF treatment during subsequent chemotherapy.

The rationale for the use of CSFs for treatment of established infections (as opposed to prophylaxis) stems from both the quantitative and qualitative effects of these agents on phagocytic cells. In neutropenic patients with life-threatening infections, survival is strongly influenced by the rapidity of neutrophil recovery. Thus, CSFs and granulocyte transfusions may be used in these settings to augment the number of circulating neutrophils. Randomized trials have not shown a benefit of the use of CSFs as adjunct therapy for uncomplicated neutropenic fever. Although the benefit of a CSF for treatment of established infections is unproven, it may be considered in the setting of profound neutropenia (absolute neutrophil count of fewer than 100/μL), uncontrolled primary disease, and serious infections such as pneumonia, infections accompanied by hypotension or multiorgan dysfunction, and invasive fungal infection.[361]

GRANULOCYTE TRANSFUSIONS

The rationale for granulocyte transfusions is to provide supportive therapy for the neutropenic patient with a life-threatening infection by augmenting the number of circulating neutrophils until autologous myeloid regeneration occurs. In the 1970s, apheresis technology for harvesting large numbers of donor granulocytes became available. Controlled trials of granulocyte transfusions as adjuvant therapy in treatment of neutropenic patients produced mixed results. In the 1980s, the enthusiasm for granulocyte transfusions waned as more effective antibiotics became available, survival from serious bacterial infections improved, and recombinant growth factors reduced the duration of neutropenia. In addition, concerns about the toxicity of granulocyte transfusions, including acute pulmonary reactions, HLA alloimmunization (which could render patients refractory to platelet transfusions and potentially impair myeloid engraftment after HSCT), and transfusion-associated infections (particularly with CMV), outweighed the perceived benefits.

Today, the impetus to reexamine the role of granulocyte transfusions stems largely from improvements in donor mobilization methods. Bensinger et al.[362] showed that G-CSF mobilization significantly increased the granulocyte yield and resulted in improved circulating neutrophil levels in neutropenic recipients. When a standard continuous-flow centrifugation apparatus is used, the mean absolute neutrophil yield per collection is typically in the range of 8×10^{10} cells when both G-CSF and dexamethasone are used in the donor preparatory regimen. Higher numbers of harvested neutrophils correlate with higher posttransfusion neutrophil counts. Furthermore, the increase in circulating neutrophils tends to be sustained for 24 to 30 hours after transfusion, as a consequence of the prolonged circulating half-life of G-CSF–mobilized granulocytes.[363] The qualitative functions of G-CSF– and steroid-mobilized neutrophils are intact based on *in vitro* observation of bactericidal activity, respiratory burst, migration to experimental skin chambers, and localization to sites of inflammation.

Successful outcomes using granulocyte transfusions have been described in patients with life-threatening fungal infections in small series and in case reports. A phase I and II trial using G-CSF–mobilized granulocyte transfusions for treatment of refractory fungal infections in neutropenic patients with hematologic malignancies reported favorable responses in 11 of 15 patients.[364] Peters et al.[365] evaluated granulocyte transfusions (G-CSF or prednisolone mobilized) in 30 patients with neutropenia and life-threatening, refractory infections. Infections cleared in 20 of 30 patients, including five of nine patients with invasive aspergillosis. No benefit of granulocyte transfusions was noted in neutropenic HSCT recipients with invasive mold infection in a retrospective series in which G-CSF donor granulocyte mobilization was not used.[366]

Price et al.[367] conducted a phase I and II study of transfusion of granulocytes derived from unrelated, non–HLA-matched, community donors after G-CSF and dexamethasone mobilization. Chills, fever, and oxygen desaturation of 3% or higher occurred in association with 7% of transfusions but did not limit therapy. Eight of 11 patients with bacterial infections or candidemia survived, but all 8 patients with invasive mold infection died. This study showed the safety and feasibility of using community donors for granulocyte apheresis donations.

In the absence of modern, prospective, randomized studies, when might granulocyte transfusion be considered? Currently, there is no justification (outside of a clinical trial) to use granulocyte transfusions either as prophylaxis or in cases of documented infections that are likely to respond to conventional therapy. The authors reserve granulocyte transfusions for patients with prolonged neutropenia and life-threatening infec-

tions refractory to conventional therapy. Filamentous fungi infections are likely to constitute the majority of such refractory infections. Infusions of amphotericin B should be separated by several hours from granulocyte transfusions to avoid pulmonary toxicity. In some highly alloimmunized patients, transfused granulocytes are rapidly consumed and are likely to produce more toxicity than benefit. In cases of allogeneic transplantation in which the donor and recipient are CMV seronegative, the use of CMV-seronegative granulocyte donors is advised.[368]

INTERFERON-γ

IFN-γ is produced by lymphocytes (CD4+, CD8+, natural killer cells) as well as macrophages and perhaps neutrophils. It is induced by a number of signals, including IL-12 and IL-18, and in turn induces hundreds of genes, including its own inducers. The antimicrobial activity induced by IFN-γ encompasses intracellular and extracellular parasites, bacteria, fungi, and viruses.

Currently, IFN-γ is licensed as a prophylactic agent for treatment of patients with chronic granulomatous disease, an inherited disorder of the phagocyte reduced nicotinamide adenine dinucleotide phosphate oxidase characterized by recurrent life-threatening bacterial and fungal infections,[369] and patients with osteopetrosis. In addition, IFN-γ in combination with antimycobacterial agents had a positive effect on patients with refractory nontuberculous mycobacterial infection resulting in defective IFN-γ production.[370] IFN-γ confers protection against a variety of experimental fungal infections in animals.[371] Adjunctive IFN-γ therapy showed promising results in a pilot study of treatment of AIDS-associated cryptococcal meningitis.[372] There is significant interest in evaluating IFN-γ as adjunctive therapy for invasive filamentous fungal infections.

ADOPTIVE IMMUNOTHERAPY IN HEMATOPOIETIC STEM CELL TRANSPLANT RECIPIENTS

Intensive preparative regimens used in allogeneic HSCT result in a profound disruption of T-cell immunity. Reconstitution of T-cell immunity occurs over several months in uncomplicated cases and is further delayed in cases of GVHD requiring high-dose steroid therapy and administration of antilymphocyte globulins. CMV and EBV establish latent infection in normal hosts, and control of reactivation is largely mediated by CD8+ CTLs.[373] CTLs recognize intracellular proteins that are presented by surface major histocompatibility complex class I molecules on antigen-presenting cells. Viral antigen–specific CD4+ T cells may be required for long-term CD8+ T-cell persistence. Over the past decade, researchers have explored whether adoptive transfer of virus-specific CTLs may be protective.

In the first study evaluating the potential of CMV-specific CTLs to restore immunity, recipients of allogeneic HSCTs from HLA-matched siblings received infusions of CD8+ CMV-specific CTL clones from their donors.[374] Such an approach led to early reconstitution of CMV-specific immunity, which persisted for at least 12 weeks after infusion, corresponding to the period of maximal risk for CMV disease. Dendritic cells and EBV-transformed cell lines transduced with a vector encoding the CMV early antigen pp65 and dendritic cells pulsed with pp65 also induce antigen-specific CTL responses.

Although withdrawal of immunosuppression is often effective in controlling EBV-induced PTLD in solid organ transplant recipients, this approach is usually insufficient to generate adequate immune recovery in allogeneic HSCT recipients to control the disease. Infusions of unfractionated peripheral blood mononuclear cells from EBV-seropositive donors have been used to treat PTLD in allogeneic HSCT recipients.[375] However, alloreactive T cells in such unfractionated preparations may induce GVHD. A potentially safer approach involves transfer of EBV-specific donor CTL clones that have been selectively enriched *in vitro*.[376,377] This method has led to persistent cellular immune responses to EBV for as long as 18 months.[377] Adoptive transfer of EBV-specific CTLs has been generally safe and effective in controlling PTLD and in preventing EBV-related PLPD when used prophylactically.

The previously described studies establish a proof of principle with regard to the feasibility of adoptive transfer of viral antigen–specific CTLs. Additional research is focused on strategies to produce antigen-presenting cells that display major antigens from multiple clinically relevant viruses to generate multispecific CTL populations.[373]

REFERENCES

1. Griffiths H, Lea J, Bunch C, Lee M, Chapel H. Predictors of infection in chronic lymphocytic leukaemia (CLL). *Clin Exp Immunol* 1992;89:374.
2. Weeks JC, Tierney MR, Weinstein MC. Cost effectiveness of prophylactic intravenous immune globulin in chronic lymphocytic leukemia [see comments]. *N Engl J Med* 1991;325:81.
3. Savage DG, Lindenbaum J, Garrett TJ. Biphasic pattern of bacterial infection in multiple myeloma. *Ann Intern Med* 1982;96:47.
4. Chapel HM, Lee M, Hargreaves R, Pamphilon DH, Prentice AG. Randomised trial of intravenous immunoglobulin as prophylaxis against infection in plateau-phase multiple myeloma. The UK Group for Immunoglobulin Replacement Therapy in Multiple Myeloma [see comments]. *Lancet* 1994;343:1059.
5. Fisher RI, DeVita VT Jr, Bostick F, et al. Persistent immunologic abnormalities in long-term survivors of advanced Hodgkin's disease. *Ann Intern Med* 1980;92:595.
6. Graham BS, Tucker WS Jr. Opportunistic infections in endogenous Cushing's syndrome. *Ann Intern Med* 1984;101:334.
7. Bodey GP, Buckley M, Sathe YS, Freireich EJ. Quantitative relationships between circulating leukocytes and infection in patients with acute leukemia. *Ann Intern Med* 1966;64:328.
8. Gerson SL, Talbot GH, Hurwitz S, et al. Prolonged granulocytopenia: the major risk factor for invasive pulmonary aspergillosis in patients with acute leukemia. *Ann Intern Med* 1984;100:345.
9. Weinberger M, Elattar I, Marshall D, et al. Patterns of infection in patients with aplastic anemia and the emergence of *Aspergillus* as a major cause of death. *Medicine (Baltimore)* 1992;71:24.
10. Anaissie E, Kontoyiannis DP, Kantarjian H, et al. Listeriosis in patients with chronic lymphocytic leukemia who were treated with fludarabine and prednisone. *Ann Intern Med* 1992;117:466.
11. O'Brien S, Kantarjian H, Beran M, et al. Results of fludarabine and prednisone therapy in 264 patients with chronic lymphocytic leukemia with multivariate analysis-derived prognostic model for response to treatment [see comments]. *Blood* 1993;82:1695.
12. Tsiodras S, Samonis G, Keating MJ, Kontoyiannis DP. Infection and immunity in chronic lymphocytic leukemia. *Mayo Clin Proc* 2000;75:1039.
13. Roy MJ, Walsh TJ. Histopathologic and immunohistochemical changes in gut-associated lymphoid tissues after treatment of rabbits with dexamethasone. *Lab Invest* 1992;66:437.
14. Hill GR, Ferrara JL. The primacy of the gastrointestinal tract as a target organ of acute graft-versus-host disease: rationale for the use of cytokine shields in allogeneic bone marrow transplantation. *Blood* 2000;95:2754.
15. Segal BH, Sneller MC. Infectious complications of immunosuppressive therapy in patients with rheumatic diseases. *Rheum Dis Clin North Am* 1997;23:219.
16. Staples PJ, Gerding DN, Decker JL, Gordon RS Jr. Incidence of infection in systemic lupus erythematosus. *Arthritis Rheum* 1974;17:1.
17. Shaukat A, Bakri F, Young P, et al. Invasive filamentous fungal infection in bone marrow transplant recipients after neutrophil count recovery: clinical, radiologic, and pathologic characteristics. In: *Focus on fungal infections*, vol 12. Phoenix, 2002.
18. Roilides E, Uhlig K, Venzon D, Pizzo PA, Walsh TJ. Prevention of corticosteroid-induced suppression of human polymorphonuclear leukocyte-induced damage of *Aspergillus fumigatus* hyphae by granulocyte colony-stimulating factor and gamma interferon. *Infect Immun* 1993;61:4870.
19. Ng TT, Robson GD, Denning DW. Hydrocortisone-enhanced growth of *Aspergillus* spp.: implications for pathogenesis. *Microbiology* 1994;140:2475.
20. Klempner MS, Noring R, Mier JW, Atkins MB. An acquired chemotactic defect in neutrophils from patients receiving interleukin-2 immunotherapy [see comments]. *N Engl J Med* 1990;322:959.
21. Kalhs P, Kier P, Lechner K. Functional asplenia after bone marrow transplantation [Letter]. *Ann Intern Med* 1990;113:805.
22. Molrine DC, Siber GR, Samra Y, et al. Normal IgG and impaired IgM responses to polysaccharide vaccines in asplenic patients. *J Infect Dis* 1999;179:513.
23. Working Party of the British Committee for Standards in Haematology Clinical Haematology Task Force. Guidelines for the prevention and treatment of infection in patients with an absent or dysfunctional spleen. *BMJ* 1996;312:430.
24. Winston DJ, Territo MC, Ho WG, et al. Alveolar macrophage dysfunction in human bone marrow transplant recipients. *Am J Med* 1982;73:859.
25. Lum LG. The kinetics of immune reconstitution after human marrow transplantation. *Blood* 1987;69:369.
26. Mackall CL, Gress RE. Pathways of T-cell regeneration in mice and humans: implications for bone marrow transplantation and immunotherapy. *Immunol Rev* 1997;157:61.
27. Winston DJ, Schiffman G, Wang DC, et al. Pneumococcal infections after human bone-marrow transplantation. *Ann Intern Med* 1979;91:835.
28. Kulkarni S, Powles R, Treleaven J, et al. Chronic graft versus host disease is associated with long-term risk for pneumococcal infections in recipients of bone marrow transplants. *Blood* 2000;95:3683.
29. Avanzini MA, Carra AM, Maccario R, et al. Antibody response to pneumococcal vaccine in children receiving bone marrow transplantation. *J Clin Immunol* 1995;15:137.
30. Storek J, Viganego F, Dawson MA, et al. Factors affecting antibody levels after allogeneic hematopoietic cell transplantation. *Blood* 2003;101:3319.
31. Sullivan KM, Dykewicz CA, Longworth DL, et al. Preventing opportunistic infections after hematopoietic stem cell transplantation: the Centers for Disease Control and Prevention, Infectious Diseases Society of America, and American Society for Blood and Marrow Transplantation Practice Guidelines and beyond. *Hematology (Am Soc Hematol Educ Program)* 2001:392.
32. Meijer E, Dekker AW, Rozenberg-Arska M, Weersink AJ, Verdonck LF. Influence of cytomegalovirus seropositivity on outcome after T cell–depleted bone marrow transplantation: contrasting results between recipients of grafts from related and unrelated donors. *Clin Infect Dis* 2002;35:703.
33. Marr KA, Carter RA, Boeckh M, Martin P, Corey L. Invasive aspergillosis in allogeneic stem cell transplant recipients: changes in epidemiology and risk factors. *Blood* 2002;100:4358.
34. Alam AR, Varma G, Hahn T, et al. Infectious complications in long-term survivors of cord blood stem cell transplantation (CBSCT): experience at Roswell Park Cancer Institute. *Blood* 2002;100:629(s).
35. Crippa F, Holmberg L, Carter RA, et al. Infectious complications after autologous CD34-selected peripheral blood stem cell transplantation. *Biol Blood Marrow Transplant* 2002;8:281.
36. Chakrabarti S, Mackinnon S, Chopra R, et al. High incidence of cytomegalovirus infection after nonmyeloablative stem cell transplantation: potential role of Campath-1H in delaying immune reconstitution. *Blood* 2002;99:4357.
37. Lundin J, Hagberg H, Repp R, et al. Phase 2 study of alemtuzumab (Anti-CD52 monoclonal antibody) in patients with advanced mycosis fungoides/Sezary syndrome. *Blood* 2003;101:4267.
38. Chakrabarti S, Avivi I, Mackinnon S, et al. Respiratory virus infections in transplant recipients after reduced-intensity conditioning with Campath-1H: high incidence but low mortality. *Br J Haematol* 2002;119:1125.
39. Marty FM, Lee SJ, Fahey MM, et al. Infliximab use in patients with severe graft-versus-host disease and other emerging risk factors for non-*Candida* invasive fungal infections in allogeneic hematopoietic transplant recipients: a cohort study. *Blood* 2003;102:2768.
40. Carpenter PA, Appelbaum FR, Corey L, et al. A humanized non-FcR-binding anti-CD3 antibody, visilizumab, for treatment of steroid-refractory acute graft-versus-host disease. *Blood* 2002;99:2712.
41. Schimpff SC, Young VM, Green WH, et al. Origin of infection in acute lymphocytic leukemia: significance of hospital acquisition of potential pathogens. *Ann Intern Med* 1972;77:707.
42. Wisplinghoff H, Seifert H, Wenzel RP, Edmond MB. Current trends in the epidemiology of nosocomial bloodstream infections in patients with hematological malignancies and solid neoplasms in hospitals in the United States. *Clin Infect Dis* 2003;36:1103.
43. Rosen AB, Fowler VG Jr, Corey GR, et al. Cost-effectiveness of transesophageal echocardiography to determine the duration of therapy for intravascular catheter-associated staphylococcal bacteremia. *Ann Intern Med* 1999;130:810.
44. Chang FY, Peacock JE Jr, Musher DM, et al. *Staphylococcus aureus* bacteremia: recurrence and the impact of antibiotic treatment in a prospective multicenter study. *Medicine (Baltimore)* 2003;82:333.
45. Tunkell AR, Sepkowitz KA. Infections caused by viridans streptococci in patients with neutropenia. *Clin Infect Dis* 2002;34:1524.
46. Elting LS, Rubenstein EB, Rolston KV, Bodey GP. Outcomes of bacteremia in patients with cancer and neutropenia: observations from two decades of epidemiological and clinical trials. *Clin Infect Dis* 1997;25:247.
47. Westling K, Ljungman P, Thalme A, Julander I. Streptococcus viridans septicaemia: a comparison study in patients admitted to the departments of infectious diseases and haematology in a university hospital. *Scand J Infect Dis* 2002;34:316.
48. van der Lelie H, Leverstein-Van Hall M, Mertens M, et al. *Corynebacterium* CDC group JK (*Corynebacterium jeikeium*) sepsis in haematological patients: a report of three cases and a systematic literature review. *Scand J Infect Dis* 1995;27:581.
49. Stamm WE, Tompkins LS, Wagner KF, et al. Infection due to *Corynebacterium* species in marrow transplant patients. *Ann Intern Med* 1979;91:167.
50. Henrickson KJ, Shenep JL, Flynn PM, Pui CH. Primary cutaneous *Bacillus cereus* infection in neutropenic children. *Lancet* 1989;1:601.
51. Cotton DJ, Gill VJ, Marshall DJ, et al. Clinical features and therapeutic interventions in 17 cases of *Bacillus* bacteremia in an immunosuppressed patient population. *J Clin Microbiol* 1987;25:672.

52. Maschmeyer G, Braveny I. Review of the incidence and prognosis of *Pseudomonas aeruginosa* infections in cancer patients in the 1990s. *Eur J Clin Microbiol Infect Dis* 2000;19:915.

53. Chatzinikolaou I, Abi-Said D, Bodey GP, et al. Recent experience with *Pseudomonas aeruginosa* bacteremia in patients with cancer: retrospective analysis of 245 episodes. *Arch Intern Med* 2000;160:501.

54. Murdoch DR. Diagnosis of *Legionella* infection. *Clin Infect Dis* 2003;36:64.

55. Bodey GP, Rodriguez S, Fainstein V, Elting LS. Clostridial bacteremia in cancer patients. A 12-year experience. *Cancer* 1991;67:1928.

56. Kurzrock R, Zander A, Vellekoop L, et al. Mycobacterial pulmonary infections after allogeneic bone marrow transplantation. *Am J Med* 1984;77:35.

57. Roy V, Weisdorf D. Mycobacterial infections following bone marrow transplantation: a 20 year retrospective review. *Bone Marrow Transplant* 1997;19:467.

58. Ip MS, Yuen KY, Woo PC, et al. Risk factors for pulmonary tuberculosis in bone marrow transplant recipients. *Am J Respir Crit Care Med* 1998;158:1173.

59. Jacobson KL, Teira R, Libshitz HI, et al. *Mycobacterium kansasii* infections in patients with cancer. *Clin Infect Dis* 2000;30:965.

60. Shah MK, Sebti A, Kiehn TE, Massarella SA, Sepkowitz KA. *Mycobacterium haemophilum* in immunocompromised patients. *Clin Infect Dis* 2001;33:330.

61. Treatment of tuberculosis. American Thoracic Society, CDC, and Infectious Diseases Society of America. *MMWR Recomm Rep* 2003;52(RR-11):1.

62. Wallace RJ, Cook JL, Glassroth J, et al. Diagnosis and treatment of disease caused by nontuberculous mycobacteria. American Thoracic Society statement. *Am J Respir Crit Care Med* 1997;156[Suppl]:S1.

63. Torres HA, Reddy BT, Raad II, et al. Nocardiosis in cancer patients. *Medicine (Baltimore)* 2002;81:388.

64. van Burik JA, Hackman RC, Nadeem SQ, et al. Nocardiosis after bone marrow transplantation: a retrospective study. *Clin Infect Dis* 1997;24:1154.

65. Moylett EH, Pacheco SE, Brown-Elliott BA, et al. Clinical experience with linezolid for the treatment of *Nocardia* infection. *Clin Infect Dis* 2003;36:313.

66. Dorman SE, Guide SV, Conville PS, et al. *Nocardia* infection in chronic granulomatous disease. *Clin Infect Dis* 2002;35:390.

67. Bow EJ, Loewen R, Cheang MS, et al. Cytotoxic therapy–induced D-xylose malabsorption and invasive infection during remission-induction therapy for acute myeloid leukemia in adults. *J Clin Oncol* 1997;15:2254.

68. Kartsonis N, DiNubile MJ, Bartizal K, et al. Efficacy of caspofungin in the treatment of esophageal candidiasis resistant to fluconazole. *J Acquir Immune Defic Syndr* 2002;31:183.

69. Ally R, Schurmann D, Kreisel W, et al. Esophageal Candidiasis Study Group. A randomized double-blind double-dummy multicenter trial of voriconazole and fluconazole in the treatment of esophageal candidiasis in immunocompromised patients. *Clin Infect Dis* 2001;33:1447.

70. Edmond MB, Wallace SE, McClish DK, et al. Nosocomial bloodstream infections in United States hospitals: a three-year analysis. *Clin Infect Dis* 1999;29:239.

71. Viscoli C, Girmenia C, Marinus A, et al. Candidemia in cancer patients: a prospective, multicenter surveillance study by the Invasive Fungal Infection Group (IFIG) of the European Organization for Research and Treatment of Cancer (EORTC). *Clin Infect Dis* 1999;28:1071.

72. Anaissie EJ, Kontoyiannis DP, O'Brien S, et al. Infections in patients with chronic lymphocytic leukemia treated with fludarabine. *Ann Intern Med* 1998;129:559.

73. Walsh TJ, Rex JH. All catheter-related candidemia is not the same: assessment of the balance between the risks and benefits of removal of vascular catheters. *Clin Infect Dis* 2002;34:600.

74. Rex JH, Bennett JE, Sugar AM, et al. Intravascular catheter exchange and duration of candidemia. NIAID Mycoses Study Group and the Candidemia Study Group. *Clin Infect Dis* 1995;21:994.

75. Rex JH, Walsh TJ, Sobel JD, et al. Practice guidelines for the treatment of candidiasis. Infectious Diseases Society of America. *Clin Infect Dis* 2000;30:662.

76. Nucci M, Anaissie E. Revisiting the source of candidemia: skin or gut? *Clin Infect Dis* 2001;33:1959.

77. Nucci M, Anaissie E. Should vascular catheters be removed from all patients with candidemia? An evidence-based review. *Clin Infect Dis* 2002;34:591.

78. Rodriguez-Adrian LJ, King RT, Tamayo-Derat LG, et al. Retinal lesions as clues to disseminated bacterial and candidal infections: frequency, natural history, and etiology. *Medicine (Baltimore)* 2003;82:187.

79. Anttila VJ, Elonen E, Nordling S, et al. Hepatosplenic candidiasis in patients with acute leukemia: incidence and prognostic implications [see comments]. *Clin Infect Dis* 1997;24:375.

80. Karthaus M, Huebner G, Elser C, et al. Early detection of chronic disseminated *Candida* infection in leukemia patients with febrile neutropenia: value of computer-assisted serial ultrasound documentation. *Ann Hematol* 1998;77:41.

81. Walsh TJ, Whitcomb PO, Revankar SG, Pizzo PA. Successful treatment of hepatosplenic candidiasis through repeated cycles of chemotherapy and neutropenia. *Cancer* 1995;76:2357.

82. Choi EH, Foster CB, Taylor JG, et al. Association between chronic disseminated candidiasis in adult acute leukemia and common IL4 promoter haplotypes. *J Infect Dis* 2003;187:1153.

83. Rex JH, Bennett JE, Sugar AM, et al. A randomized trial comparing fluconazole with amphotericin B for the treatment of candidemia in patients without neutropenia. Candidemia Study Group and the National Institute [see comments]. *N Engl J Med* 1994;331:1325.

84. Rex JH, Pappas PG, Karchmer AW, et al. A randomized and blinded multicenter trial of high-dose fluconazole plus placebo versus fluconazole plus amphotericin B as therapy for candidemia and its consequences in nonneutropenic subjects. *Clin Infect Dis* 2003;36:1221.

85. Mora-Duarte J, Betts R, Rotstein C, et al. Comparison of caspofungin and amphotericin B for invasive candidiasis. *N Engl J Med* 2002;347:2020.

86. Fukuda T, Boeckh M, Carter RA, et al. Invasive fungal infections in recipients of allogeneic hematopoietic stem cell transplantation after nonmyeloablative conditioning: risks and outcomes. *Blood* 2003;10:10.

87. Walsh TJ, Roden M, Nelson L, et al. Invasive fungal infections complicating non-myeloablative allogeneic peripheral blood stem cell transplantation (PBSCT). Paper presented at: 42nd Interscience Conference on Antimicrobial Agents and Chemotherapy; 2002; San Diego, CA.

88. Marr KA, Carter RA, Crippa F, Wald A, Corey L. Epidemiology and outcome of mould infections in hematopoietic stem cell transplant recipients. *Clin Infect Dis* 2002;34:909.

89. Anaissie EJ, Stratton SL, Dignani MC, et al. Pathogenic *Aspergillus* species recovered from a hospital water system: a 3-year prospective study. *Clin Infect Dis* 2002;34:780.

90. Caillot D, Casasnovas O, Bernard A, et al. Improved management of invasive pulmonary aspergillosis in neutropenic patients using early thoracic computed tomographic scan and surgery. *J Clin Oncol* 1997;15:139.

91. Kuhlman JE, Fishman EK, Burch PA, et al. Invasive pulmonary aspergillosis in acute leukemia. The contribution of CT to early diagnosis and aggressive management. *Chest* 1987;92:95.

92. Maertens J, Verhaegen J, Lagrou K, Van Eldere J, Boogaerts M. Screening for circulating galactomannan as a noninvasive diagnostic tool for invasive aspergillosis in prolonged neutropenic patients and stem cell transplantation recipients: a prospective validation. *Blood* 2001;97:1604.

93. Maertens J, Van Eldere J, Verhaegen J, et al. Use of circulating galactomannan screening for early diagnosis of invasive aspergillosis in allogeneic stem cell transplant recipients. *J Infect Dis* 2002;186:1297.

94. Herbrecht R, Letscher-Bru V, Oprea C, et al. *Aspergillus* galactomannan detection in the diagnosis of invasive aspergillosis in cancer patients. *J Clin Oncol* 2002;20:1898.

95. Petraitis V, Petraitiene R, Sarafandi AA, et al. Combination therapy in treatment of experimental pulmonary aspergillosis: synergistic interaction between an antifungal triazole and an echinocandin. *J Infect Dis* 2003;187:1834.

96. Boutboul F, Alberti C, Leblanc T, et al. Invasive aspergillosis in allogeneic stem cell transplant recipients: increasing antigenemia is associated with progressive disease. *Clin Infect Dis* 2002;34:939.

97. Herbrecht R, Denning DW, Patterson TF, et al. Voriconazole versus amphotericin B for primary therapy of invasive aspergillosis. *N Engl J Med* 2002;347:408.

98. Walsh TJ, Lutsar I, Driscoll T, et al. Voriconazole in the treatment of aspergillosis, scedosporiosis, and other invasive fungal infections in children. *Pediatr Infect Dis J* 2002;21:240.

99. Denning DW, Ribaud P, Milpied N, et al. Efficacy and safety of voriconazole in the treatment of acute invasive aspergillosis. *Clin Infect Dis* 2002;34:563.

100. Steinbach WJ, Benjamin DK Jr, Kontoyiannis DP, et al. Invasive aspergillosis (IA) caused by *Aspergillus terreus*: multicenter retrospective analysis of 87 cases. Paper presented at: 43rd Interscience Conference on Antimicrobial Agents and Chemotherapy; 2003; Chicago, IL.

101. Kartsonis N, Saah A, Lipka J, Taylor A, Sable C. Salvage therapy (Rx) with caspofungin (CAS) for invasive aspergillosis (IA): results from the CAS compassionate use (CU) study. Paper presented at: 43rd Interscience Conference on Antimicrobial Agents and Chemotherapy; 2003; Chicago, IL.

102. Caspofungin (Cancidas) for aspergillosis. *Med Lett Drugs Ther* 2001;43:58.

103. Gea-Banacloche JC, Peter J, Bishop M, et al. Successful treatment of invasive aspergillosis with the combination of voriconazole and caspofungin: correlation with in vitro interactions. Paper presented at: 43rd Interscience Conference on Antimicrobial Agents and Chemotherapy; 2003; Chicago, IL.

104. Kontoyiannis DP, Hachem R, Lewis RE, et al. Efficacy and toxicity of caspofungin in combination with liposomal amphotericin B as primary or salvage treatment of invasive aspergillosis in patients with hematologic malignancies. *Cancer* 2003;98:292.

105. Aliff TB, Maslak PG, Jurcic JG, et al. Refractory *Aspergillus* pneumonia in patients with acute leukemia: successful therapy with combination caspofungin and liposomal amphotericin. *Cancer* 2003;97:1025.

106. Offner F, Cordonnier C, Ljungman P, et al. Impact of previous aspergillosis on the outcome of bone marrow transplantation. *Clin Infect Dis* 1998;26:1098.

107. Marty FM, Cosimi L, Marasco WA, Rubin RH, Baden LR. Breakthrough zygomycosis in allogeneic hematopoietic stem cell transplant recipients who received voriconazole as prophylaxis or empiric therapy. Paper presented at: 43rd Interscience Conference on Antimicrobial Agents and Chemotherapy; 2003; Chicago, IL.

108. Greenberg RN, Anstead G, Herbrecht R, et al. Posaconazole (POS) experience in the treatment of zygomycosis. Paper presented at: 43rd Interscience Conference on Antimicrobial Agents and Chemotherapy; 2003; Chicago, IL.

109. Diamond RD, Bennett JE. Prognostic factors in cryptococcal meningitis: a study of 11 cases. *Ann Intern Med* 1974;80:176.

110. Dromer F, Mathoulin S, Dupont B, Brugiere O, Letenneur L. Comparison of the efficacy of amphotericin B and fluconazole in the treatment of cryptococcosis in human immunodeficiency virus–negative patients: retrospective analysis of 83 cases. French Cryptococcosis Study Group. *Clin Infect Dis* 1996;22[Suppl 2]:S154.

111. Saag MS, Cloud GA, Graybill JR, et al. A comparison of itraconazole versus fluconazole as maintenance therapy for AIDS-associated cryptococcal meningitis. National Institute of Allergy and Infectious Diseases Mycoses Study Group [see comments]. *Clin Infect Dis* 1999;28:291.

112. Walsh TJ. Trichosporonosis. *Infect Dis Clin North Am* 1989;3:43.

113. Walsh TJ, Lee JW, Roilides E, Pizzo PA. Recent progress and current problems in management of invasive fungal infections in patients with neoplastic diseases. *Curr Opin Oncol* 1992;4:647.

114. Anaissie EJ, Hachem R, Karyotakis NC, et al. Comparative efficacies of amphotericin B, triazoles, and combination of both as experimental therapy for murine trichosporonosis. *Antimicrob Agents Chemother* 1994;38:2541.

115. Martino P, Venditti M, Micozzi A, et al. *Blastoschizomyces capitatus*: an emerging cause of invasive fungal disease in leukemia patients. *Rev Infect Dis* 1990;12:570.

116. Boutati EI, Anaissie EJ. *Fusarium*, a significant emerging pathogen in patients with hema-

tologic malignancy: ten years' experience at a cancer center and implications for management. *Blood* 1997;90:999.

117. Anaissie EJ, Kuchar RT, Rex JH, et al. Fusariosis associated with pathogenic *Fusarium* species colonization of a hospital water system: a new paradigm for the epidemiology of opportunistic mold infections. *Clin Infect Dis* 2001;33:1871.

118. Raad I, Tarrand J, Hanna H, et al. Epidemiology, molecular mycology, and environmental sources of *Fusarium* infection in patients with cancer. *Infect Control Hosp Epidemiol* 2002;23:532.

119. Perfect JR, Marr KA, Walsh TJ, et al. Voriconazole treatment for less-common, emerging, or refractory fungal infections. *Clin Infect Dis* 2003;36:1122.

120. Torre-Cisneros J, Gonzalez-Ruiz A, Hodges MR, Lutsar I. Voriconazole for the treatment of *S apiospermum* and *S prolificans* infection. Paper presented at: 38th Annual Meeting of the Infectious Diseases Society of America; 2000; New Orleans.

121. Silveira F, Nucci M. Emergence of black moulds in fungal disease: epidemiology and therapy. *Curr Opin Infect Dis* 2001;14:679.

122. Deresinski SC, Stevens DA. Coccidioidomycosis in compromised hosts. Experience at Stanford University Hospital. *Medicine (Baltimore)* 1975;54:377.

123. Sepkowitz KA, Brown AE, Armstrong D. *Pneumocystis carinii* pneumonia without acquired immunodeficiency syndrome. More patients, same risk [Editorial]. *Arch Intern Med* 1995;155:1125.

124. Kovacs JA, Hiemenz JW, Macher AM, et al. *Pneumocystis carinii* pneumonia: a comparison between patients with the acquired immunodeficiency syndrome and patients with other immunodeficiencies. *Ann Intern Med* 1984;100:663.

125. Kovacs JA, Ng VL, Masur H, et al. Diagnosis of *Pneumocystis carinii* pneumonia: improved detection in sputum with use of monoclonal antibodies. *N Engl J Med* 1988;318:589.

126. Masur H, Gill VJ, Ognibene FP, et al. Diagnosis of *Pneumocystis* pneumonia by induced sputum technique in patients without the acquired immunodeficiency syndrome. *Ann Intern Med* 1988;109:755.

127. Larsen HH, Huang L, Kovacs JA, et al. Oral washes for diagnosis of *Pneumocystis* pneumonia in patients with HIV infection using quantitative touch-down PCR. Paper presented at: 43rd Interscience Conference on Antimicrobial Agents and Chemotherapy; 2003; Chicago, IL.

128. Bozzette SA, Sattler FR, Chiu J, et al. A controlled trial of early adjunctive treatment with corticosteroids for *Pneumocystis carinii* pneumonia in the acquired immunodeficiency syndrome. California Collaborative Treatment Group [see comments]. *N Engl J Med* 1990;323:1451.

129. Hughes WT, Rivera GK, Schell MJ, Thornton D, Lott L. Successful intermittent chemoprophylaxis for *Pneumocystis carinii* pneumonitis. *N Engl J Med* 1987;316:1627.

130. Ljungman P. Prevention and treatment of viral infections in stem cell transplant recipients. *Br J Haematol* 2002;118:44.

131. Saral R, Ambinder RF, Burns WH, et al. Acyclovir prophylaxis against herpes simplex virus infection in patients with leukemia. A randomized, double-blind, placebo-controlled study. *Ann Intern Med* 1983;99:773.

132. Meyers JD, Flournoy N, Thomas ED. Infection with herpes simplex virus and cell-mediated immunity after marrow transplant. *J Infect Dis* 1980;142:338.

133. Nichols WG, Boeckh M, Carter RA, Wald A, Corey L. Transferred herpes simplex virus immunity after stem-cell transplantation: clinical implications. *J Infect Dis* 2003;187:801.

134. Nguyen Q, Estey E, Raad I, et al. Cytomegalovirus pneumonia in adults with leukemia: an emerging problem. *Clin Infect Dis* 2001;32:539.

135. Hakki M, Riddell SR, Storek J, et al. Immune reconstitution to cytomegalovirus after allogeneic hematopoietic stem cell transplantation: impact of host factors, drug therapy, and subclinical reactivation. *Blood* 2003;102:3060.

136. Meijer E, Dekker AW, Verdonck LF. Influence of antithymocyte globulin dose on outcome in cytomegalovirus-seropositive recipients of partially T cell–depleted stem cell grafts from matched-unrelated donors. *Br J Haematol* 2003;121:473.

137. Nichols WG, Corey L, Gooley T, Davis C, Boeckh M. High risk of death due to bacterial and fungal infection among cytomegalovirus (CMV)-seronegative recipients of stem cell transplants from seropositive donors: evidence for indirect effects of primary CMV infection. *J Infect Dis* 2002;185:273.

138. Ljungman P, Brand R, Einsele H, et al. Donor CMV serological status and outcome of CMV seropositive recipients after unrelated donor stem cell transplantation; an EBMT Megafile analysis. *Blood* 2003;21:21.

139. Holmberg LA, Boeckh M, Hooper H, et al. Increased incidence of cytomegalovirus disease after autologous CD34-selected peripheral stem cell transplantation. *Blood* 1999;94:4029.

140. Nguyen Q, Champlin R, Giralt S, et al. Late cytomegalovirus pneumonia in adult allogeneic blood and marrow transplant recipients. *Clin Infect Dis* 1999;28:618.

141. Prentice HG, Kho P. Clinical strategies for the management of cytomegalovirus infection and disease in allogeneic bone marrow transplant. *Bone Marrow Transplant* 1997;19:135.

142. Ljungman P, Cordonnier C, Einsele H, et al. Use of intravenous immune globulin in addition to antiviral therapy in the treatment of CMV gastrointestinal disease in allogeneic bone marrow transplant patients: a report from the European Group for Blood and Marrow Transplantation (EBMT). Infectious Diseases Working Party of the EBMT. *Bone Marrow Transplant* 1998;21:473.

143. Ljungman P, Deliliers GL, Platzbecker U, et al. Cidofovir for cytomegalovirus infection and disease in allogeneic stem cell transplant recipients. The Infectious Diseases Working Party of the European Group for Blood and Marrow Transplantation. *Blood* 2001;97:388.

144. Reed EC, Wolford JL, Kopecky KJ, et al. Ganciclovir for the treatment of cytomegalovirus gastroenteritis in bone marrow transplant patients. A randomized, placebo-controlled trial. *Ann Intern Med* 1990;112:505.

145. Nichols WG, Price TH, Gooley T, Corey L, Boeckh M. Transfusion-transmitted cytomegalovirus infection after receipt of leukoreduced blood products. *Blood* 2003;101:4195.

146. Prentice HG, Gluckman E, Powles RL, et al. Impact of long-term acyclovir on cytomegalovirus infection and survival after allogeneic bone marrow transplantation. European Acyclovir for CMV Prophylaxis Study Group. *Lancet* 1994;343:749.

147. Meyers JD, Reed EC, Shepp DH, et al. Acyclovir for prevention of cytomegalovirus infection and disease after allogeneic marrow transplantation. *N Engl J Med* 1988;318:70.

148. Ljungman P, de La Camara R, Milpied N, et al. Randomized study of valacyclovir as pro-

phylaxis against cytomegalovirus reactivation in recipients of allogeneic bone marrow transplants. *Blood* 2002;99:3050.

148a. Winston DJ, Yeager AM, Chandrasekar PH, et al. Valacyclovir Cytomegalovirus Study Group. Randomized comparison of oral valacyclovir and intravenous ganciclovir for prevention of cytomegalovirus disease after allogeneic bone marrow transplantation. *Clin Infect Dis* 2003;36:749.

149. Winston DJ, Ho WG, Bartoni K, et al. Ganciclovir prophylaxis of cytomegalovirus infection and disease in allogeneic bone marrow transplant recipients. Results of a placebo-controlled, double-blind trial. *Ann Intern Med* 1993;118:179.

150. Goodrich JM, Bowden RA, Fisher L, et al. Ganciclovir prophylaxis to prevent cytomegalovirus disease after allogeneic marrow transplant. *Ann Intern Med* 1993;118:173.

151. Boeckh M, Bowden RA, Gooley T, Myerson D, Corey L. Successful modification of a pp65 antigenemia-based early treatment strategy for prevention of cytomegalovirus disease in allogeneic marrow transplant recipients [Letter]. *Blood* 1999;93:1781.

152. Einsele H, Ehninger G, Hebart H, et al. Polymerase chain reaction monitoring reduces the incidence of cytomegalovirus disease and the duration and side effects of antiviral therapy after bone marrow transplantation. *Blood* 1995;86:2815.

153. Reusser P, Einsele H, Lee J, et al. Randomized multicenter trial of foscarnet versus ganciclovir for preemptive therapy of cytomegalovirus infection after allogeneic stem cell transplantation. *Blood* 2002;99:1159.

154. Boeckh M, Nichols WG, Papanicolaou G, et al. Cytomegalovirus in hematopoietic stem cell transplant recipients: current status, known challenges, and future strategies. *Biol Blood Marrow Transplant* 2003;9:543.

155. Nichols WG, Corey L, Gooley T, et al. Rising pp65 antigenemia during preemptive anticytomegalovirus therapy after allogeneic hematopoietic stem cell transplantation: risk factors, correlation with DNA load, and outcomes. *Blood* 2001;97:867.

156. Boeckh M, Leisenring W, Riddell SR, et al. Late cytomegalovirus disease and mortality in recipients of allogeneic hematopoietic stem cell transplants: importance of viral load and T-cell immunity. *Blood* 2003;101:407.

157. Junghanss C, Boeckh M, Carter RA, et al. Incidence and outcome of cytomegalovirus infections following nonmyeloablative compared with myeloablative allogeneic stem cell transplantation, a matched control study. *Blood* 2002;99:1978.

158. Bowden RA, Rogers KS, Meyers JD. Oral acyclovir for the long-term suppression of varicella zoster virus infection after marrow transplantation. Paper presented at: 29th Interscience Conference on Antimicrobial Agents and Chemotherapy; 1989; Anaheim, CA.

159. Galil K, Lee B, Strine T, et al. Outbreak of varicella at a day-care center despite vaccination. *N Engl J Med* 2002;347:1909.

160. Hata A, Asanuma H, Rinki M, et al. Use of an inactivated varicella vaccine in recipients of hematopoietic-cell transplants. *N Engl J Med* 2002;347:26.

161. Salahuddin SZ, Ablashi DV, Markham PD, et al. Isolation of a new virus, HBLV, in patients with lymphoproliferative disorders. *Science* 1986;234:596.

162. Drobyski WR, Knox KK, Majewski D, Carrigan DR. Brief report: fatal encephalitis due to variant B human herpesvirus-6 infection in a bone marrow-transplant recipient. *N Engl J Med* 1994;330:1356.

163. Carrigan DR, Drobyski WR, Russler SK, et al. Interstitial pneumonitis associated with human herpesvirus-6 infection after marrow transplantation. *Lancet* 1991;338:147.

164. Ljungman P, Wang FZ, Clark DA, et al. High levels of human herpesvirus 6 DNA in peripheral blood leucocytes are correlated to platelet engraftment and disease in allogeneic stem cell transplant patients. *Br J Haematol* 2000;111:774.

165. Sashihara J, Tanaka-Taya K, Tanaka S, et al. High incidence of human herpesvirus 6 infection with a high viral load in cord blood stem cell transplant recipients. *Blood* 2002; 100:2005.

166. Singh N, Carrigan DR. Human herpesvirus-6 in transplantation: an emerging pathogen. *Ann Intern Med* 1996;124:1065.

167. Whimbey E, Couch RB, Englund JA, et al. Respiratory syncytial virus pneumonia in hospitalized adult patients with leukemia. *Clin Infect Dis* 1995;21:376.

168. Khushalani NI, Bakri FG, Wentling D, et al. Respiratory syncytial virus infection in the late bone marrow transplant period: report of three cases and review. *Bone Marrow Transplant* 2001;27:1071.

169. Bowden R. Respiratory virus infections after marrow transplant: the Fred Hutchinson Cancer Research Center Experience. *Am J Med* 1997;102:27.

170. Whimbey E, Champlin RE, Englund JA, et al. Combination therapy with aerosolized ribavirin and intravenous immunoglobulin for respiratory syncytial virus disease in adult bone marrow transplant recipients. *Bone Marrow Transplant* 1995;16:393.

171. Englund JA, Piedra PA, Jewell A, et al. Rapid diagnosis of respiratory syncytial virus infections in immunocompromised adults. *J Clin Microbiol* 1996;34:1649.

172. Lewinsohn DM, Bowden RA, Mattson D, Crawford SW. Phase I study of intravenous ribavirin treatment of respiratory syncytial virus pneumonia after marrow transplantation. *Antimicrob Agents Chemother* 1996;40:2555.

173. Boeckh M, Berrey MM, Bowden RA, et al. Phase 1 evaluation of the respiratory syncytial virus–specific monoclonal antibody palivizumab in recipients of hematopoietic stem cell transplants. *J Infect Dis* 2001;184:350.

174. Whimbey E, Englund JA, Couch RB. Community respiratory virus infections in immunocompromised patients with cancer. *Am J Med* 1997;102:10.

175. Nichols WG, Corey L, Gooley T, Davis C, Boeckh M. Parainfluenza virus infections after hematopoietic stem cell transplantation: risk factors, response to antiviral therapy, and effect on transplant outcome. *Blood* 2001;98:573.

176. Englund JA, Champlin RE, Wyde PR, et al. Common emergence of amantadine- and rimantadine-resistant influenza A viruses in symptomatic immunocompromised adults. *Clin Infect Dis* 1998;26:1418.

177. Hayden FG, Atmar RL, Schilling M, et al. Use of the selective oral neuraminidase inhibitor oseltamivir to prevent influenza [see comments]. *N Engl J Med* 1999;341:1336.

178. Monto AS, Robinson DP, Herlocher ML, et al. Zanamivir in the prevention of influenza among healthy adults: a randomized controlled trial [see comments]. *JAMA* 1999;282:31.

179. Machado CM, Boas LS, Mendes AV, et al. Low mortality rates related to respiratory virus infections after bone marrow transplantation. *Bone Marrow Transplant* 2003;31:695.

180. Almyroudis N, Symeonidis N, Sepkowitz KA, et al. Mortality of disseminated adenovirus (ADV) infections after allogeneic HSCT in the era of cidofovir. Paper presented at: 43rd Interscience Conference on Antimicrobial Agents and Chemotherapy; 2003; Chicago, IL.

181. Ljungman P, Ribaud P, Eyrich M, et al. Cidofovir for adenovirus infections after allogeneic hematopoietic stem cell transplantation: a survey by the Infectious Diseases Working Party of the European Group for Blood and Marrow Transplantation. *Bone Marrow Transplant* 2003;31:481.

182. Ison MG, Hayden FG, Kaiser L, Corey L, Boeckh M. Rhinovirus infections in hematopoietic stem cell transplant recipients with pneumonia. *Clin Infect Dis* 2003;36:1139.

183. Kaplan LJ, Daum RS, Smaron M, McCarthy CA. Severe measles in immunocompromised patients. *JAMA* 1992;267:1237.

184. Heegaard ED, Brown KE. Human parvovirus B19. *Clin Microbiol Rev* 2002;15:485.

185. Lok AS, Liang RH, Chiu EK, et al. Reactivation of hepatitis B virus replication in patients receiving cytotoxic therapy. Report of a prospective study. *Gastroenterology* 1991;100:182.

186. Hoofnagle JH, Dusheiko GM, Schafer DF, et al. Reactivation of chronic hepatitis B virus infection by cancer chemotherapy. *Ann Intern Med* 1982;96:447.

187. Locasciulli A, Bruno B, Alessandrino EP, et al. Hepatitis reactivation and liver failure in haemopoietic stem cell transplants for hepatitis B virus (HBV)/hepatitis C virus (HCV) positive recipients: a retrospective study by the Italian Group for Blood and Marrow Transplantation. *Bone Marrow Transplant* 2003;31:295.

188. Lau GK, Leung YH, Fong DY, et al. High hepatitis B virus (HBV) DNA viral load as the most important risk factor for HBV reactivation in patients positive for HBV surface antigen undergoing autologous hematopoietic cell transplantation. *Blood* 2002;99:2324.

189. Lau GK, He ML, Fong DY, et al. Preemptive use of lamivudine reduces hepatitis B exacerbation after allogeneic hematopoietic cell transplantation. *Hepatology* 2002;36:702.

190. Vergani D, Locasciulli A, Masera G, et al. Histological evidence of hepatitis-B-virus infection with negative serology in children with acute leukaemia who develop chronic liver disease. *Lancet* 1982;1:361.

191. Bréchot C, Degos F, Lugassy C, et al. Hepatitis B virus DNA in patients with chronic liver disease and negative tests for hepatitis B surface antigen. *N Engl J Med* 1985;312:270.

192. Dhedin N, Douvin C, Kuentz M, et al. Reverse seroconversion of hepatitis B after allogeneic bone marrow transplantation: a retrospective study of 37 patients with pretransplant anti-HBs and anti-HBc. *Transplantation* 1998;66:616.

193. Lau GK, Suri D, Liang R, et al. Resolution of chronic hepatitis B and anti-HBs seroconversion in humans by adoptive transfer of immunity to hepatitis B core antigen. *Gastroenterology* 2002;122:614.

194. Strasser SI, Myerson D, Spurgeon CL, et al. Hepatitis C virus infection and bone marrow transplantation: a cohort study with 10-year follow-up. *Hepatology* 1999;29:1893.

195. Frickhofen N, Wiesneth M, Jainta C, et al. Hepatitis C virus infection is a risk factor for liver failure from veno-occlusive disease after bone marrow transplantation [see comments]. *Blood* 1994;83:1998.

196. Strasser SI, Sullivan KM, Myerson D, et al. Cirrhosis of the liver in long-term marrow transplant survivors. *Blood* 1999;93:3259.

197. Strasser SI, McDonald GB. Hepatitis viruses and hematopoietic cell transplantation: a guide to patient and donor management. *Blood* 1999;93:1127.

198. Alter MJ, Gallagher M, Morris TT, et al. Acute non-A-E hepatitis in the United States and the role of hepatitis G virus infection. Sentinel Counties Viral Hepatitis Study Team [see comments]. *N Engl J Med* 1997;336:741.

199. Lefrere JJ, Roudot-Thoraval F, Lefrere F, et al. Natural history of the TT virus infection through follow-up of TTV DNA-positive multiple-transfused patients. *Blood* 2000;95:347.

200. Kanda Y, Tanaka Y, Kami M, et al. TT virus in bone marrow transplant recipients. *Blood* 1999;93:2485.

201. Hong DS, Jacobson KL, Raad II, et al. West Nile encephalitis in 2 hematopoietic stem cell transplant recipients: case series and literature review. *Clin Infect Dis* 2003;37:1044.

202. Israelski DM, Remington JS. Toxoplasmosis in patients with cancer. *Clin Infect Dis* 1993;17[Suppl 2]:S423.

203. Martino R, Maertens J, Bretagne S, et al. Toxoplasmosis after hematopoietic stem cell transplantation. *Clin Infect Dis* 2000;31:1188.

204. Lewis JS Jr, Khoury H, Storch GA, DiPersio J. PCR for the diagnosis of toxoplasmosis after hematopoietic stem cell transplantation. *Expert Rev Mol Diagn* 2002;2:616.

205. Igra-Siegman Y, Kapila R, Sen P, Kaminski ZC, Louria DB. Syndrome of hyperinfection with *Strongyloides stercoralis*. *Rev Infect Dis* 1981;3:397.

206. Safdar A, Papadopoulous EB, Armstrong D. Listeriosis in recipients of allogeneic blood and marrow transplantation: thirteen year review of disease characteristics, treatment outcomes and a new association with human cytomegalovirus infection. *Bone Marrow Transplant* 2002;29:913.

207. Kaplan JE, Masur H, Holmes KK, USPHS. Infectious Disease Society of America. Guidelines for preventing opportunistic infections among HIV-infected persons—2002. Recommendations of the U.S. Public Health Service and the Infectious Diseases Society of America. *MMWR Recomm Rep* 2002;51(RR-8):1.

208. Hann I, Viscoli C, Paesmans M, Gaya H, Glauser M. A comparison of outcome from febrile neutropenic episodes in children compared with adults: results from four EORTC studies. International Antimicrobial Therapy Cooperative Group (IATCG) of the European Organization for Research and Treatment of Cancer (EORTC). *Br J Haematol* 1997;99:580.

209. Sickles EA, Greene WH, Wiernik PH. Clinical presentation of infection in granulocytopenic patients. *Arch Intern Med* 1975;135:715.

210. Oude Nijhuis CS, Gietema JA, Vellenga E, et al. Routine radiography does not have a role in the diagnostic evaluation of ambulatory adult febrile neutropenic cancer patients. *Eur J Cancer* 2003;39:2495.

211. Siegman-Igra Y, Anglim AM, Shapiro DE, et al. Diagnosis of vascular catheter–related bloodstream infection: a meta-analysis. *J Clin Microbiol* 1997;35:928.

212. Schimpff S, Satterlee W, Young VM, Serpick A. Empiric therapy with carbenicillin and gentamicin for febrile patients with cancer and granulocytopenia. *N Engl J Med* 1971;284:1061.

213. Hughes WT, Armstrong D, Bodey GP, et al. 2002 guidelines for the use of antimicrobial agents in neutropenic patients with cancer. *Clin Infect Dis* 2002;34:730.

214. Pizzo PA, Hathorn JW, Hiemenz J, et al. A randomized trial comparing ceftazidime alone with combination antibiotic therapy in cancer patients with fever and neutropenia. *N Engl J Med* 1986;315:552.

215. De Pauw BE, Deresinski SC, Feld R, Lane-Allman EF, Donnelly JP. Ceftazidime compared with piperacillin and tobramycin for the empiric treatment of fever in neutropenic patients with cancer. A multicenter randomized trial. The Intercontinental Antimicrobial Study Group [see comments]. *Ann Intern Med* 1994;120:834.

216. Freifeld AG, Walsh T, Marshall D, et al. Monotherapy for fever and neutropenia in cancer patients: a randomized comparison of ceftazidime versus imipenem. *J Clin Oncol* 1995; 13:165.

217. Rolston KV, Berkey P, Bodey GP, et al. A comparison of imipenem to ceftazidime with or without amikacin as empiric therapy in febrile neutropenic patients. *Arch Intern Med* 1992;152:283.

218. Biron P, Fuhrmann C, Cure H, et al. Cefepime versus imipenem-cilastatin as empirical monotherapy in 400 febrile patients with short duration neutropenia. CEMIC (Study Group of Infectious Diseases in Cancer). *J Antimicrob Chemother* 1998;42:511.

219. Raad I, Escalante C, Hachem RY, et al. Treatment of febrile neutropenic patients with cancer who require hospitalization: a prospective randomized study comparing imipenem and cefepime. *Cancer* 2003;98:1039.

220. Cometta A, Calandra T, Gaya H, et al. Monotherapy with meropenem versus combination therapy with ceftazidime plus amikacin as empiric therapy for fever in granulocytopenic patients with cancer. The International Antimicrobial Therapy Cooperative Group of the European Organization for Research and Treatment of Cancer and the Gruppo Italiano Malattie Ematologiche Maligne dell'Adulto Infection Program. *Antimicrob Agents Chemother* 1996;40:1108.

221. Feld R, DePauw B, Berman S, Keating A, Ho W. Meropenem versus ceftazidime in the treatment of cancer patients with febrile neutropenia: a randomized, double-blind trial. *J Clin Oncol* 2000;18:3690.

222. Bow EJ, Schwarer AP, Laverdiere M, Segal BH, Anaissie E. Efficacy of piperacillin/tazobactam as initial therapy of febrile neutropenia in patients with hematologic malignancies. Paper presented at: Interscience Conference on Antimicrobial Agents and Chemotherapy; 2003; Chicago, IL.

223. Furno P, Bucaneve G, Del Favero A. Monotherapy or aminoglycoside-containing combinations for empirical antibiotic treatment of febrile neutropenic patients: a meta-analysis. *Lancet Infect Dis* 2002;2:231.

224. Feld R, Paesmans M, Freifeld AG, et al. Methodology for clinical trials involving patients with cancer who have febrile neutropenia: updated guidelines of the Immunocompromised Host Society/Multinational Association for Supportive Care in Cancer, with emphasis on outpatient studies. *Clin Infect Dis* 2002;35:1463.

225. Peacock JE, Herrington DA, Wade JC, et al. Ciprofloxacin plus piperacillin compared with tobramycin plus piperacillin as empirical therapy in febrile neutropenic patients. A randomized, double-blind trial. *Ann Intern Med* 2002;137:77.

226. Kern WV, Cometta A, De Bock R, et al. Oral versus intravenous empirical antimicrobial therapy for fever in patients with granulocytopenia who are receiving cancer chemotherapy. International Antimicrobial Therapy Cooperative Group of the European Organization for Research and Treatment of Cancer [see comments]. *N Engl J Med* 1999;341:312.

227. Furno P, Dionisi MS, Bucaneve G, Menichetti F, Del Favero A. Ceftriaxone versus beta-lactams with antipseudomonal activity for empirical, combined antibiotic therapy in febrile neutropenia: a meta-analysis. *Support Care Cancer* 2000;8:293.

228. Vancomycin added to empirical combination antibiotic therapy for fever in granulocytopenic cancer patients. European Organization for Research and Treatment of Cancer (EORTC) International Antimicrobial Therapy Cooperative Group and the National Cancer Institute of Canada Clinical Trials Group [see comments] [published erratum appears in *J Infect Dis* 1991;164(4):832]. *J Infect Dis* 1991;163:951.

229. Ramphal R, Bolger M, Oblon DJ, et al. Vancomycin is not an essential component of the initial empiric treatment regimen for febrile neutropenic patients receiving ceftazidime: a randomized prospective study. *Antimicrob Agents Chemother* 1992;36:1062.

230. National Comprehensive Cancer Network Clinical Practice Guidelines in Oncology. Fever and Neutropenia. Version 1.2002. World Wide Web URL: http://www.nccn.org. 2003.

231. Cometta A, Kern WV, De Bock R, et al. Vancomycin versus placebo for treating persistent fever in patients with neutropenic cancer receiving piperacillin-tazobactam monotherapy. *Clin Infect Dis* 2003;37:382.

232. Raad II, Whimbey EE, Rolston KV, et al. A comparison of aztreonam plus vancomycin and imipenem plus vancomycin as initial therapy for febrile neutropenic cancer patients. *Cancer* 1996;77:1386.

233. Anne S, Reisman RE. Risk of administering cephalosporin antibiotics to patients with histories of penicillin allergy. *Ann Allergy Asthma Immunol* 1995;74:167.

234. Pizzo PA, Robichaud KJ, Gill FA, et al. Duration of empiric antibiotic therapy in granulocytopenic patients with cancer. *Am J Med* 1979;67:194.

235. Pizzo PA, Commers J, Cotton D, et al. Approaching the controversies in antibacterial management of cancer patients. *Am J Med* 1984;76:436.

236. Woo PC, Wong SS, Lum PN, Hui WT, Yuen KY. Cell-wall-deficient bacteria and culture-negative febrile episodes in bone-marrow-transplant recipients. *Lancet* 2001;357:675.

237. Pizzo PA, Robichaud KJ, Gill FA, Witebsky FG. Empiric antibiotic and antifungal therapy for cancer patients with prolonged fever and granulocytopenia. *Am J Med* 1982;72:101.

238. Empiric antifungal therapy in febrile granulocytopenic patients. EORTC International Antimicrobial Therapy Cooperative Group. *Am J Med* 1989;86:668.

239. Walsh TJ, Finberg RW, Arndt C, et al. Liposomal amphotericin B for empirical therapy in patients with persistent fever and neutropenia. National Institute of Allergy and Infectious Diseases Mycoses Study Group. *N Engl J Med* 1999;340:764.

240. Cagnoni PJ, Walsh TJ, Prendergast MM, et al. Pharmacoeconomic analysis of liposomal amphotericin B versus conventional amphotericin B in the empirical treatment of persistently febrile neutropenic patients. *J Clin Oncol* 2000;18:2476.

241. Boogaerts M, Winston DJ, Bow EJ, et al. Intravenous and oral itraconazole versus intravenous amphotericin B deoxycholate as empirical antifungal therapy for persistent fever in neutropenic patients with cancer who are receiving broad-spectrum antibacterial therapy. A randomized, controlled trial. *Ann Intern Med* 2001;135:412.

242. Winston DJ, Hathorn JW, Schuster MG, Schiller GJ, Territo MC. A multicenter, randomized trial of fluconazole versus amphotericin B for empiric antifungal therapy of febrile neutropenic patients with cancer. *Am J Med* 2000;108:282.

243. Viscoli C, Castagnola E, Van Lint MT, et al. Fluconazole versus amphotericin B as empirical antifungal therapy of unexplained fever in granulocytopenic cancer patients: a pragmatic, multicentre, prospective and randomised clinical trial. *Eur J Cancer* 1996;32A:814.

244. Walsh TJ, Pappas P, Winston DJ, et al. Voriconazole compared with liposomal amphotericin B for empirical antifungal therapy in patients with neutropenia and persistent fever. *N Engl J Med* 2002;346:225.

245. Walsh T, Sable C, DePauw B, et al. A randomized, double-blind, multicenter trial of caspofungin (CS) v liposomal amphotericin B (LAMB) for empirical antifungal therapy (EAFrx) of persistently febrile neutropenic (PFN) patients (Pt). Paper presented at: 43rd Interscience Conference on Antimicrobial Agents and Chemotherapy; 2003; Chicago, IL.

246. Rubin M, Hathorn JW, Pizzo PA. Controversies in the management of febrile neutropenic cancer patients. *Cancer Invest* 1988;6:167.

247. Talcott JA, Finberg R, Mayer RJ, Goldman L. The medical course of cancer patients with fever and neutropenia. Clinical identification of a low-risk subgroup at presentation. *Arch Intern Med* 1988;148:2561.

248. Talcott JA, Siegel RD, Finberg R, Goldman L. Risk assessment in cancer patients with fever and neutropenia: a prospective, two-center validation of a prediction rule. *J Clin Oncol* 1992;10:316.

249. Klastersky J, Paesmans M, Rubenstein EB, et al. The Multinational Association for Supportive Care in Cancer risk index: a multinational scoring system for identifying low-risk febrile neutropenic cancer patients. *J Clin Oncol* 2000;18:3038.

250. Freifeld A, Marchigiani D, Walsh T, et al. A double-blind comparison of empirical oral and intravenous antibiotic therapy for low-risk febrile patients with neutropenia during cancer chemotherapy [see comments]. *N Engl J Med* 1999;341:305.

251. Talcott JA, Whalen A, Clark J, Rieker PP, Finberg R. Home antibiotic therapy for low-risk cancer patients with fever and neutropenia: a pilot study of 30 patients based on a validated prediction rule. *J Clin Oncol* 1994;12:107.

252. Rubenstein EB, Rolston K, Benjamin RS, et al. Outpatient treatment of febrile episodes in low-risk neutropenic patients with cancer. *Cancer* 1993;71:3640.

253. Malik IA, Abbas Z, Karim M. Randomised comparison of oral ofloxacin alone with combination of parenteral antibiotics in neutropenic febrile patients [published erratum appears in *Lancet* 1992;340(8811):128]. *Lancet* 1992;339:1092.

254. Malik IA, Khan WA, Karim M, Aziz Z, Khan MA. Feasibility of outpatient management of fever in cancer patients with low-risk neutropenia: results of a prospective randomized trial [see comments]. *Am J Med* 1995;98:224.

255. Rolston KV. New trends in patient management: risk-based therapy for febrile patients with neutropenia. *Clin Infect Dis* 1999;29:515.

256. Klaassen RJ, Goodman TR, Pham B, Doyle JJ. "Low-risk" prediction rule for pediatric oncology patients presenting with fever and neutropenia. *J Clin Oncol* 2000;18:1012.

257. Lucas KG, Brown AE, Armstrong D, Chapman D, Heller G. The identification of febrile, neutropenic children with neoplastic disease at low risk for bacteremia and complications of sepsis. *Cancer* 1996;77:791.

257a. Santolaya ME, Alvarez AM, Becker A, et al. Prospective, multicenter evaluation of risk factors associated with invasive bacterial infection in children with cancer, neutropenia, and fever. *J Clin Oncol* 2001;19:3415.

258. Shenep JL, Flynn PM, Baker DK, et al. Oral cefixime is similar to continued intravenous antibiotics in the empirical treatment of febrile neutropenic children with cancer. *Clin Infect Dis* 2001;32:36.

259. Freifeld A, Pizzo P. Use of fluoroquinolones for empirical management of febrile neutropenia in pediatric cancer patients. *Pediatr Infect Dis J* 1997;16:140; discussion 145.

260. Mullen CA, Petropoulos D, Roberts WM, et al. Outpatient treatment of fever and neutropenia for low risk pediatric cancer patients. *Cancer* 1999;86:126.

261. Park JR, Coughlin J, Hawkins D, et al. Ciprofloxacin and amoxicillin as continuation treatment of febrile neutropenia in pediatric cancer patients. *Med Pediatr Oncol* 2003;40:93.

262. Paganini H, Gomez S, Ruvinsky S, et al. Outpatient, sequential, parenteral-oral antibiotic therapy for lower risk febrile neutropenia in children with malignant disease: a single-center, randomized, controlled trial in Argentina. *Cancer* 2003;97:1775.

263. Engels EA, Lau J, Barza M. Efficacy of quinolone prophylaxis in neutropenic cancer patients: a meta-analysis. *J Clin Oncol* 1998;16:1179.

264. Gomez L, Garau J, Estrada C, et al. Ciprofloxacin prophylaxis in patients with acute leukemia and granulocytopenia in an area with a high prevalence of ciprofloxacin-resistant *Escherichia coli. Cancer* 2003;97:419.

265. Cruciani M, Malena M, Bosco O, et al. Reappraisal with meta-analysis of the addition of Gram-positive prophylaxis to fluoroquinolone in neutropenic patients. *J Clin Oncol* 2003; 21:4127.

266. Goodman JL, Winston DJ, Greenfield RA, et al. A controlled trial of fluconazole to prevent fungal infections in patients undergoing bone marrow transplantation [see comments]. *N Engl J Med* 1992;326:845.

267. Slavin MA, Osborne B, Adams R, et al. Efficacy and safety of fluconazole prophylaxis for fungal infections after marrow transplantation—a prospective, randomized, double-blind study. *J Infect Dis* 1995;171:1545.

268. Marr KA, Seidel K, Slavin MA, et al. Prolonged fluconazole prophylaxis is associated with persistent protection against candidiasis-related death in allogeneic marrow transplant recipients: long-term follow-up of a randomized, placebo-controlled trial. *Blood* 2000;96:2055.

269. MacMillan ML, Goodman JL, DeFor TE, Weisdorf DJ. Fluconazole to prevent yeast infections in bone marrow transplantation patients: a randomized trial of high versus reduced dose, and determination of the value of maintenance therapy. *Am J Med* 2002;112:369.

270. Marr KA, Seidel K, White TC, Bowden RA. Candidemia in allogeneic blood and marrow transplant recipients: evolution of risk factors after the adoption of prophylactic fluconazole. *J Infect Dis* 2000;181:309.

271. Bow EJ, Laverdiere M, Lussier N, et al. Antifungal prophylaxis for severely neutropenic chemotherapy recipients: a meta analysis of randomized-controlled clinical trials. *Cancer* 2002;94:3230.

272. Viscoli C, Paesmans M, Sanz M, et al. Association between antifungal prophylaxis and rate of documented bacteremia in febrile neutropenic cancer patients. *Clin Infect Dis* 2001;32:1532.

273. Rotstein C, Bow EJ, Laverdiere M, et al. Randomized placebo-controlled trial of fluconazole prophylaxis for neutropenic cancer patients: benefit based on purpose and intensity of cytotoxic therapy. The Canadian Fluconazole Prophylaxis Study Group. *Clin Infect Dis* 1999;28:331.

274. Winston DJ, Chandrasekar PH, Lazarus HM, et al. Fluconazole prophylaxis of fungal infections in patients with acute leukemia. Results of a randomized placebo-controlled, double-blind, multicenter trial [see comments]. *Ann Intern Med* 1993;118:495.

275. Kern W, Behre G, Rudolf T, et al. Failure of fluconazole prophylaxis to reduce mortality or the requirement of systemic amphotericin B therapy during treatment for refractory acute myeloid leukemia: results of a prospective randomized phase III study. German AML Cooperative Group. *Cancer* 1998;83:291.

276. Zhou H, Goldman M, Wu J, et al. A pharmacokinetic study of intravenous itraconazole followed by oral administration of itraconazole capsules in patients with advanced human immunodeficiency virus infection. *J Clin Pharmacol* 1998;38:593.

277. Menichetti F, Del Favero A, Martino P, et al. Itraconazole oral solution as prophylaxis for fungal infections in neutropenic patients with hematologic malignancies: a randomized, placebo-controlled, double-blind, multicenter trial. GIMEMA Infection Program. Gruppo Italiano Malattie Ematologiche dell' Adulto. *Clin Infect Dis* 1999;28:250.

278. Morgenstern GR, Prentice AG, Prentice HG, et al. A randomized controlled trial of itraconazole versus fluconazole for the prevention of fungal infections in patients with haematological malignancies. U.K. Multicentre Antifungal Prophylaxis Study Group. *Br J Haematol* 1999;105:901.

279. Winston DJ, Maziarz RT, Chandrasekar PH, et al. Intravenous and oral itraconazole versus intravenous and oral fluconazole for long-term antifungal prophylaxis in allogeneic hematopoietic stem-cell transplant recipients. A multicenter, randomized trial. *Ann Intern Med* 2003;138:705.

280. Marr KA, Crippa F, Leisenring W, et al. Itraconazole versus fluconazole for prevention of fungal infections in allogeneic stem cell transplant patients. *Blood* 2003;2:2.

281. Marr KA, Leisenring W, Crippa F, et al. Cyclophosphamide metabolism is impacted by azole antifungals. *Blood* 2003;22:22.

282. van Burik J, Ratanatharathorn V, Lipton J, et al. Randomized, double-blind trial of Micafungin (MI) versus fluconazole (FL) for prophylaxis of invasive fungal infections in patients (pts) undergoing hematopoietic stem cell transplant (HSCT), NIAID/BAMSG protocol 46. Paper presented at: 42nd Interscience Conference on Antimicrobial Agents and Chemotherapy; 2002; San Diego, CA.

283. Remington JS, Schimpff SC. Occasional notes. Please don't eat the salads. *N Engl J Med* 1981;304:433.

284. Hahn T, Cummings KM, Michalek AM, et al. Efficacy of high-efficiency particulate air filtration in preventing aspergillosis in immunocompromised patients with hematologic malignancies. *Infect Control Hosp Epidemiol* 2002;23:525.

285. Pizzo PA. Management of fever in patients with cancer and treatment-induced neutropenia [see comments]. *N Engl J Med* 1993;328:1323.

286. Annane D, Sebille V, Charpentier C, et al. Effect of treatment with low doses of hydrocortisone and fludrocortisone on mortality in patients with septic shock. *JAMA* 2002; 288:862.

287. Bernard GR, Vincent JL, Laterre PF, et al. Efficacy and safety of recombinant human activated protein C for severe sepsis. *N Engl J Med* 2001;344:699.

288. Muto CA, Jernigan JA, Ostrowsky BE, et al. SHEA guideline for preventing nosocomial transmission of multidrug-resistant strains of *Staphylococcus aureus* and *Enterococcus. Infect Control Hosp Epidemiol* 2003;24:362.

289. Smith TL, Pearson ML, Wilcox KR, et al. Emergence of vancomycin resistance in *Staphylococcus aureus.* Glycopeptide-Intermediate *Staphylococcus Aureus* Working Group [see comments]. *N Engl J Med* 1999;340:493.

290. Sieradzki K, Roberts RB, Haber SW, Tomasz A. The development of vancomycin resistance in a patient with methicillin-resistant *Staphylococcus aureus* infection [see comments]. *N Engl J Med* 1999;340:517.

291. Centers for Disease Control and Prevention. Vancomycin-resistant *Staphylococcus aureus* —Pennsylvania. *MMWR Morb Mortal Wkly Rep* 2002;51:902.

292. Centers for Disease Control and Prevention. *Staphylococcus aureus* resistant to vancomycin—United States. *MMWR Morb Mortal Wkly Rep* 2002;51:565.

293. Hanna H, Umphrey J, Tarrand J, Mendoza M, Raad I. Management of an outbreak of vancomycin-resistant enterococci in the medical intensive care unit of a cancer center. *Infect Control Hosp Epidemiol* 2001;22:217.

294. Donskey CJ, Chowdhry TK, Hecker MT, et al. Effect of antibiotic therapy on the density of vancomycin-resistant enterococci in the stool of colonized patients. *N Engl J Med* 2000;343:1925.

295. Eliopoulos GM. Quinupristin-dalfopristin and linezolid: evidence and opinion. *Clin Infect Dis* 2003;36:473.

296. Stevens DL, Herr D, Lampiris H, et al. Linezolid versus vancomycin for the treatment of methicillin-resistant *Staphylococcus aureus* infections. *Clin Infect Dis* 2002;34:1481.

297. Rubinstein E, Cammarata S, Oliphant T, Wunderink R. Linezolid (PNU-100766) versus vancomycin in the treatment of hospitalized patients with nosocomial pneumonia: a randomized, double-blind, multicenter study. *Clin Infect Dis* 2001;32:402.

297a. Wunderink RG, Rello J, Cammarata SK, Croos-Dabrera RV, Kollef MH. Linezolid vs vancomycin: analysis of two double-blind studies of patients with methicillin-resistant *Staphylococcus aureus* nosocomial pneumonia. *Chest* 2003;124:1789.

298. Smith PF, Birmingham MC, Noskin GA, et al. Safety, efficacy and pharmacokinetics of linezolid for treatment of resistant Gram-positive infections in cancer patients with neutropenia. *Ann Oncol* 2003;14:795.

299. Nichols RL, Graham DR, Barriere SL, et al. Treatment of hospitalized patients with complicated gram-positive skin and skin structure infections: two randomized, multicentre studies of quinupristin/dalfopristin versus cefazolin, oxacillin or vancomycin. Synercid Skin and Skin Structure Infection Group. *J Antimicrob Chemother* 1999;44:263.

300. Fagon J, Patrick H, Haas DW, et al. Treatment of gram-positive nosocomial pneumonia. Prospective randomized comparison of quinupristin/dalfopristin versus vancomycin. Nosocomial Pneumonia Group. *Am J Respir Crit Care Med* 2000;161:753.

301. Bush K, Jacoby GA, Medeiros AA. A functional classification scheme for beta-lactamases and its correlation with molecular structure. *Antimicrob Agents Chemother* 1995;39:1211.

302. National Committee for Clinical Laboratory Standards. Performance standards for antimicrobial susceptibility testing. Twelfth Informational Supplement. NCCLS document M100-S12. Wayne, PA: NCCLS, 2002.

303. Chow JW, Fine MJ, Shlaes DM, et al. *Enterobacter* bacteremia: clinical features and emergence of antibiotic resistance during therapy. *Ann Intern Med* 1991;115:585.

304. Livermore DM. Multiple mechanisms of antimicrobial resistance in *Pseudomonas aeruginosa*: our worst nightmare? *Clin Infect Dis* 2002;34:634.

305. Harris AD, Smith D, Johnson JA, Bradham DD, Roghmann MC. Risk factors for imipenem-resistant *Pseudomonas aeruginosa* among hospitalized patients. *Clin Infect Dis* 2002;34:340.

306. Linden PK, Kusne S, Coley K, et al. Use of parenteral colistin for the treatment of serious infection due to antimicrobial-resistant *Pseudomonas aeruginosa*. *Clin Infect Dis* 2003;37:E154.

307. Hamer DH. Treatment of nosocomial pneumonia and tracheobronchitis caused by multidrug-resistant *Pseudomonas aeruginosa* with aerosolized colistin. *Am J Respir Crit Care Med* 2000;162:328.

308. Khardori N, Elting L, Wong E, Schable B, Bodey GP. Nosocomial infections due to *Xanthomonas maltophilia* (*Pseudomonas maltophilia*) in patients with cancer [see comments]. *Rev Infect Dis* 1990;12:997.

309. Vartivarian SE, Papadakis KA, Palacios JA, Manning JT Jr, Anaissie EJ. Mucocutaneous and soft tissue infections caused by *Xanthomonas maltophilia*. A new spectrum. *Ann Intern Med* 1994;121:969.

310. Villers D, Espaze E, Coste-Burel M, et al. Nosocomial *Acinetobacter baumannii* infections: microbiological and clinical epidemiology [see comments]. *Ann Intern Med* 1998;129: 182.

311. Rolston K, Guan Z, Bodey GP, Elting L. *Acinetobacter calcoaceticus* septicemia in patients with cancer. *South Med J* 1985;78:647.

312. Greene JN. Catheter-related complications of cancer therapy. *Infect Dis Clin North Am* 1996;10:255.

313. Gaur AH, Flynn PM, Giannini MA, Shenep JL, Hayden RT. Difference in time to detection: a simple method to differentiate catheter-related from non–catheter-related bloodstream infection in immunocompromised pediatric patients. *Clin Infect Dis* 2003;37:469.

314. Newman KA, Reed WP, Schimpff SC, Bustamante CI, Wade JC. Hickman catheters in association with intensive cancer chemotherapy. *Support Care Cancer* 1993;1:92.

315. Press OW, Ramsey PG, Larson EB, Fefer A, Hickman RO. Hickman catheter infections in patients with malignancies. *Medicine (Baltimore)* 1984;63:189.

316. Raad II, Vartivarian S, Khan A, Bodey GP. Catheter-related infections caused by the *Mycobacterium fortuitum* complex: 15 cases and review. *Rev Infect Dis* 1991;13:1120.

317. Centers for Disease Control and Prevention. Guidelines for the prevention of intravascular catheter-related infections. *MMWR Recomm Rep* 2002;51(RR-10):1.

318. Darouiche RO, Raad II, Heard SO. A comparison of two antimicrobial-impregnated central venous catheters. Catheter Study Group. *N Engl J Med* 1999;340:1.

319. Bodey GP. Dermatologic manifestations of infections in neutropenic patients. *Infect Dis Clin North Am* 1994;8:655.

320. Harris RL, Fainstein V, Elting L, Hopfer RL, Bodey GP. Bacteremia caused by *Aeromonas* species in hospitalized cancer patients. *Rev Infect Dis* 1985;7:314.

321. Walsh TJ, Melcher GP, Rinaldi MG, et al. *Trichosporon beigelii*, an emerging pathogen resistant to amphotericin B. *J Clin Microbiol* 1990;28:1616.

322. Walmsley S, Devi S, King S, et al. Invasive *Aspergillus* infections in a pediatric hospital: a ten-year review. *Pediatr Infect Dis J* 1993;12:673.

323. Walsh TJ. Primary cutaneous aspergillosis—an emerging infection among immunocompromised patients [Editorial; Comment]. *Clin Infect Dis* 1998;27:453.

324. Mandell LA, Bartlett JG, Dowell SF, et al. Update of practice guidelines for the management of community-acquired pneumonia in immunocompetent adults. *Clin Infect Dis* 2003;37:1405.

325. Ascioglu S, Rex JH, de Pauw B, et al. Defining opportunistic invasive fungal infections in immunocompromised patients with cancer and hematopoietic stem cell transplants: an international consensus. *Clin Infect Dis* 2002;34:7.

326. Shelhamer JH, Toews GB, Masur H, et al. NIH conference. Respiratory disease in the immunosuppressed patient. *Ann Intern Med* 1992;117:415.

327. Levine SJ. An approach to the diagnosis of pulmonary infections in immunosuppressed patients. *Semin Respir Infect* 1992;7:81.

328. Shaikh ZH, Torres HA, Walsh GL, Champlin RE, Kontoyiannis DP. Open lung biopsy in bone marrow transplant recipients has a poor diagnostic yield for a specific diagnosis. *Transpl Infect Dis* 2002;4:80.

329. Walsh TJ, Bulkley BH. *Aspergillus* pericarditis: clinical and pathologic features in the immunocompromised patient. *Cancer* 1982;49:48.

330. Armstrong TS. Stomatitis in the bone marrow transplant patient. An overview and proposed oral care protocol. *Cancer Nurs* 1994;17:403.

331. Walsh TJ, Gray WC. Candida epiglottitis in immunocompromised patients. *Chest* 1987;91:482.

332. Walsh TJ, Belitsos NJ, Hamilton SR. Bacterial esophagitis in immunocompromised patients. *Arch Intern Med* 1986;146:1345.

333. Kouroussis C, Samonis G, Androulakis N, et al. Successful conservative treatment of neutropenic enterocolitis complicating taxane-based chemotherapy: a report of five cases. *Am J Clin Oncol* 2000;23:309.

334. Ibrahim NK, Sahin AA, Dubrow RA, et al. Colitis associated with docetaxel-based chemotherapy in patients with metastatic breast cancer. *Lancet* 2000;355:281.

335. Sloas MM, Flynn PM, Kaste SC, Patrick CC. Typhlitis in children with cancer: a 30-year experience. *Clin Infect Dis* 1993;17:484.

336. Kirkpatrick ID, Greenberg HM. Gastrointestinal complications in the neutropenic patient: characterization and differentiation with abdominal CT. *Radiology* 2003;226:668.

337. Shamberger RC, Weinstein HJ, Delorey MJ, Levey RH. The medical and surgical management of typhlitis in children with acute nonlymphocytic (myelogenous) leukemia. *Cancer* 1986;57:603.

338. Glenn J, Cotton D, Wesley R, Pizzo P. Anorectal infections in patients with malignant diseases. *Rev Infect Dis* 1988;10:42.

339. Barnes SG, Sattler FR, Ballard JO. Perirectal infections in acute leukemia. Improved survival after incision and débridement. *Ann Intern Med* 1984;100:515.

340. Lehrnbecher T, Marshall D, Gao C, Chanock SJ. A second look at anorectal infections in cancer patients in a large cancer institute: the success of early intervention with antibiotics and surgery. *Infection* 2002;30:272.

341. Coley SC, Jager HR, Szydlo RM, Goldman JM. CT and MRI manifestations of central nervous system infection following allogeneic bone marrow transplantation. *Clin Radiol* 1999;54:390.

342. Graus F, Saiz A, Sierra J, et al. Neurologic complications of autologous and allogeneic bone marrow transplantation in patients with leukemia: a comparative study. *Neurology* 1996;46:1004.

343. Hagensee ME, Bauwens JE, Kjos B, Bowden RA. Brain abscess following marrow transplantation: experience at the Fred Hutchinson Cancer Research Center, 1984–1992. *Clin Infect Dis* 1994;19:402.

344. Troke PF, Schwartz S, Ruhnke M, et al. Voriconazole (VCR) therapy (Rx) in 86 patients (pts) with CNS aspergillosis (CNSA): a retrospective analysis. Paper presented at: 43rd Interscience Conference on Antimicrobial Agents and Chemotherapy; Chicago, IL; 2003.

345. Sobel JD. Management of asymptomatic candiduria. *Int J Antimicrob Agents* 1999;11:285.

346. Hirsch HH, Knowles W, Dickenmann M, et al. Prospective study of polyomavirus type BK replication and nephropathy in renal-transplant recipients. *N Engl J Med* 2002;347:488.

347. American Society of Health-System Pharmacists. ASHP therapeutic guidelines on antimicrobial prophylaxis in surgery. *Am J Health Syst Pharm* 1999;56:1839.

348. Penel N, Lefebvre D, Fournier C, et al. Risk factors for wound infection in head and neck cancer surgery: a prospective study. *Head Neck* 2001;23:447.

349. Righi M, Manfredi R, Farneti G, Pasquini E, Cenacchi V. Short-term versus long-term antimicrobial prophylaxis in oncologic head and neck surgery. *Head Neck* 1996;18:399.

350. Coskun H, Erisen L, Basut O. Factors affecting wound infection rates in head and neck surgery. *Otolaryngol Head Neck Surg* 2000;123:328.

351. Norrby SR. Infection after surgery for gastrointestinal cancer. Assessing the costs. *Pharmacoeconomics* 1994;6:483.

352. Khardori N, Wong E, Carrasco CH, et al. Infections associated with biliary drainage procedures in patients with cancer. *Rev Infect Dis* 1991;13:587.

353. Kim W, Clark TW, Baum RA, Soulen MC. Risk factors for liver abscess formation after hepatic chemoembolization. *J Vasc Interv Radiol* 2001;12:965.

354. Blumberg HM, Jarvis WR, Soucie JM, et al. Risk factors for candidal bloodstream infections in surgical intensive care unit patients: the NEMIS prospective multicenter study. The National Epidemiology of Mycosis Survey. *Clin Infect Dis* 2001;33:177.

355. Eggimann P, Francioli P, Bille J, et al. Fluconazole prophylaxis prevents intra-abdominal candidiasis in high-risk surgical patients. *Crit Care Med* 1999;27:1066.

356. Heys SD, Walker LG, Smith I, Eremin O. Enteral nutritional supplementation with key nutrients in patients with critical illness and cancer: a meta-analysis of randomized controlled clinical trials. *Ann Surg* 1999;229:467.

357. Braga M, Gianotti L, Radaelli G, et al. Perioperative immunonutrition in patients undergoing cancer surgery: results of a randomized double-blind phase 3 trial. *Arch Surg* 1999;134:428.

358. Godwin JE, Kopecky KJ, Head DR, et al. A double-blind placebo-controlled trial of granulocyte colony-stimulating factor in elderly patients with previously untreated acute myeloid leukemia: a Southwest oncology group study (9031). *Blood* 1998;91:3607.

359. Heil G, Hoelzer D, Sanz MA, et al. A randomized, double-blind, placebo-controlled, phase III study of filgrastim in remission induction and consolidation therapy for adults with de novo acute myeloid leukemia. The International Acute Myeloid Leukemia Study Group. *Blood* 1997;90:4710.

360. Rowe JM, Andersen JW, Mazza JJ, et al. A randomized placebo-controlled phase III study of granulocyte-macrophage colony-stimulating factor in adult patients (>55 to 70 years of age) with acute myelogenous leukemia: a study of the Eastern Cooperative Oncology Group (E1490). *Blood* 1995;86:457.

361. Ozer H, Armitage JO, Bennett CL, et al. 2000 update of recommendations for the use of hematopoietic colony-stimulating factors: evidence-based, clinical practice guidelines. American Society of Clinical Oncology Growth Factors Expert Panel. *J Clin Oncol* 2000;18:3558.

362. Bensinger WI, Price TH, Dale DC, et al. The effects of daily recombinant human granulocyte colony-stimulating factor administration on normal granulocyte donors undergoing leukapheresis [see comments]. *Blood* 1993;81:1883.

363. Dale DC, Liles WC, Llewellyn C, Rodger E, Price TH. Neutrophil transfusions: kinetics and functions of neutrophils mobilized with granulocyte-colony-stimulating factor and dexamethasone [see comments]. *Transfusion* 1998;38:713.

364. Dignani MC, Anaissie EJ, Hester JP, et al. Treatment of neutropenia-related fungal infections with granulocyte colony-stimulating factor-elicited white blood cell transfusions: a pilot study. *Leukemia* 1997;11:1621.

365. Peters C, Minkov M, Matthes-Martin S, et al. Leucocyte transfusions from rhG-CSF or prednisolone stimulated donors for treatment of severe infections in immunocompromised neutropenic patients. *Br J Haematol* 1999;106:689.

366. Bhatia S, McCullough J, Perry EH, et al. Granulocyte transfusions: efficacy in treating fungal infections in neutropenic patients following bone marrow transplantation. *Transfusion* 1994;34:226.

367. Price TH, Bowden RA, Boeckh M, et al. Phase I/II trial of neutrophil transfusions from donors stimulated with G-CSF and dexamethasone for treatment of patients with infections in hematopoietic stem cell transplantation. *Blood* 2000;95:3302.

368. Nichols WG, Price T, Boeckh M. Cytomegalovirus infections in cancer patients receiving granulocyte transfusions. *Blood* 2002;99:3483.

369. A controlled trial of interferon gamma to prevent infection in chronic granulomatous disease. The International Chronic Granulomatous Disease Cooperative Study Group. *N Engl J Med* 1991;324:509.

370. Holland SM, Eisenstein EM, Kuhns DB, et al. Treatment of refractory disseminated non-tuberculous mycobacterial infection with interferon gamma. A preliminary report. *N Engl J Med* 1994;330:1348.

371. Stevens DA. Combination immunotherapy and antifungal chemotherapy. *Clin Infect Dis* 1998;26:1266.

372. Pappas PG, Bustamante B, Ticona E, et al. Adjunctive interferon-gamma for treatment of cryptococcal meningitis: a randomized double-blind trial. Paper presented at: 41st Interscience Conference on Antimicrobial Agents and Chemotherapy; 2001; Chicago, IL.

373. Gahn B, Hunt G, Rooney CM, Heslop HE. Immunotherapy to reconstitute immunity to DNA viruses. *Semin Hematol* 2002;39:41.

374. Walter EA, Greenberg PD, Gilbert MJ, et al. Reconstitution of cellular immunity against cytomegalovirus in recipients of allogeneic bone marrow by transfer of T-cell clones from the donor [see comments]. *N Engl J Med* 1995;333:1038.

375. Papadopoulos EB, Ladanyi M, Emanuel D, et al. Infusions of donor leukocytes to treat Epstein-Barr virus–associated lymphoproliferative disorders after allogeneic bone marrow transplantation [see comments]. *N Engl J Med* 1994;330:1185.

376. Rooney CM, Smith CA, Ng CY, et al. Use of gene-modified virus-specific T lymphocytes to control Epstein-Barr-virus–related lymphoproliferation. *Lancet* 1995;345:9.

377. Heslop HE, Ng CY, Li C, et al. Long-term restoration of immunity against Epstein-Barr virus infection by adoptive transfer of gene-modified virus-specific T lymphocytes. *Nat Med* 1996;2:551.

CHAPTER 54

Adverse Effects of Treatment

ANN M. BERGER
REBECCA A. CLARK-SNOW

SECTION **1**

Nausea and Vomiting

NATURE OF THE PROBLEM

Currently, there are many efficacious antiemetic regimens for the nausea and vomiting produced by chemotherapeutic agents. In a study conducted in 1983, cancer patients ranked nausea and vomiting as the first and second most severe side effects of chemotherapy, respectively.[1] After the emergence of new antiemetic agents and alterations in chemotherapeutic regimens, patients' perceptions of the most severe side effects were modified. In a 1993 study, 155 cancer patients receiving chemotherapy reported that they experienced an average of 20 physical and psychosocial symptoms: Nausea was ranked as the most severe symptom and vomiting as the fifth.[2] Therefore, nausea is also an important efficacy parameter when evaluating an antiemetic.

Use of these antiemetic agents has decreased the incidence and severity of nausea and vomiting induced by chemotherapy; however, these agents have not totally prevented the problem. Chemotherapy-induced nausea and vomiting continue to remain a concern for patients receiving cancer treatment. In 2002, Grunberg et al. reported that in spite of the use of modern antiemetics, chemotherapy-induced nausea and vomiting continues to be a problem for a significant number of patients receiving cancer chemotherapy. It was observed that the frequency of chemotherapy-induced nausea and vomiting, particularly delayed nausea and vomiting, is underestimated by oncology physicians and nurses.[3]

The incidence and severity of nausea or vomiting in patients receiving chemotherapy vary, depending on the type of chemotherapy given, dose, schedule, combinations of medications, and individual characteristics. The consequences of not controlling the nausea and vomiting induced by cancer treatment may lead to medical complications, a failure of the patient to comply with the cancer therapy and follow-up, and a diminished quality of life.

The supportive care of patients receiving agents with the potential to cause nausea and vomiting remains an important aspect of effective management of the oncology patient. In every treatment situation, the primary goal is prevention of chemotherapy-induced nausea and vomiting for all. However, despite an improved understanding of the pathophysiology associated with this phenomenon, the identification of predictive factors, the definition of emetic syndromes, and the development of evidence-based guidelines that incorporate the most effective antiemetic agents and regimens available to prevent and treat chemotherapy-induced emesis, there continue to be patients for whom achieving complete control (no vomiting or nausea) is problematic. To this end, patients' quality of life may be significantly compromised in the event of incomplete control.

PATHOPHYSIOLOGY OF NAUSEA AND VOMITING

The precise mechanisms by which chemotherapy induces nausea and vomiting are unknown; however, it appears probable that different chemotherapeutic agents act at different sites and that some chemotherapeutic agents act at multiple sites. The fact that different chemotherapeutic agents cause nausea and vomiting by different mechanisms and that one chemotherapeutic agent may induce nausea and vomiting by more than one mechanism helps clinicians to understand why there is no one antiemetic regimen that is effective all of the time.

Mechanisms by which chemotherapeutic agents cause nausea and vomiting are activation of the chemoreceptor trigger zone (CTZ) either directly or indirectly, peripheral stimulation of the gastrointestinal (GI) tract, vestibular mechanisms, cortical mechanisms, or alterations of taste and smell. For the majority of the chemotherapeutic agents, the most common mechanism is thought to be activation of the CTZ.

The CTZ is located in the area postrema of the brain and can be reached by emetogenic chemicals via the cerebrospinal fluid or the blood. The thought is that the mechanisms of interaction between the CTZ and chemotherapy involve the release of various neurotransmitters that activate the vomiting center. Either one or a combination of these transmitters may induce vomiting. Some of the neurotransmitters located in the area postrema of the brain that may be excited and lead to emesis include dopamine, serotonin, histamine, norepinephrine, apomorphine, neurotensin, angiotensin II, vasoactive intestinal polypeptide, gastrin, vasopressin, thyrotropin-releasing hormone, leucine-enkephalin, and substance P.[4] Other enzymes surround the CTZ, such as adenosine triphosphatase, monoamine oxidase, cholinesterase, and catecholamines; however, their role in chemotherapy-induced emesis is unknown.

Until the 1990s, the neurotransmitter that appeared to be the most responsible for chemotherapy-induced nausea and vomiting was dopamine. Many effective antiemetics are dopamine antagonists that may bind specifically to the D_2 receptor. However, there is a high degree of variation in dopamine receptor–binding affinity by these drugs. The action of some drugs that cause nausea and vomiting is affected very little or not at all by dopamine antagonists. It is known that not all the important receptors in the CTZ are dopaminergic, as the effect of dopamine antagonists is not equal to surgical ablation of the CTZ. It has also been noted that the degree of antiemetic activity of high-dose metoclopramide cannot be explained on the basis of dopamine blockade alone.

Histamine receptors are found in abundance in the CTZ; however, H_2 antagonists do not work at all as antiemetics. H_1 antagonists alleviate nausea and vomiting induced by vestibular disorder and motion sickness but not nausea and vomiting induced by chemotherapy.[5]

Knowledge that opiate receptors are found in abundance in the CTZ, as well as the facts that narcotics have mixed emetic and antiemetic effects that are blocked by naloxone and that naloxone has emetic properties, have led to the proposal of opiates or enkephalins as an antiemetic. High doses of naloxone augments emesis induced by chemotherapy, and low doses of narcotic may reduce emesis. Studies to date have shown that opiates can prevent chemotherapy-induced emesis in laboratory animals; however, both butorphanol and buprenorphine have not proven to be effective antiemetics in patients who received previous chemotherapy. One study by Lissoni et al.[6] did demonstrate that Fk-33-824 was more effective as an antiemetic in patients who received cisplatin; however, it was ineffective for patients receiving cyclophosphamide or epirubicin.

Edwards et al. found that arginine vasopressin levels rise to a greater extent in patients who vomit when they receive chemotherapy as compared with those who do not vomit.[7] It has been suggested that perhaps arginine vasopressin plays a role in nausea more than in the vomiting induced by chemotherapy. Dexamethasone, which is a known effective antiemetic, may work by reducing arginine vasopressin levels. Another mechanism of action of corticosteroids as antiemetics may be related to modulation of prostaglandin release.

Some evidence suggests that although no one neurotransmitter is responsible for all chemotherapy-induced nausea and vomiting, it appears that 5-hydroxytryptamine [serotonin (5-HT)] receptors are particularly important in the pathophysiology of acute vomiting, whereas others may be more important in the pathophysiology of nausea and delayed emesis. The role of the 5-HT type 3 (5-HT$_3$) receptor in chemotherapy-induced emesis was recognized by examining the mechanism of action of high-dose metoclopramide in decreasing cisplatin-induced emesis. High-dose metoclopramide, unlike other D_2-receptor antagonists, has an exceptionally good capacity to decrease the emesis induced by cisplatin administration. It has been recognized that metoclopramide has pharmacologic effects other than dopamine antagonism. Metoclopramide is a weak antagonist of peripheral 5-HT$_3$ receptors and can stimulate GI motility by increasing acetylcholine release from the cholinergic nerves of the GI tract. To test whether 5-HT$_3$-receptor blockade would decrease cisplatin-induced emesis, Miner et al. took a substituted benzamide, BRL 24924, which has stimulatory effects on the GI tract and is a 5-HT$_3$-receptor blocker, and demonstrated decreased emesis in ferrets that received cisplatin. This study was repeated with a nonbenzamide selective 5-HT$_3$-receptor blocker MDL 72222, which has no GI-stimulating activity. The study revealed that cisplatin-induced emesis was totally blocked by this compound.[8] The same conclusion was reached in another study using a different nonbenzamide, the selective 5-HT$_3$ antagonist ICS 205-930.[9] These studies demonstrated the role of 5-HT$_3$-receptor blockade in chemotherapy-induced emesis.

The precise mechanism of action of the 5-HT$_3$-receptor antagonists is unknown; however, the primary effect appears to be peripheral at the site of the 5-HT$_3$ receptors on the vagal afferent neurons. The GI tract contains approximately 80% of the body's supply of serotonin, and it has been suggested that perhaps chemotherapy administration causes release of serotonin from the enterochromaffin cells of the GI tract, which then stimulates emesis via both the vagus and greater splanchnic nerve as well as stimulates the area postrema of the brain. After cisplatin administration, there is an increase in urinary excretion of 5-hydroxyindoleacetic acid, the main metabolite of serotonin, and this increase parallels the number of episodes of emesis.[10] Studies have shown that the 5-HT$_3$-receptor antagonists decrease emesis from several chemotherapeutic agents, including cisplatin, cyclophosphamide, and doxorubicin.[11,12]

An important mechanism whereby chemotherapy may induce emesis is peripheral effects that are thought to arise from the pharynx and the upper GI tract. Most likely, the chemotherapy does not directly stimulate the peripheral receptors. Rather, neurotransmitters probably are released as a result of local GI irritation or damage. GI tract serotonin, dopamine, opiate, histamine, and cholinergic receptors are most likely involved in the emesis induced by chemotherapy. The peripheral effects may be abolished by vagotomy, indicating that impulses from the GI tract may reach the vomiting center via the vagus and sympathetic nerves.

In addition to serotonin, substance P has recently been identified as an important neurotransmitter involved in chemotherapy-induced nausea and vomiting. Positron emission tomography imaging of healthy human brains has demonstrated that substance P/neurokinin-1 (NK1) receptors are located centrally in the brainstem.[13] Substance P is believed to exert its effect on the emetic reflex primarily through the central mechanism of binding to the NK1 receptors in the midbrain. NK1 receptor antagonists that cross the blood–brain barrier have been shown to inhibit both acute and delayed emesis by cisplatin in animal models and human studies. Hesketh et al. analyzed data from clinical trials for the time course of cisplatin-induced emesis and demonstrated that serotonin-dependent mechanisms appeared to predominate in the first 8 to 12 hours postcisplatin, but thereafter, NK1-dependent mechanisms for emesis appeared to have relatively greater importance.[64] Specifically, early acute events responsive to 5-HT_3-receptor antagonists are likely to be mediated by peripheral serotonin release, whereas later acute and delayed events responsive to NK1 receptor antagonists are more likely to be medicated by substance P acting centrally at the NK1 receptors.[64]

Another mechanism that may be involved in chemotherapy-induced emesis could be the therapy's effect on the vestibular system. It is known that patients who have a history of motion sickness experience a greater severity, frequency, and duration of nausea and vomiting from chemotherapy than patients who do not experience motion sickness. The mechanism by which the vestibular system may lead to chemotherapy-induced emesis is unknown; however, it is postulated that sensory information that is received by the vestibular system is different from information that was expected.

Some investigators believe that taste changes induced by chemotherapy may lead to nausea and vomiting. There are two suggested mechanisms for this. First, taste is thought to inhibit some activities incompatible with eating (e.g., oral pain, gag, nausea, vomiting). Damage to taste such as that produced by some chemotherapy might release that inhibition leading to enhancement of gag, nausea, and vomiting. This is supported by a study showing taste damage in women who have suffered from hyperemesis during pregnancy.[14] Second, some chemotherapeutic agents may be tasted. For example, in a study of patients with breast carcinoma who received cyclophosphamide, methotrexate, and 5-fluorouracil, 36% reported a bitter taste in their mouth. One-third of the patients thought that the bitter taste caused vomiting.[15] The exact mechanism by which taste is changed by chemotherapy is unknown; however, it is thought that while the drugs are in the plasma or saliva, they have a direct effect on the oral mucosa or taste buds. Changes in taste may contribute both to nausea and vomiting as well as to anorexia.

Finally, chemotherapy-induced emesis may be induced by direct or indirect effects on the cerebral cortex. Animal studies have shown that nitrogen mustard partially causes emesis via direct stimulation of the cerebral cortex. Studies demonstrate that the risk of nausea and vomiting is increased when a patient's roommate is experiencing nausea and vomiting. It is also known that the amount of sleep before receiving chemotherapy may influence whether a patient develops chemotherapy-induced emesis. In addition, large differences exist in the severity and incidence of nausea and vomiting from the same chemotherapeutic agents in different countries. These studies indicate that indirect psychological effects can mediate chemotherapy-induced nausea and vomiting.

Aside from there being more than one mechanism by which each chemotherapeutic agent may induce emesis, chemotherapy induces emesis in a manner different from that of other classic emetic agents. Drugs such as apomorphine, levodopa, digitalis, pilocarpine, nicotine, and morphine cause vomiting almost immediately. Nitrogen mustard also may lead to emesis immediately; however, most chemotherapeutic agents and radiotherapy require a latency period before emesis begins. Also, most chemotherapeutic agents do not induce emesis in a monophasic way, as do the classic emetic agents. Chemotherapeutic agents induce emesis with a delayed onset, and the emesis has multiphasic time courses. When managing chemotherapy-induced emesis, one should realize that there is most likely more than one mechanism involved, suggesting that there is not one antiemetic regimen that works for all patients all of the time.

By 1991, more than 50% of patients received a serotonin antagonist antiemetic (5-HT_3) for symptom control; approximately 90% received similar treatment in 1995, with a statistically significant reduction in posttreatment vomiting. Both physicians and nurses acknowledge an improvement in patients' quality of life and treatment compliance with the use of these agents. However, trends over time have not shown an improvement in the control of nausea. In fact, data confirm that there is a significant increase in the duration of posttreatment nausea and no change in the frequency of posttreatment nausea or anticipatory symptoms.[16]

EMETIC SYNDROMES

Patients undergoing therapy for the treatment and possible cure of cancer with chemotherapy often are faced with the distressing side effects of nausea and vomiting. The goals of antiemetic therapy are as follows: (1) to achieve complete control in all settings, (2) to provide maximum convenience for patients and staff, (3) to eliminate potential side effects of the agents, and (4) to minimize the cost of treatment with antiemetic agents and drug administration.

As a result of antiemetic investigations, three major, but related emetic syndromes have been identified: acute, delayed, and anticipatory emesis. Traditionally, acute emesis is defined as occurring within the first 24 hours after administration of chemotherapy (usually within 1 to 2 hours) and is generally most severe during the initial 4 to 6 hours. Delayed emesis has been arbitrarily defined as occurring 24 or more hours after chemotherapy (range of 16 to 24 hours), with maximal risk at 48 hours. It is most commonly associated with the administration of cisplatin, carboplatin, cyclophosphamide, and doxorubicin. A study that outlines the natural history of delayed emesis concluded that although the emesis associated with this dilemma is less severe than that which is seen in the acute phase, it still poses significant problems with nutrition, hydration, and possibly a prolonged hospital course.[17]

Initial studies revealed that delayed emesis could be controlled with a regimen of metoclopramide and dexamethasone. Because of the possibility of extrapyramidal side effects such as anxiety, akathisia, restlessness, torticollis, or oculogyric crisis, with metoclopramide, patients should be given a prescription for diphenhydramine to be taken at the first sign of an extrapyramidal symptom. In the younger patient, diphenhydramine should be given prophylactically.

Early trials addressing the treatment of delayed emesis with the single-agent serotonin antagonist ondansetron were discouraging and labeled the serotonin antagonists as having low activity. Two randomized studies, one with ondansetron and one with granisetron, indicated efficacy of the serotonin antagonists for delayed emesis in patients receiving chemotherapy of intermediate emetogenicity.[18,19] New antiemetic agents have been identified and recently approved for use that are beneficial in both the prevention and treatment of delayed emesis. These agents are discussed later in New Agents.

Preventive therapy is imperative for patients to achieve the best outcome. The risk defined for acute emesis is a good predictor of delayed emesis. Patients who do not receive preventive therapy have a 70% to 90% incidence of delayed emesis with high-risk agents and a 30% to 60% risk with moderate-risk agents (Table 54.1-1).

Anticipatory emesis is a learned or conditioned response that typically occurs before, during, or after the administration of chemotherapy. In this instance, patients may be responding to a variety of stimuli that in most instances was associated with a prior experience when there was inadequate control of emesis. The corresponding psychological mechanism for anticipatory emesis is unknown and is secondary to the direct administration of the chemotherapy agent itself. Therefore, patients must be given the opportunity to receive the optimal antiemetic regimen with their initial course of chemotherapy to prevent acute and delayed emesis, and, consequently, anticipatory emesis. Treatment for the occurrence of anticipatory emesis may include the use of benzodiazepines in addition to antiemetics before and during chemotherapy. Relaxation techniques, guided visual imagery, desensitization, and hypnosis techniques may also be effective.[20,21,59,60]

In addition to hypnosis, relaxation, imagery, and desensitization, acupuncture is a nonmedicinal complementary therapy that has been shown to have benefits in chemotherapy-related nausea and vomiting. An initial trial was done with 130 patients who had a history of distressing emesis in prior chemotherapy regimens. Emesis was reduced in 97% of the subjects.[61] A National Institutes of Health consensus trial concluded that acupuncture was effective in reducing chemotherapy-induced emesis; however, placebo effect was a concern.[62] A subsequent trial that addressed the issue of placebo effect was done with women with breast cancer receiving high-dose cyclophosphamide, cisplatin, and carmustine. One hundred four women were randomly assigned to receive no needling, minimal needling at control points with mock electrostimulation, or classic antiemetic electroacupuncture once daily for 5 days. The number of emesis episodes were lower in the first 5 days for those receiving electroacupuncture compared with those receiving minimal needling at control points or no needling ($P < .001$). The effect appeared to be of limited duration in that there were no significant differences during the 9-day follow-up.[63] Clearly the data are promising; however, additional research is needed in this area.

CONTROL OF EMESIS AND RISK FACTORS

The methodology used in antiemetic trials has identified useful patient characteristics and prognostic factors that may affect antiemetic control. These indicators become important for tai-

TABLE 54.1-1. Emetic Risk of Commonly Used Chemotherapy Agents

HIGH: RISK IN NEARLY ALL PATIENTS
Cisplatin
Carmustine (>250 mg/m^2)
Cyclophosphamide (>1500 mg/m^2)
Dacarbazine (>500 mg/m^2)
Lomustine (>60 mg/m^2)
Pentostatin
Dactinomycin
Streptozotocin
Mechlorethamine

MODERATE: RISK IN $>30\%$ OF PATIENTS
Cisplatin (<50 mg/m^2)
Carmustine (<250 mg/m^2)
Cyclophosphamide (<1500 mg/m^2)
Cyclophosphamide (PO)
Doxorubicin
Epirubicin
Idarubicin
Hexamethylmelamine
Ifosfamide
Carboplatin
Irinotecan
Melphalan
Procarbazine
Mitoxantrone (>12 mg/m^2)
Cytarabine (>1 g/m^2)

LOW: RISK IN 10–30% OF PATIENTS
Methotrexate (>100 mg/m^2)
Fluorouracil (<1 g/m^2)
Doxorubicin (<20 mg/m^2)
Mitoxantrone (<12 mg/m^2)
Cytarabine (<1 g/m^2)
Temozolomide
Etoposide (PO)
Asparaginase
Gemcitabine
Mitomycin
Paclitaxel
Thiotepa
Topotecan
Docetaxel
Aldesleukin

MINIMAL: $<10\%$ RISK
Capecitabine
Vincristine
Vinblastine
Vinorelbine
Teniposide
Etoposide
Bleomycin
Rituximab
Trastuzumab
Methotrexate (<100 mg/m^2)

loring antiemetic regimens as well as designing antiemetic trials. Careful studies have identified patient-related risk factors to include prior experience with chemotherapy, alcohol intake history, age, and gender as influencing patient outcomes.

A patient's prior exposure to chemotherapy very often determines success or failure in controlling emesis with future treatment courses. As mentioned earlier in Emetic Syndromes, the administration of the appropriate antiemetic during the initial course of chemotherapy can very often eliminate the development of anticipatory emesis, in addition to decreasing the severity of delayed emesis.

Chronic and heavy alcohol usage, defined as more than 100 g of alcohol or five mixed drinks per day, whether in the past or currently, has been shown to positively affect the control of emesis.[22,23] Age as a prognostic factor cannot predict patient response to antiemetic therapy. It is, however, an important factor in determining the potential for the occurrence of acute dystonic reactions. Patients aged 30 years or younger are more prone to experience the acute dystonic reactions associated with the dopamine receptor–blocking agents such as the phenothiazines, butyrophenones, and substituted benzamides. These side effects are usually characterized by trismus or torticollis. It is also important to remember that within this population of patients, chemotherapy agents that might necessitate antiemetics often are given over several consecutive days, increasing the possibility of the occurrence of acute dystonic reactions.[23] A distinct advantage of the 5-HT$_3$ antiemetic agents is that they do not cause acute dystonic reactions, making them an especially beneficial treatment option for children and younger adults.

It has been difficult to explain the rationale for poorer control of emesis in women receiving treatment for various malignancies. A possible explanation may be that women characteristically receive chemotherapy regimens that contain highly emetogenic agents such as cisplatin and cyclophosphamide, usually given in combination, and are less likely than men to have a history of a high alcohol intake.

Other contributing factors that may affect the control of emesis include a heightened level of anxiety during the chemotherapy infusion, being prone to motion sickness, and having had severe emesis during pregnancy.[24]

ANTIEMETIC AGENTS

MOST ACTIVE AGENTS

As outlined earlier in Pathophysiology of Nausea and Vomiting, antagonism of the 5-HT$_3$ receptor is an important approach to controlling chemotherapy-induced emesis. Several agents are available that exert their efficacy in this manner. Metoclopramide, previously thought to block emesis by antagonism of a dopamine receptor (D$_2$), probably works primarily via the 5-HT$_3$ pathway at higher doses. This explains why higher doses of metoclopramide are more effective. However, metoclopramide is not selective for the 5-HT$_3$ pathway, and development of highly selective antagonists of the 5-HT$_3$ receptor allowed for good antiemetic effect with a lower side effect profile.

Several selective 5-HT$_3$ antagonists are commercially available in many countries: dolasetron, granisetron, ondansetron, and tropisetron. Other similar agents are available in individual countries or are under investigation. Multiple large, randomized clinical trials have shown no clinically significant difference among these drugs when used appropriately.[25–27] Further studies have demonstrated that a single oral dose of a 5-HT$_3$ receptor antagonist before chemotherapy has efficacy equivalent to a multiple-dosing regimen.[28–30]

Controversy remains concerning the optimal dose of the serotonin antagonists. It appears that maximal benefit occurs once all relevant receptors are saturated. No matter what the emetic source, if best results are to be achieved, an adequate dose should be given. Higher doses are not advantageous once all receptors have been saturated.[31,32] In that these are very safe and well-tolerated agents, it has been difficult to define the best dose for regimens, and different doses have been mandated in different countries. As a general rule, the lowest adequately tested dose should be assumed to be the best dose in all settings.

Although some debate persists concerning the best dose of ondansetron, the majority of trials have indicated that the lower dose (8 mg) is as effective as the higher and far more expensive dose of 32 mg.[33,34] The latter dose was superior in only one trial and was troubled by a high inadequate treatment rate, indicating a poorly conducted trial. The lower granisetron dose of 0.01 mg/kg is as effective in all circumstances as four times the dose.[35] The same recommendations continue for single-agent or combination use.

The side effect profile of the 5-HT$_3$ antagonists provides an advantage over such effective antiemetics as metoclopramide. Central nervous system effects, extrapyramidal reactions, and sedation are not observed with serotonin antagonists; this is particularly beneficial in younger patients. Common side effects include mild headaches usually not requiring treatment, transient transaminase elevations, and mild constipation with some agents.

As indicated, the antiemetic activity of metoclopramide is likely as a serotonin antagonist, although it has substantial dopamine antagonist action as well. This latter mechanism explains the potential for extrapyramidal reactions. Studies have shown that higher doses are more effective. A dose of 3 mg/kg given every 2 hours for two doses in combination with a corticosteroid has been found to be effective.[36]

Corticosteroids are valuable antiemetics. Dexamethasone is the most widely studied of all these agents in oral and parenteral preparations and in most countries is very inexpensive. Although the best dose has not been established, it appears that a single dose of 10 to 20 mg is adequate. Caution must be used when treating diabetic patients or others with a poor tolerance for corticosteroids. However, the short recommended course makes these agents very safe and easy to use. In preventing delayed emesis, adequate doses of corticosteroids are viewed as advantageous when combined with metoclopramide.

Efficacy for corticosteroids has been clearly defined for cisplatin-containing regimens as well as other types of chemotherapy with lesser emetic potential. The addition of a corticosteroid to 5-HT$_3$ antagonists significantly improves antiemetic efficacy with each of the agents. This is seen with cisplatin as well as with such drugs as anthracyclines, cyclophosphamide, and carboplatin. Therefore a corticosteroid should be added whenever the emetic source is thought to warrant a serotonin antagonist unless a clearly documented reason for not using a corticosteroid in that patient has been demonstrated.

ANTIEMETICS OF LOWER ACTIVITY

Older agents, such as phenothiazines, butyrophenones, and cannabinoids, all have some degree of antiemetic efficacy. In general, this efficacy is substantially lower than that seen with the serotonin antagonists (including high-dose metoclopramide), and the side effects are greater. When given intravenously, phenothiazines appear to be more active than when given by other routes but are associated with hypotension (especially orthostatic), which can be severe. Thus, these agents are not highly recommended. Oral forms of all three of these agents exhibit only modest activity and are of similarly low efficacy.

Several cannabinoids have been tested in chemotherapy-induced emesis and are of both historical and lay press interest. Semisynthetic agents, such as nabilone and levonantradol; tetrahydrocannabinol (or Δ9-THC), the active agent in marijuana; and inhaled marijuana, all appear to be of low and equal efficacy, with frequent autonomic side effects. These toxicities include dry mouth, hypotension, and dizziness. Dronabinol may be useful as an adjuvant to other antiemetics.

Antianxiety agents, such as the benzodiazepine lorazepam, have little efficacy as single agents in carefully conducted trials. However, they function well against anxiety in the emotionally charged atmosphere of receiving chemotherapy, although they add only a minor antiemetic effect to more active agents. They should be regarded as adjuncts to antiemetics and, in that role, can be useful for many patients. Recommended doses range from 0.5 to 1.5 mg. It is not clear that there is any advantage in giving these agents parenterally rather than orally when given with the most effective antiemetics. In addition, these drugs may be useful when given to patients with anticipatory emesis, starting 1 or more days before the next chemotherapy dosing. Side effects mainly concern sedation, which can be marked in some patients, especially if the drug is given intravenously.

TREATMENT OPTIONS BASED ON EMESIS CATEGORY

To appropriately prevent acute and delayed emesis, regimens for both syndromes should be well thought out and based on the emesis risk of the chemotherapy administered. The Antiemetic Consensus Group included representatives from several national and internationally recognized professional organizations responsible for the development of antiemetic guidelines and includes the American Society of Clinical Oncology, the American Society of Health-System Pharmacists, the Multinational Association for Supportive Care in Cancer, and the National Comprehensive Cancer Network.[25–27,37] In an attempt to simplify currently published antiemetic guidelines, the Antiemetic Consensus Group was able to reach general agreement regarding classification of emetic risk for the most commonly administered chemotherapy agents as well as a treatment algorithm that includes dosing recommendations for use by clinicians (Table 54.1-2).

The actual risk assigned to each chemotherapy agent has been classified into four categories; high, moderate, low, and minimal. Nearly all patients who receive representative agents such as cisplatin, dacarbazine and nitrogen mustard from the high-risk group experience emesis if preventive antiemetics are not given. Clinical outcomes are significantly improved with the addition of a corticosteroid such as dexamethasone.[26,38]

Therefore, for high-risk acute prevention and management of chemotherapy-induced emesis a 5-HT₃-receptor antagonist plus dexamethasone is recommended for day 1 of chemotherapy at the doses listed in Table 54.1-2. The delayed regimen in this setting should include dexamethasone with the addition of

TABLE 54.1-2. Guidelines for Antiemetic Dosing

Antiemetic	Dose: Acute Emesis	Dose: Delayed Emesis
5-HYDROXYTRYPTAMINE TYPE 3 RECEPTOR ANTAGONISTS: ADMINISTER ONCE PRECHEMOTHERAPY		
Ondansetron	0.15 mg/kg IV or 8 mg IV 12–16 mg PO	8 mg b.i.d. × 2–3 d
Granisetron	0.01 mg/kg IV or 1 mg IV 1 mg PO	
Dolasetron	1.8 mg/kg IV or 100 mg IV 100–200 mg PO	
Palonosetron	0.25 mg IV	
CORTICOSTEROID		
Dexamethasone	10–20 mg IV	High risk: 8 mg PO b.i.d. d 2–4 Moderate risk: 4–8 mg PO b.i.d. d 2–3
DOPAMINE ANTAGONISTS		
Metoclopramide	2–3 mg IV pre-chemotherapy Repeat 2 h postchemotherapy	0.5 mg/kg or 20–40 mg PO q.i.d d 2–5
Prochlorperazine	10 mg IV or PO every 3–4 h p.r.n	

a 5-HT₃-receptor antagonist, such as ondansetron, or the dopamine antagonist metoclopramide on days 2 to 4. For chemotherapy agents that are listed in the moderate-risk category, acute management includes the same recommendation as for high-risk chemotherapy; however, the delayed regimen should include dexamethasone given as a single agent, the combination of dexamethasone plus metoclopramide, or a serotonin receptor antagonist.

Guiding principles for the control of acute emesis include the following[39]:

1. Use the lowest fully effective dose.
2. Corticosteroids should be added to the regimen containing 5-HT₃ antagonists.
3. Oral antiemetics have equivalent efficacy to the intravenous formulation.
4. There is equivalence among the currently available 5-HT₃ antagonists.
5. Antiemetics may be administered as a single dose.

Patients for whom chemotherapy of low risk of emesis has been ordered benefit from receiving single-agent therapy such as dexamethasone; however, dopamine antagonists, butyrophenones, and phenothiazines may also be considered. No preventive treatment is recommended for minimally emetic chemotherapy, but clinicians are advised to provide patients with a prescription for an antiemetic to be taken on an as-needed basis.[39]

NEW AGENTS

Although substantial progress has been made in the efforts to prevent and control chemotherapy-induced emesis, it remains a significant problem, especially for patients experiencing delayed emesis and for patients undergoing high-dose chemotherapy

TABLE 54.1-3. Aprepitant Dosing for High-Risk Chemotherapy

	Day 1	Day 2	Day 3	Day 4
Aprepitant	125 mg PO	80 mg PO	80 mg PO	None
Dexamethasone	12 mg PO	8 mg PO	8 mg PO	8 mg PO
Ondansetron	32 mg IV	None	None	None

Adapted from ref. 41.

and multiple cycles of chemotherapy. Investigators have identified substance P, an 11–amino acid neuropeptide found in the GI tract and central nervous system that has been shown to elicit vomiting in animal models. Substance P exerts its effects by binding to a specific neuroreceptor, NK1. A number of compounds that selectively block the NK1 receptor have been identified.[57] These NK1 antagonists demonstrate a wide spectrum of clinical activity and have been possibly implicated in depression, bladder irritability, inflammatory bowel disease, asthma, and functional GI diseases. They also demonstrate a wide spectrum of antiemetic activity against numerous emetic stimuli.

In two large randomized, double-blind clinical trials, the combination of aprepitant (Emend), an NK1 antagonist administered with a 5-HT$_3$ antagonist and a corticosteroid, was compared with standard therapy (5-HT$_3$ plus a steroid) and was administered to patients receiving high-dose cisplatin.[40a,40b,41] Antiemetic activity was evaluated during the acute and delayed phase. In both studies, a statistically significantly higher proportion of patients receiving the aprepitant regimen had a complete response (no vomiting or rescue therapy) when compared with standard therapy. The most commonly observed side effects with this agent are mild and include fatigue, hiccups, constipation, anorexia, and headache.

Aprepitant is the first NK1 receptor antagonist of this class to be approved for the prevention of acute and delayed nausea and vomiting with initial and repeat courses of highly emetogenic chemotherapy when given in combination with a 5-HT$_3$-receptor antagonist and a corticosteroid as part of a 4-day regimen (Table 54.1-3).[41]

Aprepitant has been classified as a moderate CYP3A4 inhibitor, and clinicians have been advised to observe caution in those patients receiving concomitant medicines, including chemotherapy that is primarily metabolized via the cytochrome P-450 isoenzyme (CYP3A4), which may result in a potential drug interaction.[41]

Palonosetron (Aloxi) is a potent new second-generation 5-HT$_3$ antagonist with strong binding affinity and an extended plasma half-life of approximately 40 hours. It has demonstrated efficacy in preventing chemotherapy-induced nausea and vomiting associated with initial and repeat courses of moderately and highly emetogenic chemotherapy, as well as delayed nausea and vomiting resulting from initial and repeat courses of moderately emetogenic chemotherapy.[58] In three large phase III clinical trials,[42,43] when compared with currently available 5-HT$_3$-receptor antagonists, palonosetron provided patients with improved control during the acute and delayed phases. The side effects observed were similar in severity and frequency as the comparator agents. The most common side effects related to palonosetron were headache and constipation. This agent is currently the only approved antiemetic for the prevention of acute and delayed chemotherapy-induced nausea and vomiting for moderately emetogenic chemotherapy (see Table 54.1-2).[44]

RADIATION-INDUCED NAUSEA AND VOMITING

The etiology of radiation-induced emesis, like chemotherapy-induced emesis, is not completely understood. However, it is clear that it is a complex, multifactorial event. The incidence, severity, and onset of radiation-induced emesis appear to be related to the size of the radiation field, the dose per fraction, and the site of irradiation. Radiation-induced emesis occurs acutely in more than 90% of patients who receive total body irradiation for bone marrow transplantation, within 30 to 60 minutes in more than 80% of patients who receive single high-dose or large-field hemibody irradiation (more than 500 cGy), and within 2 to 3 weeks in approximately 50% of patients who receive conventional fractionated radiotherapy (200 cGy per fraction) to the upper abdomen.[45] Radiation-induced emesis also occurs in those patients who receive radiosurgery to the area postrema in excess of 350 to 400 cGy in a single dose. The emesis usually occurs between 1 and 12 hours after the radiosurgery.

The exact mechanism of radiation-induced emesis remains unclear. However, as with chemotherapy-induced emesis, it is thought that it most likely is due to a peripheral mechanism in the GI tract or a central mechanism involving the CTZ. It has been proposed that several substances, including dopamine, catecholamines, and prostaglandins, are released and stimulate afferent visceral fibers, an action that then initiates sensory signals to the CTZ. As a result of both preclinical and clinical studies with serotonin antagonists, it has been suggested that serotonin may be released from enterochromaffin cells of the GI tract and may mediate emesis via mechanisms involving the 5-HT$_3$ receptors, visceral afferent fibers, and the CTZ. This mechanism is most likely involved when radiation is applied to the upper abdomen, hemibody, or total body. Radiosurgery to the area postrema most likely induces emesis from the release of serotonin in the CTZ.[46]

Clinical studies in the past using metoclopramide, nabilone (cannabinoid derivative), and chlorpromazine in the treatment of radiation-induced emesis revealed a response of 50% to 58%.[47,48] In a nonplacebo trial with domperidone, a dopamine antagonist, a response of 82% was reported.[49] A nonrandomized trial comparing ondansetron with other antiemetics reported response rates of 100% for ondansetron versus 43% for other antiemetics and 19% for no antiemetic treatment for patients who received middle- to upper-hemibody irradiation.[50] A randomized study by Priestman et al.[51] of patients who received radiotherapy to the abdomen, pelvis, and thoracolumbar spine reported response rates of 45% for metoclopramide versus 97% for ondansetron. A randomized, double-blind, placebo-controlled evaluation revealed oral ondansetron to be an effective therapy for the prevention of emesis induced by total body irradiation.[52] Ondansetron has been reported to be effective in radiotherapy-induced emesis in children[53] as well as for patients who receive radiosurgery to the area postrema.[46]

Data are available from two double-blind, randomized studies in the use of oral granisetron, 2 mg once daily, in radiation-induced nausea and vomiting. In a study involving patients undergoing fractionated upper-abdominal radiation, patients who received oral granisetron had a significantly longer median time to first emesis than did those who received placebo (35 vs. 9 days, respectively) and a longer median time to first nausea (11 days vs. 1 day, respectively).[54] In another study of patients undergoing total body irradiation, patients treated with oral granisetron had significantly greater complete control compared with the historical control group over the entire 4-day treatment period (22% vs. 0%, respectively).[55]

Fauser et al.[56] reported on the use of oral dolasetron for the control of emesis during total body irradiation and high-dose cyclophosphamide in patients undergoing allogeneic bone marrow transplantation. Approximately two-thirds of the patients who received dolasetron during the irradiation and chemotherapy administration period had two or fewer episodes vomiting, and nausea was reported as mild. This trial concluded that oral dolasteron was effective and safe for the prevention of nausea and vomiting during total body irradiation.

NAUSEA AND VOMITING SECONDARY TO COMORBID CONDITIONS

A number of comorbid conditions also may lead to nausea and vomiting, even though the majority of patients with cancer develop nausea and vomiting as a result of chemotherapy or radiotherapy. Because the mechanism of the nausea and vomiting secondary to comorbid conditions is not usually well understood, it is difficult to know which antiemetics may be helpful. Controlled-release metoclopramide has been shown to be safe and effective in managing chronic nausea in patients with advanced cancer.

IMPROVING ANTIEMETIC CONTROL

The coordination of supportive care of patients with cancer involves the multidisciplinary participation of physicians, nurses, pharmacists, dietitian specialists, and, most important, patients and their families. The last two decades have seen dramatic improvements in the prevention and treatment of the side effects of cancer therapy and symptom management. With the introduction of the serotonin antagonist antiemetics and now with the more recent addition of palonosetron, a more potent second-generation serotonin antagonist, as well as aprepitant, the new NK1 antagonist, clinicians are able to provide patients with state-of-the-art therapy to prevent chemotherapy-induced emesis. This can be accomplished through the development of practical and user-friendly guidelines that incorporate precise treatment principles. Until all patients are able to achieve complete control of nausea and emesis from chemotherapy and other specific cancer treatments, investigations and clinical trials of new agents with new mechanisms of action are necessary.

REFERENCES

1. Coates A, Abraham S, Kaye SB, et al. On the receiving end. Patients' perceptions of the side-effects of cancer chemotherapy. *Eur J Clin Oncol* 1983;19:203.
2. Griffin AM, Butow PN, Coates AS, et al. On the receiving end: patients' perceptions of the side-effects of cancer chemotherapy. *Ann Oncol* 1996;7:189.
3. Grunberg SM, Hansen M, Deuson R, Mavros P. *Incidence and impact of nausea/vomiting with modern antiemetics: perception vs. reality.* Proceedings of the American Society Clinical Oncology meeting, Orlando, FL, 2002(abst).
4. Young RW. Mechanisms and treatment of radiation-induced nausea and vomiting. In: Davis CJ, Lakke-Bakaar GV, Graham-Smith DG, eds. *Nausea and vomiting: mechanisms and treatment.* Berlin: Springer-Verlag, 1986:94.
5. Fortner CL, Finley RS, Grove WR. Combination antiemetic therapy in the control of chemotherapy-induced drug emetogenic potential emesis. *Drug Intell Clin Pharm* 1985;19:21.
6. Lissoni P, Barni S, Crispino S, et al. Synthetic enkephalin analog in the treatment of cancer chemotherapy-induced vomiting. *Cancer Treat Rep* 1987;71:6665.
7. Edwards C, Carmichael J, Bayliss P, et al. Arginine vasopressin—a mediator of chemotherapy-induced emesis? *Br J Cancer* 1989;59:467.
8. Miner WD, Sanger GJ, Turner DH. Comparison of the effect of BRL 24924, metoclopramide and domperidone on cisplatin-induced emesis in the ferret. *Br J Pharmacol* 1986;88:374.
9. Costall B, Domeney AM, Nylor RJ, et al. 5-Hydroxytryptamine M-receptor antagonism to prevent cisplatin-induced emesis. *Neuropharmacology* 1986;25:959.
10. Cubeddu L, Hoffman I, Fuenmayor N, et al. Efficacy of ondansetron (GR 38032F) and the role of serotonin in cisplatin-induced nausea and vomiting. *N Engl J Med* 1990; 322:810.
11. Cubeddu L, Hoffman I, Fuenmayor N, et al. Antagonism of serotonin S3 receptors with ondansetron prevents nausea and emesis induced by cyclophosphamide-containing chemotherapy regimens. *J Clin Oncol* 1990;8:1721.
12. Bonneterre J, Chevallier B, Metz R, et al. A randomized double-blind comparison of ondansetron and metoclopramide in the prophylaxis of emesis induced by cyclophosphamide, fluorouracil, and doxorubicin or epirubicin chemotherapy. *J Clin Oncol* 1990;8:1063.
13. Hargreaves R. Imaging substance P receptors (NK1) in the living human brain using positron emission tomography. *J Clin Psychiatry* 2002;63(Suppl 11):18.
14. Sipiora ML, Murtaugh MA, Gregpire MB, Duffy VB. Bitter taste perception and severe vomiting during pregnancy. *Physiol Behav* 2000;69:259.
15. Fetting JH, Wilcox PM, Sheidler VR, et al. Tastes associated with parenteral chemotherapy for breast cancer. *Cancer Treat Rep* 1985;69:1249.
16. Roscoe JA, Morrow GR, Hickoj JT, Stern RM. Nausea and vomiting remain a significant clinical problem: trends over time in controlling chemotherapy-induced nausea and vomiting in 1413 patients treated in community clinical practices. *J Pain Manage* 2000;20:113.
17. Kris MG, Gralla RJ, Clark RA, et al. Incidence, course, and severity of delayed nausea and vomiting following the administration of high-dose cisplatin. *J Clin Oncol* 1985;3:1379.
18. Kaizer L, Warr D, Hoskins P, et al. Effect of schedule and maintenance on the antiemetic efficacy of ondansetron combined with dexamethasone in acute and delayed nausea and emesis in patients receiving moderately emetogenic chemotherapy: a phase III trial by the National Cancer Institute of Canada Clinical Trials Group. *J Clin Oncol* 1994;12:1050.
19. Guillem V, Carrato A, Rifa J, et al. High efficacy of oral granisetron in the total control of cyclophosphamide-induced prolonged emesis. *Proc Am Soc Clin Oncol* 1998;17:46a(abst).
20. Morrow GR, Morrell C. Behavioral treatment for the anticipatory nausea and vomiting induced by cancer chemotherapy. *N Engl J Med* 1982;307:1476.
21. Burish TG, Jenkins RA. Effectiveness of biofeedback and relaxation training in reducing the side effects of chemotherapy. *Health Psychol* 1992;11:17.
22. D'Acquisto RW, Tyson LB, et al. Antiemetic trials to control delayed vomiting following high-dose cisplatin. *Proc Am Soc Clin Oncol* 1986;5:257.
23. Allen JC, Gralla RJ, Reilly L, et al. Metoclopramide dose-related toxicity and preliminary antiemetic studies in children receiving cancer chemotherapy. *J Clin Oncol* 1985;3:1136.
24. Guillem V, Avanda E, Carrato A, et al. Previous history of emesis during pregnancy and motion sickness as risk factors for chemotherapy-induced emesis. *J Clin Oncol* 1999; 2280(18):590a(abst).
25. ASHP Therapeutic Guidelines on the Pharmacologic Management of Nausea and Vomiting in Adult and Pediatric Patients Receiving Chemotherapy or Radiation Therapy or Undergoing Surgery. *Am J Health Syst Pharm* 1999;56:729.
26. Gralla RJ, Osoba D, Kris MG, et al. Recommendations for the use of antiemetics: evidence-based, clinical practice guidelines. *J Clin Oncol* 1999;17:2971.
27. *Antiemesis Practice Guidelines Panel.* NCCN antiemetics practice guidelines. NCCN Proceedings. *Oncology* 1997;11:57.
28. Lofters WS, Pater JL, Zee B, et al. Phase III double-blind comparison of dolasetron mesylate and ondansetron and an evaluation of the additive role of dexamethasone in the prevention of acute and delayed nausea and vomiting due to moderately emetogenic chemotherapy. *J Clin Oncol* 1997;15:2966.
29. Audhuy B, Cappelere P, Martin M, et al. A double-blind randomized comparison of the antiemetic efficacy of two intravenous doses of dolasetron mesylate and granisetron in patients receiving high dose cisplatin chemotherapy. *Eur J Cancer* 1996;32A:807.
30. Mantovani G, Maccio A, Bianchi A, et al. Comparison of granisetron, ondansetron and tropisetron in the prophylaxis of acute nausea and vomiting induced by cisplatin for the treatment of head and neck cancer: a randomized controlled trial. *Cancer* 1996;77:941.
31. Kris MG, Gralla RJ, Clark RA, et al. Phase II trials of the serotonin antagonist GR38032F for the control of vomiting caused by cisplatin. *J Natl Cancer Inst* 1989;81:42.
32. Kris MG, Gralla RJ, Clark RA, et al. Dose ranging evaluation of the serotonin antagonist BR-C507/75 (GR38032F) when used as an antiemetic in patients receiving cancer chemotherapy. *J Clin Oncol* 1988;6:659.
33. Seynaeve C, Schuller J, Buser K, et al. Comparison of the anti-emetic efficacy of different doses of ondansetron given as either a continuous infusion or a single IV dose, in acute cisplatin-induced emesis. A multicentre, double-blind, randomized parallel group study. *Br J Cancer* 1992;66:192.
34. Ruff P, Paska W, Goedhals L, et al. Ondansetron compared with granisetron in the prophylaxis of cisplatin-induced emesis: a multicenter double-blind, randomized, parallel group study. *Oncology* 1994;5:113.
35. Navari R, Gandara D, Hesketh P, et al. Comparative clinical trial of granisetron and ondansetron in the prophylaxis of cisplatin-induced emesis. *J Clin Oncol* 1995;13:1242.
36. Kris MG, Gralla RJ, Tyson, LB, et al. Improved control of cisplatin-induced emesis with high dose metoclopramide and with combination of metoclopramide, dexamethasone and diphenhydramine. Results of consecutive trials in 255 patients. *Cancer* 1985;55:527.

37. Antiemetic Subcommittee of the Multinational Association of Supportive Care in Cancer (MASCC). Prevention of chemotherapy and radiotherapy-induced emesis: results of the Perugia Consensus Conference. *Ann Oncol* 1998;9:811.

38. Hesketh PJ, Harvey WH, Harker WG, et al. A randomized, double-blind comparison of intravenous ondansetron alone and in combination with intravenous dexamethasone in the prevention of nausea and vomiting associated with high-dose cisplatin. *J Clin Oncol* 1994;12:596.

39. Columbia Antiemetic Consensus Conference, New York, April 2001.

40a. Hesketh PJ, Grunberg SM, Gralla RJ, et al. The oral neurokinin-1 antagonist aprepitant for the prevention of chemotherapy-induced nausea and vomiting: a multinational, randomized, double blind, placebo-controlled trial in patients receiving high-dose cisplatin—the Aprepitant Protocol 052 Study Group. *J Clin Oncol* 2003;21:4112.

40b. Poli-Bigelli S, Rodrigues-Pereira J, Carides AD, et al. Addition of the neurokinin 1 receptor antagonist aprepitant to standard antiemetic therapy improved control of chemotherapy-induced nausea and vomiting. Results from a randomized, double-blind, placebo-controlled trial in Latin America. *Cancer* 2003;97:3090.

41. *Emend (aprepitant) package insert.* Whitehouse Station, NJ: Merck & Co. Inc, March 2003.

42. Rubenstein EB, Gralla RJ, Eisenberg P, et al. Palonosetron compared with ondansetron or dolasetron for prevention of acute and delayed chemotherapy-induced nausea and vomiting: combined results of two phase II trials. *Proc Am Soc Clin Oncol* 2003;22:729.

43. Labianca R, Van der Vegt SG, Mezger JM, et al. Palonosetron is a safe and well tolerated 5-HT3 receptor antagonist: safety results of a phase III trial. *Proc Am Soc Clin Oncol* 2003; 22:753.

44. *Aloxi (palonosetron HCl) injection package insert.* Minneapolis: MGI Pharma Inc, July 2003.

45. Scarantino CW, Ornitz RD, Hoffman LG, et al. Radiation-induced emesis: effects of ondansetron. *Semin Oncol* 1992;19(Suppl 15):38.

46. Bodis S, Alexander E, Kooy H, et al. The prevention of radiosurgery-induced nausea and vomiting by ondansetron: evidence of a direct effect on the central nervous system chemoreceptor trigger zone. *Surg Neurol* 1994;42:249.

47. Priestman TJ, Priestman SG. An initial evaluation of nabilone in the control of radiotherapy-induced nausea and vomiting. *Clin Radiol* 1984;35:265.

48. Lucraft HH, Palmer MK. Randomized clinical trial of levonantradol and chlorpromazine in the prevention of radiotherapy-induced vomiting. *Radiology* 1982;33:621.

49. Reyntjens A. Domperidone as an anti-emetic: summary of research reports. *Postgrad Med J* 1979;55(Suppl):50.

50. Scarantino CW, Ornitz RD, Hoffman LG, et al. Radiation-induced emesis: effects of ondansetron. *Semin Oncol* 1992;19(Suppl 15):38.

51. Priestman TJ, Roberts JT, Lucraft CH, et al. Results of a randomized double-blind comparative study of ondansetron and metoclopramide in the prevention of nausea and vomiting following high dose upper abdominal irradiation. *Clin Oncol* 1990;2:71.

52. Soitzer TR, Bryson JC, Cirenza E, et al. Randomized double-blind, placebo-controlled evaluation of oral ondansetron in the prevention of nausea and vomiting associated with fractionated total-body irradiation. *J Clin Oncol* 1994;12:2432.

53. Jurgens H, McQuade B. Ondansetron as a prophylaxis for chemotherapy and radiotherapy-induced emesis in children. *Oncology* 1992;49:279.

54. Lanciano R, Sherman DM, Michalski J, et al. The efficacy and safety of Kytril tablets (2 mg) once daily in patients receiving at least 10 fractions for malignancy. *Int J Radiat Oncol Biol Phys* 1998;42(Suppl):159(abst).

55. Spitzer TR, Friedman C, Bushnell J, et al. Oral granisetron (Kytril) and ondansetron (Zofran) in the prevention of hyperfractionated total body irradiation induced emesis: the results of a double-blind, randomized parallel group study. *Blood* 1998;92(Suppl 1):278a(abst).

56. Fauser AA, Russ W, Bischiff M. Oral dolasetron mesylate for the control of emesis during fractionated total-body irradiation and high-dose cyclophosphamide in patients undergoing allogeneic bone marrow transplantation. *Support Care Cancer* 1997;5:219.

57. Campos D, Rodrigues Pereira J, Reinhardt R, et al. Prevention of cisplatin-induced emesis by the oral neurokinin-1 antagonist, MK-869, in combination with granisetron and dexamethasone or with dexamethasone alone. *J Clin Oncol* 2002;19:1759.

58. Peschel C, Tonini G, Porcile G, et al. Single IV dose of palonosetron, a potent 5-HT3 receptor antagonist demonstrates sustained prevention of nausea and vomiting for 5 days following moderately emetogenic chemotherapy. *Proc Am Soc Clin Oncol* 2003;22:760.

59. Redd WH, Montgomery GH, DuHamel, KN. Behavioral intervention for cancer treatment side effects. *J Natl Cancer Inst* 2001;93:810.

60. Genius ML. The use of hypnosis in helping cancer patients control anxiety, pain and emesis: a review of empirical studies. *Am J Clin Hypn* 1995;37:316.

61. Dundee JW, Ghaly RG, Fitzpatrick NT, et al. Acupuncture prophylaxis of cancer chemotherapy-induced sickness. *J R Soc Med* 1989;82:268.

62. NIH Consensus Conference. Acupuncture. *JAMA* 1998;280:1518.

63. Shen J, Wenger N, Glaspy J, et al. Electroacupuncture for control of myeloablative chemotherapy-induced emesis: a randomized controlled trial. *JAMA* 2000;284:2755.

64. Hesketh PJ, Van Belle S, Aapro M, et al. Differential involvement of neurotransmitters through the time course of cisplatin-induced emesis as revealed by therapy with specific receptor antagonists. *Eur J Cancer* 2003;39:1074.

SECTION **2**

ANN M. BERGER
JANE M. FALL-DICKSON

Oral Complications

ORAL COMPLICATIONS

Effectiveness of cancer therapies designed to improve cure rates and to extend survival time, including chemotherapy, radiation therapy, and conditioning regimens used in the peripheral blood stem cell transplantation (PBSCT) setting, is tempered by side effects that may become life-threatening. Standard use of growth factors has caused a shift from hematologic to nonhematologic side effects becoming dose- and treatment-limiting. Oral complications are one such side effect category and include chemotherapy- and radiation therapy–related stomatitis and associated oropharyngeal pain, xerostomia, and oral infection and oral chronic graft-versus-host disease (cGVHD). The pathogenesis of and management strategies for these oral complications, as well as future research directions, are presented.

STOMATITIS

Stomatitis is an inflammation of the mucous membranes of the oral cavity and oropharynx characterized by tissue erythema, edema, and atrophy, often progressing to ulceration.[1] The clinical significance of chemotherapy- and radiation therapy–related stomatitis as a dose- and treatment-limiting side effect is widely recognized.[2] The frequency and severity of stomatitis are influenced by numerous patient- and treatment-related risk factors (Table 54.2-1).[3,4]

Risk factors for chemotherapy-related stomatitis are complex, and conflicting study results are seen. For example, although younger patients are considered at increased risk for stomatitis, and women have been reported to have more severe stomatitis more frequently than men, Driezen[5] reported no age or gender risk for stomatitis development. Also, although alcohol and tobacco may impair salivary function, tobacco has been associated with a decreased incidence of chemotherapy-induced stomatitis, and a study of 332 ambulatory chemotherapy patients showed no significant differences in chemotherapy-induced stomatitis incidence between outpatients who wore dental appliances, had a history of oral lesions, used diverse oral hygiene/care practices, and had a smoking history and those patients who did not.[4] Lack of stratification criteria and of clear definition of risk factors for patients entering clinical trials may contribute to conflicting study results.[3] In general, children are three times more likely than adults to develop stomatitis due to their higher proliferating fraction of basal cells. Also, drug metabolism affects stomatitis incidence and severity in patients who are unable to adequately metabolize or excrete certain chemotherapeutic agents.

Although the full spectrum of treatment-related risk factors for stomatitis remains to be defined, reported risk factors include continuous infusion therapy for breast and colon cancer [5-fluorouracil (5-FU) and leucovorin]; administration of selected anthracyclines, alkylating agents, taxanes, vinca alka-

TABLE 54.2-1. Patient- and Treatment-Related Risk Factors for Stomatitis

PATIENT-RELATED
Age older than 65 y or younger than 20 y
Gender
Poor oral health and hygiene
Periodontal diseases
Microbial flora
Chronic low-grade mouth infections
Salivary gland secretory dysfunction
Herpes simplex virus infection
Inability to metabolize chemotherapeutic agent effectively
Poor nutritional status
Exposure to oral stressors such as alcohol and smoking
Ill-fitting dental prostheses
TREATMENT-RELATED
Radiation: dose, schedule
Chemotherapy: drug, dose, schedule
Myelosuppression
Neutropenia
Immunosuppression
Reduced secretory immunoglobulin A
Oral care during treatment
Infections: bacterial, viral, fungal
Use of antidepressants, opiates, antihypertensives, antihistamines, diuretics, and sedatives
Impairment of renal and/or hepatic function
Protein or calorie malnutrition, and dehydration
Xerostomia

(Adapted from refs. 3 and 4.)

loids, antimetabolites, and antitumor antibiotics; myeloablative conditioning regimens for PBSCT or bone marrow transplantation (BMT); and radiation therapy to the head and neck.

Chemotherapy-Induced Stomatitis

Approximately 40% of chemotherapy patients develop stomatitis,[6] and approximately 50% of these patients develop severe painful lesions requiring treatment modification or parenteral analgesia.[7] In general, patients undergoing BMT have high incidence rates of stomatitis of more than 60%, and incidence rates of ulcerative stomatitis up to 78% have been reported.[8] Stomatitis may be more severe with oral infection, in particular, herpes simplex virus (HSV). There is a four times greater relative risk of septicemia in patients with stomatitis and oral infections as compared with patients without stomatitis due to the damaged mucosal barrier allowing pathogen entry. Stomatitis seen in the PBSCT setting usually begins 5 to 7 days after high-dose chemotherapy administration, with severe stomatitis usually preceding the white blood cell count nadir by 2 to 3 days. McGuire et al.[9] reported on a mixed BMT treatment sample of 47 patients that stomatitis began on average BMT day +3, lasted 9.5 days, and resolved by BMT day +12.69.

Typical oral sequelae of cytotoxic agents include epithelial hyperplasia, collagen and glandular degeneration and epithelial dysplasia, atrophy, and localized or diffuse mucosal ulceration. Nonkeratinized mucosa is most affected, including the labial, buccal, and soft palate mucosa; the floor of the mouth; and the ventral surface of the tongue. Stomatitis presents with asymptomatic erythema and progresses from solitary, white, elevated desquama-

tive patches that are slightly painful to large, contiguous, pseudomembranous, painful lesions. Histopathologically, edema of the rete pegs is noted, as well as vascular changes.

Radiation Therapy–Induced Stomatitis

Stomatitis is virtually universal when radiation therapy includes the oropharyngeal area, with the severity dependent on type of ionizing radiation, volume of irradiated tissue, dose per day, cumulative dose, and duration of radiotherapy. Stomatitis is a dose- and rate-limiting toxicity of radiation therapy for head and neck cancer and of hyperfractionated radiotherapy and chemotherapy that may improve survival time. Radiation interacts directly with DNA and damages the chromosomes and the cellular mitotic apparatus. Atrophic changes in the oral epithelium usually occur at total doses of 1600 to 2200 cGy, administered at a rate of 200 cGy per day.[10] Doses exceeding 6000 cGy are a risk factor for permanent changes in the salivary glands.[10] Pseudomembranes and ulcerations develop as stomatitis severity increases. Radiation-related dental effects do not develop from direct irradiation of the teeth but rather depend primarily on salivary changes that occur when the glands are irradiated. Direct irradiation of teeth may alter the organic or inorganic components, thus making them more susceptible to decalcification or hypocalcification. The addition of total body irradiation to PBSCT increases stomatitis severity through both direct mucosal damage and xerostomia.

Pathogenic Model for Chemotherapy- and Radiation Therapy–Induced Stomatitis

The pathogenesis of cancer treatment–related stomatitis remains incompletely elucidated.

Mucosal epithelial stem cells are located in the deep squamous epithelium superior to the basement membrane and are subjected to trauma by chemical, mechanical, and thermal factors during chewing, swallowing, and digestion. Cell population stability requires frequent replacement of oral basal epithelium cells over a 7- to 14-day cycle, thus placing them at targeted risk for cancer treatment effects. Sonis[7] proposed a hypothetical model for stomatitis development and healing that correlates a variety of clinical and laboratory data. The four interdependent phases of the model are inflammatory/vascular, epithelial, ulcerative, and healing. Each phase results from cytokine-mediated actions and the direct effect of chemotherapy or radiation therapy on the epithelium together with the patient's bone marrow status and oral bacterial flora. The relatively acute inflammatory/vascular phase occurs shortly after chemotherapy or radiation therapy administration.[7] Cytokines released from epithelial tissue include tumor necrosis factor-α, which leads to tissue damage, perhaps interleukin-6 (IL-6) and IL-1, which incites the inflammatory response and increases subepithelial vascularity, which may lead to increased local chemotherapy levels. The epithelial phase demonstrates reduced epithelial renewal and atrophy and typically begins 4 to 5 days after chemotherapy administration. Most efficient contributors to this phase are the cell-cycle S phase–specific agents, including methotrexate, 5-FU, and cytarabine.

The ulcerative/bacterial phase is the most biologically complex stage, beginning approximately 1 week after chemotherapy administration and occurring with maximum neutropenia.[7] This phase is probably not agent class–specific. During this most symptomatic phase, patients often experience acute oropharyngeal pain leading to dysphagia, decreased oral intake, and difficulty speaking. Bacterial colonization of mucosal ulceration occurs, and endotoxins produced by gram-negative organisms induce the release of IL-1 and tumor necrosis factor and production of nitric oxide that may increase local mucosal injury. Radiation therapy and chemotherapy are likely to amplify and prolong this cytokine release, thus exacerbating tissue response. Genetic expression of cytokines and enzymes critical in tissue damage may be modified by transcription factors.[7] Healing of oral lesions in the nonmyelo-suppressed patient occurs within 2 to 3 weeks and is accompanied by renewal of epithelial proliferation and differentiation, white blood cell count recovery, reestablishment of local microbial flora, and decrease in oropharyngeal pain. Sonis[10a] has recently proposed a five-phase biologic model of stomatitis that includes dynamic interactions that promote initiation, message generation, signaling and amplification, ulceration, and healing.

RADIATION THERAPY LONG-TERM EFFECTS

Long-term effects of head and neck radiation therapy include soft tissue fibrosis and obliterative endoarteritis, trismus, and non- or slow-healing mucosal ulcerations. The muscles of mastication and/or the temporal mandibular joint can become fibrotic when irradiated. Fibrosis of the masticatory muscles may occur even 1 year after radiation therapy. Extraction sites in the irradiated area usually heal slowly. Oral candidiasis is a common acute and long-term oral sequela of head and neck radiation therapy. These lesions may be removable (whitish) chronic or hyperplastic (nonremovable), may be chronic erythematous (diffuse patchy erythema), and frequently appear first as angular cheilitis. Osteoradionecrosis (ORN) is a relatively uncommon clinical entity related to hypocellularity, hypovascularity, and ischemia of tissues, with a higher incidence observed after cumulative radiation doses to the bone exceed 65 Gy.[11] This process may be spontaneous, but it is usually related to trauma such as dental extraction and can progress to pathologic fracture, infection of surrounding soft tissues, and severe pain. The risk of ORN does not diminish over time and may even increase with time after therapy. Most studies have reported ORN after tooth extractions that were not timed to allow a 10- to 14-day healing period before radiation therapy started.

CHRONIC GRAFT-VERSUS-HOST DISEASE ORAL MANIFESTATIONS

Oncology patients who have undergone allogeneic PBSCT frequently develop GVHD, an alloimmune condition derived from an immune attack mediated by donor T cells recognizing antigens expressed on normal tissues. This condition occurs in allogeneic PBSCT due to disparities in minor histocompatibility antigens between donor and recipient, inherited independently of HLA genes.[12] Acute GVHD occurs within the first 100 days after allogeneic PBSCT, and cGVHD begins as early as 70 days or as late as 15 months after allogeneic transplant. Mitchell[13] presents a comprehensive overview of treatment strategies for GVHD.

Approximately 80% of patients who have extensive cGVHD have some sort of oral involvement.[14] Oral cGVHD is a major contributing factor to the morbidity seen with allogeneic PBSCT. Although oral lesions are most common in patients with extensive cGVHD, patients may have limited disease involving only the oral cavity. Oral cGVHD presents with tissue atrophy and erythema, lichenoid changes (hyperkeratotic striae, patches, plaques, and papules), and pseudomembranous ulcerations occurring typically on buccal and labial mucosa and the lateral tongue, angular stomatitis, and xerostomia.[14] Weight loss and malnutrition remain a serious problem in the cGVHD population, and the patient's decreased oral intake related to oropharyngeal pain may be a contributing factor. Oral infection in cGVHD patients places them at risk for systemic infections, which are the primary cause of death in this population.[15]

SEQUELAE OF ORAL COMPLICATIONS

OROPHARYNGEAL PAIN

Stomatitis-related oropharyngeal pain is a complex entity. Stomatitis is the principal etiology of most pain experienced during the 3-week post-BMT time period and is often described as the most unforgettable ordeal of BMT. McGuire et al.[9] reported in a sample of autologous and allogeneic BMT patients that pain was detected before clinically observed stomatitis, that pain intensity did not correlate directly with extent of mucosal injury, and that some patients reported limited or no pain after BMT. Overall pain ratings paralleling the trend for oral tissue changes during 2 weeks after BMT have also been reported.

The sensory dimension of stomatitis-related pain includes pain intensity that has been described with general mucosal inflammation and breakdown as ranging from mild discomfort to severe and debilitating pain requiring the use of opioid analgesics.[16] Immunocompromised cancer patients with HSV infections develop larger, more painful lesions than are experienced by noncancer patients. Oral pain is associated strongly with cGVHD and has been described as severe, with patients also reporting burning, irritation, dryness, and loss of taste. Stomatitis-related oral pain seen with chemotherapy is usually of less than 3 months' duration, contrasting with the often long-lasting oral pain accompanying oral cGVHD. The affective dimension of the oral stomatitis pain experience has been demonstrated through the marked effect on the patient's psychological well-being. The behavioral dimension of pain is seen through alterations in communication and decreased oral intake. Oropharyngeal pain related to cancer treatment may lead to alteration in communication, decreased oral intake, and medication usage.

The cognitive dimension of pain refers to how pain influences the individual's thought process, self-perception, stated pain relief, and the personal meaning of the pain.[17] Patients have attached special biologic, emotional, and psychological meaning to pains in the face, head, mouth, and throat.[18] The sociocultural dimension includes demographic characteristics, cultural background, personal family and work roles, and caregiver perspectives.[17] Research has demonstrated conflicting results regarding the association between age and pain perception, and intraethnic differences in pain perception. Gender differences have been reported for pain—for example, female subjects in a pilot study testing capsaicin efficacy for stomatitis-related pain reported a higher level of pain.[19]

XEROSTOMIA

Xerostomia experienced by patients receiving radiation therapy to the head and neck region is a major sequela, with severity dependent on the radiation dosage and location, and volume of exposed salivary glands. Significant xerostomia has not been reported in patients treated with chemotherapy alone. Xerostomia can affect oral comfort, fit of prostheses, speech, and swallowing. Many of the enzymes found in patients with xerostomia contribute to the growth of caries-producing organisms, and the decrease in quantity and quality of saliva can be very harmful to the dentition.

STRATEGIES FOR PREVENTION AND TREATMENT OF ORAL COMPLICATIONS

PRETREATMENT ORAL/DENTAL STABILIZATION

Pretreatment oral/dental stabilization performed by a knowledgeable dental team in collaboration with informed patients is necessary to eliminate sites of oral infection and trauma, provide adequate cleaning, and encourage appropriate oral hygiene.[20] Patients scheduled for chemotherapy and/or head and neck radiation therapy should undergo dental screening at least 2 weeks before starting therapy. This timing allows for proper healing of any extraction sites, recovery of soft tissue manipulations, and restoration of teeth necessary for optimal mucosal health.

A panoramic radiograph, supplemented by intraoral radiographs as needed, is necessary for detection of periodontal disease, periapical infections, cyst, third molar pathology, unerupted or partially erupted teeth, and residual root tips. In general, significant problems that must be corrected include poor oral hygiene, periapical pathology, third molar pathology, periodontal disease, dental caries, defective restorations, orthodontic appliances, ill-fitting prostheses, and other potential sources of infection. It is advisable to perform a thorough root planing, scaling, and prophylaxis before any cancer treatment, with the exception of visible tumor located at the site of anticipated dental manipulation, to reduce bacteria that could lead to local infection and sepsis. Prophylactic use of acyclovir should be considered in patients who are seropositive and at high risk for reactivating HSV infection, such as those who undergo BMT or who have prolonged myelosuppression. A diagnosis of fungal, viral, or bacterial infection of mucosal lesions requires treatment to avoid the risk of systemic infection.

Oral/dental stabilization for radiation therapy is extremely important because of the potential serious sequelae. Comprehensive evaluation includes assessment of the oral mucosa and alveolar process for possible future prosthetic intervention and evaluation of ulcerations, fibromas, irritation, hyperplasia, bony spicules, and tori. Denture fit is important to assess because ill-fitting dentures are a potential source of irritation after radiation therapy exposure and there is a possibility of ulceration to underlying bone. The maximum mouth opening should be recorded at baseline to assess degree of trismus over time. Decisions by the dental team regarding extraction before radiation therapy are based on radiation exposure, type, portal field, fractionization, and total dosage; tumor prognosis and expediency of control of the cancer; and the patient's motivation to comply with the preventive regimen. As a general rule, any teeth with acute and symptomatic periodontal problems should be extracted before head and neck radiation therapy, and careful examination of extraction sites must be performed before radi-

ation therapy begins. Most studies have reported ORN after tooth extractions that did not allow 10 to 14 days of healing before starting radiation therapy. Fabrication of fluoride carriers and radiation protective mouthguards is also completed during this pretreatment time period. Generally, surgical resections of any anatomic oral or pharyngeal structure compromise oral function. Sequelae of many resections, including soft palate, tongue, hard palate, mandible, or combination, can be alleviated by intervention with maxillofacial prosthetics that restore function and cosmesis, with some limitations.

Patient and family education, counseling, and motivation are needed to promote successful preventive strategies. Communication between and among the dentist, dental hygienist, medical oncologist and/or radiation therapist, oncology nurse, and patient is critical to successful maintenance of the oral cavity. Patients often receive cancer treatment in the ambulatory setting and are responsible for their oral care at home, thus necessitating specific written instructions regarding appropriate use of oral care agents and instruments for effective daily plaque removal, use of prescribed fluoride treatments, and reportable oral cavity observations and symptoms. Numerous educational materials exist, including the comprehensive patient education packet "Oral Health, Cancer Care, and You: Fitting the Pieces Together" (http://www.nohic.nidcr.nih.gov/campaign/titlepg.htm), available through the National Oral Health Information Clearinghouse.[21]

ASSESSMENT OF THE ORAL MUCOSA

Frequent oral cavity assessment is necessary to capture clinical signs before, during, and after the treatment time course and requires a consistent approach and the use of an adequately intense white light to allow visualization of all soft and hard tissues and dentition. Although oral/dental care is provided before cancer treatment by dentists, oral assessment and treatment of oral complications is often performed by medical and nursing staff during hospitalization, thus necessitating an appropriate knowledge base regarding clinical presentation of oral complications and potential negative sequelae. Although there is no standard grading system for oral complications of cancer treatment, numerous grading tools exist that are based on two or more clinical parameters, and functional status, such as eating ability. One common tool is the National Cancer Institute Common Terminology Criteria for Adverse Events v3.0, which uses descriptive terminology and a grading scale based on severity for each reportable adverse event.[22] Other frequently used assessment tools include the following.

Oral Assessment Guide

The Oral Assessment Guide[23] was developed as a concise clinical tool to assess oral cavity changes related to stomatogenic cancer therapy using eight assessment categories (voice, swallow, lips, tongue, saliva, mucous membranes, gingiva, and teeth/dentures), each rated on three levels of descriptors: 1 equals normal findings, 2 equals mild alterations, and 3 equals definitely compromised. An overall oral assessment score is the summation of the subscale scores, giving a possible range of 8 to 24. Content-related validity, construct validity, clinical utility, and a high level of trained nurse–nurse interrater reliability (r = .912) have been reported.[23] The Oral Assessment Guide has been used frequently to assess the effect of oral care protocols, compare methods to determine the nature and prevalence of stomatitis mucositis, and to describe the incidence and severity of stomatitis in BMT patients.

Oral Mucositis Rating Scale

The Oral Mucositis Rating Scale was developed as an index to assess acute stomatitis after BMT and as "a research tool for the comprehensive measurement of a broad range of oral tissue changes associated with cancer therapy."[16] The Oral Mucositis Rating Scale was used to assess 60 patients who were 180 to 500 days post allogeneic PBSCT to determine the relationship of oral abnormalities to cGVHD.[24] Oral manifestations and sequelae most strongly associated with cGVHD included atrophy and erythema, lichenoid lesions of the buccal and labial mucosa, and oral pain.

The item pool consists of 91 items for 13 areas of the mouth that are assessed for several types of changes in seven anatomic areas: lips, labial and buccal mucosa, tongue, floor of mouth, palate, and attached gingiva. Each site is further divided into upper and lower (lips and labial mucosa), right and left (buccal mucosa), dorsal, ventral, and lateral (tongue), and hard and soft (palate). Descriptive categories include atrophy, pseudomembrane, erythema, hyperkeratosis, lichenoid, ulceration, and edema. Erythema, atrophy, hyperkeratosis, lichenoid, and edema are rated on scales of 0 to 3 (0 equals normal/no change, 1 equals mild change, 2 equals moderate change, and 3 equals severe change). Ulceration and pseudomembrane are rated on estimated surface area involved (0 equals none, 1 equals greater than 0 and 1 cm^2 or less, 2 equals greater than 1 cm^2 and 2 cm^2 or less, and 3 equals greater than 2 cm^2). The total possible score is the sum of all item scores, with a possible range of 0 to 273. The Oral Mucositis Rating Scale has demonstrated clinical and research utility.[24]

Oral Mucositis Index

The Oral Mucositis Index was developed from the Oral Mucositis Rating Scale. A downsized 20-item version of the Oral Mucositis Index (OMI-20) has been developed and validated through consensus by an expert panel of BMT oral complications specialists in the United States.[25] The OMI-20 consists of nine items measuring erythema, nine measuring ulceration, one measuring atrophy, and one measuring edema, all scored from 0 equals none to 3 equals severe, summed for a possible range of 0 to 60. The two sets of nine items measuring erythema and ulceration can be summed to produce subscale scores ranging from 0 to 27. The OMI-20 demonstrated internal consistency and test-retest and interrater reliability when evaluated in a sample of 133 adult PBSCT/BMT patients.[25]

Oral Mucositis Assessment Scale

The Oral Mucositis Assessment Scale was developed by a team of oral medicine specialists, dentists, dental hygienists, oncologists, and oncology nurses from the United States, Canada, and Europe as a scoring system for evaluating the anatomic extent and severity of stomatitis in research studies.[26,27] Oral cavity regions assessed are lip (upper and lower), cheek (right and left), right and lateral tongue, left ventral and lateral tongue, floor of mouth, soft palate/fauces, and hard palate.[26] Erythema is rated on a scale 0 to 2 (0 equals none, 1 equals not severe, and 2 equals severe), and ulceration and pseudomembrane are rated on scores based on estimated surface area involved (0 equals no lesion, 1 equals less than 1 cm^2, 2 equals 1 cm^2 to 3 cm^2, and 3 equals more than 3 cm^2), summed for a possible score range of 0 to 162.[26,27] Validity and reliability have been demonstrated for the Oral Mucositis Assessment Scale through numerous clinical research studies.[27]

World Health Organization Index

The World Health Organization Index, which gives a simple, overall rating of stomatitis, has often been used as a general comparison index to other assessment scales.[1,28] The World Health Organization Index is scaled as follows: grade 0 equals no change; grade 1 equals soreness, erythema; grade 2 equals erythema, ulcers, can eat solids; grade 3 equals ulcers, requires liquid diet only; and grade 4 equals alimentation not possible. Limitations of this tool include the lack of reliability and validity data and the inability to capture the variety of oral changes that occur with cancer treatment.[1]

ASSESSMENT OF STOMATITIS-RELATED ORAL PAIN

Oral pain related to cancer treatment is complex and often challenging to manage. Symptom management in this population is critical to avoid suffering related to symptoms such as oropharyngeal pain and psychological distress.[15] Constant communication between and among patient, physician, nurse, and caregiver regarding the oral pain experience is needed to promote effective pain management. Many valid and reliable pain intensity assessment tools exist. However, to capture the multidimensional experience of oral pain, it is necessary to use a more comprehensive pain assessment tool.

TREATMENT STRATEGIES

The optimal treatment strategies for oral complications and related sequelae have not been established. Recommended treatment strategies for stomatitis and related oropharyngeal pain are numerous but have frequently not been tested in randomized controlled clinical trials. Zlotolow and Berger[29] have presented a comprehensive review of clinical research studies focusing on treatment strategies for oral complications of cancer strategies. Conflicting study results may be related to inclusion of heterogeneous diagnosis and treatment samples, use of oral assessment tools that are unable to capture wide variations in oral cavity changes, and inappropriate timing and dose of interventions. In general, the only standard forms of care are pretreatment oral/dental stabilization, saline mouthwashes, and pain management.[30] The outcome of any oral care practice standard should be a clean, trauma-free, moist oral cavity that is maintained in a physiologic environment conducive to healing. Meticulous oral hygiene must be maintained throughout the cancer treatment process.

Responding to this need for standard treatment, a subcommittee of the Mucositis Study Section of the Multinational Association of Supportive Care in Cancer and the International Society for Oral Oncology formulated the "Clinical Practice Guidelines for the Prevention and Treatment of Cancer Therapy-

Induced Oral and Gastrointestinal Mucositis".[30a] These guidelines were derived from a comprehensive review of more than 8000 English-language publications (1966 to 2001) regarding alimentary tract mucositis using a scoring criteria that rated the studies for level of evidence and quality of research design.[31]

Direct Cytoprotectants

SUCRALFATE. Sucralfate, an aluminum salt of a sulfated disaccharide that has been used successfully to treat gastrointestinal ulceration, has been tested as a mouthwash for the prevention and treatment of stomatitis. Sucralfate's mechanism of action may be through formation of an ionic bond to proteins in an ulcer site, thereby creating a protective barrier. In addition, evidence suggests an increase in the local production of prostaglandin E_2 that leads to an increase in mucosal blood flow, mucus production, mitotic activity, and surface migration of cells.

Study results with sucralfate are conflicting and inconclusive. Solomon[32] reported a 55% objective response rate that was defined as a decrease in one grade on the Cancer and Leukemia Group B oral toxicity rating scale in 19 patients receiving chemotherapy. Pfeiffer et al.[33] found a significant reduction in edema, erythema, erosion, and ulceration in 23 of 40 evaluable patients receiving cisplatin and continuous infusion 5-FU with or without bleomycin. Patient preference favored sucralfate, although this preference was not statistically significant. Ten patients did not complete the study because swishing the sucralfate or placebo aggravated chemotherapy-induced nausea. Conversely, results from a similarly designed study, in which patients receiving remission-induction chemotherapy for acute nonlymphocytic leukemia were treated with sucralfate for stomatitis, did not support sucralfate efficacy for stomatitis.[34] This study also concluded that chronic administration of the sucralfate suspension had no effect on the incidence of gastrointestinal bleeding and ulceration, although some patients reported pain relief.[34] A North Central Cancer Treatment Group (NCCTG) phase III study of sucralfate suspension versus placebo revealed that of the 50 patients with stomatitis, the sucralfate suspension provided no beneficial reduction in the duration or severity of 5-FU–induced stomatitis and the sucralfate group had considerable additional gastrointestinal toxicity.[35] The efficacy of a sucralfate mouthwash for prevention and treatment of 5-FU–induced stomatitis was evaluated through a randomized controlled clinical trial with 81 patients with colorectal cancer, who received either sucralfate suspension or placebo four times daily during their first cycle of chemotherapy with 5-FU and leucovorin.[36] This sucralfate mouthwash did not prevent or alleviate stomatitis.

Sucralfate has also been tested in patients receiving head and neck radiation therapy. One study compared 21 patients who received standard oral care with 24 patients who received sucralfate suspension four times daily.[37] Results revealed a significant difference in mucosal edema, pain, dysphagia, and weight loss in the sucralfate group. In contrast, a double-blind placebo-controlled study with sucralfate in 33 patients who received radiation therapy to the head and neck reported no statistically significant differences in stomatitis.[38] The sucralfate group did report less oral pain and required a later start of topical and systemic analgesics throughout radiation.[38] Dodd et al.[39] evaluated the efficacy of micronized

sucralfate mouth wash versus a salt and soda mouthwash in 30 radiation therapy patients in a pilot randomized controlled clinical trial. All patients also performed a systematic oral hygiene program, the PRO-SELF Mouth Aware program. No significant difference in efficacy between the two groups was found.

GELCLAIR. Gelclair (OSI Pharmaceuticals, Melville, NY) is a concentrated, bioadherent gel indicated for the management of stomatitis-related oral pain that has recently received the 510(k) Medical Device approval by the U.S. Food and Drug Administration. Gelclair adheres to the oral surface to create a protective barrier to protect irritated tissue and exposed or sensitized nociceptors. Two open-label, prospective trials evaluated the safety and efficacy of Gelclair in patients with oral inflammatory or ulcerative lesions. Innocenti et al.[40] tested Gelclair in patients with stomatitis, severe diffuse oral aphthous lesions, and post–oral surgery pain. Results showed that oral pain was decreased 92% from baseline 5 to 7 hours after Gelclair administration. More than 50% of patients reported that the maximum effect of Gelclair lasted longer than 3 hours, and 87% of patients reported overall improvements from baseline for pain on swallowing food, liquids, and saliva after 1 week of treatment.[40] DeCordi et al.[41] administered Gelclair to patients with stomatitis three times daily before meals as a 2- to 3-minute swish and spit for 3 to 10 days. Significant improvements were reported from baseline in pain, stomatitis severity, and function.[41] There were no adverse effects reported during either trial, and patients reported that the taste, smell, texture, and ease of use of Gelclair was acceptable. Several Gelclair clinical studies are under way in the United Kingdom.

PROSTAGLANDINS, ANTIPROSTAGLANDINS, AND NONSTEROIDAL AGENTS. Prostaglandins are a family of naturally occurring eicosanoids, some of which have known cytoprotective activity. In a nonblind study, ten patients who were receiving 5-FU and mitomycin with concomitant radiation therapy for oral carcinomas were treated by Porteder et al.[42] with topical dinoprostone four times daily during treatment. The control group consisted of 14 patients who were receiving identical treatment. Eight of the ten patients who received dinoprostone were evaluable, and none developed severe stomatitis as compared with six episodes in the control arm. A second pilot study conducted with 15 patients who received radiation therapy to the head and neck reported that an inflammatory reaction in the vicinity of the tumor was detected in only five patients treated with topically applied prostaglandin E_2, and no patients developed any bullous or desquamating inflammatory lesions.[43]

Benzydamine, a nonsteroidal agent with analgesic, anesthetic, antiinflammatory, and antimicrobial properties, has been found to be efficacious for both stomatitis and radiation therapy–induced stomatitis. Epstein and Stevenson-Moore[44] reported in a double-blind, placebo-controlled trial that benzydamine hydrochloride mouth rinse produced statistically significant relief of pain from radiation-induced stomatitis and showed not only a trend toward reduction in pain but also a statistically significant reduction in the total area of ulceration.

CORTICOSTEROIDS. Two pilot studies tested the efficacy of corticosteroids for radiation therapy patients. Abdelaal et al.[45] tested a betamethasone and water mouthwash in five patients receiving radiation therapy and reported that the mucosa remained virtually ulcer-free and the patients were pain free. The proposed mechanism of action of the steroid mouthwash is inhibition of leukotriene and prostaglandin production. Another pilot study compared 21 patients receiving radiotherapy who used either an oral rinse consisting of hydrocortisone, nystatin, tetracycline, and diphenhydramine or a placebo rinse.[46] Results from the evaluable 12 patients at the end of the radiation therapy treatment showed a statistically significant difference in stomatitis with a trend toward pain reduction. No patients in the treatment group needed to interrupt radiation therapy as compared with patients in the control group, who did need to interrupt treatment.[46]

VITAMINS AND OTHER ANTIOXIDANTS. Vitamin E has been tested in chemotherapy-induced stomatitis because it can stabilize cellular membranes and may improve herpetic gingivitis, possibly through antioxidant activity. The efficacy of vitamin E was demonstrated by Wadleigh et al.[47] in 18 chemotherapy patients who were randomized to receive topical vitamin E or placebo. Statistically significant results showed that in the vitamin E group, six of nine patients had complete stomatitis resolution within 4 days of initiating therapy, whereas in the placebo group only one of nine had resolution of the lesions during the 5-day study period.[47]

Other antioxidants that have been tested include vitamin C and glutathione. Azelastine hydrochloride has been used in many allergic diseases and has been shown to be effective in the treatment of aphthous ulcers in Behçet's disease. Osaki et al.[48] reported on a study with 63 patients with head and neck tumors who received chemoradiation. Twenty-six patients received regimen 1 (vitamins C and E and glutathione), and 37 patients received regimen 2 (regimen 1 plus azelastine). Results showed that in the azelastine arm, 21 patients remained at grade 1 or 2 stomatitis, 6 patients had grade 3 stomatitis, and 10 patients had grade 4 stomatitis. In the control group, grade 3 or 4 stomatitis was observed in 6 and 15 patients, respectively, with 2 patients having grade 1 stomatitis and 2 patients having grade 2 stomatitis. Azelastine suppressed neutrophil respiratory burst both *in vivo* and *in vitro* and suppressed cytokine release from lymphocytes. The study concluded that azelastine, which suppresses reactive oxygen production and stabilizes cell membranes, may be useful to prevent chemoradiation-induced stomatitis.[48]

SILVER NITRATE. Silver nitrate, a caustic agent, has been tested for radiation therapy–induced stomatitis. Silver nitrate stimulates cell division when applied to normal mucosa, thus having potential as a preventive agent for chemotherapy-induced stomatitis. Maciejewski et al.[49] reported on 16 patients who received radiotherapy to bilateral opposing fields. Silver nitrate 2% was applied to the left side of the oral mucosa three times daily for 5 days before and during the first 2 days of radiation therapy. The right side of the oral mucosa served as the control. Patients had significantly less severe stomatitis with shorter duration in the silver nitrate group.[49] A second trial failed to confirm these results.[50] Silver nitrate needs evaluation with chemotherapy-induced stomatitis.

CRYOTHERAPY. Cryotherapy, in the form of ice chips and flavored ice pops, has been used to prevent stomatitis. The NCCTG and the Mayo Clinic reported from a controlled, randomized trial of oral cryotherapy for the prevention of 5-FU–induced stomatitis that cryotherapy reduces the severity of stomatitis.[51] A subsequent study undertaken with 178 evaluable patients who were randomized to receive 30 minutes versus 60 minutes of cryotherapy reported that both groups had similar degrees of stomatitis.[52] The conclusion was to continue to recommend the use of 30 minutes of oral cryotherapy for patients receiving bolus intensive courses of 5-FU–based chemotherapy. An additional study reported by the NCCTG and the Mayo Clinic confirmed that oral cryotherapy can reduce 5-FU–induced stomatitis.[53] Cryotherapy to induce vasoconstriction should be considered for patients who receiving 5-FU or melphalan when the agents are given over short infusion times.

LASER. The efficacy of laser treatment for oral lesion and pain control was initially studied in an animal model. A preliminary study evaluated the efficacy of laser treatment for stomatitis in 36 patients treated with diverse cancers and chemotherapy protocols.[54] Sixteen patients were treated with laser, and 20 patients served as the controls. Results revealed reduced duration of mucosal lesions, from a mean of 19.3 days in the control arm to 8.1 days in the treatment arm.[54] The efficacy of low-energy helium-neon laser was studied in 30 patients through a randomized controlled clinical trial.[55] Results demonstrated that low-energy laser reduced the severity and duration of oral mucositis in this population.[55] Further research regarding efficacy of lasers for stomatitis is needed using randomized controlled clinical trials.

MISCELLANEOUS AGENTS. A descriptive study involving 98 patients with diverse malignancies who received either chemotherapy or radiation therapy reported that Kamillosan liquid taken before and after the development of stomatitis helped to prevent and decrease the duration of stomatitis.[56] In a placebo-controlled trial conducted by the NCCTG, patients were randomized to receive chamomile or placebo plus an established oral cryotherapy regimen.[57] This study revealed that chamomile mouthwash did not reduce stomatitis associated with 5-FU.[57] Although other topical agents are used clinically for stomatitis, including kaolin and pectin (Kaopectate), diphenhydramine (Benadryl), saline, sodium bicarbonate, and gentian violet, they need to be tested in the randomized controlled clinical trial setting.

A phase III study of topical AES-14, a novel drug system designed to concentrate delivery of L-glutamine to oral mucosa for ulceration, was conducted with 121 patients at risk for stomatitis.[58] Patients were randomized to AES-14 or placebo and were treated from day 1 of chemotherapy until 2 weeks after the last chemotherapy dose or stomatitis resolution. Data suggested a potential 20% reduction of moderate to severe stomatitis with AES-14, as well as a 10% increase in grade 0 stomatitis. Currently, a more efficient replacement study is starting.

Indirect Cytoprotectants

HEMATOPOIETIC GROWTH FACTORS.
Hematologic growth factors are standard treatment for patients receiving high-dose chemotherapy, with well-established ability to decrease the duration of chemotherapy-induced neutropenia.

Effects of granulocyte-macrophage colony-stimulating factor (GM-CSF), granulocyte CSF (G-CSF), epidermal growth factor (EGF), and transforming growth factor (TGF), and cytokines such as IL-11 in the development and severity of stomatitis have been evaluated using the animal cheek pouch model in Syrian Golden hamsters. Results have demonstrated increased severity of mucosal damage in animals receiving 5-FU and EGF[59] and decreased incidence, severity, and duration of stomatitis; decreased weight loss; and increased survival in animals who received TGF-β after chemotherapy.[60] *In vitro* studies have shown that EGF is present in saliva and has the ability to affect growth, cell differentiation, cell migration, and repair mechanisms.[61] The development of increased oral toxicity or repair of the mucosa may depend on the timing of EGF administration in relation to the chemotherapy.[62] Sonis et al.[63] administered EGF or placebo to hamsters using four different treatment schedules and reported that although EGF delayed the stomatitis onset, no beneficial effects regarding stomatitis duration or severity were seen.

G-CSF has been tested as a treatment for stomatitis in numerous studies. Gabrilove et al.[64] reported on 27 patients receiving methotrexate, vinblastine, doxorubicin, and cisplatin for bladder carcinoma and escalating doses of G-CSF. The patients received the G-CSF only on their first of two cycles of chemotherapy. Although significantly less stomatitis was seen during the first cycle with the G-CSF, these results may be biased because of possible cumulative chemotherapeutic toxicity with resultant increase in stomatitis severity. Bronchud et al.[65] reported that G-CSF did not prevent severe stomatitis in a study of 17 patients with breast or ovarian carcinoma treated with escalating doses of doxorubicin with G-CSF support. In a third study, 55 patients receiving chemotherapy for non-Hodgkin's lymphoma received G-CSF, whereas 39 received chemotherapy without G-CSF. In patients who did not receive G-CSF, the main cause of treatment delay was neutropenia, whereas in those patients who did receive G-CSF, the main cause of treatment delay was stomatitis.[66]

GM-CSF has demonstrated conflicting results in patients receiving diverse treatment modalities. Saarilahti et al.[67] reported from a randomized controlled clinical trial comparing GM-CSF mouthwashes with sucralfate mouthwashes in 40 postoperative radiation therapy patients that stomatitis tended to be less severe in the GM-CSF group. In contrast to these findings, prophylaxis with GM-CSF mouthwash in a randomized trial of 90 patients undergoing high-dose chemotherapy and autologous PBSCT did not reduce frequency and duration of severe stomatitis.[68] The use of colony-stimulating factors in the treatment of stomatitis remains investigational.

TGF-β3 is an inhibitor of epithelial cell growth. In a study using Syrian hamsters conducted by Sonis et al.,[69] the topical application of TGF-β3 resulted in a decrease in chemotherapy-related stomatitis severity and duration. Spijkervet and Sonis[70] reported in an animal study with Syrian hamsters that topical application of TGF-β3 significantly reduced the severity and duration of ulcerative mucositis induced by 5-FU. Foncuberta et al.[71] reported from two phase II randomized controlled clinical trials evaluating TGF-β3 mouthwash, 10 mL (25 µg/mL), or placebo administered four times daily (or twice daily) to patients with lymphomas or solid tumors that TGF-β3 was not effective in the prevention or alleviation of chemotherapy-related stomatitis. IL-1 and IL-11 have demonstrated a cytoprotective effect.[72,73]

Keratinocyte growth factor (KGF) is a member of the fibroblast growth factor family and binds specifically to the KGF receptor.[74] KGF maintains barrier function of epithelial tissues and has potent cytoprotective and regenerative activities.[75] KGF reduced the damaging effects of radiotherapy delivered to the oral cavity in mouse models.[76,77] Meropol et al.[78] reported in a sample of 81 metastatic colon cancer patients that KGF was generally well tolerated when given at doses up to 40 µg/kg/d intravenously (IV) for 3 days before a 5-day course of fluorouracil and leucovorin. Spielberger et al.[79] reported from a clinical trial of 212 patients receiving either 60 µg/kg KGF or placebo IV for 3 days before and after a PBSCT conditioning regimen that the KGF group had a significant decrease in the mean duration of severe stomatitis and the incidence of severe stomatitis. However, Human Genome Sciences recently stopped its double-blind, crossover, dose-escalation, phase II clinical trial testing repifermin, a truncated form of recombinant human KGF-2.[80] This study conducted with 92 patients with multiple myeloma receiving PBSCT showed that the patients treated with the highest dose of repifermin, 75 µg/kg IV, had grade 2 to 4 stomatitis not significantly different from placebo treatment.[80] There is a theoretical concern regarding the potential impact of KGF on tumorigenesis. The literature is contradictory regarding this KGF effect, and therefore careful monitoring for this potential outcome should be incorporated into clinical trials testing KGF.[75]

ANTIMICROBIALS. Antimicrobial approaches have included systemic antimicrobials such as antibiotics, antivirals (acyclovir, valacyclovir, ganciclovir), and the antifungal agent, fluconazole. Donnelly et al.[81] evaluated the weight of evidence regarding the role of infection in the pathophysiology of stomatitis through a review of 31 prospective randomized trials. The authors concluded that there was no clear pattern of patient type, cancer treatment, or type of antimicrobial agent used and a lack of consistent stomatitis assessment.

Conflicting reports have been published on the use of chlorhexidine mouthwash for both alleviating stomatitis and reducing oral colonization by gram-positive, gram-negative, and *Candida* species in patients receiving radiotherapy, chemotherapy, or BMT. The majority of studies since that time have not demonstrated a reduction in stomatitis in patients receiving intensive chemotherapy and using chlorhexidine mouthwash.[82] Dodd et al.[83] tested effectiveness of the PRO-SELF Mouth Aware program in conjunction with randomization to one of two mouthwashes (0.12% chlorhexidine or sterile water) in preventing chemotherapy-related stomatitis in 222 patients. Chlorhexidine was found to be no more effective than water with regard to stomatitis incidence, days to onset, and severity, and the PRO-SELF Mouth Aware program appeared to reduce the incidence of stomatitis.[83] However, Weisdorf et al.[84] and Epstein et al.,[85] in studies evaluating effectiveness of chlorhexidine mouth rinse and chlorhexidine and nystatin mouth rinses, respectively, did show a reduction in oral colonization by *Candida* species and oral candidiasis.

Acyclovir prophylaxis is accepted treatment for HSV- and cytomegalovirus-seropositive BMT patients. A randomized controlled clinical trial comparing fluconazole with placebo conducted in BMT patients demonstrated that fluconazole prevented systemic fungal infections (7% fluconazole vs. 18% placebo) and significantly reduced the incidence of mucosal infection and oropharyngeal colonization by *Candida albicans*.[86]

Sutherland and Browman[87] reported from a review of 59 studies assessing prophylaxis of radiation therapy–induced stomatitis in head and neck cancer patients that interventions chosen on a sound biologic basis to prevent severe stomatitis are effective and that when stomatitis is assessed by clinicians, narrow-spectrum antibiotic lozenges appear to be beneficial. A study by Spijkervet et al.[88] evaluated the efficacy of lozenges containing polymyxin E, 2 mg; tobramycin, 1.8 mg; and amphotericin B, 10 mg (PTA), taken four times daily on the oropharyngeal flora for stomatitis. These researchers compared 15 radiation therapy patients using PTA and two other groups of 15 patients each, one of which was using 0.1% chlorhexidine and the other of which was using placebo. The selectively decontaminated group showed significantly reduced severity and extent of stomatitis compared with the chlorhexidine and placebo groups. In contrast, Stokman and colleagues[89] analyzed the effects of selective oral flora elimination on radiation-related stomatitis in a randomized controlled clinical trial with 65 patients with head and neck tumors who were randomized to either a lozenge of polymyxin E, 1 g; tobramycin, 1.8 mg; and amphotericin B, 13 mg or placebo. The authors concluded that selective oral flora elimination in head and neck–radiated patients did not prevent the development of severe stomatitis.

PHARMACOLOGIC MODULATION. Allopurinol mouthwash has been evaluated for the prevention and treatment of stomatitis related to 5-FU because allopurinol inhibits the enzyme orotidylate decarboxylase and formation of the metabolites of fluorodeoxyuridine monophosphate and fluorouridine.[90] A pilot study by Clark and Selvin[91] revealed that allopurinol mouthwash substantially decreased the incidence and severity of stomatitis in six patients who received bolus 5-FU. Another pilot study, involving 16 patients receiving 5-day 5-FU infusions and using allopurinol mouthwashes four to six times daily, also found that the allopurinol alleviated stomatitis in all patients.[92] Positive results of these pilot studies have led to allopurinol becoming routine practice in many institutions. However, no protective effect of allopurinol against 5-FU–induced stomatitis was seen in a randomized double-blind clinical trial conducted by the NCCTG and the Mayo Clinic.[93] The study sample consisted of 75 patients who were assigned to either allopurinol mouthwash or placebo during their first 5-day course of 5-FU with or without leucovorin.[93]

Decreased stomatitis is observed when reduced folates are given systemically after methotrexate administration. Animal studies of glutamine administration have shown a reduction in both morbidity and mortality of animals that had received a variety of chemotherapeutic agents, including methotrexate. The glutamine both preserved the morphologic structure of the gastrointestinal tract and reduced the incidence of bacteremia.[94] A randomized crossover trial tested the efficacy of oral glutamine in 24 cancer patients receiving chemotherapy who were randomized to glutamine or placebo suspension to swish and swallow on days of chemotherapy administration and at least 14 additional days.[95] Low-dose oral glutamine supplementation during and after chemotherapy significantly reduced both duration and severity of chemotherapy-related stomatitis.

Uridine has been found to protect host tissues selectively from 5-FU's toxic effects without loss of antitumor effect. A study was conducted involving 29 patients with advanced malignancies who received N-phosphonoacetyl-disodium-*l*-aspartic acid and methotrexate, each at 250 mg/m², followed 24 hours later by increasing doses of 5-FU (600 to 750 mg/m²), with a leucovorin rescue and uridine rescue for a 72-hour infusion.[96] The uridine allowed dose escalation of 5-FU to 750 mg/m², with a decrease in all toxicities of the 5-FU except stomatitis, which remained as the only significant chemotherapy-induced toxic effect.[96] A pilot study using propantheline, an anticholinergic agent that causes xerostomia, was performed to test whether stomatitis incidence from etoposide could be reduced.[97] It was hypothesized that the mucosal toxicity might be related to salivary excretion of etoposide after systemic administration. Propantheline or placebo was given to 12 patients, and there was a decrease in stomatitis incidence and severity seen in the propantheline group.[97]

Oral Chronic Graft-Versus-Host Disease

Almost all patients with extensive cGVHD require systemic immunosuppressive therapy, and there is a critical need for adjuvant therapies that are both efficacious and avoid the long-term consequences of the corticosteroid therapies. Advances in the treatment of cGVHD have been modest, and there is currently no standard therapy for cGVHD that fails to respond to initial therapy or recurs. Patients with symptomatic disease that is limited to the oral cavity benefit from topical steroids such as dexamethasone (Decadron elixir, 0.5 mg/5 mL), which has been shown to be effective therapy when used as a mouth rinse (10 mL) for 2 to 3 minutes at least four times per day.[15] Topical steroids such as fluocinonide (Lidex) have also been tried, and if local steroids alone do not control oral disease, cyclosporine swishes may be tried.[15] Systemic immunosuppressive therapy is often needed even for isolated stomatitis, and intraoral psoralen plus ultraviolet A irradiation may be needed depending on the patient's condition.[15] A topical, high-potency steroid, clobetasol (Temovate) 0.05%, may be used to decrease inflammation and oral pain three times a day for 2 to 3 weeks depending on the severity of the ulcerative oral cGVHD. However, these treatments need evaluation in a randomized controlled clinical trial setting.

LONG-TERM EFFECTS OF RADIATION THERAPY

Prevention of fibrosis of the muscles of mastication and/or the temporal mandibular joint (if in the field of radiation therapy) can be prevented or attenuated with the use of early exercises with trismus appliances after radiation therapy. Exercising using tongue depressors taped together 10 to 15 times a day for 10-minute sets can be effective in reducing trismus. Fibrosis of the masticatory muscles may occur even 1 year after radiation; thus, jaw-opening exercises should be started after stomatitis resolves and continued for more than 1 year after completion of radiation therapy.

Some authors maintain that traditional treatment of ORN with antibiotics and surgical débridement and curettage has been unsuccessful. Recent literature supports hyperbaric oxygen to boost tissue oxygenation in damaged irradiated wounds for anticipated difficult extractions and for patients with radiographic interpretation of trabecular bone pattern avascularity and telangiectasia covering mucous membranes or gingiva.[98] Most reported studies demonstrate a low incidence of ORN if

TABLE 54.2-2. Formulary of Common Treatments for Oral Complications

Complication	Directions
PREVENTION OF STOMATITIS	
Chlorhexidine gluconate 0.12% oral rinse	Rinse mouth twice daily for 30 s. Do not swallow.
NAHCO$_3$ powder, 3 tablespoons or 11.6 g	Combine all ingredients. Rinse mouth two to four times daily. Do not swallow.
NaCl powder, 3 tablespoons or 11.6 g	—
Distilled water, 1 gallon	—
Povidone iodine 0.5% oral rinse	Rinse mouth two to four times daily. Do not swallow.
TREATMENT OF STOMATITIS-RELATED PAIN	
Carafate suspension, 1 g	Rinse mouth with suspension four times daily. Do not swallow.
Diphenhydramine (Benadryl), 12.5 mg/5 mL; kaolin and pectin (Kaopectate)	Combine equal amounts of each. Rinse mouth with 10–15 mL four to six times daily. Do not swallow.
Diphenhydramine (Benadryl), 12.5 mg/5 mL: 30 mL; Maalox, 30 mL; nystatin, 100,000 U/mL: 30 mL	Combine all ingredients. Rinse mouth with 15 mL four to six times per day. Do not swallow.
Diphenhydramine (Benadryl), 12.5 mg/5 mL: 30 mL; viscous lidocaine (Xylocaine) 2%, 30 mL; Maalox, 30 mL	Combine all ingredients. Rinse mouth with 15 mL four to six times per day. Do not swallow.
Diphenhydramine (Benadryl), 12.5 mg/5 mL: 30 mL; tetracycline, 125 mg/5 mL suspension 60 mL; nystatin oral suspension, 100,000 U/mL 45 mL; viscous lidocaine (Xylocaine) 2%, 30 mL; hydrocortisone suspension, 10 mg/5 mL: 30 mL; sterile water for irrigation, 45 mL	Combine all ingredients. Rinse mouth with 15 mL four to six times per day. Do not swallow.
Gelclair	Follow manufacturer's directions for mixing contents of single-dose Gelclair packet with 40 mL or 3 tablespoons of water. Stir mixture and use at once as a mouth rinse for at least 1 minute, gargle, and spit out. Use at least t.i.d.
Opioids	May use oral or parenteral opioids, such as patient-controlled analgesia. If oral analgesics are selected, use tablets. Do not use elixir, which has alcohol and exacerbates stomatitis.
Viscous lidocaine (Xylocaine) 2% solution	Rinse mouth with 10–15 mL q2–3h. Do not swallow.
Dyclonine hydrochloride 0.5% or 1.0% solution	Rinse mouth with 10–15 mL q2–3h. Do not swallow.
XEROSTOMIA	
Xerolube, salivary substitute	Rinse mouth four to six times per day.
Salivart synthetic saliva spray	Spray mouth four to six times per day.
Biotene chewing gum	Use as needed.
Pilocarpine	5 mg PO t.i.d.
Amifostine (Ethyol)	200 mg/m^2 daily, as a 3-minute IV infusion 15–30 min before radiotherapy. Hydrate adequately, monitor blood pressure, and administer antiemetics.

NaCl, sodium chloride; NAHCO$_3$, sodium bicarbonate.
Many of the medications listed have been used alone or in combination to treat stomatitis.

preradiation dental consult and appropriate treatment (extractions) are rendered.[99] Follow-up and recall of the head and neck patient for dental preventive maintenance and treatment are essential to prevent sequelae in the oral cavity.

SYMPTOM MANAGEMENT

Oropharyngeal Pain

ANESTHETIC COCKTAILS. Several anesthetic cocktails, composed of agents such as viscous lidocaine (Xylocaine) or dyclonine hydrochloride, have been used with some success. Anesthetic agents provide only temporary relief of pain and alter taste perception, which may decrease oral intake. Other analgesics and mucosal-coating agents used for pain management include kaolin and pectin, diphenhydramine, hydrocortisone (Orabase), and Oratect Gel (benzocaine). In a prospective double-blind study involving 18 patients, viscous lidocaine with cocaine 1%, dyclonine hydrochloride 1%, kaolin and pectin solution, diphenhydramine, and saline solution were compared with a placebo.[100] The dyclonine hydrochloride 1% provided the most pain relief, and the dyclonine hydrochloride with viscous lidocaine and cocaine 1% provided the longest pain relief[100] (Table 54.2-2).

Hospital-based pharmacies commonly formulate and dispense topical mixtures containing an analgesic, an antiinflammatory agent, and a coating agent used as an oral comfort measure for oncology patients undergoing treatment. One such topical formulation recommended for use at a large clinical research center contains lidocaine viscous 2% (40 mL); diphenhydramine, 12.5 mg/5 mL (40 mL); and Maalox, 10 mg (40 mL) and is prescribed for use every 3 to 4 hours as needed. Testing these various topical formulations through randomized controlled clinical trials would promote evidence-based practice regarding these treatment recommendations.

OPIOIDS. Stomatitis-related oropharyngeal pain may be severe enough to interfere with hydration and nutritional intake and affect quality of life. Management of this severe oropharyngeal pain may be achieved by the use of opioids, often at high doses, administered by patient-controlled analgesia pumps, as well the oral, transmucosal, and parenteral routes. A recent article also reported on the successful use of topical opioids (morphine 0.08% gel, prepared with taste supplements) in treating stomatitis in a patient who was terminally ill.[101] Oral transmucosal fentanyl citrate (Actiq) was compared with morphine sulfate immediate release for treatment of breakthrough cancer pain in

134 adult ambulatory cancer patients through a randomized controlled clinical trial.[102] Study results showed that oral transmucosal fentanyl was more effective than morphine sulfate immediate release in treating breakthrough pain. Topical morphine was evaluated for stomatitis pain in 26 patients after chemoradiation for head and neck cancer.[103] Patients were randomized to morphine mouthwash (15 mL 2% morphine solution) or magic mouthwash (equal parts of lidocaine, diphenhydramine, and magnesium aluminum hydroxide). Patients in the morphine group had both significantly shorter duration and lower intensity of oral pain than the magic mouthwash group. The shift from inpatient to ambulatory care for many oncology treatments has necessitated increased use of both patient self-care activities and involvement of patient caregivers for pain management. Swisher et al.[104] described a stomatitis pain management algorithm to promote symptom management as the BMT patient transitions from inpatient to ambulatory care. A key component of this successful program was the patient self-report of oral pain to the multidisciplinary team.

CAPSAICIN. Capsaicin, the active ingredient in chili peppers, has been used for diverse pain syndromes and has potential efficacy for cancer treatment–related stomatitis.[19] Several studies support the efficacy of locally applied capsaicin in a cream vehicle for neuropathic pain syndromes such as postherpetic neuralgia and diabetic neuropathy, postmastectomy pain, stump pain, trigeminal neuralgia, reflex sympathetic dystrophy, and Guillain-Barré syndrome. Topical capsaicin has also been shown to decrease the pain associated with rheumatoid and osteoarthritis, and intranasal capsaicin spray has been shown to reduce the pain associated with cluster headaches. Topical capsaicin improves the rate of reepithelialization of wound healing in minipigs; thus, it may prove to be efficacious in wound healing in humans. Capsaicin was tested in a phase I study with chemotherapy and radiation therapy patients.[19] The capsaicin was delivered in a taffy candy vehicle (cayenne pepper candy), which the subjects were instructed to let dissolve in their mouths without chewing. After the candy had dissolved, the burn produced by the candy was allowed to fade. The patients rated their pain before and after eating the candy. Partial and temporary pain reduction was reported in 11 patients with stomatitis.[19]

Xerostomia

Sialogogues have recently been investigated as stimulants for the residual salivary parenchyma (pilocarpine, 5- and 10-mg doses), and subjective improvement has been reported in some patients. Extreme caution with the use of pilocarpine is warranted because of reported side effects of glaucoma, cardiac problems, and sweating. A randomized controlled trial of standard fractionated radiation with or without amifostine (Ethyol), administered at 200 mg/m^2 as a 3-minute IV infusion 15 to 30 minutes before each fraction of radiation, was conducted in 315 patients with head and neck cancer.[105] Patient eligibility criteria included inclusion of at least 75% of both parotid glands in the radiation field. The incidence of grade 2 or higher acute xerostomia (90 days from the start of radiotherapy) and late xerostomia (9 to 12 months after radiotherapy), as assessed by the Radiation Therapy Oncology Group Acute and Late Morbidity Score and Criteria, was significantly reduced in patients receiving Ethyol. Whole saliva collection 1

year after radiation therapy showed that more patients given Ethyol produced 0.1 g of saliva (72% vs. 49%), and the median saliva production was higher in patients who received Ethyol (0.26 vs. 0.10 g). Stimulated saliva collections did not show a difference between treatment arms. These improvements in saliva production were supported by the patients' reports of oral dryness.[105]

Artificial saliva, usually with carboxymethylcellulose as a base, has not shown increased oral cavity comfort. Patients frequently use sugarless gum and hard candies for comfort and report subjective improvement. The dental team should encourage the patient to quit or reduce the use of tobacco and alcohol. Oral hygiene regimens can reduce colonization and proliferation of oral pathogens through the use of water or saline and daily fluoride application with brushing teeth at least three times daily.

FUTURE RESEARCH DIRECTIONS

Two underlying principles of oral complications research, as presented by Peterson and Sonis,[106] are that the etiology, progression, and resolution of stomatitis have a multifactorial nature and that the human model is most appropriate for research. Also recognized is the importance of the transgenic and gene-targeted murine model to elucidate mechanisms of mucosal injury.[106] Combining the expertise of clinical researchers and basic scientists promotes formulation of novel hypotheses regarding the contributions of inflammation, sustained cytokine dysregulation, and tissue injury and repair mechanisms to the pathogenesis of oral complications.

Evaluation of the efficacy and mechanisms of systemic and topical pharmacologic agents for prevention and treatment of oral complications through experimental designs is needed and should include pediatric, geriatric, and diverse ethnic populations. Exploration of the optimal dose and timing of interventions for stomatitis and related oropharyngeal pain is needed. Clinically meaningful outcomes for the evaluation of new stomatitis treatments include oropharyngeal pain, need for opioid analgesics, inability to eat soft food, diminished quality of life and functional status, increased length of hospital stay, and inability to take medication orally.[107] Continued psychometric testing of oral cavity assessment tools is also needed. Exploration of the interrelationships among the multiple dimensions of stomatitis-related oral pain at rest and with movement may increase understanding of this complex phenomenon. Combining quantitative and qualitative research designs to study the complex symptomatology related to oral complications may yield rich results. Outcomes of these research directions include application of the best evidence at the individual patient care level.

CONCLUSION

Oral complications of cancer treatment are experienced by a large percentage of oncology patients, are biologically complex, are often challenging to treat, and lead to a cascade of negative sequelae. Oncology treatment protocols continue to be designed to examine the effect of dose-intensive treatments on clinical and survival outcomes. These vital outcomes are compromised when dose reduction or treatment cessation is necessary because of treatment-related oral complications. Although there exist numerous recommendations for prevention and treatment of oral complications and related negative sequelae, there remains a critical need to evaluate these interventions in the randomized controlled clinical trial setting using valid and reliable stomatitis assessment tools to both advance the science of oral toxicities and to improve patient care. This clinical research work requires a multidisciplinary team dedicated to both testing innovative treatment approaches and implementing appropriate findings through evidence-based practice.

REFERENCES

1. Hyland SA. Assessing the oral cavity. In: Frank-Stromborg M, Olsen SJ, eds. *Instruments for clinical health-care research.* London: Jones and Bartlett Publishers International, 1997:519.
2. National Institutes of Health Consensus Development Panel. Consensus statement: oral complications of cancer therapies. *NCI Monogr* 1989;9:3.
3. Barasch A, Peterson DE. Risk factors for ulcerative mucositis in cancer patients: unanswered questions. *Oral Oncol* 2003;39:91.
4. Dodd MJ, Miaskowski C, Shiba GH, et al. Risk factors for chemotherapy-induced oral mucositis: dental appliances, oral hygiene, previous oral lesion, and a history of smoking. *Cancer Invest* 1999;17:278.
5. Driezen S. Description and incidence of oral complications. *NCI Monogr* 1990;9:11.
6. Sonis ST. Oral complications of cancer therapy. In: DeVita VT, Hellman S, Rosenberg SA, eds. *Cancer: principles and practice of oncology,* 4th ed. Philadelphia: JB Lippincott Co, 1993:2385.
7. Sonis ST. Mucositis as a biological process: a new hypothesis for the development of chemotherapy-induced stomatotoxicity. *Oral Oncol* 1998;34:39.
8. Woo S-B, Sonis ST, Monopoli MM, et al. A longitudinal study of oral ulcerative mucositis in bone marrow transplant recipients. *Cancer* 1993;72:1612.
9. McGuire DB, Altomonte V, Peterson DE, et al. Patterns of mucositis and pain in patients receiving preparative chemotherapy. *Oncol Nurs Forum* 1993;20:1493.
10. Shih A, Miaskowski C, Dodd MJ, et al. Mechanisms for radiation-induced oral mucositis and the consequences. *Cancer Nurs* 2003;26:222.
10a. Sonis, ST. A biological approach to mucositis. *J Support Oncol.* 2004;2:21.
11. Vissink A, Jansma J, Spijkervet, et al. Oral sequelae of head and neck radiotherapy. *Crit Rev Oral Biol Med* 2003;14:199.
12. Lazarus HM, Vogelsang GB, Rowe JM. Prevention and treatment of acute graft-versus-host disease: the old and the new. A report from the Eastern Cooperative Oncology Group (ECOG). *Bone Marrow Transplant* 1997;19:577.
13. Mitchell SA. Graft versus host disease. In: Ezzone S, ed. *Hematopoietic stem cell transplantation: a manual for nursing practice.* Pittsburgh: Oncology Nursing Society, 2004:85.
14. Lloid ME. Oral medicine concerns of the BMT patient. In: Buchsel PC, Whedon MB, eds. *Bone marrow transplantation administrative and clinical strategies.* Boston: Jones and Bartlett Publishers International, 1995:257.
15. Vogelsang GB. How I treat chronic graft-versus-host-disease. *Blood* 2001;97:1196.
16. Schubert MM, Williams BE, Lloid ME, et al. Clinical scale for the rating of oral mucosal changes associated with bone marrow transplantation. Development of an oral mucositis index. *Cancer* 1992;69:2469.
17. National Institute of Nursing Research (NINR). *The nature of pain. A conceptual perspective. A report of the NINR priority expert panel on symptom management. Acute pain.* Bethesda, MD: U.S. Department of Health and Human Services, 1994:23.
18. Sessle BJ. Neural mechanisms of oral and facial pain. *Otolaryngol Clin North Am* 1989;60:493.
19. Berger A, Henderson M, Nadoolman W, et al. Oral capsaicin provides temporary relief for oral mucositis pain secondary to chemotherapy/radiation therapy. *J Pain Symptom Manage* 1995;10:243.
20. Berger AM, Kilroy, TJ. Oral complications. In: DeVita VT, Hellman S, Rosenberg SA, eds. *Cancer: principles and practice of oncology,* 6th ed. Philadelphia: JB Lippincott Co, 1997:2714.
21. U.S. Department of Health and Human Services. *Oral health, cancer care, and you: fitting the pieces together.* Bethesda, MD: U.S. Department of Health and Human Services, National Institutes of Health, National Institute of Dental and Craniofacial Research, 2002.
22. Cancer Therapy Evaluation Program. *Common terminology criteria for adverse events, version 3.0.* DCTD, NCI, NIH, DHHS June 10, 2003.
23. Eilers J, Berger AM, Petersen MC. Development, testing, and application of the oral assessment guide. *Oncol Nurs Forum* 1988;15:325.
24. Schubert MM, Sullivan KM, Morton TH, et al. Oral manifestations of chronic graft-versus-host disease. *Arch Intern Med* 1984;144:1591.
25. McGuire DB, Peterson DE, Muller S, et al. The 20 item oral mucositis index: reliability and validity in bone marrow and stem cell transplant patients. *Cancer Invest* 2002;20:893.
26. Sonis ST, Eilers JP, Epstein JB, et al. for the Mucositis Study Group. Validation of a new scoring system for the assessment of clinical trial research of oral mucositis induced by radiation or chemotherapy. *Cancer* 1999;85:2103.
27. Sonis ST, Oster G, Fuchs H, et al. Oral mucositis and the clinical and economic outcomes of hematopoietic stem-cell transplantation. *J Clin Oncol* 2001;19:2201.
28. World Health Organization. *WHO handbook for reporting results of cancer treatment,* (offset publication No. 48). Geneva: World Health Organization, 1979:15.
29. Zlotolow IM, Berger AM. Oral manifestations of cancer therapy. In: Berger AM, Portnoy RK, Weissman DE, eds. *Principles and practice of palliative care and supportive oncology,* 2nd ed. Philadelphia: Lippincott Williams & Wilkins, 2002:282.
30. Biron P, Sebban C, Gourmet R, et al. Research controversies in management of oral mucositis. *Support Care Cancer* 2000;8:68.
30a. Rubenstein, EB, Peterson, DE, Schubert, M, et al. For the Mucositis Study Section of the Multinational Association of Supportive Care in Cancer and the International Society for Oral Oncology. Clinical practice guidelines for the prevention and treatment of cancer therapy-induced oral and gastrointestinal mucositis. 2004;100:2026.
31. American Society of Clinical Oncology Classic Papers and Current Comments. 2000; 4:881.
32. Solomon MA. Oral sucralfate suspension for mucositis. *N Engl J Med* 1986;315:459.
33. Pfeiffer P, Madsen EL, Hansen O, et al. Effect of prophylactic sucralfate suspension on stomatitis induced by cancer chemotherapy. A randomized, double-blind cross-over study. *Acta Oncol* 1990;29:171.
34. Shenep JL, Kalwihsky D, Hudson PR, et al. Oral sucralfate in chemotherapy-induced mucositis. *J Pediatr* 1988;113:753.
35. Loprinzi CL, Ghosh C, Camoriani J, et al. Phase III controlled evaluation of sucralfate to alleviate stomatitis in patients receiving fluorouracil-based chemotherapy. *J Clin Oncol* 1997;15:1235.
36. Nottage M, McLachlan S-A, Brittain M-A, et al. Sucralfate mouthwash for prevention and treatment of 5-fluorouracil-induced mucositis: a randomized, placebo-controlled trial. *Support Care Cancer* 2003;11:41.
37. Scherlacher A, Beaufort-Spontin E. Radiotherapy of head-neck neoplasms: prevention of inflammation of the mucosa by sucralfate treatment. *HNO* 1990;38:24.
38. Epstein JB, Wong FLW. The efficacy of sucralfate suspension in the prevention of oral mucositis due to radiation therapy. *Int J Radiat Oncol Biol Phys* 1994;28:693.
39. Dodd MJ, Miaskowski C, Greenspan D. Radiation-induced mucositis: a randomized clinical trial of micronized sucralfate versus salt and soda mouthwashes. *Cancer Invest* 2003; 21:21.
40. Innocenti M, Moscatelli G, Lopez S. Efficacy of Gelclair in reducing pain in palliative care patients with oral lesions. Preliminary findings from an open pilot study. *J Pain Symptom Manage* 2001;24:456.
41. DeCordi SD, et al. *Gelclair: potentially an efficacious treatment for chemotherapy-induced mucositis.* Italian Anti-Tumor League III Congress of Professional Oncology Nurses. Congliano, Italy, Oct. 10–12, 2001 (abst).
42. Porteder H, Rausch E, Kment G, et al. Local prostaglandin E2 in patients with oral malignancies undergoing chemo and radiotherapy. *J Craniomaxillofac Surg* 1988;16:371.
43. Matejka M, Nell A, Kment G, et al. Local benefit of prostaglandin E2 in radiochemotherapy-induced oral mucositis. *Br J Oral Maxillofac Surg* 1990;28:89.
44. Epstein JB, Stevenson-Moore P. Benzydamine hydrochloride in prevention and management of pain in mucositis associated with radiation therapy. *Oral Surg Oral Med Oral Pathol* 1986;62:145.
45. Abdelaal AS, Barker DS, Fergusson MM. Treatment for irradiation-induced mucositis. *Lancet* 1987;1:97.
46. Rothwell BR, Spektor WS. Palliation of radiation-related mucositis. *Spec Care Dentist* 1990;10:21.
47. Wadleigh RG, Redman RS, Graham ML, et al. Vitamin E in the treatment of chemo-induced mucositis. *Am J Med* 1992;92:481.
48. Osaki T, Ueta E, Yoneda K, et al. Prophylaxis of oral mucositis associated with chemoradiotherapy for oral carcinoma by Azelastine hydrochloride (Azelastin) with other antioxidants. *Head Neck* 1994;16:331.
49. Maciejewski B, Zajusz A, Pilecki B, et al. Acute mucositis in the stimulated oral mucosa of patients during radiotherapy for head and neck cancer. *Radiother Oncol* 1991;22:7.
50. Dorr W, Jacubek A, Kummermehr J, et al. Effects of stimulated repopulation on oral mucositis during conventional radiotherapy. *Radiother Oncol* 1995;37:100.
51. Mahoud DJ, Dose AM, Loprinzi CL, et al. Inhibition of fluorouracil-induced stomatitis by oral cryotherapy. *J Clin Oncol* 1991;9:449.
52. Rocke LK, Loprinzi CL, Lee JK, et al. A randomized clinical trial of two different durations of oral cryotherapy for prevention of 5-fluorouracil-related stomatitis. *Cancer* 1993;72:2234.
53. Cascinu S, Fedeli A, Fedeli SL, et al. Oral cooling (cryotherapy), an effective treatment for the prevention of 5-fluorouracil-induced stomatitis. *Oral Oncol Eur J Cancer* 1994;30:234.
54. Pourreau-Schneider N, Soudry M, Franquin JC, et al. Soft-laser therapy for iatrogenic mucositis in cancer patients receiving high-dose fluorouracil: a preliminary report. *J Natl Cancer Inst* 1992;84:358.
55. Bensadoun RJ, Ciais G, Schubert MM, et al. Low-energy He/Ne laser in the prevention of radiation-induced mucositis. A multicenter phase III randomized study in patients with head and neck cancer. *Support Care Cancer* 1999;7:244.
56. Carl W, Emrich LS. Management of oral mucositis during local radiation and systemic chemotherapy. A study of 98 patients. *J Prosthet Dent* 1991;66:361.
57. Fidler P, Loprinzi CL, Lee JK, et al. A randomized clinical trial of chamomile mouthwash for prevention of 5-FU-induced oral mucositis. *Cancer* 1996;77:522.
58. Peterson D, Petit G. Phase III study: AES-14 in chemotherapy patients at risk for mucositis. *Proc Am Soc Clin Oncol* 2003;22:725.
59. Spijkervet FKL, Saene HKF, Panders AK, et al. Effect of chlorhexidine rinsing on the oropharyngeal ecology in patients with head and neck cancer who have irradiation mucositis. *Oral Surg Oral Med Oral Pathol* 1989;67:154.
60. Foote RL, Loprinzi CL, Frank AR, et al. Randomized trial of a chlorhexidine mouthwash for alleviation of radiation-induced mucositis. *J Clin Oncol* 1994;12:2630.
61. Sundqvist K, Liu Y, Arvidson K, et al. Growth regulation of serum free cultures of epithelial cells from normal human buccal mucosa. *In Vitro Cell Dev Biol* 1991;27A:562.
62. Sonis ST, Costa JW Jr, Evitts SM, et al. Effect of epidermal growth factor on ulcerative mucositis in hamsters that receive cancer chemotherapy. *Oral Surg Oral Med Oral Pathol* 1992;74:749.
63. Sonis ST, Tracey C, Shklar G, et al. An animal model for mucositis induced by cancer chemotherapy. *Oral Surg Oral Med Oral Pathol* 1990;69:437.
64. Gabrilove JL, Jakubowski A, Scher H, et al. Effect of granulocyte colony-stimulating factor on neutropenia and associated morbidity due to chemotherapy for transitional-cell carcinoma of the urothelium. *N Engl J Med* 1988;318:1414.

65. Bronchud MH, Howell A, Crowther D, et al. The use of granulocyte colony-stimulating factor to increase the intensity of treatment with doxorubicin in patients with advanced breast and ovarian cancer. *Br J Cancer* 1989;60:121.

66. Pettengell R, Gurney H, Radford JA, et al. Granulocyte colony-stimulating factor to prevent dose-limiting neutropenia in non-Hodgkin's lymphoma: a randomized controlled trial. *Blood* 1992;80:1430.

67. Saarilahti K, Kajanti M, Joensuu T. Comparison of granulocyte-macrophage colony-stimulating factor and sucralfate mouthwashes in the prevention of radiation-induced mucositis: a double-blind prospective randomized phase III study. *Int J Radiat Oncol Biol Phys* 2002;2:479.

68. Dazzi C, Cariello A, Giovanis P, et al. Prophylaxis with GM-CSF mouthwashes does not reduce frequency and duration of severe oral mucositis in patients with solid tumors undergoing high-dose chemotherapy with autologous peripheral blood stem cell transplantation rescue: a double blind, randomized, placebo-controlled study. *Ann Oncol* 2003;14:559.

69. Sonis ST, Lindquist L, Vugt V, et al. Prevention of chemotherapy-induced ulcerative mucositis by transforming growth factor beta 3. *Cancer Res* 1994;54:1135.

70. Spijkervet FK, Sonis ST. New frontiers in the management of chemotherapy-induced mucositis. *Curr Opin Oncol* 1998;10(Suppl 1):S23.

71. Foncuberta MC, Cagnoni CH, Brandts R, et al. Topical transforming growth factor-beta3 in the prevention or alleviation of chemotherapy-induced oral mucositis in patients with lymphomas or solid tumors. *J Immunother* 2001;24:384.

72. Zaghloul MS, Dorie MJ, Kallman RF, et al. Interleukin 1 increases thymidine labeling index of normal tissue of mice, not the tumor. *Int J Radiat Oncol Biol Phys* 1994;29:805.

73. Sonis S, Edwards L, Lucey C. The biological basis for the attenuation of mucositis: the example of interleukin-11. *Leukemia* 1999;13:831.

74. Danilenko DM. Preclinical and early clinical development of keratinocyte growth factor, an epithelial-specific tissue growth factor. *Toxicol Pathol* 1999;27:64.

75. Finch PW, Rubin JS. Keratinocyte growth factor (KGF/FGF7), a homeostatic factor with therapeutic potential for epithelial protection and repair. *Adv Cancer Res* 91 (*in press*).

76. Dörr W, Spekl K, Farrell CL. Amelioration of acute oral mucositis by keratinocyte growth factor: fractionated irradiation. *Int J Radiat Oncol Biol Phys* 2002;54:245.

77. Dörr W, Spekl K, Farrell CL. The effect of keratinocyte growth factor on healing of manifest radiation ulcers in mouse tongue epithelium. *Cell Prolif* 2002;35(Suppl 1):86.

78. Meropol NJ, Somer RA, Gutheil J. Randomized phase I trial of recombinant human keratinocyte growth factor plus chemotherapy: potential role as mucosal protectant. *J Clin Oncol* 2003;21:1452.

79. Spielberger RT, Emmanouilides C, Stiff P, et al. Use of recombinant human keratinocyte growth factor (rHuKGF) can reduce severe oral mucositis in patients with hematologic malignancies undergoing autologous peripheral blood progenitor cell transplantation (auto PBSCT) after radiation-based conditioning: results of a phase 3 trial. *Proc Am Soc Clin Oncol* 2003;22(abstr 3642).

80. *Human Genome Sciences Reports: Results Of Phase 2 Clinical Trial Of Repifermin In Patients With Cancer Therapy-Induced Mucositis.* Human Genome Sciences, Rockville, MD. World Wide Web URL: http://www.hgsi.com/news/press/04-02-02_repifermin.html, 2004.

81. Donnelly JP, Bellm LA, Epstein JB, et al. Antimicrobial therapy to prevent or treat oral mucositis. *Lancet Infect Dis* 2003;3:405.

82. Wahlin A, Wahlin BY. Effects of chlorhexidine mouthrinse on oral health in patients with acute leukemia. *Oral Surg Oral Med Oral Pathol* 1989;68:279.

83. Dodd MJ, Larson PL, Dibble SL, et al. Randomized clinical trial of chlorhexidine versus placebo for prevention of oral mucositis in patients receiving chemotherapy. *Oncol Nurs Forum* 1996;23:921.

84. Weisdorf DJ, Bostrom B, Raether D, et al. Oropharyngeal mucositis complicating bone marrow transplantation: prognostic factors and the effect of chlorhexidine mouth rinse. *Bone Marrow Transplant* 1989;4:89.

85. Epstein JB, Vickais L, Spinelli J, et al. Efficacy of chlorhexidine and nystatin rinses in prevention of oral complications in leukemia and bone marrow transplantation. *Oral Surg Oral Med Oral Pathol* 1992;73:682.

86. Slavin MA, Osborne B, Adams R, et al. Efficacy and safety of fluconazole prophylaxis for fungal infections after marrow transplantation—a prospective, randomized, double-blind study. *J Infect Dis* 1995;171:1545.

87. Sutherland SE, Browman GP. Prophylaxis of oral mucositis in irradiated head-and-neck cancer patients: a proposed classification scheme of interventions and meta-analysis of randomized controlled trials. *Int J Radiat Oncol Biol Phys* 2001;4:917.

88. Spijkervet FK, van Saene HK, van Saene JJ, et al. Effect of selective elimination of the oral flora on mucositis in irradiated head and neck cancer patients. *J Surg Oncol* 1991;46:167.

89. Stokman MA, Spijkervet FKL, Burlage FR, et al. Oral mucositis and selective elimination of oral flora in head and neck cancer patients receiving radiotherapy: a double-blind randomized clinical trial. *Br J Cancer* 2003;88:1012.

90. Schwartz PM, Dunigan JM, Marsh JC, et al. Allopurinol modification of the toxicity and antitumor activity of 5-fluorouracil. *Cancer Res* 1980;40:1885.

91. Clark PI, Selvin ML. Allopurinol mouthwash and 5-fluorouracil-induced oral toxicity. *Eur J Surg Oncol* 1985;11:267.

92. Tsarais N, Caragluris P, Kosmidus P. Reduction of oral toxicity of 5-fluorouracil by allopurinol mouthwashes. *Eur J Surg Oncol* 1998;14:405.

93. Loprinzi CI, Cianflone SG, Dose ASM, et al. A controlled evaluation of an allopurinol mouthwash as prophylaxis against 5-fluorouracil induced stomatitis. *Cancer* 1990;65:1879.

94. Fox AD, Kripe SA, Depaula JA, et al. Effect of glutamine supplemented enteral diet on methotrexate-induced enterocolitis. *JPEN J Parenter Enteral Nutr* 1988;12:325.

95. Anderson PM, Schroeder G, Skubitz KM, et al. Oral glutamine reduces the duration and severity of stomatitis after cytotoxic cancer chemotherapy. *Cancer* 1998;83:1433.

96. Seiter K, Kemeny N, Martin D, et al. Uridine allows dose escalation of 5-fluorouracil when given with N-phosphonacetyl-aspartate, methotrexate, and leucovorin. *Cancer* 1993;71:1875.

97. Ahmed T, Engelking C, Szalyga J, et al. Propantheline prevention of mucositis from etoposide. *Bone Marrow Transplant* 1993;12:131.

98. Marx RE, Johnson RP, Kline SN. Prevention of osteoradionecrosis: a randomized prospective clinical trial of hyperbaric oxygen versus penicillin. *J Am Dent Assoc* 1985;111:49.

99. Schwieger JW. Oral complications following radiation therapy: a five year retrospective report. *J Prosthet Dent* 1987;58:78.

100. Carnal SB, Blakeslee DB, Oswald SG, et al. Treatment of radiation- and chemotherapy-induced stomatitis. *Otolaryngol Head Neck Surg* 1990;102:326.

101. Krajnik M, Zylicz Z, Finlay I, et al. Potential uses of topical opioids in palliative care—report of 6 cases. *Pain* 1999;80:121.

102. Coluzzi PH, Schwartzberg L, Conroy JD, et al. Breakthrough cancer pain: a randomized trial comparing oral transmucosal fentanyl (OTFC) and morphine sulfate immediate release (MSIR). *Pain* 2001;91:123.

103. Cerchietti LC, Navigante AH, Bonomi MR, et al. Effect of topical morphine for mucositis-associated pain following concomitant chemoradiotherapy for head and neck cancer. *Cancer* 2002;95:2230.

104. Swisher ME, Scheidler VR, Kennedy MJ. A mucositis pain management algorithm: a creative strategy to enhance the transition to ambulatory care. *Oncol Nurs Forum* 1998.

105. Brizel DM, Wasserman TH, Strnad V, et al. *Final report of a phase III randomized trial of amifostine as a radioprotectant in head and neck cancer.* 41st Annual Meeting of the American Society for Therapeutic Radiology and Oncology. Texas, 1999(abst).

106. Peterson DE, Sonis S. Executive summary. *J NCI Monogr* 2001;29:3.

107. Bellum LA, Durnell L, Epstein JB, et al. Defining clinically meaningful outcomes in the evaluation of new treatments for oral mucositis: oral mucositis patients provider advisory board. *Cancer Invest* 2002;20:793.

SECTION 3

DIANE E. STOVER
ROBERT J. KANER

Pulmonary Toxicity

Pulmonary disease can be caused by a wide spectrum of pathogenetic mechanisms in patients with cancer. These include a variety of infectious agents and neoplastic disorders as well as pulmonary thromboembolic disease, pulmonary hemorrhage, pulmonary edema (cardiogenic and noncardiogenic), and leukocyte agglutinin reactions. Pulmonary toxicity caused by antineoplastic agents is being recognized more frequently, and the number of drugs known or suspected to cause lung disease is steadily increasing. Because continuing the offending agent may cause death and because withholding the agent may result in resolution of the pulmonary toxicity, it is important to recognize radiation- and drug-induced pulmonary disease. In this section, parenchymal lung disease caused by irradiation and chemotherapy is discussed. Mechanisms of lung injury, histopathologic findings, clinical and laboratory features, and diagnosis and treatment of the abnormalities produced by these agents are reviewed.

RADIATION-INDUCED PULMONARY TOXICITY

MECHANISM OF LUNG INJURY

Radiation can affect dividing and nondividing cells and can cause genetic and nongenetic damage. In the lung, a hypothetical reconstruction of radiation injury might be as follows.[1] Therapeutic radiation may result in nongenetic damage that is apparent in all cells, but capillary endothelial and type I cells (epithelial lining cells) appear most susceptible. Many of these cells, whether dividing or not, undergo early necrobiosis and slough. The apoptotic pathway appears to be an important mechanism of cellular destruction after radiation. Specific signal transduction pathways are activated by radiation, including sphingomyelin hydrolysis, which generates ceramide as a second messenger and leads to apoptotic DNA degradation. Nonlethal ionizing radiation also activates a stress response in cells, which leads to up-regulation of specific nuclear transcription factors such as nuclear factor κB and transcription of specific early-response genes such as c-abl, c-jun, Egr-1, and c-fos. This cellular activation initiates a repair process that involves cytokines and growth factors, such as basic fibroblast growth factor, vascular endothelial growth factor, and platelet-derived growth factor, as well as tumor necrosis factor-α, interleukin-1, and transforming growth factor-β (TGF-β). Prostaglandin synthesis is also up-regulated. Over time, capillaries regenerate, and the alveolar epithelium is repopulated by type II cells (surfactant-producing cells), because type I pneumocytes do not regenerate. Some of these type II cells redifferentiate into type I cells. In some animal models, bone marrow–derived stem cells also contribute to repopulation of the alveolar epithelium after radiation. If the initial injury is severe, damage to extracellular matrix components of the lung, such as basement membrane glycoproteins and proteoglycans, takes place. Consistent with this concept, ionizing radiation to lung epithelial cells *in vitro* stimulates production of matrix metalloproteinase 2, an enzyme capable of degrading the type IV basement membrane collagen.[2] This can impede reconstruction of the delicate three-dimensional structure of the alveolar-capillary unit and result in functional derangement and scar formation, even if the cellular components are able to regenerate. Genetic damage to dividing cells, such as endothelial cells or type II pneumonocytes, can also occur. Depletion of these cells may result during successive mitoses, causing a loss of integrity of pulmonary capillaries and exudation of fluid into the alveoli. At the physiologic level, loss of compliance, abnormal gas exchange, and respiratory failure can occur as a result of leakage of plasma proteins into the alveolar space. This type of genetic damage may also explain why pneumonitis can happen so late after radiation. One might speculate that some endothelial cells initially remain normal but that, in the course of the next four cell divisions, chromosomal aberrations prevent further reduplication, which leads to loss of integrity of the capillary. Alternatively or concurrently, a cellular infiltrate is observed in bronchoalveolar lavage fluid and lung tissue, which is interpreted as an inflammatory response to the radiation injury. In experimental animal models, systemic administration of corticosteroids can suppress this inflammatory response, yet does not abrogate the subsequent development of chronic fibrosis. Based on these pathophysiologic considerations, animal studies suggest that lung gene transfer of constructs encoding several superoxide dismutase genes confers protection against radiation pneumonitis. Similar protective effects have been observed with systemic administration of competitive inhibitors of nitric oxide synthase. Inhibition of endothelial cell apoptosis by therapeutic administration of basic fibroblast growth factor or vascular endothelial growth factor by protein or genetically has been beneficial in some animal models, but no human trials have been attempted.

Certain factors are critical to the development of classic radiation pneumonitis. In general, damage to the lung increases as the volume of lung tissue irradiated increases. A threshold effect also appears to occur, such that irradiation of at least 10% of the lung is required to produce significant pulmonary toxicity. This threshold may be reached in the treatment of some patients with breast cancer, depending on the specifics of their individualized treatment program. Also, the toxic effects of radiation as measured by symptoms and signs, radiographic changes, and physiologic tests are proportionate to the total amount delivered to the lung. Radiation pneumonitis after a single-dose whole lung irradiation shows a threshold level and a steep sigmoid dose-response curve. Radiation pneumonitis seldom occurs with fractionated total doses of less than 20 Gy but is highly likely when doses exceed 60 Gy. An unusual and dramatic demonstration of this principle is the use of therapeutic pneumothorax to protect the lung when high-dose external-beam radiotherapy is given for the treatment of chest-wall tumors.

Because local control of lung cancer is greater when higher doses are delivered to the tumor, methods have been devised to give high doses to the target tissue while sparing normal surrounding lung. One such technique is called *three-dimensional treatment planning*.[3] Studies have suggested that the incidence and grade of radiation pneumonitis increase in proportion to the volume of lung exposed to greater than 20 Gy, for radiation alone and for concurrent chemoradiation used to treat locally advanced lung cancer.[4] Preliminary results using these considerations to plan the radiation ports are encouraging.[5] To further spare the lung of toxicity, *in situ* isolated lung perfusion for the treatment of unresectable pulmonary tumors, preceded or followed by high-dose irradiation, soon may be available. Studies to evaluate the therapeutic activity of inhaled chemotherapeutic agents, such as doxorubicin, on metastasis to the lung are under way as well. Whether these treatment modalities will have a sparing effect on the lung or whether they will be associated with an increase in pulmonary toxicity is unknown. Besides the total radiation dose, the number of fractions into which it is divided, and, to a lesser extent, the time span over which it is delivered are important factors. The greater the number of fractions in which the radiation is given, the lower is the damaging effect. However, the incidence of radiation pneumonitis still exhibits a threshold effect and a steep sigmoidal dose-response curve. Fractionation is different from dose rate, which refers to output of the machine during radiation therapy. Dose rate certainly has an effect on lung tolerance: Radiation delivered as 5 cGy/min is less damaging than radiation delivered at 30 cGy/min, which in turn is less damaging than radiation delivered at 2 to 3 Gy/min. The incidence and severity of radiation damage to the lungs are thus related principally to the volume of lung tissue irradiated, the total dose, the fractions into which the total dose is divided, and the quality of the radiation. These considerations have allowed early investigations into the possibility of increasing the total dose of radiation to the tumor beyond what is currently considered maximum by using the three-dimensional treatment-planning strategy to reduce the risk of radiation pneumonitis in an attempt to improve local control of the cancer.

Advances in the technology of positron emission tomography scanning have improved its usefulness for diagnosis and staging of lung cancer. Combined positron emission tomography/computed tomography (CT) imaging offers some advantages in designing the radiation port and in detecting metastases not evident on CT, thus changing the intent of the radiotherapy from curative to palliative.[6] Genetic factors also influence the severity of response to lung irradiation in animals and presumably may do so in humans as well, although there is no current method to evaluate this clinically.

HISTOPATHOLOGY

The histopathologic changes of radiation-induced pulmonary toxicity can be divided into early, intermediate, and late stages based on the time course and intensity of the radiation injury. Early radiation damage (0 to 2 months after radiation) is characterized by injury to small vessels and capillaries, with the development of vascular congestion and increased capillary permeability. At this stage, a fibrin-rich exudate is present in the alveolar spaces. Hyaline membranes form on the alveoli, probably from condensation of the intraalveolar fibrin. After 1 month, there is also an inflammatory infiltrate, which may lead to a second course of increased permeability. Abnormalities in the intermediate stage (2 to 9 months after radiation) are characterized by obstruction of pulmonary capillaries by platelets, fibrin, and collagen. Alveolar-lining cells (primarily type II pneumonocytes) become hyperplastic, and the alveolar walls become infiltrated with fibroblasts and mast cells. If the radiation injury is mild, these changes may subside entirely; however, when the injury is severe, a chronic phase (9 months or more after radiation) ensues that may persist or progress for months or years. In animal models, there is marked activation of genes that encode fibrillar collagens. The histopathologic appearance is then dominated by dense fibrosis, thickening of the alveolar walls, vascular subintimal fibrosis, and luminal narrowing. In some instances, the lung may shrink to less than half its original size, with a thickened adherent pleura and scarred hilar structures.

In addition to this classic pattern of radiation pneumonitis, another syndrome of out-of-field pneumonitis, characterized by a hypersensitivity pneumonitis in areas of lung not directly radiated, has been described. This syndrome, which occurs in a minority of patients, is characterized by a bilateral lymphocytic alveolitis of activated CD4+ T lymphocytes 4 to 6 weeks after strictly unilateral lung irradiation.

CLINICAL FEATURES

Signs and Symptoms

The clinical syndrome of radiation pneumonitis develops in 5% to 15% of patients receiving high-dose external-beam radiation for treatment of lung cancer. Factors that can add to the development of radiation pneumonitis include concomitant chemotherapy, previous irradiation, and withdrawal of steroids. No significant difference is seen in the incidence of radiation pneumonitis between the young and elderly, but the pneumonitis is inclined to be more severe in the latter. Underlying chronic obstructive pulmonary disease does not appear to potentiate radiation damage.

Symptoms of acute radiation pneumonitis usually become evident 2 to 3 months after the completion of therapy; rarely, they occur within the first month and occasionally as late as 6 months after irradiation.[7] In general, the early onset of symptoms implies a more serious and more protracted clinical course. The cardinal symptom of radiation pneumonitis is dyspnea. It may be self-limited or may progress to severe respiratory distress depending on the extent and intensity of the injury. Patients may also have a nonproductive cough or a cough productive of small amounts of pinkish sputum. Frank hemoptysis early in the clinical course is distinctly uncommon; however, massive hemoptysis has been reported as a late complication of therapeutic pulmonary irradiation. Fever is unusual but can be high and spiking; in severe cases, other constitutional symptoms may occur. Chest pain, which is rarely a prominent feature, may be due to fractured ribs, pleural changes, or coughing. Symptoms of airway obstruction can occur in the first few days of radiation therapy and are usually associated with swelling of a central bronchogenic carcinoma. Severe respiratory distress can result and may be prevented by the administration of steroids the day before and several days after the initiation of radiation therapy. Hemoptysis and other manifestations of radiation pneumonitis may also occur in patients given palliative endobronchial brachytherapy or after surgical implantation of radioactive seeds.

On physical examination, signs of pulmonary involvement are minimal. Occasionally, moist rales, a pleural friction rub, or evidence of pleural fluid may be heard over the area of irradiation. In severe cases, tachypnea and cyanosis may be present, and occasionally evidence of acute cor pulmonale appears, usually predicting a fatal outcome. Finger clubbing due to radiation is distinctly unusual and, if present, is most likely caused by the underlying malignancy. Skin changes corresponding to the ports of irradiation are often present but provide no clue as to the presence or severity of the pulmonary reaction beneath.

Although patients with acute pneumonitis may show complete resolution of signs and symptoms, most develop gradual progressive fibrosis. In some cases, patients present with radiation fibrosis without a previous history of acute pneumonitis. The permanent changes of fibrosis take 6 to 24 months to evolve but usually remain stable after 2 years. Patients with fibrosis can be asymptomatic or can have varying degrees of dyspnea. The major complications of radiation pneumonitis occur late in the disease and are secondary to persistent fibrosis of a large volume of lung. These include cor pulmonale and respiratory failure.

Diagnostic Imaging

Although radiographic abnormalities are invariably found at the time clinical radiation pneumonitis is present, these changes may be seen in asymptomatic patients as well. Early radiographic changes include a ground-glass opacification, diffuse haziness, or indistinctness of the normal pulmonary markings over the irradiated area. Later, the chest radiograph may show alveolar infiltrates or dense consolidation with or without air bronchograms. As the pneumonitis progresses to fibrosis, the radiographic appearance changes to that of linear streaks radiating from the area of pneumonitis and of contraction toward the hilar, the perimediastinal, or the apical areas. Pleural effusions, if present, are usually small and always coincident with the pneumonitis. They can persist for long periods but often disappear spontaneously and never increase over a period of stability unless secondary complications occur, such as radiation-induced pericarditis. Mediastinal or hilar adenopathy and cavitation are almost always due to causes other than radiation pneumonitis. Pneumothorax is occasionally associated with radiation fibrosis but not with acute pneumonitis.

One of the most characteristic features of radiation pneumonitis and fibrosis is that the radiologic changes are confined to the outlines of the field of radiation. In a few cases, extensive changes outside the field, even in the contralateral lung, have been observed. This syndrome of out-of-field pneumonitis is thought to represent a hypersensitivity response to the radiation. Other possible explanations for this phenomenon include obstruction of lymphatic flow from radiation-induced mediastinal fibrosis and absorption of x-rays by regions outside the irradiated ports.

Some data suggest that CT scans of the chest and gallium 67 citrate imaging are more sensitive than chest radiography in the detection of radiation changes. Correlation of abnormalities seen in these tests with the development of physiologic dysfunction and clinical toxicity needs clarification.

Pulmonary Function Tests

Prediction of changes in pulmonary function after high-dose irradiation to the lung has proven to be problematic.[8] No gross physiologic changes occur in the lung until 4 to 8 weeks after completion of irradiation, usually coincident with the period of clinical pneumonitis. Then one sees a decrease in lung volumes, which can progress. These changes persist indefinitely, with little evidence of recovery. Gas exchange abnormalities, which include a decrease in diffusing capacity and arterial hypoxemia, especially with exercise, occur at approximately the same time but show some tendency toward recovery after 6 to 12 months. A fall in compliance coincident with the clinical pneumonitis is seen in most subjects. Accordingly, the elastic work of breathing is increased, and dyspnea, resulting from the increased workload, ensues. Air-flow parameters remain close to normal in most studies.

DIAGNOSIS

The diagnosis of radiation pneumonitis can sometimes be made clinically based on the timing of irradiation in relation to symptoms and the typical chest radiographic appearance (i.e., infiltrates corresponding to the margins of the irradiated portal).[8] Differentiation from recurrent malignancy or infection often poses a problem, and then lung biopsy is necessary. Although histopathologic changes are nonspecific for radiation pneumonitis, when elements of the acute stages (fibrin exudate in the alveoli) are seen adjacent to the more chronic stages (alveolar fibrosis and subintimal sclerosis), this entity can be diagnosed with reasonable certainty.

Biochemical markers that indicate radiation lung injury before the onset of clinical pathologic events would be valuable in the early diagnosis and management of patients with radiation toxicity. In irradiated animals, studies demonstrate that surfactant found in the serum may be a marker and predictor for later radiation pneumonitis. Prospective studies are needed in humans to identify the sensitivity and specificity of monitoring serum surfactant levels as an early means to diagnose clinical radiation toxicity. Although no standard tests are currently used to monitor patients for radiation pneumonitis because most methods have little predictive value, reports have suggested that soluble intercellular adhesion molecule-1 or TGF-β may be a good candidate.

TREATMENT

Three modalities of therapy have been used prophylactically and therapeutically for radiation-induced pneumonitis: corti-

costeroids, antibiotics, and anticoagulants. Of these, corticosteroid therapy is the most important.

Corticosteroid administration during irradiation in mice markedly improves the physiologic abnormalities and decreases mortality without an effect on late pulmonary fibrosis. No controlled clinical trials in humans are available on the efficacy of steroid therapy in radiation pneumonitis. Rubin and Casarett[9] collected data from eight studies on humans and categorized them according to whether corticosteroids were used prophylactically or therapeutically. Corticosteroids given prophylactically failed to prevent radiation pneumonitis, but when they were administered as clinical pneumonitis occurred, an objective response was seen. In other reports, steroid therapy failed to ameliorate severe pneumonitis. Nonetheless, it is the authors' practice to begin prednisone, 1 mg/kg, as soon as the diagnosis is reasonably certain. The initial dose is maintained for several weeks and then reduced cautiously and slowly. It has been the authors' experience that if steroids are tapered too rapidly, symptoms can be exacerbated, necessitating higher doses for longer periods. Similarly, if corticosteroids are part of a recent chemotherapeutic regimen, stopping them abruptly can precipitate clinically evident radiation pneumonitis. What parameters, if any, to follow during the tapering schedule are not known, and no studies are available. Generally, the authors follow symptoms. Most authors agree that corticosteroids have no place in the treatment of radiation fibrosis.

In experimental and clinical reports, antibiotic administration has no effect on the course or outcome of radiation pneumonitis. Although there is some rationale for the use of anticoagulants in view of the effects of irradiation on the vascular system, neither heparin injections nor oral anticoagulants have been found to be beneficial. Captopril has been shown to be effective in animal studies, but no human trials have been reported. The mechanism of action of captopril in this setting is probably not its inhibition of angiotensin-converting enzyme. Pentoxifylline also has some effects on the late phase of pneumonitis in animal models. A promising new prophylactic radioprotection agent is amifostine, which has shown significant protective effects in reducing the incidence of radiation pneumonitis in some phase I/II trials in combination with chemoradiotherapy for stage III non–small cell lung cancer, in which many of the patients were stage IIIB and required a larger radiation port.[10] Phase I/II studies of heavy ion radiotherapy, such as with a carbon beam, have begun to show promise for an improved therapeutic to toxic ratio for local treatment of primary lung cancer.

RADIATION-RELATED BRONCHIOLITIS OBLITERANS WITH ORGANIZING PNEUMONIA

Although bronchiolitis obliterans with organizing pneumonia (BOOP) is an unusual histopathologic pattern for cancer therapy–related lung injury, radiation damage resulting in BOOP has been reported.[11] Patients with lung cancer usually receive the highest doses of radiation to the largest volume of lung tissue, which makes them more susceptible to radiation pulmonary injury compared with other irradiated patients. Most of the cases of radiation-related BOOP, however, have occurred in patients receiving radiation treatment to the breast. Whether the low dose or indirect radiation that these patients receive makes them more susceptible to this type of lung injury is not known. Besides the unusual pathologic pattern in these patients, there are clinical and radiologic differences compared to conventional radiation pneumonitis. Whereas dyspnea is the hallmark of radiation-induced pneumonitis, fever and cough are the predominant features of radiation-related BOOP. Radiographically, the pulmonary infiltrates can begin in radiated areas as with radiation pneumonitis, but they always progress outside the portal, and in approximately 40% of cases, infiltrates were observed on the side contralateral to the irradiated breast. Although patients respond dramatically to corticosteroid therapy with no obvious evidence of residual damage, there is a 67% relapse rate when the drug is tapered or discontinued. Similar to conventional radiation-induced pneumonitis, there are no studies available on the minimal effective dose or duration of therapy, but in view of the high relapse rate, it seems prudent to taper corticosteroid therapy very slowly, with meticulous vigilance for clinical signs of relapse.

CHEMOTHERAPY-INDUCED PULMONARY TOXICITY

The list of chemotherapeutic agents reported to cause cytotoxic drug-induced lung disease continues to grow. A recently added agent is fludarabine.[12] An overview of the potential mechanisms of lung damage; a summary of the pathologic findings; common clinical, radiographic, and physiologic features of chemotherapy-induced pulmonary toxicity; and diagnosis and treatment are discussed in this section (Table 54.3-1).

MECHANISMS OF PULMONARY INJURY

Except for a few chemotherapeutic agents (e.g., bleomycin), the details of the pathophysiology of lung injury are unknown. Various mechanisms of pulmonary toxicity have been proposed, including a direct toxic effect on alveolar epithelial cells, the induction of an inflammatory immunologic response, and endothelial cell injury or activation causing capillary leak syndrome. These events result in clinical presentations referred to as *nonspecific interstitial pneumonitis/fibrosis, hypersensitivity pneumonitis syndrome*, and *noncardiogenic pulmonary edema.*

Certain cytotoxic drugs may induce pulmonary injury by triggering the formation of reactive oxygen metabolites, including superoxide anions,[13] hydrogen peroxide, and hydroxyl radicals, primarily from activated neutrophils. Bleomycin induces reactive oxygen radicals by forming a complex with Fe^{3+}. Consistent with a direct pathologic role for this mechanism, iron chelators ameliorate the pulmonary toxicity of bleomycin in animal models.[14] Reactive oxygen species can produce direct toxicity through participation in redox reactions and subsequent fatty acid oxidation, which leads to membrane instability.[15] Oxidants can cause other inflammatory reactions within the lung. For example, the oxidation of arachidonic acid is an initial step in the metabolic cascade that produces active mediators, including prostaglandins and leukotrienes.[16] Cytokines such as interleukin-1, macrophage inflammatory protein-1, monocyte chemoattractant protein-1, and TGF-β are released from alveolar macrophages in animal models of bleomycin toxicity resulting in fibrosis.[13,17,18] Damage or activation of alveolar epithelial cells may result in release of cytokines and growth factors that stimulate proliferation of myofibroblasts and secretion of a pathologic extracellular matrix leading to fibrosis, as has been proposed for the pathophysiology of idiopathic pulmonary fibrosis.

Cytotoxic drugs may also affect the local immune system. Because the lung is exposed to so many substances that can activate its immune system, there appears to be a pulmonary immune tolerance state to avoid overreactions.[19] This tolerance state in part may be a result of an effector and suppressor cell balance. Cytotoxic drugs can alter the normal balance, which then may cause tissue damage.[19] For example, lymphocytic alveolitis is a consistent finding in methotrexate pneumonitis, with an imbalance of the CD4/CD8 ratio.[20] As clinical improvement occurs the ratio normalizes.

Other homeostatic systems within the lung can be affected as well, such as the balance between collagen formation and collagenolysis.[19] Through modulation of fibroblast proliferation, excessive collagen deposition may result in severe, irreversible pulmonary fibrosis. Bleomycin is one cytotoxic agent that has this potential.[18] In addition, bleomycin may up-regulate collagen synthesis in fibroblasts by stimulating transcription directly through a TGF-β response element in the procollagen (I)α promoter as well as by an autocrine loop involving extracellular release of TGF-β.[21] Imbalance between the protease and antiprotease system has also been implicated in a number of pulmonary disorders, including drug toxicities.[19] Bleomycin and cyclophosphamide produce substances that can inactivate the antiprotease system, enhancing the effects of proteolytic enzymes on the lung. Bleomycin also causes profound effects on the fibrinolytic system, altering the balance between fibrin deposition and fibrinolysis on the alveolar surface, leading to fibrin deposition. Drugs may damage the lung through a variety of other mechanisms, and considerable investigation needs to be done to define and clarify the exact mechanism of lung injury for each chemotherapeutic drug.

One of the potential determinants of bleomycin toxicity is the bleomycin hydrolase, which is the major enzyme responsible for metabolizing bleomycin to a nontoxic molecule.[22] Interestingly, the two organs that are the most common targets for bleomycin toxicity (lung and skin) have the lowest levels of the enzyme. With the possibility of cloning the gene that encodes bleomycin hydrolase,[23] studies are now needed to determine if genetic variability of this enzyme accounts for individual susceptibility or immunity to bleomycin pulmonary toxicity.

HISTOPATHOLOGY

The histopathologic changes of drug-induced pulmonary toxicity show common features. Similar to radiation-induced damage, abnormalities are seen in endothelial and epithelial cells. The vascular damage is characterized by endothelial swelling with exudation of fluid into the interstitium and the intraalveolar spaces. Destruction and desquamation of type I pneumocytes occur, with delamellation and proliferation of type II pneumocytes. Mononuclear cell infiltration and fibroblast proliferation with fibrosis are common findings; the character of the inflammatory cellular infiltrate may be a feature that distinguishes the toxicity of one drug from another. Bronchoalveolar lavage studies in patients with methotrexate pulmonary toxicity have shown the presence of a T-lymphocytic alveolitis, whereas studies on some patients with bleomycin toxicity have revealed

TABLE 54.3-1. Characteristics of Pulmonary Toxicity Caused by Commonly Used Chemotherapeutic Agents

Drug	Mechanism of Injury	Histopathology	Clinical Features	Chest Roentgenogram	Diagnosis	Treatment
ALKYLATING AGENTS						
Busulfan (Myleran)[19,25,39]	No studies, but direct toxicity to epithelial lining cells is suggested	Pneumocyte dysplasia (degeneration of type I cells; atypical hyperplastic type II cells), mononuclear cell infiltration; fibrosis	4% incidence; no direct dose-dependent toxicity but may be threshold dose (>500 mg); radiation and other alkylating agents may enhance toxicity; insidious onset after 4 y (8 mo–10 y). May contribute to toxicity after bone marrow transplant. Dyspnea, cough, weight loss, weakness, fever; crepitant basilar rales; pigmentation.	Most common bibasilar reticular pattern; rarely, pleural effusion, pulmonary ossification, normal chest radiograph	Suggested by history and bizarre pneumocytes in sputum or lavage fluid. Definitive diagnosis by open lung biopsy.	Withdrawal of the drug; anecdotal reports of improvement with high-dose steroids. Prognosis poor. Mean survival after diagnosis is 5 mo.
Cyclophosphamide (Cytoxan)[19,25,40]	May be toxic through production of reactive oxygen species	Endothelial swelling; pneumocyte dysplasia; lymphocytic and histiocytic infiltration; fibrosis	<1% incidence; no direct dose dependence; synergy with oxygen and other agents possible. Acute symptoms occur early in course; subacute or chronic up to 8 y after initiation of therapy. Cough, dyspnea, fever; basilar rales.	Commonly bibasilar reticular pattern; diffuse pulmonary edema pattern also reported	As above.	Drug withdrawal; corticosteroids may hasten improvement but have no documented effect on mortality. Overall recovery approximately 65%.
Chlorambucil[19,25,41]	Unknown	Similar to busulfan; ranges from reversible interstitial to fatal fibrosis	Rare reports; subacute onset 5 mo–10 y after therapy. Cough, dyspnea, anorexia; bibasilar rales.	Bibasilar reticular pattern; rarely, normal radiograph; alveolar infiltrates not reported	As above.	Half of reported patients died despite cessation of drug and administration of steroids. Anecdotal reports of response to steroids.
Melphalan (Alkeran)[19,42]	Unknown	Similar to busulfan; pneumocyte dysplasia more common than fibrosis	Rare; appears 1–48 mo after therapy. Progressive dyspnea, productive cough, fever, malaise; bibasilar rales.	Reticular and alveolar infiltrates	As above.	Despite cessation of drug, 3 of 5 patients died of disease. In most cases, patients were receiving steroids for underlying disease.
ANTIBIOTICS						
Bleomycin[13–19,23,25,26,34]	Possible mechanisms include direct toxicity through generation of reactive oxygen metabolites and activated neutrophils; inflammation caused by alveolar macrophages producing TNF and IL-1β; increased collagen synthesis directly and via TGF-β release	Endothelial blebbing; interstitial edema, necrosis of type 1 cells and metaplastic type II cells; inflammation with polymorphonuclear cells; fibroblast proliferation and fibrosis; occasionally eosinophilic infiltration	Incidence up to 10%; common risk factors increasing age, higher doses, renal dysfunction, oxygen therapy, thoracic irradiation. Occurs during and up to 6 mo after stopping therapy. Cough, dyspnea, fever; tachypnea, crepitant rales. Hypersensitivity pneumonitis variant.	Bibasilar reticular pattern; multiple nodules similar to metastatic disease; acinar pattern, especially with hypersensitivity reaction; rarely, localized infiltrate and cavitary nodules	Bronchoalveolar lavage might suggest diagnosis (polymorphonuclear alveolitis). Transbronchial or open lung biopsy required for diagnosis, especially to rule out other causes.	Drug withdrawal. Hypersensitivity reactions, definite role for steroids; in other forms of bleomycin toxicity, efficacy less clear. Mortality between 3% and 50%.

Drug	Mechanism	Clinical Features/Incidence	Radiographic Pattern	Diagnosis	Treatment/Prognosis
Mitomycin[19,25,31,43]	Endothelial injury by alkylation of DNA; alveolar macrophage activation and cytokine release	Several patterns: similar to bleomycin; capillary leak with alveolar damage (especially with vinca alkaloid); capillary leak with thrombotic microangiopathy (related to total dose). 3–14% incidence; usually not dose related but possible synergy with oxygen, radiotherapy, and other agents. Dry cough, dyspnea; fever not seen; bibasilar rales. Acute dyspnea reaction with vinca alkaloids.	Diffuse interstitial and/or alveolar infiltrates; may be normal	Clinical picture suggestive; lung biopsy for definitive diagnosis.	Drug withdrawal; steroids may alter outcome. Mortality between 14% and 50%.
NITROSOUREAS[a]					
Carmustine (BCNU)[19,25,30]	Few studies; direct injury through generation of toxic oxidant molecules, perhaps due to depletion of the antioxidant glutathione	Similar to bleomycin; fibrosis predominates. 20–30% incidence; dose related; increased risk with preexisting lung disease and tobacco use; possible synergism with other agents; can be seen up to 17 y after drug stopped. Dry cough, dyspnea, bibasilar rales.	Bibasilar reticular pattern; >10-y posttreatment peripheral fibrosis pattern in upper lung zones; may be normal	Lung biopsy for definitive diagnosis; no bronchoalveolar lavage studies reported.	Recognition and withdrawal of the drug; steroids not beneficial if patient already on steroids for intracranial processes when toxicity develops. Mortality reported between 24% and 90%. Prognosis worse if patient treated before age 5 y. Steroids possibly beneficial acutely; after high-dose treatment.
ANTIMETABOLITES					
Methotrexate[19,20,25,44]	Direct toxic effect may play a role but mechanism not known; hypersensitivity suggested by occurrence of eosinophils and presence of increased T lymphocytes in lavage fluid	Interstitial and alveolar infiltration of lymphocytes, eosinophils, and plasma cells; occasionally poorly formed, noncaseating granuloma; fibrosis unusual. 2–8% incidence; synergism with other agents possible; occurs usually days to weeks after beginning therapy; acute: fever, chills, cough, malaise, headache; subacute: dyspnea, cough; rales common. Skin rash in 17% and blood eosinophilia in 40%; progression to fibrosis in 10%.	Early interstitial infiltrates; later, alveolar infiltrates; hilar and mediastinal adenopathy, pleural effusions described; chest radiograph can be normal	Clinical history suggestive; bronchoalveolar lavage might suggest diagnosis (increased T cells in fluid), but lung biopsy required for diagnosis.	Discontinue drug, but reports of reinstitution without recurrence of the abnormality. Dramatic responses to steroids reported. Mortality 1%; outlook favorable.
Cytosine arabinoside[45]	Unknown	Pulmonary edema; proteinaceous exudate with extravasation of red blood cells, no inflammatory cells. Abrupt onset of dyspnea; gastrointestinal toxicity coexists.	Diffuse interstitial and alveolar pattern	Clinical picture suggests diagnosis.	Supportive; no studies.
Gemcitabine[46]	—	Rare reports of diffuse alveolar damage; findings resemble ARDS. Does not appear dose dependent; dyspnea may be severe and progress to respiratory failure, chest tightness; dry cough, fine rales, low-grade fever.	Reticular nodular infiltrates or ground-glass opacities	Clinical suspicion; other causes should be excluded.	Withdraw drug; usually brisk response to corticosteroids but fatalities reported.
Fludarabine[12]	—	Rare reports of granulomas; diffuse nonspecific inflammation. Hypoxia, fever; produces decreases in CD4 cells.	Interstitial or nodular infiltrates	Associated with *Pneumocystis* so must rule out infection.	Discontinue drug; probable response to steroids.

(continued)

TABLE 54.3-1. (Continued)

Drug	Mechanism of Injury	Histopathology	Clinical Features	Chest Roentgenogram	Diagnosis	Treatment
TAXANES						
Paclitaxel (Taxol)[25,47,48]	Two types of reaction: "anaphylactoid hypersensitivity" (AH), direct mast-cell activation with histamine release; suspension vehicle (Cremophor El) causes, not the drug	No data	AH: 3–10% incidence; erythematous rash, urticaria, hypotension, dyspnea with or without bronchospasm in close proximity to infusion; rare reports and little data; no dose dependency known.	AH: normal chest radiograph	AH: clinical picture highly suggestive.	AH: slow infusion; pretreatment with corticosteroid; H₁ and H₂ histamine blockers.
	Hypersensitivity pneumonitis (HP) mechanism not known, may be due to release of histamine or other vasoactive	Little data; BAL lymphocytic alveolitis; biopsy mononuclear cells with septal thickening	HP: dyspnea and/or cough several days to weeks after treatment; fever may occur; crepitant rales or normal chest exam.	HP: patchy reticular or nodular infiltrates	HP: clinical picture should raise suspicion; other causes (e.g., infection, progression of disease) should be excluded.	HP: can resolve on its own; if severe, corticosteroids; may not recur with rechallenge.
Docetaxel (Taxotere)[25,49]	—	Little data; diffuse alveolar damage	Rare reports; fever, malaise, dyspnea.	Diffuse infiltrates	Clinical suspicion excludes other causes, especially infection.	Of four reported cases two died; two recovered with steroids.
MISCELLANEOUS						
Procarbazine (Matulane)[19,25]	Hypersensitivity	Mononuclear cell infiltration and scattered foci of eosinophils; fibrosis in one case	Acute onset within hours to days of first dose. Nausea, fever, chills, arthralgias, urticaria, dry cough, and dyspnea. Blood eosinophilia.	Interstitial infiltrates; pleural effusion	Clinical picture highly suggestive of diagnosis.	Rapid recovery after discontinuation of drug. Role of steroids not known.
Vinca alkaloids (vinblastine and vindesine)[19,31]	Unknown	Dysplasia of alveolar lining cells; interstitial and alveolar influx of inflammatory cells; fibrosis	Acute dyspnea during or shortly after the infusion, especially when given in combination with mitomycin. Wheezing may be prominent.	Diffuse interstitial and alveolar infiltrates with combination drugs; normal chest radiograph with vinca alkaloid alone	Clinical history suggests diagnosis.	Drug withdrawal; steroids probably beneficial. Prognosis poor if pulmonary infiltrates develop.
Etoposide (VP-16)[29]	Unknown	Alveolar hemorrhage	Case report of fatal toxicity after high-dose chemotherapy with bone marrow or stem cell transplant for breast cancer.	Interstitial and alveolar pattern; may be localized	Clinical picture suggestive.	Discontinue drug; some responses to steroids.

ARDS, adult respiratory distress syndrome; BAL, bronchoalveolar lavage; IL, interleukin; TGF, transforming growth factor; TNF, tumor necrosis factor.
[a]Pulmonary toxicity has been reported with all other nitrosoureas, including lomustine (CCNU), semustine (methyl-CCNU), and chlorozotocin (DCNU).

a polymorphonuclear alveolitis.[20,24] Eosinophil infiltration and granulomatous inflammation have been associated with drugs that cause apparent hypersensitivity reactions, such as methotrexate, procarbazine, and bleomycin.[19,20,22]

CLINICAL FEATURES

Table 54.3-2 lists predisposing factors associated with enhancement of drug-induced pulmonary toxicity.[19,25] Because bleomycin toxicity is relatively common, it deserves special mention. Although toxicity drastically increases with doses in excess of 450 to 500 mg, it can occur with much lower doses, especially when other risk factors are present. A study described 9 of 45 patients (20%) in whom lung toxicity developed when they received bleomycin after cisplatin infusion.[26] Renal damage after cisplatin administration, with subsequent accumulation of bleomycin, was a likely cause of the high pulmonary toxicity and mortality of 67%. Extreme caution is recommended in the administration of combined bleomycin and cisplatin chemotherapy; if possible, bleomycin should precede cisplatin infusion to minimize the risk. Some data suggest that continuous infusion of bleomycin may be associated with less pulmonary toxicity than bolus therapy[19]; however, these data are inconclusive, and further studies are warranted. Although supplemental oxygen has been a classic cofactor in bleomycin pulmonary toxicity, there are no large controlled studies.[19] An increased risk of pulmonary toxicity (4 of 12 patients, fatal in 3 of 4) was described in a small uncontrolled study of patients receiving granulocyte colony-stimulating factor in combination with bleomycin-containing chemotherapy [BACOP (bleomycin, doxorubicin, cyclophosphamide, vincristine, and prednisone)] for non-Hodgkin's lymphoma.[27] Animal studies suggest that granulocyte colony-stimulating factor may enhance migration of neutrophils to vascular spaces and promote their adhesion to already injured endothelial cells potentiating proinflammatory cytokine expression.[28]

Interest in administration of several cycles of high-dose chemotherapy followed by peripheral stem cell rescue for treatment

TABLE 54.3-2. Factors Associated with Increased Risk of Drug-Induced Pulmonary Toxicity

Risk Factors	Drugs
Total dose	Bleomycin
	Carmustine
Advanced age	Bleomycin
	Carmustine
Oxygen therapy	Bleomycin
	Cyclophosphamide
	Mitomycin
Simultaneous or prior radiation therapy to lungs	Bleomycin
	Busulfan
	Mitomycin
	Gemcitabine
Increased toxicity when given with other drugs	Carmustine
	Mitomycin
	Cyclophosphamide
	Bleomycin
	Methotrexate
	Etoposide
Preexisting pulmonary disease	Carmustine

of breast cancer and lymphoma has led to reports of pulmonary toxicity for agents not thought previously to be highly toxic to the lung, such as etoposide.[29] Importantly, careful studies of pulmonary function after high-dose chemotherapy containing cyclophosphamide/cisplatin/BCNU (carmustine) followed by autologous bone marrow transplant for treatment of breast cancer show a delayed drop in diffusing capacity averaging 30% by week 18.[30] The majority of patients were symptomatic with dyspnea and responded well to systemic corticosteroids. More of this type of toxicity can be anticipated in the future as this treatment modality becomes more common and new regimens for high-dose chemotherapy are studied.

Long intervals between drug administration and onset of clinical toxicity have been described. Late-onset pulmonary fibrosis has been reported many years after cyclophosphamide and carmustine are discontinued.[19,25]

Signs and Symptoms

The cardinal symptom of drug-induced pulmonary toxicity is dyspnea. Nonproductive cough, fatigue, and malaise are other commonly associated complaints. Other characteristics of chemotherapy-induced pulmonary disease are outlined in Table 54.3-1. Although symptoms usually develop over a period of several weeks to months, hypersensitivity drug-induced lung disease can develop over hours. Fever may be a common finding with this type of toxicity. Chest pain has been reported during infusion of bleomycin or immediately after therapy with methotrexate[19,22]; however, it is an unusual manifestation of toxicity. A syndrome of acute dyspnea, probably due to direct toxicity to the pulmonary vasculature, can occur during or shortly after vinca alkaloid infusion when given in combination with mitomycin for treatment of non–small cell lung cancer.[31] Because hemoptysis is an uncommon feature of drug-induced pulmonary toxicity, when it is present, other diagnoses should be considered. Physical examination of the lungs may be normal or may reveal end-inspiratory "velcro" rales. Finger clubbing is distinctly unusual, but it may be related to the underlying malignancy.

All-*trans*-retinoic acid treatment of leukemias can induce the retinoic acid syndrome, which consists of fever; dyspnea; weight gain; pulmonary infiltrates; pleural or pericardial effusions, or both; hypotension; renal dysfunction; and leukocytosis.[32] The pulmonary disorder is thought to be mediated by newly differentiated leukemia cells marginating into the pulmonary circulation, increasing capillary permeability and releasing cytokines that induce neutrophil migration into the interstitium. High doses of corticosteroids are the most effective treatment, and steroid prophylaxis has been reported to be useful.

Diagnostic Imaging

The most common radiographic abnormality associated with drug-induced pulmonary toxicity is a reticulonodular or interstitial pattern, or both, which may be basilar or diffuse. Pleural effusions are uncommon but have occasionally been reported in association with mitomycin, busulfan, methotrexate, and procarbazine toxicity.[19,25] Hypersensitivity lung disease associated with methotrexate and procarbazine may present with bilateral acinar infiltrates that clear rapidly.[19] In some instances, the chest radiograph is normal, even in the presence of histologically proven pulmonary infiltration and fibrosis.[19] Most commonly, methotrexate and carmustine toxicity have been reported, with normal chest radiographic findings. Hilar adenopathy is distinctly unusual and has been reported only with methotrexate toxicity.[19] Cavitating and noncavitating nodules, simulating metastatic disease, have been seen with bleomycin toxicity.[19]

High-resolution thin-section CT chest scans and gallium scintigraphy have been shown to be more sensitive techniques than chest radiography to detect pulmonary parenchymal changes in association with drug toxicity. High-resolution chest CT scans can show diffuse areas of ground-glass opacities, poorly defined areas of nodular consolidation, and centrilobular nodules.[33] Although these changes can be seen when the radiograph is normal, they are not specific for drug-induced toxicity. Magnetic resonance spectrometry may eventually be useful to differentiate among fibrosis, edema, and hemorrhage in the lung, but at present it has not been helpful to diagnose interstitial lung disorders, including drug toxicity.

Pulmonary Function Tests

The most common abnormalities associated with chemotherapy-induced pulmonary toxicity are a reduced diffusing capacity for carbon monoxide and a restrictive ventilatory defect.[19] Isolated gas transport abnormalities manifested by a decrease in the diffusing capacity or arterial hypoxemia, or both, especially with exercise, have been seen. Screening pulmonary function tests to predict which patients receiving chemotherapy are likely to develop toxicity would be helpful but have not been established. In bleomycin toxicity, changes in the diffusing capacity may be transient, whereas decreases in total lung capacity seem to correlate better with radiographic abnormalities.[33]

DIAGNOSIS

Although one might have a high clinical suspicion of drug-induced pulmonary toxicity, lung biopsy is usually necessary for a definitive diagnosis. Because pathognomonic pathologic changes associated with drug-induced pneumonitis are often not present, a biopsy is necessary to eliminate other specific diagnoses, such as opportunistic infection and malignancy. Through the use of bronchoalveolar lavage, several studies reported the presence of a characteristic or predominant cell associated with particular drugs.[20,24] Although these data might be of value in understanding the pathogenesis of drug-induced lung disorders, their usefulness in diagnosing drug toxicity is limited.

A serum marker for drug-induced pulmonary toxicity would be very useful, but none currently exists. Although elevated levels of TGF-β in plasma after high-dose chemotherapy for breast cancer predicted an increased risk of pulmonary toxicity after autologous bone marrow transplantation, its clinical applicability has been limited.[35]

TREATMENT

The most effective way to manage pulmonary toxicity associated with chemotherapeutic agents is to prevent it. Animal studies of bleomycin toxicity showed a beneficial preventative effect of dietary supplementation with taurine and niacin; no comparable human studies have been reported. If toxicity occurs, withdrawal of the offending agent is the cornerstone of therapy. Although no controlled studies in humans have systematically examined the efficacy of corticosteroids, a trial of these agents is probably warranted in most cases. The optimal dose and duration of therapy are not known; however, 1 mg/kg/d is usually initiated with a slow and careful tapering schedule because clinical deterioration after tapering has been reported. The use of lung transplant in the treatment of advanced drug-induced pulmonary fibrosis should be considered in appropriate patients. One report described the case of a 23-year-old male patient who underwent a single lung transplant because of presumed drug-induced pulmonary fibrosis 12 years after undergoing chemotherapy for acute lymphocytic leukemia.[36]

FUTURE ENDEAVORS

Several unique treatment modalities are being investigated for patients with advanced, drug-resistant, and/or surgically refractory malignancies involving the lungs. These include hyperthermic lung perfusion with high doses of cisplatin, particularly for patients with isolated lung metastasis or bronchoalveolar cancer. In one study of patients with metastatic lung sarcoma, four treated patients developed noncardiogenic pulmonary edema but survived and were disease free 13 months after treatment.[37] Delivering chemotherapeutic agents directly to the lungs by nebulization holds promise as well.[38] A few human trials have been completed and suggest that aerosol therapies have potential to shrink pulmonary metastasis from certain cancers. For example, survival in some patients with metastatic renal cell cancer has been prolonged with aerosolized chemotherapy. Although these therapies may avoid systemic toxicity, they have the potential to cause direct toxicity to the lungs. More information is needed to delineate their efficacy and toxicity in the treatment of cancer localized to the lungs.

REFERENCES

1. Hill RP, Rodemann HP, Hendry JH, et al. Normal tissue radiobiology: from the laboratory to the clinic. *Int J Radiat Oncol Biol Phys* 2001;49:353.
2. Araya J, Maruyama M, Sassa K, et al. Ionizing radiation enhances matrix metalloproteinase-2 production in human lung epithelial cells. *Am J Physiol Lung Cell Mol Physiol* 2001;280:L30.
3. Armstrong J, Burman C, Leibel S, et al. Conformal three dimensional treatment planning may improve the therapeutic ratio of high dose radiation therapy for lung cancer. *Int J Radiat Oncol Biol Phys* 1993;26:695.
4. Graham MV, Purdy JA, Emami B, et al. Clinical dose-volume histogram analysis for pneumonitis after 3D treatment for non–small cell lung cancer (NSCLC). *Int J Radiat Oncol Biol Phys* 1999;45:323.
5. Nagata Y, Takayama K, Aoki T, et al. Clinical outcome of 3-D conformal hypofractionated high-dose radiotherapy for primary and secondary lung cancer using a stereotactic technique. *Int J Radiat Oncol Biol Phys* 2003;57:S280.
6. Ciernik IF, Dizendorf E, Baumert BG, et al. Radiation treatment planning with an integrated positron emission and computer tomography (PET/CT): a feasibility study. *Int J Radiat Oncol Biol Phys* 2003;57:853.
7. McDonald S, Rubin P, Phillips TL, et al. Injury to the lung from cancer therapy: clinical syndromes, measurable endpoints, and potential scoring systems. *Int J Radiat Oncol Biol Phys* 1995;31:1187.
8. De Jaeger K, Seppenwoolde Y, Boersma LJ, et al. Pulmonary function following high-dose radiotherapy of non–small-cell lung cancer. *Int J Radiat Oncol Biol Phys* 2003;55:1331.
9. Rubin P, Casarett GW. *Clinical radiation pathology.* Philadelphia: WB Saunders, 1968.
10. Antonadou D, Throuvalas N, Petridis A, et al. Effect of amifostine on toxicities associated with radiochemotherapy in patients with locally advanced non–small-cell lung cancer. *Int J Radiat Oncol Biol Phys* 2003;57:402.
11. Stover DE, Milite F, Zakowski M. A newly recognized syndrome—radiation related bronchiolitis obliterans and organizing pneumonia. A case report and literature review. *Respiration* 2001;68:540.
12. Helman DL, Byrd JC, Ales NC, et al. Fludarabine-related pulmonary toxicity. A distinct clinical entity in chronic lymphoproliferative syndromes. *Chest* 2002;122:785.

13. Sakanashi Y, Takeya M, Yoshimura T, et al. Kinetics of macrophage subpopulations and expression of monocyte chemoattractant protein-1 (MCP-1) in bleomycin-induced lung injury of rats studied by a novel monoclonal antibody against rat MCP-1. *J Leukocyte Biol* 1994;56:741.

14. Herman EH, Hasinoff BB, Zhang J, et al. Morphologic and morphometric evaluation of the effect of ICRF-187 on bleomycin-induced pulmonary toxicity. *Toxicology* 1995;98:163.

15. Freeman BA, Crapo JD. Biology of disease: free radicals and tissue injury. *Lab Invest* 1982;47:412.

16. Lewis RA, Austen KF. The biologically active leukotrienes: biosynthesis, metabolism, receptors. functions and pharmacology. *J Clin Invest* 1984;73:889.

17. Khalil N, Whitman C, Zuo L, et al. Regulation of alveolar macrophage transforming growth factor-beta secretion by corticosteroids in bleomycin-induced pulmonary inflammation in the rat. *J Clin Invest* 1993;92:1812.

18. Chandler DB. Possible mechanisms of bleomycin induced fibrosis. *Clin Chest Med* 1990; 11:21.

19. Cooper JAD, White DA, Matthay RA. Drug-induced pulmonary disease. I. Cytotoxic drugs. *Am Rev Respir Dis* 1986;133:321.

20. White DA, Rankin JR, Stover DE, et al. Methotrexate pneumonitis: lavage findings suggest an immune mediated disorder. *Am Rev Respir Dis* 1989; 139:18.

21. King SL, Lichtler AC, Rowe DW, et al. Bleomycin stimulates pro-alpha 1 (I) collagen promoter through transforming growth factor beta response element by intracellular and extracellular signaling. *J Biol Chem* 1994;269:13156.

22. Jules-Elysee K, White DA. Bleomycin induced pulmonary toxicity. *Clin Chest Med* 1990;11:1.

23. Ferrando AA, Pendas AM, Llano E, et al. Gene characterization, promoter analysis, and chromosomal localization of human bleomycin hydrolase. *J Biol Chem* 1997;272: 33298.

24. White DA, Kris MG, Stover DE. Bronchoalveolar lavage cell populations in bleomycin-induced pulmonary toxicity. *Thorax* 1987;42:551.

25. *Drug induced pulmonary disease, 2003 UptoDate.* World Wide Web URL: http://www.uptodate.com, 2003.

26. Rabinowits M, Souhami L, Gil RA, et al. Increased pulmonary toxicity with bleomycin and cisplatin chemotherapy combinations. *Am J Clin Oncol* 1990;13:132.

27. Lei KI, Leung WT, Johnson PJ. Serious pulmonary complications in patients receiving recombinant granulocyte colony-stimulating factor during BACOP chemotherapy for aggressive non-Hodgkin's lymphoma. *Br J Cancer* 1994;70:1009.

28. Azoulay E, Herigault S, Levame M, et al. Effect of granulocyte colony stimulating factor on bleomycin-induced acute lung injury and pulmonary fibrosis. *Crit Care Med* 2003; 31:1442.

29. Crilley P, Toposlsky D, Styler MJ, et al. Extramedullary toxicity of a conditioning regimen containing busulphan, cyclophosphamide, and etoposide in 84 patients underlying autologous and allogeneic bone marrow transplantation. *Bone Marrow Transplant* 1995; 15:361.

30. Wilczynski SW, Erasmus JJ, Petros WP, et al. Delayed pulmonary toxicity syndrome following high dose chemotherapy and bone marrow transplantation for breast cancer. *Am J Respir Crit Care Med* 1998;157:565.

31. Rivera MP, Kris MG, Gralla RJ, et al. Syndrome of acute dyspnea related to combined mitomycin plus vinca alkaloid chemotherapy. *Am J Clin Oncol* 1995;18:245.

32. Vahdat I, Maslak P, Miller W, et al. Early mortality and the retinoic acid syndrome in acute promyelocytic leukemia. *Blood* 1994;87:3843.

33. Rossi SE, Erasmus JJ, McAdams HP, et al. Pulmonary drug toxicity: radiologic and pathologic manifestations. *Radiographics* 2000;20:1245.

34. Wolkowicz J, Sturgeon J, Rawji M, et al. Bleomycin-induced pulmonary function abnormalities. *Chest* 1992;101:97.

35. Anscher MS, Peters WP, Reisenbichler H, et al. Transforming growth factor beta as a predictor of liver and lung fibrosis after autologous bone marrow transplantation for advanced breast cancer. *N Engl J Med* 1993;328:1592.

36. Gossman RF, Frost A, Zamel N, et al. Results of single lung transplantation for bilateral pulmonary fibrosis. *N Engl J Med* 1990;322:727.

37. Schroder C, Fisher S, Pieck AC, et al. Technique and results of hyperthermic (41 degree C) isolated lung perfusions with high doses of cisplatin for the treatment of surgically relapsing or unresectable lung sarcoma metastasis. *Eur J Cardiothorac Surg* 2002;22:41.

38. Rao RD, Markovic SN, Anderson PM. Aerosol therapy for malignancy involving the lungs. *Curr Cancer Drug Targets* 2003;3:239.

39. Ghalie R, Reynolds J, Valentino LA, et al. Busulfan-containing pre-transplant regimens for the treatment of solid tumors. *Bone Marrow Transplant* 1994;14:437.

40. Malik SE, Myer JL, DeRemee RA, Speeks U. Lung toxicity associated with cyclophosphamide. Two distinct patterns. *Am J Respir Crit Care Med* 1996;154:1851.

41. Khong AT, McCarthy J. Chlorambucil induced pulmonary disease: a case report and review of the literature. *Am Hematol* 1998;77:85.

42. Goucher C, Rowland V, Hawkins J. Melphalan-induced pulmonary interstitial fibrosis. *Chest* 1980;77:805.

43. Linette DC, McGee KH, McFarland JA. Mitomycin induced pulmonary toxicity: case report and review of the literature. *Ann Pharmacol Ther* 1992;26:481.

44. Imokawa S, Colby TR, Leslie KO, Hemers RA. Methotrexate pneumonitis: review of the literature and histopathologic findings in nine patients. *Eur Respir J* 2000;15:373.

45. Haupt HM, Hutchins CM, Moore CW. Ara-C lung: noncardiogenic pulmonary edema complicating cytosine arabinoside therapy of leukemia. *Am J Med* 1981;70:256.

46. Gupta N, Ahmed I, Steinberg H, et al. Gemcitabine-induced pulmonary toxicity case report and review of the literature. *Am J Clin Oncol* 2002;25:97.

47. Weiss RB, Donehower RC, Wiernik PH, et al. Hypersensitivity reactions from Taxol. *J Clin Oncol* 1990;8:1263.

48. Ramanathan RK, Reddy VU, Holbert JM, et al. Pulmonary infiltrates following administration of paclitaxel. *Chest* 1996;110:289.

49. Read WL, Mortimer JE, Picus J. Severe interstitial pneumonitis associated with docetaxel administration. *Cancer* 2002;94:847.

SECTION 4

JOACHIM YAHALOM
CAROL S. PORTLOCK

Cardiac Toxicity

Many chemotherapeutic and biologic agents as well as mediastinal irradiation have been reported to have adverse effects on the heart.[1,2] The most important of these drugs [anthracyclines, mitoxantrone; cyclophosphamide (CTX), ifosfamide; paclitaxel, docetaxel; trastuzumab; and 5-fluorouracil (5-FU)] as well as mediastinal irradiation are discussed in detail. All others are listed in Table 54.4-1.

ANTHRACYCLINES

A rare, but reversible, acute cardiotoxicity and a delayed, but irreversible, dilated cardiomyopathy occur with anthracycline therapy. The acute toxicity presents as a myocarditis, with or without pericarditis, and may result in transient congestive heart failure (CHF)/arrhythmias. It is rarely a fatal complication of anthracycline therapy.

The delayed cardiomyopathy presents clinically as fatigue, dyspnea on exertion, orthopnea, sinus tachycardia, S3 gallop rhythm, pedal edema/pleural effusions, and elevated jugular venous distention. These classic features of CHF are late manifestations and may be quite subtle at onset. With awareness of the cardiac risk, anthracycline cardiomyopathy can be potentially avoided by several measures: recognizing risk factors, early detection, limiting total cumulative dose, and, more recently, using cardioprotective agents or modified and infusional drug regimens. Each of these is discussed below:

The risk of anthracycline cardiomyopathy is dependent on cumulative dose received.[3] A 5% risk is seen at 450 mg/m² for doxorubicin, 900 mg/m² for daunorubicin, 935 mg/m² for epirubicin, and 223 mg/m² for idarubicin. Cofactors for cardiotoxic risk include mediastinal irradiation, which includes the heart, older (particularly older than 70 years) or younger (younger than 15 years) age, coronary artery disease (CAD), other valvular or myocardial conditions, and hypertension. Trastuzumab appears to potentiate anthracycline cardiotoxicity, and other agents that have independent cardiac effects may be additive.

The diagnosis of anthracycline cardiac dysfunction (CD) is generally made by comparing baseline with serial left ventricular function studies using radionuclide imaging or echocardiography, or both. A left ventricular ejection fraction (LVEF) of

TABLE 54.4-1.   Uncommon Cardiovascular Toxicities

Drug	Incidence (%)	Cardiovascular Effects	Onset
Amsacrine	1	H, AR, VR, CHF	Acute, subacute
Busulfan	2	CHF	Late
Carmustine	Rare	H, AR, CP	Acute
Cisplatin	Rare	H, AR, VR, CP	Acute
Cytarabine	Rare	AR, VR, CP, P, CHF	Acute, subacute
Etoposide	1–2	H	Acute
	Rare	CP, MI	—
Interferon	Rare	H, AR, CP, MI, CHF	Acute, subacute
Interleukin-2	Dose dependent	H, AR, CP, MI	Acute, subacute
Mechlorethamine	Rare	AR	Subacute
Mitomycin[a]	10	CHF	—
Pentostatin	3–10	AR, VR, CP, MI, CHF	Subacute
Teniposide	2	H	Acute
Tretinoin[b]	14–23	H, AR	Acute, subacute
	3–6	CP, MI, P, CHF	Acute, subacute
Vinca alkaloids	10	H	Acute, subacute
	Rare	?MI	—

AR, atrial arrhythmia; CHF, congestive heart failure; CP, chest pain; H, hypotension; MI, myocardial infarction; P, pericarditis; VR, ventricular arrhythmia.
[a]In association with anthracyclines.
[b]Retinoic acid syndrome.
(From refs. 1 and 2, with permission.)

50% or greater is considered within normal range by either method. A low LVEF is a contraindication for anthracycline therapy.

Echocardiograms can also evaluate other aspects of cardiac performance as well as anatomic changes. Typical findings are left ventricular diastolic dysfunction and, later, LV systolic dysfunction, particularly affecting the septal motion. The left ventricle is initially not enlarged or only moderately enlarged; there may be a posteriorly directed mitral insufficiency jet and preservation of right ventricular function. With full development of cardiomyopathy, there is global hypokinesis and muscle wall thinning.

The electrocardiogram (ECG) findings associated with anthracycline CD include sinus tachycardia, low voltage, poor R-wave progression, and nonspecific T-wave changes. Even sinus tachycardia alone is a relatively late finding, such that serial ECGs are of little value in early detection.

In pediatrics, it is important to be aware that conduction disturbances (second-degree atrioventricular block) and arrhythmias (supraventricular and ventricular) may be detected during therapy but have no known acute/chronic consequence; subclinical CD is probably more common than in adults at comparable doses (15.5% to 27.8% at greater than 300 mg/m^2 doxorubicin). The relationship between a decrease in LVEF and the later development of dilated cardiomyopathy has not been fully established in the pediatric population, and no threshold cumulative dose has been identified below which LV dysfunction is not seen.[4–7]

Early detection of CD is important in preventing overt cardiomyopathy. Conventional methods include measurement of LVEF by radionuclide imaging or echocardiography during therapy. In a small prospective study, Nousianen et al.[8] reported that it was possible to distinguish patients likely to develop CD from others by LVEF measures at baseline and at 200 mg/m^2 doxorubicin. A fall of 10% or greater at this low cumulative dose had 72% specificity and 90% sensitivity in detecting later CD.

Mitani et al.[9] have examined the strategy of serial LVEF retrospectively and demonstrated that the overall costs of early detection were less than the medical costs of overt CHF management.

Investigational methods of CD detection include measurement of serial diastolic pressures with gated radionuclide or echocardiogram function studies; serum cardiac troponin T levels (a measure of active myocardial myocyte necrosis); and levels of brain natriuretic peptide (BNP), a peptide synthesized in the ventricles correlating with degree of heart failure.[10]

BNP levels appear to hold the greatest promise, because BNP is a simple plasma marker and may correlate with subclinical LV diastolic dysfunction. Several other methods of detection are available but are cumbersome and are rarely used; these include nuclear imaging with the labeled monoclonal antibody; indium 111 antimyosin or radiolabeled metaiodobenzyl guanidine, an analogue of norepinephrine; and percutaneous endomyocardial biopsy of the right ventricle, which may demonstrate characteristic histologic features (loss of myofibrils, distention of the sarcoplasmic reticulum, and vacuolization of the cytoplasm).[11]

In summary, anthracycline CD can be prevented by early detection. All patients should have a baseline measure of LVEF. For doxorubicin, poor-risk patients should have a repeat study at 200 mg/m^2, and all patients should have a follow-up study at 300 to 400 mg/m^2 and every 50 to 100 mg/m^2 thereafter.

Aside from early detection, other strategies that may reduce CD risk are use of anthracycline analogues (this remains controversial, as all analogues cause CD at equimolar doses), low-dose or infusional drug schedules in an attempt to reduce peak drug dose delivery, and the use of liposomal formulations. The iron-chelating cardioprotectant, dexrazoxane, decreases the risk of clinical CD in patients who have received doxorubicin doses of 300 mg/m^2 or greater.[12] The American Society of Clinical Oncology[13] recommends its use in this setting but does not advocate dexrazoxane in the adjuvant setting, when doxorubicin cumulative dose is less than 300 mg/m^2, in pediatrics, or in high-risk patients. The

American Society of Clinical Oncology also cautions dexrazoxane's use when doxorubicin therapy is anticipated to prolong survival. Clinical data are also insufficient to recommend dexrazoxane with other anthracyclines, except epirubicin in metastatic breast cancer. Other cardioprotectants under investigation are probucol, a vitamin E derivative, and melatonin. These and other candidate cardioprotectants are free radical scavengers.

The management of anthracycline CD is that of other causes of dilated cardiomyopathy.[14] Angiotensin-converting enzyme inhibitors, β-blockers, and diuretics are commonly used. As pointed out in long-term pediatric studies, these agents do not cure or permanently control the CD. Rather, the cardiomyopathy may become progressive in spite of these agents after more than 5 years. The only curative therapy at this time is cardiac transplantation.

The mechanism of anthracycline CD is not fully elucidated. It appears to be caused by the production of free radicals generated during cardiomyocyte metabolism of the anthracycline. Membrane lipid peroxidation is a consequent effect that leads to tissue damage. It is thought that free radicals are generated by enzymatic reduction of the anthracycline quinone ring and by formation of iron-anthracycline complexes. The intrinsic antioxidant defense of the cardiomyocyte is more limited than other organs, leading to its apparent selective toxicity profile.[15] Miranda et al.[16] have reported a knockout mouse model suggesting that a deficiency of the HFE gene (associated with hereditary hemochromatosis) confers increased susceptibility to doxorubicin CD. They studied wild-type, HFE (+/−), and HFE (−/−) mice that were chronically treated with doxorubicin. Survival was significantly decreased in the HFE-negative mice, and cardiac iron concentration was significantly elevated. Moreover, cardiac ultrastructural changes demonstrated iron-associated mitochondrial damage. These authors have suggested that HFE mutation screening may hold promise for identifying high-risk patients in the future.

MITOXANTRONE

Mitoxantrone is an anthracenedione, structurally related to the anthracyclines. Although it was initially thought not to be cardiotoxic, mitoxantrone is now known to cause a dose-related CD similar to anthracyclines. In cancer patients, retrospective experience reveals an incidence of CHF or decrease in LVEF (below normal or 10% or greater below baseline) in approximately 2% to 4% of patients.[17,18] Risk factors for CD include prior exposure to anthracyclines and cumulative dose of mitoxantrone. In patients with multiple sclerosis,[19] in whom mitoxantrone is used for relapsing/progressive disease, a retrospective review revealed 2 of 1378 patients with symptomatic CHF and 2.18% with asymptomatic fall of LVEF below 50%.

As a single drug in anthracycline-naive patients, mitoxantrone CD is rarely seen before 100 mg/m² cumulative dose. It is generally recommended that LVEF be monitored regularly thereafter and that a total dose of 140 mg/m² not be exceeded. When used after doxorubicin, CD is more frequent. An analysis by the Southwest Oncology Group[17] revealed a risk of 6% at 134 mg/m² prior doxorubicin and 60 mg/m² mitoxantrone, rising to a 15% risk at 120 mg/m² mitoxantrone. The mechanism of mitoxantrone CD is not fully elucidated but appears to involve iron chelates as with anthracyclines.[20]

CYCLOPHOSPHAMIDE

The classic cardiac toxicity of CTX is an acute myopericarditis associated with high-dose therapy (HDT). In the era of stem cell transplantation and vigorous hydration, irreversible hemorrhagic myonecrosis is rare. More commonly, an acute/subacute CHF develops that is generally reversible with medical management.

CTX is hepatic metabolized (cytochrome P-450 dependent) to the active drug, and it has been shown that more rapid CTX metabolism is associated with an increased risk of CHF. Ayash et al.[21] demonstrated an inverse correlation of CTX area under the curve with tumor response and CHF in the HDT of metastatic breast cancer. These investigators have suggested that CTX total dose, schedule of administration, and activation kinetics (affected by liver metabolism heterogeneity of cytochrome P-450 or concurrent drug exposures, or both) all play a role in the development of cardiotoxicity.

Prospective monitoring of 16 patients during CTX high-dose administration (7 g/m²) was reported by Morandi et al.[22] Serial enzymes (creatine phosphokinase, creatine phosphokinase–MB, and troponin I) did not become elevated using a fractionated drug administration schedule over 13 hours. The only positive findings were four cases of transient, mild diastolic and systolic LV dysfunction. Snowden et al.[23] measured serial plasma BNP in eight patients receiving CTX-based preparative regimens. Six had BNP elevations noted, beginning 1 week after treatment and recovering by week 5, and the highest BNP levels correlated with transient CHF.

Finally, Schrama et al.[24] reported their results of early and late cardiac toxicity with CTC, a CTX-based high-dose regimen used in doxorubicin-naive patients. Transient CHF developed in 6 of 100. No acute cardiotoxic fatalities occurred; late cardiotoxicity was not seen except in those who required anthracycline salvage. Thus, with current administration guidelines used with HDT, CTX cardiotoxicity is uncommon (less than 10% of patients treated), generally transient, and reversible.

IFOSFAMIDE

Ifosfamide is a congener of CTX with similar alkylating agent properties. Because of potential chemical cystitis, it is always administered with mesna. Like CTX, ifosfamide may cause a dose-related CHF, which is generally transient and reversible. Quezado et al.[25] reported no CHF at 10 g/m² (0 of 6 patients), but at 16 g/m² or greater, CHF was more common (6 of 15 patients). Clinical symptoms developed subacutely (mean, 12 days; range, 6 to 23 days) and resolved with medical management. No evidence has been shown that mesna has any cardioprotective effect for CTX or ifosfamide.

TAXANES

PACLITAXEL

The taxanes (paclitaxel and docetaxel) are important antimicrotubule agents derived from the yew tree (paclitaxel, *Taxus brevifolia*; docetaxel, *Taxus baccata*). The yew tree is known to be poisonous, and the taxine alkaloid fraction can affect cardiac conduction and automaticity. Although not fully proven, the mechanism of paclitaxel cardiotoxicity appears to be related to its taxane ring structural similarities to yew taxine.

The cardiovascular effects of paclitaxel are multiple: Asymptomatic bradycardia can be documented in almost one-third of patients, hypersensitivity reactions are associated with the cremophor EL diluent (which can be ameliorated with corticosteroids and histamine H_1- and H_2-receptor antagonists), and, most importantly, life-threatening atrial and/or ventricular rhythm disturbances and/or conduction abnormalities occur in approximately 0.5% of patients. Rare ischemic events have also been reported.

The life-threatening arrhythmias may occur acutely during infusion or subacutely up to 14 days after treatment. These tend to occur after two or more treatment exposures rather than with initial therapy. Unlike anthracyclines, paclitaxel does not appear to have a cumulative dosing threshold or limit.

In a summary review of adverse grade 4 and 5 cardiac events compiled by the National Cancer Institute,[26] atrial arrhythmias (tachycardia, flutter, and/or fibrillation) occurred in 0.24%, ventricular arrhythmias (tachycardia/fibrillation) in 0.26%, heart block in 0.11%, and ischemia in 0.29%. Paclitaxel does not appear to cause CHF. However, it has often been reported to potentiate doxorubicin-associated CHF.

Most recently, several groups have tested this question prospectively in metastatic breast cancer. Giordano et al.[27] studied 82 doxorubicin/taxane-naive patients receiving doxorubicin, 60 mg/m², followed by a 1- or 3-hour paclitaxel, 200 mg/m², infusion. This AT [doxorubicin (Adriamycin), paclitaxel (Taxol)] regimen was administered every 21 days for six to seven cycles. The LVEF fell a median of 10% (to 52.5%), with a cumulative doxorubicin dose of 310 to 360 mg/m². Biganzoli et al.[28] performed a phase III trial comparing AT [doxorubicin (60 mg/m²) followed by paclitaxel (175 mg/m² in 3-hour infusion)] versus doxorubicin/CTX (AC; 60/600 mg/m²) in 375 patients. Treatment was repeated every 3 weeks for six cycles (maximum doxorubicin, 360 mg/m²). Overt CHF was not statistically different in the two study arms (3% vs. 1%; $P = .62$). However, a fall in LVEF (10% or greater fall from baseline or 5% or greater drop below the normal range) was significantly more frequent for AT (27%) versus AC (14%). Moreover, the risk of LVEF fall was significantly greater for AT than AC at every cumulative doxorubicin dose level above 180 mg/m². In both of these studies, paclitaxel was administered within 30 minutes of preceding doxorubicin. Other groups have reported minimal cardiotoxicity when the interval between doxorubicin was 4 to 24 hours or longer.[29,30]

The enhanced cardiac toxicity of doxorubicin-paclitaxel combinations has been attributed to an interaction that reduces doxorubicin elimination, resulting in a plasma exposure of up to 30% or greater.[31] This effect on doxorubicin clearance is paclitaxel schedule dependent, occurring most prominently when paclitaxel immediately precedes doxorubicin or follows it by less than 1 hour.

More recently, Minotti et al.[32] have reported that paclitaxel also appears to facilitate the metabolic conversion of doxorubicin to the toxic metabolite doxorubicinol in a human heart *in vitro* model. The taxane, docetaxel, was also tested, and its effect on doxorubicinol generation was quite similar.

DOCETAXEL

The taxane, docetaxel, has not been associated with clinical cardiac toxicity, CHF, or enhancement of doxorubicin CD. Chan et al.[33] reported no cardiac toxicities among 161 doxorubicin-naive patients receiving docetaxel. Reversible fluid retention was detected in 60% of patients (usually edema with or without weight gain), resolving in a median of 19 weeks. Serial studies of LVEF and heart rate variability have shown no significant decreases in docetaxel-treated patients. Although docetaxel and paclitaxel increase toxic cardiomyocyte doxorubicinol production *in vitro*, only paclitaxel appears to be clinically cardiotoxic. This is explained by the lack of docetaxel effect on doxorubicin clearance and the relatively lower doses of the drug used when combined with doxorubicin.

TRASTUZUMAB

Trastuzumab is a humanized monoclonal antibody that targets p185[HER2] (erbB2 or HER2 receptor), a transmembrane receptor tyrosine kinase of the epidermal growth factor family. This receptor protein is overexpressed or amplified in 20% to 30% of breast cancers and is associated with a poor clinical outcome. Trastuzumab is an important agent in the management of metastatic breast cancer and is also under investigation in the adjuvant setting. The antibody recognizes the extracellular domain of the erbB2 receptor on the cell surface, dimerizing the receptor, with resultant internalization and down-regulation of the receptor tyrosine kinase. This mechanism plus antibody-directed cell-mediated cytotoxicity and synergistic or additive interaction with effective chemotherapy lead to tumor regression.[34–36]

It was only after U.S. Food and Drug Administration approval in 1998 that cardiac toxicity was first reported with trastuzumab, and until recently the mechanism of that toxicity was not known. It has been concluded that cardiac erbB2 is essential for normal adult cardiac function. Using cardiac erbB2-deficient conditional mutant mice, Crone et al.[37] and Ozcelik et al.[38] have reported the development of a dilated cardiomyopathy beginning in the second postnatal month and extending into adulthood of affected mice. Moreover, Crone et al.[37] have demonstrated that erbB2-deficient cardiomyocytes from this mouse model are more susceptible to anthracycline toxicity.

ErbB2 and its co-receptor erbB4 are localized to the T-tubule system of cardiomyocytes. Unfortunately, trastuzumab cannot be directly studied in the mouse because it is specific for the human erbB2 receptor. At this time it remains uncertain what molecular mechanism leads to CD in the adult heart of the cardiac erbB2-deficient mouse model. The possible roles of erbB2 in cardiomyocyte survival signaling or in the control of iron homeostasis and contractility, or both, are under investigation.

In humans, the cardiac toxicity of trastuzumab is incompletely characterized but is now a well-recognized complication of therapy.[39] The independent Cardiac Review and Evaluation Committee was established to retrospectively evaluate the available data from seven phase II and III clinical trials and reported their results in 2002.[40] This comprehensive review identified 112 patients with CD (as defined by the Cardiac Review and Evaluation Committee) among 1219 treated patients. Three studies used trastuzumab alone: 383 patients, of whom 17 had CD (4%). Among 114 patients who received single-agent trastuzumab as first therapy for metastatic disease, CD developed in 3%. In contrast, concurrent trastuzumab with anthracycline-based regimens or paclitaxel had an increased incidence of CD (27%; 13%) as compared to chemotherapy alone (11%; 1%) or antibody alone (3%).

The degree of cardiac functional impairment (New York Heart Association class III or IV) among those with CD was greatest for patients receiving trastuzumab plus concurrent anthracycline (64%), as compared to 20% receiving trastuzumab plus paclitaxel. Moreover, all patients receiving trastuzumab plus paclitaxel had functional cardiac recovery with treatment, as compared to only half the patients receiving trastuzumab plus concurrent anthracycline. Risk factors for CD included older age and cumulative doxorubicin of 300 mg/m^2 or greater. Concurrent anthracycline (doxorubicin or epirubicin) appeared to be more hazardous than temporally separated trastuzumab therapy.

The diagnosis of trastuzumab cardiac toxicity is often made by the detection of an asymptomatic fall in LVEF. Like anthracycline CD, tachycardia may be an early clinical indicator, and the late constellation of dilated, hypokinetic CD is its late manifestation. Unlike anthracyclines, trastuzumab CD does not appear to be antibody cumulative dose dependent, and it seems to be more treatable and more likely to be fully reversible.[39]

Early detection of trastuzumab CD has been prospectively studied by Burstein et al.[41] in 54 patients receiving vinorelbine (no known CD) plus trastuzumab as first treatment of metastatic breast cancer. All had 50% or greater LVEF at baseline, and 44 were rescreened at week 16. Two patients had 50% or less LVEF on rescreening with grade 2 or 3 CD. Of the 42 with normal LVEF at rescreening, none later developed greater than grade 1 CD. The authors recommend a baseline, week 16, and otherwise as needed (for symptoms of CD) LVEF for preventive detection.

It is not yet known how to prevent trastuzumab cardiac toxicity. Avoidance of concurrent anthracycline exposure and sequential chemotherapy/trastuzumab schedules are being studied. Another strategy is to identify patients at high risk, such as those with low baseline LVEF. Behr and Behe[42] have reported another interesting approach: 20 patients received a tracer dose of indium (^{111}In-DTPA)-labeled trastuzumab, and 7 of 20 had evidence of myocardial uptake. Thirteen had no myocardial uptake and no subsequent CD with trastuzumab-based therapy. All seven with myocardial uptake had later CD with antibody-containing therapy: grades 2 to 4 in six and one with arrhythmias during trastuzumab administration. A large prospective experience with this screening method is needed to determine its true predictive value; however, these preliminary results are very promising.

FLUOROPYRIMIDINES

5-FU is a synthetic pyrimidine antimetabolite and an important agent in the treatment of many common solid tumors. Its cardiac toxicity is manifested as chest pain, anginal symptoms, atrial/ventricular arrhythmias, myocardial infarction, and cardiogenic shock. Labianca et al.[43] reported the incidence of this potentially devastating complication to be 1.6% among 1083 patients. A more recent series by Tsavaris et al.[44] evaluated 427 patients, finding a 4% incidence of clinical or ECG findings, or both, among patients with no prior cardiac history. These authors found that continuous infusion had a higher incidence of cardiotoxicity (6%) as compared to other daily schedules of

administration. Moreover, the addition of leucovorin to the continuous infusion regimen appeared to further increase the cardiotoxicity risk. Schober et al.[45] did not find a higher incidence of toxicity with the addition of leucovorin in their study of 390 patients in which cardiotoxicity occurred in 3%. As others have noted, however, a prior history of cardiac disease significantly increases risk (15.1% vs. 1.5% with no history of cardiac disease).

A newer oral fluoropyrimidine, capecitabine, also appears to have associated cardiotoxicity similar to that reported for 5-FU. Van Cutse et al.[46] retrospectively reviewed the cardiotoxic adverse events reported in four large trials: 593 patients receiving 5-FU/leucovorin (Mayo Clinic regimen) for metastatic colorectal cancer and three trials of capecitabine (596 patients with metastatic colorectal cancer, 236 patients with metastatic breast cancer). In all four trials, the incidence of cardiotoxic events was 3%, with grade 3 to 4 adverse events in 1%. These authors cautioned that any fluoropyrimidine has the potential for cardiotoxicity and that treatment should be discontinued promptly for any clinical signs.

The mechanism of fluoropyrimidine cardiotoxicity is not well understood. It is speculated that this is due to vascular spasm in reaction to the parent drug and its catabolites (fluoro-beta-alanine and fluoroacetate). In an *in vitro* model, 5-FU causes vasoconstriction in smooth muscle rings that is reversible with nitrates,[47] and on electron microscopy, the changes appear to be in the small arterial endothelium.[48] Coronary angiography after the 5-FU cardiotoxic syndrome has not revealed ongoing cardiac spasm, and an autopsy evaluation of two patients has suggested myocarditis.[49] A prospective study by de Forni et al.[50] monitored 360 patients (including 9 with prior cardiac disease history) receiving 5-FU continuous-infusion therapy (96 to 120 hours). Only 2 of 28 affected patients had cardiac enzyme elevations in spite of dramatic cardiac symptomatology (in 7.6%), including angina, hypo-/hypertension, malaise, dyspnea, arrhythmia, and/or sudden death. Fatalities occurred in 8 of 360 patients (2.2%).

Predisposing factors for fluoropyrimidine cardiotoxicity include a prior history of cardiac ischemia or arrhythmia, prior mediastinal irradiation, and prior/concurrent exposure to other cardiac toxic medications. No known prophylactic regimen is available that can be provided to prevent the cardiotoxicity, and vasodilators do not necessarily relieve the symptoms once they appear. The best treatment is to discontinue the fluoropyrimidine and provide appropriate supportive measures, understanding the potential gravity of the syndrome. Preventing the potential cardiotoxicity by excluding patients with risk factors may not always be possible, and, if needed, such patients should be carefully monitored with available cardiac support.[51]

RADIATION-INDUCED HEART DISEASE

Cardiac complications resulting from mediastinal irradiation were considered rare and insignificant for a long period in the history of radiotherapy.[52,53] Since the mid-1960s, when follow-up information on a large number of patients who had been cured of Hodgkin's disease (HD) with higher doses of radiation became available, the heart has no longer been considered radioresistant.[54] Radiation-induced heart disease has now been characterized[55–57] and investigated in experimental animals,[58–62] and the pathologic features of the damage have been described with regard to the coronary arteries and all three layers of the heart.[63–68]

Pericarditis and pericardial effusion have been regarded as the most common side effects of cardiac irradiation.[55] However, modern techniques of irradiation, dose fractionation, and reduction of the heart volume irradiated in most malignancies have substantially reduced the frequency of this complication during the last decade.[69] At the same time, evidence has accumulated to suggest that ischemic heart disease resulting from radiation-induced CAD is the most concerning long-term risk of cardiac irradiation, particularly in high-risk patients.[70–74]

The clinical spectrum of radiation-induced heart disease involves most structures of the heart and is summarized as follows:

Pericardial disease
Acute pericarditis during irradiation
Delayed acute pericarditis
Pericardial effusion
Constrictive pericarditis
Myocardial dysfunction
Valvular heart disease
Electrical conduction abnormalities
CAD

Although the pathologic and clinical manifestations of radiation-induced heart disease may overlap in many patients, they are discussed separately in the following paragraphs.

PERICARDIAL DISEASE

Incidence

The risk of radiation-induced pericardial disease depends on the dose given and on the volume of the heart irradiated.[55,57,67,75–77] Even when a large volume of the heart (60% or more) is irradiated at or below 40 Gy, the risk for mild pericarditis is below 5%, and severe pericarditis is rare.[69] Smaller heart volumes (20% to 30%) may tolerate up to 60 Gy, with an expected 2% risk of mild pericarditis. The importance of volume and dose in the production of radiation pericarditis in HD was demonstrated in an analysis of mantle field radiotherapy practices at Stanford.[77] In instances in which the whole pericardium was irradiated, the pericarditis incidence was 20%, but when most of the left ventricle was excluded, it was reduced to 7%. When an additional block was implemented to shield most of the heart after 30 Gy, the incidence was reduced to only 2.5%. An update of the Stanford data corroborated this finding, demonstrating a sharp decrease in the risk of death from cardiac complications other than acute myocardial infarction for patients who received mediastinal irradiation after 1972.[71] Indeed, all series that showed a high risk of pericarditis[78–80] are of patients treated with a radiation technique, energy, and fractionation schedules that are no longer considered to be an acceptable standard of care in most centers.[74] With current radiotherapy techniques for HD and breast cancer, pericarditis is an infrequent event.[74,76,81,82]

Pathology

Clinical and pathologic changes involving the pericardium are the most common abnormalities described after cardiac irradia-

tion.[62,68] The macroscopic abnormalities consist of pericardial thickening and effusion.[55] Collagen replaces the normal adipose tissue, fibrinous exudate is present on the surface and interstitially, and proliferation of small blood vessels can be observed microscopically.[55] The pericardial fluid is protein rich and may contain strands of fibrin. The fluid ranges in appearance from serous to grossly sanguineous.[56] Over time, the fibrinous exudate may organize with the fibrotic pericardium and epicardium to develop into constrictive pericarditis. The mechanism for pericardial fibrosis and effusion is not clear. It may result from increased capillary permeability and inhibition of the local fibrinolytic mechanism.[55,83] Radiation-induced hypothyroidism should also be considered in the etiology of pericardial effusion after mediastinal irradiation.[84]

ACUTE PERICARDITIS DURING RADIATION

Acute pericarditis during the course of radiotherapy is rare. It is almost always associated with massive mediastinal tumors adjacent to the heart. The signs and symptoms are of acute nonspecific pericarditis with chest pain, fever, and often ECG abnormalities. It does not lead to a significant risk of late pericardial damage and is not an indication for interrupting the radiation course.[55,57,72]

DELAYED PERICARDITIS

Radiation-induced pericarditis typically occurs within the first year after mediastinal irradiation. The common range is between 4 months to several years after treatment.[55,57,80,85–87] Pericardial disease presents either as an acute pericarditis, as a pericardial effusion that may be asymptomatic, or as a combination of both. The symptoms of delayed acute pericarditis are indistinguishable from those of other types of pericarditis and usually consist of fever, pleuritic chest pain, pericardial friction rub, ST-T segment changes, and a decrease of the QRS voltage in the ECG.[55,56,80] Pericardial effusion may be large and manifest as an enlarged cardiac silhouette.[88] The differential diagnosis of pericardial effusion after radiation includes recurrent malignancy, idiopathic pericarditis, myxedema, and pericardial abscess.[56,89,90] It is estimated that 10% to 30% of patients with radiation-related pericardial effusion develop tamponade and require pericardiocentesis.[79,91,92] Most cases of radiation-induced pericarditis and pericardial effusion resolve spontaneously, usually within 16 months.[92] Approximately 20% of patients with delayed pericarditis progress within 5 to 10 years to develop symptomatic constriction requiring pericardiectomy.[93]

TREATMENT

Careful cardiac evaluation and monitoring with echocardiography and radionuclide ventriculography should be performed whenever radiation-induced heart disease is suspected.[85,88] Patients with mild symptoms and no hemodynamic compromise can be followed without treatment or can receive symptomatic therapy with salicylates or other nonsteroidal antiinflammatory agents.[55,56] According to reports, a few patients have received corticosteroids with apparent improvement.[94] However, relapse of symptoms or unmasking of latent radiation injury after rapid withdrawal of corticosteroid therapy has been reported.[95,96] Symptomatic pericardial effusion or clinical evidence for hemodynamic compromise warrants a drainage procedure. Pericardiocentesis with or without percutaneous placement of an indwelling catheter is successful in the majority of patients.[82,97] Failure to relieve tamponade with pericardiocentesis, recurrence of effusion, or the presence of symptomatic constrictive pericarditis requires pericardiectomy.[59,80,98] The mortality of this procedure in patients with postradiation pericarditis is high. Cameron et al.[99] report a postoperative mortality of 21%, and a review by Ni et al.[100] shows an early mortality of 22% in patients operated on for radiation-induced pericarditis and a late mortality (after 30 days or more) of 35%. The high rate of complication in previously irradiated patients is attributed to the existence of additional radiation injury to other cardiac and thoracic structures. The presence of constrictive pericarditis markedly increases the risk of patients who undergo valvular heart surgery after mediastinal irradiation.[101] Occult constrictive pericarditis requires no surgical intervention and usually has a good prognosis.[56]

MYOCARDIAL DYSFUNCTION

When myocardial dysfunction is detected after standard-dose mediastinal irradiation, it is typically mild or subclinical.[56,74,102,103] Impaired exercise capacity in asymptomatic postradiation patients has been reported.[104,105] In patients who were studied 15 days after mediastinal irradiation, a transient decrease in LVEF was observed. Complete recovery of ejection fraction 2 months after irradiation and no additional change in patients who were also receiving doxorubicin were documented in this study.[106] Noninvasive studies using echocardiography and radionuclide angiography detected subtle left ventricular dysfunction in HD patients evaluated a few years after mediastinal irradiation.[79,98,100] The majority of patients with abnormal ventricular function findings, however, do not have clinical heart failure.[96] The magnitude of the potential contribution of cardiac irradiation to the risk of doxorubicin-induced cardiomyopathy is not well established. Some data suggest potentiation of anthracycline-induced cardiotoxicity when combined with radiotherapy, however.[102–104] The histopathologies of radiation heart disease and anthracycline heart disease are different,[105] and the combined effects are probably additive rather than synergistic.[105,106] Doxorubicin-induced decrease in LVEF was aggravated with concurrent mediastinal irradiation.[107–110] In programs of combined modality therapy for HD that included relatively low doses of doxorubicin (up to 300 mg/m^2) and mediastinal irradiation of 20 to 40 Gy, no significant clinical myocardial dysfunction was detected.[111–115] However, longer follow-up is required to fully appreciate the potential risk of combined modality cardiac toxicity.[4]

Symptomatic myocardial dysfunction after a radiation dose that does not exceed 60 Gy is rare.[55] The few cases described with intractable heart failure had myocardial fibrosis as part of pancarditis, a generalized process with damage to all three layers of the heart. The hemodynamic pattern is usually of restrictive cardiomyopathy and is difficult to distinguish from constrictive pericarditis.[55,56,83] Its coexistence with pericarditis explains the poor outcome of pericardiectomy or valvular replacement when attempted under these circumstances.[55,100,101] In a pathologic analysis of cardiac tissue from patients with radiation-induced heart disease, interstitial fibrosis (of various degrees) of the myocardium was mostly pericellular and perivascular. The degree of fibrosis was proportional to the radiation dose and was not enhanced in cases in which doxorubicin therapy was also administered.[68]

VALVULAR DISEASE

Clinically significant valvular heart disease resulting from mediastinal irradiation is rare.[55,56,114,115] In a review of radiation-associated valvular disease, only ten patients with symptomatic postradiation valvular disease could be found.[114] Analysis of 635 patients treated for HD before the age of 21 years revealed 29 patients in whom new murmurs of indeterminate significance developed. Of those, 14 received mediastinal doses of 44 Gy or more, and 2 patients who received high-dose irradiation died of valvular heart disease.[71,72] When echocardiographic studies were performed in asymptomatic HD patients more than 7 years after mediastinal irradiation, valvular abnormalities were detected in 25% to 33% of the patients, although there was rarely any clinical significance. An echocardiographic study of 294 asymptomatic patients who received mediastinal irradiation disclosed moderate or severe regurgitation of the aortic valve in 5.0% of patients, of the mitral valve in 3.4%, and of the tricuspid valve in 1.4%. Four percent of the patients had aortic stenosis.[116] Valvular disease, particularly involving the aortic valve, increased with time after irradiation. Of 73 asymptomatic patients evaluated more than 20 years after mediastinal irradiation, 60% had mild or more aortic regurgitation and 16% had aortic stenosis. It is important to note that radiation dose, volumes, and technique of radiation delivery have markedly changed over the last three decades, and the lower prevalence of valvular disease in patients treated at less than 20 years may reflect those changes.[117] Of interest is a report from Norway that showed a significantly higher risk of cardiopulmonary complications for female subjects after radiation for HD.[103,118–120] Most of the changes were found in the mitral or aortic valve and consisted of thickening or regurgitation.[68,103,114,116,118,121] In one series,[104] mild pulmonary stenosis was detected in three patients 6 to 12 years after radiotherapy. Fibrous thickening of the valvular endocardium was found at autopsy in 13 of 16 young patients who received more than 35 Gy to the heart, but none of them had apparent valvular dysfunction.[63] The mean interval from irradiation to detection of valvular disease in asymptomatic and symptomatic patients was 11.5 and 16.5 years, respectively.[114] The contribution of irradiation to clinically significant valvular disease appears to be small.[68,69]

ELECTRICAL ABNORMALITIES

Many ECG abnormalities were recorded years after mediastinal irradiation, the most common clinically significant abnormality being complete atrioventricular block.[85,104,122–125] Slama et al.[126] reported that radiation-related atrioventricular block was typically infranodal and occurred at long intervals (mean of 12 years), after radiation doses above 40 Gy, most frequently in patients with abnormal conduction on ECG before the advent of complete block, and in those who had other radiation-related cardiac abnormalities.[127–129] At postmortem examination, fibrosis of the conduction system has been reported.[123,126]

Another aspect of radiation therapy and heart disease relates to the management of patients with implanted cardiac pacemakers.[131–133] Although transient interference from electromagnetic noise (with the exception of betatrons) is not a problem in properly functioning radiotherapy equipment, pacemaker-dependent patients should be closely observed during the first treatment with a linear accelerator.[131] Placing the pacemaker in an unshielded radiotherapy field may cause cumulative damage to the pacemaker components.[130] The absorbed dose to the pacemaker should be estimated before treatment. If the total dose to the pacemaker might exceed 2 Gy, the pacemaker function should be checked weekly to detect any indicator of damage that may require replacement of the device.[130]

CORONARY ARTERY DISEASE

Experiments in laboratory animals,[58–61,134–136] analysis of pathologic specimens,[63] clinical observations,[78,137–139] and, in the 1990s, long-term risk analysis in large series of patients treated for HD[70–72,140–142] all indicate that mediastinal irradiation may facilitate the development of CAD.

Studies in rabbits on an atherogenic diet and exposed to radiation showed extensive atherosclerotic coronary damage to a degree disproportionately higher than what might have been expected from the summation of the changes induced by radiation alone and by high-cholesterol diet alone.[124] Similar observations have been made in other experimental animals.[135,136]

An autopsy study in 16 young patients (aged 15 to 33 years) who received more than 35 Gy to the heart showed that 16 of 64 (25%) major coronary arteries had significant stenosis (greater than 76% obstruction), compared with only 1 of 40 (2.5%) obstructed coronary arteries in a group of age- and sex-matched controls.[63] In this study, the proximal portion of the arteries had significantly more narrowing than the distal parts. McEniery et al.[139] described coronary angiograms of 15 patients with CAD after chest irradiation. Eight of these 15 had significant narrowing (more than 50% diameter) of the left main coronary artery, and 4 had severe ostial stenosis of the right coronary artery. Stenosis at the origin of the coronary arteries appears to be a common finding for radiation-associated CAD.[73,143–146] After mediastinal irradiation, there is a greater likelihood for right coronary or left main or left anterior descending coronary artery lesions as opposed to circumflex lesions, which might be due to the fact that the former vessels, particularly at their origin, receive more radiation.[147] Coronary spasm after radiotherapy has also been documented in patients in whom acute myocardial infarction developed with patent coronary arteries.[138,148]

Reports of CAD in young patients who had received mediastinal irradiation for HD have long indicated that radiation is a facilitating factor in this multifactorial disease process.[56,63,137–139,147] However, only more recently could analyses of large databases of patients with HD demonstrate a significantly increased risk of mortality from myocardial infarction after mediastinal irradiation. These studies are summarized in Table 54.4-2. Although only approximately 1% to 2% of HD patients in these series died of myocardial infarction, the observed risk in all six series was still higher than expected.[10,70–74,81,141] Boivin et al.[140] analyzed the risk of mortality from CAD in 4665 patients treated for HD and followed for an average of 7 years. The age-adjusted relative risk of death with myocardial infarction after mediastinal irradiation was 2.6 and was even higher (relative risk, 4.0) when myocardial infarction was considered as a direct cause of death. In this study, the onset of increased risk was rapid, within the first 5 years of observation. None of the risk factors for CAD significantly altered the relative risk estimates.

Current mantle radiotherapy techniques, better fractionation schemes, and modern equipment deliver smaller doses of radiation to the coronary arteries and may have a lower risk of promoting CAD.[76] In the study by Boivin et al.,[140] the relative risk of acute myocardial infarction was reduced from 6.33 for patients treated during the years 1940 to 1966 to 1.97 (with no significant difference from unity) for patients irradiated from 1967 to 1985.

Hancock et al.[71,72] analyzed the risk of cardiac disease in patients with HD who were treated at Stanford from 1961 to 1991. The analysis that was limited to children and adolescents younger than age 21 years at the time of treatment showed that the relative risk for death from acute myocardial infarction in this age group was 41.5 (95% confidence interval, 18.1 to 82.1) and that the actuarial risk of fatal or nonfatal myocardial infarction at 22 years was 8.1%.[72] Of note, all deaths in this study occurred in patients who received relatively high doses of radiation (42 to 45 Gy) to the mediastinum. When the Stanford analysis was extended to include 2232 HD patients of all age groups, the relative risk for death from acute myocardial infarction was 3.2 (95% CI, 1.5 to 5.8).[71] This study showed that patients younger than 20 years who received high-dose irradiation had the highest relative risk, that the risk decreases with increasing age, and that patients older than 50 years of age had no increased risk. However, these results contrast with data published by other investigators,[70,73,140] suggesting an increased risk

TABLE 54.4-2.   Relative Risk of Mortality from Myocardial Infarction after Mediastinal Irradiation for Hodgkin's Disease

Study	Center	Patients (n)	Lethal Myocardial Infarctions	Relative Risk	95% Confidence Interval
Boivin et al.[140]	Multiple	4665	68	2.6	1.1–5.9
Hancock et al.[71]	Stanford	2232	55	3.2	1.5–5.8
Henry-Amar et al.[141]	European Organization for Treatment and Research on Cancer	1449	17	8.8	5.1–14.1
Mauch et al.[70]	Joint Center for Radiation Therapy (Boston)	636	15[a]	2.2[a]	1.2–3.6
Glanzmann et al.[74]	Zurich	352	8	4.2	1.8–8.3
Reinders et al.[73]	Rotterdam	258	12[b]	5.3	2.7–9.3

[a]Includes one patient who died of cardiomyopathy.
[b]Myocardial infarction or sudden death.

of acute myocardial infarction for the older age groups. The small number of patients in the Stanford study who received radiation doses of less than 30 Gy did not allow an adequate analysis of the dose effect. The average interval between HD treatment and death from acute myocardial infarction was 10.3 years, but risk was already significant during the first 5 years after treatment and remained elevated throughout the follow-up period (more than 20 years).[71]

Two European studies analyzed the ischemic heart disease in HD patients who received standard fractions and dose (30 to 42 Gy) of mediastinal irradiation.[73,74] Both studies demonstrated an increase of ischemic heart disease after mediastinal irradiation. The study from Rotterdam, with a median follow-up of 14 years, reported that 12% of the patients experienced ischemic heart disease, with a death rate of 4.7% (from myocardial infarction or sudden death).[73] When compared with expected incidence, the standardized mortality ratio was 5.3 (95% confidence interval, 2.7 to 9.3). Of importance, a multivariate analysis of risk factors in the Rotterdam study showed that increasing age, gender (male), and a pretreatment cardiac medical history were significant for developing ischemic heart disease. Treatment-related parameters did not affect the risk.[73] In a study from Zurich, a detailed analysis of the effect of other CAD risk factors on the radiation-induced risk was performed. The study showed that, although the risk of CAD after irradiation increased by 4.2 for all patients, in irradiated female patients and in all irradiated patients without other cardiovascular risk factors (smoking, hypertension, obesity, hypercholesterolemia, diabetes), the risk remained as expected in the normal population.[74]

Long-term mortality data from three trials, which randomized breast cancer patients to receive postmastectomy radiotherapy as opposed to no additional treatment, demonstrated a higher incidence of cardiac death in the irradiated group.[149–151] The excess in mortality did not appear until after 10 years posttreatment.[150–151] In one study, the increase in mortality risk was significant only in women who were irradiated for tumors in the left breast.[151] It was also increased in patients treated with orthovoltage irradiation, as opposed to those treated with more modern supervoltage equipment.[151]

These data demonstrate the risk associated with coronary artery irradiation. It should be emphasized that the old breast irradiation techniques used in these particular studies delivered high doses of radiation to the heart.[152] These techniques are no longer in use in most centers. Long-term follow-up of patients in similar randomized trials who were treated with heart-sparing techniques did not show increased cardiovascular morbidity.[153–155] Prophylactic irradiation of the internal mammary nodes using a single anterior photon beam (hockey stick technique) or large tangents, which may deliver a high dosage to the heart,[156] is not indicated in most patients irradiated for breast conservation or postmastectomy.[157,158] Techniques that reduce the risk of irradiating the coronary arteries have been developed; they include the prone breast technique[159] and use of three-dimensional CT planning and intensity-modulated radiation therapy.[160] Breast cancer patients irradiated with modern techniques are unlikely to receive a significant dose of radiation to the coronary arteries.[159–163]

Conventional-dose doxorubicin-containing chemotherapy used as an adjuvant in combination with local-regional irradiation was not associated with a significant increase in the risk of cardiac events. However, higher doses of adjuvant doxorubicin were associated with a three- to fourfold increased risk of cardiac events. This appears to be especially true in patients treated with higher dose volumes of cardiac irradiation.[164]

The radiation threshold for an increased risk of CAD has not been determined. Lederman et al.[165] reported that patients with seminoma who received a relatively low dose of mediastinal irradiation (median, 24 Gy) had more ischemic heart disease than a similar group of patients whose mediastinums were not irradiated. It should be noted, however, that the observed cardiac risk in the irradiated group did not differ significantly from the expected risk of a comparable normal population.

Monitoring and reduction of other contributing CAD factors in patients who received mediastinal irradiation should be part of the follow-up of patients who underwent mediastinal irradiation. However, the value of routine noninvasive or invasive cardiac studies in asymptomatic patients has not been determined.[74,119,166–169] Still, early detection of CAD should be encouraged, particularly in irradiated patients with other CAD risk factors,[74] because angioplastic or surgical intervention may be indicated in special anatomic or clinical situations. Successful treatment of radiation-induced coronary disease with bypass surgery and with stenting or angioplasty has been reported.[139,170,171] In some cases, surgery may be technically difficult because of mediastinal and pericardial fibrosis.[139]

CONCLUSION

It is hoped that increased awareness and knowledge about potential cardiotoxicity from chemotherapy and radiotherapy will enable physicians to adequately monitor patients and modify therapy so as to minimize serious acute and chronic cardiac sequelae. The growing information about late cardiac effects should facilitate early diagnosis and therapeutic intervention for the benefit of previously treated patients.

REFERENCES

1. Gharib MI, Burnett AK. Chemotherapy-induced cardiotoxicity: current practice and prospects of prophylaxis. *Eur J Heart Fail* 2002;4(3):235.
2. Pai VB, Nahata MC. Cardiotoxicity of chemotherapeutic agents: incidence, treatment and prevention. *Drug Saf* 2000;22(4):263.
3. Keefe DL. Anthracycline-induced cardiomyopathy. *Semin Oncol* 2001;28(12):2.
4. Steinherz LJ, Steinherz PG, Tan CT, et al. Cardiac toxicity 4 to 20 years after completing anthracycline therapy. *JAMA* 1991;266:1672.
5. Giantris A, Abdurrahman L, Hinkle A, et al. Anthracycline-induced cardiotoxicity in children and young adults. *Crit Rev Oncol Hematol* 1998;27(1):53.
6. Massin MM, Dresse MF, Schmitz V, et al. Acute arrhythmogenicity of first-dose chemotherapeutic agents in children. *Med Pediatr Oncol* 2002;39:93.
7. Kremer LCM, van der Pal HJH, Offringa M, et al. Frequency and risk factors of subclinical cardiotoxicity after anthracycline therapy in children: a systematic review. *Ann Oncol* 2002;13:819.
8. Nousiainen T, Jantunen E, Vanninen E, et al. Early decline in left ventricular ejection fraction predicts doxorubicin cardiotoxicity in lymphoma patients. *Br J Cancer* 2002;86:1697.
9. Mitani I, Jain D, Joska TM, et al. Doxorubicin cardiotoxicity: prevention of congestive heart failure with serial cardiac function monitoring with equilibrium radionuclide angiocardiography in the current era. *J Nucl Cardiol* 2003;10:132.
10. Suter TM, Meier B. Detection of anthracycline-induced cardiotoxicity: is there light at the end of the tunnel? *Ann Oncol* 2002;13(5):647.
11. Billingham ME, Mason JW, Bristow MR, et al. Anthracycline cardiomyopathy monitored by morphologic changes. *Cancer Treat Rep* 1978;62(2):865.
12. Swain SM, Whaley FS, Gerber MC, et al. Cardioprotection with dexrazoxane for doxorubicin-containing therapy in advanced breast cancer. *J Clin Oncol* 1997;15:1318.
13. Schuchter LM, Hensley ML, Meropol NJ, et al. 2002 Update of recommendations for the use of chemotherapy and radiotherapy protectants: clinical practice guidelines of the American Society of Clinical Oncology. *J Clin Oncol* 2002;20(12):2895.
14. Jessup M, Brozena S. Heart failure. *N Engl J Med* 2003;348:2007.
15. Wojtacki J, Lewicka-Nowak E, Lesniewski-Kmak K. Anthracycline-induced cardiotoxicity: clinical course, risk factors, pathogenesis, detection and prevention—review of the literature. *Med Sci Monit* 200;6(2):411.
16. Miranda CJ, Makui H, Soares RJ, et al. Hfe deficiency increases susceptibility to cardiotoxicity and exacerbates changes in iron metabolism induced by doxorubicin. *Blood* 2003;102:2574.

17. Clark GM, Tokaz LK, Von Hoff DD, et al. Cardiotoxicity in patients treated with mitoxantrone on Southwest Oncology Group phase II protocols. *Cancer Treat Symp* 1984;3:25.
18. Crossley RJ. Clinical safety and tolerance of mitoxantrone. *Semin Oncol* 1984;11[Suppl 1]:54.
19. Ghalie RG, Edan G, Laurent M, et al. Cardiac adverse effects associated with mitoxantrone (Novantrone) therapy in patients with MS. *Neurology* 2002;59:909.
20. Herman EH, Zhang J, Hasinoff BB, et al. Comparison of the structural changes induced by doxorubicin and mitoxantrone in the heart, kidney and intestine and characterization of the Fe(III)-mitoxantrone complex. *J Mol Cell Cardiol* 1997;29(9):2415.
21. Ayash LJ, Wright JE, Tretyakov O, et al. Cyclophosphamide pharmacokinetics: correlation with cardiac toxicity and tumor response. *J Clin Oncol* 1992;10(6):995.
22. Morandi P, Ruffini PA, Benvenuto GM, et al. Serum cardiac troponin I levels and ECG/echo monitoring in breast cancer patients undergoing high-dose (7 g/m²) cyclophosphamide. *Bone Marrow Transplant* 2001;28:277.
23. Snowden JA, Hill GR, Hunt P, et al. Assessment of cardiotoxicity during haemopoietic stem cell transplantation with plasma brain natriuretic peptide. *Bone Marrow Transplant* 2002;26:309.
24. Schrama JG, Holtkamp MJ, Baars JW, et al. Toxicity of the high-dose chemotherapy CTC regimen (cyclophosphamide, thiotepa, carboplatin): the Netherlands Cancer Institute experience. *Br J Cancer* 2003;88:1831.
25. Quezado ZM, Wilson WH, Cunnion RE, et al. High-dose ifosfamide is associated with severe, reversible cardiac dysfunction. *Ann Intern Med* 1993;118(1):31.
26. Arbuck SG, Strauss H, Rowinsky E, et al. A reassessment of cardiac toxicity associated with Taxol. *J Natl Cancer Inst Monogr* 1993;(15):117.
27. Giordano SH, Booser DJ, Murray JL, et al. A detailed evaluation of cardiac toxicity: a phase II study of doxorubicin and one- or three-hour-infusion paclitaxel in patients with metastatic breast cancer. *Clin Cancer Res* 2002;8:3360.
28. Biganzoli L, Cufer T, Bruning P, et al. Doxorubicin-paclitaxel: a safe regimen in terms of cardiac toxicity in metastatic breast carcinoma patients. Results from a European organization for research and treatment of cancer multicenter trial. *Cancer* 2003;97:40.
29. Gianni L, Dombernowsky P, Sledge G, et al. Cardiac function following combination therapy with paclitaxel and doxorubicin: an analysis of 657 women with advanced breast cancer. *Ann Oncol* 2001;12:1067.
30. Hudis C, Riccio L, Seidman A, et al. Lack of increased cardiac toxicity with sequential doxorubicin and paclitaxel. *Cancer Invest* 1998;16(2):67.
31. Holmes FA, Madden T, Newman RA, et al. Sequence-dependent alteration of doxorubicin pharmacokinetic by paclitaxel in a phase I study of paclitaxel and doxorubicin in patients with metastatic breast cancer. *J Clin Oncol.* 1996;14(10):2713.
32. Minotti G, Saponiero A, Licata S, et al. Paclitaxel and docetaxel enhance the metabolism of doxorubicin to toxic species in human myocardium. *Clin Cancer Research* 2001;7:1511.
33. Chan S, Friedrichs K, Noel D, et al. Prospective randomized trial of docetaxel versus doxorubicin in patients with metastatic breast cancer. *J Clin Oncol* 1999;17(8):2341.
34. Slamon DJ, Leyland-Jones B, Shak S, et al. Use of chemotherapy plus a monoclonal antibody against HER2 for metastatic breast cancer that overexpresses HER2. *N Engl J Med* 2001;344(11):783.
35. Schneider JW, Chang AJ, Garratt A. Trastuzumab cardiotoxicity: speculations regarding pathophysiology and targets for further study. *Semin Oncol* 2002;29(3):22.
36. Garratt AN, Ozcelik C, Birchmeier C. ErbB2 pathways in heart and neural diseases. *Trends Cardiovasc Med* 2003;13(2):80.
37. Crone SA, Zhao YY, Fan L, et al. ErbB2 is essential in the prevention of dilated cardiomyopathy. *Nat Med* 2002;8(5):459.
38. Ozcelik C, Erdmann B, Pilz B, et al. Conditional mutation of the ErbB2 (HER2) receptor in cardiomyocytes leads to dilated cardiomyopathy. *PNAS* 2002;99(13):8880.
39. Keefe DL. Trastuzumab-associated cardiotoxicity. *Cancer* 2002;95(7):1592.
40. Seidman A, Hudis C, Pierri MK, et al. Cardiac dysfunction in the trastuzumab clinical trials experience. *J Clin Oncol* 2002;20(5):1215.
41. Burstein HJ, Harris LN, Marcom PK, et al. Trastuzumab and vinorelbine as first-line therapy for HER2-overexpressing metastatic breast cancer: multicenter phase II trial with clinical outcomes, analysis of serum tumor markers as predictive factors, and cardiac surveillance algorithm. *J Clin Oncol* 2003;21(15):2889.
42. Behr TM, Behe M. Trastuzumab and breast cancer. *N Engl J Med* 2001;345(13):995.
43. Labianca R, Beretta G, Clerici M, et al. Cardiotoxicity of 5-FU: a study of 1083 patients. *Tumori* 1982;68:505.
44. Tsavaris N, Kosmas C, Vadiaka M, et al. Cardiotoxicity following different doses and schedules of 5-fluorouracil administration for malignancy—a survey of 427 patients. *Med Sci Monit* 2002;8(6):PI51.
45. Schober C, Papageorgiou E, Harstrick A, et al. Cardiotoxicity of 5-fluorouracil in combination with folinic acid in patients with gastrointestinal cancer. *Cancer* 1993;72(7):2242.
46. Van Cutse ME, Hoff PM, Blum JL, et al. Incidence of cardiotoxicity with the oral fluoropyrimidine capecitabine is typical of that reported with 5-fluorouracil. *Ann Oncol* 2002;13:484.
47. Mosseri M, Fingert HJ, Varticovski L, et al. In vitro evidence that myocardial ischemia resulting from 5-fluorouracil chemotherapy is due to protein kinase C–mediated vasoconstriction of vascular smooth muscle. *Cancer Res* 1993;53(13):3028.
48. Cwikiel M, Eskilsson J, Wieslander JB, et al. The appearance of endothelium in small arteries after treatment with 5-fluorouracil. An electron microscopic study of late effects in rabbits. *Scanning Micros* 1996;10(3):805;discussion, 819.
49. Sasson Z, Morgan CD, Wang B, et al. 5-Fluorouracil related toxic myocarditis: case reports and pathological confirmation. *Can J Cardiol* 1994;10(8):861.
50. de Forni M, Malet-Martino MC, Jaillais P, et al. Cardiotoxicity of high-dose continuous infusion fluorouracil: a prospective clinical study. *J Clin Oncol* 1992;10(11):1795.
51. Keefe DL, Roistacher N, Pierri MK. Clinical cardiotoxicity of 5-fluorouracil. *J Clin Pharmacol* 1993;33(11):1060.
52. Desjardins AU. Action of roentgen rays and radium on the heart and lungs. *AJR Am J Roentgenol* 1932;27:153, 303, 447.
53. Leach JEL. Effect of roentgen therapy on the heart: clinical study. *Arch Intern Med* 1943;72:715.
54. Cohn KE, Stewart JR, Fajardo LF, et al. Heart disease following radiation. *Medicine* 1967;46:281.
55. Stewart JR, Fajardo LF. Radiation-induced heart disease: an update. *Prog Cardiovasc Dis* 1984;27:173.
56. Arsenian MA. Cardiovascular sequelae of therapeutic thoracic radiation. *Prog Cardiovasc Dis* 1991;33:299.
57. Adams MJ, Lipshutz SE, Schwartz C, et al. Radiation-associated cardiovascular disease: manifestations and management. *Semin Radiat Oncol* 2003;13:346.
58. Stewart JR, Fajardo LF, Cohn KE. Experimental radiation-induced heart disease in rabbits. *Radiology* 1968;91:814.
59. Fajardo LF, Stewart JR. Experimental radiation-induced heart disease. I. Light microscopic studies. *Am J Pathol* 1970;59:299.
60. Lauk S, Kiszel Z, Buschmann J, et al. Radiation-induced heart disease in rats. *Int J Radiat Oncol Biol Phys* 1985;11:801.
61. Gillette EL, McChesney SL, Hoopes PJ. Isoeffect curves for radiation-induced cardiomyopathy in the dog. *Int J Radiat Oncol Biol Phys* 1985;11:2091.
62. Schultz-Hector S. Radiation-induced heart disease: review of experimental data on dose response and pathogenesis [Review]. *Int J Radiat Biol* 1992;61:149.
63. Brosius FC, Waller BF, Robert WG. Radiation heart disease: analysis of 16 young (aged 15 to 33 years) necropsy patients who received over 3,500 rads to the heart. *Am J Med* 1981;70:519.
64. Fajardo LF, Stewart JR, Cohn KE. Morphology of radiation-induced heart disease. *Arch Pathol* 1968;86:512.
65. Fajardo LF, Stewart JR. Pathogenesis of radiation-induced myocardial fibrosis. *Lab Invest* 1973;29:244.
66. Fajardo LF. In: Stemberg S, ed. *Pathology of radiation injury.* New York: Masson, 1982.
67. Stewart JR, Fajardo L, Gillette S, et al. Radiation injury to the heart. *Int J Radiat Oncol Biol Phys* 1995;31:1205.
68. Veinot JP, Edwards WD. Pathology of radiation-induced heart disease: a surgical and autopsy study of 27 cases. *Hum Pathol* 1996;27:766.
69. Stewart JR. Normal tissue tolerance irradiation of the cardiovascular system. *Front Radiat Ther Oncol* 1989;23:302.
70. Mauch P, Kalish L, Marcus KC, et al. Long-term survival in Hodgkin's disease. *Cancer J Sci Am* 1995;1:33.
71. Hancock SL, Tucker MA, Hoppe RT. Factors affecting late mortality from heart disease after treatment of Hodgkin's disease. *JAMA* 1993;270:1949.
72. Hancock SL, Donaldson SS, Hoppe RT. Cardiac disease following treatment of Hodgkin's disease in children and adolescents. *J Clin Oncol* 1993;1:1208.
73. Reinders JG, Heijmen BJ, Olofsen-van Acht MJ, et al. Ischemic heart disease after mantlefield irradiation for Hodgkin's disease in long-term follow-up. *Radiother Oncol* 1999;51:35.
74. Glanzmann C, Kaufmann P, Jenni R, et al. Cardiac risk after mediastinal irradiation for Hodgkin's disease. *Radiother Oncol* 1998;46:51.
75. Stewart JR, Fajardo LF. Dose response in human and experimental radiation-induced heart disease: application of the nominal standard dose (NSD) concept. *Radiology* 1971;99:403.
76. Gagliardi G, Lax I, Rutquist LE. Partial irradiation of the heart. *Semin Radiat Oncol* 2001;11:224.
77. Carmel RJ, Kaplan HS. Mantle irradiation in Hodgkin's disease. *Cancer* 1976;37:2813.
78. Appelfeld MM, Slawson RG, Spicer KM, et al. Long-term cardiovascular evaluation of patients treated by thoracic mantle radiation therapy. *Cancer Treat Rep* 1982;66:1003.
79. Appelfeld MM, Wiernik PH. Cardiac disease after radiation therapy for Hodgkin's disease: analysis of 48 patients. *Am Heart J* 1983;51:1679.
80. Ruckdeschel JC, Chang P, Martin RG, et al. Radiation-related pericardial effusions in patients with Hodgkin's disease. *Medicine* 1975;54:245.
81. Tarbell NJ, Thompson L, Mauch P. Thoracic irradiation in Hodgkin's disease: disease control and long-term complications. *Int J Radiat Oncol Biol Phys* 1990;18:275.
82. Harris JR, Recht A. In: Harris JR, Hellman S, Henderson IC, Kinne DW, eds. *Breast diseases,* 2nd ed. Philadelphia: Lippincott, 1991:406.
83. Fleming WH, Szakacs TE, King ER. The effects of gamma radiation on the fibrinolytic system of the dog lung and its modification by certain drugs: relationship to radiation pneumonitis and hyaline membrane formation in the lung. *J Nucl Med* 1962;3:34.
84. Blayney DW, Longo D. Radiation-induced pericarditis. *N Engl J Med* 1982;306:550.
85. Gottdeiner JS, Katin MJ, Borer JS, et al. Late cardiac effects of therapeutic mediastinal irradiation: assessment by echocardiography and radionuclide angiography. *N Engl J Med* 1983;308:569.
86. Totterman KJ, Personen E, Siltanen P. Radiation-related chronic heart disease. *Chest* 1983;83:875.
87. Gomm SA, Stretton TB. Chronic pericardial effusion after mediastinal radiotherapy. *Thorax* 1981;36:149.
88. Loyer EM, Delpassand ES. Radiation-induced heart disease: imaging features [Review]. *Semin Roentgenol* 1993;28:321.
89. Posner MR, Cohen GI, Skarin AT. Pericardial disease in patients with cancer. *Am J Med* 1981;71:407.
90. Carey RW, Sawicka JM, Choi NC. Cytologically negative pericardial effusion complicating combined modality therapy for localized small-cell carcinoma of the lung. *J Clin Oncol* 1987;5:818.
91. Stewart JR, Fajardo LF. Radiation-induced heart disease. *Radiol Clin North Am* 1971;3:511.
92. Martin RG, Ruckdeschel JC, Chang P, et al. Radiation-related pericarditis. *Am J Cardiol* 1975;35:216.
93. Fajardo LF, Stewart JR. Radiation-induced heart disease: human and experimental observations. In: Bristow MR, ed. *Drug-induced heart disease.* Amsterdam: Elsevier North-Holland, 1980:291.
94. Keelan MH, Rudders RA. Successful treatment of radiation pericarditis with corticosteroids. *Arch Intern Med* 1974;134:145.
95. Castellino RA, Glatstein E, Turbow MM, et al. Latent radiation injury of lungs or heart activated by steroid withdrawal. *Ann Intern Med* 1974;80:593.

96. Biran S. Corticosteroids in radiation-induced pericarditis. *Chest* 1978;74:96.
97. Krikorian JG, Hancock EW. Pericardiocentesis. *Am J Med* 1978;65:808.
98. Morton DL, Glancy L, Joseph WL, et al. Management of patients with radiation-induced pericarditis with effusion: a note on the development of aortic regurgitation in two of them. *Chest* 1973;64:291
99. Cameron J, Osterle SN, Baldwin JC, et al. The etiologic spectrum of constrictive pericarditis. *Am Heart J* 1987;113:354.
100. Ni Y, von Segesser LK, Turina M. Futility of pericardiectomy for postirradiation constrictive pericarditis? *Ann Thorac Surg* 1990;49:445.
101. Handa N, McGregor CGA, Danielson GK et al. Valvular heart operation in patients with previous mediastinal radiation therapy. *Ann Thorac Surg* 2001;71:1880.
102. Savage DE, Constine LS, Schwartz RG, Rubin P. Radiation effects of left ventricular function and myocardial perfusion in long-term survivors of Hodgkin's disease. *Int J Radiat Oncol Biol Phys* 1990;19:721.
103. Perrault DJ, Levy M, Herman JD, et al. Echocardiographic abnormalities following cardiac radiation. *J Clin Oncol* 1985;3:546.
104. Pohjola-Sintonen S, Totterman KJ, Salmo M, et al. Late cardiac effects of mediastinal radiotherapy in patients with Hodgkin's disease. *Cancer* 1987;60:31.
105. Burns RJ, Bar-Shlomo B, Druck MN, et al. Detection of radiation cardiomyopathy by gated radionuclide angiography. *Am J Med* 1983;74:297.
106. Lagrange JL, Darcourt J, Benoliel J, et al. Acute cardiac effects of mediastinal irradiation: assessment by radionuclide angiography. *Int J Radiat Oncol Biol Phys* 1992;22:897.
107. Clements IP, Davis BJ, Wiseman GA. Systolic and diastolic cardiac dysfunction early after the initiation of doxorubicin therapy: significance of gender and concurrent mediastinal radiation. *Nucl Med Commun* 2002;23:521.
108. Gomez GA, Park JJ, Panahon AM, et al. Heart size and function after radiation therapy to the mediastinum in patients with Hodgkin's disease. *Cancer Treat Rep* 1983;67:1099.
109. Merrill J, Greco FA, Zimbler H, et al. Adriamycin and radiation: synergistic cardiotoxicity. *Ann Intern Med* 1975;82:122.
110. Kinsella TJ, Ahmann DL, Giuliani ER, et al. Adriamycin cardiotoxicity in stage IV breast cancer: possible enhancement with prior left chest radiation therapy. *Int J Radiat Oncol Biol Phys* 1979;5:1997.
111. LaMonte CS, Yeh SDJ, Straus DJ. Long-term follow-up of cardiac function in patients with Hodgkin's disease treated with mediastinal irradiation and combination chemotherapy including doxorubicin. *Cancer Treat Rep* 1986;70:439.
112. Santoro A, Bonadonna G, Valagusso P, et al. Long-term results of combined chemotherapy-radiotherapy approach in Hodgkin's disease: superiority of ABVD plus radiotherapy versus MOPP plus radiotherapy. *J Clin Oncol* 1987;5:27.
113. Brice P, Tredaniel J, Monsuez JJ, et al. Cardiopulmonary toxicity after three courses of ABVD and mediastinal irradiation in favorable Hodgkin's disease. *Ann Oncol* 1991;2 [Suppl 2]:73.
114. Carlson RG, Mayfield WR, Normann S, Alexander JA. Radiation-associated valvular disease. *Chest* 1991;99:538.
115. Glanzmann C, Huguenin P, Lutolf UM, et al. Cardiac lesions after mediastinal irradiation for Hodgkin's disease. *Radiother Oncol* 1994;30:43.
116. Heidenreich PA, Hancock SL, Lee BK, et al. Asymptomatic cardiac disease following mediastinal irradiation. *J Am Coll Cardiol* 2003;42:743.
117. Byrd BF III, Mendes LA. Cardiac complications of mediastinal radiotherapy. The other side of the coin. *J Am Coll Cardiol* 2003;42:750.
118. Kadota RP, Burgert EO Jr, Driscoll DJ, et al. Cardiopulmonary function in long-term survivors of childhood Hodgkin's lymphoma: a pilot study. *Mayo Clin Proc* 1988;63:362.
119. Gustavsson A, Eskilsson J, Landberg T, et al. Late cardiac effects after mantle radiotherapy in patients with Hodgkin's disease. *Ann Oncol* 1990;1:355.
120. Lund MB, Kongerud J, Boe J, et al. Cardiopulmonary sequelae after treatment for Hodgkin's disease: increased risk in females? *Ann Oncol* 1996;7:257.
121. Warda M, Khan A, Massumi A, et al. Radiation-induced valvular dysfunction. *J Am Coll Cardiol* 1983;2:180.
122. Cohen SL, Bharati S, Glass J, et al. Radiotherapy as a cause of complete atrioventricular block in Hodgkin's disease. *Arch Intern Med* 1981;141:676.
123. Mary-Rabine L, Waleffe A, Kulbertius HE. Severe conduction disturbances and ventricular arrhythmias complicating mediastinal irradiation for Hodgkin's disease: a case report. *PACE* 1980;3:612.
124. Tzivoni D, Ratzkowski E, Biran S, et al. Complete heart block following therapeutic irradiation of the left side of the chest. *Chest* 1977;71:231.
125. Kereiakes DJ, Morady F, Ports TA. High degree atrioventricular block after radiation therapy. *Am J Cardiol* 1983;51:1233.
126. Slama M-S, LeGuludec D, Sebag C, et al. Complete atrioventricular block following mediastinal irradiation: a report of six cases. *PACE* 1991;14:1112.
127. Strender LE, Lindahl J, Larsson LE. Incidence of heart disease and functional significance of change in the electrocardiogram 10 years after radiotherapy for breast cancer. *Cancer* 1986;57:929.
128. Watchie J, Coleman CN, Raffin TA, et al. Minimal long-term cardiopulmonary dysfunction following treatment for Hodgkin's disease. *Int J Radiat Oncol Biol Phys* 987;13:513.
129. Orzan F, Brusca A, Gaita F, et al. Associated cardiac lesions in patients with radiation-induced complete heart block [Review]. *Int J Cardiol* 1993;39:151.
130. Marbach JR, Sontag MR, Van DJ, et al. Management of radiation oncology patients with implanted cardiac pacemakers: report of AAPM Task Group No. 34. American Association of Physicists in Medicine. *Med Phys* 1994;21:85.
131. Souliman SK, Christie J. Pacemaker failure induced by radiotherapy. *Pacing Clin Electrophysiol* 1994;17:270.
132. Last A. Radiotherapy in patients with cardiac pacemakers. *Br J Radiol* 1998;71:4.
133. Mouton J, Haug R, Bridier A, et al. Influence of high-energy photon beam irradiation on pacemaker operation. *Phys Med Biol* 2002;47:2879.
134. Amronim GD, Solomon RD. Production of arteriosclerosis in the rabbit: a quantitative assessment. *Arch Pathol* 1965;75:219.
135. Gold H. Production of arteriosclerosis in the rat: effect of X-ray and high-fat diet. *Arch Pathol* 1961;71:268.
136. Artom C, Lofton HB, Clarkson TB. Ionizing radiation atherosclerosis and lipid metabolism in pigeons. *Radiat Res* 1965;26:165.
137. Kopelson G, Herwig KJ. The etiologies of coronary artery disease in cancer patients. *Int J Radiat Oncol Biol Phys* 1978;4:895.
138. Yahalom J, Hasin Y, Fuks Z. Acute myocardial infarction with normal coronary arteriogram after mantle field radiation therapy for Hodgkin's disease. *Cancer* 1983;52:637.
139. McEniery PT, Dorosti K, Schiavone WA, et al. Clinical and angiographic features of coronary artery disease after chest irradiation. *Am J Cardiol* 1987;60:1020.
140. Boivin JF, Hutchison GB, Lubin JH, Mauch P. Coronary artery disease mortality in patients treated for Hodgkin's disease. *Cancer* 1992;69:1241.
141. Henry-Amar M, Hayat M, Meerwaldt JH. Causes of death after therapy for early stage Hodgkin's disease entered on EORTC protocols. *Int J Radiat Oncol Biol Phys* 1990;19:1155.
142. Cosset JM, Henry-Amar M, Meerwaldt JH. Long-term toxicity of early stages of Hodgkin's disease therapy: the EORTC experience. *Am Oncol* 1991;2[Suppl 2]:77.
143. Handler CE, Livesey S, Lawton PA. Coronary ostial stenosis after radiotherapy: angioplasty or coronary artery surgery? *Br Heart J* 1989;61:208.
144. Grollier G, Commeau P, Mercier V, et al. Post-radiotherapeutic left main coronary ostial stenosis: clinical and histological study. *Eur Heart J* 1988;9:567.
145. Om A, Ellahham S, Vetrovec GW. Radiation-induced coronary artery disease [Review]. *Am Heart J* 1992;124:1598.
146. Orzan F, Brusca A, Conte MR, et al. Severe coronary artery disease after radiation therapy of the chest and mediastinum: clinical presentation and treatment. *Br Heart J* 1993;69:496.
147. Annest LS, Anderson RP, Li W, et al. Coronary artery disease following mediastinal radiation therapy. *J Thorac Cardiovasc Surg* 1983;85:257.
148. Miller DD, Waters DD, Dangoisse V, et al. Symptomatic coronary artery spasm following radiotherapy for Hodgkin's disease. *Chest* 1983;83:284.
149. Host H, Brennhoud IO, Loeb M. Post-operative radiotherapy in breast cancer: long-term results from the Oslo study. *Int J Radiat Oncol Biol Phys* 1986;12:727.
150. Jones JM, Ribeiro GG. Mortality patterns over 34 years of breast cancer patients in a clinical trial of post-operative radiotherapy. *Clin Radiol* 1989;40:204.
151. Haybittle JL, Brinkley D, Houghton J, et al. Postoperative radiotherapy and late mortality: evidence from the Cancer Research Campaign trial for early breast cancer. *BMJ* 1989;298:1611.
152. Levitt SH, Fletcher GH. Trials and tribulations: do clinical trials prove that irradiation increases cardiac and secondary cancer mortality in the breast cancer patient? *Int J Radiat Oncol Biol Phys* 1991;20:523.
153. Wallgren A, Arner O, Bergstrom J, et al. Radiation therapy in operable breast cancer: results from the Stockholm trial in adjuvant radiotherapy. *Int J Radiat Oncol Biol Phys* 1986;12:533.
154. Stender LE, Lindahl J, Larsson LE. Incidence of heart disease and functional significance of changes in the electrocardiogram 10 years after radiotherapy for breast cancer. *Cancer* 1986;57:929.
155. Cuzick J, Stewart H, Rutqvist L, et al. Cause-specific mortality in long-term survivors of breast cancer who participated in trials of radiotherapy. *J Clin Oncol* 1994;12:447.
156. Hurkmans CW, Borger JH, Bos LJ, et al. Cardiac and lung complication probabilities after breast cancer irradiation. *Radiother Oncol* 2000;55:145.
157. Harris JR, Hellman S. Put the "hockey stick" on ice. *Int J Radiat Oncol Biol Phys* 1988;15:497.
158. Marks LB, Hebert ME, Bentel G, et al. To treat or not to treat the internal mammary nodes: a possible compromise. *Int J Radiat Oncol Biol Phys* 1994;29:903.
159. Grann A, McCormick B, Chabner ES, et al. Prone breast radiotherapy in early-stage breast cancer: a preliminary analysis. *Int J Radiat Oncol Biol Phys* 2000;47:319.
160. Landau D, Adams EJ, Webb S, Ross G. Cardiac avoidance in breast radiotherapy: a comparison of simple shielding techniques with intensity-modulated radiotherapy. *Radiother Oncol* 2001;60:247.
161. Gustavsson A, Bendahl PO, Cwikeil M, et al. No serious late cardiac effects after adjuvant radiotherapy following mastectomy in premenopausal women with early breast cancer. *Int J Radiat Oncol Biol Phys* 1999;43:745.
162. Nixon AJ, Manola J, Gelman R, et al. No long-term increase in cardiac-related mortality after breast-conserving surgery and radiation therapy using modern techniques. *J Clin Oncol* 1998;16:1374.
163. Rutqvist LE, Leidberg A, Hammar N, Dalhberg K. Myocardial infarction among women with early-stage breast cancer treated with conservative surgery and breast irradiation. *Int J Radiat Oncol Biol Phys* 1998;40:359.
164. Shapiro CL, Hardenbergh PH, Gelman R, et al. Cardiac effects of adjuvant doxorubicin and radiation therapy in breast cancer patients. *J Clin Oncol* 1998;16:3493.
165. Lederman GS, Sheldon TA, Chaffey JT, et al. Cardiac disease after mediastinal irradiation for seminoma. *Cancer* 1987;60:772.
166. Savage DE, Constine LS, Schwartz RG, et al. Radiation effects on left ventricular function and myocardial perfusion in long-term survivors of Hodgkin's disease. *Int J Radiat Oncol Biol Phys* 1990;19:721.
167. Pierga JY, Maunoury C, Valette H, et al. Follow-up thallium-201 scintigraphy after mantle field radiotherapy for Hodgkin's disease. *Int J Radiat Oncol Biol Phys* 1993;25:871.
168. Pihkala J, Happonen JM, Virtanen K, et al. Cardiopulmonary evaluation of exercise tolerance after chest irradiation and anticancer chemotherapy in children and adolescents. *Pediatrics* 1995;95:755.
169. Piovaccari G, Ferretti RM, Prati F, et al. Cardiac disease after chest irradiation for Hodgkin's disease: incidence in 108 patients with long follow-up. *Int J Cardiol* 1995;49:39.
170. Reber D, Birnbaum DE, Tollenaere P. Heart disease following mediastinal irradiation: surgical management. *Eur J Cardiothorac Surg* 1995;9:202.
171. Van Son JA, Noyez L, van Asten WN. Use of internal mammary artery in myocardial revascularization after mediastinal irradiation. *J Thoracic Cardiovasc Surg* 1992;104:1539.

ANN M. BERGER
JOYSON KARAKUNNEL

SECTION 5

Hair Loss

Hair is an important aspect of a person's self-image. Unfortunately, during many cancer treatments, hair is adversely affected. The incidence of alopecia is extremely high and is currently ranked third among the most common side effects of chemotherapy, directly behind nausea and vomiting.[5] In addition, cancer-related alopecia is not only due to chemotherapy but also to metastatic disease and presentations of different malignancies. "The loss of hair is an extremely traumatic experience precisely because it is the symbolic precursor to the loss of self. This raises the psychological terror and consequent fear that the known self will no longer exist."[1]

Hair loss can be an immense burden psychologically and physically. Currently, there are modalities to help alleviate the physical and emotional issues that are involved with alopecia. In addition, several experimental treatments are being explored. This chapter focuses on chemotherapy-induced alopecia.

ANATOMY AND PHYSIOLOGY

Normal hair is divided into three parts: the infundibulum, the isthmus, and the inferior segment (deepest area). Other structures that are attached to the hair follicle are the sebaceous gland and arrector pili muscle. The hair follicle consists of the outer and inner sheath, cuticle, hair shaft, hair matrix, dermal papilla, and follicular sheath.

Hair growth is cyclical in nature. The three separate phases during the hair life cycle are anagen, telogen, and catagen. The majority of the time most hair is in the anagen phase. Hair during this phase undergoes mitotic changes and rapid cell growth. In the telogen phase hair is dormant and mitotic activity is arrested. This phase lasts from 3 to 6 months. During the catagen phase, the hair root is separated from the hair bulb, pigment storage is terminated, and the club-shaped root end is pushed out from the bulb. Less than 1% of hair is in this phase at any time.[1]

Chemotherapy-induced alopecia frequently occurs during anagen. Hair that is exposed to chemotherapy during this phase is much thinner and more brittle because of the suppression of cell production. Chemotherapy-induced alopecia occurs within 2 to 3 weeks of chemotherapy treatment. Alopecia normally resolves within 2 to 3 months after completion or cessation of chemotherapy.[4]

Several types of alopecia are associated with problems in the transition between anagen and telogen. Hair lost during this period is called *telogen effluvium* or *hair breakage*. Normally, hair bulbs are released 4 to 6 weeks after the onset of anagen. The five functional mechanisms of telogen effluvium are immediate anagen release, delayed anagen release, short anagen syndrome, immediate telogen release, and delayed telogen release.[6] Immediate anagen release is the most important of all the mechanisms with respect to chemotherapy. The mechanism consists of hair being prematurely forced into telogen, leading to a greater amount of shedding. An example of this mechanism is seen during drug-induced alopecia and severe illness. Delayed anagen release is mainly associated with postpartum hair loss. During this time hair spends a prolonged period in anagen. This type of hair loss may occur several months after pregnancy. Short anagen syndrome is idiopathic. Hair spends a very short time in the anagen phase and then undergoes increased shedding during telogen. Immediate telogen release is when hair undergoes a shortened telogen phase but then reenters the anagen phase as a result of increased stimulation. Minoxidil mimics this phase to produce hair growth. Delayed telogen occurs when there is prolonged telogen with an immediate transition to anagen. This is usually not seen in humans but mainly in short-haired animals.

CLASSIFICATION

Classification for hair loss has been divided into several different categories. The literature has revealed several anecdotal as well as known etiologies for hair loss (Table 54.5-1). Telogen effluvium can be subdivided into three categories by the amount of time in which hair shedding occurs. These subcategories are acute telogen effluvium, chronic diffuse telogen effluvium, and chronic telogen effluvium. During acute telogen effluvium, hair loss begins to occur approximately 2 to 3 months after the insult. Some of the etiologies of this include fever, surgery, or hemorrhage. Hair growth begins again approximately 3 to 6 months after the insult has subsided. Chronic diffuse telogen effluvium is defined by shedding that is present for greater than 6 months. Some of the causes are thyroid disease, acrodermatitis enteropathica, malnutrition, iron-deficiency anemia, pancreatic disease, zinc deficiency, and drug-induced alopecia. Hair loss associated with thyroid disease, zinc deficiency, and iron-deficiency anemia begins to resolve once therapy is begun. Finally, chronic telogen effluvium is a diagnosis of exclusion once the possibilities for chronic diffuse telogen effluvium have been considered. When evaluating a patient with a possible chronic telogen effluvium, androgenetic alopecia should be excluded.

Chemically induced alopecia is due to immediate anagen release. Intravenously administered chemotherapy usually leads to greater hair loss than does orally administered chemotherapy. Hair loss generally begins approximately 2 to 4 weeks after treatment; hair usually begins to return 3 to 6 months later.[2] Some chemotherapeutic agents that have been associated with alopecia are listed in Table 54.5-2.

TABLE 54.5-1. Etiologic Classification of Alopecia

Telogen effluvium
Anagen effluvium
Follicular mucinata (anecdotal reports)
   Acute myeloid leukemia
   Squamous cell cancer of tongue
   T-cell lymphoma
   Lung cancer
Alopecia neoplastica (anecdotal reports)
   Breast cancer
   Gastric cancer
   Trophoblastic tumor
Androgenetic alopecia

TABLE 54.5-2. Chemotherapeutic Agents Associated with Alopecia

Cyclophosphamide	Nitrogen mustard	Paclitaxel
Daunorubicin	L-asparagine	Teniposide
Docetaxel	Carmustine	Topotecan
Doxorubicin	Bleomycin	Vincristine
Etoposide	Busulfan	Vinblastine
Actinomycin	Carboplatin	Ifosfamide
Amsacrine	Lomustine	Thiotepa
5-Fluorouracil	Chlorambucil	Thioguanine
Hydroxyurea	Cisplatin	Mercaptopurine
Methotrexate	Cytarabine	Vindesine
Mitomycin	Dacarbazine	Vinorelbine
Mitoxantrone	Melphalan	Hexamethylmelamine

TABLE 54.5-3. Therapeutic Interventions in Alopecia

DECREASE LOCAL DELIVERY
Scalp tourniquet
Scalp hypothermia
PROTECTION OF THE HAIR BULB
Topical minoxidil
AS101
α-Tocopherol
Inhibitors of cyclin-dependent kinase
Thiol solution
INACTIVATE CHEMOTHERAPY LOCALLY
ImuVert
Epidermal growth factor and fibroblast growth factor
Topical cyclosporine
Interleukin-1
Topical calcitriol
Liposome-entrapped monoclonal antibody
PULSED ELECTROSTATIC FIELD

In addition, some malignancies have specifically been linked to alopecia. Mixed reports have appeared of the association of prostate cancer with male-pattern baldness. Some studies have indicated that the risk of prostate cancer is as high as 50% in men who have male-pattern baldness.[7] Conversely, other studies have found no association between male-pattern baldness and prostate cancer. In addition, follicular mycosis fungoides, a rare disease associated with a poor prognosis, should be differentiated from alopecia mucinosa when considered in the setting of alopecia. These illnesses as well as others should be carefully considered when a patient presents with hair loss.

STAGING

The staging of alopecia can be very difficult, as many scales are available. Staging is further complicated by the subjectivity of many of these scales. One of the simplest scales is the National Cancer Institute Common Toxicity Criteria, which grades alopecia as absent (grade 0), mild (grade 1), or severe (grade 2).

DIAGNOSIS

The diagnosis of alopecia should begin with a thorough history and physical examination. Patients should be asked about the onset of alopecia. Drug-induced alopecia can be differentiated by considering the time elapsed since medication was initiated and alopecia started. In addition, the pattern of the hair loss should be considered as a physical finding that can help in etiology of the hair loss. Clinical examination revealing bitemporal recessions can help to narrow the diagnosis between telogen effluvium and androgenetic alopecia.

Several tests can be conducted if a diagnosis of telogen effluvium is being considered. A blood workup should include, but not be limited to, blood count, thyroid function studies, RPR (rapid plasma reagin), VDRL (Venereal Disease Research Laboratory), ANA (antinuclear antibody), and zinc and other nutritional deficiencies. In addition, several clinical tests can determine whether the patient exhibits telogen effluvium. The hair-pull test, if positive, indicates telogen effluvium; however, if the test is negative, the diagnosis cannot be ruled out. The limitations of this test are that it is extremely painful and it is unable to differentiate a specific type of hair shedding.[6] Other tests that are available are the phototrichogram and hair window tests. Both tests consist of clip-

ping hair and then monitoring for growth after a period of time. Hair growth indicates an active anagen phase.[3] The phototrichogram takes a picture of the area after the clipping. The hair is reevaluated after 3 to 5 days. The hair window test is evaluated after 3 to 30 days, without a picture. These two tests also have limitations but are used more frequently.

The most important test that helps to differentiate chronic telogen effluvium and androgenetic alopecia is the 4-mm punch biopsy. Biopsy is used in obtaining a ratio of the amount of hair that is in anagen and telogen. This test has a diagnostic accuracy of 98%.[6] In addition, a biopsy helps to differentiate between a follicular mycosis fungoides and metastatic tumor.

TREATMENT

Several treatments in varying stages of research and with varying efficacies can be used in the treatment of chemotherapy-induced alopecia (Table 54.5-3). They include scalp cooling, minoxidil, immunomodulator AS101, scalp tourniquet, α-tocopherol, pulsed electrostatic fields (ETG), and various immunomodulating compounds. The therapies fall into three general modes: decreasing blood flow to the scalp, pharmacologically protecting the hair bulb, and inactivating the chemotherapeutic agent locally.

The amount of chemotherapy that reaches the scalp can be reduced in two ways. These methods include using a scalp tourniquet or scalp hypothermia. Both methods induce vasoconstriction of superficial scalp vessels. For these methods to be effective, the chemotherapeutic agents must have short half-lives and have a rapid clearance of the drug and its metabolites.

Scalp tourniquets were first attempted in 1966. They are pneumatic devices that are placed around the hairline and inflated to a pressure greater than the systolic blood pressure while the patient is receiving the chemotherapy infusion. Several studies have been reported using scalp tourniquets that revealed their effectiveness in preventing hair loss; however, the studies are difficult to interpret because of inadequate sample size, different criteria of assessing alopecia, and differences in chemotherapy regimens. Side effects of the scalp tourniquet include nerve compression and headaches.[8,9]

Scalp hypotherapy (i.e., scalp cooling), first used in 1978, decreases blood flow to the scalp and may slow uptake of the chemotherapeutic agent by the hair follicles. Several devices, such as bags of ice, molded gel packs, and thermocirculator devices, can be used to achieve scalp hypothermia; however, it is believed that the scalp temperature must be decreased to at least 24°C to effectively prevent alopecia. Side effects include cumbersome units and patient discomfort from heavy caps. Several concerns have been raised about the use of scalp hypothermia and its use in those with liver dysfunction or in hematologic malignancies including leukemia and lymphoma, as well as a concern about the possibility of developing scalp metastases. More recent studies have found that hypothermia was effective,[10,11] and several studies found no increased incidence of scalp metastases.[12,13]

Four different medications may reduce or prevent alopecia by pharmacologically protecting the hair bulb from damaging effects of chemotherapy. These medications include AS101, topical minoxidil, α-tocopherol, thiol, and inhibitors of cyclin-dependent kinase.

AS101 (ammonium trichloro-9-dioxoethlyene-O,O'-tellurate) is a synthetic compound that is structurally similar to cisplatin. Studies initially done with mice revealed that AS101 works as an immunomodulator by stimulating production of interleukin (IL)-1, IL-2, IL-6, colony-stimulating factor, and tumor necrosis factor, thereby potentially being used to minimize cytotoxicity. The mechanism of AS101 may be due to IL-1, because there is an inverse correlation between IL-1 and alopecia.[14] An open-label prospective randomized trial done with 44 patients who had unresectable or metastatic non–small cell lung cancer and were receiving carboplatin and VP-16 revealed a significant reduction in neutropenia and thrombocytopenia as well as chemotherapy-induced alopecia.[15] Additional trials of AS101 are currently under way.

Topical minoxidil has been used for the treatment of androgenetic alopecia and alopecia areata. Two randomized trials have been performed in patients with cancer. The first trial was with 48 patients with many different solid tumors who were receiving doxorubicin-containing regimens. The minoxidil 2% twice a day did not prevent alopecia as compared to placebo.[16] Another randomized trial with 22 women being treated for breast cancer found that topical minoxidil did not prevent alopecia; however there was a statistically significant difference (favoring minoxidil) in the interval from maximal hair loss to first regrowth. Thus, the period of baldness was shortened in the minoxidil group.[17] Further studies are necessary at this time.

Oral α-tocopherol, initially tested in Angora rabbits, found that there was some degree of protection from doxorubicin-induced alopecia.[18] α-Tocopherol was tested prospectively in two trials of patients with cancer who were receiving doxorubicin. In both trials oral α-tocopherol did not prevent alopecia.[19,20]

A preclinical trial with rats revealed that inhibitors of cyclin-dependent kinase-2 applied topically reduced chemotherapy-related hair loss by 33% to 50%.[21] A preclinical trial of a thiol solution prevented ifosfamide-induced alopecia in newborn rats.[22]

Several different immunomodulators have been studied for the treatment of alopecia by inactivating the chemotherapy locally. These include ImuVert, epidermal growth factor (EGF) and fibroblast growth factor (FGF), IL-1, topical calcitriol, topical cyclosporine, and liposome-entrapped monoclonal antibodies. All of the above agents have only been studied *in vitro* and in animal models, with no translation into clinical practice.

ImuVert is a biologic response modifier that was initially developed to perform immunomodulating or immunorestorative properties for malignancies and other diseases in which immune system dysfunction is implicated. It is produced by the bacterium *Serratia marcescens*. The mechanism of action is unclear; however, it induces many cytokines, including IL-1, tumor necrosis factor, interferon-α, IL-6, granulocyte-macrophage colony-stimulating factor, and platelet-derived growth factor. In the laboratory with rats, ImuVert showed almost complete protection against Ara-C (cytosine arabinoside) and doxorubicin-induced alopecia; however, it offered no protection against cyclophosphamide-induced alopecia. Dose-limiting side effects were hypotension and flu-like symptoms. No human studies have been reported to date.[23]

Several studies in rat models have been done with other biologic response modifiers, including EGF, FGF, and IL-1. FGF given systemically only provided relief from cytarabine at the site of injection. Topical EGF provided protection in the treated area. EGF given systemically provided relief from cytarabine but not cyclophosphamide-induced alopecia.[24] Animal studies with IL-1 revealed that it is a potent inhibitor of cytarabine-induced alopecia, in an action similar to that of ImuVert; however, there was no protective effect with IL-1 and cyclophosphamide-induced alopecia.[25] These results led to the hypothesis that there may be different mechanisms for inducing alopecia depending on whether the chemotherapeutic agent is cell-cycle specific or cell-cycle nonspecific.

Cyclosporine A administered topically protected newborn rats from alopecia induced by cytarabine, etoposide, and a cyclophosphamide plus doxorubicin combination at the site of application. Cyclosporine is a potent inhibitor of P-glycoprotein, as well as a hypertrichotic agent. The mechanism of action is unknown; however, it is thought that perhaps it protects the hair follicle keratinocytes from chemotherapy by the expression of P-glycoprotein.[26]

A study done with a topical liposome-entrapped monoclonal antibody (MAD11) against doxorubicin-induced alopecia revealed that in 31 of 45 rats, alopecia was completely prevented.[27] No human studies have been done with this agent.

Topical calcitriol (1,25-dihydroxyvitamin D_3) has been evaluated in rat models and found to prevent alopecia from a cyclophosphamide-doxorubicin regimen or cyclophosphamide-etoposide regimen. At a dose of 0.2-μg topical calcitriol, the protection was noted over the entire animal and not just at the site of topical application.[28] Because there is some evidence that calcitriol can inhibit or induce differentiation of some cancer cell lines, or both, another study was undertaken with transplantable rat chloroleukemia cells from the cytotoxic effects of cyclophosphamide. The study revealed that *in vivo* pretreatment with calcitriol does not protect the rat chloroleukemia cells from the cytotoxic effect of cyclophosphamide while protecting from cyclophosphamide-induced alopecia.[29]

A pilot project using ETGs was undertaken, with 13 women receiving chemotherapy with cyclophosphamide, methotrexate, and 5-fluorouracil for breast carcinoma. All patients were treated for 12 minutes twice weekly with an ETG. Twelve of the 13 women had good hair retention throughout the chemotherapy period and afterwards. No side effects were reported. The mechanism of ETG is unknown. Randomized, double-blind control studies should be developed using ETG for chemotherapy-induced alopecia.[30]

Very few agents have been studied for radiation-induced alopecia. Tempol (4-hydroxy-2,2,6,6,-tetramethylpiperidine-1-oxyl), a stable nitroxide radical, was applied topically, with guinea pigs receiving radiation therapy. A marked increase in the extent of new hair recovery occurred.[31] Another study was done using topical or subcutaneous 16,16-demethyl prostaglandin E_2, with mice receiving radiation. The mice were protected from some degree of hair loss, particularly when they received the prostaglandin E_2 subcutaneously.[32] No human studies have been done with either of these agents.

CONCLUSION

Alopecia remains a serious problem for many patients receiving either chemotherapy or radiation therapy. One study found that some patients considered the loss of hair to be more difficult to cope with than the loss of their breasts. Another study found that alopecia was the most traumatic disease-related event apart from the initial diagnosis of the cancer and that it is a constant reminder of their disease.[5] Scalp tourniquets and scalp hypothermia are the two oldest treatments for chemotherapy-induced hair loss. Some concerns remain about scalp metastases using these techniques. Preliminary studies have shown some promise with minoxidil and AS101 for the treatment of chemotherapy-induced alopecia. In several animal studies different immunomodulators have improved alopecia; however, no human studies have been performed. Further studies are also needed to evaluate the impact of alopecia on self-image and quality of life.

Although chemotherapy and radiation cure cancer or prolong survival, health care providers also need to be concerned with the patient's quality of life. Patient education about alopecia; identification of available resources, such as the use of wigs, scarves, hats, and the American Cancer Society Look Good, Feel Better program; and supportive listening are all therapeutic interventions to help ease the burden of alopecia.

REFERENCES

1. Dorr VJ. A practitioner's guide to cancer-related alopecia. *Semin Oncol* 1998;25:562.
2. Hussein AM. Chemotherapy-induced alopecia: New developments. *South Med J* 1993; 86:489.
3. Freedberg IM, Eisen A, Wolff K, et al. *Fitzpatrick's dermatology in general medicine.* New York: McGraw-Hill, 2003:731.
4. Pickard-Holley S. The symptom experience of alopecia. *Semin Oncol Nursing* 1995; 11(4):235.
5. Munsedt K, Manthey N, et al. Changes in self-concept and body image during alopecia induced chemotherapy. *Support Care Cancer* 1997;5(2):139.
6. Harrison S, Sinclair R. Telogen effluvium. *Clin Exp Dermatol* 2002;27(5):389.
7. Hawk E, Breslow RA, Graubard BI. Male pattern baldness and clinical prostate cancer in epidemiological follow-up of the first National Health and Nutrition Examination Survey. *Cancer Epidemiol Biomarkers Prevention* 2000;9:523.
8. Hussein AM. Chemotherapy-induced alopecia: new developments. *South Med J* 1993; 86:489.
9. Wilmer Cline B. Prevention of chemotherapy induced alopecia: a review of the literature. *Cancer Nursing* 1984;7:221.
10. Katsimbri P, Bamias A, Pavlidis N. Prevention of chemotherapy-induced alopecia using an effective scalp cooling system. *Eur J Cancer* 2000;36:766.
11. Protiere C, Katrin E, Camerlo J, et al. Efficacy and tolerance of a scalp-cooling system for prevention of hair loss and the experience of breast cancer patients treated by adjuvant chemotherapy. *Support Care Cancer* 2002;10:529.
12. Ron IG, Kalmus Y, Kalmus Z, et al. Scalp cooling in the prevention of alopecia in patients receiving depilating chemotherapy. *Support Care Cancer* 1997;5:136.
13. Ridderheim M, Bjurberg M, Gustavsson A. Scalp hypothermia to prevent chemotherapy-induced alopecia is effective and safe: a pilot study of a new digitized scalp-cooling system used in 74 patients. *Support Care Cancer* 2003;11:371.
14. Sredni B, Xu RH, Albeck M, et al. The protective role of the immunomodulator AS101 against chemotherapy-induced alopecia studies on human and animal models. *Int J Cancer* 1996;65:97.
15. Sredni B, Albeck M, Tichler T, et al. Bone marrow-sparing and prevention of alopecia by AS101 in non–small-cell lung cancer patients treated with carboplatin and etoposide. *J Clin Oncol* 1995;13(9):2342.
16. Rodriguez R, Machiavelli M, Leone B, et al. Minoxidil (Mx) as a prophylaxis of doxorubicin-induced alopecia. *Ann Oncol* 1994;5:769.
17. Duvic MM, Lemak NA, Valero V, et al. A randomized trail of minoxidil in chemotherapy-induced alopecia. *J Am Acad Dermatol* 1996;35:74.
18. Powis G, Kooistra KL. Doxorubicin-induced hair loss in the Angora rabbit: a study of treatments to protect against the hair loss. *Cancer Chemother Pharmacol* 1987;20:291.
19. Martin-Jiminez M, Diaz-Rubio E, Gonzalez L, Sangro B. Failure of high-dose tocopherol to prevent alopecia induced by doxorubicin (Letter). *N Engl J Med* 1986;315:894.
20. Perez JE, Macchiavelli M, Leone BA, et al. High-dose alpha-tocopherol as a preventative of doxorubicin-induced alopecia. *Cancer Treat Rep* 1986;70:1213.
21. Davis ST, Benson BG, Bramson HN, et al. Prevention of chemotherapy-induced alopecia in rats by CDK inhibitors. *Science* 2001;291:1564.
22. Stekar J, Hilgard P, Holtei W, et al. Protection from ifosfamide-induced alopecia by topical thiols in young rats. *Cancer Chemother Pharmacol* 1990;25:306.
23. Hussein AM. Chemotherapy-induced alopecia: new developments. *South Med J* 1993;86 (5):489.
24. Jiminez JJ, Yunis AA. Protection from 1-beta-D-arabinofuranosylcytosine-induced alopecia by epidermal growth factor and fibroblast growth factor in rat model. *Cancer Res* 1992;52:413.
25. Hussein AM. Interleukin 1 protects against 1-beta-D-arabinofuranosylcytosine-induced alopecia in the newborn rat model. *Cancer Res* 1991;51:3329.
26. Hussein AM, Stuart A, Peters WP. Protection against chemotherapy induced alopecia by cyclosporine A in the newborn rat model. *Dermatology* 1995;190:192.
27. Balsari AL, Morelli D, Menard S, et. al. Protections against doxorubicin induced alopecia in rats by liposome-entrapped monoclonal antibodies. *FASEB J.* 1994;8:226.
28. Jimenenz JJ, Yunis AA. Protection from chemotherapy-induced alopecia by 1,25-dihydroxyvitamin D3. *Cancer Res* 1992;52:5123.
29. Jiminez JJ, Alvarez E, Bustamante CD, Yunis AA. Pretreatment with 1,25(OH)2D3 protects from Cytoxan-induced alopecia without protecting the leukemic cells from Cytoxan. *Am J Med Sci* 1995;310(2):43.
30. Benjamin B, Ziginskas D, Harman J, Meakin T. Pulsed electrostatic field (ETG) to reduce hair loss in women undergoing chemotherapy for breast carcinoma: A pilot study. *Psycho-Oncol* 2002;11:244.
31. Goffman T, Cuscela D, Glass J, et al. Topical application of nitroxide protects radiation-induced alopecia in guinea pigs. *Int J Radiat Oncol Biol Phys* 1992;22:803.
32. Hanson WR, Pelka AE, Nelson AK, et al. Subcutaneous or topical administration of 16,16, dimethyl prostaglandin E2 protects from radiation induced alopecia in mice. *Int J Radiat Oncol Biol Phys* 1992;23:333.

SECTION **6**

MARVIN L. MEISTRICH
RENA VASSILOPOULOU-SELLIN
LARRY I. LIPSHULTZ

Gonadal Dysfunction

For young adults who have cancer, the success of treatment with regimens that are toxic to gonadal function has made infertility an important problem. When the cancer is controlled, quality of life, which often includes the ability to have a normal child, then becomes a major issue.

Both neoplastic disease and its treatment can interfere with normal sexual and reproductive function (Table 54.6-1). Testicular and ovarian cancer directly involve the gonad, and prostate, endometrial, and cervical cancer directly involve the reproductive tract. Surgical treatment for any of these diseases results in damage or loss of these important reproductive organs. Retroperitoneal lymph node dissection (RPLND) for testicular and colon cancer, prostatectomy, and surgery involving the bladder neck may result in loss of the ability to ejaculate. Primary and metastatic tumors in the hypothalamus and pituitary can directly affect gonadotropin secretion, resulting in secondary hypogonadism. Both chemotherapy and radiation cause toxic effects on the male and female gonads. Cytotoxic therapies delivered to women during pregnancy can have teratogenic effects on the fetus. If fertility is maintained or recovers, there remains the concern about the heritability of cancer and at least a theoretical risk of mutagenic alterations to germ cells caused by cytotoxic therapies.

The reproductive consequences of cancer therapy affect many people. In the United States, 17,000 men aged 15 to 45 years are diagnosed each year with Hodgkin's disease, lymphoma, bone and soft tissue sarcomas, testicular cancer, or leukemia.[1] Of these, over 3000 are treated with doses of alkylating agents, platinum drugs, or radiation that are sufficient to induce prolonged azoospermia. Similarly, 35,000 women aged 15 to 45 years are treated for breast cancer, ovarian cancer, Hodgkin's disease, lymphoma, and leukemia; at least 80% of these patients receive radiation or alkylating agent–based cytotoxic therapies. These treatments cause not only sterility but also premature menopause in nearly 20,000 women. In addition, 12,000 children under 15 years of age are diagnosed each year with cancer, including leukemia, nervous system tumors, lymphomas, and renal and other solid tumors. Survival is approaching 80%, and because 85% of them receive chemotherapy or gonadal or pituitary irradiation, their subsequent reproductive function is a significant concern.

EFFECTS OF CYTOTOXIC AGENTS ON ADULT MEN

BIOLOGIC CONSIDERATIONS

The testis consists of the seminiferous (or germinal) epithelium arranged in tubules and endocrine components (testosterone-producing Leydig cells) in the interstitial region between the tubules. The seminiferous tubules contain the germ cells, which consist of stem and differentiating spermatogonia, spermato-

TABLE 54.6-1. Impact of Cancer and Cancer Therapy on the Reproductive System

Tumor	Direct gonadal involvement
	Reproductive tract involvement
	Hypothalamic and pituitary involvement
	Concern about heritability of cancer susceptibility
Surgery	Removal of gonad
	Genital mutilation
	Failure of emission and retrograde ejaculation
	Impotence and loss of orgasm
Radiotherapy or chemotherapy	Germ cell depletion
	Loss of gonadal hormones
	Mutagenic changes in germ cells
	Teratogenic effects on fetus
Chemotherapy	Seminal transmission of drug
Radiotherapy (cranial)	Loss of gonadotropic hormones

cytes, spermatids, and sperm, and the Sertoli cells, which support and regulate germ cell differentiation. It should be noted that drugs enter the testis by the vasculature in the interstitial region. Although the concept of a "blood–testis barrier" is found in the literature, this refers to a barrier formed by Sertoli cells to create a unique environment for the late-stage germ cells within the tubules. The testicular vasculature is permeable, and drugs can freely reach the Leydig and Sertoli cells and the spermatogonia, which are at the outer rim of the tubules. Many chemotherapeutic drugs even penetrate the Sertoli cell barrier and damage late-stage germ cells.

Among the germ cells, the differentiating spermatogonia proliferate most actively and are extremely susceptible to cytotoxic agents. In contrast, the Leydig and Sertoli cells, which do not proliferate in adults, survive most cytotoxic therapies. These cells may, however, suffer functional damage. Frequently, after cytotoxic therapies, germ cells appear to be absent and the tubules contain only Sertoli cells, a state described as *germinal aplasia*. This could be a result of killing of the spermatogenic stem cells, the loss of the ability of the somatic cells to support the differentiation of a few surviving stem cells, or a combination of the two.

After cytotoxic treatment, sperm count diminishes with a time course that depends on the sensitivities of the different spermatogenic cells and their kinetics of maturation to sperm. Because the later-stage germ cells (spermatocytes onward) are relatively insensitive to killing and progress through spermatogenesis, sperm count is not immediately affected. However, these later-stage cells are susceptible to the induction of mutagenic damage, and studies in rodents have shown they can transmit mutations induced in their DNA to the next generation.[2] The eventual recovery of sperm production depends on the survival of the spermatogonial stem cells and their ability to differentiate. Surviving stem cells can remain in the testis but fail to differentiate to sperm for several years after cytotoxic insult.[3]

The loss of germ cells has secondary effects on the hypothalamic-pituitary-gonadal axis. Inhibin secretion by the Sertoli cells declines, and because inhibin limits follicle-stimulating hormone (FSH) secretion by the pituitary, serum FSH rises. Germinal aplasia reduces testis size and testicular blood flow is consequently reduced, which results in distribution of less testosterone into the circulation.[4] Because testosterone is a nega-

TABLE 54.6-2.   Typical Clinical and Laboratory Features for Diagnosis of Male Reproductive Dysfunction

	Testis Size		Sperm Count (Millions/mL)	Serum Hormone Levels		
	Length × Width (cm)	Volume (mL)		Follicle-Stimulating Hormone (mIU/mL)	Luteinizing Hormone (mIU/mL)	Testosterone (ng/dL)
Normal men	5.0 × 3.0	15–25	20– >100	1–12	2–12	300–1200
Germinal aplasia	3.7 × 2.3	8–15	0	>20	>12	200–700

tive regulator of luteinizing hormone (LH) secretion by the pituitary and LH is the primary stimulator of testosterone synthesis by the Leydig cells, LH increases to maintain constant serum testosterone levels.

CHARACTERISTICS OF GONADAL TOXICITY

Although subnormal semen profiles, ejaculatory dysfunction, and low libido can often be results of cancer treatment, a thorough examination should be done to determine whether symptoms of these problems might have been present before treatment. A sexual and reproductive history should be taken, including information on developmental factors such as ages at testicular descent and puberty; surgery or injury to the genitals; diseases that might affect reproduction; drug, chemical, or heat exposure; and pretreatment fertility and libido status. A physical examination should consist of examination of the testicles and secondary sexual characteristics such as beard and hair distribution pattern. If there are indications, semen analysis and a hormone profile should be done and results compared with normal values (Table 54.6-2).

During the first 2 months of cytotoxic therapy, sperm counts may remain normal or be only moderately reduced. By 3 months after the initiation of therapy, which is the time required for differentiating spermatogonia to become sperm, azoospermia appears in patients given highly gonadotoxic agents. Oligospermia or even normospermia may be maintained with less toxic regimens.[5]

Germinal aplasia results in decreased levels of inhibin B and increased levels of FSH. Although FSH measurements have been used as a surrogate for sperm count, they show only an imperfect correlation, in part because of interpatient variability in baseline levels; inhibin B level would be more reliable[6] but is not routinely measured. After cytotoxic therapy, LH levels tend to be elevated and serum testosterone levels are in the low-normal range. These alterations have been ascribed to subclinical, compensated Leydig cell failure; however, changes in testicular blood flow described earlier in Biologic Considerations can also explain these observations.[4] The only treatment that produces significant Leydig cell damage and testosterone insufficiency in a high proportion of adult men is direct testicular irradiation.

The induced azoospermia can be either temporary or prolonged, depending on the survival of stem spermatogonia and their ability to proliferate, differentiate, and produce spermatozoa, which in turn depends on the nature of the cytotoxic agent and dose (Table 54.6-3). If treatment is limited to the

TABLE 54.6-3.   Effects of Different Antitumor Agents on Sperm Production in Men

Agents (Cumulative Dose for Effect)	Effect
Radiation (2.5 Gy to testis) Chlorambucil (1.4 g/m²) Cyclophosphamide (19 g/m²) Procarbazine (4 g/m²) Melphalan (140 mg/m²) Cisplatin (500 mg/m²)	Prolonged azoospermia
BCNU (1 g/m²) CCNU (500 mg/m²)	Azoospermia in adulthood after treatment before puberty
Busulfan (600 mg/kg) Ifosfamide (42 g/m²) BCNU (300 mg/m²) Nitrogen mustard Actinomycin D	Azoospermia likely, but always given with other highly sterilizing agents
Carboplatin (2 g/m²)	Prolonged azoospermia not often observed at indicated dose
Doxorubicin (Adriamycin) (770 mg/m²) Thiotepa (400 mg/m²) Cytosine arabinoside (1 g/m²) Vinblastine (50 g/m²) Vincristine (8 g/m²)	Can be additive with above agents in causing prolonged azoospermia, but cause only temporary reductions in sperm count when not combined with above agents
Amsacrine, bleomycin, dacarbazine, daunorubicin, epirubicin, etoposide, fludarabine, 5-fluorouracil, 6-mercaptopurine, methotrexate, mitoxantrone, thioguanine	Only temporary reductions in sperm count at doses used in conventional regimens, but additive effects are possible
Prednisone	Unlikely to affect sperm production
Interferon-α	No effects on sperm production

cytoxic agents that do not kill stem spermatogonia or block their differentiation, normospermia is usually restored within 3 months after the cytotoxic therapy. However, if agents that kill stem spermatogonia or affect differentiation are used, longer periods of azoospermia ensue. At lower doses of these agents, recovery to normospermic levels can occur within 1 to 3 years, but at higher doses, azoospermia can be more prolonged or even permanent. Although the probability that spermatogenesis will recover decreases with the duration of azoospermia, a few men have recovered spermatogenesis after as long as 20 years of azoospermia.[7] When sperm count recovers after cytotoxic therapy, sperm motility appears to be normal,[8] and fertility is generally restored. However, when the duration of azoospermia is long, sperm count may sometimes plateau at less than 1 million/mL,[3] and the sperm may have morphologic abnormalities[9] that are not compatible with fertility.

To evaluate the effects of cytotoxic therapy, one must consider the initial gonadal status. Men with testicular germ cell tumors have impaired semen quality even before cytotoxic therapy is instituted. Approximately 65% are oligospermic (counts less than 20 million/mL) and approximately 20% are azoospermic,[10] whereas the values are 9% and 1%, respectively, in control populations. In half of the patients with reduced semen quality, this impaired testicular function is a result of abnormalities in the remaining gonad, such as carcinoma *in situ* or a history of cryptorchidism. In the other half, it may be a result of reversible factors such as chorionic gonadotropin production by the tumor with resulting increases in estradiol levels or the trauma of the recent orchiectomy.[11] In addition, emission and ejaculation may have been compromised by earlier RPLND so that the sperm density may not accurately reflect gonadal function.[12] In contrast to the severe dysfunction seen in cases of testicular cancer, in Hodgkin's disease between 16% and 50% of patients are oligospermic, only 2% to 8% are azoospermic, and the distribution of counts in the remainder is not significantly different from normal.[13,14] Poor semen quality was more prevalent in patients with advanced than with early-stage Hodgkin's disease, but specific risk factors have not been identified. In patients with other lymphomas and sarcomas, pretreatment sperm counts tend to be normal except for similar modest increases in the incidence of oligospermia.[3,8]

Age at treatment is not a major factor in recovery from gonadal damage in men. Most studies have failed to show any age effect,[3,8] but a few have indicated increased testicular damage after cytotoxic therapy in older men.[15]

INDIVIDUAL DRUGS

The most sterilizing drugs are the alkylating agents (with the exception of dacarbazine) and cisplatin. The cumulative dose appears to be more important than the dose rate in determining whether or not sperm production will recover (see Table 54.6-3). Chlorambucil[16] and cyclophosphamide[17] induce prolonged azoospermia when given alone. The gonadal toxicities of other agents have generally been deduced from the effects of combination regimens; the doses given might be underestimates because there may be additive contributions from other drugs in the regimen. Procarbazine[18] and cisplatin in high doses[19] are also highly sterilizing. Busulfan has an additive effect on the sterility resulting from cyclophosphamide treatment.[20] Addition of high doses of ifosfamide (46 g/m^2) to cisplatin-

containing chemotherapy regimens significantly reduced the recovery of spermatogenic function.[21] Carboplatin, an analogue of cisplatin, appeared in the same combination regimens to produce less sterility than cisplatin.[10] Treatment of boys with BCNU and CCNU produced prolonged azoospermia,[22] and it is likely, but not proven, that the same would occur in adults. The agents that have only temporary effects were also identified from single-agent and combination chemotherapy regimens.

In addition to cytotoxic agents, hormonal and biologic agents are used in treatment of cancer. Although effects of hormones on adults should generally be reversible, approximately 40% of men who had more than 2 years of treatment with a gonadotropin-releasing hormone (GnRH) agonist and antiandrogen still had castrate levels of testosterone 1 year after cessation of treatment.[23] Treatment with the corticosteroid prednisone or the cytokine interferon-α has not produced any negative effects on male gonadal function.[8]

RADIATION THERAPY

The effects of radiation on the testes depend on the fractionation regimen. Whereas in all other organ systems, fractionation of radiation reduces the damage, radiation doses to the germinal epithelium of the testis given in 3- to 7-week fractionated courses cause more gonadal damage than single doses.[24] Radiation given in a few fractions before bone marrow transplantation appears to be less gonadotoxic than the same doses delivered in more fractions.

In the usual fractionated regimens, doses to the testes above 0.15 Gy are required to produce any reduction in sperm count. Doses between 0.15 and 0.5 Gy cause oligospermia. The nadir of sperm count occurs 4 to 6 months after the end of treatment, and 10 to 18 months are required for complete recovery.[25] Above 0.6 Gy, azoospermia occurs. The duration of azoospermia is dose dependent, and recovery can begin within 1 year after doses of less than 1 Gy, but not until more than 2 years after delivery of 2 Gy. Cumulative doses of fractionated radiotherapy of more than 2.5 Gy generally result in prolonged and likely permanent azoospermia. However, after a single dose of 8 Gy or fractionated doses of 10 to 13 Gy, given as total body irradiation in preparation for bone marrow transplantation, sometimes also with cyclophosphamide (4.5 g/m^2), spermatogenesis eventually recovers in 15% of the patients.[9]

Testicular androgen production is relatively resistant to irradiation: doses of over 18 Gy are required before an effect is evident, and major damage does not occur until the dose exceeds 30 Gy.[26] Gonadal scatter doses of 2 to 6 Gy from radiotherapy for prostate cancer do not produce clinically significant reductions in testosterone levels.[27] The radiation-associated impotence after such treatments is likely a result of vascular damage.

COMBINATION REGIMENS

The sterilizing potential of each combination chemotherapy or chemotherapy plus radiotherapy regimen is the additive effects of the doses of the individual agents given (see Table 54.6-3); there is no evidence for synergistic interactions between the agents. Although it is impossible to predict whether sperm production in any given man will recover, the probability of prolonged azoospermia has been determined for many combinations (Table 54.6-4). The sterilizing potential of new regimens can be predicted from

TABLE 54.6-4.   Probability of Germinal Aplasia in Men Treated with Different Combination Chemotherapy Regimens

Regimen	Disease	Courses or Dose	Patients with Prolonged Azoospermia (%)	Reference
HIGH- OR MODERATELY HIGH-DOSE ALKYLATING AGENTS				
MOPPd or MVPPd	Hodgkin's disease	≥6 Courses	85	18
CyOPPd	Hodgkin's disease	4–9 Courses	100	29
I, Pl, A, Mx	Osteosarcoma	I = 46 g/m^2	75	21
		Pl = 560 mg/m^2		
BuCy + HSCT	Leukemia, lymphoma	Cy = 4.4 g/m^2	50	9
BuTT + HSCT		Bu = 600 mg/m^2 or		
		TT = 400 mg/m^2		
BcECaMl + HSCT	Lymphoma	Bc = 300 mg/m^2	100	30
		Ml = 140 mg/m^2		
		+ Prior treatment		
MOPPd/ABVD	Hodgkin's disease	6–9 Courses	50	31
CyOPPd/ABVD, X	Hodgkin's disease	6–9 Courses	85	32
ChlVPPd/EVA	Hodgkin's disease	6–8 Courses	95	33
CyHOPd-Bleo	Lymphoma	Cy <9.5 g/m^2	17	8
		Cy >9.5 g/m^2	50	
E, Ep, B, Cy, Pd (VEBEP)	Hodgkin's disease	Cy = 8 g/m^2	40	34
CyVAD or CyAD	Sarcoma	Cy <7.5 g/m^2	30	3
		Cy >7.5 g/m^2	90	
NONALKYLATING OR LOW-DOSE ALKYLATING AGENT				
Cy, A, Mx	Sarcoma	Cy = 5.6 g/m^2	20	35
MOPPd	Hodgkin's disease	2 Courses	0	18
ABVD, X	Hodgkin's disease	6 Courses	0	5
NOVPd, X	Hodgkin's disease	3 Courses	0	13
Bc, Cy, Ca, L, Mp, TG	Leukemia	Cy = 5.1 g/m^2	0	36
PLATINUM				
PlVB	Testicular cancer	Pl ≤400 mg/m^2	10	19
		Pl >400 mg/m^2	50	
PlVB-I	Testicular cancer	Pl = 400 mg/m^2	55	37
		I = 30 g/m^2		
PlEB	Testicular cancer	Pl ≤300 mg/m^2	0	38
		Pl = 400 mg/m^2	25	
CbEB	Testicular cancer	Cb = 1.6 g/m^2	20	10
Pl, A, D	Osteosarcoma	Pl <600 mg/m^2	5	39
		Pl ≥600 mg/m^2	55	

A, doxorubicin (Adriamycin); B, bleomycin; Bc, BCNU (carmustine); Bleo, bleomycin; Bu, busulfan; Ca, cytosine arabinoside; Cb, carboplatin; Chl, chlorambucil; Cy, cyclophosphamide; D, dacarbazine; E, etoposide; Ep, epirubicin; H, doxorubicin; HSCT, hematopoietic stem cell transplantation; I, ifosfamide; L, L-asparaginase; M, mechlorethamine (nitrogen mustard); Ml, melphalan; Mx, methotrexate; Mp, 6-mercaptopurine; N, mitoxantrone (Novantrone); O, vincristine (Oncovin); P, procarbazine; Pd, prednisone; Pl, cisplatin; TG, thioguanine; TT, thiotepa; V, vinblastine; X, radiotherapy.

the information in Table 54.6-3 and the results found with similar combinations. The additive effects of agents can be seen in the case of cyclophosphamide: When cyclophosphamide is given alone, 19 g/m^2 is required to produce prolonged sterility in half the men, but only 15 g/m^2 is required when cyclophosphamide is given with a median doxorubicin dose of 450 mg/m^2 in the cyclophosphamide, doxorubicin, vincristine, and prednisone (CHOP) regimen, and only 11 mg/m^2 is required when it is given with a median doxorubicin dose of 880 mg/m^2 in the cyclophosphamide, vincristine, doxorubicin, and dacarbazine [CY(V)ADIC] regimen.[3,8] Two cycles of nitrogen mustard, vincristine, procarbazine, and prednisone (MOPP) and pelvic radiotherapy had additive effects on the induction of prolonged azoospermia,[18] but mitoxantrone, vinblastine, prednisone, and vincristine (NOVP)

chemotherapy did not enhance of the sterilizing effects of pelvic radiotherapy.[28]

EFFECTS OF CYTOTOXIC AGENTS ON ADULT WOMEN

BIOLOGIC CONSIDERATIONS

Gonadal cell kinetics in women are opposite to those in men: the germ cells are nonproliferative, whereas the somatic cells proliferate. Female germ cells only proliferate prenatally and by birth are arrested at the oocyte stage. At birth there are 1 million oocytes, which are reduced to 300,000 at puberty.

These are progressively lost by apoptosis, development, and ovulation, and fewer than 1000 oocytes remain when menopause occurs at approximately age 50 years.

Before recruitment to the process leading to ovulation, oocytes are found in primordial follicles with few pregranulosa cells, surrounded by thecal cells of the ovarian stroma. The stimulus for the initiation of follicular maturation depends on local growth factors, not the gonadotropic hormones. Once a follicle is recruited into growth, it develops until it either degenerates or ovulates. The time between recruitment of follicles and their ovulation is at least 85 days. Follicular maturation is characterized by proliferation of granulosa cells and the development of steroidogenic potential of both the thecal and granulosa cells. Estrogen production involves the stimulation of both these cell types by LH and FSH and causes the LH surge that triggers ovulation. The cyclic variations in FSH, LH, and estradiol are essential for menstrual cycles and reproduction.

Because destruction of oocytes results in loss of follicles, germ cell loss leads directly to estrogen insufficiency. Radiation and chemotherapy appear to cause this germ cell loss by direct apoptotic action on the oocytes in mouse models,[40] although primary damage to pregranulosa cells from chemotherapy was suggested in studies of human tissue.[41] When maturing follicles are destroyed by cytotoxic therapy, the result is oligomenorrhea (a reduction in the frequency of menses to between once every 40 days and once every 6 months) or temporary amenorrhea (at least 6 months without menstrual periods in a premenopausal patient). If the number of primordial follicles is reduced below the minimum necessary for menstrual cyclicity, irreversible *ovarian failure* and menopause (more than 12 months without a menstrual period) occur.

CHARACTERISTICS OF GONADAL TOXICITY

Because the size of the germ cell population in women cannot be determined, menstrual and reproductive histories are important in assessing the effects of cytotoxic therapy on ovarian function. Information on the patient's menstrual cycle during and after therapy, as well as oral contraceptive use, should be noted. Because the mechanisms of temporary and irreversible treatment-related amenorrhea are different, posttreatment follow-up must be given to evaluate the significance of the outcome. To determine if effects are related to cytotoxic therapy, pretherapy ovarian function should be evaluated from the history of menarche, menses, pregnancies, and oral contraceptive use. The symptoms of recent primary ovarian failure, including hot flashes, night sweats, insomnia, mood swings, irritability, vaginal dryness, dyspareunia, decreased libido, and bladder infection, should be recorded. Laboratory measurements of hormone levels are most definitive in the diagnosis of primary ovarian failure. FSH level is the most sensitive, but LH and estradiol levels are also useful (Table 54.6-5). The physical symptoms and the changes in hormone levels associated with ovarian failure may be masked by oral contraceptive use or hormone replacement therapy.

Cytotoxic therapy often induces temporary amenorrhea, which may occasionally last several years.[42] This temporary amenorrhea is often a result of direct ovarian damage, which causes loss of maturing follicles or failure of follicular recruitment. Alternatively, stress, malnutrition, or weight loss can cause temporary gonadal dysfunction by altering hypothalamic activity

TABLE 54.6-5. Typical Laboratory Features for Diagnosis of Ovarian Failure

Menstrual Phase	Follicle-Stimulating Hormone (mIU/mL)	Luteinizing Hormone (mIU/mL)	Estradiol (pg/mL)
Prepubertal	0–3	0–2	0–40
Follicular	3–20	2–15	10–200
Midcycle	5–16	50–150	200–700
Luteal	1–12	0.6–19.0	15–260
Ovarian failure	18–153	16–64	<50

and estrogen metabolism. Although some patients with treatment-induced temporary amenorrhea do display menopausal symptoms, these symptoms are usually indicative of permanent ovarian failure. The permanent amenorrhea may begin during chemotherapy or subsequently, after several years of oligomenorrhea.[43] Factors resulting in temporary amenorrhea during treatment appear to be age independent.[44] In contrast, the incidence of permanent treatment-induced amenorrhea (ovarian failure) dramatically and continuously increases with age at treatment (Tables 54.6-6 and 54.6-7), as expected from the decreasing number of follicles with increasing age.

If cytotoxic therapy reduces the pool of primordial follicles, premature ovarian failure should occur even in young women who continue menstruating after therapy. When women aged 13 to 19 years are treated with alkylating agent chemotherapy and radiotherapy below the diaphragm, their median age at menopause is 32 years, compared to 44 years for women treated with either radiotherapy or chemotherapy alone and 49 years for controls.[56] The degree of acceleration of menopause in these women correlates with the probability of induction of primary ovarian failure by the different therapies,[57] which indicates that loss of primordial follicles may be responsible for both effects.

Cytotoxic therapy–induced ovarian failure accelerates bone density loss. However, when only chemotherapy is used, some residual ovarian function may be present despite the menopausal state, and the rate of bone density loss is less than when pelvic radiotherapy is used.[58]

INDIVIDUAL DRUGS

In women, as in men, only alkylating agents appear to produce permanent gonadal failure (see Table 54.6-6). The cumulative dose appears to be more important than the dose rate, as evidenced by similar incidences of ovarian failure in women who received similar total doses of cyclophosphamide, given either daily over several months[48] or within 4 days.[50] High doses of cisplatin (600 mg/m² or more) also produce permanent ovarian failure.[59] Procarbazine is likely to be highly sterilizing inasmuch as permanent ovarian failure is observed after treatment with several different procarbazine-containing combinations (see Table 54.6-7).

Nonalkylating agents do not induce permanent ovarian failure. No ovarian failure was observed with 5-fluorouracil (30 g),[48] methotrexate (200 g) plus vincristine (40 g),[60] etoposide (5 g),[61] or cisplatin (less than 450 mg/m²) plus doxorubicin (less than 400 mg/m²)[59] in women 15 to 35 years of age. Doxorubicin (300 mg/m²), bleomycin, vincristine, and dacarbazine must not induce

TABLE 54.6-6. Effects of Different Cytotoxic Agents on Ovarian Function

Agent	Prepuberty	Age 20 Y	Age 35 Y	Age 45 Y	Reference(s)
CUMULATIVE DOSES TO CAUSE PERMANENT OVARIAN FAILURE					
Cyclophosphamide	>48 g	20–50 g	6–10 g	5 g	45
Melphalan	—	>240 mg/m²	>510 mg/m²	340 mg/m²	46
Busulfan	600 mg/m²	<600 mg/m²	<600 mg/m²	—	42,47
Chlorambucil	>3 g	>1.5 g	>1 g	1 g	16
Mitomycin C	—	—	≥30 g	≥30 g	48
Radiation	12 Gy	7 Gy	3 Gy	<2 Gy	49
INCIDENCE OF PERMANENT OVARIAN FAILURE					
Cyclophosphamide (7.4 g/m²)	0%	0%	60%	—	50
Radiation (pelvic) (4–5 Gy)	<10%	40%	90%	95%	51
Radiation (total body irradiation) (10 Gy)	40%	75%	100%	100%	49,50

ovarian failure, because none was observed after ABVD treatment of women up to age 41 years.[62] Although hormonal agents such as tamoxifen can produce irregular menses or amenorrhea in half the patients, the effects are largely reversible, but they can enhance development of polyps and cysts in the reproductive tract or ovaries and do have teratogenic effects.[63]

RADIATION THERAPY

Radiation therapy induces permanent ovarian failure with a marked age dependence in sensitivity (see Table 54.6-6). Irradiation of the paraaortic nodes for Hodgkin's disease results in cumulative ovarian doses of only 1.5 Gy and does not appear to interfere with menstruation in most patients.[52] Total nodal irradiation for Hodgkin's disease or pelvic radiation for cervical cancer

results in an ovarian dose of 4 to 5 Gy when proper transposition (oophoropexy) and shielding of the ovaries are performed, which preserves fertility in some younger women.[64] Total body irradiation in preparation for bone marrow transplantation delivers 8 to 12 Gy to the gonads, which destroys ovarian function in nearly all adult women.[49,50] Ovarian damage from radiation appears to be independent of whether it is given in one or six fractions.[20]

COMBINATION REGIMENS

All combinations that include procarbazine and other alkylating agents [MOPP; mechlorethamine, vinblastine, procarbazine, and prednisone (MVPP); cyclophosphamide, vincristine, procarbazine, and prednisone (COPP); and chlorambucil, vinblastine, procarbazine, and prednisone (ChlVPP)] induce ovarian failure in

TABLE 54.6-7. Probability of Ovarian Failure in Postmenarchal Females Treated with Combination Chemotherapy Regimens Containing Alkylating Agents

Regimen	Disease	Courses or Doses	Age (Y)	Incidence of Permanent Ovarian Failure (%)	Reference(s)
MOPPd or MVPPd	Hodgkin's disease	Approximately 6 courses	25	15	52
		P = approximately 6 g/m²	35	85	
MOPPd/ABVD	Hodgkin's disease	6 Courses	25	0	53
		P = 4.2 g/m²			
CyOPPd	Hodgkin's disease	Cy = 8 g/m²	<24	28	29
		P = 8 g/m²	>24	86	
ChlVPPd/EVA	Hodgkin's disease	6–8 courses	25	0	33
		P = 4 g/m²	36	100	
		Chl = 300 mg/m²			
Cy (alone) + HSCT	Aplastic anemia	Cy = 7.4 g/m²	13–58	50	20,42
BuCy + HSCT	Leukemia	Bu = 600 mg/m²	14–57	99	20
		Cy = 7.4 g/m²			
BuMl + HSCT	Various	Bu = 600 mg/m²	9–17	100	47
		Ml = 140 mg/m²			
FACy	Breast cancer	Cy = 13 g/m²	<34	0	54
			>39	100	
CyMxF	Breast cancer	Cy = 34 g/m²	<30	0	55
			>35	100	
CyAMx	Sarcoma	Cy = 5.3 g/m²	<35	0	35
			>40	100	

A, doxorubicin (Adriamycin); B, bleomycin; Bu, busulfan; Chl, chlorambucil; Cy, cyclophosphamide; D, dacarbazine; E, etoposide; F, 5-fluorouracil; HSCT, hematopoietic stem cell transplantation; M, mechlorethamine (nitrogen mustard); Ml, melphalan; Mx, methotrexate; O, vincristine (Oncovin); P, procarbazine; Pd, prednisone; V, vinblastine.

almost all older women and even in some younger ones (see Table 54.6-7). Ovarian function is maintained better by reducing the doses of these drugs through use of the MOPP/ABVD regimen.[53] Radiation and MOPP chemotherapy have additive, but not synergistic, effects, and the combination results in a higher incidence of ovarian failure than either modality alone.[65]

Similarly, regimens containing cyclophosphamide, as used in treatment of breast cancer (current average dose, approximately 3 g/m²), also produce ovarian failure; however the age dependence obscures any possible dose dependence. The treatments used for leukemia, which involve lower doses of cyclophosphamide and other agents that do not destroy primordial follicles, allow recovery of menses in women under age 35.[29] Combination chemotherapy regimens without alkylating agents do not produce ovarian failure.

EFFECTS OF CYTOTOXIC AGENTS ON CHILDREN

BIOLOGIC CONSIDERATIONS IN BOYS

In the prepubertal testis, the seminiferous tubules contain only immature Sertoli cells and spermatogonia. The Sertoli cells proliferate at an extremely low level from birth to puberty but then markedly increase in number. Spermatogonia, which are the only germ cells present in the prepubertal testis, also proliferate at a low level during the prepubertal period and transform from fetal germ cells to adult spermatogonia. Leydig cells disappear shortly after birth and are absent until puberty, when new ones are formed from mesenchymal cells already in the interstitium by a process that involves cell proliferation. The Leydig cells secrete testosterone, which, along with enhanced FSH levels, initiates spermatogenesis at a median age of 13 years.

EXTENT OF GONADAL TOXICITY IN BOYS

The germinal epithelium in the prepubertal testis is not any more resistant to cytotoxic therapy than that in adults. When chemotherapy doses to boys are expressed appropriately on a per-meter-squared basis and radiation doses are calculated, the sterilizing effects of a variety of chemotherapy[66] and radiotherapy[51] regimens can be predicted on the basis of their effects on adult testes (see Tables 54.6-3 and 54.6-4).

As in adults, radiation, alkylating agents such as procarbazine, cyclophosphamide, chlorambucil, BCNU, and CCNU, and cisplatin are the most sterilizing and produce prolonged and sometimes permanent azoospermia.[22,59] In addition, high doses of doxorubicin and cytosine arabinoside are additive with the aforementioned agents in producing gonadal damage.[67] Regimens lacking alkylating agents, such as some used for acute lymphocytic leukemia, can even allow pubertal progression of spermatogenesis during treatment[68] and do not affect subsequent sperm counts or fertility.[57]

Most chemotherapy regimens do not affect Leydig cell function, and hence the timing of pubertal development and postpubertal testosterone levels are generally normal.[69] However, busulfan plus cyclophosphamide, used in preparation for hematopoietic stem cell transplantation, appears to delay puberty in approximately 30% of boys.[42] In contrast, direct testicular irradiation, used in treatment of leukemia or sarcomas, severely damages Leydig cells. There is significant inverse age dependence:

children are more sensitive than adults, and within the prepubertal period, the youngest are most sensitive.[70] Leydig cell damage is dose dependent: 50% of boys receiving 12 Gy have extremely low testosterone levels and fail to complete puberty[42] and the figure is 75% at 24 Gy.[71]

BIOLOGIC CONSIDERATIONS IN GIRLS

Despite the low levels of circulating gonadotropins, the immature ovary is far from quiescent. Continuous development of follicles up to the antral stage begins within a few months after birth. After 6 years of age, FSH levels, the degree of follicular development, and estrogen levels all increase. Full follicular development and ovulation begin only when there is complete gonadotropin support at menarche.

EXTENT OF GONADAL TOXICITY IN GIRLS

Prepubertal girls appear to be even less susceptible than young postpubertal women to cytotoxic therapy–induced ovarian failure (see Table 54.6-6). Furthermore, girls treated with radiation or alkylating agents or both between the ages of 0 and 12 years do not experience the premature menopause during their twenties and thirties that is observed in those treated at ages 13 to 19 years.[56]

Radiation is the most damaging agent to the prepubertal ovary: 20 to 30 Gy induces permanent ovarian failure in nearly all girls.[72] Doses of 8 to 15 Gy, usually with cyclophosphamide or melphalan in preparation for bone marrow transplantation, cause failure of ovarian function and pubertal development in 50% of girls,[73] with younger girls being less sensitive than older ones.[42] Radiation doses of up to 7 Gy do not cause ovarian failure or inhibit puberty[51] but can have additive effects if chemotherapy is also given.

Most chemotherapy regimens do not cause loss of primordial follicles or failure of pubertal development and menarche. This includes high doses of cyclophosphamide of up to 48 g,[74] various combination chemotherapy regimens used to treat leukemia, and the ABVD regimen for Hodgkin's disease.[75] Even MOPP or nitrosourea chemotherapy does not affect pubertal and menstrual function development in 90% of the girls.[51,76] However, ChlVPP produces ovarian failure in 25% of girls,[77] and busulfan plus cyclophosphamide inhibits puberty in 50% of girls.[42]

Besides causing ovarian damage, irradiation for solid tumors in the abdomen (20 Gy or more for Wilms' tumor) or in preparation for hematopoietic stem cell transplantation produces irreversible damage to uterine growth and blood flow in girls. This damage affects achievement and outcome of pregnancy later in life.[78] If radiation doses are not too high (approximately 10 Gy as in total body irradiation for transplantation), sex steroid replacement can improve uterine function.

GONADAL DYSFUNCTION AFTER CRANIAL IRRADIATION

Whereas gonadal irradiation causes primary hypogonadism, cranial irradiation is associated with secondary hypogonadism due to damage to the hypothalamus or the gonadotrophs in the pituitary, or both. In patients with pituitary or suprasellar lesions, gonadotropin deficiency is often present before antineoplastic therapy; however, patients with nasopharyngeal cancer or brain

TABLE 54.6-8.   Reproductive Effects of Cranial Irradiation

Radiation Dose to Pituitary/ Hypothalamus	Disease	Reproductive Effects	Reference
CHILDHOOD CANCERS			
18–24 Gy	Leukemia	Slightly early puberty (girls) Subtle ovulatory disorder (after puberty)	83
25–49 Gy	Retinoblastoma, brain tumors, face and neck cancers	Some with precocious puberty (both genders) Higher doses: delay of puberty, gonadotropin deficiency at later times, failure of puberty	83
>50 Gy	Brain tumors, optic glioma	Some show gonadotropin deficiency (failure to undergo puberty)	83
CANCERS IN ADULTS			
10–13 Gy	Leukemia	No deficiencies at <5 y	84
20 Gy	Pituitary tumors	LH/FSH deficiency: 30% at 5 y; 40% at 10 y	85
35–40 Gy	Pituitary tumors	LH/FSH deficiency: 65% at 5 y, 90% at 10 y	85
40–70 Gy	Brain tumors	LH/FSH deficiency: 60% at 7 y	82
40–70 Gy	Nasopharyngeal, paranasal sinus tumors	LH/FSH deficiency: 15–30% at 5 y, 45% at >10 y	86

FSH, follicle-stimulating hormone; LH, luteinizing hormone.

tumors have normal hypothalamic-pituitary-gonadal axes until they receive therapeutic irradiation with fields encompassing the hypothalamic-pituitary areas. In contrast, none of the cancer chemotherapeutic drugs directly impairs hypothalamic or anterior pituitary function.

In children, prophylactic cranial irradiation with 24 Gy for leukemia does not affect LH or FSH pulsatile secretion in the first 6 years,[79] but it does produce subtle effects that appear after puberty (Table 54.6-8). Irradiation of children for cranial tumors with hypothalamic-pituitary doses in the 24- to 50-Gy range has little long-term (18-year follow-up) effect, producing only slight decreases in FSH levels and none in LH levels.[80] However, in the shorter term, they may indirectly increase LH and FSH levels and cause precocious puberty in both boys and girls.[81] Because irradiation also produces growth hormone deficiency, precocious puberty further exacerbates the risk of adult shortness. Treatment with a GnRH analogue to delay closure of the epiphysial growth plates and with growth hormone can be given to avoid growth stunting.

In adults, LH and FSH secretion decreases after cranial irradiation, and the decline becomes more severe with increasing treatment dose and time since treatment. This results in oligomenorrhea in women and low testosterone levels in men. Hyperprolactinemia might mediate the observed gonadal dysfunction in some cases.[82]

In many patients who receive multimodal treatment, the hormonal changes are complex. Although cranial irradiation may reduce LH and FSH secretion from the hypothalamus and pituitary, gonadal irradiation or chemotherapy may induce primary gonadal failure, which elevates levels of the gonadotropins.

PRESERVATION OF FERTILITY, HORMONE LEVELS, AND SEXUAL FUNCTION

CHOICE OF REGIMENS

It is sometimes possible to choose, among nearly equally curative regimens, one that minimizes the doses of the agents that are most sterilizing (see Tables 54.6-3 and 54.6-6). The use of ABVD instead of MOPP to treat Hodgkin's disease has dramatically reduced gonadal toxicity in a large group of patients.[5] In the treatment of non-Hodgkin's lymphoma, regimens that minimize the dose of cyclophosphamide, such as doxorubicin, cyclophosphamide, etoposide, vincristine, bleomycin, prednisone (VAPEC-B), produce gonadal failure less often in men than does CHOP with bleomycin.[87]

GONADAL SHIELDING

Except when the gonads must be irradiated because of actual or potential neoplastic involvement, they must be outside the field or shielded from the direct radiation beam. Nevertheless, an appreciable radiation dose from the accelerator head, collimator scatter, or internal lateral scatter may reach the gonads. Even though moderately low radiation doses may be achieved, further reductions are desirable because of the possibilities of additive effects from chemotherapy and genetic damage to the sperm.

Gonadal dose depends on distance from the field edge, field size, and photon energy. Pelvic radiation fields result in significant doses to the testis. Clamshell or other shields and beam blocking can reduce testicular doses twofold to fivefold to 2 to 3 Gy for the inverted Y field used for Hodgkin's disease and to 0.2 to 0.8 Gy for the hemipelvic field used for seminoma.[88]

To reduce ovarian dose, an oophoropexy, in which the ovaries are surgically translocated away from the direct beam, can be performed. That region is further shielded using lead blocks. Some investigators report reductions in cumulative ovarian doses to 4 to 5 Gy during total nodal irradiation,[51] which preserves fertility in younger women[64] (see Table 54.6-6).

SPERM CRYOPRESERVATION

Semen cryopreservation is an extremely important procedure for preserving the fertility potential of men after cytotoxic treatment for cancer.[89] The significance of notifying the patient of the potential risk of iatrogenic sterility as early as possible cannot be overemphasized.[90] Physicians often are aware early during the diagnostic process that the patient will most likely need to receive potentially sterilizing cytotoxic therapy, although the exact diagnosis, stage, and treatment regimen may not have yet been decided. This time should be used to initiate and complete the cryopreservation procedure. The number of samples to be banked may depend on how much time is available before starting therapy, sperm quality, and the cost of storing samples. Collection of three or four samples with approximately 48-hour periods of abstinence between sampling (a total of more than 5 days) is ideal. With current assisted reproductive technologies, however, success can be achieved with fewer samples, even with poor-quality semen. It is strongly advisable to complete sperm banking before starting therapy to avoid possible increased genetic damage in sperm collected after the start of therapy.[2] It is even possible to obtain semen with normal characteristics from 14- to 17-year-old boys by masturbation,[91] penile vibratory stimulation, or electroejaculation.[92] In addition, testicular sperm extraction is successful in 43% of pretreatment cancer patients who are azoospermic,[93] and the sperm obtained in this way can be cryopreserved and used in intracytoplasmic sperm injection (ICSI) procedures.[94] Testicular samples for sperm extraction can be obtained from orchiectomy or biopsy specimens that are routinely taken from testicular cancer patients if the surgeon is aware of the need and the processing procedures required for harvesting the sperm.

The success of *in vitro* fertilization (IVF) and ICSI makes cryopreservation of all samples containing any live sperm worthwhile. The cost of sperm banking three samples, including analysis and storage for 5 years, is between $1200 (at a university medical school clinic) and $2500 (at some private sperm banks). Intrauterine insemination is the least expensive assisted reproductive technology method (cost per cycle, $200 to $500, plus $1200 for superovulation of the female partner, if necessary), but the sperm count and quality after thawing must be high, and conception rates are low. If sperm count or motility is impaired or sample amounts are limited, IVF with or without ICSI is necessary. The average cost of IVF, including the drugs used, is $10,000 per cycle; if ICSI is included, the cost is approximately $12,000 per cycle.

OPTIMIZATION OF FERTILITY AFTER TREATMENT

If sperm count recovers after cancer therapy, it usually reaches normospermic levels, but some men remain oligospermic for extended periods. Although controlled studies have not been done, men who have recovered sperm production appear to have normal fertility, and their incidence of infertility does not appear to be any higher than the 15% rate among couples in the general population. Furthermore, cancer patients with recovered sperm counts ranging from just below 1 million to 10 million/mL are able to successfully father children.[95] Infertile patients with oligospermic counts should be managed in the same way as are those in the general population with male factor infertility, including the use of IVF and IVF with ICSI.[96]

Most women who continue to have menstrual function after cytotoxic therapy for cancer but are infertile should be treated in the same way as similar women in the general population.

One important exception is women with uterine damage from receiving more than 10 Gy of abdominal radiation in childhood. These patients have increased rates of adverse pregnancy outcomes, including fetal or neonatal death, premature delivery, and low-birth-weight babies, and hence their pregnancies must be closely monitored.[78] In women with ovarian failure, the use of donor oocytes and hormonal treatment to maintain pregnancy has been successful.[97]

ASSISTED REPRODUCTIVE TECHNOLOGIES

Assisted reproductive technologies have and still are undergoing rapid advances, providing new options for survivors of cancer with gonadal damage to achieve fertility. Previously, intrauterine artificial insemination had been the only method available, and only 30% of men who had stored high-quality semen samples were able to effect pregnancies.[98]

Currently, IVF and especially IVF with ICSI are the most successful methods for achieving pregnancies from stored semen. In IVF, 100,000 motile sperm are placed in a droplet of medium containing an oocyte; fertilization is then allowed to occur. If freezing and thawing result in severe loss of sperm motility, IVF cannot be used, but IVF with ICSI can still be used as long as the sperm are viable. In ICSI, one live spermatozoon is selected and microinjected into the cytoplasm of an oocyte.[99] With ICSI it is possible to select sperm for injection from individuals with sperm counts as low as 100 per ejaculate.[100] In both procedures, multiple oocytes are fertilized in a single cycle, the oocytes then are examined for fertilization and embryo cleavage, and several embryos are implanted into the uterine cavity. Embryos that are not transferred can be frozen for implantation at a later time. IVF, however, requires hormonal induction of multiple ovulations, and the implantation of several embryos increases the risks of fetal loss and multiple births.

Clinical pregnancy rates of 30% to 40% per cycle and delivery rates of 25% to 30% can be expected at most reproductive clinics. When three cycles are used, IVF with ICSI offers couples a success rate of 63% for having a liveborn child.[101] In one study specifically examining the use of cryopreserved sperm from cancer patients, 18% of cycles (2 of 11) resulted in complete pregnancies.[96] Furthermore, cryopreserved testicular sperm obtained by testicular sperm extraction have also been routinely used for achieving pregnancies, with pregnancies obtained in 30% of cycles of IVF with ICSI.[94] Although insemination with testicular sperm is an acceptable procedure, the use of nuclei from earlier stages (round spermatid nuclear injection) is not currently advisable.[102]

Most studies indicate no increases in congenital malformations or developmental abnormalities in the offspring from pregnancies achieved with IVF or ICSI,[103] although there are occasional reports to the contrary.[104] However, there is an increased risk of approximately 3% for chromosomal abnormalities, mostly in the numbers of sex chromosomes, in offspring of ICSI procedures.[105] Most of the chromosome abnormalities were not caused by ICSI, however, but were already present in the sperm of the infertile male parent. These abnormalities, which are common in cases of primary male infertility, would not be present in cryopreserved sperm of cancer patients.

It is also possible to cryopreserve embryos obtained by natural coitus or IVF before initiation of potentially sterilizing treatment in female cancer patients. Limitations of this method are the need for the woman to have a partner at the time, the delay in initiating cytotoxic therapy, and the contraindication of conventional ovarian stimulation protocols in cases of hormone-dependent tumors, like many breast cancers. However, some significant ovarian stimulation can be achieved by tamoxifen, which acts as an estrogen antagonist in breast tumors.[106]

FEMALE GERM CELL CRYOPRESERVATION AND DEVELOPMENT

Freezing of oocytes, unlike freezing of sperm, is currently still experimental.[107] Cryopreservation of mature (metaphase II) oocytes has resulted in successful pregnancies and birth of healthy children.[108] However, the overall frequency of success is currently very low (1% to 10%), chromosomal aneuploidy can result from freezing of metaphase cells, and conventional hormone-induced superovulation cannot be used in women with estrogen-responsive tumors.

Two alternative approaches are being investigated. The first, which involves surgical removal of ovarian tissue containing numerous primordial follicles, cryopreservation of tissue slices, and grafting back to the site of the ovary, has restored ovarian endocrine function and fertility in sheep.[109] Restoration of hormone production and follicular growth in women after transplantation of fresh or cryopreserved ovarian tissue into heterotopic (forearm) sites has been reported and lasted up to 2 years after transplantation.[110] However, what is the true long-term success rate of this technique and whether oocytes capable of IVF can be produced remain to be determined. With some cancers, particularly leukemia and neuroblastoma, but also breast and uterine carcinomas, there is also concern that malignant cells may be reintroduced with the ovarian tissue.[110]

The second approach involves cryopreservation of immature oocytes still in the germinal vesicle stage, *in vitro* maturation to meiotic metaphase II, and IVF. Although primordial follicles are most abundant in the ovary, the ability to mature and fertilize them *in vitro* and obtain normal embryo development is limited to mice.[111] In humans, cryopreserved oocytes in small antral follicles (diameter more than 5 mm) have been matured and fertilized *in vitro* and live births have been achieved, but the frequency of success is not yet any better than with cryopreserved mature oocytes.[112]

The derivation of oocytes from mouse embryonic stem cells in culture suggests the eventual power of stem cell technology and nuclear transplantation for production of oocytes, perhaps even from somatic cell nuclei.[113] However, application of such techniques to human infertility is still quite distant.

IMMATURE MALE GERM CELL CRYOPRESERVATION AND DEVELOPMENT

For restoration of spermatogenesis, the harvest and cryopreservation of spermatogonial stem cells, which are capable of proliferation, self-renewal, and repopulation of the seminiferous tubules, are under investigation. Transplantation of cryopreserved testicular germ cells from a donor mouse into the seminiferous tubules of a recipient mouse, in which endogenous stem spermatogonia were killed with busulfan, restored spermatogenesis and fertility.[114] There are preliminary indications that this technique might restore spermatogenesis in irradiated macaques.[115] Testicular cells have been harvested from men

before sterilizing cytotoxic therapy and later injected back into the testicular tubules after the completion of radiotherapy or chemotherapy. A clinical trial of this method is under way,[116] and the results are pending. This technique would be most valuable for prepubertal boys, who are too young to produce sperm but have testes enriched in spermatogonia. There is the concern, however, that cancer cells may be reintroduced into the recipients. This possibility is a contraindication in cases of leukemia or testicular cancer, but the risks with other cancers may not be high.[117]

One way to circumvent the problem of the presence of tumor cells is to first transplant the tissue into a xenogeneic host. Human spermatogonial stem cells survive and proliferate in seminiferous tubules of mice.[118] Also, subcutaneous transplantation of cryopreserved testicular tissue from immature pigs and goats into nude mice results in the production of functional sperm.[119] However, the risks of transfer of animal DNA or viruses (especially retroviruses) from the host to the human spermatogonial cells must be evaluated before such techniques could be applied.

New experimental approaches to germ cell development could some day be applied to fertility preservation in men. The *in vitro* development of human round spermatids into elongated spermatids, which were used to produce normal embryos by ICSI, has been reported.[120] Development of an *in vitro* cell line derived from genetically modified mouse spermatogonia, which proliferates to produce more spermatogonia and can be stimulated to form haploid cells,[121] holds promise as a very useful resource for optimizing proliferation of spermatogonia and production of spermatids. Furthermore, the development of sperm from mouse embryonic stem cells by a combination of induction of differentiation *in vitro* and transplantation into host testes[122] might eventually lead to methods for development of sperm from other stem cell types obtained from a cancer patient.

PHARMACOLOGIC ATTEMPTS AT PRESERVING FERTILITY

Hormone treatments have been investigated for their ability to enhance the survival of germ cells and promote recovery after cytotoxic treatments. Treatment of male rats with hormones that suppress testosterone levels or action (gonadal steroids, GnRH analogues, antiandrogens) before and during cytotoxic therapy with radiation or procarbazine enhances the subsequent recovery of spermatogenesis and fertility.[123] The original proposal that these treatments would protect the spermatogonia from killing by suppressing their proliferation is incorrect; rather, the suppression of testosterone levels protects the subsequent ability of the somatic cells of the testis to support the recovery of spermatogenesis from surviving stem spermatogonia.[124] The hormonal treatment can even be given several months after exposure to radiation or procarbazine and still restore spermatogenesis and fertility.[123]

Because stem spermatogonia are indeed present in regions of the testes of some cancer patients during prolonged periods of iatrogenic azoospermia, their recovery could possibly be stimulated. However, only one[125] out of eight clinical trials has been able to demonstrate protection of spermatogenesis in humans by hormone treatment before and during cytotoxic therapy.[126] One attempt to restore spermatogenesis by steroid hormone treatment after cytotoxic therapy was unsuccessful[127]; however, the doses of cytotoxic therapy were very high, and the hormonal suppression was given many years after the anticancer treatment. More discouraging was the failure of GnRH antagonist treatment to enhance spermatogenic recovery in a controlled primate study,[128] which suggests that there are important differences in this process in rats and in primates.

Several studies in female rats and monkeys have indicated that GnRH agonist treatments might reduce ovarian damage from cyclophosphamide.[129] Some of the apparent "protection" in the rat model could be a direct result of GnRH agonist action to decrease recruitment of primordial follicles. Clinical studies attempting to protect ovarian function in women using oral contraceptives or GnRH agonists had generally shown negative results,[130] but more recent studies with GnRH agonists reported protection of gonadal function.[131] Although these studies suggest a dramatic protective effect, they cannot be regarded as conclusive because the chemotherapy-only groups were not rigorously matched to the GnRH agonist–treated groups.

Studies have shown that the mechanism of radiation- and chemotherapy-induced apoptosis in mouse oocytes involves lipid second-messenger signaling systems, including ceramide and its metabolite sphingosine.[40] Local injection of sphingosine-1-phosphate prevented radiation-induced oocyte loss in mice, and the treated mice were able to produce normal offspring. Further studies, including the evaluation of other toxicities of sphingosine-1-phosphate, are needed before considering this approach for humans.

Even when clinical symptoms of ovarian failure are present, some residual ovarian function may remain after chemotherapy.[58] In such cases it is possible to stimulate ovulation and fertility, at least for a short time, with steroid hormones or gonadotropins or both.[132]

HORMONE REPLACEMENT THERAPY

New information that estrogen with or without progesterone given to postmenopausal women (aged 50 to 79 years) increases the cardiovascular risks[133] has led to the view that the risks of hormone replacement therapy for normal postmenopausal women (cardiovascular disease and breast cancer) outweigh the benefits (increased bone mineral density and reduced incidence of fracture). However, the physiologic replacement of ovarian hormones still remains appropriate for young, otherwise premenopausal women who have developed premature ovarian failure as a result of their malignancy or cancer treatment. This is particularly true for adolescent girls and young women in whom bone mineral density is normally increasing.[134] In these cases, it is important to test for ovarian failure shortly after treatment and, if appropriate, to start hormone replacement therapy in a timely manner. If a woman has an intact uterus, estrogen should be combined with progesterone to prevent endometrial hyperplasia and cancer.[134]

In males, germinal aplasia is often associated with testosterone levels in the low-normal range, and such individuals may experience reduced bone mineral density and a slight reduction in sexual function.[135] However, a controlled trial failed to show any benefit of testosterone treatment on bone mineral density or sexual function, which indicates that this mild hypogonadism is not of clinical importance in most men.[135] Testosterone replacement is, nevertheless, very important in cases of overt Leydig cell failure in prepubertal boys to promote secondary sexual characteristics, growth, and bone density.

PREVENTION AND MANAGEMENT OF ERECTILE AND EJACULATORY DYSFUNCTION

Ejaculation of semen first requires emission (the deposition of semen in the posterior urethra by contractions of the vas deferens, seminal vesicles, and prostate) and then antegrade ejaculation, which involves coordinated tightening of the bladder neck, relaxation of the external sphincter, and expulsion of semen. Most of these processes are controlled by trunks of nerve fibers forming the hypogastric plexus overlying the aorta and sacrum below the origin of the inferior mesenteric artery.[136] Surgery for testicular, prostate, and bladder cancer can produce neurologic dysfunction resulting in failure of emission, retrograde ejaculation, impotence, and loss of orgasm. However, improvements in surgical techniques have reduced these adverse outcomes without diminishing the efficacy of treating the cancer.

RPLND is used in the treatment of nonseminomatous testicular germ cell tumors. Based on the location of positive nodes, a modified template of dissection (unilateral dissection below the inferior mesenteric artery) that avoids disturbance of the lumbar sympathetic fibers, particularly at the hypogastric plexus, was developed.[136] The RPLND technique has been further refined by retracting postganglionic fibers from the lymph nodes over and around the aorta, which are then dissected and removed in multiple small packages, with sparing of the nerve fibers. This newer nerve-sparing modification preserves ejaculation of semen in 90% of men.[12]

Improvements have also been made in surgery for prostate and bladder cancer.[137] By avoiding damage to the nerve fibers that are located in the neurovascular bundles that innervate the penile corpora cavernosa, sexual function, including the ability to have at least a partial erection, is maintained in men undergoing radical prostatectomy or cystoprostatectomy. In cases in which the cavernous nerves cannot be spared, the technique of interposition sural nerve grafting has been shown to help preserve postoperative potency.[138] Partial or full erection returns within 18 to 24 months in more than half of men undergoing bilateral sural nerve grafting at the time of prostatectomy.

In patients who experience ejaculatory dysfunction after RPLND, use of sympathomimetic agents may enhance seminal emission and partially or completely convert the patient to antegrade ejaculation.[139] Pseudoephedrine hydrochloride, ephedrine sulfate, phenylpropanolamine hydrochloride, or imipramine hydrochloride, should be given sequentially in 2-week trials until improvements in semen volume and sperm count are observed. Natural pregnancies have been reported, but use of assisted reproductive technologies is often needed. Even when retrograde ejaculation is present, sperm may be recovered from the bladder by direct voiding into a buffering medium or by catheterization and irrigation with a somewhat alkaline solution.[140] When no ejaculation is present, electroejaculation, using a rectal probe under general anesthesia, has been successful in most patients.[141] Although patients will have some antegrade ejaculate, catheterization should always be done to collect the retrograde semen. Sperm obtained by these methods can be used with IVF-ICSI procedures to achieve 15% pregnancy rates per cycle.

For men experiencing erectile dysfunction after the afore-mentioned surgeries, phosphodiesterase type 5 inhibitors, such as sildenafil, vardenafil, and tadalafil, are clinically effective and safe treatments.[142] For patients who are not responsive to oral administration of these drugs, other treatment options for improving erectile function include intracorporeal injection therapy with a prostaglandin or a mixture of a prostaglandin, an alkaloid, and an α-adrenergic blocker, or penile prosthetic surgery. A penile prosthesis is usually not offered to patients until 2 years after radical prostatectomy to allow for tissue healing and adequate monitoring of cancer control.

GENETIC CONCERNS

BIOLOGIC CONSIDERATIONS

Many anticancer agents damage DNA and interfere with its replication and repair and with chromosome segregation in both animal and human cells. These agents induce both single-gene and chromosomal mutations in germ cells of animals,[143] both of which cause genetic disease in offspring. Mutations induced in stem spermatogonia cause continued production of mutation-carrying sperm for the lifetime of the male, whereas those induced in later stages of spermatogenesis result in production of mutation-carrying sperm for only a few months. Radiation and several alkylating agents produce single-gene mutations in murine spermatogonia, whereas other tested chemotherapeutic drugs do not.[143] Radiation is the only agent that effectively induces stable reciprocal chromosomal translocations in stem spermatogonia that can be transmitted to offspring.[144]

In male rodents, meiotic and postmeiotic germ cells are more sensitive to induction and transmission of mutations than are stem spermatogonia.[2] Therefore, mutational risks are highest when a pregnancy occurs within one spermatogenic cycle (time required for stem cells to become sperm) after the male is exposed to the damaging agent. Clinical reports of outcomes of pregnancies in which conception occurred while the father was undergoing cytotoxic therapy are too limited to evaluate the risks, but animal experiments and gamete genetic analysis show a higher risk.[2] In men, this higher-risk period extends from the start of cytotoxic therapy until 3 months after the last course. After this time, the incidence of mutations is at the lower level found in sperm that were exposed to the mutagen as stem cells.

Fewer studies of the mutagenicity of cytotoxic agents have been done in female mice, but the limited results indicate induced mutation frequencies similar to those in the male. Radiation induces single-gene and chromosomal mutations in developing oocytes.[144] Most alkylating agents and a variety of other chemotherapeutic drugs induce chromosome aberrations or other mutations in developing oocytes that result in embryonic death.[143] There are insufficient data to determine whether primordial or growing oocytes are more sensitive to induction of mutations.

PREGNANCY OUTCOME

In humans, nearly all of the case reports, small series, and a few large retrospective case studies of the outcomes of pregnancies in, or produced by, survivors of cancer indicated no significant increase in birth defects or genetic disease in offspring conceived after cytotoxic treatment above the background level in the general population of approximately 4%.[145] No increase in genetic disease was observed in 630 offspring of patients who were children or adolescents at the time of treatment and received alkylating agents or radiation proximal to the gonads.[146] A study of 368 conceptions in adult women treated previously with methotrexate alone showed no significant adverse effects,[147] as expected. In males, 70 offspring of testicular cancer patients treated with radiotherapy or chemotherapy (most received cisplatin) or both revealed no apparent increase in congenital malformations.[148] In a case-control study involving 45,000 children with congenital abnormalities, there was no higher incidence of parental exposure to alkylating agents or radiation proximal to the gonads in the parents of children with congenital abnormalities than in the parents of the control group of children.[149] The results from the atomic bomb studies in Japan also show no significant increase in genetic damage in 30,000 offspring born to radiation-exposed parents.[150] These observations should reassure those who wish to have children after treatment for cancer. However, the power of these studies can only rule out twofold or higher increases in abnormalities; the possibility remains of a small genetic risk that would increase genetic abnormalities less than twofold over background levels. Also, these long-term studies do not include many patients receiving the newer chemotherapeutic agents.

There are significant teratogenic risks from cytotoxic therapy given to a woman during pregnancy. Radiation is highly damaging; doses as low as 0.1 to 0.2 Gy in the first trimester and doses higher than 0.7 Gy in the second trimester cause microcephaly.[151] Almost all cytotoxic chemotherapeutic agents are considered teratogenic; however, some may be safely given in the second and third trimesters of pregnancy.[152] Treatment with fluorouracil, doxorubicin, and cyclophosphamide during this period did not result in any adverse effects. Methotrexate, which is a documented teratogen in the first trimester, was excluded from the combination.

GAMETE GENOMIC ANALYSIS

Because epidemiologic studies of genetic damage in humans require large numbers of offspring, direct analysis of the genetic material of gametes has huge potential advantages for identifying heritable mutations in humans. Such analyses are used only in the male because harvest of female gametes is impractical. These analyses can be used to detect both single-gene and chromosomal mutations.

Minisatellite repeat number mutations in human spermatozoa have been proposed as a useful marker for single-gene mutations. Indeed, minisatellite mutations were increased in offspring of men exposed to radiation from the Chernobyl accident.[153] However, the absence of increases in minisatellite mutations in spermatozoa from men after treatment with radiotherapy or chemotherapy indicates that the levels of such mutations are below the sensitivity of this technique.[154]

Chromosomal abnormalities are measured by sperm karyotyping after fusion with hamster eggs or by fluorescence *in situ* hybridization. Structural chromosomal aberrations were present in sperm more than 5 years after the end of MOPP or radiation therapy or both, which indicates that they are induced in stem cells.[155] Numerical aberrations (aneuploidy) can show up to a fivefold increase during and shortly after chemotherapy with

NOVP or bleomycin, etoposide, and cisplatin (BEP) and then return to baseline within 4 months or 2 years, depending on the study.[156,157] These results demonstrate that there can be significant genetic risks if conception or storage of sperm occurs during cytotoxic therapy but that this risk declines after the end of such therapy.

Numerous studies have used techniques that measure DNA or chromatin damage in human sperm, such as the comet (alkaline single-cell gel electrophoresis), sperm chromatin structure, and TUNEL (*in situ* DNA nick end labeling) assays.[158] However, these techniques only measure what might be premutational damage; knowledge of repair of such damage within the oocyte is incomplete, so no estimates of mutational risk to the offspring are yet possible from these data.

COUNSELING

Cancer patients should be informed by their physicians about the possibilities of sterility and genetic risk from their disease and its treatment. The probability that sterility will result from the planned cytotoxic therapy should be calculated from the cumulative doses of agents and combinations that cause prolonged azoospermia, ovarian failure, or pituitary damage (see Tables 54.6-3, 54.6-4, and 54.6-6 through 54.6-8). They should also be told about psychological and physical effects on sexual desire, erectile function, and the ability to achieve orgasm.

Pretreatment sperm banking must be offered to all male patients interested in having children after the completion of cytotoxic therapy. The risks of sterility from a given treatment and the probability that a different, more highly sterilizing treatment may be needed before there is another opportunity for semen storage should be considered in making the decision on sperm banking. The costs of semen cryopreservation and other assisted reproductive technologies should be presented, and the patient should be reminded that these are not standard benefits in the majority of health insurance programs in the United States. Female patients should be told that the only proven cryopreservation technique is to have some of the oocytes fertilized and to cryopreserve the embryos obtained. The cryopreservation of oocytes and the use of cryopreserved ovarian tissue are experimental at this time.

During treatment, sexual relations between partners may continue, but reliable contraceptive methods should be used. Condoms should be used when sexual intercourse occurs within 24 hours of administration of a chemotherapeutic agent to the man because of seminal transmission of chemotherapeutic drugs. The level of genetic and teratogenic risks of conception when either partner is undergoing treatment should be outlined. If conception does occur during these times, the couple should be informed of the risks and evaluate the continuation of the pregnancy. Also if a woman develops cancer during her pregnancy, the risks of treatment to the fetus should be communicated so that the appropriate decisions can be made as to when to initiate therapy, what types of therapy to use, and whether to continue or terminate the pregnancy.

It is recommended that patients wait 6 months after the end of therapy before attempting to conceive. If their fertility is preserved, the patients should be informed of the high probability of having healthy children. Although there are theoretical concerns about congenital malformations and genetic disease in offspring, the limited data for humans indicate no measurable excess risk above the background level of 4%, but small (less than twofold) increases could have escaped detection. Any pregnancy after therapy should be monitored (with ultrasonography and possibly amniocentesis) because of the potentially increased genetic risk.

Women should also be told about the risks of chemotherapy-induced premature menopause. If this does occur, it is important to present a balanced discussion of potential benefits of prompt initiation of hormone replacement therapy as well as the risks so that an individually appropriate decision may be reached.

REFERENCES

1. Ries LAG, Eisner MP, Kosary CL, et al. *SEER cancer statistics review, 1975–2000.* Bethesda, MD: National Cancer Institute, 2003.
2. Meistrich ML. Potential genetic risks of using semen collected during chemotherapy. *Hum Reprod* 1993;8:8.
3. Meistrich ML, Wilson G, Brown BW, et al. Impact of cyclophosphamide on long-term reduction in sperm count in men treated with combination chemotherapy for Ewing's and soft tissue sarcomas. *Cancer* 1992;70:2703.
4. Wang J, Galil KAA, Setchell BP. Changes in testicular blood flow and testosterone production during aspermatogenesis after irradiation. *J Endocrinol* 1983;98:35.
5. Viviani S, Santoro A, Ragni G, et al. Gonadal toxicity after combination chemotherapy for Hodgkin's disease. Comparative results of MOPP vs. ABVD. *Eur J Cancer Clin Oncol* 1985;21:601.
6. Petersen PM, Andersson AM, Rørth M, et al. Undetectable inhibin B serum levels in men after testicular irradiation. *J Clin Endocrinol Metab* 1999;84:213.
7. Marmor D, Grob-Menendez F, Duyck F, et al. Very late return of spermatogenesis after chlorambucil therapy: case reports. *Fertil Steril* 1992;58:845.
8. Pryzant RM, Meistrich ML, Wilson E, et al. Long-term reduction in sperm count after chemotherapy with and without radiation therapy for non-Hodgkin's lymphomas. *J Clin Oncol* 1993;11:239.
9. Anserini P, Chiodi S, Spinelli S, et al. Semen analysis following allogeneic bone marrow transplantation. Additional data for evidence-based counselling. *Bone Marrow Transplant* 2002;30:447.
10. Lampe H, Horwich A, Norman A, et al. Fertility after chemotherapy for testicular germ cell cancers. *J Clin Oncol* 1997;15:239.
11. Jacobsen KD, Theodorsen L, Fossa SD. Spermatogenesis after unilateral orchiectomy for testicular cancer in patients following surveillance policy. *J Urol* 2001;165:93.
12. Jacobsen KD, Ous S, Waehre H, et al. Ejaculation in testicular cancer patients after postchemotherapy retroperitoneal lymph node dissection. *Br J Cancer* 1999;80:249.
13. Meistrich ML, Wilson G, Mathur K, et al. Rapid recovery of spermatogenesis after mitoxantrone, vincristine, vinblastine, and prednisone chemotherapy for Hodgkin's disease. *J Clin Oncol* 1997;15:3488.
14. Howell SJ, Shalet SM. Effect of cancer therapy on pituitary-testicular axis. *Int J Androl* 2002;25:269.
15. Hansen PV, Trykker H, Svennakjaer IL, et al. Long-term recovery of spermatogenesis after radiotherapy in patients with testicular cancer. *Radiother Oncol* 1990;18:117.
16. Marina S, Barcelo P. Permanent sterility after immunosuppressive therapy. *Int J Androl* 1979;2:6.
17. Buchanan JD, Fairley KF, Barrie JV. Return of spermatogenesis after stopping cyclophosphamide therapy. *Lancet* 1975;2:156.
18. da Cunha MF, Meistrich ML, Fuller LM, et al. Recovery of spermatogenesis after treatment for Hodgkin's disease: limiting dose of MOPP chemotherapy. *J Clin Oncol* 1984;2:571.
19. Hansen PV, Trykker H, Helkjaer PE, et al. Testicular function in patients with testicular cancer treated with orchiectomy alone or orchiectomy plus cisplatin-based chemotherapy. *J Natl Cancer Inst* 1989;81:1246.
20. Sanders JE, Hawley J, Levy W, et al. Pregnancies following high-dose cyclophosphamide with or without high-dose busulfan or total-body irradiation and bone marrow transplantation. *Blood* 1996;87:3045.
21. Longhi A, Macchiagodena M, Vitali G, et al. Fertility in male patients treated with neoadjuvant chemotherapy for osteosarcoma. *J Pediatr Hematol Oncol* 2003;25:292.
22. Ahmed SR, Shalet SM, Campbell RHA, et al. Primary gonadal damage following treatment of brain tumors in childhood. *J Pediatr* 1983;103:562.
23. Hall MC, Fritzsch RJ, Sagalowsky AI, et al. Prospective determination of the hormonal response after cessation of luteinizing hormone–releasing hormone agonist treatment in patients with prostate cancer. *Urology* 1999;53:898.
24. Meistrich ML, van Beek MEAB. Radiation sensitivity of the human testis. *Adv Radiat Biol* 1990;14:227.
25. Gordon W, Siegmund K, Stanisic TH, et al. A study of reproductive function in patients with seminoma treated with radiotherapy and orchidectomy: (SWOG-8711). *Int J Radiat Oncol Biol Phys* 1997;38:83.
26. Petersen PM, Giwercman A, Daugaard G, et al. Effect of graded testicular doses of radiotherapy in patients treated for carcinoma-in-situ in the testis. *J Clin Oncol* 2002;20:1537.

27. Zagars GK, Pollack A. Serum testosterone levels after external beam radiation for clinically localized prostate cancer. *Int J Radiat Oncol Biol Phys* 1997;39:85.

28. Dubey P, Wilson G, Mathur KK, et al. Recovery of sperm production following radiation therapy for Hodgkin's disease after induction chemotherapy with mitoxantrone, vincristine, vinblastine and prednisone (NOVP). *Int J Radiat Oncol Biol Phys* 2000;46:609.

29. Kreuser ED, Xiros N, Hetzel WD, et al. Reproductive and endocrine gonadal capacity in patients treated with COPP chemotherapy for Hodgkin's disease. *J Cancer Res Clin Oncol* 1987;113:260.

30. Jacob A, Barker H, Goodman A, et al. Recovery of spermatogenesis following bone marrow transplantation. *Bone Marrow Transplant* 1998;22:277.

31. Viviani S, Ragni G, Santoro A, et al. Testicular dysfunction in Hodgkin's disease before and after treatment. *Eur J Cancer* 1991;27:1389.

32. Kulkarni SS, Sastry PS, Saikia TK, et al. Gonadal function following ABVD therapy for Hodgkin's disease. *Am J Clin Oncol* 1997;20:354.

33. Clark ST, Radford JA, Crowther D, et al. A comparative study of MVPP and a seven-drug hybrid regimen. *J Clin Oncol* 1995;13:134.

34. Viviani S, Bonfante V, Santoro A, et al. Long-term results of an intensive regimen: VEBEP plus involved-field radiotherapy in advanced Hodgkin's disease. *Cancer J Sci Am* 1999;5:275.

35. Shamberger RC, Sherins RJ, Ziegler JL, et al. Effects of postoperative adjuvant chemotherapy and radiotherapy on ovarian function in women undergoing treatment for soft tissue sarcoma. *J Natl Cancer Inst* 1981;67:1213.

36. Evenson DP, Arlin Z, Welt S, et al. Male reproductive capacity may recover following drug treatment with the L-10 protocol for acute lymphocytic leukemia. *Cancer* 1984;53:30.

37. Brennemann W, Stoffel-Wagner B, Helmers A, et al. Gonadal function of patients treated with cisplatin based chemotherapy for germ cell cancer. *J Urol* 1997;158:844.

38. Stephenson WT, Poirier SM, Rubin L, et al. Evaluation of reproductive capacity in germ cell tumor patients following treatment with cisplatin, etoposide, and bleomycin. *J Clin Oncol* 1995;13:2278.

39. Meistrich ML, Chawla SP, da Cunha MF, et al. Recovery of sperm production after chemotherapy for osteosarcoma. *Cancer* 1989;63:2115.

40. Tilly JL, Kolesnick RN. Sphingolipids, apoptosis, cancer treatments and the ovary: investigating a crime against female fertility. *Biochim Biophys Acta* 2002;1585:135.

41. Meirow D, Nugent D. The effects of radiotherapy and chemotherapy on female reproduction. *Hum Reprod Update* 2001;7:535.

42. Sanders JE. Growth and development after hematopoietic cell transplantation. In: Thomas ED, Blume KG, Forman SJ, eds. *Hematopoietic cell transplantation*, 2nd ed. Malden, MA: Blackwell Science, 1999:764.

43. Schilsky RL, Sherins RJ, Hubbard SM, et al. Long-term follow-up of ovarian function in women treated with MOPP chemotherapy for Hodgkin's disease. *Am J Med* 1981;71: 552.

44. Kuhajda FP, Haupt HM, Moore GW, et al. Gonadal morphology in patients receiving chemotherapy for leukemia. Evidence for reproductive potential and against a testicular tumor sanctuary. *Am J Med* 1982;72:759.

45. Boumpas DT, Austin HA III, Vaughan EM, et al. Risk for sustained amenorrhea in patients with systemic lupus erythematosus receiving intermittent pulse cyclophosphamide therapy. *Ann Intern Med* 1993;119:366.

46. Singhal S, Powles R, Treleaven J, et al. Melphalan alone prior to allogeneic bone marrow transplantation from HLA-identical sibling donors for hematologic malignancies: alloengraftment with potential preservation of fertility in women. *Bone Marrow Transplant* 1996;18:1049.

47. Teinturier C, Hartmann O, Valteau-Couanet D, et al. Ovarian function after autologous bone marrow transplantation in childhood: high-dose busulfan is a major cause of ovarian failure. *Bone Marrow Transplant* 1998;22:989.

48. Koyama H, Wada T, Nishizawa Y, et al. Cyclophosphamide-induced ovarian failure and its therapeutic significance in patients with breast cancer. *Cancer* 1977;39:1403.

49. Spinelli S, Chiodi S, Bacigalupo A, et al. Ovarian recovery after total body irradiation and allogeneic bone marrow transplantation: long-term follow up of 79 females. *Bone Marrow Transplant* 1994;14:373.

50. Sanders JE, Buckner CD, Amos D, et al. Ovarian function following marrow transplantation for aplastic anemia or leukemia. *J Clin Oncol* 1988;6:813.

51. Sy Ortin TT, Shostak CA, Donaldson SS. Gonadal status and reproductive function following treatment for Hodgkin's disease in childhood: the Stanford experience. *Int J Radiat Oncol Biol Phys* 1990;19:873.

52. Specht L, Hansen MM, Geisler C. Ovarian function in young women in long-term remission after treatment for Hodgkin's disease stage I and II. *Scand J Hematol* 1984;32:265.

53. Longo DL, Glatstein E, Duffey PL, et al. Alternating MOPP and ABVD chemotherapy plus mantle-field radiation therapy in patients with massive mediastinal Hodgkin's disease. *J Clin Oncol* 1997;15:3338.

54. Samaan NA, deAsis DN, Buzdar AU, et al. Pituitary-ovarian function in breast cancer patients on adjuvant chemoimmunotherapy. *Cancer* 1978;41:2084.

55. Dnistrian AM, Schwartz MK, Fraccia AA, et al. Endocrine consequences of CMF adjuvant therapy in premenopausal and postmenopausal breast cancer patients. *Cancer* 1983;51:803.

56. Byrne J, Fears TR, Gail MH, et al. Early menopause in long-term survivors of cancer during adolescence. *Am J Obstet Gynecol* 1992;166:788.

57. Byrne J, Mulvihill JJ, Myers MH, et al. Effects of treatment on fertility in long-term survivors of childhood or adolescent cancer. *N Engl J Med* 1987;317:1315.

58. Howell SJ, Berger G, Adams JE, et al. Bone mineral density in women with cytotoxic-induced ovarian failure. *Clin Endocrinol* 1998;49:397.

59. Wallace WHB, Shalet SM, Crowne EC, et al. Gonadal dysfunction due to cisplatinum. *Med Pediatr Oncol* 1989;17:409.

60. Shamberger RC, Rosenberg SA, Seipp CA, et al. Effects of high-dose methotrexate and vincristine on ovarian and testicular functions in patients undergoing postoperative adjuvant treatment for osteosarcoma. *Cancer Treat Rep* 1981;65:739.

61. Choo YC, Chan SYW, Wong LC, et al. Ovarian dysfunction in patients with gestational trophoblastic neoplasia treated with short intensive courses of etoposide (VP-16-213). *Cancer* 1985;55:2348.

62. Bonadonna G, Santoro A, Viviani S, et al. Gonadal damage in Hodgkin's disease from cancer chemotherapy regimens. *Arch Toxicol* 1984;Suppl 7:140.

63. Mourits MJ, DeVries EG, Willemse PH, et al. Tamoxifen treatment and gynecologic side effects: a review. *Obstet Gynecol* 2001;97:855.

64. Morice P, Juncker L, Rey A, et al. Ovarian transposition for patients with cervical carcinoma treated by radiosurgical combination. *Fertil Steril* 2000;74:743.

65. Horning SJ, Hoppe RT, Kaplan HS, et al. Female reproductive potential after treatment for Hodgkin's disease. *N Engl J Med* 1981;304:1377.

66. Jaffe N, Sullivan MP, Ried H, et al. Male reproductive function in long-term survivors of childhood cancer. *Med Pediatr Oncol* 1988;16:241.

67. Siimes MA, Dunkel L, Rautonen J. Risk factors for endocrine testicular dysfunction in adolescent and adult males who have survived malignancies in childhood. *Cancer J* 1992;5:28.

68. Muller J, Skakkebaek NE, Hertz H. Initiation of spermatogenesis during chemotherapy for leukemia. *Acta Paediatr Scand* 1985;74:956.

69. Gerres L, Bramswig JH, Schlegel W, et al. The effects of etoposide on testicular function in boys treated for Hodgkin's disease. *Cancer* 1998;83:2217.

70. Sarafoglou K, Boulad F, Gillio A, et al. Gonadal function after bone marrow transplantation for acute leukemia during childhood. *J Pediatr* 1997;130:210.

71. Blatt J, Sherins RJ, Niebrugge D, et al. Leydig cell function in boys following treatment for testicular relapse of acute lymphocytic leukemia. *J Clin Oncol* 1985;3:1227.

72. Stillman RJ, Schinfeld JS, Schiff I, et al. Ovarian failure in long-term survivors of childhood malignancy. *Am J Obstet Gynecol* 1981;139:62.

73. Couto-Silva AC, Trivin C, Thibaud E, et al. Factors affecting gonadal function after bone marrow transplantation during childhood. *Bone Marrow Transplant* 2001;28:67.

74. Watson AR, Taylor J, Rance CP, et al. Gonadal function in women treated with cyclophosphamide for childhood nephrotic syndrome: a long-term follow-up study. *Fertil Steril* 1986;46:331.

75. Fryer CJ, Hutchinson RJ, Krailo M, et al. Efficacy and toxicity of 12 courses of ABVD chemotherapy followed by low-dose regional radiation in advanced Hodgkin's disease in children: a report from the Children's Cancer Study Group. *J Clin Oncol* 1990;8:1971.

76. Clayton PE, Shalet SM, Price DA, et al. Ovarian function following chemotherapy for childhood brain tumours. *Med Pediatr Oncol* 1989;17:92.

77. Mackie EJ, Radford M, Shalet SM. Gonadal function following chemotherapy for childhood Hodgkin's disease. *Med Pediatr Oncol* 1996;27:74.

78. Critchley HO. Factors of importance for implantation and problems after treatment for childhood cancer. *Med Pediatr Oncol* 1999;33:9.

79. Mauras N, Sabio H, Rogol QD. Neuroendocrine function in survivors of childhood acute lymphocytic leukemia and non-Hodgkin's lymphoma: a study of pulsatile growth hormone and gonadotropin secretion. *Am J Pediatr Hematol Oncol* 1988;10:9.

80. Schmiegelow M, Lassen S, Poulsen HS, et al. Gonadal status in male survivors following childhood brain tumors. *J Clin Endocrinol Metab* 2001;86:2446.

81. Lannering B, Jansson C, Rosberg S, et al. Increased LH and FSH secretion after cranial irradiation in boys. *Med Pediatr Oncol* 1997;29:280.

82. Constine LS, Woolf PD, Cann D, et al. Hypothalamic-pituitary dysfunction after radiation for brain tumors. *N Engl J Med* 1993;328:87.

83. Shalet SM, Brennan BM. Puberty in children with cancer. *Horm Res* 2002;57:39.

84. Littley MD, Shalet SM, Morgenstern GR, et al. Endocrine and reproductive dysfunction following fractionated total body irradiation in adults. *Q J Med* 1991;78:265.

85. Littley MD, Shalet SM, Beardwell CG, et al. Radiation-induced hypopituitarism is dose-dependent. *Clin Endocrinol* 1989;31:363.

86. Samaan NA, Vieto R, Schultz PN, et al. Hypothalamic, pituitary and thyroid dysfunction after radiotherapy to the head and neck. *Int J Radiat Oncol Biol Phys* 1982;8:1857.

87. Radford JA, Clark S, Crowther D, et al. Male fertility after VAPEC-B chemotherapy for Hodgkin's disease and non-Hodgkin's lymphoma. *Br J Cancer* 1994;69:379.

88. Bieri S, Rouzaud M, Miralbell R. Seminoma of the testis: is scrotal shielding necessary when radiotherapy is limited to the para-aortic nodes? *Radiother Oncol* 1999;50:349.

89. Schover LR, Brey K, Lichitin A, et al. Knowledge and experience regarding cancer, infertility and sperm banking in younger male survivors. *J Clin Oncol* 2002;20:1880.

90. Schover LR, Brye K, Lichitin A, et al. Oncologists' attitudes and practices regarding banking sperm before cancer treatment. *J Clin Oncol* 2002;20:1890.

91. Kliesch S, Behre HM, Jurgens H, et al. Cryopreservation of semen from adolescent patients with malignancies. *Med Pediatr Oncol* 1996;26:20.

92. Schmiegelow ML, Sommer P, Carlsen E, et al. Penile vibratory stimulation and electroejaculation before anticancer therapy in two pubertal boys. *J Pediatr Hematol Oncol* 1998;20:429.

93. Schrader M, Muller M, Straub B, et al. Testicular sperm extraction in azoospermic patients with gonadal germ cell tumors prior to chemotherapy—a new therapy option. *Asian J Androl* 2002;4:9.

94. Park YS, Lee SH, Song SJ, et al. Influence of motility on the outcome of in vitro fertilization/intracytoplasmic sperm injection with fresh vs frozen testicular sperm from men with obstructive azoospermia. *Fertil Steril* 2003;80:526.

95. Marmor D, Duyck F. Male reproductive potential after MOPP therapy for Hodgkin's disease: a long-term survey. *Andrologia* 1995;27:99.

96. Ginsburg ES, Yanushpolsky EH, Jackson KV. In vitro fertilization for cancer patients and survivors. *Fertil Steril* 2001;75:705.

97. Larsen EC, Loft A, Holm K, et al. Oocyte donation in women cured of cancer with bone marrow transplantation including total body irradiation in adolescence. *Hum Reprod* 2000;15:1505.

98. Sanger WG, Olson JH, Sherman JK. Semen cryobanking for men with cancer-criteria change. *Fertil Steril* 1992;58:1024.

99. Palermo GD, Cohen J, Alikani M, et al. Intracytoplasmic sperm injection: a novel treatment for all forms of male factor infertility. *Fertil Steril* 1995;63:1231.

100. Rosenlund B, Sjoblom P, Tornblom M, et al. In-vitro fertilization and intracytoplasmic sperm injection in the treatment of infertility after testicular cancer. *Hum Reprod* 1998;13:414.

101. Olivius K, Friden B, Lundin K, et al. Cumulative probability of live birth after three in vitro fertilization/intracytoplasmic sperm injection cycles. *Fertil Steril* 2002;77:505.

102. Practice Committee of the Society for Assisted Reproductive Technology and the American Society for Reproductive Medicine. Round spermatid nucleus injection (ROSNI). *Fertil Steril* 2003;80:687.

103. Sutcliffe AG, Taylor B, Saunders K, et al. Outcome in the second year of life after in-vitro fertilisation by intracytoplasmic sperm injection: a UK case-control study. *Lancet* 2001;357:2080.

104. Hansen M, Kurinczuk JJ, Bower C, et al. The risk of major birth defects after intracytoplasmic sperm injection and in vitro fertilization. *N Engl J Med* 2002;346:725.

105. Retzloff MG, Hornstein MD. Is intracytoplasmic sperm injection safe? *Fertil Steril* 2003;80:851.

106. Oktay K, Buyuk E, Davis O, et al. Fertility preservation in breast cancer patients: IVF and embryo cryopreservation after ovarian stimulation with tamoxifen. *Hum Reprod* 2003;18:90.

107. Blumenfeld Z. Gynaecologic concerns for young women exposed to gonadotoxic chemotherapy. *Current Opin Obstet Gynecol.* 2003;15:359.

108. Fosas N, Marina F, Torres PJ, et al. The births of five Spanish babies from cryopreserved donated oocytes. *Hum Reprod* 2003;18:1417.

109. Baird DT, Webb R, Campbell BK, et al. Long-term ovarian function in sheep after ovariectomy and transplantation of autografts stored at −196°C. *Endocrinology* 1999;140:462.

110. Oktay K. Ovarian tissue cryopreservation and transplantation: preliminary findings and implications for cancer patients. *Hum Reprod Update* 2001;7:526.

111. O'Brien MJ, Pendola JK, Eppig JJ. A revised protocol for in vitro development of mouse oocytes from primordial follicles dramatically improves their developmental competence. *Biol Reprod* 2003;68:1682.

112. Wininger JD, Kort HI. Cryopreservation of immature and mature human oocytes. *Semin Reprod Med* 2002;20:45.

113. Hubner K, Fuhrmann G, Christenson LK, et al. Derivation of oocytes from mouse embryonic stem cells. *Science* 2003;300:1251.

114. Avarbock MR, Brinster CJ, Brinster RL. Reconstitution of spermatogenesis from frozen spermatogonial stem cells. *Nat Med* 1996;2:693.

115. Schlatt S, Foppiani L, Rolf C, et al. Germ cell transplantation into X-irradiated monkey testes. *Hum Reprod* 2002;17:55.

116. Radford J. Restoration of fertility after treatment for cancer. *Horm Res* 2003;59[Suppl 1]:21.

117. Jahnukainen K, Hou M, Petersen C, et al. Intratesticular transplantation of testicular cells from leukemic rats causes transmission of leukemia. *Cancer Res* 2001;61:706.

118. Nagano M, Patrizio P, Brinster RL. Long-term survival of human spermatogonial stem cells in mouse testes. *Fertil Steril* 2002;78:1225.

119. Honaramooz A, Snedaker A, Boiani M, et al. Sperm from neonatal mammalian testes grafted in mice. *Nature* 2002;418:778.

120. Cremades N, Sousa M, Bernabeu R, et al. Developmental potential of elongating and elongated spermatids obtained after in-vitro maturation of isolated round spermatids. *Hum Reprod* 2001;16:1938.

121. Feng LX, Chen Y, Dettin L, et al. Generation and in vitro differentiation of a spermatogonial cell line. *Science* 2002;297:392.

122. Toyooka Y, Tsunekawa N, Akasu R, et al. Embryonic stem cells can form germ cells in vitro. *Proc Natl Acad Sci U S A* 2003;100:11457.

123. Meistrich ML, Shetty G. Suppression of testosterone stimulates recovery of spermatogenesis after cancer treatment. *Int J Androl* 2003;26:141.

124. Meistrich ML, Wilson G, Kangasniemi M, et al. Mechanism of protection of rat spermatogenesis by hormonal pretreatment: stimulation of spermatogonial differentiation after irradiation. *J Androl* 2000;21:464.

125. Masala A, Faedda R, Alagna S, et al. Use of testosterone to prevent cyclophosphamide-induced azoospermia. *Ann Intern Med* 1997;126:292.

126. Howell SJ, Shalet SM. Fertility preservation and management of gonadal failure associated with lymphoma therapy. *Curr Oncol Rep* 2002;4:443.

127. Thomson AB, Anderson RA, Irvine DS, et al. Investigation of suppression of the hypothalamic-pituitary-gonadal axis to restore spermatogenesis in azoospermic men treated for childhood cancer. *Hum Reprod* 2002;17:1715.

128. Kamischke A, Kuhlmann M, Weinbauer GF, et al. Gonadal protection from radiation by GnRH antagonist or recombinant human FSH: a controlled trial in a male nonhuman primate (*Macaca fascicularis*). *J Endocrinol* 2003;179:183.

129. Ataya K, Rao LV, Lawrence E, et al. Luteinizing hormone–releasing hormone agonist inhibits cyclophosphamide-induced ovarian follicular depletion in rhesus monkeys. *Biol Reprod* 1995;52:365.

130. Waxman JH, Ahmed R, Smith D, et al. Failure to preserve fertility in patients with Hodgkin's disease. *Cancer Chemother Pharmacol* 1987;19:159.

131. Blumenfeld Z. Fertility after treatment for Hodgkin's disease. *Ann Oncol* 2002;13[Suppl 1]:138.

132. Chatterjee R, Goldstone AH. Gonadal damage and effects on fertility in adult patients with haematological malignancy undergoing stem cell transplantation. *Bone Marrow Transplant* 1996;17:5.

133. Writing Group for the Women's Health Initiative Investigators. Risks and benefits of estrogen plus progestin in healthy postmenopausal women: principal results from the Women's Health Initiative randomized controlled trial. *JAMA* 2002;288:321.

134. Mulder JE. Benefits and risks of hormone replacement therapy in young adult cancer survivors with gonadal failure. *Med Pediatr Oncol* 1999;33:46.

135. Howell SJ, Radford JA, Adams JE, et al. Randomized placebo-controlled trial of testosterone replacement in men with mild Leydig cell insufficiency following cytotoxic chemotherapy. *Clin Endocrinol* 2001;55:315.

136. Lange PH, Narayan P, Fraley EE. Fertility issues following therapy for testicular cancer. *Semin Urol* 1984;11:264.

137. Walsh PC, Mostwin JL. Radical prostatectomy and cystoprostatectomy with preservation of potency. Results using a new nerve-sparing technique. *Br J Urol* 1984;56:694.

138. Chang DW, Wood CG, Kroll SS, et al. Cavernous nerve reconstruction to preserve erectile function following non–nerve sparing radical retropubic prostatectomy: a prospective study. *Plast Reconstr Surg* 2003;111:1174.

139. Ochsenkuhn R, Kamischke A, Nieschlag E. Imipramine for successful treatment of retrograde ejaculation caused by retroperitoneal surgery. *Int J Androl* 1999;22:173.

140. Gilja I, Parazajder J, Radej M, et al. Retrograde ejaculation and loss of emission: possibilities of conservative treatment. *Eur Urol* 1994;25:226.

141. Ohl DA, Woof LJ, Menge AC, et al. Electroejaculation and assisted reproductive technologies in the treatment of an ejaculatory infertility. *Fertil Steril* 2001;76:1249.

142. Brock G, Nehra AJ, Lipshultz LI, et al. Safety and efficacy of vardenafil for the treatment of men with erectile dysfunction after radical retropubic prostatectomy. *J Urol* 2003;170:1278.

143. Witt KL, Bishop JB. Mutagenicity of anticancer drugs in mammalian germ cells. *Mutat Res* 1996;355:209.

144. Committee on the Biological Effects of Ionizing Radiation. *Health effects of exposure to low levels of ionizing radiation: BEIR V.* Washington, DC: National Academy Press, 1990.

145. Blatt J. Pregnancy outcome in long-term survivors of childhood cancer. *Med Pediatr Oncol* 1999;33:29.

146. Meistrich ML, Byrne J. Genetic disease in offspring of long-term survivors of childhood and adolescent cancer treated with potentially mutagenic therapies. *Am J Hum Genet* 2002;70:1069.

147. Rustin GJ, Booth M, Dent J, et al. Pregnancy after cytotoxic chemotherapy for gestational trophoblastic tumours. *BMJ* 1984;288:103.

148. Senturia YD, Peckham CS, Peckham MJ. Children fathered by men treated for testicular cancer. *Lancet* 1985;2:766.

149. Dodds L, Marrett LD, Tomkins DJ, et al. Case-control study of congenital anomalies in children of cancer patients. *BMJ* 1993;307:164.

150. Neel JV, Schull WJ, Awa AA, et al. The children of parents exposed to atomic bombs: estimates of the genetic doubling dose of radiation for humans. *Am J Hum Genet* 1990;46:1053.

151. Yamazaki JN, Schull WJ. Perinatal loss and neurological abnormalities among children of the atomic bomb. Nagasaki and Hiroshima revisited, 1949 to 1989. *JAMA* 1990;264:605.

152. Keleher AJ, Theriault RL, Gwyn KM, et al. Multidisciplinary management of breast cancer concurrent with pregnancy. *J Am Coll Surg* 2002;194:54.

153. Dubrova YE, Grant GR, Chumak AA, et al. Elevated minisatellite mutation rate in the post-Chernobyl families from Ukraine. *Am J Hum Genet* 2002;71:801.

154. May CA, Tamaki K, Neumann R, et al. Minisatellite mutation frequency in human sperm following radiotherapy. *Mutat Res* 2000;453:67.

155. Brandriff BF, Meistrich ML, Gordon LA, et al. Chromosomal damage in sperm of patients surviving Hodgkin's disease following MOPP therapy with and without radiotherapy. *Hum Genet* 1994;93:295.

156. Frias S, Van Hummelen P, Meistrich ML, et al. NOVP chemotherapy for Hodgkin's disease transiently induces sperm aneuploidies associated with the major clinical aneuploidy syndromes involving chromosomes X, Y, and 18 and 21. *Cancer Res* 2003;63:44.

157. Robbins WA, Meistrich ML, Moore D, et al. Chemotherapy induces transient sex chromosomal and autosomal aneuploidy in human sperm. *Nat Genet* 1997;16:74.

158. Morris ID. Sperm DNA damage and cancer treatment. *Int J Androl* 2002;25:255.

FLORA E. VAN LEEUWEN
LOIS B. TRAVIS

SECTION 7

Second Cancers

Modern chemotherapy and radiotherapy have increased substantially the survival of patients with cancer. In particular, cure rates have shown dramatic improvement for patients with Hodgkin's disease (HD), testicular cancer, and pediatric malignancies. Less impressive but nonetheless convincing improvements in survival have also been achieved for patients with breast cancer, non-Hodgkin's lymphoma (NHL), and several other tumors. Now that substantial numbers of cancer patients have such a favorable prognosis, it becomes increasingly important to evaluate the long-term complications of treatment. Because the survival benefits associated with modern treatments have been greatest for those cancers that occur at relatively young ages, cured patients are subject to long-term side effects, which may not emerge until several decades after treatment. Paradoxically, research conducted since the late 1970s has clearly demonstrated that some of the modalities used to treat cancer have the potential to induce new (second) primary malignancies. Of the many late complications of treatment, second cancers are generally considered to be the most serious, because they cause not only substantial morbidity but also considerable mortality. For example, among long-term survivors of HD, deaths from second cancers have been reported to be the largest contributor to the substantial excess mortality that these patients experience.[1] Increased risks of second cancers have been observed after radiotherapy, chemotherapy, and combined modality treatment.

In any discussion of treatment-related second malignancies, it is of primary importance to remember that not all second cancers are due to therapy. The occurrence of two primary malignancies in the same individual may reflect the operation of numerous influences. Multiple primary cancers may result from host susceptibility (genetic predisposition or immunodeficiency), common carcinogenic influences, a clustering of risk factors, treatment for the first tumor, diagnostic surveillance, a chance event, or the interaction of these factors. In view of the high prevalence of cancer in the general population and the increasing incidence of most cancers with age, it is important to exclude the role of chance in the development of second cancers. To this end, comparison with cancer incidence statistics derived from the general population is crucial. If a second malignancy is demonstrated to occur in excess, the contributions of other risk factors need to be ruled out convincingly before the increased risk can be attributed to treatment. The temporal trend of excess second cancer risk may provide an important initial clue to etiology; for example, the risk of solid tumors after radiotherapy generally increases with time since exposure. The evaluation of the carcinogenic effects of therapy, however, is complicated by the fact that therapeutic agents are frequently given in combination. Appropriate epidemiologic and statistical methods are required to quantify the excess risk and to unravel the role of treatment and other factors.

Whenever results of second cancer studies are interpreted, it must be kept in mind that the problem of treatment-induced malignancies has arisen by virtue of the success of cancer therapy. As more becomes known about the influence of various treatment factors on second cancer risk, therapies may be modified to decrease the risk while maintaining equal levels of therapeutic effectiveness.

The major aspects of second malignancy risk in relation to cancer treatment are addressed in this chapter. After a discussion of methods used for the assessment of second cancer risk, an overview of the carcinogenic effects of radiotherapy and chemotherapy is presented. Subsequently, the risk of second malignancies after treatment for HD, NHL, testicular cancer, breast cancer, ovarian cancer, and pediatric malignancies is reviewed. Emphasis is on large studies that have been published most recently.

METHODS TO ASSESS SECOND CANCER RISK

Estimates of second cancer risk after treatment of various primary malignancies derive from several sources, including population-based cancer registries, hospital-based cancer registries, and clinical trial series.[2] The epidemiologic study designs generally used are the cohort study and the case-control study.

In a cohort study, a large group of patients with a specified first malignancy (the cohort) is followed for a number of years to determine the incidence of second cancers. To evaluate whether second cancer risk in the cohort is increased compared with cancer risk in the general population, the observed number of second cancers in the cohort is compared with the number expected on the basis of age-, gender-, and calendar year–specific cancer incidence rates in the general population. The analysis takes into account the observation period of individual patients (person-years).[3] The relative risk (RR) of developing a second cancer is estimated by comparing the ratio of the observed number of second cancer cases in the cohort to the number expected. When the RR is increased, the question arises whether the excesses are due to therapy. This issue can be evaluated by comparing risks across treatment groups, preferably within specified follow-up intervals and, when possible, with a reference group of patients not treated with radiotherapy and chemotherapy. Second cancer risk in the cohort (and in different treatment groups) can also be expressed by the cumulative (actuarial estimated) risk,[4] which yields the proportion of patients alive at time t (e.g., 5 years from diagnosis) who can be expected to develop a second malignancy. When the cohort's death rate due to causes other than second malignancy is high, the assumptions underlying the actuarial method may not be valid, and competing risk techniques should be considered to estimate cumulative risk.[5,6] Because many treatment-related cancers are rare in the general population (e.g., leukemia, sarcoma), a high RR (compared to the population) may still translate into a rather low cumulative risk. Absolute excess risk (AER), which estimates the excess number of second malignancies per 10,000 patients per year, perhaps best reflects the second cancer burden in a cohort. This risk measure is also the most appropriate one by which to identify those second malignancies that contribute the most to elevated risks. Complete follow-up and valid ascertainment of second malignancies through pathology reports are critical to ensure the validity of cohort studies of second cancer risk. Overestimation of second cancer risk occurs when follow-up in the original treatment center is more complete for survivors who develop a second malignancy than those who remain healthy. This is likely to happen, because patients who remain healthy tend to lose contact with the medical system, whereas patients with a second cancer seek clinical follow-up. In view of this serious potential for bias, it is of great concern that completeness of follow-up is rarely reported in second cancer studies.

Each of the data sources used to construct a cohort has its own set of advantages and disadvantages. Population-based cancer registries frequently have large numbers of patients available, which allows the detection of even small increases in the site-specific risk of second cancers.[7] An additional advantage is that the observed and expected numbers of cancers derive from the same reference population. Disadvantages of this approach include the limited availability of treatment data, underreporting of second cancers[8,9] (in particular, hematologic malignancies and bilateral cancers in paired organs), and the use of different diagnostic criteria for second cancers. Population-based registries differ greatly in these aspects, and hence in their usefulness for second cancer studies. If treatment data are not available, it is impossible to definitively determine whether excess risk for a second malignancy is related to treatment or to shared etiologic factors with the first cancer, although temporal trends in increased risks and the examination of reciprocal risks between sites may provide preliminary clues. Despite their disadvantages, population-based registries are especially well suited to broadly evaluate which second cancers occur in excess after a wide spectrum of different first primary malignancies. They also provide a valuable starting point for case-control studies that evaluate treatment effects in detail (see later in this section).

A major strength of clinical trial databases is that detailed treatment data on all patients are available. Comparison of second cancer risk between the treatment arms of the trial controls for any intrinsic risk for a second malignancy associated with the first cancer. Limitations of most trials include the small number of patients involved and the frequent lack of data on subsequent therapy. The dearth of large numbers becomes more serious when the second cancer of interest has a low background incidence (e.g., leukemia). Furthermore, the end points of interest in the majority of clinical trials include only treatment response and survival, not the development of second cancers. Therefore, many clinical trials do not routinely collect information on second malignancies, and some do not collect any data beyond 5 years. Routine reporting and assessment of second malignancy risk should become an integral part of clinical trial research.[10]

Many large cancer treatment centers maintain registries of all admitted patients. Most of these registries have been in existence for decades and collect extensive data on treatment and follow-up. Compared with trial data, hospital registries provide larger patient numbers and a wider variety of treatments and dose levels, which may yield important information on drug and radiation carcinogenesis. Most studies of second cancer risk after HD have been based on data accrued from hospital registries.[11–15]

The cohort study is not an efficient design when examining detailed treatment factors (e.g., cumulative dose of alkylating agents) in relation to second cancer risk. Most cohorts are fairly large (to yield reliable estimates of second cancer risk),

which renders the collection of detailed treatment data for all patients prohibitively expensive and time consuming. In such instances, the nested case-control study within an existing cohort is the preferred approach. The case group consists of all patients identified with the second cancer of interest, whereas the controls are a matched sample of all patients in the cohort who did not develop the cancer concerned, although they experienced the same amount of follow-up time. Matching factors typically include age, gender, and calendar year of diagnosis of the first cancer. Even when the control group is three times as large as the case group, detailed treatment data need only be collected for a small proportion of the total cohort. In each case-control investigation, it is critical to the validity of the study that the controls be truly representative of all patients who did not contract the second cancer of interest. In data analysis, treatment factors are compared between cases and controls, and the risk associated with specific therapies is estimated relative to the risk in patients who received other treatments. The cumulative risk of developing a second malignancy cannot be derived from a case-control study. Treatment-specific AERs can be estimated, however, when the case-control study follows a cohort analysis. Several landmark studies have clearly demonstrated the strengths of case-control methodology.[8,16–23]

CARCINOGENICITY OF INDIVIDUAL TREATMENT MODALITIES

RADIOTHERAPY

The carcinogenic potential of ionizing radiation was first recognized in the mid-twentieth century,[24,25] and comprehensive reviews have been published.[26–28] Much of the data with regard to radiation effects in humans has derived from epidemiologic studies of the atomic bomb survivors in Japan,[29–31] occupationally exposed workers,[32,33] patients given large amounts of diagnostic radiation,[34,35] and patients treated with radiotherapy for malignant[16,21,22,36–38] and nonmalignant diseases.[39,40] Most types of cancer, with the exception of chronic lymphocytic leukemia, can be caused by exposure to ionizing radiation.[27,29,41] Boice et al.[26] have ranked various body tissues with regard to cancer induction by radiation; certain sites, such as the thyroid, female breast, and bone marrow, clearly are more radiosensitive than others.

The excess risk of leukemia attributable to irradiation is observed within a few years after exposure, with a peak at 5 to 9 years and a slow decline thereafter.[16,27,29,40,42] Some controversy exists as to whether, and when, leukemia risk decreases to background levels in the population.[16,27,29,43] In the atomic bomb survivors, risk declined more rapidly for those exposed earlier in life.[29] Increased risks of solid tumors have been shown to emerge much later. After a minimum induction period of 5 to 10 years,[12,14,15,40,44,45] solid tumor risk appears to conform to a time-response model consistent with a multiplicative relationship with the underlying incidence in the population—that is, risk after exposure is proportional to the background incidence of cancer over time.[27,46] Data are inconsistent as to whether the risk remains elevated throughout life. Studies in the atomic bomb survivors[30] and in women treated for benign gynecologic disorders[47] have shown that the excess RR per gray tends to be fairly stable over time for at least 30 years after irradiation. However, the last update of the mortality experience of ankylosing spondylitis patients showed that, 25 years after irradiation, risk had decreased for a number of malignancies.[40] In the few studies of second cancer risk in which the time course beyond 25 years from first treatment was evaluated, the RRs of solid tumor development tended to decrease in very long term survivors.[13,45,48,49] The most recent cancer incidence report on the Japanese atomic bomb survivors, with 42 years of follow-up, indicated that the excess RR decreased with time for the groups with younger age at exposure and remained virtually constant for the older cohorts.[30] Cancer incidence data from the atomic bomb survivors and five other groups exposed to radiation have been analyzed to specifically address the evolution of risk with increasing time since exposure in childhood.[50] Ten to 15 years after radiation exposure, the RR of solid tumors decreased with increasing follow-up time (5.7% to 6.1% per year). The excess absolute risk, however, significantly increased with time since exposure.[50]

An important part of the knowledge of radiation carcinogenesis derives from populations exposed to relatively low levels of radiation, such as the atomic bomb survivors. For solid tumors, convincing evidence for a strongly linear radiation dose-response in the lower dose ranges (up to approximately 5 Gy) has emerged.[27,30,40,46,51] The results for leukemia are less consistent, but data from most studies are compatible with a linear trend for doses of less than 1.5 to 2.0 Gy.[16,29,41] Extrapolation of radiation effects from low doses to the high-dose ranges used therapeutically cannot be done with certainty, because of the possibility of cell killing at high doses. Therefore, more recent studies of second cancer risk have focused on the shape of the radiation dose-response curve in the high-dose range.

Radiation-related leukemia risk depends on a number of parameters, such as radiation dose to the active bone marrow, dose rate, and percentage of marrow exposed. Consistent evidence indicates that the excess risk of leukemia per unit radiation dose is much higher at low doses than at the high doses administered for the treatment of malignant disease.[16,29,41,43] This phenomenon has been attributed to cell killing or inactivation of potentially leukemic cells at the higher radiation doses.[16,27] Many studies in cancer patients have shown that high radiation doses to a limited field confer very little or no increased risk of leukemia.[8,18,19,52] Both in the atomic bomb survivors and in patients who received radiotherapy for cervical cancer, leukemia risk appeared to increase with increasing average dose to the bone marrow until approximately 4 Gy, above which leukemia risk was progressively reduced with increasing dose.[16,29] However, leukemia risk in survivors of uterine cancer showed little evidence for a downturn in risk at bone marrow doses as high as 6 to 14 Gy[41]; at more than 1.5 Gy, the dose-response pattern was more or less flat, and the risk after continuous exposures from brachytherapy at comparatively low doses was similar to that after fractionated exposures at much higher doses from external-beam radiation therapy. Clearly, more research is needed into the effects of dose fractionation and portion of bone marrow irradiated. Age at exposure to irradiation does not appear to greatly influence the risk of radiation-induced leukemia,[27,29,41] although decreasing RR with increasing age at exposure has been reported for one radiogenic leukemia subtype (acute lymphoblastic leukemia, or ALL).[43]

In contrast, studies of radiogenic breast cancer have demonstrated that age at exposure is a major determinant of risk, with the greatest risk for those irradiated as children and adolescents.[13,31,45,53,54] Irradiation may thus affect cells of the mammary ducts before full organ development begins. Atomic bomb survivors who were younger than 10 years of age at the time of the bombing had an excess RR per gray five times that of women who were older than 40 years of age when exposed. A strong trend toward increasing breast cancer risk with decreasing age at exposure was also observed in patients irradiated for HD.[13,36,45] No excess breast cancer risk has been found among women irradiated at age 40 years or older.[11,17,31,36,45,46,51] In two studies, increased breast cancer risk after radiation exposure in childhood emerged at an early age (younger than 40 years), before the peak incidence in the population.[13,55] In the low-dose range, breast cancer risk increases linearly with radiation dose.[35,39,46,51,56] For a specified dose, the excess absolute rates of breast cancer were found to be remarkably similar across studies in the Japanese atomic bomb survivors and in medically irradiated populations in the United States.[46,56] Two studies have examined whether linear dose response extends to the higher dose ranges used therapeutically.[22,38] They evaluated mantle field irradiation given for HD, which results in a large dose gradient across the breast; that is, 3 to 42 Gy at a midline dose of 40 Gy. Both studies[22,38] showed increasing risk of breast cancer over this entire dose range, with eightfold increased risk for the highest dose category (median dose, 42 Gy) compared to the lowest one (less than 4 Gy) (see also Table 54.7-1 and Hodgkin's Disease, later in this chapter). However, the slope of the dose-response curve appeared to be less steep than observed in studies in the low-dose range.[46] A comparison of relative and AERs in eight irradiated cohorts showed that breast cancer risk was increased to a lesser extent after low dose-rate protracted exposures than after acute and fractionated high dose-rate exposures.[46]

Risk of lung cancer also rises with increasing radiation dose in the lower dose range[30,40] as well as in the high-dose range (see Table 54.7-1).[21,57] A leveling of risk at doses of 10 Gy or more has been observed for radiation-induced thyroid cancer.[58,59] However, even at thyroid doses of up to 60 Gy, the risk of thyroid cancer did not decrease.[58] For bone sarcoma, two studies involving survivors of childhood cancer[37,60] showed no evidence of increased risk for doses less than 10 Gy to the site of the bone tumor. Above 10 Gy, risk for bone sarcoma rose sharply with increasing dose and was more than 90-fold higher at doses of 30 to 50 Gy.[60] Importantly, studies have shown that also for solid tumors other than breast cancer, the excess RR due to radiation is much greater for children and adolescents than for adults.[12,13,15,30,45,59,61] Significantly greater RRs with younger age at radiation exposure have been reported for lung cancer,[15,45] thyroid cancer,[30,45] bone sarcoma,[12,45,61] and gastrointestinal cancer.[13,15,45] After radiation exposure in childhood, the excess RR per gray for thyroid cancer [RR, 7.7; 95% confidence interval (CI), 2.1 to 28.7] is higher than for any other solid malignancy.[30]

For radiogenic lung cancer, the interaction of radiation exposure with other risk factors, such as smoking, has been examined. Studies involving uranium and tin miners exposed to radon have indicated that smoking and radiation exposure may act multiplicatively (or at least supraadditively) in the causation of lung cancer,[62–64] which implies that the absolute risk of developing radon-induced cancer is much higher in smokers than in nonsmokers. In HD patients, the combined effects of smoking

TABLE 54.7-1. Relative Risks of Breast and Lung Cancer after Hodgkin's Disease, According to Radiation Dose to Affected Site in Breast or Lung and Number of Cycles of Chemotherapy

Radiation Dose to Affected Site in Lung (Gy)	Lung Cancer[a]			Radiation Dose to Affected Site in Breast (Gy)	Breast Cancer[b]		
	Cases/Controls	Relative Risk	95% Confidence Interval		Cases/Controls	Relative Risk	95% Confidence Interval
0	43/87	1.0	(Referent)	0–3.9	15/76	1.0	(Referent)
>0–4.9	27/84	1.6	0.5–5.2	4.0–6.9	13/30	1.8	0.7–4.5
5–14.9	14/18	4.2	0.7–21	7.0–23.1	16/30	4.1	1.4–12.3
15.0–29.9	14/22	2.7	0.2–15	23.2–27.9	9/30	2.0	0.7–5.9
30.0–39.9	60/102	8.5	3.3–24	28.0–37.1	20/31	6.8	2.3–22.3
≥40.0	31/45	6.3	2.2–19	37.2–40.4	12/31	4.0	1.3–13.4
				40.5–61.3	17/29	8.0	2.6–26.4
No. of Cycles of Alkylating Agents				*No. of Cycles of Alkylating Agents*			
0	74/188	1.0	(Referent)	0	68/132	1.0	(Referent)
1–4	22/44	4.0	1.3–12.5	1–4	10/20	0.7	0.3–1.7
5–8	58/89	6.2	2.6–17.1	5–8	17/55	0.6	0.3–1.1
≥9	28/29	13.0	4.3–45	≥9	4/29	0.2	0.1–0.7

[a]Adapted from ref. 57.
[b]Adapted from ref. 38.

and high-dose radiotherapy for HD were multiplicative in a large international study[21,57] and even stronger than multiplicative in a prior report.[65] In the latter study, the increase in lung cancer risk with increasing radiation dose was significantly greater among patients who continued to smoke after diagnosis of HD than among those who refrained from smoking. As discussed more extensively in a previous edition of this text,[66] interaction models accounting for the sequencing of radiation and smoking suggest that radiation may act as a powerful promoter of abnormal cell changes initiated by smoking.

The carcinogenic effects of therapeutic irradiation deserve much more study. Issues that need further classification include the slope of the radiation dose-response curve in the higher dose range compared to the low-dose range, and, importantly, the interaction of radiotherapy with other carcinogens (e.g., hormonal factors) and genetic susceptibility. For example, two studies found that chemotherapy-induced premature menopause strongly reduced the risk of radiation-associated breast cancer.[22,38] Increasing evidence suggests that genetic factors contribute to the development of radiation-induced cancers. This is perhaps best demonstrated in survivors of hereditary retinoblastoma who harbor a heterozygous germline mutation in the RB1 tumor suppressor gene and who have a much greater risk of developing osteosarcomas within the radiation field than children irradiated for nonhereditary retinoblastoma.[67] In addition, two studies showed that patients with a positive family history of cancer are more likely to develop radiation-associated second malignancies.[68,69] In view of the postulated radiation sensitivity of heterozygous carriers of the ataxia-telangiectasia mutated (ATM) gene, it has been speculated that AT heterozygotes (approximately 1% of the population) may have an increased risk of radiation-induced cancer, specifically breast cancer.[70,71] In two studies, however, no ATM mutations were found in a total of 56 women who had developed breast cancer after radiotherapy for HD.[69,72] Further studies should focus on the identification of other genes that may influence susceptibility to the DNA-damaging effects of

radiation. Such research will provide more insight into the mechanisms underlying radiation carcinogenesis and will also be of clinical benefit in minimizing radiation exposure to the most susceptible subgroups of the population.

CHEMOTHERAPY

The development of acute myeloid leukemia (AML) after chemotherapy for malignant disease was reported as early as 1970 by Kyle et al.[73] In the following three decades, the occurrence of this late effect increased to the extent that, in some institutions, treatment-related AML now comprises up to 10% to 20% of all AML cases.[74] Moreover, it is now established that the spectrum of treatment-related leukemia extends beyond AML. ALL, for example, is increasingly recognized as therapy related[75,76] and may comprise 5% to 10% of all secondary acute leukemia.[75] Chronic granulocytic leukemia accounts for a small percentage of secondary leukemia[76,77] and has been included in numerous analytic studies in which associations with prior chemotherapy have been evaluated,[8,18,19,23,52] although separate risk estimates have not been presented. To date only chronic lymphocytic leukemia has not been convincingly associated with prior exposure to chemotherapy.

Chemotherapy is far more potent than radiotherapy in inducing leukemia. It has become evident that at least two major syndromes of treatment-related leukemia exist,[78,79] "classic" alkylating agent–induced AML and acute leukemia related to the topoisomerase II inhibitors. Risk of alkylating agent–related leukemia typically begins to increase 1 to 2 years after the start of chemotherapy, peaks in the 5- to 10-year follow-up period, and decreases afterwards.[8,13,15,18,19,80] Even in large patient series, the number of long-term survivors has typically been too small to determine whether 15 to 20 years after chemotherapy the risk of leukemia returns to the background level of the population.[13,45]

Although two registry-based studies indicate that leukemia risk might persist among 15-year survivors of testicular cancer and HD,[45,81] it is not clear whether these late excesses might reflect the influence of salvage therapy. More than 50% of leukemias arising after alkylating agent therapy present initially as myelodysplastic syndromes (MDSs), whereas *de novo* AML is preceded by MDS much less frequently.[76] Most cases of MDS progress to AML within a year.[76] Cytogenetic studies of alkylating agent–related AML and MDS have shown unbalanced chromosome aberrations, typically with loss of whole chromosome 5 or 7 (or both), or various parts of the long arms of these chromosomes.[82] Morphologically, alkylating agent–related AML most commonly consists of French-American-British (FAB) subtypes M1 and M2, but most subtypes,[76] including erythroleukemia,[18] have been observed. Survival after secondary AML is generally quite poor, typically only several months.[83,84]

Alkylating agents with known leukemogenic effects in humans include mechlorethamine, chlorambucil, cyclophosphamide, melphalan, semustine, lomustine (CCNU), carmustine (BCNU), prednimustine, busulfan, and dihydroxybusulfan.[18,76,78,85,86] Controversial findings have been reported with regard to procarbazine,[85,87] which demonstrates an underlying mechanism of action similar to that of alkylating agents. Few studies have addressed the relative leukemogenicity of the various alkylating drugs, but a strong body of evidence to date suggests that, at doses of equal therapeutic effect, cyclophosphamide is substantially less leukemogenic than melphalan, mechlorethamine, chlorambucil, CCNU, and thiotepa.[8,18,19,85] The risk of alkylating agent–related AML has been shown to increase with increasing cumulative dose, duration of therapy, and dose-intensity.[18,85,88] Few studies have attempted to separate the effects of cumulative dose, duration of treatment, and dose intensity, which tend to be highly correlated, and the results of such analyses have been controversial (discussed later in Hodgkin's Disease and Breast Cancer).[41,85,88]

The platinating agents cisplatin and carboplatin are among the most important cytotoxic drugs introduced in the last few decades and are widely used to treat many cancers. The platinum compounds, however, demonstrate carcinogenicity *in vitro* and in laboratory animals,[10] forming intrastrand and interstrand DNA cross-links as do bifunctional alkylating agents. In a population-based study of women with ovarian cancer,[23] cisplatin-based combination chemotherapy was linked to significantly increased risks of leukemia (*P* trend for cumulative dose, <.001) in a multivariate model adjusted for other treatment parameters (discussed later in Ovarian Cancer). Future studies should evaluate whether other drug combinations that include platinum might also be linked to elevated risks of leukemia, because it is not clear whether cisplatin acts as a human leukemogen only in combination with selected cytotoxic agents.

The topoisomerase II inhibitors, especially the epipodophyllotoxins, have been implicated in the development of a clinically and cytogenetically distinct type of AML. The International Agency for Research on Cancer (IARC) concluded that the epipodophyllotoxins etoposide and teniposide are probably carcinogenic to humans.[89] Ratain and coworkers[90] were the first to recognize the potentially leukemogenic properties of etoposide-containing regimens in patients with non–small cell lung cancer, and this has also been documented for patients with other types of malignancies.[91–93] Compared with classic alkylating agent–induced AML, epipodophyllotoxin-related AML has a shorter induction period (median, 2 to 3 years) and generally lacks a preceding phase of MDS. Furthermore, this type of AML appears to be characterized by balanced translocations involving chromosome bands 11q23,

21q22, and 3q23,[89,94] as well as morphologic features consistent with acute monoblastic or myelomonocytic leukemia (M4 or M5 according to the FAB criteria).[78,95,96] However, Beaumont et al.[97] described a large series of therapy-related acute promyelocytic leukemias (M3), noting a possible association with topoisomerase II–targeted drugs and a short latency period of approximately 2 years. It is unclear whether epipodophyllotoxin-related AML has a better prognosis than classic alkylating agent–related AML, which is notoriously resistant to antileukemic treatment.[82,84]

Evidence has accumulated that the anthracyclines doxorubicin and 4-epidoxorubicin, which are intercalating topoisomerase II inhibitors, may induce a similar type of AML as the one related to epipodophyllotoxin treatment.[19,98,99] In 1987, the IARC concluded that doxorubicin was probably carcinogenic to humans, based on a review of limited data.[86] As with many cytotoxic drugs, an evaluation of the carcinogenic potential of doxorubicin is complicated, because it is typically given in combination with other chemotherapeutic agents, including alkylators.[19,61,98,100] Curtis et al.[18] found no increase in the risk of leukemia associated with doxorubicin therapy for breast cancer after adjustment for the effects of alkylating agents and radiotherapy. Although an increase in the dose of doxorubicin given to treat childhood cancer seemed weakly associated with an increased risk of leukemia after adjustment for use of alkylating agents,[52] the investigators concluded that the excess risk was almost completely attributable to alkylators. In a study of children with Wilms' tumor,[101] the RR of leukemia (six cases) after doxorubicin-containing regimens was approximately 14; however, because a relatively constant dose of doxorubicin (300 mg/m²) was used and data on treatment of relapse were incomplete, evaluation of a dose-response relation was not possible.

The relative leukemogenicity of the anthracyclines and different epipodophyllotoxins is not known. Furthermore, it is unclear whether the schedule of administration or the cumulative dose is the major determinant of leukemia risk (discussed in more detail later in Testicular Cancer and Pediatric Malignancies).[91–93,102–104] In view of the widespread use of epipodophyllotoxins and anthracyclines in curative treatments, continued evaluation of the leukemogenic potential of these agents is needed.[79,103] Detailed descriptions of molecular mechanisms involved in the development of AML after administration of these cytotoxic drugs have been provided elsewhere.[78,79,105,106] As postulated by Pedersen-Bjergaard and Rowley,[78] cytostatic drugs with different mechanisms of action [i.e., direct binding to DNA (alkylating agents) and inhibition of DNA topoisomerase II (epipodophyllotoxins and anthracyclines)] may have a synergistic effect in leukemogenesis. The topoisomerase II inhibitor mitoxantrone has also been found to induce leukemia.[97,107,108]

The antimetabolites have generally not been regarded as carcinogenic,[86] and Cheson et al.[109] observed that nucleoside analogue therapy for chronic lymphocytic leukemia did not appear to confer a significantly increased risk of second cancer. However, in a report from St. Jude Children's Research Hospital,[110] it was shown that children with ALL who received cranial irradiation and who had a wild-type thiopurine methyltransferase phenotype had an 8.3% cumulative risk of brain cancer, whereas children with ALL who received irradiation and had a defective phenotype had a 42% risk (*P* = .0077). Patients also received concurrent systemic chemotherapy with high-dose 6-

mercaptopurine (75 mg/m^2) plus high-dose methotrexate. It was hypothesized that the defective thiopurine methyltransferase activity resulted in higher exposures to thioguanine nucleotide metabolites of 6-mercaptopurine during the period of irradiation.

Just as the pharmacology of effective cancer chemotherapy is impacted by underlying principles of pharmacokinetics and pharmacodynamics (covered in Chapter 15 of this text), these influences likely contribute to the development of secondary leukemia. The possible role of polymorphisms in drug-metabolizing genes, including those coding for the cytochrome P-450 enzymes, glutathione S-transferases, and arylamine N-acetyltransferases, in chemotherapy-related leukemias has been reviewed.[111] The U.S. Children's Oncology Group is currently conducting a study of polymorphisms in drug-metabolizing enzymes and indicators of genotoxicity to possibly identify HD patients at increased risk of therapy-associated complications, including second cancer.[112] Other factors in the development of chemotherapy-related leukemias may include interindividual differences in repair of DNA damage,[113,114] germline mutations in tumor suppressor genes,[74,111] administration of concomitant medications, and interpatient variation in renal and hepatic function. Importantly, Yeoh et al.[115] suggested that gene expression profiling of pediatric ALL patients might indicate which patients are at increased risk of secondary AML, independent of treatment. Clarification of the important interrelationships between various factors is critical to a better understanding of individual susceptibility to secondary leukemia. Because cancer patients frequently receive large doses of cytotoxic drugs, interindividual differences in drug absorption, distribution, metabolism, and excretion are accentuated. Until these influences and their interrelationships are better understood, empiric end points, such as the development of acute hematopoietic toxicity after chemotherapy, might be explored for their value as possible surrogate markers of secondary leukemia risk.[85] For cytotoxic agents for which both oral and intravenous formulations are available, the route of administration in describing dose-response associations with secondary leukemia risk should also be taken into account.[23] Whether chemoprotectants such as amifostine (WR-2721), which ameliorates the myelosuppressive effects of alkylating agents[116] and platinum compounds,[117] might possibly contribute to decreased risks of second leukemias should be examined.

Many chemotherapeutic agents are known mutagens and animal carcinogens,[86] and the induction period of solid tumors may be longer than the observation period available in published research. Thus, the question of whether the increased risks of leukemia after chemotherapy may later be followed by excess risks of solid tumors is important. To date, the causal link between cyclophosphamide and bladder cancer represents one of the few established relationships between a specific cytostatic drug and a solid tumor (reviewed later in Non-Hodgkin's Lymphoma).[20,118] However, elevated risks of bone sarcomas[37,60] and lung cancer[15,21] have also been observed after alkylating agent chemotherapy (see Table 54.7-1). The contribution of chemotherapy to radiation-induced solid tumors[13,21,101,110,119,120] should also be investigated. For example, as discussed later in Pediatric Malignancies, doxorubicin was found to potentiate the development of second solid tumors after radiation for Wilms' tumor.[101] The investigators of this study[101] hypothesized that doxorubicin

may inhibit the repair of radiation-induced damage, likely through its interaction with DNA topoisomerase II.

RISK OF SECOND MALIGNANCY IN PATIENTS WITH SELECTED PRIMARY CANCERS

HODGKIN'S DISEASE

In view of the excellent cure rates that are currently achieved in the relatively young population of HD patients, it has become increasingly important to evaluate how the occurrence of second cancers affects their long-term survival. After the first reports of increased second cancer risk in HD patients in the early 1970s, an excess of AML in chemotherapy-treated patients and an increased risk of solid tumors in irradiated patients have been reported consistently in the literature.[121] The overall risk of selected second cancers compared with the general population is given in Table 54.7-2, based on the results of two large studies, one in the United Kingdom[15] and one representing a joint study conducted in the United States, Canada, Scandinavia, and the Netherlands.[45]

The largest RR (10 to 15) is observed for leukemia (with an even greater RR for AML of 22), followed by a 6- to 14-fold increased risk for NHL and 4- to 11-fold excesses for connective tissue, bone, and thyroid cancers. Moderately increased risks (twofold to fourfold) are observed for a number of solid tumors, such as cancers of the lung, stomach, esophagus, colon, breast, and cervix, and melanoma. Because leukemia and NHL are diseases with a low incidence in the population, even a high RR compared to the population may translate into a low cumulative risk. Several studies indeed show that, for the entire follow-up period, the cumulative risk of solid tumors far exceeds that of leukemia or NHL (e.g., 25-year cumulative risks of 23% and 3% for solid tumors and leukemia, respectively, in a Dutch study).[13]

AER is the best measure to judge which tumors contribute most to the second cancer burden. Table 54.7-2 shows that, compared with the general population, HD patients experience an excess of approximately 45 malignancies per 10,000 person-years of observation. Solid tumors account for the majority of excess cancers (approximately 30 per 10,000 patients per year), with lung cancer contributing 10 to 12 excess cases per 10,000 person-years. Leukemia and NHL each account for eight to nine cases per 10,000 person-years.

Temporal patterns of second cancer risk vary by tumor site. In most studies, increased leukemia risk has its peak occurrence 3 to 9 years after chemotherapy, and the risk decreases thereafter.[11,13–15,45,121,122] The RR of solid tumors is minimally elevated in the 1- to 4-year follow-up period and increases steadily with increasing follow-up time from 5 years since first treatment.[11–15,45,80] For several tumor sites (breast, thyroid), the excess risk does not become apparent until after 10 or even 15 years of observation. In studies that include data on 20-year survivors, the RR of solid tumors continued to increase through the 15- to 20-year follow-up period.[11,13–15,36,45,80,119,122,123] Only two studies to date have reported on the time course of risk 25 or more years after treatment.[13,45] In the international population-based study by Dores et al.,[45] a downturn in the RR for all solid tumors combined was observed after 25 years of follow-up, with RRs of 3.0 and 1.8 among patients in the 20- to 24-year interval and in 25-year survivors, respectively. A Dutch study[13]

TABLE 54.7-2. Relative Risk of Second Malignancies after Hodgkin's Disease: Results of Two Large Studies

Site or Type	Dores et al. (International, 2002)[45] (n = 32,591; Years of Diagnosis 1935–1994)				Swerdlow et al. (United Kingdom, 2000)[15] (n = 5519; Years of Diagnosis 1963–1993)			
	Observed Cases	Relative Risk[a]	95% Confidence Interval	Absolute Excess Risk[b] (per 10,000 Patients/Y)	Observed Cases	Relative Risk[a]	95% Confidence Interval	Absolute Excess Risk[b] (per 10,000 Patients/Y)
All malignancies	2153	2.3	2.2–2.4	47.2	322	2.9	2.6–3.2	44.5
Leukemia	249	9.9	8.7–11.2	8.8	45	14.6	10.7–19.2	8.9
Non-Hodgkin's lymphoma	162	5.5	4.7–6.4	5.2	50	14.0	10.5–18.3	9.9
Solid tumors	1726	2.0	1.9–2.0	33.1	227	2.2	1.9–2.5	25.7
Tongue, mouth, pharynx	75	3.3	2.6–4.1	2.1	6	2.8	1.1–5.8	0.8
Esophagus	29	2.8	1.8–4.0	0.7	5	2.0	0.7–4.3	0.5
Stomach	80	1.9	1.5–2.4	1.5	13	2.2	1.2–3.6	1.5
Colon	129	1.6	1.4–1.9	2.0	18	2.3	1.4–3.6	2.2
Rectum	52	1.2	0.9–1.6	0.4	7	1.3	0.5–2.5	0.3
Pancreas	40	1.5	1.1–2.0	0.5	3	1.0	0.2–2.6	0
Lung	377	2.9	2.6–3.2	9.7	8	3.4	2.7–4.2	11.7
Female breast	234	2.0	1.8–2.3	10.5	19	1.4	0.9–2.1	3.1
Uterine cervix	37	2.0	1.4–2.7	1.6	7	2.1	0.9–4.1	0.8
Prostate	98	1.0	0.8–1.2	−0.1	4	0.8	0.2–1.7	−0.3
Bladder	66	1.4	1.1–1.8	0.8	5	0.8	0.3–1.8	−0.2
Central nervous system	36	1.5	1.1–2.1	0.5	7	2.5	1.1–4.8	0.9
Thyroid	47	4.1	3.0–5.5	1.4	5	7.6	2.7–16.4	0.9
Bone	9	3.8	1.7–7.2	0.3	4	10.7	3.3–24.8	0.8
Connective tissue	32	5.1	3.5–7.2	1.0	3	3.9	1.0–10.1	0.5
Melanoma	52	1.7	1.3–2.3	0.9	6	2.3	0.9–4.6	0.7

[a]Observed cases/expected cases; expected numbers based on age-, gender-, and calendar-period specific cancer incidence in the population.
[b]Excess number of cases (observed minus expected) per 10,000 patients per year.

involving patients diagnosed with HD before age 40 years reported an RR for solid tumors of 5.3 among 25-year survivors, compared to an RR of 8.8 in the 20- to 24-year interval. This suggests that the RR may decrease in very long term survivors.

As is seen for the patterns of RRs for various second cancers with time since treatment, the AERs in long-term survivors differ greatly from those observed in the entire patient population. The AERs of solid malignancies increase at a much steeper rate than the RRs, due to the fact that, with longer follow-up, patients grow older and their background rate of cancer rises strongly. Related to this phenomenon, the AER amounts to approximately 100 excess cancer cases per 10,000 twenty-year survivors per year, compared to 45 per 10,000 per year in all HD patients (see Table 54.7-2). Based on estimates from the study by Dores and collaborators,[45] solid cancers contribute by far the most to the AER in 20-year survivors, with 92 excess cases per 10,000 patients per year, followed by NHL (8 per 10,000 per year), and AML (2 per 10,000 per year). In females, breast cancer accounts for most of the AER of solid tumors in 20-year survivors (42 per 10,000 per year).[45] Lung cancer accounts for 17 excess cases per 10,000 patients per year in 20-year survivors.

For several second cancers, the association with HD treatment factors has been investigated in more detail.

Risk Factors for Leukemia and Non-Hodgkin's Lymphoma after Hodgkin's Disease

Leukemia after HD is certainly the most studied treatment-induced malignancy, and thus extensive knowledge of its risk factors has emerged.[124] Radiotherapy alone is associated with very little or no increased risk of leukemia,[12,14,15,80] whereas alkylating agent chemotherapy is linked with greatly elevated risks. Risk of AML rises sharply with an increasing number of cycles of mechlorethamine, vincristine, procarbazine, and prednisone (MOPP) or MOPP-like regimens.[8,85] Since the 1980s, MOPP-only chemotherapy has been gradually replaced by regimens containing doxorubicin, bleomycin, vinblastine, and dacarbazine (ABVD) in many centers. Patients treated with ABVD at the Milan Cancer Institute, where this regimen was designed, were shown to have a significantly lower risk of AML than MOPP-treated patients (15-year cumulative risks of 0.7% and 9.5%, respectively).[125] Another study showed that HD patients treated with MOPP- and ABVD-containing regimens in the 1980s had substantially lower risk of AML and MDS than patients treated in the 1970s with MOPP alone (10-year cumulative risks of 2.1% and 6.4%, respectively; P = .07).[14] The German-Austrian Pediatric Hodgkin's Disease Group observed a low risk of AML (1.1% at 15 years) after treatment with regimens that contained relatively low doses of procarbazine, doxorubicin, and cyclophosphamide, without mechlorethamine.[126] Analyses of the German Hodgkin's Lymphoma Study Group also show low risks of AML after cyclophosphamide, vincristine, procarbazine, and prednisone (COPP) and ABVD (mechlorethamine replaced by cyclophosphamide) and standard BEACOPP (bleomycin, etoposide, and doxorubicin combined with COPP), whereas substantially increased risk of AML was observed for the escalated BEACOPP regimen (actuarial risk at 5 years of 2.5%).[83,127]

An important question is whether radiotherapy adds to the leukemia risk associated with chemotherapy. Evidence that combined modality treatment results in greater risk than chemotherapy alone is provided by several reports,[80,125,128] but other large series indicate that the risk of AML after combined treatment is comparable to that after chemotherapy alone.[8,12,14,15,85,122] These inconsistent results may be due partly to differences in treatment regimens among studies, but also to lack of adjustment for type and amount of chemotherapy in some reports. The interaction between radiotherapy and chemotherapy could be evaluated most rigorously in the large case-control study by Kaldor et al.,[8] which included 163 cases of leukemia after HD. When the combined effects of radiation dose to the active bone marrow and number of mechlorethamine and procarbazine-containing cycles were examined, it was found that for each category of radiation dose (less than 10 Gy, 10 to 20 Gy, and more than 20 Gy to the marrow), leukemia risk clearly increased with the number of chemotherapy cycles. In contrast, among patients receiving a given number of chemotherapy cycles, risk of leukemia did not consistently increase with higher radiation dose. Taken together, the preponderance of available data do not support the hypothesis that the combination of chemotherapy and radiotherapy confers a higher risk of leukemia than does chemotherapy alone.

Therapeutic intensification with autologous stem cell transplantation (ASCT) is increasingly used for lymphoma patients who experience relapse. Relatively high actuarial risks of AML and myelodysplasia (4% to 15% at 5 years) have been observed after ASCT for HD. Evidence suggests that much of the risk is related to intensive pretransplantation chemotherapy (see also Non-Hodgkin's Lymphoma, later in this chapter).[129–133]

The influence of host-related factors such as age on leukemia risk in HD survivors has been examined in a number of studies and has been reviewed elsewhere.[124] The reported higher cumulative risk of AML in older HD patients compared with younger ones mainly reflects the higher baseline incidence of the disease in older persons. In the few studies that have analyzed RR of leukemia by age, based on comparisons with expectations in the general population, no differences between age groups were observed,[12,13] or the RR of AML was even significantly greater at younger ages than at older ages.[8,15,45] Two studies showed, however, that the AER of leukemia increased with age at diagnosis.[15,45]

The prognosis of AML and MDS after HD treatment is extremely poor, with only 15% of patients surviving longer than 1 year and no apparent survival benefit from allogeneic stem cell transplantation.[83]

The causes of the excess risk of NHL after HD treatment are not well understood.[124] Because increased risks of NHL occur in immunosuppressed patients, such as transplant recipients,[134] and because HD may be accompanied by immunosuppression,[121] several investigators have argued that the elevated risk of NHL may be attributed to HD itself rather than to its treatment. This view is supported by several studies in which risk did not vary appreciably among treatments.[12,15] However, in other studies, the risk of NHL was found to be lowest among patients who were treated with radiotherapy alone and highest among patients who received intensive combined modality treatment, both initially and for relapse.[14,80,135,136] The inconsistent results regarding the relation to treatment may be partly attributed to diagnostic misclassification, that is, misdiagnosis of the primary tumor as HD whereas it represented NHL according to modern lymphoma classification schemes.[124,136]

In only a very few studies were diagnostic pathologic slides of the second NHL and original HD reviewed to avoid such misclassification, however, and these did not give consistent results.[14,136] Although transformation to NHL may be part of the natural history of some types of HD, the role of intensive combined modality treatment and its associated immunosuppression and of the inherent immune deficiency associated with HD should be explored further.

Risk Factors for Solid Malignancies after Treatment for Hodgkin's Disease

ROLE OF RADIATION THERAPY. Elevated risks of solid cancers after HD have generally been attributed to radiotherapy.[11–14,36,80,119,122,124,137] Nearly all sites for which excess risks have been reported (lung, breast, gastrointestinal tract, thyroid, sarcoma) are those for which elevated risks have also been described in other radiation-exposed cohorts.[27] Two case-control studies examined lung cancer risk in relation to the radiation dose to the affected lung area as well as the modifying effect of the patient's smoking habits.[21,65] In both studies, which were based on individual radiation dosimetry, it was observed that lung cancer risk rose significantly with increasing radiation dose. In the largest study, which included 227 lung cancer patients and 455 matched controls, the risk was 6.3-fold increased for patients who received 40 Gy or more (to the relevant lung area) compared to those who received no radiotherapy (see Table 54.7-1).[57] Travis and collaborators[21,57] observed that the increased RRs from smoking appeared to multiply the elevated risks from radiotherapy, which implies that there are large AERs for lung cancer among irradiated patients who smoke.

The strongly elevated risk of breast cancer after radiotherapy for HD is a major concern for female survivors.[13,45,61,138–140] Two case-control studies investigated the effect of radiation dose and other treatment factors on breast cancer risk.[22,38] The radiation dose to the area of the breast where the case's tumor had developed was estimated for each case-control set. In both studies, the risk of breast cancer increased significantly with higher radiation dose up to the highest dose levels. In the largest study[38] (105 patients with breast cancer after HD and 266 matched controls), the risk was eightfold increased for the highest dose category (median dose of 42 Gy) compared to the lowest one (less than 4 Gy) (P trend <.001) (see Table 54.7-1). In both studies, patients who received both chemotherapy and radiotherapy had significantly decreased risk (approximately halved) compared to those treated with radiotherapy alone, and the radiation-related risks appeared to be attenuated by treatment with alkylating agents or a radiation dose of 5 Gy or more delivered to the ovaries, or both.[22,38] The Dutch study clearly showed that the substantial risk reduction associated with chemotherapy was attributable to the high frequency of premature menopause in chemotherapy-treated patients (see also Role of Chemotherapy).[22] These results indicate that ovarian hormones are a crucial factor in promoting tumorigenesis once radiation has produced an initiating event.

ROLE OF CHEMOTHERAPY. A very important question is whether chemotherapy for HD can also induce solid cancers, and if so, at which sites. Several studies have indeed observed that chemotherapy significantly increased the risk of solid malignancy, in particular lung cancer risk.[15,21] The British National Lymphoma Investigation cohort study of 5519 patients[15] showed a significantly elevated risk of lung cancer after chemotherapy alone, and the RR (3.3; 95% CI, 2.2 to 4.7) compared to the general population is of similar magnitude to that observed in patients treated with either radiotherapy (RR, 2.9; 95% CI, 1.9 to 4.1) or mixed modalities (RR, 4.3; 95% CI, 2.9 to 6.2). Two large case-control studies have investigated the separate and joint roles of chemotherapy, radiotherapy, and smoking in detail.[21,141] In both reports, there was a clear trend of increasing lung cancer risk with greater number of cycles of alkylating chemotherapy (P trend <.001; see Table 54.7-1)[21] or MOPP chemotherapy (P trend <.001[21]; P trend = .07[141]). In the largest study, risk of lung cancer after therapy with alkylating agents and radiotherapy together was as expected if individual excess risks were summed, with RRs of 4.2 (95% CI, 2.1 to 8.8) for patients receiving alkylating agents alone, 5.9 (95% CI, 2.7 to 13.5) for patients receiving radiotherapy alone (more than 5 Gy), and 8.0 (95% CI, 3.6 to 18.5) for those receiving combined modality treatment, compared to patients who received no alkylating agents and had a radiation dose of 5 Gy or less.[21] Among patients treated with MOPP chemotherapy, lung cancer risk rose with increasing cumulative dose of either mechlorethamine or procarbazine.[21] Both agents are carcinogenic to rodent lungs,[86] and mustard gas is also known to cause lung cancer in humans.[142] As was observed for the joint effects of smoking and radiotherapy, the risks from smoking appeared to at least multiply risks from alkylating chemotherapy.[21,141]

In several series,[12–14,80,122] no increased risk of solid malignancy overall was observed after chemotherapy alone. However, the expected number of solid tumors 10 or more years after chemotherapy alone was less than two in nearly all negative studies, which renders it impossible to exclude a moderate increase in risk. If chemotherapy affects solid tumor risk, patients receiving combined modality treatment would be expected to have a greater RR than patients treated solely with radiotherapy, as observed in only one study.[11] No such difference was found, however, in the majority of investigations.[12,14,80,122,143] For selected sites, such as the gastrointesti-

nal tract, larger risks were observed after combined modality treatment than after radiotherapy alone.[13,15,119]

The inconsistent results with regard to the influence of chemotherapy on solid tumor risk may be partly related to the fact that most studies considered all solid tumors combined, whereas chemotherapy may differentially affect the risk of tumors at disparate sites. A study at the Netherlands Cancer Institute demonstrated that the addition of salvage chemotherapy to initial radiotherapy, compared to initial radiotherapy alone, did not influence the risk of solid cancers overall but significantly increased the risk of solid tumors other than breast cancer (RR of 9.4 vs. 4.7 for initial radiotherapy alone).[13] Conversely, patients who received salvage chemotherapy were found to experience significantly lower risks of breast cancer than patients treated with radiotherapy alone (RRs of 2.8 and 7.6, respectively), likely related to premature ovarian failure due to intensive chemotherapy.[13] Two case-control studies showed that breast cancer risk decreased with increasing number of alkylating agent cycles (see Table 54.7-1).[22,38] In the Dutch case-control study, having a chemotherapy-induced premature menopause before age 35 years was associated with a strongly reduced risk of breast cancer (RR, 0.08; 95% CI, 0.01 to 0.61).[22]

EFFECT OF AGE AT TREATMENT. Several studies have shown that the RR of solid tumors increases strongly with younger age at first treatment (Table 54.7-3).[11,13,15,45,119] The effect is most notable for breast cancer. In a Dutch study, 15-year survivors who had radiotherapy treatment before 20 years of age had an 18-fold increased risk of breast cancer; women irradiated at age 20 to 29 years had a sixfold increased risk; and a small, nonsignificant increase was observed for women irradiated at age 30 years or older (RR, 1.7).[13] These RRs translated into 25-year actuarial risk of breast cancer of 16%, both for women first treated before age 20 years and for those treated at later ages.[13] A similar trend, with even larger RRs, has been reported by researchers at Stanford University.[36] An approximately 100-fold increased risk of breast cancer has been observed after radiotherapy at ages younger than 16 years, with RRs ranging from 17 to 458.[11,36,61,122,144] This huge variation in estimated risk is likely due to large differences between series in proportion of patients irradiated, duration of follow-up, and completeness of follow-up (see Methods to Assess Second Cancer Risk, earlier in this chapter).

TABLE 54.7-3.   Relative Risks of Various Second Malignancies, According to Age at Diagnosis of Hodgkin's Disease (HD): Dores et al.[45] (International, 2002)[a]

Age at HD Diagnosis	All Second Cancers		All Solid Cancers		Female Breast	Lung	Gastrointestinal Tract	AML
	RR	AER	RR	AER	RR	RR	RR	RR
<21	7.7[b]	30.0	7.0[b]	23.8	14.2[b]	5.5[b]	10.0[b]	39.2[b]
21–30	4.3[b]	34.9	3.6[b]	25.3	3.7[b]	5.4[b]	3.9[b]	31.7[b]
31–40	2.7[b]	42.0	2.1[b]	25.4	1.2	4.0[b]	2.1[b]	35.7[b]
41–50	2.5[b]	80.5	2.1[b]	58.7	1.7[b]	3.5[b]	2.3[b]	28.6[b]
51–60	2.0[b]	107.5	1.8[b]	79.2	1.0	3.4[b]	1.6[b]	21.2[b]
≥61	1.3[b]	51.7	1.2[b]	27.0	1.1	1.5[b]	1.0	5.9[b]

AER, absolute excess risk, defined as excess number of cases (observed minus expected) per 10,000 patients per year; AML, acute myeloid leukemia; RR, relative risk, or ratio of observed cases to expected cases.
[a]n = 32,591; years of diagnosis, 1935–1994.
[b]P <.05.

Several studies have demonstrated that age at treatment for HD is also a crucial determinant of increased RRs for non-breast solid malignancies (see Table 54.7-3).[13,15,45,119] Dores and colleagues[45] reported that the RR of lung cancer decreased from a 5.5-fold increase (compared to the population) for patients diagnosed before age 21 years to a 1.5-fold excess for patients diagnosed at age 61 years or above (see Table 54.7-3). In the United Kingdom study[15] the RRs for lung cancer decreased from a 20-fold increase among those diagnosed before age 25 to a 2.2-fold excess for patients diagnosed at age 55 or above. Table 54.7-3 demonstrates that a significantly greater RR with younger age at diagnosis of HD is also observed for digestive tract cancers[13,119] and a similar age-related increase in risk is seen for cancers of the thyroid, bone, and soft tissue.[15,45] Despite the very high *relative* risks at younger ages, the *absolute excess* risks for most solid cancers are greater for those diagnosed at older age, which is related to the much higher background rate of cancer among elderly patients.[15,45] The AER from any solid malignancy increase from 24 excess cases per 10,000 patients per year in patients treated before age 21 years to 79 excess cases per 10,000 patients per year in those treated between the ages of 51 and 60 years (see Table 54.7-3). For breast cancer, however, the AER is highest among female patients treated before age 21 years.

The strongly increased RRs of solid tumors in patients treated for HD at a young age only become manifest after an extended follow-up period. This might point to a prolonged induction period, but it may also be due to this young patient group's reaching an age at which solid tumor incidence begins to rise in the general population. Only three studies distinguished the separate contributions of age at first treatment and attained age.[13,45,49] Solid tumor risk was greatest among patients treated at a young age (20 years or younger), but the largest RR emerged before the patients attained the age range at which solid tumors normally occur, which thus attenuates the AERs when survivors grew older. Among patients first treated at age 20 years or earlier in the largest study to date, the RR of developing a solid tumor at ages 40 to 59 years was significantly lower than the RR of solid tumor development before age 40 (RR, 2.3 vs. 10.5).[45] It is notable that a similar finding has been reported with regard to breast cancer risk among atomic bomb survivors in Japan.[145]

Summary

In conclusion, the occurrence of treatment-related second cancers is a major problem in survivors of HD. The substantial increase in solid tumor risk with greater follow-up time necessitates careful, lifelong medical surveillance of all patients. The greatly increased risk of NHL throughout follow-up demonstrates the importance of performing biopsies in patients with recurrent HD. Because the AER of lung cancer is much greater among smokers than nonsmokers, physicians should make a special effort to dissuade HD patients from smoking even before treatment starts. Women treated with mantle field irradiation before age 35 years are at greatly increased risk of breast cancer. The importance of regular breast examinations should be explained to them, and they should be taught breast self-examination. From 8 years after irradiation, the follow-up program for these survivors should include yearly breast palpation and mammography. There is a strong need for research to evaluate the efficacy of screening programs aimed at reduction of breast cancer mortality in these high-risk women.[146] Physicians should also be alert to the higher risk of gastrointestinal cancers in patients who have received radiation to paraaortic and pelvic fields. Thorough examination of gastrointestinal complaints is indicated. Chemotherapy also appears to increase the risk of solid malignancies, in particular lung cancer. An important question to be answered in future research is whether modern chemotherapy regimens without mechlorethamine also contribute to the risk of solid tumors, and, if so, which cytotoxic drugs are responsible for the excess risk. One of the most devastating second malignancies to occur among patients cured of HD remains chemotherapy-related leukemia. Because the poor prognosis of this complication cannot be changed by early diagnosis, it is promising that leukemia risk has decreased dramatically since the introduction of new chemotherapy regimens in the 1980s. It is hoped that current treatment protocols which limit the dose and fields of radiotherapy will similarly reduce the late risk of solid cancers.

NON-HODGKIN'S LYMPHOMA

The marked improvement in survival of patients with NHL observed in the last few decades has been due largely to the development of effective treatment regimens. The current 5-year relative survival rate is 56%,[147] which has resulted in an increasing number of long-term survivors of NHL for whom it is important to characterize second cancer risk. Several population-based studies have provided estimates of the risk of second malignancies after NHL,[148–151] with the largest series to date including 29,153 NHL patients reported to the National Cancer Institute's Surveillance, Epidemiology, and End Results (SEER) program (1973 to 1991).[151] Significantly increased risks were reported for all second cancers taken together [observed/expected (O/E) ratio, 1.2; observed, 1231; AER, 20.2 excess cancers per 10,000 NHL patients per year]. Risk increased with time, reaching 1.8 in 10-year survivors (*P* trend <.05). Significantly increased risks were observed for malignant melanoma (O/E, 2.4), AML (O/E, 2.9), and cancers of lung (O/E, 1.6), bladder (O/E, 1.3), and kidney (O/E, 1.5). A subsequent international study[150] of 6171 two-year survivors of NHL confirmed findings of the SEER program[151] and indicated that significant excesses of second cancers persisted for two decades. An update of the SEER program data (1973 to 1998) included more than 66,000 two-month survivors of NHL for whom a significantly increased 10% excess of all second cancers was evident (O/E, 1.1; AER, 19.3; observed, 4600) (L. Travis, *unpublished observations*, 2003). Increased risks of second cancers were noted at the sites reported in the previous survey of the SEER program data.[151] In addition, significant excesses were observed for several rare cancers such as Kaposi's sarcoma (O/E, 13.0) and cancers of the lip (O/E, 1.8), salivary gland (O/E, 1.8), gum and floor of the mouth (O/E, 1.4), vagina (O/E, 2.7), thyroid (O/E, 1.6), bone (O/E, 3.6), and soft tissue (O/E, 1.6). The largest AER (per 10,000 NHL patients per year) is observed for lung cancer (AER, 7.4; observed, 876; RR, 1.3) (L. Travis, *unpublished observations*, 2003). The RR of all solid tumors increased over time to reach 1.6 (95% CI, 1.2 to 2.0; AER, 84.2; *P* trend <.0001) among 20-year survivors of NHL, in whom statistically significant threefold higher risks for cancers of the colon, rectum, and bladder were apparent.

TABLE 54.7-4.   Risk of Bladder Cancer According to Cumulative Dose and Duration of Cyclophosphamide Therapy

Cyclophosphamide	Median Dose or Duration[a]	Cases (n)	Controls (n)	Matched Relative Risk[b]	95% Confidence Interval
CUMULATIVE DOSE					
<20 g[c]	10.0 g	8	22	2.4	0.7–8.4
20–49 g	34.0 g	5	6	6.3[d]	1.3–29.0
≥50 g	87.7 g	5	2	14.5[d,e]	2.3–94.0
DURATION OF THERAPY					
<1 y	6 mo	8	20	2.5	0.7–9.0
1–2 y	18 mo	3	6	3.7	0.6–22.0
>2 y	51 mo	7	4	11.8[d,e]	2.3–61.0

[a]Median cumulative dose of cyclophosphamide or median duration of therapy among all patients within the specified category.
[b]The referent group consists of 6 case subjects and 42 control subjects who were not treated with cyclophosphamide and who received a radiation dose to the bladder of 0.5 Gy or less. The multivariate model also included terms for patients who received radiotherapy without cyclophosphamide (6 case subjects and 16 control subjects).
[c]The minimum cumulative dose of cyclophosphamide in this group was 2.1 g.
[d]$P < .05$.
[e]P for trend $< .005$.
(From ref. 20, with permission.)

Analytic studies to evaluate increased risks for second cancers in relation to NHL treatment have been undertaken only for genitourinary cancers[20,152] and AML (reviewed in ref. 153). The largest study[20] of secondary genitourinary tumors to date was conducted within a cohort of 6171 two-year survivors of NHL and included 31 patients with transitional cell carcinoma of the bladder and 17 patients with kidney cancer. Detailed data on cytotoxic drugs, including cumulative dose and duration, were collected for all patients, and radiation dose to the target organ was estimated using individual daily radiotherapy logs. Cyclophosphamide-based chemotherapy was associated with a statistically significant 4.5-fold increased risk of bladder cancer, with risk strongly dependent on cumulative dose (Table 54.7-4).

A cumulative dose of cyclophosphamide of less than 20 g was associated with a nonsignificant 2.4-fold risk of bladder cancer. Doses of 20 to 50 g, and 50 g or more were followed by statistically significant elevations in risk of 6-fold and 14.5-fold, respectively (P trend = .004). Radiotherapy given without cyclophosphamide was associated with a nonsignificant 2.8-fold higher risk of bladder malignancy. The increased risk of bladder cancer after treatment with both cyclophosphamide and radiotherapy was as expected if individual risks were added together. Neither cyclophosphamide treatment nor radiotherapy was related to an increased risk of kidney cancer. The predicted absolute risk of bladder cancer among 100 NHL patients given cumulative cyclophosphamide doses of between 20 and 50 g and 50 g or more was 3 and 7 excess cancers, respectively, during the first 15 years of follow-up. The TP53 mutational spectrum of cyclophosphamide-associated bladder cancer[154] differed from patterns observed for sporadic, smoking-related, and schistosomiasis-linked tumors but not for arylamine-associated cancers.[155]

Treatment for NHL has been related to significantly increased risks of AML in several studies (reviewed in ref. 153). Because leukemic progressions of NHL (lymphocytic leukemias) are not uncommon, histopathologic verification of AML diagnosis has constituted an integral part of most series in which leukemia risk was examined. The largest study to date was the collaborative international case-control study by Travis and colleagues.[156] Among 11,386 two-year survivors of NHL, 35 cases of AML or MDS were identified. The risk of AML was only weakly related with the administration of cyclophosphamide-containing regimens (RR, 1.8; 95% CI, 0.7 to 4.9) and did not increase with increasing cumulative dose of cyclophosphamide or duration of treatment. The median total amount of cyclophosphamide, however, was only 12.5 g, which is appreciably lower than in prior studies,[14,157] which each included nine leukemia cases and reported considerably larger risks.[156,158] The weak association between cyclophosphamide therapy at lower dose levels and AML[156] is consistent with results from other studies which report that the drug has a low leukemogenic potential.[8,18,159] In terms of absolute risk, Travis et al.[156] predicted that, among 10,000 NHL patients treated for 6 months with chemotherapy regimens containing low cumulative doses of cyclophosphamide, an excess of 4 cases of AML might develop during 10 years of follow-up.[85] The importance of this conclusion is underscored by the frequent use of cyclophosphamide-containing regimens in current NHL treatment regimens.

Low-dose total body irradiation (TBI), which was used to treat NHL in the past, has been associated with substantially elevated risks of secondary leukemias.[153,160] In this treatment approach, very low individual TBI fraction sizes (most commonly 10 to 15 cGy) were administered several times a week until a total dose of approximately 150 cGy was given.[160] Higher total doses of TBI (e.g., 1000 cGy) have been used in selected conditioning regimens before bone marrow transplantation.[5] Among a cohort of 61 two-year NHL survivors given low-dose TBI as primary therapy,[153] four patients were diagnosed with AML (RR, 117 compared with population rates; 95% CI, 31.5 to 300). A fifth patient developed MDS. All five patients with secondary MDS or AML had received salvage therapy with either alkylating agents or combined modality treatment. The excess risk of AML after low-dose TBI[153] was considerably higher than the risk observed in a larger international investigation of AML after NHL,[156] although similar chemotherapy regimens were administered. The investigators[153] hypothesized that subsequent chemotherapy contributed to the elevated risk of leukemia, both directly and possibly by enhancing the effect of low-dose TBI. Data from studies of laboratory animals indicate that low-dose TBI may increase the number of bone marrow stem cells subject to potential transformation by alkylating agents.[161] Other types of NHL treatment that combine high-dose, large-field radiotherapy with alkylating agents have also been associated with very high risks of AML (100- to 1000-fold increase).[153]

Numerous studies (reviewed in ref. 133) report an increased risk of MDS and AML among patients receiving autologous bone marrow transplantation (ABMT) for lymphoma, but the individual roles of pretransplantation- and transplantation-related therapy have not been well delineated. Discrepant findings in many investigations with regard to the contributions of pretransplantation and transplantation therapies to the development of MDS and AML may reflect in part the lack of information on type, duration, and dose of cytotoxic drugs and radiotherapy given before transplantation. Many studies are also limited by sparse numbers of MDS and AML cases and a small amount of variation in transplantation conditioning regimens. Metayer et al.[133] reported the results of a large case-control study of MDS and AML conducted within a cohort of 2739 patients given ABMT for NHL or HD at 12 institutions (1989 to 1995). Detailed information was collected for all pretransplantation and posttransplantation treatment and transplantation-related procedures for 56 patients who subsequently developed MDS and AML and for 168 matched controls. Metayer et al.[133] found that the risk of MDS and AML increased significantly with the intensity of pretransplantation chemotherapy that included chlorambucil (RR, 3.8 and 8.4 for duration less than 10 months or 10 months or longer, respectively; *P* trend = .009) or mechlorethamine (RR, 2.0 and 4.3 for cumulative doses of less than 50 mg/m^2 and 50 mg/m^2 or more, respectively; *P* trend = .04), compared with the risk in patients who received cyclophosphamide-based therapy. Although conditioning regimens including TBI at doses of 12 Gy or less did not significantly increase leukemia risk (RR, 1.4) compared with non-TBI regimens, a statistically significant 4.7-fold elevated risk was observed for a TBI dose of 13.2 Gy. Metayer et al.[133] concluded that the intensity and type of pretransplantation alkylating agent chemotherapy constituted pivotal risk factors for MDS and AML after ABMT, although risk may have also been influenced by transplant-related variables. Other studies have also reported significantly increased risks of MDS and AML in association with the administration of either pretransplantation alkylating agents[162–164] or fludarabine.[165,166] In support of these results, several investigators have found chromosomal abnormalities associated with MDS and AML in pretransplantation specimens.[129,167,168] Clearly, additional work needs to be undertaken to more fully delineate the roles of the various types of prior therapy for lymphoma, the preparative regimen for transplantation, and other factors in the subsequent development of MDS and AML.

In summary, survivors of NHL are at increased risk for a number of second malignancies, although to a considerably smaller degree than are patients with HD. The excess risks of AML and bladder cancer have been shown to be treatment related. The persistent increase in the risk of all second cancers for more than 20 years after NHL treatment alerts clinicians to the importance of long-term surveillance. The elevated risk of lung cancer should encourage efforts aimed at smoking cessation for patients who use tobacco. Health care providers should also be aware of the high risk of bladder cancer among patients treated with the high-dose cyclophosphamide regimens in the past. As indicated earlier, additional research is needed to more fully delineate risk factors for MDS and leukemia after autotransplantation for NHL.

TESTICULAR CANCER

Testicular cancer patients currently experience a 5-year relative survival rate of 95%,[147] due largely to the successful introduction of cisplatin into chemotherapy protocols.[169] Thus, testicular cancer now represents the paradigm of a curable malignancy, and given the young age at diagnosis, a lifetime exists for the manifestation of late effects. Although platinum-based chemotherapy for nonseminoma and advanced seminoma was not widely given until the late 1970s, effective treatment for early-stage seminoma has included infradiaphragmatic radiotherapy for many decades. Despite the recent reductions in radiation field size and dose,[170] testicular cancer patients treated with earlier, more aggressive regimens remain at risk for possible late sequelae. Few large studies, however, have addressed the long-term risks of second cancers among testicular cancer patients[81,171–174] and also take into account the histologic type of testicular tumor.[81] The largest study to date of second malignant neoplasms after testicular cancer included 28,843 one-year survivors diagnosed with a first primary cancer of the testis between 1935 and 1993 and reported to 16 population-based cancer registries in North America and Europe.[81] More than 3300 testicular cancer patients survived longer than 20 years after diagnosis. Second cancers, excluding malignancy of the contralateral testis, were diagnosed in 1406 patients (O/E, 1.43; 95% CI, 1.36 to 1.51) (Table 54.7-5).

The absolute risk was 16 excess cancers per 10,000 men per year. Significantly elevated risks were observed for all second solid tumors (O/E, 1.4; observed, 1251), with significant site-specific excesses for ALL, acute nonlymphocytic leukemia, melanoma, NHL, and cancers of the stomach, colon, rectum, pancreas, prostate, kidney, bladder, thyroid, and connective tissue. Second cancer risk was similar after seminomas (O/E, 1.4) and nonseminomatous tumors (O/E, 1.5), with little variation in site-specific patterns. Increased risks for cancers of the small intestine (O/E, 4.4) and rectum (O/E, 1.6) were observed only for seminomas, whereas patients with nonseminomatous germ cell tumors showed twofold elevated risks for hepatobiliary cancer. Risk of solid tumors increased with time since diagnosis of testicular cancer to reach 1.5 after 20 years (*P* trend = .00002). Among 20-year survivors, 369 solid tumors (O/E, 1.5) were reported, with significant excesses for cancers of the stomach (O/E, 2.3), colon (O/E, 1.7), pancreas (O/E, 3.2), prostate (O/E, 1.4), kidney (O/E, 2.3), bladder (O/E, 2.8), and connective tissue (O/E, 4.7).[175] The actuarial risks of developing any second cancer, excluding contralateral testicular tumors, were 15.7% and 22.6% at 25 and 30 years, respectively, after testicular cancer diagnosis. The corresponding population expected risks were 9.3% and 13.1%. As shown in Figure 54.7-1, the cumulative risk of second cancer at 25 years was

TABLE 54.7-5. Observed and Expected Numbers of Selected Second Malignant Neoplasms among 1-Year Survivors of Testicular Cancer[a]

	Observed	Observed to Expected Ratio	95% Confidence Interval
All second cancers[b]	1406	1.4[c]	1.4–1.5
All solid tumors[b]	1251	1.4[c]	1.3–1.4
Esophagus	20	1.3	0.8–2.1
Stomach	93	2.0[c]	1.6–2.4
Small intestine	12	3.2[c]	1.6–5.6
Colon	105	1.3[c]	1.0–1.5
Rectum	77	1.4[c]	1.1–1.8
Liver, gallbladder	26	1.5	1.0–2.1
Pancreas	66	2.2[c]	1.7–2.8
Lung	201	1.0	0.9–1.2
Prostate	164	1.3[c]	1.1–1.5
Kidney	55	1.5[c]	1.1–2.0
Bladder	154	2.0[c]	1.7–2.4
Melanoma	58	1.7[c]	1.3–2.2
Thyroid	19	2.9[c]	1.8–4.6
Bone	6	2.4	0.9–5.3
Connective tissue	22	3.2[c]	2.0–4.8
Non-Hodgkin's lymphoma	68	1.9[c]	1.5–2.4
All leukemia	64	2.1[c]	1.6–2.7
Acute lymphoblastic leukemia	9	5.2[c]	2.4–9.9
Acute nonlymphocytic leukemia	27	3.1[c]	2.0–4.5
Chronic lymphocytic leukemia	7	0.6	0.2–1.2
Chronic granulocytic leukemia	9	0.9	0.4–1.8

[a]Includes 28,843 patients diagnosed with a first primary cancer of the testis who survived 1 or more years.
[b]Numbers exclude contralateral testicular cancers. Category of all solid tumors also excludes lympho-hematopoietic disorders.
[c]P<.05.
(From ref. 81, with permission.)

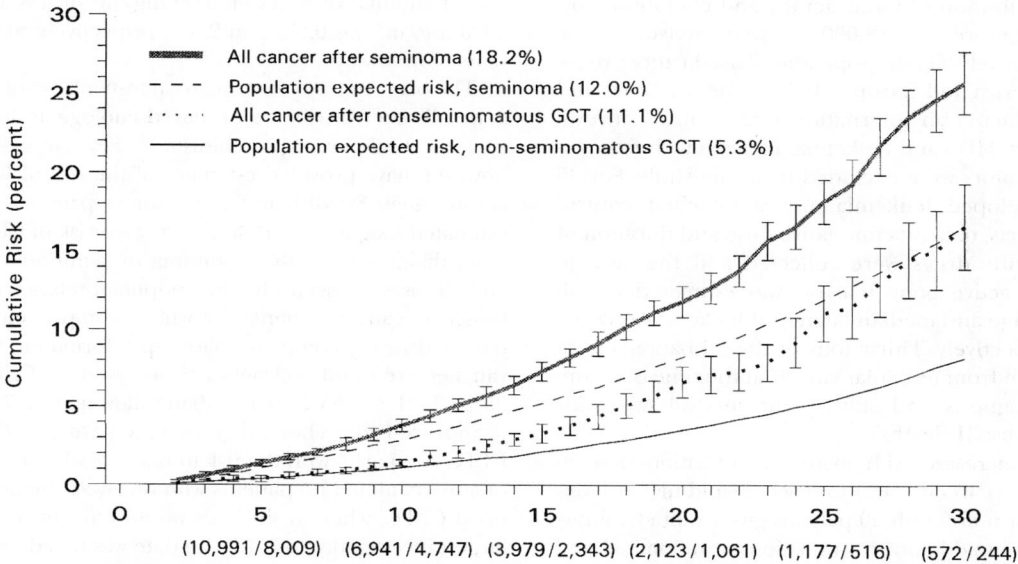

Years from Diagnosis of Testicular Cancer (No. of patients at risk: seminomas/nonseminomatous GCT)

FIGURE 54.7-1. Cumulative risk of second malignant neoplasms among 28,010 one-year survivors of testicular germ cell tumors (GCT). Percentages in parentheses indicate the actuarial risk at 25 years. Within the figure, 95% confidence intervals for point estimates are shown by vertical bars. (From ref. 81, with permission.)

higher for men with seminomas (18.2%; 95% CI, 16.8% to 19.6%) than for those with nonseminomatous tumors (11.1%; 95% CI, 9.3% to 12.9%). The differences likely reflect the younger mean age of the patients with nonseminomatous tumors, because the excess cumulative risks were comparable.

Increased risk for cancers of the stomach, bladder, and possibly pancreas were associated primarily with prior radiotherapy, whereas leukemia was linked with both antecedent radiation therapy and chemotherapy. In the past, large doses of radiation (mean, 13 to 26 Gy) could be delivered to the stomach during irradiation of the paraaortic lymph nodes.[81] In previous smaller surveys, a significant eightfold increased risk of stomach cancer was associated with infradiaphragmatic and supradiaphragmatic irradiation for testicular tumors,[173] and a fourfold to fivefold increased risk was associated with abdominal radiotherapy.[173] The international investigation by Travis et al.[81] showed for the first time that the increased risks for stomach cancer persisted for at least two decades after diagnosis of testicular cancer. After irradiation for peptic ulcer disease, significantly increased risks for stomach cancer mortality (average organ dose, 14.8) extended beyond 30 years.[176,177] A pattern of increasing risk of pancreas cancer with time in the international study,[81] with excesses mainly in testicular cancer patients who received initial radiotherapy, was also suggestive of a radiogenic effect, consistent with the location of the pancreas in the radiation field (mean organ dose, 17 to 34 Gy) during therapy for testicular cancer. The pancreas is not regarded as especially sensitive to the carcinogenic effects of ionizing radiation, however, unless very large doses are administered.[176,177]

Reports that document the increased risk of leukemia after testicular cancer have generally been based on relatively small numbers of patients[89,91,92,171,172,178,179] or lack comprehensive treatment information[81] and are thus unable to rigorously examine the contribution of radiotherapy and chemotherapy. Within a cohort of more than 18,000 one-year survivors of testicular cancer reported to eight population-based cancer registries in North America and Europe (1970 to 1993), Travis and colleagues[180] conducted an international case-control investigation of secondary MDS and leukemia. Patients with extragonadal germ cell tumors were excluded from the study. For 36 patients who developed leukemia and a matched control group of 106 subjects, data on cumulative dose and duration of all chemotherapeutic drugs were collected and the average radiation dose to active bone marrow was estimated for all patients. The average and median latency of leukemia were 6.8 and 5.0 years, respectively. Thirty four of the 36 patients were in clinical remission from testicular cancer at the time of secondary leukemia diagnosis and subsequent survival was poor (median, 8.4 months; 31 deaths).

Leukemia risk increased with increasing radiation dose to active bone marrow (*P* trend = .02) to reach 20-fold higher levels at doses of 20 Gy or more, with 20 patients given supradiaphragmatic radiotherapy in addition to irradiation of abdominal and pelvic fields accounting for much of the risk at the higher doses.[180] A nonsignificant threefold higher risk of leukemia followed pelvic-abdominal radiotherapy alone; for patients who received additional supradiaphragmatic irradiation (mean dose to bone marrow, 19.5 Gy), a significant 11-fold increased risk was apparent. Both radiation dose to active bone marrow and cumulative amount of cisplatin given (*P* trend = .001) were associated with significantly increased risks of leukemia.[180] The highly significant dose-response relation observed for total amount of cisplatin was in accordance with results in a study of women treated with platinum-based chemotherapy for ovarian cancer.[23] Although the total amount of etoposide did not add to leukemia risk when doses of cisplatin and radiation were considered, men given etoposide also received larger cumulative doses of cisplatin, which makes it difficult to separate out the component contributions to leukemia risk.[180] Moreover, the total amounts of etoposide (median, 1900 mg/m² in cases; 1600 mg/m² in controls) were relatively low. The predicted risk of leukemia at a cumulative cisplatin dose of 650 mg, given in current testicular cancer regimens, was 3.2 (95% CI, 1.5 to 8.4). Travis et al.[180] estimated that of 10,000 testicular cancer patients treated with cisplatin-based chemotherapy (cumulative dose, 650 mg), 16 excess leukemias might result during 15 years of follow-up. Although patients with mediastinal nonseminomatous germ cell tumors are inherently prone to develop secondary leukemia,[181] such a relationship has not been reported for testicular tumors.

Use of etoposide and cisplatin to treat testicular cancer has been previously linked to increased risks of leukemia in relatively small studies,[89,92,171,181,182] typically at large total amounts of etoposide (3000 mg/m² or more).[92] Considerably lower total doses of etoposide were administered in the case-control investigation reported by Travis et al.,[180] similar to the dose of less than 2000 mg/m² used in current regimens.[182] The IARC concluded that there is sufficient evidence that etoposide in combination with cisplatin and bleomycin is carcinogenic to humans.[183] The overall level of risk, however, appears relatively low.[103,184] Based on a review of selected U.S. clinical trials, Smith et al.[103] estimated that the 6-year cumulative risk of secondary leukemia is 0.7% after cumulative etoposide doses of 1500 to 2999 mg/m². Kollmannsberger et al.[184] concluded that the cumulative incidence of leukemia among testicular cancer patients given etoposide at cumulative doses of 2000 mg/m² or less and more than 2000 mg/m² was 0.5% and 2.0%, respectively, at a median of 5 years of follow-up.

The occurrence of contralateral testicular cancer (CLTC) has generally been attributed to shared etiologic influences, such as atrophic testis or cryptorchidism.[185] Few large studies,[172,174,186] however, have provided estimates of the risk of CLTC. In 2001, among 4650 Swedish testicular cancer patients, Dong et al.[174] estimated a significant 12-fold increased risk of CLTC after a primary diagnosis of either teratoma or seminoma (observed, 22 and 19 cases, respectively). In a population-based cohort of 1909 testicular cancer patients for whom comprehensive treatment data and nearly complete follow-up information were available, van Leeuwen and colleagues[172] observed 20 CLTCs (RR, 35.7; 95% CI, 21.8 to 55.2) at a median follow-up of 7.7 years. Notably, it appeared that chemotherapy may have reduced the risk of CLTC compared with the risk in patients who received radiation or surgery alone; no patients who received chemotherapy developed CLTC, whereas six cases would have been expected. The largest investigation of CLTC to date was based on 60 cases diagnosed among 2201 men with a first primary germ cell cancer at the Norwegian Radium Hospital in Oslo (1953 to 1990).[186] The cumulative risk of CLTC at 15 years of follow-up was 3.9% (95% CI, 2.8 to 5.0). Risk did not appear to be significantly influenced by treatment of the first cancer with either radiotherapy, chemotherapy, or both, but the authors pointed out that cisplatin-based chemotherapy had been administered only since 1978.[186]

In summary, patients treated for testicular cancer have less than one-third of the excess risk of second malignancy experienced by patients with HD. The increased risk of stomach cancer should alert clinicians to the importance of a careful evaluation of gastrointestinal complaints in patients who received radiotherapy to the paraaortic lymph nodes. Because reports of increased risks of gastrointestinal cancer have been based on studies in which patients were treated with high doses of radiation, it is important to determine whether smaller risks will follow the lower doses (20 to 25 Gy) that are currently used. Conventional platinum-based chemotherapy is associated with a small, but measurable, increased risk of leukemia that is linked with cumulative dose of cisplatin.[180] High-dose etoposide regimens are associated with a moderately increased leukemia risk.[89] Even though radiotherapy regimens for testicular cancer have been modified in recent decades with the introduction of smaller fields, lower doses, and elimination of prophylactic mediastinal radiation, the late effects of therapy given decades ago continue to emerge. In the future, radiation dose to second cancer sites for which risks are elevated should be estimated in individual patients along with cumulative dose of specific cytotoxic drugs to further quantify the contribution of treatment factors. Long-term follow-up studies are also needed to evaluate the risk of second solid tumors among testicular cancer patients treated with modern cisplatin-based chemotherapy.[81]

OVARIAN CANCER

Given the significant improvements in survival of ovarian cancer patients within the last 20 years,[187] the evaluation of the site-specific risk of second primary cancers has become increasingly important. The current 5-year relative survival for women diagnosed with ovarian cancer is 53%.[147] The largest follow-up study to date included more than 32,000 women with ovarian cancer, including 4402 ten-year survivors, reported to population-based cancer registries of the SEER program (1973 to 1992) and the Connecticut Tumor Registry (1935 to 1972).[153] Overall, a significantly increased risk of second cancers (O/E, 1.3; 95% CI, 1.2 to 1.4; observed, 1296) was noted. Significant excesses were observed for ocular melanoma (O/E, 4.5), and cancers of the colon (O/E, 1.3), rectum (O/E, 1.4), breast (O/E, 1.2), and bladder (O/E, 2.1), as well as leukemia (O/E, 4.2). Radiotherapy was associated with cancers of connective tissue, bladder, and possibly pancreas, whereas secondary leukemia appeared linked with prior chemotherapy. Reproductive and genetic factors predisposing to ovarian cancer may have contributed to the elevated risk of breast and colorectal neoplasms and possibly ocular melanoma. The risk of solid tumors was elevated during all follow-up intervals, including 10 to 14 years (O/E, 1.3) and 15 years or longer (O/E, 1.3), after ovarian cancer. Fifteen-year survivors experienced significant excesses of cancers of the pancreas, bladder, and connective tissue. The cumulative risk of second cancers at 20 years was 18.2%, compared with a population expected risk of 11.5%.

Latency patterns for solid tumor risk differed by type of primary therapy for ovarian cancer. After radiation therapy alone, excesses of solid tumors increased with time to reach almost twofold among long-term survivors (*P* trend = .07); an additional 88 solid tumors (O/E, 1.42) occurred after 20 or more years of follow-up. In contrast, although solid tumor risk after treatments that included chemotherapy was elevated within the 5- to 9-year

interval after ovarian cancer, nonsignificant excesses occurred in later periods. In a case-control investigation of bladder cancer after ovarian cancer, Kaldor et al.[118] reported increased risks after radiotherapy only (RR, 1.9; 95% CI, 0.8 to 4.9) compared with risks in patients treated with surgery alone. Cyclophosphamide-based chemotherapy, with or without radiotherapy, was associated with a fourfold increased risk of bladder cancer,[118] similar to the overall 4.5-fold increased risk reported after cyclophosphamide-based chemotherapy for NHL.[20]

Hemminki and colleagues[188] quantified the site-specific risk of second primary cancers among 19,400 Swedish women with ovarian cancer (1961 to 1998). New findings in this population-based survey included significantly increased risks of cancers of the stomach (O/E, 1.60; observed, 43), small intestine (O/E, 3.08; observed, 12), kidney (O/E, 1.77; observed, 44), and thyroid gland (O/E, 1.78; observed, 16). Whereas excess cancers of the kidney and thyroid were clustered within the first year after diagnosis of ovarian cancer, consistent with a surveillance effect, significantly increased risks of stomach cancer persisted among 10-year survivors. Although information on the initial course of cancer therapy was not available,[188] this latter finding may in part reflect the late sequelae of treatment, as well as the inclusion of cancers of both ovary and stomach in the constellation of tumors that comprise hereditary nonpolyposis colorectal cancer (Lynch syndrome type II).[189] The increased risk of cancers of the small intestine,[188] which was significant in the less than 1 year and 1- to 10-year period after ovarian cancer diagnosis, may similarly reflect genetic factors operant in hereditary nonpolyposis colorectal cancer–Lynch syndrome type II.[189]

Increased risks of AML and preleukemia have been reported after treatment for ovarian cancer that includes either melphalan,[159] cyclophosphamide,[19,159] or chlorambucil.[19] However, platinum-based chemotherapy is currently the most widely used regimen. In one large population-based study of more than 28,000 ovarian cancer patients in whom 96 leukemias were diagnosed, platinum-based combination chemotherapy was associated with a significant fourfold increased risk compared with risk in women who received neither alkylating drugs nor radiotherapy.[23] Leukemia risk increased with increasing cumulative platinum dose (*P* trend for dose <.001) (Table 54.7-6).

Leukemia excesses also rose with increasing duration of platinum-based chemotherapy to reach sevenfold in women treated for more than 12 months (*P* trend for duration = .001). Platinating agents were frequently given in combination with cyclophosphamide, doxorubicin, or both; however, a multivariate model that controlled for cumulative dose of these drugs produced similar results. Paclitaxel was not administered in the study.[23] Radiotherapy (average bone marrow dose, 13.4 Gy) without chemotherapy did not increase the risk of leukemia,[23] but few women received radiation only. Women who received both radiotherapy and platinum-based chemotherapy experienced a significantly higher risk of leukemia than those who received platinum-based chemotherapy alone (*P* = .006). A dose-response relationship for platinum was apparent among women treated and not treated with radiotherapy, with larger risks in the radiation-treated group; among all of the latter patients, radiotherapy was administered as part of initial treatment. Given current treatment recommendations[190] for ovarian cancer, it is unlikely that newly diagnosed women will receive both platinum and radiotherapy. Whether leukemia risk after treatment with platinum might be increased by radio-

TABLE 54.7-6. Risk of Leukemia According to the Cumulative Dose of Platinum, Duration of Therapy, and Specific Drug[a]

Dose and Duration	Number of Patients with Leukemia	Number of Matched Control Patients	Median Value in Controls[b]	Relative Risk (95% Confidence Interval)[c]
ALL PLATINUM DRUGS				
Dose[d]				
<500 mg	4	30	418 mg	1.9 (0.5–7.9)
500–749 mg	5	28	600 mg	2.1 (0.6–8.0)
750–999 mg	7	25	896 mg	4.1 (1.1–14.8)
>1000 mg	11	20	1230 mg	7.6 (2.3–25.3)[e]
Duration				
<6 mo	3	36	5.4 mo	1.2 (0.3–5.5)
6–12 mo	16	49	8.5 mo	4.3 (1.4–12.9)
>12 mo	8	18	14.2 mo	7.0 (1.8–26.6)[f]
SPECIFIC DRUG				
Cisplatin	19	85	600 mg	3.3 (1.1–9.4)
Carboplatin	3	9	3300 mg	6.5 (1.2–36.6)
Both	5	9		9.0 (2.2–37.6)
Cisplatin			720 mg	
Carboplatin			2200 mg	

[a]The data are limited to 27 patients with leukemia and 103 controls who receive platinum-based chemotherapy without melphalan.
[b]The values shown are median cumulative doses of platinum and the median duration of therapy among controls.
[c]The reference group consisted of 6 patients with leukemia and 94 controls who were not exposed to platinum derivatives of other alkylating drugs.
[d]Cumulative amounts of carboplatin were divided by 4 to convert them to cisplatin-equivalent doses.
[e]P for trend <.001.
[f]P for trend = .001.
(From ref. 23, with permission.)

therapy, however, should be examined among patients with other cancers, especially cancers of the bladder and head and neck, given therapeutic approaches to increase dose intensities of both modalities in the management of these tumors.[191,192]

In summary, survivors of ovarian cancer experience significantly increased risks of secondary leukemias and solid tumors. Even though modern platinum-based chemotherapy for ovarian cancer is associated with an increased risk of leukemia, the absolute risk is small.[23] Among 10,000 women with ovarian cancer treated for 6 months with total amounts of cisplatin of 500 to 1000 mg or 1000 mg and more and followed for 10 years, an excess of 21 and 71 leukemias, respectively, might be predicted.[23] Therefore, it is clear that the significant gains in clinical response provided by platinum-based treatment for advanced ovarian cancer, with 5-year survival rates of up to 20% to 30%,[190,193] greatly outweigh the relatively small increased risks of leukemia. Additional transdisciplinary studies should be undertaken to clarify the carcinogenic risks associated with current treatments for ovarian cancer and with shared etiologic factors, including genetic and reproductive variables. In the interim, in proposing recommendations for the follow-up of survivors of ovarian cancer,[190] it is critical to take into account their long-term predisposition to an array of second cancers.

BREAST CANCER

Numerous studies have demonstrated that women with breast cancer are at a threefold to fourfold increased risk of developing a new primary cancer in the contralateral breast.[194,195] Sig-nificant excesses relative to the general population have also been observed for cancers of the ovary,[195,196] uterus,[195–198] lung,[195,197,199–203] esophagus,[204] colon-rectum,[195,196,198] and connective tissue,[195,200,205–207] and for melanoma[195,200] and leukemia.[88,196,200] For some of these cancers, such as those of the contralateral breast, ovary, and uterus and possibly melanoma, the excesses may be fully or partly explained by a common etiology (e.g., genetic predisposition or hormonal risk factors). Other excess risks may be treatment-related or reflect the interaction of several factors. Adjuvant chemotherapy, hormonal treatment, and radiotherapy, and combinations of these modalities, are being administered to a growing proportion of breast cancer patients. In view of the proven therapeutic benefit of these treatments[208,209] and the prolonged life expectancy of those treated, it has become exceedingly important to evaluate the carcinogenic potential of adjuvant treatment.

Contralateral breast cancer accounts for 40% to 50% of all second tumors in women with breast cancer,[195] and the 15-year cumulative risk of developing contralateral disease amounts to 10% to 13%.[210,211] With this high risk, even small effects of treatment may have a large impact in terms of absolute numbers of contralateral breast cancers. The effect of radiation treatment for the initial breast cancer was evaluated in two large case-control studies in Connecticut and Denmark that involved 655 and 529 women with contralateral breast cancer, respectively. The mean radiation doses to the contralateral breast were estimated at 2.8 and 2.5 Gy, respectively.[17,212] Both studies found that radiotherapy did not contribute to the high risk of contralateral disease among women treated after the age of 45 years. However, in the Connecticut study significantly elevated risks were observed for women who underwent irradiation before the age of 45 years, with a radiation-associated RR of 1.9 among those who survived for at least 10 years.[17] Significant excess risk in women irradiated at a young age was not found in the Danish study, possibly because it included fewer women under the age of 45 years.[212] Based on results of the Connecticut study, Boice and associates[17] estimated that approximately 11% of all second breast cancers in women irradiated before age 45 years could be attributed to radiotherapy. Modern radiotherapy techniques for breast cancer deliver a lower dose to the contralateral breast than the techniques used in these studies.[17,212] It is unfortunate, therefore, that it has not been examined yet whether radiotherapy as applied from the 1980s onward affects the risk of contralateral breast cancer.

Several large studies have shown that hormonal treatment with tamoxifen reduces the risk of contralateral breast cancer by approximately 40%.[197,198,209,213,214] Data collected by the Early Breast Cancer Trialists' Collaborative Group (EBCTCG), encompassing 37,000 women in 55 trials, demonstrated that longer durations of tamoxifen use were associated with greater reductions in risk, so that 1 year, 2 years, and 5 years of treatment produced risk reductions of 13%, 26%, and 47%, respectively.[209] A 50% reduction of contralateral breast cancer risk after tamoxifen treatment was also observed among breast cancer patients with a BRCA1 or BRCA2 mutation.[215] It is not yet known whether the protective effect of tamoxifen against contralateral disease persists over prolonged follow-up periods (longer than 10 year). Some studies have provided evidence that adjuvant chemotherapy may also reduce the risk of contralateral breast cancer, a phenomenon that is likely to be mediated through drug-induced premature ovarian failure.[208,216,217]

Several studies have assessed the risk of leukemia after adjuvant chemotherapy and radiotherapy for breast cancer. The relationship between AML risk and drug dose was examined in detail in a large case-control study by Curtis and associates.[18] These investigators identified 90 cases of leukemia or MDS among 82,700 women diagnosed with breast cancer between 1973 and 1985 in five areas of the United States. Compared to patients treated without alkylating agents and irradiation, the risk of AML was significantly elevated after locoregional radiotherapy alone (RR, 2.4), after treatment with alkylating agents alone (RR, 10.0), and after treatment with alkylating agents in combination with radiotherapy (RR, 17.4). The risk of AML associated with combined modality treatment was significantly greater than that associated with the use of alkylating agents alone ($P = .02$). The study included large numbers of women who had been treated with only one alkylating agent, including cyclophosphamide. Cumulative cyclophosphamide doses of less than 20 g were associated with an approximately twofold nonsignificant increase in risk (compared to risk for women not exposed to alkylating agents), whereas women treated with 20 g or more had a 5.7-fold increased risk of AML (95% CI, 1.6 to 20.6). After adjustment for the effects of chemotherapy, the risk of AML was found to increase significantly with higher doses of radiation to the active bone marrow, with a sevenfold risk increase for patients who received 9 Gy or more (compared to risk for patients not treated with radiotherapy).

Present-day adjuvant treatment of early breast cancer is in several ways different from the treatments evaluated in this large study.[18] In the 1980s the cumulative doses of cyclophos-

phamide were reduced [12 to 15 g with six standard cycles of cyclophosphamide, methotrexate, and fluorouracil (CMF), fluorouracil, doxorubicin, and cyclophosphamide (FAC), or doxorubicin and cyclophosphamide (AC)]. Regional radiotherapy is less frequently used. On the basis of their data, Curtis and associates estimated that among 10,000 patients with breast cancer treated for 6 months with a cyclophosphamide-based regimen and followed for 10 years, an excess of only five cases of treatment-related AML would be expected to develop.[18]

The low risk of AML after CMF-based chemotherapy was confirmed by the Milan Cancer Institute[218] and the Eastern Cooperative Oncology Group,[219] who found cumulative risks of AML of 0.23% at 15 years and 0.18% at 7 years, respectively. The University of Texas M. D. Anderson Cancer Center reported a higher risk of leukemia after a standard dose-intensity FAC treatment. Fourteen cases of leukemia were observed among 1474 patients for an estimated cumulative risk of 1.5% (95% CI, 0.7 to 2.9) at 10 years. The risk of AML was significantly higher when chemotherapy was given in combination with radiotherapy (2.5% vs. 0.5%).[100]

There has been an increasing trend toward the use of dose-intensification strategies in chemotherapy protocols for breast cancer. Typically, these regimens contain high-dose cyclophosphamide in combination with one of the anthracyclines (doxorubicin or 4-epidoxorubicin) and other active drugs. The risk of AML associated with various AC regimens was quantified in six trials of the National Surgical Adjuvant Breast and Bowel Project (NSABP).[88] Based on 43 cases of AML and MDS in 8563 patients, it was found that leukemia risk strongly increased with cyclophosphamide dose intensity (rather than with cumulative dose). The 8-year cumulative incidences of AML and MDS were 1.07%, 0.49%, and 0.27% for regimens with two to four cycles containing cyclophosphamide 2400 mg/m^2/cycle and 1200 mg/m^2/cycle, and the standard AC regimen of four cycles with 600 mg/m^2/cycle, respectively. The standard-dose AC regimen was still associated with a significant sevenfold increased risk of leukemia compared to the risk in the general SEER population, and the most dose-intensive regimen was associated with a near 50-fold increased risk. Growth factor support (total dose of granulocyte colony-stimulating factor) was significantly associated with leukemia risk; however, as the authors acknowledge, this result may have no causal basis because patients receiving the higher growth factor doses may have been those who achieved the highest plasma levels of the leukemogenic drugs under study. Patients who received breast radiotherapy (after lumpectomy) had a greater risk of leukemia than those who did not (RR, 2.38; $P = .006$). The effect of doxorubicin dose could not be evaluated in this study because dose intensity was the same in all regimens (60 mg/m^2).[88] A French analysis showed low risk of AML (less than 0.2%) after a high-dose fluorouracil, epirubicin, and cyclophosphamide (FEC) regimen (100 mg/m^2/cycle of epirubicin, 500 mg/m^2/cycle of cyclophosphamide for six cycles).[220] It is noteworthy that several reports have shown very high risks of AML and MDS after chemotherapy with mitoxantrone.[89,107,108] In one study a cumulative dose effect was suggested, with 4-year cumulative rates of 0.63% and 3.89% for patients receiving cumulative doses 12 mg/m^2 or less and 56 mg/m^2 or more, respectively. Leukemia risk was significantly higher in patients treated with mitoxantrone than in those receiving anthracyclines.[107]

TABLE 54.7-7. Risk of Endometrial Cancer after Tamoxifen Therapy in Women with Breast Cancer

Study[a] and Design	No. of Breast Cancers	No. of Endometrial Cancers (No. in Tamoxifen Users)	Dose Evaluated	Duration of Tamoxifen Use	Relative Risk (95% of Confidence Interval)
Fisher et al., 1994[197]; clinical trials	4063	24 (23)	20 mg	Planned: ≥5 y	Tamoxifen vs. control: 7.5 (1.7–32.7)
					Tamoxifen vs. general population: 2.2[b]
					Tamoxifen vs. control other trial: 2.3[b]
Rutqvist et al., 1995[198]; clinical trial	4914	42 (34)	30–40 mg	48 wk–5 y	Any: 4.1 (1.9–8.9)
EBCTCG, 1998[209]; clinical trials	36,689	124 (92)	Mostly 20 mg	1, 2, or 5 y	Ever use: 2.6 (2.2–2.9)
Fisher et al., 1998[225]; prevention trial	13,388	51 (36)	20 mg	1–5 y	5 Y: 4.2 (P<.001)
					Any: 2.5 (1.4–5.0)
Curtis et al., 1996[213]; cohort (SEER based)	87,323	457 (73)	Unknown	Unknown	Any tamoxifen vs. general population: 2.0 (1.6–2.6)
					No tamoxifen vs. general population: 1.2 (1.1–1.4)
Mignotte et al., 1998[226]; case control	NA	135 (91)	20–40 mg	Varied	Ever use: 3.1 (1.1–8.7)
					≥5 Y: 10.7 (3.4–34.0)
					Trend with duration: P = .0001
Bernstein et al., 1999[224]; case control	NA	324 (146)	Mostly 20 mg	Varied	Ever use: 1.5 (1.1–2.2)
					≥5 Y: 4.1 (1.7–9.5)
					Trend with duration: P = .0002
Bergman et al., 2000[227]; case control	NA	299 (108)	20–40 mg	Varied	Ever use: 1.5 (1.1–2.0)
					≥5 Y: 6.6 (2.2–19.7)
					Trend with duration: P<.001

EBCTCG, Early Breast Cancer Trialists' Collaborative Group; NA, not available; SEER, Surveillance, Epidemiology, and End Results program.
[a]Several early reports are not presented because the dates are included in larger or updated studies presented here.[198,224,227]
[b]Because the incidence of endometrial cancer appeared to be unexpectedly low among placebo-treated women, the investigators reestimated the risk associated with tamoxifen, using population-based rates and information from another trial. However, the resulting risk estimates of 2.2 and 2.3, respectively, are less valid than the estimate based on the endometrial cancer rate in placebo-allocated controls (relative risk, 7.5) because (a) regardless of treatment, a population of breast cancer patients entered into a clinical trial may have different endometrial cancer rates than the general population; and (b) the rates used were from a different geographic area, a different period, or both.[183]
(Adapted from ref. 137.)

Patients treated with CMF-, AC-, or FAC-based chemotherapy have not been reported to be at increased risk of solid tumors.[218,221] More prolonged follow-up, however, is needed to evaluate possible carcinogenic effects 15 years or more after treatment.

Conclusive evidence has emerged that tamoxifen therapy is associated with a moderately increased risk of endometrial cancer.[197,198,209,222–225] The consistent results across studies with different designs, the duration-response relationship observed in several investigations,[224,226,227] and the established estrogen-agonist effects of tamoxifen on the endometrium[228,229] strongly support a causal relationship.[223] The individual studies, which are summarized in Table 54.7-7, show that the use of tamoxifen for 2 years is associated with an approximately twofold increased risk of endometrial cancer, whereas use for five or more years produces fourfold to eightfold excess risks. Although the risk estimates in some studies may be affected by a certain degree of detection bias as a result of gynecologic examinations in women with side effects from tamoxifen, the magnitude of the observed risk is unlikely to be explained by such bias.[223] Furthermore, the analysis of the EBCTCG not only shows increased incidence of endometrial cancer in women randomly assigned to receive tamoxifen treatment (compared to that in women not randomly assigned to receive tamoxifen) but also significantly increased mortality due to endometrial cancer.[209]

From Table 54.7-7 it is clear that elevated risks of endometrial cancer have been observed after daily tamoxifen doses of 20, 30, and 40 mg. In the Netherlands case-control study, which included different dose intensities, daily dose did not affect endometrial cancer risk in a model accounting for duration of use, and the duration-response trends were similar for daily doses of 40 mg or 30 mg and less.[227] Very few studies have addressed the risk for ex-users. In three investigations,[224,226,227] recent users and ex-users of tamoxifen were found to experience very similar increases in risk; however, only a few patients had discontinued tamoxifen more than 2 years before the diagnosis of endometrial cancer. Only two studies have addressed the combined effects of tamoxifen and other risk factors for endometrial cancer.[224,227] In the largest study conducted to date, Bernstein and colleagues[224] reported that women who previously used estrogen replacement therapy experienced greater increases in endometrial cancer risk associated with tamoxifen use than women not exposed to estrogen replacement therapy. Furthermore, the effects of tamoxifen on endometrial cancer risk were stronger among heavy women than among thin women. In the Dutch study, however, body weight did not modify the increased risk associated with tamoxifen use.[227]

An important question is whether the clinicopathologic characteristics and ultimate prognosis of endometrial cancers in women after tamoxifen treatment are different from those in patients not treated with tamoxifen. In a few early, small studies, the stage distribution and histologic features of endometrial cancers in tamoxifen-treated women were not remarkably different from those of cancers diagnosed in nontreated women.[197,213,230] Magriples and colleagues, however, reported a higher frequency of poorly differentiated and high-

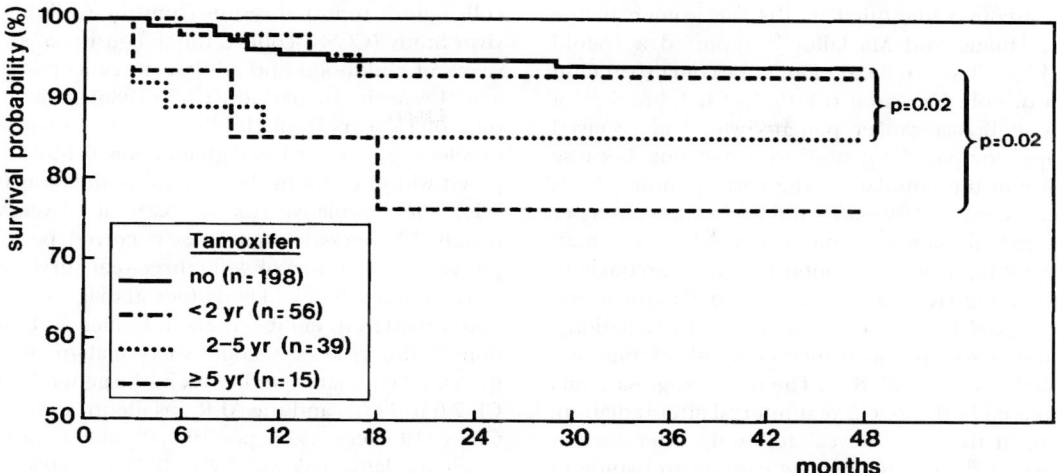

FIGURE 54.7-2. Actuarial endometrial cancer–specific survival according to duration of tamoxifen use. (From ref. 227, with permission.)

grade tumors with a poor prognosis in tamoxifen-treated patients.[231] In the Dutch study, which included 309 patients with endometrial cancer after breast cancer, endometrial tumors of International Federation of Gynecology and Obstetrics (FIGO) stages III and IV occurred more frequently among long-term tamoxifen users (two or more years) than among nonusers (17% vs. 5%; $P = .006$). Based on centralized review of diagnostic pathology slides, long-term tamoxifen users more often developed malignant mixed mesodermal tumors or sarcomas of the endometrium than did nonusers (15% vs. 3%; $P = .02$). Furthermore, the tumors diagnosed among long-term tamoxifen users were more often p53 positive and estrogen receptor negative. Figure 54.7-2 shows that the 3-year actuarial endometrial cancer–specific survival in this study was significantly worse for long-term tamoxifen users than for nonusers, largely due to the less favorable tumor characteristics associated with tamoxifen use.[227] Increased risk of generally poor-prognosis uterine sarcoma after tamoxifen use was confirmed in an analysis of NSABP trials, with 1.7 cases per 10,000 tamoxifen-treated women per year,[232] and in two other reports.[233,234]

Animal experiments have shown that tamoxifen can act as a hepatic carcinogen in rats.[235,236] However, no increased risk of hepatocellular cancer in tamoxifen-treated patents has been observed to date.[197,198,209,213] In the large metaanalysis of the EBCTCG, women randomly assigned to receive tamoxifen therapy had a slightly lower mortality from primary liver cancer than those in the control group.[209]

The joint analysis of Scandinavian tamoxifen trials showed an elevated risk of gastrointestinal cancer after tamoxifen use (RR, 1.9; 95% CI, 1.2 to 2.9)[198]; however, the excess risk was due to colorectal and stomach cancer, not to liver cancer. Further, a study from the SEER program found that tamoxifen was associated with a 50% increased risk of colorectal cancer in the period five or more years after diagnosis.[237] No such risk increase was observed in the EBCTCG data.[209]

Increased risk of lung cancer after breast cancer has been largely attributed to radiotherapy.[199,202,238–240] No appreciable risk increase has been observed within 10 years of treatment, but twofold to threefold elevated risk has been reported in 10-year survivors. treated with postmastectomy radiotherapy.[199,239,240]

The association between radiotherapy and subsequent lung cancer risk was found to be stronger for the ipsilateral lung, which supports a radiogenic effect.[199,238–240] Two studies[199,239] addressed the question of whether postlumpectomy radiotherapy is also associated with excess lung cancer risk. Radiotherapy given after breast-conserving surgery exposes the lung parenchyma to a much lower radiation dose than postmastectomy radiotherapy, because it less often involves regional radiation to the internal mammary and supraclavicular lymph nodes, and the absorbed dose from breast irradiation is reduced by the remaining breast tissue. The largest study analyzed risk factors for 475 lung cancers in 65,560 patients treated with breast-conserving surgery and 2230 lung cancers in 194,981 women treated with mastectomy in the U.S. SEER database.[239] No increased risk of lung cancer was found after postlumpectomy radiation therapy (compared with lumpectomy alone) for either lung, whereas postmastectomy radiation therapy doubled the risk of ipsilateral lung cancer 10 to 20 years after treatment.[239] Similar results (i.e., no increased risk after postlumpectomy irradiation and a 2.8-fold increased risk of ipsilateral lung cancer after postmastectomy irradiation involving chest wall and regional nodes) were found in an analysis of NSABP trial results.[199] However, in both studies[199,239] relatively few lung cancers had occurred 10 or more years after postlumpectomy radiation therapy, so that longer follow-up of patients treated in this way is needed. The AER of lung cancer after postmastectomy irradiation as estimated from these studies is approximately five excess lung cancers per 10,000 women per year, beginning 10 years after radiotherapy.[239] With current techniques for postmastectomy radiotherapy, both the volume of lung irradiated and the absorbed dose in the lung are reduced compared to the techniques used in the studies described earlier. Because lung cancer risk increases with radiation dose,[21,30] the risk of radiogenic lung cancer should be correspondingly lower. An important observation from several studies is that smokers appear to be at greater risk of radiation-associated lung cancer than nonsmokers.[201,238,241]

Radiotherapy for breast cancer is also associated with increased risk of soft tissue sarcoma,[205] and heightened concern has been expressed with regard to increased risk of angiosarcomas in the irradiated conserved breast.[207] Based on

135 soft tissue sarcomas identified in 194,798 women in the SEER database, Huang and Mackillop[205] reported a 16-fold increased risk (95% CI, 6.6 to 38.0) of angiosarcoma (based on 27 cases) and a twofold increased risk (95% CI, 1.4 to 3.3) of other sarcomas in breast cancer patients who had received radiation therapy, compared to those who had not. Because sarcomas are rare in the population, the corresponding AERs from radiation were rather low—0.75 and 0.73 excess cases per 10,000 women-years for angiosarcomas and other sarcomas, respectively. A very high risk was found for angiosarcomas in the breast or chest wall (RR, 59; 95% CI, 7.6 to 465, for irradiated patients compared to those not treated with radiation). Radiation was also associated with increased risk of angiosarcoma in the ipsilateral arm (RR, 8.3). The risk of angiosarcoma was already increased in the 2- to 5-year interval after radiation, reached its peak in the 5- to 10-year follow-up interval, and decreased thereafter.[205] In a nationwide case-control study in Sweden[206] involving 116 women with soft tissue sarcoma after a diagnosis of breast cancer between 1958 and 1992, it was found that risk of sarcomas other than angiosarcoma increased with amount of radiation, but stabilized at high doses. The study included 40 angiosarcomas (located mostly in the ipsilateral arm, with only two cases in conserved breasts). The risk of angiosarcoma was 9.5-fold increased in women with lymphedema of the arm, but radiotherapy was not a risk factor.

In conclusion, only part of the elevated risk of second malignancies after breast cancer is due to treatment. The intrinsically increased risk of developing a contralateral tumor is unlikely to be meaningfully affected by current radiotherapy for the initial breast cancer, whereas tamoxifen therapy reduces the risk of contralateral disease. Standard dose-intensity CMF treatment is associated with a low excess risk of leukemia, whereas conventional FAC treatment is associated with a slightly higher risk. Leukemia risk appears to increase with greater dose intensity of cyclophosphamide, and radiotherapy adds to this risk. Therefore, it is important to closely monitor leukemia risk associated with new dose-intensive chemotherapy regimens. Although tamoxifen use causes a moderate increase in endometrial cancer risk, the proven clinical benefit of this drug in controlling breast cancer[209] far outweighs the excess morbidity and mortality due to endometrial cancer. Clinicians should be alert to signs and symptoms in women taking tamoxifen, and long-term users should be advised to seek prompt gynecologic evaluation on the development of symptoms. The effectiveness of screening for endometrial cancer has not been demonstrated. Consequently, outside of research settings there is no basis for regular gynecologic examinations for asymptomatic patients taking tamoxifen.[242] The risk of lung cancer is approximately twofold increased after postmastectomy radiotherapy but not after postlumpectomy radiotherapy. There is ample reason to advise breast cancer patients to stop smoking when they receive radiation treatment.

PEDIATRIC MALIGNANCIES

Survival rates for children with cancer have improved substantially over the past two decades. Consequently, a rapidly growing young population is at lifelong risk for the late effects of cancer treatment. The overall pattern of second cancer risk in the population of childhood cancer survivors has been described in several large studies.[48,61,243,244] In 2001 Neglia and

colleagues[61] reported results from the Childhood Cancer Survivor Study (CCSS) cohort, which consists of 13,581 5-year survivors of childhood and adolescent cancer (diagnosed before age 21 years in the period 1970 to 1986). At a median follow-up time of 15 years from childhood cancer diagnosis, the risk of developing a second malignancy was 6.4-fold increased compared with the risk in the general population (95% CI, 5.7 to 7.1). The cumulative risk was 3.2% at 20 years, and approximately 19 excess malignancies occurred per 10,000 patients per year. In a cohort of 4400 three-year survivors of childhood cancers other than leukemia (age at diagnosis younger than 17 years) treated in eight centers in France and the United Kingdom,[48] the risk of second solid malignancies was 9.2-fold increased compared to the risk in the general population (95% CI, 7.6 to 11.0), and the AER was identical to the results in the CCSS (19 excess cases per 10,000 patients per year). The 30-year cumulative risk was 7.7% (95% CI, 5.0% to 8.2%). Olsen and collaborators[243] observed a 3.6-fold increased risk of second malignancy (95% CI, 3.1 to 4.1) in 30,880 children (age at diagnosis younger than 20 years) diagnosed with cancer and reported to the population-based cancer registries of five Nordic countries between 1943 and 1987. The cumulative risk of developing a second tumor within 28 years was 3.5%. The range in second cancer risks reported for various cohorts may be related to a population-based[243] versus hospital-based approach,[61] which may reflect treatment variation and differences between patient groups with respect to the upper age limit used for the diagnosis of childhood cancer, calendar years of diagnosis, and length and completeness of follow-up. For example, in the Nordic cohort, the overall risk of developing second cancer increased from a 2.6-fold excess in children diagnosed before 1960 to a 6.9-fold excess in children diagnosed in 1975 or later. Studies of 5-year survivors[61] likely underestimate the risk of second leukemia. A limitation of the very large and otherwise well-conducted CCSS is that second cancer risk could not be evaluated in 30% of the original cohort, due to either loss to follow-up or refusal to participate.

In all studies, the largest RRs were found for second primary bone tumors (19- and 73-fold increased risks in the CCSS[61] and French-British cohort, respectively).[48] High RRs (more than five-fold) were also observed for soft tissue sarcoma, leukemia, and cancers of the brain, thyroid, and breast (Table 54.7-8). Retinoblastoma is the initial malignancy that has been consistently associated with the largest risk of subsequent tumors,[48,243,244] although HD and sarcoma are also followed by large relative and AERs of second malignancy.[48,61] However, as shown in Table 54.7-8, all childhood cancer diagnoses are associated with an increased risk of second malignancy.[48,61]

Only a portion of the excess second cancer risk in survivors of childhood cancer is related to treatment. Retinoblastoma is the prototype of a malignancy in which genetic factors are responsible for a substantial proportion of subsequent cancers. Familial retinoblastoma is caused by inherited mutations of the RB1 tumor suppressor gene, which has been localized to chromosome region 13q14.[245,246] Approximately 80% of hereditary retinoblastoma patients have bilateral disease. In a long-term follow-up study of 1604 one-year survivors of retinoblastoma diagnosed between 1914 and 1984 (median follow-up, 20 years), the incidence of second cancers as well as risk factors for second malignancy was evaluated.[67] Overall, the risk of second malignancy was increased 17-fold compared to the expec-

TABLE 54.7-8. Comparison of Risk Indices for Second and Subsequent Malignant Neoplasms by Childhood Cancer Diagnosis in the Childhood Cancer Survivor Study Cohort[a]

	Second Malignant Neoplasms		
Childhood Cancer Diagnosis	RR (95% CI)	Cumulative Incidence 20 Y (%)	AER
All diagnoses	6.38 (5.69–7.13)	3.18	18.8
Hodgkin's disease	9.70 (8.05–11.59)	7.63	51.3
Soft tissue sarcoma	7.03 (4.92–9.73)	3.98	23.3
Neuroblastoma	6.59 (3.28–11.79)	1.87	9.5
Kidney tumor	6.03 (3.37–9.95)	1.62	10.1
Leukemia	5.66 (4.37–7.22)	2.05	12.0
Bone cancer	4.50 (2.96–6.55)	3.28	17.9
Central nervous system tumor	4.44 (2.88–6.56)	2.14	11.3
Non-Hodgkin's lymphoma	3.21 (1.76–5.39)	1.87	8.9

AER, absolute excess risk (observed cases minus expected cases per 10,000 patients per year); CI, confidence interval; RR, relative risk (ratio of observed cases to expected cases).
(Adapted from ref. 61.)

tation in the general population. The excess risk was restricted to the 961 patients with hereditary retinoblastoma (RR, 30; 95% CI, 26 to 47), with strongly increased RRs for cancers of the bone (RR, 446), soft tissue (RR, 103), nasal cavities (RR, >100), and brain (RR, 14), and for melanoma (RR, 51). No significantly increased risk of second malignancy was observed among 643 patients with nonhereditary retinoblastoma (RR, 1.6; 95% CI, 0.7 to 3.1). Fifty years after a retinoblastoma diagnosis, the cumulative risk of second primary cancer was 51.0% (±6.2%) in hereditary cases and only 5.0% (±3.0%) in nonhereditary cases. As shown in Figure 54.7-3, radiotherapy significantly increased the risk of second cancers in patients with hereditary retinoblastoma (50-year cumulative risk of 58%, vs. 27% in nonirradiated patients). Radiotherapy did not significantly affect risk in patients with nonhereditary retinoblastoma.[67] In a case-control investigation that included 52 patients with bone sarcoma, 31 with soft tissue sarcoma, and 89 controls without sarcoma, Wong and associates[67] also collected individual radiation dosimetry data. For all sarcomas combined, risk was significantly elevated at all dose levels, even at 5.0 to 9.9 Gy, and a significant increase in risk was observed with increasing radiation dose to the site of tumor (RR of 11 for doses of 60 Gy or more compared with doses of 0 to 4.9 Gy). For the first time in humans, a radiation dose-response relationship was also demonstrated for soft tissue sarcoma, with a 12-fold risk increase at doses of 60 Gy or higher. Osteosarcomas and soft tissue sarcomas that develop after hereditary retinoblastoma harbor RB1 mutations similar to those found in retinoblastoma.[247,248] Radiation is thus likely to cause somatic mutations needed to produce sarcomas in carriers of germline RB1 mutations.

Wilms' tumor is another example of an initial malignancy in which genetic predisposition contributes to the excess risk of second cancers.[249] The National Wilms' Tumor Study Group reported the second malignancy experience of 5278 patients followed for an average of 7.5 years.[101] Forty-three second malignancies were observed, with an overall RR of 8.4 (95% CI, 6.1 to 11.4). The 15- and 20-year cumulative risks of developing a second tumor were 1.6% and 3.8%, respectively. Significant excesses were observed for leukemia (RR, 7.0), lymphoma (RR, 9.0), osteosarcoma (RR, 19), soft tissue sarcoma (RR, 22), and

hepatocellular carcinoma (RR, 56)[101] (N. E. Breslow, *written communication*, April 1996). Among patients not treated with radiation or doxorubicin, the risk of second malignancy was increased threefold, which reflected genetic predisposition.[101] Each 10 Gy of abdominal irradiation was found to increase second malignancy risk by 43% in the absence of doxorubicin therapy and by 78% in its presence. Treatment with both doxorubicin and more than 35 Gy of abdominal irradiation was associated with an RR of 36 (95% CI, 16 to 72).[101] The authors hypothesized that doxorubicin might inhibit the repair of radiation-induced damage, perhaps through an effect on DNA topoisomerase II. Because the small number of second malignancies precluded an analysis by site, it is unclear whether these results apply equally for leukemia, sarcoma, and other tumors.

ALL, the most common malignancy in childhood, is also associated with an increased risk of subsequent cancer. In a series of 9720 childhood ALL patients treated in trials of the

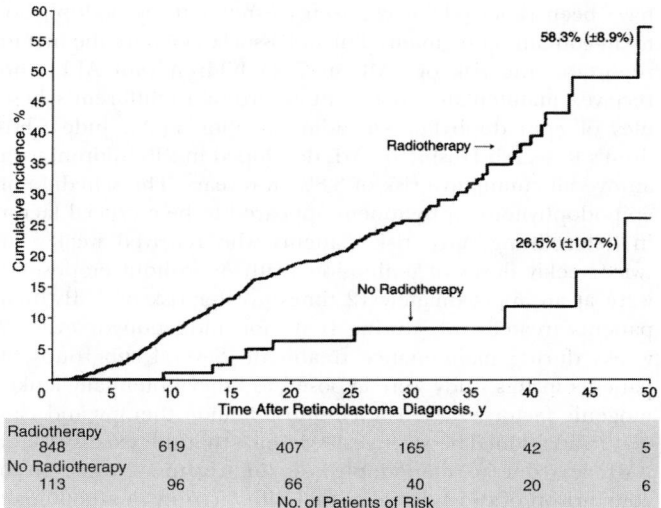

FIGURE 54.7-3. Cumulative incidence (± standard error) of second cancers after diagnosis of retinoblastoma in 961 patients with hereditary disease, by radiation treatment. (From ref. 67, with permission.)

U.S. Children's Cancer Group between 1972 and 1988, the risk of developing a second malignancy was increased 6.9-fold compared with the risk in the general population.[250] The associated 10- and 15-year cumulative risks were 1.5% and 2.5%, respectively. In a multicenter German study including 5006 ALL patients treated in the period 1979 to 1995, the RR for all second cancers was 14, with cumulative risks of 1.5% and 3.3% at 10 and 15 years, respectively, since the completion of initial treatment.[251] In both studies, the largest excess was observed for central nervous system tumors, with RRs of 22[250] and 19[251] in the two studies. Risk of second cancer was clearly associated with cranial radiation dose.[251] Most brain tumors were high-grade astrocytomas or glioblastomas, and all occurred in children who had previously received radiotherapy, mostly cranial irradiation with doses ranging from 12 to 24 Gy. A study of 1612 patients with ALL at St. Jude Children's Research Hospital, with long-term follow-up data (median follow-up, 16 years), demonstrated an excess of high-grade gliomas during the first decade of follow-up, whereas an increased risk of low-grade brain tumors was observed at later follow-up intervals.[252] The risk of second brain tumor increased significantly with increasing cranial radiation dose, with 20-year cumulative risks of 1.0%, 1.7%, and 3.2% for patients who received radiation doses of 10 to 21 Gy, 21 to 30 Gy, and more than 30 Gy, respectively. In all studies,[250–252] risk of central nervous system tumors was significantly higher in children 5 years of age or younger at first treatment.

Over the past decade, prophylactic cranial radiotherapy has been largely replaced by intrathecal methotrexate therapy. The number of intrathecal methotrexate administrations has not been found to be related to the risk of brain tumors.[252] Bhatia and colleagues[253] assessed the risk of second malignancy in a large cohort of ALL survivors (n = 8831) treated between 1983 and 1995 by the Children's Cancer Group with contemporary risk-based protocols (intensive chemotherapy, conservative use of radiation). The RR of second cancer was increased 7.2-fold, which translated into a rather low cumulative risk of 1.2% at 10 years.

Several very large studies of ALL survivors have reported negligible risks of AML after chemotherapy regimens that contain cyclophosphamide or anthracyclines or both (less than 0.5% at 10 years).[250,251,253,254] In contrast, very high risks of AML have been reported for children treated with epipodophyllotoxin-containing regimens. Pui and associates[93] were the first to report on the risk of AML in 734 children with ALL who received maintenance treatment according to different schedules of epipodophyllotoxin administration at St. Jude Children's Research Hospital. AML developed in 21 children, with an overall cumulative risk of 3.8% at 6 years. The schedule of epipodophyllotoxin treatment appeared to be a crucial factor in determining AML risk. Patients who received weekly or twice-weekly doses of teniposide (with or without etoposide) were at an approximately 12 times greater risk of AML than patients treated only during remission induction or every 2 weeks during maintenance treatment. Several subgroups of patients in this study were exposed to other potentially leukemogenic factors, such as cyclophosphamide therapy and cranial irradiation. The strongest evidence that the excess risk of AML was due to epipodophyllotoxin treatment came from comparison of two subgroups that differed only in schedule of administration. Among 84 patients who received epipodophyllotoxins weekly, the risk of AML was clearly and significantly higher (12.4% at 6 years) than the risk in 148 patients who

received the agents every other week (1.6% at 6 years; $P = .01$). Compelling evidence for a causal link between epipodophyllotoxin therapy for ALL and the development of AML was also provided by Winick and associates.[89,255]

Elevated risk of AML has also been reported after a number of other childhood malignancies, especially lymphomas.[61,102,122,243] Three case-control studies addressed the effects of radiation dose and amount of chemotherapy on the risk of AML in children treated for various malignancies.[52,102,104] A significant dose-response relationship between total dose of alkylating agents and AML risk was observed in the two early studies.[52,102] The French study, which included 61 leukemia cases diagnosed in the late 1990s,[104] found no association with alkylating agents, probably because strongly leukemogenic agents such as mechlorethamine and melphalan were infrequently used. The Late Effects Study Group[52] and the French study[104] found no association between leukemia risk and radiation dose to active bone marrow. In contrast, using similar methods of estimating bone marrow dose, Hawkins and colleagues[102] observed a highly significant trend, with an approximately 20-fold increased risk for patients receiving 15 Gy or more of radiation (compared to patients not treated with radiotherapy). These discrepant results may be explained by differences between the studies in the pattern of first cancers and in therapeutic practices. Possibly, patients in the British study received lower radiation doses to larger volumes of bone marrow, which, for a specified dose, might result in less cell killing and a greater susceptibility to leukemogenic transformation.[102]

In two case-control studies[102,104] and in the CCSS,[61] leukemia risk strongly increased with greater cumulative doses of epipodophyllotoxins. In the French study[104] leukemia risk was also associated with the cumulative dose of anthracyclines. Patients who had received 1.2 to 6.0 g/m² of epipodophyllotoxins or more than 170 mg/m² of anthracyclines had a sevenfold higher risk (95% CI, 2.6 to 19.0) compared with patients who received lower doses of these drugs or none. In patients who had received more than 6 g/m² of epipodophyllotoxins, leukemia risk was multiplied by 197 (95% CI, 19 to 2058). Schedules of administration were different from the ones used by Pui et al.[93] High risks were observed after continuous (21 consecutive days out of 28) or semicontinuous etoposide therapy, whereas low risks were observed after sequential etoposide therapy (courses lasting 3 to 5 consecutive days given every 3 to 4 weeks).[104] Unfortunately, however, the effects of cumulative dose could not be distinguished from the influence of schedule of administration because these factors were strongly correlated. It is remarkable that the British study[102] found a steep epipodophyllotoxin-associated increase in AML risk at much lower cumulative doses (only 2% of controls had more than 1.2 g/m²) than those used at St. Jude Children's Research Hospital[93] (cumulative doses of 9 g/m² or more) and in the French study.[104]

Smith and colleagues[103] reported results for patients included in trials in the United States that used epipodophyllotoxins at low (less than 1.5 g/m²), moderate (1.5 to 2.9 g/m²), or higher (3 g/m² or more) cumulative etoposide doses. The 6-year cumulative risks for AML (including MDS) in the low, moderate, and higher cumulative dose groups were 3.3%, 0.7%, and 2.2%, respectively. This result does not appear to provide support for a cumulative dose effect for the leukemogenic activity of the epipodophyllotoxins, at least not within the cumulative dose range and the treatment schedules used (cumulative etoposide dose of 5.0 g/m² or less, on daily × 2 to 5 schedules).

TABLE 54.7-9. Risk of Solid Malignancy in 4400 Three-Year Survivors of Childhood Cancer in France and the United Kingdom, According to Overall Treatment and Follow-Up Time

Treatment	Second Solid Malignancies		
	Observed/ Expected Cases	RR (95% CI)	AER per 10,000 Patient-Years
NO RT, NO CT	3/2.0	2 (0.5–4.0)	3
RT, NO CT	31/5.6	6 (4–8)	15
3–9 y	8/0.71	11 (5–21)	11
10–19 y	11/1.59	7 (4–12)	15
20–29 y	9/1.96	5 (2–8)	23
CT, NO RT	8/1.1	8 (3–14)	10
3–9 y	4/0.54	7 (2–17)	7
10–19 y	3/0.33	9 (2–24)	15
20–29 y	1/0.15	7 (0.4–29)	28
RT AND CT	71/3.8	19 (15–24)	30
3–9 y	31/1.32	23 (16–33)	24
10–19 y	31/1.71	19 (12–25)	36
20–29 y	9/0.70	13 (6–23)	54

AER, absolute excess risk (observed cases minus expected cases per 10,000 patients per year); CI, confidence interval; CT, chemotherapy; RR, relative risk (ratio of observed cases to expected cases); RT, radiotherapy. (Adapted from ref. 48.)

However, a limitation of this study is that the three treatment strata also varied with respect to the administration of radiotherapy and other cytotoxic drugs, primary tumor, and patient age, differences that were not accounted for in the analysis.[89] In view of several inconsistencies between the various studies and difficulties in disentangling the effects of cumulative dose, frequency of administration, and dose intensity, final conclusions regarding the leukemogenicity of different epipodophyllotoxin-based regimens cannot yet be drawn.

Two large studies have provided evidence that chemotherapy adds to the increased risk of solid malignancy from radiation treatment.[48,256] In the French-British study, which was based on 113 solid second malignancies in 4400 survivors, risk of solid malignancy was also significantly increased after chemotherapy alone (Table 54.7-9).[48] The RRs associated with radiotherapy alone, chemotherapy alone, and a combination of radiation and chemotherapy, were 6, 8, and 19, respectively, compared to the risk in the general population; there was no significant excess for survivors treated with either radiotherapy or chemotherapy (see Table 54.7-9).[48] A case-control study in the Nordic countries examined risk factors for 234 second malignancies identified in a very large population-based cohort and found that chemotherapy significantly potentiated the effect of radiotherapy. Although chemotherapy alone did not increase the risk, there was substantial interaction between chemotherapy and high-dose local irradiation (more than 30 Gy to the second malignancy site) and between chemotherapy and low-dose irradiation (less than 30 Gy to second malignancy site). Fewer than 10% of the second malignancies in this study were leukemias, which renders it unlikely that the findings can be attributed to associations between chemotherapy and leukemia. The CCSS also reported independent effects of chemotherapy on the risk of second malignancy overall, but did not provide information on radiation exposure.[61]

Hawkins and associates[60] addressed the quantitative relationship between radiation dose, alkylating agent therapy, and risk of bone sarcoma in a case-control study involving a British cohort of 13,175 three-year survivors of childhood cancer. Risk of bone cancer was strongly increased in all follow-up intervals beyond 3 years, with no apparent trend toward increasing or decreasing RRs up to 25 years after diagnosis of primary cancer. As in an earlier study,[37] no increased risk was observed for radiation doses to the site of the bone tumor of less than 10 Gy. For doses above 10 Gy, risk for bone sarcoma rose sharply with increasing radiation dose, with a RR of 93 for patients who received 30 to 50 Gy compared to those not treated with radiation. At higher radiation doses, however, the risk appeared to decline somewhat (Table 54.7-10). Such a downturn in RR at very high doses was also observed in a smaller case-control study of osteosarcoma after childhood cancer[257] but was not found in the large case-control investigation nested in the Late Effects Study Group cohort.[37] In the latter study, Tucker and colleagues[37] showed that the pattern of risk increase in relation to radiation dose was very similar in patients treated for retinoblastoma and in those treated for other initial malignancies. Thus, although patients with retinoblastoma have a higher intrinsic risk for sarcoma development, their RRs after radiation treatment do not appear to differ from those of patients with other childhood cancers. Importantly, the study by Hawkins and colleagues also showed that the RR of bone sarcoma increases with increasing cumulative exposure to alkylating agents, even after adjustment for radiotherapy (see Table 54.7-10). It is clear, however, that the effect of radiotherapy on sarcoma risk is stronger than that of chemotherapy. An association between chemotherapy and risk of bone sarcoma has also been observed in other studies.[37,48,61,257] An effect of alkylating chemotherapy on sarcoma risk in the absence of radiotherapy was found in two studies.[37,48] Comparative studies of children and adults irradiated for HD have shown that children have a much higher RR of developing bone sarcomas than adults, probably due to greater radiosensitivity of growing bone.[12,48,122]

The risk of thyroid cancer after radiotherapy for childhood malignancies was assessed in the Late Effects Study Group cohort.[58] High RRs compared with general population rates were observed for thyroid malignancies after treatment of neuroblastoma (RR, 350), Wilms' tumor (RR, 132), and HD (RR, 67). The RR increased significantly with time since treatment throughout the observation period (more than 20 years). In a case-control study, radiation dose to the thyroid was estimated for 23 thyroid cancer cases and 89 matched controls. Radiation doses of 2 Gy or more were associated with a 13-fold risk compared with lower doses ($P < .05$). Because all patients with thyroid cancer had been exposed to at least 1 Gy of radiation to the thyroid, the risk associated with doses less than 2 Gy could not be reliably determined in this study. However, the investigators estimated that the risk associated with doses of 2 Gy or more was approximately 130-fold increased compared with the risk in nonirradiated patients.[58] Unexpectedly, the dose-response relationship was more or less flat at radiation doses above 2 Gy; even at doses as high as 60 Gy, no decrease in thyroid cancer risk was observed. A pooled analysis of seven large studies of thyroid cancer after various radiation exposures demonstrated that the risk decreases significantly with increasing age at exposure and is highest for persons with radiation exposure before age 5 years.[59]

In conclusion, survivors of childhood cancer are at substantially elevated risk to develop new malignancies. The magnitude

TABLE 54.7-10. A Case-Control Study of Second Primary Bone Cancer in Relation to Radiation Dose and Cumulative Exposure to Alkylating Agents

| Radiation Dose (cGy) | Number of Patients | | Relative Risk (95% CI) Adjusted for Alkylating Agent Exposure | P Value |
	Cases (n = 59)	Controls (n = 220)		
0	10	61	1.0	—
1–999	13	79	0.7 (0.2–2.2)	.537
1000–2999	7	15	12.4 (0.9–163.3)	.055
3000–4999	15	7	93.4 (6.8–1285.4)	<.001
≥5000	5	6	64.7 (3.8–1103.4)	.004
Incomplete information	9	52	—	—
Test for linear trend	—	—	—	<.001

| Total Cumulative Exposure to Alkylating Agents (mg/m²) | Number of Patients | | Relative Risk (95% CI) Adjusted for Radiation Exposure | P Value |
	Cases (n = 59)	Controls (n = 220)		
0	37	164	1.0	—
1–9999	6	21	1.3 (0.3–6.0)	.698
10,000–19,999	7	20	3.0 (0.4–21.7)	.278
≥20,000	7	8	3.3 (0.8–13.8)	.107
Incomplete information	2	7	—	—
Test for linear trend	—	—	—	.080

CI, confidence interval.
(Adapted from ref. 60, with permission.)

of this risk depends on the type of the initial malignancy, because some childhood cancers, such as bilateral retinoblastoma, carry a high intrinsic risk for second cancer occurrence. Long-term survival after various types of childhood cancer has become possible through therapies introduced from the early 1970s onward. Consequently, the growing population of cured patients is just beginning to enter the ages at which adult cancers typically occur, so the full spectrum of second malignancies has not yet been encountered. It is therefore imperative that survivors of childhood cancer be carefully monitored to assess the long-term risks of various types of second cancers. Bone sarcoma has consistently been identified as the second malignancy for which the excess risk is highest. Of much interest is the potential interaction between genetic susceptibility and treatment in second cancer development. The leukemogenic potential of epipodophyllotoxin-containing regimens that vary in cumulative dose and schedule of administration should continue to be rigorously assessed, as holds true for other new chemotherapy regimens. Radiotherapy is the main risk factor for second solid tumors, although chemotherapy has been shown to add substantially to the increased risk from radiation treatment. Future studies should investigate which solid malignancies occur in excess after chemotherapy and what cytostatic drugs are involved in their etiology. Second cancers among survivors of childhood cancer are associated with a poor prognosis.[93,252] Hence, there is a pressing need to develop therapeutic strategies with less oncogenic potential, without compromising the excellent cure rates that have been achieved.

CONCLUSION

The results described in this chapter have multiple clinical implications. Knowledge of risk factors for second malignancy has made it possible to identify patient groups at high risk of devel-

oping second cancers due to treatments that they received in the past. Whenever effective screening methods are available, these should be implemented in the patients' follow-up program to improve their survival after diagnosis of second malignancy. In some cases, preventive strategies (e.g., smoking cessation) may reduce substantially the risk of developing a treatment-related cancer. The issue of treatment-induced second cancers must always be viewed in relation to the sometimes dramatic improvement in survival rates for patients with various malignancies. The risks associated with various treatments should be weighed carefully against the consequences of not using such treatments. Clinical research should focus on the development of therapeutic regimens with less carcinogenic potential. However, the arbitrary alteration of a successful therapy to mitigate second cancer risk is unwarranted. It is of the utmost importance that changes in therapy to reduce the risk of late complications be made only in the context of carefully designed clinical trials that evaluate whether the overall efficacy of treatment is maintained.

For many cancer treatments, the long-term effects on second malignancy risk are not yet known. In addition, new therapies are being introduced continuously, and the associated risks of late sequelae need to be evaluated. Whenever possible, future studies of second cancer risk should incorporate investigations at the molecular level. Results of these laboratory analyses may clarify the influence of genetic susceptibility on treatment-related risk and contribute importantly to the elucidation of mechanisms underlying drug- and radiation-induced carcinogenesis.

REFERENCES

1. Aleman BM, van den Belt-Dusebout AW, Klokman WJ, et al. Long-term cause-specific mortality of patients treated for Hodgkin's disease. *J Clin Oncol* 2003;21(18):3431.
2. Kaldor JM, Day NE, Shiboski S. Epidemiological studies of anticancer drug carcinogenicity. *IARC Sci Publ* 1986;78:189.

3. Makuch R, Simon R. Recommendations for the analysis of the effect of treatment on the development of second malignancies. *Cancer* 1979;44:250.

4. Kaplan EL, Meier P. Non-parametric estimation from incomplete observations. *J Am Stat Assoc* 1958;53:457.

5. Darrington DL, Vose JM, Anderson JR, et al. Incidence and characterization of secondary myelodysplastic syndrome and acute myelogenous leukemia following high-dose chemoradiotherapy and autologous stem-cell transplantation for lymphoid malignancies. *J Clin Oncol* 1994;12:2527.

6. Pepe MS, Mori M. Kaplan-Meier, marginal or conditional probability curves in summarizing competing risks failure time data? *Stat Med* 1993;12:737.

7. Boice JD Jr, Day NE, Andersen A, et al. Second cancers following radiation treatment for cervical cancer. An international collaboration among cancer registries. *J Natl Cancer Inst* 1985;74:955.

8. Kaldor JM, Day NE, Clarke EA, et al. Leukemia following Hodgkin's disease [see comments]. *N Engl J Med* 1990;322:7.

9. Storm HH, Prener A. Second cancer following lymphatic and hematopoietic cancers in Denmark, 1943–80. *Natl Cancer Inst Monogr* 1985;68:389.

10. Greene MH. Is cisplatin a human carcinogen? *J Natl Cancer Inst* 1992;84:306.

11. Ng AK, Bernardo MV, Weller E, Backstrand K, et al. Second malignancy after Hodgkin disease treated with radiation therapy with or without chemotherapy: long-term risks and risk factors. *Blood* 2002;100(6):1989.

12. Tucker MA, Coleman CN, Cox RS, Varghese A, Rosenberg SA. Risk of second cancers after treatment for Hodgkin's disease. *N Engl J Med* 1988;318:76.

13. van Leeuwen FE, Klokman WJ, Veer MB, et al. Long-term risk of second malignancy in survivors of Hodgkin's disease treated during adolescence or young adulthood. *J Clin Oncol* 2000;18(3):487.

14. van Leeuwen FE, Klokman WJ, Hagenbeek A, et al. Second cancer risk following Hodgkin's disease: a 20-year follow-up study. *J Clin Oncol* 1994;12:312.

15. Swerdlow AJ, Barber JA, Hudson GV, et al. Risk of second malignancy after Hodgkin's disease in a collaborative British cohort: the relation to age at treatment. *J Clin Oncol* 2000;18(3):498.

16. Boice JD Jr, Blettner M, Kleinerman RA, et al. Radiation dose and leukemia risk in patients treated for cancer of the cervix. *J Natl Cancer Inst* 1987;79:1295.

17. Boice JD Jr, Harvey EB, Blettner M, Stovall M, Flannery JT. Cancer in the contralateral breast after radiotherapy for breast cancer. *N Engl J Med* 1992;326(12):781.

18. Curtis RE, Boice JD Jr, Stovall M, et al. Risk of leukemia after chemotherapy and radiation treatment for breast cancer [see comments]. *N Engl J Med* 1992;326:1745.

19. Kaldor JM, Day NE, Pettersson F, et al. Leukemia following chemotherapy for ovarian cancer [see comments]. *N Engl J Med* 1990;322:1.

20. Travis LB, Curtis RE, Glimelius B, et al. Bladder and kidney cancer following cyclophosphamide therapy for non-Hodgkin's lymphoma. *J Natl Cancer Inst* 1995;87:524.

21. Travis LB, Gospodarowicz M, Curtis RE, et al. Lung cancer following chemotherapy and radiotherapy for Hodgkin's disease. *J Natl Cancer Inst* 2002;94(3):182.

22. van Leeuwen FE, Klokman WJ, Stovall M, et al. Roles of radiation dose, chemotherapy, and hormonal factors in breast cancer following Hodgkin's disease. *J Natl Cancer Inst* 2003;95(13):971.

23. Travis LB, Holowaty EJ, Bergfeldt K, et al. Risk of leukemia after platinum-based chemotherapy for ovarian cancer. *N Engl J Med* 1999;340(5):351.

24. Martland HS. The occurrence of malignancy in radioactive persons: a general review of data gathered in the study of the radium dial painters, with special reference to the occurrence of osteogenic sarcoma and the interrelationship of certain blood diseases. *Am J Cancer* 1931;15:2435.

25. Upton AC. Physical carcinogenesis: radiation, history and sources. In: Becker FF, ed. *Cancer: a comprehensive treatise*. New York: Plenum Press, 1975:387.

26. Boice JD Jr, Land CE, Preston DL. Ionizing radiation. In: Schottenfeld D, Fraumeni JF Jr, eds. *Cancer epidemiology and prevention*. New York: Oxford University Press, 1996:319.

27. United Nations Scientific Committee on the Effects of Atomic Radiation (UNSCEAR). UNSCEAR 2000 report to General Assembly, with scientific annexes, sources and effects of ionizing radiation. New York: United Nations, 2000.

28. Ron E. Ionizing radiation and cancer risk: evidence from epidemiology. *Pediatr Radiol* 2002;32(4):232.

29. Preston DL, Kusumi S, Tomonaga M, et al. Cancer incidence in atomic bomb survivors. Part III. Leukemia, lymphoma and multiple myeloma, 1950–1987 [published erratum appears in *Radiat Res* 1994;139(1):129]. *Radiat Res* 1994;137:S68.

30. Thompson DE, Mabuchi K, Ron E, et al. Cancer incidence in atomic bomb survivors. Part II. Solid tumors, 1958–1987. *Radiat Res* 1994;137[Suppl 2]:S17.

31. Tokunaga M, Land CE, Tokuoka S, et al. Incidence of female breast cancer among atomic bomb survivors, 1950–1985. *Radiat Res* 1994;138:209.

32. Smith PG, Doll R. Mortality from cancer and all causes among British radiologists. *Br J Radiol* 1981;54:187.

33. Wang JX, Inskip PD, Boice JD Jr, et al. Cancer incidence among medical diagnostic X-ray workers in China, 1950 to 1985. *Int J Cancer* 1990;45:889.

34. Boice JD Jr, Preston D, Davis FG, Monson RR. Frequent chest X-ray fluoroscopy and breast cancer incidence among tuberculosis patients in Massachusetts. *Radiat Res* 1991;125(2):214.

35. Miller AB, Howe GR, Sherman GJ, et al. Mortality from breast cancer after irradiation during fluoroscopic examinations in patients being treated for tuberculosis. *N Engl J Med* 1989;321:1285.

36. Hancock SL, Tucker MA, Hoppe RT. Breast cancer after treatment of Hodgkin's disease. *J Natl Cancer Inst* 1993;85(1):25.

37. Tucker MA, D'Angio GJ, Boice JD Jr, et al. Bone sarcomas linked to radiotherapy and chemotherapy in children. *N Engl J Med* 1987;317:588.

38. Travis LB, Hill DA, Dores GM, et al. Breast cancer following radiotherapy and chemotherapy among young women with Hodgkin disease. *JAMA* 2003;290(4):465.

39. Lundell M, Mattsson A, Karlsson P, et al. Breast cancer risk after radiotherapy in infancy: a pooled analysis of two Swedish cohorts of 17,202 infants. *Radiat Res* 1999;151(5):626.

40. Weiss HA, Darby SC, Doll R. Cancer mortality following X-ray treatment for ankylosing spondylitis. *Int J Cancer* 1994;59:327.

41. Curtis RE, Boice JD Jr, Stovall M, et al. Relationship of leukemia risk to radiation dose following cancer of the uterine corpus. *J Natl Cancer Inst* 1994;86:1315.

42. Boice JD Jr. Carcinogenesis—a synopsis of human experience with external exposure in medicine. *Health Phys* 1988;55:621.

43. Little MP, Weiss HA, Boice JD Jr, et al. Risks of leukemia in Japanese atomic bomb survivors, in women treated for cervical cancer, and in patients treated for ankylosing spondylitis. *Radiat Res* 1999;152(3):280.

44. Boice JD Jr, Engholm G, Kleinerman RA, et al. Radiation dose and second cancer risk in patients treated for cancer of the cervix. *Radiat Res* 1988;116:3.

45. Dores GM, Metayer C, Curtis RE, et al. Second malignant neoplasms among long-term survivors of Hodgkin's disease: a population-based evaluation over 25 years. *J Clin Oncol* 2002;20(16):3484.

46. Preston DL, Mattsson A, Holmberg E, et al. Radiation effects on breast cancer risk: a pooled analysis of eight cohorts. *Radiat Res* 2002;158(2):220.

47. Inskip PD, Monson RR, Wagoner JK, et al. Cancer mortality following radium treatment for uterine bleeding [published erratum appears in *Radiat Res* 1991;128(3):326]. *Radiat Res* 1990;123:331.

48. de Vathaire F, Hawkins M, Campbell S, et al. Second malignant neoplasms after a first cancer in childhood: temporal pattern of risk according to type of treatment. *Br J Cancer* 1999;79(11–12):1884.

49. Metayer C, Lynch CF, Clarke EA, et al. Second cancers among long-term survivors of Hodgkin's disease diagnosed in childhood and adolescence. *J Clin Oncol* 2000;18(12):2435.

50. Little MP, de Vathaire F, Charles MW, Hawkins MM, Muirhead CR. Variations with time and age in the risks of solid cancer incidence after radiation exposure in childhood. *Stat Med* 1998;17(12):1341.

51. Boice JD Jr, Preston D, Davis FG, Monson RR. Frequent chest X-ray fluoroscopy and breast cancer incidence among tuberculosis patients in Massachusetts. *Radiat Res* 1991;125:214.

52. Tucker MA, Meadows AT, Boice JD Jr, et al. Leukemia after therapy with alkylating agents for childhood cancer. *J Natl Cancer Inst* 1987;78:459.

53. Hancock SL, Tucker MA, Hoppe RT. Breast cancer after treatment of Hodgkin's disease. *J Natl Cancer Inst* 1993;85:25.

54. Hildreth NG, Shore RE, Dvoretsky PM. The risk of breast cancer after irradiation of the thymus in infancy. *N Engl J Med* 1989;321(19):1281.

55. Land CE, Hayakawa N, Machado SG, et al. A case-control interview study of breast cancer among Japanese A-bomb survivors. II. Interactions with radiation dose. *Cancer Causes Control* 1994;5:167.

56. Little MP, Boice JD Jr. Comparison of breast cancer incidence in the Massachusetts tuberculosis fluoroscopy cohort and in the Japanese atomic bomb survivors. *Radiat Res* 1999;151(2):218.

57. Gilbert ES, Stovall M, Gospodarowicz M, et al. Lung cancer after treatment for Hodgkin's disease: focus on radiation effects. *Radiat Res* 2003;159(2):161.

58. Tucker MA, Jones PH, Boice JD Jr, et al. Therapeutic radiation at a young age is linked to secondary thyroid cancer. The Late Effects Study Group. *Cancer Res* 1991;51:2885.

59. Ron E, Lubin JH, Shore RE, et al. Thyroid cancer after exposure to external radiation: a pooled analysis of seven studies. *Radiat Res* 1995;141:259.

60. Hawkins MM, Wilson LM, Burton HS, et al. Radiotherapy, alkylating agents, and risk of bone cancer after childhood cancer. *J Natl Cancer Inst* 1996;88(5):270.

61. Neglia JP, Friedman DL, Yasui Y, et al. Second malignant neoplasms in five-year survivors of childhood cancer: childhood cancer survivor study. *J Natl Cancer Inst* 2001;93(8):618.

62. Yao SX, Lubin JH, Qiao YL, et al. Exposure to radon progeny, tobacco use and lung cancer in a case-control study in southern China. *Radiat Res* 1994;138:326.

63. Moolgavkar SH, Luebeck EG, Krewski D, Zielinski JM. Radon, cigarette smoke, and lung cancer: a re-analysis of the Colorado Plateau uranium miners' data [see comments]. *Epidemiology* 1993;4:204.

64. National Research Council. Health risks of radon and other internally deposited alphaemitters. Washington, DC: National Academy Press, 1988.

65. van Leeuwen FE, Klokman WJ, Stovall M, et al. Roles of radiotherapy and smoking in lung cancer following Hodgkin's disease. *J Natl Cancer Inst* 1995;87:1530.

66. van Leeuwen FE. Second cancers. In: DeVita VT Jr, Hellman S, Rosenberg SA, eds. *Cancer: principles and practice of oncology*, 5th ed. Philadelphia: Lippincott Williams & Wilkins, 1997:2773.

67. Wong FL, Boice JD Jr, Abramson DH, et al. Cancer incidence after retinoblastoma. Radiation dose and sarcoma risk [see comments]. *JAMA* 1997;278(15):1262.

68. Kony SJ, de Vathaire F, Chompret A, et al. Radiation and genetic factors in the risk of second malignant neoplasms after a first cancer in childhood [see comments]. *Lancet* 1997;350(9071):91.

69. Nichols KE, Levitz S, Shannon KE, et al. Heterozygous germline ATM mutations do not contribute to radiation-associated malignancies after Hodgkin's disease. *J Clin Oncol* 1999;17(4):1259.

70. Easton DF. Cancer risks in A-T heterozygotes. *Int J Radiat Biol* 1994;66:S177.

71. Swift M, Morrell D, Massey RB, Chase CL. Incidence of cancer in 161 families affected by ataxia-telangiectasia [see comments]. *N Engl J Med* 1991;325:1831.

72. Broeks A, Russell NS, Floore AN, et al. Increased risk of breast cancer following irradiation for Hodgkin's disease is not a result of ATM germline mutations. *Int J Radiat Biol* 2000;76(5):693.

73. Kyle RA, Pierre RV, Bayrd ED. Multiple myeloma and acute myelomonocytic leukemia. *N Engl J Med* 1970;283:1121.

74. Smith MA, McCaffrey RP, Karp JE. The secondary leukemias: challenges and research directions. *J Natl Cancer Inst* 1996;88(7):407.

75. Hunger SP, Sklar J, Link MP. Acute lymphoblastic leukemia occurring as a second malignant neoplasm in childhood: report of three cases and review of the literature [see comments]. *J Clin Oncol* 1992;10(1):156.

76. Levine EG, Bloomfield CD. Leukemias and myelodysplastic syndromes secondary to drug, radiation, and environmental exposure. *Semin Oncol* 1992;19:47.

77. Whang-Peng J, Young RC, Lee EC. Cytogenetic studies in patients with secondary leukemia/dysmyelopoietic syndrome after different treatment modalities. *Blood* 1988;71(2):403.

78. Pedersen-Bjergaard J, Rowley JD. The balanced and the unbalanced chromosome aberrations of acute myeloid leukemia may develop in different ways and may contribute differently to malignant transformation. *Blood* 1994;83:2780.

79. Smith MA, Rubinstein L, Ungerleider RS. Therapy-related acute myeloid leukemia following treatment with epipodophyllotoxins: estimating the risks. *Med Pediatr Oncol* 1994;23:86.

80. Henry-Amar M. Second cancer after the treatment for Hodgkin's disease: a report from the International Database on Hodgkin's Disease. *Ann Oncol* 1992;3[Suppl 4]:117.

81. Travis LB, Curtis RE, Storm H, et al. Risk of second malignant neoplasms among long-term survivors of testicular cancer [see comments]. *J Natl Cancer Inst* 1997;89(19):1429.

82. Pedersen-Bjergaard J, Philip P, Larsen SO, Jensen G, Byrsting K. Chromosome aberrations and prognostic factors in therapy-related myelodysplasia and acute nonlymphocytic leukemia. *Blood* 1990;76:1083.

83. Josting A, Wiedenmann S, Franklin J, et al. Secondary myeloid leukemia and myelodysplastic syndromes in patients treated for Hodgkin's disease: a report from the German Hodgkin's Lymphoma Study Group. *J Clin Oncol* 2003;21(18):3440.

84. Neugut AI, Robinson E, Nieves J, Murray T, Tsai WY. Poor survival of treatment-related acute nonlymphocytic leukemia. *JAMA* 1990;264(8):1006.

85. van Leeuwen FE, Chorus AM, van den Belt-Dusebout AW, et al. Leukemia risk following Hodgkin's disease: relation to cumulative dose of alkylating agents, treatment with teniposide combinations, number of episodes of chemotherapy, and bone marrow damage. *J Clin Oncol* 1994;12:1063.

86. Overall evaluations of carcinogenicity: an updating of IARC Monographs volumes 1 to 42. *IARC Monogr Eval Carcinog Risks Hum Suppl* 1987;7:1.

87. Boivin JF, Hutchison GB, Zauber AG, et al. Incidence of second cancers in patients treated for Hodgkin's disease [see comments]. *J Natl Cancer Inst* 1995;87:732.

88. Smith RE, Bryant J, DeCillis A, Anderson S. Acute myeloid leukemia and myelodysplastic syndrome after doxorubicin-cyclophosphamide adjuvant therapy for operable breast cancer: the National Surgical Adjuvant Breast and Bowel Project experience. *J Clin Oncol* 2003;21(7):1195.

89. International Agency for Research on Cancer. Some antiviral and antineoplastic drugs, and other pharmaceutical agents. *IARC Monogr Eval Carcinog Risk Chem Hum* 2000;76:177.

90. Ratain MJ, Kaminer LS, Bitran JD, et al. Acute nonlymphocytic leukemia following etoposide and cisplatin combination chemotherapy for advanced non–small-cell carcinoma of the lung. *Blood* 1987;70:1412.

91. Boshoff C, Begent RH, Oliver RT, et al. Secondary tumours following etoposide containing therapy for germ cell cancer. *Ann Oncol* 1995;6:35.

92. Pedersen-Bjergaard J, Daugaard G, Hansen SW, et al. Increased risk of myelodysplasia and leukaemia after etoposide, cisplatin, and bleomycin for germ-cell tumours [see comments]. *Lancet* 1991;338:359.

93. Pui CH, Ribeiro RC, Hancock ML, et al. Acute myeloid leukemia in children treated with epipodophyllotoxins for acute lymphoblastic leukemia. *N Engl J Med* 1991;325:1682.

94. Pedersen-Bjergaard J, Pedersen M, Roulston D, Philip P. Different genetic pathways in leukemogenesis for patients presenting with therapy-related myelodysplasia and therapy-related acute myeloid leukemia. *Blood* 1995;86(9):3542.

95. Rubin CM, Arthur DC, Woods WG, et al. Therapy-related myelodysplastic syndrome and acute myeloid leukemia in children: correlation between chromosomal abnormalities and prior therapy. *Blood* 1991;78:2982.

96. Pedersen-Bjergaard J, Philip P. Balanced translocations involving chromosome bands 11q23 and 21q22 are highly characteristic of myelodysplasia and leukemia following therapy with cytostatic agents targeting at DNA–topoisomerase II [Letter]. *Blood* 1991;78:1147.

97. Beaumont M, Sanz M, Carli PM, et al. Therapy-related acute promyelocytic leukemia. *J Clin Oncol* 2003;21(11):2123.

98. Pedersen-Bjergaard J, Sigsgaard TC, Nielsen D, et al. Acute monocytic or myelomonocytic leukemia with balanced chromosome translocations to band 11q23 after therapy with 4-epi-doxorubicin and cisplatin or cyclophosphamide for breast cancer [see comments]. *J Clin Oncol* 1992;10:1444.

99. Sandoval C, Pui CH, Bowman LC, et al. Secondary acute myeloid leukemia in children previously treated with alkylating agents, intercalating topoisomerase II inhibitors, and irradiation. *J Clin Oncol* 1993;11:1039.

100. Diamandidou E, Buzdar AU, Smith TL, et al. Treatment-related leukemia in breast cancer patients treated with fluorouracil-doxorubicin-cyclophosphamide combination adjuvant chemotherapy: the University of Texas M. D. Anderson Cancer Center experience. *J Clin Oncol* 1996;14(10):2722.

101. Breslow NE, Takashima JR, Whitton JA, et al. Second malignant neoplasms following treatment for Wilms' tumor: a report from the National Wilms' Tumor Study Group. *J Clin Oncol* 1995;13:1851.

102. Hawkins MM, Wilson LM, Stovall MA, et al. Epipodophyllotoxins, alkylating agents, and radiation and risk of secondary leukaemia after childhood cancer. *BMJ* 1992;304:951.

103. Smith MA, Rubinstein L, Anderson JR, et al. Secondary leukemia or myelodysplastic syndrome after treatment with epipodophyllotoxins. *J Clin Oncol* 1999;17(2):569.

104. Le Deley MC, Leblanc T, Shamsaldin A, et al. Risk of secondary leukemia after a solid tumor in childhood according to the dose of epipodophyllotoxins and anthracyclines: a case-control study by the Societé Française d'Oncologie Pédiatrique. *J Clin Oncol* 2003;21(6):1074.

105. Davies SM. Mechanisms of cytotoxicity and leukemogenesis: topoisomerase II inhibitors and alkylating agents. In: ASCO Educational Book, American Society of Clinical Oncol-

ogy Educational Symposia, 31st annual meeting; May 20–23, 1995; Los Angeles. Los Angeles: American Society of Clinical Oncology, 1995:204.

106. Rivera GK, Pui CH, Santana VM, Pratt CB, Crist WM. Epipodophyllotoxins in the treatment of childhood cancer. *Cancer Chemother Pharmacol* 1994;34[Suppl]:S89.

107. Chaplain G, Milan C, Sgro C, Carli PM, Bonithon-Kopp C. Increased risk of acute leukemia after adjuvant chemotherapy for breast cancer: a population-based study. *J Clin Oncol* 2000;18(15):2836.

108. Saso R, Kulkarni S, Mitchell P, et al. Secondary myelodysplastic syndrome/acute myeloid leukaemia following mitoxantrone-based therapy for breast carcinoma. *Br J Cancer* 2000;83(1):91.

109. Cheson BD, Vena DA, Barrett J, Freidlin B. Second malignancies as a consequence of nucleoside analog therapy for chronic lymphoid leukemias. *J Clin Oncol* 1999;17(8):2454.

110. Relling MV, Rubnitz JE, Rivera GK, et al. High incidence of secondary brain tumours after radiotherapy and antimetabolites. *Lancet* 1999;354(9172):34.

111. Felix CA. Chemotherapy-related second cancers. In: Neugut AI, Meadows AT, Robinson E, eds. Multiple primary cancers. Philadelphia: Lippincott Williams & Wilkins, 1999:137.

112. Kelly KM, Perentesis JP. Polymorphisms of drug metabolizing enzymes and markers of genotoxicity to identify patients with Hodgkin's lymphoma at risk of treatment-related complications. *Ann Oncol* 2002;13[Suppl 1]:34.

113. Ben-Yehuda D, Krichevsky S, Caspi O, et al. Microsatellite instability and p53 mutations in therapy-related leukemia suggest mutator phenotype. *Blood* 1996;88(11):4296.

114. Zhu YM, Das-Gupta EP, Russell NH. Microsatellite instability and p53 mutations are associated with abnormal expression of the MSH2 gene in adult acute leukemia. *Blood* 1999;94(2):733.

115. Yeoh EJ, Ross ME, Shurtleff SA, et al. Classification, subtype discovery, and prediction of outcome in pediatric acute lymphoblastic leukemia by gene expression profiling. *Cancer Cell* 2002;1(2):133.

116. Alberts DS. Protection by amifostine of cyclophosphamide-induced myelosuppression. *Semin Oncol* 1999;269(2 Suppl 7):37.

117. Castiglione F, Dalla Mola A, Porcile G. Protection of normal tissues from radiation and cytotoxic therapy: the development of amifostine. *Tumori* 1999;85(2):85.

118. Kaldor JM, Day NE, Kittelmann B, et al. Bladder tumours following chemotherapy and radiotherapy for ovarian cancer: a case-control study. *Int J Cancer* 1995;63:1.

119. Birdwell SH, Hancock SL, Varghese A, Cox RS, Hoppe RT. Gastrointestinal cancer after treatment of Hodgkin's disease. *Int J Radiat Oncol Biol Phys* 1997;37:67.

120. Mauch PM, Kalish LA, Marcus KC, et al. Second malignancies after treatment for laparotomy staged IA–IIIB Hodgkin's disease: long-term analysis of risk factors and outcome. *Blood* 1996;87(9):3625.

121. Swerdlow AJ, van Leeuwen FE. Late effects after treatment for Hodgkin's disease. In: Linch DC, Degos L, Griffin JD, Loewenberg B, eds. Textbook of malignant haematology. London: Taylor & Francis, 2004.

122. Bhatia S, Robison LL, Oberlin O, et al. Breast cancer and other second neoplasms after childhood Hodgkin's disease. *N Engl J Med* 1996;334:745.

123. Foss Abrahamsen A, Andersen A, Nome O, et al. Long-term risk of second malignancy after treatment of Hodgkin's disease: the influence of treatment, age and follow-up time. *Ann Oncol* 2002;13(11):1786.

124. van Leeuwen FE, Swerdlow AJ, Valagussa P, Tucker MA. Second cancers after treatment of Hodgkin's disease. In: Mauch PM, Armitage JO, Diehl V, Hoppe RT, Weiss LM, eds. Hodgkin's disease. Philadelphia: Lippincott Williams & Wilkins, 1999:607.

125. Valagussa PA, Bonadonna G. Carcinogenic effects of cancer treatment. In: Peckham M, Pinedo H, Veronesi U, eds. Oxford textbook of oncology. Oxford: Oxford University Press, 1995:2348.

126. Schellong G, Riepenhausen M, Creutzig U, et al. Low risk of secondary leukemias after chemotherapy without mechlorethamine in childhood Hodgkin's disease. German-Austrian Pediatric Hodgkin's Disease Group. *J Clin Oncol* 1997;15:2247.

127. Diehl V, Franklin J, Pfreundschuh M, et al. Standard and increased-dose BEACOPP chemotherapy compared with COPP-ABVD for advanced Hodgkin's disease. *N Engl J Med* 2003;348(24):2386.

128. Andrieu JM, Ifrah N, Payen C, et al. Increased risk of secondary acute nonlymphocytic leukemia after extended-field radiation therapy combined with MOPP chemotherapy for Hodgkin's disease [see comments]. *J Clin Oncol* 1990;8:1148.

129. Abruzzese E, Radford JE, Miller JS, et al. Detection of abnormal pretransplant clones in progenitor cells of patients who developed myelodysplasia after autologous transplantation. *Blood* 1999;94(5):1814.

130. Andre M, Henry-Amar M, Blaise D, et al. Treatment-related deaths and second cancer risk after autologous stem-cell transplantation for Hodgkin's disease. *Blood* 1998;92(6):1933.

131. Park S, Brice P, Noguerra ME, et al. Myelodysplasias and leukemias after autologous stem cell transplantation for lymphoid malignancies. *Bone Marrow Transplant* 2000;26(3):321.

132. Traweek ST, Slovak ML, Nademanee AP, et al. Myelodysplasia and acute myeloid leukemia occurring after autologous bone marrow transplantation for lymphoma. *Leuk Lymphoma* 1996;20(5–6):365.

133. Metayer C, Curtis RE, Vose J, et al. Myelodysplastic syndrome and acute myeloid leukemia after autotransplantation for lymphoma: a multicenter case-control study. *Blood* 2003;101(5):2015.

134. Penn I. Cancers complicating organ transplantation [Editorial; Comment]. *N Engl J Med* 1990;323:1767.

135. Krikorian JG, Burke JS, Rosenberg SA, Kaplan HS. Occurrence of non-Hodgkin's lymphoma after therapy for Hodgkin's disease. *N Engl J Med* 1979;300:452.

136. Rueffer U, Josting A, Franklin J, et al. Non-Hodgkin's lymphoma after primary Hodgkin's disease in the German Hodgkin's Lymphoma Study Group: incidence, treatment, and prognosis. *J Clin Oncol* 2001;19(7):2026.

137. van Leeuwen FE, Travis LB. Second cancers. In: DeVita VT Jr, Hellman S, Rosenberg SA, eds. Cancer principles and practice of oncology, 6th ed. Philadelphia: Lippincott Williams & Wilkins, 2001:2939.

138. Goss PE, Sierra S. Current perspectives on radiation-induced breast cancer [see comments]. *J Clin Oncol* 1998;16(1):338.

139. Wolden SL, Hancock SL, Carlson RW, et al. Management of breast cancer after Hodgkin's disease. *J Clin Oncol* 2000;18(4):765.

140. Clemons M, Loijens L, Goss P. Breast cancer risk following irradiation for Hodgkin's disease. *Cancer Treat Rev* 2000;26(4):291.

141. Swerdlow AJ, Schoemaker MJ, Allerton R, et al. Lung cancer after Hodgkin's disease: a nested case-control study of the relation to treatment. *J Clin Oncol* 2001;19(6):1610.

142. Easton DF, Peto J, Doll R. Cancers of the respiratory tract in mustard gas workers. *Br J Ind Med* 1988;45(10):652.

143. Hancock SL, Hoppe RT. Long-term complications of treatment and causes of mortality after Hodgkin's disease. *Semin Radiat Oncol* 1996;6(3):225.

144. Sankila R, Garwicz S, Olsen JH, et al. Risk of subsequent malignant neoplasms among 1,641 Hodgkin's disease patients diagnosed in childhood and adolescence: a population-based cohort study in the five Nordic countries. Association of the Nordic Cancer Registries and the Nordic Society of Pediatric Hematology and Oncology. *J Clin Oncol* 1996;14:1442.

145. Land CE. Studies of cancer and radiation dose among atomic bomb survivors. The example of breast cancer [see comments]. *JAMA* 1995;274(5):402.

146. Diller L, Medeiros Nancarrow C, Shaffer K, et al. Breast cancer screening in women previously treated for Hodgkin's disease: a prospective cohort study. *J Clin Oncol* 2002;20(8):2085.

147. Ries LAG, Eisner MP, Kosary CL, et al. SEER cancer statistics review. 1975–2000. Bethesda, MD: National Cancer Institute, 2003.

148. Brennan P, Coates M, Armstrong B, Colin D, Boffetta P. Second primary neoplasms following non-Hodgkin's lymphoma in New South Wales, Australia. *Br J Cancer* 2000;82(7):1344.

149. Dong C, Hemminki K. Second primary neoplasms among 53,159 haematolymphoproliferative malignancy patients in Sweden, 1958–1996: a search for common mechanisms. *Br J Cancer* 2001;85(7):997.

150. Travis LB, Curtis RE, Glimelius B, et al. Second cancers among long-term survivors of non-Hodgkin's lymphoma. *J Natl Cancer Inst* 1993;85:1932.

151. Travis LB, Curtis RE, Boice JD Jr, Hankey BF, Fraumeni JF Jr. Second cancers following non-Hodgkin's lymphoma. *Cancer* 1991;67:2002.

152. Pedersen-Bjergaard J, Ersboll J, Hansen VL, et al. Carcinoma of the urinary bladder after treatment with cyclophosphamide for non-Hodgkin's lymphoma. *N Engl J Med* 1988;318:1028.

153. Travis LB, Weeks J, Curtis RE, et al. Leukemia following low-dose total body irradiation and chemotherapy for non-Hodgkin's lymphoma. *J Clin Oncol* 1996;14:565.

154. Khan MA, Travis LB, Lynch CF, et al. p53 mutations in cyclophosphamide-associated bladder cancer. *Cancer Epidemiol Biomarkers Prev* 1998;7(5):397.

155. Taylor JA, Li Y, He M, et al. p53 mutations in bladder tumors from arylamine-exposed workers. *Cancer Res* 1996;56(2):294.

156. Travis LB, Curtis RE, Stovall M, et al. Risk of leukemia following treatment for non-Hodgkin's lymphoma. *J Natl Cancer Inst* 1994;86:1450.

157. Pedersen-Bjergaard J, Ersboll J, Sorensen HM, et al. Risk of acute nonlymphocytic leukemia and preleukemia in patients treated with cyclophosphamide for non-Hodgkin's lymphomas. Comparison with results obtained in patients treated for Hodgkin's disease and ovarian carcinoma with other alkylating agents. *Ann Intern Med* 1985;103:195.

158. Thomas D, Pogoda J, Langholz B, Mack W. Temporal modifiers of the radon-smoked interaction [published erratum appears in *Health Phys* 1994;67(6):675]. *Health Phys* 1994;66:257.

159. Greene MH, Harris EL, Gershenson DM, et al. Melphalan may be a more potent leukemogen than cyclophosphamide. *Ann Intern Med* 1986;105:360.

160. Mendenhall NP, Noyes WD, Million RR. Total body irradiation for stage II–IV non-Hodgkin's lymphoma: ten-year follow-up. *J Clin Oncol* 1989;7(1):67.

161. Rubin P, Constine LS3, Scarantino CW. The paradoxes in patterns and mechanism of bone marrow regeneration after irradiation. 2. Total body irradiation. *Radiother Oncol* 1984;2(3):227.

162. Del Canizo M, Amigo M, Hernandez JM, et al. Incidence and characterization of secondary myelodysplastic syndromes following autologous transplantation. *Haematologica* 2000;85(4):403.

163. Harrison CN, Gregory W, Hudson GV, et al. High-dose BEAM chemotherapy with autologous haemopoietic stem cell transplantation for Hodgkin's disease is unlikely to be associated with a major increased risk of secondary MDS/AML. *Br J Cancer* 1999;81(3):476.

164. Pedersen-Bjergaard J, Pedersen M, Myhre J, Geisler C. High risk of therapy-related leukemia after BEAM chemotherapy and autologous stem cell transplantation for previously treated lymphomas is mainly related to primary chemotherapy and not to the BEAM-transplantation procedure. *Leukemia* 1997;11(10):1654.

165. Hosing C, Munsell M, Yazji S, et al. Risk of therapy-related myelodysplastic syndrome/acute leukemia following high-dose therapy and autologous bone marrow transplantation for non-Hodgkin's lymphoma. *Ann Oncol* 2002;13(3):450.

166. Micallef IN, Lillington DM, Apostolidis J, et al. Therapy-related myelodysplasia and secondary acute myelogenous leukemia after high-dose therapy with autologous hematopoietic progenitor-cell support for lymphoid malignancies. *J Clin Oncol* 2000;18(5):947.

167. Lillington DM, Micallef IN, Carpenter E, et al. Detection of chromosome abnormalities pre–high-dose treatment in patients developing therapy-related myelodysplasia and secondary acute myelogenous leukemia after treatment for non-Hodgkin's lymphoma. *J Clin Oncol* 2001;19(9):2472.

168. Mach-Pascual S, Legare RD, Lu D, et al. Predictive value of clonality assays in patients with non-Hodgkin's lymphoma undergoing autologous bone marrow transplant: a single institution study. *Blood* 1998;91(12):4496.

169. Einhorn LH. Testicular cancer as a model for a curable neoplasm: the Richard and Hinda Rosenthal Foundation Award Lecture. *Cancer Res* 1981;41(9 Pt 1): 3275.

170. Fossa SD, Horwich A, Russell JM, et al. Optimal planning target volume for stage I testicular seminoma: a Medical Research Council randomized trial. *J Clin Oncol* 1999;17(4):1146.

171. Bokemeyer C, Schmoll HJ. Treatment of testicular cancer and the development of secondary malignancies. *J Clin Oncol* 1995;13:283.

172. van Leeuwen FE, Stiggelbout AM, van den Belt-Dusebout AW, et al. Second cancer risk following testicular cancer: a follow-up study of 1,909 patients [see comments]. *J Clin Oncol* 1993;11:415.

173. Fossa SD, Langmark F, Aass N, et al. Second non-germ cell malignancies after radiotherapy of testicular cancer with or without chemotherapy. *Br J Cancer* 1990;61:639.

174. Dong C, Lonnstedt I, Hemminki K. Familial testicular cancer and second primary cancers in testicular cancer patients by histological type. *Eur J Cancer* 2001;37(15):1878.

175. Michels SD, McKenna RW, Arthur DC, Brunning RD. Therapy-related acute myeloid leukemia and myelodysplastic syndrome: a clinical and morphologic study of 65 cases. *Blood* 1985;65:1364.

176. Carr ZA, Kleinerman RA, Stovall M, et al. Malignant neoplasms after radiation therapy for peptic ulcer. *Radiat Res* 2002;157(6):668.

177. Griem ML, Kleinerman RA, Boice JD Jr, et al. Cancer following radiotherapy for peptic ulcer. *J Natl Cancer Inst* 1994;86(11):842.

178. Nichols CR, Breeden ES, Loehrer PJ, Williams SD, Einhorn LH. Secondary leukemia associated with a conventional dose of etoposide: review of serial germ cell tumor protocols. *J Natl Cancer Inst* 1993;85:36.

179. Redman JR, Vugrin D, Arlin ZA, et al. Leukemia following treatment of germ cell tumors in men. *J Clin Oncol* 1984;2(10):1080.

180. Travis LB, Andersson M, Gospodarowicz M, et al. Treatment-associated leukemia following testicular cancer. *J Natl Cancer Inst* 2000;92(14):1165.

181. Nichols CR, Roth BJ, Heerema N, Griep J, Tricot G. Hematologic neoplasia associated with primary mediastinal germ-cell tumors. *N Engl J Med* 1990;322:1425.

182. Bosl GJ, Motzer RJ. Testicular germ-cell cancer [published erratum appears in *N Engl J Med* 1997;337(19):1403]. *N Engl J Med* 1997;337(4):242.

183. International Agency for Research on Cancer. Some pharmaceutical drugs. IARC Monographs on the Evaluation of Carcinogenic Risks to Humans. Lyon, France: International Agency for Research on Cancer, 2000.

184. Kollmannsberger C, Hartmann JT, Kanz L, Bokemeyer C. Therapy-related malignancies following treatment of germ cell cancer. *Int J Cancer* 1999;83(6):860.

185. Sokal M, Peckham MJ, Hendry WF. Bilateral germ cell tumours of the testis. *Br J Urol* 1980;52:158.

186. Wanderas EH, Fossa SD, Tretli S. Risk of subsequent non-germ cell cancer after treatment of germ cell cancer in 2006 Norwegian male patients. *Eur J Cancer* 1997;33(2):253.

187. National Cancer Institute. SEER cancer statistics review, 1973–1994. Bethesda, MD: National Cancer Institute, 1997.

188. Hemminki K, Aaltonen L, Li X. Subsequent primary malignancies after endometrial carcinoma and ovarian carcinoma. *Cancer* 2003;97(10):2432.

189. Lynch HT, Lanspa S, Smyrk T, et al. Hereditary nonpolyposis colorectal cancer (Lynch syndromes I & II). Genetics, pathology, natural history, and cancer control, part I. *Cancer Genet Cytogenet* 1991;53(2):143.

190. National Institutes of Health consensus conference. Ovarian cancer. Screening, treatment, and follow-up. NIH Consensus Development Panel on Ovarian Cancer [see comments]. *JAMA* 1995;273(6):491.

191. Douple EB. Platinum-radiation interactions. *NCI Monogr* 1988;(6):315.

192. Vokes EE, Weichselbaum RR. Concomitant chemoradiotherapy: rationale and clinical experience in patients with solid tumors [published erratum appears in *J Clin Oncol* 1990;8(8):1447] [see comments]. *J Clin Oncol* 1990;8(5):911.

193. Neijt JP. New therapy for ovarian cancer [Editorial; Comment]. *N Engl J Med* 1996;334(1):50.

194. Adami HO, Bergstrom R, Hansen J. Age at first primary as a determinant of the incidence of bilateral breast cancer. Cumulative and relative risks in a population-based case-control study. *Cancer* 1985;55:643.

195. Harvey EB, Brinton LA. Second cancer following cancer of the breast in Connecticut, 1935–82. *Natl Cancer Inst Monogr* 1985;68:99.

196. Teppo L, Pukkala E, Saxen E. Multiple cancer—an epidemiologic exercise in Finland. *J Natl Cancer Inst* 1985;75:207.

197. Fisher B, Costantino JP, Redmond CK, et al. Endometrial cancer in tamoxifen-treated breast cancer patients: findings from the National Surgical Adjuvant Breast and Bowel Project (NSABP) B-14 [see comments]. *J Natl Cancer Inst* 1994;86:527.

198. Rutqvist LE, Johansson H, Signomklao T, et al. Adjuvant tamoxifen therapy for early stage breast cancer and second primary malignancies. Stockholm Breast Cancer Study Group [see comments]. *J Natl Cancer Inst* 1995;87:645.

199. Deutsch M, Land SR, Begovic M, et al. The incidence of lung carcinoma after surgery for breast carcinoma with and without postoperative radiotherapy. Results of National Surgical Adjuvant Breast and Bowel Project (NSABP) clinical trials B-04 and B-06. *Cancer* 2003;98(7):1362.

200. Ewertz M, Mouridsen HT. Second cancer following cancer of the female breast in Denmark, 1943–80. *Natl Cancer Inst Monogr* 1985;68:325.

201. Ford MB, Sigurdson AJ, Petrulis ES, et al. Effects of smoking and radiotherapy on lung carcinoma in breast carcinoma survivors. *Cancer* 2003;98(7):1457.

202. Inskip PD, Stovall M, Flannery JT. Lung cancer risk and radiation dose among women treated for breast cancer. *J Natl Cancer Inst* 1994;86:983.

203. Neugut AI, Robinson E, Lee WC, et al. Lung cancer after radiation therapy for breast cancer [see comments]. *Cancer* 1993;71:3054.

204. Ahsan H, Neugut AI. Radiation therapy for breast cancer and increased risk for esophageal carcinoma. *Ann Intern Med* 1998;128(2):114.

205. Huang J, Mackillop WJ. Increased risk of soft tissue sarcoma after radiotherapy in women with breast carcinoma. *Cancer* 2001;92(1):172.

206. Karlsson P, Holmberg E, Samuelsson A, Johansson KA, Wallgren A. Soft tissue sarcoma after treatment for breast cancer—a Swedish population-based study. *Eur J Cancer* 1998;34(13):2068.

207. Wijnmaalen A, van Ooijen B, van Geel BN, Henzen-Logmans SC, Treurniet-Donker AD. Angiosarcoma of the breast following lumpectomy, axillary lymph node dissection, and

radiotherapy for primary breast cancer: three case reports and a review of the literature. *Int J Radiat Oncol Biol Phys* 1993;26:135.

208. Early Breast Cancer Trialists' Collaborative Group. Polychemotherapy for early breast cancer: an overview of the randomised trials [see comments]. *Lancet* 1998;352(9132):930.

209. Early Breast Cancer Trialists' Collaborative Group. Tamoxifen for early breast cancer: an overview of the randomised trials [see comments]. *Lancet* 1998;351(9114):1451.

210. Chaudary MA, Millis RR, Hoskins EO, et al. Bilateral primary breast cancer: a prospective study of disease incidence. *Br J Surg* 1984;71:711.

211. Kurtz JM, Amalric R, Brandone H, Ayme Y, Spitalier JM. Contralateral breast cancer and other second malignancies in patients treated by breast-conserving therapy with radiation. *Int J Radiat Oncol Biol Phys* 1988;15:277.

212. Storm HH, Andersson M, Boice JD Jr, et al. Adjuvant radiotherapy and risk of contralateral breast cancer. *J Natl Cancer Inst* 1992;84:1245.

213. Curtis RE, Boice JD Jr, Shriner DA, Hankey BF, Fraumeni JF Jr. Second cancers after adjuvant tamoxifen therapy for breast cancer. *J Natl Cancer Inst* 1996;88(12):832.

214. O'Regan R, Jordan VC, Gradishar WJ. Tamoxifen and contralateral breast cancer [see comments]. *J Am Coll Surg* 1999;188(6):678.

215. Narod SA, Brunet JS, Ghadirian P, et al. Tamoxifen and risk of contralateral breast cancer in BRCA1 and BRCA2 mutation carriers: a case-control study. Hereditary Breast Cancer Clinical Study Group. *Lancet* 2000;356(9245):1876.

216. Bernstein JL, Thompson WD, Risch N, Holford TR. Risk factors predicting the incidence of second primary breast cancer among women diagnosed with a first primary breast cancer. *Am J Epidemiol* 1992;136:925.

217. Lavey RS, Eby NL, Prosnitz LR. Impact on second malignancy risk of the combined use of radiation and chemotherapy for lymphomas. *Cancer* 1990;66:80.

218. Valagussa P, Moliterni A, Terenziani M, Zambetti M, Bonadonna G. Second malignancies following CMF-based adjuvant chemotherapy in resectable breast cancer [see comments]. *Ann Oncol* 1994;5:803.

219. Tallman MS, Gray R, Bennett JM, et al. Leukemogenic potential of adjuvant chemotherapy for early-stage breast cancer: the Eastern Cooperative Oncology Group experience [see comments]. *J Clin Oncol* 1995;13(7):1557.

220. Benefit of a high-dose epirubicin regimen in adjuvant chemotherapy for node-positive breast cancer patients with poor prognostic factors: 5-year follow-up results of French Adjuvant Study Group 05 randomized trial. *J Clin Oncol* 2001;19(3):602.

221. Castiglione M, Goldhirsch A. Second tumours after breast cancer: is it still too soon to tell? [Editorial] [see comments]. *Ann Oncol* 1994;5:785.

222. van Leeuwen FE, Benraadt J, Coebergh JW, et al. Risk of endometrial cancer after tamoxifen treatment of breast cancer [see comments]. *Lancet* 1994;343:448.

223. International Agency for Research on Cancer. Some pharmaceutical drugs. IARC Monographs on the Evaluation of Carcinogenic Risks to Humans. Lyon, France: International Agency for Research on Cancer, 1996.

224. Bernstein L, Deapen D, Cerhan JR, et al. Tamoxifen therapy for breast cancer and endometrial cancer risk. *J Natl Cancer Inst* 1999;91(19):1654.

225. Fisher B, Costantino JP, Wickerham DL, et al. Tamoxifen for prevention of breast cancer: report of the National Surgical Adjuvant Breast and Bowel Project P-1 Study [see comments]. *J Natl Cancer Inst* 1998;90(18):1371.

226. Mignotte H, Lasset C, Bonadona V, et al. Iatrogenic risks of endometrial carcinoma after treatment for breast cancer in a large French case-control study. Fédération Nationale des Centres de Lutte Contre le Cancer (FNCLCC). *Int J Cancer* 1998;76(3):325.

227. Bergman L, Beelen ML, Gallee MP, et al. Risk and prognosis of endometrial cancer after tamoxifen for breast cancer. Comprehensive Cancer Centres' ALERT Group. Assessment of Liver and Endometrial Cancer Risk following Tamoxifen. *Lancet* 2000;356(9233):881.

228. Gottardis MM, Robinson SP, Satyaswaroop PG, Jordan VC. Contrasting actions of tamoxifen on endometrial and breast tumor growth in the athymic mouse. *Cancer Res* 1988;48:812.

229. Nayfield SG, Karp JE, Ford LG, Dorr FA, Kramer BS. Potential role of tamoxifen in prevention of breast cancer. *J Natl Cancer Inst* 1991;83:1450.

230. Fornander T, Hellstrom AC, Moberger B. Descriptive clinicopathologic study of 17 patients with endometrial cancer during or after adjuvant tamoxifen in early breast cancer. *J Natl Cancer Inst* 1993;85:1850.

231. Magriples U, Naftolin F, Schwartz PE, Carcangiu ML. High-grade endometrial carcinoma in tamoxifen-treated breast cancer patients. *J Clin Oncol* 1993;11:485.

232. Wickerham DL, Fisher B, Wolmark N, et al. Association of tamoxifen and uterine sarcoma. *J Clin Oncol* 2002;20(11):2758.

233. Lasset C, Bonadona V, Mignotte H, Bremond A. Tamoxifen and risk of endometrial cancer. *Lancet* 2001;357(9249):66.

234. Narod SA, Pal T, Graham T, Mitchell M, Fyles A. Tamoxifen and risk of endometrial cancer. *Lancet* 2001;357(9249):65.

235. Greaves P, Goonetilleke R, Nunn G, Topham J, Orton T. Two-year carcinogenicity study of tamoxifen in Alderley Park Wistar-derived rats. *Cancer Res* 1993;53:3919.

236. Williams GM, Iatropoulos MJ, Djordjevic MV, Kaltenberg OP. The triphenylethylene drug tamoxifen is a strong liver carcinogen in the rat. *Carcinogenesis* 1993;14:315.

237. Newcomb PA, Solomon C, White E. Tamoxifen and risk of large bowel cancer in women with breast cancer. *Breast Cancer Res Treat* 1999;53(3):271.

238. Neugut AI, Murray T, Santos J, et al. Increased risk of lung cancer after breast cancer radiation therapy in cigarette smokers [see comments]. *Cancer* 1994;73:1615.

239. Zablotska LB, Neugut AI. Lung carcinoma after radiation therapy in women treated with lumpectomy or mastectomy for primary breast carcinoma. *Cancer* 2003;97(6):1404.

240. Prochazka M, Granath F, Ekbom A, Shields PG, Hall P. Lung cancer risks in women with previous breast cancer. *Eur J Cancer* 2002;38(11):1520.

241. Inskip PD, Boice JD Jr. Radiotherapy-induced lung cancer among women who smoke [Editorial; Comment] [published erratum appears in *Cancer* 1994;73(9):2456]. *Cancer* 1994;73:1541.

242. Barakat RR, Gilewski TA, Almadrones L, et al. Effect of adjuvant tamoxifen on the endometrium in women with breast cancer: a prospective study using office endometrial biopsy. *J Clin Oncol* 2000;18(20):3459.

243. Olsen JH, Garwicz S, Hertz H, et al. Second malignant neoplasms after cancer in childhood or adolescence. Nordic Society of Paediatric Haematology and Oncology Association of the Nordic Cancer Registries. *BMJ* 1993;307:1030.

244. Hawkins MM, Draper GJ, Kingston JE. Incidence of second primary tumours among childhood cancer survivors. *Br J Cancer* 1987;56:339.

245. Friend SH, Bernards R, Rogelj S, et al. A human DNA segment with properties of the gene that predisposes to retinoblastoma and osteosarcoma. *Nature* 1986;323:643.

246. Knudson AG Jr, Meadows AT, Nichols WW, Hill R. Chromosomal deletion and retinoblastoma. *N Engl J Med* 1976;295:1120.

247. Brachman DG, Hallahan DE, Beckett MA, Yandell DW, Weichselbaum RR. p53 gene mutations and abnormal retinoblastoma protein in radiation-induced human sarcomas. *Cancer Res* 1991;51:6393.

248. Weichselbaum RR, Beckett M, Diamond A. Some retinoblastomas, osteosarcomas, and soft tissue sarcomas may share a common etiology. *Proc Natl Acad Sci U S A* 1988;85:2106.

249. Meadows AT, Baum E, Fossati-Bellani F, et al. Second malignant neoplasms in children: an update from the Late Effects Study Group. *J Clin Oncol* 1985;3:532.

250. Neglia JP, Meadows AT, Robison LL, et al. Second neoplasms after acute lymphoblastic leukemia in childhood. *N Engl J Med* 1991;325:1330.

251. Loning L, Zimmermann M, Reiter A, et al. Secondary neoplasms subsequent to Berlin-Frankfurt-Munster therapy of acute lymphoblastic leukemia in childhood: significantly lower risk without cranial radiotherapy. *Blood* 2000;95(9):2770.

252. Walter AW, Hancock ML, Pui CH, et al. Secondary brain tumors in children treated for acute lymphoblastic leukemia at St. Jude Children's Research Hospital. *J Clin Oncol* 1998;16(12):3761.

253. Bhatia S, Sather HN, Pabustan OB, et al. Low incidence of second neoplasms among children diagnosed with acute lymphoblastic leukemia after 1983. *Blood* 2002;99(12):4257.

254. Rosso P, Terracini B, Fears TR, et al. Second malignant tumors after elective end of therapy for a first cancer in childhood: a multicenter study in Italy. *Int J Cancer* 1994;59:451.

255. Winick NJ, McKenna RW, Shuster JJ, et al. Secondary acute myeloid leukemia in children with acute lymphoblastic leukemia treated with etoposide [see comments]. *J Clin Oncol* 1993;11:209.

256. Garwicz S, Anderson H, Olsen JH, et al. Second malignant neoplasms after cancer in childhood and adolescence: a population-based case-control study in the 5 Nordic countries. The Nordic Society for Pediatric Hematology and Oncology. The Association of the Nordic Cancer Registries. *Int J Cancer* 2000;88(4):672.

257. Le Vu B, de Vathaire F, Shamsaldin A, et al. Radiation dose, chemotherapy and risk of osteosarcoma after solid tumours during childhood. *Int J Cancer* 1998;77(3):370.

SECTION **8**

RAYMOND B. WEISS

Miscellaneous Toxicities

Chemotherapeutic agents can produce a variety of acute and chronic organ toxicities. Besides heart and pulmonary toxicities, which are discussed in other sections, damage to nerve tissue, kidneys, liver, and blood vessels may occur. In addition, hypersensitivity reactions may produce immediately life-threatening problems with hypotension and respiratory distress. Such hypersensitivity reactions may require ceasing treatment with the precipitating drug or at least finding a means to prevent or minimize the problem. Renal, hepatic, or central nervous system toxicity also may be life-threatening but usually in a less immediate manner. If the offending drug is discontinued before irreversible damage has occurred, these toxicities usually wane or resolve. For some drugs it may be possible to minimize or avert such toxicities by using toxicity protective measures or drugs. As patients live longer after receiving cancer chemotherapy, long-term toxicities such as Raynaud's phenomenon or other vascular toxicities may become evident and are sometimes debilitating and irreversible.

Antitumor drugs are often used in combination or administered with various toxicity protectants, and it may be difficult to determine which drug is most responsible for a particular form of tissue injury. Other comorbid medical conditions or the malignancy itself may cause organ damage during cancer treatment, and the antitumor agent may be blameless. Whether the toxicity is acute or chronic, awareness of the toxicity potential of each antitumor agent in use is important, and appropriate monitoring must be accomplished. This monitoring may be simple patient questioning about symptoms or serial testing, or both.

NEUROTOXICITY

VINCRISTINE, VINBLASTINE, AND VINORELBINE

The first drug class to be recognized as having neurotoxicity was the vinca alkaloids, especially vincristine. Vincristine is unique among the antitumor agents in that neurotoxicity is the sole dose-limiting problem. It causes axonal injury with relative preservation of the myelin sheath. The neurologic injury can occur in the peripheral, central, or autonomic nervous system.[1]

The most common and initial manifestations of neurotoxicity are depression of the deep tendon reflexes and paresthesias of the distal extremities.[1] The Achilles' tendon reflexes and the fingertips, respectively, are the usual initial sites of abnormalities. Loss of the tendon reflexes is usually asymptomatic. The paresthesias commonly progress proximally as vincristine therapy is continued and may involve the entire hands or feet, sometimes accompanied by burning pain. Despite the presence of peripheral paresthesias, vibration sense, position sense, pinprick sensation, and two-point discrimination are generally unaffected.

Motor dysfunction and gait disorders are initially manifested as lower extremity weakness. In rare instances there can be profound weakness, even after only modest total vincristine doses, especially if an unrecognized hereditary neuropathy such as Charcot-Marie-Tooth disease is present. In addition, when vincristine and corticosteroids are administered together, steroid myopathy may occur and cause similar symptoms of weakness, which should not be ascribed to vincristine neurotoxicity and result in a dose modification of the wrong drug. Severe bone pain (especially in the mandible) may occur acutely a few hours after drug administration but usually subsides after a few days.

Cranial nerves may be affected and cause ophthalmoplegia and facial palsy. Toxicity to the parasympathetic nervous system is manifested by constipation and difficult micturition, which can progress to paralytic ileus and bladder atony. Autonomic neuropathy can also produce orthostatic hypotension (which can be symptomatic or clinically silent) and erectile and ejaculatory dysfunction.[2] Other rare, but severe, neurotoxic manifestations observed with vincristine include cortical blindness and vocal cord paralysis (from recurrent laryngeal dysfunction) of the laryngeal nerve (with vocal cord) resulting in dysphonia and even aphonia.

Neurotoxicity from the vinca alkaloids, especially vincristine, is both an individual dose and a cumulative dose phenomenon. The usual practice in adults is to restrict individual doses of vincristine to 2 mg. Studies of higher individual vincristine dose levels have shown a very high rate of neurotoxicity.[2] Most patients will experience neuropathic symptoms after cumulative doses of 25 mg and higher. No effective prevention or treatment has been developed except to stop therapy and wait for neurologic recovery. The neuropathic symptoms may persist as long as several years after cessation of therapy, but they usually wane to a point at which they are no longer troublesome to the patient. Empiric vitamin therapy is ineffective.

Vincristine binds to the β subunit of tubulin, causing disruption of microtubule function in neuronal axons. Electrophysiologic studies indicate distal axonal dysfunction, and nerve conduction testing shows that sensory nerves are most affected, with reduced amplitude of nerve action potentials. Histologic changes are generally those of axonal degeneration.

The vincristine analogs vinblastine and vinorelbine also have neurotoxicity potential. The primary dose-limiting toxicity of both agents is myelosuppression. Neurotoxicity is less common than with vincristine. The form and range of neurotoxicity manifestations from these analogs are similar to those of vincristine, and, again, the degree of dysfunction is related to both individual and cumulative drug doses. However, vinblastine and vinorelbine seem to produce more autonomic effects, which result in frequent constipation and even paralytic ileus and obstipation.[3]

Concurrent use of two neurotoxic agents has been reported to cause enhanced neurotoxicity or no such toxicity, depending on the drug involved. The combination of vinorelbine and cisplatin seems not to be associated with increased incidence or severity of neuropathy.[4] However, when vinorelbine is used either in combination with, or sequentially after, paclitaxel there is more potential for severe neuropathy.[5] In addition, the concurrent use of vincristine and a granulocyte growth factor may precipitate a severe neuropathy involving primarily the legs.[6]

CISPLATIN AND OXALIPLATIN

Although nephrotoxicity is a major and cumulative dose-limiting toxicity of cisplatin, neurotoxicity is also a common problem and can be dose limiting for both single and cumulative doses, but primarily the latter. Cisplatin-induced neuropathy can be expressed as sensory peripheral neuropathy, Lhermitte's sign, autonomic neuropathy, grand mal or focal seizures, encephalopathy, transient cortical blindness, retrobulbar neuritis, vocal cord paralysis, and retinal injury.[7]

The incidence of neurotoxicity ranges up to 100%, depending on individual and cumulative drug dose, treatment duration, concurrent or prior neurotoxic drugs used, presence of other medical conditions also associated with neuropathies (such as diabetes), and possibly gender (women are more sensitive).[7] A cumulative cisplatin dose of 300 to 500 mg/m^2 is the range in which toxicity most commonly develops, but in rare cases single doses can also produce instances of severe toxicity.

Peripheral neuropathy similar to that induced by vincristine is the most common form of cisplatin neurotoxicity. Vincristine produces initial paresthesias in the fingers, whereas cisplatin most often affects the toes and feet. Loss of the Achilles' tendon reflexes is an early sign, and continued treatment leads to sensory ataxia and loss of proximal deep tendon reflexes and vibration sense. Although muscle cramps are a common symptom, motor function is usually not affected.

The pathophysiology of cisplatin neurotoxicity is not known, but it is probably related to the accumulation of inorganic platinum within neurons, which may be irreversible. An autopsy study[8] of platinum concentrations and histopathologic changes in the dorsal root ganglia of cisplatin-treated patients demonstrated a correlation between the tissue level of platinum and clinical neurotoxicity and neuronal histologic changes.

Treatment is cessation of therapy, but neurotoxic symptoms may last for months after cisplatin therapy is discontinued. The electrophysiologic test abnormalities may last for several years and perhaps indefinitely, especially when there is evidence of platinum retention in the circulation even years after treatment has been completed.[9] The symptoms and signs may even progress despite discontinuance of treatment. Amitriptyline has been used as treatment for the neuropathies related to administration of antitumor agents (as it has for other polyneuropathies), but no clinical trials testing its efficacy in double-blind fashion have been performed. Because treatment of cisplatin neurotoxicity is of limited benefit, prevention using protective agents has been extensively explored.[10] Amifostine, a nephrotoxicity protectant, may provide some protection against peripheral neuropathy when used in conjunction with cisplatin.[11] BNP7787 (dimesna) is a new drug with exceptional promise as a neuroprotective agent and is in advanced clinical development for this indication.[12] Supplementation with vitamin E, a cheap and readily available protectant, during cisplatin therapy has also demonstrated benefit in reducing the frequency and severity of neurotoxicity.[13]

Concurrent use of cisplatin and paclitaxel has demonstrated an enhanced potential for neurotoxicity, although there is variability, probably related to the drug doses and schedules used. At the commonly used dosages of these two drugs, more than 50% of patients may develop neuropathy, and this problem is often dose limiting.[14] When patients receiving this drug combination are closely monitored, neurotoxicity may become evident after just two cycles in some cases.

Neuropathy is the most common toxicity of the cisplatin analog oxaliplatin, and cumulative neurotoxicity in the form of peripheral neuropathy is usually dose limiting. The manifestations are peripheral or circumoral paresthesias or both, sensory ataxia, muscle cramps and fasciculations, pain in the arm where the drug is infused, jaw pain when chewing, eye pain, voice changes and slurred speech, Lhermitte's sign, and urinary bladder atony.[15] These symptoms may last only a few seconds to several hours. A neurotoxicity manifestation unique to this drug is pharyngolaryngeal dysesthesia, presenting as acute dyspnea and dysphagia that can be quite frightening to the patient. Another unusual manifestation is tetanus-like muscular contractions of the jaw or distal extremities. A characteristic aspect of any of these symptoms is that they are often precipitated or intensified by exposure to cold, including touching cold objects or drinking cold liquids, and any of them can recur with each drug dose. Patients who develop chronic peripheral neuropathy generally have near full recovery within 6 months after discontinuing therapy, in contrast to treatment with cisplatin, in which the symptoms may be enduring.

Use of neuroprotectants with oxaliplatin therapy has been studied as it has with cisplatin therapy. The only such agent to undergo the rigor of a randomized, double-blind, placebo-controlled assessment has been glutathione, which was given just before each oxaliplatin dose.[16] This agent may inhibit accumulation of the drug in the dorsal root ganglia, thus minimizing axonal injury. In a small study[16] glutathione use did reduce neurotoxicity manifestations from oxaliplatin. Infusion of calcium and magnesium just before and after oxaliplatin administration may also be of value and is undergoing further assessment.

THALIDOMIDE

Thalidomide has had a renaissance of clinical use since its release for marketing, especially in oncology. It produces a chronic peripheral sensory neuropathy in as many as 50% of patients, which often is the dose-limiting toxicity.[17,18] Extremity paresthesias (especially in the legs and feet) are the predominant manifestation. The neurotoxicity is related both to the cumulative dose (occurring after several months of daily therapy) and the daily dose, with doses of more than 75 mg posing the highest risk for problems. Sural nerve biopsies of patients taking this drug can show loss of myelinated fibers and wallerian degeneration.

CYTARABINE

Cytarabine (cytosine arabinoside, Ara-C) is given both intravenously and intrathecally, and administration by both routes can produce neurotoxicity. Manifestations include cerebellar dysfunction, seizures, peripheral neuropathy, generalized encephalopathy, necrotizing leukoencephalopathy, spinal myelopathy, basal ganglia necrosis, and pseudobulbar palsy.[19]

The highest incidence (15% to 37%) occurs in patients receiving high-dose cytarabine therapy (i.e., more than 1 g/m^2 in multiple doses).[19] The toxicity is generally acute and not related to cumulative drug doses, in contrast to the neuropathy associated with cisplatin and vincristine. Risk factors for neurotoxicity are age older than 50 years, high drug dose, prior cytarabine treatment, and renal dysfunction.[19]

Cerebellar effects (dysarthria, ataxia, and dysmetria) are the most common form of neurotoxicity. These symptoms often occur within days of first treatment and may be accompanied by headache, altered mentation, memory loss, and somnolence. Seizures have rarely occurred. Peripheral neuropathy can also occur but is rare. Symptoms range from a purely sensory neuropathy to sensorimotor polyneuropathies in a glovestocking distribution. The neuropathy can even progress to a quadriparesis with ventilatory support becoming necessary. Intrathecal cytarabine can produce an ascending myelopathy. A new sustained-release formulation of cytarabine designed for intrathecal therapy[20] allows less frequent administration but may still cause neurotoxic manifestations. All these neurologic abnormalities (even the peripheral neuropathy) rarely can progress to coma and death.

Recovery from the neurologic effects usually occurs within a few days after discontinuance of cytarabine therapy. There is no known treatment. Serial radiographic studies of the brain may show some improvement in cerebellar abnormalities after discontinuance of treatment, but progressive atrophy may also occur after a few months, associated with persistent symptoms.[21]

The mechanism of such neurotoxicity is not known. When high drug doses are used, cytotoxic concentrations of cytarabine reach the cerebrospinal fluid, but parent drug and metabolites are cleared more slowly from spinal fluid than from blood, which is a likely explanation for the dose relationship of this toxicity. Cerebellar cell death appears to be produced by cytarabine blocking of an essential deoxynucleoside.[22] Why the Purkinje cells of the cerebellum are particularly prone to injury from intravenous cytarabine, even in experimental animals, is unknown.

IFOSFAMIDE

Ifosfamide and cyclophosphamide have similar chemical structures, but ifosfamide induces neurotoxicity (as it does nephrotoxicity), whereas cyclophosphamide does not. Acute symptoms are visual and auditory hallucinations, vivid dreams, logorrhea, mutism, asterixis, incontinence, dizziness, palilalia, confusion, perseveration, agitation, personality changes, somnolence, cerebellar and cranial nerve dysfunction, hemiparesis, seizures, coma, and occasionally death.[23,24] Peripheral neuropathy and extrapyramidal abnormalities such as myoclonus and muscular spasticity have also been observed. The onset is acute up to 5 days after initiation of ifosfamide therapy, and recovery usually occurs within a few days after discontinuing therapy. Memory and affect disorders may occasionally persist. No cumulative-dose neurotoxic effects have been reported, but retreatment with ifosfamide may precipitate the same acute toxicity manifestations again.

Significant neurotoxic abnormalities occur in approximately 10% of patients treated with ifosfamide. The incidence varies depending on how carefully patients are monitored for this problem, what ifosfamide dose and method of administration are used, and whether various risk factors are present. Such risk factors are low serum albumin level, any degree of renal dysfunction, prior administration of cisplatin (which probably results in subclinical renal dysfunction), poor performance status, the presence of a central nervous system tumor, and age (children are more susceptible than adults).[23] High doses may accentuate symptoms of an underlying mild neuropathy and cause severe and painful paresthesias. For unknown reasons, oral administration of ifosfamide has more neurotoxic potential than intravenous administration.

The etiology of this neurotoxicity is probably multifactorial and is due to one or more metabolites of ifosfamide produced in high quantities.[25] Cyclophosphamide may not produce neurotoxicity because metabolites with encephalopathic potential are a minor component of its degradation. Effective treatment (besides the discontinuance of ifosfamide) is intravenous methylene blue and high-dose thiamine.[26,27] Such treatment can produce dramatic reversal of the neurotoxic manifestations. Means of prevention include use of a continuous infusion schedule of drug administration (instead of a bolus) and concurrent use of methylene blue.

5-FLUOROURACIL

5-Fluorouracil (5-FU) has been known to cause neurotoxicity since the earliest clinical trials conducted with this drug 45 years ago. Cerebellar dysfunction with findings of gait ataxia, nystagmus, dysmetria, and dysarthria is the most common form of neurotoxicity, but oculomotor palsy, confusion, somnolence, seizures, coma, and peripheral neuropathy have also been observed.[28,29] The incidence is approximately 5%, and such neurotoxicity may occur with any of the 5-FU administration schedules in common use. Neurotoxicity from this drug is acute in onset, and a cumulative dose effect has not been observed. It is now common practice to administer leucovorin in combination with 5-FU to enhance antitumor activity. Leucovorin may itself be the cause of some of the instances of seizures occurring in conjunction with administration of these two drugs.[30]

The etiology of 5-FU neurotoxicity is not well understood. 5-FU metabolites have been shown to have neuropathic action in experimental animals.[31] However, neurotoxicity is more likely due to parent drug and not metabolites, because patients have been reported who developed severe neurotoxic symptoms due to a genetic deficiency of the initial enzyme (dihydropyrimidine dehydrogenase) necessary for 5-FU catabolism.[32] Patients with complete or partial deficiency of this enzyme appear particularly susceptible to 5-FU toxicity of all kinds, including neuropathy.

METHOTREXATE

Neurotoxicity from methotrexate can be expressed as meningeal irritation, transient paraparesis, or encephalopathy. When the drug is administered intrathecally, it can cause headache, nausea and vomiting, lethargy, nuchal rigidity, and other features of meningeal irritation. Subacute abnormalities include paraparesis, hemiparesis, somnolence, cranial nerve dysfunction, cerebellar symptoms, and seizures, which can develop days to several weeks after therapy. Such encephalopathic symptoms may occur more commonly when both intrathecal and intravenous high-dose methotrexate are administered.[33] When intrathecal methotrexate is given repetitively (especially if it is administered via an intraventricular device), progressive necrotizing leukoencephalopathy may develop. The usual symptoms include initial memory loss with occasional later progression to severe dementia, gait disturbance, dysphasia, and seizures.[34] Even if serious neuropathy does not occur, subtle cognitive deficits may develop months to years later, especially in children.[35] Risk factors for such problems are cranial irradiation and the total radiation dose administered, presence of neoplastic cells in the spinal fluid, and cumulative methotrexate dose. The neurotoxic effect is probably a direct consequence of high drug dose concentrations in the cerebrospinal fluid.

Intravenous methotrexate also can produce encephalopathy, especially if high doses with leucovorin rescue are used. The manifestations and risk factors are similar to those of intrathecal methotrexate. The neurologic dysfunction may be acute and transient or delayed in onset with personality changes. Magnetic resonance imaging scans can show white matter abnormalities in asymptomatic patients that are probably subclinical manifestations of neurotoxicity. However, it has been argued that such findings do not necessarily correlate with subsequent intellectual dysfunction and therefore may be inconsequential.[36] Treatment consists of active hydration to facilitate methotrexate renal clearance and administration of leucovorin to circumvent the enzyme inhibition of methotrexate.

It has been postulated that this toxicity arises from methotrexate-related impairment of synthesis of neurotransmitters and accumulation of adenosine and homocysteine.[37] Based on this hypothesis that the neurotoxicity is related to brain accumulation of adenosine, aminophylline (an adenosine receptor antagonist) has been used successfully to reverse the neurologic effects of methotrexate.[38]

PACLITAXEL AND DOCETAXEL

The two analogues paclitaxel and docetaxel cause neurotoxicity similar to that of cisplatin and vincristine in the form of a peripheral neuropathy that can be a treatment-limiting effect.[39,40] The clinical manifestations are glove-stocking or perioral paresthesias or burning pain, loss of vibration sense, loss of deep tendon reflexes, Lhermitte's sign, and orthostatic hypotension. Transient scintillating scotomata and visual deficits due to optic neuropathy, encephalopathy with confusion and behavioral changes, and motor dysfunction with both proximal and distal extremity weakness have also been observed.[41,42] However, it is not possible to determine how much taxane-associated myopathy might be due to the antitumor drug and how much to the intermittent, but large, doses of corticosteroids that are used concurrently with the taxanes to minimize the risk of hypersensitivity reactions. A possible risk factor for initiating or enhancing the neural dysfunction from these drugs is an underlying neuropathy from comorbid conditions such as diabetes mellitus and ethanol abuse. However, one study[43] has shown that patients with diabetes may be treated with standard doses of paclitaxel and do not develop neurotoxicity to a greater degree than expected.

For paclitaxel there is both a single dose and cumulative dose relationship. Single doses larger than 175 mg/m^2 given at 3-week intervals produce a higher rate of neurotoxicity than lesser doses, and at 250 mg/m^2 neurotoxicity is dose limiting in as many as 70% of patients.[39] When paclitaxel is given weekly in 1-hour infusions, severe neurotoxicity may occur at individual doses of more than 100 mg/m^2.[44] Cumulative dosing also increases the frequency of neurotoxicity, but there is no neurotoxic dose threshold. Depending on the paclitaxel dose used, the onset of these problems can be within a few days of receiving the first dose or after several cycles of therapy. A docetaxel dose of 100 mg/m^2 also induces mild to moderate neurotoxic symptoms in as many as 50% of patients after five cycles of therapy.[40] A cumulative docetaxel dose of 400 mg/m^2 can produce severe symptoms and electrophysiologic changes in nerves, but as with paclitaxel there is no threshold dose. Concurrent or prior use of other neurotoxic agents (cisplatin, vinorelbine, or oxaliplatin) enhances the risk and degree of neurotoxicity manifestations from both taxanes.[45–48] However, in the case of the cisplatin-paclitaxel combination, most of the neurotoxicity seems to be due to cisplatin.[48]

The mechanism of taxane neurotoxicity is likely a drug effect on neuronal microtubules, causing axonal degeneration and demyelination. Neurometric testing demonstrates decreased nerve conduction velocities and absent sural nerve action potentials after use of both taxanes.

The only effective treatment, as with the other neurotoxic antitumor agents, is discontinuing therapy and allowing the symptoms to wane over time (which they usually, but not always, do). Amitriptyline may or may not provide symptom relief. Because this toxicity is so prevalent and often dose limiting with these two potent antitumor agents, development of an efficacious neuroprotectant is a high priority. Amifostine has not demonstrated efficacy as a neurotoxicity protectant for paclitaxel.[49]

There is some evidence of a benefit from glutamine,[50] available in an over-the-counter preparation, but it has not been evaluated in double-blind, placebo-controlled fashion, the only reliable means of testing. Dimesna (BNP7787) is an agent undergoing clinical development as a protectant for both paclitaxel-induced and cisplatin-induced neurotoxicity.[12]

ALTRETAMINE (HEXAMETHYLMELAMINE)

Altretamine (hexamethylmelamine) causes a variety of peripheral and central nervous system toxicities. Peripheral neuropathy is the most common form and is manifested as paresthesias, hyperesthesia, hyporeflexia, and diminished proprioception.[51] Central nervous system effects are confusion, dysphagia, personality changes, ataxia, somnolence, seizures, respiratory dyskinesia, and parkinsonian tremors.

Neurotoxicity is related to both individual and cumulative doses. Intermittent dosing schedules help reduce this side effect. The incidence varies depending on the dose but can be as high as 40%. Altretamine can be safely administered to patients who have been treated previously with cisplatin, but if significant cisplatin neuropathy is present, the neurotoxic manifestations may worsen.

PROCARBAZINE

Neurotoxicity from procarbazine has been known since it was first used clinically 40 years ago. Both central and peripheral neurotoxicity symptoms can occur. Cerebral symptoms predominate and consist of lethargy, depression, confusion, hallucinations, agitation, and rarely psychosis. Extremity paresthesias and depressed deep tendon reflexes are the manifestations of peripheral neuropathy.

This agent is most commonly used in combination with the vinca alkaloids, so it is often difficult to determine which agent is causing peripheral neuropathy symptoms. The incidence of neuropathy induced by procarbazine alone is 20% or less, but it is much higher when procarbazine and vincristine are used concurrently. Treatment is discontinuation of therapy. Cerebral symptoms usually resolve promptly, but peripheral neuropathy may last for weeks to months.

ALDESLEUKIN (INTERLEUKIN-2)

Aldesleukin (interleukin-2) is a biologic antitumor agent that produces many toxicities precipitated by increased vascular permeability. Neurotoxicity in the form of hallucinations, disorientation, agitation, combativeness, seizures, and coma may occur.[52] A neurotoxic manifestation unique to this drug is carpal tunnel syndrome, which appears to be a consequence of vascular fluid leak and resultant edema that causes pressure on the median nerve.

INTERFERON-α

Chronic encephalopathic symptoms such as decreased short-term memory and attention span, depression, sleep disturbance, mania, bipolar syndrome, and incoordination are associated with long-term use of interferon-α, an immunomodulating agent.[53] The mood disorders may be minimized by concurrent administration of paroxetine or gabapentin.

TABLE 54.8-1. Antitumor Agents That Cause Neurotoxicity

HIGH POTENTIAL FOR NEUROTOXICITY

Altretamine	Interferons (in high	Procarbazine
L-Asparaginase	doses)	Thalidomide
Carboplatin	Ifosfamide	Tretinoin
Cisplatin	Methotrexate	Vinorelbine
Cytarabine	Oxaliplatin	Vincristine
Docetaxel	Paclitaxel	Vinblastine
5-Fluorouracil	Pentostatin	

OCCASIONAL IRREVERSIBLE NEUROTOXICITY

Cisplatin	5-Fluorouracil (with	Methotrexate
Cytarabine	levamisole)	(intrathecal)
Docetaxel	Ifosfamide	Paclitaxel

ISOLATED INSTANCES OF NEUROTOXICITY

Aldesleukin (inter-leukin-2)	Dacarbazine	Irinotecan
	Gemcitabine	Melphalan (in stem
Busulfan (in stem cell transplantation doses)	Etoposide (in stem cell transplantation doses)	cell transplantation doses)
		Pegaspargase
Chlorambucil	Interferons (in low doses)	Teniposide

FLUDARABINE, CLADRIBINE, AND PENTOSTATIN

When fludarabine was tested in phase I and II trials, central nervous system toxicity was so severe that the studies had to be closed prematurely. This toxicity was clearly dose related, and at the currently recommended dose neurotoxicity symptoms are uncommon and usually no more than mild.[54] A more severe form of neurologic illness associated with fludarabine is progressive multifocal leukoencephalopathy. However, this condition is related to infection with a human polyomavirus resulting from the immunosuppression effect of this drug, rather than from a direct neurotoxicity.

Cladribine and pentostatin both can cause severe, and fatal, neurotoxicity when administered at doses producing marked myelosuppression. The manifestations are similar to those of fludarabine.[54] However, like fludarabine, drug doses in the range recommended for usual therapy produce only rare instances of severe neurotoxicity.

OTHER AGENTS AND COMBINATION THERAPIES

Table 54.8-1 lists other antitumor drugs that can produce neurotoxicity and categorizes them regarding risk for this effect. The manifestations for drug combinations are similar to those described for the individual drugs. Certain ones (e.g., melphalan and busulfan) produce problems such as generalized seizures only when very high doses are administered in the stem cell transplantation setting.

Chronic cognitive abnormalities are becoming more recognized as long-term neurotoxicity phenomena in adult patients treated with combinations of various chemotherapeutic agents. Such problems only become evident in patients who have cancers curable by chemotherapy and who thus have a long expected survival.[55]

NEPHROTOXICITY

The kidneys are the elimination pathway of many antitumor drugs and their metabolites and are thus vulnerable to injury. The entire anatomic pathway from glomerulus to distal tubule is at risk, depending on the drug involved. The symptoms vary from an asymptomatic rise in serum creatinine level or mild proteinuria to acute renal failure with anuria requiring dialysis.

CISPLATIN AND CARBOPLATIN

The nephrotoxicity of cisplatin has been well known since it was first used clinically 35 years ago. This obstacle to its clinical use has been so profound that several thousand cisplatin analogues have been synthesized in hope of finding a less nephrotoxic compound with equivalent antitumor efficacy. A means of avoiding nephrotoxicity by forcing diuresis and enhancing cisplatin excretion has allowed safer use of this drug with its wide spectrum of antitumor efficacy.

Cisplatin renal toxicity is dose related, cumulative, and manifested primarily by a decrease in the glomerular filtration rate, which is clinically approximated by increases in the serum creatinine level and decreases in creatinine clearance. Single cisplatin doses of less than 50 mg/m^2 usually cause little renal injury, but higher doses require aggressive hydration or else abrupt, irreversible renal failure may ensue. Hydration reduces cisplatin concentration and the time it is in contact with the tubular epithelium, which helps limit the injurious effect of the drug on the tubules. The hydration used most successfully is normal saline because the high chloride level inhibits cisplatin hydrolysis in the tubules, which adds to the nephrotoxicity protection effect of diuresis. Mannitol is also used to enhance diuresis, but there is no evidence mannitol is necessary. Concurrent use of furosemide to enhance diuresis further is unnecessary. A urine output of at least 100 mL/h for 2 to 4 hours before and 4 to 6 hours after cisplatin doses of 50 to 75 mg/m^2 reduces, but does not eliminate, nephrotoxicity. More intensive hydration schedules are necessary when higher cisplatin doses are used.

The pathologic lesion of cisplatin nephrotoxicity occurs primarily in the proximal and distal tubules but also may involve the collecting ducts, whereas the glomeruli are unaffected. The extent of tubular injury helps explain why electrolyte abnormalities such as hyponatremia and hypomagnesemia are so common after cisplatin administration.[56] The hypomagnesemia is symptomatic only in approximately 10% of patients, but it can last months to years after completion of therapy. Symptoms of hyponatremia include confusion and orthostatic hypotension. Hypocalcemia may also occur, resulting in tetany. Magnesium supplementation in conjunction with cisplatin administration can minimize, but does not eliminate, hypomagnesemia.[57] The mechanism of the tubular injury is not fully understood. It is not simply the tubular handling of a heavy metal, because the *trans* isomer of cisplatin is not nephrotoxic. Cisplatin produces DNA intrastrand cross-links as one of its mechanisms of antitumor effect, and the same effect probably occurs on DNA in tubule cells, causing defects in tubular (especially proximal) resorption.

A variety of substances have been evaluated for minimizing cisplatin nephrotoxicity in the hope that the cumbersome process of hydration can be circumvented. These include sodium thiosulfate, amifostine, probenecid, diethyldithiocarbamate, superoxide dismutase, hypertonic saline, glutathione, bismuth compound, and mesna.[58] Only one of these many compounds, amifostine, has provided sufficient protective benefits to become accepted for routine use. Treatment with amifostine has demonstrated statistically significant protection against cisplatin-induced nephrotoxicity, while preserving the antitumor efficacy of cisplatin,[11] and the drug is marketed for this indication. However, amifostine has its own toxicities that can be an obstacle to convenient use, such as hypotension and nausea and vomiting. The most effective means of minimizing nephrotoxicity is to be certain renal function is normal, especially in patients older than 60 years, who may have unrecognized renal dysfunction. In addition, other renal tubular toxins, such as aminoglycoside antibiotics, should be avoided whenever possible to prevent additive tubular damage.

Carboplatin was synthesized as a cisplatin alternative with less nephrotoxicity and without the requirement of hydration for safe administration. It is definitely less nephrotoxic, but it is not free of potential for renal injury, especially when administered in high doses in the stem cell transplantation setting. Carboplatin-related renal dysfunction is usually detectable only by means of sensitive kidney function tests such as urine tubular enzyme excretion or glomerular filtration rate and is transient. The serum creatinine level and creatinine clearance are rarely affected.

Life-threatening hemolytic-uremic syndrome has been reported as a rare form of acute renal dysfunction related to cisplatin. Many of the reported instances have involved combined use of cisplatin and bleomycin, so it may be unclear which drug is most culpable in initiating this fulminant toxicity.

MITOMYCIN

The capacity of mitomycin to produce nephrotoxicity has been known for many years, and the effect can be life threatening. The clinical manifestations vary from a chronic, progressive rise in serum creatinine level to fulminant onset of microangiopathic hemolytic anemia (MAHA). The latter problem has been reported in a large number of anecdotal cases.[59]

The MAHA toxicity is related to cumulative dose, but as few as several mitomycin doses can initiate it. It also can develop a few months after mitomycin therapy has been discontinued. The risk of developing MAHA increases when the cumulative mitomycin dose exceeds 60 mg.[59]

The clinical presentation of MAHA is an abrupt and often severe hemolytic anemia that usually precedes the renal dysfunction by a week or two. The peripheral blood smear shows schistocytes, and thrombocytopenia becomes apparent as renal failure develops. Other manifestations are rash, fever, arterial hypertension, central neurologic dysfunction, pericarditis, interstitial pneumonitis, pulmonary hemorrhage, hematuria, and proteinuria.[59] A high percentage of patients (65%) have noncardiogenic pulmonary edema. A prominent feature is the fact that MAHA is often precipitated or worsened by blood transfusion, which suggests that blood product administration should be avoided as much as possible when treating patients using mitomycin. The outcome is often death (more than 50% of the time), despite vigorous treatment, although some long-term survivors (who have persistent mild renal dysfunction) have been observed.[59]

Treatment includes hemodialysis and plasmapheresis. The most successful treatment has been plasma perfusion over filters containing staphylococcal protein A, a method of extracting circulating immune complexes.[60]

The pathogenesis of this acute nephropathy is uncertain. Mitomycin produces glomerular endothelial damage in experimental animals, and increases in vascular endothelial cell markers in plasma have been observed in patients who developed MAHA related to mitomycin therapy.[61] This vascular injury probably activates platelets and leads to deposition of fibrin thrombi in the microvasculature of the kidney, which thus initiates renal dysfunction and a mechanical shearing of red cells with resultant hemolysis.

METHOTREXATE

When methotrexate is administered in conventional oral or intravenous doses, nephrotoxicity is only an occasional problem. If high doses with leucovorin rescue are used, acute nephrotoxicity can pose a greater danger.

Methotrexate is excreted rapidly in the urine whether it is administered orally or parenterally. Both parent compound and the major metabolite, 7-hydroxymethotrexate, are filtered by the glomeruli and actively secreted by the tubules. At physiologic pH the drug is fully ionized, but in acidified form (pH less than 5.7), the parent drug and main metabolite are less ionized and may precipitate. During urinary excretion, drug precipitation occurs as the urine is concentrated and acidified in the tubules. The solubility of 7-hydroxymethotrexate is only one-fourth that of the parent drug, which thus provides further potential for drug precipitation within tubules and resultant acute renal dysfunction.

Acute methotrexate nephrotoxicity produces abrupt renal insufficiency. The serum creatinine level rises rapidly, and costovertebral angle pain (from renal swelling) may occur. Dehydration, oliguria, and even anuria may develop.

Methotrexate-induced renal insufficiency is primarily a physical process of tubular drug precipitation. It can be largely prevented by methods designed to hinder this drug precipitation in the tubules: hydration and urine alkalinization.[62] Whenever a drug dose high enough to require leucovorin rescue is being given, the urine should be kept alkaline (pH higher than 8) with sodium bicarbonate administration, and a urine output of 100 mL/h should be maintained. Serial serum methotrexate levels should be monitored until the drug concentration declines to 10^{-8} mol/L or less, 24 to 48 hours after administration.[62]

If methotrexate clearance is impaired by renal dysfunction already present or initiated by concurrently administered drugs, nephrotoxicity can develop or be enhanced. For example, prior therapy with cisplatin may contribute to methotrexate nephrotoxicity by causing some subclinical renal impairment, and concurrent administration of nonsteroidal antiinflammatory drugs may engender serious, and even fatal, renal dysfunction from methotrexate. Indomethacin, ketoprofen, diclofenac, and naproxen all have been reported to intensify renal dysfunction from methotrexate, whether it is being given in high or low doses. This enhanced toxicity is probably mediated by a reduction in methotrexate clearance caused by the concurrent administration of these nonsteroidal antiinflammatory drugs.

Charcoal hemofiltration, oral cholestyramine, and hemodialysis all have been used to treat acute nephrotoxicity from high methotrexate doses. A highly successful therapy has been administration of a combination of thymidine, leucovorin, and the recombinant form of the bacterial enzyme carboxypeptidase G_2,[63] which quickly converts methotrexate to a harmless metabolite. Carboxypeptidase is available on a compassionate-use basis from the National Cancer Institute for treating this life-threatening toxicity in the United States,[63] and in other countries it is available from Protherics PLC in London (http://www.protherics.com). However, simple use of high doses of leucovorin has also been beneficial.[64]

STREPTOZOCIN, CARMUSTINE, AND LOMUSTINE

Streptozocin has the most potential for nephrotoxicity in the nitrosourea drug class, and renal damage is its dose-limiting toxicity.[65] Prolonged drug administration increases the risk of such toxicity, and most patients eventually show it if therapy continues.

The kidneys are the major excretion pathway for both the parent drug and its metabolites, which is the probable main factor in the pathogenesis of the nephrotoxicity. Streptozocin injury occurs in both the glomeruli and tubules (primarily proximal), in which histologic changes have been observed, but the mechanism is unknown. Hyperphosphatemia and proteinuria are early indicators of renal effect. Renal tubular acidosis is a frequent occurrence, manifested by glycosuria, acetonuria, hyperchloremia, and aminoaciduria.[65] If streptozocin is discontinued, these effects usually resolve. A rising serum creatinine level is a later, and sometimes irreversible, sign. Hydration and diuresis during therapy may minimize the renal dysfunction.

The other two nitrosoureas in wide clinical use [carmustine (BCNU) and lomustine (CCNU)] have negligible nephrotoxicity. BCNU usually causes interstitial pneumonitis toxicity, which necessitates cessation of therapy anyway, before it affects the kidneys, and CCNU has produced only rare instances of nephrotoxicity when unusually large cumulative doses have been administered.

IFOSFAMIDE

Cyclophosphamide and ifosfamide are analogues with similar chemical structures. Both produce the metabolite acrolein, which can cause hemorrhagic cystitis during urinary excretion. Despite their similarities in chemical structure, toxicity, and antitumor efficacy, they differ significantly in their ability to cause nephrotoxicity. Cyclophosphamide produces no renal toxicity of any clinical importance, whereas ifosfamide initiates a variety of renal abnormalities that may in some instances result in death or irreversible renal failure requiring chronic hemodialysis or renal transplantation, especially in children, who are at higher risk for this problem.[66] Hypotheses regarding the mechanism of ifosfamide nephrotoxicity and the reason cyclophosphamide does not have such an effect have been formulated based on the differences in metabolism of these two drugs (ifosfamide produces much more chloracetaldehyde) and the unique effect of ifosfamide on proximal renal tubule cells.[67]

Initial clinical studies of ifosfamide showed that single high doses could precipitate acute tubular necrosis and renal failure within a few days of administration. This severe toxicity was one reason a fractionated dose schedule was developed for this drug. Administration over five consecutive days reduced both renal and bladder toxicity, but the most effective measure for reducing urinary tract problems was the development of mesna as a means of protection against the drug-induced cystitis. Mesna is now a standard accompaniment to ifosfamide use, but

it limits the cystitis, *not* the nephrotoxicity. There is no known means of preventing ifosfamide renal toxicity.

The incidence of renal toxicity varies from 5% to 30%. In addition to young age (especially younger than 5 years), risk factors are drug dose (cumulative doses of more than 60 g/m^2), unilateral nephrectomy, prior renal irradiation, presence of retroperitoneal masses, and prior or concurrent cisplatin treatment (i.e., anything that has compromised renal function).[68] Clinical manifestations include tubular dysfunction, Fanconi's syndrome, and a rising serum creatinine level. The tubular injury is indicated by aminoaciduria, glycosuria, renal tubular acidosis, hypokalemia, proteinuria, and phosphaturia with hypophosphatemia. These abnormalities can even result in renal rickets and growth retardation in children and osteomalacia in adults, which require long-term therapy.[68] Once acute renal dysfunction from this drug becomes evident, it may or may not be reversible, so frequent monitoring of renal and tubular function during ifosfamide therapy is important so that treatment can be initiated promptly when dysfunction occurs. Progression to renal failure is generally not a problem in children,[68,69] but such progression may occur in adults, even with only moderate cumulative doses of ifosfamide. Renal abnormalities also may not become evident until long after ifosfamide therapy has been completed, and in children the manifestations of nephrotoxicity can still be present as long as a decade later.[70]

GEMCITABINE

The fluorine-substituted pyrimidine gemcitabine does not produce any meaningful acute or chronic nephrotoxicity, but it does have the capacity to precipitate acute manifestations of the hemolytic-uremic syndrome, which can be fatal.[71] The only predisposing risk factor for this condition is the duration of gemcitabine therapy. The median interval of treatment before onset was approximately 6 months in the largest reported series.[71]

OTHER AGENTS

Table 54.8-2 lists the antitumor agents that have been reported to cause renal injury. They are classified according to the risk of such toxicity, from those drugs with high risk for producing

TABLE 54.8-2. Antitumor Agents That Cause Nephrotoxicity

HIGH POTENTIAL FOR NEPHROTOXICITY	
Aldesleukin (interleukin-2)	Ifosfamide
Azacitidine	Methotrexate (in high doses)
Cisplatin	Mitomycin
Gallium nitrate	Streptozocin
AZOTEMIA WITHOUT NEPHROTOXICITY	
L-Asparaginase	Dacarbazine
OCCASIONAL IRREVERSIBLE NEPHROTOXICITY	
Cisplatin	Lomustine (CCNU)
Gallium nitrate	Mitomycin
Fludarabine	Pentostatin
Ifosfamide	Streptozocin
Interferons	
ISOLATED INSTANCES OF NEPHROTOXICITY	
Carboplatin	6-Mercaptopurine
Gemcitabine	Methotrexate (in low doses)

severe damage to those for which damage has been described in only an occasional anecdotal report.

HEPATOTOXICITY

A number of antitumor agents cause hepatic toxicity (Table 54.8-3). This toxicity takes three main forms: hepatocellular dysfunction and chemical hepatitis, venoocclusive disease (VOD), and chronic fibrosis.

HEPATOCELLULAR DYSFUNCTION

Hepatic injury manifesting as hepatocellular dysfunction is usually due to a direct effect of either the parent drug or a metabolite and is an acute event. Serum hepatic enzyme levels rise as cellular damage occurs. Steatosis and cholestasis may occur as the toxic effect progresses. Hepatic metastases, viral hepatitis, and drugs administered for other therapeutic purposes (e.g., antiemetics) can cause similar enzymatic abnormalities. Thus, the clinical picture, findings of appropriate laboratory and radiologic studies, and the pattern of abnormal results on liver function tests must be analyzed to identify the cause of the hepatic changes.

The drugs most likely to cause enzymatic abnormalities and rises in serum bilirubin level are L-asparaginase, BCNU in high doses, cytarabine, dactinomycin, etoposide, gemcitabine, 6-mercaptopurine, methotrexate in high doses, streptozocin, and vincristine.

L-Asparaginase causes the widest spectrum of liver abnormalities and is associated with the highest incidence of hepatotoxicity. It produces changes in liver enzymes and in hepatic protein synthesis, which results in low plasma levels of albumin, globulins, lipoproteins, and clotting factors. Prolongation of the prothrombin and thrombin times is one result. Acute hepatic failure has also been reported.[72] Fatty metamorphosis is commonly seen,[72] and these changes may persist for several months after discontinuing treatment.

Cytarabine hepatotoxicity is a common event in the treatment of acute leukemia, especially when high doses are used.[73]

TABLE 54.8-3. Antitumor Agents That Cause Hepatotoxicity

HIGH POTENTIAL FOR HEPATOTOXICITY	
L-Asparaginase	Interferons (in high doses)
Cytarabine	Methotrexate (long-term therapy)
Gemtuzumab ozogamicin	Streptozocin
HIGH POTENTIAL FOR HEPATOTOXICITY WITH HIGH DOSES	
Busulfan	Dactinomycin
Carmustine (BCNU)	Methotrexate
Cyclophosphamide	Mitomycin
Cytarabine	
OCCASIONAL IRREVERSIBLE HEPATOTOXICITY	
Busulfan (in high doses)	Gemcitabine
Carmustine (in high doses)	Methotrexate
Cytarabine	Mitomycin
Dacarbazine	
ISOLATED INSTANCES OF HEPATOTOXICITY	
Dacarbazine	6-Mercaptopurine
Chlorambucil	Pentostatin
Hydroxyurea	6-Thioguanine
Interferons (in low doses)	Vincristine

Patients with acute leukemia are subject to severe sepsis and transfusion-related hepatitis and receive a variety of potentially hepatotoxic drugs, so it is always difficult to isolate cytarabine as the sole hepatotoxin. However, hyperbilirubinemia developing in temporal relation to cytarabine administration, accompanied by histologic abnormalities in liver biopsy specimens, has confirmed the hepatotoxic potential of this drug.[73]

The agent 6-mercaptopurine has been known for over 40 years to cause hepatotoxicity, which in rare cases may even be fatal.[74] Intrahepatic cholestasis is the most common abnormality, and liver function usually returns to normal with discontinuation of therapy.

Hepatic dysfunction may occur in up to 10% of patients with Wilms' tumor treated with dactinomycin, but it is very uncommon when this drug is used for treatment of other malignancies. Hepatomegaly, enzyme abnormalities, and jaundice may occur.[75] Fever is also common, and thrombocytopenia may occur. Most cases appear to be associated with Wilms' tumors occurring in the right kidney, so the tumor mass effect present in the liver region may play a contributing role in this toxic manifestation.[76]

Acute and severe (even fatal) hepatocellular dysfunction has been reported in isolated instances from gemcitabine, pentostatin, thalidomide, raltitrexed, and chlorambucil.

VENOOCCLUSIVE DISEASE

VOD results from blockage of outflow in the small centrilobular and sublobular hepatic vessels. Antitumor drugs known to produce this form of hepatotoxicity are dactinomycin, cyclophosphamide, cytarabine, dacarbazine, 6-mercaptopurine, mitomycin, and 6-thioguanine. In addition, high doses of busulfan, BCNU, cyclophosphamide, and mitomycin given in the stem cell transplant setting can cause VOD. The combination of dactinomycin, vincristine, and moderately increased doses of cyclophosphamide has also been observed to cause VOD in children.[77]

The clinical features of VOD are painful hepatomegaly, ascites, peripheral edema, marked elevations in serum enzyme and bilirubin levels, and hepatic encephalopathy. The onset is often abrupt, occurring during the first week after transplantation, and the clinical course is fulminant. It is caused by damage to endothelial cells, sinusoids, and hepatocytes in the area of the liver surrounding the central vein.[78] Thrombosis is precipitated, causing ischemia and hepatocellular necrosis. There also may be a component of direct hepatocellular injury related to the high doses of drugs and not mediated by thrombosis. VOD occurring in the transplantation setting may be irreversible and lead to death with multiorgan failure in 20% to 65% of the patients developing it.[79] All the drugs reported to induce VOD at high doses have been alkylating agents. This situation may not be due to any unusual tendency of alkylating agents to cause VOD, but rather to the fact these are the drugs used in very large doses in the stem cell transplantation setting.

A drug with the capacity to produce hepatocellular dysfunction commonly[80] and VOD rarely[81] is the monoclonal antibody gemtuzumab ozogamicin. There may be a greater risk for the latter toxicity when the patient has previously undergone stem cell transplantation.

Conventional doses of certain antitumor agents (e.g., dacarbazine, gemcitabine, 6-mercaptopurine, and 6-thioguanine) have also been reported to initiate hepatic VOD in isolated cases. Why only sporadic patients develop this life-threatening complication is unknown. It may be some sort of idiosyncratic or hypersensitivity reaction.

CHRONIC FIBROSIS

Methotrexate used for cancer treatment can produce acute and reversible hepatocellular injury and elevation of serum enzyme levels that is only rarely a clinical problem requiring cessation of treatment.[82] The potential for acute hepatic toxicity is greater when high-dose methotrexate is being administered. Chronic hepatotoxicity from this drug in the oncologic setting is generally avoided by the use of intermittent dosing schedules. However, long-term use of methotrexate for the treatment of nonmalignant diseases (e.g., rheumatoid arthritis) poses a hazard for the development of irreversible hepatic fibrosis. Patients with autoimmune diseases may already have underlying liver abnormalities, so methotrexate may not be the sole etiologic factor in development of this chronic toxicity.

HYPERSENSITIVITY REACTIONS

Most of the available antitumor agents can produce hypersensitivity reactions, and as new agents are approved for marketing, sporadic reports of hypersensitivity to the new drug begin to appear in the medical literature. A substantial minority of the antitumor agents in use cause such reactions in 5% or more of patients treated. There are several drugs (e.g., L-asparaginase and the taxanes) for which hypersensitivity reactions are frequent enough to be a major treatment-limiting toxicity. Most of the other antitumor drugs produce such reactions only sporadically. The mechanism of these reactions is often unknown or evaluated only in a single patient. Premedication regimens designed to prevent or minimize reactions from the taxanes and a new formulation of L-asparaginase (pegaspargase) created to minimize reactions from this drug have been successful in reducing the frequency and the severity of this toxicity.

L-Asparaginase produces hypersensitivity reactions in 10% to 30% of patients treated, and the reactions can be immediate and life threatening with all the components of anaphylaxis. This high rate is related to the fact L-asparaginase is a polypeptide of bacterial origin, displaying multiple antigenic sites that can stimulate production of immunoglobulin E or other immunoglobulins. These immunoglobulins can then mediate an acute anaphylactic reaction.

The clinical manifestations are typical of type I hypersensitivity reactions with acute onset of agitation, wheezing, pruritus, extremity pain, rash, angioedema, and hypotension.[83] L-Asparaginase reactions appear to be mediated by an immunoglobulin E antibody in at least some cases. Complement activation also occurs, perhaps induced by specific immunoglobulin G or immunoglobulin M antibodies. A number of factors increase the risk for hypersensitivity reactions, including a history of atopy or other drug allergy, prior L-asparaginase therapy (including even several years previously), high drug doses, and intravenous administration of the drug. Intramuscular administration often reduces the severity of reactions, but they can still occur and may do so several hours after the drug is given. Concurrent treatment with prednisone and vincristine (for the

acute leukemia being treated) also appears to reduce the risk of reactions.

No reliable method has been found to identify who will have a reaction from any one dose of L-asparaginase. Intradermal skin testing may give either false-negative or false-positive results, and test doses of the drug are valueless. The development of L-asparaginase antibodies after repeated drug exposure is associated with a higher risk for reactions, and the greater the antibody concentration, the greater the risk. One must approach each dose of L-asparaginase as the one that could initiate a hypersensitivity reaction and be prepared to treat it. Antianaphylactic medication must be at hand, and the patient should be observed for approximately 1 hour after the drug is administered.

When a hypersensitivity reaction occurs to the *Escherichia coli* source of L-asparaginase, one can substitute the *Erwinia chrysanthemi* form. This drug form is immunologically distinct, and it may allow continued asparaginase therapy. Patients may still sustain a hypersensitivity reaction to the substitute; however, most (more than 75%) do not and can complete the planned therapy. *Erwinia* asparaginase has been used as part of the initial leukemia therapy, instead of the *E coli* version, but the antileukemia efficacy appears inferior, whereas allergy toxicity is identical.[84] Precautions for treating anaphylaxis are necessary no matter the origin of the L-asparaginase. A third form of L-asparaginase (pegaspargase) provides another alternative for the patient who is reactive to either of the other forms of asparaginase. This form is a conjugate of polyethylene glycol with the enzyme.[85] It may be the least immunogenic of all three forms of this drug, but hypersensitivity reactions are still possible.

Paclitaxel has a high potential for initiating hypersensitivity reactions, and because of this fact, it is necessary to administer prophylaxis therapy before each dose.[86] The Cremophor EL excipient used to maintain solubility of paclitaxel has long been suspected of being the initiator of these reactions. When docetaxel was first evaluated in clinical trials, it was assumed that premedication to prevent hypersensitivity reactions was unnecessary, because docetaxel is formulated with Tween 80 (instead of Cremophor EL), and thus reactions would be unlikely to occur. This assumption proved incorrect, because docetaxel can initiate hypersensitivity reactions with the same manifestations and with approximately the same frequency (5%) as paclitaxel.[87] The signs and symptoms can occur despite premedication with antihistamines and corticosteroids in adequate doses.

Either the cause of such reactions is the two taxanes themselves or Cremophor EL and Tween 80 are equally capable of causing reactions. One patient who reacted to paclitaxel also reacted to docetaxel used as a substitute,[88] so at least in this instance the reactant was the taxane rather than the excipient. Although uncertainty remains regarding which component of these drugs causes the reactions, a taxane that is free of Cremophor EL has been developed that appears not to produce hypersensitivity reactions and does not require corticosteroid premedication.[89] The mechanism of such reactions to the taxanes has not been well studied. Although a few reported cases of hypersensitivity reactions have occurred in later drug cycles, the fact that they occur most often with the first taxane dose[86,87] suggests a nonimmunologic mechanism.

The clinical manifestations are those of any type I hypersensitivity reaction and include bronchospasm and wheezing, agitation, chest and back pain, rash, angioedema, and hypotension. The onset is usually within a few minutes of starting a drug infusion, and even very small drug doses are capable of initiating a reaction. Another manifestation of apparent hypersensitivity is pulmonary infiltrates typical of a hypersensitivity pneumonitis that may resolve either spontaneously or after corticosteroid therapy.[90]

To prevent or assuage the hypersensitivity reactions, paclitaxel is usually infused over 1 to 3 hours. Infusion over any interval shorter than 1 hour may precipitate an unacceptable frequency of reactions.[91] Premedication with corticosteroids and antihistamines is standard procedure. Docetaxel is given over 1 hour, and premedications must also be used. Such measures reduce the frequency and perhaps the intensity of reactions but do not fully prevent them. If the patient does not experience a reaction after the first dose of a taxane, it may be possible to cease further use of premedications and minimize the side effects of the corticosteroids, especially during taxane therapy given weekly.[92]

In contrast to L-asparaginase and the taxanes, hypersensitivity reactions from carboplatin rarely occur before a number of doses (a reported median of ten) have been administered.[93] The incidence of hypersensitivity reactions from this agent has been reported to be as high as 12% in patients with ovarian cancer,[93] for whom prolonged treatment with platinum agents is common. Desensitization may be successful and allow further carboplatin administration after a hypersensitivity reaction has occurred.[94] Oxaliplatin is also known to produce hypersensitivity reactions after a number of doses (again, a median of approximately ten) at a rate of slightly over 10%.[95]

Many other chemotherapeutic agents (Table 54.8-4) are known to produce hypersensitivity reactions in at least sporadic instances. Most of these reactions have the features of a type I hypersensitivity, whether mediated by immunoglobulin E or due to nonimmunologic causes. Hemolytic anemia (a type II reaction) is an uncommon form of such toxicity. Some drugs, such as methotrexate, can produce acute episodes that are typical of a type III reaction and cause interstitial pneumonitis and vasculitis.

TABLE 54.8-4. Antitumor Agents That Cause Hypersensitivity Reactions

HIGH POTENTIAL FOR HYPERSENSITIVITY REACTIONS EARLY IN TREATMENT

L-Asparaginase	Paclitaxel
Docetaxel	Teniposide

HIGH POTENTIAL FOR HYPERSENSITIVITY REACTIONS LATE IN TREATMENT

Carboplatin	Oxaliplatin

OCCASIONAL INSTANCES OF HYPERSENSITIVITY REACTIONS

Anthracyclines	Cytarabine	Melphalan
Aldesleukin (interleukin-2)	Dacarbazine	6-Mercaptopurine
Bleomycin	Etoposide	Methotrexate
Capecitabine	Fludarabine	Mitomycin
Carboplatin	5-Fluorouracil	Mitoxantrone
Chlorambucil	Hydroxyurea	Pegaspargase
Cisplatin	Ifosfamide	Pentostatin
Cyclophosphamide	Interferons	Procarbazine
	Mechlorethamine	Vinca alkaloids

In most instances of hypersensitivity reaction to antitumor drugs, only isolated cases are studied adequately to define the cause of the reaction, and it is not possible to exclude the excipients used in drug formulation (e.g., benzyl alcohol, dimethyl acetamide) or other drugs given concurrently (e.g., mesna, mannitol, white cell growth factors, antiemetics, amifostine, and even corticosteroids) as the source of the reactivity. When hypersensitivity reactions occur from one drug, it is often possible to continue therapy by either substituting another drug in the same class or by premedication with prophylactic agents.

VASCULAR TOXICITY

Five main forms of vascular toxicity can be produced by anticancer agents: VOD, thrombotic microangiopathy with hemolytic-uremic syndrome, venous or arterial thrombosis, vascular ischemia (involving cerebral, myocardial, or extremity arterial vessels), and bleeding (a recent addition to this list with the development of antiangiogenic agents). VOD of hepatic vessels is discussed in the section Hepatotoxicity, and microangiopathy is discussed in the section Nephrotoxicity: Mitomycin.

Venous thrombosis in association with metastatic cancer has long been recognized (Trousseau's syndrome). Irinotecan is one drug that may potentiate the tendency for venous thromboses to develop in the presence of metastatic tumor.[96] Antitumor agents can also induce venous thrombosis in the form of pulmonary emboli and extremity thromboses, even in the absence of demonstrable metastatic cancer.[97,98] Although they are less common, thromboses of cerebral, coronary, and extremity arteries can also be initiated by chemotherapy, again in the absence of demonstrable cancer.[99] These events are not limited to one form of cancer. They have occurred in a variety of cancers as disparate as early-stage breast cancer, testicular cancer, and lymphomas. One drug associated, more than others, with such thrombotic episodes is cisplatin,[100] and a combination of chemotherapy with tamoxifen can produce a higher rate of such thrombotic episodes than either treatment alone.[98] Thalidomide given in conjunction with chemotherapy also contributes to a risk of venous thromboses.[101] Arterial ischemia without thrombosis can be induced by chemotherapy in major coronary or cerebral vessels and in the small vessels of the extremities. Myocardial ischemia and infarction may occur in patients who receive continuous infusions of 5-FU, and precipitous heart failure and sudden death have been reported.[102] Such events may occur in patients who have no known underlying coronary vessel disease and develop a few days after the start of the first infusion of 5-FU. The pathogenesis seems to be 5-FU induction of coronary spasm, but the physiologic mechanism is not known. Anginal symptoms are often a precursor and can be relieved by discontinuing the 5-FU therapy. Transient ischemic attacks of cerebral vessels may occur from cisplatin, which may be a vasospastic phenomenon related to electrolyte disturbance from the renal effects of this drug.[103]

Raynaud's phenomenon occurs as a chronic toxicity in approximately 40% of young men treated with cisplatin-bleomycin regimens for testicular cancer.[104] Cigarette smoking increases the risk for this toxicity. Clinical manifestations are painful digits and paresthesias, which may last indefinitely years after the chemotherapy is completed. The mechanism appears to be vasospasm, without thrombosis, in the terminal arterioles of the fingers due to impaired smooth muscle function. Whether this problem is related to the cisplatin or bleomycin (or both) used in treating testicular cancer is uncertain, because such events have been reported in isolated cases in which the patient received only one of these agents. A continuous infusion of 5-FU may also engender digital arterial spasm and Raynaud's phenomenon, similar to the vasospasm it can cause in coronary arteries.[105]

With the advent of antiangiogenesis agents, a new vascular toxicity of anticancer therapy has become evident in the form of bleeding diathesis. This toxicity is presumably due to drug effects on microscopic blood vessels. The bleeding may be minor in the form of transient epistaxis or major with gastrointestinal hemorrhage.[106] In opposite fashion one such agent, bevacizumab, may also contribute to the development of thrombotic episodes in conjunction with chemotherapy.[106]

REFERENCES

1. Pal PK. Clinical and electrophysiological studies in vincristine-induced neuropathy. *Electromyogr Clin Neurophysiol* 1999;39:323.
2. Haim N, Epelbaum R, Ben-Shahar M, et al. Full dose vincristine (without 2-mg dose limit) in the treatment of lymphomas. *Cancer* 1994;73:2515.
3. Lonardi F, Pavanato G, Ferrari V, et al. Neurotoxicity after chemotherapy with vinorelbine. *Eur J Cancer* 1993;29A:1794.
4. Le Chevalier T, Brisgand D, Douillard J-Y, et al. Randomized study of vinorelbine and cisplatin versus vindesine and cisplatin versus vinorelbine alone in advanced non–small-cell lung cancer: results of a European multicenter trial including 612 patients. *J Clin Oncol* 1994;12:360.
5. Fazeny B, Zifki U, Meryn S, et al. Vinorelbine-induced neurotoxicity in patients with advanced breast cancer pretreated with paclitaxel—a phase II study. *Cancer Chemother Pharmacol* 1996;39:150.
6. Weintraub M, Adde MA, Venzon DJ, et al. Severe atypical neuropathy associated with administration of hematopoietic colony-stimulating factors and vincristine. *J Clin Oncol* 1996;14:935.
7. Cersosimo RJ. Cisplatin neurotoxicity. *Cancer Treat Rev* 1989;16:195.
8. Gregg RW, Molepo JM, Monpetit VJA, et al. Cisplatin neurotoxicity: the relationship between dosage, time, and platinum concentration in neurologic tissues, and morphologic evidence of toxicity. *J Clin Oncol* 1992;10:795.
9. Gietema JA, Meinardi MT, Messerschmidt J, et al. Circulating plasma platinum more than 10 years after cisplatin treatment for testicular cancer. *Lancet* 2000;355:1075.
10. Cavaletti G, Zanna C. Current status and future prospects for the treatment of chemotherapy-induced peripheral neurotoxicity. *Eur J Cancer* 2002;38:1832.
11. Kemp G, Rose P, Lurain J, et al. Amifostine pretreatment for protection against cyclophosphamide-induced and cisplatin-induced toxicities: results of a randomized control trial in patients with advanced ovarian cancer. *J Clin Oncol* 1996;14:2101.
12. Verschraagen M, Boven E, Ruijter R, et al. Pharmacokinetics and preliminary clinical data of the novel chemoprotectant BNP7787 and cisplatin and their metabolites. *Clin Pharmacol* 2003;74:157.
13. Pace A, Savarese A, Picardo M, et al. Neuroprotective effect of vitamin E supplementation in patients treated with cisplatin chemotherapy. *J Clin Oncol* 2003;21:927.
14. Berger T, Malayeri R, Doppelbauer A, et al. Neurological monitoring of neurotoxicity induced by paclitaxel/cisplatin chemotherapy. *Eur J Cancer* 1997;33:1393.
15. Grothey A. Oxaliplatin—safety profile: neurotoxicity. *Semin Oncol* 2003;30(4 Suppl 15):5.
16. Cascinu S, Catalano V, Cordella L, et al. Neuroprotective effect of reduced glutathione on oxaliplatin-based chemotherapy in advanced colorectal cancer: a randomized, double-blind, placebo-controlled trial. *J Clin Oncol* 2002;20:3478.
17. Bastuji-Garin S, Ochonisky S, Bouche P, et al. Incidence and risk factors for thalidomide neuropathy: a prospective study of 135 dermatologic patients. *J Invest Dermatol* 2002;119:1020.
18. Chaudhry V, Cornblath DR, Corse A, et al. Thalidomide-induced neuropathy. *Neurology* 2002;59:1872.
19. Baker WJ, Royer GL, Weiss RB. Cytarabine and neurologic toxicity. *J Clin Oncol* 1991;9:679.
20. Glantz MJ, Jaeckle KA, Chamberlain MC, et al. A randomized controlled trial comparing intrathecal sustained-release cytarabine (DepoCyt) to intrathecal methotrexate in patients with neoplastic meningitis from solid tumors. *Clin Cancer Res* 1999;5:3394.
21. Miller L, Link MP, Bologna S, Parker BR. Cerebellar atrophy caused by high-dose cytosine arabinoside: CT and MR findings. *AJR Am J Roentgenol* 1989;152:343.
22. Wallace TL, Johnson EM. Cytosine arabinoside kills postmitotic neurons: evidence that deoxycytidine may have a role in neuronal survival that is independent of DNA synthesis. *J Neurosci* 1989;9:115.
23. Weiss RB. Ifosfamide vs cyclophosphamide in cancer therapy. *Oncology (Huntingt)* 1991;5:67.
24. Merimsky O, Inbar M, Reider-Grosswasser I, Scharf M, Chaitchik S. Ifosfamide-related acute encephalopathy: clinical and radiological aspects. *Eur J Cancer* 1991;27:1188.
25. Chatton J-Y, Idle JR, Vågbø CB, Magistretti PJ. Insights into the mechanisms of ifosfamide encephalopathy: drug metabolites have agonistic effects on α-amino-3-hydroxy-5-methyl-4-isoxazolepropionic acid (AMPA)/kainate receptors and induce cellular acidification in mouse cortical neurons. *J Pharmacol Exp Ther* 2001;299:1161.
26. Kupfer A, Aeschlimann C, Wermuth B, Cerny T. Prophylaxis and reversal of ifosfamide encephalopathy with methylene-blue. *Lancet* 1994;343:763.
27. Buesa JM, García-Teijido P, Losa R, Fra J. Treatment of ifosfamide encephalopathy with intravenous thiamin. *Clin Cancer Res* 2003;9:4636.
28. Bygrave HA, Geh JI, Jani Y, Glynne-Jones R. Neurological complications of 5-fluorouracil chemotherapy: case report and review of the literature. *Clin Oncol (R Coll Radiol)* 1998;10:343.
29. Pirzada NA, Ali II, Dafer RM. Fluorouracil-induced neurotoxicity. *Ann Pharmacother* 2000;34:35.
30. Meropol NJ, Creaven PJ, Petrelli NJ, White RM, Arbuck SG. Seizures associated with leucovorin administration in cancer patients. *J Natl Cancer Inst* 1995;87:56.
31. Okeda R, Shibutani M, Matsuo T, et al. Experimental neurotoxicity of 5-fluorouracil and its derivatives is due to poisoning by the monofluorinated organic metabolites, monofluoroacetic acid and α-fluoro-β-alanine. *Acta Neuropathol* 1990;81:66.
32. Milano G, Etienne MC, Vierrefate V, et al. Dihydropyrimidine dehydrogenase deficiency and fluorouracil-related toxicity. *Br J Cancer* 1999;79:627.
33. Rubnitz JE, Relling MV, Harrison PL, et al. Transient encephalopathy following high-dose methotrexate treatment in childhood acute lymphoblastic leukemia. *Leukemia* 1998;12:1176.
34. Mahoney DH, Shuster JJ, Nitschke R, et al. Acute neurotoxicity in children with B-precursor acute lymphoid leukemia: an association with intermediate-dose intravenous methotrexate and intrathecal triple therapy—a Pediatric Oncology Group study. *J Clin Oncol* 1998;16:1712.
35. Iuvone L, Mariotti P, Colosimo C, et al. Long-term cognitive outcome, brain computed tomography scan, and magnetic resonance imaging in children cured of acute lymphoblastic leukemia. *Cancer* 2002;95:2562.
36. Bleyer WA. Leukoencephalopathy detectable by magnetic resonance imaging: much ado about nothing? *Int J Radiat Oncol Biol Phys* 1995;32:1251.
37. Quinn CT, Griener JC, Bottiglieri T, et al. Elevation of homocysteine and excitatory amino acid neurotransmitters in the CSF of children who receive methotrexate for the treatment of cancer. *J Clin Oncol* 1997;15:2800.
38. Peyriere H, Poiree M, Cociglio M, et al. Reversal of neurologic disturbances related to high-dose methotrexate by aminophylline. *Med Pediatr Oncol* 2001;36:662.
39. Postma TJ, Vermoken JB, Liefting AJM, Pinedo HM, Heimans JJ. Paclitaxel-induced neuropathy. *Ann Oncol* 1995;6:489.
40. Hilkens PHE, Verweij J, Vecht CJ, Stoter G, van den Bent MJ. Clinical characteristics of severe peripheral neuropathy induced by docetaxel (Taxotere). *Ann Oncol* 1997;8:187.
41. Ziske CG, Schöttker B, Gorschlüter M, et al. Acute transient encephalopathy after paclitaxel infusion: report of three cases. *Ann Oncol* 2002;13:629.
42. Freilich RJ, Balmaceda C, Seidman AD, Rubin M, DeAngelis LM. Motor neuropathy due to docetaxel and paclitaxel. *Neurology* 1996;47:115.
43. Gogas H, Shapiro F, Aghajanian C, et al. The impact of diabetes mellitus on the toxicity of therapy for advanced ovarian cancer. *Gynecol Oncol* 1996;61:22.
44. Seidman AD, Hudis CA, Albanel J, et al. Dose-dense therapy with weekly 1-hour paclitaxel infusions in the treatment of metastatic breast cancer. *J Clin Oncol* 1998;16:3353.
45. Parimoo D, Jeffers S, Muggia FM. Severe neurotoxicity from vinorelbine-paclitaxel combinations. *J Natl Cancer Inst* 1996;88:1079.
46. Faivre S, Kalla S, Cvitkovic E, et al. Oxaliplatin and paclitaxel combination in patients with platinum-pretreated ovarian carcinoma: an investigator-originated compassionate-use experience. *Ann Oncol* 1999;10:1125.
47. Hilkens PHE, Pronk LC, Verweij J, et al. Peripheral neuropathy induced by combination chemotherapy of docetaxel and cisplatin. *Br J Cancer* 1997;75:417.
48. Cavaletti G, Bogliun G, Crespi V, et al. Neurotoxicity and ototoxicity of cisplatin plus paclitaxel in comparison to cisplatin plus cyclophosphamide in patients with epithelial ovarian cancer. *J Clin Oncol* 1997;15:199.
49. Gelman K, Eisenhauer E, Bryce C, et al. Randomized phase II study of high-dose paclitaxel with or without amifostine in patients with metastatic breast cancer. *J Clin Oncol* 1999;17:3038.
50. Vahdat L, Papadopoulos K, Lange D, et al. Reduction of paclitaxel-induced peripheral neuropathy with glutamine. *Clin Cancer Res* 2001;7:1192.
51. Weiss RB. The role of hexamethylmelamine in advanced ovarian carcinoma treatment. *Gynecol Oncol* 1981;12:141.
52. Siegel JP, Puri RK. Interleukin-2 toxicity. *J Clin Oncol* 1991;9:694.
53. Kirkwood JM, Bender C, Agarwala S, et al. Mechanisms and management of toxicities associated with high-dose interferon alfa-2b therapy. *J Clin Oncol* 2002;20:3703.
54. Cheson BD, Vena DA, Foss FM, Sorenson JM. Neurotoxicity of purine analogs: a review. *J Clin Oncol* 1994;12:2216.
55. Ahles TA, Saykin AJ, Furstenberg CT, et al. Neuropsychologic impact of standard-dose systemic chemotherapy in long-term survivors of breast cancer and lymphoma. *J Clin Oncol* 2002;20:485.
56. Lajer H, Daugaard G. Cisplatin and hypomagnesemia. *Cancer Treat Rev* 1999;25:47.
57. Evans TRJ, Harper CL, Beveridge IG, Wastnage R, Mansi JL. A randomized study to determine whether routine intravenous magnesium supplements are necessary in patients receiving cisplatin chemotherapy with continuous infusion 5-fluorouracil. *Eur J Cancer* 1995;31A:174.
58. Pinzani V, Bressolle F, Haug IJ, et al. Cisplatin-induced renal toxicity and toxicity-modulating strategies: a review. *Cancer Chemother Pharmacol* 1994;35:1.
59. Lesesne JB, Rothschild N, Erickson B, et al. Cancer-associated hemolytic-uremic syndrome: analysis of 85 cases from a national registry. *J Clin Oncol* 1989;7:781.
60. Snyder HW, Mittelman A, Oral A, et al. Treatment of cancer chemotherapy-associated thrombotic thrombocytopenic purpura/hemolytic uremic syndrome by protein A immunoadsorption of plasma. *Cancer* 1993;71:1882.

61. Nagaya S, Wada H, Oka K, et al. Hemostatic abnormalities and increased vascular endothelial cell markers in patients with red cell fragmentation syndrome induced by mitomycin C. *Am J Hematol* 1995;50:237.

62. Ackland SP, Schilsky RL. High-dose methotrexate: a critical reappraisal. *J Clin Oncol* 1987;5:2017.

63. Widemann BC, Balis FM, Murphy RF, et al. Carboxypeptidase-G$_2$, thymidine, and leucovorin rescue in cancer patients with methotrexate-induced renal dysfunction. *J Clin Oncol* 1997;15:2125.

64. Flombaum CD, Meyers PA. High-dose leucovorin as sole therapy for methotrexate toxicity. *J Clin Oncol* 1999;17:1589.

65. Weiss RB. Streptozocin: a review of its pharmacology, efficacy, and toxicity. *Cancer Treat Rep* 1982;66:427.

66. Loebstein R, Atanackovic G, Bishai R, et al. Risk factors for long-term outcome of ifosfamide-induced nephrotoxicity in children. *J Clin Pharmacol* 1999;39:454.

67. Rossi R. Nephrotoxicity of ifosfamide—moving towards understanding the molecular mechanisms. *Nephrol Dial Transplant* 1997;12:1091.

68. Marina NM, Poquette CA, Cain AM, et al. Comparative renal tubular toxicity of chemotherapy regimens including ifosfamide in patients with newly diagnosed sarcomas. *J Pediatr Hematol Oncol* 2000;22:112.

69. Rossi R, Pleyer J, Schafers P, et al. Development of ifosfamide-induced nephrotoxicity: prospective follow-up in 75 patients. *Med Pediatr Oncol* 1999;32:177.

70. Skinner R. Chronic ifosfamide nephrotoxicity in children. *Med Pediatr Oncol* 2003;41:190.

71. Fung MC, Storniolo AM, Nguyen B, et al. A review of hemolytic uremic syndrome in patients treated with gemcitabine therapy. *Cancer* 1999;85:2023.

72. Sahoo S, Hart J. Histopathological features of L-asparaginase-induced liver disease. *Semin Liver Dis* 2003;23:295.

73. Pizzuto J, Aviles A, Ramos E, Cervera J, Aguirre J. Cytosine arabinoside induced liver damage: histopathologic demonstration. *Med Pediatr Oncol* 1983;11:287.

74. Laidlaw ST, Reilly JT, Suvarna SK. Fatal heptotoxicity associated with 6-mercaptopurine therapy. *Br J Haematol* 1999;105:316.

75. Raine J, Bowman A, Wallendszus K, Pritchard J. Hepatopathy-thrombocytopenia syndrome—a complication of dactinomycin therapy for Wilms' tumor: a report from the United Kingdom Childrens Cancer Study Group. *J Clin Oncol* 1991;9:268.

76. Davidson A, Pritchard J. Actinomycin D, hepatic toxicity, and Wilms' tumor—a mystery explained? *Eur J Cancer* 1998;34:1145.

77. Ortega JA, Donaldson SS, Ivy SP, et al. Venoocclusive disease of the liver after chemotherapy with vincristine, actinomycin D, and cyclophosphamide for the treatment of rhabdomyosarcoma. A report of the Intergroup Rhabdomyosarcoma Study Group. *Cancer* 1997;79:2435.

78. Bearman SI. Avoiding hepatic veno-occlusive disease: what do we know and where are we going? *Bone Marrow Transplant* 2001;27:1113.

79. Carreras E, Bertz H, Arcese W, et al. Incidence and outcome of hepatic veno-occlusive disease after blood or marrow transplantation: a prospective cohort study of the European Group for Blood and Marrow Transplantation. *Blood* 1998;92:3599.

80. Sievers EL, Larson RA, Stadtmauer EA, et al. Efficacy and safety of gemtuzumab ozogamicin in patients with CD33-positive acute myeloid leukemia in first relapse. *J Clin Oncol* 2001;19:3244.

81. Cohen AD, Luger SM, Sickles C, et al. Gemtuzumab ozogamicin (Mylotarg) monotherapy for relapsed AML after hematopoietic stem cell transplant: efficacy and incidence of hepatic veno-occlusive disease. *Bone Marrow Transplant* 2002;30:23.

82. van Outryve S, Schrijvers D, van den Brande J, et al. Methotrexate-associated liver toxicity in a patient with breast cancer: case report and literature review. *Neth J Med* 2002;60:216.

83. Woo MH, Hak LJ, Storm MC, et al. Hypersensitivity or development of antibodies to asparaginase does not impact treatment outcome of childhood acute lymphoblastic leukemia. *J Clin Oncol* 2000;18:1525.

84. Duval M, Suciu S, Ferster A, et al. Comparison of *Escherichia coli*-asparaginase with *Erwinia*-asparaginase in the treatment of childhood lymphoid malignancies: results of a randomized European Organization for Research and Treatment of Cancer—Children's Leukemia Group phase 3 trial. *Blood* 2002;99:2734.

85. Ettinger LJ, Kurtzberg J, Voute PA, Jürgens H, Halpern SL. An open-label, multicenter study of polyethylene glycol-L-asparaginase for the treatment of acute lymphoblastic leukemia. *Cancer* 1995;75:1176.

86. Weiss RB, Donehower RH, Wiernik PH, et al. Hypersensitivity reactions from taxol. *J Clin Oncol* 1990;8:1263.

87. Tyson LB, Kris MG, Corso DM, Choy E, Timoney JP. Incidence, course, and severity of taxoid-induced hypersensitivity reaction in 646 oncology patients. *Proc Am Soc Clin Oncol* 1999;18:585a.

88. Denman JP, Gilbar PJ, Abdi EA. Hypersensitivity reaction (HSR) to docetaxel after a previous HSR to paclitaxel. *J Clin Oncol* 2002;20:2760.

89. Ibrahim NK, Desai N, Legha S, et al. Phase I and pharmacokinetic study of ABI-007, a Cremophor-free, protein-stabilized, nanoparticle formulation of paclitaxel. *Clin Cancer Res* 2002;8:1038.

90. Khan A, McNally D, Tutschka PJ, Bilgrami S. Paclitaxel-induced acute bilateral pneumonitis. *Ann Pharmacother* 1997;31:1471.

91. Tsavaris NB, Kosmas C. Risk of severe acute hypersensitivity reactions after rapid paclitaxel infusion of less than 1-h duration. *Cancer Chemother Pharmacol* 1998;42:509.

92. Quock J, Dea G, Tanaka M, et al. Premedication strategy for weekly paclitaxel. *Cancer Invest* 2002;20:666.

93. Markman M, Kennedy A, Webster K, et al. Clinical features of hypersensitivity reactions to carboplatin. *J Clin Oncol* 1999;17:1141.

94. Rose PG, Fusco N, Smrekar M, Mossbruger K, Rodriguez M. Successful administration of carboplatin in patients with clinically documented carboplatin hypersensitivity. *Gynecol Oncol* 2003;89:429.

95. Brandi G, Pantaleo MA, Galli C, et al. Hypersensitivity reactions related to oxaliplatin (OHP). *Br J Cancer* 2003;89:477.

96. Rothenberg ML, Meropol NJ, Poplin EA, Van Cutsem E, Wadler S. Mortality associated with irinotecan plus bolus fluorouracil/leucovorin: summary findings of an independent panel. *J Clin Oncol* 2001;19:3801.

97. Weiss RB, Tormey DC, Holland JF, Weinberg VE. Venous thrombosis during multimodal therapy of primary breast carcinoma. *Cancer Treat Rep* 1981;65:677.

98. Pritchard KI, Paterson AHG, Paul NA, et al. Increased thromboembolic complications with concurrent tamoxifen and chemotherapy in a randomized trial of adjuvant therapy for women with breast cancer. *J Clin Oncol* 1996;14:2731.

99. Wall JG, Weiss RB, Norton L, et al. Arterial thrombosis associated with adjuvant chemotherapy for breast carcinoma: a Cancer and Leukemia Group B study. *Am J Med* 1989;87:501.

100. Czaykowski PM, Moore MJ, Tannock IF. High risk of vascular events in patients with urothelial transitional cell carcinoma treated with cisplatin based chemotherapy. *J Urol* 1998;160:2021.

101. Zangaro M, Siegel E, Barlogie B, et al. Thrombogenic activity of doxorubicin in myeloma patients receiving thalidomide: implications for therapy. *Blood* 2002;100:1168.

102. Meyer CC, Calis KA, Burke LB, Walawander CA, Grasela TH. Symptomatic cardiotoxicity associated with 5-fluorouracil. *Pharmacotherapy* 1997;17:729.

103. King M, Fernando I. Vascular toxicity associated with cisplatin. *Clin Oncol (R Coll Radiol)* 2003;15:36.

104. Berger CC, Bokemeyer C, Schneider M, Kuczyk MA, Schmoll H-J. Secondary Raynaud's phenomenon and other late vascular complications following chemotherapy for testicular cancer. *Eur J Cancer* 1995;31A:2229.

105. Papamichael D, Amft N, Slevin ML, D'Cruz D. 5-fluorouracil-induced Raynaud's phenomenon. *Eur J Cancer* 1998;34:1983.

106. Kabbinavar F, Hurwitz HI, Fehrenbacher L, et al. Phase II, randomized trial comparing bevacizumab plus fluorouracil (FU)/leucovorin (LV) with FU/LV alone in patients with metastatic colorectal cancer. *J Clin Oncol* 2003;21:60.

CHAPTER 55

Supportive Care and Quality of Life

SECTION **1**

KATHLEEN M. FOLEY

Management of Cancer Pain

Advances in the diagnosis and treatment of cancer, coupled with advances in understanding of the anatomy, physiology, pharmacology, and psychology of pain perception, have led to improved care of the patient with pain of malignant origin.[1] Specialized methods of cancer diagnosis and treatment provide the most direct approach to treating cancer pain by treating the cause of the pain. However, before the introduction of successful antitumor therapy, when treatment of the cause of the pain has failed, or when injury to bone, soft tissue, or nerve has occurred as a result of therapy, appropriate pain management is essential. Patients with cancer are managed most effectively by a multidisciplinary approach that draws on the expertise of a wide range of health care professionals. The goal of pain therapy for patients receiving active treatment is to provide them with sufficient relief to tolerate the diagnostic and therapeutic approaches required to treat their cancer. For patients with advanced disease, pain control should be sufficient to allow them to function at a level they choose and to die relatively free of pain.[2] The management of the symptom of pain is only one component of a broad palliative care approach for cancer patients.[3] Control of other symptoms, treatment of psychological distress, and attention to the religious, spiritual, and existential dimensions of the patient's illness experience should be concurrently addressed to maintain the patient's quality of life throughout the cancer illness course from diagnosis to death.

EPIDEMIOLOGY

Existing studies based on numerous national and international surveys and World Health Organization (WHO) estimates suggest that moderate to severe pain is experienced by one-third of cancer patients receiving active therapy and by 60% to 90% of patients with advanced disease.[3–9] There are 17 million new cases of cancer diagnosed worldwide each year and 5 million cancer deaths, which account for large numbers of patients who suffer from cancer pain.[4] Pain associated with direct tumor involvement is the most common cause of cancer pain, occurring in as many as 85% of patients reported from a pain service study, to 65% from an outpatient cancer center pain clinic survey.[3] Bone pain is the most common type, with tumor infiltration of nerve and hollow viscus as the second and third most common pain sources. Cancer therapy causes pain in 15% to 25% of patients receiving chemotherapy, surgery, or radiation therapy. Three percent to 10% of patients with cancer have pain caused by non–cancer-related problems, with pain syndromes reflecting the common causes of pain in the general population.

Patients with cancer often have multiple causes of pain and multiple sites of pain.[4–10] Based on a variety of survey data, up to one-third of patients had more than one pain and 81% of patients reported two or more distinct pain complaints; 34% reported three pains. Cross-cultural studies from India, Thailand, Vietnam, Germany, France, Taiwan, the Philippines, and China report a similar prevalence of cancer pain in patients in active therapy and advanced disease.[10]

Studies have focused not only on the prevalence of pain but on its intensity, the degree of pain relief, and the effect of pain on quality of life in patients with various cancers, including lung, colon, ovarian, and pancreatic cancers.[11–16] These studies point out the fact that pain is prevalent in ambulatory patients, as well as hospitalized patients, and compromises function in approximately one-half of the patients who experience it.

A series of studies have focused on the seriously ill and nursing home cancer population and have identified a high prevalence of pain in these populations. The Study to Understand Prognoses and Preferences for Outcomes and Risks of Treatments (SUPPORT) showed that 50% of adults who die in the hospital experience moderate to severe pain in the last 3 days of life.[17] A study of 4000 elderly nursing home residents with cancer revealed that 24%, 29%, and 38% of those over age 85 years, 75 to 84 years, and 65 to 74 years, respectively, reported daily pain.[18] Twenty-six percent in daily pain did not receive any medication. Those older than 85 years who reported pain were most likely to receive no analgesic. Similar studies of children report that 54% to 85% of pediatric inpatients and 26% to 35% of pediatric outpatients experience pain. Up to 62% to 90% of children experience pain at the end of life.[19]

Such studies have led to an assessment of the factors that influence the prevalence of cancer pain. Primary tumor type is one factor. Tumors that commonly metastasize to bone such as breast or prostate are associated with a higher incidence of pain (60% to 80%) than lymphoma and leukemia. Stage of disease is a contributing factor, with increasing pain prevalence with disease progression. For example, fewer than 15% of patients with nonmetastatic disease report pain. Tumors that occur in close proximity to neural structures also produce a higher incidence of pain. Patient variables such as anxiety, depression, and history of previous substance abuse influence the patient's report and experience of pain.[20]

Several studies have detailed the characteristics of patient populations followed by pain services and palliative and hospice care programs, providing further data on the magnitude of the cancer pain problem.[16,21–26] The 10-year experience of a German anesthesiology-based pain service associated with a palliative care program reported on the course of treatment of 2118 patients over a period of 140,478 treatment days.[26] In their survey, gastrointestinal and head and neck cancers were the most common types, with the majority of pain (85%) caused by tumor involvement. Pain intensity data were collected throughout the course of treatment. Eighty-two percent of patients had moderate to very severe pain at the beginning of treatment, but only 7% reported pain of such high intensity at the completion of treatment.

Several studies have also addressed the epidemiology and ethnography of pain treatment. In a study to assess the effect of a comprehensive medical and neurologic evaluation of pain in the cancer patient, 64% of patients had a lesion newly identified by the pain consultant.[27] Of note, more than 50% were neurologic in origin, and in 19% of patients further anticancer therapy combined with analgesic approaches was recommended. Further studies have observed that neurologic lesions make up a substantial portion of painful lesions in the cancer population. In a prospective study of neurologic symptoms, neurologic diagnoses, and primary tumors in all patients with a history of systemic cancer referred to the Memorial Sloan-Kettering Cancer Center Neurology Consultation Service, the three most common symptoms in 851 patients were back pain (18.2%), altered mental status (17.1%), and headache (15.4%).[28] The most common neurologic diagnosis was brain metastases (15.9%), followed by metabolic encephalopathy (10.2%), pain associated

with bone metastases only (9.9%), and epidural extension or metastases of tumor (8.4%).[29]

In studies of patients with far-advanced disease cared for in palliative care programs, pain is the most common physical symptom. Of note, pain management significantly reduced this symptom, but several other prominent symptoms, including anxiety, fatigue, weakness, anorexia, nausea and vomiting, and dyspnea, were less effectively managed.[29] This observation indicates the critical need to evaluate, prioritize, and treat all symptoms to improve cancer pain patients' quality of life.

BARRIERS TO CANCER PAIN MANAGEMENT

Numerous barriers to effective pain management have been identified using various methodologies to survey health care professionals and the public. In a study by Cleeland et al., 56% of cancer patients followed by the Eastern Cooperative Oncology Group reported moderate to severe pain 50% of the time.[16] Studies performed in connection with the Eastern Cooperative Oncology Group's survey of physicians' knowledge and attitudes regarding cancer pain management demonstrated that 86% of physicians felt that the majority of patients were undermedicated. Only 51% of physicians believed pain control in their setting was good or very good, and 31% would wait until the patient's expected survival was 6 months or shorter before starting maximal analgesia. These barriers have been categorized as physician related, patient related, and institutionally related and are detailed in Table 55.1-1.[30] Numerous strategies and interventions have been developed to specifically address each of the barriers.[31–33] For example, patient reluctance to take pain medication can be overcome through effective patient education and coaching.[31] Physician management can be improved through specific use of guidelines and nursing interventions.[32] The implementation of pain management standards by the Joint Commission for the Accreditation of Healthcare Organizations requires all health care organizations accredited by the commission to implement policies and procedures that make pain assessment and effective management strategies a routine part of every patient's care.[33]

Systematic efforts to identify and address regulatory barriers have evolved in the last 10 years. Joranson and Gilsin have worked to complete a criteria-based analysis of state policies identifying numerous impediments that are inconsistent with current knowledge and practices in pain management.[34] The U.S. Drug Enforcement Administration collaborated with 21 health care organizations on a joint consensus statement to promote a balanced policy which recognizes that clinicians and regulators share the responsibility for ensuring that approaches to diversion are balanced with appropriate prescription of analgesic medications.[35] Three Institute of Medicine reports have called attention to the need to educate health care professionals in pain management and more broadly in palliative care.[8,36,37] *Improving Palliative Care for Cancer*, the report of the Institute of Medicine's National Cancer Policy Board, specifically recommends that comprehensive cancer centers develop "centers of excellence to advance pain research and training."[8] The American Society of Clinical Oncology and the European Society of Medical Oncology have strongly supported health care professional training and continuing education in pain management

TABLE 55.1-1.   Barriers to Cancer Pain Management

PROFESSIONAL BARRIERS
Inadequate knowledge of pain mechanisms
Inadequate knowledge of pain assessment
Inadequate knowledge of the appropriate use of pain medications
Fear of producing iatrogenic addictions
Concern about analgesic side effects
Concern about the development of tolerance
Inability to differentiate between tolerance, physical dependence, and psychological addiction
Fear of regulatory scrutiny
Time and reimbursement pressures that prohibit effective pain assessment and management
PATIENT BARRIERS
Reluctance to report pain
Reluctance to take pain medications as prescribed
Concerns about addiction
Belief that pain is inevitable and not treatable
Lack of access to cancer pain management professionals
Inability to effectively manage the side effects of pain medications
Fear of masking symptoms
Cost of pain medications
Inadequate knowledge of how to adjust the dose of pain medications
Lack of comprehensive insurance coverage for pain management
SYSTEM BARRIERS
Failure to make pain management a high priority
Failure to recognize the importance of pain management in patient care
Lack of a systematic and collaborative approach to pain assessment and management
Lack of organized pain management teams
Inadequate reimbursement for pain management
Regulations that restrict the prescription and dispensing of controlled substances

(Adapted from ref. 30.)

in their professional organizations.[38,39] The American Cancer Society has supported national educational programs for health care professionals and the public. These efforts point up the importance of broad national initiatives to address these barriers and emphasize the fundamental principles of cancer pain management and the importance of institutional commitment to provide improved pain management.

DEFINITION OF PAIN

The definition of pain proposed by the International Association for the Study of Pain is "an unpleasant sensory and emotional experience associated with actual or potential tissue damage or described in terms of such damage."[40] Because pain is a subjective complaint, there is no definitive way to distinguish pain occurring in the absence of tissue damage from pain resulting from such damage. Pain as a somatic delusion or masked depression is rare in cancer patients, and the presence of pain usually implies a pathologic process.

ANATOMY AND PHYSIOLOGY OF PAIN

Extensive investigations over the last 30 years have expanded knowledge of the ascending and descending central nervous system pathways that process and modulate nociceptive information. These advances provide a scientific rationale for the use of new and improved methods of cancer pain treatment.[1,2,5,6] A brief review of the neuroanatomy, physiology, and pharmacology of pain provides a background for the later discussions of specific drug, anesthetic, and neurosurgical approaches. Detailed information now supports the theory that activation of peripheral receptors in both superficial and deep structures and viscera by mechanical and chemical stimuli excites afferent discharges. Nonnociceptive messages are transmitted through rapidly conducting A-beta fibers and nociceptive information is signaled through slowly conducting A-delta and C-fiber afferents. The receptor endings of A-delta fibers most often respond to one sensory stimulus, whereas most C-fiber receptors are multimodal and respond to multiple high-threshold stimuli. These C-fiber nociceptors contain a series of specific proteins called *transducers* that are released in response to various noxious thermal, mechanical, or chemical stimuli. Studies have identified both the vanilloid receptor that is the target protein associated with tissue inflammation and the voltage-gated sodium channel NAV1.8 that is involved in the mechanism of both inflammation and neuropathic pain. These proteins are the focus of pharmacologic approaches to block their actions and, in turn, block pain.[41,42] The primary sensory afferents have their cell bodies in the dorsal root ganglion, and their axons enter the spinal cord via the dorsal root. The synaptic connections of these primary afferents with the corresponding second-order nociceptive neurons in the spinal dorsal horn are the initial site of processing for sensory information and act as a relay in transmitting noxious signals to the central nervous system.[43]

They ascend or descend from one or two segments in Lissauer's tract and synapse in specific laminae in the dorsal horn, lamina I and lamina II. Evidence suggests that myelinated nociceptors project to laminae I and V and unmyelinated nociceptors to lamina II and possibly lamina I, and that nonnociceptive myelinated afferents project to only deep laminae. The dorsal horn is a critical site for modulating sensory input. Sensory transmission is mediated through excitatory amino acids (EAAs), predominantly glutamate.[44] The EAA aspartate and the neuropeptide substance P and calcitonin gene-related peptide are also involved. Excitatory synaptic transmission from the primary afferent is also modulated by the N-methyl D-aspartate (NMDA) receptor as well as non-NMDA receptors. After EAA-NMDA receptor interaction, intracellular calcium influx and mobilization of intracellular calcium lead to subsequent changes in second-messenger systems. One second-messenger system activated after EAA-NMDA receptor interaction is the generation of nitric oxide via the enzyme nitric oxide synthase. There is also an increase in transcription of immediate early gene c-fos, which may regulate the subsequent expression of endogenous opioid genes, preproenkephalin, and preprodynorphin. NMDA receptor activation initiates and maintains central sensitization and the component known as *windup*. These phenomena are manifestations of persistent signaling from primary sensory afferents. Central sensitization is thought to be the major mechanism underlying neuropathic pain and accounts for the hyperpathia and enlarged cutaneous receptor fields that occur after nerve injury.

At the level of the second-order neurons in the dorsal horn, sensory processing occurs through interactions among neurochemical transmitters released by primary afferents, including gamma-aminobutyric acid, glycine, adenosine, bombesin, cholecystokinin, dynorphin, enkephalin, neuropeptide Y, neurotensin, substance P, somatostatin, and vasoactive intestinal polypeptide.

Several ascending pathways arise from these second-order neurons and decussate in the central gray of the spinal cord to become the neospinothalamic and paleospinothalamic tracts. These tracts project to discrete regions of the thalamus and cortex. The neospinothalamic pathway subserves pain intensity and localization, whereas the phylogenetically older paleospinothalamic pathway subserves the arousal and emotional component of pain. Descending pathways, the most important of which originate from the periaqueductal gray nuclei of the midbrain, synapse in the raphe magnus nucleus of the medulla. From this nucleus, a medial pathway, the dorsal longitudinal fasciculus, projects to the dorsal horn to modulate pain transmission. This pathway represents an important descending inhibitory pathway. A more laterally placed descending pathway from the locus ceruleus to the dorsal horn also plays a role in pain modulation at the spinal cord level.

Opiate receptors, stereospecific binding sites on the end of free nerve endings that bind exogenous opioids, are localized in the ascending and descending pain pathways. These receptors mediate the multiple pharmacologic effects of the opioid analgesics. Subpopulations of opioid receptors, including high-affinity and low-affinity μ receptors and γ, κ, and δ receptors, are localized to specific areas of the brain and spinal cord. More recently, several opioid receptor subtypes have been cloned and quantitative changes in the messenger RNA for these receptors determined in experimental models. The cloning of these subtypes of receptors that mediate different pharmacologic effects and then are located in specific cerebral and spinal sites offers the possibility of developing new analgesics targeted for specific receptors. For example, μ receptors modulate predominantly supraspinal analgesia, whereas δ and κ receptors are important in modulating analgesia at the spinal cord level. The periaqueductal gray region in the midbrain and dorsal horn in the spinal cord are rich in these receptors and are the supraspinal and spinal sites that mediate opioid analgesia. The use of brainstem stimulation and the administration of opioid analgesics directly into the cerebrospinal fluid bathing the selective opioid sites in animals and cancer patients with pain are procedures based on this knowledge. Pain transmission at the spinal cord level can be inhibited by the direct application of morphine, and these studies have led to the use of spinal opioid analgesia in clinical pain states.[46–49] The genetic variation in opioid receptor populations in experimental animals suggests a similar variation in humans. Such data may partially explain the wide interindividual differences among patients and their response to opioid analgesia and tolerance.[45] There is now increasing information about the molecular basis of opioid tolerance development. A variety of NMDA receptor antagonists have been demonstrated both to attenuate and to reverse experimental opioid analgesic tolerance.[44] Therefore, the confluence of NMDA receptors in pain transmission and their role in the development of tolerance have provided new insights into the role of opioid receptors in analgesia.

These advances in the understanding of pain-modulatory systems and their neuroanatomic and neuropharmacologic correlates have had a major effect on the management of patients with pain. A better understanding of the molecular biology of both nociceptive and neuropathic pain is facilitating the wide application of a variety of agents, including NMDA antagonists, vanilloid receptor antagonists, sodium and calcium channel agonists and antagonists, specific neurotoxins, and topical and local systemic anesthetics and opioids.

TYPES OF PAIN

Three types of pain have been described based on the neuroanatomy and the neurophysiology of pain pathways: somatic, visceral, and neuropathic pain. Each type results from activation and sensitization of nociceptors and mechanoreceptors in the periphery by either mechanical stimuli (e.g., tumor compression or infiltration) or chemical stimuli (e.g., epinephrine, serotonin, bradykinin, prostaglandin, or histamine).

SOMATIC PAIN

When nociceptors are activated in cutaneous or deep tissues, somatic pain results, typically characterized by a dull or aching but well-localized pain. Metastatic bone pain, postsurgical incisional pain, and myofascial and musculoskeletal pain are common examples of somatic pain.

VISCERAL PAIN

Visceral pain results from activation of nociceptors from infiltration, compression, extension, or stretching of the thoracic, abdominal, or pelvic viscera. This typically occurs in patients with intraperitoneal metastases and is common with pancreatic cancer. This type of pain is poorly localized; is often described as deep, squeezing, and pressure-like; and when acute is often associated with significant autonomic dysfunction, including nausea, vomiting, and diaphoresis. Visceral pain is often referred to cutaneous sites that may be remote from the site of the lesion (e.g., shoulder pain with diaphragmatic irritation). It may be associated with tenderness in the referred cutaneous site. Increasing data have demonstrated the role of κ opioid receptors in modulating visceral pain.[50]

NEUROPATHIC PAIN

Neuropathic pain results from injury to the peripheral or central nervous system as a consequence of tumor compression or infiltration of peripheral nerves or the spinal cord, or from chemical injury to the peripheral nerve or spinal cord caused by surgery, radiation therapy, or chemotherapy. Examples of neuropathic pain include both metastatic and radiation-induced brachial and lumbosacral plexopathies, chemotherapy-induced peripheral neuropathies, paraneoplastic peripheral neuropathies, and postmastectomy, postthoracotomy, and phantom limb pain.[51] Pain from nerve injury is often severe and is described as burning or dysesthetic, with a vise-like quality. The pain is typically most common in the site of sensory loss and may be associated with hypersensitivity to nonnoxious (allodynia) and noxious stimuli. Intermittently, patients complain of paroxysms of burning or electric shock–like sensations. The latter symptoms result from the phenomenon of central sensitization.

These three types of pain may occur alone or combined in the same patient. Experimental models of bone and nerve pain have provided greater insight into the mechanisms underlying these clinical pain states. For example, Clohisy and Manyth have developed a bone tumor model and demonstrated multiple pain mechanisms and their molecular biologic correlates.[52] Their studies suggests that bone pain is a mixed pain, both somatic and neuropathic. These correlative studies with animal models provide the opportunity to test bone pain model responses to clinical treatments. For example, opioids, gabapentin, nonsteroidal antiinflammatory agents produce analgesic efficacy in this bone tumor model.[52]

TEMPORAL ASPECTS OF PAIN

ACUTE PAIN

Acute pain is characterized by a well-defined temporal pattern of pain onset, generally associated with subjective and objective physical signs and with hyperactivity of the autonomic nervous system. These signs provide the physician with objective evidence that substantiates the patient's complaint of pain. Acute pain is usually self-limited and responds to treatment with analgesic drug therapy and to treatment of its precipitating cause. This type of pain can be further subdivided into subacute and episodic. Subacute pain comes on over several days, often with increasing intensity, and represents a pattern of progressive pain symptomatology. Episodic or intermittent pain occurs during confined periods of time on a regular or irregular basis. All of the pains in this category of acute pain have associated autonomic hyperactivity.

CHRONIC PAIN

Chronic pain is the persistence of pain for more than 3 months, with a less well-defined temporal onset. The autonomic nervous system adapts, and chronic pain patients lack the objective signs common to those with acute pain. Chronic pain leads to significant changes in personality, lifestyle, and functional ability. Treatment of chronic pain in the cancer patient is especially challenging because it requires a careful assessment of not only the intensity of the pain but its broad multidimensional aspects. Evidence suggests that the persistence of pain has a major negative effect on the quality of life of patients with pain and cancer.

Investigators have developed a nomenclature to describe a series of specific pains in cancer patients with both acute and chronic pain states. *Baseline pain* is the average pain intensity experienced for 12 or more hours during a 24-hour period. *Breakthrough pain* is a transient increase in pain to greater than moderate intensity occurring on a baseline pain of moderate intensity or less. Various epidemiologic studies provide a range of prevalence of breakthrough pain from 23% to as high as 90% of cancer patients. [53–56] In a study of 70 adult inpatient cancer patients, 65% reported breakthrough pain.[54] The median number of reported pains was four, with a wide range. Most pains had a rapid onset and a brief duration. Breakthrough pain has a diversity of characteristics. Some authors have detailed the prevalence of such transitory flares of pain. In a study of 613 consecutively treated cancer patients, 39%

reported transitory flares that were severe or worse in 92% of patients.[53] There were no correlations with gender, age, tumor site, stage, or therapy. The pain was somatic in 39%, visceral in 22%, and neuropathic in 36%. In this and other series, the transitory increase in pain marks the onset or worsening of pain at the end of the dosing interval or the regularly scheduled analgesic. In other patients, it is caused by an action of the patient, referred to as *incident pain*. Sometimes the incident pain has a nonvolitional precipitant, such as flatulence. Most breakthrough or transitory pains are thought to be associated with a known malignant cause from direct tumor infiltration. Clinical trials of an oral transmucosal fentanyl preparation have focused attention on the clinical management of such episodes of worsening pain.[55]

INTENSITY OF PAIN

Pain may also be defined on the basis of intensity, but there are limitations to a concept of pain based solely on intensity. Specific categoric scales of pain intensity have been used in which patients are asked to describe their pain as mild, moderate, severe, or excruciating.[57] Visual analog scales (VASs) have also been used. These are often a 10-cm line anchored on either end by two points, signifying *no pain* and *worst possible pain*. The patient is asked to mark the intensity of the pain on the line. Numeric scales are also commonly used, and patients are asked to rate their pain between 1 (no pain) and 10 (worst possible pain). These scales have their limitations, but they are part of a series of validated instruments that include a measure of pain intensity as one of the components of the pain experience to be defined.

MEASUREMENT OF PAIN

Multidimensional pain assessment is the recommended approach to the study of pain prevalence and pain intervention. Several validated instruments for pain measurement attempt to look at it in a multidimensional way. The use of such methods can provide rapid evaluation in clinical settings of the major aspects of the pain experienced by cancer patients. Mandates of the Joint Commission for the Accreditation of Healthcare Organizations require the use of pain scales in routine clinical care.[33]

BRIEF PAIN INVENTORY

The Wisconsin Brief Pain Inventory (BPI) is a self-administered, easily understood, brief method to assess pain.[58] It addresses the relevant aspects of pain (history, intensity, location, and quality) and the ability of the pain to interfere with the patient's activities and helps to provide an understanding of its cause. The history of pain and its relation to the patient's disease are assessed initially. If the patient admits to pain in the last month, he or she answers questions about current manifestations of pain. If the patient has no pain, he or she skips to the end of the questionnaire to complete demographic information. For patients with pain, a human figure drawing is provided on which the patients shades the area corresponding to the pain. Patients are asked to rate their pain at its worst, their usual pain, and their pain at the time they are completing the questionnaire. The pain scales consist of numbers from 0 to 10; 0 is labeled *no pain* and 10 is labeled *pain as bad as you can imagine.* Patients are asked to report the medications or treatments they receive for pain, the percentage relief that these medications or treatment provide, and their belief about the cause of their pain. Finally, they are asked to rate how much the pain interferes with their mood, relations with other people, and functional ability (walking, sleeping, working, enjoying life). All patients, including those without pain, are asked for basic demographic information about marital status, education, occupation, spouse's occupation, and months since diagnosis.

This inventory has been translated into numerous languages and has been used to assess pain in cancer patients in such diverse settings as Vietnam, Mexico, the Philippines, China, and the University of Wisconsin Cancer Center. Data from these studies suggest that cancer pain patients from widely different cultural and linguistic backgrounds respond in a similar fashion in rating the severity of their cancer-related pain and the interference caused by the pain.

MCGILL PAIN QUESTIONNAIRE

The McGill Pain Questionnaire (MPQ) is an extensively used pain assessment instrument that produces scores on four empirically derived dimensions, as well as several summary scores.[59] The instrument consists of 78 adjectives that cluster in 20 categories. Within each category, the adjectives are arranged in order of intensity from low to high. The categories are divided into four dimensions: sensory, affective, evaluative, and miscellaneous. The patient is asked to choose one adjective from each applicable category that describes an aspect of his or her current pain, and the score for each dimension is obtained by adding the rank values of the selected adjectives. A total summary score is derived by adding the scores across the four dimensions, and a total word count is also obtained. Finally, a rating of present pain intensity is made on a five-point scale. Studies with this instrument have demonstrated that the factors derived reflect specific sensory qualities and combined emotional and sensory dimensions. This tool has also been used to assess distinct score profiles according to the nature of pain. For instance, patients with acute pain tend to use more sensory words, but patients with chronic pain tend to use more affective and reaction word subgroups. The MPQ offers a methodologic approach to assess the sensory, affective, and evaluative components of pain, but it may be more difficult and cumbersome for patients to understand and complete than some other pain assessment tools and may be limited by its language constraints.

MEMORIAL PAIN ASSESSMENT CARD

The Memorial Pain Assessment Card (MPAC) (Fig. 55.1-1) was initially developed by the Analgesic Studies Section of the Memorial Sloan-Kettering Cancer Center to assess the relative potency of new and standard analgesic drugs. In that context, this method was found repeatedly to be a valid, reliable, efficient, and sensitive measure.[60] The MPAC consists of three VASs that measure pain intensity, pain relief, and mood, and a set of pain severity descriptors adapted from the Tursky rating scale. The card is 8.5 in. × 11.0 in. and is folded in the middle

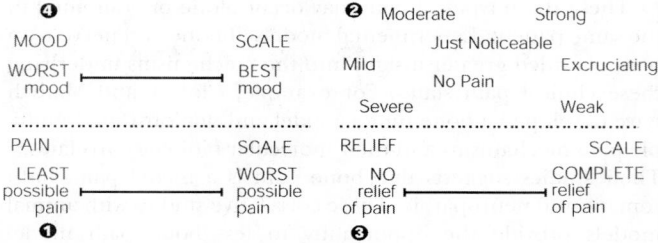

FIGURE 55.1-1. Memorial Pain Assessment Card, front (1 and 4) and back (2 and 3) sides. The card is folded along the broken line, and each measure is presented to the patient separately, in the numbered order. (1) Visual analog scale (VAS) for pain intensity; (2) modified Tursky pain descriptors scale; (3) VAS for pain relief; and (4) VAS for mood. (From ref. 52, with permission.)

so that the four sides can be quickly presented to the patient. Three sides are imprinted with the 100-mm-long VAS scale; the fourth side is the set of Tursky adjectives. The pain intensity VAS is anchored by the terms *least possible pain* and *worst possible pain.* The patient is asked to place a mark along the line to indicate his or her subjective judgment of pain intensity. The score on this and the other VASs is obtained by measuring the distance in millimeters between the left end of the line and the patient's mark. The Tursky pain adjective scale is a categorical measure of pain intensity. Eight intensity descriptors, ranging from *no pain* to *excruciating*, are printed in a random arrangement and the patient is asked to circle the adjective that describes his or her subjective experience of pain severity. Side 3 of the MPAC is a pain-relief VAS. Patients are asked to indicate with a mark the degree of pain reduction they experienced after the most recent intervention, which is usually the administration of an analgesic drug. On side 4, the VAS measures the subjective experience of mood; on this side patients are asked to rate their current feeling, from *worst* to *best.* The instructions for administration of these scales are simple and readily understood, and an experienced patient can complete the four ratings in less than 20 seconds.

The MPAC has been compared with the MPQ, the Profile of Mood States Questionnaire (a standardized self-report instrument that measures six dimensions of mood, reflecting degree and type of psychological distress), the Hamilton Rating Scale for Depression (an interviewer-rated scale evaluating the presence and severity of 17 symptoms typical of clinical depression), and the Zung Anxiety Scale (a standardized self-report scale that evaluates the presence and severity of various symptoms of anxiety). The MPAC and the MPQ provide reasonably equivalent assessments of the intensity dimension of pain. However, scores on the evaluative scales of the MPQ did not correlate significantly with any of the measures of the MPAC, which suggests that the cognitive-judgmental dimension of pain may be independent of the experiences of intensity, relief, and mood. None of the MPQ subscale ratings correlated significantly with the VAS ratings of mood and pain relief.

These observations have led to the conclusion that the VAS mood scale on the MPAC represents a much more global assessment of general psychological distress rather than a specific pain-related affect. This would suggest that the MPAC provides a broader assessment of the patient by its use of the mood scale, whereas the MPQ has a more narrow focus of simply representing pain-related emotional distress. What was particularly impressive was that, through the use of any of the available scales, patients could differentiate pain and mood when they were explicitly asked. The perceptions of pain intensity and pain relief have different weights as components of psychological distress. The existence of such distinctions has important clinical and theoretical significance. Although the perception of pain intensity was found to contribute significantly to subjective distress, the perception of inadequate pain relief was a more important factor. The MPAC provides valid, multidimensional information for the evaluation of pain and distress in cancer patients. It can distinguish pain intensity from pain relief and from global suffering, and it can be used to study the subtle interactions of these factors. With repeated administration it has now been demonstrated to be valid, reliable, easy to use, and nondisruptive. The MPAC and the BPI are the tools recommended for use in the clinical evaluation of individual patients and as an outcome measure in clinical trials.

MEMORIAL SYMPTOM ASSESSMENT SCALE

The Memorial Symptom Assessment Scale (MSAS) is a validated, patient-rated measure that provides multidimensional information about a diverse group of common symptoms.[61] Thirty-two physical and psychological symptoms are characterized in terms of intensity, frequency, and distress. The MSAS provides a Global Distress Index (MSAS-GDI), a ten-item subscale that reflects global symptom distress and separate subscales that measure physical (MSAS-Phys) and psychological (MSAS-Psych) symptom distress. Ongoing studies have confirmed its value in patients with various types of cancer, and studies of its reliability and validity with repeated administration are currently under way. The use of the MSAS allows the concurrent measurement of pain and various other symptoms, psychological distress, and psychological factors and represents overall a useful, patient-accepted method to measure the multidimensional issues facing cancer patients with pain. Newer studies have identified the usefulness of a short form for rapid assessment.[62]

EUROPEAN ORGANIZATION FOR RESEARCH AND TREATMENT OF CANCER QUALITY OF LIFE QUESTIONNAIRE-C30

The European Organization for Research and Treatment of Cancer has included specific pain questions in its Quality of Life Questionnaire-C30 (QLQ-C30) quality-of-life scale. The pain scale measures pain intensity and interference with function. The pain scale has a four-level verbal rating scale (*not at all, a little, quite a bit, very much*) measuring the presence of pain and pain interference with daily activities. The responses are summed to a composite score and transformed to a 0 to 100 pain scale of severity. The pain severity composite score better represents the cancer pain experience than the intensity score alone. In published studies, it has been shown to reliably predict functional status, toxicity, and chemotherapy response. Because of its multiple scales, the QLQ-C30 requires more time, attention, and cooperation on the part of patients, which makes it less useful as a routine measurement tool.[63]

CLASSIFICATION OF PATIENTS WITH CANCER PAIN

Five types of cancer pain patients can be identified, exemplifying the distinctions between acute and chronic pain (Table 55.1-2). Although these categories are fluid, they serve as a useful preamble for discussion of the specific therapeutic approaches to the management of cancer patients.

GROUP I: PATIENTS WITH ACUTE CANCER-RELATED PAIN

Group I, patients with acute cancer-related pain, can be subdivided further according to etiology.

Group IA: Tumor-Associated Pain

For group IA patients, those with tumor-associated pain, pain is the major symptom prompting medical consultation and the diagnosis of cancer. In addition, pain has a special significance as the harbinger of the patient's illness. Recurrent pain during the course of the illness or after successful therapy has the immediate implication of recurrent disease. Defining the cause of the pain may present a diagnostic problem, but effective treatment of its cause (e.g., radiation therapy for bone metastases) is usually associated with dramatic pain relief in most patients.

Group IB: Pain Associated with Cancer Therapy

Group IB patients have postoperative pain, pain secondary to oral ulceration from chemotherapy, or myalgias secondary to corticosteroid withdrawal. The cause of the pain is readily identifiable, and its course is predictable and self-limited (Table 55.1-3). These patients do not represent difficult diagnostic problems. Pain treatment directed at the cause of the pain is used to manage the transient symptoms. These patients endure significant pain for the promise of a successful outcome.

GROUP II: PATIENTS WITH CHRONIC CANCER-RELATED PAIN

Group II patients, those with chronic cancer-related pain, represent difficult diagnostic and therapeutic problems, in contrast to patients with acute cancer-related pain. They can be

TABLE 55.1-2.   Types of Patients with Pain from Cancer

I. Patients with acute cancer-related pain
  a. Associated with the diagnosis of cancer
  b. Associated with cancer therapy (surgery, chemotherapy, or radiation)
II. Patients with chronic cancer-related pain
  a. Associated with cancer progression
  b. Associated with cancer therapy (surgery, chemotherapy, or radiation)
III. Patients with preexisting chronic pain and cancer-related pain
IV. Patients with a history of drug addiction and cancer-related pain
  a. Actively involved in illicit drug use
  b. In methadone maintenance program
  c. With a history of drug abuse
V. Dying patients with cancer-related pain

TABLE 55.1-3. Cancer-Related Acute Pain Syndromes

ACUTE PAIN ASSOCIATED WITH DIAGNOSTIC AND THERAPEUTIC INTERVENTIONS

Acute pain associated with diagnostic interventions

Lumbar puncture headache
Arterial or venous blood sampling
Bone marrow biopsy
Lumbar puncture
Colonoscopy
Myelography
Percutaneous biopsy
Thoracocentesis

Acute postoperative pain

Acute pain caused by other therapeutic interventions

Pleurodesis
Tumor embolization
Suprapubic catheterization
Intercostal catheter
Nephrostomy insertion

Acute pain associated with analgesic techniques

Injection pain
Opioid headache
Spinal opioid hyperalgesia syndrome
Epidural injection pain

ACUTE PAIN ASSOCIATED WITH ANTICANCER THERAPIES

Acute pain associated with chemotherapy infusion techniques

Intravenous infusion pain
Venous spasm
Chemical phlebitis
Vesicant extravasation
Anthracycline-associated flare reaction
Hepatic artery infusion pain
Intraperitoneal chemotherapy abdominal pain

Acute pain associated with chemotherapy toxicity

Mucositis
Corticosteroid-induced perineal discomfort
Corticosteroid pseudorheumatism
Painful peripheral neuropathy
Headache
   Intrathecal methotrexate meningitic syndrome
   L-Asparaginase–associated dural sinus thrombosis
   Trans-retinoic acid headache
Diffuse bone pain
   Trans-retinoic acid
   Colony-stimulating factors
5-Fluorouracil–induced anginal chest pain
Postchemotherapy gynecomastia

Acute pain associated with hormonal therapy

Luteinizing hormone–releasing factor tumor flare in prostate cancer
Hormone-induced pain flare in breast cancer

Acute pain associated with immunotherapy

Interferon-induced acute pain

Acute pain associated with radiotherapy

Incident pain associated with positioning
Oropharyngeal mucositis
Acute radiation enteritis and proctocolitis
Early-onset brachial plexopathy
Subacute radiation myelopathy

ACUTE PAIN ASSOCIATED WITH INFECTION

Acute herpetic neuralgia

(From ref. 71, with permission.)

divided for discussion purposes into two groups: those with chronic pain from tumor progression, and those with chronic pain related to cancer treatment. Both groups share the characteristic of a pain symptom that has persisted for more than 3 months.

Group IIA: Chronic Pain from Tumor Progression

In patients with chronic pain associated with progression of disease (e.g., patients with carcinoma of the pancreas, metastatic melanoma to bone, or Pancoast's syndrome), the pain escalates in intensity secondary to tumor infiltration of adjacent bone, nerve, or soft tissue. Combinations of antitumor therapy, analgesic drug therapy, anesthetic blocks, and behavioral approaches are applied with varying degrees of success. Psychological factors play a significant role in this group of patients, in whom palliative cancer therapy may be of little value and is physically debilitating. The sense of hopelessness and fear of impending death may further add to and exaggerate the pain complaint; pain then becomes an aspect of the global *suffering* component.[65] Identifying both the pain and the suffering component is essential to the development of adequate therapy for these patients. Management approaches must be directed to controlling the pain and identifying and developing treatment strategies for each of the components of the patient's symptoms and psychological distress. Analgesic therapy combined with a wide range of alternative approaches is necessary to provide adequate analgesia. Such patients are appropriate candidates for palliative care programs to address the broader aspects of symptom management and psychological support.

Group IIB: Chronic Pain Associated with Cancer Therapy

Group IIB includes patients with chronic pain associated with cancer therapy, such as patients who develop pain after mastectomy, thoracotomy, or limb amputation (phantom limb). The pain in these patients is secondary to nerve injury (neuropathic pain) with the development of a traumatic neuroma. Treatment of the pain for these patients is limited by the lack of available methods to remove the cause of the pain. Again, treatment is directed at the symptoms, not the cause. These patients closely parallel those in the general population with chronic intractable pain syndromes. Psychological factors play a significant role in how these patients adapt to and function with chronic pain. Defining this group is imperative: identifying the cause of the pain as not directly related to tumor markedly alters the patient's therapy, prognosis, and psychological state. Each of the primary modalities of cancer therapy is associated with a series of specific chronic pain syndromes with characteristic pain patterns and clinical presentations (Tables 55.1-4 through 55.1-6). Although it is consoling to both the patient and the physician to realize that the pain does not represent recurrent or progressive disease, the persistence of the pain is a constant reminder of the previous diagnosis of cancer.

In these patients, all approaches aimed at maintaining the patient's functional status should be used. Alternative methods of therapy, in contrast to drug therapy, represent the major management approach. This group of patients with neuropathic pain is increasing in number and accounts for 15% to 25% of patients referred to medical pain clinics.

TABLE 55.1-4. Treatment-Related Chronic Pain Syndromes

POSTCHEMOTHERAPY PAIN SYNDROMES
Chronic painful peripheral neuropathy
Avascular necrosis of femoral or humeral head
Plexopathy associated with intraarterial infusion
CHRONIC PAIN ASSOCIATED WITH HORMONAL THERAPY
Gynecomastia with hormonal therapy for prostate cancer
CHRONIC POSTSURGICAL PAIN SYNDROMES
Postmastectomy pain syndrome
Postradical neck dissection pain
Postthoracotomy pain
Postoperative frozen shoulder
Phantom pain syndromes
   Phantom limb pain
   Phantom breast pain
   Phantom anus pain
   Phantom bladder pain
Stump pain
Postsurgical pelvic floor myalgia
CHRONIC POSTRADIATION PAIN SYNDROMES
Plexopathies
   Radiation-induced brachial and lumbosacral plexopathies
   Radiation-induced peripheral nerve tumors
Chronic radiation myelopathy
Chronic radiation enteritis and proctitis
Burning perineum syndrome
Osteoradionecrosis

(From ref. 71, with permission.)

TABLE 55.1-5. Tumor-Related Chronic Pain Syndromes

BONE PAIN
Multifocal or generalized bone pain
   Multiple bony metastases
   Marrow expansion
Vertebral syndromes
   Atlantoaxial destruction and odontoid fractures
   C-7 to T-1 syndrome
   T-12 to L-1 syndrome
   Sacral syndrome
Back pain and epidural compression
Pain syndromes of the bony pelvis and hip
   Hip joint syndrome
HEADACHE AND FACIAL PAIN
Intracerebral tumor
Leptomeningeal metastases
Base of skull metastases
   Orbital syndrome
   Parasellar syndrome
   Middle cranial fossa syndrome
   Jugular foramen syndrome
   Clivus syndrome
   Sphenoid sinus syndrome
Painful cranial neuralgias
   Glossopharyngeal neuralgia
   Trigeminal neuralgia
TUMOR INVOLVEMENT OF THE PERIPHERAL NERVOUS SYSTEM
Tumor-related radiculopathy
   Postherpetic neuralgia
Cervical plexopathy
Brachial plexopathy
   Malignant brachial plexopathy
   Idiopathic brachial plexopathy associated with Hodgkin's disease
Malignant lumbosacral plexopathy
Tumor-related mononeuropathy
Paraneoplastic painful peripheral neuropathy
   Subacute sensory neuropathy
   Sensorimotor peripheral neuropathy
PAIN SYNDROMES OF THE VISCERA AND MISCELLANEOUS TUMOR-RELATED SYNDROMES
Hepatic distention syndrome
Midline retroperitoneal syndrome
Chronic intestinal obstruction
Peritoneal carcinomatosis
Malignant perineal pain
   Malignant pelvic floor myalgia
Ureteric obstruction
PARANEOPLASTIC NOCICEPTIVE PAIN SYNDROMES
Tumor-related gynecomastia

(From ref. 71, with permission.)

GROUP III: PATIENTS WITH PREEXISTING CHRONIC PAIN AND CANCER-RELATED PAIN

Group III includes patients with a history of chronic nonmalignant pain who develop cancer and pain. Psychological factors play a significant role in this group of patients, whose psychological and functional status is already compromised by their chronic nonmalignant pain state. These patients are at high risk of developing further functional incapacity and escalating chronic pain symptoms. However, their history should not be used in a punitive way to minimize or deny their complaints. Identifying this group of patients as a high-risk group helps to improve psychological assessment and intervention.

GROUP IV: PATIENTS WITH A HISTORY OF DRUG ADDICTION AND PAIN

Group IV includes patients with a history of drug addiction who have cancer-related pain. Three subgroups can be identified: patients actively involved in illicit drug use and drug-seeking behavior, those receiving methadone in a maintenance program, and those who have not used drugs for several years. Undertreatment with analgesic drugs occurs most commonly in this group of patients. Assessment of reported pain by physicians and nurses is colored by the fact that the pain symptoms are confused with drug-seeking behavior. Attention to the medical and psychological needs of these patients requires individualized assessment and consultation with experts in drug-related problems. The first subgroup represents a major management problem that strains the most tolerant of medical care systems. Pain in the other two subgroups is readily managed, with the recognition that the psychological stresses consequent to the pain and cancer may place the patient at a high risk for recidivism. There is increasing expertise to address the need of this patient population, with experts in addiction medicine and cancer pain working together to provide a coordinated system of care.[66]

GROUP V: DYING PATIENTS WITH PAIN

In dying patients with pain, diagnostic and therapeutic considerations are directed at maintaining the patient's comfort. This group is distinguished from group II patients, because the psy-

TABLE 55.1-6. Causes of Brachial Plexopathy in Patients with Breast Cancer: Distinguishing Clinical Features

Feature	Tumor Infiltration	Radiation Fibrosis	Transient Radiation Injury	Acute Ischemic Injury
Incidence of pain	80%	18%	40%	Painless
Location of pain	Shoulder, upper arm, elbow, fourth and fifth fingers	Shoulder, wrist, hand	Hand, forearm	Hand, forearm
Nature of pain	Dull ache in shoulder, lancinating pains in elbow and ulnar aspect of hand; occasional paresthesias and dysesthesias	Ache in shoulder; prominent paresthesias in C-5 to C-6 distribution of hand and arm	Ache in shoulder; prominent paresthesias in C-5 to C-6 distribution of hand and arm	Paresthesias in C-5 to C-6 distribution of hand and arm
Severity	Moderate to severe (severe in 98%)	Usually mild to moderate (severe in 20–30%)	Mild	Mild
Course	Progressive neurologic dysfunction: atrophy and weakness in C-7 to T-1 distribution; persistent pain; occasional Horner's syndrome	Progressive weakness; panplexus or upper plexus distribution; Horner's syndrome uncommon	Transient weakness with complete resolution	Acute nonprogressive weakness and sensory loss
Study findings				
Magnetic resonance imaging	High-signal intensity mass on T2-weighted images; may enhance with gadolinium	Low-signal intensity lesion on T2-weighted images; generally nonenhancing with gadolinium	No data	Normal
Computed tomography	Mass: circumscribed or diffuse tissue infiltration	Diffuse tissue infiltration	Normal	Angiography demonstrates subclavian artery
Electromyography	Segmental slowing	Diffuse myokymia	Segmental slowing	Segmental slowing

From Cherny NI, Foley KM. Brachial plexopathy in patients with breast cancer. In: Harris JR, Hellman S, Henderson IC, Kinne D, eds. *Diseases of the breast*, 2nd ed. Philadelphia: Lippincott, 1996:796, with permission.

chological factors further compound adequate pain management. The issues of hopelessness and coping with death and dying become more prominent, and the suffering component must be addressed.[67–69] Inadequate control of pain in the dying patient exacerbates the suffering component and demoralizes the family and the caregivers, who feel that they have failed in treating the patient's pain at a time when adequate treatment may matter the most. Rapid escalation of analgesic drug therapy, usually by the parenteral route (intravenous, subcutaneous, or transdermal), and amelioration of psychological symptoms should be attempted. The risk to benefit ratios in analgesic approaches become less of an issue when the goal of pain therapy is the patient's comfort. It is now widely recognized that it is the role and the responsibility of the physician to treat pain and suffering in this population of patients. Defined guidelines for the care of the dying have been published.[68,69] Good physician–patient communication, which includes issues of truth telling and the assault of truth; respect for patients' religious, cultural, and spiritual needs; and clear definition of the goals of care can improve the care of this population of patients.[68–70]

COMMON PAIN SYNDROMES

Pain in the cancer patient results from direct tumor infiltration and from the various cancer treatments and can occur unrelated to the cancer and cancer therapy. Tables 55.1-3 through 55.1-5 list the common acute and chronic pain syndromes that occur in patients with cancer. These lists are a compendium of various sources but serve to summarize the broad and now well-recognized pain syndromes that occur often uniquely in this population of patients.[3,5,6,51,71,72]

CLINICAL ASSESSMENT OF PAIN

Certain general principles should be followed in evaluating cancer patients who complain of pain. Lack of attention to these general principles is the major cause for misdiagnosis of a specific pain syndrome. Adequate assessment is a critical component for defining the appropriate therapeutic strategy for each patient. The general principles are the following:

Believe the patient's complaint of pain.
Take a careful history of the patient's pain complaint.
Evaluate the patient's psychological state.
Perform a careful medical and neurologic examination.
Order the appropriate diagnostic studies and personally review the results.
Treat the pain to facilitate the appropriate workup.
Reassess the patient's response to therapy.
Individualize the diagnostic and therapeutic approaches.
Clearly define the goals of care.
Discuss advance directives with the patient and family.

BELIEVE THE PATIENT'S COMPLAINT OF PAIN

Critical to the management of the patient with cancer pain is the establishment of a trusting relationship with the physician. The complaint of pain is a symptom, not a diagnosis. Pain perception is not simply a function of the amount of physical injury sustained by the patient but is a complex state determined by multiple factors. The diagnosis of a specific pain syndrome and a complete understanding of the patient's psychological state is not always accomplished during the initial evaluation. In fact, it may take several weeks to define its nature because of the lack of radiologic or pathologic verification. It may take a similar period to fully comprehend each patient's psychological makeup. Numerous examples in the assessment of patients with pain and cancer highlight the limitation of the diagnostic process. It is not uncommon for patients with tumor infiltration of the brachial plexus from either lung or breast cancer to have pain for several weeks or months before the onset of objective radiologic and neurologic findings. A comprehensive evaluation involves taking a careful history; performing a detailed medical, neurologic, and psychological evaluation; developing a series of diagnosis-related hypotheses; and ordering the appropriate diagnostic studies.

TAKE A CAREFUL HISTORY OF THE PATIENT'S PAIN COMPLAINT

A careful history of the patient's pain complaint should include the patient's description of site of pain, quality of pain, exacerbating and relieving factors, temporal pattern, exact onset, associated symptoms and signs, interference with activities of daily living, effect on the patient's psychological state, and response to previous and current analgesic therapies. Patients should be asked to describe the intensity, frequency, and severity of their baseline pain and episodes of breakthrough pain. Routine pain assessment tools should be provided to patients and families to record the patient's pain experience and provide easy recording of analgesic drug use and the use of rescue medications. Multiple pain complaints are common in patients with advanced disease and must be ranked, classified, and recoded.

EVALUATE THE PATIENT'S PSYCHOLOGICAL STATE

The patient's current level of anxiety and depression must be clarified and his or her past history of such symptoms must be defined. Knowledge of the patient's previous psychiatric history and need for past hospitalization for psychiatric care helps to clarify the patient's potential psychological risk. Information on how the patient has handled previous painful events may provide insight into whether the patient has demonstrated chronic illness behavior or has a past history of a chronic pain syndrome. It is important to know about a personal or family history of alcohol or drug dependence, to understand why the patient may be fearful of taking or refuse to take opioid drugs.

Because each patient has his or her own understanding of the meaning of pain, it is useful to have the patient elaborate this meaning.[65,73,74] Does he or she think it represents recurrent tumor, or is he or she convinced it is simply arthritis? Evidence suggests that when patients have a clear understanding of the meaning of their pain as representing recurrent tumor, they have increased psychological distress.

The importance of defining the psychological makeup of the patient with pain is supported by a variety of studies that have focused on the effect of suffering in patients with pain.[2,57] Psychological factors play a significant role in accounting for the differences in pain experiences in cancer patients. A series of psychiatric syndromes have been described for cancer

patients, with depression occurring in as many as 25% of patients.[20,74] The depression presents either as an acute stress response or as a major depression. Awareness of the common psychiatric syndromes when evaluating the pain complaint expands the physician's understanding of such a complaint.

Although it is critical to know as much as possible about each patient with pain, some information may not be readily available in the first interview; in some instances it may never be available because of the lack of intellectual competence on the patient's part to define clearly the various components of the pain complaint. It is often necessary to verify the history by consulting a family member who may provide information that the patient is unable or unwilling to provide. The family may be more objective in assessing a disability of a patient who underreports his or her symptoms. Similarly, in a patient who is a poor historian, the family member may be able to provide essential information that may alter the diagnostic approach. All attempts should be made to compile a careful history and define the medical, neurologic, and psychological profile of the pain complaint. In geriatric patients with compromised cognitive function, the use of geriatric pain and symptom scales should be integrated.[18]

It is also useful to define for the patient the goal of treatment. Some patients may have unreasonable expectations for adequate pain control, whereas others fail to critically consider the various options available to them. Before starting any new procedure, review carefully with patients the risks and benefits to provide them with their expectation of the potential outcome of the therapeutic approach. As patients become more active in defining advance directives and as they focus on the quality of life, it is critical to ask patients to define what they would do if the pain were intractable or intolerable.[74] Did the patient have a family member who died a painful death? In the author's experience, patients who have had such an experience are particularly fearful of their own deaths. Does the patient have suicidal thoughts or a pact with a family member? Does the patient have a family history of suicide? Does the patient have drugs in reserve or a gun in the house that he or she might use in desperation?[74] In a study by Chochinov et al., pain alone did not correlate with patients' suicidal ideation.[74] Significant depression appeared to be the major correlating factor, although pain clearly played a role in the development of depression in some patients. This series of questions allows patients to discuss openly their fears of death and their intention to take matters into their own hands rather than trust the health care professional. Such open discussions can allow the physician to better define for the patient the options for care and to reassure the patient of the physician's commitment to care. Because patients rarely offer this information unless requested, it is critical to develop specific questions that can be readily integrated into the initial history taking by the physician. Discussing with the patient how he or she would die and engaging the patient in a discussion of his or her concerns and desires can address the commonly heard comment of patients, "I have never died before, how do I do it?"

PERFORM A CAREFUL MEDICAL AND NEUROLOGIC EXAMINATION

A medical and neurologic examination helps provide the necessary data to substantiate the history. It also provides a direct assessment of the cognitive status of the patient. Knowledge of the referral patterns of pain and the common cancer pain syndromes can direct the examination. The commonly described pain syndromes in cancer patients associated with postmastectomy pain can readily be defined as separate from tumor infiltration of the brachial plexus[51,75] (see Table 55.1-6).

The physical and neurologic examination allows the physician to visually inspect and palpate the site of pain and to look for the associated physical and neurologic signs that might help to better define the nature of the pain symptom. Defining the degree of motor or sensory changes can help identify the specific site in the nervous system that may be involved. Similarly, in patients with sensory loss, the presence of allodynia and hyperesthesia can further identify the nature of the sensory problem and define a neuropathic pain syndrome. Moreover, the degree of muscle spasm, gait instability, and impaired coordination can only be fully assessed by such an evaluation. In patients with neuropathic pain, the use of quantitative sensory testing can help define the underlying mechanism and determine selection of drug therapy.

ORDER THE APPROPRIATE DIAGNOSTIC STUDIES AND PERSONALLY REVIEW THE RESULTS

Diagnostic studies confirm the diagnosis and define in patients with metastatic disease the site and extent of tumor infiltration. Computed tomography and magnetic resonance imaging (MRI) are the most useful diagnostic procedures in evaluating cancer patients with pain. Positron emission tomography helps to further define tumor and differentiate tumor from radiation injury and postsurgical injury. The bone scan is a useful screening device and is more sensitive for demonstrating abnormalities in the bone before changes appear on a plain radiograph. However, a negative finding on bone scan does not rule out bony metastatic disease, nor does a positive finding on bone scan confirm the diagnosis of metastatic tumor. In patients with collapsed vertebral bodies, MRI can distinguish osteoporotic from tumor-induced bony changes. The physician should review the results personally with the radiologist to correlate any pathologic change with the site of pain.

Evaluation of the extent of metastatic disease may help to discover the relation of the pain complaint to possible recurrent disease. The measurement of tumor markers such as carcinoembryonic antigen, cancer antigen 125, cancer antigen 15-3, and prostate-specific antigen can be useful in a patient in whom recurrent tumor is suspected. The use of radiolabeled carcinoembryonic antigen to scan for tumor recurrence may be helpful to differentiate recurrent colon and other gastrointestinal tumors and recurrent lung tumors from postoperative changes. In certain pain syndromes, the presence of recurrent disease is closely associated with the onset of pain (e.g., the appearance of late postthoracotomy pain syndrome in a patient after initial resolution of the postoperative pain).

TREAT THE PAIN TO FACILITATE THE APPROPRIATE WORKUP

No patient should be evaluated inadequately because of a significant pain problem. Early management of the pain while the source is investigated markedly improves the patient's ability to participate in the necessary diagnostic procedures. Table 55.1-7

TABLE 55.1-7. Reasons for Referral to the Pain Service (n = 100)

Reason for Referral[a]	No. of Referrals
Uncontrolled chronic pain despite analgesic therapy	73
Excessive side effects without adequate analgesia	24
Difficulties in assessment	22
Uncontrolled acute pain despite analgesic therapy	12
Change route of opioid administration	8
Concern regarding drug-seeking behavior or possibility of addiction	8
Excessive side effects with adequate analgesia	5
Manage preexistent route of drug administration	2
Concern that the patient's analgesic regimen involves too many pills	2
Concern that pain is disproportionate for extent of disease	1
Concern that patient is using excessive opioid therapy	1

[a]Physicians were asked to record one or more reasons for referral. The three reasons that were never cited included uncontrolled pain in a patient not on analgesic therapy, concern that the patient is receiving too many drugs, and concern that the treatment is too expensive. (From ref. 25, with permission.)

lists the reasons identified for seeking a pain consultation at Memorial Sloan-Kettering Cancer Center. During the initial evaluation of the pain complaint, early consideration of the use of alternative methods of pain control, including anesthetic and neurosurgical approaches, should be considered (e.g., the temporary use of a local anesthetic via an epidural catheter to manage sacral pain).

REASSESS THE PATIENT'S RESPONSE TO THERAPY

Continual reassessment of the response of the patient's pain complaint to the prescribed therapy provides the best method to validate the initial diagnosis as correct. If relief is less than predicted or if the pain worsens, reassessment of the treatment approach or a search for a new cause of the pain should be considered. A common example is the patient with epidural cord compression who develops a second block proximal to the one being radiated, with neurologic signs mimicking those of the original one.[76]

INDIVIDUALIZE THE DIAGNOSTIC AND THERAPEUTIC APPROACHES

Evaluation of the patient must be closely linked to the patient's level of function, ability to participate in the diagnostic workup, willingness to undergo the necessary diagnostic approaches, objective evidence that treatment approaches may be beneficial, and life expectancy. Careful judgment is required to select diagnostic approaches that will have a direct effect on the choice of the therapeutic strategy or will answer a specific question. The random use of diagnostic procedures in these patients, particularly those with advanced cancer and significant pain, is inappropriate because it may have an adverse effect on their quality of life. Open discussion with the patient about the need for assessment as well as the therapeutic options is critical to allow the patient to be part of the decision-making process. For some patients, diagnostic procedures such as MRI are inappropriate because they simply confirm the existence of a disease for which no treatment is available or for which the treatment would be a major surgical procedure (e.g., vertebral body resection) that would be inappropriate for a dying patient. Patient refusal of evaluation or treatment must be respected when the physician has fully explained the options and is convinced that the patient has an accurate understanding of the implications of undertaking no further workup or treatment.[77]

DISCUSS ADVANCE DIRECTIVES WITH THE PATIENT AND FAMILY

When approaches for treatment are being developed, there must be an open discussion about advance directives so that the physician has a clear understanding of the patient's goal for therapy or his or her ambivalence in developing a therapeutic strategy. The physician must have unconditional positive regard for the patient, placing the control of symptoms of pain and treatment of psychological distress in the highest regard. Knowledge of the patient's decisions about resuscitation, living wills, and symptom management should he or she become incompetent improves the physician's ability to appropriately and humanely care for the dying patient with advanced disease.[69] In a study of patients at Memorial Sloan-Kettering Cancer Center evaluated by the Pain and Palliative Care Service, patients reported reluctance to discuss end-of-life care issues with their physicians, preferring to discuss their concerns with family and friends. Patients often fear that if they express ambivalence about a treatment strategy suggested by the oncologist, the oncologist will withdraw the suggestion for antitumor approaches.[78] Such data emphasize the need for education of families regarding the continuum of cancer care, including issues of pain management and the role of sedation in patients whose lives are ending.

MANAGEMENT OF CANCER PAIN

The management of cancer pain combines treatment of the primary disease with analgesic drug therapy and anesthetic, neurosurgical, rehabilitative, psychological (cognitive-behavioral), psychiatric, and complementary and alternative methods. Individualization of the treatment strategy and titration to effective pain relief are the hallmarks of this therapeutic approach. Increasing sophistication in the use of analgesic drugs, coupled with advances in research on the underlying mechanisms of pain, has provided the scientific rationale for the more effective use of standard analgesic drug therapy (nonopioid, opioid, and adjuvant drugs), including the use of novel means of drug administration (transdermal and transmucosal), the use of novel methods (bisphosphonates and calcitonin for bone pain, antidepressants and anticonvulsants for neuropathic pain), and the use of anesthetic, neurosurgical, psychological, and psychiatric approaches concurrently applied in the overall continuum of care.

Pain management is only one aspect of a broad palliative care approach, but it serves as a model for the scientific rigor and clinical trials that have defined cancer pain treatment as a specific strategic focus. The full impact of such a comprehensive approach has not been fully determined. Data evaluating the use of analgesic drug therapy for cancer pain alone indicate that 70% to 90% of patients report adequate analgesia.

Studies at various pain services, hospices, and palliative care programs report results showing that as many as 95% of patients receive effective analgesia.

To develop appropriate outcome assessment methods and to provide a basis for comparison of treatment strategies, Dr. Bruera[64] has developed the Edmonton Staging System for cancer pain, patterning it on the various staging systems for different primary tumors. Stage I (good prognosis), stage II (intermediate prognosis), and stage III (poor prognosis) are based on five prognostic features, including the presence or absence of neuropathic pain, incident pain, psychological distress, rapid tolerance development, and a history of drug addiction or alcohol abuse.[6] This methodology, in preliminary studies, has been validated as a way to compare different patient populations with different primary tumors in clinical trials and outcome assessments of cancer pain therapy.

ANALGESIC DRUG THERAPY

Numerous guidelines for the management of cancer pain have been issued by various organizations and researchers.[2,30,79–81] All of these guidelines have emphasized that analgesic drug therapy is the mainstay of treatment and have focused on the aims of drug therapy to achieve adequate pain relief safely within an acceptable time frame, minimize side effects of treatment, and provide ongoing analgesic therapy by the most convenient and least noxious means available. More recently, detailed descriptions of the decision-making process implemented during the treatment of patients with pain have provided further data on the rationale for and outcomes of specific decisions and have detailed a series of principles in the selection of opioid drug and route of administration. Reasons for cancer pain consultation and guidelines for the rational use of analgesics in the management of cancer pain are detailed later. These guidelines are based on clinical pharmacologic principles, clinical trials, available metaanalyses of analgesic studies, and the clinical experience of the Pain Service at Memorial Sloan-Kettering Cancer Center. Table 55.1-7 lists the reasons why patients with pain were referred to an inpatient consultation service at Memorial Sloan-Kettering Cancer Center. These reasons for referral point out the complexity that is now faced in providing individualized pharmacotherapy for patients with pain. These data also point out the need for physicians and nurses to be knowledgeable in the use of these guidelines to provide patients with effective analgesia. These data, from 100 consecutively treated inpatients who were referred over a 14-week period to the Memorial Sloan-Kettering Cancer Center Pain Service, show 158 reasons for referral.[25] The two most common reasons were uncontrolled chronic pain, which occurred in 73 patients, and excessive side effects without adequate analgesia despite analgesic therapy, which occurred in 24 patients. The most common reasons included difficulties in pain assessment and poorly controlled acute pain. At the time of initial evaluation, 77 patients had a pain intensity of 7 out of 10, and 18 patients had a pain intensity of 4 to 6 out of 10. After initial evaluation by the Pain Service physicians, the therapeutic intent of analgesic therapy was to provide comfort and function for 87 patients and comfort only for 13 patients. Comfort and function were the therapeutic intent of analgesic therapy for 75 of the patients discharged (92%), and comfort only was the goal for 17 of the patients who died (94%). After initial evaluation, the Pain

Service physicians changed the opioid drug, the route of administration, or both for 58 patients. Of 42 patients whose regimens were not changed, 17 were discharged, 3 died, and 22 required subsequent changes in either drug or route of administration. In short, a total of 80 patients required changes in opioid therapy before death or discharge. Sixty-four patients required more than one change in therapy. Forty-four patients required one or more changes, and 20 patients required two or more changes. These data are particularly important in indicating the complexity of analgesic drug therapy in this population of patients. Side effects were problematic in providing patients with a balance between adequate analgesia and excessive side effects. It is critical, then, that the goals of care for an individual patient be recognized and help provide the essential context for therapeutic decision making. When patients give equal priority to optimal comfort and function, the therapeutic attempt is to achieve an adequate degree of relief without compromising cognitive and physical function. When comfort is the overriding goal of care, there is a willingness to use whatever analgesic therapy is necessary to achieve relief, even if function is diminished in the process. To achieve the goal of care when both comfort and function are to be maximized, substantial effort is necessary to achieve an optimal balance between relief and side effects through dosage adjustment, sequential trials of opioid drugs, coadministration of adjuvant medications, and the use of spinal analgesic techniques. Increasing attention has been focused on the need to switch patients from one opioid to another. Several studies have outlined the need for opioid rotation and substitution.[82–87]

In the section World Health Organization Three-Step Analgesic Ladder that follows, detailed guidelines for the rational use of analgesics in the management of cancer pain are provided (Table 55.1-8). The use of drug therapy should be within the armamentarium of any physician or nurse who cares for cancer patients with pain. Similarly, some of the psychological and psychiatric approaches should be widely available for integration. The use of specific anesthetic and neurosurgical techniques often requires the services of trained medical personnel who have clinical experience in managing cancer pain, but such approaches may require referral to a specialty center. The widespread use of alternative and complementary therapies and the development of integrative medical programs within cancer centers point to the increasing role of such approaches to reduce suffering in the cancer patient.

WORLD HEALTH ORGANIZATION THREE-STEP ANALGESIC LADDER

As part of a global program of the WHO, the Cancer and Palliative Care Unit has created a Cancer Pain Relief Program and, through a series of expert panels, has developed guidelines for the treatment of cancer pain.[4,88] This program has achieved a broad international consensus, based on the concept that analgesic drug therapy is the mainstay for the majority of patients with cancer pain. Field testing of the WHO guidelines, in conjunction with clinical experience, has shown that 70% to 90% of cancer patients' pain can be controlled using a simple and inexpensive method described as the *three-step analgesic ladder*.[88] This approach is based on the use of a combination of nonopioid, opioid, and adjuvant drugs, titrated to meet the individual needs of the patient according to the severity of pain and its pathophysiology (Tables 55.1-9 through

TABLE 55.1-8. Guidelines for the Rational Use of Analgesics in the Management of Cancer Pain

START WITH A SPECIFIC DRUG FOR A SPECIFIC TYPE OF PAIN
KNOW THE PHARMACOLOGY OF THE DRUG PRESCRIBED
Know the relative potency of the drug
Know the duration of the analgesic effect
Know the pharmacokinetics of the drug
Know the equianalgesic doses for the drug and its route of administration
ADMINISTER ANALGESIC ON A REGULAR BASIS
GEAR THE ROUTE OF ADMINISTRATION TO THE PATIENT'S NEEDS
Oral
Buccal
Rectal
Subcutaneous
Intrathecal
Sublingual
Transmucosal
Transdermal
Intravenous
Intraventricular
USE A COMBINATION OF DRUGS TO PROVIDE ADDITIVE ANALGESIA
Narcotic plus nonnarcotic (aspirin, acetaminophen, nonsteroidal antiinflammatory drugs)
Narcotic plus adjuvants
ANTICIPATE AND TREAT SIDE EFFECTS
Sedation
Respiratory depression
Nausea and vomiting
Constipation
Multifocal myoclonus and seizures
MANAGEMENT OF THE TOLERANT PATIENT
Use combinations of nonopioid and opioid drugs
Use combinations of drug therapy, anesthetic, and neurosurgical procedures
Switch to an alternative opioid analgesic, starting with one-half the equianalgesic dose
Use epidural local anesthetics
Reassess the nature of the pain
PREVENT AND TREAT ACUTE WITHDRAWAL
Taper drugs slowly
ANTICIPATE COMPLICATIONS
Overdose
Psychological dependence

55.1-11). Implementation of the analgesic guidelines, assurance of drug availability (specifically opioids), the education of health care professionals, and designation of cancer pain as a priority for all national cancer control programs are the major goals of the WHO effort.[89]

Step 1

Step 1 of the analgesic ladder focuses on analgesic drug therapy for patients with mild to moderate cancer pain. Such patients should be treated with a nonopioid analgesic that may or may not be combined with an adjuvant drug, depending on the specific pain pathophysiology. For example, in a patient with mild pain from bone metastases, the use of acetaminophen, aspirin, or one of the other nonsteroidal antiinflammatory drugs (NSAIDs) would be appropriate. In a patient with mild pain from a peripheral neuropathy, the combination of a

TABLE 55.1-9.   Nonopioid Analgesics for Mild to Moderate Pain

Class	Generic Name	Half-Life (h)	Dosing Schedule	Recommended Starting Dose (mg)	Maximum Starting Dose (mg)
Salicylates	Aspirin	3–12	q4–6h	2600	6000
	Choline magnesium trisalicylate	9–17	q12h	200	600
	Diflunisal	8–12	q12h	1500 mg × 1, then 1000 q12h	4000
p-Aminophenol derivative	Acetaminophen (paracetamol)	2–4	q4–6h	2600	4000
Propionic acids	Ibuprofen	1.8–2	q4–8h	1200	3200
	Fenoprofen	2–3	q4–6h	800	3200
	Ketoprofen	2–3	q6–8h	150	300
	Naproxen	13	q12h	550	1100
	Naproxen sodium	13	q12h	550	1100
Acetic acids	Etodolac	7	q6–8h	600	1200
	Ketorolac	4–7	q6h	15–30 q6h IV, IM; 10 q6h PO	120 IV, IM; 40 PO
Fenamates	Meclofenamic acid	1.3	q6–8h	150	400
	Mefenamic acid	2	q6h	500 × 1, then 250 q6h	1000

nonopioid with a tricyclic antidepressant drug, such as amitriptyline, would be appropriate.

Step 2

Step 2 focuses on patients with moderate pain who failed to achieve adequate relief after a trial of a nonopioid analgesic. They are candidates for a combination of a nonopioid [e.g., aspirin, acetaminophen, cyclooxygenase-2 (COX-2) inhibitors, other NSAIDs] and an opioid such as codeine, oxycodone, propoxyphene, buprenorphine, or tramadol. Depending on the pain pathophysiology, adjuvant drugs should be used as well.

Step 3

Step 3 is for those patients who report severe pain or who report moderate pain that is inadequately managed after appro-

priate administration of drugs at the second step of the ladder. Nonopioids are often used in combination with opioids to spare the opioid effect, and adjuvants are used depending on the pain pathophysiology or the need to control other concurrent symptoms in the individual patient.

In short, the analgesic drug ladder of the WHO simply defines a method for using drug combinations and is based on previously well-tested pharmacologic principles. What continues to be controversial in the application of the WHO ladder is the choice of the analgesic drug for the individual patient. Such controversies are discussed within the framework of the current application of the guidelines for rational use.[82,90–92] Critical assessment of the WHO ladder has raised challenging questions to the selection of specific drugs. For example, a metaanalysis of the role of NSAIDs in bone pain did not define them as any more or less effective than opioids.[93]

TABLE 55.1-10.   Opioid Drugs Commonly Used in Cancer Pain Management

Drug[a]	Intramuscular (mg)	Oral (mg)	Half-Life (h)	Duration of Action (h)
Codeine	130	200	2–3	2–4
Dihydrocodeine		200	2–3	2–4
Oxycodone	15	30	2–3	2–4
Propoxyphene	50	100	2–3	2–4
Morphine	10	30 (repeated dose) 60 (single dose)	2–3	3–4
Hydromorphone	1.5	7.5	2–3	2–4
Methadone	10	20	15–190	4–8
Meperidine	75	300	2–3	2–4
Oxymorphone	1	10 (per rectum)	2–3	3–4
Levorphanol	2	4	12–15	4–8
Fentanyl (parenteral)	0.1	—	1–2	1–3
Fentanyl (transdermal system)[b]	—	—	—	48–72
Fentanyl (transmucosal)	—	—	1–2	1–2

[a]Oxycodone, hydromorphone, and morphine available in slow-release preparations.
[b]Transdermal fentanyl, 100 μg/h; morphine, 4 mg/h.

TABLE 55.1-11. Adjuvant Analgesics in the Management of Cancer Pain

ADJUVANT DRUGS FOR NEUROPATHIC PAIN
Antidepressants
Anticonvulsants
Oral and cutaneous local anesthetics
Corticosteroids
Clonidine
Benzodiazepines
Neuroleptics
α_2-Adrenergic agonist drugs
N-methyl D-aspartate antagonists
Calcitonin
ADJUVANT DRUGS FOR BONE PAIN
Bisphosphonates
Gallium nitrate
Calcitonin
Strontium 89
ADJUVANTS TO TREAT SIDE EFFECTS
Antiemetics
   Compazine
   Metoclopramide
   Ondansetron
Psychostimulants
   Caffeine
   Methylphenidate
   Dextroamphetamine
Laxatives
   Senna
ADJUVANTS TO ENHANCE ANALGESIA
Acetaminophen
Nonsteroidal antiinflammatory drugs
Hydroxyzine

CLASSES OF DRUGS

NONOPIOID ANALGESICS

The nonopioid analgesics include acetaminophen and the NSAIDs, of which aspirin is the prototypic agent. These compounds are most commonly used orally, and their analgesia is limited by a ceiling effect, so that increasing the dose beyond a certain level (900 to 1300 mg/dose of aspirin) produces no increase in peak effect. Tolerance and physical dependence do not occur with repeated administration. Aspirin and the other NSAIDs have analgesic, antipyretic, antiinflammatory, and antiplatelet actions. Some NSAIDs, such as choline magnesium trisalicylate, lack the antiplatelet effects of aspirin. Others (e.g., ibuprofen) appear to produce fewer gastrointestinal side effects than aspirin. The COX-2 inhibitors are agents that offer the unique advantage of less gastrointestinal and renal toxicity and no effect on platelet function. Three drugs are currently marketed as COX-2 inhibitors—rofecoxib, celecoxib, and valdecoxib—but they have not been studied in cancer patients to define their particular role. Medications currently available for use are based on U.S. Food and Drug Administration approval: rofecoxib for acute pain management and osteoarthritis, and celecoxib for osteoarthritis and rheumatoid arthritis. Acetaminophen, which is equipotent to aspirin, is an analgesic and antipyretic. It is much less effective as an antiinflammatory agent but does not interfere with platelet function.

In general, this class of drugs is thought to produce analgesia by inhibiting activation of peripheral nociceptors through their prevention of the formation of prostaglandin E_2, a known sensitizer of peripheral receptors to nociceptive stimulation from tissue injury. Evidence suggests that central mechanisms augment the peripheral effects of these drugs via inhibition of neural activity induced by EAAs such as glutamate or tachykinins such as substance P. The NSAIDs differ both in duration of analgesic action and in their pharmacokinetic profile. Ibuprofen and fenoprofen have short half-lives and the same duration of action as aspirin, whereas diflunisal and naproxen have longer half-lives and are longer acting. These drugs are thought to have a special role to play in the management of bone pain because numerous studies have shown that aspirin inhibits tumor growth in an animal model of metastatic bone tumor. A metaanalysis of studies using NSAIDs to treat bone pain did not demonstrate them to be more effective than weak opioids such as codeine, oxycodone, and propoxyphene.[93] From clinical experience, some patients respond better to one NSAID than to another, and each patient should be given an adequate trial of one drug on a regular basis before switching to another. Survey data from the WHO demonstration projects suggest that 20% to 40% of patients obtain pain relief with the use of nonopioid analgesics alone.[94]

Numerous studies have elucidated the major risk factors for gastrointestinal toxicity associated with NSAID use. Various factors contribute to the high risk of ulcer complications, including advanced age, use of higher doses, concomitant administration of corticosteroids, and a history of either ulcer disease or previous gastrointestinal complications from NSAIDs. The empiric use of various prophylactic therapies to prevent gastrointestinal complications is controversial. Except for misoprostol, there is no evidence that any of these approaches reduces the risk of serious gastrointestinal toxicity. The empiric approach at this time is to administer misoprostol to all patients who have significant risk factors for gastrointestinal complications.[95] Many of these data have been accumulated in the general literature and have not been specifically analyzed for patients with cancer. Several NSAIDs have been approved by the U.S. Food and Drug Administration for use as analgesics for mild to moderate pain and are listed in Table 55.1-9. Guidelines for the use of NSAIDs in patients with cancer are largely empiric. This class of drugs represents the first-line approach, but the choice and use of the nonopioid need to be individualized. Each patient should be given an adequate trial of one nonopioid analgesic before switching to an alternative one. Such a trial should include administration of the drug to maximum levels at regular intervals. Because there is a great variability among patient responses to different drugs, patients may require trials with several NSAIDs before finding an effective drug and dose regimen. If pain relief is not obtained, adding an opioid to a nonopioid provides additive analgesia. Combinations containing codeine, oxycodone, and propoxyphene are available, but these combinations often contain less than the full dose of 650 mg of aspirin or acetaminophen. Prescribing each drug separately provides a better method for individualizing pain control. This is particularly important when the patient requires escalation of the combination to provide analgesia, in which case the additional amount of the NSAID or acetaminophen may become excessive.

OPIOID DRUGS

The opioid analgesics, of which morphine is the prototype, vary in potency, efficacy, and adverse effects. These drugs produce their analgesic effects by binding to discrete opiate receptors in the peripheral and central nervous systems. This group also includes a series of heterogeneous substances with varying chemical structures. In contrast to the nonopioid analgesics, opioid analgesics, at least the opioid pure agonists, do not appear to have a ceiling effect (i.e., as the dose is escalated on a log scale, the increment in analgesia is linear to the point of loss of consciousness). There are also series of drugs that are pure antagonists (i.e., they block the effect of morphine at the receptor). The antagonist drug most commonly used in clinical practice is naloxone, which is administered to reverse respiratory depression and other complications associated with opioid overdose.

Effective use of the opioid drugs requires the balancing of the most desirable effects of pain relief with the undesirable effects of nausea, vomiting, mental clouding, sedation, constipation, tolerance, and physical dependence. These undesirable effects impose a practical limit on the dose useful for a particular patient and have led to the concept of opioid responsiveness (see Principles of Opioid Drug Therapy, later in this chapter).

The use of opioids in the management of cancer pain remains a controversial issue.[82,90,92,96,97] Some of the controversies include their role in the management of neuropathic pain, which has been suggested to be *opioid resistant*, the specific choice of opioid drug, the use of sequential trials of opioids, routes of administration, development of tolerance, risk of addiction, economic factors influencing these controversies, and the concern that opioids are agents of physician-assisted suicide and euthanasia.[98-100] When appropriate, these controversies are addressed in the following discussion of the principles of opioid drug therapy.

Principles of Opioid Drug Therapy

START WITH A SPECIFIC DRUG FOR A SPECIFIC TYPE OF PAIN. As defined by the three-step analgesic ladder, the specific drug chosen is dependent in part on the degree of pain intensity. As previously noted, cancer patients commonly have multiple sites and types of pain. It has been suggested that neuropathic pain, which accounts for 15% to 20% of pain problems that are difficult to manage, is opioid resistant and that opioid drugs should not be used in this patient population.[92] Studies involving cancer patients with both nociceptive and neuropathic pain, as well as controlled studies of nonmalignant neuropathic pain, demonstrate the variable responsiveness of neuropathic pain to opioid analgesics. A continuum of opioid responsiveness, rather than an all-or-none quantal phenomenon, has been clearly observed. *Opioid responsiveness* is defined as the degree of analgesia achieved during dose escalation to either intolerable side effects or adequate analgesia. Patient characteristics and pain-related factors, as well as drug-selective effects, influence this variable response.

A wide range of adjuvant analgesics has been suggested to provide analgesia alone or in combination with opioid drug therapy, and there are specific adjuvants for bone pain and neuropathic pain. The choice of a specific drug is dictated not only by pain intensity and type of pain, but also by the patient's prior opioid exposure, history of allergy, and history of side effects.

The WHO cancer pain guidelines designated morphine as the drug of choice in its Cancer Pain Relief Program. The choice was based on practical, not scientific, considerations. The introduction of the WHO program rapidly demonstrated the limited availability of morphine worldwide for oral treatment of chronic cancer pain.[4] Morphine consumption worldwide is now used as an indicator of the success of the WHO Cancer Pain Relief Program. The Pain and Policy Center at the University of Wisconsin tracks changes in morphine consumption worldwide and has demonstrated that increases in consumption correspond to expansion of national pain and palliative care programs.[101] For example, in Japan, after a nationwide program to improve cancer pain management, a 17-fold increase in morphine consumption has been reported. The expanded use of morphine, combined with new formulations and new information about the analgesic activities of its metabolites, focuses renewed attention on its clinical pharmacology with recognition of morphine-6-glucuronide (M6G) as an active metabolite.[102] Human studies have shown that M6G is analgesic in humans and appears in the plasma and cerebrospinal fluid of patients receiving morphine systemically.[103] In renal dysfunction, M6G has an increased elimination half-life and decreased clearance, which confirm a true delay in elimination of the compound and lead to an increase in the ratio of M6G to morphine during chronic therapy.[104] Adverse effects (nausea and respiratory depression) have been attributed to plasma concentration of the metabolite, particularly in patients with renal failure.[105] However, attempts to correlate M6G to morphine ratio or M6G to morphine-3-glucuronide (M3G) ratio with side effects such as cognitive impairment or myoclonus have not been successful. Various factors may influence the levels of both M6G and M3G, including route (increased M6G after oral administration), age (increased M3G and M6G if older than 70 years), male gender (decreased morphine and M6G plasma concentrations), concurrent use of tricyclic antidepressants (increased M3G), and use of ranitidine (increased morphine). Studies have described polymorphism in the morphine gene and variability in patient responses to morphine and M6G.[106] Controlled-release oral morphine is currently available in a wide range of doses from 50 to 200 mg for every 8-, 12-, and 24-hour administration. These preparations provide analgesia comparable to that of immediate-release forms and offer increased convenience, improved compliance, and a reduction in duration of pain.

The increasing need for a wide range of opioids to manage cancer pain has led to the widespread use of a series of opioid alternatives to morphine, including hydromorphone, oxycodone, oxymorphone, and levorphanol, all congeners of morphine. Hydromorphone has poor oral availability and a short half-life. It is highly soluble and available in a high-potency parenteral form (10 mg/mL), which makes it a useful choice for chronic subcutaneous administration. Because of its short half-life, it is commonly used in the elderly patient. Myoclonus has been reported after high doses, possibly due to accumulation of its metabolites (3-0 methyl glucuronide and hydromorphone-6-glucuronide).[107] When compared in a double-blind trial of patient-controlled analgesia, no differences in analgesia or side effects were noted between morphine and hydromorphone.[108] Although cognitive performance was poorer in the hydromorphone group, patients reported better mood than those receiving morphine. Hydromorphone is available in slow-release preparations.

Oxycodone, which is commonly administered in a 5-mg dose at the second step of the WHO analgesic ladder, can also be used in the third step at higher doses. It is now available in a slow-release preparation.[109] Its half-life is 3 to 4 hours. Oxymorphone is its active metabolite. Oxymorphone is currently available in intravenous and rectal preparations and serves as an alternative to morphine and its other congeners. Oral preparations are in development. Oxymorphone has a reduced histamine effect and may be of use in patients who complain of headache or itch after administration of other opioids.

Levorphanol has high bioavailability but a long plasma half-life (12 to 16 hours). It should be used cautiously because, with repeated administration, accumulation may occur.

The role of methadone in managing cancer pain also remains controversial.[83–87,110] Methadone represents a second-line drug for cancer pain patients who have had prior exposure to opioids. It is a relatively inexpensive oral analgesic, but its name has negative connotations for cancer patients, who view methadone as a drug used to treat addicts. The bioavailability of methadone is higher than that of morphine (85% vs. 35%, respectively). Its analgesic potency also differs, with a parenteral to oral ratio of 1:2 in contrast to 1:6 for morphine. Moreover, the plasma half-life of methadone is 17 to 24 hours, with reports of up to 50 hours in some cancer patients, but with a duration of analgesia of only 4 to 8 hours. Significant adverse effects have been reported in cancer patients receiving methadone by various routes. The discrepancy between the analgesic duration and plasma half-life of methadone has made it a difficult drug to use in the naive patient because of the need for careful titration.

A number of case reports have highlighted the possibly greater analgesic potency of methadone than the often quoted 1:1 equivalency with morphine.[83–87] Studies of interindividual differences in response to opioid analgesics have demonstrated that dramatically reduced dosages of methadone are required to produce analgesia in patients chronically taking morphine or hydromorphone. Several authors have shown marked reductions in the equianalgesic dose of methadone when patients with either uncontrolled pain or extreme side effects were switched to methadone. These clinical survey studies suggested up to a 75% reduction in the methadone equianalgesic dose when switching from hydromorphone to methadone. In the only prospective study, Ripamonti et al. developed a specific dose ratio based on the patients' morphine doses.[84] For patients taking 30 to 90 mg of morphine, the dose ratio is 4:1; for those taking 90 to 300 mg daily, the dose ratio is 6:1; and for those taking 300 mg or more, the dose ratio is 8:1. Bruera et al. developed a similar ratio for hydromorphone based on survey data.[83] In patients receiving more than 330 mg of hydromorphone, the dose ratio is 1.6:1.0; and in those receiving less than 300 mg, the dose ratio is 0.95:1.0.

Studies of the use of methadone by experienced clinicians in caring for advanced cancer patients at home report fewer dose escalations and good pain control, which supports the use of methadone in home settings.[85] Methadone can be administered by a variety of routes, but the subcutaneous route is associated with adverse effects, including cutaneous hypersensitivity.[110] Due to its long half-life, some offer the suggestion that methadone be administered every 8 to 12 hours, whereas others have demonstrated analgesic efficacy and safety in acute 3- to 4-hour dosing intervals. Ongoing studies are attempting to elucidate better the clinical pharmacology of methadone to facilitate its broader use.

Meperidine is a drug that should not be used chronically in the management of patients with cancer pain. Meperidine has a poor parenteral to oral ratio (1:4). It is available in oral and intramuscular preparations, but repetitive intramuscular administration is associated with local tissue fibrosis and sterile abscess. Repetitive dosing of meperidine (more than 250 mg/d) can lead to accumulation of normeperidine, an active metabolite that can produce central nervous system hyperexcitability.[111] This hyperirritability is characterized by subtle mood effects followed by tremors, multifocal myoclonus, and occasional seizures. It occurs most commonly in patients with renal disease but can also occur after repeated administration in patients with normal renal function. Naloxone does not reverse meperidine-induced seizures, and its use in meperidine toxicity is controversial. There have been some case reports that the use of naloxone has precipitated generalized seizures in individual patients. In rare instances, central nervous system toxicity characterized by hyperpyrexia, muscle rigidity, and seizure has been reported after the administration of a single dose of meperidine to patients receiving treatment with monoamine oxidase inhibitors.

With the development of a novel transdermal patch for administration, fentanyl is an opioid analgesic used effectively in cancer pain patients for management of both acute and chronic pain.[112] The half-life of fentanyl is 1 to 2 hours. Manfredi's group have drafted guidelines for fentanyl use summarizing all of the current data.[87] In chronic cancer pain management, relative potency comparisons have not been fully established, but the common dosing guideline is that 4 mg of intravenous morphine is equivalent to 100 μg of intravenous fentanyl. The uniqueness of this preparation facilitates the management of patients who are unable to take drugs by mouth by providing them with continuous opioid analgesia. Patches are currently available in 25 to 100 μg/h doses and are changed every 72 hours. When a patient is started on the fentanyl patch, there is up to a 12- to 15-hour delay in the onset of analgesia, and alternate approaches must be used to maintain patients' pain control during this period. Specific guidelines for switching to the fentanyl patch after an intravenous infusion of fentanyl have been developed and are based on use of a 1:1 conversion ratio. Fentanyl can also be used as an anesthetic premedication, as well as intravenously and epidurally for pain control. Oral transmucosal formulations have demonstrated effectiveness in treating breakthrough pain in cancer patients.[55] Oral transmucosal fentanyl (Actiq) is available in a range of doses from 200 to 1600 μg. Twenty-five percent of the preparations in a lozenge formulation in a stylet is absorbed transmucosally over a 15-minute period and an additional 25% is absorbed via the gastrointestinal tract over the following 90 minutes. Onset of relief occurs in 5 minutes. Oral transmucosal fentanyl citrate in dose-titration trials has been shown to be safe and effective, with the effective dose being a variable requiring titration in the majority of patients.

KNOW THE EQUIANALGESIC DOSE OF THE DRUG AND ITS ROUTE OF ADMINISTRATION. Knowing the equianalgesic dose can ensure more appropriate drug use. Lack of attention to these differences in drug dose is the most common cause of undermedication of pain patients. These equianalgesic doses have been derived from assessment of the relative analgesic potency of a drug. *Relative potency* is the ratio of the doses of two analgesics required to produce the same effect. Estimates of relative potency allow calculation of the equianalgesic dose, which provides the basis for selecting the appropriate dose when switching drugs or route of administration of the same drug. The values in Table 55.1-10 are based on studies in which 10 mg of morphine was the standard dose.[112] The equianalgesic dose is the recommended starting dose, with the optimal dose for each patient determined by dose adjustment. There is now evidence to suggest that relative potency may differ in single-dose and repeated-dose studies. For example, for morphine, a 1:6 relative analgesic potency ratio should be used for patients with acute pain, whereas a 1:2 or 1:3 ratio is more appropriate in patients treated with repeated doses on a chronic basis. For methadone, the equianalgesic dose ratios vary with the degree of prior exposure, as previously discussed earlier in the section Start with a Specific Drug for a Specific Type of Pain.[83,84]

ADMINISTER ANALGESICS REGULARLY AFTER INITIAL TITRATION. Medication should be given regularly to maintain the plasma level of the drug above the minimum effective concentration for pain relief. In the initial titration, patients should be advised to take their medication as needed to determine their total 24-hour requirements. This is also the time frame for reaching the steady-state level of drug, which depends on the drug's half-life. For morphine, steady state can be reached in 24 hours; with methadone, it may take up to 5 to 7 days to reach steady state. In patients on a fixed schedule, rescue medications equivalent to one-half of the standing dose should be available for breakthrough pain.

Continuous intravenous and subcutaneous opioid infusions to manage both acute and chronic cancer pain are commonly administered using a patient-controlled analgesic pump programmed to the patient's need with a set *lock-out time* to prevent overdosing. This method of drug administration is especially useful in managing patients with breakthrough pain. It is a significant advance in facilitating adequate titration of analgesics in chronic cancer patients, allowing discharge to home and hospice settings.

GEAR THE ROUTE OF ADMINISTRATION TO THE PATIENT'S NEEDS. Various methods of drug delivery of opioids have been developed in an attempt to maximize pharmacologic effects and minimize side effects. Most patients require at least two routes of drug administration and 20% need up to four approaches during the course of their cancer pain treatment, from diagnosis to death.

The oral route is preferable and easy. Orally administered drugs have a slower onset of action, delayed peak time, and longer duration of effect. Drugs given parenterally have a rapid onset of action but a shorter duration of effect. Slow-release preparations of morphine, hydromorphone, and oxycodone allow more convenient dosing of cancer pain patients every 8 to 12 hours or every 24 hours.

For cancer pain management by the sublingual route, there are drugs that are well absorbed sublingually, including both fentanyl and methadone.[114] As discussed in Start with a Specific Drug for a Specific Type of Pain, there is now an oral transmucosal fentanyl citrate preparation that has been widely studied for the management of breakthrough pain and is absorbed transmucosally.

For the rectal route, oxymorphone, hydromorphone, and morphine are available in suppository form. Oxymorphone suppositories produce analgesia equivalent to 10 mg of parenteral morphine. Slow-release oxycodone and morphine preparations have also been demonstrated to be effective rectally, and ongoing studies with rectal methadone suggest that this drug is well absorbed by the rectal route.

The transdermal route is a convenient way to deliver a potent short-acting opioid on a continuous basis. Drug is released through the skin patch at a nearly constant amount per unit time with a concentration gradient from patch to skin. Serum fentanyl concentrations increase and steady-state levels are approached at 12 to 24 hours.[113] After patch removal, the drug persists in the skin, with falling blood levels over 24 hours. For calculation of the equianalgesic dose, 4 mg of intravenous morphine is equivalent to 100 µg of fentanyl transdermally. Innovative transdermal delivery systems are in development, which include systems for immediate-dose delivery using iontophoresis and drug reservoirs. Iontophoresis is the transfer of ionic solutes through biologic membranes under the influence of an electric field. It offers an alternative system for parenteral administration and has been shown to allow for comparatively rapid achievement of fentanyl dose levels using a transdermal system.

Various parenteral routes include intermittent and continuous subcutaneous, intravenous, epidural, intraventricular, and intrathecal infusions. The use of intermittent and continuous subcutaneous infusions is most useful in patients who cannot tolerate oral analgesics because of gastrointestinal obstruction or intractable nausea and vomiting and do not have intravenous access. The usefulness of this technique has been demonstrated using morphine, heroin, hydromorphone, levorphanol, and fentanyl. Administration of methadone by this route is associated with the development of a cutaneous hypersensitivity syndrome.[110]

Patient-controlled analgesic pumps designed to infuse continuously but with options for bolus administration are connected to a 27-gauge butterfly needle that the patient can insert into a new subcutaneous site every third to sixth day. Limited pharmacokinetic studies have demonstrated that, for example, systemic absorption of the drug at steady state reaches 87% bioavailability from subcutaneous infusion of hydromorphone.[115]

Intermittent and continuous intravenous infusions are used if intravenous access is available and more commonly in patients who are hospitalized. Specific guidelines for the use of continuous infusions have been developed.[116]

Use of intermittent and continuous epidural and intrathecal opioid infusions is based on the demonstration of opioid receptors in the dorsal horn of the spinal cord and the availability of opioid drugs to suppress noxious stimuli at the spinal cord level.[45,48] Localized selective analgesia is produced without motor or sensory blockade. Analysis of the pharmacokinetics of epidural opioid administration demonstrate that there is significant systemic uptake after epidural injection, comparable with that after an intramuscular injection of the same drug and dose. However, distribution of the drug directly into the cerebrospinal fluid is 10 to 100 times greater. Existing studies demonstrate that this approach is used with approximately 10% of cancer patients to maximize analgesia and minimize side effects. This technique is commonly used in patients who have mixed nociceptive neuropathic pain syndromes and in whom combinations of local anesthetics and opioids are administered epidurally. A 3-year retrospective outcome study of the use of epidural catheters in the management of chronic cancer pain identified the occurrence of technical problems and infection, including epidural abscesses, in a significant number of patients. The study suggests that epidural catheters be used in patients with limited life expectancy.[117]

Smith et al. completed a randomized clinical trial in which an implantable drug delivery system was compared to comprehensive medical management of refractory cancer pain.[118] The patients using the implantable system reported better pain relief with fewer drug side effects and improved survival. Cost-effectiveness studies have not been done, but there is clearly the added cost of the pump, and the costs of the system need to be compared to the costs of nonpump medicines and the potential savings from prevention of hospitalizations for pain management analyzed.[118] Rarely, intraventricular opioid infusion has been used to manage patients with pain in the cervical and craniofacial region from tumor infiltration.[119] Dosages between 1.0 and 7.5 mg/24 h have been used, and excellent results have been reported in 70% of patients. At present, there is not a clear indication that this intraventricular route offers special advantages over systemic approaches.[119]

USE A COMBINATION OF DRUGS. The use of a combination of drugs enables a physician to increase analgesic effects without escalating the opioid dose. Combinations that produce additive analgesic effects include an opioid plus a nonopioid, an opioid plus an antihistamine (100 mg of intramuscular hydroxyzine), and an opioid plus an amphetamine (10 mg of intramuscular dextroamphetamine).[120–124] Trials of opioids combined with dextromethorphan demonstrate additive analgesia.

ANTICIPATE AND TREAT SIDE EFFECTS. The side effects of the opioid analgesics often limit their effective use. The most common side effects are sedation, respiratory depression, nausea, vomiting, constipation, and multifocal myoclonus and seizures.

Sedation and drowsiness vary with the drug and dose and may occur after both single and repeated administration. They are mediated through activation of opiate receptors in the reticular formation and diffusely throughout the cortex. Management of these effects includes reducing the individual drug dose but giving the drug more frequently or switching to an analgesic with a shorter plasma half-life. As mentioned in the section Use a Combination of Drugs, trials of opioids combined with the NMDA antagonist dextromethorphan demonstrate additive analgesia as well. In controlled trials, amphetamine, methylphenidate, and caffeine have been demonstrated to counteract opioid-induced sedative effects. Anecdotal data for pemoline suggest that starting doses of 18.5 mg may be useful. Modafinil, currently approved for the treatment of narcolepsy in doses starting at 100 mg twice daily, has been reported to be useful in managing sedation, and donepezil (Aricept), which is U.S. Food and Drug Administration approved for treatment of Alzheimer's disease, has been suggested as clinically useful in treating opioid-induced sedation.[125–127] It is important to discontinue all other drugs that might exacerbate the sedative effects of the opioid analgesic, including a wide variety of medications such as cimetidine, barbiturates, and other anxiolytic medications.

Respiratory depression is the most serious adverse effect of the opioid drugs. It occurs most commonly after short-term administration of an opioid and is usually associated with other signs of central nervous system depression, including sedation and drowsiness. The opioid agonist drugs act on brainstem respiratory centers to produce, as a function of dose, increasing respiratory depression to the point of apnea. Tolerance to this effect develops rapidly with repeated drug administration, which allows prolonged use without significant risk of respiratory depression.

Respiratory depression can be reversed by giving the short-acting opioid antagonist naloxone (suggested dose, 0.4 mg/mL). Repeated administration, including an intravenous drip, may be necessary to prevent respiratory arrest in such patients. In patients receiving opioids for prolonged periods who develop respiratory depression, diluted doses of naloxone (0.4 mg in 10 mL of saline) should be titrated carefully to prevent the precipitation of severe withdrawal symptoms while reversing the respiratory depression. A useful dosing normogram for continuous intravenous infusion of naloxone has been developed in which two-thirds of the initial bolus is started on an hourly basis and titrated against the patient's symptoms.[128]

In some patients, the use of naloxone to reverse drug-induced respiratory depression can be dangerous. An endotracheal tube should be placed in the comatose patient before giving naloxone to prevent aspiration from excessive salivation and bronchial spasm induced by naloxone administration. In patients receiving meperidine over a longer period, naloxone may precipitate seizures by lowering the seizure threshold and by allowing the convulsant activity of the active metabolite, normeperidine, to become evident. In this instance, special attention must be given to the potential seizure effect of naloxone. If naloxone is used, diluted doses, slow titration, and appropriate seizure precautions are advised. There is insufficient clinical evidence to make more specific recommendations. If respiratory support can be effected by other means (i.e., continuous stimulation to maintain the patient's wakefulness), such an approach may place the patient at less risk and clearly in less discomfort.

The opioid analgesics produce nausea and vomiting by an action limited to the medullary chemoreceptor trigger zone. The incidence of nausea and vomiting is markedly increased in ambulatory patients. Tolerance develops to these side effects with repeated administration. The occurrence of nausea with one drug does not mean that all drugs will produce it. Switching to alternative opioid analgesics and using an antiemetic together with the opioid analgesic are ways to obviate this effect. Lack of controlled trials to identify a specific first-line agent has supported the practice of using sequential trials of agents beginning with prochlorperazine concurrently with the opioid to clarify a useful regimen. Droperidol has also been noted to be effective against opioid-induced nausea and vomiting.

Constipation results from the action of these drugs at multiple sites in the gastrointestinal tract and in the spinal cord to produce a decrease in the intestinal secretions and peristalsis, which leads to a dry stool and constipation. When opioid analgesics are started, a regular bowel regimen, including use of cathartics and stool softeners, should also be instituted. Several bowel regimens have been suggested because of their specific ability to counteract the effects of the opioid drugs, but none has been studied in a controlled way.[129] Anecdotal surveys suggest that doses far above those used for routine bowel management are needed, that senna derivatives are effective, and that careful attention to dietary factors along with the use of a bowel regimen can reduce patient complaints dramatically. Tolerance to this effect develops over time, but relatively slowly. Oral naloxone has been shown to be effective in treating constipation, but its use is variable depending on the degree of opioid exposure of the patient. Clinical trials of the orally effective opioid antagonist methylnatrexone suggest that this agent works as a targeting drug to counteract constipation.[130]

Multifocal myoclonus may occur with high doses of all of the opioid drugs. Multifocal myoclonus and seizures have been reported in patients receiving multiple doses of meperidine (250 mg or more per day), although signs and symptoms of central nervous system hyperirritability may occur with toxic doses of all the opioid analgesics. In a series of cancer patients receiving meperidine, accumulation of the active metabolite normeperidine was associated with these neurologic signs and symptoms. However, in a similar group of cancer patients with pain, subtle mood effects were noted after meperidine administration, which suggests a spectrum of central nervous system effects. Management of this hyperirritability includes discontinuing the meperidine, using intravenous diazepam if seizures occur, and substituting morphine to control the persistent pain. Because the half-life of normeperidine is 16 hours, it may take 2 or 3 days for the signs of central nervous system hyperirritability to clear completely. Meperidine use is contraindicated in patients with chronic renal disease, but these complications noted in cancer pain treatment occurred in patients with normal renal function.[111] Morphine and hydromorphone at high doses produce myoclonus, which has not been directly associated with their known active metabolite such as M6G and hydromorphone-6-glucuronide. In dying patients with myoclonus, the use of benzodiazepines or barbiturates has been reported anecdotally to suppress this sign, improving the patient's comfort.

Opioid hyperexcitability and hyperalgesia have been reported with the use of increasing opioid doses by the parenteral acute and epidural routes. They have most often been observed in patients on high doses of morphine and hydromorphone and are characterized by uncontrolled pain, hypervigilance, total body hyperalgesia, and allodynia. They are best managed by rapid dose reduction and substitution with an alternative opioid such as methadone. The mechanism of action is unclear.

In animal studies of morphine use, the mechanism of action is thought to be related to M3G, which in animals is associated with allodynia and hyperalgesia after intracerebroventricular administration. This action of M3G is mimicked by strychnine, a glycine agonist. Glycine mediates postsynaptic inhibition on dorsal horn neurons. It is suggested that high doses of morphine or its metabolites may act via a spinal antiglycinergic effect, reducing postsynaptic inhibition and thus causing allodynia and myoclonus.

MANAGE TOLERANCE. The earliest sign of the development of tolerance is the patient's complaint that the duration of effective analgesia has decreased. For reasons not yet understood, the rate of development of tolerance varies greatly among cancer patients. Some demonstrate tolerance within days of initiating opioid therapy; others experience pain control for many months on the same dosage. Studies in an outpatient clinic population, a hospitalized population, and a home care population revealed three patterns of drug use: rapid increase in opioid requirements, stabilization at one dose for several weeks or months, and decrease or elimination of opioids.[131] Increased opioid requirements are most commonly associated with disease progression rather than with tolerance alone. With the development of tolerance, increases in the frequency of the dose of the opioid are required to provide continued pain relief. Because the analgesic effect is a logarithmic function of the dose of opioid, a doubling of the dose may be needed to restore full analgesia. There appears to be no limit to the development of tolerance, and with appropriate dose adjustments patients can continue to obtain pain relief. Tolerance to the respiratory effects of opioid doses occurs. This degree of tolerance makes it safe for patients to increase their opioid doses for analgesia.

Tolerance to one opioid does not lead to complete tolerance to another opioid. This phenomenon of incomplete cross-tolerance is best exemplified in the dramatic reduction in dosages needed to provide analgesia when patients are switched from, for example, morphine or hydromorphone to methadone, as previously discussed in Start with a Specific Drug for a Specific Type of Pain.[83–86] Further data elucidating the mechanism of opioid tolerance demonstrate that the NMDA receptor plays a critical role in opioid tolerance in analgesia.[44] In animal models of neuropathic pain, NMDA antagonists block the development of tolerance without blocking morphine analgesia. Of interest, methadone is a racemic mixture of D and L isomers and the D isomer is a noncompetitive antagonist to the NMDA receptor. These findings have focused new attention on methadone's opioid and nonopioid mechanisms of action and its potential role in the management of neuropathic pain. The use of analgesic combinations can reduce the amount of opioid required. Similarly, the use of bolus or continuous epidural local anesthetics in patients with perineal pain can dramatically reduce the need for systemic opioids and reverse tolerance.

TAPER DRUGS SLOWLY. The long-term administration of opioid analgesics is associated with the development of physical dependence, a state in which the sudden cessation of the opioid analgesic produces signs and symptoms of withdrawal: agitation, tremors, insomnia, fear, marked autonomic nervous system hyperexcitability, and exacerbation of pain. Slowly tapering the dose of the opioid analgesic prevents such symptoms. The appearance of abstinence symptoms from the time of drug withdrawal is related to the elimination half-life for the particular drug. The type of abstinence syndrome similarly varies with the drug. For example, with morphine, withdrawal symptoms occur within 6 to 12 hours after drug cessation. Reinstituting the drug in doses of approximately 25% of the previous daily dose suppresses these symptoms.

ANTICIPATE COMPLICATIONS. Overdose with opioid analgesics occurs either intentionally, when a patient takes an excessive amount of drug in a suicide attempt, or unintentionally, when the recommended dosage accidentally produces excessive sedation and respiratory depression. In both instances, the complication can be treated effectively with naloxone. Intentional overdose in cancer patients occurs rarely, and concern for this is overemphasized. Overdose in patients previously stabilized on an opioid regimen for cancer pain rarely is caused by drug intake alone. More commonly, the cause is the medical deterioration of the patient with a superimposed metabolic encephalopathy. Eagel et al. studied the use and misuse of naloxone and found that sedation was the most common reason for naloxone use.[132] Of note, in this study of naloxone use in 34 patients over 1 year at a cancer center, 71% of patients had a medical reason other than opioid dose escalation as an explanation for the change in medical condition prompting naloxone use. After naloxone administration, 64% of patients experienced significant side effects; 42% had increased pain and 14% had increased agitation. Intravenous boluses of 0.4 mg of naloxone were given rather than titrated doses of diluted naloxone as has been recommended.[133] Reducing the opioid drug dosage and carefully assessing the patient's metabolic status usually provide the differential diagnosis. Patients who have taken an unintentional drug overdose should be scrutinized carefully to rule out other causes of excessive sedation, confusion, or respiratory depression. In such cases, a reversal of these effects with naloxone is more therapeutic than diagnostic.

Psychological dependence or addiction is characterized by a concomitant behavioral pattern of drug abuse evidenced by craving a drug for other than pain relief and overwhelming involvement in the use and procurement of the drug. This is a state distinct from tolerance and physical dependence, which are responses to the pharmacologic effects of long-term opioid administration. The profound fear of causing psychological dependence plays a major role in a physician's reluctance to prescribe opioid analgesics, particularly in cancer patients in the early phase of their disease. Patients may share this fear, consistently taking less analgesic drug than is effective to control their pain. Increasing evidence suggests that cancer patients with pain can take opioid analgesics for prolonged periods but can discontinue such drugs when adequate pain relief is achieved using other approaches. In almost all instances, dramatic escalation of drug intake is associated with progression of disease and subsequent death. Few patients with cancer and pain become psychologically dependent on the drugs and participate in drug seeking and illicit drug use. Careful evaluation of patients who might be at risk for this complication is necessary, but such concern should not be punitive to the patient with severe cancer pain.

Out-of-control aberrant drug taking among oncology patients with or without a prior history of substance abuse represents a serious and complex clinical occurrence. Passik and Portenoy have developed guidelines for management of such patients.[66] The most difficult situations present themselves in the patient who is actively abusing illicit or prescription drugs or alcohol while concurrently receiving medical therapies. Such patients need a multidisciplinary approach usually focused on a harm-reduction concept that attempts to enhance social support for the patient to maximize treatment compliance. Passik and Portenoy have outlined a series of approaches to maximize a number of strategies for promoting compliance, including the consideration of a written contract between the team and patient, the inclusion of spot urine toxicology screens to assess compliance, set expectations regarding attendance at the clinic, and the patient's management of medication supplies. It is often most useful to see the patient on a regular basis, often every several days, and to limit prescribing of opioids to that basis until the patient has demonstrated his or her willingness to be compliant and to follow an appropriate drug regimen. Other approaches include encouraging the patient to attend a 12-step program and engaging the patient's family members and friends to further bolster social support and functioning. Such approaches can be helpful in an outpatient setting, but in an inpatient setting when patients demonstrate manipulative behaviors in the inappropriate use of medication, direct discussion with the patient about the drug use in an open manner is a first step. Providing the patient with a private room near the nurses' station to monitor the patient and discourage attempts to leave the hospital for purchase of illicit drugs and requiring visitors to check in with the nursing staff before visitation are additional steps. The daily testing of urine specimens is another method to evaluate compliance. Underlying all of this is the attempt to provide the patient with a supportive environment that respects the patient's pain symptomatology and serious medical illness and attempts to limit harm to the patient or others by the aberrant drug use and behaviors.

ADJUVANT DRUGS

Adjuvant drugs are used to enhance opioid analgesia, provide analgesia for certain types of pain (e.g., neuropathic pain, bone pain, and visceral pain), and treat opioid side effects or other symptoms associated with pain.[134] They are an integral part of the WHO three-step analgesic ladder. Because of the lack of well-defined guidelines for their use, sequential drug trials are necessary to identify the most useful drug and dose titration to find a safe and effective dose. Table 55.1-11 lists the commonly used adjuvants and their therapeutic categories.

Adjuvants to Enhance Analgesia

Adjuvants to enhance analgesia have been previously discussed in the section Use a Combination of Drugs earlier in this chapter. Acetaminophen, NSAIDs, hydroxyzine, and dextromethorphan have been demonstrated to provide additive analgesia to patients chronically receiving opioids.

Adjuvant Analgesics for Neuropathic Pain

The common neuropathic pain syndromes in patients with cancer include injury to peripheral nerves and plexus by tumor invasion, chemotherapy, surgery, or viral agents. Depending on the intensity of pain, nonopioid and opioid analgesics are the first-line agents. However, as previously discussed in Start with a Specific Drug for a Specific Type of Pain, there is evidence to suggest that neuropathic pain has a variable responsiveness to opioid drug regimens. Neuropathic pain is less responsive to nonopioid and opioid approaches. Some of the commonly used adjuvant drugs for managing this population of patients are described in the following sections.

Antidepressants

The tricyclic antidepressants may be the most useful group of psychotropic drugs applied in pain management.[135–137] Their analgesic effects are mediated by enhancement of serotonin activity. Data from controlled trials indicate that both the tertiary amine tricyclic antidepressants (amitriptyline, doxepin, imipramine, and clomipramine) and the secondary amine compounds (desipramine and nortriptyline) have analgesic effects. More recently, one of the serotonin selective reuptake inhibitors, paroxetine, has also been shown to have analgesic properties in patients with neuropathic pain.[137] These drugs have been reported to be effective in treating continuous dysesthesias as well as intermittent lancinating dysesthetic pain. The doses used for analgesia are far below those needed to produce an antidepressant effect. The analgesic properties of these drugs appear to be independent of their mood-altering effects. Patients should be started on low doses of 10 to 25 mg and the dose titrated up to achieve adequate analgesia in a 2- to 4-week trial. Blood levels should be measured to determine both patient compliance and drug absorption, because of wide individual variation. Patients who are unable to tolerate amitriptyline or who are predisposed to experiencing its sedative, anticholinergic, or hypotensive effects should be considered for a trial with a secondary amine tricyclic antidepressant or a serotonin selective reuptake inhibitor such as paroxetine. In the management of cancer patients with pain, the antidepressant drugs are the first-line therapeutic approach for neuropathic pain, and every attempt should be made to provide the patient with a several-week trial before discontinuing these drugs.

Anticonvulsants

The role of anticonvulsants in the management of patients with neuropathic pain is based, in part, on the fact that the mode of action is to stabilize membranes and alter sodium and calcium influx.[138] Many patients with neuropathic pain complain of paroxysmal, brief, lancinating pains. To date, clinical experience with the anticonvulsants has been positive. The drugs most commonly used include gabapentin, carbamazepine, and phenytoin. Survey studies have suggested the usefulness of valproic acid, clonazepam, lamotrigine, topiramate, and oxycarbazepine.[139] Gabapentin is considered the first-line anticonvulsant to manage neuropathic pain. Controlled trials in patients with diabetic neuropathy, postherpetic neuralgia, and acquired immunodeficiency syndrome neuropathy demonstrate the effectiveness of this agent in reducing pain. Dosages range from 900 to 1800 mg/d.[131] The major drug side effect is sedation. Patients should be started at 300 mg/d and rapidly titrated to 900 mg/d. Pain relief in up to 30% to 50% of patients has been suggested. Clinical studies with carbamazepine demonstrate efficacy, but the usefulness of this drug in the cancer population is limited by its potential to produce bone marrow suppression, particularly leukopenia. The dosing guidelines used for the treatment of seizures are suggested in managing neuropathic pain. Each of the drugs should be initiated at low doses and gradually titrated upward. There is anecdotal experience to suggest that administering intravenous loading doses of phenytoin to patients in an acute crisis with severe lancinating pain may be of clinical value. Both valproate and clonazepam have been reported anecdotally to be useful in managing neuropathic pain, but these are considered third-line agents in this patient population. Currently, there are no data to relate the plasma level and pain relief for any of these drugs. As previously stated in Start with a Specific Drug for a Specific Type of Pain, sequential trials are necessary to identify the most useful agent.

Local Anesthetics

The use of both brief intravenous local anesthetic infusions (lidocaine) and maintenance oral anesthetic drugs has demon-strated some efficacy in the management of chronic neuropathic pain, particularly in those patients with both lancinating and continuous dysesthesias. Mexiletine is the oral local anesthetic for which there are pilot data to support its analgesic efficacy.[140] The initial dosage of mexiletine is low, at 150 mg/d, with gradual upward dose titration. Electrocardiograms should be monitored at higher doses, and measurement of blood levels of mexiletine may be useful to prevent toxicity. Currently, there are no good data available to predict which patients might respond to the use of oral local or intravenous anesthetics, such as have been compiled on the use of brief local anesthetic infusions, to determine control of cardiac arrhythmias.

Epidural local anesthetics (bupivacaine, lidocaine) have been most widely used to manage neuropathic pain, either alone or in combination with an opioid. Alternatively, the use of brief intravenous infusions of lidocaine may be helpful in patients who have an opioid-refractory continuous dysesthesia that has not responded to an antidepressant or anticonvulsant.[141] These drugs clearly serve as a second-line approach, with individualized therapy the rule.

Cutaneous Local Anesthetics

The use of cutaneous anesthesia has been suggested to be most helpful in patients who have significant allodynia and marked hyperesthesia. The topical application of a local anesthetic, such as a eutectic mixture of local anesthetics, has been demonstrated to be efficacious in patients with postherpetic neuralgia.[142] The cream should be applied under an occlusive dressing to increase skin penetration and augment analgesic efficacy. The use of high-concentration lidocaine (5% and 10%) has also been reported to be effective in patients with significant allodynia associated with postherpetic neuralgia. Current indications for its use include peripheral nerve injury, peripheral neuropathy, ischemic pain, peripheral vascular disease, and unstable angina. Few cancer patients have been treated using this approach, and therefore it is not possible to fully assess its role in cancer pain management. [143]

Corticosteroids

A series of controlled and uncontrolled surveys have demonstrated that the use of chronic corticosteroid therapy to reduce pain in patients with breast and prostate cancer improves quality of life.[144,145] In a controlled study of corticosteroid use in patients with far-advanced disease, transient improvement in appetite, analgesia, and mood were noted, but they were not sustained after the initial effect. The major indications for corticosteroid use include refractory neuropathic pain, bone pain, pain associated with capsular expansion or duct obstruction, and headache due to increased intracranial pressure. In certain cancer pain syndromes, such as epidural cord compression, 85% of patients receiving 100 mg of dexamethasone as part of their radiation therapy protocol reported significant pain relief associated with marked reduction in analgesic requirements.[76] Similarly, in patients with tumor infiltration of the brachial and lumbosacral plexus, corticosteroids provided additive analgesic effects. The risk of adverse effects associated with corticosteroid therapy varies with the duration. Long-term use may be associated with gastrointestinal toxicity and acute psychosis. A wide range of dosages have been suggested, including dosages of 30 mg/d in patients with prostate cancer, which was effective in providing improved quality of life and reduced pain. As stated, with epidural cord compression, initial doses of 100 mg with maintenance doses of 16 mg have been associated with effective analgesia. In the author's experience, the use of 16 mg as a loading bolus and rapid titration to lower dosages of approximately 4 mg/d is one approach commonly used in the management of refractory chronic pain in patients with advanced disease.

Other Adjuvant Drugs

A wide variety of other drugs have been used to manage neuropathic pain, including benzodiazepines, neuroleptics, α_2-adrenergic agonist drugs, NMDA antagonists, and peptides. Of the benzodiazepines, clonazepam is commonly used in patients with lancinating or paroxysmal pain. The use of these drugs must be balanced with their potential to cause somnolence and cognitive impairment. They serve as second- to third-line therapy in patients who have not responded to antidepressant or anticonvulsant drug therapy. Of the neuroleptics, pimozide has been reported to be analgesic in patients with trigeminal neuralgia.[146] Methotrimeprazine has been demonstrated to have analgesic properties comparable to those of morphine.[147] This drug has sedative, anxiolytic, and antiemetic properties and is commonly used in patients who have excessive opioid side effects. It provides analgesia by a nonopioid mechanism.

Coadministration of these drugs with opioids can often be effective in patients with neuropathic pain. Of the α_2-adrenergic agonist drugs, clonidine has been demonstrated to be analgesic in controlled trials.[148] It can be administered by either the oral or transdermal route and has been reported to be specifically effective in patients with dysesthetic pain, who demonstrate sympathetic hyperactivity. After intrathecal administration, clonidine was reported to improve pain in patients with intolerable neuropathic pain. Dextromethorphan and ketamine are two commercially available NMDA antagonists. Both have been shown to have analgesic effects in controlled studies. The mechanism of action relates to the fact that the NMDA receptor reduces the development of the windup phenomenon, which occurs as a result of changes in the response of central dorsal horn neurons with neuropathic pain. Case reports have suggested that dextromethorphan has been beneficial in selected patients, although a controlled trial of low-dose dextromethorphan produced negative results. The use of ketamine infusions have been previously well established to produce analgesia, and they have been reintroduced into clinical use as brief infusions for the management of patients with refractory neuropathic pain. Further studies are necessary to demonstrate the safety and efficacy of these treatment approaches in long-term management of chronic neuropathic pain. Oral ketamine in case reports has demonstrated efficacy in cancer patients with pain uncontrolled by other approaches.[149,150]

Calcitonin has been reported to provide analgesia in patients with sympathetically maintained pain and in patients with acute phantom pain.[151] The mechanism underlying these analgesic effects is unknown, but it has suggested the empiric use of calcitonin in patients with refractory neuropathic pain. The clinical, anecdotal literature suggests that patients be treated initially at low dosage after initial skin testing to rule out hypersensitivity to this agent, with gradual escalation to a range of 100 to 200 IU/d. Its use chronically has not been assessed, and further studies are necessary to define its place in the treatment of patients with neuropathic pain.

Adjuvant Drugs for Bone Pain

Metastatic disease to bone is the most common cause of pain in patients with cancer. Analgesic drug therapy is commonly used to manage the pain during the initial treatment with either chemotherapy or radiation therapy. Numerous investigators have identified a management approach for bone pain, which includes the use of specific surgical palliative approaches, radiotherapeutic approaches, hormonal therapies, and bone resorption inhibitors. Multifocal metastatic bone disease that is refractory to routine treatments may benefit from the use of a series of agents, including the bisphosphonate compounds, gallium nitrate, calcitonin, and strontium 89. The current bisphosphonate drugs pamidronate, zoledronate, clodronate, and etidronate bind to bone hydroxyapatite, inhibiting osteoclast activity, and are highly effective in the management of bony metastatic disease and in multiple myeloma.[152–154] Pamidronate is usually administered as a brief infusion in a starting dose of 60 to 120 mg. Analgesia, if it occurs, usually appears within days but may accrue for many weeks with repeated infusions. In two studies, pamidronate at dosages of 30 to 60 mg every 2 weeks produced relief of pain in 30% to 60% of patients. The analgesic effect of bisphosphonates appears to be dose dependent. Current recommendations include a regimen of intravenous pamidronate, 60 mg every 2 weeks for at least two or three treatments. If no response is obtained, therapy can be discontinued. If the drug is effective, a biweekly regimen can be continued. A study of pamidronate, 120 mg intravenously, versus placebo in patients with painful bone metastases revealed a correlation between analgesic response and collagen cross-links, which suggests that the presence of such peptide cross-links may be used to select those patients more likely to achieve improvement in pain with bisphosphonate therapy. The major indication for these drugs is to prevent skeletal morbidity, with data in breast cancer patients and patients with multiple myeloma showing efficacy in reduction of fractures and reduction in bone pain. Clodronate may be administered orally and has been demonstrated to be efficacious in patients with breast cancer and multiple myeloma.

Calcitonin has also been reported anecdotally to be useful in patients with malignant bone pain, but the appropriate dose and dosing frequency have not been well defined.[155] Gallium nitrate has also been used with some efficacy in patients with metastatic bone pain, but the limited experience has not well defined the appropriate dosing guidelines, and nephrotoxicity has been reported.[156] Strontium 89 is a bone-seeking radiopharmaceutical, recognized as useful in the treatment of bone pain secondary to metastatic disease.[157,158] Its use is indicated in patients with refractory multifocal pain due to osteoblastic lesions who have a life expectancy of longer than 3 months, who have sufficient bone marrow reserve (i.e., a platelet count above 60,000 and a white blood cell count above 2400), and for whom there is no further planned myelosuppressive chemotherapy. The onset of effect is slow and may require several weeks, with peak effects at 2 to 3 months. Bone marrow suppression is the major adverse effect, with irreversible thrombocytopenia.

The selection of any one of these treatments to manage metastatic bone pain needs to be individualized, and there is evidence that both the bisphosphonates and strontium 89 have clearly demonstrated efficacy in certain patients.

Adjuvants to Treat Side Effects

Nausea and vomiting, confusion, sedation, and constipation are common opioid-induced side effects. The use of drugs to manage these effects has been discussed previously in Anticipate and Treat Side Effects. The use of caffeine, methylphenidate, and dextroamphetamine have all been demonstrated in clinical trials to reduce opioid-induced sedation. Haloperidol is the treatment of choice to manage hallucinations and agitated delirium in patients receiving opioid analgesics. The use of bowel regimens to manage depressed gastrointestinal motility has also been discussed in Anticipate and Treat Side Effects.

PSYCHOLOGICAL APPROACHES

Psychological approaches should be an integral part of the care of the cancer patient with pain. A series of psychological variables contribute to the cancer pain experience and suffering, such as perception of control, the meaning of pain, fear of death, depressed mood, and hopelessness. The level of psychological distress experienced by each patient varies depending on personality, coping ability, social support, and medical factors. Pain has a profound effect on levels of emotional distress, and psychological factors such as depression and anxiety intensify the pain experience. Measures of emotional disturbance have been reported to be predictors of pain in advancing later stages of cancer. The incidence of pain, depression, and delirium increases with high levels of physical debilitation in advanced disease. Approximately 25% of all cancer patients experience severe depressive symptoms, with the prevalence increasing to 77% in those with advanced illness. Uncontrolled pain is a major factor in suicide of cancer patients.

Various psychological interventions have been advocated for patients with cancer pain. Optimal treatment is multimodal and requires pharmacologic, psychotherapeutic, and cognitive-behavioral approaches. The roles of the psychiatrist, psychologist, and social worker in cancer pain management are well described in the literature.

The goals of short-term psychotherapy are to provide emotional support, continuity, and information and to assist patients in adapting to the crisis. Communication skills are of paramount importance for patient and family, particularly regarding pain and analgesic issues. The needs of the patient and family must be addressed. Psychotherapy in the cancer pain setting is primarily nonanalytic and focuses on current issues and exploration of reactions to cancer, which often provides insight into other life issues. Group interventions may also be helpful.

A specialized approach called cognitive-behavioral therapy has been used to treat pain disorders, including cancer pain.[159] This approach uses short-term therapeutic interventions based on theoretically and empirically derived principles that can be adapted to each patient's problems and needs. It includes a set of systematic mental and behavioral techniques designed to modify specific emotional, behavioral, and social problems as well as the global experience of pain and distress. Its major goal is to enhance the sense of personal control or self-efficacy. In a multidisciplinary approach to cancer pain, not every patient needs referral for this therapy, but it is useful if all members of the pain team follow a cognitive-behavioral model. Because cognitive-behavioral therapy is a commonsense psychological approach consisting of specific techniques, it can be learned and practiced by any interested clinician, nurse, or social worker, who can gain practical training in the use of these techniques and apply them effectively.

Various intervention methods have been developed and are arbitrarily divided into behavioral and cognitive methods for discussion purposes. These approaches must be targeted to each patient's needs.

Behavioral techniques include ways to modify physiologic pain reactions and pain behaviors. Relaxation training can be used by all caregivers who manage patients with pain and cancer. Its mechanism of action includes the reduction of muscle tension, and it can provide the patient with a sense of improved self-control and a calming diversion of attention, breaking the associated pain-anxiety-tension cycle. Techniques range from simple deep-breathing exercises to more specialized methods of biofeedback and hypnosis. Contingency management is another behavioral approach designed to modify dysfunctional pain behaviors and replace them with well behaviors.

Cognitive techniques are designed to modify dysfunctional mental processes or to teach adaptive coping strategies. Cognitive coping and cognitive modification are approaches in which distraction, focusing, and perception and interpretation of the meaning of pain are assessed.

ANESTHETIC AND NEUROSURGICAL APPROACHES

Anesthetic and neurosurgical approaches are most effective in treating patients with well-defined localized pain. Tables 55.1-12 and 55.1-13 outline the indications for their use. Ten percent to 20% of cancer pain patients require these approaches, together with pharmacologic approaches, to obtain adequate analgesia.

In a prospective study, Ventafridda and colleagues evaluated two groups of patients for 3 months who presented with intractable cancer pain not responsive to specific anticancer therapies.[21] One group was treated with sequential pharmacologic approaches using the analgesic ladder. The second group was treated with a multimodal approach of analgesic therapy followed by the use of neurolytic blocks or chronic spinal opioid administration. Patients treated with neurolytic procedures combined with pharmacologic therapy showed a statistically significantly greater degree of pain relief than those treated with drugs alone by the third week of therapy. However, by 6 weeks, there was no statistical difference between the two groups. Complete pain relief without the need for analgesic drug therapy persisted to 3 months in 29% of the patients who received spinal opiates, 25% treated with celiac ganglion neurolytic block, 24% undergoing percutaneous cordotomy, 12% treated with chemical rhizotomy, and 7% receiving gasserian thermorhizotomy. This study demonstrated that, although analgesic therapy is the mainstay of treatment, anesthetic and neurosurgical procedures provide an important, but limited, contribution to adequate analgesia. Cherny

TABLE 55.1-12. Types of Anesthetic Procedures Commonly Used in Cancer Pain

Type of Procedure	Most Common Indications
Inhalation therapy with nitrous oxide	Breakthrough pain, incidental pain in patients with diffuse poorly controlled pain
Intravenous barbiturates (sodium pentobarbital)	Diffuse body pain and suffering inadequately controlled by systemic opioids
Local anesthetic by intravenous, subcutaneous, or transdermal application	Neuropathic pain in any site with local application to the area of hyperesthesia or allodynia
Trigger point injections	Focal muscle pain
Nerve block	
Peripheral	Pain in discrete dermatomes in chest and abdomen or in distal extremities
Epidural	Unilateral lumbar or sacral pain; midline perineal pain; bilateral lumbosacral pain
Intrathecal	Midline perineal pain; bilateral lumbosacral pain
Autonomic	
Stellate ganglion	Reflex sympathetic dystrophy
Lumbar sympathetic	Reflex sympathetic dystrophy of the lower extremities; lumbosacral plexopathy; vascular insufficiency of the lower extremity
Celiac plexus	Midabdominal pain from tumor infiltration
Intermittent or continuous epidural infusion with local anesthetics	Unilateral and bilateral lumbosacral pain; midline perineal pain; neuropathic pain from the midthoracic region down
Intermittent or continuous epidural or intrathecal with local opioid analgesics	Unilateral and bilateral pain below the midthoracic region; often combined with local anesthetics
Intermittent or continuous intraventricular infusions with opioid analgesics	Head and neck pain and upper chest pain
Chemical hypophysectomy	Diffuse bone pain

et al. reported that 17% of patients in a prospective study of 100 cancer patients treated at Memorial Sloan-Kettering Cancer Center were evaluated for anesthetic and neurosurgical approaches, with 10% requiring such approaches. One study assessed attitudes of oncologists toward interventional cancer pain treatments. Eighty-one percent of oncologists reported patient referral to pain specialists, yet their familiarity with intrathecal therapy was low, with only 46% referring patients for intrathecal therapy in the previous 6 months. The invasive nature of device placement was cited as a drawback by 42% of physicians.[25]

Several factors are important in selecting the appropriate procedure for each patient. Because diffuse pain problems are common in cancer patients and most of the procedures are useful for management of well-defined localized pain, the role of these approaches is limited at best. Further complicating their use is the limited number of professionals who have expertise in these procedures. As patients become more cognizant of their disease and treatment options, they are often hesitant to undergo neurodestructive procedures. Patients often consider their pain to be an important marker for their disease and are frightened of the potential, although unlikely, complications of these procedures. As a result, these procedures are

often performed late in the illness, and full evaluation of their effectiveness and duration of action is limited by patients' overriding medical problems.

Except for the use of local anesthetics, these procedures are often not very effective in managing neuropathic pain and are most helpful in managing most types of somatic and visceral pain. However, cancer patients often have a mixed somatic, visceral, and neuropathic pain syndrome. The author advocates early consideration of the use of some of these anesthetic and neurosurgical procedures in patients to improve their quality of life through adequate pain management.

LOCAL ANESTHETICS

Anecdotal reports and several controlled studies support the use of cutaneous, subcutaneous, intravenous, intrapleural, and epidural local anesthetics in the management of patients with somatic, visceral, and neuropathic pain.[160]

Intravenous lidocaine should be considered as both a diagnostic and therapeutic approach in patients with neuropathic pain.[161] If such patients obtain an analgesic response, a trial of oral mexiletine or the use of continuous subcutaneous lidocaine should be considered to determine whether prolonged relief may be possible. Although no studies have confirmed that the response to lidocaine predicts a response to mexiletine for pain, a comparable predictive value exists in the cardiac literature, in which the effectiveness of intravenous lidocaine in controlling ventricular arrhythmias predicts the usefulness of mexiletine for this same disorder.

Brose and Cousins reported the use of continuous subcutaneous infusions in two patients with cancer-related neuropathic pain, advocating this approach as an alternative for patients who do not respond to standard opioid and adjuvant treatments as well as anesthetic approaches for neuropathic pain.[141]

Intrapleural local anesthetics have been used for acute pain in the chest wall and have been adapted for the management of chronic cancer pain.[162] Anesthetic delivered via a subcutaneously tunneled intrapleural catheter offered long-term relief of right upper quadrant pain from hepatic metastases in a patient with significant pain from tumor infiltration of the liver. This novel method offers an alternative approach for patients with local or regional pain in the pleural and abdominal regions.

Epidural local anesthetics are used to manage localized pain syndromes, usually below the waist. Intermittent and continuous epidural infusions of local anesthetics have been used to manage the difficult chronic pain associated with metastatic disease below the waist, often involving the sacrum and lumbosacral plexus.[163] This method consists of infusing a local anesthetic via a subcutaneous infusion pump or Ommaya reservoir to a catheter, temporarily or permanently placed in the epidural space. If the amount and concentration of the anesthetic are varied, effective pain relief can be achieved without interrupting significant motor or autonomic function. The risk of infection is minimized because local anesthetics have antimicrobial effects. The use of continuous low-dose infusions of local anesthetics is associated with minimal systemic side effects. Further studies on the use of this technique in comparison with standard therapies are needed to define its place in the management of the cancer patient. Its major advantages are that the resultant analgesia is not cross-tolerant with the analgesia produced by the opioid analgesics and

TABLE 55.1-13.   Neuroablative and Neurostimulatory Procedures for Relief of Pain from Cancer

Site	Procedure	Indications
NEUROABLATIVE PROCEDURES		
Nerve root	Rhizotomy	Useful in somatic and neuropathic pain from tumor infiltration of the cranial and, rarely, intercostal nerves.
Spinal cord	Dorsal root entry zone lesion	Useful in unilateral neuropathic pain from brachial, intercostal, and lumbosacral plexopathy and postherpetic neuralgia.
	Cordotomy	Useful in unilateral pain below the waist. Often combined with local neurolytic blocks in perineal and bilateral lumbosacral plexopathy; may be performed bilaterally.
	Myelotomy	Useful in midline pain below the waist but rarely used because it involves extensive surgery.
Brainstem	Mesencephalic tractomy	Useful in pain in the nasopharynx and trigeminal region.
Thalamus	Thalamotomy	Useful in unilateral neuropathic pain in the chest and lower extremity.
Cortex	Cingulotomy	Useful through a stereotactic approach for diffuse pain.
Pituitary	Transsphenoidal hypophysectomy	Useful in pain control of bone metastases in endocrine-dependent tumors, breast, and prostate.
NEUROSTIMULATORY PROCEDURES		
Peripheral nerve	Transcutaneous and percutaneous electrical nerve stimulation	Useful in reducing painful dysesthesias from tumor infiltration of nerve or trauma (e.g., neuroma).
Spinal cord	Dorsal column stimulation	Of limited use in neuropathic pain in the chest, midline, and lower extremities.
Thalamus	Thalamic stimulation	Of rare use in neuropathic pain in the chest, midline, or lower extremity.

that temporary use of this technique allows for reducing the amount of systemic opiate drugs and therefore partially reversing tolerance. This has been a useful preliminary approach in patients for whom the use of spinal opiate analgesia is considered but who have developed tolerance from large doses of systemic opiates. Because tolerance develops to these analgesic effects, this approach is temporary (days to weeks) rather than long-term. This approach is most useful in patients who experience an acute pain crisis, such as the patient with a pathologic hip fracture who is not a surgical candidate; this approach would allow the patient to move about in bed. In patients with chronic cancer neuropathic pain, local anesthetics combined with opioids are used.

PERIPHERAL NERVE BLOCK

Peripheral nerve blocks are used both diagnostically to localize the nerve distribution and therapeutically to interrupt pain transmission within a determined nerve distribution. This technique is limited to areas of the body in which the interruption of both motor and sensory function will not interfere with the patient's functional status. This approach is most commonly used in patients who have pain in the head, chest, or abdomen.[164,165] This technique is also limited by the fact that each peripheral nerve subserves sensory function over many levels, and usually several nerves must be blocked to provide adequate analgesia. These techniques are most useful in patients with somatic pain; neuropathic pain is rarely controlled by peripheral nerve blocks alone. Examples of successful blocks include gasserian ganglion block for craniofacial pain, intercostal blocks for chest wall infiltration from tumor, and paravertebral blocks for radicular pain.

In patients with somatic pain who respond to a local anesthetic block, neurolytic blockade with either alcohol or phenol may provide more prolonged relief. A block produced by phenol tends to be less profound and of shorter duration than that produced by alcohol. Phenol has local anesthetic as well as neurolytic effects.

The most common peripheral neurolytic block is a paravertebral block for localized intercostal pain. Based on experience in treating patients with chest wall pain, the author advises that this procedure be performed using fluoroscopic control or computed tomographic localization to accurately interrupt the individual intercostal nerve.

Epidural and intrathecal neurolytic blocks have been used primarily to manage patients with far-advanced disease whose pain is either unilateral in the chest or abdomen or midline in the perineum. These approaches are less useful in managing upper and lower limb pain associated with brachial and lumbosacral plexopathy because of the high risk of motor weakness associated with effective neurolytic blockade by this route. Epidural phenol blocks are useful in management of chest wall pain over several dermatomes. Such an approach obviates the need for multiple paravertebral injections. Phenol is injected in small increments (1 to 2 mL/segment) over 2 or 3 days by an epidural catheter, and preliminary data demonstrate 80% pain relief in patients with documented somatic pain. Epidural and intrathecal phenol blocks have been used to manage perineal pain, but no studies have delineated the superiority of one approach over the other.[163]

A review of a large number of cases of alcohol subarachnoid block reports an average of 60% of patients experiencing good relief, 21% achieving fair relief, and 18% obtaining poor relief.[163–165] Because the duration of pain relief has seldom been documented in careful follow-up studies, the overall estimate for relief of pain with both subarachnoid alcohol and phenol blocks suggests a mean duration of pain relief of between 2 weeks and 3 months.

Complications are of two kinds. With intrathecal injection, a self-limiting spinal headache may occur. Complications that result from the action of neurolytic substances on nerve fibers include motor paresis, loss of sphincter function, impairment of touch and proprioception, and troublesome dysesthesias. Injection in the thoracic region has a low complication rate. In the author's experience, many cancer patients already have both motor and autonomic dysfunction before the use of neurolytic blockade; these often remain the same or may worsen. Patients should be informed of the risk of these procedures, with particular attention given to the fact that they may develop motor paresis and bladder dysfunction, specifically incontinence, after the blockade.

The selection of patients for management with epidural or intrathecal neurolytic agents should be based on the following criteria: exhaustion of appropriate antitumor approaches; clear clinical and radiologic definition of the pain; poor candidacy for percutaneous cordotomy; failure of nonopioid, opioid, and adjuvant analgesics to produce adequate analgesia without significant side effects; a favorable response to diagnostic or epidural or intrathecal blocks, producing at least 75% pain relief; and MRI of the spine or myelography done before the procedure that rules out tumor infiltration of the subarachnoid space.

AUTONOMIC NERVE BLOCK

Sympathetic block is effective in conditions with vasomotor or visceromotor hyperactivity. This hyperactivity accompanies many of the cancer-related pain syndromes such as visceral pain or plexopathies. The most commonly used sympathetic block is that of the celiac ganglion for pain due to abdominal malignancy, including cancer of the pancreas, stomach, duodenum, liver, gallbladder, adrenal gland, and colon. Nociceptive fibers of the splanchnic, sympathetic, vagal, phrenic, and somatic nerves converge on the celiac ganglion, which is amenable to a regional block that is successful in 70% to 85% of patients treated.[164]

Standardized approaches for the use of this technique have been described using computed tomographic monitoring or fluoroscopic control. After placement of the needle, 25 mg of absolute alcohol mixed with local anesthetic and contrast is injected. Bilateral needle placement has been reported to provide the best results, but anecdotal reports suggest that unilateral needle placement on the right provides comparable analgesia.[166] The major side effect of the procedure is transient hypotension, and patients must be well hydrated and monitored carefully during the procedure and for 4 to 6 hours afterward. Significant neurologic complications occur in fewer than 1% of patients if proper technique is used. Complications include paraparesis, postural hypotension, and urinary difficulties.

Although there has been debate about the usefulness of this procedure in patients with pancreatic cancer, it should be considered as one option, together with pharmacologic approaches, in managing these patients. The use of thoracic endoscopy to perform sympathetic blockade in patients with cancer may replace the standard celiac plexus approach.

Lumbar sympathetic block may provide significant relief of intractable urogenital pain or pain due to carcinomatous invasion of local nerves and plexus in the perineum and lower extremity.[165] This ganglion conveys visceral nociceptive afferents from the pelvic viscera. Pain caused by cancer of the sigmoid colon or rectum may be relieved by bilateral lumbar

sympathetic block if the disease is confined to those viscera. Pain caused by cancer of the seminal vesicles or prostate may sometimes be relieved by bilateral lumbar sympathetic block. Similarly, pain caused by uterine cancer may be relieved if the disease is confined to the body of the uterus. In many instances, however, the block must be extended to the T-12 ganglion. Good evidence suggests that lumbar sympathetic block alone is not useful in patients with lumbosacral plexopathy; therefore, the role of this procedure is limited to management of pain at specific anatomic sites.

Stellate ganglion block may sometimes be useful for pain in the face, upper neck, ear, and hemicranium. However, the potential complications of stellate ganglion block limit the use of neurolytic solution with this technique, because there is a high risk of spillage of the neurolytic material into the brachial plexus, with secondary nerve injury and focal pain.

NEUROADENOLYSIS OF THE PITUITARY

Chemical hypophysectomy is a special use of a neurolytic method. Several early studies suggest that 35% to 95% of patients undergoing this procedure report pain relief, with a median duration of 6 to 7 weeks and a maximum duration of 20 weeks.[167] The mechanism by which analgesia is produced may be alcohol tracking up the pituitary stalk into the hypothalamus, with consequent disruption of the hypothalamic-thalamic endorphinergic pain pathways. Side effects include diabetes insipidus, cranial nerve palsies, cerebrospinal fluid leakage, and, rarely, meningitis. The lack of detailed clinical data limits critical assessment of these studies. This technique is rarely, if ever, used in patients with diffuse pain.

NEUROSURGICAL APPROACHES

Neurosurgical approaches for cancer pain can be divided into two major categories: antitumor and antinociceptive. These approaches are often used alone or in combination by neurosurgeons to provide improved pain relief.[168,169]

Antitumor Approaches

Antitumor approaches are often more acceptable to patients because they focus on cancer treatment, offering the hope of prolonged survival. The major procedures are listed in Table 55.1-13 and include tumor removal from the spine, epidural space, or adjacent plexus; stabilization procedures for spinal fracture, instability, and subluxation; and implantation of regional delivery devices for epidural, intrathecal, and intraventricular opioid drugs.

Tumor removal through resection of spinal metastases is associated with dramatic improvements in pain in 70% to 90% of patients.[170,171] With the use of improved methods of internal fixation with methyl methacrylate and improved stabilizing procedures, the use of this approach has increased in patients with intractable continuous or incidental back and neck pain. Patients may also have an associated segmental instability associated with a pathologic fracture of the vertebral body or subluxation, syndromes that place patients at significant risk for neurologic dysfunction. Careful radiologic workup is necessary to define the specific anatomic basis for the spinal pain, but aggressive surgical approaches have improved the quality of life for many patients bedridden by uncontrolled pain. In patients with epidural cord compression, the indications for surgery include uncontrolled pain in a patient with a pathologic fracture or a solitary relapse in the epidural space or vertebral body from a radioresistant tumor. In patients with radiosensitive tumors who relapse after radiation therapy, spinal surgery should be considered as a reasonable approach and is specifically indicated in the patient with an acute neurologic deterioration during radiation therapy. When percutaneous or open vertebral body biopsy is impossible, surgical resection should be strongly considered to define the primary tumor type in patients with undiagnosed lesions; this serves as both a diagnostic and a therapeutic procedure.

In patients with paraspinal tumor or tumor infiltration of the plexus, *en bloc* resection of tumor has successfully provided pain relief and has served as a debulking antitumor procedure. Among patients with Pancoast's syndrome, invasion of the spine or epidural extension is present in 20% at initial presentation and is associated with a significant morbidity in up to 50% of patients when local treatment is ineffective. For the good-risk patient with plexopathy and spinal invasion, Sundaresan et al. recommend surgery in which tumor is removed from the lower plexus, C-8 to T-1, and the vertebral body is resected, with brachytherapy to provide further tumor control.[171]

In patients with tumor invasion of the paraspinal area (specifically the psoas and iliacus muscles), radical resection of these tumor masses concurrent with spinal surgery, followed by brachytherapy, combines antitumor and antinociceptive therapies.

When the use of these neurosurgical procedures is contemplated to provide palliative surgery with an antinociceptive component, the patient's extent of disease, performance score, prognosis, and ability to tolerate the surgery must be weighed.

Antinociceptive Procedures

Antinociceptive procedures include neuroablative, neurostimulatory, and neuropharmacologic approaches.

NEUROABLATIVE PROCEDURES. Neuroablative procedures involve the production of a surgical or radiofrequency lesion along the nociceptive neural pathway. Section of the posterior roots (rhizotomy), lesioning of the lateral dorsal horn (dorsal root entry zone lesion), and interruption of the ascending neospinothalamic pathway (cordotomy) or the crossing interneuronal fibers (myelotomy) in the spinal cord are examples of neuroablative procedures performed for pain relief.

Cordotomy, either percutaneous or open, is the most common neuroablative procedure used to manage cancer pain.[172–174] It is the neurosurgical procedure of choice for patients with unilateral pain below the waist and with a relatively short life expectancy. Cordotomy is usually effective for 1 to 3 years, with dysesthesias substituting for analgesia in patients living longer than 3 years. Pain in the chest wall or upper extremity may be successfully treated initially with cordotomy, but extensive data demonstrate that, with time, the level of analgesia drops, which limits the effectiveness of this approach. Somatic pain appears to be the most responsive to cordotomy; visceral and neuropathic pain are less responsive for reasons that are not fully understood.

Percutaneous cordotomy is performed in a supine, awake patient through a lateral C-1 to C-2 approach.[169,172] A needle is advanced under fluoroscopic control until cerebrospinal fluid is obtained. A minimyelogram is recorded to identify the dentate ligament. A cordotomy electrode is passed through the spinal needle and the spinal cord is punctured with the aid of impedance monitoring. Electrophysiologic stimulation is performed to identify the spinothalamic tract and then a radiofrequency lesion is made in the appropriate painful site. Such a lesion interrupts pain and temperature sensation on the contralateral side of the lesioned site. Patients typically report spontaneous relief of pain in the area corresponding to the lesion.

The anatomic area at the lesion site includes fibers mediating respiration and autonomic function. These fibers are adjacent to the anterior horn and the cervical spinothalamic fibers. Near the lumbar spinothalamic tract are the fibers governing the intercostal muscles. This quadrant of the spinal cord also contains the sacral fibers to and from the bladder, which are closer to the spinothalamic fibers. These anatomic relations explain some of the complications associated with cordotomy: bladder dysfunction, respiratory compromise, and ipsilateral motor weakness.

From the literature, which does not provide comparative studies in cancer patients with pain, pain relief can be obtained in 60% to 80% of patients immediately after cordotomy; results at 6 to 12 months are 40% to 50%.[169–174] In a retrospective survey of 40 percutaneous cordotomies in patients with predominantly unilateral pain below the waist, 70% of patients obtained complete relief with continued use of some supplemental analgesics, 16% had moderate relief, and 13% did not benefit from this procedure.[174] In another study, Arbit reported that 16% of patients referred for percutaneous cordotomy could not undergo the procedure because of difficulty in positioning or in participating in the procedure, even with the use of increased analgesic drug doses and anesthetic assistance.[169] Careful patient selection is necessary for this procedure.

Open cordotomy is usually done below the cervicothoracic junction through a hemilaminectomy or full laminectomy. Open cordotomy should be reserved for the patient who cannot tolerate a percutaneous approach or for the patient with limited motor or sensory dysfunction from tumor infiltration below the waist in whom bilateral cordotomy is to be done for bilateral or midline pain.

The complications of cordotomy vary with the type of procedure (percutaneous or open) and are also strongly influenced by the patient's premorbid neurologic condition. Many patients have borderline bladder function and mild paresis from tumor infiltration that is transiently or permanently exacerbated by these procedures. In a series at Memorial Sloan-Kettering Cancer Center, 45% of patients had transient or permanent urinary retention.[174] After cordotomy, there is often an unmasking of pain ipsilateral to the cordotomy site. This pain was reported in 22% of patients in one series.[169] In some patients it was difficult to clarify if this nerve pain was caused by unidentified tumor and really represented mirror pain or was caused by the unmasking of tumor-related pain. In 60% of patients in the Arbit series, unmasking of pain on the contralateral side occurred because of bilateral lumbosacral plexopathy. Dysesthesias characterized by burning pain in the area of sensory loss are reported in 1%

to 2% of patients after a delay of several months to 2 years after the procedure. Ipsilateral motor weakness results from an inadvertent anterior extension of the lesion to involve the corticospinal tract. In the author's series, 7% of patients had transient paresis and 22% had permanent paresis. Most series report motor paresis in 10% to 20% of patients.

Respiratory complications occur in patients with a dysfunctional lung contralateral to the site of the cordotomy. This is a predictable risk when patients undergo cordotomy on the same side as their only functioning lung: interruption of the reticulospinal fibers controlling the intercostal muscles and of the phrenic nerve may occur because of their proximity to the lateral spinothalamic tract in this spinal cord quadrant.

Several other complications, including headache, fever, and meningismus, are associated with the percutaneous procedure, as well as a Horner's syndrome because of interruption of the sympathetic tract.

In the author's series, 30% of patients demonstrated a profound depressive syndrome associated with significant pain relief.[174] Patients should be warned about this complication, but the factors contributing to its development have not been fully clarified. Rapid reduction in opioids, realization that with pain relief they must face their terminal illness, and other factors, including exhaustion, depression, and preexisting psychopathology, may all play a role in the appearance of this problematic complication. Psychological intervention and the use of tricyclic antidepressants have been effective in managing these patients.

Dorsal rhizotomy is the next most common neuroablative procedure used for cancer pain. It is performed by sectioning the posterior sensory rootlets, and a specific localized dermatomal pain level can be identified. It can be performed by an operative section of the nerve or peripheral nerve block by a neurolytic block. Among patients with chest wall pain from tumor invasion, improved analgesia in 50% to 80% has been reported with dorsal rhizotomy.[175] Arbit et al. have adapted this procedure to manage patients with significant chest wall pain.[176]

Rhizotomies of the trigeminal nerve, nervus intermedius, glossopharyngeal nerve, and portions of the vagus nerve are effective in controlling pain from head and neck tumors that invade the base of the skull.[177] Bilateral sacral rhizotomy has been reported to treat sacral or perineal pain involving the sacral plexus at the S-2 and S-3 levels. However, these patients have often had extensive radiation therapy, and wound closure in the irradiated skin over the sacrum may complicate recovery and increase the risk to benefit ratio. A neurolytic, epidural, or subarachnoid block is usually considered before surgical sacral rhizotomy.

The use of a dorsal root entry zone lesion is based on the recognition that nociceptive fibers enter laminae I and II at the dorsal horn; interruption of this anterior lateral site has been associated with reduction in neuropathic pain in experimental animals. This approach has been used most commonly in cases of avulsion of the brachial plexus, postherpetic neuralgia, and postradiation plexopathy. Because this approach has not been widely used to treat cancer pain, its usefulness for brachial and lumbosacral plexopathy is not established, but it is an interesting approach for such patients.[178] The procedure requires a laminectomy of several levels to provide an adequate approach to this anatomic site, and this may be too extensive a procedure

for the cancer patient with advanced disease. Further studies are necessary to determine its usefulness.

The midline commissural myelotomy approach has been used in patients with midline perineal or coccygeal pain or bilateral pain in the lower extremities. Using a limited midline myelotomy, Gildenberg and Hirschberg reported satisfactory pain relief in 10 to 14 patients with midline pain below the waist from cancer.[179] This procedure is based on the fact that nociceptive fibers cross in the anterior commissure from the dorsal horn to the contralateral spinothalamic pathway. This approach is used rarely, if ever, in patients with bilateral pain.

Cingulotomy using a stereotactic procedure with MRI to permit creation of a radiofrequency lesion has received attention in the treatment of some patients with cancer pain. Four patients with pain from widely metastatic, diffuse bone disease who were receiving opioid analgesics reported immediate pain relief with bilateral cingulate lesions.[180] The pain relief persisted until death in 2 to 6 weeks. This procedure was previously used to treat psychiatric illness and has a long history of use in management of severe chronic pain from a variety of neuropathic syndromes. The literature suggests that up to 50% of cancer patients have had moderate, marked, or complete pain relief for 3 months after the procedure. The extent to which the development of this improved method will alter the use of this technique needs to be clarified.

NEUROSTIMULATORY PROCEDURES. Neurostimulatory procedures involving the peripheral nerve and spinal cord are generally based on the gate theory of pain. The original theory suggests that there is a neurophysiologic gating mechanism in the spinal cord, probably within the substantia gelatinosa. Noxious sensation is conducted via small-diameter peripheral nerve fibers and nonnoxious sensation via large-diameter fibers, and both send collaterals to the substantia gelatinosa and up the spinal dorsal columns. Stimulation of the small fibers tends to promote pain, or *open the gate*, whereas stimulation of the large fibers tends to inhibit pain or *close the gate*. Because the large nerve fibers ascend in a compact bundle through the dorsal columns, they are accessible to selected electric stimulation. Retrograde firing of the large fibers ensues, and pain sensation is inhibited at multiple levels of the spinal cord below that being stimulated.

Based on reports that high-frequency (50- to 100-Hz) percutaneous electrical nerve stimulation relieved chronic neurogenic pain, transcutaneous electrical nerve stimulation (TENS) was used to treat neuropathic pain and was reported effective. Although control studies are lacking, numerous clinical surveys suggest that this approach is useful for nociceptive and neuropathic pain. With the advent of sophisticated electronic devices, various patterns of electric stimulation are currently in use transcutaneously, including pulsed (burst), modulated (ramped), random, and complex waveforms, all designed to improve efficacy. Patients are instructed on proper electrode placement in a dermatomal pattern and are instructed to try both intermittent and continuous stimulation. By trial and error, analgesic effects should be observed either immediately or, in some cases, after the stimulation is discontinued.

TENS is used for a wide variety of pains and serves as a safe, noninvasive approach. Clinical experience suggests its usefulness in some patients with peripheral nerve pain. Several investigators have reported that it is useful in cancer pain for a wide variety of tumor-related and neuropathic pain syndromes.[181]

Further studies are necessary to define the usefulness of TENS in the cancer patient with pain.

The dorsal column stimulation technique involves introducing an electrode into the epidural or intrathecal space and advancing it to the appropriate level overlying the dorsal columns. The main indications for placement of a dorsal column stimulator are intractable dysesthetic or deafferentation pain of the limbs or trunk, such as radiation-induced brachial or lumbosacral plexopathy. This procedure is effective in 43% to 75% of patients and carries a low morbidity. The most common complication is failure of the device itself, which occurs in approximately 10% of patients annually. Other complications include infection, cerebrospinal fluid fistula, allergic or rejection response to the device material, and changes in stimulation over time, which may be related to cellular changes around the electrode or shifts in its position.

Thalamic stimulation involves the placement of electrodes in the medial thalamus and has been reported to be most useful for managing neuropathic pain from lesions in the central and peripheral nervous system. There is a series of reports on the usefulness of this technique in patients with head and neck cancer and prominent cranial neuropathic pain, but the limited use of this technique in these patients makes it difficult to define its specific role.[182,183]

NEUROPHARMACOLOGIC APPROACHES

Epidural and intraspinal analgesia using opioids alone or in combination with local anesthetics, clonidine, or both, or with experimental agents is used to manage chronic cancer pain in patients with a reasonable (1-year) expected survival.[184] In all instances, patients should have a trial of an epidural or intraspinal drug combination before permanent implementation is considered. It is advised that patients have a continuous intrathecal trial lasting as long as possible before permanent implementation. A wide array of external and implantable catheters and pumps is available with specific indications and uses. Both computer-controlled battery-operated pumps and continuous fixed-infusion pumps are used. Cost of the pump, the patient's psychosocial status and social support systems, and the patient's ability to care for the pump and port are important considerations in the decision to use such devices. As discussed previously in the section Gear the Route of Administration to the Patient's Needs, a randomized clinical trial of intrathecal opioids compared to comprehensive medical management reported improved pain relief, less drug toxicity, and improved survival.[118]

TRIGGER POINT INJECTION AND ACUPUNCTURE

The use of trigger point injections is within the scope of the practicing physician.[185] Patients with significant musculoskeletal pain often identify specific tender trigger point areas, and injection of these trigger points with either saline or local anesthetic is associated with significant pain relief. Effective relief of pain from trigger point injections is not by itself diagnostic of musculoskeletal pain, however, and an evaluation of the cause of the pain is still necessary to rule out other specific sources.

Acupuncture has been used to treat both acute and chronic pain. The selected acupuncture points are manually or electrically stimulated with a needle until the patient feels the sensation. A wide variety of acupuncture techniques is available, ranging from a traditional Chinese approach to a Western adaptation. Laser acupuncture with external laser probes has also been used. The studies involving cancer patients with pain represent large, uncontrolled, retrospective surveys. Minimal stimulation in manual acupuncture was used in all cases, and three acupuncture treatments represented an adequate trial. Fifty-two percent of patients reported some pain improvement for at least 7 days; an additional 30% and 22% had pain relief for 2 days or less or reported increased mobility alone, respectively.[186] A lack of detailed pain assessment in specific acupuncture techniques and lack of a critical review of the patient population make it difficult to interpret these observations. Based on its current empiric use, this approach is relatively safe, but its benefit in cancer patients with pain remains undefined.

PHYSIATRIC APPROACHES

Rehabilitation medicine plays an important role in the multidisciplinary approach to the patient with cancer pain. Physiatrists are concerned with a patient's physical functioning and provide expertise in assessing how impairment in a patient's physical capacity affects his or her ability to function. A wide variety of interventions are available, including TENS, diathermy (heating pads, ultrasound treatments, hydrotherapy), and cryotherapy (ice and vapocoolants). Assistive devices and braces, as well as therapeutic exercise and massage, are important. Trigger point injections and acupuncture have also been used. These interventions are commonly used in combination with other pain therapy approaches, particularly behavioral and pharmacologic approaches. Rehabilitation approaches are discussed throughout the text specific to cancer patients' needs.

A large body of data supports the use of rehabilitative interventions in acute and chronic nonmalignant pain, but similar studies have not addressed the rehabilitation needs of the cancer pain patient. From the author's experiences, neurologic dysfunction is one of the common components in patients with cancer pain, and aggressive neurorehabilitation is necessary to promote ambulation in these patients and provide them with functional independence.

SEDATION IN THE IMMINENTLY DYING

NITROUS OXIDE

Nitrous oxide has analgesic properties and has been used in the management of patients with far-advanced disease to provide added analgesia. It is administered with oxygen through a nonrebreathing face mask in concentrations from 25% to 75%. Its use in combination with systemic opioid analgesics is associated with improvement of symptoms of pain and anxiety and a demonstrable improvement in alertness.[187] This anesthetic approach should be considered in patients with breakthrough pain or incident pain to provide adequate analgesia to facilitate their care.

INTRAVENOUS BARBITURATES

The use of intravenous barbiturates has been advocated to manage dying patients who have inadequate analgesia or uncontrolled symptoms and who ask to be maintained in a sedated state. Intravenous thiopental titrated to a level of sedation was the approach advocated in a series involving 17 terminally ill patients.[188] The authors suggested that the value of this approach is based on the use of one agent to treat both physical and psychological symptoms. This approach may be seen as a more generalized one than palliative care and should be considered only if the standard approaches using opioid analgesics and adjuvant drugs fail to provide adequate analgesia with minimum side effects. However, because it is the physician's responsibility to manage not only pain but also suffering, this may be a reasonable approach, particularly in the dying patient with profound dyspnea, myoclonus, or agitation. Further studies are needed to clarify the usefulness of this approach. In the published study, 13 of 17 patients developed somnolence and died. The somnolence lasted from 2 hours to 4 days, with an average of 23 hours. Four patients died without being somnolent.

Several problematic symptoms often arise in the management of the dying patient, including intractable vomiting, profound dyspnea, extreme agitation and anxiety, and uncontrolled pain. Several authors have reported that most cancer patients have crescendo symptoms before death, requiring initiation of somnolence.[189–191] This approach offers one method to manage patient care in these difficult situations.

Whatever pain management techniques are used, the physician is responsible for providing continuing care, constantly reassessing both the diagnosis and the treatment to achieve optimal relief of pain and suffering for both patient and family.

The care of patients with cancer and chronic pain strains the resources of a single physician, especially after the patient's discharge from the hospital. Various supportive care and continuing care programs have been developed to manage dying patients, both in the hospital and at home. In these patients, the focus of treatment shifts to symptom control and palliative comfort care. Palliative care services, home- and hospital-based hospice care, and high-technology home care programs are some of the approaches to care for patients with terminal illness.

The program at Memorial Sloan-Kettering Cancer Center centers on the patient and family and is coordinated by a nurse, physician, and social worker.[192] The nurse is responsible for day-to-day management of the patient's pain and works with the patient, family, and community physicians and nurses on symptom control and supportive care. Community health professionals work with the patient at home, and the team is available to the patient, family, and community health workers on a 24-hour-a-day basis.

ALGORITHM FOR CANCER PAIN MANAGEMENT

An algorithm has been developed that integrates all of these management approaches for cancer pain. It attempts to integrate assessment techniques, drug therapy, behavioral approaches, and anesthetic and neurosurgical approaches and stresses continuity of care. Treatment begins with a diagnostic evaluation that addresses the medical, psychological, and social components of pain. A plan is developed to treat the cancer and pain. If the anticancer treatment is effective, pain relief usually occurs and the drugs used for analgesia can be discontinued without difficulty. Pain treatment begins with the use of analgesic drugs, starting with nonopioid drugs alone or in combination. If these drugs are successful, no further therapy is necessary. If severe persistent pain does not respond to analgesic drugs or if the side effects of the drugs are not tolerated, the physician should consider switching analgesics (e.g., from oral morphine to methadone), changing the route of administration (e.g., from oral to subcutaneous), or performing a cordotomy for localized pain. A trial of an adjuvant drug together with the opioid and nonopioid drug would also be appropriate. In patients with excessive sedation or confusion, the use of a neurostimulant or haloperidol provides adequate treatment of the side effects of the opioid drugs and maintains the patient's analgesia while markedly reducing concurrent side effects. Alternatively, epidural or intrathecal opioids may be considered if systemic analgesics produce excessive side effects such as confusion or sedation. If the pain is localized (e.g., intercostal pain from tumor infiltration of the chest wall), neurolytic blocks are indicated. If the pain is unilateral and below the waist, cordotomy should be considered. For diffuse pain, nitrous oxide inhalation may be tried. Cognitive-behavioral approaches must be integrated from the onset of treatment and should be used along with the medical and surgical approaches.

FUTURE DIRECTIONS

The study of pain in cancer patients offers a unique opportunity to use clinical observations to advance our biologic knowledge. There is a critical need to expand both the research and educational efforts in cancer pain to improve the control of pain in these patients. Information on the basic mechanisms of pain modulation can be culled only from a careful study of these clinical pain problems. These patients can teach us the physiologic and psychological differences between acute and chronic pain problems, the importance of the evolution of psychological factors, the difference between pain and suffering, the clinical pharmacology of analgesic drugs, and the behavioral mechanisms humans use to suppress pain. The use of innovative approaches based on sound scientific principles and advances in research technology offers the opportunity to understand the complex phenomenon of pain.

REFERENCES

1. Foley KM. Advances in cancer pain. *Arch Neurol* 1999;56:413.
2. Foley KM. Clinical crossroads: a 44-year old woman with severe pain at the end of life. *JAMA* 1999;281:1937.
3. Foley KM. Pain assessment and cancer pain syndromes. In: Doyle D, Hanks GWC, Calman K, Cherny N, eds. *Oxford textbook of palliative medicine*, 3rd ed. New York: Oxford University Press, 2003.
4. World Health Organization. *Cancer pain relief*, 2nd ed. Geneva: World Health Organization, 1996.
5. Levy MH. Pharmacologic treatment of cancer pain. *N Engl J Med* 1996;335(15):1124.
6. Bruera E, Kim HN. Cancer pain. *JAMA* 2003;290(18):2476.
7. Sepulveda C, Marlin A, Yoshida T, Ulrich A. Palliative care: the World Health Organization's global perspective. *J Pain Symptom Manage* 2002;24(2):91.
8. Foley KM, Gelband H, eds. Institute of Medicine. National Cancer Policy Board. *Improving palliative care for cancer*. Washington, DC: National Academies Press, 2001.
9. Ingham J, Portenoy RK. Symptom assessment. *Hematol Oncol Clin North Am* 1996;10(1):21.
10. Cleeland CS, Ladinsky JL, Serlin RC, Thuy NC. Multidimensional measurement of cancer pain: comparisons of US and Vietnamese patients. *J Pain Symptom Manage* 1988;3:23.
11. Portenoy RK, Miransky J, Thaler HT, et al. Pain in ambulatory patients with lung or cancer: prevalence, characteristics and impact. *Cancer* 1992;70:1616.
12. Portenoy RK, Thaler HT, Kornblith AB, et al. Pain in ovarian cancer: prevalence, characteristics, and associated symptoms. *Cancer* 1994;74:907.
13. Kelsen D, Portenoy RK, Thaler HT, et al. Pain and depression in patients with newly diagnosed pancreas cancer. *J Clin Oncol* 1995;13:748.

14. Schuit KW, Sleijfer DT, Meijler WJ, et al. Symptoms and functional status of patients with disseminated cancer visiting outpatient departments. *J Pain Symptom Manage* 1998;16:290.

15. Weber M, Huber C. Documentation of severe pain, opioid doses, opioid related side effect with patients with cancer: a retrospective study. *J Pain Symptom Manage* 1999;17:49.

16. Cleeland CS, Gonin R, Hatfield AK, et al. Pain and its treatment in outpatients with metastatic cancer. *N Engl J Med* 1994;330:592.

17. The SUPPORT principal investigators. A controlled trial to improve care for seriously ill hospitalized patients: the Study to Understand Prognosis and Preferences for Outcomes and Risks of Treatments. *JAMA* 1995;274:1591.

18. Bernabei R, Gambassi G, Lapane K, et al. Management of pain in elderly patients with cancer. *JAMA* 1998;279:1877.

19. Ellis JA, McCarthy P, Herson L, et al. Pain practices: a cross-Canada survey of pediatric oncology centers. *J Pediatr Oncol Nurs* 2003;20(1);26.

20. Chochinov HM, Breithart WS, eds. *Handbook of psychiatry in palliative medicine.* New York: Oxford University Press, 1999.

21. Ventafridda V, DeConno F, Riparnonti C, Gamba A, Tamburini M. Quality-of-life assessment during a palliative care programme. *Ann Oncol* 1990;1:415.

22. Coyle N, Adelhardt J, Foley KM, Portenoy RK. Character of terminal illness in the advanced cancer patient: pain and other symptoms during the last 4 weeks of life. *J Pain Symptom Manage* 1990;5:83.

23. Ventafridda V, Ripamonti C, DeConno F, Tamburini M. Symptom prevalence and control during cancer patients' last days of life. *J Palliat Care* 1990;6:7.

24. Moulin DE, Foley KM. A review of a hospital-based pain service. In: Foley KM, Bonica JJ, Ventafridda V, eds. *Advances in pain research and therapy.* New York: Raven Press, 1990:413.

25. Cherny NI, Chang V, Frager G, et al. Opioid pharmacotherapy in the management of cancer pain. *Cancer* 1995;76:1283.

26. Zech DL, Grond S, Lynch J, Hertel D, Lehman KA. Validation of World Health Organization guidelines for cancer pain relief: a 10-year prospective study. *Pain* 1995;63:65.

27. Gonzales GR, Elliott KJ, Portenoy RK, Foley KM. Impact of a comprehensive evaluation in the management of cancer pain. *Pain* 1991;47:141.

28. Clouston P, DeAngelis L, Posner JB. The spectrum of neurologic disease in patients with systemic cancer. *Ann Neurol* 1992;31:268.

29. Portenoy RK, Thaler HT, Kornblith AB, et al. Symptom prevalence, characteristics and distress in a cancer population. *Qual Life Res* 1994;3:183.

30. American Pain Society Quality of Care Committee. Quality improvement guidelines for the treatment of acute pain and cancer pain. 2004 (*in press*).

31. Miaskowski C, Dodd M, West C, et al. Randomized clinical trial of the effectiveness of a self-care intervention to improve cancer pain management. *J Clin Oncol* 2004;22:1713.

32. DuPenn S, DuPenn AR, Pulissar N, et al. Implementing guidelines for cancer pain management: results of a randomized controlled clinical trial. *J Clin Oncol* 1999;17(1):361.

33. Berry PH, Dahl JL. The new JCAHO pain schedule: implications for pain management nurses. *Pain Manag News* 2000;1(1):3.

34. Joranson DE, Gilsin AM. Regulatory barriers to pain management. *Semin Oncol Nurs* 1998;14(2):158.

35. Joranson DE, Gilson AM, Ryan KM, Maurer MA, Joranby JP. *Achieving balance in federal and state pain policy: a guide to evaluation,* 2nd ed. Madison, WI: Pain and Policy Studies Group, University of Wisconsin Comprehensive Cancer Center, 2000.

36. Fields MJ, Cassel CK, Committee on Care at the End of Life. *Approaching death: improving care at the end of life.* Washington, DC: National Academies Press, 1997.

37. Fields MJ, Behrman RE. *When children die. Improving palliative care and end-of-life care for children and their families.* Washington, DC: National Academies Press, 2003.

38. Cancer care during the late phase of life. *J Clin Oncol* 1998;16:1986.

39. Cherny NI. European Society of Medical Oncology (ESMO) joins the palliative care community [Editorial]. *Palliat Med* 2003;17:475.

40. IASP Subcommittee on Taxonomy. Pain terms: a list with definitions and notes on usage. *Pain* 1980;8:249.

41. Caterina MJ, Jaluss D. The vanilloid receptor: a molecular gateway to the pain pathway. *Annu Rev Neurosci* 2001;24:487.

42. Gold MS. Sodium channels and pain therapy current opinion. *Anesthesiology* 2000;13(5):565.

43. Besson JM. The neurobiology of pain. *Lancet* 1999;353:1610.

44. Gorman AL, Elliott KJ, Inturrisi CE. The D- and L-isomers of methadone bind to the non-competitive site on the N-methyl-D-aspartate (NMDA) receptor in rat forebrain and spinal cord. *Neurosci Lett* 1997;223:5.

45. Pasternak GW. Incomplete cross tolerance and multiple mu opioid peptide receptors. *Trends Pharmacol Sci* 2001;22:67.

46. Max MB, Inturrisi CE, Kaiko RF, et al. Epidural and intrathecal opiates: distribution in CSF and plasma and analgesic effects in patients with cancer. *Clin Pharmacol Ther* 1985;38:631.

47. Onofrio BM, Yaksh TL. Long-term pain relief: intrathecal morphine infusion in 53 patients. *J Neurosurg* 1990;72:200.

48. Yaksh TL. Spinal opiate analgesia: characteristic and principles of action. *Pain* 1981;11:293.

49. Bennett G, Burchiel K, Buchser E, et al. Clinical guidelines for intraspinal infusion report of an expert panel. Polyanalgesic Consensus Conference. *J Pain Symptom Manage* 2000;20(2):S37.

50. Cervero F, Laird JMA. Pain: visceral pain. *Lancet* 1999;353:2145.

51. Elliott K, Foley KM. Neurologic pain syndromes in patients with cancer. *Crit Care Clin* 1990;6:393.

52. Clohisy DR, Mantyh PW. Bone cancer pain. *Cancer* 2003;97(3):866.

53. Portenoy RK, Hagen NA. Breakthrough pain: definition, prevalence, and characteristics. *Pain* 1990;41:273.

54. Petzke F, Radbruch L, Zech D, Loick G, Grong S. Temporal presentation of chronic cancer pain: transitory pains on admission to a multidisciplinary pain clinic. *J Pain Symptom Manage* 1999;17:391.

55. Portenoy RK, Payne R, Coluzzi P, et al. Oral transmucosal fentanyl citrate (OTFC) for the treatment of breakthrough pain in cancer patients, a controlled dose titration study. *Pain* 1999;79:303.

56. Davis MP. Guidelines for breakthrough pain dosing. *Am J Hosp Palliat Care* 2003;20(5):229.

57. Wallenstein SL. Measurement of pain and analgesia in cancer patients. *Cancer* 1984;53:2217.

58. Daut RL, Cleeland CS, Flanery RC. The development of the Wisconsin Brief Pain Questionnaire to assess pain in cancer and other diseases. *Pain* 1983;1:197.

59. Graham C, Bond SS, Gertrovitch MM, Cook MR. Use of the McGill Pain Questionnaire in the management of cancer pain—replicability and consistency. *Pain* 1980;8:377.

60. Fishman B, Pasternak S, Wallenstein SL, et al. The Memorial Pain Assessment Card: a valid instrument for the assessment of cancer pain. *Cancer* 1986;60:1151.

61. Chang VT, Hwang SS, Feuerman M, et al. Symptom and quality of life survey of medical oncology patients at a Veterans Affairs Medical Center. A role for symptom assessment. *Cancer* 2000;88:1175.

62. Hwang SS, Chang VT, Fairclough DL, Kasimis B. Development of a cancer pain prognostic scale. *J Pain Symptom Manage* 2002;24(4):366.

63. Aaronson NK, Ahmedzai S, Bergman B, et al. The European Organization for Research and Treatment of Cancer QLQ-C30: a quality-of-life instrument for use in international clinical trials in oncology. European Organization for Research and Treatment of Cancer. *J Natl Cancer Inst* 1993;85:365.

64. Chang VT, Hwang SS, Feuerman M. Validation of the Edmonton symptom assessment scale. *Cancer* 2000;88:2164.

65. Cherny NI, Coyle N, Foley KM. Suffering in the advanced cancer patient. Part I: a definition and taxonomy. *J Palliat Care* 1994;10:57.

66. Passik SD, Portenoy RK. Substance abuse issues in palliative care. In: Berger A, et al., eds. *Principles and practices of supportive oncology.* Philadelphia: Lippincott–Raven Publishers, 1998.

67. Foley KM. The relationship of pain and symptom management to patient requests for physician-assisted suicide. *J Pain Symptom Manage* 1991;6:289.

68. Cherny NI, Coyle N, Foley KM. Guidelines in the care of the dying cancer patient. *Hematol Oncol Clin North Am* 1996;10:261.

69. Cassem NH. The dying patient. In: Cassem NH, ed. *Massachusetts General Hospital handbook of general hospital psychiatry.* St. Louis: Mosby Year Book, 1991:343.

70. Block SD. Perspectives on care at the close of life. Psychological considerations, growth, and transcendence at the end of life: the art of the possible. *JAMA* 2001;285(22):2898.

71. Cherny NI, Portenoy RK. Cancer pain: principles of assessment and syndromes. In: Wall PK, Melzack R, eds. *Textbook of pain.* London: Churchill Livingstone, 1994:787.

72. Foley KM. The treatment of cancer pain. *N Engl J Med* 1985;313:84.

73. Cassell EJ. The nature of suffering and the goals of medicine. *N Engl J Med* 1982;306:639.

74. Chochinov HM, Wilson KG, Enns M, et al. Desire for death in the terminally ill. *Am J Psychiatry* 1995;152:1185.

75. Cherny NI, Foley KM. Brachial plexopathy in patients with breast cancer. In: Harris JR, Hellman S, Henderson IC, Kinne D, eds. *Breast diseases,* 2nd ed. Philadelphia: Lippincott, 1996:796.

76. Posner JB. *Neurologic complications of cancer.* Philadelphia: FA Davis, 1995.

77. Emmanuel EJ. Pain and symptom control: patient rights and physician responsibilities. *Hematol Oncol Clin North Am* 1996;10:41.

78. Constantini-Ferrando M, Foley KM, Rapkin BD. Communicating with patients about advanced cancer. *JAMA* 1998;280:1403.

79. Benedetti C, Brock C, Cleeland C, et al.; National Comprehensive Cancer Network. NCCN practice guidelines for cancer pain. *Oncology* 2000;14(11A):135.

80. American Pain Society. *Principles of analgesic use in the treatment of acute pain and cancer pain,* 3rd ed. Skokie, IL: American Pain Society, 1992.

81. Management of Cancer Pain Guideline Panel. Management of cancer pain: clinical practice guideline. Rockville, MD: U.S. Public Health Service, Agency for Health Care Policy and Research, 1994. AHCPR Pub. No. 94-0592.

82. McQuay H. Opioids in pain management. *Lancet* 1999;353:2229.

83. Bruera E, Pereira J, Watanabe S, et al. Opioid rotation in patients with cancer pain. A retrospective comparison of dose ratios between methadone, hydromorphone, and morphine. *Cancer* 1996;78:852.

84. Ripamonti C, Groff L, Bernelli C, et al. Switching from morphine to oral methadone in treating cancer pain: what is the equianalgesic dose ratio? *J Clin Oncol* 1998;16:3216.

85. Mercadante S, Casuccio A, Aguello A, et al. Morphine versus methadone in the pain treatment of advanced cancer patients followed up at home. *J Clin Oncol* 1998;16:3656.

86. Mercadante S, Casuccio A, Calderone L. Rapid switching from morphine to methadone in cancer patients with poor response to morphine. *J Clin Oncol* 1999;17:3307.

87. Kornick CA, Santiago-Palma J, Schulman G, et al. A safe and effective method for converting patients from transdermal to intravenous fentanyl for the treatment of acute cancer-related pain. *Cancer* 2003;97(12):3121.

88. Ventafridda V, Caraceni A, Gamba A. Field-testing of the WHO Guidelines for Cancer Pain Relief: summary report of demonstration projects. In: Foley KM, Bonica JJ, Ventafridda V, Callaway MV, eds. *Second International Congress on Cancer Pain. Advances in pain research and therapy,* vol. 16. New York: Raven Press, 1990:451.

89. Stjernsward J. Palliative medicine: a global perspective. In: Doyle D, Hanks G, Cherny N, eds. *Oxford textbook of palliative medicine,* 3rd ed. New York: Oxford University Press, 2003.

90. Foley KM. Controversies in cancer pain: medical perspective. *Cancer* 1989;63:2266.

91. Jadad AR, Bowman GP. The WHO analgesic ladder for cancer pain management. Stepping up the quality of its evaluation. *JAMA* 1996;274:1870.

92. Portenoy RK, Foley KM, Inturrisi CE. The nature of opioid responsiveness and its implications for neuropathic pain: new hypotheses derived from studies of opioid infusions. *Pain* 1990;43:273.

93. Eisenberg E, Berkey CS, Carr DB, Mosteller F, Chalmers TC. Efficacy and safety of nonsteroidal antiinflammatory drugs for cancer pain: a meta-analysis. *J Clin Oncol* 1994; 12:2756.

94. Ventafridda V, DeConno F, Panerai AE, et al. Nonsteroidal anti-inflammatory drugs as the first step in cancer pain therapy; double-blind, within-patient study comparing nine drugs. *J Int Med Res* 1990;18:21.
95. Langman MJS. Treating ulcers in patients receiving anti-arthritic drugs. *QJM* 1989;73:1089.
96. Foley KM. Changing concepts of tolerance to opioids. What the cancer patient has taught us. In: Chapman CR, Foley KM, eds. *Current and emerging issues in cancer pain: research and practice.* New York: Raven Press, 1993:331.
97. Ferrell BR, Griffith H. Cost issues related to pain management: report from the cancer pain panel of the Agency for Health Care Policy and Research. *J Pain Symptom Manage* 1994;9:221.
98. Foley KM. Competent care for the dying instead of physician-assisted suicide. *N Engl J Med* 1997;336:54.
99. Foley KM. For more rhetoric and less regulation. *Pain Forum* 1995;4:197.
100. Foley KM. Opioids and chronic neuropathic pain. *N Engl J Med* 2003;348(13):1279.
101. Joranson DE, Ryan KM, Gilson AM, Dahl JL. Trends in medical use and abuse of opioid analgesics. *JAMA* 2000;283(13):1710.
102. Paul D, Standifier KM, Inturrisi CE, Pasternak GW. Pharmacological characterization of morphine-6-glucuronide, a very potent morphine metabolite. *J Pharmacol Exp Ther* 1989;251:477.
103. Portenoy RK, Thaler HT, Inturrisi CE, Friedlander-Klar H, Foley KM. Metabolite, morphine-6-glucuronide, contributes to the analgesia produced by morphine infusion in pain patients with normal renal function. *Clin Pharmacol Ther* 1992;51:422.
104. Portenoy RK, Foley KM, Stuhnan J, et al. Plasma morphine and morphine-6-glucuronide during chronic morphine therapy for cancer pain: plasma profiles, steady-state concentrations and the consequences of renal failure. *Pain* 1991;47:13.
105. Hagen N, Foley KM, Cebrone DJ, Portenoy RK, Inturrisi CE. Chronic nausea and morphine-6-glucuronide. *J Pain Symptom Manage* 1991;6:125.
106. Chicurel ME, Dalma-Weiszhausz DD. Microarrays in pharmacogenomics—advances and future promise. *Pharmacogenomics* 2002;3:589.
107. Babul N, Darke AC, Hagen N. Hydromorphone metabolite accumulation in renal failure. *J Pain Symptom Manage* 1995;10:184.
108. Moulin DE, Kreeft JH, Murray-Parsons N, et al. Comparison of continuous subcutaneous and intravenous hydromorphone infusions for management of cancer pain. *Lancet* 1991;337:465.
109. Kaiko BF, Benziger DP, Fitzmartin RD, et al. Pharmacokinetic-pharmacodynamic relationships of controlled-release oxycodone. *Clin Pharmacol Ther* 1995;59:50.
110. Bruera E, Fainsinger R, Moore M, et al. Local toxicity with subcutaneous methadone. *Pain* 1991;45:141.
111. Kaiko RR, Foley KM, Grabinski PY, et al. Central nervous system excitatory effects of meperidine in cancer patients. *Ann Neurol* 1983;13:180.
112. Houde RW. Methods for measuring clinical pain in humans. *Acta Anaesthesiol Scand* 1982;74[Suppl]:25.
113. Portenoy RK, Southam MA, Gupta SK, et al. Transdermal fentanyl for cancer pain: repeated dose pharmacokinetics. *Anesthesiology* 1993;78:36.
114. Weinberg DS, Inturrisi CE, Reidenberg B, et al. Sublingual absorption of selected opioid analgesics. *Clin Pharmacol Ther* 1988;44:335.
115. Moulin DE, Kreeft JH, Murray-Parsons N, Bouquillon AL. Comparison of continuous subcutaneous and intravenous hydromorphone infusions for management of cancer pain. *Lancet* 1991;337:465.
116. Portenoy RK, Moulin DE, Rogers A, Inturrisi CE, Foley KM. Infusion of opioids in cancer pain: clinical review and guidelines for use. *Cancer Treat Rep* 1985;70:575.
117. Devulder J, Ghys L, Dhondt W, Rolly G. Spinal analgesia in terminal care: risk versus benefit. *J Pain Symptom Manage* 1994;9:75.
118. Smith TJ, Staats PS, Deer T, et al. Randomized clinical trial of an implantable drug delivery system compared with comprehensive medical management for refractory cancer pain: impact on pain, drug-related toxicity, and survival. *J Clin Oncol* 2002;20(19):4040.
119. Dennis CG, DeWitty RL. Long-term intraventricular infusion of morphine for intractable pain in cancer of the head and neck. *Neurosurgery* 1990;26:404.
120. Beaver WT. Comparison of analgesic effects of morphine sulfate, hydroxyzine and other combinations in patients with postoperative pain. In: Bonica JJ, Ventafridda V, eds. *Advances in pain research and therapy.* New York: Raven Press, 1976:553.
121. Forrest WH, Brown B, Brown C, et al. Dextroamphetamine with morphine for the treatment of postoperative pain. *N Engl J Med* 1977;296:712.
122. Bruera E, Chadwich S, Brenneis C, et al. Methylphenidate associated with narcotics for the treatment of cancer pain. *Cancer Treat Rep* 1987;71:67.
123. Mercandante S, Casuccio A, Genovese G. Ineffectiveness of dextromethorphan in cancer pain. *J Pain Symptom Manage* 1998;16:317.
124. Laska EM, Sunshine A, Mueller F, et al. Caffeine as an analgesic adjuvant. *JAMA* 1984;251:1711.
125. Branas P, Jordan R, Fry-Smith A, Burls A, Hyde C. Treatments for fatigue in multiple sclerosis: a rapid and systematic review. *Health Technol Assess* 2000;4(27):1.
126. Birks JS, Harvey R. Donepezil for dementia due to Alzheimer's disease. *Cochrane Database Syst Rev* 2000;(4):CD001190.
127. Breitbart W, Rosenfeld B, Kaim M, Funesti-Esch J. A randomized, double-blind, placebo-controlled trial of psychostimulants for the treatment of fatigue in ambulatory patients with human immunodeficiency virus disease. *Arch Intern Med* 2001;161(3):411.
128. Goldfrank L, Weisman RS, Enick JK, Lo MW. A normogram for continuous intravenous naloxone. *Ann Emerg Med* 1986;1:566.
129. Derby S, Portenoy RK. Assessment and management of opioid-induced constipation. In: Portenoy RK, Bruera E, eds. *Topics in palliative care*, vol. 1. New York: Oxford University Press, 1997;1:95.
130. Yuan CS, Foss JF, O'Connor M, et al. Methylnaltrexone for reversal of constipation due to chronic methadone use: a randomized controlled trial. *JAMA* 2000;283:367.
131. Kanner RM, Foley KM. Patterns of narcotic drug use in a cancer pain clinic. *Ann N Y Acad Sci* 1981;362:161.
132. Eagel B, Portnoy R, Foley KM. Use and misuse of naloxone. *J Pain Symptom Manage* 2000 (*in press*).
133. Manfredi PL, Ribeiro S, Chandler SW, Payne R. Inappropriate use of naloxone in cancer patients with pain. *J Pain Symptom Manage* 1996;11:131.
134. Portenoy RK. Adjuvant analgesic agents. *Hematol Oncol Clin North Am* 1996;10:103.
135. Max MB, Culnane M, Schafer SC, et al. Amitriptyline relieves diabetic neuropathy pain in patients with normal or depressed mood. *Neurology* 1987;37:589.
136. Max MB, Schafer SC, Culnane M, et al. Association of pain relief with drug side effects in postherpetic neuralgia: a single dose study of clonidine, codeine, ibuprofen, and placebo. *Clin Pharmacol Ther* 1988;43:363.
137. Sindrup SH, Gram LF, Brosen K, et al. The selective serotonin reuptake inhibitor paroxetine is effective in the treatment of diabetic neuropathy symptoms. *Pain* 1990;42:135.
138. Backonja M, Beydoun A, Edwards KR, et al. Gabapentin for the symptomatic treatment of painful neuropathy in diabetes mellitus, a randomized controlled trial. *JAMA* 1998;280:1831.
139. Stute P, Soukup J, Menzel M, Sabatowski R, Grond S. Analysis and treatment of different types of neuropathic cancer pain. *J Pain Symptom Manage* 2003;26(6):1123.
140. Dejgard A, Petersen P, Kastrup J. Mexiletine for treatment of chronic painful diabetic neuropathy. *Lancet* 1988;1:9.
141. Brose WG, Cousins MJ. Subcutaneous lidocaine for treatment of neuropathic cancer pain. *Pain* 1991;45:141.
142. Ehrenstrom GME, Reiz SLA. EMLA—a eutectic mixture of local anesthetics for topical anesthesia. *Acta Anaesthesiol Scand* 1982;26:596.
143. Rowbotham MC, Davies PS, Fields HL. Topical lidocaine relieves postherpetic neuralgia. *Ann Neurol* 1995:37:246.
144. Tannock I, Gospodarowicz M, Meakin W, et al. Treatment of metastatic prostate cancer with low-dose prednisone: evaluation of pain and quality of life as prognostic indices of response. *J Clin Oncol* 1989;7:590.
145. Bruera E, Roca E, Cedaro L, Carraro S, Chacon R. Action of oral methylprednisolone in terminal cancer patients: a prospective randomized double-blind study. *Cancer Treat Rep* 1985;69:751.
146. Lechin F, vander Dijs B, Lechin ME, et al. Pimozide therapy for trigeminal neuralgia. *Arch Neurol* 1989;9:960.
147. Beaver WT, Wallenstein SM, Houde RW, et al. A comparison of the analgesic effects of methotrimeprazine and morphine in patients with cancer. *Clin Pharmacol Ther* 1966;7:436.
148. Eisenach JC, Dewan DM, Rose JC, et al. Epidural clonidine produces antinociception, but not hypotension, in sheep. *Anesthesiology* 1987;66:496.
149. Persson J, Axelsson G, Hallin RG, et al. Beneficial effects of ketamine in a chronic pain state with allodynia, possibly due to central sensitization. *Pain* 1995;60:217.
150. Slatkin NS, Rhiner M. Ketamine in the treatment of refractory cancer pain. *J Support Oncol* 2003;14:287.
151. Jaeger H, Maier C. Calcitonin in phantom limb pain: a double blind study. *Pain* 1992;48:21.
152. Ernst DS, MacDonald RN, Paterson AH, et al. A double-blind, crossover trial of intravenous clodronate in metastatic bone pain. *J Pain Symptom Manage* 1992;7:4.
153. Glover D, Lipton A, Keller A, et al. Intravenous pamidronate disodium treatment: bone metastases in patients with breast cancer. *Cancer* 1994;74:2949.
154. Bloomfield DJ. Should bisphosphonates be part of the standard therapy of patients with multiple myeloma or bone metastases from other cancers? An evidence based review. *J Clin Oncol* 1998;16:1218.
155. Roth A, Kolaric K. Analgesic activity of calcitonin in patient with painful osteolytic metastases of breast cancer: results of a controlled randomized study. *Oncology* 1986;43:283.
156. Warrel RP, Lovett D, Dilmanian FA, et al. Low-dose gallium nitrate for prevention of osteolysis in myeloma: results of a pilot randomized study. *J Clin Oncol* 1993;11:2443.
157. Porter AT, McEwan AJ, Powe JE, et al. Results of a randomized phase-III trial to evaluate the efficacy of strontium-89 adjuvant to local field external beam irradiation in the management of endocrine resistant metastatic prostate cancer. *Int J Radiat Oncol Biol Phys* 1993;25:805.
158. Berna L, Carrio J, Alinso C, et al. Bone pain palliation with strontium 89 in breast cancer patients with bone metastases with refractory bone pain. *Eur J Nucl Med* 1995;22:1101.
159. Loscalzo M, Amendola J. Psychosocial and behavioral management of cancer pain: the social work contribution. In: Foley KM, Bonica JJ, Ventafridda V, eds. *Advances in pain research and therapy.* New York: Raven Press, 1990:429.
160. Kalso E, Tramer MR, McQuay HJ, Moore RA. Systemic local anesthetic type drugs in chronic pain. A systematic review. *Eur J Pain* 1998;2(1):3.
161. Edwards WT, Habib F, Burney RG, Begin G. Intravenous lidocaine in the management of various chronic pain states. *Reg Anesth* 1985;10:1.
162. Waldman SD, Cronen MC. Thoracic epidural morphine in the palliation of chest wall pain secondary to relapsing polychondritis. *J Pain Symptom Manage* 1989;4:38.
163. Cherny NI, Arbit E, Jain S. Invasive techniques in the management of cancer pain. *Hematol Oncol Clin North Am* 1996;10:121.
164. Patt R. Peripheral neurolysis and the management of cancer pain. In: Patt R, ed. *Cancer pain.* Philadelphia: Lippincott, 1993:359.
165. Robertson DH. Transsacral neurolytic nerve block. An alternative approach to intractable perineal pain. *Br J Anaesth* 1983;55:873.
166. Rossi M, Zaninotto G, Finco C, Codello L, Ancona E. Thoracoscopic bilateral splanchnicotomy for pain control in unresectable pancreatic cancer. *Chir Ital* 1995;47(2):55.
167. Gianasi C. Neuroadenolysis of the pituitary: an overview of development, mechanisms, technique and results. In: Benedetti C, Chapman CR, Moricca G, et al., eds. *Advances in pain research and therapy.* New York: Raven Press, 1984:647.
168. Sundaresan N, DiGiacinto GV, Hughes EO. Neurosurgery in the treatment of cancer pain. *Cancer* 1989;63:2365.

169. Arbit E. Neurosurgical management of cancer pain. In: Foley KM, Bonica JJ, Ventafridda V, eds. *Advances in pain research and therapy.* New York: Raven Press, 1990:289.

170. Sundaresan N, Galicich JH, Lane JM, Scher H. Stabilization of the spine involved by cancer. In: Dunsker DB, Schmidek HH, eds. *The unstable spine.* Orlando, FL: Grune & Stratton, 1986:249.

171. Sundaresan N, Hilaris BS, Martini N. The combined neurosurgical-thoracic management of superior sulcus tumors. *J Clin Oncol* 1987;5:1739.

172. Lahuerta T, Lipton SA, Wells JD. Percutaneous cervical cordotomy: results and complications in a recent series of 100 patients. *Ann R Coll Surg Exp* 1985;67:41.

173. Ischia S, Luzzani A, Ischia A, et al. Subarachnoid neurolytic block (L5, S1) and unilateral percutaneous cervical cordotomy for the treatment of neoplastic vertebral pain. *Pain* 1984;19:123.

174. Macaluso C, Arbit E, Foley KM. Cordotomy for lumbosacral, pelvic, and lower extremity pain of malignant origin: safety and efficacy. *Neurology* 1988;38:110.

175. Barrash JM, Milan EL. Dorsal rhizotomy for the relief of pain of malignant tumor origin. *J Neurosurg* 1973;38:755.

176. Arbit E, Galicich JH, Burt M, et al. Modified open thoracic rhizotomy for treatment of intractable chest wall pain of malignant etiology. *Ann Thorac Surg* 1989;48:820.

177. Giorgi C, Broggi G. Surgical treatment of glossopharyngeal neuralgia and pain from cancer of the nasopharynx. *J Neurosurg* 1984;61:952.

178. Nashold BS, Ostdahl RH. Dorsal root entry zone lesions for pain relief. *J Neurosurg* 1979;51:59.

179. Gildenberg PL, Hirschberg RM. Limited myelotomy for the treatment of intractable cancer pain. *J Neurol Neurosurg Psychiatry* 1984;47:94.

180. Hassenbusch SJ, Pillay PK, Barnett GH. Radiofrequency cingulotomy for intractable cancer pain using stereotaxis guided by magnetic resonance imaging. *Neurosurgery* 1990;27:220.

181. Thompson JW, Filshie J. In: Doyle D, Hanks G, MacDonald N, eds. *Transcutaneous electrical nerve stimulation and acupuncture in palliative care medicine.* New York: Oxford University Press, 1992.

182. Levy RM, Lamb S, Adams JE. Treatment of chronic pain by deep brain stimulation: long-term followup and review of the literature. *Neurosurgery* 1987;21:885.

183. Young RF, Brechner T. Electrical stimulation of the brain for relief of intractable pain due to cancer. *Cancer* 1986;57:1266.

184. Staats P. Neuraxial infusion for pain control: when, why and what to do after the implant. *Oncology* 1999;13:58.

185. Travell JG, Simons DG. *Myofascial pain and dysfunction: the trigger-point manual.* Baltimore: Williams & Wilkins, 1983.

186. Filshle J. Acupuncture and malignant pain problems. *Acupunct Med* 1990;8:38.

187. Fosburg MT, Crone RK. Nitrous oxide analgesia for refractory pain in the terminally ill. *JAMA* 1983;250:511.

188. Green VFR, David WH. Titrated intravenous barbiturates in the control of symptoms in patients with terminal cancer. *South Med J* 1991;84:332.

189. Cherny NI, Portenoy RK. Sedation in the management of refractory symptoms: guidelines for evaluation and treatment. *J Palliat Care* 1994;10:31.

190. Roy D. Need they sleep before they die? *J Palliat Care* 1990;6:3.

191. Ventafridda V, Ripamonti C, De Conno F, et al. Symptom prevalence and control during cancer patients' last days of life. *J Palliat Care* 1990;6:7.

192. Coyle N. A model of continuity of care for cancer patients with chronic pain. *Med Clin North Am* 1987;71:24.

J. STANLEY SMITH
DAVID FRANKENFIELD
WILEY W. SOUBA

SECTION 2

Nutritional Support

Patients with cancer, due either to the disease itself or its treatment, often lose appetite, weight, and energy. Malnutrition in these patients becomes common and is a true malnutrition syndrome, differing from the protein-calorie malnutrition seen in pure starvation because of an inflammatory component (Table 55.2-1). The etiology of this vexing and clinically obvious problem is not completely clear, although newer studies are shedding more light on its causes and proposing newer avenues of treatment.

The goals of nutritional support in cancer are to increase functional capacity and quality of life, even in advanced cases. Patients may be much more concerned with their ability to function as nearly normal as possible or to maintain a good quality of life than with their ultimate mortality. When lean body mass is lost, function and quality of life suffer. Nearly all cancer patients lose weight; the challenge is to keep them from losing their lean body mass as well.

Cancer treatments, including surgery, drugs, and radiation, may interfere with the patient's ability to taste, ingest, swallow, or digest food. Surgery and radiation of the gastrointestinal tract may affect the digestion or absorption of nutrients, or both. Drugs may cause nausea, diarrhea, and anorexia. Although many new agents have been developed to combat these side effects, patients still suffer through treatment. One of the major side effects presenting a significant challenge to the cancer patient is alteration of taste, or dysgeusia.

DYSGEUSIA

To be effective, chemotherapeutic drugs must be distributed throughout the body and may be secreted or excreted in tears, saliva, sweat, bile, or urine. Drugs in the saliva may markedly alter taste (dysgeusia), leading to food revulsion and avoidance.[1] After early satiety, dysgeusia is the most common challenge in patients on chemotherapy. Not only may certain tastes be affected, but food consistency or texture may factor as well, requiring more chewing that may increase saliva production, resulting in the rotten taste. Dysgeusia may induce nutritional disorders and protein wasting in chronic disorders, such as liver disease, AIDS, or cancer. Multiple other mechanisms may be involved in dysgeusia besides drug effects, including zinc deficiency, morphologic changes in the lingual papillae, and even a neuropathy.[2] Dysgeusia may also be caused by depression, which may initially be unrecognized in cancer patients. Some of the newer antidepressants may have an effect here.[3]

The two main types of dysgeusia are loss of taste acuity and distortion of taste.[1] Loss of taste acuity comes from drug inhibition of taste receptor function. Taste distortion results from drugs activating the taste receptor in an abnormally persistent fashion or preventing activation of the receptor.

Various attempts at treatment of dysgeusia have been made, but when a drug makes a food taste awful, there is not much relief. Each patient must experiment through trial and error to find the foods that are best consumed with the least alteration in taste. Different tastes can be tested using sugar for sweet, lemon juice for sour, salt (for salt), and aspirin or quinine for bitter. By testing, a patient may find the least repulsive tastes.

Usually, soft, fatty, or greasy foods are tolerated best because they can be swallowed with little chewing and therefore little saliva production. Attempts at dietary supplementation with elements such as zinc, folic acid, α-lipoic acid, and vitamins of the "B" class may alleviate some of the metallic taste but are only mildly helpful.[4–6] Zinc seems to work best with a "sweet" dysgeusia, but drugs often give a more metallic taste. Drugs such as vincristine and the taxanes may have the worst associated dysgeusia. These seem to be secreted in the saliva and, after the first bite or chew, often produce a horrible taste sensation. The best treatment remains withdrawal of the offending drug, but this may not be possible with chemotherapy. After drug cessation, the taste returns toward normal over a 2-month period.[7]

TABLE 55.2-1. Metabolic Differences between the Response to Simple Starvation and Advanced Malignant Disease

Parameter	Simple Starvation	Advanced Malignant Disease
Basal metabolic rate	– or decreased	–, increased, or decreased
Presence of mediators	–	+++
Hepatic ureagenesis	+	+++
Negative nitrogen balance	+	+++
Gluconeogenesis	+	+++
Muscle proteolysis	+	+++
Hepatic protein synthesis	+	+++
Lipolysis	+	+++

–, normal; +, slightly increased; +++, a substantial increase.

TABLE 55.2-2. Metabolic Abnormalities in Animal and Human Cancer Cachexia

Substrate	Clinical Parameter	Observation
Water	Total body water	Increased
Energy	Energy balance	Negative
	Energy stores	Diminished
Lipid	Body fat mass	Decreased
	Lipoprotein lipase activity	Decreased
	Fat breakdown	Increased
	Serum lipid levels	Increased
Carbohydrate	Gluconeogenesis	Increased
	Insulin resistance	Present
	Body glucose consumption	Increased
	Hepatic glucose production	Increased
Protein	Muscle mass	Diminished
	Muscle proteolysis	Increased
	Muscle amino acid release	Increased
	Hepatic protein synthesis	Increased
	Hepatic amino acid transport	Increased
	Nitrogen balance	Negative

Perhaps a more effective regimen is nutrition counseling to give a patient a goal protein and calorie intake that allows him or her to force enough food past the taste to avoid weight loss and muscle depletion. Even foods that taste "OK" one day may be revolting the next. Furthermore, once a menu of "OK" foods is found to work, it may become boring during prolonged treatment. The patient, with the aid of caregivers, must continually experiment to find the foods that are palatable and provide the necessary amounts of nutrients.

Examples of some soft, greasy-type, protein-rich foods that may be palatable include spare ribs, a rare juicy steak, mussels, clams, oysters, and chicken wings or thighs (dark meat). A rich salty sauce such as barbecue or teriyaki may help as well. Sweets may be worse than salt. Other food choices include pasta with tangy sauces such as marinara.

Patients with dysgeusia may need to avoid dense meats, such as chicken breast, pork loin or chops, and lamb chops. These require more chewing and elicit a marked salivary response, bringing out the unpleasant taste. Another suggestion for the patient with dysgeusia is ground meats. This solves the texture problem and allows some protein-rich food to be added to pastas and soups that need little, if any, chewing.

Treatments aimed at improvement of dysgeusia may certainly improve the patient's quality of life. This is an area where more research is desperately needed.

WEIGHT LOSS AND CANCER CACHEXIA

The amount of weight loss with cancer varies with the type of cancer. Pancreatic cancer may be the worst, with many patients suffering a critical weight loss within a short period of time. More than 10% of the patient's usual weight lost within 6 months is defined as critical.[8] Weight loss occurs as a result of two main causes. The first is the tumor itself and its treatment, and the second is the body's metabolic/inflammatory response to the tumor. Tumors or tumor treatment may cause gastrointestinal tract obstruction, dysphagia, dysgeusia, early satiety, fatigue, or pain, leading to starvation or semistarvation. These issues can be addressed and resolved with proper nutrition counseling and support. More difficult to manage are the inflammatory changes brought about by the tumor's presence. Direct effects of cytokines and other inflammatory mediators,

the acute-phase response, and proteolysis are difficult to reverse with traditional nutritional support because they are not a result of starvation or semistarvation. This syndrome is known as *cancer cachexia.*

Cancer cachexia is a profound destructive process characterized by lean tissue breakdown of skeletal muscle and harmful abnormalities in fat and carbohydrate metabolism in spite of adequate energy and nutrient intake[9] (Table 55.2-2). Cachexia arises when the cancer creates a generalized inflammatory state, and, although these patients look starved, the condition does not respond to short-term nutritional repletion.[10] The diagnosis depends on a history of substantial weight loss accompanied by physical evidence of muscle wasting and demonstration of an acute-phase response such as an increase in the level of C-reactive protein.[11]

Multiple substances interact to produce cancer cachexia, including tumor products, hormones, and inflammatory mediators. This interaction promotes gluconeogenesis, limits anabolism, and increases catabolism.

The body's response to cancer has many parallels to inflammation of acute illness or injury. The cytokines, tumor necrosis factor-α, IL-1, IL-6, and interferon-γ, appear to have a significant role.[12] The n-6 fatty acid–derived eicosanoids have also been implicated in cachexia. Administration of many of these mediators into healthy volunteers leads to anorexia, weight loss, an acute-phase protein response, protein and fat breakdown, rises in the levels of cortisol and glucagons, falls in insulin, insulin resistance, anemia, fever, and elevated energy expenditure. Because elevated levels of these cytokines are rarely found in the blood of cancer patients, the effect may be more from local than from systemic production or from other mediators activated by an early burst of cytokine activity.

An additional mediator for the cachexia syndrome is a 24-kD glycoprotein described as proteolysis-inducing factor (PIF), which has been found in the urine of patients with pancreatic cancer.[13] PIF activates the ubiquitin proteolytic pathway, resulting in proteolysis and cytokine and acute-phase protein synthesis.[14] PIF has been found to be expressed in patients with significant weight loss.[15] This may be the common proteolytic pathway for muscle breakdown in cancer patients. Glickman and Ciechanover[16] have provided a biochemical review of the ubiquitin-proteasome system. Enzymes link ubiquitin onto proteins targeted for destruction by the proteasome, a large protease complex. This is a normal process of muscle breakdown that goes haywire in cachexia.

Eicosanoids seem to be involved with cytokine and with PIF activation of ubiquitin.[17] Perhaps manipulating the eicosanoid milieu may attenuate catabolism. Hussey and Tisdale[18] showed that pretreatment for 3 days with the n-3 fatty acid eicosapentaenoic acid (EPA) attenuated the effect of PIF. Multiple other studies have shown that the n-3 fatty acids have antitumor and anticachectic effects.[19–22] Inhibition of tumor growth, antiinflammatory effects, and preservation of skeletal muscle appear to result from the use of supplemental fish oil capsules; this is the rationale for use of the n-3 fatty acids in nutritional supplementation. For patients with cachexia who can tolerate oral feeding, the authors recommend a high-protein diet rich in essential amino acids (EAAs), branched-chain amino acids (BCAAs), and omega-3 fatty acids.

NUTRITION SUPPORT FOR WEIGHT LOSS AND CANCER CACHEXIA

Because weight loss due to starvation/semistarvation is mediated differently than weight loss from inflammatory response (cancer cachexia), the approach to feeding the cancer patient is also different depending on the cause of the weight loss. A fundamental concept to remember is that, because muscle mass is key to functions of daily living, lean body mass must be maintained for quality of life. Increase in body weight is only important insofar as the gain is in the lean body mass.

A study by Ovesen et al.[23] found that dietary counseling and use of supplements increased food intake by 30%, but the patients failed to gain weight. Even though the dietary intakes increased, they were still below the estimated energy requirements for those patients. Therefore, calorie support alone does not seem to support weight gain in cancer cachexia. Perhaps weight maintenance is more desirable than gain.

Pharmacologic agents such as the steroid megestrol acetate have been used to increase appetite but seem to cause fat gain rather than lean body mass.[24] Likewise, corticosteroids may also increase appetite but are catabolic agents that induce muscle breakdown, especially in fatigued cancer patients who are inactive.[25]

Nutritional interventions become valuable to cancer patients when they are easily applied, promote preservation of lean body mass, and aim to maintain function and quality of life. Several new reports have examined supplements and additives for use in cancer patients to maintain weight and lean body mass. Importantly, nutrition counseling must be the foundation of any supplement or additive program designed to raise energy or protein intake.

Much of the recent interest involves fish oil. The omega-3 fatty acids found in fish, mainly EPA at a dose of 3 g/d, seem to stabilize weight, reverse negative nitrogen balance, promote lean body mass gain, and improve functional capacity when provided with a protein and calorie supplement compared to a similar protein/calorie intake without the EPA. Such supplements provide approximately 300 kcal plus 1 g EPA in 250-mL volume. Appetite also improved with consumption of the supplement.[26–28]

Another area of supplementation involves amino acids and creatine. EAAs have been shown to stimulate more protein synthesis than a combination of EAA and nonessential amino acid (NAA), such as is found in the high-quality whey protein. The body maintains the concentration of NAAs, and their intake is not needed to stimulate muscle synthesis.[29]

More recently, the role of leucine (i.e., an essential branched-chain amino acid, EAA and BCAA) in maintaining muscle and lean body mass has emerged.[30,31] Leucine seems to have numerous metabolic roles for protein synthesis. It appears to activate factors that promote muscle formation. Leucine may be an important additive to maintain muscle mass in cancer but needs further study.

BCAAs in general have also been studied for their effects on anorexia and early satiety. Cangiano et al.[32] demonstrated that tryptophan competitively decreases hypothalamic uptake of BCAA, leading to the sensation of early satiety. Because this is a competitive uptake, an increase in BCAA may help resolve it.

Arginine has been found to modulate tumorigenesis and cancer spread in the rat as well as improve survival when supplemented to patients with head and neck cancer.[33,34] Glutamine supplementation improved nitrogen retention and increased protein synthesis in tumor-bearing rats without affecting the size or protein synthesis of the tumor in the same animal.[35] An amino acid mixture containing arginine, glutamine, and β-hydroxy β-methylbutyrate (a metabolite of leucine) promoted deposition of lean body mass in lung cancer patients without reported side effects.[36]

Creatine has become a favorite supplement of athletes and body builders because it is purported to increase muscle mass and muscle energy.[37] The use of creatine in sports and for muscle performance makes it a target for possible supplementation in cancer patients, but there have been no studies yet. In general, creatine is a safe supplement unless renal impairment is present.

Anabolic agents have also been tried in cancer to increase muscle mass and weight gain. Older studies have had conflicting results, but a more recent report using oxandrolone concluded that weight-losing cancer patients not only gained weight with this agent but increased lean body mass and functional performance as well.[38]

Based on the evidence above, the authors recommend that advanced cancer patients add to their food intake a high-protein supplement, 3 g fish oil, and perhaps some amino acids, especially BCAA. The high-protein supplements are readily available at any grocery store, and vitamin shops sell fish oil capsules (1 g each) and amino acids. These can easily be incorporated into a daily routine with appropriate nutrition counseling.

Drinking may often be easier for a patient than chewing: It requires less energy, stimulates less saliva, rarely causes gagging, and may speed gastric emptying. Two commercial products, Pro-Sure (Ross Products, Abbott Laboratories, Abbott Park, IL) and Resource Support (Novartis Nutrition Corp, Minneapolis, MN), are also available that provide energy, protein, EPA, and amino acids in a ready-to-drink can.

NUTRITION AND TUMOR GROWTH

With the introduction of specialized enteral and parenteral feeding regimens into clinical medicine, aggressive nutritional support can be provided to cancer patients who previously could not or would not eat. However, concerns over the stimulation of tumor growth have existed for many years. This forces a clinical dilemma as to whether the tumor growth may be significant. Multiple trials have investigated this, but there is much heterogeneity and numbers are small. The largest human trial confirmed that parenteral nutrition support stimulated DNA replication of tumor cells.[39] Because nutrition repletion might stimulate tumor growth, it was postulated that nutrition support in addition to aggressive chemotherapy would provide enhanced effectiveness in killing tumor cells. However, even when chemotherapy was combined with parenteral nutrition, the DNA replication of tumor cells was above baseline values, indicating tumor growth in the face of therapy.[39] Perhaps the cachexia syndrome is partly protective by limiting the growth of the tumor and, if the nutrient intake is artificially increased, tumor growth would be accelerated.

NUTRITIONAL ASSESSMENT OF THE CANCER PATIENT

To determine the best strategies for treatment of the cancer patient, the nutritional status must first be determined. The goal is to decide whether deficiencies are due to impaired intake or inflammatory changes. This determination is done by a careful history and physical examination followed by additional tests to confirm the clinical impression. The history should include inquiries about appetite, taste changes, swallowing or digestive problems, preferred foods, and weight loss. The Patient-Generated Subjective Global Assessment is a form including prognostic components of patient and clinical history that is very sensitive for predicting the risk of malnutrition in cancer patients.[40]

The physical examination can establish the diagnosis of muscle wasting and specific nutrient deficiencies. Hollowing of the temporal fossae, prominent scapulae, and emaciated limbs are reliable signs of loss of lean body mass. Anthropometric measurements should be done, including measurement of body weight and height, skinfold thickness, and a 24-hour urine collection for the measurement of nitrogen. Measurements of albumin (a negative acute-phase protein and nutritional marker if inflammation is not present) and C-reactive protein (a positive acute-phase protein and marker of inflammation) can help identify traditional malnutrition versus cachexia due to the inflammatory response. At the authors' institution, albumin is an $11 test and C-reactive protein is $47 (similar to the cost of prealbumin). These tests have an approximately 4-hour turnaround time.

Peripheral blood lymphocyte counts and skin testing to common antigens for assessment of delayed hypersensitivity have been used as indicators of immunocompetence in the cancer patient. Altered immunologic responses are not specific for nutritional deficiencies and are often observed even in patients with advanced malignant disease who are well nourished. Serum albumin and transferrin are the most common serum proteins measured, but C-reactive protein should be measured to assess the acute-phase response. Other laboratory studies useful in nutritional assessment include red blood cell indices to determine iron and micronutrient deficiencies, plasma glucose to assess insulin resistance, blood urea nitrogen to determine renal status, and liver function tests to evaluate hepatic function.

A clear indication for malnutrition is weight loss greater than 10% of usual body weight in the past 6 months. Decreased levels of absolute lymphocyte counts, serum proteins, and function scores are confirmatory. An elevated C-reactive protein level confirms the presence of the acute-phase response of inflammation.

INDICATIONS FOR NUTRITION SUPPORT

Once a cancer patient has been determined to be malnourished, some form of nutrition support should be recommended. A consensus statement recommends that nutrition support for malnourished preoperative patients could reduce postoperative complications by 10%.[41] Furthermore, provision of the proper amount and type of calories and nutrients increases functionality and quality of life for these patients. Even in very advanced stages, cancer patients and their families will want nutrition support as one of the few quality-of-life components that they can control in their final days.

Although it seems apparent that provision of nutrition support to the malnourished cancer patient would be beneficial, evidence that the malnutrition could be reversed is lacking. Instead, the goal is to preserve lean body mass as much as possible. A consensus regarding the role and efficacy of nutrition support in patients with cancer is lacking. Nonetheless, cancer patients represent one of the largest patient populations to receive nutrition support in hospital, nursing home, or home environments. Therefore, most physicians and surgeons are using aggressive nutrition support under specific circumstances.

PARENTERAL VERSUS ENTERAL NUTRITION IN CANCER PATIENTS

Numerous clinical trials have evaluated the use of aggressive nutritional support as adjunctive therapy during the administration of antineoplastic regimens to cancer patients, but well-designed studies make up a small fraction of these. Past trials do not demonstrate any consistent benefits of the nutrition, perhaps because they were not well randomized. A trial by Braga et al.[42] did randomize patients into three groups: One was a control group that was supplemented before and after surgery with standard enteral formula, the second was a group supplemented with an immunoenriched formula before surgery but with a standard formula after surgery, and the third was given the immunoenriched formula before and after surgery. The group with the enriched formula before and after surgery had fewer complications and a shorter hospital stay than the other two groups. This may be the first study to show that provision of specific key substrates (omega-3 fatty acids and amino acids) is beneficial to outcome.

Enteral nutrition encompasses not only tube feeding but oral nutrition as well. Patients who can maintain adequate oral intake through food and food supplements may be able to avoid feeding tube placement, but much guidance and monitoring are essential so that the patient can make the necessary food choices and adaptations in texture and preparation. Close monitoring is also necessary to detect failure of oral feeding early so that tube feeding can begin in a timely manner. Many liquid supplements and food bars are available to help the

TABLE 55.2-3.   Proposed Benefits of Oral and Enteral Nutrition versus Parenteral Nutrition

Maintain gut mucosal mass
Maintain brush border enzyme activity
Support gut immune function
Preserve gut mucosal barrier function
Maintain a balanced luminal microflora environment
Improve outcome after chemotherapy and radiation therapy

patient maintain adequate oral intake. Additionally, many vitamin, mineral, amino acid, herbal, and omega-3 oil supplements are widely available over the Internet and in local stores. Because the U.S. Food and Drug Administration does not regulate these supplements or their claims, the physician should inquire frequently about their use to avoid interactions and the development of false hopes by the patient.

Several randomized, controlled trials[26–28] have investigated the combination of calorie and protein support with n-3 fatty acids (usually fish oil) to modulate the inflammatory signals that lead to cancer cachexia while providing adequate building blocks for repletion of body cell mass. These trials have shown that such an approach does indeed promote body weight gain principally as body cell mass and that the patient's sense of well-being is improved. The n-3 fatty acid supplementation is 3 g/d. Protein/calorie supplements are now available that provide this level of supplementation, or the same amount can be obtained from three fish oil gelcaps, 3-oz Siskowet lake trout, 4-oz mackerel, or 5.5-oz farmed Atlantic salmon.

Most authorities agree, because of the greater incidence of complications with parenteral nutrition, that enteral nutrition is always the preferred route of feeding cancer patients if the gastrointestinal tract is functional (Table 55.2-3). Using in-between meal supplements; inserting soft, comfortable nasogastric feeding tubes; or inserting gastrostomy or jejunostomy feeding catheters can accomplish this. Consideration of tube feeding must be thought of early before falling blood counts make tube passage risky.

Commonly used enteral formulas are listed in Table 55.2-4. A physician order form for enteral nutrition is presented in Figure 55.2-1.

SPECIFIC INDICATIONS FOR THE USE OF TOTAL PARENTERAL NUTRITION IN THE CANCER PATIENT

See Table 55.2-5.

PATIENTS WITH ENTEROCUTANEOUS FISTULAS

In patients with cancer who undergo major gastrointestinal surgery, enterocutaneous fistulas occasionally develop that preclude the use of the gastrointestinal tract for nutritional support. In such patients, enteral nutrition may stimulate fistula output and can result in metabolic disturbances and dehydration. Total parenteral nutrition (TPN) can affect the course of disease in cancer patients with gastrointestinal fistulas. Studies indicate that TPN increases the spontaneous closure rate of enterocutaneous fistulas, although fistulas that originate from

radiated or neoplastic bowel have a much lower rate of spontaneous closure. In such patients, aggressive early surgical treatment is generally indicated. Provision of TPN maintains the nutritional status of the cancer patient who develops an enterocutaneous fistula such that he or she better tolerates operative intervention if closure does not occur. Perhaps insulin-like growth factor or a progestogen may help in this situation.

PATIENTS WITH HEPATIC OR RENAL FAILURE

Liver failure occasionally develops in patients with cancer after major surgery or from cytotoxic chemotherapy. Because of liver damage and portasystemic shunting, these patients develop derangements in their circulating levels of amino acids. The plasma aromatic to BCAA ratio is increased. Transport of amino acids across the blood–brain barrier favors the aromatic amino acids such as tryptophan, precursors for false neurotransmitters such as serotonin, which contribute to lethargy and encephalopathy. Treatment of individuals with liver failure with solutions enriched in BCAA and deficient in aromatic amino acids may result in improved tolerance to the administered protein and clinical improvement in the encephalopathic state. BCAA preparations are also available for oral or enteral use if TPN is not otherwise indicated.

TPN with amino acids of high biologic value may also be useful in patients with acute renal failure. Presumably, provision of only EAAs allows the body to maximally reuse nitrogen for the synthesis of NAAs and thereby helps prevent rapid increases in blood urea nitrogen. If the hypermetabolic cancer patient is receiving dialysis, there appears to be no advantage to using an EAA solution, and therefore a balanced standard amino acid formulation is recommended. Solutions containing BCAAs or just EAAs are expensive and probably not worth the cost except in specific patients in whom adjusted standard formulas are not tolerated.

ACUTE RADIATION AND CHEMOTHERAPY ENTERITIS

Cancer patients who receive abdominal or pelvic irradiation or chemotherapy may develop severe and prolonged mucositis and enterocolitis, precluding use of the gastrointestinal tract for nutritional support. Under these circumstances, TPN should be provided to malnourished patients until the enteritis resolves and oral feeding can be resumed. Moreover, under circumstances in which chemotherapy has been contraindicated secondary to severe malnutrition, TPN may be beneficial in optimizing nutritional status and allowing the initiation of the chemotherapeutic regimen. When enteral nutrition is feasible in such patients, TPN has not demonstrated a treatment advantage. When studies have been performed using well-nourished patients, the effects of TPN predictably have not been beneficial.

Patients undergoing radiation treatment may also develop malnutrition secondary to inadequate nutritional intake from an inability to eat. The potential side effects from radiotherapy are broad and include nausea, vomiting, mucositis, xerostomia, dysphagia, diarrhea, and anorexia. Whenever possible, the enteral route is preferable for nutritional support. However, in cases involving severe dysfunction of the gastrointestinal tract, TPN is indicated. TPN can be useful in allowing the malnourished, poor-risk patient to complete radiotherapy with less morbidity. Patients undergoing irradiation of the head, neck, or

TABLE 55.2-4. Adult Nutrition: Enteral Formulary

Tube Feedings	Standard isotonic with fiber	High protein with fiber	Very high protein with fiber	High-calorie fiber-free	High-calorie limited electrolytes	High-protein peptide-based	Standard peptide-based	Elemental	*Modular Supplements* Carbohydrate	Fat-MCT	Fat-LCT	Protein
Brand name	Ultracal	Fiber source HN	Isosource VHN	Nutren 1.5	Nutren 2.0	SandoSource peptide	Peptamen	Vivonex TEN	Polycose	MCT oil	Microlipid	ProMod
Manufacturer	Mead Johnson	Novartis	Novartis	Nestle	Nestle	Novartis	Nestle	Novartis	Ross Labs	Mead Johnson	Mead Johnson	Ross Labs
Calories/mL	1.06	1.2	1.0	1.5	2.0	1.0	1.0	1.0	2	7.7	4.5	6/scoop
Protein (g/L)	45	53	62	60	80	50	40	38	0	0	0	5/scoop
Carbohydrate (g/L)	142	160	130	170	196	160	127	210	0.5/mL	0	0	0.7/scoop
Fiber (g/L)	14	10	10	0	0	0	0	0	0	0	0	0
Fat (g/L)	39	39	29	68	76	17	39	3	0	0.93/mL	0.5/mL	0
Protein source	Milk protein concentrate, casein	Soy isolate and concentrate	Sodium and calcium caseinate	Calcium-potassium caseinate	Calcium-potassium caseinate	Casein hydrolysate, free amino acids, casein	Hydrolyzed whey protein	Free amino acids	None	None	None	Whey
Carbohydrate source	Maltodextrin	Corn syrup, hydrolyzed cornstarch	Hydrolyzed cornstarch	Maltodextrin sucrose	Corn syrup, maltodextrin, sucrose	Hydrolyzed cornstarch	Maltodextrin, cornstarch	Maltodextrin, modified cornstarch	Hydrolyzed cornstarch	None	None	Lactose
Fiber source	Cellulose, soy fiber, acacia	Partially hydrolyzed guar gum	Partially hydrolyzed guar gum	None	None	None	None	None	None	None	None	None
Fat source	Canola, MCT, sunflower, corn oil	Canola, MCT oil	Canola, MCT oil	MCT, canola, corn oil, soy lecithin	MCT, canola oil, soy lecithin, corn oil	MCT, soy oil, lecithin	MCT, sunflower oil, soy lecithin	Safflower oil	None	MCT oil	Safflower oil	None
MCT:LCT	40:60	50:50	50:50	50:50	75:25	54:46	70:30	0:100	0	100:0	0:100	0
Volume to meet RDI	1120	1165	1250	1000	750	1750	1500	2000	NA	NA	NA	NA
Sodium (mEq/L)	59	52	60	51	56	52	22	26	0.02/mL	0	0	1/scoop
Potassium (mEq/L)	47	51	46	48	49	41	32	24	0.03/mL	0	0	2/scoop
Phosphorus (mM/L)	32	32	26	32	43	18	22	16	0.03/mL	0	0	1/scoop
Magnesium (mEq/L)	33	28	26	33	44	19	33	17	0	0	0	0
Vitamin K (μg)	80	80	64	75	100	46	80	40	0	0	0	0
% Free water	83	81	85	78	70	84	85	85	70	0	44	0

	High-protein lactose-free	High-protein high-calorie lactose-free	High-calorie milkshake (lactose)	Renal (lactose-free)	High-protein sugar-free (lactose)	High-calorie (lactose)	Clear liquid supplement	Gelatin (clear liquid)	Pudding (full liquid)
Osmolality (mOsm/kg water)	360	490	300	430–530	720	490	270–380	630	630
Brand name	Boost High Protein	Boost Plus	Mighty Shake	ReNeph	Instant Breakfast	Scandi-shake	NuBasics	Hi-Pro Gelatin	Magic Cup
Manufacturer	Mead Johnson	Mead Johnson	Diamond Crystal	Nutra Balance	Nestle	Scandi-pharm	Nestle	Novartis	Diamond Crystal
Serving size (mL)	240	240	180	120	270	360	163	120	120
Calories/mL	1.0	1.5	1.6	2.1	0.8	1.7	163	1.5	2.3
Protein (g/svg)	15	14	9	8	12	13	6.5	12	8
Carbohydrate (g/svg)	33	45	48	32	24	69	34	33	36
Fiber (g/svg)	0	0	0	0	0	0	0	0	1
Fat (g/svg)	6	14	6	10	8	29	0	0	11
Protein source	Milk protein, casein	Milk protein, casein	Milk protein	Whey	Milk protein	Milk protein casein	Whey isolate	Egg white gelatin	Milk protein
Carbohydrate source	Corn syrup, sucrose	Corn syrup, sucrose	Corn syrup, lactose, sucrose, Maltodex	Maltodex, fructose, corn syrup solids	Maltodextrin, lactose, Aspartame	Maltodextrin, sucrose, lactose, corn syrup solids	High-fructose corn syrup	Sucrose, maltodextrin	Corn syrup
Fiber source	None	None	None	None	None	None	None	None	Guar gum
Fat source	Canola, sunflower, corn oil	Canola, sunflower corn oil	Milk fat	Canola oil	Milk fat	Vegetable, MCT oil, lecithin	None	None	Soybean, cottonseed oil
Volume to meet RDI	946	946	NA	NA	1065	NA	NA	NA	NA
Sodium (mEq/svg)	7.4	7.4	7.4	4	4	8	2.2	4.3	7
Potassium (mEq/svg)	9.7	9.7		0.26	9	17	1.3	2.6	5
Phosphorus (mM/svg)	10	10	10	0.8	17	18	0.7	5	NA
Magnesium (mEq/svg)	8.7	8.7	3	3	11	0	1	0	NA
Vitamin K (µg/svg)	32	32	0	Trace	20	<10	4.7	Trace	NA

LCT, long chain triglyceride; MCT, medium chain triglyceride; NA, not available; RDI, relative dose intensity; TEN, total enteral nutrition; svg, serving.

Note: 2002–2003 Adult Nutrition Enteral Products Formulary, Pennsylvania State University, M. S. Hershey Medical Center, Prepared by the Clinical Nutrition Department and the Parenteral and Enteral Nutrition Subcommittee of the Pharmacy and Therapeutics Committee.

PENNSTATE
Milton S. Hershey Medical Center
College of Medicine

ADULT ENTERAL NUTRITION:
PHYSICIAN ORDER FORM (TUBE FEEDING)

Instructions to physician:

- Complete this form to initiate tube feedings or to change formula type. Changes in rate or strength can be made directly on the physician order form.
- Composition of formulas are listed on the Adult Nutrition Enteral Formulary Card (see nutrition support dietitian for a copy). Formulary also available on the Infoweb at the Clinical Nutrition Department site. Nutrition support algorithms are likewise available on the infonet (Guidelines/Pathway section of Patient Care).

Orders

1. Verify tube placement before use via KUB (complete x-ray form for KUB). Limit 2 KUB's per attempt at placement.

2. Consult nutrition support for assessment.

3. Check as needed:

☐ Aspiration precautions (especially for gastric and duodenal feedings): Residual check every 4 hours. If residual > 150 mL, hold feeding for one hour and resume when residual < 150 mL. Elevate head of bed 30-40 degrees or place in reverse Trendelenberg position.

☐ Flush feeding tube with 15 mL tap water before and after medication administration via feeding tube and before and after residual checks and bolus feedings.

☐ Tap water boluses _________ mL, _________ times per day.

☐ If patient receiving enteral Dilantin, hold tube feeding for one hour before and after each Dilantin dose.

4. Formula (or equivalent formulary substitution)

☐ **Isosource VHN** (1.0 cal/mL, 62 g pro/L, fiber-containing. Typical Use: Standard acute care/severe malnutrition formula in ICU and ward)

☐ **Fibersource HN** (1.2 cal/mL, 54 g pro/L, fiber-containing. Typical Use: Moderate malnutrition/inflammatory stress)

☐ **Nutren 2.0** (2.0 cal/mL, 80 g pro/L, fiber-free. Typical Use: Volume and electrolyte restrictions such as renal or hepatic failure)

☐ **Ultracal** (1.06 cal/mL, 44 g pro/L, fiber-containing. Typical Use: Maintenance feeding or mild malnutrition)

☐ **Nutren 1.5** (1.5 cal/mL, 60 g pro/L, fiber-free. Typical Use: Moderately volume-limited, moderate malnutrition, fiber-free intake needed)

☐ **Peptamen** (1.0 cal/mL, 40 g pro/L, fiber-free, peptide. Typical Use: Moderate malnutrition with impaired digestive function)

☐ **Peptinex DT** (1.0 cal/mL, 50 g pro/L, fiber-free, peptide. Typical Use: Malnutrition/stress with impaired digestive function)

☐ **Vivonex TEN** (1.0 cal/mL, 38 g pro/L, fiber-free, elemental. Typical Use: Maldigestion or when fat-free intake is needed)

☐ 1:1 mix of two formulas selected above (Typical Use: If one product alone does not meet the patient's nutrient profile)

5. Formula Strength (diluted strength generally not recommended or needed)

☐ Full Strength ☐ 3/4 strength ☐ 1/2 strength

6. Additives:

_____ scoops Promod/L feeding (5 g protein/scoop) _____ mL MCT Oil/day (8 calories/mL)

_____ mL Polycose Liquid/day (2 calories/mL) _____ mL Microlipid/day (4.5 calories/mL)

7. Infusion Route and Method:

☐ Naso/orogastric Continuous _______ mL/hour over ________ hours/day

☐ Naso/orojejunal Bolus ________ mL ________ times/day (circle pump or syringe)

☐ Gastrostomy Gravity Drip _______ mL over ______ hours _______ times/day

☐ Jejunostomy

8. Fax order to Nourishment Room (x0076)

Physician Signature Beeper No. Date Time

FIGURE 55.2-1. Adult enteral nutrition physician order form (tube feeding).

chest need to be considered for early tube placement so that enteral nutrition can be used.

USE OF PERIOPERATIVE TOTAL PARENTERAL NUTRITION IN CANCER PATIENTS

One of the best studies to date evaluating the effects of preoperative TPN was published by the Veterans Affairs Total Parenteral Nutrition Cooperative Study Group.[43] Three hundred ninety-five patients, many of whom had cancer, were entered into and completed this prospective randomized trial. The patients were divided into one of four groups: well-nourished, borderline malnourished, moderately malnourished, or severely malnourished. Patients in each malnourished category were randomized to at least 7 days of preoperative TPN or immediate operation. Patients randomized to receive TPN received 1000 kcal/d in excess of calculated caloric requirements. Lipid was provided on a daily basis. One criticism of this study was that patients were allowed to eat in addition to receiving parenteral feedings. Another criticism was that the greater incidence of hyperglycemia in the TPN group might have influenced the results. Analysis of the data from this study indicated that there was no difference in short-term or long-term survival among groups. Infectious complications, including pneumonia, abscess, and

TABLE 55.2-5. Indications for the Use of Total Parenteral Nutrition (TPN) in the Cancer Patient

---

A. TPN for brief, in-hospital periods (7–10 d)
  1. TPN is not indicated:
    a. In well-nourished or mildly malnourished patients undergoing chemotherapy, radiation therapy, or surgery.
    b. In patients with rapidly progressive malignant disease who fail to respond to treatment and in those patients who have evidence of terminal disease and are not candidates for further antitumor therapy.
  2. TPN is indicated:
    a. In severely malnourished patients who are responding to chemotherapy or in those in whom gastrointestinal or other toxicities preclude adequate enteral intake for 7–10 d or a longer period. Available evidence would suggest that patients who are candidates for TPN under these circumstances should, when feasible, receive TPN before or in conjunction with the institution of therapy.
B. Prolonged periods of inhospital TPN or home TPN
  1. TPN is not indicated:
    a. In patients with rapidly progressive tumor growth that is unresponsive to therapy.
  2. TPN is indicated:
    a. In those patients for whom treatment-associated toxicities preclude the use of enteral nutrition and represent the primary impediment to the restoration of performance status. Such patients usually respond to antitumor therapy.
    b. In selected malnourished cancer patients in whom the natural history of the disease can be expected to permit a period of normal or near normal performance status. Such patients should be receiving antitumor therapy with a reasonable anticipation of response, or the natural history of the untreated tumor is such that a reasonable quality of life can be expected (survival longer than 6–12 mo).

---

line sepsis, were statistically significantly higher in borderline or mildly malnourished patients receiving TPN, but not in severely malnourished patients. Noninfectious complications (impaired wound healing) were significantly lower only in those patients receiving TPN who were in the severely malnourished group (greater than 15% weight loss and serum albumin less than 2.8 mg%). This study strongly suggests that preoperative TPN should be limited to the severely malnourished patient and particular attention should be paid to close monitoring of blood glucose. Therefore, contraindications to the use of preoperative TPN should include patients requiring emergency operation and those who are only mildly or moderately malnourished.

In the few patients who are candidates for preoperative nutritional support, the authors recommend instituting TPN only if the gastrointestinal tract cannot be used for tube feedings. In most patients undergoing major abdominal surgery, feeding tubes can be placed intraoperatively if resumption of oral feedings is not anticipated for relatively lengthy periods of time (7 to 10 days) after surgery. TPN may also be required in the well-nourished cancer patient in whom a postoperative complication develops that precludes enteral support. For example, some cancer patients develop a prolonged ileus after an abdominal procedure that precludes the use of the intestinal tract as a route of feeding. Such an occurrence is generally unpredictable, and the cause of the ileus is often not demonstrated. If the patient is unable to eat by postoperative day 7, TPN should be considered. The ileus may persist for several weeks, especially in gastric or pancreatic cancer

patients. Although provision of TPN does not influence the disease process per se, it is beneficial because it prevents further erosion of lean body mass.

Two prospective studies have helped to further clarify the indications and contraindications for the use of TPN in the surgical patient with cancer. Brennan et al.[44] examined the use of routine postoperative TPN after major pancreatic resection. In patients randomized to receive TPN starting on postoperative day 1, the investigators found a statistically significant increase in the incidence of intraabdominal abscesses as well as a tendency toward an increased incidence of peritonitis and bowel obstruction. The control group received a peripheral infusion of dextrose rather than luminal nutrition, suggesting that the increase in complications was not due to the absence of luminal nutrients but rather to some toxic effect of the TPN. The authors concluded that routine use of postoperative TPN was not indicated and may in fact have harmful side effects. It should be noted that many surgeons would elect to place a feeding jejunostomy in such patients.

In contrast to the Brennan study, Fan et al.[45] studied the use of perioperative (starting 7 days before the planned procedure) TPN for patients undergoing hepatectomy for hepatocellular carcinoma. They found that patients randomized to receive perioperative TPN had a statistically significant reduction in infectious complications and a decreased diuretic requirement compared with similar patients who did not receive TPN. The significance of this study is that it is only one of two studies that show a benefit to the use of routine perioperative TPN in patients not experiencing severe malnutrition. In addition, it establishes a distinct group of patients in whom routine perioperative TPN may be of benefit. The mechanism by which TPN is of value in these patients is not known.

PATIENTS WITH SHORT BOWEL SYNDROME

Short bowel syndrome may develop in cancer patients secondary to multiple bowel resections or massive resection of infarcted bowel. Most of these individuals, if cured of their cancer, can now survive for long periods on home TPN. Due to the duration of therapy involved, these patients are at risk for development of long-term problems, such as micronutrient deficiency, bone demineralization, or line sepsis. Studies by Wilmore et al.[46] have demonstrated that the requirement for TPN could be decreased or even eliminated in patients with short gut syndrome by providing a nutritional regimen consisting of supplemental glutamine, growth hormone, and a modified oral high-carbohydrate, low-fat diet. A marked improvement was seen in the absorption of nutrients with this combination therapy and a decrease in stool output. In addition, TPN requirements were reduced by 50%, as were the costs associated with care of these individuals. Discontinuation of the growth hormone did not increase TPN needs in these patients once they had undergone successful gut rehabilitation.

COMPOSITION OF TOTAL PARENTERAL NUTRITION FORMULATIONS

TPN solutions are administered through a central venous catheter that is generally inserted into the subclavian vein. TPN solutions are hyperosmolar and calorie dense (1 kcal/mL or greater). The addition of minerals, vitamins, and electrolytes completes the basic composition of the solution. Solutions must be prepared under sterile conditions. Because of the hyperosmolarity of such solutions, they must be delivered into a high-flow system to prevent venous sclerosis. In the past, as a general rule, 65% of total nonprotein calories were provided as dextrose and 35% in the form of an intravenous fat emulsion. However, we should rethink this in light of the more recent data about n-6 fatty acids and inflammation. A lipid formulation of n-3 fatty acids would be more beneficial; however, one is not available in the United States. Patients receiving TPN should be monitored regularly by measuring blood sugar, serum electrolytes, triglycerides, and liver function test results. The amounts of the various electrolytes provided to cancer patients receiving TPN may vary depending on factors such as previous nutritional and hydration status. Careful monitoring is critical because severe hypokalemia or hypophosphatemia can develop with aggressive feedings. Hypophosphatemia may develop in the chronically malnourished cachectic cancer patient given dextrose infusion who uses phosphate to make adenosine triphosphate. This is referred to as the *refeeding syndrome* and was originally seen in starved refugees suddenly given a high caloric diet. These electrolyte disturbances can develop rapidly and are much more life threatening than hyponatremia. Critical drops in serum phosphate levels below 1.5 mmol/dL can lead to an irreversible cardiac arrest.

POTENTIAL COMPLICATIONS OF TOTAL PARENTERAL NUTRITION

Advances in technology, monitoring, and catheter care have greatly reduced the incidence of complications associated with the use of TPN. The establishment of a nutritional support team (physician, dietitian, nurse, and pharmacist) and the recognition of such a team as an important part of overall patient care have also been key factors in reducing complications. Complications of TPN that occur in cancer patients can be divided into four types: (1) mechanical (pneumothorax, laceration of the subclavian artery, air embolism, catheter embolism), (2) metabolic (hyperglycemia, electrolyte abnormalities, abnormalities in liver enzymes), (3) infectious (catheter sepsis), and (4) thrombotic (catheter occlusion, superior vena caval thrombosis). Catheter sepsis is a frequent cause of febrile neutropenia and must be excluded as a cause in these patients.

EFFECTS OF TOTAL PARENTERAL NUTRITION ON THE GASTROINTESTINAL TRACT

Although the intestinal tract had long been considered an organ of inactivity in critically ill patients, this concept has clearly been shown to be invalid. Disuse of the gastrointestinal tract, either via starvation or nutritional support by TPN, may lead to numerous physiologic derangements as well as changes in gut microflora, impaired gut immune function, and disruption of the integrity of the mucosal barrier. Thus, maintaining gut function in the cancer patient who is receiving vigorous therapy may be essential to minimize septic complications and organ failure.

The majority of studies that have examined the effects of TPN on intestinal function and immunity have been done in animals. These studies clearly demonstrate that TPN is detrimental and related to intestinal disuse. In rats receiving TPN, villous atrophy develops and there appears to be a breakdown in the gut mucosal barrier. TPN results in significant disruption

of the intestinal microflora and bacterial translocation from the gut lumen to the mesenteric lymph nodes. In addition, when insults such as chemotherapy or radiation are introduced into these models, animals on TPN have a much higher mortality. This body of literature suggests that under certain circumstances, TPN may predispose patients to an increase in gut-derived infectious complications. Whether these are related to bacterial translocation or just absorption of endotoxins or cytokines is still debated. TPN supplemented with glutamine may play a role in preventing the morphologic changes in the gut and lead to reduced infection rate.

IMPROVING THE EFFICACY OF CURRENT FEEDING REGIMENS

ROLE OF AMBULATION

Patients with cancer may be bedridden but should be encouraged to ambulate or exercise as much as is feasible. Exercise can increase functional aerobic capacity, stimulate skeletal muscle amino acid uptake, and reduce proteolysis in normal individuals even if receiving TPN. It is unclear whether higher exercise thresholds are necessary to induce anabolism in nutritionally depleted cancer patients, although a higher threshold does seem to reduce fatigue.

PHARMACOLOGIC AND HORMONAL THERAPY

Insulin, the primary anabolic hormone in the body, may have potential beneficial effects because of its role in stimulating muscle amino acid uptake and protein synthesis. Studies indicate that treatment with insulin stimulates food intake and nitrogen retention without stimulating tumor growth. Likewise, administration of insulin in combination with antineoplastic drugs to tumor-bearing rats on TPN preserved lean body mass and retarded tumor growth. Whether these observations can be extrapolated to the clinical arena is unknown.

The availability of recombinant human growth hormone has led investigators to examine its role as an anabolic agent in patients. The present data indicate that growth hormone is capable of promoting accrual of lean body mass in healthy individuals. It is unclear whether this anabolism will be observed in cachectic cancer patients. A potential downside to the use of growth hormone in patients is its association with the development of lymphoid malignancies. In tumor-bearing rats, treatment with exogenous growth hormone has been shown to increase carcass weight and improve the host immune response. Additional studies that examine the effects of growth hormone on tumor growth parameters are necessary before clinical use of this drug is justifiable.

Additional research using the progestogens, megestrol acetate and medroxyprogesterone acetate, as well as melatonin, is needed to assess the value of their use in treating or preventing cancer cachexia. Current recommendations for megestrol acetate are 480 mg/d in addition to nutritional support.

USE OF GLUTAMINE AND ARGININE

The classification of glutamine as a nonessential or nutritionally dispensable amino acid implies that, in its absence from the diet, it can be synthesized in adequate quantities from other amino acids and precursors. For this reason, and because of the relative instability and short shelf life of parenteral glutamine compared with other amino acids, it has not been considered necessary to include glutamine in nutritional formulas. Glutamine is present in oral and enteral diets only at the relatively low levels characteristic of its concentration in most dietary proteins. Based on our knowledge of the changes in glutamine metabolism that are characteristic of the host with cancer, this categorization of glutamine as an NAA may be misleading. Several studies in the tumor-bearing host suggest that supplemental glutamine may benefit the cancer patient. One of the best studies to date evaluating the effects of glutamine-enriched TPN in cancer patients is a randomized, double-blind, controlled trial in adults receiving allogeneic bone marrow transplants for hematologic malignancies.[47] Patients received a standard, glutamine-free TPN solution or an experimental isonitrogenous, isocaloric solution supplemented with L-glutamine (0.57 g/kg body weight per day). Patients received the diets for approximately 4 weeks after transplantation. Individuals receiving glutamine-supplemented parenteral nutrition after bone marrow transplant had improved nitrogen balance, a diminished incidence of clinical infections, less fluid accumulation, and a shortened hospital stay. In a more recent study, glutamine-enriched TPN was shown to prevent the increase in gut mucosal permeability that develops with the administration of commercially available glutamine-free TPN. Van der Hulst et al.[48] randomized surgical patients requiring parenteral feedings to either receive standard TPN or glutamine-enriched TPN for 10 to 14 days. Duodenal mucosal biopsies and gut permeability studies were performed at the start and completion of TPN. The investigators found no change in either villous height or gut permeability in the group receiving glutamine-enriched TPN, whereas the control group showed loss of villous height and increased gut permeability. This study provides strong evidence in favor of a gut-protective effect of glutamine. Similarly, arginine, because of its immunomodulatory properties, may be useful as a dietary supplement in cancer patients, but further work is necessary to more clearly define the potential role of these two amino acids in the nutritional care of the cancer patient.

TECHNIQUES OF PROVIDING NUTRITIONAL SUPPORT

TRANSNASAL (NASOGASTRIC AND NASODUODENAL) FEEDING CATHETERS

The use of transnasal feeding catheters for intragastric feeding or for duodenal intubation is a popular adjunct for providing nutritional support by the enteral route. The stomach is easily accessed by the passage of a soft flexible [8-French (Fr.)] feeding tube. Intragastric feedings provide several advantages for the patient. The stomach has the capacity and reservoir for bolus feedings that more closely mimic human meal patterns. Feeding into the stomach results in the stimulation of biliary-pancreatic axis, which is probably trophic for the small bowel, and gastric secretions have a dilutional effect on the osmolarity of the feedings, reducing the risk of diarrhea. The major risk of intragastric feeding is the regurgitation of gastric contents,

resulting in aspiration into the tracheobronchial tree. This risk is highest in patients who have an altered mental sensorium or who are paralyzed.

The placement of the feeding tube through the pylorus into the fourth portion of the duodenum reduces the risk of regurgitation and aspiration of feeding formulas. To place a transnasal intraduodenal feeding catheter, the patient should be in the sitting position with the neck slightly flexed. This allows for the passage of a lubricated 8-Fr. polyurethane feeding catheter (with a stylet in place) through the patient's nose in a posterior and inferior direction, bringing the catheter to the level of the pharynx. The head is brought back to a neutral position, and the patient is instructed to swallow while the feeding catheter is simultaneously passed down into the esophageal lumen. The advancement of the catheter is continued for a distance of approximately 45 to 50 cm. Once the catheter is confirmed to be in the stomach by injecting air while listening over the epigastrium, the patient is laid on the right side and the tube is advanced another 15 to 20 cm. This should position the tube into the duodenum and can be confirmed by listening over the right upper quadrant while advancing the tube. A newer tube-positioning system is also available using a magnet to drag the tube to and around the duodenum. The stylet is removed, and the position of the catheter is confirmed radiographically before the initiation of feedings. Tubes can be positioned fluoroscopically if necessary.

Gastric feedings are initiated by a bolus test volume of saline, representing the hourly feeding volume infused over 1 hour, into the stomach. The tube is clamped for 30 minutes and then checked for residual volume. If less than 50% of the volume load returns, the selected volume is appropriate. In general, duodenal feedings can be started at 30 to 50 mL/hr at full-strength concentration unless the patient has been at bowel rest for several days, in which case the feed may need to be slowed or diluted to avoid bloating or diarrhea. In such patients, the authors generally increase the rate of infusion before increasing the concentration. Despite these precautions, some degree of diarrhea develops in approximately 10% to 20% of patients receiving enteral feedings secondary to malabsorption and the osmotic load of the feedings. When this occurs, the rate of feeding should be decreased by 50% rather than stopping the feedings altogether. The rate of feedings is then increased as tolerated over the next 3 to 4 days.

GASTROSTOMY TUBE FEEDINGS

A feeding gastrostomy should be considered in patients who require long-term enteral nutrition and in those with unresectable carcinomas of the head and neck or esophagus. In patients with an unresectable esophageal carcinoma who are not surgical candidates or in individuals who are unable to maintain caloric needs, a permanent gastrostomy should be considered. A temporary Stamm gastrostomy is a popular method for access to the gastric lumen that can be performed at the time of any major abdominal procedure. The surgical technique is relatively simple and straightforward.[49] After placement, the gastrostomy tube is placed to gravity drainage for 24 hours and then feeds are started. If the patient tolerates them, the authors advance enteral feedings, as described earlier in Transnasal (Nasogastric and Nasoduodenal) Feeding Catheters.

Percutaneous endoscopic gastrostomy (PEG) to provide access for gastric feedings can be performed without a laparotomy or general anesthesia. This technique involves the safe passage of an endoscope into the stomach. The stomach is then dilated by the insufflation of air via the endoscope. Transabdominal illumination with the endoscopic light source selects an area on the anterior abdominal wall, usually halfway between the costal margin and the umbilicus. Local anesthesia is injected over the site followed by the insertion of an Angiocath percutaneously into the stomach. A wire is passed through the Angiocath, grabbed by a snare that has been passed through the endoscope, and pulled back with the endoscope out of the mouth. A standard percutaneous gastrostomy tube with a wire loop is attached to the guidewire and pulled back down the esophagus and out through the abdominal wall. Extending the snare down the lumen of PEG tube allows the endoscope to be passed back with the tube as the PEG is pulled under direct visualization into the stomach to confirm placement. The PEG is pulled taut with the stomach to the abdominal wall and then sutured. Inability to pass the endoscope safely or to identify the transabdominal illumination of the endoscope tip within the dilated stomach is a contraindication to the procedure. Ascites, coagulopathies, and intraabdominal infections are relative contraindications as well.

FEEDING CATHETER JEJUNOSTOMY PLACEMENT AND WITZEL JEJUNOSTOMY

A feeding catheter jejunostomy should be placed after any major upper abdominal oncologic procedure if prolonged enteral nutrition support is anticipated, especially after gastric or pancreatic cancer surgery. The simplest method is a needle catheter jejunostomy, which can be performed fairly quickly at the end of the definitive operation. The entire length of a 14-gauge needle is used to create a subserosal tunnel approximately 30 to 40 cm distal to the ligament of Treitz, and then the needle tip is introduced into the jejunal lumen. A 16-gauge feeding catheter is inserted through the needle and advanced 30 to 40 cm distally into the bowel lumen, and the needle is withdrawn. The catheter is secured to the jejunal wall with sutures, and then a 2-cm length of the wall of the loop of jejunum is anchored to the parietal peritoneum. The catheter is then secured to the skin with nylon sutures. The needle catheter jejunostomy is generally removed 2 to 4 weeks postoperatively when no longer needed.

A more permanent form of feeding jejunostomy uses a 14-Fr. red rubber catheter for feeding. The placement technique is construction of a simple Witzel tunnel and takes only 10 to 15 minutes. Jejunal feeding catheters can be used immediately for feeding purposes after the operation. Catheter care is essential to maintain patency, and the nursing staff needs to flush the catheter with saline every 8 hours to ensure adequate patency. The catheter can be removed at the patient's bedside at the desired time by simple traction, and the resulting fistula should close quickly. Gastrostomies and jejunostomies can now be done by laparoscopic techniques using anchors inserted across the abdominal wall to secure the wall of the stomach or jejunum to the parietal peritoneum.

CENTRAL VENOUS TOTAL PARENTERAL NUTRITION

The preferred method of access to the superior vena cava is by percutaneous cannulation of the subclavian vein. Alternate sites include the internal and external jugular vein, but with the catheter exiting in the neck region this makes it more difficult to secure and maintain a sterile dressing site. Thus, long-term indwelling catheters should be down over the chest wall because of the increased risk of catheter infections. Percutaneous catheters and subcutaneous "ports" can be placed over the pectoral area of the chest for ease of access and repeated use.

An individual who is experienced in the placement of a central venous catheter should perform the technique. To reduce the risk of hemorrhagic complications, patients with a platelet count below 50,000/mL should receive fresh platelets before catheter insertion. The procedure is performed using aseptic technique; the surgeon should wear a hat, mask, gown, and gloves. The patient is placed in Trendelenburg's position with both arms at the sides and the head turned away from the site of insertion. The chest is shaved, prepped, and draped in a sterile fashion. Local anesthesia is infiltrated near the insertion site at the junction of the middle and medial thirds of the clavicle as well as the underlying tissues along the inferior border of the clavicle. A standard subclavian insertion tray is used for catheter insertion via the Seldinger technique. The tip of the needle is inserted into the skin and subcutaneous tissues at the midpoint of the clavicle, aiming for the suprasternal notch. The needle is directed parallel to the patient's bed, inserting beneath the clavicle, with negative pressure applied at all times to the syringe. The prompt inflow of blood into the syringe indicates entrance into the subclavian vein, and the needle is advanced a few millimeters to ensure that the bevel is within the lumen of the vessel. The patient is instructed to perform a gentle Valsalva maneuver to prevent an air embolism, the syringe is disconnected from the needle, the guidewire is passed through the needle lumen, and the needle is then withdrawn over the guidewire. The passage of the wire through the needle should be met with minimal resistance, and the needle should be removed only after 15 cm of the wire has been passed into the vessel. A small incision is made at the guidewire exit site, and a dilator is passed over the wire. The dilator is then removed and is replaced by the catheter that is advanced to 20 cm. The wire is withdrawn, and the catheter is flushed with sterile saline. The catheter is then sutured into position, the insertion site is cleaned, and a sterile dressing is placed. A portable chest radiograph is taken to confirm placement of the catheter. Chest films are inspected for location of the catheter tip and to search for evidence of pneumothorax or hemothorax.

Now with peripherally inserted central catheters, central TPN can be administered even if the subclavian or jugular veins are unavailable for use. Peripherally inserted central catheter lines are usually inserted through an antecubital location and threaded into the central veins. The technical problems of placement are much less, but long-term use may be complicated by decreased mobility of the arm, thrombosis, or infection.

Complications from long-term central venous catheterization in the cancer patient population include venous thrombosis and catheter-related infections. Thrombosis of the central vessels is a complication that may often be overlooked. The clinical suspicion of subclavian vein thrombosis is only approximately 3%, whereas studies that use phlebography or radionuclide venography indicate that the incidence is as high as 35%. With increased use of the internal jugular veins for long-term indwelling catheters and ports, more patients are presenting with the signs of a superior vena caval syndrome (swelling in the head, neck, and arms). Low-dose warfarin (Coumadin) may help prevent thrombosis.

Febrile episodes are not uncommon in the cancer patient population, particularly in the neutropenic individual. Blood culture may or may not show a pathogen, but if primary catheter sepsis is confirmed, the catheter must be removed immediately. The tip of the catheter is sent to the laboratory for culture and compared with the blood cultures drawn from the patient. Appropriate antibiotics are administered, and a new catheter is inserted when the patient's repeat blood culture results are negative. If the patient has an indwelling port or long-term percutaneous catheter, an attempt to clear the catheter with antibiotics can be made, although results are variable.

CONCLUSION

Multiple causes may be responsible for anorexia and weight loss in the cancer patient. Changes in taste, swallowing, digestion, and absorption may all affect the way a patient desires or appreciates food. These changes most often come from the cancer treatment, not the tumor itself. However, the tumor or the body's response to the tumor produces changes in metabolism that bring about the cachexia syndrome.

Every patient with advanced cancer needs nutritional support, whether it is in the form of nutrition counseling for better dietary choices or supplemental nutrients. Some cancer patients need to be provided complete nutrition to overcome complications in their treatment. Much research is now focused on the effect of specific nutrients to address metabolic alterations that can make the cancer patient resistant to the usual effects of feeding. This research has the capacity to completely change the way in which nutrition is provided to the cancer patient. The practitioner must remember that the goal of nutrition support for cancer patients is to increase functionality and improve quality of life.

REFERENCES

1. Henkin RI. Drug-induced taste and smell disorders. *Drug Saf* 1994;11:318.
2. Kettaneh A, Fain O, Stirnemann J, Thomas M. Taste disorders. *Rev Med Interne* 2002;23:622.
3. Maina G, Vitalucci A, Gandolfo S, Bogetto F. Comparative efficacy of SSRI's and amisulpride in burning mouth syndrome: a single-blind study. *J Clin Psychiatry* 2002;63:38.
4. Heyneman CA. Zinc deficiency and taste disorders. *Ann Pharmacother* 1996;30:186.
5. Yukawa M, Naka H, Murata Y, et al. Folic acid responsive neurological diseases in Japan. *J Nutr Sci Vitaminol* 2001;47:181.
6. Femiano F, Scully C, Gombos F. Idiopathic dysgeusia; an open trial of alpha lipoic acid therapy. *Int J Oral Maxillofac Surg* 2002;31:625.
7. Osaki T, Ohshima M, Tomita Y, et al. Clinical and physiological investigations in patients with taste abnormality. *J Oral Pathol Med* 1996;25:38.
8. Blackburn GL, Bistrian BR, Maini BS, et al. Nutritional and metabolic assessment of the hospitalized patient. *JPEN* 1977;1:11.
9. MacDonald N, Easson AM, Mazurak V, et al. Understanding and managing cancer cachexia. *JACS* 2003;197:144.
10. Barber MD. The pathophysiology and treatment of cancer cachexia. *Nutr Clin Pract* 2002;17:203.
11. Tisdale MJ. Biology of cachexia. *J Natl Cancer Inst* 1997;89:1763.
12. Argiles JM, Lopez-Soriano FJ. The role of cytokines in cancer cachexia. *Med Res Rev* 1999;19:223.
13. Todorov P, Cariuk P, McDevitt T, et al. Characterization of a cancer cachectic factor. *Nature* 1996;379:739.
14. Lorite MJ, Smith HJ, Arnold JA, et al. Activation of ATP-ubiquitin-dependent proteolysis in skeletal muscle in vivo and murine myoblasts in vitro by a proteolysis-inducing factor. *Br J Cancer* 2001;85:297.
15. Cabal-Manzano R, Bhargava P, Torres-Duarte A, et al. Proteolysis-inducing factor is expressed in tumours of patients with gastrointestinal cancers and correlates with weight loss. *Br J Cancer* 2001;84:1599.
16. Glickman MH, Ciechanover A. The ubiquitin-proteasome proteolytic pathway: destruction for the sake of construction. *Physiol Rev* 2002;82:373.
17. Ross JA, Fearon KC. Eicosanoid-dependent cancer cachexia and wasting. *Curr Opin Clin Nutr Metab Care* 2002;5:241.
18. Hussey HJ, Tisdale MJ. Effect of a cachectic factor on carbohydrate metabolism and attenuation by eicosapentaenoic acid. *Br J Cancer* 1999;80:1231.
19. Jho D, Babcock TA, Helton WS, et al. Omega-3 fatty acids: implications for the treatment of tumor-associated inflammation. *Am Surg* 2003;69:32.
20. Hardman WE. Omega-3 fatty acids to augment cancer therapy. *J Nutr* 2002;132:3508S.
21. Jho DH, Babcock TA, Tevar R, et al. Eicosapentaenoic acid supplementation reduces tumor volume and attenuates cachexia in a rat model of progressive non-metastasizing malignancy. *JPEN* 2002;26:291.
22. Sauer LA, Dauchy RT, Blask DE. Mechanism for the antitumor and anticachectic effects of n-3 fatty acids. *Cancer Res* 2000;60:5289.
23. Ovesen L, Allingstrup L, Hannibal J, et al. Effect of dietary counseling on food intake, body weight, response rate, survival, and quality of life in cancer patients undergoing chemotherapy: a prospective randomized study. *J Clin Oncol* 1993;11:2043.
24. Loprinzi CL, Schaid DJ, Dose AM, et al. Body composition changes in patients who gain weight while receiving megestrol acetate. *J Clin Oncol* 1993;11:152.
25. Ferrando AA, Stuart CA, Sheffield-Moore M, et al. Inactivity amplifies the catabolic response of skeletal muscle to cortisol. *J Clin Endocrinol Metab* 1999;84:3515.
26. Barber MD, McMillan DC, Preston T, et al. The metabolic response to feeding in weight-losing pancreatic cancer patients and its modulation by a fish oil–enriched nutritional supplement. *Clin Sci* 2000;98:389.
27. Fearon KCH, von Meyenfeldt M, Moses AGW, et al. An energy and protein dense, high n-3 fatty acid oral supplement promotes weight gain in cancer cachexia. *Eur J Cancer* 2001;37[Suppl 6]:s27.
28. Capra S, Bauer J, Davidson W, et al. Nutritional therapy for cancer-induced weight loss. *Nutr Clin Pract* 2002;17:210.
29. Tipton KD, Ferrando AA, Phillips SM, et al. Post-exercise net protein synthesis in human muscle from orally administered amino acids. *Am J Physiol* 1999;276:E628.
30. Layman DK. The role of leucine in weight loss diets and glucose homeostasis. *J Nutr* 2003;133:261S.
31. Anthony JC, Anthony TG, Kimball SR, et al. Orally administered leucine stimulates protein synthesis in skeletal muscle of postabsorptive rats in association with eIF4F production. *J Nutr* 2000;130:139.
32. Cangiano C, Laviano A, Meguid MM, et al. Effects of administration of oral branched-chain amino acids on anorexia and caloric intake in cancer patients. *J Natl Cancer Inst* 1996;88:550.
33. Liepa GU, Alford B, Van Beber AD. Arginine: the neglected amino acid. *Inform* 1994;111:1276.
34. Van Bokhorst-DeVander Schueren MA, Quak JJ, VonBlomberg-VanderFlier BM, et al. Effect of perioperative nutrition, with and without arginine supplementation, on nutritional status, immune function, postoperative morbidity, and survival in severely malnourished head and neck cancer patients. *Am J Clin Nutr* 2001;73:323.
35. Souba WW. Glutamine and cancer. *Ann Surg* 1993;218:715.
36. May PE, Barber A, D'Olimpio JT, et al. Reversal of cancer-related wasting using oral supplementation with a combination of beta-hydroxy-beta-methylbutyrate, arginine, and glutamine. *Am J Surg* 2002;183:471.
37. Izquierdo M, Ibanez J, Gonzalez-Badillo JJ, et al. Effects of creatine supplementation on muscle power, endurance, and sprint performance. *Med Sci Sports Exerc* 2002;34:332.
38. Von Roenn J, Tchekmedyian S, Ottery FD. Oxandrolone increases weight, lean tissue, performance status and quality of life scores in cancer related weight loss. *Support Care Cancer Abstract* 2002.
39. Jin D, Phillips M, Byles JE. Effects of parenteral nutrition support and chemotherapy on the phasic composition of tumor cells in gastrointestinal cancer. *JPEN* 1999;23:237.
40. McMahon C, Decker G, Ottery FD. Integrating proactive nutritional assessment in clinical practices to prevent complications and cost. *Semin Oncol* 1998;25[2 Suppl 6]:20.
41. Klein S, Kinney J, Jeejeebhoy K, et al. Nutritional support in clinical practice: review of the published data and recommendation for future research directions. *JPEN* 1997;21:133.
42. Braga M, Gianotti L, Nespoli L, et al. Nutritional approach in malnourished surgical patients. *Arch Surg* 2002;137:174.
43. Buzby GP. The Veterans Affairs Total Parenteral Nutrition Cooperative Study Group. Perioperative total parenteral nutrition in surgical patients. *N Engl J Med* 1991;325:525.
44. Brennan MF, Pisters PWT, Posner M, et al. A prospective randomized trial of total parenteral nutrition after major pancreatic resection for malignancy. *Ann Surg* 1994;220:436.
45. Fan ST, Lo CM, Lai ECS, et al. Perioperative nutritional support in patients undergoing hepatectomy for hepatocellular carcinoma. *N Engl J Med* 1994;331:1547.
46. Wilmore DW, Byrne TA, Young LS, et al. A new treatment for patients with the short bowel syndrome: growth hormone, glutamine, and a modified diet. *Ann Surg* 1995;222:243.
47. Ziegler TR, Young LS, Benfell K, et al. Glutamine-supplemented parenteral nutrition improves nitrogen retention and reduces hospital mortality versus standard parenteral nutrition following bone marrow transplantation: a randomized, double-blind trial. *Ann Intern Med* 1992;116:821.
48. van der Hulst RRWJ, van Kreel BK, von Meyenfeldt MF, et al. Glutamine and the preservation of gut integrity. *Lancet* 1993;341:1363.
49. Hautamaki RD, Souba WW. Principles and techniques of nutritional support in the cancer patient. In: Karakousis CP, Copeland EM, Bland KI, eds. *Atlas of surgical oncology*. Philadelphia: WB Saunders,1995:740.

PATRICIA A. GANZ
MARK S. LITWIN
BETH E. MEYEROWITZ

SECTION 3

Sexual Problems

To understand the impact of a cancer diagnosis and its treatment on sexual health and functioning, it is useful to have some knowledge about what is "normal," as well as the range of sexual problems that occur in the general population not affected by cancer. Table 55.3-1 describes a broad range of factors that influence sexual functioning before a cancer diagnosis (e.g., age, gender, anxiety, chronic disease) and after a cancer diagnosis. Other naturally occurring age-related events often coincide with cancer (e.g., erectile dysfunction and menopause). Cancer treatments, however, cause unique side effects not usually experienced in other patient populations (e.g., body image changes, infertility, fatigue, and pain). Sexual problems can also be exacerbated by the uncertain prognosis associated with a cancer diagnosis. In this chapter, some background about normal sexual health and functioning is provided to give a context for the changes associated with a cancer diagnosis. General changes in sexuality associated with cancer as well as treatment and site-specific changes are then discussed.

SEXUAL HEALTH AND PHYSIOLOGY

HUMAN SEXUAL RESPONSE CYCLE

The human sexual response cycle, as detailed by Masters and Johnson,[1] involves the physiologic changes that occur when individuals receive adequate sexual stimulation. The human sexual response cycle consists of four, somewhat arbitrary, phases—excitement, plateau, orgasm, and resolution. Although Masters and Johnson's research advanced the knowledge of the psychophysiology of human sexual response, the four-phase model of the human sexual response cycle has been criticized on both conceptual and methodologic grounds.[2,3] In a triphasic model of human sexuality, Kaplan[4] addressed two of the primary concerns—the characterization of the phases of sexual responding as sequential and interdependent and the inattention to motivational aspects of sexuality. The triphasic model is characterized by separate desire, excitement, and orgasm phases. Kaplan proposed that these are discrete phases controlled by distinct neurophysiologic mechanisms. Thus, she suggested that different etiologic factors and treatment approaches should be considered, depending on the phase in which difficulties occur.[5]

SEXUAL DYSFUNCTIONS AND PROBLEMS

The official nomenclature for diagnosing sexual dysfunctions[6] uses the triphasic model of sexuality—involving disturbances in desire, excitement, or orgasm or by pain associated with sexual intercourse. For patients to be diagnosed with a sexual dysfunction, their disturbance or pain must cause marked

TABLE 55.3-1. Factors Affecting Sexual Functioning before and after a Cancer Diagnosis

Before Cancer	After Cancer
DEMOGRAPHIC FACTORS	Unchanged
Age	
Gender	
Ethnicity	
PSYCHOLOGICAL STATUS	Unchanged, better, or worse; new
Anxiety disorders	fear of recurrence, increased
Depressive disorders	sense of vulnerability
CHRONIC HEALTH PROBLEMS	Unchanged or worse
Diabetes	
Hypertension	
Cardiovascular disease	
Arthritis	
PARTNERSHIP FACTORS	Better, worse, or unchanged
Availability of a partner	
Quality of the relationship	
Partner's health and physical	
problems	
BODY IMAGE	Likely to change, probably worse
Sexual attractiveness	
Self-esteem	
GENDER-SPECIFIC FACTORS	
Menopause-related changes	Likely to change, probably worse,
(women)	especially if estrogen is prohib-
Vaginal dryness	ited; premature menopause
Decreased sexual interest	
Erectile dysfunction (men)	Unchanged or worse, especially if
Age-related	pelvic surgery or androgen-
Psychogenic	ablative therapy performed
Neurovascular changes	
CANCER-SPECIFIC FACTORS	Cancer-related symptoms: pain,
Occasionally may precede diag-	fatigue, nausea; treatment toxici-
nosis	ties; infertility; severity and degree
	of influence related to stage of
	disease and treatment goals

distress or interpersonal difficulties, must be persistent or recurrent, and cannot be due to another psychiatric disorder (e.g., mood or personality disorders). The diagnosis also includes reference to etiologic factors. If only one set of factors is associated with dysfunction (psychological causes, general medical conditions, or substance use), then the diagnosis so indicates. For many cancer patients, sexual dysfunctions are diagnosed as "due to combined factors," indicating a more complex etiology in which multiple causes contribute to the dysfunction.

In addition to diagnosable disorders, many patients experience disruptions that are less intense in nature but that nonetheless cause decreases in previously enjoyable sexual activities and reduce global satisfaction with sexuality. The subjective experience of a satisfying sex life may or may not be associated with the ability to progress through the phases of the human sexual response cycle. Some individuals with no diagnosable dysfunction can be dissatisfied with factors such as the frequency or variety of sexual behavior, whereas some individuals with organically based dysfunctions can enjoy other forms of sexual and intimate contact. Also, as indicated in Table 55.3-1, cancer can have an indirect influence on sexuality through disruptions in partnership factors, body image, and overall psychological well-being.

SEXUAL PROBLEMS AND THEIR PREVALENCE AMONG THE GENERAL POPULATION

PREVALENCE OF SEXUAL DYSFUNCTIONS AND PROBLEMS

Sexual problems are common.[7,8] In a large and extensive national survey of sexuality of 18- to 59-year-olds in the United States, 43% of women and 31% of men reported dysfunction in one of the diagnostic categories during the previous year.[9] Among men, premature ejaculation was the most common complaint (28.5%), followed by anxiety about performance (17.0%), lack of interest in sex (15.8%), and inability to keep an erection (10.4%).[7] Women most frequently reported lack of interest in sex (33.4%), inability to reach orgasm (24.1%), not finding sex pleasurable (21.2%), difficulty becoming lubricated (18.8%), and pain during intercourse (14.4%). Individuals who experienced emotional or stress-related problems or who were victims of adult–child sexual contact were significantly more likely to report sexual dysfunction. Other predictors varied somewhat between men and women, with poor health being particularly salient for men and falling household income and low sexual activity being important for women. Despite these difficulties, most respondents indicated that sex was emotionally satisfying and was associated with very positive feelings.

Although specific prevalence rates vary somewhat in other studies,[10–13] depending on study sample and methodology, the general conclusions are similar. Sexual dysfunction is a common experience, but it need not result in dissatisfaction with sexuality or loss of intimacy. Sexuality after cancer should be viewed within this larger context.

SEXUALITY AND AGING

Normal aging is associated with decreases in both physiologic functioning and behavioral aspects of sexuality. For example, vasocongestion during arousal occurs more slowly, extending the time required for penile erection and vaginal lubrication. More intense and direct tactile stimulation typically is required for arousal and orgasm than is needed in younger men and women. As most men age, erections are less rigid, ejaculation is less forceful, and the refractory period lasts longer. In addition to the anatomic changes associated with menopause, women experience decreased lubrication and, in some cases, reduced intensity of orgasm. Chronic medical conditions and general ill health can exacerbate the natural slowing of sexual response.[14]

Sexual desire and the frequency of sexual thoughts appear to decline with age, particularly for men, although sexual interest does remain present.[2,9,15] Researchers consistently have found that erectile functioning also worsens with age, with increases in dysfunction beginning in middle age and increasing gradually over the rest of the life span.[9,16,17] For women, the prevalence of arousal disorders, as indicated by difficulty lubricating, increases with age.[2,9]

Sexual activity decreases with age for both women and men.[7,16,18] In some cases, this decrease results from the absence of a partner, coupled with an unwillingness to engage in self-pleasuring activities, especially among very old women.[9,18] Even among older married couples, rates of intercourse decrease.[7,16] Nonetheless, many older individuals consider sex an important part of their lives and have satisfying sex lives.[7] Age alone is not an adequate explanation for serious sexual dysfunction or inactivity among interested older adults.

MENOPAUSE AND SEXUAL FUNCTIONING

Menopause occurs when a previously menstruating woman with an intact uterus and ovaries has had amenorrhea for at least 12 months. The average age of menopause in North American women is 51 years.[19] Endocrine disorders or conditions can lead to secondary amenorrhea. Cancer treatment-induced secondary amenorrhea is the most relevant consideration in this chapter. The menopausal transition is characterized by decreased responsiveness of the ovaries to luteinizing hormone and follicle-stimulating hormone. Gradually, over time, the estradiol levels fall as the ovarian follicles are depleted and there is no further response to luteinizing hormone and follicle-stimulating hormone. Clinical symptoms of estrogen deficiency begin to occur with these changes. Lowered levels of estradiol affect various target tissues, including the vagina, skin, bone, vascular endothelium, and smooth muscle, as well as the hypothalamic temperature-regulating centers.[20] The ovaries are the primary source of androgens in women, persisting into postmenopause, and decreased production of ovarian androgens may account for changes in libido during this time.[21] Symptoms associated with estrogen deficiency include vasomotor symptoms (hot flashes, sweats, palpitations), urinary incontinence, and vaginal dryness. Vasomotor symptoms are most frequent (up to 75% of menopausal women) and are among the earliest symptoms of menopause, with the more gradual onset of urinary incontinence and vaginal dryness in the later postmenopausal years.[20]

The impact of menopause on sexual health is controversial because many women remain sexually active into old age. Several population-based studies of perimenopausal and menopausal women have documented that most women who have partners are sexually active[22]; however, changes can occur in sexual functioning (desire, arousal, orgasm) that are age-related[18,20,23] and to which menopause may contribute. Research suggests that in postmenopausal women, a variety of factors are potential moderators of the components of sexual functioning (e.g., psychological distress, quality of the partner relationship, physical activity, body mass index).[22] Without sufficient levels of endogenous estrogen, the vaginal epithelium becomes atrophic, leading to clinical symptoms of vaginal dryness and dyspareunia. With chronic or untreated symptoms of vaginal dryness, postmenopausal women often choose to avoid sexual intercourse completely. Hormone replacement therapy is effective in managing menopausal symptoms, such as hot flashes and vaginal dryness, but does not appear to improve sexual functioning.[24,25] Untreated vaginal dryness can contribute to dyspareunia, thus affecting both desire and arousal in women with cancer (discussed later in Chemotherapy). If one adds to this the variety of physical, psychosocial, and treatment-related factors associated with cancer treatment, a menopausal woman may certainly experience sexual dysfunction. Nevertheless, the menopause per se may not be the culprit.

ERECTILE DYSFUNCTION IN HEALTHY AGING MEN

As healthy men age, androgen levels begin to decline.[26,27] Although these changes do not occur as precipitously as in menopause, a steady, age-related diminution is noted in most men. This can result in declining libido, which in turn tends to decreased erectile function; however, it is not uncommon for men to remain libidinous and potent well into advanced years. Peripheral circulatory problems and degenerative neuromuscular conditions also become more common, both increasing the incidence of vasculogenic and neurogenic erectile dysfunction (see Table 55.3-1).[28]

IMPACT OF CANCER AND ITS TREATMENT ON SEXUAL HEALTH

PSYCHOLOGICAL DISTRESS

Symptoms of anxiety or depression are common among cancer patients.[29-32] Patients with higher levels of psychological distress experience more sexual dysfunction.[29-34] For example, in a study of 227 newly diagnosed breast cancer patients, women who were identified as being "at-risk" for psychosocial distress had more sexual difficulties than a comparison "low-risk" group, both at 1 month after surgery and 1 year later.[29] Sexual problems that were increased in frequency were lack of interest in having sex, difficulty with arousal, and difficulty reaching orgasm.[29] In a comprehensive follow-up study of Hodgkin's disease and acute leukemia survivors, higher levels of distress were found in the Hodgkin's disease survivors, which was associated with significantly poorer sexual functioning than in the acute leukemia survivors.[32] In patients with early-stage cervical cancer, psychological as well as physical problems were highly correlated with sexual outcome.[34] Thus, psychological distress, is an important variable that influences sexual outcomes, both acutely and chronically, in cancer patients.

BODY IMAGE CHANGES

The body changes associated with cancer and its treatment are often dramatic, ranging from surgical defects and deformities (e.g., limb amputation, loss of a breast, radical neck dissection) to total body alopecia from chemotherapy (e.g., loss of scalp hair, eyebrows, eyelashes, pubic and axillary hair) to more subtle changes (e.g., weight loss secondary to disease or treatment, weight gain from corticosteroids). All of these alterations can influence the patient's sense of sexual attractiveness and self-esteem.[35]

For women with breast cancer, the major advantage of breast-conserving surgery is the preservation of body image.[36-38] Patients with head and neck cancer often experience a range of physical and psychosocial problems related to disfiguring surgery, with consequent effects on sexual functioning.[39] Patients with colorectal cancer and stomas experience more body image problems than nonstoma patients and have poorer sexual functioning.[40] Thus, contemporary organ preservation treatments or those that provide immediate reconstructive surgery may spare cancer patients the added burden of poorer body image. In one study, more favorable body image was a significant predictor of sexual interest in breast cancer survivors.[41] Nevertheless, the complexity of contemporary combined modality treatment (surgery, radiation therapy, and chemotherapy) aimed at organ preservation may also contribute to poorer body image through weight loss and hair loss, which

may have a temporary or long-term adverse effect on body image.[32,42,43] For some patients, weight gain is an important consequence of treatment that can interfere with body image. This effect has been particularly noted for women receiving adjuvant chemotherapy for breast cancer.[44]

DETERIORATING PHYSICAL FUNCTION, FATIGUE, AND PAIN

Declining physical functioning and the symptoms of fatigue and pain negatively influence sexual functioning. In a cross-sectional evaluation of 779 patients with colorectal, lung, and prostate cancers at all phases of disease, sexual functioning was poorest for patients with advanced metastatic disease, who concomitantly experienced more frequent and severe physical problems associated with the cancer.[45] This finding was most significant for the patients with colorectal and lung cancer, whereas sexual problems were important for prostate cancer patients independent of stage and physical symptoms.[45]

Fatigue is an important symptomatic problem for cancer patients and survivors.[46,47] Although this may be the result of clinical problems, such as anemia, which can be managed medically with transfusions or growth factors, chronic fatigue after cancer treatment may be multifactorial and represent late effects of chemotherapy and radiation, as well as be manifestations of both pain and depression.[48] Fatigue has been most dramatically noted in patients treated for Hodgkin's disease,[43,47,49] in which the impact of fatigue on quality of life is multifaceted, including sexual dysfunction.

Uncontrolled pain can contribute to sexual dysfunction through its association with psychological distress, poor appetite, and lack of sleep, all of which can decrease sexual interest. Surprisingly, little empiric research has been conducted in this area. However, one study demonstrated the association of pain with decreased sexual functioning after high-dose chemotherapy and autologous bone marrow support.[50] Another study that examined breast cancer patients with upper extremity lymphedema found that the presence of associated pain predicted psychological distress, but it did not independently predict sexual dysfunction.[51]

PARTNER RELATIONSHIPS

The literature suggests that the presence of a partner plays an important role in the maintenance of an active sex life for both men and women.[7,9,18,22] Problems in the marital relationship after cancer usually reflect preexisting stresses and strains, such that marital dissolution as a result of cancer is probably less common than once thought.[52] Often, cancer patients cite improvement in their love relationships rather than deterioration.[53] In a study of prostate cancer survivors compared with aged-matched healthy controls, marital function did not differ between treatment groups and controls.[54] The presence of a spouse or partner is invaluable for patients facing the possibility of sexual dysfunction from cancer or its treatments. Partners provide much needed emotional support and may also contribute to the clinical decision-making process.

In addressing the partner relationship, it is also important never to assume that the patient is heterosexual. The astute clinician should probe in a nonjudgmental way about the patient's partnership status and ensure that a same-gender partner is included, as appropriate, in medical decision making. Some gay and lesbian couples may fear being honest, even with their physicians. A few words of candid support may go a long way in allowing patients to feel better about involving their same-gender partner.

The literature suggests that survivors of childhood and adolescent cancers are at increased risk for marital difficulties. In a large study of long-term survivors of childhood cancers compared with sibling controls, both male and female survivors were less likely to marry than sibling controls, and the marriage deficit was particularly pronounced for survivors of brain and central nervous system tumors.[55] In addition, the average length of first marriages was shorter for survivors than controls.[55] Men who had survived central nervous system tumors before the age of 10 years and male survivors of retinoblastoma had substantially higher divorce rates than controls. These findings have largely been confirmed in a preliminary report from the Childhood Cancer Survivor Study, in which rates of marriage have been compared with U.S. population census data and are found to be reduced.[56] These findings may have important long-term implications for the sexual functioning of these long-term survivors.

SPECIFIC TREATMENTS

SURGERY IN GENERAL AND PELVIC SURGERY

Surgical treatment usually involves hospitalization, general or local anesthesia, and exploration of body cavities (thoracic, abdominal, pelvic), with adjacent organ dysfunction and the need to recover from the treatment insult. Postoperative pain and fatigue are important factors that limit recovery of sexual functioning for several weeks after surgery. Surgical treatments with the most significant impact on sexual functioning are those involving the pelvis, such as radical prostatectomy, radical cystectomy, abdominal-perineal resection for rectal cancer, and radical hysterectomy for gynecologic cancers. When radiation is added to surgical treatments, additional nerve and tissue injury may occur, with fibrosis and occasional pelvic pain syndromes. Changes in body image may occur as a result of surgery, especially when it is disfiguring and visible to others, but even hidden body scars may present a difficulty for some patients.

In men, pelvic surgery for prostate, bladder, or rectal cancer can easily damage the parasympathetic sacral fibers that are responsible for penile erection. These nerves course posterolateral to the prostate and anterolateral to the rectum and are intimately associated with both structures, especially at the apex of the prostate just anterior to the rectal wall. Although techniques have been developed for identification and preservation of these neurovascular bundles during radical prostatectomy[57] and radical cystectomy,[58] such preservation is much more difficult during abdominal-perineal resection of the rectum.[59] These nerves do not need to be cut to disrupt their function. The trauma of dissection to separate them from the prostate or rectum may also lead to their permanent failure. The effect is immediate, and neuronal recovery is slow, often lasting months or years.[60] Pelvic surgery for bladder or rectal cancer may also result in female sexual dysfunction, largely due to scarring, shortening, and stenosis of the vagina.[61] Despite initial dyspareunia, many women who are treated for bladder cancer with sur-

gery and radiation ultimately do enjoy a return of sexual function.[62]

Retroperitoneal lymphadenectomy in men with testis cancer does not interfere with erections, but it may cause retrograde ejaculation. The primary landing site for lymphatic spread from the testes is located in the interaortocaval region for right-sided tumors and in the paraaortic region for left-sided tumors. From here, metastatic deposits can extend cephalad or caudad alongside the great vessels. Intertwined with these lymphatic channels are the lumbar sympathetic fibers that are responsible for normal antegrade ejaculation. If these are damaged during surgery, patients may experience a failure of both seminal emission and bladder neck closure. This in turn results in retrograde ejaculation. Although the patient is able to enjoy the pleasure of orgasm, it is dry and fluidless. Techniques to preserve these nerve fibers by using template dissections have been popularized and are largely successful at maintaining antegrade ejaculation in most men undergoing retroperitoneal lymphadenectomy.[63,64]

The effects of pelvic and genital surgery on sexual response in men and women vary depending on the organs involved and are summarized in Tables 55.3-2 and 55.3-3. Schover and Fife[65] have provided an excellent overview of the components of the sexual response that are affected by these various surgical procedures. The amount of dysfunction depends on the extent of injury to the sacral plexus (especially for erectile functioning in men), and for women, vaginal lubrication is influenced by oophorectomy and the loss of estrogen, as well as the prohibition against estrogen replacement therapy. Dry orgasms occur in men after radical prostatectomy and radical cystectomy through surgical removal of the prostate and seminal vesicles. For women, vaginal shortening and anatomic changes that result from several of the surgical procedures lead to dyspareunia and the need to use lubricants and vaginal dilators.

With contemporary multimodal therapy, the extent of surgery can be limited through the addition of chemotherapy and radiation to control local and distant disease. Specific examples are primary radiation therapy for prostate cancer, bladder-conserving surgery with radiation and chemotherapy, and sphincter preservation treatment of anal and rectal cancer. These approaches still have associated sexual dysfunctions, but the time course and specific problems differ from surgery alone.

CHEMOTHERAPY

The effects of systemic chemotherapy on sexual functioning can be conceptualized as acute and chronic, with somewhat different risks for men and women. Acutely, and dependent on the type of chemotherapeutic agent, many patients experience nausea, vomiting, fatigue, hair loss, and mucositis. All of these factors contribute to a decrease in well-being and diminished interest in sexual activity. Women may experience vaginal and perineal mucositis from some agents, with some data suggesting decreased vaginal lubrication as a late effect of chemotherapy.[66,67] Loss of body hair decreases sexual attractiveness for most individuals. All of these effects are intensified in those receiving high-dose chemotherapy regimens.[68] Protracted fatigue may be a significant contributor to sexual dysfunction in bone marrow transplantation survivors.[50]

For women, one of the most dramatic consequences of chemotherapy treatment is the development of premature meno-

TABLE 55.3-2. Effects of Surgery for Pelvic or Genital Cancer on Male Sexual Physiology

Procedure	Desire	Pleasure from Touch	Ability to Have Erection	Orgasm	Ejaculation	Pain with Intercourse
Radical prostatectomy	No change	No change	Decreased functioning that is age-dependent	No change or some decreased intensity	Dry orgasm	Rare
Radical cystectomy	No change	No change	Decreased functioning that is age-dependent	No change or some decreased intensity	Dry orgasm	Rare, but more likely after complete urethrectomy
Abdominoperineal resection	No change	No change	Some impairment but less than radical prostatectomy	No change or some decreased intensity	Dry orgasm	Rare, but some perineal pain or phantom rectal sensations
Total pelvic exenteration	No change	No change	Almost always impaired	No change or some decreased intensity	Dry orgasm	Rare; possible genital edema from groin dissection
Partial penectomy	No change	Erotic sensation in remaining genital area	No change	No change	No change	Rare; possible genital edema from groin dissection
Total penectomy	No change	Erotic sensation in remaining genital area	Not possible	No change; need to identify erotic zones	No change; semen comes out perineal urethrostomy	Occasional; genital edema from groin dissection

(Adapted from ref. 31.)

pause, with the consequent loss of fertility.[69,70] In a prospective study of a cohort of 183 early-stage breast cancer patients receiving no adjuvant therapy, either chemotherapy or tamoxifen adjuvant therapy, or both chemotherapy and tamoxifen,[71] age and systemic chemotherapy were the strongest predictors of menopause in women with locoregional disease, with tamoxifen making a small contribution (Fig. 55.3-1). As Figure 55.3-1 demonstrates, the probability of menopause with chemotherapy begins to rise at approximately 35 years of age, with more than 40% of women at age 40 years predicted to become amenorrheic. The closer a woman was to the age of natural menopause (age 51), the greater her risk of amenorrhea.[71] Women in this study were only followed for 1 year after treatment, and some may have subsequently resumed menstruating. Because some evidence suggests that amenorrhea may be beneficial in preventing breast cancer recurrence, it may be an acceptable consequence of treatment for some women. Nevertheless, the effects

of menopause on sexual functioning (discussed earlier in Menopause and Sexual Functioning), especially vaginal dryness, may contribute to sexual dysfunction in breast cancer survivors.[41]

Preservation of fertility is very important for younger patients treated for leukemia, testicular cancer, lymphoma, and Hodgkin's disease. Although current regimens for Hodgkin's disease that avoid alkylating agent therapy [e.g., doxorubicin (Adriamycin), bleomycin, vinblastine, and dacarbazine] may spare ovarian and testicular function in terms of fertility and premature menopause, their value in preservation of sexual functioning may be more limited.[31] In a study comparing survivors of advanced-stage Hodgkin's disease and acute leukemia survivors treated on a variety of chemotherapy protocols, Hodgkin's disease survivors experienced significantly poorer sexual relationships than the leukemia survivors.[32] Thus, the specific type of chemotherapy regimen and its duration can have differing effects on sexual functioning.

TABLE 55.3-3. Effects of Surgery for Pelvic or Genital Cancer on Female Sexual Physiology

Procedure	Desire	Pleasure from Touch	Vaginal Lubrication	Ease of Orgasm	Orgasm	Pain with Intercourse
Radical hysterectomy	No change	No change	May need ERT	No change	No change	Rare; shorter vagina
Radical cystectomy	No change	No change	Reduced, may need ERT	No change	No change	Frequent, but can be treated
Abdominoperineal resection	No change	No change	May need ERT	Probably no change	No change	Frequent, but can be treated
Total pelvic exenteration and vaginal reconstruction	No change	Some loss of erotic zones	Lost	Need to relearn how to reach orgasm	No change or mild decreased intensity	Occasional
Radical vulvectomy	No change	Some loss of erotic zones	No change	Need to relearn how to reach orgasm	?	Frequent, but can be treated

ERT, estrogen replacement therapy.
(Adapted from ref. 31.)

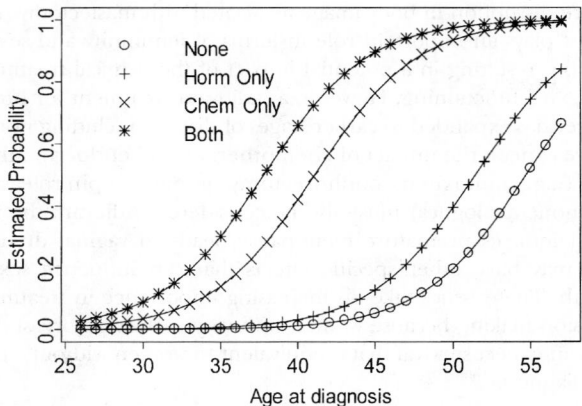

FIGURE 55.3-1. Probability of menopause during the first year after the diagnosis and adjuvant treatment of breast cancer. Chem, chemotherapy; Horm, hormone. (From ref. 44, with permission.)

RADIATION THERAPY

The acute effects of radiation include fatigue, nausea, skin changes, and hair loss, with local changes limited to the radiation port area. Fatigue can interfere with sexual functioning, and hair loss and skin changes can affect sexual functioning through changes in body image. Long-lasting effects on skin and hair may occasionally occur, especially when combined-modality therapies are used. Radiation injury to the pelvis can lead to fibrosis of soft tissue, as well as nerve damage, with loss of sexual functioning attributable to treatment. This is especially an issue when high-dose primary therapy is given, as for prostate cancer, bladder-conservation treatment, cervical cancer, and rectal cancers. In addition, injury to adjacent normal tissues (rectum, bladder, vagina) can lead to symptomatic problems (proctitis, cystitis, vaginal stenosis) that can detract from sexual activities.

Primary pelvic irradiation for prostate or bladder cancer may be as damaging to the erectile nerves as surgery. Radiation also damages the small blood vessels that supply and drain the corpora cavernosa.[72] The primary difference is the time course over which the effect is seen. Whereas surgical nerve injury reveals itself immediately, radiation injury to the nerves and vessels often does not manifest itself for many months. Because the mechanism of radiation tissue damage is to induce cell death and scarring over time, the pelvic vessels and erectile nerves may retain normal function initially and then decline fairly rapidly as long as 18 to 36 months after the completion of treatment.[73] Three-dimensional conformal and intensity-modulated radiation therapy have improved the radiation oncologist's ability to focus the beam at the center of the prostate and decrease the dose delivered to its periphery, where the nerves are located.[74,75] To treat prostate cancer effectively, however, an adequate dose must be administered to the entire gland, and this can certainly cause subsequent nerve damage. Proton beam therapy, a variation of external-beam radiotherapy, is heavily marketed as causing fewer erectile complications in prostate cancer patients; however, no published evidence supports this claim.

Brachytherapy, the implantation of radioactive seeds into the prostate, has gained national prominence because it, too, is reputed to cause fewer complications than external-beam ther-

apy.[76] However, longitudinal measurements of sexual function after brachytherapy suggest that patients fare no better than those undergoing external-beam radiation.[77] In addition, brachytherapy is often administered with androgen ablation and external-beam radiation, combinations that may further compromise sexual function.

ENDOCRINE TREATMENTS

Treatments used in the management of endocrine-sensitive cancers have important effects on sexual functioning. Tamoxifen, an antiestrogen, increases the rate of vaginal discharge and vasomotor symptoms in a proportion of breast cancer patients[66] and in those women taking this therapy for breast cancer prevention.[78,79] Although rates of sexual activity did not appear to differ between the women taking tamoxifen and those taking a placebo in the Breast Cancer Prevention Trial, subtle differences in sexual functioning for women taking tamoxifen were noted (see Breast Cancer, later in this chapter).[78] A small study examined the effect of tamoxifen and sexual functioning in patients with breast cancer and found that the desire, arousal, and orgasmic problems were not increased; however, more than one-half of patients complained of pain, burning, or discomfort with intercourse and the majority of those with these symptoms routinely used a vaginal lubricant with intercourse.[80]

Weight gain is an important side effect of megestrol acetate, sometimes used in the treatment of metastatic breast and endometrial cancers. Weight gain contributes to a poorer body image and potentially affects sexual functioning.[81] There is renewed interest in ovarian ablation as adjuvant therapy for breast cancer, either with surgical oophorectomy or with use of gonadotropin-releasing hormone analogues.[82,83] The precipitation of premature menopause in these women may cause substantial disruption in sexual functioning. Aromatase inhibitors are the newest class of endocrine therapy for breast cancer.[84] These agents are given to postmenopausal women and lower the estrogen level to undetectable levels. Primarily studied in advanced breast cancer patients thus far, only limited data are available on sexual functioning in the adjuvant setting, but these agents are likely to contribute to vaginal dryness.

For men with advanced prostate cancer, the mainstay of therapy is androgen ablation,[85] using either surgical or medical castration. Chemical castration is achieved with gonadotropin-releasing hormone blockers with or without the addition of antiandrogens to eliminate the effect of adrenal androgens. Other agents, such as aminoglutethimide or ketoconazole, may also be used for the same effect. The primary sexual side effect of androgen ablation is loss of libido. Many men report the ability to have erections and ejaculations despite the absence of testosterone, although decline in libido is universal. As a result, men who are sexually active and asymptomatic from the cancer (e.g., those who have a rising prostate-specific antigen level without documented metastatic disease) often choose to delay hormone therapy. For men who are experiencing clinical progression of metastatic prostate cancer, sexual function may already have declined or disappeared as their constitutional symptoms have advanced. For these individuals, androgen ablation may not have a great impact on erectile function, which is already greatly reduced.[86] Bicalutamide monotherapy has recently gained popularity because it preserves many aspects of sexual function in many men with early metastatic prostate cancer.[87]

CONCERNS ABOUT FERTILITY

Preservation of fertility is an important aspect of treatment, especially for those who have not had children, and a special concern for survivors of childhood cancer and young adults treated with curative-intent therapy. Byrne and colleagues[88] estimated the risk of infertility after treatment in a retrospective cohort study of childhood cancer survivors and controls. The survivors, diagnosed before the age of 20 years, were treated between 1945 and 1975 at five cancer centers in the United States. Married survivors were less likely than their sibling controls to have ever begun a pregnancy. Infradiaphragmatic radiation therapy decreased fertility in both sexes by approximately 25%, and chemotherapy with alkylating agents, with or without radiation, was associated with a fertility deficit of approximately 60% in men. Among women, no effect of alkylating agents alone was found in this young group of patients; however, a moderate fertility deficit was noted when alkylating agents were combined with infradiaphragmatic radiation.[88]

More detailed studies of gonadal function tend to confirm these general observations, with evidence of preserved Leydig cell function in young boys receiving treatment, but also of increased germ cell dysfunction and decreased spermatogenesis.[89,90] Female childhood cancer survivors do not exhibit significant changes in gonadal function with contemporary treatments.[90] Even in young women treated for ovarian dysgerminoma, reproductive function can be preserved with conservative surgery and contemporary chemotherapy treatment regimens.[91]

For young adults with cancer, strategies to conserve fertility are often used and are highly dependent on the type of cancer and available treatments.[92] The regimen of doxorubicin, bleomycin, vinblastine, and dacarbazine has largely replaced other alkylating agent–containing regimens for Hodgkin's disease because of a more limited risk of infertility.[93] In general, however, diseases that require treatment with alkylating agents are likely to put both men and women at risk for infertility.[92] The risk for women begins to rise after 30 years of age, and for men the risk is present at any age. Cryopreservation of sperm is a strategy used to preserve fertility in men.[94,95] Newer approaches to ovarian tissue preservation and subsequent reimplantation are on the horizon for women.[96,97]

A past history of cancer, uncertainty related to reproductive potential, and changes in sense of self-esteem and attractiveness may impair dating and sexual function in young adults with a history of cancer. Often, childhood cancer survivors have limited awareness of their past treatment, and they often confront this aspect of their health for the first time as they marry and attempt to start a family. Importantly, these individuals can be reassured that their offspring are unlikely to experience adverse consequences as a result of past parental treatments for cancer.[98,99]

SEXUAL PROBLEMS ASSOCIATED WITH SPECIFIC CANCERS

BREAST CANCER

Breast cancer is one of the most frequently studied cancer sites regarding sexual functioning due to the breast surgery and the severe disruption in body image associated with mastectomy. The breast plays an important role in terms of femininity and sexual identity, resulting in a potential impact of the surgical treatment on sexual functioning. However, as adjuvant treatment for breast cancer has expanded to earlier stages of disease, including noninvasive cancer, the impact of chemotherapy and endocrine therapy (e.g., tamoxifen, oophorectomy, gonadotropin-releasing hormone analogues) must also be considered. Adjuvant therapy often induces premature menopause, leads to vaginal dryness, and may have other specific effects that can influence sexual health. These issues take on increasing importance in treatment decision making because women with very early-stage breast cancer can expect survival that is equivalent to women without a cancer diagnosis.[100]

One of the most investigated questions in breast cancer patients has been the impact of type of surgery on sexual health and quality of life.[36–38,101–103] There is consensus that breast-conserving surgery offers a better sense of body image to women but only limited differences in other dimensions of quality of life (physical, emotional, or social functioning). In only a few studies were women randomly assigned to the type of surgical treatment; most have been observational cohort studies in which patient choice or preference for treatment likely occurred. Thus, some bias could be influencing the results. Nevertheless, the consistency of findings across so many studies and countries suggests that the findings are real. In studies that have specifically addressed sexual functioning,[38,102–104] little difference was found between the two types of surgery, although in the one randomized treatment trial,[104] there was a suggestion of better sexual functioning in women with conservation surgery.

In a study comparing women with breast conservation treatment to those receiving mastectomy with reconstruction, Schover[105] found that the two groups did not differ in body image, satisfaction with relationships, or sexual life. However, the authors did find that women with breast reconstruction experienced less caressing of the breast in lovemaking than women with partial mastectomy.[105] In a study of sexual health and functioning in breast cancer survivors,[67] body image influenced sexual interest, but the type of surgery did not predict any aspect of sexual health after breast cancer. In a large study of almost 2000 breast cancer survivors,[106] those who had received mastectomy with reconstruction reported the greatest negative impact of breast cancer on their sex lives. Although mastectomy negatively affects body image, it does not necessarily impact sexual health and functioning. As has been shown in healthy women without breast cancer[22] and in breast cancer survivors,[41] other factors may play a more important role in influencing sexual health in middle-aged women (e.g., presence of a partner, vaginal dryness, emotional well-being, quality of the partnered relationship).

The etiology of sexual dysfunction in breast cancer survivors has not been well studied. Multiple predisposing factors are involved, including preexisting sexual problems, negative sexual self-schemas, and normal age-related changes in sexual functioning.[107–110] In addition, induction of premature menopause by chemotherapy contributes to estrogen deficiency with associated vasomotor symptoms and poor vaginal lubrication that may contribute to sexual dysfunction.[69,111,112] These symptoms may be exacerbated by tamoxifen adjuvant therapy.[113] However, the results from two placebo-controlled trials of tamoxifen in high-risk women did not find that tamoxifen affected sexual functioning.[78,79] Multiple studies suggest an important role for chemotherapy in increasing sexual dysfunction in women with breast cancer.[66,67,112,114] This effect may be working through the precipitation of premature menopause and loss of both estrogens and androgens from the ovary,[114] or possibly through a direct effect on the vaginal epithelium, causing vaginal dryness.[67]

Sexual functioning in long-term survivors of breast cancer has been compared with information on women without a cancer diagnosis.[67,115,116] Overall, the breast cancer survivors reported fairly high levels of satisfaction with their sexual relationships and functioning that are similar to noncancer comparison groups.[67,116] Nevertheless, in a more detailed analysis, approximately one-third of women reported that breast cancer had a negative impact on their sex life, and most reported negative changes in at least some areas (e.g., frequency of sexual activity, awareness of decreased lubrication in vagina with sexual activity, pain in genital area during sexual activity, discomfort when touching breast cancer surgery area).[116] Women who were most likely to report a negative impact were significantly more likely to report relationship difficulties, to have experienced changes in hormonal levels because of breast cancer (premature menopause or discontinuation of hormone replacement), and to be bothered by vaginal dryness.[116] These findings are similar to those obtained in smaller samples of breast cancer survivors.[115,117]

PROSTATE CANCER

The effect of erectile dysfunction on sexual functioning after treatment for prostate cancer has been studied extensively with a variety of experimental designs. All studies have shown that men undergoing radical prostatectomy or pelvic irradiation have more sexual impairment than age-matched controls.[118,119] Despite consistent reports of better outcomes with nerve-sparing techniques in centers of excellence, rates of sexual dysfunction in random national population-based samples reveal that erectile dysfunction remains common after surgery[120,121] or radiation[122] for early-stage prostate cancer.

Talcott[123] found that patients who underwent nerve-sparing surgery had low levels of sexual function that were not significantly different from men who underwent non–nerve-sparing procedures. However, those who had bilateral nerve-sparing reported significantly better potency at 1 year than did those who underwent unilateral or non–nerve-sparing surgery. In a longitudinal follow-up study, Talcott et al.[73] also published the first prospective cohort study of patients treated with either surgery or radiotherapy, using validated quality-of-life instruments before treatment and at 3 and 12 months afterward. Initially, surgery patients had more impotence; however, over time, sexual function declined in the radiotherapy group and improved in the surgery group. Hence, with longer follow-up, treatment group differences in sexual function continued to narrow. Other studies also have shown that the incidence of impotence increases to approximately 40% during the 2 to 3 years after radiation therapy for localized prostate cancer.[124,125]

In another longitudinal study of men treated with surgery or radiation for early-stage prostate cancer,[126] sexual function steadily improved. Although sexual function was significantly better in radiation than surgery patients immediately after treatment, by 2 years later, radiation patients began to show modest declines in sexual function, whereas surgery patients continued to improve. Older men were much less likely than younger men to regain sexual function after treatment.

TESTIS CANCER

Therapy for testicular cancer, including orchiectomy, retroperitoneal lymphadenectomy, and radiation therapy, can cause a variety of physical and psychological sequelae.[127] Rieker et al.[128,129] showed that these patients express distress over poor sexual performance and infertility, although not with decreased libido. Those with ejaculatory dysfunction noted more strained intimate relationships and more psychological problems. Compared with healthy controls, testis cancer patients do not report more difficulty with relationships, employment, divorce, or overall mental outlook. In a recent study of patients with early stage seminoma,[130] treatment-induced body image changes and concerns about fertility were noted, but sexual problems detected did not differ from healthy controls.

A metaanalysis of 36 empirical studies between 1975 and 2000 found that problems with ejaculatory function were reported most frequently, which were related to retroperitoneal surgery; however, erectile dysfunction was related to irradiation and was reported least frequently.[131] Other sexual problems were not related to treatment modality.

BLADDER CANCER

Most men who undergo cystectomy for bladder cancer either report erectile dysfunction before treatment or develop it after treatment. Despite this observation, at least 50% of these patients continue to enjoy some form of sexual stimulation other than coitus after recuperation from surgery.[132] For women, changes in vaginal lubrication may occur if women are estrogen deficient.[65] In a study that examined quality of life and sexual functioning in patients undergoing cystectomy, reconstruction by continent cutaneous ileocecal diversion, or simple conduit diversion, the authors found equivalent declines in quality of life related to sexual problems, disturbed partner relationships, and emotional dysfunction in all three surgical groups.[133] In another similarly designed study, patients with ileal conduit had the poorest self-image, as defined by a decrease in sexual desire and in all forms of physical contact (sexual and nonsexual).[134] Those who later underwent conversion from ileal conduit diversions to continent cutaneous Kock pouches were the most physically and sexually active. Gerharz et al.[135] found that, after cystectomy, patients diverted with an ileal conduit had worse scores than continent reservoir patients in sexual activity and general quality-of-life domains. Hart et al.[136] reported more optimistic findings, showing that general quality of life was not differentially affected by the choice of urinary diversion method after cystectomy in either women or men.

GYNECOLOGIC CANCERS

Cancer involving the female genital organs immediately evokes concerns about sexual dysfunction. Sexual problems can predate the diagnosis and are usually exacerbated by cancer treatments.[137] Cancers of the uterine corpus and cervix make up the majority of gynecologic cancers (roughly 70%), and these primarily localized cancers are treated with surgery, radiation therapy, or both. Rarer cancers, such as vulvar cancer, may be treated with a variety of local or extensive surgical modalities, with some use of topical therapies. Other gynecologic cancers (ovarian cancer, trophoblastic disease, uterine sarcomas) are treated with combinations of chemotherapy, surgery, and sometimes radiotherapy. The more disseminated nature of these cancers and the severity of the disease lead to different patterns of sexual dysfunction. For all gynecologic cancers, the age, partnership status, menopausal status, and preexisting sexual functioning of a woman play an important role in her sexual rehabilitation after cancer treatment (see Table 55.3-1 and review by Andersen[138]).

In a comparison of healthy control subjects and women with early-stage cervical and uterine cancer, Andersen et al.[137] found few differences in aspects of the sexual response cycle reported before the onset of signs or symptoms of the cancer. However, a substantial number of the gynecologic cancer patients reported a disruption in sexual responsiveness with the onset of symptoms, including changes in desire, excitement, orgasm, and resolution and a global deterioration in sexual functioning.[137] These changes were most often associated with symptoms of fatigue, postcoital bleeding, and multiple other signs and symptoms.

Sexual functioning outcomes in patients with gynecologic cancers often have been reported in small case series. Andersen and colleagues[139] prospectively studied 47 women with early-stage gynecologic cancers (cervix, n = 33; endometrium, n = 9; ovary, n = 5) and benign gynecologic disease before treatment and then interviewed them again at 4, 8, and 12 months posttreatment. Whether women had benign or malignant disease, they reported similar declines in frequency of intercourse, decreased sexual excitement, and a less positive global evaluation of their sexual life. In addition, a three- to sixfold increase in the incidence of sexual dysfunction diagnoses was found in comparison to the rates in healthy women.[139] Pain with intercourse, prominent early in the recovery period in treated women, improved with time but remained more frequent in the cancer patients. Although both treated groups experienced increased sexual dysfunctions posttreatment, the cancer patients experienced a higher incidence of inhibited excitement. As discussed by Andersen et al.,[139] these particular changes can be a manifestation of increased anxiety associated with the cancer diagnosis.

In a study of cervical cancer patients, Schover[140] examined sexual frequency, function, and behavior in 61 women with early-stage invasive carcinoma of the cervix in relation to type of treatment. Sexual satisfaction, capacity for orgasm, and frequency of masturbation remained stable over 12 months of observation posttreatment; however, frequency of sexual activity with a partner and the range of sexual practices decreased significantly over the course of the year of follow-up. Although at 6 months, few differences were noted between those who had received irradiation and those who had not, at the 12-month assessment, the women receiving radiotherapy had more dyspareunia (as well as an abnormal vaginal examination) and had more problems with sexual desire and arousal.[140] Treatment modality had no effect on marital happiness or stability.

These findings suggest an additional complication from irradiation of the pelvis, which is vaginal stenosis or foreshortening. Several other studies have documented this problem,[141,142] with levels of sexual activity being lowest at the completion of radiotherapy. The finding of progressive dyspareunia and vaginal shortening[140] suggests the need for active intervention in these women, with the need for early use of vaginal lubricants, resumption of sexual activity, or use of dilators

to maintain vaginal length and elasticity. A recent study of a psychoeducational group intervention found improved use of vaginal dilatation and less fear about sex after cancer treatment in those who received the intervention.[143]

These small descriptive studies shed some light on the mechanisms of sexual dysfunction and the range of sexual problems in the first year after treatment for cervical cancer. However, the late sexual effects of treatment for cervical cancer are important because this is a group of women who are likely to be cured of their disease and be long-term cancer survivors. A report by Bergmark et al.[144] provides important new information on vaginal changes and sexuality in a large sample of Swedish cervical cancer survivors (n = 256) and a concurrent control sample (n = 350). The cancer survivors had been treated, on average, approximately 5 years earlier and were a mean age of 51 years at the time they responded to the study questionnaire. Significant differences were found between the two groups in problems with vaginal lubrication (26% of the women with cancer vs. 11% of the controls), reporting of a short vagina (26% of the women with cancer vs. 3% of the controls) and decreased vaginal elasticity (23% of the women with cancer vs. 4% of the controls). In spite of these significant changes associated with the treatment of cervical cancer, no differences were noted in sexual interest, desire, frequency of vaginal intercourse, or orgasm; however, there was more distress related to the frequency of vaginal intercourse and problems during vaginal intercourse among the women with a history of cervical cancer.[144]

Treatment with surgery alone was associated with decreased vaginal lubrication, vaginal shortness, and decreased vaginal elasticity.[144] When surgery was combined with radiotherapy or when radiotherapy was given alone, no apparent differences in these vaginal outcomes were found when compared with surgery alone, except for some decreased sexual interest among those treated with radiotherapy alone. Interestingly, treatment for cervical cancer negatively influenced feelings of femininity and attractiveness among the cervical cancer survivors but did not seem to influence sexual satisfaction.[144] Finally, it should be noted that the use of a healthy control group in this study was important, in that 41% of both patients and controls reported little or no interest in sex in the previous 6 months, with more than 50% reporting reduced sexual desire in the previous 5 years. Without a control group, these findings might have been attributed to the history of cancer.

In spite of being diagnosed with the third most common gynecologic cancer, ovarian cancer patients have been less frequently studied.[145] These patients experience all of the physical changes associated with the treatment of uterine and cervical cancer due to surgical removal of the uterus and ovaries. However, their treatment is often dominated by the use of systemic or intraperitoneal chemotherapy and the side effects of this treatment, especially decreased physical functioning, fatigue, pain, and abdominal discomfort. Symptoms of advanced cancer significantly impact sexual functioning in these women.

Sexual functioning after vulvar cancer has been examined in two series.[146,147] In a comparison of women with *in situ* vulvar cancer and a matched sample of gynecologically healthy women, a higher rate of inhibited sexual excitement and inhibited orgasm was found among the women with cancer, as well as an increasing rate of sexual inactivity over time, compared with the healthy women.[146] The wider the surgical excision, the greater the magnitude of sexual disruption.[146] In a prospective study of ten couples, with the women being treated for vulvar cancer with radical vulvectomy, there was a postoperative decline in functioning with gradual recovery over 2 years.[147] However, genital symptoms of sexual arousal and satisfaction were diminished in the cancer group and did not return to levels of those found in the control group,[147] and general satisfaction with sexual interaction with the partner hardly changed over a 2-year period of observation.

HODGKIN'S DISEASE

Hodgkin's disease survivors have been found to have elevated levels of psychological distress, on average, compared with healthy controls, and those survivors in greater distress reported more problems in other areas of functioning, including sexual problems.[30] When survivors rated their overall current sexual satisfaction, the median scores were similar to healthy subjects. However, when asked to consider the effect of cancer on their sexual life, 37% reported one or more sexual problems, primarily because of decreased sexual satisfaction (31%), interest (21%), and activity (18%). Of these survivors, 26% had been tested and were told they were infertile, and an additional 27% believed that they were infertile.[30] In addition, all survivors who were not currently married experienced higher distress than those who were married, and 56% of those who were separated or divorced attributed their marital status to having had cancer.[30] In a comparative study of survivors of Hodgkin's disease and acute leukemia,[31] substantially more psychological distress and poorer sexual functioning were noted among the Hodgkin's disease survivors. A recent prospective longitudinal clinical trial in early-stage Hodgkin's disease found a decline in sexual functioning with treatment that improved by 1 year after diagnosis.[49]

COLORECTAL CANCER

Colorectal cancer most often occurs in persons older than 60 years of age. The limited literature available on sexual dysfunction in this disease focuses on the consequences of abdominoperineal resection and ostomies. After radical surgery for rectal cancer in women,[61] prospective studies of small samples suggest a decline in sexual activity postoperatively, with decreased interest, lubrication, and orgasmic activity. In a study comparing abdominoperineal resection with colostomy and low anterior resection, sexual functioning was preserved at a higher rate with low anterior resection. Overall, the prognostic variables most influencing posttreatment sexual functioning include the woman's age at surgery, the magnitude of the surgical intervention, handmade versus stapled anastomoses, and the number of autonomic nerves present in the surgical specimen.[61]

For men, similar issues pertain; however, erectile dysfunction is a more salient issue.[148] A study of 60 sexually active men surgically treated for colorectal cancer found that sexual activity was decreased in 32%.[148] The distribution of difficulties among those affected were dry ejaculate (25%), erection not firm enough for penetration (45%), and complete absence of erection (25%). The decreases in sexual functioning occurred in all groups of patients, from high anterior resection to low anterior resection to abdominoperineal resection, but were most frequent in those with abdominoperineal resection.[148]

A review of quality of life in colorectal cancer relative to sphincter-preserving procedures found that stoma patients reported higher levels of psychological distress than nonstoma patients and that sexual functioning of male and female stoma patients were consistently more impaired than that of patients with intact sphincters.[40] Both groups were troubled by frequent and unpredictable bowel function that increases psychological distress and can affect sexual functioning.[40]

STRATEGIES FOR ASSESSMENT AND INTERVENTION

ASSESSMENT

A comprehensive assessment of sexual difficulties requires an interdisciplinary and multifaceted approach, which is often beyond the scope of the oncology team's activities. Depending on the particular problem(s), it can be important to consider hormonal, physiologic, anatomic, psychological, cognitive, behavioral, relational, and cultural factors in a biopsychosocial model (see Table 55.3-1).[149] To provide a differential diagnosis, it also is necessary to assess for psychopathology, medical conditions, substance abuse, and relationship difficulties as primary etiologic factors. Modes of assessment include open-ended conversations, structured diagnostic interviews, standardized self-report questionnaires, medical examination, and laboratory studies. Several resources are available for readers who wish to learn about specific assessment procedures.[2,4,13,150,151]

Although a comprehensive assessment is unrealistic within the constraints of an oncology practice, a preliminary review of sexual difficulties is essential to providing optimal care to the cancer patient. Patients regularly report that they would like to discuss sexual issues with their physicians but feel reluctant to do so.[111,152] In parallel, it is clear that health care professionals feel uncomfortable discussing these issues with patients.[153] Therefore, it is up to the medical team to broach the issue and open lines of communication.[154] Straightforward questions about each of the four categories of sexual dysfunction—desire, arousal, orgasm, and pain—and questions about sexual activity and satisfaction generally provide sufficient information to determine the need for further testing or referral.[10] One member of the team should be identified as a primary resource for assessment and referral.

COUNSELING, INTERVENTION, AND REFERRAL

After a member of the oncology team has raised the issue of sexuality and made a preliminary assessment of reported problems, a decision must be made regarding the level and type of intervention that is needed.[155] In some cases, the specific concerns that arise can be addressed directly by a member of the team who has developed expertise in sexuality and cancer. Providing patients and their partners (when appropriate) with information about sexual functioning, aging, and sexual problems related to the cancer experience can help to normalize many concerns. Patients also can benefit from receiving written materials, such as those available from the National Cancer Institute and the American Cancer Society or produced by other experts.[156] They may also benefit from learning about local resources for cancer patients and survivors. For limited problems, specific suggestions or a brief course of sexual counseling may be sufficient. For example, for a woman with vaginal dryness who cannot use estrogen, a vaginal lubricant or moisturizer might be extremely effective. Schover and colleagues[12] found that 63.5% of cancer patients who received brief sexual counseling within a cancer center reported improvement; however, those who were depressed or in conflicted marriages were least likely to benefit.

For patients with more complex problems, referral to a mental health professional with special training in sex therapy, marital therapy, or individual psychotherapy with cancer patients should be considered. The oncologist plays a pivotal role in ensuring successful treatment by making appropriate referrals that normalize the need for therapy. In addition, specific medical interventions such as those detailed in the next two sections may be helpful.

MEDICAL INTERVENTIONS FOR WOMEN

One of the most important targets for intervention in women is vaginal dryness. This problem is common for women as they age,[23] independent of cancer treatment, and is usually managed with some form of estrogen therapy. In women who can receive estrogen therapy after cancer, this treatment is the most effective therapeutic remedy, and it can be used topically or systemically. A study of the prevalence and predictors of sexual dysfunction in long-term survivors of bone marrow transplantation found that early intervention with hormone therapy after transplant substantially decreased reports of dyspareunia and improved sexual satisfaction.[157] Changing hormone replacement therapy after 1 year, either by starting therapy or electing to stop hormone therapy, did not show a measurable influence on reported sexual satisfaction at 3 years.[157] This suggests that once sexual problems are established early after cancer treatment (vaginal dryness, dyspareunia), it may be more difficult to restore satisfactory sexual activity. Hormonal therapy early on should be considered for patients receiving chemotherapy in this setting if it is not otherwise contraindicated.

Vaginal dryness can be managed with lubricants and moisturizers,[158,159] but far more effective are topical estrogen preparations. Recently, the use of an estradiol-impregnated ring, which slowly releases estradiol and is not systemically absorbed, has gained popularity for relief of symptoms of vaginal dryness in healthy women and women with cancer.[160] This therapy has now been accepted for concomitant use in prevention and treatment trials for breast cancer.

In a study addressing menopausal symptoms in breast cancer survivors, Ganz et al.[161,162] found that most of the women who wanted some form of treatment were highly symptomatic, with more than 80% having two of three symptoms (hot flashes, vaginal dryness, urinary incontinence). Using education, counseling, lifestyle modifications, and several pharmacologic agents, after a 4-month period of intervention, a significant improvement in the target menopausal symptoms and sexual functioning was demonstrated in the women assigned to treatment, compared with a no-treatment control group. Unlike the single-agent pharmacologic trials, this study tried to address all three symptoms simultaneously, as well as tailor the treatment strategies to the individual's needs and her willingness or unwillingness to take a medication.[162]

Although less well studied for safety and benefit,[21] androgen-replacement therapy should be considered in women with complaints of decreased libido and absent or severely diminished levels of free testosterone. Various preparations of testosterone are available, and a patch for women may soon be approved for marketing. Testosterone cream can also be compounded and used in sparing amounts, with dramatic improvement in libido in many women. For breast cancer patients, there are theoretical concerns about the risk of metabolic conversion of testosterone to estrogen, which may limit its use.

Other important strategies to consider are the treatment of psychological distress and marital or partner difficulties. In both healthy women and women with breast cancer,[22,41] distress in these domains has been shown to influence sexual functioning and satisfaction. Control of pain and other symptoms may also be critical for ensuring sufficient relaxation to allow women to engage in meaningful sexual activities.

MEDICAL AND SURGICAL INTERVENTIONS FOR MEN

The clinical management of cancer patients with erectile dysfunction should follow the same algorithms used in other men presenting for evaluation of impotence. However, brief sexual counseling in the primary oncology setting plays a critical role in the care of the patient, even when other interventions are prescribed.[163] The model currently used in the management of patients with erectile dysfunction involves a stepwise approach. First-line therapies are selected based on their ease of administration, reversibility, and noninvasiveness. Oral erectogenic agents, such as sildenafil, vardenafil, tadalafil, yohimbine (often considered a placebo), trazodone, and phentolamine, have gained widespread popularity, largely because of the convenience and effectiveness of sildenafil.[164] Sildenafil, vardenafil, and tadalafil work in most forms of erectile dysfunction and have few side effects. They are selective type 5 phosphodiesterase inhibitors, which increase penile cyclic guanosine monophosphate, thus enhancing the effect of nitric oxide in response to sexual stimulation. In the penis, the effect of these agents is to increase cavernosal smooth muscle dilation, a requisite component of erection. Doses of 25, 50, or 100 mg (for sildenafil) or 5, 10, or 20 mg (for vardenafil) taken 1 hour before sex are successful in approximately 70% of impotent men and last for 4 to 6 hours. Tadalafil may be taken in doses of 10 or 20 mg, has a more rapid onset, and lasts for 24 to 36 hours in a similar proportion of men. If both cavernosal nerves are severed during radical prostatectomy, the phosphodiesterase inhibitors are not effective. If only one nerve is spared, the pharmacologic effect is moderated,[165] but further study is needed in this population. In patients on androgen-ablation therapy, they are also less effective, primarily because libido is so low. Because the cavernosal nerves are typically damaged by external-beam or interstitial seed radiation, erectile dysfunction is common after either.[167] Men undergoing these therapies may also benefit from the phosphodiesterase inhibitors. In small studies of men receiving conformal radiation[167,168] or brachytherapy,[169] sildenafil is reported to be effective in the majority of the men.

Side effects with all three are minor and may include mild headache, facial flushing, rhinitis, dyspepsia, or blue-hued vision.[170] Sildenafil, vardenafil, and tadalafil may not be used concomitantly with therapeutic or recreational nitrates. Sildenafil may not be taken with food. Vardenafil may not be used in men with long QT syndrome or in those taking α blockers;

lower doses are required in men taking ritonavir or indinavir. Tadalafil may be taken with food and with tamsulosin, an α blocker commonly prescribed for men with benign prostatic hyperplasia. Any erectogenic agent should be used with caution in men with a history of sickle cell disease, multiple myeloma, leukemia, or other conditions that may predispose to priapism.

Another noninvasive technique is the penile vacuum erection device.[171,172] Although it is somewhat more cumbersome and requires training, a substantial minority of patients prefer the vacuum erection device for its simplicity, safety, and effectiveness. A clear, plastic cylinder is placed around the penis and sealed at the skin with lubricant. A small handheld pump, attached by a rubber tube to the tip of the cylinder, is activated, creating a vacuum around the penis within the cylinder. This draws blood into the erectile bodies and creates an erection. Once the penis becomes tumescent, a rubber constriction band is placed around the base of the penis to retain the erection, and the cylinder is removed. After sex, the band is removed, allowing the penile blood to drain. Few risks are associated with use of the vacuum erection device.

Second-line therapies involve the administration of pharmacologic vasodilators, either by direct intracavernosal needle injection[173] or by intraurethral suppository.[174] Injections typically include prostaglandin E_1 alone or in combination with papaverine or phentolamine. Both methods function by producing dilation of the cavernosal smooth muscle, enhancing the vascular component of penile erection. Intracavernosal injection is much more effective than intraurethral administration, but it also carries a greater short-term risk of priapism or pain and a small long-term risk of corporal scarring at the injection sites. With intracavernosal medication, the patient is trained to draw up the drug in a tuberculin syringe and inject it into the penis. He must take care to insert the needle perpendicular to the long axis of the penis and advance it all the way through the fat and fascial layers into the corpus cavernosum. Because of intercavernosal vascular connections, only one corpus needs to be injected to induce erection. The patient must be careful to avoid the nerve bundle dorsally and the urethra ventrally. He must also rotate injection sites and apply 2 to 3 minutes of pressure after injection to avoid bruising. The less effective intraurethral medication is sold as a suppository loaded into a small applicator that the patient inserts into his urethral meatus. Once in position, he pushes the medicated pellet out by advancing a small probe. The medication is packaged with pictorial instructions that facilitate patient teaching. With either penile vasodilator, the dose must be individually titrated.

Third-line therapies include the surgical implantation of semirigid or inflatable penile prostheses.[175] This outpatient surgical procedure involves a single, small dorsal or ventral incision at the base of the penis. After dissecting and entering the corpora cavernosa, their internal spongy tissue is compressed with dilators and their size calibrated. The appropriate length prostheses are inserted into both corpora. Semirigid prostheses may contain malleable metal rods encased in silicone, or they may be made of solid silicone. After recovery from surgery, the semirigid penile prosthesis requires no training and is ready for use approximately 8 to 12 weeks postoperatively. Inflatable prostheses contain pliable hollow tubes that are filled with saline from a nearby reservoir by activating a pump. In the three-piece versions, the reservoir is implanted through the groin in the perivesical space, and the pump is implanted subcutaneously in the scrotum. These components are connected to each other and to the cylinders with silicone tubing. A two-piece version is also available, in which the pump and reservoir are combined into one scrotal component. Self-contained inflatable prostheses have the cylinders, reservoir, and pump all located in one structure. These have become the preferred choice because of easier surgical implantation. After recovery, the inflatable prosthesis requires detailed training before the patient becomes comfortable with its use. The primary advantage of the inflatable version is that it appears flaccid when not in use; however, it is also associated with a greater chance of mechanical problems, which may require further surgery. Both semirigid and inflatable prostheses carry some risk of infection, but this complication is uncommon. Placement of a penile prosthesis is an invasive maneuver, in which any residual spontaneous erectile capacity is lost. This option is reserved for refractory cases of erectile dysfunction. If the devices ever require removal, natural erections are unlikely to return.

CONCLUSION

Sexual problems are prevalent in the general population, and age-related changes in sexual interest and responsiveness occur naturally. Adding a cancer diagnosis and its treatments to this background can exacerbate existing sexual problems, and an active sex life may cease for some cancer patients. Understanding the natural history of sexual problems associated with specific treatments and cancers can enhance the ability of clinicians to detect sexual problems in their patients. Because patients seldom directly express sexual concerns to their health care provider, either before or after cancer treatment, the treating oncologist needs to take the initiative by finding a comfortable way to ask, "How is your sex life going?" Often, a good time to ask this question is somewhere in the middle or toward the end of a treatment course. This can serve as a "check-in" to let the patient know the clinician is willing to talk about these issues. If the patient has no problems or is not interested in talking, the conversation ends there. However, patients know that they can bring up the topic in the future if they wish. Similarly, patients who want to discuss their concerns about sexual functioning appreciate the opportunity to discuss the specific problems. The clinician can readily provide normative information, reassurance, referrals, and specific remedies (e.g., treatment for vaginal dryness, medication of erectile dysfunction, treatment of pain).

Special situations, such as the young adult with cancer, with or without his or her spouse, or the teenager with cancer, require a special effort on the part of the clinician to address sexual concerns. With less experience and self-confidence, these individuals may be even shyer about bringing up the topic of sexuality with their oncologists. For the young adult with cancer, it is especially incumbent upon the clinician to talk about sex during and after treatment. In these situations, the difficult questions may be, for example, "Should I tell a new romantic interest about the cancer on the first date, or should I wait?" Of course, these problems are relevant for the single patient at any age.

With the increasing media attention given to sexual health in the general population, patients now expect their physicians to be well informed and receptive to discussing these issues. The very privileged relationship that oncologists have with their patients, guiding them through treatment decisions for a life-threatening condition, should permit the physician to assist the patient with this aspect of health and recovery. Physicians are fortunate that a growing body of research on sexual health after cancer now exists that can inform and guide those discussions.

REFERENCES

1. Masters WH, Johnson VE. *Human sexual response*. Boston: Little, Brown and Company, 1966.
2. Bancroft J. *Human sexuality and its problems*. Edinburgh, Scotland: Churchill Livingstone, 1989.
3. Tiefer L. The medicalization of women's sexuality. *Am J Nurs* 2000;100:11.
4. Kaplan HS. *Disorder of sexual desire: the new sex therapy*. New York: Brunner/Mazel, 1979.
5. Kaplan HS. *The evaluation of sexual disorders: psychological and medical aspects*. New York: Brunner/Mazel, 1983.
6. American Psychiatric Association. *Diagnostic and statistical manual of mental disorders*, 4th ed. Washington, DC: American Psychiatric Association, 1994.
7. Laumann EO, Gagnon JH, Michael RT, Michaels S. *The social organization of sexuality: sexual practices in the United States*. Chicago: University of Chicago Press, 1994.
8. Frank E, Anderson C, Rubinstein D. Frequency of sexual dysfunction in "normal" couples. *N Engl J Med* 1978;299:111.
9. Laumann EO, Paik A, Rosen RC. Sexual dysfunction in the United States: prevalence and predictors. *JAMA* 1999;281:537.
10. Ackerman MD, Carey MP. Psychology's role in the assessment of erectile dysfunction: historical precedents, current knowledge, and methods. *J Consult Clin Psychol* 1995;63:862.
11. Beck JG. Hypoactive sexual desire disorder: an overview. *J Consult Clin Psychol* 1995;63:919.
12. Schover LR, Evans RB, von Eschenbach AC. Sexual rehabilitation in a cancer center: diagnosis and outcome in 384 consultations. *Arch Sex Behav* 1987;16:445.
13. Wincze JP, Carey MP. *Sexual dysfunction: a guide for assessment and treatment*. New York: Guilford Press, 1991.
14. Bachmann GA. Sexual function in the perimenopause. *Obstet Gynecol Clin North Am* 1993;20:379.
15. Schiavi RC, Schreiner-Engel P, Mandeli J, Schanzer H, Cohen E. Healthy aging and male sexual function. *Am J Psychiatry* 1990;147:766.
16. Diokno AC, Brown MB, Herzog AR. Sexual function in the elderly. *Arch Intern Med* 1990;150:197.
17. Feldman HA, Goldstein I, Hatzichristou DG, Krane RJ, McKinlay JB. Impotence and its medical and psychosocial correlates: results of the Massachusetts Male Aging Study. *J Urol* 1994;151:54.
18. Thirlaway K, Fallowfield L, Cuzick J. The Sexual Activity Questionnaire: a measure of women's sexual functioning. *Qual Life Res* 1996;5:81.
19. McKinlay SM. The normal menopause transition: an overview. *Maturitas* 1996;23:137.
20. Greendale GA, Lee NP, Arriola ER. The menopause. *Lancet* 1999;353:571.
21. Braunstein GD. Androgen insufficiency in women: summary of critical issues. *Fertil Steril* 2002;77:94.
22. Greendale GA, Hogan P, Shumaker S. Sexual functioning in postmenopausal women: the postmenopausal estrogen/progestin interventions (PEPI) trial. *J Womens Health* 1996;5:445.
23. Ganz PA, Day R, Ware JE Jr, Redmond C, Fisher B. Base-line quality-of-life assessment in the National Surgical Adjuvant Breast and Bowel Project Breast Cancer Prevention Trial. *J Natl Cancer Inst* 1995;87:1372.
24. Myers LS, Dixen J, Morrissette D, Carmichael M, Davidson JM. Effects of estrogen, androgen, and progestin on sexual psychophysiology and behavior in postmenopausal women. *J Clin Endocrinol Metab* 1990;70:1124.
25. Sherwin BB. The impact of different doses of estrogen and progestin on mood and sexual behavior in postmenopausal women. *J Clin Endocrinol Metab* 1991;72:336.
26. Morales A, Tenover JL. Androgen deficiency in the aging male: when, who, and how to investigate and treat. *Urol Clin North Am* 2002;29:975.
27. Tenover JL. Testosterone and the aging male. *J Androl* 1997;18:103.
28. Helgason AR, Adolfsson J, Dickman P, et al. Factors associated with waning sexual function among elderly men and prostate cancer patients. *J Urol* 1997;158:155.
29. Schag CA, Ganz PA, Polinsky ML, et al. Characteristics of women at risk for psychosocial distress in the year after breast cancer. *J Clin Oncol* 1993;11:783.
30. Kornblith AB, Anderson J, Cella DF, et al. Hodgkin disease survivors at increased risk for problems in psychosocial adaptation. The Cancer and Leukemia Group B. *Cancer* 1992;70:2214.
31. Kornblith AB, Anderson J, Cella DF, et al. Comparison of psychosocial adaptation and sexual function of survivors of advanced Hodgkin disease treated by MOPP, ABVD, or MOPP alternating with ABVD. *Cancer* 1992;70:2508.
32. Kornblith AB, Herndon JE, Zuckerman E, et al. Comparison of psychosocial adaptation of advanced stage Hodgkin's disease and acute leukemia survivors. Cancer and Leukemia Group B. *Ann Oncol* 1998;9:297.
33. Cull A, Cowie VJ, Farquharson DI, et al. Early stage cervical cancer: psychosocial and sexual outcomes of treatment. *Br J Cancer* 1993;68:1216.
34. Mumma GH, Mashberg D, Lesko LM. Long-term psychosexual adjustment of acute leukemia survivors: impact of marrow transplantation versus conventional chemotherapy. *Gen Hosp Psychiatry* 1992;14:43.
35. Wood JD, Tombrink J. Impact of cancer on sexuality and self-image: a group program for patients and partners. *Soc Work Health Care* 1983;8:45.
36. Kiebert GM, de Haes JC, van de Velde CJ. The impact of breast-conserving treatment and mastectomy on the quality of life of early-stage breast cancer patients: a review. *J Clin Oncol* 1991;9:1059.
37. Moyer A. Psychosocial outcomes of breast-conserving surgery versus mastectomy: a meta-analytic review. *Health Psychol* 1997;16:284.
38. Ganz PA, Schag AC, Lee JJ, Polinsky ML, Tan SJ. Breast conservation versus mastectomy. Is there a difference in psychological adjustment or quality of life in the year after surgery? *Cancer* 1992;69:1729.
39. De Boer MF, McCormick LK, Pruyn JF, Ryckman RM, van den Borne BW. Physical and psychosocial correlates of head and neck cancer: a review of the literature. *Otolaryngol Head Neck Surg* 1999;120:427.
40. Sprangers MA, Taal BG, Aaronson NK, te Velde A. Quality of life in colorectal cancer. Stoma vs. nonstoma patients. *Dis Colon Rectum* 1995;38:361.
41. Ganz PA, Desmond KA, Belin TR, Meyerowitz BE, Rowland JH. Predictors of sexual health in women after a breast cancer diagnosis. *J Clin Oncol* 1999;17:2371.
42. Gritz ER, Wellisch DK, Wang HJ, et al. Long-term effects of testicular cancer on sexual functioning in married couples. *Cancer* 1989;64:1560.
43. Fobair P, Hoppe RT, Bloom J, et al. Psychosocial problems among survivors of Hodgkin's disease. *J Clin Oncol* 1986;4:805.
44. Goodwin PJ, Ennis M, Pritchard KI, et al. Adjuvant treatment and onset of menopause predict weight gain after breast cancer diagnosis. *J Clin Oncol* 1999;17:120.
45. Ganz PA, Schag CA, Lee JJ, Sim MS. The CARES: a generic measure of health-related quality of life for patients with cancer. *Qual Life Res* 1992;1:19.
46. Andrykowski MA, Curran SL, Lightner R. Off-treatment fatigue in breast cancer survivors: a controlled comparison. *J Behav Med* 1998;21:1.
47. Loge JH, Abrahamsen AF, Ekeberg O, Kaasa S. Hodgkin's disease survivors more fatigued than the general population. *J Clin Oncol* 1999;17:253.
48. Bower JE, Ganz PA, Desmond KA, et al. Fatigue in breast cancer survivors: occurrence, correlates, and impact on quality of life. *J Clin Oncol* 2000;18:743.
49. Ganz PA, Moinpour CM, Pauler DK, et al. Health status and quality of life in patients with early-stage Hodgkin's disease treated on Southwest Oncology Group Study 9133. *J Clin Oncol* 2003;21:3512.
50. Winer EP, Lindley C, Hardee M, et al. Quality of life in patients surviving at least 12 months following high dose chemotherapy with autologous bone marrow support. *Psychooncology* 1999;8:167.
51. Passik SD, Newman ML, Brennan M, Tunkel R. Predictors of psychological distress, sexual dysfunction and physical functioning among women with upper extremity lymphedema related to breast cancer. *Psychooncology* 1995;4:255.
52. Dorval M, Maunsell E, Taylor-Brown J, Kilpatrick M. Marital stability after breast cancer. *J Natl Cancer Inst* 1999;91:54.
53. Andrykowski MA, Curran SL, Studts JL, et al. Psychosocial adjustment and quality of life in women with breast cancer and benign breast problems: a controlled comparison. *J Clin Epidemiol* 1996;49:827.
54. Litwin MS, Hays RD, Fink A, et al. Quality-of-life outcomes in men treated for localized prostate cancer. *JAMA* 1995;273:129.
55. Byrne J, Fears TR, Steinhorn SC, et al. Marriage and divorce after childhood and adolescent cancer. *JAMA* 1989;262:2693.
56. Rauck AM, Green DM, Yasui Y, Mertens A, Robison LL. Marriage in the survivors of childhood cancer: a preliminary description from the Childhood Cancer Survivor Study. *Med Pediatr Oncol* 1999;33:60.
57. Walsh PC, Donker PJ. Impotence following radical prostatectomy: insight into etiology and prevention. *J Urol* 1982;128:492.
58. Venn SN, Popert RM, Mundy AR. "Nerve-sparing" cystectomy and substitution cystoplasty in patients of either sex: limitations and techniques. *Br J Urol* 1998;82:361.
59. Kinn AC, Ohman U. Bladder and sexual function after surgery for rectal cancer. *Dis Colon Rectum* 1986;29:43.
60. Litwin MS, Melmed GY, Nakazon T. Life after radical prostatectomy: a longitudinal study. *J Urol* 2001;166:587.
61. van Driel MF, Weymar Schultz WC, van de Wiel HB, Hahn DE, Mensink HJ. Female sexual functioning after radical surgical treatment of rectal and bladder cancer. *Eur J Surg Oncol* 1993;19:183.
62. Schover LR, von Eschenbach AC. Sexual function and female radical cystectomy: a case series. *J Urol* 1985;134:465.
63. Coogan CL, Hejase MJ, Wahle GR, et al. Nerve sparing post-chemotherapy retroperitoneal lymph node dissection for advanced testicular cancer. *J Urol* 1996;156:1656.
64. Donohue JP, Foster RS. Retroperitoneal lymphadenectomy in staging and treatment. The development of nerve-sparing techniques. *Urol Clin North Am* 1998;25:461.
65. Schover LR, Fife M. Sexual counseling of patients undergoing radical surgery for pelvic or genital cancer. *J Psychosoc Oncol* 1985;3:21.
66. Ganz PA, Rowland JH, Meyerowitz BE, Desmond KA. Impact of different adjuvant therapy strategies on quality of life in breast cancer survivors. *Recent Results Cancer Res* 1998;152:396.
67. Ganz PA, Rowland JH, Desmond K, Meyerowitz BE, Wyatt GE. Life after breast cancer: understanding women's health-related quality of life and sexual functioning. *J Clin Oncol* 1998;16:501.
68. Neitzert CS, Ritvo P, Dancey J, et al. The psychosocial impact of bone marrow transplantation: a review of the literature. *Bone Marrow Transplant* 1998;22:409.
69. Bines J, Oleske DM, Cobleigh MA. Ovarian function in premenopausal women treated with adjuvant chemotherapy for breast cancer. *J Clin Oncol* 1996;14:1718.
70. Knobf MK, Mullen JC, Xistris D, Moritz DA. Weight gain in women with breast cancer receiving adjuvant chemotherapy. *Oncol Nurs Forum* 1983;10:28.

71. Goodwin PJ, Ennis M, Pritchard KI, Trudeau M, Hood N. Risk of menopause during the first year after breast cancer diagnosis. *J Clin Oncol* 1999;17:2365.

72. Goldstein I, Feldman MI, Deckers PJ, Babayan RK, Krane RJ. Radiation-associated impotence. A clinical study of its mechanism. *JAMA* 1984;251:903.

73. Talcott JA, Rieker P, Clark JA, et al. Patient-reported symptoms after primary therapy for early prostate cancer: results of a prospective cohort study. *J Clin Oncol* 1998;16:275.

74. Beard CJ, Propert KJ, Rieker PP, et al. Complications after treatment with external-beam irradiation in early-stage prostate cancer patients: a prospective multiinstitutional outcomes study. *J Clin Oncol* 1997;15:223.

75. Zelefsky MJ, Fuks Z, Leibel SA. Intensity-modulated radiation therapy for prostate cancer. *Semin Radiat Oncol* 2002;12:229.

76. Merrick GS, Wallner KE, Butler WM. Permanent interstitial brachytherapy for the management of carcinoma of the prostate gland. *J Urol* 2003;169:1643.

77. Valicenti RK, Bissonette EA, Chen C, Theodorescu D. Longitudinal comparison of sexual function after 3-dimensional conformal radiation therapy or prostate brachytherapy. *J Urol* 2002;168:2499.

78. Day R, Ganz PA, Costantino JP, et al. Health-related quality of life and tamoxifen in breast cancer prevention: a report from the National Surgical Adjuvant Breast and Bowel Project P-1 Study. *J Clin Oncol* 1999;17:2659.

79. Fallowfield L, Fleissig A, Edwards R, et al. Tamoxifen for the prevention of breast cancer: psychosocial impact on women participating in two randomized controlled trials. *J Clin Oncol* 2001;19:1885.

80. Mortimer JE, Boucher L, Baty J, et al. Effect of tamoxifen on sexual functioning in patients with breast cancer. *J Clin Oncol* 1999;17:1488.

81. Kornblith AB, Hollis DR, Zuckerman E, et al. Effect of megestrol acetate on quality of life in a dose-response trial in women with advanced breast cancer. The Cancer and Leukemia Group B. *J Clin Oncol* 1993;11:2081.

82. Berglund G, Nystedt M, Bolund C, Sjoden PO, Rutquist LE. Effect of endocrine treatment on sexuality in premenopausal breast cancer patients: a prospective randomized study. *J Clin Oncol* 2001;19:2788.

83. Nystedt M, Berglund G, Bolund C, Fornander T, Rutqvist LE. Side effects of adjuvant endocrine treatment in premenopausal breast cancer patients: a prospective randomized study. *J Clin Oncol* 2003;21:1836.

84. Smith IE, Dowsett M. Aromatase inhibitors in breast cancer. *N Engl J Med* 2003;348:2431.

85. Huggins C, Hodges CV. Studies in prostate cancer. I. The effects of castration, of estrogen and androgen injection on serum phosphatases in metastatic carcinoma of the prostate. *Cancer Res* 1941;1:293.

86. Cassileth BR, Soloway MS, Vogelzang NJ, et al. Quality of life and psychosocial status in stage D prostate cancer. Zoladex Prostate Cancer Study Group. *Qual Life Res* 1992;1:323.

87. Anderson J. The role of antiandrogen monotherapy in the treatment of prostate cancer. *BJU Int* 2003;91:455.

88. Byrne J, Mulvihill JJ, Myers MH, et al. Effects of treatment on fertility in long-term survivors of childhood or adolescent cancer. *N Engl J Med* 1987;317:1315.

89. Sklar CA, Robison LL, Nesbit ME, et al. Effects of radiation on testicular function in long-term survivors of childhood acute lymphoblastic leukemia: a report from the Children Cancer Study Group. *J Clin Oncol* 1990;8:1981.

90. Muller HL, Klinkhammer-Schalke M, Seelbach-Gobel B, Hartmann AA, Kuhl J. Gonadal function of young adults after therapy of malignancies during childhood or adolescence. *Eur J Pediatr* 1996;155:763.

91. Brewer M, Gershenson DM, Herzog CE, et al. Outcome and reproductive function after chemotherapy for ovarian dysgerminoma. *J Clin Oncol* 1999;17:2670.

92. Kreuser ED, Hetzel WD, Billia DO, Thiel E. Gonadal toxicity following cancer therapy in adults: significance, diagnosis, prevention and treatment. *Cancer Treat Rev* 1990;17:169.

93. Viviani S, Santoro A, Ragni G, et al. Gonadal toxicity after combination chemotherapy for Hodgkin's disease. Comparative results of MOPP vs ABVD. *Eur J Cancer Clin Oncol* 1985;21:601.

94. Schover LR, Brey K, Lichtin A, Lipshultz LI, Jeha S. Oncologists' attitudes and practices regarding banking sperm before cancer treatment. *J Clin Oncol* 2002;20:1890.

95. Schover LR, Brey K, Lichtin A, Lipshultz LI, Jeha S. Knowledge and experience regarding cancer, infertility, and sperm banking in younger male survivors. *J Clin Oncol* 2002;20:1880.

96. Opsahl MS, Fugger EF, Sherins RJ, Schulman JD. Preservation of reproductive function before therapy for cancer: new options involving sperm and ovary cryopreservation. *Cancer J Sci Am* 1997;3:189.

97. Oktay K, Newton H, Gosden RG. Transplantation of cryopreserved human ovarian tissue results in follicle growth initiation in SCID mice. *Fertil Steril* 2000;73:599.

98. Janov AJ, Anderson J, Cella DF, et al. Pregnancy outcome in survivors of advanced Hodgkin disease. *Cancer* 1992;70:688.

99. Mulvihill JJ, McKeen EA, Rosner F, Zarrabi MH. Pregnancy outcome in cancer patients. Experience in a large cooperative group. *Cancer* 1987;60:1143.

100. Lippman ME, Hayes DF. Adjuvant therapy for all patients with breast cancer? *J Natl Cancer Inst* 2001;93:80.

101. Maunsell E, Brisson J, Deschenes L. Psychological distress after initial treatment for breast cancer: a comparison of partial and total mastectomy. *J Clin Epidemiol* 1989;42:765.

102. Wolberg WH, Romsaas EP, Tanner MA, Malec JF. Psychosexual adaptation to breast cancer surgery. *Cancer* 1989;63:1645.

103. Fallowfield LJ, Hall A. Psychosocial and sexual impact of diagnosis and treatment of breast cancer. *Br Med Bull* 1991;47:388.

104. Schain WS, d'Angelo TM, Dunn ME, Lichter AS, Pierce LJ. Mastectomy versus conservative surgery and radiation therapy. Psychosocial consequences. *Cancer* 1994;73:1221.

105. Schover LR, Yetman RJ, Tuason LJ, et al. Partial mastectomy and breast reconstruction. A comparison of their effects on psychosocial adjustment, body image, and sexuality. *Cancer* 1995;75:54.

106. Rowland JH, Desmond KA, Meyerowitz BE, et al. Role of breast reconstructive surgery in physical and emotional outcomes among breast cancer survivors. *J Natl Cancer Inst* 2000;92:1422.

107. Hawton K, Gath D, Day A. Sexual function in a community sample of middle-aged women with partners: effects of age, marital, socioeconomic, psychiatric, gynecological, and menopausal factors. *Arch Sex Behav* 1994;23:375.

108. Rosen RC, Taylor JF, Leiblum SR, Bachmann GA. Prevalence of sexual dysfunction in women: results of a survey study of 329 women in an outpatient gynecological clinic. *J Sex Marital Ther* 1993;19:171.

109. Sarrel PM. Sexuality and menopause. *Obstet Gynecol* 1990;75(4 Suppl):26S.

110. Cyranowski JM, Andersen BL. Schemas, sexuality, and romantic attachment. *J Pers Soc Psychol* 1998;74:1364.

111. Kaplan HS. A neglected issue: the sexual side effects of current treatments for breast cancer. *J Sex Marital Ther* 1992;18:3.

112. Schover LR. The impact of breast cancer on sexuality, body image, and intimate relationships. *CA Cancer J Clin* 1991;41:112.

113. Ganz PA. Impact of tamoxifen adjuvant therapy on symptoms, functioning, and quality of life. *J Natl Cancer Inst Monogr* 2001;(30):130.

114. Schover LR. Sexuality and body image in younger women with breast cancer. *J Natl Cancer Inst Monogr* 1994;(16):177.

115. Dorval M, Maunsell E, Deschenes L, Brisson J, Masse B. Long-term quality of life after breast cancer: comparison of 8-year survivors with population controls. *J Clin Oncol* 1998;16:487.

116. Meyerowitz BE, Desmond KA, Rowland JH, Wyatt GE, Ganz PA. Sexuality following breast cancer. *J Sex Marital Ther* 1999;25:237.

117. Lindley C, Vasa S, Sawyer WT, Winer EP. Quality of life and preferences for treatment following systemic adjuvant therapy for early-stage breast cancer. *J Clin Oncol* 1998;16:1380.

118. Widmark A, Fransson P, Tavelin B. Self-assessment questionnaire for evaluating urinary and intestinal late side effects after pelvic radiotherapy in patients with prostate cancer compared with an age-matched control population. *Cancer* 1994;74:2520.

119. Fransson P, Widmark A. Self-assessed sexual function after pelvic irradiation for prostate carcinoma. Comparison with an age-matched control group. *Cancer* 1996;78:1066.

120. Fowler FJ Jr, Barry MJ, Lu-Yao G, et al. Patient-reported complications and follow-up treatment after radical prostatectomy. The National Medicare Experience: 1988–1990 (updated June 1993). *Urology* 1993;42:622.

121. Fowler FJ Jr, Barry MJ, Lu-Yao G, et al. Effect of radical prostatectomy for prostate cancer on patient quality of life: results from a Medicare survey. *Urology* 1995;45:1007.

122. Fowler FJ Jr, Barry MJ, Lu-Yao G, Wasson JH, Bin L. Outcomes of external-beam radiation therapy for prostate cancer: a study of Medicare beneficiaries in three surveillance, epidemiology, and end results areas. *J Clin Oncol* 1996;14:2258.

123. Talcott JA. Quality of life in early prostate cancer. Do we know enough to treat? *Hematol Oncol Clin North Am* 1996;10:691.

124. Crook J, Esche B, Futter N. Effect of pelvic radiotherapy for prostate cancer on bowel, bladder, and sexual function: the patient's perspective. *Urology* 1996;47:387.

125. Turner SL, Adams K, Bull CA, Berry MP. Sexual dysfunction after radical radiation therapy for prostate cancer: a prospective evaluation. *Urology* 1999;54:124.

126. Litwin MS, Flanders SC, Pasta DJ, et al. Sexual function and bother after radical prostatectomy or radiation for prostate cancer: multivariate quality-of-life analysis from CaPSURE. Cancer of the Prostate Strategic Urologic Research Endeavor. *Urology* 1999;54:503.

127. Schover LR. Sexuality and fertility in urologic cancer patients. *Cancer* 1987;60(Suppl 3):553.

128. Rieker PP, Edbril SD, Garnick MB. Curative testis cancer therapy: psychosocial sequelae. *J Clin Oncol* 1985;3:1117.

129. Rieker PP, Fitzgerald EM, Kalish LA, et al. Psychosocial factors, curative therapies, and behavioral outcomes. A comparison of testis cancer survivors and a control group of healthy men. *Cancer* 1989;64:2399.

130. Incrocci L, Hop WCJ, Wijnmaalen A, Slob AK. Treatment outcome, body image, and sexual functioning after orchiectomy and radiotherapy for stage I–II testicular seminoma. *Int J Radiat Oncol Biol Phys* 2002;53:1165.

131. Jonker-Pool G, van de Wiel HB, Hoekstra HJ, et al. Sexual functioning after treatment for testicular cancer—review and meta-analysis of 36 empirical studies between 1975–2000. *Arch Sex Behav* 2001;30:55.

132. Schover LR, Evans R, von Eschenbach AC. Sexual rehabilitation and male radical cystectomy. *J Urol* 1986;136:1015.

133. Mansson A, Johnson G, Mansson W. Quality of life after cystectomy. Comparison between patients with conduit and those with continent caecal reservoir urinary diversion. *Br J Urol* 1988;62:240.

134. Boyd SD, Feinberg SM, Skinner DG, et al. Quality of life survey of urinary diversion patients: comparison of ileal conduits versus continent Kock ileal reservoirs. *J Urol* 1987;138:1386.

135. Gerharz EW, Weingartner K, Dopatka T, et al. Quality of life after cystectomy and urinary diversion: results of a retrospective interdisciplinary study. *J Urol* 1997;158(3 Pt 1):778.

136. Hart S, Skinner EC, Meyerowitz BE, et al. Quality of life after radical cystectomy for bladder cancer in patients with an ileal conduit, cutaneous or urethral Kock pouch. *J Urol* 1999;162:77.

137. Andersen BL, Lachenbruch PA, Anderson B, deProsse C. Sexual dysfunction and signs of gynecologic cancer. *Cancer* 1986;57:1880.

138. Andersen BL. Sexual functioning complications in women with gynecologic cancer. Outcomes and directions for prevention. *Cancer* 1987;60(Suppl 8):2123.

139. Andersen BL, Anderson B, deProsse C. Controlled prospective longitudinal study of women with cancer: I. Sexual functioning outcomes. *J Consult Clin Psychol* 1989;57:683.

140. Schover LR, Fife M, Gershenson DM. Sexual dysfunction and treatment for early stage cervical cancer. *Cancer* 1989;63:204.

141. Bruner DW, Lanciano R, Keegan M, et al. Vaginal stenosis and sexual function following intracavitary radiation for the treatment of cervical and endometrial carcinoma. *Int J Radiat Oncol Biol Phys* 1993;27:825.

142. Flay LD, Matthews JH. The effects of radiotherapy and surgery on the sexual function of women treated for cervical cancer. *Int J Radiat Oncol Biol Phys* 1995;31:399.

143. Robinson JW, Faris PD, Scott CB. Psychoeducational group increases vaginal dilation for younger women and reduces sexual fears for women of all ages with gynecological carcinoma treated with radiotherapy. *Int J Radiat Oncol Biol Phys* 1999;44:497.

144. Bergmark K, Avall-Lundqvist E, Dickman PW, Henningsohn L, Steineck G. Vaginal changes and sexuality in women with a history of cervical cancer. *N Engl J Med* 1999;340:1383.

145. Ganz PA. Overview—quality of life assessment and issues. In: Sharp F, Blackett T, Berek J, Bast R, eds. *Ovarian cancer 5.* Oxford: Isis Medical Media, 1998:409.

146. Andersen BL, Turnquist D, LaPolla J, Turner D. Sexual functioning after treatment of in situ vulvar cancer: preliminary report. *Obstet Gynecol* 1988;71:15.

147. Weijmar Schultz WC, van de Wiel HB, et al. Psychosexual functioning after the treatment of cancer of the vulva. A longitudinal study. *Cancer* 1990;66:402.

148. Koukouras D, Spiliotis J, Scopa CD, et al. Radical consequence in the sexuality of male patients operated for colorectal carcinoma. *Eur J Surg Oncol* 1991;17:285.

149. Rosen RC, Leiblum SR. Treatment of sexual disorders in the 1990s: an integrated approach. *J Consult Clin Psychol* 1995;63:877.

150. Schover LR, Jensen SB. *Sexuality and chronic illness: a comprehensive approach.* New York: Gilford Press, 1988.

151. Daker-White G. Reliable and valid self-report outcome measures in sexual (dys)function: a systematic review. *Arch Sex Behav* 2002;31:197.

152. Loehr J, Verma S, Seguin R. Issues of sexuality in older women. *J Womens Health* 1997;6:451.

153. Stead ML, Brown JM, Fallowfield L, Selby P. Lack of communication between healthcare professionals and women with ovarian cancer about sexual issues. *Br J Cancer* 2003;88:666.

154. Read S, King M, Watson J. Sexual dysfunction in primary medical care: prevalence, characteristics and detection by the general practitioner. *J Public Health Med* 1997;19:387.

155. Annon J. *Behavioral treatment of sexual problems.* Honolulu, HI: Enabling Systems, 1974.

156. Schover LR. *Sexuality and fertility after cancer.* New York: John Wiley & Sons, 1997.

157. Syrjala KL, Roth-Roemer SL, Abrams JR, et al. Prevalence and predictors of sexual dysfunction in long-term survivors of marrow transplantation. *J Clin Oncol* 1998;16:3148.

158. Nachtigall LE. Comparative study: Replens versus local estrogen in menopausal women. *Fertil Steril* 1994;61:178.

159. Loprinzi CL, Abu-Ghazaleh S, Sloan JA, et al. Phase III randomized double-blind study to evaluate the efficacy of a polycarbophil-based vaginal moisturizer in women with breast cancer. *J Clin Oncol* 1997;15:969.

160. Holmgren PA, Lindskog M, von Schoultz B. Vaginal rings for continuous low-dose release of oestradiol in the treatment of urogenital atrophy. *Maturitas* 1989;11:55.

161. Ganz PA, Greendale GA, Petersen L, et al. Managing menopausal symptoms in breast cancer survivors: results of a randomized controlled trial. *J Natl Cancer Inst* 2000;92:1054.

162. Zibecchi L, Greendale GA, Ganz PA. Continuing education: comprehensive menopausal assessment: an approach to managing vasomotor and urogenital symptoms in breast cancer survivors. *Oncol Nurs Forum* 2003;30:393.

163. Schover LR. Sexual rehabilitation after treatment for prostate cancer. *Cancer* 1993;71(Suppl 3):1024.

164. Meinhardt W, Kropman RF, Vermeij P. Comparative tolerability and efficacy of treatments for impotence. *Drug Saf* 1999;20:133.

165. Lowentritt BH, Scardino PT, Miles BJ, et al. Sildenafil citrate after radical retropubic prostatectomy. *J Urol* 1999;162:1614.

166. Incrocci L, Slob AK, Levendag PC. Sexual (dys)function after radiotherapy for prostate cancer: a review. *Int J Radiat Oncol Biol Phys* 2002;52:681.

167. Incrocci L, Hop WC, Slob AK. Efficacy of sildenafil in an open-label study as a continuation of a double-blind study in the treatment of erectile dysfunction after radiotherapy for prostate cancer. *Urology* 2003;62:116.

168. Valicenti RK, Choi E, Chen C, et al. Sildenafil citrate effectively reverses sexual dysfunction induced by three-dimensional conformal radiation therapy. *Urology* 2001;57:769.

169. Raina R, Agarwal A, Goyal KK, et al. Long-term potency after iodine-125 radiotherapy for prostate cancer and role of sildenafil citrate. *Urology* 2003;62:1103.

170. Goldstein I, Lue TF, Padma-Nathan H, et al. Oral sildenafil in the treatment of erectile dysfunction. Sildenafil Study Group. *N Engl J Med* 1998;338:1397.

171. Earle CM, Seah M, Coulden SE, Stuckey BG, Keogh EJ. The use of the vacuum erection device in the management of erectile impotence. *Int J Impot Res* 1996;8:237.

172. Turner LA, Althof SE, Levine SB, et al. Treating erectile dysfunction with external vacuum devices: impact upon sexual, psychological and marital functioning. *J Urol* 1990;144:79.

173. Godschalk MF, Chen J, Katz PG, Mulligan T. Treatment of erectile failure with prostaglandin E1: a double-blind, placebo-controlled, dose-response study. *J Urol* 1994;151:1530.

174. Padma-Nathan H, Hellstrom WJ, Kaiser FE, et al. Treatment of men with erectile dysfunction with transurethral alprostadil. Medicated Urethral System for Erection (MUSE) Study Group. *N Engl J Med* 1997;336:1.

175. Montague DK. Penile prostheses. An overview. *Urol Clin North Am* 1989;16:7.

SECTION 4

ELLEN T. MATLOFF

Genetic Counseling

Clinically based genetic testing has become widely available in the past decade and has brought with it a growing demand for accurate risk assessment and cancer genetic counseling. Extensive coverage of this topic by the media and widespread advertising by commercial testing laboratories has further fueled the demand for counseling and testing.

The field of cancer genetic counseling is evolving rapidly to meet the newfound needs of patients and the medical community. Cancer genetic counseling is a communication process between a health care professional and an individual concerning cancer occurrence and risk in his or her family.[1] The process, which may include the entire family through a blend of genetic, medical, and psychosocial assessment and intervention, has been described as a bridge between the fields of traditional oncology and genetic counseling.[1]

The goals of this process include providing the client with an assessment of individual cancer risk, while offering the emotional support needed to understand and cope with this information.[2] It also involves deciphering whether the cancers in a family are likely to be caused by a mutation in a cancer gene and, if so, which one. To achieve the informed consent crucial to the testing process, each patient is thoroughly counseled about the associated risks, benefits, and limitations of testing. If the patient is interested in pursuing testing, the counselor identifies a laboratory that offers appropriate genetic testing and facilitates sample collection and shipping and interpretation of test result. The result disclosure session includes detailed counseling about medical management options for early detection and risk reduction and may include referrals to prevention trials, surveillance programs, and medical specialists.

Counselors find that this process differs from "traditional" genetic counseling in several ways. Clients seeking cancer genetic counseling are rarely concerned with the reproductive decisions and risks that are often the primary focus in traditional genetic counseling but are instead seeking information about their own and other relatives' chances of developing cancer.[3] In addition, the risks given are not absolute but change over time as the family and personal history changes and the patient ages. The risk reduction options available are often radical (e.g., chemoprevention or prophylactic surgery) and are not appropriate for every patient at every age. The ultimate goal of cancer genetic counseling is to help the patient reach the decision best suited to his or her personal situation, needs, and circumstances.

WHY IS CANCER GENETIC COUNSELING NECESSARY?

Advances in genetic testing have brought new opportunities for tailoring a patient's medical management to the patient's risks, but also new challenges. There are complex medical and psychological consequences of cancer genetic testing that affect the patient and the entire family. Potential clients must be made aware of these risks *before* testing and, when possible, assisted in avoiding pitfalls. Commercial genetic testing companies are campaigning actively to sell test kits both to medical providers and directly to consumers.[4] These marketing campaigns have been called misleading and manipulative and have the potential to persuade providers and patients to order tests that may not be appropriate or that they do not have the ability to interpret accurately.[4] Therefore, the need for accurate genetic counseling—by qualified professionals who do not have a conflict of interest in selling test kits—is more important than ever.

There are a limited number of referral centers across the country specializing in cancer genetic counseling, but the numbers are growing. Graduate programs in genetic counseling are actively integrating this new body of knowledge into their curricula and are producing more counselors who can provide cancer services. However, some experts insist that the only way to keep up with the overwhelming demand for counseling is to educate more physicians and nurses in cancer genetics.[5] The feasibility of adding another specialized and time-consuming task to the clinical burden of these professionals is questionable. A more practical goal may be to better educate primary care providers in the area of generalized risk assessment so that they can screen their patient populations for individuals at high risk for hereditary cancer and refer them on to comprehensive counseling and testing programs.

WHO IS A CANDIDATE FOR CANCER GENETIC COUNSELING?

Only 5% to 10% of most cancers are due to mutations within inherited cancer susceptibility genes.[6] The key for the clinician is to determine which patients are at greatest risk of carrying a hereditary mutation. There are six risk factors that are common in hereditary cancer syndromes (Table 55.4-1). The first is early age of cancer onset. This risk factor, even in the absence of a family history, has been shown to be associated with an increased frequency of germline mutations in many types of cancers.[7,8] The second risk factor is the presence of the same cancer in multiple relatives on the same side of the pedigree. These cancers do not need to be of similar histologic type to be caused by a single mutation. The third risk factor is the clustering of cancers known to be caused by a single gene mutation in one family (e.g., breast and ovarian cancers or colon, ovarian, and uterine cancers). The fourth risk factor is the occurrence

TABLE 55.4-1. Risk Factors for Hereditary Cancer Syndromes

Early age of onset (e.g., <45 y for breast cancer; <50 y for colon cancer)

Multiple family members on the same side of the pedigree with the same cancer

Clustering of cancers in the family known to be caused by a single gene mutation (e.g., breast and ovarian cancers; colon, uterine, and ovarian cancers)

Multiple primary cancers in one individual (e.g., breast and ovarian cancer; multiple primary colon cancers)

Ethnicity (e.g., Jewish ancestry for breast and ovarian cancer syndrome)

Unusual presentation of cancer (e.g., breast cancer in a male)

of multiple primary cancers in one individual. This includes multiple primary breast and colon cancers as well as separate cancers known to be caused by a single gene mutation (e.g., breast and ovarian cancer in a single individual). Ethnicity also plays a role in determining who is at greatest risk for carrying a hereditary cancer mutation. Individuals of Jewish ancestry are at increased risk to carry three specific BRCA1/2 mutations[9] and the I1307K APC allele.[10] The final risk factor for a hereditary cancer syndrome is the presence of a cancer that presents unusually, the prime example of which is breast cancer in a male. These risk factors should be viewed in the context of the entire family history and must be weighed in proportion to the number of individuals who have not developed cancer.

A less common, but extremely important, finding is the presence of birth defects or unusual physical findings that are known to be associated with rare hereditary cancer syndromes. Examples include benign skin findings and thyroid disorders in Cowden disease, sebaceous skin tumors in Muir-Torre syndrome, and desmoid tumors or dental abnormalities in familial adenomatous polyposis (FAP).[11]

At the present time, breast-ovarian cancer syndrome referrals account for the majority of patients seen in the average cancer genetic counseling clinic. In this chapter, the breast-ovarian cancer counseling session will serve as a paradigm that all other sessions may follow broadly.

COMPONENTS OF THE CANCER GENETIC COUNSELING SESSION

PRECOUNSELING INFORMATION

Before coming in for genetic counseling, the counselee should be given some basic information about the process. This information, which can be imparted by telephone or in the form of written material, should outline what the counselee can expect at each session and what information he or she should collect before the first visit. The counselee can then begin to collect medical and family history information and pathology reports that will be essential for the genetic counseling session.

FAMILY HISTORY

An accurate family history is undoubtedly one of the most essential components of the cancer genetic counseling session. Optimally, a family history should include at least three generations; however, patients do not always have this information. For each individual affected with cancer, it is important to document the exact diagnosis, age at diagnosis, treatment strategies, and environmental exposures (i.e., occupational exposures, exposure to cigarettes or other agents).[11] The current age of the individual and the laterality and occurrence of any other cancers must also be documented.[3] Individuals should be asked if there are any consanguineous (inbred) relationships in the family, if any relatives were born with birth defects or mental retardation, and whether other genetic diseases run in the family, because these pieces of information could prove important in reaching a diagnosis. Cancer diagnoses should be confirmed with pathologic reports whenever possible. A study by Love et al.[12] revealed that individuals accurately reported the primary site of cancer only 83% of the time in their first-degree relatives with cancer and

67% and 60% of the time in second- and third-degree relatives, respectively. It is common for patients to report a uterine cancer as an ovarian cancer or a colon polyp as an invasive colorectal cancer. These differences, although seemingly subtle to the patient, can make a tremendous difference in risk assessment.

The most common misconception in family history taking is that somehow a maternal family history of breast, ovarian, or uterine cancer is more significant than a paternal history. Conversely, many still believe that a paternal history of prostate cancer is more significant than a maternal history. Few cancer genes discovered thus far are located on the sex chromosomes, and therefore both maternal and paternal histories are significant and must be explored thoroughly. Patients should be encouraged to report changes in their family history over time (e.g., new cancer diagnoses, genetic testing results in relatives), because this may change their risk assessment and counseling.

DYSMORPHOLOGY SCREENING

Congenital anomalies, benign tumors, and unusual dermatologic features occur in a large number of hereditary cancer predisposition syndromes. Examples include osteomas of the jaw in FAP, palmar pits in Gorlin's syndrome, and papillomas of the lips and mucous membranes in Cowden disease. Obtaining an accurate past medical history of benign lesions and birth defects, and screening for such dysmorphology can greatly impact diagnosis and counseling. For example, BRCA1/2 testing is inappropriate in a patient with breast cancer who has a family history of thyroid cancer and the orocutaneous manifestations of Cowden disease.

RISK ASSESSMENT

Risk assessment is one of the most complicated components of the genetic counseling session. It is crucial to remember that risk assessment changes over time as the person ages and as the health statuses of their family members change.[3]

Risk assessment can be broken down into three separate components:

1. What is the chance that the counselee will develop the cancer observed in his or her family (or a genetically related cancer)?
2. What is the chance that the cancers in this family are caused by a single gene mutation?
3. What is the chance that the gene mutation in this family can be identified with current knowledge and laboratory techniques?

Cancer clustering in a family may be due to genetic or environmental factors or both, or may be coincidental, because some cancers are very common in the general population. Although inherited factors may be the primary cause of cancers in some families, in others, cancer may develop because an inherited factor increases the individual's susceptibility to environmental carcinogens.[13] It is also possible that members of the same family may have similar environmental exposures, due to shared geography or patterns in behavior and diet, that may increase the risk of cancer.[14] Therefore, it is important to distinguish the difference between a familial pattern of cancer (due to environmental factors or chance) and a hereditary pattern of cancer (due to a shared genetic mutation).

Several models are available to calculate the chance that a woman will develop breast cancer. Each model has its strengths and weaknesses, and the counselor must decide which model is most appropriate for each individual family. The Gail model takes into account current age, age at first menses, age at first live birth, and number of previous biopsies when calculating risk.[15] Although this model is useful in determining entry into clinical trials, its use is *not appropriate* in families in which there is a question of a hereditary cancer syndrome. The Gail model considers only first-degree relatives in its calculations and therefore does not take into account paternal family history and extended family members. It does not weigh age at breast cancer diagnosis, occurrence of ovarian cancer, Jewish ancestry, occurrence of male breast cancer, and other factors essential in hereditary risk assessment and is therefore not the appropriate tool when hereditary cancer is in question.

The Claus model allows calculation of a woman's empiric chance of developing breast cancer, by decade and lifetime, based on some aspects of maternal and paternal family history.[16] This model does not take into account ancestry, occurrence of ovarian cancer, or extended family history, and is therefore not useful in families in which there appears to be a genetic mutation. Of course, all empiric risks become moot in families in which DNA testing has revealed a mutation for cancer predisposition.

Several other models, including a computer-based model, are available that help to determine the chance that a BRCA mutation will be found in a family.[17] These models can be helpful in determining the probability that a mutation will be found but cannot factor in other risks that may be essential in hereditary risk calculation (e.g., presence of a sister who was diagnosed with breast cancer after radiation treatment for Hodgkin's disease).

DNA TESTING

DNA testing is now available for a variety of hereditary cancer syndromes. However, despite misrepresentation by the media,[18] testing is feasible for only a small percentage of individuals with cancer. DNA testing offers the important advantage of presenting clients with *actual risks* instead of the empiric risks derived from risk calculation models. DNA testing can be very expensive (full BRCA1/2 testing currently costs more than $2900); therefore, insurance authorization should be obtained before testing is ordered. Obtaining this authorization often requires submission of a letter of medical necessity and a pedigree, and the process can take several weeks or months to complete.

The results of DNA testing are generally provided in person in a result disclosure session. It is recommended that patients bring a close friend or relative with them to this session who can provide them with emotional support and who can help them listen to and process the information provided.

One of most crucial aspects of DNA testing is accurate result interpretation. One study found that test results for the hereditary colon cancer syndrome FAP were misinterpreted more than 30% of the time by those ordering the testing.[19] More recent data have shown that many medical providers have difficulty interpreting even basic pedigrees and genetic test results.[20] This is particularly concerning in an era in which testing companies are canvassing physicians' offices and are encouraging them to perform their own counseling and testing. The potential impact of test results on the patient and his or her family is great, and therefore accurate interpretation of the results is paramount.

Results of genetic testing fall into four categories:

1. *True positive:* An individual is found to carry a mutation that is known to be deleterious.
2. *True negative:* An individual is found not to carry the deleterious mutation found in his or her family, and therefore the individual's cancer risks are reduced to the population risks.
3. *Uninformative:* A mutation cannot be found in affected family members of a family in which the cancer pattern appears to be hereditary; there is likely an undetectable mutation within the gene, or the family carries a mutation in a gene different from the ones tested. These results are not "true negative" and do *not* mean that the cancers are not hereditary.
4. *Variant of uncertain significance:* A genetic change is identified whose significance is unknown. It is helpful to test other affected family members to see if the mutation segregates with disease in the family. If it does not segregate, the variant is less likely to be significant. If it does, the variant is more likely to be significant. It is rarely helpful (and can be detrimental) to test unaffected family members for such variants.

To pinpoint the mutation in a family, an affected individual most likely to carry the mutation should be tested first, whenever possible. This is most often a person affected with the cancer in question. Test subjects should be selected with care, because it is possible for a person to develop sporadic cancer in a hereditary cancer family. For example, in a family with early-onset breast cancer it would not be ideal to first test a woman diagnosed with breast cancer at age 65 years, because she may represent a sporadic case.

If a mutation is detected in an affected relative, other family members can be tested for the same mutation with a great degree of accuracy. Family members who do not carry the mutation found in their family are deemed "true negative." Those who are found to carry the mutation in their family have more definitive information about their risks to develop cancer. This information can be crucial in assisting patients in decision making regarding surveillance and risk reduction.

If a mutation is not identified in the affected relative, it usually means that either the cancers in the family (1) are not hereditary or (2) are caused by an undetectable mutation or a mutation in a gene different from the ones tested. A careful review of the family history and the risk factors will help to decipher whether interpretation (1) or (2) is more likely. In cases in which the cancers appear hereditary and no mutation is found, DNA banking should be offered to the proband for a time in the future when improved testing may become available. A notarized letter indicating exactly who in the family has access to the DNA should accompany the banked sample.

The penetrance of mutations in cancer susceptibility genes is also difficult to interpret. Initial estimates derived from high-risk families indicated very high cancer risks for BRCA1 and BRCA2 mutation carriers.[21] More recent studies done on populations that were not selected for family history have revealed lower penetrances.[22] Some have interpreted these population-based data as being "more accurate" and have suggested that they apply to all families. In fact, the higher range of risk may be more accurate for families who present with strong histories of breast and ovarian cancer. Because exact penetrance rates cannot be determined for individual families at this time, it is prudent to provide patients with a range of cancer risk and to explain that their risk probably falls somewhere within this spectrum.

Female carriers of BRCA1/2 mutations have a 50% to 85% lifetime risk to develop breast cancer and between a 15% and 60% lifetime risk to develop ovarian cancer.[9,21,22] It is important to note that the classification *ovarian cancer* also includes cancer of the fallopian tubes and primary peritoneal carcinoma.[23,24] Carriers of hereditary nonpolyposis colorectal cancer (HNPCC) gene mutations have a 65% to 85% lifetime risk to develop colon cancer, and female carriers have at least a 30% to 40% lifetime risk of uterine cancer and as high as a 10% risk of ovarian cancer.[25,26]

OPTIONS FOR SURVEILLANCE AND RISK REDUCTION

The cancer risk counseling session is a forum to provide counselees with information, support, options, and hope. Mutation carriers can be offered earlier and more aggressive surveillance, chemoprevention plus surveillance, or prophylactic surgery.

It is recommended that individuals at increased risk for breast cancer have annual mammograms beginning between the ages of 25 and 35 and annual or semiannual clinical breast examinations, and perform monthly breast self-examinations.[27] BRCA1/2 carriers may take tamoxifen in hopes of reducing their risks of developing breast cancer. Tamoxifen has proven effective in women at risk due to a positive family history of breast cancer, and there are limited data to suggest that it may reduce risk in BRCA1/2 carriers, although this requires further investigation.[28–30] Prophylactic bilateral mastectomy appears to reduce the risk of breast cancer by more than 90% in women at high risk for the disease.[31] Before genetic testing was available, it was not uncommon for entire generations of cancer families to have their at-risk organs removed without individuals' knowing if they were *personally* at increased risk for their familial cancer. Fifty percent of individuals in hereditary cancer families will *not* carry the inherited predisposition gene and can be spared prophylactic surgery or invasive high-risk surveillance regimens. Therefore, it is clearly not appropriate to offer prophylactic surgery until a patient is referred for genetic counseling and, if possible, testing (Table 55.4-2).[32]

Women who carry BRCA1/2 mutations are also at increased risk to develop second contralateral and ipsilateral primaries of the breast.[33] These data bring into question the option of breast-conserving surgery in women at high risk to develop a second primary within the same breast. For this reason, BRCA1/2 carrier status can have a profound impact on surgical decision making.[32]

Women who carry BRCA1/2 mutations are also at increased risk to develop ovarian, fallopian tube, and primary peritoneal cancer, even if no one in their families has developed these cancers. Surveillance for ovarian cancer is complex, with the recommended interventions being annual transvaginal ultrasonography and measurement of cancer antigen 125 levels beginning between the ages of 25 and 35 years.[27] The effectiveness of such surveillance in detecting ovarian cancers at early, more treatable stages has not been proven in any population. Some data have indicated that oral contraceptive use reduces the risk of ovarian cancer in women carrying BRCA mutations.[34] The impact of this intervention on breast cancer risk is not known. However, it is possible that, given the difficulties in screening and treatment of

TABLE 55.4-2.   Cancer Genetic Counseling and Testing Resources

---

CANCERNET
(800) 4-CANCER
(800) 422-6237
http://www.cancer.gov/search/geneticsservices/
A free service designed to aid in locating providers of cancer risk counseling and testing services.

FORCE (FACING OUR RISK OF CANCER EMPOWERED)
(866) 824-RISK
(866) 824-7475
http://www.facingourrisk.org/
A nonprofit organization that offers education and support to individuals who are at risk for, or are known to carry, BRCA mutations.

GENETESTS
(206) 616-4033
http://www.genetests.org
A genetic testing resource offering current information on laboratories and testing availability for specific conditions.

NATIONAL SOCIETY OF GENETIC COUNSELORS
(610) 872-7608
http://www.nsgc.org
Offers a listing of genetic counselors in user's area who specialize in cancer.

---

ovarian cancer, a risk-benefit analysis would favor the use of oral contraceptives in carriers of BRCA1/2 mutations.[14] Prophylactic bilateral salpingo-oophorectomy (BSO) is currently the most effective means to reduce the risk of ovarian cancer, but even women who have had this procedure may develop primary peritoneal carcinoma.[23,35] There has been some debate about whether BRCA1/2 carriers should opt for total abdominal hysterectomies or BSO due to the fact that small stumps of the fallopian tubes remain after BSO alone. The question of whether or not BRCA carriers are at increased risk for uterine serous papillary carcinoma has also been raised.[36–38] If a relationship does exist between BRCA mutations and uterine cancer, the risk appears to be low and not elevated over that of the general population.[39] Removing the uterus may make it possible for a BRCA carrier to take unopposed estrogen or tamoxifen in the future without risk of uterine cancer, but this surgery is associated with a longer recovery time and has more side effects than does BSO. Each patient should be counseled about the pros and cons of each procedure.

Data indicate that BRCA carriers who opt for prophylactic oophorectomy also have a reduced chance to develop a subsequent breast cancer, particularly if they have this surgery before menopause.[40,41] Healthy premenopausal women who opt for oophorectomy and therefore experience premature surgical menopause may be candidates for hormone replacement therapy with the lowest dose of estrogen possible.[14] This may provide some of the benefits of hormone replacement therapy while minimizing the potential breast cancer–related risks. Preliminary data suggest that premenopausal BRCA1 carriers who have oophorectomies followed by hormone replacement therapy still have a reduced risk of future breast cancers.[42]

The standard surveillance method in carriers of HNPCC mutations is full colonoscopy to the cecum every 1 to 3 years beginning between the ages of 20 and 25 years.[43] Although several studies are investigating chemopreventive options for colorectal cancer, no agents are currently approved for clinical use. Prophylactic subtotal colectomy with ileorectal anastomosis is an option for HNPCC carriers, and a decision analysis revealed that this procedure may offer slightly greater gains in life expectancy for young HNPCC carriers than surveillance alone.[44]

Options for endometrial cancer surveillance include endometrial aspiration and transvaginal ultrasonography beginning between the ages of 25 and 35 years. The efficacy of such surveillance in HNPCC carriers is unknown. Oral contraceptive use is known to reduce the risk of endometrial cancer in the general population,[45] but the impact of this intervention in HNPCC carriers is currently unknown. Prophylactic transabdominal hysterectomy is also an option. Although this option is likely to reduce risk of uterine cancer significantly, long-term prospective studies of the impact of this intervention on HNPCC carriers have not been performed. Women who carry HNPCC mutations are also at risk for ovarian cancer and should therefore be offered the surveillance and risk reduction options discussed earlier for ovarian cancer.

Genetic counseling and testing are also available for many rare cancer syndromes, including von Hippel-Lindau syndrome, multiple endocrine neoplasias, and FAP. Surveillance and risk reduction for patients who are known mutation carriers for such conditions may decrease the associated morbidity and mortality of these syndromes.

FOLLOW-UP

A follow-up letter to the patient is a concrete means of documenting the information conveyed in the sessions so that the patient and his or her family members can review it over time. It is crucial that this letter be sent only to the patient and health care professionals to whom the patient has granted access to this information, and in most cases it should not be placed in the patient's general medical records. A follow-up phone call is also helpful, particularly in the case of a positive test result. Some programs provide patients with an annual or biannual newsletter updating them on new information in the field of cancer genetics. A small proportion of patients may return for a follow-up counseling session months, or even years, after their initial consult to discuss the emergence of new family history data or new clinical issues, or because they are now ready to move forward with genetic testing.

ISSUES IN CANCER GENETIC COUNSELING

PSYCHOSOCIAL ISSUES

The psychosocial impact of cancer genetic counseling cannot be underestimated. Just the process of scheduling a cancer risk counseling session may be quite difficult for some individuals with a family history of cancer who are not only frightened about their own cancer risk but are reliving painful experiences associated with the cancer of their loved ones.[2] Counselees may be faced with an onslaught of emotions, including anger, fear of developing cancer, fear of disfigurement and dying, grief, lack of control, negative body image, and a sense of isolation.[11] Some counselees are wrestling with the fear that insurance companies, employers, family members, and even future partners will react negatively to their cancer risks. For many, it is a double-edged sword as they balance their fears and apprehensions about dredging up these issues with the possibility of obtaining reassuring news and much-needed information.

Individuals' perceived cancer risk is often dependent on many "nonmedical" variables. They may estimate that their risk is higher if they look like an affected individual or share some of that individual's personality traits.[11] Their perceived risks vary depending on whether their relatives were cancer survivors or died painful deaths from the disease. Many people wonder not "if" they are going to get cancer, but "when."

The counseling session is an opportunity for individuals to express why they believe they have developed cancer or why their family members have cancer. Some explanations may revolve around family folklore, and it is important to listen to and address these explanations rather than dismiss them.[11] In doing this the counselor allows the clients to alleviate their greatest fears and to give more credibility to the "medical" theory. Understanding a patient's perceived cancer risk is important, because that fear may *decrease* surveillance and preventive health care behaviors.[46] For patients and families who are moving forward with DNA testing, a referral to a mental health care professional is often very helpful. Genetic testing has an impact not only on the patient but also on his or her children, siblings, parents, and extended relatives. This can be overwhelming for an individual and the family, and should be discussed in detail before testing.

To date, studies conducted in the setting of before and after genetic counseling have revealed that, at least in the short term, most patients do not experience adverse psychological outcomes after receiving their test results.[47,48] In fact, preliminary data have revealed that individuals in families with known mutations who seek testing seem to fare better psychologically at 6 months than those who avoid testing.[49] Although these data are reassuring, it is important to recognize that genetic testing is an individual decision and is not right for every patient or every family.

PRESYMPTOMATIC TESTING OF CHILDREN

Presymptomatic testing of children has been widely discussed, and most concur that it is appropriate only when the onset of the condition regularly occurs in childhood or there are useful interventions that can be applied.[50] For example, DNA-based diagnosis of children and young adults at risk for hereditary medullary thyroid carcinoma has improved the management of these patients.[51] DNA-based testing for RET mutations is virtually 100% accurate and allows at-risk family members to make informed decisions about prophylactic thyroidectomy. FAP is a disorder that occurs in childhood and in which mortality can be reduced if detection is presymptomatic.[52] Testing is clearly indicated in these instances.

Questions have been raised about parents' right to demand testing of children for adult-onset diseases. Parents may have a constitutionally protected right to demand that unwilling physicians order this testing, but there is little risk of liability for damages for refusal unless the child suffers physical harm as a direct result of this refusal.[50] The child's right *not* to be tested must be considered. Whenever childhood testing is not medically indicated, it is preferable that testing decisions be postponed until the child is an adult and can decide for himself or herself whether or not to be tested.

CONFIDENTIALITY

The level of confidentiality surrounding cancer genetic testing is paramount due to concerns of genetic discrimination. Many programs are opting to keep shadow files separate from the general hospital charts. Patient-identifying data are generally not entered into computer databases that are accessible by modem or a network of users. Some counseling programs are submitting DNA samples to laboratories coded by number only, in an attempt to increase the level of confidentiality. Special precautions should be taken to protect confidentiality when leaving voice mail messages at home and at work regarding patient appointments. Conversations with patients or other colleagues via e-mail that include patients' names are discouraged, because the Internet is not secure. In addition, genetic counseling summary letters are often sent directly to patients and are copied to the referring physicians only with the explicit permission of the patient. These measures are taken because confidentiality and genetic discrimination are a grave concern for many of the patients seen in the cancer genetic counseling clinic.[53]

Confidentiality of test results within a family can also be an issue, because genetic counseling and testing often reveal the risk statuses of family members other than the patient. Under confidentiality codes, the patient needs to grant permission before at-risk family members can be contacted. It has been questioned whether or not a family member can sue a health care professional for negligence if the individual is identified to be at high risk yet is not so informed.[54] Most recommendations have stated that the burden of confidentiality lies between the provider and the patient. However, more recent recommendations state that confidentiality *should* be violated if the potential harm of not notifying other family members outweighs the harm of breaking a promise of confidentiality to the patient.[55] There is no easy solution for this difficult dilemma, and situations must be considered on a case-by-case basis with the assistance of the in-house legal department and ethics committee.

Patients should be counseled about the benefits to other family members of knowing testing results, but, at the present time, the decision to inform them is ultimately the patient's. Extended family members who are notified, with the patient's consent, may not always be grateful to receive this information and may feel that their privacy has been invaded by being contacted.

INSURANCE AND DISCRIMINATION ISSUES

When genetic testing for cancer predisposition first became widely available, the fear of health insurance discrimination—felt by both patients and providers—was one of the most common concerns.[53,56] It appears that the risks of health insurance discrimination were overstated and that almost no discrimination by health insurers has been reported.[57] More and more patients are choosing to submit their genetic counseling and testing charges to their health insurance companies. In the past few years, more insurance companies have agreed to pay for counseling and testing,[58] perhaps in light of decision analyses that show these services and subsequent prophylactic surgeries to be cost effective.[59]

The risk of life insurance discrimination, however, is more realistic. Patients should be counseled about such risks before they pursue genetic testing. Laws relevant to genetic discrimination can be found at http://www.ncgbc.org/pdffiles/geneticdiscrimination.pdf.

FUTURE DIRECTIONS

The field of cancer genetic counseling and testing has grown tremendously over the past decade. Although cancer genetic counseling is currently targeted at individuals with strong family histories of cancer, this focus has begun to broaden. Genetic testing is now offered to patients diagnosed with early-onset breast and colon cancer to guide surgical decision making, because the risk of new primaries is greater in individuals who carry germline mutations.[32,33] U.S. Food and Drug Administration approval of tamoxifen therapy as a method of breast cancer risk reduction for women at moderately increased risk of the disease has increased the number of genetic counseling referrals. These patients need to be counseled about their personal risks of developing breast cancer, and the counseling session should include a discussion of the risks of osteoporosis, coronary heart disease, menopausal symptoms, and cognitive deficiencies, and the pros and cons of hormone replacement therapy versus use of selective estrogen receptor modulators such as tamoxifen.

The finding of microsatellite instability (MSI) in colon tumors has long been recognized as a marker of increased risk for hereditary colon cancer that warrants further genetic testing.[60] More recent data indicate that fluorouracil-based chemotherapy may decrease survival in patients with high-frequency MSI tumors.[61] If these data are correct, MSI status will become very important in guiding chemotherapy decision making and MSI detection may become a standard test performed on every colon tumor. If so, many more patients at high risk for hereditary colon cancer will be identified and will be referred for genetic counseling and testing.

Genetic testing for high-prevalence, low-penetrance mutations, such as the APC mutation I1307K, may become more widespread in the future. I1307K is a common mutation among Ashkenazi Jews and is associated with an increased, but relatively modest, risk of colorectal cancer.[10] The usefulness of such testing among Jews with a family history of colon cancer has been questioned, because increased surveillance is recommended due to the family history, regardless of the test result. Gruber et al. contend that Ashkenazi Jewish individuals with *no* family history of colon cancer may actually derive the most benefit from such testing, because a positive test result would elucidate which patients in that population would benefit from increased colorectal surveillance.[62] This shift in emphasis from rare, high-risk mutation screening to broad screening for lower-penetrance mutations could change the face of the field of cancer genetic counseling.

The combination of technologic advances in genetic testing, new pharmacologic developments for cancer risk reduction, and increased usefulness of testing in high- and moderate-risk populations will result in a significant expansion in the field of cancer genetic counseling. Direct-to-consumer marketing campaigns by commercial testing companies will likely flood physicians with requests for testing, many of which will be inappropriate.[63]

Maintenance of high standards for thorough genetic counseling, informed consent, and accurate result interpretation will be paramount in reducing potential risks and maximizing the benefits of this technology in the next century.

REFERENCES

1. Peters J. Breast cancer genetics: relevance to oncology practice. *Cancer Control* 1995;195.
2. Kelly PT. Informational needs of individuals and families with hereditary cancers. *Semin Oncol Nurs* 1992;8:288.
3. Peters JA. Familial cancer risk part 1: impact on today's oncology practice. *J Oncol Manage* 1994;18.
4. Hull SC, Prasad K. Reading between the lines: direct-to-consumer advertising of genetic testing. *Hastings Cent Rep* 2001;3:33.
5. Collins FS. Preparing health professionals for the genetic revolution. *JAMA* 1997;278 (15):1285.
6. Claus EB, Schildkraut JM, Thompson WD, et al. The genetic attributable risks of breast and ovarian cancer. *Cancer* 1996;77:2318.
7. Loman N, Johannsson O, Kristoffersson U, et al. Family history of breast and ovarian cancers and BRCA1 and BRCA2 mutations in a population-based series of early-onset breast cancer. *J Natl Cancer Inst* 2001;93:1215.
8. Farrington SM, Lin-Goerke J, Ling J, et al. Systematic analysis of hMSH2 and hMLH1 in young colon cancer patients and controls. *Am J Hum Genet* 1998;63:749.
9. Struewing JP, Hartge P, Wacholder S, et al. The risk of cancer associated with specific mutations of BRCA1 and BRCA2 among Ashkenazi Jews. *N Engl J Med* 1997;336:1401.
10. Gryfe R, Nicola ND, Lal G, Gallinger S, Redston M. Inherited colorectal polyposis and cancer risk of the APC I1307K polymorphism. *Am J Hum Genet* 1999;64:378.
11. Schneider KA. *Counseling about cancer: strategies for genetic counseling*, 2nd ed. New York: Wiley-Liss, 2002.
12. Love RR, Evan AM, Josten DM. The accuracy of patient reports of a family history of cancer. *J Chron Dis* 1985;38:289.
13. Hodgson SV, Maher ER. *A practical guide to human genetics*. Cambridge: Cambridge University Press, 1993.
14. Olopade OI, Weber BL. Breast cancer genetics: toward molecular characterization of individuals at increased risk for breast cancer: Part II. *PPO Updates* 1998;12(11):1.
15. Gail MH, Brinton LA, Byar DP, et al. Projecting individualized probabilities of developing breast cancer for white females who are being examined annually. *J Natl Cancer Inst* 1989;81:1879.
16. Claus EB, Risch N, Thompson WD. Autosomal dominant inheritance of early-onset breast cancer. *Cancer* 1994;73:643.
17. Parmigiani G, Berry DA, Aguilar O. Determining carrier probabilities for breast cancer susceptibility genes BRCA1 and BRCA2. *Am J Hum Genet* 1998;62:145.
18. Richards MPM, Hallowell N, Green JM, Murton F, Statham H. Counseling families with hereditary breast and ovarian cancer: a psychosocial perspective. *J Genet Couns* 1995; 4:219.
19. Giardiello FM, Brensinger JD, Petersen GM, et al. The use and interpretation of commercial APC gene testing for familial adenomatous polyposis. *N Engl J Med* 1997;336:823.
20. Brierley K, Kim K, Matloff E, et al. Obstetricians' and gynecologists' knowledge, interests, and current practices with regard to providing breast and ovarian cancer genetic counseling. *J Genet Couns* 2001;10:438.
21. Ford D, Easton DF, Bishop DT, et al. Risks of cancer in BRCA1-mutation carriers. *Lancet* 1994;343:692.
22. Antoniou A, Pharoah PDP, Narod S, et al. Average risks of breast and ovarian cancer associated with BRCA1 or BRCA2 mutations detected in case series unselected for family history: a combined analyses of 22 studies. *Am J Hum Genet* 2003;72:1117.
23. Piver MS, Jishi MF, Tsukada Y, et al. Primary peritoneal carcinoma after prophylactic oophorectomy in women with a family history of ovarian cancer. *Cancer* 1993;71:2751.
24. Aziz S, Kuperstein G, Rosen B, et al. A genetic epidemiological study of carcinoma of the fallopian tube. *Gynecol Oncol* 2001;80:341.
25. Marra G, Boland CR. Hereditary nonpolyposis colorectal cancer. *J Natl Cancer Inst* 1995;87:1114.
26. Aarnio M, Mecklin J-P, Aaltonen LA, et al. Lifetime risk of different cancers in hereditary non-polyposis colorectal cancer (HNPCC) syndrome. *Int J Cancer* 1995;64:430.
27. Burke W, Daly M, Garber J, et al. Recommendations for follow-up care of individuals with an inherited predisposition to cancer. II. BRCA1 and BRCA2. *JAMA* 1997;277:997.
28. Fisher B, Costantino JP, Wickerman DL, et al. Tamoxifen for the prevention of breast cancer: report of the National Surgical Adjuvant Breast and Bowel Project P-1 study. *J Natl Cancer Inst* 1998;90:1371.
29. King M-C, Wieand S, Hale K, et al. Tamoxifen and breast cancer incidence among women with inherited mutations in BRCA1 and BRCA2. *JAMA* 2001;286:2251.
30. Narod SA, Brunet J-S, Ghadirian P, et al. Tamoxifen and risk of contralateral breast cancer in BRCA1 and BRCA2 mutation carriers: a case-control study. *Lancet* 2000;356:1876.
31. Hartmann LC, Schaid DJ, Woods JE, et al. Efficacy of bilateral prophylactic mastectomy in women with a family history of breast cancer. *N Engl J Med* 1999;340:77.
32. Matloff ET. The breast surgeon's role in BRCA1 and BRCA2 testing. *Am J Surg* 2000;180:294.
33. Turner BC, Harold E, Matloff E, et al. BRCA1/BRCA2 germline mutations in locally recurrent breast cancer patients after lumpectomy and radiation therapy: implications for breast-conserving management in patients with BRCA1/BRCA2 mutations. *J Clin Oncol* 1999;Oct:3017.
34. Narod SA, Risch H, Moslehi R, et al. Oral contraceptives and the risk of hereditary ovarian cancer. *N Engl J Med* 1998;339:424.
35. American College of Obstetrics and Gynecology. Committee opinion: breast-ovarian cancer screening. *Am J Obstet Gynecol* 1996;176:1.
36. Hornreich G, Beller U, Lavie O, et al. Is uterine serous papillary carcinoma a BRCA1-related disease? Case report and review of the literature. *Gynecol Oncol* 1999;75:300.
37. Levine DA, Lin O, Barakat RR, et al. Risk of endometrial carcinoma associated with BRCA mutation. *Gynecol Oncol* 2001;80:395.
38. Goshen R, Chu W, Elit L, et al. Is uterine papillary serous adenocarcinoma a manifestation of the hereditary breast-ovarian cancer syndrome? *Gynecol Oncol* 2000;79:477.
39. Boyd J. BRCA: the breast, ovarian, and other cancer genes. *Gynecol Oncol* 2001;80:337.
40. Rebbeck TR, Lynch HT, Neuhausen SL, et al. Prophylactic oophorectomy in carriers of BRCA1 or BRCA2 mutations. *N Engl J Med* 2002;346:1616.
41. Kauff ND, Satagopan JM, Robson ME, et al. Risk-reducing salpingo-oophorectomy in women with a BRCA1 or BRCA2 mutation. *N Engl J Med* 2002;346:1609.

42. Rebbeck TR, Levin AM, Eisen A, et al. Breast cancer risk after bilateral prophylactic oophorectomy in BRCA1 mutation carriers. *J Natl Cancer Inst* 1999;91(17):1475.

43. Burke W, Petersen G, Lynch P, et al. Recommendations for follow-up care of individuals with an inherited predisposition to cancer. Hereditary nonpolyposis colon cancer. *JAMA* 1997;277:915.

44. Syngal S, Weeks JC, Schrag D, et al. Benefits of colonoscopic surveillance and prophylactic colectomy in patients with hereditary nonpolyposis colorectal cancer mutations. *Ann Intern Med* 1998;129:787.

45. Silverberg SG, Makowski EL. Endometrial carcinoma in young women taking oral contraceptive agents. *Obstet Gynecol* 1975;46:503.

46. Kash KM, Holland JC, Halper MS, Miller DG. Psychological distress and surveillance behaviors of women with a family history of breast cancer. *J Natl Cancer Inst* 1992;84:24.

47. Lerman C, Narod S, Schulman K, et al. BRCA1 testing in families with hereditary breast-ovarian cancer: a prospective study of patient decision making and outcomes. *JAMA* 1996;275(24):1885.

48. Croyle RT, Smith KR, Botkin JR, et al. Psychological responses to BRCA1 mutation testing: preliminary findings. *Health Psychol* 1997;16:63.

49. Lerman C, Hughes C, Lemon SJ, et al. What you don't know can hurt you: adverse psychologic effects in members of BRCA1-linked and BRCA2-linked families who decline genetic testing. *J Clin Oncol* 1998;16:1650.

50. Clayton EW. Removing the shadow of the law from the debate about genetic testing of children. *Am J Med Genet* 1995;57:630.

51. Ledger GA, Khosia S, Lindor NM, Thibodeau SN, Gharib H. Genetic testing in the diagnosis and management of multiple endocrine neoplasia type II. *Ann Intern Med* 1995;122:118.

52. Rhodes M, Bradburn DM. Overview of screening and management of familial adenomatous polyposis. *Gut* 1992;33:125.

53. Bluman LG, Rimer BK, Berry DA, et al. Attitudes, knowledge, and risk perceptions of women with breast and/or ovarian cancer considering testing for BRCA1 and BRCA2. *J Natl Cancer Inst* 1999;17:1040.

54. Tsoucalas CL. Legal aspects of cancer genetics—screening, counseling, and registers. In: Lynch HT, Kullander S, eds. *Cancer genetics in women*, vol I. Boca Raton, FL: CRC Press, 1987:9.

55. The American Society of Human Genetics Social Issues Subcommittee on Familial Disclosure. ASHG statement: Professional disclosure of familial genetic information. *Am J Hum Genet* 1998;62:474.

56. Matloff ET, Shappell H, Brierley K, et al. What would you do? Specialists' perspectives on cancer genetic testing, prophylactic surgery and insurance discrimination. *J Clin Oncology* 2000;18(12):2484.

57. Hall MA. *Genetic discrimination.* North Carolina Genomics and Bioinformatics Consortium, Research Triangle Park, NC. World Wide Web URL: http://www.ncgbc.org/pdffiles/geneticdiscrimination.pdf, 2003.

58. Manley SA, Pennell RL, Frank TS. Insurance coverage of BRCA1 and BRCA2 sequence analysis. *J Genet Couns* 1998;7(6):A462.

59. Grann VR, Whang W, Jacobson JS, et al. Benefits and costs of screening Ashkenazi Jewish women for BRCA1 and BRCA2. *J Clin Oncol* 1999;17:494.

60. Lindor NM, Burgart LJ, Leontovich O, et al. Immunohistochemistry versus microsatellite instability testing in phenotyping colorectal tumors. *J Clin Oncol* 2002;20:1043.

61. Ribic CM, Sargent DJ, Moore MJ, et al. Tumor microsatellite-instability status as a predictor of benefit from fluorouracil-based adjuvant chemotherapy for colon cancer. *N Engl J Med* 2003;95:2422.

62. Gruber SB, Petersen GM, Kinzler KW, Vogelstein B. Cancer, crash sites, and the new genetics of neoplasia. *Gastroenterology* 1999;116(1):210.

63. Gray S, Olopade OI. Direct-to-consumer marketing of genetic tests for cancer: buyer beware. *J Clin Oncol* 2003;21:3191.

SECTION 5

BETH L. DINOFF
JOHN L. SHUSTER

Psychological Issues

"Not life, but good life, is to be chiefly valued." —Socrates

A landmark epidemiologic study by Derogatis and colleagues[1] revealed that 47% of a broad sample of cancer patients qualified for at least one psychiatric diagnosis using diagnostic criteria of the *Diagnostic and Statistical Manual of Mental Disorders, Third Edition*. If 2003 cancer incidence data[2] are used, this prevalence rate would mean that roughly 627,000 of the patients diagnosed with cancer each year suffer with clinically significant comorbid psychological disorders or symptoms. If those who bear the burden of subclinical suffering and distress are included, an even greater overall number of cancer patients might benefit from intervention.

Psycho-oncology is a clinical subspecialty focusing on the psychological, behavioral, and social aspects of cancer. Dimensions of psycho-oncology include the psychological consequences that patients experience at various stages of disease and the possible effect that psychological, behavioral, and social responses have on morbidity and mortality.[3] Entire textbooks and chapters on this subject are available to the interested reader.[4–6] Psychiatrists and psychologists working in psycho-oncology assist patients in adapting to life after a cancer diagnosis, coping with medical interventions, adjusting to survivorship, and facing disease progression or terminal illness. This chapter on psychological issues in oncology focuses on the phases of cancer-related illness and the psychological complications associated with each illness phase. The presentation, diagnosis, and practical first-line management of psychological and psychiatric complications of cancer and its treatment are also addressed.

PHASES OF ILLNESS

INITIAL DIAGNOSIS

Approximately 90% of the observed psychiatric disorders in the Derogatis et al.[1] study were reactions to the cancer diagnosis or treatment. Given the threat to life and well-being that cancer represents, most people experience stress in response to the diagnosis. *Stress* refers to any event in which the internal or external demands are perceived as taxing or exceeding the adaptive resources of an individual.[7] Every potentially stressful event is filtered through this cognitive appraisal process, and, thus, no two people experience any event in the same way. Responses to the cancer diagnosis vary widely based on disease-related factors, such as the type, stage, and location of cancer, the treatment selected, and treatment outcomes. Furthermore, the individual's age, sex, and education moderate levels of distress. Finally, reactions to the cancer diagnosis are mediated by previous experience with cancer patients, social support, hope, and use of coping strategies.

Coping entails efforts to master the condition that is stressful, which often requires a novel response from the individual. Coping responses can be divided into two main categories: problem-focused coping and emotion-focused coping.[7] Problem-focused coping includes efforts to improve the situation by taking action to change things. Problem-focused coping is particularly useful in situations in which the person's efforts can actually modify the stressor. Pursuing all options to eliminate disease is an example of problem-focused coping. On the other hand, emotion-focused coping involves strategies that are used to relieve the emotional impact of stress. Examples include talking about fears, joking, distancing, relaxation, and distraction. These actions are designed not to change the situation but to make the person feel better about the event. Emotion-focused coping strategies tend to be more effective than problem-focused coping strategies when the stressor itself is outside the individual's control, as is the case with many illness-related stressors.

The most difficult time for patients is likely to be at the time of diagnosis, with distress typically decreasing after the first year. In addition to the external stressors of a cancer diagnosis (e.g., complicated terminology, invasive medical procedures, increased doctor visits), patients must face their own internal fears about existential issues that may have been avoided before, such as feeling out of control, feeling that life is unfair, or feeling that they are doomed to die a difficult death. The just-world hypothesis explores the idea that people have a strong need to believe that the world is a just and orderly place in which people get what they deserve. Therefore, maintaining perception of control is vital for patients who experience cancer as a threat to well-being. Research on control perception indicates that women who are given a choice of medical treatments experience fewer depressive symptoms than women not given treatment options.[8] Concerns about social isolation are common, particularly in women with breast or gynecologic cancers.[9] Many of these concerns stem from the stigma associated with a cancer diagnosis. As might be expected, body image perceptions of control are prominent in patients after head and neck cancer surgery.[10]

Significant adjustment is likely to be required from each patient with a new diagnosis of cancer. Patients may temporarily complain of emotional instability, irritability, nervousness, concentration problems, rumination, fatigue, sadness, and tearfulness.[4] Typically, this period, which can be consumed by shock, disbelief, fear, anxiety, emotional trauma, or denial, is brief as people begin to focus on treatment selection and use of coping strategies. It may take weeks to months for people to incorporate new information about their medical condition. When emotional, psychological, or behavioral symptoms begin to interfere with the patient's ability to formulate a comprehensive management plan, a psychiatric referral is warranted.

Denial is a coping strategy that has been associated with adjustment in cancer patients. Denial should be viewed as a normal coping mechanism that people use when facing an overwhelming situation.[11] In the short term, such as the weeks and months after initial diagnosis, denial offers people emotional detachment from the effects of the shock. This detachment permits psychological preservation and allows people to adjust in a gradual way to decrease levels of arousal and anxiety that could significantly impair treatment participation. Over time, as arousal in response to the disease decreases, people gradually confront cancer and its consequences. When denial becomes a long-term strategy of avoidance, however, negative outcomes, including loneliness and increased medical complications, may ensue.[12]

TREATMENT PHASE

Adapting to cancer is not a single, isolated event. Continuous coping efforts are required, and when coping efforts are ineffective, people are at risk for developing distress. Previously well-defined roles of parent, spouse, employee, and so on, are subject to dramatic alterations as people enter difficult treat-ment regimens and begin to see themselves as cancer patients or people with illnesses. As people transition from the initial shock of the diagnosis, they enter a phase of requiring long-term coping skills.

While participating in treatment, patients often experience fear of pain, death, and iatrogenic complications. Psychological complaints may mimic treatment effects and thereby complicate medical management. Grief reactions to the loss of a body part or function are not uncommon. As patients gain more experience with the demands of their medical regimens, most garner the psychological resources needed to navigate a steady course. These individuals demonstrate adequate psychological adjustment. However, a substantial proportion of cancer patients experience depressive symptoms associated with their disease or suffer anxiety symptoms, which indicates that, for a significant minority of individuals, the demands of being a cancer patient are psychologically taxing.

Given current cancer survival rates, many patients will experience cancer as a chronic rather than an acute illness. Therefore, quality of life becomes an important determinant of treatment outcome. Cancer is a risk factor for acquired psychological disorders. During the initial treatment phase, cancer patients may be undergoing surgical resection, radiotherapy, and adjuvant chemotherapy or a combination of interventions.[4] In cancer patients, comorbid depression has been associated with poor quality of life and functional impairment. Even though depression among cancer patients has decreased as life expectancy has increased, a significant proportion of patients experience mood disorders. Depression is associated with increased morbidity and mortality in cancer patients. Stommel and colleagues[13] found that patients with a history of depression were 2.6 times more likely to die from cancer within the 19 months after diagnosis. Patients in pain are twice as likely to experience depressive symptoms as are patients who are not in pain.

Hope has been defined as a cognitive process in which people are focused on goals and the necessary planning to meet those goals.[14] Pursuing goals should produce positive emotions, and experiencing barriers to goals may produce negative feelings. Initially after diagnosis, cancer patients may experience barriers to reaching important life goals and associated negative feelings. However, over time, new goals accompanied by positive feelings can develop. Hope has been associated with positive psychological adjustment. For example, people who are high in hope feel invigorated and think positively about achieving goals,[14] and they also feel good about themselves. Hope in relation to cancer can be thought of as a confident expectation that good will come to one in the future. Focusing on concrete goals that one can reasonably count on reaching and look forward to accomplishing may increase feelings of hope in cancer patients. Post-White and colleagues[15] outline five themes influencing hope in cancer patients. They are finding meaning, relying on inner resources, affirming relationships, living in the present, and anticipating survival.

SURVIVORSHIP

Long-term survival rates for many types of cancer have improved substantially due to early detection and treatment advances. In fact, more than half of patients diagnosed with cancer can expect to live 20 or more years.[16] Nevertheless, the psychological and physical consequences of cancer remain long after treatment has been completed and the patient is assured that there is "no evidence of disease." Unfortunately, cancer survivorship is not a guarantee that life will return to precancer normalcy. Many patients report that they were a different person before cancer than they are currently or after-cancer. Alterations in mental status can occur as a result of chemotherapy or radiation treatment. Neurobehavioral side effects of treatment may impair attention, concentration, and functional abilities.[17] Furthermore, cancer survivors can experience subsyndromal levels of psychological distress in association with the end of treatment, chronic fatigue, changes in body image, and personal relationships.

Survivors must cope with both waiting and monitoring their bodies for recurrences. For some patients the decline in medical surveillance is particularly difficult. Such experiences, can cause tremendous suffering in cancer patients. Research on bone marrow transplant recipients[18] indicates that they experience numerous psychosocial "late effects" in the following domains: physical (fatigue, feelings of physical damage), psychological (fears about the future, loss of control, feelings of isolation), and community reintegration (separation from family and friends, stigmatization, difficult in resuming social relationships). Use of social support, a type of coping strategy, has been associated with adjustment in people with cancer. Social support or lack thereof can influence both the physical and psychological outcomes of medical illnesses. Social support affects individuals in two ways. First, social support can have a direct, beneficial impact on health. For example, a person with cancer may be more disposed to attend therapy sessions if a family member attends as well. Second, social support can buffer or protect an individual from the negative effect of serious health problems. For example, visits from family and friends may help prevent serious depressive symptoms.

ADVANCED DISEASE

People are usually assigned a diagnosis of advanced cancer or terminal disease when they have a life expectancy of 3 to 6 months or when care becomes palliative rather than curative.[19] People with advanced disease can have unresolved physical, psychological, and spiritual concerns, which may impair remaining quality of life. As cure becomes unlikely, the focus of treatment should shift to symptom management and palliative care. Prompt recognition, assessment, and treatment of the patient's symptoms are critically important to maintaining comfort and dignity and allowing the patient to die well.[20]

Twycross and Wilcock[21] recommend that care of the dying individual extend well beyond pain and symptom management. Providers are encouraged to support patients as they cope with decreasing physical abilities and as they experience anticipatory grief over the future loss of family, friends, and everything that is familiar. Care and support of the family are essential in treating the dying person. In other words, to be maximally effective, the provider should demonstrate care for the suffering individual and not solely for physical symptoms. Chochinov[22] describes this model as dignity-conserving care. The provider is encouraged to interview the individual using thoughtful questions such as, "Can you tell me a little about your life history, particularly those parts that you think are

most important?" and "What are your hopes and dreams for your loved ones?" In this way, the clinician may begin to understand the sources of distress and suffering for each individual dying person.

Suffering depends on personal loss of meaning and purpose.[12] Thus, suffering is connected subjectively to the value a person places on what is lost. Suffering is a two-sided coin. It can breed great isolation and conflict as described earlier. However, it is important to note that the end of life can and often does foster deep personal or spiritual growth. Byock[23] has outlined five things that are related to finding peace with one's own impending death. People who are dying should be afforded the opportunity to express these thoughts: Please forgive me; I forgive you; Thank you; I love you; and Goodbye. When people are allowed to resolve these five issues, dying can be completed with a sense of peace and closeness with loved ones.

PSYCHOLOGICAL COMPLICATIONS OF CANCER

Emotional and psychological consequences of cancer are common and can become significant sources of suffering. Although not all psychological distress among cancer patients meets diagnostic criteria for mental disorder, all distress should be evaluated and treatment offered if indicated and desired. The National Comprehensive Cancer Network has published a useful guideline for the assessment and management of psychological distress in the setting of a cancer diagnosis.[24] A brief description of presentation, assessment, and management of common psychological complications of cancer follows.

ADJUSTMENT DISORDERS

Adjustment disorders are an intermediate state between severe psychological distress (i.e., mood or anxiety disorders) and "normal" reactions to stressful events. Such stress-related disorders must be viewed within the context of the patient's coping skills and the timing of the stressful event(s). Adjustment disorders result when emotional or behavioral symptoms emerge within 3 months of the onset of an identifiable stressor, causing marked distress or significant impairment in functioning.[25]

Adjustment disorder may manifest itself in the cancer setting as poor coping—patients seem to be in a tailspin as they struggle to adapt to the reality of being given a cancer diagnosis, the life adjustments required to participate in cancer therapy, the side effects of therapy, and the existential unease precipitated by confrontation with serious illness. Complaints of feeling "out of control" are common, as are reports of distress at the "unfairness" of cancer. The need for restoration of a sense of control and emotional equilibrium is usually obvious.

Derogatis et al.[1] reported that adjustment disorders accounted for 68% of all psychiatric diagnoses in their study. Despite the apparent significance of this clinical problem, further details regarding the epidemiology of adjustment disorders in cancer patients are unclear. Randomized clinical trials have not been used to determine appropriate treatment modalities in this population. Intervention for adjustment disorder should include provision of emotional support and monitoring for the emergence of more serious disorders, and the choice of intervention should be guided by prevailing symptoms and comorbidities.

ANXIETY

To some extent, anxiety in the setting of a cancer diagnosis is universal. However, when a patient's functioning, participation in care planning, or quality of life becomes impaired, anxiety is considered pathologic. Anxiety symptoms tend to appear at crisis or transition points in cancer diagnosis and treatment, such as at initial diagnosis, the beginning or completion of therapy, or the detection of advancing disease.[26,27]

Anxiety may be described by the patient as fear, jitteriness, hypervigilance, insomnia, shortness of breath, increased heart rate, worry, numbness, or muscle tension. These symptoms are related to the arousal that accompanies perceptions of threat or harm. Such arousal may lead patients to interpret anxiety symptoms as manifestations of cancer or, alternatively, to unduly minimize attention to (and reporting of) these or unrelated physical symptoms for fear of being told that cancer is the source of the symptom. Patients with anxiety also have diminished capacity to understand information about their disease, are less tolerant of interventions, and less likely to continue with treatment.[27]

Symptoms of cancer and its treatment may mimic the symptoms of anxiety (Table 55.5-1). Poorly controlled pain, hypoxia, sepsis, withdrawal, and adverse drug reactions (i.e., akathisia from antiemetic drugs) may present as anxiety.[28] Patients with preexisting diagnoses of anxiety disorder (including panic disorder, obsessive-compulsive disorder, and generalized anxiety disorder) are at risk for symptom reemergence or exacerbation in situations provoking heightened arousal. Because these disorders tend to be chronic and recurrent, patients with preexisting anxiety disorder diagnoses are likely to benefit from formal psychiatric consultation.

A substantial proportion of cancer survivors exhibit symptoms of posttraumatic stress disorder (PTSD).[29] PTSD can result when a person has been exposed to a traumatic event and responds with intense fear, feelings of helplessness, or horror. PTSD symptoms are more likely to occur when there is a sudden event (e.g., complication of cancer treatment) that is overwhelming, life threatening, uncontrollable, and unpredictable. Early intervention with debriefing and symptom reduction is essential to the prevention of chronic problems associated with PTSD.[30,31]

Cancer-related anxiety is initially managed with efforts to reduce fears and restore a sense of control, coupled with treatment with anxiolytic drugs (Table 55.5-2), as needed. Cognitive-

TABLE 55.5-1. Differential Diagnosis of Anxiety in Medical Illness

---

Anxiety disorders (panic disorder, generalized anxiety disorder, posttraumatic stress disorder)
Coping and personality style (avoidant, dependent)
Delirium
Fear
Side effects (akathisia from antiemetics)
Spiritual and existential concerns
Undertreated pain
Other undertreated physical complications (dyspnea, sepsis)
Withdrawal states (opiates, sedatives)

(From ref. 28, with permission.)

TABLE 55.5-2. Anxiolytic Medications Commonly Used to Treat Cancer Patients

Drug	Usual Dosage Range (mg)	Dose Route(s)
BENZODIAZEPINES		
Short acting		
Alprazolam	0.25–2.0 b.i.d to q.i.d	Oral, sublingual
Lorazepam	0.5–2.0 b.i.d to q.i.d	Oral, sublingual, intravenous, intramuscular, subcutaneous
Long acting		
Diazepam	5–10 b.i.d to q.i.d	Oral, sublingual, intravenous
Clonazepam	0.5–2.0 b.i.d. or t.i.d.	Oral
NONBENZODIAZEPINES		
Buspirone	5–20 t.i.d.	Oral
ANTIDEPRESSANTS		
Fluoxetine	20–80 daily	Oral
Paroxetine	10–60 daily	Oral
Sertraline	50–200 daily	Oral
Desipramine	12.5–150 daily	Oral
Imipramine	12.5–150 daily	Oral
Nortriptyline	10–125 daily	Oral
NEUROLEPTICS	See Table 55.5-5	

behavioral techniques are also helpful for managing anxiety in the long term. Techniques such as relaxation, diaphragmatic breathing, and hypnosis have been effective in decreasing the sympathetic arousal that occurs with anxiety. Chronic anxiety may also benefit from anxiolytic pharmacotherapy.

DEPRESSION

Depression in the setting of illness such as cancer is a complex concept, encompassing problems ranging from temporary sadness and discouragement to an adjustment disorder with depressed features to an episode of major depression. Although lesser degrees of depression and dysphoria may merit clinical attention depending on concurrent suffering and distress or impairments in quality of life, depression that exceeds the criteria for a major depressive episode[25] always merits attention. A depressive episode is characterized by the presence of five or more of the following symptoms for a period of at least 2 weeks: depressed mood most of the day, markedly diminished interest in pleasurable activities, significant weight loss or decrease in appetite, insomnia or hypersomnia, psychomotor agitation or retardation, fatigue or loss of energy, feelings of worthlessness or excessive guilt, diminished ability to think or concentrate, and pervasive thoughts of death or suicide. The presentation of depression in cancer patients is complicated by the fact that many of the neurovegetative signs of depression (e.g., anorexia, fatigue, weight loss, insomnia) are not specific to depression and could be attributed to cancer. Thus, the affective and cognitive symptoms of hopelessness, guilt, worthlessness, and suicidal ideation may solidify the diagnosis.

Evaluation of depressed patients should include a search for medical conditions or drugs that may produce depressive symptoms in cancer patients (Table 55.5-3). Depression should be assessed using the criteria of the *Diagnostic and Statistical Manual of Mental Disorders,* fourth edition,[25] listed earlier. Evaluation for these symptoms is useful not only for initial diagnosis

TABLE 55.5-3. Differential Diagnosis of Depression in Medical Illness

Mood disorders (major depression, dysthymia, bipolar disorder)
Anger
Anxiety
Coping and personality style (avoidant, schizoid)
Delirium ("quiet" type)
Dementia
Emotional numbing (adjustment disorder)
Interpersonal problems
Narcissistic injury
Side effects of treatment
Spiritual and existential concerns
Strong feelings of loss of control or autonomy
Undertreated nausea and vomiting
Undertreated pain
Other undertreated physical complications

(From ref. 28, with permission.)

TABLE 55.5-4. Antidepressant Medications Commonly Used to Treat Cancer Patients

Drug	Usual Starting Dose (mg/d)	Usual Therapeutic Dose (mg/d)
SEROTONIN REUPTAKE INHIBITORS		
Citalopram	20	40–60
Fluoxetine	20	20–40
Paroxetine	10	20–30
Sertraline	25–50	50–200
TRICYCLIC ANTIDEPRESSANTS[a]		
Desipramine	12.5–50.0	100–200
Imipramine	50	100–200
Nortriptyline	10–25	75–150
OTHERS		
Bupropion[b]	75–100	100–300
Mirtazapine	15	30–45
Venlafaxine[b]	75	150–225

[a]Dosages can be guided by serum levels, especially for nortriptyline.
[b]Usually administered in divided doses; sustained-release form available.

but also for monitoring the effectiveness of treatments.[32] Intervention is also indicated for subthreshold symptoms judged to be the cause of substantial suffering and distress.[28,33]

Goals of therapeutic intervention for depression include restoration of a sense of control, maintenance of morale, and preservation of a "fighting spirit" to combat cancer if curative therapies are indicated. Attention to repair and maintenance of important relationships, strengthening of other sources of social support, and meaningful expression of religion and spirituality are often very helpful in reversing or averting depression. Symptom reduction and reversal of full clinical depression is best achieved with antidepressant medications (Table 55.5-4), either alone or in combination with psychotherapies [e.g., cognitive-behavioral therapy (CBT)] with demonstrated benefit for depressed patients.

DELIRIUM

Delirium is a disturbance in consciousness and cognition that develops as a consequence of global cerebral dysfunction.[25,34] The disturbances that can lead to delirium typically develop over a relatively short period of time (hours to days) and in the setting of a physical, toxic, or metabolic derangement that affects cerebral functioning and metabolism. Delirium is common in patients with serious illness, and its prevalence is greater in populations with more acute or advanced disease. A number of other problems can cause agitation that mimics (or is comorbid with) delirium, and the apparently delirious patient should be screened for the presence of these factors.[35]

Goals of treatment for delirium in the cancer patient include maximization of patient comfort, minimization of patient and family distress, resolution (when possible) of the underlying problem driving the delirium, and optimization of the patient's cognitive functioning.[36] Nonpharmacologic approaches include establishing a soothing physical environment, titrating reassuring contact with others to avoid both overstimulation and understimulation, and providing frequent calm reorientation of the patient. Judicious use of antipsychotic medications, as outlined in Table 55.5-5, is the mainstay of pharmacologic therapy for delir-

ium.[35] Antipsychotics have been shown to speed resolution of depression, not just mask symptoms.[37] Antipsychotics should be tapered to discontinuation soon after stable resolution of delirium. Patients and families need information about the cause, course, treatment, and likely outcome of a delirious episode (although patient education obviously needs to be deferred until after the delirium clears).

SUICIDAL IDEATION

The rate of completed suicides among cancer patients is low. Severely depressed or acutely intoxicated patients are at highest risk. Suicide risk is somewhat elevated among cancer patients who have poorly controlled symptoms, head and neck cancers, advanced disease, delirium, or a history of alcoholism. Loss of hope is a strong risk factor for suicide.[38]

Contemplation of suicide as a possibility, on the other hand, is relatively common among cancer patients. As long as such suicidal ideation does not approach a plan of action, it does not pose a significant threat to life. Many cancer patients voice suicidal ideations as a contingency plan (e.g., "If my suffering gets too awful to bear, I can always end my life"). Although

TABLE 55.5-5. Neuroleptic Medications Commonly Used to Treat Cancer Patients

Drug	Usual Dose (mg)	Dose Route(s)
Haloperidol	0.5 b.i.d. to 5.0 q.i.d.	Oral, intramuscular, intravenous, subcutaneous
Chlorpromazine	25–50 b.i.d. to 100 q.i.d.	Oral, intramuscular
Risperidone	0.5 b.i.d. to 16.0 q.d.	Oral
Olanzapine	2.5 q.d. to 20.0 q.d.	Oral
Quetiapine	25–200 b.i.d.	Oral
Ziprasidone	20–80 b.i.d.	Oral, intramuscular

Note: Parenterally administered benzodiazepines (or sometimes opiates) can be used to manage the symptoms of delirium and agitation when the therapeutic goal is to provide calm and sedation rather than resolution of delirium and restoration of cognitive functioning.

such conditional ideation necessitates serial monitoring and screening for complications, such as depression, it is not as serious as a statement of suicidal intent (e.g., "I can't take it anymore—killing myself is my only way out").

Assessments of suicide risk should include questions about suicidal ideation; the nature, intensity, and duration of the thoughts; any plan, intent, or current access to lethal means; the degree to which the patient has come to peace about any plan considered; any possible prior attempt(s), especially any attempts in the recent past; and any comorbid alcohol or drug use.[39] If the patient answers in the affirmative to any questions about suicidal ideation, the assessment elements listed here (especially the presence of a suicide plan) should be explored. There is little risk that such an assessment will introduce the possibility of suicide as a previously unconsidered option for a distressed patient. In fact, most patients who have not come to peace with a plan to kill themselves are relieved to receive caring attention for their distress and to discuss plans to relieve the depression and despair that cause such painful restriction of any view of possible alternatives and a future.

Patients judged to be at high risk for suicidal behavior should be protected from self-harm. Clinicians should have a low threshold for psychiatric referral if a patient is judged to be at high risk of a suicide attempt.[39] Patients who are unambivalent about enacting a plan for suicide, as well as those whose behavior is driven by delusions or hallucinatory commands to kill themselves, are difficult to manage safely without hospitalization.

THERAPIES

PHARMACOTHERAPIES

Safe and effective first-line pharmacotherapy in the setting of severe medical illness requires basic knowledge of properties of the drugs prescribed and familiarity with a relatively small number of "broad-spectrum" drugs.[40] This section briefly outlines the agents commonly used to manage psychiatric symptoms in cancer patients. Patients with symptoms refractory to first-line management or those requiring complicated drug regimens (e.g., combination therapies or regimens with high potential for drug interactions) can benefit from psychiatric consultation.

Selective Serotonin Reuptake Inhibitors

Among the antidepressants, selective serotonin reuptake inhibitors (SSRIs) are the most commonly used for cancer patients. Their proven effectiveness, ease of administration, and general tolerability make them the most widely prescribed class of agents for depression among cancer patients. The side effect profile of SSRIs is generally benign, with nausea, jitteriness, and headache most common.[40] Sexual side effects often emerge with long-term treatment. Clinically significant drug interactions, mediated by inhibition or induction of cytochrome P-450 isoenzmes, are a possibility with SSRI therapy. As with all standard antidepressants, the lag time for treatment onset to full therapeutic benefit is usually measured in weeks. SSRIs have been linked to abnormal bleeding in thrombocytopenic patients in several reports.

Stimulants

Psychostimulants (e.g., methylphenidate, dextroamphetamine) are effective in reducing depressive symptoms in the medically ill.[41] They are particularly useful when the patient has a limited life expectancy, because they do not have the lag time to onset of effect characteristic of other antidepressants. Stimulants can help reverse the sedation caused by opiates and have also demonstrated synergistic analgesia when coadministered with opiates. Tolerance to the beneficial effects of stimulants on mood develops with prolonged use, which limits their usefulness as a primary agent in most patients. In addition, stimulants may worsen or precipitate delirium and may induce intolerable side effects (e.g., insomnia, hypertension, tachycardia, hallucinations) at higher doses. Table 55.5-6 outlines a dosing protocol for use of psychostimulants in medically ill patients.

Other Antidepressants

In addition to SSRIs and stimulants, a number of other antidepressant drugs are useful in treating cancer patients. All have the typical lag time to onset of effect. Tricyclic antidepressants (e.g.,

TABLE 55.5-6. Use of Psychostimulants to Treat Depression

ADVANTAGES
Well tolerated and effective
No lag time to effect
Rapid clearance
Paradoxically improve appetite
Pemoline comes in chewable form
DISADVANTAGES
Can only be given by the oral route
May worsen or precipitate delirium
Side effects include insomnia, hypertension, tachycardia, restlessness, hallucinations
May induce tolerance, withdrawal depression with prolonged use
AGENTS
Dextroamphetamine (Dexedrine)
    Starting dose: 2.5–5.0 mg/d (a.m.)
    "High" dose: 20 mg/d
Methylphenidate (Ritalin)
    Starting dose: 2.5–5.0 mg b.i.d. (a.m. and noon)
    "High" dose: 40 mg/d
Pemoline (Cylert)
    Starting dose: 18.75–37.5 mg b.i.d. (a.m. and noon)
    "High" dose: 100 mg/d
PROTOCOL
Begin with starting dose.
Check response daily.
Raise dose by smallest increments until one of the following occurs:
    Resolution of depression
    Emergence of intolerable side effects
    "High" dose approached or exceeded[a]

[a]"High" dose is not an absolute dose ceiling but exceeds the dose usually required for treatment of depression in terminal illness; reaching this dose should serve as a flag to reassess diagnosis and response before continuation or further dose increases.
(From Shuster JL, Chochinov HM, Greenberg BD. Psychiatric aspects and psychopharmacologic strategies in palliative care. In: Stoudemire A, Fogel BS, Greenberg DB, eds. *Psychiatric care of the medical patient*, vol. 2. New York: Oxford University Press, 2000:315, with permission.)

imipramine, nortriptyline, desipramine) are reliably effective and relatively inexpensive, but have more side effects (e.g., constipation, tachycardia, orthostasis, sedation, dry mouth) than more commonly used drugs. Tricyclics are particularly useful when their sedative, appetite-stimulating, or adjuvant analgesic properties can be beneficial to the depressed cancer patient.

Bupropion is a stimulating agent without serotonergic activity, so it is often of particular use in treating depressed cancer patients with prominent fatigue or thrombocytopenia. The strong sedative and appetite-stimulating properties of mirtazapine are often used to advantage in the setting of cancer. Trazodone is commonly used in low doses as an aid to promote sleep.

Anxiolytics

As outlined in Table 55.5-2, benzodiazepines are the mainstay of pharmacotherapy for acute anxiety symptoms. Shorter-acting agents may require frequent dosing (three or four times daily), whereas longer-acting agents pose a higher risk of accumulation of metabolites with frequent or prolonged use. Patients with chronic or recurrent anxiety symptoms often benefit from first-line therapy with an antidepressant (e.g., SSRI) at standard doses for treatment of depression, with or without a short-acting benzodiazepine for breakthrough anxiety symptoms. Neuroleptics (also known as major tranquilizers) are helpful for anxiety with extreme agitation or acute anxiety in patients intolerant of benzodiazepines.

Antipsychotics

Other indications for use of antipsychotic agents in the cancer setting include primary treatment of psychotic symptoms and delirium. Butyrophenone antipsychotics (e.g., haloperidol) are also very effective as antiemetics.

PSYCHOTHERAPIES

Psychological problems may be alleviated through a variety of psychosocial techniques.[42] This section briefly describes the major interventions that are available for people coping with cancer.

Cognitive-Behavioral Therapy

CBT for the treatment of depression and anxiety is based on the assumption that thoughts or cognitions are directly related to behaviors and emotions.[43] These cognitions may be identified and altered, particularly when they are no longer adaptive (cognitive distortions), and changes in thinking can then produce changes in feelings and behaviors. Central to CBT is identifying the particular cognitive distortions that each individual uses. CBT also stresses that positive thoughts, feelings, and attitudes can be acquired through skills training and practice. CBT skills may be taught to individuals or in groups and may include diversion of attention or distraction, relaxation, reframing of the painful experience, positive affirmation, increase of activity, humor, and prayer. CBT techniques have been found to be effective in reducing cancer-related depression and other symptoms of distress.[44] Specific

techniques have been described for reducing anger, guilt feelings, and fear of death.

Behavioral and Relaxation Therapies

Behavioral and relaxation techniques are typically introduced to cancer patients explicitly for the treatment of fears and anxiety or for pain control. They are considered appropriate adjuvant therapies for the management of stress-related disorders. These interventions are based on the premise that emotions and behaviors are learned or reinforced and may therefore be unlearned or extinguished. Most behavioral techniques begin with teaching relaxation strategies such as deep breathing (an anxiety-inhibiting response) that may be paired with an anxiety-provoking stimulus such as a doctor's appointment, needles, or chemotherapy. With continued pairing the relaxation response is expected to supplant the anxiety response. Turk and Feldman[45] recommend the use of behavioral techniques in the cancer patient who has become increasingly preoccupied with monitoring disease progression, because this can lead to hypervigilance and hyperarousal. In addition, relaxation training has been found to be beneficial in reducing anticipatory nausea. Behavioral interventions are usually brief, concrete, and highly structured.

Supportive (Supportive-Expressive) Therapies

Classen et al.[46] use the term supportive-expressive treatment strategies to describe interventions designed to provide an environment through which cancer patients may feel free to express all their concerns and receive emotional support. In this type of setting, patients may ventilate their feelings as well as engage in problem-solving efforts. Thus, supportive-expressive treatments emphasize using both problem- and emotion-focused coping strategies. One new area of research is exploring the benefits of emotional disclosure on physical and psychological health. Stanton and colleagues[47] used a writing paradigm and found that women with breast cancer who wrote about their deepest thoughts and feelings about breast cancer and women who wrote about the positive effects of cancer had fewer medical appointments for cancer-related morbidities than did women in a control group.

Meaning-Based Psychotherapy

Coping research has demonstrated the psychological and physical benefits of finding meaning when confronting illness. Breitbart[48] recommends that two main components of spirituality be addressed in distressed patients: faith and religious beliefs, and meaning and spiritual well-being. Greenstein and Breitbart[49] have developed a group intervention to help people with advanced disease find meaning in their lives. Sessions focus on aspects of meaning such as responsibility to others, creativity, transcendence, and determination of one's unique values and priorities. The intervention also focuses on developing goals that may be related to connecting with others or reintegration with one's own life. This treatment is offered in a brief and semistructured format.

Group Therapy

Many of the same skills that are taught in individual therapies are effectively communicated via group interventions. Group therapies are an effective means of helping selected patients cope with cancer. In a pivotal study, Spiegel and colleagues[50] found that women with metastatic breast cancer who participated in weekly supportive group therapy had significantly higher survival rates than women who did not participate. Subsequent research on alteration of survival rates with group interventions has been equivocal, and much further research is necessary before such therapies should be recommended as life extending.

Support Groups

Self-help and support groups along with educational programs provide additional resources for cancer patients and their families. During these encounters patients are allowed to express their concerns and listen to the experience of others in similar circumstances. Often support groups are coordinated by non-professional volunteers who may be cancer survivors themselves. Nevertheless, these settings can help individuals feel that they are not alone and that others understand their experiences. Support groups provide a sense of belonging as well as meeting some of the psychoeducational needs of cancer patients.

REFERENCES

1. Derogatis LR, Morrow GR, Fetting J, et al. The prevalence of psychiatric disorders among cancer patients. *JAMA* 1983;249(6):751.
2. *Statistics for 2003.* American Cancer Society. World Wide Web URL: http://www.cancer.org/docroot/STT/stt_0_2003.asp?sitearea=STT&level=1, 2003.
3. Holland JC. Societal views of cancer and the emergence of psycho-oncology. In: Holland JC, ed. *Psycho-oncology.* New York: Oxford University Press, 1998:3.
4. Fawzy FI, Servis ME, Greenberg DB. Oncology and psychooncology. In: Wise MG, Rundell JR, eds. *The American Psychiatric Publishing textbook of consultation-liaison psychiatry: psychiatry in the medically ill.* Washington, DC: American Psychiatric Publishing, 2002:657.
5. Holland JC, ed. *Psycho-oncology.* New York: Oxford University Press, 1998.
6. Chochinov HM, Breitbart W. *Handbook of psychiatry in palliative medicine.* New York: Oxford University Press, 2000.
7. Lazarus R. *Psychological stress and the coping process.* New York: McGraw-Hill, 1966.
8. Fallowfield L, Hall A, Maguire GP et al. Psychological outcomes of different treatment policies in women with early breast cancer outside a clinical trial. *BMJ* 1990;301(6752):575.
9. Bottomly A. Depression in cancer patients: a literature review. *Eur J Cancer* 1998;7:181.
10. Dropkin MJ. Body image and quality of life after head and neck cancer surgery. *Cancer Pract* 1999;7(6):309.
11. Fichtenbaum J, Kirshblum S. Psychological adaptation to spinal cord injury. In: Kirshblum S, Campagnolo D, DeLisa JA, eds. *Spinal cord medicine.* Philadelphia: Lippincott Williams & Wilkins, 2002:300.
12. Houldin AD. *Patients with cancer: understanding the psychological pain.* Philadelphia: Lippincott Williams & Wilkins, 2000.
13. Stommel M, Given BA, Given CS. Depression and functional status as predictors of death among cancer patients. *Cancer* 2002;94:2719.
14. Snyder CR, Cheavens J, Michael ST. Hoping. In: Snyder CR, ed. *Coping: the psychology of what works.* New York: Oxford University Press, 1999:205.
15. Post-White J, Ceronsky C, Kreitzer MJ, et al. Hope, spirituality, sense of coherence, and quality of life in patients with cancer. *Oncol Nurs Forum* 1996;23(10):1571.
16. Brenner H. Long-term survival rates of cancer patients achieved by the end of the 20th century: a period analysis. *Lancet* 2002;360:1131.
17. Myers CA. Neuropsychological aspects of cancer and cancer treatment. *Cancer Rehabilitation, Physical Medicine and Rehabilitation: State of the Art Reviews* 1994;8(2):229.
18. Baker F, Zabora J, Polland A, et al. Reintegration after bone marrow transplantation. *Cancer Pract* 1999;7(4):190.
19. Breitbart W, Levenson JA, Passik SD. Terminally ill cancer patients. In: Breitbart W, Holland JD, eds. *Psychiatric aspects of symptoms management in cancer patients.* Washington, DC: American Psychiatric Press, 1993:173.
20. Breitbart W, Jaramillo JR, Chochinov HM. Palliative and terminal care. In: Holland JC, ed. *Psycho-oncology.* New York: Oxford University Press, 1998:437.
21. Twycross R, Wilcock A. *Symptom management in advanced cancer,* 3rd ed. Oxon, England: Radcliffe Medical Press, 2001.
22. Chochinov HM. Dignity-conserving care—a new model for palliative care: helping the patient feel valued. *JAMA* 2002;287(17):2253.
23. Byock I. *Dying well.* New York: Riverhead Books, 1997.
24. *NCCN clinical practice guidelines in oncology. Distress management.* National Comprehensive Cancer Network. World Wide Web URL: http://www.nccn.org.
25. American Psychiatric Association. *Diagnostic and statistical manual of mental disorders,* 4th ed. Washington, DC: American Psychiatric Association, 1994.
26. Maguire P. Late adverse psychological sequelae of breast cancer and its treatment. *Eur J Surg Oncol* 1999;25:317.
27. Noyes R Jr, Holt CS, Massie MJ. Anxiety disorders. In: Holland JC, ed. *Psycho-oncology.* New York: Oxford University Press, 1998:548.
28. Shuster JL, Jones GR. Approach to the patient receiving palliative care. In: Stern TA, Herman J, eds. *The MGH guide to psychiatry in primary care.* New York: McGraw-Hill, 1998:147.
29. Jacobsen PT, Sadler IJ, Booth-Jones M, et al. Predictors of posttraumatic stress disorder symptomatology following bone marrow transplantation for cancer. *J Consult Clin Psychol* 2002;70(1):235.
30. Widows MR, Jacobsen PT, Fields KK. Relation of psychological vulnerability factors to posttraumatic stress disorder symptomatology in bone marrow transplant recipients. *Psychosomatic Med* 2000;62(6):873.
31. Mundy EA, Blanchard EB, Cirenza E, et al. Posttraumatic stress disorder in breast cancer patients following autologous bone marrow transplantation or conventional cancer treatments. *Behav Res Ther* 2000;38(10):1015.
32. Spitzer RL, Williams JB, Kroenke K, et al. Utility of a new procedure for diagnosing mental disorders in primary care: the PRIME-MD 1000 study. *JAMA* 1994;272:1749.
33. Chochinov HM, Wilson KG, Enns M, Lander S. "Are you depressed?" Screening for depression in the terminally ill. *Am J Psychiatry* 1997;154:674.
34. Lipowski ZJ. Delirium: acute confusional states. New York: Oxford University Press, 1990.
35. Shuster JL. Confusion, agitation, and delirium at the end of life. *J Palliat Med* 1998;1:177.
36. American Psychiatric Association. Practice guideline for the treatment of patients with delirium. *Am J Psychiatry* 1999;156(5 Suppl):1.
37. Breitbart W, Marotta R, Platt MM, et al. A double-blind trial of haloperidol, chlorpromazine, and lorazepam in the treatment of delirium in hospitalized AIDS patients. *Am J Psychiatry* 1996;153:231.
38. Chochinov HM, Wilson KG, Enns M, Lander S. Depression, hopelessness, and suicidal ideation in the terminally ill. *Psychosomatics* 1998;39(4):366.
39. Shuster JL, Lagomasino IT, Stern TA. Suicide. In: Irwin RS, Cerra FB, Rippe JM, eds. *Intensive care medicine,* 4th ed. Philadelphia: Lippincott–Raven Publishers, 1999:2415.
40. Brown TM, Stoudemire A, Fogel BS, Moran MG. Psychopharmacology in the medical patient. In: Stoudemire A, Fogel BS, Greenberg DB, eds. *Psychiatric care of the medical patient,* 2nd ed. New York: Oxford University Press, 2000:329.
41. Masand PS, Tesar GE. Use of stimulants in the medically ill. *Psychiatr Clin N Am* 1996;19:515.
42. Sheard T, Maguire P. The effect of psychological interventions on anxiety and depression in cancer patients: results of two meta-analyses. *Br J Cancer* 1999;80(11):1770.
43. Beck AT. *Cognitive therapy and the emotional disorders.* New York: International Universities Press, 1976.
44. Lovejoy NC, Tabor D, Matteis M, et al. Cancer-related depression: part I—neurologic alterations and cognitive-behavioral therapy. *Oncol Nurs Forum* 2000;27(4):667.
45. Turk DC, Feldman CS. A cognitive-behavioral approach to symptom management in palliative care. In: Chochinov HM, Breitbart W, eds. *Handbook of psychiatry in palliative medicine.* Oxford: Oxford University Press, 2000:223.
46. Classen C, Abramson S, Angell A. Effectiveness of a training program for enhancing therapists' understanding of the supportive-expressive treatment model for breast cancer groups. *J Psychother Pract Res* 1997;6(3):211.
47. Stanton AL, Danoff-Burg S, Sworowski LA, et al. Randomized, controlled trial of written emotional expression and benefit finding in breast cancer patients. *J Clin Oncol* 2002;20(20):4160.
48. Breitbart W. Spirituality and meaning in supportive care: spirituality- and meaning-centered group psychotherapy interventions in advanced cancer. *Support Care Cancer* 2002;10(4):272.
49. Greenstein M, Breitbart W. Cancer and the experience of meaning: a group psychotherapy program for people with cancer. *Am J Psychother* 2000;54(4):486.
50. Spiegel D, Kraemer H, Bloom J, et al. Effect of psychosocial treatment on survival of patients with metastatic breast cancer. *Lancet* 1989;2(8668):888.

BONNIE A. INDECK

Community Resources

The impact of continuous changes in the health care system has persisted in causing greater numbers of patients to be treated in ambulatory settings. Services in these settings range from maintenance of central lines to chemotherapy, nutritional support, pain control, intravenous antibiotics, and blood support. Patients are admitted to the hospital only if their condition is so serious that it necessitates an acute level of care or they require chemotherapy protocols available only in an inpatient setting. Ever-changing reimbursement issues along with an ever-increasing number of cancer survivors[1] have placed yet a greater burden on the community to provide services for this often chronically ill population.

Community resource directories are regularly updated to include the latest evolving information, although this can be a challenge due to frequency of change. Cancer Care is just one source that publishes a comprehensive listing of services.[2] In addition, access to personal computers and the Internet have allowed individuals to gather information with unprecedented ease. Although, theoretically, this easy access to the most current information should allow the patient to acquire the assistance needed to live with this illness, a gap still remains between availability of these resources and the needs of the individual. This gap in the availability of services occurs in many communities and within many insurance carriers.

The individual diagnosed with cancer undergoes an experience that is intensely personal, that calls into question basic assumptions and expectations about life, and that somehow must be integrated into a sense of self and thus involves the complexities of individual personalities. Those who are working with this population must understand the adaptation that occurs to deliver effective service. This adaptation involves incorporating a new sense of self after living through the crisis of diagnosis, initial treatment, potential side effects, and emotional impact on one's self and one's family. In addition to discussing individual adjustment, this chapter addresses different types of support and resources that may be beneficial to the patient and family, the impact of the Internet, the effect of an evolving health care delivery and reimbursement system and survivorship issues and concludes with a list of available resources.

INITIAL DIAGNOSIS OF CANCER

Cancer is the second major cause of mortality in the United States.[3] More than 1.36 million people will be diagnosed with cancer in 2004, and the 5-year relative survival rate has steadily increased.[1] Although these statistics present an increase in survivorship, the reality of living with cancer represents something quite different. Concerns must be broadened to view cancer as a chronic or curable illness. The majority of the million-plus people who are diagnosed with cancer view their own mortality but move from focusing on their mortality to dealing with their illness. It is incumbent on medical providers to help the patient participate in a plan to develop adequate internal and external resources for living with cancer.

The spectrum of reactions include fear, shock, despair, anger, and anxiety, and/or total insensibility.[4] More than 20 years ago, Weisman and Worden identified the immediate coping response of denial as appropriate, albeit temporarily.[5] This is still valid today, but given the changing nature of today's medical delivery system, the patient may need to be helped to progress from denial to mastery in a more expeditious fashion. Although today's cancer patients suffer distress that is often not considered or reflected in the economics of treatment, they still desire and need psychosocial intervention to cope with their cancer. The medical system has resources that can address these emotions and enable a person to function more effectively. The physician may call on members of the team such as the oncology social worker or oncology nurse to assist in presenting the diagnosis, giving "bad" news, or aiding in the transition from curative to palliative care. These team members can facilitate the understanding of the diagnosis in many distinct ways. The professional oncology team helps the patient move toward a sense of mastery over the situation. Assistance is provided so that a patient moves along a continuum through which control is gained and progress is made from a passive to an active state. This progression promotes an active course of treatment. The team encourages the patient to choose options that are in synchrony with his or her value system, thus ensuring the highest quality of life (QOL) for the patient in the continuum of his or her illness.

SOCIAL SUPPORT NETWORK

Recent literature has identified and recognized the importance of a social support network. Research has consistently found that people coping with cancer have difficulty with interpersonal relationships and that one's social support system can alleviate these stressors.[6] Although this network may not prolong the life of a cancer patient, it has been shown to enhance the QOL one experiences. The providers in a social support network may be professionals from the community, family, friends, significant others, organizations, and/or agencies. These providers enable cancer patients to enhance their coping skills so that they may function in an effective, competent, and proficient manner. The literature continues to report that this social support network has a strong positive impact on the psychological well-being of the cancer patient.[7,8] The constructs of the social support system, identified as emotional, informational, or instrumental, defined by Wortman are the structure in which support and resources for the person with cancer are defined.[9]

EMOTIONAL SUPPORT

Psychosocial interventions have consistently contributed to a positive outcome on the emotional adjustment of a person coping with cancer, and emotional support is frequently considered to be one of the most essential interventions. Dunkel-Schetter surveyed 79 cancer patients and found that 81% defined emotional support as most helpful, followed by informational support (41%) and instrumental aid (6%).[10]

ASSESSMENT AND EVALUATION OF COPING SKILLS

Individuals deal with problems in diverse ways. It is important that the medical team identifies an individual's ability to cope with stress so there is some indication of how the patient will deal with his or her cancer. An assessment of other crises endured and how those were handled is particularly helpful in an assessment and evaluation. Studies have led to development of a profile of predictors of poor coping skills.[11] Some indicators of the ability to cope with crises are character traits such as rigidity of behavior or morose outlook on life. This type of patient may not be amenable to the support received or may need more intense intervention. Substance abuse, recent losses, social isolation, or other debilitating illnesses may be warning signs that an individual may be emotionally overwhelmed. Cancer causes a significant level of emotional distress, and disruptions in routine functioning are commonplace. Some of these disruptions may have lingering effects and cause enduring problems. In these cases, specialized or individualized support may be necessary for this person to cope with his or her diagnosis.

FAMILY AS EMOTIONAL SUPPORT

As the newly diagnosed person enters the health care system, it is important for the professionals to recognize that this person rarely functions alone. He or she usually summons his or her closest family to become the immediate support system. Health care professionals must recognize the significance of including the family at times of diagnosis, recurrence, change in treatment plans, and terminal illness. The family system changes when the diagnosis is made. All members who interact with the patient should be aware of the potential changes and the subsequent impact on the family.

The family value and belief system must be understood so that help can be provided within the context of the sociocultural system. Fears are minimized and coping skills enhanced if understanding is provided within a familiar context. One needs to recognize that cancer is not openly discussed in all cultural groups. Certain cultural groups may need special assistance to contend with a health care system where the patient is expected to be an active participant. Roles within the family frequently change when a diagnosis of cancer is made. Family members may need help in evaluating whether these role changes are comfortable for them. In addition, a family member who is also a health care professional, and particularly an oncology health care professional, may need help in maintaining the role of a family member rather than becoming the resource person. The alacrity to help is frequently seen during the initial crisis of diagnosis. This is the time a family pulls itself together and offers whatever resources it can provide for the newly diagnosed patient. As the illness extends over time and sometimes becomes chronic, family support may wane and become difficult to sustain. It is therefore imperative that psychosocial support be provided to the family members, allowing them to continue to support the patient. It is often at this time that patients and families may need to find resources outside the immediate family system.

EMOTIONAL SUPPORT OUTSIDE THE FAMILY SYSTEM

The social support network includes friends, neighbors, both self-help and professionally facilitated support groups, religious groups, community agencies, and health care professionals.[11] A review of the literature has indicated that using emotional support, whether informal or formal, can relieve distress.[12] It is important that there be some commonality perceived in the support system. People undergoing similar experiences may find it easier to relate to each other. The cancer is accepted more easily. If the perception is that a situation is understood, empathy can be accepted, and emotional support to the patient becomes positive. The validity of the cancer patient's experiences must be recognized by the support system for support to be effective. A member of a support system who truly does not understand the trauma cannot minimize the anxieties and fears of the cancer patient. Support is not effective in a situation in which real feelings are not recognized.

Visitation Groups

The American Cancer Society has many groups maintained by volunteers who have had cancer experiences. Reach to Recovery, CanSurmount, and the ostomy programs all have volunteers who have undergone some type of cancer experience. In the past, these volunteers were able to visit with newly diagnosed patients in the hospital. Today, due to shortened hospital stays, these volunteers must be creative in finding the appropriate time to see the patient—often after the patient has been discharged. Therefore, health care professionals need to take special care in providing patients with information about these groups, and patients need to be encouraged to become proactive and make the first contact themselves. The health care professional that one meets in the hospital is an invaluable source of information.

Self-Help Groups

An extensive network of self-help groups exists for the cancer patient. Self-help groups are frequently formed by people with similar interests or concerns, and many of these groups are disease-specific. This is not a professionally led group, but rather a gathering led by the peer participants, although medical professionals may be invited to present their particular expertise. Information about self-help groups can be accessed through the National Self-Help Network. This organization is listed individually in each state. Often, self-help groups are offspring of professionally facilitated groups that have come to conclusion.

Support Groups

Traditional support groups are available in most communities and are facilitated by health care professionals. The professional has the responsibility of establishing a group that is cohesive and has the goals of providing educational and emotional support. Groups may be established for patients, for family members and significant others, or for patients and family together. Although emotional support and social support are separated for descriptive purposes here, they are frequently intertwined and often inseparable. The family member who transports a cancer patient for daily radiation treatments is both part of the social support system and also provides necessary emotional support.

Role of Medical Team in Emotional Support

The medical team is composed of numerous people who can assist the cancer patient. Social workers, clinical nurse specialists, nurse practitioners, chaplains, psychologists, psychiatrists, and nutritionists are often available to provide services. Although these professionals may not be immediately available in every setting, referrals can be made for consultation. Ancillary personnel have become more important in today's system of health care delivery due to increased time constraints physicians incur. Specialized health care professionals can also help a patient navigate the health care system with greater ease and less stress.

INFORMATION SUPPORT

It is axiomatic that knowledge is power and that cancer patients and families who know more about their illness and are actively involved in treatment decisions cope better than those who are more passive do. It is this demand for knowledge and information that helps those individuals to feel less powerless and more in control of the situation. The need for information depends not only on individual desire for control, but also on a person's educational, cultural, and financial background.[13] In the past, initial cancer information was obtained in the physician's office or hospital, often in a unilateral direction from provider to recipient.[14] Alarmingly, in a study performed by Chapman et al. in the United Kingdom, it was discovered that a significant proportion of the lay public did not understand phrases often used in cancer conversations, that knowledge of basic anatomy could not be assumed, and that asking patients if they understood was likely to overestimate comprehension.[15] Today, there is a greater demand for dialogues that are occurring through questioning and challenging.

According to Fernsler and Cannon,[16] "patients with cancer benefit from education in terms of their ability to care for themselves, enhanced self-image and self-esteem, improved symptom management, reduced anxiety and reduced disruption in daily life." Other benefits of education include increased participation in treatment decisions and improved understanding. There may be some inherent differences for some individuals with obtaining information due to personality style. Too much information can increase anxiety for some people and cause greater difficulty in coping. It is therefore important to first assess a person's readiness to receive information by reviewing his or her culture, literacy, educational level, psychological adjustment, socioeconomic background, and personal preferences for control.

As culture influences the very meaning of the disease to that individual, it is imperative to understand that person's background, values, and beliefs. Communities also vary by culture, implying that culturally sensitive material must be developed. Providers must explore the patient's educational level and determine how to maximize both comprehension and retention of material while encouraging greater patient participation in decisions and greater dialogue with the health care team. "The ability to read, understand and act on information is often dangerously low. More than 40% of patients with chronic illnesses are functionally illiterate."[17] Almost one-fourth of all adult Americans read at or below fifth-grade level, and according to the 2000 census, 19 million people have limited proficiency in English.[17] The Commonwealth Fund has shown that minorities who have low health literacy report problems such as not understanding medical instructions or not being treated respectfully. This can result in poor compliance, confusion in understanding the medical system, and medical errors.[18] Can-

cer patients who are deficient in literacy skills may experience different outcomes due to disparities in care or barriers to care. To ensure that patients understand, offer small amounts of information at a time, make sure all written material is at a fifth-grade level or below, develop language-appropriate material, and verify that patients understand the information by asking what they understand, not if they understand. Various high-tech devices are also being tested on the market, such as talking prescription-recording devices for instructions and electronic pill organizers.[19] In a study by Hahn et al.,[19] an ethnically diverse group of 126 patients with a range of literacy skills and computer experience reported that a "talking touchscreen" was easy to use and understand when exploring self-reported QOL information. The talking touchscreen may also assist providers and organizations in delivering more effective communication for this population, increase the understanding of health problems, and provide necessary information for decision making, thereby improving health outcomes.[20]

Print materials are often helpful, particularly those endorsed by the physician; however, screening for low-literacy populations is mandatory. Social workers can often remove barriers that may hinder education by facilitating communication or by connecting to community resources whose main goal it is to educate the public.

INTERNET

Few technologies have expanded as quickly and have had such a significant impact on society as computers and, more specifically, the Internet. In September 2001, 66% of the population (174 million) used computers, and 54% of the population (143 million Americans) were on-line as of the same date. The rate of growth of Internet use in the United States is close to 10% in 1 year. In 2000, 41.5% of households had access, and, in 2001, the number jumped to 50.5%.[21] Use of the Internet is increasing regardless of income, education, age, race, ethnicity, or gender.[21]

In the past, information was unidirectional from health professionals to patients; now, many patients are seeking out this information for themselves, often coming to the appointment with information in hand. For those who are less knowledgeable, some organizations include lessons on learning how to use a computer and navigate the Internet, as do many local libraries. One study reports that in follow-up interviews, participants attributed a great deal of their well-being to becoming more computer-savvy, hence more knowledgeable and more active in maintaining their health.[22] A recent study showed that 45% of adults turn to the Internet for numerous health care–related purposes. Pandey et al. explored different models to explain Internet use for obtaining health information. They found that it served to supplement information received from traditional sources and particularly that women who have significant demands on their time are more likely to use the Internet.[23] Fogel et al. reported that use of the Internet for information on breast health issues is associated with greater social support and less loneliness for these women. This social support differs by race and ethnicity.[24] However, there are data that suggest that oncologists disagree on the impact of patient Internet use, reporting both advantages and disadvantages with this technology because of misinformation and potential increased levels of anxiety.[25]

Although access to Internet information is vital, accurate, reliable information is not always easy to obtain, as Web sites are not regulated or reviewed by a governing body. It is therefore imperative that one knows how to evaluate for credible sources of information. One should initially try using government and medical association sites, as well as the following:

- Look for the author's and publisher's name, professional standing, and contact information.
- All information should be current, with the last update of the site noted.
- Look for references. Is there a medical advisory board?
- The information should be well organized so that it is logical and easy to follow.
- Disclaimers should be used (i.e., the information provided is not a substitute for visiting a physician).
- Commercial sponsorship should be clearly noted.
- More than one source should be used to ensure that the information is consistent.
- Above all, be cautious!

A new trend is emerging whereby some patients are now e-mailing their physicians to facilitate communication, particularly between office visits. According to the American Medical Association, approximately 25% of physicians contact at least some of their patients by e-mail. Some doctors use patient e-mail in their practices, but most aren't ready to log on.[26] The benefits are efficiency and convenience, but the downsides may be liability, being reimbursed, and lack of patient privacy. Some suggestions include discussion of nonclinical or nonurgent matters only on-line, such as prescription refills and appointments, and using this technology judiciously.

COMPUTER GROUPS

Groups are an effective means of providing psychosocial support to individuals with cancer. These groups also provide information and education, but, today, often the strain of diagnosis and the rigors of treatment combined with concerns about confidentiality may discourage patients from attending these groups. Until recently, people had to physically leave their homes and go to hospitals, physician offices, or other community locations to attend a support group. With increasing use of computers, Internet support groups have become more popular.[27] The ability to use this technology has assisted individuals in overcoming barriers, such as groups held at inconvenient times, barriers to access, ill health, or the stigma that may be associated with attending the group. Benefits achieved include increased control of time of participation and of information disclosed or obtained, safety to discuss difficult issues, availability of information, and subsequent support. These groups also benefit individuals with hearing or speech disabilities. Logistical obstacles such as time spent in the assembly of the group or in travel, cost of transportation, facility costs, and scheduling problems are overcome. An additional important benefit is anonymity, which may lead to greater self-disclosure, honesty, and intimacy while allowing specific issues to be more quickly discussed, along with a discussion of taboo topics that may otherwise not arise. One of the major disadvantages noted is decreased interpersonal relationships. Although anonymity may be an advantage, the inability to see individuals,

hear their voices, or read their body language may encourage isolation or interfere with empathy. The Wellness Community and Cancer Care are just two organizations that offer on-line support groups. Owen et al. found that Internet-based psychological therapy can complement face-to-face psychological care.[28] It has also been demonstrated in a study by Lieberman et al.[29] that after 16 weeks of intervention, patients with breast cancer reported decreased depression symptoms, decreased reaction to pain, and an ability to "express more zest for life" and deepen their spiritual lives. Sixty-seven percent of these women reported being helped by the experience.

INSTRUMENTAL SUPPORT

Most medical care is provided on an outpatient basis, which can create additional stressors for the patient and support system. Transportation can sometimes emerge as a barrier to quality treatment. Medications that were previously administered in the hospital are now given on an outpatient basis and may not be covered by insurance. Home care and medical equipment needs may be intensified as hospital stays have become abbreviated.

FINANCES

The cost of the illness and the impact on the patient and family have been well documented. The direct cost of the illness as well as the incidental expenses such as transportation, parking, and child care can be overwhelming to patients. Of people with cancer, it was found that 87% had experienced a significant increase in monthly expenses directly related to the disease.[34] Wang et al. indicated that minorities had more concerns about finances than Caucasians.[30] For the elderly and others on fixed incomes, the uninsured, and the unemployed, these expenses become significant barriers to continuing treatment.

Patients are often reluctant to discuss their finances with the physicians and may feel more comfortable with another member of the medical team. A social worker can do an in-depth financial assessment, including a full discussion of insurance coverage and subsequent referral to available resources. Constant reevaluation of insurance coverage is necessary, as insurance changes with employment changes, managed care providers differ in services offered, and family income changes. Patients may feel pressure, either self-imposed or by hospital and physician offices, for prepayment and/or payment of outstanding bills, all adding to the stress of contending with cancer.

Coverage for medical care costs in the United States comes from four main sources: the federal government, employers and private health insurance, state and local government, and private households. Exploration of privately funded sources should be made with the assistance of the social worker. Cancer Care and The Leukemia & Lymphoma Society are two agencies that frequently assist with finances. Hospital and communities may have funds established from donations that help with finances for the cancer patient.

The federal government funds the Medicare program and the Social Security Disability program. Eligibility is governed by age, permanent disability, and work history. Eligibility for Medicaid and local welfare programs always involves a means test, although this differs regionally. Application for Medicaid is made through the state department of social services.

TRANSPORTATION

Frequently, patients live at great distances from treatment centers or are too debilitated to drive themselves. Family members, although well meaning and caring, may not be able to devote as much time as they wish to provide transportation, which is rarely covered by insurance.

The American Cancer Society, the American Red Cross, Cancer Care, and The Leukemia & Lymphoma Society are agencies that can assist in funding or transporting patients to medical care. In many areas, local towns or regional districts provide transportation to medical appointments. Resources change frequently, and it is necessary to investigate local services to assess availability.

HOME HEALTH CARE

Home health care provides for those patients who do not require hospitalization and is the most rapidly expanding segment of the health care industry today. Agencies, visits, and services have multiplied exponentially due to several major influences: demographic changes, managed care, and the patient's desire to remain at home. The older population is expected to more than double by the year 2030. Combined with steadily increasing pressure from insurance companies and managed care programs to search for the least expensive treatment method and to emphasize the lowest appropriate level of care, low-cost alternatives, and early discharge from hospitals and other health care facilities, one can see the impact on all patients regardless of the demographics. Advanced technologies have been developed in many areas to allow those in this population to be maintained in their own home. Sensors that can confirm specific activity without infringing on a person's rights under the Health Insurance Portability and Accountability Act can issue medication reminders, enable close monitoring, and support patient compliance, thereby enabling increased independence at home.[31]

To be eligible for home care services, a patient must be homebound and require skilled nursing services. Short-term custodial services may be provided after the above criteria are met. Home health care also provides for continuity of care between physician visits.

HOSPICE

Hospice home care is available for patients living at home and requiring nursing care who have a prognosis of 6 months or less. The first hospice was organized in Connecticut in 1974, and currently there are approximately 3000 hospice programs in the United States providing care for close to one-half million dying patients. In addition to providing nursing care, emphasis is also placed on support of patient and family. Physicians, nurses, social workers, clergy, volunteers, aides, and other ancillary personnel work together to provide services to patient and family from diagnosis through bereavement. This continuum of support can be invaluable for those dealing with a terminal illness. Data indicate, however, that although most people with advanced cancer could benefit from hospice care, they do not use this resource, and if they do, it is often too close to the time of death to enable them to take full advantage of the benefits.[32]

BARRIERS TO EFFECTIVE HOME CARE

Home care should provide the support, reassurance, and medical assistance necessary to help the patient function while remaining in the comfort of his or her own home. The success of a good home care plan depends on the skills of the professional responsible for planning for this service before discharge from the hospital. A serviceable home care plan also relies heavily on family support and family caregivers. Most insurance companies follow Medicare guidelines and usually provide for a maximum of 2 to 3 hours of home care daily.

The burden of home care usually becomes the responsibility of the primary caregiver who, although frequently willing to provide care on a time-limited basis, cannot continue to do so for an extended period. Patients may lack knowledge regarding the available services or may be unable to afford services to supplement insurance-covered home care. In some areas, there are geographic limitations, and not all services are available in all areas. There are added limitations at this time due to nursing shortages that restrict the ability of many agencies to accept referrals as quickly as the patient may need.

In caring for a patient at home, the caregivers must provide various levels of support. Needs may range from the highly technical to simple companionship and monitoring for safety. Technical support can be received from a home health care agency; the less technical type of support such as house cleaning, shopping, or cooking may be available from church or synagogue groups or senior center groups.

MEDICAL EQUIPMENT

At various times during the course of treatment for cancer, a patient may need special medical equipment or require modification to his or her home. Before discharge from the hospital or during the course of treatment, the medical team can make this assessment. Home health care personnel can also complete a safety evaluation. Insurance may cover these items, but only when prescribed by a physician. It is critical that the patient and those providing care be given ample instruction in the care and use of any equipment.

TRENDS AFFECTING DEMAND FOR COMMUNITY SERVICES

Continual changes in the health care environment affect the need for specific resources. The maelstrom of public debate in the 1990s swirled around the concerns of escalating medical spending and suboptimal care, along with increasing awareness that there is a significant contingent of Americans with no or inadequate insurance.[33] Uninsured Americans have more limited access to health care services, and 30% to 55% forego or postpone care.[34] Employers have continued to streamline choices of health plans while shifting the costs to the employee and sometimes terminating coverage due to the high cost of premiums. Employees are paying 48% more than they did in 2000, an average of $2790 annually.[35] Some plans limit benefits such as prescription coverage or charge higher copays and deductibles. In addition, "casual" employees and part-time workers rarely receive insurance. The rising unemployment rate has also contributed to this picture.

The 1985 Consolidated Omnibus Budget Reconciliation Act allows people to leave their jobs and pay privately for their insurance, but it does not consider the expense involved. Although the Health Insurance Portability and Accountability Act prohibits denial of those with preexisting conditions, this cost is so exorbitant that it becomes self-limiting, protecting only a few hundred thousand instead of the millions who have lost insurance.

Prescription costs are increasing exponentially. Often state programs do not cover the most costly drugs that people undergoing cancer treatment may require. Although there may be assistance through pharmaceutical companies, the process is often tedious, and criteria for eligibility are not always known preceding the application process. Patients who cannot afford medications and are therefore noncompliant with prescribed regimens cost the United States between $13 and $15 billion annually due to additional office visits and hospitalization.[36] Twenty-five percent of the uninsured population report unfilled prescriptions and are also less likely to receive preventative services such as mammograms, Pap smears, and prostate examinations. Thirty-six percent had difficulty paying medical bills, and 17% had to alter their life significantly to do so.[34] Those who are uninsured may develop a pattern of "learned helplessness" in response to barriers to health care and may internalize the stigma of being uninsured, blaming themselves.

Hospitals have experienced billions of dollars in reduced Medicare payments, and these reductions potentially compromise a hospital's standard of care. As individuals are now hospitalized for shorter periods of time, the multidisciplinary team is often no longer able to help patients adjust to a new diagnosis while anticipating the next phase of the illness and adapting to its demands. Often a social worker or discharge planner works with the patient and family to plan for transition to the community while assessing the barriers to care and subsequent plan for appropriate intervention. Although reimbursable services are obtainable, there is a wide gap for patients without adequate coverage. These concerns support the demand for a universal health policy that would allow greater access for a majority of Americans.

SURVIVORSHIP

The National Coalition for Cancer Survivorship defines survivors as living through and beyond a cancer diagnosis.[37] Today there are approximately 10 million cancer survivors,[38] and for the first time since the 1930s, the death rate has steadily decreased and is leveling off or declining in all major sites. These statistics are mainly true for the nonminority community. African Americans continue to have higher incidence rates and are at greater risk of dying from cancer than any other racial or ethnic group, although certain racial/ethnic groups experience higher rates for specific cancers than other groups.[1]

QOL issues for survivors include fatigue and pain, menopausal symptoms, and reproductive and fertility concerns as well as fears related to recurrence and immobility after treat-

ment. There have also been cases of discrimination in the workplace, with consequent economic burdens. The American Cancer Society and The Leukemia & Lymphoma Society direct part of their mission toward the needs of cancer survivors. Continuing assessment of QOL issues along with appropriate interventions in the community can enhance the lives of the ever-increasing number of survivors. New and creative resources must be developed to meet the needs of this growing population. "Satisfaction with treatment is an important early indicator of medical outcome for cancer patients."[39] Patient satisfaction may be enhanced when hospital staff attend to and provide for the psychosocial needs of a person with a cancer. This lesson can be used in any setting that provides for the medical care of such a patient.

APPENDIX: COMMON COMMUNITY RESOURCES

This appendix lists the most commonly used and helpful resources. Some may change without notice. Therefore, please check before giving this information to patients and family members. This is not an all-inclusive list because of the plethora of resources available.

The following health literacy resources may be helpful in simplifying communication and learning:

Firstfind.info	http://www.firstfind.info
Harvard School of Public Health	http://www.hsph.harvard.edu/healthliteracy
Literacy Volunteers of America	http://www.literacyvolunteers.org/home/
U.S. Department of Health and Human Services	http://www.usability.gov
National Institute for Literacy	http://www.nifl.gov
Plain Language Action & Information Network	http://www.plainlanguage.gov

BONE MARROW/STEM CELL TRANSPLANTATION

- Blood & Marrow Transplant Information Network: 1-888-597-7674; http://www.bmtinfonet.org. Provides a newsletter, resource directory, and support services via e-mail or telephone and access to a list of attorneys who advocate for patients who have insurance difficulties.
- BMT Support Online: http://www.bmtsupport.org. Provides support and education on-line.
- Caitlin Raymond International Registry: 1-800-726-2824; http://www.crir.org. An international search coordinating center that assists individuals in finding compatible donors.
- Cancer Care: 1-800-813-HOPE; http://www.cancercare.org. Provides information, counseling, and support in addition to limited financial aid.
- Children's Organ Transplant Association: 1-800-366-2682; http://www.cota.org. Provides fundraising assistance and promotes organ, marrow, and tissue donation.
- International Bone Marrow Transplant Registry: 1-414-456-8325; http://www.IBMTR.org. Provides statistical information on transplantation.

- National Bone Marrow Transplant Link: 1-800-LINK-BMT; http://www.nbmtlink.org. For those considering transplants, it provides publications to help cope with logistics, finances, and medical insurance as well as providing peer support.
- The National Children's Cancer Society: 1-314-241-1600; http://www.nationalchildrenscancersociety.com. Provides financial assistance for children diagnosed before 18 years of age as well as emotional support, education information, and advocacy in addition to a parents' network.
- National Marrow Donor Program: 1-800-627-7692; http://www.marrow.org. Central registry facilitating searches and matches of unrelated donors and recipients.
- National Transplant Assistance Fund: 1-800-642-8399; http://www.transplantfund.org. Helps individuals raise funds for medically related transplant expenses and offers financial grants to eligible patients.
- The Leukemia & Lymphoma Society: 1-888-282-9465; http://www.lls.org. Provides publications, support, education, and limited financial aid.
- The Marrow Foundation: 1-202-638-6601; http://www.themarrowfoundation.org. Assists patients with uninsured financial needs and increases understanding and diversity of the National Marrow Donor Program's registry of unrelated donors.

CHILDREN'S CAMPS

- Camps for siblings who are grieving a loss, often organized through a local hospice. Examples are Camp Begin-Again (1-703-538-2043) and Camp Starfish (1-202-895-0124).
- National Cancer Institute: 1-800-4-CANCER; http://www.cancer.gov. Helps guide patients to local resources.
- Candlelighters Childhood Cancer Foundation: 1-800-366-2223; http://www.candlelighters.org. Provides a list of camps.
- Children's Oncology Camping Association International: http://www.coca-intl.org. Provides a list of all registered camps categorized by state.
- KidsCamps.com: http://www.kidscamps.com. Provides a directory for "special needs" camps, including cancer/oncology camps.
- KOA Care Camps: 1-205-824-0022; http://www.koacare-camps.com. Provides financial support to camps that are designed for children who have cancer, are in remission, or have siblings who would like to attend. A list of camps categorized by state is available.
- Therapy/Respite Camps for Kids: http://www.wmoore.net/therapy.html. Provides information about camps with children with special needs and/or respite, categorized by region.

CARE FACILITIES

Care facilities provide for the continuous health-related care of patients who are temporarily or permanently unable to manage living at home. Different levels of care are available, and patients should explore these services with a member of the health care team to ascertain the appropriate level needed. Patients should also confer with their insurance company to determine coverage.

- Hospice: Provides supportive, palliative, and terminal care physically and emotionally.

- Rehabilitation: Provides services to patients with the goal of restoring them to an optimal level of functioning. This may include both subacute or acute rehabilitation services.
- Skilled nursing facility: A nursing facility with the staff and equipment to give skilled nursing care and other health-related services. Go to http://www.medicare.gov or http://www.ahca.org to begin a search.

CHILDHOOD RESOURCES

- Candlelighters Childhood Cancer Foundation: 1-800-366-2223; http://www.candlelighters.org. Provides an annual bibliography and resource guide, quarterly newsletter, youth newsletter, and handbooks.
- Children's Hospice International: 1-800-2-4-CHILD; http://www.chionline.org. Ensures medical, psychological, social and spiritual support to children with life-threatening conditions and their families.
- Children's Organ Transplant Association: 1-800-366-2682; http://www.cota.org. Provides fundraising assistance and promotes organ, marrow, and tissue donation.
- CureSearch National Childhood Cancer Foundation: 1-800-458-6223; http://www.nccf.org. Provides information on new treatments and psychosocial support as well as a newsletter.
- Famous Fone Friends: 1-310-204-5683. Links children who are confined to the home or hospital by telephone with entertainers and athletes.
- Starbright Foundation: 1-800-315-2580; http://www.starbright.org. Creates media-based programs that help seriously ill children and teenagers better cope with their disease and enhance their QOL.
- The Compassionate Friends: 1-877-969-0010; http://www.compassionatefriends.org. Assists families toward the positive resolution of grief after the death of a child and provides information to help others be supportive.

EMOTIONAL SUPPORT

Many patients experience emotional distress when diagnosed and treated for cancer. Although adaptation begins shortly after the diagnosis, it may continue with varying intensity through the continuum of an illness depending on the psychological, social, and medical variables that occur. To adequately cope with the impact of the diagnosis, emotional support is essential for the patient, family, and/or caregiver. Many individuals rely on community resources to procure that support, which may include self-help and/or professional individual or group modalities. Many ambulatory and hospital-based settings may provide social work, psychiatric services, and pastoral care.

This section lists common agencies, although most of the organizations that provide support are listed later in Internet.

American Cancer Society: 1-800-ACS-2345; http://www.cancer.org.
   Cancer Survivors Network: Individuals supporting one another and sharing personal experiences with cancer.
   I Can Cope: Support group for individuals with cancer and their families.
   Look Good . . . Feel Better: A free service for women with cancer that teaches beauty techniques to help enhance appearance and self-image during treatment.

Look Good . . . Feel Better for Teens: A free program that assists teenaged patients with the effects of cancer.

Man to Man: Helps men and their families cope with prostate cancer by providing education and support.

Reach to Recovery: Support, information, and comfort provided by trained volunteers before, during, and after breast cancer treatment.

Taking Charge of Money Matters: A workshop for patients and families regarding financial concerns that arise during or after cancer treatment.

Cancer Care: 1-800-813-HOPE; http://www.cancercare.org. Provides free professional help through counseling, education, information, referral, and direct financial assistance.

Coping Magazines: 1-615-790-2400; http://www.copingmag.com. Provides practical tips for living with cancer.

Family service agencies: Provide information, emotional support, and psychological assistance.

Mental health centers: Provide emotional support and psychological interventions.

National Cancer Institute: http://www.cancer.gov.

Databases

PDQ (Physician Data Query): Cancer information—updated monthly—that summarizes the latest advances in treatment, supportive care, screening, prevention, and genetics. Includes clinical trials, organizations, and physicians active in cancer care.

CANCERLIT: searchable bibliographic database, updated monthly, from the 1960s to the present

General education

Site-specific materials

Complementary and alternative medicine options

Clinical trial information

Nutrition

Cancer facts

Internet resources

National Cancer Institute Web site (http://www.cancer.gov)

CancerNet

CancerTrials

National Cancer Institute publications locator

LiveHelp instant messaging service

CancerMail

Cancer information service: 1-800-4-CANCER

Office of Cancer Survivorship

Teaching modules

Office of Cancer Complementary and Alternative Medicine

National Coalition for Cancer Survivorship: 1-877-622-7937; http://www.canceradvocacy.org.

Private practitioners: Provide emotional support and psychological interventions often partially covered through insurance reimbursement.

Religious organizations: Provide emotional support, pastoral care, and spiritual guidance.

Su Familia: The National Hispanic Family Health Helpline: 1-866-783-2645. Provides basic information to help prevent and manage chronic conditions and refers patients to local health providers and federally supported programs.

The Leukemia & Lymphoma Society: 1-888-282-9465; http://www.lls.org. Funds blood cancer research, education, and patient services for leukemia, lymphoma, Hodgkin's disease, and myeloma.

Well Spouse Foundation: 1-800-838-0879; http://www.wellspouse.org. Provides support to the spouses and partners of the chronically ill through groups and newsletters.

Y-ME National Breast Cancer Organization: 1-800-221-2141 (English), 1-800-986-9505 (Spanish); http://www.yme.org. Provides information, empowerment, and peer support for people with breast cancer.

FERTILITY

Often the chances of having children may be decreased or eliminated from the effects of cancer treatment. There are several medically assisted ways that may keep patient options open, but insurance coverage should be explored, as these services are not always reimbursable.

- Sperm banking: Cryopreservation allows men to bank their sperm before undergoing cancer treatment.
- Intrauterine insemination: In this process, frozen sperm are inserted into the woman's uterus.
- Freezing embryos: Cryopreservation of a woman's eggs fertilized by sperm before the beginning of cancer treatment (it is not always possible to freeze eggs). However, this process may take time and is not always possible, as it causes a treatment delay.
- Cryopreservation of ovaries: The procedure is still in early stages and not yet proven effective.
- *In vitro* fertilization: The process assists the natural reproductive process by combining the sperm and egg outside the body.
- Donor sperm, eggs, and embryos: Donors can be used for insemination or for the *in vitro* process.
- Medications: Medications that preserve ovarian function by "shutting down" the ovaries during chemotherapy are being offered but are thus far unproven.
- American Society for Reproductive Medicine: 1-205-978-5000; http://www.asrm.org.
- Fertile Hope: 1-888-994-HOPE; http://www.fertilehope.org.
- RESOLVE: The National Infertility Association: 1-888-623-0744; http://www.resolve.org.
- The Organization of Parents through Surrogacy: 1-847-782-0224; http://www.opts.com.
- Adoptive Families: 1-800-372-3300; http://www.adoptive-families.com.

FINANCIAL ASSISTANCE

Heavy financial burdens for patients and families are often related to a diagnosis of cancer. These concerns should be discussed with a member of the patient's health care team who can help inform and guide the patient through the process.

Income-Related

Food stamps are designed to assist eligible individuals or families to purchase food.

Short-term disability income is sometimes offered through an employer. The patient should explore this with the benefits office.

U.S. Social Security Administration: 1-800-772-1213; http://www.ssa.gov. The governmental agency that oversees the following:

Supplemental Security Income: Supplements income for individuals who are aged, blind, or disabled with limited income.

Social Security Disability: Pays benefits for the long-term totally disabled person who has worked enough "quarters" and certain family members.

Treatment-Related

Avon Foundation Breast Cancer Crusade: http://www.avoncompany.com/women/avoncrusade. A special assistance fund for underserved women who are in need of diagnostic services and/or treatment for cancer.

Cancer Care: 1-800-813-HOPE; http://www.cancercare.org. Provides limited grants for some people in need in some regions.

Cancer Fund of America: 1-800-578-5284; http://www.cfoa.org. Assists patients by sending products such as Boost, adult diapers, bed pads, gloves, and hygiene kits.

General assistance: Provides for medical expenses for those individuals with limited income and assets. The patient should contact his or her local Department of Social Services for eligibility criteria.

Hill-Burton program: 1-800-638-0742; http://www.hrsa.gov/osp/dfcr. Health facilities that provide free or low-cost care to individuals who cannot afford to pay. Eligibility is based on income and assets.

Internal Revenue Service: 1-800-829-1040; http://www.irs.ustreas.gov. Medical costs that are not covered by insurance can sometimes be deducted from taxes.

The Leukemia & Lymphoma Society: 1-888-282-9465; http://www.lls.org. Provides limited financial aid to patients with leukemia, lymphoma, Hodgkin's disease, and myeloma for specific items.

Medicaid: http://www.cms.gov/medicaid. A jointly funded, federal-state health insurance program for certain low-income and needy people. The patient should call his or her local department of social services for more information.

Pharmaceutical assistance programs

Pharmaceutical companies offers drugs at no or low cost to eligible individuals. Application can be made directly to the company or access can be through Pharmaceutical Research and Manufacturers of America (http://www.phrma.org).

Some states offer programs that assist with the cost of prescription drugs for the elderly or disabled who meet financial eligibility. The patient should look in the blue pages of his or her telephone book or refer to http://www.medicare.gov.

Together Rx: 1-800-865-7211; http://www.togetherrx.com. A prescription savings program for eligible Medicare enrollees.

Transportation: Some agencies may provide services through a volunteer program such as the American Cancer Society or the patient's local church or synagogue. Or reimbursement may be obtained through various agencies such as The Leukemia & Lymphoma Society or Cancer Care.

YWCA EncorePlus: 1-800-953-7587. Aids women in need of early detection education and breast and cervical cancer screening and support services. Also provides women recovering from breast cancer with peer group support and an exercise program.

HOME HEALTH CARE

Resource guidance can be provided through the patient's physician's office or through hospital departments of social work or discharge planning. The following require physician orders and, often, preauthorization.

- Durable medical equipment: Equipment that is available through certified local suppliers, such as wheelchairs or walkers.
- Hospice: Provides comprehensive home care services to individuals with a limited prognosis.
- Visiting nurse/public health nurse: Provides skilled care, aides, and ancillary services to eligible individuals for limited periods of time.
- Proprietary home care agencies: Provide highly technical care at home such as intravenous antibiotics or chemotherapy.

For those who require a nursing home level of care but prefer to remain in their own home with the help of family, friends, community services, and professional care agencies, Medicare (http://www.medicare.gov) offers limited access to two unique programs to eligible enrollees who need a comprehensive medical and social service delivery system:

- Program of All Inclusive Care for the Elderly
- Social Health Maintenance Organization

HOUSING

- American Cancer Society: 1-800-ACS-2345; http://www.cancer.org. Provides a resource list of free housing opportunities in various geographic locations.
- National Association of Hospital Hospitality Houses: 1-800-542-9730; http://www.nahhh.org. Provides a resource list of hospitality houses in the area in which the patient is receiving medical care.
- Ronald McDonald House: http://www.rmhc.com. Provides housing for families of out-of-town pediatric patients. The patient should contact his or her physician's office or hospital social work department.

INTERNET RESOURCES

The following is a list of common, but not all-inclusive, Internet sites for people with cancer, their families, and caregivers. Resource books that list Internet sites, such as *"A Helping Hand,"* by Cancer Care, may also be helpful.

Alliance for Lung Cancer Advocacy, Support, and Education	http://www.alcase.org
American Brain Tumor Association	http://hope.abta.org
American Cancer Society	http://www.cancer.org
American Institute for Cancer Research	http://www.aicr.org
American Pain Society	http://www.ampainsoc.org
American Society of Clinical Oncology	http://www.asco.org
Association of Cancer Online Resources	http://www.acor.org
Blood and Marrow Transplant Information Network	http://www.bmtnews.org
cancerandcareers.org (women)	http://www.cancerandcareers.org
Brain Tumor Society	http://www.tbts.org
Cancer Care	http://www.cancercare.org
CancerGuide	http://www.cancerguide.org
Cancer Hope Network	http://www.cancerhopenetwork.org
Cancer News on the Net	http://www.cancernews.com
Candlelighters Childhood Cancer Foundation	http://www.candlelighters.org
Chemocare.com	http://www.chemocare.com
Children's Hospice International	http://www.chionline.org
Choice in Dying	http://www.caregiver.ca/cgddddcd.html
Colon Cancer Alliance	http://www.ccalliance.org
Colorectal Cancer Network	http://www.colorectal-cancer.net
Corporate Angel Network	http://www.corpangelnetwork.org
Cure for Lymphoma Foundation	http://cfl.healthology.com
CureSearch National Childhood Cancer Foundation	http://www.nccf.org
Dream Foundation	http://www.dreamfoundation.com
Gilda's Club International	http://www.gildasclub.org
Hospice Education Institute	http://www.hospiceworld.org
International Association of Laryngectomees	http://www.larynxlink.com
International Myeloma Foundation	http://www.myeloma.org
Lance Armstrong Foundation	http://www.laf.org
Living Beyond Breast Cancer	http://www.lbbc.org
Lymphoma Research Foundation	http://www.lymphoma.org
Make-A-Wish Foundation	http://www.wish.org
Multiple Myeloma Research Foundation	http://www.multiplemyeloma.org
National Association for Home Care & Hospice	http://www.nahc.org
National Bone Marrow Transplant Link	http://www.nbmtlink.org
National Brain Tumor Foundation	http://www.braintumor.org
National Breast Cancer Coalition	http://www.natlbcc.org
National Cancer Institute	http://www.cancer.gov
National Center for Complementary and Alternative Medicine	http://nccam.nih.gov
National Coalition for Cancer Survivorship	http://www.canceradvocacy.org
National Hospice and Palliative Care Organization	http://www.nhpco.org
National Kidney Cancer Association	http://www.nkca.org
National Lymphedema Network	http://www.lymphnet.org
National Marrow Donor Program	http://www.marrow.org
National Organization for Rare Disorders	http://www.raredisorders.org
National Ovarian Cancer Coalition	http://www.ovarian.org
National Patient Travel Helpline	http://www.npath.org
National Prostate Cancer Coalition	http://www.4npcc.org
National Self Help Clearinghouse	http://www.selfhelpweb.org
Office of Complementary and Alternative Medicine	http://www3.cancer.gov/occam
Ovarian Cancer National Alliance	http://www.ovariancancer.org
Pancreatic Cancer Action Network	http://www.pancan.org
Patient Advocate Foundation	http://www.patientadvocate.org
Pediatric Oncology Resource Center	http://www.acor.org/diseases/ped-onc
People Living with Cancer	http://www.plwc.org
Prostate Cancer Foundation	http://www.prostatecancerfoundation.org
RadiologyInfo	http://www.radiologyinfo.org
Ronald McDonald House	http://www.rmhc.com
Society of Gynecologic Oncologists	http://www.sgo.org
Support for People with Oral and Head and Neck Cancer	http://www.spohnc.org
Susan G. Komen Breast Cancer Foundation	http://www.komen.org
The Compassionate Friends	http://www.compassionatefriends.org
The Oral Cancer Foundation	http://www.oralcancerfoundation.org
The Skin Cancer Foundation	http://www.skincancer.org
The Wellness Community	http://www.thewellnesscommunity.org

ThyCa: Thyroid Cancer Survivors' Association	http://www.thyca.org
United Ostomy Association	http://www.uoa.org
Us TOO	http://www.ustoo.com
Vital Options International	http://www.vitaloptions.org
Y-ME National Breast Cancer Organization	http://www.yme.org

Proprietary Internet Resources

http://www.cancereducation.com
http://www.cancerfacts.com
http://www.cancergroup.com
http://www.cancerhelp.com
http://www.cancer-info.com
http://www.cancernews.com
http://www.cancerpage.com
http://www.cancerresources.com
http://www.cancersource.com
http://www.nocr.com
http://www.oncology.com
http://www.oncolink.com

PALLIATIVE CARE

Palliative care focuses on the prevention and relief of physical, emotional, and spiritual pain and suffering, often occurring toward the end of life.

American College of Physicians	http://www.acponline.org
Cancer Care	http://www.cancercare.org
Choice in Dying	http://www.caregiver.ca/cgddddcd.html
Growth House	http://www.growthhouse.org
Hospice Patients Alliance	http://www.hospicepatients.org
Last Acts	http://www.lastacts.org

TRANSPORTATION

- Angel Flight America: 1-800-446-1231; http://www.angelflightamerica.org. Volunteer pilots provide transportation to those in medical and financial need on general aviation aircraft, within 1000 miles.
- Corporate Angel Network: 1-866-328-1313; http://www.corpangelnetwork.org. Provides free air transportation for cancer patients traveling to treatment using empty seats on corporate jets.
- Midwest Miracle Miles: 1-414-570-3644; http://www.midwestairlines.com/frequentflyer/programs/miraclemiles.asp. Provides medical transportation for those in medical and financial need through a registered organization; for example, a hospital or cancer center.
- Miracle Flights for Kids: 1-702-261-0494; http://www.miracleflights.org. Provides medical air transportation to those in medical and financial need.
- National Patient Travel Helpline: 1-800-296-1217; http://www.npath.org. Provides information and referrals about all forms of charitable long-distance medical air transportation.

- Northwest Airlines KidCares: 1-612-726-4206; http://www.nwa.com/corpinfo/aircares/about/kidcares.shtml. Provides free air travel for a child aged 18 and younger using donated miles.
- Operation Liftoff: 1-888-354-5757; http://www.operation-liftoff.com. Provides medical transportation to those children 18 and younger with a life-threatening illness. One person may accompany the child and a discount may be given for the second adult.

WISH FOUNDATIONS

- A Wish with Wings: 1-817-469-9474; http://www.awishwithwings.com. Grants wishes to children with life-threatening diseases.
- Dream Foundation: 1-805-564-2131; http://www.dreamfoundation.com. Grants dreams to terminally ill adults.
- Make-A-Wish Foundation: 1-800-722-9474; http://www.wish.org. Grants wishes to children with life-threatening illnesses.
- Sunshine Foundation: 1-800-767-1976; http://www.sunshinefoundation.org. Grants wishes to chronically or terminally ill children whose families are under financial strain due to the illness.

REFERENCES

1. American Cancer Society. Cancer statistics, 2004. World Wide Web URL: http://www.cancer.org, 2004.
2. Cancer Care Inc. *"A helping hand": the resource guide for people with cancer*, 2nd ed. New York: Cancer Care Inc., 2002.
3. Minino AM, Smith BL. *Deaths: Preliminary Data for 2000. National Vital Statistics Report.* Centers for Disease Control, Atlanta. World Wide Web URL: http://www.cdc.gov/nchs/data/nvsr/nvsr49/nvsr49_12.pdf, Oct. 9, 2001.
4. Zabora JR, Blanchard CG, Smith ED, et al. Prevalence of psychological distress among cancer patients across the disease continuum. *J Psychosoc Oncol* 1997;15:73.
5. Weisman AD, Worden JW. The existential plight in cancer: significance of the first 100 days. *Int J Psychiatry Med* 1976;7:1.
6. Holland J. Historical overview. In: Holland JC, Rowland JH, eds. *Handbook of psychooncology.* New York: Oxford University Press, 1989:3.
7. Gotay CC, Wilson MG. Social support and screening in African American, Hispanic and Native American women. *Cancer Pract* 1998;6:31.
8. Guidry JJ, Aday LA, Zhang D, et al. The role of informal and formal social support networks for patients with cancer. *Cancer Pract* 1997;5:241.
9. Wortman CB. Social support and the cancer patient. *Cancer* 1984;5(Suppl):2339.
10. Dunkel-Schetter C. Social support and cancer: findings based on patient interviews and their implications. *J Soc Issues* 1984;40:77.
11. Rowland JH. Intrapersonal resources: coping. In: Holland JC, Rowland JH, eds. *Handbook of psychooncology.* New York: Oxford University Press, 1989:58.
12. Cwikel JG, Behar LC, Zabora JR. Psychosocial factors that affect the survival of adult cancer patients: a review of research. *J Psychosoc Onc* 1997;15:1.
13. Harris KA. The informational needs of patients with cancer and their families. *Cancer Pract* 1998;6:39.
14. Lee RG, Garvin T. Moving from information transfer to information exchange in health and health care. *Social Sci Med* 2003;56:449.
15. Chapman K, Abraham C, Jenkins V, et al. Lay understanding of terms used in cancer consultations. *Psychooncology* 2003;12:557.
16. Fernsler JI, Cannon CA. The whys of patient education. *Semin Oncol Nurs* 1991;7:79.
17. *To Promote Understanding, Assume Every Patient Has a Literacy Problem.* Institute for Safe Medication Practices, Huntingdon Valley, PA. World Wide Web URL: http://www.ismp.org/MSAarticles/promote.html, Oct. 31, 2001.
18. Collins KS, Hughes DL, Doty MM, et al. *Diverse Communities, Common Concerns: Assessing Health*

Care Quality for Minority Americans. The Commonwealth Fund, New York. World Wide Web URL: http://www.cmwf.org, March 2002.

19. Hahn EA, Cella D, Dobrez D, et al. The talking touchscreen: a new approach to outcomes assessment in low literacy. *Psychooncology* 2004;13:86.

20. Hodge FS, Toms FD, Guillermo T. Achieving cultural competency and responsive health care delivery. *Cancer Suppl* 1998;83:1714.

21. *A Nation Online. How Americans Are Expanding Their Use of the Internet.* U.S. Department of Commerce, Economics and Statistics Administration. World Wide Web URL: http://www.esa.doc.gov/ANationOnLineEXSFeb02.cfm, 2002.

22. Edgar L, Greenberg A, Remmer J. Providing Internet lessons to oncology patients and family members: a shared project. *Psychooncology* 2002;11:439.

23. Pandey SK, Hart JJ, Tiwary S. Women's health and the Internet: understanding emerging trends and implications. *Social Sci Med* 2003;56:179.

24. Fogel J, Albert SM, Schnabel F, et al. Racial/ethnic differences and potential psychological benefits in use of the Internet by women with breast cancer. *Psychooncology* 2003;12:107.

25. Oncologists disagree on impact of patient Internet use. *CA Cancer J Clin* 2003;53:135.

26. Kritz FL. Uncertainty @dr-mail.com. *The Washington Post* 2003 April 1.

27. Smith J. "Internet patients" turn to support groups to guide medical decisions. *J Natl Cancer Inst* 1998;90:1695.

28. Owen JE, Klapow JC, Roth DL, et al. Improving the effectiveness of adjuvant psychological treatment for women with breast cancer: the feasibility of providing online support. *Psychooncology* 2004;13:281.

29. Lieberman M, Golant M, Glese-Davis J, et al. Electronic support groups for breast carcinoma: a clinical trial of effectiveness. *Cancer* 2003;97:920.

30. Wang X, Cosby LG, Harris MG, Liv T. Major concerns and needs of breast cancer patients. *Cancer Nurs* 1999;22:157.

31. Fordahl M, Associated Press. "Technology is starting to help senior citizens." *New Haven Register* 2003 Sept. 21.

32. Medicare managed care patients more likely to use hospice. *CA Cancer J Clin* 2003;53:202.

33. Pear R. "New study finds 60 million uninsured during a year." *The New York Times* 2003 May 12.

34. Van Loon RA, Borkin JR, Steffen JJ. Healthcare experiences and preferences of uninsured workers. *Health Soc Work* 2002;27:17.

35. Freudenheim M. "Employees paying ever-bigger share for healthcare." *The New York Times* 2003 Sept. 10.

36. Parker-Oliver D, Crandall L. Medication assistance program: University of Missouri Health Care Department of Social Services. *Health Soc Work* 2002;27:303.

37. Clark EJ, Stovall E, Leigh S, et al. *Imperatives for quality cancer care: access, advocacy, action and accountability.* Silver Spring, MD: National Coalition for Cancer Survivorship, 1996.

38. Deimling GT, Kahana B, Bowman KF, et al. Cancer survivorship and psychological distress in later life. *Psychooncology* 2002;11:479.

39. Walker MS, Risvedt SL, Haughey BH. Patient care in multidisciplinary cancer clinics: does attention to psychosocial needs predict patient satisfaction? *Psychooncology* 2003; 12:291.

SECTION 7

JANET L. ABRAHM

Specialized Care of the Terminally Ill

Providing expert care to patients who are terminally ill offers new challenges to the oncology team.* When patients are receiving antineoplastic therapy, they, their families, and their oncology teams know the roles that they are to play. The demands of the chemotherapy regimen and the life-threatening nature of its side effects are the primary priority. When patients' tumors progress through multiple therapies, the team's challenge becomes how to integrate more palliative care principles into their care. They must learn about their patients' goals and values and how they want to spend the time they have left, and they must help them die in a manner that is consistent with their wishes. To do this, the team engages in new types of conversations with patients and their families and among themselves and broadens their assessments to be able to ensure physical comfort, address psychological needs, and identify social and spiritual sources of distress.

These conversations are made more difficult by the reversal in the usual roles played by the team and the patient and family. As von Gunten et al.[1] state: "To provide palliative care, practitioners must shift their focus to the patient's point of view. The patient becomes the expert on suffering, and the physician becomes the consultant. Often, health care professionals find this to be a striking contrast to providing therapy with curative or remissive intent: In that paradigm, practitioners' knowledge of the science of medicine and the management of disease is paramount."

To succeed, oncology teams have to overcome significant attitudinal barriers, including their own beliefs about death,[2] and the public's "belief that prolongation of life is the predominant goal of medicine."[3] These barriers lead to fewer discussions about dying, appointing health care proxies, or completing advance directives. The unfortunate result has been that families report they feel isolated, misinformed, and unprepared about the expected prognosis of the patient and about the course in which the disease is likely to run.[4]

DISCUSSING PROGNOSIS

When the disease is far advanced but the patient is still receiving antineoplastic therapy, the team faces a difficult choice: impart the best estimate of prognosis, which is usually only months, or continue therapy without "the talk." The cultural "norms" of medicine mitigate against offering realistic prognoses, and they support optimism (Table 55.7-1).[5] Even physicians referring patients to a hospice program do not usually tell them the likeliest prognostic estimate.[6] Twenty percent never communicated a survival estimate, even to a patient who requested the information; 37% communicated the same estimate they formulated; and 40% communicated a different estimate, being optimistic 70% of the time. In one study, patients' actual median survival was 26 days, but the physicians' median formulated prognosis of survival was 75 days, and what they would have told the patient was 90 days. More experienced clinicians favored no disclosure. Females and physicians who referred more often to hospice programs were more likely to favor pessimistically discrepant disclosure.

Physicians may assume that patients who want to know their prognoses will raise the subject with them. No data are available, however, on how often patients with advanced refractory disease ask about their prognosis. One study suggests that patients would rather tell the house staff than their oncologist their preferences about resuscitation (58% vs. 32%).[7]

Discussions of prognosis can be very painful for clinicians, because they may cause feelings of guilt, failure, or sadness. These talks take not only time but also skills that are not developed in standard oncology fellowship training: conducting family meetings, counseling patients who are in psychological

---

Oncology team here refers to an oncologist, physician assistant, or nurse (Bachelor's-prepared or Master's-prepared clinical nurse specialist or nurse practitioner) and social worker, when available.

TABLE 55.7-1.   Medical Norms

Avoid making predictions
Keep the predictions you do make to yourself
Keep them from patients unless they ask
Do not be specific
Do not be extreme
BE OPTIMISTIC

(Adapted from ref. 5.)

---

distress, and helping people cope with grief and anger. Practical educational handbooks[8,9] and CD-ROMs[10] for clinicians interested in improving their skills are available. A study of the efficacy of intensive education in such communication for oncology fellows is currently under way.[11]

Potential benefits of having a discussion of prognosis with relatively asymptomatic patients whose prognosis is likely to be limited include enabling them to make truly informed decisions regarding participation in experimental trials and in advance care planning. It can be easiest to raise these issues during the consent discussion for the third or fourth palliative chemotherapy or for a phase I study. For support, most patients bring to these discussions the family member(s) or friends, or both, involved in their treatment. The team can use the review of potentially serious side effects of the therapy or trial being offered to help patients understand the need to identify a health care proxy. They can raise a previous experience with a life-threatening complication, if necessary, to reinforce educating the proxy in the patient's wishes.

Paradoxically, the discussion is likely to lessen fears of abandonment and strengthen the trust patients have in the oncology team. It will not eliminate their hope, although it may significantly alter what they were hoping for. Knowing they have only months to live, they can identify remaining goals and redirect their hope into accomplishing these.

ADVANCE CARE PLANNING

Patients' beliefs about their likelihood of successful resuscitation and about the quality and length of their survival have a significant impact on their wishes regarding do-not-resuscitate orders. Resuscitation has very limited efficacy for patients with advanced malignancy. Those who have had bone marrow transplant for hematologic malignancies and who have required mechanical ventilation and more than 4 hours of pressor support or have had renal or hepatic failure did not survive the intensive care unit stay.[12] Patients with metastatic cancer who have an observed arrest in the hospital have a 13% to 50% chance of being successfully resuscitated, but all died during the hospitalization.[13,14]

Patients who think they have as little as a 10% chance of surviving 6 months often want resuscitation and ongoing life-prolonging care.[15] Not until they think the odds of surviving 6 months are less than 10% do patients overwhelmingly choose comfort care and decline resuscitation.[15] Therefore, until patients know their true prognosis, their do-not-resuscitate decisions are likely to be informed more by hope than fact. Patients are also concerned about returning to their previous functional and cognitive status and decline resuscitation if there is a high likelihood of residual impairment.[16] Imparting an accurate prognosis and estimate of likelihood of impairment does, therefore, help patients make reasonable choices for themselves about resuscitation.

Discussion about resuscitation should begin with the larger exploration of the patients' hopes and fears, goals for their remaining life, and values about how they want to live that life.[17] Reviewing the patients' activities at home, their coping mechanisms (e.g., faith, friends, physical exercise), their fears and hopes, and the core components of what quality of life means to them naturally leads into a discussion of resuscitation and reliance on life-support machines. Knowing what kind of life would be minimally acceptable and what would be worse than dying, the oncology team can decide whether they can even recommend resuscitation.

Phrasing the questions clearly can also help patients give answers that reflect their feelings accurately. Advance directive discussions that begin "Do you want everything done?" almost always lead to an affirmative response. Rephrasing to ask, rather, "If you DIED, would you want to be resuscitated?" may lead to a very different answer, especially if, in preparation for the discussion, the oncologist reviews the data about the efficacy of resuscitation discussed above.

Conversations that include these subjects give patients and families a better appreciation of their role in the collaboration between themselves and the oncology team. Groundwork is laid for later explorations of patient and family fears about what will happen as the disease progresses or if the patient has a serious complication from the disease or the treatment. Without a discussion when the patient's condition is stable, oncologists are likely to find themselves in the difficult position of trying to determine the patient's wishes during a medical crisis. Alternatively, their families may have to try to determine what the patient would have wanted, without ever having had a chance to discuss this with them. For some patients, intubation during their last days may be worse than dying. Their families and oncology teams need to know this to act as true surrogates when the need arises.

Before beginning this difficult conversation, clinicians may find it helpful to examine their own feelings about the news they have to impart and identify any feelings of frustration, grief, or sadness they may be experiencing. Support from the entire team during the talk, for the patient and family and for the person delivering the news, is also useful. After the meeting, other team members can remain behind to help patients and their families cope with the news and answer questions not previously raised.

HOPE

Discussions like the ones outlined above need not eliminate hope. Most patients with advanced disease do not hope for a cure. They hope that their lives will be prolonged as much as possible, and they also hope that they will be healthy enough to enjoy the remaining time they have. Most patients hope for a pain-free death, one that is in accord with their wishes.[18] They want time to say their goodbyes, bring closure to their lives, and leave their legacies. Sadly, however, the demands of chemotherapy may have caused them to focus all their hopes on disease remission. They may have forgotten how to hope for anything else.

Before they began treatment, most patients had a variety of plans for the future that filled up the "calendars" by which they ran their lives.[19] The calendars include the public calendar (e.g., holidays, such as Thanksgiving, Christmas, and Passover), personal calendar (e.g., birthdays, anniversaries, weddings, and graduations), and daily calendar (e.g., work, church, soccer practice, and play dates).[19] After the initiation of chemotherapy, however, all these were superseded by the treatment calendar, in which patients vest magical powers to bring about a cure.

Any disruption in the treatment calendar therefore can provoke anxiety for patients and their families, who strive to complete the treatments "on time." When blood counts are too low, for example, patients ask the nutritionist what they should eat "to get back on schedule." Oncologists know that the dates are not so important for palliative treatment regimens but patients do not, and they never ask to delay a treatment to feel better for an important event. The proposal of a delay of chemotherapy until after Thanksgiving, for example, is usually met with a puzzled refusal.

Oncology teams can help patients with advanced disease develop new kinds of hope by deemphasizing the treatment calendar and encouraging patients to reintegrate into activities that were meaningful before treatment began. They can reassure them that minor alterations in the schedule will not affect the efficacy of the treatment. Patients and families can participate with the oncology team in scheduling treatment sessions to accommodate important family celebrations or holidays.

Despite refractory disease, however, some patients cling to the hope of further treatment "should their counts recover." The oncology team need not, if they believe it would be harmful, dash that hope. However, they can help these patients and families enlarge the scope of their goals by encouraging them to work on projects and valued relationships while they are waiting for the next therapy. If the patient is unlikely to survive long enough to meet the goal (e.g., a child's wedding or graduation, the birth of a grandchild), he or she can be urged to make videotapes, create a scrapbook and narrate it, write letters or buy presents for children or grandchildren for events far into the future, or create cradles or blankets that will embody their love and ensure that they will be there in spirit. Scrapbooks are particularly useful, because they are a form of life review.

As disease progresses despite ongoing treatment, patients who have begun to reengage in non–treatment-related activities and who have developed a broader relationship with their oncology team are more likely to understand that the oncologist is not abandoning them when he or she says that the burden of another therapy is much greater than the potential benefit. Such patients do not complain that stopping treatment is "waiting around to die," because they have other activities to fill their days. The oncology team members are seen as allies in maximizing the life they have left and as partners to the end.

BARRIERS THAT INHIBIT ADVANCE CARE PLANNING DISCUSSIONS

For a number of reasons, physicians are reluctant to talk about anything beyond the next planned therapy with patients who have refractory disease.[20] Physicians may share with patients a fear of dying and may not themselves have designated a health care proxy or completed a living will. Many have never grieved for the many deaths experienced during training and in the practice of oncology.[21] They may not have asked themselves the questions their patients with advanced disease are forced to ask: What is the meaning of my life? Who will remember me? What legacy will I leave? If something happens to me tomorrow, is there anything that would be left undone?

After completing their own advance care plans, oncologists may find that discussions with patients about advance directives become an exploration of the ways to help another person down this difficult path. Having grieved, physicians may find it easier to meet with compassion the intense feelings that arise in patients and families facing great losses, understanding that the pain will lessen. After answering the questions patients ask themselves, physicians may more easily initiate discussions with patients and families about prognosis, advance care planning, or progression of disease.

CURIOSITY

Questions that will help physicians discover their patients' hopes, goals, and fears come less from the taking of a medical history than from the physician's own natural curiosity.[9] Physicians might ask themselves: Who is this person sitting across from me? What is the story of his life/his work/his family? Of what is she most proud? What does he regret the most? What most surprised her? What does he do for fun? Would that be possible if she gets weaker or is unable to think as clearly? What does he worry most about losing? Who will she find it hardest to leave? The answers to these questions will lead naturally to others that will deepen the understanding and the trust between them. The questioning should continue until the physician feels that he or she could responsibly serve as a surrogate for the patient in making health-related decisions.

HEALING VERSUS CURING

In discussing their lives, their hopes, and their fears with the oncology team, patients begin to understand that they are cared for as people, not just patients. Some may reveal fears that the team can dispel, such as a fear of dying in uncontrolled pain, of suffocating, or of being abandoned. Others identify problems best addressed by chaplains, social workers, and psychiatrists, and the team can make these referrals. Healing (i.e., a return to wholeness that includes body, mind, and spirit) can still occur, therefore, even if the patient never achieves another remission.

HOW TO TELL THE CHILDREN

In addition to school counselors, the oncology team can play an important role in helping parents tell their children about their illness, their prognosis, and even that they expect to die. The following are the recommended principles and techniques[22]:

1. Learn about the children. Ask parents to tell you about their children, including their ages and how they coped with problems in the past.
2. Maximize the child's support system. Help parents determine who among their family and friends can help

keep the children's schedules as close to normal as possible, including sleeping, eating, school, friends, and out-of-school activities. Explain that it may be necessary to overcome children's resistance to forming relationships with nonparental friends for fear of seeming disloyal to their parents.

3. Facilitate honest communication about the illness. Parents need to take the time that their children need to answer all their questions in an age-appropriate manner. Children from 3 to 7 years old need to ask them what they think caused the cancer. Children of this age may believe that they caused their parent's illness and feel guilty about it. These very young children do not understand that death is permanent, however, and therefore it does not help to prepare them for the death itself ahead of time. Older children (7 to 12 years) may also fear that their behavior contributed to the cancer and also need to be reassured that they cannot catch it and that their parent did not necessarily do anything to acquire it. They do know that death is permanent, and therefore they may need to discuss their fears and concerns about their parent leaving them. Children should be encouraged to share any stories they have heard but do not understand and to ask whatever questions occur to them. Parents, however, have to be careful to understand what the real question is and should feel free not to answer every question right away. Saying "That is an important question. Let me think about it," is acceptable, provided that the question is answered at a later time.

4. Address common questions. Parents should avoid euphemisms and name the cancer specifically. Calling cancer a "boo-boo" or bump, for example, may scare and confuse children, who themselves have had many a boo-boo or bump. In response to "How much should we share with the children?," Dr. Rauch recommends, "Everything." Assume that children will hear what adults are discussing and that they will feel more frightened by being left to interpret the information alone than if they are present and able to be comforted should they show distress. Although it is very important to let them know a parent is available to talk if they want to, Rauch advises parents to let their children initiate the discussions. "Are you going to die?" is the question parents most commonly fear.[22] In reply, ask about particular concerns, such as whom they will live with. While including in their answer that they might die, parents need to add that they are doing all they can to live as long and as well as possible.

5. Prepare for hospital visits. Children should be allowed to visit the hospital if they want to, except when a parent is confused or agitated, which a young child is unlikely to understand. Children need special preparation for what they are about to see, however, including a discussion of their fears and expectations. They should be taken by someone who can leave when the child is ready to leave. After the visit, the child should be asked to discuss any parts that were difficult or enjoyable or were different from what they expected. Children who do not want to visit can be helped to communicate by preparing letters, drawings, or other gifts, making tapes or videotapes, or talking on the phone or videophone.

6. Saying goodbye. Rauch writes, "If one's children know they are loved, and why they are loved, there is usually no need to say the word *goodbye.*" However, she encourages parents and their children to say a last "I love you" in person whenever possible. If necessary, it can happen when the parent is in a coma or after the parent has died. Children should also be given "a road map for the grief process ahead"[22] and be helped to feel all right about going on with school and other activities after the death by asking about them.

Using these guidelines, clinicians can often help parents make the plans needed for care of their children when they are gone. Although they face their deaths with undiminished sadness, parents may be able to say what their children need to hear. Some parents with refractory cancer will be able to understand that not being resuscitated, far from betraying their children, is actually a last gift.

CULTURAL/RELIGIOUS CONSIDERATIONS

Ethnicity, culture, socioeconomic status, religion, and religious background all affect the ways that patients experience illness and face death.[23–25] The best way to show respect for patient and family views is to individualize the approach to each patient and family. Table 55.7-2 provides questions that can help clinicians in their explorations in all the relevant areas: language, religious beliefs/concerns, cultural context, health beliefs, decision-making patterns, and social support and resources.[23,26]

TABLE 55.7-2. Questions to Assess Individual Patient and Family Needs

---

Which language do you wish to use to discuss your illness?

Is it appropriate to discuss the diagnosis, the prognosis, and the possibility of death with the patient?

Religious beliefs/concerns

   Do you have a religious affiliation? How important is this religion to you?

   Do you and your family think life is sacred? How do you think about death?

   Do you believe in miracles?

   Do you believe in life after death?

   Are there any special ways the person should be handled after death?

Cultural context

   Do any of the following affect how you think about illness, death, or dying: your role and importance in your family; your country of origin; a personal experience with poverty, being a refugee, discrimination, or not having enough access to medical care?

Health beliefs

   What do you think causes illness? How do these things cause someone to die?

Decision-making patterns

   Who makes the important decisions in your family?

   Do you and your family think you don't have much chance to change the course of your illness, or do you think that there are things you can do to change what will happen?

Social support and resources

   Would it be helpful for us to speak with community or religious leaders or family members or anyone else to help us understand things that are important to you as we care for you?

(Adapted from ref. 23.)

CARE WITHOUT CHEMOTHERAPY

In some patients, the oncologist may believe that treatment would do more harm than good. How can this be expressed to patients? The key is in the words used and their implications, not just their literal meanings. If the oncologist says, "I could offer you a 5-FU [5-fluorouracil]-containing regimen," the patient and family think it would be of benefit. However, if the oncologist adds, "...but it is very unlikely to help you live longer or better," he or she clearly understands that the physician does not want to continue treatment. Most patients who hear, "There is nothing more I can offer you," feel hopeless and abandoned. What the oncologist actually means, however, is more likely to be conveyed by saying, "There are no other treatments against the cancer that would help you live longer or more comfortably. But there are many ways I can care for you and help you achieve your other goals. And I will work hard to be sure that no symptoms such as pain get in your way."

Even saying "I'm sorry" can be misinterpreted to be an apology. Using the phrase "I wish things were different" conveys more clearly the oncologist's meaning.[27] "I wish..." can be used in a number of clinical scenarios, including, "...delivering very bad news; responding to unrealistic hopes from a patient or family; responding to expressions of loss, grief, and hopelessness; responding to disappointment in medicine or the physician; responding to demands for aggressive treatment when prognosis is very poor; responding to medical complications or errors."[27]

PALLIATIVE CARE PROGRAM

Families who were otherwise very satisfied with the care the patient received have complained that they never knew the patient was dying until the patient was no longer able to speak with them. They suffer from ongoing grief at having had no opportunity to tie up the loose ends of their relationship. It may be very difficult, however, for the oncology team to encourage the fight for life and at the same time let the patient and family know that unless something extraordinary happens, the patient is likely to die soon. Oncology teams who can hold both these contradictory feelings within themselves are likely to be able to help patients and their families hold them as well. They can make sure that patients and families have had a chance to come to closure before the patient dies from the disease or a treatment-related side effect.

Most oncologists and their nursing colleagues have not been trained, either in medical or nursing school or in postgraduate training, to help dying patients and their families make these transitions.[28] For particularly complex situations, therefore, the primary oncology team can consult a palliative care team. Palliative care teams usually include a specially trained nurse (often a clinical specialist or a nurse practitioner) and a physician. Some also have nurses skilled in complementary therapy, social workers, chaplains, and pharmacists. Teams assist with symptom management; advance care planning; emotional, psychological, spiritual, or existential suffering; closure and legacies; and care during the last days.[28] They provide patient and family education and family counseling, problem solving, and support. Although some palliative care teams are involved only with patients near the end of life, others work with individuals at any point along their disease trajectory (diagnosis, relapse, or terminal care). Teams provide consultation as well as primary clinical care.

Palliative care teams can also help with the decision to stop chemotherapy, when the oncologist believes that the burden has become greater than the benefit. Oncologist Dr. Timothy Gilligan[29] describes such a partnership:

> As oncologists go, I have great respect for the limitations of what chemotherapy can accomplish, yet I have found many patients to be very difficult to dissuade from receiving chemotherapy when I did not think it was a good idea. While sometimes I can also be their palliative care doctor, I have found it extremely helpful for some patients to have the palliative care service come in—sometimes with me, sometimes on their own—to have a "it's time to change the course" conversation (in addition to helping with symptom management).... I...think that the value of palliative care providers is not just that they are better at these conversations, but that they're not burdened by the history of a "we're going to fight your cancer together" relationship. Clearly, many patients do want to have end-of-life discussions with the oncologist with whom they have built a relationship of trust over the months or years: one has to make decisions based on the individual patient. And I certainly do not mean to imply that the oncologist should exit when the palliative care team arrives. The palliative care team is an addition, not a substitution.

The efficacy of these teams has been reported in mostly uncontrolled prospective, retrospective, observational, or cross-sectional studies.[30] A metaregression and metaanalysis of these studies of the effect of palliative care on end-of-life experiences of patients and their caregivers confirmed a small benefit on patient outcomes, including pain and other symptoms, and a nonsignificant trend toward benefits for satisfaction and therapeutic intervention.[30] The review revealed wide variations in the services offered by the teams.

A comparison group study of a home-based palliative care service in the Kaiser Permanente system showed significant advantages of the service for patients at a significant cost saving for the health system.[31] The intervention patients (i.e., enrolled in the palliative care program) were patients who had a life-threatening disease [usually chronic obstructive pulmonary disease (COPD), congestive heart failure (CHF), or cancer] and a prognosis of approximately 1 year or less to live. They were not required to forgo curative therapy or their primary care physician, but home visits were made by the palliative care physician. Comparison group patients (who received usual care) were drawn from patients with a diagnosis of COPD, CHF, or cancer; two or more emergency department visits or hospitalizations in the past year; and a prognosis of 24 months. Analysis was performed on the 300 patients who died during the 2-year study. As compared with the group receiving usual care, the group cared for in the palliative care program had increased satisfaction with services ($P < .001$) and significantly fewer emergency room visits ($P < .001$), days in the hospital ($P < .001$), days in skilled nursing facilities ($P = .005$), and outpatient physician visits ($P = .001$). They had significantly more home visits from all disciplines ($P < .001$) and deaths at home (90% vs. 57%). Controlling for days on service, severity of illness, and CHF, the cost per patient of the group receiving home palliative care was significantly less ($7990 vs. $14,570; $P < .001$). Studies in England[32] and Canada[33] showed similar savings by decreasing inpatient days. In-hospital deaths in the Canadian study decreased from 84% to 55%.

Some of the palliative care programs include inpatient units that can decrease hospital costs and resource utilization.[34] A case-control study was done in a closed unit run by palliative care specialists who developed and used a standardized palliative care order set. The study found that daily charges were 59% lower (*P* = .005), as were total costs (57%; *P* <.009) for patients who died within the unit compared with patients matched for diagnosis and age who died outside the unit.[35]

Palliative care teams also offer less quantifiable but equally valuable benefits to the institutions within which they operate.[34] They increase staff morale, decrease staff turnover, and enhance expertise in palliative and end-of-life care. Through consultations and formal and informal teaching sessions, the teams instruct staff and physicians in the palliative care needs of patients undergoing active therapies and those making the transition off chemotherapy. Palliative care teaching rounds and seminars also demonstrate how to work within an interdisciplinary group and how to provide comprehensive care across care sites (inpatient, outpatient, home) using joint problem solving.[28]

The majority of hospitals and academic centers do not have palliative care services.[34] Of teaching hospitals in the United States (26% of which were part of or associated with a medical school; 53% had only residency training programs), only 18% have a palliative care consultation service, 19% an inpatient unit, and 22% a hospice affiliation.[36] Although 49% have a pain service, only 23% that had a pain service had either a palliative care consultation service or an inpatient unit. An additional 20% were planning palliative care programs.[36]

Currently, there are two training programs for palliative care nurse practitioners and approximately 25 palliative care fellowship programs that train one to two fellows a year. To increase the number of trained personnel to deliver these services to their aging veteran population, the Veterans' Administration also funds six sites, each offering two fellowship slots for physicians and two for other health care personnel. Until sufficient numbers of comprehensively trained palliative care nurse practitioners and physicians exist, clinicians with portions of the training (e.g., an anesthesia pain specialist or nurse practitioner specializing in pain management without additional palliative care experience or training or a family physician serving as a hospice medical director) might serve as supervising physicians for the palliative care team.

Establishing a palliative care program involves identifying clinicians (usually nurse practitioners and physicians) who have the core palliative care skills, are willing to provide palliative care consultation, and have the time and the financial backing to do so. A variety of models exist for providing the services. Most palliative care teams in acute care facilities are hospital supported,[36] and they are seeing significant numbers of patients.[34] Hospitals may fund only a nurse practitioner to be the core of the team, supervised either by a palliative care physician on the staff of a hospice (through a contractual relationship) or a staff physician with appropriate expertise. Effective billing techniques have been developed that help insurers understand and pay for the service the teams provide.[37] Full-risk health organizations, such as Kaiser Permanente and the Veterans' Administration, support palliative care teams that for them are cost effective.[31]

Hospice organizations are increasingly embracing palliative care. Medicare now allows for a hospice medical director to do a single consultation before patient enrollment in the hospice program. Some hospice organizations are adding palliative care consultation teams to their organizations. The teams see patients at home or in long-term care or rehabilitation facilities or may provide inpatient consultation on a contractual basis.[34]

Hospitals or health care organizations wishing to start a palliative care team can obtain the logistical and financial information needed from the Center for Advancing Palliative Care (CAPC). CAPC offers 3-day training courses (e.g., "Planning, Funding, and Sustaining a Hospital-Based Palliative Care Program"), operations manuals that include, but are not limited to, "Planning a Hospital-Based Palliative Care Program: A Primer for Institutional Leaders," "CAPC How-To Manual," "Hospital-Hospice Partnerships in Palliative Care," and "Palliative Care and JCAHO [Joint Commission on Accreditation of Healthcare Organizations] Standards" and a Web site (http://www.capc.org). Also, six CAPC Palliative Care Leadership Centers throughout the country offer on-site training with their palliative care programs. Per the CAPC Web site: "The Centers represent diverse care delivery settings, including academic medical centers, cancer centers, health systems, and community-based organizations. They will provide visitors with an in-depth, individualized curriculum and ongoing mentoring to help fast-track visitors' own palliative care programs. The Palliative Care Leadership Center initiative is funded by the Robert Wood Johnson Foundation and led by the Center to Advance Palliative Care." Site visit curricula include hospital needs assessment, financing, and business planning; how to choose organizational and service models; staffing; measuring clinical and financial impact; strategies for ensuring and managing growth; hospice-hospital collaborations; and marketing palliative care to clinicians and patients. The Palliative Care Leadership Centers also provide ongoing mentoring to the visiting programs.

HOSPICE PROGRAMS

The Medicare Hospice Benefit was established in 1982 as part of the Tax Equity and Fiscal Responsibility Act.[38,39] Then, as now, the attending physician and the hospice medical director were both required to certify that the patient was terminally ill when the prognosis was 6 months or less, if the disease followed its usual course. No other criteria have been mandated for cancer patients. A number of misconceptions delay and prevent referrals to the hospice, however (Table 55.7-3).

Hospice teams (including nurses, medical directors, social workers, chaplains, and volunteers) are especially valuable as partners in caring for patients who are dying from cancer. Hospice programs seek neither to prolong life nor to hasten death but to provide comfort and dignity and enhance the quality of the time that remains.[38] Hospice programs support the patient and the family, help them identify their remaining hopes and goals, and assist them in realizing them. In addition to assessing and managing the patient's physical problems, the hospice team is a source of patient and family education, practical support, and psychological and spiritual counseling.[40,41]

Hospice programs also prepare families for their losses and offer bereavement programs after the death. Bereavement counselors can provide support for family members experiencing anticipatory grief before the patient's death and communicate regularly with the bereaved for the year after the death.

TABLE 55.7-3. Common Misconceptions about Hospice Care

Misconception: *Patients enrolling in hospice must choose not to be resuscitated.*

Misconception: *Patients enrolled in hospice lose their primary physicians.* The referring primary care physician or oncologist continues to direct and approve all of the patient's care. If the patient requires either inpatient hospice admission for symptom control or routine admission for a diagnosis unrelated to the terminal illness, the physician may bill Medicare under Part B for any visits.

Misconception: *Hospice patients cannot be hospitalized and remain enrolled in hospice.*

Misconception: *Hospice patients cannot participate in research projects while enrolled in hospice.* Yes they can, so long as the project is consistent with the mission of hospice.

Misconception: *Hospice nursing personnel do not provide sophisticated care.* The palliative care delivered by hospice nurses requires astute assessment and expert intervention tailored to the patient and family goals. Tube feedings, intravenous hydration or nutrition, or intravenous medications to control symptoms may be included in the hospice plan of care.

Misconception: *Patients can "use up" their hospice eligibility.* Patients who live longer than 6 months will continue to receive services, so long as they continue to meet eligibility criteria for hospice care. Patients who choose to revoke the hospice benefit to seek life-prolonging therapies may choose to reenroll if their goals change.

Misconception: *Patients must have a live-in caregiver to enroll in hospice.* Hospices that care for "live-alone" patients have special protocols to enhance their safety.

Survivors receive letters containing advice and expressing concern and are invited to memorial services. They are also informed about drop-in support groups and bereavement groups designed to meet special needs (e.g., parents who have lost young children, teenagers who have lost a parent).

TABLE 55.7-4. Levels of Clinical Care Provided

	Routine	*Continuous*[a]	*Inpatient*[b]	*Respite*[c]
24-h "on call"	✓	✓	✓	✓
HHA	≤2 h/d	—	—	—
RN visits	≤3/wk + prn	—	—	—
SW visits	q2wk	—	—	—
Chaplain visits	q2–4wk	—	—	—
Volunteer	2–4 h/wk	—	—	—
MD	prn	—	—	—
OT/PT/RT	prn	—	—	—
Continuous nursing	—	≥8 h RN/d	—	—
Inpatient care	—	—	prn	—
Respite care	—	—	—	5 d/mo

HHA, home health aide; OT/PT/RT, occupational therapy/physical therapy/radiation therapy; prn, as needed; RN, registered nurse; SW, social worker.
[a]Continuous home care. Patients with, for example, refractory cough, dyspnea, pain, or delirium can receive 24-h nursing and home health aide services.
[b]Inpatient care. Rarely used. For refractory symptoms that cannot be controlled at home, even with continuous care. The referring physician admits the patient and may bill for his/her services under Medicare Part B.
[c]Respite care. The goal of the respite (in a community skilled or intermediate nursing facility) is either to provide a rest for the caregiver or to remove the patient to an adequate facility when the home is temporarily inadequate to meet the patient care needs.

TABLE 55.7-5. Hospice Services

PERSONNEL
Medical director, nurses, social workers, home health aides, chaplains, volunteers, administrative personnel, medical consultations, occupational therapy, physical therapy, speech therapy, bereavement counseling
ITEMS NEEDED FOR PALLIATION OF TERMINAL ILLNESS
Prescription medications
Durable medical equipment and supplies
Oxygen
Radiation and chemotherapy
Laboratory and diagnostic procedures
OTHER
Transportation when medically necessary for changes in level of care
When needed, continuous care at home or in a skilled nursing facility or inpatient setting
Respite care (care in a nursing facility that provides a "respite" for the caregivers)

Hospice programs provide a continuum of care, from home to the inpatient setting. Although, by law, 80% of days of patient care must take place in the home, all Medicare-certified hospices are required to provide four levels of care: routine home care, continuous home care, respite care in nursing homes, and inpatient care[39] (Table 55.7-4).

The services provided by hospice are listed in Table 55.7-5. Hospice provides 95% of the cost of prescription drugs related to the terminal diagnosis and necessary for its palliative treatment (and many waive the other 5% if there is no insurance coverage). Hospice programs provide all durable medical equipment, supplies, and oxygen for needs related to the terminal diagnosis; laboratory and diagnostic procedures related to the terminal diagnosis; and transportation when medically necessary for changes in the patient's level of care.

The manner in which hospices are financed, however, can limit the palliative services that they can afford to provide. The Medicare hospice benefit is a capitated reimbursement program that reimburses a hospice a *per diem* based on the patient's level of care (approximately $130/d for routine or respite care, approximately $500/d for inpatient acute care). Benefits offered by other forms of insurance are modeled on Medicare's hospice program. Aggressive palliation, including transfusion, palliative radiation, and chemotherapeutic or hematopoietic agents can be provided by large hospices (i.e., with an average daily census of greater than 300 patients). Given this reimbursement schedule, however, such care is often prohibitively expensive for small to moderately sized hospices (i.e., an average daily census of less than 50). Cancer patients who are eligible for enrollment may decline because they would have to relinquish helpful therapies. Hospices can work with insurers other than Medicare, however, to "carve out" provision of the more costly therapies while allowing patients to receive hospice services.

RELIEF OF SUFFERING

Patients report that the components of a "good death" include (1) optimizing physical comfort, (2) maintaining a sense of continuity with one's self, (3) maintaining and enhancing relationships, (4) making meaning of one's life and death, (5) achieving a sense of control, and (6) confronting and preparing for death.[42] Control of physical and psychological suffering is a

TABLE 55.7-6. Physical Sources of Distress Near the End of Life

Source	Medication(s)	Dose and Route (PO/SL/IV/SC/PR)
Fatigue	Methylphenidate	2.5–5.0 mg PO 8 a.m./noon; can increase as needed
Insomnia	Temazepam	7.5–30.0 PO hs (lower dose in elderly)
	Zolpidem	5–10 mg PO hs
	Trazodone	25–100 mg PO hs
Pain (continuous)	Opioid (morphine, oxycodone)	Oral concentrates or IV or SC infusion
	Fentanyl	Transdermal
Pain (intermittent)	Morphine, oxycodone	SL oral concentrates
	Hydromorphone	PR
Depression	Methylphenidate	2.5–5.0 mg PO q.a.m. or q.a.m. and noon
Anxiety	Lorazepam	0.5–2.0 mg SL q2h
	Clonazepam	0.5–2.0 mg PO b.i.d.
Delirium	Haloperidol	1–5 mg PO, SC, IV, PR q2–12h
	Chlorpromazine	12.5–50.0 mg PO, IV, PR q4–8h
	Olanzapine wafer	2.5–5.0 mg SL qhs or b.i.d.; 2.5 mg SL prn q4h prn
Agitated delirium	Midazolam	1.0–2.5 mg IV/SC load; 0.5–1.5 mg/h IV/SC or 25% of loading dose; increase as needed
Dyspnea (anxiety)	Lorazepam	1 mg PO, SL q2h
Dyspnea (other)	Opioid	For example, morphine, 5–10 mg PO, IV, or by nebulizer q2h
	Chlorpromazine	25–50 mg PO, PR q4–12h
Cough	Opioid	Nebulized with dexamethasone, e.g., morphine, 5–10 mg PO, IV, or by nebulizer q2h
	Lidocaine	2 mL 2% lidocaine in 1 mL normal saline for 10 min
	Albuterol/terbutaline	Nebulized
Hiccups	Baclofen	10–20 mg PO t.i.d.
	Metoclopramide	10–20 mg PO/IV/SC/PR q.i.d.
	Nifedipine	10–20 mg PO t.i.d.
	Haloperidol	1–4 mg PO/SC/PR t.i.d.
	Chlorpromazine	25–50 mg PO/IV qd–qid
"Death rattle"	Scopolamine	Transdermal scopolamine patch 1–3 q3d
	Hyoscyamine	0.125–0.25 SL t.i.d.–q.i.d.
	Glycopyrrolate	0.2–0.6 mg PO/SC/IV t.i.d.
Nausea	Olanzapine	2.5–5.0 mg SL hs–b.i.d.
	Lorazepam, metoclopramide, dexamethasone, or haloperidol	IV or compounded suppositories with desired agents (depending on presumed cause of nausea) q6 PR
Palliative sedation	Midazolam	1.0–2.5 mg IV/SC load; 0.4 mg/h IV/SC drip; increase as needed
For refractory symptoms	Pentobarbital	2–3 mg/kg IV load; 1–2 mg/kg/h IV drip
	Lorazepam	0.5–1.0 mg/h IV
	Propofol	2.5–5.0 µg/kg/min IV

hs, at bedtime; PR, per rectum; SL, sublingual.
(Adapted from refs. 59 and 88.)

prerequisite to allowing patients and caregivers to address these social and spiritual/existential dimensions of their lives and to minimize the suffering of bereaved survivors.

In the last days to week before death, a significant percentage of people exhibit or experience fatigue or pain (70%), restlessness/agitation/delirium or noisy or moist breathing (60%), urinary incontinence or retention (50%), dyspnea (20%), or nausea and vomiting (10%).[43] Most patients will have stopped eating by then, and many will have stopped drinking as well.[44] Most of the physical problems experienced by dying patients can be controlled using a limited number of medications given by the oral, rectal, transdermal, or, if necessary, parenteral route (Table 55.7-6).

FATIGUE

Pain, anxiety, depression, and insomnia are important causes of generalized weakness and fatigue and should be minimized when-

ever possible (see Insomnia, Pain, and Psychological Disorders, later). In the last weeks of life, diminished oral intake and the metabolic effects of progressive disease also contribute, and refeeding does not ameliorate the weakness. In patients for whom fatigue is problematic, the psychostimulant methylphenidate may be effective.[45] A preliminary report of patient-adjusted dosing in a nonrandomized trial suggested benefit in a majority of patients within 7 days and no serious side effects. Patients used up to 20 mg/d in divided doses.[46] Modafinil (Provigil), an agent approved for narcolepsy, has not yet been assessed for its effect on fatigue. It is recommended for opioid-induced sedation.[47]

INSOMNIA

Insomnia in dying patients may result from undertreated pain, depression, anxiety, delirium, dyspnea, nocturnal hypoxia, nausea and vomiting, or, rarely, pruritus. Medications that can cause insomnia include corticosteroids and antiemetics (prochlorperazine, metoclopramide, 5-HT$_3$-receptor antagonists).[48] In addition, patients' sleep-wake cycle may be reversed because they are inactive and napping much of the day.

Data from controlled trials indicate that benzodiazepines [oxazepam (Serax), 10 to 20 mg, or temazepam (Restoril), 15 to 30 mg], antidepressants, and zolpidem (Ambien) are effective agents. Trazodone [25 to 100 mg PO at bedtime (hs)] may be useful for patients with paradoxical reactions to benzodiazepines. For patients with nighttime delirium, oral quetiapine (Seroquel), 25 to 50 mg PO qhs (for elderly patients); olanzapine (Zyprexa), 2.5 to 5.0 mg PO qhs; or haloperidol (e.g., Haldol; beginning at 0.5 to 2.0 mg PO and increasing as needed to 5 mg) are needed. Clonazepam (Klonopin), 0.5 to 1.0 mg PO, should be used for patients with restless legs syndrome. Patients who resist taking these medications may fear that they will not reawaken. Exploring these concerns can help patients use the therapy to be alert and less fatigued during daylight hours.

PAIN CONTROL

Pain is one of the most distressing and disabling problems faced by patients with terminal illness and by their families.* However, using World Health Organization guidelines for cancer pain relief, 50% of cancer patients near death will have no pain, 25% mild to moderate pain, and only 3% severe pain.[49] Even in the last months or weeks, interventional anesthetic and neurolytic techniques, described elsewhere, should be considered for that small minority of patients whose pain cannot be relieved by any other method short of sedation[50] (see Chapter 55.1).

When patients have not previously received opioids, patient and family misconceptions about opioids must often be overcome: becoming an addict, "feeling high," "using up" the effective agents and having nothing left if the pain gets worse, and developing refractory constipation. Even families who want the patient to be comfortable may be worried that the opioid is "killing" the patient. They may need reassurance that a declining respiratory rate is normal as patients die.

Frequent pain assessment, including the patient's satisfaction with the pain level, remains the cornerstone of an effective management strategy (see Chapter 55.1). Some patients who lose the ability to use the numerical scales to describe their pain may be able to use the scales designed for children, such as the Wong-Baker faces scale (see Chapter 55.1). If the patient has an impaired memory or poor concentration but can still report pain accurately, repeat assessments should be done when the peak pain relief is expected (e.g., 15 minutes after a parenteral dose, 60 minutes after an oral dose). If the patient becomes nonverbal, it may be necessary to monitor for expressions of apparent discomfort when the patient is moved or when a part of the body known to have been painful in the past is touched. Behavioral scales have been developed for nonverbal demented patients,[51] but they have not been validated for nonverbal dying patients.

Not all patients who exhibit distress are in pain. Delirium may present as pain. Patients who moan without any apparent provocation, or in response to nonpainful stimuli such as having their lips moistened, may be delirious. Delirium is espe-

cially likely in patients with these behaviors who have not reported pain before they became nonverbal. The assessment and management of delirium in this population are discussed further below in the section Delirium.

Even in patients on stable drug regimens, physiologic changes at the end of life make it necessary to monitor them carefully for the appearance of opioid-related side effects such as myoclonus or delirium. With decreasing renal function, for example, patients taking sustained-release preparations of morphine or oxycodone may develop these side effects from decreased clearance of the drugs and their metabolites. If the respiratory rate declines to less than 6 and opioids are thought to be the cause, opioid doses should be decreased 25% and the patient should be monitored carefully for increasing discomfort. Naloxone is almost never indicated. If a sedated patient has a dangerous reduction of the respiratory rate, both thought to be caused by opioids, naloxone can be diluted in 10 mL and given 1 mL at a time until the respiratory rate recovers to greater than 6. If the naloxone is given undiluted, the patient is likely to experience severe opioid withdrawal.

If the patient becomes unable to take pills, a liquid, transmucosal,[52] rectal,[53,54] transdermal, or pelleted opioid should be substituted. Kadian and Avinza are morphine sustained-release pellets packaged into capsules that can be opened. The pellets can be sprinkled on food or suspended in liquid and either swallowed or placed into feeding tubes every 12 to 24 hours. A subcutaneous (SC) or intravenous (IV) opioid infusion is required for patients whose opioid dose is too large to be delivered by sublingual, transdermal, or rectal routes. Parenteral opioid administration is also useful in those patients who would benefit from the patient-controlled analgesia option.

Changes in opioid route or agent require meticulous calculations using a table (see Chapter 55.1) or a conversion program (e.g., http://www.hopkinskimmelcancercenter.org/specialtycenters/index.cfm). Anesthesia pain or palliative care teams or clinical pharmacists can assist in performing these conversions if questions arise. First, the total daily dose of the current opioid being taken is calculated. Next, that dose is converted to the equianalgesic dose of the new opioid given in the new route. For patients with well-controlled pain, that equianalgesic dose of the new opioid is reduced by 25% to 33% because of incomplete cross-tolerance among opioids. If the patient has uncontrolled pain, no dose reduction should be taken. Finally, the total daily dose is divided into the desired oral or parenteral schedule.

For example, a patient with well-controlled pain on 300 mg morphine sulfate (MS Contin) PO q8h develops hallucinations and becomes unable to take pills. The hospice nurse suggests replacing the oral morphine with a parenteral (SC) hydromorphone (Dilaudid) infusion. Oral morphine (900 mg/24 h) is equivalent to [900/30 = x/1.5] or 45 mg/24 h hydromorphone, because 30 mg oral morphine is equivalent to 1.5 mg IV/SC hydromorphone. Decreasing by one-third for incomplete cross-tolerance results in the total daily hydromorphone dose of 30 mg. The SC infusion rate is [30 mg/24 h] or 1.25 mg/h hydromorphone. If the patient had uncontrolled pain, the daily hydromorphone dose would be 45 mg and the infusion rate of hydromorphone would be [45 mg/24 h] or 1.8 mg/h SC.

Adjuvants for bone and nerve pain should be continued if they have been effective. For bone pain, a liquid (e.g., ibuprofen) and a rectal nonsteroidal antiinflammatory drug (NSAID;

---

*Pain assessment and management are extensively reviewed by Dr. Foley in Chapter 55.1. This discussion is limited to issues of pain assessment and management particular to patients who are dying.

e.g., indomethacin)[53] are available. In addition, parenteral ketorolac tromethamine (Toradol) offers the pain-relieving potency of parenteral morphine (30-mg parenteral ketorolac is approximately equal to 12 mg parenteral morphine). Ketorolac has all the side effects of the NSAIDs, however, and is not recommended for long-term use. Adjuvants for neuropathic pain can also be given SC (e.g., dexamethasone) or rectally (e.g., doxepin to replace an oral tricyclic antidepressant).

Therapy to prevent and treat constipation in dying patients should be continued because constipation can cause delirium in this population. All patients on opioids should receive a scheduled, not an as-needed (prn) stool softener and laxative [e.g., dioctyl sodium sulfosuccinate (Colace) + senna] with a prn osmotic agent (e.g., sorbitol) while they can still take oral medications. Patients who are nonverbal but appear uncomfortable and have not had a stool for longer than 72 hours should be assessed for impaction and treated with appropriate enemas (e.g., mineral oil retention enema for an impacted patient), disimpaction when needed, and suppositories.

PSYCHOLOGICAL DISORDERS

Depression

Depression is an important, reversible cause of distress in terminally ill patients. It can be due to poorly controlled pain, drugs (e.g., opioids, corticosteroids), central nervous system tumor, metabolic abnormalities (e.g., hypercalcemia, hyponatremia), vitamin deficiency, or anemia. It may recur in patients with past histories of depression. Many of the usual somatic signs of depression (e.g., anorexia, sleep disturbances, fatigue, or weight loss) are not specific enough to make the diagnosis in this population.

Symptoms and signs that are specific for depression include feelings of sadness, crying, anhedonia, or feelings of worthlessness, guilt, hopelessness, or helplessness.[55] Comprehensive evaluation of terminally ill patients who answered, "Yes," to "Are you depressed?" is very likely to confirm that the patients are depressed.[56] Clinicians wishing to explore further can ask their patients, "How do you see your future? What do you imagine is ahead for yourself with this illness? What aspects of your life do you feel most proud of? Most troubled by?"[55]

Treatment of depression is worthwhile even when patients have only weeks to live. Pain control must be optimized, because uncontrolled pain is a major risk factor for depression and for suicide.[55] Counseling can provide emotional support and help patients find meaning and pride in the lives they have led and purpose for the time remaining. Most dying patients also require an antidepressant. The psychostimulants dextroamphetamine and methylphenidate (2.5 to 5.0 mg at 8 a.m. and noon; maximum dose, 60 to 90 mg) often act within a few days.[57] If the patient is expected to live longer than weeks to a few months, a trial of a stimulant and a selective serotonin reuptake inhibitor should be initiated (see Chapter 55.5 for suggested agents and starting doses). If the regimen is effective, the stimulant can be titrated off several weeks later. Tricyclic antidepressants are less useful in patients with advanced disease because of their side effect profile. One should consult psychiatrists for patients who do not respond to first-line agents, when unsure of the diagnosis, when the patient previously had a major psychiatric disorder, when there are compli-

cating psychiatric disorders or the patient is suicidal or requesting assisted suicide, or when there are dysfunctional family dynamics.[55]

Anxiety

Anxiety in this population is often situational, involving concerns related to the terminal illness.[58] Fear of death, impairment, or pain and concerns about the past all contribute. Hospitalization can add a sense of isolation, loneliness, a sense of uselessness, and concerns about lack of information or misinformation about what is happening.[59] Other causes include drugs (corticosteroids, metoclopramide, opioid neurotoxicity, withdrawal from benzodiazepines or alcohol), uncontrolled pain or other symptoms, hypoxia, dyspnea, metabolic abnormalities (sepsis, hypoglycemia), insomnia, and preexisting psychiatric disorders.[59]

Anxious patients may present with uncontrolled worry, a sense of impending doom, motor tension, restlessness, autonomic hyperactivity (e.g., palpitations, sweating, dry mouth, tightness in the chest), nausea/vomiting/diarrhea, feeling on edge, difficulty concentrating or relaxing, insomnia, or irritability. They often feel out of control and helpless. Some patients with severe anxiety are actually suffering from a delirium. If, in addition to being anxious, the patient has hallucinations or extreme psychomotor agitation, or is disoriented or paranoid, the anxiety is likely to be part of a delirium.

Finding a physiologic cause of the anxiety (e.g., hypoxia) in a dying patient should not stop the search for additional contributing psychological, social, or spiritual problems. Counseling from social work, psychiatry, or chaplaincy may be needed to identify and, when possible, allay the underlying cause(s).[42,58] For dying patients, empiric therapy with lorazepam (0.5 to 2.0 mg sublingually q3h prn) or clonazepam (0.5 to 2.0 mg PO b.i.d.) may offer significant benefit. A more complete discussion of the assessment and management of anxiety is found in Chapter 55.5.

Delirium

Delirium has been reported in up to 80% of dying patients.[60] Etiologies of delirium include medications (especially opioids, NSAIDs, and high-dose corticosteroids), metabolic abnormalities (hypercalcemia, hyperglycemia, uremia), constipation, bladder outlet obstruction, dehydration, hypoxia, fever, infection, uncontrolled pain, hepatic failure, brain tumors, and brain metastases.[61–63] Opioid-related central nervous system toxicities occur more frequently in patients with renal dysfunction, with impaired cognition before starting the opioids, on high doses of opioids for long periods of time, with dehydration, or taking other psychoactive drugs.[64]

Delirious patients may appear agitated or hypoactive or vacillate between these states.[61] Symptoms of delirium include insomnia and daytime somnolence, nightmares, restlessness or agitation (which mimics uncontrolled pain), irritability, distractibility, hypersensitivity to light and sound, anxiety, difficulty in concentrating or marshaling thoughts, fleeting illusions, hallucinations and delusions, emotional lability, attention deficits, and memory disturbances.

Patients can be screened for delirium by physicians and nurses using a validated screening instrument.[64] For patients who are not actively dying, a comprehensive psychiatric evaluation may be appropriate to confirm the diagnosis, evaluate for likely contributing factors, and exclude other psychiatric disorders, such as anxiety, minor depression, anger, dementia, or psychosis.[61] The exact cause of delirium is found in only approximately 43% of cases,[62] and the etiology is often multifactorial.[60–65] In dying patients, however, the burden of the evaluation may exceed the benefit of finding a specific reversible cause. Empiric therapy may be sufficient. Discussion with the patient's health care proxy can help clarify the issue.

Treatment for delirium should be initiated as soon as the diagnosis is made, even in patients who are undergoing efforts to eliminate the underlying cause(s). One should ask family members, friends, or well-known caregivers to be present. The patient's surroundings should be made as familiar as possible; hearing aids and glasses should be restored, and the patient should be reoriented frequently. Medications should be begun from those listed in Table 55.7-6. Olanzapine, 2.5 to 5.0 mg PO b.i.d. and prn q4h, and haloperidol, 1 mg IV or 2 mg PO/PR q4h and q2h prn (up to 20 mg in 24 hours), are most commonly used. Olanzapine is available in a wafer that dissolves in the mouth (Zydis).

RESPIRATORY DISORDERS

Dyspnea

The prevalence of cancer-related dyspnea in dying patients is approximately 70%.[66] Causes include anxiety, tumor infiltration, underlying cardiac and pulmonary conditions, anemia, and pleural and pericardial effusions. Pericardial effusions and tamponade are particularly subtle causes of dyspnea in cancer patients. Dyspnea is often present in the absence of tachypnea in the hospice population: 77% of patients reported dyspnea, but only 39% had tachypnea charted.[67]

When they have a reversible process, terminally ill patients benefit from the same specific therapies recommended for patients with less advanced disease. For panic due to perceived breathlessness, an oral opioid, chlorpromazine, or, for refractory panic, midazolam may be needed (see Table 55.7-6). For patients with less anxiety, empiric opioids and anxiolytics are also used (see Table 55.7-6).

Patients with continuous dyspnea often benefit from sustained-release opioid preparations, with immediate-release rescue doses every 2 hours being useful. For patients unable to take oral medications, nebulized opioids,[68] furosemide,[69] or opioid drips with a patient-controlled analgesia option can be very effective. If an opioid drip is begun for dyspnea, however, hospital staff, patients, and families must be carefully educated that the purpose is to control the symptom of dyspnea, not to hasten death. Patients who resist use of the opioid may fear going to sleep and not reawakening. Exploring these concerns can help patients use the medication to improve alertness and energy during daylight hours.

Cough

Cough, which is present in approximately 40% of patients with advanced cancer, is caused by postnasal drip, infection, heart failure, asthma/COPD, esophageal reflux, angiotensin-converting enzyme inhibitors, obstruction of the airway, and disorders of swallowing. Patients respond to oral opioids, sweet elixirs containing dextromethorphan, opioid elixirs, or methadone syrup. For more resistant coughs, higher doses of oral or nebulized opioids (morphine or hydromorphone, often combined with dexamethasone every 4 hours through a nebulizer using room air or oxygen through an open face mask) may be helpful. In addition, nebulized anesthetics (e.g., 2 mL 2% lidocaine in 1 mL normal saline for 10 minutes) can be given up to three times a day.[59] For patients who have tenacious mucus, nebulized saline, albuterol (0.5 mg in 2.5 mg normal saline), or terbutaline is helpful,[59] whereas expectorants and mucolytics are not. Ipratropium exacerbates this problem and should be discontinued when possible.

Hiccups

Hiccups are embarrassing and exhausting and interfere with a patient's ability to eat, drink, and sleep. In patients with cancer, they are most commonly caused by gastric compression, injury to vagus or phrenic nerves, uremia, hyponatremia, hypocalcemia, benzodiazepines, barbiturates, IV corticosteroids, or rarely ear infections, pharyngitis, esophagitis, or pneumonia. Pharmacologic therapies are listed in Table 55.7-6. Chlorpromazine is effective but causes significant postural hypotension, which may not be a problem in this population. Metoclopramide, baclofen, haloperidol, and nifedipine are probably equally effective and safer in older more ambulatory patients.[70] Valproate or phenytoin (Dilantin) can be tried for refractory hiccups. If sedation is not a concern, midazolam can be used.[71]

Massive Hemoptysis

Massive hemoptysis, such as hematemesis, hematochezia, or exsanguination from a tumor eroding into a major vessel, is rare but can be horrifying to observe for professional caregivers or family or friends. If such a complication is likely to develop, dark-colored sheets, towels, and blankets can be used to mask the blood. One should consider insertion of a peripherally inserted central catheter line for patients without an indwelling venous access device to provide emergency IV access for patient sedation. For patients at home in hospice programs, hospice nurses provide instruction to those family members who feel able to administer an IV infusion of morphine and a benzodiazepine IV [e.g., midazolam (Versed), 1.0- to 2.5-mg load followed by 0.4 mg/h IV initial infusion] or per rectum [diazepam (e.g., Valium), 10 mg, or lorazepam (e.g., Ativan), 2 mg] while waiting for the nurse to arrive. Inpatients must have these medications available on the hospital unit to be used immediately when needed. When the event occurs, the patient is placed bleeding side down, in Trendelenburg's position if possible, and the medications are given.

GASTROINTESTINAL DISORDERS

Anorexia and Xerostomia

Families may fear that patients who take little nourishment will suffer from hunger pangs or from thirst. However, patients at the end of life are unlikely to be thirsty or hungry,[72] even if they voluntarily refuse food and fluids to hasten their deaths.[73] Families may equate not eating with "giving up" and may urge

TABLE 55.7-7.   Nausea/Vomiting

Etiology	Drug	Initial Dose[a]
Initiation or escalation of opioid therapy	Prochlorperazine	10 mg PO or 25 mg PR b.i.d./t.i.d.
	Olanzapine	2.5–5.0 mg PO/SL once daily
CNS disease	Dexamethasone	2–4 mg PO/PR b.i.d.
Vertigo	Hyoscyamine	0.125–0.25 mg PO/SC t.i.d.
	Scopolamine	Transdermal patch
Candidal mucositis	Fluconazole	100 mg PO qd
Liver/renal failure	Haloperidol	1.5–5.0 mg PO/PR IV t.i.d.
	Olanzapine	2.5–5.0 mg PO/SL b.i.d.
Constipation	Senna; polyethylene; glycol; bisacodyl (Dulcolax)	—
Gastritis	Proton pump inhibitor	20 mg PO qd
Delayed gastric emptying	Metoclopramide	10–20 mg PO/PR b.i.d. to q.i.d.; 1–3 mg/h IV/SC
Bowel obstruction[b]	Octreotide	150–300 mg SC b.i.d.–t.i.d.

CNS, central nervous system; PR, per rectum; SL, sublingual.
[a]For nausea, initial steps should be (1) treat cause, if identified; (2) consider changing to a different opioid agent.
[b]For symptomatic therapy when surgery is not indicated.
(Adapted from refs. 59, 75, and 76.)

placement of a feeding tube or parenteral nutrition or hydration. One should explore what they hope the intervention would accomplish ("What do you hope you/he will be able to do if we give him nutrition through a feeding tube/through his vein?"). Their answers are likely to reveal that either the patient or the family has an unrealistic expectation of how much the intervention will improve the patient's function or enable achievement of goals.

Clinicians can help families realize that not only will patients not recover function but that they may experience additional distress. Parenteral hydration in dying patients, for example, causes nausea and vomiting from increased gastric secretions; dyspnea from ascites, upper airway secretions, and pulmonary edema; and pain from ascites and peripheral edema.[72] Feeding tubes may leak and lead to aspiration. When they understand the burdens and risks of these interventions, families often stop requesting them and realize that nothing valuable is being withheld.

The xerostomia that is common in this population is usually due to opioids, not to dehydration.[74] No correlation has been found between reports of thirst or dry mouth and hydration status,[74] and no controlled studies have shown that rehydration is effective. Moistening the mouth with swabs or offering sips of water, ice chips, or fruit-flavored ice usually ameliorates the xerostomia.

Nausea/Vomiting/Diarrhea

Nausea and vomiting in the dying patient are due to initiation or escalation of opioids, disease of the central nervous system or the inner ear, oral infections, hepatic or renal failure, metabolic abnormalities (hypercalcemia, hyponatremia, hyper- or hypoglycemia), constipation, gastritis, and functional or mechanical obstruction of the gastrointestinal tract. Therapy should be directed at the underlying etiology[59,75,76] (Table 55.7-7). Diarrhea can persist in end-stage patients' graft-versus-host disease, and octreotide (300 to 600 mg SC t.i.d.) may be as helpful as it is in acute graft-versus-host disease.[77] If the octreotide controls the

diarrhea, one should consider using its depot (LAR) formulation monthly (20 to 30 mg/mo).

SOCIAL SOURCES OF DISTRESS

Among social sources of distress are financial concerns and the many changes in roles and relationships that accompany advanced illness. With increasing debility, patients lose their roles in the community, their roles in the workplace, and even their roles in the family.[78] They may have concerns about who will care for their parents or children when they have died and who will provide financially. Worries about burdening the family or that the family will fail them when they really need them may lead patients to request physician-assisted suicide.[79] Social workers are the key team members who can help alleviate or at least ameliorate these sources of distress and can help the caregivers cope.

Caregivers of patients with advanced disease are themselves at increased risk of physical and psychological deterioration. Virtually all caregivers are family members (96%), most of them women (72%). Spouses are at the greatest risk, with increased mortality and suicide rates after the spouse's death.[80] Caregivers at the highest risk for deterioration are in the lower socioeconomic groups,[81] are ill themselves, have a prior history of depression, are people of color,[81] or have been caring for patients for longer periods of time (greater than 6 months).[82] Unrelieved symptoms and high physical caregiving needs also increase caregiver burden.[81] Caregiver education; communication among the health care team, patient, and family; and web, print, and telephone-based resources of support and information (e.g., Cancer Care, Inc., http://www.cancercare.org) all can address caregiver needs and ease caregiver burden.[83]

Ongoing communication with the oncology team, even when the patient can no longer come to see the physician, is crucial to the success of a home care program for the dying patient. Although families previously monitored patients for early warning signs as they rode the roller coaster typical of chemotherapy treatments, they need to know that now they can relinquish those tasks without exposing the patient to danger.

If the patient is not enrolled in hospice, the oncology team needs to explain to the family what to expect as the patient dies and how to recognize when the patient's last days are approaching. Some family members may want to change their focus from "cheerleader" to companion. Others may have limited support from someone who will care for their own family while they support the dying patient or limited vacation, sick, and family leave days.

The family also needs help locating additional home care resources or, if the patient and caregiver prefer, an acceptable nursing facility. For family members planning to give the care at home, hospital beds, commodes, and home health aides may be among the equipment and services required. The subject of hospice enrollment should be reexplored at this time. As the patient weakens, the implications of being cared for by hospice may be less frightening and the advantages more apparent.

SPIRITUAL/EXISTENTIAL DISTRESS

Spiritual or existential concerns of dying patients include making meaning of their lives, wondering whether they are loved by family and friends, asking for or giving forgiveness, and wondering how to say goodbye or thank you.[84] Some patients want to reconnect with religious traditions and carry out the rituals that surround dying in their culture or religion.[25] Clinicians can help patients find solace and closure at the end of life by exploring religious and spiritual beliefs and listening empathetically.[42,85] When patients are still able to do so, physicians can urge them to talk more about their lives, using some of the same questions listed above in the section Curiosity. In the telling, patients prioritize, order, celebrate, and mourn.

Physicians can encourage the patient and family to review their concerns together, validate the need for religious or spiritual counseling, and obtain psychiatric or social work counseling for the patient or to help the family resolve troubling issues. For some patients and families, discussing "The Five Things" together brings healing and closure. The Five Things are: "Forgive me; I forgive you; Thank you; I love you; and Goodbye." [84] When patients are unable to speak or are spending a great deal of time sleeping, oncologists can encourage their families to tell each other what they remember about the patient. For many patients and families, this difficult period can become a time of growth and healing, resolution, remembrance of good times together, and transmission of a legacy.[42]

PALLIATIVE SEDATION

Palliative sedation is "the monitored use of medications to relieve refractory and unendurable symptoms by inducing varying degrees of unconsciousness but not death."[86] It is considered when, despite expert multidisciplinary evaluation and management, a patient who is near death continues to experience intolerable physical, psychological, or spiritual/existential symptoms.[87] Fewer than 5% of patients fall into this category. Those who do most commonly experience refractory pain, cough, dyspnea, seizures, or delirium. The doses of opioid, benzodiazepine, or neuroleptic needed to control the symptom(s) sedate the patient or cause other intolerable side effects (e.g., myoclonus). In other cases, the request for sedation for refractory symptoms arises when psychological or spiritual/existential concerns coexist with physical problems.

The goal of palliative sedation is to relieve intractable distress, not to hasten death. The median time of death after initiation of palliative sedation is 1.3 to 3.2 days.[88] Palliative sedation is not euthanasia or physician-assisted suicide. Euthanasia is a deliberate action that, to relieve suffering, directly leads to the death of a patient.[86] Euthanasia can be accomplished rapidly (e.g., with high-dose potassium infusion) or slowly by continually increasing the dose of an opioid or sedative with the intent of stopping the patient's breathing. Euthanasia is illegal in the United States. Physician-assisted suicide is the provision by a physician of medications that can end a person's suffering and his or her life, but the patient him- or herself chooses to take the medication. Physician-assisted suicide is legal at the time of this writing only in Oregon.

Palliative sedation, by contrast, is legal throughout the United States. It is in concert with nursing[86] and medical codes of ethics and with the 1997 Supreme Court decision that reaffirmed using whatever was necessary to relieve the suffering of a dying patient.[86] When using palliative sedation for symptom control, the physician and nursing staff collaborate to titrate the medications to deliver the lowest dose that provides patient comfort. Palliative sedation can be used whether or not the patient has chosen to receive IV or enteral nutrition or hydration. It is not used, however, unless patients have declined cardiopulmonary resuscitation, mechanical ventilation, and dialysis.

Expert palliative care and pastoral consultation, evaluation by a psychiatrist, and discussions among the health care team, the patient, and the family members should be undertaken before sedation is administered. Most often, all concerned reach a consensus on the need for and the acceptability of sedation as a means of achieving symptom control. Obtaining formal informed consent either from the patient or from the health care proxy is recommended. Medications used to produce the sedation that relieves the distressing symptom(s) include opioids, neuroleptics, IV benzodiazepines, and SC or IV barbiturates (see Table 55.7-6).[89]

THE FINAL DAYS

Signs that the patient is entering the last 10 to 14 days include:[90]

Dehydration, tachycardia, followed by decrease in heart rate and blood pressure

Perspiration, clammy skin, cool extremities; just before death, mottling

Diminished breath sounds, irregular breathing pattern with periods of apnea or full Cheyne-Stokes respiration; grunting or moan with exhale

Mouth droop; difficulty swallowing; loss of gag reflex with pooling of secretions causing "death rattle"

Incontinence of bladder or rectum

Agitation ± hallucinations; stillness, difficult to arouse

COMFORT MEASURES ONLY

For many such patients, orders are placed for "comfort measures only." "Comfort care" can be misunderstood by the patient and family as a withdrawal of what were in the past effective measures. House staff can be confused about how to deliver care in these circumstances. Care, to them and to families, means meticulous attention to the patient's metabolic balance, hemoglobin and platelet levels, and hydration status, along with evaluation and treatment for life-threatening complications such as infections or pulmonary emboli.

When a patient is no longer improving from antibiotics, gets no further energy from transfusions, and is in the last weeks of life, neither families nor house staff intuitively understand that these formerly effective manifestations of care are now no longer relevant or useful. Statements such as "We are going to stop the antibiotics" or "Transfusions are not indicated" suggest that the treatment would be effective but is being withheld for an unclear reason. Openly acknowledging this misunderstanding and offering other models of care obviate unnecessary interventions while maintaining the satisfaction of all the caregivers in their roles.

When patients are receiving comfort care, therefore, it is important to help families understand that therapies that are no longer working will be discontinued and that every effort will be made to provide the greatest possible comfort. House staff can be redirected to make frequent daily visits to monitor for comfort. They should assess for pain, dyspnea, delirium, urinary retention, constipation, myoclonus, and excessive upper airway secretions ("death rattle"). Family and friends who are present should also be invited to report their observations and encouraged to ask questions. Family and visitors need to be encouraged to feel free to touch and speak with the patient. They may be afraid to do so, particularly when the patient is in an intensive care unit attached to a number of machines and IV lines.

Discussions should also begin with the family to learn whether their religious or cultural tradition has any specific requirements for the days immediately preceding or immediately after the death. The family can then begin to assemble the group who are to perform the rituals and begin to explain to the unit staff what they will need.

SUPPORT FOR HOUSE STAFF

House staff rarely review with the medical team their reactions to the care of dying patients and to the death itself.[91] Interns are in special need of emotional support after a patient's death.[92] Senior attending staff may not be seen as an important source of support.[92] It may be helpful to offer a forum for interns that is staffed by members of the palliative care team or psychosocial oncology to help them debrief. The author's group offers an hour weekly to biweekly for this purpose. The conference is well attended by interns on the oncology services, who willingly share with each other their experiences, challenges, and feelings about caring for dying patients and their families (J. L. Abrahm, S. D. Block, *personal communication*, 2003).

AFTER THE DEATH

After the patient dies, the nurses usually wash the body and remove IV lines, catheters, or any other equipment, unless the case will be reviewed by the medical examiner or such care is inconsistent with the family's religious or cultural practices.[89,93] Physicians called to confirm the death should first confer with the nurses regarding the circumstances of the death and the advisability of inviting a hospital chaplain to support the family or unit staff. After the physician verifies that the patient has died (i.e., there are no heart sounds, pulse, respirations, or pupillary light reflex), he or she documents the death in the medical record and completes a death certificate. The family should not be asked to leave the room during the confirmation of death. The physician then requests permission for an autopsy and, if appropriate, organ donation and informs the primary oncologist of the time of death and the circumstances surrounding it.

The physicians who are present at the death, or who have been asked to verify the patient's death, should offer condolences to the others present. If invited to participate in a prayer, it is perfectly appropriate to do so. Allowing those present to spend as much time as they need to, to say or do whatever they feel they need to do, including touching the body, improves their ability to cope with their acute grief.[92] One should answer the family's questions and, if the family was not present at the death, review the dying process with them. They should be reassured about pain control or other concerns they had about the patient's suffering before the death. Such thorough explanations can improve the ability of the bereaved survivors to cope and can minimize anger directed at the physician.[94] Expressions of comfort, such as hugging, or expressions of emotion, such as tears, are not inappropriate, so long as the manifestations are moderated to the extent that the family does not feel called on to comfort the physician.

Condolences should be offered as well to the nurses and other staff who have cared for the patient. One should share with them compliments the family has offered about the care the patient received, for example, "Her family told me they were so appreciative of the wonderful care you gave her." Receiving support and comfort from the unit staff and appreciation for the professional way the physician cared for the patient is also appropriate.

The death should be discussed with the team at the next scheduled attending rounds or sooner if the circumstances surrounding the death warrant. The inpatient team and the primary oncology team can both send a condolence note or card, which the family usually welcomes.[94] In the note, one should offer recollections and admiration for the patient and comfort the family. One should include the patient's name, something memorable to the physician about them, praise for the family's involvement in the care, an offer to answer any remaining questions about the death, and, at the end, an expression of sympathy for their loss. When possible and it feels appropriate, clinicians can attend the wake, funeral, or memorial service, which may facilitate closure for them.[93]

GRIEF AND BEREAVEMENT

Even before the patient dies, family members and loved ones may suffer from anticipatory grief, which can include "anger, guilt, anxiety, irritability, sadness, feelings of loss, and decreased ability to function at usual tasks."[95] Openly acknowledging their grief and providing counseling and support through social work, psychiatry, or chaplaincy staff are recommended.[95] Patients, similarly, may need help grieving for their losses.

After the patient's death, the grief of the survivors has been described as a "process of experiencing the psychological, behavioral, social, and physical reactions to the perception of loss."[96]

TABLE 55.7-8. Common Manifestations of Grief

COMMON FEELINGS/BEHAVIORS	COMMON PHYSICAL SYMPTOMS
Fear and anxiety	Changes in appetite
Anger and guilt	Decreased energy; weakness
Depression and despair	Nausea and diarrhea
Separation and longing	Changes in sex drive
Sudden wave of psychic pain	Inability to sleep or sleeping too much
Confusion	Feeling something stuck in the throat
Inability to concentrate or make decisions	Tightness in chest, breathlessness
Tearfulness and crying	Oversensitivity to noise
Sighing	Restlessness
Yearning	Dry mouth
Helplessness	Vivid dreams
Relief	**COMMON THOUGHTS**
COMMON SPIRITUAL RESPONSES	Preoccupation with "if only," "what if"
Hope	Preoccupation with memories
Faith may be strengthened, altered, or abandoned	Sense of his/her presence
	"Who am I now?"
	Disbelief

(From ref. 98, with permission.)

Their initial grief may manifest as "denial, intense crying spells, anxiety, numbness,"[95] and the other physical, psychological, emotional, and spiritual manifestations listed in Table 55.7-8.

The intensity of a survivor's grief is predicated on a number of factors relating to the deceased and the survivor's relationship with the deceased, characteristics of the mourner him- or herself, the nature of the death, and societal and cultural factors. Sudden or accidental death, suicide, or homicide also magnifies the grief experienced, but a good support system and religious rituals can lessen it. Families of cancer patients may experience increased grief if the death is sooner than they were led to expect. A pulmonary embolus coming early in the course of a patient with locally advanced prostate cancer or late in the course of a patient bedridden from metastatic pancreatic cancer can cause the same intensity of grief for families who were not prepared for the possibility.

Six months or so after the death, most survivors find they are suffering less from the problems described in Table 55.7-8.[94] They accept the reality of the death, they are able to be involved emotionally with family and friends, and they accommodate to the new demands of life without the person who has died.[94,96] "Pangs of grief," which are "intrusive, time-limited intense yearning and pining for the deceased,"[94] can occur at anniversaries or when an unexpected reminder of the deceased appears and may continue to occur for years.

Clinicians can help identify those families who need help through this process by contacting the family several weeks to a month after the death to ask about (1) how they have been responding to their loss ("Is there anything that has been especially troubling to you?"), (2) their current social support and coping strategies, and (3) practical concerns, such as finances.[95] Psychologists, social workers, and hospice bereavement counselors can be consulted for families who are not coping well in the months after the death.

Patients enrolled in hospice programs receive regular bereavement services for a year after the patient's death. These include the calls and cards after the death, assessment of need for individual bereavement counseling,[97] invitations to bereavement support groups and memorial services, and letters at regular intervals offering practical advice. Oncology practices can offer similar bereavement programs, with letters at 3 and 6 months, at the anniversary of the death, before the winter holiday season, and at a year after the death. Such programs are well received by the bereaved survivors.[98]

For a minority of bereaved survivors, the acute grief symptoms do not diminish for 6 months after the death, and they develop what has been termed *complicated grief*.[94–96,99] In one taxonomy, patterns of complicated grief include (1) chronic grief, which is a normal grief reaction that persists much longer than expected; (2) delayed grief, in which the normal grief reactions are postponed after being suppressed; (3) exaggerated grief, which is characterized by self-destructive behaviors; and (4) masked grief, in which survivors do not recognize that their loss is affecting their behavior.[93] A validated diagnostic algorithm for complicated grief suggests that patients must have "separation distress" ("intrusive, intermittent yearning and thoughts about the deceased") and extreme levels of at least four of eight "traumatic distress" symptoms: ("purposelessness, feeling that life is meaningless, numbness, feeling that part of oneself has died, shattered world view, assuming symptoms of the deceased, disbelief, or bitterness") for at least 6 months, and they must cause significant functional impairment.[94] People suffering from complicated grief have a markedly increased risk of medical, psychological, social, and substance abuse problems.[94]

It can sometimes be challenging to distinguish between manifestations of grief and those of depression.[42] Block explains that, although survivors with grief have "somatic distress, sleep and appetite disturbances, decreased concentration, social withdrawal, and sighing," they do not express "hopelessness, helplessness, feelings of worthlessness, guilt, or suicidal ideation." People with grief can still get pleasure at times, have only passive wishes "for death to come quickly," and look forward to the future, whereas for those with depression, "nothing is enjoyable" and the feelings are "constant, unremitting." Some may have "intense and persistent suicidal ideation and no sense of a positive future."

Depression may be more responsive to pharmacologic therapy than grief. Methylphenidate, selective serotonin reuptake inhibitors, tricyclic antidepressants, and bupropion SR all improved depression.[42,94,99] Randomized trials of patients with complicated grief indicate that tricyclic antidepressants and interpersonal psychotherapy do not ameliorate complicated grief.[94] These patients may respond, however, to crisis intervention, "guided mourning," or brief dynamic psychotherapy.[94] Paroxetine (Paxil) was effective in reducing symptoms by approximately 50% in an open-label trial.[94]

CONCLUSION

Specialized care of the terminally ill patient requires proficiency in communication skills, willingness to share realistic prognoses with patients and families, and a commitment to understanding the patient's goals, values, hopes, and fears. As death approaches, the oncology team is called on to expand the care that it offers. In addition to chemotherapy, that care encompasses the physical, psychological, social, spiritual, and existential needs of patients and their families. Palliative care and hospice teams can assist, but the oncology team often remains central, directing the plan of care and, later, supporting bereaved families. It is a privilege and an honor to care for those who die. Those who do so must care for themselves as well and grieve for the losses that a career in oncology inevitably entails. Along with these costs, however, they can take comfort in the knowledge that they did their best to provide safe passage to all their patients and that, although they did not always cure them, the patients often were healed.

REFERENCES

1. von Gunten CF, Neely KJ, Martinez J. Hospice and palliative care: program needs and academic issues. *Oncology* 1996;10:1070.
2. Seravalli E. The dying patient, the physician, and the fear of death. *N Engl J Med* 1988;319:1728.
3. Meier DE, Morrison RS, Cassel CK. Improving palliative care. *Ann Intern Med* 1997;127:225.
4. Zuckerman C. Project Director, Hospital Palliative Care Initiative, United Hospital Fund. Speech "Dying in New York City Hospitals" delivered June 17,1997 at "Care for Dying Patients: building palliative care programs." sponsored by the United Hospital Fund, New York.
5. Christakis N. *Death foretold: prophecy and prognosis in medical care.* Chicago: University of Chicago Press, 1999.
6. Lamont EB, Christakis NA. Prognostic disclosure to patients with cancer near the end of life. *Ann Intern Med* 2001;134:1096.
7. Lamont EB, Siegler M. Paradoxes in cancer patients' advance care planning. *J Palliat Med* 2000;3:27.
8. Buckman RR. *How to break bad news: a guide for health care professionals.* Baltimore: Johns Hopkins University Press, 1992.
9. Faulkner A, Maguire P. *Talking to cancer patients and their relatives.* Oxford: Oxford Medical Publications, 1994.
10. Buckman R, Baile WF. *A practical guide to communication skills in cancer care.* 3-CD ROM set; University of Calgary. 2001
11. Back AL, Arnold RM, Tulsky JA, et al. Teaching communication skills to medical oncology fellows. *J Clin Oncol* 2003;21:2433.
12. Rubenfeld GD, Crawford SW. Withdrawing life support from mechanically ventilated recipients of bone marrow transplants: a case for evidence-based guidelines. *Ann Intern Med* 1996;125:625.
13. Faber-Langendoen K. Resuscitation of patients with metastatic cancer. Is transient benefit still futile?[see comments]. *Arch Intern Med* 1991;151:235.
14. Schapira DV, Studnicki J, Bradham DD, et al. Intensive care, survival, and expense of treating critically ill cancer patients. *JAMA* 1993;269:783.
15. Weeks JC, Cook EF, O'Day SSJ, et al. Relationship between cancer patients' predictions of prognosis and their treatment preferences [see comments]. *JAMA* 1998;279:1709.
16. Fried TR, Bradley EH, Towle VR, Allore H. Understanding the treatment preferences of seriously ill patients. *N Engl J Med* 2002;346:1061.
17. Quill TE. Initiating end-of-life discussions with seriously ill patients: addressing the "elephant in the room." *JAMA* 2000;284:2502.
18. Curtis JR, Patrick DL. How to discuss dying and death in an ICU. In: Curtis JR, Rubenfeld GD, eds. *Managing death in the intensive care unit.* Oxford: Oxford University Press, 2001:85.
19. Schou KC, Hewison J. *Experiencing cancer: quality of life in cancer treatment.* Buckingham, England: Open University Press, 1999.
20. Levy MM. Making a personal relationship with death. In: Curtis JR, Rubenfeld GD, eds. *Managing death in the intensive care unit.* Oxford: Oxford University Press, 2001:31.
21. Block SD. Helping the clinician cope with death in the ICU. In: Curtis JR, Rubenfeld GD, eds. *Managing death in the intensive care unit.* Oxford: Oxford University Press, 2001:183.
22. Rauch PK, Muriel AC, Cassem NH. Parents with cancer: who's looking after the children. *J Clin Oncol* 2002;20:4399.
23. Danis M. The roles of ethnicity, race, religion, and socioeconomic status in end-of-life care in the ICU. In: Curtis JR, Rubenfeld GD, eds. *Managing death in the intensive care unit.* Oxford: Oxford University Press, 2001:215.
24. Crawley LM, Marshall PA, Lo B, Koenig BA. Strategies for culturally effective end-of-life care. *Ann Intern Med* 2002;136:673.
25. Bigby JA, ed. *Cross-cultural medicine.* Philadelphia: American College of Physicians, 2003.
26. Koenig B, Gates-Williams J. Understanding cultural differences in caring for dying patients. *West J Med* 1995;163:244.
27. Quill TE, Arnold RM, Platt F. "I wish things were different": expressing wishes in response to loss, futility, unrealistic hopes. *Ann Intern Med* 2001;135:551.
28. Abrahm JL. The palliative care consultation team as a model for palliative care education. In: Portenoy RK, Bruera E, eds. *Topics in palliative care,* vol 4. Oxford: Oxford University Press, 2000:147.
29. Gilligan T. When do we stop talking about curative care? *J Palliat Med* 2003;6:657.
30. Higginson IJ, Finlay IG, Goodwin DM, et al. Is there evidence that palliative care teams alter end-of-life experiences of patients and their caregivers? *J Pain Symptom Manage* 2003;25:150.
31. Brumley RD, Enguidanos S, Cherin DA. Effectiveness of a home-based palliative care program for end-of-life. *J Palliat Med* 2003;6:715.
32. Raftery JP, Addington-Hall JM, MacDonald LD, et al. A randomized controlled trial of the cost-effectiveness of a district co-ordinating service for terminally ill cancer patients. *J Palliat Med* 1996;10:151.
33. Bruera E, Neumann C, Gagnon B, et al. The impact of a regional palliative care program on the cost of palliative care delivery. *J Palliat Med* 1999;3:181.
34. Abrahm JL. Care without chemotherapy: the role of the palliative care team. *CA* 2002;8:357.
35. Smith TJ, Coyne P, Cassel B, et al. A high volume specialist palliative care unit and team may reduce in-hospital end-of-life care costs. *J Palliat Med* 2003;6:699.
36. Billings JA, Pantilat S. Survey of palliative care programs in the United States. *J Palliat Med* 2001;4:309.
37. von Gunten CF, Ferris FD, Kirschner C, Emanuel L. Coding and reimbursement mechanisms for physician services in hospice and palliative care. *J Palliat Med* 2000;3:157.
38. Saunders C. The founding philosophy. In: Saunders C, Summers DH, Teller N, eds. *Hospice: the living idea.* Philadelphia: W.B. Saunders, 1981:4.
39. 42 Codes of Federal Regulations, Part 418. Medicare Hospice Regulations, 1993.
40. Lynn J. Serving patients who may die soon and their families: the role of hospice and other services. *JAMA* 2001;85:925.
41. National Hospice Organization. *Standards of a hospice program of care.* Arlington, VA: National Hospice Organization, 1993.
42. Block SD. Psychological considerations, growth, and transcendence at the end of life: the art of the possible. *JAMA* 2001;285:2898.
43. Coyle, N, Adelhardt J, Foley KM, Portenoy RK. Character of terminal illness in the advanced cancer patient: pain and other symptoms during the last four weeks of life. *J Pain Symptom Manage* 1990;5:83.
44. Ferris FD, von Gunten CF, Emanuel LL. Competency in end-of-life care: last hours of life. *J Palliat Med* 2003;6:605.
45. The NCCN clinical practice guidelines in oncology: cancer-related fatigue. *J NCCN* 2003;1:308.
46. Bruera E, Driver L, Barnes E, et al. Patient-controlled methylphenidate for cancer-related fatigue: a preliminary report. *Proc ASCO* 2003;22:737.
47. American Pain Society: *Principles of analgesic use in the treatment of acute pain and cancer pain,* 5th ed. Glenview, IL: American Pain Society, 2003.
48. Savard J, Marin CM. Insomnia in the context of cancer: a review of a neglected problem. *J Clin Oncol* 2001;19:895.
49. Grond S, Zech D, Schug SA, et al. Validation of World Health Organization guidelines for cancer pain relief during the last days and hours of life. *J Pain Symptom Manage* 1991;6:411.
50. Saberski LR. Interventional approaches in oncology pain management. In: Berger AM, Portenoy RK, Weissman DE, eds. *Principles and practice of supportive oncology.* Philadelphia: Lippincott–Raven, 1998.
51. AGS Panel on Persistent Pain in Older Persons. The management of persistent pain in older persons. *JAGS* 2002;50:S205.
52. Payne R, Coluzzi P, Hart L, et al. Long-term safety of oral transmucosal fentanyl citrate for breakthrough cancer pain. *J Pain Symptom Manage* 2001;22:575.
53. Davis MP, Walsh D, LeGrand SB, Naughton M. Symptom control in cancer patients: the clinical pharmacology and therapeutic role of suppositories and rectal suspensions. *Support Care Cancer* 2002;10:117.
54. Kaiko RF, Fitzmartin RD, Thomas GB, et al. The bioavailabilty of morphine in controlled-release 30 mg tablets. *Pharmacotherapy* 1992;12:107.
55. Block SD. Assessing and managing depression in the terminally ill patient. *Ann Intern Med* 2000;132:209.
56. Chochinov HM, Wilson KG, Enns M, Lander S. "Are you depressed?" Screening for depression in the terminally ill. *Am J Psychiatry* 1997;154:674.
57. Rozans M, Dreisbach A, Lertora JJL, Kahn MJ. Palliative uses of methylphenidate in patients with cancer: a review. *J Clin Oncol* 2002;20:335.

58. Stark D, Kiely M, Smith A, et al. Anxiety disorders in cancer patients: their nature, associations, and relation to quality of life. *J Clin Oncol* 2002:20:3137.

59. Storey P, Knight CF, Schonwetter RS. *Pocket guide to hospice/palliative medicine*. Glenview, IL: American Academy of Hospice and Palliative Medicine, 2003.

60. Massie MJ, Holland J, Glass E. Delirium in terminally ill cancer patients. *Am J Psychiatry* 1983:140:1048.

61. Abrahm JL. Advances in pain management for older patients. *Clin Geriatr Med* 2000;16:(2):269.

62. Casarett D, Inouye S, for the American College of Physicians End of Life Task Force. Diagnosis and management of delirium near the end of life. American College of Physicians consensus paper. *Ann Intern Med* 2001;135:32.

63. Bruera E, Miller L, McCallion J, et al. Cognitive failure in patients with terminal cancer. *J Pain Symptom Manage* 1992;7:192.

64. Lawlor PG, Gagnon B, Mancini IL, et al. Occurrence, causes, and outcome of delirium in patients with advanced cancer: a prospective study. *Arch Intern Med* 2000;160:786.

65. Pereira J, Bruera E. Emerging neuropsychiatric toxicities of opioids. *J Pharmaceut Care Pain Symptom Control* 1997;5:3.

66. Ruben DB, Mor M. Dyspnea in terminally ill cancer patients. *Chest* 1986;89:234.

67. Thomas JR, von Gunten CF. Management of dyspnea. *Support Oncol* 2003;1:23.

68. Coyne PJ, Viswanathan R, Smith TJ. Nebulized fentanyl citrate improves patients' perception of breathing, respiratory rate, and oxygen saturation in dypsnea. *J Pain Symptom Manage* 3002;23:157.

69. Kohara H, Ueoka H, Aoe K, et al. Effect of nebulized furosemide in terminally ill cancer patients with dyspnea. *J Pain Symptom Manage* 2003;26:962.

70. Smith HS, Busracamwongs A. Management of hiccups in the palliative care population. *Am J Hospice Palliat Care* 2003;20:149.

71. Wilcock A, Twycross R. Midazolam for intractable hiccup. *J Pain Symptom Manage* 1996;12:59.

72. McCann RM, Hall WJ, Groth-Juncker A. Comfort care for terminally ill patients; the appropriate use of nutrition and hydration. *JAMA* 1994;272:1263.

73. Ganzini L, Goy ER, Miller LL, et al. Nurses' experiences with hospice patients who refuse food and fluids to hasten death. *N Engl J Med* 2003;349:359.

74. Ellershaw JE, Sutcliffe JM, Saunders CM. Dehydration and the dying patient. *J Pain Symptom Manage* 1995;10:192.

75. Srivastava M, Brito-Dellan N, Davis MP, et al. Olanzapine as an antiemetic in refractory nausea and vomiting in advanced cancer. *J Pain Symptom Manage* 2003;25:578.

76. Ripamonti C, Twycross R, Baines M, et al. Clinical-practice recommendations for the management of bowel obstruction in patients with end-stage cancer. *Support Care Cancer* 2001;9:223.

77. Ippoliti C, Champlin R, Bugozia N, et al. Use of octreotide in the symptomatic management of diarrhea induced by graft-versus-host disease in patients with hematologic malignancies. *J Clin Oncol* 1997;15:3330.

78. Cassell E. *The nature of suffering and the goals of medicine*. New York: Oxford University Press, 1991.

79. Block SD, Billings JA. Patient requests to hasten death: evaluation and management in terminal care. *Arch Intern Med* 1994;154:2039.

80. Jagger C, Sutton CJ. Death after marital bereavement: is the risk increased? *Stat Med* 1991;10:395.

81. Lev EL, McCorkle R. Loss, grief, and bereavement in family members of cancer patients. *Semin Oncol Nurs* 1998;14:145.

82. Kristjanson L, Leis A, Koop PM, et al. Family members' care expectations, care perceptions, and satisfaction with advanced care: results of a multi-site pilot study. *J Palliat Care* 1997;134:5.

83. Levine C. The loneliness of the long-term care giver. *N Engl J Med* 1999;340:1587.

84. Byock I. *Dying well: the prospect of growth at the end of life*. New York: Riverhead Books, 1997.

85. Lo B, Ruston D, Kates LW, et al. Discussing religious and spiritual issues at the end of life; a practical guide for physicians. *JAMA* 2002;287:749.

86. Lynch M. Palliative sedation. *Clin J Oncol Nurs* 2003;7:653.

87. Cowan JD, Walsh D. Terminal sedation in palliative medicine—definition and review of the literature. *Support Care Cancer* 2001;9:403.

88. Cowan JD, Palmer TW. Practical guide to palliative sedation. *Curr Oncol Rep* 2002;4:242.

89. Truog RD, Berde CB, Mitchell C, Grier HE. Barbiturates in the care of the terminally ill. *N Engl J Med* 1992;327:1678.

90. Pitorak EF. Care at the time of death: how nurses can make the last hours of life a richer, more comfortable experience. *AJN* 2003;103:42.

91. Ferris TGG, Hallward JA, Ronan L, Billings JA. When the patient dies: a survey of medical housestaff about care after death. *J Palliat Med* 1998;1:231.

92. Redinbaugh EM, Sullivan AM, Block SD, et al. Doctors' emotional reactions to recent death of a patient: cross sectional study of hospital doctors. *BMJ* 2003;327:185.

93. Ferris FD, von Gunten CF, Emanuel LL. Competency in end-of-life care: last hours of life. *J Palliat Med* 2003;6:605.

94. Prigerson HG, Jacobs SC. Caring for bereaved patients: "All the doctors just suddenly go." *JAMA* 2001;286:1369.

95. Casarett D, Kutner JS, Abrahm J. Life after death: a practical approach to grief and bereavement. *Ann Intern Med* 2001;134:208.

96. Rando TA. *Treatment of complicated mourning*. Champaign, IL: Research Press, 1993.

97. Parkes CM. Bereavement in adult life. *BMJ* 1998;316:856.

98. Abrahm JL, Cooley ME, Ricacho L. Efficacy of an educational bereavement program for families of veterans with cancer. *J Cancer Ed* 1995;10:207-212.

99. Zisook S, Shuchter SR, Pedrelli P, et al. Bupropion sustained release treatment for bereavement: results of an open trial. *J Clin Psychiatry* 2001;62:227.

Lynn H. Gerber
Mary M. Vargo
Rebecca G. Smith

CHAPTER **56**

Rehabilitation of the Cancer Patient

The most recent demographic data suggest that more than 60% of the 1.2 million people diagnosed annually with cancer will survive longer than 5 years.[1,2] These data help define cancer as a chronic disease that is likely to be associated with disability or a change in functional status during the course of the illness.

Function is a term that is broadly defined as the ability to perform daily routines and includes elements from physical, psychological, social, and vocational domains. The rehabilitation model describes a continuum in which anatomic and physiologic abnormalities (impairments) are related to functional limitations, which may produce disability.[3,4] Not all impairments cause functional limitation or disability (e.g., "silent infarcts," "osteochondroma," etc.), and disability does not necessarily imply that an individual is handicapped or limited in his or her ability to carry out various individual roles (e.g., student, worker, etc.). The relationships among impairment, disability, and handicap are neither linear nor unidirectional. For example, because disability can cause impairments (e.g., disuse atrophy and weakness), rehabilitation interventions may help reverse impairments as well as improve function.

It is the role of rehabilitation specialists to help patients establish and maintain good function. These specialists include physiatrists (physicians trained in physical medicine and rehabilitation), physical and occupational therapists, speech language pathologists (who evaluate language, cognition and articulation, and swallowing and assist in tracheostomy care), and recreation (leisure management) therapists.

Rehabilitative evaluations of patients with cancer diagnoses concentrate on the neuromusculoskeletal system and the impact that it has on function. Assessment usually uses standardized and validated instruments that evaluate all domains for possible rehabilitation interventions: impairments, functional limitation, disability, and handicap (societal limitation). Quality-of-life measures, designed to assess an individual's relative satisfaction with his or her life, are often used. Quality of life may be independent of level of performance or function. Examples of outcome measures are available.[5-7] Two of the most frequently used scales are compared in Table 56-1.

Management of patients with cancer diagnoses is very complex. Contributing to this complexity is that cancer patients are frequently older than the seventh decade, have other chronic illnesses, and take a variety of medications. Cancer is usually a multisystem disease, whose multimodal treatments are often toxic to the musculoskeletal system [e.g., radiation-induced fibrosis, cardiotoxic chemotherapy such as doxorubicin (Adriamycin), steroid-induced myopathy, etc.]. The trajectory of the disease passes through a variety of stages, whose duration and severity are unpredictable and often disrupt the stability of daily work/school/leisure routines.

The functional problems of each stage differ, but each may benefit from treatment. Even during transition from disease-free or stable disease to recurrence (from stage 3 to 4), life expectancy after recurrence can be substantial. For example, it is greater than 24 months in breast cancer patients with bony metastatic disease.[8] This period is likely to require treatment to maximize function and life quality and warrants preventive and restorative rehabilitation. Features of each of the stages, symptoms, and typical interventions are presented in Table 56-2.

Cancer and its treatment can cause significant impairments to many organ systems. These impairments may impart functional limitations. A list of the commonly seen impairments, associated symptoms related to cancer, and their treatments are summarized in Table 56-3.

The degree of limitation resulting from impairment may range from changing societal roles and ability to function in the

TABLE 56-1. Comparison of Two Functional Outcomes

Eastern Cooperative Oncology Group	Karnofsky
0: Fully active, able to carry on all predisease performance without restriction	100: Normal, no complaints, no evidence of disease
1: Restricted in physically strenuous activity but ambulatory and able to carry out a light sedentary nature routine (e.g., light housework, office work)	90: Able to carry on normal activity, minor signs or symptoms of disease
	80: Normal activity with effort, some signs and symptoms of disease.
2: Ambulatory and capable of all self-care but unable to carry out any work activities; up and about >50% of waking hours	70: Cares for self, unable to carry on normal activity or do active work.
	60: Requires occasional assistance but is able to care for most of his/her needs
3: Capable of only limited self-care, confined to bed or chair >50% of waking hours	50: Requires considerable assistance and frequent medical care
	40: Disabled, requires special care and assistance
4: Completely disabled; cannot carry on any self-care, totally confined to bed or chair	30: Severely disabled, hospitalization indicated; death not imminent
	20: Very sick, hospitalization indicated; death not imminent
	10: Moribund fatal processes progressing rapidly

TABLE 56-2. Phases of Cancer

Phase of Cancer	Possible Symptoms	Frequent Rehabilitation
I: Staging/pretreatment	Anxiety, pain, functional loss	Education about functional impact of treatment(s), fit for mobility aids, if needed
II: Primary treatment	Pain, anxiety, decreased mobility, wound care, mild edema, decreased strength, fatigue	Education about prevention of loss of motion and strength; lymphedema management; ROM, strengthening, pain management; relaxation/sleep, hygiene
III: Posttreatment/intercurrent	Mobility, edema, fatigue, weakness, deconditioning, weight gain, ± pain	Education about fitness and healthy lifestyle; exercise to improve strength, stamina; possible wrapping of limb, good nutrition/weight control
IV: Recurrence	See II, also possible bony metastatic disease, CNS, other organ system involvement, fatigue	See II; orthotics, gait aids, adaptive equipment, aerobic exercise
V: End of life	Fatigue, decreased mobility, possible dependence in self-care	Education about energy conservation; support, leisure, family counseling

CNS, central nervous system; ROM, range of motion.

community to being unable to stand, walk, or care for oneself independently. The first step to restoring lost function or preventing functional decline is to determine if there are deficits in strength, endurance, limb motion, mobility, and safety; as well as general level of cognition and interest in life activities. Communication skills and oral motor function can be assessed during the interview: once identified, treatment begins.

Special consideration should be given to the prescription of medications that may reduce fatigue and improve cognitive awareness and spasticity; treat depression or anxiety; and prevent or treat osteoporosis. Complimentary strategies, such as relaxation techniques, yoga, Tai Chi, stress management, and acupuncture may have a role in improving function and lessening the side effects of nausea and pain. The efficacy of several of these complementary strategies is still unknown. Recreational therapy is helpful in promoting desired activity that is usually performed outside the medical environment and may promote hopefulness, self-esteem, and community reintegration.

IMPACT OF CANCER TREATMENT ON FUNCTION

CHEMOTHERAPY TOXICITIES

Many chemotherapeutic agents produce fatigue, anemia, and other systemic effects that can lead to physical deconditioning. This is compounded by commonly seen symptoms, including anorexia, nausea and vomiting, and mucositis (glossitis, stomatitis, pharyngitis). Specific nutritional problems include vitamin B_1 deficiency from prolonged vomiting and mucositis from folic acid deficiency (common with methotrexate).[9] Antimetabolites such as 5-fluorouracil and 6-mercaptopurine result in thiamine deficiency, producing lip and oral cavity changes. Other common deficiencies are of vitamins B_2 and K. Edema may result

from hypoproteinemia. Extravasation of chemotherapeutic agents, especially anthracyclines, can produce severe soft tissue reaction, leading to chronic contracture and induration.

Peripheral polyneuropathy may be produced by some agents, most notably vincristine, and also paclitaxel (Taxol). Intrathecal regimens may produce central nervous system (CNS) abnormalities, especially when unusually high doses are given. This has been most often noted with methotrexate. High doses of corticosteroids can produce weakness due to myopathy as well as mental status changes. Reproductive side effects may occur, including early menopause in women and detrimental effects on sperm production in men. Hormonal therapies for prostate cancer result in a decrease in serum testosterone and a decrease in sexual function in a majority of cases.

RADIATION-INDUCED TISSUE DAMAGE

Radiation therapy can produce acute side effects, as well as subacute or late effects with the potential to impact functional performance. Although systemic effects such as fatigue may be attributed to radiation therapy, the majority of the adverse effects are localized to the site being radiated. Patients receiving combined chemotherapy and radiation therapy are at risk for additive toxicities.

A concern regardless of the site being radiated, but especially over a joint, is progressive soft tissue fibrosis with risk of contracture. A range of motion (ROM) program is essential in preserving joint motion, especially after higher doses have been administered. Pentoxifylline (Trental) shows promise in decreasing the effects of chronic radiation-induced fibrosis.[10]

TABLE 56-3.   Organ Systems: Sequelae of Cancer and Its Treatment

Organ System and Impairments	Symptoms/Impairments and Limitations	Prevention/Treatment
SKIN		
Decubiti	Pain, discomfort	Repositioning q2h; air mattress, chemical or mechanical débridement. Optimize skin care, plastic surgery for flaps.
Fibrosis	Contracture, pain	—
Contracture	Loss of joint ROM, pain	Prevention: ROM exercises 2–3 times/d, proper positioning in bed, splinting to maintain a functional position of hands and feet, early mobilization. Treatment: passive ROM with terminal stretch, physical modalities such as heat to promote prolonged stretching; treat spasticity with stretching, modalities, and pharmacologic intervention; surgical interventions (tendon lengthening, myotendinous transfers, osteotomies)
MUSCULOSKELETAL		
Muscle atrophy, myopathy	Weakness, fatigue, difficulty in ambulating, impaired ability to perform ADLs	Based on type of myopathy (see below)
Paraneoplastic syndrome	—	Isometric exercise
Carcinomatous: neuropathy/myopathy	—	No exercise
Steroid myopathy	—	Isometric exercise
Osteopenia/osteoporosis	Fracture of hip, long bone, vertebrae, ribs; pain	ADLs and ambulatory aids, calcium, vitamin D, and bisphosphonates
Pathologic fractures		
Long bone, hip	Pain that increases with weight bearing, tenderness, joint or extremity swelling, ambulatory and ADL dysfunction	Pain management, appropriate ADLs and ambulatory devices; determine stability of bone and extent of metastatic involvement
Vertebrae, ribs	Pain, vertebrae tenderness; pain that is worsened when taking deep breaths, chest-wall tenderness	Pain management, abdominal binder or corset for acute and subacute pain management, PT as tolerated. ROM exercises 2–3 times/d; active ambulation 1–2 times/d.
Amputations	Pain: postsurgical, phantom, and/or neuropathic, phantom sensation; loss of ability to perform ADLs and/or mobilize, poor body image	Preamputation and postamputation education and counseling, pain management, including medications, desensitization techniques, and physical modalities. Prostheses, ambulatory aids, and assistive devices; PT for residual limb care, preprosthetic and prosthetic training, generalized strengthening and endurance exercise program.
CARDIOVASCULAR		
Deconditioning, fibrosis, cardiomyopathy	Fatigue, dyspnea, generalized weakness, poor exercise tolerance	Consult cardiologist to assess cardiac stability. PT that may include progressive ambulation, stair climbing, wheelchair activities, and progressive exercise; also, teach energy conservation techniques.
LYMPHATIC		
Axial lymphedema	Swelling, pain, paresthesias of face, chest wall, abdominal and pelvic walls	Prevention, precautions, and education; complex decongestive therapy; bandages during acute treatment
Peripheral lymphedema	Swelling, pain, weakness, and/or paresthesias of the affected limb	Compression garments during maintenance phases
PULMONARY		
Fibrosis, lung resection, pulmonary toxic drugs	Dyspnea, fatigue, generalized weakness and deconditioning	Oxygen therapy, pharmacologic therapy, PT to promote improved endurance and strength, as well as use of ambulatory aids as required. OT to teach breathing and energy conservation techniques, as well as use of assistive devices.
GASTROINTESTINAL		
Complications of tumor: invasion and sequelae of surgery (i.e., colostomy, ileostomy, prolonged immobilization)	Bowel obstruction, constipation, nausea, vomiting, loss of appetite, fatigue, generalized weakness, deconditioning. Poor body image, fatigue, deconditioning, decubiti.	Surgical and pharmacologic intervention to treat underlying condition and symptoms; patient and family education on ostomy care; PT to promote improved ambulation, strength, and endurance; OT to promote ADLs with appropriate assistive devices
Side effects of drugs: gastritis, ulcers; nausea, vomiting; constipation	Pain, nausea, vomiting, loss of appetite, fatigue, generalized weakness, deconditioning	Pharmacologic intervention to treat symptoms; PT to promote improved ambulation, strength, and endurance; OT to promote ADLs with appropriate assistive devices

(continued)

TABLE 56-3. *(Continued)*

Organ System and Impairments	Symptoms/Impairments and Limitations	Prevention/Treatment
Neurogenic bowel		
Upper motor neuron	Constipation	Bowel program: minimize medications that cause constipation (e.g., narcotics, tricyclic antidepressants); increase fiber and fluid intake; daily stool softener; daily bowel motility agent; use recto-colic reflex with manual stimulation and/or suppository in sitting position; use gastrocolic reflex and plan defecation after a meal
Lower motor neuron	Fecal incontinence	—
UROGENITAL		
Neurogenic bladder		
Lower motor neuron	Varied presentation: urinary incontinence or urinary retention	Urodynamic studies: female—indwelling catheter; male—condom catheter; female/male—ICP
Upper motor neuron	Urinary retention with associated incontinence	Urodynamic studies: female/male—ICP; medications with anticholinergic properties such as imipramine and oxybutynin may decrease detrusor tone
Detrusor sphincter dyssynergia	Urinary retention with associated incontinence	—
Prostatectomy[1]	Urinary incontinence	PT for pelvic floor reeducation
Sexual dysfunction	Poor body image and fear of rejection due to altered anatomy	Sexual and body image counseling
Cervical cancer[1]	Pain with penetration due to stenosis/fibrosis and reduced lubrication	Vaginal dilators, artificial lubricants, and changes in sexual positions may minimize discomfort
Testicular, prostate, and colon cancer[1]	Hormonal changes, infertility, diarrhea, dermatologic manifestations status postorchiectomy and/or pelvic and abdominal radiation. These changes can lead to erectile dysfunction, painful and/or retrograde ejaculation, loss of libido, changes in male self-image. Injured vascular and nerve innervation to sexual organs may cause incontinence, impotence, ejaculatory dysfunction.	Erectile dysfunction: topical intraurethral therapies, oral medication, intracavernosal injection therapy, vacuum-assisted devices, and penile prosthesis
Spinal cord injuries		
Women	Lack of sensation at typical erogenous areas, decreased vaginal lubrication, decreased libido; reflex and psychogenic stimulation may produce lubrication	Artificial lubricants, stimulation of nontraditional erogenous zones (i.e., ear, neck, skin) at level of injury
Men	Lack of sensation at typical erogenous areas; reflex erections and psychogenic erections may occur; varied degrees of impotence, inability to maintain an erection, ejaculatory dysfunction	Stimulation of nontraditional erogenous zones (i.e., ear, neck, skin) at level of injury. Treatments for erectile dysfunction as summarized above.
CNS: BRAIN[3]		
Stroke/tumor		
Motor weakness	Difficulty ambulating and performing ADLs	PT and OT to promote improved mobility and ADLs; orthoses, assistive devices
Sensory loss	Impaired balance and proprioception, making it difficult to ambulate and/or perform ADLs	PT and OT to promote improved mobility and ADLs; skin care education to prevent decubiti, burns, and other soft tissue injuries
Dysphagia	Difficulty eating, fear of choking, loss of appetite, weight loss	ST to promote improved swallowing by postural changes, dietary modifications, thermal stimulation, and oral-motor exercises
Dysarthria	Difficulty communicating and being understood due to oral motor weakness	ST to promote improved communication with oral-motor exercises, communication boards, and other compensatory techniques
Aphasia	Difficulty communicating verbal and/or written language due to poor comprehension and/or ability to express one's thoughts	Speech/cognitive therapy to promote improved comprehension and expression by various remediation, compensation, and education strategies
Apraxia	Inability to execute purposeful movement (commonly of a limb) unexplained by motor, sensory, or proprioception loss	PT, OT, and ST (if oral apraxia) to improve ADLs, mobility, and/or communication by strategies, including cueing and reeducation

(continued)

TABLE 56-3.   (*Continued*)

Organ System and Impairments	Symptoms/Impairments and Limitations	Prevention/Treatment
CNS: SPINAL CORD		
SCI		
Paraplegia	Varied ability to stand, transfer, and ambulate due to varied lower extremity weakness	PT and OT to promote highest level of function possible in transfers, mobility, and ADLs. These may include wheelchair mobility, ambulation with lower extremity orthoses and assistive devices, transfers using transfer boards, and performance of upper extremity ADLs, including eating and performing bowel and bladder program with various upper extremity orthoses. Customized wheelchair prescription to maximize mobility and prevent decubiti.
Tetraplegia	Generally, unable to independently stand and ambulate. Varied ability to perform ADLs and transfer due to varied upper extremity weakness. May be independent with wheelchair mobility.	—
Sensory loss	Decubiti, pain	PT and OT to teach weight shift techniques (q20min when sitting, q2h when in bed); education regarding skin care, wheelchair cushions, air/foam mattresses
Neurogenic bowel	See Gastrointestinal section	See Gastrointestinal section
Neurogenic bladder	See Urogenital section	See Urogenital section
Sexual dysfunction	See Urogenital section	See Urogenital section
PNS		
Cervical radiculopathy	Upper extremity, neck and/or shoulder pain, paresthesias, sensory loss and/or weakness in a dermatomal or myotomal distribution	Rule out tumor invasion/progression. Surgery consult if progressive neurologic decline, vertebral column instability, and/or associated bowel or bladder dysfunction. Pain management: OT to help centralize pain, improve posture and poor body biomechanics; upper extremity orthoses to help perform ADLs.
Lumbar radiculopathy	Lower extremity, back, and/or buttocks pain; paresthesias, sensory loss, and/or weakness in a dermatomal or myotomal distribution	Rule out tumor invasion/progression. Surgery consult if progressive neurologic decline, vertebral column instability, and/or associated bowel or bladder dysfunction. Pain management: PT to help centralize pain, improve posture and poor body biomechanics; upper extremity orthoses to help perform ADLs.
Brachial plexopathy	Upper extremity, neck and/or shoulder pain, paresthesias, sensory loss and/or weakness in multiple dermatomes and/or myotomes	Rule out tumor invasion/progression. Pain management: OT to promote improved ADLs by reducing pain, promoting strengthening and stretching exercises as tolerated, prefabricating upper extremity orthoses and providing assistive devices. Rule out tumor invasion/progression.
Lumbosacral plexopathy	Lower extremity, back, or buttocks pain; paresthesias; sensory loss, and/or weakness in multiple dermatomes and/or myotomes	Pain management: PT to promote improved mobility and ADLs by reducing pain, promoting strengthening and stretching exercises as tolerated, prefabricating lower extremity orthoses, and providing assistive devices to aid in ambulation and ADLs
Peripheral neuropathy: sensory, motor, sensorimotor	Upper and/or lower extremity pain, paresthesias, sensory loss and/or weakness (distal more than proximal) in a nondermatomal and/or nonmyotomal distribution	Pain management: orthoses, upper and/or lower. Education regarding insensate skin care to prevent decubiti, burns, and other soft tissue injuries. PT to promote improved balance and proprioception and provide appropriate ambulatory aids. OT to promote improved ADLs with appropriate assistive devices.
PSYCHIATRY		
Depression	Depressed mood, disinterested in ADLs, loss of hope, increased or decreased appetite and/or sleep	Pharmacologic intervention, behavioral therapy to promote improved coping skills, relaxation techniques and self-esteem; regular exercise, community activities
Anxiety/psychosis	Agitation, fear, restlessness	—

ADLs, activities of daily living; CNS, central nervous system; ICP, intermittent catheterization program; OT, occupational therapy; PNS, peripheral nervous system; PT, physical therapy; ROM, range of motion; SCI, spinal cord injury; ST, speech therapy.

After radiation therapy of 3000 to 5000 rads to bony metastatic lesions, remineralization is noted within 2 months and maximal at 3 months, and remodeling is completed at 6 months to 1 year.[11] Because of this protracted time course, protected weight bearing may be indicated during the first several months after radiation to long bone or, in lesions meeting instability criteria, surgical operative stabilization before radiation therapy. If the epiphysis is irradiated, growth will be arrested.

Brain effects can include acute changes, which are usually transient and more common with single doses greater than 300 rads; early delayed encephalopathy, presenting within several months due to demyelination; and, rarely,[12] late delayed encephalopathy, caused by irreversible white matter necrosis.[13] Early delayed encephalopathy responds well to corticosteroids; however, with late delayed encephalopathy the response is less consistent. Memory loss or cognitive dysfunction may result from brain atrophy after whole brain irradiation.[13]

Myelopathic complications of radiation range from Lhermitte's syndrome (onset 1 to 4 months, lasting weeks to months), which can be seen in patients undergoing radiation for head and neck tumors, to transverse myelitis or delayed radiation myelopathy. The latter usually has its onset at 9 to 18 months, generally after more than 5000 rads, often presenting as a Brown-Séquard syndrome or with radicular pain. Deficits usually progress slowly, then stabilize without improvement. Radiation-induced plexopathies generally present in delayed fashion months to years after completion of treatment, typically when more than 6000 rads has been given.[13]

Radiation for head and neck cancer malignancies can produce a variety of complications. Hyposalivation often results and can interfere with swallowing. This can be addressed in a variety of ways, including the use of products designed to relieve oral dryness (gums, toothpastes, rinses), medications such as pilocarpine or bromhexine to promote increased salivary flow,[9] and nutritional counseling for strategies for maximizing oral intake, usually involving plenty of fluids and moist foods. Medications with anticholinergic side effects should be avoided. Radiation-induced dental disease can occur largely because of decreased salivary flow and, to a lesser extent, a direct effect on the teeth and surrounding soft tissues. Because the saliva becomes sticky,[23] the patient converts to a soft, high-carbohydrate diet, but this further promotes dental caries. Mechanical débridement of the tongue with a soft toothbrush and use of a spray mister before meals maximize taste bud access. A sodium fluoride gel should be used daily, and dilute peroxide, saline rinses, or salt and baking soda (1 tsp of each in 1 qt water)[15] can be used during the course of treatment to cleanse the mouth.

Other head and neck effects of radiation therapy include tongue sensitivity, which is temporary; reduced taste sensation, which usually improves over time; and limited jaw motion. Fibrosis of the base of the tongue after radiation therapy produces dysphagia, but aspiration is rare. Trismus may result from high radiation doses to the buccinator, pterygoid, or masseter muscles. Radiation to the neck can produce soft tissue fibrosis and laryngeal edema. Voice changes such as change in quality or reduced volume may be most prominent at the end of the day. Treatment of nasal cavity and paranasal sinus tumors can produce CNS complications, including radiation-induced encephalopathy, and a delayed, transient vertiginous syndrome. Radiation can also cause palsy of cranial nerves IX through XII as a delayed complication.

Radiation to the stomach or small intestine may produce nausea, vomiting, and the sensation of fullness. Over the long term, intestinal obstruction, perforation, bleeding, malabsorption, or fistulas may occur. Bowel rest and total parenteral nutrition may be needed in cases of severe radiation enteritis.

Patients with radiation-induced skin damage should avoid sun exposure, rubbing (such as straps, belts, or collars), or tape or chemical irritants (such as perfumes or deodorants) to the affected site.[12,15] For mild cases, improvement may be obtained with lotions such as baby oil or topical "vitamin A&D" ointment or cornstarch in intertriginous areas. For more severe cases, options can include a topical corticosteroid (1% hydrocortisone), cleansing with half-strength peroxide, or application of specialized wound care preparations.[15]

Radiation therapy to the prostate or testicles can produce erectile dysfunction, possibly as a result of acceleration of preexisting atherosclerosis from postradiation fibrotic changes. In women, radiation therapy to the pelvis produces premature menopause, with a dose of as low as 600 to 1000 rads permanently destroying ovarian function. Radiation also produces damage to the vaginal epithelium, and the fibrotic process can continue over years, leading to stenotic changes and dyspareunia. Vaginal dilators can preserve the integrity of the vagina. Estrogen therapy also may be of some benefit, as well as vaginal lubricants.

Thoracic (mantle) radiation therapy may be complicated by radiation pneumonitis, cardiac abnormalities (constrictive pericarditis, cardiomyopathy), and hypothyroidism.[12] Aseptic necrosis of the femoral heads is described in 10% of long-term survivors of inverted Y-field (abdominopelvic) irradiation and MOPP [mechlorethamine (Mustargen), vincristine (Oncovin), procarbazine, and prednisone].[12,16,17]

SURGICAL COMPLICATIONS

Surgical treatment of cancer can also lead to deconditioning, the severity of which is proportionate to the duration of postoperative immobility. For each week of immobility, approximately 10% to 20% of muscle mass is lost. Other postsurgical impairments depend on the anatomic site of the procedure. Surgical sites often associated with postoperative rehabilitation needs include the head and neck, brain, spine, limbs, and lymph node dissections. Usually, these require physical and occupational interventions to restore limb mobility and treat soft tissue pain.[18] Surgery to the chest or abdomen, impacting vital visceral structures, may be associated with limited chestwall excursion and chest-wall pain. Chest physical therapy to promote diaphragmatic breathing and good respiratory management may help.

Complications of mastectomy or lumpectomy with axillary lymph node dissection include wound complications, loss of strength and motion to the arm, dysesthesias, axillary web syndrome,[19] phantom breast sensations, and arm edema. Rarely, nerve injury occurs, including stretch injury to the long thoracic nerve supplying the serratus anterior muscle, resulting in scapular winging, and injury to the dorsal scapular nerve to the latissimus dorsi muscle.[20] Patients undergoing immediate reconstruction with TRAM (transverse rectus abdominis myocutaneous) flap make similar gains in ROM as non-TRAM patients.[21]

BIOLOGICS

Side effects of biologic agents, such as interferons, tumor necrosis factor, interleukins, and granulocyte-stimulating factors, may produce acute, local inflammatory reactions; limb edema; and ischemia. Severe fatigue is a frequent concomitant of interferon treatment, which may limit patients' tolerance of rehabilitation therapies. Colony-stimulating factors may cause bone pain. In recent years, newer techniques such as monoclonal antibody therapy (rituximab) and radioactive monoclonal antibodies show promise of effectiveness, with a minimum of side effects.

REHABILITATION INTERVENTIONS

NONPHARMACOLOGIC PAIN MANAGEMENT

The reader is referred to Chapter 55.1 for an in-depth discussion of cancer pain management, including pharmacologic strategies. The role for rehabilitation typically emphasizes nonpharmacologic interventions, as well as adjunctive medications to address musculoskeletal or neuritic overlay syndromes. Pain evaluation includes determination of whether the pain is due to tumor, treatment factors, or other reasons. Chronicity of symptoms, and pattern of the pain (localized or generalized, constant or intermittent), also affect the approach. The orientation is also toward determining the impact that pain has on limiting function.

Direct tumor spread accounts for most cancer pain (65% to 75%), and antitumor therapy can be highly effective in controlling it.[22] However, the cancer population tends to be elderly and pain management is challenging in them. They may not tolerate pain medication well, and comorbid painful conditions may compound the problems. Medications and other strategies to impact fatigue, sleep/wake, and mood also can favorably impact pain control. Pain management strategies designed to totally relieve symptoms are strongly encouraged by the World Health Organization. Because some necessary rehabilitation interventions such as passive stretching or various forms of active exercise may induce pain, strategies for pain control should be used surrounding such interventions and other predictable triggers for pain.

The appropriate strategy depends on the nature and pattern of the pain. Psychological strategies, such as guided imagery, hypnotherapy, biofeedback, and deep breathing, can be performed for various pain etiologies, although controlled studies are lacking in the cancer population. Soft tissue pain may respond to physical therapy strategies, including strengthening of surrounding musculature, and physical modalities. Deep heat modalities are customarily avoided to an area where active regional malignancy exists,[23] and heat over insensate areas should also be avoided to prevent burn injury. General aerobic exercise has been shown to improve mental outlook and may result in an improved ability to cope with pain. Pain of muscle or bone etiology is usually worse on weight bearing or other mechanical stress and improves with relative rest to the affected part. Splinting or assistive devices may be required to achieve protected weight bearing (see Management of Bony Metastases, later). Neuritic pain, on the other hand, is often worse at rest. The patient may benefit from desensitization strategies such as vibration or tapping. Topical agents such as anesthetic (lidocaine) or analgesic (nonsteroidal antiinflammatory medication) patches or chili pepper extract–based ointments (capsaicin) can be tried (the latter should not be applied to the face). Local injection with anesthetic or cortico-steroid can be considered when the pain generator is determined to be inflammation of tendon, muscle, bursa, or joint.

Electrical stimulation and nontraditional therapy such as acupuncture are gaining in acceptance to relieve acute pain in patients with cancer diagnoses. In severe cases, neurosurgical procedures, such as implantation of dorsal column stimulators, and neuroablative procedures (neurectomy, rhizotomy, cordotomy) can be considered. Comprehensive pain treatment centers offer cognitive and behavioral management strategies as adjuvant treatment for cancer-related pain.

Some conditions benefit from specialized pain control strategies. For example, whirlpool treatment may be of benefit for the intractable pruritus and widespread skin scaling that can occur with mycosis fungoides. A rib belt can relieve pain in individuals with rib metastasis or fracture. However, because it may have the effect of inhibiting full chest expansion, the rib belt should be removed at intervals. The patient's status after chest surgery best tolerates coughing with the knees flexed and the incision splinted by firm pressure from a pillow or towel roll. As the patient recovers, he or she should be instructed in techniques to promote maximal chest expansion, including coughing, pursed-lip breathing (inhalation through the nose, exhalation through pursed lips), diaphragmatic breathing (the patient places the hands over the abdomen to consciously promote expansion with inspiration), and segmental breathing (hand over upper or lower portion of the rib cage during inhalation).[24]

EXERCISE FOR THE CANCER PATIENT: GENERAL ASPECTS

The most immediate rationale that patients with cancer should exercise is to avoid effects of deconditioning, which include muscle weakness and atrophy, loss of cardiorespiratory fitness, and decreased efficiency of energy metabolism at a cellular level. Exercise can also affect immune parameters, including effects on macrophages, natural killer cells, neutrophils, and regulating cytokines; however, the clinical impact of these effects is not well understood.[25] Appropriate precautions should be incorporated into the exercise program (Table 56-4). As with all individuals, when possible, the form of exercise should be one that is enjoyable for the cancer patient.

Most studies examining effects of exercise in cancer (Table 56-5) fall into two groups, those with physical performance end points and those assessing potential quality-of-life or psychological benefits. The effect of exercise on various other factors, including body weight, fatigue, cellular function, cell counts, and hospital length of stay, has also been examined. All studies measuring physical performance show benefit in parameters such as exercise time, functional capacity, heart rate, workload intensity, and 12-minute walk distance. Aerobic exercise, at moderate levels, has been most thoroughly studied. Effect on fatigue is favorable but variable.[26–28] Reported levels of depression and anxiety are improved,[29,30] as well as quality-of-life scores.[30–32] Some studies that have examined group exercise programs, whose formats have a social dimension and therefore may have social and psychological benefits, but it is not clear from available literature whether the group format has any advantages in terms of compliance or fitness outcomes.

A strong justification for exercise in cancer patients is weight reduction. Body mass index is directly proportional to tumor recurrence rates and all-cause mortality.[33] Obesity is also a risk fac-

TABLE 56-4. Exercise Precautions for Cancer Patients

Medical Problem	Laboratory Values	Recommendations
THROMBOCYTOPENIA Normal values: platelets 150,000–450,000/m³	30,000–50,000/m³	Active exercise/ROM, light weights (1–2 lb; no heavy resistance/isokinetics); ambulation
	20,000–30,000/m³	Self-care activity, gentle exercise (passive or active)
	<20,000/m³	Ambulation and self-care with assistance as needed for endurance/balance safety; minimal or cautious exercise/activity; essential ADLs only
ANEMIA Normal values: hematocrit 37–47%; hemoglobin 12–16 g/dL	Hematocrit <25%, hemoglobin <8 g/dL	Light ROM exercise, isometrics; avoid aerobic or progressive programs
	Hematocrit 25–35%; hemoglobin 8–10 g/dL	Essential ADLs, assistance as needed for safety; light aerobics, light weights (1–2 lb)
	Hematocrit >35%; hemoglobin >10 g/dL	Ambulation and self-care as tolerated; resistance exercise, ambulation, self-care as tolerated
BONY METASTASIS Plain x-ray findings: high risk indicated by following: cortical lesions >2.5–3.0 cm; >50% cortical involvement; painful lesions; unresponsive to radiation	>50% cortex involved	No exercises; touch down: not weight bearing, use crutches, walker; active ROM exercise (no twisting)
	25–50% cortex involved	No stretching; partial weight bearing; light aerobic activity; avoid lifting/straining activity
	0–25% cortex involved	Full weight bearing
PULMONARY DYSFUNCTION Pulmonary function tests, chest radiograph	<50% of predicted FEV₁ or diffusion capacity	No aerobic exercise
	50–75% of predicted FEV₁ or diffusion capacity	Light aerobic exercise
	75%+ of predicted FEV₁ or diffusion capacity	Most programs fine
	Large plural effusions or pericardial effusions or multiple metastases to lungs	ROM; few submaximal isometrics; consult cardiologist and oncologist
CARDIAC DYSFUNCTION Ejection fraction, electrocardiogram	Low	Low aerobics
	Recent PVCs; fast atrial arrhythmia; ventricular arrhythmia; ischemic pattern	No aerobics; consult cardiologist
ELECTROLYTE ABNORMALITIES Na	Below 130	No exercise
K⁺	Below 3.0 (hyperkalemia) requires treatment	No exercise
Calcium	Above 6.0 (hyperkalemia) requires treatment	
ENDOCRINE Diabetes on insulin	Monitor carefully, as exercise may potentiate the response to insulin	

ADLs, activities of daily living; FEV₁, forced expiratory volume in 1 second; PVCs, premature ventricular contractions; ROM, range of motion.

tor for lymphedema.[34] Weight control and weight reduction require limitation of caloric intake, but exercise can help maintain weight loss and help prevent deconditioning and dependence. Patients in the active treatment phase may have side effects that interfere with adequate nutrition, and in this setting, treating fatigue is likely to be critical and promoting increased caloric intake may be an integral part of management. Such patients may experience food aversions, mucositis, poor appetite, dysphagia, and postsurgical barriers to adequate nutrition. Such nutritional factors should be addressed to promote optimal activity tolerance and healing. This often requires a multifactorial approach, emphasizing food that the patient prefers and can handle safely, oral preparations for mucositis, and, at times, appetite stimulants. The use of anabolic steroids such as oxandrolone has been described to augment weight gain and the building of muscle mass; however, it is just beginning to be studied in the cancer population.[35] Attention must also be paid to ensure adequate hydration to prevent orthostatic hypotension. The issue of an appropriate exercise program should be visited in all cancer patients, with the exception of those with cachexia.[36] Cachexia is defined as greater than 25% loss of lean bone mass or a body mass index less than or equal to 10% below normal range. Most cachectic patients are not consuming adequate amounts of protein or calories to meet basal needs and should focus on maintaining basic functional skills and quality-of-life priorities.[36]

Multiple factors can be causative or contributory to fatigue, and thus the problem of fatigue must be approached in an individualized manner. Common problems include cytokine effects (either endogenous or due to treatment), anemia, pain, depression, medication side effects, poor nutrition, and coexisting endocrine disturbances such as hypothyroidism. Addressing such factors to the extent possible will optimize exercise performance. Physical deconditioning itself leads to fatigue, with activities that had been customary for the patient becoming more effortful. Therefore, exercise itself is considered important in the treatment and prevention of fatigue. Treatment of anemia with recombinant erythropoietin has been found to result in improved preservation of exercise capacity compared to controls in patients with cachexia due to gastrointestinal tumors.[37] Use of stimulant medication has also been considered to counteract fatigue and may have the added benefit of mitigating the amount of opioid medication required.[22]

Special concerns in the bone marrow transplant population include high potential for deconditioning and social isolation and the need for precautions over a prolonged period of time due to low blood counts and medical complications. During periods of low exercise tolerance, emphasizing sitting or recumbent exercise facilitates compliance. Standing should be encouraged, at least for brief periods, to avoid gastrocnemius and soleus tightness. Exercises can include ROM, deep breathing,

TABLE 56-5. Efficacy of Exercise Studies

Author	Population	Controlled?	Intervention	Outcome
MacVicar et al., 1989[42]	45 breast cancer patients receiving noncardiotoxic chemotherapy	Yes, placebo (stretching) and no-exercise groups	3 times/wk, 10-wk aerobic interval training	40% gain in functional capacity in the aerobic exercise group, with longer work periods, improved heart rate parameters, and ability to tolerate a higher-intensity workload
Berglund et al., 1993[45]	60 (mostly) breast cancer patients s/p radiation or chemotherapy	Yes, matched comparison group	Group exercise: 4 sessions mixed training (strength, aerobic, aquatic); education in coping strategies	Improved self-reported strength in the study group
Sharkey et al., 1993[43]	12 children and young adults s/p anthracycline treatment for cancer	No	Aerobic conditioning 2 times/wk for 12 wk supervised; 1 time/wk home session added at wk 7	8–14% increase in exercise time, peak oxygen uptake, ventilatory anaerobic threshold; no change in exercise heart rate or stroke volume
Dimeo et al., 1996[38]	20 bone marrow transplant patients with stabilized platelet counts	Yes	Aerobic (treadmill) exercise 30 min/d for 6 wk	Improved physical performance, improved heart rate parameters, and decreased lactate formation with exercise
Dimeo et al., 1997[41]	70 solid tumor patients undergoing high-dose chemotherapy and autologous peripheral blood stem cell transplant	Yes	Supervised daily supine bicycle ergometry (bed ergometer) for 30 min	Decreased decrement in performance, pain, duration of neutropenia, and thrombocytopenia; shorter hospitalization
Segal et al., 2001[44]	24 breast cancer survivors	Yes; 3 groups: exercise only, exercise plus behavior modification, and neither (data for both exercise groups considered together in the results because findings were similar); also, partial crossover component with 5 patients crossing over	Unsupervised 4 d/wk, 10-wk aerobic exercise at home or exercise facility	Exercise groups with decreased levels of depression and anxiety, no effect of exercise on self-esteem scores; improved compliance when physicians had recommended exercise
Courneya, 2003[31]	25 cancer patients (breast, multiple myeloma, lymphomas) undergoing autologous bone marrow transplant	No	"Encouraged" walking and cycle ergometry, tracking mode, frequency and duration of exercise	Mean exercise time <8 min/d; 24% no exercise at all. Duration of exercise positively correlates with quality-of-life scores.
Na et al., 1999[a]	35 postoperative patients with stomach cancer ("curative" surgery)	Yes	Arm and bicycle ergometry 2 times/d, 5 d/wk for 14 d, starting after operative day 2	Increased measurable natural killer cell activity at day 14 in the exercise group
Porock, 2000[b]	9 home hospice patients with life expectancy of at least 2 mo	No	Duke Energizing Exercise plan (various activities over the course of a day)	Improved quality-of-life scores, no change in fatigue scores
Schwartz, 2000[28]	27 newly diagnosed breast cancer patients undergoing chemotherapy	No randomized controls; patients self-selected into exercise or not. Patients considered exercisers by log data and if 12-min walk time improved.	8-wk home-based program 15–30 min 3–4 d/wk; exercise quantified via accelerometry and log; fatigue scores also logged	12-min walk improved 10% in exercisers, decreased 16% in nonexercisers; variable fatigue data; improved worst daily fatigue scores in exercisers
Schwartz, 2000[28]	71 newly diagnosed non-metastatic breast cancer patients beginning chemotherapy	No randomized controls; patients considered exercisers if doing at least a 15-min session 4 d/wk	8-wk home-based progressive aerobic program, 4 d/wk; exercise quantified via accelerometry and log. Body weight, fatigue scores, and side effect checklist logged.	Exercisers maintain body weight, nonexercisers gain weight (also weigh more at baseline); improved 12-min-walk test in exercisers (15% increase vs. 23% decrease in controls). No difference in nausea or anorexia. Lower posttest fatigue in exercisers.

(continued)

TABLE 56-5. (*Continued*)

Author	Population	Controlled?	Intervention	Outcome
Wall, 2000[102]	104 preoperative lung cancer patients	Yes	7- to 10-d program of breathing, arm and leg exercises, walking, and stair climbing	Psychologically, increased power (capacity to knowingly participate in change) in exercisers; physical parameters not assessed
Adamsen et al., 2001[46]	17 men with cancer (various)	No	13 2-h sessions over 16 wk; 1st hour with exercise (various forms), 2nd hour with educational session	Improved reported energy level and self-confidence
Blanchard et al., 2001[29]	34 breast cancer survivors	High-anxiety and low-anxiety groups compared	Acute bout of cycle ergometer exercise to target heart rate 150–160	Improved anxiety scores in patients with high initial anxiety
Schwartz et al., 2001[26]	72 breast cancer patients receiving chemotherapy	No randomized controls; self-selected into exercisers or not	Low to moderate intensity (15–30 min, 3–4 d/wk) home-based aerobic exercise	Improved short-term (same day) fatigue
Segal et al., 2001[44]	123 breast cancer patients receiving adjuvant therapy	Yes. Randomized into supervised exercise, self-directed exercise, and usual care groups. Data also analyzed by chemotherapy vs. other adjuvant care.	Walking program to 50–60% VO_2 max over 26 wk	Increased reported physical function per SF-36 in both exercise groups. Aerobic capacity gains only in the supervised-exercise, nonchemotherapy patients.
Courneya et al., 2003[30]	53 postmenopausal breast cancer survivors s/p surgery and radiotherapy and/or chemotherapy	Yes	Recumbent or upright cycle ergometry 3 times/wk for 15 wk	Exercise group with increased peak oxygen consumption and increased overall quality-of-life scores

s/p, status post.
[a]Na YM, Lee JS, Park JS, et al. Early rehabilitation program in post mastectomy patients: a prospective clinical trial. *Yonsei Med J* 1999;40:1.
[b]Porock D, Kristjanson LJ, Tinnelly K, Duke T, Blight J. An exercise intervention for advanced cancer patients experiencing fatigue: a pilot study. *J Palliat Care* 2000;16:30.

aerobic activity, and light resistive exercise, such as bridging or use of light weights.[37] Even if the patient is feeling poorly, a brief session, if only for passive ROM or massage, maintains a habit of activity and builds trust with the therapist for future sessions.[38] One study of treadmill training in bone marrow transplant patients with stabilized platelet counts resulted in improved physical performance. Patients were able to exercise 30 minutes daily, under an interval pattern (incorporating rest periods) for 6 weeks, with exercise intensity titrated to 80% of calculated maximum heart rate or lactate concentration of 3 mmol/L in capillary blood.[38] Rehabilitation strategies for children with graft-versus-host disease (GVHD) have also been reported.[40]

The complication of chronic GVHD can lead to skin rash and erythema, fasciitis, limb edema, and joint contractures. Protective padding should be applied, including over the soles of the feet during exercise. Other treatments include active assisted ROM and nighttime splinting of the hands and feet.[39] Adjunctive medication, such as quinine, carbamazepine, or baclofen, can be considered for cramping, and etretinate in the setting of contractures. The high-dose steroids used to treat GVHD can lead to complications, including myopathy, aseptic necrosis, and osteoporosis. To counteract potential adverse effects of corticosteroids, the exercise program should emphasize proximal muscle strengthening, back extension, posture, and upper limb weight bearing.[16]

Response to exercise is generally favorable (see Table 56-5). Patients receiving cardiotoxic chemotherapy do not show improved cardiac parameters but exhibit improved performance as a result of peripheral adaptation. A controlled study of patients performing daily supine bicycle ergometry, to a heart rate of 50% of calculated cardiac reserve while receiving high-dose chemotherapy (nonanthracycline) followed by autologous peripheral blood stem cell transplantation for solid tumors, found multiple benefits in the exercise group, including less decrement in performance per treadmill testing, less pain, and even decreased duration of neutropenia and shorter hospitalization.[41] Another aerobic training program in women undergoing a noncardiotoxic chemotherapy regimen for breast cancer found 40% improvement in functional capacity, improved heart rate, longer work periods, and higher-intensity workload attainable than in controls. This study also had a placebo group doing only stretching exercises, and the aerobic training group performed better in the above parameters except for heart rate.[42] However, cancer patients treated with cardiotoxic agents such as anthracyclines (in doses of greater than 100 mg/m[2]) sustain permanent cardiac damage, resulting in reduced maximal oxygen uptake, lack of improved heart rate and stroke volume responses, ST- and T-wave changes, and exercise-induced hypotension.[43] Aerobic exercise in this population can nevertheless improve exercise time, peak oxygen uptake, and ventilatory anaerobic threshold.[43] Another study of breast cancer patients receiving adjuvant therapy, stratified by chemotherapy (approximately two-thirds receiving anthracyclines) or no chemotherapy (radiation or hormonal treatment), found gains in patient-reported physical function whether the exercise program is self-directed (6 months, 5 times/wk progressive walking program, with use of an exercise diary) or supervised (similar program, 3 times/wk supervised, and twice weekly at home) and may be greater with the self-directed approach. However, measured gains in functional capacity were significant only in the supervised exercise group of patients who were not receiving chemotherapy.[44] Thus, it remains unclear to what extent patient-reported function correlates with outcome measures such as functional capacity. Low- to moderate-intensity, home-based aerobic exercise is associated with reduced fatigue in women receiving chemotherapy for breast cancer; however, the effect of exercise on fatigue appears to be more immediate (same day) than sustained.[26]

Models have been developed for group exercise therapy combined with educational sessions, such as training in coping strategies, or education about specific aspects of malignancy. Findings have included improved self-report of physical strength[45] in a group of primarily breast cancer patients after radiation or chemotherapy, or both; and improved energy level and self-confidence in a group of men with malignancy of various forms and stages.[46] Functional parameters were not measured in either group, however.

Attention should be paid to any weight-bearing restrictions (see Tables 56-3 and 56-4). Although evidence-based support is scant, in general, exercise should emphasize low bony impact, such as isometric strengthening, and low-impact aerobic conditioning activities, such as swimming, riding a stationary bicycle, or walking. The patient should also be advised on good body mechanics (in particular, avoiding sudden spine or limb torsions) and fall prevention strategies (including environmental modifications). Climbing steps in a step-to-step pattern instead of step-over-step minimizes the period of single-limb support.

Studies have shown efficacy of bisphosphonates such as pamidronate and clodronate in preventing or delaying complications of bony metastatic disease, such as pain and pathologic fractures, due to inhibition of osteolysis. Pamidronate has been advocated for breast cancer patients with metastatic bone pain, concurrently with chemotherapy or hormonal therapy.[47]

The above sections have dealt largely with deconditioning. Some cancer patients have specific exercise needs based on the extent or treatment of tumor, such as those with head and neck malignancies, neurologic tumors, postmastectomy impairments, or sarcomas. The reader is referred to subsequent sections in this chapter that address specific tumors. The primary purpose of exercise, as with deconditioning, is to maintain or improve function and general fitness and also to facilitate normal movement patterns and prevent painful musculoskeletal complications that can develop in individuals with long-standing biomechanical derangements (e.g., shoulder-hand syndrome in a hemiplegic patient). In the setting of these conditions, exercise is often combined with other strategies such as use of appropriate equipment and therapeutic modalities. Although lifestyle modifications are often necessary, the patient should be encouraged to assume the fullest possible range of activities, including recreational interests.

Moderate exercise is believed to be beneficial for individuals with cancer.[39,43,48] The basic program includes exercises to maintain independence and quality of life through interventions designed to improve ROM and strength, endurance, and flexibility. The program should be individualized to focus on reducing functional limitations. Specific precautions must be considered when prescribing exercises in individuals with cancer. These include hematologic, cardiac, pulmonary, skeletal, electrolyte, and endocrine conditions. The specific guidelines are summarized in other sections of this chapter and in Table 56-4.

MODALITIES OF HEAT, COLD, AND ELECTRICITY

Physical modalities are nonpharmacologic agents used to produce a therapeutic effect in tissues. They include heat, cold, and electrotherapy. They are frequently used to reduce pain, facilitate stretch, aid in wound care, and introduce medications such as corticosteroids. Heat includes superficial and deep heating modalities. Superficial heat is applied to the surface of the skin to achieve the maximum tissue temperatures in skin and subcutaneous fat. Superficial heat is applied using heating pads, moist compresses, Hydrocollator packs, paraffin baths, and whirlpool baths. Deep heat is directed to heat muscle, tendons, ligaments, or bone. It is most commonly applied using ultrasound waves. Medication such as 1% lidocaine or corticosteroids can be applied using ultrasound. This technique is known as *phonophoresis*. The ultrasound waves facilitate the diffusion of the medication into the deeper tissue zones. Phonophoresis is often used to treat tendonitis, bursitis, scar tissue, neuromas, and adhesions that may be complications associated with cancer or its treatments.[49]

Cold modalities, also known as *cryotherapy*, are often used to treat acute pain and inflammation associated with musculoskeletal disorders, as well as myofascial pain, spasticity, and emergent care of minor burns. Cryotherapy should not be used in cold-intolerant patients or those with cryoglobulins, cold hypersensitivity, and Raynaud's disease.[49]

Transcutaneous electrical nerve stimulation (TENS) is the most common form of electroanalgesia. It has been used to help reduce neuropathic and nociceptive pain conditions, depending on the type of TENS unit and parameters chosen. It is applied by placing one to four electrode pads surrounding the area of pain. A small stimulating unit is connected, and specific frequency, pulse width, and amplitude settings are selected based on the type of pain and the patient's response. The analgesic effect of TENS may be due to a combination of mechanisms, including acting as a counterirritant in the CNS to inhibit activity of dorsal horn nociceptive neurons, activating the production of endogenous opioids, and possibly activating other neurotransmitter systems, including the serotonergic and substance P systems.[50] The TENS unit should not be applied over or near a malignancy unless it is being used in patients with terminal cancer.[49]

Precautions should be considered when prescribing modalities. Heat should not be applied to an area of acute trauma and inflammation and in patients with bleeding diatheses, edema, peripheral vascular disease, large scars, impaired sensation, or cognitive or communication deficits that impair their ability to report pain. The use of all heat forms and electricity is contraindicated over malignancies because of their potential for increasing the rate of local tumor growth or hyperemia spread. This may be overlooked in the terminally ill patient if modalities are to be used as adjuvants to improve pain relief or reduce inflammation.[49,50] Cryotherapy is the treatment of choice for acute trauma and inflammation. It can also be used in patients with bleeding diathesis and large scars. Otherwise, the above precautions apply.

LYMPHEDEMA MANAGEMENT

Lymphedema or a sense of fullness in the limb even without circumferential changes is frequently reported by patients who have undergone lymph node dissection. Findings tend to develop over a protracted period of time, and the median interval between treatment and onset is 39 months.[51] Risk factors for lymphedema include extent of surgery, receipt of axillary radiation, and obesity.[34,52] Lymphedema can result from lymphatic obstruction and thrombophlebitis from extrinsic compression on adjacent veins (lymphomas). The severity of lymphedema can fluctuate, making surveillance of this condition difficult, and also complicates the ability to perform research on outcomes of specific strategies. Nonetheless, numerous treatment strategies have been developed and are in common use. It is not known whether some of these strategies will prevent lymphedema in at-risk individuals; however, a number of simple precautions are routinely advised.

Comorbid impairments, including ROM deficits, reduced strength, neurologic deficits, pain, and impaired self-care, are common.[53] Needle sticks should be avoided in the affected limb, but if considered necessary, as for diagnostic or therapeutic procedures for comorbid conditions, they should be kept to a minimum and performed with strict aseptic technique and an increased intensity of the patient's usual lymphedema control regimen.[54] Prevention of lymphedema depends on two factors: (1) promoting lymph outflow, hence elevating the limb; exercising; using specialized wraps or massage techniques; or avoiding constriction and protecting from infection, scarring, and burns; and (2) limiting lymph production by using compression garments and avoiding vasodilation through heat exposure (sun, sauna, and steam). Use of a compression garment that uses 30 to 50 mm Hg also is effective. Typically, garments of 30/20 or 40/30 (with higher pressure distally) are sufficient for upper limb lymphedema. The usefulness of compression pumps, either single or multichannel machines, is controversial. Some efficacy has been shown for this approach,[55] and it is often advocated, especially in severe cases or when other measures have had only limited success. Other studies have not shown significant benefit, however.[34] Manual lymph drainage has been shown to be effective. The technique requires training in the use of a special manual drain using a delicate massage technique, compression bandaging, and a series of exercises.[56] Better compliance appears to produce better results, although gains can be partially maintained even in noncompliant patients. Use of multilayer bandaging produces better results than use of a garment alone.[57] Various techniques or schools for massage and exercise exist, and a modified manual lymph drainage program using devices such as sticks and rollers has been described. Long-term efficacy of surgical treatments for this problem is considered questionable. The role of medications such as coumarins is controversial,[58] and diuretics do not have benefit. The threshold for initiation of antibiotics for suspicion of cellulitis should be low. Dietary measures such as avoiding excess salt (to minimize fluid retention) and emphasizing flavonoid-containing fruits and vegetables (which enhance macrophage function in breaking down excess proteins) are advisable. Lymphedema management entails a daily lifelong regimen, and thus obtaining adequate control represents a significant commitment for the affected person. Involvement of a physical therapist or occupational therapist with specialized expertise in lymphedema management techniques is crucial.

MANAGEMENT OF BONY METASTASES

Patients with bony metastatic disease or soft tissue impairments involving the spine or limbs may require protected weight bearing, either to avoid further bony injury (for example, in the healing phase after radiation therapy and/or surgical stabilization of pathologic fracture) or to assist in pain control. Various radiologic parameters have been developed to assess risk of pathologic fracture in long bone and in the spine. When metastatic bone lesions are present, 90% of the time the lesions are multiple, and 20% of the time this includes upper limb involvement. Thus, if management is to include assistive devices, the patient should be assessed as to bony integrity at sites beyond those of known clinical involvement. Size criteria for pathologic fracture risk in long bone include lesions measuring greater than 2.5 cm in the lower limb and more than 3.0 cm in the upper limb, involvement of more than 50% of the cortex, intramedullary lesions of more than 50% to 60% cross-sectional diameter, involvement of cortical length equal to or greater than the cross-sectional diameter at that level, or, in the case of the femoral neck, cortical destruction of greater than 1.3 cm. In practice, the actual size may be difficult to delineate, due to infiltrative, permeating pattern and surrounding osteopenia. Factors such as histology (with highly vascular or lytic lesions perhaps at highest risk) and location (importance to weight bearing) are also considerations.[59] In the spine, the three-column model of Denis is often used in assessing stability,[60] with the spine divided into anterior (anterior longitudinal ligament, anterior half of vertebral body and disk), middle (posterior half of vertebral body and disk and posterior longitudinal ligament), and posterior (posterior elements) columns. The lesion is considered unstable if two or more columns are involved or, in some cases, if the middle column alone is involved. The criteria of Harrington also incorporate neurologic involvement into the model as follows:

1. No significant neurologic involvement
2. Bone involvement without instability/collapse
3. Major neurologic involvement without bone involvement
4. Bony collapse without neurologic compromise
5. Major neurologic compromise and vertebral collapse

Those in categories I to III can benefit from rehabilitation treatment designed to relieve pain and promote function. These patients benefit from light weight, easily donned corsets that offer pain relief, as does the use of superficial heat and TENS units. Patients who have stage IV and V involvement, when not responsive to radiation and chemotherapy for their bony or neurologic problems, require surgical stabilization.

A walker or crutches are needed for complete non–weight bearing of a lower limb. A single cane can be used in cases of smaller, but painful, lesions. For somewhat larger or more symptomatic lesions, a forearm crutch permits approximately 25% more force transmission through the device than a conventional cane (Fig. 56-1). In the thoracic spine where there is anterior or middle column involvement, prevention of spinal flexion is the bracing goal. A thoracolumbar orthosis in a two-piece clamshell design (Fig. 56-2) or a Jewett-type brace affords stability in all directions. Of particular concern are the atlantoaxial and thoracolumbar junctions, due to significant bending and torquing moments at these interfaces. Cervical spine stability requires the use of a two-poster (Fig. 56-3), four-poster, or halo design orthosis. For cervical spine pain, without instability or luxation of more than a few millimeters, a Philadelphia collar is well tolerated and appropriate (Fig. 56-4).

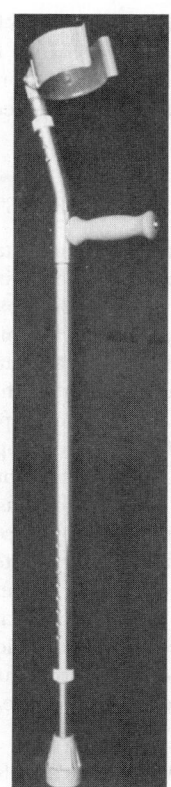

FIGURE 56-1.   Forearm crutch.

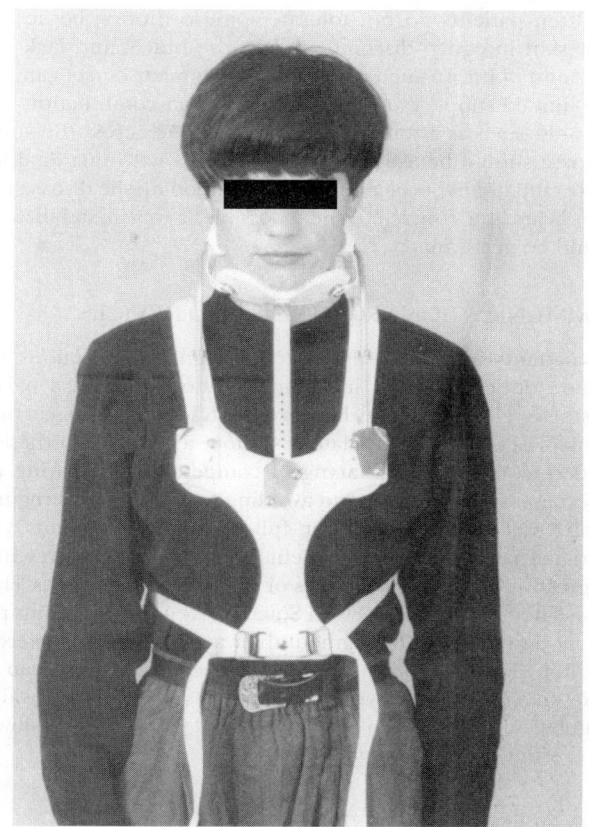

FIGURE 56-3.   Two-poster cervical orthosis for stabilization of flexion/extension.

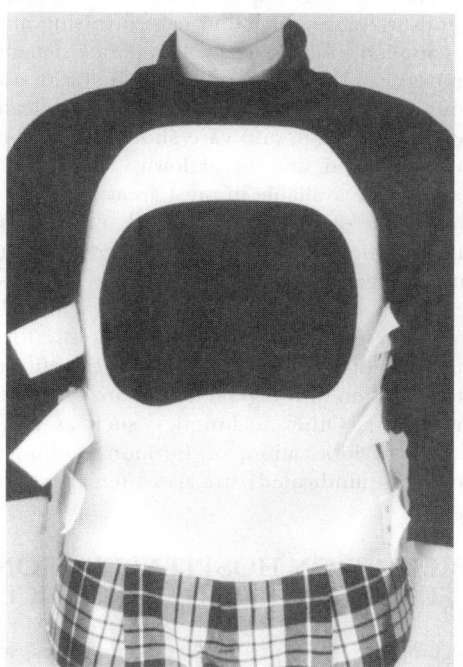

FIGURE 56-2.   Molded body jacket for thoracolumbar spinal support.

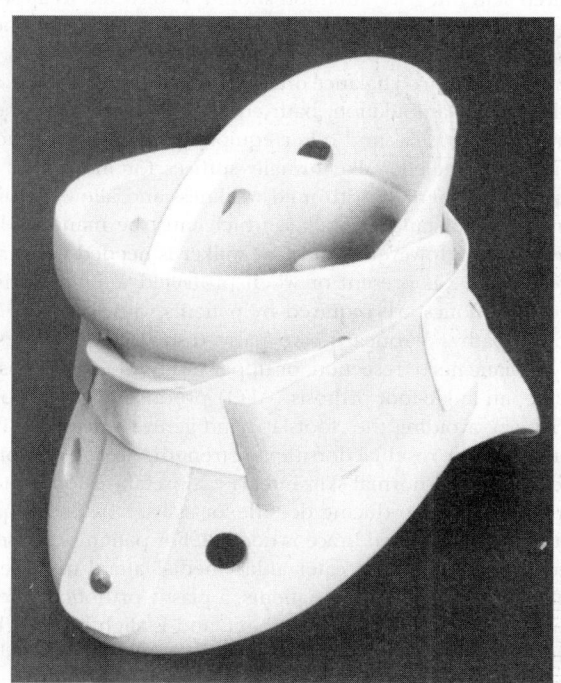

FIGURE 56-4.   Philadelphia collar.

Often patients do not tolerate spine orthotics, because of poor skin integrity, discomfort from the brace, and lack of a clear end point. In such cases a thoracolumbar corset can provide limited support and pain relief. Use in combination with gait aids, such as a walker, minimizes torque across the spine. Bed rest should be avoided because additional functional loss will occur, and hypocalcemia and thromboembolic disease may complicate the course.[61] When possible, surgical stabilization should be performed.

COMMUNICATION PROSTHESIS AND DEVICES

For patients with head and neck malignancies, options can include devices to assist in communication, such as a palatal prosthesis, electronic speech devices, or tracheoesophageal prosthesis (TEP). After soft palate resection, a palatal prosthesis is needed to restore velopharyngeal competence, improving the hypernasal speech quality and avoiding nasopharyngeal regurgitation. (See Chapter 26.3 for full discussion.) Patients with restricted jaw motion may benefit from mechanical stretching progressively with tongue blades or other devices (such as Therabite, Therabite Corp., Newton Square, PA) and continuous passive motion devices[62] to augment their active stretching exercise program. For patients with feeding issues, oral transit can be achieved with use of a syringe or pusher spoon. If the residual tongue tissue is unable to contact the hard palate, a palate-lowering prosthesis should be offered.[63]

MANAGEMENT OF PERIPHERAL NEUROPATHY

For all patients who are exercising, but in particular those with peripheral polyneuropathies or with other risk factors for impaired skin integrity, attention should be directed to appropriate nonconstrictive footwear to minimize the likelihood of ulceration resulting from poor sensory feedback. Patients with weakness or impaired balance often need equipment such as assistive devices for ambulation, bath equipment such as tub bench and raised toilet seat, and other equipment for self-care such as reachers. A wheeled walker usually suffices for individuals with balance impairment or with mild weakness and allows a quicker cadence than a standard walker, which must be manually lifted between steps. However, a standard walker is needed when more severe weakness is present or when protected weight bearing is needed. Orthotics are required by patients with footdrop from polyneuropathy, peroneal nerve palsy (usually due to pressure injury), sciatic nerve resection, or upper motor neuron disease. In this case, an ankle-foot orthosis (AFO) produces a more normal gait pattern, avoiding the "footslap" and genu recurvatum. If the patient has some residual dorsiflexor strength, a relatively normal-shaped limb, and normal skin integrity, a prefabricated posterior leafspring device, producing dorsiflexor assist, may be adequate. If not, a custom molded brace is needed. For patients with severe weakness, this includes greater ankle medial-lateral trimlines for increased stability. For most patients, a plastic orthotic is preferable, as it is considered more aesthetic and is slightly more lightweight than metal and can be used with different pairs of shoes; however, double metal upright braces may be advantageous for those with poor skin integrity or those for whom extensive future adjustments are anticipated.

Equipment often of benefit for individuals performing self-care tasks include one-handed sock donners, elastic shoelaces, and specialized eating devices such as a high-rimmed plate and rocking knife. Those with ataxia may benefit from weighted utensils. In all such cases, occupational therapy referral is essential to assure the strategies and equipment that are the best fit for the particular patient.

AMPUTATION AND LIMB SPARING

For cancer patients undergoing amputation, prosthesis fitting and prescription are similar to those without cancer. Although cancer amputees tend to have more proximal amputations than noncancer amputees, the average age of the amputee with cancer is younger than that of other amputees, most of whom are older individuals with severe vascular disease and, often, other medical problems.[64] Thus, the cancer patient is often a "good user" and a candidate for prosthetic options that are durable and technically up to date. Socket adaptations can be made by adding and subtracting stump socks, using a series of flexible sockets, or padding the lining to adapt the fit. For proximal upper limb resections, such as forequarter amputation or shoulder disarticulation, prosthesis use proves cumbersome and the patient often prefers to focus on one-handed function with the remaining limb, with provision of a molded shoulder prosthesis for cosmesis. After limb-sparing procedures, patients often benefit from specialized bracing and footwear.

EQUIPMENT FOR BOWEL, BLADDER, AND SEXUAL IMPAIRMENTS

Patients with gastrointestinal or genitourinary malignancies may receive ostomy placement and require training in its care. A variety of ostomy collection systems are available, including one-piece collection bags applied directly to the skin using an adhesive and two-piece collection bags involving an occlusive seal that is applied to the skin and a separate detachable bag. Collection bags can be closed and disposed of with each use, or open, allowing for drainage and reuse. Proper cleaning technique prevents infection, and care should be applied to prevent skin maceration and breakdown. Support groups for ostomy patients are available in most areas. Patients unable to achieve oral intake due to head and neck, esophageal, or neurologic malignancies require training in feeding via tube.

Patients with genitourinary malignancies may also experience an effect on sexual function. In men, vacuum devices for erectile function can be considered, especially for those in whom pharmacologic measures are not of benefit or are contraindicated. Women with vaginal fibrosis may benefit from use of dilator devices. Other techniques, such as psychological strategies, use of lubrication, or hormonal adjunctive treatment (if not contraindicated), are also often appropriate.

REHABILITATION HOSPITALIZATION AND BASIC FUNCTIONAL INDEPENDENCE

With widespread use of functional outcome scales, such as the 126-point Functional Independence Measure (FIM) in inpatient rehabilitation centers, multiple studies in recent years have uniformly demonstrated the capacity for patients with cancer to benefit from intensive multidisciplinary rehabilitation. The Karnofsky scale improves in parallel with FIM but, as a 10-

point scale, does not appear to offer the level of discrimination needed for identifying more subtle but potentially significant gradations in motor, self-care, and cognitive function. It has been suggested, however, that the Karnofsky scale, given its widespread use by oncologists, helps in the identification of patients with possible rehabilitation needs. In one study, all patients admitted to rehabilitation had Karnofsky scores of 40 to 60.[65] Several studies, all using FIM, have included control groups of patients with "equivalent" impairments, such as stroke or traumatic brain injury, comparing to brain tumor, and traumatic spinal cord injury (SCI), comparing to neoplastic SCI. These studies have found a shorter average rehabilitation length of stay and lower total FIM gains in the cancer patients but comparable FIM efficiency (amount of functional gain per day of rehabilitation). Studies including postdischarge follow-up information (ranging from 3 months to 1 year) have all found that the preponderance of cancer patients able to be contacted maintain or even improve their functional status. Some studies show a high rate of transfer back to acute care,[65] but not all.[66] This underscores the need for excellent communication and relationships between rehabilitation, primary care, and oncology staff, as well as the need for the rehabilitation staff to be attuned to the medical needs of the cancer population. These complications are often related to the treatment regimen and can include infection as a result of myelosuppression, neurologic complications of chemotherapy, and inanition.

Studies do not agree on whether brain tumor patients receiving radiation therapy during rehabilitation do better[65] or worse[67] than their peers. No difference in functional gain appears to be present between patients with primary versus metastatic brain tumor.[68] For brain tumor patients, favorable factors may include first presentation to rehabilitation (as opposed to subsequent rounds of rehabilitation for tumor recurrence),[69] meningioma, and left-sided brain lesions.[67] For spinal cord cases, favorable factors include incomplete neurologic lesion, primary spinal lesion (as opposed to metastatic lesion), or radiation myelitis. One study[77] found more pronounced gains in orthopedic and postoperative cases compared to CNS or asthenia cases. Reassuringly, virtually all studies have found the discharge-to-home rate to be high, comparable to percentages seen in noncancer patients.

Although research clearly shows that cancer patients benefit from acute rehabilitation, it is not yet clear, as is evident from above, which subgroups show the greatest gains, and it is not clear what percentage of hospitalized cancer patients will meet acute rehabilitation criteria. The latter probably depends on the patient mix in any particular facility. It is generally accepted that hospitalized cancer patients, especially those with head and neck, neurologic, breast, and lung malignancies, have significant rehabilitation needs; distinction was not made between rehabilitation goals that could be met on an inpatient versus outpatient basis. In recent years, skilled nursing facilities are also an increasingly common discharge site, especially for those patients unable to tolerate acute rehabilitation or those whose needs are not great enough to justify the intensity of acute rehabilitation. It must be remembered that all acute rehabilitation patients, including those in the studies cited above, are not randomly admitted but rather are preselected according to criteria including (1) presence of realistic functional goals, (2) projected ability to tolerate 3 hours of rehabilitation therapy per day, (3) presence of multidisciplinary rehabilitation needs, and (4) level of need that exceeds mere "fine tuning" of function (generally with an admission FIM score of 85 or less). Physiatry consultation during acute cancer care assists with decision making about the setting for future rehabilitation efforts and provides ongoing evaluation and treatment of issues, including mobility, self-care, cognition, communication, swallowing, pain control, and prosthetics-orthotics. Rehabilitation for the terminal cancer patient should be aimed at symptom control and supporting quality-of-life issues.[70]

VOCATIONAL ISSUES

Although the individual with cancer can face barriers in the workplace, studies have shown some favorable aspects.[71] Statistics regarding return to work after diagnosis and treatment for cancer are variable, ranging from 30% to 93% of cases across 14 studies, with a mean of 62%. Factors negatively associated with return to work include nonsupportive work environment, manual labor job, and head and neck cancer.

An early study from a life insurance company looking at its own experience of employees with a history of cancer found good employment records (performance, absence rate) and normal turnover.[72] In one postal survey from the Netherlands, of patients considered to have cured cancer (7 to 9 years after diagnosis, at least 5 years without relapse), 44% of individuals who were working at the time of diagnosis with cancer maintained employment. Those with head and neck tumors were least likely to return to work, although it was unclear whether this related to physical limitations or the fact that this group was on average older than the other responders. Among all employed patients in this study, 50% continued to experience physical symptoms. Most subjects (53%) maintained an optimistic attitude about possible promotion or better income, which was more optimistic than the general population, and current absenteeism in these long-term survivors did not differ from the rate before diagnosis. However, mean income increased less for the cancer survivors than for the population as a whole; 11% reported feeling hampered because others knew about the cancer, and 5% were in "adapted work or special working conditions." More were working part-time (24% of those remaining employed vs. 14% before diagnosis). Eighty-nine percent of patients attempting to modify or take out new insurance (life, medical, or funeral) experienced difficulty.[72] Of survivors of cancer diagnosed during adolescence, employment parameters were comparable to those of age-matched controls, with the cancer patients reporting a higher average income. Applying for health, life, or disability insurance was frequently problematic. Another study of 253 long-term (5 to 7 years after initial presentation) cancer survivors found that 67% maintained employment and that 86% of them were able to return to their prior schedules. The lowest employment rate was seen in those with prostate cancer; however, this was believed to be explained by age rather than disability. Of those who had stopped working, only 24% cited poor health or disability as the reason.[73] Of note, this population consisted of insured individuals who were believed to have had early diagnosis. Although, historically, concerns of employer discrimination abound, these authors raise the possibility that some patients with cancer actually work longer than originally planned so that they can maintain their insurance.

Resources for cancer patients include the appropriate rehabilitation services to facilitate return to employment, including vocational services. Legal rights are present under the Rehabilitation Act (1973), which prohibits discrimination by employers receiving federal funding, the Americans with Disability Act, and state regulations. For those with residual disability, vocational support for job placement or retraining may be available via state Vocational Rehabilitation bureaus. The Job Accommodation Network (1-800-ADA-WORK) provides information on accommodation options. The Family Medical Leave Act of 1993 provides additional protections for individuals who require an interrupted work schedule because of sickness or treatment appointments.

REHABILITATION TREATMENTS OF SPECIFIC TUMORS

SPINAL CORD TUMORS

Patients with SCI either as a result of tumor, its treatment, or pre-existing conditions present a management challenge. Symptomatic SCI due to spinal metastasis occurs in up to 5% of all cancer patients.[74] It can cause significant disability. Spinal cord injuries may result from malignant invasion, tumor compression, trauma, syrinx or hematoma formation, vascular events, radiation myelitis, or high-dose intrathecal chemotherapy.[75] Radiation myelitis does not develop until years after application of therapy and is directly dependent on the dose of radiation.

Spinal cord injuries are classified according to the level of the motor and sensory injury, as well as the completeness of injury. A complete SCI, level A, describes an injury that results in the loss of all motor function and sensation at the lowest level of spinal cord and is described in patients without anal sphincter sensation and motor tone. If sensation or motor function is preserved at the sacral level, an incomplete injury has occurred and is classified as level B through D, depending on the degree of motor function or sensation, or both, that is present.[76]

Special syndromes are also related to the area of spinal cord injured. These include the anterior, central, and cauda equina syndrome and the Brown-Séquard syndrome. The central cord syndrome is often caused by an intramedullary tumor, syrinx, or vascular event. The central cord is injured, and the peripheral cord is generally intact. Thus, persons have more upper extremity involvement with relative sparing of the lower extremities. Persons with a Brown-Séquard syndrome present with unilateral weakness below the level of injury and contralateral sensory loss. Persons with a cauda equina syndrome classically present with urinary retention, constipation, varied lower extremity weakness, and hyporeflexia or areflexia. The presence of a cauda equina syndrome is a surgical emergency. The presence of these symptoms and signs requires a surgical consultation.

The neurologic level of injury is described as the most distal level at which motor function or sensation is preserved. For example, the distal motor level is considered preserved if the manual muscle testing grade of that muscle is 5 and the one immediately below that level is equal to or less than 3. In another example, a neurologic level with a manual muscle testing grade 4 is considered preserved if all motor levels above that level are 5. The sensory level is considered preserved if light touch and sharp sensations are intact, 2/2.[76]

The level of injury significantly affects function. Persons with a C3 injury or above usually require long-term ventilation.

Those with a C4 level may be able to wean off the ventilator. Persons with a C5 level of injury may be partially independent, with skills such as feeding and grooming with the aid of orthoses. A C6 injury maintains active wrist extension, and, thus, these patients can use tenodesis to improve their grasp. Persons with a C6 level of injury are usually independent, with feeding, grooming, and upper extremity hygiene after assistance with setting up the utensils. They also have the potential to independently transfer with a transfer board. The C7 injury is the key level for becoming independent in most activities at the wheelchair level. Persons with a C7 level of injury should be able to transfer without a transfer board and drive a custom-adapted van or car. Those with C8 and T1 injuries have improved hand function. The preserved thoracic levels provide the ability to maintain trunk stability. They should all be independent, with activities of daily living (ADLs) and mobility skills at the wheelchair level. Persons with thoracic levels of injury have the potential to stand with the aid of orthoses and assistive devices for therapeutic benefit. The people with lower thoracic and high lumbar levels of injury may be able to stand and ambulate with lower extremity orthoses and assistive devices. This is generally for therapeutic endeavors and short household distances only, due to the high cost of energy required to perform these activities. Persons with injuries at the L3 level or lower have the potential to ambulate in the community with the use of orthoses and assistive devices such as canes or walkers.[77] Thus, the more distal the level of injury, the greater the potential for functional independence.

Orthoses are fabricated devices used to provide support or improve function of a moveable body part.[78] They are commonly prescribed to people with SCIs and include upper and lower extremity devices. The upper extremity devices may permit gravity-eliminated movements of the arm to aid in function of someone with injury at the C5 level. The static wrist splints protect the joint and facilitate use of a weakened grasp in those with no or weak wrist extension. They can also be used to reduce spasticity or prevent contracture. Dynamic wrist splints, including the tenodesis splint, are used to enhance or create a functional grip.[78]

Lower extremity orthoses are used to stabilize and protect the joints, as well as aid in therapeutic standing and therapeutic and functional ambulation. The type of lower extremity orthoses is influenced by the level of injury. Persons with thoracic or high lumbar lesions require a hip-knee-ankle-foot orthosis to promote more hip support and control. A reciprocating gait orthosis is a type of hip-knee-ankle-foot orthosis that enables people with these levels of injury to ambulate. The knee-ankle-foot orthoses are used in people with weak quadriceps but intact thigh flexors. They lock the knee in extension while ambulating. A lesion at L4 or lower provides good thigh strength and varying degrees of leg and foot strength. Thus, control at the ankle is provided by an AFO. The AFO provides support and assistance with dorsiflexion or plantar flexion of the ankle, or both.[78]

The care of patients with acute SCI includes maintenance of ventilation in those with high levels of injury. It also includes treatment of pain, autonomic dysregulation, and bowel and bladder dysfunction. Patients are at risk of developing deep venous thrombosis (DVT), pulmonary emboli (PE), pulmonary and urinary tract infections, fecal impaction, decubiti, immobilization hypocalcemia, spasticity and contractures, and osteoporosis. A comprehensive treatment plan includes DVT and PE prophylaxis, spirometry and chest physiotherapy; initiation of intermittent urinary catheterization every 4 to 6 hours when urine volumes are less than 2000 mL/d; initiation of a bowel program, turning every 2 hours; and use of high airflow mattresses, use of heel protectors, and daily ROM and physical therapy.[76]

The use of low-molecular-weight heparin is currently recommended for DVT and PE prophylaxis during the acute management phase of SCI. The independent use of low-dose unfractionated heparin, elastic compression stockings, and intermittent pneumatic compression devices is not recommended. When used alone, they appear to be relatively ineffective. It is recommended that low-molecular-weight heparin be continued or converted to full-dose oral anticoagulation for a minimum of 3 months or at least until completion of the rehabilitation phase.[79]

Patients with injuries above the T6 level are at risk of developing autonomic dysreflexia, which is defined as an increase in blood pressure of greater than 20 mm Hg above baseline. It results from stimulation of the splanchnic division of the sympathetic nervous system by a noxious stimulus below the level of the lesion and causes the sympathetic responses of vasoconstriction and hypertension. The body's autoregulation mechanisms are interrupted due to the spinal cord lesion, and the uncontrolled blood pressure continues. Classically, the patient's heart rate decreases because of the intact response of the parasympathetic nervous system via the vagus nerve. The patient may develop a severe headache, experience an increase in spasticity, and describe a vague discomfort. This is a medical emergency, and immediate treatment must be initiated, including sitting the person upright, loosening tight-fitting clothing, checking for bladder distention, and either checking an indwelling catheter for kinks or initiating urinary catheterization. A urine sample should be sent for analysis and culture. A rectal examination should be performed to evaluate for and treat fecal impaction, and an inspection for ingrown toenails and infected decubiti should be made. If the source of the autonomic stimulation is not found or the blood pressure continues to be elevated, or both, nitroglycerin paste can be applied.[80] Oral or sublingual nifedipine is no longer indicated for the treatment of this hypertensive emergency due to the risk of profound hypotension, myocardial infarction, and death. If the source of the stimulus is not found or the blood pressure continues to be elevated, or both, the patient should be transferred to the intensive care unit for treatment with intravenous nitroprusside.

Once the patient has undergone necessary surgery for tumor resection and medical stability is obtained, further assessment by the oncology and rehabilitation teams is made to determine the patient's prognosis and potential to restore function by participating in a rehabilitation program. Chemotherapy or radiation therapy, or both, can be initiated simultaneously. The patient's ability to participate in rehabilitation therapies while undergoing further treatments must be considered when an acute or subacute inpatient rehabilitation program is sought. Rehabilitation programs for those with SCI due to spinal tumors have been shown to improve mobility and self-care.[81] Research indicates that clinical and functional status is a valuable prognostic factor for survival of those with SCI due to metastatic tumor disease.[82] Thus, selection of patients who have potential to improve func-

tion may improve survivability as well as quality of life and ability to perform ADLs and mobility.

BRAIN TUMORS

Brain tumors vary widely in aggressiveness and in prognosis. Even a benign or relatively low-grade lesion may have severe functional consequences depending on location and the extent to which excision is feasible. The most common neurologic deficits in brain tumor patients undergoing acute rehabilitation include impaired cognition (80%), weakness (78%), and visual-perceptual impairment (53%). Most patients have multiple impairments.[68] Although prognosis (for life expectancy) may be a factor, most rehabilitation disposition decisions are guided by the patient's neurologic status, clinical course, and activity tolerance. A patient whose neurologic status is actively worsening will likely not benefit from intensive rehabilitation.

Relatively favorable prognostic factors are solitary brain lesion and ambulatory status. Presence of headache, visual disturbance, or impaired consciousness (related to increased intracranial pressure) at presentation is a poor prognostic factor.

Specific rehabilitation interventions depend on the combination of deficits and are generally comparable to measures used for patients with other etiologies of brain disorders, such as traumatic brain injury or stroke. Rehabilitation measures include attention to bed mobility, transfer, self-care and ambulation skills (if necessary, incorporating wheelchair use), strategies to promote functional cognition, clear communication, bowel and bladder continence, safe swallowing, adequate nutritional intake, optimal sensory input (including vision and hearing), and adequate nighttime sleep. Attention must be paid to prevention of complications of immobility (DVT, skin breakdown) and to potential for complications related to the tumor (pain, neurologic decline, seizure, depression). The hemiplegic patient will benefit from gait training with assistive device and a brace such as an AFO when appropriate. Proper arm positioning, with support of the shoulder to prevent pain in a flaccid limb, should be used. A variety of adaptive equipment items are available for individuals who must perform tasks one-handed, such as reachers, sock donners, and elastic shoelaces. Cognitive strategies often rely on compensations such as keeping a regular routine and maintaining a journal or "memory notebook." The patient's insight into cognitive deficits may be impaired, and education regarding these deficits can allow the patient to more effectively compensate and allow the family, friends, and caregivers to have appropriate expectations. In some cases, especially those in which cognitive status is anticipated to remain fairly stable, where functional expectations are high, or where conflict or confusion exists about the patient's abilities, neuropsychological testing is useful to more fully define the extent of cognitive deficits and also to elucidate cognitive strengths. For example, determining whether an individual learns best with auditory, written, or nonverbal presentations can facilitate the most efficient compensation for cognitive deficits. Pharmacologic and nonpharmacologic therapies to address pain, spasticity, mood, bowel/bladder, and sleep/wake issues are often indicated.

A wide range of tumor types have been treated in acute rehabilitation, including, but not limited to, glioblastoma multiforme, meningioma, astrocytoma, metastatic lesions of various types, oligodendrogliomas, craniopharyngiomas, acoustic neuromas, and pituitary tumors.[65,67] In one study of adult patients, frontal lobe involvement was the most common location. It is unclear to what extent tumor type or location has an impact on rehabilitation prognosis; however, one study found a tendency for better gains in meningioma patients and in those with left hemispheric lesions.[67]

Although the shorter length of stay in brain tumor patients compared to individuals with other brain disorders may relate to better initial functional status, other possible contributing factors include fewer behavioral sequelae, better social supports, and expedited discharge planning due to prognostic factors.[83] In one study, although functional status improved during rehabilitation, quality-of-life scores did not improve until discharge home. The FIM and the disability rating scale are more sensitive than the Karnofsky performance status scale in detecting change in functional status.[84]

Often, brain tumor patients are undergoing radiation therapy concurrent with the rehabilitation. Due to potential for fatigue, radiation sessions should be scheduled for late in the day, after the rehabilitation therapies.[84] Corticosteroids should be maintained while the patient is undergoing radiation treatment, as edema resulting from the radiation can produce lethargy. Anticonvulsant therapy is appropriate in patients with a history of seizure and probably for short-term use perioperatively. Efficacy of seizure prophylaxis for brain tumor patients without a history of seizure is unclear. Measures for prophylaxis of DVT, such as intermittent pneumatic compression with or without low-dose heparin, are warranted. Incidence of postoperative DVT may be highest in meningioma patients (72%) and lower in brain metastasis (20%).[84] Although there may be concern about the risk of bleeding into the brain tumor with systemic anticoagulation, the risks of inferior vena cava filter may outweigh the risks of anticoagulation in this population, and therefore anticoagulation is usually not contraindicated. Seizure management is the most frequent medical problem encountered during rehabilitation in the brain tumor population, followed by cardiac disease, diabetes, DVT, and genitourinary problems.[85]

HEAD AND NECK TUMORS

Head and neck cancers involve body parts that are highly visible, structurally complex, and crucial to survival, requiring close integration of oncology and rehabilitation care. Tobacco and alcohol habits must be addressed. Oral resections may produce deficits in speech and swallowing that can be addressed by exercises and prosthetic management. Mandibulectomy can affect cosmesis and the ability to chew, especially anterior mandible (arch) resections.[86] A partial laryngectomy can result in severe swallowing difficulties but only mild problems with speech and voice. Total laryngectomy patients need training in new voice production techniques or augmentative communication systems. Patients with lesions affecting facial or cranial structures may experience cranial nerve involvement (most notably facial nerve involvement in the case of salivary tumors and 25% incidence of cranial nerve involvement with nasopharyngeal tumors). See Chapter 26.3 for a detailed discussion of communication and deglutition issues.

Pretreatment

The individual must be assessed for potential needs, including swallowing, communication, maxillofacial prosthetics (with base-line impressions made when appropriate), hearing, and oral care. A system should be in place to indicate basic needs after surgery, including a buzzer or bell for general alerting, writing supplies (i.e., pad and pencil, magic slate), or an alphanumeric picture board. Electronic communication devices can be demonstrated. Visits from cancer survivors who have undergone successful speech rehabilitation or viewing of films and literature from the American Cancer Society are beneficial. Screening for cognitive dysfunction and personality or affective disorders assists treatment planning.

Postsurgery

As soon as feasible, oral-motor and jaw exercises are initiated, focusing on ROM, strength, speed, flexibility, and sensory awareness of the involved structures. After unilateral mandibular resections, strengthening of masticatory muscles helps to prevent drift to the nonsurgical side.[14,86] Lingual, labial, and velar exercises are important in retraining speech articulation and often involve teaching compensatory movement patterns. Sensory stimulation and massage can be useful adjuncts to exercise in preventing fibrosis.

Nutrition and Swallowing Management

Nutrition is often provided nonorally at first (percutaneous endoscopic gastrostomy or nasogastric tube). Before oral intake is resumed, evaluation of oropharyngeal function is needed. Patients who have undergone supraglottic laryngectomy have the greatest risk of aspiration, because bilateral protective structures have been removed, followed by those with bilateral superior laryngeal nerve excision or extensive oral resections, especially sacrifice of the tongue base.[87] Oral resections can produce aspiration risk because the impaired propulsive force weakens pharyngeal transit. Total laryngectomy is not expected to result in aspiration risk, because the airway and food pathway are fully separated by this procedure. In most cases, even in 85% of supraglottic laryngectomy patients,[87] a functional swallow is reattained as the patient recovers from the treatment intervention. However, delayed deterioration in swallowing, although probably rare, has been described. Patients with total laryngectomy may experience difficulty with bolus transit due to cricopharyngeal muscle (upper esophageal sphincter) hypertrophy.[88] This has been treated by such measures as mechanical dilatation or botulinum toxin injection.

Use of various tastes, spices, textures, or olfactory input can be used to stimulate salivary flow in postradiation patients. Moist, soft, or smooth foods, such as buttered noodles, puddings, yogurts, ices, hot or cold soups, juice, purees, liquids, and dietary supplements (shakes), should be presented. Various medicinal preparations are also available to counteract pain or dryness. (See Radiation-Induced Tissue Damage, earlier.)

Swallowing strategies focus on safety (prevention of aspiration) and efficiency (ease and adequacy of oral intake). Common interventions include modifying food texture, head-positioning maneuvers (such as chin tuck to prevent laryngeal penetration or neck extension for gravity assist of oral transit), and behavioral techniques (double swallow or alternating textures to reduce pharyngeal residue; supraglottic swallow technique of breath-hold–swallow–cough sequence for aspiration risk). In some cases, adaptive equipment, such as long-handled utensils, syringe, or shortened straw (when suck is weak), facilitate oral intake. The strategies often require strict compliance and, therefore, intact cognition.

Communication

The performance status scale measures understandability of speech, diet factors, and eating in public.[89] This scale can be administered by untrained professionals, is reliable, and can discriminate across the broad range of head and neck cancers.

Initially, individuals rely on written communication and nonverbal mechanisms such as gestures and eye contact. Artificial speaking devices (electrolarynxes) are widely recommended, are relatively inexpensive ($200 to $600), are reimbursable through most insurance policies, and require just a few training sessions. Battery-powered tone generators convey sound through tissue of the neck or directly into the mouth by catheter, to be articulated into speech. Inability to obtain a good neck seal or localized soreness may preclude early use of the neck model. A third type of device, the pneumatic external-reed larynx, diverts air from the tracheostomy site past a vibrating membrane into the mouth by rubber tubing and is not commonly used in the United States. Voice and telephone amplifiers can enhance whispered or dysphonic speech.

Speech synthesizers and other communication aids with digital displays and paper printouts are also available. One inexpensive device allows the user to request basic needs, spell words, generate simple questions and statements, and phone for emergency services (Vocaid, Texas Instruments, Dallas, TX). A variety of more sophisticated computer-based synthetic speech systems have been developed for the severely speech- and motor-handicapped person. The use of text telephones (TT) and fax machines may also be helpful for electronic communication in the work setting.

Postlaryngectomy options include esophageal speech and TEP speech. In esophageal speech, air is swallowed into the esophagus, then released volitionally through the pharyngoesophageal segment, and articulated in a normal manner. The pharyngoesophageal segment substitutes for the vocal cords as a vibratory source for production of voice. Barriers include tissue scarring, nerve damage, poor sphincter relaxation, hearing loss, limited trained instructors, and learning difficulties. The combination of pharyngectomy and esophagectomy makes learning esophageal speech impossible. Partial glossectomy or base of tongue resection also limits its feasibility. TEP speech is easier to learn and is considered to produce the best voice quality. Patients must learn to coordinate timing of speech with exhalation. A tape about voice reconstruction after total laryngectomy for patients and professionals is available from Cine-Med (Woodbury, CT).

Musculoskeletal Management

Complications of radical neck dissection include facial lymphedema; wound infection and dehiscence; injury to cranial nerves VII, X, and XII; and carotid injury. Asymmetric neck motion results from removal of the sternocleidomastoid, platysmas, and other muscles and shoulder dysfunction from sacrifice of the spinal accessory nerve.[14,87,90] Loss of trapezius function results in shoulder depression and protraction, and this malalignment produces incomplete and painful active excursion of the shoul-

der, often with range of abduction of less than 90 degrees. The rhomboids and levator scapula become overstretched and the pectoralis major shortened. The sternoclavicular joint bears increased weight, leading to clavicle subluxation and arthritic changes. When the spinal accessory nerve is not involved, a modified radical neck dissection can be performed, sparing shoulder function. Treatment should emphasize maintenance of neck and shoulder ROM and avoidance of excessive internal rotation at the shoulder and scapular protraction (the "sling" position). Strengthening of the remaining scapular stabilizer muscles should be pursued. Immediate postsurgical rehabilitation after radical neck dissection and other surgeries for head and neck cancer should involve guidance from the surgeon, taking into account skin, vascular, and bone integrity. In general, however, the therapy involves passive neck ROM, emphasizing flexion and rotation, beginning when the sutures are removed, to the limits of graft or suture line stretch, progressing to active ROM and isometric strengthening by week 4. Some patients may experience dyspnea due to loss of the sternocleidomastoid and platysmas muscles for accessory respiration and benefit from instruction in breathing exercises and energy conservation techniques.

PROSTATE CANCER

Prostate cancer is the most common cancer in men and the second leading cause of cancer deaths in men.[91] For those with bony metastasis, issues to address include bone pain, fracture, and impaired mobility (see earlier in Management of Bony Metastases). Survival may be quite prolonged even after onset of bony metastatic disease. Metastatic lesions are typically blastic, and although it is commonly stated that blastic metastasis produces less risk of fracture than lytic lesions, pathologic fracture does occur in prostate cancer patients. Surrounding or generalized osteopenia may contribute to the fracture risk. Men who have undergone radical prostatectomy or radiation therapy are prone to incontinence and impotence. In addition, antiandrogen therapy is often associated with loss of muscle mass, strength, and endurance, and fatigue may ensue. Early intervention with strengthening and aerobic conditioning may be helpful. Inguinal or pelvic lymphadenopathy can result in lymphedema or DVT. Pain, fatigue, and urinary dysfunction are most likely to have a negative impact on quality of life in patients with prostate cancer. Strategies for managing incontinence can include frequent voiding and use of incontinence garments. The patient should be screened for urinary retention and for infection.

Treatments for erectile dysfunction include sildenafil (especially with mild erectile dysfunction), bupropion, penile prosthesis, and, when appropriate, testosterone replacement.[92] Physical changes may interfere with the patient's concept of his sexual attractiveness. Depression may result in low sexual drive. Psychological distress with impact on sexual function may be more common in younger adults with cancer than in older individuals. Sexual dysfunction in cancer patients may persist long after treatment is completed, and thus it is important for the practitioner to inquire about it.[92]

GRAFT-VERSUS-HOST DISEASE

Chronic GVHD occurs 3 to 14 months after hematopoietic stem cell transplantation in 20% of matched sibling and 40%

of matched nonsibling recipients of allogeneic bone marrow. GVHD is considered chronic if its duration is 90 days or more.

The most frequent sequelae of chronic GVHD (cGVHD) are erythema and blistering of skin and mucous membranes. Skin involvement develops in approximately 85% of patients. A substantial percentage of those with cGVHD develop soft tissue involvement or neurologic complications, or both. These include myositis, fasciitis, lymphedema, and, rarely, polyneuropathy, myasthenia gravis, and transverse myelitis.

Several reports identify problems of associated steroid-related complications, in particular, steroid myopathy with loss of type of two fibers and muscle weakness and atrophy. Vertebral collapse and avascular necrosis of bone (mainly hips and knees) are also thought to be secondary to steroid use.[93] Sleep cycles are often disrupted. Sequelae of these effects may include decreased stamina, fatigue, weakness, and dysphoria. Treatment for steroid myopathy includes decreasing the steroid dose and providing strengthening exercises. To restore bone health, decreasing steroid dose, adding a bisphosphonate to reduce osteoclastic activity, and reintroducing weight bearing to assist in bone remineralization may be helpful.

Myositis has been associated with electromyographic findings consisting of polyphasics, elevated creatine phosphokinase, and positive muscle biopsy. Patients have had proximal shoulder and hip girdle weakness and, sometimes, chest-wall weakness.[94] These impairments are associated with fatigue, functional loss, and dependence in daily routines. The myositis usually responds to better control of cGVHD.

Fasciitis is characterized by a sudden, painful swelling of the skin associated with acute GVHD, with edema being significant and leading to sclerosis. It can involve the trunk or the upper or lower extremities. In a substantial proportion of cases, it is associated with strenuous exercise, but this is not a necessary antecedent. The rehabilitative treatments should be started early and directed toward maintaining joint ROM and controlling lymphedema. Fasciitis appears to be unresponsive to steroids.

Patients undergoing bone marrow transplantation report reduced functional level and increased fatigue, psychological distress, and diminished sexual function.[95] Data suggest that aerobic exercise mitigates fatigue, accelerates discharge from the hospital after bone marrow transplantation, and results in a more rapid rise in hemoglobin in patients who receive aerobic training compared to those who do not.[41]

EXTREMITY SARCOMA

Local control of sarcomas is achieved with limb-sparing procedures that minimize disability without compromising life expectancy. Success is reported to be 95%.[96] Decisions about whether amputation is needed are usually made based on whether local control can be obtained; whereas tumor location, involvement of neurologic tissue, and size often are the better predictors of function.

Improvement in function after limb-sparing procedures has been the result of (1) surgical techniques that maximally preserve unaffected tissue, often determined by quantitative imaging; (2) use of endoprostheses, which have an 88% 10-year survival rate[97] and which have replaced allografts; (3) reconstructive procedures involving soft tissue; (4) refined radiotherapy procedures; and (5) efficacy of chemotherapy in controlling

local and distant spread. Amputation is occasionally needed for those with large, proximal tumors and in children who have not reached skeletal maturity. This latter group may be ineligible because of possible growth plate arrest on the operative side and significant leg length discrepancy as growth continues on the nonoperative side.

The most frequent site for endoprosthetic placement is the distal femur, followed by the proximal tibia. The latter remains more challenging surgically because of the relative superficial position of the tibia. Proximal humeral, scapular, and elbow endoprostheses have also been placed with success. Hemipelvic replacement has been performed, with poor results, but iliofemoral arthrodesis for proximal lesions is associated with good functional outcome.[98]

The rehabilitation specialists provide patient evaluations that help identify the functional level of the patient preoperatively and what the likely functional needs after treatment will be. Instruction in the use of mobility aids, orthotic use to assist in joint stabilization, and strengthening and aerobic exercise prescription and supervision are provided preoperatively and postoperatively in conjunction with the operating surgeon. Patients with sarcoma are likely to be young, recently active, and impatient about resuming activity. Education concerning the recovery process and possible need for a brace if nerve or a major muscle group, or both, has been sacrificed should be undertaken.

Endoprosthetic loosening may occur, depending on the amount of wear and tear from activities, but endoprostheses can last for up to 10 years. For long-term survivors, endoprosthetic replacement will be needed. Replacement reconstructions are generally limited to two to three. Reconstructions are also necessary for prosthetic dislocation, bone fracture, and loosening. Removal of the prosthesis is often necessary for serious bony infection. Infections with some organisms (*Staphylococcus epidermidis*) have been successfully treated with 3 months of appropriate intravenous antibiotics. Therefore, some patients who initially underwent limb-sparing procedures require amputations later in their life. They need to be aware of the possibility of these problems preoperatively when choosing a limb-sparing surgery.

If the patient needs an amputation, the most functional level should be selected. A very short above-knee amputation (AKA) can be fitted with a prosthesis and is much more functional and energy efficient than a hip disarticulation. In some cases, a hip disarticulation can be converted to a short AKA by use of a custom-made short femoral endoprosthesis. A short below-elbow and below-knee amputation can be fitted appropriately with a prosthesis and is much more functional than its counterpart (above-elbow and AKA).

Preprimary and Postprimary Treatment Phases

Most commonly, pain, weakness, joint motion abnormalities, deconditioning, and mobility are the major management problems facing the rehabilitation team. In general, for soft tissue sarcoma (STS) patients, early treatment begins with correct positioning in bed to reduce joint swelling and maintain support and alignment for a reconstructed limb. A posterior splint or sling may be needed. Passive ROM by a physical or occupational therapist is performed for joints distal to the resection, and active motion is performed by the patient in joints proximal to the resection. On day 2, the patient is allowed to transfer out of bed with assistance and sit in a chair with proper limb positioning. For lower limb procedures, non–weight-bearing gait with crutches or a walker and posterior knee splint are initiated; if the upper extremity is the operative site, an appropriate sling or splint is used. After drains are removed, gait progresses with toe touch and partial weight bearing, and active motion is begun to the affected joint, advancing as the wound heals. The patient may be fully weight bearing after the staples are removed.

Procedures such as the Tikhoff-Lindberg technique for shoulder STSs that require extensive soft tissue reconstruction may progress more slowly and usually require a sling or shoulder harness for support. The goal is to develop adequate strength and function in the hand as rapidly as possible and to control edema using soft wraps.

Bony reconstruction usually has a longer postoperative rehabilitation course, and the progression of treatment is highly dependent on the type and extent of the excision and the development of complications. Skin breakdown or infection at the initial closure site and soft tissue or joint infection may delay rehabilitation.

If no complications occur, patients with humeral excisions can be given passive hand ROM on day 2 and actively use their hand 2 weeks postoperatively. Passive ROM is performed on the elbow for 3 weeks postoperatively. Patients usually lack approximately 40 degrees of extension. Use of moist heat over the elbow followed by gentle stretching can be started at approximately 4 weeks after a reconstructive procedure involving the shoulder if the wound is sufficiently healed and can withstand the tension of biceps lengthening. The therapist performs progressive passive ROM of the shoulder beginning with 20 degrees flexion-extension, then adding abduction and internal-external rotation. Close contact with the surgeon is maintained in increasing the degree of ROM. Usually, passive ROM in abduction and internal-external ROM attained is approximately 60 degrees. Active ROM is not expected to be functional.

Patients with distal femoral endoprosthetic replacements generally wear a knee immobilizer for 3 weeks. The therapist performs passive ROM of distal joints and begins limited-arc passive knee ROM of the involved joint between 2 to 3 weeks, carefully observing the wound closure for any signs of potential breakdown from increased tension with ROM. When the sutures are removed, active assistive ROM is performed, and the ROM arc is gradually increased. The patient should be able to perform some isometric exercises in the immobilizer on day 3 and begin active ROM at 1 month. Quadriceps strengthening to assure knee stability is very important. Exercise intensity is advanced with addition of a few pounds of resistance at 6 weeks. Patients walk non–weight bearing with crutches and a knee immobilizer until the staples are removed. They are advanced to toe touching and increased weight bearing to tolerance, while monitoring pain and looking for development of any knee effusion. If an effusion should occur, less weight bearing is initiated. When the quadriceps is sufficiently strengthened to support the knee (2 to 3 months later), patients may ambulate with a cane, followed by no cane when stable.

Patients with proximal tibial resections have a slower course. One main reason for this is that the surgical procedure requires quadriceps reconstruction with a gastrocnemius flap and reattachment of the quadriceps mechanism to the metal endoprosthesis. Healing of the reconstruction takes longer. The limb is elevated for 10 days. Quadriceps isometrics are started on day 2. ROM and weight bearing are introduced at a slower pace. The patient wears a bivalved cast for a month. Knee ROM begins when the cast is removed. Active motion exercise starts when the patient is able to extend the knee. Often, the patient wears a long leg brace for an additional 2 months, which allows 30 degrees of flexion. Full weight bearing with a cane is not expected before 4 to 5 months. The quadriceps mechanism is initially weaker than with the distal femoral procedure due to the quadriceps reconstruction. A more significant knee extension lag can occur. More intensive quadriceps strengthening is needed to help to reduce knee extension lag, allow for active knee extension, and ensure safe gait. Usually, the final outcome is pain-free, independent ambulation without a cane and independence in ADLs 6 to 8 months after surgery.

Early rehabilitation for amputees begins with fitting the residual limb with an immediate postoperative cast placed in the operating room, to shape the residual limb and control edema and pain. This is recommended for above- and below-elbow amputation, AKA, and below-knee amputation levels. Those undergoing higher-level amputation are treated with elastic wraps. These are less efficient in reducing swelling, phantom limb sensation, and pain, and treatment may require TENS or medication.

Below-knee, above-knee, above-elbow, and below-elbow amputees are fitted with an immediate postoperative cast after the suture line is closed, and a temporary pylon and foot are added at day 10 postoperatively for the below-knee and above-knee amputees. A permanent limb is ordered when the residual limb is well shaped and the patient does not have fluid and weight shifts from chemotherapy. If no chemotherapy is involved, a permanent prosthesis is made 6 weeks postoperatively. For chemotherapy patients, this may be delayed by 3 months.

Two main types of prostheses are used: endoskeletal and exoskeletal. Endoskeletal prostheses have an internal metal support system and an external molded, soft skin-color cover. They are more cosmetically acceptable to many and are lighter in weight than exoskeletal prostheses. However, they tear when subjected to contact sports or even walking in the woods. Exoskeletal prostheses have a hard durable shell, can be used for sports activities, and are heavier.

New components using graphite for joint components have lessened the weight of prostheses. The choice of the particular types of components, such as knees and ankles, and strength of cables for an upper extremity prosthesis depend on the activities in which the patient is engaged. Young amputees [common in the case of osteosarcoma (OS)] prefer hydraulic knees that facilitate such activities as dancing, and ankles that are flexible, which facilitate push-off in the gait cycle and render gait more propulsive. These are useful for sports activities.

Better form-fitting, more naturally aligned prosthetic sockets are routinely used. More sporty socket suspensions and prostheses are available, including swim legs and adaptations for skiing. Myoelectric upper extremity prostheses with switches are sometimes used but are very expensive. They are more cosmetic, but the hand component can lift only light objects.

Management of pain postoperatively is essential. Pharmacologic treatment with narcotics is vital in the first postoperative week. Rehabilitation treatments begin with proper limb positioning to reduce edema and avoid contracture. Immobilization of operative sites using splints and TENS is a common adjunct. Acupuncture may also be useful to reduce pain.

Edema can cause pain and interfere with function. Significant lymphedema commonly occurs with STS resections involving the adductor and hamstring, anterior compartment muscle groups, and breast sarcoma. This lymphedema is controlled by proper positioning and the use of a compression garment. With these four excisions, edema is often chronic and needs to be treated long term with combined modalities of massage, wrapping, and pumping. It can usually be well controlled or reduced. A new technique of nonelastic wrapping has proved very effective in management.

In the immediate postoperative phase, crutches and walkers are often needed. Frequently, patients do not require these devices at 6 months. Orthoses are needed after some soft tissue resections to replace lost function. The most common brace used is for knee control after excision of the quadriceps, for ankle control after gastrocnemius with peroneal nerve removal, and for wrist extension after radial nerve or forearm extensor removal. For knee control, an AFO with 5-degree plantar flexion is often used. This creates an extension movement to stabilize the knee. The peroneal nerve brace is a plastic AFO to correct equinovarus of the foot. A cock-up splint is used to maintain wrist extension, or a dynamic outrigger brace is used to restore finger extension if the long extensors have been resected.

Cosmesis is very important to cancer patients. Wide local excision of STS often causes soft tissue deficits. Some of these can be ameliorated by soft, contoured fillers. Some examples of these are a buttock prosthesis for buttectomies, a gastrocnemius prosthesis, a shoulder prosthesis for forequarter amputations and after the Tikhoff-Lindberg procedure, and a foot prosthesis after partial-ray resection. Breast prostheses made of various materials (gels, fluff, etc.) are used for mastectomies secondary to sarcoma.

Fatigue results from inactivity, the disease itself, depression, and chemotherapy [doxorubicin(Adriamycin)]. Exercise to increase strength and joint motion is an important component in facilitating and maintaining the regaining of function in limb-spared patients. Often, low-intensity, low-impact aerobic programs are prescribed. Frequently, particular muscles are targeted for exercise (e.g., quadriceps in distal femoral and proximal tibial limb-sparing procedures for OS and partial quadriceps removal for STS). General strengthening and ROM exercises are performed for uninvolved muscles. Isometrics and isotonic strengthening with weights to 2 lb using a short lever arm are permitted in patients with endoprostheses. Isokinetic machine exercise is not permitted.

Maintaining at least critical joint motion for function is important. It is not necessary that the joint motion be completely normal for adequate function.

Intercurrent Phase

Patients are generally independent either with or without assistive devices and braces. Some patients may need a change in vocational status. OS limb-spared patients generally have good to excellent function, as judged by the Enneking assessment and gait analysis.[98] Some, however, fall into the poor to fair cat-

egories. Gait analysis reveals that such patients may have slower cadence and uneven stride lengths. They often use substitutive muscle strategies.[98] These vary widely. For instance, in the presence of a weak quadriceps, such patients strike their toe first on stance rather than heel strike. This creates an extension moment at the knee to help to stabilize it and, therefore, to improve gait safety. Limb-spared procedures require a reconstruction if there is dislocation, fracture at the bone cement interface, serious infection unresponsive to intravenous antibiotics, or worn-out components. Studies of these reconstructions are limited to case reports but indicate good to excellent function.

The function of limb-spared patients versus amputees has been addressed. Some amputees may be more functional than limb-spared patients and vice versa. Because some prosthetic limbs are durable, participation in contact sports, running, high-impact dances, tennis, and golf are no problem. However, amputees with cosmetic limbs, humeral OS, or lower limb sparing should have more restriction in sport activities. Limited sport may be needed to preserve endoprostheses. However, an upper extremity Tikhoff-Lindberg procedure for humeral OS is much more functional than a forequarter amputation.

STS can occur in all age groups, but the median age tends to be midlife and later. This places people in that part of their lives when they are working and supporting families. As a result, some may need to change their vocation, although many remain in their jobs with reasonable accommodation. OS occurs in children and young adults. Often, they are faced with career choices influenced by their level of physical as well as cognitive abilities. Career counseling is advised.

Recreational and social activities are important to cancer patients. Individuals with wide local excision often can continue their premorbid recreational and social activities. With resections that require bracing, some activities are not possible. Patients with STS and radiated bone and OS with endoprostheses must avoid contact sports and activities that cause torquing. In addition, impact activities (running, some dances) are not appropriate for limb-spared OS patients. These more aggressive activities can result in bony fracture, bone-prosthetic interface fracture, endoprosthetic dislocation, and early breakdown of prosthetic components.

Education of the patient about which activities are appropriate is important in preventing complications. Adaptive methods of participating in some sports are appropriate. For instance, modification of stance, position, and swing may reduce torque and allow some lower limb–spared patients to play golf. Doubles tennis played at less aggressive levels may also be appropriate. A young teenager going to the prom can dance but needs to avoid torquing and high-impact dances.

Limb-spared patients should be followed up from a rehabilitation standpoint to ensure that no long-term radiotherapy problems (motion loss, radiculopathy, and cord syndromes) are developing that would decrease function. Any new development of pain should signal local reoccurrence or fracture at the endoprosthetic junction. Amputees generally need new prostheses every 4 to 5 years, depending on level of use.

Recurrence

When metastases occur with OS, they are most commonly to the lung or other bones. Often, it is a single metastasis or a few, possibly amenable to local resections. With STS, lung metastases occur. Patients may have multiple surgical procedures over time, usually a median sternotomy or thoracotomy with pleura and chest-wall resections. A newer procedure allows for removal of lung metastases without major chest surgery. These surgical treatment interventions often are associated with postoperative chest pain and deconditioning. Patients become fatigued and anxious, may lose weight during chemotherapy, and may require rehabilitation interventions much as they did in the initial phase. Vocational and educational endeavors are disrupted. Rehabilitation strategies to relieve postoperative pain (TENS) and reduce fatigue (assistive devices, energy conservation techniques) and anxiety (stress management, relaxation techniques, and imagery) are helpful. Referral to a dietitian is made to support good nutrition.

End of Life

If metastases return and are inoperable, patient safety remains the major concern. Preservation of function is the goal, as long as bony integrity can be assured. If not, partial or non–weight bearing may have to be initiated. At this stage, emotional support, comfort, and education about problem solving to promote and preserve independence can be provided by the rehabilitation team.

MELANOMA

In advanced or recurrent melanoma, oncologists have reported the efficacy of isolated limb perfusion with various chemotherapeutic agents (e.g., melphalan) and biologic response modifiers (e.g., tumor necrosis factor and interferon) where mild to moderate limb toxicity has been reported. Complications resulting from these procedures include transient peripheral neuropathy, edema, skin breakdown, and vascular compromise with tissue necrosis. As a result of these complications, rehabilitation of these patients is often protracted and requires careful daily monitoring of the skin for areas of pressure combined with an active program of exercises and progressive ambulation. Management of edema, using compression garments and inelastic wraps, may be achieved for symptom relief and control. Amputation rarely must be performed to treat complications of limb perfusion. Prosthetic fitting and training can be undertaken.

Metastatic disease to bone may occur, jeopardizing long bone and spinal stability. Treatment should be undertaken only after the extent of bony involvement and risk of fracture have been determined. Patients in whom metastases to the brain develop should be assessed for cognitive function as well as problems of mobility. (See earlier in Brain Tumors.)

GASTROINTESTINAL MALIGNANCIES

Colorectal cancer is the fourth most prevalent carcinoma in the United States, the second leading cause of cancer death, and the only major malignancy that affects men and women almost equally. Efforts in recent years have focused on screening for early detection, as Dukes A disease (tumor limited to the mucosa) is 85% to 95% curable. Almost 40% remain who do not survive 5 years, suggesting that disability or symptoms can result from tumor or its treatment, which will require management. Pancreatic cancer remains among the most refrac-

tory to cure of all malignancies, and favorable prognostic indicators have not been delineated. Patients with this diagnosis often present with severe weight loss, sometimes cachexia, and depression. Those with esophageal, liver, and stomach malignancies, which carry a poor prognosis, also may present in this way. In general, when liver metastasis occurs, the clinical state deteriorates rapidly.

Most often, rehabilitation is indicated for acute postoperative management after abdominal surgery. The most frequently seen functional problem is mobilization, and then mobility. Patients with bony involvement need careful review of x-rays and scans to determine extent of disease to protect weight-bearing bones using gait aids or spinal orthotics, or both. Good pain control is essential. Tolerance to active therapy and overall medical stability determine whether this is done in an acute, subacute, or rehabilitation setting. In postsurgical cases, close communication with the referring surgeon is important for management of drains and potential complications.

A very common problem seen in this population is fatigue, often attributable to loss of muscle mass, or, for some, cachexia. The phenomenon is also known as *cancer fatigue*, which is thought to be secondary to the presence of inflammatory cytokines. Treatment of this fatigue has been quite refractory to traditional rehabilitation interventions, and exercise in the presence of cachexia is contraindicated. Calorie intake is usually below even basal metabolic needs, and the ability to generate needed energy through gluconeogenesis is markedly impaired. If the precachectic state can be identified, it may be possible to maintain muscle mass and delay cachexia.

Conversely, data suggest that obesity is a risk factor for cancer, and, furthermore, it is a risk factor for cancer recurrence. Gastrointestinal tract tumors are among the tumor types most likely to develop or recur, or both, in association with obesity.[33] Fitness programs, designed to improve aerobic capacity, have been shown to result in improved function, better work performance, and overall satisfaction on a number of parameters.

LUNG CANCER

Lung cancer and its sequelae lead to significant morbidity and mortality. The most common symptoms associated with lung cancer and its surgical, chemotherapy, and radiation treatments include fatigue, pain, dyspnea, cough, and insomnia.[99] The results of a study indicate that the impact of dyspnea, pain, and fatigue on daily life activities in ambulatory patients with advanced lung cancer is significant.[100] Clearly, rehabilitative interventions that reduce these symptoms and improve independence in function can enhance one's quality of life.

Lung cancer rehabilitation has classically been described in two phases, a preoperative or pretreatment phase and a postoperative phase. The preoperative phase includes a thorough medical, social, and functional assessment. Having information regarding the patient's pretreatment cancer type and stage; hematologic status; electrolytes; cardiopulmonary function, including chest-wall expansion; and musculoskeletal status, as well as vocational status and family support, helps identify pretreatment impairments and improve posttreatment care. Patients are given breathing exercises to perform before their surgery to improve air entry, increase efficiency of respiratory muscles, increase chest mobility, and decrease the risk of pneumonia. Patients are instructed to perform these exercises before and after surgery. The use of nonpharmacologic interventions, including special breathing and relaxation techniques, activity pacing, counseling, and/or positive thinking, can help reduce the sense of dyspnea in lung cancer patients.[99–102] Additional exercises, including daily stretches, walking, and stair climbing, as tolerated, should be encouraged. These activities may improve cardiopulmonary status and reduce symptoms. They may also improve a patient's sense of well-being and generate a restored sense of hope and power because of their ability to focus on doing something positive for their health.[99,100]

The initial postoperative phase involves relieving postoperative pain and preventing the complications of immobility by initiating passive ROM exercises, skin care including pressure relief techniques, and prevention of thromboemboli. The patient is instructed to perform breathing exercises and use incentive spirometry after extubation. He or she should be mobilized and encouraged to ambulate with appropriate assistive devices as soon as possible. Patients with lung cancer also experience sequelae imposed by metastatic disease. These commonly affect the central nervous, peripheral nervous, and musculoskeletal systems. Table 56-3 summarizes these impairments and provides treatment strategies to improve cognition, communication, mobility, and ADLs.

Consideration of the patient's postoperative treatment plan and functional potential should be made to facilitate appropriate referral for inpatient or outpatient rehabilitation, skilled nursing care, or a home rehabilitation program. Counseling regarding the patient's prognosis, functional limitations, and changing functional and social roles helps facilitate the patient's and family's adjustment and understanding of his or her condition. Palliative care issues may also need to be addressed.

BREAST CANCER

The 5-year survival rates of women with breast cancer are 81.6% and 65.8% for white and black women, respectively.[1] The median life expectancy for those with bony metastases is greater than 24 months.[8] Lifestyle-related factors that contribute to obesity increase the likelihood of recurrence and mortality in those with breast cancer.[33] Breast cancer survivors experience long-term functional limitations and poor economic outcomes.[103] These factors imply that women with breast cancer need rehabilitation to promote and preserve function.

Using the model described earlier in this chapter (see Table 56-2), initial contact with the rehabilitation team centers around education about what to expect in terms of the impact of surgery, radiation, and/or chemotherapy on function. This helps patients plan for return to work/home routines or establish new ones and ameliorate stress through relaxation and guided imagery.

The second phase of treatment is in response to the variety of clinical problems resulting from primary cancer treatment that may have functional impact. Treatments are designed to reduce impairments, relieve symptoms, and promote the best functional outcomes. Educational and interventional strategies are summarized in Table 56-6. The efficacy of rehabilitation interventions has been documented for hospitalization, arm mobility and weakness, lymphedema management, fatigue mitigation, efficacy of exercise, and improvement in quality of life.[44,104,105]

TABLE 56-6. Treatment/Education Checklist for Breast Surgery Patients

PATIENT EDUCATION
Lymphedema precautions
Posture realignment
Shoulder movement guidelines
Lifting precautions (<5 lb for 2 wk; <10 lb for 6 wk)
Exercise guidelines if receiving radiation treatment
Breast self-examination and its importance
Weight control
Relaxation techniques for stress reduction

PATIENT TAUGHT AND PERFORMED
Lymphedema monitoring: circumferential measurements
Elevation/positioning of involved upper extremity
Pumping exercises
Deep-breathing exercises (emphasizing upper chest and rib cage expansion)
Cervical range of motion exercises
Shoulder shrugs/retractions
Elbow flexion/extension/supination/pronation
Active shoulder range of motion exercises (avoid incisional stretch pain)
Aerobic exercise program including ergometry
Other

(Adapted from Gerber L, et al. In: Harris JR, et al., eds. *Disease of the breast*, 3rd ed. Philadelphia: Lippincott Williams & Wilkins, 2004.)

Common problems seen in this phase of rehabilitation include arm swelling, breast/chest-wall swelling, and tenderness. ROM deficits in the shoulder and neck; stiffness and pain in the shoulder, trapezius, and neck; weakness in hand grip strength; scapular winging; and medial arm numbness are commonly seen. Many of these symptoms respond easily and quickly to standard rehabilitation interventions. Associated symptoms often include depression, anxiety, and fatigue and functional limitations in ADLs, such as dressing, bathing, and grooming. Delays in returning to work or leisure activity may follow. Some of these delays occur because patients are fearful about injuring their arms. Data from one study suggest that vigorous upper extremity exercise does not result in an increased amount of limb edema in women with breast cancer.[106] Studies indicate that early postoperative rehabilitation intervention improves functional outcomes.

At one institution (National Institutes of Health), all patients undergoing a mastectomy or axillary dissection, or both, are referred to rehabilitation. Those undergoing radiation therapy are seen frequently to help patients maintain ROM and review strategies for fatigue management and skin care as part of routine management. Routine approaches to postaxillary dissection shoulder mobilization are presented in Table 56-7.

Patients undergoing radiation therapy are treated throughout their course of treatment and are encouraged to maintain a ROM program for the rest of their lives. Close monitoring is needed to prevent potential sequelae of radiation, which include local erythema and possible burn, local edema in the radiation field, limb edema, and soft tissue fibrosis. In addition, shoulder mobility may be influenced by the radiation field and dosimetry.[107] All patients who undergo radiation therapy for breast cancer should be instructed in a daily home exercise program to maintain their shoulder ROM and strength. (Patients require at least 110 degrees of shoulder abduction to receive radiation to the axilla.) Without this daily stretching

TABLE 56-7. Recommended Postoperative Shoulder Mobilization Schedule[51]

Postoperative Day	Flexion (Degrees)	Abduction (Degrees)	Internal and External Rotation (Degrees)
1–2[a]	40	40	To tolerance
3[a]	45	45	To tolerance
4–6[a]	45–90	45	To tolerance
7	To tolerance	To tolerance	To tolerance
Drains out[b]	To tolerance	To tolerance	To tolerance

[a]Gentle accessory mobilization of glenohumeral joint may also be included.
[b]Active assistive range of motion exercises are added, or an overhead pulley is used at this time when needed.

program, radiation-induced fibrosis can occur and cause contractures, resulting in permanent physical disability.

Ideally, the patient should be seen for instruction in a program of functional exercise, including daily stretching, often with use of an overhead pulley system. The authors are cautious about scheduling exercise within 1 hour of radiation. It is thought that increased blood flow induced by exercise, through a radiated field, may enhance the radiation effect. Data on this are scant. Because it is often difficult to regain full ROM if there has been significant loss of shoulder ROM due to immobilization after axillary dissection and radiation, early mobilization is strongly encouraged. Patient education before discharge from rehabilitation is extremely important in empowering the patient to be independent in self-management, in mitigating fatigue, and in reducing the risk of cardiovascular disease.

All patients receive encouragement and education regarding the benefits of continuing to live a healthy lifestyle and maintain aerobic fitness.[9] Table 56-8 represents a summary of the authors' approach to comprehensive rehabilitation for the patient diagnosed with breast cancer. Before discharge, all patients who have undergone mastectomy are fitted for a temporary breast prosthesis.

Possible complications resulting from axillary dissection include trauma to the long thoracic nerve, producing weakness of the serratus anterior muscle, and scapular winging. Exercise to the shoulder girdle should be done in the supine position to stabilize the scapula until the serratus anterior muscle has regained functional strength. Recovery is usually complete.[20]

The development of superficial cord-like structures along the medial aspect of the upper arm and over the anterior elbow can develop after axillary lymphadenectomy or sentinel lymph node dissection.[19] These fibrous bands are believed to be sclerosing lymphatics. They can cause pain and limit shoulder flexion and abduction when the elbow is fully extended or may limit elbow extension. These symptoms are self-limited. The cords can break spontaneously or during a treatment session when the therapist gently applies manual traction to them. Often a popping sound can be heard when the cords break, and consequently an increase in shoulder ROM will be noted. These are avascular structures and do not bleed when ruptured.

Pain is a common symptom, and several patterns of pain are observed in this population. Acutely, there is incisional pain, which usually resolves within 2 weeks. It is not uncommon for patients to experience medial arm pain and paresthesias

because the intercostobrachial and medial brachial cutaneous nerves can be damaged during axillary lymphadenectomy. Although the intensity of these symptoms subsides over time, the medial arm numbness may be permanent and may be experienced as discomfort. Younger women (younger than 45 years) appear to have an approximately six times higher risk of numbness of the arm than older women (65 years or older).[107] Shoulder pain may be present as the arm is mobilized and range is gained. This pain usually resolves as functional ROM is achieved (flexion, 135 degrees; abduction, 110 degrees; external rotation, 65 degrees; and internal rotation, 45 degrees).

Lymphedema may develop in 25% to 33% of breast cancer survivors within their lifetime. Irradiation of the axilla after level one or two dissection increases the risk of lymphedema by 3.57-fold.[107] Early detection and intervention are likely to minimize the adverse effects of lymphedema. Often the patient identifies heaviness or fullness of the arm or remaining breast tissue, or both, before it is ever visible by simple observation. Pre- and postoperative assessments by girth measurements, water displacement, or use of the perometer (Fig. 56-5) of the upper extremities provide the best method of assessment.[108] Initial treatment may consist of patient education, elevation, and a compression sleeve. More refractory edema may require manual lymphatic drainage massage, low-stretch compression bandaging, compression pumps using low pressure, and exercises.[56,57]

The third phase, or intercurrent phase of cancer rehabilitation, is that time when primary treatment is completed and tumor is eradicated or controlled. The goals are to help patients reestablish life routines, return to home and work activity, adopt a healthy lifestyle, and resolve some of the anxiety of the earlier phases. Ongoing chemotherapy may increase weight (a serious concern for prognosis),[109] cause a rapid onset of fatigue,[110] and produce cardiac dysfunction,[111] cognitive impairment that may be long term,[112] and osteoporosis.[113] Radiation therapy often produces fatigue even without concomitant chemotherapy.[114] Radiation therapy to the mediastinum and for treatment of left-sided breast cancer may lead to cardiopulmonary dysfunction and atherosclerosis. Treatment during this phase should include introduction into aerobic conditioning to support functional activity. This type of exercise may help with weight maintenance, if not weight reduction.

Should the tumor recur, this introduces phase four, which combines the approach described for phases 1 and 2. Tumor recurrence usually produces heightened anxiety and substantial disruption of daily routines, which require a great deal of support and assistance in problem solving to maintain function. A practical approach, addressing one problem at a time, is often most successful. With successful treatment, the intercurrent phase resumes. Should breast cancer treatment be unsuccessful in tumor eradication, rehabilitation treatment is aimed at maintenance or restoration of function or substitution through use of adaptive equipment. If the disease progresses, it may enter a terminal phase in which patients have different needs. Metastatic bone disease is associated with an average survival rate of 2 years.[8] It is often treated with radiation, which may produce some fatigue and may have long-term sequelae if lung, gastrointestinal tract, and muscle/nerve are in the radiation field. Pulmonary and muscle fibrosis and esophagitis may occur and require additional therapies. For the long bones of the lower extremity, if more than 50% of the cortex or two-thirds of the medullary canal is involved, fracture risk is high. Non–weight-bearing is recommended. Vertebral body collapse poses a sub-

TABLE 56-8. Summary of Recommendations for Rehabilitation Treatments

Problem	Preoperative Evaluation	Postoperative Evaluation				
		0–2 Wk	2–12 Wk	3–6 Mo	6–12 Mo	>1 Y
Edema	Obtain baseline measurements. If edema present, determine cause.	Instruct in preventive arm care. If edema present, 2–4 cm, without erythema: Treat and instruct patient in MLD; low-stretch compression bandaging, exercises; fit with ready-made compression sleeve. If edema present, >4 cm, without erythema: Same as 2–4 cm; use compression pump after MLD with pressures ≤45 mm Hg. Any, with erythema, Rx: antibiotics.	Same as 0–2 wk	Same as 0–2 wk. Depending on severity, patient may require custom-made compression sleeve. Instruct patient to bandage at night and wear compression sleeve during the day and when flying.	Same as 3–6 mos. With pain, rule out metastasis.	Same as 3–6 mo. With pain, rule out metastasis.
Shoulder motion	Obtain baseline measurements. If <145 degrees flexion or abduction <60 degrees of ER/IR, Rx: heat and ROM exercise. Precautions must be taken for proper arm position intraoperatively.	—	Begin use of pulley. If <145 degrees of flexion or abduction <60 degrees of ER/IR, Rx: use heat, ice (except when patient is being actively irradiated). Active and passive stretch. If no progress by wk 8, add NSAIDs to regimen and check monthly.	Determine ROM. If <160 degrees of flexion, 145 degrees of abduction, or 60 degrees of ER/IR, Rx: ROM exercises with assistance from physical therapist.	Determine ROM. If <160 degrees of flexion, 145 degrees of abduction, or 60 degrees of ER/IR, and if ROM exercises not effective, Rx: scan, NSAIDs, intraarticular steroids.	Same as 6–12 mo
Muscle strength	Obtain baseline measurement of shoulder complex strength, particularly stabilizers of scapula	Evaluate strength. If weakness, especially serratus anterior, support scapula with patient in supine position during exercises.	Evaluate strength of shoulder girdle muscle. Strength should be returning by end of this period. Maintain ROM. If weakness, continue to support scapula during exercises.	Evaluate strength of shoulder girdle muscles. If abnormal strength, determine cause. Postoperative weakness should be resolved by 6 mo.	Same as 3–6 mo	Same as 3–6 mo
Prosthesis	NA	Fluff or, when wound heals, permanent prosthesis	Same as 0–2 wk	Consider reconstruction	Same as 3–6 mo	Same as 3–6 mo
Psychological support	Orientation to surgery, radiation, and common postoperative problems	Support group and relaxation techniques, if appropriate	Same as 0–2 wk	Same as 0–2 wk	Same as 3–6 mo	Same as 3–6 mo

ER, external rotation; IR, internal rotation; MLD, manual lymph drainage; NA, not applicable; NSAIDs, nonsteroidal antiinflammatory drugs; ROM, range of motion; Rx, therapy.
(From Gerber L, et al. In: Harris JR, et al., eds. *Diseases of the breast*, 3rd ed. Philadelphia: Lippincott Williams & Wilkins, 2004, with permission.)

stantial risk for pain, and if the segment is unstable, root or cord compression may result. Corseting is helpful for pain relief in those without spinal instability. Spinal instability with cord compromise should be surgically stabilized. Bracing can help reduce vertebral instability and works well in the thoracic vertebrae; but it is usually inadequate to control lower thoracic/lumbar instability. Reports suggest that the use of methylmethacrylate provides bony stabilization for long bones and vertebrae.[115]

CNS involvement or pulmonary/pleural involvement often requires substantial amounts of intervention to help reduce tumor burden using radiation or chemotherapy, or both. These may produce a fatigue syndrome for which exercise training may not be feasible. In that case, substituting physical activity such as walking or recreational activity may be effective in promoting function while offering quality. Patients with metastatic disease to the lung and CNS may require inpatient rehabilitation hospi-

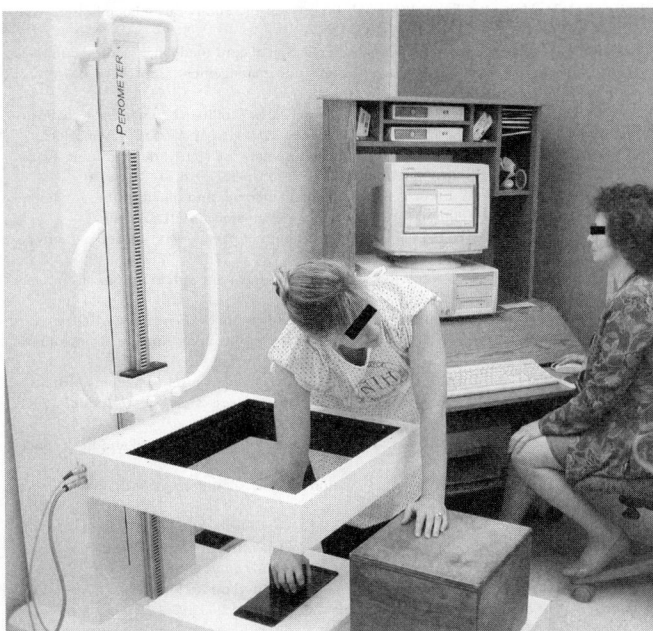

FIGURE 56-5. Upper extremity girth measurement using the perometer. (See Color Fig. 56-5 in the CD-ROM.)

talization. Data suggest that this is effective and often restores patients to a higher functional level, similar to CNS or pulmonary diseases that are not a result of cancer.[65,66] It is important to identify cachexia, the loss of greater than 10% of lean mass. Aerobic exercise of patients during this phase should not be done unless protein calorie nutrition is adequate to support basal metabolic needs plus what is needed for daily functional activity. In an average-sized person, 3.5 mL/min/kg oxygen (this equals 1 metabolic equivalent test) is needed to circulate to tissues during the resting state. Two to three times that is needed for daily routines, and exercise may require that a considerably higher volume be delivered. No additional contraindications to therapy should be present (see Table 56-4). Resistance exercise and nutritional supplementation may be a useful adjunct when the metabolic conditions are stable.

This is yet another phase of management in which independence may be lost, irretrievably so, and the rehabilitation goals are likely to shift toward symptom relief and maintenance of quality. Family support may be one of the most important aspects of care. If cachexia is present, exercise may be counterproductive because nutritional requirements may be greater than consumption. In the terminal phase patients often report good quality of life.[116]

REFERENCES

1. American Cancer Society. *Cancer Stat* 1999;49:41.
2. SEER database. World Wide Web URL: http://www.SEER.cancer.gov/publicdata, 1973–2001.
3. Nagi SZ. A study in the evaluation of disability and rehabilitation potential. Concepts, methods and procedures. *Am Pub Health* 1964;54:1568.
4. *Disability in America.* Washington, DC: National Academy Press, 1991:9.
5. McDowell I, Newell C. *Measuring health,* 2nd ed. New York: Oxford University Press, 1996:404.
6. Cella DF, Tulsky DS, Gray G, et al. The Functional Assessment Cancer Therapy Scale: development validation of the general measure. *J Clin Oncol* 1993;11:570.
7. Kemmler G, Holzner B, Kopp M, et al. Comparison of two QOL instruments for cancer patients. *J Clin Oncol* 1999;17:2932.
8. Mundey GR, Guise TA, Yoneda T. In: Harris JR, Lippman ME, Morrow M, Osborne CK, eds. *Biology of bone metastases in diseases of the breast,* 2nd ed. Philadelphia: Lippincott Williams & Wilkins, 2000:911.
9. Spence R. Nutritional concerns in cancer patients. *PM&R State Art Rev* 1994;8:404.
10. Dion MW, Hussey DH, Doornbos JF, et al. Preliminary results of a pilot study of pentoxifylline in the treatment of late radiation soft tissue necrosis. *Int J Radiat Oncol Biol Phys* 1990;19:401.
10a. Okunieff P, Augustine E, Hicks JE, et al. Pentoxifylline in the treatment of radiation-induced fibrosis. *J Clin Oncol* 2004;22:2207.
11. Matsubayashi T, Koga H, Nishiyama Y, et al. The reparative process of metastatic bone lesions after radiotherapy. *Jpn J Clin Oncol Suppl* 1981;11:253.
12. Casciato DA, Lowitz BB. *Manual of clinical oncology,* 4th ed. Philadelphia: Lippincott Williams & Wilkins, 2000.
13. DeLattre JY, Posner JB. Neurological complications of chemotherapy and radiation therapy. In: Aminoff MJ, ed. *Neurology and general medicine.* New York: Churchill-Livingstone 1989:365.
14. Dudgeon BJ, DeLisa JA, Miller RM. Head and neck cancer: rehabilitation approach. *Am J Occup Ther* 1980;34:243.
15. Shank B. *Radiotherapy: implications for general patient care.* In: Wittes RE, ed. *Manual of oncologic therapeutics.* Philadelphia: JB Lippincott Co, 1991:60.
16. Holtzman L, Chesey K. Rehabilitation of the leukemia/lymphoma patient. In: McGarvey CL, ed. *Physical therapy for the cancer patient.* New York: Churchill-Livingstone, 1990:85.
17. Skarin AT, Dorfman DM. Non-Hodgkin's lymphomas: current classification and management. *CA Cancer J Clin* 1997;47:351.
18. Vandenborne K, Elliot MA, Walter GA, et al. Longitudinal study of skeletal muscle adaptations during immobilization and rehabilitation. *Muscle Nerve* 1998;21:1006.
19. Moskovitz AH, Anderson BO, Yeung RS. Axillary web syndrome after axillary dissection. *Am J Surg* 2001;181:434.
20. Duncan MA, Lotze MT, Gerber LH, et al. Incidence, recovery, and management of serratus anterior muscle palsy after axillary node dissection. *Phys Ther* 1983;63:1243.
21. Guo Y, Truong AN. Functional outcome after physical therapy of breast cancer patients status post modified radical mastectomy versus mastectomy and transverse rectus abdominis myocutaneous flap. *Arch Phys Med Rehabil* 1998;79:1157.
22. Cheville AL. Pain management and cancer rehabilitation. *Arch Phys Med Rehabil* 2000;82(1):S84.
23. Sicard-Rosenbaum L, Lord D, Danoff JV, et al. Effects of continuous therapeutic ultrasound on growth and metastasis of subcutaneous murine tumors. *Phys Ther* 1995;75:3.
24. Shea BD, Vlad G. Rehabilitation of the lung cancer patient. In: McGarvey CL, ed. *Physical therapy for the cancer patient.* New York: Churchill-Livingstone 1990:29.
25. Shephard RJ, Shek PN. Cancer, immune function, and physical activity. *Can J Appl Physiol* 1995;20(1):1.
26. Schwartz AL, Mori M, Gao R, et al. Exercise reduces daily fatigue in women with breast cancer receiving chemotherapy. *Med Sci Spts Exerc* 2001;33:718.
27. Winningham ML. Strategies for managing cancer-related fatigue syndrome. *Cancer Suppl* 2001;92:988.
28. Schwartz AL. Daily fatigue patterns and effect of exercise in women with breast cancer. *Cancer Pract* 2000;8(1):16.
29. Blanchard CM, Courneya KS, Laing D. Effects of acute exercise on state anxiety in breast cancer survivors. *Oncol Nurs Forum* 2001;28(10):1617.
30. Courneya KS, Mackey JR, Bell GJ, et al. Randomized controlled trial of exercise training in postmenopausal breast cancer survivors: cardiopulmonary and quality of life outcomes. *J Clin Oncol* 2003;21(9):1660.
31. Courneya KS, Friedenreich CM, Sela RA, et al. Group psychotherapy and home-based physical exercise trial in cancer survivors. *Psycho Oncol* 2003;12:357.
32. Fairey AS, Courneya KS, Field CS, et al. Physical exercise and immune system function in cancer survivors; a comprehensive review and future directions. *Cancer* 2002;94:539.
33. Calle EE, Rodriguez C, Walker-Thurmond K, et al. Overweight, obesity, and mortality from cancer in a prospectively studied cohort of U.S. adults. *N Engl J Med* 2003; 348(17):1625.
34. Johansson K, Lie E, Ekdahl C, et al. A randomized study comparing manual lymph drainage with sequential pneumatic compression for treatment of postoperative arm lymphedema. *Lymphology* 1998;31:56.
35. Langer CL, Hoffman JP, Ottery FD. Clinical significance of weight loss in cancer patients: rationale for the use of anabolic steroid agents in the treatment of cancer-related cachexia. *Nutrition* 2001;17(1):S1.
36. Daneryd P, Svanberg E, Korner U, et al. Protection of metabolic and exercise capacity in unselected weight-losing cancer patients following treatment with recombinant erythropoietin: a randomized prospective study. *Cancer Res* 1998;58:5374.
37. Gillis TA, Donovan ES. Rehabilitation following bone marrow transplantation. *Cancer* 2001;92:998.
38. Dimeo F, Bertz H, Finke J, et al. An aerobic exercise program for patients with haematological malignancies after bone marrow transplantation. *Bone Marrow Transplant* 1996;18:1157.
39. Smelz JK, Schlicht LA. Rehabilitation of the cancer patient after bone marrow transplantation. *PM&R State Art Rev* 1994;8:321.
40. Trovato MK, Pidcock FS, Christensen JR, et al. Chronic graft versus host disease in children: a review of function and rehabilitative needs. *Arch Phys Med Rehabil* 1998;79:1157.
41. Dimeo F, Fetscher S, Lange W, et al. Effects of aerobic exercise on the physical performance and incidence of treatment-related complications after high-dose chemotherapy. *Blood* 1997;90:3390.

42. MacVicar MG, Winningham ML, Nickel JL. Effects of aerobic interval training on cancer patients' functional capacity. *Nurs Res* 1989;38:348.

43. Sharkey AM, Carey AB, Heise CT, et al. Cardiac rehabilitation after cancer therapy in children and young adults. *Am J Cardiol* 1993;71:1488.

44. Segal R, Evans W, Johnson D, et al. Structured exercise improves physical functioning in women with stages I and II breast cancer: results of a randomized controlled trial. *J Clin Oncol* 2001;19(3):657.

45. Berglund G, Bolund C, Gustavsson U-L. Starting again—a comparison study of a group rehabilitation program for cancer patients. *Acta Oncol* 1993;32:15.

46. Adamsen L, Rasmussen JM, Pedersen LS. Brothers in arms: how men with CA experience a sense of comradeship through group intervention. *J Clin Nurs* 2001;10:528.

47. Hillner BE, Ingle JN, Berenson JR. American Society of Clinical Oncology guideline on the role of bisphosphonates in breast cancer (exercise). *J Clin Oncol* 2000;18:1378.

48. Dimeo F, Rumberger BG, Keul J, et al. Aerobic exercise as therapy for cancer fatigue. *Med Sci Spts Exerc* 1998;30:475.

49. Weber, David C, Brown, et al. Physical agent modalities. In: Braddom L. *Physical medicine and rehabilitation.* Philadelphia: Saunders, 1996:449.

50. James MC. Physical therapy for patients after bone marrow transplantation. *Phys Ther* 1987;67(6):947.

51. Gerber LH, Lampert M, Wood C, et al. Comparison of pain, motion and edema after modified radical mastectomy versus local excision with axillary, dissection and radiation. *Breast Cancer Res Treat* 1992;21:139.

52. Aitken RJ, Gaze MN, Rodger A, et al. Arm morbidity within a trial of mastectomy and either nodal sample with selective radiotherapy or axillary clearance. *Br J Surg* 1989; 76:568.

53. Carson CJ, Coverly K, Lasker-Hertz S, et al. The incidence of co-morbidities in the treatment of lymphedema. *J Oncol Manage* 1999;8:13.

54. Armstrong M, Vargo MM. Safety of diagnostic or therapeutic needle interventions in lymphedema patients. *Arch Phys Med Rehabil* 2001;82:1305.

55. Bastien MR, Goldstein BG, Lesher JL Jr, et al. Treatment of lymphedema with a multi-compartment pneumatic compression device. *J Am Acad Dermatol* 1989;20:853.

56. Foldi E, Foeldi M, Weissleder H. Conservative treatment of lymphedema of the limbs. *Angiol J Vasc Dis* 1985;36:171.

57. Badger CMA, Peacock JL, Mortimer PS. A randomized, controlled, parallel-group clinical trial comparing multilayer bandaging followed by hosiery versus hosiery alone in the treatment of patients with lymphedema of the limb. *Cancer* 2000;88:2832.

58. Loprinzi CL, Kugler JW, Sloan JA, et al. Lack of effect of coumarin in women with lymphedema after treatment for breast cancer. *N Engl J Med* 1999;340:346.

59. Vargo MM. Orthopedic management of malignant bone lesions. *PM&R State Art Rev* 1994;8:363.

60. Denis F. Spinal instability as defined by the three-column spine concept in acute spinal trauma. *Clin Orthop* 1984;189:65.

61. Boland PJ, Billings J, Healey JH. The management of pathologic fractures. *J Back Musculoskel Rehabil* 1993;3:27.

62. Buchbinder D, Currivan RB, Kaplan AJ, et al. Mobilization regimens for the prevention of jaw hypomobility in the radiated patient. *J Oral Maxillofac Surg* 1993;51:863.

63. Logemann JA. Rehabilitation of head and neck cancer patients. *Cancer Treat Res* 1999;100:91.

64. King JC, Williams RP, McAnelly RD, et al. Rehabilitation of tumor amputees and limb salvage patients. *PM&R State Art Rev* 1994;8(2):297.

65. O'Toole DM, Golden AM. Evaluating cancer patients for rehabilitation potential. *West J Med* 1991;155:3847.

66. Marciniak CM, Sliwa JA, Heinemann AW. Functional outcomes of persons with brain tumors after inpatient rehabilitation. *Arch Phys Med Rehabil* 2001;82:457.

67. Cole RP, Scialla SJ, Bednarz L. Functional recovery in cancer rehabilitation. *Arch Phys Med Rehabil* 2000;81:623.

68. O'Dell MW, Barr K, Spanier D, et al. Functional outcome of inpatient rehabilitation in persons with brain tumors. *Arch Phys Med Rehabil* 1998;79:1530.

69. Mukand JA, Blackinton DD, Crincoli MG, et al. Incidence of neurologic deficits and rehabilitation of patients with brain tumors. *Am J Phys Med Rehabil* 2001;80:346.

70. Yoshioka H. Rehabilitation for the terminal cancer patient. *Am J Phys Med Rehabil* 1994;73:199.

71. Spelten ER, Sprangers MAG, Verbeek JHAM. Factors reported to influence the return to work of cancer survivors: a literature review. *Psychooncology* 2002;11:124.

72. Wheatley GM, Cunnick WR, Wright BP, et al. The employment of persons with a history of treatment for cancer. *Cancer* 1974;33:441.

73. Van der Wouden JC, Greaves-Otte JGW, Greaves J, et al. Occupational reintegration of long term cancer survivors. *J Occup Med* 1992;34(11):1084.

74. Parsch D, Mikut R., Abel R. Post acute management of patients with spinal cord injury due to metastatic tumour disease: survival and efficacy of rehabilitation. *Spinal Cord* 2003; 41:205.

75. Werner RA. Paraplegia and quadriplegia after intrathecal chemotherapy. *Arch Phys Med Rehabil* 1988;69:1054.

76. Kirshblum SC, Groah SL, McKinley WO, et al. Spinal cord medicine. Etiology, classification and acute medical management. *Arch Phys Med Rehabil* 2002;83(3):S50.

77. Gittler MS, McKinley WO, Stiens SA, et al. Spinal cord injury medicine: rehabilitation outcomes. *Arch Phys Med Rehabil* 2002;3(3):S65.

78. Dietz MA, Aisen M. Spinal cord injury. In: Aisen M, ed. *Orthotics in neurologic rehabilitation.* New York: Demos Publications, 1992:97.

79. Geerts WH, Heit JA, Clagett PG, et al. Prevention of venous thromboembolism. *Chest* 2001;119:132S.

80. McKinley WO, Gittler MS, Kirshblum SC, et al. Spinal cord medicine. Medical complications after spinal cord injury: identification and management. *Arch Phys Med Rehabil* 2002;83(3S-1):S58, S90.

81. McKinley WO, Conti-Wyncken AR, Volac CW, et al. Rehabilitative functional outcome of patients with neoplastic spinal cord compressions. *Arch Phys Med Rehabil* 1996;77:892.

82. New PW, Rawicki HB, Bailey MJ. Nontraumatic spinal cord injury: demographic characteristics and complications. *Arch Phys Med Rehabil* 2002;83(7):996.

83. Huang ME, Wartella JE, Kreutzer JS. Functional outcomes and quality of life in patients with brain tumors: a preliminary report. *Arch Phys Med Rehabil* 2001;82:1540.

84. Kirshblum S, O'Dell MW, Ho C, et al. Rehabilitation of persons with central nervous system tumors. *Cancer Suppl* 2001;92:1029.

85. Bell K, O'Dell MW, Barr K, et al. Rehabilitation of the patient with brain tumor. *Arch Phys Med Rehabil* 1998;79:S37.

86. Shah JP, Lydiatt W. Treatment of cancer of the head and neck. *Cancer J Clin* 1995;45:352.

87. Beckhardt RN, Murray JG, Ford CH, et al. Factors influencing functional outcome in supraglottic laryngectomy. *Head Neck* 1994;16:232.

88. Meesala S, Vargo M. Dysphagia: a markedly delayed complication in patients with a history of head and neck carcinoma: a report of three cases. *Arch Phys Med Rehabil* 2003; 82(3):243.

89. List MA, Ritter-Sterr C, Lansky SB. A performance status scale for head and neck cancer patients. *Cancer* 1990;66(3):564.

90. Saunders WH, Johnson EW. Rehabilitation of the shoulder. *Radical Neck Dissection* 1975;84:812.

91. Ries LAG, Eisner MP, Kosary CL, et al. SEER cancer statistics review. NCI, Bethesda, MD: NCI, 1973–1999. World Wide Web URL: http://seer.cancer.gov/csr/1975_2001/, 2004.

92. McKee AL, Schover LR. Sexuality rehabilitation. *Cancer Suppl* 2001;92:1008.

93. Tauchmanova L, DeRosa G, Serio D, et al. Avascular necrosis in long-term survivors after allogeneic or autologous stem cell transplantation. *Cancer* 2003;97:2453.

94. Stephenson AL, Mackenzie IRA, Levy RD, et al. Myositis association graft versus host disease presenting as respiratory weakness. *Thorax* 2001;56:82.

95. Neitzert CS, Ritvo P, Dancey J, et al. The psychosocial impact of bone marrow transplantation: a review of the literature. *Bone Marrow Transplant* 1998;22:409.

96. Wadajo FM, Bickels J, Wittig J, et al. Complex reconstruction in the management of extremity sarcomas. *Curr Opin Oncol* 2003;15:304.

97. Bickels J, Wittig JC, Kollender Y, et al. Distal femur resection with endoprosthetic reconstruction: a long-term follow-up study. *Clin Orthop* 2002;400:225.

98. Fuchs B, O'Connor MI, Kaufman KR, et al. Iliofemoral arthrodesis and pseudoarthrosis: a long-term function outcome evaluation. *Clin Orthop* 2002;402:220.

99. Fialka-Moser V, Crevenna R, Korpan M, et al. Cancer rehabilitation. Particularly with aspects of physical impairments. *J Rehabil Med* 2003;35:153.

100. Hately J, Laurence V, Scott A, et al. Breathlessness clinics within specialist palliative care settings can improve the quality of life and functional capacity of patients with lung cancer. *Palliat Med* 2003;17:410.

101. Tanaka K, Tatsuo A, Okuyama T, et al. Impact of dyspnea, pain, fatigue on daily life activities in ambulatory patients with advanced lung cancer. *J Pain Symptom Manage* 2002; 23(5):417.

102. Wall LM. Changes in hope and power in lung cancer patients who exercise. *Nurs Sci Q* 2000;13:234.

103. Chirikos TN, Russell-Jacobs A, Cantor AB. Indirect economic effects of long-term breast cancer survival. *Cancer Pract* 2002;10(5):248.

104. Burnham TR, Wilcox A. Effects of exercise on physiological and psychological variables in cancer survivors. *Med Sci Spts Exerc* 2002;34:1863.

105. Harris SR, Niesen-Vertommen SL. Challenging the myth of exercise-induced lymphedema following breast cancer: a series of case reports. *J Surg Oncol* 2000;74:95.

106. Ververs JM, Roumen RM, Vingerhoets AJ, et al. Risk, severity and predictors of physical and psychological morbidity after axillary lymph node dissection for breast cancer. *Eur J Cancer* 2001;37:991.

107. Mandelblatt JS, Edge SB, Meropol NJ, et al. Sequelae of axillary lymph node dissection in older women with stage I and II breast carcinomas. *Cancer* 2002;95:2445.

108. Stanton AW, Northfield JW, Holroyd B, et al. Validation of an optoelectronic limb volumeter (perometer). *Lymphology* 1997;30:77.

109. Chlebowski RT, Aiello E, McTiernan A. Weight loss in breast cancer patient management. *J Clin Oncol* 2002;20(4):1128.

110. Jacobsen PB, Hann DM, Azzarello LM, et al. Fatigue in women receiving adjuvant chemotherapy for breast cancer: characteristics, course, and correlate. *J Pain Symptom Manage* 1999;18(4):233.

111. Seidman A, Hudis C, Pierri MK, et al. Cardiac dysfunction in the trastuzumab trials experience. *J Clin Oncol* 2002;20:1215.

112. Phillips KA, Bernhard J. Adjuvant breast cancer treatment and cognitive function: current knowledge and research directions. *J Natl Cancer Inst* 2003;95(3):190.

113. Mincey BA. Osteoporosis in women with breast cancer. *Curr Oncol Rep* 2003;5(1):53.

114. Jereczek-Fossa BA, Marsiglia HR, Orecchia R. Radio therapy related fatigue. *Crit Rev Oncol Hematol* 2002;41:317.

115. Mazanec DJ, Podichetty VK, Mompoint A, et al. Vertebral compression fractures: manage aggressively to prevent sequelae. *Cleve Clin J Med* 2003;70(2):147.

116. Justice B. Why do women treated for breast cancer report good health despite disability. *Psycho Rep* 1999;84:392.

CHAPTER **57**

Societal Issues in Oncology

SECTION **1**

CHRISTOPHER K. DAUGHERTY

Ethical Issues

This chapter examines several important ethical issues, primarily in medical oncology, related to both clinical care and clinical research involving cancer patients. With regard to clinical care, an effort has been made to cover those topics of greatest importance to the cancer physician: informed consent and decision making; prognosis determination and communication; and ethical issues in the care of patients with life-threatening and life-ending disease, including palliative care and specific dilemmas related to providing end-of-life care. In examining clinical research in oncology, the chapter focuses on ethical principles that ought to guide such research; the issues surrounding the concept and practice of informed consent for clinical trials; and the specific ethical issues and dilemmas associated with phase I, II, and III trials in oncology. Wherever possible, available empiric research is highlighted in an attempt to address, and even resolve, the ethical issues and dilemmas that arise within the cancer care and research settings.

ETHICAL ISSUES IN CLINICAL CARE IN ONCOLOGY

MEDICAL ETHICS AND ONCOLOGY

To practice medicine competently and to provide high-quality care for cancer patients and others, physicians require both scientific and technical proficiency as well as a working knowledge of medical ethics.[1] It is within the dynamic relationship between doctor and patient where medical ethics takes shape and creates the issues and challenges faced in medical care. Furthermore, most day-to-day ethical problems that arise in patient care, whether in oncology or elsewhere, arise and are resolved within this relationship. As well, beyond the day-to-day problems, the most significant and challenging issues also typically arise within the context of this relationship. Crucial components in the analysis of any ethical issue include an understanding by both parties of the medical and scientific facts; the preferences, values, and goals of both patient and the physician; and the external constraints such as cost, limited resources, legal duties, and other social and/or cultural forces that shape or restrict choices.[2] For instance, in the cancer setting, physicians often have an excellent opportunity to cement trust and reduce the chances of future conflict regarding end-of-life care decisions by communicating clearly and compassionately with patients about prognosis and treatment goals.

For a variety of reasons, ethical issues arise in oncology practice either more frequently or more intensely than in the past. Frequently unprecedented ethical problems have arisen as a result of (1) the medical and social forces of the last quarter century that have raised an appropriate level of awareness of the need to respect patient autonomy and (2) the ever-accelerating development of scientific advances and new technologies. Such problems have raised multiple questions, including the following: When should efforts to prolong or improve life with chemotherapy be stopped? To what populations of patients should potentially life-saving or life-prolonging (but highly toxic) therapies that use significant clinical resources, such as stem cell transplantation, be applied? How does one effectively respect a patient's stated preference for prognostic information when it also challenges either the best efforts of the clinician's communication skills or the clinician's ability to respect a perceived need to empower the patient with information and make him or her an autonomous decision maker? Although less than in the recent past, managed care continues to give rise to new ethical issues such as limitations on decision-making freedom for patients and physicians and potential financial conflicts of interest associated with limiting the use of health care resources. In addition, several ethical issues continue to challenge cancer clinicians regardless of the presence, or use, of modern technology. These specifically include such issues as informed consent, decision making, information preferences, prognosis communication, and those issues that arise in the care of patients with life-ending cancer diagnoses (i.e., those with terminal illness).

INFORMED CONSENT AND SHARED DECISION MAKING

The process by which physicians and patients make decisions together is often summarized in the phrase *informed consent.* This doctrine, which reflects respect for patients and their moral authority to make decisions for themselves, is at the heart of the relationship between physician and patient. The doctrine is based on the ethical principles of respect for individual autonomy, dignity, and self-determination.[3] Informed consent has three key components: disclosure; competency, or the ability to understand; and voluntariness.

Disclosure means that physicians discuss with their patients the medical diagnosis, prognosis, and risks and benefits associated with possible treatment options. Patients are entitled to enough information to permit them to ask reasonable questions about the diagnosis and the options that are available. *Competency* means that patients are capable of understanding the relevant information, appreciating their own needs and values, manipulating information rationally, and communicating a treatment choice. *Voluntariness* means that a patient makes a choice freely, without coercion or other unfair inducements from the physician or anyone else.

Informed consent is a process of ongoing communication and dialogue between doctor and patient. In this process, physicians can help to empower patients to act in an autonomous manner by educating them about the nature of their medical problems and the reasonable medical alternatives to resolve (or cope with) them. Patients are then in a position to choose treatment based on their own personal preferences, values, and goals. This subsequently enables them to directly exercise their autonomy or control over treatment decisions. It is specifically worth noting that no cancer patient can make a truly informed decision about a particular plan of care until he or she has been made aware of, and understands, the potential alternatives. For cancer patients and others, either in clinical research or receiving clinical care, disclosure by the patient's health care provider of all available and reasonable treatment alternatives is one of the central components of the informed consent process.[1,3,4]

As described earlier, disclosure is essential if shared decision making is to occur.[3,5] In addition to the strong ethical arguments that support patient participation in medical decision making, patient participation is also advocated because it has been linked to better health outcomes, including decreased

anxiety, increased patient satisfaction, and improved compliance.[6–10] Many practitioners believe that improvement in overall quality of life can occur only when patients are fully informed of all reasonable alternatives and become equal partners in the decision-making process. With particular regard to care involving cancer patients with progressive disease—where potential medical treatment options may run the full spectrum from hospice care to stem cell transplantation—informing patients about available treatment options can only improve any subsequent communication encounters where the need to either use or forgo such alternatives may become necessary.[11] Although challenges may exist as to how a clinician can effectively and meaningfully disclose such alternatives and still make timely and relevant clinical decisions without overwhelming patients and families, the ethical argument of the need to disclose still persists.

INFORMATION PREFERENCES AND DECISION MAKING

It is important to recognize treatment decision making and information seeking as distinctive and separate components of the medical encounter.[12,13] Traditionally, the link between patients' desire for decision-making control has been assumed to be directly related to their information-seeking patterns.[14–17] It has also been assumed that patients are unable to achieve more involvement in treatment decision making because they have insufficient information, and it has been assumed that patients who want more control also want more information about their treatment options.[15] Conversely, those who are information seekers are assumed to prefer involvement in decision making because of their proactive approach to maintaining their health. However, increasing evidence suggests that, although patients generally express *preferences* for information about their illness and treatment,[7,14–17] they might not necessarily engage in information-*seeking* behaviors.[18,19] Furthermore, their preferences for participating in treatment decision may vary and may not be linked to their wish for information, especially as it relates to preferences for prognostic information.[15,17,20] Some studies have shown little correlation between patients' overall information-seeking behaviors and their actual level of desire for participation in treatment decisions.[14,17,18,21,22]

PROGNOSIS DETERMINATION AND COMMUNICATION

Overview of the Challenge

Considering the life-threatening severity of their illness, it is not unreasonable to assume that prognostic information would play a pivotal role in shaping the overall medical decision-making process of cancer patients and help them make the most appropriate treatment decisions. In fact, from an ethical perspective, a discussion of prognosis is an integral and necessary part of the communication and treatment decision-making processes for cancer patients. This is the case, in part, because prognostic information has been shown to be significantly associated with cancer patients' treatment choices.[23] Nevertheless, several studies have suggested that advanced-cancer patients have an inadequate understanding of their prognoses,[24–27] with patients generally overestimating the probability of their long-term survival. As well, many terminally ill cancer patients may state that the purpose of their treatment is to cure them.[24,27,28] Despite this available empiric data, it should be recognized that this issue (i.e., awareness of prognosis) remains a difficult one to study because patient anxiety, fear, and the need to maintain hope in the face of a grave prognosis may affect advanced-cancer patients' stated understanding of their prognoses. In addition, this research may be limited because from a methodologic standpoint, these same emotions may affect their measured responses to queries about their awareness of when they believe they are going to die. Thus, these *measured responses* may not necessarily be an accurate reflection of cancer patients' *true awareness* of their prognoses. Moreover, it is unknown what effect a physician's own anxiety and/or his or her own desire to help patients maintain hope has on actual physician communication of prognoses to cancer patients.

Physician Prognosis-Disclosure Practices

Early research examining physician communication with cancer patients, some of which dates from the 1940s and 1950s, clearly documented a great reluctance to disclose a cancer diagnosis and virtually no willingness to discuss prognosis.[29–34] The evidence strongly suggests that it was not that cancer physicians did not wish to tell a *diagnosis*, but rather that they did not want to give what would otherwise have then been an implied (or assumed) terminal *prognosis*.[29,30] By the late 1970s, however, full disclosure of a cancer diagnosis had become the norm.[35] This is a result of multiple factors, including community and public health education efforts toward early cancer detection and the fact that the perceived threat of a cancer diagnosis as a fatal disease had lessened, the U.S. government's declaration of the "war on cancer," and the ever-increasing range of treatment options available—including many with high rates of success.[36]

Considering (and even in spite of) these events, it is still not difficult to imagine that physicians would remain reluctant to want to give a terminal prognosis. In fact, with regard to current practices toward disclosure of prognosis to cancer patients, the available empiric data document that physicians withhold information.[20,37–41] Physicians would appear to be reluctant to disclose grim prognostic information for the same ethical and psychological reasons they traditionally withheld a diagnosis.[34,41] Physicians may fear that the revelation of a grim prognosis will psychologically damage patients' hope to survive.[38–43] Physicians may also feel discomfort when placing odds on survival, recurrence, and cure.[39] Thus, although the behavior of physicians has changed regarding disclosure of diagnosis, only limited information is available regarding how they have changed with regard to practices of disclosure of prognosis.

Although physicians have ethical obligations to disclose a terminal prognosis, questions remain as to how such prognostic information ought to be provided. Some cancer patients may better understand their prognosis when it is discussed through the use of numeric descriptors, whereas others understand their prognoses when it is conveyed in a qualitative manner. Patients may also discern important information about their prognoses based on physicians' use of euphemisms; vague estimations; and nonverbal or nonlinguistic cues—for example, tone of voice, word choice, extent of eye contact, and so forth. Last, some variable proportion of the population may (even overtly) state that they simply do not want prognostic information. Complicating all of this, quantitative research has shown that patients generally have inaccurate estimates of their prognoses.[23–26] From the cancer physicians' perspective, situational factors, including the seriousness of the disease, patient characteristics, and seniority of the physician, have been shown to influence the extent to which physicians disclose prognostic information.[39,43] Although not uniformly, most studies investigating how physicians foresee cancer patients' prognoses reveal that physicians themselves are often overly and incorrectly optimistic in their predictions of individual cancer patient survival.[44–46] Yet, how physician communication, and/or lack thereof, contributes to patient misunderstanding remains unknown.[47]

How oncologists themselves make decisions about presenting prognostic information is undoubtedly a complex process, potentially influenced by multiple factors, including the patient's clinical condition and sociodemographics. As well, the physician's own sociocultural background may influence the depth and style of presenting prognostic information. In addition, the strength of the personal relationships between particular oncologists and patients, the perceived patient desire for control over medical decisions, and a patient's information-seeking preferences may influence a physician's information-giving practices.[39] An oncologist may provide more information about a patient's prognosis when a patient requests it or may present little information based on his or her understanding of a patient's psychological state.

In the end, cancer physicians cannot rely on their own unproven assumptions about what they think are their patients' preferences for information. As in all settings of medical care, cancer physicians should base their communications with patients on evidence. Thus, they must *specifically elicit their patients' preferences* for the kinds of information that are vital for ethically appropriate decision making. As well, this elicitation of preferences must be explored with individual patients, particularly if patients are making specific requests to not receive particular kinds of information—for example, prognostic information. It may, in some circumstances, eventually be ethically justifiable to withhold (or postpone the disclosure of) such information to some patients for cultural or psychological reasons. However, before this can be done, cancer physicians must fulfill their moral obligations by further exploring and defining the personal justifications of individual patients for not wanting information that is otherwise considered vital for ethically sound medical decision making.

ETHICAL ISSUES IN THE CARE OF CANCER PATIENTS WITH LIFE-THREATENING AND LIFE-ENDING DISEASE

Oncologists deal almost exclusively with patients with serious and life-threatening diseases, many who are terminally ill. It is therefore essential that oncologists have a working knowledge regarding the ethical issues and overt dilemmas present in end-of-life cancer care, including specific issues surrounding implementation of palliative and hospice care and potential requests for physician-assisted suicide (PAS).

Ethical Dilemmas in End-of-Life Cancer Care: Referral to Hospice

As mentioned, in the cancer care setting where prognosis is known to result in eventual death (i.e., advanced cancer), how and when such prognoses should be communicated remain matters of concern and controversy. In addition, several equally important concerns arise regarding how and when palliative care that specifically involves no further anticancer agents may be exclusively implemented. For advanced-cancer patients who, by definition, have a life-ending diagnosis for which an anticancer standard of care has failed them, it remains unclear what factors actually influence their decisions to receive any particular form of care. For the more than 500,000 advanced-cancer patients who die each year in the United States, from both societal and medical perspectives, it is accepted that the ideal alternatives of care would include receiving state-of-the-art palliative care, as available in hospice. But it would also include participation in clinical research involving an experimental agent (e.g., phase I trials). Because of the complexities related to predicting time to death in those with advanced cancer, it may be difficult for oncologists to know when referral to hospice is appropriate or when it is still medically appropriate to continue attempts at anticancer therapy, including experimental agents.

For advanced-cancer patients to formally receive hospice care in the United States through Medicare and insurance hospice benefits, they must be documented by their physician as having a prognosis of 6 months or less. As it is currently provided within third-party payer systems, hospice care remains greatly underused for advanced-cancer patients. Only approximately 20% to 30% of cancer patients die each year while under hospice care.[48–51] In addition, even among those referred to hospice, their survival times strongly suggest that many of these patients do not receive the full palliative benefits that can be gained from hospice enrollment, with the median survival of cancer patients in hospice to be on the order of 2 to 3 weeks.[50,51] It has been argued that one of the obstacles to providing appropriate palliative care is a result of physician inaccuracy in predicting time to death.[46,50] Although this undoubtedly plays some role in many physicians' hesitancy (and even unwillingness) to refer cancer patients to hospice, it does not provide a complete explanation for the apparent underuse of hospice services. Other reasons clearly exist for this hesitancy and unwillingness, including perceived dilemmas related to physicians' desire to effectively communicate terminal prognoses to cancer patients and their families and still be able to facilitate the maintenance of hope; patients' and families' hesitancy or unwillingness to accept such prognoses; physician concerns regarding loss of control over their patients' medical care; and concerns about the methods by which the majority of hospice care is paid for in the United States, which may be insufficient to meet the needs of the dying.

Perceptions about damaging patient's and family's hope in the face of communicating a terminal prognosis remain a matter of concern among many clinicians. In fact, some clinicians believe that if they were to *effectively* communicate a terminal prognosis to a patient, they would essentially destroy the patient's hope.[39,41] Many physicians maintain that regardless of how sensitively or compassionately a terminal diagnosis is communicated, the ability of patients to sustain any meaningful hope is compromised. Although many clinicians within the palliative care community might argue that such hope can still be maintained in the face of effective (yet compassionate) prognosis disclosure, the impact of this physician belief on creating obstacles to quality end-of-life care should not be underestimated.

In addition, for patients and families to accept referral to hospice, they presumably must in some way accept (or at least acknowledge) a terminal prognosis. This may not necessarily have to be the case in every single instance, but patients or family members often must sign consent forms for hospice care documenting that the terminal prognosis of the patient has been disclosed (even understood) and that they wish to receive no further treatment aimed at reversing their cancer. In addition, they must typically sign an advance directive stating that they wish no life-sustaining interventions be used in their care at some point after (or before) hospice enrollment. Physicians often perceive that such disclosure of a terminal prognosis, and the requirements associated with signing such forms, may also severely damage a patient's and family members' hopes. As well, physicians may believe, with patients and family members often sharing this belief, that to agree to such care is to essentially "give up." Patients are known to deny their terminal prognoses even in the face of explicit physician disclosure.[39,46] If this is the case, it obviously is more difficult, perhaps even unethical, to refer such patients to hospice who willingly choose not to accept their terminal prognoses.

Some physicians and patients may also have fears or concerns regarding patient abandonment if and when they are referred to hospice. This may be the case in settings in which a cancer patient has been receiving significant amounts of anticancer therapy for several months or years before the recognition of a terminal prognosis. Now, with the introduction of the potential for hospice care, the care environment may be perceived as changing in dramatic ways. For example, such patients no longer receive chemotherapy or no longer undergo their previous pattern of physician and nursing visits. This may be particularly true for those patients who have received their cancer care almost exclusively at hospitals or medical centers some distance from their homes or communities. Traditionally, when patients are referred to hospice in the United States, they typically undergo fewer (if any) physician office visits, receiving the vast majority of care in the home. Thus, patients may feel as though they are being abandoned by their physicians and health care providers. Some physicians may even perceive this threat of abandonment (real or otherwise) within patients or family members and, as a result, do not pursue the option of hospice care.

Even further complicating matters, physicians may develop conflicts of interests when the appropriate time comes for when adequate palliative care could be provided within hospice. These conflicts can be due to financial and/or psychological reasons. For example, consider a patient who is appropriate for referral to hospice yet a physician continues to make medical decisions that involve chemotherapy—and receives reimbursement for such care. Although difficult for oncologists to acknowledge, a physician may have financial conflicts of interest that unknowingly influence treatment decisions and result in an unwillingness to refer to hospice for fear of lost income. Another more common (and perhaps more acceptable) example is that physicians may perceive referral to hospice as implying loss of either decision control or loss of a significant personal relationship. As a result, they may be psychologically unable to refer because they have emotional needs to maintain decision control or maintain (understandable) attachments to their patients.

A final example of the dilemmas present in providing end-of-life care to advanced-cancer patients relates to the Medicare and insurance benefits that exist to provide reimbursement for hospice care in the United States.[48] Currently, such care is paid for through a per diem benefit, with the Medicare per diem being approximately $120 a day (the actual rate depending on the region of the country in which the care is provided). A clear dilemma arises for some cancer patients, whose prognoses are undoubtedly terminal (i.e., consistent with less than 6 months of life) but who may have an otherwise excellent performance status and show evidence for continuing to benefit from rather expensive or aggressive palliative interventions. These might include such interventions as antibiotics, blood transfusions, and possibly even chemotherapy in some specific circumstances (e.g., palliative chemotherapy for pancreatic carcinoma, indolent breast cancer, hormone-refractory prostate cancer, and hematologic malignancies). In these advanced-cancer patient examples, the hospice benefit per diem would not cover the costs of aggressive palliative care. As a result, physicians may not ever refer certain populations of patients to hospice. Or, they may perceive that hospices are not particularly interested in caring for such patients because of the high cost of such palliative interventions. Indeed, many hospices do have practical and appropriate concerns about cost containment. Thus, for a hospice that is attempting to maintain its solvency and continue to care for many terminally ill patients, many aggressive interventions may be financially prohibitive.

Some of the dilemmas present in providing end-of-life cancer care in the United States might be eliminated, or at least reduced in magnitude, by increasing or restructuring the Medicare hospice benefit. As well, continuing medical education programs designed at improving communication techniques among oncologists may be effective in improving the ability of cancer physicians to communicate a terminal prognosis without perceptions, real or otherwise, of destroying patient and family hope.[52] Cancer physicians themselves could greatly benefit from having a better understanding as to how hospice care is provided and paid for. For instance, physicians would do well to recognize the significant amount of clinical decision control most hospices are more than willing to allow physicians to maintain over their patients, including helping patients to continue to make clinic visits. As well, many physicians are often surprised to learn that they can continue to bill for such clinical services, as allowed by the hospice benefit. Physicians would also do well if they had a better understanding as to how the 6-month prognostic milestone for hospice enrollment can be interpreted—that is, with a great deal of flexibility allowed and no penalties for honest inaccuracies in prognosis predictions. Last, with regard to the use of written forms that involve the disclosure of a terminal prognosis or the use of advance directives, physicians may be surprised to learn that many hospices may be willing to at least temporarily forgo the need to sign such forms early in the enrollment process if there is a perception that such forms may only lead to an increase in the emotional suffering of patients and families. In the meantime, however, as long as perceptions and beliefs (appropriate or otherwise) exist among physicians, patients, and families that to accept (or disclose) a terminal cancer prognosis is equivalent to giving up hope,[53] there will likely always be hesitancy, resistance, and even unwillingness to accept end-of-life care as it has been traditionally provided.

Physician-Assisted Suicide

Oncologists must be informed about PAS so that they are prepared to discuss this controversial issue if patients or their families raise it. Clinicians must also be able to distinguish among PAS, the withdrawal (or forgoing) of life-sustaining treatment, and euthanasia. *PAS* is defined as a physician prescribing a lethal dose of medication and sometimes providing technical advice to a patient, who subsequently commits suicide without further assistance from the physician.[54] The distinction between PAS and euthanasia is generally based on who administers the lethal dose: the patient (in PAS) or the physician (in euthanasia). PAS also differs from a competent adult patient's right to decline life-sustaining treatment in terms of the actual cause of death, the class of patients potentially affected by the practice, and the legality of the action. For example, PAS is currently illegal except in Oregon, whereas the right of patients to decline or forgo life support is clinically, ethically, and legally the standard of care throughout the United States.[1] The final distinction is the most subtle one (i.e., between PAS and aggressive pain management as occurs when a morphine drip is hung). Essentially, if the morphine drip is being used to palliate the patient's symptoms of pain, nausea, anxiety, and so forth, its use does not represent PAS; whereas, if the morphine drip is being used deliberately to hasten the patient's death or kill the patient, it probably represents euthanasia rather than PAS.

A request for PAS is obviously a sign that significant suffering, physical and/or emotional, is taking place. Such a request should never be ignored, deferred, or downplayed. Whenever PAS is raised in the clinical context, oncologists should be certain that the patient's suffering in all its myriad of forms is being addressed. Given the degree of suffering that is represented by a request for PAS, oncologists should become adept at distinguishing the degree to which such a request is a result of unaddressed, yet still reversible, suffering. The oncologist should make every effort to ensure that pain is being controlled; that symptoms other than pain such as depression, dyspnea, pruritus, and constipation are adequately managed; that advance care planning has been done; and that—perhaps most important—the patient is given every possible opportunity to maintain control over his or her situation (e.g., by being permitted to make medical choices). Recognizing that suffering is both physical and emotional is extremely important because of the fact that depression, rather than physical pain, is often associated with patient requests for PAS. Studies have found that 25% of cancer patients meet criteria for major or minor depression,[55,56] and suicide rates among cancer patients are substantially higher than those among the general public.[57] Despite the prevalence of potentially treatable mood disorders, data from the Netherlands suggest that only 3% of requests for PAS resulted in a psychiatric consultation.[58]

Two studies of physicians in the state of Washington have been published to help characterize the current status of PAS in the United States. In a 1994 survey study by Cohen and colleagues of 938 physicians (69% response rate),[59] 54% thought that euthanasia should be legal in some situations, but nearly one-half agreed with the statement that euthanasia is never ethically justified. Hematologists and oncologists were most likely to oppose PAS. Two years later, more research from Washington reported on actual requests for PAS.[60] The major finding of this 828-physician survey study was that 12% had received one or more explicit requests for PAS, and 4% for euthanasia, in the past year. The requests were generally from patients with cancer, neurologic disorders, and acquired immunodeficiency syndrome. Patients' requests were most often perceived as being based on concerns about loss of control, being a burden to others, and loss of dignity. Physicians reported providing PAS in 24% of cases in which it had been requested and described providing PAS more often to patients with physical symptoms. The authors note that physicians did not consult their colleagues in many cases.

A report commissioned by the Dutch government to empirically evaluate the practice of euthanasia reported that there were approximately 2300 cases of euthanasia per year (1.8% of all deaths) and 400 cases of PAS per year (0.3% of all deaths) in the Netherlands.[61] In addition, there were 1000 cases (0.8% of all deaths) in which patients received euthanasia either without explicitly requesting it or while deemed incompetent to make such a request.[62] In 56% of these cases, the patient was no longer competent when euthanasia was performed. Overall, 27% of Dutch physicians who were interviewed indicated that they had performed euthanasia at least once without an explicit voluntary request for euthanasia by the patient. Dutch experiences also document a high complication rate (23%) associated with efforts to perform PAS in 114 cases.[63] In 21 of these cases (18%), the physician decided to administer a lethal medication, which thus transformed the situation from PAS to actual direct euthanasia. These data suggest that in the Netherlands, a slippery slope has developed in which euthanasia has been extended from competent adults who voluntarily request it to incompetent patients (both adults and children) who have never made such a request.

Further information regarding attitudes and practices regarding PAS in the United States is available from an empiric, vignette-based study, by Emanuel et al. The investigators examined the experiences of the public, cancer patients, and oncologists.[64] In the hypothetical setting of unremitting pain, approximately two-thirds of cancer patients and the public found both euthanasia and PAS acceptable. They found it less acceptable in the setting of existential suffering or in the setting in which there was the potential for a patient to be a "burden on the family." Among patients actually experiencing pain, they were more likely to find euthanasia and PAS unacceptable. Among oncologists, more than one-half stated they had had a request for either euthanasia or PAS, and one in seven said they had performed either practice at least once. In a related set of data, nearly one-half of these oncologists could imagine a situation in which they would want PAS or euthanasia for themselves.[65] These oncologists were more than twice as likely to find euthanasia or PAS acceptable for their patients, as compared with oncologists who could not imagine a situation in which they would want PAS or euthanasia for themselves (86% vs. 42%, respectively). Many oncologists (42%) who would find PAS or euthanasia unacceptable for themselves still found these practices ethical for their patients. These data suggest that there is significant, although not majority support, for the use of PAS—and even euthanasia in at least some cancer care cases—and that as many as 15% of oncologists have carried out such practices at least once in their professional careers. Interestingly, in subsequent research, Emanuel found that some oncologists appeared to have suffered adverse consequences (emotional or psychological) from having performed PAS or euthanasia.[66] Further research is undoubtedly needed to better understand oncologists' attitudes to PAS and their perception of pain and suffering and their perceived obligations in helping cancer patients to end their lives.

Another data source that is being closely scrutinized derives from the experience in the state of Oregon, which legalized PAS on October 27, 1997. During the first 2 years of PAS activity, 56 persons requested lethal medications, and 41 died after taking the medication.[67,68] The most common underlying diagnosis was cancer, and the most common reasons for PAS were not physical pain but rather "loss of autonomy due to illness, loss of control of bodily functions," and a wish to determine and control the manner of one's death. Based on these two reports, the use of PAS in Oregon occurs infrequently and has generally involved patients who were well-insured, educated, and already in hospice programs.

In the end, cancer clinicians should at least recognize that some patients may benefit from knowing that PAS is not an option that their physician would typically contemplate, and this reassurance may strengthen the trust that cancer patients place in their doctors. Alternatively, many patients may greatly benefit from knowing that their physicians are willing to at least discuss the concept of a request for PAS and acknowledge the suffering it represents. These patients may even further benefit from an open and honest discussion specifically exploring PAS as a viable possibility, for no more reason than that it may have beneficial effects due to the meaningful acknowledgment of a patient's deepest thoughts and the sense of control it allows them to exercise over their lives. These benefits may extend to the point of a patient even forgoing further efforts to actively seek out requests for PAS.

ETHICAL ISSUES IN CANCER CLINICAL TRIALS

This section of the chapter examines the ethical issues that arise from clinical research involving cancer patients, beginning with a brief overview of specific principles that guide the ethical conduct of clinical research. Further discussion and background pertaining to the concept and process of informed consent as it specifically relates to cancer patients and clinical research, including the use of consent forms for research, follow. The ethical issues of clinical trials in oncology, including phase I, II, and III studies, are then examined. Wherever possible, empiric information is incorporated into these discussions from research on the informed consent and clinical trial process in cancer.

ETHICAL PRINCIPLES GUIDING CLINICAL RESEARCH

The main objective of clinical research in oncology is to improve medical care for future cancer patients. From both a societal and ethical perspective, this is viewed as a laudable and important goal. As such, no meaningful criticisms can be made against the need and desire to better care for those with cancer. However, when one examines the methods by which this goal is pursued, problematic issues can be found. As is discussed, it is the process of using current patients as research subjects to achieve this goal in which several ethical dilemmas are created.

Whether in the context of clinical practice or clinical research, several specific principles guide the management of patients by physicians.[69] The first such principle worthy of mention in this context is that one ought not to use others as means to an end. In the process of clinical research, this general ethical principle is, in many ways, allowed to be violated.

However, to allow violation of this principle, it is expected that no patient can participate as a research subject unless there is the potential for benefit and unless they have provided adequate informed consent. No doubt, in considering what is an acceptable degree of potential benefit, this safeguard is in place for a great proportion of clinical research. (Here, benefit is implied as it is traditionally measured in oncology—i.e., as a specific anticancer response or improvement in a patient–subject's symptoms.) However, as is discussed later in Ethical Issues in Phase I Trials, ethical dilemmas that challenge this safeguard are created in the early drug development process in which the potential for such benefit may be exceedingly small.

A second related ethical principle that must guide behavior in the research setting is that one should not allow harm to come to others. Certainly, oversimplification or generalization of this principle would lead to the prohibition of specific patterns of behavior in the clinical (nonresearch) setting of cancer care, where the harm from toxicities is deemed acceptable because of the known benefits to be achieved. Thus, as with the first principle mentioned, the specific issue of harm cannot truly be weighed without consideration of the relative benefit that may be achieved for cancer patients. However, when cancer patients participate as research subjects in early clinical trials of anticancer agents (i.e., phase I and II trials), there is a greater relative potential for harm to come to patients as a result of the specific methodologies and research objectives used in these trials. In addition to the recognition that benefit is not likely, there is even an expectation that harm will come. In fact, it may even be a goal of a clinical trial to produce harm. In addition to the need for subjects to provide adequate informed consent, the safeguard that must also be in place to allow violation of this principle is that the potential for harm to participating subjects must be warranted either as a result of the potential benefits to be achieved or (more commonly) that, given the circumstances of many advanced-cancer patients participating in such trials, there are perceived to be no other available meaningful anticancer alternatives.

A third ethical principle that guides behavior in this context is that one ought never to deceive others. Within clinical research, several safeguards are in place that are designed to prevent the deception of patients who become the subjects of research. The informed consent process itself and other federal and institutional regulations provide mechanisms in which oversight of both specific research protocols and the methods of information provision are present to prevent any intentional deception of patients. More important, the conscientious communication efforts of participating physician–investigators are also relied on to prevent deception. However, in the setting of early trials of investigational agents in which research subjects are most often those with far-advanced disease, many have wondered about the potential vulnerability of these subjects and the potential for them to be unintentionally deceived.[68] Indeed, the very fact that the agents under study in early drug trials have shown promise in preclinical models creates a variety of stated or unstated inducements that may play on some advanced-cancer patients, potentially overwhelming desire for therapeutic benefit and lead to a process akin to deception—albeit unintentional.

In a final principle worthy of mention, medical ethics itself teaches that the interests of an individual physician's patient should be placed above the interests of others. One can easily argue that placing cancer patients in a clinical trial involving a new investigational agent does not at all compromise their interest in receiving state-of-the-art care. However, one must keep in mind that the overall goal of clinical research (improving care for future patients) remains intact whenever a patient enters a clinical trial. Thus, at the very least, other interests beyond the individual care of a patient are present when a patient enters a clinical trial.

INFORMED CONSENT FOR CLINICAL RESEARCH

The concept of informed consent, which acknowledges the rights of patients to voluntarily participate in health care, applies both to clinical practice and clinical research.[3,70] Informed consent in clinical research is related to, but recognized as being more stringent than, informed consent outside the context of clinical trials.[70,71] This heightened consent standard exists for at least two reasons. First, from an ethical perspective, a patient considering clinical trial participation is always viewed as *potentially* vulnerable.[72] As a result, he or she may have great difficulty in appreciating the distinctions between the therapeutic and research aspects of any given alternative of care or treatment. The informed consent process and the ethics of clinical research require that such a clear distinction be made.[4,73] Second, the physician–investigator is seen as having an intrinsic conflict of interest in his or her role as both a physician for an individual patient and as a scientific investigator attempting to develop improved methods of medical care and treatment.[69,71,73] As previously mentioned, within the context of a relationship that is solely therapeutic, the physician places his or her patients' interests above all else.[1] However, within the context of clinical research, investigators have additional interests that may not be relevant to their patients' interests and may cloud investigators' judgment as to what information is important for adequate consent.

A definition of informed consent for clinical research that encompasses all relevant aspects of the process remains somewhat elusive, with varying definitions having been described.[3,69,70–72] Generally, it is viewed as a process of communication between a patient–subject and a clinician–investigator regarding an investigational or experimental treatment. Within this communication process, several elements must be disclosed. These include the disclosure of the type of research to be performed, the risks and benefits of the treatment or research, the unproven nature of the research, the alternatives other than participation in the clinical trial, and, finally, disclosure of the subject's freedom to withdraw or not to participate in the research without any detrimental effect on the patient's continued access to adequate health care. Separate from the issue of disclosure, there is the issue of actual understanding on the part of the patient with regard to these disclosed elements. How much of an understanding of these elements is required for adequate informed consent to take place remains a matter of controversy.[3,69,74] However, from an ethical standpoint, it is accepted that the process of informed consent requires a *meaningful* attempt on the part of clinician–investigators to help patients understand those aspects of the consent process that have been disclosed so that patients may autonomously and voluntarily decide to participate in research.[69] Other elements that have been described as important parts of the informed consent process include maintaining the confidentiality of a research subject's participation and, controversially, possible disclosure of potential conflicts of interest (financial and otherwise) on the part of the clinician–investigator.

In an attempt to emphasize the importance of the distinctions between research and therapy, most ethical regulations governing clinical research and the subsequent review processes that are guided by these regulations have focused on the informed consent process as a means of protecting potentially vulnerable research subjects from physical and psychological harm.[71,72,74] These regulations have relied heavily on written informed consent documents to achieve full disclosure of the important elements of consent, including the risks of research participation, the nature of the research, and alternatives to research participation. Thus, informed consent is currently and most commonly viewed as a means of protection of a potentially vulnerable research subject from harm.[71,72] However, from the inception of these regulations to the present day, many critics have recognized the imperfect nature of the methods used to regulate the informed consent process.[75–79] More recent empiric research on informed consent, a great proportion of which has been conducted in the cancer setting, has been helpful in attempting to objectively identify the current problems and deficiencies associated with written consent documents and their oversight. As reviewed elsewhere, several studies reported since 1978 have increasingly demonstrated that, although regulations are being followed, informed consent documents have become increasingly unreadable, lengthy, and uninformative.[80–84] Indeed, they may actually be interfering with what might otherwise be an ethically appropriate informed consent process for patients, including not only those with cancer, but any patient considering therapeutic clinical trial participation.

In considering the available empiric data, one is certainly left to wonder about the usefulness and value of the current consent process for therapeutic clinical trials. Particular concerns develop when one recognizes that great emphasis continues to be placed on consent forms and their content. Such concerns become even more challenging in areas either in which consent forms detail investigational therapies with relatively extreme toxicities or in which the therapeutic goals of the alternatives to clinical trial participation may be quite different from the inherent or perceived goals of investigational therapy—that is, early phase trials where alternatives to trial participation are not uncommonly palliative, or even hospice, care.

ETHICAL ISSUES IN PHASE I TRIALS

It is in the specific setting of cancer trials involving new agents (i.e., phase I trials) in which the general concerns about informed consent in therapeutic clinical trials become especially troubling and challenging.[69,72,83,85] This is because phase I trials typically involve patients with advanced, eventually life-ending disease in a research endeavor where the chance of meaningful, objective, therapeutic benefit has traditionally been described as being quite low, less than 5%.[86–89] As a result of the dose-escalation methods in these trials,[85] a more specific dilemma is the relative ratio of toxicity and benefit for patients who participate. Further complicating this is the need to adequately inform patients about these particular issues and then allow them to willingly and freely consent to participate in such studies. The complexities of the consent process for advanced-cancer patients in phase I trials relate both to what degree such patients should be viewed as vulnerable and to what extent a participating physician's own expectations and interests play a role in guiding patients to decide to participate. This unique form of clinical research creates an intense environment of medical decision making in which, arguably, many patients may not benefit from the traditional informed consent process.

If patients were to participate in phase I trials solely for altruistic reasons—in other words, to help forward cancer research and potentially help future cancer patients—phase I trials would probably carry less ethical conflict. As well, this would imply that the traditional informed consent process might more readily achieve the desired ideal outcome of understanding all elements of consent, including an understanding of the nature of phase I research and the alternatives to trial participation, as these less vulnerable patients would not necessarily be seeking benefit for themselves. However, the objective information available regarding the informed consent process for patients participating as research subjects in phase I trials shows that altruism is not the primary motivating factor for patients participating in such clinical research. As reviewed in this section, the empiric studies examining the phase I consent process highlight the true ethical dilemmas associated with this early stage of clinical research.

In the first studies of patients surrounding these issues, European investigators evaluated the quality of informed consent among small numbers of patients with advanced cancer who were offered participation in phase I trials.[90,91] The majority of patients who gave their consent were motivated by hope for improvement of their condition, pressure exerted by relatives and friends, or simply feeling they had "no choice." Some patients did mention the desire to contribute to the progress of medicine. Encouragement by relatives or friends appeared to be a powerful force in motivating some patients to participate in phase I trials.

Investigators at the University of Chicago conducted several in-depth survey studies of advanced-cancer patients who have given informed consent to participate in phase I trials at their institution.[27,92–94] In addition, the oncologists identified by the surveyed patients as responsible for their care and consent have been surveyed as well.[27] In these studies, the vast majority of patients stated that they decided to participate in a phase I trial for reasons of possible therapeutic benefit, with other reasons cited as the advice or trust of physicians and because of family pressure. Altruistic feelings, although perhaps present, appeared to have a limited role in motivating patients to participate in these trials. Although nearly all surveyed subjects said that they understood all or most of the information provided to them about the trial in which they had decided to participate, generally speaking, only approximately 25% to 35% were able to state the purpose of the trial in which they were participating (with patients able to state the purpose of phase I trials as dose-escalation or dose-finding studies being more educated). Given some of these results, it may not be surprising that several studies have repeatedly shown that the expectations of benefit among advanced-cancer patients enrolled in phase I trials greatly exceed what can be feasibly and realistically expected from a medical or research point of view.[27,92,93,95–97] Although surveyed oncologists have had wide-ranging beliefs regarding expectations of possible benefits and toxicities for their patients participating in a phase I trial, their expectations have never exceeded those of their subjects. Thus, patients who participate in phase I trials are almost exclusively motivated by the hope of therapeutic benefit. Many patients may be unaware of the research purposes of phase I trials and are unable to recall whether alternatives to clinical trial participation, including palliative care or other nonexperimental therapies, were either discussed with or disclosed to them.[92]

These data regarding patient understanding exist despite the fact that all surveyed patients in these studies had signed consent forms detailing the research purpose of phase I trials and the alternatives to trial participation. In fact, in in-depth analyses of hundreds of consent forms used for phase I trials, Horng and colleagues have more recently shown that the content of these forms is accurate and appropriate in the descriptions of risks, the low likelihood of benefits, the research purpose of the trials, and alternatives to trial participation.[98] Furthermore, Tomamichel and colleagues, in an analysis of the communication process involved in informed consent for cancer patients agreeing to participate in phase I trials, found that informed consent communications with patients was satisfactory from a quantitative point of view and that the most important items of information were acceptably communicated to patients.[95]

The information gained from this research strongly supports the argument that the current process of obtaining informed consent for phase I trials may be inadequate to appropriately ensure that such advanced-cancer patients understand both the nature of the research in which they are participating and the alternatives to trial participation. In addition, despite recognizing the existence of their potential vulnerability, it is not known how that vulnerability specifically affects an advanced-cancer patient's ability to give what is otherwise perceived to be adequate informed consent. Some have argued that to even assume that the population of advanced-cancer patients participating in phase I trials is vulnerable is ethically unacceptable and that patients should be allowed to hold whatever beliefs they choose either about their disease and/or the potential for benefit to be gained from investigational agents.[99] However, such arguments give short shrift to the research data outlined earlier and also completely ignore the fact that many of these patients are vulnerable to a variety of stated and unstated inducements within the research setting, creating an environment of potentially coercive situations. Further research is required to better understand and delineate these issues and their importance on the informed consent process in this difficult and highly charged setting. As well, innovative and meaningful interventions designed to improve patient understanding and decision making are needed to fulfill physicians' obligations of ensuring that the best consent process possible occurs for the advanced-cancer patients enrolling in these often nontherapeutic research studies.[100]

ETHICAL ISSUES IN PHASE II TRIALS

Phase II trials of new agents create ethical issues quite similar to those in phase I trials, most notably because they also typically involve the participation of human subjects with otherwise incurable illnesses in biomedical research. Thus, the potential vulnerability of these patients in seeking therapy comes into play in their decisions to participate in trials with a similarly low likelihood of therapeutic benefit. Although still troubling, however, issues in phase II trials can be viewed as potentially less complex for several reasons. In the phase II setting, there is less of the unknown for both oncologist–investigator and patient, as all agents studied in phase II trials have at least completed toxicity-finding and dose-determination (phase I) studies. Thus, there may be greater attitudes of certainty with regard to expected toxicities. There may also be greater hope or expectations of benefit, in part because these agents are being administered at or near the maximum tolerated dose. Therefore, one unique issue in the phase II trial is the higher likelihood of toxicity developing for all patients in a trial. The intentions and motivations of a participating oncologist in the role of physician–healer or physician–investigator are central issues in both phase I and II trials. Yet, for better or for worse, expectations or hope of benefit for their patients may be greater in the phase II setting. This may translate into greater therapeutic intent and subsequently be communicated to patients, resulting in greater expectations or hopes on their part as well.

Although these issues may be less complex and more easily examined in the phase II setting involving new agents, they are still troubling because of an overall low probability of benefit with regard to tumor responses in these trials.[101] In fact, this concern may actually increase even as a phase II study is accruing patient–subjects. This relates to the accepted statistical requirements of phase II trials of new agents that are present to exclude, with an accepted amount of certainty or confidence, a low level of efficacy for a new agent.[85] Traditional stopping rules for many phase II trials would allow as many as 14 consecutive nonresponders to accrue to a trial before concluding that the agent lacks disease-specific efficacy. Yet, physician–investigators' attitudes and beliefs may change significantly with regard to an agent under study as early-response data accumulate that would suggest a lack of clinical efficacy to most clinicians but the trial remains open to reach the statistically required accrual.

How should evolving data be handled during a phase II trial that suggest a lack of efficacy but are not sufficiently substantiated from a statistical standpoint? In a study of even a small number of patients, if an agent is given to initial patient–subjects without apparent benefits or tumor responses—but not enough patients have been involved to satisfy statistical requirements— what information should be provided to prospective patient– subjects? For example, in a simple phase II single-agent study seeking to accrue 14 to 20 patients, if six evaluable patient– subjects have been administered the agent and are known to have not received any apparent benefits, what should the informed consent process consist of for prospective patient–subjects with regard to risks and benefits?

Oncologists' attitudes, perceptions, and biases toward clinical trial chemotherapy may substantially affect clinical trial accrual. Thus, it is appropriate to assume that these factors are likely to have some effect on clinicians' willingness to accrue to phase II trials. How oncologists assimilate information and communicate it to prospective cancer patient–subjects likely changes over the course of a trial. As well, oncologists' enthusiasm or beliefs toward the potential efficacy of an agent may decline as information is acquired regarding nonresponders, or even as other, newer trials begin. Yet, the consent forms for such trials are almost always static—that is, not significantly different than when the trial first began, potentially leading to subjects receiving conflicting information. What is troubling about this is that, quite often, accrual will continue (albeit perhaps slower) using the same consent process and/or form until the statistical requirements for accrual have been satisfied. This may well be justified from a scientific and statistical standpoint to establish confidence regarding lack of efficacy of a new agent in a specific disease, but the potential dilemma remains and is no less troubling. Some might argue that as nonresponse information accumulates, such declining enthusiasm for a new agent should be allowed to affect accrual and should be uniformly communicated to prospective patient–subjects. However, traditionally, after the initiation of a phase II trial, subsequent patients are accrued with little formal response or toxicity information available to prospective subjects about prior evaluable patients in the trial. Interestingly, if such information could be fully and appropriately withheld from involved clinician–investigators, some of the described dilemmas in phase II trials might resolve themselves. As well, if one could guarantee an unprecedented quick rate of accrual of all the subjects necessary to meet the statistical requirements for a phase II trial, these dilemmas could potentially be less challenging, as there would not be an opportunity for significant response (or nonresponse, as the case may be) data to be generated before accrual was completed. Practically speaking, these actions are not likely to be routinely achievable. Research on these issues in the phase II setting is needed to better delineate their resolvable components. More progressive trial designs should also be considered.

ETHICAL ISSUES IN PHASE III TRIALS

Although ethical issues are present throughout all phases of clinical research, and early trials of new agents certainly present troubling dilemmas, it is randomized phase III trials that have undergone the most intense scrutiny. Indeed, much of this scrutiny has centered on the randomized trial process specifically in *cancer* clinical research. The overall informed consent process in phase III trials and, more specifically, how disclosure to potential subjects regarding the randomization process itself should be conducted remain issues of controversy. An even more basic and primary ethical concern is the application of the phase III trial design itself, with much debate and controversy focused on when, rather than if, it is ethically appropriate to perform randomized comparative trials.[102–107] Such concerns deal with a perceived dilemma for the treating physician of a specific patient and whether the physician's therapeutic responsibilities to that individual patient overwhelm any responsibilities to clinical research and the needs to improve medical care for future patients.[105,106] Supporters of this view have argued that the responsibilities of the physician as healer carry far greater moral weight than those of the physician as investigator, to the extent that it becomes unethical to allow a random process to be the determining factor in what therapy a patient receives. Complicating this further is the fact that in the phase III setting, the lines separating research from therapy are sometimes less clear.[4,73,108]

Much of the debate regarding ethical issues in phase III trials has centered around the issue of equipoise. As originally defined by Fried,[109] *equipoise* is viewed as a state of genuine uncertainty on the part of a clinical investigator or treating physician regarding the comparative merits of different treatments for a patient's specific disease process, such as cancer. For an individual investigator or physician caring for a particular patient, some have argued that equipoise must exist for the clinician that he or she can ethically ask (or encourage) that patient to participate in an appropriately designed phase III

trial. Others have argued that a broader definition of equipoise be accepted to justify randomized phase III trials; specifically, that clinical equipoise need not exist for an individual physician or investigator but need only exist within a specified medical community.[110,111] Thus, in community equipoise, some physicians may have a great deal of certainty regarding what is the best therapy for their patients, but an equal proportion of physicians have an opposing viewpoint regarding what is the best therapy. Finally, more recent arguments have sought to place specific constraints on these two types of equipoise and to argue that both community and clinical equipoise must be in evidence for phase III trials to be justified.

In the cancer setting, clinicians, researchers, and ethicists have debated this issue of equipoise (whether it should be applied as an individual vs. a community standard) and even whether randomized studies are ethical at all.[105] The empiric research available from the cancer setting strongly suggests that the issue of equipoise remains quite unresolved for investigators, clinicians, and even patients.[112–120] As well, many oncologists view the informed consent process requirements within randomized clinical trials as too cumbersome or potentially threatening to the patient and/or to the relationship between doctor and patient, to the extent that they are a significant obstacle to patient accrual to phase III trials.[112,113,118,120] More recently, some bioethicists have argued that, because concepts of clinical equipoise conflate the necessary distinctions between research and therapy, equipoise should be abandoned entirely within discussions regarding the ethics of phase III trials.[108]

Keeping this issue of equipoise in mind and returning to the process of informed consent in phase III trials, Freedman has quite rationally argued that an *individual* physician or investigator is not the sole arbiter of appropriate or acceptable medical practice.[110] Rather, the medical community as a whole determines equipoise, and an individual physician can remain ethically and morally justified in consenting patients to participate in a phase III trial if he or she recognizes that the medical community at large is uncertain as to what is the best standard of care, even if the physician him- or herself is not in equipoise. Royall extended this argument, noting that in situations involving an autonomous patient, the decision to participate in a randomized study does not rest with the physician but with the patient.[121] This is certainly the case as long as an adequate (perhaps ideal) process of informed consent can be carried out. Royall argued that what is needed for randomized trials to be justifiably conducted, beyond the presence of medical uncertainty (or equipoise) regarding particular therapies, is not physicians without preferences. Rather, it is patients who are informed of the uncertainty (i.e., the existence of perceived equipoise) and are autonomously willing to consent to randomization. Thus, within the context of phase III trials, the informed consent process becomes one of utmost importance.

Given the issues surrounding equipoise and the known obstacles that the consent process for randomized trials creates, some efforts have been undertaken to examine alternatives to the conventional methods of informed consent for phase III trials.[122–126] The alternatives to this conventional method of consent and randomization include so-called preconsent randomization, where subjects are first randomized to one arm of the trial and then asked to consent to participation. Such methods were specifically proposed to make the informed consent process less cumbersome and threatening for a participating physician–investigator.

The common theme of such designs is that patients are asked to consent to a specific treatment rather than to participate in a randomized trial. Many statistical difficulties arise with such randomized consent designs, including an inability to blind subjects to the treatment. As well, such designs create both an underestimation and a dilution of possible differences in treatment effects, resulting in larger (and even unpredictable) accrual goals. Significant ethical issues also arise with such designs, including the fact that many subjects would likely receive biased information from the participating physician–investigator approaching them for inclusion in the trial about the particular treatment to which they had already been prerandomized, which actually would challenge whether equipoise any longer could exist for the involved physician–investigator and patient–subject.

Interestingly, even considering such criticisms, nearly a dozen cancer clinical trials have used these or similar consent designs.[125,126] Most of these trials had been originally initiated with conventional consent designs but were then modified to include randomized consent designs to improve on slow patient accrual. Several of these trials increased their accrual rates substantially, some by a factor of three to six times the initial accrual rates.[127–129] Despite these improvements in accrual, these consent designs remain controversial. Gallo and colleagues examined the use of such trial designs, comparing different preconsent procedures for a hypothetical randomized trial among more than 2000 healthy subjects.[122] The investigators concluded that preconsent randomization methods are highly inefficient with regard to improving accrual, as subjects knowingly randomized to receive standard treatment would be likely to refuse clinical trial entry. In general, the ethical and statistical difficulties have prevented their implementation on a routine basis, and they have not been recommended for such use.

CONCLUSION

If cancer physicians and investigators are to provide high-quality cancer care and conduct clinical research according to the highest possible standards, they must maintain a heightened sensitivity to the ethical issues discussed. Continued study and debate regarding these complex issues are unquestionably needed if the dilemmas present in cancer care and research are to be addressed and, it is to be hoped, resolved. Considering their long-standing awareness, cancer physicians and investigators remain well qualified to continue to provide guidance in shaping this future study.

REFERENCES

1. Jonsen AR, Siegler M, Winslade WJ. *Clinical ethics*, 4th ed. New York: McGraw-Hill, 1998.
2. Siegler M. The physician–patient accommodation: a central event in clinical medicine. *Arch Intern Med* 1982;142:1899.
3. Faden RR, Beauchamp TL, King NMP. *A history and theory of informed consent*. New York: Oxford University Press, 1986.
4. Bok S. Shading the truth in seeking informed consent for research purposes. *Kennedy Inst Ethics J* 1995;5:1.
5. Vetch RM. Abandoning informed consent. *Hastings Cent Rep* 1995;25:5.
6. Tarlov AL, Ware JE, Greenfield S, et al. The Medical Outcomes Study: an application of methods for monitoring the results of medical care. *JAMA* 1989;262:925.
7. Sutherland HJ, Llewellyn-Thomas HA, Lockwood GA, Tritchler DL, Till JE. Cancer patients: their desire for information and participation in treatment decisions. *J Royal Soc Med* 1989;82:260.
8. Margalith I, Shapiro A. Anxiety and patient participation in clinical decision-making: the case of patients with ureteral calculi. *Soc Sci Med* 1997;45:419.
9. Hall JA, Roter DL, Katz NR. Meta-analysis of correlates of provider behavior in medical encounters. *Med Care* 1988;26:657.
10. Waitzkin H, Stoeckle JD. The communication of information about illness: clinical, sociological, and methodological considerations. *Adv Psychosomat Med* 1972;8:180.
11. Orona CJ, Koenig BA, Davis AJ. Cultural aspects of nondisclosure. *Camb Q Healthcare Ethics* 1994;3:338.
12. Ong LM, De Haes JCJM, Hoos AM, Lammes FB. Doctor–patient communication: a review of the literature. *Soc Sci Med* 1995;40:903.
13. Turner S, Maher EJ, Young T, Hudson GV. What are the information priorities for cancer patients involved in treatment decisions? An experienced surrogate study in Hodgkin's disease. *Br J Cancer* 1996;73:222.
14. Cassileth BR, Zupkis RV, Sutton-Smith K, March V. Information and participation preferences among cancer patients. *Ann Intern Med* 1980;92:832.
15. Hack TF, Degner LF, Dyck DG. Relationship between preferences for decisional control and illness information among women with breast cancer: a quantitative and qualitative analysis. *Soc Sci Med* 1994;39:279.
16. Strull WM, Lo B, Charles G. Do patients want to participate in medical decision making? *JAMA* 1984;252:2990.
17. Blanchard CG, Labrecque MS, Ruckdeschel JC, Blanchard EB. Information and decision-making preferences of hospitalized adult cancer patients. *Soc Sci Med* 1988;27:1139.
18. Beisecker AE, Beisecker TD. Patient information-seeking behaviors when communicating with doctors. *Med Care* 1990;28:19.
19. Ende J, Kazis L, Ash A, Moskowitz MA. Measuring patients' desire for autonomy: decision making and information-seeking preferences among medical patients. *J Gen Intern Med* 1989;4:23.
20. Hagerty RG, Butow PN, Ellis P, et al. Cancer patient preferences for communication of prognosis in the metastatic setting. *J Clin Oncol* 2004;22:1721.
21. Charles C, Redko C, Whelan T, Gafni A, Reyno L. Doing nothing is no choice: lay constructions of treatment decision-making among women with early-stage breast cancer. *Sociol Health Illness* 1998;20:71.
22. Turk-Charles S, Meyerowitz BE, Gatz M. Age differences in information seeking among cancer patients. *Intl J Aging Hum Dev* 1997;45:85.
23. Weeks JC, Cook F, O'Day SJ, et al. Relationship between cancer patients' predictions of prognosis and their treatment preferences. *JAMA* 1998;279:1709.
24. Eidinger RN, Schapira DV. Cancer patients' insight into their treatment, prognosis, and unconventional therapies. *Cancer* 1984;53:2736.
25. Mackillop WJ, Stewart WE, Ginsburg AD, Stewart SS. Cancer patients' perceptions of their disease and its treatment. *Br J Cancer* 1988;58:355.
26. Sulmassy DP, Terry PB, Weisman CS, et al. The accuracy of substituted judgments in patients with terminal diagnoses. *Ann Intern Med* 1998;128:621.
27. Daugherty C, Ratain MJ, Grochowski E, et al. Perceptions of cancer patients and their physicians involved in phase I trials. *J Clin Oncol* 1995;13:1062.
28. Cohen L, deMoor C, Amato RJ. The association between treatment specific optimism and depressive symptomatology in patients enrolled in phase I cancer clinical trials. *Cancer* 2002;91:1949.
29. Fitts WT, Ravdin IS. What Philadelphia physicians tell patients with cancer. *JAMA* 1953;153:901.
30. Oken D. What to tell cancer patients: a study of medical attitudes. *JAMA* 1961;175:1120.
31. Kelley WD, Friesen SR. Do cancer patients want to be told? *Surgery* 1950;27:822.
32. Koenig RR. Anticipating death from cancer: physician and patient attitudes. *Mich Med* 1969;68:899.
33. Gerle B, Lunden G, Sandlom P. The patient with inoperable cancer from the psychiatric and social standpoints. *Cancer* 1960;13:1206.
34. McIntosh J. Processes of communication, information seeking and control associated with cancer: a selective review of the literature. *Soc Sci Med* 1974;8:167.
35. Novack DH, Plumer R, Smith RL, et al. Changes in physicians' attitudes toward telling the cancer patient. *JAMA* 1979;241:897.
36. Patterson JT. *The dread disease: cancer and modern American culture*. Cambridge, MA: Harvard University Press, 1987.
37. Seale C. Communication and awareness about death: a study of a random sample of dying people. *Soc Sci Med* 1991;32:943.
38. Miyaji N. The power of compassion: truth-telling among American doctors in the care of dying patients. *Soc Sci Med* 1993;36:249.
39. Gordon EJ, Daugherty CK. "Hitting you over the head:" oncologists disclosure of prognosis to advanced cancer patients. *Bioethics* 2003;17:142.
40. Miller M. Phase I cancer trials: a collusion of misunderstanding. *Hastings Cent Rep* 2000;30:34.
41. Kodish E, Post SG. Oncology and hope. *J Clin Oncol* 1995;13:1817.
42. DelVecchio Good MJ, Good B, Schaffer C, et al. American oncology and the discourse on hope. *Cult Med Psychiatry* 1990;14:59.
43. Amir M. Considerations guiding physicians when informing cancer patients. *Soc Sci Med* 1987;24:741.
44. Heyse-Moore LH, Johnson-Bell VE. Can doctors accurately predict the life expectancy of patients with terminal cancer? *Palliat Med* 1987;1:165.
45. Mackillop WJ, Quirt CF. Measuring the accuracy of prognostic judgments in oncology. *J Clin Epidemiol* 1997;50:21.
46. Christakis N. *Death foretold: prophecy and progress in medical care*. Chicago: University of Chicago Press, 2000.
47. The SUPPORT Principal Investigators. A controlled trial to improve care for seriously ill hospitalized patients. The Study to Understand Prognoses and Preferences for Outcomes and Risks of Treatments (SUPPORT). *JAMA* 1995;274:1591.
48. Foley KM, Gelbard H, eds. *Institute of Medicine report: improving palliative care for cancer*. Washington, DC: National Academy Press, 2001.
49. Virnig BA, Kind S, McBean M, et al. Geographic variation in hospice use prior to death. *J Am Geriatric Soc* 2000;48:1117.

50. Christakis NA, Escarce JJ. Survival of Medicare patients after enrollment in hospice programs. *N Engl J Med* 1996;355:172.
51. McCarthy EP, Burns RB, Ngo-Metzger Q, Davis RB, Phillips RS. Hospice use among Medicare, managed care, and fee-for-service patients dying with cancer. *JAMA* 2003;289:2238.
52. Fallowfield L, Lipkin M, Hall A. Teaching senior oncologists communication skills: results from phase I of a comprehensive longitudinal program in the United Kingdom. *J Clin Oncol* 1998;16:1961.
53. Hinton J. How reliable are relatives' retrospective reports of terminal illness? Patients' and relatives' accounts compared. *Soc Sci Med* 1996;43:1229.
54. Quill TE, Cassel CK, Meier DE. Care of the hopelessly ill. Proposed clinical criteria for physician-assisted suicide. *N Engl J Med* 1992;327:1380.
55. Bukberg J, Penman D, Holland JC. Depression in hospitalized cancer patients. *Psychosom Med* 1984;46:199.
56. Chochinov HM, Wilson KG, Enns M, et al. Prevalence of depression in the terminally ill: effects of diagnostic criteria and symptom threshold judgments. *Am J Psychiatry* 1994;151:537.
57. Allebeck P, Bolund C, Ringback G. Increased suicide rate in cancer patients. A cohort study based on the Swedish Cancer-Environment Register. *J Clin Epidemiol* 1989;42:611.
58. Groenewould JH, Van Der Maas J, Van Der Wal G, et al. Physician-assisted death in psychiatric practice in the Netherlands. *N Engl J Med* 1997;336:1795.
59. Cohen JS, Fihn SD, Boyko EJ, et al. Attitudes toward assisted suicide and euthanasia among physicians in Washington state. *N Engl J Med* 1994;331:89.
60. Back AL, Wallace JI, Starks HE, et al. Physician-assisted suicide and euthanasia in Washington State. Patient requests and physician responses [see comments]. *JAMA* 1996;275:919.
61. Van Der Maas PJ, Van Delden JJ, Pijnenborg L, et al. Euthanasia and other medical decisions concerning the end of life [see comments]. *Lancet* 1991;338:669.
62. Pijenborg L, van der Maas PJ, van Delden JJM, Looman CWN. Life terminating acts without explicit request of the patient. *Lancet* 1993;341:1196.
63. Groenewould JH, van der Heide A, Onwuteaka-Philipsen BN, et al. Clinical problems with performance of euthanasia and PAS in the Netherlands. *N Engl J Med* 2000;348:551.
64. Emanuel EJ, Fairclough DL, Daniels ER, et al. Euthanasia and physician-assisted suicide: attitudes and experiences of oncology patients, oncologists, and the public [see comments]. *Lancet* 1996;347:1805.
65. Howard OM, Fairclough DL, Daniels ER, et al. Physician desire for euthanasia and assisted suicide: would physicians practice what they preach? [see comments]. *J Clin Oncol* 1997;15:428.
66. Emanuel EJ, Daniels ER, Fairclough DL, et al. The practice of euthanasia and physician-assisted suicide in the United States: adherence to proposed safeguards and effects on physicians [see comments]. *JAMA* 1998;280:507.
67. Chiu AE, Hedberg K, Higgison GK, Fleming DW. Legalized physician-assisted suicide in Oregon—the first year's experience. *N Engl J Med* 2000;340:577.
68. Sullivan AD, Itedberg K, Fleming DW. Legalized physician-assisted suicide in Oregon—the second year. *N Engl J Med* 2000;342:598.
69. *The final report of the Advisory Committee on Human Radiation Experiments.* New York: Oxford University Press, 1996.
70. Applebaum PS, Lindz CN, Meisel A. *Informed consent: legal theory and clinical practice.* New York: Oxford University Press, 1987.
71. Levine RJ. *Ethics and regulation of clinical research*, 2nd ed. Baltimore: Urban and Schwarzenburg, 1986.
72. National Commission for the Protection of Human Subjects of Biomedical and Behavioral Research. *Belmont Report: ethical principles and guidelines for the protection of human subjects of research.* Publication number (05) 78-0012. Washington, DC: U.S. Government Printing Office, 1978.
73. Freedman B, Fuks A, Weijer C. Demarcating research in treatment: a systematic approach for the analysis of the ethics of clinical research. *Clin Res* 1992;40:655.
74. The President's Commission for the Study of Ethical Problems in Medicine and Biomedical and Behavioral Research. *Implementing human research regulations: the adequacy and uniformity of federal rules and their implementation.* Publication number 040-000-00471-8. Washington, DC: U.S. Government Printing Office, 1983.
75. Epstein LC, Lasagna L. Obtaining informed consent, form or substance. *Arch Intern Med* 1969;123:682.
76. Gray BH, Cooke RA, Tannebaum AS. Research involving human subjects. The performance of institutional review boards is assessed in this empirical study. *Science* 1978;201:1094.
77. Hammerschmidt DE, Keanse MA. Institutional review board review lacks impact on the readability of consent forms for research. *Am J Med Sci* 1992;304:341.
78. Edgar H, Rothman DJ. The institutional review board and beyond: future challenges to the ethics of human experimentation. *Milbank Q* 1995;73:489.
79. Redshaw ME, Harris A, Baum JD. Research ethics committee audit: differences between committees. *J Med Ethics* 1996;22:78.
80. Kent G. Shared understandings for informed consent: the relevance of psychological research on the provision of information. *Soc Sci Med* 1996;43:1517.
81. Verheggen FWSM, van Wijmen FCB. Informed consent in clinical trials. *Health Policy* 1996;36:131.
82. Simes RJ, Tattersal MHN, Coates AS, et al. Randomized comparison of procedures for obtaining informed consent in clinical trials of treatment for cancer. *BMJ* 1986;293:1065.
83. Daugherty CK. Impact of therapeutic research on informed consent and the ethics of clinical trials: a medical oncology perspective. *J Clin Oncol* 1999;17:1601.
84. Edwards SJL, Lilford RJ, Thornton J, et al. Informal consent for clinical trials: in search of the "best" method. *Soc Sci Med* 1998;47:1825.
85. Ratain MJ, Mick R, Schilsky R, Siegler M. Statistical and ethical issues in the design and conduct of phase I and II clinical trials of new anticancer agents. *J Natl Cancer Inst* 1993;85:1637.
86. Von Hoff DD, Turner J. Response rates, duration of response, and dose response effect in phase I studies in antineoplastics. *Invest New Drugs* 1991;9:115.
87. Decoster G, Stein G, Holdener EE. Responses and toxic deaths in phase I clinical trials. *Ann Oncol* 1990;2:175.
88. Estey E, Hoth D, Wittes R, et al. Therapeutic responses in phase I trials of antineoplastic agents. *Cancer Treat Rep* 1986;70:1105.
89. Smith TL, Lee JJ, Kantarjian HM, et al. Design and results of phase I cancer clinical trials: 3 year experience at MD Anderson Cancer Center. *J Clin Oncol* 1996;14:287.
90. Rodenhuis S, van-den Heuvel WJ, Annyas AA, et al. Patient motivation and informed consent in a phase I study of an anticancer agent. *Eur J Cancer Clin Oncol* 1984;20:457.
91. Willem Y, Sessa C. Informing patients about phase I trials—how should it be done? *Acta Oncol* 1989;28:106.
92. Daugherty CK, Banik DM, Janisch L, Ratain MJ. Quantitative analysis of ethical issues in phase I trials: a survey interview study of 144 advanced cancer patients. *IRB* 2000;22:6.
93. Daugherty CK, Ratain MJ, Minami H, et al. Study of cohort-specific consent and patient control in phase I cancer trials. *J Clin Oncol* 1998;16:2305.
94. Gordon DJ, Daugherty CK. Referral and decision making among advanced cancer patients participating in phase I trials at a single institution. *J Clin Ethics* 2001;12:31.
95. Tomamichel M, Sessa C, Herzig S, et al. Informed consent for phase I studies: evaluation of quantity and quality of information provided to patients. *Ann Oncol* 1995;6:321.
96. Yoder LH, O'Rourke TJ, Ethyre A, Spears DT. Expectations and experiences of patients with cancer participating in phase I clinical trials. *Oncol Nurs Forum* 1997;24:891.
97. Itoh K, Sasaki Y, Fuji H, et al. Patients in phase I trials of anti-cancer agents in Japan: motivation, comprehension and expectations. *Br J Cancer* 1997;76:107.
98. Horng S, Emanuel EJ, Wilfond B, et al. Descriptions of benefits and risks in consent forms for phase I oncology trials. *N Engl J Med* 2003;347:2134.
99. Agrawal M, Emanuel EJ. Ethics of phase I oncology studies. Reexamining the data. *JAMA* 2003;290:1075.
100. Daugherty CK, Kass N, Fogarty L, Sugarman J, Hlubock FJ. Effects of a CD-ROM educational intervention on understanding among advanced cancer patients enrolled in early phase clinical trials. *Proc Am Soc Clin Oncol* 2003;(abst).
101. Marsoni S, Hoth D, Simon R, et al. Clinical drug development: an analysis of phase II trials. *Cancer Treat Rep* 1987;71:80.
102. Schafer A. The ethics of the randomized clinical trial. *N Engl J Med* 1982;307:719.
103. Kodish E, Lantos JD, Siegler M. Ethical considerations in randomized controlled clinical trials. *Cancer* 1990;65(Suppl):2400.
104. Marquis D. Leaving therapy to chance: an impasse in the ethics of clinical trials. *Hastings Cent Rep* 1983;13:40.
105. Hellman S, Hellman DS. Of mice but not men. Problems of the randomized clinical trial. *N Engl J Med* 1991;324:1585.
106. Markman M. Ethical difficulties with randomized clinical trials involving cancer patients: examples from the field of gynecologic oncology. *J Clin Ethics* 1992;3:193.
107. Emanuel EJ, Peterson WB. Ethics of randomized clinical trials. *J Clin Oncol* 1998;16:365.
108. Miller FG, Brody J. A critique of clinical equipoise: therapeutic misconception in the ethics of clinical trials. *Hastings Cent Rep* 2003;33:19.
109. Fried C. *Medical experimentation: personal integrity and social policy.* Amsterdam: North Holland Publishing, 1974.
110. Freedman B. Equipoise and the ethics of clinical research. *N Engl J Med* 1987;317:141.
111. Freedman B. A response to a purported ethical difficulty with randomized clinical trials involving cancer patients. *J Clin Ethics* 1992;3:231.
112. Taylor KM, Margolese RG, Soskolne CL. Physicians' reasons for not entering eligible patients in a randomized clinical trial of surgery for breast cancer. *N Engl J Med* 1984;310:1363.
113. Taylor KM, Shapiro M, Soskolne CL, et al. Physician response to informed consent regulations for randomized clinical trials. *Cancer* 1987;60:1415.
114. Fetting JH, Simonoff LA, Piantodosi S, et al. The effects of patients' expectations of benefit with standard breast cancer adjuvant chemotherapy on participation in a randomized clinical trial: a clinical vignette study. *J Clin Oncol* 1990;8:1476.
115. Silverman WA, Altman DG. Patients' preferences and randomized trials. *Lancet* 1996;347:171.
116. Cassileth BR, Lusk ES, Hurwitz S, et al. Attitudes towards clinical trials among patients and the public. *JAMA* 1982;248:968.
117. Slevin MJ, Stubb L, Plant HJ, et al. Attitudes to chemotherapy: comparing views of patients with cancer with those of doctors, nurses, and the general public. *BMJ* 1990;300:1458.
118. Taylor KM, Feldstein ML, Skeel RT, et al. Fundamental dilemmas of the randomized clinical trial process: results of a survey of 1,737 Eastern Cooperative Oncology Group investigators. *J Clin Oncol* 1994;12:1796.
119. Lynoe N, Sandland M, Jacobson L. Cancer clinical research—some aspects on doctors' attitudes to informing participants. *Acta Oncol* 1996;35:749.
120. Ellis PM. Attitudes towards and participation in randomized clinical trials in oncology: a review of the literature. *Ann Oncol* 2000;11:939.
121. Royall RM. Ignorance and altruism. *J Clin Ethics* 1992;3:229.
122. Gallo C, Perrone F, Deplando S, Giust C. Informed versus randomized consent to clinical trials. *Lancet* 1995;346:1060.
123. Simel DL, Feussner JR. A randomized controlled trial comparing quantitative informed consent formats. *J Clin Epidemiol* 1991;44:771.
124. Baum M. New approach for recruitment into randomized controlled trials. *Lancet* 1993;341:812.
125. Altman DG, Whitehead J, Parman MK, et al. Randomized consent designs in cancer clinical trials. *Eur J Cancer* 1995;31A:1934.
126. Zelen M. Strategy and alternate randomized designs in cancer clinical trials. *Cancer Treat Rep* 1982;66:1095.
127. Riethmuller G, Schneider-Gadicke E, Schilmok G, et al. Randomized trial of monoclonal antibody for adjuvant therapy of resected Dukes' C colorectal carcinoma. *Lancet* 1994;343:1177.
128. Mansour EG, Gray R, Shatila AH, et al. Efficacy of adjuvant chemotherapy of high-risk node-negative breast cancer. *N Engl J Med* 1989;320:485.
129. Fisher B, Redmond C, Poisson R, et al. Eight-year results of a randomized clinical trial comparing total mastectomy and lumpectomy with or without irradiation in the treatment of breast cancer. *N Engl J Med* 1989;320:822.

Economic Issues

ALBERT B. EINSTEIN, JR.

Since the signing of the 1971 National Cancer Act, cancer care delivery has evolved into a very sophisticated, complex system. Modern cancer care programs involve multiple physician specialists, private practice and hospital-based services, and a growing number of supportive care services. With the patient as the focal point, health care institutions have developed comprehensive, multidisciplinary, coordinated cancer care programs that emphasize quality and service.[1] The cancer product line has become one of the top two or three most economically important clinical programs for many academic and community medical centers.

As health care enters the 21st century, the economic issues relevant to health care in general are threatening to dismember the existing cancer care delivery system. All of the key stakeholders in providing cancer care are threatened by the rapid rise in health care costs and the decline in adequate reimbursement for their services. The economic challenge for cancer care providers is how to continue to provide high-quality care with an increasing price tag in a society that is committed to limiting health care expenditures and that does not provide universal health care coverage for its citizens.

U.S. HEALTH CARE ECONOMY

In 1997, health care expenditures in the United States were $1.1 trillion, 14% of the gross national product.[2] Total U.S. expenditures for cancer care accounts for approximately 5% of the total health care expenditures and approximately 10% of all Medicare expenditures.[3] Health care expenditures as a percentage of the gross national product have been rapidly rising (7% in 1970 and 12% in 1990) and are estimated to reach 26% by 2030.[2] Waldo et al.[4] propose that this rapid rise can be explained by multiple factors: (1) the proliferation and cost of new medical technology; (2) the rapid rise in Medicare- and Medicaid-related government spending; (3) the Americans' lack of sensitivity to health care costs with the current insurance programs; (4) the increase in the aged population; and (5) the general lack of incentive in the fee-for-service reimbursement system to enhance efficiency and productivity.

In the early 1990s, the drain of high health care costs reached an intolerable level for employers and government. Per capita health care costs had increased from $750 in 1970 to $2500 in 1990. The 1992 federal budget included $838 billion for health care, compared with $430 billion for education and $270 billion for defense. Medicare's share of the federal budget in 1990 was 7.5% and was projected to be 15% by 2010. Despite the United States' health care expenditure being significantly greater than other Western countries, clinical outcomes data indicated inferior life expectancy and increased infant mortality in the United States.[5] Faced with these economic challenges, both federal and state governments as well as major employers made many efforts on a number of different fronts to reduce the rate of rise of health care spending.

In the 1992 presidential election campaign, health care reform became the major issue with the goals of cost control,

universal health coverage, and continuing high-quality care. Shortly after Bill Clinton's inauguration as president, a major policy planning effort, led by his wife, Hillary Rodham Clinton, produced a managed competition model, a hybrid of government regulation and free-market forces.[6] In this plan, employers and other health care consumers would form health insurance–purchasing cooperatives, and insurance companies would competitively bid for the health care business. A basic benefits package was defined, and health benefits paid for by business would be extended to the uninsured. After extensive debate and lobbying, Congress failed to pass appropriate legislation in 1993 and the Clinton plan died.

Although Congress wrestled with the health care reform issues, a number of states initiated their own efforts at health care reform.[7] Oregon uniquely established a commission that prioritized all medical services and procedures, determined the available state funding, and drew a funding line and thereby established a basic health benefits package for its Medicaid beneficiaries.[8]

In 1994, the Republicans regained control of Congress and many of the state legislatures. They successfully squelched health care reform in favor of using market forces to allocate medical resources.[9] Health care reform was replaced by health care cost control. The majority party pursued significant cost reduction measures in both the Medicare and Medicaid programs to slow the rate of growth of per capita health expenditures. In addition, the federal government encouraged the development of Medicare health maintenance organization (HMO) models (Medicare Plus) to provide a market-driven means of achieving significant cost reductions.

MEDICARE COST-CONTAINMENT EFFORTS

With a significant budget deficit and rising health expenditures, Congress passed the Balanced Budget Act (BBA) of 1997. The BBA limited Medicare expenditures by reforming the Medicare payment system with caps on reimbursement rates and further movement away from cost-based reimbursement. Medicare introduced the hospital outpatient prospective payment system with the use of ambulatory payment categories (APCs) similar to the inpatient prospective payment diagnosis-related group program. The BBA did significantly slow the Medicare spending rate to 1.5% in 1998, with a proposed reduction of $116.4 billion between 1998 and 2002 and $393.8 billion between 1998 and 2007.[10] The majority of reductions were in fee-for-service payments to hospitals, home health agencies, rehabilitation hospitals, and Medicare Plus contractors through the outpatient prospective payment system.

The cost savings of $103 billion to $191.5 billion over the first 5 years exceeded congressional expectations to the detriment of the health care system. These drastic cuts in reimbursement caused significant reduction in hospital and physician profitability, forcing elimination of many nonprofitable services and staff reductions. Some small rural hospitals and home health agencies declared bankruptcy. Academic hospitals experienced marked decreases in graduate medical education expenses and disproportionate share payments. Pressured by inadequate reimbursement, Medicare Plus contractors reduced benefits, adopted enrollment strategies to avoid adverse risk, or withdrew entirely from the program. In 2000, 15% of Medicare beneficiaries withdrew from the Medicare Plus program, 65 insurers failed to renew, and 53

HMOs reduced their coverage benefits.[10] The BBA's negative economic impact was more severe than expected, and some relief was needed.

In 1999, Congress passed the Medicare Balanced Budget Refinement Act, which restored $8.4 billion in reimbursement reductions through adjustments in the update factor of the reimbursement formula. Despite this attempt to lessen the BBA's impact, the American Hospital Association–Lewin Group report predicted that the already thin hospital margins would still be further reduced by 1.6% to 6.6%.[10]

Most recently, after several years of debate and negotiations, Congress passed the Medicare Prescription Drug Improvement and Modernization Act (MMA) of 2003, which implemented prescription drug benefits for seniors as well as many other significant changes that affected cancer care reimbursement. Estimates state that the new law will increase Medicare expenditures by at least $400 billion between 2004 and 2014. However, although trying to increase prescription drug benefits to senior citizens, Congress still has failed to address the fundamental economic issues of U.S. health care: the financing of Medicare for the future, the beneficiaries' basic benefits package, universal health care coverage, and Medicare administrative reform.

MEDICARE REIMBURSEMENT FOR CANCER SERVICES

In addition to the broad negative impact of the BBA, both academic and community cancer care programs have had to cope with additional unique Medicare reimbursement issues, the most significant being chemotherapy reimbursement. The dramatic rise in drug costs, especially cancer chemotherapeutic agents, has been a major problem for Medicare, as well as other payers.

Medicare's initial benefit covered the cost of drugs administered in a hospital inpatient or outpatient setting or incident to a physician visit. Successful lobbying by the oncology community has subsequently resulted in the expansion of this benefit to include reimbursement for (1) oral forms of chemotherapy drugs for which intravenous forms are also available and (2) indications for U.S. Food and Drug Administration–approved chemotherapy drugs other than those for which they were originally approved ("off-label") that are documented in one of the two major drug compendia or peer-reviewed medical literature published in selected publications.

Halbert et al.[11] analyzed claims data to ascertain the specific components of drug spending for cancer care. They concluded that chemotherapy administered in the clinic or office setting was the single most important cost driver compared with supportive therapy and chemotherapy adjuncts. The rapid rise in drug costs (76%) over 3 years was primarily due to a shift in treatment patterns to newer, more expensive antineoplastic agents.

Medicare chemotherapy reimbursement has been based on a drug's average wholesale price (AWP), which is defined by the drug industry and unregulated by law or federal policy. Hospital inpatient drug costs are rolled into the diagnosis-related group payment, and the outpatient costs are either paid individually or bundled into an APC. Physician office drug costs are reimbursed individually as a percentage of AWP. Both hospitals and physicians charge a separate drug administrative fee to cover the costs of supplies, staff, and overhead. Providers have argued that any profit in the drug cost reimbursement goes to offset the losses from the under reimbursement of the drug administration costs and that the two need to be considered together to account for the total cost of chemotherapy.

To help balance the budget in 1997, Congress reduced chemotherapy drug reimbursement from 100% to 95% AWP. More recently, the Centers for Medicare and Medicaid Services (CMS) and some congressional leaders have come to believe that medical oncologists and hospitals were making an inappropriate profit on drugs at Medicare's expense. In 1999 and 2000, Government Accounting Office studies of Medicare's payments for drugs and practice expenses in the private oncologists' practice setting concluded that a wide disparity often existed between a drug's actual acquisition cost (AWP minus 13% to 34%) and Medicare's payment for the drug. The discounts resulted in Medicare paying at least $532 million more than the provider's acquisition cost in 2000.[12] In 2003, CMS used the rules making process to significantly reduce chemotherapy drug reimbursement in the hospital outpatient setting without appropriate readjustment for the costs of drug administration. High-cost drug payment rates were reduced, and all drugs costing less than $150 were bundled into the chemotherapy APC rate.

Congress's most recent attempt to "fix" the chemotherapy reimbursement problem was included in the very complicated 2003 MMA, effective Jan. 1, 2004. The major changes for the office-based oncology practices include the following:

- In 2004, chemotherapy drug reimbursement will decline from 95% to 85% of AWP, but the decline will be partially offset by a one-time 50% to 90% increase in drug administration reimbursement.
- In 2005, the one-time 32% increase in drug administration reimbursement will be eliminated.
- In 2006, Congress has required that CMS enact a new drug payment methodology other than AWP, possibly based on average manufacturers price, widely available market price, manufacturers average sales price, or wholesale acquisition cost.
- In 2006, oncologists may have to choose between purchasing drugs with a reimbursement rate of average sales price plus 6% or obtaining the drugs through a competitive acquisition program contractor, who would manage the Medicare payment.
- The potential reimbursement for oral chemotherapy drugs will be determined after a 2-year demonstration project, with a report to congress by January 1, 2006.

The Congressional Budget Office predicts that government savings in drug acquisition will reach $4.2 billion over 10 years, most of the savings involving cancer chemotherapy drugs.[13] Dr. Margaret Tempero, former president of the American Society of Clinical Oncology, expressed the concerns of many that "the impacts on practices will be far-reaching and severe . . . Some practices will have to cut back on the number of Medicare patients they treat, or stop treating Medicare patients all together."[14]

For hospital-based cancer programs, the 2003 MMA improved chemotherapy drug reimbursement by $150 million compared with the significant reductions created in 2003 by CMS rule making. Important hospital reimbursement changes effective January 2004 included the following:

- New drugs and biologics on the 2003 pass-through payment schedule will be paid at 85% of AWP if they were approved by the U.S. Food and Drug Administration before April 1, 2003, or 95% of AWP if approved after April 1, 2003.

- Sole-source drugs and biologicals will have a payment floor of 88% of AWP in 2004 and 83% in 2005 and a payment ceiling of 95% of AWP.
- Innovator multiple-source drugs will have a payment ceiling of 68% of AWP without a payment floor, and noninnovator multiple-source drugs, a ceiling of 46% of AWP.
- New drugs and biologicals will be paid at 95% of AWP immediately after U.S. Food and Drug Administration approval until a Healthcare Common Procedure Coding System code is assigned.
- Only drugs costing less than $50 will be bundled into the administration APC compared with the previous $150 level.
- Multiple pushes of drugs will be paid for with a once-daily limitation.

The law also requires two Government Accounting Office surveys in 2004 and 2005 of the true hospital drug acquisition costs so that drugs can be reimbursed based on acquisition cost beginning in 2006. An additional study will be performed by the Medicare Payment Advisory Commission with a report to Congress by January 1, 2006 to evaluate the costs of pharmacy, handling, and overhead in the hospital setting.[13] Clearly, future changes in chemotherapy reimbursement are to be anticipated, with potential significant impact on patient access to care, site of care, medical oncology manpower, and the introduction of new exciting chemotherapeutic and biologic agents.

Historically, radiation therapy, especially intensity-modulated radiation therapy, has been relatively well reimbursed by Medicare. Cancer programs have used the revenues from radiation therapy to offset the losses of other essential cancer services. Beginning in 2004, however, CMS has implemented reductions as high as 30% in many APC payments for common radiation therapy procedures. The 2003 MMA does require that all devices of brachytherapy consisting of a seed or seeds (or radioactive source) be paid based on the hospital's charge for each device adjusted to cost rather than a fixed amount for the procedure.[13] However, the complexity of radiation therapy coding with the new APC system has resulted in many hospitals not adequately reporting their radiation therapy charges to Medicare. Medicare's reimbursement rates are based on the charges reported by the hospitals. Accurate and complete charge reporting is essential for Medicare to appropriately reimburse for any service. The challenge of managing radiation therapy programs continues to be the high cost of capital investment with changing, unpredictable payment rates.

MEDICAID COST-CONTAINMENT EFFORTS

Medicaid also has experienced significant growth and funding problems during the 1990s and early 2000s. In 2002, 51 million persons, or one in seven, were on a Medicaid program, more than Medicare. The federal government provided $259 billion, 57% of total funding for Medicaid and $2 billion more than Medicare. With the economic recession of the early 2000s, states have experienced a marked decline in revenues and double-digit increases in their health care expenditures. The 2002 growth rate of Medicaid expenditures was 12.1% compared with the 8.8% annual growth predicted for 2002 to 2012 and the average 7.1% annual growth rate for all health care expenditures.[15] States have attempted to limit the costs of prescrip-

tion drugs, reduce or delay reimbursement for providers, limit program eligibility, reduce the number of beneficiaries, or in the case of Oregon, ration health care. In response to Medicaid's declining reimbursement and increasing paperwork, many physicians have elected not to participate in their state's Medicaid program. As a result, Medicaid beneficiaries' access to primary care providers and to specialists has become limited. Many beneficiaries delay getting health care early and seek urgent health care at hospital emergency departments only when absolutely necessary. In turn, hospital emergency departments are facing a crisis in managing the increased patient volumes and finding physicians willing to care for the Medicaid patients. This social and health care dilemma awaits Congress and the administration's determination of the amount and mechanisms of federal support for Medicaid programs during this time of economic recession,

INSURANCE INDUSTRY COST-CONTAINMENT EFFORTS

After the failure of the national health care reform plan in 1993, the insurance industry and large employers emerged as the driving forces to reduce the cost of health care. Managed care plans replaced the traditional indemnity plans. Investor-owned health plans, hospitals, and health care companies began to flourish and became the "darlings of Wall Street." Insurers gained control of large populations of patients, limited the size of their physician provider panels, and used primary care gatekeepers and preauthorization controls to limit use of expensive medical specialists and procedures. The insurers negotiated marked reductions in hospitalization costs in exchange for access to patients. Capitated insurance plans that provided a fixed payment per patient regardless of costs were implemented.

In response to perceived opportunities, insurance plans initially proliferated. As profits subsequently failed to materialize, consolidation created fewer, larger, and more powerful insurance corporations. The large HMOs became models for standardizing care, increasing efficiency and reducing costs. The goals of the insurance industry were to reduce their costs, offer lower premiums to employers, limit their high-risk liability, and increase their profits.

Many managed care plans enthusiastically contracted with Medicare to manage its beneficiaries and offered additional benefits such as outpatient prescription drug coverage to lure enrollees (Medicare Plus program). However, the inadequate federal payments resulting from the BBA forced many companies to reduce benefits or withdraw altogether from the program. Many beneficiaries were forced to return to the standard Medicare program and seek gap coverage.[10]

The managed care model has remained strong in states such as Florida and California, whereas more open discounted fee-for-service contracts with preferred provider organizations have become more common in other geographic areas. After a period of severe reductions in reimbursement and significant cost cutting, the more powerful provider organizations have forced renegotiations of reimbursement rates to recover their true costs. Some hospitals and physician groups have refused to contract with individual insurance plans rather than provide services for rates below their costs. In addition, consumer demand has forced insurers to once again offer patient choice of providers and direct access to specialty care. The era of severe ratcheting down of provider reimbursement and control of patient choice seems to have passed. Many insurers are now looking at standardization of care, quality measures, and provider report cards as means of directing patients to quality, efficient providers.

HOSPITAL ECONOMIC ISSUES

During the managed care era of the 1990s, hospitals were forced to accept lower reimbursement, reduce costs, and develop new organizational and network strategies to remain economically viable and competitive. Hospitals in many areas consolidated into integrated health care systems or networks to become more cost-efficient, control capital expenditures, and command larger market shares. Antitrust laws, fraud and abuse issues, and taxation concerns created significant obstacles in developing these relationships. For-profit hospital management companies purchased many struggling smaller rural hospitals as well as some highly inefficient urban medical centers to develop large, bottom-line–driven organizations.

To improve their financial situation, many hospitals have strategically emphasized their more profitable clinical programs and deemphasized or eliminated entirely their nonprofitable services. Cancer services, along with cardiovascular, are usually one of the largest and more profitable clinical areas for full-service hospitals. Hospital-based cancer care programs have evolved since the early 1970s into very sophisticated, well-coordinated multidisciplinary services dedicated to optimizing both disease management and quality of life.[1] Many hospitals have developed cancer product or service line management structures. The product line's strategic goals usually are to increase efficiency and coordination in a high-volume program, increase patient volumes, enhance the community reputation, and attract medical and nursing expertise. Hospitals are investing significant capital in new cancer facilities and technology to support the service lines in this very competitive market segment.

While trying to maintain the economic viability of their cancer programs with rapidly changing reimbursement, some cancer programs have found themselves in competition with members of their own medical staff or for-profit service organizations for the more profitable ambulatory services. In some communities, radiation oncologists have built their own freestanding radiation therapy centers in direct competition with and to the disadvantage of their local hospital. Private practice medical oncologists, who have traditionally administered chemotherapy in their offices, have added additional services such as diagnostic positron emission tomography scanners as new profit centers. Outpatient administration of chemotherapy and management of associated complications have become more sophisticated, reducing the need for hospital admissions. In response to the competition from office-based oncologists, some hospitals are employing oncologists to keep their cancer program and related revenues intact. Approximately 60% to 70% of hospital cancer program revenues is now generated in the outpatient setting.

Continued analysis of the cancer product line is essential for optimal management and justification for its existence and investment of new capital resources. An evaluation of the economic impact of a hospital's comprehensive cancer program should include cancer screening, the standard inpatient and outpatient treatment services (radiation therapy, medical oncology, chemotherapy drugs and administration, and surgery) as well as related ancillary and supportive care services. A cancer-related diagnosis-related group analysis provides a limited data set and misses many legitimate cases. A cancer-related *International Classification of Diseases*, ninth revision procedure code analysis including primary, secondary, and tertiary codes is preferable. This model provides a more inclusive data set representative of the scope of cancer services to best understand the program's true economic value.

With decreasing reimbursement, however, hospitals continue to struggle to maintain comprehensive programs. Many essential nonreimbursable services that enhance the cancer patient's quality of life are economically threatened because they are not directly reimbursable, and their costs are paid for by the more profitable treatment services. Operational revenues have historically funded continued capital investments in new emerging technology and staff support for clinical research. Many health care institutions are now appealing to their communities for more philanthropic support for new facilities, new technology, clinical research, and patient supportive care services and programs. Although some have had a long tradition for philanthropic support, many have only recently initiated or reenergized their development programs. However, the economic recession of the early 2000s has made development efforts even more challenging.

PHYSICIAN ECONOMIC ISSUES

In the 1990s, independent practicing physicians had difficulty coping with the pressures of decreasing reimbursement, the controls and contractual complexities of managed care, the increasing practice overhead costs, and the rise in malpractice insurance premiums. Some formed independent physicians' associations and/or joined physician provider organizations, physician–hospital alliances, and HMOs to compete for managed care contracts and preserve a flow of patients. Others abandoned private practice to become employed physicians of hospitals, insurance corporations, or for-profit physician management corporations. For-profit practice management companies, such as Texas Oncology and American Oncology Resources, later to merge into US Oncology, initially bought medical oncology practices to form a national network. Physicians sought professional security and predictability by being part of larger organizations.[16]

The penetration and impact of managed care contracting on physicians vary significantly from one area of the United States to another. Managed care has initially reduced the professional costs of cancer care in the larger population areas. However, patient pressures for access to physicians of their choice, especially specialists, have forced managed care organizations to open their physician panels and allow direct patient access to specialists and hospitals of their choice.

Medicare reimbursement policies are critical to the practicing oncologists because 30% or more of their patients are likely to be Medicare beneficiaries and the private insurance industry often adapts its policies to mimic Medicare. Practice overhead, including the costs of compliance with payer and regulatory requirements and malpractice insurance, continues to increase. Caring for the needs of cancer patients is more time-consuming and resource-intensive than managing primary care or general internal medicine patients. The medical oncologists' challenges are convincing the payers to recognize the uniqueness of their practices, obtaining adequate reimbursement for their services and continuing to be able to provide chemotherapy profitably in the office setting.

NATIONAL CANCER INSTITUTE–DESIGNATED AND UNIVERSITY CANCER CENTERS ECONOMIC ISSUES

Academic medical centers were also forced to undergo radical changes in their culture and practice to survive in the managed care world. They have had to develop clinical programs that economically compete with the private practice sector to produce clinical revenue for faculty support and to ensure patient access for their primary missions: education and research. Although academic institutions traditionally have represented excellence, managed care organizations have not seen them as adding value or improving their margin or market share. The payers believe that academic centers have not been cost-competitive and do not understand health care economics.[17,18]

Reorganization strategies were pursued by academic medical centers in the 1990s to retain economic viability. Tulane University sold its hospital to a for-profit hospital management corporation and used the proceeds of the sale to support its academic mission.[19] The University of Oregon Health Sciences Center legislatively separated itself from the University of Oregon to enable it to be more competitive in the health care environment.[20] The University of Arizona's clinical faculty and the community physicians in Tucson, AZ, formed a network to secure primary care patients for the academic physicians and to preserve self-determination for the community physicians.[21] The University of Pennsylvania purchased and allied itself with other hospitals and medical practices.[22] Academic medical centers also had to provide more service-oriented, accessible, cost-efficient clinical group practices to be more competitive and generate funding for their faculties. Many have developed networks of primary care practices that feed patients into academic specialty clinics and the academic medical center. The nature of "town-and-gown" relations has become more economically determined, hence more competitive rather than collegial.

The BBA of 1997 substantially reduced payments for graduate medical education to teaching hospitals. Medicare has always recognized the greater cost of teaching hospitals through the direct graduate medical education and the indirect graduate medical education payments. In 1997, the total direct graduate medical education payment was $2.3 billion and the indirect graduate medical education payment, $5.1 billion.[23] Many members of Congress believed that the teaching hospitals were too expensive and "fat." The BBA proposed to reduce the indirect graduate medical education by 29% over 5 years. At the same time, the private insurance industry reduced its reimbursement rates to academic centers because it did not believe it was its role to subsidize medical education. The result was a freezing of resident physician positions in many specialties and cancellation of educational program expansion plans.

In addition, the BBA reduced disproportionate care payments, which helped to offset the cost of charity care, by 5% over 5 years, then revised to 3% in 2001 and 4% in 2002.[23] Many academic hospitals had a significant charity care mission in their communities. Hence, this reduction in funding coupled with the reductions in Medicaid reimbursement had particularly deleterious economic impact on the teaching hospitals.

In the 1990s, a number of academic institutions had additional economic problems related to Medicare fraud and abuse charges. The Investigator General's Office and the Federal Bureau of Investigation initiated a substantial Medicare fraud investigation of selected academic institutions regarding improper or absence of documentation of services for which Medicare was billed. For the initial institutions audited, documentation was found to be lacking, which resulted in multimillion dollar settlements. These investigations forced academic institutions to revise their documentation and coding and billing practices and policies to ensure compliance with Medicare regulations. Corporate compliance programs were established at significant cost. Faculty physicians were forced to ensure their presence, in addition to the resident physicians, at the time that billable services were provided and had to appropriately document their involvement. These changes significantly increased the time faculty physicians spent on clinical services rather than relying extensively on the resident physicians to perform many of these functions.

With declining clinical revenue and increased competition for research funding, academic cancer center faculties have been forced to expand clinical revenues in support of faculty salaries. Some have developed clinical faculty tracks to recognize and appropriately promote primarily clinical faculty. However, the increased emphasis on clinical practice potentially diminishes faculties' academic performance, particularly for junior faculty members. In addition, the academic cancer centers' increased clinical visibility in their communities has in many cases positioned them to be in competition with the private practice of oncology, frequently their major source of referrals for research protocols. Many National Cancer Institute (NCI)–designated centers, such as the H. Lee Moffitt Cancer Center & Research Institute, have developed community affiliate networks that promote collaborative research-based relationships with the private oncology community.

CLINICAL RESEARCH

The federally funded NCI has been the major funding source for the U.S. cancer research effort since the 1971 National Cancer Act. The NCI has been instrumental in supporting through its peer-review evaluation process individual research projects, intramural research, the cancer center program, cancer control research, special research programs, and the clinical trial infrastructure. Since 1999, the president and Congress have been committed to doubling the funding for the National Institutes of Health, including the NCI. The Y2005 NCI requested budget is $6.211 billion, with $626 million for research project grants, $59 million for intramural research, $120 million for cancer centers, $225 million for clinical trials infrastructure, and $63 million for Special Programs of Research Excellence.[24]

Clinical trial research has been an integral part of private oncology practice, as well as academic practice, and has been instrumental in developing new cancer therapies. The funding for these trials generally comes from federal government grants and from pharmaceutical and medical technology industry contracts. Accrual to clinical trials has been problematic in the managed care and cost reduction environment due to the payers' perception that care in a clinical trial was more expensive than standard care and not proven treatment. Managed care organizations often had blanket policies denying reimbursement for services provided for patients on a research trial, or they considered them on a case-by-case basis. Whether insurance companies should pay patient care costs on expensive clinical trials such as autologous stem cell transplant for metastatic breast cancer has been extremely controversial, with some patients suing their insurance companies to gain access to the investigational therapy.[25]

The question whether medical care on a sponsored clinical research trial costs significantly more than standard care has been studied. The Congressional Budget Office[26] estimated that clinical trial costs would be 25% higher than standard care. A Mayo Clinic study[27] showed the costs to be 3% to 13% higher depending on the clinical trial. A Kaiser HMO study[28] reported a 10% higher mean 1-year direct patient care cost for clinical trial enrollees compared with matched controls treated with standard therapy, with the major difference being the cost of the chemotherapy, especially for patients on a bone marrow transplant protocol. A Memorial Sloan-Kettering study[29] found that care in a clinical trial was 17% less than standard care. An American Association of Cancer Institutes pilot study[30] failed to show any significant difference in charges between study patients and control patients. Hence, the available data indicate that clinical trial participation does not significantly increase patient care costs, if at all, compared with standard care except for bone marrow transplant protocols.

In the late 1990s, patient advocacy groups and the oncology professional community exerted significant pressure on government and private payers to provide funding for patient care costs in clinical trials. As of August 2001, 14 states had passed comprehensive clinical trial legislation mandating the coverage of routine patient care costs for patients in approved clinical trials. The Institute of Medicine[31] in its 2000 report on the quality of cancer care recommended that Medicare reimburse for the "routine care for patients in clinical trials in the same way it reimburses for routine care for patients not in clinical trials." In 2000, President Bill Clinton ordered Medicare to reimburse for medical care expenses incurred as part of clinical trials funded or conducted by governmental agencies as well as those meeting qualifying criteria. With the federal government having taken the lead, the NCI has negotiated similar coverage with many of the major private insurers.

In spite of improved funding for patient care costs and sponsor funding of individual trials, conducting a major clinical trials research program as part of a comprehensive cancer program is still expensive. Funding for research infrastructure costs from the NCI Community Clinical Oncology Program, clinical research organizations, and the pharmaceutical industry has facilitated community clinical research efforts, producing a significant increase in accrual to cooperative group and industry sponsored clinical trials. Decreasing patient care reimbursement, however, has sufficiently stressed both the physicians and health care institutions to weaken support for clinical research programs. Increasing governmental regulations and industry sponsor requirements have significantly increased the indirect costs of clinical research. Practicing oncologists, pressured to see an increasing number of patients, have less time to devote to discussing clinical trials with their patients. Most community clinical research programs are unable to cover total costs through grants and contracts and need to supplement funding with operational revenues or philanthropy. In spite of these impediments, many private practice oncologists continue to justify clinical research as an essential component of oncology practice and an important resource for new patient referrals.

Evaluating the economic impact of new therapies has become an important component of many clinical trials. The NCI has provided procedures and guidelines for performing economic evaluations alongside cancer clinical trials.[32] These analyses have been important in choosing between two or more treatments that yield clinically similar outcomes, as in the case of non–small cell lung cancer.[33] Expensive cancer supportive care drugs such as the colony-stimulating factors, erythropoietin, and antiemetics have undergone significant economic analysis to clarify and substantiate their value in reducing complications of chemotherapy.[34,35] Cancer Care Ontario, a provincial agency mandated to integrate and coordinate the cancer control services in Ontario, Canada, systematically evaluates each new drug based on clinical evidence and cost in deciding about purchasing a new drug for its regional cancer care network.[36] With the high cost of new drugs, many hospital pharmacy and therapeutics committees and insurance carriers now consider both clinical benefit and cost in introducing new agents to their formularies.

IMPACT OF GENOMICS

One of the major milestones in biologic discovery has been the decoding of the human genome.[37] This remarkable feat has contributed immensely to the understanding of cancer as a genetic disease and the identification of specific genetic abnormalities associated with the development of specific types of cancer. Genetic testing is now a standard of practice for evaluating individuals believed to be at high risk for breast, ovarian, hereditary nonpolyposis colon, hereditary polyposis colon, and medullary thyroid cancers. Five percent to 10% of people with common cancers have family histories of cancer, some representing a genetic predisposition to the cancer.[38]

The economic consideration of genetic screening for hereditary cancers is a significant issue, given its relatively low frequency in the overall population and the fact that currently many insurers do not pay for testing. Brown and Kessler[39] explored the economic implications of screening for hereditary nonpolyposis colon. They concluded that genetic testing should be preserved for patients with known family histories that suggest the syndrome and not be applied to the overall population in order to contain its associated cost.

Genomics has the potential to transform the management of cancer through identifying high-risk patients, initiating prevention strategies, diagnosing cancer earlier, identifying individual cancer susceptibility to various treatments, and predicting an individual patient's likelihood of response or complications from treatment. The knowledge of an individual's health care risks potentially will increase their health insurance cost, which may influence employers regarding hiring the individual and/or providing benefits. The identification of high-cancer-risk individuals and early institution of effective cancer prevention strategies will lead to the elimination of significant health care costs associated with the treatment of the disease. Insurers and employers, it is hoped, will recognize the economic benefits of this strategy and support it.

COMPLEMENTARY AND ALTERNATIVE MEDICINE

Complementary and alternative methods (CAMs) include many different services and therapies ranging from generally accepted supportive care services to non–evidenced-based treatments touted to be "natural" and an alternative to evidence-based allopathic medicine. Eisenberg et al.[40] first reported in 1993 that 34% of cancer patients used at least one CAM therapy in the previous year. In 1997, patients spent $27 billion of out-of-pocket expenses for CAMs, an amount comparable to all U.S. physician services.[41] A telephone survey[42] of western Washington cancer patients revealed that 70.2% used at least one form of CAMs, 16.6% were seeing alternative providers, 19.1% were using mind relaxation therapies, and 64.6% used dietary supplements. Expenditures for CAMs averaged $68 per user per year, with a range of $4 to $14,659. Expense estimates for dietary and herbal supplements have ranged from $4 to $2861 per year. CAM usage has been correlated with younger age, female gender, higher education status, and higher income.

Insurance coverage for CAMs varies considerably from state to state and from plan to plan. Some states such as Washington mandate that insurers cover a large number of these services and license CAM providers. Most herbal medications and CAM services are generally out-of-pocket expenses based on lack of evidence of efficacy.

The realization that CAMs are popular and a major economic factor has forced allopathic medicine to strategize how to cope with it. The federal government has established the NCI Office of Cancer Complementary and Alternative Medicine and the National Center for Complementary and Alternative Medicine to promote and support research on the efficacy and safety of alternative therapies. Several NCI-designated cancer centers such as Memorial Sloan-Kettering Cancer Center, the Dana-Farber Cancer Institute, and the M. D. Anderson Cancer Center have established research programs in complementary therapies.[43] Many community medical centers have embraced CAM services as part of their comprehensive cancer program, and some emphasize it to differentiate their program from the competition.[44] New outpatient cancer centers are being designed with dedicated space for spas and CAM services. Experience, however, demonstrates that cancer programs should consider CAM services to enhance the quality of a cancer patient's life, not as a significant profit center.

STANDARDIZATION OF PRACTICE

Unnecessary variability in medical care has accounted for a significant amount of economic waste and created quality-of-care issues. Many organizations have resorted to clinical guidelines and pathways to better manage cancer care, reduce practice variability, and promote cost efficiency. The Institute of Medicine[45] has defined practice guidelines as "systematically developed statements to assist practitioner and patient decisions about appropriate health care for specific clinical circumstances." Credible guidelines are evidence-based, although consensus development plays an important role where evidence is lacking. They should apply to 60% of the cases in a given category. Forty percent variability is to be expected and accepted. A pathway differs from a guideline in being a detailed step-by-step description of optimal management for a particular clinical procedure. National level oncology guidelines have been developed by the National Comprehensive Cancer Network, American Society of Clinical Oncology, NCI consensus development conferences, the Agency for Healthcare and Quality Research, and many specialty professional societies. Although they do not directly address the cost of cancer care, guidelines have been used by hospitals, medical practices, and insurers as a benchmark for standardization and judging the appropriateness of clinical practices with economic implications. Smith and Hillner[46] reported that documented improvement in compliance rates, lengths of stay, complication rates, and financial outcomes are linked to provider accountability and incentives for the process and outcomes. Many insurers work with clinical practitioners to define guidelines to facilitate appropriate reimbursement decisions.

Individual hospitals have effectively reduced costs by implementing clinical pathways and case management systems that standardize equipment, procedures, supplies, drug use, and nursing practices. Chemotherapy and supportive care drug use have been prime targets for these pathways because of their relatively high cost and susceptibility to variability of physician practice. Reducing the variability of supplies, equipment, drugs, and clinical practice has become a potent tool for reducing costs in the hospital setting.

HEALTH ECONOMICS AND THE ECONOMIC BURDEN OF CANCER

The scholastic field of health care economics has gained prominence as the financial resources for health care have become constrained. Its application to cancer care is still in the earliest phases. Government, private payers, the pharmaceutical industry, and even health care providers all recognize the growing need to consider costs and outcomes when making public policy and clinical decisions. Economic analyses provide insight into the costs to be considered when making these decisions.[45]

A common economic analysis in oncology focuses on the economic burden for society of a particular type of cancer or on comparing costs and benefits of two or more different procedures or treatment regimens.[47] The *economic burden* of a particular type of cancer is defined as the costs of the resources directly used in treatment and care plus the value of the loss of production and other useful activities caused by the illness or its treatment. Economic analyses assume that the goal of health care policy makers is to maximize the total aggregate health care benefits obtained. The overall direct health care cost of cancer comprises only 5% to 7% of the total U.S. costs of illness.

Economic studies that focus on the long-term costs of cancer care at the individual patient level are more useful as inputs to cost-effectiveness studies or to estimate capitation payments for cancer cases. The Surveillance, Epidemiology, and End Results program (SEER)–Medicare linked database has become an important resource for cost-of-care–related data.[48] The SEER program tumor registry is used to identify individual cases with a particular type and stage of disease, and the Medicare database provides the direct costs for the identified cases by both Part A and Part B reimbursement.

Brown et al.[49] reported the estimated total cost of illness from cancer in 1990 to be $96.126 billion, of which $27.458 billion was direct cost of care, $9.895 billion was cost of loss of work, and $58.773 billion was lost income due to death. From 1963 to 1995, the direct cost of cancer care as a percentage of all health care costs has been relatively stable at approximately 5% in spite of an increase from $1.279 billion to $41.2 billion. Brown et al. provides an excellent discussion of the hazards of this kind of analysis.

Brown et al.[49] also reported the cancer site–specific direct cost estimates per case according to stage at diagnosis using the SEER-Medicare linked database. One of the advantages of this analysis is the ability to estimate costs for different phases of the illness. The national direct costs for Medicare beneficiaries in 1996 for all sites was $42.39 billion, for breast cancer $5.98 billion, for colorectal cancer $5.71 billion, for prostate cancer $4.61 billion, and for lung cancer $4.68 billion. In 1996, the average Medicare payments per individual with breast cancer in the first year after diagnosis for breast cancer was $9230, with colorectal cancer $21,608, with lung cancer $20,340, and with prostate cancer $8869.[50] The higher first-year costs in part related to the inadequate screening for colorectal and lung cancers, resulting in higher percentages of patients presenting with more advanced disease and requiring more expensive treatment. The SEER database has also been linked to HMO cost-of-care databases for cost analyses of patients younger than age 65 with different types of cancer to provide similar analyses.[51] The methodology for developing estimates of the indirect costs of cancer care has not been as well developed as for the direct costs.

Brown et al.[49] believe that the value and purposes of these economic evaluations are to (1) provide one component of the overall economic burden associated with cancer morbidity and mortality; (2) help understand the magnitude of financial and productive resources that must be mobilized to effectively care for cancer patients; (3) provide inputs to cost-effectiveness evaluations of cancer control strategies; and (4) evaluate the societal benefit–cost returns on investments in cancer research and control. Economic analyses are important to governmental agencies and HMOs that need to rationally allocate limited resources and make decisions between alternative policies and interventions.

THE FUTURE

Contemporary society faces the immense problems of rising health care costs, limited resources for health care, and the lack of universal health care. America needs to decide whether health care is a human right or an economic privilege and how many resources should be committed to it in an era of competing economic demands. Leadership is required to establish a framework for the health care system of the future, toward which society can move in a stepwise manner.

Neither Congress nor the presidency has to date shown the willingness or ability to address major health care reform. Rather, government and employers have decided they can afford only a specific amount of health care expenditure and, since 1997, have chosen a cost-containment health care strategy. The congressional debate over the 2003 omnibus Medicare bill has revealed the marked differences in visions for the Medicare of the future. Both the House and Senate envision a greater participation of private health plans in Medicare. The House version directs Medicare to compete with private insurance plans.[52] Congress is obviously seeking ways to shift some of the burden of Medicare to the private sector and to its beneficiaries.

Under the pressure of limited reimbursement over the past decade, health care providers have been forced to reduce their costs and limit their services. At the same time, citizens are increasingly demanding and using health care services. Each individual faced with a medical crisis wants the very best care possible as rapidly as possible. This cost-containment strategy can work only short-term before the cancer care delivery system is severely damaged to the detriment of quality patient care. Piecemeal changes such as reducing reimbursement for the cost of chemotherapy drugs without adjusting the rest of the system will produce highly deleterious effects on the availability and quality of cancer care services. The economic forces at work will potentially make providing cancer care so difficult for hospitals and physicians that the entire system that has been developed over the past 30 years will be destroyed. The ultimate loser is the patient, who is in desperate need of high-quality, comprehensive cancer care.

REFERENCES

1. Einstein Jr AB. Societal issues in oncology: Health care reform. In: DeVita Jr VT, Hellman S, Rosenberg SA, eds. *Cancer, principles and practice of oncology*, 5th ed. Philadelphia: Lippincott–Raven Publishers, 1997:2957.
2. Smith S, Heffler S, Freeland M, et al. The next decade of health spending: a new outlook. *Health Aff (Millwood)* 1999;18:86.
3. Hodgson TA, Cohen AJ. Medical expenditures for major diseases. *Health Care Financ Rev* 1999;21:119.
4. Waldo DR, Sonnefeld ST, Lemieux JA, et al. Health spending through 2030: three scenarios. *Health Aff (Millwood)* 1991;10:231.
5. Everson LK. Cancer program development in the 1990s. *Oncol Issues* 1993;8:8.
6. Clinton B. The Clinton health care plan. *N Engl J Med* 1992;327:804.
7. Rogal DL, Helm WD. State models: tracking states' efforts to reform their health systems. *Health Aff (Millwood)* 1993;12:27.
8. Fox DM, Leichter HM. The ups and downs of Oregon's rationing plan. *Health Aff (Millwood)* 1993;12:66.
9. Iglehart JK. Republicans and the new politics of health care. *N Engl J Med* 1995;332:972.
10. Rivers PA, Tsai KL. The impact of the Balanced Budget Act of 1997 on Medicare in the USA: the fallout continues. *Int J Health Care Qual Assur Inc Leadersh Health Serv* 2002;15:249.
11. Halbert RJ, Zaher C, Wade S, et al. Outpatient cancer drug costs: changes, drivers, and the future. *Cancer* 2002;94:1142.
12. Iglehart JK. Health policy report: Medicare and drug pricing. *N Engl J Med* 2003;348:1590.
13. Association of Community Cancer Centers. The issues: historic changes to Medicare will affect cancer programs. *Oncol Issues* 2004;19:8.
14. American Society of Clinical Oncology news release. ASCO criticizes cuts to cancer care included in medicare bill. Nov. 25, 2003.
15. Iglehart JK. Health policy report: the dilemma of Medicaid. *N Engl J Med* 2003;348:2140.
16. Bodenheimer T. The American health care system: physicians and the changing medical marketplace. *N Engl J Med* 1999;340:584.
17. Golembesky HE. New market forces are special challenge to academic health centers. *Physician Exec* 1995;21:18.
18. Iglehart JK. The American health care system: teaching hospitals. *N Engl J Med* 1993;329:1052.
19. Pope J. Tulane: rocking the gentle South. *GFP Notes* 1995;8:10.
20. Kertesz L. Oregon academic medical center breaks state tie. *Mod Healthc* 1995;30:20.
21. Montague J. Southwest symbiosis. *Hosp Health Netw* 1994;20:40.
22. Iglehart JK. Academic medical centers enter the market: the case of Philadelphia. *N Engl J Med* 1995;333:1019.
23. Dickler R, Shaw G. The Balanced Budget Act of 1997: its impact on US teaching hospitals. *Ann Intern Med* 2000;132:820.

24. von Eschenbach. The nation's investment in cancer research. A plan for fiscal year 2005. NIH publication No. 30-5446. October 4, 2003.

25. Peters WP, Rogers MC. Variation in approval by insurance companies of coverage for autologous bone marrow transplantation for breast cancer. *N Engl J Med* 1994;330: 473.

26. *Congressional Budget Office Cost Estimate, G.G. 3605/S: 1980, Patients' Bill of Rights Act of 1998.* Congressional Budget Office, U.S. Congress, Washington D.C. World Wide Web URL: http://www.cbo.gov. July 16, 1998.

27. Wagner JL, Alberts SR, Sloan JA, et al. Incremental costs of enrolling patients in clinical trials: a population based study. *J Natl Cancer Inst* 1999;91:847.

28. Fireman BH, Fehrenbacher L, Gruskin EP, et al. Cost of care for patients in cancer clinical trials. *J Natl Cancer Inst* 2000;92:136.

29. Quirk J, Schrag D, Radzylner M, et al. Clinical trial costs are similar to and may be less than standard care and inpatient (INPT) charges at an academic medical center (AMC) are similar to major, minor, and non-teaching hospitals. *Proc Am Soc Clin Oncol* 2000;19:433a(abstr 1696).

30. Bennett CL, Stinson TJ, Vogel V, et al. Evaluating the financial impact of clinical trials in oncology: results from a pilot study from the Association of American Cancer Institutes/ Northwestern University clinical trials costs and charges project. *J Clin Oncol* 2000;18:2805.

31. Aaron HJ, Gelband H, eds. *Extending Medicare reimbursement in clinical trials: Committee on Routine Patient Care Costs in Clinical Trials for Medicare Beneficiaries.* Washington D.C.: National Academy Press, 2000.

32. Schulman KA, Boyko Jr WL. Evaluating cancer costs in NCI trials. *Cancer Treat Res* 1998;97:37.

33. Saristan JA, Kennedy-Martin T, Rosell R, et al. Economic evaluation in a randomized phase III clinical trial comparing gemcitabine/cisplatin and etoposide/cisplatin in non-small cell lung cancer. *Lung Cancer* 2000;28:97.

34. Stewart DJ, Dahrouge S, Coyle D, Evans WK. Costs of treating and preventing nausea and vomiting in patients receiving chemotherapy. *J Clin Oncol* 1999;17:344.

35. Lyman GH, Kuderer NM, Balducci L. Cost-benefit analysis of granulocyte colony-stimulating factor in the management of elderly cancer patients. *Curr Opin Hematol* 2002;9:207.

36. Evans WK, Nefsky M, Pater J, et al. Cancer Care Ontario's new drug funding program: controlled introduction of expensive anticancer drugs. *Chronic Dis Can* 2002;23:152.

37. Collins FS. Shattuck lecture—medical and societal consequences of the Human Genome Project. *N Engl J Med* 1999;341:28.

38. Ponder BAJ. Costs, benefits and limitations of genetic testing for cancer risk. *Br J Cancer* 1999;80 (Suppl 1):46.

39. Brown ML, Kessler LG. The use of gene test to detect hereditary predisposition to cancer: economic considerations. *J Natl Cancer Inst* 1995;87:1131.

40. Eisenberg DM, Kessler RC, Foster C, et al. Unconventional medicine in the United States. *N Engl J Med* 1993;328:246.

41. Eisenberg DM, Davis RB, Etiner SL, et al. Trends in alternative medicine use in the United States, 1990–1997. *JAMA* 1998;280:1569.

42. Patterson RE, Neuhouser ML, Henderson MM, et al. Types of alternative medicine used by patients with breast, colon, or prostate cancer: predictors, motives and costs. *J Altern Complement Med* 2002;8:477.

43. Richardson MA, Sanders T, Palmer JL, et al. Complementary/alternative medicine use in a comprehensive cancer center and the implications for oncology. *J Clin Oncol* 2000;18:2505.

44. Shapiro DA, Safer M. Integrating complementary therapies into a traditional oncology practice. *Oncol Issues* 2002;17:35.

45. Field MJ, Lohr KN, eds. *Clinical practice guidelines: directions for a new program. Institute of Medicine, Committee on Clinical Practice Guidelines.* Washington D.C.: National Academy Press, 1990.

46. Smith TJ, Hillner BE. Ensuring quality cancer care by the use of clinical practice guidelines and critical pathways. *J Clin Oncol* 2001;19:2886.

47. Neymark N. Techniques for health economics analysis in oncology: Part 1. *Crit Rev Oncol Hematol* 1999;30:1.

48. Brown ML, Riley GF, Schussler BS, et al. Estimation of health care costs related to cancer treatment from SEER-Medicare data. *Med Care* 2002;40:IV,104.

49. Brown ML, Lipscomb J, Snyder C. The burden of illness of cancer: economic cost and quality of life. *Ann Rev Public Health* 2001;22:91.

50. National Cancer Institute. *National Cancer Institute 2001 Cancer Progress Report.* World Wide Web URL: http://progressreport.cancer.gov/2001, 2004.

51. Taplin SH, Barlow W, Urban N, et al. Stage, age, comorbidity and direct costs of colon, prostate, and breast cancer care. *J Natl Cancer Inst* 1995;87:417.

52. Iglehart JK. Prescription-drug coverage for Medicare beneficiaries. *N Engl J Med* 2003;349:923.

GRANT A. WILLIAMS
PATRICIA KEEGAN
NEIL R. P. OGDEN
RICHARD PAZDUR
ROBERT TEMPLE
MARK MCCLELLAN

SECTION 3

Regulatory Issues

The U.S. Food and Drug Administration (FDA) plays important roles in the development and approval of drugs, biologics, and devices for treating cancer. These roles vary with the stage of product development and include subject protection, guidance on clinical trial design, verification of results in marketing applications, and determining whether products should be marketed. Cancer therapies are regulated by FDA centers. The Center for Drug Evaluation and Research (CDER) regulates drugs and biotechnology-derived biologic products, the Center for Biologics Evaluation and Research (CBER) regulates vaccines and cell-derived biologic products, and the Center for Devices and Radiological Health (CDRH) regulates medical devices. The regulatory requirements for cancer drugs and biologics are similar and are summarized together throughout this chapter. Cancer device regulation is discussed separately in a later section, Regulation of Devices for Cancer Treatment and Diagnosis.

HISTORY OF U.S. FOOD AND DRUG ADMINISTRATION REGULATION OF DRUGS AND BIOLOGICS

The FDA's responsibility for regulating new drugs is derived largely from three laws. The Pure Food and Drug Act of 1906 authorized the FDA to regulate drugs only with regard to labeled claims of strength and purity. Two medical catastrophes led to FDA regulation of drug safety and efficacy. The Federal Food, Drug and Cosmetic Act of 1938 (FD&C Act), passed in response to deaths caused by a toxic vehicle in a sulfonamide elixir, required demonstration of drug safety before marketing. The effectiveness requirement was added in 1962 after birth defects were associated with the use of thalidomide. This law required substantial evidence of effectiveness and specified that this evidence must be derived from "adequate and well-controlled clinical investigations." Separate laws that pertain to medical devices are discussed later in the section Regulation of Devices for Cancer Treatment and Diagnosis.

The regulation of biologic products began with the 1902 Biologics Control Act, which was passed in response to the deaths of children from contaminated antitoxins and vaccines. This law provided federal authority to regulate all aspects of commercial production of vaccines, serums, toxins, and antitoxins and similar products with the objective of ensuring their safety, purity, and potency. The Biologics Control Act was subsequently incorporated into the 1944 Public Health Services Act, which defined biologic products as "any virus, therapeutic serum, toxin, antitoxin, vaccine, blood, blood component or derivative, allergenic product or analogous product, or arsphenamine." Regulatory oversight of biologic products was formally transferred from the National Institutes of Health to the FDA Bureau of Biologics in 1972. Appropriate provisions of the Biologics Control Act and the 1938 FD&C Act are used to guide the regulation of biologic products.

Detailed regulations published in the *Federal Register* and codified in the Code of Federal Regulations (CFR) outline the regulatory requirements for investigational drugs and biologic products (21 CFR 312), licensure of biologic products under a Biologics License Application (BLA; 21 CFR 601), and drug marketing for New Drug Applications (NDA; 21 CFR 314). Several regulations were specifically intended to improve or speed development of drugs for serious and life-threatening diseases such as cancer. In 1988, Subpart E of the Investigational New Drug (IND) regulations set the philosophic tone for cancer drug regulation to "exercise the broadest flexibility in applying the statutory standards, while preserving appropriate guarantees for safety and effectiveness." Subpart E also outlines procedures to improve communication and facilitate early meetings between the FDA and drug sponsors. In 1992, the accelerated approval (AA) regulations (Subpart H of the NDA regulations or Subpart E of the BLA regulations) outlined standards for early approval of drugs for serious and life-threatening disease when they provide an advantage over available therapy, allowing reliance on surrogate end points reasonably likely to predict clinical benefit.

U.S. FOOD AND DRUG ADMINISTRATION OVERSIGHT OF CLINICAL TRIALS FOR DRUGS AND BIOLOGICS

Investigational drugs must be administered under an IND application submitted to the FDA. The regulations describe two parties involved in IND submission: the *sponsor*, who is responsible for reporting to the FDA, and the *investigator*, who performs the trial. The sponsor may be a pharmaceutical company, an academic institution, or an individual (e.g., the sponsor/investigator). Sponsors are to select only investigators "qualified by training and experience as appropriate experts to investigate the drug." For a cancer drug IND, one of the investigators is generally a licensed physician with training and experience in treating cancer.

INITIAL INVESTIGATIONAL NEW DRUG SUBMISSION

When an IND is submitted to the FDA, a team of scientific reviewers evaluate the safety data from animals or other sources, evaluate the proposed phase I study, and judge whether patients would be exposed to an unreasonable and significant risk. These issues are discussed individually in the following sections.

Need to Submit an Investigational New Drug Application

All studies of nonapproved drugs must be done under an IND. For approved drugs, however, some studies require an IND and some are exempt from the IND requirement. To determine that an IND is not needed, the investigator and sponsor must find that the study meets all of the five exemption requirements: The study (1) is not intended to support approval of a new indication or a significant change in the product labeling, (2) is not intended to support a significant change in advertising, (3) does not involve a route of administration or dosage level or use in a patient population or other factor that significantly increases the risks (or decreases the acceptability of the risks) associated with the use of the drug product, (4) is conducted in compliance with Institutional Review Board (IRB) and informed consent regulations, and (5) will not be used to promote unapproved indications. A cancer drug guidance clarifies the FDA's interpretation of the IND exemption regulations with regard to what constitutes a significant increase in risk from use of approved cancer drugs in clinical studies. Oncologists frequently use cancer drugs in doses and in combinations not yet described in the label. Such "off-label" use, when safety has been demonstrated by published data or past clinical experience, is not considered an increased risk and would not require an IND for study. The cancer IND exemption guidance provides examples to clarify FDA interpretation.[1]

Investigational New Drug Application Process

The IND process spans the entire time of drug investigation. It includes the initial IND application and later IND amendments to provide safety reports or submit additional protocols. The initial IND application usually consists of a phase I clinical protocol and data to support the safety of the proposal. The latter would include *in vitro*, animal, and/or human evidence describing drug toxicity and allowing prediction of a safe starting dose and manufacturing data describing the composition, manufacture, and control of the drug substance and drug product. After the FDA receives the initial IND, sponsors are required to wait 30 days before initiating the proposed study unless they request and receive a waiver of the 30-day review period from the FDA. A multidisciplinary team of FDA scientists, including oncologists, animal toxicologists, chemists, and clinical pharmacologists, determine whether it is safe to proceed with the study. The FDA may put an IND "on hold" if it believes subjects would be exposed to unreasonable and significant risk of injury or if there is insufficient information to assess the risks. The most common reason for a hold is insufficient information to support the safety of the proposed dose or regimen.

The FDA frequently meets with sponsors and investigators in PreIND meetings to review proposed IND plans and to clarify IND requirements. The FDA has provided guidance on the design of preclinical studies needed to support the proposed phase I study. For oncology drugs, at least two studies are usually needed, one in a rodent and one in a nonrodent species. Animal studies should use the same schedule and administration proposed for the phase I clinical study. The starting dose for investigational drugs used in human studies is usually one-tenth of the mouse STD_{10} (dose at which 10% of animals have severe toxicity) calculated on a milligrams per meter squared basis, provided this dose does not cause irreversible toxicity in nonrodents. If this dose results in irreversible toxicity, one-sixth of the highest dose that does not produce irreversible toxicity is selected for the starting dose.[2] The approach to establishing safe starting doses for biologic products differs and is described further in Biologic Drug Products: Special Considerations, later. Phase I oncology trials are seldom performed in healthy volunteers. Oncology drugs are usually toxic (often genotoxic), and phase I oncology studies generally escalate until the occurrence of severe toxicities. Limited phase I or pharmacokinetic studies can be performed in healthy volunteers for oncology drugs that are relatively nontoxic.

Phase I Trial Design

The FDA has accepted a variety of phase I trial designs for cancer drugs. In the 1980s and early 1990s, the modified Fibonacci scheme was commonly used. Pharmacologically guided dosing was evaluated in the early 1990s with some success but was difficult logistically. Beginning in the early and mid-1990s, the FDA allowed investigators to use a variety of new methods for accelerating dose escalation.[3]

U.S. FOOD AND DRUG ADMINISTRATION INVOLVEMENT IN CLINICAL TRIAL DESIGN

The FDA meets frequently with commercial IND sponsors throughout drug development. Before IND submission, the FDA and sponsor discuss the adequacy of preclinical studies and the design of proposed phase I clinical studies in "PreIND meetings." A critical FDA role in drug development is to meet with sponsors to provide advice on the design of phase III (and sometimes phase II) clinical trials that will support NDA or BLA marketing applications. The multidisciplinary FDA team attending these meetings includes oncologists, statisticians, clinical pharmacologists, and usually external expert consultants. FDA chemists also meet to discuss manufacturing and quality control issues. Legislation now allows sponsors to submit protocols subsequent to these meetings and request a Special Protocol Assessment (SPA) that provides for a binding agreement.[4] After the clinical trials have been conducted and trial results are available, sponsors again meet with the FDA in PreNDA meetings to discuss whether an NDA may be warranted and, if so, to discuss details of an NDA submission.

U.S. FOOD AND DRUG ADMINISTRATION AND THE DRUG APPROVAL PROCESS

After clinical trials have been completed and an NDA has been submitted, the FDA verifies data quality and judges whether trial results demonstrate that the drug is safe and effective for the proposed use. After approval, the FDA continues to evaluate drug safety and regulate drug marketing.

The package insert describes clinical trial results from data that have been carefully reviewed and validated by FDA review teams. Regulations require that NDAs contain all relevant information about manufacturing, preclinical pharmacology and toxicology, human pharmacokinetics and bioavailability, clinical data, and statistical analyses. NDA applicants must submit detailed financial disclosure information about investigators. FDA review of the NDA involves a multidisciplinary team of chemists, toxicologists, clinical pharmacologists, oncologists, statisticians, microbiologists, site inspectors, and a project manager. FDA reviewers evaluate the primary data, available in the form of case report forms or electronic data; verify analyses; and, where appropriate, perform additional analyses. FDA field inspectors verify that information on case report forms is supported by source data, such as hospital charts. This NDA review process leads to a high level of confidence in the information that supports NDA approval and that is described in the package insert. This information not only documents the basis of drug approval but can be used in drug marketing, which is an incentive for manufacturers to submit additional NDA applications (supplemental NDAs) to update their labels.

Applications are prioritized for review according to their importance. Based on the Prescription Drug User Fee Act (PDUFA), the FDA performs NDA review with either a 6-month or a 10-month goal. Applications representing a significant improvement compared to marketed products are assigned *priority* status and a 6-month review goal, whereas *standard* applications have a 10-month review goal.

The FDA routinely seeks external advice on the design, analysis, and interpretation of clinical trials. Consultants are screened to exclude conflict of interest. Individual consultants advise the FDA during the design of clinical trials and early stages of NDA review. After initial NDA review, the FDA presents selected NDAs to the Oncologic Drugs Advisory Committee (ODAC). This group is composed of oncologists, statisticians, patient advocates, consumer representatives, and a nonvoting industry representative. At the public meetings of ODAC, the NDA applicant summarizes the results in an initial presentation, the FDA presents review findings, ODAC discusses the issues, and ODAC votes on questions submitted by the FDA. The FDA is not obligated to adhere to the advice provided. Information about ODAC meetings (including background packages, presentation slides, and meeting transcripts) and on drug approvals (including FDA review documents and approved labeling) can be found on the FDA Internet site.[5,6]

After reviewing the NDA, the FDA takes an action, which is communicated to the company by one of three types of letters: an approval letter that allows the sponsor to market the drug, an approvable letter that identifies deficiencies that must be corrected before drug marketing, or a not approvable letter, which identifies more serious deficiencies that cause ultimate approval to be relatively unlikely.

BASIS FOR CANCER DRUG APPROVAL

When determining whether to approve an NDA, the FDA evaluates whether the overall evidence supporting safety and efficacy meets the regulatory requirements for drug approval. In the following sections, the regulatory requirements, study end points [in the context of regular approval (RA) or AA], trial designs, and number of studies needed for the approval of cancer drugs are discussed.

REGULATORY REQUIREMENTS FOR NEW DRUG APPROVAL

Sponsors must demonstrate that drugs are safe and must provide substantial evidence of effectiveness from "adequate and well-controlled clinical investigations." Such effects could include important clinical outcomes (e.g., survival), symptomatic improvement, or effects on established surrogate end points, such as blood sugar, blood pressure, or blood cholesterol, and all of these end points have often been used as a basis for approval.[7] In 1992, new regulations allowed AA for drugs that were intended for serious or life-threatening diseases and showed an improvement over available therapy. In this setting, the FDA may grant marketing approval based on an effect on a surrogate end point that is reasonably likely ("based on epidemiologic, therapeutic, pathophysiologic, or other evidence") to predict clinical benefit. These surrogates were explicitly less well established than the ones in regular use (blood pressure, cholesterol). A drug is approved under the AA rule on condition that the manufacturer conduct clinical studies to verify and describe the actual benefit. If the postmarketing studies fail to demonstrate clinical benefit or if the applicant does not demonstrate due diligence in conducting the required studies, the drug can be removed from the market under an expedited process. In the following discussions, the term *regular approval* is used to designate the usual route of drug approval to distinguish it from AA associated with a postmarketing commitment to demonstrate clinical benefit. End points for RA and AA are described in the following sections.

End Points for Regular Approval of Cancer Drugs

RA requires evidence of clinical benefit or improvement in an established surrogate of benefit. In oncology, survival is obviously the gold standard for clinical benefit, but the FDA has accepted other end points for cancer drug approval. In the 1970s, the FDA usually approved cancer drugs based on objective response rates (ORRs). In the early 1980s, after discussion with ODAC, the FDA determined that ORR was generally not sufficient evidence for approval.[8] Given the toxicity of cancer drugs, approval needed evidence of improvement in survival or in a patient's quality of life—for example, improved physical functioning or improved tumor-related symptoms. Potentially acceptable end points were described in a 1991 FDA/National Cancer Institute (NCI) publication.[9] Disease-free survival was accepted as an adequate end point for adjuvant cancer treatment when a large proportion of patients with recurrence were symptomatic. Durable complete response was considered an acceptable end point in testicular cancer and acute leukemia because the untreated conditions were quickly lethal or even in some chronic leukemias and lymphomas, where it was clear that remission would lead to less infection, bleeding, and blood product support. The authors proposed that ORR alone might sometimes support drug approval but that response duration, relief of tumor-related symptoms, and drug toxicity should also be evaluated. As discussed in the following sections, ORR alone with an adequate response duration has sometimes supported both RA and AA, especially in patients with heavily pretreated or refractory disease.

Survey of End Points Supporting Regular Approval of Cancer Drugs, 1990 to 2002

A report summarized the end points supporting cancer drug approval by the FDA's Division of Oncology Drugs from 1990 through 2002.[10] As summarized in Table 57.3-1, 68% (39 of 57) of the cancer drug RAs for new drugs or for new treatment indications were based on nonsurvival end points. Tumor measurements played an important role, serving as primary or secondary evidence supporting 47% (27 of 57) of RAs. Ten of these 27 approvals were based on ORR alone, 9 on tumor response and effects on tumor-specific symptoms, 7 on ORR and time to progression (TTP), and one on TTP alone. Prolonged complete

TABLE 57.3-1. Summary of End Points for Regular Approval of Oncology Drug Marketing Applications, January 1, 1990, to November 1, 2002

TOTAL	57
Survival	18
Response rate	10
Time to progression	1
Response rate and time to progression	7
↓ Tumor-specific symptoms	4
Response rate and ↓ tumor-specific symptoms	9
Disease-free survival	2
Recurrence of malignant pleural effusion	2
Occurrence of breast cancer	2
↓ Impairment creatinine clearance	1
↓ Xerostomia	1

↓, decreased.

responses led to approval of five drugs for treatment of leukemic disorders. In these settings, patients with complete responses were expected to have fewer symptoms associated with bleeding, anemia, and infection and perhaps to have improved survival. Partial response rates and TTP were the primary evidence supporting the approval of numerous hormonal agents for breast cancer, including anastrazole, exemestane, letrozole, toremifene, and fulvestrant. This evidence was derived from randomized trials comparing the new agent to approved hormonal drugs (e.g., tamoxifen) that allowed at least a preliminary comparison of other end points such as survival.

Improvement in tumor-related symptoms supported approval in several clinical settings. The mitoxantrone approval for patients with symptomatic prostate cancer metastases was based on improvement in patients' bone pain. Approvals of two bisphosphonate drugs (pamidronate and zoledronate) were based on a composite bone morbidity end point (skeletal-related events). In several clinical settings, tumor-related symptoms plus objective tumor responses provided mutually supportive evidence leading to drug approval. In diseases with cutaneous manifestations, such as Kaposi's sarcoma and cutaneous T-cell lymphoma, improvements in cosmesis, cutaneous signs, and cutaneous symptoms have provided such evidence. Similarly, in cancers obstructing esophageal or bronchial passages, approvals were based on improvement in symptoms of luminal obstruction and objective responses of intraluminal tumors. Such evidence supported the approval of photodynamic therapy for palliation of obstructing esophageal and endobronchial cancers.[11]

Several commonly used end points have not supported cancer drug approval. Cancer drugs have to date not been approved based on changes in health-related quality of life (HRQOL) because of flaws in design and conduct of studies evaluating HRQOL. Future HRQOL studies need to avoid problems with HRQOL data by blinding observers, minimizing missing data, providing detailed analysis plans, validating instruments in the intended population, and defining clinically meaningful differences on HRQOL instruments. Time to treatment failure (TTF) has not supported drug approval. TTF is a composite end point measuring time from randomization to discontinuation of treatment for any reason (including for progression of disease, treatment toxicity, and death). Because it combines elements of safety and efficacy, TTF is not an acceptable end point for documenting effectiveness. Tumor marker end points also have not led to any cancer drug approvals, although prostate-specific antigen changes provided supportive evidence for the approval of mitoxantrone for prostate cancer.

Accelerated Approval of Cancer Drugs

The intent of the 1992 AA regulations was to speed access to promising new drugs for patients with serious or life-threatening disease who lacked satisfactory treatment. The AA regulations allow approval based on a surrogate end point "reasonably likely to predict clinical benefit." Because of the long-accepted role of tumor responses in guiding cancer treatment, ORR has been the main surrogate end point supporting cancer drug AA. Drugs approved under AA regulations must provide a benefit over available therapy. To satisfy this requirement, most sponsors have designed single-arm studies in patients with tumors that are refractory to available therapy. In the refractory setting, where, by definition, no available therapy exists, an acceptable ORR and response duration have served as evidence of benefit over available therapy and thus the basis for AA. AA can also be achieved by demonstrating an improvement in a surrogate end point compared to a standard drug in a randomized trial. This approach tests drug activity in less refractory tumors and provides a toxicity comparison relative to standard therapy.

The FDA has concluded that more than one drug could be approved under AA for a given indication. Drugs approved only under AA will not be considered to be "available therapy." Thus, if a new drug (Drug A) receives AA in a "refractory setting," that setting would still be considered a refractory setting until Drug A wins RA.[12]

The AA initiative has clearly been successful in making cancer drugs available. Since the first cancer AA in 1995, AA has been the initial approval mechanism for 16 new cancer drugs and biologics (Table 57.3-2). AA has also enabled eight new indi-

cations for previously marketed drugs. New approvals under AA have predominantly relied on confirmed responses as surrogate end points, including tumor response, hematologic response, cytogenetic response, and cytologic response.

After gaining AA based on a surrogate end point, the drug manufacturer is responsible for completing phase IV (postmarketing) commitments to determine whether the drug provides clinical benefit. The regulations allow the FDA to remove the drug from the market if sponsors do not demonstrate "due diligence" in completing these commitments or if the drug does not provide clinical benefit. In oncology, phase IV studies have often targeted a slightly different population than the AA indication; for example, AA may be for refractory colon cancer and the confirmatory study for first-line treatment of colon cancer. In 2003, a special session of ODAC discussed how the planning and conduct of oncology AA confirmatory studies could be improved. The ODAC consensus was that phase IV trials need to be planned early in oncology drug development, consistent with the AA regulations, which state that phase IV trials are generally expected to begin before drug approval. One strategy that may ensure completion of the confirmatory study is to target AA based on an interim analysis of a surrogate end point (e.g., response rate or TTP) in a randomized trial, with the ultimate clinical benefit (e.g., survival) to be demonstrated at the trial's completion. This design led to the AA of oxaliplatin in combination with 5-fluorouracil/leucovorin for advanced colorectal cancer.

CLINICAL TRIALS SUPPORTING DRUG APPROVAL

Evidence from clinical trials is central to cancer drug approval. By law, the FDA must base approval decisions on substantial evidence of efficacy from adequate and well-controlled investigations. Regulations describe the meaning of "adequate and well-controlled investigations" (21 CFR 314.126). Studies must

TABLE 57.3-2. Cancer Drugs and Biologics Initially Approved by Accelerated Approval

Product	Year	Indication	Surrogate End Point
Liposomal doxorubicin (Doxil)	1995	2nd-line Kaposi's sarcoma	RR
Dexrazoxane (Zinecard)	1995	Reduction of doxorubicin cardiomyopathy	Cardiac benefit proven; ultimate outcome uncertain
Irinotecan (Camptosar)	1996	2nd-line colon Ca	RR
Docetaxel (Taxotere)	1996	2nd-line breast Ca	RR
Capecitabine (Xeloda)	1998	Refractory breast Ca	RR
Denileukin diftitox (Ontak)	1999	Relapsed/refractory CTCL	RR, response duration
Liposomal cytarabine (DepoCyt)	1999	Lymphomatous meningitis	Cytologic response
Temozolomide (Temodar)	1999	Refractory anaplastic astrocytoma	CR, CR duration
Gemtuzumab ozogamicin (Mylotarg)	2000	AML 2nd line, elderly	CR and CRp
Alemtuzumab (Campath)	2001	3rd-line B-CLL	RR, response duration
Imatinib mesylate (Gleevec)	2001	CML in BC, AC, or CP after interferon failure	Hematologic and cytogenetic response
Oxaliplatin (Eloxatin)	2002	2nd-line colorectal Ca	RR and TTP
Ibritumomab (Zevalin)	2002	Relapsed/refractory follicular NHL	RR, durable responses
Gefitinib (Iressa)	2003	3rd-line NSCLC	RR
Bortezomib (Velcade)	2003	3rd-line multiple myeloma	RR, durable responses
Tositumomab (Bexxar)	2003	Refractory low-grade and follicular NHL	RR

AC, accelerated phase; AML, acute myelogenous leukemia; BC, blast crisis; B-CLL, B-lineage chronic lymphocytic leukemia; Ca, cancer; CML, chronic myelogenous leukemia; CP, chronic phase; CR, complete response; CRp, complete response with decreased platelets; CTCL, cutaneous T-cell lymphoma; NHL, non-Hodgkin's lymphoma; NSCLC, non–small cell lung cancer; RR, response rate; TTP, time to progression.

allow a valid comparison to a control and must provide a quantitative assessment of the drug's effect. In this section, the type of evidence (clinical trial design) and the amount of evidence (number of trials) that have been required for cancer drug approval are discussed.

Single-Arm Studies

The most reliable method for demonstrating efficacy is to show a statistically significant improvement in a clinically meaningful end point in blinded, randomized, controlled trials. Other approaches have also been successful in certain settings. In single-arm studies, in which major tumor regressions occur infrequently in the absence of treatment (a kind of historic control), ORR and response duration have sometimes been accepted as substantial evidence supporting AA or even RA in settings in which there is no effective alternative therapy. In contrast to the success of this approach, evidence from historically controlled trials attempting to show improvement in survival or TTP have seldom been adequate to support drug approval. These outcomes vary among study populations in ways that cannot always be predicted; for example, changes in concomitant supportive care may differ by location or may change over time.[13] Consequently, comparisons of time-to-event end points such as TTP or survival generally need a direct comparison to a control in a randomized trial, unless the effect is very large (e.g., testicular cancer or acute leukemia).

Studies Designed to Demonstrate Superiority

Placebo control (i.e., no treatment at all) is often considered unethical in cancer trials but, in some settings, may be acceptable. For instance, in early-stage cancer when standard practice is to give no treatment, comparing a relatively nontoxic treatment to a placebo would be reasonable. Placebo controls are not an ethical problem if a new treatment is compared to placebo, each added to standard therapy, a so-called add-on study. It is also possible to compare new therapy to standard therapy where the benefit of standard therapy is unknown or marginal. In that case, the new therapy would need to show superiority.

Studies Designed to Demonstrate Noninferiority

The goal of noninferiority (NI) trials is to demonstrate that a new drug is effective by showing that it is not less effective, by some defined amount, than a standard drug. NI studies involve direct comparison to a control but are based on historic assumptions about the control drug's efficacy and usually assume that at least a substantial fraction of the control drug's historically documented effect is retained by the new drug. Difficulties are found with NI trials. These trials need to rely on historic data to establish the expected size of treatment effect of the active control. A critical assumption is that the treatment effect of the active control that was observed historically will also be observed in the current population in the new study. This assumption is difficult to support, as results of trials are almost never identical. Optimally, the estimated size of the treatment effect of the active control will be based on a comprehensive metaanalysis of historic studies that reproducibly demonstrate the effectiveness of the control agent. The variability in the metaanalysis will be reflected in the choice of the NI margin.[13] NI designs generally require many patients to provide meaningful results. Given the complex issues involved, sponsors designing NI trials should consult early with the FDA.[14,15]

Isolating Drug Effect in Combinations

Because marketing approval is for a drug product rather than for a drug combination, trials supporting regulatory approval need to isolate the effectiveness of the proposed agent. Evidence is needed showing not only the effectiveness of the regimen but also establishing the contribution of the new drug to that regimen. The simplest way to demonstrate the individual contribution of a new drug in a regimen is using an "add-on" design, as discussed above in the section Studies Designed to Demonstrate Superiority. In exceptional cases, an effect of a combination may be so dramatic that studies to isolate each component's contribution would be difficult or impossible to conduct. Approval of the component might nonetheless be possible if there were support for a contribution of each component (animal data, other human data, etc.).

Trial Designs for Radiotherapy Protectants and Chemotherapy Protectants

Radiotherapy protectants and chemotherapy protectants are drugs designed to ameliorate the toxicities of radiotherapy or chemotherapy. Trials to evaluate these agents usually have two objectives. The first objective is to assess whether the protecting drug achieves its intended purpose of ameliorating the cancer treatment toxicity. Unless the mechanism of protection is clearly unrelated to the mechanism of antitumor activity (e.g., antinausea agents that ameliorate nausea via central nervous system receptors), a second trial objective is to determine whether anticancer efficacy is compromised by the protectant. Because the comparison of antitumor activity between the two arms of the trial is an NI comparison, a large number of patients may be required to achieve this objective.[16]

Independent Substantiation of Clinical Trial Results

The legal basis for FDA efficacy requirements is the 1962 efficacy amendment to the FD&C Act requiring substantial evidence of effectiveness derived from "adequate and well-controlled clinical investigations." This led to the FDA's interpretation, supported by judicial decisions, that at least two studies are generally required for drug approval.[7] Results from a single trial may provide a false impression for reasons that include unrecognized trial bias and chance (associated with occasional spurious findings when trials are repeated multiple times). In most cases, the FDA has required at least two well-controlled clinical trials. At other times, it has found that evidence from a single trial was sufficient, but "generally only in cases in which a single multicenter study of excellent design provided highly reliable and statistically strong evidence of an important clinical benefit, such as an effect on survival, and a confirmatory study would have been difficult to conduct on ethical grounds." In many cases, however, the FDA has relied on one study of a specific condition, together with other studies of different stages of disease or in other populations.[17] Thus, as detailed in an FDA guidance document, for approved cancer drugs, often only a single study may be needed to support additional marketing indications.[18] The legal basis for drug approval based on a single trial plus other supporting evidence was written into law in the 1997 Food and Drug Administration Modernization Act (FDAMA).

DRUG SAFETY REPORTING AND EVALUATION

For studies conducted under an IND, investigators are required to promptly report drug-associated adverse experiences to the IND sponsor. Sponsors subsequently must report in writing to the FDA within 15 days events that are serious and unexpected (e.g., events not described in the investigators' brochure) and to notify the FDA by telephone or facsimile within 7 days for fatal or life-threatening drug-associated events. At the time of drug approval, safety information collected during IND investigations is summarized in the package insert. After drug approval, additional drug safety information is collected through a mandatory system for drug manufacturers and a voluntary system for health providers and patients (MEDWatch). Manufacturers must promptly report information to the FDA about adverse experiences that are serious and unexpected (events not described in the package insert). MEDWatch reports can be submitted via the Internet.[19] Through the MEDWatch program, the FDA solicits information on serious adverse events, defined as those that involve death, a life-threatening condition, hospitalization, disability, a congenital anomaly, or medically important events that require an intervention to prevent one of these serious outcomes. These postmarketing reports are useful for identifying rare adverse events not detected in clinical trials. They are less useful for evaluating known toxicities, because a precise toxicity event rate cannot be determined.

ACCESS TO INVESTIGATIONAL DRUGS

The FDA strongly endorses participation in clinical trials; however, situations exist in which investigational drugs are made available under an IND primarily to treat a disease or condition rather than to study the drug's safety and effectiveness. The FDAMA of 1997 codified long-standing FDA practices by providing guiding criteria for treatment access. The FDAMA states that a physician may seek to obtain a drug for an individual patient for treatment use when the patient's physician has determined that no comparable or satisfactory alternative therapy exists. The FDA must then determine (1) that there is sufficient evidence of safety and effectiveness to support use of the investigational drug; (2) that provision of the investigational drug will not interfere with the initiation, conduct, or completion of clinical investigations to support marketing approval; and (3) that the sponsor or clinical investigator has submitted information sufficient to satisfy the IND requirements. Treatment use of experimental drugs can be grouped into two broad categories according to the number of people treated: expanded access (large numbers) and single patient treatment, including small studies of similarly situated patients. Regardless of the category of treatment use, all applications for investigational treatment require an investigator, informed consent, a sponsor who accepts responsibility for the study and

communicates with the FDA, a drug supplier (who may also be the sponsor), and oversight by an IRB.

Expanded access protocols outline a treatment regimen to be used for a predefined patient group. Since the early 1970s, the FDA has facilitated access to drugs under investigation for serious and life-threatening diseases, including cardiovascular, antiviral, and oncology drugs, to thousands of patients. Two specific mechanisms for expanded access are the Treatment IND and NCI-sponsored Group C programs. The 1987 Treatment IND regulations permit widespread access to an investigational drug if there is no comparable or satisfactory alternative, if the sponsor is pursuing marketing approval with due diligence, if the drug is nearing the end of its development, and if the data support the conclusion that the drug may be effective for the intended use in the intended population. Through an agreement with the FDA, in the past NCI has provided expanded access to approximately 20 investigation agents through a mechanism called *Group C*.

The FDA has granted single patient use of experimental drugs by several mechanisms. It can grant a single patient exception to receive a drug under an existing IND when a patient is ineligible for the specified protocol. Under a single patient exception, the existing commercial IND sponsor provides the drug and is responsible for reporting to the FDA. If the commercial sponsor is unwilling to assume responsibility for a special exception, an investigator can perform the role of sponsor for a single patient treatment use. The investigator must obtain the drug from a manufacturer and apply directly to the FDA for an IND. This application should include completed 1571 and 1572 forms, an outline of the patient's history, a treatment plan, and a commitment to obtain informed consent and IRB approval.[20] Although these mechanisms for single patient use provide access to investigational drugs, the preferred mechanism for access is participation in a clinical trial or in an expanded access protocol where useful data are more likely to be collected.

BIOLOGIC DRUG PRODUCTS: SPECIAL CONSIDERATIONS

Biologics, in contrast to drugs that are chemically synthesized, are derived from living sources (e.g., human or animal cells or tissues, microorganisms). Many biologics are complex mixtures and are not easily identified or characterized. These features explain differences in the regulatory approach to biologic products. For example, certain testing requirements, such as potency and general safety tests, are unique to biologic products because sponsors cannot fully characterize the products or, despite rigorous manufacturing and controls, ensure freedom from contamination with infectious agents.

The early development and testing of biologic products may be different from that of drugs. Biologic products may elicit an immune response in animals or may, if human source derived, have a different level of activity in animal species. Therefore, preclinical testing may rely more heavily on *in vitro* testing or require testing only in relevant animal species, such as nonhuman primates. The basis for establishing the starting dose may differ from the standard approach used for cancer drugs. The primary mechanism of action may not be direct cytotoxicity; therefore, the clinical starting dose and dose range are frequently based on the anticipated biologic activity (optimal biologic dose) rather than a tolerable toxicity level. Because most biologic products cause an immune response in human subjects, immunogenicity testing is needed. For tumor vaccines, the induction of an immune response is intended and central to the mechanism of activity. The goal is to optimize dose and schedule to overcome host tolerance to tumor antigens without inducing an immune response against normal human tissues. Unfortunately, proteins, toxins, and cell/tissue therapies may induce unintended immune responses. The clinical development plan for most biologic therapies includes an assessment of the presence, incidence, and clinical impact of an immune response to the investigational biologic product.

Despite some differences in the FDA's regulatory approach to product characterization and early clinical development of cancer drugs and cancer biologics, the goals and ultimate regulatory requirements for demonstrating safety and efficacy (including trial designs and end points) are similar. FDA programs to facilitate development of cancer treatments (described later in U.S. Food and Drug Administration Initiatives and Guidances Expediting Approval of Cancer Drugs, Biologics, and Devices), such as the use of SPAs, priority review, and Fast Track designation, apply to biologics as well as drugs.

REGULATION OF DEVICES FOR CANCER TREATMENT AND DIAGNOSIS

Many of the laws and regulations for medical devices differ from those guiding the regulation of drugs and biologics. The following sections review the history of medical device regulation, the types of investigational device applications, and CDRH review of device marketing applications.

HISTORY OF U.S. FOOD AND DRUG ADMINISTRATION DEVICE REGULATION

The medical device laws were enacted after a catastrophe associated with a female contraceptive implant. Congress gave the FDA the authority for premarket regulation of devices on May 26, 1976, by passing the Medical Device Amendments (the 1976 amendments) to the FD&C Act. Under section 513 of the FD&C Act, the FDA must classify devices into one of three regulatory classes: class I, class II, or class III. FDA classification of a device is determined by the amount of regulatory oversight needed to provide reasonable assurance of safety and effectiveness. The devices are classified as follows:

- Class I (general controls): Sufficient information exists showing that the general controls described in the Act are sufficient.
- Class II (special controls): General controls by themselves are insufficient, but there is sufficient information to establish special controls to provide such assurance. The Safe Medical Devices Act of 1990 broadened the definition of class II devices to include devices for which special controls can provide such assurance, including performance standards, postmarketing surveillance, patient registries, development and dissemination of guidelines, recommendations, and any other appropriate actions the agency deems necessary.

- Class III [premarket approval (PMA)]: Information is insufficient to qualify for class I or class II, and the device meets one of the following conditions:
  - It is life sustaining or life supporting.
  - Its use is of substantial importance in preventing impairment of human health.
  - The proposed use presents a potentially unreasonable risk of illness.

In the late 1970s, the FDA held expert panel meetings to assist in classifying medical devices marketed in the United States. Subsequently, most preamendment devices (devices marketed before May 28, 1976, the date of the 1976 amendments) were classified by the FDA through regulations into one of the three regulatory classes. Devices introduced into interstate commerce for the first time on or after May 28, 1976, are classified through the premarket notification or 510(k) process. Section 510(k) of the FD&C Act provides that persons who intend to market a new device without submitting a PMA (because they believe the device is "substantially equivalent" to a legally marketed predicate device) must submit a premarket notification ("a 510k" application), which allows the FDA to verify whether the new device is substantially equivalent to a legally marketed device.[21] In 1998, based on the FDAMA, the FDA published in the *Federal Register* (63 FR 3142) a list of each type of class II device that does not require a 510(k). Many devices were exempted from 510(k) requirements by this law. In summary, devices can be regulated as class I (exempt from any specific controls), class I reserved and class II requiring a 510(k), class II exempt from 510(k) requirements with special controls, and class III requiring a PMA.

Congress charged the FDA with developing and implementing Mammography Quality Standards Act (MQSA) regulations in 1992. Interim regulations, issued in December, 1993, became effective in February, 1994. In 1995, the FDA began enforcing MQSA when it initiated an inspection program. Congress enacted MQSA to ensure that all women have access to quality mammography for the detection of breast cancer in its earliest, most treatable stages.

U.S. FOOD AND DRUG ADMINISTRATION OVERSIGHT OF DEVICE INVESTIGATIONS

The investigational device exemption (IDE) allows sponsors to ship their devices in interstate commerce for the purposes of investigational human use.[21] IDEs are required for studies of devices that are not yet marketed for use by the medical specialty that would use the device and when the studies involve significant risks to subjects. Alternatively, investigation of a new use by the same medical specialty would only require IRB approval but would not necessitate an IDE.[22] The IDE does not provide marketing approval or clearance for a device. The focus of the IDE is to protect subjects participating in studies of investigational devices. The IDE is analogous to the IND required for drug investigations, with similar requirements for reporting adverse events.[23] The CDRH actively participates in device clinical trial design with the PreIDE program. PreIDE submissions can be submitted to the CDRH for consultation and for review of proposed clinical trials. CDRH reviewers work with the sponsor to define reasonable inclusion and exclusion criteria, outcome measures, follow-up details, and statistical analysis plans.[24]

Several mechanisms exist for use of investigational devices outside of an approved IDE. These include emergency use of unapproved medical devices, individual patient access to investigational devices intended for serious diseases, treatment use of investigational devices, continued access to investigational devices, and expanded access mechanisms for unapproved devices. Additional information is available at CDRH Internet sites.[21-23]

U.S. FOOD AND DRUG ADMINISTRATION REVIEW OF DEVICE MARKETING APPLICATIONS FOR CANCER

Device applications are reviewed by two CDRH offices, the Office of *In Vitro* Diagnostic Device Evaluation and Safety (OIVD) and the Office of Device Evaluation (ODE). OIVD was created in 2003 to regulate *in vitro* diagnostic devices, including the marketing of devices that detect and diagnose cancer. OIVD uses the same general review mechanisms, regulations, and criteria as ODE to review and approve devices (21 CFR Parts 862, 864, and 866). The ODE in the CDRH conducts the premarket reviews for all other devices. Most devices labeled for cancer treatments are marketed through the 510(k) process (class II) or PMA process (class III).

510(k) Submission: Equivalence to a Predicate Device

Under the 510(k) process, the applicant compares testing, design, and labeling of a new device to a predicate device.[25] On review of the application, the FDA can find the new device to be equivalent to the predicate device based solely on technical comparisons. One problem encountered in device review is the broad indications for use previously cleared for some predicate devices. For example, before the 1976 amendments, cryosurgery devices were cleared for uses such as for "oncology," "tumor destruction," or "prostate tumors." Thus, 510(k) applications approved based on technical arguments that the new device has the same performance characteristics as cryosurgery devices may have the same broad labeling indications previously granted for cryosurgery devices.

Devices for cancer treatment can be labeled in two ways: as a tool (e.g., to cut, coagulate, or ablate) or as a specific treatment (e.g., to treat melanoma). For example, a scalpel, a laser, and an electrosurgical device all cut soft tissues in surgery. However, if the applicant plans to market these devices for a specific use, then a specific equivalent predicate (with labeling) or clinical data demonstrating that capability would be required.

Premarket Approval Process and Product Development Plan

For devices requiring a PMA or product development plan (PDP), the applicant must establish with valid scientific evidence that there is reasonable assurance the device is safe and effective under the conditions of use prescribed, recommended, or suggested in the proposed labeling (21 USC 360e). Effectiveness is to be determined with respect to the persons for whose use the device is represented or intended with respect to the conditions of use prescribed, recommended, or suggested in the labeling of the device, and weighing any probable benefit to health from the use of the device against probable risk of injury or illness from such use. PMAs are to be reviewed in 180 days after FDA receipt of a PMA that meets established content requirements. Typically, the PMA review includes a detailed analysis of the device (including device design, performance, and manufacture) and a detailed analysis of the clinical study.[26] The amount of evidence necessary to establish that a device is safe and effective for its intended use depends on the particular study, the types of data involved, and the other evidence available to support the indication for use. PMA submissions rarely involve a comparison to other marketed devices and usually compare the performance of the new device to no treatment or to standard of care in a randomized prospective study, or both. The PMA and PDP review processes are similar to the NDA review process described in the section FDA and the Drug Approval Process. The PDP is similar to the PMA process except that the clinical data and other information required for approval are prospectively agreed on.[27] The PDP describes the agreed on details of design and development activities, the outputs of these activities, and acceptance criteria for these outputs. The requirement for approval is the same as for a PMA.

Humanitarian Device Exemptions and Humanitarian Use Designations

Humanitarian device exemptions (HDEs) and humanitarian use designations (HUDs) are mechanisms for early marketing of devices. HUD is determined by the Office of Orphan Products and is defined as a device intended to benefit patients in the treatment and diagnosis of diseases or conditions that affect fewer than 4000 individuals in the United States per year.[28] After the HUD is granted, the sponsor may submit an HDE application to ODE for review of safety and probable benefit in the target patient population. No comparable device may be available to treat the disease or condition other than devices available under an HDE or being studied under an IDE. The agency has 75 days from the date of receipt to review an HDE application.[29]

EVIDENCE NEEDED FOR CANCER-SPECIFIC DEVICE APPLICATIONS

In vitro diagnostic devices (reviewed by OIVD) and treatment and *in vivo* diagnostic devices (reviewed by ODE) are critical to the care of cancer patients. Devices are regulated according to the use(s) for which they are labeled and according to device design. An electrosurgical device can be labeled for cutting soft tissues, for coagulation necrosis of tumors, or for treating lung cancer. An x-ray machine can be for diagnostic or therapeutic use. The amount of evidence needed to support each indication is different, based on the predicate devices available, the degree of similarity of the new device to the predicate device(s), and the risks to the patients associated with the indication for use and the technology involved. For a surgical device with a "cutting soft tissues" indication for use, ODE requires that the applicant demonstrate substantially equivalent performance of their device. Typically, if a surgical device is not marketed in the United States, *ex vivo* tissue comparison data are required to show equivalence. For a "coagulation necrosis of tumor indication," sufficient information is required to show that the device can reliably cause necrosis of a given volume of tumor tissue. For an indication for treatment of cancer or for the necrosis of a cancer that is not typically managed with necrosis, clinical evidence of benefit would be expected. The burden of demonstrating safety and effectiveness or substantial equivalence remains with the sponsor.

INVESTIGATIONS OF DEVICES IN COMBINATION WITH DRUGS OR BIOLOGICS

Studies evaluating drugs or biologics used in combination with medical devices are usually regulated primarily by one FDA review center (CDRH, CDER, or CBER) with consultation to another center(s). The determination of primary regulatory and review authority can be a complex judgment depending on the products' primary mechanism of action, whether they are "copackaged," whether they will be used exclusively together, and whether the labels for existing products must be changed when the combination use is approved. The FDA has established the Office of Combination Products to address such issues. A formal Request for Designation can be obtained to clarify regulatory jurisdiction.[30] Regardless of which center has primary regulatory responsibility, experts from both centers usually participate in the review process to provide needed expertise. Such collaboration resulted in simultaneous approvals of NDAs for photofrin (drug) and PMAs for lasers (devices) to allow photodynamic therapy for lung cancer and esophageal cancer.

U.S. FOOD AND DRUG ADMINISTRATION INITIATIVES AND GUIDANCES EXPEDITING APPROVAL OF CANCER DRUGS, BIOLOGICS, AND DEVICES

Discussed above are initiatives to expedite the development and approval of cancer drugs including AA under Subpart H of the IND regulations. Other regulatory initiatives for cancer or other life-threatening diseases are discussed below.

- Subpart E: Codified in 1988, Subpart E of the IND drug regulations (21 CFR 312 Subpart E) outlines special procedures to expedite the development, evaluation, and marketing of new therapies for life-threatening diseases, such as cancer. These procedures reflected the recognition that physicians and patients are generally willing to accept greater risks or side effects from products that treat life-threatening illnesses in view of the possible benefits of therapy. Subpart E recommends early and frequent meetings with the agency at PreIND, end-of-phase II, and PreNDA meetings to address potential problems in drug development or clinical trial design. Other recommendations that for many years have been incorporated into cancer drug regulation are consideration of the severity of disease and the availability of other therapy when making regulatory judgments and consultation with outside scientific consultants and advisory committees.
- Orphan drug: Cancer drug development has benefited from the Orphan Drug Act of 1983. This law provides for financial incentives to promote the development of drugs for rare diseases. For drugs intended to treat rare cancers (affecting fewer than 200,000 U.S. patients), sponsors can apply for Orphan Drug designation, which affords the potential for 7 years of marketing exclusivity on drug approval, tax incentives, and eligibility for orphan drug research grants.[31]

- Decreased NDA review times: FDA NDA review time, as well as time to approval after application submissions, for cancer drugs and for all drug times have decreased in recent years. The PDUFA provided resources that allowed the FDA to increase the number of drug reviewers. Under the PDUFA, the review goal for a priority NDA (an NDA appearing to provide an advantage over existing therapy) is 6 months.
- Multiple accelerated approvals: As noted earlier, in Basis for Cancer Drug Approval, the FDA made it clear that more than one drug could be approved under AA for a given indication.
- Guidance documents: Several FDA guidance documents have specifically addressed cancer drug development issues. Previously discussed were guidance documents on clinical study requirements for new treatment indications and on cancer drug IND exemptions. Another guidance document on cancer data collection provides guidelines for minimizing unnecessary data collection.[32]
- Interagency task force: The FDA has embarked on a process to provide detailed guidance on clinical trial end points for cancer drug approval. It is working with the NCI and cancer professional organizations to hold public workshops for each of the major cancer treatment indications. After further discussion of these issues before ODAC, the FDA plans to write a series of guidance documents on end points for the most common cancer treatment settings.
- FDAMA and Fast Track: The FDAMA attempted to facilitate the review process by the "Fast Track" program. The FDA designates development plans as Fast Track if the drug is intended to treat a serious or life-threatening condition and if it demonstrates the potential to address an unmet medical need.[33] An advantage of Fast Track designation is that sponsors may submit portions of an application early, such as the chemistry section or the animal toxicology section, before submission of the complete NDA. FDA review could provide early feedback on application deficiencies, thus speeding the overall process.
- SPAs: FDAMA also introduced the SPA to improve the quality of final protocols. The SPA, usually submitted after an end-of-phase II meeting, provides for a 45-day FDA protocol review. FDA responses to protocol-related SPA questions are binding unless new unrecognized public health issues emerge. The FDA strongly encourages oncology sponsors to request a SPA when submitting phase III protocols.
- Clinical Trials Data Bank: FDAMA also established a Clinical Trials Data Bank for serious or life-threatening diseases. This requires submission of information about all clinical trials evaluating efficacy.[34]
- Pediatrics: Recent initiatives have sought to improve drug development in children. The pediatric exclusivity program, first described in FDAMA, is a voluntary program that provides incentives for doing pediatric studies. The FDA generates a written request for studies to be done. If sponsors perform and report on the studies, the FDA can grant 6 months of marketing exclusivity extension for all indications. The Best Pharmaceuticals for Children Act describes a similar program to encourage pediatric development of drugs that are off patent.
- Cancer device advisory panels: The CDRH has convened meetings of general and plastic surgery advisory panels to discuss clinical trial design issues for lung tumor coagulation necrosis devices and for breast tumor coagulation necrosis.[35,36]

REFERENCES

1. Guidance for Industry: IND exemptions for studies of lawfully marketed drug or biological products for the treatment of cancer, September 2003. Available at World Wide Web URL: http://www.fda.gov/cder/guidance/5459.htm.
2. DeGeorge J, Ahn C, Andrews P, et al. Regulatory considerations for preclinical development of anticancer drugs. *Cancer Chemother Pharmacol* 1998;41:173.
3. Simon R, Freidlin B, Rubinstein L, et al. Accelerated titration designs for phase I clinical trials in oncology. *J Natl Cancer Inst* 1997;89:1138.
4. Guidance for Industry: Special protocol assessment, May 2002. Available at World Wide Web URL: http://www.fda.gov/cder/guidance/3764.htm.
5. Oncologic Drugs Advisory Committee materials are available at: World Wide Web URL: http://www.fda.gov/cder/audiences/acspage/oncologicmeetings1.htm.
6. New drug approval information is available at World Wide Web URL: http://www.fda.gov/cder/foi/nda/.
7. Temple R. Development of drug law, regulations, and guidance in the United States. In: Munson PL, Mueller RA, Breese GR, eds. *Principles of pharmacology: basic concepts and clinical applications*. New York: Chapman & Hall, 1996:1643.
8. Johnson JR, Temple R. Food and Drug Administration requirements for approval of anticancer drugs. *Cancer Treat Rep* 1985;69:1155.
9. O'Shaughnessy J, Wittes R, Burke G, et al. Commentary concerning demonstration of safety and efficacy of investigational anticancer agents in clinical trials. *J Clin Oncol* 1991;9:2225.
10. Johnson JR, Williams G, Pazdur R. End points and United States Food and Drug Administration approval of oncology drugs. *J Clin Oncol* 2003;21:1404.
11. Williams G, Pazdur R, Temple R. Assessing tumor-related signs and symptoms to support cancer drug approval. *J Biopharm Stat* Feb 2004;14:5.
12. Guidance for industry: available therapy, 2004. Available at World Wide Web URL: http://www.fda.gov/cder/guidance/5244fnl.pdf, 2004.
13. Guidance for Industry: International Conference on Harmonization (ICH) Topic E10, Choice of control group and related issues in clinical trials, 1999. Available at World Wide Web URL: http://www.fda.gov/cder/guidance/4155fNL.htm.
14. Rothmann M, Li N, Chen G, et al. Design and analysis of non-inferiority mortality trials in oncology. *Stat Med* 2003;22(2):239.
15. Ibrahim A, Scher N, Williams G, et al. Approval summary for zoledronic acid in treatment of multiple myeloma and cancer bone metastases. *Clin Cancer Res* 2003;9(7):2394.
16. Williams G, Cortazar P, Pazdur R. Developing drugs to decrease the toxicity of chemotherapy. *J Clin Oncol* 2001;19(14):3439.
17. Guidance for Industry: Providing clinical evidence of effectiveness for human drug and biological products, 1998. Available at World Wide Web URL: http://www.fda.gov/cder/guidance/1397fnl.pdf, 2004.
18. Guidance for Industry: FDA approval of new cancer treatment uses for marketed drug and biological products. Available at World Wide Web URL: http://www.fda.gov/cder/guidance/1484fnl.htm, 2004.
19. MEDWatch information available at World Wide Web URL: http//www.fda.gov/medwatch/, 2004.
20. Information available at World Wide Web URL: http://www.fda.gov/cder/cancer/singleind.htm, 2004.
21. Food, Drug & Cosmetic Act, section 513(I).
22. IDE regulation information available at World Wide Web URL: http://www.fda.gov/cdrh/devadvice/ide/index.shtml and at 1-800-638-2041, 2004.
23. Information on IDE policy available at World Wide Web URL: http://www.fda.gov/cdrh/ode/idepolcy.html, 2004.
24. Information on PIDEs available at World Wide Web URL: http://www.fda.gov/cdrh/ode/d99-1.html, 2004.
25. Information on 510(k)s available at World Wide Web URL: http://www.fda.gov/cdrh/manual/510kprt1.html, 2004.
26. Information on the PMA review process available at World Wide Web URL: http://www.fda.gov/cdrh/devadvice/pma/, 2004.
27. Information on PDP available at World Wide Web URL: http://www.fda.gov/cdrh/pdp/420.html, 2004.
28. Information on HUD available at World Wide Web URL: http://www.fda.gov/cdrh/ode/hdeinfo.html, 2004.
29. Information on HDE available at World Wide Web URL: http://www.fda.gov/cdrh/ode/guidance/1381.html, 2004
30. Information on combination products available at World Wide Web URL: http://www.fda.gov/oc/combination, 2004.
31. Information available at World Wide Web URL: http://www.fda.gov/orphan/, 2004.
32. Guidance for Industry: Cancer drug and biological products—clinical data in marketing applications, November 2001. Available at World Wide Web URL: http://www.fda.gov/cder/guidance/4332fnl.htm, 2004.
33. Guidance for Industry: Fast Track drug development programs—designation, development, and application review, 1998. Available at: http://www.fda.gov/cder/guidance/2112fnl.htm, 2004.
34. Guidance for Industry: Clinical trials for serious or life-threatening diseases; establishment of a data bank, March 2000. Available at World Wide Web URL: http://www.fda.gov/cder/guidance/3585fnl.htm, 2004.
35. General and Plastic Surgery Advisory Panel. Tumor coagulation necrosis devices, February 28, 2003. Summary available at World Wide Web URL: http://www.accessdata.fda.gov/scripts/cdrh/cfdocs/cfAdvisory/details.cfm?mtg=385, 2004.
36. General and Plastic Surgery Advisory Panel. Clinical trial design issues for breast tumor coagulation necrosis devices, July 24, 2003. Summary available at World Wide Web URL: http://www.accessdata.fda.gov/scripts/cdrh/cfdocs/cfAdvisory/details.cfm?mtg=385, 2004.

SECTION 4

RICHARD M. SATAVA
JONATHAN D. LINKOUS
JAY H. SANDERS

Telemedicine

The Institute of Medicine has defined *telemedicine* as "the use of electronic information and communications technologies to provide and support health care when distance separates the participants."[1] This all-inclusive definition allows for many of the information age technologies to be included within the domain of telemedicine, such as the electronic medical record, distributed computing, picture archiving and communication system, and even the simple use of the telephone for follow-up consultation.[2] However, the most common concept of telemedicine is remotely providing care to a patient with a direct physician–physician or physician–patient contact. In many instances, the physician care is substituted by a nurse or other physician extender. Yet, the overall intent is to bring some level of care through the use of telecommunication technology to a patient in a remote area who does not have access to health care.[3] The most frequently used technology is two-way audio and video over terrestrial (telephone lines or fiber optic cable) or satellite communication, although the use of newer wireless technologies with personal digital assistants is being rapidly introduced.[4]

Numerous systems have been developed over the years, from the simple combinations of camera and closed-circuit television with a telephone to sophisticated integrated "solutions" that contain high-definition cameras and monitors and high-bandwidth audio and multiple peripherals devices, such as electronic stethoscope, electrocardiogram, ultrasound,[5] handheld digital video cameras (for skin and dermatology), digital spirometer (for pulmonary function studies),[6] and noninvasive laboratory tests (pulse oximeter, blood sugar).[7,8] The list of devices that can bring the patient closer to the health care provider continues to expand, yet the one most requested—the sense of touch—has eluded a simple, accurate, reliable, and practical device.

There are two main forms of telemedicine—real-time and store-and-forward. In real-time, there is a direct communication between the generalist physician and a physician–consultant (usually for teleconsultation on a difficult problem or for second opinion) or between physician and patient. In store-and-forward, a diagnostic study is usually performed (e.g., x-ray, pathology slide, photograph of a skin lesion), and the image is sent to a receiving site, where it is stored until the physician views the image. Most images should have a text consultation request, although there is some use of simple e-mailing of consultations.[9] Store-and-forward has the advantage of being asynchronous, meaning available to the consulting physician at any convenient time, whereas real-time requires scheduling of time so both parties are available at the same time. Thus, store-and-forward has been very successful, principally for the reasons of ease of use and the additional fact that store-and-forward services are reimbursable (discussed later in Barriers and Challenges).

Telemedicine using real-time audio and video consultation is most often used by primary care physicians and physician extenders to provide the most basic of health care needs to underserved areas or for special circumstances. The most successful implementation of this telemedicine is in the rural populations, such as Bureau of Indian Affairs reservations for the Indian Nations[10] and isolated farming communities, or for dangerous circumstances such as Bureau of Prisons detention facilities[11,12] or military battlefield operations.[13,14] The largest network of telemedicine today is the combined U.S. Department of Defense and Department of Veterans Affairs (VA), which connects all the military and VA hospitals and clinics worldwide. This is greatly enhanced by a single electronic medical record (frequently referred to as the *government computerized patient record* or *GCPR*).[15] During the recent military operations in Afghanistan and Iraq, more than 3000 military medics carried handheld personal digital assistants with a computerized medical record (the Battlefield Medical Information System—Telemedicine),[16] which was connected through many portals to the Internet and virtually any military hospital. There have also been pilot demonstrations of the extreme capability of telemedicine, such as the Everest Extreme Expeditions in 1998 and 1999, which relayed over 18,000 miles in real time the vital signs of climbers while they climbed through the dangerous Khumbu Icefall to Camp 2 at 23,000 feet on Mount Everest.[17]

APPLICATIONS OF TELEMEDICINE

The spread of telemedicine to the specialties has been variable. There has been great success with teleradiology, telepathology, telecardiology, and teledermatology, all of which can be accomplished using the store-and-forward mode. For direct physician-to-patient care, one of the most successful has been telepsychiatry,[18] although virtually every specialty has had pilot studies in telemedicine, including teleoncology. The Association of Telehealth Service Providers has documented telemedicine services in more than 40 clinical specialties areas.

Telemedicine encompasses different types of programs and services provided for the patient. The types of services have been categorized as specialist referral services, patient consultations, patient monitoring, medical education, and consumer medical and health information.

Specialist referral services typically involve a specialist assisting a more general practitioner in rendering a diagnosis. This may involve a patient "seeing" a specialist over a live, remote consult or the transmission of diagnostic images and/or video along with patient data to a specialist for viewing later. Recent surveys have shown a rapid increase in the number of specialty and subspecialty areas that have successfully used telemedicine. The 1999 survey by the Association of Telehealth Service Providers showed that the 40 clinical services were being provided from more than 40 different clinical facilities. Radiology continues to make the greatest use of telemedicine, with thousands of images "read" by remote providers each year.

Of particular interest to oncology is telepathology, which has been enhanced by the introduction of the "virtual slide"—an entire histologic section that is scanned into the computer.[19] This permits the slide to be viewed on a computer monitor at any resolution (rather than the fixed resolutions of a standard microscope) and can be seen simultaneously by many pathologists in many different cities. Molnar et al.[20] demonstrated that the overall concordance of virtual slide and the standard microscope has a consensus diagnosis of 95.1% and 97.0%, respectively. Clinically important concordance was 96.1% and 98.0% for virtual and standard, respectively. The two methods showed concordance in 92.0% of cases and clinically important concordance in 94.1% of cases. Of those diagnoses that were not in agreement, all except one were due to a difference of interpretation that was not due to the quality of the image. Thus, as the new direct histologic scanners become available, the use of digital pathology slides should follow the pathway of radiology, in which many hospitals no longer have any film because all images are digital.

Another trend in specialty teleconsultation is first emerging in radiology, where the use of computer-aided diagnosis and sophisticated decision support systems have been shown to have a diagnostic accuracy approaching that of expert radiologists.[21] This is particularly relevant for screening of "normal" x-rays or cytology to detect a first-order approximation for suspicious abnormalities that are then brought to the attention of the expert consultant. Another leveraging of technology is presaged by the "grid computing," where massive numbers of computers are linked together into a single network that allows many institutions to participate in a megadatabase and share images among all physicians to improve the accuracy of radiologic diagnosis.[22] Thus, information age technologies based on telemedicine are coming together to dramatically improve the quality, speed, and efficacy of providing care.

The most common service provided through telemedicine is patient consultations, such as using audio, video, and medical data between a patient and a primary care physician (or physician extender) for use in determining a diagnosis and treatment plan. This might originate from a remote clinic to a physician's office using a direct transmission link or may include communicating to a physician over the Web. The most rapidly growing use of telemedicine is in home health care[23] and hospice[24] care. The implementation of home health care can significantly change the pattern of the provision of health care and has the potential to decrease the cost.

Home telemedicine is facilitated by patient monitoring services that use various devices to remotely collect and send data to a monitoring station for interpretation. Such "home telehealth" applications might include a specific vital sign, a laboratory test such as blood glucose,[8] an electrocardiogram, or a variety of indicators for homebound patients. Although these patient-monitoring devices require that the patient assist in taking the desired study and transmitting the data, an interesting new development is "intelligent clothing," such as the "smart T-shirt,"[25] with embedded sensors that can automatically monitor vital signs and transmit them to a central monitoring facility. Such services can be used to supplement the use of visiting nurses or provide continuous updating of data rather than infrequent periodic testing.

Medical education has become a very large industry that is exploiting the power of telemedicine. This provides continuing medical education credits for health professionals and special medical education seminars for targeted groups in remote locations. The earliest uses of telesurgery in surgical education were the transmitting of live surgery during conferences and then quickly spread to providing courses, seminars, and video (when the compression technologies became available) over the Internet. Numerous Web sites have become available, one of which is specifically for surgery called WebSurg (http://www.websurg.com) under the direction of Professor Jacques Marescaux, M.D., of the European Institute for TeleSurgery in Strasbourg, France.[26] This remarkable Web site provides an enormous range of educational opportunities for the medical student to surgical oncologist, including the concept of preoperative planning of surgical resection of liver tumors.

Consumer medical and health information includes the use of the Internet for consumers to obtain specialized health information and on-line discussion groups to provide peer-to-peer support. Most of these sites are not under the direct control of the medical profession, and many have been developed by cancer patients and their families, providing important information and emotional support. Although of value to cancer patients, many are not from "trusted sources" and can be a source of victimization of patients.

TELEMEDICINE IN OTHER COUNTRIES

The delivery of remote patient services in other countries is growing rapidly, in some countries much faster than in the United States. In countries with socialized medicine, a national policy that encourages the use of remote patient services can spur significant initial investments. Two examples include Canada and United Kingdom, although the Scandinavian countries, Italy, Greece, Australia, China, and Japan all have implemented national telemedicine efforts. In 2000, Health Canada launched the Canada Health Infostructure Partnerships Program, a 2-year, $80 million (Canada) program to support the implementation of innovative applications of information and communications technologies in the health sector that has continued support by the national and regional governments.[27] In the United Kingdom, there are currently 120 telemedicine projects and 135 United Kingdom companies involved in telemedicine. The United Kingdom government, realizing the need for innovative technology in the National Health Service, has placed a heavy emphasis on funding advanced technologies. An investment of $1.6 billion has been committed by the government to further push forward this modernization. The National Health Service plan is committed to ensure that all local health services will have facilities for telemedicine by 2005.[28]

TELEMEDICINE IN ONCOLOGY CARE— CURRENT PRACTICES

Applications of telemedicine in oncology are growing and expanding the horizons of clinical care. The following are examples of implementation in oncology on a state (Kansas), regional (Washington, Wyoming, Alaska, Montana, and Idaho; or WWAMI), and international (United States, Brazil, and Chile) basis.

In Kansas, a statewide program using telemedicine for tele-oncology was established in 1996.[29] Working as a team with the local primary care provider and where available, local medical and radiation oncologists, a consultant oncologist provides hematologic/oncologic diagnoses. Other specialists provide support services, including pain management, telepsychiatry, remote hospice support, and access to cancer support groups. Controlled scientific studies of patient satisfaction, efficacy, and cost have demonstrated the positive results in all three areas. Although the average cost per consultation is still high (approximately $600 per visit), there has been a significant reduction in costs since 2000 with reduced technology and connectivity expenses. Increased use during the first decade of the 21st century, projected over the next few years, will yield a positive cash flow for the oncology program.

The Veterans Administration hospital facility in Seattle provides medical oncology, radiation, and surgery for a large region, including Washington, Wyoming, Alaska, Montana, and Idaho (the WWAMI region). The center uses telemedicine for tumor boards, referring patients from local sites to the Veterans Hospital (Seattle), as well as multidisciplinary discussions and treatment recommendations for the entire clinical spectrum of malignant disease. Sixty-two percent of the patients were treated at their closest facility; 38% were referred to the cancer center for treatment and/or additional diagnostic studies. Preliminary clinical results demonstrate the program is feasible and provides improved access for multidisciplinary cancer care, improved referral coordination, and minimization of patient travel and treatment delays. The program has been found to increase patient access to oncology specialists and increase specialty education of local providers throughout the service area.[30]

A unique multinational effort providing pediatric oncology care using telemedicine was undertaken, with sites in the United States, Brazil, and Chile. The effort is driven by the need for specialized surgeons trained in the treatment complexity of pediatric oncology. The primary aim of the effort is ongoing training of local surgeons involving weekly consults, proctored telesurgery, and educational conferences. Posttest evaluation results indicated a 26% improvement in overall patient care, with even more increases in patient care at the more distant sites.[31]

TELESURGERY

Advances in technological applications in surgical oncology and telemedicine come together in robotic surgery. The grist of science fiction in 1996, robotic surgery, guided by a surgeon located miles away, has now become a reality. Used for surgical training as well as remotely controlled, minimally invasive laparoscopic surgery, such systems are now widely in use, with more than 1000 robotic surgical systems worldwide (data concerning number of sales of da Vinci surgical robotic system obtained from Intuitive Surgical, 950 Kifer Road, Sunnyvale, CA 94086). Most robotic surgical systems are currently operated with the surgeon located in the same room as the robot to improve surgeon dexterity. Remote robotic surgery, initially demonstrated in 2001 by Marescaux et al., in a trans-Atlantic cholecystectomy between New York City and Strasbourg, France, proved that the fundamental principles of robotic surgery could be transitioned to clinical practice.[32] Because of limitations related to practicality, experience, cost, and reimbursement, only a few investigators have been successful in using telesurgery on patients many miles away. Those circumstances in which telesurgery is routine practice are all in a single-payer system, where the reimbursement issues do demonstrate a cost–benefit advantage. For example, in Canada, Mehran Anvari, M.D., has been performing weekly routine true telesurgery from McMaster University Medical Center in Hamilton, Ontario, to North Bay, Ontario, for advanced minimally invasive abdominal procedures (M. Anvari, *personal communication*, January 2004). This initiative will be expanded to multiple centers in Canada, which will be able to operate on patients in multiple remote locations. Until the issue of reimbursement for remote telesurgery is addressed on a more comprehensive level to provide incentive to more routine use of telesurgery, there are a number of efforts to bring telemedicine into (instead of sending out of) the operating room. Rosser et al.[33] has been using telementoring and teleproctoring to help surgeons who have learned a new procedure to be mentored through their first few cases at their home institutions. On a more mundane level, access to teleconsultation and/or information during a surgical procedure is being studied by many hospitals that are building their "operating room of the future."[34] One of the most important advances has been the innovative concept of the "perioperative systems design," which uses all information sciences, including telemedicine, to revolutionize and integrate the entire process of a surgical event, from the moment the patient is brought into the preoperative holding area until discharge from the hospital.[35]

TELEMEDICINE IMPACT ON NATIONAL MEDICAL POLICY

The areas discussed earlier are on the leading edge of remote oncology services and advanced technology in surgery today. Their application is being demonstrated in medical centers and in the laboratory, with efficiencies and efficacy evaluated in clinical trials to improve individual patient care. Another aspect of clinical trials is to improve, in a global sense, the outcomes of oncologic surgery. Telemedicine's contribution is through the facilitation of multi-institutional trials. Perednia[36] proposed a national effort of the Clinical Telemedicine Cooperative Group, which is based on the successful use of collaborative research by clinical oncology research groups, such as the Southwest Oncology Group.

Other areas in which telemedicine addresses national problems include improving geographic access, responding to the challenges of an aging society, and improving consumer access through Web-based telemedicine.

People living in rural and remote areas throughout the world struggle to access quality specialty medical care in a timely manner. Telemedicine allows many elements of medical practice to be accomplished when the patient and health care provider are geographically separated. This separation could be across town, across a region, or even across the world. Health providers in a growing number of medical specialties use telemedicine, including dermatology, oncology, radiology, surgery, cardiology, psychiatry, and home health care.

With the aging of the population in most developing nations, tele–home care has probably one of the greatest potentials for rapid growth worldwide. In 1994, the U.S.-based National Association for Home Care estimated that 15,000 providers delivered care to 7 million individuals requiring in-home services because of acute illness and long-term health conditions. Throughout the decade, the home-monitoring industry developed electronic and telecommunication equipment that enables medical care to be provided using telemedicine techniques rather than relying on in-person care to patients in their homes. Increasingly, hospital technology is relocating to the home. Home care creates advantages in terms of cost savings, but it also presents challenges for device manufacturers, untrained users, and patients. With more technologies moving into home care and more and sicker patients being treated outside the hospital, the home care approach to health care is here to stay. Aging patterns across Europe closely resemble the U.S. trend, and in Asia, the rapidly changing demographic characteristics and the tradition for caring for elders at home create a challenge and a unique opportunity for the implementation of tele–home care.

A rapidly emerging presence in telemedicine is the use of the Internet as a vehicle for the delivery of medical care. It is poised to become a major factor in the delivery of health care during the first decade of the 21st century, challenging the traditional structure in the delivery of health care around the world. Numerous companies are investing in telecommunications delivery services and health care systems in an effort to emerge as a major player in providing consultations, diagnoses, treatment, and delivery of prescription medications all on-line, usually with the consumer paying for the services by credit card. This opens the potential for horizontal monopolies for health care—the virtual on-line medical system. These services will be primarily in general medical treatment at first but will eventually include specialty care services as well. This has created a challenge in regulating the safe delivery of health care for nations with established medical systems as well as international bodies. It also places much greater power in the hands of the consumer to obtain information, purchase medical products, and even arrange for virtual consultations with providers.

The emergence of Web-based telemedicine provides many challenges to the existing structure for regulating health and medical services, to the authority of local and regional providers, to nations and individuals without adequate access to advanced communications services and the Internet, and to the traditional relationships that exist between doctor and patient. These are both challenges and opportunities and will inevitably alter the current delivery systems in most countries.

BARRIERS AND CHALLENGES

There are some real and perceived barriers to more widely implementing telemedicine for oncology. On the scientific side, there is a resistance to accept the new technology, with some evidence indicating telemedicine is not as safe as conventional practice (e.g., the telediagnosis of cancer on frozen section). Moser et al.[37] compared the accuracy of telepathology diagnosis and conventional diagnosis of frozen sections, using paraffin-embedded tissue as the gold standard. Out of a total of 270 cases, there was a correct diagnosis by remote frozen section in 227 cases (84.1%) and an incorrect diagnosis in 23 cases (8.5%). There was an equal amount of false-positive (12 cases, or 4.4%) and false-negative diagnoses (11 cases, or

4.1%). By comparison, the conventional frozen-section diagnosis was incorrect in only one case (0.4%) of a false-negative diagnosis. Other studies have shown comparability with tele-diagnosis; therefore, it is critical to ensure a rigid clinical trial to establish efficacy.

The second most difficult barrier is reimbursement or cost-effectiveness.[38] There are niche markets where the government is willing to pay for the provision of telemedicine, such as rural Native American health care or prisons; however, it will be much more difficult to establish cost-effectiveness until telemedicine is recognized by third-party payers.

Barriers to the institution of a telemedicine cancer program usually relate to social acceptance and practicality.[39] However, there is some evidence that telemedicine has the potential to relieve some very difficult problems, not the least of which is the nursing shortage.[40]

CONCLUSION

Significant hurdles remain, including legal and regulatory barriers and acceptance of the use of telemedicine by health care professionals' medical institutions. The number of areas that have been successful, such as expert consultation, better access to specialty care, distant education, facilitating multidisciplinary consultations, and multi-institutional trials, are seeds that need to grow. Barriers are slowly starting to come down, and there is a growing body of research data that indicate how telemedicine can improve patient outcomes and reduce health care costs. Telemedicine is in a transition that is indicative of an industry, service, or technology that is maturing. The long-term outlook for telemedicine is very good, and all indications point to this being a huge market, resulting in expanded access for individuals throughout the world. The question does not appear to be if, but when.

REFERENCES

1. Institute of Medicine. *Telemedicine: a guide to assessing telecommunications in healthcare.* Washington, DC: National Academy Press, 1996:16.
2. Wronski I. Rural and remote medicine comes of age. *Aust J Rural Health* 2003;11:161.
3. Kim HS, Oh JA. Adherence to diabetes control recommendations: impact of nurse telephone calls. *J Adv Nurs* 2003;44:256.
4. Fontelo P, Ackerman M, Kim G, Locatis C. The PDA as a portal to knowledge sources in a wireless setting. *Telemed J E Health* 2003;9:141.
5. Fuentes A. Remote interpretation of ultrasound images. *Clin Obstet Gynecol* 2003;46:878.
6. Bruderman I, Abboud S. Telespirometry: novel system for home monitoring of asthmatic patients. *Telemed J* 1997;3:127.
7. Luethi U, Risch L, Korte W, Bader M, Huber AR. Tele-hematology: critical determinants for successful implementation. *Blood* 2004;103:486.
8. Rohrscheib M, Robinson R, Eaton RP. Non-invasive glucose sensors and improved informatics—the future of diabetes management. *Diabetes Obes Metab* 2003;5:280.
9. Ortolon K. E-mail medicine. *Tex Med* 2002;98:41.
10. McNeill KM, Weinstein RS, Holcomb MJ. Arizona Telemedicine Program: implementing a statewide health care network. *J Am Med Inform Assoc* 1998;5:441.
11. Doty E, Zincone LH Jr, Balch DC. Telemedicine in the North Carolina prison system. A cost-benefits analysis. *Stud Health Technol Inform* 1996;29:239.
12. Brecht RM, Gray CL, Peterson C, Youngblood B. The University of Texas Medical Branch—Texas Department of Criminal Justice Telemedicine Project: findings from the first year of operation. *Telemed J* 1996;2:25.
13. Navein J, Hagmann J, Ellis J. Telemedicine in support of peacekeeping operations overseas: an audit. *Telemed J* 1997;3:207.
14. Satava RM. Virtual reality and telepresence for military medicine. *Comput Biol Med* 1995;25:229.
15. Fitzmaurice JM. A new twist in US health care data standards development: adoption of electronic health care transactions standards for administrative simplification. *Int J Med Inf* 1998;48:19.
16. Morris T. Battlefield Medical Information System—Telemedicine. Telemedicine and Advanced Technology Research Center. World Wide Web URL: http://www.projectmesa.org/ftp/SSG_SA/SA06_Ottawa_2003/BMIS-T.ppt, 2004.
17. Satava R, Angood PB, Harnett B, Macedonia C, Merrell R. The physiologic cipher at altitude: telemedicine and real-time monitoring of climbers on Mount Everest. *Telemed J E Health* 2000;6:303.
18. Hilty DM, Marks SL, Urness D, Yellowlees PM, Nesbitt TS. Clinical and educational telepsychiatry applications: a review. *Can J Psychiatry* 2004;49:12.
19. Costello SS, Johnston DJ, Dervan PA, O'Shea DG. Development and evaluation of the virtual pathology slide: a new tool in telepathology. *J Med Internet Res* 2003;5:e11.
20. Molnar B, Berczi L, Diczhazy C, et al. Digital slide and virtual microscopy based routine and telepathology evaluation of routine gastrointestinal biopsy specimens. *J Clin Pathol* 2003;56:433.
21. Mendez AJ, Souto M, Tahoces PG, Vidal JJ. Computer aided diagnosis for breast masses detection on a telemammography system. *Comput Med Imaging Graph* 2003;27:497.
22. Amendolia SR, Brady M, McClatchey R, et al. MammoGrid: large-scale distributed mammogram analysis. *Stud Health Technol Inform* 2003;95:194.
23. Kaufman DR, Patel VL, Hilliman C, et al. Usability in the real world: assessing medical information technologies in patients' homes. *J Biomed Inform* 2003;36:45.
24. Doolittle GC, Yaezel A, Otto F, Clemens C. Hospice care using home-based telemedicine systems. *J Telemed Telecare* 1998;4[Suppl 1]:58.
25. Lymberis A, Olsson S. Intelligent biomedical clothing for personal health and disease management: state of the art and future vision. *Telemed J E Health* 2003;9:379.
26. Malassagne B, Mutter D, Leroy J, et al. Teleeducation in surgery: European Institute for Telesurgery experience. *World J Surg* 2001;25:1490.
27. Health Infostructure in Canada, Health Canada, Office of Health and the Information Highway. World Wide Web URL: http://www.hc-sc.gc.ca/ohih-bsi/chics/inve.html, 2004.
28. The NHS plan: A plan for investment. A plan for reform. Section 4. Investing in NHS facilities. World Wide Web URL: http://www.nhs.uk/nationalplan/npch4.htm, 2004.
29. Doolittle GC, Allen A. Practicing oncology via telemedicine. *J Telemed Telecare* 1997;3:63.
30. Billingsley KG, Schwartz DL, Lentz S, et al. The development of a telemedical cancer center within the Veterans Affairs Health Care System: a report of preliminary clinical results. *Telemed J E Health* 2002;8:123.
31. Razzouk BI. Distance training of a pediatric oncology surgeon through a three site international collaboration. Presented at: American Telemedicine Association Meeting; June 5, 2001; Fort Lauderdale, FL.
32. Marescaux J, Leroy J, Gagner M, et al. Transatlantic robot-assisted telesurgery. *Nature* 2001;413:379.
33. Rosser JC Jr, Herman B, Giammaria LE. Telementoring. *Semin Laparosc Surg* 2003;10:209.
34. Doarn CR. Telemedicine in tomorrow's operating room: a natural fit. *Semin Laparosc Surg* 2003;10:121.
35. Sandberg WS, Ganous TJ, Steiner C. Setting a research agenda for perioperative systems design. *Semin Laparosc Surg* 2003;10:57.
36. Perednia DA. Telemedicine system evaluation and a collaborative model for multi-centered research. *J Med Syst* 1995;19:287.
37. Moser PL, Lorenz IH, Sogner P, et al. The accuracy of telediagnosis of frozen sections is inferior to that of conventional diagnosis of frozen sections and paraffin-embedded sections. *J Telemed Telecare* 2003;9:130.
38. Subirana Serrate R, Ferrer-Roca O, Gonzalez-Davila E. A cost-minimization analysis of oncology home care versus hospital care. *J Telemed Telecare* 2001;7:226.
39. Whitten P, Adams I. Success and failure: a case study of two rural telemedicine projects. *J Telemed Telecare* 2003;9:125.
40. Felder R. Medical automation—a technologically enhanced work environment to reduce the burden of care on nursing staff and a solution to the health care cost crisis. *Nurs Outlook* 2003;51:S5.

OLIVIER RIXE
PETER HARPER
DAVID KHAYAT

SECTION 5

International Differences in Oncology

National resources obviously result in differences in the management of all diseases, and this is also the case in the diagnosis, staging, and treatment of cancers. What is more surprising is how great the differences are between supposedly similar developed nations, even within the same geographic areas, and those differences are amplified when one looks across continents, despite similar socioeconomic positions. The disparity between westernized developed nations and the "developing" nations is even greater.[1]

The geographic variations in cancer incidence depend on the patient's characteristics (genetic and cultural) and environmental issues (for instance, the very high rate of melanoma in Australia and New Zealand essentially due to the western population immigrating to these areas),[2] and these variations are then altered by social changes (for instance, time of first pregnancy in North America and obesity).[3] Even within the westernized nations, there are differences in the collection and collation of statistics related to cancer, and yet it is on these statistics that many decisions are being made. Finally, the development of care systems, screening, and ethical considerations add to the difficulties of analyzing these figures.

In developing countries, malnutrition and infectious disease remain the major health problems. A new challenge is the overwhelming incidence of human immunodeficiency virus in Africa that places cancer in a relatively modest position of priorities. Nevertheless, more than 50% of the world's cancer burden, in terms of cases and deaths, are occurring in developing countries.[4]

The population demands for treatment will also change rapidly in those nations undergoing enormous economic change. China and India are predicted to be the first and third largest economies in the world within 50 years. Such changes in wealth will be reflected in changes in health care needs.

DEVELOPING NATIONS

A lack of comprehensive information is available on incidence and mortality data within the majority of developing nations. In many, the information available has followed a localized initiative of research-orientated clinicians and pathologists. The authors have reviewed the cancer mortality data from ten Asian countries, eight in South America, and a single country in Africa in the target year of 1995.[5] The data, such as it is, support a lower cancer incidence in many of the developing nations when compared to westernized nations. The global cancer incidence in 1990 in Vietnam and Venezuela were 133 and 104.1 per 100,000 males, compared to an incidence in the United States in males of 161.8. Lower incidences were seen in females, 91.7 and 91.8, respectively, than in the United States in a similar period (160.4). Compared to international data, the incidence of breast and prostate cancers remains low in developing countries.[6]

Cancer rates between ethnic groups within the same nation also differ. In South Africa, breast cancer incidence is low in black women (11.3 per 100,000), whereas the rate is 65 per 100,000 in black women in the United States. By contrast, the breast cancer incidence in white women in South Africa is identical to that of those in westernized nations. Within the black community there is high parity and a higher proportion of breast feeding, and the population is younger at the time of first birth. Even within the ethnic group, differences are found. In blacks and mixed-race women in South Africa under the age of 55, the rate was 16.3 for those living in villages and 26.6 per 100,000 for those living in urban areas.[7]

CANCERS AND MORTALITY: DIFFERENCES IN THE MORE DEVELOPED COUNTRIES

The EUROCARE project and the National Institute Programme in the United States are based on similar registrational programs.[8] Predominant cancers are colorectal, lung, breast, and prostate. In Australia and New Zealand, where population migration from European countries has occurred, melanoma has a particularly high incidence. As one looks over nations of the widened European community, again using the 1995 figures, the overall western European "cancer" rate is 420.9 per 100,000. Austria is the only nation with a rate under 400 per 100,000. Hungary has a reported a rate of 566.6 and the Czech Republic 480.5. The lowest male all-cancer rates are documented in the northern European countries (Sweden and the United Kingdom), and the highest rates in women were observed in Denmark.[9]

National screening and national treatment programs and access to care via health services vary from nation to nation. What is clear is that over two decades cancer survival has improved. In the case of testicular cancer, this was clearly due to the development of the platinum-based chemotherapy regimens, and in pediatric oncology it was a result of the development of comprehensive treatment protocols and strategies as a result of an ongoing clinical trials program that has proved very effective.

Educational and socioeconomic issues have shown a dramatic change in the incidence and the outcome of the treatment of lung cancer. Eastern European lung cancer rates continue to remain very high. However, the rate in North American men continues to fall. Within North America, where tobacco consumption has not continued to decline, lung cancer incidence in women has been at a plateau since the mid-1990s (female lung cancer incidence, 27.2 per 100,000). In eastern Europe, rates remain high across the population group with the continuing dominance of smoking and heavy industry.[8]

The incidence of prostate cancer has risen since the 1960s, particularly in North America, the United Kingdom, Austria, and France. Survival rates are undoubtedly increasing in the United States, with the introduction of prostate-specific antigen (PSA) testing in the mid-1990s and early surgical and radiotherapeutic intervention. The incidence in the U.S. black population is 50 to 60 times higher than rates in China. This is also seen in the black ethnic minority groups within western Europe.[10]

SCREENING

It is clear that within the developed nations the prognosis of some tumors is changing. Improved survivals have been achieved for breast cancer and colon cancer and, most recently, for prostatic cancer in the United States. It is apparent that the majority of these differences are due to earlier-stage patients being diagnosed and that those earlier-stage tumors are being detected by screening and by earlier presentation by an informed population.

MAMMOGRAPHIC SCREENING

In the most developed nations, breast cancer screening is considered routine in women aged 50 to 70 years. Clinical breast examination and mammography are generally recommended every 1 to 3 years, depending on the medical organization. Differences are found between mammography rates and subsequent interventions between the United States and the United Kingdom. Between 1996 and 1999, the results of 5.5 million mammograms in women older than 40 years were identified. Recall and negative open surgery biopsy rates were twice as high in the United States as in the United Kingdom.[11,12] High-volume and centralized mammography screening programs have been adopted in the United Kingdom, where the change is apparent in the stage of patients being treated.

The early detection of breast cancer in countries with limited resources was reviewed by Anderson et al.[13] Here the focus is not only on public education and awareness but on the necessity to expand early detection efforts to include mammographic screening. In a review by Katz et al.,[14] disparities in screening between social economic strata were seen in Western countries such as the United States and Canada. The screening rate was higher in the United States in 1984 than in Canada (47.0% vs. 38.8%). In both countries, women with higher education and income were more likely to seek screening.[14] In a further review of 17 cancer registries in six European countries in 1990 to 1991, the earliest stage cancers were found in France, followed by Italy and the Netherlands, and contrasted with England and Spain, which at that time had the most advanced stages at the time of diagnosis.[15]

SCREENING FOR COLON CANCER

The general recommendations for the screen of colon cancer normally include annual fecal blood testing combined with sigmoidoscopy at 5- to 10-year intervals in patients older than 50 years,[16] exploring the differences in stage at presentation, and trying to relate this to a credible explanation of reported differences in survival of patients with colorectal cancer.[17] Significant differences for 5-year relative survival rates were found for rectal carcinoma: 35% in the Spanish registry and 48% in French and Swiss registries. In this study, "stage" at diagnosis was the only independent prognostic factor and appeared to be the main determinant of survival inequalities.[18] In France over the last 20 years, there has been a significant improvement in overall survival, and this does appear to be correlated with the proportion of patients with stage I and II disease who have been diagnosed in that time.[19] An identical observation was made with rectal cancer.[20]

Despite these figures, there is a great variability in screening procedures for colorectal cancer between nations. Attitudes and practices are not homogeneous between nations and between physicians. In the United States, 80% of physicians indicated that they would recommend colorectal screening with fecal occult blood and flexible sigmoidoscopy. However, only 29% performed this latter procedure.[21]

Screening is now considered without doubt to be an effective method of reducing colorectal cancer incidence and mortality. The United States Preventive Services Task Force reviewed the evidence and gave a grade A recommendation that all men and women older than 50 years should be screened for colorectal cancer.[22] In the United Kingdom, the Department of Health has demonstrated its commitment to colorectal cancer screening by funding a national demonstration pilot to assess the feasibility and acceptability of fecal occult blood testing in the general population.[23] Together with the Medical Research Council, it is also funding a randomized trial of a single flexible sigmoidoscopy screen offered at approximately age 60 years with colonoscopy for those found at flexible sigmoidoscopy to have a high risk of adenoma. The trial has reported that flexible sigmoidoscopy was acceptable, feasible, and safe but has yet to report on the magnitude and duration of efficacy.[24]

PROSTATIC SCREENING

Cooper et al.[25] have reviewed the disagreement between clinical guidelines and the use of the PSA. These vary from the American Cancer Society recommendation of 2001: "The PSA test should be offered annually beginning at age 50 to men who have a life expectancy of at least 10 years. Men at high risk should begin testing at age 45. Prior to testing, men should have an opportunity to learn about the benefits and limitations of testing for early prostate cancer detection and treatment."[26] The American College of Physicians in 1997 gave a contrary review: "Rather than screening all men for prostate cancer as a matter of routine, physicians should describe the potential benefits and known harms of screening, diagnosis, and treatment; listen to the patient's concerns; and then individualize the decision to screen."[27] In 1998, the American College of Preventive Medicine recommended against routine population screening with the PSA test.[28] In 1999, the American Urological Association said, "The decision to use PSA for the early detection of prostate cancer should be individualized. Patients should be informed of the known risks and the potential benefits . . . Early detection of prostate cancer should be offered to asymptomatic men, 50 years of age or older with an estimated life expectancy of more than 10 years."[29] A Canadian task force on the periodic health examination in 1994 stated, "There is insufficient evidence to include prostatic specific antigen screening in the period health examination of men over 50 years of age. Exclusion of PSA from routine medical examination is recommended on the basis of low positive predictive value and the known risk of adverse effects associated with therapies of unproven effectiveness."[30] In 2002, the United States Preventive Services Task Force stated, "The evidence is insufficient to recommend for or against routine screening for prostate cancer using prostate-specific antigen testing . . . ."[31]

The study by Cooper et al. showed two practice patterns. Most participants recommended regular PSA screening beginning at the age of 50 for asymptomatic men with no known risk factors and at least a 10-year life expectancy. These routine "screeners" attributed their approach to experience that "supported" the benefit of PSA screening and to patient "demand" for the test. Other physicians discussed the implications of PSA screening with patients before offering the test but neither recommended for nor against it. The approach of these nonroutine screeners was primarily guided by the lack of scientific evidence documenting the benefit of PSA screening.

ANTICANCER DRUG DEVELOPMENT THROUGHOUT THE WORLD

Genetic polymorphisms within different populations can result in greatly differing toxicity and outcome data when similar protocols are used across nations and continents. Awareness of these issues is vital. Clinical trials are undertaken within clearly defined groups in terms of performance status, age, and comorbidity factors, and yet once a drug is licensed, it is used on the general population, in whom very little data are available.

The drug development of CPT-11 is a case in point.[32] The active cytotoxic metabolite (SN-38) of this topoisomerase I inhibitor is detoxified by the enzyme UGT1A1. Significant variations of the UGT1A1 promoter allele were demonstrated among individuals of European and Asian origin. In Japan, hyperbilirubinemia was associated with individuals with a single nucleotide polymorphism in UGT1A1 exon 1. Direct correlations made between SN-38 metabolism and the UGT1A1 promoter genotype in Europe and Japan were clearly related to differences in CPT-11–induced leukopenia in phase I and II trials. This has resulted in differences in recommended dose and schedule for this camptothecin derivative in those nations (weekly vs. every 3 weeks).

P-glycoprotein has also shown important polymorphisms. The variability of the MDR-1G in coding for the transmembrane transporter protein between white, Japanese, and African Americans influences drug detoxification (hence toxicity) and activity.[33]

Thymidylate synthase is the enzyme target of the fluoropyrimidine agents. Significant polymorphism of thymidylate synthase exists, and these levels can be correlated to differences of toxicity and activity in different ethnic groups.[34]

DRUG APPROVAL PROCESS

The drug approval process differs among national groups. Within the United States (the largest pharmaceutical market in the world), the U.S. Food and Drug Administration centralizes the drug submission process.[35] Within Europe, the European Medicines Evaluation Agency (EMEA) coordinates drug authorization procedures, including scientific evaluation, efficacy, and quality issues. The data submitted for approval by the EMEA are evaluated by the CPME (Comité Permanent des Médecins Européens), and if approved, this results in a single market authorization, valid for the European Union. A decentralized option can also be taken by which the drug may be licensed in one or two nations. Most anticancer drugs following the EMEA procedures are approved within 18 months. Since the introduction of this procedure in 2002, 24 oncologic agents have been approved.[36]

CANCER TREATMENT STRATEGY: EUROPEAN AND UNITED STATES DIFFERENCES

Colorectal cancer is in the top three cancer presentations in the United States and in Europe. The difference in how it is treated in the two continents is instructive.

In 1988 and 1989, two large U.S. trials performed within a cooperative group setting demonstrated a significant advantage for adjuvant chemotherapy in stage III colon cancer. This was subsequently confirmed by European studies. Based on the intergroup and NSABP (National Surgical Adjuvant Breast and Bowel Project) C-04 trials, 5-fluorouracil (5-FU) with low-dose leucovorin given for 6 months became the accepted standard treatment in the United States. By contrast, protracted 5-FU with leucovorin was used in France and some European countries, based on the results of original phase II and phase III studies (de Gramont regimen).[37]

In the metastatic setting, chemotherapy strategies have differed between the United States and Europe because of the earlier introduction of oxaliplatin into Europe. Building on the short infusion 5-FU with leucovorin (de Gramont regimen), Europe developed two protocols using additional oxaliplatin or additional irinotecan (FOLFOX and FOLFIRI). The combination with irinotecan in the United States is largely given on a weekly basis as the Rottenberg schedule and typically biweekly with 5-FU and leucovorin in Europe using the Douillard regimen.[38]

Similar differences in practice occur in T3N1 rectal cancer. In T3 or lymph node–positive rectal cancer, or both, postoperative chemoradiotherapy is considered in the United States to be the treatment of choice, following trials run under the NSABP and intergroup organization. By contrast, most European physicians have a policy of preoperative radiotherapy, followed by total mesorectal excision.[37]

DIFFERENCES IN CANCER SURVIVAL

It may be quite interesting to look at differences in cancer survival across nations using breast and lung cancers as models. In breast cancer, the prognostic factors are increasingly well defined. Nevertheless, across nations there are large variations in treatment policy and in survival. In addressing the survival issues, the Eurocare Study has analyzed data from 22 countries in Europe, covering 42 kinds of cancer. The study looked at 5-year survival in 1.8 million adult cancer patients and 24,000 children diagnosed between 1990 and 1994 and followed until 1999. Sweden, Finland, and France have the best 5-year survivals for breast cancer: 82.6%, 81.4%, and 81.3%, respectively. Poland has the worst 5-year survival at 63.1%. Within the United Kingdom, the rates for England, Scotland, and Wales are 73.6%, 72.3%, and 69.5%, respectively.[8]

As we look across continents, 5-year survival is 84.9% in Japan (however, breast cancer incidence is low) and 83.8% in the United States according to an OECD (Organisation for Economic Co-operation and Development) study. Whether these indicators can effectively assess the performance of a given health care system remains a complex issue, but these figures do not appear to be related to the number of mammography or radiotherapy machines. In the United Kingdom, within the time points concerned there were far fewer specialized staff and equipment in place than in the other nations discussed above. The same variability is also observed when one looks at the percentage of women diagnosed with breast cancer who receive breast-conserving surgery. This figure ranges between 60% for Sweden to 93% for France. Differences are also seen in the proportion of women receiving breast-conserving surgery, who will then receive local irradiation (43% in the United States, 93% in France, and 90% in Belgium). Surveys in the United States have confirmed that treatment differences are related to access to specialized centers and radiotherapy equipment.[39] The OECD study does not agree with this but suggests that the method of payment, that is, global budget versus the DRG (diagnosis-related group) payment methods may play a significant role in the quality of care in breast cancer.[40]

Survival rates in lung cancer are very poor, and even the very best of 1-year survival does not equal the 5-year breast cancer survival outlined above. Despite improvements in the diagnosis and treatment, the overall prognosis of a patient with non–small cell lung cancer has hardly improved over time. In small cell lung cancer, the dramatic sensitivity of this tumor has changed at least the short-term survival dramatically, although 3-year survival has not altered greatly.

The EUROCIM (European Cancer Incidences and Mortality) database allows geographic variation and changes in incident data to be reviewed. Survival can be derived from the EUROCARE database. Although the incidence of lung cancer among men in Denmark, Finland, Germany, Italy, the Netherlands, Switzerland, and the United Kingdom has been decreasing since the 1980s, the age-adjusted rate for men in other European countries increased at least until the mid-1990s. Among women, the peak in incidence was not reached in the 1990s. The proportion of adenocarcinoma has been increasing, probably due to the increased smoking of low-tar filter cigarettes. Within Europe, survivals vary greatly—for example, France (1-year survival, 42%; 5-year survival, 13%) and Poland (1-year survival, 25%; 5-year survival, 6%).[41]

ACCESS TO CANCER CARE IN DEVELOPED NATIONS

Outcome in the treatment of cancer is clearly related to stage at the time of diagnosis. Rapid access of patients to the appropriate specialist is, therefore, essential. Equally, the facilities have to be available immediately downstream of that initial referral to enable completion of all investigations and biopsies, with a definitive treatment planned and thereafter appropriate access to the treatment modality, surgery, radiotherapy, or chemotherapy.

The developed countries have universal health care systems in place, and initial stage at the time of presentation could be a specific end point to evaluate their efficiency. Looking across the three continents—United States, Europe, and Japan—we find very different health care systems. However, all offer the population universal medicare coverage. How does this compare within a nation when comparing rural with urban populations? In Canada, residing in a region where the socioeconomic status is low does not significantly affect access to elective surgery. Twenty-two common procedures were reviewed, and the only difference found was that relating to a radical prostatec-

tomy.[42] Even within this group, there was only a 4.4-day difference in time to surgery. The difference across the groups is quite acceptable.

By contrast, numerous studies have reported differences in the United States in time to diagnosis, time to complete cancer staging, and survival between black and white patients with breast cancer. Income, as a variable, was marginally associated with stage of disease for the white population—that is, within that group the socioeconomic factors were not found to be important ($P = .06$).[43] Between nations, rather than within nations, is more difficult to compare.

A review of access to radiotherapy was based on number of machines and radiation oncologists. In 1989 to 1990, a comparison was made between the United States and Japan. The number of external megavoltage treatment machines was 2397 in the United States and 494 in Japan. Full-time equivalent radiation oncologists were 2335 and 366, respectively. The ratio of patients to full-time equivalent radiation oncologists was 151 to 200 in the United States and 51 to 100 in Japan. Interestingly, 49% of American patients were treated with radiation therapy, whereas only 15% of Japanese patients had radiation as a prime modality of treatment. Overall, there were fewer treatment simulators, fewer treatment-planning computers, and fewer support personnel.[44]

In 1995, a report was published comparing access to radiotherapy between Canada and the United States, based on replies to a questionnaire from 97 centers. Median waiting times to start radiotherapy for carcinoma of the lung, larynx, prostate, and breast were significantly longer in Canada. However, the emergency treatment of spinal cord compression was similar in the two nations. The prolonged waiting times in Canada for routine radical treatment were considered by the majority of oncologists in both countries to be "medically unacceptable."[45]

A series of surveys also looked at the satisfaction of medical staff with the facilities available to them. In 1993, looking at the United States, Canada, and the former West Germany, 50% of doctors in Canada cited the lack of well-equipped medical facilities as a problem, compared to 14% in the United States and 20% in the former West Germany.[46]

Nevertheless, the situation in North America is not without its difficulties. It is expensive! In Canada, the average cost of treating a patient with non–small cell lung cancer in 1996 ranged from $6333 to $17,889 Canadian dollars.[47] In France in 2001, the figure appeared to be 13,969 Euros.[48] The cost of terminal care is significant and is up to 51% of the total cost in France. Of U.S. physicians, 70% report that the patient's inability to afford necessary treatment is a serious problem, as compared to 25% in Canada and 15% in the former West Germany. The availability of appropriate treatment for poor and uninsured patients is clearly serious.[46]

Life expectancy among the elderly has been improving for many decades, and there is evidence that health among the elderly is also improving. This is associated with significant costs, and these have been reviewed in the United States. Lubitz et al.[49] used the 1992 to 1998 Medicare Current Benefits Survey and classified persons' health according to functional status and whether or not they were institutionalized, and by their self-reported health. A person with no functional limitations at 70 years of age had a life expectancy of 14.3 years and an expected cumulative health care expenditure of approximately $136,000. A person with limitation in at least one activity of daily living had a life expectancy of 11.6 years and expected cumulative expenditure of approximately $145,000. For those who were institutionalized, cumulative expenditures were much higher.[49]

Entry to clinical trials is seen as the gold standard in terms of developing evidence-based treatment. Barriers to enrollment of minority patient groups exist within developed countries (physician lack of information, patient fears, distrust of the health care system), and within developing nations only a few percent of patients are entered onto clinical trials.

TRAINING AS AN ONCOLOGIST

Marked differences are found across nations in the number of medical oncologists and the separation of medical oncology from radiation oncology. The medical oncology subspecialty began in the 1970s in the United States and over the last 30 years[50] has evolved due to the introduction of increasingly complex treatments. In the meantime, clinical hematologists have also developed the subspecialty of hematooncology. Within Europe, only four countries—Great Britain, Portugal, the Republic of Ireland, and Spain since 1992—officially recognize medical oncology as a subspecialty. Italy and France offer a specific training program in medical oncology. Training in medical oncology in Germany is linked to that of hematology, and quite considerable chemotherapy is delivered by surgeons.[51] For example, the gynecologist also undertakes the chemotherapy of gynecologic tumors and the surgical and chemotherapeutic management of breast cancer. The time taken to become a specialist varies across nations; this can be 4 to 9 years from graduation. Most recently, the European Society of Medical Oncology has designed a program of certification, with standard requirements over the European Union, giving a total training period of 6 years, with a common internship in internal medicine of at least 2 years. Thereafter, there is a training program in oncology for 3 or 4 years.[52]

RESEARCH

Support for research and for clinical trials differs across the continents and between nations. The large cooperative groups in the United States have proved over decades to be extremely effective in completing trials and publishing appropriately. The well-known U.S. cooperative groups include NSABP, Southwest Oncology Group, Gynecologic Oncology Group, and Eastern Cooperative Oncology Group. These have a central core funding administered from the National Cancer Institute, are reviewed in terms of the effectiveness of the organization, and are audited in terms of their efficiency.

In Europe, the predominant organization crossing all nations is the European Organization for Research and Treatment of Cancer, which is centrally funded.[53] Interested clinicians and organizations apply for membership of the various subgroups, and continuing membership of those subgroups is dependent on accrual to studies. Most recently, groups trying to span all continents have developed, and these have included the International Gynaecological-Gynae Cancer Society and, in breast cancer, the Breast Cancer International Research Group,

offering international collaboration regardless of the nation of origin. A new initiative in the United Kingdom, the National Cancer Research Network, has been developed with the intention that, by 2005, 10% of all cancer patients will be entered onto relevant clinical trials. This exciting concept is being watched with interest.

"TRUTH TELLING": DIFFERENCES BETWEEN NATIONS

Differences are found in what patients want to know and what doctors wish to "tell" between nations and between different ethnic groups within nations. In a study by Blackhall et al.,[54] senior citizens from California were questioned regarding whether they wished to know about a terminal disease. The four ethnic groups (European American, African American, Korean American, Mexican American) significantly differed in what they felt they wanted to know. Korean Americans and Mexican Americans (respectively, 47% and 65%) were significantly less likely than European Americans and African Americans to believe that the patient should be told the diagnosis. Similar differences in these groups were reported regarding the extent of the truth that should be shared in the case of a terminal prognosis. Korean Americans and Mexican Americans were more likely to hold a "family-centered model" of medical decision making rather than one of "patient autonomy," as supported by the European Americans and African Americans.

Doctors' attitudes in what to tell the patient about this prognosis also differ. In 1993, 260 gastroenterologists from all parts of Europe undertook a structured questionnaire[55] concerning their attitudes to telling patients of their "poor prognosis." Gastroenterologists in northern Europe would normally be explicit as to the diagnosis to the patient and the patient's spouse, whereas gastroenterologists from southern and eastern European countries usually concealed the diagnosis from the patients, even after being asked to tell the patient the truth. Adenis et al.[56] reviewed how gastroenterologists, surgeons, and oncologists in northern France delivered the diagnosis and prognosis of colon cancer. They found the attitudes almost midway between that of northern Europe (tell everything) and the Mediterranean and eastern European countries, where little was discussed.

In Japan, physicians are more likely to give patients an optimistic account of their prognosis, whereas they are inclined to give the family a more pessimistic view.[57] In a further survey in Japan of 35 physicians, 21 nurses, and 63 patients, Seo et al.[58] found that just over half the patients who had expressed a wish to be told the diagnosis had in fact been told it. Thirty-one of the 35 Japanese physicians thought overall that telling a correct diagnosis had a positive effect. It was stressed in their answers that medical staff and family members should respect the patient's point of view.

It is clear that in Western countries, there is an increasing cultural pressure to give the correct diagnosis and, as near as possible, the correct prognosis.[59] In 1987, Holland et al.[60] reviewed the words used by 90 physicians from 20 nations in discussing the diagnosis of cancer. At that time, fewer than 40% of oncologists in Africa, France, Hungary, Italy, Spain, and Japan used the word *cancer* in their discussion, whereas greater than 80% of doctors in Austria, northern Europe, and Switzerland were comfortable using the word *cancer*.[60]

The authors believe that a tremendous change has taken place throughout the world. Virtually all cancer doctors now discuss the prognosis openly with the patient and with the family. While respecting that some individuals do not want information, it is generally accepted that the majority of patients are fully informed as to the nature, treatment options, and prognosis of their diseases.

CANCER IN THE ELDERLY

A leader in the *Journal of Clinical Oncology* by Hyman Muss[61] is entitled "Paris and New York—More in Common Than You Think!" This editorial discussed the study of Extermann et al.[62] to compare the willingness of older French and American patients to receive cancer chemotherapy. They undertook this review to test their perception that "elderly" European cancer patients were less likely to accept chemotherapy than "elderly" American cancer patients. Extermann et al. sent an anonymous questionnaire to 320 French and American outpatients aged 70 to 95. The cancer patients were seen at the Moffitt Center in Florida and the Centre Leon Berard in Lyon, France. Participants were asked to review two different scenarios describing "strong" and "mild" chemotherapy regimens and to define the minimum benefits for which they would accept chemotherapy, including curing the cancer, prolonging survival, and reducing symptoms. American and French cancer patients had similar acceptance rates for strong chemotherapy (a platinum/taxane regimen) and mild chemotherapy (a vinorelbine-based regimen). French noncancer patients were significantly less likely to accept any chemotherapy, strong or mild. For prolongation of survival, the minimal threshold for French and for American cancer patients accepting chemotherapy treatment averaged approximately 20 months, and approximately 70% of both cancer patient groups would accept chemotherapy to reduce symptoms. Nevertheless, the actual diagnosis of cancer does seem to concentrate the mind. For the noncancer patient theoretically discussing the situation of chemotherapy, only 52% of French patients but 68% of American patients would accept strong chemotherapy. For a milder chemotherapy, there was less "tradeoff" and less variation between the nations.[61]

The cultural differences among French and American patients and physicians and that relationship to medical care have been discussed.[63] The differences in recommendations suggested that French physicians were more likely to be resistant to "patient autonomy" in making medical decisions than the American physicians and that individuals in the United States are urged to assume greater responsibility for their own health. The editorial by Muss[61] brought attention to this because in numerous studies the physician's recommendation is the most important factor in patients accepting treatment, especially in older patients. He comments that in western Europe and the United States, the majority of patients desire precise information—whether good or bad—concerning their cancer diagnoses, and they allocate the major role in treatment decisions to their physicians.[64] Muss also points out in his editorial that ageism represents a cultural bias that commonly results in the undertreatment of older patients with cancer.[65] We must clearly inform all our patients with cancer about the benefits and risks of treatment and make sure that they understand the treatment options available to them.

CONCLUSION

Important differences exist in access to specialist care to specialist facilities between nations and even within nations. The position of ethnic minority groups needs continuous review and continuous improvement. Access to appropriate treatment protocols, which may include newer and more expensive drugs or techniques (intensity-modulated radiotherapy and brachytherapy), needs to be continually assessed, and protocols should be appropriately validated.

It is absolutely necessary to cooperate in terms of clinical practice guidelines across the world, helping the less developed countries to fight cancer ethically and appropriately within their own needs and priorities. As ever, information is the best method of achieving change, and a standardization of data collation across nations and continents is needed.

REFERENCES

1. Jemal A, Thomas A, Murray T, Thun M. Cancer statistiques, 2002. *CA Cancer J Clin* 2002;52(1):23.
2. Garbe C, McLeod GR, Buettner PG. Time trends of cutaneous melanoma in Queensland, Australia and Central Europe. *Cancer* 2000;89(6):1269.
3. Kelsey JL, Bernstein L. Epidemiology and prevention of breast cancer. *Annu Rev Public Health* 1996;17:47.
4. Parkin DM, Bray F, Ferlay J, Pisani P. Estimating the world cancer burden: Globocan 2000. *Int J Cancer* 2001;4(2):153.
5. Sankaranarayanan R, Black RJ, Parkin DM, eds. *Cancer survival in developing countries.* IARC Scientific Publication No. 145. Lyon: IARC Press, 1998.
6. Levi F, Lucchini F, Negri E, La Vecchia C. Worldwide patterns of cancer mortality, 1990–1994. *Eur J Cancer Prev* 1999;8(5):381.
7. Vorobiof DA, Sitas F, Vorobiof G. Breast cancer incidence in South Africa. *J Clin Oncol* 2001;19[18 Suppl]:125S.
8. Sant M, Capocaccia R, Coleman MP, et al., EUROCARE Working Group. Cancer survival increases in Europe, but international differences remain wide. *Eur J Cancer* 2001;37(13):1659.
9. Bray F, Sankila R, Ferlay J, Parkin DM. Estimates of cancer incidence and mortality in Europe in 1995. *Eur J Cancer* 2002;38(1):99.
10. Quinn M, Babb P. Patterns and trends in prostate cancer incidence, survival, prevalence and mortality. Part I: International comparisons. *BJU Int* 2002;90(2):162.
11. Smith-Bindman R, Chu PW, Miglioretti DL, et al. Comparison of screening mammography in the United States and the United Kingdom. *JAMA* 2003;290(16):2129.
12. Esserman L, Cowley H, Eberle C, et al. Improving the accuracy of mammography: volume and outcome relationships. *J Natl Cancer Inst* 2002;94(5):369.
13. Anderson BO, Braun S, Lim S, et al. Early detection of breast cancer in countries with limited resources. *Breast J* 2003;9[Suppl 2]:S51.
14. Katz SJ, Zemencuk JK, Hofer TP. Breast cancer screening in the United States and Canada, 1994: socioeconomic gradients persist. *Am J Public Health* 2000;90(5):799.
15. Sant M. Eurocare Working Group. Differences in stage and therapy for breast cancer across Europe. *Int J Cancer* 2001;15;93(6):894.
16. Zoorob R, Anderson R, Cefalu C, Sidani M. Cancer screening guidelines. *Am Fam Physician* 2001;63(6):1101.
17. Woodman CB, Gibbs A, Scott N, et al. Are differences in stage at presentation a credible explanation for reported differences in the survival of patients with colorectal cancer in Europe? *Br J Cancer* 2001;14;85(6):787S.
18. Monnet E, Faivre J, Raymond L, Garau I. Influence of stage at diagnosis on survival differences for rectal cancer in three European populations. *Br J Cancer* 1999;81(3):463.
19. Faivre-Finn C, Bouvier-Benhamiche AM, Phelip JM, et al. Colon cancer in France: evidence for improvement in management and survival *Gut* 2002;51(1):60.
20. Finn-Faivre C, Maurel J, Benhamiche AM, et al. Evidence of improving survival of patients with rectal cancer in France: a population based study. *Gut* 1999;44(3):377.
21. Klabunde CN, Frame PS, Meadow A, et al. A national survey of primary care physicians' colorectal cancer screening recommendations and practices. *Prev Med* 2003;36(3):352.
22. United States Preventive Services Task Force. Screening for colorectal cancer: recommendations and rationale. *Ann Intern Med* 2002;137:129.
23. Steele R, Parker R, Patnick J, et al. A demonstration pilot trial for colorectal cancer screening in the United Kingdom; a new concept in the introduction of healthcare strategies. *J Med Screen* 2001;8:197.
24. UK Flexible Sigmoidoscopy Screening Trial Investigators. Single flexible sigmoidoscopy screening to prevent colorectal cancer; baseline findings of a UK multicentre randomised trial. *Lancet* 2002;359:1591.

25. Cooper CP, Merritt TL, Ross LE, et al. To screen or not to screen, when clinical guidelines disagree: primary care physicians' use of the PSA test. *Prev Med* 2004;38:182.

26. Smith RA, von Eschenbach AC, Wedner R, et al. American Cancer Society guidelines for the early detection of cancer: update of early detection guidelines for prostate, colorectal and endometrial cancers. *CA Cancer J Clin* 2001;51:38.

27. American College of Physicians. Screening for prostate cancer. *Ann Intern Med* 1997;126:450.

28. Ferrini R, Woolf S. American College of Preventive Medicine practice policy: screening for prostate cancer in American men. *Am J Prev Med* 1998;15:81.

29. American Urological Association. Prostate-specific antigen (PSA) best practice policy. *Oncology* 2000;14:267.

30. Canadian Task Force on the Periodic Health Examination. *The Canadian guide to clinical preventive health care.* Canadian Task Force on the Periodic Health Examination: Ottawa, Canada, 2003.

31. U.S. Preventive Services Task Force. Screening for prostate cancer: recommendations and rationale. *Ann Intern Med* 2002;1379:15.

32. Innocenti F, Iyer L, Ratain MJ. Pharmacogenetics of anticancer agents: lessons from amonafide and irinotecan. *Drug Metab Dispos* 2001;29(4 Pt 2):596.

33. Ameyaw MM, Regateiro F, Li T, et al. MDR1 pharmacogenetics: frequency of the C3435T mutation in exon 26 is significantly influenced by ethnicity. *Pharmacogenetics* 2001;11(3):217.

34. Pullarkat ST, Stoehlmacher J, Ghaderi V, et al. Thymidylate synthase gene polymorphism determines response and toxicity of 5-FU chemotherapy. *Pharmacogenomics J* 2001;1(1):65.

35. Hirschfeld S, Pazdur R. Oncology drug development: United States Food and Drug Administration perspective. *Crit Rev Oncol Hematol* 2002;42(2):137.

36. Schwartsmann G, Ratain MJ, Cragg GM, et al. Anticancer drug discovery and development throughout the world. *J Clin Oncol* 20[18 Suppl]:47S.

37. Wils J, O'Dwyer P, Labianca R. Adjuvant treatment of colorectal cancer at the turn of the century: European and US perspectives. *Ann Oncol* 2001;12(1):13.

38. Wilke H. An international, multidisciplinary approach to the management of advanced colorectal cancer. International Working Group in Colorectal Cancer. *Anticancer Drugs* 1997;8[Suppl 2]:S27.

39. Sant M; Eurocare Working Group. Differences in stage and therapy for breast cancer across Europe. *Int J Cancer* 2001;93(6):894.

40. Hugues M. *Summary of results from breast cancer disease study.* In: *A disease-based comparison of health systems.* Paris: OECD, 2003:79.

41. Janssen-Heijnen ML, Coebergh JW. The changing epidemiology of lung cancer in Europe. *Lung Cancer* 2003;41(3):245.

42. Shortt SE, Shaw RA. Equity in Canadian health care: does socioeconomic status affect waiting times for elective surgery? *CMAJ* 2003;168(4):413.

43. Hunter CP, Redmond CK, Chen VW, et al. Breast cancer: factors associated with stage at diagnosis in black and white women. Black/White Cancer Survival Study Group. *J Natl Cancer Inst* 1993;85(14):1129.

44. Teshima T, Owen JB, Hanks GE, et al. A comparison of the structure of radiation oncology in the United States and Japan. *Int J Radiat Oncol Biol Phys* 1996;34(1):235.

45. Mackillop WJ, Zhou Y, Quirt CF. A comparison of delays in the treatment of cancer with radiation in Canada and the United States. *Int J Radiat Oncol Biol Phys* 1995;32(2):531.

46. Blendon RJ, Donelan K, Leitman R, et al. Physicians' perspectives on caring for patients in the United States, Canada, and West Germany. *N Engl J Med* 1993;328(14):1011.

47. Evans WK, Will BP, Berthelot JM, Wolfson MC. The economics of lung cancer management in Canada. *Lung Cancer* 1996;14(1):19.

48. Braud AC, Levy-Piedbois C, Piedbois P, et al. Direct treatment costs for patients with lung cancer from first recurrence to death in France. *Pharmacoeconomics* 2003;21(9):671.

49. Lubitz J, Cai L, Kramarow E, Lentzner H. Health, life expectancy, and health care spending among the elderly. *N Engl J Med* 2003;349(11):1048.

50. Kennedy BJ. Medical oncology: its origin, evolution, current status, and future. *Cancer* 1999;85(1):1.

51. Ashele C, Sobrero A, Lombardo C, Santi L. How uniform are post-graduate training programs in medical oncology in the European Union? *Ann Oncol* 1995;6(5):441.

52. Wagener DJ, Vermorken JB, Hansen HH, Hossfeld DK. The ESMO programme of certification and training for medical oncology. *Ann Oncol* 1998;9(6):585.

53. Zurlo A, Therasse P. Addressing the challenge of intergroup studies in oncology: the EORTC experience. European Organisation for Research and Treatment of Cancer. *Eur J Cancer* 2002;38[Suppl 4]:S169.

54. Blackhall LJ, Murphy ST, Frank G, et al. Ethnicity and attitudes toward patient autonomy. *JAMA* 1995;13;274(10):820.

55. Thomsen OO, Wulff HR, Martin A, Singer PA. What do gastroenterologists in Europe tell cancer patients? *Lancet* 1993;341(8843):473.

56. Adenis A, Vennin P, Hecquet B. What do gastroenterologists, surgeons and oncologists tell patients with colon cancer? Results of a survey from the northern France area. *Bull Cancer* 1998;85(9):803..

57. Akabayashi A, Kai I, Takemura H, Okazaki H. Truth telling in the case of a pessimistic diagnosis in Japan. *Lancet* 1999;354(9186):1263.

58. Seo M, Tamura K, Shijo H, et al. Telling the diagnosis to cancer patients in Japan: attitude and perception of patients, physicians and nurses. *Palliat Med* 2000;14(2):105.

59. Mitchell JL. Cross-cultural issues in the disclosure of cancer. *Cancer Pract* 1998;6(3):153.

60. Holland JC, Geary N, Marchini A, Tross S. An international survey of physician attitudes and practice in regard to revealing the diagnosis of cancer. *Cancer Invest* 1987;5(2):151.

61. Muss HB. Paris and New York: more in common than you think! *J Clin Oncol* 2003;21(17):3189.

62. Extermann M, Albran G, Chen H, et al. Are older French patients as willing as older American patients to undertake chemotherapy? *J Clin Oncol* 2003;21:3214.

63. Eisinger F, Geller G, Burke W, et al. Cultural basis for differences between United States and French clinical recommendations for women at increased risk of breast and ovarian cancer. *Lancet* 1999;353:919.

64. Aaronson NK. Assessing the quality of life of patients with cancer: East meets West. *Eur J Cancer* 1998;34:767.

65. Yellen SB, Cella DF, Leslie WT. Age and clinical decision making in oncology patients. *J Natl Cancer Inst* 1994;86:1766.

SECTION 6

ANDREW C. VON ESCHENBACH

The National Cancer Program*

Today's rapid advances in biomedical research will usher in an era when annual physical examinations include screening procedures that evaluate patients' genetic, environmental, and lifestyle risks for cancer. Serum genomic and proteomic patterns and advanced imaging technologies will be used to detect incident cancers at the earliest stages. Integrated targeted mechanistic-based interventions will modulate the behavior of the malignant tumor and its host environment. This is not a glimpse of the future but a view from the threshold of the new era of molecular oncology—an era in which the preemption of cancer will largely eliminate the suffering and death caused by this devastating disease.

Since the days of Hippocrates, physicians have dedicated their lives to relieving suffering and prolonging life, while sci-

entists have pursued the quest for knowledge to understand life itself. The passage of the National Cancer Act in 1971 focused these noble human endeavors on a commitment to conquer cancer. The National Cancer Institute (NCI) is dedicated to nurturing the investment that we committed to over 30 years ago, an investment that has led us to an exponential expansion of our understanding of the cancer process at the genetic, molecular, and cellular levels. The elucidation of the biologic mechanisms that determine susceptibility, transformation, proliferation, invasion, and metastasis has brought us to a thrilling threshold—a strategic inflection point at which knowledge of cancer equates with power over cancer. We can now see clearly a future in which we will eliminate the suffering and death due to cancer by 2015. This is not a prediction that we will "cure" or eliminate all cancer. Rather we now have the power to create a future in which no one will suffer and die as a result of the disease. We have set a mission with a purpose and a timeline. The path to the future is clear, and the NCI is committed to focusing its resources and to integrating and galvanizing the efforts of our myriad partners in the National Cancer Program to make that future a reality at the earliest possible date.

The expansion of knowledge is occurring exponentially, as evidenced by the volume of scientific discoveries and their applica-

---

*Portions of this chapter have appeared in previous articles.

tions. However, we are still in the earliest realization of this goal and must secure further expansion and application of resources and tools. Information technologies and other advanced technologies, such as genomic and proteomic microarray analyses, molecular imaging, and high-throughput screening, are providing the ability to identify many of the complex mechanisms responsible for cancer's lethal phenotype. As we understand more completely the steps of the carcinogenic process—the oncogenes, the tumor suppressor genes, transduction pathways, and cell-signaling mechanisms—we will identify the targets in that process that are vulnerable to interruption, modulation, and control. Our strategy is based on preempting the outcome of the disease process using a comprehensive approach to integrated, targeted, mechanistic-based interventions. This will be accomplished by preventing the disease from occurring or progressing, by finding new methods for early detection and elimination, by modulating malignant pathways, and by precisely predicting which treatment regimens will succeed or fail.

This construct of *cancer preemption* portends a powerful strategy to prevent, eliminate, and modulate cancer's progression. The success of preemption depends on continuing to advance a discovery, development, and delivery paradigm. *Discovery* will be grounded in striving to further understand and unravel the complexity of the genetic, molecular, cellular, and micro- and macroenvironmental mechanisms involved in the process of malignant transformation and progression. Preemption strategies will focus on identifying and disrupting these mechanisms. *Development* will use molecularly targeted drugs and biologics for detection, prevention, and treatment. Novel combinations of anticancer agents combined with imaging and molecular biosensors will be applied. *Delivery* will put into practice effective prevention, early detection, prediction, and treatments for defined, at-risk populations with defined outcomes and measures and opportunities to observe and study the dynamic expression of the cancer process in patients.

Not only do we have a clear goal, but we are already accelerating the pace of progress. The genomic and proteomic revolutions are allowing us to detect a handful of cancers earlier, make more accurate diagnoses, and consequently make better treatment decisions. Similarly, technology-dependent, individualized, molecularly targeted therapies, based on a patient's disease-specific profile of markers, are being used to manage the disease. We have moved beyond a hoped-for vision to an expected outcome. What follows are specific initiatives that are building the path to the day when we will reduce the cancer burden and allow patients to enjoy a better quality of life.

NATIONAL CANCER INSTITUTE AS STEWARD OF THE NATIONAL CANCER PROGRAM

The NCI is currently operating with far more intellectual capital, financial resources, and technological capability than ever before. Certain pervasive system-wide barriers, however, currently hinder the rate at which we are able to discover, develop, and deliver the interventions needed to preempt all cancer deaths. For example:

- Cancer research teams tend to have great depth in a given area of expertise but insufficient breadth across the related areas of expertise that are needed to move beyond "reductionist" models of disease process. To move toward integrative or systems models of cancer biology and to harvest the preemption opportunities that will arise from such models, we must assemble transdisciplinary teams of investigators with varying mixtures of biologists, chemists, clinicians, physicists, mathematicians, materials scientists, and bioengineers.

- Our current strategic inflection point in cancer research—at which progress can be accelerated exponentially—is due in part to the advanced state of our knowledge about cancer as a disease process and in large measure to the transformational nature of advanced technologies for cancer research and care. Advanced technology development and deployment efforts, however, have not yet been optimally integrated with cancer research and patient care. As a result, most cancer researchers and care providers are not yet able to take full advantage of the transformational nature of these advanced technologies, such as information technologies and nanotechnology. A coordinated national effort in this area has the potential to dramatically accelerate the progress of cancer research and improve the outcomes of patient care.

- Cancer research data tend to exist in tightly controlled databases and repositories in ways such that relatively few cancer researchers have access to them. Implementing bioinformatics systems that improve cancer researchers' access to extant data and annotated biorepositories will enable them to answer their research questions better, more rapidly, and more efficiently. Systemic improvements of this type will likely also stimulate the creativity of researchers and enable them to pose innovative research questions.

- Currently, a serious disconnect exists between cancer research and regulatory processes such that the development, testing, and approval of new interventions are needlessly slow. Systems solutions are needed to bridge the points of disconnect and move the best ideas from discovery to development to delivery.

While continuing to support investigator-initiated research and long-standing priority programs across the discovery, development, and delivery continuum, we are also focused on removing impediments to progress that are common to many members of the cancer research community, in areas from basic science to clinical research to implementation and delivery of health care. Seven areas of cross-cutting strategic relevance to cancer preemption are our current highest priorities: molecular epidemiology; integrative cancer biology; prevention, early detection, and prediction; interventions; bioinformatics; designing an integrated clinical trials system; and overcoming cancer health disparities.[1]

HARNESSING THE POWER OF MOLECULAR EPIDEMIOLOGY

Merging the insights of the genomic revolution with those of population sciences holds one important key to better understanding the causes of cancer. On our immediate horizon is the opportunity to identify and quantify the role of nongenetic causes of cancer—including diet, obesity, exercise, and energy balance; tobacco and alcohol; ionizing, solar, and other radiation; viruses and other infectious agents; hormones and metabolic processes; and chemicals in the occupational and general environment—and to do so in the context of the influence of host genetic factors. This includes the high-penetrance genes responsible for inherited cancers and common low-penetrance genes in the population that produce susceptibility to cancer and may be involved in a high proportion of all cancers. By understanding the behavioral, environmental, genetic, and epigenetic causes of cancers in human populations, we can identify important new avenues to improve cancer prevention and treatment.

By its nature, molecular epidemiology is a transdisciplinary team-based approach that is dependent on emerging technologies and population-based databases. In addition to important investments in advanced technologies to harness the full power of molecular epidemiology, we are focused on developing strategic partnerships that enable transdisciplinary science and data sharing. One important example is the Consortium of Cohorts,[2] an international collaboration of investigators who are tracking 23 independently funded population cohorts totaling more than 1.2 million people. These investigators are breaking new ground in many areas, including understanding the contribution of hormone- and growth factor–related genes and their interactions with risk factors and circulating levels of hormones and growth factors, in breast and prostate cancers. Other important examples are the Case-Control Consortia,[3] the Cancer Family Registries,[4] and the Cancer Genetics Network.[5]

DEVELOPING AN INTEGRATIVE UNDERSTANDING OF CANCER BIOLOGY

The wealth of knowledge harvested from recent advances in cancer research provides us the opportunity to integrate this knowledge to understand the higher-order, complex, interactive, dynamic, and spatial relationships of networks within cancer cells and between cancer cells and their environment. Although molecular signatures of cancer provide the foundation, we now have the opportunity—and the need—to move beyond our understanding of cancer at the level of a single molecule, pathway, or cell and move toward developing an integrative understanding of cancer biology. This requires research in the areas of intracellular networks, cell–cell interactions, tumor microenvironment, and the effect on carcinogenesis by organism extrinsic factors, such as chemical carcinogens, viruses, and bacteria. The objective of the research is to generate *in silico* (i.e., computer-based) models that recapitulate the complex systems, including the roles of the microenvironment and macroenvironment, in cancer initiation and progression.

Developing an integrative understanding of cancer biology requires collaborative research, interdisciplinary researchers, novel bioinformatics and laboratory technologies, and advanced training programs. NCI's new Integrative Cancer Biology Program[6] is an important step toward integrating knowledge in a higher order to understand the complex, interactive, dynamic, and spatial relations of cancer cell systems. By establishing training and outreach programs, hosting high-level "think tanks," and funding extramural research, we hope to make integrative cancer biology a key instrument in fostering the growth of predictive and preventive cancer care.

Understanding the complex networks that exist within and between cancer cells, tumors, and the micro- and macroenvi-

ronments will lead to the development of novel, rationally designed, predictive, and prognostic tools, and targets for intervention. Understanding extrinsic factors in the context of integrative cancer biology will further advance our ability to eliminate suffering and death from cancer.

PROVIDING BIOINFORMATICS INFRASTRUCTURE

To increase the integration of data and information, NCI has created the cancer Biomedical Informatics Grid (caBIG),[7] a bioinformatics platform that will ultimately enable cancer researchers across the country—and around the world—to easily share data in a manner that will enhance the synthesis and integration of data into information that will create knowledge. NCI and its designated cancer centers formed the first group of codevelopers and adopters of caBIG, allowing direct input and participation from the cancer research community and ensuring that it directly addresses their needs. However, it is not limited to the designated cancer centers, as researchers from around the world will have open-source, voluntary access to the common platform of caBIG. By using common tools, research teams will pursue new collaborative efforts and leverage their findings and expertise across the cancer research community and redefine how cancer research is conducted and shared.

DEVELOPING PREVENTION, EARLY DETECTION, AND PREDICTION APPROACHES

Because of its critical importance to the achievement of our goal, we are focusing on many other important prevention, early detection, and prediction strategies in addition to integrative cancer biology. One strategic priority is the development of multiple validated biomarkers for exposure assessment and as surrogate end points for incidence and precancer detection, based on an understanding of the interplay between genetic and environmental risk factors. The Early Detection Research Network[8] is an investigator-driven consortium that is establishing a national infrastructure to move promising biomarkers and technology into clinically validated tools for early prediction of cancer and to identify individuals at risk for cancer before the disease develops. Other promising areas of research include new immunologic agents for cancer, such as the human papillomavirus vaccine for cervical cancer, not only for the treatment of cancer but also as a prophylactic measure by vaccinating populations to prevent the disease.

Current areas of high priority in smoking and tobacco cessation include the development of products and programs that prevent smoking and promote smoking cessation among high-risk populations, especially children and young adults. Nicotine replacement products and other medication development products for smoking cessation are being pursued. As future aids in smoking cessation, research is being supported on small, portable devices to deliver a "smoking dose" of nicotine in a reliable manner, as well as devices that affect the pulmonary delivery of nicotine.

Another important opportunity being aggressively pursued by the NCI is the dissemination of evidenced-based cancer prevention and early detection programs, through the development and full implementation of evidence-based public health campaigns to reduce smoking, encourage healthy eating behaviors, and increase physical activity across populations, including underserved populations. Coordinated public health approaches at the federal, state, and local levels, with active involvement by voluntary health agencies and other nonprofit organizations, and by the private sector, will greatly enhance the success of these activities.

FACILITATING THE DEVELOPMENT OF CANCER INTERVENTIONS

Developing effective interventions to prevent, detect, and treat cancer, in partnership with the cancer community at large, must be our highest priority if we are to achieve our goal. This will require renewed attention to, and investment in, activities pivotal to translating discoveries into proven "products," and ensuring that those products are rapidly moved into the marketplace.

The NCI plans to facilitate the development of cancer interventions by integrating the various phases of cancer drug discovery, development, and delivery through active partnerships with the communities of biomedical science research, technology development, commercial organizations, and other federal agencies. The NCI Cancer Nanotechnology Plan[9] is being developed to initiate dialogue and encourage the development of cross-disciplinary teams among cancer research communities and technology developers to focus on the potential of nanotechnology for cancer prevention, diagnosis, and treatment. The National Biospecimens Network[10] proposes to establish a national resource that standardizes key aspects of tissue collection, processing, annotation, access, and distribution to facilitate comparison of genomic and proteomic data derived from biospecimens collected at different institutions. Public–private partnerships are being developed to rapidly validate targets for new tests and therapeutics. The NCI has established strategic partnerships with the U.S. Food and Drug Administration[11] to discover and develop surrogate end points of cancer and to improve the effectiveness and efficiency of the regulatory process for new cancer drugs. The current development of strategic partnerships of NCI with the Centers for Medicare and Medicaid Services is designed to provide mutual understanding between the organizations so that they can work together to create opportunities for enhanced cancer care delivery.

CREATING AN INTEGRATED CLINICAL TRIALS SYSTEM

Clinical trials have brought us to a point of success in many malignancies, such as childhood leukemia and testicular cancer and are our *de facto* mechanisms of continuous quality improvement. They were widely implemented in an era when very little was available for therapeutic application and a linear process of phases I, II, and III served to test safety, efficacy, and then comparison to current standards. The process is also pyramidal, with small numbers of patients for phases I and II and often with very large numbers of patients for phase III. Success

is often defined and measured by a statistical level of confidence that the intervention being tested has resulted in improved survival or observed tumor reduction. Certain minor variations have been introduced into these themes over the years, but the clinical trials process remains the fundamental paradigm and, over the years, has been institutionalized by the development of infrastructures such as the Cooperative Groups and Community Clinical Oncology Program.

To accelerate progress in intervention development, the United States needs a clinical trials system capable of addressing the full range of clinically relevant questions—including prevention, early detection, and treatment—with diverse population subgroups. The system must be easily accessible to a wide range of cancer patients and populations at risk, to the broad investigator and clinical care communities, and to the government agencies involved in the research and regulatory processes. Finally, the system must be supported by bioinformatics.

The clinical trials program for the future needs to accommodate interventions that are developed according to and directed to specific genetic, molecular, and cellular mechanisms. Cross-category integration and biologic end points will define the conduct of the trials. Designed interventions for defined populations at risk with profiling of the patient and the tumor will become the standard of care. The need for long-term monitoring of safety and applications at the earliest stages of disease will impact risk-benefit management. The question now confronting us is whether we are optimally configured to facilitate these new functions. We have embarked on an analysis of what would constitute an ideal system, and we have partnered with the U.S. Food and Drug Administration to ultimately apply new principles into practical enhancements for clinical research.

Establishing a seamless national clinical trials infrastructure across the spectrum of NCI-supported extramural and intramural clinical trials research groups will increase participation in and accelerate the completion of trials, increase patient safety and security, and accelerate the development and delivery of novel detection and intervention technologies. Improved communications among regulatory agencies and clinical trials groups will enable the design of updated policies and new technologies that optimize resources and minimize time to deliver new interventions through the regulatory process. Instituting mechanisms for two-way communication among clinical researchers and the broader community of health care providers will improve the adoption of new standards of practice, the design of new trials, and the postapproval evaluation of new interventions.

OVERCOMING HEALTH DISPARITIES

The unequal burden of cancer that is borne by various population groups within the United States is unacceptable. We must effectively intervene in ways that lower cancer morbidity and mortality in all communities regardless of race, ethnicity, gender, age, sexual orientation, and socioeconomic status, and especially in those communities that have suffered the greatest cancer burden. This requires reducing exposures to preventable causes of cancer and increasing access to evidence-based cancer detection, diagnosis, treatment, and survivorship services.

The movement toward molecular medicine and the dependence on advanced technology and the role of centers of excellence could widen the gap and increase disparities in outcomes. Much remains to be learned about how to accomplish these objectives. We are working aggressively to identify and understand the numerous and multifaceted factors that cause and contribute to cancer health disparities, as well as to understand how to tailor and apply what we know about modifiable risk factors, prevention, screening, early detection, treatment, survivorship, and end-of-life care to the diverse cultural, racial, and socioeconomic population groups across the United States. Overcoming barriers in accessing cancer information and services and providing policy makers with appropriate information and effective alternative interventions will lead to a sustainable impact on cancer health disparities.

Committed to eliminating the unequal burden of suffering and death due to cancer, the Department of Health and Human Services has issued recommendations designed to harness the energies and resources of the federal government so that cancer health disparities will become a thing of the past. The NCI was instrumental in developing these priorities. Included in the recommendations are plans to assemble a Federal Leadership Council on Cancer Health Disparities led by the Health and Human Services Secretary with the secretaries of other appropriate federal departments to mobilize a comprehensive national effort to evaluate, develop, and implement programs that will ultimately ensure unbiased access to continuous quality preventive care, early detection, and treatment of cancer for every American.

A CRITICAL "ENTERPRISE-WIDE" OPPORTUNITY: TECHNOLOGY DEVELOPMENT AND INTEGRATION

One of the long-range ways in which the NCI plans to reduce obstacles and accelerate progress across the strategic areas to reach the 2015 goal is to encourage and support enterprise-wide opportunities for advanced technology development. This will provide critical, future tools to integrate our scientific knowledge with the incredible advances made in computing power, sophisticated analytic software, hardware development, and networking that enables collaboration on a global scale. It would serve to provide a coordinated infrastructure to create new advanced biomedical technologies, provide training that facilitates interdisciplinary collaboration, and offer exceptional opportunities to integrate advanced technologies into biomedical research.

The NCI has identified five broad areas of potential focus for opportunities in technology development. Continued input from the extramural community and our advisors is further defining and developing these areas, which include integrative computational biology and bioinformatics, advanced imaging, bioengineering and advanced prototyping, development and preclinical testing of prevention and therapeutic agents, and research resources.

INTEGRATIVE COMPUTATIONAL BIOLOGY AND BIOINFORMATICS

To improve connectivity and synthesis of data among cancer researchers from all sectors, this effort will support further development of integrative computational biology and bioinformat-ics. Data and image archiving and ultra–high-capacity services to support complex analysis of vast amounts of genomic and proteomic data are needed in this critical area. The development of new analytic approaches, integrating progress made in commercial and government applications of computer science, is also being considered. To bridge the divergent expertise needed for large, multidisciplinary team approaches to cancer research and care, programs for advanced training in computation and other biomedical technology applications are critical and necessary to accomplish our goal.

ADVANCED IMAGING

To improve nearly all areas of cancer research, especially in the diagnosis of cancer and in monitoring the impact of cancer therapies *in vivo* in real time, advanced imaging programs are needed. As currently envisioned, a broad array of imaging modalities, such as high-energy-force magnetic resonance imaging, nuclear imaging prototypes, positron emission tomography, optical imaging, ultrasonography, and others could be intensely developed. To better understand functional interactions and foster molecularly designed biopharmaceutical product development, new technologies could facilitate the development of molecular imaging reagents and support the use of these reagents in the dynamic assessment of cell function and interactions at the subcellular and macromolecular level.

BIOENGINEERING AND ADVANCED PROTOTYPING

To develop novel technological advances in areas such as nanotechnology and high-throughput screening, coordinated bioengineering programs are being considered. Specific areas of research and development include material device construction, nanoscale fabrication, sensor development, and delivery systems. These technologies could be housed in dedicated facilities to develop models and prototypes of revolutionary diagnostic platforms to accelerate product development and dramatically enhance our ability to effectively detect cancer, deliver targeted therapeutics, and monitor the effectiveness of interventions.

DEVELOPMENT AND PRECLINICAL TESTING OF PREVENTION AND THERAPEUTIC AGENTS

To enable the development and preclinical testing of new therapeutic and preventive agents, broad access to unique resources and critical facilities is needed for all investigators. Comprehensive and rapid screening programs for molecular targets using biomarkers are critically needed to optimize chemical design and future testing modules. Chemical genomics programs could provide established libraries of new molecular entities, support a range of activities including the identification of effector activities, and establish safety profiles among combinations of molecules. To produce custom biopharmaceuticals for proof-of-principle clinical trials, a national state-of-the-art biopharmaceutical development program, including current Good Manufacturing Practices production facilities, is being considered.

SHARED RESEARCH RESOURCES

Availability of research resources such as novel animal models and biologic repositories to the entire research community is critical and will be pivotal to accelerating scientific discoveries through development to delivery to the patient. Activities such as the production of mouse models of disease and vivarium facilities and the acquisition, archiving, and distribution of chemical libraries, biologic compounds, tissues, and collections of natural products could be provided as a service to investigators as part of the national resource. High-throughput screening and testing facilities serviced by robotics could be used to rapidly speed the identification of molecular targets.

Technology development schemes must be based on innovation, translational application, commercialization, and bridging the gap between discovery and delivery. The inclusion of partnerships between academic and research institutes, the biotechnology and pharmaceutical industries, and other government agencies is needed to catalyze and accelerate research, development, and application of new diagnostic approaches and treatments.

An advanced biomedical technology development plan is an example of cross-cutting, long-range NCI initiatives designed to support the key strategies defined to reach our goal. These initiatives, taken together, will greatly accelerate the progress of cancer care and research and greatly benefit all members of the cancer research community. Most importantly, these initiatives will create extraordinary opportunities to improve human health by creating revolutionary new products to conquer disease.

CONCLUSION

The destination for our journey has become clear—to end suffering and death from cancer—and the path by which to reach the destination is rapidly revealing itself. We must now foster programs that accelerate the discovery, development, and delivery of successful new prevention, detection, diagnostic, and treatment interventions to preempt the cancer process.

Our progress in understanding and intervening to preempt the cancer process will inevitably pay enormous dividends, in terms of reducing the cancer burden and in other areas of health and health care. While we are studying disease processes in the context of cancer, the knowledge gained and the resulting preemption strategies that are developed will have broad relevance to many of the major diseases that afflict the peoples of the world. The successful preemption of cancer will transform all areas of health care. By developing and providing evidence-based interventions to all individuals in need, we will produce a cost-effective health care system and, most importantly, a society of healthy, productive people.

REFERENCES

1. Web site link to NCI Strategic Priority Areas. World Wide Web URL: http://www.cancer.gov/directorscorner/directorsupdate-08-27-2003, 2004.
2. Web site link to NCI Consortium of Cohorts. World Wide Web URL: http://epi.grants.cancer.gov/Consortia/cohort.html, 2004.
3. Web site link to NCI Case-Control Consortia. World Wide Web URL: http://epi.grants.cancer.gov/Consortia/casecontrol.html, 2004.
4. Web site link to NCI Cancer Family Registries. World Wide Web URL: http://epi.grants.cancer.gov/CFR/, 2004.
5. Web site link to the NCI Cancer Genetics Network. World Wide Web URL: http://epi.grants.cancer.gov/CGN/, 2004.
6. Web site link to the NCI Integrative Cancer Biology Program (ICBP). World Wide Web URL: http://dcb.nci.nih.gov/newsdetail.cfm?ID=12, 2004.
7. Web site link to the NCI cancer Biomedical Informatics Grid (caBIG). World Wide Web URL: http://cabig.nci.nih.gov/, 2004.
8. Web site link to the NCI Early Detection Research Network (EDRN). World Wide Web URL: http://www3.cancer.gov/prevention/cbrg/edrn/, 2004.
9. Barker A. Nanotechnology: building cross-disciplinary research teams to enable advanced technologies. *NCI Cancer Bull* 2004;1:101.
10. Web site link to the National Biospecimen Network (NBN). World Wide Web URL: http://www.cancer.gov/directorscorner/directorsupdate-11-18-2003, 2004.
11. Web site link to NCI-FDA Joint Program to Streamline Cancer Drug Development. World Wide Web URL: http://www.cancer.gov/newscenter/pressreleases/NciFdaCollab, 2004.

Daniel R. Masys

CHAPTER **58**

Information Systems in Oncology

In an era when the amount of information relevant to clinical medicine far exceeds the capacity of any individual to absorb it and the rate of change in health sciences knowledge makes textbooks out of date before they are printed, electronic information sources have become an essential tool of scientists, health care providers, and patients and their families. Data networks, of which the global Internet is the largest and most pervasive, form conduits for "just in time" access to information from thousands of public and private sources. Information access devices ranging from desktop computers to handheld "personal digital assistants" to Internet-enabled cell phones and television sets form an increasingly ubiquitous infrastructure that is used by professionals and the lay public alike. This chapter provides a survey of some of the types and sources of information systems relevant to clinical oncology, including online resources and electronic medical records (EMR) systems that provide guidance to avoid medical errors.

The words *data, information,* and *knowledge* are often used interchangeably as if roughly synonymous in the context of the systems used to manage them. However, it is useful in a health care context to make a distinction between these terms, because the types of technologies that acquire, store, and present each vary substantially. For purposes of this chapter, data are those primary facts and observations acquired in the course of providing health care services, such as the numeric value of a blood pressure measurement, a hemoglobin value, or the relating of a family history that a parent died of cancer. Data contribute to and in some cases become information when they inform an assessment or action, such as the diagnosis of an individual case of cancer or the calculation of risk that the same kind of cancer will develop in an

individual as his or her parent experienced. In turn, information can be systematically organized and analyzed to produce knowledge, which is the accumulated understanding of real-world objects and ideas. In this context, knowledge is the framework on which practitioners base their decisions about individuals, comparing the person-specific data and information with the science base of what is believed to be generally true about human health and disease. The discipline called *medical informatics* addresses the conceptual organization of data, information, and knowledge and the computer and communications technologies that support research, health professions education, and clinical care. The related discipline of bioinformatics is focused on technologies and analytic methods related to molecular sequence, structure, and function in support of molecular biology, genetics, and newer data-intensive life science methods such as genomics and proteomics.

Electronic knowledge sources can be divided into two general categories. The first, familiar to anyone who has searched the biomedical literature or used an Internet search engine to find information, is intended for viewing, reading, and/or printing by a human user. The second category of knowledge is less obvious but growing significantly in importance. It has been termed *embedded knowledge* and is represented in computers as sets of "if-then" rules that run in the background of clinical information and EMR systems. These "event monitors" continuously compare patient-specific laboratory results, diagnoses, medications, and provider orders to an internal set of rules representing knowledge for optimal care, such as chemotherapy dose guidelines in the setting of cytopenias or prescribing limits based on drug allergies and drug–drug interactions. When the conditions of a rule are met, such as the finding that digoxin has just been ordered in a patient who is hypokalemic, the system generates an alert to the provider that an adverse event may occur if the drug order is completed without correcting the physiologic abnormality.

This chapter presents an overview of both categories of knowledge management systems, provides a basis for assessing the quality of online information, gives examples of Internet-accessible oncology resources, and provides guidelines for selecting an EMR system for an oncology practice. Specific online sources and characteristics of systems have been verified as of this writing, but nothing is so constant as change in the world of electronic information. For this reason, specific references to information services and products are supplemented with more general principles that apply to all examples of a particular class of resources (e.g., oncology Web sites for patients) or systems.

THE INTERNET

The information technology most emblematic of present times is the Internet, which is a global "network of networks" built on a set of common rules for the communication of data between computers. These relatively simple rules, called *TCP/IP* for Transmission Control Protocol/Internet Protocol, enable computing devices from thousands of different manufacturers in hundreds of different countries worldwide to communicate with one another.[1] The standards of the Internet were first developed in the 1970s and were the province primarily of universities, government agencies, and military installations. In the 1990s, these communications technologies saw explosive, exponential growth propelled by the development of HTTP (Hypertext Transport Protocol), which underpins the World Wide Web, now so familiar that it is simply referred to as *the Web* throughout the world.

The number of Internet users has been growing steadily over the past two decades, and 54% of Americans used the Internet in 2002.[2] The number of persons with access to the Internet is projected to rise to 80% of those in the United States, Canada, and the industrialized countries of the world by 2005, with more than a billion users worldwide by the end of the decade.[3,4] In the United States, an estimated 93 million persons, representing 80% of Internet users surveyed by the Pew Internet and American Life Survey, have searched for health information online.[5] The strongest predictor of online health information use is educational level, regardless of race or ethnicity. Other factors that affect the use of the Internet for health information include gender (women more commonly seeking health information than men), prior experience with online searching (those with 4 or more years of experience seeking health information more than those with 1 year or less), presence of a chronic illness (those with chronic illnesses seeking information more commonly than those without), and mode of access (broadband users seeking information more frequently than dial-up users). Internet use by health professionals has been estimated to be 100% for physicians and 72% for nurses, and 90% of health care professionals report that patients have brought to them information accessed from the Internet for their consideration.[6]

Use of the Internet to access health information has been negatively affected by two issues: the impediments to access for persons in disadvantaged groups within society, which has been

TABLE 58-1. Quality Criteria for Health-Related Web Sites

Criteria	Elements
Authorship	Explicit authorship is noted, along with credentials and affiliations of authors. Authors are qualified health professionals.
Attribution	Sources for content are noted with specific references and attribution of copyright where appropriate. Health claims are supported with references to research results and/or published articles.
Disclosure	Funding for the Web site and its content is clearly stated. Sponsorship is noted, and advertisements are explicitly labeled as advertising.
Currency	Dates of posting and most recent update are indicated. Contact information for the Web editor and/or system administrator is provided.
Links	Accurate descriptions for the content of all hyperlinked sites is provided, respecting legal requirements and privacy where applicable. Links are tested for correctness, and the information from the linked site is valid.
Peer review	Site uses a formal peer review process and/or editorial board.

(Adapted from ref. 11.)

termed the *digital divide*, and the variable quality of health information available online. Although the difference between information "haves" and "have nots" has been portrayed as lack of equipment or personal awareness,[7] it appears to be better characterized and predicted by differences in education, literacy, and language barriers.[8,9] Variable quality of health information available on the Internet is a persistent concern of health care professionals and patients, with health professionals having a higher frequency of negative opinions about the value of online information than patients.[5,10] Criteria have been developed and published by advocacy organizations such as HON (Health on the Net Foundation), by which quality and reliability of health information can be explicitly assessed, as shown in Table 58-1. These include credentials and affiliations of authors, appropriate attribution and references, financial disclosure, currency of updates, valid links to other sites, and peer review of information presented on the site.[11] Not surprisingly, only a small fraction of patients use any formal set of criteria for evaluating health-related Web sites, but the general principle of finding consensus among Web sites and not exclusively trusting any single source of information (including one's own physician) is an increasingly common mode of information seeking by patients and their families.[5,12]

ONCOLOGY-RELATED WEB SITES

Table 58-2 provides a sample of some widely used Web sites related to oncology, with notation of whether they contain information directed to clinicians (C), patients (P), or both. These sites have been provided by their host organizations for 3 or more years and as of this writing state that they adhere to HON criteria. *Caveat emptor* (buyer beware) applies to this list and any list of URLs (Uniform Resource Locators), however, because of the changeable nature of Internet site identifiers, the potential for previously high-quality sites to become stale with outdated information, and the propensity of successful health Web sites to change hands among owner organizations with differing corporate philosophies.

TABLE 58-2. Oncology-Related Web Sites

Category	Site Name	Target Audience: Clinician (C), Patient (P)	URL
COMPREHENSIVE: MANY TOPICS	American Cancer Society	C, P	http://www.cancer.org
	CancerEducation.com	C, P	http://www.cancereducation.com
	Cancer Care	C, P	http://cancercare.org
	Cancer Information Service, U.S. National Cancer Institute (NCI)	C, P	http://cis.nci.nih.gov
	CancerGuide: Steve Dunn's cancer information page	P	http://cancerguide.org
	CancerNet (NCI)	C, P	http://cancernet.nci.nih.gov
	CancerSource.com	C, P	http://www.cancersource.com
	National Coalition for Cancer Survivorship	P	http://canceradvocacy.org
	Healthfinder, U.S. Dept. of Health and Human Services (DHHS)	P	http://www.healthfinder.gov
	MEDLINE*plus*, U.S. National Library of Medicine	P	http://www.nlm.nih.gov/medlineplus/cancers.html
	OncoLink	C, P	http://oncolink.upenn.edu
	TeleSCAN Telematics Services in Cancer (European)	C, P	http://telescan.nki.nl/
SITE-SPECIFIC CANCER INFORMATION			
Brain cancer	American Brain Tumor Association	C, P	http://www.abta.org/
	National Brain Tumor Foundation	P	http://www.braintumor.org
Breast cancer	Breast Cancer and Environmental Risk Factors Project	C	http://envirocancer.cornell.edu
	Breast Cancer Online	C, P	http://www.bco.org
	Community Breast Cancer Health Project	P	http://www.cbhp.org/
	ENCORE	P	http://www.smywca.org/encore.html
	Inflammatory Breast Cancer Research Foundation	P	http://www.ibcresearch.org
	National Breast Cancer Coalition	P	http://www.natlbcc.org
	Susan G. Komen Breast Cancer Foundation	P	http://www.komen.org/bci/
	Y-ME National Breast Cancer Organization	P	http://www.y-me.org
Eye cancer	Eye Cancer Network	P	http://www.eyecancer.com
Genitourinary cancers	American Foundation for Urologic Disease	C, P	http://www.afud.org
	Kidney Cancer Association	C, P	http://kidneycancerassociation.org
Gynecologic cancers	American College of Obstetricians and Gynecologists	C, P	http://www.acog.org
	National Cervical Cancer Coalition	P	http://www.nccc-online.org
	National Ovarian Cancer Coalition	P	http://www.ovarian.org
Head and neck cancer	Support for People with Oral and Head and Neck Cancer, Inc.	P	http://www.spohnc.org
Leukemia	Leukemia and Lymphoma Society of America	C, P	http://www.leukemia.org
Lung cancer	Alliance for Lung Cancer	P	http://www.alcase.org
	Lung Cancer.org	C, P	http://www.lungcancer.org
Lymphoma	Leukemia and Lymphoma Society of America	C, P	http://www.leukemia.org
	Lymphoma Information Network	P	http://www.lymphomainfo.net
	Lymphoma Research Foundation of America	C, P	http://lymphoma.org
Multiple myeloma	International Myeloma Foundation	C, P	http://myeloma.org
	Multiple Myeloma Research Foundation	C, P	http://multiplemyeloma.org
Pediatric cancers	Miami Children's Hospital: Children's Brain & Spinal Cord Tumors	P	http://www.mch.com/clinical/neurosurgery/parents_starting/tumors.htm
	Candlelighters Childhood Cancer Foundation	P	http://www.candlelighters.org
	Children's Hospice International	P	http://www.chionline.org
	National Childhood Cancer Foundation	P	http://www.nccf.org
	Outlook: Life Beyond Childhood Cancer	P	http://www.outlook-life.org
	Children's Oncology Group	C	http://www.childrensoncologygroup.org/
	National Children's Cancer Society	P	http://www.children-cancer.com
Prostate cancer	US TOO International	P	http://www.ustoo.com
Skin cancer	Melanoma Patients' Information	P	http://www.mpip.org
	Melanoma Education Fund	P	http://www.skincheck.com

(continued)

TABLE 58-2.   *(Continued)*

Category	Site Name	Target Audience: Clinician (C), Patient (P)	URL
TREATMENT-ORIENTED SITES			
Bone marrow transplantation	BMT Support Online	P	http://www.bmtsupport.org
	National Bone Marrow Transplant Link	C, P	http://www.nbmtlink.org/
	National Marrow Donor Program	C, P	http://www.marrow.org
Clinical guidelines for cancer treatment	Agency for Healthcare Research and Quality	C	http://www.ahcpr.gov
	Cancer Care Ontario	C, P	http://www.cancercare.on.ca/
	National Guideline Clearinghouse	C	http://www.guideline.gov
Treatment centers	U.S. National Cancer Institute Cancer Centers	C, P	http://www.cancer.gov/cancercenters/
Genetics	Cancer Family Registries	C	http://epi.grants.cancer.gov/CFR/
	Cancer Genetics Network	C	http://epi.grants.cancer.gov/CGN/
	Genetics of Cancer	P	http://www.cancergenetics.org
	Mendelian Inheritance in Man	C	http://ncbi.nlm.nih.gov/omim
Prevention	American Institute for Cancer Research	P	http://www.aicr.org
	Cancer Research Foundation of America	C, P	http://www.preventcancer.org
	Harvard Center for Cancer Prevention	C, P	http://www.hsph.harvard.edu/cancer
	NCI/CDC 5 A Day Diet Guidance	C, P	http://5aday.gov
	Tobacco-Related Disease Research	C	http://www.trdrp.org
Testing for cancer	Cancer Imaging Research	C, P	http://www.bccancer.bc.ca/research/imaging
	FDA list of mammography screening sites	C, P	http://www.fda.gov/cdrh/mammography/certified.html
Coping with cancer	CancerSymptoms	P	http://cancersymptoms.org
	Hospice Link	C, P	http://hospiceworld.org
	National Hospice Organization	C, P	http://www.nho.org
	National Lymphedema Network	P	http://lymphnet.org
	Oral Complications of Cancer	P	http://www.nohic.nidcr.nih.gov/campaign/pubslisting.asp
	Hospice Web	P	http://www.hospiceweb.com
	United Ostomy Association, Inc.	P	http://www.uoa.org
	Washington-Alaska Cancer Pain Initiative	P	http://www.wacpi.org
Support and resources	Association of Cancer Online Resources	C, P	http://www.acor.org
	Cancer Care	P	http://www.cancercare.org
	Cancer Hope Network	P	http://www.cancerhopenetwork.org
	Cancer Supportive Care Programs	P	http://www.cancersupportivecare.com
	Corporate Angel Network	C	http://www.corpangelnetwork.org
	Gilda's Club, Inc.	P	http://www.gildasclub.org
	NCI Office of Cancer Survivorship	C, P	http://dccps.nci.nih.gov/ocs
	National Coalition for Cancer Survivorship	P	http://www.canceradvocacy.org
	Patient Advocate Foundation	P	http://www.patientadvocate.org
	R. A. Bloch Cancer Foundation	P	http://www.blochcancer.org
	Support for People with Oral and Head and Neck Cancer	P	http://www.spohnc.org
	National Children's Cancer Society	P	http://children-cancer.com
	The Wellness Community	P	http://www.wellnesscommunity.org
	Vital Options	P	http://www.vitaloptions.org
Cancer literature	American Association for Cancer Research	C	http://www.aacr.org
	American Society of Clinical Oncology	C, P	http://www.asco.org
	Cancer Literature in PubMed	C	http://cancernet.nci.nih.gov/search/pubmed
	Cancer News on the Net	P	http://www.cancernews.com
	Electronic Journal of Oncology	C	http://www.elecjoncol.org
	NCI Publications Locator	C	https://cissecure.nci.nih.gov/ncipubs/
	MEDLINE via PubMed	C	http://www.nlm.nih.gov
Statistics	American Cancer Society Statistics	C	http://www.cancer.org
	CDC National Program of Cancer Registries	C	http://www.cdc.gov/cancer/npcr
	NCI Surveillance, Epidemiology and End Results (SEER) Registry	C	http://seer.cancer.gov

(continued)

TABLE 58-2. (*Continued*)

Category	Site Name	Target Audience: Clinician (C), Patient (P)	URL
OTHER RESOURCES			
Minority health	Intercultural Cancer Council	C, P	http://icc.bcm.tmc.edu
	National Asian Women's Health Resource Center	P	http://www.nawho.org
	Office of Minority Health Resource Center	C, P	http://www.omhrc.gov
Spanish language information	NCI Cancernet	C, P	http://cancernet.nci.nih.gov
	Cancer Care	P	http://www.cancercare.org
	NOAH: New York Online Access to Health	P	http://www.noah-health.org
	Y-ME National Breast Cancer Coaltion	P	http://www.y-me.org
Associations and societies	American Association for Cancer Research	C	http://www.aacr.org
	American Society for Clinical Oncology	C, P	http://www.asco.org
	Association of Community Cancer Centers	C, P	http://www.accc-cancer.org
	Oncology Nursing Society	C	http://www.ons.org
	Society of Surgical Oncology	C	http://www.surgonc.org
U.S. government health agencies	Agency for Healthcare Research and Quality	C	http://www.ahcpr.gov
	Centers for Disease Control and Prevention	C, P	http://www.cdc.gov
	ClinicalTrials.gov	C, P	http://www.clinicaltrials.gov
	Food and Drug Administration	C, P	http://www.fda.gov
	Healthfinder	P	http://www.healthfinder.gov
	National Cancer Institute	C, P	http://www.cancer.gov
	National Center for Complementary and Alternative Medicine	C, P	http://www.nccam.nih.gov
	National Institutes of Health	C, P	http://www.nih.gov
	National Library of Medicine	C, P	http://www.nlm.nih.gov
	National Women's Health Information Center	P	http://www.4women.gov

(Adapted from ref. 13.)

Cancer information from government sources has historically been the most comprehensive and trusted. The U.S. National Cancer Institute (NCI) has developed and made available online a wide variety of cancer-related data, information, and knowledge over the past 25 years. Most NCI services use formal peer review of content and a process of regular revision to accommodate recent findings from the scientific literature. The substantial resources provided by government funding contribute to a more elaborate infrastructure for promoting accuracy, balance, breadth, and currency of these oncology resources. Included among them is PDQ, the Physician Data Query database that includes literature-based, full-text summaries of current-consensus best evidence for cancer prevention, diagnosis, staging, treatment, and prognosis. Also included within PDQ are summaries of cancer clinical trials by cancer type, treatment modality, and geographic location and directories of physicians and other health professionals who provide oncology-related services.[14] The NCI's CANCER-LIT database contains more than 1.5 million citations and abstracts from greater than 4000 different sources, along with preformulated search "digests" for more than 90 commonly searched clinical topics.

CANCER INFORMATION BY PHONE AND FAX

A computer with Internet access is not the sole access mechanism for topic-specific oncology information. The NCI also supports a nationwide network of regional offices as part of its Cancer Information Services (CIS) program that responds to inquiries made via a nationwide toll-free number: 1-800-4-CANCER. CIS staff accepts disease-specific inquiries from patients, family members, health professionals, and the general public and responds to those inquiries with customized searches and distribution of approximately 600 publications on cancer prevention, diagnosis, treatment, supportive care, community services, and oncology-related research findings. Information is also available through automated fax-back technologies via Cancer Fax and an automated e-mail–based service. Of note is that nearly 20% of the 900,000 callers who contact the CIS program via phone each year have found the toll-free phone number on the Internet.[13]

ELECTRONIC MEDICAL RECORDS

A well-designed and implemented EMR system is arguably the most powerful tool an oncologist can use to optimize the quality and efficiency of care delivered, but the process of choosing and implementing the technology is neither easy nor inexpensive. The remainder of this chapter reviews features of EMRs that are relevant to oncology, discusses the issues to be considered in the decision to implement an EMR, and provides an overview of trends that are guiding the continued evolution of EMR technologies for the future.

Early EMR systems (and the most primitive of current systems) were not much more than passive receptacles of demographic data, problem lists, clinic notes, and laboratory tests. In this aspect, the EMR is simply an electronic replacement for paper charts, capable of storing and retrieving manually entered data in a fashion fully analogous to the manual recording, storage, and retrieval of physical records. Modern EMR designs provide this basic function but in addition facilitate the use of the EMR as a channel of communication for coordination of care and provision of patient-specific clinical decision support via alerts and reminders triggered by elements of a particular patient's disease, medications, and current laboratory findings. Well-designed EMRs also support secondary aggregation and analyses of data, such as health outcomes assessment among specific groups of patients, resource utilization analysis and management, practice profiling, optimization of billing and justification of third-party charges, and an increasing amount of external reporting in electronic format to payers, regulators, and accreditation organizations.

These analytic and reporting tasks generally require that the contents of the EMR be organized and retrievable using standardized coding of elements such as symptoms, signs, diagnoses, procedures, and services provided. For example, to analyze how many patients have been seen in a particular time period who have acute myelogenous leukemia or one of its variants, a system needs to have standard numeric diagnostic codes for types of leukemia or consistent use of the same words used to describe the condition, or both. A computerized search for "myelogenous" will not retrieve records of those patients whose diagnosis is "acute myeloid leukemia," "acute nonlymphocytic leukemia," or "myeloblastic leukemia" unless the system has some technical provision for uniform coding or an underlying dictionary that can supply possible synonyms for the term being searched. Free narrative text, whether typed via a keyboard or created via automated techniques such as voice-recognition software, usually lacks the structure necessary to support automated alerts, coding, and systematic outcomes analysis.

Just as health-related Web sites are transforming the information-gathering behaviors of physicians and patients, the Internet is profoundly influencing the design of best-of-breed EMR systems. The ubiquity of the Internet lends itself to anywhere, anytime access to EMR information by clinicians and also portends new models of shared information management among providers and their patients. Legal factors such as the Privacy Rule of the Health Insurance Portability and Accountability Act of 1996 (HIPAA) give patients a uniform right to inspect, copy, and request amendments to their medical records. In response to this set of federal regulations, many major vendors of EMR systems are creating products that include the ability to give patients secure Web-accessible views of their medical records.

FUNCTIONAL COMPONENTS OF ELECTRONIC MEDICAL RECORD SYSTEMS

A functional view of the requirements for EMR systems was provided by the 1991 Institute of Medicine report entitled "The Computer-Based Patient Record: An Essential Technology for Health Care."[15] It defined 12 key characteristics of an effective EMR:

1. Supports problem lists
2. Measures health status and function levels
3. Documents clinical reasoning and rationale
4. Provides longitudinal and timely linkages with other patient records
5. Guarantees confidentiality and provides audit trails
6. Provides reliable and continuous authorized user access
7. Supports simultaneous user views of the record
8. Provides timely access to local and remote information resources
9. Facilitates clinical problem solving
10. Supports direct data entry by physicians
11. Supports practitioners in measuring and managing costs and improving quality
12. Provides flexibility to support existing and evolving clinical needs within a specialty area

From a clinician's point of view, the functionality of EMRs can be organized into clinical care processes that occur constantly throughout the day (although not necessarily in any predictable order). These include[16]

1. Time management and scheduling
2. Reviewing of diagnostic test results, previous encounter notes, and other patient-specific documents such as procedure and consultant reports
3. Diagnostic test ordering
4. Documentation of patient encounters, with attention to evaluation and management requirements to support precertification and reimbursement for services provided
5. Medication prescribing and administration; in oncology settings this often includes infusion chemotherapy management
6. Electronic approval for documentation and orders
7. Context-specific knowledge access and clinical decision support; in oncology practices, this may include support for standard therapy and for research therapy protocols, with automated eligibility checking and patient-specific treatment calendars, as well as access to the relevant medical literature and online databases; also relevant to oncology are support for staging and standardized toxicity reporting
8. Data analysis and report generation
9. Message-based communications with other systems and providers and with patients
10. Patient education

General-purpose EMR systems can be configured to support these clinical care processes, and a variety of oncology-specific EMR systems are available. The importance of each of these processes to an individual practice setting will vary widely, and there is no "one size fits all" or simple evaluation metric to judge whether any given EMR feature is necessary or even useful.

The ability to send and receive patient data to and from other computer systems is a key feature of modern EMR systems, and standards exist for how individual pieces of information such as an individual laboratory test result or a narrative discharge summary can be communicated among EMR systems connected by networks. Health Level 7 (HL7) is the most widely used and generally accepted standard for what might be thought of as the electronic envelopes by which EMR information can be exchanged by computers. Compliance with HL7 standards for communication often makes the difference between an EMR that requires the user to manually enter every

TABLE 58-3. Electronic Medical Records (EMRs) System Vendors

Vendors	Notes
ONCOLOGY-SPECIFIC EMRS	
IknowMed: 1608 Fourth St., Third Floor, Berkeley, CA 94710; Phone: 510-558-4500; Fax: 510-525-3640; Web site: http://www.iknowmed.com	Primarily designed for medical oncology practices; includes automatic evaluation and management coding, clinical decision support, clinical trials screening at point of care, chemotherapy library
IMPAC Medical Systems, Inc.: 100 West Evelyn Ave., Mountain View, CA 94041; Phone: 888-464-6722; Fax: 650-988-1834; Web site: http://www.impac.com	Primarily designed for radiation oncology practices; includes practice management but does not include patient-specific clinical decision support
Intellidose: IntrinsiQ Data Corp., 800 South St., Suite 190, Waltham, MA 02453-9912; Phone: 800-565-2279; Fax: 781-647-9242; Web site: http://www.intellidose.com	Automates chemotherapy order writing; includes safety checking algorithms for route-of-administration errors, errors of omission, body surface area limitations, patient allergies, and out-of-range lab results
OPTX: 1610 Wynkoop St., Suite 300, Denver, CO 80202; Phone: 303-623-7700; Fax: 303-623-7900; Web site: http://www.healthierpractices.com	Provides authoring tools for creating clinical therapy protocols with decision support rules
GENERAL-PURPOSE EMRS WITH ONCOLOGY FEATURES	
Eclipsys Corp.: 1750 Clint Moore Rd., Boca Raton, FL 33487; Phone: 561-322-4321; Fax: 561-322-4320	Sunrise Clinical Manager is a general-purpose EMR that has modules for oncology practices
Cerner Corp.: 2800 Rockcreek Pkwy., Kansas City, MO 64117; Phone: 816-201-1024; Fax: 816-474-1742; Web site: http://www.cerner.com	EMR systems for medium and large practices, including inpatient and outpatient modules
Epic Systems Corp.: 5301 Tokay Blvd., Madison, WI 53711-1027; Phone: 608-271-9000; Fax: 608-271-7237; Web site: http://www.epicsystems.com	Primary focus in ambulatory systems; integrates with voice-recognition systems for data input, includes practice analysis tools and clinical decision support

piece of information from the keyboard and an EMR where patient information can be automatically received from sources such as clinical laboratories and automatically inserted into the patient's record.

HL7 is an important communications standard, but the ability to communicate information with other systems also depends on the use of standard names and codes for symptoms, signs, diagnoses, services, and procedures. Figuratively, HL7 defines the envelope and how it is addressed for sending, whereas naming and coding systems define the language used in the messages put in the electronic envelope. Most clinicians are familiar with Current Procedural Terminology (CPT) and International Classification of Diseases (ICD) coding that supports billing functions, but there are more comprehensive naming and coding systems that have the capability to represent many more of the concepts that occur in clinical care and are recorded in the medical record. Most prominent among these are the Systematized NOmenclature of MEDicine (SNOMED) developed by the College of American Pathologists and the Unified Medical Language System (UMLS) maintained by the U.S. National Library of Medicine.

Adherence to communications and coding standards may not always be a visible part of an EMR, but it is an essential component of the behind-the-scenes data management machinery. EMR systems that use these nationally and internationally recognized naming and coding systems will more easily be able to exchange clinical information in an automated fashion as "interoperability" becomes an increasingly important feature of clinical computing systems in an Internet-connected world.

A comprehensive guide to the process of planning, acquiring, and implementing an EMR system would occupy many more pages than a single chapter can cover, and books devoted entirely to the subject of EMR implementation are available to assist in understanding in detail how to proceed.[17,18] More than 200 companies have EMR products. A sampling is provided in Table 58-3 of vendors who currently have EMR products specifically designed for oncology or general-purpose EMR systems with oncology-specific modules or features. Special-purpose EMRs are more likely to have unique features for one subspecialty but are also more likely to be produced by small companies with relatively few customers. This list is offered as a sampler, with the caveat that in the world of information technologies, acquisitions, and mergers, company and product names and features are constantly changing. No endorsement of the products provided by these vendors is expressed or implied by inclusion in this listing.

Healthy skepticism can be a valuable tool in the process of deciding which EMR, if any, to acquire and implement. No regulatory body or certifying organization exists that tests vendor claims or independently proves that software performs as advertised. It can often be difficult to distinguish "vaporware" that will appear in a future release from features that actually exist and are in use by current customers. For this reason, the product acquisition process should include time spent visiting at least two locations where the product one is considering is in everyday use. As well, cost is a major issue in the implementation of a sophisticated EMR. A long-recognized relationship exists between the size of the practice and the difficulty of implementing an EMR. Solo practitioners have the luxury of choosing nearly any system that suits them but generally have limited resources relative to the entry-level costs for full-featured EMR systems. Groups of 50 or more physicians often have the combined resources to purchase high-end systems (so-called enterprise-level EMRs costing hundreds of thousands to millions of dollars) but find that achieving consensus among providers to adopt the changes in clinical workflow that accompany deployment of an EMR is the rate-limiting step in moving forward.

FUTURE TRENDS

The published literature of medical informatics has demonstrated convincingly that EMRs can improve the quality and consistency of care delivered. In inpatient settings, EMRs with patient-specific alerts and reminders can reduce length of stay, decrease redundant test ordering, reduce the time to effective therapy for critical laboratory abnormalities, and decrease medical errors, such as preventable adverse drug interactions.[19,20] In outpatient settings EMRs have been shown to improve efficiency and productivity of practice and consistency of care in a variety of ways, including such widely differing activities as compliance with preventive medicine guidelines, establishment of advance directives, and speed of diagnostic test ordering.[21,22] From the perspective of cognitive science, this improvement occurs for a simple reason. Humans are superb at recognizing patterns within complex sets of information, and this is the special talent of experienced diagnosticians. At the same time, however, humans are ill suited to remembering long lists of facts, such as possible drug–drug interactions and the exact timing of complex multidrug and multimodality therapies. Modern health care is built on a foundation of decision making that requires pattern recognition and consideration of multiple lists and rules for optimal care. Computerized logic can quickly and effortlessly evaluate tens of thousands of rules and possible conditions, and thus it is a natural "intellectual amplifier" to complement the cognitive skills of the health care provider.

This truth has not been lost on scientific review groups and policy makers. In 2001, the Institute of Medicine of the National Academy of Sciences issued a report entitled *Crossing the Quality Chasm: A New Health System for the 21st Century,* noting the beneficial effects of EMRs and establishing a national goal of the elimination of handwritten medical records within 10 years.[23] Whether that goal is achieved remains to be seen, but other forces at work in the science of human biology and health care may make the computer an indispensable tool for optimally managing an individual patient's care. The completion of the human genome sequence has spawned development of new diagnostics and new drugs with novel forms of action that are appropriate for certain genotypes but not others. Gene expression microarray data derived from simultaneous measurement of the activation state of thousands of genes simultaneously is proving to be a diagnostic predictor in certain forms of cancer and portends a data-intensive health care environment. Molecular diagnosis will likely reveal that common disorders such as hypertension and diabetes have dozens of molecular variants for which specific treatments will be indicated. This world of increasing diagnostic complexity and increasing therapeutic choices will benefit substantially from the power of clinical decision support within EMR systems.

Innovations in computing and communications will continue to lower the barrier to use of EMR systems as well. Current palm-top computers (also called *personal digital assistants,* or *PDAs*) are limited in memory, speed, and display capability and are not well suited as a facile data entry device for most clinicians. The emerging generation of thin and lightweight tablet computers will provide touch screen pointing capability, improved handwriting recognition, and high-resolution color graphics, combined with wireless networking capability in a package similar to a thick tablet of standard writing paper.

EMRs will also be enhanced with a shared view of access and ownership of the medical record. Although health care institutions and providers will continue to have the statutory obliga-

tion to create and maintain health care records, the HIPAA Privacy Rule has given patients a uniform right of access to their medical records nationwide and the right to request amendments and corrections to the record. Several early pilot studies have tested the notion of providing patients access to their medical records via the Internet[24,25] and have found that it is technically feasible to do so with adequate security and that it improves patient satisfaction and understanding of their personal health conditions. Current EMR systems often have a Doctor's Notes section and a Nurse's Notes section; future EMRs will also commonly have a Patient's Notes section for the information they contribute to their own care records. Some physicians see this as a lamentable erosion of and threat to their authority in the area of clinical care; others perceive it as a natural evolution of shared responsibility and consumer empowerment. The message with respect to choosing an EMR is to make sure it has flexibility for future adaptation to accommodate changes in the scientific, administrative, and regulatory aspects of health care delivery.

CONCLUSION

The continued growth of data, information, and knowledge in oncology and pressures to implement a systems approach to health care delivery to minimize errors and maximize efficiency will make computing and communications technologies central to the effective practice of oncology. Knowledge represented in human readable formats available via large numbers of Web sites will increasingly be complemented by knowledge embedded in computerized clinical decision support functions of EMR.

REFERENCES

1. Masys DR. Internet technologies. In: Carter J. Electronic patient records: a guide for clinicians and administrators. Philadelphia: American College of Physicians, 2001.
2. National Telecommunications and Information Administration (NTIA). A nation online: how Americans are expanding their use of the Internet. World Wide Web URL: http://www.ntia.doc.gov, accessed September 29, 2003.
3. Schement J, Curtis T. Tendencies and tensions of the information age. New Brunswick, NJ: Transaction Publications, 1997.
4. NUA Internet Surveys. How many online? World Wide Web URL: http://www.nua.ie/surveys/how_many_online/, accessed September 20, 2003.
5. Pew Internet & American Life Project. Internet health resources, health searches and e-mail have become more commonplace, but there is room for improvement in search and overall Internet access. World Wide Web URL: http://pewinternet.org, accessed September 1, 2003.
6. Jadad A, Sigouin C, Cocking L, et al. Internet use among physicians, nurses and their patients. *JAMA* 2001;286(12):1451.
7. Dickerson SS, Brennan PF. The Internet as a catalyst for changing power in patient/provider relationships. *Nursing Outlook* 2002;50(5):195.
8. Easton MS, LaRose R. Internet self-efficacy and the psychology of the digital divide. *JCMC* 200;6(1). World Wide Web URL: http://www.ascusc.org/jcmc/vol6/issue1/eastin.html, accessed September 20, 2003.
9. Children's Partnership. Online content for low-income and underserved Americans. World Wide Web URL: http://www.childrenspartnership.org, accessed September 29, 2003.
10. Eysenbach G, Powell J, Kuss O, Sa E. Empirical studies assessing the quality of health information for consumers on the World Wide Web: a systematic review. *JAMA* 2002;287(20):2691.
11. Health on the Net Foundation. HON code of conduct for medical and health Web sites. World Wide Web URL: http://www.hon.ch/HONcode/, accessed September 1, 2003.
12. Berland GK, Elliott MN, Morales LS, et al. Health information on the Internet: accessibility, quality, and readability in English and Spanish. *JAMA* 2001;285(20):2612.
13. Hubbard SM. Information systems in oncology. In: DeVita VT, Hellman S, Rosenberg SA, eds. *Cancer: principles and practice of oncology,* 6th ed. Philadelphia: Lippincott Williams & Wilkins, 2001:3135.
14. Hubbard SM, Thurn A. The National Cancer Institute's CancerNet: a reliable source of current cancer information on the Internet. *Health Care Internet* 1997;1:15.

15. Dick RS, Steen EB, Detmer DE. *The computer-based patient record: an essential technology for health care*. Washington, DC: The Institute of Medicine. National Academy Press, 1991.

16. Adapted from Morgan MW. Identifying and understanding clinical care processes. In: Carter JH, ed. *Electronic medical records*. Philadelphia: American College of Physicians, 2001.

17. Carter JH, ed. *Electronic medical records: a guide for clinicians and administrators*. Philadelphia: American College of Physicians–American Society of Internal Medicine, 2001.

18. Kissinger K, ed. *Information technology for integrated health systems: positioning for the future*. New York: John Wiley and Sons, 1995.

19. Bates DW, Cohen M, Leape LL, et al. Reducing the frequency of errors in medicine using information technology. *J Am Med Inform Assoc* 2001;8(4):299.

20. Balas EA. Information systems can prevent errors and improve quality. *J Am Med Inform Assoc* 2001;8(4):398.

21. Overhage JM, Perkins S, Tierney WM, McDonald CJ. Controlled trial of direct physician order entry: effects on physicians' time utilization in ambulatory primary care internal medicine practices. *J Am Med Inform Assoc* 2001;8(4):361.

22. Chin HL, McClure P. Evaluating a comprehensive outpatient clinical information system: a case study and model for system evaluation. *Proc 19th Annu Symp Comput Appl Med Care* 1995:717.

23. Institute of Medicine. *Crossing the quality chasm: a new health system for the 21st century*. Washington, DC: National Academy Press, 2001.

24. Masys D, Baker D, Butros A, Cowles KE. Giving patients access to their medical records via the Internet: the PCASSO experience. *J Am Med Inform Assoc* 2002;9(2):181.

25. Cimino JJ, Patel VL, Kushniruk AW. The patient clinical information system (PatCIS): technical solutions for and experience with giving patients access to their electronic medical records. *Int J Med Inf* 2002;68(1–3):113.

Ethan M. Basch
Catherine E. Ulbricht

CHAPTER **59**

Complementary, Alternative, and Integrative Therapies in Cancer Care

BACKGROUND

DEFINITIONS

The term *complementary and alternative medicine* (CAM) has been variably defined but is generally regarded as encompassing a broad group of healing philosophies, diagnostic approaches, and therapeutic interventions that do not belong to the politically dominant (conventional) health system of a particular society.[1,2] Some authors separately define alternative therapies as those used in place of conventional practices, whereas complementary or integrative medicine can be combined with mainstream approaches.[2,3] Other terms used to refer to CAM include *folkloric, holistic, irregular, nonconventional, non-Western, traditional, unconventional, unorthodox,* and *unproven medicine.*

In the United States and other Western nations, CAM therapies are often defined functionally as interventions neither taught in medical schools nor available in hospital-based practices.[4] Examples include dietary supplements (amino acids, herbal products/botanicals, minerals, vitamins, and substances that increase total dietary intake),[5] modalities (manipulative therapies, mind–body medicine, and energy/bioelectromagnetic-based approaches), spiritual healing, and nutritional/dietary alteration.

Boundaries between CAM and conventional therapies are not always clear and often change over time. Scientific evidence has led to broader mainstream acceptance of some CAM therapies and rejection of others.

COMPLEMENTARY AND ALTERNATIVE MEDICINE RESEARCH

The safety and efficacy of many CAM approaches are not well studied, although the body of research is growing. In 1992, the U.S. Congress established the Office of Alternative Medicine within the National Institutes of Health, with a budget of $2 million to "investigate and evaluate promising unconventional medical practices." In 1998, Congress elevated the status of the Office of Alternative Medicine to a National Institutes of Health center, becoming the National Center for Complementary and Alternative Medicine (NCCAM). The budget of NCCAM has progressively increased, from $50 million in fiscal year 1999 to $114 million in 2003, toward its mission to "support rigorous research on CAM, to train researchers in CAM, and to disseminate information to the public and professionals on which CAM modalities work, which do not, and why."

PREVALENCE

In the United States, an estimated 44% of the population used at least one CAM therapy in 1997.[4,6–8] Surveys published since

1999 suggest that between 25% and 83% of U.S. cancer patients have used CAM therapies at some point after diagnosis, with variations in utilization rates depending on geographic area and type of cancer (Table 59-1).[9–24] These reports suggest the use of high-dose vitamins among cancer patients to be 21% to 81%, herbs and supplements 9% to 60%, combination herbal teas (e.g., Essiac) 7% to 25%, and lifestyle diets (such as vegan or macrobiotic) 9% to 24%. Earlier studies generally report lower overall prevalence of CAM use (9% to 54%), possibly due to increasing rates of use or to broadening of the definition of CAM in survey questionnaires and in the views of respondents.[25,26]

Initial studies of CAM prevalence were conducted in children during the 1970s and 1980s and focused on concerns around use of the toxic therapy Laetrile. Reported prevalence was 9% to 16%,[26] but more recent research in children reports higher rates of use, similar to that of adults.[27,28]

CAM use appears to be more common among those with higher educational level, higher income, female sex, younger age, use of chemotherapy or surgery, or history of CAM use before diagnosis. Overall, surveys vary in terms of definitions of CAM and of specific types of therapy included in questionnaires, complicating assessment of overall prevalence.

Use of CAM is also prevalent among cancer patients outside of the United States, including Canada, Europe, South America, and Asia, with overall prevalence of use greater than 30%.[29] Therapies used vary significantly between regions.

SAFETY CONCERNS

QUALITY OF LIFE

In some studies, use of CAM therapies is independently associated with worse quality of life (greater depression, fear of recurrence, more symptoms)[12,30] and shorter survival.[31] These observations are often interpreted as reflecting increased use of alternative therapies in response to psychological symptoms or distress or as coping behavior.[32] However, the possibility that some CAM therapies may cause adverse outcomes is sometimes considered as a cause of these observed results.

Significant potential morbidity and cost have been indirectly associated with herb/supplement–drug interactions, including increased emergency room visits, outpatient clinic visits, and perioperative complications.[33–35] However, the true direct and indirect costs, morbidity, and mortality associated with CAM-related interactions or adverse effects are not known or well studied.

ANTIOXIDANT INTERFERENCE WITH CHEMOTHERAPY OR RADIATION

Because oxidative damage to cells may increase the risk of cancer, the use of antioxidant herbs and vitamins has been proposed for cancer treatment or prevention. Examples include vitamins A, C, and E, as well as lycopene, green tea, soy, grape seed extract, melatonin, and selenium (a component of the antioxidant glutathione peroxidase). Concern has been raised that antioxidants may interfere with radiation therapy or some chemotherapy agents (e.g., alkylating agents, anthracyclines, or platinums), which themselves can depend on oxidative damage to tumor cells for cytotoxicity. Studies of the effects of anti-oxidants on cancer therapies yield mixed results, with some reporting antagonistic effects, others noting synergism, and most suggesting no significant interaction.[36,37] This remains an area of study and controversy.

DRUG INTERACTIONS

Limited published data are available regarding potential interactions between specific herbs/vitamins and prescription drugs.[38–46] Therefore, it is often recommended that patients refrain from regular use of high-dose agents during chemotherapy, unless they are demonstrated in studies not to result in significant interactions.

St. John's wort (*Hypericum perforatum*) is of particular concern, with multiple well-documented drug interactions. This herb appears to inhibit the hepatic enzyme cytochrome P-4503A4 acutely, then induce it with repeated administration. A study of individuals given irinotecan (CPT-11) reports a greater than 50% reduction in serum levels of the active metabolite SN-38 after concomitant administration of St. John's wort.[47] St. John's wort should be used cautiously in combination with other drugs with similar modes of metabolism.

Based on preclinical data, other herbs that may induce P-4503A4 include hops (*Humulus lupuli*), chasteberry (*Vitex agnus-castus*), bloodroot (*Sanguinaria canadensis*), oregano [*Oregano* species (spp.)], damiana (*Turnera* spp.), and yucca (*Yucca* spp.). Agents that may inhibit P-4503A4 include cannabinoids, grapefruit juice, milk thistle (*Silybum marianum*), the chaparral component nordihydroguaiaretic acid (NDGA), goldenseal (*Hydrastis canadensis*), cat's claw (*Uncaria tomentosa, Uncaria guianensis*), *Echinacea angustifolia* root, wild cherry (*Prunus serotina*), chamomile (*Matricaria chamomilla*), and licorice (*Glycyrrhiza glabra*).

BLEEDING

Multiple herbs and supplements carry an increased risk of bleeding. Multiple case studies have reported clinically significant bleeding with the use of *Ginkgo biloba* (either alone or with aspirin or warfarin) and isolated case reports of bleeding with the use of saw palmetto (*Serenoa repens*) and garlic (*Allium sativum*). These agents should be discontinued before surgical procedures and should be used cautiously with other agents that increase the risk of bleeding. Numerous other herbs and vitamins may increase bleeding risk based on known constituents, preclinical data, or traditional use (Table 59-2).

PHYTOESTROGENS

Phytoestrogens are plant-based compounds structurally similar to estradiol, capable of binding to estrogen receptors as agonists or antagonists. Multiple popular herbs contain phytoestrogens, such as black cohosh (*Cimicifuga racemosa*), red clover (*Trifolium pratense*), and soy (*Glycine max*) (Table 59-3). Effects of these agents in hormone-sensitive cancers remain unclear, and use in patients with estrogen receptor–positive breast cancer is particularly controversial. It is generally recommended that these agents be cautiously used in this population, although some authors assert that antagonistic effects of some herbs may actually be beneficial. Preliminary study of soy for control of hot flashes in women with breast cancer suggests possible safety, although the pending

TABLE 59-1. Prevalence of Complementary and Alternative Medicine (CAM) Use in U.S. Cancer Patients (Results Published since 1999)

Study	Sample Size	Study Location	Population	Cancer Type	Most Common CAM Treatments	Overall Prevalence of CAM Use
Adler and Fosket, 1999[10]	86	San Francisco	Adult women	Breast	Not specified	69–72%
Bernstein and Grasso, 2001[11]	100	South Florida	Adults	Mixed	Vitamins/antioxidants (81%), herbs (54%), relaxation techniques (30%), massage (20%)	80%
Burstein et al., 1999[12]	480	Massachusetts	Adult women seen in hospitals	Breast	Relaxation techniques (32%), megavitamins (21%), self-help groups (28%), herbs (20%), spiritual healing (18%), massage (15%), lifestyle diets (11%)	Total: 67% (started CAM since diagnosis: 28%)
Friedman et al., 1997[27]	161 (81 with cancer)	Gainesville, FL	Children seen in university hospital outpatient clinic	Mixed	Prayer (64%), spiritual healing (16%), relaxation techniques (11%), herbs (9%), massage (7%), megavitamins (7%), imagery (5%)	Cancer patients: 65%; controls: 40%
Gotay et al., 1999[13]	343	Hawaii	Adults	Mixed	Prayer (50%), herbs (33%), mind–body therapies (20%)	36%
Kao and Devine, 1999[14]	50	Philadelphia	Men undergoing radiation at tertiary care center	Prostate	Herbs (60%), megavitamins (41%), chiropractic/massage (18%), relaxation/meditation (18%), special diets (18%)	37%
Kelly et al., 2000[28]	78	New York, NY	Children seen in academic health center clinic	Mixed	Dietary modification, herbs, mind–body approaches	84%
Lee et al., 2002[15]	543	San Francisco	Men in state tumor registry	Prostate	Herbs (16%), counseling/support groups (10%), lifestyle diets (9%), spiritual/faith healing (4%), megavitamins (4%), relaxation methods (3%)	30%
Lippert et al., 1999[16]	190	Charlottesville, VA	Men seen at academic health center	Prostate	Vitamins (34%), prayer/religious practices (25%), herbs (13%)	43%
Maskarinec et al., 2000[17]	1168	Hawaii	Adults in state tumor registry	Mixed	Spiritual healing, vitamins, herbs, dietary alterations	25%
Morris et al., 2000[18]	617	Portland, OR	Adults in community hospital cancer registry	Breast and "other"	Nutrition (63%), massage (53%), herbs (44%)	Breast: 84%; other: 66%
Patterson et al., 2002[19]	356	Western Washington	Adults	Breast, colorectal, prostate	Vitamins/minerals (64%), herbs (38%), meditation/prayer/group support (19%)	70%
Richardson et al., 2000[20]	453	Houston, TX	Adults seen in tertiary cancer care center	Mixed	Spiritual practices (79%), vitamins (60%), herbs (38%), massage (33%), chiropractic/osteopathic treatments (23%), yoga (10%), Tai Chi/Qi Gong (8%)	83%
Shumay et al., 2002[21]	143	Hawaii	Adults in state tumor registry	Mixed	Herbs/supplements (58%), vitamins/minerals (50%), spiritual healing (48%), special diets (48%), meditation (28%), massage/body work (25%), guided imagery (24%), support groups (17%), relaxation (17%), acupuncture (17%), healing touch (17%), yoga (13%)	80%
Sparber et al., 2000[22]	100	Bethesda, MD	Adults enrolled in clinical trials	Mixed	Spiritual healing (36%), relaxation (26%), lifestyle diet (24%), megavitamins (22%)	63%
Swisher et al., 2002[23]	113	St. Louis, MO	Adult women seen at academic health center	Gynecologic	Faith healing/therapeutic touch (26%), visualization/psychic therapy (15%), relaxation techniques/meditation/yoga (12%), herbs (11%), megavitamins (11%), medicinal teas (7%), shark cartilage (6%)	50%
VandeCreek et al., 1999[24]	112	Midwestern U.S.	Adult women seen at academic health center	Breast	Prayer (76%), spiritual healing (29%)	74%

TABLE 59-2. Herbs and Supplements That May Increase the Risk of Bleeding or Clotting

---

AGENTS REPORTED TO CAUSE CLINICALLY SIGNIFICANT BLEEDING IN CASE REPORT(S)
Garlic (*Allium sativum*), *Ginkgo biloba*, saw palmetto (*Serenoa repens*)

AGENTS THAT MAY INCREASE THE RISK OF BLEEDING, BASED ON MECHANISM OF ACTION, PRECLINICAL DATA, OR TRADITIONAL USE
Alfalfa (*Medicago sativa*),[a] American ginseng (*Panax quinquefolium*), angelica (*Angelica archangelica*),[a] anise (*Pimpinella anisum*),[a] arginine (L-arginine), asafetida (*Ferula asafetida*),[a] asafetida (*Ferula foetida*),[b] aspen bark, bilberry (*Vaccinium myrtillus*), birch (*Betula barosma*),[c] black cohosh (*Cimifuga racemosa*),[b] bladderwrack (*Fucus vesiculosus*), bogbean (*Menyanthes trifoliata*), boldo (*Peumus boldus*), borage seed oil, bromelain (*Anas comosus*), capsicum, cat's claw (*Uncaria tomentosa*), celery (*Apium graveolens*),[a] chamomile (*Matricaria recutita*),[a] chaparral [*Larrea tridentate* (DC) Coville, *Larrea divaricata* Cav] clove (*Eugenia aromatica*), coleus (*Coleus forskohlii*), cordyceps (*Cordyceps sinensis*), danshen (*Salvia miltiorrhiza*), devil's claw, dong quai (*Angelica sinensis*), EPA (eicosapentaenoic acid), evening primrose oil (*Oenothera biennis*),[c] fenugreek (*Trigonella foenum-graecum*),[a] feverfew (*Tanacetum parthenium*),[c] fish oil, flaxseed/flax powder (not a concern with flaxseed oil), garlic (*Allium sativum*),[c] ginger (*Zingiber officinalis*),[c] ginkgo (*Ginkgo biloba*),[c] ginseng,[c] grapefruit juice, grape seed (*Vitis vinifera*), green tea (*Camellia sinensis*), guggul (*Commiphora mukul*), gymnestra, horse chestnut (*Aesculus hippocastanum*),[a] horseradish (*Radicula armoracia*), leopard's bane (*Arnica montana*), licorice (*Glycyrrhiza glabra*),[c] lovage root, male fern (*Dryopteris filix-mas*), meadowsweet (*Spirea/Filipendula ulmaria*),[b] nordihydroguaiaretic acid (NDGA), omega-3 fatty acids, onion, papain, *Panax ginseng*,[c] parsley (*Petroselinum crispum*), passion flower (*Passiflora incarnata*), poplar,[b] prickly ash (*Zanthoxylum* spp.),[a] propolis, quassia (*Picrasma excelsa*),[a] red clover (*Trifolium pratense*),[a] reishi (*Ganoderma lucidum*), rue, saw palmetto (*Serenoa repens*), Siberian ginseng (*Eleutherococcus senticosus*), soy,[c] Spanish bayonet (*Yucca* spp.), sweet birch,[b] sweet clover (*Melilotus* spp.),[a] turmeric (*Curcuma longa*), vitamin C,[c] vitamin E,[c] willow bark (*Salix* spp.),[b] wild carrot, wild lettuce, wintergreen[b]

POSSIBLE PROCOAGULANT AGENTS
Coenzyme Q10, DHEA (dihydroepiandrosterone), *Panax ginseng*

---

[a]Agents with coumarin constituents.
[b]Agents with salicylate constituents.
[c]Agents that inhibit platelets.
(From http://www.naturalstandard.com, with permission.)

---

results of ongoing research in this area may provide more definitive safety data.[48] Potentially estrogenic agents have been used in prostate cancer, although evidence remains inconclusive.

HEPATOTOXICITY

Multiple herbs and supplements may cause hepatotoxicity or transaminitis, based on human research or known hepatotoxic constituents, and should be used cautiously in combination with other hepatotoxic agents (Table 59-4).

STANDARDIZATION

Preparation of herbs and supplements may vary from manufacturer to manufacturer and from batch to batch within one manufacturer. Because the active components of a product are often not clear, standardization may not be possible, and the clinical effects of different brands may not be comparable.

PATIENT–CLINICIAN COMMUNICATION

Some research reports that neither adult[23] nor pediatric[27] patients receive sufficient information or discuss CAM therapies with a physician, pharmacist, nurse, or CAM practitioner, whereas other studies find that more than 60% of patients discuss CAM with their physician.[20] These discrepancies likely reflect an overall heterogeneity in clinicians' styles of managing patients who use CAM.

Most physicians do not receive formal training regarding the safety and effectiveness of CAM and have limited knowledge in

---

TABLE 59-3. Herbs with Potential Estrogenic or Progestational Activity

---

Potential phytoestrogenic herbs (contain constituents reported to act as estrogen receptor agonists and/or to exhibit estrogenic properties in basic science studies, animal research, or human trials)
    Alfalfa (*Medicago sativa*), black cohosh (*Cimicifuga racemosa*),[a] bloodroot (*Sanguinaria canadensis*), burdock (*Arctium lappa*), hops (*Humulus lupulus*),[b] kudzu (*Pueraria lobata*),[c] licorice (*Glycyrrhiza glabra*),[b] pomegranate (*Punica granatum*),[b] red clover (*Trifolium pratense*),[c] soy (*Glycine max*),[c] thyme (*Thymus vulgaris*), white horehound (*Marrubium vulgare* L.), yucca (*Yucca* spp.)
Potential phytoprogestational herbs (contain constituents reported to exhibit progestin-like activity in basic science and/or animal studies)
    Chasteberry (*Vitex agnus-castus*), bloodroot (*Sanguinaria canadensis*), oregano (*Oregano* spp.), damiana (*Turnera* spp.), yucca (*Yucca* spp.)

---

[a]Estrogen and isoflavone constituents.
[b]Estriol, estrone, estradiol, or estrogen constituents.
[c]Isoflavone constituents.
(From http://www.naturalstandard.com, with permission.)

TABLE 59-4. Herbs and Supplements with Potential Hepatotoxic Effects

---

Ackee (*Blighia sapida*), bee pollen, birch oil (*Betula lenta*), blessed thistle (*Cnicus benedictus*),[a] borage (*Borago officinalis*), bush tea (*Crotalaria* spp.),[b] butterbur (*Petasites hybridus*), chaparral (*Larrea tridentate*), coltsfoot (*Tussilago farfara*), comfrey (*Symphytum* spp.), dihydroepiandrosterone (DHEA), *Echinacea purpurea, Echium* spp.,[c] germander (*Teucrium chamaedrys*), *Heliotropium* spp., horse chestnut parenteral preparations (*Aesculus hippocastanum*), Jin-bu-huan (*Lycopodium serratum*), kava (*Piper methysticum*), lobelia (*Lobelia inflata*), L-tetrahydropalmatine (THP), mate (*Ileus paraguayensis*),[b] niacin (vitamin B$_3$), niacinamide, Paraguay tea (*Ilex paraguayensis*), periwinkle (*Catharanthus roseus*), *Plantago lanceolata*,[a] pride of Madeira (*Echium fastuosum*),[b] rue (*Ruta graveolus*), sassafras (*Sassafras albidum*), skullcap (*Scutellaria lateriflora*), *Senecio* spp./groundsel (*Senecio jacobea, Senecio vulgaris, Senecio spartioides*),[b] tansy ragwort (*Senecio jacobea*),[b] turmeric (*Curcuma longa*), Tu-san-chi (*Gynura segetum*),[b] uva ursi (*Arctostaphylos uva-ursi* Spreng), valerian (*Valeriana officinalis*), white chameleon (*Atractylis gummifera*)

---

[a]Contains tannins and may be hepatotoxic in large quantities.
[b]Contains pyrrolizidine alkaloids.
(From http://www.naturalstandard.com, with permission.)

TABLE 59-5. Evidence-Based On-Line Complementary and Alternative Medicine (CAM) Resources (for Clinicians and Patients)

Natural Standard Research Collaboration: http://www. naturalstandard.com	An international multidisciplinary research collaboration that maintains an online database of systematic reviews of CAM therapies, as well as patient information and monthly news briefs
M. D. Anderson Complementary/Integrative Medicine Education Resources (CIMER): http://www.mdanderson.org/ departments/CIMER	An informational site maintained by M. D. Anderson Cancer Center with information on CAM therapies relevant to cancer patients and access to other resources
CancerSource: http://www. cancersource.com	A patient-oriented site that includes information on selected CAM therapies
National Center for Complementary and Alternative Medicine (NCCAM): http:// nccam.nih.gov	A site maintained by NCCAM, the National Institutes of Health center dedicated to primary CAM research
Office of Dietary Supplements: http://ods.od.nih.gov/ index.aspx	A federal agency that supports research and disseminates research results in the area of dietary supplements
Cochrane Collaboration: http:/ /www.cochrane.org	An international collaboration that prepares systematic reviews of numerous medical therapies, including many CAM approaches
ConsumerLab and Consumer Reports: http://www. consumerlab.com; http:// www.consumerreports.org	Organizations that evaluate commercially available products and adulterants for constituents and publish online lists of these test results

this area.[49] There appears to be significant concern among practitioners about potential safety risks and patient out-of-pocket expenses associated with CAM use.[50,51] Surveys suggest a desire by clinicians for access to quality CAM information, to improve quality of care and to enhance communication with patients.[52,53] Due to potential adverse effects and interactions associated with CAM use, clinicians are often encouraged to ask patients about CAM use, although it is not known if beneficial outcomes result from this practice. Recommended approaches for clinicians to patients who use CAM have been published[37,54] and generally include suggestions to encourage patients to discuss their reasons for seeking CAM, to provide patients with evidence-based information about specific CAM therapies (or explain when there is insufficient available evidence), to explain known safety concerns noting that "natural" does not always equate with safety, to support patients emotionally and psychologically even if they choose a CAM therapy with which the clinician does not agree, and to provide close clinical follow-up of patients using CAM therapies. Several evidence-based CAM informational resources are available online for clinicians and patients and can be used as a starting point for discussions in this area (Table 59-5).

SPECIFIC COMPLEMENTARY AND ALTERNATIVE MEDICINE THERAPIES

Surveys report a wide variety of CAM approaches used by cancer patients, as treatment or supportive care. Many therapies used are the same as those used in the general population for common noncancer indications, such as St. John's wort (*Hypericum perforatum*) for depression, kava (*Piper methysticum*) for anxiety, *Echinacea purpurea* for common cold symptoms, or yoga/massage/Tai Chi for nonspecific well-being. A number of therapies are particularly popular among cancer patients, with variable levels of available scientific research.

THERAPIES USED FOR CANCER TREATMENT AND SECONDARY PREVENTION

MAITAKE MUSHROOM EXTRACT (*GRIFOLA FRONDOSA*) AND BETA-GLUCANS

Maitake mushroom extract has been used traditionally in Japan as a food and medicine. This agent has become popular among cancer patients in North America, Europe, and Asia despite limited scientific evidence, based on purported immunomodulatory properties. In preclinical research, polysaccharide constituents of maitake, such as beta-glucans, have been associated with proposed host-mediated antitumor mechanisms, such as induction of nitric oxide synthase by maitake D fraction, increased macrophage tumor necrosis factor, and antiangiogenesis.[55]

In a small 2002 case series, therapy with maitake powder and beta-glucan MD fraction was associated with tumor regression in greater than 50% of patients with stage II to IV breast, lung, and liver cancer, whereas no improvements were observed in leukemia, gastric cancer, or brain tumors.[56] This series was not well described, with limited information regarding patient baseline characteristics.

Although maitake is not well studied, a long history of dietary use suggests safety in low doses. Possible adverse effects of concentrated extracts, based on animal research, include hypoglycemia and hypotension. It is not clear if this agent interacts with chemotherapy regimens.

SHIITAKE MUSHROOM EXTRACT (*LETINULA EDODES*)

Shiitake is used traditionally in Japan as a food and medicine. Preclinical evidence has been obtained of cellular immunity potentiation and tumor growth inhibition by the polysaccharide compounds lentinan and krestin. Limited human evidence includes a negative case series in 62 men with locally advanced or metastatic prostate cancer, who were administered shiitake mushroom extract for 6 months.[57] Progression of disease was reported in 38% of men, with no response in others, and a mean prostate-specific antigen (PSA) increase of 6.4% overall. Multiple reports have been published of allergy with contact or ingestion, including rash, toxic epidermal necrolysis, and photodermatitis.

SOY (*GLYCINE MAX*)

Therapeutic use of soy has received widespread press coverage due to its proposed use as a hormone replacement therapy. Strong evidence has been shown supporting the benefits of soy for cholesterol reduction and as a source of dietary protein and good evidence for alleviation of menopausal hot flashes or for diarrhea in young children/infants.

Isoflavonoids in soy act as mixed estrogen receptor agonists/antagonists and as such are labeled *phytoestrogens*. These constituents compete with estradiol for binding sites. A dose effect has been reported, with antagonism at lower doses and agonistic properties in higher doses. Isoflavonoids may also possess antioxidant activity. Laboratory and animal studies of the soy isoflavonoid genistein note tyrosine kinase inhibition, antiangiogenic properties, and induction of apoptosis. However, genistein has also been reported to increase growth of pancreatic tumor cells *in vitro*. Currently, there is no reliable human research of soy or isoflavones for the treatment of malignancies. Ongoing research is being conducted in patients with prostate cancer.

Due to concerns regarding estrogenic effects, soy supplement use is generally discouraged in patients with breast cancer. Preliminary study of soy for control of hot flashes in women with breast cancer suggests possible safety, although the pending results of ongoing research in this area may provide more definitive safety data.[48] Preliminary human research reports that short-term use of soy isoflavones does not elicit endometrial hypertrophy.

In theory, soy supplements may interfere with the effects of some chemotherapy regimens or radiation therapy because of antioxidant properties. Caution with anticoagulants may be advisable due to animal evidence of platelet aggregation inhibition.

CHAPARRAL TEA AND NORDIHYDROGUAIARETIC ACID

Chaparral (*Larrea tridentata, Larrea divaricata*) is derived from a shrub found in desert regions of the southwestern United States and Mexico and has been used in Native American medicine. There is preclinical evidence of antioxidant properties of chaparral and its component NDGA.[58]

In a 1970 case series, 59 patients with advanced malignancies (types not documented) were treated with 16 to 24 oz of chaparral tea or 250 to 3000 mg of NDGA daily for 4 weeks.[59] Although 25% tumor regression was noted in four patients, no improvement or tumor progression was reported in other subjects. Adverse effects included nausea, vomiting, diarrhea, abdominal cramps, rash, stomatitis, and fever.

Multiple reports have been published of serious adverse reactions associated with chaparral, including liver cirrhosis/failure, kidney cysts/failure, and kidney cancer. Chaparral was removed from the U.S. Food and Drug Administration GRAS (generally recognized as safe) list in 1970. Chaparral and NDGA are generally considered unsafe and are not recommended for use.

LAETRILE

Laetrile is an alternative cancer agent marketed in Mexico and other countries outside of the United States. It is derived from amygdalin, which is found in the pits of fruits and nuts such as bitter almond (*Prunus amygdalus*). Multiple cases of cyanide poisoning, including deaths, have been associated with treatment.[60–62]

Based on a 1982 phase II trial, the U.S. National Cancer Institute (NCI) concluded that Laetrile is not a beneficial chemotherapeutic agent.[63] This study included 178 non–end-stage patients with mixed tumor types, including gastric, colon, breast, and lung. One-third of patients had not received any prior chemotherapy. For 21 days, intravenous Laetrile was administered, combined with "metabolic therapy" (pancreatic enzymes, vitamins). After treatment, one subject with gastric cancer was classified as improved, based on measurable tumor

regression. However, 95 patients experienced tumor progression, and all evaluable subjects experienced disease progression within 7 months of treatment. Adverse effects included nausea, vomiting, headache, dizziness, mental obtundation, dermatitis, and cyanide toxicity. Despite this risk–benefit profile, many patients still travel outside of the United States to receive this therapy.

MISTLETOE (*VISCUM ALBUM*)

Once considered a sacred herb in Celtic tradition, mistletoe has been used for centuries for diverse medical conditions. Beginning in the early twentieth century, mistletoe came into use in Europe as a cancer therapy and is currently one of the most commonly used herbs for cancer in Germany.

Preclinical studies report immunomodulatory properties of lectins isolated from mistletoe, including increased macrophage tumor necrosis factor production and increased interleukin-1 and interleukin-6 levels,[64] as well as direct cytotoxic effects of viscotoxin constituents and stimulation of natural killer cell–mediated cytotoxicity.[65] Multiple case series, retrospective analyses, and prospective trials of mistletoe extracts in humans have been published, largely conducted in Europe, including subjects with breast, lung, cervical, colorectal, gastric, ovarian, and pancreatic cancer, and renal cell carcinoma and glioma. A 1994 systematic review included 11 controlled clinical trials, not all randomized, and concluded that overall methodologic quality of studies was poor and results indeterminate.[66] Subsequent publications have not provided definitive evidence of efficacy,[67–69] except for negative results in patients with melanoma.[70] Mistletoe products that have been used in clinical trials include Abnoba viscum, Eurixor, Helixor, Iscador (with added copper, mercury, and silver), Isorel, and Vysorel.

ESSIAC HERBAL COMBINATION TEA

Essiac is a combination herbal tea originally developed in the 1920s by the Canadian nurse Rene Caisse ("Essiac" is Caisse spelled backwards). The original proprietary formula contained burdock root (*Arctium lappa*), sheep sorrel (*Rumex acetosella*), slippery elm inner bark (*Ulmus fulva*), and Turkish rhubarb (*Rheum palmatum*). The recipe is said to be based on a traditional Ojibwa (Native American) remedy. Later formulations added other herbs, including blessed thistle (*Cnicus benedictus*), red clover (*Trifolium pratense*), kelp (*Laminaria digitata*), and watercress (*Nasturtium officinale*).

Caisse administered the formula orally and parenterally to numerous cancer patients during the 1920s and 1930s. No reliable research of Essiac has been published. Mouse studies at Memorial Sloan-Kettering Cancer Center in the 1970s were never formally published, and 86 human case reports collected retrospectively in 1988 by the Canadian Department of National Health and Welfare yielded unclear results.[71] Despite this lack of evidence, Essiac and Essiac-like products (which may add additional herbs) remain popular among cancer patients.

HOXSEY FORMULA

The original "Hoxsey formula" was developed in the mid-1800s, when a horse belonging to John Hoxsey was observed to recover from cancer after feeding in a field of wild plants. These herbs were collected and used to treat ill animals. The "formula" was passed down in the Hoxsey family, and John Hoxsey's great-grandson Harry Hoxsey, an Illinois coal miner, marketed an herbal mixture based on the formula as a cancer treatment.

The first Hoxsey clinic opened in the 1920s in Illinois, and Hoxsey therapy became popular for cancer in the United States during the 1940s and 1950s, with clinics operating in multiple states. At that time, the Dallas Hoxsey clinic was one of the largest private cancer hospitals in the world. However, after legal conflicts with the American Medical Association and U.S. Food and Drug Administration, the last U.S. clinic closed in the 1950s. The formula was passed to Mildred Nelson, a nurse in the clinic, who used the formula to open and operate a Hoxsey clinic in Tijuana, Mexico.

The modern Hoxsey formula consists of a tonic taken by mouth, preparations placed on the skin, and other supportive therapies. The tonic is individualized for each patient according to cancer type and medical history. An ingredient often present is potassium iodide. Other ingredients are then added and may include licorice, red clover, burdock, stillingia root, berberis root, pokeroot, cascara, aromatic USP 14, prickly ash bark, and buckthorn bark. A caustic red paste can be used and contains antimony trisulfide, zinc chloride, and bloodroot. A topical yellow powder can also be used and contains arsenic sulfide, talc, sulfur, and a "yellow precipitate." A clear solution can be administered and contains trichloroacetic acid.

No well-designed human studies have evaluated the safety or effectiveness of Hoxsey formula. A small number of individual human cases and case series have reported miraculous cancer cures,[72,73] but many included patients appearing not to have had biopsy-proven cancer, patients who were treated with concomitant therapies, or patients who experienced progressive disease.

PC-SPES

PC-SPES is a proprietary herbal combination that was produced until early 2002 by BotanicLab, Inc. for use in prostate cancer patients ("PC" stands for prostate cancer, and *spes* is Latin for hope). The formula purportedly contained eight herbs, including *Serenoa repens* (saw palmetto), *Chrysanthemum morifolium* (chrysanthemum, mum, Chu-hua), *Ganoderma lucidum* (reishi mushroom, Ling Zhi), *Glycyrrhiza glabra* (licorice), *Isatis indigotica* Fort (Da Qing Ye, dyer's wood), *Panax pseudoginseng* (San Qi), *Rabdosia rubescens* (rubescens, Dong Ling Cao), and *Scutellaria baicalensis* (skullcap, Huang-chin).

Multiple early-phase studies produced promising results in androgen-dependent and -independent tumors, including greater than 50% PSA reduction in most patients, improved bone scan findings, and improved pain/quality-of-life scores.[74–78] Initial proposed mechanisms included inhibition of aromatase, 12-lipoxygenase, or 5α-reductase by the skullcap flavone *baicalin* and estrogenic effects. However, PC-SPES was removed from the U.S. market in early 2002 after the U.S. Food and Drug Administration reported adulteration with prescription drugs. Different lots were found to contain variable amounts of warfarin, indomethacin, and the estrogen DES (diethylstilbestrol).[79]

It is recommended that patients dispose of any PC-SPES from original lots, which may be adulterated. Currently, there are numerous "copy-cat" products on the market with similar names but unknown effectiveness or safety.

SHARK CARTILAGE AND AE-941

Use of shark cartilage by cancer patients became popular in the 1980s after several reported miracle cures,[80] many of which were reported by a single manufacturer. Early justifications for use of shark cartilage in cancer patients stemmed from accounts that cancer does not develop in sharks (subsequently reported not to be true).

Preclinical studies demonstrating antiangiogenic properties,[81,82] case reports, and early-phase human research have been reported,[83] but no published, randomized, controlled trials of shark cartilage use in cancer patients. In 2000, two manufacturers settled with the U.S. Federal Trade Commission for $1 million over false claims made in product marketing.

Shark cartilage preparations are not standardized, and testing of products has found some to contain largely filler or water. Shark cartilage contains up to 25% calcium and has been associated with hypercalcemia.[83] These supplements can be expensive, costing patients up to hundreds of dollars out-of-pocket each week. The most common adverse effects reported are mild to moderate stomach upset and nausea. In several studies, 5% to 10% of patients stopped taking shark cartilage because of gastrointestinal distress (nausea, vomiting, constipation, dyspepsia), and 20% to 40% experienced milder symptoms of cramping or bloating.

A proprietary shark cartilage derivative called *AE-941* (*Neovastat*), a matrix metalloproteinase inhibitor, has been evaluated in a phase II trial including 144 patients.[84] In 22 patients with renal cell carcinoma, a significant survival advantage was observed in those receiving 240 mL/d versus 60 mL/d (16.3 vs. 7.1 months). In addition, two objective responses were seen in the higher-dose group. Based on these results, there is an ongoing phase III trial in patients with renal call carcinoma and lung cancer.

ANTINEOPLASTONS

Antineoplastons are a group of naturally occurring peptide fractions that were observed by Stanislaw Burzynski, MD, PhD, in the late 1970s to be absent in the urine of cancer patients. He hypothesized that these substances may have antineoplastic properties. In the 1980s, Burzynski identified chemical structures for several of these antineoplastons and developed a process to prepare them synthetically.

The use of antineoplastons in the treatment of various cancer types has been reported in laboratory and animal studies and in limited preliminary human research.[85–88] In 1991, the Cancer Therapy Evaluation Program of the NCI examined records of seven patients with brain tumors treated at the Burzynski Clinic in Texas. Based on these findings, the NCI sponsored a clinical trial in patients with brain tumors. However, due to difficulty recruiting patients and a disagreement over study design, this research was canceled. The results in nine patients included before cancellation were reported but were not conclusive. In 1997, Dr. Burzynski experienced legal troubles for permitting antineoplastons to be shipped out of Texas.

Scientific evidence is inconclusive regarding the effectiveness of antineoplastons in the treatment of cancer. Several preliminary human studies (case series, phase I/II trials) have examined antineoplaston types A2, A5, A10, AS2-1, and AS2-5 for a variety of cancer types. It remains unclear whether antineoplastons are effective or what doses may be safe.

HYDRAZINE SULFATE

Hydrazine sulfate is an industrial chemical that serves as an intermediate in the synthesis of several pharmaceutical agents. Based on tumor regression in mouse models and promising early-phase human data, the NCI sponsored three randomized placebo-controlled trials of hydrazine sulfate in lung cancer (added to platinum-based chemotherapy)[89,90] and in colon cancer.[91] In 1994, these studies reported no significant improvements in survival associated with hydrazine. The results were met with controversy and criticism by some authors, including suggestions that concomitant use of other drugs may have altered the efficacy of hydrazine. As a result, the General Accounting Office launched a formal investigation of the trial results and concluded that they were properly conducted and reported.[92] Hydrazine sulfate has been associated with hepatotoxicity, nausea, vomiting, fatigue, neuropathy, and reduced quality of life in cancer patients.

GERSON THERAPY AND COFFEE ENEMAS

Developed in the 1930s by Max Gerson, a German-born physician, the Gerson approach aims to alter electrolyte "imbalances" that are believed to promote tumor progression. Therapy involves a lactovegetarian diet low in sodium and high in potassium, fruit juices, vitamins, and coffee enemas. This treatment is administered at a clinic in Tijuana, Mexico, and is coordinated by the Gerson Institute U.S. office in California.

Limited study has been conducted on this therapeutic approach. A briefly described retrospective analysis of melanoma patients treated between 1975 and 1990 has been published, with favorable reported results compared to historic controls.[93] However, prospective data are not available. Coffee enemas may carry a risk of caffeine toxicity due to systemic absorption, infection from mucosal damage, or bowel perforation.

OTHER THERAPIES

Many other agents are used by cancer patients as possible treatments but are not well studied. Preliminary evidence suggests that flaxseed is not beneficial in patients with prostate cancer.[94] Other herbs and supplements that are used without reliable evidence include aloe, barley, bitter melon, bladderwrack, bromelain, burdock, calendula, chamomile, clay, coenzyme Q10, danshen, DHEA (dihydroepiandrosterone), echinacea, evening primrose oil, eyebright, ginger, ginseng, ginkgo, goldenseal, guggul, gymnema, hops, horsetail, kava, *Lactobacillus*, lavender, marshmallow, milk thistle, oleander, passion flower, pennyroyal, peppermint, propolis, red clover, sorrel, St. John's wort, sweet almond, turmeric, and white horehound.

THERAPIES USED FOR SUPPORTIVE CARE

CHEMOTHERAPY TOXICITY

Several CAM therapies have been used or evaluated for prevention or alleviation of chemotoxicity, although clear benefits have not been demonstrated. Coenzyme Q10 has been studied for the prevention of anthracycline cardiotoxicity, based on purported antioxidant effects, without conclusive results.[95] Omega-3 fatty acids have also been suggested for this indication, as have antioxidant vitamins (vitamins A and C), without

reliable scientific evaluation. An initial human study of vitamin E for prevention of cisplatin neuropathy is promising but inconclusive due to large dropout (43%).[96] In China, danshen (*Salvia miltiorrhiza*) and dong quai (*Angelica sinensis*) have been used to treat bleomycin pulmonary toxicity, without available scientific research. Other approaches used but not studied for chemotoxicity include astragalus (*Astragalus membranaceus*), *Ginkgo biloba*, Essiac tea, and *Panax ginseng*, as well as acupressure, hypnotherapy, relaxation therapy, polarity therapy, and spiritual healing.

CACHEXIA

No CAM therapy has been demonstrated as beneficial for weight loss, wasting, or appetite suppression associated with malignancy. Two randomized, controlled trials report no significant benefits of supplementation with omega-3 fatty acids or fish oil in cancer patients with cachexia.[97,98]

NAUSEA AND VOMITING

Initial supportive evidence has been shown for the use of ginger (*Zingiber officinale*)[99,100] or P6 (wrist) acupuncture[101] and acupressure[102] in the management of chemotherapy-related nausea and vomiting. These approaches have not been compared to prescription antiemetics. Other CAM approaches used but not well studied include black tea (*Camellia sinensis*), calendula (*Calendula officinalis*), clove (*Eugenia aromatica*), elder (*Sambucus nigra*), lavender (*Lavandula angustifolia*), marshmallow (*Althaea officinalis*), oleander (*Nerium oleander, Thevetia peruviana*), peppermint (*Mentha x piperita*), valerian (*Valeriana officinalis*), white horehound (*Marrubium vulgare*), and wild yam (*Dioscoreaceae*), as well as aromatherapy, guided imagery, hypnotherapy, massage, polarity therapy, and transcutaneous electrical nerve stimulation.

CONSTIPATION

Numerous natural derivatives are used for constipation and are often recommended by physicians. Strong evidence supports the laxative effects of oral senna or *Aloe vera* latex, and there is good evidence for psyllium (*Plantago ovata, Plantago isphagula*) and flaxseed (*Linum usitatissimum*). Numerous other natural sources of fiber are used by patients for this indication.

WELL-BEING

Multiple therapies have been evaluated for their effects on general well-being, quality of life, and other symptoms, including pain.[101–110]

RADIOTHERAPY: ADVERSE EFFECTS

Prunus amygdalus dulcis, Medicago sativa, bladderwrack (*Fucus vesiculosus*), *Panax ginseng*, milk thistle (*Silybum marianum*), spirulina, ozone therapy, polarity treatment, or Reiki has been used for nonspecific symptoms related to radiation. *Salvia miltiorrhiza* has been used in cases of radiation pneumonitis. Topical preparations have been applied to try and minimize radiation skin reactions, including chamomile (for which there is inconclusive evidence) and aloe (which evidence suggests is not beneficial in this situation).[111–114]

THERAPIES USED FOR PRIMARY CANCER PREVENTION

Numerous herbs and vitamins have been proposed as cancer prevention agents, for use in healthy individuals or those at high risk for development of malignancies due to genetic predisposition or environmental exposures. Most evidence is epidemiologic, based on large surveys or case-control studies, with only rare cohort or randomized, controlled trials. Many proposed agents contain antioxidants, based on the premise that preventing oxidative damage may decrease the risk of cancer.

LYCOPENE

Lycopene is a carotenoid, present in human serum, liver, adrenal glands, lungs, prostate, colon, and skin, at higher levels than other carotenoids. Most dietary lycopene is derived from tomatoes and tomato-based products. Lycopene is also present in apricots, pink grapefruit, guava, rose hip, palm oil, and watermelon. Antioxidant and antiproliferative properties have been reported in preclinical research, and there are more than 75 case-control or cohort studies of the association between increased tomato/tomato-based product intake or serum lycopene levels with cancer risk. Approximately two-thirds of these studies suggest benefits in the range of 40% risk reduction, although fewer than half of the studies are statistically significant, and numerous studies provide negative results.[115] No prospective controlled data are available and there is only limited study of concentrated lycopene supplements.

SELENIUM

Selenium is a trace mineral found in soil, water, and some foods. It is an essential element in several metabolic pathways, including the glutathione-peroxidase pathway. Selenium appears to promote antioxidant activity in the body via glutathione peroxidase, a selenium-dependent enzyme.

Initial evidence has suggested that selenium supplementation reduces the risk of developing prostate cancer in men with normal baseline PSA levels and low selenium blood levels. This is the subject of large, well-designed studies, including the Nutritional Prevention of Cancer Trial (NPC), and the ongoing Selenium and Vitamin E Cancer Prevention Trial (SELECT),[116–131] as well as prior population and case-control studies. [132,133]

The NPC was conducted in 1312 Americans and reported that 200 mg of daily selenium reduces the overall incidence of prostate cancer, although these protective effects only occurred in men with baseline PSA levels less than or equal to 4 ng/mL and those with low baseline blood selenium levels (less than 123.2 ng/mL).[116,121,125,134] The NPC trial was primarily designed to measure the development of nonmelanoma skin cancers and not other types of cancers, and, therefore, these prostate cancer results cannot be considered definitive. To settle this question, further study is underway: The SELECT trial is in progress, with a goal to include 32,400 men with serum PSA levels less than or equal to 4 ng/mL. SELECT was started in 2001, with results expected in 2013.

Laboratory studies have reported several potential mechanisms for selenium's beneficial effects in prostate cancer, including decrease in androgen receptors and PSA production,[135,136] antioxidant effects, angiogenesis inhibition, or apoptosis.[137–142]

It is not known whether selenium is helpful in men who already have been diagnosed with prostate cancer to prevent progression or recurrence of disease.[143] It does appear that selenium may not be beneficial in those with elevated PSA levels or with normal to high selenium levels. It remains unclear whether men at risk (or all men) should have their serum selenium values measured; results of the SELECT study may provide additional guidance. There is evidence that low selenium levels are associated with an increased risk of prostate cancer,[132] and several mechanisms for the beneficial effects of selenium supplementation have been suggested.[137,144,145]

In the NPC trial, no benefits were seen in reducing the risk of colorectal or lung cancers. Although an overall reduction in cancer risk was observed, it is not clear which specific types of cancer, besides prostate cancer, may be affected.

GREEN TEA

Green tea is produced from the dried leaves of *Camellia sinensis*, a perennial evergreen shrub from which black tea and oolong tea are also derived. Animal and laboratory research reports that tea components such as polyphenols possess antioxidant, antiangiogenic, and proapoptotic properties, as well as reduce serum estrogen levels. Several large case-control and cohort studies have been published, largely focused on gastrointestinal and breast cancers.[146–150] Results are variable, with some suggesting chronic tea consumption may decrease cancer risk but others reporting no benefits. Studies have been observational, and other lifestyle choices of tea drinkers may confound these results.

One cup of green tea contains approximately 50 mg caffeine, and excessive tea consumption may lead to adverse effects or toxicity. Green tea supplement capsules usually contain less caffeine (approximately 5 mg of caffeine in 500 mg).

VITAMIN A

Vitamin A is comprised of retinol and its carotenoid precursors. All-*trans* retinoic acid, a retinol analogue, is well established as a differentiation agent in patients with acute promyelocytic leukemia. However, there is little evidence for the use of nonprescription vitamin A supplements for cancer treatment or prevention. Proposed use is based on antioxidant activity. Trials have yielded variable results, suggesting no reduction in prostate cancer risk[151] and possible increased risk of lung cancer in high-risk patients.[152] Due to the possibility of hypervitaminosis A with supplementation of this fat-soluble vitamin, chronic intake of large doses is discouraged.

VITAMIN C (ASCORBIC ACID)

Limited clinical research has been conducted on vitamin C for cancer prevention. In the 1980s, there was initial excitement over epidemiologic evidence correlating high dietary vitamin C intake with reduced rates of cancer, although use of vitamin C in observed populations may have correlated with other healthy lifestyle choices (diet, exercise) that confounded findings. A subsequent prospective trial found no reduction in rates of breast cancer.[153] Preclinical evidence of reduced platelet aggregation suggests that risks may outweigh potential benefits. Patients may experience scurvy symptoms after abrupt withdrawal of chronic megadoses.

VITAMIN E (α-TOCOPHEROL)

Vitamin E is a fat-soluble vitamin with antioxidant properties. Epidemiologic studies suggest possible reduced breast, lung, and prostate cancer risk. However, prevention trials report no reduction in risk of lung,[154] breast,[155] or colon[156] cancer. Initial research suggests slowed progression of prostate cancer in one trial using three-times the recommended daily allowance.[157] Therefore, further study is warranted in patients with existing prostate cancer, but efficacy for prevention is not established. Preclinical evidence of reduced platelet aggregation has been shown.

OTHER THERAPIES

Numerous other therapies are used for cancer prevention but are not well studied. These include aloe, black tea, bromelain, cranberry, eucalyptus oil, ginseng, grape seed extract, *Lactobacillus acidophilus* (colon cancer risk reduction), milk thistle, oleander, omega-3 fatty acids/fish oil, psyllium (colon cancer risk reduction), red clover, and spirulina.

REFERENCES

1. Panel on Definition and Description, Office of Alternative Medicine, National Institutes of Health, CAM Research Methodology Conference, Bethesda, MD, April 1995.
2. Zollman C, Vickers A. ABC of complementary medicine: what is complementary medicine? *BMJ* 1999;319:693.
3. Cassileth BR. "Complementary" or "alternative?" It makes a difference in cancer care. *Comp Ther Med* 1999;44:22.
4. Eisenberg DM, Davis, RB, Ettner SL, et al. Trends in alternative medicine use in the United States, 1990–1997. Results of a follow-up national survey. *JAMA* 1998;280(18):1569.
5. Dietary Supplement Health and Education Act of 1994 (DSHEA), Public Law 103-417, October 25, 1994 (103rd Congress).
6. Wolsko PM, Eisenberg DM, Davis RB, et al. Insurance coverage, medical conditions, and visits to alternative medicine providers. Results of a national survey. *Arch Intern Med* 2002;162:281.
7. Astin JA. Why patients use alternative medicine: results of a national survey. *JAMA* 1998;279:1548.
8. Druss B. Association between use of unconventional therapies and conventional medical services. *JAMA* 1999;282:651.
9. White JD. The National Cancer Institute's perspective and agenda for promoting awareness and research on alternative therapies for cancer (keynote address). *J Alt Comp Med* 2002;8(5):545.
10. Adler SR, Fosket JR. Disclosing complementary and alternative medicine use in the medical encounter: a qualitative study in women with breast cancer. *J Fam Pract* 1999;48:453.
11. Bernstein BJ, Grasso T. Prevalence of complementary and alternative medicine use in cancer patients. *Oncology (Huntington)* 2001;15(10):1267.
12. Burstein HJ, Gelber S, Guadagnoli E, at al. Use of alternative medicine by women with early-stage breast cancer. *N Engl J Med* 1999;340(22):1733.
13. Gotay CC, Hara W, Issel BF, et al. Use of complementary and alternative medicine in Hawaii cancer patients. *Hawaii Med J* 1999;58(4):94.
14. Kao GD, Devine P. Use of complementary health practices by prostate carcinoma patients undergoing radiation therapy. *Cancer* 2000;88(3):615.
15. Lee MM, Chang JS, Jacobs B, et al. Complementary and alternative medicine use among men with prostate cancer in 4 ethnic populations. *Am J Public Health* 2002;92(10):1606.
16. Lippert MC, McClain R, Boyd JC, et al. Alternative medicine use in patients with localized prostate carcinoma treated with curative intent. *Cancer* 1999;86(12):2642.
17. Maskarinec G, Shumay DM, Kakai H, et al. Ethnic differences in complementary and alternative medicine use among cancer patients. *J Alt Comp Med* 2000;6(6):531.
18. Morris KT, Johnson N, Homer L, et al. A comparison of complementary therapy use between breast cancer patients and patients with other primary tumor sites. *Am J Surg* 2000;179:407(abst).
19. Patterson RE, Neuhouser ML, Hedderson MM, et al. Types of alternative medicine used by patients with breast, colon, or prostate cancer: predictors, motives, and costs. *J Alt Comp Med* 2002;8(4):477.
20. Richardson MA, Sanders T, Palmer JL, et al. Complementary/alternative medicine use in a comprehensive cancer center and the implications for oncology. *J Clin Oncol* 2000;18(13):2505.
21. Shumay DM, Maskarinec G, Gotay CC, et al. Determinants of the degree of complementary and alternative medicine use among patients with cancer. *J Alt Comp Med* 2002;8(5):661.
22. Sparber A, Bauer L, Curt G, et al. Use of complementary medicine by adult patients participating in cancer clinical trials. *Oncol Nurs Forum* 2000;27(4):623.
23. Swisher EM, Cohn DE, Goff BA, et al. Use of complementary and alternative medicine among women with gynecologic cancers. *Gyn Oncol* 2002;84:363.
24. VandeCreek L, Rogers E, Lester J. Use of alternative therapies among breast cancer outpatients compared with the general population. *Alt Ther Health Med* 1999;5(1):71.
25. Ernst E, Cassileth BR. The prevalence of complementary/alternative medicine in cancer. A systematic review. *Cancer* 1998;83(4):777.
26. Sparber A, Wooten JC. Surveys of complementary and alternative medicine: Pt II. Use of alternative and complementary cancer therapies. *J Alt Comp Med* 2001;7(3):281.
27. Friedman T, Slayton WB, Allen LS, et al. Use of alternative therapies for children with cancer. *Pediatrics* 1997;100(6):E1(2–6).
28. Kelly KM, Jacobson JS, Kennedy DD, et al. Use of unconventional therapies by children with cancer at an urban medical center. *J Pediatr Hematol Oncol* 2000;22(5):412.
29. Ernst E, Cassileth BR. The prevalence of complementary/alternative medicine in cancer: a systematic review. *Cancer* 1998;83:777.
30. DiGianni LM, Garber JE, Winer EP. Complementary and alternative medicine use among women with breast cancer. *J Clin Oncol* 2002;20(18s):34s.
31. Risberg T, Vickers A, Bremnes RM, et al. Does use of alternative medicine predict survival from cancer? *Eur J Cancer* 2003;39(3):372.
32. Sollner W, Maislinger S, DeVries A, et al. Use of complementary and alternative medicine by cancer patients is not associated with perceived distress or poor compliance with standard treatment but with active coping behavior. *Cancer* 2000;89(4):873.
33. Rogers EA, Gough JE, Brewer KL. Are emergency department patients at risk for herb-drug interactions? *Acad Emerg Med* 2001;8(9):932.
34. Farah MH, Edwards R, Lindquist M, et al. International monitoring of adverse health effects associated with herbal medicines. *Pharmacoepidemiol Drug Safety* 2000;9:105.
35. Ang-Lee MK, Moss J, Yuan CS. Herbal medicines and perioperative care. *JAMA* 2001;286:208.
36. Seifried HE, McDonald SS, Anderson DE, et al. The antioxidant conundrum in cancer. *Cancer Res* 2003;63:4295.
37. Weiger WA, Smith M, Boon H, et al. Advising patients who seek complementary and alternative medical therapies for cancer. *Ann Intern Med* 2002;137(11):889.
38. Palmer ME, Haller C, McKinney PE, et al. Adverse events associated with dietary supplements: an observational study. *Lancet* 2003;361(9352):101.
39. Fugh-Berman A. Herb-drug interactions. *Lancet* 2000;355(9198):134.
40. Abebe W. Herbal medication: potential for adverse interactions with analgesic drugs. *J Clin Pharm Ther* 2002;27(6):391.
41. Ernst E. Possible interactions between synthetic and herbal medicinal products. Pt 1: A systematic review of the indirect evidence. *Perfusion* 2000;13:4.
42. Ernst E. Interactions between synthetic and herbal medicinal products. Pt 2: A systematic review of the direct evidence. *Perfusion* 2000;13:60.
43. Piscitelli SC, Burstein AH. Herb-drug interactions and confounding in clinical trials. *J Herb Pharmacother* 2002;2(1):23.
44. Izzo AA, Ernst E. Interactions between herbal medicines and prescribed drugs: a systematic review. *Drugs* 2001;61(15):2163.
45. Hardy ML. Herb-drug interactions: An evidence-based table. *Alt Med Alert* 2000;June:64.
46. Lambrecht J, Hamilton W, Rabinovich A. A review of herb-drug interactions: documented and theoretical. *US Pharmacist* 2000;25(8):1.
47. Mathijssen RHJ, Verweij J, De Bruijn P, et al. Modulation of irinotecan (CPT-11) metabolism by St. John's wort in cancer patients. American Association for Cancer Research, 93rd Annual Meeting, San Francisco, April 6–10, 2002.
48. Quella SK, Loprinzi CL, Barton DL, et al. Evaluation of soy phytoestrogens for the treatment of hot flashes in breast cancer survivors: A North Central Cancer Treatment Group Trial. *J Clin Oncol* 2000;18(5):1068.
49. Jonas WB. Alternative medicine—learning from the past, examining the present, advancing to the future. *JAMA* 1998;280:1616.
50. Angell M. Alternative medicine—the risks of untested and unregulated remedies. *N Engl J Med* 1998;339(123):839.
51. Studdert DM. Medical malpractice implications of alternative medicine. *JAMA* 1998;280(18):1610.
52. Winslow LC, Shapiro H. Physicians want education about complementary and alternative medicine to enhance communication with their patients. *Arch Intern Med* 2002;162(10):1176.
53. Kroll DJ. Concerns and needs for research in herbal supplement pharmacotherapy and safety. *J Herb Pharmacother* 2001;1(2):3.
54. Eisenberg DM. Advising patients who seek alternative medical therapies. *Ann Intern Med* 1997;127:61.
55. Adachi K, Nanba H, Kuroda H. Potentiation of host-mediated antitumor activity in mice by beta-glucan obtained from *Grifola frondosa* (maitake). *Chem Pharm Bull (Tokyo)* 1987; 35(1):262.
56. Kodama N, Komuta K, Nanba H. Can maitake MD-fraction aid cancer patients? *Alt Med Rev* 2002;7(3):236.
57. deVere White RW, Hackman RM, Soares SE, et al. Effects of a mushroom mycelium extract on the treatment of prostate cancer. *Urology* 2002;60:640.
58. Birkenfeld S, Zaltsman YA, Krispin M, et al. Antitumor effects of inhibitors of arachidonic acid cascade on experimentally induced intestinal tumors. *Dis Colon Rectum* 1987;30(1):43.
59. Smart CR, Hogle HH, Vogel H, et al. Clinical experience with nordihydroguaiaretic acid—"chaparral tea" in the treatment of cancer. *Rocky Mt Med J* 1970;67(11):39.
60. Ortega JA, Creek JE. Acute cyanide poisoning following administration of Laetrile enemas. *J Pediatr* 1978;93(6):1059.
61. Beamer WC, Shealy RM, Prough DS. Acute cyanide poisoning from laetrile ingestion. *Ann Emerg Med* 1983;12(7):449.
62. Smith FP, Butler TP, Cohan S, et al. Laetrile toxicity: a report of two patients. *Cancer Treat Rep* 1978;62(1):169.
63. Moertel CG, Fleming TR, Rubin J, et al. A clinical trial of amygdalin (Laetrile) in the treatment of human cancer. *N Engl J Med* 1982;306(4):201.

64. Stein GM, Edlund U, Pfuller U, et al. Influence of polysaccharides from *Viscum album* L. on human lymphocytes, monocytes and granulocytes in vitro. *Anticancer Res* 1999;19(5B):3907.
65. Schink M. Mistletoe therapy for human cancer: the role of the natural killer cells. *Anticancer Drugs* 1997;8[Suppl 1]:S47.
66. Kleijnen J, Knipschild P. Mistletoe treatment for cancer: review of controlled trials in humans. *Phytomedicine* 1994;1:255.
67. Grossarth-Maticek R, Kiene H, Baumgartner SM, et al. Use of Iscador, an extract of European mistletoe (*Viscum album*), in cancer treatment: prospective nonrandomized and randomized matched-pair studies nested within a cohort study. *Alt Ther Health Med* 2001;7(3):57.
68. Lenartz D, Schierholz JM, Menzel J, et al. Influence of complementary mistletoe lectin therapy in the treatment of malignant glioma. *Zeitschrift für Onkologie* 1999;31(2):44.
69. Schaefermeyer G, Schaefermeyer H. Treatment of pancreatic cancer with *Viscum album* (Iscador): a retrospective study of 292 patients 1986–1996. *Comp Ther Med* 1998;6(4):172.
70. McNamee D. Mistletoe extract ineffective in melanoma. *Lancet* 1999;354:1101.
71. Kaegi E. Unconventional therapies for cancer: 1. Essiac. The Task Force on Alternative Therapies of the Canadian Breast Cancer Research Initiative. *CMAJ* 1998;158(7):897.
72. Austin S, Baumgartner E, DeKadt S. Long term follow-up of cancer patients using Contreras, Hoxsey and Gerson therapies. *J Naturopathic Med* 1995; 5(1):74.
73. Gebland H. *The Hoxsey treatment. Unconventional cancer treatments.* Washington, DC: U.S. Government Printing Office, 1990:75.
74. de la Taille A, Buttyan R, Hayek O, et al. Herbal therapy PC-SPES: in vitro effects and evaluation of its efficacy in 69 patients with prostate cancer. *J Urol* 2000;164(4):1229.
75. DiPaola RS, Zhang H, Lambert GH, et al. Clinical and biologic activity of an estrogenic herbal combination (PC-SPES) in prostate cancer. *N Engl J Med* 1998;339(12):785.
76. Oh WK, George DJ, Hackmann K, et al. Activity of the herbal combination, PC-SPES, in the treatment of patients with androgen-independent prostate cancer. *Urology* 2001; 57(1):122.
77. Pfeifer BL, Pirani JF, Hamann SR, et al. PC-SPES, a dietary supplement for the treatment of hormone-refractory prostate cancer. *BJU Int* 2000;85(4):481.
78. Small EJ, Frohlich MW, Bok R, et al. Prospective trial of the herbal supplement PC-SPES in patients with progressive prostate cancer. *J Clin Oncol* 2000;18(21):3595.
79. Reynolds T. Contamination of PC-SPES remains a mystery. *J Natl Cancer Inst* 2002;94(17):1266.
80. Mathews J. Media feeds frenzy over shark cartilage as cancer treatment. *J Natl Cancer Inst* 1993;85(15):1190.
81. Brem H, Folkman J. Inhibition of tumor angiogenesis mediated by cartilage. *J Exp Med* 1975;141(2):427.
82. Langer R, Brem H, Falterman K, et al. Isolations of a cartilage factor that inhibits tumor neovascularization. *Science* 1976;193(4247):70.
83. Miller DR, Anderson GT, Stark JJ, et al. Phase I/II trial of the safety and efficacy of shark cartilage in the treatment of advanced cancer. *J Clin Oncol* 1998;16(11):3649.
84. Batist G, Patenaude F, Champagne P, et al. Neovastat (AE-941) in refractory renal cell carcinoma patients: report of a phase II trial with two dose levels. *Ann Oncol* 2002; 13(8):1259.
85. Buckner JC, Malkin MG, Reed E, et al. Phase II study of antineoplastons A10 (NSC 648539) and AS2-1 (NSC 620261) in patients with recurrent glioma. *Mayo Clin Proc* 1999;74(2):137.
86. Burzynski SR, Kubove E. Initial clinical study with antineoplaston A2 injections in cancer patients with five years' follow-up. *Drugs Exp Clin Res* 1987;13[Suppl 1]:1.
87. Sugita Y, Tsuda H, Maruiwa H, et al. The effect of antineoplaston, a new antitumor agent on malignant brain tumors. *Kurume Med J* 1995;42(3):133.
88. Tsuda H, Sata M, Kumabe T, et al. Quick response of advanced cancer to chemoradiation therapy with antineoplastons. *Oncol Rep* 1998;5(3):597.
89. Kosty MP, Fleishman SB, Herndon JE, et al. Cisplatin, vinblastine, and hydrazine sulfate in advanced, non–small-cell lung cancer: a randomized placebo-controlled, double-blind phase III study of the Cancer and Leukemia Group B. *J Clin Oncol* 1994;12(6):1113.
90. Loprinzi CL, Goldberg RM, Su JQ, et al. Placebo-controlled trial of hydrazine sulfate in patients with newly diagnosed non–small-cell lung cancer. *J Clin Oncol* 1994;12(6):1126.
91. Loprinzi CL, Kuross SA, O'Fallon JR, et al. Randomized placebo-controlled evaluation of hydrazine sulfate in patients with advanced colorectal cancer. *J Clin Oncol* 1994;12 (6):1121.
92. Nadel MV. Contrary to allegation, NIH hydrazine sulfate studies were not flawed. Report to the Chairman and Ranking Minority Member, Human Resources and Intergovernmental Relations Subcommittee, House Committee on Government Reform and Oversight, 1995:1.
93. Hildenbrand GL, Hildenbrand LC, Bradford K, et al. Five-year survival rates of melanoma patients treated by diet therapy after the manner of Gerson: a retrospective review. *Alt Ther Health Med* 1995;1:29.
94. Demark-Wahnefried W, Price DT, Polascik TJ, et al. Pilot study of dietary fat restriction and flaxseed supplementation in men with prostate cancer before surgery: exploring the effects on hormonal levels, prostate-specific antigen, and histopathologic features. *Urology* 2001;58(1):47.
95. Eaton S, Skinner R, Hale JP, et al. Plasma coenzyme Q(10) in children and adolescents undergoing doxorubicin therapy. *Clin Chim Acta* 2000;302(1–2):1.
96. Pace A, Savarese A, Picardo M, et al. Neuroprotective effect of vitamin E supplementation in patients treated with cisplatin chemotherapy. *J Clin Oncol* 2003;21(5):927.
97. Bruera E, Strasser F, Palmer JL, et al. Effect of fish oil on appetite and other symptoms in patients with advanced cancer and anorexia/cachexia: a double-blind, placebo-controlled study. *J Clin Oncol* 2003;21(1):129.
98. Fearon KC, Von Meyenfeldt MF, Moses AG, et al. Effect of a protein and energy dense n-3 fatty acid enriched oral supplement on loss of weight and lean tissue in cancer cachexia: a randomised double blind trial. *Gut* 2003;52(10):1479.
99. Pace J, Conlin DS. Oral ingestion of encapsulated ginger and reported self-care actions for the relief of chemotherapy-associated nausea and vomiting. *Dissertation Abstracts Int* 1987;47(8):3297-B.
100. Ernst E, Pittler MH. Efficacy of ginger for nausea and vomiting: a systematic review of randomized clinical trials. *Br J Anaesth* 2000;84(3):367.
101. Dundee JW, Ghaly RG, Fitzpatrick KT, et al. Acupuncture prophylaxis of cancer chemotherapy-induced sickness. *J R Soc Med* 1989;82:268.
102. Williams CJ, Price H, Serious K. A randomized trial of acupressure for chemotherapy induced emesis. *Proc Annu Meet Am Soc Clin Oncol* 1992;1394(abst).
103. Corner J, Cawley N, Hildebrand S. An evaluation of the use of massage and essential oils on the well-being of cancer patients. *Int J Palliat Nurs* 1995;2(1):67.
104. Kolcaba K, Fox C. The effects of guided imagery on comfort of women with early stage breast cancer undergoing radiation therapy. *Oncol Nurs Forum* 1999;26(1):67.
105. Corner J, Cawley N, Hildebrand S. An evaluation of the use of massage and essential oils on the well-being of cancer patients. *Int J Palliat Nurs* 1995;1:67.
106. Ferrell-Torry AT, Glick OJ. The use of therapeutic massage as a nursing intervention to modify anxiety and the perception of cancer pain. *Cancer Nurs* 1993;16(2):93.
107. Risberg T, Wist E, Kaasa S, et al. Spiritual healing among Norwegian hospitalised cancer patients and patients' religious needs and preferences of pastoral services. *Eur J Cancer* 1996;32A(2):274.
108. Fellowes D, Gambles M, Lockhart-Wood K, et al. Reflexology for symptom relief in patients with cancer. *Cochrane Database of Systematic Reviews*, 2002, vol. 2.
109. Olson K, Hanson J. Using Reiki to manage pain: a preliminary report. *Cancer Prev Control* 1997;1(2):108.
110. Giasson M, Bouchard L. Effect of therapeutic touch on the well-being of persons with terminal cancer. *J Holist Nurs* 1998;16(3):383.
111. Olsen DL, Raub W Jr, Bradley C, et al. The effect of aloe vera gel/mild soap versus mild soap alone in preventing skin reactions in patients undergoing radiation therapy. *Oncol Nurs Forum* 2001;28(3):543.
112. Williams MS, Burk M, Loprinzi CL, et al. Phase III double-blind evaluation of an aloe vera gel as a prophylactic agent for radiation-induced skin toxicity. *Int J Radiat Oncol Biol Phys* 1996;36(2):345.
113. Maiche A. Effect of chamomile cream and almond ointment on acute radiation skin reaction. *Acta Oncol* 1991;30(3):395.
114. Balzarini A, Felisi E, Martini A, et al. Efficacy of homeopathic treatment of skin reactions during radiotherapy for breast cancer: a randomised, double-blind clinical trial. *Br Homeopath J* 2000;89(1):8.
115. Giovannucci E. Tomatoes, tomato-based products, lycopene, and cancer: review of the epidemiologic literature. *J Natl Cancer Inst* 1999;91(4):317.
116. Combs GF. Status of selenium in prostate cancer prevention. *Br J Cancer* 2004;91:195.
117. Huff J. Re: Selenium supplementation and secondary prevention of nonmelanoma skin cancer in a randomized trial. *J Natl Cancer Inst* 2004;96:333.
118. Whanger PD. Selenium and its relationship to cancer: an update dagger. *Br J Nutr* 2004;91:11.
119. Finley JW. Reduction of cancer risk by consumption of selenium-enriched plants: enrichment of broccoli with selenium increases the anticarcinogenic properties of broccoli. *J Med Food* 2003;6:19.
120. Klein EA, Lippman SM, Thompson IM, et al. The selenium and vitamin E cancer prevention trial. *World J Urol* 2003;21:21.
121. Duffield-Lillico AJ, Dalkin BL, Reid ME, et al. Selenium supplementation, baseline plasma selenium status and incidence of prostate cancer: an analysis of the complete treatment period of the Nutritional Prevention of Cancer Trial. *BJU Int* 2003;91:608.
122. Klein EA, Thompson IM, Lippman SM, et al. SELECT: the selenium and vitamin E cancer prevention trial. *Urol Oncol* 2003;21:59.
123. Vinceti M, Malagoli C, Bergomi M, et al. Correspondence re: Duffield-Lillico et al., Baseline characteristics and the effect of selenium supplementation on cancer incidence in a randomized clinical trial: a summary report of the Nutritional Prevention of Cancer Trial. *Cancer Epidemiol Biomarkers Prev* 2003;12:77.
124. Klein EA. Clinical models for testing chemopreventative agents in prostate cancer and overview of SELECT: the Selenium and Vitamin E Cancer Prevention Trial. *Recent Results Cancer Res* 2003;163:212.
125. Duffield-Lillico AJ, Slate EH, Reid ME, et al. Selenium supplementation and secondary prevention of nonmelanoma skin cancer in a randomized trial. *J Natl Cancer Inst* 2003;95:1477.
126. Moyad MA. Selenium and vitamin E supplements for prostate cancer: evidence or embellishment? *Urology* 2002;59(4 Suppl 1):9.
127. Reid ME, Duffield-Lillico AJ, Garland L, et al. Selenium supplementation and lung cancer incidence: an update of the nutritional prevention of cancer trial. *Cancer Epidemiol Biomarkers Prev* 2002;11:1285.
128. Combs GF Jr, Clark LC, Turnbull BW. An analysis of cancer prevention by selenium. *Biofactors* 2001;14(1–4):153.
129. Clark LC, Dalkin B, Krongrad A, et al. Decreased incidence of prostate cancer with selenium supplementation: results of a double-blind cancer prevention trial. *Br J Urol* 1998;81(5):730.
130. Clark LC, Combs GF Jr, Turnbull BW, et al. Effects of selenium supplementation for cancer prevention in patients with carcinoma of the skin. A randomized controlled trial. Nutritional Prevention of Cancer Study Group. *JAMA* 1996;276(24):1957.
131. Clark LC, Dalkin B, Krongrad A. Decreased incidence of prostate cancer with selenium supplementation: results of a double-blind cancer prevention trial. *J Am Nutraceutic Assoc* 1999;2(1):14.
132. Li H, Stampfer MJ, Giovannucci EL, et al. A prospective study of plasma selenium levels and prostate cancer risk. *J Natl Cancer Inst* 2004;96(9):696.
133. Hartman TJ, Albanes D, Pietinen P, et al. The association between baseline vitamin E, selenium, and prostate cancer in the alpha-tocopherol, beta-carotene cancer prevention study. *Cancer Epidemiol Biomarkers Prev* 1998;7(4):335.

134. Duffield-Lillico AJ, Reid ME, Turnbull BW, et al. Baseline characteristics and the effect of selenium supplementation on cancer incidence in a randomized clinical trial: a summary report of the nutritional prevention of cancer trial. *Cancer Epidemiol Biomarkers Prev* 2002;11(7):630.

135. Dong Y, Zhang H, Hawthorn L, et al. Delineation of the molecular basis for selenium-induced growth arrest in human prostate cancer cells by oligonucleotide array. *Cancer Res* 2003;63(1):52.

136. Dong Y, Lee SO, Zhang H, et al. Prostate specific antigen expression is down-regulated by selenium through disruption of androgen receptor signaling. *Cancer Res* 2004;64(1):19.

137. Fleming J, Ghose A, Harrison PR. Molecular mechanisms of cancer prevention by selenium compounds. *Nutr Cancer* 2001;40(1):42.

138. Zu K, Ip C. Synergy between selenium and vitamin E in apoptosis induction is associated with activation of distinctive initiator caspases in human prostate cancer cells. *Cancer Res* 2003;63(20):6988.

139. Kim YS, Milner J. Molecular targets for selenium in cancer prevention. *Nutr Cancer* 2001;40(1):50.

140. Lu J. Apoptosis and angiogenesis in cancer prevention by selenium. *Adv Exp Med Biol* 2001;492:131.

141. Stewart MS, Spallholz JE, Neldner KH, et al. Selenium compounds have disparate abilities to impose oxidative stress and induce apoptosis. *Free Radic Biol Med* 1999;26(1-2):42.

142. Tapiero H, Townsend DM, Tew KD. The antioxidant role of selenium and seleno-compounds. *Biomed Pharmacother* 2003;57(3-4):134.

143. Stratton MS, Reid ME, Schwartzberg G, et al. Selenium and inhibition of disease progression in men diagnosed with prostate carcinoma: study design and baseline characteristics of the 'Watchful Waiting' Study. *Anticancer Drugs* 2003;14(8):595.

144. Ganther HE. Selenium metabolism and mechanisms of cancer prevention. *Adv Exp Med Biol* 2001;492:119.

145. Lamson DW, Brignall MS. Antioxidants in cancer therapy; their actions and interactions with oncologic therapies. *Altern Med Rev* 1999;4(5):304.

PART 4

NEWER APPROACHES IN CANCER TREATMENT

Patrick Hwu

CHAPTER **60**

Gene Therapy

With increased understanding of the molecular nature of cancer, investigators are now focused on developing methods for using this knowledge to design novel therapeutics. Gene therapy, which can be defined as the introduction of new genetic material into cells for therapeutic intent, is a tool that may aid in the development of novel cancer therapies based on important basic scientific advances in the understanding of the immune system and the molecular biology of cancer.

Gene therapy encompasses a broad array of experimental cancer therapies, including immunization with cytokine or tumor antigen genes as well as the introduction of toxic genes directly into tumors (Table 60-1). Since the first gene transfer trial in 1989, a large number of gene therapy clinical trials have been initiated (Table 60-2). Forty-nine gene marking studies have now been initiated involving over 270 patients. Investigational therapeutic studies involving gene transfer have largely been conducted in cancer patients, representing 403 of the 636 clinical trials that have been initiated worldwide (see Table 60-2). The vast majority of these cancer clinical trials have focused on enhancing the immune response against the tumor using cytokine, costimulatory, tumor antigen, or lymphocyte receptor genes (n = 241) or on directly targeting the tumor using suicide, tumor suppressor, or antisense genes (n = 122; Table 60-3). Despite this significant effort, few clinical responses have been reported, which underscores the need for alternative strategies and improved vector development.

Two requirements exist for successful genetic manipulation of a eukaryotic cell. First, a method must exist to provide successful gene insertion into the correct cell type with adequate efficiency for a particular therapeutic purpose. Some therapeutic approaches may require permanent gene transfer, whereas for others, transient activity may suffice. Second, the inserted gene must be adequately expressed by that cell. For some purposes a high level of expression is required, whereas for others a low level of gene expression is sufficient. Constitutive or regulated expression may be necessary depending on the specific application.

METHODS OF GENE TRANSFER

Numerous techniques are available for gene transfer into mammalian cells (Table 60-4). The choice of a particular gene transfer technique depends on the biologic requirements of the specific therapeutic strategy. For example, to protect hematopoietic stem cells from the toxic effects of systemic chemotherapy, often given for several cycles, the multidrug resistance gene (MDR) must be stably integrated into stem cells, using gene transfer techniques that include use of retroviral vectors. However, to immunize patients against tumors, it is possible that only transient expression of antigen genes by viral vectors such as adenovirus will be sufficient.

Many techniques of gene transfer use viruses to introduce genetic material, because viruses in most cases can deliver genes to cells with higher efficiencies compared to nonviral methods.

RETROVIRAL VECTORS

Retroviruses are RNA viruses that are capable of stably integrating DNA within the host cell genome. The replication cycle of a retrovirus begins with viral attachment to a cell by a specific receptor. The virus enters the cell and the viral RNA is reverse transcribed to DNA by the virally encoded reverse transcriptase.

TABLE 60-1. Cancer Gene Therapy Approaches

Strategies	Examples of Potential Experimental Approaches
Genetic modification of the immune response	
Active immunization	
Modification of tumor cells with genes that enhance tumor immunogenicity	Patient immunization with tumor cells modified by the introduction of cytokine genes (e.g., IL-2 or GM-CSF) or costimulatory molecules (e.g., B7-1). Gene transfer into tumor cells can be performed in the laboratory (*ex vivo*) or directly into the patient (*in vivo*).
Immunization with genes encoding tumor antigens	Patient immunization with genes encoding melanoma antigens recognized by T cells, such as MART-1. Immunization can be accomplished by direct injection of DNA or by injection of viral vectors encoding tumor antigens, such as vaccinia, fowlpox, or adenoviral or retroviral vectors. Immunization can be performed directly *in vivo* or by transduction of antigen-presenting cells (e.g., dendritic cells) with tumor antigen genes, followed by administration to the patient.
Genetic modification of immune effector cells	
Enhance survival of immune cells	Transduction of tumor-specific lymphocytes with the IL-2 gene to enhance their survival *in vivo*.
Increase tumor recognition	Use of novel receptor genes to allow lymphocytes to recognize new targets on tumor cells.
Increase antitumor efficacy of immune cells	Retroviral transduction of tumor infiltrating lymphocytes with the TNF gene in an attempt to deliver large quantities of TNF to the tumor site.
Decrease toxicity of effector cells	Treatment of BMT patients with donor T cells containing suicide gene to eliminate the cells before the development of graft-versus-host disease.
Modification of tumors with genes that have direct antitumor effects	
Tumor suppressor genes	Replace mutated or absent tumor suppressor genes to decrease tumor growth.
Antisense, ribozymes, and RNA interference	Decrease expression of products of activated oncogenes.
Suicide genes	Kill tumor cells by introduction of genes that produce toxic products. Tumor-specific promoters or tumor-specific delivery can be used to decrease systemic toxicity.
Selective replication of virus in tumor	Use of E1B-defective adenovirus capable of replicating only in tumors lacking functional p53.
Introduction of genes into normal tissues to protect them from chemotherapy or radiotherapy	Transduce bone marrow cells with multidrug resistance gene to decrease hematopoietic toxicity from subsequent chemotherapy.
Antiangiogenic gene therapy	Express genes that have antiangiogenic properties or inhibit proangiogenic cytokines.

BMT, bone marrow transplantation; GM-CSF, granulocyte-macrophage colony-stimulating factor; IL-2, interleukin-2; TNF, tumor necrosis factor.

The viral DNA is then transported to the nucleus, where it integrates into the host cell genome. The integrated viral DNA, termed the *provirus*, is transcribed, and then both spliced and unspliced transcripts are translated to form the viral proteins. Some of the unspliced transcripts are packaged, via a packaging signal sequence (ψ), into viral capsids. The mature viruses then bud from the host cell membrane.

Retroviral vectors for gene transfer have been constructed by substituting the gene of interest in place of the viral protein coding regions,[1,2] which, thus, makes these vectors replication incompetent (Fig. 60-1). These vectors are packaged into retro-

TABLE 60-2. Gene Therapy and Gene Marking Clinical Studies

	Protocols		Patients	
Diseases	Number	%	Number	%
Cancer	403	63.4	2392	68.4
Monogenic diseases	78	12.3	309	8.8
Infectious diseases	41	6.4	408	11.7
Vascular diseases	51	8	86	2.5
Other diseases	12	1.9	21	0.6
Gene marking	49	7.7	274	7.8
Healthy volunteers	2	0.3	6	0.2
Total	**636**	**100**	**3496**	**100**

(From the *Journal of Gene Medicine*, with permission.)

TABLE 60-3. Cancer Gene Therapy Trials

Approach	Gene	No. of Trials
Immune enhancement	Antigen or costimulatory molecules[a]	104
	Cytokine[b]	126
	Lymphocyte receptor	9
	Antibody	2
Direct tumor killing	Suicide	60
	Tumor suppressor	56
	Antisense	12
Bone marrow protection	Drug resistance	12
Other		22
Total		**403**

[a]Includes combinations of antigens and costimulatory molecules.
[b]Includes combinations of cytokines and costimulatory molecules.
(Summarized from the *Journal of Gene Medicine*, with permission.)

TABLE 60-4. Comparison of Gene Transfer Methods

Profile	Gene Transfer Method						
	Retrovirus[a]	Lentivirus	Adenovirus	Adeno-Associated Virus	Vaccinia	Fowlpox	Nonviral
Efficiency of gene transfer	Moderate	Moderate	High	Moderate	High	High	Low
Stable vs. transient	Stable	Stable	Transient	Stable	Transient	Transient	Transient
Gene expression	Variable[b]	Variable[b]	Variable[b]	Variable[b]	High	High	Variable[b]
Immunogenicity[c]	Low	Low	Moderate	Low	High	High	Low
In vitro toxicity	Low	Low	Low	Low	High	Low	Low
Titer	Low[d]	Low[d]	High	See comments	High	High	NA
Comments	Requires replicating cells	Stable gene transfer to nondividing cells	New vector design should lead to decreased immunogenicity	High-titer preparations difficult to produce; production requires replication-competent adenovirus	Most infected cells die within 24 h; replication competent	—	Easy to produce clinical-grade material; fewer safety issues compared with viral methods

NA, not applicable.
[a]Murine leukemia virus–based vectors.
[b]Gene expression depends on specific promoter and cell type.
[c]Immunogenicity from expression of normal viral proteins.
[d]Can be concentrated to high titer with ultracentrifugation.

viral particles using helper, or packaging, cell lines that contain the structural viral protein genes in *trans* (i.e., from another site in the packaging cell genome). Because the retroviral vector contains the ψ sequences, it is packaged into the mature virus and is capable of infecting target cells but incapable of replication due to the absence of the retroviral protein coding regions. The viral structural genes provided in *trans* are not packaged due to the absence of the ψ sequences.

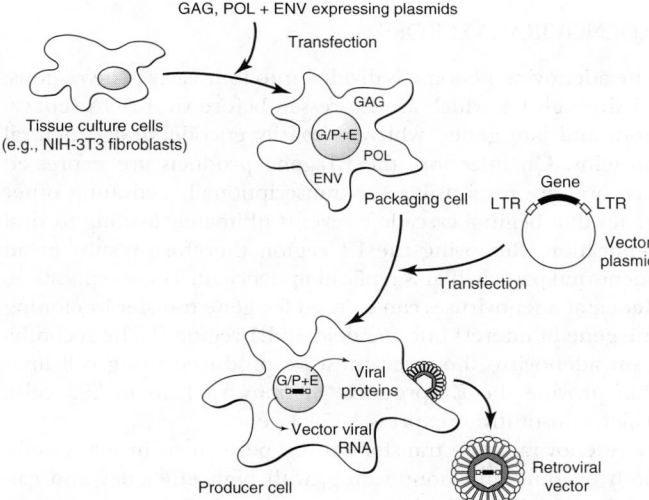

FIGURE 60-1. Production of retroviral vectors with packaging cells. The gene of interest is cloned into a retroviral vector and then transfected into a helper cell line, which provides the retroviral structural genes in *trans*. The retroviral structural genes cannot be packaged due to the absence of a packaging sequence (ψ), whereas the retroviral vector can be packaged, which thereby produces a replication-incompetent retrovirus. LTR, long terminal repeats. (From ref. 194, with permission.)

Use of retroviral vectors is one of the most common methods of gene transfer in currently approved gene therapy protocols. Its advantages include the ability to stably integrate into the host genome and the absence of viral protein expression. Current disadvantages of retroviral vectors include low titers resulting in low levels of gene transfer efficiency, although new methods have been described to concentrate retroviral supernatants using ultracentrifugation.[3]

Retroviral packaging cells can use a variety of envelope genes from other viruses. Because the envelope protein is the primary determinant of the host range of the retrovirus, the particular envelope, or pseudotype, used can have a profound impact on transduction efficiencies.[4] Table 60-5 lists a number of envelope genes along with their relative host ranges. The recent development of packaging cell lines using alternative envelope genes has resulted in significant advances in the ability to transduce primary lymphocytes. Retroviral vectors produced from the PG13 packaging cell line,[5] which uses the gibbon ape leukemia virus envelope (GALV), are capable of transducing B cells[6] and T cells[7] with significantly higher efficiencies than are those derived from amphotropic packaging cell lines. By combining the use of PG13-packaged vectors with a 1-hour centrifugation at 1000 g, Bunnell et al. were able to obtain transduction efficiencies of primary T cells in the 40% range.[8]

TABLE 60-5. Envelopes Used for Retroviral Vectors

Envelope Source	Host Range
Ecotropic	Mouse, rat
Amphotropic	Human, mouse, rat, rabbit, cat, dog, monkey
Gibbon ape leukemia virus	Human, rat, rabbit, cat, dog, monkey (not mouse)
Vesicular stomatitis virus G protein	All

The vesicular stomatitis virus (VSV) G glycoprotein can also be used to pseudotype retroviral vectors.[9] Unlike other envelope proteins, the VSV-G protein confers enhanced physical stability to retroviral particles, which allows concentration with ultracentrifugation to titers of 10^9 or higher. VSV-G pseudotyped retroviral vectors have a wide host range and have been used successfully to transduce primary T cells.[10]

In addition, future retroviral vectors may contain improved promoters for higher and regulatable levels of gene expression.

RISK OF INSERTIONAL MUTAGENESIS FROM RETROVIRAL VECTORS

Because retroviral vectors insert into the genome in a relatively random fashion, gene transfer can potentially activate an oncogene and thereby induce transformation of the target cell. There are a number of potential mechanisms for this activation, including integration of an enhancer element that can enhance transcription of the oncogene, direct transcription of the oncogene from the retroviral promoter, or disruption of a gene-silencing element. Although wild-type replication-competent retroviruses are known to be leukemogenic, due to the ability to insert multiple times into the genome, until recently this was only a theoretical concern for replication-incompetent retroviral vectors.

In a study by Cavazzana-Calvo et al., ten infants with X-linked severe combined immunodeficiency (SCID), characterized by an absence of the common chain (γc), received hematopoietic stem cells gene-modified with a retroviral vector containing γc.[11] Although this was one of the first gene therapy trials to demonstrate efficacy, with recovery of hematopoietic cells in all but one patient, two of the ten patients developed T-cell leukemia 2.5 years after cell infusion. The leukemic cells in both patients demonstrated retroviral insertion around the LMO2 oncogene, which suggests that the leukemia was induced by retroviral insertion. In one patient, the leukemic cells expressed multiple T-cell receptor (TCR) clonotypes, which indicates that a prethymic progenitor cell was transformed. The delay in the development of leukemia after stem cell infusion suggests that other factors besides gene insertion were required for transformation.[12]

It is not clear why leukemia was seen in a significant number of patients in this trial, whereas no leukemia has been reported in more than 250 patients treated with retrovirally transduced hematopoietic stem cells over the past decade. It is possible that the immunodeficient state of the patients with X-linked SCID allowed selective proliferation of the transformed cells. In addition, the transgene, γc, is a common chain in a number of cytokine receptors, including interleukin (IL)-7 and IL-15, which are known to regulate T-cell proliferation. Gene transfer to hematopoietic stem cells is also more efficient in infants than in adults, which may have increased the likelihood of an insertion in a particular oncogene.[13]

Further study is required to determine the risk of leukemogenesis in patients with other diseases receiving retrovirally transduced hematopoietic stem cells containing other transgenes. Improvements in vector design, such as the use of tissue-specific promoters, the incorporation of suicide genes, or the development of vectors with more predictable integration patterns, will increase the safety of this technology. However, leukemia has not been reported in more than 100 other clinical trials using retroviral vectors, and thus this complication remains infrequent.

LENTIVIRAL VECTORS

Stable gene transfer using vectors based on murine retroviruses is possible only in dividing cells. Human immunodeficiency virus (HIV) can infect and integrate into the genome of nonproliferating cells due to the presence of proteins that mediate the active transport of the lentiviral preintegration complex through the nucleopore. These proteins—integrase, matrix, and *vpr*—interact with the nuclear import machinery to transport the HIV preintegration complex from the cytoplasm to nucleus.

Naldini et al. designed lentiviral vectors based on HIV that are capable of stably infecting nondividing cells. A packaging construct was used to express HIV proteins in *trans*. To avoid production of wild-type HIV, the construct is defective for the production of viral envelope and the accessory protein Vpu and has deletions in the 5' signal sequence. To make defective lentiviral vectors, packaging cells are transiently transfected with the packaging construct along with a separate plasmid encoding a heterologous envelope protein, such as VSV-G protein. A third plasmid, the transfer vector, encodes the gene of interest along with the packaging signal and other *cis*-acting sequences of HIV required for packaging, reverse transcription, and integration.[14] Lentiviral vectors are currently being refined to enhance safety, transduction efficiency, and convenience.[15] HIV-based lentiviral vectors have been shown to be efficient vehicles of gene transfer into postmitotic cells, including brain, liver, muscle, CD34+ hematopoietic cells, and retina.[14,16–20] Current efforts are focused on the use of lentiviral vectors in the transduction of hematopoietic stem cells in an attempt to enhance long-term engraftment of gene-modified cells.[17]

ADENOVIRAL VECTORS

The adenoviral genome is divided into four early gene regions, E1 through E4, which are expressed before viral DNA replication, and late genes, which primarily encode viral structural proteins. On infection, the E1 gene products are expressed first and are responsible for transcriptionally activating other genes that begin a cascade of events ultimately leading to viral replication. Removing the E1 region therefore results in an adenoviral particle that is replication deficient. These replication-deficient adenoviruses can be used for gene transfer by cloning the gene of interest into the deleted E1 region.[21] The recombinant adenovirus, however, must be produced using cell lines that provide the E1 products in *trans*, such as in 293 cells, which constitutively express Ad5 E1 genes.

Adenoviral gene transfer can be performed in many cells, both dividing and nondividing, with high efficiency and can result in high levels of gene expression. Cell entry is a multistage process, using the coxsackie and adenovirus receptor (CAR), which is widely expressed on many cell types. This is followed by interactions with avb3 and avb5 integrins on host cells.[22]

Adenoviral vectors can be produced at high titers and are capable of infecting some tissues directly *in vivo*, such as pulmonary epithelial cells.[23] However, because adenoviral DNA exists episomally, with little or no incorporation into the host cell genome, expression of the transgene is transient and is lost as the infected cell divides. For some therapeutic strategies, this high-level, transient expression may be adequate, whereas other treatment approaches may require more prolonged gene expression.

One potential problem with *in vivo* administration of current adenoviral vectors is their ability to trigger a host immune response. Both neutrophilic and lymphocytic inflammatory infiltrates can be seen histologically at sites of injection of adenoviral vectors.[24] In addition, antibody responses to adenoviral vectors have been demonstrated in a variety of animal models, and gene expression with repeated dosing is inversely proportional to the antibody response in some systems.[25] Nude mice expressing adenoviral vectors in the liver exhibit transgene expression for 60 days compared to 21 days in normal mice, which implies that the absence of T cells can lead to longer gene expression. Cytotoxic T-lymphocyte (CTL) responses against adenoviral proteins have also been reported.[26] It has been postulated that late gene products, such as adenoviral hexon and fiber proteins, may be the cause of the T-cell response.

The effect of neutralizing antibodies on current clinical efforts with recombinant adenovirus is not clear. In a clinical trial using recombinant adenoviruses containing tumor antigen genes, high levels of neutralizing antibody were found in the pretreatment sera of patients, which may have impaired the ability of these viruses to immunize patients.[27] However, in another study, intratumoral administration of an adenoviral vector expressing β-galactosidase resulted in β-galactosidase–specific T-helper, CTL, and antibody responses in three of four patients.[28]

Improvements in adenoviral pharmacokinetics are important in the development of this vector as a systemic delivery agent. The half-life of adenovirus in mice is less than 2 minutes. Due to a tropism for the liver, perhaps secondary to high hepatic levels of CAR and α_v integrins, intravenous injections of low titers of adenovirus are sequestered in the liver. Use of higher doses of adenovirus can partially overcome this sequestration, but continued uptake by Kupffer cells in the liver reduces the circulating levels of the virus. This is illustrated in studies in which the hepatic circulation is bypassed by clamping the portal vein and hepatic artery. When the clamp is removed, circulating adenoviral levels fall.[29]

Hepatic tropism and the induction of inflammation may lead to toxicity from adenoviral vectors in predisposed patients. One treatment-related death has been reported, possibly due to a systemic inflammatory response initiated by adenoviral vector infusion. The patient was an 18-year-old male with ornithine transcarbamylase deficiency who received intrahepatic recombinant adenovirus type 5, deleted in E1 and E4, expressing the human ornithine transcarbamylase complementary DNA. This was associated with a systemic inflammatory response with high serum levels of IL-6 and IL-10, disseminated intravascular coagulation, and multiple organ system failure leading to death within 98 hours of the adenovirus infusion.[30] This case highlights the need to further study the immune response against viral vectors.

Much work in vector development remains to be done for adenoviral vectors to be fully used in effective gene therapy strategies.

ADENO-ASSOCIATED VIRUS VECTORS

Adeno-associated virus (AAV), a member of the parvovirus family, can replicate only in the presence of a helper virus, such as an

adenovirus. The virus is nonenveloped and consists of a single-stranded linear DNA of 4.7 kb, which contains two major open reading frames. The left-hand open reading frame encodes the Rep proteins, which are responsible for AAV replication. The right-hand open reading frame encodes the Cap proteins, which form the structural proteins of the viral capsid. In the absence of a helper virus, such as an adenovirus, AAV cannot replicate but instead integrates into the host genome, through the AAV inverted terminal repeats present on each end of the AAV genome. This ability to integrate makes AAV an attractive vehicle for gene transfer.

To provide room for a transgene, the majority of the AAV genome between the inverted terminal repeats can be removed and replaced with a gene of interest driven by an appropriate promoter.[31] Once packaged, the replication-incompetent AAV vector has been shown to be capable of infecting and integrating into a target cell genome.

The use of alternative serotypes of AAV is also under investigation. Currently, the majority of vectors use AAV serotype 2. However, some cells, such as hepatocytes and hematopoietic cells, are difficult to infect with this serotype. In addition, many people have been exposed to wild-type AAV-2 and therefore have circulating, neutralizing antibodies. Consequently, efforts are under way to construct vectors with one of the five other serotypes of AAV or to use capsids from these serotypes ("pseudotyping").[32]

POX VECTORS

The poxviruses are a family of DNA viruses characterized by a large enveloped virion containing enzymes for messenger RNA (mRNA) synthesis, a genome composed of a single linear double-stranded DNA molecule of 130 to 300 kb, and the ability to replicate within the cytoplasm of the infected cell. The poxvirus genome encodes 150 to 200 genes, which can be divided into early and late genes. Early genes are expressed before viral DNA replication, and late genes are expressed after DNA replication.

Several properties of poxviruses make them attractive vectors for the introduction of foreign genes.[33] Because of the large size of the poxvirus genome, large amounts of foreign DNA can be incorporated without adversely effecting viral infectivity. Several silent or nonessential regions of the genome have been identified for the insertion of foreign DNA by homologous recombination. Plasmids that provide viral promoters as well as regions to facilitate homologous recombination into nonessential sites, such as the viral thymidine kinase (TK) region, have been constructed to produce recombinant vaccinia vectors. Multiple genes can be inserted each at a different site in the virus. Screening methods have been designed to isolate and expand recombinant clones containing the genes of interest.

A primary advantage of recombinant poxviruses is the large amount of gene expression that is possible due to the use of vaccinia transcription factors. Because gene expression is entirely cytoplasmic and does not rely on host-cell transcriptional machinery, it is not dependent on potential regulatory mechanisms of the host cell, and hence high levels of gene expression have been observed in a wide variety of cell types.

Disadvantages of poxviruses are the transient nature of gene expression and the cell lysis that results after infection. Some attenuated vaccinia strains[33] have been developed that result in delayed lysis of infected human target cells. Avipox viruses, such as fowlpox or canarypox, or swine poxviruses can infect human cells but do not result in cell lysis.[34] Another problem with recombinant poxviruses is that up to 200 viral gene products are expressed, many of which may be immunogenic or may adversely interact with the target cell or the gene product of interest.

NONVIRAL METHODS OF GENE TRANSFER

Cationic lipids, complexed to DNA, have been developed that are capable of mediating high gene transfer efficiencies *in vitro* for some cell types. Cationic lipids[35] such as DOTMA (1,2-dioleyloxypropyl-3-trimethyl ammonium bromide), the prototype cationic lipid, along with a neutral lipid such as DOPE (dioleoyl-phosphatidyl-etanolamine) can be complexed with DNA and added to cultured cells. New formulations of lipids are currently under development that may allow improved *in vitro* gene transfer as well as *in vivo* administration. Cationic lipid formulations have already been used to deliver genes to the lung *in vivo*[36] as well as intratumorally.[37-39] More recently, DNA-gelatin nanospheres have been used to allow the slow release of DNA *in vivo*. In a murine model, intramuscular injection of nanospheres containing the β-galactosidase marker gene led to higher expression levels than injection with naked DNA or DNA-lipid complexes.[40]

Physical methods of gene transfer include the "gene gun,"[41] which propels gold beads coated with DNA into cells. Although this method results in low transfection efficiencies, gene transfer to epithelial cells can be performed *in vivo*, which gives it a potential role in immunization strategies.

The direct *in vivo* injection of DNA alone into selected tissues, such as muscle[42] and thyroid,[43] can result in gene transfer. This approach, termed *naked DNA*, has been used primarily in studies attempting to immunize against the products of the encoded genes.

Nonviral methods of gene delivery are more convenient and have obvious safety advantages over viral methods. However, the majority of current nonviral gene transfer methods result in transient gene expression, and the efficiency of gene transfer is lower than with most viral methods. To address these issues, several strategies are being studied. Ultrasonography has been demonstrated to enhance cell membrane permeability to DNA. Increased gene expression was seen with application of ultrasound to tissue after DNA injection.[44] Gene delivery may also be enhanced by complexing DNA to peptides or polymers. To obtain prolonged gene expression, stable integration of plasmid DNA by incorporating transposons or integrases is being evaluated.[45]

HYDRODYNAMIC GENE TRANSFER

New techniques are emerging that allow efficient systemic expression of naked DNA constructs in murine models. Wolff's group has demonstrated that high levels of DNA expression in hepatocytes, and to a lesser extent in other organs, can be obtained after the rapid intravenous injection of plasmid DNA in a large volume (10% of body weight). Gene expression was dependent on the speed of injection as well as the injection volume. Expression of specific genes was promoter dependent and could be detected for several days. This technique, termed *hydrodynamic gene transfer*, has proven useful for studies requiring gene expression in the liver.[46] In addition, studies of secreted proteins, in which the liver is used as an ectopic site to produce large amounts of material for continuous systemic delivery, have been performed.[47] This allows the study of novel proteins such as new cytokines without the need to produce large amounts of recombinant material. With dependence on such large volumes, this technique is confined to use in animal models. However, it is conceivable that this technique could be used in patients with delivery of lower volumes via occlusion catheters introduced into the portal vein.

GENE MARKING STUDIES

The first human gene transfer study in 1989 was designed to assess the safety and feasibility of gene transfer in humans, using a marker gene, neomycin phosphotransferase (NeoR), for an enzyme that inactivates neomycin and neomycin analogs.[48]

Subsequent goals of gene marking studies were to understand the biology of cancer and cancer treatments. For example, because a unique, foreign gene was introduced into cells, the fate of these cells could be followed *in vivo*. Adoptively transferred T cells could be followed for their survival *in vivo*, and patients receiving autologous bone marrow transplants transduced with marker genes could be followed to see whether subsequent recurrences were in part due to the presence of viable tumor cells in the transferred bone marrow.

T-CELL MARKING STUDIES

The first gene transfer study in humans was performed in 1989 at the Surgery Branch of the National Cancer Institute.[48] Tumor-infiltrating lymphocytes (TILs) were genetically modified with a marker gene encoding NeoR. The goals of the study were to evaluate the safety and feasibility of using gene-modified cells in humans. In addition, because a unique, foreign gene was placed into the TIL, survival and distribution studies of the infused cells could be done using polymerase chain reaction (PCR) assays on DNA from peripheral blood lymphocytes and tumor biopsy specimens.

Because this was the first study of its kind, issues of safety for the patients and the public were a major concern of regulatory agencies, such as the Recombinant DNA Advisory Committee (RAC). Consequently, many safety studies were required before approval of this and subsequent clinical trials. Ultimately, ten patients were treated, and there were no safety or toxicity problems associated with the gene transfer. Using PCR analysis, TILs were found in tumor biopsy specimens up to 64 days after infusion and in peripheral blood up to 189 days after infusion[48] (Fig. 60-2). Since this initial study, there have been over 300 human gene transfer and therapy studies approved by the RAC, and research in this field throughout the world has tremendously expanded.

T-cell marking studies have been performed using melanoma TILs,[49] renal TILs,[50] bone marrow stem cells,[51] and anti-HIV CTLs.[52] Using gene-marked Epstein-Barr virus (EBV)–specific CTLs in immunocompromised patients, Heslop et al. found that EBV precursors could proliferate in response to *in vivo* or *ex vivo* viral challenge for as long as 18 months[53] (Fig. 60-3).

Researchers at the University of Washington in Seattle have used NeoR-marked, HIV-1 Gag-specific CD8+ CTL clones to treat HIV-infected individuals.[54] When PCR amplification for

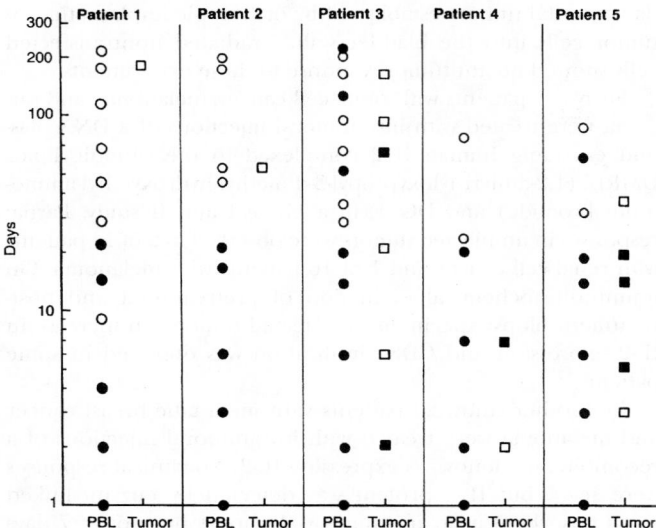

FIGURE 60-2. Results of polymerase chain reaction assays of peripheral blood mononuclear cells (PBL; *circles*) and tumor biopsy specimens (*squares*) obtained from patients at various intervals after the infusion of gene-transduced tumor-infiltrating lymphocytes. Open symbols denote negative results, and solid symbols denote positive results. All results were corroborated in at least two separate Southern blot assays. The assays were performed and assessed in a blinded fashion. (From ref. 48, with permission.)

the neo gene followed by *in situ* hybridization with fluorescein-labeled neo-specific oligonucleotides was used, the percentage of circulating transduced cells could be quantitated by flow cytometry. One day after cell infusion, 2.0% to 3.5% of CD8+ cells circulating in the periphery were neo positive. The frequency of neo-modified CTLs was found to correlate inversely with the percentage of HIV-infected cells in the peripheral blood after cell infusion. In addition, neo-positive CTLs were found to accumulate in lymph node biopsy specimens obtained 4 days after cell infusion (2.2% to 7.9%) when compared to the concurrent percentages of neo-positive CTLs circulating in the periphery (0.5% to 0.7%). Interestingly, neo-positive

CTL aggregates were found in the parafollicular regions of the lymph node near cells that were productively infected with HIV. This illustrates the usefulness of cell marking to determine not only the overall traffic and survival of infused cells but also their microanatomic localization.

HEMATOPOIETIC STEM CELL MARKING STUDIES

The ability to label stem cells with unique, integrated DNA sequences has enabled investigators to track stem cells and their differentiated progeny.[55] This has allowed studies such as the comparison of bone marrow stem cells with peripheral blood stem cells for their ability to reconstitute the host. In addition, because microscopic tumor deposits present within the marrow are marked by retroviral vectors as well, attempts have been made to assess the source of disease recurrence after autologous bone marrow transplantation therapy in patients with acute myeloid leukemia and neuroblastoma. In one study, bone marrow was harvested during complete remission and retrovirally transduced with the Neo[R] gene before reinfusion. Three of 12 acute myeloid leukemia patients experienced relapse, and in 2 of these patients, tumor cells from the relapse contained the Neo[R] gene. Of nine neuroblastoma patients studied, three experienced relapse, and in all three cases, the Neo[R] gene was found in the recurrent tumor cells.[56] Analysis of neuroblastoma DNA for discrete integration sites revealed that at least 200 malignant cells were introduced with the autologous marrow transplant and contributed to the relapse.[57]

In a similar study using Neo[R]-transduced autologous CD34 cells in patients with chronic myelogenous leukemia (CML), two patients experiencing relapse were studied and both had leukemic cells that were positive for the Neo[R] gene.[58] Thus, it is clear that remission marrow can contribute to disease relapse.

Using similar techniques, a variety of bone marrow purging regimens can be evaluated within the same patient to assess their success in eliminating tumor cells from the marrow.[59] This allows recurrent tumor cells to be analyzed genetically to determine if they had previously been exposed to a particular purging regimen.

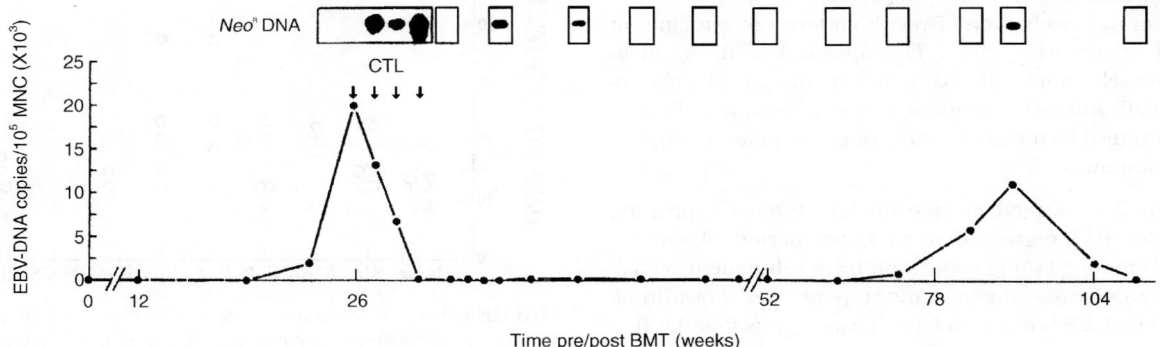

FIGURE 60-3. Recruitment of gene-marked, Epstein-Barr virus (EBV)–specific cytotoxic T lymphocytes (CTL) by antigenic stimulation *in vivo*. DNA was obtained from peripheral blood mononuclear cells (MNC) of a patient between 0 and 108 weeks after bone marrow transplantation (BMT) and divided into two portions. One was analyzed by polymerase chain reaction amplification using EBV-specific primers, whereas the second was amplified using neo-specific primers. The figure shows the relationship between levels of EBV-DNA and the presence of neomycin phosphotransferase (Neo[R])–marked, EBV-specific, gene-positive T cells. (From ref. 53, with permission.)

Finally, gene transfer itself is being investigated as a purging technique, using antisense oligodeoxynucleotides against activated oncogenes as a means to eliminate tumor cells within the autologous marrow.[60]

GENETIC MODIFICATION OF THE IMMUNE RESPONSE

Several approaches have been proposed for cancer gene therapy (see Table 60-1). One strategy that has been pursued is an attempt to enhance the immune response against cancer using gene transfer techniques.

ACTIVE IMMUNIZATION

In the past few years, much has been learned concerning the nature of the T-cell response to human cancers. Tumor antigens recognized by T cells have been cloned from melanoma cells.[61,62] These antigens have been shown to be nonmutated melanocyte differentiation antigens, nonmutated proteins expressed only in selected tissues such as testes, or mutated intracellular proteins. Despite the expression of known antigens on tumor cells, however, these tumors grow in their hosts, seemingly unopposed by any antitumor immune response. This lack of an adequate immune response could be due to a number of factors, including deficient tumor antigen processing and presentation, lack of immune costimulation, production of inhibitory factors by the tumor cell, and insufficient helper activity from CD4 cells. In an attempt to bypass these potential deficiencies and stimulate a stronger antitumor response in the host, tumor cells have been genetically modified with a variety of cytokine genes and costimulatory molecules, and these modified tumor cells have been used as antitumor vaccines.

Modification of Tumor Cells with Genes That Enhance Tumor Immunogenicity

CYTOKINE GENES. In contrast to the systemic administration of cytokines, which results in low concentrations *in vivo*, the introduction of genes encoding cytokines into tumor cells can result in the production of very high levels of cytokines in the tumor microenvironment. This approach is designed to more accurately mimic the paracrine nature by which cytokines normally interact to regulate immune responses. Tumors have been transduced with a variety of genes in an attempt to enhance immunogenicity.

Interleukin-2. In several murine models, tumors expressing the gene for IL-2 regress after an initial period of growth, which leads to long-lasting protection from subsequent rechallenge.[63] In some cases, the immune response was shown to be dependent on CD8 but not on CD4. This suggests that the IL-2 released by the tumor cells was bypassing the need for help from CD4 cells. In many studies, however, it was not clear whether systemic immunity was enhanced to levels greater than that which could be achieved using irradiated, nonmodified tumor cells.

In another study,[64] intraperitoneal, irradiated IL-2–transduced murine bladder cancer cells were capable of treating 7-day parental tumors established by orthotopic implantation of tumor cells into the bladder wall. Irradiated nontransfected cells showed no antitumor response in these experiments.

Forty-five patients with renal cell cancer, melanoma, and sarcoma were treated with intratumoral injections of a DNA plasmid encoding human IL-2 complexed to the cationic lipids DMRIE (1,2-dimyristyloxypropyl-3-dimethyl-hydroxyethyl ammonium bromide) and DOPE in a phase I and II study. Partial responses in uninjected tumors were observed in 2 of 14 patients with renal cell cancer and 1 of 16 patients with melanoma. On immunohistochemical evaluation of pretreatment and posttreatment biopsy specimens of injected tumors, an increase in IL-2 expression and CD8+ infiltration was observed in some patients.[37]

In another study, 23 patients with metastatic breast cancer and melanoma were treated with intratumoral injections of a recombinant adenovirus expressing IL-2. No clinical responses were seen, but IL-2 protein was detected by enzyme-linked immunosorbent assay in tumor at 48 hours but not at 7 days after injection. This demonstrated that some transgene expression could be detected despite the presence of preexisting neutralizing antibodies against adenovirus.[65] Other trials have used autologous tumor or fibroblasts, or both, expressing IL-2 in melanoma[66] and colorectal cancer patients,[67] but no clinical responses have been reported.

Granulocyte-Macrophage Colony-Stimulating Factor. Granulocyte-macrophage colony-stimulating factor (GM-CSF) is a cytokine with the unique ability to stimulate the differentiation of hematopoietic progenitor cells into dendritic cells, potent antigen-presenting cells. This property may allow increased presentation of tumor antigens on dendritic cells after immunization with tumors that express GM-CSF. In a comparative study,[68] mice were immunized with irradiated B16 melanoma cells that were transduced with either IL-2, IL-4, IL-5, IL-6, GM-CSF, interferon-γ (IFN-γ), tumor necrosis factor-α (TNF-α), intracellular adhesion molecule-1 (ICAM-1), or CD2. Only mice immunized with GM-CSF–transduced tumor cells were significantly protected against a subsequent tumor challenge (Fig. 60-4). IL-4– and IL-6–trans-

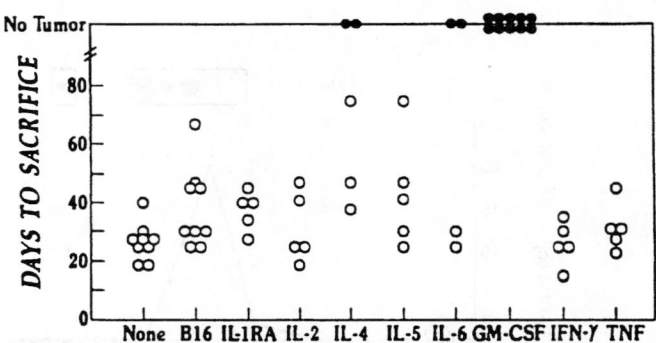

FIGURE 60-4. Comparative analysis of vaccine efficacies of a poorly immunogenic murine tumor transduced with different cytokine genes. Syngeneic C57BL/6 mice were vaccinated subcutaneously with 5×10^5 irradiated (3500 rad) B16 melanoma cells transduced with eight different cytokine genes using the MFG retroviral vector. Animals were challenged 14 days later with 1×10^6 live nontransduced B16 cells subcutaneously. Open circles, animal succumbed to tumor challenge; filled circles, animal protected from tumor challenge; GM-CSF, granulocyte-macrophage colony-stimulating factor; IFN-γ, interferon-γ; IL, interleukin; TNF, tumor necrosis factor. (From ref. 68, with permission.)

duced tumor cells were minimally protective, but none of the other transduction agents produced a significant systemic antitumor response. GM-CSF–transduced B16 melanoma cells were also capable of significantly impacting 3-day subcutaneous implants of a small inoculum of nontransduced B16 cells.[68] Immunization with GM-CSF–transduced tumor generated long-lasting systemic antitumor immunity that was dependent on both CD4+ and CD8+ T cells. Further studies have demonstrated that GM-CSF–transduced tumor vaccines activate bone marrow–derived antigen-presenting cells to process and present tumor antigens to both CD4+ and CD8+ T cells.[69] Activated, tumor-specific CD4+ T cells were in turn shown to express both Th1 and Th2 cytokines that recruited other effector cells to the tumor, including eosinophils and macrophages. In addition, antitumor activity of GM-CSF–transduced vaccines were found to depend on the production of IFN-γ, IL-4, and IL-5.[70]

Three clinical studies have been reported using GM-CSF–transduced tumors in renal cell cancer,[71] melanoma,[72] and prostate cancer.[73] In a phase I, randomized, double-blind dose-escalation study, patients with metastatic renal cell cancer were immunized with intradermal and subcutaneous injections of either nontransduced or GM-CSF–transduced autologous, irradiated renal cancer cells. Biopsy specimens from patients receiving GM-CSF–transduced vaccines demonstrated infiltrates of macrophages, dendritic cells, eosinophils, neutrophils, and T cells consistent with preclinical studies. Delayed-type hypersensitivity responses using nontransduced autologous tumor cells revealed eosinophil infiltrates in only those patients who previously received GM-CSF–transduced vaccines. One partial response was seen in nine patients treated with GM-CSF–transduced vaccines.[71]

In a phase I trial for patients with metastatic melanoma, 21 patients were immunized intradermally and subcutaneously with autologous melanoma cells transduced to express GM-CSF. Again, immunization sites were found to be infiltrated with T lymphocytes, dendritic cells, macrophages, and eosinophils in all 21 patients. Although only 1 of 21 patients had an objective partial response, 11 of 16 patients evaluated had T-lymphocyte and plasma cell infiltrates in tumor biopsy specimens after immunization.[72] In a phase I trial evaluating GM-CSF–transduced prostate cancer vaccination, delayed-type hypersensitivity reactions against nontransduced autologous tumor cells were positive in two of eight patients before vaccination and in seven of eight patients after vaccination. However, no clinical responses were reported.[73]

Interferon-γ. The introduction of the IFN-γ gene into tumor cells can lead to the up-regulation of major histocompatibility complex (MHC) class I and class II gene products.[74] Although this can lead to decreased tumorigenicity,[75] it is unclear whether systemic immunity is enhanced. However, in some tumor systems with low class I expression or antigen-processing defects, IFN-γ–transduced tumor allowed the isolation of CD8+ lymphocytes capable of treating established pulmonary metastases from the parental, nontransduced tumor.[76] Thus, for some cancers, immunization with IFN-γ–transduced tumor cells may allow the isolation of T cells capable of impacting established, systemic disease.

Other Cytokine Genes. The introduction into tumor cells of a variety of other cytokine genes, such as TNF,[77] IL-1,[78] IL-4,[79] IL-6,[80] IL-7,[81] IL-13,[82] granulocyte colony-stimulating factor,[83] monocyte chemoattractant protein,[84] and RANTES (regulated upon activation, normal T cell expressed and secreted),[85] can

lead to decreased tumorigenicity. There is no evidence, however, that these manipulations can increase systemic immunity above that which can be elicited from irradiated tumor cells.

Tahara et al. introduced the IL-12 gene into murine MCA207 tumor cells (MCA207-IL-12), which resulted in decreased tumorigenicity. In addition, mice were injected with 3×10^5 MCA207 cells in the left flank on day 0, followed by treatment on day 3 with saline, MCA207-Neo^R, or MCA207-IL-12. Thirty-three percent of mice were free of tumor by day 21 when treated with MCA207-IL-12 tumor, compared to no animals free of tumor when treated with saline or MCA207-Neo^R tumor.[86] However, it is not clear whether these effects were due to the paracrine secretion of IL-12 or to a systemic effect of secreted IL-12.

Although the transduction of tumor cells with a variety of cytokine genes can result in decreased tumorigenicity in murine models, few studies have demonstrated that this leads to an enhanced immune response against the parental, nontransduced tumor compared to immunization with irradiated, nontransduced tumor cells. In one study, Hock et al. demonstrated that tumor cells modified with different cytokine genes (IL-2, IL-4, IL-7, TNF, or IFN-γ) were only slightly superior to irradiated parental cells as immunogens. Moreover, parental cells admixed with the classical adjuvant *Corynebacterium parvum* were found to be superior to the cytokine-modified tumors in their ability to immunize mice against the tumor.[87]

NONCYTOKINE GENES

B7-1 (CD80). The activation of T lymphocytes requires that they come in contact with a specific antigen and a costimulatory signal. One potential reason that some cancers develop and evade the immune system is that T lymphocytes are not adequately costimulated to become activated. The adhesion molecules B7-1 (CD80) and B7-2 (CD86) can bind to the CD28 receptor on T cells to provide costimulation.[88] Several groups have demonstrated that tumor cells transfected with B7-1 locally regress and lead to protection against subsequent tumor challenge with the parental tumor.[89,90] In one study,[91] regression of B7-transduced tumors was dependent on the intrinsic immunogenicity of the parental tumor. Further studies are needed to assess the potency of B7 in the ability to stimulate an antitumor response.

HLA-B7. Several clinical trials have been performed using intratumoral injection with plasmid DNA encoding HLA-B7 in HLA-B7–negative patients in the hopes of generating a stronger immune response against unmodified tumor cells, based on murine models.[92] Intratumoral injection of HLA-B7 plasmid DNA in a cationic lipid vector resulted in RNA or protein expression at the injection site in some patients,[39] but no tumor regression was seen in noninjected sites.

Immunization with Genes Encoding Tumor Antigens

RECOMBINANT VACCINES. Whole tumor cells have been used as immunogens because the specific antigens recognized by T cells have been largely unknown. However, the cloning of several melanoma antigens recognized by T cells[61,93] has opened new possibilities for active immunization strategies for cancer. Studies in murine models have demonstrated that antigens expressed at high levels in recombinant adenoviral, fowlpox, and vaccinia vector systems can induce a significant antitumor immune response against tumors bearing the same antigen.[94,95] Recombinant viral vaccines can result in the *in vivo* production of high quantities of heterologous proteins. However, expression of native viral proteins by these vectors can also result in a host immune response against the vector itself, which thereby diminishes the effectiveness of repeated immunizations.

Immunization studies with naked DNA given intramuscularly or DNA administered on gold beads using the gene gun technique have resulted in significant antitumor effects. Because these methods do not use viral vectors, no irrelevant viral proteins are expressed, which thus allows repeated immunizations.

Current efforts are focused on enhancing immune responses through adjuvant exogenous cytokine administration or introduction of genes encoding cytokines or costimulatory molecules into the recombinant vectors.

DENDRITIC CELLS. Another strategy to actively immunize a patient against cancer is to use potent antigen-presenting cells, such as dendritic cells. These cells are capable of stimulating immune responses from quiescent lymphocytes. Dendritic cells pulsed with tumor peptide or protein antigens have been shown to have significant antitumor effects in murine models[96] and were reported to be effective in one study of patients with lymphomas. Nestle and colleagues treated 16 patients with metastatic melanoma with intranodal injections of dendritic cells pulsed with tumor lysates or peptides derived from known tumor antigens. Eleven of 16 patients demonstrated a positive delayed-type hypersensitivity reaction to peptide-pulsed dendritic cells, and clinical responses were observed in 5 patients.[97]

Although antitumor responses can be obtained in murine models by administering dendritic cells pulsed with peptide antigens or whole proteins, this approach limits immune responses to specific defined MHC-binding epitopes within a given antigen or requires the production of recombinant proteins. For many tumor antigens, though, multiple epitopes have been described that bind to a variety of MHC molecules. One strategy that may enable the presentation of multiple, even undefined epitopes within a given tumor antigen is the introduction of an antigen gene into the dendritic cell. This may allow multiple epitopes to be presented in the context of both class I and class II molecules as well as the constitutive expression of these antigens in transduced dendritic cells. Several strategies have been proposed to genetically modify dendritic cells with tumor antigens. One is to transduce bone marrow cells and differentiate the cells *in vitro* into dendritic cells, using GM-CSF.[98,99] Another is the transient transfection of dendritic cells using cationic lipids,[100] gene gun, adenovirus,[101] or recombinant influenza virus.[102]

GENETIC MODIFICATION OF IMMUNE EFFECTOR CELLS

There are several lines of evidence indicating that adoptively transferred T cells can be therapeutically effective. TILs have been shown to mediate significant responses in patients with melanoma, even in those for whom previous therapy with IL-2 has failed.[103] Adoptively transferred cytomegalovirus (CMV)-specific T cells have been shown to prevent CMV infections in patients after allogeneic bone marrow transplantation.[104] Infusion of donor T cells has been effective in treating the EBV-driven lymphoproliferative disease that sometimes complicates

allogeneic bone marrow transplantation.[56] Patients with CML recurrence after allogeneic bone marrow transplantation can experience remission after transfer of donor T cells.[105] Several strategies for the genetic modification of transferred T cells attempt to increase their effectiveness.

Enhancing Survival of Immune Cells

For T cells to be functional against a tumor, they must survive *in vivo*, recognize the target, and then execute an adequate antitumor effector mechanism, either by direct cell lysis or by release of cytokines that may attract and stimulate other immune cells. There are several ways to potentially enhance these steps. T cells grow in response to stimulation by various cytokines, such as IL-2. On adoptive transfer of TILs in murine models, the administration of systemic IL-2 potentiates the antitumor effect, presumably by maintaining growth and viability of the administered TILs.[106] By inserting the gene for IL-2, TILs may become able to stimulate themselves in an autocrine fashion, as demonstrated by Yamada et al. and Karasuyama et al. in CTLL and murine HT-2 T cells, respectively.[107,108] Treisman et al. demonstrated that a T-cell clone transduced with the IL-2 gene could grow in an IL-2–independent fashion while maintaining antigen specificity.[109] Liu and Rosenberg demonstrated that IL-2 transduction of primary T cells recognizing melanoma tumor antigens resulted in proliferation after antigen stimulation in the absence of exogenous cytokines.[110] This approach is currently being evaluated in a clinical trial for patients with advanced melanoma.

Increasing Tumor Recognition by Using Novel Receptor Genes

CHIMERIC ANTIBODY/T-CELL RECEPTOR GENES. Although adoptive immunotherapeutic strategies have been developed for some cancers, tumor-reactive T cells are difficult to isolate and expand from most types of cancer. A variety of monoclonal antibodies have been developed that bind to specific cancers, although cancer therapy with antibodies has been largely disappointing, partially due to the lack of an adequate effector mechanism to destroy tumor cells on binding. By combining the antigen-recognition domains from antibodies with the intracellular signaling chains of T cells, chimeric receptors can be generated that activate T cells based on antibody-like recognition. This approach, which uses the antigen-binding capabilities of antibodies with the potent antitumor activity of T cells, would allow the production of specific T cells against any antigen for which a monoclonal antibody exists. This strategy could widely generalize the use of adoptive immunotherapy for cancer and infectious diseases.

The successful combination of antibody variable regions with T-cell signaling chains has been established for several model antigens, such as phosphorylcholine, digoxin, and trinitrophenyl.[111–113] These initial approaches, however, required the use of two genes, because the antibody variable region is encoded by a combination of light and heavy chains. This two-gene strategy, however, is impractical to apply in clinical trials using primary T cells. Therefore, chimeric receptors encoded on a single gene[114] were designed by using single-chain antibody variable (scFv) regions in which the light- and heavy-chain variable regions are connected by a flexible linker.[115,116]

TABLE 60-6. Effect of Ganciclovir Treatment on Elimination of Herpes Thymidine Kinase–Modified Donor Lymphocytes and on Graft-Versus-Host Disease (GVHD)

Patient	GVHD (Grade)	Preganciclovir	24 H after Ganciclovir	Clinical Outcome of GVHD
		Proportion of Transduced PBL (%)		
1	Acute skin (II/III)	13.4	$<10^{-4}$	CR
2	Acute liver (III)	2.0	$<10^{-4}$	CR
8	Chronic lung, skin, gastrointestinal tract	11.9	2.8	PR

CR, complete remission of GVHD; PBL, peripheral blood lymphocytes; PR, partial remission of GVHD. (Adapted from ref. 124.)

These scFv fragments were joined to TCR ζ or Fc receptor γ chains, both of which are closely related and have been demonstrated to be capable of mediating TCR signal transduction.[117]

Besides triggering direct T-cell activation with γ and ζ chains, antibody variable regions can be coupled to other signaling chains, such as the intracellular portion of CD28, an important T-cell costimulatory receptor. This approach has been found to enhance T-cell survival and proliferation *in vitro*.[118]

These strategies have the potential of widely generalizing the use of adoptive immunotherapy. Investigators have constructed scFv-γ and scFv-ζ receptors against ovarian cancer using an anti-α folate receptor monoclonal antibody,[114] against breast cancer using an anti-HER2 monoclonal antibody,[119] against colon cancer using an anti-GA733 monoclonal antibody,[120] and against HIV using an anti-gp41 monoclonal antibody.[121] This strategy could be applied to a wide range of cancer histologic types or infectious diseases for which appropriate monoclonal antibodies exist.

NATIVE T-CELL RECEPTOR GENES. T-cell specificity can also be altered by the introduction of genes encoding native TCRs. The TCR consists of an α- and β-chain heterodimer that confers the ability to specifically recognize peptide–MHC complexes on antigen-presenting cells and target cells. TCRs derived from melanoma-specific CTLs have now been identified, cloned, and characterized.[122] Clay et al.[123] transduced primary lymphocytes with a TCR gene specific for the MART-1 melanoma tumor rejection antigen. Because the TCR consists of two individual chains, a retroviral vector was constructed that used internal ribosomal entry sites (IRES sequences) that allow the translation of multiple genes from a single transcript. Primary T cells transduced with this construct were capable of specifically recognizing tumor cells expressing the MART-1 melanoma tumor antigen in the context of HLA-A2. As more TCRs recognizing specific tumor antigens are characterized and cloned, this strategy may generalize the use of adoptive immunotherapy and circumvent the need to isolate T cells with specific reactivities from each individual patient.

Transducing T Cells and Donor Lymphocytes with Suicide Genes

Adoptively transferred T cells have been safely administered to many patients over the last 10 years. However, in specific situations, the adoptively transferred cells may be toxic to the host, such as in the treatment of immunocompromised HIV patients. In the setting of allogeneic bone marrow transplantation for hematologic malignancies, donor lymphocyte infusions can be highly effective against tumor as well as EBV-induced lymphoma but may also incite graft-versus-host disease. In an attempt to increase the therapeutic index of adoptively transferred cells in these situations, "suicide" genes can be introduced into lymphocytes to specifically delete the transduced cells should they become toxic to patients *in vivo*. The gene for herpes TK (hTK) has been used for this purpose, because it specifically sensitizes cells to the antiviral agent ganciclovir.

In one study using hTK-transduced donor lymphocytes, three of eight patients receiving donor lymphocytes after allogeneic bone marrow transplantation for hematologic malignancies developed acute or chronic graft-versus-host disease. In these patients, ganciclovir administration significantly diminished the number of circulating hTK-transduced cells within 24 hours, which resulted in complete or partial remission of the graft-versus-host disease[124] (Table 60-6).

In another study, anti-HIV CTLs were transduced with a fusion gene encoding hTK and the selectable marker hygromycin before administration into HIV-infected patients.[125] Because HIV patients are immunocompromised, the CTLs could be irradiated with ganciclovir should the transduced cells become toxic. However, initial results of the trial revealed that the patients were developing cellular immune responses against the hTK-hygromycin fusion protein, which thus demonstrates that foreign genes, including selectable markers, can themselves become targets of the host immune response.

Increasing Antitumor Efficacy of Immune Cells

TNF has potent antitumor activity against large tumor burdens in some murine models.[126] However, humans can only tolerate 2% of the systemic TNF dose (by weight) required in mice, due to dose-limiting hypotension.[127] High doses of TNF, administered locally via direct tumor injection[128,129] or isolated limb perfusion,[130] can result in dramatic tumor regressions in some cancer patients. At the National Cancer Institute Surgery Branch, regressions of liver metastases have been seen in patients treated with TNF administered as a component of an isolated hepatic perfusion.[131] Therefore, tumor regressions seem possible in patients when adequate local concentrations of TNF can be achieved. Because TILs have been demonstrated to accumulate at sites of tumor,[132–134] the transduction of TILs with the TNF gene may allow high concentrations of TNF to be delivered locally in the absence of systemic toxicity.[135]

Twelve patients were treated with TNF-transduced TILs in a phase I trial using escalating doses of TILs and IL-2. No safety problems or toxicity have been detected. However, primary lymphocytes transduced with the TNF gene probably do not produce high enough levels of TNF, and migration to tumor may not be sufficient for this approach to be clinically effective.

In an alternative strategy, studies have been performed using mesenchymal stem cells as a vehicle to traffic to tumors *in vivo*.[136] Finally, another approach to increase TNF delivery to tumors that has been attempted has involved the use of an adenoviral vector expressing TNF under control of the radiation-inducible Egr-1 promoter. After intratumoral injection of this recombinant adenovirus and concomitant radiation treatment, 21 of 30 patients demonstrated an objective tumor response. In four of five patients with synchronous lesions, enhanced responses were seen in patients receiving adenovirus plus radiation therapy compared to those receiving radiation therapy alone. However, the actual amount of gene transfer was not assessed, and it is not clear whether the radiation therapy upregulated promoter activity. In addition, this approach is confined to tumors amenable to local therapy and would not be applicable to patients with systemic disease.[137]

MODIFICATION OF TUMORS WITH GENES THAT HAVE DIRECT ANTITUMOR EFFECTS

The gene therapies that have been discussed thus far have all focused on the stimulation of the immune system to react against tumor cells. Another approach to cancer gene therapy is to introduce into tumor cells genes that have direct antiproliferative or toxic effects on that cell. This approach, however, requires techniques to directly administer genes into tumor cells *in vivo* with high efficiencies. Currently, this is not technically possible. However, as vector development continues, the direct administration of genes into patients may play a more important role. Some preliminary studies have been initiated that use direct *in vivo* administration of genes into tumor cells.

TUMOR SUPPRESSOR GENES

Cancer can result from the abnormal expression of genes that control the cell cycle. Some genes, termed *tumor suppressor genes*, regulate cell growth, and their absence by mutation or deletion results in the malignant phenotype. One approach to treat tumors with deleted or mutated tumor suppressor genes is to replace these genes by *in vivo* gene transfer. Currently, gene transfer techniques do not exist that are capable of efficiently delivering these genes systemically to all tumor cells in the body, and significant technical improvements are required if this is to become a practical approach.

Because of this limitation in systemic delivery, several groups have attempted local gene delivery of tumor suppressor genes.[138] Swisher and colleagues treated 28 patients with non–small cell lung cancer with intratumoral administration of an adenovirus vector containing wild-type p53 complementary DNA. Reverse transcriptase–PCR analysis of posttreatment biopsy specimens were positive for the presence of vector-specific p53 mRNA in 12 of 26 patients. Partial response of the injected lesion was observed in 2 of 25 evaluable patients (8%).[139] Because local therapy is of limited usefulness in the face of metastatic

disease, these studies highlight the need for improved vectors that would allow efficient, systemic gene delivery.

ANTISENSE AND RIBOZYMES

Oncogenes are genes that cause uncontrolled cell growth when mutated or overexpressed, and neutralization of these genes can reverse the malignant phenotype. One approach to inactivate genes uses antisense oligodeoxynucleotides,[140] which are short sequences that are complementary to target RNA transcripts and can induce mRNA degradation through endogenous cellular nucleases, such as RNase H. Antisense oligonucleotides can also inhibit gene expression by modulating splicing or inhibiting translation of the RNA into protein. Numerous modifications can be made to the oligonucleotides to increase their resistance to nucleases and to enhance their potency and pharmacokinetics. The most common modification is to substitute one of the nonbridging oxygen atoms with sulfur to produce phosphorothioate oligodeoxynucleotides. A number of other modifications are being evaluated to improve oligonucleotide function *in vivo*.

Oligonucleotides have been shown to enter cells by at least two pathways—endocytosis and pinocytosis—and significant activity of antisense constructs has been observed *in vitro* using tissue culture cell lines. *In vitro* growth suppression has been demonstrated using antisense oligonucleotides against Bcl-2[141] in leukemia cells, BCR-ABL[142] in CML cells, MYC[143] in lymphoma cell lines, and MYB[144,145] in adenocarcinoma and leukemia cell lines.

Several studies have been performed in mice demonstrating *in vivo* efficacy of antisense oligonucleotides against tumors. Antisense inhibition of c-myb mRNA increased survival of SCID mice bearing human K562 leukemia cells.[146] In another study, antisense against the p65 subunit of nuclear factor κB inhibited the growth of the murine fibrosarcoma K-BALB and the murine melanoma B16.[147]

One antisense oligonucleotide, a 21-nucleotide sequence complementary to the immediate early region 2 of CMV mRNA, has been approved by the U.S. Food and Drug Administration for local administration to treat CMV retinitis. A number of other agents are being studied in clinical trials. Webb and colleagues treated nine patients with non-Hodgkin's lymphoma with daily subcutaneous Bcl-2 antisense oligonucleotide for 2 weeks. Bcl-2 overexpression can promote tumorigenesis by causing resistance to programmed cell death (apoptosis). A complete response was observed in one of nine patients with resolution of left axillary lymphadenopathy.[148] For patients with advanced melanoma, a randomized phase III multicenter trial has been conducted using dacarbazine alone compared with dacarbazine plus a phosphorothioate antisense molecule that targets the first six codons of the open reading frame of Bcl-2 mRNA. Analysis of data for all patients on an intent-to-treat basis (n = 771) revealed a median survival of 9.1 months for patients treated with the combination compared to 7.9 months for patients treated with dacarbazine alone (P = .18). Analysis of results for patients who had at least 12 months of follow-up (n = 480) demonstrated a median survival of 10.1 months for those receiving the combination compared to 8.1 months for those receiving dacarbazine alone (P = .035).[149] Further follow-up and repeat trials are required to fully evaluate use of this agent in treatment of patients with melanoma. A number of other

TABLE 60-7. Antisense Oligonucleotides Currently in Clinical Trials for Cancer Treatment

Oligonucleotide	Molecular Target	Disease Indication	Chemistry	Status	Sponsor
LY900003 (Affinitak, ISIS 3521)	Protein kinase C-α	Cancer	Phosphorothioate oligodeoxynucleotide	Phase III/II	Lilly/ISIS Pharmaceuticals
Oblimersen (Genasense, G3139)	Bcl-2	Cancer	Phosphorothioate oligodeoxynucleotide	Phase III/II	Aventis Pharmaceuticals/Genta
ISIS 2503	Ha-*ras*	Cancer	Phosphorothioate oligodeoxynucleotide	Phase II	ISIS Pharmaceuticals
GTI-2040	Ribonucleotide reductase, R1 subunit	Cancer	Phosphorothioate oligodeoxynucleotide	Phase II	Lorus Therapeutics
GT1-2501	Ribonucleotide reductase, R2 subunit	Cancer	Phosphorothioate oligodeoxynucleotide	Phase II	Lorus Therapeutics
LErafAON	c-raf kinase	Cancer—radiosensitization	Liposome formulation of phosphorothioate oligodeoxynucleotide	Phase I/II	NeoPharm
AP12009	TGF-β2	Malignant glioma	Phosphorothioate oligodeoxynucleotide	Phase I/II	Antisense Pharma
Gem-231	Protein kinase A	Cancer	Phosphorothioate 2'-*O*-methyl/oligodeoxynucleotide chimera	Phase II	Hybridon
MG98	DNA methyltransferase	Cancer	Phosphorothioate 2'-*O*-methyl/oligodeoxynucleotide chimera	Phase II	MethyGene/MGI Pharma/British Biotech
OGX-011 (ISIS 112989)	Clusterin	Cancer	Phosphorothioate 2'-*O*-methoxyethyl/oligodeoxynucleotide chimera	Phase I/II	Oncogenix/ISIS Pharmaceuticals
Oncomyc-NG	c-myc	Cancer	Morpholino	Phase I/II	AVI BioPharma
Angiozyme	VEGF	Cancer	Ribozyme	Phase I/II	Sirna Therapeutics

TGF-β2, transforming growth factor-β2; VEGF, vascular endothelial growth factor.
(From ref. 150), with permission.)

clinical trials of cancer treatment using antisense oligonucleotides are currently under way (Table 60-7). A number of genes are being targeted in these trials, including protein kinase C-α, Ha-ras, vascular endothelial growth factor (VEGF), c-myc, c-raf kinase, and transforming growth factor-β2.[150]

A current limitation to this approach is the inability to successfully deliver antisense constructs to tumor cells *in vivo* with adequate efficiency. In addition, studies of antisense oligonucleotides must be interpreted carefully, due to the possibility of nonspecific effects. For example, because charged oligonucleotides are polyanions, they can bind nonspecifically to growth factors, such as basic fibroblast growth factor.[151]

Another potential method to target activated oncogenes is through the use of ribozymes. These are RNA enzymes that catalyze endoribonucleolytic cleavage of RNA.[152] Several investigators have reported cleavage of the bcr-abl transcript, involved in the pathogenesis of CML, by specific hammerhead ribozymes. Anti-fos and anti-ras ribozymes have also been reported.[152] Currently, a clinical trial is under way to evaluate a ribozyme against vascular endothelial growth factor receptor-1 (VEGFR-1, also known as Flt-1) in patients with advanced malignancies. As with other tumor-targeting gene therapy approaches, a major challenge remains to efficiently deliver ribozymes to target cells *in vivo*.

SUICIDE GENES

Because retroviral vectors integrate preferentially into dividing cells, replicating tumor cells might be targeted with relative specificity compared to normal tissues. To test this hypothesis, Culver et al.[153] implanted cell lines producing recombinant retrovirus containing the hTK gene into brain tumors in rats and then delivered systemic ganciclovir therapy. Ganciclovir is a nucleotide analog that is converted into a cytotoxic molecule by hTK but is a poor substrate for mammalian TK. When this method was used, tumors regressed, and significant toxicity to surrounding normal tissues was not observed. Because the hTK gene can only be delivered locally *in vivo*, this treatment approach is limited to those cancers whose primary morbidity is due to local, unresectable disease. Over 30 clinical trials using suicide gene therapy have been approved by the RAC and include studies involving patients with brain tumors, mesothelioma, prostate cancer, head and neck cancer, ovarian cancer, and colorectal cancer. These trials use retroviral and adenoviral gene transfer techniques to deliver the herpes simplex virus TK (HSV-TK) or cytosine deaminase suicide genes, followed by systemic therapy with ganciclovir (for HSV-TK) or 5-fluorocytosine (for cytosine deaminase).

A major limitation in the current application of *in vivo* gene therapy approaches for cancer, such as suicide gene strategies, is the absence of an adequate delivery system that can transfer the suicide gene to all cancer cells within a patient's body. Despite a potential "bystander effect" that may mediate the destruction of tumor cells surrounding those expressing the suicide gene, current gene transfer technology is too inefficient to allow the application of this strategy for the treatment of disseminated metastatic cancer. A second limitation to the use of suicide genes is that of specificity. For any cancer therapy to be effective, there must be greater toxicity for the tumor cells than for normal tissues. Retroviral vectors may theoretically be more selective for tumor cells than for normal tissues because retroviruses only infect proliferating cells. However, retroviruses are suboptimal for *in vivo* administration because of their low efficiency of transduction. Adenoviral vectors, on the other hand, show no selectivity for tumor cells, although a number of groups are attempting to modify surface receptors to engineer specificity.

Enhanced tumor specificity might also be accomplished by using tumor-specific promoter and enhancer regions to direct transcription of the suicide genes. For example, the α-fetoprotein promoter is primarily active in hepatoma cells,[154] whereas the tyrosinase promoter is specifically active in melanocytes and melanoma cells.[155] This approach has also been suggested to target tumor vasculature, using promoters that are relatively specific for endothelial cells, such as the E-selectin, vascular cell adhesion molecule, and CD31 promoters.[156] The use of tumor- or tumor-vasculature–specific promoters might decrease destruction of normal cells, because the latter would not express the suicide gene product. Yet, for these approaches, the fundamental problem of inadequate gene delivery still remains.

SELECTIVE REPLICATION OF VIRUS IN TUMORS

In vivo gene delivery to tumors using replication-defective viral systems is presently inadequate to obtain sufficient transduction efficiency. The design of a virus that could specifically replicate in and destroy tumor cells would be of obvious value. Some efforts[157] have used E1B-defective adenoviruses capable of specifically replicating and destroying tumor cells that lack p53 tumor suppressor function. The p53 protein is a transcription factor that acts as a potent tumor suppressor by its ability to induce cell-cycle arrest and apoptosis. Functional p53 is present in normal cells but absent in over 50% of the common solid tumors. Normally, on viral infection, p53 triggers early apoptosis of the cell and thereby limits viral replication and spread. However, many viruses have evolved proteins, such as the adenoviral E1B 55-kD protein, that inhibit normal p53 function and thus allow maximal viral replication. E1B-defective adenoviruses, therefore, cannot fully replicate in normal tissues expressing p53 but can replicate in tumor cells that lack functional p53.

Bischoff et al. found that an E1B-deleted adenovirus (ONYX-015) could lyse p53-deficient human tumor cells but not cells with functional p53.[157] Intratumoral injection of ONYX-015 caused regression of human cervical carcinomas grown in nude mice. Heise and colleagues reported augmentation of antitumor effects of ONYX-015 by chemotherapy,[158] as well as the efficacy of intravenously administered ONYX-015 in nude mice with subcutaneous human tumor xenografts.[159] Clinical trials are ongoing to test this approach in patients with head and neck cancer. Systemic delivery of ONYX-015 by the intravenous route has been studied in patients with metastatic lung cancer and delivery of ONYX-015 by hepatic artery infusion has been studied in patients with metastatic colorectal cancer.[160,161] Side effects included fevers, rigors, and a dose-dependent transient transaminitis. No clinical responses were seen. For systemic delivery to be effective, hepatic uptake must be addressed. In murine models, 80% of ONYX-015 is taken up by the liver after intravenous injection.

Studies have questioned whether the tumor specificity of ONYX-015 is strictly related to p53 expression by the tumor cells. Rothmann et al. found that replication of ONYX-015 was independent of p53 status in tumor cells[162] and Hall and colleagues reported that productive adenovirus infection was dependent on the p53 pathway.[163] Therefore, much needs to be determined regarding the host range and mechanism of action of ONYX-015.

A related approach, oncolytic virotherapy, uses viruses that propagate more efficiently in tumors than in normal cells. Examples include attenuated strains of a number of RNA viruses, such as the mumps virus, Newcastle disease virus, measles virus, VSV, human reovirus, poliovirus, and influenza virus. A variety of mechanisms may explain the specificity for some viral strains for tumor. For example, double-stranded RNA from RNA viruses induces protein kinase R, a protein kinase that limits viral spread through induction of apoptosis. Tumors are often defective in the protein kinase R pathway and therefore are more permissive for replication of RNA viruses. In addition, specificity may be secondary to specific receptor usage or specific activity of a viral IRES. In addition, genetic engineering of RNA viruses to redirect viral entry to receptors highly expressed on tumor cells or to introduce genes to enhance tumor killing, such as suicide genes, may enhance the specificity of this approach.[164] Development of the next generation of tumor-specific "smart viruses" must address enhanced specificity and systemic delivery as well as methods to prevent humoral and cellular host immune responses against the virus.

INTRODUCTION OF GENES INTO NORMAL TISSUES TO PROTECT THEM FROM CHEMOTHERAPY OR RADIOTHERAPY

MULTIDRUG RESISTANCE GENE THERAPY

Expression of the MDR gene decreases the toxicity from certain chemotherapy drugs, such as paclitaxel (Taxol), doxorubicin (Adriamycin), vincristine, and dactinomycin, by encoding for a transmembrane molecule that actively pumps these cytotoxic agents out of the cell.[165] Expression of the MDR gene in tumor cells is commonly associated with tumor resistance to these cytotoxic agents. Sorrentino et al.[166] transplanted MDR-transduced bone marrow cells into mice and substantially enriched for these cells after treatment with paclitaxel. Several clinical trials are now under way that attempt to genetically modify bone marrow cells with the MDR gene, followed by their reinfusion into the patient in an attempt to decrease hematopoietic toxicity from subsequent chemotherapy. However, clinical trials involving patients who received transduced bone marrow have shown that only a small percentage of hematopoietic cells are gene modified.[167] This limitation has been confirmed by several groups attempting to decrease chemotherapy toxicity with MDR-transduced hematopoietic progenitor cells. Cowan et al. found low levels of short-term engraftment of MDR-transduced cells in three of four patients treated,[168] and Hesdorffer and colleagues had similar results in two of five patients.[169] Hanania et al. found that the method of transduction was important and compared a 3-day transduction method on a stromal monolayer to a 4- to 6-hour transduction procedure in a culture bag. Three to 4 weeks after transplantation, zero of ten patients receiving cells transduced using the supernatant method had MDR-positive cells, whereas five of eight patients receiving cells transduced using the stromal method had MDR-positive cells.[170] However, the percentage of positive cells was not quantified and was presumably low because sensitive PCR methods were required for detection.

Therefore, the success of this strategy may depend on whether the levels of gene transfer are sufficient to allow the administration of higher doses of chemotherapy. If this approach is to have a significant impact in cancer therapy, an effective chemotherapeutic regimen must exist that can eradicate tumor before the development of significant nonhematopoietic toxicities, such as liver failure.

RADIOPROTECTIVE GENE THERAPY

To increase the therapeutic ratio of cancer radiotherapy, genes that decrease toxicity can be introduced into normal tissues. In a strategy to protect the lung from radiation damage, Epperly et al. introduced the gene encoding the antioxidant manganese superoxide dismutase into the lungs of mice by intratracheal injection of recombinant adenovirus[171] or plasmid and liposome.[172] Expression of manganese superoxide dismutase resulted in decreased expression of inflammatory cytokines. Increased survival and decreased irradiation-induced organizing alveolitis were observed. No bystander protection to thoracic tumors (orthotopic Lewis lung carcinoma) was seen in this murine model. Thus, this approach may be helpful to decrease radiation-induced toxicity but is dependent on the ability to deliver genes to normal tissues.

ANTIANGIOGENIC GENE THERAPY

The discovery by Folkman[173] in the 1970s that tumors produce substances which stimulate the growth of their vasculature has led to intensive investigation into methods to inhibit tumor neovessel formation. Production of proangiogenic cytokines, including VEGF and fibroblast growth factor, results in angiogenesis, which is required for tumor growth.[174] One gene therapy strategy, therefore, has been to inhibit the production or function of proangiogenic cytokines. A second strategy involves the delivery of genes that encode inhibitors of angiogenesis.[175] A number of endogenous proteins have been described that are capable of inhibiting angiogenesis, and their expression *in vivo* may result in antitumor activity through interference with tumor blood supply.

GENES THAT INHIBIT PROANGIOGENIC CYTOKINES

VEGF is a proangiogenic cytokine that can bind to two high-affinity receptors (VEGFR-1 or Flt-1, and VEGFR-2 or KDR) expressed on vascular endothelial cells. An endogenous, alternatively spliced soluble form of Flt-1 (sFlt-1) has been identified[176] that is capable of inhibiting the effects of VEGF on vascular endothelial cells *in vitro*. Systemic administration of recombinant adenovirus expressing sFlt-1 resulted in tumor inhibition in mice with preexisting lung or liver metastases.[177] In another preclinical model using GS-9L gliosarcoma cells in rats, intracerebral or subcutaneous intratumoral injection of retrovirus-producing cells encoding a dominant-negative VEGFR-2 resulted in tumor inhibition that was associated with decreased vessel density within tumors.[178]

Antisense approaches are also being tested as a means to inhibit VEGF. Use of a recombinant adenovirus encoding antisense VEGF for intratumoral injection of subcutaneous human gliomas in nude mice resulted in the inhibition of tumor growth.[179] The von Hippel-Lindau (VHL) gene[180] has been shown to down-regulate VEGF production by human renal cancer cells.[181] Therefore, gene therapy by introducing the VHL gene into tumors is a potential strategy to down-regulate VEGF expression *in vivo*. As with other approaches that depend on *in vivo* gene delivery into tumor cells, this approach is limited by the requirement for an efficient system that allows gene transfer to a majority of cancer cells *in vivo*.

Urokinase-type plasminogen activator (uPA) is a fibroblast growth factor that can result in endothelial cell proliferation. Soluble N-terminal fragments of uPA have been used to competitively inhibit the binding of endogenous uPA with its receptor. Systemic administration of recombinant adenovirus encoding a competitor fragment of uPA has been shown to inhibit liver metastases in an experimental model of human colon cancer in nude mice.[182]

Tie-2 is an endothelium-specific receptor tyrosine kinase that plays an important role in angiogenesis of embryonic vasculature through the interaction with its ligand, angiopoietin 1.[183] Systemic administration of a recombinant adenovirus expressing a soluble Tie-2 receptor (sTie-2) capable of blocking Tie-2 activation resulted in growth inhibition of subcutaneous murine mammary (4T1) and melanoma (B16F10.9) cells. In addition, the sTie-2 recombinant adenovirus inhibited the development and neovascularization of pulmonary metastases.[184]

GENES WITH ANTIANGIOGENIC PROPERTIES

A number of endogenous inhibitors of angiogenesis have been described and include antiangiogenic proteolytic fragments, interleukins, IFNs, thrombospondins, and tissue inhibitors of matrix metalloproteinases (TIMPs). Angiostatin is a 38-kD internal fragment of plasminogen, and endostatin is a 20-kD fragment derived from the C-terminal noncollagenous domain of the basement membrane constituent collagen XVIII.[185] Administration of angiostatin and endostatin can lead to tumor dormancy and regression in murine models.[185] However, these proteins have been difficult to produce in large quantities for clinical use due to instability. Because it may be necessary to administer antiangiogenic agents chronically to maintain long-term tumor suppression, other strategies besides administration of recombinant protein may be required for these approaches to be effective. Gene therapy using genes encoding these proteolytic fragments may be an attractive alternative to exogenous dosing.

Systemic administration of recombinant adenovirus-expressing angiostatin resulted in dose-dependent inhibition of the establishment and growth of C6 rat gliomas in nude mice.[186] Using intravenous delivery of complexes of cationic liposomes and plasmid DNA encoding angiostatin, Liu et al.[187] demonstrated reduced B16F10 melanoma metastases in a 7-day tumor model.

Feldman et al. demonstrated inhibition of subcutaneous MC38 murine colon adenocarcinomas using intravenous administration of recombinant adenovirus expressing the endostatin gene. In this model, circulating levels of endostatin were as high as 2038 ng/mL in nude mice after injection of adenovirus.[188]

Preclinical gene therapy approaches have been investigated using genes encoding a number of other antiangiogenic agents, including IL-4, IL-10, IL-12, IFN-β, thrombospondin-1, TIMP-1, TIMP-2, and platelet factor-4. In addition, the combination of ionizing radiation and intratumoral administration of a recombinant adenovirus expressing TNF-α resulted in tumor suppression in a murine xenograft model mediated by the destruction of tumor microvasculature.[189]

MOLECULAR IMAGING OF GENE-MODIFIED CELLS

To evaluate the effectiveness of gene transfer, the ability to measure expression *in vivo* would be valuable. New technologies are under development to follow the expression of novel genes *in vivo*, especially when the transgene either can be detected directly or has enzymatic activity that allows a detectable substrate to be modified such that it accumulates intracellularly. Bioluminescent imaging techniques capable of detecting light-emitting enzymes are useful in small animal models of gene transfer. This technique has been used in a number of murine gene therapy studies. For example, in a model of experimental autoimmune encephalomyelitis Costa et al. studied migration of adoptively transferred myelin basic protein–reactive CD4+ T cells that were retrovirally transduced with a luciferase–green fluorescent protein fusion protein.[190] Using bioluminescent imaging, they found that T cells migrated to the central nervous system of symptomatic animals. In an orthotopic rat glioma model, Rehemtulla et al. imaged gene expression after intratumoral injection of an adenoviral vector expressing both a suicide gene (yeast cytosine deaminase) and the luciferase reporter gene. Diffusion-weighted magnetic resonance imaging was used to determine tumor cell killing, whereas bioluminescent imaging was used to follow gene expression *in vivo*. This approach allowed multiple time points to be observed in a noninvasive fashion.[191]

Due to lack of sensitivity of bioluminescent imaging in larger animals, other techniques will be required to evaluate transgene expression in patients. For example, radiolabeled 2'-fluoro-2'-deoxy-1-β-D-arabinofuransyl-5-iodouracil (FIAU) crosses cell membranes and is phosphorylated by HSV-TK. In the phosphorylated form, FIAU no longer crosses cell membranes, and therefore it accumulates in HSV-TK–expressing cells. This accumulation can be imaged by a gamma camera or positron emission tomography. Hackman et al. demonstrated that HSV-TK–expressing tumor cells, implanted subcutaneously, could be imaged by positron emission tomography after administration of [[124]I]FIAU.[192] This technique can be valuable for evaluating *in vivo* migration of T cells. Koehne et al. evaluated the *in vivo* migration of [^{131}I]FIAU-labeled HSV-TK–transduced T cells using a gamma camera. T cells initially accumulated in the lung (1 hour), but then migrated to an EBV-positive lymphoma xenograft (Fig. 60-5A). Migration was observed to an autologous (matched) tumor but not to an allogeneic (unmatched) tumor (see Fig. 60-5B). Quantitation of tumor infiltration by transduced T cells using flow cytometry correlated with the amount of accumulated label.[193] Therefore, this can be an important noninvasive method to measure T-cell migration *in vivo*.

CONCLUSION

The ability to introduce genetic material into mammalian cells has allowed us to begin to envision new strategies to treat cancer. However, many challenges lie ahead before these new approaches become clinically useful. Progress in gene therapy is dependent on the techniques of gene transfer. Continued

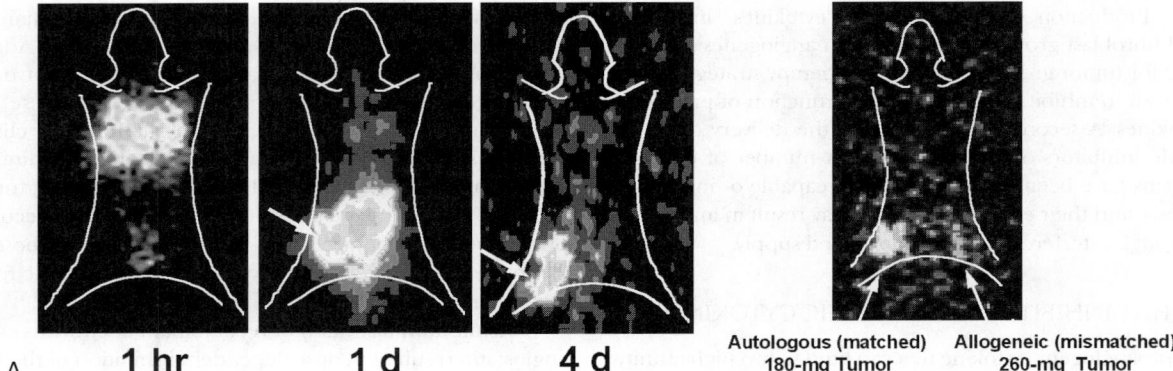

A   **1 hr**   **1 d**   **4 d**   Autologous (matched) 180-mg Tumor   Allogeneic (mismatched) 260-mg Tumor   B

FIGURE 60-5. **A:** Representative serial planar gamma camera images of severe combined immunodeficiency (SCID) mice bearing a human Epstein Barr virus (EBV) lymphoma xenograft at 1 hour, 1 day, and 4 days after tail vein injection of 3 × 10⁷ autologous, EBV-specific T cells transduced with NIT (i.e., dicistronic retoviral vector encoding herpes simplex virus–thymidine kinase and a mutated human low-affinity nerve growth factor receptor) and isolated on the basis of nerve growth factor receptor expression). These T cells were then labeled *in vitro* with [^{131}I]2'-fluoro-2'-deoxy-1-β-D-arabinofuransyl-5-iodouracil ([^{131}I]FIAU). For anatomic orientation, manually drawn body contours of the mouse are shown. The arrows in the 1-day and 4-day images identify the tumor. **B:** Selective accumulation of adoptively transferred NIT+ human autologous EBV-specific T lymphocytes in autologous EBV lymphoma xenografts. Planar gamma camera image and manually drawn body contour of an SCID mouse bearing a 180-mg autologous (matched) and a 260-mg allogeneic (mismatched) human EBV lymphoma xenograft at 4 days after tail vein injection of 3 × 10⁷ [^{131}I]FIAU-labeled NIT-transduced autologous EBV-specific T cells. The image contrast between the autologous NIT+ and allogeneic tumors is consistent with threefold activity concentration ratio between these tumors. (From ref. 193, with permission.) (See Color Fig. 60-5 in the CD-ROM.)

advances in vector biology to enhance the efficiency, safety, and specificity of gene transfer will be essential to develop improved cancer therapies. The initial clinical trials in gene therapy have demonstrated the feasibility and safety of manipulating genetic material in patients and have focused attention on the areas that require further research.

REFERENCES

1. Miller AD, Miller DG, Garcia JV, et al. Use of retroviral vectors for gene transfer and expression. *Methods Enzymol* 1993;217:581.
2. Danos O, Mulligan RC. Safe and efficient generation of recombinant retroviruses with amphotropic and ecotropic host ranges. *Proc Natl Acad Sci U S A* 1988;85:6460.
3. Burns JC, Friedmann T, Driever W, et al. Vesicular stomatitis virus G glycoprotein pseudotyped retroviral vectors: concentration to very high titer and efficient gene transfer into mammalian and nonmammalian cells [see comments]. *Proc Natl Acad Sci U S A* 1993;90:8033.
4. Miller AD. Cell-surface receptors for retroviruses and implications for gene transfer. *Proc Natl Acad Sci U S A* 1996;93:11407.
5. Miller AD, Garcia JV, von Suhr N, et al. Construction and properties of retrovirus packaging cells based on gibbon ape leukemia virus. *J Virol* 1991;65:2220.
6. Bauer TR Jr, Miller AD, Hickstein DD. Improved transfer of the leukocyte integrin CD18 subunit into hematopoietic cell lines by using retroviral vectors having a gibbon ape leukemia virus envelope. *Blood* 1995;86:2379.
7. Lam JS, Cowherd R, Rosenberg SA, Hwu P. Improved gene transfer into lymphocytes using retroviruses that express the gibbon ape leukemia virus envelope. *Hum Gene Ther* 1996;7:1415.
8. Bunnell BA, Muul LM, Donahue RE, Blaese RM, Morgan RA. High-efficiency retroviral-mediated gene transfer into human and nonhuman primate peripheral blood lymphocytes. *Proc Natl Acad Sci U S A* 1995;92:7739.
9. Yee JK, Friedmann T, Burns JC. Generation of high-titer pseudotyped retroviral vectors with very broad host range. *Methods Cell Biol* 1994;43(Pt A):99.
10. Gallardo HF. Recombinant retroviruses pseudotyped with the vesicular stomatitis virus G glycoprotein mediate both stable gene transfer and pseudotransduction in human peripheral blood lymphocytes. *Blood* 1997;90:952.
11. Cavazzana-Calvo M, Hacein-Bey S, de Saint BG, et al. Gene therapy of human severe combined immunodeficiency (SCID)-X1 disease. *Science* 2000;288:669.
12. Hacein-Bey-Abina S, Von Kalle C, Schmidt M, et al. LMO2-associated clonal T cell proliferation in two patients after gene therapy for SCID-X1. *Science* 2003;302:415.
13. Kohn DB, Sadelain M, Glorioso JC. Occurrence of leukaemia following gene therapy of X-linked SCID. *Nat Rev Cancer* 2003;3:477.
14. Naldini L, Blomer U, Gallay P, et al. In vivo gene delivery and stable transduction of non-dividing cells by a lentiviral vector [see comments]. *Science* 1996;272:263.
15. Kafri T, van Praag H, Ouyang L, Gage FH, Verma IM. A packaging cell line for lentivirus vectors. *J Virol* 1999;73:576.
16. Naldini L, Blomer U, Gage F, Trono D, Verma I. Efficient transfer, integration, and sustained long-term expression of the transgene in adult rat brains injected with a lentiviral vector. *Proc Natl Acad Sci U S A* 1997;93:11382.
17. Case SS, Price MA, Jordan CT, et al. Stable transduction of quiescent CD34(+)CD38(−) human hematopoietic cells by HIV-1–based lentiviral vectors. *Proc Natl Acad Sci U S A* 1999;96:2988.
18. Kane S, Pastan I, Gottesman M. Genetic basis of multidrug resistance of tumor cells. *J Bioenerg Biomembr* 1990;22:593.
19. Miyoshi H, Smith KA, Mosier DE, Verma IM, Torbett BE. Transduction of human CD34+ cells that mediate long-term engraftment of NOD/SCID mice by HIV vectors. *Science* 1999;283:682.
20. Miyoshi H, Takahashi M, Gage FH, Verma IM. Stable and efficient gene transfer into the retina using an HIV-based lentiviral vector. *Proc Natl Acad Sci U S A* 1997;94:10319.
21. Berkner KL. Expression of heterologous sequences in adenoviral vectors. *Curr Top Microbiol Immunol* 1992;158:39.
22. Green NK, Seymour LW. Adenoviral vectors: systemic delivery and tumor targeting. *Cancer Gene Ther* 2002;9:1036.
23. Rosenfeld MA, Yoshimura K, Trapnell BC, et al. In vivo transfer of the human cystic fibrosis transmembrane conductance regulator gene to the airway epithelium. *Cell* 1992;68:143.
24. Yei S, Mittereder N, Wert S, et al. In vivo evaluation of the safety of adenovirus-mediated transfer of the human cystic fibrosis transmembrane conductance regulator cDNA to the lung. *Hum Gene Ther* 1994;5:733.
25. Yei S, Mittereder N, Tank K, O'Sullivan C, Trapnell BC. Adenovirus-mediated gene transfer for cystic fibrosis: quantitative evaluation of repeated in vivo vector administration to the lung. *Gene Ther* 1994;1:192.
26. Yang Y, Nunes FA, Berencsi K, et al. Cellular immunity to viral antigens limits E1 deleted adenoviruses for gene therapy. *Proc Natl Acad Sci U S A* 1994;91:4407.
27. Rosenberg SA, Zhai Y, Yang JC, et al. Immunizing patients with metastatic melanoma using recombinant adenoviruses encoding MART-1 or gp100 melanoma antigens. *J Natl Cancer Inst* 1998;90:1894.
28. Gahery-Segard H, Molinier-Frenkel V, Le Boulaire C, et al. Phase I trial of recombinant adenovirus gene transfer in lung cancer. Longitudinal study of the immune responses to transgene and viral products. *J Clin Invest* 1997;100:2218.

29. Ye X, Jerebtsova M, Ray PE. Liver bypass significantly increases the transduction efficiency of recombinant adenoviral vectors in the lung intestine, and kidney. *Hum Gene Ther* 2000;11:621.
30. Raper SE, Chirmule N, Lee FS, et al. Fatal systemic inflammatory response syndrome in an ornithine transcarbamylase deficient patient following adenoviral gene transfer. *Mol Genet Metab* 2003;80:148.
31. Muzyczka N. Use of adeno-associated virus as a general transduction vector for mammalian cells. *Curr Top Microbiol Immunol* 1992;158:97.
32. Grimm D. Production methods for gene transfer vectors based on adeno-associated virus serotypes. *Methods* 2002;28:146.
33. Moss B. Poxvirus expression vectors. *Curr Top Microbiol Immunol* 1992;158:25.
34. Wild F, Giraudon P, Spehner D, Drillien R, Lecocq JP. Fowlpox virus recombinant encoding the measles virus fusion protein: protection of mice against fatal measles encephalitis. *Vaccine* 1990;8:441.
35. Felgner PL, Ringold GM. Cationic liposome-mediated transfection. *Nature* 1989;337:387.
36. Stribling R, Brunette E, Liggitt D, Gaensler K, Debs R. Aerosol gene delivery in vivo. *Proc Natl Acad Sci U S A* 1992;89:11277.
37. Galanis E, Hersh EM, Stopeck AT, et al. Immunotherapy of advanced malignancy by direct gene transfer of an interleukin-2 DNA/DMRIE/DOPE lipid complex: phase I/II experience. *J Clin Oncol* 1999;17:3313.
38. Stopeck AT, Hersh EM, Akporiaye ET, et al. Phase I study of direct gene transfer of an allogeneic histocompatibility antigen, HLA-B7, in patients with metastatic melanoma. *J Clin Oncol* 1997;15:341.
39. Nabel GJ, Gordon D, Bishop DK, et al. Immune response in human melanoma after transfer of an allogeneic class I major histocompatibility complex gene with DNA-liposome complexes. *Proc Natl Acad Sci U S A* 1996;93:15388.
40. Truong-Le VL, August JT, Leong KW. Controlled gene delivery by DNA-gelatin nanospheres. *Hum Gene Ther* 1998;9:1709.
41. Yang NS, Burkholder J, Roberts B, Martinell B, McCabe D. In vivo and in vitro gene transfer to mammalian somatic cells by particle bombardment. *Proc Natl Acad Sci U S A* 1990;87:9568.
42. Wolff JA, Malone RW, Williams P, et al. Direct gene transfer into mouse muscle in vivo. *Science* 1990;247:1465.
43. Sikes M, O'Malley BW, Finegold MJ, Ledley FD. In vivo gene transfer into rabbit thyroid follicular cells by direct DNA injection. *Hum Gene Ther* 1994;5:827.
44. Amabile PG, Waugh JM, Lewis TN, et al. High-efficiency endovascular gene delivery via therapeutic ultrasound. *J Am Coll Cardiol* 2001;37:1975.
45. Niidome T, Huang L. Gene therapy progress and prospects: nonviral vectors. *Gene Ther* 2002;9:1647.
46. Zhang G, Budker V, Wolff JA. High levels of foreign gene expression in hepatocytes after tail vein injections of naked plasmid DNA. *Hum Gene Ther* 1999;10:1735.
47. Wang G, Tschoi M, Spolski R, et al. In vivo antitumor activity of interleukin 21 mediated by natural killer cells. *Cancer Res* 2003;63:9016.
48. Rosenberg SA, Aebersold P, Cornetta K, et al. Gene transfer into humans—immunotherapy of patients with advanced melanoma, using tumor-infiltrating lymphocytes modified by retroviral gene transduction. *N Engl J Med* 1990;323:570.
49. Lotze MT. The treatment of patients with melanoma using interleukin-2, interleukin-4 and tumor infiltrating lymphocytes. *Hum Gene Ther* 1992;3:167.
50. Miller AR, Skotzko MJ, Rhoades K, et al. Simultaneous use of two retroviral vectors in human gene marking trials: feasibility and potential applications. *Hum Gene Ther* 1992;3:619.
51. Brenner SA, Rill DR, Holladay MS, et al. Gene marking to determine whether autologous marrow infusion restores long-term haematopoiesis in cancer patients. *Lancet* 1993;342:1134.
52. Riddell SR, Greenberg PD, Overell RW, et al. Phase I study of cellular adoptive immunotherapy using genetically modified CD8+ HIV-specific T cells for HIV seropositive patients undergoing allogeneic bone marrow transplant. The Fred Hutchinson Cancer Research Center and the University of Washington School of Medicine, Department of Medicine, Division of Oncology. *Hum Gene Ther* 1992;3:319.
53. Heslop HE, Ng CY, Li C, et al. Long-term restoration of immunity against Epstein-Barr virus infection by adoptive transfer of gene-modified virus-specific T lymphocytes. *Nat Med* 1996;2:551.
54. Brodie SJ, Lewinsohn DA, Patterson BK, et al. In vivo migration and function of transferred HIV-1-specific cytotoxic T cells [see comments]. *Nat Med* 1999;5:34.
55. Brenner MK, Rill DR, Moen RC, et al. Gene marking and autologous bone marrow transplantation. *Ann N Y Acad Sci* 1994;716:204; discussion 214.
56. Brenner MK, Rill DR, Heslop HE, et al. Gene marking after bone marrow transplantation. *Eur J Cancer* 1994;30A:1171.
57. Rill DR, Santana VM, Roberts WM, et al. Direct demonstration that autologous bone marrow transplantation for solid tumors can return a multiplicity of tumorigenic cells. *Blood* 1994;84:380.
58. Deisseroth AB, Zu Z, Claxton D, et al. Genetic marking shows that Ph+ cells present in autologous transplants of CML contribute to relapse after autologous bone marrow in CML. *Blood* 1994;83:3068.
59. Brenner M, Krance R, Heslop HE, et al. Assessment of the efficacy of purging by using gene marked autologous marrow transplantation for children with AML in first complete remission. *Hum Gene Ther* 1994;5:481.
60. Gewirtz AM. Potential therapeutic applications of antisense oligodeoxynucleotides in the treatment of chronic myelogenous leukemia. *Leuk Lymphoma* 1993;11[Suppl 1]:131.
61. Kawakami Y, Eliyahu S, Delgado CH, et al. Cloning of the gene coding for a shared human melanoma antigen recognized by autologous T cells infiltrating into tumor. *Proc Natl Acad Sci U S A* 1994;91:3515.
62. Brichard V, Van Pel A, Wölfel T, et al. The tyrosinase gene codes for an antigen recognized by autologous cytolytic T lymphocytes on HLA-A2 melanomas. *J Exp Med* 1993;178:489.

63. Fearon E, Pardoll D, Itaya T, et al. Interleukin-2 production by tumor cells bypasses T helper function in the generation of an antitumor response. *Cell* 1990;60:397.
64. Connor J, Bannerji R, Saito S, et al. Regression of bladder tumors in mice treated with interleukin 2 gene-modified tumor cells [published erratum appears in *J Exp Med* 1993;177(6):following 1831]. *J Exp Med* 1993;177:1127.
65. Stewart AK, Lassam NJ, Quirt IC, et al. Adenovector-mediated gene delivery of interleukin-2 in metastatic breast cancer and melanoma: results of a phase 1 clinical trial. *Gene Ther* 1999;6:350.
66. Palmer K, Moore J, Everard M, et al. Gene therapy with autologous, interleukin 2-secreting tumor cells in patients with malignant melanoma. *Hum Gene Ther* 1999;10:1261.
67. Sobol RE, Shawler DL, Carson C, et al. Interleukin 2 gene therapy of colorectal carcinoma with autologous irradiated tumor cells and genetically engineered fibroblasts: a Phase I study. *Clin Cancer Res* 1999;5:2359.
68. Dranoff G, Jaffee E, Lazenby A, et al. Vaccination with irradiated tumor cells engineered to secrete murine granulocyte-macrophage colony-stimulating factor stimulates potent, specific, and long-lasting anti-tumor immunity. *Proc Natl Acad Sci U S A* 1993;90:3539.
69. Huang AY, Golumbek P, Ahmadzadeh M, et al. Role of bone marrow-derived cells in presenting MHC class I-restricted tumor antigens. *Science* 1994;264:961.
70. Hung K, Hayashi R, Lafond-Walker A, et al. The central role of CD4(+) T cells in the antitumor immune response. *J Exp Med* 1998;188:2357.
71. Simons JW, Jaffee EM, Weber CE, et al. Bioactivity of autologous irradiated renal cell carcinoma vaccines generated by ex vivo granulocyte-macrophage colony-stimulating factor gene transfer. *Cancer Res* 1997;57:1537.
72. Soiffer R, Lynch T, Mihm M, et al. Vaccination with irradiated autologous melanoma cells engineered to secrete human granulocyte-macrophage colony-stimulating factor generates potent antitumor immunity in patients with metastatic melanoma. *Proc Natl Acad Sci U S A* 1998;95:13141.
73. Simons JW, Mikhak B, Chang JF, et al. Induction of immunity to prostate cancer antigens: results of a clinical trial of vaccination with irradiated autologous prostate tumor cells engineered to secrete granulocyte-macrophage colony-stimulating factor using ex vivo gene transfer. *Cancer Res* 1999;59:5160.
74. Ogasawara M, Rosenberg SA. Enhanced expression of HLA molecules and stimulation of autologous human tumor infiltrating lymphocytes following transduction of melanoma cells with gamma-interferon genes. *Cancer Res* 1993;53:3561.
75. Watanabe Y, Kuribayashi K, Miyatake S, et al. Exogenous expression of mouse interferon gamma cDNA in mouse neuroblastoma C1300 cells results in reduced tumorigenicity by augmented anti-tumor immunity. *Proc Natl Acad Sci U S A* 1989;86:9456.
76. Restifo NP, Spiess PJ, Karp SE, et al. A nonimmunogenic sarcoma transduced with the cDNA for interferon-gamma elicits CD8+ T cells against the wild-type tumor: correlation with antigen presentation capability. *J Exp Med* 1992;175:1423.
77. Asher AL, Mule JJ, Kasid A, et al. Murine tumor cells transduced with the gene for tumor necrosis factor-alpha. Evidence for paracrine immune effects of tumor necrosis factor against tumors. *J Immunol* 1991;146:3227.
78. Douvdevani A, Huleihel M, Zöller M, Segal S, Apte RN. Reduced tumorigenicity of fibrosarcomas which constitutively generate IL-1 alpha either spontaneously or following IL-1 alpha gene transfer. *Int J Cancer* 1992;51:822.
79. Tepper R, Pattengale P, Leder P. Murine interleukin-4 displays potent anti-tumor activity *in vivo*. *Cell* 1989;57:503.
80. Porgador A, Tzehoval E, Katz A, et al. Interleukin 6 gene transfection into Lewis lung carcinoma tumor cells suppresses the malignant phenotype and confers immunotherapeutic competence against parental metastatic cells. *Cancer Res* 1992;52:3679.
81. McBride WH, Thacker JD, Comora S, et al. Genetic modification of a murine fibrosarcoma to produce interleukin 7 stimulates host cell infiltration and tumor immunity. *Cancer Res* 1992;52:3931.
82. Lebel-Binay S, Laguerre B, Quintin-Colonna F, et al. Experimental gene therapy of cancer using tumor cells engineered to secrete interleukin-13. *Eur J Immunol* 1995;25:2340.
83. Colombo MP, Ferrari G, Stoppacciaro A, et al. Granulocyte colony-stimulating factor gene transfer suppresses tumorigenicity of a murine adenocarcinoma *in vivo*. *J Exp Med* 1991;173:889.
84. Rollins BJ, Sunday ME. Suppression of tumor formation *in vivo* by expression of the JE gene in malignant cells. *Mol Cell Biol* 1991;11:3125.
85. Mule JJ, Custer MC, Averbook B, et al. RANTES secretion by gene-modified tumor cells results in loss of tumorigenicity *in vivo*: role of immune cell subpopulations. *Hum Gene Ther* 1996;7:1545.
86. Tahara H, Zitvogel L, Storkus W, et al. Effective eradication of established murine tumors with IL-12 gene therapy using a polycistronic retroviral vector. *J Immunol* 1995;154:6466.
87. Hock H, Dorsch M, Kunzendorf U, et al. Vaccinations with tumor cells genetically engineered to produce different cytokines: effectivity not superior to a classical adjuvant. *Cancer Res* 1993;53:714.
88. Linsley PS, Clark EA, Ledbetter JA. T-cell antigen CD28 mediates adhesion with B cells by interacting with activation antigen B7/BB-1. *Proc Natl Acad Sci U S A* 1990;87:5031.
89. Chen L, Ashe S, Brady WA, et al. Costimulation of antitumor immunity by the B7 counterreceptor for the T lymphocyte molecules CD28 and CTLA-4. *Cell* 1992;71:1093.
90. Townsend SE, Allison JP. Tumor rejection after direct costimulation of CD8+ T cells by B7-transfected melanoma cells [see comments]. *Science* 1993;259:368.
91. Chen L, McGowan P, Ashe S, et al. Tumor immunogenicity determines the effect of B7 costimulation on T cell-mediated tumor immunity. *J Exp Med* 1994;179:523.
92. Plautz GE, Yang ZY, Wu BY, et al. Immunotherapy of malignancy by *in vivo* gene transfer into tumors [see comments]. *Proc Natl Acad Sci U S A* 1993;90:4645.
93. Van Der Bruggen P, Traversari C, Chomez P, et al. A gene encoding an antigen recognized by cytolytic T lymphocytes on a human melanoma. *Science* 1991;254:1643.
94. Wang M, Bronte V, Chen PW, et al. Active immunotherapy of cancer with a non-replicating recombinant fowlpox virus encoding a model tumor-associated antigen. *J Immunol* 1995;154:4685.
95. Bronte V, Tsung K, Rao J, et al. IL-2 enhances the function of recombinant poxvirus-based vaccines in the treatment of established pulmonary metastases. *J Immunol* 1995;154:5282.
96. Celluzzi CM, Mayordomo JI, Storkus WJ, et al. Peptide-pulsed dendritic cells induce antigen-specific CTL-mediated protective immunity. *J Exp Med* 1996;183:283.
97. Nestle FO, Alijagic S, Gilliet M, et al. Vaccination of melanoma patients with peptide- or tumor lysate-pulsed dendritic cells. *Nat Med* 1998;4:328.
98. Specht J, Wang G, Do M, et al. Dendritic cells retrovirally transduced with a model antigen gene are therapeutically effective against established pulmonary metastases. *J Exp Med* 1997;186:1213.
99. Reeves ME, Royal RE, Lam JS, Rosenberg SA, Hwu P. Retroviral transduction of human dendritic cells with a tumor-associated antigen gene. *Cancer Res* 1996;56:5672.
100. Alijagic S, Moller P, Artuc M, et al. Dendritic cells generated from peripheral blood transfected with human tyrosinase induce specific T cell activation. *Eur J Immunol* 1995;25:3100.
101. Song W, Kong HL, Carpenter H, et al. Dendritic cells genetically modified with an adenovirus vector encoding the cDNA for a model antigen induce protective and therapeutic antitumor immunity. *J Exp Med* 1997;186:1247.
102. Bhardwaj N, Bender A, Gonzalez N, et al. Influenza virus-infected dendritic cells stimulate strong proliferative and cytolytic responses from human CD8+ T cells. *J Clin Invest* 1994;94:797.
103. Rosenberg SA, Packard BS, Aebersold PM, et al. Use of tumor infiltrating lymphocytes and interleukin-2 in the immunotherapy of patients with metastatic melanoma. Preliminary report. *N Engl J Med* 1988;319:1676.
104. Walter EA, Greenberg PD, Gilbert MJ, et al. Reconstitution of cellular immunity against cytomegalovirus in recipients of allogeneic bone marrow by transfer of T-cell clones from the donor. *N Engl J Med* 1995;333:1038.
105. Drobyski WR, Keever CA, Roth MS, et al. Salvage immunotherapy using donor leukocyte infusions as treatment for relapsed chronic myelogenous leukemia after allogeneic bone marrow transplantation: efficacy and toxicity of a defined T-cell dose. *Blood* 1993;82:2310.
106. Shu S, Chou T, Rosenberg SA. *In vitro* sensitization and expansion with viable tumor cells and interleukin-2 in the generation of specific therapeutic effector cells. *J Immunol* 1986;136:3891.
107. Yamada G, Kitamura Y, Sonoda H, et al. Retroviral expression of the human IL-2 gene in a murine T cell line results in cell growth autonomy and tumorigenicity. *EMBO J* 1987;6:2705.
108. Karasuyama H, Tohyama N, Tada T. Autocrine growth and tumorigenicity of interleukin 2-dependent helper T cells transfected with IL-2 gene. *J Exp Med* 1989;169:13.
109. Treisman J, Hwu P, Minamoto S, et al. Interleukin-2-transduced lymphocytes grow in an autocrine fashion and remain responsive to antigen. *Blood* 1995;85:139.
110. Liu K, Rosenberg SA. Interleukin-2-independent proliferation of human melanoma-reactive T lymphocytes transduced with an exogenous IL-2 gene is stimulation dependent. *J Immunother* 2003;26:190.
111. Kuwana Y, Asakura Y, Utsunomiya N, et al. Expression of chimeric receptor composed of immunoglobulin-derived V regions and T-cell receptor-derived C regions. *Biochem Biophys Res Comm* 1987;149:960.
112. Gross G, Waks T, Eshhar Z. Expression of immunoglobulin-T-cell receptor chimeric molecules as functional receptors with antibody-type specificity. *Proc Natl Acad Sci U S A* 1989;86:10024.
113. Hwu P, Schwarz S, Custer M, et al. Use of soluble recombinant TNF receptor to improve detection of TNF secretion in cultures of tumor infiltrating lymphocytes. *J Immunol Methods* 1992;151:139.
114. Hwu P, Shafer GE, Treisman J, et al. Lysis of ovarian cancer cells by human lymphocytes redirected with a chimeric gene composed of an antibody variable region and the Fc receptor gamma chain. *J Exp Med* 1993;178:361.
115. Huston JS, Levinson D, Mudgett-Hunter M, et al. Protein engineering of antibody binding sites: recovery of specific activity in an anti-digoxin single-chain Fv analogue produced in *Escherichia coli*. *Proc Natl Acad Sci U S A* 1988;85:5879.
116. Bird RE, Hardman KD, Jacobson JW, et al. Single-chain antigen-binding proteins. *Science* 1988;242:423.
117. Romeo C, Seed B. Cellular immunity to HIV activated by CD4 fused to T cell or Fc receptor polypeptides. *Cell* 1991;64:1037.
118. Krause A. Antigen-dependent CD28 signaling selectively enhances survival and proliferation in genetically modified activated human primary T lymphocytes. *J Exp Med* 1998;188:619.
119. Stancovski I, Schindler DG, Waks T, et al. Targeting of T lymphocytes to Neu/HER2-expressing cells using chimeric single chain Fv receptors. *J Immunol* 1993;151:6577.
120. Daly T, Royal RE, Kershaw M, et al. Recognition of human colon cancer by T cells transduced with a chimeric receptor gene. *Cancer Gene Ther* 2000;7:284.
121. Finer MH, Dull TJ, Qin L, et al. kat: a high-efficiency retroviral transduction system for primary human T lymphocytes. *Blood* 1994;83:43.
122. Cole DJ, Weil DP, Shilyansky J, et al. Characterization of the functional specificity of a cloned T-cell receptor heterodimer recognizing the MART-1 melanoma antigen. *Cancer Res* 1995;55:748.
123. Clay TM, Custer M, Sachs J, et al. Efficient transfer of a tumor antigen-reactive TCR to human peripheral blood lymphocytes confers anti-tumor reactivity. *J Immunol* 1999;163:507.
124. Bonini C, Ferrari G, Verzeletti SS, et al. HSV-TK gene transfer into donor lymphocytes for control of allogeneic graft-versus-leukemia [see comments]. *Science* 1997;276:1719.
125. Riddell SR, Elliott M, Lewinsohn DA, et al. T-cell mediated rejection of gene-modified HIV-specific cytotoxic T lymphocytes in HIV-infected patients [see comments]. *Nat Med* 1996;2:216.
126. Haranaka K, Satomi N, Sakurai A. Antitumor activity of murine tumor necrosis factor (TNF) against transplanted murine tumors and heterotransplanted human tumors in nude mice. *Int J Cancer* 1984;34:263.
127. Spriggs D, Sherman M, Michie H, et al. Recombinant human tumor necrosis factor administered as a 24-hour intravenous infusion. A phase I and pharmacologic study. *J Natl Cancer Inst* 1988;80:1039.
128. Bartsch H, Pfizenmaier K, Schroeder M, Nagel G. Intralesional application of recombinant human tumor necrosis factor alpha induces local tumor regression in patients with advanced malignancies. *Eur J Cancer Clin Oncol* 1989;25:287.

129. Kahn J, Kaplan L, Ziegler J, et al. Phase II trial of intralesional recombinant tumor necrosis factor alpha (rTNF) for AIDS associated Kaposi's sarcoma (KS). *Proc Am Soc Clin Oncol* 1989;8:4(abst).
130. Lienard D, Ewalenko P, Delmotte J, Renard N, Lejeune F. High-dose recombinant tumor necrosis factor alpha in combination with interferon gamma and melphalan in isolation perfusion of the limbs for melanoma and sarcoma. *J Clin Oncol* 1992;10(1):52.
131. Fraker DL, Alexander HR. The use of tumour necrosis factor (TNF) in isolated perfusion: results and side effects. The NCI results. *Melanoma Res* 1994;4[Suppl 1]:27.
132. Fisher B, Packard B, Read E, et al. Tumor localization of adoptively transferred indium-111 labeled tumor infiltrating lymphocytes in patients with metastatic melanoma. *J Clin Oncol* 1989;7:250.
133. Griffith KD, Read EJ, Carrasquillo JA, et al. *In vivo* distribution of adoptively transferred indium-111 labeled tumor infiltrating lymphocytes and peripheral blood lymphocytes in patients with metastatic melanoma. *J Natl Cancer Inst* 1989;81:1709.
134. Pockaj BA, Sherry RM, Wei JP, et al. Localization of 111-indium-labelled tumor infiltrating lymphocytes to tumor in patients receiving adoptive immunotherapy. *Cancer* 1994;73:1731.
135. Hwu P, Yannelli J, Kriegler M, et al. Functional and molecular characterization of TIL transduced with the TNFα cDNA for the gene therapy of cancer in man. *J Immunol* 1993;150:4104.
136. Studeny M, Marini FC, Champlin RE, et al. Bone marrow-derived mesenchymal stem cells as vehicles for interferon-beta delivery into tumors. *Cancer Res* 2002;62:3603.
137. Senzer N, Mani S, Rosemurgy A, et al. TNFerade biologic, an adenovector with a radiation-inducible promoter, carrying the human tumor necrosis factor alpha gene: a phase I study in patients with solid tumors. *J Clin Oncol* 2004;22:592.
138. Roth JA, Nguyen D, Lawrence DD, et al. Retrovirus-mediated wild-type p53 gene transfer to tumors of patients with lung cancer [see comments]. *Nat Med* 1996;2:985.
139. Swisher SG, Roth JA, Nemunaitis J, et al. Adenovirus-mediated p53 gene transfer in advanced non–small-cell lung cancer. *J Natl Cancer Inst* 1999;91:763.
140. Mercola D, Cohen JS. Antisense approaches to cancer gene therapy. *Cancer Gene Ther* 1995;2:47.
141. Reed JC, Stein C, Subasinghe C, et al. Antisense-mediated inhibition of BCL2 protooncogene expression and leukemic cell growth and survival: comparisons of phosphodiester and phosphorothioate oligodeoxynucleotides. *Cancer Res* 1990;50:6565.
142. Szczylik C, Skorski T, Nicolaides NC, et al. Selective inhibition of leukemia cell proliferation by BCR-ABL antisense oligodeoxynucleotides. *Science* 1991;253:562.
143. McManaway ME, Neckers LM, Loke SL, et al. Tumour-specific inhibition of lymphoma growth by an antisense oligodeoxynucleotide. *Lancet* 1990;335:808.
144. Melani C, Rivoltini L, Parmiani G, Calabretta B, Colombo MP. Inhibition of proliferation by c-myb antisense oligodeoxynucleotides in colon adenocarcinoma cell lines that express c-myb. *Cancer Res* 1991;51:2897.
145. Anfossi G, Gewirtz AM, Calabretta B. An oligomer complementary to c-myb-encoded mRNA inhibits proliferation of human myeloid leukemia cell lines. *Proc Natl Acad Sci U S A* 1989;86:3379.
146. Ratajczak MZ, Kant JA, Luger SM, et al. *In vivo* treatment of human leukemia in a scid mouse model with c-myb antisense oligodeoxynucleotides. *Proc Natl Acad Sci U S A* 1992;89:11823.
147. Higgins KA, Perez JR, Coleman TA, et al. Antisense inhibition of the p65 subunit of NF-kappa B blocks tumorigenicity and causes tumor regression. *Proc Natl Acad Sci U S A* 1993;90:9901.
148. Webb A, Cunningham D, Cotter F, et al. BCL-2 antisense therapy in patients with non-Hodgkin lymphoma. *Lancet* 1997;349:1137.
149. Millward M. Bcl-2 antisense therapy for melanoma. Paper presented at: Perspectives in Melanoma VI; November 13, 2003; Miami, FL (abst).
150. Dean NM, Bennett CF. Antisense oligonucleotide-based therapeutics for cancer. *Oncogene* 2003;22:9087.
151. Stein CA. Antisense oligodeoxynucleotides. In: DeVita VT, Hellman S, Rosenberg SA, eds. *Biologic therapy of cancer*, 2 ed. Philadelphia: JB Lippincott, 1995:759.
152. Poeschla E, Wong-Staal F. Antiviral and anticancer ribozymes. *Curr Opin Oncol* 1994;6:601.
153. Culver K, Ram Z, Wallbridge S, et al. *In vivo* gene transfer with retroviral vector-producer cells for treatment of experimental brain tumors. *Science* 1992;256:1550.
154. Huber BE, Richards CA, Krenitsky TA. Retroviral-mediated gene therapy for the treatment of hepatocellular carcinoma: an innovative approach for cancer therapy. *Proc Natl Acad Sci U S A* 1991;88:8039.
155. Vile RG, Hart IR. *In vitro* and *in vivo* targeting of gene expression to melanoma cells. *Cancer Res* 1993;53:962.
156. Bicknell R. Vascular targeting and the inhibition of angiogenesis. *Ann Oncol* 1994;5[Suppl 4]:S45.
157. Bischoff JR, Kirn DH, Williams A, et al. An adenovirus mutant that replicates selectively in p53-deficient human tumor cells [see comments]. *Science* 1996;274:373.
158. Heise C, Sampson-Johannes A, Williams A, et al. ONYX-015, an E1B gene-attenuated adenovirus, causes tumor-specific cytolysis and antitumoral efficacy that can be augmented by standard chemotherapeutic agents [see comments]. *Nat Med* 1997;3:639.
159. Heise CC, Williams AM, Xue S, Propst M, Kirn DH. Intravenous administration of ONYX-015, a selectively replicating adenovirus, induces antitumoral efficacy. *Cancer Res* 1999;59:2623.
160. Nemunaitis J, Cunningham C, Buchanan A, et al. Intravenous infusion of a replication-selective adenovirus (ONYX-015) in cancer patients: safety, feasibility and biological activity. *Gene Ther* 2001;8:746.
161. Reid T, Galanis E, Abbruzzese J, et al. Intra-arterial administration of a replication-selective adenovirus (dl1520) in patients with colorectal carcinoma metastatic to the liver: a phase I trial. *Gene Ther* 2001;8:1618.
162. Rothmann T, Hengstermann A, Whitaker NJ, Scheffner M, Zur HH. Replication of ONYX-015, a potential anticancer adenovirus, is independent of p53 status in tumor cells. *J Virol* 1998;72:9470.
163. Hall AR, Dix BR, O'Carroll SJ, Braithwaite AW. p53-dependent cell death/apoptosis is required for a productive adenovirus infection [see comments]. *Nat Med* 1998;4:1068.
164. Russell SJ. RNA viruses as virotherapy agents. *Cancer Gene Ther* 2002;9:961.
165. Gottesman M. How cancer cells evade chemotherapy: sixteenth Richard and Hinda Rosenthal Foundation award lecture. *Cancer Res* 1993;53:747.
166. Sorrentino BP, Brandt SJ, Bodine D, et al. Selection of drug-resistant bone marrow cells *in vivo* after retroviral transfer of human MDR1. *Science* 1992;257:99.
167. Dunbar CE, Kohn DB, Schiffmann R, et al. Retroviral transfer of the glucocerebrosidase gene into CD34+ cells from patients with Gaucher disease: *in vivo* detection of transduced cells without myeloablation. *Hum Gene Ther* 1998;9:2629.
168. Cowan KH, Moscow JA, Huang H, et al. Paclitaxel chemotherapy after autologous stem-cell transplantation and engraftment of hematopoietic cells transduced with a retrovirus containing the multidrug resistance complementary DNA (MDR1) in metastatic breast cancer patients [see comments]. *Clin Cancer Res* 1999;5:1619.
169. Hesdorffer C, Ayello J, Ward M, et al. Phase I trial of retroviral-mediated transfer of the human MDR1 gene as marrow chemoprotection in patients undergoing high-dose chemotherapy and autologous stem-cell transplantation. *J Clin Oncol* 1998;16:165.
170. Hanania EG, Giles RE, Kavanagh J, et al. Results of MDR-1 vector modification trial indicate that granulocyte/macrophage colony-forming unit cells do not contribute to post-transplant hematopoietic recovery following intensive systemic therapy [published erratum appears in *Proc Natl Acad Sci U S A* 1997;13;94(10):5495]. *Proc Natl Acad Sci U S A* 1996;93:15346.
171. Epperly MW, Bray JA, Krager S, et al. Intratracheal injection of adenovirus containing the human MnSOD transgene protects athymic nude mice from irradiation-induced organizing alveolitis. *Int J Radiat Oncol Biol Phys* 1999;43:169.
172. Epperly MW, Travis EL, Sikora C, Greenberger JS. Manganese [correction of Magnesium] superoxide dismutase (MnSOD) plasmid/liposome pulmonary radioprotective gene therapy: modulation of irradiation-induced mRNA for IL-I, TNF-alpha, and TGF-beta correlates with delay of organizing alveolitis/fibrosis. *Biol Blood Marrow Transplant* 1999;5:204.
173. Folkman J. Tumor angiogenesis: therapeutic implications. *N Engl J Med* 1971;285:1182.
174. Folkman J. What is the evidence that tumors are angiogenesis dependent? [Editorial]. *J Natl Cancer Inst* 1990;82:4.
175. Feldman AL, Libutti SK. Progress in antiangiogenic gene therapy of cancer. *Cancer* 2000;89:1181.
176. Kendall RL, Thomas KA. Inhibition of vascular endothelial cell growth factor activity by an endogenously encoded soluble receptor. *Proc Natl Acad Sci U S A* 1993;90:10705.
177. Kong HL, Hecht D, Song W, et al. Regional suppression of tumor growth by *in vivo* transfer of a cDNA encoding a secreted form of the extracellular domain of the flt-1 vascular endothelial growth factor receptor. *Hum Gene Ther* 1998;9:823.
178. Machein MR, Risau W, Plate KH. Antiangiogenic gene therapy in a rat glioma model using a dominant-negative vascular endothelial growth factor receptor 2. *Hum Gene Ther* 1999;10:1117.
179. Im SA, Gomez-Manzano C, Fueyo J, et al. Antiangiogenesis treatment for gliomas: transfer of antisense-vascular endothelial growth factor inhibits tumor growth *in vivo*. *Cancer Res* 1999;59:895.
180. Linehan WM, Lerman MI, Zbar B. Identification of the von Hippel-Lindau (VHL) gene. Its role in renal cancer. *JAMA* 1995;273:564.
181. Gnarra JR, Zhou S, Merrill MJ, et al. Post-transcriptional regulation of vascular endothelial growth factor mRNA by the product of the VHL tumor suppressor gene. *Proc Natl Acad Sci U S A* 1996;93:10589.
182. Li H, Lu H, Griscelli F, et al. Adenovirus-mediated delivery of a uPA/uPAR antagonist suppresses angiogenesis-dependent tumor growth and dissemination in mice. *Gene Ther* 1998;5:1105.
183. Suri C, Jones PF, Patan S, et al. Requisite role of angiopoietin-1, a ligand for the TIE2 receptor, during embryonic angiogenesis [see comments]. *Cell* 1996;87:1171.
184. Lin P, Buxton JA, Acheson A, et al. Antiangiogenic gene therapy targeting the endothelium-specific receptor tyrosine kinase Tie2. *Proc Natl Acad Sci U S A* 1998;95:8829.
185. O'Reilly MS, Boehm T, Shing Y, et al. Endostatin: an endogenous inhibitor of angiogenesis and tumor growth. *Cell* 1997;88:277.
186. Griscelli F, Li H, Bennaceur-Griscelli A, et al. Angiostatin gene transfer: inhibition of tumor growth *in vivo* by blockage of endothelial cell proliferation associated with a mitosis arrest. *Proc Natl Acad Sci U S A* 1998;95:6367.
187. Liu Y, Thor A, Shtivelman E, et al. Systemic gene delivery expands the repertoire of effective antiangiogenic agents. *J Biol Chem* 1999;274:13338.
188. Feldman AL, Restifo NP, Hwu P, Libutti SK. Antiangiogenic gene therapy of cancer utilizing a recombinant adenovirus to elevate systemic endostatin levels in mice. *Cancer Res* 2000;60:1503.
189. Staba MJ, Mauceri HJ, Kufe DW, Hallahan DE, Weichselbaum RR. Adenoviral TNF-alpha gene therapy and radiation damage tumor vasculature in a human malignant glioma xenograft. *Gene Ther* 1998;5:293.
190. Costa GL, Sandora MR, Nakajima A, et al. Adoptive immunotherapy of experimental autoimmune encephalomyelitis via T cell delivery of the IL-12 p40 subunit. *J Immunol* 2001;167:2379.
191. Rehemtulla A, Hall DE, Stegman LD, et al. Molecular imaging of gene expression and efficacy following adenoviral-mediated brain tumor gene therapy. *Mol Imaging* 2002;1:43.
192. Hackman T, Doubrovin M, Balatoni J, et al. Imaging expression of cytosine deaminase-herpes virus thymidine kinase fusion gene (CD/TK) expression with [^{124}I]FIAU and PET. *Mol Imaging* 2002;1:36.
193. Koehne G, Doubrovin M, Doubrovina E, et al. Serial *in vivo* imaging of the targeted migration of human HSV-TK-transduced antigen-specific lymphocytes. *Nat Biotechnol* 2003;21:405.
194. Eglitis MA, Anderson WF. Retroviral vectors for introduction of genes into mammalian cells. *Biotechniques* 1988;6:608.

CHAPTER 61

Cancer Vaccines

SECTION 1

DOUGLAS R. LOWY
JOHN T. SCHILLER

Preventive Vaccines

High morbidity and mortality from cancer have stimulated concerted efforts to understand the causes of cancer and to prevent cancer from developing. The recognition that environmental factors may account for the majority of cancers has encouraged researchers to identify the exogenous factors that trigger the carcinogenic process, to define their role in tumorigenesis, and to develop approaches to interfere with this process. Infectious agents make up one important class of environmental factors implicated in tumor development, and prophylactic vaccines have a long history of success in preventing nonmalignant diseases induced by infectious agents.[1-3] This section of the chapter discusses efforts to use this approach to prevent malignant disease induced by infectious agents implicated in cancer etiology and pathogenesis.

BACKGROUND

Although the oncogenic potential of some infectious agents, such as hepatitis B virus (HBV), was recognized three decades ago, many of the infectious agents now believed to be oncogenic were discovered after 1975 (Table 61.1-1).[2] These latter include the oncogenic human papillomaviruses (HPV), hepatitis C virus, herpesvirus type 8, and *Helicobacter pylori*. It seems likely that further research will result in the attribution of addi-

tional forms of cancer to infectious agents. The expanded list will arise by demonstrating that infectious agents already recognized as oncogenic may be causally involved in additional forms of cancer or by attributing these additional cancers to other infectious agents not yet recognized as oncogenic.

Identification of an infectious agent in the etiology of a malignant process implies that timely interference with the infection could prevent the tumor from arising.[4] The development of effective vaccines against infectious carcinogenic agents represents a potentially powerful form of intervention. The prototype for this approach is the HBV vaccine, which can protect immunized individuals against both acute disease and the malignant consequences attributable to the virus.[5,6] More recently, a candidate papillomavirus vaccine has also been shown to prevent HPV infection in a proof-of-principle efficacy trial.[7]

This section briefly considers how infectious oncogenic agents lead to cancer, discusses general issues related to the development of vaccines against these agents, and presents individual discussions of the three agents that account for the most cancers worldwide: *H pylori*, HBV, and HPV.

INFECTIOUS AGENTS AND CANCER

Reducing exposure to an identified carcinogen represents the principal approach to decreasing the carcinogenic effects of many environmental carcinogens. For carcinogens such as cigarette smoke, entrenched human behavior and conflicting economic interests may present considerable obstacles to reducing or eliminating exposure. By contrast, a vaccine against an infectious carcinogen does not require modification of the behavior that leads to exposure because the vaccine attenuates the oncogenic activity

TABLE 61.1-1. Oncogenic Infectious Agents

Agent	Tumor Types	Annual Cases Worldwide (Estimate)
BACTERIA		
Helicobacter pylori	Stomach cancer, gastric lymphoma	505,000
VIRUSES		
Human papillomavirus	Cervical, anal, vaginal, other cancers	447,000
Hepatitis B virus	Liver cancer	285,000
Hepatitis C virus	Liver cancer	113,000
Human immunodeficiency virus	Kaposi's sarcoma, non-Hodgkin's lymphoma	52,000
Human herpesvirus type 8	Kaposi's sarcoma	44,000
Epstein-Barr virus	Lymphomas (Hodgkin's, non-Hodgkin's, Burkitt's)	30,000
Human T-cell lymphotropic virus-1	Adult T-cell leukemia	3000
PARASITES		
Schistosomes	Bladder cancer	10,000
Liver flukes	Cholangiocarcinoma	800

(Adapted from ref. 2.)

of the infectious agent by reducing or preventing infection of target tissue.[8,9] Furthermore, the induction of *herd immunity* via the widespread use of an effective vaccine offers the possibility of reducing the risk of nonimmunized individuals to exposure to the infectious agent. Vaccination also offers the long-term possibility of eliminating the agent from the environment.

Before vaccination itself is considered, it is worthwhile to review some features of oncogenic infectious agents, because

their characteristics may have implications for vaccine development, testing, and implementation. Viruses, bacteria, and parasites have been implicated in the pathogenesis of human cancer (see Table 61.1-1). Investigators at the International Agency for Research on Cancer estimated that in 1990 approximately 15% of cancers worldwide could be attributed to infectious agents (Table 61.1-2).[2] In the United States and other developed countries, a smaller proportion of cancers (approximately 9%) are associated with these agents, whereas they account for a higher proportion (approximately 20%) in developing countries.

Several factors probably account for these regional differences. Some of the infectious agents, such as parasites with oncogenic potential, are extremely uncommon in the United States or the rate of infection varies greatly, as with HBV.[10] For others, such as HPV, infection in the United States is common, but screening such as Papanicolaou (Pap) smear testing for premalignant lesions in the cervix leads to effective treatment before carcinomas develop.[11] In still other instances, strain differences or the interaction between the infectious agent and environmental factors, host factors, or both might help determine the rate of carcinogenic progression.[10]

The identified oncogenic infectious agents share at least four characteristics: the ability to establish chronic infection, the actual establishment of chronic infection in those individuals destined to develop malignancy attributable to the infection, an interval of many years between the initial infection and the development of malignancy, and a benign (i.e., nonmalignant) outcome for most infected individuals. These characteristics imply that cancer attributable to infectious agents develops only after prolonged infection and that a malignant outcome arises only after the development of infection-dependent changes in the host.

Consistent with current concepts of the multistep nature of carcinogenesis, the changes in the host probably involve genetic alterations in potential target cells, impairment of the immune system, or both. Because not all infectious agents that establish a

TABLE 61.1-2. Cancers Attributable to Infection: Estimate of Worldwide Distribution According to Type (Annual Number of Cases in Thousands)[a]

Tumor Type	Developed Countries	Developing Countries	World	Percentage of Tumor Type Attributable to Infection
Stomach cancer	202	294	497	56
Cervical cancer	80	336	416	88
Liver cancer	47	352	399	81
Kaposi's sarcoma in acquired immunodeficiency syndrome	16	28	44	—
Vulvar cancer	10	21	31	88
Hodgkin's disease	12	18	30	49
Bladder cancer	0	10	10	3
Non-Hodgkin's lymphoma in acquired immunodeficiency syndrome	4	4	9	—
Gastric lymphoma	3	5	8	76
Burkitt's lymphoma	0	8	8	81
Leukemias	1	2	3	—
Cholangiocarcinoma	0	1	1	—

[a]Figures in each column represent the estimated number of cases of that tumor type attributed to infection, except for the column on the right, which represents the percentage of all cancers of that type worldwide attributed to an infectious cause.
(Adapted from ref. 2.)

chronic infection are carcinogenic, chronic infection with agents not implicated in carcinogenesis must be much less efficient in inducing the types of changes that lead to cancer than are those agents that are implicated in carcinogenesis.

Infection seems to induce tumors by three main mechanisms, either singly or in combination, depending on the agent. In some instances, such as with HPV, the agent infects the potential target cell population and induces a series of changes from within those cells that lead to cancer.[12] Some of the changes may include alterations in the agent itself, so that only a subset of its genetic information is expressed. The viral genes that continue to be expressed contribute directly to the tumorigenic phenotype by, for example, inactivating the activity of tumor suppressor genes.

In a second scenario, as occurs with *H pylori*, the infectious agent is present in the target tissue and induces cancer by local effects, usually chronic inflammation, but the agent remains outside the tumor cells.[13,14] By the time the tumor is capable of distant metastasis, if not sooner, its growth becomes independent of the infectious agent.

The third mechanism, which is more indirect, results in increased tumor risk secondary to suppression of the host immune system. This process has been identified in tumors that arise as a consequence of infection with the human immunodeficiency virus (HIV), which predisposes infected individuals to a variety of tumors.[15] Because the immunosuppression associated with HIV renders patients much more susceptible to chronic infection with other agents, including those with oncogenic potential, many of the tumors result from the combined effects of coinfection with HIV and these other agents.

PROPHYLACTIC VERSUS THERAPEUTIC VACCINATION

Vaccination against an infectious oncogenic agent can be contemplated in three possible clinical settings: as a prophylactic vaccine to prevent infection or acute disease, as a therapeutic vaccine to treat an established infection before a malignancy has been induced, and as a therapeutic vaccine to treat the infection after the malignant tumor has developed, as long as the tumor still depends on the presence of the infectious agent. The use of vaccines in the treatment of cancer is covered in Chapter 61.2.

An ideal vaccine would be effective both in preventing and in treating premalignant disease, as well as in reducing the likelihood of transmission of the agent to uninfected individuals. The long interval between the initial infection and cancer development means that there is a relatively long opportunity to identify and treat the infected population. In addition, it is usually easier to carry out therapeutic clinical trials that determine efficacy than to conduct prophylactic trials. A therapeutic vaccine trial can limit its enrollment to infected individuals at a particular stage of disease, and the response to vaccine can be evaluated, usually within a short period, by suppression of infection and of the disease. A vaccine with therapeutic efficacy would also have the advantage of reducing the incidence of malignant disease much sooner than a prophylactic vaccine, because the ability to target people with active infection intervenes much later in the infectious process than a purely prophylactic vaccine, which must be given before exposure to

the agent. These considerations underscore the potential usefulness of determining whether successes with therapeutic vaccines in experimental animal systems, such as vaccines against *H pylori*[16,21] and papillomaviruses,[17,18] can be achieved in people.

Despite these theoretical advantages of vaccines with therapeutic efficacy, the challenge to develop such vaccines remains formidable. It has proven easier to develop prophylactic vaccines against infectious agents than therapeutic ones. Of the more than 20 approved vaccines in the United States, all are approved for prevention, rather than treatment, of established infection.[19]

The comparative ease with which prophylactic vaccines can be developed, relative to the continuing difficulties of therapeutic vaccine development, makes prophylactic vaccination an important approach for cancer vaccines. Another advantage of prophylactic vaccines is that they do not depend on identifying individuals with premalignant disease. Furthermore, worldwide public health vaccine efforts are designed primarily for the administration of prophylactic vaccines, and this vaccine approach has been extremely successful and highly cost-effective in combating many infectious diseases. In addition, the primary disease induced by some oncogenic infectious agents, such as HBV and HBC, can provide sufficient rationale for development of a prophylactic vaccine, in addition to the long-term prevention of cancer.

Several theoretical and practical concerns arise in developing a prophylactic vaccine. Safety is especially important for a vaccine whose primary goal is to prevent cancer, because many individuals will never be infected by the agent, the majority of infected individuals will never develop malignancy, and malignancy only develops many years after infection. In addition, many years are required to determine whether a candidate prophylactic vaccine can prevent cancer. The minimum theoretical duration of efficacy trials whose end point is prevention of malignancy is the length of the latent period between infection and malignancy. Thus, although many studies have shown that HBV vaccination is highly effective in preventing acute disease (hepatitis), there is much less documentation that this vaccine actually reduces the frequency of hepatocellular carcinoma.[5,10]

Although cancer prevention might appear to be a necessary end point for establishing the efficacy of a cancer vaccine, there can be serious ethical obstacles to using this clinical end point. For those clinical situations in which the standard of care involves the treatment of premalignant lesions to prevent the development of malignancy, as with cervical abnormalities identified on Pap smear screening, it may be unethical to delay treatment until cancer develops. In addition, once a vaccine has been shown to be effective in preventing infection, it might be considered unethical to withhold the vaccine from the control group, despite the possible ambiguities such vaccination might create for efforts to determine directly whether the vaccine could reduce cancer frequency.

For those oncogenic infectious agents (see Table 61.1-1) that induce nonmalignant diseases which carry significant morbidity and economic cost long before they cause cancer, it may be more practical to use a nonmalignant end point in efforts to demonstrate efficacy, with the effect on cancer being determined, directly or indirectly, by follow-up studies. This was the approach taken with the HBV vaccine, which has been approved for use in the United States because of its ability to prevent acute hepatitis. However, the presumption that the vaccine would prevent many liver cancers attributable to HBV infection was also considered in recommending widespread use of the vaccine.

The most critical information for vaccine development is the knowledge of which antigens can induce protective immunity. For HBV, many aspects of its immunology and its role in carcinogenesis remain incompletely understood, but identification of a *protective* viral antigen was able to lead to development of an effective vaccine.[10,20]

It appears to be easier to develop vaccines against agents such as HBV and HPV whose natural history in most individuals is characterized by self-limited infection and long-term resistance to reinfection. A successful vaccine can induce protective immunity against these agents by mimicking key aspects of the effective immune response to natural infection. By contrast, it is much more challenging to develop vaccines against agents such as *H pylori*[13,16,21] and hepatitis C virus,[22] for which infection is commonly lifelong and resolution of the infection is not associated with long-term resistance to reinfection. A successful vaccine against these agents, therefore, has the added burden of inducing an immune response that is substantially more effective than the response to natural infection.

In natural infection, the cellular and humoral arms of the immune system generally function together either to interfere with the initial phases of infection or to eradicate established infection. Antibodies capable of neutralizing the infectious agent appear to be the prime effectors in preventing infection, whereas CD8+ T cells usually serve more critical roles in the resolution of established infection.[9,23] The success of prophylactic vaccines in inducing long-term protection against infection probably lies primarily in their ability to induce neutralizing antibodies, although other immune components probably also contribute to their overall effectiveness.

HEPATITIS B VIRUS

The identification of HBV in the 1960s led to epidemiologic studies that have clarified its worldwide role in hepatocellular cancer.[10,20,24–26] Although infection with this DNA virus can cause acute hepatitis, its most serious global consequences are chronic hepatitis, cirrhosis, and hepatocellular carcinoma, all of which are associated with chronic HBV infection. It is estimated that there are more than 1 million chronic HBV carriers in the United States and more than 300 million carriers throughout the world. The virus is believed to account for approximately 1 million deaths per year worldwide, about one-half of them secondary to hepatocellular carcinoma.

In highly endemic areas, the lifetime risk of exposure may exceed 50%, and most HBV infections occur perinatally or in early childhood. In areas of low endemicity, HBV transmission occurs mainly in adults, often via sexual exposure or parenteral exposure from infected shared needles used with illicit drugs. The risk of medical exposure to infected blood products has been greatly reduced by systematic screening of these materials for HBV.

The HBV carrier state, which is a measure of persistent infection, is a critical determinant of the long-term risk for hepatocellular carcinoma. HBV carrier rates vary dramatically in different populations, from less than 0.5% in the United States and many other countries with high standards of living to 10% to 20% in parts of Africa, Asia, and the South Pacific. The relative incidence of cancer attributable to HBV follows a similar geographic distribution, with many studies consistently showing that chronic HBV infection is an important risk factor for hepatocellular carcinoma.

The frequency with which persistent HBV infection is established varies inversely with the age at exposure. The highest risk by far occurs during the perinatal period and the first year of life. More than 70% of neonates born to infected mothers become chronic carriers, compared with around 8% of those exposed at 3 years of age and an even lower proportion in immunocompetent adults.[10]

Conversely, HBV is much more likely to induce acute hepatitis in older age groups, whereas acute infection is usually asymptomatic when exposure occurs in the perinatal period. This difference occurs because the acute hepatic disease results from the immune response to infection, as HBV does not directly induce hepatocellular damage. Thus, the relative immunoincompetence of infants probably accounts for their lack of symptoms and for the high frequency with which the virus establishes persistent infection in this age group.

The precise role of the virus in the development of hepatocellular carcinoma has not been fully determined. Persistent infection appears to lead to cancer mainly as the result of chronic inflammation and repeated cellular regeneration, and some evidence implicates the viral X gene, which encodes a transcription factor, in this process.[27] Most cases of liver cancer associated with HBV infection arise after chronic hepatitis has led to cirrhosis. Hepatocellular carcinoma may develop after as few as 5 to 10 years of infection, but it does not usually occur until an individual has been infected for at least 20 to 30 years. Ongoing infection continues to be a risk factor for carcinoma, with an estimated cumulative risk of 15% for an individual who has had persistent infection for 50 years.[10]

The rate of hepatocellular carcinoma attributable to HBV is at least three times higher in males than in females, even when a similar proportion of males and females are exposed to HBV. The difference is explained in part by the higher frequency with which the HBV carrier state is established in males (close to 2:1) and the greater likelihood of females to eliminate the carrier state.

The HBV vaccine is the prototype prophylactic vaccine against an oncogenic infectious agent. A key to HBV vaccine development was the recognition that the neutralizing antibodies were directed against the hepatitis B surface antigen (HB$_s$Ag), and that there is only one HBV serotype. The HB$_s$Ag is expressed in relatively pure form as circulating enveloped virus-like particles (VLPs) in the blood of infected HBV carriers. The HB$_s$Ag particles do not carry the viral genome and are not infectious. It was possible to purify the particles, inactivate possibly contaminating infectious virus with formalin (which should also have inactivated other viruses), and test the particles as a subunit vaccine in human clinical trials, which were initiated in 1975.

The HB$_s$Ag vaccine was well tolerated, induced an immune response in almost all those receiving it, and reduced the infection rate in adults by at least 95% and in neonates by at least 85%. The protection rates in neonates may be further increased by giving hepatitis B immunoglobulin in addition to the vaccine. The vaccine was licensed in the United States in 1981.

An analogous HB$_s$Ag particle vaccine has been produced in yeast by recombinant DNA technology, and it was licensed in the United States in 1986. The recombinant vaccine has replaced the blood-derived vaccine, although the immunogenic properties of the latter product are somewhat superior to those of the recombinant material. Efficacy trials have shown that the recombinant vaccine confers a similar rate of protection against HBV as the blood-derived vaccine.[10] In addition, the recombinant vaccine is less expensive to manufacture and does not have the theoretical concern of contaminating infectious material, although extensive analysis of the blood-derived vaccine recipients failed to document excess exposure to infectious agents.

The initial series of immunizations with either vaccine preparation confers protection against infection for at least several years. In instances in which breakthrough infection has occurred, it has not been associated with development of a chronic carrier state. Routine revaccination is not recommended at this time by vaccine advisory groups in the United States. Further studies, in progress, should determine whether this policy should remain in place or be modified.

The long interval between HBV infection and the development of hepatocellular carcinoma means that only limited data thus far indicate directly that vaccination can actually decrease the incidence of cancer attributable to HBV. Data from an HBV vaccination program in Taiwan, an area with high HBV endemicity where universal vaccination was instituted in 1984, do show such a reduction in children.[5,6] From 1990 to 1994, the incidence of cancer in children aged 6 to 14 years was one-half the rate before vaccination was implemented, and that for children aged 6 to 9 years was only one-fourth the rate of the earlier period.

These results indicate that HBV vaccination can achieve the long-term goal of cancer reduction. However, such a reduction will occur only if the populations most at risk are given the vaccine in a timely manner. Even in such a setting, reduction in cancer among adults, in whom the incidence is highest, would not be expected to be seen until these children reach adulthood.

HUMAN PAPILLOMAVIRUS

Papillomaviruses are epitheliotropic agents that induce benign papillomas of the skin and mucous membranes.[12,28] In contrast to HBV, there are more than 100 HPV genotypes (types).[29] A subset of HPV types that are almost always transmitted sexually is the main cause of human cervical cancer. Infection with these HPV types is a strong risk factor for cervical cancer, and HPV DNA from one or more of these types is found in virtually all cervical tumors.[30–32] The virus encodes oncoproteins that appear to be required both for the induction and the maintenance of the cancer.[12]

HPV infection has also been linked to the majority of anal cancers, in which the molecular pathogenesis seems to be similar to that of cervical cancer, as well as to other anogenital malignancies and to tumors of the upper aerodigestive tract.[33,34] The precise relationship between HPV infection and the development of some of these cancers is not as firmly established as that between HPV infection and cervical cancer.

As with HBV, cancer attributable to HPV develops only after many years of persistent HPV infection and is an infrequent outcome of infection. Cervical HPV infection is remarkably common, with sensitive polymerase chain reaction assays indicating prevalence rates of 20% to 40% among young sexually active women. Most infections are self-limited, and clinical cures are associated with resistance to reinfection. The antigenic divergence between HPV types is such that protection appears to be largely type specific.

The HPVs associated with cervical and anal cancer are usually designated as high-risk types, as contrasted with the low-risk types, which also participate in anogenital infection but are almost never found in cervical or anal cancers.[12,35] Although there are several high-risk HPV types, HPV-16 is the most common type, being present in more than one-half of cervical cancers worldwide. HPV-18 is second in frequency. The viral E6 and E7 genes of the high-risk types are preferentially retained and expressed in the tumors, where they inactivate the p53 and Rb tumor suppressor proteins, respectively.

In principle, cervical cancer is already a largely preventable disease. In countries in which Pap smear screening reaches most women, the incidence of cervical cancer has decreased markedly.[36] In the United States, for example, the rate of cervical cancer has decreased several-fold since the 1950s, from more than 50 in 100,000 to less than 10 in 100,000. This decrease in cancer rates is even more impressive because it has occurred during a period in which increased sexual promiscuity has been associated with an increased frequency of genital HPV infection.

The cost of Pap smear screening and follow-up is high (estimated to be more than $5 billion annually in the United States), however, and Pap smear screening is not routinely available in many less well-developed countries. This situation has made cervical cancer the leading cancer among women in many developing countries, and it remains the third most common female cancer worldwide.[37]

Establishing the etiologic link between HPV infection and cervical cancer (and other tumors) has focused interest on developing an HPV vaccine.[38,39] The main goal would be to reduce the incidence of cervical cancer, which accounts for approximately 75% of the cancers worldwide attributable to HPV infection (see Table 61.1-1).[2] Because cervical cancer is especially prevalent in developing countries, such a vaccine would potentially have its greatest public health effect in these populations. In the United States, an effective HPV vaccine might reduce the incidence of cervical cancer below its current level by reaching populations that do not receive adequate Pap screening. In addition, widespread vaccine use in the United States would be expected to decrease the frequency of genital HPV infection and thereby reduce the number of cervical dysplasias requiring treatment and the overall cost of cervical cancer screening programs. Thus, fewer women would need to deal with the personal, social, medical, and economic issues associated with a diagnosis of genital HPV infection and the conditions it causes.

Because papillomaviruses contain oncogenes, and a prophylactic vaccine would be directed toward healthy young individuals, efforts to develop a prophylactic vaccine have emphasized a subunit approach, analogous to that used for HBV vaccine.[38,39] Indeed, constitutive high-level expression of the L1 major structural viral protein, even in nonmammalian cells, leads to its efficient self-assembly into VLPs that resemble authentic viral capsids structurally and antigenically. Preparative amounts of VLPs can be synthesized in insect cells or yeast. Such VLPs are suitable immunogens that, as is true of authentic virions, possess the immunodominant conformational epitopes capable of raising high titers of neutralizing antibodies.

Because papillomaviruses are species-specific, animal papillomavirus models have been used preclinically to evaluate VLPs as a candidate subunit prophylactic vaccine.[38] Excellent results (90% to 100% protection, even without adjuvant, against high-dose virus challenge) have been obtained with systemic immunization in three models, one cutaneous and two oral mucosal. The neutralizing antibodies induced by the vaccine appear to be largely responsible for the protection, which can last at least 1 year. Excellent protection was also reported in the cutaneous animal model when a vaccinia vector was used to express L1 or when the L1 gene was injected as naked DNA. However, administration of protein seems more likely to be readily accepted by regulatory authorities in developed countries.

Early safety and immunogenicity trials in which healthy human volunteers were injected intramuscularly with HPV-11 and HPV-16 L1 VLPs showed that the vaccines, with or without adjuvant, were well tolerated and induced antibody titers comparable with the protective levels induced in animals.[40,41] Vaccine-induced antibodies have also been demonstrated at the cervix, with relatively constant levels seen at that site in women taking hormonal contraceptives but with substantial fluctuation in titer during the menstrual cycle in ovulating women.[42]

These encouraging findings have been greatly extended by a double-blind, placebo-controlled, proof-of-principle efficacy trial of a candidate HPV-16 L1 VLP vaccine (manufactured by Merck) given intramuscularly with alum as an adjuvant, in which the vaccine conferred complete protection against persistent HPV-16 infection.[7] The reported interim analysis encompassed approximately 1500 young women, divided equally between the placebo group (alum alone) and the group that received the vaccine. The women in both groups, who were HPV DNA negative before vaccination and remained HPV DNA negative throughout the vaccination period, were monitored for the acquisition of genital HPV DNA during an average of 17.4 months after vaccination. Among the placebo group during this postvaccination period, there were 41 cases of acquired persistent HPV-16 infection (defined primarily as positive HPV-16 DNA test results on genital samples taken at least 4 months apart). By contrast, there were no cases of persistent HPV-16 infection in the vaccinated group. Because persistent HPV infection is closely related to the development of high-grade cervical dysplasia, these impressive results are believed to represent strong presumptive evidence that the vaccine will eventually be able to reduce the incidence of cervical cancer attributable to HPV-16.

If the efficacy of the HPV-16 L1 VLP vaccine is attributable to neutralizing antibodies, the type-specific nature of these antibodies implies that one potential disadvantage of the L1 VLP vaccine is that protection is also likely to be type-specific. This question was not addressed in the interim analysis of the efficacy trial, which did not report the incidence of infection by HPV types other than HPV-16. However, the observed distribution of (mainly low-grade) cervical dysplasia cases between the placebo group and the vaccinated group is consistent with the vaccine protection being largely type-specific. Although each of the 9 cases of cervical dysplasia associated with HPV-16 infection was found in the placebo group, the 44 cases of cervical dysplasia not associated with HPV-16 were divided evenly between the placebo and vaccine groups. Interim analysis of an independent

double-blind, placebo-controlled, proof-of-principle trial of a bivalent vaccine composed of HPV-16 and HPV-18 VLPs with AS04 as adjuvant (manufactured by GlaxoSmithKline) also reported complete protection against persistent infection of the two HPV types targeted by the vaccine.

The positive results with both proof-of-principle trials are being followed up with large-scale phase III efficacy trials of candidate polyvalent HPV L1 VLP vaccines that will be given to thousands of women, who will be followed for several years. One trial tests the GlaxoSmithKline bivalent HPV-16 and HPV-18 vaccine with AS04 adjuvant. The other trial tests a quadrivalent vaccine manufactured by Merck, composed of VLPs for HPV-16, HPV-18, HPV-6, and HPV-11 with alum as an adjuvant. It therefore targets the two HPV types responsible for the majority of genital warts, HPV-6 and HPV-11, in addition to the cervical cancer–causing types HPV-16 and HPV-18. The goals of each trial include determining whether the candidate vaccine can reduce the incidence of precancerous lesions (moderate- and high-grade cervical dysplasia) attributable to HPV-16 and HPV-18, in addition to protecting against persistent infection by these HPV types. The duration of protection will also be assessed. In addition, the quadrivalent vaccine might be found to confer protection against genital infection attributable to HPV-6 and HPV-11.

As noted earlier in Prophylactic versus Therapeutic Vaccination, cervical cancer cannot be used as an end point for the trials, because it is unethical to allow cervical lesions arising in women in a vaccine study population to progress to malignancy. A cancer end point would also require more than 20 years to establish, given the long interval between infection and cancer. Fortunately, the surrogate end points of persistent HPV infection and high-grade cervical dysplasia have been shown to be tightly linked to the risk of progression to invasive cancer.[32,36]

If the phase III vaccine trials produce positive results that lead to licensure by the U.S. Food and Drug Administration, it will be important to develop policies regarding the appropriate age for vaccination of women and to determine whether men should also be vaccinated. It is likely that young adolescent girls will be the main target group to receive the vaccine. For males, it would be useful to document that administering the vaccine to men actually reduces their incidence of infection with the targeted HPV types, because such evidence would support the rationale for widespread vaccination of males.

The anticipated type specificity of protection will probably lead vaccine manufacturers to broaden the HPV coverage of the vaccines by adding VLPs from more HPV types to the vaccine, if the vaccines being tested in the phase III trials currently are eventually licensed. It will presumably be necessary to show that such additions do not impair the immunogenicity of the VLPs in the parent vaccine.

Despite the promise of the VLP vaccines, alternative approaches are being considered.[17,18,39] Some approaches, such as mucosal immunization with purified VLPs or use of nonpathogenic enteric bacteria that express L1 protein, might be easier to deliver as a prophylactic vaccine in the developing world. It should also be noted that the current candidate prophylactic vaccines are not expected to benefit the approximately 5 million women with existing HPV infection who are destined over the next 20 years to develop cervical cancers from which they will die. For these women, it will be necessary to develop an effective therapeutic vaccine, ideally one that might also have prophylactic activity. Vaccines composed of nonstructural viral proteins, with or without VLPs, have been shown to prevent and, in some cases, treat animal papillomavirus infection, in addition to working in tumorigenic models with cells that express a papillomavirus protein. Some purely therapeutic candidates are currently undergoing trials.

HELICOBACTER PYLORI

H pylori, which was discovered in 1982, induces chronic gastric infection in almost one-half of the world population. Infection with *H pylori* is associated with a variable proportion of several disorders, including duodenal ulcer, gastric ulcer, gastric carcinoma (which is the second most common cancer worldwide), and gastric mucosa–associated lymphoid tissue lymphoma.[2,13,14,43]

H pylori infection is usually acquired in childhood. It disproportionately affects people of lower socioeconomic status, and the majority of adults from developing countries are infected. The bacterium is found less frequently among individuals in developed countries such as the United States, and the low rate of infection in children in developed countries suggests that the proportion in adults will continue to fall.

Most *H pylori* infections are asymptomatic and have a benign outcome. When infection does lead to stomach cancer, it usually takes decades. In this process, bacterially induced chronic gastritis is believed to progress to atrophic gastritis and metaplasia, and then to cancer. The bacterium appears to be required only until atrophic gastritis develops. Experimental *H pylori* infection of Mongolian gerbils can induce these sequential pathologic changes, including gastric adenocarcinoma.[44]

Gastric mucosa–associated lymphoid tissue lymphoma is much less common than gastric carcinoma and has a distinct pathogenesis.[14] This B-cell lymphoma arises from *H pylori*–dependent chronic stimulation of Peyer's patches in the gastric mucosa. Localized mucosa-associated lymphoid tissue tumors often remain dependent on continued stimulation by bacterial antigens, and eradication of the bacteria with antibiotic treatment may frequently be associated with lymphoma regression at this stage. However, the growth of more invasive tumors, which may become widely disseminated, is usually autonomous, and these tumors typically do not respond to antibacterial therapy.

Several bacterial virulence factors account for the ability of *H pylori* to colonize and persist in the gastric mucosa.[13,16,21] Although different isolates of *H pylori* are closely related antigenically, those associated with carcinoma contain a cassette of genes that are designated as a pathogenicity-associated island whose marker is a cytotoxin-associated antigen (CagA).

In principle, *H pylori* infection can be eradicated by combined treatment with several antimicrobial agents plus proton pump inhibitors. However, the high cost of treatment and the emergence of antibiotic resistance make this approach poorly suited for bacterial eradication from whole populations. These limitations have fostered efforts to develop *H pylori* vaccines.[13,16] However, although humoral and cellular immune responses develop in most infected individuals, it is uncommon for these infections to disappear spontaneously, and reinfection may occur after successful antibiotic treatment. These characteristics of *H pylori* infection, combined with imperfect animal models, pose a challenge to successful vaccine development. However, in preclinical vaccine studies, responses have been obtained with animal models. Mucosal immunization with bacterial lysates, purified bacterial antigens, or attenuated salmonellae encoding *H pylori* antigen can all prevent experimental infection. Some of these vaccines have also had some success in eradicating established infection in the animal models. It remains to be determined which of these approaches will prove efficacious in human vaccine trials. Thus far, results of clinical trials of single antigens have been disappointing, and efforts are under way to test vaccines consisting of several antigens. The most desirable outcome would be development of a cost-effective vaccine that could eradicate established infection while also protecting against new infections. Such a vaccine would have the long-term benefits of a purely prophylactic vaccine while reducing the incidence of gastric cancer after a much shorter interval.

REFERENCES

1. Ames BN, Gold LS. The prevention of cancer. *Drug Metab Rev* 1998;30:201.
2. Pisani P, Parkin DM, Munoz N, Ferlay J. Cancer and infection: estimates of the attributable fraction in 1990. *Cancer Epidemiol Biomarkers Prev* 1997;6:387.
3. Montesano R, Hall J. Environmental causes of human cancers. *Eur J Cancer* 2001;37[Suppl 8]:S67.
4. Persing DH, Prendergast FG. Infection, immunity, and cancer. *Arch Pathol Lab Med* 1999;123:1015.
5. Chang MH, Chen CJ, Lai MS, et al. Universal hepatitis B vaccination in Taiwan and the incidence of hepatocellular carcinoma in children. Taiwan Childhood Hepatoma Study Group [see comments]. *N Engl J Med* 1997;336:1855.
6. Lee CL, Hsieh KS, Ko YC. Trends in the incidence of hepatocellular carcinoma in boys and girls in Taiwan after large-scale hepatitis B vaccination. *Cancer Epidemiol Biomarkers Prev* 2003;12:57.
7. Koutsky LA, Ault KA, Wheeler CM, et al. A controlled trial of a human papillomavirus type 16 vaccine. *N Engl J Med* 2002;347:1645.
8. Hilleman MR. Overview of viruses, cancer, and vaccines in concept and in reality. *Recent Results Cancer Res* 1998;154:345.
9. Murphy BR, Chanock RM. Immunization against viral diseases. In: Knipe DM, Howley PH, eds. *Fields virology*. Philadelphia: Lippincott Williams & Wilkins, 2001:435.
10. Hollinger FB, Liang TJ. Hepatitis B viruses. In: Knipe DM, Howley PH, eds. *Fields virology*. Philadelphia: Lippincott Williams & Wilkins, 2001:2971.
11. Rinas AC. The gynecological Pap test. *Clin Lab Sci* 1999;12:239.
12. Lowy DR, Howley PH. Papillomaviruses. In: Knipe DM, Howley PH, eds. *Fields virology*. Philadelphia: Lippincott Williams & Wilkins, 2001:2231.
13. Sutton P, Doidge C. *Helicobacter pylori* vaccines spiral into the new millennium. *Dig Liver Dis* 2003;35:675.
14. Du MQ. Molecular biology of gastric MALT lymphoma: application in clinical management. *Hematology* 2002;7:339.
15. Scadden DT. AIDS-related malignancies. *Annu Rev Med* 2003;54:285.
16. Ruggiero P, Peppoloni S, Rappuoli R, Del Giudice G. The quest for a vaccine against *Helicobacter pylori*: how to move from mouse to man? *Microbes Infect* 2003;5:749.
17. Fausch SC, Da Silva DM, Eiben GL, Le Poole IC, Kast WM. HPV protein/peptide vaccines: from animal models to clinical trials. *Front Biosci* 2003;8:s81.
18. Stanley MA. Progress in prophylactic and therapeutic vaccines for human papillomavirus infection. *Expert Rev Vaccines* 2003;2:381.
19. Plotkin SA, Orenstein WA, Offit PA, eds. *Vaccines.* Philadelphia: WB Saunders, 2004.
20. Blumberg BS. Hepatitis B virus, the vaccine, and the control of primary cancer of the liver. *Proc Natl Acad Sci U S A* 1997;94:7121.
21. Prinz C, Hafsi N, Voland P. *Helicobacter pylori* virulence factors and the host immune response: implications for therapeutic vaccination. *Trends Microbiol* 2003;11:134.
22. Forns X, Bukh J, Purcell RH. The challenge of developing a vaccine against hepatitis C virus. *J Hepatol* 2002;37:684.
23. Kaech SM, Wherry EJ, Ahmed R. Effector and memory T-cell differentiation: implications for vaccine development. *Nat Rev Immunol* 2002;2:251.
24. Beasley RP. Hepatitis B virus. The major etiology of hepatocellular carcinoma. *Cancer* 1988;61:1942.
25. International Agency for Research on Cancer. Hepatitis viruses. IARC Monographs, vol. 59. Lyon, France: IARC, 1995.
26. El-Serag HB. Hepatocellular carcinoma: an epidemiologic view. *J Clin Gastroenterol* 2002; 35:S72.
27. Chen PJ, Chen DS. Hepatitis B virus infection and hepatocellular carcinoma: molecular genetics and clinical perspectives. *Semin Liver Dis* 1999;19:253.
28. International Agency for Research on Cancer. Human papillomaviruses. IARC Monographs, vol. 64. Lyon, France: IARC, 1995.
29. de Villiers EM. Papillomavirus and HPV typing. *Clin Dermatol* 1997;15:199.

30. Bosch FX, Manos MM, Munoz N, et al. Prevalence of human papillomavirus in cervical cancer: a worldwide prospective. *J Natl Cancer Inst* 1995;87:796.

31. Walboomers JM, Jacobs MC, Manos MM, et al. Human papillomavirus is a necessary cause of invasive cervical cancer worldwide. *J Pathol* 1999;189:12.

32. Bosch FX, Lorincz A, Munoz N, Meijer CJ, Shah KV. The causal relation between human papillomavirus and cervical cancer. *J Clin Pathol* 2002;55:244.

33. Melbye M, Frisch M. The role of human papillomaviruses in anogenital cancers. *Semin Cancer Biol* 1998;8:307.

34. Gillison ML, Shah KV. Human papillomavirus–associated head and neck squamous cell carcinoma: mounting evidence for an etiologic role for human papillomavirus in a subset of head and neck cancers. *Curr Opin Oncol* 2001;13:183.

35. Lazo PA. The molecular genetics of cervical carcinoma. *Br J Cancer* 1999;80:2008.

36. Schiffman MH. New epidemiology of human papillomavirus infection and cervical neoplasia. *J Natl Cancer Inst* 1995;87:1345.

37. Parkin DM, Pisani P, Ferlay J. Estimates of worldwide incidence of 25 cancers in 1990. *Int J Cancer* 1999;80:827.

38. Lowy DR, Schiller JT. Papillomaviruses: prophylactic vaccine prospects. *Biochim Biophys Acta* 1999;1423:M1.

39. Schiller JT, Lowy DR. Human papillomavirus vaccines for cervical cancer prevention. In: Plotkin SA, Orenstein WA, Offit PA, eds. *Vaccines.* Philadelphia: WB Saunders, 2004:1259.

40. Evans TG, Bonnez W, Rose RC, et al. A phase 1 study of a recombinant viruslike particle vaccine against human papillomavirus type 11 in healthy adult volunteers. *J Infect Dis* 2001;183:1485.

41. Harro CD, Pang YY, Roden RB, et al. Safety and immunogenicity trial in adult volunteers of a human papillomavirus 16 L1 virus-like particle vaccine. *J Natl Cancer Inst* 2001;93:284.

42. Nardelli-Haefliger D, Wirthner D, Schiller JT, et al. Specific antibody levels at the cervix during the menstrual cycle of women vaccinated with human papillomavirus 16 virus-like particles. *J Natl Cancer Inst* 2003;95:1128.

43. Uemura N, Okamoto S, Yamamoto S, et al. *Helicobacter pylori* infection and the development of gastric cancer. *N Engl J Med* 2001;345:784.

44. Watanabe T, Tada M, Nagai H, Sasaki S, Nakao M. *Helicobacter pylori* infection induces gastric cancer in mongolian gerbils. *Gastroenterology* 1998;115:642.

NICHOLAS P. RESTIFO
JONATHAN J. LEWIS

SECTION 2

Therapeutic Vaccines

A decade ago, it seemed rational that the burgeoning knowledge of the molecular identities of tumor antigens and a deeper understanding of basic immunology would point the way to an effective therapeutic cancer vaccine. Significant progress has been made, and objective responses after immune-based treatments are observed in a small number of patients—even in those with bulky, metastatic disease. Notwithstanding this progress, however, we do not yet have in hand a cancer vaccine that can reliably and consistently induce tumor destruction or improve patient survival.

This chapter reviews some of the observations made in the research laboratory and the translation of these results to the clinic. The focus is on the challenges of clinical trials and the development of cancer vaccines.

ELICITATION OF TUMOR-SPECIFIC IMMUNE RESPONSES

The principle that T cells are critically important in the immune response against cancer was confirmed originally in mice with methylcholanthrene-induced tumors.[1,2] In some human and mouse malignancies, T cells within the mass of a tumor have been shown to specifically recognize autologous tumor cells *in vitro* and to proliferate and specifically secrete cytokines, chemokines, and lytic factors in response to stimulation with autologous tumor cells.[3–5] Antitumor T cells can be grown to large numbers *in vitro* and transferred adoptively to treat even substantial tumor burdens in both humans and mice.[6] Finally, tumor antigens recognized by autologous human T cells have been identified by the use of molecular cloning techniques.[7–11]

T cells use structures on their surfaces called *T-cell receptors* (TCRs) that recognize peptide fragments of antigens, termed *epitopes*, that are noncovalently complexed with major histocompatibility complex (MHC) molecules. Early mouse studies suggested that tumor rejection is largely dependent on CD8+, cytolytic T cells (CTLs). In addition, adoptive transfer of pure populations of CD8+ T lymphocytes has been shown to mediate tumor regression in humans and in mice.[12,13] Thus, most efforts to develop therapeutic anticancer vaccines have focused on CD8+ T lymphocytes. It is important to recognize, however, that CD4+ T cells play a potentially enormous role in the antitumor response in their roles as both helper cells and regulatory cells.

CD8+ T cells recognize MHC class I molecules presenting peptide epitopes that are generally 8 to 10 residues in length. These epitopes are processed from intracellular proteins and then presented on the surface of the cell by MHC molecules (Fig. 61.2-1). Antigen processing involves the cleaving of peptides from proteins within the cell, usually by a large multicatalytic structure called the proteasome. Peptides are then transported into the endoplasmic reticulum by a heterodimeric molecule called the *transporter associated with antigen processing*. In the endoplasmic reticulum, peptides form stable complexes with MHC class I molecules. After a complex of antigen and MHC completes its journey through the Golgi apparatus to the cell surface, it is potentially recognizable by a T cell.

MHC molecules (also called *HLA molecules* in humans) are very polymorphic. HLA diversity is what makes the job of the transplant surgeon so difficult—this diversity must be taken into account by the cancer immunotherapist. Many vaccine studies use patients expressing a common HLA molecule known as HLA-A*0201 (expressed in approximately 40% of the population).

IDENTIFICATION OF TUMOR-ASSOCIATED ANTIGENS SUITABLE FOR THERAPEUTIC TARGETING

A variety of techniques have been applied to identify tumor antigens recognizable by tumor-specific T cells. None has been more successful than an approach that uses transient transfection of pools of genes from a tumor-derived complementary DNA library to confer recognition on a target cell and thus identify the gene encoding the target epitope.[14,15] Although cloning efforts have been prodigiously successful, protein chemists have also made inroads into the identification of target antigens by pushing the limits of high-performance liquid chromatography and tandem mass spectrometry. Peptides can be eluted from MHC complexes derived from tumor cell membranes and characterized directly.[16] In addition, candidate tumor antigens can

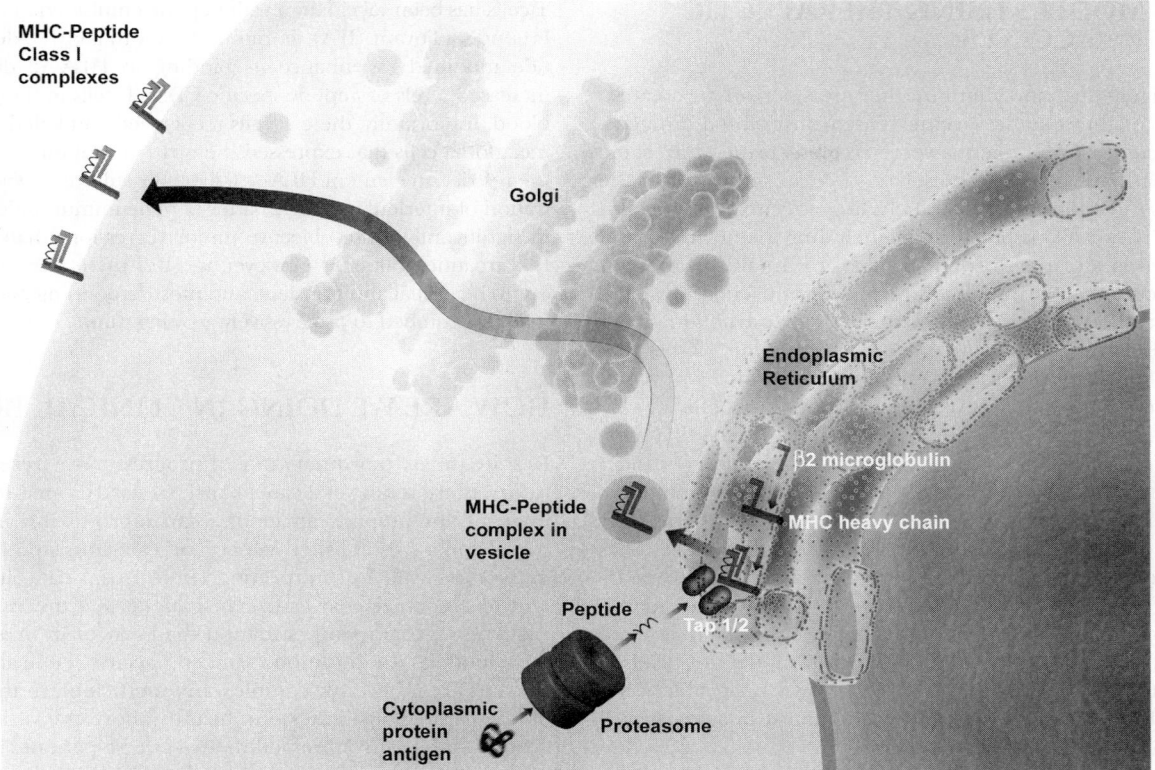

FIGURE 61.2-1. The processing and presentation of cytoplasmic antigens in the major histocompatibility complex (MHC) class I pathway (see text).

be tested by the reverse immunology method, specifically by sensitizing immune cells with the candidate antigen and then testing the ability of sensitized cells to kill tumor cells that are known to express the antigen.

To date, dozens of MHC class I (and class II)–associated tumor antigens have been discovered. It is difficult to know from merely reading the available literature how many of these candidate tumor antigens are actually suitable targets for tumor immunotherapy. A valid target antigen for T-cell–based therapy must be processed and presented in the context of MHC molecules. Given the low numbers of available MHC molecules on a cell's surface and the large numbers of possible peptides in the proteome, the chances that any given peptide will be presented on the tumor cell surface are low (probably less than 1%).[17] Therefore, it is clearly not enough to assume that the mere identification of the expression of a mutated candidate antigen will result in the MHC-restricted presentation of that antigen on the tumor cell surface.

The need for positive and negative control tumor lines is often overlooked. Rigorous (and numerous) controls are needed to convincingly demonstrate that a candidate antigen is a suitable target for use in an immunotherapy trial. This antigen must also be expressed with some specificity by the tumor, either because tumors express the antigen at levels sufficiently higher than in vital organs or because the antigen is differentially processed and presented by the tumor.

Despite these practical and theoretical concerns, there are many antigens that have been convincingly shown to be valid targets for immunotherapy.[18] The success of tumor antigen identification approaches put to rest the notion that spontaneous human tumors—unlike their experimental mouse counterparts—simply lacked the expression of antigens recognizable by the immune system.

ENHANCEMENT OF TUMOR ANTIGEN IMMUNOGENICITY BY MODIFICATION OF EPITOPE SEQUENCES

Tumor antigens in their original form generally bind poorly to their restricting MHC molecules. In addition, peripheral autoreactive T-cell precursors recognize their cognate peptide–MHC complexes with low affinity. Thus, most tumor antigens identified so far are poorly immunogenic *in vivo*. Dramatic increases in the magnitude of T-cell responses and sensitivity to antigen stimulation have been observed in both human and mouse models using agonistic altered peptide ligands. These altered peptides are capable of enhancing the stability of a peptide–MHC complex because of modifications in the MHC anchor residues[19] or because of favorable and generally conservative changes to peptide at the interface with the TCR.[20] Most importantly, the enhanced T-cell responses can retain their specificity to the native antigen, which allows them to kill target tumor cells measured by *ex vivo* assays. In a clinical trial using anchor-modified gp100 peptide immunization in melanoma patients, a dramatic increase of tumor-reactive T-cell response was seen.[21] Thus, antigenic peptide modified on the basis of these ideas could be of significant value in vaccination against tolerant or weakly immunogenic tumor cells.

EARLY MODELS USING THERAPEUTIC CANCER VACCINES

With antigens in hand, immunotherapists set off to create a new class of therapeutic vaccines based on defined antigens. Recombinant immunogens were created using the same viruses that have proven themselves to be so successful in the realm of infectious diseases, including vaccinia, polio, and influenza A, as well as some others, including adenoviruses and bird poxviruses (canarypox and fowlpox).[22] In animal models, these vaccines can prime T-cell responses and elicit powerful immune responses that lead to tumor cell destruction. However, when these viruses were tried in the clinic, it became apparent that experiments in animal models failed to predict key aspects of recombinant vaccine function in people.

One reason for these disappointing results may be that most of the preclinical animal data relied on prevention-of-cancer designs (i.e., the vaccine is given before the tumor is even established). In those animal studies that employ a therapeutic design, the tumors used are often tiny, even microscopic. Studies with a therapeutic design often "treat" tumors that are established for a very brief period of time (generally a few days). Experimental tumors treated shortly after transplantation are generally not vascularized and thus do not model any realistic clinical situation, in which even a small tumor imageable using computed tomography or magnetic resonance imaging is well vascularized.

Another potential problem that has been uncovered in early clinical trials is immunity to an antigenically complex vaccine that is immunodominant over a response to a transgene-encoded weak tumor antigen. This problem was not adequately studied in early experimental animal models, and it remains exceedingly difficult to model in ongoing preclinical work. This problem may be summarized as follows: Vectors may interfere with the induction of reactivity to the encoded tumor antigen through the poorly understood mechanisms of immunodominance. T-cell responses elicited by protein immunization tend to focus on one or a few sites in the antigen. Whether this phenomenon is driven by the predetermined TCR repertoire or the competition among T cells based on their affinity to antigenic determinants or the characteristics of antigen processing is not known. In viral vector–based vaccines, self-antigens are coexpressed with viral proteins. If the immunodominant sites reside in the viral components, the vaccine will fail to elicit the desired immune responses.

CONSISTENT INCREASES IN TUMOR-SPECIFIC T CELLS WITHOUT CONSISTENT CLINICAL RESPONSES

There is now incontrovertible evidence that the frequencies of precursors of tumor-specific T cells can be increased after immunization using several different tumor-associated antigens, including those antigens that are nonmutated "self" tissue differentiation antigens.[21] The presence of increased antitumor T-cell precursors after vaccination has been convincingly demonstrated in both mice and humans, using tetramer or enzyme-linked immunospot (ELISPOT) analysis or real-time reverse transcriptase-polymerase chain reaction, among other techniques.

Thus far, in patients with advanced melanoma studied at the National Cancer Institute, the strategy most effective for increasing T cells has been vaccination with peptide emulsified in incomplete Freund's adjuvant (IFA). Immunization with a gp100-derived peptide modified to enhance its binding to HLA-A2 dramatically increased levels of peptide-specific CD8+ T cells in the peripheral blood. Importantly, these T cells recognized and killed a variety of melanoma cells that expressed the gp100 melanoma antigen and the restriction element HLA-A*0201 after culture *ex vivo*. Administration of interleukin-2 (IL-2) after peptide immunization resulted in significantly more objective tumor regressions than seen after IL-2 treatment alone.[21] However, most of these responses turned out to be partial and transient, and most responding patients eventually succumbed to progressively growing tumor.

HOW ARE WE DOING IN CLINICAL TRIALS?

Despite the extraordinary rate of progress in the research laboratory, there is not yet a cancer vaccine used alone for the treatment of any human cancer that can reproducibly induce the regression of established cancer or can consistently prolong patient survival. In interpreting clinical trial data, it is important to recognize that cancer in patients is a much more heterogeneous therapeutic situation than cancer in *in vitro* and *in vivo* models. In addition, cancer vaccine clinical trials in patients are inherently complex and inefficient. In the absence of clinical response rates significantly above the variable background rate that is observed in any diverse patient cohort, it is often difficult to accurately interpret data. Furthermore, any end point other than objective clinical response or patient survival in a randomized trial should be used with caution.

There are several differences between therapeutic cancer vaccines and chemotherapeutic agents that have important implications for the design of early clinical trials.[23] Most vaccines are innately safe and do not require phase I dose-finding trials. Many investigators maintain that it is more practical to treat patients with intact immune systems and cancers that are likely to recur but that are not clinically evident (adjuvant setting) with either single or escalating doses of the candidate vaccine. Others argue that the treatment of patients with no measurable disease unnecessarily lengthens the evaluation of a clinical response and that induction of objective responses in patients with measurable disease is a more efficient way to evaluate the effectiveness of a cancer vaccine.

Due to human heterogeneity, clinical trials are less efficient than laboratory studies. Because of this inefficiency, animal models may be useful in the optimization of vaccine schedule, mode of delivery, adjuvants, and cofactor molecules. Unfortunately, there are no good, consistent models in which large, established, nonimmunogenic tumors can be induced to regress using a cancer vaccine given alone.[12] Most successful cancer vaccine models in mice are based on the prevention of challenge or the treatment of tiny tumor burdens.

Comparison of results for a new vaccine regimen with results for a control group from a previous trial is hazardous, especially when historical control groups are used. This is because changes in disease patterns, diagnoses, staging precision, and treatments can bias the end points of a patient cohort over time. In rare circumstances, large series of control patients are available from contemporaneous protocols at the same institution, with the same eligibility criteria and response assessment as in the new protocol. Even in these unusual circumstances, careful evaluation of comparability should be performed and results of the comparison used for limited phase II purposes, rather than for claiming treatment effectiveness.

The major challenge in developing cancer vaccines and interpreting cancer vaccine trials is to determine early on whether there is efficacy or futility. The most valuable end point is survival, but use of this end point is impractical in most studies. Immune response measurement is now highly refined but often difficult to correlate with clinical outcome. Techniques for measuring antibody response have become relatively well established. T-cell responses are more difficult to quantify and interpret. They can be measured through biologic assays, for example, a skin test for delayed-type hypersensitivity (DTH); by assessment of number and function of antigen-specific T cells in peripheral blood; and by assessment of histologic changes and antigen-specific T-cell number and function within the tumor. How to correlate measurements in the peripheral blood with those in the tumor is not yet known.

DTH is commonly used to measure responses to autologous and allogeneic cell vaccines. Application of appropriate controls for DTH testing is often difficult, and it may be impossible to know that a positive reaction truly indicates response to a relevant tumor antigen and not, for example, to serum or other components of the cell-based vaccine, such as proteins contained in the growth medium. Detection of antigen-specific T cells in blood or tumor can be measured by structure (e.g., presence of a particular TCR) or function (production of cytokine in response).

If the peptide to which the immune response is directed is known, peptide–MHC complexes in the form of tetramers can be used to detect T cells bearing the appropriate TCR using fluorescence-activated cell sorting. By this technique, the number of peptide-specific T cells in a bulk population can be enumerated, and after sorting, the functional capacity of the T cells can be characterized. The tetramer technique is promising but is still limited by the sensitivity of the flow cytometer. Common measures of function include chromium-release cytotoxicity assays and the assessment of cytokine release in supernatants or by ELISPOT.

Clinical benefit or response must be measured objectively. The response of residual tumor to vaccination is certainly best measured by rigorous criteria such as the response evaluation criteria in solid tumors (RECIST). It can be difficult or impossible to measure statistically significant increases in survival or disease-free survival or in time to progression in small phase I and II studies. The use of surrogate variables is also complex, in that there is frequently no correlation between measured immune response and tumor response.[21] After vaccination with defined tumor antigens that are recognized by T cells, a proportion of cancer patients may manifest an immune response as measured by a variety of methods (e.g., by assessment of T-cell function or by expression of staining with tetramers loaded with tumor-associated antigens). It appears that some patients express large numbers of tumor-specific T cells and have tumor progression, whereas others display tumor regression with an absence or low frequency of antivaccine T cells.[21,24,25]

LESSONS FROM MELANOMA

Much experimental work with cancer vaccines is done in patients with metastatic melanoma. There are valuable lessons in three examples of treatments for melanoma that seemed to show clear clinical benefit in early phase trials but were unable to be proven efficacious in large, phase III randomized studies. The first is the Dartmouth regimen [dacarbazine, cisplatin, carmustine (BCNU), and tamoxifen] for stage IV melanoma. Several single-institution phase II trials reported that the Dartmouth regimen can induce major tumor responses in 40% to 50% of patients with stage IV melanoma.[26,27] In a large phase III randomized study[28] involving 231 patients, there was no difference in survival time between patients treated with the Dartmouth regimen and those treated with dacarbazine alone.

The second is the addition of immunotherapy to chemotherapy (biochemotherapy). Several phase II trials with biochemotherapy have shown encouraging response rates in metastatic melanoma, and metaanalyses and one small, single-institution, phase III trial suggested survival benefit.[29–31] A large phase III study was conducted by the U.S. Intergroup (Eastern Cooperative Oncology Group, Southwest Oncology Group, and Cancer and Leukemia Group B) to determine the relative efficacy of biochemotherapy.[32] Patients were randomly assigned to receive cisplatin, vinblastine, and dacarbazine (CVD) either alone or concurrently with IL-2 and interferon (biochemotherapy). In this study 405 patients were evaluated. Of note, grade 4 toxicity occurred in 37% of patients given CVD alone versus 63% given CVD plus and IL-2 interferon. The overall response rate was 17.1% in the biochemotherapy group and 11.4% in the group given CVD alone. This did not translate into a survival advantage: The median survival for the biochemotherapy group was 8.4 months and for the CVD-alone group was 8.7 months. Thus, although biochemotherapy produces a slightly higher response rate and progression-free survival than CVD alone, this does not appear to be associated with either improved quality of response or overall survival.

The third example is the G_{M2} ganglioside vaccine. The G_{M2} ganglioside is a serologically well-defined melanoma antigen and the most immunogenic ganglioside expressed on melanoma cells. Several studies conducted at Memorial Sloan-Kettering Cancer Center have demonstrated that administration of G_{M2} in combination with bacille Calmette-Guérin (BCG) induced immunoglobulin (Ig) M anti-G_{M2} antibodies in the majority of patients and that these antibody responses were correlated with improved recurrence-free survival and overall survival in patients with stage III melanoma. A variety of G_{M2} vaccine formulations were studied, and a commercial vaccine preparation was selected consisting of G_{M2} coupled to keyhole limpet hemocyanin (KLH) and combined with the QS-21 adjuvant. Immunization of melanoma patients with the GMK vaccine has been shown to induce high titers of IgM antibodies in more than 80% of patients as well as IgG antibodies that had not been previously observed with administration of G_{M2} plus BCG. These induced anti-G_{M2} antibodies have been reported to mediate complement-dependent cytotoxicity and antibody-dependent cellular cytotoxicity of melanoma cell lines *in vitro*.[33–37] A large randomized study was conducted by the Intergroup, Intergroup trial E1694.[32] In this study, 880 patients with stage III melanoma were randomly assigned to treatment conditions. The trial was closed after interim analysis indicated inferiority of GMK compared with high-dose interferon.

Thus, findings in early-stage clinical trials are often not borne out in later-phase studies. In the absence of significant numbers of patients who experience objective responses, claims for cancer vaccine efficacy are likely to be reliable only if demonstrated in large, randomized studies.

CLINICAL TRIAL DATA

Dozens of clinical trials using varieties of cancer vaccines in cancer treatment have been completed and dozens more are ongoing. These are reviewed extensively elsewhere.[38] Later, data from selected cancer vaccine studies are reviewed.

WHOLE CELL AND LYSED CELL VACCINES

Whole cell tumor vaccines have been studied in the clinic for several decades. Personalized whole cell autologous tumor vaccines are likely to contain relevant shared and mutated tumor antigens; however, it is technically difficult to prepare a whole cell vaccine for each individual patient. Allogeneic tumor cell vaccines, formulated as lysates of laboratory cell lines containing shared tumor antigens, are much easier and practical to manufacture.[39,40] Autologous and allogeneic whole cell tumor vaccines stimulate limited immune responses. Although some nonrandomized studies have reported clinical benefit,[41,42] no randomized clinical trial using this class of tumor vaccine has been able to show clear objective clinical response or superiority in other measures of clinical benefit.[39,40,43,44]

Melacine (Corixa Corp., Seattle, WA) is an allogeneic melanoma tumor cell lysate combined with the adjuvant Detox. In early studies, it showed rare antitumor activity in metastatic melanoma (5% to 10%). Its efficacy was tested in a study involving patients with intermediate-thickness (1.5- to 4.0-mm) melanoma (Southwest Oncology Group trial 9035) in the largest randomized controlled trial (n = 689) of vaccine therapy for human cancer reported to date. Patients with completely resected intermediate-thickness melanoma randomly assigned to receive Melacine had a relapse-free survival that was not significantly different from that of patients randomly assigned to receive observation without further therapy. The observed hazard ratio, when adjusted for all recognized stratification and prognostic variables, was 0.97 (P_2 = .83).[40]

Canvaxin (CancerVax Corp., Carlsbad, CA) is an irradiated preparation of whole melanoma cells from three allogeneic melanoma cell lines given together with BCG.[41] Its use was studied in the treatment of 150 patients with stage IV melanoma in whom complete surgical resection could be done. In this nonrandomized study the 5-year overall survival rate was 39% for patients receiving the vaccine and 19% for patients not receiving a vaccine, as estimated from a historical database. Survival after vaccine administration was significantly correlated with the DTH immune response to vaccine but not with response to a control antigen, as previously reported.[41] In a separate, nonrandomized study of patients with stage III melanoma, 935 patients received Canvaxin in the adjuvant setting, and results for these patients were comparatively analyzed with results for 1667 patients who did not receive vaccine. The 5-year overall survival rate was 49% for those who received the vaccine and 37% for those who did not.[42] Although the number of patients in these studies is large, these nonrandomized data are difficult to evaluate precisely. A much more definitive answer will come from ongoing, large, randomized phase III trials comparing Canvaxin vaccine to a control regimen (BCG alone) in patients with stage III and IV melanoma.

Other whole cell or lysate cancer vaccines are being studied in the setting of non-Hodgkin's lymphoma, acute lymphoblastic leukemia, gastrointestinal cancer, brain cancer, and cervical cancer, using adjuvants that include IL-2, KLH, granulocyte-macrophage colony-stimulating factor (GM-CSF), BCG, and haptenization with dinitrophenol.

GENE-MODIFIED TUMOR VACCINES

Gene-modified tumor vaccines are frequently composed of autologous tumor cells that have been transfected with an immunostimulatory gene. Comparison of the antitumor effects in preclinical models has suggested that GM-CSF expressed in tumor cells is the most active in stimulating immune response and giving antitumor activity.[45] Several cytokine-modified autologous tumor cell vaccines have been tested in clinical trials.[45–54] All of these trials have been phase I and II studies.

In one study, patients with metastatic non–small cell lung cancer were vaccinated with irradiated autologous tumor cells engineered to secrete GM-CSF.[54] The vaccines reportedly elicited dendritic cell, macrophage, granulocyte, and lymphocyte infiltrates and reportedly stimulated the development of DTH reactions to irradiated, dissociated, autologous, nontransfected tumor cells in most patients. Metastatic lesions were resected after vaccination and reportedly showed T-lymphocyte and plasma cell infiltrates with tumor necrosis in three of six patients. Stable disease was reported in a subset of patients, and one mixed response was observed. Although interesting, these clinical data are soft signs of activity.

GM-CSF–transfected allogeneic cell lines were tested in pancreatic cancer in a phase I study.[55] Fourteen patients with stage I, II, or III pancreatic adenocarcinoma were enrolled. Eight weeks after pancreaticoduodenectomy, patient cohorts received escalating doses of vaccine cells. Twelve of 14 patients then went on to receive a 6-month course of adjuvant radiation and chemotherapy. One month after completing adjuvant treatment, six patients still in remission received up to three additional monthly vaccinations with the same vaccine dose that they had received originally without toxicity. Vaccination induced increased DTH responses to autologous tumor cells in three patients who also reportedly had an increased disease-free survival time. Because of the limited number of patients, and because correlation does not indicate causality, it is difficult to accurately evaluate these data. Patients with the best immune responses may survive longer because they are inherently healthier. Thus, the apparent increase in the DTH response may be due to the fact that those patients capable of making immune responses have the least aggressive tumor burdens and thus survive longer.

Other ongoing trials include studies in neuroblastoma, acute myelogenous leukemia, and prostate, ovarian, and renal cell cancers using tumor cells modified with IL-2, B7-1, CD40L, and transforming growth factor-β antisense in addition to GM-CSF.

HEAT-SHOCK PROTEINS

Heat-shock proteins (HSPs) have many important functions as demonstrated by studies *in vitro* and *in vivo*.[56,57] They have been demonstrated to activate CD8+ and CD4+ lymphocytes, induce innate immune response including natural killer cell activation and cytokine secretion, and induce maturation of dendritic cells. In addition, they have a fundamental biologic role in chaperoning antigenic peptides in cells.[58-67] The first autologous HSP vaccine introduced in clinical trials was Oncophage or, HSPPC-96 (HSP–peptide complex 96; Antigenics, Inc., Woburn, MA), produced from surgically resected cancer tissue and formulated for intradermal or subcutaneous injection. HSPPC-96 trials started with a phase I pilot study involving patients with advanced cancers and a phase I study involving patients with resected pancreatic adenocarcinoma.[68-71] Subsequently, nine phase I and II clinical studies were performed to further define the profile of the vaccine, to characterize immune responses, and to evaluate clinical activity.

In a study of patients with metastatic melanoma,[72] 64 patients underwent surgical resection of metastatic tissue required for vaccine production, 42 patients were vaccinated without experiencing toxicity, and 39 were evaluable. Antigen-specific antimelanoma T-cell response was assessed by ELISPOT assay on peripheral blood mononuclear cells obtained before and after vaccination. Of 28 patients with measurable disease, 2 had objective responses (complete responses of 559+ and 703+ days). An additional three had stable disease at the end of follow-up. Immune responses were increased after vaccination as measured using the ELISPOT assay on peripheral blood mononuclear cells in approximately half of the patients tested (11 of 23). Similar levels of detectable immune response were also seen in a phase II trial involving colon cancer patients who were vaccinated with autologous HSPPC-96.[73,74] Although there seemed to be a correlation between detectable immune response and survival, healthier patients who survive longer may have the best immune responses.

The effects of autologous HSP vaccination have also been studied in 61 patients with stage IV renal cell carcinoma.[75] Subcutaneous IL-2 was given to those patients who showed disease progression while on HSP vaccine. Two patients had partial responses, and one had a complete response. The objective response rate of 5% is similar to that seen as part of the background response variability in this disease.

Other vaccines being tested in ongoing clinical efforts using HSPs are Javelin by Mojave Therapeutics (Hawthorne, NY) and Oncocine HspE7 by Stressgen Biotechnologies (Victoria, BC, Canada). HSPs are in trials involving cancer types as diverse as chronic myelogenous leukemia, non-Hodgkin's lymphoma, and breast, gastric, gastrointestinal, and pancreatic cancer. Multicenter large, randomized phase III trials are now under way in both adjuvant settings (renal cell carcinoma with high risk for recurrence after nephrectomy) and metastatic disease settings (metastatic melanoma) to ultimately define the magnitude of clinical efficacy of this autologous HSP vaccine used as a monotherapy.

PEPTIDE-BASED VACCINES

Peptide antigens that contain the appropriate HLA-restricted amino acid sequence can be relatively easily manufactured and administered. Peptides alone are usually nonimmunogenic. They are frequently given together with an immunologic adjuvant and sometimes modified in structure to change binding characteristics. Many immunodominant epitopes from tumor antigens have a low to intermediate binding affinity for the MHC molecule and are subdominant epitopes recognized by low-affinity T cells that have evaded central tolerance selection in the thymus. This low binding affinity usually is due to lack of optimal amino acids at the peptide anchoring sites. Preclinical studies and studies in humans have demonstrated that tumor-derived peptides engineered to have an enhanced ability to bind to MHC molecules by substitution of amino acids at anchor positions (known as *fixed-anchor analogues*) lead to enhanced immune responses.[21,76-80]

Peptide-based vaccines require knowledge and matching of the exact HLA haplotype and antigen to provide the appropriate peptide epitope for each individual. For example, the most common HLA molecule in the general population is HLA-A*0201 (or HLA-A2.1), which accounts for 30% to 40% of the major ethnicities. An HLA-A*0201 peptide-based approach would therefore only be suitable for slightly more than one-third of the patients whose tumors express a certain tumor antigen for which the immunodominant HLA-binding epitope has been defined, which is currently limited to few cancers.

Many different peptides have been tested in the clinic.[38,81-98] Melanoma peptides were the first to be tested in phase I and phase II studies for active immunization of patients with metastatic melanoma.[21,99-103] Clinical responses have been observed in 0% to 30% of vaccinated patients. In one of the first studies, 16 patients were vaccinated with Melan-A/MART-1$_{27-35}$ and IFA. In this trial, 15 of 16 patients developed a CTL-specific response in their blood but showed no concomitant clinical effect.[102] In contrast, 42% of patients receiving a modified gp100 peptide [gp100-209(2M)] and a high systemic dose of IL-2 demonstrated a clinical response.[21] Patients who received the peptide alone showed no response. Ten of 22 patients with resected stage III and IV melanoma who were treated with Melan-A/MART-1$_{27-35}$ peptide with IFA developed immune responses, and there was a suggestion of a prolonged time to relapse.[104]

Recombinant IL-12 has been used in combination with vaccination with both gp100-209(2M) and tyrosinase in IFA in patients with resected melanoma.[92] Recurrence-free and overall survival of these vaccinated subjects compared favorably with that of historical groups, although the small numbers of patients and use of historical controls prohibit the determination of clinical benefit. Vaccination of patients with metastatic melanoma with the MAGE-3.A1 peptide without adjuvant reportedly resulted in induction of regression of cutaneous disease to a disease-free state in 2 patients of an initial patient cohort of 39.[98] Immunization using peptides administered without adjuvant (in saline) was ineffective in human trials using the gp100-209(2M) peptide at the National Cancer Institute (*S. A. Rosenberg*).

Peptide vaccines have been administered with GM-CSF. In a very small study, Jäger et al.[105] treated three patients with metastatic melanoma with a mixture of Melan-A/MART-1$_{27-35}$/gp100/tyrosinase peptides and GM-CSF and reported CTL induction and transient tumor regression in all three patients. In a study in which metastatic melanoma patients were vaccinated with tyrosinase peptides and GM-CSF, there was one mixed clinical response.[106] Three different peptides from the cancer-testis antigen NY-ESO-1 were given to 12 HLA-A2–positive cancer patients with progressing NY-ESO-1–expressing tumors of different histologic types.[107] First, the patients received the peptides without GM-CSF. After 50 days, patients with no evidence of disease progression then received the peptides with GM-CSF. In those who could be tested, an induction of peptide-specific CTL responses (observed in four of seven patients) was associated with disease stabilization and objective regression of some but not other metastases (mixed responses).

Peptides have also been used to immunize patients with several other cancers, including those of the pancreas, breast, and ovary. More than 90% of pancreatic adenocarcinomas have a specific mutation in the twelfth, thirteenth, or sixty-first codon of the K-ras oncogene. In a study using vaccination with K-ras peptides and GM-CSF, there was an association between immune response and patient survival.[108] These data are interesting, but again it is very difficult to draw definitive conclusions, given the small number of patients, low response rates, and use of historical controls.

Patients with Her-2/neu–positive breast and ovarian cancers were vaccinated with class II HLA-restricted Her-2/neu peptides together with GM-CSF. All patients reportedly developed Her-2/neu peptide–specific T-cell responses measured by DTH reactions to the peptide.[89,90] Epitope spreading was reportedly observed in 84% of patients and significantly correlated with the generation of a HER-2/neu protein-specific T-cell immunity. Objective clinical responses were not reported in these studies.

More than a dozen other peptide vaccination trials are ongoing using a large number of different peptides with several different adjuvants to treat cancer histologic types that include cancers of the prostate, ovary, cervix, liver, and lung. Ongoing cancer vaccine trials include the use of whole proteins as well (MAGE-3 and NY-ESO-1 proteins).

NAKED DNA

Intramuscular injection of naked plasmid DNA results in gene expression and possible immune responses against the expressed protein. DNA plasmid immunogens consist of an antigen gene regulated by a promoter with constitutive activity that can also be conjugated with gold particles and propelled into the skin using a helium gas "gene gun."[78,109,110] The protein antigen produced by the target cells is taken up by host antigen-presenting cells, processed, and cross-presented to the immune system in the draining lymph nodes, although direct transfection of rare antigen-presenting cells residing at the injection site has also been demonstrated. Naked DNA plasmids have low immunologic potency in animal models[111] and were weak immunogens in humans in a study using plasmid encoding a modified version of human gp100.[112] Clinical trials of naked DNA are under way using plasmids encoding tyrosinase and MART-1. Other trials use plasmid DNA to encode an immunostimulatory molecule such as HLA-B7 or IL-2.

One approach to improving the efficacy of naked DNA immunization is the use of xenoantigen vaccination.[113] One experimental trial in dogs with melanoma immunized with human tyrosinase plasmid DNA has provided the experimental background for planned xenoimmunization of patients with melanoma.[114] Another future direction for enhancing the function of naked nucleic acid immunization includes the use of self-replicating RNA vaccines[115] or DNA vaccines encoding Alphavirus replicons.[116]

VIRAL VECTORS

A variety of viral vectors have been used in cancer immunotherapy. Tumor antigen DNA sequences can be inserted into atten-

uated pox viruses that are unable to replicate in mammalian hosts (including modified vaccinia Ankara, fowlpox, or canarypox).[22,117] Other vectors include recombinant replication-incompetent viral vectors (adenovirus, retrovirus, lentivirus), which are modified viruses that have been specifically mutated to be incapable of self-replication.[38,118]

A study was performed in which recombinant adenoviruses expressing either MART-1 or gp100 were used to immunize patients with metastatic melanoma.[119] In this phase I study, 54 patients received escalating doses of recombinant adenovirus encoding either MART-1 or gp100 melanoma antigen administered either alone or followed by IL-2. One of 16 patients with metastatic melanoma receiving the recombinant adenovirus MART-1 alone experienced a complete response. Other patients achieved objective responses, but they had received IL-2 along with an adenovirus, and their responses could be attributed to the cytokine. Immunologic assays showed no consistent immunization to the MART-1 or gp100 transgenes expressed by the recombinant adenoviruses. High levels of neutralizing antibody present in patients' sera before treatment may have impaired the ability of these viruses to immunize patients against melanoma antigens.

Enhancing the immune potency of recombinant poxvirus-based vectors can be reportedly achieved by the coexpression of cytokines or costimulatory molecules in the viral vector. Poxviruses have a large capacity to carry and express multiple genes. Several of these are in clinical trial development. Several costimulatory molecules using recombinant orthopox vectors (replication-competent vaccinia recombinants and replication-defective avipox recombinants) as a backbone have been studied. These include B7.2, intracellular adhesion molecule-1 (ICAM-1), lymphocyte function–associated antigen-3 (LFA-3), and CD70. One vector contains antigen [carcinoembryonic antigen (CEA) or prostate-specific antigen (PSA)], and B7.1, ICAM-1, and LFA-3, designated by the acronym TRICOM, which synergize to enhance T-cell responses to levels far greater than that achieved by any one or two costimulatory molecules. These vaccines are being studied in the clinic and a phase I trial was reviewed.[120] Sequential vaccinations with fowlpox–CEA (6D)–TRICOM (B7.1/ICAM-1/LFA-3) alone and sequentially with vaccinia–CEA (6D)–TRICOM and GM-CSF were administered to 58 patients with advanced CEA-expressing carcinomas. Significant CEA-specific T-cell responses were reportedly observed in all patients tested, with a higher increase in those cohorts receiving GM-CSF. Based on published evidence, it does not appear that objective clinical partial or complete responses as judged by traditional criteria were observed; however, one patient was reportedly found to be disease free after death from an unrelated cause on postmortem examination.

EX VIVO DENDRITIC CELL VACCINES

Different antigen loading procedures have been used for dendritic cell antigen presentation. Synthetic HLA-binding peptide epitopes or the complete DNA sequence in a viral vector can be used to load the dendritic cell vaccines. Several methods of loading dendritic cells with uncharacterized tumor antigens have also been tested. These include using tumor lysates, messenger RNA (mRNA), or apoptotic bodies fed to dendritic cells that are then taken up by macropinocytosis or endocytosis. *Ex vivo* dendritic cell–based strategies have been used in clinical trials and occasional responses in patients have been reported. Because these studies are early, it is not possible to critically evaluate the magnitude or benefit of these clinical responses.

In one study of patients with melanoma,[121] dendritic cells were pulsed with Mage-3A1 tumor peptide and a recall antigen, tetanus toxoid or tuberculin. Mixed responses were reported in some patients. The magnitude and effectiveness of this type of vaccine may become clearer in larger studies. In another study, patients with metastatic melanoma received a CD34–dendritic cell vaccine pulsed with MART-1, tyrosinase, MAGE-3, gp100, and Flu-MP peptides, and KLH. Enhanced immunity was correlated with increased patient survival.[122] In another study, 20 patients with pancreatic, hepatocellular, cholangiocellular, or medullary thyroid carcinoma were treated with tumor lysate–pulsed dendritic cells.[123] None of the patients had objective clinical responses by standard criteria, although several immunologic parameters were measured.

Several studies have tested the ability to generate response when transfecting dendritic cells with mRNA.[124–126] In one phase I and II study, patients with resected hepatic metastases of colon cancer were treated with autologous dendritic cells loaded with CEA mRNA.[124] Of the 24 evaluable patients in the dose-escalation phase, one patient reportedly experienced the disappearance of a tumor marker. In another study of patients with metastatic renal cell carcinoma, renal tumor RNA–transfected dendritic cells were administered to ten evaluable patients.[125] Expansion of tumor-specific T cells with reactivities to a broad set of renal tumor-associated antigens, including telomerase reverse transcriptase, G250, and oncofetal antigen, but not against self-antigens expressed by normal renal tissues, was detected after immunization in some patients. Most patients received secondary therapies after vaccination, but tumor-related mortality of study subjects was reportedly unexpectedly low. In another study, PSA mRNA–transfected dendritic cells were administered to patients with metastatic prostate cancer.[126] Induction of PSA-specific T-cell responses was reportedly obtained in all patients, but clinical responses as measured by standard criteria were not reported in this study.

One study by the Dendreon Corporation (Seattle, WA) used an antigen-presenting cell vaccine loaded with an antigen called *prostatic acid phosphatase* linked to GM-CSF to treat men with hormone-refractory prostate cancer.[127] In a retrospective subset analysis, limited clinical efficacy was claimed. Numerous other *ex vivo* protocols are reported to be under way using dendritic cells pulsed with tumor lysates and dendritic cell–cancer cell hybrids (see ref. 38).

IMMUNE RESPONSES DO NOT ALWAYS TRANSLATE INTO CLINICAL RESPONSES— PROPOSED MECHANISMS OF TUMOR ESCAPE

The current notion that tumor cells must escape immune recognition is based largely on the idea that neoantigens expressed by tumor cells as a consequence of their genetic instability will be immunogenic. There is little doubt that the tumor contains a large number of mutations that can potentially generate new antigens recognizable by the immune system, but there is considerable doubt about what the immunologic response to these

potential immunogens will be. A number of groups have conducted experiments in which highly immunogenic foreign antigens, such as the hemagglutinin protein from influenza, the β-galactosidase enzyme from *Escherichia coli*, and the ovalbumin (OVA) protein from the chicken are expressed in tumor cells. The results are fairly uniform: tumors tend to grow progressively, retaining their lethality despite the expression of a foreign and highly immunogenic protein by the tumor cell.

Proposed mechanisms for tumor escape include those relating to the inherent genetic instability of tumor cells and others that might be shared by many normal cells in the body. The latter include the lack of expression of costimulatory molecules (B7-1/CD80, B7-2/CD86, and CD40L), the induction of suppressor cell activity, and the production of immunoinhibitory substances such as transforming growth factor-β or IL-10. Many of these proposals are intuitively appealing but lack direct experimental evidence or consistent results. For example, Fas ligand has been proposed as a mediator of the tumor "counterattack." However, controlled experiments show that expression of Fas ligand in animal tumor models results not in escape but in more rapid rejection.[128] Several groups have proposed the loss of β_2-microglobulin as a mechanism of immune escape.[129] Clearly, similar arguments can be advanced with regard to other events that decrease or eliminate MHC class I expression on the surface, such as loss of the MHC class I heavy chain or of TAP or LMP complex components.[130]

A greater understanding of the interactions of costimulatory molecules with negative regulatory molecules, such as CTL-associated antigen-4 (CTLA-4) may enable more direct interventions.[131] CTLA-4 is an activation-induced receptor with affinity for the costimulatory molecules B7-1 and B7-2 CTLA-4 recognition of B7 costimulatory molecules by activated lymphocytes provides an off switch for the immune response. Monoclonal antibodies that block CTLA-4 prevent its engagement by B7 costimulatory molecules and inhibit this off switch. Multiple animal models have shown that CTLA-4 antibodies enhance antitumor responses, either alone or in combination with cancer vaccines. Clinical trials using an anti–CTLA-4 antibody (MDX-010) have now been reported.[132]

FUTURE DIRECTIONS: FOCUS ON T-CELL ACTIVATION AND DEATH

Significant evidence indicates that the central reasons for the failed antitumor immune response may be deficiencies in the maintenance of sustained tumor-specific T-cell activation. It is now clear that there are many ways in which triggering a TCR can result in the ultimate inactivation or even demise of the T cell bearing it. The difference between antigen presentation in the tumor environment and in a virally infected tissue is likely the activation of resident antigen-presenting cells, the scavengers and danger sensors of the immune system. The lack of proinflammatory mediators that induce maturation of dendritic cells, in conjunction with the abundant antigen presentation by noncostimulatory, tolerance-producing tumor cells, is the factor that may tip the T-cell activation–inactivation balance in favor of tumor-specific T-cell tolerance. On the other hand, overstimulation can terminate an otherwise effective T-cell response through activation-induced cell death, fratricide, or exhaustion.[133]

Although new antigen discovery and epitope mapping continue to be an important part of tumor immunology, few would argue that several excellent targets expressed on a range of tumor histologic types are now available. The next important breakthrough in cancer immunotherapy may come from an understanding of how to enhance T-cell avidity, how to maintain T-cell activation while preventing T-cell apoptosis, and how to reduce or eliminate the effects of negative regulatory factors.

In animal research, a number of new transgenic mouse models are now available, which allow for a reductionistic study of tumor interactions with elements of the innate and adaptive immune system. One particularly fruitful area currently under development involves the use of TCR transgenic mice. It is now clear that very large numbers of tumor-specific transgenic CD8+ and CD4+ T cells have little effect on the growth rate or lethality of syngeneic tumor cells that express the antigens targeted by these transgenic T cells. These transgenic mouse systems model key aspects of the increased tumor-specific T cells found in some patients with cancer after active immunization. Using these models, the authors and others are evaluating cellular and molecular mechanisms in T-cell activation, death, and anergy as they relate to the development of more effective cancer vaccines.

CONCLUSION

There are sufficient data to support the notion that cancer vaccines can induce antitumor immune responses in humans with cancer. How best to translate this increase in immune responsiveness to consistent and reproducible objective cancer regression or increased survival remains unclear at this time. Despite monumental advances in the understanding of molecular and cellular immunology, researchers have thus far been unable to translate this into clearly defined and measurable clinical benefit.

REFERENCES

1. Gross L. Intradermal immunization of C3H mice against a sarcoma that originated in an animal of the same line. *Cancer Res* 1943;3:326.
2. Foley EJ. Antigenic properties of methylcholanthrene-induced tumors in mice of the strain of origin. *Cancer Res* 1953;13:835.
3. Rabinowich H, Cohen R, Bruderman I. Functional analysis of mononuclear cells infiltrating into tumors: lysis of autologous human tumor cells by cultured infiltrating lymphocytes. *Cancer Res* 1987;47:173.
4. Barth RJ Jr, Mule JJ, Spiess PJ, et al. Interferon gamma and tumor necrosis factor have a role in tumor regressions mediated by murine CD8+ tumor-infiltrating lymphocytes. *J Exp Med* 1991;173:647.
5. Toes RE, Ossendorp F, Offringa R, et al. CD4 T cells and their role in antitumor immune responses. J Exp Med 1999;189:753.
6. Topalian S, Solomon D, Avis FP, et al. Immunotherapy of patients with advanced cancer using tumor infiltrating lymphocytes and recombinant interleukin-2: a pilot study. *J Clin Oncol* 1988;6:839.
7. Boon T, Cerottini JC, Van den Eynde B, et al. Tumor antigens recognized by T lymphocytes. *Annu Rev Immunol* 1994;12:337.
8. Boon T, Gajewski TF, Coulie PG. From defined human tumor antigens to effective immunization? *Immunol Today* 1995;16:334.
9. Rosenberg SA. A new era for cancer immunotherapy based on the genes that encode cancer antigens. *Immunity* 1999;10:281.
10. Boon T, Old LJ. Cancer tumor antigens. *Curr Opin Immunol* 1997;9:681.
11. Boon T, Coulie PG, Van den Eynde B. Tumor antigens recognized by T cells. *Immunol Today* 1997;18:267.
12. Overwijk WW, Theoret MR, Finkelstein SE, et al. Tumor regression and autoimmunity after reversal of a functionally tolerant state of self-reactive CD8+ T cells. *J Exp Med* 2003;198:569.
13. Dudley ME, Wunderlich JR, Robbins PF, et al. Cancer regression and autoimmunity in patients after clonal repopulation with antitumor lymphocytes. *Science* 2002;298:850.
14. van der Bruggen P, Traversari C, Chomez P, et al. A gene encoding an antigen recognized by cytolytic T lymphocytes on a human melanoma. *Science* 1991;254:1643.
15. Van den Eynde B, Lethe B, Van Pel A, et al. The gene coding for a major tumor rejection antigen of tumor P815 is identical to the normal gene of syngeneic DBA-2 Mice. *J Exp Med* 1991;173:1373.
16. Cox AL, Skipper J, Chen Y, et al. Identification of a peptide recognized by five melanoma-specific human cytotoxic T cell lines. *Science* 1994;264:716.
17. Yu ZY, Restifo NP. Cancer vaccines: progress reveals new complexities. *J Clin Invest* 2002;110:289.
18. Rosenberg SA. Progress in human tumour immunology and immunotherapy. *Nature* 2001;411:380.
19. Parkhurst MR, Salgaller ML, Southwood S, et al. Improved induction of melanoma-reactive CTL with peptides from the melanoma antigen gp100 modified at HLA-A*0201-binding residues. *J Immunol* 1996;157:2539.
20. Dyall R, Bowne WB, Weber LW, et al. Heteroclitic immunization induces tumor immunity. *J Exp Med* 1998;188:1553.
21. Rosenberg SA, Yang JC, Schwartzentruber DJ, et al. Immunologic and therapeutic evaluation of a synthetic peptide vaccine for the treatment of patients with metastatic melanoma. *Nat Med* 1998;4:321.
22. Restifo NP. Developing recombinant and synthetic vaccines for the treatment of melanoma. *Curr Opin Oncol* 1999;11:50.
23. Simon RM, Steinberg SM, Hamilton M, et al. Clinical trial designs for the early clinical development of therapeutic cancer vaccines. *J Clin Oncol* 2001;19:1848.
24. Coulie PG, van der BP. T-cell responses of vaccinated cancer patients. *Curr Opin Immunol* 2003;15:131.
25. Coulie PG, Karanikas V, Lurquin C, et al. Cytolytic T-cell responses of cancer patients vaccinated with a MAGE antigen. *Immunol Rev* 2002;188:33.
26. McClay EF, Berd D, Mastrangelo MJ. The Dartmouth regimen: gone or going strong? *Cancer Invest* 1998;16:421.
27. Nathan FE, Mastrangelo MJ. Systemic therapy in melanoma. *Semin Surg Oncol* 1998;14:319.
28. Chapman PB, Einhorn LH, Meyers ML, et al. Phase III multicenter randomized trial of the Dartmouth regimen versus dacarbazine in patients with metastatic melanoma. *J Clin Oncol* 1999;17:2745.
29. Eton O, Legha SS, Bedikian AY, et al. Sequential biochemotherapy versus chemotherapy for metastatic melanoma: results from a phase III randomized trial. *J Clin Oncol* 2002;20:2045.
30. Legha SS, Ring S, Eton O, et al. Development of a biochemotherapy regimen with concurrent administration of cisplatin, vinblastine, dacarbazine, interferon alfa, and interleukin-2 for patients with metastatic melanoma. *J Clin Oncol* 1998;16:1752.
31. Legha SS, Ring S, Eton O, et al. Development and results of biochemotherapy in metastatic melanoma: the University of Texas M. D. Anderson Cancer Center experience. *Cancer J Sci Am* 1997;3[Suppl 1]:S9.
32. Atkins, Lee S, Flaherty L, et al. A prospective randomized phase III trial of concurrent biochemotherapy (BCT) with cisplatin, vinblastine, dacarbazine (CVD), IL-2 and interferon alpha-2b (IFN) versus CVD alone in patients with metastatic melanoma (E3695): an ECOG-coordinated intergroup trial. *Proc Am Soc Clin Oncol* 2003;22:708.
33. Chapman PB, Morrisey D, Panageas KS, et al. Vaccination with a bivalent G(M2) and G(D2) ganglioside conjugate vaccine: a trial comparing doses of G(D2)-keyhole limpet hemocyanin. *Clin Cancer Res* 2000;6:4658.
34. Chapman PB, Morrissey DM, Panageas KS, et al. Induction of antibodies against G_{M2} ganglioside by immunizing melanoma patients using G_{M2}-keyhole limpet hemocyanin + QS21 vaccine: a dose-response study. *Clin Cancer Res* 2000;6:874.
35. Zhang S, Cordon-Cardo C, Zhang HS, et al. Selection of tumor antigens as targets for immune attack using immunohistochemistry: I. Focus on gangliosides. *Int J Cancer* 1997;73:42.
36. Yao TJ, Begg CB, Livingston PO. Optimal sample size for a series of pilot trials of new agents. *Biometrics* 1996;52:992.
37. Livingston PO, Wong GY, Adluri S, et al. Improved survival in stage III melanoma patients with G_{M2} antibodies: a randomized trial of adjuvant vaccination with G_{M2} ganglioside. *J Clin Oncol* 1994;12:1036.
38. Ribas A, Butterfield LH, Glaspy JA, et al. Current developments in cancer vaccines and cellular immunotherapy. *J Clin Oncol* 2003;21:2415.
39. Fisher RI, Terry WD, Hodes RJ, et al. Adjuvant immunotherapy or chemotherapy for malignant melanoma. Preliminary report of the National Cancer Institute randomized clinical trial. *Surg Clin North Am* 1981;61:1267.
40. Sondak VK, Liu PY, Tuthill RJ, et al. Adjuvant immunotherapy of resected, intermediate-thickness, node-negative melanoma with an allogeneic tumor vaccine: overall results of a randomized trial of the Southwest Oncology Group. *J Clin Oncol* 2002;20:2058.
41. Hsueh EC, Essner R, Foshag LJ, et al. Prolonged survival after complete resection of disseminated melanoma and active immunotherapy with a therapeutic cancer vaccine. *J Clin Oncol* 2002;20:4549.
42. Morton DL, Hsueh EC, Essner R, et al. Prolonged survival of patients receiving active immunotherapy with Canvaxin therapeutic polyvalent vaccine after complete resection of melanoma metastatic to regional lymph nodes. *Ann Surg* 2002;236:438.
43. Mitchell MS. Perspective on allogeneic melanoma lysates in active specific immunotherapy. *Semin Oncol* 1998;25:623.
44. Wallack MK, Sivanandham M, Balch CM, et al. Surgical adjuvant active specific immunotherapy for patients with stage III melanoma: the final analysis of data from a phase III, randomized, double-blind, multicenter vaccinia melanoma oncolysate trial. *J Am Coll Surg* 1998;187:69.
45. Dranoff G, Jaffee E, Lazenby A, et al. Vaccination with irradiated tumor cells engineered to secrete murine granulocyte-macrophage colony-stimulating factor stimulates potent, specific, and long-lasting anti-tumor immunity. *Proc Natl Acad Sci U S A* 1993;90:3539.

46. Shawler DL, Bartholomew RM, Garrett MA, et al. Antigenic and immunologic characterization of an allogeneic colon carcinoma vaccine. *Clin Exp Immunol* 2002;129:99.

47. Sobol RE, Shawler DL, Carson C, et al. Interleukin 2 gene therapy of colorectal carcinoma with autologous irradiated tumor cells and genetically engineered fibroblasts: a Phase I study. *Clin Cancer Res* 1999;5:2359.

48. Freeman SM, McCune C, Robinson W, et al. The treatment of ovarian cancer with a gene modified cancer vaccine: a phase I study. *Hum Gene Ther* 1995;6:927.

49. Sobol RE, Royston I, Fakhrai H, et al. Injection of colon carcinoma patients with autologous irradiated tumor cells and fibroblasts genetically modified to secrete interleukin-2 (IL-2): a phase I study. *Hum Gene Ther* 1995;6:195.

50. Jaffee EM, Hruban RH, Biedrzycki B, et al. Novel allogeneic granulocyte-macrophage colony-stimulating factor-secreting tumor vaccine for pancreatic cancer: a phase I trial of safety and immune activation. *J Clin Oncol* 2001;19:145.

51. Soiffer R, Lynch T, Mihm M, et al. Vaccination with irradiated autologous melanoma cells engineered to secrete human granulocyte-macrophage colony-stimulating factor generates potent antitumor immunity in patients with metastatic melanoma. *Proc Natl Acad Sci U S A* 1998;95:13141.

52. Jaffee EM, Abrams R, Cameron J, et al. A phase I clinical trial of lethally irradiated allogeneic pancreatic tumor cells transfected with the GM-CSF gene for the treatment of pancreatic adenocarcinoma. *Hum Gene Ther* 1998;9:1951.

53. Dranoff G, Soiffer R, Lynch T, et al. A phase I study of vaccination with autologous, irradiated melanoma cells engineered to secrete human granulocyte-macrophage colony stimulating factor. *Hum Gene Ther* 1997;8:111.

54. Salgia R, Lynch T, Skarin A, et al. Vaccination with irradiated autologous tumor cells engineered to secrete granulocyte-macrophage colony-stimulating factor augments antitumor immunity in some patients with metastatic non–small-cell lung carcinoma. *J Clin Oncol* 2003;21:624.

55. Jaffee EM, Hruban RH, Biedrzycki B, et al. Novel allogeneic granulocyte-macrophage colony-stimulating factor–secreting tumor vaccine for pancreatic cancer: a phase I trial of safety and immune activation. *J Clin Oncol* 2001;19:145.

56. Basu S, Binder RJ, Ramalingam T, et al. CD91 is a common receptor for heat shock proteins gp96, hsp90, hsp70, and calreticulin. *Immunity* 2001;14:303.

57. Binder RJ, Han DK, Srivastava PK. CD91: a receptor for heat shock protein gp96. *Nat Immunol* 2000;1:151.

58. Rivoltini L, Castelli C, Carrabba M, et al. Human tumor-derived heat shock protein 96 mediates *in vitro* activation and *in vivo* expansion of melanoma- and colon carcinoma-specific T cells. *J Immunol* 2003;171:3467.

59. Mazzaferro V, Coppa J, Carrabba MG, et al. Vaccination with autologous tumor-derived heat shock protein gp96 after liver resection for metastatic colorectal cancer. *Clin Cancer Res* 2003;9:3235.

60. Hoos A, Levey DL. Vaccination with heat shock protein-peptide complexes: from basic science to clinical applications. *Expert Rev Vaccines* 2003;2:369.

61. Belli F, Testori A, Rivoltini L, et al. Vaccination of metastatic melanoma patients with autologous tumor-derived heat shock protein gp96-peptide complexes: clinical and immunologic findings. *J Clin Oncol* 2002;20:4169.

62. Srivastava P. Roles of heat-shock proteins in innate and adaptive immunity. *Nat Rev Immunol* 2002;2:185.

63. Manjili MH, Wang XY, Park J, et al. Immunotherapy of cancer using heat shock proteins. *Front Biosci* 2002;7:d43.

64. Sato K, Torimoto Y, Tamura Y, et al. Immunotherapy using heat-shock protein preparations of leukemia cells after syngeneic bone marrow transplantation in mice. *Blood* 2001;98:1852.

65. Udono H, Levey DL, Srivastava PK. Cellular requirements for tumor-specific immunity elicited by heat shock proteins: tumor rejection antigen gp96 primes CD8+ T cells in vivo. *Proc Natl Acad Sci U S A* 1994;91:3077.

66. Blachere NE, Udono H, Janetzki S, et al. Heat shock protein vaccines against cancer. *J Immunother* 1993;14:352.

67. Udono H, Srivastava PK. Heat shock protein 70–associated peptides elicit specific cancer immunity. *J Exp Med* 1993;178:1391.

68. Lewis JJ, Janetzki S, Livingston PO, et al. Pilot trial of vaccination with autologous tumor-derived gp96 heat shock protein-peptide complex (HSPPC-96) in patients with resected pancreatic adenocarcinoma. *Proc Am Soc Clin Oncol* 1999;17:1687.

69. Janetzki S, Palla D, Rosenhauer V, et al. Immunization of cancer patients with autologous cancer-derived heat shock protein gp96 preparations: a pilot study. *Int J Cancer* 2000; 88:232.

70. Lewis JJ, Janetzki S, Schaed S, et al. Evaluation of CD8(+) T-cell frequencies by the Elispot assay in healthy individuals and in patients with metastatic melanoma immunized with tyrosinase peptide. *Int J Cancer* 2000;87:391.

71. Maki RJ, Lewis JJ, Janetzki S, et al. Phase I study of HSPPC-96 (Oncophage®) vaccine in patients with completely resected pancreatic adenocarcinoma. *Eur J Cancer* 2003;1:(5 Suppl)19.

72. Belli F, Testori A, Rivoltini L, et al. Vaccination of metastatic melanoma patients with autologous tumor-derived heat shock protein gp96-peptide complexes: clinical and immunologic findings. *J Clin Oncol* 2002;20:4169.

73. Mazzaferro V, Coppa J, Carrabba MG, et al. Vaccination with autologous tumor-derived heat-shock protein gp96 after liver resection for metastatic colorectal cancer. *Clin Cancer Res* 2003;9:3235.

74. Rivoltini L, Castelli C, Carrabba M, et al. Human tumor-derived heat shock protein 96 mediates *in vitro* activation and *in vivo* expansion of melanoma- and colon carcinoma-specific T cells. *J Immunol* 2003;171:3467.

75. Assikis VJ, Daliani L, Pagliaro C, et al. Phase II study of an autologous tumor derived heat shock protein-peptide complex vaccine (HSPPC-96) for patients with metastatic renal cell carcinoma (mRCC). *Proc Am Soc Clin Oncol* 2003;22:386.

76. Gold JS, Ferrone CR, Guevara-Patino JA, et al. A single heteroclitic epitope determines cancer immunity after xenogeneic DNA immunization against a tumor differentiation antigen. *J Immunol* 2003;170:5188.

77. Overwijk WW, Tsung A, Irvine KR, et al. gp100/pmel 17 is a murine tumor rejection antigen: induction of "self"-reactive, tumoricidal T cells using high-affinity, altered peptide ligand. *J Exp Med* 1998;188:277.

78. Hawkins WG, Gold JS, Dyall R, et al. Immunization with DNA coding for gp100 results in CD4 T-cell independent antitumor immunity. *Surgery* 2000;128:273.

79. Ross HM, Weber LW, Wang S, et al. Priming for T-cell-mediated rejection of established tumors by cutaneous DNA immunization. *Clin Cancer Res* 1997;3:2191.

80. Dyall R, Bowne WB, Weber LW, et al. Heteroclitic immunization induces tumor immunity. *J Exp Med* 1998;188:1553.

81. Noguchi M, Kobayashi K, Suetsugu N, et al. Induction of cellular and humoral immune responses to tumor cells and peptides in HLA-A24 positive hormone-refractory prostate cancer patients by peptide vaccination. *Prostate* 2003;57:80.

82. Cebon J, Jager E, Shackleton MJ, et al. Two phase I studies of low dose recombinant human IL-12 with Melan-A and influenza peptides in subjects with advanced malignant melanoma. *Cancer Immun* 2003;3:7.

83. Phan GQ, Touloukian CE, Yang JC, et al. Immunization of patients with metastatic melanoma using both class I- and class II-restricted peptides from melanoma-associated antigens. *J Immunother* 2003;26:349.

84. Peterson AC, Harlin H, Gajewski TF. Immunization with Melan-A peptide-pulsed peripheral blood mononuclear cells plus recombinant human interleukin-12 induces clinical activity and T-cell responses in advanced melanoma. *J Clin Oncol* 2003;21:2342.

85. Smith JW, Walker EB, Fox BA, et al. Adjuvant immunization of HLA-A2-positive melanoma patients with a modified gp100 peptide induces peptide-specific CD8+ T-cell responses. *J Clin Oncol* 2003;21:1562.

86. Bettinotti MP, Panelli MC, Ruppe E, et al. Clinical and immunological evaluation of patients with metastatic melanoma undergoing immunization with the HLA-Cw*0702-associated epitope MAGE-A12:170-178. *Int J Cancer* 2003;105:210.

87. Scheibenbogen C, Schadendorf D, Bechrakis NE, et al. Effects of granulocyte-macrophage colony-stimulating factor and foreign helper protein as immunologic adjuvants on the T-cell response to vaccination with tyrosinase peptides. *Int J Cancer* 2003;104:188.

88. Parmiani G, Castelli C, Dalerba P, et al. Cancer immunotherapy with peptide-based vaccines: What have we achieved? Where are we going? *J Natl Cancer Inst* 2002;94:805.

89. Disis ML, Gooley TA, Rinn K, et al. Generation of T-cell immunity to the HER-2/neu protein after active immunization with HER-2/neu peptide-based vaccines. *J Clin Oncol* 2002;20:2624.

90. Knutson KL, Schiffman K, Cheever MA, et al. Immunization of cancer patients with a HER-2/neu, HLA-A2 peptide, p369-377, results in short-lived peptide-specific immunity. *Clin Cancer Res* 2002;8:1014.

91. Slingluff CL Jr, Yamshchikov G, Neese P, et al. Phase I trial of a melanoma vaccine with gp100(280-288) peptide and tetanus helper peptide in adjuvant: immunologic and clinical outcomes. *Clin Cancer Res* 2001;7:3012.

92. Lee P, Wang F, Kuniyoshi J, et al. Effects of interleukin-12 on the immune response to a multipeptide vaccine for resected metastatic melanoma. *J Clin Oncol* 2001;19:3836.

93. Gajewski TF, Fallarino F, Ashikari A, et al. Immunization of HLA-A2+ melanoma patients with MAGE-3 or MelanA peptide-pulsed autologous peripheral blood mononuclear cells plus recombinant human interleukin 12. *Clin Cancer Res* 2001;7:895s.

94. Gilewski T, Adluri S, Ragupathi G, et al. Vaccination of high-risk breast cancer patients with mucin-1 (MUC1) keyhole limpet hemocyanin conjugate plus QS-21. *Clin Cancer Res* 2000;6:1693.

95. Pinilla-Ibarz J, Cathcart K, Korontsvit T, et al. Vaccination of patients with chronic myelogenous leukemia with bcr-abl oncogene breakpoint fusion peptides generates specific immune responses. *Blood* 2000;95:1781.

96. Lee KH, Wang E, Nielsen MB, et al. Increased vaccine-specific T cell frequency after peptide-based vaccination correlates with increased susceptibility to *in vitro* stimulation but does not lead to tumor regression. *J Immunol* 1999;163:6292.

97. Schaed SG, Klimek VM, Panageas KS, et al. T-cell responses against tyrosinase 368-376(370D) peptide in HLA*A0201+ melanoma patients: randomized trial comparing incomplete Freund's adjuvant, granulocyte macrophage colony-stimulating factor, and QS-21 as immunological adjuvants. *Clin Cancer Res* 2002;8:967.

98. Marchand M, van Baren N, Weynants P, et al. Tumor regressions observed in patients with metastatic melanoma treated with an antigenic peptide encoded by gene MAGE-3 and presented by HLA-A1. *Int J Cancer* 1999;80:219.

99. Slingluff CL Jr, Petroni GR, Yamshchikov GV, et al. Clinical and immunologic results of a randomized phase II trial of vaccination using four melanoma peptides either administered in granulocyte-macrophage colony-stimulating factor in adjuvant or pulsed on dendritic cells. *J Clin Oncol* 2003;21:4016.

100. Stewart JH, Rosenberg SA. Long-term survival of anti-tumor lymphocytes generated by vaccination of patients with melanoma with a peptide vaccine. *J Immunother* 2000;23:401.

101. Lewis JJ, Janetzki S, Schaed S, et al. Evaluation of CD8(+) T-cell frequencies by the Elispot assay in healthy individuals and in patients with metastatic melanoma immunized with tyrosinase peptide. *Int J Cancer* 2000;87:391.

102. Cormier JN, Salgaller ML, Prevette T, et al. Enhancement of cellular immunity in melanoma patients immunized with a peptide from MART-1/Melan A. *Cancer J Sci Am* 1997;3:37.

103. Salgaller ML, Marincola FM, Cormier JN, et al. Immunization against epitopes in the human melanoma antigen gp100 following patient immunization with synthetic peptides. *Cancer Res* 1996;56:4749.

104. Wang F, Bade E, Kuniyoshi C, et al. Phase I trial of a MART-1 peptide vaccine with incomplete Freund's adjuvant for resected high-risk melanoma. *Clin Cancer Res* 1999;5:2756.

105. Jager E, Ringhoffer M, Dienes HP, et al. Granulocyte-macrophage-colony-stimulating factor enhances immune responses to melanoma-associated peptides *in vivo*. *Int J Cancer* 1996;67:54.

106. Scheibenbogen C, Schmittel A, Keilholz U, et al. Phase 2 trial of vaccination with tyrosinase peptides and granulocyte-macrophage colony-stimulating factor in patients with metastatic melanoma. *J Immunother* 2000;23:275.

107. Jäger E, Gnjatic S, Nagata Y, et al. Induction of primary NY-ESO-1 immunity: CD8+ T lymphocyte and antibody responses in peptide-vaccinated patients with NY-ESO-1+ cancers. *Proc Natl Acad Sci U S A* 2000;97:12198.

108. Gjertsen MK, Buanes T, Rosseland AR, et al. Intradermal ras peptide vaccination with granulocyte-macrophage colony-stimulating factor as adjuvant: clinical and immunological responses in patients with pancreatic adenocarcinoma. *Int J Cancer* 2001;92:441.

109. Irvine KR, Rao JB, Rosenberg SA, et al. Cytokine enhancement of DNA immunization leads to effective treatment of established pulmonary metastases. *J Immunol* 1996;156:224.

110. Ross HM, Weber LW, Wang S, et al. Priming for T-cell-mediated rejection of established tumors by cutaneous DNA immunization. *Clin Cancer Res* 1997;3:2191.

111. Leitner WW, Ying H, Restifo NP. DNA and RNA-based vaccines: principles, progress and prospects. *Vaccine* 1999;18:765.

112. Rosenberg SA, Yang JC, Sherry RM, et al. Inability to immunize patients with metastatic melanoma using plasmid DNA encoding the gp100 melanoma-melanocyte antigen. *Hum Gene Ther* 2003;14:709.

113. Bowne WB, Srinivasan R, Wolchok JD, et al. Coupling and uncoupling of tumor immunity and autoimmunity. *J Exp Med* 1999;190:1717.

114. Bergman PJ, McKnight J, Novosad A, et al. Long-term survival of dogs with advanced malignant melanoma after DNA vaccination with xenogeneic human tyrosinase: a phase I trial. *Clin Cancer Res* 2003;9:1284.

115. Ying H, Zaks TZ, Wang RF, et al. Cancer therapy using a self-replicating RNA vaccine. *Nat Med* 1999;5:823.

116. Leitner WW, Hwang LN, deVeer MJ, et al. Alphavirus-based DNA vaccine breaks immunological tolerance by activating innate antiviral pathways. *Nat Med* 2003;9:33.

117. Restifo NP. The new vaccines: building viruses that elicit antitumor immunity. *Curr Opin Immunol* 1996;8:658.

118. Ribas A, Butterfield LH, Economou JS. Genetic immunotherapy for cancer. *Oncologist* 2000;5:87.

119. Rosenberg SA, Zhai Y, Yang JC, et al. Immunizing patients with metastatic melanoma using recombinant adenoviruses encoding MART-1 or gp100 melanoma antigens. *J Natl Cancer Inst* 1998;90:1894.

120. Marshall J, Odogwu L, Hwang J, et al. A phase I study of sequential vaccinations with fowlpox-CEA (6D)-TRICOM (B7.1/ICAM-1/LFA-3) alone, and sequentially with vaccinia-CEA (6D)-TRICOM and GM-CSF in patients with CEA-expressing carcinomas. *Proc Am Soc Clin Oncol* 2003;22:165.

121. Thurner B, Haendle I, Roder C, et al. Vaccination with mage-3A1 peptide-pulsed mature, monocyte-derived dendritic cells expands specific cytotoxic T cells and induces regression of some metastases in advanced stage IV melanoma. *J Exp Med* 1999;190:1669.

122. Banchereau J, Fay J, Pascual V, et al. Dendritic cells: controllers of the immune system and a new promise for immunotherapy. *Novartis Found Symp* 2003;252:226; discussion 235.

123. Stift A, Friedl J, Dubsky P, et al. Dendritic cell-based vaccination in solid cancer. *J Clin Oncol* 2003;21:135.

124. Morse MA, Nair SK, Mosca PJ, et al. Immunotherapy with autologous, human dendritic cells transfected with carcinoembryonic antigen mRNA. *Cancer Invest* 2003;21:341.

125. Su Z, Dannull J, Heiser A, et al. Immunological and clinical responses in metastatic renal cancer patients vaccinated with tumor RNA-transfected dendritic cells. *Cancer Res* 2003;63:2127.

126. Heiser A, Coleman D, Dannull J, et al. Autologous dendritic cells transfected with prostate-specific antigen RNA stimulate CTL responses against metastatic prostate tumors. *J Clin Invest* 2002;109:409.

127. Rini BI. Technology evaluation: APC-8015, Dendreon. *Curr Opin Mol Ther* 2002;4:76.

128. Restifo NP. Not so Fas: re-evaluating the mechanisms of immune privilege and tumor escape. *Nat Med* 2000;6:493.

129. Restifo NP, Marincola FM, Kawakami Y, et al. Loss of functional beta(2)-microglobulin in metastatic melanomas from five patients receiving immunotherapy. *J Natl Cancer Inst* 1996;88:100.

130. Restifo NP, Esquivel F, Kawakami Y, et al. Identification of human cancers deficient in antigen processing. *J Exp Med* 1993;177:265.

131. Van Elsas A, Sutmuller RPM, Hurwitz AA, et al. Elucidating the autoimmune and antitumor effector mechanisms of a treatment based on cytotoxic T lymphocyte antigen-4 blockade in combination with a B16 melanoma vaccine: comparison of prophylaxis and therapy. *J Exp Med* 2001;194:481.

132. Phan GQ, Yang JC, Sherry RM, et al. Cancer regression and autoimmunity induced by cytotoxic T lymphocyte-associated antigen 4 blockade in patients with metastatic melanoma. *Proc Natl Acad Sci U S A* 2003;100:8372.

133. Overwijk WW, Restifo NP. Creating therapeutic cancer vaccines: notes from the battlefield. *Trends Immunol* 2001;22:5.

Mark E. Dudley
Steven A. Rosenberg

CHAPTER **62**

Cell Transfer Therapy

BACKGROUND

An expanding understanding of cellular immunology combined with rapid advances in molecular genetics is opening new opportunities for immunotherapy for cancer patients. Adoptive cell transfer (ACT) therapy currently represents the most effective means for manipulating the human immune system to reject invasive metastatic cancer. ACT therapy involves the isolation of antitumor T cells from a patient with cancer, their *ex vivo* expansion and activation, and their autologous infusion back into the patient along with appropriate growth factors. Cell transfer therapy has shown promising results in recent clinical trials for treatment of patients with metastatic melanoma and lymphoma. Also, new methods for the *in vivo* identification of transferred cells are revealing the functional characteristics of T cells and the molecular nature of antigens relevant to successful immune-mediated tumor destruction.

The cellular basis of tumor destruction mediated by antitumor lymphocytes has been firmly established in preclinical models, and many tumor antigens that confer immune recognition and mediate tumor destruction have been characterized. Tumor-reactive CD8+ cytotoxic T lymphocytes (CTLs) are required for effective tumor immunity and treatment in mouse tumor models.[1,2] In some tumor models, transfer of CD4+ helper cells is also required for the establishment or maintenance of tumor immunity.[3,4] In general, the antigens recognized by CTLs consist of nine– or ten–amino acid peptides derived from intracellular proteins, noncovalently bound in the major groove of a class I major histocompatibility molecule.[5] In mouse tumor models and in patients, expression cloning methods have taken advantage of tumor-reactive CTLs to clone and identify tumor antigens and the genes encoding them.[6] Dozens of tumor antigens have been identified, including cancer-testes antigens that may be expressed in tumors of multiple histologic types, overexpressed tissue differentiation antigens that may be expressed by many tumors of specific histologic origin, or unique tumor antigens that may be expressed only by an individual tumor.

The abundance of target antigens has led to a proliferation of clinical trials with the aim of vaccinating patients against the antigens expressed by their tumors. A variety of vaccine vehicles delivering numerous tumor antigens have been investigated[1] and are described in Chapter 61. Many of these vaccine approaches have greatly increased the number of tumor-reactive lymphocytes in the circulation, but only rare and sporadic tumor regressions have been seen. These results emphasize the need for a clearer understanding of the interaction of the immune system with growing tumors and have motivated the investigation of alternate treatment approaches for patients with cancer.

Many hypotheses have been proposed to explain the failure of vaccine-induced or endogenous immune cells to eliminate tumors.[7] Tumors may fail to fully activate tumor-reactive lymphocytes, which leads to a low number or aberrant activation status of antitumor effector cells. Alternately, normal immune regulatory mechanisms could prevent the accumulation of sufficient numbers of cells with sufficient avidity against tumor antigens to mount an effective antitumor immune response. These (and many other) potential mechanisms of immune evasion by tumors can be overcome by the application of ACT methods for cancer treatment. ACT combines three conceptual elements to overcome some of the potential shortfalls of vaccine therapies (Fig. 62-1). First, cell transfer therapy calls for the *ex vivo* generation of effector lymphocyte cultures. Theoretically, this allows

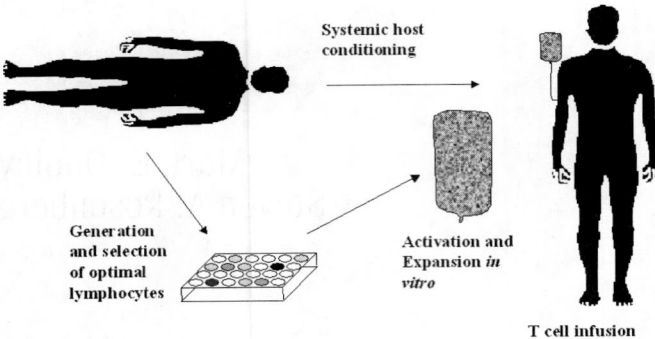

Systemic host conditioning

Generation and selection of optimal lymphocytes

Activation and Expansion *in vitro*

T cell infusion and IL-2 therapy

FIGURE 62-1. Adoptive cell transfer therapy for patients with cancer involves (1) the generation and selection of lymphocyte cultures with desired characteristics, (2) the *in vitro* expansion and activation of the T cells, and (3) the conditioning of the patient for optimum treatment efficacy before infusion of the cells and interleukin-2 (IL-2) support.

the investigator to select T cells with the optimal antigen specificities, functions, and phenotypes. Second, the selected T cells are activated and expanded to large numbers *ex vivo*. This *in vitro* growth and activation eliminates any potentially immunosuppressive influences of the tumor and circumvents normal immune regulatory mechanisms. Third, antitumor chemotherapy or systemic immune-modulatory agents can be administered to the patient while the effector cells are sequestered outside the body, so that any deleterious effects of those treatments are avoided. Different clinical trials investigating ACT therapies have capitalized on these three strategic elements to different extents.

PRECLINICAL STUDIES OF ADOPTIVE CELL TRANSFER

T-cell transfer approaches in mouse models have been optimized to investigate not only the specific aspects of the cell transfer approach but also the basic principles of tumor immunity. Although early efforts focused on transferring resistance to challenge by transplanted tumors, current work is aimed at solving the more difficult but more relevant problems of treating vascularized, established tumors. The description of a murine model using transfer of transgenic T cells reactive against the gp100 melanoma antigen has demonstrated the potency of ACT for the destruction of large invasive murine tumors and has helped elucidate the requirements for effective therapy.[8] Numerous antigens of diverse genetic origin, including tumor-unique antigens,[9] tissue differentiation antigens,[10,11] and antigens derived from overexpressed oncogenes,[12] can target established tumors for rejection in adoptive transfer systems in mouse models. In each of these mouse models of effective ACT, the specificity of the transferred lymphocytes for an antigen that is expressed by the tumor cells is a critical component for successful tumor treatment.

Other characteristics of the transferred cells that can dramatically impact their function have been defined and quantified in mouse models. The number of transferred cells is often directly correlated with treatment efficacy. Similarly, the avidity of CTLs for their cognate antigen is correlated with efficacy,

and CTLs with high avidity are more effective than low-avidity cells.[11] The tumor-specific cytokine secretion of the cells is often the best correlate of their *in vivo* therapeutic potential.[13,14] Studies using transgenic mice as well as gene knockout mice promise to provide further insights into the mechanisms of tumor destruction and the features of tumor-reactive T cells that can influence therapeutic efficacy.

Mouse models have also revealed that the host immune environment can dramatically impact the persistence and activity of transferred lymphocytes, and thus the efficacy of ACT therapy. Several adjuvant systemic treatments can strongly impact the effectiveness of transferred cells, including the administration of IL-2 or other cytokine administration after cell transfer.[15–17] A report with significant potential to impact the clinical practice of cell therapy demonstrated that concomitant vaccination is required with cell transfer for effective tumor destruction and the onset of antigen-specific autoimmunity.[8]

In several tumor treatment models in mice, immunosuppression before ACT was highly effective for increasing the impact of the transferred cells.[16,18–20] The role of immune suppression before ACT therapy and the mechanism(s) responsible for this effect are currently the subject of intense investigation and have important implications for the practice of ACT therapy in patients. North and others described a CD4+ lymphocyte population that suppressed the antitumor effects of ACT therapy.[18,21] More recently, Sakaguchi's group described a regulatory T-cell population consisting of CD4+ and CD25+ cells and demonstrated that their elimination could greatly improve the efficacy of adoptive immunotherapy.[22] These results support the investigation of lymphodepletion and its effects on potential suppressor cell populations in cancer patients.

Other hypotheses have been proposed to explain the dramatic impact of immunosuppression on ACT in mouse models. Depletion of endogenous lymphocytes may boost the survival or activation of transferred T cells by providing access to homeostatic lymphocyte survival and proliferative signals such as IL-7.[23,24] Ma et al. have demonstrated in a mouse tumor treatment model that homeostatic activation can nonspecifically enhance vaccination and tumor treatment effectiveness.[25] These studies support the further investigation of homeostatic T-cell regulation and its effects on tumor-specific lymphocytes in patients.

CLINICAL TRIALS

NONSPECIFIC LYMPHOCYTE CULTURES

The most difficult impediment to the wider application of ACT therapy for patients with cancer is the difficulty in generating large numbers of tumor-reactive cells for treatment. Because unselected peripheral blood lymphocytes (PBLs) are readily obtainable from most patients, extensive efforts have been invested in generating tumor-reactive cells from PBLs. T cells and natural killer cells can be highly activated *in vitro* with superphysiologic levels of IL-2. These lymphokine-activated killer (LAK) cells exhibited selective lysis of tumor cells compared with normal cells in culture and mediated antitumor effects in some mouse models.[26] These preclinical findings were translated into clinical trials to investigate the efficacy of LAK cells for treatment of patients with tumors of several different histologic types. Some sporadic reports of successful treatment in small clinical trials with nonspecific cells were made, but the concurrent use of systemic IL-2 therapy or chemotherapy with the transfer of cells confounded the interpretation of response rates. Larger, randomized studies failed to demonstrate a benefit of LAK treatment together with high-dose IL-2 therapy compared with IL-2 treatment alone for solid tumors.[27,28] The use of LAK cells for treatment of patients with some hematologic malignancies, as well as their use in combination with antitumor antibodies in which the natural killer component of transferred LAK cells may exhibit antibody-dependent cellular cytotoxicity, continues to be investigated.

Another approach to the use of PBLs in cell transfer therapy involves the *ex vivo* activation of enriched T-cell populations with low concentrations of IL-2 (or other cytokines) combined with nonspecific T-cell receptor stimulation through the CD3 molecule, often in combination with CD28 costimulation. As a stand-alone therapy for solid malignancies, this treatment has not been effective.[29] Research is continuing to define the potential role for CD3/CD28–stimulated PBLs as targets for gene transfer and some hematologic malignancies. In general, no clinical trial has demonstrated a reproducible therapeutic effect of ACT using nonspecific lymphocytes for treatment of solid malignancies. Results of these clinical and preclinical efforts emphasize the critical role of tumor rejection antigens and the specific CTLs that recognize them in successful immunotherapy for patients with cancer.

IN VITRO–GENERATED TUMOR-REACTIVE LYMPHOCYTES

The application of ACT therapy for patients is limited by the logistical and practical difficulties inherent in the *in vitro* generation of large numbers of tumor-reactive lymphocytes. Although this goal can be achieved in mice by vaccination and harvesting of whole immune spleens, in clinical trials the problem is more vexing. Despite technical difficulties, some tumor histologic types, including metastatic melanoma and posttransplant lymphoproliferative disorder, have been successfully treated with ACT therapy in clinical trials. Posttransplant lymphoproliferative disorder is a paradigmatic example of ACT therapy because methods have been established for the rapid and predictable generation of tumor-specific lymphocyte cultures.

Epstein-Barr virus (EBV)–associated lymphoproliferative disease is a complication of immunosuppression and occurs at a significant frequency in patients undergoing allogeneic bone marrow or solid organ transplantation (see Chapter 48.2). More than 90% of healthy adults harbor cryptic EBV infections, which are held in check by virus-specific T cells. In the posttransplantation immunosuppressed state, reactivation of latent EBV can result in the transformation and unchecked proliferation of B-cell lineage lymphocytes and the subsequent evolution of overt lymphoma. Many EBV-induced B-cell tumors express EBV-derived viral antigens and thus are highly immunogenic. Infusions of bulk, uncultured lymphocytes from donors of allogeneic bone marrow transplants were sufficient to restore anti-EBV immunity and to eliminate EBV-associated lymphoma from some transplant recipients with posttransplant lymphoproliferative disorder.[30] However, in this setting, the donor lymphocyte

infusions could initiate or exacerbate graft-versus-host disease. A more specific lymphocyte population was obtained by repetitive stimulations of PBLs *in vitro* with EBV-transformed lymphoblastic cell lines.[31] These lymphoblastic cell line cells efficiently presented viral antigens and costimulation necessary to activate and expand T cells *in vitro*. The resulting EBV-specific T-cell cultures contained both CD8+ HLA class I–restricted lymphocytes and CD4+ HLA class II–restricted lymphocytes that could recognize EBV-derived antigens. Transfer of the cultured EBV-specific lymphocytes was capable of eliminating lymphoma and establishing persistent anti-EBV immunity in the recipients.

The absolute limit of antigen specificity has been achieved in the use of cloned T cells for ACT therapy for cytomegalovirus (CMV) infections, which constitute a significant medical problem for immunosuppressed patients, including transplant recipients. The transfer of T-cell clones was first reported for the prevention of CMV infection after bone marrow transplantation.[32] CMV-specific CD8+ T-cell clones were readily isolated and expanded *in vitro* from seropositive marrow donors. The transfer of the virus-specific clones to marrow recipients was effective in preventing acute CMV infections in the posttransplantation period. These encouraging results with anti-CMV clones motivated the investigation of cloned tumor-reactive T cells for treatment of patients with cancer, including patients with melanoma.

The results of clinical trials with cloned lymphocytes for the treatment of patients with solid malignancies have been disappointing. No objective clinical responses to treatment with cloned melanoma-reactive T cells were seen in several clinical trials, regardless of whether clones were transferred without cytokine support or with IL-2 administration.[33,34] Sensitive fluorescence cytometry or polymerase chain reaction methods were used in these studies to monitor the persistence of the cloned T cells.[35] The transferred lymphocytes rapidly disappeared from the peripheral blood. In a study by Yee et al., extended administration of low-dose IL-2 enhanced the clonal lymphocyte survival at low levels *in vivo* for a few weeks but was not sufficient to induce any objective tumor response.[34] It thus appeared that highly avid recognition of tumor antigen by the transferred lymphocyte cultures was not sufficient for the *in vivo* regression of established solid tumors. Several explanations could account for the lack of therapeutic efficacy in these ACT trials with cloned lymphocytes. Full inflammatory immunity may include a requirement for antigen-specific CD4+ cells, or destruction of bulky tumors may require the long-term persistence of transferred cells. Alternately, cloned T cells might fail *as therapy* due to proliferative exhaustion, aberrant trafficking, or selection of antigen-loss tumor variants.

Other methods have been investigated for the generation of tumor antigen–specific cells for ACT treatment of solid tumors of nonviral etiology. Chang et al. have attempted to generate lymphocyte cultures that specifically recognize renal cell cancer or melanoma by a strategy of *in vivo* vaccination with irradiated autologous tumor, followed by harvesting of the vaccine-draining lymph node. The vaccine-draining lymph node cells were enriched in tumor-reactive T cells and were activated and expanded using nonspecific T-cell receptor stimulation and IL-2 *in vitro*.[36,37] Patients with advanced renal cell cancer were treated with tumor-draining lymph node lymphocytes and IL-2 therapy, and 9 patients of 34 treated were reported to exhibit an objective response (26%), although it was difficult in this study to distinguish these responses from those expected from IL-2 therapy alone.[38]

Other approaches for generating tumor antigen–specific cultures build on the molecular identification of tumor antigens by driving cell expansions *in vitro* with synthetic antigens. For instance, in a pilot trial involving eight patients, dendritic cells were pulsed with immunogenic peptides from melanoma antigens to stimulate patients' PBLs.[39] Antigen-specific cultures were obtained and expanded, and ACT with these cells was found to be safe and well tolerated. Some persistence of the transferred T cells was detected, and one objective partial response to treatment was reported. The use of dendritic cells for repetitive stimulations has not been widely attempted because it is logistically difficult to generate sufficient numbers of dendritic cells to drive the expansion of large numbers of lymphocytes. A similar strategy proposes the replacement of dendritic cells with artificial antigen-presenting cells.[40–43] The antigen-driven expansion of tumor-specific lymphocytes would simplify and extend the use of ACT for tumor therapy and deserves further investigation.

TUMOR-INFILTRATING LYMPHOCYTES

Tumor-infiltrating lymphocytes (TILs) represent an alternate source of exquisitely tumor-specific lymphocytes available for treatment of some patients with melanoma. In preclinical models, TILs from immunogenic, transplantable sarcomas of mice were easily generated and expanded *in vitro* and routinely demonstrated specific lytic activity toward their cognate tumor cells. TILs from mouse tumors were highly effective in treating mice with established hepatic or lung metastases.[16] Some human tumors, including melanoma,[44–48] renal cell carcinoma,[49,50] and glioma,[51] can also generate TILs that are suitable for use in ACT therapy. In contrast, TILs from other common tumor histologic types rarely produce CD8+ T cells that recognize their autologous tumors.[52,53]

Melanoma lesions seem particularly suited to this approach, and TILs from melanoma lesions often contain both CD4+ and CD8+ cells that recognize HLA-matched lesions as well as their autologous tumors.[54–57] In fact, melanoma lesions appear to be a repository for tumor-reactive T cells, and, in one study, refinements in the methods for growing TIL cultures resulted in the generation of autologous tumor-reactive lymphocytes from 78% of assessable TILs.[45] Most importantly, *in vitro* expanded TILs from melanoma lesions were active *in vivo*. In a series of 89 consecutively treated patients who were given autologous TILs and high-dose IL-2 at the Surgery Branch of the National Cancer Institute, 34% achieved an objective clinical response.[58] Clinical response of treated patients correlated with lysis of autologous tumor cells[56] and autologous tumor-specific secretion of cytokines.[59] Many of these responses were transient, however, and little persistence of the transferred cells was seen.[60] Some of the antigens that are recognized by effective TILs and potentially mediate tumor regression *in vivo* have been characterized at the molecular level (see Chapter 61.2). These clinical and immunologic results provide some of the most compelling evidence that cell transfer therapy can mediate the regression of metastatic cancer in humans and support the further evaluation of TILs as a source of lymphocytes for adoptive transfer studies.

ADOPTIVE CELL TRANSFER THERAPY AFTER LYMPHODEPLETING CHEMOTHERAPY IN PATIENTS WITH MELANOMA

An effective ACT immunotherapy capable of mediating sustained regression of bulky invasive cancers in approximately 45% of patients with metastatic melanoma was reported.[61] This treatment involved chemotherapy-induced lymphodepletion followed by TIL transfer and IL-2 administration. Patients received a reduced-intensity conditioning regimen with cyclophosphamide (60 mg/kg for 2 days) followed by 5 days of fludarabine (25 mg/m^2) that caused a moderate and transient myelosuppression and an almost complete but transient depletion of circulating lymphocytes. Most patients recovered endogenous marrow function, and circulating neutrophils were reconstituted to normal levels within 2 weeks.[33] Normal lymphocyte recovery occurred as well, although, as previously reported for this dose and schedule of fludarabine,[62] some patients experienced delayed recovery of CD4+ cells. The day after the last dose of fludarabine, when lymphocyte counts were negligible, patients received highly activated and expanded tumor-reactive TIL cultures, as well as high-dose IL-2 therapy (720,000 IU/kg IL-2 every 8 hours to tolerance).

A summary of results for the first 13 HLA-A2–positive patients treated with this regimen is given in Table 62-1. Six patients demonstrated objective clinical responses with greater than 50% reduction of metastatic disease, and four others had significant mixed responses. All patients had disease refractory to prior treatment with IL-2 alone and three of the responding patients had previously received the same chemotherapy with cloned cells and had not responded. The treatment caused substantial tumor regression of metastatic deposits in the lung, liver, brain, adrenal gland, muscle, cutaneous and subcutaneous tissue, and lymph nodes (Fig. 62-2). Since that report, an additional 22 patients have received similar treatments, and the response rate for this heavily pretreated group of melanoma patients is 51%, including four repeat responses. Some patients who responded to treatment also demonstrated autoimmune skin depigmentation (vitiligo in 14 patients) or autoimmune inflammation of the eye (uveitis in 5 patients). The correlation between tumor regression and the onset of autoimmunity raises interesting questions about the immune mechanisms of solid tumor destruction. This linkage has been noted previously in patients receiving immunotherapy.[63,64] These immune phenomena have also been linked in mouse models of tumor therapy with ACT or vaccination approaches[10,65] and in melanoma patients treated with CTL-associated antigen-4 blockade.[66] These results suggest that autoimmunity and tumor rejection share some underlying mechanisms or require a magnitude of immune response that is rarely achieved by other approaches. The association of tumor immunity and autoimmunity in patients treated with ACT therapy emphasizes the need for aiming these responses to antigens unique to tumors or expressed only on normal tissues that are dispensable for survival.

The tumor regressions observed in some patients responding to lymphodepletion and ACT therapy were accompanied by dramatic *in vivo* activation and proliferation of the transferred cells. Several patients demonstrated a dramatic but transient lymphocytosis comprised of the transferred cells with antitumor activity approximately a week after cell transfer (Fig. 62-3A). Lymphocytes from the patients' peripheral blood had a highly activated phenotype for several weeks after transfer. These hematologic features

TABLE 62-1. Response Rate and Rate of Onset of Autoimmunity in HLA-A2–Positive Patients Treated with Nonmyeloablative but Lymphodepleting Chemotherapy and Transfer of Rapidly Expanded Tumor-Infiltrating Lymphocytes

Patient	Age/Sex	Cells ($\times 10^{-10}$)	Antigens[a]	Sites of Evaluable Metastases	Response (Mo)	Autoimmunity
1	18/M	2.3	A	Axillary, mesenteric, pelvic lymph nodes	PR (29)	None
2	30/F	3.5	G, M	Cutaneous, subcutaneous	PR (8)	Vitiligo
4	57/F	3.4	G, M	Cutaneous, subcutaneous	PR (2)	None
6	37/F	9.2	A	Lung, intraperitoneal, subcutaneous	PR (23)	None
9	57/M	9.6	M, A	Cutaneous, subcutaneous	PR (11)	Vitiligo
10	55/M	10.7	M	Lymph nodes, cutaneous, subcutaneous	PR (14)	Uveitis
3	43/F	4.0	G, A	Brain, cutaneous, liver, lung	NR	None
5	53/M	3.0	G, A	Brain, lung, lymph nodes	NR (mixed)	None
7	44/M	12.3	M, A	Lymph nodes, subcutaneous	NR (mixed)	Vitiligo
8	48/M	9.5	G	Subcutaneous	NR	None
11	29/M	13.0	M	Liver, pericardial, subcutaneous	NR (mixed)	Vitiligo
12	37/F	13.7	M	Liver, lung, gallbladder, lymph nodes	NR	None
13	41/F	7.7	M	Subcutaneous	NR	None
Total	6F, 7M	Average: 7.8			6 PR, 7 NR	5+, 8–

F, female; M, male; NR, no objective response; NR (mixed), regression of some tumor nodules with progression at other sites; PR, partial response with more than 50% reduction of tumor volume and no progression at any site and no new disease.
Note: Patients 2, 4, 5, 7, 8, 11, and 12 received more than one course of treatment. Patients' conditioning chemotherapy consisted of 2 days of cyclophosphamide (60 mg/kg) followed by 5 days of fludarabine (60 mg/m^2), and the indicated number of lymphocytes were infused on the following day. High-dose interleukin-2 therapy (720,000 IU/kg every 8 hours) was started the day of cell infusion and continued to patient tolerance or a maximum of 15 doses.
[a]Infused cells were reactive against the HLA-A2 gp100:209-217 epitope, the HLA-A2 MART-1:27-36 epitope, or another epitope expressed by the patient's autologous tumor cells (G, M, and A, respectively).

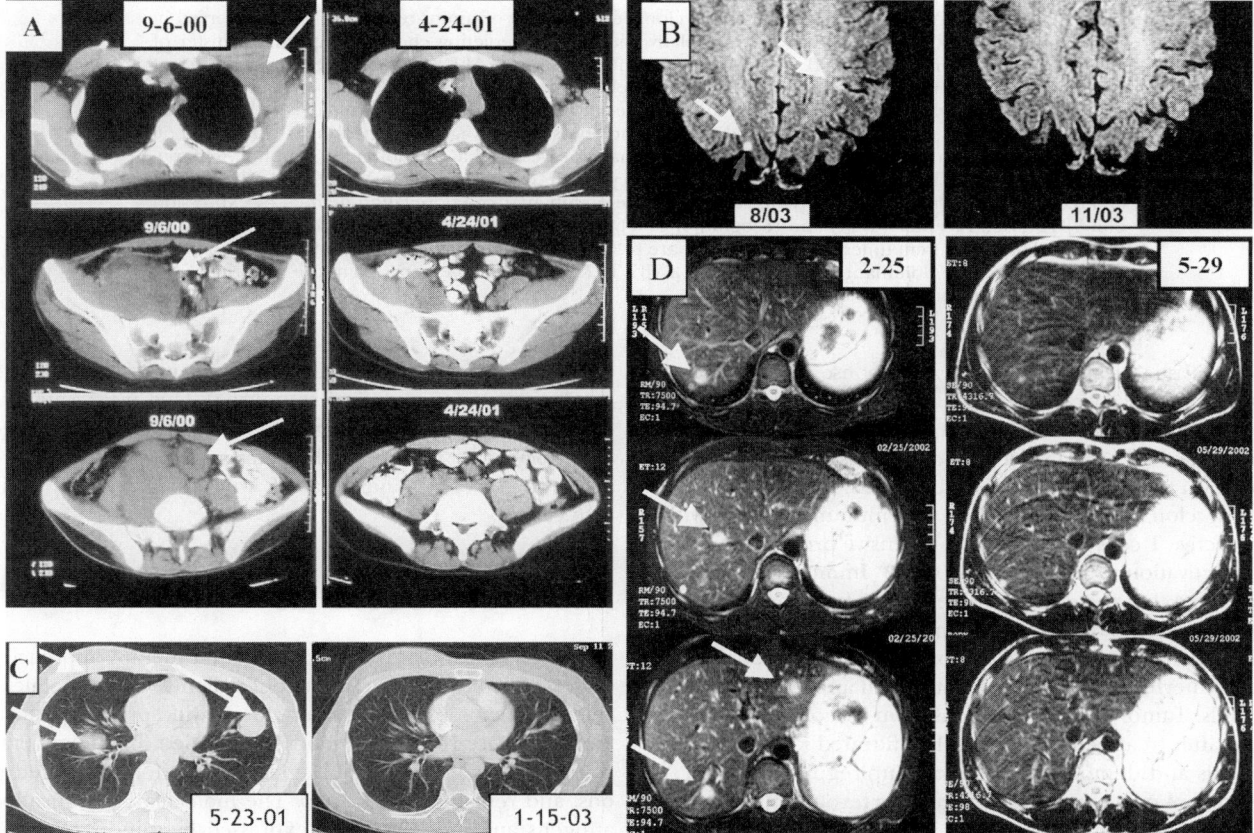

FIGURE 62-2. Adoptive cell transfer therapy after nonmyeloablative but lymphodepleting chemotherapy results in the regression of tumors in some patients. Arrows point to metastatic lesions in pretreatment scans that are substantially reduced or absent in posttreatment scans. **A:** Regression of bulky nodal disease in the axilla (*top*), pelvis (*middle*), and mesentery (*lower*) visualized by computed tomography (CT) scans. **B:** Regression of multiple brain metastases visualized by CT scans. **C:** Regression of multiple lung metastases visualized by CT scans. **D:** Regression of multiple liver metastases shown by magnetic resonance imaging scans.

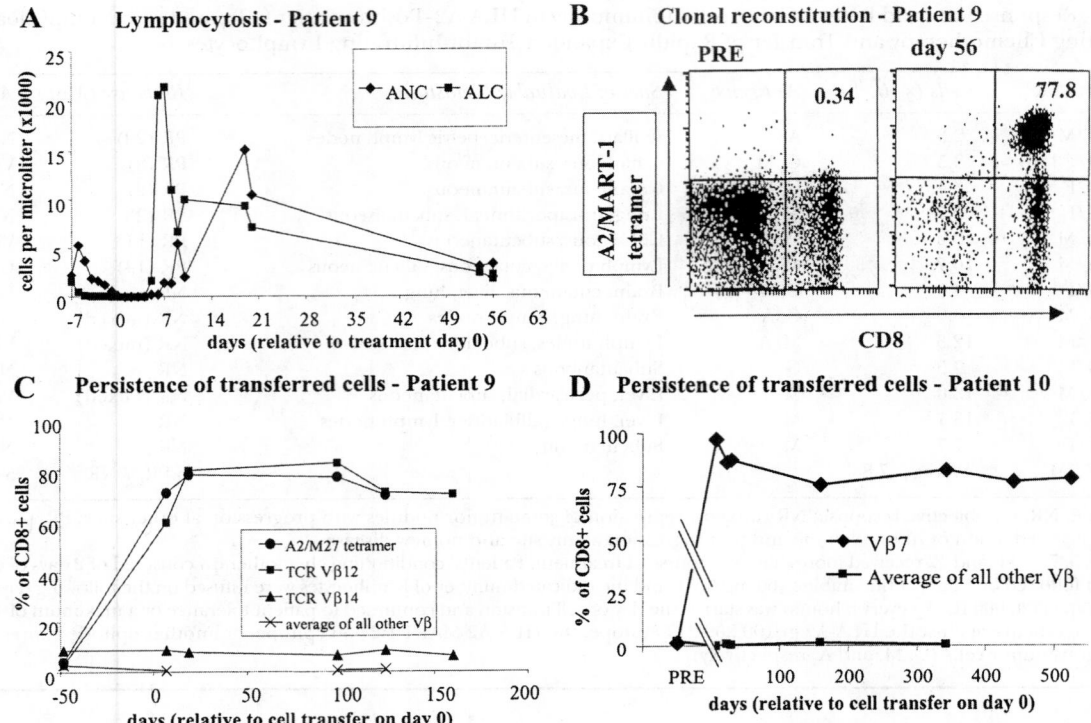

FIGURE 62-3.   Transient lymphocytosis and clonal engraftment of tumor-reactive cells was observed in some patients after treatment with nonmyeloablative but lymphodepleting chemotherapy and transfer of tumor-infiltrating lymphocytes (TILs). **A:** Absolute lymphocyte count (ALC) and absolute neutrophil count (ANC) are graphed for the period immediately after cell transfer for patient 9. The upper limit of normal ALC is around 4000 lymphocytes/mm³. **B:** Fluorescence-activated cell sorter (FACS) analysis with HLA-A2/MART-1:26-35(27L) tetramer demonstrated background levels of staining before treatment (PRE), but 56 days following TIL administration to patient 9, FACS analysis revealed that the dominant lymphocyte population consisted of CD8+ cells reactive with the melanocyte differentiation antigen MART-1. **C:** The peripheral blood lymphocytes of patient 9 consisted of a single dominant T-cell population defined by expression of a Vβ12 T-cell receptor (TCR) and recognition of tetramerized HLA-A2/MART-1:26-35(27L). Results of FACS analysis at different times after TIL transfer are plotted. **D:** Peripheral blood lymphocytes of patient 10 consisted of a single dominant clone expressing a Vβ7 TCR, and the clone persisted as the majority of the circulating T cells for more than 500 days.

are characteristic of an acute immune response such as occurs during clearance of a viral infection.

Using fluorescence cytometry, reverse transcriptase-polymerase chain reaction, and DNA sequence analysis, the lymphocytosis was shown to derive from the infused TILs. Each patient had an almost clonal repopulation of the immune system with tumor-reactive T cells resulting from extensive proliferation as a result of activation *in vivo* (see Fig. 62-3*B*). Immunologic assays demonstrated that the circulating cells were functional directly *ex vivo* and caused the lysis of tumor cells and the antigen-specific secretion of high levels of inflammatory cytokines, including interferon-γ, when stimulated with antigen-expressing tumor cells. Tumor biopsy specimens from responding patients obtained after treatment were densely infiltrated with the transferred cells and demonstrated striking up-regulation of HLA expression, a known consequence of interferon-γ stimulation. Concurrent with tumor regression and the onset of autoimmune manifestations in these patients, the clonal populations of tumor-reactive cells repopulated the patients' immune systems and stably persisted as the major lymphocyte population in the blood for months after TIL administration (see Fig. 62-3*C,D*). In a study examing the persistence of transferred cells in the peripheral blood of 25 patients receiving this treatment, the

persistence of transferred TIL clonotypes was statistically correlated with objective clinical response.[77] This *in vivo* activation, clonal engraftment, and long-term persistence of tumor-specific lymphocytes in patients with metastatic cancer represent the achievement of a major goal of immunotherapy for patients with cancer.

ADDITIONAL STUDIES

Cell transfer is the most effective immunotherapy approach currently available for the treatment of patients with metastatic cancer, although obstacles remain to its widespread application. Simpler, more reliable methods are needed for the generation of tumor-specific cells that engraft, persist for prolonged periods, and remain active *in vivo*. The molecular identification of antigens and T-cell epitopes expressed by tumors provides an opportunity to use repetitive *in vitro* stimulations with defined tumor antigens to generate tumor-specific cells for patient treatment. Patients who have received vaccination before lymphocyte harvest could be ideal candidates for this approach, and clinical trials to evaluate the combination of *in vivo* vaccination and *ex vivo* T-cell expansion are currently accruing patients.

Genetic engineering is providing other approaches for generating T cells with a defined antitumor specificity, including the redirection of T-cell specificity by transfer of genes encoding a tumor antigen–specific T-cell receptor or antibody combining site-receptor signaling chimera.[67–70] Clinical trials with T-cell receptor–engineered lymphocytes are in progress to assess the usefulness of this approach. Ultimately, the wider application of cell transfer strategies may require the identification of additional tumor antigens, including antigens expressed by tumors of diverse histologic origins, as well as a better understanding of the T-cell receptors that mediate *in vivo* tumor recognition and the proliferation and persistence of the transferred cells.

The tumor antigen specificity of infused cells is a well-established requirement for treatment efficacy in mouse models and clinical trials, but there is mounting evidence that additional characteristics of lymphocytes have a decisive impact on treatment efficacy. Characteristics of T cells such as the ability to traffic, *in vivo* proliferation, and maintenance of inflammatory activation may all play important roles in mediating tumor regression. In CD8+ lymphocytes, many of these characteristics are known to be affected by the maturation state of the cells[71,72] and can be influenced by the cytokine milieu.[73] Translation of these findings to clinical-scale culture for ACT treatment of patients is proceeding, as is genetic engineering of lymphocytes to constitutively express their own growth factors to enhance survival after cytokine withdrawal *in vivo*.[74] Lymphocytes transduced with the gene encoding IL-2 can proliferate for months *in vitro* with repetitive antigen stimulation in the absence of added IL-2, and those cells are currently being evaluated in ACT clinical trials. A more detailed understanding of these and other factors influencing CD8+ T-cell persistence *in vivo* could be translated into improved lymphocyte cultures for ACT therapy.

Similarly, the optimal manipulation of the host immune environment to enhance *in vivo* antitumor activities remains to be determined. For instance, understanding and exploiting the dual roles of CD4+ cells in tolerance, autoimmunity, and tumor immunity have important clinical implications. A requirement for CD4+ cells in the persistence of CD8+ cells underscores the need to incorporate CD4+ cells in ACT therapies.[75,76] Confounding this aim is the identification in mice and humans of a CD4+/CD25+ T-cell compartment that exhibits potent immune-suppressive effects *in vivo*. The need to eliminate these suppressor cells as well as provide "space" in the immune system constitutes a strong rationale for continued investigation of lymphodepleting conditioning for ACT therapy. Finally, the role of concurrent vaccination after T-cell transfer is well established in mouse models, and T-cell–mediated antigen-specific immunity in humans is also likely affected by the context and quantity of the antigen. Identifying optimal vaccination strategies for tumor antigens recognized by the transferred cells and combining them with cell transfer therapy approaches may improve clinical antitumor immune responses. The optimal combination of a permissive host immune environment, tumor antigen specificity, and T cells with the appropriate function and phenotype could lead to more widely applicable ACT protocols and effective immunotherapy for patients with cancer.

REFERENCES

1. Rosenberg SA. Progress in human tumour immunology and immunotherapy. *Nature* 2001;411:380.

2. Dudley ME, Rosenberg SA. Adoptive-cell-transfer therapy for the treatment of patients with cancer. *Nat Rev Cancer* 2003;3:666.

3. Rosenstein M, Eberlein TJ, Rosenberg SA. Adoptive immunotherapy of established syngeneic solid tumors: role of T lymphoid subpopulations. *J Immunol* 1984;132:2117.

4. Sakai K, Chang AE, Shu S. Effector phenotype and immunologic specificity of T-cell-mediated adoptive therapy for a murine tumor that lacks intrinsic immunogenicity. *Cell Immunol* 1990;129:241.

5. Shastri N, Schwab S, Serwold T. Producing nature's gene-chips: the generation of peptides for display by MHC class I molecules. *Annu Rev Immunol* 2002;20:463.

6. Renkvist N, Castelli C, Robbins PF, Parmiani G. A listing of human tumor antigens recognized by T cells. *Cancer Immunol Immunother* 2001;50:3.

7. Khong HT, Restifo NP. Natural selection of tumor variants in the generation of "tumor escape" phenotypes. *Nat Immunol* 2002;3:999.

8. Overwijk WW, Theoret MR, Finkelstein SE, et al. Tumor regression and autoimmunity after reversal of a functionally tolerant state of self-reactive CD8+ T cells. *J Exp Med* 2003;198:569.

9. Barth RJ Jr, Bock SN, Mule JJ, Rosenberg SA. Unique murine tumor-associated antigens identified by tumor infiltrating lymphocytes. *J Immunol* 1990;144:1531.

10. Overwijk WW, Lee DS, Surman DR, et al. Vaccination with a recombinant vaccinia virus encoding a "self" antigen induces autoimmune vitiligo and tumor cell destruction in mice: requirement for CD4(+) T lymphocytes. *Proc Natl Acad Sci U S A* 1999;96:2982.

11. Zeh H, Perry-Lalley D, Dudley ME, Rosenberg SA, Yang JC. High avidity CTLs for two self-antigens demonstrate superior *in vitro* and *in vivo* antitumor efficacy. *J Immunol* 1999;162:989.

12. Ercolini AM, Machiels JP, Chen YC, et al. Identification and characterization of the immunodominant rat HER-2/neu MHC class I epitope presented by spontaneous mammary tumors from HER-2/neu-transgenic mice. *J Immunol* 2003;170:4273.

13. Aruga A, Shu S, Chang AE. Tumor-specific granulocyte/macrophage colony-stimulating factor and interferon gamma secretion is associated with *in vivo* therapeutic efficacy of activated tumor-draining lymph node cells. *Cancer Immunol Immunother* 1995;41:317.

14. Barth RJ Jr, Mule JJ, Spiess PJ, Rosenberg SA. Interferon gamma and tumor necrosis factor have a role in tumor regressions mediated by murine CD8+ tumor-infiltrating lymphocytes. *J Exp Med* 1991;173:647.

15. Cheever MA, Greenberg PD, Fefer A, Gillis S. Augmentation of the anti-tumor therapeutic efficacy of long-term cultured T lymphocytes by *in vivo* administration of purified interleukin 2. *J Exp Med* 1982;155:968.

16. Rosenberg SA, Spiess P, Lafreniere R. A new approach to the adoptive immunotherapy of cancer with tumor-infiltrating lymphocytes. *Science* 1986;233:1318.

17. Klebanoff CA, Finkelstein SE, Surman DR, et al. IL-15 enhances the *in vivo* anti-tumor activity of tumor-reactive CD8+ T cells. *Proc Natl Acad Sci U S A* 2004;101(7):1969.

18. North RJ. Cyclophosphamide-facilitated adoptive immunotherapy of an established tumor depends on elimination of tumor-induced suppressor T cells. *J Exp Med* 1982;155:1063.

19. Berenson JR, Einstein AB Jr, Fefer A. Syngeneic adoptive immunotherapy and chemoimmunotherapy of a Friend leukemia: requirement for T cells. *J Immunol* 1975;115:234.

20. Antony PA, Restifo NP. Do CD4+CD25+ immunoregulatory T cells hinder tumor immunotherapy? *J Immunother* 2002;25:202.

21. Dye ES, North RJ. T cell–mediated immunosuppression as an obstacle to adoptive immunotherapy of the P815 mastocytoma and its metastases. *J Exp Med* 1981;154:1033.

22. Shimizu J, Yamazaki S, Sakaguchi S. Induction of tumor immunity by removing CD25+CD4+ T cells: a common basis between tumor immunity and autoimmunity. *J Immunol* 1999;163:5211.

23. Fry TJ, Mackall CL. Interleukin-7: master regulator of peripheral T-cell homeostasis? *Trends Immunol* 2001;22:564.

24. Maine GN, Mule JJ. Making room for T cells. *J Clin Invest* 2002;110:157.

25. Ma J, Urba WJ, Si L, et al. Anti-tumor T cell response and protective immunity in mice that received sublethal irradiation and immune reconstitution. *Eur J Immunol* 2003;33:2123.

26. Rosenberg SA. Immunotherapy of cancer by systemic administration of lymphoid cells plus interleukin-2. *J Biol Response Mod* 1984;3:501.

27. Rosenberg SA, Lotze MT, Yang JC, et al. Prospective randomized trial of high-dose interleukin-2 alone or in conjunction with lymphokine-activated killer cells for the treatment of patients with advanced cancer [published erratum appears in *J Natl Cancer Inst* 1993;85(13):1091]. *J Natl Cancer Inst* 1993;85:622.

28. Dillman RO, Oldham RK, Tauer KW, et al. Continuous interleukin-2 and lymphokine-activated killer cells for advanced cancer: a National Biotherapy Study Group trial. *J Clin Oncol* 1991;9:1233.

29. Lum LG, LeFever AV, Treisman JS, Garlie NK, Hanson JP Jr. Immune modulation in cancer patients after adoptive transfer of anti-CD3/anti-CD28-costimulated T cells—phase I clinical trial. *J Immunother* 2001;24:408.

30. O'Reilly RJ, Small TN, Papadopoulos E, et al. Biology and adoptive cell therapy of Epstein-Barr virus–associated lymphoproliferative disorders in recipients of marrow allografts. *Immunol Rev* 1997;157:195.

31. Rooney CM, Smith CA, Ng CY, et al. Infusion of cytotoxic T cells for the prevention and treatment of Epstein-Barr virus–induced lymphoma in allogeneic transplant recipients. *Blood* 1998;92:1549.

32. Walter EA, Greenberg PD, Gilbert MJ, et al. Reconstitution of cellular immunity against cytomegalovirus in recipients of allogeneic bone marrow by transfer of T-cell clones from the donor. *N Engl J Med* 1995;333:1038.

33. Dudley ME, Wunderlich JR, Yang JC, et al. A phase I study of nonmyeloablative chemotherapy and adoptive transfer of autologous tumor–specific T lymphocytes in patients with metastatic melanoma. *J Immunother* 2002;25:243.

34. Yee C, Thompson JA, Byrd D, et al. Adoptive T cell therapy using antigen-specific CD8+ T cell clones for the treatment of patients with metastatic melanoma: *in vivo* persistence, migration, and antitumor effect of transferred T cells. *Proc Natl Acad Sci U S A* 2002;99:16168.

35. Yee C, Greenberg P. Modulating T-cell immunity to tumours: new strategies for monitoring T-cell responses. *Nat Rev Cancer* 2002;2:409.

36. Chang AE, Aruga A, Cameron MJ, et al. Adoptive immunotherapy with vaccine-primed lymph node cells secondarily activated with anti-CD3 and interleukin-2. *J Clin Oncol* 1997;15:796.

37. Chang AE, Li Q, Jiang G, et al. Phase II trial of autologous tumor vaccination, anti-CD3-activated vaccine-primed lymphocytes, and interleukin-2 in stage IV renal cell cancer. *J Clin Oncol* 2003;21:884.

38. Yang JC, Sherry RM, Steinberg SM, et al. Randomized study of high-dose and low-dose interleukin-2 in patients with metastatic renal cancer. *J Clin Oncol* 2003;21:3127.

39. Meidenbauer N, Marienhagen J, Laumer M, et al. Survival and tumor localization of adoptively transferred Melan-A-specific T cells in melanoma patients. *J Immunol* 2003;170:2161.

40. Maus MV, Thomas AK, Leonard DG, et al. *Ex vivo* expansion of polyclonal and antigen-specific cytotoxic T lymphocytes by artificial APCs expressing ligands for the T-cell receptor, CD28 and 4-1BB. *Nat Biotechnol* 2002;20:143.

41. Oelke M, Maus MV, Didiano D, et al. *Ex vivo* induction and expansion of antigen-specific cytotoxic T cells by HLA-Ig-coated artificial antigen-presenting cells. *Nat Med* 2003;9:619.

42. Tham EL, Jensen PL, Mescher MF. Activation of antigen-specific T cells by artificial cell constructs having immobilized multimeric peptide-class I complexes and recombinant B7-Fc proteins. *J Immunol Methods* 2001;249:111.

43. Sili U, Huls MH, Davis AR, et al. Large-scale expansion of dendritic cell-primed polyclonal human cytotoxic T-lymphocyte lines using lymphoblastoid cell lines for adoptive immunotherapy. *J Immunother* 2003;26:241.

44. Arienti F, Belli F, Rivoltini L, et al. Adoptive immunotherapy of advanced melanoma patients with interleukin-2 (IL-2) and tumor-infiltrating lymphocytes selected *in vitro* with low doses of IL-2. *Cancer Immunol Immunother* 1993;36:315.

45. Dudley ME, Wunderlich JR, Shelton TE, Even J, Rosenberg SA. Generation of tumor-infiltrating lymphocyte cultures for use in adoptive transfer therapy for melanoma patients. *J Immunother* 2003;26:332.

46. Itoh K, Tilden AB, Balch CM. Interleukin 2 activation of cytotoxic T-lymphocytes infiltrating into human metastatic melanomas. *Cancer Res* 1986;46:3011.

47. Yannelli JR, Hyatt C, McConnell S, et al. Growth of tumor-infiltrating lymphocytes from human solid cancers: summary of a 5-year experience. *Int J Cancer* 1996;65:413.

48. Topalian SL, Muul LM, Solomon D, Rosenberg SA. Expansion of human tumor infiltrating lymphocytes for use in immunotherapy trials. *J Immunol Methods* 1987;102:127.

49. Belldegrun A, Muul LM, Rosenberg SA. Interleukin 2 expanded tumor-infiltrating lymphocytes in human renal cell cancer: isolation, characterization, and antitumor activity. *Cancer Res* 1988;48:206.

50. Figlin RA, Pierce WC, Kaboo R, et al. Treatment of metastatic renal cell carcinoma with nephrectomy, interleukin-2 and cytokine-primed or CD8(+) selected tumor infiltrating lymphocytes from primary tumor. *J Urol* 1997;158:740.

51. Quattrocchi KB, Miller CH, Cush S, et al. Pilot study of local autologous tumor infiltrating lymphocytes for the treatment of recurrent malignant gliomas. *J Neurooncol* 1999;45:141.

52. Hom SS, Rosenberg SA, Topalian SL. Specific immune recognition of autologous tumor by lymphocytes infiltrating colon carcinomas: analysis by cytokine secretion. *Cancer Immunol Immunother* 1993;36:1.

53. Dadmarz R, Sgagias MK, Rosenberg SA, Schwartzentruber DJ. CD4+ T lymphocytes infiltrating human breast cancer recognise autologous tumor in an MHC-class-II restricted fashion. *Cancer Immunol Immunother* 1995;40:1.

54. Markus NR, Rosenberg SA, Topalian SL. Analysis of cytokine secretion by melanoma-specific CD4+ T lymphocytes. *J Interferon Cytokine Res* 1995;15:739.

55. Robbins PF, el Gamil M, Li YF, et al. Multiple HLA class II-restricted melanocyte differentiation antigens are recognized by tumor-infiltrating lymphocytes from a patient with melanoma. *J Immunol* 2002;169:6036.

56. Topalian SL, Solomon D, Rosenberg SA. Tumor-specific cytolysis by lymphocytes infiltrating human melanomas. *J Immunol* 1989;142:3714.

57. Wang RF, Wang X, Rosenberg SA. Identification of a novel major histocompatibility complex class II–restricted tumor antigen resulting from a chromosomal rearrangement recognized by CD4(+) T cells. *J Exp Med* 1999;189:1659.

58. Rosenberg SA, Yannelli JR, Yang JC, et al. Treatment of patients with metastatic melanoma with autologous tumor-infiltrating lymphocytes and interleukin 2. *J Natl Cancer Inst* 1994;86:1159.

59. Schwartzentruber DJ, Hom SS, Dadmarz R, et al. *In vitro* predictors of therapeutic response in melanoma patients receiving tumor-infiltrating lymphocytes and interleukin-2. *J Clin Oncol* 1994;12:1475.

60. Rosenberg SA, Aebersold P, Cornetta K, et al. Gene transfer into humans—immunotherapy of patients with advanced melanoma, using tumor-infiltrating lymphocytes modified by retroviral gene transduction. *N Engl J Med* 1990;323:570.

61. Dudley ME, Wunderlich JR, Robbins PF, et al. Cancer regression and autoimmunity in patients after clonal repopulation with antitumor lymphocytes. *Science* 2002;298:850.

62. Cheson BD. Infectious and immunosuppressive complications of purine analog therapy. *J Clin Oncol* 1995;13:2431.

63. Phan GQ, Attia P, Steinberg SM, White DE, Rosenberg SA. Factors associated with response to high-dose interleukin-2 in patients with advanced melanoma. *J Clin Oncol* 2001;19:3477.

64. Yee C, Thompson JA, Roche P, et al. Melanocyte destruction after antigen-specific immunotherapy of melanoma. Direct evidence of T cell–mediated vitiligo. *J Exp Med* 2000;192:1637.

65. van Elsas A, Hurwitz AA, Allison JP. Combination immunotherapy of B16 melanoma using anti-cytotoxic T lymphocyte–associated antigen 4 (CTLA-4) and granulocyte/macrophage colony-stimulating factor (GM-CSF)-producing vaccines induces rejection of subcutaneous and metastatic tumors accompanied by autoimmune depigmentation. *J Exp Med* 1999;190:355.

66. Phan GQ, Yang JC, Sherry RM, et al. Cancer regression and autoimmunity induced by cytotoxic T lymphocyte–associated antigen 4 blockade in patients with metastatic melanoma. *Proc Natl Acad Sci U S A* 2003;100:8372.

67. Clay TM, Custer MC, Sachs J, et al. Efficient transfer of a tumor antigen-reactive TCR to human peripheral blood lymphocytes confers anti-tumor reactivity. *J Immunol* 1999;163:507.

68. Morgan RA, Dudley ME, Yu YY, et al. High efficiency TCR gene transfer into primary human lymphocytes affords avid recognition of melanoma tumor antigen glycoprotein 100 and does not alter the recognition of autologous melanoma antigens. *J Immunol* 2003;171:3287.

69. Parker LL, Do MT, Westwood JA, et al. Expansion and characterization of T cells transduced with a chimeric receptor against ovarian cancer. *Hum Gene Ther* 2000;11:2377.

70. Walker RE, Bechtel CM, Natarajan V, et al. Long-term *in vivo* survival of receptor-modified syngeneic T cells in patients with human immunodeficiency virus infection. *Blood* 2000;96:467.

71. Wherry EJ, Teichgraber V, Becker TC, et al. Lineage relationship and protective immunity of memory CD8 T cell subsets. *Nat Immunol* 2003;4:225.

72. Geginat J, Lanzavecchia A, Sallusto F. Proliferation and differentiation potential of human CD8+ memory T-cell subsets in response to antigen or homeostatic cytokines. *Blood* 2003;101:4260.

73. Schluns KS, Lefrancois L. Cytokine control of memory T-cell development and survival. *Nat Rev Immunol* 2003;3:269.

74. Liu K, Rosenberg SA. Transduction of an IL-2 gene into human melanoma-reactive lymphocytes results in their continued growth in the absence of exogenous IL-2 and maintenance of specific antitumor activity. *J Immunol* 2001;167:6356.

75. Sun JC, Bevan MJ. Defective CD8 T cell memory following acute infection without CD4 T cell help. *Science* 2003;300:339.

76. Shedlock DJ, Shen H. Requirement for CD4 T cell help in generating functional CD8 T cell memory. *Science* 2003;300:337.

77. Robbins PF, Dudley ME, et al. Persistence of transferred lymphocyte clonotypes correlates with cancer regression in patients receiving cell transfer therapy. *Cutting Edge J Immunol* (in press).

Judah Folkman

CHAPTER **63**

Antiangiogenesis Agents

Sustained angiogenesis is a process critical to the continued growth of solid tumors, their metastases, and leukemias.[1] Microvascular endothelial cells are usually recruited to human tumors at an early stage of tumorigenesis—for example, *in situ* carcinoma in a breast duct[2] or horizontal melanoma in the epidermis. Tumor cells per se and/or stromal cells and inflammatory cells (i.e., macrophages, mast cells, and T cells) are the source of angiogenic factors.[3,4]

ANGIOGENIC SWITCH

These angiogenic factors are mainly proteins, such as vascular endothelial growth factor (VEGF), basic fibroblast growth factor, (bFGF), platelet-derived growth factor-BB, placental growth factor, pleiotrophin, transforming growth factor-β, platelet-derived endothelial cell growth factor, and others. These positive regulators of angiogenesis mediate endothelial cell migration and proliferation and microvessel formation in tumors undergoing the switch to the angiogenic phenotype, also called the "angiogenic switch."[5] The source of endothelial cells during the angiogenic switch can be either from preexisting microvasculature (i.e., formation of new sprouts, or tumor cell co-option of preexisting microvessels leading to apoptosis of preexisting endothelial cells and then induction of new vessel sprouts)[6] or from circulating endothelial stem cells.[7–9] The term "switch to the angiogenic phenotype" was first used to describe the phenomenon in which hyperplastic islets in transgenic mice (RIP-Tag), switch from small (less than 1 mm), white microscopic dormant tumors to red, rapidly growing tumors.[5] The morphologic and molecular events of the angiogenic switch are still being elucidated. However, preliminary data from nonangiogenic human tumors implanted into immunodeficient mice in the Folkman laboratory reveal discrete events in which blind sprouts form, but without a lumen. After lumen formation, the sprouts may fill with blood, but there is a period of no flow and little or no leakage of blood from the tip of the sprout. It is unclear what prevents hemorrhage from the tip of these sprouts. Sprouts connect with each other and blood flow follows, giving the previously white microtumor a red, hyperemic appearance.

ANGIOGENIC SWITCH—AN UNCOMMON EVENT

Autopsies of individuals who died of trauma often reveal microscopic-sized *in situ* cancers.[10] Approximately 39% of women aged 40 to 50 years who did not have cancer in their lifetime were found at autopsy to harbor *in situ* cancers in their breast. But breast cancer is diagnosed in only 1% of women in this age range. In men between age 60 and 70 years, *in situ* prostate cancer was found in 46% of autopsies, but only 1% of men are diagnosed clinically in this age range. Virtually all autopsied individuals aged 50 to 70 years present with *in situ* carcinomas in the thyroid gland, whereas only 0.1% of individuals in this age group are diagnosed with thyroid cancer during this period of life. Histologic sections of *in situ* carcinomas of the thyroid showed that those tumors less than 0.5 mm in diameter were not neovascularized, whereas those more than 4 mm in diameter were generally highly neovascularized (J. Folkman, L. Andersson, *unpublished data*) (Fig. 63-1).

ONCOGENES DRIVE ANGIOGENIC SWITCH

Many oncogenes are proangiogenic, and this appears to play a major role in their tumorigenic activity. The proangiogenic oncogenes listed in Table 63-1 up-regulate a tumor cell's expression of angiogenic proteins and/or down-regulate inhibitors of angiogenesis.[11–15]

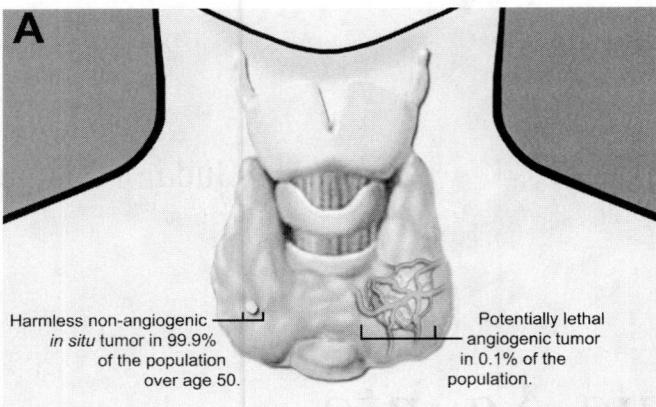

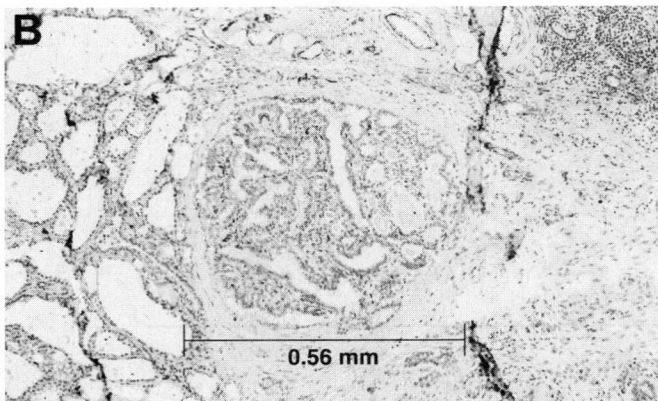

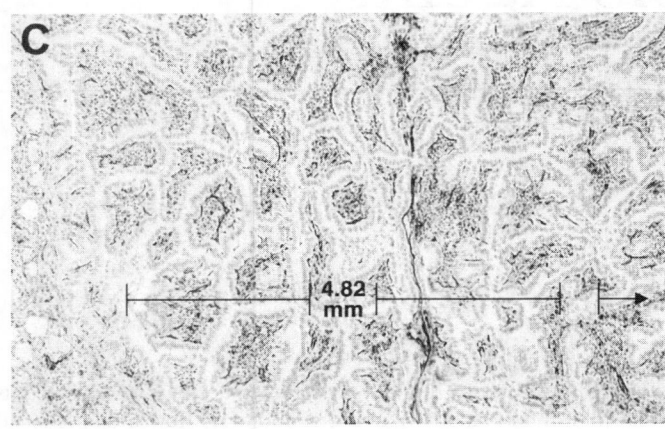

FIGURE 63-1. Papillary adenocarcinoma *in situ* in human thyroid gland found at autopsy of an individual who died of trauma. **A:** Diagram of nonangiogenic versus angiogenic papillary carcinomas of the thyroid gland. **B:** Microsection stained with antibody to CD31 to show vascular endothelium (brown), 0.56-mm diameter. Before the angiogenic switch, a few dilated microvessels are seen at the periphery. No blood vessels are observed within the lesion, but a few endothelial cells have migrated into the tumor. **C:** A more than 5-mm papillary adenocarcinoma of the thyroid gland after the angiogenic switch in a different individual. (Courtesy of Dr. Lief Andersson, Helsinki Central Hospital, Helsinki, Finland.) (See Color Fig. 63-1 in the CD-ROM.)

Clear evidence that oncogenes also increase angiogenic activity by the tumor cell comes from transfection of the bcl-2 oncogene into prostate cancer cells that are already capable of forming angiogenic tumors.[15] VEGF production was significantly increased, and angiogenic activity was significantly increased as quantified by increased microvessel density. Therefore, drugs that target oncogenes, their products, or the receptors of these products not only inhibit proliferation of tumor cells or increase their apoptotic rate (the two usual end points used in the screening process to discover such anticancer drugs), but *these drugs also inhibit tumor angiogenesis.* Thus, both gefitinib (Iressa)[16] and cetuximab (Erbitux),[17] which block the EGF receptor tyrosine kinase, also potently inhibit angiogenesis. It may be helpful for an oncologist to know this because such a drug, on the basis of its antiangiogenic activity, may be active against more tumors than only the tumor for which it was originally approved. Furthermore, although it is customary to discontinue conventional chemotherapy in the presence of drug resistance, drugs that also have antiangiogenic activity may be continued and a second angiogenesis inhibitor added to cover a tumor's expression of redundant angiogenic proteins.

SWITCH TO THE ANGIOGENIC PHENOTYPE

These autopsy studies suggest that the vast majority of microscopic, *in situ* cancers never switch to the angiogenic phenotype during a normal lifetime and that such nonangiogenic tumors are harmless. After the angiogenic switch, however, tumors can

metastasize and are potentially lethal. The hypothesis that tumors are angiogenesis-dependent was first proposed in 1971.[18] Since then, this hypothesis has been supported by hundreds of studies of biologic and pharmacologic evidence reported in the

TABLE 63-1.   Examples of Tumor Angiogenesis Driven by Oncogenes or Potential Oncogenes

Oncogene	Implicated Proangiogenic Activity
EGFR	VEGF, bFGF, IL-8 up-regulation
K-ras, H-ras	VEGF up-regulation, TSP down-regulation
v-rc	VEGF up-regulation, TSP down-regulation
c-myb	TSP-2 down-regulation
N-myc	Angiogenic properties in neuroblastomas
c-myc	Cooperates with ras to down-regulate TSP-1
HER-2	VEGF up-regulation
PyMT	TSP-1 down-regulation
c-fos	VEGF expression
HPV-16	Secretion of VEGF and interferon-α
v-p3k	VEGF production and angiogenesis
PTTG1	VEGF and bFGF up-regulation
bcl-2	VEGF up-regulation

bFGF, basic fibroblast growth factor; IL, interleukin; TSP, thrombospondin; VEGF, vascular endothelial growth factor.
Note: Many different oncogenes code for increased expression of positive regulators of angiogenesis and decreased expression of negative regulators of angiogenesis.
(Adapted from refs. 11 and 15.)

1970s and 1980s and has been proven by genetic evidence reported in the 1990s (for review, see reference 1). Genetic evidence provides the most compelling proof that tumors and their metastases are angiogenesis-dependent. The basis of these experiments and some examples are the following: (1) transfection of dominant-negative receptors for a proangiogenic protein into endothelial cells in the tumor bed,[19] (2) transfection of angiogenic oncogenes into normal cells,[20] (3) transfection of genes for antiangiogenic proteins into tumor cells,[21] and (4) manipulation of developmental genes.[22,23]

ENDOGENOUS ANGIOGENESIS INHIBITORS

The infrequency of microscopic *in situ* tumors that actually undergo the angiogenic switch (less than 1%) suggests that naturally occurring endogenous inhibitors exist in the body that counteract or resist angiogenesis under physiologic conditions.[24] At least 12 such endogenous angiogenesis inhibitors have been discovered to date (Table 63-2).

What is the evidence that these endogenous angiogenesis inhibitors are functional at the physiologic concentrations found in blood or tissues? In thrombospondin-null mice, implanted tumors grow significantly faster than the same tumors in wild-type mice.[25] The most compelling evidence has been reported by Raghu Kalluri's laboratory.[25,26] Tumstatin, a peptide fragment of 232 amino acids, residing in the α_3 chain of collagen type IV,[28] is a potent angiogenesis inhibitor that binds to the $\alpha_v\beta_3$ integrin expressed by proliferating endothelial cells. Its normal blood level is 336 ± 28 ng/mL. When the α_1 chain is knocked out, tumstatin blood levels fall to 0, and implanted tumors grow up to four times faster than their counterparts in wild-type mice. However, when recombinant tumstatin is administered to the mice at a dose just sufficient to raise tumstatin to the physiologic level of 336 ng/mL, the tumor slows down to its growth rate in wild-type mice. Higher doses further inhibit tumor growth. Therefore, tumors growing in wild-type mice are growing more slowly than their potential ceiling rates. In the future, as other endogenous inhibitors are demonstrated to function at physiologic levels, it is possible that they may act as an orchestra of tumor suppressors.[29,30] It is also likely that additional endogenous angiogenesis inhibitors will be discovered. When the autopsy findings of *in situ* cancers in the majority of adults,[10] the author's and others' findings that the majority of these microscopic *in situ* tumors are nonangiogenic (Folkman et al., *unpublished data*), and the demonstrations[25,28] that deletion

TABLE 63-2. Examples of Endogenous Angiogenesis Inhibitors

Angiostatin
Cleaved antithrombin III
Canstatin
Endostatin
Interferon-α/-β
Platelet factor-4
2-Methoxyestradiol
Tetrahydrocortisol-S
Thrombospondin-1
Tumstatin
Vitamin D–binding protein-macrophage activating factor

of endogenous angiogenesis inhibitors increase tumor growth are taken together, an interesting speculation is that the majority of individuals are constantly protected from the angiogenic or potentially lethal form of cancer by their own endogenous angiogenesis inhibitors.[29]

RATIONALE FOR ANTIANGIOGENIC THERAPY OF CANCER

For more than 50 years, the cancer cell has been virtually the sole target of anticancer therapy. However, the cancer cell is genetically unstable, and mutations accumulate (Fig. 63-2).[30] For example, a human colorectal cancer cell may have as many as 11,000 total genomic alterations. In contrast, although there may be significant differences in gene expression between an endothelial cell in a tumor bed and its counterpart in normal tissue, genomic alterations in human endothelial cells in the tumor bed have not been reported. The genetic stability of endothelial cells may make them less susceptible to acquired drug resistance.[32] Furthermore, endothelial cells in the microvascular bed of a tumor may support 50 to 100 tumor cells. When this amplification potential is taken together with the lower toxicity of most angiogenesis inhibitors, it has been predicted that antiangiogenic therapy should be significantly less toxic than conventional cytotoxic. Therefore, it has become feasible to propose that treating the endothelial cell in a tumor, or the endothelial cell and the cancer cell, may be more effective than treating the cancer cell alone. As a result, the microvascular endothelial cell recruited by a tumor has become an important second target in cancer therapy, and angiogenesis inhibitors are emerging as a new class of therapeutic agents.

EXCLUSIVE AND INCLUSIVE ANGIOGENESIS INHIBITORS

At this writing, there are more than 30 angiogenesis inhibitors in clinical trials in the United States for patients with advanced cancer in addition to others in other countries (Table 63-3).

For some of these drugs, antiangiogenic activity is the only known function. They are *exclusively* antiangiogenic. Bevacizumab (Avastin), endostatin, angiostatin, VEGF-Trap, and TNP-470 are examples. For other angiogenesis inhibitors, the antiangiogenic activity is *included* with other functions of the drug. In many cases, antiangiogenic activity was discovered after the drug received U.S. Food and Drug Administration approval for a different function. For example, celecoxib (Celebrex) was found to be an angiogenesis inhibitor after it was already in wide use for arthritis as a cyclooxygenase-2 inhibitor.[35] For some angiogenesis inhibitors in this group, the drug is known to clinicians only by the activity for which it received U.S. Food and Drug Administration approval, but its antiangiogenic activity is relatively unknown except to the scientific community. An example is bortezomib (Velcade), a proteasome inhibitor the U.S. Food and Drug Administration approved for the treatment of multiple myeloma in the spring of 2003. However, Velcade was previously reported to be a potent angiogenesis inhibitor by scientists from the National Cancer Institute,[36] the M. D. Anderson Cancer Center,[37] and the Dana-Farber Cancer Institute.[38] The result of this incomplete diffusion of knowledge through the clinical community is that Velcade, because of its antiangio-

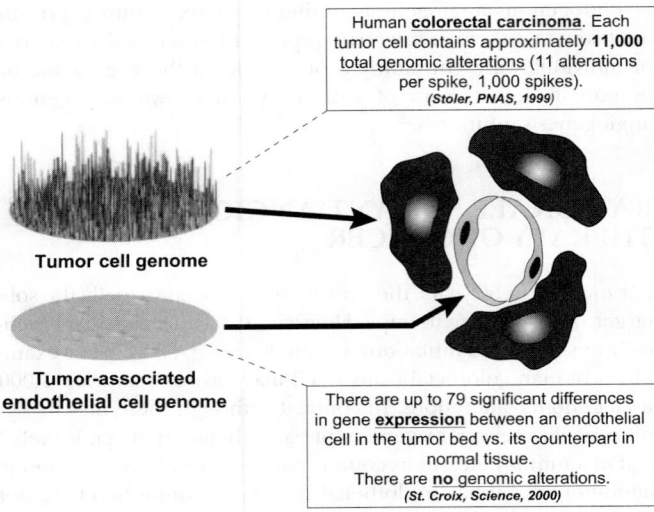

FIGURE 63-2. Angiogenesis inhibitors target genetically stable endothelial cells. There are temporary differences in gene expression between an endothelial cell in the tumor bed and its counterpart in normal tissue. In contrast, each cancer cell contains numerous genomic alterations that accumulate with each mutation. (From ref. 31, with permission.) (See Color Fig. 63-2 in the CD-ROM.)

genic activity, may have a much wider spectrum of anticancer activity than just multiple myeloma.

Thalidomide presents a different example of the difficulty of understanding the clinical applications of an angiogenic inhibitor when the drug has other functions. Thalidomide was first reported to be an angiogenesis inhibitor in 1994 by D'Amato et al.[39] Thalidomide inhibited angiogenesis induced by either bFGF or VEGF in rabbits. It entered phase II clinical trials for solid tumors and especially for brain tumors. At Folkman's suggestion, it was first used for multiple myeloma by Barlogie and showed significant inhibitory activity in patients who had failed conventional chemotherapy.[40] However, because microvessel density in the bone marrow did not decrease coincident with remission of the disease, some clinicians assumed that the efficacy of thalidomide in multiple myeloma was not based on its antiangiogenic activity.[41] Other mechanisms of action were sought. Thalidomide weakly suppresses the production of tumor necrosis factor-α (TNF-α), but other, more potent inhibitors of TNF-α have little or no antiangiogenic activity. Thalidomide also has some direct antiproliferative activity against multiple myeloma cells *in vitro*, but very high concentrations are required (for review, see reference 1). Nevertheless, it would be an advantage if thalidomide could inhibit both endothelial cells and cancer cells in multiple myeloma. Subsequently, it was demonstrated that, although quantification of microvessel density in many different tumor types is a reproducible prognostic marker for the risk of future metastasis and mortality, it is not a good indicator of efficacy of antiangiogenic therapy. This is best explained by data from experimental tumors that reveal that during tumor regression induced by an angiogenesis inhibitor, microvessel density can decrease if capillary dropout exceeds tumor cell dropout (autolysis), increase if tumor cell dropout exceeds capillary dropout, or remain the same if disappearance of capillaries and tumor cells parallels each other.[42] Therefore, because microvessel density is dictated by intercapillary distance, detec-

TABLE 63-3.   Examples of Angiogenesis Inhibitors for Cancer Therapy

Drugs That Are Exclusively Antiangiogenic	*Drugs That Include Antiangiogenic Activity*
In clinical trial	U.S. Food and Drug Administration–
Angiostatin	approved
Bevacizumab (Avastin)	Celecoxib (Celebrex)
Endostatin	Trastuzumab (Herceptin)
Tetrahydrocortisol	Gefitinib (Iressa)
TNP-470	Rosiglitazone
ABT 510 (thrombospondin-1	Taxol
peptide)	Bortezomib (Velcade)
Vascular endothelial growth	Zoledronic acid (bisphosphonate)
factor-Trap	Interferon-α
Vitaxin	In clinical trial
Not yet in clinical trial	AGO 13736
Arresten	BAY 43-9006
Canstatin	CP547632
Cleaved antithrombin III	C225 (Erbitux)
Vitamin D–binding protein-	Combretastatin
macrophage activating factor	NM-3
Platelet-derived growth factor	OS1774 (Tarceva)
Tumstatin	PTK787
	SU-11248
	Thalidomide (and 3-amino tha-
	lidomide)
	2-Methoxyestradiol

Note: Some of the more than 30 angiogenesis inhibitors currently in clinical trial in the United States. Those drugs that are exclusively antiangiogenic have no other function, such as bevacizumab (left column). Those drugs that have other functions and are also potent angiogenesis inhibitors are listed in the right column.
(From ref. 34, with permission.)

tion of a decrease in microvessel density during treatment with an angiogenesis inhibitor indicates that the agent is active. However, the absence of a drop in microvessel density does not indicate that the agent is ineffective.[42] Also since the report of the efficacy of thalidomide for multiple myeloma, numerous papers have shown that efficacy of thalidomide in multiple myeloma is based mainly on its antiangiogenic activity and not on its anti–TNF-α activity.[39,43] Other reports show that receptors for VEGF are expressed in multiple myeloma and that interference with VEGF signaling can block myeloma. At this writing, thalidomide is being used in more than 160 clinical trials at more than 70 medical centers, and more than 120,000 patients are being treated. Oncologists around the world have confirmed Barlogie's finding that thalidomide causes a 50% reduction in tumor burden in approximately a third of patients with refractory disease.[44] Australia has become the first country to approve thalidomide for multiple myeloma, where it is considered to be "the best treatment advance in the past 25 years."[44]

DIRECT AND INDIRECT ANGIOGENESIS INHIBITORS

When an angiogenesis inhibitor is used in a patient, it may be helpful for oncologists to consider whether a "direct" or "indirect" inhibitor is being administered (Fig. 63-3).[34]

A direct angiogenesis inhibitor blocks vascular endothelial cells from proliferating, migrating, or increasing their survival

Types of Angiogenesis Inhibitors

	Indirect	Direct
Inhibitor	*Iressa*	*Endostatin*
Mechanism	Inhibits synthesis by tumor cells of angiogenic proteins: **bFGF, VEGF,** and **TGF-α**.	Inhibits endothelial cells from responding to multiple angiogenic proteins, e.g., **bFGF, VEGF, IL-8, PDGF**.

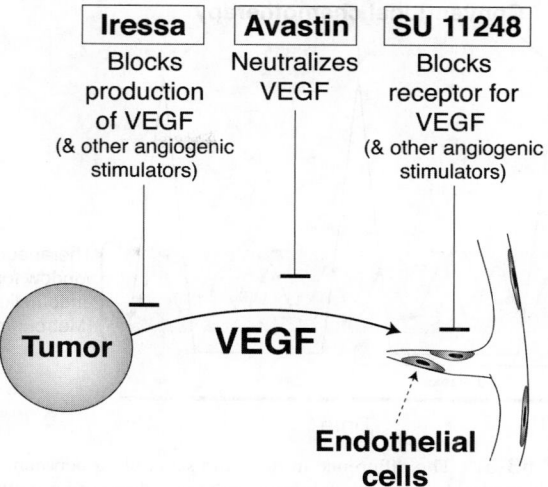

FIGURE 63-3. **A:** An "indirect" angiogenesis inhibitor blocks synthesis of an angiogenic protein by a tumor cell, neutralizes the angiogenic protein, or blocks the endothelial receptor for that protein. Several drugs designed to block oncogene expression or to block the signal transduction pathway of an oncogene block expression of the angiogenic proteins that were induced by the oncogene (e.g., Iressa blocks the epidermal growth factor receptor tyrosine kinase). A "direct" angiogenesis inhibitor prevents endothelial cells from responding to a wide spectrum of angiogenic stimuli (e.g., endostatin). (From ref. 34, with permission.) **B:** Three examples of "indirect" angiogenesis inhibitors. (From ref. 1, with permission.) bFGF, basic fibroblast growth factor; IL, interleukin; PDGF, platelet-derived growth factor; TGF, transforming growth factor; VEGF, vascular endothelial growth factor.

in response to a spectrum of proangiogenic proteins, including VEGF, bFGF, platelet-derived growth factor, interleukin-8, and others (Table 63-4). It remains to be determined whether the set of proangiogenic proteins inhibited by a given angiogenesis inhibitor may depend on the specific integrin on endothelial cells to which that inhibitor binds. For example, tumstatin binds to $\alpha_v\beta_3$ and endostatin binds to $\alpha_5\beta_1$.[29,45] Nevertheless, direct angiogenesis inhibitors are less likely to induce acquired drug resistance. In contrast, indirect angiogenesis inhibitors decrease or block expression of a tumor cell product, neutralize the tumor product itself, or block its receptor on endothelial cells. Figure 63-3 illustrates three indirect angiogenesis inhibitors. Most indirect angiogenesis inhibitors block the activity of one or two proangiogenic proteins—for example, VEGF. If over time, tumor cell mutations lead to increased expression of other proangiogenic proteins, not blocked by the indirect inhibitor, this may give the appearance of drug resistance. For example, in women diagnosed with breast cancer for the first time, immunohistologic analysis of the tumors showed that 60% were producing only VEGF (Fig. 63-4).[46]

TABLE 63-4. Examples of Direct and Indirect Angiogenesis Inhibitors

Direct	Indirect
Angiostatin	Bevacizumab (Avastin)
Arresten	C225 (Erbitux)
Canstatin	Trastuzumab (Herceptin)
Endostatin	Interferon-α
Thrombospondin-1 (and -2)	Gefitinib (Iressa)
Tumstatin	NM-3
2-Methoxyestradiol	PTK787
Vitaxin	SU-11248

However, in other patients or in patents with tumor recurrences, up to six different proangiogenic proteins were being produced. VEGF was only one of these.

ANTIANGIOGENIC (METRONOMIC) CHEMOTHERAPY

Conventional cytotoxic chemotherapy must pass through microvascular endothelium before it reaches tumor cells. Therefore, endothelial cells should also be a target for chemo-

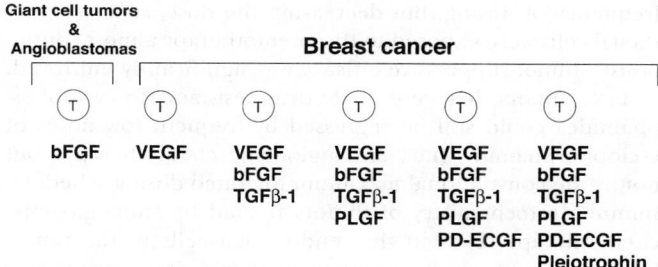

FIGURE 63-4. Production of proangiogenic proteins by human tumors. In women presenting with the first diagnosis of breast cancer, approximately 60% of the tumors express only vascular endothelial growth factor (VEGF). However, breast cancers in some patients may express up to six angiogenic proteins. High-grade giant cell tumors and angioblastomas (*left*) produce predominately basic fibroblast growth factor (bFGF) as their main angiogenic stimulator. Because these tumors rarely express redundant angiogenic proteins, interferon-α, which decreases expression of bFGF, has been used successfully for 3 to 5 years in patients without the development of drug resistance and with complete and durable tumor regression. PD-ECGF, platelet-derived endothelial cell growth factor; PLGF, placental growth factor; TGF, transforming growth factor. (From ref. 191, with permission.) (Drawn from data in refs. 46 and 184.)

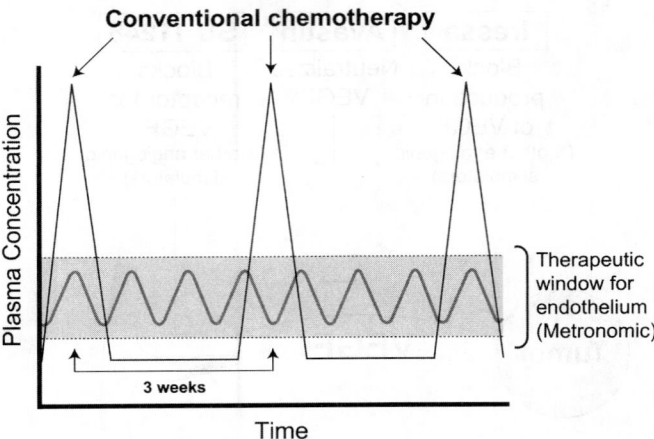

FIGURE 63-5.   The difference in dose and scheduling between *conventional chemotherapy*, in which maximum tolerated doses are separated by drug holidays of weeks to allow rescue of the bone marrow, versus low-dose frequent *metronomic* therapy, which continuously exposes vascular endothelium to chemotherapy. (See Color Fig. 63-5 in the CD-ROM.)

therapy. If so, then why is acquired drug resistance so commonly associated with chemotherapy? Endothelial cells are diploid, nonmutating normal cells and should not become resistant to chemotherapy[32] for the same reason that bone marrow does not develop acquired drug resistance. Furthermore, because one endothelial cell can support the growth of approximately 50 tumor cells, why doesn't endothelium exposed to cytotoxic chemotherapy continue to restrict tumor growth even after the tumor cells per se have become drug-resistant? Browder et al. solved this conundrum by suggesting that, because traditional administration at maximum tolerated dosing requires an off-therapy period (drug holiday) of 2 to 3 weeks to rescue bone marrow, endothelial cells may resume growth during this period when they are not exposed to chemotherapy (Fig. 63-5).[47] In fact, the return of bone marrow proliferation may depend on the resumption of endothelial cell proliferation. Browder et al. demonstrated that if the prolonged off-therapy intervals of chemotherapy were eliminated by increasing the frequency of dosing, but decreasing the dose, so that endothelial cells were exposed to the chemotherapy almost continuously, tumor-suppressive efficacy was significantly improved. In fact, tumors that were made drug-resistant (to cyclophosphamide) could still be regressed by frequent low doses of cyclophosphamide (i.e., antiangiogenic chemotherapy) but not by the conventional maximum tolerated dosing schedule. Immunohistochemistry of tumors treated by antiangiogenic chemotherapy revealed that endothelial cells in the tumor bed underwent apoptosis approximately 4 days *before* tumor cells (which had been proliferating) subsequently became apoptotic.

Browder and Folkman discussed these results with Robert Kerbel approximately 2 years before submitting them for publication. Kerbel's laboratory in Toronto reproduced these results and extended them to different types of chemotherapy.[48] Papers from both laboratories were published the same month because Kerbel graciously delayed publication of his paper so that it would not precede Browder's paper. In an accompanying editorial, Hanahan suggested the name "metronomic" therapy.[49] Recently, "ultra-low" low doses of paclitaxel have been reported to be highly antiangiogenic without any direct cytotoxic effect on tumor cells.[50]

METRONOMIC CHEMOTHERAPY UP-REGULATES EXPRESSION OF THROMBOSPONDIN-1, AN ENDOGENOUS INHIBITOR OF ANGIOGENESIS

Kerbel's laboratory fed tumor-bearing mice with low-dose cyclophosphamide in their drinking water and found a significant rise in circulating thrombospondin-1, a potent endogenous angiogenesis inhibitor.[51,52] There was concomitant tumor inhibition. However, in thrombospondin-null mice, the metronomic cyclophosphamide had no antitumor effect. The important implications of this experiment are that (1) chemotherapy may be, in part, endothelial cell–dependent; (2) metronomic chemotherapy can induce the increased expression of an endogenous angiogenesis inhibitor; and (3) drug resistance is bypassed by optimizing chemotherapy dose and frequency for its antiangiogenic effect. Furthermore, this experiment raises the question of whether other chemotherapeutic agents can induce the expression of either thrombospondin-1 or other endogenous angiogenesis inhibitors.

OTHER SMALL MOLECULES CAN UP-REGULATE EXPRESSION OF ENDOGENOUS ANGIOGENESIS INHIBITORS

Doxycycline (but not tetracycline) has been reported to restore expression of thrombospondin-1 in tumor cells harboring mutant *ras* oncogenes.[53] Rosiglitazone[54] and other peroxisome proliferator–activated receptor γ ligands improve the antiangiogenic and antitumor activity of thrombospondin-1 by increasing the expression of its receptor, CD36.[55] Administration of celecoxib to rats (and to patients) increases circulating levels of endostatin, an endogenous angiogenesis inhibitor that is a cryptic fragment of collagen XVIII.[56] Celecoxib appears to release endostatin from platelets, where it is normally sequestered. This mechanism may contribute to the antiangiogenic and antitumor activity of Celebrex.[35]

Taken together, these reports imply that a set of small molecules can be used as therapeutic agents to up-regulate expression of proteins in the body that themselves are angiogenesis inhibitors (Fig. 63-6). It is possible that additional such low-molecular-weight inducers of endogenous angiogenesis inhibitors may be discovered in the future.

ENDOSTATIN: AN ARCHETYPIC ENDOGENOUS ANGIOGENESIS INHIBITOR

Endostatin is a 20-kD cryptic fragment of collagen XVIII.[57,58] It is discussed in detail in this section because it is the first endogenous angiogenesis inhibitor to be discovered as a cryptic fragment of a basement membrane protein. Also, it has been extensively studied by many laboratories. Endostatin was reviewed in reference 1, when, at the beginning of 2003, there were more than 350 publications on endostatin. As of 2004, there are more than 600 publications. Highlights of these reports include new findings on mechanism of action, physiologic function, structure–activity relationships, experimental therapeutics including gene therapy, and early clinical studies. These new data are summarized later and updated from reference 1.

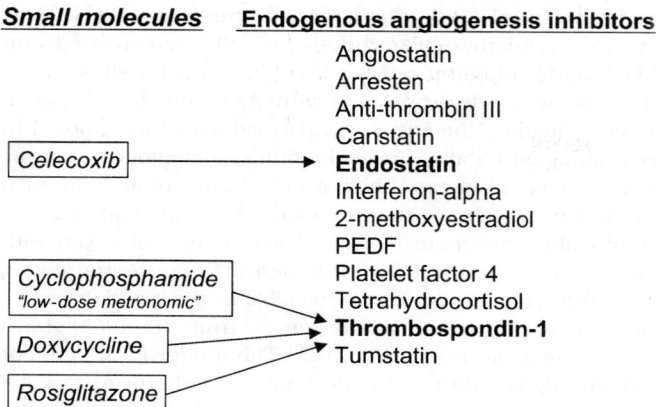

FIGURE 63-6. Illustration of recent data that shows that low-molecular-weight compounds that can be taken orally can induce increased expression of endogenous angiogenesis inhibitors in the body. PEDF, pigment epithelium-derived factor.

Only type IV and XVIII collagens are found in all vertebrates down to worms (*Caenorhabditis elegans*). Therefore, endostatin is approximately 600 million years old. Recombinant endostatin produced in yeast is a potent angiogenesis inhibitor with antitumor activity against a wide spectrum of human and animal tumors in mice. A functional receptor for endostatin has been identified as the $\alpha_5\beta_1$ integrin on endothelial cells.[29,45,57–60]

Discovery of Endostatin

Endostatin was first isolated and sequenced from conditioned medium of murine hemangioendothelioma based on the same strategy used for the discovery of angiostatin.[113] Surgical removal or irradiation[61] of a primary tumor often suppresses growth of metastases or of other tumors at remote sites. A primary tumor can be angiogenic because it is expressing and secreting angiogenic stimulators (i.e., VEGF) in excess of its ability to generate certain angiogenesis inhibitors by enzymatic cleavage of larger proteins (i.e., angiostatin).[21] In the circulation, however, an angiogenic stimulator, such as VEGF, has a short half-life (minutes), in contrast to the longer half-life of an angiogenesis inhibitor (hours). As a result, the blood in a tumor-bearing animal or individual inhibits angiogenesis in remote metastases. A murine hemangioendothelioma that generated endostatin led to the discovery of this angiogenesis inhibitor.[57] Subsequently, many other tumors have been found to generate endostatin. High-resolution crystal structures have been reported for murine[62] and human[63] endostatin (Fig. 63-7). An elastase[64] and a cathepsin[65] are required to cleave endostatin from collagen XVIII.

Structure–Activity Relationships

Endostatin is derived from the nontriple helical C-terminal non–collagenous-1 domain of collagen XVIII. Endostatin is present in basement membranes and vessel walls. Elastic fibers of the aorta and sparse elastic fibers of veins are especially rich in collagen XVIII.[66] Some, but not all, capillaries or arterioles show weak labeling for endostatin. Within the elastic fibers, endostatin is colocalized and/or binds to fibulin-1 and fibulin-2, nidogen-1 and nidogen-2, laminin-1, and perlecan.[67] Recombinant murine endostatin binds to heparin with a K_d of 0.3 µM.[68] A major site of four clustered arginines, 155, 158, 184, and 270, and a second site (R193, R194) are essential for binding to heparin as well as to heparan sulfate and sulfatides, but not to fibulin-1 and fibulin-2. A minimum heparin size of 12-mer (dodecasaccharide) is necessary for efficient binding, and there is a crucial role for 2-O and 6-O sulfation. A synthetic arginine-rich dendrimer that mimics the surface of endostatin and has high affinity for heparin has similar antiangiogenic activity in the chick embryo. This experiment demonstrates the important role of heparin affinity for the inhibitory activity of endostatin.[69] The affinity of endostatin for heparin or heparan sulfate is zinc-dependent.[70,71] Although two subsequent reports with murine-soluble recombinant endostatin concluded that zinc binding was not necessary for endostatin's antiangiogenic and antitumor activity,[68,72] it is now clear that zinc binding is critical for endostatin's antiangiogenic and antitumor activi-

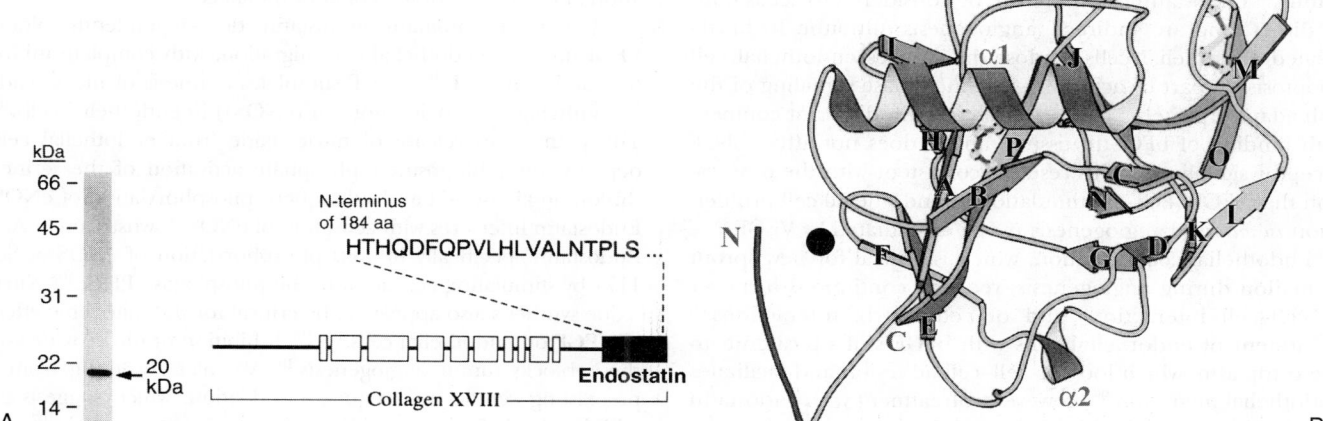

FIGURE 63-7. **A:** N-terminal amino acid sequence of human endostatin. (From ref. 57, with permission.) **B:** Three-dimensional crystal structure of human endostatin. (From ref. 63, with permission.) (See Color Fig. 63-7*B* in the CD-ROM.)

ties. Kashi Javaherian and Robert Tjin in the Folkman laboratory have shown that a short peptide of endostatin has equivalent antiangiogenic and antitumor activity as full-length endostatin if the zinc-binding N-terminal histidines are present, but not if a histidine is substituted by a different amino acid (K. Javaherian et al., *submitted*, 2004).

Interestingly, other peptides of endostatin have recently been reported to mimic the antiangiogenic and antitumor activity of endostatin.[73-75]

Of the 20 collagen isoforms that have been identified so far in mammalian species, collagens IV, XV, and XVIII (which possess C-terminal globular domains) have been implicated in regulation of angiogenesis.[76] Of interest is that homologues of these three collagens have also been identified in the worm *C elegans*, where the endostatin domain of type XVIII collagen controls migration of neuronal cells and axon guidance instead of vascular endothelial cells.[77] The evolutionary age of endostatin of approximately 600 million years may be responsible in part for its lack of toxicity in animals and patients.[78,79] Of interest is that certain regulators of endothelial cell migration have (or had) control of axon migration—for example, endostatin, neuropilin,[80] semaphorins, and ephrins,[81,82] among others (Bielenberg et al.[193]). This relationship provides insight into how development of nerves and blood vessels may be coordinated.

Mechanisms of Endostatin Activity

Novel mechanisms are beginning to be revealed for the antiangiogenic action of endostatin. The $\alpha_5\beta_1$ integrin binds endostatin and is a functional receptor.[29,45] Tumor cells induce the up-regulation of $\alpha_5\beta_1$ integrin. This finding suggests that endostatin may be more effective against those tumors that induce the up-regulation of $\alpha_5\beta_1$ integrin.

Endostatin blocks the binding of $VEGF_{121}$ and $VEGF_{165}$ to the KDR/Flk-1 receptor; blocks tyrosine phosphorylation of this receptor; and blocks activation of its intracellular signaling events,[83] extracellular signaling–regulated kinase, p38 mitogen-activated protein kinase, and p125FAK.[84] This receptor mediates endothelial cell motility and proliferation. Although endostatin does not bind to VEGF,[84] it does down-regulate VEGF expression in tumor cells (similar to the effect of angiostatin).[85] Endostatin can therefore be considered to act as both a "direct" and an "indirect" angiogenesis inhibitor. In bFGF-treated endothelial cells, endostatin induces endothelial cell apoptosis, in part by activating tyrosine kinase signaling of the Shb adaptor protein.[86] However, endostatin does not compete with binding of bFGF to tissues, and it does not affect bFGF receptor signaling.[87] This result is consistent with the observation that bFGF (FGF-2) stimulation of endothelial cell proliferation *in vitro* and angiogenesis *in vivo* is mediated by VEGF.[88]

Endothelial cell migration, which is critical for new sprout formation during angiogenesis, requires continuous turnover of cell–cell interactions and of cell–matrix interactions.[89] Treatment of endothelial cells with bFGF shifts β-catenin to the cytoplasm, which loosens cell–cell adhesion and facilitates endothelial migration.[90] However, cotreatment with endostatin transiently blocks this shift. Cell–matrix interactions are maintained in part by formation of focal adhesions and actin stress fibers. Either bFGF or endostatin alone induces tyrosine phosphorylation of focal adhesion kinase and paxillin, which leads

to formation of focal adhesions and actin stress fibers. However, when microvascular endothelial cells are cotreated with bFGF and endostatin, focal adhesion and actin stress fibers decrease, which decreases migration of endothelial cells. In an *in vivo* situation, the entire vascular bed would be exposed to circulating endostatin. But endostatin's antiangiogenic activity would affect only areas of high growth factor stimulation, such as those present in the tumor associated endothelium.[90] These results also contribute to lack of side effects observed with endostatin in clinical trials. Although high concentrations of administered endostatin are detectable in the vasculature of a tumor bed, normal vasculature remote from the tumor shows no increased endostatin reactivity.[91] This unique localization of systemically administered endostatin to newly formed angiogenic microvessels appears to reverse the loosening of endothelial cells to each other and to their basement membrane. Endothelial migration is also inhibited. Both events are necessary for the initial formation of angiogenic sprouts.

Formation of new angiogenic sprouts is also associated with up-regulation of the urokinase plasminogen activator system on the surface of endothelial cells. Proangiogenic proteins, such as bFGF, increase the secretion of urokinase plasminogen activator and plasminogen activator inhibitor (PAI-1), leading to an overall increase in proteolytic activity of migrating endothelial cells. Endostatin treatment of endothelial cells markedly decreases their production of urokinase plasminogen activator and PAI-1.[92]

Endostatin also binds and inhibits the catalytic activity of specific metalloproteinases,[93,94] further contributing to inhibition of endothelial cell migration and possibly secondary inhibition of tumor cell invasion. Tumor progression and angiogenesis are reduced in matrix metalloproteinase (MMP)-2–deficient mice, and MMP-2 is required for the switch to the angiogenic phenotype.[95-98]

Endostatin also binds to glypicans on the endothelial cell surface at concentrations that suggest that glypicans may behave as low-affinity endostatin receptors.[99] Endostatin causes G_1 arrest in endothelial cells by decreasing the hyperphosphorylated retinoblastoma gene product and down-regulating cyclin D1 messenger RNA (mRNA) and protein.[100] Transcription through the LEF1 site in the cyclin D1 promoter is essential for endostatin's inhibitory activity. Others report that endostatin arrests proliferation and causes apoptosis of endothelial cells.[101,102]

Human recombinant endostatin dose-dependently blocks VEGF-induced endothelial cell migration, with complete inhibition at 100 ng/mL.[103] VEGF stimulates synthesis of nitric oxide [endothelial nitric oxide isoform (eNOS)] in endothelial cells.[104] The pathway to release of nitric oxide from endothelial cells depends on sphingosine-1 phosphate activation of the serine/threonine kinase Akt and subsequent phosphorylation of eNOS. Endostatin interferes with activation of eNOS downstream of Akt. Endostatin specifically inhibits phosphorylation of eNOS at Ser 1177 by stimulating activation of the phosphatase PP2A.[103] Nitric oxide synthesis also appears to be critical for the mitogenic effect of VEGF on endothelial cells.[105-107] Inhibition of nitric oxide synthesis blocks tumor angiogenesis.[108] Vascular sprouting from a preexisting venule may require vasodilation, which suggests an additional role for nitric oxide production in angiogenesis.[107]

Endostatin binds and increases the phosphorylation of two proteins that regulate cytoskeletal function in endothelial cells, heat-shock protein 27 (hsp 27) and cofilin.[109] The angiogenesis inhibitors thrombospondin-1 and TNP-470, as well as fumagillin, also operate through this common pathway, which appears to prevent endothelial cell migration.

Hypoxia and Endostatin

During hypoxia, production of endostatin is significantly decreased, in part by the degradation of endostatin in pericytes as well as in endothelial cells.[110] Exogenous endostatin is more rapidly degraded when incubated with conditioned media from hypoxic endothelial cells, although the mechanism is unclear. Nevertheless, endostatin degradation in the hypoxic tumor may facilitate the switch to the angiogenic phenotype. Furthermore, the treatment of a patient with a large hypoxic tumor may require higher doses of endostatin because of endostatin degradation. Of interest from a therapeutic standpoint is that endostatin incubation with microvascular endothelial cells *in vitro* leads to down-regulation of gene expression of hypoxia-inducible factor-1 alpha (HIF-1 alpha) and up-regulation of an endogenous inhibitor of HIF-1 alpha.[111]

Endostatin in Development

During eye development, hyaloid vessels supply the vitreous and the lens. Subsequently, these vessels regress so that the vitreous and lens become transparent. Endostatin appears to be required for regression of the hyaloid vessels because they fail to regress in endostatin's absence. In a rare disease called *Knobloch syndrome*, the hyaloid vessels fail to regress, retinal vasculature fails to develop, and patients suffer retinal degeneration and blindness, among other abnormalities.[112-114] In this syndrome, a splice mutation in human collagen XVIII leads to a truncated protein lacking the endostatin fragment. A proposed mechanism of retinal degeneration is that persistent hyaloid vessels increase oxygen in the retina, which suppresses HIF-1 and VEGF, both of which drive normal vascular growth in the normal developing retina. Retinal vasculature also fails to develop in a collagen XVIII–deficient mouse model.[115] Thus, a pathologic deficiency of endostatin in humans and mice provides experimental and clinical evidence that endostatin is an endogenous inhibitor of angiogenesis under normal conditions.

Platelets Contain Endostatin

Platelets contain at least 14 positive regulators and approximately 12 negative regulators of angiogenesis (Fig. 63-8).[116] The positive regulators include VEGF-A, VEGF-C, bFGF, hepatocyte growth factor, angiopoietin 1, platelet-derived growth factor, heparanase, and sphingosine-1 phosphate, among others. The negative regulators include endostatin, platelet factor-4, thrombospondin, plasminogen (angiostatin), high-molecular-weight kininogen (domain 5), and α_2-antiplasmin, among others. These stimulators and inhibitors of endothelial cell migration and proliferation may be released into a blood clot in a wound in an orchestrated sequence to regulate neovascularization.[117] For example, thrombin induces the release of the proangiogenic protein VEGF from platelets.[118] Thrombin also induces the release of endostatin from platelets.[119] Thrombin induction of endostatin release is mediated by proteinase-activated receptor-4, independent of platelet aggregation and of the action of adenosine diphosphate. It is possible that endostatin is one of

the physiologic mechanisms restricting wound angiogenesis to a finite time period (approximately 12 to 14 days in mice) and location.

Endostatin is released from platelets *in vitro* and *in vivo* by administration of the nonsteroidal antiinflammatory drugs celecoxib and flurbiprofen or HCT 1026 (a nitric oxide–releasing derivative of flurbiprofen). They also release endostatin from platelets[56] and elevate the plasma level of endostatin. From these findings, one can ask whether the antiangiogenic activity of celecoxib is in part endostatin-dependent. It is not clear at this writing whether the antiangiogenic activity of celecoxib is dependent on cyclooxygenase-2. There are other unanswered questions. What is the turnover rate of endostatin in platelets? Do cancer patients on long-term celecoxib therapy deplete their platelet stores of endostatin? Can platelets be loaded with endostatin that is administered systemically or by incubating platelets with endostatin *in vitro*? Would cancer patients treated with celecoxib benefit from periodic endostatin therapy? Would patients on long-term endostatin benefit from celecoxib therapy? Taken together, these findings indicate that endostatin is normally distributed among three compartments: (1) sequestered as a cryptic fragment in collagen XVIII in basement membranes, (2) stored in platelets, and (3) circulating as low levels of free endostatin.

Endostatin and Vascular Permeability

Endostatin decreases vascular permeability. bFGF treatment increases permeability of [^{3}H] insulin through confluent monolayers of capillary endothelial cells in a Transwell assay, an effect that is counteracted by cotreatment with endostatin.[90] In mice that have received an intravenous injection of Evans blue dye, a large blue stain appears at the site of a subcutaneous injection of VEGF or platelet-activating factor (Miles test). Pretreatment with endostatin blocks the permeability induced by these proteins. Endostatin pretreatment prevented the opening of interendothelial junctions and pericyte detachment caused by VEGF injection *in vivo*.[119a] Endostatin treatment of endothelial cells *in vitro* increased membrane-bound localization of zonula occludens (ZO-1) and decreased endothelial permeability. These results imply that systemic administration of endostatin to patients may decrease edema in brain tumors or decrease ascites in ovarian cancer, but these speculations remain to be demonstrated.

Systemic Administration of Endostatin

Systemic administration of endostatin inhibits tumor growth or regresses different tumors. The first recombinant endostatin was from *Escherichia coli* in an insoluble form because this had previously been successful with angiostatin[120] and because refolding of the inclusion body to a soluble form by urea guanidine-hydrochloride and glutathione gave a low yield (1%).[57,58] When this endostatin preparation was administered subcutaneously every day for prolonged periods of time in mice (185 days for Lewis lung carcinoma, 160 days for T241 fibrosarcoma, and 80 days for B-16 murine melanoma), there was no drug resistance. After discontinuation of endostatin at these time periods, tumors did not recur. They remained dormant at a microscopic size.[58] This was determined not to be due to an immunologic mechanism. Another possibility is preferential storage of endostatin in the

A

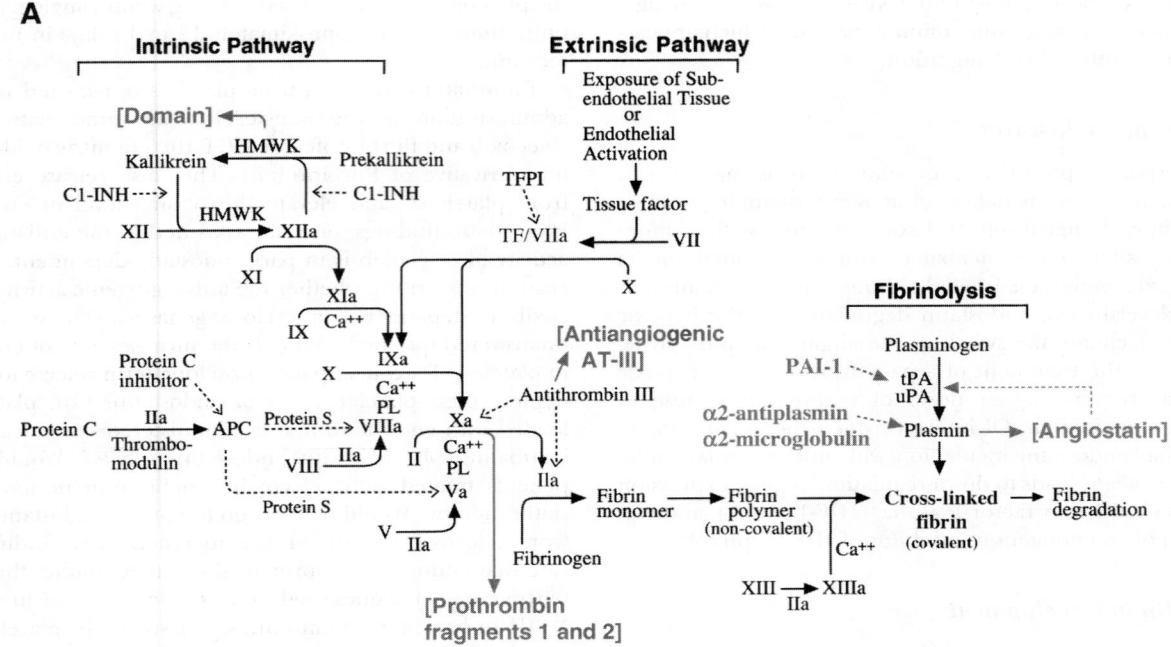

B

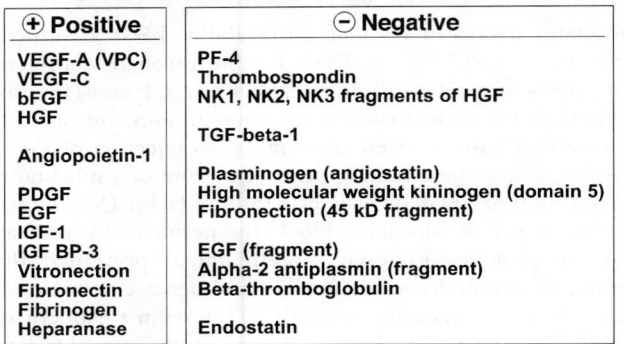

FIGURE 63-8.   Angiogenesis inhibitor proteins in platelets and in the hemostatic system. **A:** Cryptic fragments derived from coagulation and fibrinolytic proteins that suppress angiogenesis are indicated in bold red. Fibrinolytic pathway inhibitors that regulate angiogenesis are also printed in red. Coagulation factors are depicted by Roman numerals, and activation is indicated by a small a. Coagulation cascade and fibrinolytic pathway inhibitors are indicated by a dashed arrow. **B:** Positive and negative regulators of angiogenesis carried by platelets. APC, antigen-presenting cell; AT-III, antithrombin III; bFGF, basic fibroblast growth factor; C1-INH, complement factor-1 esterase inhibitor; EGF, epidermal growth factor; HGF, hepatocyte growth factor; HMWK, high-molecular-weight kininogen; IGF BP, insulin-like growth factor binding protein; NK, natural killer (cell); PAI, plasminogen activator inhibitor; PDGF, platelet-derived growth factor; PF-4, platelet factor 4; PL, anionic phospholipids; TF, tissue factor; TFPI, tissue factor pathway inhibitor; TGF, transforming growth factor; tPA, tissue-type plasminogen activator; uPA, urokinase plasminogen activator; VEGF, vascular endothelial growth factor. (From ref. 116, with permission.) (See Color Fig. 63-8*A* in the CD-ROM.)

matrix at the site of the regressed tumor.[121] This same dormancy has been observed after 40 days of endostatin therapy of rat mammary cancer induced by oral carcinogen.[122] Other investigators have reported successful tumor inhibition with insoluble endostatin from *E coli*.[123]

Soluble endostatin from *E coli* also inhibits tumor growth.[124] Soluble recombinant mouse endostatin and human endostatin produced in yeast (*Pichia pastoris*) are the most widely used preparations of endostatin for therapeutic studies and have demonstrated a wide spectrum of antitumor activity (Table 63-5). However, in contrast to insoluble endostatin from *E coli*, which appears to provide *sustained release* of endostatin, soluble preparations of endostatin demonstrate the most optimal antitumor activity when they are administered continuously.[125] When endostatin was administered to severe combined immunodeficient mice bearing human pancreatic carcinoma (p53$^{-/-}$), 24-hour continuous parenteral administration was tenfold more effective than the same dose administered as a bolus once every day.[125] Tumor growth was inhibited in a dose-dependent manner, but only continuous administration caused tumor regression (Fig. 63-9). Even endothelial cells growing *in vitro* were

inhibited more effectively by continuous administration of endostatin (from a floating microosmotic pump in 24-well plates) than by endostatin added to the wells once every day.[125] Continuous administration of endostatin is more effective than intermittent administration for other tumors.[126] These experiments illustrate what may be a general characteristic of optimal antiangiogenic therapy: *Angiogenesis inhibitors are most effective when endothelial cells in a tumor bed are constantly exposed to therapeutic levels of the inhibitor.* This is because endothelial cells in the vascular bed of a tumor are constantly exposed to proangiogenic stimuli from the tumor cells and from local stroma. To inhibit tumor growth or to regress tumors, the continuous angiogenic output of a tumor needs to be continuously counteracted by angiogenesis inhibitors in the blood. An analogy would be titration of blood glucose by insulin. It is easier to understand how to design effective antiangiogenic therapy by thinking of it in terms of a process of *titration* of inhibitor or inhibitors against angiogenic stimulators and not as maximum tolerated dosing, which requires prolonged off-therapy intervals, or "drug holidays."

A wide variety of other tumors in many different laboratories have been inhibited by endostatin in mice and rats without

TABLE 63-5. Examples of Endostatin Activity Against a Spectrum of Different Tumors

Fibrosarcoma, Lewis lung, B-16 murine melanoma	O'Reilly et al., *Cell* 1997[57]; *Nature* 1997[191]
Spontaneous pancreatic islet cancer	Bergers et al., *Science* 1999[135]
Spontaneous mammary carcinoma	Yokoyama et al., *Cancer Res* 2000[134]
Gliosarcoma	Sorensen et al., *Neuro-oncol* 2002[136]
Spontaneous murine breast cancer	Perletti et al., *Cancer Res* 2000[122]
Ovarian cancer	Yokoyama et al., *Cancer Res* 2000[134]
SQ20B radioresistant cancer (with or without short radiotherapy)	Hanna et al., *Cancer J* 2000[140]
Human pancreatic cancer	Kisker et al., *Cancer Res* 2001[175]
Lewis lung carcinoma	Huang et al., *Cancer Res* 2001[123]
Human neuroblastoma	Kuroiwa et al., *Int J Mol Med* 2001[132]
Human lung cancer	Boehle et al., *Int J Cancer* 2001[131]
Lymphoma (with or without angiostatin)	Scappaticci et al., *Angiogenesis* 2001[137]
Murine neuroblastoma (with or without green fluorescent protein)	Davidoff et al., *Cancer Gene Ther* 2001[188]
Murine gliomas (released from cells in beads)	Read et al., *Nature Biotechnol* 2001[149]
Glioblastoma (released from cells in beads)	Joki et al., *Nature Biotechnol* 2001[150]
Colon carcinoma	Ye et al., *Endocrinology* 2002[128]
Leukemia	Iversen et al., *Leukemia* 2002[130]
Liver metastases (with or without chemotherapy)	te Velde et al., *Br J Surg* 2002[189]
Rat malignant glioma	Sorensen et al., *Neoplasia* 2002[190]

Note: A few of more than 600 publications on endostatin to show the broad spectrum of antitumor activity, as described in the text.

evidence of toxicity or drug resistance. These include lung adenocarcinoma, thyroid carcinoma, colon carcinoma, leukemia, human non–small cell lung cancer, human pancreatic cancer, human neuroblastoma, mammary cancer (soluble endostatin from *E coli*), colon cancer metastases to liver, spontaneous mouse mammary carcinoma (delayed onset, decreased tumor burden, and prolonged survival), and spontaneous pancreatic islet carcinomas (see Table 63-5).[127–135]

Mammary carcinomas were more potently inhibited by a mutated form of endostatin in which an alanine residue was substituted for a proline at position 125 (P125A) than by the wild-type endostatin. Gliosarcoma both orthotopic and ectopic in rats was markedly inhibited (approximately 50%) after only 10 days of treatment by a relatively low dose of murine endostatin (0.3 mg/kg). Inhibition of tumor growth persisted after cessation of therapy.[136]

Endostatin Administered Together with Angiostatin

Reports of endostatin administered in combination with angiostatin, whether as separate proteins, as separate genes, or as a fusion protein of angiostatin and endostatin in tumor-bearing animals, all show a synergistic increase in efficacy.[137–139] Although the mechanism of synergy is unclear at this writing, one possibility is that endostatin and angiostatin each upregulate thrombospondin-1 expression or protect it from enzymatic destruction.

Potentiation of Radiotherapy

Endostatin (and angiostatin) potentiates radiotherapy in tumor-bearing mice when the inhibitor is administered at the same time as the ionizing radiation.[140] Tumors regress when treated with a combination of ionizing radiation and endostatin but not with either agent alone. It can be speculated that repair of radiation damage to active endothelium in a tumor bed may be retarded in the presence of an angiogenesis inhibitor. This experiment also suggests that radiotherapy may be in part endothelial-dependent. It is also possible that antiangiogenic therapy combined with radiotherapy replaces an angiogenesis inhibitor (e.g., angiostatin) generated by an intact primary tumor, but is decreased when the primary tumor regresses.[61] The optimal schedule of radiotherapy and antiangiogenic therapy for cancer patients is unclear.

Endostatin Gene Therapy in Animals

Endostatin gene therapy in tumor-bearing mice has generally been successful when administered locally, but it has been problematic when administered systemically.

In an example of local gene therapy, mouse liver tumor cells transfected with a retroviral vector containing the murine endostatin gene were injected subcutaneously or into the peritoneal cavity.[141] After 63 days, tumors arising from endostatin transduced tumor cells were inhibited by 99% of the control

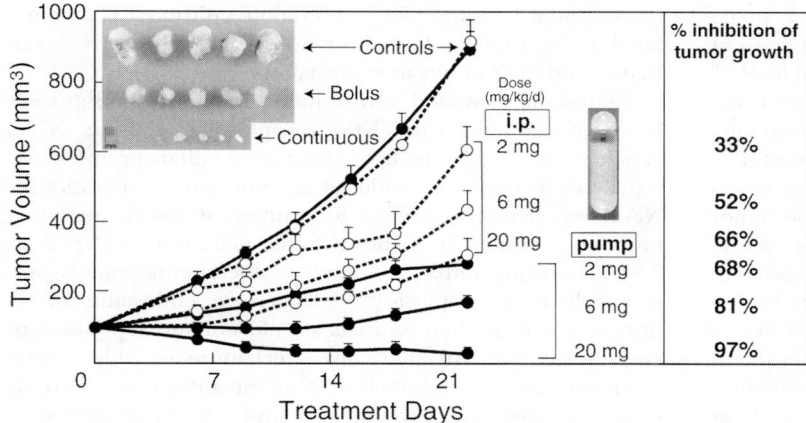

FIGURE 63-9. Endostatin administered to severe combined immunodeficiency mice bearing human pancreatic cancer (which is p53[−/−]). Endostatin therapy is administered either as a once-daily bolus by intraperitoneal injection or continuously from a microosmotic pump (Alzet) implanted in the peritoneal cavity. It pumps 1 μL/h and provides the same total dose as the bolus but spread out over 24 hours. All doses inhibit tumor growth, but only the continuous dosing causes tumor regression. (From ref. 125, with permission.)

tumors (P <.001). Survival for endostatin-transduced tumors was 91% compared with 0% for untreated controls.[142] Other reports of local gene therapy with endostatin show effective tumor inhibition in animals bearing human hepatic carcinoma, renal cell carcinoma, and mouse melanoma.[143–145] Gliomas were inhibited by gene transfers to tumor cells that were then implanted into rat brains.[146] Gliomas were also inhibited by intratumoral implantation of alginate-encapsulated beads containing packaging cells transfected with endostatin.[148–150]

A human breast carcinoma, MDA-MB435, was markedly inhibited when the cells were transduced with endostatin, but another breast cancer, MCF7, was not inhibited.[147]

Also, intratumoral gene transfer of endostatin inhibited mouse mammary tumors (MidT2-1) but had a minimal effect in human breast cancer (MDA-MB435) in severe combined immunodeficiency disease mice.[151,152] Despite many successes of endostatin gene transfer into tumor cells, unsolved problems remain. In another report, endostatin gene transfer into a human breast cancer (MDA-MBA335), significantly inhibited growth of the tumor but not when the breast cancer was MCF7. In contrast, angiostatin gene transfer into MCF7 breast cancer was very inhibitory but had only minimal effect on MDA-MB435 breast cancer cells.[146] A different type of breast cancer (MCA-4) transduced with endostatin was significantly inhibited.[152] The basis for these differences is unclear. It remains to be determined if different breast cancers induce up-regulation of different endothelial integrins and whether any of these would differ from the integrin that binds endostatin.[45,29]

Systemically administered gene therapy (by an intravenous or intramuscular vector in mice or rats) significantly inhibited tumor growth in renal cell carcinoma, Lewis lung carcinoma, adenocarcinoma MC38, hemangioendothelioma, spontaneous breast cancer and its metastases, and colon cancer [when the gene was injected intramuscularly and endostatin serum levels were only moderately elevated (35 to 40 ng/mL)].[153–158] Adenoviral gene transfer of endostatin delayed growth of breast cancer implants and retarded their growth by 67% after the tumors appeared.[155]

However, other reports of systemically administered endostatin gene therapy failed to inhibit tumor growth. For example, either local or systemic endostatin gene therapy failed to inhibit rat tumors despite the achievement of serum levels more than 10 to 200 times above normal levels of endostatin.[159] Kuo et al. also were unable to demonstrate significant inhibition of tumor growth and only 23% to 33% (P <.002 and P <.0001, respectively) inhibition of corneal angiogenesis when viruses encoding angiostatin or endostatin were administered as a single intravenous injection, despite the fact that peak serum levels of endostatin reached 400 to 599 times above the normal level.[160] In contrast, viruses encoding soluble forms of Flk1 or Flt1, the receptors for VEGF, resulted in approximately 80% growth inhibition of the same tumor and strong inhibition of corneal neovascularization (74% to 80%; P <.001). A strong correlation was observed between the effects of the different viruses on tumor growth and the activity of the viruses in the inhibition of corneal micropocket angiogenesis. It is unclear why angiostatin and endostatin delivered by systemically administered gene therapy should be so ineffective as tumor inhibitors, whereas soluble VEGF receptors administered by the same viruses and in the same tumor models should inhibit tumor growth so effectively. However, three speculations may be considered as a basis

for future research. Antiangiogenic and antitumor activity of endostatin are dose-dependent, but recent experiments reveal a U-shaped curve of efficacy (see later in Biphasic Effect of Some Angiogenesis Inhibitors) analogous to interferon-α.[161] In one tumor system, human recombinant endostatin protein administered at 50 mg/kg/d inhibited tumor growth by 47%; 100 mg/kg by 84%, and 1000 mg/kg by 37%. Therefore, it is possible that super high levels of endostatin above an optimum level lose activity *in vivo*. A second speculation is that endostatin may aggregate at very high serum levels or that its folding may be affected. A third speculation is that serum plasmin levels may be increased by certain viruses or by high viral titers. Other authors subsequently have reported failure of endostatin gene transfer to significantly inhibit a murine leukemia when endostatin was transduced into hematopoietic stem cells and serum endostatin levels of 300 ng/mL were reached, or to inhibit metastases from a fibrosarcoma when serum endostatin levels of up to 700 ng/mL were obtained.[162,163] Of interest is that these authors previously reported in collaboration with Folkman and O'Reilly enhanced antitumor activity with an endostatin–angiostatin fusion protein engineered in hematopoietic stem cells.[164]

Gene Expression in Human Endothelial Cells Induced by Endostatin

To determine how the endothelial cell genome and proteome react to endostatin treatment, Abdollahi et al. used a genome-wide expression profile covering 95% of the human genome and phosphorylation analysis on antibody arrays.[111] In a study of the effect of human endostatin on primary isolated human microvascular endothelial cells growing *in vitro*, array-based gene expression was analyzed in approximately 75,000 human genes. Endostatin significantly down-regulated expression of HIF-1 alpha. Endostatin also down-regulated many upstream activators of HIF-l alpha, including c-jun/Fos, Ets, and EGFR. Endostatin also down-regulated the Id transcription factors (Fig. 63-10). These genes are proangiogenic, and deletion of three alleles of Id1 and Id3[22,23] results in healthy mice that cannot mount an angiogenic response to implanted tumor cells. Endostatin substantially down-regulated MMP-2 and $\alpha_v\beta_3$ integrin. Ephrin signaling is down-regulated by endostatin. The ephrin/Eph family has recently been shown to participate in the regulation of angiogenesis. Both ephrin B1 and ephrin B2 induce sprouting angiogenesis *in vitro* to an extent similar to the angiogenic activity of VEGF or angiopoietin 1.[165] Endostatin also down-regulated ephrin A1. Although ephrins generally do not induce endothelial proliferation, ephrin A1 is up-regulated during capillary tube formation.[166] Kuo et al. have shown that endostatin inhibits tube formation *in vitro*.[167]

Endostatin inhibited TNF-α–induced angiogenic signaling by down-regulating the TNF-α receptor. In addition, NFκB (nuclear factor of kappa light chain gene enhancer in B cells) was down-regulated by endostatin. Endostatin inactivation of NFκB was demonstrated by four different assays, including immunochemistry. It is thought that activation of NFκB by TNF-α, ionizing radiation, or chemotherapeutic agents protects cells from apoptosis.[168,169] Therefore, endostatin inhibition of NFκB in these settings should enhance apoptosis of endothelial cells. An alternative mechanism by which endostatin may mediate endothelial cell arrest and apoptosis is by its down-regulation of activator protein-1. Activator protein-1,

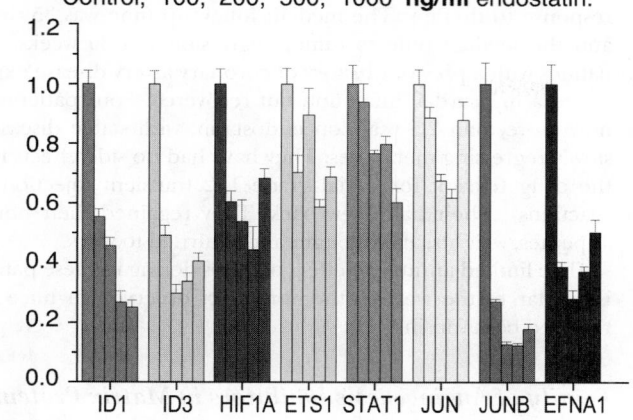

Dose dependence of mRNA expression at **4 hours**:
Control, 100, 200, 500, 1000 **ng/ml** endostatin.

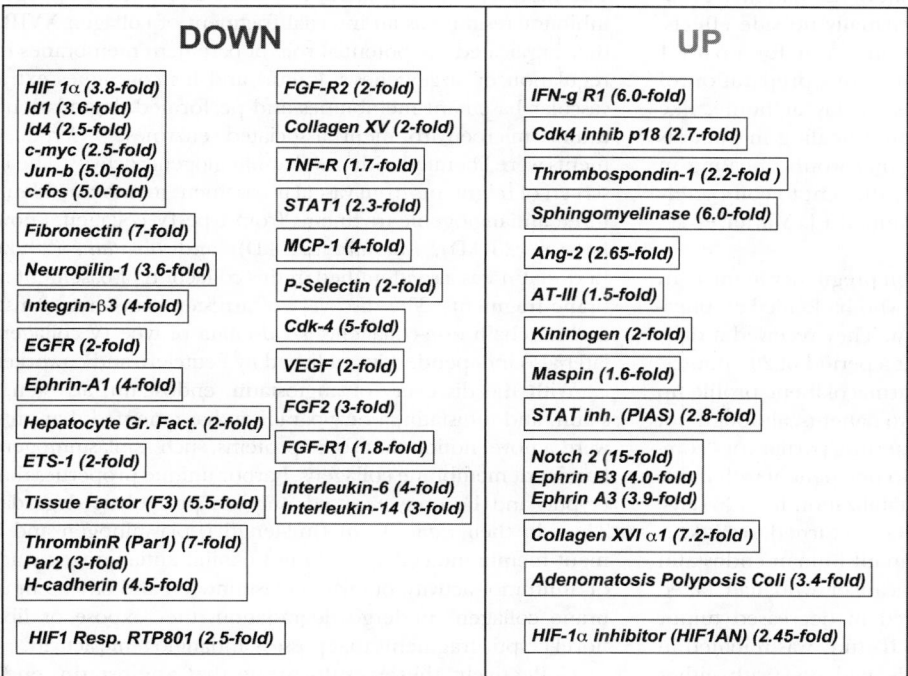

DOWN		UP
HIF 1α (3.8-fold) Id1 (3.6-fold) Id4 (2.5-fold) c-myc (2.5-fold) Jun-b (5.0-fold) c-fos (5.0-fold)	FGF-R2 (2-fold)	IFN-g R1 (6.0-fold)
	Collagen XV (2-fold)	Cdk4 inhib p18 (2.7-fold)
Fibronectin (7-fold)	TNF-R (1.7-fold)	Thrombospondin-1 (2.2-fold)
Neuropilin-1 (3.6-fold)	STAT1 (2.3-fold)	Sphingomyelinase (6.0-fold)
Integrin-β3 (4-fold)	MCP-1 (4-fold)	Ang-2 (2.65-fold)
EGFR (2-fold)	P-Selectin (2-fold)	AT-III (1.5-fold)
Ephrin-A1 (4-fold)	Cdk-4 (5-fold)	Kininogen (2-fold)
Hepatocyte Gr. Fact. (2-fold)	VEGF (2-fold)	Maspin (1.6-fold)
ETS-1 (2-fold)	FGF2 (3-fold)	STAT inh. (PIAS) (2.8-fold)
Tissue Factor (F3) (5.5-fold)	FGF-R1 (1.8-fold)	Notch 2 (15-fold) Ephrin B3 (4.0-fold) Ephrin A3 (3.9-fold)
ThrombinR (Par1) (7-fold) Par2 (3-fold) H-cadherin (4.5-fold)	Interleukin-6 (4-fold) Interleukin-14 (3-fold)	Collagen XVI α1 (7.2-fold)
HIF1 Resp. RTP801 (2.5-fold)		Adenomatosis Polyposis Coli (3.4-fold)
		HIF-1α inhibitor (HIF1AN) (2.45-fold)

FIGURE 63-10. **A:** A few examples of gene expressions in human microvascular endothelial cells after treatment with human endostatin. Dose dependence of messenger RNA (mRNA) expression at 4 hours. Note, for example, that ID1, ID3, and HIF1A are all significantly down-regulated with increasing endostatin concentrations but that there is a U-shaped curve with increasing concentrations. **B:** Examples of sets of genes that are down-regulated or up-regulated in endothelial cells. Endostatin resets these endothelial genes en masse toward a quiescent nonproliferating, nonmigrating state. (From ref. 111, with permission.) (See Color Fig. 63-10*A* in the CD-ROM.)

consisting of c-Fos and c-Jun, normally prevents apoptosis. Of interest is that the promoter regions of VEGF, VEGFR2, and HIF-1 alpha contain several activator protein-1–binding elements. These networks define a potential network of targets by which endostatin may exert its antiangiogenic effect. STAT1 and STAT3 were down-regulated twofold in endothelial cells treated by endostatin. STATs (signal transducers and activators of transcription factors) up-regulate genes that encode inhibitors of apoptosis (e.g., Bcl-2), inducers of angiogenesis (e.g., VEGF), and cell cycle regulators (e.g., cyclins D1/D2 and c-myc).[170] After endostatin treatment of endothelial cells, most of the genes downstream of STAT were strongly down-regulated. These include the apoptosis inhibitor Bcl-2 and the cell cycle regulators cyclins D1/D2 and c-myc.

Thrombin receptors (proteinase-activated receptor-1 and proteinase-activated receptor-2) were also significantly down-regulated by endostatin. Several factors contribute to the proan-

giogenic activity of thrombin. Thrombin is a potent stimulus for release of VEGF by transcriptional regulation activation of HIF-1 alpha.[171] Thrombin also up-regulates expression of VEGF receptors on endothelial cells.[172] In a positive loop, VEGF accelerates thrombin generation, another proangiogenic event.[173] This loop has implications for cancer patients. The majority of cancer deaths are directly attributable to thrombosis or bleeding. Another link between angiogenesis and thrombin is that cleaved or latent conformations of antithrombin III (ATIII) potently inhibit angiogenesis.[174] It was found that endostatin significantly up-regulates ATIII. The enzymatic degradation of ATIII (58 kD) to the antiangiogenic form (53 kD) appears to be by tumor-generated enzymes.[175] This observation emphasizes that endostatin down-regulates proangiogenic genes and simultaneously up-regulates genes that lead to inhibition of angiogenesis.

Endostatin directly down-regulated Ets-1 in endothelial cells in a time-dependent manner and decreased the mRNA level of most of the Ets-1 target genes, such as MMP-1 and integrin-β_3. Ets positively regulates angiogenesis by inducing several target genes, including uPA, MMP-1, MMP-3, MMP-9, and integrin-β_3, and the elimination of the Ets-1 activity by a dominant negative molecule inhibits angiogenesis *in vivo*.[176–180] A striking finding is that several pathways thought to be distinct in fact intercommunicate to bring about a focused antiangiogenic response in the tumor bed, directly as a result of endostatin treatment. It is not clear whether many of the small molecular angiogenesis inhibitors produce such a focused antiangiogenic response at the genetic level as endostatin does.[116,117,181]

Preclinical and Clinical Applications of Endostatin

Several interesting characteristics of endostatin make it advantageous for clinical use in cancer patients. First, it is not toxic. At this writing, endostatin is in phase I/II clinical trials, and to date it has only been used in approximately 120 patients. However, all centers report that there are virtually no side effects, even in patients who have been on endostatin for up to 1 year.[192] Patients who receive the subcutaneous preparation of endostatin take their own injections each day at home, like insulin. (Endostatin does not delay wound healing in patients or in animals.) It has been confirmed that wound healing in mice is not delayed by endostatin doses sufficient to completely inhibit growth of tumors in the same animal (J. Marler et al., *unpublished data*, 2000).

Endostatin appears to have no effect on pregnancy in mice. In a phase I trial of endostatin, 25 patients who had failed all previous therapy were treated with endostatin. They received a daily intravenous bolus dose of endostatin over a period of 20 minutes. Endostatin was safe and had a linear pharmacokinetic profile up to 599 mg/m^2/d. Tumors regressed in two patients, although not sufficiently to satisfy the criteria for the terms "partial" or "complete" response used for chemotherapy. In one patient with metastatic melanoma, there was prolonged stabilization for 426 days, with a much improved quality of life, and he returned to work.

In phase I safety studies[78] of recombinant human endostatin in patients with metastatic progressive cancer who had failed conventional therapy, treatment resulted in decreased tumor size in two patients. Therefore, a phase II study was initiated in this patient population. In 37 evaluable patients (with either metastatic carcinoid or metastatic islet cell carcinoma of the pancreas) self-administered by subcutaneous injection of dosages of 60 to 90 mg/m^2/d according to World Health Organization criteria, two (5%) experienced minor responses; one of these patients experienced a more than 50% decrease in tumor marker

(chromogranin A) levels. Twenty-three (62%) had stable disease, and 12 (32%) had progressive disease as their best response to therapy. The median follow-up time was 35 weeks, and the median time to tumor regression was 39 weeks. One patient with a previous history of coronary artery disease experienced a myocardial infarction but recovered. Four patients are now more than 2.5 years on endostatin, with stable disease or slowly regressing metastases. They have had no side effects from the drug (except for initial grade 1/2 transient injection site reactions). Their hair grew back. They regained their normal appetites, weights, and strength and returned to work.

The limited antitumor effect of bolus dosing in these patients is similar to the weak antitumor effect observed in mice that received bolus dosing.

Family of Angiogenesis Inhibitors in Matrix Proteins

The discovery of endostatin, a specific and potent angiogenesis inhibitor residing as an internal fragment of collagen XVIII, further implicated the potential role of basement membranes in the regulation of angiogenesis. Kalluri and his colleagues extracted vascular basement membranes and performed degradation with tumor microenvironment associated enzymes.[28] Cryptic fragments were liberated with novel antiangiogenic activity. The initial screen of fragments from vascular basement membrane identified three antiangiogenic fragments from type IV collagen, known as *arresten* (26 kD), *canstatin* (24 kD), and *tumstatin* (28 kD).[27] Endostatin was also identified in this collection of basement membrane fragments. The discovery of arresten, canstatin, tumstatin, and α3 chain non-collagenous-1 domain of type IV collagen was later also independently published by Petitclerc and coworkers.[28]

With the discovery of angiostatin, endostatin, arresten, canstatin, and tumstatin, a new paradigm has emerged that puts forward a novel notion that some proteins, such as plasminogen and basement membrane collagens, harbor unique properties that are cryptic and become exposed only on proteolytic degradation. Thus, in their intact form (full-length), plasminogen and basement membrane collagens do not exhibit antiangiogenic activity or antitumor activity, but when plasminogen and basement membrane collagens undergo degradation, they expose or liberate novel cryptic fragments that possess antiangiogenic activity.

Collectively, these results argue that angiostatin, endostatin, tumstatin, canstatin, and arresten may function as cryptic tumor suppressor proteins, offering an additional line of defense *against* tumor progression by blocking angiogenesis switching. When taken together with the findings that a change in amino acid sequence of endostatin due to a polymorphism corre-

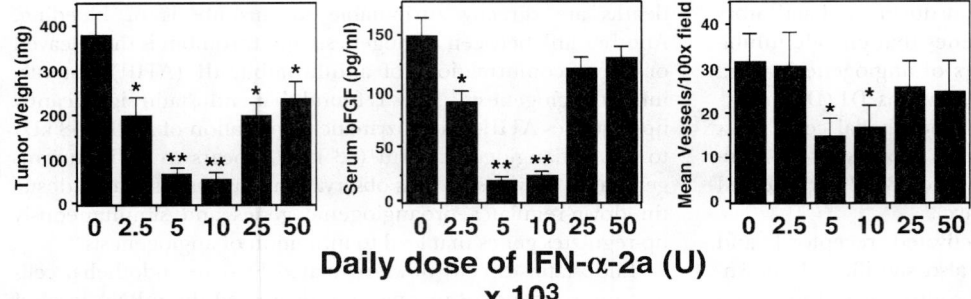

FIGURE 63-11. U-shaped efficacy curve in tumor-bearing mice treated with murine interferon-α (IFN-α). There is an optimum low dose of IFN-α that is more effective than the high dose for decreased tumor weight (*left panel*), for decreased serum basic fibroblast growth factor (bFGF) (*middle panel*), and for decreased mean vessel density in the tumors (*right panel*). (From ref. 161, with permission.)

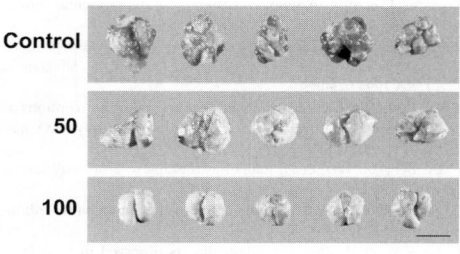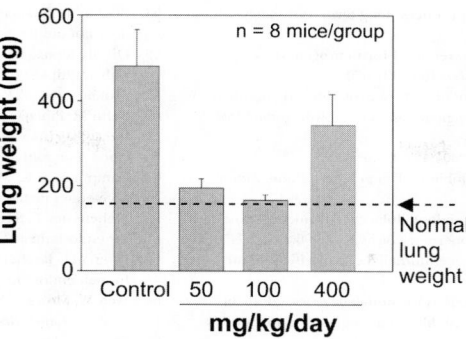

FIGURE 63-12. The antiangiogenic and antitumor efficacy of rosiglitazone, a peroxisome proliferator–activated receptor γ ligand, follows a U-shaped curve analogous to interferon-α and inhibits angiogenesis and tumor growth. (From ref. 54, with permission.) (See Color Fig. 63-12 in the CD-ROM.)

lates with an increased susceptibility to prostate cancer, and that, conversely, an increase in physiologic levels of endostatin results in less propensity for emergence of solid tumors in individuals with Down syndrome (associated with an extra copy of type XVIII collagen), these results suggest that endogenous angiogenesis inhibitors act as tumor suppressors that are orchestrated to prevent a focus of angiogenesis under normal conditions.

BIPHASIC EFFECT OF SOME ANGIOGENESIS INHIBITORS

The antiangiogenic activity and antitumor activity of certain angiogenesis inhibitors follow a U-shaped curve. This was first demonstrated experimentally with interferon-α.[161] Lower doses were more effective than higher doses in suppressing tumor growth, microvessel density, and circulating bFGF in tumor-bearing animals (Fig. 63-11). A similar biphasic response has been observed with rosiglitazone (a peroxisome proliferator–activated receptor γ ligand)[54] (Fig. 63-12). Also, endostatin therapy in animals follows a U-shaped curve when administered as a protein (I. Celik et al., *unpublished data*, 2004) or as gene therapy. The mechanism of this biphasic effect remains to be elucidated. Nevertheless, it may provide a partial explanation for the efficacy of low-dose (metronomic) chemotherapy.

FUTURE DIRECTIONS

Angiogenesis inhibition is being validated as an anticancer therapy in an increasing number of clinical trials. The most compelling results have been reported for patients with advanced colon cancer treated with Avastin.[182] Other validations include the successful durable complete regression of recurrent high-grade giant cell tumors in the maxilla or mandible by low-dose interferon-α[183–186] and also long-term (up to 5 years) complete remissions of multiple myeloma.[187]

There remains an urgent need for surrogate biomarkers of efficacy of angiogenesis inhibitors because their general paucity of side effects precludes the use of "maximum tolerated dose" as a guide to dosing and because some of them follow a U-shaped dose-response curve.

Antiangiogenic therapy is a new modality for which many traditions for cytotoxic chemotherapy do not apply. For example, "maximum tolerated dosing" is often not applicable with angiogenesis inhibitors. Also, prolonged "stable" disease (years) without side effects can be a useful goal of certain angiogenesis inhibitors. Furthermore, several misperceptions have not held up in the face of data that seem at first glance to

be counterintuitive—this is, that "p53$^{-/-}$ tumors would not be responsive to angiogenesis inhibitors"[194] or that "angiogenesis inhibitors would be defeated by tumor hypoxia."[195]

There is increasing evidence that angiogenesis inhibitors may be used in combination with each other or in combinations with low-dose (metronomic) chemotherapy.

It is also possible that, in the future, antiangiogenic therapy may be used as preventive therapy before the appearance of a tumor or to prevent recurrence after surgical removal of a tumor, but, in both cases, guided by molecular or cellular biomarkers in the blood or urine.

REFERENCES

1. Folkman J, Kalluri R. Medicine. Tumor angiogenesis. In: Kufe DW, Pollock RE, Weichselbaum RR, et al., eds. *Cancer medicine*, 6th ed. Hamilton, Ontario: BC Decker, 2003:161.
2. Weidner N, Semple JP, Welch WR, et al. Tumor angiogenesis and metastasis—correlation in invasive breast carcinoma. *N Engl J Med* 1991;324:1.
3. Carmeliet P, Jain RK. Angiogenesis in cancer and other diseases. *Nature* 2000;407:249.
4. Bergers G, Brekken R, McMahon G, et al. Matrix metalloproteinase-9 triggers the angiogenic switch during carcinogenesis. *Nature Cell Biol* 2000;2:737.
5. Hanahan D, Folkman J. Patterns and emerging mechanisms of the angiogenic switch during tumorigenesis. *Cell* 1996;86:353.
6. Holash J, Maisonpierre PC, Compton D, et al. Vessel cooption, regression, and growth in tumors mediated by angiopoietins and VEGF. *Science* 1999;284:1994.
7. Asahara T, Murohara T, Sullivan A, et al. Isolation of putative progenitor endothelial cells for angiogenesis. *Science* 1997;275:964.
8. Shi Q, Rafii S, Wu MH-D, et al. Evidence for circulating bone marrow-derived endothelial cells. *Blood* 1998;92:362.
9. Hatzopoulos AK, Folkman J, Vasile E, et al. Isolation and characterization of endothelial progenitor cells from mouse embryos. *Development* 1998;125:1457.
10. Black WC, Welch HG. Advances in diagnostic imaging and overestimations of disease prevalence and the benefits of therapy. *N Engl J Med* 1993;328:1237.
11. Rak J, Yu JL, Klement G, Kerbel RS. Oncogenes and angiogenesis: signaling three-dimensional tumor growth. *J Invest Dermatol Symp Proc* 2000;5:24.
12. Kerbel RS, Viloria-Petit A, Okada F, Rak J. Establishing a link between oncogenes and tumor angiogenesis. *Mol Med* 1998;4:286.
13. Rak J, Yu JL, Kerbel RS, Coomber BL. What do oncogenic mutations have to do with angiogenesis/vascular dependence of tumors? *Cancer Res* 2002;62:1931.
14. Petit AM, Rak J, Hung MC, et al. Neutralizing antibodies against epidermal growth factor and ErB-2/neu receptor tyrosine kinases down-regulate vascular endothelial growth factor production by tumor cells in vitro and in vivo: angiogenic implications for signal transduction therapy of solid tumors. *Am J Pathol* 1997;151:1523.
15. Fernandez A, Udagawa T, Schwesinger C, et al. Angiogenic potential of prostate carcinoma cells overexpressing bcl-2. *J Natl Cancer Inst* 2001;93:208.
16. Ciardiello F, Caputo R, Bianco R, et al. Inhibition of growth factor production and angiogenesis in human cancer cells by ZD1839 (Iressa), a selective epidermal growth factor receptor tyrosine kinase inhibitor. *Clin Cancer Res* 2001;7:1459.
17. Karashima T, Sweeney P, Slaton JW, et al. Inhibition of angiogenesis by the antiepidermal growth factor receptor antibody ImClone C225 in androgen-independent prostate cancer growing orthotopically in nude mice. *Clin Cancer Res* 2002;8:1253.
18. Folkman J. Tumor angiogenesis: therapeutic implications. *N Engl J Med* 1971;285:1182.
19. Millauer B, Shawver LK, Plate KH, et al. Glioblastoma growth inhibited in vivo by a dominant-negative Flk-1 mutant. *Nature* 1994;367:576.
20. Arbiser JL, Moses MA, Fernandez CA, et al. Oncogenic H-ras stimulates tumor angiogenesis by two distinct pathways. *Proc Natl Acad Sci U S A* 1997;94:861.
21. Cao Y, O'Reilly MS, Marshall B, et al. Expression of angiostatin cDNA in a murine fibro-

sarcoma suppresses primary tumor growth and produces long-term dormancy of metastases. *J Clin Invest* 1998;101:1055.

22. Lyden D, Young AZ, Zagzag D, et al. Id1 and Id3 are required for neurogenesis, angiogenesis and vascularization of tumour xenografts. *Nature* 1999;401:670.

23. Lyden D, Hattori K, Dias S, et al. Impaired recruitment of bone-marrow-derived endothelial and hematopoietic precursor cells blocks tumor angiogenesis and growth. *Nature Med* 2001;7:1194.

24. Folkman J, Kalluri R. Cancer without disease. *Nature* 2004;427:787.

25. Lawler J. Thrombospondin-1 as an endogenous inhibitor of angiogenesis and tumor growth. *J Cell Mol Med* 2002;6:1.

26. Maeshima Y, Colorado PC, Kalluri R. Two RGD-independent alpha vbeta 3 integrin binding sites on tumstatin regulate distinct anti-tumor properties. *J Biol Chem* 2000;275:23745.

27. Maeshima Y, Sudhakar A, Lively JC, et al. Tumstatin, an endothelial cell-specific inhibitor of protein synthesis. *Science* 2002;295:140.

28. Petitclerc E, Boutaud A, Prestayko A, et al. New functions for non-collagenous domains of human collagen type IV. Novel integrin ligands inhibiting angiogenesis and tumor growth in vivo. *J Biol Chem* 2000;275:8051.

29. Sudhakar A, Sugimoto H, Yang C, et al. Human tumstatin and human endostatin exhibit distinct antiangiogenic activities mediated by alphav beta3 and alpha5 beta1 integrins. *Proc Natl Acad Sci U S A* 2003;100:4766.

30. Hamano Y, Zeisberg M, Sugimoto H, et al. Physiological levels of tumstatin, a fragment of collagen IV alpha3 chain, are generated by MMP-9 proteolysis and suppress angiogenesis via alphaVbeta3 integrin. *Cancer Cell* 2003;3:589.

31. Folkman J, Hahnfeldt P, Hlatky L. Cancer: looking outside the genome. *Nat Rev Mol Cell Biol* 2000;1:76.

32. Kerbel RS. Inhibition of tumor angiogenesis as a strategy to circumvent acquired resistance to anti-cancer therapeutic agents. *Bioessays* 1991;13:31.

33. Modzelewski RA, Davies P, Watkins SC, et al. Isolation and identification of fresh tumor-derived endothelial cells from a murine RIF-1 fibrosarcoma. *Cancer Res* 1994;54:336.

34. Kerbel R, Folkman J. Clinical translation of angiogenesis inhibitors. *Nat Rev Cancer* 2002;2:727.

35. Masferrer JL, Leahy KM, Koki AT, et al. Antiangiogenic and antitumor activities of cyclooxygenase-2 inhibitors. *Cancer Res* 2000;60:1306.

36. Sunwoo JB, Chen Z, Dong G, et al. Novel proteasome inhibitor PS-341 inhibits activation of nuclear factor-kappa B, cell survival, tumor growth, and angiogenesis in squamous cell carcinoma. *Clin Cancer Res* 2001;7:1419.

37. Nawrocki ST, Bruns CJ, Harbison MT, et al. Effects of the proteasome inhibitor PS-341 on apoptosis and angiogenesis in orthotopic human pancreatic tumor xenografts. *Mol Cancer Ther* 2002;1:1243.

38. LeBlanc R, Catley LP, Hideshima T, et al. Proteasome inhibitor PS-341 inhibits human myeloma cell growth in vivo and prolongs survival in a murine model. *Cancer Res* 2002;62:4996.

39. D'Amato RJ, Loughnan MS, Flynn E, et al. Thalidomide is an inhibitor of angiogenesis. *Proc Natl Acad Sci U S A* 1994;91:4082.

40. Singhal S, Mehta J, Desikan R, et al. Antitumor activity of thalidomide in refractory multiple myeloma. *N Engl J Med* 1999;341:1565.

41. Raje N, Anderson K. Thalidomide—a revival story. *N Engl J Med* 1999;341:1606.

42. Hlatky L, Hahnfeldt P, Folkman J. Clinical application of antiangiogenic therapy: microvessel density, what it does and doesn't tell us. *J Natl Cancer Inst* 2002;94:883.

43. Bertolini F, Mingrone W, Alietti A, et al. Thalidomide in multiple myeloma, myelodysplastic syndromes and histiocytosis. Analysis of clinical results and of surrogate angiogenesis markers. *Ann Oncol* 2001;12:987.

44. Habeck M. Australia approves thalidomide. *Lancet Oncol* 2003;4:713.

45. Wickstrom SA, Alitalo K, Keski-Oja J. Endostatin associates with integrin alpha5beta1 and caveolin-1, and activates Src via a tyrosyl phosphatase-dependent pathway in human endothelial cells. *Cancer Res* 2002;62:5580.

46. Relf M, LeJeune S, Scott PA, et al. Expression of the angiogenic factors vascular endothelial cell growth factor, acidic and basic fibroblast growth factor, tumor growth factor beta-1, platelet-derived endothelial cell growth factor, placenta growth factor, and pleiotrophin in human primary breast cancer and its relation to angiogenesis. *Cancer Res* 1997;57:963.

47. Browder T, Butterfield CE, Kraling BM, et al. Antiangiogenic scheduling of chemotherapy improves efficacy against experimental drug-resistant cancer. *Cancer Res* 2000;60:1878.

48. Klement G, Baruchel S, Rak J, et al. Continuous low-dose therapy with vinblastine and VEGF receptor-2 antibody induces sustained tumor regression without overt toxicity. *J Clin Invest* 2000;105:R15.

49. Hanahan D, Bergers G, Bergsland E. Less is more, regularly: metronomic dosing of cytotoxic drugs can target tumor angiogenesis in mice. *J Clin Invest* 2000;105:1045.

50. Wang J, Lou P, Lesniewski R, et al. Paclitaxel at ultra low concentrations inhibits angiogenesis without affecting cellular microtubule assembly. *Anticancer Drugs* 2003;14:13.

51. Bocci G, Francia G, Man S, et al. Thrombospondin 1, a mediator of the antiangiogenic effects of low-dose metronomic chemotherapy. *Proc Natl Acad Sci U S A* 2003;100:12917.

52. Streit M, Riccardi L, Velasco P, et al. Thrombospondin-2: a potent endogenous inhibitor of tumor growth and angiogenesis. *Proc Natl Acad Sci U S A* 1999;96:14888.

53. Kalas W, Gilpin S, Yu JL, et al. Restoration of thrombospondin 1 expression in tumor cells harbouring mutant ras oncogene by treatment with low doses of doxycycline. *Biochem Biophys Res Commun* 2003;310:109.

54. Panigrahy D, Singer S, Shen LQ, et al. PPARgamma ligands inhibit primary tumor growth and metastasis by inhibiting angiogenesis. *J Clin Invest* 2002;110:923.

55. Huang H, Campbell S, Nelius T, et al. PPAR-gamma ligands improve anti-tumorigenic and anti-angiogenic efficacy of thrombospondin-1 through modulating its receptor CD36. New directions in angiogenesis research. *Am Assoc Cancer Res* 2003;(abstrA15).

56. Ma L, del Soldato P, Wallace JL. Divergent effects of new cyclooxygenase inhibitors on gastric ulcer healing: Shifting the angiogenic balance. *Proc Natl Acad Sci U S A* 2002;99:13243.

57. O'Reilly MS, Boehm T, Shing Y, et al. Endostatin: an endogenous inhibitor of angiogenesis and tumor growth. *Cell* 1997;88:277.

58. Boehm T, Folkman J, Browder T, et al. Antiangiogenic therapy of experimental cancer does not induce acquired drug resistance. *Nature* 1997;390:404.

59. Oh SP, Kamagata Y, Muragaki Y, et al. Isolation and sequencing of cDNAs for proteins with multiple domains of Gly-Xaa-Yaa repeats identify a distinct family of collagenous proteins. *Proc Natl Acad Sci U S A* 1994;91:4229.

60. Rehn M, Pihlajaniemi T. Alpha1(XVIII), a collagen chain with frequent interruptions in the collagenous sequence, a distinct tissue distribution, and homology with type XV collagen. *Proc Natl Acad Sci U S A* 1994;91:4234.

61. Camphausen K, Moses MA, Beecken WD, et al. Radiation therapy to a primary tumor accelerates metastatic growth in mice. *Cancer Res* 2001;61:2207.

62. Hohenester E, Sasaki T, Olsen BR, Timpl R. Crystal structure of the angiogenesis inhibitor endostatin at 1.5 A resolution. *EMBO J* 1998;17:1656.

63. Ding Y-H, Javaherian K, Lo K-M, et al. Zinc-dependent dimers observed in crystals of human endostatin. *Proc Natl Acad Sci U S A* 1998;95:10443.

64. Wen W, Moses MA, Wiederschain D, et al. The generation of endostatin is mediated by elastase. *Cancer Res* 1999;59:6052.

65. Felbor U, Dreier L, Bryant RA, et al. Secreted cathepsin L generates endostatin from collagen XVIII. *EMBO J* 2000;19:1187.

66. Miosge N, Sasaki T, Timpl R. Angiogenesis inhibitor endostatin is a distinct component of elastic fibers in vessel walls. *FASEB J* 1999;13:1743.

67. Sasaki T, Larsson H, Tisi D, et al. Endostatins derived from collagens XV and XVIII differ in structural and binding properties, tissue distribution and anti-angiogenic activity. *J Mol Biol* 2000;301:1179.

68. Sasaki T, Larsson H, Kreuger J, et al. Structural basis and potential role of heparin/heparan sulfate binding to the angiogenesis inhibitor endostatin. *EMBO J* 1999;18:6240.

69. Kasai S, Nagasawa H, Shimamura M, et al. Design and synthesis of antiangiogenic/heparin-binding arginine dendrimer mimicking the surface of endostatin. *Bioorg Med Chem Lett* 2002;12:951.

70. Ricard-Blum S, Feraud O, Lortat-Jacob H, et al. Characterization of endostatin binding to heparin and heparan sulfate by surface plasmon resonance and molecular modeling: role of divalent cations. *J Biol Chem* 2004;279:2927.

71. Boehm T, O'Reilly MS, Keough K, et al. Zinc-binding of endostatin is essential for its antiangiogenic activity. *Biochem Biophys Res Commun* 1998;252:190.

72. Sim BKL, Fogler WE, Zhou XH, et al. Zinc ligand-disrupted recombinant human endostatin: potent inhibition of tumor growth, safety and pharmacokinetic profile. *Angiogenesis* 1999;3:41.

73. Cho H, Kim WJ, Lee YM, et al. N-/C-terminal deleted mutant of human endostatin efficiently acts as an anti-angiogenic and anti-tumorigenic agent. *Oncol Rep* 2004;11:191.

74. Wickstrom SA, Alitalo K, Keski-Oja J. An endostatin-derived peptide interacts with integrins and regulates actin cytoskeleton and migration of endothelial cells. *J Biol Chem* 2004;279:20178.

75. Chillemi F, Francescato P, Ragg E, et al. Studies on the structure-activity relationship of endostatin: synthesis of human endostatin peptides exhibiting potent antiangiogenic activities. *J Med Chem* 2003;46:4165.

76. Marneros AG, Olsen BR. The role of collagen-derived proteolytic fragments in angiogenesis. *Matrix Biol* 2001;20:337.

77. Ackley BD, Crew JR, Elamaa H, et al. The NC1/endostatin domain of *Caenorhabditis elegans* type XVIII collagen affects cell migration and axon guidance. *J Cell Biol* 2001;152:1219.

78. Eder JP Jr, Supko JG, Clark JW, et al. Phase I clinical trial of recombinant human endostatin administered as a short intravenous infusion repeated daily. *J Clin Oncol* 2002;20:3772.

79. Kulke M, Bergsland E, Ryan DP, et al. A phase II, open-label, safety, pharmacokinetic, and efficacy study of recombinant human endostatin in patients with advanced neuroendocrine tumors. *Proc Am Soc Clin Oncol* 2003;22:239 (abst. 958).

80. Miao H-Q, Lee P, Lin H, et al. Neuropilin-1 expression by tumor cells promotes tumor angiogenesis and progression. *FASEB J* 2000;14:2532.

81. Shin D, Garcia-Cardena G, Hayashi S, et al. Expression of ephrinB2 identifies a stable genetic difference between arterial and venous vascular smooth muscle as well as endothelial cells, and marks subsets of microvessels at sites of adult neovascularization. *Dev Biol* 2001;230:139.

82. Wang HU, Chen ZF, Anderson DJ. Molecular distinction and angiogenic interaction between embryonic arteries and veins revealed by ephrin-b2 and its receptor Eph-B4. *Cell* 1998;93:741.

83. Wickstrom SA, Alitalo K, Keski-Oja J. Endostatin associates with lipid rafts and induces reorganization of the actin cytoskeleton via down-regulation of RhoA activity. *J Biol Chem* 2003;278:37895.

84. Kim YM, Hwang S, Kim YM, et al. Endostatin blocks vascular endothelial growth factor-mediated signaling via direct interaction with KDR/Flk-1. *J Biol Chem* 2002;277:27872.

85. Hajitou A, Grignet C, Devy L, et al. The antitumor effect of endostatin and angiostatin is associated with a down-regulation of vascular endothelial growth factor expression in tumor cell. *FASEB J* 2002;16:1802.

86. Dixelius J, Larsson H, Sasaki T, et al. Endostatin-induced tyrosine kinase signaling through the Shb adaptor protein regulates endothelial cell apoptosis. *Blood* 2000;95:3403.

87. Chang Z, Choon A, Friedl A. Endostatin binds to blood vessels in situ independent of heparan sulfate and does not compete for fibroblast growth factor-2 binding. *Am J Pathol* 1999;155:71.

88. Seghezzi G, Patel S, Ren CJ, et al. Fibroblast growth factor-2 (FGF-2) induces vascular endothelial growth factor (VEGF) expression in the endothelial cells of forming capillaries: an autocrine mechanism contributing to angiogenesis. *J Cell Biol* 1998; 141:1659.

89. Shuster CB, Herman IM. The mechanics of vascular cell motility. *Microcirculation* 1998;5:239.

90. Dixelius J, Cross M, Matsumoto T, et al. Endostatin regulates endothelial cell adhesion and cytoskeletal organization. *Cancer Res* 2002;62:1944.

91. Strik HM, Schluesener HJ, Seid K, et al. Localization of endostatin in rat and human gliomas. *Cancer* 2001;91:10130.

92. Wickström S, Veikkola T, Rehn M, et al. Endostatin-induced modulation of plasminogen activation with concomitant loss of focal adhesions and actin stress fibers in cultured human endothelial cells. *Cancer Res* 2001;61:6511.
93. Kim Y-M, Jang J-W, Lee O-H, et al. Endostatin inhibits endothelial and tumor cellular invasion by blocking the activation and catalytic activity of matrix metalloproteinases 2. *Cancer Res* 2000;60:5410.
94. Lee SJ, Jang JW, Kim YM, et al. Endostatin binds to the catalytic domain of matrix metalloproteinase-2. *FEBS Lett* 2002;519:147.
95. Fang J, Shing Y, Wiederschain D, et al. Matrix metalloproteinase-2 (MMP-2) is required for the switch to the angiogenic phenotype in a novel tumor model. *Proc Natl Acad Sci U S A* 2000;97:3884.
96. Itoh T, Tanioka M, Yoshida H, et al. Reduced angiogenesis and tumor progression in gelatinase A-deficient mice. *Cancer Res* 1998;58:1048.
97. Bergers G, Brekken R, McMahon G, et al. Matrix metalloproteinase-9 triggers the angiogenic switch during carcinogenesis. *Nature Cell Biol* 2000;2:737.
98. Coussens LM, Tinkle CL, Hanahan D, et al. MMP-9 supplied by bone marrow-derived cells contributes to skin carcinogenesis. *Cell* 2000;103:481.
99. Karumanchi SA, Jha V, Ramchandran R, et al. Cell surface glypicans are low-affinity endostatin receptors. *Mol Cell* 2001;7:811.
100. Hanai J, Dhanabal M, Karumanchi SA, et al. Endostatin causes G1 arrest of endothelial cells through inhibition of cyclin D1. *J Biol Chem* 2002;277:16464.
101. Dhanabal M, Ramchandran R, Waterman MJF, et al. Endostatin induces endothelial cell apoptosis. *J Biol Chem* 1999;274:11721.
102. Xu R, Yao ZY, Xin L, et al. NC1 domain of human type VIII collagen (alpha 1) inhibits bovine aortic endothelial cell proliferation and causes cell apoptosis. *Biochem Biophys Res Commun* 2001;289:264.
103. Urbich C, Reissner A, Chavakis E, et al. Dephosphorylation of endothelial nitric oxide synthase contributes to the anti-angiogenic effects of endostatin. *FASEB J* 2002;16:706.
104. Morales-Ruiz M, Lee M-J, Zollner S, et al. Sphingosine 1-phosphate activates akt, nitric oxide production, and chemotaxis through a Gi protein/phosphoinositide 3-kinase pathway in endothelial cells. *J Biol Chem* 2001;276:19672.
105. Ziche M, Morbidelli L, Choudhuri R, et al. Nitric oxide synthase lies downstream from vascular endothelial growth factor-induced but not basic fibroblast growth factor-induced angiogenesis. *J Clin Invest* 1997;99:2625.
106. Papapetropoulos A, Garcia-Cardena G, Madri JA, Sessa WC. Nitric oxide contributes to the angiogenic properties of vascular endothelial growth factor in human endothelial cells. *J Clin Invest* 1997;100:3131.
107. Garcia-Cardena G, Folkman J. Is there a role for nitric oxide in tumor angiogenesis? *J Natl Cancer Inst* 1998;90:560.
108. Gallo O, Masini E, Morbidelli L, et al. Role of nitric oxide in angiogenesis and tumor progression in head and neck cancer. *J Natl Cancer Inst* 1998;90:587.
109. Keezer SM, Ivie SE, Krutzsch HC, et al. Angiogenesis inhibitors target the endothelial cell cytoskeleton through altered regulation of heat shock protein 27 and cofilin. *Cancer Res* 2003;63:6405.
110. Wu P, Yonekura H, Li H, et al. Hypoxia down-regulates endostatin production by human microvascular endothelial cells and pericytes. *Biochem Biophys Res Commun* 2001;288:1149.
111. Abdollahi A, Hahnfeldt P, Maercker C, et al. Gene regulation by endostatin amplifies anti-angiogenic function. *Mol Cell* 2004;13:649.
112. Sertie AL, Sossi V, Camargo AA, et al. Collagen XVIII, containing an endogenous inhibitor of angiogenesis and tumor growth, plays a critical role in the maintenance of retinal structure and in neural tube closure (Knobloch syndrome). *Hum Mol Genet* 2000;9:2051.
113. Suzuki OT, Sertie AL, Der Kaloustian VM, et al. Molecular analysis of collagen XVIII reveals novel mutations, presence of a third isoform, and possible genetic heterogeneity in Knobloch syndrome. *Am J Hum Genet* 2002;71:1320.
114. Menzel O, Bekkeheien RC, Reymond A, et al. Knobloch syndrome: novel mutations in COL18A1, evidence for genetic heterogeneity, and a functionally impaired polymorphism in endostatin. *Hum Mutat* 2004;23:77.
115. Fukai N, Eklund L, Marneros AG, et al. Lack of collagen XVIII/endostatin results in eye abnormalities. *EMBO J* 2002;21:1535.
116. Folkman J, Browder T, Palmblad J. Angiogenesis research: guidelines for translation to clinical application. *Thromb Haemost* 2001;86:23.
117. Browder T, Folkman J, Pirie-Shepherd S. The hemostatic system as a regulator of angiogenesis. *J Biol Chem* 2000;275:1521.
118. Möhle R, Green D, Moore MAS, et al. Constitutive production and thrombin-induced release of vascular endothelial growth factor by human megakaryocytes and platelets. *Proc Natl Acad Sci U S A* 1997;94:663.
119. Ma L, Hollenberg MD, Wallace JL. Thrombin-induced platelet endostatin release is blocked by a proteinase activated receptor-4 (PAR4) antagonist. *Br J Pharmacol* 2001;134:701.
119a. Nomi M, et al. Endostatin reduces vascular leakage by promoting vascular integrity. *J Clin Invest* 2004; (*submitted*).
120. O'Reilly MS, Holmgren L, Shing Y, et al. Angiostatin: a novel angiogenesis inhibitor that mediates the suppression of metastases by a Lewis lung carcinoma. *Cell* 1994;79:315.
121. Black WR, Agner RC. Tumour regression after endostatin therapy. *Nature* 1998;391:450.
122. Perletti G, Concari P, Giardini R, et al. Antitumor activity of endostatin against carcinogen-induced rat primary mammary tumors. *Cancer Res* 2000;60:1793.
123. Huang X, Wong MK, Zhao Q, et al. Soluble recombinant endostatin purified from *Escherichia coli*: antiangiogenic activity and antitumor effect. *Cancer Res* 2001;61:478.
124. He ZY, Chen ZY, Qiu CP, et al. Cloning, expression and tumor suppression of human endostatin. *Sheng Wu Hua Xue Yu Sheng Wu Wu Li Xue Bao (Shanghai)* 2000;32:333.
125. Kisker O, Becker CM, Prox D, et al. Continuous administration of endostatin by intraperitoneally implanted osmotic pump improves the efficacy and potency of therapy in a mouse xenograft tumor model. *Cancer Res* 2001;61:7669.
126. Kuroiwa M, Takeuchi T, Lee JH, et al. Continuous versus intermittent administration of human endostatin in xenografted human neuroblastoma. *J Pediatr Surg* 2003;38:1499.
127. Liu DL, Wen JX, Tong WC, Ben LH. Inhibition of lung adenocarcinoma LA795 in mice by recombinant human endostatin. *Di Yi Jun Yi Da Xue Xue Bao* 2001;21:917.
128. Ye C, Feng C, Wang S, et al. Antiangiogenic and antitumor effects of endostatin of follicular thyroid carcinoma. *Endocrinology* 2002;143:3522.
129. Solaun MS, Mendoza L, De Luca M, et al. Endostatin inhibits murine colon carcinoma sinusoidal-type metastases by preferential targeting of hepatic sinusoidal endothelium. *Hepatology* 2002;35:1104.
130. Iversen PO, Sorensen DR, Benestad HB. Inhibitors of angiogenesis selectively reduce the malignant cell load in rodent models of human myeloid leukemias. *Leukemia* 2002;16:376.
131. Boehle AS, Kurdow R, Schulze M, et al. Human endostatin inhibits growth of human non-small-cell lung cancer in a murine xenotransplant model. *Int J Cancer* 2001;94:420.
132. Kuroiwa M, Ikeda H, Hongo T, et al. Effects of recombinant human endostatin on a human neuroblastoma xenograft. *Int J Mol Med* 2001;8:391.
133. Calvo A, Yokoyama Y, Smith LE, et al. Inhibition of the mammary carcinoma angiogenic switch in C3(1)/SV40 transgenic mice by a mutated form of human endostatin. *Int J Cancer* 2002;101:224.
134. Yokoyama Y, Green JE, Sukhatme VP, Ramakrishnan S. Effect of endostatin on spontaneous tumorigenesis of mammary adenocarcinoma in a transgenic mouse model. *Cancer Res* 2000;60:4362.
135. Bergers G, Javaherian K, Lo KM, et al. Effects of angiogenesis inhibitors on multistage carcinogenesis in mice. *Science* 1999;284:808.
136. Sorensen DR, Read TA, Porwol T, et al. Endostatin reduces vascularization, blood flow, and growth in a rat gliosarcoma. *Neuro-oncol* 2002;4:1.
137. Scappaticci FA, Contreras A, Smith R, et al. Statin-AE: a novel angiostatin-endostatin fusion protein with enhanced antiangiogenic and antitumor activity. *Angiogenesis* 2001;4:263.
138. Scappaticci FA, Smith R, Pathak A, et al. Combination angiostatin and endostatin gene transfer induces synergistic antiangiogenic activity in vitro and antitumor efficacy in leukemia and solid tumors in mice. *Mol Ther* 2001;3:186.
139. Yokoyama Y, Dhanabal M, Griffioen AW, et al. Synergy between angiostatin and endostatin: inhibition of ovarian cancer growth. *Cancer Res* 2000;60:2190.
140. Hanna NN, Seetharam S, Mauceri HJ, et al. Antitumor interaction of short-course endostatin and ionizing radiation. *Cancer J* 2000;6:287.
141. Feldman AL, Alexander HR, Hewitt SM, et al. Effect of retroviral endostatin gene transfer on subcutaneous and intraperitoneal growth of murine tumors. *J Natl Cancer Inst* 2001;93:1014.
142. Wang X, Liu F, Li X, et al. Inhibitory effect of endostatin mediated by retroviral gene transfer on human liver carcinoma SMMC7721 in vivo. *Zhonghua Wai Ke Za Zhi* 2002;40:692.
143. Cichon T, Jamrozy L, Glogowska J, et al. Electrotransfer of gene encoding endostatin into normal and neoplastic mouse tissues: inhibition of primary tumor growth and metastatic spread. *Cancer Gene Ther* 2002;9:771.
144. Szary J, Szala S. Intra-tumoral administration of naked plasmid DNA encoding mouse endostatin inhibits renal carcinoma growth. *Int J Cancer* 2001;91:835.
145. Yamanaka R, Zullo SA, Ramsey J, et al. Induction of therapeutic antitumor antiangiogenesis by intratumoral injection of genetically engineered endostatin-producing Semliki Forest virus. *Cancer Gene Ther* 2001;8:796.
146. Indraccolo S, Gola E, Rosato A, et al. Differential effects of angiostatin, endostatin and interferon-alpha(1) gene transfer on in vivo growth of human breast cancer cells. *Gene Ther* 2002;9:867.
147. Peroulis I, Jonas N, Saleh M. Antiangiogenic activity of endostatin inhibits C6 glioma growth. *Int J Cancer* 2002;97:839.
148. Read TA, Farhadi M, Bjerkvig R, et al. Intravital microscopy reveals novel antivascular and antitumor effects of endostatin delivered locally by alginate-encapsulated cells. *Cancer Res* 2001;61:6830.
149. Read TA, Sorensen DR, Mahesparan R, et al. Local endostatin treatment of gliomas administered by microencapsulated producer cells. *Nat Biotechnol* 2001;19:29.
150. Joki T, Machluf M, Atala A, et al. Continuous release of endostatin from microencapsulated engineered cells for tumor therapy. *Nat Biotechnol* 2001;19:35.
151. Jin X, Bookstein R, Wills K, et al. Evaluation of endostatin antiangiogenesis gene therapy in vitro and in vivo. *Cancer Gene Ther* 2001;8:982.
152. Ding I, Sun JZ, Fenton B, et al. Intratumoral administration of endostatin plasmid inhibits vascular growth and perfusion in MCa-4 murine mammary carcinomas. *Cancer Res* 2001;61:526.
153. Sacco MG, Cato EM, Ceruti R, et al. Systemic gene therapy with anti-angiogenic factors inhibits spontaneous breast tumor growth and metastasis in MMTVneu transgenic mice. *Gene Ther* 2001;8:67.
154. Feldman AL, Restifo NP, Alexander HR, et al. Antiangiogenic gene therapy of cancer utilizing a recombinant adenovirus to elevate systemic endostatin levels in mice. *Cancer Res* 2000;60:1503.
155. Sauter BV, Martinet O, Zhang WJ, et al. Adenovirus-mediated gene transfer of endostatin in vivo results in high level expression and inhibition of tumor growth and metastases. *Proc Natl Acad Sci U S A* 2000;97:4802.
156. Shi W, Teschendorf C, Muzyczka N, Siemann DW. Adeno-associated virus-mediated gene transfer of endostatin inhibits angiogenesis and tumor growth in vivo. *Cancer Gene Ther* 2002;9:513.
157. Wen XY, Bai Y, Stewart AK. Adenovirus-mediated human endostatin gene delivery demonstrates strain-specific antitumor activity and acute dose-dependent toxicity in mice. *Hum Gene Ther* 2001;12:347.
158. Blezinger P, Wang J, Gondo M, et al. Systemic inhibition of tumor growth and tumor metastases by intramuscular administration of the endostatin gene therapy. *Nature Biotechnol* 1999;17:343.

159. Lefesvre P, Attema J, van Bekkum D. Adenoviral gene transfer of angiostatic ATF-BPTI inhibits tumour growth. *BMC Cancer* 2002;2:17.

160. Kuo CJ, Farnebo F, Yu EY, et al. Comparative evaluation of the antitumor activity of anti-angiogenic proteins delivered by gene transfer. *Proc Natl Acad Sci U S A* 2001;98:4605.

161. Slaton JW, Perotte P, Inoue K, et al. Interferon alpha mediated down-regulation of angio-genesis-related genes and therapy of bladder cancer are dependent on optimization of biological dose and schedule. *Clin Cancer Res* 1999;5:2726.

162. Eisterer W, Jiang X, Bachelot T, et al. Unfulfilled promise of endostatin in a gene ther-apy-xenotransplant model of human acute lymphocytic leukemia. *Mol Ther* 2002;5:352.

163. Pawliuk R, Bachelot T, Zurkiya O, et al. Continuous intravascular secretion of endostatin in mice from transduced hematopoietic stem cells. *Mol Ther* 2002;5:345.

164. Bachelot T, Pawliuk R, Treilleux I, et al. Retrovirus-mediated gene transfer of an angio-statin-endostatin fusion protein with enhanced anti-tumor properties in vivo. *Proc Am Assoc Cancer Res* 1998;39:271(abst 1856).

165. Brantley DM, Cheng N, Thompson EJ, et al. Soluble Eph A receptors inhibit tumor angiogenesis and progression in vivo. *Oncogene* 2002;21:7011.

166. Gehling UM, Ergun S, Schumacher U, et al. In vitro differentiation of endothelial cells from AC133-positive progenitor cells. *Blood* 2000;95:3106.

167. Kuo CJ, LaMontagne KR Jr, Garcia-Cardena G, et al. Oligomerization-dependent regula-tion of motility and morphogenesis by the collagen XVIII NC1/endostatin domain. *J Cell Biol* 2001;152:1233.

168. Wang CY, Mayo MW, Baldwin AS Jr. TNF- and cancer therapy-induced apoptosis: potenti-ation by inhibition of NF-kappaB. *Science* 1996;274:784.

169. Beg AA, Baltimore D. An essential role for NF-kappaB in preventing TNF-alpha-induced cell death. *Science* 1996;274:782.

170. Buettner R, Mora LB, Jove R. Activated STAT signaling in human tumors provides novel molecular targets for therapeutic intervention. *Clin Cancer Res* 2002;8:945.

171. Carmeliet P. Biomedicine. Clotting factors build blood vessels. *Science* 2001;293:1602.

172. Tsopanoglou NE, Maragoudakis ME. On the mechanism of thrombin-induced angiogen-esis. Potentiation of vascular endothelial growth factor activity on endothelial cells by up-regulation of its receptors. *J Biol Chem* 1999;274:23969.

173. Zucker S, Mirza H, Conner CE, et al. Vascular endothelial growth factor induces tissue factor and matrix metalloproteinases production in endothelial cells: conversion of pro-thrombin to thrombin results in progelatinase A activation and cell proliferation. *Int J Cancer* 1998;75:780.

174. O'Reilly MS, Pirie-Shepherd S, Lane WS, Folkman J. Antiangiogenic activity of the cleaved conformation of the serpin antithrombin. *Science* 1999;285:1926.

175. Kisker O, Onizuka S, Banyard J, et al. Generation of multiple angiogenesis inhibitors by human pancreatic cancer. *Cancer Res* 2001;61:7298.

176. Sharrocks AD. The ETS-domain transcription factor family. *Nat Rev Mol Cell Biol* 2001;2:827.

177. Chen Z, Fisher RJ, Riggs CW, et al. Inhibition of vascular endothelial growth factor-induced endothelial cell migration by ETS1 antisense oligonucleotides. *Cancer Res* 1997;57:2013.

178. Nakano T, Abe M, Tanaka K, et al. Angiogenesis inhibition by transdominant mutant Ets-1. *J Cell Physiol* 2000;184:255.

179. Oda N, Abe M, Sato Y. ETS-1 converts endothelial cells to the angiogenic phenotype by inducing the expression of matrix metalloproteinases and integrin beta 3. *J Cell Physiol* 1999;178:121.

180. Iwasaka C, Tanaka K, Abe M, Sato Y. Ets-1 regulates angiogenesis by inducing the expres-sion of urokinase-type plasminogen activator and matrix metalloproteinases-1 and the migration of vascular endothelial cells. *J Cell Physiol* 1996;269:522.

181. Daly ME, Makris A, Reed M, et al. Hemostatic regulators of tumor angiogenesis: a source of antiangiogenic agents for cancer treatment? *J Natl Cancer Inst* 2003;95:1660.

182. Hurwitz H, Fehrenbacher L, Cartwright T, et al. Bevacizumab (a monoclonal antibody to vascular endothelial growth factor) prolongs survival in first-line colorectal cancer (CRC): results of a phase III trial of bevacizumab in combination with bolus IFL (irinote-can, 5-fluorouracil, leucovorin) as first-line therapy in subjects with metastatic CRC. *Proc Am Soc Clin Oncol* 2003;(abst 3646).

183. Kaban LB, Mulliken JB, Ezekowitz RA, et al. Antiangiogenic therapy of a recurrent giant cell tumor of the mandible with interferon alfa-2a. *Pediatrics* 1999;103:1145.

184. Marler JJ, Rubin JB, Trede NS, et al. Successful antiangiogenic therapy of giant cell angio-blastoma with interferon alfa 2b: report of 2 cases. *Pediatrics* 2002;109:E37.

185. Kaban LB, Troulis MJ, Ebb D, et al. Antiangiogenic therapy with interferon alpha for giant cell lesions of the jaws. *J Oral Maxillofac Surg* 2002;60:1103.

186. Folkman J. Discussion. Antiangiogenic therapy with interferon alpha for giant cell lesions of the jaws. *J Oral Maxillofac Surg* 2002;60:1111.

187. Ng SS, Brown M, Figg WD. Thalidomide, an antiangiogenic agent with clinical activity in cancer. *Biomed Pharmacother* 2002;56:194.

188. Davidoff AM, Leary MA, Ng CY, et al. Autocrine expression of both endostatin and green fluorescent protein provides a synergistic antitumor effect in a murine neuroblastoma model. *Cancer Gene Ther* 2001;8:537.

189. te Velde EA, Vogten JM, Gebbink MF, et al. Enhanced antitumour efficacy by combining conventional chemotherapy with angiostatin or endostatin in a liver metastasis model. *Br J Surg* 2002;89:1302.

190. Sorensen DR, Leirdal M, Iversen PO, et al. Combination of endostatin and a protein kinase Calpha DNA enzyme improves the survival of rats with malignant glioma. *Neoplasia* 2002;4:474.

191. Folkman J. Angiogenesis in breast cancer. In: Bland KI, Copeland EM III, eds. *The breast: comprehensive management of benign and malignant disorders*, vol. 1, 3rd ed. St. Louis: WB Saunders, 2004:563.

192. *A critical review of endostatin and its biology*. Endostatin Banbury Conference. Cold Spring Harbor Laboratories, NY, March 10–13, 2002.

193. Bielenberg DR, Hida Y, Shimizu A, et al. Semaphorin 3F, a chemorepulsant for endothe-lial cells, induces a poorly vascularized, encapsulated, non-metastatic tumor phenotype. *J Clin Invest* 2004; (*in press*).

194. Browder T, Folkman J, Hahnfeldt P, et al. Antiangiogenic therapy and p53. *Science* 2002;297:471a.

195. Kieran MW, Folkman J, Heymach J. Angiogenesis inhibitors and hypoxia. *Nat Med* 2003;9:1104.

Ferenc A. Jolesz
Kullervo H. Hynynen

CHAPTER **64**

Focused Ultrasound

Even though the primary application of ultrasound in medicine is in diagnostic imaging, therapeutic use of acoustic energy has been routinely practiced in the treatment of cancer since the 1930s. Indeed, it was recognized several decades ago that converging, high-intensity, focused ultrasound (FUS) beams can be applied as a "surgical" technique to treat neoplastic tissue, particularly deeply embedded soft tissue tumors. In FUS surgery, the localized high temperature induces cell damage due to protein denaturation and capillary bed destruction, causing subsequent coagulation necrosis that occurs without injuring the surrounding normal tissue.

Despite this obvious benefit, widespread acceptance of FUS as a noninvasive thermal ablation method did not take place until magnetic resonance imaging (MRI) was developed. MRI, a noninvasive imaging system that provides accurate targeting of focused sound waves by detecting tumor margins with high sensitivity and by depicting the surrounding anatomy in exquisite detail, can also monitor temperature distribution in real time, effectively generating "temperature maps" of the targeted surgical field during treatment. These powerful imaging features, in turn, enable the FUS delivery of thermal energy at doses that are both safe and therapeutically effective. As numerous studies suggest, the integration of MRI and FUS creates an imaging environment in which a *real-time*, image-controlled, noninvasive soft tissue coagulation system is feasible and from which a wide range of clinical applications in cancer therapy may ultimately benefit.

FUNDAMENTAL PRINCIPLES OF FOCUSED ULTRASOUND SURGERY

Sound waves are defined as pressure waves that propagate by cyclic compression and decompression of the substance (the media) through which sound waves pass. When an ultrasound wave propagates through media, various interactions occur such as interference, diffraction, reflection, absorption, and scattering, the extent of which depends on the frequency of ultrasound, the velocity of ultrasound, the number of scattering sites (tissue interfaces), and tissue density. All of these factors, taken separately or in combination, may contribute to the attenuation of the pressure waves.

FUS systems direct concentrated ultrasonic pressure waves that travel through the body to a designated depth without depositing a substantial amount of energy along the beam path. At the focal point, the acoustic energy is then converted to thermal energy resulting in local tissue heating. Because the ultrasound beam is transmitted from a transducer that is several centimeters in diameter, the ultrasound intensity at the millimeter-sized focal spot can be several hundred times greater than in the overlying tissues. Similarly, the ultrasound exposure drops off rapidly across the focus, thus limiting the high ultrasound exposure to the focal volume. As a result, the induced temperature field is also tightly focused. Although this point of convergence is predictable in homogeneous media, the exact location of the focal spot and the associated heat distribution are less unpredictable in the presence of tissue boundaries with acoustic interfaces. MRI, therefore, is essential in targeting and monitoring FUS to provide feedback of the actual effects *in vivo*.

Using the concave, geometric shape of a single piezoelectric transducer, pressure waves can be directed to a tightly focused point (approximately 1 to 10 mm in diameter) within the body. Similar focusing can be achieved with phased arrays driven by electric signals phased to obtain a common focal point—that is, on-line control of the ultrasound wave front. Phased arrays have several attractive characteristics that are particularly desirable for image-controlled FUS: (1) the ability to focus at variable depths; (2) the ability to control focal size during a treatment requiring multiple sonications; (3) the ability to modify the driving signals, effectively compensating for the effects of overlying tissues on the focal location; and (4) the ability to electrically move the focal spot (beam steering) *without* physically moving the transducer. Large tissue volumes can thus be exposed with optimized, energy-deposition patterns.

INTERACTION BETWEEN TISSUE AND THE ULTRASOUND BEAM

In hyperthermia, selective tumor killing is achieved by uniform temperature distribution at a narrow therapeutic range (42° to 46°C) that is maintained for approximately an hour within a relatively large volume. In FUS, the temperature in the focal zone is raised above 56°C and is held for a few seconds until coagulation is achieved. Because thermal ablation above this critical level is not selective, FUS is more comparable to surgery than to hyperthermia. If temperature exceeds 60°C for 1 second or more, the heated tissue undergoes irreversible thermal coagulation necrosis. In adjacent tissue volumes, where only a limited temperature rise has occurred, normal conduction and perfusion quickly cool the tissue after the application of the energy, leaving no residual effect.

The rapid deposition of thermal energy for tumor treatment is especially important because of unpredictable tumor vascularity. That is, sharp focusing and rapid energy deposition lead to a relatively narrow temperature gradient and a peak temperature rise of between 60° to 80°C that is independent on cooling by blood flow. Longer exposure times on the order of minutes, on the other hand, increase heat transfer via blood flow and perfusion. In other words, *the more shallow the temperature gradients, the more variable the thermal effects.* Based on theoretical models in *in vivo* animal experiments and in ongoing patient studies, exposures of approximately 10 to 12 seconds and less can reduce the irregular variations caused by heterogeneous tissue vascularity.[1]

During FUS sonications, energy concentration gain factors of several hundred can be achieved in the focal spot versus energy deposited in tissue along the beam path. After this relatively brief FUS treatment at the focal spot, the thermal damage zones are condensed with sharp demarcation between live and dead cells at the edges.[2] From the hotter center to the cooler periphery, the thermal damage zones include denatured structural proteins and denatured or inactivated enzymes. Evidence of thermal damage, moreover, can be detected in surrounding tissues just peripheral to the central coagulation zone. Thermal damage typically includes a complex series of physiologic vascular responses that produce hemostasis, hemorrhage, and hyperthermia. Other heat-related changes are due to the release of lytic enzymes from ruptured cells, the discharge of proteases and lipases from reactive inflammatory cells, and ischemia related to occlusive intravascular thrombosis in thermally damaged blood vessels. Heat can also trigger apoptosis, a series of events leading to cellular and nuclear fragmentation in specifically genetically programmed cells.[3]

High-intensity FUS beams can also be distorted into shock waves at the focus. When pressure amplitudes are increased, another mechanism of ultrasound tissue interaction—cavitation—results. *Cavitation* refers to the collapse (implosion) of rapidly developed gas microbubbles at the focal zone due to extremely intense ultrasound excitation. If the pressure amplitude is great enough, the bubbles expand to their resonant size and then implode. This collapse has the potential to microscopically generate high pressures, propagating shock waves, and high temperatures. This action may also contribute to the direct mechanical effects of tissue. This mechanism has the potential to influence cell membrane and blood–brain barrier (BBB) permeability, can activate chemicals, and may offer new therapeutic options for targeted drug delivery and gene therapy.[4–6]

MAGNETIC RESONANCE IMAGING GUIDANCE FOR THERMAL ABLATIONS

Tumor ablation, when executed at high temperatures, constitutes a minimally invasive alternative to surgery and radiation therapy, but it requires accurate targeting and *real-time* control of energy deposition. Although thermal ablations have been performed under image guidance by ultrasound, computed tomography, and x-ray, MRI offers the most sensitive tumor localization and, at the same time, provides three-dimensional control of energy deposition and detection of thermally induced tissue changes. The integration of MRI with thermal ablation provides "closed-loop" feedback as a means of planning, targeting, guiding, monitoring, and most importantly, controlling therapy. MRI-based monitoring, moreover, has been shown to enhance the effectiveness of thermal ablations such as those performed by laser, radiofrequency, microwave, and cryosurgery.[7] Real-time temperature-sensitive imaging can measure temperature elevations over time to enable the calculation of the total thermal dose delivered to the target tissue. At the same time, it can prevent unwanted heating of surrounding normal tissue. Indeed, MRI not only defines tumor margins and temperature distributions, it can depict critical anatomic structures such as nerves and blood vessels—features that clearly enhance safety and effectiveness.

Temperature-sensitive MRI sequences can also be used to detect temperature elevations at levels that do not induce any histologic or physiologic tissue damage.[8] Thus, the location of the focus can be detected at powers sufficiently low to verify accurate targeting without any tissue damage. Several MRI parameters are temperature-sensitive enough to detect temperature changes in the range of 2° to 3°C above body temperature and identify energy deposition *before* irreversible tissue damage is induced. Temperature-sensitive MRI sequences, especially those based on water proton frequency shift, are useful in ensuring that the target volume is adequately treated and the critical temperature that guarantees cell death (higher than 56°C) is achieved.[9] Moreover, the tissue injury induced by the thermal exposure can also be detected immediately after treatment by multiparametric MR images and by an intravenous contrast agent that may demonstrate decreased or absent enhancement due to the occlusion of the microvasculature.[10]

Temperature sensitivity and high sensitivity to tissue integrity make MRI an ideal imaging modality to accurately target, monitor, and control FUS. MRI-based *quantitative imaging*, moreover, can be used to optimize and control energy delivery during thermal ablations. The feasibility of MRI-derived dosimetry for predicting the size of lesions produced during FUS therapy has been demonstrated.[11] Closed-loop control, however, requires the complete integration of the imaging and the therapy delivery systems.

MAGNETIC RESONANCE IMAGING–GUIDED FOCUSED ULTRASOUND THERAPY DELIVERY SYSTEMS

The successful implementation of MRI guidance for the control of several thermal ablation methods[7] has resulted in the integration of MRI with FUS.[12,13] After promising, early studies that showed the feasibility of MRI-guided FUS, General Electric Medical Systems, in collaboration with the MRI division of the Brigham and Women's Hospital, manufactured the first prototype clinical MR-guided ultrasound for breast tumor FUS in 1994. In this initial application, the ultrasound fields were generated by a single, focused transducer mounted on a standard MRI table. A computer-controlled positioning device activated transducer movement.[14] A functionally similar device for breast cancer treatments (with a different mechanical transducer positioning system) was subsequently developed by Siemens.[15] InSightec Ltd. (Tirat Carmel, Israel), in collaboration with the Brigham and Women's MRI division, designed and implemented the first MRI-monitored and *MRI-controlled* FUS system. In this system, real-time MRI thermometry has been used to control treatment parameters to achieve the desired outcome. A second-generation system has incorporated phased-array technology for electronic focusing, tissue aberration correction, and steering. Specifically, a FUS phased-array transducer with more than 200 elements and a 120-mm diameter transducer has been developed and is in current use. The integration of the treatment system with the MR scanner enables coordination of both energy delivery and treatment monitoring in a single system (Fig. 64-1).

The first commercial MRI-guided FUS system (InSightec's ExAblate 2000) achieves target definition (localization) in three dimensions and is now used commercially and in clinical research for various tumor treatments at multiple sites. Monitoring is also accomplished with a near real-time, temperature-sensitive MRI sequence. Rapid image acquisition throughout the sonications ensures temporal resolution matched to the time constant of thermal effects. The thermometry data are used by the physician to control treatment parameters to achieve the desired results. Such control is based on the quantification of temperature elevation and on the deposited thermal dose.

Once the patient is positioned on the MRI table, the physician acquires a set of MR images, identifies the target volume of tissue to be treated, and draws the treatment contours.

During the treatment, a series of small, bean-shaped volumes of FUS energy (approximately 20 mm × 8 mm) is directed into the target for less than 20 seconds, heating the tissue to between 65° and 85°C to induce thermal coagulation. MR images taken continuously during the sonications provide both diagnostic and quantitative quality images of the target tissue; a real-time temperature map overlays to confirm the therapeutic effect of the treatment. The thermal map is then used to monitor the treatment in progress and confirm that the ablation is going according to plan, thus closing the therapy loop.

The physician uses the MR system to identify the appropriate target volume in three dimensions. Therapy planning software (using a real-time three-dimensional ultrasound simulator) calculates the number, size, and placement of sonications needed to cover the entire treatment volume. After approval of the treatment plan, the user performs a series of verification sonications. A first geometric verification is performed using very low energy, sonications, generating a relatively small temperature rise in the tissue that is *below* the threshold of ablation. The location of the focal point is detected by the temperature-sensitive MRI phase sequence, and its position relative to the planned target point is verified. Any errors in the mechanical alignment of the system or variations in the location of the focal spot can be corrected by the user at this point (Fig. 64-2). The second phase of monitoring and controlling treatment entails verifying the energy required to deliver a therapeutic dose. In this step, a sonication at the full dose level is delivered, and it is monitored by MRI phase shift–based, temperature-sensitive imaging. The ExAblate 2000 system allows the user to compare the actual thermal dose with that predicted and make adjustments where necessary.

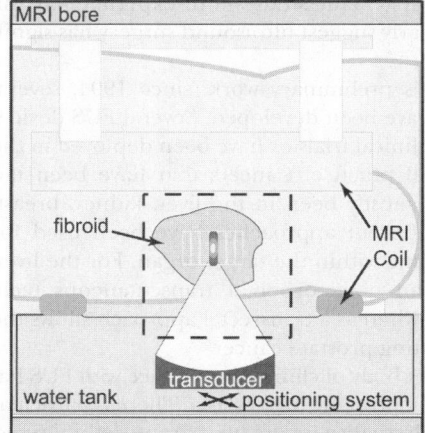
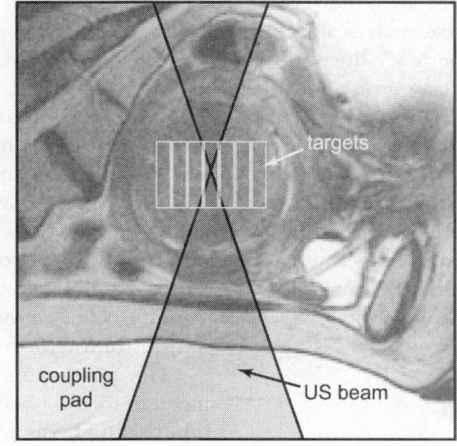
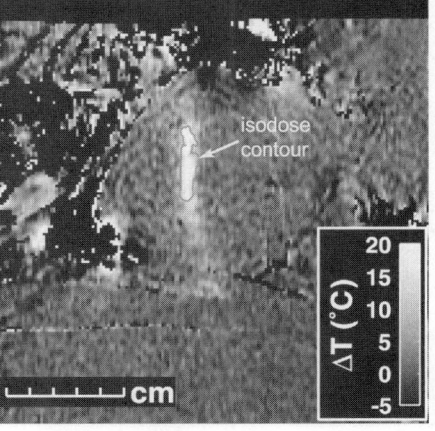

A–C

FIGURE 64-1. **A:** A diagram of the magnetic resonance imaging (MRI)–guided ultrasound (US) system. **B:** A focused US beam outline over a T2-weighted image for treatment planning purposes. **C:** A temperature-sensitive image showing the focal temperature elevation in a fibroid. (See Color Fig. 64-1 in the CD-ROM.)

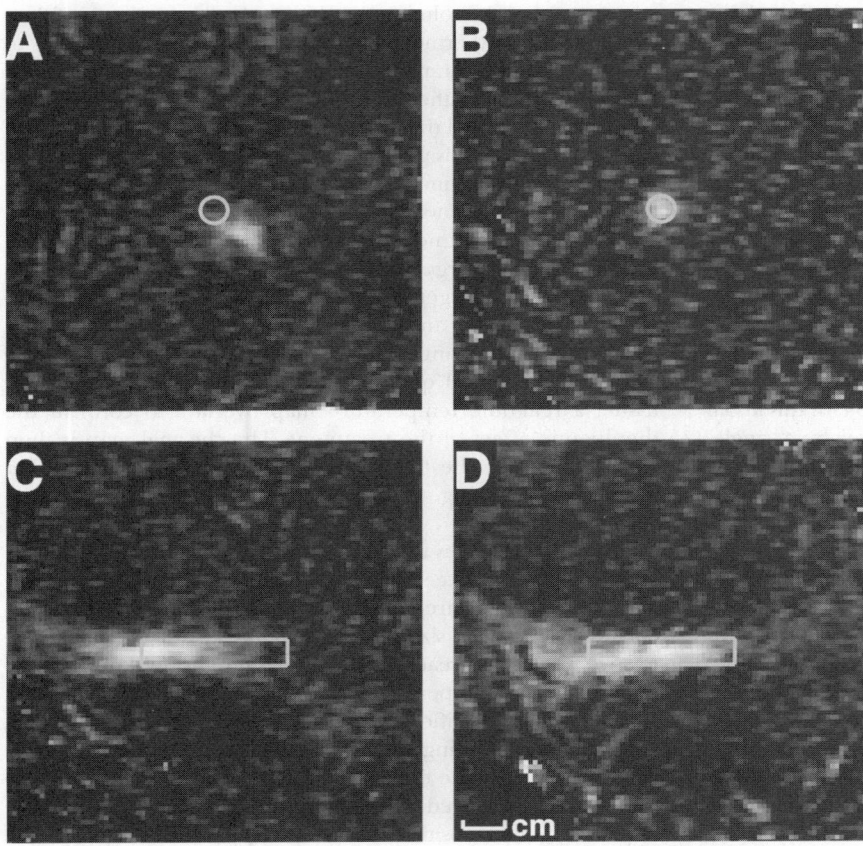

FIGURE 64-2. Magnetic resonance imaging–derived temperature images of four sonications used to verify the focal coordinate during a focused ultrasound treatment of a uterine fibroid. The image in **A** shows the initial low-power sonication. The heating is located a few millimeters away from the target (indicated by a *circle*). The user indicates the location of the heating with the mouse pointer, and when the sonication is repeated, the heating is at the correct location (**B**). The coronal images in **A** and **B** were perpendicular to the direction of the ultrasound beam. This procedure is then repeated to verify that the focus is targeted at the correct depth (**C,D**) by monitoring the temperature rise along the direction of the ultrasound beam. (See Color Fig. 64-2 in the CD-ROM.)

During the treatment process, points are treated in a sequential manner: Once a single point is treated, the transducer focal point and scan plane are moved to an adjacent location and the process repeated until the entire targeted volume is covered. A variable number of adjacent focal spots can be combined to cover a three-dimensional therapy volume of an arbitrary shape (Fig. 64-3). Treatment volumes of up to 4 cm in diameter can be treated in a single 90-minute session. Discrete areas in the tumor are consecutively treated at operator-controlled time intervals to prevent significant heat accumulation in surrounding tissue. Because the beam is focused on the treatment area, there is no significant heating effect on pain-sensitive areas such as adjacent normal tissue or skin. If the patient does experience discomfort, treatment parameters can be modified or intravenous analgesia can be applied.

After the final sonication, the physician can evaluate the accumulated dose map. At that point, the user may decide to add additional points to complete the layer or to end the treatment. After the treatment is completed, the volume ablated is verified by an appropriate, contrast-enhanced MRI scan. However, because the treatment has ablated the tissue and coagulated the small blood vessels in the target volume, the treated volume does not enhance.

CLINICAL APPLICATIONS

HISTORY

The use of ultrasound in cancer treatments began in the 1930s and since has continued. The first proposed use of FUS beams to induce noninvasive deep tissue destruction was proposed by Lynn et al.[16] This technique was subsequently developed by the Fry brothers, who used FUS to destroy small tissue volumes in the central nervous system in animals and in humans.[17] Burov[18] used high-intensity pulsed ultrasound and produced resorption of rabbit carcinomas as well as resorption of human malignant melanomas. This high-intensity approach was subsequently tested in the treatment of human breast[19] and in brain tumors.[19] Although the tumor responses achieved were promising, the phase I clinical feasibility studies described earlier were not conclusive. However, systematic studies with experimental animal tumor models clearly suggest ultrasound surgery has significant potential.[20]

Encouraged by this preliminary work, since 1994, several commercial systems have been developed. Several FUS devices are in current use in clinical trials or have been deployed in the early stages of clinical practice. Cancers that have been targeted with FUS have mostly been in the liver, kidney, breast, and prostate. Two different approaches have been used for placing the focal volume within the target organ. For the liver, kidney, and breast, an extracorporeal transcutaneous technique has been used, whereas a transrectal approach shows the most promise for treating prostate cancer.

The most significant body of clinical experience with FUS has been in treating benign prostatic hyperplasia. There is particular interest in FUS as an alternative treatment to transurethral resection of the prostate for debulking enlarged prostates[21] and for the treatment of prostate and bladder carcinomas.[22] Although thermal ablation of the gland with a transrectal approach has been demonstrated, the clinical results have been disappointing

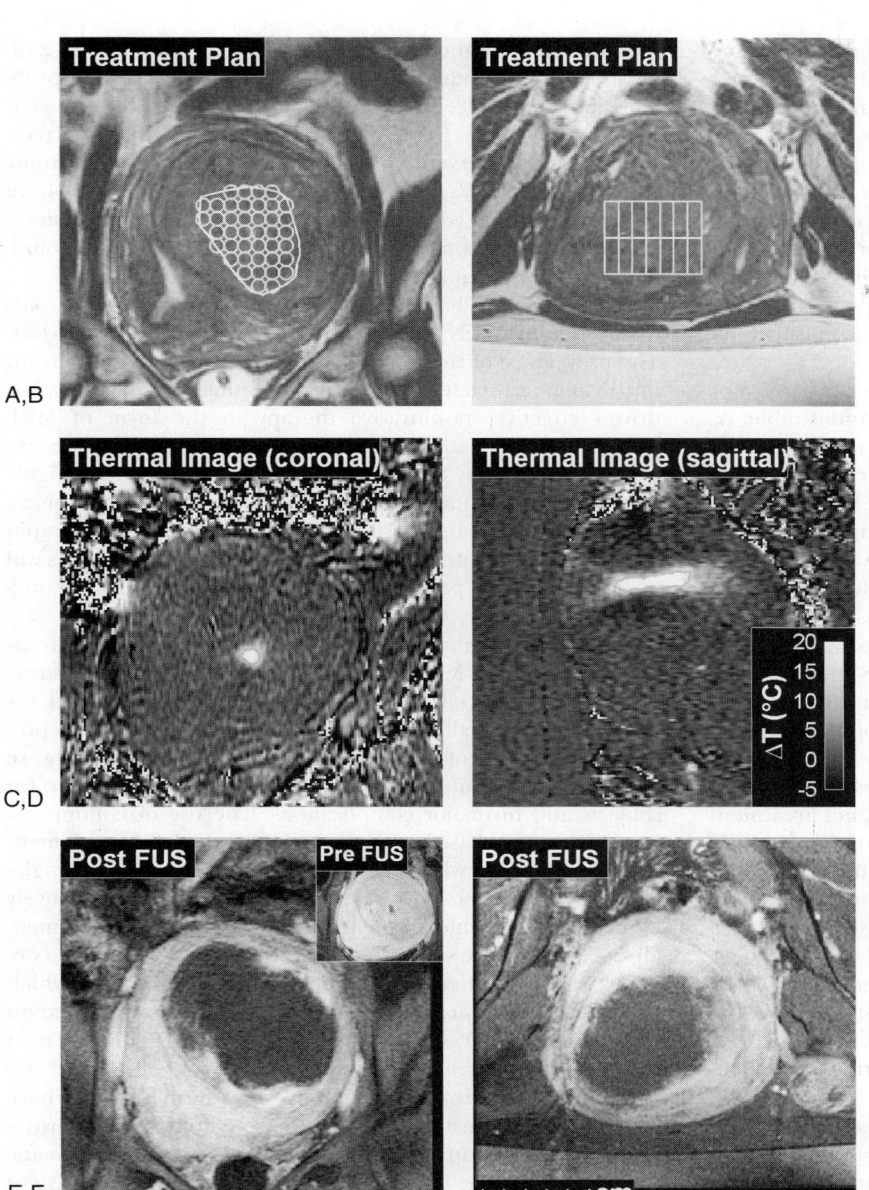

FIGURE 64-3. Magnetic resonance images acquired before, during, and after focused ultrasound (FUS) surgery in a uterine fibroid. **A,B:** T2-weighted images used for treatment planning. The individual target locations are shown. **C,D:** Temperature maps acquired during two sonications. The contours indicate the regions that reached a thermal dose of at least 240 equivalent minutes at 43°C and were used to guide the treatment. **E,F:** Contrast-enhanced T1-weighted images acquired immediately after the treatment. The coronal images on the left were perpendicular to the direction of the US beam. The axial and sagittal images on the right were acquired along the beam direction. The image in the inset in **E** shows a contrast-enhanced T1-weighted image acquired several days before the treatment. (See Color Fig. 64-3 in the CD-ROM.)

and have not matched those of the "gold standard" transurethral resection of the prostate procedure. The reason for this is not clear but most likely due to the lack of appropriate image guidance, monitoring, and control. Several clinical trials using the single-focus system for prostate cancer have used two different devices manufactured by Focus Surgery (Sonablate, Indianapolis)[23] and EDAP (Ablatherm, Lyon, France).[24] Both devices use a spherically curved transducer that combines both ultrasound imaging and therapy capability. The transducer is positioned in the rectum to allow sonications of the prostate tissue through the rectal wall. The imaging capability of this system is used to map the prostate and to guide the therapy beam, but it does not aid in temperature-sensitive imaging or in making thermal dose calculations.

FUS probes have been developed for the ablation of liver.[25,26] FUS can also be used experimentally for hemostasis and for occluding blood vessels.[27,28] Because FUS not only occludes capillaries but also larger arteries and veins, it can effectively interrupt blood flow to a tumor and may serve as an adjuvant to chemotherapy or radiation therapy.

MAGNETIC RESONANCE IMAGING–GUIDED FOCUSED ULTRASOUND SURGERY CLINICAL TRIALS

The first clinical application of FUS centered on the treatment of fibroadenomas of the breast.[29] Fibroadenomas are well-circumscribed benign tumors easily distinguishable from adjacent normal breast tissue on MR images with and without contrast enhancement. The breast is ideally suited to FUS because of its relatively external position and the ease with which it can be immobilized. Targeting is straightforward, and thermal therapy is well monitored by MRI. The initial phase I trial established the feasibility and safety of FUS; most important, the treatment was well tolerated by patients. The majority of fibroadenomas were successfully treated with the prototype single element transducer with a series of overlapping lesions. Follow-up MRI showed complete or partial lack of contrast uptake, indicating tumor devascularization and necrosis by thermal coagulation.[29]

Fibroadenoma represents a well-defined and a clinically meaningful target for MRI-guided FUS, and as a logical next step, this novel treatment approach has been applied to breast malignancies. Although MRI has poor specificity as a diagnostic tool for breast cancer, it has very high sensitivity in detecting tumor margins. Because the tumor has been histologically identified before treatment, the lack of specificity is irrelevant. MRI's high sensitivity, on the other hand, is especially helpful in correctly targeting breast cancers, where the sensitivity of MRI is as high as 90% to 98%.[30]

Although conventional surgical lumpectomy is not a major procedure, it is still invasive and cosmetically undesirable. As an incisionless, scarless, noninvasive, ablative tumor debulking method, FUS may have a great appeal for patients who want to preserve the integrity of the breast. Moreover, the tumor definition using MRI is superior to using direct surgical visualization or any other imaging modality. Clearly, MRI-guided FUS has the potential to serve as a safe, noninvasive debulking procedure for the treatment of breast cancer.

In a phase I clinical trial, 15 patients with invasive breast carcinomas were treated with MRI-guided FUS before their planned surgical resection. The effectiveness of the treatment was determined by histopathologic analysis of the resected mass quantifying the volumes of necrosed and residual tumor.[31] Although there was substantial *undertreatment* with the prototype single-element transducer, much higher treatment efficiency was achieved in subsequent sonications with the closed-loop, temperature-controlled, multielement, phased-array transducer because of its ability to monitor the temperature and dose. Because breast tumors can be close to the skin, a skin cooling system was added. With these added capabilities, the pathology findings showed that on average, 98% of the tumor volume was effectively targeted and nearly 95% of the targeted breast cancer was necrosed.

In early cases, residual tumor was identified predominantly at the periphery of the tumor mass, indicating the need to increase the total targeted area with a corresponding increase in sonications. In a second series, patients with a single biopsy-proven breast carcinoma who either were considered at increased surgical risk or who had refused surgery underwent MRI-guided FUS as an adjunct to therapy with tamoxifen.[32] Percutaneous biopsy was performed after 6-month follow-up, and if residual tumor was present, a second MRI-guided FUS treatment session was performed, followed by repeat biopsy. In each of these cases, lack of contrast enhancement was used as an indicator of tumor destruction. Residual enhancement suggested untreated tumor deposits. Nineteen of 24 patients had negative biopsy results after one or two treatment sessions.

These results clearly demonstrate MRI-guided FUS as a precise, noninvasive method of targeting and treating breast carcinomas. Indeed, as technology advances and more treatment experience is acquired, even more compelling outcomes are expected. Whether MRI-guided FUS can replace open surgery in some breast cancer patients or will be used as palliative or adjuvant local therapy modality remains an open question, however.

So far the most successful application of MRI-guided FUS is the treatment of uterine leiomyoma (fibroid), the most common neoplasm of the female pelvis. They occur in 20% to 25% of women of reproductive age and can cause a variety of problems, including bleeding, pelvic pain, infertility, compression symptoms, urinary frequency, and bowel obstruction. Traditional surgical interventions typically entail either hysterectomy or myomectomy. Various minimally invasive alternatives have also been introduced, including endometrial ablation, hysteroscopic or laparoscopic myomectomy, uterine artery embolization, and thermal ablation with laser or radiofrequency.

FUS treatment has the potential to ablate uterine fibroids totally noninvasively while preserving fertility (see Fig. 64-3). The prevalence of these tumors, combined with the significant impairment associated with current treatment alternatives, has driven effective, noninvasive therapy in the form of MRI-guided FUS. Indeed, the advantages of MRI-guided FUS are clear: Not only has thermal mapping proven safe and highly accurate, but this mode of treatment is also performed on an outpatient basis, and with fewer complications, and rapid recoveries, the treatment of these common, benign tumors will no longer pose a painful and debilitating condition for millions of women.

The already completed feasibility multicenter clinical trials demonstrates that MRI-guided FUS provides targeted destruction with an excellent safety profile.[10,33] Initially, patients underwent planned hysterectomy after treatment, which provided pathologic correlation of treatment. All treatments were conducted in an outpatient setting with minimal discomfort for subjects and no major complications. The use of continuous-wave ultrasonic phased-array technology reduced the treatment time significantly when compared with the previous, single-element transducer. This has made the treatment of relatively large fibroids possible. In the phase II safety study of 55 women, all except one were successfully treated as outpatients with conscious sedation. There were no injuries to other organs, which would suggest improper targeting, and no postembolization syndrome. Only 10% of the patients took over-the-counter pain medications posttreatment.

To date, more than 500 patients with uterine fibroids have been treated. Almost 90% have reported symptomatic improvement after 3 months, and 95% have reported symptomatic improvement after 6 months—empiric evidence consistent with the posttreatment shrinkage of the tumor verified with follow-up MRIs. Although these fibroids were partially treated, there is a direct relationship between treatment volume and shrinkage as well as between volume reduction and symptomatic relief. Improvements in treatment methods may further improve future results.

Current, although still limited, clinical applications of MRI-guided FUS have enabled physicians, moreover, to demonstrate long-range potential to impact a broad spectrum of benign and malignant soft tissue tumors. MRI-guided FUS's promise for cancer treatment is clear, and indeed, may ultimately replace open surgeries such as lumpectomy, especially when tumor margins are barely visible to the surgeon's eye or absent altogether (but are generally more evident on MRI). Obviously, MRI targeting can be further improved if the procedure is performed at higher-field strength and tumor-seeking contrast agents are applied. Improved thermal mapping and dosimetry can also result in better treatment efficiency within the targeted tissue volumes. FUS is clearly superior to other methods of thermal ablation because of the absence of invasive probes and the lack of wide thermal gradients during energy deposition. Only FUS can guarantee homogenous treatment effects in heterogeneous tissues and the full coverage of tumors with complex shapes and configurations. Nevertheless, MRI-guided FUS is essentially a debulking method, and, like surgery, it should be part of a comprehensive treatment strategy.

FUTURE APPLICATIONS

The noninvasive nature of FUS has special appeal in the brain, where the ability to treat or destroy deep tissue volumes without injuring the overlying tissues is essential. However, substantial absorption by the bony skull is a daunting problem. The bone has a very high absorption and acoustic impedance compared with soft tissues. These features not only create unwanted thermal effects near the skull, but also interfere with the planned energy distribution at the targeted deep tissue. Nevertheless, numerous studies have shown that the brain can be effectively ablated through bone, especially at lower ultrasound frequencies. Large, hemispherical phased arrays can be constructed that deliver adequate energy through human skull sample to coagulate brain tissue *in vivo* without excessive temperature elevation on the skull surface.[34] To optimize the treatment, acoustic aberrations of the ultrasonic beam caused by the uneven thickness of the skull must be overcome. The correction is accomplished automatically by planning software based on a set of previously acquired computed tomographic images.[35] The computed tomography–corrected sonications were tested in animal brains *in vivo*, effectively producing focal coagulation without overheating the skull, thereby demonstrating the basic feasibility of performing transskull ultrasound focusing and treatments. This system, the ExAblate 3000 (InSightec, Ltd.), will be ready in 2005 for conducting experiments on large animals and for clinical tests on brain tumor coagulation. This same system is planned for other applications such as the targeted BBB opening.

In addition to coagulating brain tissue, the sharply demarcated FUS lesions reveal leakage of large molecules through the BBB. This method, however, should not be used to open the BBB because damage to brain tissue may occur and is unpredictable. FUS energy delivered above the cavitation threshold can also induce focal BBB opening without causing thermal effects or damaging neurons in the sonicated area.[4] There are several challenges in using ultrasound exposures to open the BBB: Chief among these is ensuring that targeted energy delivery is localized only to the capillary walls without damaging the adjacent neural elements. The BBB can be reproducibly opened by localizing the cavitation-generated mechanical stresses to the blood vessel walls by injecting preformed gas bubbles (routinely used as ultrasound imaging contrast agents) into the blood stream just before the sonications.[4] Because the bubbles are intravascular, any adverse effects to the adjoining brain tissue should be minimal. The opening is reversible, and the power levels used are orders of magnitude lower than that required for generating thermal effects and tissue ablation. Because this technique allows the procedure to be performed in a clinical MRI scanner, the images can be used on-line to aim and monitor the ultrasound exposures. Thus, MRI-guided FUS can target an image-specified tissue volume anywhere in the brain—a feature very desirable for both molecular targeting and molecular imaging of the brain. This controlled opening of the BBB at a desired location would permit novel, noninvasive methods of treating brain tumors. Specifically, it would provide targeted access for chemotherapy and gene therapy and allow the use of large, molecular-sized peptides, neuroactive proteins, and various antibodies. It could even provide a vascular route for implanting cells in the brain.[36]

Preformed microbubbles can also be used for targeted drug delivery and gene therapy elsewhere in the body. FUS-induced collapse of gas-filled microspheres produces powerful microstreaming that can enable the diffusion of drugs through otherwise impenetrable cell membranes. Low-intensity FUS-induced increase of cell permeability can be used to increase drug uptake into cells and improve gene transfection. It may prove, moreover, a potential method for targeted drug delivery, nontoxic chemotherapy, and safe, nonviral gene therapy; ultimately it may offer additional new therapeutic options.[6]

CONCLUSION

There is an ongoing effort to explore novel therapies that treat the tumor without causing harm to normal tissues. Image-controlled thermal ablations may provide just such a therapy. Among methods of thermal ablations, noninvasive FUS has demonstrated the most potential. Introducing and integrating the temperature-sensitive MRI-guidance into the targeting and energy delivery process have effectively revived this relatively old ablation method.[37] Indeed, successful clinical trials suggest MR-guided FUS may eventually replace invasive surgeries and ionizing radiation–based radiotherapies.

MR-guided FUS surgery has several key advantages:

- Real-time MR thermal imaging provides real-time feedback and treatment verification; in effect, it is used in a "closed loop" to control the deposited dose and confirm treatment coverage.
- A nondestructive "test" pulse can be used to confirm targeting.
- Spatial control is precise, predictable, and reproducible.
- There is an ability to treat tumors of arbitrary shapes within the body.
- The energy source is nonincisional; therefore, there is no destructive entry track.
- The method results in nonhemorrhagic, sharply demarcated lesions.
- The treatment effects are instantaneous and localized, and systemic side effects are minimal.
- There is no cumulative dose, and the treatments are repeatable multiple times (as opposed to radiosurgery).

MRI-guided FUS unquestionably has a future not only in cancer treatment, but also in several other areas of medicine. Vascular occlusion, targeted drug delivery, and gene therapy are extremely exciting potential applications. Further technology developments will definitely improve both energy delivery and image-based control. Initial clinical trials strongly suggest FUS may offer a viable alternative to conventional surgery and radiation therapy. Its efficacy and safety have been demonstrated in a variety of animal models and in preliminary clinical studies in neoplasms (breast cancer) and benign tumors (uterine fibroids and fibroadenoma). These studies have established, moreover, that the FUS treatment has a low incidence of side effects and is a low-risk procedure for patients.

REFERENCES

1. Billard BE, Hynynen K, Roemer RB. Effects of physical parameters on high temperature ultrasound hyperthermia. *Ultrasound Med Biol* 1990;16:409.
2. Fry WJ, Barnard JW, Fry FJ, Krumins RF, Brennan JF. Ultrasonic lesions in the mammalian central nervous system. *Science* 1955;122:517.
3. Vykhodtseva N, McDannold N, Martin H, et al. Apoptosis in ultrasound-produced threshold lesions in the rabbit brain. *Ultrasound Med Biol* 2001;27:111.
4. Hynynen K, McDannold N, Vykhodtseva N, et al. Noninvasive MR imaging-guided focal opening of the blood-brain barrier in rabbits. *Radiology* 2001;220:640.
5. Umemura SI, Kawabata KI, Sasaki K. In vitro and in vivo enhancement of sonodynamically active cavitation by second-harmonic superimposition. *J Acoust Soc Am* 1997;101:569.
6. Unger EC, Matsunaga TO, McCreery T, et al. Therapeutic applications of microbubbles. *Eur J Radiol* 2002;42:160.
7. McDannold, NJ, Jolesz, FA. Magnetic resonance image-guided thermal ablations. *Top Magn Reson Imaging* 2000;11:191.
8. Hynynen K, Vykhodtseva NI, Chung A, et al. Thermal effects of focused ultrasound on the brain: determination with MR Imaging. *Radiology* 1997;204:247.
9. Landry J, Marceau N. Rate-limiting events in hyperthermic cell killing. *Radiat Res* 1978;75:573.
10. Tempany CM, Stewart EA, McDannold N, et al. MR imaging-guided focused ultrasound surgery of uterine leiomyomas: a feasibility study. *Radiology* 2003;226:897.
11. Chung A, Jolesz FA, Hynynen K. Thermal dosimetry of a focused ultrasound beam in vivo by MRI. *Med Phys* 1999;26:2017.
12. Jolesz FA, Jakab PD. Acoustic pressure wave generation within an MR imaging system: potential medical applications. *J Magn Reson Imaging* 1991;1:609.
13. Cline HE, Schenck JF, Hynynen K, et al. MR-guided focused ultrasound surgery. *J Comput Assist Tomogr* 1992;16:956.
14. Hynynen K, Freund W, Cline HE, et al. A clinical noninvasive MRI monitored ultrasound surgery method. *Radiographics* 1996;16:185.
15. Huber PE, Jenne JW, Rastert R, et al. A new noninvasive approach in breast cancer therapy using magnetic resonance imaging-guided focused ultrasound surgery. *Cancer Res* 2001;61:8441.
16. Lynn JG, Zwemer RL, Chick AJ, et al. A new method for the generation and use of focused ultrasound in experimental biology. *J Gen Physiol* 1942;26:179.
17. Fry WJ, Barnard JW, Fry FJ. Ultrasonically produced localized selective lesions in the central nervous system. *Am J Phys Med* 1955;34:413.
18. Burov AK. High intensity ultrasonic oscillations for the treatment of malignant tumors in animal and man. *Dokl Akad Nauk SSSR* 1956;106:239.
19. Oka M. Surgical application of high-intensity focused ultrasound. *Clin All Round (Jpn)* 1960;13:1514.
20. Kishi M, Mishima T, Itakura T, et al. *Experimental studies of effects of intense ultrasound on implantable murine glioma.* Amsterdam: Exerpta Medica. Proceedings of the 2nd European Congress on Ultrasonics in Medicine. 1975:28.
21. Sanghvi NT, Fry FJ, Bihrle R, et al. Noninvasive surgery of prostate tissue by high -intensity focused ultrasound. *IEEE Trans Ultrason Ferroelectr Freq Contr* 1996;43:1099.
22. Gelet A, Chapelon JY, Bouvier R, et al. Local control of prostate cancer by transrectal high intensity focused ultrasound therapy: preliminary results. *J Urol* 1999;161:156.
23. Sanghvi NT, Hawes RH. High-intensity focused ultrasound. *Gastrointest Endosc Clin N Am* 1994;4:383.
24. Chapelon JY, Ribault M, Vernier F, et al. Treatment of localized prostate cancer with transrectal high intensity focused ultrasound. *Eur J Ultrasound* 1999;9:31.
25. Visioli AG, Rivens IH, ter Haar GR, et al. Preliminary results of a phase I dose escalation clinical trial using focused ultrasound in the treatment of localised tumours. *Eur J Ultrasound* 1999;9:11.
26. Uchida T, Sanghvi NT, Gardner TA, et al. Transrectal high-intensity focused ultrasound for treatment of patients with stage T1b-2n0m0 localized prostate cancer: a preliminary report. *Urology* 2002;59:394.
27. Hynynen K, Colucci V, Chung A, et al. Noninvasive artery occlusion using MRI guided focused ultrasound. *Ultrasound Med Biol* 1996;22:1071.
28. Vaezy S, Marti R, Mourad P, Crum L. Hemostasis using high intensity focused ultrasound. *Eur J Ultrasound* 1999;9:79.
29. Hynynen K, Pomeroy O, Smith D N, et al. MR imaging-guided focused ultrasound surgery of fibroadenomas in the breast: a feasibility study. *Radiology* 2001;219:176.
30. Schnall MD. Breast MR imaging. *Radiol Clin North Am* 2003;41:43.
31. Gianfelice D, Khiat A, Amara M, et al. MR imaging-guided focused US ablation of breast cancer: histopathologic assessment of effectiveness—initial experience. *Radiology* 2003;227:849.
32. Gianfelice D, Khiat A, Boulanger Y, Amara M, Belblidia A. Feasibility of magnetic resonance imaging-guided focused ultrasound surgery as an adjunct to tamoxifen therapy in high-risk surgical patients with breast carcinoma. *J Vasc Interv Radiol* 2003;14:1275.
33. Stewart EA, Gedroyc WM, Tempany CM, et al. Focused ultrasound treatment of uterine fibroid tumors: safety and feasibility of a noninvasive thermoablative technique. *Am J Obstet Gynecol* 2003;189:48.
34. Hynynen K, Clement G, McDannold N, et al. A 500 element ultrasound phased array system for noninvasive focal surgery of the brain—a preliminary rabbit study with ex vivo human skulls. *Magn Reson Med* 2004;52:100.
35. Clement GT, Hynynen K. A non-invasive method for focusing ultrasound through the human skull. *Phys Med Biol* 2002;47:1219.
36. Visted T, Lund-Johansen M. Progress and challenges for cell encapsulation in brain tumor therapy. *Expert Opin Biol Ther* 2003;3:551.
37. Jolesz FA, Hynynen K. Magnetic resonance image-guided focused ultrasound surgery. *Cancer J* 2002;8(Suppl 1):S100.

C. A. Stein
Luba Benimetskaya
Sridhar Mani

CHAPTER **65**

Antisense Inhibition of Gene Expression

For many decades, the field of cytotoxic chemotherapy has been dominated either by small organic or organometallic molecules. Although, depending on tumor type, these species are more or less effective, and they are almost universally toxic. This toxicity is a direct consequence of their nonspecificity; although they "attack" targets that are important to the maintenance of the neoplastic phenotype, they "attack" another set of targets that are ultimately responsible for the viability of normal cells as well. Furthermore, except in some highly unrepresentative cases, there is virtually no way of avoiding this problem in biologic systems because the interactions of small molecules with their protein or DNA targets are essentially defined by a series of often overlapping (as a function of concentration) dissociation constants.

How then can the specificity of chemotherapy be increased and hence the nonspecific toxicity decreased? Because it is true, for example, that the use of small molecules to target protein-protein interactions leads to toxicity, consideration has to be given to other technologies that can more specifically block or eliminate the function of the targeted protein. One of the more conceptually elegant ways of accomplishing this is to target, rather than the protein itself, the messenger RNA (mRNA) that encodes the nucleic acid sequence that will be translated by the ribosome into a specific protein (or proteins, if mRNA splicing variants are considered). If that protein is ultimately responsible for the growth and/or viability of a tumor cell, a knockdown in its expression may lead to either sensitization of the cell to cytotoxic chemotherapy or to outright cellular death (Fig. 65-1). The targeting of the bcl-2 mRNA, which is discussed later in Mechanism of Action of the Antisense Effect, is an example of such a strategy that has found clinical application.

In targeting the mRNA that encodes the protein rather than the protein itself, advantage can be taken of the exquisite specificity generated by the Watson-Crick base pair interaction to, at least in theory, produce a highly specific therapy. All that is required is to know the sequence of the mRNA, and a small piece of DNA, or small interfering (siRNA), can be chemically synthesized complementary to it. A simple calculation demonstrates that an oligodeoxynucleotide of 15 to 17 mer in length is sufficiently long so that its sequence is represented only once in the entire human genome.[1] siRNAs are always at least 21 mer in length, so Watson-Crick specificity with respect to the entire genome is also ensured.[2]

Because the mRNA sequence is defined as "sense," the complementary oligodeoxyribonucleotide is therefore "antisense." The binding of the antisense oligodeoxyribonucleotide (from now on abbreviated as *oligonucleotide*) to its target mRNA forms a hybrid mRNA–DNA duplex species. The formation of this duplex leads, as described in Mechanism of Action of the Antisense Effect, to the inhibition of translation of that mRNA into protein. For all intents and purposes, this is also true of siRNAs, although their mechanism of translation inhibition appears to be much more complex than that of antisense oligonucleotides,[3] and at the time of this writing is not as well understood. However, because of the current lack of clinical data with siRNAs, these molecules are not further discussed in this chapter.

Therefore, in theory, antisense biotechnology provides a highly specific way of eliminating the activity of a protein because of the specificity of the Watson-Crick base pair interaction. In practice, however, despite its intellectual elegance and relative conceptual simplicity, it has been far more difficult to

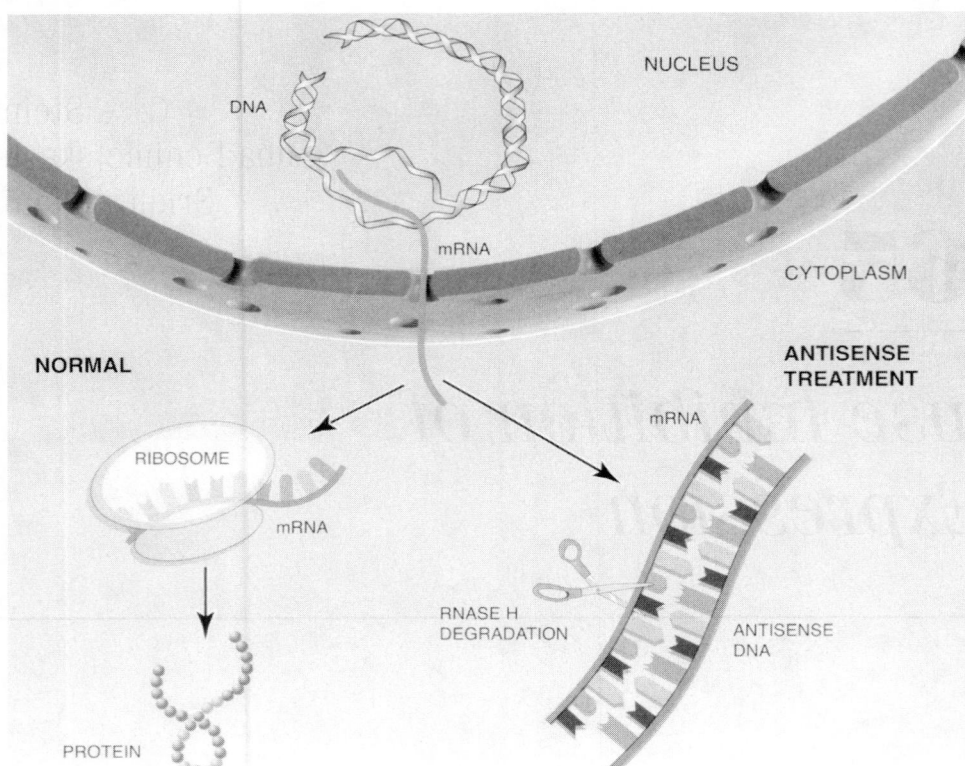

FIGURE 65-1. The theoretical basis of antisense technology. DNA is found in the nucleus, which is transcribed to messenger RNA (mRNA), seen here as a red line exiting the nucleus. mRNA is normally translated by the ribosome into protein in the cytoplasm. The figure depicts an antisense DNA oligodeoxyribonucleotide binding to mRNA by virtue of Watson-Crick complementary between bases on the opposite strands. The mRNA is then cleaved by the ubiquitous enzyme RNase H at the site of oligonucleotide binding. A minor error in this illustration is that it depicts RNase H degradation as occurring in the cytoplasm, when in fact it most likely occurs predominately in the nucleus. In addition, antisense oligonucleotides may also block translation by RNase H–independent mechanisms, although the concentrations required to accomplish this may be much higher than those of oligonucleotides, which elicit an RNase H–dependent mechanism. (From Stein CA. Antisense inhibition as cancer therapy. *Sci Med* 2002;8:313, with permission.) (See Color Fig. 65-1 in the CD-ROM.)

obtain clinical successes with antisense oligonucleotides than was ever considered at the time extensive research on this method began, now almost 25 years ago.[4] Nevertheless, it should be recognized that the clinical development of monoclonal antibodies as therapeutic agents have also followed a difficult and lengthy path, and that this will undoubtedly be true for virtually any new technology, despite the often irrational exuberance greeting its inception.

OLIGONUCLEOTIDE STABILITY AND EFFICACY: THE ROLE OF PHOSPHOROTHIOATES

By the early 1980s, it had been recognized that normal DNA, which contains phosphodiester linkages bridging the deoxyribose sugars in the oligonucleotide chain, could not be used as antisense effector molecules (although, as described later, they may yet have use as drugs). This is because they are digested quite rapidly in human plasma, mostly by exonuclease activity.[5] This fact prompted chemists to devise oligonucleotides that were more nuclease-resistant than phosphodiesters, and their initial studies focused on methylphosphonate oligonucleotides, where a methyl group replaced an oxygen atom at each phosphorus atom in the oligonucleotide chain (Fig. 65-2). This substitution preserved the sequence of the nitrogenous nucleobases and did in fact generate highly nuclease-resistant oligonucleotides that were able to hybridize quite well with their targeted mRNAs. Phosphorothioate oligonucleotides have been widely used as antisense reagents in tissue culture, having been targeted successfully against genes such as c-raf kinase,[6] ICAM-1,[7] Ha-ras,[8] and many others. However, oligonucleotides are also chemicals,

and the methylphosphonate substitution changed the fundamental chemical nature of the oligonucleotide and in doing so generated a host of insoluble problems.

One of these problems is that the substitution of an uncharged methyl group for a charged oxygen atom at each phosphorus atom produced a molecule with no charge. Phosphodiester oligonucleotides are polyanions (contain many negative charges) and as a result are highly water-soluble, in contrast to methylphosphonates, which are sparingly soluble. Initially, the reduction in charge was thought to be a major positive attribute of the methylphosphonates, as it was not believed that charged oligonucleotides could efficiently penetrate hydrophobic, lipidic cell membranes. Although this is true, because of the polarity of the nucleobases, neither do methylphosphonates, or in fact, any other class of oligonucleotide.[9,10] In addition, the lack of charge, and thus the lack of aqueous solubility, led to significant formulation problems. Finally, when oligonucleotides are charged, it is the charge rather than its sequence that governs its physicochemical behavior in solution. When oligonucleotides are uncharged, as is the case with the methylphosphonates and other classes of oligonucleotide as well, it is the sequence, which is different for each target, that dominates its solution behavior. This fact has, in part, led to the endless difficulties that have been faced with uncharged oligonucleotides and to a degree explains why they are not being extensively used in clinical cancer-related trials. However, as is discussed later in Mechanism of Action of the Antisense Effect, several other reasons mitigate against the success of uncharged oligonucleotides for such indications.

The class of oligonucleotide that is currently used in the clinic is the phosphorothioate (see Fig. 65-2). This type of molecule, first synthesized by Wojciech Stec and colleagues in

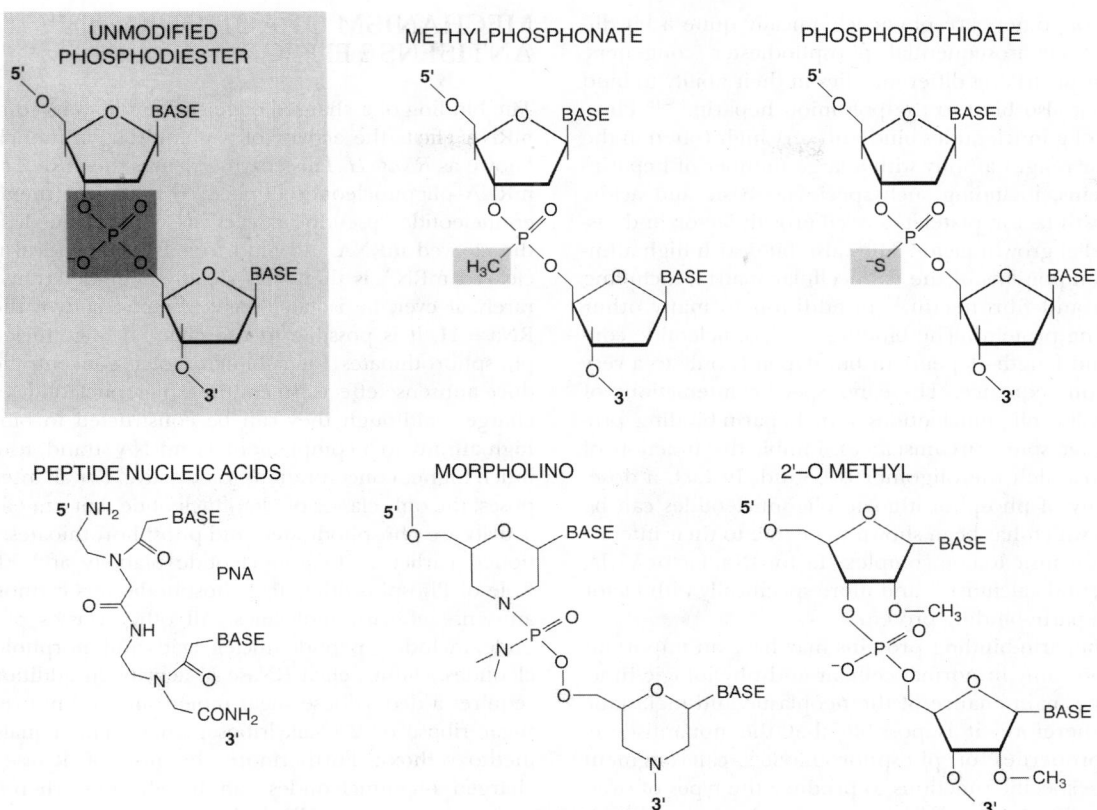

FIGURE 65-2. Chemical modifications of the natural phosphodiester oligonucleotide structure. Phosphodiester oligonucleotides cannot be used as antisense drugs because they are degraded by nucleases. The phosphorothioate backbone modification is the modification that is virtually universally used in the clinic (e.g., phosphorothioate is the backbone of G3139) because of its properties of relative nuclease resistance, aqueous solubility, ease of manufacture, relatively favorable hybridization properties with its target messenger RNA, and ability to elicit RNase H activity. On the other hand, phosphorothioate oligonucleotides also produce significant nonsequence specificity. Methylphosphonates and morpholino and peptide nucleic acids are not highly soluble, do not absorb to cell membranes, and do not elicit RNase H activity, although their hybridization properties are highly favorable. 2-O-methyloligoribonucleotides are useful in gap-mers. (From Stein CA. Antisense inhibition as cancer therapy. *Sci Med* 2002;8:313, with permission.) (See Color Fig. 65-2 in the CD-ROM.)

1984[11] takes advantage of the fact that sulfur is directly underneath oxygen in the periodic table and that the two are thus isoelectronic. In a phosphorothioate oligonucleotide, a sulfur atom replaces an oxygen atom at a nonbridging position at each phosphorus in the chain, but the charge, and thus the property of aqueous solubility, is retained. Phosphorothioate oligonucleotides are also much more nuclease-resistant than phosphodiesters,[12] but they are not nuclease-proof. Rather, they are relatively slowly digested to nucleotide monothiophosphates, which are then eliminated. Phosphorothioates also form relatively stable duplexes with a targeted mRNA, but the melting temperature of the duplex is somewhat lower than what would be found for the corresponding isosequential phosphodiester oligonucleotide. This diminution is due to the fact that the phosphorothioate linkage is chiral—that is, it is bound to four different substituents—unlike the phosphodiester linkage, where each phosphorus is bound to two, identical, nonbridging oxygen atoms. Depending on the orientation of the sulfur atoms, the phosphorothioate linkage can exist in one of two mirror images, called the *Rp and Sp diastereomers*. When a phosphorothioate oligonucleotide is synthesized by a

DNA synthesizer (machines that are now capable of producing kilogram quantities of oligonucleotide), each phosphorothioate linkage is produced as an approximately equal mixture of Rp and Sp diastereomers (mirror images). This in turn means that for a phosphorothioate oligomer of length n, there are approximately 2^n different diastereomers that can be formed, a very large number indeed considering that the antisense bcl-2 oligomer, for example, is 18 bases in length. However, the sulfur atom in the Sp diastereomer points into the major groove of the duplex formed between the oligomer and its targeted mRNA, and because sulfur is a larger atom than oxygen, this destabilizes the duplex (i.e., lowers its melting temperature).[13] On the other hand, the Rp linkage is not duplex-destabilizing, but unlike the nuclease-resistant Sp linkage, it is about as nuclease-sensitive as a phosphodiester linkage. Nevertheless, the diminution in melting temperature due to the presence of Sp phosphorothioate linkages is not sufficient to rule out their use as antisense effector molecules.

As mentioned earlier, synthetic oligonucleotides are chemicals. In fact, despite the favorable property of aqueous solubility and adequate hybridization to a complementary mRNA, phosphorothioate oligomers are physicochemically quite a bit different from their isosequential phosphodiester congeners. Perhaps the most striking difference lies in their ability to bind to proteins that also bind to the polyanion heparin.[14–16] Phosphorothioate oligonucleotides bind with very high (often in the low nanomolar range) affinity with a large number of heparin-binding proteins, including such species as basic and acidic fibroblast growth factor, platelet-derived growth factor, and vascular endothelial growth factor. They also bind with high affinity to many components of the extracellular matrix, including both laminin and fibronectin,[17] in addition to many other heparin-binding proteins. The binding is oligonucleotide concentration– and length–dependent but depends only to a very small extent on sequence. These nonspecific interactions of phosphorothioate oligonucleotides with heparin-binding proteins may, under some circumstances, inhibit the function of the protein to which the oligomer is bound. In fact, a dose-limiting toxicity of phosphorothioate oligonucleotides can be coagulopathy, which has been shown to be due to their interaction with the intrinsic tenase complex (factor IXa, factor VIIIa, phospholipid, and calcium),[18] and more specifically with factor IX,[19] itself a heparin-binding protein.

However, heparin-binding proteins may have an important role to play, not only in normal cellular and physiologic function, but in the maintenance of the neoplastic and metastatic phenotype. Therefore, it is possible that the nonantisense, nonspecific properties of phosphorothioates can augment their sequence specific functions to produce the types of overall anticancer effects that have been commonly observed both *in vitro* and *in vivo*. In fact, at the present time, the authors believe that a much stronger statement can be made, which is that absolute specificity is, for all intents and purposes, unattainable when phosphorothioate oligonucleotides are used. Virtually two decades of experience have all too frequently demonstrated that there is frequently only a two- to fourfold difference in oligonucleotide concentration between a specific and nonspecific down-regulation of protein expression. These relatively small differences make it very difficult to control for nonsequence specificity, both in tissue culture and in experimental animals. As a result, it is difficult, if not impossible, to state with any certainty that an observed phenotype is produced as a direct result of a specific knockdown. (This may not be the case when siRNAs are used because of their ostensibly higher specificity.) Rather, as described, the observed phenotype obtained after treatment of cells with phosphorothioate oligonucleotides is invariably the result of a combination of antisense plus nonantisense effects.

What does this fact imply for the field in general and for the use of antisense oligonucleotides as anticancer therapeutics? Although unquestionably adding to its complexity while at the same time diminishing the property absolute specificity on which it was initially predicated, the authors believe that the combination of antisense plus nonantisense effects on tumor cell phenotype can only augment clinical efficacy. In fact, it is possible that antisense interventions that are too specific (e.g., siRNAs) may produce little, except in certain well-defined but relatively rare instances, in the way of durable clinical responses. This is due to the highly redundant network of signaling pathways in clinical human tumors, entities that, although frequently lost sight of, behave very differently from human tumor cell line xenografts in immunosuppressed mice.

MECHANISM OF ACTION OF THE ANTISENSE EFFECT

The binding of a charged oligonucleotide to its complementary mRNA elicits the activity of a ubiquitous intranuclear enzyme known as *RNase H*. This enzyme cleaves the mRNA strand of the mRNA–oligonucleotide duplex,[20,21] rendering the antisense oligonucleotide "pseudocatalytic," as it can then dissociate from the cleaved mRNA and bind to another identical mRNA. The cleaved mRNA is then very rapidly degraded, and in fact can rarely, if ever, be isolated. As a direct result of the activity of RNase H, it is possible to use charged oligonucleotides (e.g., phosphorothioates) at submicromolar concentrations to produce antisense effects. In contrast, oligonucleotides that are not charged, although they can be constructed to bind with very high affinity to a complementary mRNA strand, usually require much higher concentrations to be active. For all intents and purposes, the only classes of oligonucleotide that can elicit RNase H activity are phosphodiesters and phosphorothioates, but as mentioned earlier in Oligonucleotide Stability and Efficacy: The Role of Phosphorothioates, phosphodiesters cannot be used as antisense effector molecules. All other classes of oligonucleotide, including peptide nucleic acids and morpholino oligonucleotides, cannot elicit RNase H activity. In addition, RNase H requires a deoxyribose sugar moiety and will not recognize the sugar ribose or 2'-O-alkylribose, where alkyl equals methyl or methoxyethoxy. Furthermore, because of RNase H activity, charged oligonucleotides can be effective when targeted to many sites on the mRNA, including 3' downstream regions. Uncharged oligonucleotides, on the other hand, tend to be active only when targeted to the initiation codon region.[22] When targeted further downstream, they are relatively easily dissociated from their targets by the unwinding activity of the 80S ribosome.[23] Although the activity of RNase H is important for the submicromolar efficacy of antisense phosphorothioate oligonucleotides, a problem arises because the enzyme is not "stringent." For example, although G3139, the anti-bcl-2 phosphorothioate oligonucleotide now completing several phase III clinical trials, is 18 mer in length, RNase H does not require an intact 18 mer mRNA–G3139 duplex for it to cleave the bcl-2 mRNA. Rather, it may require a duplex region of only 6 to 10 mer[24] in length to cleave the target. However, in any 18 mer, there are a relatively large number of nested 6- to 10-mer sequences, although these short sequences are not necessarily unique to the bcl-2 mRNA. In fact, these short sequences may be scattered throughout the entire human transcriptome, although admittedly, many of these sites on nontargeted mRNAs are not accessible to the oligonucleotide, RNase H, or both. Nevertheless, this lack of stringency can, at least in theory, give rise to the RNase H cleavage of nontargeted mRNAs, or "irrelevant cleavage."[25,26] Similar to other forms of nonsequence specificity, and for mostly the same reasons, irrelevant cleavage may not necessarily be detrimental to clinical efficacy, but *a priori* it is impossible to predict just what targets might be cleaved. Paradoxically, the lack of stringency of RNase implies that the longer the oligonucleotide, the less specific it becomes, as the number of nested sequences contained within it also increases. Oligonucleotides that are too short (i.e., fewer than 15 mer) are not unique, and, especially when the backbone is phosphorothioate, they tend to have melting temperatures that are too low for use as antisense molecules. Predominately for these reasons, the optimum length of a phosphorothioate oligonucleotide is 18 to 20 mer; G3139 is an 18 mer; and Isis 3521, which was unsuccessful in a large trial non–small cell lung cancer, is 20 bases in length.

Many attempts have been made to reduce or eliminate irrelevant cleavage, the most successful being the use of so-called gapmers. These are oligonucleotides designed so that the backbone consists of all phosphorothioate linkages but that in addition contain non–RNase H-sensitive substituents at both the 3' and 5' termini.[27] These are usually four or more 2'-O-alkyl (methyl or methoxyethoxy) residues, which increase melting temperature while diminishing irrelevant cleavage, although other species such as locked nucleic acids have also been used.[28] 2'-O-methoxyethoxy substituents also dramatically alter oligonucleotide pharmacokinetics. The central region of the molecule, or gap, remains deoxyribonucleotide to preserve at least some RNase H activity, which is vital for 3' mRNA targeting and submicromolar antisense efficacy. In one variation of this strategy, an inverted (3'-3' or 5'-5') deoxythymidine residue is also linked to both the 3' and 5' termini to further increase nuclease resistance. In addition to increasing specificity and melting temperature, the use of the gap mer strategy can produce antisense effector molecules that are effective in the low nanomolar range,[29] or at about the same concentrations at which siRNAs are frequently effective. However, as discussed earlier in Oligonucleotide Stability and Efficacy: The Role of Phosphorothioates, whether or not extremely high specificity is a beneficial or deleterious property of an effective anticancer drug, at least for the major solid tumors of adulthood

(breast, lung, prostate, gastrointestinal), is very much an open question at the present time. To date, however, almost all clinical trials using phosphorothioate oligonucleotides have used non–gap-mer molecules.

DELIVERY OF OLIGONUCLEOTIDES INTO CELLS

Charged, and indeed uncharged, oligonucleotides cannot pass through hydrophobic lipid bilayers. Rather, charged oligonucleotides adsorb, most likely by binding to heparin-binding proteins, to the protein component of cell membranes. As the cell membrane is endocytosed, the adsorbed oligonucleotides come to be localized into intracellular vesicles known as *endosomes* (Fig. 65-3). Uncharged oligonucleotides, on the other hand, cannot adsorb to the cell surface and can only be internalized from the bulk, or fluid, phase by the process of pinocytosis, whereby they too come to reside in endosomes.[30] However, the pinocytotic process is quite inefficient compared with adsorptive endocytosis, which is another reason that uncharged oligonucleotides are difficult to use as antisense molecules—that is, it is extremely difficult for cells to internalize them in sufficient concentration.

However, even after "internalization," charged oligonucleotides are found predominately in endosomes, an intracellular compartment in which neither mRNA nor RNase H are ever located. In fact, the fate of phosphorothioate oligonucleotides

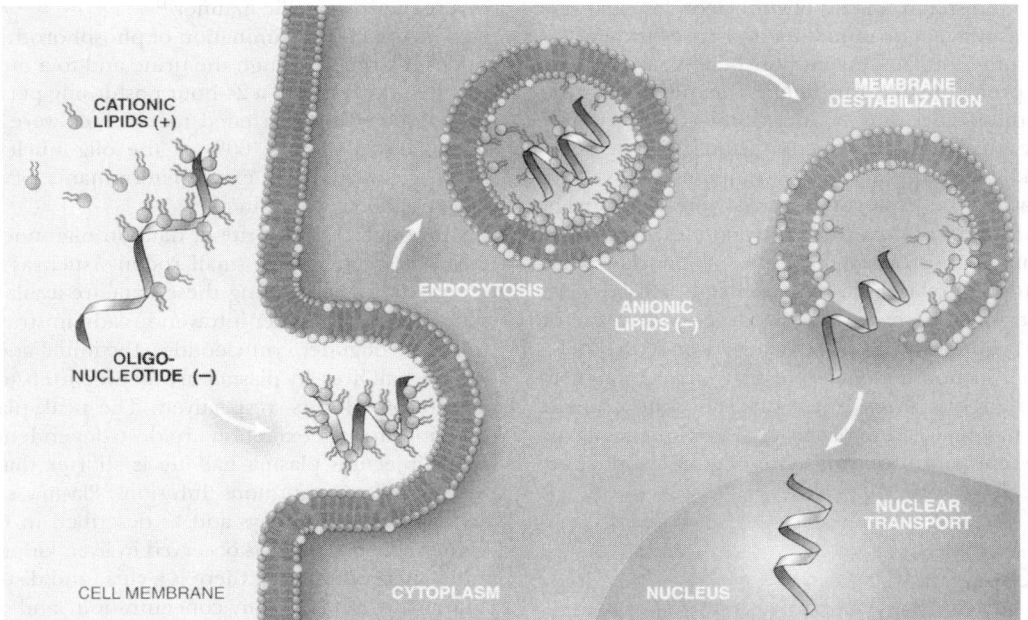

FIGURE 65-3. The delivery of polyanionic oligonucleotides to cells via cationic lipids. Shown in the left part of the figure are cationic lipids (e.g., lipofectin), noncovalently binding to negatively charged oligonucleotides. These complexes adsorb to anionic lipids on the cell membrane, which invaginates to form an endosome. Within the liposome, the cationic lipid and oligonucleotide dissociate, and the lipid inserts into and destabilizes the endosomal membrane. This leads to endosomal rupture, and the entrapped oligonucleotide is then carried, probably by active processes, into the nucleus. Antisense activity is believed to occur predominately in the cell nucleus, as this is the site of RNase H activity. In contrast, small interfering RNA activity is believed to occur in the cytoplasm. Although it is believed that endogenous carriers exist *in vivo*, this has never rigorously been demonstrated. (From Stein CA. Antisense inhibition as cancer therapy. *Sci Med* 2002;8:313, with permission.) (See Color Fig. 65-3 in the CD-ROM.)

is to be either entrapped in the endosomes, which will fuse with lysosomes and in which the oligomers will be digested, or alternatively, to be slowly exocytosed.[30] The process vital to antisense efficacy is rupture of the endosome and release of its oligonucleotide contents, which then, by active but poorly understood processes, travel to the cell nucleus. However, the rate of spontaneous endosomal rupture is far too slow for antisense purposes, and because nuclear localization is the sine qua non of antisense efficacy, endosomal localization is a dead end for naked oligonucleotides.

To promote nuclear delivery, at least in tissue culture experiments, synthetic oligonucleotides must be delivered with carriers[30,31] (see Fig. 65-3). These carriers are usually cationic lipids, but a wide variety of other polycations have also been used. Cationic lipids form complexes with charged (but not uncharged) oligonucleotides. These complexes also adsorb to the cell surface and are also endocytosed into endosomes.[1] However, once within the endosome, the cationic lipid dissociates from the oligonucleotide[32,33] and inserts into the endosomal membrane lipid bilayer. This causes a change in the lipid phase of the membrane and leads to a much higher rate of endosomal rupture and, hence, nuclear localization of the oligonucleotide and antisense efficacy.[34]

For experiments in tissue culture, some form of carrier is an absolute requirement for efficacy at submicromolar oligonucleotide concentrations. For *in vivo* studies, on the other hand, it has long been a dogma that no external carrier is required because there exist natural, intrinsic carrier molecules. However, the nature of such molecules has never been defined, nor, in fact, has it ever been rigorously and reproducibly proven in the clinic that naked phosphorothioate oligonucleotides can enter human tumors in sufficient quantities for antisense efficacy.[35,36]

This conundrum is, in fact, the authors believe, at the heart of many of the problems that this field has experienced over the years, and these questions of intracellular delivery have never been truly adequately addressed. It should also be noted that the same kinds of problems will undoubtedly exist for experiments that can be performed with any class of nucleic acid, be they phosphorothioate oligonucleotides or siRNAs. The apparent inability of oligonucleotides of any class whatever to penetrate lipid bilayers in the absence of a carrier has in many ways served as a brake on the development of the entire area of DNA medicines. Nevertheless, despite this problem and questions of nonsequence specificity, irrelevant cleavage, and a myriad of other issues, one phosphorothioate oligonucleotide has emerged as of this writing as the lead candidate to be the first anticancer antisense oligonucleotide, the anti–bcl-2 molecule G3139.

PHARMACOKINETICS

Phosphorothioate oligonucleotides of varied length and base composition bind serum proteins (albumin and α_2-macroglobulin) in a species-dependent manner.[37,38] Protein binding is saturable, a fact that greatly impacts on *in vivo* pharmacokinetics and stability. Tissue distributions of varying phosphorothioate oligonucleotide base and length compositions have been extensively investigated in mice, rats, and monkeys after intradermal, intravenous, intraperitoneal, and subcutaneous administration. After intravenous administration, there is a rapid clearance of these oligomers, with distribution half-lives of less than 1 hour. Plasma clearance is biphasic, and the terminal elimination half-life ranges between 40 and 60 hours based on radioactivity assays performed on labeled oligonucleotides. Notably, at 12 to 24 hours after administration, the presence of intact oligonucleotides and metabolites can be demonstrated in plasma. In rats, saturable protein binding is observed at intravenous doses of between 15 and 20 mg/kg.

However, intratumoral kinetics are understood much less.[39] In one human tumor model, the Walker 256 tissue-isolated tumor preparation, Nakajima et al.[40] demonstrated that an important determinant of intratumoral uptake of oligonucleotide is the unbound plasma concentration of the parent molecule. However, it is unclear what specific intratumoral characteristics result in optimal antisense effects.

Although the distribution of phosphorothioate oligonucleotides to tumor cells is critical, normal tissue distribution and clearance are also vital in determining overall efficacy. Phosphorothioate oligonucleotides distribute to highly perfused organ tissues such as the liver, kidney, bone marrow, and spleen. The rates of tissue absorption and elimination also vary by organ site. The largest site of accumulation of phosphorothioate oligonucleotides is the liver (an intravenous dose of 30 mg/kg in rats yields liver area under the curve values of between 1432.5 and 6538.2 $\mu g/mL/h$). Accumulation may be greatest in the Kupffer's cells within the liver. Phosphorothioate oligonucleotides also accumulate in kidneys, especially in the proximal tubular lumen and within intratubular epithelial cells. There, they suppress renal Na^+/Pi cotransport, perhaps in a sequence-specific manner.[41]

The total body elimination of phosphorothioate oligonucleotides is largely through the urine and to a much lesser extent through the feces. In a 24-hour postdosing period, 40% of both intact and chain-shortened metabolites were excreted in the urine. By 240 hours, 60% of the oligonucleotide was eliminated. However, the exact determinants of renal clearance have not been determined.[41]

Although the majority of data on oligonucleotide pharmacokinetics come from small rodents such as mice and rates, fewer studies confirming these data are available in mammals such as monkeys. After intravenous administration of phosphorothioate oligodeoxynucleotides, the initial and terminal elimination half-lives in plasma are between 0.6 to 1.0 hours and 42.2 to 56.3 hours, respectively. The peak plasma concentration and urinary excretion are dose-dependent. In monkeys, a single-injection plasma half-life is shorter than that achieved with a 4-day continuous infusion. Plasma steady states are achieved in 4 to 9 days and as described in rodents; a much higher concentration is observed in liver, kidney, heart, spleen, and pancreas. Notably, there is a clear and distinct relationship among dose, maximum concentration, and activated partial thromboplastin time changes such that prolonged infusion with lower maximum concentration resulted in reduced activated partial thromboplastin time elevations.[41]

CLINICAL STUDIES

Phosphorothioate oligonucleotide pharmacokinetics have been well described in humans. In these studies, the plasma concentration has been linearly proportional to dose. Plasma concentrations reached steady state within 24 to 48 hours of dosing, and in the case of a 20-mer complementary to the p53 mRNA, 60% of the administered dose was cleared in the urine. Administration of ^{35}S-labeled GEM91, an anti–human immunodeficiency virus oligonucleotide that did not succeed in clinical trials, at a dose of 0.1 mg/kg in six human immunodeficiency virus–infected individuals, resulted in peak plasma concentrations of 295 ng/mL by the end of the infusion. The plasma disappearance of GEM91-derived radioactivity was described as the sum of two exponentials with half-life values of 0.18 and 26 hours. Analysis of the radioactivity in plasma revealed intact oligonucleotide up to 2 hours after dosing. Urinary excretion represented 49% and 70% of the total administered dose at 24 and 96 hours, respectively, with most of the compound being degraded. Multiple dosing did not result in cumulative effects on plasma pharmacokinetic parameters.[39]

Extensive pharmacokinetic studies have also been performed on G3139. Rapid distribution and elimination from plasma were observed, with low blood levels reached after 6 hours. Triexponential clearance kinetics from the plasma were observed, with α, β, and γ half-lives of 5 minutes, 37 minutes, and 11 hours, respectively. Most of the oligonucleotide was protein-bound (98% after 5 minutes). In tissues, the highest accumulations were found in the kidneys and liver. Pretreatment renal function was the only factor identified by multivariate analysis to significantly affect the rate of plasma clearance.[42]

CLINICAL TRIALS OF G3139

Many different reviews describe the ability of bcl-2 to prevent apoptosis induced by cytotoxic chemotherapy.[43–46] In fact, bcl-2 protein has been demonstrated to promote resistance to a wide variety of agents, including cisplatin, topoisomerase II inhibitors, alkylating agents, antimetabolites, and radiation.[47–52] Down-regulation of bcl-2 protein expression by G3139 has been demonstrated in a large number of tumor cell lines both *in vitro* and *in vivo*.[53–55] In particular, DoHH2 lymphoma cells, which bear a t(14:18) translocation, appear to be particularly sensitive to G3139 treatment. In a SCID mouse–human tumor xenograft model, virtual complete abolition of tumor growth was demonstrated in 83% of the treated animals (50 of 60) after an infusion of 100 μg/d $\times$ 14 days.[54] If the treatment was extended for 3 weeks, the xenografted lymphoma was eliminated in all the animals, even at the level of polymerase chain reaction. However, this particular cell line is somewhat unusual in that bcl-2 protein appears to be necessary for cellular viability. This is not necessarily true in other cell lines.

Nevertheless, Webb et al.[56] initiated a phase I trial with G3139 in nine patients with lymphoma in whose cell bcl-2 protein was "elevated." All patients had failed at least two therapeutic interventions. Patients were treated at two doses, 4.6 and 73.6 mg/m[2]/d. The maximum tolerated dose was not achieved. There was one complete response, three patients with stable disease, and five with progressive disease. A subsequent study administered G3139 via continuous infusion to 21 patients at doses of 4.96 to 196 mg/m[2]/d $\times$ 2 weeks. There was one patient with a complete response, there were two patients with minor response (MR), there were nine with stable disease, and the remaining nine had progressive disease. In seven of 16 evaluable patients, bcl-2 protein was diminished in cells derived from lymph nodes (two patients) or in samples of peripheral blood or bone marrow (five patients).

The trials that have generated the most interest in oblimersen sodium (Genasense) are those (phases II and III) that have recently been completed in advanced melanoma. It was clear from studies on the 518A2 melanoma cell line that G3139 could down-regulate the expression of bcl-2 protein and mRNA.[57] In SCID mice, when G3139 was combined with dacarbazine, perhaps the currently most active agent in this disease, tumors were entirely eliminated in three of six animals. Based on these data, a phase I trial of the combination of G3139 plus dacarbazine was initiated in 14 patients,[35] the majority of whom had failed previous interferon-α therapy. The oligonucleotide was administered via continuous infusion using an ambulatory pump, and dacarbazine (200 mg/m[2]) was administered on days 5 through 9 of a 28-day cycle. A "clear reduction" in the expression of bcl-2 protein expression, derived from biopsy samples of cutaneous melanoma lesions, was observed in 83% of patients (10 of 12 evaluable) who achieved plasma levels of G3139 less than 1 μg/mL. The patient who achieved the complete response demonstrated the greatest decrease in bcl-2 expression (70%), but except for this one individual, no patient with as much as a 60% decrease achieved even a partial response, and patients who achieved a 40% decrease did so.

Chemotherapy-related toxicity has been relatively modest. At doses of more than 4.1 mg/kg/d, transient fever was observed in seven patients, and grade 3 increases in bilirubin and hepatic enzymes, perhaps more related to the dacarbazine, have been observed in four patients. Fatigue was frequent; grade 1 rash was seen in four; and grade 2 lymphopenia, thrombocytopenia, and neutropenia were observed in seven, two, and two patients, respectively.

Strikingly, evidence of antitumor activity was observed in 6 of 14 patients. This consisted of one complete response, two partial responses, and two MRs, with disease stabilization lasting for at least 1 year. Overall survival exceeds 17 months, which represents more than a doubling of historical survivals. These data led to the initiation and completion of a phase III, multicenter, randomized, global registration trial of dacarbazine plus G3139 versus dacarbazine, which accrued its target of 771 patients to each arm and closed in January 2003. This trial is now the largest ever conducted in advanced melanoma. The progression-free survival (estimated median, days) is 78 for the combination versus 49 for the single agent (P = .001). The response rate was 11.7% for the combination versus 6.8% for dacarbazine alone (P = .019). The overall median survival for the patients (intent to treat) who have been followed on the protocol for at least 12 months is 10.1 versus 8.1 months, an increase of 25%.[58] The overall survival of all patients is at the time of this writing (September 2003) still pending but is expected to approximate the median survival of the approximately 530 patients already determined after 1 year. These results are highly encouraging in an extremely refractory disease that has hitherto been very difficult to treat by any therapeutic intervention attempted in the last 40 years. Moreover, trials in the adjuvant setting, in which greater activity may be anticipated, will probably commence in the near future. In addition to these data, the results of phase III trials of G3139 in myeloma and chronic lymphocytic leukemia are also thought to be imminent.

But even should these trials be successful in the clinic, many scientific issues remain unsolved. Can phosphorothioate oligonucleotides truly behave as antisense effector molecules in tumor cells, or does their apparent clinical activity depend predominately on nonspecific mechanisms? Phrased differently, is G3139 the first or the last member of a novel class of antineoplastic therapeutic agents? Given the redundancy of cellular signaling, is it even possible that highly specific antisense effector molecules, such as siRNAs ostensibly are, can be clinically successful? How can the pharmacokinetic profile, cellular delivery and targeting, and lipid-bilayer penetrating ability of charged antisense-type molecules be improved to decrease the cost of goods, increase efficacy, and decrease toxicity? For the field of DNA medicines to advance, these issues will form a focus of intense scrutiny in the years to come.

REFERENCES

1. Stein CA, Cheng YC. Antisense oligonucleotides as therapeutic agents—is the bullet really magical? *Science* 1993;261:1004.
2. Tuschl T. Expanding small RNA interference. *Nat Biotechnol* 2002;20:446.
3. Nykanen A, Haley B, Zamore PD. ATP requirements and small interfering RNA structure in the RNA interference pathway. *Cell* 2001;107:309.
4. Stephenson ML, Zamecnik PC. Inhibition of Rous sarcoma viral RNA translation by a specific oligodeoxyribonucleotide. *Proc Natl Acad Sci U S A* 1978;75:285.
5. Eder PS, De Vine RJ, Dagle JM, et al. Substrate specificity and kinetics of degradation of antisense oligonucleotides by a 3' exonuclease in plasma. *Antisense Res Dev* 1991;1:141.
6. Monia BP. First- and second-generation antisense inhibitors targeted to human c-raf kinase: in vitro and in vivo studies. *Anticancer Drug Des* 1997;12:327.
7. Chiang MY, Chan H, Zounes MA, et al. Antisense oligonucleotides inhibit intercellular adhesion molecule I expression by two distinct mechanisms. *J Biol Chem* 1991;266:18162.
8. Cowsert LM. In vitro and in vivo activity of antisense inhibitors of ras: potential for clinical development. *Anticancer Drug Des* 1997;12:359.
9. Tonkinson JL, Stein CA. Patterns of intracellular compartmentalization, trafficking and acidification of 5'-fluorescein labeled phosphodiester and phosphorothioate oligodeoxynucleotides in HL60 cells. *Nucleic Acids Res* 1994;22:4268.
10. Akhtar S, Basu S, Wickstrom E, et al. Interactions of antisense DNA oligonucleotide analogs with phospholipid membranes (liposomes). *Nucleic Acids Res* 1991;19:5551.
11. Stec W, Zon G, Egan V. Automated solid-phase synthesis, separation and stereochemistry of phosphorothioate analogues of oligodeoxyribonucleotides. *J Am Chem Soc* 1984;106:6077.
12. Stein CA, Subasinghe C, Shinozuka K, et al. Physicochemical properties of phosphorothioate oligodeoxynucleotides. *Nucleic Acids Res* 1988;16:3209.
13. LaPlanche L, James TL, Powell C, et al. Phosphorothioate modified oligodeoxy-nucleotides III. NMR and UV spectroscopic studies of the Rp-Rp, Sp-Rp, and Sp-Sp duplexes [d(GGsAATTCC)]2 derived from diastereoisomeric O-ethyl phosphorothioate. *Nucleic Acids Res* 1986;14:9081.
14. Guvakova MA, Yakubov LA, Vlodavsky I, et al. Phosphorothioate oligodeoxynucleotides bind to basic fibroblast growth factor, inhibit its binding to cell surface receptors, and remove it from low affinity binding sites on extracellular matrix. *J Biol Chem* 1995;270:2620.
15. Fennewald SM, Rando RF. Inhibition of high affinity basic fibroblast growth factor binding by oligonucleotides. *J Biol Chem* 1995;270:21718.
16. Rockwell P, O'Connor WJ, King K, et al. Cell-surface perturbations of the epidermal growth factor and vascular endothelial growth factor receptors by phosphorothioate oligodeoxynucleotides. *Proc Natl Acad Sci U S A* 1997;94:6523.
17. Khaled Z, Benimetskaya L, Zeltser R, et al. Multiple mechanisms may contribute to the cellular anti-adhesive effects of phosphorothioate oligodeoxynucleotides. *Nucleic Acids Res* 1996;24:737.
18. Sheehan JP, Lan H-C. Phosphorothioate oligonucleotides inhibit the intrinsic tenase complex. *Blood* 1998;92:1617.
19. Sheehan JP, Phan TM. Phosphorothioate oligonucleotides inhibit the intrinsic tenase complex by an allosteric mechanism. *Biochemistry* 2001;40:4980.
20. Walder RY, Walder JA. Role of RNase H in hybrid-arrested translation by antisense oligonucleotides. *Proc Natl Acad Sci U S A* 1988;14:6433.
21. Minshull J, Hunt T. The use of single-stranded DNA and RNase H to promote quantitative "hybrid arrest of translation" of mRNA/DNA hybrids in reticulocyte lysate cell-free translations. *Nucleic Acids Res* 1986;14:6433.
22. Dias N, Dheur S, Nielsen PE, et al. Antisense PNA tridecamers targeted to the coding region of Ha-ras mRNA arrest polypeptide chain elongation. *J Mol Biol* 1999;294:403.
23. Liebhaber SA, Cash FE, Shakin SH. Translationally associated helix-destabilizing activity in rabbit reticulocyte lysate. *J Biol Chem* 1984;259:15597.
24. Monia BP, Lesnik EA, Gonzalez C, et al. Evaluation of 2'-modified oligonucleotides containing 2'-deoxy gaps as antisense inhibitors of gene expression. *J Biol Chem* 1993;268:14514.
25. Stein CA. Is irrelevant cleavage the price of antisense efficacy? *Pharmacol Ther* 2000;85:231.
26. Giles RV, Tidd DM. Enhanced RNase H activity with methylphosphonodiester/phosphodiester chimeric antisense oligodeoxynucleotides. *Anticancer Drug Des* 1992;7:37.
27. Sewell KL, Geary RS, Baker BF, et al. Phase I trial of ISIS 104838, a 2'-methoxyethyl modified antisense oligonucleotide targeting tumor necrosis factor-alpha. *J Pharmacol Exp Ther* 2002;903:1334.
28. Grunweller A, Wyszko E, Bieber B, et al. Comparison of different antisense strategies in mammalian cells using locked nucleic acids, 2'-O-methyl RNA, phosphorothioates and small interfering RNA. *Nucleic Acids Res* 2003;31:3185.
29. Vickers TA, Koo S, Bennett CF, et al. Efficient reduction of target RNAs by small interfering RNA and RNAs H-dependent antisense agents. *J Biol Chem* 2003;278:7108.
30. Lebedeva I, Benimetskaya L, Stein CA, et al. Cellular delivery of antisense oligonucleotides. *Eur J Pharm Biopharm* 2000;50:101.
31. Zabner J, Fasbender AJ, Moninger T, et al. Cellular and molecular barriers to gene transfer by a cationic lipid. *J Biol Chem* 1995;270:18997.
32. Benimetskaya L, Takle GB, Vilenchik M, et al. Cationic porphyrins: novel delivery vehicles for antisense oligodeoxynucleotides. *Nucleic Acids Res* 1998;26:5310.
33. Marcusson EG, Bhat B, Manoharan M, et al. Phosphorothioate oligodeoxyribonucleotides dissociate from cationic lipids before entering the nucleus. *Nucleic Acids Res* 1998;26:2016.
34. Zelphati O, Szoka Jr FC. Mechanism of oligonucleotide release from cationic liposomes. *Proc Natl Acad Sci U S A* 1996;93:11493.
35. Cunningham CC, Holmlund JT, Geary RS, et al. A Phase I trial of H-ras antisense oligonucleotide ISIS 2503 administered as a continuous intravenous infusion in patients with advanced carcinoma. *Cancer* 2001;92:1265.
36. Jansen B, Wacheck V, Heere-Ress E, et al. Chemosensitisation of malignant melanoma by BCL2 antisense therapy. *Lancet* 2000;356:1728.
37. Srinivasan SK, Iversen P. Review of in vivo pharmacokinetics and toxicology of phosphorothioate oligonucleotides. *J Clin Lab Anal* 1995;9:129.
38. Zhang R, Iyer RP, Yu D, et al. Pharmacokinetics and tissue disposition of a chimeric oligodeoxynucleoside phosphorothioate in rats after intravenous administration. *J Pharmacol Exp Ther* 1996;278:971.
39. Agrawal S, Temsamani J, Galbraith W, et al. Pharmacokinetics of antisense oligonucleotides. *Clin Pharmacokinet* 1995;28:7.
40. Nakajima S, Koshino Y, Nomura T, et al. Intratumoral pharmacokinetics of oligonucleotides in a tissue-isolated tumor perfusion system. *Antisense Nucleic Acid Drug Dev* 2000;10:105.
41. Crooke ST. Potential roles of antisense technology in cancer chemotherapy. *Oncogene* 2000;19:6651.
42. Waters JS, Webb A, Cunningham D, et al. Phase I clinical and pharmacokinetic study of bcl-2 antisense oligonucleotide therapy in patients with non-Hodgkin's lymphoma. *J Clin Oncol* 2000;18:1812.
43. Reed JC. Bcl-2 and the regulation of programmed cell death. *J Cell Biol* 1994;124:1.
44. Reed JC. Bcl-2: prevention of apoptosis as a mechanism of drug resistance. *Hematol Oncol Clin North Am* 1995;9:451.
45. Reed JC, Jurgensmeier JM, Matsuyama S. Bcl-2 family proteins and mitochondria. *Biochim Biophys Acta* 1998;1366:127.
46. Dias N, Stein CA. Potential roles of antisense oligonucleotides in cancer therapy. The example of Bcl-2 antisense oligonucleotides. *Eur J Pharm Biopharm* 2002;54:263.
47. Miyashita T, Reed JC. Bcl-2 oncoprotein blocks chemotherapy-induced apoptosis in a human leukemia cell line. *Blood* 1993;81:151.
48. Kamesaki S, Kamesaki H, Jorgensen TJ, et al. Bcl-2 protein inhibits etoposide-induced apoptosis through its effects on events subsequent to topoisomerase II-induced DNA strand breaks and their repair. *Cancer Res* 1993;53:4251.
49. Baffy G, Miyashita T, Williamson JR, et al. Apoptosis induced by withdrawal of interleukin-3 (IL-3) from an IL-3-dependent hematopoietic cell line is associated with repartitioning of intracellular calcium and is blocked by enforced Bcl-2 oncoprotein production. *J Biol Chem* 1993;268:6511.
50. Walton MI, Whysong D, O'Connor PM, et al. Constitutive expression of human Bcl-2 modulates nitrogen mustard and camptothecin induced apoptosis. *Cancer Res* 1993;53:1853.
51. Fisher TC, Milner AE, Gregory CD, et al. Bcl-2 modulation of apoptosis induced by anticancer drug: resistance to thymidylate stress is independent of classical resistance pathways. *Cancer Res* 1993;53:3321.
52. Tang C, Willingham MC, Reed JC, et al. High levels of p26BCL-2 oncoprotein retard Taxol-induced apoptosis in human pre-B leukemia cells. *Leukemia* 1994;8:1960.
53. Kitada S, Miyashita T, Tanaka S, et al. Investigations of antisense oligonucleotides targeted against bcl-2 RNAs. *Antisense Res Dev* 1993;3:157.
54. Cotter FE, Corbo M, Raynaud F, et al. Bcl-2 antisense therapy in lymphoma: in vitro and in vivo mechanisms, efficacy, pharmacokinetics and toxicity studies. *Ann Oncol* 1996;7:32.
55. Gleave ME, Miayake H, Goldie J, et al. Targeting bcl-2 gene to delay androgen-independent progression and enhance chemosensitivity in prostate cancer using antisense bcl-2 oligodeoxynucleotides. *Urology* 1999;54:36.
56. Webb A, Cunningham D, Cotter F, et al. BCL-2 antisense therapy in patients with non-Hodgkin lymphoma. *Lancet* 1997;349:1137.
57. Jansen B, Schlagbauer-Wadl H, Brown BD, et al. bcl-2 antisense therapy chemosensitizes human melanoma in SCID mice. *Nat Med* 1998;4:232.
58. Genta press release. September 10, 2003.

INDEX

Index

Page numbers followed by *f* indicate figures; those followed by *t* indicate tables.

A

Abandonment concerns in referral to hospice care, 2750
ABC transporters, 330
  in estramustine resistance, 408
  in kidney cancer, 1155–1156
  in platinum drug therapy, 350
  in taxane resistance, 400
  in vinca alkaloid resistance, 394
Abdomen
  infections of, 2503
    postoperative, 2506
  tumors of
    in Burkitt's lymphoma, 1951, 1952
    in Hodgkin's disease, 2035
    in Mediterranean lymphoma, 1974
    postoperative infections in, 2506
    in rhabdomyosarcoma, 1917
Abdominoperineal resection
  in anal cancer, 1133, 1135
  in rectal cancer, 1114–1115
  sexual function after, 2666t, 2671
Abducens nerve in nasopharyngeal cancer, 711, 712
ABL (abl), 53t
  fusion with *BCR. See BCR-ABL*
  as target in imatinib therapy, 70, 313
ABO compatibility in transfusions, 2400–2401
  and hemolytic reactions, 2406
  of platelets, 2403

Abscess
  of brain, 2504
    intracranial pressure increase in, 2282, 2286
  drainage techniques, 631
  periurethral, 2301
Absorption
  of chemotherapy drugs, 319
  of radiation, 277, 277f, 278f
ABV chemotherapy
  in Hodgkin's disease, 2042, 2043t, 2043–2044
    in advanced stage, 2049t, 2050, 2054, 2055t
    in early stage with unfavorable progno-sis, 2046t, 2047, 2047t
  in Kaposi's sarcoma, 2251, 2251t
ABVD chemotherapy in Hodgkin's disease, 338, 1954–1955, 2037, 2044
  in advanced stage, 2048, 2050, 2052, 2053, 2054, 2055
    clinical trials on, 2049t
    dose, schedule, and cycle length in, 2051t
    results of, 2055t
  in children, 1954–1955
  in early stage, 2042, 2043t, 2044
    with unfavorable prognosis, 2045, 2046, 2046t, 2047, 2047t
  in elderly, 2061
  fertility concerns in, 2064, 2566, 2567

  in HIV infection and AIDS, 2062
  in pregnancy, 2061
  in salvage regimen for relapse, 2057
  second cancer risk in, 2063, 2581
ABX-EGF, 304, 313
  in colorectal cancer, 1101
AC chemotherapy in breast cancer
  in early-stage, 1446, 1447, 1448t, 1449, 1450
  metastatic, 1460, 1461
  in pregnancy, 1463, 1464
  second cancers associated with, 2591, 2592
Academic medical centers, 2763
Acanthamoeba infections, 2485–2486
Acanthosis nigricans, 2198, 2198t
Acetabulum, metastatic disease of, 2379f, 2379–2380
Acetaminophen in pain management, 2629t, 2630, 2636
Acetic acid therapy, percutaneous, 634
  in liver cancer, 634, 998
N-Acetylcysteine
  in cystitis prevention, 2303
  in lung cancer prevention, 529
N-Acetyltransferase
  in carcinogen metabolism, 189t
  in drug metabolism, 321
Achalasia, esophageal cancer risk in, 865
α_1-Acid glycoprotein levels in docetaxel ther-apy, 402–403

Amsterdam criteria on hereditary nonpolyposis colorectal cancer, 560, 1064, 1064t
Amyloidosis, 2200, 2200t
  cutaneous lichen, 1491, 1493, 1515t
  in plasma cell neoplasms, 2163, 2170
Amyotrophic lateral sclerosis, 2205
Anal cancer, 1125–1136
  in adenocarcinoma, 1126, 1135
  advanced disease, 1134–1135
  of anal canal, 1129–1135
    in adenocarcinoma, 1135
    anatomy in, 1125–1126
    natural history in, 1127
  anatomy in, 1125–1126
  chemotherapy in
    in adenocarcinoma, 1135
    in advanced disease, 1134t, 1134–1135
    in early-stage disease, 1130
    in HIV infection and AIDS, 1136
    in intermediate-stage disease, 1130–1133, 1131t, 1132t
    in perianal cancer, 1135
    in regional lymph node involvement, 1133–1134
    in small cell cancer, 1135
  early-stage, 1130, 1130t
  epidemiology of, 1126
  in HIV infection and AIDS, 1126–1127, 1136, 2259–2260
    prognosis in, 1129
    screening for, 1129, 2259
  incidence of, 1126
  intermediate-stage, 1130–1133
  metastasis of, 1133–1135
    chemoradiation in, 1131
    natural history in, 1127–1128
    from perianal skin, 1135
    prognosis in, 1129
    to regional lymph nodes, 1133–1134
    in small cell cancer, 1135
    stage IV, 1134–1135
    staging of, 1128t, 1128–1129, 1129t
  natural history in, 1127–1128
  papillomaviruses in, 178, 1126–1127, 2843
    in HIV infection and AIDS, 2259, 2260
  pathology in, 1126
  of perianal skin (anal margin), 1135
    anatomy in, 1125, 1126
    natural history in, 1128
    pathology in, 1126
    staging of, 1129, 1129t
  prognostic factors in, 1129
  radiation therapy in
    in adenocarcinoma, 1135
    in advanced disease, 1134t, 1134–1135
    complications of, 1132–1133
    contraindications to, 1133
    dose and duration in, 1132, 1132t
    in early-stage disease, 1130, 1130t
    in HIV infection and AIDS, 1136
    in intermediate-stage disease, 1130–1133, 1131t, 1132t
    in perianal cancer, 1135
    in regional lymph node involvement, 1133–1134
    in small cell cancer, 1135

risk factors and etiology in, 1126–1127
small cell, 1126, 1135
squamous cell, 1126, 1127, 1129–1135
    natural history in, 1127, 1128
    of perianal skin, 1135
    staging of, 1128t, 1128–1129, 1129t
surgery in
    in early-stage disease, 1130
    in HIV infection and AIDS, 1136
    in intermediate-stage disease, 1130, 1133, 1133t
    in perianal cancer, 1135
    radial resection in, 1133
    reconstructive, 1133
    in regional lymph node involvement, 1133, 1134
    salvage, 1133, 1133t
  in tobacco use, 1127
Anal infections, 2503–2504
Anal intraepithelial neoplasia, 1126, 1127, 1129
Anal sphincters
  anatomy of, 1110, 1125–1126
  in fecal continence, 1110, 1125–1126
  in rectal cancer surgery, 1110
    and radiation therapy, 1118, 1121, 1122
    in stage I disease, 1113
    in stage II and III disease, 1114–1115
Analgesics, 2627–2636, 2645
  in addiction history and pain, 2623
  adjuvant drugs used with, 2630t, 2636–2639
  barriers to effective use of, 2616–2617
  in bone sarcoma, perioperative, 1648
  equianalgesic dose of, 2632–2633
  guidelines on use of, 2628t, 2628–2629
  nonopioid, 2628–2629, 2629t, 2630
  opioid, 2629t, 2630–2636. *See also* Opioid therapy
  in pancreatic cancer, locally advanced, 970
  patient-controlled, 2633, 2634
    in bone sarcoma, 1648
  relative potency of, 2632–2633
  routes of administration, 2632–2634
  side effects of, 2630, 2634–2635
    nephropathy in, 1139–1140
  in terminal illness, 2624
  World Health Organization guidelines on, 2628–2629
Analytic epidemiologic studies, 217, 219–222
Anaphase in mitosis, 84
  transition to, 86, 87f
Anaphase-promoting complex, 85, 86, 87, 87f
Anaphylaxis in transfusion reactions, 2407, 2407t
Anaplastic cancer
  of salivary glands, 723
  of thyroid. *See* Thyroid tumors, anaplastic
Anastomosis
  in colorectal cancer resection, 1077, 1078, 1115
  in prostatectomy, 1217, 1217f
    stricture of, 1220

Anastrozole
  in breast cancer, 462–463, 1445, 1445t
    bilateral, 1465
    in ductal carcinoma *in situ,* 1431
    in elderly, 1470
    metastatic, 1457t, 1458, 1458t
    prediction of response to, 1425
    and tamoxifen therapy, 459, 1445, 1445t
  pharmacology of, 462–463
Androgens and androgen receptors
  and pharmacology of antiandrogen therapy, 464–465
  in prostate cancer, 464–465, 1200–1201, 1203
    altered profile of receptor coregulators, 1201
    and antiandrogen therapy, 464–465, 1231, 1232f, 1235–1241
      duration of response to, 1237
      indications for initiation of, 1238–1239, 1239f
      long-term, 1248
      with radiation therapy, 1239–1241, 1240t
      with radical prostatectomy, 1239
      sexual function in, 2667–2668
      side effects of, 1235, 1238, 1241
      with watchful waiting, 1239
    and castration resistance, 1200, 1201
    ligand-independent activation of receptor, 1200
    mutations in receptor, 1201
    signaling alterations, 1200, 1201f
Andropause, 1235
Anemia, 2194
  in androgen ablation therapy for prostate cancer, 1235
  aplastic, interleukin-11 therapy in, 2456
  of cancer, 2451
  in cervical cancer, 1305
  in chemotherapy, 2194, 2448–2450
    in testicular germ cell tumors, 1288
    erythropoietin therapy in, 2448–2450. *See also* Erythropoietin, therapy with
  Fanconi's, 42t, 2201t
  hemolytic. *See* Hemolytic anemia
  in interferon therapy, 426
  in leukemia
    chronic lymphocytic, 2137, 2138, 2449t, 2450
    chronic myelogenous, 2123
  in lymphoma, 2449t
  in myelodysplastic syndromes, 2148, 2449t, 2450
    supportive care in, 2150
    treatment of, 2151
  in myeloma, 2449t, 2450
  in paraneoplastic syndromes, 2194
  pernicious, surveillance for gastric cancer in, 638
  in plasma cell neoplasms, 2163
  pure red cell aplasia, 2194
  in radiation therapy, 2194
    erythropoietin therapy in, 2448–2450, 2449t

Tamm-Horsfall protein, 2163
Tamoxifen, 457–459
  in breast cancer, 457–459
    in adjuvant therapy, 296–297
    and anastrozole therapy, 1445, 1445t
    bilateral, 1465
    in BRCA1 and BRCA2 mutations, 561,
        1411, 1428, 2682
    in chemoprevention, 1427–1428,
        2591, 2682
    in ductal carcinoma *in situ*, 1431,
        1432t
    in early-stage disease, 1443t, 1443–
        1444, 1444f
      preoperative, 1436
      recurrence and mortality rates in,
        1450t
    in elderly, 1470, 1471f
    estrogen and progesterone receptor
        status affecting, 1424, 1443
    interaction with other drugs, 459
    in lobular carcinoma *in situ*, 1434
    in male, 1465
    metastatic, 1456–1457, 1457t, 1458,
        1458t, 1459
    ovarian ablation compared to, 1444
    prediction of response to, 1424, 1425
    recurrent, 1469
    resistance to, 1404, 1412
    second cancers associated with, 457,
        458
      endometrial, 2592t, 2592–2593,
        2593f
      gastrointestinal, 2593
    sexual function in, 2666, 2667, 2667f
    toremifene compared to, 459
  in cerebral astrocytoma, 1853–1854
  chemical structure of, 458, 458f
  and drug interactions, 459
  endometrial cancer associated with, 457,
      1342, 2592t, 2592–2593, 2593f
  in endometrial cancer therapy, 1352,
      1352t
  in kidney cancer, 1153
  in liver cancer, 1001t, 1002, 1002t
  in melanoma, 1799t, 1799–1800, 2849
  in meningioma, 1864
  metabolism of, 458f, 458–459
  in ovarian cancer, recurrent, 1386
  pharmacology of, 457–459
  in stomach cancer, postoperative, 932
  toxicity of, 457, 458
Tamponade, cardiac, 2387
TAP (transporter associated with antigen pro-
      cessing), 144, 144f, 425, 2846
TaqMan assay, 3
Tar and nicotine content of cigarettes, 190,
      198, 495–496, 753–754
Taste sensations
  chemotherapy affecting, 2649
    nausea and vomiting in, 2517
  in dysgeusia, 2649–2650
  evaluation of changes in, 738
  radiation therapy for oral tongue cancer
      affecting, 682
Tax protein in HTLV-1 leukemogenesis, 168–
      169

Taxanes, 398–407
  administration of, 406–407
  discovery and development of, 398
  interaction with other drugs, 403
  mechanism of action, 399–400
  pharmacokinetics of, 401t, 401–403
  resistance to, 400–401
  structure of, 398, 399f
  toxicity of, 401t, 403–406
    pulmonary, 2542t
Taxes on tobacco products, 500–501, 754
Taxol. *See* Paclitaxel
Taxus brevifolia, paclitaxel derived from, 308–
      309, 398
Tea preparations
  chaparral tea, 2810
  Essiac formulations, 2810
  green tea, 1249, 2813
Technetium 99m scans, 592, 593f, 593t
Teeth
  plaque removal, 2502
  radiation exposure affecting, 2524, 2526,
      2724
  stabilization and hygiene measures for,
      2526
  xerostomia affecting, 2526
Tegafur, 362
  and uracil
    in cholangiocarcinoma, 1021t, 1022
    in colorectal cancer, 1082–1083,
        1093
    in lung cancer, 782
    in pancreatic cancer, metastatic or
        recurrent, 975t, 976, 977t
    in stomach cancer, 929t, 935t, 936
TEL gene fusions, 1941, 2078t, 2086
  with *AML1*, 54, 2079, 2086
    in lymphoblastic leukemia, acute, 15,
        17
  and prognosis in leukemia, 1944, 2079
Telangiectasia and ataxia, 2201t
  and *ATM* gene. *See ATM*
Telemedicine, 2777–2781
  barriers and challenges to, 2780–2781
  equipment used in, 2777
  impact on national medical policy,
      2780
  international uses of, 2779
  in military, 2778
  in oncology care, 2779
  real-time, 2777, 2778
  store-and-forward services, 2777–2778
  in surgery, 2779–2780
Telephone support services
  of National Cancer Institute, 2799
  in smoking cessation programs, 498
Teletherapy, 276
  cobalt 60 megavoltage units in, 278, 279
Telogen effluvium, 2556, 2557
Telomerase, 35, 90, 93, 105–111
  as biomarker in cancer, 109
  in esophageal cancer, 867t, 869
  in head and neck cancer, 659
  in lung cancer, 746t, 749
  in pancreatic cancer, 951, 954–955
  in prostate cancer, 1199–1200
  reactivation of, 106, 107, 108

  structure, regulation, and function of, 35,
      106
  as therapy target in cancer, 35, 109–111,
      110f
Telomerase reverse transcriptase, 93, 106, 109
  in breast cancer, 1410
  in lung cancer, 749
  in pancreatic cancer, 954–955
  in pheochromocytoma, 1538
  as therapy target, 110f, 110–111
Telomere loop, 105f
  phosphorylation of, 77, 78, 85, 85f
Telomeres, 35–36, 90, 105–111
  alternative lengthening mechanism, 106,
      109f, 111
  attrition or shortening of, 109f
    in carcinogenesis, 107, 107f, 108–109,
        109f
    in cellular senescence, 90, 93, 106,
        109f
  as biomarker in cancer, 109
  in cirrhosis and hepatocellular carci-
      noma, 108
  in esophageal cancer, 869
  genomic instability in dysfunction of, 107,
      107f, 108
    radiation-induced, 210–211
  length determination in peripheral blood
      lymphocytes, 109
  in lung cancer, 749
  and menin interactions, 1490–1491
  in pancreatic cancer, 951
  structure and function of, 35, 105f, 105–
      106
    G-quadruplex structure in, 110
    as therapy target, 110
  as therapy target in cancer, 109–111, 110f
    clinical trial designs on, 111
  in ulcerative colitis, 108, 109
Telomeric repeat amplification protocol, 35,
      109
Telophase in mitosis, 84
Temazepam in insomnia, 2709t, 2710
Temozolomide, 337, 338, 338f
  in adrenocortical carcinoma, 1534
  in brainstem glioma, 1855–1856
  carcinogenic and toxic effects of, 339
  in cerebellar astrocytoma, 1856
  in cerebral astrocytoma, 1851–1852
    and radiation therapy, 1849, 1852–
        1853
    recurrent, 1853
  DNA damage from, 339f
  in melanoma, 1798, 1798t, 1801
  in oligodendroglioma, 1859, 1860
Temporal bone tumors, 720–721
  treatment of, 721–722
Temporal lobe
  herniation in intracranial tumors, 1837,
      1841, 2281, 2283
  tumors of, 1836–1837
Temporomandibular joint
  radiation therapy affecting, 2525, 2531
  synovial sarcoma of, 1595f
Teniposide, 382t
  clinical use of, 383
  discovery and development of, 382